MW01091691

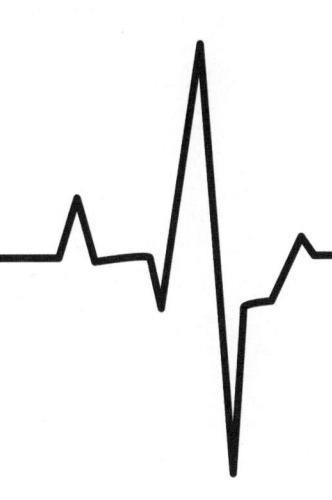

FUHRMAN & ZIMMERMAN'S

PEDIATRIC
CRITICAL CARE

FUHRMAN & ZIMMERMAN'S
PEDIATRIC
CRITICAL CARE

FIFTH EDITION

BRADLEY P. FUHRMAN, MD, FCCM

Professor and Chair, Department of Pediatrics, Texas Tech University – Paul L. Foster School of Medicine, Physician-in-Chief, El Paso Children's Hospital, El Paso, Texas

Robert S.B. Clark, MD

Professor and Chief, Pediatric Critical Care Medicine, Medical Director, Brain Care Institute, Children's Hospital of Pittsburgh of UPMC, Associate Director, Safar Center for Resuscitation Research, University of Pittsburgh, School of Medicine, Pittsburgh, Pennsylvania

Monica Relvas, MD, FAAP, FCCM, MSHA

Medical Director, Pediatric Critical Care Medicine, Covenant Women and Children's Hospital, Associate Clinical Professor, Texas Tech University, Lubbock, Texas

Alexandre T. Rotta, MD, FCCM

Linsalata Family Chair in Pediatric Critical Care and Emergency Medicine, Chief, Division of Pediatric Critical Care Medicine, UH Rainbow Babies and Children's Hospital, Professor, Department of Pediatrics, Case Western Reserve University School of Medicine, Cleveland, Ohio

JERRY J. ZIMMERMAN, MD, PhD, FCCM

Professor of Pediatrics and Anesthesiology, Faculty, Pediatric Critical Care Medicine, Seattle Children's Hospital, Harborview Medical Center, University of Washington School of Medicine, Seattle, Washington

Ann E. Thompson, MD, MHCPM

Professor, Critical Care Medicine, Vice Dean, University of Pittsburgh School of Medicine, Pittsburgh, Pennsylvania

Joseph D. Tobias, MD

Chief, Department of Anesthesiology and Pain Medicine, Nationwide Children's Hospital, Professor of Anesthesiology and Pediatrics, The Ohio State University, Columbus, Ohio

ELSEVIER

ELSEVIER

1600 John F. Kennedy Blvd.
Ste 1800
Philadelphia, PA 19103-2899

PEDIATRIC CRITICAL CARE, FIFTH EDITION   ISBN: 978-0-323-37839-0
Copyright © 2017 by Elsevier, Inc. All rights reserved.

No part of this publication may be reproduced or transmitted in any form or by any means, electronic or mechanical, including photocopying, recording, or any information storage and retrieval system, without permission in writing from the Publisher. Details on how to seek permission, further information about the Publisher's permissions policies and our arrangements with organizations such as the Copyright Clearance Center and the Copyright Licensing Agency, can be found at our website: www.elsevier.com/permissions.

This book and the individual contributions contained in it are protected under copyright by the Publisher (other than as may be noted herein).

Notices

Knowledge and best practice in this field are constantly changing. As new research and experience broaden our understanding, changes in research methods, professional practices, or medical treatment may become necessary.

Practitioners and researchers must always rely on their own experience and knowledge in evaluating and using any information, methods, compounds, or experiments described herein. In using such information or methods they should be mindful of their own safety and the safety of others, including parties for whom they have a professional responsibility.

With respect to any drug or pharmaceutical products identified, readers are advised to check the most current information provided (i) on procedures featured or (ii) by the manufacturer of each product to be administered, to verify the recommended dose or formula, the method and duration of administration, and contraindications. It is the responsibility of practitioners, relying on their own experience and knowledge of their patients, to make diagnoses, to determine dosages and the best treatment for each individual patient, and to take all appropriate safety precautions.

To the fullest extent of the law, neither the Publisher nor the authors, contributors, or editors assume any liability for any injury and/or damage to persons or property as a matter of products liability, negligence or otherwise, or from any use or operation of any methods, products, instructions, or ideas contained in the material herein.

Previous editions copyrighted 2011, 2006, 1998, 1992.

Library of Congress Cataloging-in-Publication Data

Names: Fuhrman, Bradley P., editor.
Title: Pediatric critical care / [edited by] Bradley P. Fuhrman, Jerry J. Zimmerman, Joseph A. Carcillo,
    Robert S.B. Clark, Monica Relvas, Alexandre T. Rotta, Ann E. Thompson, Joseph D. Tobias.
Other titles: Pediatric critical care (Fuhrman)
Description: Fifth edition. | Philadelphia, PA : Elsevier, [2017] | Includes bibliographical references and index.
Identifiers: LCCN 2016034617 | ISBN 9780323378390 (hardcover : alk. paper)
Subjects: | MESH: Critical Care | Child | Infant
Classification: LCC RJ370 | NLM WS 366 | DDC 618.92/0028—dc23 LC record available at
    https://lccn.loc.gov/2016034617

Legends for Cover Figures:

Figures from left to right:
Schematic depiction of gram-negative bacteremia.
Schematic depiction of Toll-like receptor 4, an element of innate immunity that binds lipopolysaccharide of the gram-negative cell wall (endotoxin), initiating a cascade of intracellular signaling to promote a proinflammatory host response.
Host mRNA expression of the most affected genes in a child with bacterial sepsis. Red, upregulation; blue, downregulation. Courtesy, Hector Wong.
Alterations in microvascular flow and effective capillary density of the buccal mucosa using orthogonal polarization spectral imaging in a patient with bacterial sepsis.

Senior Content Strategist: Sarah Barth
Senior Content Development Specialist: Laura Schmidt
Publishing Services Manager: Patricia Tannian
Senior Project Manager: Sharon Corell
Book Designer: Patrick Ferguson

Printed in China.

Last digit is the print number: 9   8   7   6   5   4   3   2   1

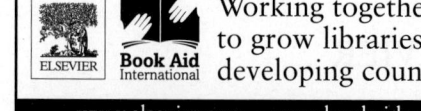

Working together to grow libraries in developing countries

www.elsevier.com • www.bookaid.org

Contributors

Isaac Josh Abecassis, MD

Resident Physician
Department of Neurological Surgery
University of Washington
Seattle, Washington

Rachel S. Agbeko, MD, PhD, FRCPCH, FFICM

Consultant in Paediatric Intensive Care
Department of Paediatric Intensive Care
Great North Children's Hospital
The Newcastle upon Tyne Hospitals NHS Foundation Trust
Associate Clinical Lecturer
Institute of Cellular Medicine
Newcastle University
Newcastle upon Tyne
United Kingdom

P. David Adelson, MD, FACS, FAAP

Director
Barrow Neurological Institute at Phoenix Children's Hospital
Diane and Bruce Halle Chair of Pediatric Neurosciences
Chief
Pediatric Neurosurgery
Phoenix Children's Hospital
Phoenix, Arizona

Matthew N. Alder, PhD, MD

Instructor of Pediatrics, University of Cincinnati College of Medicine
Division of Critical Care Medicine
Cincinnati Children's Hospital Medical Center
Children's Hospital Research Foundation
Cincinnati, Ohio

Omar Al Ibrahim, MD

Director
Cutaneous Laser and Cosmetic Surgery
Mohs Micrographic and Reconstructive Surgery
Dermatology
University of Connecticut
Farmington, Connecticut

Melvin C. Almodovar, MD

Medical Director
Cardiac Intensive Care Unit
Department of Cardiology
Boston Children's Hospital
Boston, Massachusetts

Alexandra R. Aminoff, MD

Pediatric Rheumatology
The Permanente Medical Group
Kaiser Permanente Northern California
Oakland, California

Catherine Amlie-LeFond, MD

Director
Pediatric Vascular Neurology Program
Professor
Seattle Children's Hospital/University of Washington
Seattle, Washington

Derek C. Angus, MD, MPH, FRCP

Distinguished Professor and Mitchell P. Fink Endowed Chair
Department of Critical Care Medicine
Professor of Critical Care Medicine, Medicine, Health Policy and Management, and Clinical and Translational Science
University of Pittsburgh Schools of the Health Sciences
Pittsburgh, Pennsylvania

Joan C. Arvedson, BS, MS, PhD

Program Coordinator, Feeding and Swallowing Services
Speech Pathology and Audiology
Children's Hospital of Wisconsin
Milwaukee, Wisconsin

Francois Aspesberro, MD

Pediatric Critical Care Medicine
Seattle Children's Hospital/University of Washington
Seattle, Washington

John E. Baatz, PhD

Professor
Pediatrics - Neonatology
Medical University of South Carolina
Charleston, South Carolina

Harris P. Baden, MD

Professor & Chief
Pediatric Cardiac Critical Care
Seattle Children's Hospital/University of Washington
Seattle, Washington

Srinivasarao Badugu, MD

Assistant Professor
Department of Pediatrics
Texas Tech University
El Paso, Texas

Adnan M. Bakar, MD

Assistant Professor of Pediatrics
Section Head
Pediatric Cardiac Critical Care
Hofstra Northwell School of Medicine
Pediatric Critical Care Medicine
Pediatric Cardiology
Cohen Children's Medical Center of New York
New Hyde Park, New York

Katherine Banker, MD

Clinical Assistant Professor
Pediatrics
Critical Care
Seattle Children's Hospital/University of Washington
Seattle, Washington

John L. Bass, MD

Professor of Pediatrics
Director
Pediatric Interventional Catheterization
University of Minnesota/Masonic Children's Hospital
Minneapolis, Minnesota

Hülya Bayir, MD

Safar Center for Resuscitation Research
Department of Critical Care Medicine
University of Pittsburgh School of Medicine
Children's Hospital of Pittsburgh of UPMC
Pittsburgh, Pennsylvania

Pierre Beaulieu, MD, PhD, FRCA

Professor
Departments of Medicine and Anesthesiology
Faculty of Medicine
Université de Montréal
Montreal, Quebec, Canada

Lance B. Becker, MD

Director
Center for Resuscitation Science
Perelman School of Medicine at the University of
Pennsylvania
Philadelphia, Pennsylvania

Michael J. Bell, MD

Professor of Critical Care Medicine, Neurological Surgery,
and Pediatrics
Director
Pediatric Neurocritical Care
Director
Pediatric Neurotrauma Center
Associate Director
Safar Center for Resuscitation Research
University of Pittsburgh School of Medicine
Pittsburgh, Pennsylvania

M.A. Bender, MD, PhD

Associate Professor
University of Washington
Fred Hutchinson Cancer Research Center
Seattle, Washington

Wade W. Benton, PharmD

Executive Director
Medical Affairs
Relypsa
Redwood City, California

Robert A. Berg, MD

Russell Raphaely Endowed Chair
Division Chief
Critical Care Medicine
Professor of Anesthesiology
Critical Care and Pediatrics
The Children's Hospital of Philadelphia
Perelman School of Medicine at the University of
Pennsylvania
Philadelphia, Pennsylvania

Katherine V. Biagas, MD, FCCM, FAAP

Director
Pediatric Critical Care Medicine Fellowship
Associate Professor of Pediatrics
Columbia University Medical Center
New York, New York

Naomi B. Bishop, MD

Assistant Professor
Pediatrics
Director
Quality and Patient Improvement
Pediatric Critical Care Medicine
Weill Cornell Medicine
New York, New York

Julie Blatt, MD

Professor
Pediatric Hematology Oncology
University of North Carolina
Chapel Hill, North Carolina

Douglas L. Blowey, MD

Associate Professor
Pediatrics and Pharmacology
Pediatric Nephrology
University of Missouri—Kansas City/ Children's Mercy
Hospital
Kansas City, Missouri

Jeffrey L. Blumer, PhD, MD

Professor of Pediatrics
University of Toledo
College of Medicine and Life Sciences
Toledo, Ohio

Robert H. Bonow, MD

Resident Physician
Department of Neurological Surgery
University of Washington
Seattle, Washington

Barbara W. Brandom, MD

North American MH Registry of MHAUS
Adjunct Professor of Nurse Anesthesia
Retired Professor of Anesthesiology
University of Pittsburgh
Pittsburgh, Pennsylvania

Richard J. Brilli, MD, FAAP, MCCM

Division of Critical Care Medicine
Department of Pediatrics
Nationwide Children's Hospital
The Ohio State University College of Medicine
Columbus, Ohio

Thomas V. Brogan, MD

Professor
Department of Pediatrics
Seattle Children's Hospital/University of Washington
Seattle, Washington

Ronald A. Bronicki, MD, FCCM, FACC

Critical Care Medicine and Cardiology
Texas Children's Hospital and Baylor College of Medicine
Houston, Texas

Samuel R. Browd, MD, PhD, FAANS, FAAP

Professor
Department of Neurological Surgery
Seattle Children's Hospital/University of Washington
Seattle, Washington

Timothy E. Bunchman, MD

Professor and Director Pediatric Nephrology
Children's Hospital of Richmond
Virginia Commonwealth University School of Medicine
Richmond, Virginia

Jeffrey P. Burns, MD, MPH

Chief and Shapiro Chair of Critical Care Medicine
Boston Children's Hospital
Professor of Anesthesia
Harvard Medical School
Boston, Massachusetts

Derya Caglar, MD

Assistant Professor
Pediatrics
Attending Physician
Pediatric Emergency Medicine
Seattle Children's Hospital/University of Washington
Seattle, Washington

Sally Campbell, BS

Haematology Registrar
Clinical Haematology
Royal Children's Hospital
Melbourne, Victoria, Australia

Joseph A. Carcillo, MD

Associate Professor of Critical Care Medicine and Pediatrics
Children's Hospital of Pittsburgh of UPMC
University of Pittsburgh School of Medicine
Pittsburgh, Pennsylvania

Hector Carrillo-Lopez, MD

Professor of Pediatric Critical Care and Pediatrics
Hospital Infantil de Mexico Federico Gomez
Universidad Nacional Autonoma de Mexico
Mexico City, Mexico

Katherine Cashen, DO

Pediatric Intensivist
Children's Hospital of Michigan
Assistant Professor
Division of Critical Care Medicine
Department of Pediatrics
Wayne State University School of Medicine
Detroit, Michigan

Antonio Cassara, MD

Visiting Assistant Professor
University of Pittsburgh School of Medicine
Pittsburgh, Pennsylvania

John R. Charpie, MD, PhD

Professor and Division Director, Pediatric Cardiology
Pediatrics and Communicable Diseases
University of Michigan Medical School
Ann Arbor, Michigan

Adrian Chavez, MD

Director
Pediatric Intensive Care
Hospital Infantil de Mexico Federico Gomez
Head Professor of Pediatric Critical Care and Pediatrics
Facultad de Medicina
Universidad Nacional Autonoma de Mexico
Mexico City, Mexico

Robert H. Chun, MD

Associate Professor
Department of Otolaryngology
Division of Pediatric Otolaryngology
Medical College of Wisconsin
Milwaukee, Wisconsin

Jonna Derbenwick Clark, MD, MA

Assistant Professor
Pediatrics, Critical Care Medicine
Affiliate Faculty
Treuman Katz Center for Pediatric Bioethics
Department of Pediatrics
Seattle Children's Hospital/University of Washington
Seattle, Washington

Robert S.B. Clark, MD

Professor and Chief
Pediatric Critical Care Medicine
Medical Director
Brain Care Institute
Children's Hospital of Pittsburgh of UPMC
Associate Director
Safar Center for Resuscitation Research
University of Pittsburgh School of Medicine
Pittsburgh, Pennsylvania

Katherine C. Clement, MD

Assistant Professor of Pediatrics
UNC School of Medicine
Chapel Hill, North Carolina

Thomas Conlon, MD

Director of Pediatric Critical Care Ultrasound
Assistant Professor
Department of Anesthesiology and Critical Care Medicine
The Children's Hospital of Philadelphia
University of Pennsylvania Perelman School of Medicine
Philadelphia, Pennsylvania

Edward E. Conway, Jr., MD, MS

Chairman and Pediatrician-in-Chief
Milton and Bernice Stern Department of Pediatrics
Beth Israel Medical Center
Professor of Pediatrics
Icahn School of Medicine at Mount Sinai
New York, New York

Craig M. Coopersmith, MD

Professor of Surgery
Department of Surgery
Emory University School of Medicine
Atlanta, Georgia

Seth J. Corey, ME

Professor in Pediatrics and Cell and Molecular Biology
Northwestern University Feinberg School of Medicine
Evanston, Illinois

Peter N. Cox, MD

Professor
Critical Care Medicine
Hospital for Sick Children
Toronto, Ontario, Canada

Martha A.Q. Curley, RN, PhD, FAAN

Ellen and Robert Kapito Professor in Nursing Science
School of Nursing/Anesthesia and Critical Care Medicine
University of Pennsylvania
Nurse Scientist
Critical Care and Cardiovascular Program
Boston Children's Hospital
Boston, Massachusetts

Marek Czosnyka, PhD

Professor of Clinical Neuroscience
University of Cambridge Clinical School
Department of Neurosurgery
Addenbrooke's Hospital
Cambridge, United Kingdom

Heidi J. Dalton, MD, MCCM

Professor of Pediatrics
Virginia Commonwealth University
Clinical Professor of Surgery
George Washington University
Director
Adult and Pediatric ECLS
INOVA Fairfax Medical Center
Falls Church, Virginia

Mihaela Damian, MD, MPH

Clinical Assistant Professor
Department of Pediatrics
Stanford University
Palo Alto, California

Peter J. Davis, MD

Dr. Joseph H. Marcy Endowed Chair in Pediatric Anesthesia
University of Pittsburgh School of Medicine
Anesthesiologist-in-Chief
Children's Hospital of Pittsburgh of UPMC
Department of Anesthesia
Pittsburgh, Pennsylvania

Nicolas de Prost, MD, PhD

Service de Réanimation Médicale
Hôpital Henri Mondor
Assistance Publique
Groupe de Recherche Clinique CARMAS
Université Paris Est Créteil
Créteil, France

Clifford S. Deutschman, MD

Professor of Anesthesiology and Critical Care
Director
Sepsis Research Program
Perelman School of Medicine at the University of Pennsylvania
Philadelphia, Pennsylvania

Cameron Dezfulian, MD

Safar Center for Resuscitation Research
Department of Critical Care Medicine
University of Pittsburgh School of Medicine
Children's Hospital of Pittsburgh of UPMC
Pittsburgh, Pennsylvania

Douglas S. Diekema, MD, MPH

Professor of Pediatrics and Bioethics
Treuman Katz Center for Pediatric Bioethics
Seattle Children's Hospital/University of Washington
Seattle, Washington

Allan Doctor, MD

Professor of Pediatrics and Biochemistry
Washington University School of Medicine
St. Louis, Missouri

Meaghan Doherty, MD

Pediatric Cardiology Fellow
Cardiology
Children's Hospital of Pittsburgh
Pittsburgh, Pennsylvania

Molly V. Dorfman, MD, PhD

Pediatric Critical Care
Valley Children's Hospital
Madera, California

John J. Downes, MD

Department of Anesthesiology and Critical Care Medicine
The Children's Hospital of Philadelphia
Perelman School of Medicine at the University of
Pennsylvania
Philadelphia, Pennsylvania

Didier Dreyfuss, MD

Professor of Medicine
Hospital of Paris
Paris, France

Christine Duncan, MD

Assistant Professor
Pediatric Hematology Oncology
Dana-Farber Cancer Institute
Boston, Massachusetts

Phylicia D. Dupree, MD

Resident Physician
General Surgery
University of Cincinnati
Cincinnati, Ohio

Howard Eigen, MD

Professor of Pediatrics (ret.)
Indiana University School of Medicine
President
Inspire Foundation
Indianapolis, Indiana

Nahed El-Hassan, MD

Associate Professor of Pediatrics
University of Arkansas for Medical Sciences
Arkansas Children's Hospital
Little Rock, Arkansas

Carl O. Eriksson, MD

Assistant Professor
Pediatric Critical Care
Department of Pediatrics
Oregon Health and Science University
Portland, Oregon

Kate Felmet, MD

Assistant Professor
Departments of Critical Care Medicine and Pediatrics
University of Pittsburgh School of Medicine
Pittsburgh, Pennsylvania

Jeffrey R. Fineman, MD

Professor of Pediatrics
University of California, San Francisco
San Francisco, California

Ericka L. Fink, MD, MS

Associate Professor
Safar Center for Resuscitation Research
Department of Critical Care Medicine
University of Pittsburgh School of Medicine
Children's Hospital of Pittsburgh of UPMC
Pittsburgh, Pennsylvania

Frank A. Fish, MD

Professor
Pediatrics
Vanderbilt Medical Center
Nashville, Tennessee

Tamara N. Fitzgerald, MD, PhD

Assistant Professor
Department of Surgery
Texas Tech University – Paul L. Foster School of Medicine
El Paso, Texas

Joseph T. Flynn, MD

Professor of Pediatrics
Chief - Division of Nephrology
Seattle Children's Hospital/University of Washington
Seattle, Washington

J. Julio Pérez Fontán, MD

Robert L. Moore Chair in Pediatrics
Professor and Chairman, Department of Pediatrics
University of Texas Southwestern Medical Center
Physician-in-Chief, Children's Medical Center, Dallas
Dallas, Texas

Michael J. Forbes, MD, FAAP

Director
Clinical Research and Outcomes Analysis
Pediatric Intensive Care Unit
Fellow
American Academy of Pediatrics Society of Critical Care
Medicine
Akron, Ohio

Joseph M. Forbess, MD

Director
Cardiothoracic Surgery
Co-Director
Heart Center
Children's Health, Dallas
Professor of Thoracic and Cardiovascular Surgery
Pogue Distinguished Chair in Pediatric Cardiac Surgery
Research
University of Texas Southwestern Medical Center
Dallas, Texas

Deborah E. Franzon, MD

Clinical Professor of Pediatrics
Division of Critical Care Medicine
University of California, San Francisco
San Francisco, California

W. Joshua Frazier, MD

Division of Critical Care Medicine
Department of Pediatrics
Nationwide Children's Hospital
The Ohio State University College of Medicine
Columbus, Ohio

F. Jay Fricker, MD

UF Health Congenital Heart Center
Gainesville, Florida

Bradley P. Fuhrman, MD, FCCM

Professor and Chair
Department of Pediatrics
Texas Tech University – Paul L. Foster School of Medicine
Physician-in-Chief
El Paso Children's Hospital
El Paso, Texas

Xiomara Garcia-Casal, MD

Associate Professor of Pediatrics
University of Arkansas for Medical Sciences
Arkansas Children's Hospital
Little Rock, Arkansas

Rebecca Gardner, MD

Assistant Professor
Pediatrics
University of Washington
Seattle, Washington

Eli Gilad, MD

Pediatric Critical Care
Alberta Children's Hospital and the University of Calgary
Calgary, Alberta, Canada

Richard M. Ginther, Jr., CCP, FPP

Faculty Associate
Pediatric Perfusionist
Pediatric Cardiothoracic Surgery
University of Texas Southwestern Medical Center
Children's Health Dallas
Dallas, Texas

Nicole Glaser, MD

Professor
Pediatric Endocrinology
UC Davis Children's Hospital
Sacramento, California

Denise M. Goodman, MD, MS

Attending Physician
Division of Critical Care Medicine
Medical Director
Case Management and Care Coordination (Physician Advisor)
Ann and Robert H. Lurie Children's Hospital of Chicago
Professor
Northwestern University Feinberg School of Medicine
Chicago, Illinois

Ana Lía Graciano, MD, FAAP, FCCM

Department of Pediatrics
Critical Care Medicine
Medical Director
Pediatric Cardiac Intensive Care
University of Maryland School of Medicine
Baltimore, Maryland

Kristin C. Greathouse, PhD(c), MS, BSN, CPNP-AC

The Heart Center
Nationwide Children's Hospital
Columbus, Ohio

Bruce M. Greenwald, MD, FAAP, FCCM

Professor of Clinical Pediatrics
Executive Vice-Chairman
Department of Pediatrics
Chief
Division of Pediatric Critical Care Medicine
Weill Cornell Medicine
New York, New York

Björn Gunnarsson, MD

Department of Research
Norwegian Air Ambulance Foundation
Drøbak, Norway
SAR Helicopter
Ørland Main Air Station, Norway

Punkaj Gupta, MBBS

Associate Professor of Pediatrics
University of Arkansas for Medical Sciences
Arkansas Children's Hospital
Little Rock, Arkansas

Mark W. Hall, MD, FCCM

Associate Professor of Pediatrics
Chief
Division of Critical Care Medicine
Nationwide Children's Hospital
The Ohio State University
Columbus, Ohio

Yong Y. Han, MD

Physical Scientist
NOAA/NESDIS
Center for Satellite Application and Research
College Park, Maryland

Cary O. Harding, MD

Professor
Molecular and Medical Genetics
Oregon Health and Science University
Portland, Oregon

Mary E. Hartman, MD, MPH, FRCP

Assistant Professor of Pediatrics
Pediatric Critical Care Medicine
Department of Pediatrics
Washington University School of Medicine
St. Louis, Missouri

Silvia M. Hartmann, MD

Assistant Professor
Pediatric Critical Care Medicine
Seattle Children's Hospital/University of Washington School
of Medicine
Seattle, Washington

Christopher M.B. Heard, MB, ChB, FRCA

Clinical Professor of Anesthesiology Pediatrics
Pediatric and Community Dentistry
The State University of New York at Buffalo
Buffalo, New York

Lynn J. Hernan, MD

Associate Professor
Pediatrics
Texas Tech University—Paul L. Foster School of Medicine
El Paso, Texas

Mark J. Heulitt, MD, FCCM

Medical Director of Pediatric Intensive Care Unit
Spence and Becky Wilson Baptist Children's Hospital
Memphis, Tennessee

Julien I. Hoffman, MD

Professor (Emeritus)
Pediatrics
University of California, San Francisco
San Francisco, California

Simon Horslen, MD

Professor
Pediatrics
University of Washington School of Medicine
Seattle, Washington

Agnes I. Hunyady, MD

Attending Anesthesiologist
Seattle Children's Hospital/University of Washington
Assistant Professor
University of Washington School of Medicine
Seattle, Washington

Laura Marie Ibsen, MD

Professor
Pediatrics and Anesthesiology
Oregon Health and Science University
Portland, Oregon

Hanneke IJsselstijn, MD, PhD

Pediatric Surgery and Intensive Care
Erasmus MC - Sophia Children's Hospital
Rotterdam, The Netherlands

Andrew Inglis, Jr., MD

Associate Professor
Department of Otolaryngology
Seattle Children's Hospital/University of Washington
Seattle, Washington

Gretchen A. Linggi Irby, PharmD

Pharmacist
Seattle, Washington

Olivia K. Irby, MD

Assistant Professor of Pediatrics
University of Arkansas for Medical Sciences
Arkansas Children's Hospital
Little Rock, Arkansas

Gisele E. Ishak, MD

Associate Professor
Department of Radiology
University of Washington
Seattle Children's Hospital/University of Washington
Seattle, Washington

Travis C. Jackson, PhD

Research Assistant Professor
Department of Critical Care Medicine
Associate Director of Cell Signaling
Safar Center for Resuscitation Research
Pittsburgh, Pennsylvania

Susan Jacob, PharmD

Investigational Drug Service
Seattle Children's Hospital/University of Washington
Seattle, Washington

Shelina M. Jamal, MD

Clinical Assistant Professor
Pediatric Critical Care
Seattle Children's Hospital/University of Washington
Seattle, Washington

David Jardine, MD

Associate Professor
Department of Otolaryngology
Seattle Children's Hospital/University of Washington
School of Medicine
Seattle, Washington

Alberto Jarillo, MD

Head
Respiratory Therapy Service
Associate Professor of Pediatric
Critical Care and Pediatrics
Hospital Infantil de Mexico Federico Gomez
Mexico City, Mexico

Alison M. Jeziorski, MD, MBA

Assistant Professor
Department of Anesthesia and Perioperative Medicine
Medical University of South Carolina
Charleston, South Carolina

Umesh Joashi, MD

Consultant Paediatric Intensivist
Leeds Teaching Hospitals NHS Trust
Leeds, United Kingdom

Prashant Joshi, MD

Associate Professor
Pediatrics
University of Nebraska Medical Center
Omaha, Nebraska

Richard J. Kagan, MD

Professor
Surgery
University of Cincinnati College of Medicine
Cincinnati, Ohio

Prince J. Kannankeril, MD

Associate Professor
Pediatrics
Vanderbilt Children's Hospital
Nashville, Tennessee

Robert K. Kanter, MD†

Adjunct Senior Research Scientist
National Center for Disaster Preparedness
Columbia University
New York, New York

Oliver Karam, MD

Associate Professor
Pediatric Intensive Care Unit
Geneva University Hospital
Geneva, Switzerland

Cristin D. W. Kaspar, MD

Pediatric Nephrology Fellow
Children's Hospital of Richmond
Virginia Commonwealth University School of Medicine
Richmond, Virginia

Robinder G. Khemani, MD, MsCI

Associate Director of Research
Department of Anesthesiology and Critical Care
Critical Care Medicine
Children's Hospital Los Angeles
Associate Professor of Pediatrics
University of Southern California Keck School of Medicine
Los Angeles, California

Mary A. King, MD

Professor of Genome Sciences and of Medicine
University of Washington
Seattle, Washington

Christa C. Jefferis Kirk, PharmD

Clinical Staff Pharmacist
Critical Care
Seattle Children's Hospital
Seattle, Washington

Niranjan (Tex) Kissoon, MD

Professor in Acute and Critical Care—Global Child Health
Pediatrics and Surgery (EM)
The University of British Columbia and BC Children's Hospital
Vancouver, British Columbia, Canada

Patrick M. Kochanek, MD, MCCM

Ake N. Grenvik Professor and Vice Chair of Critical Care Medicine
Professor of Anesthesiology, Pediatrics and Bioengineering, and Clinical and Translational Science
Director
Safar Center for Resuscitation Research
University of Pittsburgh School of Medicine
Pittsburgh, Pennsylvania

Keith C. Kocis, MD, MS

Director
Pediatric Cardiac Intensive Care
Interim Director
Pediatric Critical Care Medicine
Sidra Medical and Research Center
Doha, Qatar

Samuel A. Kocoshis, MD

Professor
Pediatrics
University of Cincinnati College of Medicine
Cincinnati, Ohio

Tsingyi Koh, PharmD, BCPS

Principal Clinical Pharmacist Pediatrics/Solid Organ Transplant
Department of Pharmacy
National University Hospital
Singapore

†Deceased

Ada Kong, PharmD

Research Pharmacist
Seattle Children's Hospital/University of Washington
Seattle, Washington

Ildiko H. Koves, MD, FRACP

Associate Professor
Endocrinology and Diabetes
Seattle Children's Hospital/University of Washington
Seattle, Washington

Thomas J. Kulik, MD

Senior Associate in Cardiology
Cardiology
Boston Children's Hospital
Boston, Massachusetts

Vasanth H. Kumar, MD

Associate Professor
Department of Pediatrics
Director
Neonatal-Perinatal Medicine Fellowship Program
The State University of New York at Buffalo
Women and Children's Hospital of Buffalo
Buffalo, New York

Jacques Lacroix, MD

Professor
Division of Pediatric Intensive Care
Department of Pediatrics
Sainte-Justine Hospital
Université de Montréal
Montreal, Quebec, Canada

Satyan Lakshminrusimha, MD

Professor of Pediatrics
Chief
Division of Neonatology
Women and Children's Hospital of Buffalo
Director
Center for Developmental Biology
The State University of New York at Buffalo
Buffalo, New York

Thomas J. Lee, MD

Major
United States Air Force
San Antonio, Texas

Marie Leiner, PhD

Research Associate Professor
Pediatrics
Texas Tech University Health Sciences Center
El Paso, Texas

Daniel L. Levin, MD

Professor Emeritus
Departments of Pediatrics and Anesthesia
Children's Hospital at Dartmouth
Geisel School of Medicine
Lebanon, New Hampshire

Mithya Lewis-Newby, MD, MPH

Associate Professor
Departments of Pediatrics and Bioethics and Humanities
Treuman Katz Center for Pediatric Bioethics
Seattle Children's Hospital/University of Washington School
of Medicine
Seattle, Washington

Mary W. Lieh-Lai, MD, FAAP, FCCP

Senior Vice President for Medical Accreditation
Accreditation Council for Graduate Medical Education
Professor of Pediatrics (Vol)
Wayne State University School of Medicine
Chicago, Illinois

Catherine Litalien, MD, FRCPC

Associate Professor
Division of Pediatric Intensive Care
Department of Pediatrics
Director
Clinical Pharmacology Unit
CHU Sainte-Justine
Université de Montréal
Montreal, Quebec, Canada

Alejandro Lopez-Magallon, MD

Assistant Professor
Critical Care Medicine
University of Pittsburgh
Pittsburgh, Pennsylvania

Robert Lynch, MD

Critical Care—Pediatric
Mercy Clinic
St. Louis, Missouri

John D. Lyons, MD

Research Resident
Emory University School of Medicine
Atlanta, Georgia

Sitratullah Maiyegun, MD, FAAP

Associate Professor
Pediatrics
Texas Tech University—Paul L. Foster School of Medicine
Health Sciences Center
El Paso, Texas

Amy T. Makley, MD

Assistant Professor of Surgery
University of Cincinnati
Cincinnati, Ohio

Alfredo Maldonado, MS, MD

Assistant Professor
Department of Pediatrics
Division of Pediatric Emergency Medicine
Texas Tech University Health Sciences Center
El Paso, Texas

Barry Markovitz, MD

Professor
Anesthesiology and Pediatrics
USC Keck School of Medicine
Los Angeles, California

Paula M. Mazur, MD

Associate Clinical Professor of Pediatric Emergency
Medicine and Child Abuse Pediatrics
University Pediatrics Associates
John R. Oishei Children's Hospital
Buffalo, New York

Jennifer McArthur, MD

Associate Professor of Pediatrics
Pediatric Critical Care
Medical College of Wisconsin
Milwaukee, Wisconsin

Gwenn E. McLaughlin, MD, MSPH, FAAP, FCCM

Professor of Clinical Pediatrics
Division of Pediatric Critical Care Medicine
University of Miami Miller School of Medicine
Attending Physician
Miami, Florida

Susan F. McLean, MD, FACS

Associate Professor of Surgery
Texas Tech University Health Sciences Center El Paso
Surgical Intensive Care Unit Director and Associate Trauma
Medical Director
University Medical Center of El Paso
El Paso, Texas

Nilesh M. Mehta, MD

Associate Professor of Anesthesia
Harvard Medical School
Senior Associate
Director of Critical Care Nutrition
Department of Anesthesiology, Perioperative
and Pain Medicine
Boston Children's Hospital
Boston, Massachusetts

Renuka Mehta, MS

Medical College of Georgia Medical Center
Augusta, Georgia

Ann J. Melvin, MD

Associate Professor
Pediatric Infectious Diseases
Seattle Children's Hospital/University of Washington School
of Medicine
Seattle, Washington

Ayesa N. Mian, MD

Pediatric Nephrology
University of Rochester School of Medicine
Rochester, New York

Rohit Mittal, MD

Research Resident
Emory University
Atlanta, Georgia

Patricia A. Moloney-Harmon, RN, MS, CCNS, CCRN, FAAN

Clinical Nurse Specialist
Children's Services
Sinai Hospital
Baltimore, Maryland

Paul Monagle, MBBS, MD, MSC

Professor
Stevenson Chair
Head of Department
Paediatrics
University of Melbourne
Melbourne, Victoria, Australia

Chet Moorthy, MD

Medical Director of Radiology
El Paso Children's Hospital
El Paso, Texas

Wynne Morrison, MD, MBE

Assistant Professor
Department of Anesthesiology and Critical Care
Director
Pediatric Advanced Care Team
The Children's Hospital of Philadelphia
Perelman School of Medicine at the University of
Pennsylvania
Philadelphia, Pennsylvania

Ricardo Munoz, MD

Chief
Pediatric Cardiac Critical Care
Children's Hospital of Pittsburgh of UPMC
Pittsburgh, Pennsylvania

Raj Munshi, MD

Nephrology
Seattle Children's Hospital/University of Washington
Seattle, Washington

Srinivas Murthy, MD

Assistant Professor of Critical Care
Pediatrics
BC Children's Hospital
University of British Columbia
Vancouver, British Columbia, Canada

Jennifer A. Muszynski, MD

Assistant Professor of Pediatrics
Division of Critical Care Medicine
Department of Pediatrics
Nationwide Children's Hospital
The Ohio State University College of Medicine
Columbus, Ohio

Vinay M. Nadkarni, MD, MS

Endowed Chair
Pediatric Critical Care Medicine
Professor of Anesthesiology
Critical Care and Pediatrics
The Children's Hospital of Philadelphia
Perelman School of Medicine at the University of
Pennsylvania
Philadelphia, Pennsylvania

Thomas A. Nakagawa, MD

Professor and Section Head
Pediatric Critical Care Medicine
Anesthesiology and Pediatrics
Wake Forest School of Medicine
Winston-Salem, North Carolina

Navyn Naran, MD

Niagara Falls, Ontario, Canada

Tara M. Neumayr, MD

Instructor of Pediatrics
Division of Pediatric Critical Care Medicine
Washington University School of Medicine
St. Louis, Missouri

Akira Nishisaki, MD, MSCE

The Children's Hospital of Philadelphia
Department of Anesthesiology and Critical Care Medicine
Philadelphia, Pennsylvania

Victoria F. Norwood, MD

Robert J. Roberts Professor of Pediatrics
Chief of Pediatric Nephrology
University of Virginia
Charlottesville, Virginia

Daniel A. Notterman, MA, MD, FAAP, FCCM

Professor
Department of Molecular Biology
Princeton University
Princeton, New Jersey
Clinical Professor of Pediatrics
Rutgers—Robert Wood Johnson Medical School
New Brunswick, New Jersey

Alan W. Nugent, MBBS

Associate Professor
Pediatrics
University of Texas Southwestern Medical Center
Director
Cardiac Catheterization
Children's Medical Center
Dallas, Texas

Peter Oishi, MD

Associate Professor of Pediatrics
Medical Director
Pediatric Intensive Care Unit, Transport and Access,
Transitional Care Unit
Director
Pediatric ECLS Program
UCSF Beinoff Children's Hospital, San Francisco
San Francisco, California

Jeffrey Ojemann, MD

Division Chief of Neurosurgery
Director of Epilepsy Surgery
Co-Director
Epilepsy Program
Richard G. Ellenbogen Endowed Chair in Pediatric
Neurosurgery
Seattle Children's Hospital/University of Washington
College of Medicine
Seattle, Washington

Richard A. Orr, MD, FCCM

Professor
Critical Care Medicine and Pediatrics
Staff
Cardiac Intensive Care Division
University of Pittsburgh Medical Center
Pittsburgh, Pennsylvania

Yves Ouellette, MD, PhD

Assistant Professor of Pediatrics
Mayo Clinic
Rochester, Minnesota

Daiva Parakininkas, MD

Associate Professor of Pediatrics
Divisions of Critical Care/Pulmonary and Sleep Medicine
Medical College of Wisconsin
Children's Hospital of Wisconsin
Milwaukee, Wisconsin

Robert I. Parker, MD

Professor and Vice Chair for Academic Affairs
Director
Pediatric Hematology/Oncology
Stony Brook Long Island Children's Hospital
Associate Director
Stony Brook University Cancer Center
State University of New York at Stony Brook
Stony Brook, New York

Sanjiv Pasala, MD

Assistant Professor of Pediatrics
University of Arkansas for Medical Sciences
Arkansas Children's Hospital
Little Rock, Arkansas

Tony Pearson-Shaver, MD

Medical Education—Pediatrics
Children's Hospital Navicent Health
Macon, Georgia

Jesus Peinado, MD

Assistant Professor
Pediatrics
Texas Tech University Health Sciences Center
El Paso, Texas

Mark J. Peters, MBChB, MRCP, FRCPCH, PhD

Professor of Paediatric Intensive Care
UCL Great Ormond Street Institute of Child Health
Honorary Consultant
Paediatric and Neonatal Intensivist
Great Ormond Street Hospital NHS Foundation Trust
London, United Kingdom

Brent J. Pfeiffer, MD, PhD, FAAP

Assistant Professor of Clinical Pediatrics
Division of Pediatric Critical Care Medicine
University of Miami Miller School of Medicine
Attending Physician
Holtz Children's Hospital
Miami, Florida

Carrie A. Phillipi, MD, PhD

Professor
Pediatrics
Oregon Health and Science University
Portland, Oregon

Maury N. Pinsk, MD, MSc, FRCPC, FASN

Professor
Pediatrics and Child Health
Director of Northern and Rural Pediatric Education
Winnipeg Children's Hospital
Health Sciences Centre
College of Medicine
University of Manitoba
Winnipeg, Manitoba, Canada

Murray M. Pollack, MD

Critical Care Medicine
Children's National Health System
Professor of Pediatrics
George Washington University School of Medicine and
Health Sciences
Washington, DC

Steven Pon, MD

Associate Director Pediatric Critical Care
Pediatrics
Weill Cornell Medical College
New York, New York

Tom Preston, CCP

Innovative ECMO Concepts, Inc.
Arcadia, Oklahoma

Prakad Rajapreyar, MD

Pediatric Critical Care
Milwaukee, Wisconsin

Samiran Ray, MBBChir, MA

Research Fellow
Respiratory
Critical Care and Anaesthesia Section
UCL Great Ormond Street Institute of Child Health
London, United Kingdom

Erin P. Reade, MD, MPH, FAAP

Associate Professor of Pediatrics
The University of Tennessee College of Medicine
Chattanooga
Pediatric Intensivist
The Children's Hospital at Erlanger
Chattanooga, Tennessee

Kenneth E. Remy, MD, MHSc

Assistant Professor of Pediatrics
Division of Pediatric Critical Care Medicine
Department of Pediatrics
Washington University School of Medicine
St. Louis, Missouri

Eileen Rhee, MD

Assistant Professor
Division of Pediatric Critical Care Medicine
Attending Physician
Pediatric Advanced Care Team
Seattle Children's Hospital/University of Washington
Seattle, Washington

Jean-Damien Ricard, MD

Paris Diderot University
Paris, France

Nicole L. Richardson, PharmD

Pediatric Critical Care Pharmacist
Seattle Children's Hospital/University of Washington
Seattle, Washington

Joan S. Roberts, MD

Associate Professor
Pediatrics/Critical Care
Seattle Children's Hospital/University of Washington
Seattle, Washington

Stephen Rogers, PhD

Staff Scientist
Pediatric Critical Care Medicine
Washington University School of Medicine
St. Louis, Missouri

Kimberly R. Roth, MD, MPH

Physician Director
Prehospital and Emergency Care Services
Assistant Professor
Pediatric Emergency Medicine
University of Pittsburgh School of Medicine
Pittsburgh, Pennsylvania

Alexandre T. Rotta, MD, FCCM

Linsalata Family Chair in Pediatric Critical Care and
Emergency Medicine
Chief
Division of Pediatric Critical Care Medicine
UH Rainbow Babies and Children's Hospital
Professor
Department of Pediatrics
Case Western Reserve University School of Medicine
Cleveland, Ohio

Mark E. Rowin, MD

Associate Professor of Pediatrics
University of Tennessee College of Medicine, Chattanooga
Pediatric Intensivist
The Children's Hospital at Erlanger
Chattanooga, Tennessee

Lewis P. Rubin, MD

Emeritus Professor
Department of Medicine
University of California - San Diego
La Jolla, California

Randall Ruppel, MD

Assistant Professor of Pediatrics
Virginia Tech Carilion School of Medicine
Medical Director
Neonatal/Pediatric Transport Team
Carilion Clinic Children's Hospital
Roanoke, Virginia

Rita M. Ryan, MD

Chair and Professor
Department of Pediatrics
Medical University of South Carolina
Pediatrician-in-Chief
MUSC Children's Hospital
Charleston, South Carolina

Ahmed Said, MD, PhD

Instructor of Pediatrics
Pediatric Critical Care Medicine
Washington University School of Medicine
St. Louis, Missouri

Nagela Sainte-Thomas, BS, MS, MD

Pediatric Emergency Medicine
El Paso Children's Hospital
El Paso, Texas

Rosanne Salonia, MD

Department of Pediatric Critical Care
University of Pittsburgh Medical Center
Pittsburgh, Pennsylvania

Devaraj Sambalingam, MD, MRCPCH(UK)

Assistant Professor
Division of Neonatology
Department of Pediatrics
Texas Tech University Health Sciences Center
El Paso, Texas

L. Nelson Sanchez-Pinto, MD

Assistant Professor, Section of Critical Care
Department of Pediatrics
University of Chicago
Chicago, Illinois

Mary Sandquist, MD

Fellow
Division of Critical Care Medicine
Cincinnati Children's Hospital Medical Center
Cincinnati, Ohio

Ajit A. Sarnaik, MD

Assistant Professor of Pediatrics
Wayne State University
Critical Care Medicine
Children's Hospital of Michigan
Detroit, Michigan

Ashok P. Sarnaik, MD

Professor of Pediatrics
Wayne State University
Critical Care Medicine
Children's Hospital of Michigan
Detroit, Michigan

Georges Saumon, MD

UFR de Medecine
University of Paris
Paris, France

Robert Sawin, MD

Surgeon-in-Chief
General Surgery, Oncology, and Transplantation
Professor of Surgery
Seattle Children's Hospital/University of Washington
Seattle, Washington

Matthew C. Scanlon, MD, CPPS

Pediatric Critical Care Specialist
Children's Hospital of Wisconsin
Professor
Medical College of Wisconsin
Milwaukee, Wisconsin

Kenneth A. Schenkman, MD, PhD

Associate Professor
Department of Pediatrics
Pediatric Critical Care Medicine
Seattle Children's Hospital/University of Washington
School of Medicine
Seattle, Washington

Stephen M. Schexnayder, MD

Professor of Pediatrics and Internal Medicine
University of Arkansas for Medical Sciences
Chief of Staff
Arkansas Children's Hospital
Little Rock, Arkansas

Charles L. Schleien, MD, MBA

Philip Lanzkowsky Professor and Chair of Pediatrics
Cohen Children's Medical Center
Hofstra Northwell School of Medicine
New Hyde Park, New York

George J. Schwartz, MD

Professor and Chief
Pediatric Nephrology
University of Rochester Medical Center
Rochester, New York

Steven M. Schwartz, MD, MS, FRCPC

Head
Division of Cardiac Critical Care Medicine
The Hospital for Sick Children
Toronto, Ontario, Canada

Hayden T. Schwenk, MD, MPH

Clinical Assistant Professor
Pediatric Infectious Diseases
Stanford School of Medicine
Palo Alto, California

Gabrielle Douthitt Seibel, ARNP

Odessa Brown Sickle Cell Program
Seattle Children's Hospital/University of Washington
Seattle, Washington

Dennis W.W. Shaw, MD

Professor of Radiology
Department of Radiology
University of Washington
Seattle, Washington

Steven L. Shein, MD

Pediatric Critical Care Medicine
UH Rainbow Babies and Children's Hospital
Assistant Professor of Pediatrics
Case Western Reserve University School of Medicine
Cleveland, Ohio

Charles W. Shepard, MD

Pediatric Cardiology
Children's Heart Clinic
Minneapolis, Minnesota

Michael Shoykhet, MD, PhD

Assistant Professor of Pediatrics
Pediatric Critical Care Medicine
The Mallinckrodt Department of Pediatrics
Washington University School of Medicine
St. Louis, Missouri

Dennis W. Simon, MD

Assistant Professor
University of Pittsburgh School of Medicine
Pittsburgh, Pennsylvania

V. Ben Sivarajan, MD, MS, FRCPC

Associate Professor
Pediatrics
Pediatric Cardiac Intensive Care Unit
Division of Pediatric Critical Care
Department of Pediatrics
Stollery Children's Hospital and University of Alberta
Hospitals
Faculty of Medicine
University of Alberta
Edmonton, Alberta, Canada

Peter Skippen, MD

Clinical Professor
BC Children's Hospital
University of British Columbia
Vancouver, British Columbia, Canada

Lincoln S. Smith, MD

Associate Professor of Pediatrics
Pediatric Critical Care Medicine
Seattle Children's Hospital/University of Washington
Seattle, Washington

Michael C. Spaeder, MD, MS

Assistant Professor
Pediatric Critical Care
University of Virginia School of Medicine
Charlottesville, Virginia

Richard H. Speicher, MD

Medical Director
Pediatric Intensive Care Unit
UH Rainbow Babies and Children's Hospital
Associate Professor of Pediatrics
Case Western Reserve University School of Medicine
Cleveland, Ohio

Philip C. Spinella, MD

Associate Professor, Department of Pediatrics
St. Louis Children's Hospital
Washington University School of Medicine
St. Louis, Missouri

Stephen Standage, MD

Assistant Professor
Pediatrics
University of Washington School of Medicine
Seattle, Washington

David M. Steinhorn, MD

Professor of Pediatrics
Children's National Medical Center
Washington, DC

Claire Stewart, MD

Clinical Fellow
Division of Critical Care Medicine
Cincinnati Children's Hospital Medical Center
Cincinnati, Ohio

Elizabeth A. Storm, MD

Assistant Professor of Pediatrics
University of Arkansas for Medical Sciences
Arkansas Children's Hospital
Little Rock, Arkansas

Michael H. Stroud, MD

Assistant Professor of Pediatrics
University of Arkansas for Medical Sciences
Arkansas Children's Hospital
Little Rock, Arkansas

Erik Su, MD

Director of Critical Care Ultrasound
Division of Pediatric Anesthesiology and Critical Care
The Johns Hopkins University School of Medicine
Baltimore, Maryland

Robert M. Sutton, MD, MSCE

Associate Professor of Anesthesiology
Critical Care and Pediatrics
The Children's Hospital of Philadelphia
Perelman School of Medicine at the University of
Pennsylvania
Philadelphia, Pennsylvania

Jordan M. Symons, MD

Professor of Pediatrics
Department of Pediatrics
University of Washington School of Medicine
Seattle, Washington

Julie-An Talano, MD

Associate Professor
Children's Hospital of Wisconsin
Milwaukee, Wisconsin

Robert T. Tamburro, Jr., MD

Program Officer
Pediatric Trauma and Critical Illness Branch
National Institute of Child Health and Human Development
Rockville, Maryland

Robert C. Tasker, MBBS, MD, FRCP

Professor of Neurology and Anaesthesia (Pediatrics)
Harvard Medical School
Senior Associate Physician
Department of Anesthesiology, and Perioperative Pain
Medicine
Division of Critical Care Medicine
Boston Children's Hospital
Boston, Massachusetts

Ann E. Thompson, MD, MHCPM

Professor
Critical Care Medicine
Vice Dean
University of Pittsburgh School of Medicine
Pittsburgh, Pennsylvania

Ann H. Tilton, MD

Professor of Neurology and Pediatrics
Section Chair
Child Neurology
Louisiana State University Health and Sciences Center
Co-Director
Children's Hospital Rehabilitation Center
Children's Hospital of New Orleans
New Orleans, Louisiana

Joseph D. Tobias, MD

Chief
Department of Anesthesiology and Pain Medicine
Nationwide Children's Hospital
Professor of Anesthesiology and Pediatrics
The Ohio State University
Columbus, Ohio

I. David Todres, MD†

Department of Anesthesia and Critical Care Medicine
Massachusetts General Hospital
Harvard Medical School
Boston, Massachusetts

Troy Torgerson, MD, PhD

Associate Professor
Pediatrics
University of Washington
Seattle, Washington

Chani Traube, MD, FAAP, FCCM

Associate Professor of Clinical Pediatrics
Division of Pediatric Critical Care Medicine
Weill Cornell Medicine
New York, New York

Marisa Tucci, MD

Professor
Division of Pediatric Intensive Care
Department of Pediatrics
Sainte-Justine Hospital
Université de Montréal
Montreal, Quebec, Canada

David A. Turner, MD, FCCM, FCCP

Associate Director
Graduate Medical Education
Duke University Hospital and Health System
Associate Professor
Department of Pediatrics
Duke Children's Hospital/Duke University School of
Medicine
Durham, North Carolina

†Deceased

Alan H. Tyroch, MD, FACS, FCCM

Professor and Founding Chair of Surgery
Texas Tech University Health Sciences Center El Paso
Chief of Surgery and Trauma Medical Director
University Medical Center of El Paso
El Paso, Texas

Alisa Van Cleave, MD

Assistant Professor
Division of Pediatric Critical Care Medicine
Attending Physician
Pediatric Advanced Care Team
Seattle Children's Hospital/University of Washington
Seattle, Washington

Meredith G. van der Velden, MD

Associate in Critical Care Medicine
Boston Children's Hospital
Instructor of Anesthesia
Harvard Medical School
Boston, Massachusetts

David J. Vaughan, MD

Executive Director of Quality and Safety
Hamad Medical Corporation
Doha, Qatar

Erika Vazquez, MD

Pediatric Emergency Medicine
El Paso, Texas

Shekhar T. Venkataraman, MD

Professor
Critical Care Medicine
University of Pittsburgh School of Medicine
Pittsburgh, Pennsylvania

Mihaela Visoiu, MD

Assistant Professor of Anesthesiology
Children's Hospital of Pittsburgh
Pittsburgh, Pennsylvania

Amélie von Saint André-von Arnim, MD

Assistant Professor
Department of Pediatrics
Division of Pediatric Critical Care Medicine
Department of Global Health (Adjunct)
Seattle Children's Hospital/University of Washington
Seattle, Washington

Surabhi B. Vora, MD, MPH

Assistant Professor
Pediatric Infectious Diseases
Seattle Children's Hospital/University of Washington
Seattle, Washington

Alpana Waghmare, MD

Assistant Professor
Pediatric Infectious Diseases
Seattle Children's Hospital/University of Washington
Seattle, Washington

Mark S. Wainwright, MD, PhD

Founders' Board Chair in Neurocritical Care
Professor of Pediatrics and Neurology
Northwestern University Feinberg School of Medicine
Evanston, Illinois
Director
Ann and Robert H. Lurie Children's Hospital of Chicago
Chicago, Illinois

Martin Wakeham, MD, FAAP

Pediatric Critical Care
Children's Hospital of Wisconsin
Assistant Professor
Medical College of Wisconsin
Milwaukee, Wisconsin

Carol A. Wallace, MD

Professor
Pediatrics
Seattle Children's Hospital/University of Washington
Seattle, Washington

Jessica S. Wallisch, MD

Pediatric Critical Care Fellow
Critical Care Medicine
University of Pittsburgh
Pittsburgh, Pennsylvania

R. Scott Watson, MD, MPH

Professor
Department of Pediatrics
Pediatric Critical Care Medicine
Seattle Children's Hospital/University of Washington
Seattle, Washington

Ashley N. Webb, MSc, PharmD, DABAT

Director
Kentucky Regional Poison Control Center of Kosair
Children's Hospital
Louisville, Kentucky

Scott L. Weiss, MD, MSCE

Assistant Professor of Critical Care and Pediatrics
Department of Anesthesia and Critical Care
The Children's Hospital of Philadelphia
Perelman School of Medicine at the University of
Pennsylvania
Philadelphia, Pennsylvania

Jesse Wenger, MD

Assistant Professor of Pediatrics
Critical Care
Seattle Children's Hospital/University of Washington
Seattle, Washington

Derek S. Wheeler, MD, MMM
Chief of Staff
Professor and Associate Chair
Clinical Affairs
Division of Critical Care Medicine
Cincinnati Children's Hospital Medical Center
Cincinnati, Ohio

Harry Wilson, MD
Associate Professor
Pathology
Texas Tech University Health Sciences Center
El Paso, Texas

Hector R. Wong, MD
Professor of Pediatrics
Director
Critical Care Medicine
Cincinnati Children's Hospital Medical Center
Cincinnati, Ohio

Ellen Glenn Wood, MD
Professor of Pediatrics
Division of Pediatric Nephrology
Pediatrics
Saint Louis University
Cardinal Glennon Children's Medical Center
St. Louis, Missouri

Alan D. Woolf, MD, MPH
Associate Chief Medical Education Officer
Director, Pediatric Environmental Health Center
Boston Children's Hospital
Professor of Pediatrics
Harvard Medical School
Boston, Massachusetts

Beryl F. Yaghmai, MD
Pediatrics
Wesley Healthcare
Wichita, Kansas

Ofer Yanay, MD
Associate Professor
Department of Pediatrics
Division of Critical Care
Seattle Children's Hospital/University of Washington
Seattle, Washington

Danielle M. Zerr, MD, MPH
Professor
Pediatric Infectious Diseases
Seattle Children's Hospital/University of Washington
Seattle, Washington

Hengqi (Betty) Zheng, MD
Fellow
Gastroenterology and Hepatology
Seattle Children's Hospital/University of Washington
Seattle, Washington

Jerry J. Zimmerman, MD, PhD, FCCM
Professor of Pediatrics and Anesthesiology
Faculty
Pediatric Critical Care Medicine
Seattle Children's Hospital
Harborview Medical Center
University of Washington School of Medicine
Seattle, Washington

Preface

Wandering through the exhibit hall of the Toronto Convention Center and the 8th World Congress of Pediatric Critical and Intensive Care Medicine, I am beginning to compose the text of these forward comments in my head. Although pediatric critical care medicine has embraced a global perspective from the beginning, the international flavor of this meeting is particularly striking. Perhaps this reflects the fact that the pediatric critical care medicine fellowship training program at the Hospital for Sick Children has always been a melting pot for trainees around the world. Poster presentations and associated rich discussions here suggest that all pediatric critical care practitioners face similar challenges. Without a doubt the fifth edition embodies the spirit of pediatric critical care medicine as I am experiencing it in person here in Toronto.

At the Elsevier booth I spot a mock-up of the fifth edition of *Pediatric Critical Care*. Even though I know that one should not judge a book by its cover, I must say, the cover looks pretty good, and moreover, I know the contents of the book are outstanding. Once again, all of the effort involved in this revision appears worthwhile. This notion is affirmed by colleagues from all over the world who take time from their busy schedules to make a point of telling me that they are anxious to receive their copy of the latest edition later this year. Meanwhile, I am aware that authors and section editors continue to review final proofs of their chapters, and Monica Relvas continues to encourage contributors to provide board review questions in the correct format. Subsequently I travel back to Chicago where Brad Fuhrman and I first met to design the first edition of *Pediatric Critical Care* in 1990. At that time, just 3 years after the first board certification exam, our field was considerably less mature than what I witness daily in the Seattle Children's Hospital intensive care units and at national and international meetings.

From the beginning, pediatric critical care medicine has embraced the concept of multidisciplinary care including engagement of the family in the care plan, but brief review of the contents of Section I of the fifth edition documents how far we have come. The vision espoused by the Institute for Patient and Family Centered Care—engagement of patients and families in the critical care plan—took shape around the same time as the first edition of this textbook. Neonatal and pediatric intensive care units were understandably early adaptors of this philosophy. Now, multiinstitutional quality improvement initiatives like ICU Liberation and the Patient-Centered Outcomes Research-Intensive Care Unit Collaborative endeavor to enhance family engagement, not because of some ethical imperative but because this practice improves clinically meaningful, long-term outcomes. In order to maximize the benefits of family engagement, the patient must be awake enough to participate. Accordingly, the evolved approach to analgesia and anxiolysis now focuses on comfort and pain control while minimizing sedation.

Basic research scientists in translational collaboration with bedside critical care providers have enhanced our understanding of organs, cells, molecular biology, and now genetics with the ever-present goal of making the critically ill child whole again. Advances in our understanding of cardiovascular, pulmonary, neurologic, renal, gastrointestinal, metabolic, endocrine, and hematologic disorders, infectious diseases, and traumatic injury are chronicled throughout the fifth edition. Such understanding reflects a marked increase in the traditional research and quality improvement productivity of our specialty.

Two centuries ago Ignaz Semmelweis was ridiculed for his radical views on care provider handwashing. Two decades ago handwashing was regarded as important but was not regularly practiced. Today hand cleansing before and after patient contact is considered a mandatory quality measure and, as one element of a bundle of practices, validated with collaborative, multiinstitutional data, has been associated with a sustained plummet in catheter-related bloodstream infections and hospital-acquired infections in general. Like our hematology-oncology colleagues, pediatric intensivists need to develop a culture of a learning health care system, where clinical care and research are so intertwined that each cannot be separated from the other and each continuously informs the other. Every child in an intensive care unit should be a potential candidate for enrollment into a clinical investigation that ideally has been informed by translated basic research.

Although computer technology and the electronic medical record have enhanced care of our patients in many ways, an unanticipated consequence has been the movement of critical care practitioners away from the bedside and into a room with multiple computer stations. Even though modern care providers may have a wealth of information at their fingertips, if not at the bedside, the provider is missing the essence of critical care medicine: continuous titration and advancement of care, particularly weaning of support when it is no longer indicated; serial physical and ultrasonographic examinations; discussion with other care providers; sitting on the bed, holding the patient's hand, if only for a moment or two. Sir Samuel Luke Fildes captured the basic nature and quality of (critical care) medicine in his 1891 painting, *The Doctor*. It is worth taking a look to reconnect with what is ultimately the most important aspect of our specialty.

Years ago Peter Safar reminded us that critical illness begins and ends outside of the intensive care unit and hospital. Thanks in part to our neonatology colleagues and to our own success, children with chronic, comorbid conditions increasingly comprise the majority of admissions to pediatric intensive care units. As mortality associated with pediatric critical illness has steadily declined over the past several decades, critical care practitioners are acknowledging and addressing the substantial and enduring morbidity burden that many children and families surviving critical illness "take home." Almost certainly, the next large clinical interventional trial in pediatric critical care will need to examine a composite outcome measure that includes both mortality and morbidity.

With this fifth edition of *Fuhrman and Zimmerman's Pediatric Critical Care,* we are proud to deliver a contemporary, comprehensive overview of the discipline. New and updated text, extensive figures and tables, electronic supplemental information, board review questions, and Expert Consult online all enhance the effectiveness of this latest edition. We are indebted to our families and colleagues for condoning our

absence or inattentiveness to other matters, to the many dedicated authors who collaboratively have once again composed a gold standard textbook for the field of pediatric critical care medicine, and to the staff of Elsevier whose patience and expertise ultimately brought all things together.

Jerry J. Zimmerman, MD, PhD
Bradley P. Fuhrman, MD
Co-editors, *Pediatric Critical Care*

Contents

| Section I | Pediatric Critical Care: The Discipline |

1 History of Pediatric Critical Care Medicine 3
Daniel L. Levin, John J. Downes, and I. David Todres[†]

2 High-Reliability Pediatric Intensive Care Unit: Role of Intensivist and Team in Obtaining Optimal Outcomes 19
Derek S. Wheeler and Richard J. Brilli

3 Subspecialization Within Pediatric Critical Care Medicine 25
Ann E. Thompson

4 Critical Communication in the Pediatric Intensive Care Unit 35
Shelina M. Jamal, Katherine Banker, and Harris P. Baden

5 Professionalism in Pediatric Critical Care 40
Bradley P. Fuhrman

6 Nurses in Pediatric Critical Care 43
Patricia A. Moloney-Harmon and Martha A.Q. Curley

7 Research in Pediatric Critical Care 52
Robinder G. Khemani and Martha A.Q. Curley

8 Proving the Point: Evidence-Based Medicine in Pediatric Critical Care 61
R. Scott Watson, Mary E. Hartman, and Derek C. Angus

9 Prediction Tools for Short-Term Outcomes Following Critical Illness in Children 66
Michael C. Spaeder and Murray M. Pollack

10 Long-Term Outcomes Following Critical Illness in Children 73
Francois Aspesberro, Jerry J. Zimmerman, and R. Scott Watson

11 Safety and Quality Assessment in the Pediatric Intensive Care Unit 82
Matthew C. Scanlon and Martin Wakeham

12 Information Technology in Critical Care 90
L. Nelson Sanchez-Pinto, Steven Pon, and Barry Markovitz

13 Building Partnerships: Patient- and Family-Centered Care in the Pediatric Intensive Care Unit 104
Jonna Derbenwick Clark

14 Ethics in Pediatric Intensive Care 112
Mithya Lewis-Newby and Douglas S. Diekema

15 Ethical Issues in Death and Dying 122
Meredith G. van der Velden and Jeffrey P. Burns

16 Palliative Care in the Pediatric Intensive Care Unit 127
Alisa Van Cleave, Eileen Rhee, and Wynne Morrison

17 Process of Organ Donation and Pediatric Donor Management 135
Thomas A. Nakagawa

18 Pediatric Transport: Shifting the Paradigm to Improve Patient Outcome 149
Kate Felmet, Richard A. Orr, Yong Y. Han, and Kimberly R. Roth

19 Pediatric Vascular Access and Centeses 158
Sanjiv Pasala, Elizabeth A. Storm, Michael H. Stroud, Punkaj Gupta, Nahed El-Hassan, Thomas J. Lee, Olivia K. Irby, Xiomara Garcia-Casal, and Stephen M. Schexnayder

20 Emerging Role of Ultrasonography in the Pediatric Intensive Care Unit 181
Erik Su, Akira Nishisaki, and Thomas Conlon

21 Pediatric Critical Care in Resource-Poor Settings 201
Amélie von Saint André-von Arnim and Niranjan (Tex) Kissoon

22 Educating the Intensivist 208
Mary W. Lieh-Lai, Denise M. Goodman, David A. Turner, and Katherine Cashen

23 Lifelong Learning 219
Carrie A. Phillipi and Laura Marie Ibsen

24 Public Health Emergencies and Emergency Mass Critical Care 226
Robert K. Kanter,[†] Carl O. Eriksson, and Mary A. King

| Section II | Cardiovascular System |

25 Structure and Function of the Heart 235
V. Ben Sivarajan and Steven M. Schwartz

[†]Deceased

26 Regional Peripheral Circulation 254
    Peter Oishi, Julien I. Hoffman, Bradley P. Fuhrman, and
    Jeffrey R. Fineman

27 Endothelium and Endotheliopathy 270
    Yves Ouellette

28 Principles of Invasive Monitoring 279
    Molly V. Dorfman and Kenneth A. Schenkman

29 Assessment of Cardiovascular Function 292
    Melvin C. Almodovar, Thomas J. Kulik,
    and John R. Charpie

30 Myocardial Dysfunction, Extracorporeal Life
    Support, and Ventricular Assist Devices 302
    Ana Lía Graciano, Umesh Joashi, and Keith C. Kocis

31 Echocardiographic Imaging: Noninvasive Cardiac
    Diagnostics 325
    John L. Bass and Charles W. Shepard

32 Diagnostic and Therapeutic Cardiac
    Catheterization 341
    Alan W. Nugent

33 Pharmacology of the Cardiovascular System 352
    Naomi B. Bishop, Bruce M. Greenwald,
    and Daniel A. Notterman

34 Cardiopulmonary Interactions 380
    Bradley P. Fuhrman and Ronald A. Bronicki

35 Disorders of Cardiac Rhythm 392
    Frank A. Fish and Prince J. Kannankeril

36 Shock States 417
    Lincoln S. Smith, Srinivasarao Badugu,
    and Lynn J. Hernan

37 Pediatric Cardiopulmonary Bypass 430
    Richard M. Ginther, Jr., and Joseph M. Forbess

38 Critical Care After Surgery for Congenital
    Cardiac Disease 447
    V. Ben Sivarajan and Alexandre T. Rotta

39 Cardiac Transplantation 480
    F. Jay Fricker

40 Acute and Chronic Heart Failure 488
    Meaghan Doherty, Alejandro Lopez-Magallon, and
    Ricardo Munoz

41 Physiologic Foundations of Cardiopulmonary
    Resuscitation 499
    Adnan M. Bakar, Kenneth E. Remy,
    and Charles L. Schleien

42 Performance of Cardiopulmonary Resuscitation in
    Infants and Children 526
    Robert M. Sutton, Robert A. Berg, and Vinay M. Nadkarni

| Section III | Respiratory System |

43 Structure and Development of the Upper
    Respiratory System in Infants and Children 539
    Robert H. Chun and Joan C. Arvedson

44 Structure and Development of the Lower
    Respiratory System in Infants and Children 547
    John E. Baatz and Rita M. Ryan

45 Physiology of the Respiratory System 556
    Mark J. Heulitt and Katherine C. Clement

46 Noninvasive Respiratory Monitoring and
    Assessment of Gas Exchange 567
    Beryl F. Yaghmai and Kenneth A. Schenkman

47 Overview of Breathing Failure 577
    Katherine V. Biagas, Robert K. Kanter,[†] Navyn Naran,
    and Bradley P. Fuhrman

48 Ventilation/Perfusion Inequality 589
    Thomas V. Brogan and David J. Vaughan

49 Mechanical Dysfunction of the Respiratory
    System 595
    J. Julio Pérez Fontán

50 Specific Diseases of the Respiratory System:
    Upper Airway 612
    David Jardine, Andrew Inglis, Jr., and Agnes I. Hunyady

51 Pediatric Acute Respiratory Distress Syndrome 627
    Lincoln S. Smith and Robinder G. Khemani

52 Ventilator-Induced Lung Injury 636
    Jean-Damien Ricard, Nicolas de Prost, Alexandre T. Rotta,
    Georges Saumon, and Didier Dreyfuss

53 Asthma 646
    Steven L. Shein, Richard H. Speicher, Howard Eigen, and
    Alexandre T. Rotta

54 Neonatal Respiratory Disease 662
    Devaraj Sambalingam and Lewis P. Rubin

55 Pneumonitis and Interstitial Disease 682
    Daiva Parakininkas

56 Diseases of Pulmonary Circulation 706
    Satyan Lakshminrusimha and Vasanth H. Kumar

57 Mechanical Ventilation and Respiratory Care 734
    Shekhar T. Venkataraman

58 Noninvasive Ventilation: Concepts
    and Practice 770
    Shekhar T. Venkataraman

[†]Deceased

59 Extracorporeal Life Support 785
    Heidi J. Dalton, Tom Preston, and Hanneke IJsselstijn

Section IV   Central Nervous System

60 Structure, Function, and Development of the
    Nervous System 809
    Michael Shoykhet and Robert S.B. Clark

61 Brain Malformations 832
    Robert H. Bonow, Isaac Josh Abecassis, and Samuel R. Browd

62 Neurologic Assessment and Monitoring 842
    Mark S. Wainwright

63 Neuroimaging 857
    Gisele E. Ishak and Dennis W.W. Shaw

64 Pediatric Neurocritical Care 877
    Michael J. Bell and Mark S. Wainwright

65 Coma and Depressed Sensorium 883
    Tony Pearson-Shaver and Renuka Mehta

66 Intracranial Hypertension and Brain
    Monitoring 897
    Robert C. Tasker and Marek Czosnyka

67 Status Epilepticus 913
    Edward E. Conway, Jr.

68 Hypoxic-Ischemic Encephalopathy:
    Pathobiology and Therapy of the
    Postresuscitation Syndrome in Children 929
    *Ericka L. Fink, Robert S.B. Clark, Hülya Bayir,
    Cameron Dezfulian, and Patrick M. Kochanek*

69 Pediatric Stroke and Intracerebral
    Hemorrhage 951
    Catherine Amlie-Lefond and Jeffrey Ojemann

70 Central Nervous System Infections and Related
    Conditions 965
    Erin P. Reade, Dennis W. Simon, and Mark E. Rowin

71 Acute Neuromuscular Diseases and Disorders 984
    Ann H. Tilton

Section V   Renal, Fluids, Electrolytes

72 Renal Structure and Function 997
    Maury N. Pinsk and Victoria F. Norwood

73 Fluid and Electrolyte Issues in Pediatric Critical
    Illness 1007
    Robert Lynch, Ellen Glenn Wood, and Tara M. Neumayr

74 Tests of Kidney Function in Children 1026
    Ayesa N. Mian and George J. Schwartz

75 Glomerulotubular Dysfunction and Acute
    Kidney Injury 1040
    Cristin D.W. Kaspar and Timothy E. Bunchman

76 Acid-Base Disorders 1061
    Hector Carrillo-Lopez, Adrian Chavez, and Alberto Jarillo

77 Renal Pharmacology 1098
    Douglas L. Blowey

78 Pediatric Renal Replacement Therapy in the
    Intensive Care Unit 1105
    Raj Munshi and Jordan M. Symons

79 Acute Severe Hypertension 1114
    Joseph T. Flynn

**Section VI   Metabolism, Endocrinology,
and Nutrition**

80 Cellular Respiration 1131
    *Scott L. Weiss, Clifford S. Deutschman,
    and Lance B. Becker*

81 Biology of the Stress Response 1145
    Stephen Standage and Jerry J. Zimmerman

82 Inborn Errors of Metabolism 1151
    Cary O. Harding

83 Genetic Variation in Health and Disease 1168
    David Jardine

84 Molecular Foundations of Cellular Injury:
    Apoptosis and Necrosis 1173
    Rohit Mittal, John D. Lyons, and Craig M. Coopersmith

85 Common Endocrinopathies in the Pediatric
    Intensive Care Unit 1178
    Ofer Yanay and Jerry J. Zimmerman

86 Diabetic Ketoacidosis 1196
    Ildiko H. Koves and Nicole Glaser

87 Nutrition in the Critically Ill Child 1205
    Nilesh M. Mehta

Section VII   Hematology-Oncology

88 Structure and Function of Hematopoietic
    Organs 1225
    Seth J. Corey and Julie Blatt

89 Erythron in Critical Illness 1234
    Ahmed Said, Stephen Rogers, and Allan Doctor

90 Hemoglobinopathies 1246
    M.A. Bender and Gabrielle Douthitt Seibel

91 Coagulation and Coagulopathy in Critical Illness 1261
    Robert I. Parker

92 Thrombosis in Pediatric Intensive Care 1282
    Sally Campbell and Paul Monagle

93 Transfusion Medicine in the Pediatric Intensive
    Care Unit 1295
    Jacques Lacroix, Marisa Tucci, Oliver Karam, and
    Philip C. Spinella

94 Hematology and Oncology Problems in the
    Intensive Care Unit 1312
    Jesse Wenger, Rebecca Gardner, and Joan S. Roberts

95 Critical Illness Involving Children Undergoing
    Hematopoietic Cell Transplantation 1325
    Jennifer McArthur, Christine Duncan, Prakad Rajapreyar,
    Julie-An Talano, and Robert T. Tamburro, Jr.

Section VIII   Gastrointestinal System

96 Gastrointestinal Structure and Function 1345
    David M. Steinhorn

97 Disorders and Diseases of the Gastrointestinal
    Tract and Liver 1358
    Claire Stewart and Samuel A. Kocoshis

98 Applications of Gastrointestinal
    Pharmacology 1372
    Susan Jacob, Silvia M. Hartmann, Ada Kong, and
    Nicole L. Richardson

99 Acute Liver Failure, Liver Transplantation, and
    Extracorporeal Liver Support 1382
    Simon Horslen and Hengqi (Betty) Zheng

100 Acute Abdomen 1394
    Robert Sawin and Derya Caglar

Section IX   Immunity and Infection

101 Innate Immune System 1403
    Samiran Ray, Rachel S. Agbeko, and Mark J. Peters

102 Adaptive Immunity 1413
    W. Joshua Frazier, Kristin C. Greathouse, and
    Jennifer A. Muszynski

103 Congenital Immunodeficiency 1422
    Troy Torgerson

104 Acquired Immune Dysfunction 1440
    Gwenn E. McLaughlin and Brent J. Pfeiffer

105 Immune Balance in Critical Illness: SIRS, CARS, and
    Immunoparalysis 1454
    Mark W. Hall

106 Pediatric Rheumatic Disease: Diagnosis, Treatment,
    and Complications 1462
    Alexandra R. Aminoff and Carol A. Wallace

107 Bacterial and Fungal Infections, Antimicrobials,
    and Antimicrobial Resistance 1475
    Deborah E. Franzon, Hayden T. Schwenk, and
    Mihaela Damian

108 Life-Threatening Viral Diseases and Their
    Treatment 1485
    Surabhi B. Vora, Alpana Waghmare, Danielle M. Zerr, and
    Ann J. Melvin

109 Infectious Syndromes in the Pediatric Intensive
    Care Unit 1497
    Srinivas Murthy and Peter N. Cox

110 Hospital-Acquired Infection in the
    Pediatric Intensive Care Unit: Epidemiology
    and Control 1506
    Srinivas Murthy and Peter Skippen

111 Sepsis 1520
    Matthew N. Alder, Mary Sandquist, and Hector R. Wong

112 Multiple Organ Dysfunction/Failure Syndrome in
    Children 1541
    Joseph A. Carcillo

Section X   Environmental Hazards

113 Bites and Stings 1553
    Alfredo Maldonado, Nagela Sainte-Thomas,
    and Erika Vazquez

114 Heat Injury 1562
    Ofer Yanay and Eli Gilad

115 Accidental Hypothermia 1567
    Björn Gunnarsson and Christopher M.B. Heard

116 Drowning 1572
    Ajit A. Sarnaik, Mary W. Lieh-Lai, and Ashok P. Sarnaik

117 Burn and Inhalation Injuries 1582
    Phylicia D. Dupree, Amy T. Makley, and Richard J. Kagan

Section XI   Pediatric Trauma

118 Evaluation, Stabilization, and Initial Management
    After Multiple Trauma 1599
    Alan H. Tyroch, Susan F. McLean, and Chet Moorthy

119 Severe Traumatic Brain Injury in Infants
    and Children 1613
    Patrick M. Kochanek, Michael J. Bell, Hülya Bayir,
    Travis C. Jackson, Jessica S. Wallisch, Michael J. Forbes,
    Randall Ruppel, P. David Adelson, and Robert S.B. Clark

120 Thoracic Injuries in Children 1638
     Tamara N. Fitzgerald

121 Abdominal Trauma in Pediatric Critical Care 1644
     Susan F. McLean and Alan H. Tyroch

122 Child Abuse 1655
     *Paula M. Mazur, Lynn J. Hernan, Sitratullah Maiyegun, and
     Harry Wilson*

123 Violence-Associated Injury Among
     Children 1663
     Jesus Peinado and Marie Leiner

Section XII   Pharmacology and Toxicology

124 Principles of Drug Disposition in the
     Critically Ill Child 1673
     Jeffrey L. Blumer

125 Molecular Mechanisms of Drug Actions: From
     Receptors to Effectors 1689
     Catherine Litalien and Pierre Beaulieu

126 Adverse Drug Reactions and Drug-Drug
     Interactions 1707
     *Wade W. Benton, Christa C. Jefferis Kirk, Tsingyi Koh, and
     Gretchen A. Linggi Irby*

127 Principles of Toxin Assessment
     and Screening 1728
     Alan D. Woolf

128 Toxidromes and Their Treatment 1736
     Ashley N. Webb and Prashant Joshi

**Section XIII   Anesthesia Principles for the Pediatric
Intensive Care Unit**

129 Airway Management 1751
     Ann E. Thompson and Rosanne Salonia

130 Anesthesia Effects and Organ System
     Considerations 1776
     Alison M. Jeziorski, Antonio Cassara, and Peter J. Davis

131 Anesthesia Principles and Operating Room
     Anesthesia Regimens 1786
     Joseph D. Tobias

132 Malignant Hyperthermia 1801
     *Mihaela Visoiu, Ericka L. Fink,
     and Barbara W. Brandom*

133 Neuromuscular Blocking Agents 1810
     Joseph D. Tobias

134 Sedation and Analgesia 1827
     Christopher M.B. Heard and Omar Al Ibrahim

135 Tolerance, Withdrawal, and Dependency 1862
     Joseph D. Tobias

136 Pediatric Delirium 1869
     Chani Traube and Bruce M. Greenwald

Pediatric Critical Care: The Discipline

History of Pediatric Critical Care Medicine*

Daniel L. Levin, John J. Downes, and I. David Todres[†]

"In critical care, it strikes one that the issues are three: realism, dignity, and love."

Jacob Javitz, 1986 (inspirational award honoree, Society of Critical Care Medicine, posthumously)

PEARLS

- The evolution of pediatric critical care medicine reflects long progress in anatomy, physiology, resuscitation and ventilation, anesthesia, anesthesiology, neonatology, pediatric general and cardiac surgery, and pediatric cardiology.
- The role of nursing is absolutely central to the evolution of critical care units.
- Until the 1950s and 1960s, intensive care units were organized by grouping patients with similar diseases, but in the 1960s neonatal intensive care units grouped children according to age and severity of illness, and pediatric intensive care units followed this example.
- Sophisticated interhospital transfer services proved significant in reducing morbidity and mortality of critically ill children starting in the1970s. This *retrieval medicine* holds great promise for future improvements in care.
- In pediatric critical care medicine there have been remarkable achievements in the ability to understand and treat critical illness in children as well as progress in the organization of pediatric critical care medicine, education, and research in the field.
- Increasing use of improved technology has advanced the care of critically ill children but has not eliminated errors, complications, or potentially long-term sequelae, and it is associated with a need for greater focus on establishing a humane, caring environment for the patients and their families.

*The work is supported, in part, by the Susan J. Epply Endowment, Children's Hospital at Dartmouth (DLL).
†Deceased.

Evolution of Modern Medicine

The evolution of pediatric critical care medicine (PCCM) reflects a long series of contributions from anatomy, physiology, resuscitation and ventilation, anesthesia, anesthesiology, neonatology, pediatric general and cardiac surgery, pediatric cardiology and the many individuals responsible for the discoveries and innovations.[1,2] Intensive care units were originally organized by grouping together patients with the same or similar diseases but, when neonatologists grouped children according to age and severity of illness, pediatric intensive care units (PICUs) followed their example. Transport or *retrieval medicine* developed and nurses took on a major role in providing care to critically ill and injured children.

Anatomy and Physiology

What seems simple and obvious today took a great deal of time, effort, and insight to understand. This section discusses some of the contributions that advanced medicine, enabled the development of cardiorespiratory support, and, eventually, led to the establishment of intensive care.

Andreas Vesalius (1514–1564), the Flemish anatomist, corrected many previous mistakes in anatomy and provided positive pressure ventilation via a tracheotomy tube to asphyxiated fetal lambs. Michael Servetus of Spain (1511–1553) correctly described the pumping action of the heart's ventricles and the circulation of blood from the right heart through the lungs to the left heart. Unfortunately he was burned at the stake at the hands of the radical Calvinists in Geneva for his published theologic views. Matteo Realdo Columbo (1515–1559) described pulmonary circulation and the concept that the lungs added a spirituous element to the blood by the admixture of air. William Harvey (1578–1657), with his genius, published *De Motu Cordis*[3] (On the Motion of the Heart) in 1628. Because he did not yet have the microscope, he could not see the capillaries and thus could not include the mechanism for transfer of blood from the arterial to the venous system of the pulmonary circulation. Capillaries were first described by Marcello Malpighi (1628–1694, Italian) in *De Pulmonibus* (On the Lungs) in 1661. Thomas Willis (1611–1675) and, eventually, William Cullan (1710–1790) led the way to our understanding of the role of the nervous system as the site for consciousness and the regulation of vital phenomena. Richard Lower (1631–1691) proved it was the passage of blood through the lungs, ventilation of the lungs, and gas exchange with blood that vivified the blood and turned it red. Stephen Hales (1677–1761) measured blood pressure with a brass tube connected to a 9-foot glass tube in a horse. Joseph Black (1728–1799) identified carbon dioxide as a gas expired from human lungs.

Karl Wilhelm Scheele (1742–1785) isolated oxygen, as did Joseph Priestley (1733–1804), who named it dephlogisticated air and determined its vital role in supporting combustion. Antoine Laurent Lavoisier (1743–1794) identified oxygen as the vital element taken up by the lungs that maintains life and gave it its name (literally *acidgenerator*). Oxygen's essential role in physiology and biochemistry was not clarified until the late 19th century when Felix Hoppe-Seyler (1825–1895) described the transportation of oxygen in blood by hemoglobin.

Giovannni Morgagni (1682–1771) initiated the field of anatomic pathology in his classic book *De Sedibus et causis morborum per anatomen indagatis* published in 1761. He described in detail his observations of the diseased organs in more than 700 autopsies of persons with a wide variety of disorders and made correlations with the patient's appearance and symptoms, the initial clinical-pathologic basis of medicine. In 1842 Crawford Long in Georgia and in 1846 William Morton in Boston demonstrated the efficacy and safety of ether anesthesia, thereby opening the era of modern surgery. Joseph Lister (1827–1912), one of the founders of modern surgery, reasoned that bacteria were the source of pus in rotten organic material and in 1865 used carbolic acid in surgical fields to eliminate bacteria. This technique dramatically improved patient outcomes from surgical wounds and after surgery. Along with the discovery of antibiotics, antiseptic technique was an important step in patient care. Nonetheless, imperfect antiseptic technique, sepsis, inflammation, and the consequences of multiorgan failure still represent a major portion of what pediatric intensivists deal with today. Robert Koch (1843–1910) developed his postulates in 1882 in order to attribute the etiology of a disease to a particular microorganism in a logical, scientific manner. He also identified the tubercle bacillus as the cause of tuberculosis and was awarded the Nobel Prize in 1905. Wilhelm Konrad von Röntgen (1845–1923) discovered x-rays in 1895. Scipione Riva-Rocci (1863–1937), in 1896, measured blood pressure using the sphygmomanometer, and Nikolai Korotkoff introduced his auscultation method of determining systolic and diastolic pressure in 1905.[1]

Resuscitation and Ventilatory Support

The key to understanding the present practice of intensive care for children lies in knowing the history of scientific study of cardiorespiratory anatomy and physiology and the discovery of techniques to support ill patients. Although one could think our current practice suddenly emerged with the late 20th century, technical discoveries and accomplishments in the development of resuscitation and ventilation taken for granted today date back to the Bible, and numerous events and contributions led to current practice. In a biblical story,[1,4,5] Elisha resurrected a young boy who was dead when "he climbed onto the bed and stretched himself on top of the child, putting his mouth to his mouth, his eyes to his eyes, and his hands to his hands, and as he lowered himself onto him the child's flesh grew warm.... Then the child sneezed and opened his eyes."

In 117 CE, Antyllus performed tracheotomies for patients with upper airway obstruction.[6] Paracelsus, a sixteenth-century Swiss alchemist and physician, first provided artificial ventilation to both animals and dead humans using a bellows,[6] and Andreas Vesalius, a Flemish professor of anatomy, in De Humani Corporis Fabrica, reported ventilating open-chest dogs, fetal lambs, and pigs using a tracheostomy and fireplace bellows in 1543.[7-9]

The French obstetrician Desault, in 1801, described how to successfully resuscitate apneic or limp newborns by digital orotracheal intubation with a lacquered fabric tube and then blowing into the tube.[1] In 1832 Dr. John Dalziel in Scotland developed a bellows-operated intermittent negative pressure device to assist ventilation.[8] In 1864 Alfred F. Jones, of Lexington, Kentucky, built a body-enclosing tank ventilator, and in the 1880s Alexander Graham Bell developed a so-called vacuum jacket driven by hand-operated bellows.[8] In 1876 Woillez, in Paris, built what was probably the first workable iron lung, which was strikingly similar to the respirator introduced by McKhann and Drinker in 1929 and manufactured for widespread use by Emerson in 1931.[10] Braun developed an infant resuscitator, as described by Doe in 1889, which was used successfully in 50 consecutive patients. A respirator developed by Steuart in Cape Town, South Africa, in 1918 apparently successfully treated a series of polio patients, but he did not report it.[8]

In 1888 Joseph O'Dwyer, a physician working at the New York Foundling Hospital who was concerned about the high death rate in croup and laryngeal diphtheria, instituted the manual method of blind oral laryngeal intubation using short tapered brass tubes that entered the subglottic lumen. Despite severe criticism from associates and the other practitioners, he persisted assembling a series of various diameter tubes for the palliation of severe adult and pediatric laryngeal edema due to infections, including diphtheria.

George Fell, another New York physician, devised a method of ventilation with a foot-operated bellows and exhalation valve connected by rubber tubing to the O'Dwyer tube (Fig. 1.1).[8] In 1898 Rudolph Matas of New Orleans adapted the

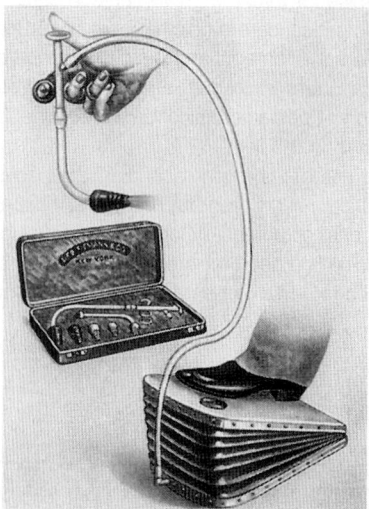

Fig. 1.1. Fell-O'Dwyer respiratory apparatus. (Reproduced with permission, Blackwell Scientific Publications, Oxford.)

Fell-O'Dwyer technique to perform chest wall surgery and, in the early 1900s, George Morris Dorrance of Philadelphia used the technique to perform resuscitations.[8] In 1910, at the Trendelenburg Clinic in Leipzig, two thoracic surgeons, A. Lawen and R. Sievers, developed a volume-preset, positive pressure, electrically powered piston-cylinder ventilator with a draw-over humidifier. It was used with a tracheotomy tube during and after thoracic surgery and for a variety of disorders causing respiratory failure.[1]

Over a long career, Chevalier Jackson (1858–1955), a surgeon at Temple University in Philadelphia, developed techniques for laryngoscopy, bronchoscopy, and tracheotomy.[1] He revolutionized the procedure of tracheotomy and developed a detailed protocol of airway care. His design of tubes, made of silver, for patients of all ages set the standard for tracheotomy tubes for more than the first half of the 20th century.

In 1958 Peter Safar, then at the Baltimore City Hospital, published studies proving that the long-standing pulmonary resuscitation technique of chest-pressure arm lift was virtually worthless. In effect, he went back to Elisha and proved jaw thrust and mouth-to-mouth resuscitation superior.[11] Soon after, W.B. Kouwenhoven and James Jude at Johns Hopkins published work on the effectiveness of closed-chest cardiac massage.[12] Beck and his team, in 1946, had demonstrated open-chest electrical defibrillation. In 1952 Zoll and coworkers proved the efficacy of external defibrillation and, in 1956, the effectiveness of external cardiac pacing.[13]

Contributions of Specific Disciplines
Pediatric Anesthesiology
PCCM developed initially through the efforts of pediatric anesthesiologists, as well as pediatric general and cardiac surgeons and neonatologists. In fact, most of the original PICUs were founded by pediatric anesthesiologists (Table 1.1).[1,4,14-24] Before discrete, geographically separate, intensive care units evolved, critically ill children often received close monitoring, intensive nursing care, and pulmonary support in the postanesthetic recovery room. There the anesthesiologists were the attending physicians with the requisite knowledge and skills for this effort. In addition to those PICUs noted in Table 1.1, there were certainly others that were not as well documented.

Pediatric General and Cardiac Surgery
Dr. William E. Ladd (1880–1967) at Boston Children's Hospital (BCH) pioneered the development of many techniques to operate on non-cardiac congenital malformations. His protégé, Dr. Robert Gross, first successfully operated on patent ductus arteriosus in 1937 and later on other congenital cardiac lesions.

Dr. C. Crawfoord in Sweden and Dr. Gross in Boston both successfully repaired a coarctation of the aorta in 1945. In the same year, at Johns Hopkins, Drs. Alfred Blalock (surgeon) and Helen Taussig (cardiologist) with Mr. Vivien Thomas (laboratory assistant) created the subclavian-to-pulmonary artery shunt for tetralogy of Fallot. Dr. John Gibbon at Jefferson Medical College Hospital in Philadelphia performed the first successful open-heart surgery using cardiopulmonary bypass for closure of an atrial septal defect in an adolescent girl in 1953.[1] These advances in pediatric surgery created the need for excellent and often complex postoperative care.

Dr. C. Everett Koop, who had completed surgical residency at the University of Pennsylvania in 1945, then trained in Boston with Dr. Gross for 6 months. He returned to the University of Pennsylvania and the Children's Hospital of Philadelphia (CHOP) in 1946. With the help of Dr. Leonard Bachman, director of anesthesiology, and the nursing staff, Dr. Koop developed the first neonatal surgical intensive care unit in 1962. Dr. Bachman and his young associate, John J. Downes, subsequently set up the first full PICU in North America in 1967 at CHOP.

Neonatology
Pediatric critical care owes a great debt to neonatologists and their special care nurseries.[1,4,25] The first and most prominent of these was established in the 1880s in Paris by obstetrician Etienne Tarnier and his young associate Pierre Budin at the Hospital la Charitre with a unit that had a full-time dedicated nursing staff, incubators, gavage feeding of breast milk, and aseptic practices. These practices reduced hospital preterm infant mortality in less than a decade from 197/1000 live births to 46/1000 live births. Their work presaged the development of modern neonatal intensive care in the 20th century. In 1914 the first premature infant center in the United States was opened at Michael Reese Hospital in Chicago by Dr. Julius Hess (1876–1955). Canadian pediatrician Dr. Alfred Hart performed exchange transfusions involving peripheral artery cannulation in 1928. In 1932 Drs. Louis Diamond, Kenneth Blackfan, and James Batey at BCH determined the pathophysiology of hemolytic anemia and jaundice of erythroblastosis fetalis, and in 1948 they described exchange transfusions using a feeding tube inserted in the umbilical vein.

In the 1950s and 1960s Dr. Geoffrey Dawes at the Nuffield Institute for Medical Research at Oxford University, using fetal and newborn lambs, described for the first time the fetal and transitional circulation of mammalian newborns. In the late 1950s, Columbia University's obstetrical anesthesiologist Virginia Apgar, who had devised the Apgar score for assessing birth asphyxia, recruited Dr. L. Stanley James to develop animal and human investigation of the transitional pulmonary-cardiovascular adaptation during labor, delivery, and the postnatal period. Dr. James and his team at Columbia, and Dr. Abraham Rudolph, a South African pediatric cardiologist, and his team at Albert Einstein Medical Center in New York City and subsequently at the Cardiovascular Research Institute in San Francisco, performed extensive studies in fetal lambs, rhesus monkeys, and term and preterm human newborns that defined the human cardiopulmonary adaptation to delivery and postnatal life. They also determined the biochemical factors and time course of birth asphyxia and recovery. In 1959 a research fellow at Harvard, Dr. Mary Ellen Avery (with mentor Dr. Jere Mead), discovered deficiency of alveolar surfactant in lungs of newborns dying from respiratory distress syndrome (RDS). This discovery led to a better understanding of neonatal pulmonary disorders and eventually led to the intratracheal instillation of surfactant in newborn preterm infants to prevent or mitigate the severity of respiratory distress syndrome. In the 1960s state-of-the-art neonatal ICUs were established at Colombia-Presbyterian Hospital (Dr. Silverman), University of Pennsylvania (Dr. Boggs), Vanderbilt University (Dr. Stahlman), Toronto Hospital for Sick Children (Dr. Swyer), and the University of California at San Francisco (Dr. Tooley).

TABLE 1.1	Some Early Pediatric Intensive Care Units and Programs[a]		
Year	**Institution/Location**	**Medical Director(s)**	**Director(s) Specialty[b]**
1955	Children's Hospital, Göteborg, Sweden	G. Haglund	Ped Anesth.
1961	St. Goran's Children's Hospital, Stockholm, Sweden	H. Feychting	Ped Anesth.
1961	Great Ormond Street Children's Hospital, London, England	W. Glover	Ped Anesth.
1963	Hospital St. Vincent de Paul, Paris, France	J. B. Joly G. Huault	Neonatology Neonatology
1963	Royal Children's Hospital, Melbourne, Australia	I. H. McDonald J. Stocks	Ped Anesth. Ped Anesth.
1963	Adelaide Children's Hospital, Adelaide, Australia	T. Allen I. Stevens	Ped Anesth. Ped Anesth.
1964	Alden Hey Children's Hospital Liverpool, England	G. J. Rees	Ped Anesth.
1967	Children's Hospital of Philadelphia, Philadelphia, Pennsylvania	J. J. Downes	Ped Anesth.
1967	Children's Memorial Hospital, Chicago, Illinois	D. Allen F. Seleny J. Cox	Ped Anesth. Ped Anesth. Ped Anesth.
1968[c]	Children's Hospital District of Columbia, Washington, DC[d]	C. Berlin	Ped.
1968	Children's Hospital Calvo Mackenna, Santiago de Chile	E. Bancalari	Ped.
1969	Children's Hospital of Pittsburgh, Pittsburgh, Pennsylvania	S. Kampschulte	Ped Anesth.
1969	Yale-New Haven Medical Center, New Haven, Connecticut	J. Gilman N. Talner	Ped Anesth. Ped Cardiol.
1970[e]	Hospital for Sick Children, Toronto, Canada	A. Conn	Ped Anesth.
1971	Massachusetts General Hospital, Boston, Massachusetts	D. Shannon I. D. Todres	Ped Pulm. Ped. & Ped. Anesth.
1971	Long Island Jewish Hospital, New York	B. Holtzmann	Ped Pulm.
1971	Montefiore Hospital, New York	R. Kravath	Ped Pulm.
1972	Sainte Justine Hospital, Montreal, Canada	M. Weber A. Lamarre	Ped. Ped Pulm.
1972	Children's Hospital "Dr. R. Guiterrez," Buenos Aires, Argentina	J. Sasbon	Ped.
1972	Children's Hospital "Pedro Elizade," Buenos Aires, Argentina	C. Bonno	Ped.
1972	Hospital for Sick Children, Edinburgh, Scotland	H. Simpson	Pulmonology
1974	Red Cross Children's War Memorial Hospital, Cape Town, South Africa	M. Klein	Ped Pulm.
1975	Private Hospital, Uruguay	M. Gajer	Ped.
1975	Children's National Hospital Medical Center, Washington, DC	P. R. Holbrook A. Fields	Ped. Ped.
1975	Children's Medical Center, Dallas, Texas	D. Levin F. Morriss	Ped. Ped. & Ped Anesth.
1976	Hospital Infantil La Paz, Madrid, Spain	F. Ruza	Ped.
1977	Johns Hopkins Medical Center, Baltimore, Maryland	M. C. Rogers S. Nugent	Ped. & Ped Anesth.
1977	Sheba Medical Center, Israel	F. Barzilay	Ped.
1977	Children's Hospital of San Diego, San Diego, California	B. Peterson	Ped. & Ped Anesth.
1977	Hospital de Clinicas, Sao Paulo, Brazil	A. Wong	Ped.
1978	Hospital Sãa Lucas da Puers, Porto Alegre, Brazil	P. Celiny R. Garcia	Ped.
1978	Sophia's Children's Hospital, Rotterdam, Netherlands	E. van der Voort H. van Vught	Ped. Ped.
1978	Children's Hospital of Los Angeles, Los Angeles, California	E. Arcinue	Ped.
1979	University of Minnesota Hospital, Minneapolis, Minnesota	B. Fuhrman	Ped.
1979	Hospital de Clinicas de Porto Alegre, Brazil	P. R. Carvhalho	Ped.
1980	Moffett Hospital, San Francisco, California	G. Gregory	Ped Anesth.
1980	Children's Hospital Boston, Boston, Massachusetts	R. Crone	Ped. & Ped. Anesth.

[a]This is not intended to be an absolutely complete list. It is primarily comprised of units well documented in the literature and personally known to the authors.
[b]Primary specialties (not all inclusive).
[c]Although conceptual development of unit started in 1965, Dr. Berlin states the first year of operation of the present ICU was in 1969 (opened December 1968).
[d]Columbia Hospital District of Columbia was a precursor of Children's National Hospital Medical Center.
[e]This 20-bed state-of-the art unit followed an experience with four designated beds in the PACU beginning in 1964.
Adapted from references 1, 4, 14–24.

Pediatric Cardiology

As previously indicated, the vision of Dr. Taussig in devising a method to treat *blue babies* and successful cardiac operations led to infants and children who survived surgery and needed postoperative intensive care. Advances in technology, especially for imaging, have allowed clinicians to "see" into living patients with astounding accuracy. Increased understanding of anatomy and physiology has led to improved surgical and nonsurgical care for children with complex cardiopulmonary problems. Developments in cardiac catheterization and interventional radiology have enabled clinicians to treat many lesions without open-heart surgery and potentially difficult postoperative intensive care. This concept was introduced in 1968 by Dr. William Rashkind at CHOP with the introduction of the balloon atrial septostomy for infants with transposition of the great arteries. Growth of techniques that allow effective intervention in many complex cardiac conditions, both nonsurgical and surgical, has resulted in many pediatric centers creating specific cardiac intensive care units often run by pediatric cardiac intensivists. Cognitive impairment in some infants with complex lesions or chromosomal abnormalities and the occasional development of chronic respiratory failure with dependence on mechanical ventilation for months or years are two of the occasional major sequelae of these highly successful endeavors. The value of PCCM for these cardiac patients and other critically ill children has been well documented by Dr. Jacqueline Noonan who noted, "Much success of the surgery can be attributed to a group of pediatric intensivists, pediatric intensive care units, improved ventilatory support, and trained respiratory therapists."[26]

Early Use of Mechanical Ventilation in Neonates and Children

The first series of carefully observed infants and children with respiratory failure was published in 1959. In that year, Drs. P.M. Smythe (pediatrician) and Arthur Bull (anesthesiologist) reported the first real success in mechanical ventilation of a series of neonates with respiratory failure caused by neonatal tetanus. These infants were paralyzed with curare to relax the tetanic muscle spasms and ventilated for 4 to 14 days using tracheotomy and a modified Radcliff adult ventilator.[27] Up until that time, infants or children were rarely given ventilator support for more than a few hours, with either adult ventilators or manual ventilation. Neither specifically designed pediatric ventilators nor small volume blood gas analysis was available. Dr. Smythe had to overcome these obstacles by innovation. Due to local cultural practices, Bantu children from tribal areas were particularly prone to develop tetanus. On July 13, 1957, at Groote Schuur Hospital, he performed a tracheostomy and began intermittent positive pressure ventilation for these infants with the assistance of anesthesiologist Dr. Bull. This was truly a landmark event in the evolution of PCCM. Although considered a success story in that it was the first time infants survived up to several weeks of positive pressure mechanical ventilation, the first seven of nine patients died. Eventually their survival rate reached 80% to 90%. They commented, "No praise can be too high for the nursing staff, who were all student nurses and without any special training." David Todres, a medical student at that time, was giving curare to and observing these infants, sparking his interest in critical care.

In 1963–1964 in Toronto, Drs. Paul Swyer, Maria Delivoria-Papadopoulos, and Henry Levison were the first to successfully treat a series of moribund premature infants with RDS and respiratory failure. They used positive pressure mechanical ventilation and supportive care[28] and emphasized the importance of a full-time team, including dedicated nurses and therapists as well as physicians. In 1968 Dr. George Gregory and colleagues at the University of California at San Francisco demonstrated improved survival with early use of continuous positive airway pressure (CPAP) without assisted ventilation or with positive end-expiratory pressure (PEEP) added to the mechanical ventilation regimen.[29] A prerequisite for successful long-term mechanical ventilation was the ability to maintain an endotracheal tube. An important contribution to the development of intensive care and long-term mechanical ventilation was the use of plastic endotracheal tubes for prolonged intubation and ventilation. Dr. Bernard Brandstater, an Australian trained in Adelaide, Philadelphia, London, and San Francisco and working at the American Hospital in Beirut, Lebanon, reported prolonged nasotracheal intubation as an alternative to the tracheostomy at the First European Congress of Anesthesia in Vienna in 1962.[30]

Progress in treating a disorder leads to unforeseen complications and new disorders. Successful treatment of RDS led to some survivors with chronic lung disease (bronchopulmonary dysplasia [BPD]), retinopathy of prematurity, and hypoxic brain injury, conditions that remain significant today. Pediatric intensive care allows successful treatment of disorders previously considered hopeless, but it also results in small numbers of infants and children with long-term problems that require study, clinical commitment, and long-term advocacy for them and their families.

Poliomyelitis and Creation of the First Intensive Care Units

Poliomyelitis epidemics occurred worldwide in the early 20th century but seemed especially severe in Western Europe and North America. There was no treatment and, until the late 1920s, no effective life support for those victims with respiratory failure. Fortunately, the confluence of great scientific and clinical minds and the organizational efforts of physicians, nurses, and therapists addressing the needs of polio patients led to the creation of dedicated polio respiratory care units for patients of all ages. In 1929 Philip Drinker, an engineer, with pediatricians Louis Shaw and Charles F. McKhann at BCH published their experience with an electrically powered negative pressure, body-enclosing mechanical ventilator, later termed the *iron lung* (Fig. 1.2).[10,31]

Polio outbreaks occurred in the summer months worldwide in the 1930s and 1940s. The polio epidemics of the early 1950s were very severe in Los Angeles and Copenhagen. In 1952 Dr. H. C. Lassen, the chief epidemiologist at Blegdam Hospital in Copenhagen, described treating 2772 patients with polio. Of these, 316 were in respiratory failure and initially received assisted ventilation with iron lungs in a large respiratory care unit. During that summer, they had a census of as many as 70 patients in respiratory failure in that unit. Unfortunately the mortality of patients supported by an iron lung ventilator was nearly 90%, with the cause of death frequently being unrecognized upper airway obstruction. When the census of patients

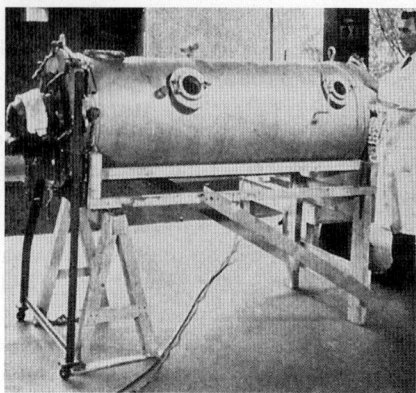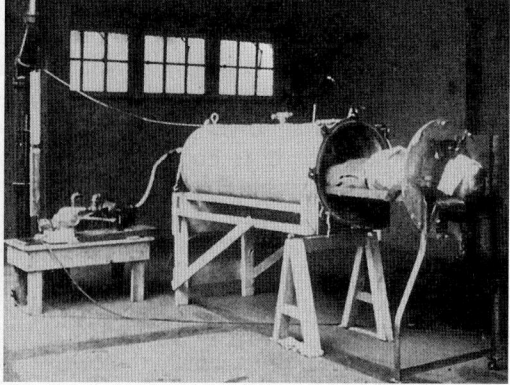

Fig. 1.2. Drinker negative pressure mechanical ventilator. (Reproduced with permission, Blackwell Scientific Publications, Oxford.)

in respiratory failure exceeded the available number of iron lung ventilators, Bjorn Ibsen, the chief of anesthesiology at the hospital, with the help of his medical staff and nurse anesthetists, performed tracheal intubation and then tracheostomy along with manual positive pressure ventilation with 50% oxygen and tracheal suctioning. This care was carried out in 200 patients with respiratory failure. To provide continuous manual ventilation on a 24-hour basis, Ibsen recruited, trained, and used 200 nursing students and aides along with 200 medical students each working 8-hour shifts to provide manual ventilation, as well as 27 technicians per day to care for the patients. The mortality in patients receiving this care decreased from 90% to 40%.[32-34]

At that time, patients from outlying areas were sent in ambulances without sufficient attendants or airway care and arrived moribund. Lassen and Ibsen started to send so-called retrieval teams in ambulances out to pick up the patients in the countryside, with marked improvement in status on arrival. They also started passing stomach tubes early on for nutrition, and the rubber-cuffed tracheostomy tubes were replaced with a silver cannula that caused less tracheal mucosal damage. Even with all these improvements Dr. Ibsen noted, "Naturally we ran into a lot of complications."[34]

Drs. Ibsen and Lassen also received help from other people who were focusing their efforts on treating polio. The clinical biochemist Dr. Poul Astrup developed a micro method to measure capillary arterialized pH and PCO_2 in infants, children, and adults. C.G. Engstrom, a Swedish anesthesiologist, designed and clinically tested the first modern volume-preset positive pressure mechanical ventilator. This spectacular and thrilling story culminated in a cohort of patients with respiratory failure being treated in a single geographic area and cared for by full-time physicians, nurses, and technicians: *the first modern intensive care unit*. Although these units tended to disband after the summer-fall polio season, they led to the creation of full-time respiratory care units at the Radcliff Infirmary of Oxford University and elsewhere in Europe and North America in the 1950s.

Soon after these events, in 1958, Peter Safar led development of the first multidisciplinary ICU in North America at Baltimore City Hospital in 1958.[35] In 1960 Barrie Fairley and colleagues created the ICU at Toronto General Hospital followed in 1962 with the ICU at Massachusetts General Hospital under Drs. Henning Pantoppidan and Henrik Bendixen.

Definitions

Some of the difficulty in telling the history of pediatric critical care medicine is defining a PICU and a pediatric intensivist. The current definitions are as follows.

Pediatric Intensive Care Unit

An ad hoc committee of the American Academy of Pediatrics, Diseases of the Chest Section established Guidelines for the Organization of Children's Intensive Care Units in July 1975.[36] In 1983 the American Academy of Pediatrics and Society of Critical Care Medicine published Joint Guidelines for Pediatric Intensive Care Units (PICUs),[37] which were updated in 1993[38] and 2004[39] and then retired in 2013.[40] The committee defined a PICU as "a hospital unit which provides treatment to children with a wide variety of illnesses of life-threatening nature including children with highly unstable conditions and those requiring sophisticated medical and surgical treatment."

Pediatric Intensivist

Randolph and coworkers[41] defined a pediatric intensivist (in the United States) as "any one of the following: (a) a pediatrician with subspecialty training in PCCM and subspecialty certification from the American Board of Pediatrics (ABP); (b) a pediatric anesthesiologist with special competency in critical care with subspecialty certification from the American Board of Anesthesiology; (c) a pediatric surgeon with special competency in critical care with subspecialty certification from the American Board of Surgery; (d) a physician (as above) eligible for subspecialty certification by the appropriate respective board." Similar requirements for training exist or are in development elsewhere in the world.

First Pediatric Intensive Care Units

In 1955 Dr. Goran Haglund at the Children's Hospital of Göteborg, Sweden,[18] developed the first PICU, which he called a pediatric emergency ward. The patient who inspired Dr. Haglund to organize the unit was a 4-year-old boy who was operated on in 1951 for a ruptured appendix. Postoperatively, he lapsed into a coma and the surgeon declared he had done all he could and the boy would die of *bacteriotoxic coma*. The anesthesiologist offered to help and the boy was intubated, given manual positive pressure respiration with generous oxygen, tracheostomized, and given a large blood transfusion. After about 8 hours, the bowels started to function, and 4 hours later he was out of coma. After 20 hours, he had spontaneous respiration and had been successfully treated for respiratory insufficiency and shock.

This new unit had seven acute care beds with full-time nurses and nursing assistants providing 24-hour coverage. In the first 5 years, the team treated 1183 infants and children, with a mortality rate of 13.6%. Haglund went on to state, "But what we did was something else. It was the application of the basic physiology to clinical practice. Our main purpose was not to heal any disease; it was to forestall the death of the patient. The idea was—and is—to gain time, time so that the special medical or surgical therapy can have desired effects."[18] Haglund was also careful to point out that "There are few jobs more exciting, demanding, and taxing than emergency nursing. Our nurses and nurse assistants are tremendous. They must be!"[18]

Central Role of Critical Care Nursing

Although many sources emphasize the role of advanced technology in the creation of adult, neonatal, and pediatric critical care,[1,19] skilled nursing care was even more important in this evolving process. Porter[42] and others remind us of the vital role of nursing in triage and organization of care for patients by degree of illness. Long before the organizational efforts of the 20th century, Florence Nightingale (1820–1920) organized a volunteer service with 20 nurses and created a clean environment at the British military hospital at Skutari, Turkey, in 1854 during the Crimean War. Although the care consisted mostly of hygiene and nutrition, within 6 months of her arrival the mortality rate dropped from 40% to 2%.[43] Nightingale provided the definition of nursing as "helping the patient to live."[43] These efforts were continued in the United States by Dorothea Dix (1802–1887) and Clara Barton (1821–1912), the "Angel of the Battlefield," during the American Civil War. Barton also brought the Red Cross to America in 1882.

As the complexity of medical and surgical care evolved in the late 19th and early 20th century, the need to cohort sick patients and provide skilled nursing care became apparent, especially for the premature newborn and for the victims of poliomyelitis as cited earlier. Then, as now, the recovery of the critically ill pediatric or adult patient depended on the skilled nurse at the bedside who was trained to use the life support and monitoring equipment at hand but to remain focused on the stability and comfort of the person in the bed.

In the mid-to-late 1970s, as pediatric cardiovascular surgery for more complex lesions in infants was developing, nurses provided postoperative care in designated units. Children with Reye syndrome suddenly appeared, requiring complex multisystem care. In addition, in the 1980s emergency medical services (EMS) systems began transporting severely injured children to hospitals, where they required rapid assessment and intervention by nurses and physicians and initiation of cardiorespiratory and neurologic support.[44]

Pediatric critical care nurses joined the Society of Critical Care Medicine and the American Association of Critical Care Nurses emphasizing the care of children. In the mid-1990s, pediatric critical care nurses founded their own society and established a peer-reviewed journal. Also in the 1990s,

advanced practice nurses and nurse practitioners began to specialize in pediatric critical care. They continue to function as important critical care team members to augment both physician and nursing care as well as conduct clinical research.[44,45]

Role of Pediatric Anesthesiologists and Pediatricians in Founding Pediatric Critical Care Medicine

An important, early physician-directed multidisciplinary PICU in North America was established at CHOP in 1967 as an outgrowth of a hospital-wide respiratory intensive care service.[1,46] The unit consisted of an open ward of six beds equipped with bedside electronic monitoring and respiratory support capabilities and an adjacent intensive care chemistry laboratory staffed 24 hours per day. The nurses were assigned full-time to the unit, and most had previously served in the recovery room, the infant ICU, or the cardiac surgery postoperative ward. Dr. John Downes was the medical director and worked closely with two other anesthesiologists, Dr. Leonard Bachman, chief of anesthesiology, and Dr. Charles Richards, and a pediatric allergist/pulmonologist, Dr. David Wood. Four pediatric anesthesiology/critical care fellows provided 24-hour in-unit service. Dr. C. Everett Koop (chief of surgery), Dr. William Rashkind (the father of interventional pediatric cardiology), Dr. John Waldhausen (one of the nation's few full-time pediatric cardiac surgeons and a creative thinker), Dr. Sylvan Stool (a pioneer in pediatric otolaryngology), and other staff and residents provided close, collaborative patient care, education, and clinical research.

In 1969 Dr. Peter Safar and his trainee, Stephen Kampschulte, developed a 10-bed PICU at the Children's Hospital of Pittsburgh. That same year, James Gilman, a pediatric anesthesiologist, and Norman Talner, a pediatric cardiologist, established a six-bed PICU at the Yale-New Haven Medical Center.

In 1970 at the Hospital for Sick Children in Toronto, Dr. Alan Conn resigned as director of the Department of Anesthesiology to become director of a new multidisciplinary 20-bed PICU, by the far the largest and most sophisticated unit in North America. During the prior decade Dr. Conn and his colleagues had cohorted critically ill infants and children in a sequestered area of the postanesthesia care facility where they had developed considerable expertise in critical care. This new state-of-the-art PICU was the forerunner of units developed in major pediatric centers throughout North America throughout the 1970s and beyond. Dr. Geoffrey Barker, who went on to develop one of the largest multinational fellowship training programs in the world, followed Dr. Conn.

Also in 1971 Dr. David Todres, an anesthesiologist and pediatrician, and Dr. Daniel Shannon, a pediatric pulmonologist, founded a 16-bed multidisciplinary unit for pediatric patients of all ages at the Massachusetts General Hospital.[1,4] The units in Philadelphia, Toronto, and Boston established vibrant training programs in critical care medicine and conducted clinical research. Among their numerous accomplishments, Dr. Conn became a noted authority on the management of near-drowning victims, and Dr. Todres and Dr. Downes pioneered long-term mechanical ventilation for children at home with chronic respiratory failure. These early PICUs and their training programs had a favorable impact on mortality and morbidity rates, particularly those associated with acute respiratory failure, leading to the development of similar units and programs in most major pediatric centers in North America, Western Europe, and Japan during the 1970s and early 1980s.

The development of the PICU at Children's Memorial Hospital (CMH), Northwestern University Medical School, Chicago, illustrates how many of the early PICUs evolved. The unit was first started as a four-bed area set in one of the postoperative care wards by pediatric anesthesiologists David Allen and Frank Seleny. Anesthesiologist Dr. John Cox arrived in August of 1964 and was named director. He states the unit never formally opened. It "sort of started" in the four-bed unit in the postoperative ward in 1964 and became a 14-bed separate designed unit in late 1967. Dr. Cox was the director until 1975 when he was succeeded by Dr. Richard Levin. During this time, Dr. Hisashi Nikaidoh, who was a surgery resident in 1966–1967, remembers taking care of a renal transplant patient, and the care was provided by nephrology, general surgery, and immunology without a centralized PICU service. Dr. Zehava Noah, who was educated in Israel and trained in the UK, did a critical care fellowship in anesthesia at CMH, developed a closed medical-surgical PICU in 1979, and was named the director in 1981. There was also an associate surgical director.[47-50]

Some of the early PICUs were directed by pediatricians. In 1966 Dr. Max Klein joined Drs. H. de V. Heese and Vincent Harrison in a two-bed neonatal research unit at the Groote Shuur Hospital in Cape Town. Their research resulted in many significant papers, not the least of which was "The Significance of Grunting in Hyaline Membrane Disease,"[51] demonstrating that oxygen tensions fell when infants were not allowed to grunt. By 1969, at Red Cross War Memorial Children's Hospital in Cape Town, South Africa, pediatric patients with respiratory failure (eg, Guillain-Barré) were ventilated on the general wards, and although outcomes improved, deaths were still common. Dr. Max Klein encouraged Dr. Malcolm Bowie (consultant) to start a six-bed ICU, or "high-care ward." After further training in South Africa and at the University of California San Francisco, in 1974, Dr. Klein returned to Cape Town where he combined the neonatal tetanus ward of Dr. Smythe and the six-bed ICU of Dr. Bowie into the first full-time PICU in South Africa.[52] It took Dr. Klein 25 years of persistent effort to create a nonsegregated PICU.

The path for pediatricians providing care for the sickest patients on a full-time basis remained unclear for an extended period. Subsequent early leaders in the field each carved out their own path. Dr. Daniel Levin completed pediatric cardiology and neonatology fellowships to learn the care of sick children. However he found few Chairs of Pediatrics interested in hiring an "intensivist." Then, in 1975 Drs. Levin and Frances Morriss (trained in pediatrics and pediatric anesthesia) were recruited to start a PICU at Children's Medical Center of Dallas.

There were so few of this new breed of intensivists that many became directors upon completion of residency and fellowship. At the beginning, few other physicians wanted to be responsible for pediatric intensive care.[23] Eventually more pediatricians decided to devote their careers to being members of a multidisciplinary team taking care of the sickest children in hospitals on a full-time basis. In 1975 the CHOP program started to accept PCCM trainees who were pediatricians without anesthesia training.

In 1967 Dr. Peter Holbrook as a medical student at the University of Pennsylvania began a part-time job in the PICU at CHOP and developed a strong interest in PCCM. Informed at the time that one needed anesthesia training to successfully work in the PICU, Holbrook shelved the idea and entered pediatric residency training at Johns Hopkins. When the PCCM idea resurfaced he found that many still felt a physician needed anesthesia training to function in the PICU. Disagreeing with the reasoning behind such a requirement, he pursued critical care training with Dr. Peter Safar in Pittsburgh who welcomed him as a fellow in critical care medicine. In 1975 Dr. Holbrook and pediatrician Dr. Alan Fields, who also trained in Pittsburgh, were recruited to the new, modern Children's Hospital National Medical Center (Washington, DC), as pediatricians in the Department of Anesthesia to direct the PICU.

Dr. Bradley Peterson,[53] after pediatric and neonatology training and an anesthesiology residency at Stanford University, became director of the new PICU at Children's Hospital of San Diego in 1977. Dr. Bradley Fuhrman, following pediatric cardiology and neonatology fellowships, started the first PICU at University of Minnesota Hospital in 1979.[54]

Dr. George Lister,[55] after a pediatric residency at Yale and a fellowship in cardiopulmonary physiology at the University of California San Francisco (UCSF), in 1977 joined the staff at the UCSF Moffitt Hospital San Francisco, as an attending in its combined adult-pediatric ICU. Due to the director's illness, he quickly found himself the co-director of the unit.[55] He eventually returned to Yale as an attending in the PICU and chief of the section of critical care.

Dr. Mark Rogers, after completion of pediatric residency at BCH and anesthesiology residency at Massachusetts General Hospital and pediatric cardiology fellowship at Duke, in 1975 became director of the first PICU at Johns Hopkins Hospital.[56] Subsequently, in 1980 Dr. Rogers became chair of the Department of Anesthesiology and Critical Care Medicine at Johns Hopkins and chief editor of a major textbook of pediatric intensive care (Table 1.2).

Growth of Pediatric Critical Care Medicine

The field of PCCM grew rapidly in the late 1970s and 1980s. However, there was a struggle for authority in both adult and pediatric units. The culture of intensive care was changing from one in which each specialty service cared for its part of the patient to one in which a full-time critical care service cared for the whole patient, with help of consulting specialties.[22,89]

For PCCM to achieve its full potential, it required several elements: a national organization to provide a venue in which to meet and communicate, acceptance and validation of pediatric critical care as a subspecialty, nationally approved training requirements, and academic credibility with meaningful research.

A small group of interested physicians met at the Society of Critical Care Medicine (SCCM) National Meeting in 1979 and decided to petition the SCCM to form a section on pediatrics. The society had no subsections, but the petition was successful, and the pediatric section with Dr. Russell Raphaely as chair was formed in 1980.[1] In 1983 a committee of the SCCM developed guidelines for organization of PICUs,[37] which were

TABLE 1.2   Textbooks in Pediatric Critical Care Medicine

Year First Edition	Title	Editors	Reference
1971	The Care of the Critically Ill Child	R. Jones, J. B. Owen-Thomas	57
1971	Pediatric Intensive Care: Manual	K. Roberts, J. Edwards	58
1972	Nelson's, The Critically Ill Child: Diagnosis and Medical Management	J. Dickerman, J. Lucey	59
1977	Pediatrie d'urgence	G. Huault, H. Labrune	60
1979	A Practical Guide to Pediatric Intensive Care	D. Levin, F. Morriss, G. Moore	61,62,63,64
1980	Tratado de Cuidados Intensivos Pediatrucos (Textbook of Pediatric Intensive Care)	F. J. Ruza	65
1980	Core Curriculum for Pediatric Critical Care Nursing	M. C. Slota	66
1983	Pediatric Critical Care	J. Bloedel Smith	67
1984	Nursing Care of the Critically Ill Child	M. F. Hazinski	68
1984	Textbook of Critical Care	W. K. Shoemaker, W. L. Thompson, P. R. Holbrook	69
1984	Pediatric Intensive Care	E. Nussbaum	70
1985	Temas em Terapia Intensiva (Issues in Pediatric Intensive Care)	J. Piva, P. Carvalho, P. Celiny Garcia	71
1985	Critical Care Pediatrics	S. Zimmerman, J. Gildea	72
1987	Pediatric Intensive Care	J. P. Morray	73
1987	Textbook of Pediatric Intensive Care	M. C. Rogers	74
1992	Pediatric Critical Care	B. P. Fuhrman, J. J. Zimmerman	75
1993	Textbook of Pediatric Critical Care	P. R. Holbrook	76
1994	Urgences & Soins Intensif Pediatriques	J. Lacroix, M. Gauthier, P. Hubert, F. Leclenc, P. Gaudreault	77
1995	Critical Heart Disease in Infants and Children	D. G. Nichols, D. E. Cameron, W. J. Greeley, D. W. Lappe, R. M. Ungerleider, R. C. Wetzel	78
1996	Critical Care of Infants and Children	I. D. Todres, J. H. Fugate	79
1996	Critical Care Nursing of Infants and Children	M. A. Curley, J. Bloedel-Smith, P. A. Moloney Harmon	80
1997	Illustrated Textbook of Pediatric Emergency & Critical Care Procedures	R. A. Dieckmann, D. H. Fiser, S. M. Selbst	81
1997	Pediatric Intensive Care	N. S. Morton	82
2001	Manual de Cuidados Intensivos Pediatricos	J. Lopez-Herce Cid, C. Calvo Rey, M. J. Lorente Acosta, A. Baltodano Aquero	83
2004	Medicinia Intensiva em Pediatria	J. Piva, P. Celiny Garcia	84
2005	Cuidudo Intensivo Pediatrico y Neonatal	J. Forero, J. Alarcon, G. Cassalett	85
2006	Pediatric Critical Care Medicine	A. D. Slonim, M. M. Pollack	86
2006	Manual de Cuidado Intensivo Pediatrico	G. Cassalett, M. C. Patarroyo	87
2007	Pediatric Critical Care Medicine: Basic Science and Clinical Evidence	D. S. Wheeler, H. R. Wong, T. P. Shanley	88

regularly updated[38,39] until January 2013, after which time they were retired.[40]

In 1984, after petitions by pediatric intensivists, a Section of Critical Care Medicine was established in the American Academy of Pediatrics (AAP) with Dr. Russell Raphaely as chair.[90] These organizations then petitioned for recognition of PCCM fellowships from the American College of Graduate Medical Education (ACGME) and for the subspecialty of PCCM by the American Board of Pediatrics (ABP). Legitimization of the subspecialty was achieved with establishment of a new sub-board of Pediatric Critical Care Medicine of the ABP in 1985 and the first certifying examination in 1987, at which time 182 subspecialists were certified.[90] Certification provided a clear basis for hospital credentialing of PCCM physicians.[91] In addition to certification by the ABP, the American Board of Anesthesiology and the American Board of Surgery confer subspecialty certification with special competency in critical care. In 1989 special requirements for training in PCCM were developed by the ACGME with formally accredited programs first recognized in 1990.[92]

Growth in Numbers of Pediatric Intensive Care Units

In 1979 there were 150 PICUs of four or more beds identified, and another 42 thought to exist.[93] Most were just special care nursing units, and only 40% had a pediatric intensivist available at all times. Forty percent of the units had fewer than seven beds and only one half had affiliated transport systems. By 1995, there were 306 and in 2001 there were 349 general PICUs. Of these, 94% had a pediatric intensivist on staff. Pediatric ward beds *decreased* by 22.4% between 1980 and 1989—by 10.8% between 1990 and 1994, and by 15.7% between 1995 and 2000. During the same three time periods, PICU beds *increased* by 26.2%, 19.0%, and 12.9%, respectively.[41]

Growth in Training Programs and Education

In 1983–1984 there were 32 PCCM training programs, and the ACGME accredited 28 of them in 1990. By 2013–2014 the number had increased to 64 accredited training programs with 489 enrolled fellows, of whom about 56% are women.[94] Eighty-five percent of applicants for subspecialty board certification in 2006 intended to work exclusively as intensivists.[94]

Educational programs in PCCM have progressed considerably at the annual SCCM, AAP, Pediatric Academic Societies (PAS), American Thoracic Society (ATS), and American College of Chest Physicians meetings, as well as at independent meetings such as the Pediatric Critical Care Colloquium (PCCC) and the World Federation of Pediatric Intensive Critical Care Societies (WFPICCS). Dr. Barker had the vision of the need to bring together pediatric intensive care from many parts of the world. This led to his founding directorship of the WFPICCS, which has done much to foster development of pediatric critical care around the world, bringing vital critical care skills and experience to benefit multiple countries. Numerous textbooks on PCCM have appeared in many languages (see Table 1.2), and the journal *Pediatric Critical Care Medicine* was launched in 2000.[95]

Academic credibility that results from meaningful scientific research has come slowly. In the early days, intensivists were mostly consumed by clinical and administrative responsibilities, but high-quality science, addressing a broad range of problems, has gradually emerged. Multiinstitutional organizations have allowed studies that require more patients than can be drawn from a single institution to be designed, funded, and completed. In the early 1990s, the Pediatric Critical Care Study Group (PCCSG) was formed.[96] It was followed by the Pediatric Acute Lung Injury and Sepsis Investigators (PALISI) network,[97-99] which employed the successful programmatic model of research developed by the Canadian Critical Care Trials Group (CCCTG).[100-102] PALISI has grown and prospered through the voluntary collaboration of more than 70 North America member PICUs.

The virtual PICU was started in 1997 to bring data management technologies to critical care. In 2004 Virtual PICU Systems (VPS) was formed by Drs. Thomas Rice and Ramesh Sachdeva (Children's Hospital and Health System of Milwaukee) and Dr. Randall Wetzell (Children's Hospital Los Angeles) in conjunction with the National Association of Children's Hospitals and Related Institutions (NACHRI) to develop a PICU registry to facilitate quality improvement and research. VPS currently has more than 125 members and a massive database describing more than 1 million critical care admissions.[103,104]

In April 2004, the *Eunice Kennedy Shriver* National Institute of Child Health and Human Development (NICHD) established funding for the first federally supported network for pediatric critical care research, the Collaborative Pediatric Critical Care Research Network (CPCCRN). The Network is a multicentered program designed to investigate the safety and efficacy of treatment and management strategies to care for critically ill children, as well as the pathophysiologic basis of critical illness and injury in childhood.[105-108]

NICHD has also supported research in PCCM by developing and supporting young investigators in the field through the Pediatric Critical Care and Trauma Scientist Development Program (PCCTSDP), a K-12 research training program. The PCCTSDP, which began in 2004 as the Pediatric Critical Care Scientist Development Program (PCCSDP), entered its third project period in 2014 under the continuing direction of Dr. Michael Dean at the University of Utah and has now expanded to include pediatric trauma physicians as well.[105]

Perhaps most notably, in 2013 NICHD created an independent branch, the Pediatric Trauma and Critical Illness Branch, to further support research in pediatric critical illness and injury. The mission of the new branch is to prevent and reduce all aspects of childhood trauma and critical illness to enhance healthy outcomes for all children across the continuum of care.[105,107,108]

The growth of education and research in PCCM has coincided with, and presumably resulted in, better care for children as reflected in the decrease in mortality from septic shock. During the period from 1958 to 1966, in patients younger than 16 years of age at the University of Minnesota, mortality in septic shock was 95%; now with PICU care it is less than 10%.[109] Drs. Murray Pollack and Timothy Yeh established the basis for studying severity-adjusted mortality in pediatrics and demonstrated that patients do better when cared for by pediatric intensivists.[110] Although many would attribute these improvements to technology and scientific advances, Dr. Yeh and others remind us that the presence of a full-time nursing and medical team and attention to basic principles rather than exotic high technology improve outcomes.[111] This is echoed by Dr. Shann's two rules of PCCM: rule 1 is "the most important thing is to get the basics exactly right all of the time"; rule 2 is "organizational issues are crucially important."[23] In addition, Yeh as well as Ibsen[34] and Orr have emphasized the important contributions of regionalization and the quality of PCCM transport teams in improving outcomes.[112,113]

Organizations, although important, are created, developed, and nurtured by people who devote a great deal of time and effort to their success. Many pediatric intensivists have contributed to these efforts and have been rightfully recognized for that. Some of the individuals from organizations in the United States are listed in Tables 1.3 through 1.6.

Cost of Success in Pediatric Critical Care Medicine

Everything comes at a cost. In the field of PCCM, as in many others, advances have led to increased financial cost, survivors with chronic disease, medical errors, and occasional dehumanization of patients. Accurate estimates of the extraordinary but often necessary financial costs of modern care of the

TABLE 1.3	Chairs, Pediatric Critical Care Medicine Subboard, American Board of Pediatrics[a]
1985-1987	Peter Holbrook, MD
1988-1990	Bradley Fuhrman, MD
1991-1992	Thomas Green, MD
1993-1996	Ann Thompson, MD
1997-1998	Daniel Notterman, MD
1999-2000	David Nichols, MD
2001-2002	Jeffrey Rubenstein, MD
2003-2004	Alice Ackerman, MD
2005-2006	Donald Vernon, MD
2007-2008	Karen Powers, MD
2009-1010	M. Michele Mariscalco, MD
2011-2012	Laura Ibsen, MD
2013-2014	Susan Bratton, MD
2015-2016	James Fortenberry, MD

[a]Medical Editor, 1985-2004, George Lister, MD; 2004, Jeffrey Rubenstein, MD

TABLE 1.4	Pediatric Intensivists Serving as President of Society of Critical Care Medicine
1982	George Gregory, MD
1984	Dharampuri Vidyasagar, MD
1988	Peter Holbrook, MD
1992	Russell Raphaely, MD
2001	Ann Thompson, MD
2004	Margaret M. Parker, MD

TABLE 1.5	Chairs, Executive Committee, Section on Critical Care Medicine, American Academy of Pediatrics
1984-1987	Russell Raphaely, MD
1987-1990	Fernando Stein, MD
1990-1992	J. Michael Dean, MD
1992-1996	Kristan Outwater, MD
1996-2000	Timothy Yeh, MD
2000-2004	M. Michele Moss, MD
2004-2008	Alice Ackerman, MD
2008-2012	Donald Vernon, MD
2012-2014	Edward Conway, Jr., MD

TABLE 1.6	Chairs, Pediatric Section, Society of Critical Care Medicine
1980-1981	Russell Raphaely, MD
1981-1983	Peter Holbrook, MD
1983-1984	Bernard Holtzman, MD
1984-1985	Bradley Furhman, MD
1985-1986	Frank Gioia, MD
1986-1987	Timothy Yeh, MD
1987-1988	Fernando Stein, MD
1988-1989	Thomas Rice, MD
1989-1991	Ann Thompson, MD
1991-1994	J. Michael Dean, MD
1994-1996	Debra Fiser, MD
1996-1998	Tom Green, MD
1998-2000	Daniel Notterman, MD
2000-2002	Richard Brilli, MD
2002-2004	M. Michele Moss, MD
2004-2006	Stephanie Storgion, MD
2006-2008	Edward Conway, Jr., MD
2008-2010	Vicki Montogmery, MD
2010-2012	Jeffrey Burns, MD
2012-2014	Ken Tegtmeyer, MD
2014-2016	Derek Wheeler, MD

did not survive in the 1960s and early 1970s. Although we return many very sick children to complete health, a small number, often with associated complex disorders, survive but live with chronic neurologic, respiratory, cardiac, or renal disease. These children and their families usually require extraordinary medical and social support, and advocacy in order to thrive.

As PICUs have evolved, intensivists have developed greater sophistication in dealing with individual family concerns, pain management, ethical issues, palliative care, social and spiritual needs,[116] cultural differences, and the value of involving families as members of the team by including them on daily rounds.[117] These issues are described in more detail elsewhere in this text.

Since the inception of PCCM, members of the team have experienced long hours of stressful work and occasional feelings of despair and frustration that their efforts are not making a difference. This can lead to emotional distress and a sense of loss of fulfillment in their professional lives. Understanding of this problem by local medical and nursing leaders helps the team members realize they are making an important difference through their efforts and dedication, thereby reducing burnout and enhancing staff morale.[118-120]

Around the World

People around the world have made many contributions to the evolution of PCCM, through innovative treatment of specific diseases, creating PICUs (see Table 1.1), and advancing

critically ill child are difficult to obtain but are frequently high.[114,115]

Children with preexisting chronic disease and an acute critical illness have prolonged PICU stays, frequent readmissions, and the need for intensive care at home or in the rare pediatric subacute facility. Most patients with these conditions education (see Table 1.2[121]). The following discussion highlights the global origins of PCCM but is not intended to be all inclusive.

Canada

As described earlier, Dr. Alan Conn, anesthetist-in-chief at the Hospital for Sick Children, Toronto, envisioned and successfully opened a multidisciplinary PICU for medical and surgical patients in 1971.[122] At the Children's Hospital of Montreal, a medical PICU was created in 1972 by a pediatrician, Dr. Michel Weber, and pulmonologist Dr. Andre Lamarre. Drs. Marie Gauthier, Jacques Lacroix (Universite de Montreal), and John Gordon (McGill University) in 1992 were active in the development and implementation of a fellowship program in PCCM supervised by the Royal College of Physicians and Surgeons of Canada.[123]

South Africa

As noted earlier, in 1959 Drs. P.M. Smythe and Arthur Bull conceived a brilliant therapeutic plan to treat infants afflicted with neonatal tetanus from infected umbilical cord stumps,[27] and Dr. Max Klein continued their tradition at Red Cross Children's War Memorial Hospital, opening a special unit for critically ill children in 1974 with full-time intensivists Dr. Max Klein and Drs. Louis Reynolds, Jan Vermeulen, Paul Roux, and later Andrew Argent.[4,5,124]

Japan

In the 1960s Dr. Seizo Iwai, chief of anesthesia at the National Children's Hospital in Tokyo, was the first Japanese physician to introduce mechanical ventilation and arterial blood gas analysis of critically ill infants, fostering a tradition of anesthesiologists taking care of critically ill infants and children outside of the operating room. He was a strong force in developing a close relationship with other Asian countries and invited trainees from those countries to promote teaching and pediatric critical care development in their homeland. His close working relationship with Drs. Conn and Barker in Toronto paved the way for Dr. Katsuyuki Miyasaka to study in Toronto with Dr. Conn and in Philadelphia with Dr. Downes. Dr. Miyasaka returned to Japan in 1977 and, in October 1994, opened the first geographically distinct PICU in Japan at the National Children's Hospital and helped to found the Japanese Society of Pediatric Intensive Care. He continues to foster the development of a new generation of pediatric intensivists as a hospital director and plays a major role in facilitating this process.[125]

India

Neonatal intensive care units (NICUs) in India were established in the 1960s, first at the All India Institute of Medical Sciences, Delhi, and subsequently at teaching hospitals in other major cities.[126-128]

The first PICUs were established at major postgraduate centers (Delhi, Chennai, Chandigarh, Mumbai, and Lucknow).[129] Growth of PICUs had been mainly in the private sector, although major government teaching hospitals are also improving the PICUs in their locations. An intensive care chapter of the Indian Academy of Pediatrics (IAP) was formed in 1997, and the Pediatric Section of Intensive Care of the Indian Society of Critical Care Medicine (ISCCM) was formed in 1998.[130] Currently, 24 recognized PICUs are accredited for

providing training.[131] Prompt access to the available services is critical for pediatric patients. A study at a children's hospital in Hyderabad, Andhra Pradesh, India, has shown that patients travel long distances (up to 500 km) to seek pediatric critical care, with survival inversely proportional to the distance traveled.[132] To overcome these difficulties, a bold and innovative statewide patient transport program, the Emergency Management and Research Institute (EMRI), was launched in 2005 with a fleet of 70 ambulances deployed in the state of Andhra Pradesh.[132] The public-private collaborative organization has 2500 staff including emergency medical technicians (EMTs), support staff, and associates and a call center in the capital city of Hyderabad.[133]

Australia and New Zealand

As in the United States and Canada, Australian PICUs started forming in the early 1960s, arising from wards that performed postoperative recovery care for children following congenital heart surgery,[134-141] with continuing development of PICUs in major cities. There was creative development in many centers throughout Australia, some of which are Melbourne, Adelaide, Camperdown, Brisbane, and Perth. We will present some of the history and refer the reader to a more detailed account with *AUSPIC News* edited by Frank Shann in 1993.[134]

At the Free Hospital for Sick Children Melbourne, pediatric anesthesiologists Jan H. McDonald and John Stocks developed a 10-bed multidisciplinary PICU. They conducted clinical studies, including a large study demonstrating the safety and efficacy of oral and nasal plastic endotracheal tubes for airway management of children requiring mechanical ventilation.[142]

In Adelaide Children's Hospital, Adelaide, Australia, in the early 1960s, Tom Allen and Ian Steven from the Department of Anesthesia began treating upper airway obstruction with prolonged oral and then nasal intubation.[144] Long-term mechanical ventilation using Bird ventilators commenced in 1963.[143]

Pediatric intensive care was established at Princess Margaret Hospital in Perth by Nerida Dilworth (anesthesia) in the early 1960s. Prolonged nasal intubation was first performed in September 1963. In May 1969, a dedicated area in one of the medical wards was set aside for the care of critically ill children. The first full-time intensivists were appointed in 1986 (Alan Duncan, director, and Paul Swan, specialist). The modern 10-bed pediatric intensive care unit was opened in April 1987.[145]

Matthew Spence, an anesthesiologist, originally from Glasgow, pioneered critical care medicine for adults and children in Auckland Hospital, New Zealand, opening the first adult and pediatric ICU in 1958. Cardiac surgery for children in New Zealand started at Green Lane Hospital, Auckland, in the 1950s, and a dedicated intensive care was established there in 1963, led by the cardiac surgeon Sir Brian Barrett-Boyes and anesthesiologists Drs. Marie Simpson and Eve Scelye. The first specialized pediatric emergency transport service commenced in Victoria in 1980.[146-150]

In March 1991, Elizabeth Segedin was appointed as a full-time pediatric intensivist (with no PICU!) to plan for the development of a pediatric unit. With the building of the new hospital for children in Auckland, intensive care for children was reorganized to a single pediatric intensive care unit at the Starship, which opened on December 2, 1991, with Dr. Segedin as director.

Europe

In Europe, pediatric intensive care followed shortly after the poliomyelitis epidemic in Denmark in 1952. As described previously, in 1955 Dr. Goran Haglund, a pediatric anesthesiologist, established the first medical-surgical PICU for infants and children at the Children's Hospital in Göteborg in Sweden.[28] In 1961 Dr. Hans Feychting, also a pediatric anesthesiologist, established the first PICU at St. Goran's Children's Hospital in Stockholm, Sweden, and became recognized as a pioneer in the development of pediatric intensive care in Europe.

In France, in 1963, a newborn presented with tetanus and was admitted to l'Hôpital des Enfants Malades of Paris. Shortly afterward, Dr. Gilbert Huault and JB Joly, both neonatologists, opened the first multidisciplinary PICU in France at Saint Vincent de Paul Children's Hospital. This unit was the first pediatrician-directed PICU in Europe; it soon became a major influence on the development of PICUs. Drs. Francois Beaufils, Jean Christophe Mercier, and Denis Devictor were to play an important role in further development of European pediatric critical care medicine.[151]

In London, a pediatric anesthesiologist, William Glover, opened a unit for care of postoperative cardiac patients in 1961 at the Hospital for Sick Children in Great Ormond Street. Soon all patients needing ventilator care were admitted to that unit.[152] In 1964 a well-designed discrete 13-bed PICU was developed by Dr. G. Jackson Rees, a pediatric anesthesiologist, at the Alder Hey Children's Hospital in Liverpool. Other units soon followed, essentially serving as areas allowing prolonged postoperative support.[153]

In Spain, pediatrician Dr. Francisco Ruza started working in neonatal surgical intensive care in 1969. In 1976 he opened a multidisciplinary medical-surgical PICU for older infants and children at Hospital Infantil La Paz in Madrid. This center, directed by Dr. Ruza, has served as a major training center for pediatric intensivists not only from Spain but from South America as well.[154] From this center, Dr. Ruza has also promoted the teaching and high-quality research related to pediatric critical pathology.

The first PICUs in the Netherlands were established in the late 1970s and early 1980s at Rotterdam's Sophia Children's Hospital under Edwin van de Voort and Hans van Vught in Rotterdam. PICUs were also developed at Wilhelmina Children's Hospital in Utrecht and Emma Children's Hospital at the Academic Medical Center in Amsterdam.[155] These PICUs are multidisciplinary, and all are part of university teaching hospitals. In 1995 the Dutch Pediatric Association established a section on Pediatric Intensive Care Medicine that certifies training of nearly all Dutch pediatric intensivists. A nationwide transport system connects this centralized care system of pediatric critical care. Units were opened in Germany[156] and Slovakia[157] as well as in Krakow, Poland, and many other European locations.

Israel

Although located in the Middle East, Israel has traditionally been part of European scientific organizations, and most pediatric intensivists in Israel trained in North America. The first PICU in Israel was established in 1977 by Dr. Zohar Barzilay as a five-bed facility located within Children's Hospital at Sheba. Israel now has 12 PICUs and two cardiac PICUs. Extracorporeal membrane oxygenation services as well as cardiac transplantation are provided nationwide as part of the national health insurance program. About 30% of the patients in many of the PICUs in Israel come from the Palestinian Authority. Palestinian physicians trained in PCCM in Israel established the first PICU in Gaza.[158,159]

Latin America

The first PICU in Latin America was established in Argentina at the Dr. Ricardo Gutierrez Children's Hospital in Buenos Aires in 1969 as part of a general surgery ward. In 1972 Dr. Jorge Sasbon became first staff director of the PICU. In 1972 a PICU was set up in Pedro de Elizalde Children's Hospital, Buenos Aries, under guidance of Dr. Clara Bonno.[23]

In Brazil in the 1970s, epidemics of polio and meningococcal disease, with a high mortality, led to the creation of small units for care of these patients. These units were precursors of PICUs later established at Hospital das Clínicas São Paolo by Dr. Anthony Wong (1977), at Hospital São Lucas in Porto Alegre by Dr. Pedro Celiny (1978), at Hospital de Clinicas de Porto Alegre (1979) by Paulo R. Carvalho, and in Rio de Janeiro. In 1982 Dr. Jefferson Piva opened a 13-bed PICU at Hospital da Criança Santo Antonio in Porto Alegre.[160]

One of the pediatric critical care pioneers in Latin America was Dr. Mauricio Gajer, a dedicated physician from Uruguay. Dr. Gajer traveled to France where he worked with Professors Huault and Beaufils. After returning to Uraguay he created the first private PICU in Montevideo, Uruguay, in 1975.

In Colombia, pediatric intensive care started in the early 1960s with postoperative care of cardiovascular patients in Clínica Shaio of Bogotá, with adult cardiologists in charge. Then in the 1970s Dr. Merizalde, a pediatrician with training in pediatric cardiology, provided care for pediatric cardiovascular patients.[161]

In 1956 at Luis Calvo Mackenna Children's Hospital, in Santiago, Chile, a single-bed postoperative care unit was started by Drs. Helmut Jager (cardiac surgeon) and Fernando Eimbecke (cardiologist). In 1968 this evolved into a five-bed PICU led by Dr. Eduardo Bancalari, a neonatologist. He was later joined by pediatricians Drs. Patricio Olivio and Jaime Cordero. In the 1980s additional PICUs developed, including one with Dr. Carlos Casar at Roberto del Rio Children's Hospital in Santiago, Chile, later directed by Dr. Bettina von Dessauer (pediatrician).[162,163] Intensivists there have devoted great effort toward developing a network and transport systems to overcome the impact of Chile's challenging geography.

Similarly, the first intensive care unit in San Jose, Costa Rica, was opened in 1969 at Hospital Nacional de Niños "Dr. Carlos Sáenz H" as a postoperative cardiac care unit. It was initially a nine-bed unit run by anesthesiologists and surgeons. Eventually pediatricians, without special PCCM training, became involved. In 1982 Dr. Aristides Baltodano trained in PCCM in Toronto, becoming the first pediatric intensivist in Costa Rica at Hospital Nacional de Niños "Dr. Carlos Sáenz H." The hospital now has a 22-bed multidisciplinary unit with more than 1000 admissions per year.[164]

Over time a critical care network throughout Latin America has improved access, transport, and specific critical care knowledge in all countries. However, there is still work to do to facilitate access to critical care and achieve results comparable to those in high-resource countries. Sociedad Latin Americana de Cuidados Intensivos Pediatricos (SLACIP) has

TABLE 1.7   Accessibility to Pediatric Critical Care Medicine in High-Mortality Countries

Organization	Program	Purposes	References
SCCM	Pediatric Fundamental Critical Care Support (PFCCS)	1. Prioritize needs 2. Appropriate tests 3. Identify and respond to changing vital signs 4. Need for transport	178,179
BCH	OPEN Pediatrics	Free online educational platform	180,181
AAP	Helping Babies Breathe (HBB)	Neonatal resuscitation	182,183
AHA	Saving Children's Lives and Pediatric Emergency Assessment Programs (PEARS)	Resuscitation training	184
WHO	Integrated Management of Childhood Illness (IMCI)	Identify sick children early	185

played a crucial role. Every 2 years a Latin American Pediatric Intensive Care Congress takes place. A SLACIP symposium prior to each WFPICCS World Congress has become a tradition since the first world congress in Baltimore in 1992. The common language among more than 70 countries with many culture and challenges forms a common bond.

High-Mortality Countries

In 2013 6.3 million children died before age 5 years.[165] Over 95% of these deaths occurred in high-mortality countries, and 52% were caused by infections—especially pneumonia, diarrhea, and malaria—that could be prevented or treated at low cost.[166] Asia, for example, is the world's hot spot for the emergence and reemergence of infectious diseases that threaten the world (ie, severe acute respiratory syndrome [SARS] and influenza) but still has huge burdens of the traditional infectious diseases (malaria, tuberculosis, HIV, diarrhea, dengue, etc.). Asia also leads the world in the emerging and global export of drug resistance to many pathogens, despite undergoing a period of unprecedented economic growth. Approximately 96% of children in the world live and die in resource-poor countries. Replicating success demonstrated in many countries more broadly in India and elsewhere will have an immense impact on national resources. For example, in India, because of the high birth rates (annual births of 25 million) and large pediatric population (35% of total or approximately 300 million), as well as the need for trained people and material resources to service them, the required number of NICU and PICU beds will be enormous. It would therefore seem prudent for all district hospitals (750 in the country) to be upgraded to provide level II services that will meet the needs of rural communities.[167] Increased access to PCCM for those at all economic levels should improve survival and eventually decrease the birth rate once people are more confident their children will live.

Although the development of PICUs is essential for the overall improvement of child survival in developing countries, the high cost of intensive care limits patients' access to PICU services.[168,169] Basic and cost-effective care have proved to have a major impact on improving the survival of infants and children. For example, a study in New Guinea demonstrated that the systematic use of pulse oximetry and supplemental oxygen reduced mortality from pneumonia by 35%.[170] However, the cost was $51 for each child, which is beyond the means for many low-income countries where a high proportion of child

TABLE 1.8   International Pioneer Awards World Federation of Pediatric Intensive Critical Care Societies[a]

Name	Country
Alan Conn, MD	Canada
John Downes, MD	United States
Hans Feychting, MD	Sweden
Maurico Gajer, MD	Uruguay
Gilbert Huault, MD	France
Seigo Iwai, MD	Japan
Max Klein, MD	South Africa
John Stocks, MD	Australia

[a]Awarded Montreal, 2000.

deaths occur.[171] Because hospital care is often not available to children in high-mortality countries, several authors have emphasized the need for preventive measures and improved primary health care.[172-177] It is therefore important to train health care personnel and families in early detection of infants and children at high risk for mortality from infections and sepsis, which lead to critical disorders such as respiratory failure. Prompt initiation of treatment can reduce the need for critical care services (Table 1.7).

Summary

The evolution of PCCM has been long and complex. It owes a great deal to innovations in anatomy, physiology, ventilation and resuscitation, anesthesia, anesthesiology, neonatology, pediatric general and cardiac surgery, pediatric cardiology, and nursing as well as to the many individuals who advanced these fields around the world. Any attempt to relate the history of PCCM is inherently incomplete. Several individuals have been recognized for their contributions to PCCM in general, and we recognize them now (Tables 1.8, 1.9, and 1.10).

Acknowledgments

We thank the following individuals and organizations for gathering material for this chapter and especially for trying to help us get facts and dates correct: Andrew Argent, Aristides

TABLE 1.9	Distinguished Career Awardees, Section on Critical Care, American Academy of Pediatrics

Year	Name
1995	I. David Todres, MD
1996	John Downes, MD
1997	Peter Holbrook, MD
1998	George Gregory, MD
1999	George Lister, MD
2000	Russell Raphaely, MD
2001	Murray Pollack, MD
2002	Daniel Levin, MD
2003	Ann Thompson, MD
2004	Bradley Fuhrman, MD
2005	J. Michael Dean, MD
2006	David Nichols, MD
2007	Ashok Sarnaik, MD
2008	Patrick Kochanek, MD
2009	Jerry Zimmerman, MD
2010	M. Michele Moss, MD
2011	Timothy Yeh, MD
2012	Niranjan Kissoon, MD
2013	Vinay Nadkarni, MD
2014	Barry Markovitz, MD
2015	Thomas Rice, MD

TABLE 1.10	Pediatric Award Recipients, Society of Critical Care Medicine

ASMUND S. LAERDAL MEMORIAL AWARD LECTURE	
2012	Robert A. Berg, MD
SHUBIN-WEIL MASTER CLINICIAN/TEACHER: EXCELLENCE IN BEDSIDE TEACHING AWARD	
1990	John J. Downes, MD
1993	Alan I. Fields, MD
2011	Arno Zaritsky, MD
2013	Robert Truog, MD
2014	Madelyn Kahana, MD
2015	David Nichols, MD
GRENVIK FAMILY AWARD FOR ETHICS	
1993	Robert D. Truog, MD
1999	I. David Todres, MD
2013	Wynne Morrison, MD
2015	Jeffrey Burns, MD
DISTINGUISHED SERVICE AWARD	
2002	Patrick M. Kochanek, MD
2004	Ann E. Thompson, MD
2007	Margaret M. Parker, MD
2009	Richard J. Brilli, MD
2009	Alan I. Fields, MD
2012	Edward Conway, Jr., MD
2012	Timothy Yeh, MD
2013	M. Michele Moss, MD
AMERICAN COLLEGE OF CRITICAL CARE MEDICINE DISTINGUISHED INVESTIGATOR AWARD	
2002	Murray M. Pollack, MD
2007	Patrick M. Kochanek, MD
BARRY A. SHAPIRO MEMORIAL AWARD FOR EXCELLENCE IN CRITICAL CARE MANAGEMENT	
2010	M. Michele Mariscalco, MD
2014	Ann E. Thompson, MD
2015	Richard J. Brilli, MD
LIFETIME ACHIEVEMENT AWARD	
2010	John J. Downes, MD
NORMA J. SHOEMAKER AWARD FOR CRITICAL CARE NURSING EXCELLENCE	
2011	Lauren Sorce, RN
DHARMAPUNI VIDYASAGAR AWARD FOR EXCELLENCE IN PEDIATRIC CRITICAL CARE MEDICINE	
2015	Patrick Kochanek, MD

Baltonado, Geoffrey Barker, John Beca, Jeffrey Burns, Gabriel Cassalett, Edward E. Conway, Jr., Mark Coulthard, John Cox, Peter Cox, Robert Crone, Martha Curley, J. Michael Dean, Bettina von Dessauer, Denis Devictor, Alan Duncan, Gideon Eshel, Alan Fields, Ericka Fink, Bradley Fuhrman, Jonathan Gillis, William Glover, Denise Goodman, Thomas Green, George Gregory, David Hatch, Mary Fran Hazinski, Peter Holbrook, Robin Horak, Hector James, Tamara Jenkins, Niranjan (Tex) Kissoon, Max Klein, Patrick Kochanek, Jacques LaCroix, Jos Latour, George Little, George Lister, Kathryn Maitland, Barry Markowitz, Neil Matthews, M. Michele Mariacalo, Peter Meaney, M. Michele Moss, David Nichols, Hisashi Nikaidoh, Zehava Noah, John Pearn, Carol Pendergast, Bradley Peterson, Jefferson Piva, Arnold Platzker, Bala Ramachandran, Adrienne Randolph, Russell Raphaely, Thomas Rice, Mark Rogers, Francisco Ruza, Hiro Sakai, David Schell, Frank Shann, Janice Bloedel Smith, Gregory Stidham, Robert Tumburro, Sue Tellez, James Thomas, Ann Thompson, Ron Trubuhovich, Edwin vander Voort, Amir Vardi, Dharmapuri Vidyasagar, Randall Wetzel, Gary Williams, Douglas Willson, Timothy Yeh, the American Academy of Pediatrics (AAP), the Subboard of the American Board of Pediatrics (ABP), the American College of Graduate Medical Education (ACGME), the Society of Critical Care Medicine (SCCM), the World Federation of Pediatric Intensive and Critical Care Societies (WFPICCS), and the National Institutes of Health (NIH).

In Memoriam: Professor Max Klein (1941–2015).

Key References

1. Downes JJ. Development of pediatric critical care medicine: how did we get here and why? In: Wheeler DS, Wong HR, Shanley TP, eds. *Pediatric Critical Care Medicine: Basic Science and Clinical Evidence*. London: Springer; 2007:3-30.
7. Grenvik A, Eross B, Powers D. Historical survey of mechanical ventilation. *Int Anesthesiol Clin*. 1980;18:1-10.
8. Somerson SJ, Sicilia MR. Historical perspectives on the development and use of mechanical ventilation. *J Am Assoc Nurse Anesth*. 1992;60:83-94.
10. Drinker PA, McKhann CF III. The iron lung. *JAMA*. 1986;255:1476-1480.
11. Safar P, Escarraga LA, Elam JO. A comparison of the mouth-to-mouth and mouth-to-airway methods of artificial respiration with the chest-pressure arm-lift methods. *N Engl J Med*. 1958;258:671-677.
13. Safar P. On the history of modern resuscitation. *Crit Care Med*. 1996;24(suppl):S3-S11.
16. Downes JJ. Historic origins and role of pediatric anesthesiology in child health care. *Pediatr Clin North Am*. 1994;41:1-14.
18. Haglund G, Werkmaster K, Ekstrom-Jodal B, McDougall DH. The pediatric emergency ward-principles and practice after 20 years. In: Stetson JB, Swyer PR, eds. *Neonatal Intensive Care*. St. Louis: WH Green; 1976:73-87.
23. Rogers MC. The history of pediatric intensive care around the world. In: Nichols DG, ed. *Roger's Textbook of Pediatric Intensive Care*. Philadelphia: Lippincott Williams & Williams; 2008:3-17.
26. Noonan JA. A history of pediatric specialties: the development of pediatric cardiology. *Pediatr Res*. 2004;56:298-306.
27. Smythe PM, Bull A. Treatment of tetanus neonatorum with intermittent positive-pressure respiration. *Br Med J*. 1959;2:107-113.
28. Delivonia-Papadopoulos M, Swyer PR. Assisted ventilation in terminal hyaline membrane disease. *Arch Dis Child*. 1964;39:481-484.
29. Gregory G, Kitterman J, Phibbs R, et al. Treatment of the idiopathic respiratory distress syndrome with continous positive airway pressure. *N Engl J Med*. 1971;284:1333-1340.
30. Brandstater B. *Prolonged intubation an alternative to tracheostomy in infant procedures*. Vienna: First European Congress of Anesthesiology; 1962:106.
31. Drinker P, McKhann CF. The use of a new apparatus for the prolonged administration of artificial respiration. I. A fatal case of poliomyelitis. *JAMA*. 1929;92:1658-1660. (Reprinted *JAMA* 1986; 225: 1473-1475).
32. Ibsen B. Treatment of respiratory complications in poliomyelitis: the anesthetist's viewpoint. *Dan Med J*. 1954;1:9-12.
33. Lassen HCA. A preliminary report on the 1952 epidemic of poliomyelitis in Copenhagen: with special reference to the treatment of acute respiratory insufficiency. *Lancet*. 1953;1:37-41.
34. Ibsen B. The anesthetist's viewpoint on the treatment of respiratory complications in poliomyelitis during the epidemic in Copenhagen, 1952. *Proc R Soc Med*. 1954;42:72-74.
41. Randolph AG, Gonzales CA, Cortellini L, Yeh TS. Growth of pediatric intensive care units in the United States from 1995 to 2001. *J Pediatr*. 2004;144:792-798.
51. Harrison VC, Heese H de V, Klein M. The significance of grunting in hyaline membrane disease. *Pediatrics*. 1968;41:549-559.
61. Levin D, Morriss F, Moore G. *A Practical Guide to Pediatric Intensive Care*. St. Louis: CV Mosby; 1979.
63. Levin D, Morriss F, eds. *Essentials of Pediatric Intensive Care*. St. Louis: Quality Medical Publications; 1990.
74. Rogers MC, ed. *Textbook of Pediatric Intensive Care*. Philadelphia: Williams & Wilkins; 1988.
90. Lister G. Pediatric critical care medicine. In: Pearson HA, ed. *The American Board of Pediatrics 1933-2008*. Chapel Hill, NC: American Board of Pediatrics; 2008:168-172.

High-Reliability Pediatric Intensive Care Unit: Role of Intensivist and Team in Obtaining Optimal Outcomes

Derek S. Wheeler and Richard J. Brilli

PEARLS

- A modern pediatric intensive care unit (PICU) is a complex system, operating in conjunction with other complex systems (inpatient units, operating room, and emergency department) within and between hospitals.
- Incorporating principles of highly reliable organizations is necessary to bring about system changes that will lead to further improvements in PICU outcomes.
- As multidisciplinary PICU team leaders, pediatric intensivists should understand and manage all system aspects, not just clinical care.
- PICU structure, processes, and outcomes are key system components requiring skilled management for PICUs to achieve high reliability.
- A current and ongoing pediatric intensivist shortage is expected to influence future staffing models for physicians and nonphysician caregivers.
- Anticipated future changes in reimbursement methodology will likely influence the value proposition of current diagnostic and treatment models in an increasingly high-tech PICU world.
- Despite inherent challenges, severity-adjusted comparative data for PICU outcomes are available and useful for assessing outcomes within and between hospitals.

Introduction

An often repeated quotation states, "Every system is perfectly designed to achieve the results it gets." This is certainly true of pediatric intensive care units (PICUs). If PICU leaders intend to achieve better outcomes, then they must change the system. The Institute of Medicine's report, *Crossing the Quality Chasm,*[1] raised significant concerns about health care quality in the United States and called for a fundamental redesign of the US health care delivery system. Since that time, the health care industry has begun to adopt practices of other industries

such as nuclear power, commercial aviation, and US Navy aircraft carrier flight deck operations that operate nearly accident free within inherently dangerous environments.[2] Organizations using these principles are referred to as high-reliability organizations (HROs), and we posit that ICUs must become HROs if outcomes are to improve further (Table 2.1).

Studying HROs has yielded five interrelated principles that characterize how individuals in these organizations behave and think—greatly decreasing the likelihood of error and enhancing an organization's ability to quickly recover when an error occurs (Table 2.2).[2,3] "Preoccupation with failure" means treating even minor errors as potential catastrophes and learning opportunities. "Sensitivity to operations" implies that leaders pay attention to operations at all levels, especially at the front line, relying heavily on transparent, nonpunitive information dissemination to everyone. "Reluctance to simplify" recognizes dangers of oversimplification in complex systems, and HROs actively look for differing viewpoints when analyzing events. "Deference to expertise" implies that in traditionally hierarchical organizations like hospitals, understanding of operational details for any process may reside within frontline staff. When possible, shifting operational responsibility to the front line may optimize results. Recently, greater recognition has been given to parents by including them in the frontline team.[4] "Commitment to resilience" specifies that when unforeseen events occur, HROs adapt swiftly, communicate rapidly, and solve problems creatively.

To date, high-reliability care in the US health care system remains elusive. Data from pediatric hospitals suggest recommended care is delivered only 55% of the time.[5] However, three pediatric hospital systems have reported significant harm reduction by applying HRO principles as part of robust quality improvement (QI) programs.[6-8] Further, pediatric hospitals have banded into statewide[9] and national collaboratives[10] using HRO principles and quality improvement science to lower serious safety event (SSE) rates and various hospital-acquired conditions (HACs).

TABLE 2.1   System Characteristics as They Relate to Differing Levels of Reliability

Low Reliability (Generally More Basic & Inconsistent) ←	Reliability →	High Reliability (Generally More Robust & Effective)
Individual preference prevails	Personnel informed by reliability science	Sophisticated organizational design
Intent to perform well	Implementation of human factors	Integrated hierarchies, processes, teams
Individual excellence rewarded	Standardization of processes is norm	Error-proofing: forced function, shutdown
Human vigilance for risk, error, harm	Ambiguities in standard work eliminated	Failure modes & effects analysis
Hard work, trying harder after failures	"Work-around" solutions eliminated	Routine simulation for training/reinforcing
Codified policies, procedures, guidelines	Reminders & decision support built in	Strong teamwork climate
Personal checklists	Standard checklists (real-time compliance)	Strong safety culture
Retrospective performance feedback	Good habits/behaviors leveraged	Staff perception of psychologic safety
Didactic training/retraining	Error-proofing: warnings, sensory alerts	Preoccupation with failure
Awareness raising	Deliberate redundancy in critical steps	Reluctance to simplify interpretations
Basic standardization (equipment, brands, forms)	Key tasks scheduled/assigned	Sensitivity to operations
	Some simulation training for emergencies	Deference to expertise
	Real-time performance feedback	Commitment to resilience

Modified from Weick KE, Sutcliffe KM. Managing the Unexpected: Resilient Performance in an Age of Uncertainty. San Francisco, CA: Jossey-Bass; 2007:194; Nolan T, Resar R, Haraden C, Griffin FA. Improving the reliability of health care, IHI Innovation Series white paper, 2004; AHRQ: Becoming a high reliability organization: operational advice for hospital leaders, AHRQ Publication No. 08-0022. Rockville, MD: Agency for Healthcare Research and Quality; 2008. http://www.ahrq.gov/qual/hroadvice/.
Table copied with permission from Niedner MF, Muething SE, Sutcliffe KM. The high-reliability pediatric intensive care unit. Pediatr Clin North Am. 2013;60:563-580.

TABLE 2.2   High-Reliability Organizations: Contexts and Adaptive Characteristics

Contexts	Characteristics
Marked complexity in systems, processes, technology, and work	Preoccupation with failure
Environment is socially and/or politically unforgiving	Reluctance to simplify interpretations
Consequences for failure are potentially catastrophic	Sensitivity to operations
Cost of failure precludes learning through trial and error or traditional experimentation	Deference to expertise
	Commitment to resilience

Table copied with permission from Niedner MF, Muething SE, Sutcliffe KM. The high-reliability pediatric intensive care unit. Pediatr Clin North Am. 2013; 60:563-580.

PICUs are an essential, rapidly expanding part of hospital systems. Critically ill patients receive care in a PICU and, in some cases, from the PICU team "outside" the PICU. Niedner and colleagues[11] recently described the current state of US PICUs and their journey toward high reliability. They concluded that although progress has been made and many PICUs are on the journey, currently no hospital or PICU truly fulfills all of the HRO criteria. Aside from these challenges, physician leaders in the PICU must also pay attention to other aspects of the system, well beyond clinical care (eg, education of trainees, coordination of care with other disciplines), which adds challenges.[12] This chapter's purpose is to equip pediatric intensivists, as leaders of multidisciplinary PICU teams, with an enhanced understanding of the PICU as a system within the hospital system, including how to manage and evaluate PICU functioning and ultimately optimize outcomes. Integrated into this discussion are specific challenges to attaining high-reliability care delivery that exist in the current milieu. It is through implementation of this administrative

knowledge, combined with clinical expertise, that a highly reliable PICU may soon develop.

PICU as System

Industrial engineering and operations research would describe hospitals and PICUs as "emergent" systems.[13] Emergence is a phenomenon in which larger systems arise from combined interactions of smaller systems in such a way that the whole is greater than the sum of the individual components or parts. The PICU is a system with inputs and outputs. PICU inputs include critically ill patients admitted from all units within the health care system, and outputs include patients transferred back to those same units, including home. Therefore overall quality of care in the PICU cannot be viewed in isolation. Indeed, the "whole" system ("critical care") is greater than the sum of the individual components (eg, emergency department, operating room, hospital inpatient unit, interhospital transport, rehabilitation unit). Improvements at the whole system level will only occur if the PICU is viewed in its entirety, rather than as a collection of multiple, individual components. This concept has fostered a relatively new way of thinking about the modern ICU as an "ICU without walls" rather than as a distinct, geographic unit. As McQuillan stated years ago, "the greatest impact on the outcome for intensive care units may come from improvements in the input to intensive care, particularly in the quality of acute care. …"[14] The "PICU without walls" concept is perhaps best understood with the reduced morbidity and mortality that has been associated with implementation of rapid response systems and enhanced situation awareness.[15-17]

Models of Critical Care Delivery

Avedis Donabedian, an early "systems thinker" in health care, stated that health care quality should be based on three dimensions—structure, processes, and outcomes (Fig. 2.1).[18] In this model, processes are effective (1) when the right

DONABEDIAN'S MODEL

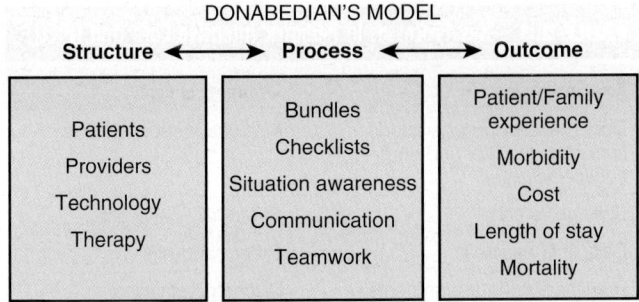

Fig. 2.1. Donabedian's model for quality. (Reproduced with permission from Donabedian A. Evaluating the quality of medical care. Milbank Mem Fund Q. 1966;44:166-206.)

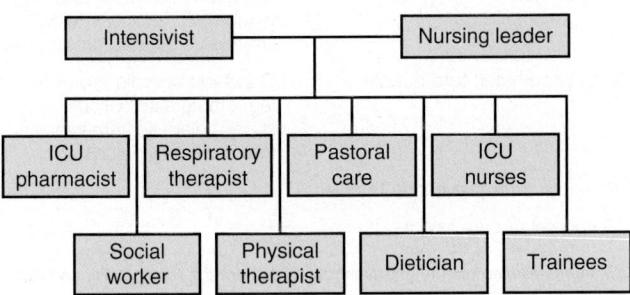

Fig. 2.2. Typical pediatric intensive care unit (PICU) team structure incorporating high-reliability organization principles. Co-leading the team with a physician and nurse together signals both "deference to expertise" and "reluctance to simplify." Inclusion of all other disciplines serving the PICU population at the same level incorporates the concept of "sensitivity to operations."

structures are in place to support them and (2) when outcomes are measured so that these processes can be evaluated for effectiveness and modified to produce better results. *Structure* refers to the setting in which care is delivered, whose elements include patients, providers, technology, and therapy.[13] Providers include the entire PICU team. When organized according to HRO principles, the team is optimally co-led by a physician and a nurse and is inclusive of all disciplines that touch the patient (Fig. 2.2). A recent trend is greater subspecialization of PICUs based on specific subpopulations of critically ill children (eg, neurointensive care, cardiac intensive care). These subspecialty PICUs are discussed elsewhere in this textbook. Structure also encompasses the physical design of the ICU, monitoring and support equipment, and information systems often equipped with decision support.[19,20] The PICU is a technical environment in which the interface between technology and humans can both improve care, as well as increase error risk. For example, computerized physician order entry (CPOE) can significantly improve quality of care provided in the ICU setting,[21] but it may also increase the risk of errors if not properly implemented or used.[22] These structural elements interact with key *processes* in the ICU to drive improved outcomes. *Processes* refer specifically to how care is provided in the ICU setting, including incorporation of high-reliability principles into daily functioning. *Outcomes* refer to end points of care, including commonly used quality and safety measures, as well as other key outcomes such as length of stay, patient/family experience, and cost/value.

Structure

The critical care team is perhaps the most important structural component driving quality of care in the PICU. Unfortunately, there is a growing shortage of fully trained critical care providers.[23,24] These shortages are particularly relevant to various PICU physician staffing models, including high-intensity staffing and 24/7 physician coverage[25] (described later). The exact number of physicians practicing pediatric critical care medicine is unknown. A 2011 survey by the American Board of Pediatrics reported 1881 board-certified pediatric intensivists in the United States but did not account for physicians no longer practicing critical care or others (cardiologists, anesthesiologists) staffing PICUs. It also noted that pediatric intensivists are aging (average age of 49), with 25% of board-certified pediatric intensivists 56 or older.[26] Importantly, critical care physicians are retiring at an earlier age, and less than 1% of medical school graduates choose to enter critical care medicine, suggesting that these shortages will continue to worsen.[24,27] Early retirement is particularly concerning given the many studies reporting burnout as a common occurrence in critical care medicine.[28] Staffing models that incorporate more advanced practice nurses,[29,30] physician assistants,[31] and hospitalists,[32] as well as telemedicine[33] and care regionalization,[26] have been proposed as potential solutions to the critical care physician shortage.[13]

The American College of Critical Care Medicine (ACCM) Task Force on Models of Critical Care Delivery summarized relevant literature on ICU staffing models in 2001 and again in 2015.[25] The Task Force recommended that all critically ill patients should be cared for by a multidisciplinary team of critical care providers led by an intensivist, including a critical care pharmacist.[34] In adult ICUs high-intensity staffing (previously called a "closed" model), wherein a dedicated team is directly responsible for all aspects of ICU care, is associated with better outcomes than a low-intensity staffing model (previously called an "open" model), in which patients are admitted and cared for by their primary care or subspecialty physician, often with limited input from a critical care team.[13,25,27,35]

Optimal physician coverage and direct presence in the PICU remains unclear. Several studies comparing ICUs with and without 24/7 attending critical care physician coverage have been published with a variety of results.[36] The ACCM Task Force on Models of Critical Care Delivery did not provide guidance on this issue.[25] Full 24/7 in-hospital intensivist staffing is uncommon. A 2001 study examining pediatric ICUs revealed that only 17% of all PICUs had 24/7 in-hospital intensivist physician staffing, and PICUs with more than 20 ICU beds were much more likely to provide 24/7 in-hospital intensivist staffing.[26] In a more recent study limited to pediatric and adult ICUs at academic medical centers, 33% of survey respondents indicated their hospital provided 24/7 intensivist in-house coverage.[37] Currently, evidence to support 24/7 in-hospital attending physician staffing is not compelling. A study in adults[38] suggested that a 24/7 attending coverage model was not associated with improved outcomes in ICUs with high-intensity daytime staffing. However, in those ICUs with low-intensity daytime staffing, 24/7 in-hospital intensivist presence was associated with significantly improved outcomes. Although data regarding optimal physician staffing in PICUs are limited, Arias and colleagues,[39] in a retrospective review, demonstrated a higher risk-adjusted mortality rate for critically ill children admitted to the ICU during evening hours compared with those admitted during daytime hours. Differential attending coverage between day and night was cited as a concern. Conversely, Peeters and colleagues[40] failed to demonstrate any significant differences in outcomes during off-hours admission to their PICU. Coverage at night in this PICU was provided by a resident physician, with attending physicians living close (<15 minutes) to the hospital. Others have reported similar findings.[41] Finally, Nishisaki and colleagues[42] reported that 24/7 in-hospital intensivist coverage decreased duration of mechanical ventilation and PICU length of stay but did not affect risk-adjusted mortality. For now, the issue of 24/7 in-hospital intensivist coverage and improved outcomes remains unresolved.

Optimal physician-to-patient staffing ratio in the ICU is also unclear. A study in adult ICUs[43] did not show a relationship between staffing ratios and mortality. Several studies have demonstrated an association between nursing workload and nurse retention, burnout, patient safety, and outcomes in ICUs.[28,44] We found no specific data in PICUs related to either nurse or physician staffing. The Society of Critical Care Medicine published guidelines regarding how to address this important issue but did not recommend specific physician-to-patient ratios.[45]

Process

Process refers specifically to how care is delivered in the ICU setting. The aforementioned structural elements interact with key processes to drive outcomes. It is important to emphasize that structural elements cannot compensate for the lack of an appropriate institutional climate that supports standardized, reliable, evidence-based processes[13,25,46] and uses high-reliability principles. To illustrate, a retrospective analysis involving more than 101,000 critically ill patients receiving care at 123 ICUs in US hospitals showed that risk- and severity-adjusted mortality rates were higher for patients receiving care exclusively by critical care physicians compared with patients cared for entirely by non–critical care physicians.[47] The conclusion was *not* that intensivists were the problem but rather that there was a need for reliable processes in the ICU setting.[48] For example, intensivists may have used their personal judgment for clinical decision making instead of following a standardized protocol that may be associated with better outcomes. Given the technical and procedural-based nature of the specialty of critical care medicine, perhaps intensivists performed more invasive procedures, which could have adversely impacted outcome. Adequate structure and optimal processes, accompanied by rigorous use of high-reliability principles, are essential to drive improved outcomes. Optimal nurse and physician staffing structure will not consistently prevent an adverse drug event from causing harm if rigorous medication double-check techniques are not practiced with every medication administration.

Multiple studies have shown significant reductions in various types of patient harm in PICUs through implementing standardized, reliable processes including the use of *bundles* (Table 2.3). A *bundle* is a relatively short list of standardized, generally evidence-based or best practice interventions for a patient population or disease that, when implemented consistently, lead to improved outcomes. It is the combination of elements performed reliably and in aggregate that drive the improvement. *Checklists* have also been used to

TABLE 2.3	Key Processes in Pediatric Intensive Care Unit (PICU)
Rounding Process	**Transitions of Care**
Daily multidisciplinary rounds (including medical and surgical subspecialists)	Medication reconciliation
Daily goals sheet	OR-to-ICU hand-offs
Daily shift huddles	Other hand-offs
Primary nursing assignments	Discharge planning
PICU leadership walk rounds	
Bundles	**Protocols**
Central line insertion bundle	Clinical pathways
VARI bundle	Standard care protocols (eg, extubation readiness testing, sedation/analgesia protocols)
Urinary catheter care bundle	Condition-specific protocols (eg, status asthmaticus, sepsis, diabetic ketoacidosis, traumatic brain injury)
Pressure ulcer prevention bundle	
Peripheral IV care bundle	

ICU, intensive care unit; IV, intravenous; OR, operating room; VARI, ventilator-associated respiratory infection.
Modified from Riley C, Poss WB, Wheeler DS. The evolving model of pediatric critical care delivery in North America. Pediatr Clin North Am. 2013;60: 545-562.

improve overall care of critically ill children admitted to the PICU. Gawande and Pronovost advocate using checklists in the ICU.[49,50] Daily goals improve communication and collaboration between team members and different disciplines of the critical care team.[51] Finally, structured communication during multidisciplinary rounds[52] and hand-offs[53,54] are additional key processes driving quality and improved outcomes in the PICU.

When all these elements have come together successfully, a unit has begun to function like an HRO. Several PICUs have adopted some of the characteristics of HROs to drive improvements in safety and quality.[11,55] To the degree that these principles are operational, errors and adverse events should dramatically decrease and outcomes should improve.

Outcomes

It is a challenge to compare outcomes between PICUs given the marked heterogeneity in case mix and illness severity. Although the American Academy of Pediatrics commissioned a working group to identify a list of quality measures for the pediatric ICU, it is not yet finalized. Multiple measures have been proposed,[56,57] though no single measure is likely sufficient to adequately summarize overall quality of care that a critically ill child receives in a particular PICU. It is likely that a panel of metrics, which includes both process and outcome measures, will be necessary. Similar panels, albeit without process measures, are already in use. The Preventable Harm Index is currently used to aggregate total events of harm over a given time for hospitals or groups of hospitals[9,10,58,59] and can be customized to specific units such as a PICU. Wetzel and colleagues[60] described methods to compare PICU effectiveness and efficiency. Using a data collecting network, Virtual

Pediatric Systems, severity-adjusted comparisons among PICUs for LOS, efficiency, and mortality are possible.

An outcome in Donabedian's construct that deserves further mention is value. Value, at least in the current context, is a function of improving outcomes and the overall patient and family experience, while minimizing the costs of care to the patient and the health care system. We have previously emphasized that structure and process are important drivers of outcomes, which is probably true for the overall patient and family experience as well. The key in today's health care climate is to improve outcomes and family experience without incurring increased or excessive costs. Schleien has documented many financial aspects related to PICU care delivery and discusses ways to enhance revenue and decrease cost in a system, which in this country is largely fee-for-service based.[61] He anticipates that over time, it is likely that the overall payment system will shift to capitation and many incentives currently in place for overutilization of various diagnostic and therapeutic resources may shift. If this results in limitations on use of expensive unproven technologies and medications, when these services and products would have been available previously, it may present challenges for pediatric intensivists to provide high-quality care with optimal value-based outcomes.

Further impacting the cost of care is the previously described shortage in pediatric intensivists. Simple laws of supply and demand are relevant here. As the supply of adequately trained pediatric intensivists decreases, hospitals will have to pay more to recruit them. This factor, in addition to higher staffing demands on intensivists, growth of specialized ICUs (eg, CICU, NICU), and changes in duty hour requirements for trainees, will affect the professional cost of providing pediatric intensive care.

Summary

A modern PICU is a complex system interacting with multiple other complex systems. To attain, or even approach, HRO level performance, the pediatric intensivist will need more than just clinical expertise. As leader of a multidisciplinary PICU team, he or she must consistently reinforce and model HRO principles, understand and manage delivery of optimal clinical care, and deal with realities of specialist shortage, rapidly changing reimbursement mechanisms, and ever-increasing expectations of parents and patients to be team members. Intensivists have risen to great challenges in the past, and there is every reason to expect that spirit to continue.

Key References

1. Institute of Medicine, ed. *Crossing the Quality Chasm: A New Health System for the Twenty-first Century.* Washington, DC: National Academy Press; 2001.
2. Weick KE, Sutcliffe KM. *Managing the Unexpected: Resilient Performance in an Age of Uncertainty.* San Francisco, CA: Jossey-Bass; 2007.
3. Weick KE, Sutcliffe KM, Obstfeld D. Organizing for high reliability: processes of collective mindfulness. In: Sutton R, Staw B, eds. *Research in Organizational Behavior.* Greenwich, CT: JAI Press; 1999:81-124.
4. Kuhlthau KA, Bloom S, VanCleave J, et al. Evidence for family-centered care for children with special health care needs: a systematic review. *Acad Pediatr.* 2011;11:136-143.
5. Mangione-Smith R, DeCristofaro AH, Setodji CM, et al. The quality of ambulatory care delivered to children in the United States. *N Engl J Med.* 2007;357:1515-1523.
6. Muething SE, Goudie A, Schoettker PJ, et al. Quality improvement initiative to reduce serious safety events and improve patient safety culture. *Pediatrics.* 2012;130:e423-e431.
7. Peterson T, Teman S, Connors R. A safety culture transformation: its effects at a children's hospital. *J Patient Saf.* 2012;8:125-130.
8. Brilli RJ, McClead RE Jr, Crandall WV, et al. A comprehensive patient safety program can significantly reduce preventable harm, associated costs, and hospital mortality. *J Pediatr.* 2013;163(6):1638-1645.
9. Lyren A, Brilli R, Bird M, et al. Ohio Children's Hospitals' Solution for Patient Safety: a framework for pediatric patient safety improvement. *J Healthc Qual.* 2013; doi:10.1111/jhq.12058; <http://www.onlinelibrary.wiley.com/doi/10.1111/jhq.12058/abstract>; Accessed 23.04.15.
10. CMS.gov, Centers for Medicare & Medicaid Services. Welcome to the Partnership for Patients. July 7, 2014. <http://www.partnershipforpatients.cms.gov> Accessed 23.04.15.
11. Niedner MF, Muething SE, Sutcliffe KM. The high-reliability pediatric intensive care unit. *Pediatr Clin North Am.* 2013;60:563-580.
12. St. Andre A. The formation, elements of success, and challenges in managing a critical care program: part I. *Crit Care Med.* 2015;43:874-879.
13. Riley C, Poss WB, Wheeler DS. The evolving model of pediatric critical care delivery in North America. *Pediatr Clin North Am.* 2013;60:545-562.
14. McQuillan P, Pilkington S, Allan A, et al. Confidential inquiry into quality of care before admission to intensive care. *BMJ.* 1998;316:1853-1858.
15. Sharek PJ, Parast LM, Leong K, et al. Effect of a rapid response team on hospital-wide mortality and code rates outside the ICU in a Children's Hospital. *JAMA.* 2007;298:2267-2274.
16. Tibballs J, Kinney S. Reduction of hospital mortality and of preventable cardiac arrest and death on introduction of a pediatric medical emergency team. *Pediatr Crit Care Med.* 2009;10:306-312.
17. Brady PW, Muething S, Kotagal U, et al. Improving situation awareness to reduce unrecognized clinical deterioration and serious safety events. *Pediatrics.* 2013;131:e298-e308.
18. Donabedian A. Evaluating the quality of medical care. *Milbank Mem Fund Q.* 1966;44:166-206.
19. Bartley J, Streifel AJ. Design of the environment of care for safety of patients and personnel: does form follow function or vice versa in the intensive care unit? *Crit Care Med.* 2010;38:S388-S398.
20. Valentin A, Ferdinande P. Improvement EWGoQ. Recommendations on basic requirements for intensive care units: structural and organizational aspects. *Intensive Care Med.* 2011;37:1575-1587.
21. Maslove DM, Rizk N, Lowe HJ. Computerized physician order entry in the critical care environment: a review of current literature. *J Intensive Care Med.* 2011;26:165-171.
22. Han YY, Carcillo JA, Venkataraman ST, et al. Unexpected increased mortality after implementation of a commercially sold computerized physician order entry system. *Pediatrics.* 2005;116:1506-1512.
23. Krell K. Critical care workforce. *Crit Care Med.* 2008;36:1350-1353.
24. Grover A. Critical care workforce: a policy perspective. *Crit Care Med.* 2006;34:S7-S11.
25. Weled BJ, Adzhigirey LA, Hodgman TM, et al. Critical care delivery: the importance of process of care and ICU structure to improved outcomes. An update from the American College of Critical Care Medicine Task Force on Models of Critical Care [epub ahead of print]. *Crit Care Med.* 2015;Mar 23.
26. Randolph AG, Gonzales CA, Cortellini L, et al. Growth of pediatric intensive care units in the United States from 1995 to 2001. *J Pediatr.* 2004;144:792-798.
27. Pronovost PJ, Angus DC, Dorman T, et al. Physician staffing patterns and clinical outcomes in critically ill patients: a systematic review. *JAMA.* 2002;288:2151-2162.
28. Embriaco N, Papazian L, Kentish-Barnes N, et al. Burnout syndrome among critical care healthcare workers. *Curr Opin Crit Care.* 2007;13:482-488.
29. Verger JT, Marcoux KK, Madden MA, et al. Nurse practitioners in pediatric critical care: results of a national survey. *AACN Clin Issues.* 2005;16:396-408.
30. Sorce L, Simone S, Madden M. Educational preparation and postgraduate training curriculum for pediatric critical care nurse practitioners. *Pediatr Crit Care Med.* 2010;11:205-212.
31. Mathur M, Rampersad A, Howard K, et al. Physician assistants as physician extenders in the pediatric intensive care unit setting—A 5-year experience. *Pediatr Crit Care Med.* 2005;6:14-19.
32. Siegal EM, Dressler DD, Dichter JR, et al. Training a hospitalist workforce to address the intensivist shortage in American hospitals: a position paper

from the Society of Hospital Medicine and the Society of Critical Care Medicine. *Crit Care Med*. 2012;40:1952-1956.

33. Yager PH, Clark ME, Heda RD, et al. Reliability of circulatory and neurologic examination by telemedicine in a pediatric intensive care unit. *J Pediatr*. 2014;165:962-966.

34. Horn E, Jacobi J. The critical care clinical pharmacist: evolution of an essential team member. *Crit Care Med*. 2006;34:S46-S51.

35. Kim MM, Barnato AE, Angus DC, et al. The effect of multidisciplinary care teams on intensive care unit mortality. *Arch Intern Med*. 2010; 170:369-376.

36. Cavallazzi R, Marik PE, Hirani A, et al. Association between time of admission to the ICU and mortality: a systematic review and metaanalysis. *Chest*. 2010;138:68-75.

37. Diaz-Guzman E, Colbert CY, Mannino DM, et al. 24/7 in-house intensivist coverage and fellowship education: a cross-sectional survey of academic medical centers in the United States. *Chest*. 2012;141:959-966.

38. Wallace DJ, Angus DC, Barnato AE, et al. Nighttime intensivist staffing and mortality among critically ill patients. *N Engl J Med*. 2012;366: 2093-2101.

39. Arias Y, Taylor DS, Marcin JP. Association between evening admissions and higher mortality rates in the pediatric intensive care unit. *Pediatrics*. 2004;113:e530-e534.

40. Peeters B, Jansen NJG, van Vught AJ, et al. Off-hours admission and mortality in two pediatric intensive care units without 24-h in-house senior staff attendance. *Intensive Care Med*. 2010;36:1923-1927.

41. Numa A, Williams G, Awad J, Duffy B. After-hours admissions are not associated with increased risk-adjusted mortality in pediatric intensive care. *Intensive Care Med*. 2008;34:148-151.

42. Nishisaki A, Pines JM, Lin R, et al. The impact of 24-hr, in-hospital pediatric critical care attending physician presence on process of care and patient outcomes. *Crit Care Med*. 2012;40:2190-2195.

43. Dara SI, Afessa B. Intensivist-to-bed ratio: association with outcomes in the medical ICU. *Chest*. 2005;128:567-572.

44. Carayon P, Gurses AP. A human factors engineering conceptual framework of nursing workload and patient safety in intensive care units. *Intensive Crit Care Nurs*. 2005;21:284-301.

45. Ward NS, Afessa B, Kleinpell R, et al. Intensivist/patient ratios in closed ICUs: a statement from the Society of Critical Care Medicine Taskforce on ICU staffing. *Crit Care Med*. 2013;41:638-645.

46. Gajic O, Afessa B. Physician staffing models and patient safety in the ICU. *Chest*. 2009;135:1038-1044.

47. Levy MM, Rapoport J, Lemeshow S, et al. Association between critical care physician management and patient mortality in the intensive care unit. *Ann Intern Med*. 2008;148:801-809.

48. Nguyen YL, Wunsch H, Angus DC. Critical care: the impact of organization and management on outcomes. *Curr Opin Crit Care*. 2010;16: 487-492.

49. Scales DC, Dainty K, Hales B, et al. A multifaceted intervention for quality improvement in a network of intensive care units: a cluster randomized trial. *JAMA*. 2011;305:363-372.

50. Hales BM, Pronovost PJ. The checklist—a tool for error management and performance improvement. *J Crit Care*. 2006;21:231-235.

Subspecialization Within Pediatric Critical Care Medicine

Ann E. Thompson

PEARLS

- The tremendous expansion of scientific and medical knowledge and efforts to combine different disciplinary perspectives has led to new approaches to investigating and understanding a variety of phenomena. New fields that cross traditional boundaries between disciplines have emerged from this work.
- Interdisciplinary knowledge and research bring multiple perspectives to thought surrounding topics of interest or concern and help avoid some of the blind spots of a single discipline.
- Trends toward subsubspecialization within critical care, usually focused on patients with disorders specific to one organ system, must balance the potential for improved patient care that results from in-depth knowledge of the disorders of that system with potential loss of more general multisystem expertise.
- We seek to avoid the extremes; neither the "Jack of all trades and master of none" nor "people who know more and more about less and less, until they know everything about nothing" serves us or our patients well.
- Subsubspecialists have an obligation to develop new knowledge in their areas of critical care, identify best practices relevant to the management of disorders studied, and demonstrate improved outcomes for their patients.

Early History

Efforts to repair injury and treat diseases, often seen as possession by evil spirits or punishments by the gods, are nearly as old as humankind. Ancient artifacts include items that resemble surgical instruments, and writings from ancient Egyptian, Babylonian, and Chinese periods demonstrate efforts to understand and relieve a broad range of ailments; included are mentions of children and their illnesses. Hippocratic physicians recognized that illnesses of younger and older children differed and were not the same as those in adults. Perhaps the first pediatric specialist was Soranus of Ephesus, who addressed infant nutrition, made recommendations about appropriate child rearing, and described symptoms of common childhood disorders. Pediatric textbooks became available in the 1400s, but even in the European[1,2] colonies of the New World where children were victims of the usual epidemics of infectious diseases as well as other illness and injury, there were essentially no physicians willing to care for them for lack of training and expertise. Care was left to family members and midwives.[3] Although there were modest advances through the 18th century, most notably the beginnings of immunization with cowpox to prevent the more deadly smallpox, rather little changed in the care of children.

Modern attention to diseases of childhood can be considered to have begun with recognition of the appalling mortality rates in childhood, largely related to infectious process, poor nutrition, and filthy living conditions, all closely related for a large majority of children. Forty percent of the deaths in Boston from 1840 to 1845 occurred in children younger than 5 years.[3] Oddly, even though neonatology would emerge as an early subspecialty of pediatrics, concern about the very high infant mortality in the late 19th century was not an immediate focus of the emerging specialty of pediatrics. Infant deaths were viewed as expected and similar to high neonatal losses in other animal species. Its emergence was an unsurprising outgrowth of pediatrics' focus on infants from its start.

In the second half of the 19th century pediatrics began to truly emerge as a distinct specialty of medicine. Advances in medical science, primarily in Europe, including among others the germ theory of disease, further understanding of biochemistry and physiology, and recognition of the cell as a basic unit of life, began to provide a footing for understanding and treating disease more as it is conducted today. In the United States, two key figures in the development of pediatrics as a specialty were Job Lewis Smith and Abraham Jacobi. Together they formed the American Pediatric Society, which was not only the first independent pediatric professional society but also the first medical specialty society in the United States. Jacobi coined the term *pediatrics* and changed fundamentally the way children were treated.

In the first quarter of the 20th century advances in medical science that defined important differences between children and adults gradually led to the recognition and acceptance of pediatrics as a distinct specialty. Attention to child welfare grew in Europe and eventually reached the United States, along with the importance of preventive aspects of medicine. A fracas between the pediatric section and the governing body of the American Medical Association (AMA) over providing health services for mothers and children led to the formation of the American Academy of Pediatrics in 1930 and the American Board of Pediatrics in 1933. The first step toward specialization in the care of children was complete.

As the 20th century progressed, effective prevention or cure of numerous infectious diseases allowed increased attention to congenital anomalies, chronic diseases, and malignancies, and technologic advances allowed new surgical procedures and extended life support, initially for neonates and subsequently for older infants and children as extensively described in Chapter 1.

The history of pediatrics and medicine in general in the 20th century was one of progressive divisions into specialty and subspecialty areas of expertise and, increasingly, into sub-subspecialization. In the United States, following the 1910 Flexner report and its emphasis on research-based education, which reflected the growing understanding of the physiologic and biochemical basis of human disease, pursuit of new knowledge increased dramatically. As physicians and scientists focused more narrowly and developed expertise around specific areas of medicine, many generalists began to devote significant portions of their practice to these more limited areas and consider themselves specialists. In 1917 ophthalmology was the first specialty area to create its own assessment board. For the remainder of the 20th century specialties proliferated; by the end of the century there were 24 specialty boards within the American Board of Medical Specialties (ABMS). Additional specialization occurred within the specialties, leading to current recognition by the ABMS of nearly 130 subspecialties.[4] In addition, it is estimated there are more than 100 self-designated specialty boards outside the ABMS.[5] As biomedical science has advanced further, there have been requests for the recognition of additional subspecialties and, increasingly, for subsubspecialties. As has occurred in other disciplines within and outside of medicine, some of these subsubspecialties have emerged from a single large subspecialty, such as cardiology (eg, interventional cardiology, cardiac electrophysiology, heart failure, and transplant cardiology), whereas others combine elements from and cross multiple disciplines such as palliative care, sports medicine, or sleep medicine (American boards of internal medicine, family medicine, pediatrics, psychiatry and neurology, otolaryngology, and anesthesiology).

Throughout recorded human history there have been evolving ways of perceiving the world and structuring ways of evaluating phenomena, discussing them, and developing solutions to perceived problems. No single perspective sees all aspects of a phenomenon or can necessarily lay claim to the correct or complete view. However, development of disciplines of thought, organized around problems and theories and ways of investigating them, have helped people conceptualize the world and communicate those concepts. One definition of discipline is "a scientific domain that uses a specific methodology, as well as a specific vocabulary … and generally constitutes the teaching domain of science" and other academic fields.[6] Over time disciplines evolve; their perceived significance changes; and they may interact in new ways, as new social or scientific needs and professions emerge.

With the tremendous expansion of scientific and medical knowledge, particularly in the last century, new approaches to investigating and understanding a variety of phenomena have resulted from combining different disciplinary perspectives. From these studies have grown new interdisciplinary theoretic and methodological identities, new fields that cross traditional boundaries between disciplines. Although there has been extensive academic discussion about somewhat confusing concepts of multidisciplinarity, interdisciplinarity, and transdisciplinarity, a definition that will suffice for the purposes of this chapter is that interdisciplinarity brings together distinctive components of knowledge, research, education, and theory of two or more disciplines. Interdisciplinary knowledge and research bring multiple perspectives to thought surrounding topics of interest or concern and help avoid some of the blind spots of a single discipline. Moreover, many complex problems require interdisciplinary approaches and yield to methods of research that combine those of multiple disciplines. Throughout modern science, and increasingly within fields of medicine, new hybrid disciplines have emerged from division and recombination of mature specialties (Fig. 3.1A and B). As knowledge continues to increase, specialization is inevitable, because no single theory or conceptual framework can encompass all that is known, nor can any human being know all there is to know. The long-recognized field of biochemistry, providing the basis for much of our understanding of human disease, is a hybrid of biology and chemistry. Biomedical engineering, combining knowledge and research methods from biology, medicine, and engineering, is a more recent hybrid discipline. There are many more.

Within medicine, specialization often occurs within a specialty, as was the case for cardiology, endocrinology, critical care medicine, and other subspecialties of pediatrics. However, some subspecialties cross numerous specialty lines, including sleep medicine, palliative care, sports medicine, and others, combining knowledge from dissimilar groups.

Rational progressive subspecialization requires advances in medical science and technology, professional interest, and a number of economic factors.[7] There must be a large enough patient population for subspecialists to maintain their skills. Care by a physician with additional, but potentially narrow, expertise should not result in patient care that is progressively more fragmented, with no coordination of services necessary to meet a patient's broader needs. Care by multiple specialists must at least be accompanied by excellent communication among them, significantly better than commonly occurs at present. This is important for all patients, but it is particularly critical for the children with multiple complex problems who constitute an increasing fraction of pediatric intensive care patients.

There are significant social policy considerations as well. Does the benefit to the public of clear standards for new areas of medical knowledge outweigh the costs of training and certification that burden physicians and are likely passed on to patients? How much does increased specialization increase the cost of care? If there is increased cost, is it offset by gains in health outcomes? In addition to the highest health expenditures as a share of the gross domestic product, the United States has the largest number of specialties and subspecialties in the world—40 more than in Canada, for example—but health outcomes are not among the best.[7,8] Part of the reason for more specialties is likely the larger US population, which leads to larger numbers of patients with specific diseases and related needs, perhaps best treated by a specialist, and perhaps generating a need to relieve a generalist of a portion of the demand for care. However, the need for a sizable population to care for to maintain competence leads to a concentration of these subspecialists in large population centers and may decrease the availability of adequate expertise in small communities.[9] An additional factor that encourages specialization is that reimbursement for care provided by a specialist or

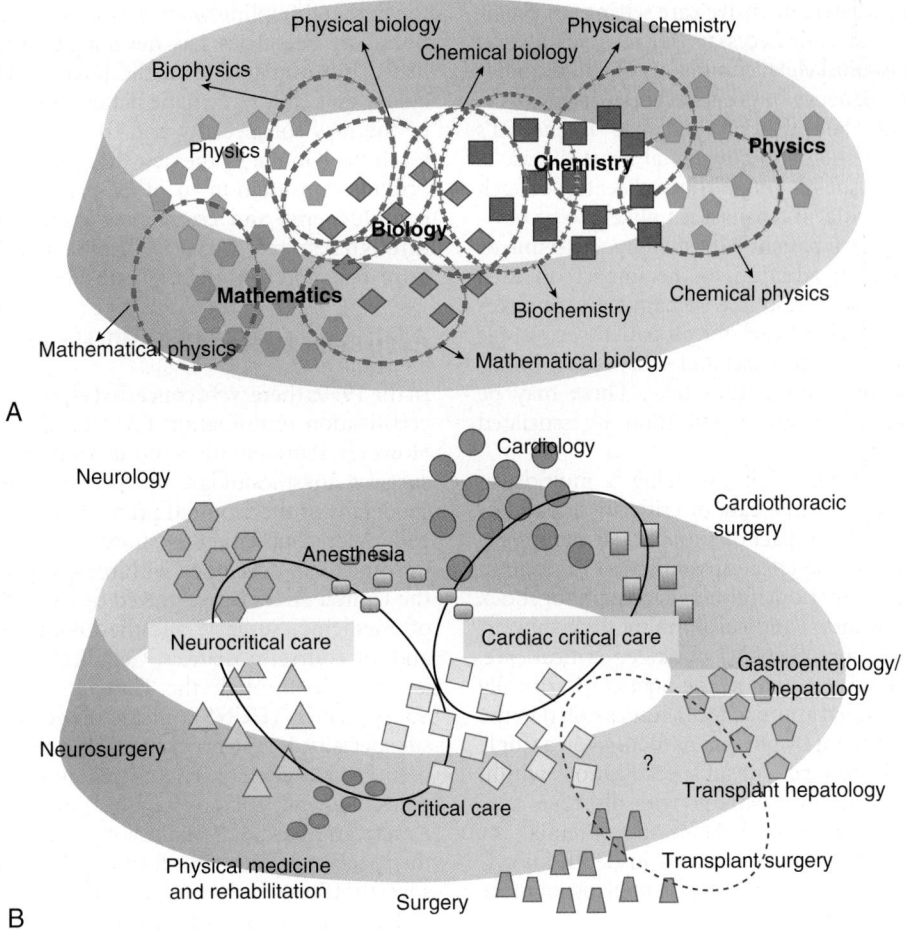

Fig. 3.1. Emergence of New Fields of Science and Medicine. (A) Development of new disciplines from the classical mathematics, physics, chemistry, and biology. (B) Emerging subsubspecialty fields of pediatric critical care.

subspecialist is often more generous than that provided to generalists. When that is the case, it is particularly important to be able to demonstrate improved outcomes and not simply greater expense.

Nearly every specialty board in the ABMS has grappled with the idea of specialization and its impact on the represented field as a whole and on subsequent education.[9-17] Does focus on a subset of patients lead to the specialist's loss of more general knowledge? Does the generalist lose the opportunity and skill required to care for a subset of patients? What is the impact on patient care during hours and days when one or the other is not available? Is there a need to provide duplicate physician coverage?

Arguments favoring subsubspecialization as well as board certification include the existence of a large enough and well-defined population to support specific practice, the value of setting standards and defining core competencies that define the knowledge and skill set of practitioners who label themselves specialists, reassurance to the public that the practitioner has appropriate expertise, and recognition for the work these subspecialists have done and the expertise they have developed. Opposing views include the observations that there are often multiple training pathways that lead to expertise and great difficulty merging the requirements of each (as seen in early efforts to develop unified certification in the

parent field of critical care medicine); competence in managing other problems often encountered in the subspecialty population may develop through some, but not all, of these pathways; the cost of certification and its maintenance is significant; requiring subsubspecialty certification may exacerbate existing physician shortages in the field; and the data supporting improved outcome when care is provided by these practitioners are yet to be generated. These arguments were well stated in the proceedings of the 10th International Conference of the Pediatric Cardiac Intensive Care Society, but they are virtually identical to those that have been made by one specialty after another.[18]

What is the impact on education? If a resident or fellow is primarily exposed to a series of relatively short subspecialty rotations, does he or she have an opportunity to develop competence in even the basic elements of practice? If there is little experience caring for patients not already diagnosed with a subspecialty problem, can a resident develop adequate diagnostic and problem-solving skills?

On the one hand, there is evidence from numerous walks of life that it takes many hours of practice to master a skill, whether technical or cognitive. Medicine is no exception. An intensivist becomes far more adept than does a fellow at assessing the adequacy of resuscitation from shock after caring for hundreds of patients. On the other hand, after years of practice limited to a pediatric intensive care setting, an intensivist is likely to have lost skills necessary for recognizing and treating common musculoskeletal complaints of childhood. It is likely that a similar sequence of events occurs with progressive subspecialization. The general pediatric intensivist's capacity to care for patients with congenital heart disease is likely to atrophy if he or she no longer routinely cares for such patients, whereas the cardiac intensivist is unlikely to be optimally skilled in managing a patient with meningococcemia or fulminant liver failure. In addition to the impact on each person's skill set, the human resource demands must be recognized. To maintain excellent care for all patients, coverage by both general pediatric intensivists and subspecialty intensivists must be available around the clock. These may be acceptable consequences of subspecialization if associated with improved outcome.

Intensive care has prided itself on being a multiorgan system specialty that assures that care of critically ill patients includes recognition of the impact of support for one system on others. Understanding the effect of ventilation for injured lungs on cardiovascular function; fluid management for shock on heart, lungs, and kidneys; and cardiopulmonary support on brain perfusion are core elements of skilled critical care. This expertise is believed to differ, to the benefit of critically ill patients, from the blinded approach sometimes noted in the assessment and management by physicians focused on a single organ system. Trends toward subsubspecialization within critical care, usually focused on patients with disorders specific to one organ system, must balance the potential for improved patient care that results from an in-depth knowledge of the disorders of that system with potential loss of more general multisystem expertise.

A a number of the specialty boards have addressed the question of what constitutes a subspecialty. The American Board of Internal Medicine has developed a set of criteria by which applications for subspecialty status are considered[19] (Box 3.1). In particular, a new subspecialty should include the existence of a unique body of knowledge, contribute new information and advance research, reflect a social need and improve outcomes, and outweigh any negative impact on the practice of the parent discipline or an existing subspecialty. The American Board of Pediatrics has developed similar criteria, unpublished but available from the board.[20] These criteria seek to assure that children will be better served by the establishment of the new subspecialty and that the new subspecialists will teach the content of the new discipline to learners at all levels, provide consultation to other practitioners, provide special complex care, and create new knowledge in the discipline through research (Box 3.2). These criteria would also apply to *third-tier subcertification,* or subsubspecialty certification.

Adult Subspecialization Within Critical Care

In the 1970s there were concerted efforts to establish a common certification examination for critical care medicine (CCM). However, representatives of the American boards of medicine, surgery, anesthesiology, and pediatrics were unable to agree on details of the required prerequisite training, and the effort collapsed.[21] Subsequently subspecialization with certification in some form developed within each specialty. Critical care in the United States is recognized by the ABMS as a subspecialty of medicine, surgery, anesthesiology, emergency medicine, and, of course, pediatrics. Certification in neurocritical care is available through the United Council for Neurological Subspecialties (UCNS) outside the ABMS and as an enfolded subspecialty 1-year program within the standard 7-year neurosurgical residency. There is interest within obstetrics and gynecology as well, and certification is available through the American Board of Anesthesiology. To date, however, none of the specialty boards have formally recognized further subsubspecialization within critical care.

The large volume of critically ill or injured adult patients meets one of the criteria for subsubspecialization. Particularly in large general hospitals, intensivists, surgeons and surgical subspecialists, internal medicine and medical subspecialists, along with nurses and hospital administrators have responded to the large population by setting up intensive care units that serve patients who suffer primarily from disorders of specific organ systems. In addition to general medical and general surgical ICUs, cardiac and cardiothoracic surgery ICUs have become common, particularly in the United States, although less so elsewhere in the world. Increasingly, units dedicated to trauma, primary pulmonary disease, neurologic disorders, and transplantation are also being established in adult facilities. In some settings intensivists spend time in several

---

BOX 3.1   Criteria for Recognition as a Subspecialty

- There exists a unique body of knowledge not fully incorporated into the *parent* discipline.
- The discipline has clinical applicability to be practiced in a form distinct from the parent discipline.
- The discipline must contribute scholarly generation of new information and advance research in the field.
- There must be a social need for the discipline and evidence that its practice improves patient care.
- The discipline requires formal training with supervision and direct observation.
- Commonly the discipline involves complex technology or site-of-care opportunities for learning.
- The positive value of certification in the discipline outweighs any negative impact on the parent discipline or on basic education in its core competencies.

Adapted from the American Board of Internal Medicine. The final report of the Committee on Recognizing New and Emerging Disciplines in Internal Medicine (NEDIM)-2; http://www.abim.org/~/media/ABIM%20Public/Files/pdf/report/nedim-2-report.pdf

---

BOX 3.2   Guidelines for Establishing a New Subspecialty in Pediatrics

- Children will be better served by the establishment of the new subspecialty.
- The subspecialist will not replace the general pediatrician in providing continuity of care.
- New subspecialists will do the following:
  - Teach the discipline to medical students, residents, trainees in the subspecialty, and other health professionals
  - Provide consultation in the subspecialty to general pediatricians and others
  - Provide complex (usually tertiary) care and perform procedures that are special to the subspecialty
  - Create new knowledge in the field through research
- The new subspecialty has a unique body of knowledge and a scientific basis.

different subspecialty-focused ICUs; in others they work in a single unit.

Subspecialized Pediatric Intensive Care Units

Traditionally, pediatric intensive care units (PICUs) have been general medical-surgical units. Care models have typically included a pediatric intensivist leading a team of nurses, other ICU professionals, and often residents or fellows in collaboration with pediatric medical and surgical specialists. The degree of management control afforded the PICU team varies, but the basic structure is fairly consistent. Aside from neonatal units, ICUs developed for patients with congenital and acquired heart diseases are the only common subspecialty units, although there have been a small number of units focused on the care of burned children. Sine the early 2000s, there has been an increased focus on developing neurointensive care units.

There is evidence from adult medicine that cohorting patients with similar conditions may have a positive impact on outcome. Patients with acute myocardial infarction benefit from care in a coronary care unit and patients with stroke are more likely to be alive, independent, and living at home 1 year later if treated in acute stroke units.[22-25] A number of retrospective studies provide evidence of improved outcome and decreased resource consumption for adult patients treated in neurocritical care units for intracerebral hemorrhage and traumatic brain injury.[26-30] The explanation for improved outcome is not entirely certain, but the presence of a neurointensivist-led team and use of evidence-based standardized protocols for management appear to be important factors.[31-33] Proponents of neurointensive care attribute improved outcome to optimal application of neuromonitoring and therapeutic advances, as well as the presence of dedicated neurointensivists,[33,34] similar to the impact of the high-intensity involvement of intensivists in general ICU outcome.[35]

In pediatrics the data are more limited. Several studies demonstrate improved outcome for children with cancer treated in specialized centers.[36-38] A study of patients admitted to a specialized unit for exacerbations of asthma may also be noteworthy.[39] These children received protocol-based care by specially trained staff, with case managers who coordinated care with the child's primary care physician and communication with families. Although not all of the outcome measures of interest (reduced length of stay, emergency department visits, and readmissions) might be directly relevant to critical care, the organization of care and communication strategies employed may be entirely applicable.

Cardiac Intensive Care

In many children's hospitals and perhaps larger pediatric services in general hospitals, infants and children with congenital or acquired heart disease constitute one of the largest PICU patient populations. In addition to the usual respiratory and cardiovascular monitoring, those with congenital heart disease, in particular, benefit from expertise regarding their hearts' structure, function, and physiology both before and after surgery, as well as skilled application of echocardiography. In the first decades of pediatric intensive care, physician care teams composed of cardiothoracic surgeons and

intensivists, with intermittently involved cardiologists, provided postoperative care for these patients. Typically, surgeons maintained strong control over patient management, even when not able to be present in the PICU. The perception was that intensivists lacked sufficient cardiac expertise to provide optimal postoperative management, whereas pediatric cardiologists as a group lacked general intensive care skills and usually only rounded on patients once or twice daily or when called to evaluate specific concerns. Strong pressure from surgeons for units dedicated to the care of these patients without the distractions of other patients, along with a perception that optimal postoperative care requires special expertise that combines the skills of pediatric intensivists with those of pediatric cardiologists (as well as elements of those of neonatologists, cardiac surgeons, and cardiac anesthesiologists), resulted in what can be considered the hybrid discipline of pediatric cardiac intensive care (Fig. 3.2).

As is the case with other hybrid disciplines, there are several pathways for training. At present, these include an additional year of cardiac intensive care training for pediatric critical care–trained intensivists, an additional 9 to 12 months of intensive care training for cardiologists,[40] or combined fellowships in both pediatric cardiology and pediatric critical care medicine of 5 to 6 years.[41] Although the American Board of Pediatrics does not formally recognize this further subspecialization, at least 19 children's hospitals in the United States and Canada offer additional training to meet these guidelines, nearly all for 1 year.[42] The Society of Pediatric Cardiology Training Program Directors, the American Academy of Pediatrics, the American Heart Association, and the American College of Cardiology approved guidelines that focused on the development of specific competencies in 2015.[43] This document describes the knowledge and skills the fellow must develop, rather than defining the amount of time that needed to be spent on a subspecialty service or performing a certain number of procedures in order to complete training.

At present, many children's hospitals have distinct cardiac intensive care units, perhaps as many as half or even two-thirds of those with congenital cardiac surgery programs. Many of the remainder have dedicated cardiac beds within a general PICU.[44,45] Although staffing varies, most include specifically trained cardiac intensivists or identify a group of general intensivists who elect to spend all or most of their clinical time in the cardiac intensive care unit (CICU). Similarly, there is a growing focus on developing a nursing staff devoted to this group of patients.[44,46]

Mortality in children undergoing congenital heart surgery has improved dramatically. There is evidence that higher patient volume is associated with decreased mortality following congenital heart surgery,[47-52] and larger volume centers are more likely to have dedicated CICUs. (It should be noted that the volume-outcome relationship is strong, but not perfect; there are smaller programs that have excellent outcomes.)[53] Admission to a dedicated CICU rather than the neonatal intensive care unit has been associated with decreased resource use in infants with prenatally diagnosed congenital heart disease.[54] To date, however, evidence does not demonstrate improved survival based on the CICU versus PICU model of postoperative care. The only studies to date examining the relationship between models of postoperative intensive care and outcome[55,56] found no relationship overall between mortality, length of stay or complications (including cardiac arrest,

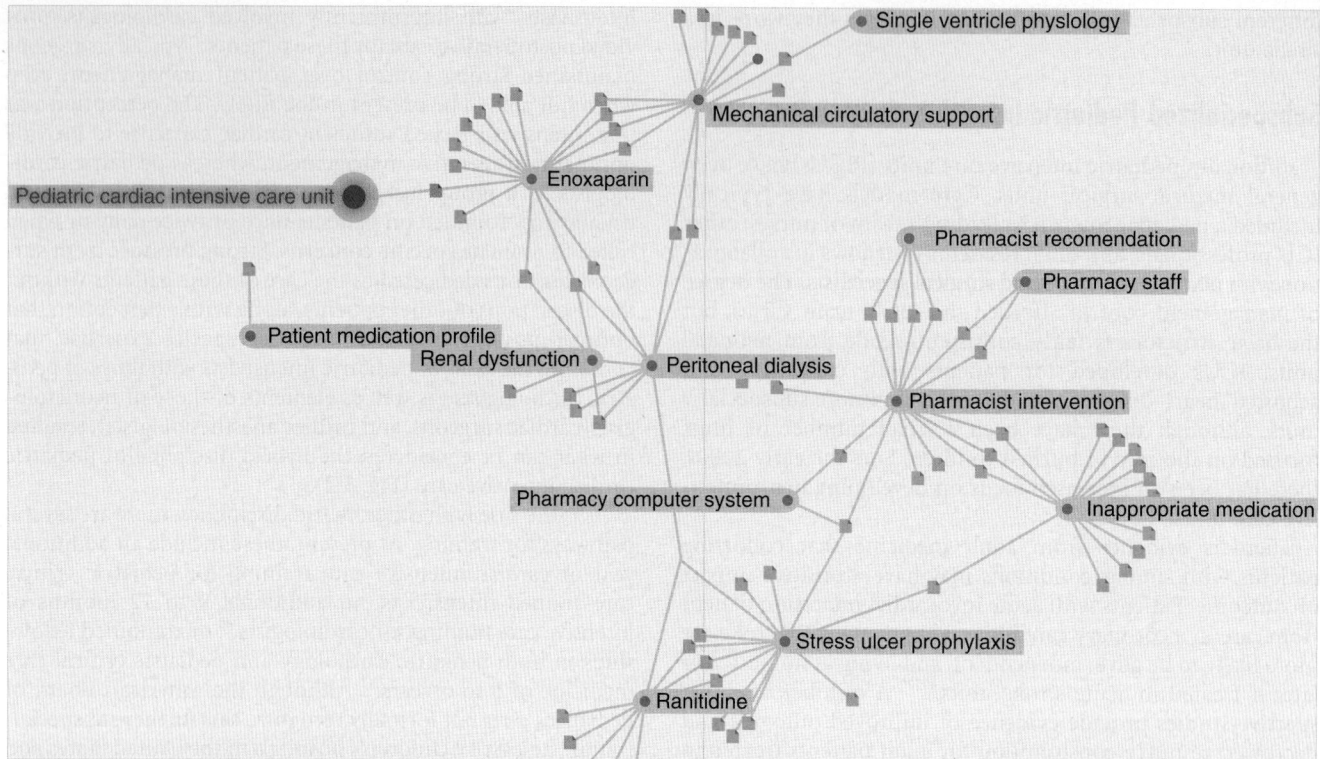

Fig. 3.2. Multidisciplinary Strands in CICU Treatment Decisions. A single simple example of the multidisciplinary input that contributes to the practice of cardiac critical care. Many more complex examples could be generated.

mechanical circulatory support, arrhythmias acute, respiratory insufficiency requiring reintubation or prolonged mechanical ventilation, renal failure requiring renal replacement therapy, new seizures or neurologic deficit, or infection), and the model of care. The Society of Thoracic Surgeons and the European Association for Cardio-Thoracic Surgery (STS-EACTS) category 3 patients, primarily including children undergoing complete atrioventricular canal repair and arterial switch for transposition of the great vessels, was the only subgroup in which a survival benefit was noted.

The volume-outcome relationship has also been demonstrated for PICUs, with larger units reporting a lower mortality.[57] Although larger centers with larger PICUs are more likely to have a separate CICU, more than a quarter of CICUs are in low-volume centers. There are currently no data that describe the volume-outcome relationship in CICUs, other than through their association with cardiac surgery programs. It is possible that outcome for these patients, whether cared for in a CICU or a PICU, is related to the organization of care in each setting. CICUs are more likely to be staffed with fellows and midlevel practitioners than with residents and attending physicians with combined cardiology and critical care expertise, but these factors have not yet been shown to impact outcome.[45] Although adequate nurse staffing has been shown to be important in many settings,[58] no clear relationship between nurse staffing and skill mix and outcome has been demonstrated for CICUs.[46] One study did identify increased risk of an unsuccessful resuscitation if the patient's primary nurse had less than a year's CICU experience. It is possible that units dedicated to the care of a specific subset of ICU patients might be characterized by greater esprit de corps, having a smaller team of physicians, nurses, and others with

a special identity and dedication to a specific goal. On the other hand, many ICU nurses share critical care's multiorgan system focus, and relatively few indicate preparedness and a willingness to care for a limited population. Developing a cadre of specially trained nurses well prepared to care for these patients is a likely requirement; if accomplished it may contribute to both patient safety and esprit de corps.[59,60] In addition to well-trained staff, excellent interprofessional collaboration may be a defining characteristic of units with the best outcomes.[58,61-64]

Management of most conditions treated in ICUs varies substantially between and within institutions, and data regarding best practices are sparse. Although CICUs and other subspecialty units might be ideal settings for defining best evidence-based practices, developing treatment guidelines around them, and streamlining care, there is only limited evidence so far that this is occurring. A survey exploring hypoplastic left heart syndrome management described widely varying practices in virtually every aspect of care, regardless of the ICU model.[65] The National Pediatric Cardiology Quality Improvement Collaborative has demonstrated further variations.[66,67] Individual institutions are beginning to develop clinical process guidelines for patients undergoing and recovering from specific procedures, and these do demonstrate improved outcome, including decreased ICU and hospital length of stay and decreased resource utilization and cost.[68-72] There are ongoing efforts to standardize practices, but comparative outcome studies have not been reported.

Of particular note to this discussion is the recognition that infants and children with congenital heart disease are at very high risk for neurodevelopmental deficits. Identifying causes of these problems, particularly those that may be responsive to treatment, is a high priority for everyone caring for these patients.[73-79] The opportunity to collaborate with other intensivists and neonatologists, especially those particularly focused on neurocritical care, represents a chance to bring together again the best skills and diverse perspectives of a variety of intensive care subspecialists.

Neurocritical Care

As outcome for nearly all critically ill infants and children has improved over the past several decades, brain injury has been left as the major cause of PICU mortality and long-term morbidity.[80] Children with neurologic disorders are more than three times more likely to die than those without, and their care is significantly more costly.[81,82] The etiology of brain injury is variable and includes patients with seizures, CNS infection, spinal cord injury, and those following neurosurgery for hydrocephalus, tumors, and epilepsy, but patients with stroke and trauma have mortality rates far in excess of those with other disorders. Patients with severe traumatic brain injury (TBI) constitute less than 1% of patients with neurologic disorders admitted to PICUs but account for nearly 30% of the mortality in this group. There are more deaths in childhood from TBI than from all childhood cancers combined or from heart disease.[80] Significantly improving mortality and morbidity in critically ill pediatric patients will require making progress with these patients.

In addition to primary neurologic disorders that prompt admission to the PICU, neurologic injury complicates the course and outcome of many other critical illnesses. Incorporating optimal care of the nervous system is an essential component in the management of shock, liver failure, sepsis, and

cardiac disease, among others. Neonatologists have also begun to develop a focus on neurologic injury in their patients and have taken steps toward what might evolve as a subspecialty within their field. Infants with extreme prematurity, perinatal asphyxia, neonatal seizures, status epilepticus, and multisystem disease are all at risk for neurologic morbidity, which mars much of the dramatically improved survival in this population.[83-85] Similarly, as long-term survival has improved following repair or palliation of complex congenital heart abnormalities, it has become apparent, as noted earlier, that significant neurologic dysfunction is present in many patients.[75,76] They are at increased risk for cognitive impairment as well as impairment of gross and fine motor skills, language and communication deficits, visual perceptual deficits, and behavioral and psychologic abnormalities. Some of these deficits are related to coexisting congenital brain abnormalities, but others are acquired as secondary effects of cardiopulmonary bypass, hypoxemia, and hypoxic-ischemic events. A question arises: Should there be a subsubspecialty of critical care or neurology that focuses on all of these disorders? (See Fig. 3.3.) Or should clinician-investigators in neurocritical care identify best practices and new treatments that can be adapted to other pediatric intensive care settings?

Efforts toward improving neurologic morbidity and mortality can be considered to be as old as PICUs in general, but the first defined pediatric neurocritical care service was probably the neurocritical care consultation service at Boston Children's Hospital, established in 1996.[87] In 2009 the first primary pediatric neurocritical care service was established at Children's Hospital of Pittsburgh. By 2015, there were nearly 30 pediatric neurocritical care services in the United States, mostly following a consultation model. The consultation

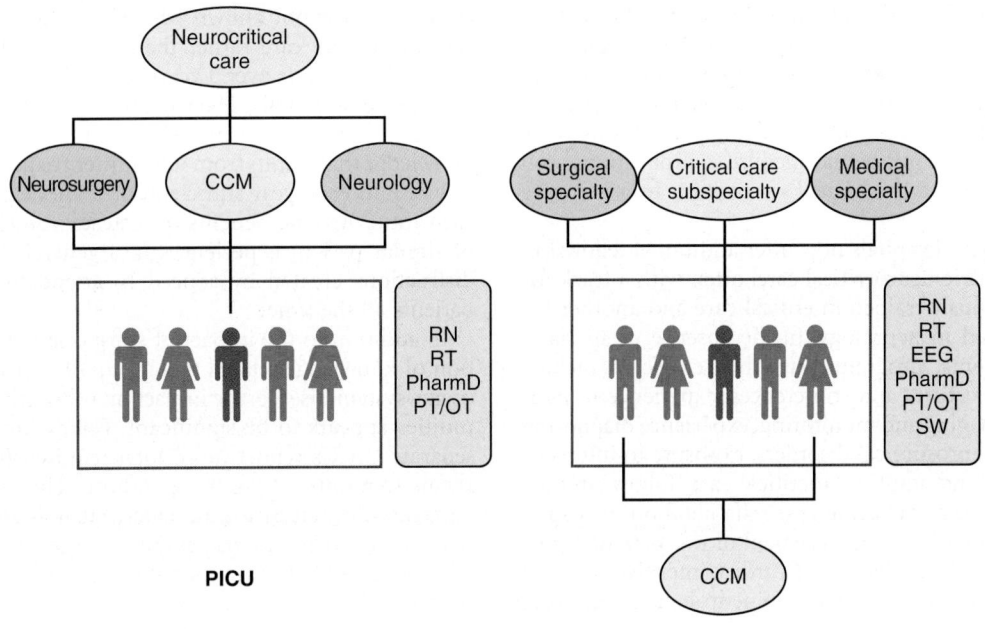

Consultation model   Integrated primary service

Fig. 3.3. Models of Neurocritical Care. The consultation service combines a dedicated neurology team with the general PICU team. No new CCM resources are required, but managing variations in care is challenging. Night and weekend coverage is provided by neurology fellows on that service. The integrated neurocritical care team is led by the attending intensivist who directs a separate PICU team, with coattending physicians from neurology or neurosurgery as appropriate. Adherence to evidence-based protocols are more readily achieved. Attending level expertise is available 24/7.

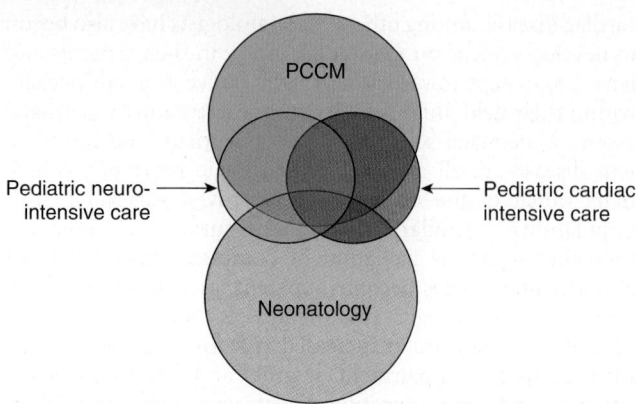

Fig. 3.4. Intersection of Intensive Care Interests and Research Opportunities. Shared concerns related to, in particular, residual neurologic morbidity provide an opportunity to collaborate with other intensivists and neonatologists and a chance to bring together again the best skills and diverse perspectives of a variety of intensive care subspecialists.

model typically involves a core group of rotating pediatric neurologists with neurocritical care clinical and research interests who provide a consistent ICU presence. The service typically includes neurology residents who are dedicated to ICU consultation for a set period and provide round-the-clock in-house coverage. This team works with the general PICU team of attending intensivist, pulmonary and critical care medicine (PCCM) fellows, and rotating pediatric residents (Fig. 3.4A).[86] The alternative neurocritical care service model includes a pediatric neurocritical care attending (one of a defined subset of the PCCM attendings, with a subspecialty focus on neurologic illness and injury) on service daily and available at night, with a PCCM fellow and pediatric resident on service 24 hours a day (Fig. 3.4B). A neurologist or neurosurgeon serves as a coattending representative for relevant patients. Regardless of the model, the goal is to "resuscitate and support the acutely ill neurologic patient, minimize secondary neurologic injury and medical complications, and expedite and facilitate the patient's transition to a recovery environment."[87,88]

Several children's hospitals now offer additional fellowship training in pediatric neurocritical care, often with a track for physicians previously trained in critical care and another for physicians trained in neurology. In the absence of specialty board requirements, programs vary, but curricula include regular focused lectures and conferences, experience in neurophysiologic imaging and monitoring, experience diagnosing and managing neurosurgical disorders, exposure to interventional radiology and adult neurocritical care, follow-up outpatient care, physical medicine and rehabilitation exposure, and research related to the management of this patient population. Some include an element of cardiac intensive care and neonatology with a focused interest in neurologic monitoring and neuroprotection.

As is the case with cardiac critical care, evidence for improved outcome following establishment of a pediatric neurocritical care unit is sparse. Efforts are being made to identify risk factors related to outcome in these patients.[89,90] However, a retrospective review of outcome following severe TBI before and after a neurocritical care service demonstrated

risk-adjusted increased discharge home without assistance and decreased mortality.[91]

Adequate "Dose" of Subsubspecialty Training

An additional question that needs to be addressed is that of the appropriate "dose" of education around the management of patients with cardiac or neurologic dysfunction or any other subset of PICU patients if they are treated separately from the general population. The Residency Review Committee (RRC) for Pediatrics of the American Council on Graduate Medical Education (ACGME) has set requirements for PCCM fellowships. There must be "an affiliated cardiac surgical program with a volume of at least 100 cases per year," and, if there is a separate CICU, "provision must be made for fellows to have substantial patient care experience in the pediatric cardiac surgical ICU, and such rotations should be considered mandatory rather than elective experiences."[92]

No such requirements have been set for any other subset of patients to date. The RRC has limited the time that can be spent in a CICU to 6 months of the 3-year PCCM fellowship. Although other intensive care experiences (examples provided include patients from outside the usual PICU population such as adult medical and neonatology) may be part of the program, these must be limited to 4 months overall and must not replace time in the PICU.[93] These requirements predate the emergence of neurocritical care or any other potential subsubspecialty population.

Although the minimum number of patients (at least for cardiac surgery) and the maximum time devoted to them in settings outside the PICU are included in program requirements, these requirements are based on expert opinion. There are currently no data that define the number of patients or location of their care that results in optimal or even adequate education. It is not known whether "bolus" doses of focused subsubspecialty care rather than a steady infusion of caring for similar patients over 3 years results in a better retention of knowledge and skills. Even if both have the potential to be similarly effective in achieving a steady state, the half-life of knowledge that results from intermittent exposure is unknown. Is 1 month each year sufficient, or is the fellow starting over each time? Are the benefits of a steady infusion over 3 years of similar patient experiences in a general PICU lost in the distractions created by a need to attend to many types of patients all the time?

In addition to the impact of subspecialty ICUs on acquisition of knowledge related to a group of patients with specific organ-system disease, the impact on other educational opportunities appears to be significant. Fellowship programs with separate CICUs report more total required ICU months (16 versus 13 months) than those without. The impact appears to be greatest on elective experiences such as adult or neonatal ICU time, pain management service, toxicology/poison control center exposure, or interventional radiology, among others.[94]

Impact on Research

Pediatric critical care medicine is a young subspecialty, and research addressing topics of major interest is even younger. However, since the late 1990s, there has been substantive progress in training investigators and conducting both basic and clinical studies (see also Chapter 7). In every area of medicine most new knowledge has been generated by physicians and scientists who devote themselves to a field full time. In addition to the impact of focused clinical practice that subspecialization may bring, there is an opportunity to advance our understanding of the biology underlying specific disease processes and develop new management strategies. There is early evidence that this is occurring.

The Pediatric Heart Network (PHN), supported by the National Heart, Lung, and Blood Institute, was formed following recognition that although the incidence of congenital heart disease is at least triple that of childhood cancer, there has been little related research. The network is intended to allow multi-institutional studies to overcome the small number of patients with specific diagnoses at any given studies. The PHN also supports nursing, health services, and quality improvement research, as well as a program of clinical research mentoring. Relatively few of the studies to date have addressed CICU aspects of care, but others are ongoing.[95]

The Pediatric Neurocritical Care Research Group[96] is a group of investigators from multiple disciplines, including pediatric critical care, pediatric neurology, pediatric neurosurgery, pediatric anesthesia, and pediatric rehabilitation medicine, from more than 30 institutions in four countries. The group is dedicated to performing studies focused on optimizing functional outcomes for critically ill children with neurologic conditions. Current investigations address multiple aspects of traumatic brain injury, nonconvulsive status epilepticus in children, and biomarkers of brain injury in extracorporeal membrane oxygenation patients, among others.

At present it is not possible to draw an adequately informed conclusion about the value of further subspecialization within pediatric critical care medicine or even to affirm the value of existing "almost" subsubspecialties. Data related to their current impact or their likely future impact on patient outcomes or educational results remain limited. From a health policy perspective, whether the trend toward further subspecialization advances the goals of improving medical care, impacting population health, and managing cost remains to be determined.[9] It does appear that the existing subsubspecialty groups are facilitating research by bringing problems of particular importance for certain patient groups into clearer focus and drawing interested investigators into more coherent groups (eg, Pediatric Heart Network (PHN), the Pediatric Neurocritical Care Research Group) that are able to address them. It may be that identification of best practices and results of this research disseminated to the pediatric critical care medicine community as a whole will be the most important outcome of limited additional subspecialization.

Key References

7. Detsky AS, Gauthier SR, Fuchs VR. Specialization in medicine: how much is enough? *JAMA*. 2012;307:463-464.
10. Cassel DK, Reuben DB. Specialization, subspecialization, and subsubspecialization in internal medicine. *N Engl J Med*. 2011;364:1169-1173.
18. Anand V, Kwiatkowski DM, Ghanayem N, et al. Training pathways in pediatric cardiac intensive care. Proceedings from the 10th International Conference of the Pediatric Cardiac Intensive Care Society. *World J Pediatr Congenit Heart Surg*. 2016;7:81-88.
19. *Final report of the Committee on Recognizing New and Emerging Disciplines in Internal Medicine (NEDIM) — 2*. Philadelphia: American Board of Internal Medicine; 2006 <http://www.abim.org/pdf/nedim-2-report.pdf>.

20. American Board of Pediatrics. Guidelines for establishing a new subspecialty. Approved by ABP Board of Directors February 1994. Revised June 2006. Personal communication (G. McGuinness) Unpublished.
26. Diringer MN, Edwards DF. Admission to a neurologic/neurosurgical intensive care unit is associated with reduced mortality rate after intracerebral hemorrhage. *Crit Care Med*. 2001;29:635-640.
29. Mirski MA, Chang CWJ, Cowan R. Impact of a neuroscience intensive care unit on neurosurgical patient outcomes and cost of care: evidence-based support for an intensivist-directed specialty ICU model of care. *J Neurosurg Anesthes*. 2001;13:83-92.
31. Elf K, Nilsson P, Enblad P. Outcome after traumatic brain injury improved by an organized secondary insult program and standardized neurointensive care. *Crit Care Med*. 2002;30:2129-2134.
33. Suarez JI. Outcome in neurocritical care: advances in monitoring and treatment and effect of a specialized neurocritical care team. *Crit Care Med*. 2006;34(suppl):S232-S238.
34. Kurtz P, Fitts V, Sumer Z. How does care differ for neurological patients admitted to a neurocritical care unit versus a general ICU? *Neurocrit Care*. 2011;15:477-480. doi:10.1007/s12028-011-9539-2.
35. Pronovost PJ, Angus DC, Dorman T, et al. Physician staffing patterns and clinical outcomes in critically ill patients: a systematic review. *JAMA*. 2002;288:2151-2162.
40. Kulik T, Giglia TM, Kocis KC, et al. Task force 5: requirements for pediatric cardiac critical care. *J Am Coll Cardiol*. 2005;46:1396-1399.
43. Ross RD, Brook M, Koenig P, et al. 2015 SPCTPD/ACC/AAP/AHA Training Guidelines for Pediatric Cardiology Fellowship Programs (Revision of the 2005 Training Guidelines for Pediatric Cardiology Fellowship Programs): introduction. *Circulation*. 2015;132:e43-e47.
44. Hickey PA, Gauvreau K, Tong E, et al. Pediatric cardiovascular critical care in the United States: nursing and organizational characteristics. *Am J Crit Care*. 2012;21:242-250.
46. Hickey P, Gauvreau K, Connor J, et al. The relationship of nurse staffing, skill mix, and Magnet recognition to institutional volume and mortality for congenital heart surgery. *J Nurs Adm*. 2010;40:226-232.
47. Welke KF, O'Brien SM, Peterson ED, et al. The complex relationship between pediatric cardiac surgical case volumes and mortality rates in a national clinical database. *J Thorac Cardiovasc Surg*. 2009;137: 1133-1140.
54. Johnson JT, Tani LY, Puchalski MD, et al. Admission to a dedicated cardiac intensive care unit is associated with decreased resource use for infants with prenatally diagnosed congenital heart disease. *Pediatr Cardiol*. 2014;35:1370-1378.
55. Burstein DS, Jacobs JP, Li JS, et al. Care models and associated outcomes in congenital heart surgery. *Pediatrics*. 2011;127:e1482-e1489.
56. Hilvers PS, Thammasitboon S. Does ICU structure impact patient outcomes after congenital heart surgery? A critical appraisal of "care models and associated outcomes in congenital heart surgery" by Burstein et al (Pediatrics 2011; 127: e1482-1489). *Pediatr Criti Care Med*. 2014; 15:77-81.
57. Tilford JM, Simpson PM, Green JW, et al. Volume-outcome relationships in pediatric intensive care units. *Pediatrics*. 2000;106(2 Pt 1):289-294.
58. Shortell SM, Zimmerman JE, Rousseau DM, et al. The performance of intensive care units: does good management make a difference? *Med Care*. 1994;32:508-525.
60. Kane JM, Preze E. Nurses' perception of subspecialization in pediatric cardiac intensive care unit; quality and patient safety implications. *J Nurs Care Qual*. 2009;24:354-361.
61. Zimmerman JE, Shortell SM, Rousseau DM, et al. Improving intensive care: observations based on organizational case studies in nine intensive care units: a prospective, multicenter study. *Crit Care Med*. 1993;21: 1443-1451.
62. Baggs JG, Schmitt MH, Mushlin AI, et al. Association between nurse-physician collaboration and patient outcomes in three intensive care units. *Crit Care Med*. 1999;27:1991-1998.
63. Wheelan SA, Burchill CN, Tilin F. The link between teamwork and patients' outcomes in intensive care units. *Am J Crit Care*. 2003;12: 527-534.
64. Shekelle PG. Nurse-patient ratios as a patient safety strategy: a systematic review. *Ann Intern Med*. 2013;158:404-409.
65. Wernovsky G, Ghanayem N, Ohye RG, et al. Hypoplastic left heart syndrome: consensus and controversies in 2007. *Cardiol Young*. 2007;17(suppl 2):75-86.
66. Slicker J, Hehir DA, Horsley M, et al. Nutrition algorithms for infants with hypoplastic left heart syndrome; birth through the first interstage period. *Congenit Heart Dis*. 2013;8:89-102.

67. Anderson JB, Iyer SB, Schidlow DN, et al. Variation in growth of infants with a single ventricle. *J Pediatr.* 2012;161:16-21.e1, quiz 21.e2-3.

68. Davis JT, Allen HD, Cohen DM. Fiscal impact of a practice pattern for secundum atrial septal defect repair in children. *Am J Cardiol.* 1994;74: 512-514.

69. Srinivasan C, Sachdeva R, Morrow WR, et al. Standardized management improves outcomes after the Norwood procedure. *Congenit Heart Dis.* 2009;4:329-337.

70. Gaies MG, Clarke NS, Donohue JE, et al. Personnel and unit factors impacting outcome after cardiac arrest in a dedicated pediatric cardiac intensive care unit. *Pediatr Crit Care Med.* 2012;13:583-588.

71. Bhakta RT, Stockwell DC. Transitions of care in the pediatric cardiac intensive care unit. *Crit Care Med.* 2012;40:2245-2246.

72. Agarwal HS, Saville BR, Slayton JM, et al. Standardized postoperative handover process improves outcomes in the intensive care unit: a model for operational sustainability and improved team performance. *Crit Care Med.* 2012;40:2109-2115.

76. Gaynor JW, Stopp C, Wypij D, et al. Neurodevelopmental outcomes after cardiac surgery in infancy. *Pediatrics.* 2015;135:816-825.

77. Tabbutt S. How to improve neurodevelopmental and quality of life outcomes following early surgery for congenital heart disease? *Dev Med Child Neurol.* 2013;55:1072-1073.

78. Marino BS, Lipkin PH, Newburger JW. Neurodevelopmental outcomes in children with congenital heart disease: evaluation and management: a scientific statement from the American Heart Association. *Circulation.* 2012;126:1143-1172.

79. Tabbutt S, Gaynor JW, Newburger JW. Neurodevelopmental outcomes after congenital heart surgery and strategies for improvement. *Curr Opin Cardiol.* 2012;27:82-91.

80. Kilbaugh TJ, Huh JW, Berg RA. Neurological injuries are common contributors to pediatric intensive care unit deaths: a wake-up call. *Pediatr Crit Care Med.* 2011;12:601-602.

81. Moreau JF, Fink EL, Hartman ME, et al. Hospitalizations of children with neurologic disorders in the United States. *Pediatr Crit Care Med.* 2013;14:801-810.

82. Au AK, Carcillo JA, Clark RSB, et al. Brain injuries and neurological system failure are the most common proximate causes of death in children admitted to a pediatric intensive care unit. *Pediatr Crit Care Med.* 2010;12:566-571.

84. Hannah C, et al. Neurocritical care for neonates: pediatric neurology. *Curr Treat Options Neurol.* 2011;13:574.

85. Bonifacio SL, Glass HC, Peloquin S, et al. A new neurological focus in neonatal intensive care. *Nat Rev Neurol.* 2011;7:485-494.

86. LaRovere KL, Graham RJ, Tasker RC, et al. Pediatric neurocritical care: a neurology consultation model and implication for education and training. *Pediatr Neurol.* 2013;48:206-211.

87. LaRovere KL, Riviello JJ. Emerging subspecialties in neurology: building a career and a field: pediatric neurocritical care. *Neurology.* 2008;70: e89-e91.

88. Murphy S. Pediatric neurocritical care. *Neurother.* 2012;9:3-16.

89. Friess SH, Naim MY, Helfaer MA. Is pediatric neurointensive care a legitimate programmatic advancement to benefit our patients and our trainees, or others? *Pediatr Crit Care Med.* 2010;11:758-760.

91. Pineda JA, Leonard JR, Mazotas IG, et al. Effect of implementation of a paediatric neurocritical care programme on outcomes after severe traumatic brain injury: a retrospective cohort study. *Lancet Neurol.* 2013;12:45-52.

94. Morrison WE, Helfaer MA, Nadkarni VM. National survey of pediatric critical care medicine fellowship clinical and research time allocation. *Pediatr Crit Care Med.* 2009;10:397-399.

95. Kaltman JR, Andropoulos DB, Checchia PA. Report of the pediatric heart network and national heart, lung, and blood institute working group on the perioperative management of congenital heart disease. *Circulation.* 2010;121:2766-2772.

96. Pediatric Neurocritical Care Research Group. Available at <http://www.pncrg.org>. Accessed 20.03.16.

Critical Communication in the Pediatric Intensive Care Unit

Shelina M. Jamal, Katherine Banker, and Harris P. Baden

PEARLS

- Recognition of a high rate of medical errors resulting from ineffective communication and teamwork compelled development of strategies and tools to promote situational awareness and a shared mental model in the health care setting.
- Using specific design elements in the intensive care unit (ICU) can enhance patient surveillance and nonverbal communication.
- Applying standardized work such as organized huddles, checklists, and structured rounds can result in less variability and more consistent communication within multidisciplinary ICU care teams.
- Intentional and ongoing education and assessment of communication skills, such as closed-loop communication, and using techniques such as simulation and debriefing are vital.
- Implementation of interdisciplinary team training provides skills that improve teamwork, enhance communication, and contribute to patient safety.

"Safety first" is the mantra of 21st century American health care since the Institute of Medicine's 1999 publication, "To Err Is Human: Building a Safer Health System."[1] That groundbreaking report drew attention to the high rate of medical errors resulting from ineffective communication and teamwork and compelled an industry-wide effort to transform health care delivery systems and practices. Contemporary pediatric intensive care units (ICUs) are highly technical and data-rich environments, with specialized, multidisciplinary care teams that are ever rotating to provide 24/7 coverage. Accordingly, establishment of an effective and reliable system of communication is imperative in every ICU.

Various schemes and tools are available to optimize communication and mitigate risk. Common to all is the focus on ensuring that every member of the health care team, including the patient, is "on the same page." For example, borrowing from the US Department of Defense and other high-reliability industries, the Agency for Healthcare Research and Quality

developed TeamSTEPPS, a collection of strategies and tools to promote "situational awareness" and development of a "shared mental model" by fostering communication, leadership, situation monitoring, and mutual support, all rooted in team structure and dynamics.[2] Dr. Mica Endsley, Chief Scientist of the US Air Force, pioneered the development and evaluation of systems to support human situation awareness and decision making, which she defined as "the perception of elements in the environment within a volume of time and space, the comprehension of their meaning, and the projection of their status in the near future."[3] Kenneth Craik, philosopher and psychologist, first described the concept of mental models as an explanation of an individual's thought process about a particular situation that can be influenced by the surrounding circumstances, team member dynamics, and a person's intuitive perception.[4] Mental models shape behavior and set an approach, a personal algorithm, to solving problems. In the team setting, it is imperative that all individual members share the same mental model.

This chapter describes communication tools and other techniques to enhance situational awareness and the development of a shared mental model as ways of improving patient safety in the critical care setting. Comprehensive efforts encompass ICU design, monitoring systems, electronic medical records, patient flow schemes, closed-loop communication, staffing models, and team training. The authors discuss verbal and visual communication strategies that have been deployed in the medical setting with successful and sustainable results.

Intensive Care Unit Design

According to the 2012 Society of Critical Care Medicine's Guidelines, optimal ICU design can help reduce medical errors, improve patient outcomes, reduce length of stay, increase social support for patients, and play a role in reducing patient cost.[5] Private rooms enhance the patient and family experience, and minimizing noise and disturbances can promote the healing process.[6-8] On the other hand, published reports describe a correlation between lower ICU visibility and increased mortality.[9] As a consequence, reliable monitoring systems are crucial to patient safety and quality of care. This includes not only bedside monitoring but also remote monitoring of patients from central workstations and throughout the ICU. Several design elements can enhance situational awareness, patient surveillance, and nonverbal communication in the ICU.

In patient rooms:
- Monitoring should be visible from the door and the care team's workspace.
- Display boards in the room can be used for daily care plans, patient and family questions, and family contact information.
- Signage in the room can convey information to care team members, ancillary staff, and families (eg, isolation requirements, fracture risk, fall risk, difficult airway, or an open chest).
- Boards outside the patient's room identify the nurse, responsible physician, and contact information.

Within the ICU:
- Remote centralized monitoring should be in place so that even when not in the vicinity of the patient, their monitoring is visible (eg, monitors at various places in the unit itself, conference rooms, call rooms).
- A central board near the main workstation shows the physical layout of the unit, patient location, nursing assignment, admits and transfers for the day, the care team, and their contact information.
- Signage denoting a sterile procedure is in progress creates a physical barrier to encourage nonessential personnel to avoid the area, as well as promoting situational awareness within the greater ICU team.
- Remote access to operating room boards or intraoperative cameras allows the ICU team to follow a patient's progress and be prepared for the patient arrival.

Medical Record

Extracting useful information from the electronic medical record can be challenging. Alerts and notifications regarding code status, medication allergies, or important social issues allow rapid orientation to the patient's status and care plan. In development are monitoring and prediction models that take patient data (ie, from the telemetry monitors) and identify patterns that might warn of impending clinical deterioration. Likewise, these techniques may be helpful in retrospective reviews for quality improvement purposes.

Huddles

Huddles are brief gatherings that bring team members together to create a shared mental model regarding a distinct procedure or event, or a status update across the entire ICU.[10-12] They should include team introductions, review of planned activities, anticipation of problems that may arise, and creation of contingency plans. Huddles serve to activate teams, empowering each team member to share responsibility in the completion of the task, while encouraging openness and trust among the team, facilitating communication, and improving overall situational awareness.[10]

Keys to successful implementation of huddles in a medical setting include these criteria[13-15]:
- Designation of a leader
- Mandatory participation of *all* team members
- Incorporation into standard work practice

- Time limits of 10 minutes or less
- Occurrence in a central location

Huddles can be used in these and other scenarios:
- Admission, to facilitate communication to review events, create a care plan, and highlight risks/concerns
- Periprocedure to orient the team, define roles, and identify potential pitfalls and contingency plans
  - ICU day/night shift changes to review expected procedures, admissions, transfers, discharges, and high-acuity patients
  - ICU workflow management to discuss planned ICU admissions and discharges, as well as their impact on staffing, bed availability, and hospital census
  - Daily check-in (a health care performance initiative),[16] for a focused and directed conversation to address safety/quality issues from the past 24 hours, anticipated safety/quality issues in the next 24 hours, and status reports on issues identified that day or day prior

Checklists

Checklists have been widely adopted by the health care industry, with demonstrated reductions in morbidity, mortality, and preventable errors.[17-20] A commonly used checklist is the Universal Protocol, created in 2004 by The Joint Commission Board of Commissioners, to address the wrong-site, wrong-procedure, and wrong-person surgery and other procedures.[21-22] A 2010 survey found more than 90% of respondents agreed or strongly agreed that there was benefit in using the Universal Protocol in hospital units where invasive procedures are performed.

Well-constructed checklists serve as follows:
- Function as communication tools with demonstrated benefit in routine procedures (eg, extubation, procedural sedation, MRI screening, and preoperative screening) and less frequent occurrences (eg, extracorporeal membrane oxygenation [ECMO] cannulation, computer downtime).[23-28]
- Increase the reliability of care processes. Checklists performed at the end of rounds have been shown to reduce central line–associated bloodstream infections, optimize nutrition, enhance sedation weaning, etc.[29-32]
- Serve as evaluation/audit tools.

Though creation and implementation of checklists are important, shifting the culture and behaviors of those using the checklist is what determines success. Implementing mandatory checklists with limited focus on transformation of attitudes can result in no change in outcomes.[33]

Rounds

Performance of daily rounds in a standardized format results in less variability and more consistent communication within the team. To ensure a shared mental model and optimize situational awareness, all team members (eg, physicians, nurses, pharmacists, nutritionists, family members) should participate on rounds in preassigned roles. Structured reporting of data and presentation of information ensures that no issues are missed and all concerns are addressed. Daily rounds conclude with review of safety checks and order read-back: closed-loop communication with all team members that re-enforces the shared mental model.

Closed-Looped Communication

Deficiencies in verbal communication impair the development of team structure, collaboration, and task performance.[34-35] Standardized methods of communication have been developed to promote safety and efficiency, thereby reducing the risk of team breakdowns.[36-37] A common method used in health care settings is closed-loop communication, which involves three steps:

1. Sender transmits a message using standardized terminology
2. Receiver accepts the message and verbally acknowledges receipt and understanding
3. Sender verifies that the message has been received and interpreted correctly

Transitions of Care

Reliable communication is essential at times of transitions of care. Duty-hour restrictions for physicians in training have led to increased hand-offs and the potential for discontinuity in patient care.[38] Consistent use of a hand-off tool (eg, I-PASS: *I*llness Severity, *P*atient Summary, *A*ction List, *S*ituation Awareness and Contingency Plans, *S*ynthesis by Receiver) has been associated with reductions in medical errors and preventable adverse events, as well as improvements in communication, without a negative effect on workflow.[39] Transfers between hospitals to the ICU can be especially high risk as they involve transport of critically ill patients, variable team members and skillsets, and resources limited by space and mobility. Transmission of clear, concise, and accurate information is imperative (see also Chapter 18).

Creation of a "Communication Center" can facilitate this process by doing the following:

- Using a single phone number for all referring hospitals and providers wishing to initiate transfer of a patient
- Recording phone conversations to clarify information transmitted, as well as quality improvement initiatives
- Conferencing simultaneously with multiple team members
- Ensuring prompt and reliable access to the transport team while en route

Medical Training

The *Accreditation Council for Graduate Medical Education* requires that Pediatric Critical Care Medicine fellows "demonstrate interpersonal and communication skills that result in the effective exchange of information and collaboration with patients, their families, and health professionals."[40] Communication is also a cornerstone of effective team leadership and is a key feature of Pediatric Advanced Life Support training.[41] Staff perceptions of teamwork and team behavior are related to the quality and safety of patient care and identify aspects of communication and teamwork that lead to safer patient care.[42] Additionally, evaluation of a trainee's ability to communicate is changing with the development of clinical competencies and milestones (see also Chapter 22). Intentional education and assessment of communication skills are a growing expectation.[43]

Incorporating communication into medical training comprises these and many other ways:

- A longitudinal curriculum during undergraduate or graduate medical training
- Strategies specific to a certain rotation or environment
- Focus on communication as a marker for ongoing quality improvement

One effective means of teaching and evaluating communication in the ICU is through the use of simulation.[44] Simulation scenarios focused on closed-loop communication skills, such as clarity of roles and responsibilities, order repeat-backs, clarifying questions, knowledge sharing, reevaluation and summarizing, and mutual respect, give ICU staff the opportunity to practice in a high-fidelity, low-risk environment.[45-49] Some scenarios, like an ECMO cannulation, allow for incorporation of multiple disciplines (eg, physicians, trainees, nurses, respiratory therapists) leading to more realistic simulation of infrequent, high-risk events that require precise teamwork.[50-51] Simulation is further enhanced with thorough debriefing.

Debriefing

"Debriefing" originated in the military (analyzing a mission after it is completed) and gained traction in critical incident reviews (mitigating stress following critical events).[52] According to Kolb, the process of reflective observation is a cornerstone of lifelong adult learning.[53] In medical simulation, debriefing is facilitated reflection that leads participants to analyze and learn from an event.[52] Debriefing is also helpful after high-risk, infrequent events and after any event team members find particularly challenging. Effective debriefing can improve skill acquisition and retention, as well as staff satisfaction.[41,54-57]

In general, debriefing includes the following[58-65]:

- Structure: Phases include description, analogy/analysis, and application. A communication tool ensures that key points are addressed and the process is standardized.
- Content: Focus can include communication, medical management processes, and logistics.
- Participation: Team members should be active participants in self-reflection.
- Action items: Development of reliable method for follow-up is essential.

Team Training

The Institute of Medicine calls for interdisciplinary team training programs for critical care settings.[1] Extensive team training curricula based on concepts central to Crew Resource Management (CRM) exist and continue to evolve.[66-71] Examples include TeamSTEPPS and Veterans Affairs Medical Team Training (VA MTT).

Common themes among these programs emerge[67]:

- Developing communication strategies that flatten hierarchy and encourage team member assertiveness
- Cross-training to tasks, duties, and responsibilities of all team roles
- Simulating errors and contingencies
- Conducting facilitated debriefings
- Creating shared mental models and situational awareness
- Encouraging closed-loop communication

Deliberate and ongoing team training and evaluation are imperative to sustaining improvement in patient safety.[72-75]

Conclusion

Intensive care units are high-stake, high-risk environments. Reliable and accurate communication are essential to optimizing patient care and safety. An ICU focused on safety is characterized by thoughtful design, reliable organizational systems of communication, and unwavering commitment to teamwork. These elements foster a shared mental model and improve situational awareness among all team members, leading to greater efficiency and safer health care delivery.

Key References

1. *Front matter. To Err Is Human: Building a Safer Health System*. Washington, DC: The National Academies Press; 2000.
2. *TeamSTEPPS 2.0: Core Curriculum*. Rockville, MD: Agency for Healthcare Research and Quality; 2014: http://www.ahrq.gov/professionals/education/curriculum-tools/teamstepps/instructor/index.html.
5. Thompson DR, Hamilton DK, Cadenhead CD, et al. Guidelines for intensive care unit design. *Crit Care Med*. 2012;40(5):1586-1600.
8. Xie H, Kang J, Mills GH, et al. Clinical review: the impact of noise on patients' sleep and the effectiveness of noise reduction strategies in intensive care units. *Cochrane Database Syst Rev*. 2009;(13).
9. Leaf DE, Homel P, Factor PH, et al. Relationship between ICU design and mortality. *Chest*. 2010;137:1022-1027.
10. *Meeting tools: huddles*. Cambridge, MA: Institute for Healthcare Improvement; 2015: http://www.ihi.org/resources/Pages/Tools/Huddles.aspx.
11. *Use regular huddles and staff meetings to plan production and to optimize team communication*. Cambridge, MA: Institute for Healthcare Improvement; 2015: http://www.ihi.org/resources/Pages/Changes/UseRegularHuddlesandStaffMeetingstoPlanProductionandtoOptimizeTeamCommunication.aspx.
15. No authors listed. Medication huddles slash adverse drug events, promote safety culture across all hospital units, including the ED. *ED Manag*. 2014;26(3):suppl 1-suppl 4.
16. Stockmeier C, Clapper C. *Daily Check-In for Safety: From Best Practice to Common Practice. HPI White Paper Series*. 1st ed. Virginia Beach, VA: Healthcare Performance Improvement, LLC; 2010: http://hpiresults.com/publications/HPI%20White%20Paper%20-%20Daily%20Check-In%20REV%200%20SEP%202010.pdf.
17. Bergs J, Hellings J, Cleemput I, et al. Systematic review and meta-analysis of the effect of the WHO surgical safety checklist on postoperative complications. *Br J Surg*. 2014;101(3):150-158.
18. Haynes AB, Weiser TG, Berry WR, et al. A surgical safety checklist to reduce morbidity and mortality in a global population. *N Engl J Med*. 2009;360(5):491-499.
19. Hales BM, Pronovost PJ. The checklist—a tool for error management and performance improvement. *J Crit Care*. 2006;21(3):231-235.
20. Bosk CL, Dixon-Woods M, Goeschel CA, et al. Reality check for checklists. *Lancet*. 2009;374:444-445.
21. *Universal Protocol*. Oakbrook Terrace, IL: The Joint Commission; 2015: http://www.jointcommission.org/standards_information/up.aspx.
23. Li S, Rehder KJ, Giuliano JS Jr, et al. Development of a quality improvement bundle to reduce tracheal intubation-associated events in pediatric ICUs. *Am J Med Qual*. 2014;[epub ahead of print].
24. Davis DA, Mazmanian PE, Fordis M, et al. Accuracy of physician self-assessment compared with observed measures of competence: a systematic review. *JAMA*. 2006;296:1094-1102.
25. Pronovost PJ, Goeschel CA, Colantuoni E, et al. Sustaining reductions in catheter related bloodstream infections in Michigan intensive care units: observational study. *BMJ*. 2010;340:c309.
26. Haynes AB, Weiser TG, Berry WR, et al. Changes in safety attitude and relationship to decreased postoperative morbidity and mortality following implementation of a checklist-based surgical safety intervention. *BMJ Qual Saf*. 2011;20:102-107.
27. Berenholtz SM, Pham JC, Thompson DA, et al. Collaborative cohort study of an intervention to reduce ventilator-associated pneumonia in the intensive care unit. *Infect Control Hosp Epidemiol*. 2011;32:305-314.
28. Lipitz-Snyderman A, Steinwachs D, Needham DM, et al. Impact of a statewide intensive care unit quality improvement initiative on hospital mortality and length of stay: retrospective comparative analysis. *BMJ*. 2011;342:d219.
31. Sharma S, Peters MJ, PICU/NICU Risk Action Group. "Safety by DEFAULT": introduction and impact of a pediatric ward round checklist. *Crit Care*. 2013;17(5):R232.
32. Centofanti JE, Duan EH, Hoad NC, et al. Use of daily goals checklist for morning ICU rounds: a mixed-methods study. *Crit Care*. 2014;42(8):1797-1803.
33. Urbach DR, Govindarajan A, Saskin R, et al. Introduction of surgical safety checklists in Ontario, Canada. *NEJM*. 2014;370:1029-1038.
38. DeRienzo CM, Frush K, Barfield ME, et al. Hand-offs in the era of duty hours reform: a focused review and strategy to address changes in the Accreditation Council for Graduate Medical Education Common Program Requirements. *Acad Med*. 2012;87(4):403-410.
39. Starmer AJ, Spector ND, Srivastava R, et al. Changes in medical errors after implementation of a hand-off program. *N Engl J Med*. 2014;371:1803-1812.
40. ACGME Program Requirements for Graduate Medical Education in Pediatric Critical Care Medicine. ACGME Approved: September 12, 2006; Effective: July 1, 2007: https://www.acgme.org/acgmeweb/Portals/0/PFAssets/2013-PR-FAQ-PIF/323_critical_care_peds_07012013.pdf.
41. Cheng A, Rodgers DL, van der Jagt E, et al. Evolution of the Pediatric Advanced Life Support course: enhanced learning with a new debriefing tool and web-based module for PALS instructors. *Pediatr Crit Care Med*. 2012;13(5):589-595.
42. Manser T. Teamwork and patient safety in dynamic domains of healthcare: a review of the literature. *Acta Anaesthesiol Scand*. 2009;53:143-151.
43. Turner DA, Mink RB, Lee KJ, et al. Are pediatric critical care medicine fellowships teaching and evaluating communication and professionalism? *Pediatr Crit Care Med*. 2013;14(5):454-461.
44. McGaghie WC, Issenberg SB, Cohen ER, et al. Does simulation-based medical education with deliberate practice yield better results than traditional clinical education? A meta-analytic comparative review of the evidence. *Acad Med*. 2011;86(6):706-711.
45. Steadman RH, Coates WC, Huang YM, et al. Simulation-based training is superior to problem-based learning for the acquisition of critical assessment and management skills. *Crit Care Med*. 2006;34(1):151-157.
47. Allan CK, Thiagarajan RR, Beke D, et al. Simulation-based training delivered directly to the pediatric cardiac intensive care unit engenders preparedness, comfort, and decreased anxiety among multidisciplinary resuscitation teams. *J Thorac Cardiovasc Surg*. 2010;140(3):646-652.
49. Cuoto TB, Kerrey BT, Taylor RG, et al. Teamwork skills in actual, in situ, and in-center pediatric emergencies: performance levels across settings and perceptions of comparative educational impact. *Simul Healthc*. 2015;10(5):76-84.
52. Fanning RM, Gaba DM. The role of debriefing in simulation-based learning. *Simul Healthc*. 2007;2(2):115-125.
53. Kolb D. *Experiential Learning: Experience as a Source of Learning and development*. Upper Saddle River, NJ: Prentice Hall; 1984.
54. Percarpio KB, Harris FS, Hatfield BA, et al. Code debriefing from the Department of Veterans Affairs (VA) Medical Team Training program improves the cardiopulmonary resuscitation code process. *Jt Comm J Qual Patient Saf*. 2010;36(9):424-429, 385.
57. Cheng A, Hunt EA, Donoghue A, et al. Examining pediatric resuscitation education using simulation and scripted debriefing. *JAMA Pediatr*. 2013;167(6):528-536.
58. Eppich W, Cheng A. Promoting excellence and reflective learning in simulation. Development and rationale for a blended approach to health care simulation debriefing. *Simul Healthc*. 2015;10(2):106-115.
60. Raemer D, Anderson M, Cheng A, et al. Research regarding debriefing as part of the learning process. *Simul Healthc*. 2011;6(7):S52-S57.
61. Edelson DP, LaFond CM. Deconstructing debriefing for simulation-based education. *JAMA Pediatr*. 2013;167(6):586-587.
65. Kolbe M, Weiss M, Grote G, et al. TeamGAINS: a tool for structured debriefings for simulation-based team trainings. *BMJ Qual Saf*. 2013;22:541-553.
67. Weaver SJ, Dy SM, Rosen MA, et al. Team-training in healthcare: a narrative synthesis of the literature. *BMJ Qual Saf*. 2014;23:359-372.
68. Thomas EJ. Improving teamwork in healthcare: current approaches and the path forward. *BMJ Qual Saf*. 2011;20(8):647-650.
69. Buljac-Samardzic M, Dekker-van Doorn CM, van Wijngaarden JDH, et al. Interventions to improve team effectiveness: a systematic review. *Health Policy (New York)*. 2010;94:183-195.
70. Cumin D, Boyd MJ, Webster CS, et al. A systematic review of simulation for multidisciplinary team training in operating rooms. *Simul Healthc*. 2013;8(3):171-179.

71. Weaver SJ, Lyons R, DiazGranados D, et al. The anatomy of health care team training and the state of practice: a critical review. *Acad Med.* 2010;85(11):1746-1760.

72. Eppich WJ, Brannen M, Hunt EA. Team training: implications for emergency and critical care pediatrics. *Curr Opin Pediatr.* 2008;20:255-260.

73. Mayer CM, Cluff L, Lin W, et al. Evaluating efforts to optimize TeamSTEPPS implementation in surgical and pediatric intensive care units. *Jt Comm J Qual Patient Saf.* 2011;37(8):365-374.

74. Van Schaik SM, Plant J, Diane S, et al. Interprofessional team training in pediatric resuscitation: a low-cost, in situ simulation program that enhances self-efficacy among participants. *Clin Pediatr (Phila).* 2011;50(9): 807-815.

75. Stocker M, Allen M, Pool N, et al. Impact of an embedded simulation team training programme in a pediatric intensive care unit: a prospective, single centre, longitudinal study. *Intensive Care Med.* 2012;38:99-104.

Professionalism in Pediatric Critical Care

Bradley P. Fuhrman

PEARLS

- The medical profession is largely self-regulated and confers many benefits on its members.
- To sustain these professional benefits, physicians must honor their contract with society.
- Professionalism is, in its simplest form, putting the patient first, placing altruism before self-interest.
- Beyond that, professionalism is a more complete charter that ties altruism to the concrete realities of the doctor-patient relationship and the marketplace in which doctors practice.
- The Physician Charter is grounded in the principles of altruism, patient autonomy, and social justice. It represents the physician's contract with society.

Pediatric critical care medicine (PCCM) is a profession. To be certified and practice as a pediatric intensivist, individuals must master several bodies of special knowledge, complete apprenticeships in pediatrics and pediatric critical care, earn various educational certificates, pass examinations (the culmination of which is the American Board of Pediatrics certifying examination in pediatric critical care), and be granted a license by a state medical board. PCCM as a profession oversees that process much as a guild controls its members and membership. As a profession, pediatric intensivists train themselves, test themselves, credential themselves, and discipline themselves. Pediatric intensivists derive many benefits from their status as professionals. They are paid as professionals, respected as professionals, and valued by society as professionals.

There exist contracts between professions and society. In exchange for the benefits "professionalism" confers and the autonomy, self-governance, and control of licensure that physicians are granted, society expects physicians to meet its needs within the boundaries of their expertise. Physicians gain the advantages listed earlier because they provide the quality of service that society requires.

Professionalism is, in the end, the set of responsibilities and behaviors that fulfill physicians' contract with society. These characteristics exemplify the good and virtuous doctor because that is the model society would hold physicians to, not because virtue has intrinsic value (which it does), but because deviation from virtue breaks the contract.

The Virtuous Doctor

Most would agree as to which characteristics exemplify the good and virtuous doctor. Society has watched doctors portrayed on television for decades in the persons of James Kildare, Konrad Styner, David Zorba, Ben Casey, Meredith Grey, and Marcus Welby. These are the characters that physicians' parents, as well as the rest of society, expect physicians to emulate. But over the past 15 to 20 years the professional organizations of medicine have obsessed over defining, teaching, assessing, and understanding professionalism. The reader might ask, "why is that?"

The Stakes

Health care now consumes (produces) about 17% of the US gross domestic product.[1] It has become increasingly technology intense and engages financial giants in the form of pharmaceutical companies, device/equipment manufacturers, and information storage/management enterprises. It employs about 14,000,000 workers.[2] Two of the largest third-party payers are Medicare and Medicaid, which together expend 4.7% of the gross domestic product on health care. Those payments flow from the general (tax) coffers to individual physicians among other recipients. We now live in a "medical marketplace"[3] and hear patients referred to by administrators as "customers" or by insurers as "covered lives." How physicians manage patients in this context is of great financial import, so it should be no surprise that many of the traits characterized as professionalism have financial implications.

The Great Paradox of the Medical Profession

A constant tension pervades medicine where principles of "self-interest" and "altruism" coexist.[4] In most human endeavors, it is considered appropriate to identify individuals' best interests and make decisions accordingly. It is in one's best interest to obey the law, brush one's teeth, and work for a living. Yet it is in the best interest of society for physicians to treat patients altruistically. The physician's pledge to society is to be altruistic in dealing with patients, to put the patient first, before oneself. These two principles, self-interest and altruism, are polarized and often conflict. With each medical decision come these questions: "Was this for the patient or for the doctor? Whose interest did this serve?" In its simplest sense, professionalism in medicine comes down to putting the patient first.

The reader may consider a concrete example: It is 4 am. A pediatric intensivist hasn't slept a wink and is hard at work in the pediatric intensive care unit (PICU) trying to finish his documentation so that he can catch some shuteye. The emergency department (ED) resident calls. He has a child with a fever who looks sick. He asks if the intensivist would mind taking a look to see if the child needs to come to the PICU. What should the pediatric intensivist do?
1. Go take a look at the child.
2. Have the child admitted to general pediatrics.
3. Hold the child in the ED until 7 am when relief arrives for the day shift.
4. Just bring the child up to the PICU.
5. Send the child home; it's just a fever.

Altruism says that the intensivist should go take a look. That would be best for the patient. It could improve the quality of the triage decision and optimize patient care.

Self-interest suggests options 2, 3, or 5 because the child is not the intensivist's immediate problem and addresses the intensivist's exhaustion.

So the professionalism issue here is altruism, "patient first," but there is also the issue of financial overlay. The PICU provides expensive care and is a costly resource. A decision to admit to the PICU should not be made casually. General pediatrics may not be able to safely care for the patient, and a bad outcome means a lawsuit. Hospitalization should be avoided unless really necessary. It costs money. However, holding the patient in the ED is a dissatisfier and will damage the hospital in the eyes of the community.

Professionalism is a larger issue than merely resolving the "patient first" medical paradox, and it received a much more thorough examination in the late 1990s and first decade of the new millennium. Many of the groups that regulate medicine on physicians' behalf weighed in. Among them were the American Board of Internal Medicine Foundation, the American College of Physicians–American Society of Internal Medicine, and the European Federation of Internal Medicine, who worked together to draft the document *Medical Professionalism in the New Millennium: A Physician Charter.*[5]

Professionalism, the Physician Charter

The Charter adopted three principles and made 10 commitments to fulfill the medical profession's contract with society:

Principle 1: *Primacy of Patient Welfare.* Altruism demands that the patient's needs be given precedence over self-interest, market forces, societal pressure, and administrative exigency.
Principle 2: *Patient Autonomy.* Physicians must be honest with their patients and, whenever possible, empower them to make informed decisions.
Principle 3: *Social Justice.* There should be fair distribution of health care resources.

Commitment 1: *Professional Competence.* Each individual physician must assure his or her own, and the profession as a whole must assure its members', competence. Professionals are responsible for putting mechanisms in place to assure lifelong learning and competence.
Commitment 2: *Honesty with Patients.* Patients must be completely and honestly informed. Medical errors must be acknowledged. Mistakes must be analyzed to improve the quality of health care.
Commitment 3: *Patient Confidentiality.* Patient trust demands that confidences be protected. Trust is essential to the doctor-patient (patient-doctor) relationship.
Commitment 4: *Appropriate Relations to Patients.* Patients are inherently vulnerable. Professionalism demands that they not be exploited.
Commitment 5: *Improve Quality of Care.* Physicians must not only maintain clinical competence but also work collaboratively to reduce medical errors, increase patient safety, minimize overuse of health care resources, and optimize outcomes of care.
Commitment 6: *Improve Access to Care.* Physicians must strive to reduce barriers to equitable health care and foster uniform and adequate standards of care.
Commitment 7: *Just Distribution of Finite Resources.* The physician must make wise and cost-effective use of limited resources.
Commitment 8: *Scientific Knowledge.* Where possible, care should be evidence based.
Commitment 9: *Manage Conflicts of Interest.* To maintain patient trust, physicians must recognize, disclose, and deal with conflicts of interest that arise in the course of their professional activities.
Commitment 10: *Assure the Integrity of Professional Responsibilities.* The profession must define, organize, and assure the standards of its current and future members.

The PICU as a Site for Medical Education and Lifelong Learning

The renaissance of interest in professionalism has created an endeavor to weave the topic into medical education, build it into curricula, and focus on it in coursework.[6] Despite that interest, medical student altruism, social interest, and other qualities of positive social value have been noted to decline as the student progresses through medical school and the early phase of clinical training.[7-11] The altruistic freshman is transformed by clinical experiences into the cynical senior. It has been argued that this growth of cynicism reflects the gap between what physicians say as teachers (the formal curriculum) and what physicians do as practitioners (the hidden curriculum).[12] When physicians do not "walk the talk," they plant the seeds of cynicism and nonprofessionalism.

For example: Dr. Blunt and an impressionable medical student are suturing in place a central line. Their patient is in a chemically induced coma, from self-medication, compounded by subsequent hypoxia. His story is tragic, and the student knows that the teenager deserves sympathy and respect. As Dr. Blunt ties the last knot, she comments, "It would have been easier if he weren't so fat." A lesson about sympathy and respect has gone array.

In the PICU, doctors, students, and nurses are compressed into a small, tense space. They are all engaged in lifelong learning as they play their separate roles in patient care. So, throughout their development and maturation as professionals, care providers in the PICU are continuously learning professionalism and cynicism from their colleagues.

All PICU care providers should clean up their acts, take care that their words and actions reflect the formal curriculum, fulfill their contract with society, and behave toward their patients as the professionals they set out to be.

References

1. World Health Organization. Global health expenditure database. 2015; <http://data.worldbank.org/indicator/SH.XPD.TOTL.ZS>.
2. Congressional Budget Office. Federal spending and the government's major health care programs is projected to rise substantially relative to GDP. 2013; <http://www.cbo.gov/publication/44582>.
3. Frankford DM, Konrad TR. Responsive medical professionalism: integrating education, practice and community in a market-driven era. *Acad Med*. 1998;73:138-145.
4. Jonsen AR. Watching the doctor. *N Engl J Med*. 1983;308:1531-1535.
5. ABIM Foundation, ACP-ASIM Foundation and EFIM. Medical professionalism in the new millennium: a physician charter. *Ann Intern Med*. 2002;136(3):243-246.
6. Inui TS. *A flag in the wind: educating for professionalism in medicine*. Association of American Medical Colleges, 2003 <https://members .aamc.org/eweb/upload/A%20Flag%20in%20the%20Wind%20 Report.pdf>.
7. Wear D. Professional development of medical students: problems and promises. *Acad Med*. 1997;72:1056-1062.
8. Testerman JK, Morton KR, Loo LK, et al. The natural history of cynicism in physicians. *Acad Med*. 1996;71:S43-S45.
9. Feudtner C, Christakis DA, Christakis NA. Do clinical clerks suffer ethical erosion? Students' perceptions of their ethical environment and personal development. *Acad Med*. 1994;69:670-679.
10. Marcus ER. Empathy, humanism, and the professionalization process of medical education. *Acad Med*. 1999;74(11):1211-1215.
11. Crandall SJS, Volk RJ, Loemker V. Medical students' attitudes toward providing care for the underserved. *J Amer Med Assoc*. 1993;269: 2519-2523.
12. Coulehan J. Today's professionalism: engaging the mind but not the heart. *Acad Med*. 2005;80(10):892-898.

Nurses in Pediatric Critical Care

Patricia A. Moloney-Harmon and Martha A.Q. Curley

PEARLS

- Along with other members of the multidisciplinary team of dedicated intensive care experts, nursing navigates safe passage for patients and families during critical illness.
- Nurses coordinate the patient's and family's experiences by their continuous attention to the person who exists underneath all the advanced technology that is being employed.
- Building a humanistic environment that endorses parents as unique individuals capable of providing essential elements of care to their children constitutes the foundation for family-centered care.
- Caring practices include a constellation of nursing activities that are responsive to the uniqueness of the patient/family and create a compassionate and therapeutic environment with the aim of promoting comfort and preventing suffering.
- Excellence in a pediatric critical care unit is achieved through a combination of many factors and is highly dependent on a healthy work environment.
- Studies have demonstrated that a stable, established, and proficient nursing workforce improves patient outcomes.
- A successful critical care professional advancement program recognizes varying levels of staff nurse knowledge and expertise and fosters advancement through a wide range of clinical learning and professional development experiences.
- Technical training alone is insufficient for meeting patient and family needs in the critical care environment.

Pediatric critical care nursing has evolved tremendously over the years. The nurse plays a vitally important role in the pediatric intensive care unit (PICU) in fostering an environment in which critically unstable, highly vulnerable infants and children benefit from vigilant care and the highly coordinated actions of a skilled team of patient-focused health care professionals. Pediatric critical care nursing practice encompasses staff nurses who provide direct patient care, nursing leaders who facilitate an environment of excellence, professional staff development that ensures continued nursing competence and professional growth, and nurse scientists who generate knowledge to support the practice of pediatric critical care nursing. This chapter discusses the essential components of pediatric critical care nursing practice.

Describing What Nurses Do: The Synergy Model

The Synergy Model describes nursing practice based on the needs and characteristics of patients and their families.[1] The fundamental premise of this model is that patient characteristics drive required nurse competencies. When patient characteristics and nurse competencies match and synergize, optimal patient outcomes result. The major components of the Synergy Model encompass patient characteristics of concern to nurses, nurse competencies important to the patient, and patient outcomes that result when patient characteristics and nurse competencies are in synergy.

Patient Characteristics of Concern to Nurses

Every patient and family member brings unique characteristics to the PICU experience. These characteristics—stability, complexity, predictability, resiliency, vulnerability, participation in decision making, participation in care, and resource availability—span the continuum of health and illness. Each characteristic is operationally defined as follows.

Stability refers to the person's ability to maintain a steady state (see also Chapter 81). Complexity is the intricate entanglement of two or more systems (eg, physiologic, family, and therapeutic). Predictability is a summative patient characteristic that allows the nurse to expect a certain trajectory of illness. Resiliency is the patient's capacity to return to a restorative level of functioning using compensatory and coping mechanisms. Vulnerability refers to an individual's susceptibility to actual or potential stressors that may adversely affect outcomes. Participation in decision making and participation in care are the extents to which the patient and family engage in decision making and in aspects of care, respectively. Resource availability refers to resources that the patient/family/community bring to a care situation and include personal, psychologic social, technical, and fiscal resources.

These eight characteristics apply to patients in all health care settings. This classification allows nurses to have a common language to describe patients that is meaningful to all care areas. For example, a critically ill infant in multisystem organ failure might be described as an individual who is unstable, highly complex, unpredictable, highly resilient, and vulnerable, whose family is able to become involved in decision making and care but has inadequate resource availability.

Each of these eight characteristics forms a continuum, and individuals fluctuate around different points along each continuum. For example, in the case of the critically ill infant in multisystem organ failure, stability can range from high to low, complexity from atypical to typical, predictability from uncertain to certain, resiliency from minimal reserves to generous reserves, vulnerability from susceptible to safe, family participation in decision making and care from no capacity to full capacity, and resource availability from minimal to extensive. Compared with existing patient classification systems, these eight dimensions better describe the needs of patients that are of concern to nurses.

Nurse Competencies Important to Patients and Families

Nursing competencies, which are derived from the needs of patients, also are described in terms of essential continua: clinical judgment, clinical inquiry, caring practices, response to diversity, advocacy/moral agency, facilitation of learning, collaboration, and systems thinking.

Clinical judgment is clinical reasoning that includes clinical decision making, critical thinking, and a global grasp of the situation coupled with nursing skills acquired through a process of integrating formal and experiential knowledge. Clinical inquiry is the ongoing process of questioning and evaluating practice, providing informed practice on the basis of available data, and innovating through research and experiential learning. The nurse engages in clinical knowledge development to promote the best patient outcomes. Caring practices are a constellation of nursing activities that are responsive to the uniqueness of the patient/family and create a compassionate and therapeutic environment with the aim of promoting comfort and preventing suffering. Caring behaviors include, but are not limited to, vigilance, engagement, and responsiveness. Response to diversity is the sensitivity to recognize, appreciate, and incorporate differences into the provision of care. Differences may include, but are not limited to, individuality, cultural practices, spiritual beliefs, gender, race, ethnicity, disability, family configuration, lifestyle, socioeconomic status, age, values, and alternative care practices involving patients/families and members of the health care team. Advocacy/moral agency is defined as working on another's behalf and representing the concerns of the patient/family/community. For example, the nurse serves as a moral agent in identifying and helping to resolve ethical and clinical concerns within the clinical setting. Facilitation of learning is the ability to use the process of providing care as an opportunity to enhance the patient's and family's understanding of the disease process, its treatment, and its likely impact on the child and family. Collaboration is working with others (ie, patients, families, and health care providers) in a way that promotes and encourages each person's contributions toward achieving optimal and realistic patient goals. Collaboration involves intradisciplinary and interdisciplinary work with colleagues. Systems thinking is appreciating the care environment from a perspective that recognizes the holistic interrelationships that exist within and across health care systems.

These competencies illustrate a dynamic integration of knowledge, skills, experience, and attitudes needed to meet patients' needs and optimize patient outcomes. Nurses require competence within each domain at a level that meets the needs of their patient population. Logically, more compromised patients have more severe or complex needs; this in turn requires the nurse to possess a higher level of knowledge and skill in an associated continuum. For example, if a patient is stable but unpredictable, minimally resilient, and vulnerable, primary competencies of the nurse center on clinical judgment and caring practices (which include vigilance). If a patient is vulnerable, unable to participate in decision making and care, and has inadequate resource availability, the primary competencies of the nurse focus on advocacy/moral agency, collaboration, and systems thinking. Although all the eight competencies are essential for contemporary nursing practice, each assumes more or less importance depending on a patient's characteristics. Optimal care is most likely when there is a match between patient needs/characteristics and nurse competencies.

Clinical Judgment

Clinical judgment—that is, skilled clinical knowledge, use of discretionary judgment, and the ability to integrate complex multisystem data and understand the expected trajectory of illness and human response to critical illness—defines competent nursing practice. In critical care, the novice nurse focuses on individual aspects of the patient and the environment. As expertise develops, the nurse develops a global understanding of the situation. The expert nurse is much better able to anticipate the needs of patients, predict the patient's trajectory of illness, and forecast the patient's level of recovery. The best nursing care often is invisible, as it should be, because untoward effects and complications are prevented. Along with other members of the dedicated team of PICU health care professionals, nurses, when exhibiting all key nursing competencies, facilitate the safest passage for patients and families through critical illness. Safe passage may include helping the patient and family move toward a greater level of self-awareness, knowledge, or health; transition through the acute care environment or stressful events; or a peaceful death.

Clinical Inquiry

Clinical inquiry optimizes the delivery of evidence-based care. Studying the clinical effectiveness of care and how it influences patient outcomes provides information that helps balance cost and quality. Quality improvement methods include use of multidisciplinary teams that work together to help systems operate in a way that promotes the best interests of patient care (see Chapter 11). Collaborative practice groups working with clinical practice guidelines (CPGs) provide the opportunity to initiate evidence-based and expert consensus-based interventions.

CPGs—that is, patient-centered multidisciplinary and multidimensional plans of care—help the team provide evidence-based practice and improve the process of care delivery. Effective CPGs are driven by patient needs and help provide evidence linking interventions to patient outcomes. Evidence-based guidelines can help to eliminate interventions that are steeped in tradition and opinion but do not actually benefit patients.

Caring Practices

Caring practices bring clinical judgment into view. Caring practices are activities that are meaningful to the patient and family and enhance their feelings that the health care team cares about them. Families equate caring behaviors with competent behaviors. Families trust that nurses will be vigilant. Vigilance, which includes alert and constant watchfulness, attentiveness, and reassuring presence, is essential to limit the complications associated with a patient's vulnerabilities.[1]

Nurses coordinate the patient's and family's experiences by their continuous attention to the person who exists underneath all the advanced technology that is employed. This steady attention can make an important difference by helping patients and their families better tolerate the experience of critical illness. This aspect of practice, near continuous presence with patients, is unique to the profession of nursing.[1] For example, in working with patients with head injuries, caring nurses acknowledge the patients by surrounding them with their possessions, such as family pictures and cards from friends and their favorite music. Nurses talk with their unresponsive patients, orienting them and telling them what is going on, which preserves the patient's humanness. Occasionally a patient responds, as evidenced by an increase in heart rate or blood pressure, a decrease in intracranial pressure, or the shedding of a tear. Nurses take this level of communication one step further by teaching this process to family members so they too can interact with their critically ill loved one.

Pediatric and neonatal critical care nurses have provided leadership by integrating family-centered care into the practice of critical care. Building a humanistic environment that endorses parents as unique individuals capable of providing essential elements of care to their children lays the foundation for family-centered care. Family-centered care is more than just providing parents with unlimited access to their children.[1]

Nursing research ascertains that parents have the need for hope, information, and proximity; they must believe that their loved one is receiving the best care possible; and they seek the opportunity to be helpful, to be recognized as important, and to talk with other parents who have similar issues. Pediatric critical care nurses have gone beyond the identification of family needs to illustrating interventions that patients and families find helpful[1] and providing families with what they need to help their child. Parents believe the most important contribution pediatric critical care nurses make is to serve as the interpreter by translating their critically ill child's responses to others within the PICU environment.

Response to Diversity

Response to diversity honors the differences that exist among people and individuals. At a minimum, it requires that care be delivered in a nonjudgmental, nondiscriminatory manner. Effective communication with patients and families at their level of understanding may require customizing the health care culture to meet the diverse needs and strengths of families. Skilled nurses foresee differences and beliefs within the team and negotiate consensus in the best interest of the patient and family.

Advocacy/Moral Agency

Moral agency acknowledges the particular trust inherent within nurse-patient relationships, a trust gained from the nursing profession's long history of speaking on the patient's behalf in an effort to preserve a patient's *lifeworld* (Hooper, personal communication, 1996). The holistic view of the patient that nurses often possess is a reflection of moral awareness.

When a cure is no longer possible, nurses turn their focus to ensuring that death occurs with dignity and comfort. Nurses help "orchestrate" death by supporting parents and family members through the death of their loved one (see also Chapters 15 and 16). Nurses often coordinate the experience for patients and families when death is imminent.[2]

Pediatric critical care nurses support the practice of family presence during procedures and resuscitation. Including family members during pediatric resuscitation is not a universal practice. However, a systematic review of family presence during resuscitation in the PICU supports the belief that parents who are able to be present are better able to adjust to their child's death and better able to cope.[3] Parents who were not able to stay described more anguish. Local guidelines and education have been developed to facilitate parental presence during resuscitation. Importantly, physicians and nurses report increased comfort with parental presence when they, the professionals, are prepared to help support parent presence.[4]

Facilitation of Learning

Nurses facilitate learning so that patients and their families can become knowledgeable about the health care system and make informed choices. Teaching is an almost continuous process that involves helping the patient and family understand the critical care environment and therapies involved in critical care. Also essential is reinforcement of the patient's experience and how, most likely, the infant or child will cope with the ICU experience. This education provides patients with the capacity to help themselves manage the experience and for parents to help their infants and children.

Collaboration

Collaboration requires commitment by the entire multidisciplinary team. A classic study by Knaus and associates[5] found an inverse relationship between actual and predicted patient mortality and the degree of interaction and coordination of multidisciplinary intensive care teams. Hospitals with good collaboration and a lower mortality rate had a comprehensive nursing educational support program that included a clinical nurse specialist and clinical protocols that staff nurses can independently initiate. A study published in 2015 examined the relationship between nurse-physician collaboration and the development of hospital-acquired infections in critically ill adults. These results demonstrated that nurse-physician collaboration was inversely related to the incidence of ventilator-associated pneumonia and central line–associated infections.[6]

Systems Thinking

Nurses are constantly challenged to design, implement, and evaluate whole programs of care, manage units where programs of care are provided, and determine whether the health care system is meeting patient needs.[7] These vital components require a patient-centered culture that stresses strong leadership, coordination of activities, continuous multidisciplinary communication, open collaborative problem solving, and conflict management.[8] For many years nurses have learned to manipulate the system on behalf of their patients; however, systems thinking[9]—that is, the ability to understand and effectively manipulate the complicated relationships involved in complex problem solving—is a new but necessary skill in taking overall responsibility for the caregiving environment.

Managing complex systems is essential to creating a safe environment. Nurse-patient relationships commonly occur around transitional periods of instability brought about by the demands of the health care situation. Helping patients make transitions between elements of the health care system—for example, into and out of the community, or even into and out of the PICU—requires systems knowledge and intradisciplinary collaboration.

Optimal Patient Outcomes

According to the Synergy Model, optimal patient outcomes result when patient characteristics and nurse competencies synergize. A *nurse-sensitive outcome*, a term first coined by Johnson and McCloskey,[10] defines a dynamic patient or family caregiver state, condition, or perception that is responsive to nursing interventions. Brooten and Naylor[11] noted, "The current search for 'nurse-sensitive patient outcomes' should be tempered in the reality that nurses do not care for patients in isolation and patients do not exist in isolation." Outcomes have been described at three levels: patient, provider, and system.

Patient-Level Outcomes

Major patient-level outcomes of concern to pediatric critical care nurses include hemodynamic stability and the presence or absence of complications. Outcomes related to limiting iatrogenic injury and complications of therapy demonstrate the potential hazards present in illness and in the critical care environment. Patient/family satisfaction ratings are subjective measures of health or the quality of health services. Patient satisfaction measures involving nursing care typically include technical/professional factors, trusting relationships, and education experiences. Patient-perceived functional status and quality of life are multidisciplinary outcome measures. Linking patient satisfaction, functional status, and quality of life is important because the three factors often are related.

Provider-Level Outcomes

Provider-level outcomes include the extent to which care/treatment objectives are attained within a predicted time period. For example, providers are frequently interested in minimizing the duration of shock and organ dysfunction in general. Nurses coordinate the day-to-day efforts of the entire multidisciplinary team. The nurse's role as the coordinator of numerous services is essential for optimal patient outcomes and shorter lengths of stay. As discussed, nurse-physician collaboration and positive interaction is associated with lower mortality rates, high patient satisfaction with care, and low hospital-acquired complications.[5,6]

System-Level Outcomes

Critical care units must manage resources and maintain quality as collaboratively defined by both users and providers in the system. The goal is high-quality care at appropriate cost for the greatest number of people who need it. Important patient-system outcome data include recidivism and costs/resource utilization. Recidivism—that is, readmission—is repeated work that adds to the personal and financial burden of receiving/requiring and providing care. In addition to patient and system factors, nurses can decrease the patient's length of stay through coordination of care, prevention of complications, timely discharge planning, and appropriate referral to community resources. Reducing length of stay while tracking emergency department visits and rehospitalization helps to ensure that cost shifting is not occurring.

Nightingale Metrics

One population-specific approach to measurement of nurse-sensitive outcomes is the Nightingale Metrics.[12] This program

---

BOX 6.1 Pediatric Intensive Care Unit: Example of Nightingale Metrics

- State Behavioral Scale (SBS) scores every 4 hours
- In patients with a central venous line, changing the dressing every 7 days
- Development of an enteral feeding guideline
- Mouth care every 4 hours
- Venous thromboembolism (VTE): Risk factors, central line removal, prophylactic medications
- Parental presence
- Pressure ulcer bundle: If patient is immobile, documentation of position change every 2 hours and positioning of heels off the bed; if not on bed rest, documentation of patient being out of bed or held in parent's or nurses' arms in previous 24 hours
- Ventilator-associated pneumonia bundle: Head of bed elevation at 30 to 45 degrees; documentation of oral hygiene twice in 24 hours; peptic ulcer prophylaxis (in patients not receiving tube feedings); discussion of extubation readiness test on rounds; daily holiday from sedation or chemical paralysis
- "Time to critical intervention": response to panic laboratory value, the time intervals from sending specimen to laboratory to first intervention to correct laboratory value

---

was developed so that bedside nurses could be actively involved in identifying nurse-sensitive metrics important to their unique patient and family practice. Nurses give care in an environment that should support the capacity of the patient and family to heal. In addition to supportive care, a large aspect of nursing is preventive care that often is not measured; thus care is often invisible. When measuring outcomes, it is important to account for the invisible aspects of nursing that have a tremendous impact on patients. This might include steps taken, according to the best understanding of what works, to prevent a particular complication. For example, invisible are the large numbers of pressure ulcers that never develop because of good nursing care. The Nightingale Metrics reflect current standards of care, are based on evidence, and are measurable (Box 6.1).

Leadership

Excellence in a pediatric critical care unit is achieved through a combination of many factors and is highly dependent on effective leadership.[13] Numerous studies have demonstrated the importance of leadership in creating an environment where both nurses and patients can flourish.

Specialized units such as PICUs require staff with the expert knowledge and skill required to meet the multifaceted needs of patients and families. A healthy work environment should improve retention and recruitment. An evidence-based practice working group at one facility piloted several leadership proposals to enrich the nursing work environment. The criteria instituted by the American Association of Critical Care Nurses Standards for Establishing and Sustaining Healthy Work Environments—which include skilled communication, true collaboration, effective decision making, appropriate staffing, meaningful recognition, and authentic leadership—were the basis for the proposals. When these standards were integrated with qualities of the staff such as clinical proficiency, personal values, and management experience, the results showed improvement in absenteeism, patient and staff satisfaction, and nursing quality indicators.[14]

The literature demonstrates that an established and proficient workforce improves patient outcomes. A study conducted by Aiken and colleagues[15] observed the effect of nurse staffing levels on patient outcomes and factors affecting nurse retention. A total of 10,184 nurses from 168 hospitals were surveyed. After adjusting for patient and hospital characteristics, each additional patient per nurse was associated with a 7% increase in the likelihood of dying within 30 days of admission and a 7% increase in the odds of failure to rescue (death subsequent to a complication that develops during the hospital stay). In addition, after adjusting for nurse and hospital characteristics, each additional patient per nurse was associated with a 23% increase in the odds of burnout and a 15% increase in the odds of job dissatisfaction.

Aiken and colleagues[16] have continued their work by assessing the net effects of work environments on nurse and patient outcomes. Using data from the same hospitals and nurses, they investigated whether better work environments were related to lower patient mortality and better nurse outcomes independent of nurse staffing and the education of the registered nurse workforce in hospitals.[16] Work environments were evaluated according to the practice environment scales of the Nursing Work Index. Three of the five subscales studied were nursing foundations for quality of care; nurse manager ability, leadership, and support; and collegial registered nurse/physician relationships. Outcomes studied included job satisfaction, burnout, intent to leave, quality of care, mortality, and failure to rescue. They found that a greater percentage of nurses working in hospitals with unsupportive care environments reported higher burnout levels and dissatisfaction with jobs. They also found that work environment had a significant effect on nurses' plans to leave their units. When all patient and nurse factors were taken into account, the likelihood of patients dying within 30 days of admission was 14% lower in hospitals with healthier care environments. These findings support the observation that nursing leaders have at least three major opportunities to boost nurse retention and patient outcomes. These opportunities include increasing nurse staffing, using a more highly educated nurse workforce, and enhancing the work environment.

Work conducted by the same investigators validated their previous findings. An observational study using discharge data for 422,730 patients aged 50 years or older who underwent common surgeries in 300 hospitals in nine European countries demonstrated that an increase in a nurses' workload boosted the probability of inpatient mortality by 7%. In addition, a greater number of nurses with bachelor's degrees was associated with a 7% lower risk of mortality.[17]

One of the best examples of a work environment that champions the nurse at the bedside is the magnet hospital designation. Data demonstrate that hospitals that use the structure for magnet designation achieve significant improvements in their work environments.[16] Hospitals that have even some of the magnet characteristics illustrate improved nurse and patient outcomes. Characteristics of magnet hospitals that have the most impact on nurse and patient outcomes are investments in staff development, superior management, frontline manager supervisory skill, and good nurse/physician collaboration.[16]

Nurses who work in magnet hospitals do identify their environments as healthy. A study of 12,233 nurses confirmed healthy work environments in 82% of 540 clinical units and provided evidence that applying structures that support inter- and intradisciplinary collaboration and decision making promote the development of healthy work environments.[18] The importance of a healthy work environment cannot be stressed enough as the means to ensure a viable, competent, and caring workforce. Nurses look for a culture that respects the nurse's experience, skills, abilities, and unique contributions.

Beacon Award

The Beacon Award for Critical Care Excellence, created by the American Association of Critical-Care Nurses (AACN), distinguishes adult critical care, adult progressive care, and pediatric critical care units that attain high-quality outcomes. This prestigious award provides the critical care community with a means of recognizing achievements in professional practice, patient outcomes, and the health of the work environment.

A pediatric critical care unit can achieve the Beacon Award by meeting several criteria in the areas of recruitment and retention; education, training, and mentoring; evidence-based practice and research; patient outcomes; healing environment; and leadership and organizational ethics. Together these characteristics provide a comprehensive view of any given ICU. To date, 25 pediatric critical care units have received the Beacon Award for Critical Care Excellence (M. Sanchez, personal communication, 2015).

Professional Development

A critical aspect of development for the nurse is the ability to advance and be recognized professionally. A successful critical care professional advancement program recognizes varying levels of staff nurse knowledge and expertise and fosters advancement through a wide range of clinical learning and professional development experiences. Essential components of this program include an orientation program, a continuing education plan, and an array of other opportunities for clinical and professional development. Unit-based advancement programs are most effective when they are linked to the nursing department's professional advancement program.

A professional advancement program that recognizes and rewards evolving expertise contains elements of both clinical and professional development strategies. The Synergy Model's ability to describe a patient-nurse relationship that optimizes patient and family outcomes illuminates the various dimensions of critical care nursing practice that require attention from a development perspective.[1,19] The impact of these contributions can be measured based on the nurse's level of expertise, and professional development strategies can be focused to have an impact on patient care.

By combining the nurse competencies identified in the Synergy Model and the behaviors identified in Benner's levels of practice,[20] a continuum of expertise can be described that matches behavior with practice levels. It focuses recognition and reward on clinical practice. The impact of expert nurses on patient outcomes is presented in quantitative and financial terms that can be understood throughout the health care system. The model links clinical competencies to patient outcomes.

Nurses require a broad body of knowledge to meet patient and organizational needs. This requirement necessitates a lifelong process of professional development targeted to specific levels of clinical practice. Nurses can choose from many learning options, such as academic education, continuing education programs, participation in research, collaborative learning, case studies, and simulations. Nurses view the availability of continuing education, both as learning in the unit and in-service education, as very important.[21]

Staff Development

The goal of nursing staff development programs is safe, competent practice. Comprehensive programs provide the critical resources to support and promote practice. In addition, professional nursing standards of practice, health care laws, regulations, and accreditation requirements focus on the components of competent patient care to protect the health care consumer. The establishment of a staff development program that is linked to clinical practice is key to the success of professional nurse development.

Technical training alone is no longer sufficient to meet the care delivery needs of the nurse in the critical care environment. In addition to knowledge about disease processes and physiologic instability associated with them, critical care nurses require broad knowledge and expertise in areas such as communication, critical thinking, and collaboration.[8] They need to attain the diverse skills necessary to meet the complex needs of their patients and families.

The theory and science required to meet the synergy competencies include topics such as specific disease processes, nursing procedures, cultural awareness, moral and ethical principles and reasoning, research principles, and learning theories. This information can be presented using a variety of methods, including lectures, written information, posters, self-studies, or computer-based technology. However, it is essential that the information be related to realistic clinical situations. Clinical scenarios, case studies, and simulations that represent the dynamic and ambiguous clinical situations nurses encounter daily are most effective.[21]

Bedside teaching is particularly helpful in the development of clinical judgment and caring practice skills. Expert nurses are role models of many of the competencies delineated by the Synergy Model. Novice nurses learn by watching these expert nurses and emulating their behaviors. Clinical teaching also enables the novice practitioner to gain experience with unfamiliar interventions in a safe and protected environment. Communicating and demonstrating clinical knowledge focuses learning, positively affects patient outcomes, and adds to the total body of nursing knowledge.[22]

Simulation-based learning has been incorporated with increased frequency into pediatric critical care nursing practice as a state-of-the-art educational approach. Simulation serves several purposes, such as enhancing patient safety, increasing clinical competence, and promoting effective teamwork. Simulation provides a nonthreatening environment where participants can integrate cognitive, psychomotor, and affective skill attainment without fear of hurting patients.[23]

Information about research and research use builds clinical inquiry and system thinking skills. Demystifying research, outcome, and quality processes contributes to the development of these key skills. The use of journal club formats and supporting staff involvement in research helps develop clinical inquiry skills. Building knowledge in the areas of health care trends and political action expands system thinking skills. The development of critical thinking skills and problem solving skills also assists with the development of system thinking.

Developing excellent communication skills is an essential part of nurses' professional development plans. In addition to their value in enhancing relationships with patients, families, and colleagues, good communication skills are critical for teaching less experienced staff. Presenting clinical teaching strategies and helping staff to determine learner readiness and to assess understanding will facilitate learning. The importance of developing patience, flexibility, and a nonconfrontational style is reinforced. Negotiation, conflict resolution, time management, communication, and team building are components of collaboration skills. Role playing, role modeling, and clinical narratives are methodologies that have been used to develop collaboration skills.

Nurses learn technical skills and scientific principles in many ways, but caring practices and advocacy are developed only through relationships that evolve over time.[20] Nurturing, professional relationships with experienced staff allow novices to integrate their evolving perspectives into practice. Expert nurses who share their clinical knowledge and coach other nurses have a tremendous impact on novice nurses. Nurses who coach do so because they are able to clinically persuade and guide less experienced staff in challenging situations. They demonstrate expert skills and expedite the ongoing clinical development of others.

A variety of staff development programs exist, but most fall into three general categories: orientation, in-service education, and continuing education programs.

Orientation

Orientation programs help acclimate new staff to unit-based policies, procedures, services, physical facilities, and role expectations in a work setting. A specific type of orientation that has developed in response to the nursing shortage is the critical care internship program. These programs have been developed as a mechanism to recruit and train entry-level nurses. They are designed to integrate nurses with little or no nursing experience into the complex critical care environment. They provide extended clinical support for novice nurses and introduce new knowledge more deliberately than do traditional orientation programs. Basic information and skill acquisition are the core features of these programs. This foundation builds on the knowledge and skills acquired in nursing school programs. Teaching usually is under the direction of a hospital educator and generally involves less senior staff members as preceptors. Typically, the novice nurse starts with providing care to the least complex patients. The program establishes a foundation on which the novice can develop into a competent clinician.[24]

AACN has partnered with the Child Health Corporation of America to release the Essentials of Pediatric Critical Care Orientation program. This program provides a bridge for the knowledge gap between what nurses learn in their basic education program and what they need to know in order to achieve initial clinical competence with critically ill pediatric patients. The program consists of an interactive eight-module course that provides case scenarios and practice activities that augment knowledge and improve job satisfaction. This program provides flexibility because it is a self-paced didactic e-learning course that can be incorporated into a blended learning environment that combines traditional educational activities such as preceptorships, discussion groups, workshops, and simulation experiences.

In-Service Education

In-service education programs, which are the most frequent type of staff development activity, involve workplace learning experiences that help staff to perform assigned functions and maintain competency.[21] These programs usually are informal and narrow in scope. They often are spontaneous sessions resulting from new situations on the unit in settings such as patient rounds or staff meetings. Examples of planned in-service sessions are demonstrations of new equipment, procedure reviews, and patient care conferences.

Continuing Education

New medical developments, legislation, regulations, professional standards, and expectations of health care consumers help determine the need for continuing education.

Continuing nursing education includes planned, organized learning experiences designed to expand knowledge and skills beyond the level of basic education.[21] The focus is on knowledge and skills that are not specific to one institution and that build on previously acquired knowledge and skills. Examples of continuing education programs include formal conferences, seminars, workshops, and courses.

Certification in Pediatric Critical Care Nursing

In 1975, the AACN Certification Corporation was established to formally recognize the professional competence of critical

---

TABLE 6.1   Pediatric Critical Care Registered Nurse Test Plan

I. Clinical Judgment (80%)

A. Cardiovascular (14%)
1. Acute pulmonary edema
2. Cardiac surgery (eg, Norwood, Blalock-Taussig shunt, tetralogy of Fallot repair, arterial switch)
3. Cardiogenic shock
4. Cardiomyopathies (eg, hypertrophic, dilated, restrictive, idiopathic)
5. Dysrhythmias
6. Heart failure
7. Hypovolemic shock
8. Interventional cardiology (eg, catheterization)
9. Myocardial conduction system defects
10. Structural heart defects (acquired and congenital, including valvular disease)

B. Pulmonary (18%)
1. Acute lung injury (eg, acute respiratory distress syndrome, respiratory distress syndrome)
2. Acute pulmonary embolus
3. Acute respiratory failure
4. Acute respiratory infections (eg, acute pneumonia, croup, bronchiolitis)
5. Air leak syndromes (eg, pneumothorax, pneumopericardium)
6. Aspiration (eg, aspiration pneumonia, foreign body, meconium)
7. Asthma, chronic bronchitis
8. Bronchopulmonary dysplasia
9. Congenital anomalies (eg, diaphragmatic hernia, tracheoesophageal fistula, choanal atresia, pulmonary hypoplasia, tracheal malacia, tracheal stenosis)
10. Pulmonary hypertension
11. Status asthmaticus
12. Thoracic surgery
13. Thoracic trauma (eg, fractured ribs, lung contusions, tracheal perforation)

C. Endocrine (5%)
1. Acute hypoglycemia
2. Diabetes insipidus
3. Diabetic ketoacidosis
4. Inborn errors of metabolism
5. Syndrome of inappropriate secretion of antidiuretic hormone (SIADH)

D. Hematology/Immunology (3%)
1. Coagulopathies (eg, idiopathic thrombocytopenic purpura, disseminated intravascular coagulation, heparin-induced thrombocytopenia)
2. Oncologic complications

E. Neurology (14%)
1. Acute spinal cord injury
2. Brain death (irreversible cessation of whole brain function)
3. Congenital neurologic abnormalities (eg, myelomeningocele, encephalocele, atrioventricular malformation)
4. Encephalopathy (eg, anoxic, hypoxic-ischemic, metabolic, infectious)
5. Head trauma (eg, blunt, penetrating, skull fractures)
6. Hydrocephalus
7. Intracranial hemorrhage/intraventricular hemorrhage (eg, subarachnoid, epidural, subdural)
8. Neurologic infectious disease (eg, congenital, viral, bacterial)
9. Neuromuscular disorders (eg, muscular dystrophy, Guillain-Barré syndrome, myasthenia gravis)
10. Neurosurgery
11. Seizure disorders
12. Space-occupying lesions (eg, brain tumors)
13. Spinal fusion
14. Stroke (eg, ischemic, hemorrhagic)

F. Gastrointestinal (6%)
1. Acute abdominal trauma
2. Acute gastrointestinal hemorrhage
3. Bowel infarction/obstruction/perforation (eg, necrotizing enterocolitis, mesenteric ischemia, adhesions)
4. Gastroesophageal reflux
5. Gastrointestinal abnormalities (eg, omphalocele, gastroschisis, volvulus, Hirschsprung disease, malrotation, intussusception)
6. Gastrointestinal surgeries
7. Hepatic failure/coma (eg, portal hypertension, cirrhosis, esophageal varices, biliary atresia)
8. Malnutrition and malabsorption

G. Renal (6%)
1. Acute renal failure
2. Chronic renal failure
3. Life-threatening electrolyte imbalances

H. Multisystem (11%)
1. Asphyxia
2. Distributive shock (eg, anaphylaxis)
3. Hemolytic uremic syndrome
4. Multiorgan dysfunction syndrome (MODS)
5. Multisystem trauma
6. Near drowning
7. Sepsis/septic shock
8. Systemic inflammatory response syndrome (SIRS)
9. Toxic ingestions/inhalations (eg, drug/alcohol overdose)
10. Toxin/drug exposure

I. Behavioral/Psychosocial (3%)
1. Abuse/neglect
2. Developmental delays
3. Failure to thrive

II. Professional Caring and Ethical Practice (20%)

A. Advocacy/Moral Agency (2%)

B. Caring Practices (4%)

C. Collaboration (4%)

D. Systems Thinking (2%)

E. Response to Diversity (2%)

F. Clinical Inquiry (2%)

G. Facilitation of Learning (4%)

Data from Pediatric CCRN Test Plan, Aliso Viejo, CA, 2015, American Association of Critical-Care Nurses.

care nurses. The mission of the AACN Certification Corporation is to certify and promote critical care nursing practice that optimally contributes to desired patient outcomes. The program establishes the body of knowledge necessary for critical care registered nurse (CCRN) certification, tests the common body of knowledge needed to function effectively within the critical care setting, recognizes professional competence by granting CCRN status to successful certification candidates, and assists and promotes the continual professional development of critical care nurses.

In 1997 the unique competencies of pediatric, neonatal, and adult critical care nurses were rearticulated using the Synergy Model[1] as a conceptual framework. AACN has published the new test plan (Table 6.1). To date more than 4000 pediatric critical care nurses hold CCRN–Pediatric certification (C. Hartigan, personal communication, 2015), and more than 50 hold the Pediatric CCRN-K credential. This is the new knowledge-based CCRN credential for nursing professionals who do not work at the bedside but apply knowledge in a way that enhances the positive impact of patients, nurses, or organizations on acutely or critically ill adult, pediatric, or neonatal patients. CCRN-K certification may be obtained by completing an initial exam or as a renewal option for CCRN and CCRN-E (Tele-ICU Acute/Critical Care Nursing) certificants who no longer do traditional bedside care. AACN also provides clinical nurse specialist certifications in pediatric critical care.

Nursing Research

Pediatric critical care nursing is a science as well as an art. It is vital that nursing interventions supporting the care of the critically ill child and his or her family be grounded in high-quality evidence generated though pediatric-specific research. Whereas knowledge generated in the larger neonatal and adult populations can inform pediatric practice, the developmental and maturational differences in our unique patient population may require independent study. A group of nurse scientists convened to summarize the state of the science in pediatric critical care nursing and to prioritize a list of nursing research topics for future focus. The group identified four top research priorities as described in Table 6.2.[25]

TABLE 6.2	Four Top Research Priorities Identified by Nurse Scientists in Pediatric Critical Care Nursing

1. Facing death: end-of-life care and decision making: What nursing interventions directly impact the child and family's experience during withdrawal of support in the PICU?
2. Caring for patient's families: Evaluate the long-term psychosocial impact of a child's critical illness on family outcomes.
3. Making a case: Communicating clinical assessments and improving teamwork: Can effective team communication models improve patient and family outcomes in pediatric critical care?
4. Diagnosing and managing life-sustaining physiologic functions: Articulate core nursing competencies that prevent unstable situations from deteriorating into crises in pediatric critical care.

From Tume LN, Coetzee M, Dryden-Palmer K, et al. Pediatric critical care nursing research priorities—initiating international dialogue. Pediatr Crit Care Med. 2015;16:e174-182.

Summary

Pediatric critical care nursing has evolved into a specialty in its own right. Pediatric critical care nurses make significant and unique contributions to the health care of children. A pediatric critical care nurse requires knowledge and skills in both the art and science of nursing. A supportive, empowered environment and support for professional advancement are essential to the development of knowledge and skills.

References

1. Curley MAQ. Patient-nurse synergy: optimizing patients' outcomes. Am J Crit Care. 1998;7:64-72.
2. Curley MAQ. The essence of pediatric critical care nursing. In: Curley MAQ, Moloney-Harmon PA, eds. Critical Care Nursing of Infants and Children. Philadelphia: WB Saunders; 2001.
3. McAlvin SS, Carew-Lyons A. Family presence during resuscitation and invasive procedures in pediatric critical care. Am J Crit Care. 2014;23:477-485.
4. Curley MAQ, Meyer EC, Scoppettuolo LA, et al. Parent presence during invasive procedures and resuscitation: evaluating a clinical practice change. Am J Respir Crit Care Med. 2012;186:1133-1139.
5. Knaus WA, Draper EA, Wagner DP, et al. An evaluation of the outcome from intensive care in major medical centers. Ann Intern Med. 1985;104:410-418.
6. Boev C, Xia Y. Nurse-physician collaboration and hospital-acquired infections in critical care. Crit Care Nurs. 2015;35:66-72.
7. O'Grady TP. A new age for practice: creating the framework for evidence. In: Malloch K, O'Grady TP, eds. Introduction to Evidence-Based Practice in Nursing and Healthcare. 2nd ed. Sudbury, MA: Jones and Bartlett; 2009.
8. American Association of Critical-Care Nurses. AACN standards for establishing and sustaining healthy work environments: a journey to excellence. Am J Crit Care. 2005;14:187-197.
9. Senge PM. The Fifth Discipline: The Art and Practice of the Learning Organization. New York: Doubleday; 1990.
10. Johnson M, McCloskey JC. Quality in the nineties. In: Series on Nursing Administration. Vol. 3. Delivery of Quality Health Care. St. Louis: Mosby Year Book; 1992.
11. Brooten D, Naylor MD. Nurses' effect on changing patient outcomes. Image (IN). 1995;7:95-99.
12. Curley MA, Hickey PA. The nightingale metrics. Am J Nurs. 2006;106:66-70.
13. Dent RL, Armstead C, Evans B. Three structures for a healthy work environment. AACN Adv Crit Care. 2014;25:94-100.
14. Nayback-Beeb AM, Forsythe T, Funari T, et al. Using evidence-based leadership initiatives to create a healthy nursing work environment. Dimen Crit Care Nurs. 2013;32:166-173.
15. Aiken LH, Clarke SP, Sloane DM, et al. Hospital nurse staffing and patient mortality, nurse burnout, and job dissatisfaction. JAMA. 2002;288:1987-1993.
16. Aiken LH, Clarke SP, Sloane DM, et al. Effects of hospital care environments on patient mortality and nurse outcomes. JONA. 2008;38:223-229.
17. Aiken LH, Sloane DM, Bruyneel L, et al. Nurse staffing and education and hospital mortality in nine European countries: a retrospective observational study. Lancet. 2014;383:1824-1830.
18. Kramer M, Maquire P, Brewer BB. Clinical nurses in Magnet hospitals confirm productive, healthy unit work environments. J Nurse Manag. 2011;19:5-17.
19. Micheli A, Curley MAQ. Using the synergy model to describe nursing work and progressive levels of practice. In: Curley MAQ, ed. Synergy: The Unique Relationship Between Nurses and Patients, Indianapolis. Sigma Theta Tau International; 2007.
20. Benner P, Tanner C, Cheslea C. Expertise in Nursing Practice: Caring, Clinical Judgment, and Ethics. 2nd ed. New York: Springer Publishing; 2009.
21. Skees J. Continuing education: a bridge to excellence in critical care nursing. Crit Care Nurs Q. 2010;33:104-116.

22. Guilhermino MC, Inder KJ, Sundin D, et al. Nurses' perceptions of education on invasive mechanical ventilation. *J Contin Educ Nurs*. 2014;45: 225-232.

23. Roh YS, Lee WS, Chung HS, et al. The effects of simulation-based resuscitation training on nurses' self efficacy and satisfaction. *Nurs Educ Today*. 2011;33:123-128.

24. Welding N. Creating a nurse residency: decrease turnover and increase clinical competence. *Med Surg Nurs*. 2011;20:37-40.

25. Tume LN, Coetzee M, Dryden-Palmer K, et al. Pediatric critical care nursing research priorities—initiating international dialogue. *Pediatr Crit Care Med*. 2015;16:e174-182.

Research in Pediatric Critical Care

Robinder G. Khemani and Martha A.Q. Curley

PEARLS

- Pediatric critical care is an ideal venue for research because of the rapid progression of disease and resulting ability to observe change, few comorbid conditions compared with adult critical care, the breadth of subspecialty care, the developmental spectrum, abundant existing data, the interprofessional nature of PICUs, and a collaborative research infrastructure.
- Pediatric critical care research is challenged by limited understanding of the interplay between development and critical illness, imprecise short-term outcomes, limited bench-to-bedside translations, perceptions of cherry-picking good ideas from adults rather than generating novel ideas, the complex interaction between the evolution of disease and management, the relative value of research in our specialty, and variability in management.
- Opportunities for growth of pediatric critical care research lie in big data and informatics, precision science approaches, novel medical devices designed with children in mind, and adaptive methods in clinical trials.
- The future of pediatric critical care research is threatened by limited extramural funding, the academic focus of discovery, confusion about the role of our specialty, segmentation of the pediatric critical care market, consent rates for pediatric studies, and the perception of a "small pediatric market."

Strengths, Weaknesses, Opportunities, and Threats to Pediatric Critical Care Research

Pediatric critical care research is at an exciting crossroad. There has been tremendous growth in the number of investigators engaging in research related to pediatric critical care, with an increasing number of high-impact discoveries and publications.[1-5] While there has historically been a divide between clinical and laboratory research, the bench-to-bedside to bench translational models have enabled modern scientists to bring breakthrough understanding to the care of critical illness. It is now common that pediatric critical care researchers have "feet" in both domains or collaborate extensively with others outside their own domain.

This chapter is meant to describe the current state of pediatric critical care research. Using a strengths, weaknesses, opportunities, and threats (SWOT) approach, we highlight the factors related to conducting clinical research in our subspecialty. The following sections are in no way exhaustive; instead, they highlight broad areas and issues related to pediatric critical care research.

Strengths of Pediatric Critical Care Research

Many factors make pediatric critical care an ideal venue for research and discovery. These include the rapid progression of disease and resulting ability to determine the impact of experimental measures, few comorbid conditions compared with adult critical care, the breadth of subspecialty care, the developmental spectrum, abundant existing data, the interprofessional nature of pediatric ICUs (PICUs), and a collaborative research infrastructure.

Rapid Progression of Disease and Short-Term Outcomes

A distinct advantage of critical care research in general is that patient response to treatment can be measured quickly. Frequently, the critical phase of disease evolves over minutes or days, rather than months or years. Therapeautic decisions often have an immediate, measurable, physiologic response. Although short-term improvements in physiology may not impact long-term outcomes,[3,4,6-15] the immediate changes have led to fundamental discoveries to better understand the pathophysiology and develop new therapies. Some of the early discoveries regarding cardiopulmonary interactions and pulmonary hypertension, which are crucial for management of ventilated patients, for example, were derived from studies on children or animal models of pediatric disease.[16-21]

Moreover, while there is a growing evidence about the long-term impact of ICU management, many therapies have immediate impact on short-term outcomes like mortality, length of mechanical ventilation, length of ICU or hospital stay, and functional status at ICU or hospital discharge.[22,23] In general, clinical research studies in critical care are less subject to loss of patients to follow-up. These characteristics have helped advance clinical care through more detailed understanding of, for example, the importance of early goal-directed therapy for sepsis,[24] timely administration of antibiotics for septic shock,[25] and mechanical ventilation strategies and adjuvant therapies for patients with acute respiratory distress syndrome (ARDS).[9,26] Although the rapidity of the disease states leads to some advantages, particularly with regards to measuring short-term outcomes, it introduces a set of challenges regarding timing of interventions (see weakness later), which may partially explain negative trials in pediatric critical care.

Fewer Comorbid Conditions

Management of critically ill patients is a complex interplay between the severity and evolution of acute critical illness and a patient's usual health status. Two critically ill children with similar etiology and initial severity of pediatric acute respiratory distress syndrome (PARDS) may have markedly different outcomes based on the presence or absence of preexisting chronic lung disease or immunodeficiency.[3,27] Chronic illness is a major consideration in pediatric critical care, with recent estimates that over 50% of all PICU patients have complex chronic conditions on admission to the PICU, which are associated with higher severity of illness-adjusted mortality.[28] However, these rates are still significantly lower than those published in adults (65%–80%).[29] Furthermore, the current landscape of many adult ICUs has an increasing number of elderly and extremely elderly patients, who have stepwise increases in mortality risk as a function of age.

Although higher mortality rates in adult critical care may allow the use of mortality as a viable outcome variable in adult critical care research, preexisting comorbidities make it difficult to test the efficacy of new therapeutic interventions. For example, severity of illness is a less robust predictor of outcome in adults than in children. This finding is highlighted in the ARDS literature, where markers of oxygenation are more clearly associated with mortality in pediatric ARDS than in adult ARDS.[30-32] While death from ARDS in both adults and children is frequently from multiple organ failure, and not refractory hypoxemia, the hypoxemia metrics likely capture the severity of the initial insult, as well as the inflammatory response seen in ARDS. This common response may ultimately explain the development of multiple organ dysfunction that leads to death in both adult and pediatric ARDS. The presence of preexisting comorbidities modifies this response, as a less severe insult in an elderly patient or someone with immunodeficiency may be more likely to result in death than the same insult in a previously healthy individual. Furthermore, the presence of multiple comorbidities amid a lifetime of chronic illness confounds the potential benefits of therapeutic interventions. Even reversal of the acute pathophysiology with a therapy does not reverse the progressive organ dysfunction because previous insults to those organs from a lifetime of chronic disease prevent recovery.

Pediatric Intensive Care Clinicians as Generalists

The modern era of pediatric critical care training mandates general pediatric training first. Although there has been some separation into specialty ICUs (eg, cardiac, neurologic), patients in most PICUs represent nearly every pediatric specialty and subspecialty. The range of disorders facilitates transfer of knowledge and discovery and encourages collaborative relationships among specialties. Hence, pediatric critical care research can be disease or organ specific, with partnership with subspecialists. It is through such collaborative relationships, for example, that the importance of acute kidney injury and the utility of renal replacement therapy have come to the forefront of research in recent years. This has led to the development of standardized criteria to define kidney injury, a wealth of new methodologies and equipment for renal replacement services applicable for the smallest children, and overall improvements in mortality and morbidity for children who develop kidney injury.[33-42] Similar results are seen in the realm of neurocritical care, with partnerships among intensivists, neurologists, and neurosurgeons to develop, test, and implement more advanced neuro-monitoring techniques and treatments.

Developmental Spectrum

A distinct challenge but also a strength of pediatric critical care research stems from the age and development spectrum seen in PICUs. Pulmonary and cardiac physiology, for example, change as a function of age and maturation. Although there is no clear population-based cut point at which a child becomes an adult, lung growth and development are often complete by the time the child reaches adult height.[43,44] As a consequence, the development of new research techniques related to respiratory support or monitoring can be developed in the PICU, tested on adolescents, and translated to adults. The opposite may be more problematic, as devices developed for adults are often difficult to scale to pediatrics. Even modern pulmonary function equipment, which is standard in many adult ICUs or pulmonary function laboratories, will not work on young children who are unable to cooperate with the testing process. Moreover, the size of the device (eg, the dead space of many pneumotachometers) potentially leads to physiologic instability in pediatric patients. On the other hand, if children form the basis for the creation of a technique to measure lung volumes, in which careful attention is paid to overcoming developmental or size-based limitations, these techniques can be successfully used immediately in adults, even in those who are not cooperative.[45-47]

Several commonly used therapies have been developed for use in critically ill children and subsequently applied to adults. Surfactant was developed for, and has had dramatic impact on, premature infants and has been the subject of numerous trials in adult and pediatric ARDS, albeit with generally negative benefit to date. High-frequency oscillatory ventilation (HFOV) was developed in children, and although recent adult trials have curbed the enthusiasm of the applicability of HFOV for the early management of adult ARDS,[48,49] HFOV is still applicable and often used for adults with severe ARDS. Finally, the cystic fibrosis (CF) drug Kalydeco (Ivacaftor), which targets the underlying protein defect in CF for patients with the G551D mutation, underwent its first phase III clinical trial in patients 12 years of age and older and demonstrated significant sustained improvement in short-term lung function, nutrition, and fewer pulmonary exacerbations.[50] These studies, admittedly involving children most similar to adults, but without the consequences of longer-standing disease, introduced a new paradigm in CF research targeting drug development specific for the genetic mutations responsible for the disease, with more personalized approaches to therapies.

Wealth of Existing Data to Analyze

Critical care research benefits from the large amount of existing medical data available for secondary analysis. Electronic health care records and monitoring systems in modern ICUs allow storage and potentially ready access to large amounts of physiologic data. Although one needs to be cautious regarding the quality of data stored with inadequate annotation of important clinical events, important associations among physiologic events, treatments, and outcomes can be identified. Advancements in statistical and machine learning techniques have refined our ability to use these data in meaningful ways (see also Chapter 12).

The degree of granularity of existing data often dictates its usefulness for answering specific questions.[51] Many datasets created for other purposes, such as claims or billing, quality improvement, and other research studies, can be accessed for secondary analysis. The accessibility and cost varies, but these resources offer the opportunity for investigators to determine the existing process of care or examine the strength of the association between a variable of interest and a given outcome before engaging in subsequent studies,[52] generate hypotheses, or engage in predictive modeling. Moreover, with advancements in statistical techniques, it is possible to link deidentified databases using probabilistic models, without violating any issues related to patient privacy. Observational data have been key to developing and refining of global and disease-specific severity of illness scores and characterizing variables associated with outcome for critically ill children with head injury, asthma, acute respiratory distress syndrome, sepsis, and trauma, among others.[53-57] Existing data can also help monitor the postmarketing surveillance of new drugs, identifying higher rates of intussusception from certain types of rotavirus vaccination.[58] Moreover, reanalysis of existing data has led to the development of more advanced and new developments in critical care monitoring, which can improve short-term morbidity or mortality.[59]

Interprofessional Care

Intensive care research, particularly in pediatrics, benefits from the interprofessional nature of the care team. Each critically ill child interacts with a multitude of intensive care clinicians (physicians, nurses, respiratory therapists, pharmacists, social workers, physical and occupational therapists, nutritionists, etc). Pediatric critical care has embraced a team-based approach for patient care, which facilitates research. This multidisciplinary team approach introduces new lines of research that may target aspects of the patient experience and morbidity not often considered when clinicians remain in their disciplinary silos. These interprofessional collaborations have led to some of the most innovative research in pediatric critical care, highlighting the importance that each of these disciplines has on the science of critical care, and developing methods to improve outcomes for children.[1,2,4,60-63] In many ways, pediatric critical care has taken the lead in knowledge development related to the importance of interprofessional care for the critically ill patient.

Collaborative Research Networks

Pediatric critical care is advantaged by collaborative research. There are now several research networks in place. Some research networks do not have funding but provide a vehicle for investigators to have their science reviewed critically and enlist collaborating sites that have some existing research infrastructure. The Pediatric Acute Lung Injury and Sepsis Investigator (PALISI) network[27] is an example of such a network. With the benefit of PALISI networking, numerous investigators have been able to secure extramural funding for large clinical trials or simply get a group of collaborating institutions together to voluntarily conduct unfunded but important research. The list of publications from networks like PALISI continues to grow, and the organization provides opportunities for the training and future development of pediatric critical care researchers. Similar collaborative research networks exist internationally and have pediatric sections, including the Canadian Critical Care Trials Group (CCCTG), the Australian and New Zealand Intensive Care Society (ANZICS), and the European Society of Pediatric and Neonatal Intensive Care (ESPNIC).[27] Other research networks

have resources available for conducting research projects, but participation is often limited on the basis of competitive applications. Such an example is the National Institutes of Health[64] Collaborative Pediatric Critical Care Research Network (CPCCRN).[65]

Weaknesses of Pediatric Critical Care Research

While there is much strength in the current state of pediatric critical care research, some of the same strengths can be perceived as weaknesses. Some of these weaknesses relate to the complex interplay between development and critical illness, challenges with short-term outcomes, limited bench-to-bedside translations, perceptions of cherry-picking good ideas from adults rather than generating novel ideas, the complex interplay between the evolution of disease and management, the relative value of research in our specialty, and variability in management with lack of equipoise.

Patient Development Intersecting With Critical Illness

While the age spectrum of critically ill children in PICUs can be a strength when translating findings back to adults, the complex interplay between the pathophysiology of critical illness and age (eg, developmental process, immune response, epidemiology of diseases) complicates research. Researchers have to consider age-based stratifications, as the expected response to therapies or pathophysiology may be different in the infant compared with the older child or adolescent. A simple example relates to normalization of vital signs for severity of illness scoring, where a heart rate of 120 may be normal in an infant but abnormal in an adolescent. More complicated examples relate to potential differences in response to therapy as a function of age, such as prone positioning for ARDS, where age may be an imperfect surrogate for chest wall elastance, which may ultimately influence the recruitabilty of the lung when turning a patient from the supine to prone position.[4,10] Furthermore, the risks of some therapies may be quite different across the age spectrum. For example, administration of surfactant to an infant with ARDS may be easier (less volume to distribute, easier to position the patient to get more equal distribution throughout the lung) than to a 70-kg adolescent. This heterogeneity in potential treatment effect (based on age or other factors) ultimately affects the design of clinical trials, requiring alternative types of randomization or stratification a priori, or planned subgroup analysis.

There are also differences in disease etiology and epidemiology for which age is an imperfect surrogate. For example, a subdural hematoma in a 3-month-old with inflicted trauma secondary to child abuse is very different from a subdural hematoma in a 13-year-old in a motor vehicle accident. Some studies report lower mortality rates for younger children with ARDS compared with older children.[66] There are multiple potential explanations for such observations including different clinical triggers for ARDS (higher incidence of respiratory viral infections in younger children), developmental responses to mechanical ventilation and different rates of ventilator-induced lung injury (VILI), and potentially different inflammatory responses.

Most research studies and clinical trials in pediatrics are designed to include a representative sample of the children, but the study protocols may need to be different to account for these age and developmental differences, and ultimately subgroups may need to be considered to evaluate the risk-benefit profile as a function of age group. Moreover, the subgroupings can be somewhat arbitrary and need to be linked to the individual research question on the basis of the proposed relationship between age and the outcome and intervention being studied. This is an important limitation in pediatric critical care research.

Short-Term Outcomes

Over the past several decades, mortality rates for critically ill infants and children have decreased.[67,68] Although this speaks to the evolution of our specialty and translates into important benefits for our patients, mortality as a primary outcome measure in PICU clinical trials is now rarely useful because even some of the highest-risk diagnoses (eg, ARDS, septic shock) have mortality rates below 10%. A clinical trial would require enrollment of more than 2000 patients per arm to demonstrate a statistically significant 25% relative risk reduction in mortality.

Other patient-centered, clinically meaningful outcome measures such as residual morbidity affecting functional status and quality of life, as well as cost of care, are available, but clinical researchers frequently employ surrogate outcome measures such as length of stay, length of mechanical ventilation, ventilator-free days, new or progressive organ dysfunction, or organ failure–free days. Imprecision in measurement introduces potential for bias. For example, length-of-stay variables are subject to practice variation by providers or institutions and organ dysfunction variables may be subject to interpretation or incomplete data (eg, Glasgow Coma Scale). Moreover, there has been a trend to create composite variables like ventilator-free days (ie, days in 28 days in which a patient is alive and not on a ventilator) to reduce the sample size needed for clinical trials by combining "bad outcomes"—death and prolonged ventilation. Limitations with these composite variables relate to potential opposite effects of the intervention (eg, results in improved mortality but longer time on a ventilator); imprecise or variable definitions (eg, how to handle noninvasive ventilation), which limit generalizability; and potential limited importance to the patient.

It is also unclear if these surrogate short-term outcomes truly measure patient morbidity. It is critical that surrogate outcome measures relate in a meaningful way to patient-centered outcomes. Does longer length of time on a ventilator translate into more functional disability for patients after they leave the hospital, or several years later? Short- and longer-term measures of morbidity are increasingly being used for clinical research studies (ie, functional status at hospital discharge, neurodevelopmental outcome at 12 or 18 months), which are clearly relevant and important. However, these studies are challenging as well: There is variability in the instruments used to assess long-term outcomes along the developmental spectrum, and the studies are expensive and difficult to conduct. Most are labor intensive, and patients may be lost to follow-up. On the other hand, there exists at least the opportunity to follow patients for decades after the initial event, to truly understand the lifetime of consequences that may result from critical illness or injury.

Limited Translation From Bench to Bedside

The complexities of critical illness pose big challenges to bench models for disease progression and therapy. Despite many excellent animal models for sepsis, therapeutic strategies that have targeted specific factors in the causal pathway for sepsis have nearly all been negative. When moving to pediatric sepsis, the additional factors related to the variable immune response as a function of maturation and development add further complexity to this picture. Although there have been several successes, the difficulty in creating animal or in vitro models that account for the developmental components of a disease process has limited relevant bench research.[69] For example, while there are a multitude of pediatric researchers concentrating on animal models related to developmental aspects of the lung, there are still little data that characterize how the inflammation seen in ARDS may differ on the basis of age or development.[70] Although most theorize that there is indeed a relationship between the pathophysiology of ARDS and lung growth and development, sparse bench data support this, perhaps related to complexities in creating appropriate models. Certainly there are success stories of pediatric critical care investigators who have translated findings from bench to bedside, but most major successes have occurred in fields outside of critical care.

Perceptions of Cherry-Picking and Haphazard Borrowing From Adults

For a variety of reasons, pediatric critical care often looks to adult critical care for day-to-day patient management and research. Many of the large pediatric clinical trials have first been conducted in adults.[1,4,61] Such studies are much more readily conducted in adult ICUs because of the larger volume of patients and researchers in adult critical care compared with pediatrics, but some view pediatric critical care research as less novel in identifying new questions. Of course, there can be extraordinary innovation in pediatric critical care research, such as the initial approach to surgical palliation for single-ventricle physiology or use of veno-venous in preference to veno-arterial extracorporeal life support. Translation of adult research protocols to the pediatric setting in and of itself requires careful consideration and innovation. Many examples of research interventions that have been successful in adults exist, but they do not have the same results in children.[4,9] The differing results may be the consequence of many factors such as disease severity, physiologic development, and comorbidities. Nevertheless, there are still other studies and principles that are almost universally embraced, without pediatric-specific evidence. Even with evidence, there may be differences in pediatrics.[71,72] Finally, and conversely, there are a host of therapies and management strategies that pediatric practitioners use routinely, despite adult evidence indicating that they may not be beneficial.[48,49,73,74] These actually provide opportunity for investigation.

Complex Interplay Between Disease Progression and Therapy

One of the unique challenges to critical care research is that nearly all disease processes have been altered by therapy by the time the patient reaches the ICU. One can truly understand the potential therapeutic benefits for antibiotics for otitis media because patients can be randomized to receive antibiotics or no antibiotics. We could then understand the natural history of the disease and what would be expected if the patient was not treated. However, the inherent nature of most acute care physicians, especially intensivists operating in the setting of immediately threatening instability, is to intervene. When patients arrive with severe asthma, within hours they may receive steroids, inhaled and possibly IV beta agonists, magnesium, anticholinergics, Heliox, aminophylline, and bilevel positive pressure ventilation. Each of these interventions has an expected time to therapeutic effect, but it is rare to wait for the intervention to take full effect before adding the next therapy. The result is lack of clarity regarding what made the patient better.

Determining the impact of specific elements of treatment is further complicated because patients appear in the ICU at various points in the disease process, having received different treatments before arrival. A child who is 5 days into a case of ARDS who has an oxygenation index of 40 may be very different from a child who shows up in the emergency department with 6 hours of the onset of symptoms and proceeds to require intubation for ARDS related to pneumonia, with the same oxygenation index of 40. The first child has been exposed for 5 days to medical therapies intended to support her severe lung disease, while the second has received limited medical intervention. They are also, of course, in very different stages of the disease process, and therapies may need to be tailored to these differences. Early administration of some therapies is crucial to successful outcome (ie, antibiotics at the first sign of sepsis), while others may be instituted for persistent disease that has been unresponsive to other therapies (ie, high-frequency oscillatory ventilation). Research studies must address or control for patient characteristics that include timing and evolution of disease, as well as previous therapies through careful consideration of the expected physiology, inclusion and exclusion criteria, etc.

Relative Value of Research as a Specialty

In general, pediatric training programs place some value on research, as scholarly work is required by the American Board of Pediatrics and for academic promotion. Although all pediatric critical care fellows are trained in some aspect of research, most will not go on to generate new knowledge in their career. In pediatric critical care nursing, formal research training occurs at the doctorate (ie, Ph.D.) level. This is not unique to pediatric critical care, yet motivated and well-trained researchers are essential for the growth and advancement of any field. Financial pressure on clinical departments may increase demands on even some of the most qualified and experienced junior investigators to assume very large clinical workloads. Factors contributing to these demands include the reimbursement mix of individual hospitals, 24/7 coverage models, the value of research to an institution or department, the rates of extramural or intramural funding, extent of philanthropic support, administrative or service duties, and need for work-life balance. Increasingly, research is marginalized by these other factors, and investigators initially motivated and excited to do research become discouraged or lack adequate support or recourses to be successful.

Variable Management Strategies

Among common themes to management of critically ill patients, there is significant interinstitution and intrainstitution variability in management strategies for a variety of disease states and even for routine management of sedation, fluid status, antibiotics, ventilator support, vasoactive-inotropic support, and so on. There are few systematic,

agreed-upon protocols that are used within institutions and even fewer across institutions. In many ways, practice variability has some advantages, as therapies can be best tailored to the individual patient. In addition, if we can analyze the practice variability with advanced mathematics and statistics approaches, it may be possible to discover best practices. This approach is the focus of the ongoing ADAPT trial (http://www.adapttrial.org/) that is attempting to identify best practices for pediatric traumatic brain injury. However, for most clinical research studies, this practice variability introduces bias and the variability may dilute the treatment effect of a proposed intervention. For example, in considering the relationship between a variable of interest and ventilator-free days, it is readily apparent that the results of the intervention might be confounded by variable management of sedation or extubation practices. This has been well illustrated in previous pediatric critical care studies.[75] For example, a PALISI investigation found no difference in length of ventilation among three modes of ventilator weaning, but the biggest confounder and determinant of length of ventilation was the level of sedation.[75] Without specifically controlling for sedation, which was variable across and within institutions, it was difficult to draw firm conclusions about whether weaning strategy affects length of ventilation.

ICU Stay Is Not the Patient's or Family's Entire Experience

Critical care research is increasingly complicated by preexisting comorbidities and experiences, as well as long-term effects of ICU-based therapies. As researchers increasingly consider patient-centered outcomes beyond mortality (eg, functional status, cognitive impairment) (see also Chapter 8), it is even more important to consider the status of the patient before ICU admission in evaluating the effect of ICU interventions. There are limited tools available to control for the preexisting state of the patient, and many of them are subject to recall bias of caregivers who are often asked to fill out developmental questionnaires at times of high stress and anxiety. Limited ability to evaluate pre-ICU function complicates assessment of the attributable change in functional status as a consequence of an ICU intervention. Moreover, some scales cannot differentiate significant changes in functional impairment for subsets of children with severe preexisting disability,[2] resulting in potential exclusion of a large subset of patients from research studies. Furthermore, findings of decrements in long-term function after ICU admission may not be attributable to ICU specific therapies, as there are a multitude of additional complex confounders related to new chronic illness or disability, family dynamics and changes, and psychosocial or posttraumatic stress from critical illness or the events leading to the ICU stay. To that end, several outcome meaures are uniquely important to pediatric critical care, particularly related to the effects of the child's critical illness on the family or caregiver, the child's neurodevelopment, school function, learning, attention, behavior, and functional status.

Opportunities for Pediatric Critical Care Research

Many of the aforementioned strengths and weaknesses can be turned into opportunities for the future. Some of the biggest opportunities lie in the realms of big data and informatics; precision science approaches; novel medical devices designed with children in mind, which can be translated back to adults;

secondary use of existing data; and adaptive methods to overcome some of the biggest hurdles in pediatric critical care clinical trials.

Informatics and Big Data

The ICU is a natural environment for big data applications and informatics research. The amount of ICU patient data stored in the electronic health records, physiologic monitors, custom databases, and laboratory feeds is massive (see also Chapter 12). Much of these data are available for secondary analysis and research and are enticing for computer scientists and machine learning researchers looking for clinical partners who can help interpret findings. There have been numerous examples of successful collaborations among intensivists, engineers, and computer scientists that have not only resulted in interesting publications but also informatics-based solutions to critical care problems.[59,76-81] Such collaborations have potential to translate into smarter solutions for patient monitoring, predictive analytics to prevent complications or suggest therapies that may benefit an individual patient, and precision science approaches based simply on existing data. The ICU is a natural environment for these endeavors because outcomes can be objective and measured quickly, with an abundance of supporting data. The analytic techniques may be complicated given that most ICU data are inconsistently sampled. Repeated time series analysis, which mandates specific mathematic techniques, may be useful in this setting.[78] Computer scientists want to tackle these problems in concert with clinical partners.

Precision Science (e.g., Genomics, Proteomics)

Critical illness provides a fascinating framework to understand the complex interplay between the development or severity of critical illness and genetic- or biomarker-based risk stratification. Numerous examples of genes have been implicated in susceptibility to certain types of critical illness, and more and more data are emerging about using serum- or plasma-based biomarkers to risk stratify adult and pediatric patients with some of the most common and lethal critical illnesses such as sepsis and ARDS.[5,82-92] Although these analyses were initially limited to only the most sophisticated research laboratories, point-of-care testing is now becoming a reality. Access to this information may be helpful in therapy decisions on the basis of a priori risk from genetic factors or biomarker expression. These may form the basis of new, smarter clinical trials targeting therapies designed to benefit specific subgroups of patients, rather than treating all patients perceived to have the same clinical syndrome (such as sepsis or ARDS) as if they comprise a homogeneous population.[5,83,93-96] This approach has revolutionized cancer therapeutic trials and has great promise for future research in critical care.

Novel Diagnostic and Therapeutic Approaches to Deal With the Developmental Spectrum

Children cared for in ICUs present special challenges because of age, size, and developmental ability. Because they are frequently viewed as vulnerable populations, children are often excluded during the creation of new medical devices, drugs, or diagnostics. When these drugs or diagnostics are designed for adults, adapting them for children may be difficult, requiring significant reengineering and substantial cost, often resisted by device or drug manufacturers because of the marginal gain anticipated from the "small" pediatric market. However, if the innovation starts with children in mind, it is likely that a formulation of drug or medical device will be adaptable for adults, as has been done with surfactant (see earlier). This drives innovative solutions that can ultimately be translated back to older children and adults.

Existing Data Approaches

As mentioned in the strength section, there is an increasing amount of existing data related to pediatric critical care readily available for research, which can be used to generate or test hypotheses. Although many of these data sources used individually have limitations, newer analytic techniques enable linking discrete datasets, even without patient identifiers. This significantly increases the number and type of data elements available to control for potential confounding variables and answer a question, allowing for more robust conclusions. There are increasing numbers of pediatric critical care investigators with specific training or interest in techniques to analyze existing data, and it is an exciting new area for young investigators with few barriers to entry. Training or knowledge of appropriate analytic techniques is essential,[51] but this research is generally inexpensive, can be accomplished quickly, and requires limited equipment.

Smart Clinical Trial Design

Many therapies have been shown to be beneficial in adults but lack evidence of efficacy in children. Newer statistical approaches may facilitate designing more feasible clinical trials in children, particularly when adult data are supportive of a therapy. Pediatric critical care researchers often struggle to design trials that are feasible and have important clinical outcomes, given the overall better outcome of critically ill children compared with critically ill adults. Approaches such as Bayesian clinical trials afford the opportunity to adapt the trial to information that accrues during the trial.[97] This can allow the design of the trial to be modified, change accrual targets, drop or add treatment arms, or focus the recruitment on subpopulations of patients who are responding to the treatment. Bayesian trials also allow for using historical information (such as adult data) to synthesize results of relevant trials. These approaches seem well suited for pediatric critical care research, in which researchers are often burdened with relatively rare diseases and a heterogeneous patient population and treatment effect.[98]

Threats to Pediatric Critical Care Research

Unfortunately, there are many challenges to the continued success of pediatric critical care researchers. Some have been outlined in the weaknesses section, but there are additional major threats. These challenges include limited extramural funding, the academic focus of discovery, confusion about the role of our subspecialty, the segmentation of the pediatric critical care market away from research intensive institutions, consent rates for pediatric studies, and the perception of a "small pediatric market," as discussed later.

Extramural Funding

Federal funding for research has decreased in real terms since 1998, making it challenging for all but the most experienced of investigators to develop sustainable programs of funded research. The home for pediatric critical care research in the NIH is the Eunice Kennedy Shriver National Institute of Child Health and Development (NICHD), which has a specific Pediatric Trauma and Critical Care branch but a limited budget compared with other institutes, making it difficult for NICHD to fund many studies that have the potential to change clinical practice. Pediatric critical care investigators often seek funding from other agencies within the NIH (eg, NHLBI, NINDS), where there may be limited experience with or knowledge about pediatric diseases.[1,2] Moreover, the substantially smaller burden of pediatric critical illness compared with either acute or chronic disease in adults makes it more challenging to fund large-scale studies in pediatric critical care. While there are opportunities through private philanthropy, foundations, and intramural funding, the missions of each of these funding sources may limit the focus of investigator-initiated research and discovery. Limited funding makes it difficult to obtain preliminary data resulting in few pediatric first-in-human studies. Funding agencies are often unwilling to take risks on investigators or ideas with high potential for reward if the risks of failure have not been minimized. This reality can crush innovation.

Academic Approach to Science

The classic paradigm of a single-academic physician who excels as clinician, investigator, and educator (the "three-legged-stool") is no longer realistic for the vast majority of intensivists. Instead, it is increasingly common for critical care clinicians (and other subspecialists) to develop strength or expertise in one or two domains. It is particularly difficult to be successful as an investigator without substantial protected time for research. Protecting the time of junior investigators until they secure extramural funding can be an expensive proposition and may not be possible without significant ongoing departmental commitment or intramural funds. The difficult funding environment exacerbates this problem: Investigators may become discouraged when excellent proposals, which would have previously been funded, are not successful. More and more, departments provide protected time only to investigators with special training or established track records of funding. Increasingly, the importance of obtaining funding to support one's research has been reallocated solely to those holding research-tract appointments.

Confusion About the Role of Our Specialty

Ultimately, pediatric critical care is a supportive specialty and a service line for most hospitals. While philanthropists often visit the critical care environment, patients infrequently come to a particular hospital because of the ICU services. They may come to see a particular surgeon or other pediatric subspecialist who is an expert for their disease condition. When a patient develops ARDS, parents rarely request transfer to one ICU over another because the ICU has an ARDS expert. More commonly, transfer occurs only when the complexity of care becomes too great for a smaller ICU or specific technologic support is only available at another center. Hence, from the viewpoint of many administrators, investing resources in the ICU (especially for research) may be harder to justify as the ICU itself is not bringing in patients and generating revenue. Moreover, there is often little understanding, particularly with the public or potential philanthropists, about what types of patients are treated in PICUs. While the public may have experience or understanding of neonatal ICUs with premature babies or adult ICUs because of family members who have had heart attacks or strokes, most people never have any interaction with the PICU. This makes fundraising for research in pediatric critical care even more challenging because the PICU is an unknown entity for so many. Making a clear case to administrators and the general public about the central role of critical care in modern health care, enabling effective management of children with disorders as varied as respiratory failure from asthma or common viruses, cancer, congenital heart disease, transplantation, and trauma, is essential if critical care is to receive its share of resources needed to improve outcomes.

Segmentation of the Pediatric Critical Care Market Away From Research Institutions

An increasing number of smaller hospitals are developing pediatric critical care services to retain patients within their hospital system and attract specialists who are likely to generate revenue for the hospital. Depending on the market or city, there may be dozens of hospitals that have PICUs, with selective referral patterns based on perceived acuity of the patient, insurance type or status, or family preference. The resulting dilution or modification of the patient population at academic research institutions limits the opportunity to conduct research, particularly on the most common disorders, and limits the generalizability of research findings. For example, if 90% of patients enrolled in a research study about a new therapy for pediatric sepsis have significant preexisting comorbidities including cancer or immunosuppression, the results may not be applicable to a child who is previously healthy and develops sepsis. Increasingly, there is a discrepancy between the types of patients seen in academic research centers and other community-based ICUs. If these community-based ICUs do not participate in research studies (because they have no infrastructure for research), researchers may not be effectively testing generalizable research hypotheses.

Consent Practices for Clinical Trials in Children

In general, consent rates for pediatric critical care research trials are lower than for adults. Probably more importantly, because children are considered vulnerable populations, the risk-benefit profiles are often more heavily scrutinized by both institutional review boards and parents. It is therefore often difficult to get consent for pediatric critical care studies when there is limited or no potential benefit for the child. This changes the design of many research studies and may affect the ability to definitively answer the research question. Issues related to patient assent are also complicated. Ascertaining whether the child is of appropriate developmental ability to assent may be subjective. Obtaining assent or consent from many of the children who are of appropriate age or developmental status may not be possible because they are critically ill, often sedated, and intubated. Moreover, practices related to assent are highly variable across institutions and institutional review boards.[23,60,99]

With the limited number of pediatric institutions engaging in clinical research, there is frequently overlap of investigations within a single institution, with multiple research studies competing for the same patients. Parents and families can develop "study fatigue" and become resentful of requests for consent perceived to be excessive. Investigators must be aware of all the other studies the families may be approached to participate in and whether the studies can allow for coenrollment. If not, prioritization of the studies becomes necessary, which ultimately may result in inadequate recruitment and loss of funding for some otherwise meritorious investigations.

Perception of Pediatrics as a Small Market

Maintaining solvency in the medical technology and pharmaceutical industry is challenging. While there has been incredible growth in the number of medical devices and drugs on the market in recent years, there is also intense competition. Smaller companies are frequently bought by large multinational organizations only after their products have become profitable and achieved adequate market share. For the most part, pediatric indications and devices do not drive these profits. As a result, a large company is unlikely to make a significant investment in a pediatric-specific product. Smaller companies may be more willing but still may be reluctant if there is no clear adult market potential, as they will not be able to sell their business to a larger company. While there have been some federally funded initiatives to foster research and development into pediatric specific devices and drugs, academic partnership with industry for the development of a pediatric specific device or drug is still extremely difficult.

Conclusions

Despite multiple threats, there are reasons to be optimistic about the future of pediatric critical care research. Research paradigms are changing, and increasingly there are new applications, data sources, methods and techniques that will revolutionize the way researchers approach scientific problems. Researchers in pediatric critical care have taken the lead in how best to interact and involve families in clinical care and complex decision making. Using adaptive clinical trial design that may make working with smaller populations more successful is becoming more common. Most pediatric intensivists are eager to participate in multi-institutional trials and most exhibit increasing sophistication regarding the design and value of research. More intensivists and Ph.D.-prepared nurse scientists with specialized research training (T-32, K-08, K-23, and K-12 programs) are required to justify protected time. In the past, pediatric intensivists were nearly entirely devoted to keeping the child alive in the moment, but over the past 10 to 15 years, there has been significant development of clinician-scientists in pediatric critical care focused on answering important questions about mechanisms and treatment of disease. As a community of pediatric critical care practitioners, we will need to continue to embrace innovation and stimulate the newer generation of clinician scientists to not be afraid of breaking the traditional mold of the academic-scientist to discover new knowledge regarding the care of critically ill children.

Key References

1. Curley MA, Wypij D, Watson RS, et al. Protocolized sedation vs usual care in pediatric patients mechanically ventilated for acute respiratory failure: a randomized clinical trial. *JAMA*. 2015;313:379-389.
2. Moler FW, Silverstein FS, Holubkov R, et al. Therapeutic hypothermia after out-of-hospital cardiac arrest in children. *N Engl J Med*. 2015;372: 1898-1908.
3. Willson DF, Thomas NJ, Markovitz BP, et al. Effect of exogenous surfactant (calfactant) in pediatric acute lung injury: a randomized controlled trial. *JAMA*. 2005;293:470-476.
4. Curley MA, Hibberd PL, Fineman LD, et al. Effect of prone positioning on clinical outcomes in children with acute lung injury: a randomized controlled trial. *JAMA*. 2005;294:229-237.
5. Wong HR, Lindsell CJ, Pettila V, et al. A multibiomarker-based outcome risk stratification model for adult septic shock. *Crit Care Med*. 2014;42: 781-789.
14. Afshari A, Brok J, Moller AM, Wetterslev J. Inhaled nitric oxide for acute respiratory distress syndrome (ARDS) and acute lung injury in children and adults. *Cochrane Database Syst Rev*. 2010;(7):CD002787.
17. Fuhrman BP, Smith-Wright DL, Kulik TJ, Lock JE. Effects of static and fluctuating airway pressure on intact pulmonary circulation. *J Appl Physiol*. 1986;60:114-122.
20. Gordon JB, Tod ML, Wetzel RC, et al. Age-dependent effects of indomethacin on hypoxic vasoconstriction in neonatal lamb lungs. *Pediatr Res*. 1988;23:580-584.
21. Wetzel RC, Martin LD. Pentobarbital attenuates pulmonary vasoconstriction in isolated sheep lungs. *Am J Physiol*. 1989;257:H898-H903.
22. Pollack MM, Holubkov R, Glass P, et al. Functional Status Scale: new pediatric outcome measure. *Pediatrics*. 2009;124:e18-e28.
23. Khemani RG, Newth CJL. The design of future pediatric mechanical ventilation trials for acute lung injury. *Am J Respir Crit Care Med*. 2010; 182:1465-1474.
24. de Oliveira CF. Early goal-directed therapy in treatment of pediatric septic shock. *Shock*. 2010;34(suppl 1):44-47.
26. Douglas SL, Daly BJ, O'Toole EE, et al. Age differences in survival outcomes and resource use for chronically critically ill patients. *J Crit Care*. 2009;24:302-310.
27. Santschi M, Jouvet P, Leclerc F, et al. Acute lung injury in children:therapeutic practice and feasibility of international clinical trials. *Pediatr Crit Care Med*. 2010;11:681-689.
28. Edwards JD, Houtrow AJ, Vasilevskis EE, et al. Chronic conditions among children admitted to U.S. pediatric intensive care units: their prevalence and impact on risk for mortality and prolonged length of stay. *Crit Care Med*. 2012;40:2196-2203.
30. Flori HR, Glidden DV, Rutherford GW, Matthay MA. Pediatric acute lung injury: prospective evaluation of risk factors associated with mortality. *Am J Respir Crit Care Med*. 2005;171:995-1001.
31. Trachsel D, McCrindle BW, Nakagawa S, Bohn D. Oxygenation index predicts outcome in children with acute hypoxemic respiratory failure. *Am J Respir Crit Care Med*. 2005;172:206-211.
32. Khemani RG, Conti D, Alonzo TA, et al. Effect of tidal volume in children with acute hypoxemic respiratory failure. *Intensive Care Med*. 2009;35: 1428-1437.
33. Alkandari O, Eddington KA, Hyder A, et al. Acute kidney injury is an independent risk factor for pediatric intensive care unit mortality, longer length of stay and prolonged mechanical ventilation in critically ill children: a two-center retrospective cohort study. *Crit Care*. 2011;15:R146.
41. Schneider J, Khemani R, Grushkin C, Bart R. Serum creatinine as stratified in the RIFLE score for acute kidney injury is associated with mortality and length of stay for children in the pediatric intensive care unit. *Crit Care Med*. 2010;38:933-939.
42. Selewski DT, Cornell TT, Blatt NB, et al. Fluid overload and fluid removal in pediatric patients on extracorporeal membrane oxygenation requiring continuous renal replacement therapy. *Crit Care Med*. 2012;40:2694-2699.
45. Hammer J, Newth CJ. Infant lung function testing in the intensive care unit. *Intensive Care Med*. 1995;21:744-752.
46. Hammer J, Newth CJ. Effect of lung volume on forced expiratory flows during rapid thoracoabdominal compression in infants. *J Appl Physiol*. 1995;78:1993-1997.
48. Ferguson ND, Cook DJ, Guyatt GH, et al. High-frequency oscillation in early acute respiratory distress syndrome. *N Engl J Med*. 2013;368: 795-805.
50. Ramsey BW, Davies J, McElvaney NG, et al. A CFTR potentiator in patients with cystic fibrosis and the G551D mutation. *N Engl J Med*. 2011; 365:1663-1672.
51. Bennett TD, Spaeder MC, Matos RI, et al. Existing data analysis in pediatric critical care research. *Front Pediatr*. 2014;2:79.
55. Benneyworth BD, Gebremariam A, Clark SJ, et al. Inpatient health care utilization for children dependent on long-term mechanical ventilation. *Pediatrics*. 2011;127:e1533-e1541.
57. Odetola FO, Clark SJ, Freed GL, et al. A national survey of pediatric critical care resources in the United States. *Pediatrics*. 2005;115:e382-e386.

58. Yih WK, Lieu TA, Kulldorff M, et al. Intussusception risk after rotavirus vaccination in U.S. infants. *N Engl J Med*. 2014;370:503-512.

59. Moorman JR, Carlo WA, Kattwinkel J, et al. Mortality reduction by heart rate characteristic monitoring in very low birth weight neonates: a randomized trial. *J Pediatr*. 2011;159:900-906.e901.

60. Curley MA, Arnold JH, Thompson JE, et al. Clinical trial design—effect of prone positioning on clinical outcomes in infants and children with acute respiratory distress syndrome. *J Crit Care*. 2006;21:23-32.

61. Meert KL, Eggly S, Berg RA, et al. Feasibility and perceived benefits of a framework for physician-parent follow-up meetings after a child's death in the PICU. *Crit Care Med*. 2014;42:148-157.

64. Coghill M, Ambalavanan N, Chatburn RL, et al. Accuracy of a novel system for oxygen delivery to small children. *Pediatrics*. 2011;128:e382-e387.

65. Khemani RG, Sward K, Morris A, et al. Variability in usual care mechanical ventilation for pediatric acute lung injury: the potential benefit of a lung protective computer protocol. *Intensive Care Med*. 2011;37:1840-1848.

66. Zhu YF, Xu F, Lu XL, et al. Mortality and morbidity of acute hypoxemic respiratory failure and acute respiratory distress syndrome in infants and young children. *Chin Med J*. 2012;125:2265-2271.

67. PALICC. Recommendations from the Pediatric Acute Lung Injury Consensus Conference. *Pediatr Crit Care Med*. 2015;16:428-439.

68. Yehya N, Servaes S, Thomas NJ. Characterizing degree of lung injury in pediatric acute respiratory distress syndrome. *Crit Care Med*. 2015;43:937-946.

70. Smith LS, Zimmerman JJ, Martin TR. Mechanisms of acute respiratory distress syndrome in children and adults: a review and suggestions for future research. *Pediatr Crit Care Med*. 2013;14:631-643.

72. de Jager P, Burgerhof JG, van Heerde M, et al. Tidal volume and mortality in mechanically ventilated children: a systematic review and meta-analysis of observational studies. *Crit Care Med*. 2014;42:2461-2472.

73. Arnold JH, Anas NG, Luckett P, et al. High-frequency oscillatory ventilation in pediatric respiratory failure: a multicenter experience. *Crit Care Med*. 2000;28:3913-3919.

75. Randolph AG, Wypij D, Venkataraman ST, et al. Effect of mechanical ventilator weaning protocols on respiratory outcomes in infants and children: a randomized controlled trial. *JAMA*. 2002;288:2561-2568.

80. Saria S, Rajani AK, Gould J, et al. Integration of early physiological responses predicts later illness severity in preterm infants. *Sci Transl Med*. 2010;2:48ra65.

82. Wong HR. Genetics and genomics in pediatric septic shock. *Crit Care Med*. 2012;40:1618-1626.

83. Wong HR, Cvijanovich NZ, Allen GL, et al. Validation of a gene expression-based subclassification strategy for pediatric septic shock. *Crit Care Med*. 2011;39:2511-2517.

84. Sapru A, Curley MAQ, Brady S, et al. Elevated PAI-1 is associated with poor clinical outcomes in pediatric patients with acute lung injury. *Intensive Care Med*. 2009;36:157-163.

86. Dahmer MK. Critical genetic variations in critical illness. *Crit Care Med*. 2011;39:1826-1827.

87. Dahmer MK, O'Cain P, Patwari PP, et al. The influence of genetic variation in surfactant protein B on severe lung injury in African American children. *Crit Care Med*. 2011;39:1138-1144.

94. Nguyen TC, Carcillo JA. Therapeutic plasma exchange as a strategy to reverse multiple organ dysfunction syndrome in patients receiving extracorporeal life support. *Pediatr Crit Care Med*. 2015;16:383-385.

97. Kalil AC, Sun J. Bayesian methodology for the design and interpretation of clinical trials in critical care medicine: a primer for clinicians. *Crit Care Med*. 2014;42:2267-2277.

98. Berry DA. Bayesian clinical trials. *Nat Rev Drug Discov*. 2006;5:27-36.

99. Randolph AG, Meert KL, Neil ME, et al. The feasibility of conducting clinical trials in infants and children with acute respiratory failure. *Am J Respir Crit Care Med*. 2003;167:1334-1340.

Proving the Point: Evidence-Based Medicine in Pediatric Critical Care

R. Scott Watson, Mary E. Hartman, and Derek C. Angus

"Not all clinicians need to appraise evidence from scratch, but all need some skills."[1]

PEARLS

- Physicians have an ethical and clinical obligation to use the best available evidence whenever applicable.
- The evidence base for critical care is growing rapidly.
- Practicing evidence-based medicine is straightforward, and keeping up with relevant evidence is becoming easier and less time consuming.
- PubMed includes research methodology filters (found under the "Clinical Queries" heading) that enhance the efficiency of searching the literature.
- Multiple evidence-based medicine–related resources can be found on the Internet.

Evidence-based medicine (EBM) is simply the integration of the best available evidence with individual clinical expertise and patient preferences.[1,2] One could easily make the incorrect assumption that its practice is, and always has been, ubiquitous. However, proven interventions are often misapplied, and striking variations in clinical practice (not attributable to patient differences) occur even when high-quality evidence is available.[3-8] Practicing EBM in critical care in general and pediatric critical care in particular poses unique challenges. Decisions that can have profound implications for a child and his or her family must be made quickly and, until recently, with little good external evidence. However, pediatric critical care and EBM both have matured to the point that EBM is an indispensable and realistic component of optimal practice.

Despite decades of international support and growth, the practice of EBM continues to be hindered by misconceptions. It is not "cookbook medicine" that suppresses the individual freedom of practitioners.[9] It is not a cost-cutting tool. Treatments found to be effective may be more expensive than the previous standard of care. It is also realistic to think that physicians in the "real world" can practice it. Advances in literature search engines and the increasing availability of EBM resources make it accessible and applicable for busy clinicians.

This chapter provides an overview of the steps in practicing EBM, including definitions of selected terms used in EBM (Appendix A, available online at http://www.expertconsult.com). Critical care is in the midst of a groundswell of outstanding clinical research that is improving the outcome of critically ill patients. Our goal is to demystify the process of EBM so that pediatric intensivists can incorporate it as a fundamental element in their practice.

Evidence-Based Medicine Process

The steps in the EBM process are straightforward: (1) define the problem, (2) search for relevant evidence, (3) evaluate the evidence, and (4) apply the evidence.

1. Define the problem.

The practice of EBM always begins and ends with a patient. Defining the problem in EBM terms requires the provider to frame the problem in a way that will ultimately inform care.[10] The key components to a focused EBM question include:

    a. The patient (or population) with a specific disease, demographic characteristics, or risk factors

    b. The intervention or exposure in need of greater understanding (eg, a medication, test, disease, environmental exposure)

    c. The comparison or main alternative to whatever one wishes to do (there may not always be one)

    d. The outcomes of greatest interest

Ultimately, clinical EBM questions will fall into one of four categories: (1) diagnosis, (2) therapy, (3) prognosis, or (4) etiology or harm. The category of clinical question, in turn, dictates the kinds of studies that are most relevant. For example, questions about therapy are usually best answered with a randomized controlled trial (RCT) or systematic review. On the other hand, to determine the prevalence of a disease or risk factors for its development, observational studies are necessary (see "Types of Studies" later).

2. Search for relevant evidence.

Medical subject headings (MeSH) are descriptive terms assigned to each bibliographic reference in Medline by the National Library of Medicine. There are 27,149 descriptors in the 2014 MeSH, organized into a hierarchical structure (http://www.nlm.nih.gov/pubs/factsheets/mesh.html). At the top level are broad headings such as "Diseases" or "Organisms." More specific headings are found at more narrow levels of the 12-level hierarchy, such as "Sepsis" and *Neisseria meningitidis.*"

There are also more than 218,000 cross-reference entry terms that assist users in finding the most appropriate MeSH (eg, "MODS, see Multiple Organ Failure"). An online, searchable list of the entire MeSH vocabulary and suggestions for key words is available at the National Library of Medicine (http://www.nlm.nih.gov/mesh/meshhome.html). Online search engines have incorporated many of these terms into easy-to-use research methodology filters for clinicians. PubMed, for example, allows searchers to select filters for studies of etiology, diagnosis, therapy, and prognosis. Similar filters can be found in Ovid Technologies' search engine, in addition to filters on clinical prediction guides, qualitative studies, costs, and economics. In both, the choices are presented under the "Clinical Queries" heading. Highly sensitive searches produce comprehensive retrievals (particularly useful for subjects in which little work has been done), highly specific searches retrieve only the most rigorous studies and little nonrelevant material (for subjects in which much work has been published), and optimized searches maximize the tradeoff between sensitivity and specificity.[11-13]

In addition to Medline, other specialized databases and Internet-based resources are available that can yield relevant results quickly. Table 8.1 lists a sample of these resources. One of the best known is the Cochrane Library, which contains a large collection of peer-reviewed systematic reviews of health care interventions.[14] It is thoroughly indexed and easily searched. In addition, the PedsCCM Evidence-Based Journal Club posts critical reviews of studies related to pediatric critical care.

3. **Evaluate the evidence.**

Study Types

Interventional Studies

Interventional studies are clinical experiments, the strongest of which is the RCT, the gold standard in the assessment of the efficacy of an intervention.[15,16] Randomization minimizes the risk of an unequal distribution of known and unknown factors (confounders) that may influence patient outcome. The presence of a control group helps distinguish changes in outcome that result from the therapy in question from changes that otherwise would have occurred. Because of their high cost, RCTs are usually designed to maximize the likelihood of finding a positive effect. Therefore they tend to be efficacy studies, with highly selected patient populations treated by experienced providers. The effectiveness of a therapy as used in general practice (rather than in the specific, carefully controlled setting of an RCT) often requires additional study, usually through subsequent observational studies.[17] See Box 8.1 for factors to consider in appraising the quality and applicability of interventional studies.

Observational Studies

The principal alternative to experimental studies involves observation. Observational studies are powerful tools for addressing many questions that RCTs cannot and for generating hypotheses that can be tested in interventional trials. They can elucidate epidemiologic characteristics and prognosis of diseases or effects of organizational characteristics on outcome. They can provide information on a treatment's effectiveness (vs. efficacy) and determine cost-effectiveness. They have become increasingly sophisticated, but, as with all study types, they have limitations. Confounding may be difficult to control. Even if known confounders are well controlled, unknown or unmeasured confounders may influence results. Selection of an appropriate control group is crucial but can be difficult. Different kinds of observational studies address different types of questions.

In **case-control studies,** researchers compare subjects with a particular outcome (cases) with subjects who do not have the outcome (controls). Ideally, the case and control subjects are identical except for (1) the outcome of interest and (2) the risk factor or exposure that leads to the outcome of interest. With such a study, risk factors or exposures that are responsible for the outcome (eg, smoking as a risk factor for lung cancer) can be identified. Of course, finding groups of patients that are so nearly identical is impossible. However, well-done case-control studies that include rigorously selected cases and controls can be extremely informative. They often are the only feasible study method for uncommon outcomes or when the lag time between an exposure and outcome is long.

Cross-sectional studies provide a snapshot of a population at one point in time. They can identify the prevalence of a condition, such as of sepsis among patients in an ICU. They are relatively inexpensive and can be conducted in a short time. Cross-sectional studies usually establish only association, not causality.

In **cohort studies,** researchers follow a group of subjects through time, recording exposures and outcomes. Cohort studies have a number of strengths, including the ability to establish the timing and sequence of events and provide population-based results. The best cohort studies measure exposures and outcomes in a blinded, objective manner; have long and complete follow-up; and identify known confounders.

Case reports may be the only available information in support of a therapeutic strategy, especially for extremely rare or fatal conditions. The difficulty generalizing from case reports makes them among the weakest forms of clinical evidence.

Research Summaries

Research summaries that provide a standardized, thorough critique of studies are particularly valuable for busy clinicians. Single studies can be presented in a standardized format called a *critically appraised topic.*[18] Multiple studies of a single topic can be summarized in several different ways. **Narrative reviews** include traditional review articles and textbooks. A knowledgeable author reviews the literature, formulates an opinion, and disseminates this opinion along with references to support it. Narrative reviews can provide a detailed qualitative discussion that is easy to comprehend, is well organized, and synthesizes tremendous amounts of information. Unfortunately, the literature is rarely searched and evaluated in an organized, reproducible manner. Inherent lags in publishing times can make them an unreliable source of current information. For example, in 1988, pooled data from nearly 9000 patients with acute myocardial infarction in 15 studies on the use of prophylactic lidocaine in patients showed that the practice was useless at best. Nonetheless, in 1990, narrative review articles and textbooks still contained more recommendations for its use than against it.[19]

A **systematic review** combines the results of multiple studies through the systematic search, assembly, and appraisal

TABLE 8.1   Partial List of EBM Resources on the Internet

Resource	Website
EBM Websites	
Centre for EBM, Oxford	www.cebm.net
Centre for Evidence-Based Child Health	http://www.ich.ucl.ac.uk/ich/academicunits/Centre_for _evidence_based_child_health/Homepage
EBM Toolkit, University of Alberta	http://www.ebm.med.ualberta.ca/
User's Guide to Evidence-Based Practice, Centre for Health Evidence	http://www.cche.net/usersguides/main.asp
University of Washington EBM Internet resources	http://healthlinks.washington.edu/ebp
Netting the Evidence: Database of EBM Websites	http://www.sheffield.ac.uk/~scharr/ir/netting/
Health Information Research Unit, McMaster University	http://hiru.mcmaster.ca
Up to Date	http://www.uptodate.com/
Introduction to Evidence-Based Practice (online tutorial published by Duke University and the University of North Carolina at Chapel Hill)	www.hsl.unc.edu/services/tutorials/ebm/index.htm
MEDLINE Searches	
PubMed	www.pubmed.org
Systematic Reviews	
Cochrane Collaboration	http://www.cochrane.org/
AHRQ Evidence-Based Practice	http://www.ahrq.gov/clinic/epcix.htm
National Guideline Clearinghouse (AHRQ)	http://www.guidelines.gov/
Clinical Evidence (from the *British Medical Journal*)	http://www.clinicalevidence.com/ceweb/conditions/index.jsp
Best Evidence Topics	http://www.bestbets.org
Centre for Reviews and Dissemination, University of York	http://www.york.ac.uk/inst/crd
Critical Care Journal Clubs	
Critical Care Journal Club, Critical Care Forum	http://ccforum.com/articles/browse.asp?sort=Journal%20 club%20critique
PedsCCM Evidence-Based Journal Club	http://pedsccm.org/EBJournal_Club_intro.php
American Thoracic Society, Evidence-Based Critical Care	http://www.thoracic.org/sections/clinical-information/ critical-care/evidence-based-critical-care/index.html
Online EBM Journals	
ACP Journal Club	http://www.acpjc.org/
Bandolier	http://www.medicine.ox.ac.uk/bandolier/
Evidence-Based Medicine	http://ebm.bmjjournals.com/
Journals	
Pediatric Critical Care Medicine	http://www.pccmjournal.com
Critical Care Medicine	http://www.ccmjournal.com
Critical Care Forum	http://ccforum.com/
Pediatrics	http://pediatrics.aappublications.org/
Journal of Pediatrics	http://www.jpeds.com/
Archives of Pediatrics and Adolescent Medicine	http://archpedi.ama-assn.org/
JAMA	http://www.jama.com
New England Journal of Medicine	http://www.nejm.com
British Medical Journal	http://www.bmj.com
The Lancet	http://www.thelancet.com

of primary research. Search criteria are predefined, including the inclusion and exclusion criteria for individual studies. The methods section provides search terms and key words to establish reproducibility. They can provide an excellent summary of the literature up to the date of the review. The main disadvantage is that they are only as good as the studies they include. However, even when the studies are weak, systematic reviews can be an important means by which to identify gaps in evidence and thus outline a research agenda.

In a **meta-analysis,** data are combined from multiple studies to yield a quantitative summary. If the combined studies use similar methodology and are of high quality,

BOX 8.1 Critical Appraisal of a Study of Therapy

Are the Results of the Study Valid?
1. Were patients effectively randomized?
2. Were all the patients accounted for?
3. Was follow-up complete?
4. Were patients analyzed according to how they were randomized (ie, intention to treat)?
5. Were all people involved in the study blinded?
6. Were the groups similar at the start?
7. Were the groups treated equally apart from the experimental intervention?

Are the Results Clinically Useful?
- How large was the treatment effect?
- How precise was the estimate of the treatment effect?
- Are the patients similar to the "norm"?
- Were all clinically important outcomes considered?
- Was a cost-to-benefit analysis performed?

Adapted from Sackett DL, Straus SE, Richardson WS, et al. *Evidence-Based Medicine: How to Practice and Teach EBM.* 2nd ed. London: Harcourt; 2000.

meta-analyses can increase the power to find an effect. However, difficulties in interpretation of summary statistics arise when meta-analyses combine studies that vary in quality, population, or intervention.

Levels of Evidence

One of the most widely used taxonomies for classifying evidence and clinical recommendations comes from the Oxford Centre for Evidence-Based Medicine (Appendix 8B, available online at http://www.expertconsult.com). Each study can be assigned a level of evidence based on its design and quality. For a given topic, the quality of the entire body of evidence forms the basis for the strength (or grade) of a clinical recommendation. The best studies are level 1a evidence (systematic reviews of studies using similar methods), and the weakest studies are level 5 evidence (expert opinion). Clinical recommendations are then graded from A (consistent level 1 evidence) to D (level 5 evidence or troublingly inconsistent or inconclusive studies).

4. Apply the evidence.

The strongest evidence is useless unless it is effectively applied (Box 8-1). Clinicians must use their knowledge and experience to understand how the results of studies can be applied to individual patients. With evidence in hand, a clinician practicing EBM will place it in the context of the specific clinical circumstances and the patient's (or guardian's) preferences.[20] Patient characteristics or preferences may be sufficiently uncommon to render even good evidence inapplicable.

EBM can be implemented on a larger scale through clinical practice guidelines and clinical pathways, which can disseminate and promote best practice at institutional, regional, or national levels. They are especially useful for common illnesses and procedures, and they allow implementation of EBM even when individual physicians are unable to incorporate evidence by themselves because of a lack of either time or expertise. The most compelling guidelines contain a summary of the evidence both for and against the guideline and how to apply the recommendations to specific clinical situations.[18]

Challenges to Evidence-Based Medicine

Until recently, a paucity of strong evidence existed to support particular care paradigms in the critically ill, with even less evidence related to critically ill children. A basic tenet of EBM is that a lack of evidence that an intervention is effective is *not* proof that an intervention is ineffective (ie, "Absence of evidence is not evidence of absence"). This issue is particularly relevant to pediatric critical care, in which numerous therapies are used without proven efficacy, and the evidence base for many other therapies is from studies of adults. Whether unproven therapies should be used depends on (1) whether proven alternatives are available, (2) the likelihood and magnitude of potential harm from the therapy, (3) the natural history of the disease or condition being treated, (4) in the case of prophylaxis, the risk of developing disease, and (5) the cost of treatment (as well as the cost of not treating the patient).

Conclusion

The practice of critical care is changing constantly, but studies documenting remarkable practice variation suggest that the change is much too inconsistent. Intensivists tend to be resourceful, creative, efficient, experts in pathophysiology and comfortable with applying clinical skills to desperate circumstances amidst a paucity of evidence. Although critical care physicians often have both the predilection and facility for making important decisions quickly and independently, that same temperament may impede the acquisition and application of a growing body of evidence related to critical illness and critical care.

All physicians have an ethical responsibility to apply EBM. Meticulously designed and executed clinical research is expensive and difficult to perform. Society expends scarce resources on it. Subjects in clinical trials face significant personal risks in hopes of a better outcome and for the advancement of knowledge. Our responsibility extends beyond individual patients, for whom the benefits of using the best available treatment are usually clear. We owe it to subjects of prior trials, researchers who carried out the trials, and the society that supported them to use and build on the knowledge gained. The unique vulnerability of critically ill patients, with their significant risk of death or long-term morbidity, creates perhaps an even stronger ethical imperative for intensivists to use evidence whenever it is available. When evidence is inadequate, we are left to do our best with our clinical expertise for our current patient and to generate the evidence needed for future patients.

References

1. Guyatt GH, Meade MO, Jaeschke RZ, et al. Practitioners of evidence based care. Not all clinicians need to appraise evidence from scratch but all need some skills. *BMJ.* 2000;320:954.
2. Sackett DL, Rosenberg WM, Gray JA, et al. Evidence based medicine: what it is and what it isn't. *BMJ.* 1996;312:71.
3. Bungard TJ, McAlister FA, Johnson JA, et al. Underutilisation of ACE inhibitors in patients with congestive heart failure. *Drugs.* 2001;61:2021.
4. Bungard TJ, Ghali WA, Teo KK, et al. Why do patients with atrial fibrillation not receive warfarin? *Arch Intern Med.* 2000;160:41.
5. Sim I, Cummings SR. A new framework for describing and quantifying the gap between proof and practice. *Med Care.* 2003;41:874.

6. Bickell NA, McEvoy MD. Physicians' reasons for failing to deliver effective breast cancer care: a framework for underuse. *Med Care*. 2003; 41:442.

7. McAlister FA, Teo KK, Lewanczuk RZ, et al. Contemporary practice patterns in the management of newly diagnosed hypertension. *Can Med Assoc J*. 1997;157:23.

8. Eisenberg MJ, Califf RM, Cohen EA, et al. Use of evidence-based medical therapy in patients undergoing percutaneous coronary revascularization in the United States, Europe, and Canada. Coronary Angioplasty Versus Excisional Atherectomy Trial (CAVEAT-I) and Canadian Coronary Atherectomy Trial (CCAT) investigators. *Am J Cardiol*. 1997;79:867.

9. Reinertsen JL. Zen and the art of physician autonomy maintenance. *Ann Intern Med*. 2003;138:992.

10. Doig GS, Simpson F. Efficient literature searching: a core skill for the practice of evidence-based medicine. *Intensive Care Med*. 2003;29:2119.

11. Davidoff F, Haynes B, Sackett D, et al. Evidence based medicine. *BMJ*. 1995;310:1085.

12. Evidence-Based Medicine Working Group. Evidence-based medicine. A new approach to teaching the practice of medicine. *JAMA*. 1992;268: 2420.

13. Haynes RB, Wilczynski NL. Optimal search strategies for retrieving scientifically strong studies of diagnosis from Medline: analytical survey. *BMJ*. 2004;328:1040.

14. Sackett DL, Straus SE, Richardson WS, et al. *Evidence-Based Medicine: How to Practice and Teach EBM*. 2nd ed. London: Harcourt; 2000.

15. Ware JH, Antman EM. Equivalence trials. *N Engl J Med*. 1997;337:1159.

16. Lamas GA, Pfeffer MA, Hamm P, et al. Do the results of randomized clinical trials of cardiovascular drugs influence medical practice? The SAVE investigators. *N Engl J Med*. 1992;327:241.

17. Rubenfeld GD, Angus DC, Pinsky MR, et al. Outcomes research in critical care: results of the American Thoracic Society Critical Care Assembly Workshop on Outcomes Research. *Am J Respir Crit Care Med*. 1999; 160:358.

18. Sackett DL, Haynes RB, Tugwell P. *Clinical Epidemiology: A Basic Science for Clinical Medicine*. Boston: Little, Brown & Co; 1985.

19. Mulrow CD. Rationale for systematic reviews. In: Chalmers I, Altman DG, eds. *Systematic Reviews*. London: BMJ Publishing Group; 1995.

20. Cook DJ, Hebert PC, Heyland DK, et al. How to use an article on therapy or prevention: pneumonia prevention using subglottic secretion drainage. *Crit Care Med*. 1997;25:1502.

Prediction Tools for Short-Term Outcomes Following Critical Illness in Children

Michael C. Spaeder and Murray M. Pollack

PEARLS

- Physiologic instability is a key factor in the prediction of short-term outcomes in critically ill patients.
- Prediction tools are central to controlling for severity of illness in studies and unit-based quality assessments for both internal and external benchmarking.
- Regression analysis is typically the central technique for the construction of outcomes prediction tools.
- Assessment of the validity of prediction tools centers on two statistical measures: discrimination and calibration.
- Although mortality has historically been the predicted outcome, prediction tools for morbidity have recently been developed.

Introduction

Current efforts to provide high-quality, error-free care require the evaluation of complex systems and the assessment of quality of care. Outcomes research is an important aspect of both requirements. Scoring systems add objectivity to these assessments, especially in critical care units. Controlling for population differences such as differences in severity of illness enables both the inclusion of different health care systems in a single investigative effort and contrasting individual health care systems in quality of care assessments. Mortality adjusted for physiologic status and other case mix factors has been the core methodology of adult, pediatric, and neonatal intensive care assessments for decades. Scoring systems are basic to controlling for severity of illness in studies and unit-based quality assessments for both internal and external benchmarking.

However, mortality rates in most pediatric intensive care units (PICUs) have decreased since these methods were developed. Medical therapies are increasingly focused on reducing morbidity in survivors. Unfortunately, quantitative outcome assessment methods continue to focus on the dichotomous outcome of survival and death. Recently, there has been a new appreciation of the importance of patient outcomes other than mortality, including discharge functional status, and better understanding of its determinants. The future will most likely see a diversity of patient outcomes of interest, methods

to associate risk factors with these outcomes, and use of these risk factors for outcome prediction.

Historical Perspective

The "modern" history of intensive care unit (ICU) scoring systems started with the Clinical Classification Scoring (CCS) system, a subjective categorization of a patient's anticipated clinical needs ranging from routine inpatient care (Category 1) to frequent physician and nursing assessments and therapeutic interventions (Category 4) and the Therapeutic Intervention Scoring System (TISS).[1] Although simple, the CSS system established the basis of severity of illness as a concept related to both physiologic instability and amount and intensity of therapy. The TISS was based on the concept that as patients got sicker, they received more therapy such as mechanical ventilation or vasoactive agent infusions; thus the number and sophistication of therapies, which could be expressed numerically, served as a proxy for severity of illness. Initially, 76 therapies and monitoring techniques were graded from 1 to 4 on the basis of complexity, skill, and cost required to provide these modalities. The TISS score still exists today, although the number of therapies has been reduced and objectivity has been added to the score.[2]

The concepts of sequential or multiple organ system failures (MOSFs) were also important in the development of concepts of severity of illness. Mortality rates increased as the number of failed organ systems increased. The MOSF syndrome was initially described in children in 1986.[3] Although there have been numerous minor adjustments to the definition of an organ system failure, they continue to be based on the initial concepts of failure defined as extreme physiologic dysfunction or use of a therapy preventing that dysfunction. Organ system failures have also been proposed as an outcome measure; since death is uncommon in PICUs, it is appealing to postulate that the number of organ failures or the temporal resolution of these organ failures could be a practical outcome.

Physiologic status is the underlying foundational concept for MOSF and the TISS score. Conceptually, severity of illness may be considered a continuous variable with extremes of outcomes (survival, death) occurring at low and high values. The threshold value determining survival or death is unknown and may vary from patient to patient. Physiologic instability has been an exceptionally productive concept expressed in multiple scoring systems in pediatric, neonatal, and adult intensive care with scores such as the Pediatric Risk of Mortality (PRISM) score, Score for Neonatal Acute Physiology (SNAP), Acute Physiology and Chronic Health Evaluation (APACHE), and many others.

Recently, the development of new morbidity during critical illness has also been related to physiologic instability, with the morbidity risk rising as the instability increases until, at higher states of instability, high morbidity risk transitions to mortality. The interest and investigations of morbidity have been hindered by the lack of measurement methods that are reliable, relevant, and practical for large studies. The recent development of the Functional Status Scale and its use in a national study of more than 10,000 critically ill children hold promise that morbidity will be a more important and relevant outcome in critical care assessments.[4]

Methods

Conceptual Framework

When possible, the severity method should include variables fundamental to the issues being assessed. The fundamental role of pediatric critical care has been to monitor and treat physiologic instability. The development of severity measures has mirrored this role, first as descriptive categories, then as quantification of therapy designed to treat physiologic instability, and finally as physiologic instability itself as the foundational concept. As databases become larger and more data are available digitally, availability of descriptive, categorical, and diagnostic data contained in administrative and clinical databases has increased. These data can also be associated with severity of illness and are being used for quality measures such as standardized mortality ratios and measures of severity of illness in academic studies. However, variables such as diagnosis and operative status are proxy variables whose risk estimation is, at least in part, one or more steps removed from physiologic status. Therefore they are indirect measures of severity. One must be aware that data such as diagnosis are subject to "gaming" to alter an individual site's results. Methods based on primarily categorical data often do not perform well in all critical care environments.

Statistical Issues

Regression analysis is typically the central technique for the construction of outcomes prediction tools. The type of outcome variable (eg, continuous, dichotomous) is one determinant of the type of regression analysis used. Multiple linear regression analysis is most often used for models that seek to predict outcomes that are continuous variables (eg, length of stay). Logistic regression analysis is most often used for models that seek to predict outcomes that are categorical variables (eg, survival/death).

The assessment of the validity of a prediction tool centers on two statistical measures: discrimination and calibration.[5] Discrimination is the accuracy of a model in differentiating outcomes groups and is most often assessed by the area under the receiver operating characteristic (AUC) curve. An AUC = 1 represents a model with perfect accuracy while an AUC = 0.5 represents a model with no apparent accuracy. A rough guide for model discriminatory performance is as follows:

AUC = 0.9–1 (excellent), 0.8–0.9 (good), 0.7–0.8 (fair), 0.6–0.7 (poor), and 0.5–0.6 (fail). Calibration refers to the ability of a model to assign the correct probability of outcome to patients over the entire range of risk prediction. In practical terms for an outcome like mortality, calibration assesses whether the model-estimated probability of mortality for patients with a particular covariate pattern agrees with the actual observed mortality rate. The most accepted method for measuring calibration is the Hosmer Lemeshow goodness-of-fit test.

An important issue in developing and evaluating severity methods is the population used to derive the method. The methods are models based on the populations used to develop them. In the following examples, the Vermont Oxford Neonatal outcome predictor was developed in a large population from inborn nurseries and has been criticized for its lack of applicability to referral centers. The Paediatric Index of Mortality (PIM) has been developed in predominantly Australian and European populations where the relationship of categorical and physiologic variables to outcome may be different from in the United States or a developing country.

Prediction Tools for Assessment of Mortality Risk

Neonatal Intensive Care Unit Prediction Methods

Three well-established prediction methods are used for the assessment of severity of illness and mortality risk in neonates: the Clinical Risk Index for Babies II (CRIB II),[6] SNAP-II,[7] and the Vermont Oxford Network risk adjustment.[8] All scores can be calculated during the first 12 hours of life.

CRIB II is the second-generation of CRIB (Cockburn 1993), which was developed on 812 neonates born less than 1500 gm or at less than 31 weeks' gestation in the United Kingdom.[9] CRIB II is a simplified version of CRIB, validated on 3027 neonates born at 32 weeks' gestation or less. It is a five-item score composed of sex, gestation, birth weight, admission temperature, and worst base excess in first 12 hours of life.

SNAP-II is the second-generation of SNAP (Richardson 1993), which was a physiology-based severity of illness score with 34 variables for babies of all birth weights from the United States and Canada.[10] SNAP-II simplified SNAP to six physiologic variables: mean blood pressure, lowest temperature, PaO_2/FiO_2 ratio, lowest serum pH, seizure activity, and urine output. In an effort to improve the predictive capabilities of SNAP-II for mortality, three additional variables were added: birth weight, small for gestation age, and Apgar (appearance, pulse, grimace, activity, and respiration) score less than 7 at 5 minutes. The resulting nine-variable score for prediction of mortality risk was named Score for Neonatal Acute Physiology with Perinatal Extension (SNAPPE-II).

The Vermont Oxford Network is a network of more than 800 institutions worldwide that maintains databases on interventions and outcomes for infants cared for at member institutions. The Vermont Oxford Network risk adjustment model includes terms for gestational age, race, sex, location of birth, multiple birth, 1-minute Apgar score, small for gestational age, major birth defect, and mode of delivery.

Revalidation efforts of these tools employing a variety of data sources have demonstrated largely similar discriminatory abilities among the tools. Using data from the Vermont Oxford Network, Zupancic et al. validated SNAPPE-II on nearly 10,000 infants with similar performance to the Vermont

TABLE 9.1   Pediatric Risk of Mortality (PRISM) Score III

For computation of mortality and morbidity risk, physiologic variables are measured only in the first 4 hours of pediatric intensive care unit (PICU) care and laboratory variables are measured in the time period from 2 hours before PICU admission through the first 4 hours. See references for the appropriate time periods to assess cardiovascular surgical patients younger than 3 months of age. The neurologic PRISM III consists of the mental status and pupillary reflex parameters. Only the first PICU admission is scored. Please check publications for the most up-to-date prediction algorithms.

CARDIOVASCULAR AND NEUROLOGIC VITAL SIGNS		
Systolic Blood Pressure (mm Hg)	Score = 3	Score = 7
Neonate	40-55	<40
Infant	45-65	<45
Child	55-75	<55
Adolescent	65-85	<65
Temperature	Score = 3 <33°C or >40°C	
Mental status	Score = 5 Stupor/coma or GCS <8	
Heart Rate (beats per minute)	Score = 3	Score = 4
Neonate	215-225	>225
Infant	215-225	>225
Child	185-205	>205
Adolescent	145-155	>155
Pupillary reflexes	Score = 7 One fixed	Score = 11 Both fixed

ACID-BASE, BLOOD GASES		
Acidosis (pH or total CO$_2$)	Score = 2	Score = 6
pH	7.0-7.28	<7.0
CO$_2$	5-16.9	<5
PCO$_2$ (mm Hg)	Score = 1 50-75	Score = 3 >75
Alkalosis: total CO$_2$ (mmol/L)	Score = 4 >34	
PaO$_2$ (mm Hg)	Score = 3 42-49	Score = 6 <42

CHEMISTRY TESTS		
Glucose	Score = 2 >200 mg/dL or >11 mmol/L	
Potassium (mmol/L)	Score = 3 >6.9	
Blood urea nitrogen	Score = 3	
Neonate	>11.9 mg/dL or >4.3 mmol/L	
All other ages	>14.9 mg/dL or >4.3 mmol/L	
Creatinine	Score = 2	
Neonate	>0.85 mg/dL or >75 mmol/L	
Infant	>0.90 mg/dL or >80 mmol/L	
Child	>0.90 mg/dL or >80 mmol/L	
Adolescent	>1.30 mg/dL or >115 mmol/L	

HEMATOLOGY TESTS		
White Blood Cell Count (cells/mm^3)	Score = 4	
	<3000	
Platelet count (×103 cells/mm^3)	Score = 2 100-200	Score = 4 Score = 5 50-99 <50
Prothrombin time (PR) or		
Partial thromboplastin (time) (PTT)	Score = 3	
Neonate	PT >22 or PTT >85	
All other ages	PT >22 or PTT >57	

GCS, Glasgow Coma Scale.

Oxford Network risk adjustment.[11] Within this study cohort, the addition of congenital anomalies to SNAPPE-II improved discrimination significantly. Reid et al. compared CRIB-II and SNAPPE-II in a cohort of Australian preterm infants and found similar performance between the tools and good overall discriminatory ability.[12]

Pediatric Intensive Care Unit Prediction Tools

The prediction of mortality in the PICU has centered primarily on the use of two different acuity scoring systems, the PRISM III score[13] and the PIM3.[14]

PRISM III (Table 9.1) is a third-generation physiology-based score for quantifying physiologic status and mortality prediction. The original tool was developed on 11,165 patients

from 32 different PICUs in the United States and includes 21 physiologic variables. The mortality predictions are routinely updated, the last update being completed on 19,000 patients. Among PRISM III's strengths are its flexibility to extend beyond mortality prediction to provide risk-adjusted PICU length-of-stay estimates.[15] Historically, PRISM III mortality risk assessments were made using physiologic data from the initial 12 hours of PICU care. Notably, PRISM quantifies physiologic status and uses categorical variables to facilitate accurate estimation of mortality risk.

Recently, PRISM III underwent improvements to reduce bias and potential sources of error in more than 10,000 patients collected by the Collaborative Pediatric Critical Care Research Network (CPCCRN) of the National Institute of

Child Health and Human Development.[16] Initially, PRISM used PICU outcome and subsequent PICU admissions in the same hospitalizations with additional mortality risk. But discharge decision making is an important aspect of quality of care. For example, an inappropriately discharged PICU patient with a subsequent PICU readmission during the same hospitalization was previously credited as a good outcome for the first admission, while the subsequent admission had an additional mortality risk credited to the subsequent PICU admission mortality risk. Therefore the subsequent PICU admission mortality risk was inflated even though it was associated with the premature or inappropriate discharge. The new version of PRISM III uses only the first PICU admission, and hospital outcome is predicted. Second, the PRISM observation time period has changed from the sampling period for the first 12 hours of care to a significantly shorter time period (2 hours before admission to 4 hours after admission for laboratory data and the first 4 hours of PICU care for other physiologic variables) since this better separates the PRISM score from therapies.[17] Third, admission of cardiovascular patients for "optimizing" therapy or observation before their intervention is now common in many institutions, and this necessitated a new definition of the PRISM observation period. An objective method to determine the PRISM III observation for cardiovascular patients is now available. Finally, when PRISM was initially developed, the scores for physiologic derangements for each variable were calibrated to mortality odds ratios, so the PRISM III score for each variable represented equivalent risk. Over time, new therapies have evolved and these equivalencies could have changed. This was tested and adjustments were made by partitioning PRISM into its five major subcategories. The new PRISM III algorithm partitions PRISM III into the neurologic and non-neurologic components for outcome prediction.

The PIM3 mortality prediction model was developed from 53,112 patients from 60 PICUs in Australia, New Zealand, Ireland, and the United Kingdom (Table 9.2). PIM3 requires 10 variables collected from the time of initial patient contact to 1 hour after arrival in the PICU. In contrast with PRISM III, PIM3 employs only four physiologic variables but includes six categorical variables that classify patients on the basis of reason for admission, use of mechanical ventilation in the first hour, and diagnostic risk strata. PIM3 has not been extensively tested in the United States.

Numerous obvious differences distinguish PRISM III from PIM3 (eg, interval for data collection, number of physiologic variables, inclusion of nonphysiologic data). The impact that these differences have on mortality prediction in the form of bias must be considered.[5,18] Foundationally, PRISM quantifies physiologic instability (PRISM III score) and uses categorical variables to facilitate accurate estimation of mortality risk while PIM only estimates mortality risk. PIM has not performed well in cardiovascular surgical populations where outcome is strongly associated with postoperative physiologic status.[18a] PIM3 uses a 1-hour (vs. 4 hours for PRISM III) PICU observation time, and this might imply it is potentially less affected by PICU therapies. However, the variable observation period before PICU admission could impose significant institution-level bias on the basis of the percent of patients transported to the PICU from other locations and the involvement of the PICU team in the transport or emergency department care. PIM3 includes a therapeutic intervention

| **TABLE 9.2** | Paediatric Index of Mortality 3 (PIM3) Variables and Model Coefficients |

Score calculated based on variables collected from the time of initial patient contact to 1 hour after arrival in the pediatric intensive care unit.

Variable	Coefficients
Pupils fixed to light? (yes/no)	3.8233
Elective admission (yes/no)	−0.5378
Mechanical ventilation in the first hour (yes/no)	0.9763
Absolute value of base excess (mmol/L)	0.0671
SBP at admission (mm Hg)	−0.0431
$SBP^2/1000$	0.1716
$100 \times FiO_2/PaO_2$ (mm Hg)	0.4214
Recovery post procedure?	
Yes, recovery from a bypass cardiac procedure	−1.2246
Yes, recovery from a nonbypass cardiac procedure	−0.8762
Yes, from a noncardiac procedure	−1.5164
Very high-risk diagnosis (yes/no)	1.6225
Cardiac arrest preceding ICU admission	
Severe combined immunodeficiency	
Leukemia or lymphoma after first induction	
Bone marrow transplant recipient	
Liver failure is main reason for ICU admission	
High-risk diagnosis (yes/no)	1.0725
Spontaneous cerebral hemorrhage	
Cardiomyopathy or myocarditis	
Hypoplastic left heart syndrome	
Neurodegenerative disease	
Necrotizing enterocolitis is main reason for ICU admission	
Low-risk diagnosis (yes/no)	−2.1766
Asthma is main reason for ICU admission	
Bronchiolitis is main reason for ICU admission	
Croup is main reason for ICU admission	
Obstructive sleep apnea is main reason for ICU admission	
Diabetic ketoacidosis is main reason for ICU admission	
Seizure disorder is main reason for ICU admission	
Constant	−1.7928

ICU, intensive care unit; SBP, systolic blood pressure.

(mechanical ventilation) as a predictor variable that introduces bias from the prehospital and emergency department settings and introduces a therapy into the score when the use of the score to evaluate quality of care is closely related to the provision of therapy.

New Algorithms in the Public Domain

It should be clear to any practitioner of critical care that severity of illness and mortality risk are dynamic variables subject to a variety of influences such as therapies provided, presence of comorbidities, and evolution of the disease process. Although not designed to specifically predict mortality risk, there are severity of illness scores obtained over the course of PICU care that correlate with mortality risk. The Paediatric Logistic Organ Dysfunction (PELOD) score quantifies degree of organ dysfunction among six different organ systems—neurologic, cardiovascular, respiratory, renal, hematologic, and hepatic.[19] The score was developed from 594 patients and subsequently validated on 1806 patients demonstrating good discrimination of mortality (AUC = 0.91).[20]

Among the subgroup of infants admitted to the PICU or cardiac ICU following repair or palliation of congenital heart disease, efforts have been taken to ascribe risk of mortality based on surgical procedure and patient covariates. The Society for Thoracic Surgeons and European Association for Cardiothoracic Surgery (STS-EACTS) Congenital Heart Surgery Mortality Score was introduced in 2009. The score was developed on 77,294 procedures entered into the STS and EACTS Congenital Heart Surgery databases and validated on an additional 27,700 procedures.[21] Procedure-specific relative risks of in-hospital mortality were estimated for more than 140 congenital heart disease procedures. To combine procedure-specific risks with patient-specific factors, the patient's age, weight, and preoperative hospital length of stay were added to the model. The STS-EACTS score has good discrimination for in-hospital mortality (AUC = 0.816) and outperformed both the Risk Adjustment for Congenital Heart Surgery (RACHS-1) and the Aristotle Basic Complexity score in this cohort of more than 100,000 congenital heart disease procedures.

Next Generation: Morbidity and Mortality Prediction—Trichotomous Outcome

Morbidity Assessment

Although mortality adjusted for physiologic status and other case mix factors has been the core methodology of adult, pediatric, and neonatal intensive care assessments for decades, mortality for most pediatric critical illnesses has decreased since these methods were developed. More important, therapies are increasingly focused on reducing morbidity in survivors. However, most quantitative outcome assessment methods continue to focus on the dichotomous outcome of survival versus death.

A major challenge of pediatrics is the development of well-defined morbidity measures that are rapid, reliable, and objective; measure the child's status at the time of testing; and are applicable to a broad range of ages in a variety of environments. In-depth testing such as neuropsychologic methods will remain the clinical standard, but other methods applicable to all pediatric ages and sufficiently rapid to be used in large samples are necessary. The Glasgow Outcome Scale score was adapted to children in the Pediatric Cerebral and Overall Performance Category scores (PCPC/POPC), but sufficient inter-rater reliability was only achievable when neighboring categories were combined[22]; therefore using these scores in outcome studies risked requiring very large sample sizes to detect significant differences. The history of outcome studies in adult medicine demonstrated the value of scales such as the activities of daily living scale. Such a functional status measure would enable researchers to track the trajectory of disease and recovery and might enable us to project future functional status, resource needs, economic impact, and other effects of illness in large numbers of patients. Thus the foundation of the Functional Status Scale (FSS) was to adapt the concepts of activities of daily living to pediatrics in a manner that met the criteria described earlier.[4]

The FSS was developed through a formal consensus process by pediatric health care specialists from 11 institutions, including pediatricians, neurologists, developmental psychologists, physiatrists, nurses, respiratory therapists, and intensivists. The FSS is composed of six domains including respiratory status, feeding, motor functioning, communication, sensory functioning, and mental status. Each domain is objectively assessed from normal to very severe dysfunction. The score was composed to enable it to be assessed from the parents' or caregivers' reports or medical records. It was validated on more than 800 patients from seven institutions against an adaptive behavior scale, has very good inter-rater reliability, and has been used in numerous studies including a study of more than 10,000 pediatric patients. Comparisons with the POPC and PCPC demonstrated FSS increases with each higher POPC and PCPC category. However, the dispersion of the FSS scores indicated a lack of precision in the POPC/PCPC system when compared with the more objective and granular FSS system.[23]

A recent multisite study of more than 5000 pediatric ICU patients demonstrated the importance of the development of new functional status morbidities during intensive care.[24] The rate of new functional status morbidities assessed by an increase of 3 or greater in the FSS score was 4.8%, twice as high as the rate of hospital deaths. On hospital discharge, the good category decreased from a baseline of 72% to 63%, mild abnormality increased from 10% to 15%, moderate abnormality status increased from 13% to 14%, severe status increased from 4% to 5%, and very severe was unchanged at 1%. The highest new morbidity rates were in the neurologic diagnoses (7.3%), acquired cardiovascular disease (5.9%), cancer (5.3%), and congenital cardiovascular disease (4.9%). New morbidities occurred in all ages, especially in those younger than 12 months of age. New morbidities involved all FSS domains with the highest proportions involving respiratory, motor, and feeding dysfunction.

The recent data compared with historical data suggest that pediatric critical care may have exchanged mortality for morbidity over the past several decades. Although it is not possible to precisely compare the rates over time because of the different research methods, data from the 1990s demonstrated a PICU mortality rate of 4.6% and a PICU morbidity rate of 3.1% (based on a ≥2 POPC change) while the current demonstrated a hospital mortality rate of 2.4% and morbidity rate of 4.8%. Thus the "morbidity and mortality rate" decreased from only 7.7% to 7.2% as the mortality rated decreased and the new morbidity rate increased. Because these rates are not severity or risk adjusted, the changes in admission criteria and other factors that have occurred in the past several decades could have also significantly influenced this comparison.

Recently the Collaborative Pediatric Critical Care Research Network multisite study demonstrated that new functional status morbidities associated with PICU stays present on hospital discharge are associated with many of the same factors as mortality, including physiologic status measured by the PRISM III score, age, admission source, and diagnostic factors.[25] Importantly, these new morbidities when measured with the FSS score can be modeled simultaneously with mortality. Critical care mortality is usually associated with physiologic abnormalities in the cardiovascular, respiratory, neurologic, and hematologic systems. It appears that new morbidity significantly affecting functional status is often an event along the path toward mortality as both outcomes are strongly associated with the degree of physiologic alterations. Trichotomous modeling uncovered the phasic association of morbidity risk with physiologic status; morbidity risk increases with physiologic instability but then decreases as patients with potential morbidity die. Recent studies indicate that trichotomous logistic regression can produce a well-performing model for simultaneous prediction of both morbidity and mortality suitable for risk adjustment in research, quality, and other studies.

The inclusion of morbidity and mortality in outcome prediction has wide implications for research trials and quality programs, especially those currently based on internal or external benchmarking of standardized mortality ratios. Care assessments that focus on morbidity and mortality will have wide appeal and relevance. Potentially, evaluations of, and improvements in, the structure and process of care analogous to those resulting from the investigations of the variability of standardized mortality ratios could result from the inclusion of this important new outcome. Initiatives that monitor standardized mortality ratios could find relevance in the inclusion of standardized morbidity ratios as well.

Application of Prediction Tools in Pediatric Intensive Care

Prediction tools can be applied at both the population and individual patient levels. At the population level, prediction tools are used in benchmarking, which is a process in which the performance of entities (eg, individuals, PICUs, institutions) is observed and then compared with internal or external standards. Clinical scoring systems (eg, PRISM III) are used to control for severity of illness and other factors, thus allowing for standardized comparisons. The two most common standardized comparisons used in pediatric intensive care are the standardized mortality ratio (observed mortality rate divided by the expected mortality rate) and the standardized length-of-stay ratio (observed length of stay divided by the expected length of stay).

Internal benchmarking is distinguished from external benchmarking as it relates to the comparison of performance within the entity. For example, an individual PICU may want to compare the impact of a new care protocol on length of stay as compared with the current internal standard of care for a particular illness. Calculating a standardized ICU length-of-stay ratio would allow for the comparison of practices while accounting for differences in patients' severity of illness between the two groups. External or competitive benchmarking allows for the direct comparisons between individual hospitals or PICUs by controlling for differences in case mix.

At the individual patient level, the uses of prediction tools for short-term outcome are varied. Clinical scoring systems are often employed in clinical trials and outcomes analyses to control for patient severity of illness or in measuring changes in physiologic status after a novel therapy has been initiated.[5]

Future Directions—Prediction Tools for Decision Support

The use of computerized decision support in adult, pediatric, and neonatal ICUs has grown considerably over the past several years. The integration of alerts, reminders, and protocols into computer order entry systems can help in guiding therapy and the reduction of medication errors.[26] There is, however, still a paucity of effective and validated decision support tools to guide the critical care practitioner in making real-time decisions that affect short-term patient outcomes. The use of continuous monitoring data in the ICU to predict clinical deterioration is a recent subject of great interest. Moorman and colleagues[27] developed a predictive algorithm for clinical deterioration in very-low-birth-weight infants employing heart rate characteristics monitoring and demonstrated, in a randomized clinical trial of 3003 patients, a 20% relative reduction of mortality with a number needed to monitor of 48. Efforts to develop predictive monitoring algorithms in older children and adults are under way.

The increasing availability of large pediatric critical care datasets potentially provides the foundation for the creation of decision support tools. The various pediatric critical care data sources in the United States and worldwide vary greatly as they relate to accessibility/cost, clinical detail, and represented population.[28] The expectation of the National Institutes of Health that federally funded investigators make their data widely and freely available to the public will only increase the amount of available data. Currently, datasets generated from research conducted by the CPCCRN and the Pediatric Emergency Care Applied Research Network are available to researchers. The Pediatric Existing Data Analysis group of the Pediatric Acute Lung Injury and Sepsis Investigators maintains a regularly updated list of pediatric critical care data sources (http://pedal.vpicu.net/datasources.html).

References

1. Cullen DJ, Civetta JM, Briggs BA, Ferrara LC. Therapeutic intervention scoring system: a method for quantitative comparison of patient care. *Crit Care Med.* 1974;2(2):57-60.
2. Lefering R, Zart M, Neugebauer EA. Retrospective evaluation of the simplified Therapeutic Intervention Scoring System (TISS-28) in a surgical intensive care unit. *Intensive Care Med.* 2000;26(12):1794-1802.
3. Wilkinson JD, Pollack MM, Ruttimann UE, et al. Outcome of pediatric patients with multiple organ system failure. *Crit Care Med.* 1986;14(4):271-274.
4. Pollack MM, Holubkov R, Glass P, et al. Functional Status Scale: new pediatric outcome measure. *Pediatrics.* 2009;124(1):e18-e28.
5. Marcin JP, Pollack MM. Review of the methodologies and applications of scoring systems in neonatal and pediatric intensive care. *Pediatr Crit Care Med.* 2000;1:20-27.
6. Parry G, Tucker J, Tarnow-Mordi W. CRIB II: an update of the clinical risk index for babies score. *Lancet.* 2003;361:1789-1791.
7. Richardson DK, Corcoran JD, Escobar GJ, et al. SNAP-II and SNAPPE-II: simplified newborn illness severity and mortality risk scores. *J Pediatr.* 2001;138:92-100.
8. Horbar JD, Soll RF, Edwards WH. The Vermont Oxford Network: a community of practice. *Clin Perinatol.* 2010;37:29-47.
9. Cockburn F, Cooke RWI, Gamsu HR, et al. The CRIB (clinical risk index for babies) score: a tool for assessing initial neonatal risk and comparing performance of neonatal intensive care units. *Lancet.* 1993;342:193-198.
10. Richardson DK, Gray JE, McCormick MC, et al. Score for neonatal acute physiology: a physiologic severity index for neonatal intensive care. *Pediatrics.* 1993;91:617-623.
11. Zupancic JAF, Richardson DK, Horbar JD, et al. Revalidation of the score for neonatal acute physiology in the Vermont Oxford Network. *Pediatrics.* 2007;119:e156-e163.
12. Reid S, Bajuk B, Lui K, et al. Comparing CRIB-II and SNAPPE-II as mortality predictors for very preterm infants. *J Paediatr Child Health.* 2014;e-pub ahead of print.
13. Pollack MM, Patel KM, Ruttimann UE. PRISM III: an updated Pediatric Risk of Mortality score. *Crit Care Med.* 1996;24(5):743-752.

14. Straney L, Clements A, Parslow RC, et al. Paediatric index of mortality 3: an updated model for predicting mortality in pediatric intensive care. *Pediatr Crit Care Med.* 2013;14:673-681.

15. Ruttimann UE, Pollack MM. Variability in duration of stay in pediatric intensive care units: a multiinstitutional study. *J Pediatr.* 1996;128(1):35-44.

16. Pollack MMHR, Funai T, Berger JT, et al. The Pediatric Risk of Mortality (PRISM) Score III. *Update.* 2015;*Submitted.* 2015.

17. Pollack MM, Dean JM, Butler J, et al. The ideal time interval for critical care severity-of-illness assessment. *Pediatr Crit Care Med.* 2013;14(5):448-453.

18. Tibby SM, Taylor D, Festa M, et al. A comparison of three scoring system for mortality risk among retrieved intensive care patients. *Arch Dis Child.* 2002;87:421-425.

18a. Czaja AS, Scanlon MC, Kuhn EM, Jeffries HE. Performance of the Pediatric Index of Mortality 2 for pediatric cardiac surgery patients. *Pediatr Crit Care Med.* 2011;12(2):184-189.

19. Leteurtre S, Martinot A, Duhamel A, et al. Development of a pediatric multiple organ dysfunction score: use of two strategies. *Med Decis Making.* 1999;19:399-410.

20. Leteurtre S, Martinot A, Duhamel A, et al. Validation of the paediatric logistic organ dysfunction (PELOD) score: prospective, observational, multicentre study. *Lancet.* 2003;362:192-197.

21. O'Brien SM, Clarke DR, Jacobs JP, et al. An empirically based tool for analyzing mortality associated with congenital heart surgery. *J Thorac Cardiovasc Surg.* 2009;138:1139-1153.

22. Fiser DH. Assessing the outcome of pediatric intensive care. *J Pediatric.* 1992;121:69-74.

23. Pollack MM, Holubkov R, Funai T, et al. Relationship between the functional status scale and the pediatric overall performance category and pediatric cerebral performance category scales. *JAMA Pediatrics.* 2014;168(7):671-676.

24. Pollack MM, Holubkov R, Funai T, et al. Pediatric intensive care outcomes: development of new morbidities during pediatric critical care. *Pediatr Crit Care Med.* 2014;15(9):821-827.

25. Pollack MM, Holubkov R, Funai T, and the CPCCRN Network. Simultaneous prediction of new morbidity, mortality, and survival without new morbidity from pediatric intensive care: a new paradigm for outcomes assessment. *Crit Care Med.* 2015;43:1699-1709.

26. Williams CN, Bratton SL, Hirshberg EL. Computerized decision support in adult and pediatric critical care. *World J Crit Care Med.* 2013;2:21-28.

27. Moorman JR, Carlo WA, Kattwinkel J, et al. Mortality reduction by heart rate characteristic monitoring in very low birth weight neonates: a randomized trial. *J Pediatr.* 2011;159:900-906.

28. Bennett TD, Spaeder MC, Matos RI, et al. Existing data analysis in pediatric critical care research. *Front Pediatr.* 2014;2:79.

Long-Term Outcomes Following Critical Illness in Children

Francois Aspesberro, Jerry J. Zimmerman, and R. Scott Watson

PEARLS

- Development of specialized pediatric intensive care has contributed to substantially reduced mortality for critically ill children.
- Publications suggest that pediatric critical care may have "exchanged" decreased mortality for increased long-term morbidity, with children struggling to perform at their premorbid levels following a PICU stay.
- The post–intensive care syndrome, first described in adults, may also occur in this vulnerable population of children.
- Research has identified physical, cognitive, and mental health domains as the major areas of impairment in survivors of critical illness.
- There is an urgent need for additional research to better characterize post–intensive care morbidity and its risk factors with the goal of minimizing adverse sequelae associated with critical illness.

As pediatric intensive care has become progressively more effective at sustaining life during hospitalization for critical illness, a wide range of long-term detrimental sequelae among survivors is becoming apparent. For intensivists, a comprehensive understanding of the long-term effects of critical illnesses and critical care therapies is essential for the design of interventions to improve care and enhance the lives of patients and their families who experience life-threatening illness and injury.

Mortality Reduction: The First Frontier for Critical Care Medicine

Mortality reduction was the first frontier of critical care medicine and remains the most commonly used measure of outcome following critical illness. Fortunately, the subspecialty of pediatric critical care has matured considerably, and mortality rates have decreased substantially (Fig. 10.1).[1-4] Mortality rates as low as 3% were reported for 80,739 children included in the Virtual Pediatric Intensive Care Unit (PICU) Systems database, who were admitted to PICUs between 2005 and 2008.[5] Despite low overall short-term mortality, some children surviving critical illness remain at increased risk of death following hospitalization. Most notably, children *surviving* hospitalization for severe sepsis have mortality rates 2 to

50 times greater than that of the general population, depending on age and gender.[6]

Mitigating Long-Term Morbidity: The Next Frontier for Pediatric Critical Care Medicine

Unfortunately, many children surviving critical illness struggle to perform at their preillness levels. Thus, improvements in mortality have not necessarily led to concomitant reductions in morbidity. Increases in survival and morbidity have suggested to some that pediatric critical care has exchanged mortality for morbidity.[7,8] Although this may have been an unavoidable consequence of initial success in improving survival from life-threatening illness, the next frontier for the field is to understand the antecedents of this morbidity so that it can be prevented whenever possible and minimized when it does occur.

Post–Intensive Care Syndrome

Post–intensive care syndrome (PICS) is defined as new or worsened problems in cognitive, psychiatric, or physical function in a patient following a critical illness that persist beyond acute care hospitalization.[9] In addition to patients, family members themselves are also at risk of developing a variant of this syndrome, PICS-Family, with psychiatric symptoms, such as depression, posttraumatic stress, anxiety, or complicated grief. PICS has been described in adults surviving critical illness, but research in the area of pediatric PICS is currently lacking, and its incidence in children remains unknown. Nonetheless, it provides a useful conceptual framework for morbidity among pediatric survivors of critical illness, who, like adult survivors, are at risk of long-term impairment in multiple domains, including physical, cognitive, social, and emotional functioning[10] (Fig. 10.2).

Impact of Pediatric Critical Illness on Health-Related Quality of Life

Children surviving critical illness incur elevated risk of postdischarge mortality and morbidity, with impairment in physical, cognitive, emotional, and social function, as well as overall health-related quality of life (HRQL) (Table 10.1).[1,11-16] Patients' families also suffer emotional, financial, and social strains, which, in turn, can make it more difficult for them to support the recovery of their children. The assessment of HRQL has gained increased consideration in patients surviving after critical illness.[17,18] Baseline HRQL[19] is determined by genetics[20]; parent, family, and home characteristics[21]; and chronic, comorbid conditions.[22,23] In addition to the effects of acute illness,[24] these same variables likely impact HRQL recovery following critical illness. In assessing HRQL among a generalized sample of US children >6 years of age (60,031 children included in the 2003/2004 National Survey of Children's Health), lower HRQL was noted for children in lower socioeconomic status groups, those with health care access barriers, adolescents compared with children, and individuals with chronic medical conditions.[25]

In 1995, Wilson and Cleary published a conceptual model of patient outcomes linking clinical variables with HRQL (Fig. 10.3).[26] Individual characteristics include personality traits, chronic comorbid conditions, and genetics. Environmental characteristics include parental stress, family dynamics, and home demographics. Critical illness includes the intensity and duration of organ system dysfunction.

As early as 1948, the concept of maximizing quality of life as a fundamental right was included as one of the basic principles in the World Health Organization's Constitution

through the statements, "Health is a state of complete physical, mental and social well-being and not merely the absence of disease or infirmity" and "The enjoyment of the highest attainable standard of health is one of the fundamental rights of every human being" (World Health Organization, 1949, p. 1).[27,28] Quality of life is defined as an individual's perception of his or her position in life, in the context of the culture, environment, and value systems in which the person lives and in relation to the individual's goals, expectations, standards, and concerns.[11,29] HRQL is defined as quality of life in which

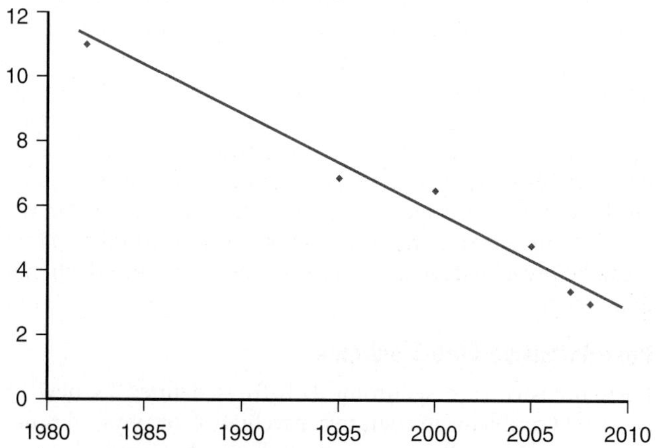

Fig. 10.1. Historical decline of PICU mortality.

TABLE 10.1	Domains of Long-Term Outcomes and Examples of Morbidity Following PICU Discharge
Domain	**Morbidity Example**
Physical	Neuromuscular weakness ICU-associated polyneuropathy Pain Disturbed sleep patterns and nightmares Pulmonary morbidity
Cognitive	Executive function Processing speed Memory Attention Academic performance (lifelong effects)
Mental health	Anxiety Depression Acute stress disorder Posttraumatic stress disorder (PTSD)
Family	Mental health of parents and siblings Divorce
Social	Reduced ability to interact with peers Missed school Family Isolation from friends and family members
Economic	Costs of care Loss of income due to missed work or job loss

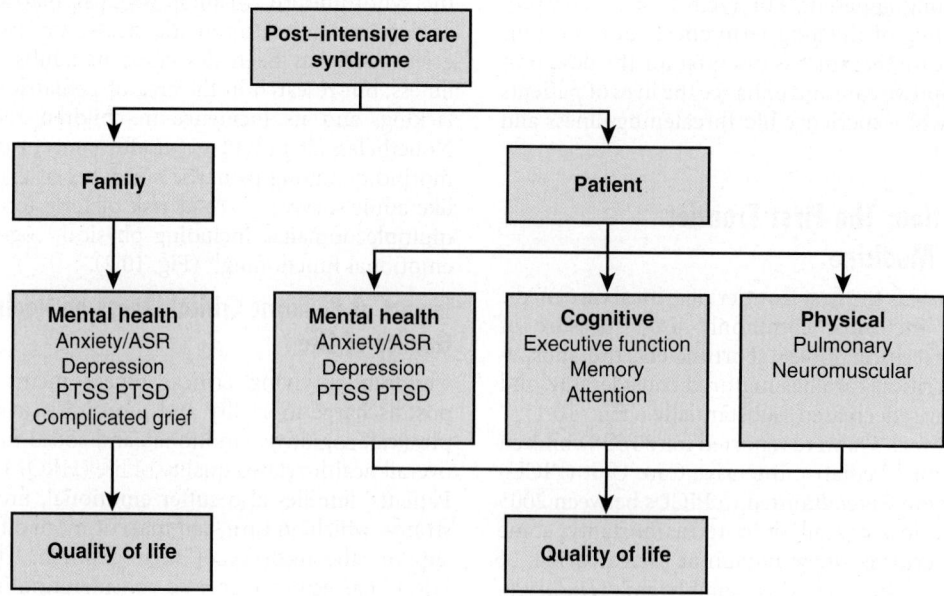

Fig. 10.2. Post–intensive care syndrome.

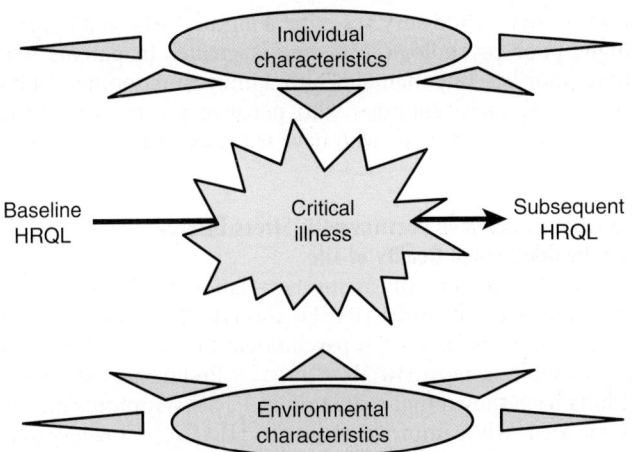

Fig. 10.3. Individual characteristics and environmental characteristics.

a dimension of personal judgment over one's health and disease is added.[30,31] In the case of children, HRQL is influenced by factors such as the ability to participate in peer groups and the ability to keep up with developmentally appropriate activities. It provides a broad view of child health, encompassing aspects of perceived health, health behavior, and well-being.[27,25,32]

Outcomes Following Cardiopulmonary Resuscitation

Ebrahim and colleagues reviewed the effects of resuscitation intensity, illness severity, and baseline disease on adaptive behavior and functional outcomes on HRQL of children urgently admitted to a PICU.[33] This study found that more intense modes of resuscitation and increasing severity of illness were independently associated with the development of acquired brain injury and reduced HRQL. Higher severity of illness was found to correlate with worsening HRQL 6 months after discharge but not at 2 years.[34] However, not all the studies are in agreement; some have not found an association between measures of severity of illness and HRQL among survivors of pediatric intensive care.[14,35]

Outcomes for Long-Stay Pediatric Intensive Care Unit Patients

Since the mid-1990s, the demographics of children admitted to PICUs have changed, with admission of more children with multiple chronic problems, increased readmission rates, and a growing number of children who stay in the PICU for longer periods of time.[36] Conlon and associates assessed HRQL 2 to 10 years after PICU discharge for 193 children who required at least 28 days of pediatric intensive care.[1] Impaired HRQL was found in 43% of the PICU survivors, of whom 20% had poor HRQL with persistent disabling health problems.

Outcomes Following Pediatric Severe Infection

Severe infections such as meningococcemia and other forms of sepsis are associated with high morbidity. Children surviving meningococcemia exhibit impaired HRQL, especially within the physical domain, up to 3 years after discharge from a PICU.[37,38] In meningococcal septic shock, less favorable scores on behavioral and emotional measurement scales were significantly also associated with poorer HRQL.[38] Similarly, in

a cohort of children in urban Senegal surviving bacterial meningitis, HRQL scores were significantly lower than controls.[39]

Als and coworkers published a prospective neuropsychologic function study of school-aged children who survived meningoencephalitis, sepsis, and other disorders.[40] Admission to PICUs was followed by deficits in neuropsychologic performance and educational difficulties, with more severe difficulties noted following meningoencephalitis and septic illness. Their results show that in the 3 to 6 months following discharge from intensive care, school-aged children significantly underperform on measures of neuropsychologic function. Analysis of the effect of illness type on outcome revealed that aspects of neuropsychologic function, such as memory function, and teacher-rated academic performance were most reduced in children with meningoencephalitis and septic illness. Multivariable linear regression revealed that worse performance on a composite score of neuropsychologic impairment was more prevalent when children were younger, from a lower social class, and had experienced seizures during their admission (p <0.02).

Farris and colleagues reviewed the functional outcome of 384 children who survived severe sepsis employing the Pediatric Overall Performance Category score.[41] Thirty-four percent of survivors had a decline in their functional status at 28 days, and 18% had poor functional outcome. Clinical factors associated with increased risk of poor outcome included central nervous system infections, intraabdominal infection, a history of recent trauma, requirement for cardiopulmonary resuscitation, and high PRISM III score. Decline in functional status 28 days after onset of severe sepsis is a frequent and potentially clinically meaningful patient-centered outcome. The duration of follow-up in this particular cohort was relatively short. Longer duration of follow-up would provide an improved sense of the severity and duration of morbidity experienced by survivors of pediatric sepsis. It would also provide an indication of the proportion of patients that return to their baseline functional status and how much time is required to achieve this result.

Outcomes Following Pediatric Acute Respiratory Distress

Children with acute respiratory distress (ARDS) continue to have high short-term mortality, especially those with comorbid conditions such as an immunocompromised state or sepsis.[40] Little knowledge of long-term outcomes exists for children who survive pediatric ARDS. Significant long-term effects reported in adult ARDS survivors include diminished lung function, decreased exercise tolerance, and reduced neurocognitive function that impact daily living and decrease quality of life.[42-47]

Pediatric Traumatic Brain Injury: A Model for Multidisciplinary Outcomes Assessment

Pediatric traumatic brain injury is an example of the need for multidisciplinary outcomes assessment and intervention after pediatric critical care. A leading cause of death in childhood, major trauma also leads to long-term morbidity among the 80% who survive the acute hospitalization.[32,48-50] Parent proxy reports 2 years after injury showed that injured children and adolescents continue to have significantly worse motor functioning, autonomy, cognition, and social functioning, and significantly fewer positive emotions than the normative sample, even after controlling for age, gender, and maternal socioeconomic status.[27] Child self-reports showed fewer physical complaints but more motor function and autonomy deficits. Holbrook and coworkers found that a high proportion of adolescents hospitalized with an injury screened positive for acute stress disorder, and this negatively impacted HRQL outcomes during the first 2 years after injury.[51] More attention has been focused on the psychosocial effects of injury on a child's health and well-being. Not only is it important to measure the impact an injury has on the child's psychosocial health during a defined period after the injury, but it is also important to analyze the developmental implications of the injury on the child's future well-being. HRQL measurements can play a valuable role in documenting the recovery trajectory after different types of injuries, including traumatic injury.

Antecedents and Variables Associated With Outcomes

Effect of Chronic Comorbid Conditions on Outcomes Following Critical Illness

Chronic conditions are common among children admitted to US PICUs, occurring in up to 52% of admissions.[52] Children with preexisting comorbid conditions may be particularly vulnerable to long-term adverse outcomes, as such children demonstrate greater risk for PICU admission in general, greater injury from a given insult, and increased lasting morbidity following illness.[22,34,37,53-59] Such children are at increased risk for multiple organ dysfunction syndrome (MODS) and increased PICU mortality. Nonetheless, children with chronic diagnoses seem to be just as likely as previously healthy children to return to their baseline functional status after MODS. Of note, return to baseline functional status varies by chronic illness category. Patients with congenital heart disease and those who receive solid organ transplants have higher rates of functional outcomes improvement than their healthy counterparts. This initially counterintuitive finding is most likely due to resolution of chronic organ dysfunction following operative cardiac repair or organ transplantation.

Effect of Parent, Family, and Home Characteristics on Outcomes Following Critical Illness

Children are dependent on their families for their physical, emotional, and social needs, and family characteristics can significantly influence children's HRQL. Multiple contextual factors related to the home environment influence outcomes following illness. Higher maternal education has been shown to contribute significantly to better child HRQL,[60] whereas lower paternal education resulted in lower child HRQL.[27] Socioeconomic status (SES) has repeatedly been demonstrated as an important determinant of health and mortality: The lowest SES is associated with the poorest outcomes.[61-67] In addition it is important to note that SES may change during the evaluation period of a longitudinal study as the family copes with lost work time and expenses related to medical care.

Parents of PICU survivors may have psychologic sequelae affecting their own quality of life.[11] Reduced parental physical and psychosocial well-being has been shown to consistently predict poorer child adjustment.[67-71] Among ICU survivors, psychologic morbidity, including anxiety and depression among family members, affects patient outcomes, including critical decision making by the patients.[72] Not surprisingly, highly functioning, adaptive families have better

HRQL after a child survives critical illness.[48] Also not surprisingly, poor psychologic outcome is greater in parents who have poor baseline mental health, family functioning, coping skills, and social support, who perceive greater severity of illness in their child, or who have witnessed their child being injured.

Association Between Posttraumatic Stress Disorder and Health-Related Quality of Life

Multiple studies identify an inverse relationship between posttraumatic stress disorder (PTSD) and HRQL following critical illness, demonstrating the psychologic impact of illness and injury on long-term HRQL.[13,14,27,51,73-82] Preliminary studies in adults have shown that reduction in PTSD symptoms may be associated with improvements in HRQL.[83] Consideration should be given to providing psychologic support for children, adolescents, and parents after PICU admission. Reliable diagnosis and efficacious treatments for PTSD are available and could potentially lead to beneficial interventions for children and adolescents at risk.[84,85]

Exposure to Invasive Technology

Children hospitalized in PICUs are subjected to highly invasive interventions often necessary to overcome the critical period of their illness, yet little is known about their subsequent psychologic adjustment.[86] Rennick and colleagues followed 120 children for 6 months after PICU and ward discharge.[74] Children who were younger, most severely ill, and who endured more invasive procedures had significantly more medical fears, a lower sense of control of their health, and ongoing posttraumatic stress responses for 6 months postdischarge. These findings indicate that invasiveness coupled with length of stay and severity of illness in young children may have adverse long-term effects. Newburger and associates showed that increased length of stay in infants during hospitalization for arterial switch was independently associated with decreased intelligence quotient (IQ) at 8 years of age (1.4 IQ points lower for each additional day in the ICU between 3 and 13 days).[87]

Metrics for Patient-Centered Outcomes: Functional Status and Health-Related Quality of Life

With improved survival, new disease patterns have emerged related to long-term complications of critical illness and its treatment. As noted earlier, historically, the management of pediatric critical illness focused on survival as the primary goal, and it is still the most commonly used determinant in outcome studies after intensive care.[1,27] Once survival rates improved, the physical, mental, and HRQL sequelae of critical illness began to appear.[1,2,26-28,48] HRQL and functional status (FS) represent clinically meaningful outcome measures for children surviving critical illness. Validated pediatric HRQL and functional status measures are now available and should be used in research that examines how pediatric critical care practitioners can maximize recovery among children surviving critical illness.[88]

Ideal Health-Related Quality of Life Outcome Measure

HRQL instruments should provide reliable and valid measures that can quickly and easily be used to quantify morbidity or disability after a child's critical illness or injury. These tools need to be multidimensional and include, at a minimum, the physical, mental, and social health domains outlined by the World Health Organization.[1,89] Ideal HRQL questionnaires should measure all the health dimensions relevant to the studied patient population and preferably be completed by the children themselves (≥6–8 years of age).

When selecting an HRQL instrument, it is important to consider the following six factors[32,48,90]:

- *Psychometric properties.* Reliability consists of internal consistency and reproducibility. Validity assesses the extent to which an instrument measures the construct it is intended to measure.
- *Responsiveness or sensitivity to change.* Does the instrument detect change after an intervention over time? Responsiveness is examined in longitudinal studies that compare the outcomes of a group expected to change to another group that is not.
- *Interpretability of HRQL scores.* It is important to be able to translate a quantitative score or change in scores to a qualitative category or to an external measure that has a familiar meaning. An instrument's interpretability is enhanced when there are normative data from a representative sample of the general population or data from patients with specific clinical conditions.
- *Response burden.* The time, effort, and other demands that are placed on the respondent who is completing the instrument will affect the outcome. Completing the instrument should not create undue physical or emotional strain on the respondent.
- *Mode of administration.* Self-report is considered the gold standard in HRQL measurement, and children are assumed to have unique awareness of their own health. Most of the HRQL instruments have both child and proxy versions; however, the age at which self-report is available varies among the instruments. Proxy investigation is second best because proxy reports do not always correspond with self-evaluations, particularly with regard to internal factors, such as emotions.
- *Instrument adaptation.* Practitioners should consider if the instrument has been adapted or translated for use with children who differ from the original population for which it was developed in terms of culture or language.

Performance and Shortcomings of Health-Related Quality of Life Tools

Table 10.2 (eSupplement) contains a list of 22 HRQL measures that have been used in the pediatric critical care studies.[88] This table summarizes the most important psychometric properties of these tools. The majority of the referenced studies used HRQL assessment tools that are far from ideal. Although most of these studies reported construct validity, only a few included the most important characteristics, such as proxy report, age range, time/effort burden, and sensitivity to change over time. Some of the best instruments for assessing HRQL that are currently available are the PedsQL 4.0 generic core scales, KIDSCREEN-27, the 28-item short child health questionnaire parent form (CHQ-PF28), and KINDL. These tools are offered as both self and proxy reports, cover a wide age range of children, are brief with a low response burden, are multidimensional, and have been shown to have internal consistency and test-retest reliability, as well as sensitivity to change over time, and content and construct validity.

Novel Approaches to Improving Long-Term Outcomes for PICU Survivors

Pediatric intensivists must lead the effort to better understand and optimize long-term outcomes through clinical practice, research, and advocacy. All pediatric critical care practitioners should actively acknowledge and address the long-term physical, cognitive, and mental health impact of critical care on their patients. To better understand and optimize long-term outcomes, critical care practitioners must engage in clinical research in these areas. Such research should include information about the ICU course, as well as surrounding events, such as preexisting comorbidities, reason for admission, and illness severity. There is an urgent need for follow-up programs to study the intensity and duration of the morbidity burden following critical illness, as well as to develop novel interventions aimed at maximizing long-term outcomes.

Outcomes Assessment Program

In January 2010, Seattle Children's Hospital (SCH) developed and launched one of the first outcomes assessment programs (OAPs) in the United States. The OAP is designed to measure patient- and family-centered outcomes of care on all children admitted to SCH. The program accomplished this goal by assessing two key patient-centered outcomes: HRQL and family experiences with care. Families and patients are asked to score HRQL and functional status[91] at the time of admission and then again 4 to 12 weeks after discharge. The National Research Corporation (NRC) Picker Family Experience Survey (FES) is administered at the time of discharge to assess family experience with care.[92] The main objective of conducting these measurements is to allow the hospital to better understand and improve on the HRQL and care experiences of the populations it serves. The OAP was developed with multistakeholder input and has a steering committee that includes quality of care researchers, physicians, nurses, and an ethicist, as well as families and interpreters. Although no direct benefit of the program has yet been established, Dasai and colleagues demonstrated that HRQL measurement was associated with a more traditional, objective outcomes commonly used to measure the effectiveness of quality improvement interventions.[93]

Follow-Up Programs for ICU Survivors

Aside from recommendations from the Pediatric Acute Lung Injury Consensus Conference for the care of children after pediatric ARDS,[94] there is currently no other specific guidance in place for follow-up of survivors of pediatric critical illness. Long-term outcomes assessment should be incorporated in follow-up programs of PICU survivors, and it should form part of the gold standard of critical care delivery. Pediatric intensivists and psychologists should be involved as core members of follow-up teams. In 2011, the Indiana University School of Medicine opened one of the first collaborative care clinics aimed at meeting the recovery needs of adult ICU survivors in the United States.[95] The mission of the clinic is to maximize the cognitive, physical, and psychologic recovery of ICU survivors via patient and caregiver needs assessment and a follow-up visit that includes a family conference. Preliminary data from 53 patients showed that only 12% had normal cognition. The three most common diagnoses at follow-up were ICU-acquired cognitive impairment,

TABLE 10.2 Performance and Shortcomings of Health Related Quality of Life (HRQL) Assessment Tools (eSupplement)

HRQOL Instrument	Name/Country of Origin	Age Range	No. Items	No. Domains	Time in Minutes	Report	Reliability	Validity	Sensitivity to Change	Physical	Emotional	Social Behavioral	Role (School)	References of Studies
CHIP-AE	Child Health & Illness Profile—Adolescent Edition (United States)	11-17	183	6	45	Self	ICC Test-retest	Content construct criterion		x	x	x	x	7,9,18,45
CHIP-CE	Child Health & Illness Profile—Child Edition (United States)	6-11	76 (proxy) 45 (self)	5	20	Proxy or self	ICC Test-retest	Content construct criterion		x	x	x	x	7,9,18,45
CHQ-CF87	Child Health Questionnaire—Child Form (United States)	10-18	87	13	20	Proxy or self (10+)	ICC Test-retest	Content construct criterion	x	x	x	x	x	7,9,28,29,69
CHQ-PF50	Child Health Questionnaire—Parent Form (United States)	5-18	50	13	20	Proxy or self (5+)	ICC Test-retest	Content construct criterion	x	x	x	x	x	7,9,28,29
CHQ-PF28	Child Health Questionnaire—Parent Form (United States)	5-18	28	13	5-10	Proxy or self (5+)	ICC Test-retest	Content construct criterion	x	x	x	x	x	7,9,28,29
COOP	Dartmouth COOP Charts (United States)	8-18	6	6		Self	Test-retest	Construct		x	x	x	x	7,9
DISABKIDS		4-16	37	6	10	Proxy or self	ICC Test-retest	Content construct		x	x	x		7,9
EQ-5D	EuroQOL (Europe)	5-18	5	6		Proxy or self	Test-retest	Construct		x	x	x	x	7,9
FIM/ WEEFIM	Functional Independence Measure	0-18	18			Proxy	Test-retest	Content construct		x		x		7,9
FS IIR	Functional Status II Revised (United States)	0-16	14	8	10	Proxy	ICC Test-retest	Content construct		x	x	x		7,9
HUI 3	Health Utilities Index Mark 3 (Canada)	2-18	45	8	<5	Proxy or self	Test-retest	Construct		x	x			4,7,9,23,27, 30,36,51

Abbrev.	Instrument	Age range	No. items	No. domains	Time (min)	Respondent	Reliability	Validity						References
ITQOL	Infant & Toddler QOL Questionnaire	2mo-5	103	10		Proxy	ICC Test-retest	Content construct criterion	x	x	x		x	7,9,28
KIDSCR-52	Kidscreen (International)	8-18	52	10	15-20	Proxy or self	ICC	Content construct	x	x	x	x	x	7,9
KIDSCR-27	Kidscreen (International)	8-18	27	5	10-15	Proxy or self	ICC Test-retest	Content construct	x	x	x	x	x	7,9
KINDL	(Germany)	8-16 4-7	24 12	6 4	5-10	Proxy or self	ICC	Content construct	x	x	x	x	x	7,9
PEDI	Pediatric Evaluation & Disability Inventory	0-8	237			Proxy	ICC Test-retest	Content construct criterion		x	x		x	7,9
PedsQL 4.0	Pediatric Quality of Life Inventory (United States)	2-18	23	4	5-10	Proxy or self (5+)	ICC Test-retest	Content construct predictive	x	x	x	x	x	1,7,9,21,22,30, 34,41,72,76,77
QWD	Quality of Well-Being Scale	4-18	29			Proxy or self (11+)	Test-retest	Construct		x	x		x	7,9,39
TACQOL	TNO-AZL Child QOL TNO-AZL Parent QOL (Netherland)	6-15	108	7	10	Proxy or self (8+)	ICC	Content construct		x	x	x	x	7,9,67,68
TA PQOL	(Netherland)	1-5	43	4	10	Proxy				x	x	x	x	7,9,10
YQOL-R	Youth Quality of Life Instrument—Research Version (United States)	11-18	56	4	10-15	Self	ICC Test-retest			x	x	x	x	7,9
VSP-A	Vecu et Sante Percue de l'Adolescent (France)	11-17	37	9		Self	ICC Test-retest	Content construct		x	x	x	x	7,9

ICC, internal consistency.

depression, and dyspnea. The average time between visits was 2.5 months. Significant core improvements were seen in functional and cognitive domains but not in the behavioral-psychologic domain.

Innovative Trichotomous Outcome Model

Assessment of longer-term mortality, morbidity, and patient-centered outcomes is increasingly necessary.[96] Pollack and coworkers developed a new tool that combines the Functional Status Scale (FSS) and components of the Pediatric Risk of Mortality (PRISM) III score to determine if death and important nonmortal short-term outcomes can be predicted simultaneously, based on physiologic and other data available shortly after PICU admission.[96] This trichotomous outcome model is unique in that it has the potential to provide a benchmark for in-hospital morbidity as well as mortality. It might be expanded in the future to include long-term outcome. It predicts three possible outcomes: death, intact survival, and survival with new functional disability. Although the FSS was not designed for use in individual patients, further studies of the wider patient and family impact of a change in FSS score, including the relationships of FSS to HRQL, future health care use, and postdischarge function and recovery, will be essential to understand the full implications of new morbidity identified with the FSS.[97]

Research Aims[98]

The traditional 28-day mortality outcome used in clinical trials of sepsis, ARDS, trauma, and many other critical illnesses does not account for important long-term sequelae of critical illness. Some studies have examined children's outcomes during the first year following PICU discharge, but relatively little is known about their long-term outcomes. Future trials should include long-term outcome measurements, as well as mortality and HRQL/functional status, to truly understand the full impact of critical illness in children. There is a need for well-designed, prospective, longitudinal studies with serial assessments that will satisfy the following objectives:

- Identify PICU survivors most at risk.
- Characterize long-term outcomes.
- Generate recovery curves for various illnesses.
- Identify factors associated with long-term morbidity and recovery.
- Define potential targets for intervention.

Potential Targets for Interventions

Many adverse sequelae of critical illness and critical care are amenable to intervention. Acute loss of skeletal muscle mass, which is greatest in patients with multiorgan failure, contributes to the ongoing physical disability common among survivors of critical illness.[99,100] Early and more aggressive physical therapy and passive range of motion introduced in the ICU may reduce ICU neuropathy and other musculoskeletal complications, but the ability to stratify risks and tailor programs to individual needs requires further study. As sleep is known to be severely disturbed in the hospital, interventions that improve the quality of sleep may reduce cognitive and psychiatric sequelae.[101,102] Delusional memories are reported by almost a third of children surviving critical illness. These can be exacerbated by exposure to opiates and benzodiazepines, and they are associated with an increased risk of PTSD.[13] The

pharmacologic milieu encountered during critical illness is a blend of potent neurologically active drugs that may facilitate transition to delirium. Interventions such as memory books and journals kept by family members may facilitate reintegration into life after critical illness.[103-106]

Psychologic impairments such as depression are prominent and important features of PICS.[107] Critical illness and its outcomes affect not only critically ill children but also their families. There is an increased risk of mental health disorders, such as anxiety, depression, and posttraumatic stress disorder, in the families and caregivers of PICU survivors.[108-112] Psychologic support may improve outcomes in children and parents alike. There is a need to understand the risk factors of increased care provider burden and worsened family dynamics that PICU survivor families face. Further research is essential to establish the optimal timing, extent, and type of psychologic support for these children and families.

Conclusions

Critical care practitioners are classically trained in resuscitation science that is detailed throughout this textbook. Historically this has been associated with a marked decrease in mortality associated with childhood critical injury and illness (see Fig. 10.1). There has been greater recognition that critical care begins and ends outside the walls of the intensive care unit. Intensivists and their care-provider colleagues are increasingly aware of the impact of genetics, family dynamics, home environment, and preexisting comorbidities on the intensity, duration, and outcome of critical illness. Although the critical care team may be acutely interested in duration of shock, length of mechanical ventilator and dialysis support, new or progressive organ dysfunction, and PICU and hospital resource utilization, these are surrogate outcomes that may or may not be associated with durable, clinically meaningful, patient-centered outcomes.[113] With maturation of the field of pediatric critical care medicine, critical care practitioners now have the opportunity as well as the obligation to look beyond PICU discharge with a goal of minimizing not only mortality but also the burden of long-term morbidity in accordance with patients' and families' expectations. Ultimately, maximizing long-term functional status and health-related quality of life should be the most important goals of critical care medicine.

Key References

1. Conlon NP, Breatnach C, O'Hare BP, et al. Health-related quality of life after prolonged pediatric intensive care unit stay. *Pediatr Crit Care Med.* 2009;10:41-44.
2. Typpo KV, Petersen NJ, Hallman M, et al. Day 1 multiple organ dysfunction syndrome is associated with poor functional outcome and mortality in the pediatric intensive care unit. *Pediatr Crit Care Med.* 2009;10:562-570.
6. Czaja AS, Zimmerman JJ, Nathens AB. Readmission and late mortality after pediatric severe sepsis. *Pediatrics.* 2009;123:849-857.
7. Pollack MM, Holubkov R, Funai T, et al. Pediatric intensive care outcomes: development of new morbidities during pediatric critical care. *Pediatr Crit Care Med.* 2014;15:821-827.
8. Rennick JE, Childerhose JE. Redefining success in the PICU: new patient populations shift targets of care. *Pediatrics.* 2015;1354(2):e289-e291.
11. Knoester H, Grootenhuis MA, Bos AP. Outcome of pediatric intensive care survivors. *Eur J Pediatr.* 2007;166:1119-1128.
13. Colville G, Kerry S, Pierce C. Children's factual and delusional memories of intensive care. *Am J Respir Crit Care Med.* 2008;117:976-982.

26. Wilson IB, Cleary PD. Linking clinical variables with health-related quality of life. *JAMA*. 1995;273:59-65.

29. Knoester H, Bronner MB, Bos AP, Grootenhuis MA. Quality of life in children three and nine months after discharge from a paediatric intensive care unit: a prospective cohort study. *Health Qual Life Outcomes*. 2008;6:1-9.

37. Buysse CM, Raat H, Hazelzet JA, et al. Surviving meningococcal septic shock: health consequences and quality of life in children and their parents up to 2 years after pediatric intensive care unit discharge. *Crit Care Med*. 2008;36:596-602.

40. Als LC, Nadel S, Cooper M, et al. Neuropsychologic function three to six months following admission to the PICU with meningoencephalitis, sepsis, and other disorders: a prospective study of school-aged children. *Crit Care Med*. 2013;41:1094-1103.

51. Holbrook TL, Hoyt DB, Coimbra R, et al. Trauma in adolescents causes long-term market deficits in quality of life: adolescent children do not recover preinjury quality of life or function up to two years postinjury compared to national norms. *J Trauma*. 2007;62:577-583.

74. Rennick JE, Johnson CC, Dougherty G, et al. Children's psychological responses after critical illness and exposure to invasive technology. *J Dev Behav Pediatr*. 2002;23:133-144.

77. Holbrook TL, Hoyt DB, Coimbra R, et al. Long-term posttraumatic stress disorder persists after major trauma in adolescents: new data on risk factors and functional outcome. *J Trauma*. 2005;58:764-769.

81. Colville G, Pierce C. Patterns of post-traumatic stress symptoms in families after paediatric intensive care. *Intensive Care Med*. 2012;38:1523-1531.

87. Newburger JW, Wypij D, Bellinger DC, et al. Length of stay after infant heart surgery is related to cognitive outcome at age 8 years. *J Pediatr*. 2003;143:611-616.

88. Aspesberro F, Mangione-Smith R, Zimmerman JJ. Health-related quality of life following pediatric critical illness. *Intensive Care Med*. 2015;41:1235-1246.

94. Quasney MW, Lopez-Fernandez YM, Santschi M, Watson RS, for the Pediatric Acute Lung Injury Consensus Conference Group. The outcomes of children with pediatric acute respiratory distress syndrome: proceedings from the Pediatric Acute Lung Injury Consensus Conference. *Pediatr Crit Care Med*. 2015;16(5 suppl 1):S23-S40.

96. Pollack MM, Holubkov R, Funai T, et al. Simultaneous prediction of new morbidity, mortality, and survival without new morbidity from pediatric intensive care: a new paradigm for outcomes assessment. *Crit Care Med*. 2015;43:1699-1709.

Safety and Quality Assessment in the Pediatric Intensive Care Unit

Matthew C. Scanlon and Martin Wakeham

PEARLS

- The six domains of quality in the pediatric intensive care unit are safety, effectiveness, patient centeredness, timeliness, efficiency, and equity.
- Research demonstrates that errors in health care are often caused by poorly designed systems of care.
- Three essential activities of a patient safety program include risk identification, risk analysis, and risk reduction.
- Safety science distinguishes between the reactive, people-focused Safety I (akin to quality assurance work) and the proactive, systems-focused Safety II.

Recognition of the importance of quality improvement and patient safety for pediatric intensive care units (PICUs) has been steadily increasing, and there have been some provocative and important additions to the world of safety and quality that have particular relevance for PICUs. Of note, increasingly it appears that the worlds of patient safety, quality improvement (QI), and safety science are divergent. This statement may seem counterintuitive, if not even heretical. This chapter articulates the rationale for this statement and explores the implications for pediatric critical care.

Brief Consideration of the Relationship Between Safety and Quality

Both the Institute of Medicine (in its report *Crossing the Quality Chasm*) and conventional wisdom suggest that quality and patient safety are related, with the latter being one of the six domains of the former (Table 11.1). Based on this report, safety is a prerequisite to achieving quality. That is, it is impossible to achieve true quality without improving safety. Those who argue that attention to other aspects of quality beyond safety is critical still confirm this observation.[1] For the pediatric critical care provider, the important point is that safety is a necessary prerequisite for quality, but improving safety is insufficient to achieve quality.

Although the fundamental relationship between quality and safety remains unchanged, there appear to be important differences between the methods necessary for QI and those necessary for achieving safety, depending on the context of care. Because the PICU is one of the settings where this distinction may have tremendous impact, it is imperative that intensivists understand the differences. These will be discussed in the section titled "Fundamentals of Patient Safety With an Introduction to Safety I and Safety II."

State of Safety and Quality in Pediatric Intensive Care Units

Since 1999 when the Institute of Medicine's report *To Err Is Human* drew recognition to the scope of preventable medical harm,[2] there have been dramatic changes in how quality and safety are managed in PICUs. These include the continued existence of PICU-specific quality measures endorsed by the National Quality Forum (Table 11.2), a dramatic reduction in central venous catheter–associated bloodstream infections (CA-BSIs), and engagement of intensivists in the work of the Solutions for Patient Safety (SPS) collaborative[3,4] Although data on the SPS collaborative do not provide PICU-specific results, the self-reported data indicate that, since 2012, the collaborative has saved more than 4700 children from serious harm while saving greater than $92 million. PICU-related areas of improvement include ventilator-associated pneumonia (VAP), CA-BSI, catheter-associated urinary tract infections (CAUTIs), and venous thromboembolism. These results reflect the creation of standardized bundles of care, which then were implemented at participating children's hospitals.

Although the SPS work has focused on what can be described as the creation of topic-specific improvement bundles, implementation of the bundles, and then quality assurance work, it largely does not reflect either a systems-focused approach or what will be described as Safety II.

Fundamentals of Quality Improvement and Patient Safety: Systems Thinking

To understand patient safety and quality in health care, one first must recognize the importance of systems to the way care is delivered. The Institute of Medicine, drawing from James Reason's studies of errors, defines a system as "a set of interdependent elements interacting to achieve a common aim."[2] One model of systems in health care consists of five interaction components: (1) people (2) use tools and technologies (3) to perform tasks (4) within an environment (5) in the context of an organization.[5] Each of these five components interacts with the others to yield the emergent properties (greater than the sum of the parts) of safety and quality.

TABLE 11.1 The Institute of Medicine's Six Domains of Quality

Domain	Definition	PICU Example
Safety	Freedom from preventable harm during care[2]	Prevention of central line–associated infections
Effectiveness	Providing services based on the best available scientific knowledge in order to achieve the best outcome	Following American College of Critical Care Medicine guidelines for hemodynamic support of pediatric and neonatal patients in septic shock[72]
Patient/family centered	Provision of care in a manner that is respectful of and responsive to individual patient preferences, needs, and values	The presence and involvement of parents on rounds[73]
Timeliness	The reduction of waiting and potentially harmful delays for both those who give and receive care	Timely administration of antibiotics and fluids in septic shock
Efficiency	Achieve adequate outcomes while keeping resource utilization appropriate, thus minimizing cost	Reduction of length of stay without increasing unplanned readmissions
Equity	Quality of care provided in the PICU should be independent of characteristics such as gender, ethnicity, geographic location, and socioeconomic status	Risk-adjusted mortality and resource utilization for critically ill children did not differ according to race, gender, or insurance status; however, uninsured children had significantly greater physiologic derangement at time of PICU admission[74]

TABLE 11.2 Endorsed Pediatric Intensive Care Unit Measures

Measure	Description
PICU standardized mortality ratio	The ratio of actual deaths over predicted deaths for PICU patients, adjusted using an accepted risk of mortality tool
PICU severity-adjusted length of stay	The number of days between PICU admission and discharge for patients, adjusted using an accepted risk of mortality tool
PICU rate of unplanned readmissions within 24 hours of PICU discharge	The total number of patients requiring unscheduled readmission to the PICU within 24 hours of discharge or transfer, over the number of discharges and transfers

Several essential implications follow from this model. First, no matter how safe any component is (eg, an intensivist who never makes mistakes), it is the five components and their interactions that determine if care is safe and of high quality. Second, if one changes any of these components, it will have

impact on the other components and their interactions. This is illustrated through the routine practice of cannulation for extracorporeal membrane oxygenation (ECMO) in the PICU. Merely changing the environment from the PICU to the hospital parking lot would have dramatic implications for the people, their tasks, the tools, and the organization's culture and liability. A third implication of this model is that changes to one or more of the five components will inevitably impact their emergent properties of safety and quality. This is illustrated by the growing literature that suggests that safety technologies may actually cause errors and harm.[6-11] Thus for critical care providers, understanding the role of systems in the work done in an intensive care unit (ICU) is crucial to improving quality or reducing harm.

Additional characteristics of systems that are important to intensivists are their complex adaptive nature[12] and the concept of tight coupling.[13] A complex adaptive system is one with several characteristics. First, complex adaptive systems have multiple similar agents that are autonomous entities that observe and act on their environment (such as PICU providers). More important, these multiple agents are adaptive, allowing for a high degree of resilience to system changes. The complex adaptive nature of the PICU is illustrated by sudden, unpredicted events such as codes, an unplanned extubation, or even multiple simultaneous admissions. In each of these scenarios, the future was unpredictable, the response was adaptive, and order is emergent rather than predetermined.

A tightly coupled system has events that must occur sequentially; it does not tolerate variation in supplies or inputs without creating delays and may tolerate failures less well than systems with slack designed into them. An example of tight coupling in the PICU is the common challenge of patient flow. An unplanned admission from the operating room (OR) requires a PICU bed postoperatively. The OR team is under pressure to transfer the patient to the PICU as soon as possible to free up the OR and prevent delays in the surgical schedule. However, the patient who could leave the PICU cannot be transferred because there is no floor bed. There are no floor beds because there is a delay in paperwork and the need for a parent to drive the floor patient home. In this process, failure at any step leads to delay, the steps allow for little variation in process, and the majority of steps must occur sequentially. These features of complex, tightly coupled systems are endemic in health care settings.

Quality Improvement and Value

Quality has been defined as "the degree to which health services for individuals and populations increase the likelihood of desired health outcomes and are consistent with current professional knowledge."[14] This definition, which comes from the Institute of Medicine, draws from the work of Donabedian.[15] In his work, quality was defined in the context of structure, process, and outcomes. In other words, to measure quality, one should consider the structure or capacities of health care, the process or interactions between patients and care providers, and the outcomes or evidence of changes in a patient's health condition. Ideally, considerations of quality should incorporate all three components.

The Institute of Medicine has identified six essential domains for achieving health care quality.[16] These areas include safety, effectiveness, patient-centeredness, timeliness, efficiency, and equity. Based on these and Donabedian's components of quality, efforts to improve quality should consider improvement of process, structure, or outcome focused on one of the six areas identified by the Institute of Medicine. The six domains, their definitions, and PICU-relevant examples are displayed in Table 11.1.

A discussion of the definition of quality should include potential shifts in thinking. Of note, there is literature suggesting that beyond quality, the issue of value is important to health care. In this context, value is defined as a measure of quality per unit cost.[17] This can be illustrated by considering what automobile the reader drives. Whether an entry-level compact car or a loaded luxury vehicle, for each consumer there is some determination of both the quality of the vehicle and whether that quality is worth the cost. Although robust measures of quality and true costs remain elusive in health care, critical care providers could improve value to patients by improving quality, reducing cost, or both.

Quality Improvement Methods

QI seeks to improve the quality of care. To improve care, one must first define the process of care that needs improvement. Ideally, a goal is set to define what is desired in terms of the outputs of the process. Then data are obtained to understand the process, and finally interventions are made with follow-up measurement to assess the change, positive or negative.[18]

Several important components are included in the previous paragraph. First, one must define and understand a specific process or system. This is critical to making improvement feasible. For example, a hospital may identify that its length of stay (LOS) for patients with diabetic ketoacidosis is prolonged compared with peer organizations. However, efforts to improve all the elements involved in the hospital course simultaneously likely will fail because of the magnitude of the efforts. Instead, by identifying the components included in the hospitalization and contributing to the LOS, it may be possible to focus on manageable segments of the care process and make incremental changes (Table 11.2).

A second important concept is understanding variation in the data and the value of data over time (see the section titled "Variation and Display of Data Over Time"). As data are understood, goals can be set and interventions made. Continuing data acquisition allows assessment of the impact of the interventions. The establishment of goals provides a target for interventions and a context for measuring data. To paraphrase a QI cliché, changing a process through an intervention is not the same as improving a process. Instead, measurement of data and comparison to set goals allow for assessment of improvement.

Ideally, these changes and reevaluations are done in an iterative manner. This method has been labeled as the "plan, do, study, act (PDSA) cycle."[18] The Institute for Healthcare Improvement (www.IHI.org) has advocated use of a PDSA method over a short period to create what it calls "rapid cycle improvement." With either model, changes often are introduced quickly and sometimes multiple changes are introduced simultaneously. This method has evoked pushback from some physicians because of an apparent lack of scientific and statistical rigor. From a QI standpoint, many improvements are achieved without the need to meet a given P value. Ironically, the resistance to QI methodology because of lack of statistical rigor is inconsistent with much clinical practice in the PICU. There does not exist a standard of care that every intervention

performed in resuscitating a patient be accompanied by evaluation for statistical significance. In fact, resuscitations may involve multiple interventions (endotracheal intubation, chest compressions, administration of medications) in a rapidly sequential or simultaneous manner. With a successful resuscitation, an intensivist may be unable to identify which of numerous interventions was responsible for the improvement. Arguably, if improvement occurred, neither the patient nor the family necessarily cares which intervention resulted in the positive change. Such is the QI mindset. If a given intervention can be identified and causation established for a specific improvement, this information may be applied to different settings. However, the goal is improvement, and improvement without clear identification of the causative factor remains an improvement.

Variation and Display of Data Over Time

If an intensivist watches a physiologic monitor for any length of time, it is normal to view variability in heart rate and other vital signs. This reflects the dynamic nature of physiologic systems and processes. Similarly, health care processes vary within certain ranges under normal circumstances. Reacting to changes within normal variation may lead to interventions that increase variation rather than reduce it.[19] However, the range within which the variation is occurring may be outside the desired goal. Thus improvement may address the amount of variation associated with an existing system or fundamental redesign of the system.

Again, understanding the normal variation in a process is critical. The PICU provides physiologic illustrations of this concept. A patient who is doing reasonably well in the PICU has a normal range of heart rate variability, and loss of heart rate variability has been associated with increased risk of death in certain populations.[20] Similarly, a relatively well patient in the PICU who acutely develops either tachycardia or bradycardia merits evaluation for new or worsened pathology. In this case, the heart rate variation that normally occurs does so within certain parameters. This variation is called *common cause variation* in the QI literature. When the variation crosses either the upper parameter (tachycardia) or lower parameter (bradycardia), then something is amiss. The same holds true for processes and systems within health care. Variation that crosses certain thresholds or is an abnormal outlier is called *special cause variation.*

Plotting data over time allows for an understanding of this variation, normal or abnormal, in data. When data points (eg, length of stay) are placed on a chart with time (eg, in days) plotted on the ordinate, this is called a *run chart. Control charts,* or statistical process control charts, also plot data over time. However, control limits are added that help define the limits of normal variation. Control limits, first described by Walter Shewart in the 1920s, are calculated in a variety of statistical manners, in part depending on the type of control chart. The type and distribution of data determine the choice of control[21]; methods for choosing a control chart are beyond the scope of this chapter. At the most basic limit, control levels are set at three times the standard deviation of the data, around the line of central tendency.

In general, when data exist within the control limits, a process is said to be in control. Data that either extend beyond the control limits or demonstrate one of several patterns suggest either an unstable process or a process that is responding to a change. This change may be an intentional effort to alter a process or may represent the effect of an unknown cause. Returning to the heart rate analogy, a patient who becomes bradycardic from hypoxia would demonstrate deviation of the normal heart rate variation in response to the special cause (hypoxia). Correction of the hypoxia ideally returns the heart rate (process) to its normal range of variation. An example of a control chart is displayed in Fig. 11.1, which illustrates the rates of codes outside the ICU relative to the introduction of rapid response teams.

Other Quality Improvement Tools

Interested readers are directed to one of the numerous QI primers available for a thorough discussion of tools used in QI. However, several of these tools bear at least some mention. A Pareto chart is simply a histogram used to identify the major contributors to a problem or variation. For example, if PICU length of stay (LOS) is of concern, it may be beneficial to identify which, if any, diagnosis categories contribute to the prolonged LOS. By plotting LOS in days on the abscissa against diagnosis on the ordinate, those diagnoses that contribute to the greatest portion of the length of hospitalization might be identified.

Root cause analysis (RCA) is another tool used to attempt to identify the root cause for an event or problem. In its simplest form, RCA is performed by asking the question "why?" five times. Often used in conjunction with a cause-and-effect or Ishikawa diagram, the process of root cause investigation seeks to identify what caused a failure in a process (safety related or quality related) by defining the contributing factors. From each of the five categorical branches, smaller branches are added that answer the question "why?" and in turn the same question of "why?" is asked again. The resultant diagram often is described as a fishbone, explaining the third name for this diagram: a fishbone diagram.

By asking "why?" repeatedly, the belief is that the root cause of a problem can be identified. This leads to three limitations of RCA. First, there is the great danger of introducing hindsight bias. The investigators' beliefs of what happened may lead them to identify only those things on the cause-and-effect diagram. A second, related limitation is that RCAs may restrict problem solving and brainstorming to only those factors that are known. Because one only knows what one knows and, similarly, one doesn't know what one doesn't know, there is the potential for missing important factors. Finally, the most important limitation of RCA as a tool is the suggestion that there is a single root cause. This is a dangerous belief. Usually there are multiple causes of events. To limit thinking to one or two causes oversimplifies the situation and may preclude meaningful improvement. The use of RCA should be tempered with the knowledge of these limitations and the potential for drawing incorrect conclusions. For an excellent and sobering discussion of the limitations of RCA, readers are encouraged to read works by Nemeth, Wu, and Nicolini.[22-24]

Fundamentals of Patient Safety With an Introduction to Safety I and Safety II

Traditionally, patient safety is defined as freedom from preventable injury, an adaptation of the definition used by the Institute of Medicine.[2] This definition is in keeping with what is now known as Safety I, with an associated goal of minimizing the number of times when things go wrong. Safety I views the causes of things going wrong as human, organizational, and technical failures. Further, it presumes systems of care to be well understood, highly predictable and reliable—with the exception of the human element.[25,26] An alternative viewpoint is that safety is when things go right under a variety of circumstances. This Safety II approach understands that not only are people part of systems but safety primarily occurs from people adapting to suboptimal systems in the face of changing situations (Table 11.3).

TABLE 11.3 Contrasting Safety I and Safety II

Characteristics	Safety I	Safety II
Defined by:	Its opposite: failure	Its goal: success
Systems are:	Well designed, well understood	Poorly understood, dynamic
Procedures are:	Correct and complete	Incomplete, underspecified, and based on imagined concept of how work is done, not on how work is actually done
People:	Are flawed, prone to violations, and thus a liability Should behave as expected and trained	Adjust behavior and interpret procedures based on the context
Accidents come from:	Failures in human compliance, malfunctions, and variation in human behavior	Incomplete adaptation to situations
Safety management approach	Reactive, responding to events	Proactive, seeking to anticipate and prevent events

Adapted from Hollnagel E, Leonhardt J, Licu T, et al. From Safety I to Safety II: a white paper, 2013. Available at www.eurocontrol.int; Hollnagel E. A tale of two safeties. Nuclear Safety and Simulation, 2013;4:1-9; and Robert Wears (personal communication).

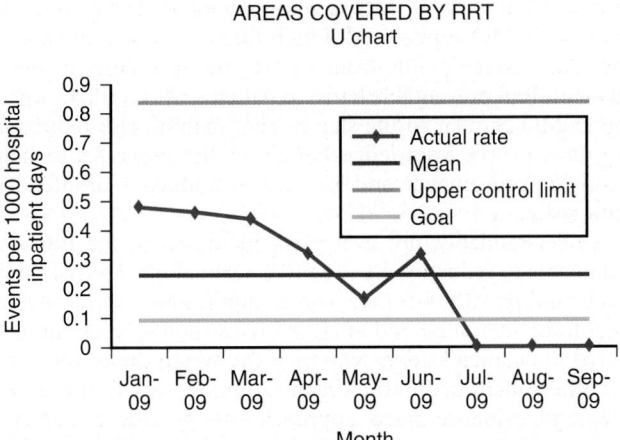

Fig. 11.1. Control chart demonstrating codes outside the pediatric intensive care unit in areas covered by a rapid response team (RRT).

Safety I can be compared to quality assurance (QA) in health care. QA was the predecessor to QI and largely focused on assuring compliance with policies and reactively finding fault when something went wrong.[27] However, although flawed, not all aspects of Safety I are bad. For instance, variation from following the central venous catheter insertion bundle is an example of a nonvalue added variation that largely poses risk without benefit.

Errors, Injuries, Systems, Hazards, and Risks

A central goal of all health care is to provide care without causing harm. Unfortunately, the identified harm in health care is often incorrectly attributed to a problem with errors, instead of understanding that both errors and harm are the result of poorly designed systems of care that either promote errors or allow harm to occur in the face of errors. This is manifested through such statements as "We wouldn't have this safety problem if we could stop people from making so many errors." This, in turn, suggests that to achieve safety, we simply need to urge people to follow policies and be careful. However, people make errors; as long as there are people in PICUs, there will be errors. To that end, there are numerous safety improvement efforts that focus on people that can be seen by the following solutions: warning labels, signs and posters exhorting staff to "be careful" and to "do this" or "do not do that," repeated educational campaigns, and reliance on policies and procedures. None of these activities is bad per se, and in fact they can be part of an effective safety effort. However, they are not sufficient to provide safety. In each of those "solutions," the goal is to error-proof the people, despite the inherent property of people to err. No amount of rules, education, or warnings will prevent errors from occurring.

In contrast, the science of human factors engineering (HFE) supports the belief that efforts to improve patient safety that depend on requiring people to be infallible are misguided, wasteful, and potentially harmful. The previous section on systems thinking clearly identified patient safety and quality as emergent properties of systems. Not surprisingly, there is research that demonstrates that errors often are caused by poorly designed systems, or design-induced errors.[28] Therefore if an error occurs, one should not ask "why did the person make the mistake" but rather "what caused the mistake to occur?"

A clinical example that is relevant to PICU care is the restriction of the availability of high-risk medications. Sources of medication errors include the storage of look-alike vials or medications of the same name but differing concentrations in the same area for use in the PICU. In this case, the look-alike medications represent hazards, which may or may not lead to errors and injuries. An incorrect look-alike medication can be given in error, potentially resulting in harm. A safety program focused on people would solve this problem through educating staff to pay more attention to look-alike vials and to make the labels on the medications appear more distinct. In contrast, an HFE or system-based approach would involve elimination of the hazard by removing the high-risk medications to another area, making it impossible to confuse medications or concentrations. In others words, by redesigning the systems for medication storage and access, the opportunity for error (and harm) decreases or even vanishes. Central to this solution is the characteristic of using system redesign to reduce the risk of errors and harm. Consistent with epidemiologic and public health models that attempt to identify, understand, and reduce risk factors for disease or injury, the risk-reduction approach described here is a standard HFE and safety science approach.[29-31]

Improvement in the Pediatric Intensive Care Unit

The thought of improving safety in the PICU is daunting. The number and complexity of care processes seem overwhelming, and it is reasonable to wonder how to even begin. Building on the concepts of systems and risk reduction, a simple approach to improving patient safety in the PICU involves three steps: risk identification, risk analysis, and risk reduction.[32]

The process of risk identification is relatively straightforward. Drawing on reported events, chart reviews, concerns identified by staff, patients, and families, as well as issues identified in other units in a hospital, one can compile a list of potential risks that may be relevant to the patients cared for in the PICU. Of note, both errors and injuries inform the identification of risks. However, rather than focusing exclusively on trying to reconstruct prior events, the idea is to use past events to guide proactive improvement efforts to prevent future risks.

As the list of identified potential risks is generated, the next step is to systematically analyze the risks. This analysis involves three major steps. First, ask: "Is our PICU at risk for this happening?" If the identified risk was related to a published report of ECMO pump failure and ECMO is not performed in your PICU, then you can safely conclude that this risk does not apply. In contrast, if your PICU does perform ECMO, then the second step involves gathering more information to inform the risk assessment. This step might involve understanding what brand or type of pump was failing and whether this pump is in your center. Finally, after all available data are gathered (or perhaps new data are collected), the final step in risk analysis is to provide clinical interpretation by clinical experts familiar with the process. In the case of the ECMO pump scenario, a group of surgeons, intensivists, nurses, and perfusionists would weigh available data to determine the extent of risk for their PICU population.

The last step of improving safety would be performing risk reduction, which would involve pulling together a team to brainstorm improvements and the potential unintended consequences of each potential improvement. The latter portion of this step is critical. A simple but potentially hazardous solution to the ECMO scenario would be electing to cease all new ECMO support. Although this solution would surely prevent adverse events from ECMO pump failure, it might also result in preventable harm to patients who could be saved by ECMO. Similar to the step of risk analysis, risk reduction requires people knowledgeable about the processes to help guide improvements and prevent introducing unintended new risks.

Understandably, not every risk identified in the PICU is amenable to reduction by the PICU team alone. For risks that cross multiple units or may require significant resource investment, the identified and analyzed risks should be communicated to hospital leaders who then can weigh these risks with all others identified in the organization. However, this proactive and evidence-based approach can provide a standard framework for safety improvement. Additionally, this risk-based safety improvement approach lends itself readily to risk-based safety metrics.[75-77]

Culture

As attention shifts from individuals to systems, inevitably the issue of accountability is raised. Commonly expressed concerns center on whether focusing on systems rather than individuals somehow absolves health care providers from responsibility. In part, this concern arises from a well-intended (but misguided) effort to move from a punitive culture in health care to a blame-free environment. The intention was not to create systems lacking individual accountability but to avoid blaming individuals for situations beyond their control or that resulted from human error to which anyone would be vulnerable.

One solution that represents a system focus has been described as a *just culture*.[33] Under this model, systems problems and human error are considered. The model promotes efforts to learn from errors without punishing individuals involved. Systems problems that create situations in which individuals are "set up" to make errors also are treated as learning opportunities. When individuals violate policies, often because of normalization of deviance, the response again is not punitive but instead focused on making it easier to do the right thing. In the PICU, this can be seen when workload constraints make performing required double checks on pump programming unrealistic. Staff members may fail to perform double checks daily without event, and no action is taken to stop the behavior. However, when a neglected double check leads to an error or harm, the traditional mindset is to punish the involved parties, despite a systematic acceptance of this behavior. In a just culture model, rather than punish the individual, efforts are made to again make it easier or more desirable to do the right thing.

Systems thinking and a just culture are consistent with punishment. This may occur in the face of willful or reckless behaviors that place patients at risk. If a physician provides patient care while intoxicated, this is an example of reckless behavior that would be unacceptable in a just culture. When behaviors show a pattern of violations that individually may not represent reckless behavior but collectively demonstrate a high-risk pattern, the just culture model proposes two considerations.[34] First, the person may work in a high-risk situation where such patterns are inevitable. Alternatively, the person involved may have individual characteristics, such as marital stress or deteriorating physical abilities, which would require removing the person from that situation in a nonpunitive manner. It should be noted that, on rare occasions, individuals may be viewed as out of control because of mental health problems, substance abuse, or even patterns of behavior. As mentioned previously, a just culture would require prompt intervention to help or remove these individuals to prevent harm to patients and other providers.

Importantly, the SPS adoption of Healthcare Performance Improvement (HPI)'s framework for serious safety events (SSEs), though presented along with a just culture framework, promotes blaming people. The HPI (and thus SPS) framework for prioritizing safety events focuses on "deviations from generally accepted practice standards."[35] According to HPI, these are either due to human error or to equipment failure. Beyond ignoring all science related to socio-technical systems, the HPI framework also shows a lack of understanding of the ubiquitous nature of deviations and violations by providers to compensate for otherwise unworkable systems of care delivery.[36-38,75-77] As a result, the patient safety efforts have largely shifted to a reactive, people-focused version of "whack a mole," chasing the last safety event while searching for the root cause to blame.

Teams and Teamwork

The need for improved teamwork is a recurring theme in patient safety. This is certainly true in the PICU environment. However, there are important differences in how critical care physicians and nurses perceive what is meant by teamwork and how well their teams perform.[39] One conclusion by the authors is that these differences might be due to training, gender, or role-related culture. Another potential explanation may be a poor understanding of the sciences of teams and team performance.[40-47]

In PICUs, there are a variety of teams. There is the patient's care team comprising the nurses, respiratory therapists, pharmacists, attending physicians, and perhaps trainees such as residents and fellows. There are also the within-discipline clinical teams, such as the nursing or physician team that cares for a given patient over shifts, days, and weeks. A nurse and his or her nursing assistant might also be a team, as might all of the nurses on a given shift in a given ICU. However, despite that fact that we might call each of these *teams*, that does not mean that they identify themselves or perform as teams.

Teams are "two or more individuals with specialized roles and responsibilities who must interact dynamically and interdependently and are organized hierarchically to achieve common goals and objectives."[46] But more than that, according to HFE evidence, high-performing teams are those that have been trained to have, and have demonstrated proficiency in, specialized knowledge, skills, and attitudes that support teamwork.[33] For example, in high-performing teams, all team members have the following knowledge: They share the same mental model of what needs to get done, they all know the team mission, and they all know each others' roles and expectations. Similarly, in high-performing teams all team members have been trained and have demonstrated proficiency in the following skills: backup behavior, team leadership, conflict resolution, and closed-loop communication, among others. However, few health care organizations train their staff to have that knowledge or those skills. Until that happens, HFE research suggests that there will not be high-functioning teams in health care (including PICUs).[47]

Technology

PICUs are full of technology. Not surprisingly, there is a perception that additional technologies may enhance safety. This perception exists despite the fact that *fallible humans* design the technologies used to prevent human error. Specific technologies attributed with improving safety include electronic health records, clinical decision support, computer provider order entry (CPOE), bar-coded medication administration, and "smart" infusion pumps. These technologies have been linked to a reduction in errors, even though little evidence exists that they reduce harm to patients. There is also evidence that these technologies can introduce new types of errors, violations, and harm.[6-11,48-54]

That technologies intended to improve safety may create added errors, rule violations, and risks may seem counterintuitive. However, the systems model described previously helps explain this seeming paradox. For instance, CPOE does not exist in a vacuum within the ICU. Instead, people (physicians, nurses, pharmacists) must use the CPOE system to perform tasks (ordering, modifying, and managing medications) within a busy and often distracting ICU environment. Independent of whether the CPOE system works as intended, the interactions among technology and people, tasks and environment, not to mention how the technology was implemented and supported, will ultimately determine whether the CPOE improves or sometimes worsens medication safety.[55] Health information technologies intended to improve safety may have usability problems[56-61] that increase the likelihood of user errors, provide misleading feedback, lead to high rates of false alarms, or cause difficulties interpreting data. Examples of usability problems include CPOE systems that preselect a patient, increasing the likelihood of entering orders on the incorrect patient, and defibrillators that have unclear displays resulting in failed attempts of patient cardioversion. If such usability problems exist, they can lead to the previously mentioned design-induced errors.

The issue of alarm and alert fatigue (the latter from electronic health records [EHR]) is an increasingly problematic issue. Both stem from fundamental problems with how monitors, devices, and EHRs are designed. The result is whole-scale desensitization of providers because of the poor signal-to-noise ratio. Perhaps what is most worrisome about this issue is that there exists no literature on resensitizing providers.[62-64]

As with team training, there is a rich body of non–health care literature and a growing body of health care–specific literature that can guide the design, selection, and implementation of technologies to yield the best results.[65-68] Without leveraging this knowledge, PICU providers risk the unintended but foreseeable consequences of suboptimal technology adoption and potential harm to their patients.

Patient Safety in the Pediatric Intensive Care Unit: Past, Present, and Future

The body of health care safety science has grown dramatically since the previous edition of this text. Now, patient safety is the subject of its own textbooks, with numerous national and international meetings devoted to expanding knowledge and improving solutions (Table 11.4). With this in mind, it is impossible to provide a complete discussion of all topics for the PICU audience. It is important to know that there are many important topics worthy of additional consideration. These include fatigue and performance in the PICU, the potential for simulation, and the importance of leadership and the culture of safety in the PICU.

There is an evolution in the approach to patient safety within a clinical environment, including the PICU. The most basic approach that still exists in health care is one of denial (ie, the belief that a PICU has no safety issues). However, in the absence of concrete evidence that harm such as CABSIs or decubitus ulcers do not occur in that unit, this approach resembles that of the Flat Earth Society: unfounded disbelief.

Beyond denial is the reactive approach, characterized by error counting, blame finding, and people-based solutions. One example of organizational implementation of a reactive approach is the previously discussed HPI framework adopted by SPS.[35] Unfortunately, this approach may be well intended but harmful because of the impact on care providers and the culture of safety. Next is a proactive approach in which PICU

TABLE 11.4 Sampling of Major Patient Safety Meetings and References

Meeting or Text Title	Annotation
National Patient Safety Foundation Annual Patient Safety Congress	Annual national conference focused on patient safety improvement
Agency for Research and Quality Annual Conference	Annual national conference focused on the science of patient safety
Institute for Healthcare Improvement's Annual National Forum on Quality Improvement in Health Care	Annual national meeting focused on quality with some emphasis on safety
National Initiative for Child Healthcare Quality's Annual Forum on Improving Children's Healthcare and Childhood Obesity Congress	Annual national meeting focused on pediatric quality with limited emphasis on safety
To Err Is Human: Building a Safer Health System	Seminal publication addressing the patient safety problem in the United States
Handbook of Human Factors and Ergonomics in Health Care and Patient Safety	Authoritative text providing the basic science of patient safety
Internal Bleeding: The Truth Behind America's Terrifying Epidemic of Medical Mistakes	Despite sensational title, an excellent introduction to patient safety issues

teams seek to identify, understand, and reduce risks in their environment. However, nothing about this approach assures that variation will not undermine safety improvement efforts.

The desire to eliminate unwanted and harmful variation is central to the standardization-based approach to safety. In these aspiring "high-reliability organizations," there is a focus on standardization of processes in the care environment. For processes such as preparing and dispensing a medication, handoff communications, or placing a central venous catheter, standardization will reduce unwanted variation and potentially reduce waste while improving quality and safety. At the same time, the practice of standardization can be overused. Standardizing the ordering, dispensing, and administration processes of aminoglycosides in septic PICU patients would be beneficial; standardizing to a single dose of aminoglycosides regardless of patient age, weight, or renal function would be potentially dangerous.

If standardization of a process will support the needs of ICU providers in all or nearly all cases, HFE supports its use, allowing exceptions for the few cases where a standard process does not apply. If, on the other hand, standardization will only support the needs of the providers some of the time, then standardization may be problematic. After all, if a standardized process does not fit many typical situations, then standardizing will simply create more "violators."

The goal of safety programs both in and out of the PICU is resilience. "Resilience is the ability of systems to mount a robust response to unforeseen, unpredicted, and unexpected demands and to resume or even continue normal operations."[69] Any PICU faced with a mass casualty or even simultaneous cardiac arrests in patients understands the challenge of unanticipated demands on the system of care delivery. What is less clear is whether the PICU team can rise to meet these demands while still providing care to the other patients in the PICU. Safety science has revealed that it is the people in the complex systems that provide resilience or the ability of the system to function safely despite the inherent complexity and the risks.[70,71] Thus when PICUs are provided resources and designed such that they can meet these demands while providing care to the other patients and assure safe and high-quality outcomes, then the goal of resilience is met.

Conclusions

The issues of patient safety and quality have proved to be more than a fad. Patients, their families, payers, regulatory bodies, and a growing number of health care professionals are all focusing on these issues. As is true with any complex system, there are no easy answers to improvement, and improvements targeted at fixing people are destined to fail. Instead, by learning and applying quality and safety science, there is the opportunity to enhance the historically good outcomes achieved in the PICU.

Key References

2. Kohn LT, Corrigan JM, Donaldson MS. Why do errors happen? In: Kohn LT, Corrigan JM, Donaldson MS, eds. *To Err Is Human: Building a Safer Health System*. Washington, DC: National Academy Press; 1999.
5. Carayon P, Hundt AS, Karsh B-T, et al. Work system design for patient safety: the SEIPS model. *Qual Saf Health Care*. 2006;15(suppl 1):i50-i58.
6. Koppel R, Metlay JP, Cohen A, et al. Role of computerized physician order entry systems in facilitating medication errors. *JAMA*. 2005;293:1197-1203.
7. Nebeker JR, Hoffman JM, Weir CR, et al. High rates of adverse drug events in a highly computerized hospital. *Arch Intern Med*. 2005;165:1111-1116.
8. Han YY, Carcillo JA, Venkataraman ST, et al. Unexpected increased mortality after implementation of a commercially sold computerized physician order entry system. *Pediatrics*. 2005;116:1506-1512.
9. Thompson DA, Duling L, Holzmueller CG, et al. Computerized physician order entry, a factor in medication errors: descriptive analysis of events in the intensive care unit safety reporting system. *J Clin Outcomes Manage*. 2005;12:407-412.
12. Zimmerman B, Lindberg C, Plsek P. *Edgeware: Insights from Complexity Science for Health Care Leaders*, Irving, TX, 1988, VHA.
13. Perrow C. *Normal Accidents: Living With High-Risk Technologies*. 2nd ed. New York: Basic Books; 1984.
16. Committee on Quality of Health Care in America. *Crossing the Quality Chasm: A New Health System for the 21st Century*. Washington, DC: National Academy Press; 2001.
19. Wheeler DJ. *Understanding Variation: The Key to Managing Chaos*. Knoxville, TN: SPC Press; 1993.
21. Kelley DL. *How to Use Control Charts for Healthcare*. Milwaukee, WI: ASQ Quality Press; 1999.
22. Wu WA, Lipshutz AK, Pronovost PM. Effectiveness and efficiency of root cause analysis in medicine. *JAMA*. 2008;299:685-687.
23. Nicolini D, Waring J, Mengis J. Policy and practice in the use of root cause analysis to investigate clinical adverse events: mind the gap. *Soc Sci Med*. 2011;73:217-225.
24. Nemeth CP, Cook RI, Donchin Y, et al. Learning from investigation: experience with understanding healthcare adverse events, Proceedings of the Human Factors and Ergonomics Society Annual Meeting. 50: 914-917, 2006.
25. Hollnagel E, Leonhardt J, Licu T, et al. From Safety I to Safety II: a white paper. 2013. Available at <www.eurocontrol.int>.
26. Hollnagel E. A tale of two safeties. *Nuclear Safety and Simulation*. 2013;4:1-9.
27. Wiseman B, Kaprielian VS, Contrasting QI and QA. 2016. Available at <http://patientsafetyed.duhs.duke.edu/module_a/introduction/contrasting_qi_qa.html>.
35. Throop C, Stockmeier C, HPI SEC & SSER Patient Safety Measurement System for Healthcare, HPI White Paper Series Revision 2-May. 2011. Available at <https://hpiresults.com/publications/HPI%20White%20Paper%20-%20SEC%20&%20SSER%20Measurement%20System%20REV%202%20MAY%202011.pdf>.
36. Alper SJ, Holden RJ, Scanlon MC, et al. Self-reported violations during medication administration in two paediatric hospitals. *BMJ Qual Saf*. 2012;21:408-415.
37. Koppel R, Wetterneck T, Telles JL, et al. Workarounds to barcode medication administration systems: their occurrences, causes and threats to patient safety. *J Am Med Inform Assoc*. 2008;15:408-423.
38. Dekker S. *Patient Safety: A Human Factors Approach*. New York: CRC Press; 2011.
40. Burke CS, Salas E, Wilson-Donnelly K, Priest H. How to turn a team of experts into an expert medical team: guidance from the aviation and military communities. *Qual Saf Health Care*. 2004;13:I96-I104.
44. Salas E, Cannon-Bowers JA. The science of training: a decade of progress. *Ann Rev Psychol*. 2001;52:471-499.
47. Salas E, Wilson KA, Murphy CE. What crew resource management training will not do for patient safety unless. *J Patient Saf*. 2007;3:62-64.
48. Karsh BT, Weiner MB, Abbott PA, et al. Health information technology: fallacies and sober realities. *J Am Med Inform Assoc*. 2010;17:617-623.
49. Koppel R, Metlay JP, Cohen A, et al. Role of computerized physician order entry systems in facilitating medication errors. *JAMA*. 2005;293:1197-1203.
62. Landrigan CP. Crying wolf: false alarms and patient safety. *J Hosp Med*. 2015;10:409-410.
69. Nemeth C, Wears R, Woods D, et al. Minding the gaps: creating resilience in healthcare. In: Henricksen K, Battles JB, Keyes MA, Grady ML, eds. *Agency for Healthcare Research and Quality's Advances in Patient Safety: New Directions and Alternative Approaches*. Vol. 3. Performance and Tools. Rockville, MD: AHRQ; Publication No. 08-0034-1. 2008.
70. Hollnagel E, Woods DD. *Joint Cognitive Systems: Foundations of Cognitive Systems Engineering*. New York: CRC Press; 2005.
71. Hollnagel E, Woods DD, Leveson N, eds. *Resilience Engineering: Concepts and Precepts*. Surrey: Ashgate; 2006.
73. Latour JM, van Goudoever JB, Hazelzet JA. Parent satisfaction in the pediatric ICU. *Pediatr Clin North Am*. 2008;55:779-790.

Information Technology in Critical Care

L. Nelson Sanchez-Pinto, Steven Pon, and Barry Markovitz

PEARLS

- Health care organizations around the world are adopting digital infrastructures, opening the door to a data-driven and evidenced-based transformation of the way we take care of our patients. However, the road ahead is long and not without hurdles.
- Physicians must learn about the evolving information technologies in health care to develop realistic expectations, maximize their benefit, ensure patient safety, and avoid pitfalls.
- In most institutions, administrators and nurses drive the advancement of various information technologies. Physicians, especially intensivists, must become involved in the selection and development of these technologies if their needs and concerns are to be adequately addressed.
- Organizations and clinicians must ensure the security and confidentiality of personally identifiable protected health information. They must understand the legislated privacy rules and safeguard the security and confidentiality of patient data.
- As each incremental phase of implementation of an electronic health record is approached, the focus should be on overcoming specific barriers to care rather than on the nebulous goal of "creating a paperless process."
- Health care organizations that take full advantage of their digital infrastructures and data assets in an organized, systematic, and attentive manner will stand to benefit the most in coming years.

Medicine is an information service. From the bits of data that stream out of the patients' monitors and the stories the patients recount to the signs and symptoms identified by clinicians and the diagnoses they formulate, medical information is wielded to protect life and shepherd death. Compassion, judgment, and technical skill may distinguish excellence in the discipline, but information defines the science of medicine.

Health care systems around the world are undergoing a digital revolution, and the adoption of electronic health records (EHRs) is just one of the early steps. This digitalization, along with the extraordinary advances in the biomedical sciences, is contributing to the remarkable expansion of medical information. This deluge of "big data" threatens to drown even the most conscientious clinician, who devotes every waking hour of every day to collecting, cataloguing, assimilating, and applying the information that will help his or her patients. Fortunately, advances in health information technology (IT) can also facilitate this task. Health IT gives us immediate access to vast knowledge and decision support while streamlining the tedious chores of searching and collating information. It has changed the way we practice medicine, and it continues to evolve every day.

Demonstrations of the potential of health IT typically inspire awe and admiration. However, when the technology migrates from demonstration to actual use, awe and admiration sometimes give way to disappointment. The novel features that users think they need are either impossible to achieve or require significant reengineering of the original product. Health IT is continually improving, but understanding its limitations is as important as envisioning its promise.

Health IT has a long road ahead of it to achieve its full potential. Physicians, especially intensivists, should help chart that road and keep the focus on the most important of our tasks: improve the care we provide to our patients.

Digital Infrastructure in Health Care

Great effort has been devoted in the past decade to digitalizing health care in the United States and around the world. The US federal government has been especially active in this purpose by incentivizing the adoption of EHRs and accelerating the data utility across the country.[1] One of the major advantages of a digitalized health care system is the potential to analyze the electronic information of health care transactions, both clinical and nonclinical, in order to learn what practices improve care and reduce costs. This so-called "learning health system" has been hailed as the way to continuously improve health care.[2,3] It is estimated that, if the US health care system were to make use of its electronic data in an effective way, it could save up to $300 billion per year.[4]

HITECH Act and Meaningful Use of EHRs

The Health Information Technology for Economic and Clinical Health (HITECH) Act was enacted under the Title XIII of the American Recovery and Reinvestment Act of 2009 and carries a commitment of up to $27 billion to improve the US health information technology infrastructure.[1] The HITECH Act outlined plans to encourage implementation and meaningful use of EHRs through the Centers for Medicare & Medicaid Services (CMS) EHR Incentive program. This program has evolved to include three stages, each with its own goals and priorities and with different incentive dollars depending on the year of adoption of each stage by hospitals and providers.

The EHR meaningful use criteria stages are:
- *Stage 1* (which began in 2011), which focuses on electronically capturing health information in a standardized format, tracking key clinical conditions, and sharing clinical quality measures;
- *Stage 2* (2014), which focuses on rigorous health information exchange, e-prescribing, and increased emphasis on patient-controlled data; and
- *Stage 3* (2016), which focuses on improving quality, safety, and efficiency in order to improve health outcomes.

In addition to the CMS Medicare and Medicaid EHR Incentive program, the HITECH Act created programs to regionally support the implementation of EHRs, support state-level health information exchange (HIE) projects, create health IT workforce training programs, fund health IT research through the strategic health information technology advanced research projects (SHARP), develop interoperability standards and specifications, and create the Nationwide Health Information Network (NHIN)—a common national platform for health information exchange (Fig. 12.1).[5]

Learning Health System

The Institute of Medicine, sponsored by the US Office of the National Coordinator for Health Information Technology, published a report in 2011 that explored strategies to accelerate the implementation of a digital infrastructure in health care and the development of a learning health system.[2] They defined the learning health system as a system "designed to generate and apply best evidence for collaborative health choices of each patient and provider; to drive the process of discovery as a natural outgrowth of patient care; and to ensure innovation, quality, safety, and value in health care." Information technology is the functional engine of such a system, and hence the development of the digital infrastructure is a natural prerequisite (Fig. 12.2).

The need for a learning health system in the United States stems from the paradox in which the health system finds itself. The rapid growth of molecular diagnostics, genetics, proteomics, imaging, and therapeutics is overwhelming clinicians and patients who have to sift through more and more information with each decision. At the same time, we lack of evidence of which approaches are the most beneficial, cost-efficient, and safe. The impact of all this is compounded by the fact that health care costs continue to rise, exhausting the purchasing power of consumers and reducing the competitiveness edge of US employers, yet patient outcomes are less than optimal when compared with other large health care systems around the world.

The Institute of Medicine expanded this topic in 2012 with the report *Best Care at Lower Cost* in which it makes 10 recommendations to radically improve the US health care system.[3] The first three recommendations are in direct relationship with the learning health system and the use of clinical decision support (CDS):
- *Recommendation #1: The Digital Infrastructure.* Improve the capacity to capture clinical, care delivery process, and financial data for better care, system improvement, and generation of new knowledge.
- *Recommendation #2: The Data Utility.* Streamline and revise research regulations to improve care, promote capture of clinical data, and generate knowledge.
- *Recommendation #3: Clinical Decision Support.* Accelerate integration of best clinical knowledge into care decisions. Decision support tools and knowledge management systems should be routine features of health care delivery

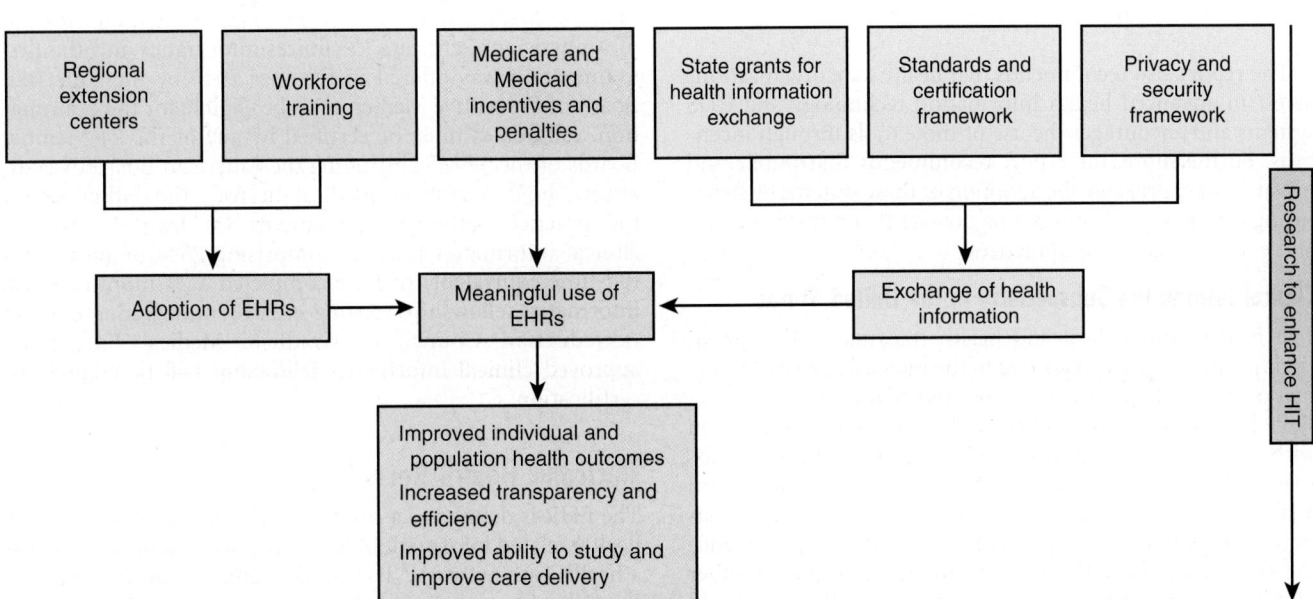

Fig. 12.1. The Health Information Technology for Economic and Clinical Health Act's framework for meaningful use of electronic health records. *EHR,* electronic health record; *HIT,* health information technology. (From Blumenthal D. Launching HITECH. N Engl J Med. 2010;362:382-385.)

Internal   **External**

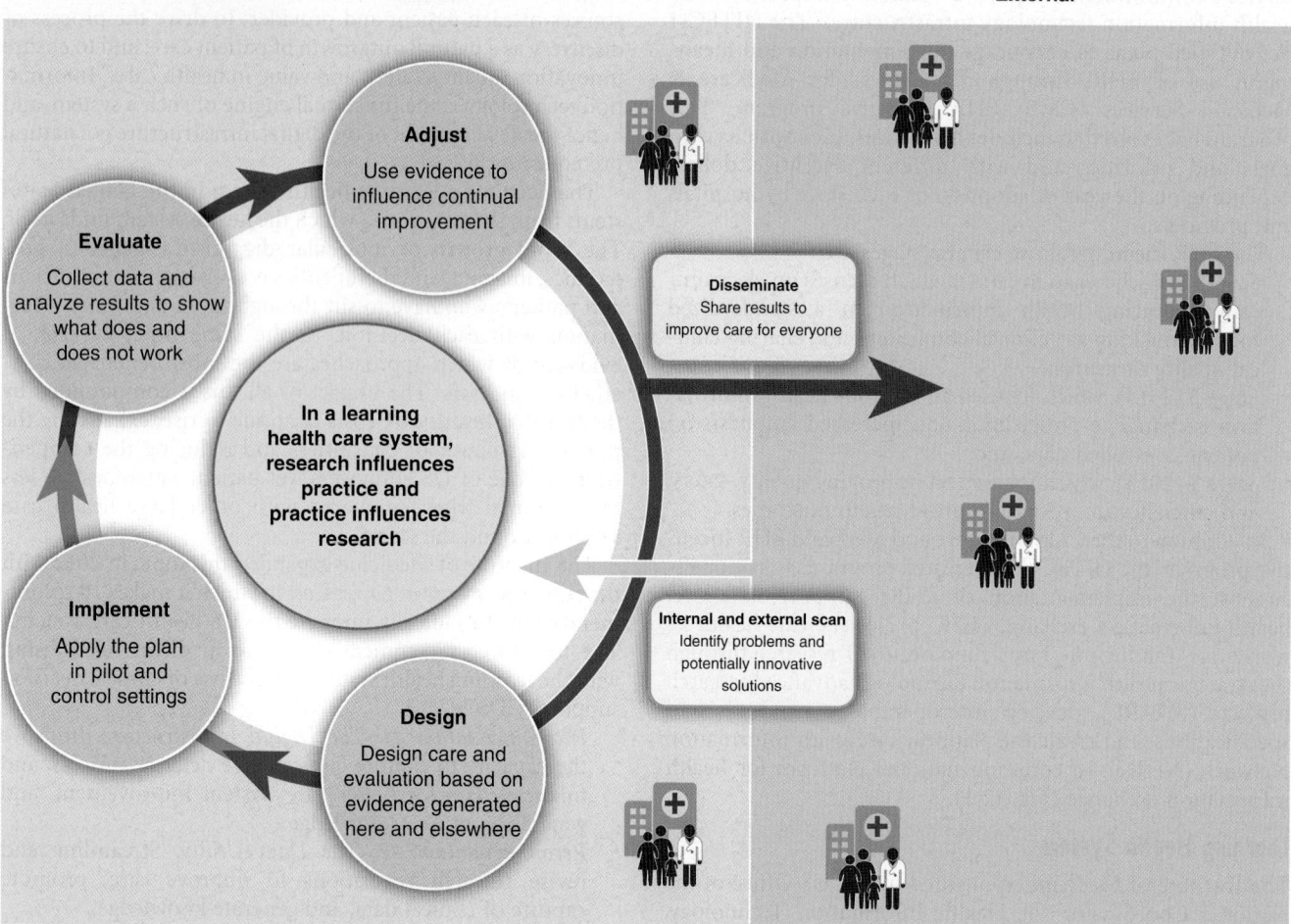

Fig. 12.2. Phases of the learning health system, as proposed by the Group Health Cooperative, Seattle, WA. (From Greene SM, Reid RJ, Larson EB. Implementing the learning health system: from concept to action. Ann Intern Med. 2012;157:207-210.)

to ensure that decisions made by clinicians and patients are informed by current best practice.

The report also recommends that health care organizations invest in advanced health information technology and CDS systems and encourages the use of these tools through incentives. Furthermore, the report recommends that public and private payers promote the adoption of these systems by structuring payments and contracting policies that reward effective and evidence-based care practices.

Clinical Informatics Subspecialty in the United States

The field of biomedical and health informatics has grown significantly in recent years due to the increasing role of information technology in health care and higher demand for a skilled workforce that can bridge the science of information with the reality of clinical care.[6] Clinical informatics is a subspecialty of biomedical and health informatics that focuses on analyzing, designing, implementing, and evaluating information systems that improve care, reduce cost, and/or enhance the experience of health care consumers. There are a number of graduate-level courses, master's degrees, fellowships, and doctorate programs designed to train health care professionals in the field of clinical informatics. In 2011, the American

Board of Medical Specialties (ABMS) announced the creation of a physician certificate in clinical informatics and the first examination was offered in October 2013 by the American Board of Preventive Medicine. To be eligible for the examination, candidates must be certified by any of the 24 Member Boards of the ABMS (including the American Board of Pediatrics), hold a current medical license, and either satisfy the practice pathway requirements (at least 3 years of clinical informatics practice comprising 25% or more of a full-time equivalent) or have completed a 24-month clinical informatics fellowship. Starting in 2018, only graduates of an Accreditation Council of Graduate Medical Education–approved clinical informatics fellowship will be eligible for certification.[7]

Electronic Health Record

The EHR is defined as a comprehensive database of personal, health-related information that is accessed and updated across a health care network.[8] Its potential and real benefits include the following:

- Improved quality of care through more timely, more complete, and better-organized information delivery to the health care provider, with decision support and clinical pathways.

- Cost savings through elimination of duplicate testing, shorter lengths of stay, and more efficient data collection and review.
- Higher productivity by structuring patient care tasks to improve continuity of care and reduce practice variation by facilitating the creation of more consistent and more comprehensive content and by making the medical records more readily accessible to more users simultaneously.
- Facilitation of research, education, quality improvement, outcomes assessment, and strategic planning.

The three principal functions of such a database, like any database, are data acquisition, data access, and data storage.

Data Acquisition

The complete EHR acquires data from a variety of sources, including hospital registration, nursing and physician input, laboratory services, radiology and other test interpretations, therapist and nutrition services, monitoring devices, and physicians' orders. The most important system that feeds the database is the "enterprise-wide master patient index," which ensures that each patient is identified properly and uniquely. All other systems must have the correct identifier in order to deliver their data to the correct patient record. A multimedia database can include images such as radiographs, electrocardiograms, fetal monitoring, sonography, magnetic resonance images, computerized tomograms, and even paper-based documents such as consent forms, living wills, questionnaires, and, sometimes, handwritten notes and hand-drawn diagrams. Data acquisition is organized in a manner that minimizes duplicative effort and maximizes data consistency.

One of the significant challenges to any implementation of an EHR is engineering the various interfaces between it and the host of systems that feeds it data. Some of the feeder systems, such as laboratory services, have their own established validation protocols that are applied before transmission to the EHR.

Data originating from bedside devices such as cardiopulmonary monitors, pulse oximeters, ventilators, and intravenous infusion pumps represent critical elements of the patient care record. Manual capture and entry of these data into the EHR by nurses and other health care practitioners are associated with inefficiency and transcription errors. Technology is currently available to connect devices to the EHR through bedside medical device interfaces (BMDIs). BMDI allows properly formatted data from a medical device to flow into and update the patient's EHR.

One of the challenges in BMDI relates to the diversity of medical devices and EHRs, which makes it impractical for most vendors to directly connect. Often, biomedical device integration systems are required to extract, read, interpret, and forward data to the EHR in order for it to be useful. Basic physiologic data including heart rate, blood pressure, and respiratory rate are generally the first to be targeted for EHR integration. Other monitoring data that can be integrated with the EHR include temperature, pulse oximetry, end-tidal CO_2, and cardiac output measurements. Other devices that can be connected via BMDI include intravenous infusion pumps, ventilators, dialysis, hemofiltration systems, cerebral oxygenation monitors, and extracorporeal membrane oxygenation systems.

One of the clear benefits associated with BMDI is the improved efficiency associated with not having to manually retrieve and record the data. The increased efficiency therefore allows the nurse to spend more time at the patient's bedside or in other important activities. Though this time saving is minimal for any one piece of patient data, when the aggregated data for each patient and for the entire facility are considered, the opportunity for cost saving likely exceeds the cost of the initial investment. Another potential benefit is improved completeness and accuracy of the data in the EHR. BMDI increases data-sampling frequency possibilities, which is particularly important in a dynamic patient situation where data may be changing rapidly. Providers may request higher data sampling frequencies without impacting the need for additional patient care resources. In addition, reading and manually recording data into an EHR are often associated with transcription errors, the likelihood of which is reduced with BMDI. Having said that, inaccurate data can also be sampled from the bedside monitors, such as when an electrocardiographic lead comes loose from the patient, and if this is not corrected by bedside providers, erroneous data can be introduced into the EHR.

Considering that a data element passes from one of several feeder systems through different computers, with possible transformations of that data element along the way, and considering the possibilities of lost transmissions, computer down-times, and network interruptions, consistent error-free data feeding would seem almost impossible. In a high-volume environment, a centralized interface engine that routes and converts transaction messages from disparate feeder systems, such as an enterprise service bus,[9] can solve many of the interface issues efficiently and in a timely fashion, with the added value of being able to perform streaming analytics and complex event detection using these electronic messages.[10]

The capture of textual information, such as progress notes, nursing assessments, or even radiology reports, presents particular challenges for several reasons. For the most part, text is entered via a keyboard hard-wired to the system but may be through voice or handwriting recognition or via handheld and wireless devices. Text entry with menu systems feeding structured and unstructured forms has been met with some success. Although these solutions do not have the same expressivity of free text, they lend themselves to the capture of text as structured data. Collecting structured data facilitates future analysis, but despite this significant advantage over collecting free text, it tends to be rigid, can make documenting the unusual impossible, generally requires more time to collect, and may be a significant source of frustration for the clinician. Another strategy is to allow free text entries but to apply natural language processing (NLP) to extract data from it for analysis. Even with the significant promise that NLP analytics represents in other care settings, one of the unique characteristics of the critical care environment is the abundance of structured data (vital signs, fluid inputs and outputs, medications administered, etc.) that remain underanalyzed.[11]

Data Access

The EHR serves as the focal point for most health care professionals. It might be accessed at inpatient sites but also in emergency departments, nursing facilities, continuing care centers, physician offices, clinics, laboratory facilities, treatment centers, and, in the case of home health services, the patient's home. An ideal EHR should be available when and where it is needed. However, databases with sensitive information must be controlled to prevent unauthorized use or alteration. These systems must satisfy five requirements:

1. Access control: Only authorized persons are allowed access for authorized uses.
2. Authentication: Some confirmation that a person granted access is, in fact, who he or she purports to be.
3. Confidentiality: No unauthorized disclosure of information is allowed.
4. Integrity: Information content is unalterable except under authorized circumstances.
5. Attribution/nonrepudiation: Actions taken (access, data entry, and data modification) are reliably traceable.

The interface through which most health care providers interact with the EHR should be user-friendly and intuitive. Most clinicians have little time or patience to sit through tedious training sessions, and, once trained, few clinicians will recall more than a minimum required to complete their immediate, routine tasks.

The system should be capable of providing a full, seamless view of the patient over time and across points of care. Views should be configurable so that a given user's information needs and workflow can be accommodated. Both detailed and summary views that juxtapose relevant data allow the clinician to acquire the information required to optimize expedient decision making. Displays should be configured to highlight key information while suppressing clutter but making all pertinent data readily accessible. Dynamic linkages should exist between the electronic health record and supporting functions such as expert systems, clinical pathways, protocols, policies, reference material, and the medical literature.

Response times must be sufficiently speedy, and workstations should be conveniently accessible to the point of care. Mobile connections are a bonus. Access to patient data via wireless connections with portable devices is an attractive alternative for users but must overcome usability and security hurdles before it can be fully implemented.

The patient database also supports many areas of research, education, decision support, and external reporting. Thus data in aggregate can be accessed by administration, finance, quality assurance, and research areas.

Data Storage

Multimedia data of the comprehensive EHR are stored on media that allow for long-term storage while allowing searches and rapid retrieval of enormous volumes of data. The database must be updated in a way that ensures it is current, complete, and consistent. Data, once entered, should be modifiable only in accordance with strict rules that ensure data integrity.

The architecture of the database can be centralized or distributed, replicated or not. A centralized database is stored at a single site, whereas a distributed database is a single logical database with segments that are spread across multiple locations connected by a network. A replicated database has the advantage over a nonreplicated database by having at least one copy of all records in case the primary copy is inaccessible because of computer or network failure. The challenge of replication is maintaining consistency among all the copies, which requires, in turn, timely, automatic synchronization of the original database and its replicas. More and more health

care organizations are moving their EHR data to cloud-based computing systems as the federal regulatory, security, and privacy issues resolve.[12]

Once stored, the data should have a time stamp. Although data can be modified, both the original and revised versions should be maintained with appropriate time stamping. Appropriate safeguards must ensure database integrity so that its pieces do not lose their links and the data are not subject to unauthorized modification. Supplanting the paper record with the EHR as the official medical record requires thoughtful consideration of the limitations of paper copies to reflect accurately the electronic record. Sanctioned hard copies of the patient record will be necessary for sharing with other health care institutions or with the legal system.

Whereas a clinical data repository is a database optimized to retrieve data on individual patients, a clinical data warehouse (CDW) is a database designed to support data analysis across individuals. This function can be distinguished from a simple archival function. The CDW structure is designed to support a variety of analyses, including elaborate queries on large amounts of data. The data are generally static and updated intermittently in batches rather than continuously.

Hospitals can use CDWs to perform financial analyses or quality assessments. With decision support tools, they can be useful in negotiating managed care contracts or distributing resources to clinical or ancillary services. Subsets of a CDW that are structured to support a single department or function are "data marts." These subsets are designed to perform periodic analyses or to produce standard reports run repeatedly, such as monthly financial statements or quality measures. Data mining applications can sift through mountains of data in the CDW and run complex algorithms to find obscure patterns (see section on Health Analytics).

Limitations and Pitfalls

Information technology in the form of an EHR promises improved patient care.[13,14] Potential benefits of information technology include providing rapid access to integrated clinical data and extant medical knowledge, eliminating illegibility, improving communication, and issuing applicable reminders and checks for appropriate medical actions.

A number of studies show that clinical information systems can provide various benefits, including increasing adherence to guidelines and decreasing medication errors.[15] However, any benefit may be outweighed by new problems introduced by the systems themselves. In effect, one set of problems may be traded for another.

The medical information space is vastly more complicated than it seems at first. EHR software programs are enormously complex, are built by large teams of programmers with input by numerous clinicians, demand high-speed processors and high-bandwidth networks, and rely on often fragile interfaces with other hospital systems. Implementation currently requires tremendous effort by both clinicians and technical specialists to configure these systems according to the specific needs of an institution and in ways that will enhance care rather than impede it. An often unappreciated complicating factor is that the technology does not simply replace paper; it also reengineers care—deliberately or not.

Errors can and do occur in programming or configuration. Many programming deficiencies can be detected and corrected with thorough testing, preferably in a development environment that does not affect real patients; however, some of these problems will only become apparent under unique circumstances that are presented by patient care. Indefatigable vigilance for these errors is essential.

Numerous other unintended consequences result from implementing an EHR, including the creation of new kinds of errors, an increase in work for clinicians, an untoward alteration of workflow and change in communication patterns, an increase in system demands, a persistence of paper use, and the fostering of potential overdependence on the technology.[16] Examples of unintended consequences are the "illusion of communication," where the user of the EHR is under the illusion that entering information in the system is enough to communicate to the appropriate person who needs to act on that information, and juxtaposition errors, where a user might click on the adjacent name in a list and inadvertently enter the wrong information.

The benefit of legibility in electronically written notes can be outweighed by novel problems. Overuse of copy-paste functions can result in repetitive, monotonous, and loquacious notes punctuated by the sin of propagating erroneous text verbatim. Automatic transcription of data such as laboratory results or vital signs often bypasses cognition, something that is much less likely when data are transcribed by hand.

Documentation in a structured format rather than as free text can enhance completeness and facilitate later data retrieval; however, it can also increase work by forcing the clinician to find ways to fit round pegs into square holes. Similarly, rigidly structured order input can force clinicians to waste time trying different ways to order nonstandard tests or therapies.

Clinical alerts can help clinicians make decisions (eg, when penicillin is mistakenly ordered for an allergic patient), but persistent interruptions of work by alerts can increase the cognitive load of the clinician, who must decipher their meaning and assess the risk in each specific circumstance. The frequency of these alerts can become intolerable when they are not delivered to the right clinician, with the right information, and at the right time and place, leading to the so-called "alert fatigue" phenomenon.[17] When these alerts become too frequent and too predictable, clinicians often adapt by dismissing them automatically, which both diminishes the alert effectiveness and may ultimately harm the patient.[18]

Many care providers blame clinical information systems for unsatisfactory reductions in face-to-face communication. Some users complain that the EHR creates an "illusion of communication,"[16] where users believe that information entered into the system will be somehow communicated to the relevant personnel. This assumption can result in missed or delayed execution of orders or failure to appreciate the recommendations of a consultant. Users may erroneously assume that allergies entered into the system will adequately protect patients from receiving offending food or drugs.

No installed EHR can remain static for long. Maintenance, revisions, and upgrades of both software and hardware contribute to constant flux. Consequences should be expected with every change, and many changes require testing that can become onerous. Although minor changes can occur without supplemental training of personnel, failure to provide training for some changes can cause significant user frustration and errors. Some configuration changes requested by one group may also adversely affect other users in unexpected ways. Mechanisms must be developed to resolve conflicts of this nature. As clinicians become increasingly dependent on the system, pressure to keep the system operational mounts, requiring around-the-clock technical support.

Human Factors Engineering

Cognitive science, computer science, and human factors engineering are among many disciplines that can facilitate development of a successful EHR system. Human factors engineering investigates human capabilities and limitations and applies that knowledge in the design of systems, software, environments, training, and personnel management. Application of human factors considerations in developing an EHR can maximize successful design and implementation of these systems. Some human factors principles may seem self-evident but can be overlooked when not approached systematically. Developers must understand the users, undertake detailed task analyses, and assess computer-supported cooperative work—the study of how people work within organizations and how technology affects them and their work. Three principles that may improve clinical information systems are accounting for incentive structures, understanding workflow, and promoting awareness of the activities of other group members. Institutional and personal incentives for using an EHR differ, but only the latter will effectively influence use. Awareness of the roles played by other team members enhances collaboration. Improving collaboration may decrease the incidence of medical errors.[19]

Another important area of human factors engineering relates to interface design. Interfaces should be simple and consistent, with important data highlighted, such as the patient name or weight. "Progressive disclosure" means that commonly used and important functions should be presented first and in a logical order, whereas infrequently used functions should be hidden but available. Minimizing the clinicians' cognitive load can be accomplished by displaying all relevant information together on one screen rather than relying on the user to remember critical bits of data from different parts of the chart. Potential user errors should be anticipated, and easy error recovery should be designed into the system. Error messages should be informative and could include advice about error recovery. Other feedback should be provided to acknowledge user actions, particularly when the system appears frozen. Given the chaotic health care environment, the interface should also be designed to forgive interruptions, allowing work to be saved and facilitating task resumption.

User satisfaction is an important predictor of system success. Satisfaction is enhanced when the systems are designed with the users' needs and preferences in mind. Peers who serve as advocates for their groups during development and subsequently teach other users generally increase acceptance of the systems. Ease of use, rapid response times, flexibility and customizability, mobile workstations, implementation of effective decision support tools, access to reference information, and adequate training and support are all important factors in enhancing both user satisfaction and system success.[20]

Implementation

Implementation of an EHR system requires an investment of additional staff, hardware, software, and an expanded communications infrastructure or network. For large hospital networks, the costs can be extremely high.

Developing an EHR requires careful planning and phased implementation. The specific needs of the institution must be examined, particularly with regard to the existing technology and practices. The process should be viewed as an opportunity to enhance care, rather than simply to replace the paper, and requires reassessment of existing practices and reengineering of health care delivery. As each incremental phase of implementation is approached, the focus should be on overcoming specific barriers to care rather than on the nebulous goal of "creating a paperless process."[21]

Ensuring that the EHR satisfies every need involves considerable planning, designing, and testing. Even well-designed, off-the-shelf EHR systems can satisfy only 80% of the complex requirements of any multipractitioner organization. The remainder must be either adapted from other content or created from scratch. Substantial "expert" direction from teams of physicians, nurses, other allied health care providers, and medical records and financial staff is required to assist in developing the design and implementation of all EHRs.[22] If clinicians abdicate their responsibility in participating in this process, they are virtually ensuring that the resulting system will fail to satisfy their needs. Physician acceptance and participation can be enhanced by acknowledging the importance of physicians in the process, training them early and often, frequently and routinely eliciting their feedback, and demonstrating responsiveness to their needs and concerns.

Clinical Decision Support

According to the American Medical Informatics Association definition, "clinical decision support systems provide clinicians, staff, patients, or other individuals with knowledge and person-specific information, intelligently filtered or presented at appropriate times, to enhance health and health care." They further specify: "It encompasses a variety of tools and interventions such as computerized alerts and reminders, clinical guidelines, order sets, patient data reports and dashboards, documentation templates, diagnostic support, and clinical workflow tools."[23] These systems are not intended to make clinical decision but to provide context-specific knowledge and enable the ultimate decision makers, who are the clinicians, patients, and health care organizations, to make better decisions.[24]

As discussed earlier, there is currently a disconnect in the US health care system between the growth of medical knowledge and the increasing concerns about suboptimal care and rising costs.[23,24] The implementation of CDS systems has been proposed as the tool to close the gap between the generation of new knowledge and its application to practice in order to optimize care while reducing unnecessary costs.[25] However, most CDS systems currently in use are associated with vendor EHRs and have a limited scope. The greatest adoption has been in the form of simple alerts, order sets, prescription templates, drug-allergy, and drug dose checks. This type of basic CDS has had a modest impact on quality of care and reduction of errors,[15] highlighting the importance of investing in the development and adoption of advanced CDS systems. The Institute of Medicine recommends that health care providers and organizations invest in CDS systems and make them a routine feature of health care delivery.[3] It is indeed the responsibility of clinicians and the organizations in which they work to promote the optimal use of knowledge and best

practices in the clinical decision-making process, and CDS systems hold the potential to make such practice a seamless part of patient care.

CDS systems can be generally categorized into three different types[24]:
- Alerts, reminders, and recommendations
- Medical knowledge databases and "infobuttons"
- Dashboards, data visualization, and templates

Alerts, Reminders, and Recommendations

Alerts, reminders, and recommendations are the most widely used type of CDS, most of them integrated in EHRs or computerized provider order entry (CPOE) systems. Drug-drug interaction, drug-allergy, and drug dose checks are some examples of these basic CDS, which are usually triggered by one or two pieces of patient-related information. Reminders such as immunizations due or age-based health screenings also fall into this category. Recommendations such as order sets and order sentences are also included in this category. Order sets have received much attention in the CDS literature, mainly because they provide straightforward CDS within CPOE systems, they are easy and faster to use than writing single orders, and they deliver just-in-time, evidence-based prompts.[26] A prospective study looking at the effect of CPOE with CDS implementation in a pediatric ICU found a 99.4% reduction in prescribing errors and a 40.9% reduction in potential adverse drug events.[27]

Another type of alerting system that is starting to make its way into clinical practice is the application of real-time algorithms on physiologic monitoring data to predict events and alert clinicians. In neonatal medicine, the most prominent of these is the analysis of heart rate variability and changes over time to predict sepsis, which has been subject to a large randomized control trial showing a significant reduction in mortality.[28] A study of this scope has not yet been performed in the pediatric critical care setting, but this type of physiologic waveform analysis and algorithm development is currently an active area of research with a lot of promise in the field of critical care.[11]

Medical Knowledge Databases

Medical knowledge databases have flourished with the advent of widespread Internet access in patient care. These databases might be connected to EHRs and have the capability of retrieving highly relevant online documents through the so-called "infobuttons." An example of this is the Lexicomp Drug database that can be accessed from many EHRs to find information about a specific drug. Another example of this type of resource is UpToDate, an online database with almost 10,000 peer-reviewed medical articles with diagnostic and management recommendations, which can be used as a stand-alone resource or through an EHR interface. When these resources are accessed from an EHR, it is often through an infobutton, which, when clicked, performs a patient- or condition-specific query of the knowledge database. Health Level Seven International (HL7), the standard development organization, has created a standard for "context-aware knowledge retrieval," which has been implemented in many commercial EHRs as an infobutton manager. Full-text electronic resources have seen increased use among trainees,[29] but their success at meeting knowledge needs and supporting clinical decisions has not been systematically studied. The reality is that clinicians continue to have many informational needs in everyday practice and those needs are frequently unmet.[30]

Dashboards, Data Visualization, and Templates

Dashboards, data visualization, and templates have not received much attention in the CDS literature until recently, but they represent an upcoming area of research. The principle behind the use of these tools is that good decisions are not only based on having the right information but also in how the information is consumed. CDS systems that take into account the increasingly important aspect of human-computer interaction and make use of data visualization tools and information displays in an optimal way can make a significant impact in the clinical decision-making process.[24]

An interesting area of research that focuses on information consumption in the ICU is the redesign of electronic interfaces to support and improve clinical decision making. Researchers at Mayo Clinic have shown that in a simulated scenario of critically ill patients, the use of an interface containing only highly relevant information organized around organ systems was associated with reductions in task load, time to task completion, and errors of cognition when compared with a standard EHR interface (Fig. 12.3).[31]

CDS Effectiveness

The study of CDS effectiveness, along with other health information systems and applications, such as CPOE, has always been limited by variability in the quality of the systems. Having said that, a large systematic review of 148 randomized controlled trials that evaluated the effectiveness of CDS systems of both locally developed and commercial systems showed moderate to strong evidence that CDS can reduce morbidity, reduce cost of care, increase the rate of ordering recommended treatments and other services, and increase health care provider satisfaction.[15] The review did not show an overall impact on length of stay, mortality, efficiency, or health care provider acceptance. Another review of CDS systems, this time in the pediatric ICU, also found some studies showing a positive impact of these systems in the process of care but noted the importance of human factors, implementation, and usability aspects of these systems as key factors in their success.[32]

Within the literature there are also many examples of CDS systems that have fallen short of the intended goals or have resulted in unintended consequences.[16] An example of this is a study that showed using a hard stop alert for changing prescribing behavior within a CPOE in which the order was blocked from further execution when the alert was triggered was effective at preventing the order from being placed, but it also delayed the treatment of patients who needed immediate drug therapy.[33]

It is clear that much more research and development needs to occur in order for CDS systems to fulfill their role in the transformation of our health care system, as has been proposed by the Institute of Medicine and other organizations. More rigorous research to support the content and deployment of these systems, more robust and controlled development and validation methodologies, and better dissemination and implementation practices are all necessary steps before CDS systems will achieve their full potential.

Patient Safety and Technology in the ICU

Patient safety concerns remain paramount in any hospital system, including clinical information systems.[34] To the extent possible, redundant systems should be in place to minimize the effect of the failure of a single component. Robust downtime contingency plans must be developed should the clinical information systems cease normal function in either planned or unplanned situations. These contingency plans must account for continued data acquisition and retrieval and provide for mechanisms for communication among health care providers and services. Users should be informed about recovery procedures and what they mean to the clinical database. Do backlogged data generated during the down time ever enter the system? How are they timed? Or is there a gap in the clinical information that the clinicians must fill in for themselves if they want the whole picture?

Many anomalous circumstances related to the EHR can threaten patient safety. Data, such as a laboratory value or a physician order, can be entered into the wrong patient record and prompt the clinician to respond appropriately but on the wrong patient. Similarly, data can be displayed in ways that are so confusing that they are interpreted incorrectly.

Default behaviors of portions of the EHR should be designed carefully because busy or distracted clinicians may accept the default without understanding what they are accepting or without considering the consequences. For example, default drug dosing options for renally cleared medications, which might be appropriate for most patients, might not be safe for neonates and patients with renal dysfunction.

Automated Adverse Event Detection

Children are at significant risk for adverse events. By an estimate, every day a child spends in a pediatric ICU in the United States, his or her cumulative risk for an adverse event increases by almost 7%.[35] Traditional methods used to detect adverse events in children included manual chart review and voluntary incident reporting. These detection systems are inefficient and significantly underestimate the number and prevalence of adverse events.[36]

Another detection strategy relies on trigger methodology where an occurrence, found on manual chart review, triggers further investigation to determine the presence of an adverse event.[37] For example, the administration of flumazenil may trigger the detection of benzodiazepine-induced respiratory depression. Automated adverse event detection relies on the generation of a trigger report from the EHR, which indicates the possibility that an adverse event has occurred, requiring further investigation. This methodology has been proven an efficient and cost-effective way to detect adverse events. Other more advanced algorithms for detection of adverse events have been tested, and even though some have been successful, further research and development are necessary in this area.[38]

Smart Infusion Pumps

Errors related to intravenous infusions are often associated with significant harm in the pediatric ICU. A study involving pediatric inpatients noted that intravenous infusions were associated with 54% of potential adverse drug events.[39] Furthermore, adverse drug events associated with intravenous infusion devices generally result from incorrect programming. Smart infusion pumps represent an improved form of pumps,

Problem list:

#1 Septic shock
#2 Respiratory failure
#3 Cauda equina syndrome
#4 History of alcohol abuse
#5 History of Marfan syndrome

Heart

Procedures/Notes: CATH Procedure

Problems - Updated:

ST III	0.2	ECG	13:26	
HR	76	ECHO	N/A	
MBP	59	Troponin T0	N/A	
		Hb	10.9	
		Lactate	0.5	
		SvO2	N/A	
Fluids In [2 hours]	108.41	Hct	33.1	
Phenylephrine	0.1	Active Type	N/A	
Vasopressin	0.03	Blood Loss 4 hr	N/A	
Digoxin	125 MCG	Int Dev#1	Forearm R 20G	
		Int Dev#2	Forearm R	
		Int Dev#3	Hand L 20G	
		Int Dev#4	UppArm R 19/18G	

CVS - Updated: 16:50

Kidney

UOP [4 hours]	790	Na	135	
UOP [24 hours]	3983	Cl	110	
Net Fluids [from mL]	2135	K+	52	
Admission Weight	89	Mg2+	1.9	
Daily Weight	89	Ca2+	3.69	
		PO4–	3.7	
		Arion Gap	10	
		BUN	42	
		CK	N/A	

RENAL - Updated: 16:50

GI

Diet Type	NPO	Albumin	N/A	
Abd. Assmt	Soft	Amylate	N/A	
Bowel Sounds	Hypoactive	Lipase	N/A	
		Bilirubin	N/A	
		Glucose	130.0	
		CT Abdomen	N/A	

GI - Updated: 16:50

Infectious Diseases

Active Meds: Meropenem, levofloxacin

ToC	38.1	Meropenem	500 MG
WCC	18.7		
Microbiology	4		

INFX - Updated: 16:50

Lung

RR	21	Pa02	80	
SpO2	97	pH	7.25	
PF ratio	133	PCO2	39	
Secretions	Large White	HC03	17	
		CXR	14:10	
		CT Chest	N/A	
Ventilator Mode	CMV			
PEEP	5			
TV	410			
P Plat	12			
02%	50			

RESP - Updated: 16:50

Brain

Active Meds: Fentanyl, midazolam, acetaminophen, lorazepam

Procedures/Notes: Consult

GCS	14	CT Brain	N/A
RASS	+3/VAgitated	MRI Brain	N/A
Pain Score #1	0	CNS Angio	N/A
		EEG	N/A
Fentanyl	25		

CNS - Updated: 16:50

Hematology

Hemoglobin	10.9	RBC	N/A
Platelets	233	Platelets	N/A
Hct	33.1	FFP	N/A
APTT	32	Cryoprecipitate	N/A
Heparin	1750		

HEM - Updated: 16:50

Fig. 12.3. Interface with highly relevant information organized around organ systems designed by the research team at Mayo Clinic. (From Ahmed A, Chandra S, Herasevich V, et al. The effect of two different electronic health record user interfaces on intensive care provider task load, errors of cognition, and performance. Crit Care Med. 2011;39:1626-1634.)

and a recent systematic review showed that they significantly reduced programming errors.[40]

Most intravenous infusion pumps in use today have the flexibility and capacity to deliver a wide range of infusion rates and volumes. In an effort to standardize pump systems throughout an organization, the same device may be used to deliver medications to an infant or adolescent. Therefore significant dosing errors can be easily programmed by a bedside provider if there are no double checks or electronic decision-support systems in place. Smart infusion pumps contain sophisticated software that allows for programming medication safety libraries within each pump. In addition, these devices may be queried to allow aggregation and analysis of data regarding infusion practices for quality improvement purposes. Furthermore, some pump vendors offer the ability to connect the device via a wireless network to allow bidirectional flow of information to and from the pumps.

Smart infusion pump medication libraries include drug name, usual concentrations, and dose range checking to avoid high or low dosing for both infusion and bolus dosing. Generally these libraries are created for a given patient care unit, patient population, or provider group. Providers who attempt to program the pump beyond the limits set in the library will encounter an alert that may either be overridden (soft alert) or not overridden (hard alert). The impact of smart infusion pump technology on patient safety is not completely clear at this time. These devices must be paired with optimal design and process change in order to achieve meaningful outcomes.[40]

Medication Bar Coding

In 2004, the FDA published a "Bar Code Rule" mandating manufacturers and repackagers to have a bar code of the National Drug Code on the immediate drug containers label.[41] An integrated system that includes bar coding of medications focuses on preventing errors in drug administration, which may represent up to 38% of medication errors.[42] The essential components for safe medication administration using bar code technology revolve around the "five rights": the right patient, right drug, right dose, right route, and right time. In bar code medication administration, the nurse uses a bedside scanning device to scan the medication, patient's wristband, and nurse's identification. A query is then sent to the EHR to the patient's medication orders. A match on the five rights then signals the nurse that the medication may be administered. Though bar code medication administration systems have been associated with error prevention, they have also been associated with new types of errors, such as those introduced when a busy nurse has to select a medication from a list and document the administration time using a keyboard and mouse.[43] Proper implementation is key to achieving value with these systems.

Privacy and Security of Health Information
Privacy of Health Information

Ensuring the privacy of personal health information has always been a concern, but the availability of this information in electronic form raises new concerns because securing it is not a simple matter of putting it under lock and key. In legislating the Health Insurance Portability and Accountability Act (HIPAA) to protect health insurance coverage for workers and their families when they change or lose their jobs, Congress also sought to alleviate some of the administrative burdens on health care providers by mandating standards for electronic data interchange. Because electronic transactions between providers and insurers would become easier, and more personal health information would become available in electronic form, privacy and security rules were incorporated into the legislation. These rules apply specifically to protected health information (PHI), which is any health information that can be linked to an individual (Box 12.1).

BOX 12.1   Elements Considered Protected Health Information

Names
   All elements of dates (except year) for dates directly related to an individual, including:
      Birth date
      Admission date
      Date of procedure
      Discharge date
      Date of death
   Telephone numbers, fax numbers
   Electronic mail addresses
   Social Security numbers
   Medical record numbers
   Health plan beneficiary numbers
   Account numbers
   Certificate/license numbers
   Vehicle identifiers and serial numbers
   Device identifiers and serial numbers
   Web URLs
   IP address numbers
   Biometric identifiers, including fingerprints and voiceprints
   Full-face photographic images and any comparable images
   All geographic subdivisions smaller than a state, including:
      Street address
      City
      County
      Zip code, and their equivalent geocodes
   Any other unique identifying number, characteristic, or code

---

The privacy rule applies to protected health information whether it is stored in electronic form or not. The rule limits the nonconsensual use or release of protected health information, gives patients new rights to access their medical records and to know who accessed them, restricts most disclosures of health information to the minimum needed for the intended purpose, establishes penalties for improper use or disclosure, and establishes new requirements for access to records by researchers and others. The impact of HIPAA on research relates to consent paperwork that safeguards the privacy of patients participating in research, simplified guidelines regarding the limited circumstances where patient health information can be used for research purposes without authorization by the research subject, and clarifying methods by which protected patient health information can be de-identified so that such information can be disclosed freely.[44]

With regard to health data integration and sharing, the concept of privacy can be considered a double-edged sword: too much risks blocking progress and limiting research; too little risks loss of public trust and confidence and potentially undermines a well-intended effort.[45] Both overregulation and underregulation have their problems, and striking a balance is essential. In a survey for clinical scientists on patient privacy and its effects on research, most of the respondents felt that the HIPAA Privacy Rule did not enhance privacy for patients and resulted in increased difficulty to complete research studies.[46] For these and other reasons, the Institute of Medicine recommended in their *Best Care at Lower Cost* report to "streamline and revise research regulations to improve care, promote the capture of clinical data, and generate knowledge."[3] The Institute proposed two strategies to achieve this goal: 1) to expand and accelerate the review of HIPAA and institutional review board policies and address the potential impediments they might be causing to research and 2) to engage patients, clinicians, health care organizations and other stakeholders to develop strategies that improve the understanding of the benefits of using clinical data in meaningful ways.

Security of Health Information

The security of a networked system involves at least three components: physical security, prevention of unauthorized access, and protection from malicious software.

Physical access to sensitive portions of the system must be secure. Servers should be in locked rooms with controlled access. Networking closets with wiring and hubs should be locked. Sensitive equipment must be protected from extreme temperatures, fire, and water damage. Backup power sources are required. Workstations, wherever possible, should be in open areas where their use can be monitored but not so open that unauthorized persons can peer over a user's shoulder to steal a user name and password or see sensitive information. Physical security also involves ensuring that the data are backed up and readily accessible whenever they are needed.

Preventing unauthorized electronic access involves blocking attacks from the outside and authenticating legitimate users before allowing them access. Wireless networks must be configured to minimize the risk of intruders tapping into the system. Systems can be attacked by malicious software, loosely labeled as viruses. Securing systems from these threats is becoming increasingly challenging.

The HIPPA Security Rule attempts to provide a uniform level of protection of all protected health information that is housed or transmitted electronically. These standards mandate safeguards for physical storage and maintenance of equipment that contains patient data. Network closets and servers should be locked up, and data must be backed up. The displays of computers in public areas should be turned away from open view, and screens should be installed to limit the viewing angle. Storing protected health information on computers in unlocked offices, on laptops, or on removable media such as flash drives is prohibited unless the data are encrypted. Users should log out of applications that access PHI when those applications are no longer needed. Access to data must be limited to authorized personnel on an as-needed basis with clear administrative policies for granting and revoking those privileges. There must also be technical safeguards to prevent unauthorized intrusion into networks or interception of transmissions over open networks. Firewalls should protect hospital networks, particularly if there are wireless access points. PHI should never be sent by email without encryption because standard email is inherently insecure.

Telemedicine

Telemedicine in pediatrics refers to use of electronic communications technology to provide health care for infants, children, adolescents, and young adults when geographic distance separates the clinician from the patient, caretaker, or referring practitioner.[47] Pediatric subspecialties, including critical care, have experimented in telemedicine for decades, and evidence suggests that such care is both clinically and cost-effective. Although many technical, legal, and financial hurdles remain, telemedicine remains a viable and valuable care delivery model for critical care.[48]

Even though intensivist coverage in ICUs is associated with a reduction in mortality and resource utilization,[49] the cost and shortage of intensivists can preclude hospitals in areas of need from providing these services. Despite the fact that "tele-ICU" care cannot replace on-site expert care, studies have shown that the use of telemedicine can result in higher quality of care, more efficient resource utilization, and higher satisfaction by patients and providers.[48,50]

The cost of implementation of a telemedicine program in an ICU can be substantial—in the order of tens of thousands of dollars per monitored bed—which can play a significant role in its cost-effectiveness.[51] Many programs use fixed cameras and microphones in patient rooms and remote connections to physiologic monitors and EHRs.[50] Robots can even roam between patient's rooms.[52] Using today's advances in technology, it is also possible to implement it inexpensively with a mobile computer configured with a web cam and wireless connection[53] or even by staff members armed with a smartphone.

"Big Data" in Critical Care

The digitalization of health care is opening the door to an era of big data in medicine. Larger and larger datasets of biomedical information will become available to researchers in every field of health care, providing an opportunity to gain tremendous insight from them. Data from genomic, proteomic, physiologic monitoring, imaging, operational, and financial datasets are starting to enrich clinical data warehouses everywhere, but much of that data still remains underanalyzed.[54] If we develop the appropriate infrastructure to learn from these data and use it to improve care, we could benefit from the disruptive phenomenon of big data, much like the retail, manufacturing, and financial industries have done.[4]

Biomedical advances and the availability of massive amounts of patient-related data also come with an inevitable consequence: a growing knowledge gap. While medical knowledge continues to grow exponentially, the cognitive capacity of a human brain remains fixed. David Eddy, one of the fathers of evidenced-based medicine, eloquently said that "the complexity of modern medicine exceeds the inherent limitations of the unaided human mind,"[55] and that was more than a quarter of a century ago. The reality is that clinicians, like other human beings, are excellent at pattern recognition but significantly underperform with complex information processing tasks.[54] Evidence shows that the human brain cannot simultaneously consider more than about four pieces of information at one time in order to make a decision, something that is increasingly misaligned with today's health care environment. Advanced analytic algorithms and decision support systems could bridge this knowledge gap by sifting through the deluge of data, performing complex processing tasks, and presenting the bedside clinician with the most relevant pieces of information about the patient in order to enhance the decision-making process. Whether this will become a reality of everyday medicine remains to be seen.

Critical care medicine could especially benefit from big data–driven research. On the one hand, we routinely use many interventions and practices in the ICU that lack evidence to support them in an evermore complex clinical environment and on the other hand, we have a tremendous amount of structured data being generated by a myriad of monitoring devices, laboratory tests, and clinician charting that could be analyzed to improve our understanding of critical illness and the therapies we use. Some experts advocate the development of highly detailed critical care databases in order to inform the design of clinical investigations, develop decision support systems, and test clinical algorithms using real-world data.[11]

Health Analytics

A health analytics program, also known as health data mining or data science program, is a data-driven research and development program within a health care organization. While the emphasis of such a program might range from the purely clinical to a more business/financial focus, the common goal of health analytics programs is to exploit the data resources in an organization to improve processes, reduce costs, and provide better care.[54] A health analytics program requires competencies in several areas of the data life cycle, and a multidisciplinary team composed of clinicians, engineers, statisticians, and other stakeholders is most likely to produce the most beneficial program. Three key areas of a health analytics program are:

1. *Data management.* This includes data capturing, aggregation, and structuring for analysis, as well as the overarching competencies of data governance and quality assurance. Data management is probably the most resource intensive of the components of a health analytics program and requires a significant institutional commitment.
2. *Statistical learning.* The analysis of large biomedical data can be performed using traditional biostatistical analyses, as well as machine learning algorithms, which become necessary with more complex, multidimensional datasets. The goal of the statistical learning is to apply mathematical principles to the data in order to describe past events, understand current trends, and build prediction models.
3. *Information and knowledge delivery.* The final step in a health analytics program is possibly the most critical step. How effectively the insight gained from the data is delivered to the decision makers can determine the success of a program. Less sophisticated modes of information delivery such as reports or alerts will likely have a lower impact than more advanced forms of clinical decision support, predicative modeling, or systems optimization.

Clinical Data Research Networks

As the advanced analytic capabilities of individual health care organizations are developing, there is another important trend in health care: the aggregation of clinical data across institutions. Integrating data from multiple databases to form repositories for new discovery is not an easy task. Several barriers, both technical and nontechnical, such as security, interoperability, privacy, and data ownership, can limit the scope of these projects, but there are promising new initiatives taking place.

One of the most notable initiatives is the clinical research network proposed by the Patient-Centered Outcomes Research Institute (PCORI).[56] PCORI was created under the Affordable Care Act of 2010 to promote comparative effectiveness research across the United States. PCORnet, the National Patient-Centered Clinical Research Network, is a PCORI-based initiative to create a large, highly representative network for conducting clinical outcomes research. PCORnet's proposed infrastructure is composed of 11 health system–based

networks and 18 patient group–based networks, and its goal is to generate interoperable datasets to support multinetwork observational and randomized clinical studies.[57]

The pediatric community has long made use of the Pediatric Health Information System (PHIS), a clinical-financial claims database with more than 6 million cases. PHIS is currently embarking on a proof-of-concept project called PHIS+ with the specific aim of developing the infrastructure to link laboratory results and radiologic reports from six large children's hospitals in the United States to the administrative data from PHIS in order to enhance its granularity and facilitate research.[58]

The true value of these clinical data research networks cannot yet be predicted, but there can be no argument that the limitation of most studies in pediatrics and critical care is currently the paucity of data available from single institutions. In aggregate, who knows what we may learn?

MIMIC Database

The Multi-parameter Intelligent Monitoring in Intensive Care (MIMIC) database is a public-access database containing clinical data for more than 40,000 adult and neonatal ICU patients from Beth Israel Deaconess Medical Center in Boston, Massachusetts, and is hosted by the Laboratory of Computational Physiology at the Massachusetts Institute of Technology.[11] MIMIC, which is now on its second version, also contains physiologic waveform data from monitoring devices for about a fourth of its patients. In addition, researchers from around the world routinely contribute series of patients to the database with physiologic waveform data from devices such as electroencephalograms, near-infrared spectroscopy monitors, and fetal electrocardiograms. The clinical data in MIMIC is de-identified and has been shared with more than 600 researchers from more than 32 countries, and it has been used to produce hundreds of peer-reviewed papers. MIMIC is offered along with numerous open-access toolkits to facilitate tasks such as query building, data visualization, and time-series analysis. It is an excellent research resource for the critical care community, and even though it does not contain any pediatric ICU patients at this point, there are plans on making that addition in future versions of the database.[59]

Virtual Pediatric ICU Systems

In collaboration with the National Association of Children's Hospitals and Related Institutions, Child Health Corporation of America (now the Children's Hospital Association), and the National Outcomes Center located at Milwaukee Children's Hospital and Medical System, the Virtual PICU, funded by the Children's Hospital Los Angeles and the L.K. Whittier Foundation, developed a data collection tool specifically designed to understand pediatric critical care, the distribution of demographics, diagnoses, and outcomes and to form a basis for clinical research, quality improvement, and, ultimately, comparative data analysis. Over the years, there has been a significant expansion of the database, and it has evolved into a comprehensive tool for quality improvement and benchmarking.[60]

As of 2014, there are 119 PICUs participating in the web-based application of Virtual PICU Systems (VPSs) that now includes more than 1 million patient admissions. Affiliated institutions participate in an advisory committee, a users' group organization with annual meetings, and a research committee. They also receive periodic comparative quality reports detailing the performance of their ICUs along multiple axes, modeled on the Institute of Medicine's "Six Dimensions of Quality."

The VPS database has been used extensively to inform pediatric critical care research. Merely providing demographics and descriptions and diagnostic patterns in critical care has aided the design of multiple national research projects and National Institutes of Health–funded projects. However, the core purpose of the prospective data collection is quality improvement, allowing comparative data reporting against comparable but unidentified institutions. These reports enable intensivists to objectively demonstrate the quality of the care they provide.

Conclusion and Future Directions

Medicine is an information service, and critical care is perhaps the most information-intensive medical subspecialty. It is no accident that many intensivists have a particular interest in health IT, but every practitioner will be more effective if he or she obtains the skills to better manage the flow of information. Furthermore, as physician leaders focusing on health IT, intensivists can lead the way in creating a safer environment for all patients. Understanding the limitations and pitfalls of the technology and exercising caution as it is implemented is of paramount importance for success.

As everyday users of health IT, intensivists should understand the threats to privacy and security, not only for our patients but also for ourselves. Systems are as vulnerable as their weakest link. Sustained vigilance and safe computing practices are essential to avoid calamitous data loss or exposure to exploitation.

The wider adoption of health IT is also fueling new trends in data sharing, analytics, and collaborative research, at a scale never before seen in health care. The impact that this can have in the practice of medicine has yet to be determined, but as frontline care providers of the most vulnerable and information-intensive patients, intensivists must continue to play a central role in the development and use of information technologies in our field.

Acknowledgments

We gratefully acknowledge the contribution of Carl Weigle, MD, and Brian Jacobs, MD, FCCM, who authored this chapter in previous editions.

References

1. Office of the National Coordinator for Health Information Technology. 2014; Available at: www.HealthIT.gov.
2. Grossman C, McGinnis JM. *Digital Infrastructure for the Learning Health System: The Foundation for Continuous Improvement in Health and Health Care: Workshop Series Summary.* Washington, DC: National Academies Press; 2011.
3. Smith M, Saunders R, Stuckhardt L, McGinnis JM. *Best Care at Lower Cost: the Path to Continuously Learning Health Care in America.* Washington, DC: National Academies Press; 2013.
4. Brown B, Chui M, Manyika J. *Are You Ready for the Era of "Big Data"?* New York City, NY: McKinsey Global Institute; 2011.
5. Blumenthal D. Launching HIteCH. *N Engl J Med.* 2010;362:382-385.
6. Deleted in review.
6. Hersh W. The health information technology workforce: estimations of demands and a framework for requirements. *Appl Clin Inform.* 2010;1:197-212.
7. Gardner RM, Safran C. *Clinical Informatics Subspecialty Certification and Training. Informatics Education in Healthcare.* New York, NY: Springer; 2014:43-58.
8. Lehmann HP. *Aspects of Electronic Health Record Systems.* New York, NY: Springer; 2006.
9. Towards a Service-Oriented Architecture for Interconnecting Medical Devices and Applications. *High Confidence Medical Devices, Software, and Systems and Medical Device Plug-and-Play Interoperability, 2007.* HCMDSS-MDPnP. Joint Workshop. New York, NY: IEEE; 2007.
10. Wang D, Rundensteiner EA, Wang H, Ellison RT III. Active complex event processing: applications in real-time health care. *Proceedings VLDB Endowment.* 2010;3:1545-1548.
11. Anthony Celi L, Mark RG, Stone DJ, Montgomery RA. "Big data" in the intensive care unit. Closing the data loop. *Am J Respir Crit Care Med.* 2013;187:1157-1160.
12. Schweitzer EJ. Reconciliation of the cloud computing model with US federal electronic health record regulations. *J Am Med Inform Assoc.* 2012;19:161-165.
13. Amarasingham R, Pronovost PJ, Diener-West M, et al. Measuring clinical information technology in the ICU setting: application in a quality improvement collaborative. *J Am Med Inform Assoc.* 2007;14:288-294.
14. Amarasingham R, Plantinga L, Diener-West M, et al. Clinical information technologies and inpatient outcomes: a multiple hospital study. *Arch Intern Med.* 2009;169:108-114.
15. Bright TJ, Wong A, Dhurjati R, et al. Effect of clinical decision-support systems: a systematic review. *Ann Intern Med.* 2012;157:29-43.
16. Ash JS, Sittig DF, Dykstra R, et al. The unintended consequences of computerized provider order entry: findings from a mixed methods exploration. *Int J Med Inf.* 2009;78:S69-S76.
17. Kesselheim AS, Cresswell K, Phansalkar S, et al. Clinical decision support systems could be modified to reduce 'alert fatigue' while still minimizing the risk of litigation. *Health Aff (Millwood).* 2011;30:2310-2317.
18. Carspecken CW, Sharek PJ, Longhurst C, Pageler NM. A clinical case of electronic health record drug alert fatigue: consequences for patient outcome. *Pediatrics.* 2013;131:e1970-e1973.
19. Harrison MI, Koppel R, Bar-Lev S. Unintended consequences of information technologies in health care—an interactive sociotechnical analysis. *J Am Med Inform Assoc.* 2007;14:542-549.
20. Johnson CM, Johnson TR, Zhang J. A user-centered framework for redesigning health care interfaces. *J Biomed Inform.* 2005;38:75-87.
21. Scott JT, Rundall TG, Vogt TM, Hsu J. Kaiser Permanente's experience of implementing an electronic medical record: a qualitative study. *BMJ.* 2005;331:1313-1316.
22. Schulman J, Kuperman GJ, Kharbanda A, Kaushal R. Discovering how to think about a hospital patient information system by struggling to evaluate it: a committee's journal. *J Am Med Inform Assoc.* 2007;14:537-541.
23. Osheroff JA, Teich JM, Middleton B, et al. A roadmap for national action on clinical decision support. *J Am Med Inform Assoc.* 2007;14:141-145.
24. Musen MA, Middleton B, Greenes RA. *Clinical Decision-Support Systems. Biomedical Informatics.* New York, NY: Springer; 2014:643-674.
25. Bates DW, Kuperman GJ, Wang S, et al. Ten commandments for effective clinical decision support: making the practice of evidence-based medicine a reality. *J Am Med Inform Assoc.* 2003;10:523-530.
26. Bobb AM, Payne TH, Gross PA. Viewpoint: controversies surrounding use of order sets for clinical decision support in computerized provider order entry. *J Am Med Inform Assoc.* 2007;14:41-47.
27. Potts AL, Barr FE, Gregory DF, et al. Computerized physician order entry and medication errors in a pediatric critical care unit. *Pediatrics.* 2004;113:59-63.
28. Moorman JR, Carlo WA, Kattwinkel J, et al. Mortality reduction by heart rate characteristic monitoring in very low birth weight neonates: a randomized trial. *J Pediatr.* 2011;159:900-906. e1.
29. Duran-Nelson A, Gladding S, Beattie J, Nixon LJ. Should we Google it? Resource use by internal medicine residents for point-of-care clinical decision making. *Acad Med.* 2013;88:788-794.
30. Hersh WR. *Information Retrieval: A Health and Biomedical Perspective.* New York NY: Springer; 2009.
31. Ahmed A, Chandra S, Herasevich V, et al. The effect of two different electronic health record user interfaces on intensive care provider task load, errors of cognition, and performance. *Crit Care Med.* 2011;39:1626-1634.

32. Mack EH, Wheeler DS, Embi PJ. Clinical decision support systems in the pediatric intensive care unit. *Pediatr Crit Care Med.* 2009;10:23-28.

33. Strom BL, Schinnar R, Aberra F, et al. Unintended effects of a computerized physician order entry nearly hard-stop alert to prevent a drug interaction: a randomized controlled trial. *Arch Intern Med.* 2010;170:1578-1583.

34. Karsh BT. Beyond usability: designing effective technology implementation systems to promote patient safety. *Qual Saf Health Care.* 2004;13:388-394.

35. Agarwal S, Classen D, Larsen G, et al. Prevalence of adverse events in pediatric intensive care units in the United States. *Pediatr Crit Care Med.* 2010;11:568-578.

36. Ferranti J, Horvath MM, Cozart H, et al. Reevaluating the safety profile of pediatrics: a comparison of computerized adverse drug event surveillance and voluntary reporting in the pediatric environment. *Pediatrics.* 2008;121:e1201-e1207.

37. Rozich JD, Haraden CR, Resar RK. Adverse drug event trigger tool: a practical methodology for measuring medication related harm. *Qual Saf Health Care.* 2003;12:194-200.

38. Forster AJ, Jennings A, Chow C, et al. A systematic review to evaluate the accuracy of electronic adverse drug event detection. *J Am Med Inform Assoc.* 2012;19:31-38.

39. Kaushal R, Bates DW, Landrigan C, et al. Medication errors and adverse drug events in pediatric inpatients. *JAMA.* 2001;285:2114-2120.

40. Ohashi K, Dalleur O, Dykes PC, Bates DW. Benefits and risks of using smart pumps to reduce medication error rates: a systematic review. *Drug Safety.* 2014;37:1011-1020.

41. Food and Drug Administration, HHS. Bar code label requirement for human drug products and biological products. Final rule. *Fed Regist.* 2004;69:9119-9171.

42. Leape LL, Bates DW, Cullen DJ, et al. Systems analysis of adverse drug events. *JAMA.* 1995;274:35-43.

43. Poon EG, Keohane CA, Yoon CS, et al. Effect of bar-code technology on the safety of medication administration. *N Engl J Med.* 2010;362:1698-1707.

44. Nosowsky R, Giordano TJ. The Health Insurance Portability and Accountability Act of 1996 (HIPAA) privacy rule: implications for clinical research. *Annu Rev Med.* 2006;57:575-590.

45. McGraw D, Dempsey JX, Harris L, Goldman J. Privacy as an enabler, not an impediment: building trust into health information exchange. *Health Aff (Millwood).* 2009;28:416-427.

46. Ness RB, Joint Policy Committee, Societies of Epidemiology. Influence of the HIPAA Privacy Rule on health research. *JAMA.* 2007;298:2164-2170.

47. Spooner SA, Gotlieb EM. Telemedicine: pediatric applications. *Pediatrics.* 2004;113:e639-e643.

48. Marcin JP. Telemedicine in the pediatric intensive care unit. *Pediatr Clin North Am.* 2013;60:581-592.

49. Wilcox ME, Chong CA, Niven DJ, et al. Do intensivist staffing patterns influence hospital mortality following ICU admission? A systematic review and meta-analyses. *Crit Care Med.* 2013;41:2253-2274.

50. Thomas EJ, Lucke JF, Wueste L, et al. Association of telemedicine for remote monitoring of intensive care patients with mortality, complications, and length of stay. *JAMA.* 2009;302:2671-2678.

51. Kumar G, Falk DM, Bonello RS, et al. The costs of critical care telemedicine programs: a systematic review and analysis. *CHEST J.* 2013;143:19-29.

52. Garingo A, Friedlich P, Tesoriero L, et al. The use of mobile robotic telemedicine technology in the neonatal intensive care unit. *J Perinatol.* 2012;32:55-63.

53. Yager PH, Cummings BM, Whalen MJ, Noviski N. Nighttime telecommunication between remote staff intensivists and bedside personnel in a pediatric intensive care unit: a retrospective study. *Crit Care Med.* 2012;40:2700-2703.

54. Burke J. *Health Analytics: Gaining the Insights to Transform Health Care.* Hoboken, NJ: John Wiley & Sons; 2013.

55. Eddy DM. Clinical decision making: from theory to practice. Practice policies—what are they? *JAMA.* 1990;263:877-878, 880.

56. Selby JV, Beal AC, Frank L. The Patient-Centered Outcomes Research Institute (PCORI) national priorities for research and initial research agenda. *JAMA.* 2012;307:1583-1584.

57. Selby JV, Lipstein SH. PCORI at 3 years—progress, lessons, and plans. *N Engl J Med.* 2014;370:592-595.

58. Keren R. *PHIS: Augmenting the Pediatric Health Information System with Clinical Data.* Philadelphia, PA: Children's Hospital of Philadelphia; 2013.

59. MIMIC II Databases. Available at: <http://physionet.org/mimic2/>. Accessed 24.02.15.

60. Virtual PICU Systems LLC. 2015; Available at: <http://www.myvps.org>.

Building Partnerships: Patient- and Family-Centered Care in the Pediatric Intensive Care Unit

Jonna Derbenwick Clark

" 'Intensive care unit.' Wow, those are scary words for parents to hear! … We viewed the intensive care unit as a place people went when their medical situation was desperate or where they were likely to die."[2]

PEARLS

- Patient- and family-centered care (PFCC) uses an "innovative approach to the planning, delivery, and evaluation of health care that is grounded in a mutually beneficial partnership among patients, families, and providers."[1]
- Fundamental principles of PFCC include:
  - Honoring differences and respecting each individual patient and family
  - Maintaining flexibility in practice, policies, and procedures to fully accommodate the needs of patients and families
  - Sharing honest and consistent information using collaborative communication
  - Using a transdisciplinary approach to provide optimal support for the family unit
  - Developing a partnership built on mutual respect among health care providers, patients, and families
  - Empowering patients and families to participate in shared medical decision making
- Incorporating PFCC into practice improves patient and family satisfaction, reduces stress and anxiety, fosters the parent-child relationship, and ultimately increases the quality, efficacy, efficiency, and safety of health care delivered.
- Overcoming real and perceived barriers to incorporating PFCC into practice requires an explicit, collaborative, and transparent approach involving all stakeholders to identify creative solutions.

Many parents share this perspective when faced with the hospitalization of a critically ill child.[2] These families not only face the extreme crisis of having a sick child whose life may be threatened; they are forced into a foreign environment and culture that can be intimidating, overwhelming, and perceived as unwelcoming. Families in the ICU are at one of the worst moments in their lives and suffer from an extreme level of stress, where they may feel powerless and out of control. This level of stress creates short- and long-term consequences, as many parents and children face severe emotional distress, which may result in posttraumatic stress disorder (see also Chapter 10).[3-7]

In order to mitigate the severity of this stress response and optimize the quality of medical care provided, patient- and family-centered care (PFCC) is a philosophy that highlights the importance of including the patient, when possible, and family in the provision of health care. The American Academy of Pediatrics (AAP) acknowledges that the "family is the primary source of a child's strength and support" and defines PFCC as "an innovative approach to the planning, delivery, and evaluation of health care that is grounded in a mutually beneficial partnership among patients, families, and providers."[1] PFCC can be incorporated across the spectrum of health care, from home to outpatient to inpatient, and is essential for the provision of high-quality care in the intensive care unit. Ongoing research in this area demonstrates that parent participation in the care of a hospitalized child directly benefits the child by reducing anxiety, improving cooperation, improving activity level, and reducing the length of stay.[8] Additional data reveal more effective utilization of health care resources, reduced health care costs, and improved provider satisfaction.[1]

Definition of "Family"

In the delivery of PFCC, patients and families, rather than health care providers or the legal system, define their families.[9,10] Because family structures are heterogeneous and evolve over time within a variety of cultural contexts, the term *family* requires a broad definition, referring to "two or more persons who are related in any way—biologically, legally, or emotionally."[9,10] A wide variety of family structures exist, including blended families, single-parent households, adoptive homes, same-sex couples, and transgenerational models where extended family members, such as grandparents, aunts, uncles, or siblings, serve as the primary caretakers.[7,9,10] Although health care providers and institutions have a legal obligation to respect the law regarding surrogate decision making for minors, they also have an ethical and professional obligation to respect the broader definition of family in practice, acknowledging that the family is the primary source of strength and support for the child.[1,8]

Historical Evolution of Patient- and Family-Centered Care

The conceptual aspects of PFCC date back to the 1950s, when studies demonstrated a negative impact of maternal-child separation, leading to a shift toward encouraging parent participation in the care of the hospitalized child.[1,8,10,11] In 1983, the Committee on Hospital Care and Pediatric Section of the Society of Critical Care Medicine published *Guidelines for Pediatric Intensive Care Units,* highlighting that, "Parents should be allowed to stay with the critically ill child as much as possible."[12] These guidelines explained that the presence of parents may lead to faster recovery, stating, "The familiar face and voice of a parent may reach a child who appears comatose but is beginning to respond to stimuli."[12] In the following 2 decades, there was extensive research in the value and benefit of PFCC in health care communities. Several national organizations were founded, including Family Voices, an organization that advocates for family-centered, community-based services for children with special needs, in addition to the Institute for Patient- and Family-Centered Care, an organization that helps foster partnerships among health care professionals, patients, and families to advance family-centered care in health care settings.[1] More recently, several national organizations including the Institute of Medicine (2001), Maternal and Child Health Bureau (2005), American College of Critical Care Medicine (ACCCM) Task Force (2007), and American Academy of Pediatrics (2012) have furthered this approach by developing guidelines and endorsing that PFCC is essential to the provision of high-quality care.[1,13]

Fundamental Needs of Patients and Families in the ICU

Because of the complexity and intensity of the pediatric intensive care unit (PICU), families' needs are high. Although specific needs of the individual patient and family are important to consider, there is consensus that most families share similar needs including: 1) honest, accurate, and up-to-date information; 2) close proximity to the patient; 3) timely notification of any changes in the patient's condition; 4) assurance that the health care team cares about the child and that the patient is receiving excellent care; 5) access to resources to meet basic physiologic needs; and 6) feeling that there is hope.[7,14-17] Research demonstrates that provider perceptions often underestimate the needs of families. Furthermore, when families' needs *are* known, they are not adequately addressed in practice. Unfortunately, when families' needs are not met, there is a negative impact on satisfaction with care, in addition to a greater amount of stress and anxiety.[6,7,17]

Core Principles of Patient- and Family-Centered Care[1,11]

The practice of PFCC, in which patients and families are treated as integral partners with the health care team, is now

---

BOX 13.1   Core Principles of Patient- and Family-Centered Care

- Honor differences and demonstrate respect for each individual child and her family
- Maintain flexibility in procedures, policies, planning, and delivery of health care
- Share information using collaborative communication through a variety of approaches, including written information, bedside updates, family-centered rounds, and transdisciplinary care conferences
- Provide informal and formal support for the child and family using a transdisciplinary model of practice
- Collaborate with patients and families through the development of a partnership at all levels of health care
- Empower patients and families to participate in shared medical decision making

Adapted from American Academy of Pediatrics. Patient- and family-centered care and the pediatrician's role. Pediatrics. 2012;129:394-404.

---

recognized as the standard of care in pediatric critical care medicine.[1,11] Borrowing from the framework established by the AAP, the following discussion highlights each of the fundamental principles of PFCC within the context of the pediatric intensive care unit[1] (Box 13.1).

1. Honoring Differences and Respecting Each Child and Family

One of the most fundamental aspects of developing a "mutually beneficial partnership" with patients and their families requires a relationship of mutual respect, in which differences among the stakeholders are honored.[1] The AAP states, "Listen to and respect … each child and family's innate strengths and cultural values. Honor racial, ethnic, cultural, and socioeconomic background and patient and family experiences."[1] Recognizing that one individual cannot be an expert on all cultures, faiths, ethnicities, spirituality, or religious practices, practicing cultural humility is crucial, acknowledging biases and assumptions.[18] All admissions to the ICU are extremely distressing, whether a child suffers from acute respiratory failure due to respiratory syncytial virus or has multiple organ dysfunction syndrome following a bone marrow transplant. Patients and families demonstrate a wide range of responses within their own social construct, using a variety of coping mechanisms to overcome the distressing state.

In the ICU, where major medical decisions regarding life, death, and quality of life are often made in a short time frame, differences in beliefs and value systems may be accentuated among health care providers and families. Furthermore, in an environment of extreme stress, where patients and families are in state of crisis, tensions between the stakeholders may be exacerbated. Taking the time to listen to different perspectives and understand how knowledge, past experiences, and value systems impact decisions is essential. In the majority of situations, families and health care providers desire what is in the best interest for the child. Acknowledging that values and belief systems affect perceptions of what actions are in the best interest for the child can be helpful when navigating challenging circumstances. For example, parents of a beloved child who suffers from a life-threatening illness with a poor prognosis may choose to prolong life as long as possible, treasuring and valuing each day they have with their child alive, while health care providers may view prolonging life as merely prolonging suffering. Developing a collaborative relationship ensures that differences in opinion are respected.

For non–English-speaking patients and families, where fundamental communication and language barriers exist, developing a partnership built on trust and understanding may be especially difficult. The use of in-person language interpreters and cultural navigators who serve as health care guides for the family and cultural guides for the health care providers is essential to building this relationship. Optimizing additional means for communication with non–English-speaking families, such as a video interpreter service, can also be beneficial.

2. Maintaining Flexibility in Practice and Procedures to Deliver Health Care Within the Context of the Family

The PICU is a highly complex environment that requires a systematic approach to policies and protocols to ensure the delivery of efficient, effective, and safe health care. When developing these policies and protocols, it is essential to recognize how these systems and processes impact patients and families. Hospital systems and organizations need to "ensure flexibility in organizational policies, procedures, and provider practices so services can be tailored to the needs, beliefs, and cultural values of each child and family."[1] Practices and procedures should "facilitate choice … about approaches to care."[1]

Historically, hospitals were designed as sterile environments that restricted visitation, with fear of spread of infection and the breach of confidentiality.[10] However, with the evolution of PFCC, many health care organizations and institutions are making the effort to better accommodate patients' and families' needs by including them in the planning and delivery of care. When a child is hospitalized in the ICU, the needs of the family are extremely high.[7,16,17] Addressing many of these needs can be approached considering the following categories: 1) visitation policies and physical accommodations for families, 2) family-centered rounds, 3) family presence during cardiopulmonary resuscitation and other invasive procedures, and 4) collaborative communication.[13,19] When assessing the potential benefits and harms of policies, procedures, and delivery of health care in these areas, open dialogue and transparency regarding the needs of all the stakeholders are essential, allowing for creative solutions when conflicts arise.

Geography of ICU

In planning and designing an ICU, the geography of the unit needs to accommodate both health care providers and patients and families. For example, a unit that allows for effective and efficient management of multiple critically ill patients is essential for health care providers, while patients and families need privacy, space in close proximity to their child, and access to an area where they may find respite from the intensive environment to build strength and repose.[12,20]

Admission Process and Visiting Hours

Parents and family members should be treated as partners, rather than visitors, within the ICU. They should feel welcomed into the foreign environment through the use of a variety of communication styles, both spoken and written, and remain well informed of processes and procedures. In general, visiting hours for parents and primary caretakers should be nonrestrictive in order to optimize parent and child bonding.[13] However, maintaining flexibility in these visiting policies is important as there may be unique circumstances when limiting visitation by family members is necessary to create a calm and healing environment for the child.

Creating a "Personalized" Room

Patients and families should have the liberty to create an environment that mimics home, with decorations, photographs, favorite toys, and blankets as long as the modifications do not place the child at risk and do not interfere with the provision of medical care.[12,13] Although the ICU is a place of work for the health care providers, it is the bedroom for a critically ill child and potentially may be the last place a dying child spends time.[21] Creating a home environment is beneficial to not only the child but also the health care team in that it helps providers gain insight into who the child is as a person, enabling them to address the needs of the child more appropriately.

Sibling Participation

Siblings of critically ill children are severely affected and need to be supported according to the values of the family.[7,22] Siblings need maintenance of a familiar lifestyle, including family cohesion, distraction from the immediate crisis, hospital visitation, and developmentally appropriate information.[7] The transdisciplinary team, including child life specialists and social workers, can help educate parents and caregivers about anticipated questions and emotional responses that may occur and provide appropriate referral services and support systems.[22]

Parental Presence During Cardiopulmonary Resuscitation and Invasive Procedures

Numerous professional organizations, including the American Heart Association and ACCCM, endorse offering families the option to remain in close proximity to their loved ones during cardiopulmonary resuscitation and invasive procedures.[23,24] Allowing family presence has direct benefits for parents and caregivers, including improved satisfaction, better understanding, reduced anxiety, better coping, more emotional stability, and improved adjustment to a child's death.[24-26] Despite these potential benefits, the practice remains controversial. Clinicians raise concerns that parental presence may increase the risk for litigation and may impact technical performance, clinical decision making, and the ability to teach.[24,25] In a large single-center study, using formal practice guidelines and interprofessional education to prepare clinicians for parental presence, "few clinicians reported that parent presence affected their technical performance (4%), therapeutic decision making (5%), or ability to teach (9%)."[25] By developing protocols, institutional policies, education, and dedicated staff resources to allow parental choice and provide support for parental presence during invasive procedures and cardiopulmonary resuscitation, these concerns can be minimized.[24]

Transition Points and Follow-Up Care, Including Bereavement

Once adjusted to the ICU, many families ultimately appreciate the high level of physician supervision and nursing presence, making transitions to the acute care floor potentially difficult. Supporting families through these transitions during the course of an illness is necessary.[27] For families who spend an especially long period of time in the ICU, providing families with realistic expectations and allowing the family to visit the acute care floor before transfer can be beneficial. In addition to providing additional support for transitions between different geographic locations in the hospital, developing a framework to help families transition through different approaches to care, from curative to life prolonging to comfort care, is important.[19] Furthermore, using a systematic approach to follow up with families following the death of child, with condolence letters and formal follow-up meetings, is also necessary to reduce the perception of abandonment and improve the bereavement process. (See also Chapters 15 to 16.)[16,28,29,30]

Sharing Information Using Collaborative Communication

High-quality communication with families is essential in the ICU where medical information is complex and detailed, high stakes decisions are required, and multiple teams of health care providers are involved.[31] While there is a spectrum of preferred decision-making roles of families, ranging from an independent and autonomous approach to delegating decisions to clinicians, most families need to be well informed.[5] Optimizing communication with families reinforces the development of a partnership with families, acknowledging the important role of parents and caregivers and their unique knowledge of their child. The AAP recommends, "sharing complete, honest, and unbiased information with patients and their families on an ongoing basis so that they may effectively participate in care and decision making."[1]

Over the past 2 decades, there has been extensive research in optimizing communication among health care providers, particularly in the ICU and surrounding end-of-life care decision making. (See also Chapter 16.)[30,32,33] In the ICU, information is shared using three different verbal models, including individual updates at the bedside, family-centered rounds, and formal care conferences. Written information may also be provided. Often a combination of all these approaches is necessary to optimize communication with patients and families. Depending on the educational, social, and cultural backgrounds of patients and families, in addition to different provider styles, a variety of approaches to communication may be used.

Elements of High-Quality Communication

Sharing medical information is complex and requires a high level of skill among health care providers (see also Chapter 4). Although using a variety of means to communicate with patients and families is necessary, the language used and other specific elements are also important. According to parents, high-quality elements of communication include: "comprehensive and complete information; clarity of information with the use of clear language; ease of access to caregivers and their explanations through the course of care; pacing of information, soliciting of parents' emotional responses, and addressing their questions; consistency of information; honesty; lack of false hope; empathy as demonstrated verbally and nonverbally; effective communication; summary statements; and next steps."[22,33,34] A useful tool is the VALUE mnemonic, where family statements are *Valued*, family emotions are *Acknowledged*, the family is *Listened* to, the patient is *Understood* as a person, and family questions are *Elicited*.[35] This mnemonic

emphasizes the importance of using collaborative communication, or a form of communication in which interpersonal communication and the relationship between the parties are "inexorably entwined."[19] Collaborative communication can accomplish at least five important tasks in PFCC including: 1) establishing a set of goals that guides collaborative efforts; 2) exhibiting mutual respect and compassion for each other; 3) developing sufficiently complete understanding of differing perspectives; 4) ensuring maximum clarity and correctness of what is communicated; and 5) managing intrapersonal and interpersonal processes that affect how information is sent, received, and processed.[19]

Particularly in the setting of the ICU, optimizing these elements of high-quality communication may be difficult due to the number of health care team providers involved and the short time frame in which news must be delivered. Therefore adequate training for all health care providers who interact with families is essential. In addition, when patients spend prolonged periods of time within the ICU, or have multiple subspecialty services involved, the identification of a continuity provider whose role is to maintain consistency in the health care plan while ensuring adequate communication with the family can be beneficial. Furthermore, using a team approach with respectful and excellent communication among team members, including physicians and nurses, ensures that clear, consistent, and comprehensive information is shared in an empathetic manner. Collaboration within the health care team results in improved overall outcomes in critical care including increased patient survival, decreased length of stay, and decreased readmission rates, in addition to improved patient and family satisfaction, decreased symptoms of anxiety and depression among family members, and reduced ICU nurse and physician burnout.[35]

Family-Centered Rounds

Rounds in the ICU serve several purposes including: 1) providing a setting for decision making related to the management of the child's care, 2) ensuring adequate communication among health care team members, and 3) allowing for teaching of medical students, residents, and other trainees.[36] Aligning with a patient- and family-centered approach, incorporating the patient, when possible, and family into these rounds fosters a partnership with the family. Although larger and more extensive studies are necessary to fully determine the benefits and potential barriers to this approach, many professional organizations endorse it. According to several pediatric studies, this approach improves family satisfaction, improves communication between all stakeholders, increases family trust in the medical team, and potentially improves the quality of medical care provided, leading to shorter lengths of stay.[37-39] Several potential barriers and health care provider concerns regarding this approach include: 1) prolongation of rounds, 2) breach of confidentiality of protected health information, 3) reduced opportunities for teaching, and 4) concern for undermining trust of the health care team when different opinions are shared or teaching is done.[36,38,40] Although all of these concerns are valid, current evidence does not support them. On the contrary, family-centered rounds have demonstrated improved efficiency and communication because family concerns are addressed with clarity, preventing communication gaps and confusion. In addition, family presence usually lends itself to additional teaching opportunities.[38,40] Finally, when surveyed, the majority of parents are not concerned about privacy issues and therefore this concern can easily be discussed with parents on an individual basis.[36,38,40] To remain effective and efficient, using a family-centered approach to rounding requires thoughtful planning and following specific guidelines to streamline the process. Highlighting the purpose of rounds to all stakeholders and identifying explicit roles before rounds can help prevent misunderstandings.[36]

Structured Transdisciplinary Care Conferences

In critical care, where illnesses are life threatening and changes occur rapidly, sharing information with frequent updates at the bedside is crucial. Furthermore, in circumstances where medical decision making is highly complex, multiple subspecialties and disciplines are involved, or the severity of illness may lead to the demise of the patient, proactive and timely structured transdisciplinary care conferences may also be beneficial.[35] Although there is variability in the approach and style of these conferences, the palliative care and adult critical care literature provide a general framework for the facilitation of these conferences and highlight several tools.[19,35,41-43] In adult critical care, specific aspects of these conferences are associated with increased quality of care, decreased family psychologic symptoms, improved family ratings of communication, and improved outcomes. These aspects include timeliness (occur within 72 hours of ICU admission), private location for the conference, consistent communication by all members of the health care team, increased proportion of time spent listening to families speak, the use of empathetic statements, assurance that the loved one will not suffer, and providing explicit support for decisions made by the family.[35,41] Although additional research is needed to detail the benefits and potential negative aspects of this format for communication in the pediatric patient population, this approach should be considered as a potentially useful approach to optimize communication with families.

Providing Transdisciplinary Support for the Family Unit

Fundamental to PFCC is this mantra: "providing and ensuring formal and informal support for the child and family for each phase of the child's life."[1] Due to the complex nature of pediatric critical illness and the high level of emotional distress triggered by hospitalization, a transdisciplinary team approach is necessary to provide full support for the patient and family, including siblings, who are at high risk for feeling abandoned and neglected. Acknowledging that patients and families enter the ICU with varying degrees of internal coping mechanisms in addition to external support systems is critical to optimizing support.

Recognizing that all members of the health care team have different expertise, teams from a multitude of disciplines should be incorporated, when appropriate, demonstrating the value in providing a holistic approach to care. Nurses at the bedside play a crucial role in recognizing family coping strategies, identifying unmet family needs, and bridging gaps in communication.[7] Consultations with subspecialists in palliative care and ethics should be considered early in the course of hospitalization to improve communication, prevent conflict, identify important goals through eliciting patient values and preferences, and ultimately optimize shared medical decision making.[5] Physical therapy, occupational therapy, and rehabilitation medicine should be incorporated into the patient's care using a systematic approach to assist with functional recovery and potentially improve long-term quality of life. Specialists in music, art, and pet therapy; psychology; child life; and educational services can improve the quality of life in the ICU and reduce ICU-related morbidities, such as anxiety, depression, delirium, psychosis, and posttraumatic stress disorder.[4,7] Social workers can provide assistance to reduce both emotional distress and stressors that arise from practical aspects of having a child hospitalized, such as food, transportation, and employment, while chaplains can address the spiritual needs of the patient and family.[5,12,44] With the multitude of providers involved, excellent communication is necessary, as different messages can contribute additional stress to families.

In addition to incorporating health care providers from multiple disciplines, peer-to-peer support can also be highly beneficial.[1] Families may choose to serve on patient advocacy committees, share their experiences with other families through family support groups, and volunteer to serve as consultants to other families who are affected by similar disease processes or experiences. Allowing families who are in a crisis mode to contact and access other families who have shared similar experiences may broaden coping mechanisms and may help guide families through their journey, particularly when they are faced with making difficult decisions.

Collaborating and Building Partnerships With Patients and Families

Developing a partnership with families is essential to fulfilling the fundamental principles of PFCC. A partnership requires an "interpersonal relationship between two or more people who work together to achieve a mutually defined purpose," which, in the PICU, is, "providing the best possible care for the child from a holistic perspective."[45] The holistic approach requires inclusion of the family, as the center of strength for the child. When partnering with parents and caregivers who know the child best and provide invaluable information regarding who the child is as a person, health care providers treat the child more effectively and address the needs more appropriately.[45] This partnership, when developed effectively, allows parents and health care providers to contribute their own expertise to achieve a common goal, leading to a relationship in which the power differential between health care providers and families is diminished.[10]

Although building a partnership with patients and families at the bedside is essential, optimizing PFCC also requires collaboration, "at all levels of health care: in the delivery of care to the individual child; in professional education, policy making, program development, implementation, and evaluation; and in health care facility design."[1] Encouraging families to participate in all the dimensions of health care through serving on family advisory councils, quality improvement projects, and developing research protocols is critical.[1] Furthermore, building this partnership requires a transdisciplinary approach and is "grounded in collaboration among patients, families, physicians, nurses, and other professionals in clinical care."[1] In order to optimize these relationships, clarity and transparency regarding the roles, boundaries, and expertise of each stakeholder are critical.

Empowering Patients and Families to Facilitate Shared Medical Decision Making

PFCC is optimized through "recognizing and building on the strengths of individual children and families and empowering them to discover their own strengths, build confidence, and participate in making choices and decisions about their health care."[1] Empowering the patient and family to participate in shared decision making is fundamental because "the perspectives and information provided by families, children, and young adults are essential components of high-quality clinical decision making."[1] In the ICU setting, complex and high-stakes decisions are made in a short time frame. In many circumstances, there is a high degree of uncertainty in outcomes, making these decisions even more difficult. The majority of these clinical decisions are based on the medical expertise, empirical evidence, experience of the health care providers and consultants, and most importantly, the values and perspectives of the patient and family.

By definition, shared decision making occurs when the physician, patient (if possible), and family "share their opinions and jointly reach a decision."[35] Dimensions of shared decision making include (1) providing medical information and eliciting patient values, preferences, and goals; (2) exploring the family's preferred role in decision making; and (3) deliberation and decision making.[35,46] Collaborative communication, as discussed earlier in this chapter, is required to adequately fulfill the first dimension. In regards to dimension 2, multiple studies demonstrate that families have varying decision-making preferences, particularly regarding limitation of life support or other aggressive interventions.[5,35] Therefore before making assumptions, exploring the family's preferential role in decision making is important. Furthermore, shared decision making should not be interpreted as allowing the family to decide without support from the providers, or giving families increased responsibility or autonomy, as, "there is a fine balance between supporting and guiding a family while allowing the family appropriate space to make their own decisions."[11,22] Most families do not want to feel alone when making difficult decisions. Recommendations and guidance from providers may help alleviate potential burdens associated with making difficult decisions. Finally, shared decision making does not mean that families should exclusively drive medical care or be empowered to make decisions that are not medically sound. The key aspect of shared decision making is that the process is collaborative and incorporates the opinions and expertise of all stakeholders. "Finding the right balance" among stakeholders to achieve "goal-oriented patient care" through established frameworks for shared decision making is necessary to provide optimal PFCC.[46]

There are multiple benefits associated with shared decision making. When patients and families become active participants in their health care, there is improved understanding and more motivation to follow through with care. In addition, for parents and caregivers who lose their sense of control with the hospitalization of a critically ill child, participating in decisions can provide a great source of strength. As one mother explains, "I was able to still be her mom."[47] By "encouraging them to continue actively in their parental role by promoting shared decision making and helping the family to retain their responsibilities throughout hospitalization," parents and caregivers retain their identities, which fosters the integrity of the parent-child relationship, maintains cultural and family traditions, and demonstrates respect for and value of the child as a person.[45,47] Although further studies are necessary to elucidate the important driving factors for parental decision making, parents overall want to be "good parents."[48] Understanding what parents value as important factors in "being a good parent" potentially may improve the quality of PFCC.[48]

Patient- and Family-Centered Care Improves Outcomes for All Stakeholders

Over the past 2 decades, PFCC has improved outcomes in the provision of high-quality patient care. According to the AAP, "patient- and family-centered care can improve patient and family outcomes, improve the patient's and family's experience, increase patient and family satisfaction, build on child and family strengths, increase professional satisfaction, decrease health care costs, and lead to more effective use of healthcare resources."[1]

According to numerous studies, patients and families directly benefit from the incorporation of the fundamental principles into practice. Patients and families have reduced anxiety, better cooperation, improved satisfaction, reduced emotional distress, better adjustment to hospitalization, and faster recovery from illness and surgery.[1,8] Because the needs of families are addressed more explicitly, families also have improved functioning, increased confidence in providing ongoing care to their child, greater willingness to seek help from health care providers, a greater degree of trust, and improved competence in problem-solving and making complicated health care decisions.[1,8] When families receive clear and consistent communication and actively participate in the care of their child, they experience a greater sense of control, resulting in preservation of the parent-child relationship, with reduced anxiety, posttraumatic stress, and complicated grief.[8]

Health care providers, institutions, and the health care systems also directly benefit from PFCC. When health care providers gain important insights into the needs and values of patients and their families, they establish trusting relationships and improve the quality, efficiency, and safety of the care they provide. As a result, providers have improved work satisfaction, which leads to improved job performance, reduced burnout, and decreased staff turnover.[1] With the provision of higher-quality care, health care institutions and systems benefit with reduced health care costs, improved patient and family satisfaction, and reduced risk for litigation, and they potentially gain a more competitive position in the marketplace.[1]

Overcoming Barriers and Challenges to Patient- and Family-Centered Care in the ICU

Although significant progress has been made in incorporating PFCC into the ICU, there remains a gap between current and proposed practice. Ongoing research reveals that families continue to express that their needs are not always met.[2,8,14,16,21] The reasons for this gap in practice are likely multifactorial, but several barriers are extremely challenging to overcome (Box 13.2). First, there is a fundamental difference in perceiving the ICU as a "bedroom" versus an "office."[21] For families,

BOX 13.2	Potential Barriers to Patient- and Family-Centered Care in the ICU

- Dichotomy in patient, family, and provider needs of the ICU as a "bedroom" versus an "office"
- Emotional intensity of life-altering and life-threatening circumstances
- High-stakes nature and complexity of medical decision making, requiring explicit value-based decisions
- Implicit and explicit power differential among health care providers, patients, and families
- Exaggeration of cultural and language barriers in the fast-paced, emotionally intense, and complex setting
- Health care provider misperception of increased risk for litigation, distraction, and the inability to teach trainees with greater family involvement
- Increased complexity of patient population, lending to medically and technologically savvy families who have different needs and potentially require different models of care

BOX 13.3	Overcoming Barriers to Patient- and Family-Centered Care in the ICU

- Provide formal training in cultural humility; develop a robust interpreter service and hire cultural navigators
- Provide formal training in collaborative communication and goal-oriented, shared medical decision making
- Include patient and family input for ICU policies, procedures, planning, and delivery of health care
- Acknowledge and maintain transparency regarding implicit and explicit values and practices in the ICU
- Support and engage in patient- and family-centered care research to identify and overcome additional barriers
- Develop adequate support systems for health care providers who suffer from compassion fatigue and vicarious trauma

the ICU needs to serve as a "bedroom," where a sick child can experience warmth, comfort, and a healing environment. On the other hand, critical care providers need an "office" equipped with computers, monitors, alarms, and advanced technology. This dichotomy fundamentally inhibits the creation of a "bedroom" and reinforces the role of "the visitor" and "the patient" rather than fostering a collaborative partnership.[21] Second, the emotional intensity of the life-altering and life-threatening circumstances is unavoidable. The impact of this emotional intensity on patients and families, requiring extensive coping mechanisms, and the complexity of the medical care provided creates an implicit power differential among health care providers, patients, and families, furthermore reducing the ability to develop a partnership. Finally, the necessity to make high-stakes decisions wrought with uncertainty exposes fundamental differences in belief and value systems that are potentially challenging to overcome. Even under ideal circumstances with the most advanced communication systems and extensive training in cultural humility, these differences can create intense barriers and conflict, rooted in different perceptions of what is in the best interest of the patient, further impeding the development of partnership. Overcoming these fundamental barriers requires acknowledgement, transparency, and further research to identify both the explicit and implicit practices and values within the ICU[21] (Box 13.3). Using a model of PFCC, this research requires using a collaborative approach in which all stakeholders have an equal voice in order to develop creative solutions.

In addition to these fundamental barriers, the patient population that requires pediatric intensive care is increasingly complex. Accommodating the needs of parents of medically complicated children who are medically and technologically savvy may require different models of care.[49] PICUs need to be able to fully accommodate the "skills and expertise" of families of chronically ill and medically complex patients, and "there is a clear need for research that identifies what constitutes success to these families, along with the challenges faced by staff who care for them ... [in order to] change practice and foster a culture of supportive care inside the PICU."[49] PFCC is not equivalent to family-driven care, in which families exclusively direct the medical care, dominating the relationship. The establishment of professional boundaries and specific roles is critical in the development of mutually respectful and collaborative partnerships.

Finally, the development of compassion fatigue and secondary traumatization experienced by health care providers who are witnesses to extreme suffering of children and families in this complex environment can also lead to disengagement from patients and families.[50] High clinical workloads and demanding extraneous professional obligations can lead to provider burnout and the loss of the ability to maintain an empathetic approach to patients and families. Therefore the needs of health care providers also should be explicitly recognized and addressed by institutions and health care systems in order to improve the quality of PFCC delivered.

Summary

The pediatric critical care unit is a complex environment that creates a high level of stress for patients and families. Incorporating PFCC into practice improves patient and family satisfaction, reduces stress and anxiety, fosters the parent-child relationship, and ultimately increases the quality, efficacy, efficiency, and safety of care delivered. Developing a partnership with patients and families built on mutual respect, using collaborative communication, providing extensive support for the family unit, and encouraging patient and family participation in all aspects of care, including shared medical decision making, are fundamental principles essential to the practice of patient- and family-centered care. Overcoming real and perceived barriers to incorporating PFCC into practice requires a collaborative and transparent approach involving all stakeholders to identify creative solutions, while providing adequate support to health providers who are at risk for compassion fatigue, secondary traumatization, and burnout.

References

1. American Academy of Pediatrics. Patient- and family-centered care and the pediatrician's role. *Pediatrics*. 2012;129:394-404.
2. Merk L, Merk R. A parents' perspective on the pediatric intensive care unit: our family's journey. *Pediatr Clin North Am*. 2013;60:773-780.
3. Atkins A, Coleville G, John M. A "biopsychosocial" model for recovery: a grounded theory of families' journeys after a pediatric intensive care admission. *Intensive Crit Care Nurs*. 2012;28:133-140.
4. Colville G, Darkins J, Hesketh J, et al. The impact of parents on a child's admission to intensive care: integration of qualitative findings from a cross-sectional study. *Intensive Crit Care Nurs*. 2009;25:72-79.
5. Doorenbos A, Lindhorst T, Starks H, et al. Palliative care in the pediatric ICU: challenges and opportunities for family-centered practice. *J Soc Work End Life Palliat Care*. 2012;8:297-315.

6. Nelson L, Gold J. Posttraumatic stress disorder in children and their parents following admission to the pediatric intensive care unit: a review. *Pediatr Crit Care Med.* 2012;13:1-10.
7. Shudy M, Lihinie de Almeida M, Landon C, et al. Impact of pediatric critical illness and injury on families: a systematic literature review. *Pediatrics.* 2006;118(suppl 3):S203-S218.
8. Just AC. Parent participation in care: bridging the gap in the pediatric ICU. *Newborn Infant Nurs Rev.* 2005;5:179-187.
9. <http://www.ipfcc.org/faq.html> Institute for Patient- and Family-Centered Care: Frequently Asked Questions; 2010 Accessed 02.04.15.
10. Frazier A, Frazier H, Warren NA. A discussion of family-centered care within the pediatric intensive care unit. *Crit Care Nurs Q.* 2010; 33:82-86.
11. Kuo D, Houtrow A, Arango P, et al. Family-centered care: current applications and future directions in pediatric health care. *Matern Child Health J.* 2012;16:297-305.
12. Bergeson PS, Holbrook PR. Committee on Hospital Care and Pediatric Section of the Society of Critical Care Medicine. Guidelines for pediatric intensive care units. *Pediatrics.* 1983;72:364-372.
13. Meert K, Clark J, Eggly S. Family-centered care in the pediatric intensive care unit. *Pediatr Clin North Am.* 2013;60:761-772.
14. Coyne I, Cowley S. Challenging the philosophy of partnership with parents: a grounded theory study. *Int J Nurs Stud.* 2007;44:893-904.
15. Foster MJ, Whitehead L, Maybee P, et al. The parents', hospitalized child's, and health care providers' perceptions and experiences of family centered care within a pediatric critical care setting: a metasynthesis of qualitative research. *J Fam Nurs.* 2013;19:431-468.
16. Latour J, van Goudoever J, Schuurman BE, et al. A qualitative study exploring the experiences of parents of children admitted to seven Dutch pediatric intensive care units. *Intensive Care Med.* 2011;37:319-325.
17. Wong P, Liamputtong P, Koch S, et al. Families' experiences of their interactions with staff in an Australian intensive care unit (ICU): a qualitative study. *Intensive Crit Care Nurs.* 2015;31:51-63.
18. Juarez JA, Marvel K, Brezinski KL, et al. Bridging the gap: a curriculum to teach residents cultural humility. *Fam Med.* 2006;38(2):97-102.
19. Feudtner C. Collaborative communication in pediatric palliative care: a foundation for problem-solving and decision-making. *Pediatr Clin North Am.* 2007;54:583-607.
20. Beck SA, Weis J, Griesen G, et al. Room for family-centered care—a qualitative evaluation of a neonatal intensive care unit remodeling project. *J Neonatal Nurs.* 2009;15:88-99.
21. MacDonald ME, Liben S, Carnevale FA, et al. An office or a bedroom? Challenges for family centered care in the pediatric intensive care unit. *J Child Health Care.* 2012;16:237-249.
22. Jones BL, Contro N, Koch KD. The duty of the physician to care for the family in pediatric palliative care: context, communication, caring. *Pediatrics.* 2014;133(suppl 1):S8-S15.
23. Carroll DL. The effect of intensive care unit environments on nurse perceptions of family presence during resuscitation and invasive procedures. *Dimens Crit Care Nurs.* 2013;33:34-39.
24. Dingeman RS, Mitchell EA, Meyer EC, et al. Parent presence during complex invasive procedures and cardiopulmonary resuscitation. *Pediatrics.* 2007;120:842-854.
25. Curley M, Meyer E, Scoppettuolo L, et al. Parent presence during invasive procedures and resuscitation: evaluating a clinical practice change. *Am J Respir Crit Care Med.* 2012;186:1133-1139.
26. McAlvin SS, Carew-Lyons A. Family presence during resuscitation and invasive procedures in pediatric critical care: a systematic review. *Am J Crit Care.* 2014;23:477-484.
27. Berube K, Fothergill-Bourbonnais F, Thomas M, et al. Parents' experience of the transition with their child from a pediatric intensive care unit to the hospital ward: Searching for comfort across transitions. *J Pediatr Nurs.* 2014;29:586-595.
28. Davis R. A small kindness. *J Hosp Med.* 2010;5:569-570.
29. Kean S. A framework for a physician-parent follow-up meeting after a child's death in a PICU and why this family-centered care approach should interest us all. *Crit Care Med.* 2014;42:214-216.
30. Meert K, Eggly S, Berg R, et al. Feasibility and perceived benefits of a framework for physician-parent follow-up meetings after a child's death in the PICU. *Crit Care Med.* 2014;42:148-157.
31. Walter J, Benneyworth B, Housey M, et al. The factors associated with high quality communication for critically ill children. *Pediatrics.* 2013;131(suppl 1):S90-S95.
32. de Vos M, Bos A, Plotz F, et al. Talking with parents about end of life decisions for their children. *Pediatrics.* 2015;135:e465-e476.
33. Meert K, Eggly S, Pollack M, et al. Parents' perspectives on physician-parent communication near the time of a child's death in the pediatric intensive care unit. *Pediatr Crit Care Med.* 2008;9:2-7.
34. Orioles A, Miller VA, Kersun LS, et al. "To be a phenomenal doctor you have to be the whole package": physician's interpersonal behaviors during difficult conversations in pediatrics. *J Pall Med.* 2013;16:929-933.
35. Curtis JR, White DB. Practical guidance for evidence-based ICU family conferences. *Chest.* 2008;134:835-843.
36. McPherson G, Jefferson R, Kissoon N, et al. Toward the inclusion of parents on pediatric critical care unit rounds. *Pediatr Crit Care Med.* 2011;12:e255-e261.
37. Drago M, Aronson P, Madrigal V, et al. Are family characteristics associated with attendance at family centered rounds in the PICU? *Pediatr Crit Care Med.* 2013;14:e93-e97.
38. Ingram T, Kamat P, Coopersmith C, et al. Intensivist perceptions of family-centered rounds and its impact on physician comfort, staff involvement, teaching, and efficiency. *J Crit Care.* 2014;29:915-918.
39. Walker-Vischer L, Hill C, Mendez S. The experience of Latino parents of hospitalized children during family-centered rounds. *J Nurs Adm.* 2015;45:152-157.
40. Davidson J. Family presence on rounds in neonatal, pediatric, and adult intensive care unit. *Ann Am Thorac Soc.* 2013;10:152-156.
41. Lautrette A, Darmon M, Megarbane B, et al. A communication strategy and brochure for relatives of patients dying in the ICU. *N Engl J Med.* 2007;356:469-478.
42. McDonagh JR, Elliott TB, Engelberg RA, et al. Family satisfaction with family conferences about end-of-life care in the intensive care unit: increased proportion of family speech is associated with increased satisfaction. *Crit Care Med.* 2004;32:1484-1488.
43. Scheunemann L, McDevitt M, Carson S, et al. Randomized, controlled trials of interventions to improve communication in intensive care: a systematic review. *Chest.* 2011;139:543-554.
44. Majdalani M, Doumit M, Rahi A. The lived experience of parents of children admitted to the pediatric intensive care unit in Lebanon. *Int J Nurs Stud.* 2014;51:217-225.
45. Ames K, Rennick J, Baillargeon S. A qualitative interpretive study exploring parents' perception of the parental role in the paediatric intensive care unit. *Intensive Crit Care Nurs.* 2011;27:143-150.
46. Quill T, Holloway R. Evidence, preferences, recommendations—finding the right balance in patient care. *N Engl J Med.* 2012;366:1653-1655.
47. McGraw S, Truog R, Solomon M, et al. "I was able to still be her mom"—parenting at end of life in the pediatric intensive care unit. *Pediatr Crit Care Med.* 2012;13:e350-e356.
48. October T, Fisher K, Feudtner C, et al. The parent perspective: "being a good parent" when making critical decisions in the intensive care unit. *Pediatr Crit Care Med.* 2014;15:291-298.
49. Rennick J, Childerhose J. Redefining success in the PICU: new patient populations shift targets of care. *Pediatrics.* 2015;135:e289-e291.
50. Meadors P, Lamson A. Compassion fatigue and secondary traumatization: provider self-care on intensive care units for children. *J Pediatr Health Care.* 2008;22:24-34.

Ethics in Pediatric Intensive Care

Mithya Lewis-Newby and Douglas S. Diekema

PEARLS

- Ethical issues in the pediatric intensive care unit (PICU) include high-visibility crises, as well as subtle everyday ethical issues that stem from values and biases that infuse daily decisions.
- Critical care clinicians should develop an approach to ethical issues that includes (1) recognition and clarification, (2) information gathering, (3) ethical analysis, (4) communication of recommendations, and (5) support of the patient, family, and medical team.
- Autonomy to make choices in medical decisions is embodied in the requirements of the Doctrine of Informed Consent: disclosure, understanding, competency, and voluntariness.
- Adolescents designated as emancipated or mature minors may be considered competent to make independent medical decisions. Clinicians should strongly consider including adolescents in medical decisions even if they do not possess the legal right to do so.
- Surrogate decision making is common in the PICU. For previously competent patients, surrogates should make decisions consistent with the patient's previously expressed values ("substituted judgment standard"). For patients who have not previously been competent, surrogates must decide what is in the best interest of the patient from the patient's perspective ("best interest standard").
- Except in emergencies, clinicians must obtain legal permission to override parental refusals of recommended medical services. Clinicians must establish that the intervention will benefit the child and that forgoing the intervention places the child at significant risk of serious harm. Mediation and negotiation toward finding a mutually acceptable solution should be attempted before seeking legal intervention.
- Disputes regarding potentially inappropriate or "futile" services in cases where there is a lack of consensus about what constitutes accepted medical practice should be resolved through a fair process-based approach.

Defining Bioethics

"Bioethics is the discipline devoted to the identification, analysis, and resolution of value-based problems and competing moral claims that arise in medicine between patients, families, healthcare professionals, healthcare institutions, and society at large."[1]

Examples of Ethical Issues in the PICU

Critical care clinicians (including physicians, nurses, respiratory therapists, and other staff) face issues every day in the practice of pediatric critical care medicine. Some ethical issues occur daily (everyday ethics) in the pediatric intensive care unit (PICU) but may be subtle and difficult to recognize, such as how rounds are prioritized or how implicit biases are infused into clinician communication and decision making. Other ethical issues, such as a heated disagreement between the medical team and a family about the best course of action for a critically ill child (crisis ethics), are typically more obvious to everyone involved. The following are examples of ethical issues that may arise in the PICU:

- Prioritizing rounds to address the sickest first (prioritarianism and scarce resource allocation)
- Advising a family to withdraw life-sustaining therapies in the setting of a severe brain injury (value-based judgment)
- Transfusing a hemorrhaging child against the wishes of his parents who are of the Jehovah's Witness faith (best interest standard and harm principle)
- Treating an air-hungry dying child with morphine to the point of unconsciousness and bradypnea (doctrine of double effect)
- Lifting sedation on an 18-year-old on extracorporeal membrane oxygenation (ECMO) to discuss the possible limitation of life support (doctrine of informed consent)

Domains of Bioethics

The practice of bioethics encompasses many different domains. These domains may be present to varying degrees in individual ethical issues.

Value-Based Decision Making

In pluralistic societies (such as the United States) where moral diversity is prevalent, individuals or groups may have competing or conflicting moral claims. These moral claims are based on differing values that are not easily compared. For example, some individuals may place great value on the extension of life even if it entails significant burdens, whereas other individuals may value the quality of life more highly than life extension. The clinician should make every effort to identify and understand the moral values that underlie the positions of different stakeholders.

State and National Laws and Legal Precedence

The law interacts frequently with bioethics in several important ways. First, the answer to many questions that are framed as ethical issues is based on the law (eg, age of competency for decision making). Second, at times legal action may be required for the resolution of ethical issues (eg, a court-appointed decision maker may be required in certain cases of medical neglect). Finally, legal precedent may help inform analogous bioethics cases (eg, previous cases regarding emergent blood transfusions or the prolongation or withdrawal of life support).

Professional Codes and Health Care Organization Policies and Regulations

Most medical disciplines adhere to a professional "code of ethics."[1,2] These codes should be considered in ethical analysis. Additionally, health care organizations issue various policies around ethics (eg, allocation of resources, conscientious objection, or disclosure of medical error) with which the ethicist and clinician must be familiar. Finally, national health care organizations such as Medicaid and Medicare, as well as insurance companies, may have regulations that impact ethical practice (such as the Centers for Medicare and Medicaid Services [CMS] requirement that all patients older than 18 be asked about an advanced directive on admission to the hospital).

Communication, Negotiation, and Mediation

A large portion of ethical issues stems from communication that has broken down. In many cases, what may seem like an intractable dispute can be resolved by repairing communication between parties. Resolving some communication problems may be facilitated by the ethicist, a role in which expert conflict mediation skills prove valuable. For example, staff distress may be addressed with a staff-only meeting to better understand the roots of the distress and allow a venue in which differences of opinion can be aired. Another example includes a family who feels that their goals are unheard or misunderstood and who may benefit from a series of facilitated care conferences with the medical team at which a common understanding of the situation and goals of care might be achieved.

Prevailing Ethical Theories and Norms

Certainly, the ethicist should be knowledgeable about prevailing ethical theories and norms and adept at applying them to bioethical dilemmas (see later section for more details about specific ethical theories). There is no overarching ethical theory that can resolve all ethical dilemmas. Instead, ethical dilemmas are often examined under the lens of several theories in order to come to a "best possible" recommendation. It is important to recognize that these ethical theories and norms are not static, and that they are society and culture dependent.

Who Should Address Ethical Issues in the PICU?

A wide variety of ethical issues arise in the PICU. Different ethical issues may require different levels of analysis and resolution. Some issues may be resolved with relatively basic skills, while the resolution of other issues may require significantly advanced skills. Some ethical issues may be resolved easily and quickly by the critical care clinician, others may require the advanced skills of an ethics consultant, and others may require review by a multimember ethics committee.

Critical Care Team

Many ethical issues can and should be addressed by the intensivist or the PICU team. Just as pediatric intensivists are trained to provide primary cardiology, neurology, nephrology, palliative, and other specialized care with subspecialty consultation in complex cases, the same should be true for bioethics. All pediatric intensivists should be trained in and pursue continuing education in bioethics. Ethical issues are common in the PICU, and all intensivists should have a solid understanding of the basic aspects involved in identifying, analyzing, and resolving bioethical dilemmas. This will require an understanding of the basics of the domains mentioned earlier, as well as comfort with a basic tool set for approaching ethical issues. Routinely addressing basic ethical issues may resolve simpler bioethical issues quickly, help in deescalating more complex conflicts before they become intractable, and in some cases prevent issues from arising in the first place.

Ethics Consultant

For more complex bioethical dilemmas, pediatric bioethics specialists may be consulted. Ethicists come from a variety of disciplines, training, and experiences. Ethics consultants should have advanced skills in ethical assessment and analysis, ethical and hospital processes, and interpersonal skills in negotiation, communication, and facilitation. Additionally, ethics consultants should be experienced in advanced moral reasoning and ethical theory, be facile with advanced bioethical concepts, and have a strong knowledge base about how health care systems, clinical context, institutional policies, and health law impact ethical decisions.[3] The *pediatric* bioethics consultant should additionally be knowledgeable about the unique ethical issues that arise in the pediatric setting.

Ethics Committee

Some ethical issues may require resolution or final recommendation from a full ethics committee, composed of members from a wide variety of disciplines and representing a diverse set of values, experiences, and perspectives. Ideally, ethics committees should promote a fair process and reduce the risk of arbitrariness.[3,4] Examples of issues that are optimal for an ethics committee review include cases involving an intractable conflict of values, potentially high-visibility cases, and institutional ethics issues. Ethics committees may also perform post-hoc review of cases handled by ethics consultants for purposes of quality improvement.

Approach to Bioethics Dilemmas in the PICU

Critical care clinicians should learn and become competent with a basic organized analytic approach to ethical dilemmas. Several approaches have been published, and most contain the same basic elements.[5-7] In general, a systematic approach to ethical issues will involve five elements: recognition and clarification, information gathering, analysis of issues, communication of recommendations, and support (Fig. 14.1, Tables 14.1 and 14.2).

Recognition and Clarification of Ethical Issues

The first step in approaching any ethical issue is to recognize that the situation raises a question related to ethics. Some issues may be more appropriately handled by a child protection team (when neglect or abuse is obviously the issue) or a palliative care team (when there is no conflict over the appropriateness of palliative care but help is required in transitioning to a palliative care plan) (see also Chapter 16). During this

Clinical reasoning   **Clinical ethical reasoning**

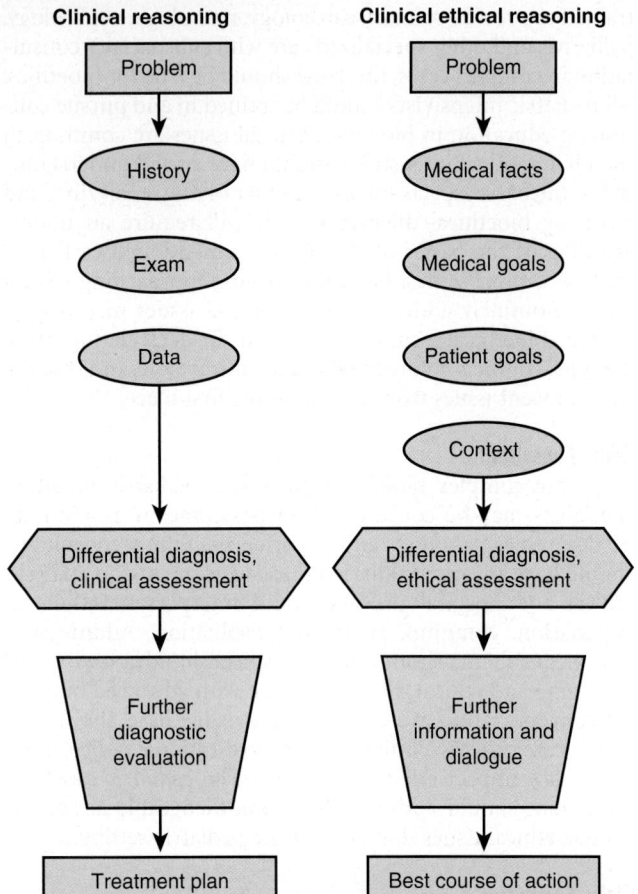

Fig. 14.1. Comparison between clinical reasoning and clinical ethical reasoning. (From Kaldjian L, Weir R, Duffy T. A clinician's approach to clinical ethical reasoning. J Gen Intern Med. 2005;20:306-311.)

TABLE 14.1	CASES—A Step-by-Step Approach to Ethics Consultation
C	**C**LARIFY THE CONSULTATION REQUEST • Characterize the type of consultation request • Obtain preliminary information from the requester • Establish realistic expectations about the consultation process • Formulate the ethics questions
A	**A**SSEMBLE THE RELEVANT INFORMATION • Consider the types of information needed • Identify the appropriate sources of information • Gather information systematically from each source • Summarize the case and the ethics questions
S	**S**YNTHESIZE THE INFORMATION • Determine whether a formal meeting is needed • Engage in ethical analysis • Identify the ethically appropriate decision maker • Facilitate moral deliberation about ethically justifiable options
E	**E**XPLAIN THE SYNTHESIS • Communicate the synthesis to key participants • Provide additional resources • Document the consultation in the health record • Document the consultation in consultation service records
S	**S**UPPORT THE CONSULTATION PROCESS • Follow up with participants • Evaluate the consultation • Adjust the consultation process • Identify underlying systems issues

From http://www.ethics.va.gov/integratedethics/ecc.asp. Ethics Consultation: Responding to Ethics Questions in Health Care, p. 25.

first stage, it is also appropriate to assess and optimize communication. Communication that has broken down is frequently a contributor, if not the basis of ethical disputes. At a minimum, improving communication commonly will help to diffuse a crisis so that the issue can be addressed productively. At times, improved communication between parties may be sufficient to resolve the issue all together. Finally, once an ethical issue has been identified, the next step is to try to articulate, as precisely as possible, the nature of the ethical question.

Information Gathering

"Good ethics requires good facts" is a common saying in bioethics circles. Sound bioethical recommendations can only arise from a solid understanding of the facts involved in the case. Facts include medical facts, such as the mortality rate for a procedure or condition both at the institution and nationally, alternate medical options, or an accurate assessment of the child's medical condition. Facts also include relevant contextual details such as family culture and religion, family circumstances, available resources and support, etc. A useful tool for gathering facts surrounding an ethical issue is the "four categories" method (Table 14.2).[7]

During this phase, it is important to seek to understand the perspectives, values, and goals of the patient (if possible), the family or other surrogates, and various involved members of the medical team (including primary physicians, consulting physicians, nurses, and other staff). When possible, these perspectives should be obtained firsthand to avoid the inevitable misunderstandings that result from second- or third-hand information. It is important to understand stakeholders' opinions, but also the goals and values behind their opinions. Often, a better understanding of the stakeholders' underlying values and deeper goals can help to clarify stated requests and open a path to resolution.

Finally, identifying or refining the core ethical dilemma or primary conflict may be easier once the appropriate data have been collected and the voices of those with a stake in the situation have been heard. It is an important skill and part of the assessment to be able to identify and clarify the ethical dimensions to the dilemma.

Analysis of Ethical Issues

Once the ethical question has been clarified, the facts have been gathered, and the voices of the stakeholders heard, the next step is to begin an ethical analysis of the case. Relevant institutional policies, health care regulations, and legal standards should be applied to the case.

In value-based ethical dilemmas a variety of ethical theories may be applied to assist in determining the recommended course of action. It is important to understand that there is no consensus about a predominant ethical theory. All ethical theories have benefits and limitations. They can and should be used in combination to help analyze the situation and assist

TABLE 14.2	A Case-Based Approach to Ethical Decision Making

MEDICAL INDICATIONS
Principles of Beneficence and Nonmaleficence
1. What is the patient's medical problem? Is the problem acute? Chronic? Critical? Reversible? Emergent? Terminal?
2. What are the goals of treatment?
3. In what circumstances are medical treatments not indicated?
4. What are the probabilities of success of various treatment options?
5. In sum, how can this patient be benefited by medical and nursing care, and how can harm be avoided?

PATIENT PREFERENCES
Principles of Respect for Autonomy
1. Has the patient been informed of benefits and risks, understood this information, and given consent?
2. Is the patient mentally capable and legally competent, and is there evidence of incapacity?
3. If mentally capable, what preferences about treatment is the patient stating?
4. If incapacitated, has the patient expressed prior preferences?
5. Who is the appropriate surrogate to make decisions for the incapacitated patient?
6. Is the patient unwilling or unable to cooperate with medical treatment? If so, why?

QUALITY OF LIFE
Principles of Beneficence, Nonmaleficence, and Respect for Autonomy
1. What are the prospects, with or without treatment, for a return to normal life, and what physical, mental, and social deficits might the patient experience even if treatment succeeds?
2. On what grounds can anyone judge that some quality of life would be undesirable for a patient who cannot make or express such a judgment?
3. Are there biases that might prejudice the provider's evaluation of the patient's quality of life?
4. What ethical issues arise concerning improving or enhancing a patient's quality of life?
5. Do quality-of-life assessments raise any questions regarding changes in treatment plans, such as forgoing life-sustaining treatment?
6. What are the plans and rationale to forgo life-sustaining treatment?
7. What is the legal and ethical status of suicide?

CONTEXTUAL FEATURES
Principles of Justice and Fairness
1. Are there professional, interprofessional, or business interests that might create conflicts of interest in the clinical treatment of patients?
2. Are there parties other than clinicians and patients, such as family members, who have an interest in clinical decisions?
3. What are the limits imposed on patient confidentiality by the legitimate interests of third parties?
4. Are there financial factors that create conflicts of interest in clinical decisions?
5. Are there problems of allocation of scarce health resources that might affect clinical decisions?
6. Are there religious issues that might affect clinical decisions?
7. What are the legal issues that might affect clinical decisions?
8. Are there considerations of clinical research and education that might affect clinical decisions?
9. Are there issues of public health and safety that affect clinical decisions?
10. Are there conflicts of interest within institutions or organizations (eg, hospitals) that may affect clinical decisions and patient welfare?

Adapted from Jonsen AR, Siegler M, Winslade W. Clinical Ethics. 7th ed. New York, NY: McGraw-Hill; 2010. https://depts.washington.edu/bioethx/tools/4boxes.html.

in coming to the "best possible" set of recommendations. The following is a limited example of ethical theories that may be applied to the analysis of ethical dilemmas:

Consequentialism

A consequentialist approach to moral decisions will focus primarily on the predicted outcomes of various choices. Of reasonable options available, the best choice will be the one most likely to provide the most favorable balance of benefit versus burden. Generally in bedside decision making, a consequentialist approach is based in the principle of beneficence, focusing the analysis on the benefits and burdens *to the patient*.[8]

Deontology

A deontologic approach to moral decisions will focus on moral duties, rights of others, and ethical rules and principles, regardless of the ultimate outcome of the decision. A deontologist might, for example, insist on the application of a rule to always tell the truth, rather than attempting to assess whether telling the truth would result in a good or a bad outcome.

Principalism

Most medical ethicists agree on a small number of principles that should generally guide medical behavior. These include respect for autonomy, beneficence, nonmaleficence, and justice. The principle of **respect for autonomy** places the desires and decisions of the competent patient as the most important consideration in deciding on a course of action. Because individual values about benefits and harms differ, individual wishes should be respected, and the clinician's primary duty is to assure that the patient has the information required to make a decision and understands that information. Some have argued for a broader principle of respect for persons, on the basis that there are ways of respecting persons that are important even for nonautonomous individuals (like children). The principle of **beneficence** requires that clinicians take positive steps to help their patients, and medical interventions should ultimately benefit the patient. This principle demands that the primary consideration in all therapeutic decisions be the good of the patient. Closely related to the principle of beneficence is the principle of nonmaleficence. **Nonmaleficence** holds that clinicians have a duty to avoid causing unnecessary harm to patients. In the PICU, many medical therapies (such as intubation) inadvertently cause suffering or are burdensome, and the principle of nonmaleficence requires that the benefit of these procedures justify the harm, burden, or suffering that may occur as a result of their use. The **principle of double effect** (see Chapter 15 for further details) is sometimes used in determining whether an action that causes both benefit and harm can be justified. At its core, this principle requires that clinicians always consider the suffering of the patient when making medical recommendations. Finally, the principle of *justice* is a complicated principle that seeks fairness when competing claims exist. Among other things, the principle requires that scarce resources be distributed fairly and not based on irrelevant factors. One limitation of principalism is that it lacks guidance about how to prioritize these principles when they are in conflict with one another in an individual case.[9]

Virtue-Based Ethics

Virtue-based theories of ethics emphasize the moral character of the individual clinician. In other words, the clinician who possesses desirable, virtuous characteristics is more likely to make the best ethical choice most consistently. Virtue-based approaches tend to be most helpful when addressing boundary issues, conscientious objection, or other issues related to professionalism and are often less helpful in the more typical conflicts that occur in the patient care setting.

Casuistic Ethics

A casuistic approach to ethical issues analyzes the current ethical issue by comparing it with prior similar cases and others' past experiences and previous outcomes to help determine the best decision. It is similar to the reasoning used in legal cases, where key precedential cases may be used as "anchors" for appropriate resolutions. The analysis then seeks to explore similarities and differences between the current situation and those precedential cases in determining whether similar or different resolutions would be most appropriate.

Care Ethics

Ethics of care shifts the moral question from "what is just?" to "how should we respond?" Instead of basing decisions on universal standards and impartiality, the ethics of care argues that caring for others and preserving relationships are the foundations of morality.

Narrative Ethics

Narrative approaches to ethical issues emphasize the importance of understanding cases in all of their details and complexities and seek to avoid reducing cases to essential elements and then applying a rule or principle. In this approach, details matter and the resolution of a specific situation may be determined by how each of the possible options will best fit the narrative of the patient's life (or death).

During the process of ethical analysis and consideration of recommendations, it may be helpful to consider whether a solution exists that has not yet been considered by the different stakeholders. Initially, in a conflict, stakeholders may strongly advocate for their specific requests. Through a thorough examination of the case, optimization of communication, and a deeper understanding of the underlying goals and values of the stakeholders, an alternative solution that may satisfy all of the stakeholders, at least to some degree, may become apparent. Clinical ethicists should always seek to identify these alternate, often creative, solutions.

Communication of Recommendations

Once an ethical analysis has occurred, the resulting recommendations must be communicated to the parties with a stake in the outcome. This may include a note or notes in the patient's chart and may involve discussions with the patient, family, and staff involved in the care of the patient. Care should be taken to fully and transparently disclose the rationale behind the recommendations. Stakeholders should have the opportunity for appeal, a process that may be facilitated by the ethics committee, a patient advocate, or some other institutional mechanism. Importantly, the recommendations of ethics consultants and committees are just that—recommendations to the clinical team. Support for the recommendations and ultimate decision making may require hospital administration or even the courts in some cases.

Support

Even after a decision has been made about how to proceed, patients, families, and staff often require additional support.

Address Staff Distress

Medical staff distress is often an important component of ethical issues. Staff may experience moral distress from continuing or not pursuing a particular plan for a patient. Addressing staff distress through individual conversations or staff-only meetings may help to deescalate the conflict. Failure to address staff distress may contribute to burnout, job dissatisfaction, and compassion fatigue.[10]

Support the Patient and Family

Patients and families involved in an ethical dilemma are often under a tremendous amount of stress. This is in addition to the stresses that result simply from having a child admitted to the PICU. Families may perceive a lack of power and support in the PICU environment and even the ethics consultants and committees may be seen as part of the power structure of the hospital. It is important to identify advocates and support mechanisms for patients and families under these conditions (see also Chapter 13).

Ethics of Patient and Surrogate Decision Making

Although the concept of patient autonomy seems obvious to all who practice medicine in this era, it was only a little over 60 years ago when the trend was for doctors to be more paternalistic and directive about medical decisions and for patients to accept these decisions. In the 1960s, a patient movement began to advocate for more patient autonomy in decision making. In that era, the predominant ethical cases surrounded the right to die. A landmark case in 1975 involved Karen Ann Quinlan, whose parents wanted the right to remove the ventilator from their daughter who was in a persistent vegetative state. The physicians refused, believing they would be killing her and fearful of homicide charges. The beginning of the patient autonomy movement was focused on the right to *refuse* treatments. Generally speaking, these trends toward autonomy and personal choice became embodied in the ***doctrine of informed consent.*** Over the past several decades the pendulum has continued to shift beyond "right to die" cases. More recent trends in the patient autonomy movement surround the "right to live" and "right to demand treatments."

Patient Decision Making

Patients are given a tremendous amount of latitude to accept or refuse offered medical treatments if the patient is deemed competent for decision making.

Doctrine of Informed Consent

The doctrine of informed consent applies to both medical decisions and research. Informed consent must satisfy four requirements that apply when surrogates provide permission, as well as when consent is obtained directly from patients. *Disclosure* means the clinician should supply the patient with sufficient information that a "reasonable person" would desire to be able to make an informed medical decision. *Understanding* means the clinician should assess the patient's understanding of the proposed course of action, the risks and benefits of that course of action, and any available alternatives along with the risks and benefits associated with those. Understanding may be particularly impaired in the critical care setting, where the high stakes and time pressures can impact the ability to achieve optimal understanding. *Capacity* means the patient must meet legal requirements for competency, be able to understand the medical decision, form a reasonable judgment based on the consequences of the decision, and be able to communicate that decision to others. Legally, children younger than the age of 18 are not considered competent for medical decision making with the exception of emancipated and mature minors. *Emancipated minors* are considered competent on the basis of characteristics that are defined by state law but which may include pregnancy, parenthood, or establishing financial independence. *Mature minors* represent another category that is defined by state law whereby a minor, usually above a certain age, can be judged competent to make certain medical decisions. Most states require a judge to make these determinations, and the judge may restrict the determination to the medical decisions at hand. *Voluntariness* means decisions must be voluntary and not subject to coercion, manipulation, or undue influence. Importantly, physicians should not withhold or deemphasize information in an effort to manipulate patients.[11]

Emergency Exception to Informed Consent

Under specific emergent circumstances, informed consent may be forgone in order to provide necessary lifesaving medical interventions. The emergency exception requires that the medical care in question is required emergently, the patient is incompetent, that no surrogates are readily available, and that medical intervention is needed to save the patient's life or prevent permanent disability.

Advance Directives

Advanced directives allow formerly competent patients to document their values and medical decision-making preferences ahead of time.[12] *Living wills* document values and desires in writing, and *health care durable power of attorney* designates a surrogate who presumably understands the patient's values and desires. The Patient Self-Determination Act requires all Medicare/Medicaid participating institutions to inform patients older than the age of 18 of their rights to formulate advance directives on admission. Advanced directives for children can also be developed by parents or other guardians with input from children as appropriate.[13]

Child and Adolescent Decision Making

Children younger than the age of 18 are generally considered not competent to make medical decisions unless they meet criteria for emancipation or mature minor status. However, most agree that the opinions of children and adolescents should not simply be disregarded. Adolescents should be involved in discussions about their health care and should be offered the opportunity to voice their feelings, opinions, and concerns, and they should be provided reasonable opportunities to make choices and have those choices respected.[14] On the other hand, there is no consensus as to whether any adolescent is truly mature enough to refuse lifesaving treatment in situations where there is likely to be a good prognosis with a proven intervention. Although adolescents older than the age of 13 are generally capable of making rational decisions, they are less likely to do so under conditions of high emotion or intense pressure. They are more likely than adults to act impulsively without full consideration of consequences, and they tend to weigh current rewards and harms more strongly than future consequences of a decision.

Many factors would be relevant in determining whether an adolescent possesses sufficient maturity to make a life-altering medical decision. Minimally, however, judges and clinicians should require a high level of psychosocial maturity and consider the adolescent's ability to understand and reason, project meaningfully into the future, express a relatively settled set of values and beliefs, and demonstrate that his or her decision is driven more by long-term interests than short-term concerns. The chances of a good outcome with treatment and the burden of the proposed interventions are also relevant considerations. In general, it would be unusual to allow an adolescent to refuse interventions in a situation where the parents would not be allowed to make that decision for him or her.[15]

Shared Decision Making

The patient autonomy movement that began in the 1960s moved us away from a predominantly paternalistic approach. There has been some concern that the pendulum has swung too far and that patients are all too frequently provided with a menu of options without sufficient guidance in decision making. The middle ground is shared decision making. Shared decision making should combine the clinician's expert knowledge and experience with the patient's values and preferences. Even though patients are rightfully granted autonomy to give informed consent, clinicians should not abdicate responsibility for recommending a course of action and guiding the patient through the decision-making process (see Chapter 13 for additional discussion).

Surrogate Decision Making

In critical care medicine (adult and pediatric), it is not uncommon for patients to lack decision-making capacity. In these situations, a surrogate decision maker is required to participate in medical decision making. Surrogate decision making falls into two categories: decision making for patients who were previously recognized as competent under the law (eg, a 22-year-old) and patients who have never been competent (eg, a 4-month-old). Surrogates must adhere to different standards in each of these two categories.

Surrogate Decision Making for Previously Competent Patients

In this category of the formerly competent patient, the surrogate decision maker (parent, spouse, etc.) must adhere to the *substituted judgment standard*. In other words, the surrogate is asked to make decisions most consistent with what the patient would have wanted. This is an attempt to preserve the patient's autonomy and honor the patient's values. There may be some cases in the PICU where this standard applies, such as older adolescents who have been living with chronic disease or young adults who have been admitted to the unit.

Surrogate Decision Making for Never-Competent Patients

In this category of the not previously competent patient (which includes the majority of patients in the PICU), surrogates are held to a different standard—that of the *best interest standard*. In theory, most children have not yet developed stable values and beliefs, and therefore these values cannot be known and cannot be used for surrogate decision making. The best interest standard attempts to maximize the benefit-to-burden ratio for the patient, from the patient's perspective. This, of course, is open to interpretation (and conflict) regarding how to calculate and weigh the various "benefits" and "burdens" as they would be experienced by the patient. "Quality of life" is a phrase that arises commonly in conversations about a patient's best interest. It is important to keep in mind that "quality of life" is a subjective and value-based assessment. Clinicians should be aware of their own biases, and caution should be used when applying this concept to the best interest standard.

Parents as Surrogate Decision Makers

Parents (or guardians) are generally empowered to make health care decisions on behalf of their children and, with few exceptions, have the legal authority to do so. From an ethical perspective, parents are generally considered the default surrogate decision makers for their children because they are most likely to understand the unique needs of each child and are presumed to desire what is best for the child. Additionally, some degree of family autonomy is considered an important social value. Finally, in settings of uncertainty, family values and competing family interests may be considered.

Limits of Parental Refusals

In most situations, parents are granted wide latitude in the decisions they make on behalf of their children, and the law has respected those decisions except when they place the child's health, well-being, or life in jeopardy.[16] Parental authority is not absolute, however, and when a parent or guardian fails to adequately guard the interests of a child, the decision may be challenged and the state may intervene. A clinician's authority to interfere with parental decision making is limited. Except in emergency situations where a child's life is threatened imminently, or a delay would result in significant suffering or risk to the child, the physician cannot do anything to a child without the permission of the child's parent or guardian. Touching (physical examination, diagnostic testing, or administering a medication) without consent is generally considered a battery under the law. The clinician's options include either tolerating the parents' decision (while continuing to try to convince them to act otherwise) or involving a state agency to assume medical decision-making authority on behalf of the child.

Only the state can order a parent to comply with medical recommendations. This can take different forms but most frequently either includes involvement of child protective services (under a claim of medical neglect) or a court order. Both of these represent a serious challenge to parental authority and will generally be perceived as disrespectful and adversarial by parents. Such action interferes with family autonomy, can adversely affect the family's future interactions with medical professionals, and can negatively impact the emotional well-being of the child. Neither should be undertaken without serious consideration. Before initiating involvement of state agencies to limit parental authority and override parental refusal, the clinician must establish that (1) the recommended course of action is likely to benefit the child in an important way; (2) the treatment is of proven efficacy with a reasonable likelihood of success; (3) the parent or surrogate's decision to refuse intervention places the child at *significant* risk of *serious* harm in comparison with the recommendations of the health care team (applying the *harm principle*); and that (4) all attempts at mediation and negotiation to find a mutually acceptable solution have been exhausted (Box 14.1).[17]

Limits of Parental Demands

There are also limits to a parent's ability to *demand* medical therapies that are not recommended by the medical team. Clinicians need not always accede to parental requests. Health care professionals have an independent obligation to apply their knowledge and skills in a way that meets professional standards of care and benefits the patient. For example, clinicians can refuse parental requests for medical therapies for their children that clearly are not medically indicated, such as antifungal medications for a bacterial pneumonia or an appendectomy for acute gastroenteritis.

There are other circumstances, however, when parents and the medical team have value-based disagreements about medical therapies. A classic example is that of parents who demand ongoing mechanical ventilation for their child in a persistent vegetative state against the recommendation of the medical team. These cases involving requests or demands for potentially inappropriate or nonbeneficial treatments (previously known as "futility" cases) require special consideration primarily because it is difficult to prioritize conflicting values in our pluralistic society. To resolve these value-based disagreements, most major medical societies recommend the use of what is called a "fair process-based approach." Once

---

BOX 14.1	Conditions for Justified State Interference with Parental Decision Making

1. By refusing to consent, are the parents placing their child at significant risk of serious harm?
2. Is the harm imminent, requiring immediate action to prevent it?
3. Is the intervention that has been refused necessary to prevent the serious harm?
4. Is the intervention that has been refused of proven efficacy and therefore likely to prevent the harm?
5. Does the intervention that has been refused by the parents not also place the child at significant risk of serious harm, and do its projected benefits outweigh its projected burdens significantly more favorably than the option chosen by the parents?
6. Would any other option prevent serious harm to the child in a way that is less intrusive to parental autonomy and more acceptable to the parents?
7. Can the state intervention be generalized to all other situations?
8. Would most parents agree that the state intervention was reasonable?

Diekema DS. Parental refusals of medical treatment: the harm principle as threshold for state intervention. Theor Med Bioeth. 2004;25:243-264.

again, optimizing early intrateam and team-family communication, as well as attempts at early conflict resolution, may prevent many of these cases from reaching a "crisis" level.[18] (For a complete discussion of this complicated topic, see Chapter 15.)

Other Ethical Issues in the PICU
Research Ethics

On the quest for continual improvement of the delivery of critical care, children admitted to the PICU are often participants in research. Clinicians should be familiar with the basic ethical and regulatory aspects of clinical research in children.[19,20] The doctrine of informed consent applies to most research. Child assent is generally required for research involving children unless an institutional review board (IRB) has waived the regulatory requirement for child assent because the child lacks the capacity for assent or the research offers a prospect of *direct* benefit to the child that is not available outside of the research. In healthy children, only research that poses no more than minimal risk to the child is acceptable. In children with disease, more than minimal risk may be acceptable only if there is a prospect of direct benefit to the individual child or if the research is likely to yield generalizable knowledge that is vital to understanding the child's condition *and* the research exposes the child to no more than a minor increase over minimal risk. All research requires approval of an IRB.

There are additional ethical considerations regarding research in the PICU. First, patients and families in the PICU are commonly under tremendous duress, are particularly vulnerable due to critical illness, and may have difficulty truly engaging in the informed consent process.[21] Second, PICU clinicians and researchers are often one and the same, and families may feel conflicted about declining research and may worry about how their lack of research participation may influence the clinical care their child receives. Researchers should be cautious to avoid undue influence or pressure on families when approaching them about enrollment in PICU research.

Resource Allocation

Resource allocation is pertinent in the PICU in two ways. Planning for disasters and other surges in the need for critical care requires careful consideration of how scarce resources will be allocated when demand exceeds resources. Additionally, one of the greatest ethical dilemmas facing our current generation is the need to control resource consumption and allocate health care resources in a sustainable way on a daily basis. As technology advances at breathtaking speeds, there is more and more we can do to prolong life. What is our individual or collective role in controlling the use of technology and practicing stewardship of our resources? National experts have thus far been unable to come to consensus on an ethical approach to fairly allocate resources during disasters or how to consistently and fairly balance cost, quality of care, and quality of life in the critical care setting. Importantly, resource allocation policies should be addressed at the policy level, NOT at the bedside by individual clinicians. Individual institutions should have clear protocols about allocation of limited resources (eg, PICU beds, ventilators, ECMO circuits, diversion policies) that may occur during times of surge so that individual clinicians make triage decisions using the same standardized criteria in order to avoid variability as much as possible. ICU clinicians should engage at the institutional, regional, and national level to affect public policy regarding the allocation of resources. Finally, any resource allocation strategy should be developed with broad social input and should be transparent[22-25] (see also Chapter 24).

Ethical Issues at the End of Life

Many ethical dilemmas arise at the end of life. These issues, which include withdrawing and withholding life support, analgesia, and sedation at the end of life and the *doctrine of double effect,* definitions of death, and organ donation, are covered in other chapters (see also Chapters 15-17).

Limits to Clinician Refusals

Generally, clinicians have no legal duty to provide illegal therapies, therapies for which the physician is not qualified or competent to provide, therapies that are considered "unnecessary" or "nonindicated" (such as antifungals for a bacterial pneumonia), or any therapy that is disallowed by institutional or legal decision. However, clinicians may not refuse to provide accepted medical care to patients on the basis of invidious discrimination (eg, race, gender).

There is ongoing debate, however, about the extent to which a clinician can refuse to provide accepted medical care based on personal moral beliefs, also known as *conscientious objections.*[26,27] Generally, these types of refusals should only be accommodated if the refusal will not harm the patient and the refusal will not create undue burdens for colleagues or the institution. Providing a personal exemption under these circumstances typically requires that another clinician take over the care of the patient in a timely manner. Accommodation may not be possible in all cases; in such instances the clinician would be required to provide the service or face institutional or legal consequences.

Importantly, a conscientious objection is not sufficient justification for unilaterally forgoing life-sustaining therapies against the wishes of a patient or surrogates. A conscientious objection should only be used to request a personal exemption from providing a service (a shield), not to impose the clinician's moral values onto the patient (a sword). A fair process-based approach should be used to resolve such conflicts, as discussed previously.

Medical Training

Many PICUs are located within pediatric teaching hospitals. Nursing students, medical students and residents, and other professional trainees may rotate through PICUs, learning valuable critical care medicine. There are also a fair number of PICUs nationally that have established pediatric critical care medicine fellowships, and these training programs are essential to continuing to train the next generation of pediatric intensivists. The balance of benefits to the trainee (and potentially patient and family) must be weighed against the potential risks and burdens to the patient and family from receiving care from an inexperienced clinician, particularly in the setting of a critically ill child. To mitigate the risks and burdens to the child and the family, other teaching methods (such as simulation) should be optimized, strict standards for supervision should be applied until competency is established, and the level of training should always be disclosed to the family[28] (see also Chapter 22).

Use of Unproven Medical Therapies

In the often dramatic and emotionally charged fight to save a child's life, the medical team may consider employing medical therapies that are new, have little to no evidence, or can be considered truly experimental outside of a conventional research setting. Typically, clinicians only consider these options when all other conventional options have failed and the outcome without them is near certain death. The potential benefits to using unproven medical therapies include prolonging the child's life, "pushing the envelope" for the development of new therapies and technologies over time, and adding to the fund of knowledge about the therapy. Because childhood critical illness is relatively rare, large randomized controlled trials may be unrealistic. On the other hand, although idealistically applied, use of these unproven therapies or technologies may burden patients, families, staff, and health care systems with little gain. An earnest attempt to consider the balance of benefit and burden of unproven therapies must be undertaken before they are offered to families. Clinicians should be aware of any conflict of interest or self-benefit they may receive from use of the therapy. The lack of evidence for the therapy should be carefully disclosed to the family.[20] Finally, attempts should be made to enroll in ongoing trials of the therapy or, if this is not available, at the very least details of the case should be carefully documented and published if possible. Finally, clinicians should be aware of when an innovative therapy, device, or procedure is regulated by the FDA because additional requirements exist in these situations.

Global Health

It is increasingly common for pediatric critical care clinicians to be intertwined with global heath delivery in resource-limited settings in several ways: (1) clinicians may participate in medical missions or disaster relief efforts; (2) U.S. fellowships may train clinicians from other countries; and (3) pediatric critical care clinicians may engage in helping to develop PICUs or training programs in other countries. Certainly, much can be gained from sharing knowledge and experience and developing these relationships. As always, clinicians should be careful to not impose U.S. cultural values and norms onto other cultures and societies. Importantly, ethical principles familiar to the US critical care clinician are not necessarily universal and should not be applied indiscriminately to other cultures. US clinicians may be emotionally challenged by practicing under different ethical norms (particularly when caring for critically ill children) and should be prepared to refrain from judging unfamiliar values. Systems developed to provide critical care in other countries should meet the needs of the people who use them and should be developed to be self-sustaining[29,30] (see Chapter 21). Finally, ethical dilemmas may arise for patients and families from other countries who require critical care in the United States. It is important to engage in learning about the family's values and cultural norms when addressing ethical issues in this setting. Incorporating these sometimes unfamiliar values and norms into an ethical analysis may be challenging, particularly when they do not coincide with Western notions of patient autonomy, patient-centered best interests, or the appropriateness of disclosure of medical information to the patient.

Medical Errors

With rare exception, medical errors of all types should be disclosed to patients and families.[31,32] Truthfulness with patients and surrogates can be considered part of the fiduciary duty of a clinician. Any determination that an error should not be disclosed to a patient or family should be reviewed by a third party or a larger committee. If a clinician witnesses another's error, the clinician is similarly obligated to take steps to ensure the error is disclosed.

Relationship Boundaries

Clinicians in the PICU form relationships with patients and families at a stressful time in their lives. At times, intense, deep, caring relationships may develop; these can be meaningful and therapeutic for the clinician, as well as the patient or family. The long-standing medical culture of training clinicians to maintain emotional distance from patients and families may not only be unrealistic in the emotionally charged PICU but also contribute to career dissatisfaction and burnout. Additionally, families consistently report desiring clinicians who genuinely care about them and their child. Deep, genuine, caring relationships between clinicians and patients and families may be beneficial.[33] Care should be taken, however, to avoid nonbeneficial or harmful relationships. Romantic or overly intimate relationships should be avoided. Caution should be exercised when considering a relationship that extends beyond the walls of the PICU and boundaries of the medical relationship, including social media contact.[34]

Preventive Ethics

Many ethical dilemmas have recurring themes and common triggers and may be predicted before the conflict reaches a state of crisis. A proactive, as opposed to a reactive, approach may address, deescalate, or even prevent crisis ethics situations from arising. This would clearly be of benefit to the patient, family, staff, and institution alike. One approach is to embed an ethicist in the PICU to make rounds and identify ethical issues to be addressed proactively. Another approach is to create PICU systems to address common triggers, such as assigning continuity physicians to chronic patients. However it is accomplished, it is in everyone's interest to avoid intractable crisis ethical dilemmas.[35]

Goals for the Ethical Practice of the Intensivist

It is essential for critical care clinicians to understand the basis for complex ethical decisions and actions so that intensivists' patient care remains morally and ethically sound in the setting of high stakes, high pressures, competing needs, great uncertainty, and diverse perspectives and values. There are few absolutes in bioethics. By its nature it is a continually shifting field, to which intensivists must constantly adjust and to which intensivists must actively contribute. Despite changes and advances in this field, critical care clinicians can continually provide the best, most ethical care by understanding the history of ethical standards and current debate. Intensivists must continue to focus on compassionate and empathetic care, which will nearly always identify the right course of

| BOX 14.2 | Goals for Ethical Practice of the Intensivist |

Focus on compassionate and empathetic care
- Value collaboration with patients, families, and colleagues
- Hone relational techniques and communication and mediation skills
- Continually explore self-values and values of others
- Develop a basic approach to ethical dilemmas
- Understand the history and meaning of prevailing ethical norms applicable in the ICU
- Stay up to date on current ethical controversies applicable in the ICU
- Know when to involve experts in ethics, conflict resolution, and family and staff support

action. The critical care team must value collaboration and constantly work to improve their communication and mediation skills. Critical care clinicians should open their hearts to deep relationships and be willing to explore the values of others and their own. Finally, intensivists should always be open to incorporating the expertise of others who can add to their practice. An intentional focus on these qualities will promote ethically sound care even in a rapidly changing and inherently uncertain environment (Box 14.2).

References

1. American Medical Association Council on Ethical and Judicial Affairs. *Code of Medical Ethics: Current Opinions with Annotations, 2012-2013.* Chicago, IL: American Medical Association; 2013.
2. American Nurses Association. *Code of Ethics for Nurses with Interpretive Statements.* Silver Spring, MD: ANA; 2008.
3. ABSH. *ASBH Core Competencies for Health Care Ethics Consultation.* 2nd ed. Glenview, IL: American Society for Bioethics and Humanities; 2011.
4. American Academy of Pediatrics. Committee on Bioethics. Institutional ethics committees. *Pediatrics.* 2001;107:205-209.
5. Kaldjian L, Weir R, Duffy T. A clinician's approach to clinical ethical reasoning. *J Gen Intern Med.* 2005;20:306-311.
6. Fox E, Berkowitz KA, Chanko BL, Powell T. Ethics Consultation: Responding to Ethics Questions in Health Care. <www.ethics.va.gov/IntegratedEthics>. Accessed 30.04.15.
7. A Case-Based Approach to Ethical Decision-Making. adapted from Jonsen AR, Siegler M, Winslade W, eds. In: *Clinical Ethics.* 7th ed. New York: McGraw-Hill; 2010 <https://depts.washington.edu/bioethx/tools/4boxes.html>.
8. Pellegrino ED, Thomasma DC. *For the Patient's Good: The Restoration of Beneficence in Health Care.* New York, NY: Oxford University Press; 1988.
9. Beauchamp TL, Childress JF. *Principles of Biomedical Ethics.* 5th ed. New York, NY: Oxford University Press; 2001.
10. Rushton CH. Defining and addressing moral distress: tools for critical care nursing leaders. *AACN Adv Crit Care.* 2006;17:161-168.
11. Berg JW, Appelbaum PS, Lidz CW, Parker LS. *Informed Consent: Legal Theory and Clinical Practice.* 2nd ed. Fair Lawn, NJ: Oxford University Press; 2001.
12. Field MJ, Cassel CK, eds. *Institute of Medicine, Committee on Care at the End of Life: Approaching Death: Improving Care at the End of Life.* Washington, DC: National Academies Press; 1997.
13. American Academy of Pediatrics, Committee on Bioethics. Guidelines on foregoing life-sustaining medical treatment. *Pediatrics.* 1994;93: 532-536.
14. American Academy of Pediatrics, Committee on Bioethics. Informed consent, parental permission, and assent in pediatric practice. *Pediatrics.* 1995;95:314-317.
15. Diekema DS. Adolescent refusals of life-saving treatment: are we asking the right questions? *Adolesc Med State Art Rev.* 2011;22:213-228.
16. American Academy of Pediatrics, Committee on Bioethics. Religious objections to medical care. *Pediatrics.* 1997;99:279-281.
17. Diekema DS. Parental refusals of medical treatment: the harm principle as threshold for state intervention. *Theor Med Bioeth.* 2004;25: 243-264.
18. Bosslet GT, White DB, Au D, et al. An official ATS/AACN/ACCP/ESICM/SCCM policy statement: responding to requests for futile and potentially inappropriate treatments in intensive care units. *Am J Respir Crit Care Med.* 2015;191:1318-1330.
19. Field MJ, Berman RE, eds. *Institute of Medicine: Ethical Conduct of Clinical Research Involving Children.* Washington, DC: National Academies Press; 2004.
20. Diekema DS. Conducting ethical research in pediatrics: a brief historical overview and review of pediatric regulations. *J Pediatr.* 2006;149: S3-S11.
21. Hulst JM, Peters JW, van den Bos A, et al. Illness severity and parental permission for clinical research in a pediatric ICU population. *Intensive Care Med.* 2005;31:880-884.
22. Persad G, Wertheimer A, Emanuel EJ. Principles for allocation of scarce medical interventions. *Lancet.* 2009;373:423-431.
23. Christian MD, Toltzis P, Kanter RK, et al. Treatment and triage recommendations for pediatric emergency mass critical care. *Pediatr Crit Care Med.* 2011;12:S109-S119.
24. Sinuff T, Kahnamoui K, Cook DJ, et al. Rationing critical care beds: a systematic review. *Crit Care Med.* 2004;32:1588-1597.
25. Truog RD, Brock DW, Cook DJ, et al. Rationing in the intensive care unit. *Crit Care Med.* 2006;34:958-963.
26. Lewis-Newby M, Wicclair M, Pope T, et al. Managing conscientious objections in intensive care medicine: an official policy statement of the American Thoracic Society. *Am J Respir Crit Care Med.* 2015;191: 219-227.
27. Committee on Bioethics. Policy statement—physician refusal to provide information or treatment on the basis of claims of conscience. *Pediatrics.* 2009;124:1689-1693.
28. Ziv A, Wolpe PR, Small SD, Glick S. Simulation-based medical education: an ethical imperative. *Simul Healthc.* 2006;1:252-256.
29. Hyder AA, Pratt B, Ali J, et al. The ethics of health systems research in low- and middle-income countries: a call to action. *Glob Public Health.* 2014;9:1008-1022.
30. Riviello ED, Letchford S, Achieng L, Newton MW. Critical care in resource-poor settings: lessons learned and future directions. *Crit Care Med.* 2001;39:860-867.
31. O'Connor E, Coates HM, Yardley IE, Wu AW. Disclosure of patient safety incidents: a comprehensive review. *Int J Qual Health Care.* 2010;22: 371-379.
32. Boyle D, O-Connell D, Platt FW, Albert RK. Disclosing errors and adverse events in the intensive care unit. *Crit Care Med.* 2006;34:1532-1537.
33. Remen RN. Practicing a medicine of the whole person: an opportunity for healing. *Hematol Oncol Clin North Am.* 2008;22:767-773.
34. Committee on Bioethics. Policy statement—pediatrician-family-patient relationships: managing the boundaries. *Pediatrics.* 2009;124:1685-1688.
35. US Department of Veterans Affairs. *National Center for Ethics in Health Care, Preventive Ethics: Addressing Ethics Quality Gaps on a Systems Level.* 2nd ed. Washington, DC: VA; 2014. Available at: <http://www.ethics.va.gov/PEprimer.pdf>.

Ethical Issues in Death and Dying

Meredith G. van der Velden and Jeffrey P. Burns

PEARLS

- Although decision making at the end of life most commonly rests with a child's parents, there may be times when a parent requests therapies that are deemed inappropriate by the clinical team. These therapies need not and should not be delivered.
- As truly futile treatment is difficult and rare to define, deliberation over these possible inappropriate therapies should focus on intensive communication and negotiation with hospital processes available for support and deliberation when this fails.
- Rationing decisions should be considered but not ad hoc for an individual patient when evaluating the appropriateness of a treatment at the end of life.
- The majority of deaths that occur in the pediatric intensive care unit do so following a decision to withdraw or withhold life-sustaining treatments.
- There is no legal or moral distinction between withdrawing and withholding treatment.
- The doctrine of double effect supports the use of aggressive treatment for comfort at the end of life including analgesia and sedation.

Many of the ethical issues that emerge in the care of the critically ill child do so at the end of life. Although many controversies still exist and new ethical dilemmas continually surface when facing death in the pediatric intensive care unit (PICU), significant progress toward a degree of consensus has been made over the years. This chapter provides an overview of ethical concerns that arise at the end of life in the PICU, including decision making near the end of life, the ethics of withdrawal and withholding of life-sustaining treatments, issues around death determination, and issues that arise after death has been declared. Much of the discussion of the delivery of end-of-life care can be found in the chapter on palliative care (see also Chapter 16).

Decision Making at the End of Life

As addressed in Chapter 14, there is little debate that decision-making authority for infants and children, particularly those in the PICU who are unable or too young to make decisions, rests with the parents.[1] In light of the diversity of individual and family values and the complexity of the decisions being made, parents are justifiably provided wide discretion in these health care decisions for their children.[2] There is, however, similar consensus that physicians have an obligation to protect their patients in a way that may involve challenging the wishes of the parents on behalf of a child's "best interests" when this rare situation arises.[3]

More than 30 years ago, the President's Commission for the Study of Ethical Problems in Medicine and Biomedical Research[3] produced the original guiding documents for most of these issues. In addition to addressing the determination of "best interests" when approaching treatment options, the commission also discussed an approach to decision making with parents. It concluded that although decision-making authority should rest with the parents under most circumstances, there may be times when it is appropriate for the physician to act against the parents' wishes, specifically when parents choose to forgo clearly beneficial treatment and when parents prefer to provide futile treatment (Table 15.1).

Although most physicians agree, and ethics and the law support, the opinion that delivering treatment that is "futile" is inappropriate, the concept of futility has been so controversial that it is rarely an effective support for a physician in overriding a parent's wishes. Regardless, most major societies including the American Academy of Pediatrics (AAP), Society of Critical Care Medicine (SCCM), and American Medical Association (AMA) do support the physician in withholding futile treatments from patients when it can be so determined.[1,4,5] The problem still rests in determining when care is "futile."

While much progress has arguably been made in our approach to cases of "futility," as practitioners in the intensive care unit (ICU), situations continue to arise in which parents wish to administer treatments and support that are deemed inappropriate and nonbeneficial by the providers. In these scenarios, how do practitioners balance the interests of the patient, family, society, and themselves? Is determining "futility" in these situations possible or even appropriate?

Burns and Truog address the concept of futility and these questions by describing historical and generational accounts of the notion of futility and, in doing so, suggest a practical approach to resolving questions of medical futility.[6] The first generation describes attempts at defining futility in order to resolve disputes with family members. These have included attempts to quantitatively (eg, treatment has been useless in the past 100 cases), qualitatively (eg, "treatment that merely preserves permanent unconsciousness"),[7] and physiologically (eg, treatment unable to achieve its physiologic goal) define the concept. All of these definitional approaches have been largely unsuccessful in actually resolving questions of disputed therapies between families and care providers as a result of flaws inherent in the definitions, along with failure to reach consensus on the definition in the background of a pluralistic society.[8]

TABLE 15.1	Decision Making in the Pediatric Intensive Care Unit	
Physician's Assessment of Treatment Options	**Parents Prefer to Accept Treatment**	**Parents Prefer to Forgo Treatment**
Clearly beneficial	Provide treatment	Provide treatment (during review process)
Ambiguous/ Uncertain	Provide treatment	Forgo treatment
Futile	Provide treatment	Forgo treatment

Following recognition that attempts to define futility failed, generation two describes the subsequent period, which attempted to address disputed cases through the use of procedures aimed at resolution. These have taken the form of individual hospital policies outlining processes to be followed in cases where the appropriateness of a therapy was brought into question and attempts at consensus between the family and clinicians failed. In general, these policies aim to represent all parties involved and most often include an ethics consultation with possible courses of action if resolution of the dispute is not achieved by mere involvement of this third party. The possible actions include further attempts at resolution, transfer of care, or judicial involvement for the purpose of, or hospital endorsement of, unilateral action on behalf of the clinical team. Ultimately, the policies transfer the decision-making authority from the bedside clinicians and family to this third party. With these processes, the major concern that arises focuses on the neutrality of the committee on behalf of the disputed parties.[9] A survey on attitudes and practices of pediatric critical care providers showed that despite most hospitals having these policies, providers do not make unilateral decisions to forgo treatment against the wishes of the family but rather provide the requested support until consensus is reached.[10] While this reports practice rather than preference, another survey demonstrated that the majority of pediatric intensivists questioned are not in support of limiting therapies against the wishes of families,[11] giving further support to the notion that even with policies in place, acting against the wishes of the family is not likely.

The final generation focuses on enhancement of early communication and negotiation with families when anticipating and making decisions about the use of life-sustaining treatments. In concert, this involves clinicians supporting each other while they respect the wishes of the family and deliver care with which they may disagree. This final generation, while not the easiest or most straightforward, may represent the approach that is most aligned with the underpinnings of dedicated critical care—to provide support for patients *and* their families through illness and death.

A final issue relevant to the discussion of decision making around the use of life-sustaining therapies in a critically ill patient is the rationing medical care. While it can be tempting to consider cost control in these discussions, as it is a pressing consideration in health care today, it should be separated from the decision of the appropriateness of a medical treatment for an individual patient. The questions of cost and appropriateness, although both important, are fundamentally

different, and the approaches to answering them should reflect this. Furthermore, ICU care is known to be costly, but the limitation of its use at the end of life is not certain to result in significant cost savings.[12] Rationing at the bedside can be complicated,[13] and for this reason, the AAP has supported the separation of rationing decisions and bedside decision making for any individual patient.[14]

A multisociety statement from 2015 including the American Thoracic Society, American Association of Critical Care Nurses, American College of Chest Physicians, European Society of Intensive Care Medicine, and Society of Critical Care Medicine provides consensus recommendations for responding to requests for potentially inappropriate treatments in ICUs. Their recommendations are grounded in shared decision-making authority between the patients and families and their clinicians. They include the following: (1) implementation of strategies to prevent intractable conflicts; (2) recommendation for use of the term *potentially inappropriate* over *futile* to describe treatments that may accomplish an effect (i.e., are not futile) but are not justifiable to provide on the basis of other considerations; (3) delineation of a process of conflict resolution in cases that remain intractable despite communication and negotiation; (4) restriction of the term *futile* to those rare cases when the treatment can be physiologically so determined; and (5) pursuit of efforts led by the medical profession at the level of policy and legislation to determine when life-prolonging treatments should not be used.[15]

Withholding and Withdrawing of Life-Sustaining Treatments

While disagreements about the use of life-sustaining treatment do arise on occasion, it is far more common that a family and the medical team reach consensus about a decision to withdraw life-sustaining therapies. Furthermore, a majority of deaths in the PICU occur after the withdrawal of life-sustaining therapies.[16,17] While there may be regional, national, and international variability in the number and percentage of patients who have a decision made to withdraw life-sustaining therapies,[17] the ethics of the process of withdrawing life-sustaining treatments remain the same.

At this stage, the difference between withdrawing and withholding treatment may come into question. Although the actions of withdrawing and withholding a therapy may feel undeniably different to families and the care team, there is no true moral or legal distinction between the two.[3] Any treatment not directed at comfort may be withdrawn or withheld if agreed upon by the family and clinical team, including, but not limited to, mechanical circulatory or ventilatory support, medications supporting the circulation, renal replacement therapy, antibiotic therapy, and hydration and nutrition. Although clinicians and families may make morally and legally defensible decisions to limit such treatments, it is never acceptable to limit care directed at providing comfort and emotional support for the patient and his or her family.[18]

Once the decision is made to focus on comfort rather than life-sustaining therapies, whether these are being withdrawn or withheld going forward, the aggressiveness of and attention to care cannot dissipate. The doctrine of double effect remains the guiding principle when considering therapies to be used

BOX 15.1 Four Conditions of the Doctrine of Double Effect

The action itself must be good or at least morally neutral
The good effect and not the bad effect must be intended
The good effect must be a result of the action itself and not by
    means of the bad effect
The good effect must proportionally outweigh the bad effect

at the end of life when the focus has transitioned from sustenance of life to comfort. While a contentious topic related in part to concerns of oversimplification and misplaced focus on physician intent, it remains relevant and supportive when drawing the line between possibly unacceptable (eg, euthanasia) and acceptable (eg, aggressive palliative therapy) treatment courses.[18]

As alluded to, the doctrine relies on a distinction between what is intended and what is merely foreseen by the clinician. It states that for any action that has two effects, one good and one bad, it is justifiable if the following four conditions are met (Box 15.1): (1) the action itself must be morally good or neutral; (2) the good and not the bad effect must be intended; (3) the good effect must be a result of the action and not by means of the bad effect; and (4) the good effect must proportionally outweigh the bad effect.[19]

As clinicians address a number of therapies considered when treating pain and suffering at the end of life, this doctrine supports many, such as the use of analgesia and sedation. It falls short in justifying actions such as the administration of neuromuscular blockade to a dying patient, as well as other courses of treatment that might fall under the distinction of active euthanasia.

Both the American College of Critical Care Medicine of the Society of Critical Care Medicine and the American Thoracic Society provide guidelines on the delivery of care at the end of life with specific recommendations on management of symptoms.[18,20] Among other topics, the guidelines provide a framework for consideration of withdrawing, withholding, or administering therapies. In general, whether deciding to continue or stop a therapy (eg, antibiotics, mechanical ventilation) or considering the initiation of a new therapy for symptom management (eg, analgesia), the decisions should center around the patient's needs and should incorporate ongoing patient assessment and consideration of established guidelines.[18]

Analgesia

Along with the avoidance of painful interventions, it is well accepted that pharmacologic interventions aimed at pain relief are indicated when withdrawing life-sustaining treatments. The goal for a patient who has had life-sustaining treatments withheld or withdrawn is to treat any signs of discomfort or pain. Consistent with the doctrine of double effect, the focus of analgesic medications, including opioids with their known side effect of respiratory depression, should be directed at this perceived pain and not to directly cause death. This is best accomplished by careful patient assessment and use of objective scales when appropriate and available, as well as attention to the appropriate dosing titrated to effect, based on a patient's prior exposure to the medications being considered. The medication dosing will vary patient to patient, and any guidelines or procedures should reflect this

anticipated variability. To reiterate, the goal of administering these therapies is only to treat patient discomfort and not to hasten the dying process or treat concerns of family members with medication for the patient. The latter concern can and should be dealt with in other ways. In addition to emotional and psychologic support for family members, anticipatory guidance on the process can help avoid the situation when a family may perceive discomfort and request medications without objective signs from the patient.[18]

Sedation

Most sedative agents lack analgesic properties, but their role in symptom management at the end of life is no less relevant. In addition to treating symptoms such as anxiety and agitation, they may also have a role in the treatment of refractory pain and suffering not relieved by analgesic medications. This latter indication works by lowering patient consciousness until symptoms are relieved. Sedation used in this manner has been labeled terms such as *palliative sedation, total sedation,* and *terminal sedation,* the last of which has received much criticism.[21] While critics of the practice claim a slide toward active euthanasia, the dominant view is that when intended and titrated to relieve symptoms, not to achieve unconsciousness or death, this does not represent euthanasia and is a key component in the delivery of quality end-of-life care.[22] As with titration of analgesics, the doctrine of double effect remains the principle that puts intent as central and defends the process. In a survey of US physicians, there exists broad support for the acceptance of unconsciousness as a side effect of sedation to treat suffering and refractory pain.[23] In its statement on palliative care in children, the AAP endorses the use of adequate analgesia and sedation to treat pain and other symptoms in patients with terminal conditions, while explicitly not supporting the practice of physician-assisted suicide or euthanasia.[24]

Neuromuscular Blockade

Neuromuscular blocking agents have no analgesic or sedative properties. Furthermore, while the pharmacologic activity of these agents may give the *appearance* to others (ie, family members) that a patient is without distress, in doing so they actually mask many of the objective signs of suffering we use when titrating medications for such symptoms. There is, thus, no role for the initiation of neuromuscular blockade at the end of life.[18,25] The more challenging question arises when determining what to do with existing neuromuscular blocking agents when the team and family have come to the decision to withdraw mechanical ventilation. With the principal goal being to adequately treat a patient's discomfort at the end of life when life-sustaining treatments have been withdrawn, attempts should be made to restore neuromuscular function, including delay in withdrawal when reasonable, in order to regain access to many of the signs and symptoms used to titrate medications for pain and discomfort. There may be times, however, when the restoration of function cannot be accomplished in a reasonable time period due to factors such as altered drug metabolism and clearance resulting from organ dysfunction and length of treatment with such agents. In such cases, the benefit of delaying withdrawal of mechanical ventilation may be outweighed by the burden on the family that comes with this delay. In these rare cases, withdrawing mechanical ventilation without restoration of neuromuscular function is justifiable but must be balanced with extra attention to ensuring patient comfort in the absence of typical signs and symptoms of pain or anxiety.[25] This is reflected in the SCCM recommendations for end-of-life care in the ICU.[18]

Artificial Hydration and Nutrition

As mentioned earlier, any treatment that is not directed at comfort may be withdrawn or withheld at the end of life if the family so chooses and the care team is in agreement. This no less true for the administration of artificial hydration and nutrition. Although withholding or withdrawing these therapies may be more psychologically distressing for caregivers and family, it is important to be clear that ethics and the law do not distinguish between these and other life-sustaining treatments. Guidelines of the AAP and SCCM[18,26,27] provide support for such decisions based on the same considerations of benefit and burden as with the withdrawal and withholding of other life-sustaining therapies.[1] In recognition of the unique distress that withdrawing or withholding this therapy may present, the AAP strongly recommends the involvement of ethics committees when these decisions are considered.[27]

Death Determination

The death of a patient in the ICU can occur in one of three ways: (1) following the withholding or withdrawal of life-sustaining treatments, (2) following unsuccessful resuscitation, and (3) brain death. The former two paths lead to the more widely accepted cardiorespiratory death, while the latter is a concept that has engendered controversy despite its steady legal standing.[28] According to the language of the Uniform Determination of Death Act drafted by the President's Commission for the Study of Ethical Problems in Medicine and Biomedical and Behavioral Research in 1981, death itself can be determined by either the "irreversible cessation of circulatory and/or respiratory functions" or "the irreversible cessation of all function of the entire brain, including the brain stem."[29] Despite the criticism of the determination of death by neurologic criteria, which centers mainly around questions of its biological validity,[28] it remains a widely recognized determination both legally and clinically and has been well accepted in pediatrics.[30,31] Furthermore, its existence allows for the possibility of organ donation in these patients in accordance with "the dead-donor rule," which states that vital organs can only be taken from someone who is dead.[32] These paradigms around organ donation are being questioned now more than ever, however, as a response to the burgeoning controversy with the notion of brain death as true biological death and with the limitation in opportunities for organ donation this requirement affords.[28,32] The details of organ donation itself are addressed in the chapter on organ donation (see also Chapter 17).

References

1. American Academy of Pediatrics Committee on Bioethics. Guidelines on foregoing life-sustaining medical treatment. *Pediatrics.* 1994;93:532-536.
2. Informed consent, parental permission, and assent in pediatric practice. Committee on Bioethics, American Academy of Pediatrics. *Pediatrics.* 1995;95:314-317.
3. President's Commission for the Study of Ethical Problems in Medicine and Biomedical and Behavioral Research. *Deciding to Forego Life-Sustaining Treatment: A Report on the Ethical, Medical, and Legal Issues in Treatment Decisions.* Washington, DC: US Government Printing Office; 1983.
4. Consensus statement of the Society of Critical Care Medicine's Ethics Committee regarding futile and other possibly inadvisable treatments. *Crit Care Med.* 1997;25:887-891.
5. American Medical Association. *Opinion 2.035 Futile care. Code of Medical Ethics.* Chicago, IL: American Medical Association; 2006. Available at: http://www.ama-assn.org/apps/pf_new/pf_online?f_n=resultLink&doc=policyfiles/HnE/E-2.035.HTM&s_t=2.035&catg=AMA/HnE&catg=AMA/BnGnC&catg=AMA/DIR&&nth=1&&st_p=0&nth=1&.
6. Burns JP, Truog RD. Futility: a concept in evolution. *Chest.* 2007;132:1987-1993.
7. Schneiderman LJ, Jecker NS, Jonsen AR. Medical futility: its meaning and ethical implications. *Ann Intern Med.* 1990;112:949-954.
8. Truog RD, Brett AS, Frader J. The problem with futility. *N Engl J Med.* 1992;326:1560-1564.
9. Truog RD. Tackling medical futility in Texas. *N Engl J Med.* 2007;357:1-3.
10. Burns JP, Mitchell C, Griffith JL, Truog RD. End-of-life care in the pediatric intensive care unit: attitudes and practices of pediatric critical care physicians and nurses. *Crit Care Med.* 2001;29:658-664.
11. Morparia K, Dickerman M, Hoehn KS. Futility: unilateral decision making is not the default for pediatric intensivists. *Pediatr Crit Care Med.* 2012;13:e311-315.
12. Luce JM, Rubenfeld GD. Can health care costs be reduced by limiting intensive care at the end of life? *Am J Respir Crit Care Med.* 2002;165:750-754.
13. Truog RD, Brock DW, Cook DJ, et al. Rationing in the intensive care unit. *Crit Care Med.* 2006;34:958-963; quiz 71.
14. Ethics and the care of critically ill infants and children. American Academy of Pediatrics Committee on Bioethics. *Pediatrics.* 1996;98:149-152.
15. Bosslet GT, Pope TM, Rubenfeld GD, et al. An official ATS/AACN/ACCP/ESICM/SCCM policy statement: responding to requests for potentially inappropriate treatments in intensive care units. *Am J Respir Crit Care Med.* 2015;191:1318-1330.
16. Burns JP, Sellers DE, Meyer EC, et al. Epidemiology of death in the PICU at five U.S. teaching hospitals. *Crit Care Med.* 2014;42:2101-2108.
17. Moore P, Kerridge I, Gillis J, et al. Withdrawal and limitation of life-sustaining treatments in a paediatric intensive care unit and review of the literature. *J Paediatr Child Health.* 2008;44:404-408.
18. Truog RD, Campbell ML, Curtis JR, et al. Recommendations for end-of-life care in the intensive care unit: a consensus statement by the American College [corrected] of Critical Care Medicine. *Crit Care Med.* 2008;36:953-963.
19. Beauchamp TL, Childress JF. *Principles of Biomedical Ethics.* 7th ed. New York, NY: Oxford University Press; 2012.
20. Lanken PN, Terry PB, Delisser HM, et al. An official American Thoracic Society clinical policy statement: palliative care for patients with respiratory diseases and critical illnesses. *Am J Respir Crit Care Med.* 2008;177:912-927.
21. Papavasiliou ES, Brearley SG, Seymour JE, et al. From sedation to continuous sedation until death: how has the conceptual basis of sedation in end-of-life care changed over time? *J Pain Symptom Manage.* 2013;46:691-706.
22. ten Have H, Welie JV. Palliative sedation versus euthanasia: an ethical assessment. *Journal of pain and symptom management.* 2014;47:123-136.
23. Putman MS, Yoon JD, Rasinski KA, Curlin FA. Intentional sedation to unconsciousness at the end of life: findings from a national physician survey. *J Pain Symptom Manage.* 2013;46:326-334.
24. American Academy of Pediatrics. Committee on Bioethics and Committee on Hospital Care. Palliative care for children. *Pediatrics.* 2000;106:351-357.
25. Truog RD, Burns JP, Mitchell C, et al. Pharmacologic paralysis and withdrawal of mechanical ventilation at the end of life. *N Engl J Med.* 2000;342:508-511.
26. Truog RD, Cist AF, Brackett SE, et al. Recommendations for end-of-life care in the intensive care unit: the Ethics Committee of the Society of Critical Care Medicine. *Crit Care Med.* 2001;29:2332-2348.
27. Diekema DS, Botkin JR, Committee on B. Clinical report—forgoing medically provided nutrition and hydration in children. *Pediatrics.* 2009;124:813-822.

28. Truog RD, Miller FG. Changing the conversation about brain death. *Am J Bioethics*. 2014;14:9-14.
29. Guidelines for the determination of death. Report of the medical consultants on the diagnosis of death to the President's Commission for the Study of Ethical Problems in Medicine and Biomedical and Behavioral Research. *JAMA*. 1981;246:2184-2186.
30. American Academy of Pediatrics Task Force on Brain Death in Children. Guidelines for the determination of brain death in children. *Pediatrics*. 1987;80:298-300.
31. Nakagawa TA, Ashwal S, Mathur M, et al. Clinical report—guidelines for the determination of brain death in infants and children: an update of the 1987 task force recommendations. *Pediatrics*. 2011;128:e720-740.
32. Truog RD, Miller FG, Halpern SD. The dead-donor rule and the future of organ donation. *N Engl J Med*. 2013;369:1287-1289.

Palliative Care in the Pediatric Intensive Care Unit

Alisa Van Cleave, Eileen Rhee, and Wynne Morrison

PEARLS

- Pediatric intensivists must have a high level of competency in core palliative care skills, including communication, shared decision making, appropriate limitation of interventions, pain and symptom management, and end-of-life care.
- Medical and technologic advancements have led to a growing number of children living with complex, chronic, life-limiting illnesses. These children should receive high-quality palliative care alongside curative and life-extending therapies.
- Mastery of communication skills is a vital part of critical care training. When in doubt, talk less and listen more.
- When considering the limitations of interventions, clinicians should focus on eliciting a family's values, goals, and hopes for their child and develop recommendations for care aimed toward achieving those goals, rather than presenting a "menu" of interventions from which the family chooses.
- *Do not attempt resuscitation* (DNAR) is more appropriate terminology than *do not resuscitate* (DNR) because it does not assume that resuscitation will be successful.
- Compassionate extubation is an important ICU skill that requires meticulous planning and preparation for both family members and staff.
- When the goals of care shift toward comfort, pain and symptom management must be prioritized, using both pharmacologic and nonpharmacologic interventions.
- Care of the family extends beyond the child's death and includes bereavement services and follow-up visits with ICU staff if the family desires.
- Indications for consultation by a specialty palliative care team include complex decision making and communication support, symptom management, and transition to hospice.

Introduction

Caring for children with life-limiting illnesses is an important role for the pediatric intensivist. Over the past 2 decades, the overall mortality rate of pediatric intensive care units (PICUs) in US teaching hospitals has decreased by half, due in part to medical and technologic advancements.[1] These advancements have increased the longevity of children with diagnoses that were previously uniformly fatal and have resulted in a growing number of children who live with chronic, life-limiting conditions, many of whom are technology dependent. Children with complex, chronic illnesses represent an increasing proportion of hospitalized pediatric patients, many of whom require frequent care in the PICU.[2] In this population of patients, the intensivist must consider the child's illness trajectory, quality of life, symptom burden, and family preferences for care during each admission. Due to the broad spectrum of illnesses with variable trajectories and prognoses that characterize pediatric patients, flexible models of the balance between curative and palliative care must be employed, as depicted in Fig. 16.1.[3]

In order to adequately care for children with chronic, life-limiting conditions, as well as those who are near the end of life, pediatric intensivists must have a high degree of competency in core palliative care skills, including communication, shared decision making, appropriate limitation of interventions, and pain and symptom management. This chapter explores the practice of palliative care in the PICU by intensivists, palliative care providers, and the interdisciplinary team.

Palliative Care Consults in the PICU

The compelling need for family-centered care and the broad range of pathophysiologies that exist in ICUs demand a mixed model of integrative and consultative palliative care, which allows for a wider distribution of a limited subspecialty resource.[4,5] *Primary* palliative care is an integrative model that focuses on maximizing and standardizing palliative care practices that clinicians routinely incorporate into the care of their patients.[6,7] *Secondary* palliative care uses consultation of a palliative care team for complex, subspecialty-level problems. Secondary palliative care helps ensure that there is adequate assessment and management of symptoms, as well as attention to emotional and psychologic distress, practical and financial concerns, and spiritual and cultural needs, as part of comprehensive patient- and family-centered care.[4] (For more on patient and family-centered care, see Chapter 13.)

Indications for specialty palliative care consultation include complex decision making and communication support (for either the medical team or family), symptom management, optimization of quality of life, hospice transition, and end-of-life care that extends beyond usual care practices. Parents of

Key ☐ Curative ■ Palliative

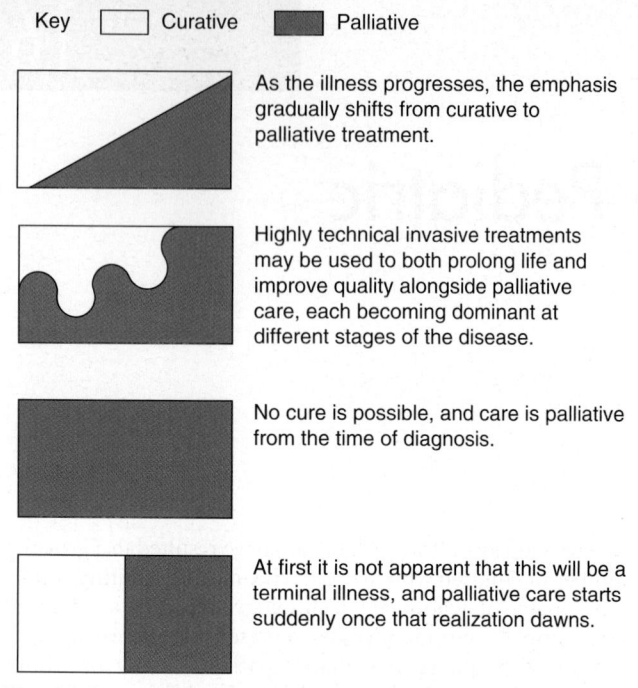

As the illness progresses, the emphasis gradually shifts from curative to palliative treatment.

Highly technical invasive treatments may be used to both prolong life and improve quality alongside palliative care, each becoming dominant at different stages of the disease.

No cure is possible, and care is palliative from the time of diagnosis.

At first it is not apparent that this will be a terminal illness, and palliative care starts suddenly once that realization dawns.

Fig. 16.1. A graphical representation of the balance between curative and palliative therapies in various clinical contexts. (From Sourkes B, Frankel L, Brown M, et al. Food, toys, and love: pediatric palliative care. Curr Probl Pediatr Adolesc Health Care. 2005;35:350-386.)

critically ill children often face difficult, value-laden decisions amid bewildering amounts of information and an "irreducible amount of uncertainty."[8] Communication expertise around eliciting patient and family preferences and translating those preferences into decision making are part of the core set of skills for intensivists. Palliative care specialists can provide additional support and guidance in particularly complex situations to help elucidate goals of care for patients and families.[9]

Epidemiology of Pediatric Death in the PICU

Deaths occur in several different ways for children in the PICU. Most deaths in the United States follow a decision to limit or discontinue life-sustaining interventions, rather than failed resuscitative efforts.[1,10-15] In a recent US multi-institutional prospective study, 70% of PICU deaths occurred after withholding or withdrawing life-sustaining treatments, 16% occurred after brain death, and 14% occurred after an unsuccessful resuscitation attempt.[1]

Although there are limited data characterizing the timing of death for PICU patients, the same study revealed two distinct profiles of death in the PICU: one in which death occurred within 7 days of admission to the PICU and another in which death occurred following a longer length of hospitalization. The children in the first group were more likely to have been previously healthy and died following failed resuscitation events, whereas those who died later in their hospitalization tended to have preexisting diagnoses and DNAR orders and died in the context of withdrawal of life-sustaining technology.[1]

In many cases, particularly for children whose death occurs later in a hospitalization, there is uncertainty around the exact timing of death following the removal of life-sustaining therapies or a decision to limit escalation of life-prolonging therapies. Preparing the team and family for this uncertainty will allow an opportunity for dialogue to ensure that symptom management is appropriately addressed and that comfort is prioritized. To that end, a question may arise regarding whether the patient should remain in the PICU, be transferred to the primary inpatient ward service, or possibly be discharged home. Many factors are involved in this question, including the complexity of symptom management, need for technologic support, a strong relationship between the patient and a specific care team, as well as provider and family comfort level with the provision of care in various locations.

Hospice Support in the Home

For a number of families, allowing their child to die at home is a great source of comfort. Hospice agencies are invaluable partners specifically skilled to coordinate and facilitate such a care plan. Hospices provide comfort-oriented medical care and psychosocial support to patients with life-limiting illnesses and their families. US hospices are independent agencies structured to be compliant with Medicare guidelines.[16,17] Hospice agencies typically provide care to adults, and few are dedicated specifically to the care of children. However, many adult hospices will care for children if a pediatric medical team advises their care. Notably, hospices do not provide shift-based home nursing care for patients. Hospice nurses visit patients on a regular basis (from biweekly to monthly, depending on their needs) to help caregivers assess symptoms and manage changes in clinical status. They are also on call 24 hours a day for support by phone and, in special circumstances, can provide continuous in-home care for up to 72 hours for patients who are actively dying. Although hospital-based palliative care teams and community-based hospices are distinct, pediatric palliative care teams work closely with hospices to help ensure a seamless transition from hospital to home.[18,19]

Communication

The importance of communication in the intensive care setting has become abundantly clear over the past 2 decades (see also Chapter 4). Health care providers communicate with families in many ways in the ICU, but the hallmark of ICU communication is the family meeting. In a typical family meeting, members of the medical team sit down with the patient's family away from the bedside to formally discuss the patient's care. Commonly, these meetings are organized by the medical team to facilitate difficult conversations, including the delivery of bad news, discussions regarding goals of care, and end-of-life care preferences.

Suboptimal Communication in the ICU

Excellent bidirectional communication between providers and families is an essential part of providing comprehensive, family-centered care in the intensive care unit.[20-22] In fact, some families deem the quality of a physician's communication skills more important than their clinical skills.[23] Failure to provide adequate communication puts patients and families at risk for poor outcomes, including anxiety, depression, and posttraumatic stress disorder.[24]

Despite its importance, studies continue to reveal that communication between families and providers in the ICU is suboptimal.[25-29] In a recent study,[30] researchers interviewed parents of children who died in the PICU regarding the communication that occurred around their child's end-of-life care. More than 70% of parents gave constructive feedback to physicians regarding the way information was conveyed during their child's terminal illness. The most common issue raised in this study was physician availability and attentiveness to the families' informational needs. Other concerns included honesty, withholding of information, use of complex language, pacing of information delivery, providing false hope, body language, and affect during bad news delivery.

Families with Limited English Proficiency

Families with limited English proficiency (LEP) are at even greater risk of receiving poor communication from health care providers, despite using trained medical interpreters. Patients with LEP are less satisfied with physician communication than English-speaking patients, including the degree to which physicians listen, answer questions, explain concepts, and provide support.[31-35] A recent study compared the quality of communication during interpreted and noninterpreted PICU family meetings.[36] Interpreted meetings had fewer elements of shared decision making and a greater imbalance between physician and family speech. In fact, LEP families spoke for less than 4 minutes during meetings that lasted 43 minutes on average. Though this finding may be cultural to some degree, it is difficult to argue that effective, bidirectional communication can occur with so little family participation, especially when discussing such complex issues as the care of a critically ill child.

The Family Meeting as an ICU "Procedure"

Complex, value-laden decisions, such as the decision to withhold or withdraw life-sustaining therapies, are typically made during ICU family meetings. For that reason, conducting a family meeting with clear, compassionate, bidirectional communication is a critical ICU "procedure" that must be effectively taught to all trainees.[37] Importantly, because ICU family meetings are frequently organized when the medical team wants to discuss limiting or withdrawing life-sustaining measures, it is possible to foster a hidden agenda that implies that, when family meetings are conducted well, families choose to limit or withdraw interventions. In actuality, a successful family meeting is one in which the medical team elicits the patient's and family's goals and values, and a care plan is crafted that achieves their goals and honors their values.

Communication Pearls

Palliative care specialists receive extensive training on conducting difficult conversations, and they can be called on as a resource for both the medical team and family. However, effective communication of difficult and complex information is a core competency for all intensivists, and these skills must be learned early in training and honed throughout one's career. A number of strategies exist to assist clinicians in conducting these conversations,[38] one of which is the SPIKES protocol,[39] summarized in Table 16.1.

Phrases to Avoid

Several antiquated phrases remain in the vernacular of health care providers and must be eliminated, such as "withdrawal of care," "Nothing more can be done," and "There is no hope." Care is *never* withdrawn from a patient in the ICU. There is

TABLE 16.1 SPIKES: A Protocol for Delivering Bad News

Set up: Find a private space with adequate seating. Never conduct a conversation of this nature without sitting down.
Patient perspective: Begin by allowing the patient or family to share their understanding, concerns, and goals for the meeting. Always listen before you talk.
Invitation: Obtain the family's permission to give them the information you want to share. This can also be an opportunity for a "warning shot," or a phrase that prepares the family for difficult news. As an example, one could say, "Unfortunately, I have some difficult information to share with you. Is it all right if I talk about that during this meeting?"
Knowledge: Deliver the information clearly and compassionately. Go slowly, and allow for silence. Families may only hear the first piece of bad news delivered before their emotional response prevents further comprehension. Resist the temptation to continue delivering information if the family is having an emotional response. Instead, acknowledge and validate their emotions.
Emotions: Though some providers may feel uncomfortable addressing emotions, families consistently report the importance of empathy from health care providers. The presence or absence of empathy can leave indelible marks on family members for years to come. If unsure how to respond, listening with empathic statements is always appropriate.
Summary: Provide a brief summary of the meeting, ensuring that you have addressed the goals and concerns laid out by the family at the start of the meeting. State the next steps, and plan for future conversations.

Adapted from Baile WF, Buckman R, Lenzi R, et al. SPIKES—A six-step protocol for delivering bad news. Oncologist. 2000;5:302-311.

always more that can be done to help ensure comfort, provide support, maintain dignity, and create meaning. Allowing families to maintain hope is important.[40] Providers may worry that preserving hope and truth-telling are mutually exclusive. However, research suggests the opposite: truthful disclosure of prognostic information, even in the setting of poor prognosis, is associated with increased parental hope.[41] This may be because hope is not solely defined by a particular medical outcome. Truthful prognostic information, when delivered compassionately, can allow parents to focus on achievable hopes, such as comfort, quality of life, and meaningful relationships. Eliminating these phrases will help ensure that families do not feel abandoned by the medical team.

Though protocols and guidelines can be helpful, all providers will encounter situations in which it is difficult to know what to say or how to proceed. When this occurs, we are reminded by Elaine Meyer of the importance of "being present, not perfect."[42] Connecting with patients and families on a human level by bearing witness to their suffering will facilitate continued collaboration amid even the most difficult circumstances.

Limitation of Interventions

One of the most difficult options for a family and the medical team to consider when a child may be dying is whether advanced technologic supports offer any benefit. Such supports can include invasive or noninvasive mechanical ventilation, medical or mechanical support of the circulation, surgical interventions, renal replacement therapy, intravenous medications, or medically administered nutrition and hydration. Forgoing such interventions requires that the family and medical team agree that such therapies offer little chance of benefit, that the pain or suffering they cause is not worth the hoped-for benefit, that the therapies no longer provide a reasonable quality of life, or that they otherwise do not help to achieve important goals for the child and family. (For more on medical ethics and decision making, please see Chapter 14.)

Do Not Attempt Resuscitation Orders

An important tool when determining desired goals is the do not attempt resuscitation (DNAR) order. Such orders historically became necessary when medical care advanced to such a degree that many "intensive care" interventions, such as mechanical ventilation or cardiopulmonary resuscitation (CPR), became the default pathway to appropriately prolong life in most circumstances.[43,44] Such orders are unique in medical care, since having the order in place is necessary to avoid performing an intervention, rather than to request it.

DNAR is becoming a more commonly used term than *do not resuscitate* as DNAR does not presuppose that resuscitation attempts will be successful. Some centers have shifted terminology for DNAR orders even further by calling them *allow natural death* (AND) orders.[45,46] The general public may have an inflated perception of the success of CPR, based somewhat on media depictions.[47] A physician's willingness to share his or her medical opinion regarding the likelihood of success of CPR, especially if that likelihood is low, may be helpful in a family's decision making. Using phrases that focus on what will be provided (eg, comfort) rather than on what will be withheld (eg, resuscitation) may help families understand the reasoning behind such choices. How choices are presented, or "framed," may affect patient and family decisions.[48-50]

In discussions with the patient and family, it is imperative that the clinician elicit the family's overall goals rather than presenting a list of all possible interventions and asking for a yes/no answer to each. Once the family has articulated their goals (eg, "going home," "avoiding painful procedures," or "waiting to see if he can get back to baseline"), then the clinician can focus on determining which specific interventions might help achieve those goals. DNAR orders are not "all or none," and a range of interventions could make sense depending on the clinical circumstances. Clarity in the orders is important, however, for team communication and consistency, especially if multiple transitions in care providers may occur.

During these discussions, it is important to avoid phrases such as "Do you want us to do everything for him?" Such phrases are nonspecific and imply that "doing" is the right course of action,[51] because the converse is to "do nothing." In circumstances where a clinician feels strongly that invasive technologic support will not lead to long-term benefit, it is acceptable to recommend against CPR or intubation as a way to protect the child from interventions that won't help.[52] Making a recommendation is an important part of shared decision making, and recommendations should be based on the goals and values articulated by the patient and family.[53] Although the ethical justification for withholding a therapy is exactly the same for withdrawing a therapy, it may be psychologically more difficult for some families to stop interventions that are already in place than it is to forgo pursuing new ones. Limitations of interventions may often therefore begin as "nonescalation" plans, with consideration of withdrawal of an intervention only if the trajectory becomes clear.

Compassionate Extubation

Discontinuing mechanical ventilation (now called *compassionate extubation*) is an important skill for all intensivists. It requires meticulous planning and symptom management. Preparing the family is an important first step. This includes determining whom should be present, asking if they would like to hold their child during extubation, and distinguishing between expected signs that are part of the dying process (eg, color change, noisy breathing) versus signs that would be treated with additional medication. A quiet, private location is preferable in which the medical team is immediately available. Care providers should avoid overly precise predictions of how quickly a patient will die following compassionate extubation, as some patients may breathe better on their own than anticipated. Providing a range of time, such as "minutes to hours" or "days to weeks," gives families a general idea of expected time course. Preparing medications ahead of time to treat anticipated symptoms is important, and having a titration plan in place may help staff assess and respond to distress.[54] It is sometimes helpful to decrease ventilatory support shortly before extubation to assess whether the patient develops dyspnea. If the patient appears uncomfortable on lower ventilatory settings, additional doses of medication can be given before extubation. Although medication for dyspnea and agitation is essential, neuromuscular blockade should not be administered if a ventilator is being withdrawn. Neuromuscular blockade may hasten death and also makes it difficult to assess distress or determine whether additional medications for comfort are needed.[55,56] It is certainly possible to discontinue other interventions, such as vasoactive infusions, extracorporeal circulatory support, or supplementary oxygen, while awaiting resolution of neuromuscular blockade before extubation.

Pain and Symptom Management

When the goals of care shift to comfort, it is important to pay close attention to medication management and symptom control. Common symptoms at the end of life include pain, dyspnea, anxiety, and agitation. Many medications that treat these symptoms are part of routine ICU care (Table 16.2). Medication choices may differ significantly depending on how long a child is expected to live following removal of ICU interventions, what sources of pain exist, or how neurologically intact the patient is, although there is likely large variability between different centers.[57] Table 16.2 includes typical starting doses, but doses will need to be a significantly higher level if a patient has developed tolerance. Medications should be titrated to effect, with the maximum dose dictated only by side effects. For opioids and benzodiazepines, bolus doses and infusion rates may be repeatedly increased by 20% to 50% until symptoms are controlled, which typically occurs before respiratory depression. In patients without intravenous access, other routes of medication administration (transdermal, sublingual, rectal, subcutaneous) can be considered rather than increasing discomfort by necessitating needle sticks and procedures to maintain venous access.

Medication Management
Opioids
Several commonly used opioids are listed in Table 16.2. Opioids treat both pain and dyspnea and may also have sedating effects.

TABLE 16.2 Medications Commonly Used for Pain and Distress at the End of Life[a]

Medication	Routes	Starting Dose	Notes
Opioids			
Morphine	PO, SL, PR, SQ, IV	0.05-0.1 mg/kg every 3-4 h Infusion: 0.01-0.03 mg/kg/h	Renally excreted; causes histamine release
Hydromorphone	PO, IV, SQ, SL	0.015 mg/kg every 3-4 h Infusion: 0.003 mg/kg/h	
Fentanyl	IV, SQ, buccal, nasal, patch	0.5-1 mcg/kg every 30 min Infusion: 1 mcg/kg/h	Transdermal patches available in 12.5, 25, 50, 75 and 100 mcg/h
Methadone	PO, IV	0.05-0.1 mg/kg every 6-12 h initially, then decrease frequency	Long acting and may accumulate; may be adjunctive for neuropathic pain via NMDA effects; prolongs QT interval; multiple drug interactions
Benzodiazepines			
Midazolam	PO, IV, SC	0.05-0.1 mg/kg every 2-4 h Infusion: 0.03-0.1 mg/kg/h	Onset of action within minutes when given IV
Lorazepam	PO, IV, IM	0.025-0.1 mg/kg every 4-8 h	Less hypotension than midazolam, slightly slower onset
Diazepam	PO, PR	0.05-0.2 mg/kg every 6-12 h	IM and IV formulations available but rarely used due to pain/phlebitis; IV form may also be given PO or PR
Other Sedatives and Adjuncts			
Ketamine	PO, IM, IV	0.2-0.5 mg/kg/dose	May be adjunctive for neuropathic pain via NMDA effects
Gabapentin	PO	10 mg/kg/day	For neuropathic pain; increase daily until 30 mg/kg/day, then reassess
Amitriptyline	PO	5 mg	For neuropathic pain; target dose 0.5-1 mg/kg/day

[a]All doses are starting doses for patients not previously exposed and may need to be escalated to much higher levels.
IV, intravenous; kg, kilogram; mcg, microgram; mg, milligram; NMDA, N-methyl-D-aspartate; PO, oral; PR, per rectum; SL, sublingual; SQ, subcutaneous; n/a, not applicable.

They work via central nervous system μ-receptors. Potential side effects include constipation, nausea, pruritus, urinary retention, and respiratory depression.[58,59] Side effects should be anticipated and prevented if possible (eg, with a bowel regimen). Intractable side effects can sometimes be managed by rotating to another agent in the class.[60] Some side effects, such as nausea and vomiting, may resolve over time.

Distinguishing features of specific opioids are important to mention. Codeine should be avoided because approximately 10% of the general population lacks the hepatic enzyme necessary to convert it to morphine, and up to 35% of children demonstrate inadequate conversion to morphine.[61] Meperidine should also be avoided because its metabolite, normeperidine, can accumulate and cause seizures. Fentanyl is commonly used in ICUs because of its rapid onset and titratability, but it can be problematic at the end of life if used for longer than brief periods because tolerance can develop rapidly. However, the transdermal (patch) form is often useful for patients who are unable to tolerate enteral medications and no longer have IV access. Morphine leads to histamine release, which can cause pruritus, and hypotension, which may improve with rotation to hydromorphone. At very high doses, morphine has neuroexcitatory effects that cause hyperalgesia, delirium, and myoclonus. Morphine should also be avoided in renal failure, as accumulation of its metabolites causes myoclonus.

Methadone
Methadone differs from other opioids and therefore bears special mention. It is a μ-receptor agonist, as well as an N-mNethyl-D-aspartate (NMDA) receptor antagonist. It has a long and highly variable half-life. Its NMDA effects can sometimes improve pain control in patients who have become tolerant to high doses of other opioids, and it may also be effective in treating neuropathic pain. Its long half-life can lead to drug accumulation, which may cause late-onset side effects such as obtundation. Careful adjustment of dosing schedules is required. Methadone has many drug-drug interactions that require careful review. It can also prolong the QT interval, so it is prudent to screen patients with an electrocardiogram before its initiation.

Other Pharmacologic Agents
Acetaminophen or NSAIDs (eg, ibuprofen, naproxen, ketorolac) may be useful adjuncts to the medications listed in Table 16.2. However, doses of these medications cannot be escalated because of the risk of toxicity. Combination agents, such as acetaminophen with oxycodone, should be avoided because acetaminophen limits the ability to escalate the opioid component.

Ketamine is a dissociative anesthetic that also has NMDA effects. It offers excellent pain control and may have opioid-sparing benefits. However, it can cause disturbing hallucinations. Similar to methadone, it may have advantages for neuropathic pain.

Other useful techniques to achieve pain control include regional nerve blocks, lidocaine patches, and occasionally treatment with steroids.

Symptom Management
Pain
A multitude of agents are available for the treatment of pain, many of which are discussed earlier (see also Chapters 134 and

135). Neuropathic pain may be treated by methadone, gabapentin, or amitriptyline. Steroids and IV bisphosphonates are useful adjuncts for pain relief due to malignant bone pain. Nonpharmacologic adjuncts to pain control may also be useful. Research suggests that integrative therapies, such as art and music therapy, can be effective adjuncts for pain treatment in children with cancer.[62]

Dyspnea

Opioids are the mainstay of treatment for dyspnea. Nebulized opioids are sometimes used, although they have not shown consistent benefit in controlled trials.[63,64] In addition to opioids, dyspnea may be improved with a fan blowing in the face. Other respiratory support such as supplementary oxygen or noninvasive positive pressure can be considered if they enhance comfort, but there is no mandate to use them if they add to distress or prohibit patient disposition to another location (eg, home or outside of the ICU) that would be preferable to the family. If noninvasive ventilation is used, excessive positive pressure should be avoided as it is more likely to lead to discomfort and skin breakdown.

Agitation and Anxiety

Benzodiazepines are often useful to treat agitation or anxiety at the end of life and may also help decrease opioid requirement.[65] Low doses may be sufficient, but some patients may require escalation to sedating doses. A calm, quiet environment can be helpful, but so can distracting or enjoyable activities.

Nausea and Vomiting

Several agents are available for the treatment of nausea and vomiting. Ondansetron or metoclopromide are often effective. Benzodiazepines are also useful. Phenothiazines, such as promethazine and prochlorperazine, are efficacious but can be very sedating. They may also cause extrapyramidal side effects, which diphenhydramine can help mitigate. Olazapine or haloperidol can be used when other agents are ineffective.[66]

Seizures

Seizures can also occur at the end of life, for which benzodiazepines are a good first-line agent. Levetiracetam or valproate is sometimes used to prophylax against seizures in patients at high risk (eg, with brain tumors).[65]

Bowel Obstruction

Bowel obstruction is a particularly difficult situation to manage. Decompression with nasogastric drainage may improve symptoms. Relieving constipation is often important. Steroids may be beneficial if the obstruction is due to a mass. Motility agents can be helpful, but they may also increase pain. Octreotide (intravenous or subcutaneous) has been used to decrease intestinal secretions and may improve symptoms such as vomiting.[67] Palliative surgery can be considered, but the degree and duration of benefits versus burdens should be carefully weighed.[66]

Palliative Sedation

Rarely, symptoms may remain uncontrolled at the end of life despite maximal medical management. In such circumstances, palliative sedation may be considered. *Palliative sedation* is "the use of sedative medications to relieve intolerable suffering from refractory symptoms by a reduction in patient consciousness."[68,69] Benzodiazepines, barbiturates, dexmedetomidine, or propofol can be used. Additionally, propofol has advantageous effects against nausea, pruritus, seizures, and myoclonus, while dexmedetomidine is useful because it does not cause respiratory depression. Sedation to unconsciousness can be justified when symptoms cannot be managed by other means and death is considered "imminent" (eg, within hours to days). Protocols have been published that guide the implementation of palliative sedation, which include prerequisite consensus by an interdisciplinary team that symptoms are truly refractory and that the patient is imminently dying of a terminal illness.[70]

Practical Aspects of Care at the End of Life

As the death of a patient is anticipated, several practical aspects of care must be accomplished in a timely and sensitive manner (see also Chapter 15). Specific issues to address with family and staff before the patient's death include notification of an organ procurement organization (OPO), discussion of expected signs or symptoms the child may exhibit, cultural or spiritual needs during or after the dying process, sibling support, and autopsy. Hospitals are required to notify the local OPO when the death of any patient is anticipated so that the OPO may determine whether the patient could be a potential organ or tissue donor. Generally, the OPO must be contacted before the patient's death to determine candidacy. If the patient is a suitable donor, the clinical team then notifies the family that a representative from the OPO will meet with them to answer questions about organ donation and determine whether the family wants to participate. A timely discussion about organ donation is particularly crucial when donation after circulatory death (DCD) is considered. (For more on organ donation, please refer to Chapter 17.)

The exact timing and trajectory of symptoms are often difficult to predict at the end of life. Therefore conversations should generally focus on how to identify discomfort and the medications and techniques (eg, oxygen, positioning, massage) that will be provided to relieve suffering. Frequent communication between the medical team and family optimizes care for the dying child, and it may help alleviate anxiety for both staff and family. Further, addressing a family's specific cultural or spiritual needs around death is an important way to provide additional support. Using child life specialists to help siblings comprehend the death of their brother or sister is an invaluable source of support for the family during the end-of-life process.

Addressing the family's wishes regarding autopsy before the child's death will allow time for thoughtful consideration and appropriate planning. The physician who discusses obtaining an autopsy ideally should know the patient and family well, and the physician must know the indications for and limitations of autopsy in order to advise the family. Some families choose autopsy to obtain more information on the etiology of death, if it is unclear, or potentially to provide reassurance that the underlying disease was irreversible. On occasion, an autopsy may disclose an unrecognized genetic disorder that may have clinical implications for the family.[71] An autopsy could also answer questions that may arise in the future. Some families are motivated to pursue autopsy because the findings could contribute to medical knowledge and possibly help another child and family. If a family elects to pursue an autopsy, a designated physician must offer a follow-up visit to review the results.

After the declaration of death, families may desire privacy with their child. During this time, essential documentation can be performed. The death summary note includes a brief description of the patient's medical history and the events that led to death. The rationale used to titrate sedation and analgesia, if administered, is important to document. The death certificate, which is separate from the death summary note, must be completed promptly. The coroner or medical examiner must be notified to determine whether a forensic autopsy is indicated, which typically occurs in cases of trauma or abuse but varies with jurisdiction, and families should be informed if such a decision is made. Notification of other providers from different care teams, including subspecialty teams, referring providers, and primary care providers, is important. If the child attended school or day care, or had home nursing or hospice support, the agencies should be notified, with the parents' permission.

Care of Family and Staff After a Child's Death

The death of a child is a tragic event that affects all who are touched by it. Grief support is a crucial part of the ongoing care that bereaved families need after their child dies, and these services are typically provided by referral to a community or hospital-based bereavement program. Such programs provide ongoing support and frequent assessments to identify complicated grief when it occurs. Bereaved families of chronically ill children often describe a sense of "double loss," both for their child and for their medical team, who cared for them over the course of months or years.[72] Family members may also grieve the same child in very different ways and on different timelines, which may cause distress for some providers, but is actually a normal phenomenon. In addition, sibling grief is sometimes overlooked due to the varying ways that children in different developmental stages express emotion. Parents often try to protect siblings from the trauma of the ill child's end-of-life care, though studies show that this strategy leaves siblings feeling excluded and abandoned, which persists long into bereavement.[73]

Staff members in the ICU are also impacted by the death of a child and are at risk for compassion fatigue and burnout due to repeated exposure to secondary trauma.[74] The American College of Critical Care Medicine Task Force guidelines for support of the patient and family in the ICU setting recommend structured support mechanisms for staff, such as debriefing sessions,[75] which can be facilitated by social work, spiritual care, or palliative care. For some individuals, these sessions provide a safe forum to discuss their feelings about a particular patient or experience, which can help process grief. Others may benefit from developing personalized ways to process stress or grief, which can include any number of activities, such as exercise, reflective writing, outdoor activities, engaging in a spiritual practice, or meeting with a counselor or therapist regularly. In addition, some staff members choose to send condolence letters or attend memorial services for children as a way to further support the family, honor the memory of the child, and process their own grief. Research suggests that these gestures are positively received by families[76]

and can be beneficial for some providers. Finally, recent studies suggest that follow-up meetings between bereaved parents and critical care physicians are beneficial to both parties and are crucial to providing family-centered care.[77]

Key References

1. Burns JP, Sellers DE, Meyer EC, et al. Epidemiology of death in the PICU at five US teaching hospitals. *Crit Care Med.* 2014;42:2101-2108.
2. Davies D, Hartfield D, Wren T. Children who "grow up" in hospital: inpatient stays of six months or longer. *Paediatr Child Health.* 2014;19: 533-536.
3. Sourkes B, Frankel L, Brown M, et al. Food, toys, and love: pediatric palliative care. *Curr Probl Pediatr Adolesc Health Care.* 2005;35:350-386.
4. von Gunten CF. Secondary and tertiary palliative care in US hospitals. *JAMA.* 2002;287:875-881.
7. Boss R, Nelson J, Weissman D, et al. Integrating palliative care into the PICU: a report from the Improving Palliative Care in the ICU Advisory Board. *Pediatr Crit Care Med.* 2014;15:762-767.
8. Renjilian CB, Womer JW, Carroll KW, et al. Parental explicit heuristics in decision-making for children with life-threatening illnesses. *Pediatrics.* 2013;131:e566-e572.
9. Dahlin CM, ed. *The National Consensus Project for Quality Palliative Care: Clinical Practice Guidelines for Quality Palliative Care.* 3rd ed. Pittsburgh, PA: The National Consensus Project for Quality Palliative Care; 2013.
12. Lee KJ, Tieves K, Scanlon MC. Alterations in end-of-life support in the pediatric intensive care unit. *Pediatrics.* 2010;126:e859-e864.
18. Feudtner C, Feinstein JA, Satchell M, et al. Shifting place of death among children with complex chronic conditions in the United States, 1989-2003. *JAMA.* 2007;297:2725-2732.
19. Feudtner C. Epidemiology and the care of children with complex conditions. In: Wolfe J, Hinds P, Sourkes B, eds. *Textbook of Interdisciplinary Pediatric Palliative Care.* Philadelphia, PA: Elsevier; 2011:7-18.
20. Curtis JR, White DB. Practical guidance for evidence-based ICU family conferences. *Chest.* 2008;134:835-843.
22. Meyer EC, Ritholz MD, Burns JP, et al. Improving the quality of end-of-life care in the pediatric intensive care unit: parents' priorities and recommendations. *Pediatrics.* 2006;117:649-657.
26. Azoulay E, Chevret S, Leleu G, et al. Half the families of intensive care unit patients experience inadequate communication with physicians. *Crit Care Med.* 2000;28:3044-3049.
30. Meert KL, Eggly S, Pollack M, et al. Parents' perspectives on physician-parent communication near the time of a child's death in the pediatric intensive care unit. *Pediatr Crit Care Med.* 2008;9:2-7.
33. Guerrero AD, Chen J, Inkelas M, et al. Racial and ethnic disparities in pediatric experiences of family-centered care. *Med Care.* 2010; 48:388-393.
36. Van Cleave AC, Roosen-Runge MU, Miller AB, et al. Quality of communication in interpreted versus noninterpreted PICU family meetings. *Crit Care Med.* 2014;42:1507-1517.
37. Hurd CJ, Curtis JR. The intensive care unit family conference. Teaching a critical intensive care unit procedure. *Ann Am Thorac Soc.* 2015;12: 469-471.
39. Baile WF, Buckman R, Lenzi R, et al. SPIKES-A six-step protocol for delivering bad news: application to the patient with cancer. *Oncologist.* 2000;5:302-311.
40. Orioles A, Miller VA, Kersun LS, et al. "To be a phenomenal doctor you have to be the whole package": physicians' interpersonal behaviors during difficult conversations in pediatrics. *J Palliat Med.* 2013;16:929-933.
41. Mack JW, Wolfe J, Cook EF, et al. Hope and prognostic disclosure. *J Clin Oncol.* 2007;25:5636-5642.
42. Meyer EC. July 7, 2014. On being present, not perfect [video file]. Available at: <http://vector.childrenshospital.org/2014/07/communication-and-the-patient-experience-on-being-present-not-perfect/>.
43. Burns JP, Edwards J, Johnson J, et al. Do-not-resuscitate order after 25 years. *Crit Care Med.* 2003;31:1543-1550.
44. Morrison W, Berkowitz I. Do not attempt resuscitation orders in pediatrics. *Pediatr Clin North Am.* 2007;54:757-771, xi-xii.
46. Venneman SS, Narnor-Harris P, Perish M, et al. "Allow natural death" versus "do not resuscitate": three words that can change a life. *J Med Ethics.* 2008;34:2-6.

48. Barnato AE, Arnold RM. The effect of emotion and physician communication behaviors on surrogates' life-sustaining treatment decisions: a randomized simulation experiment. *Crit Care Med.* 2013;41:1686-1691.

50. Halpern SD, Ubel PA, Asch DA. Harnessing the power of default options to improve health care. *N Engl J Med.* 2007;357:1340-1344.

51. Feudtner C, Morrison W. The darkening veil of "do everything." *Arch Pediatr Adolesc Med.* 2012;166:694-695.

52. Clark JD, Dudzinski DM. The culture of dysthanasia: attempting CPR in terminally ill children. *Pediatrics.* 2013;131:572-580.

53. Kon AA. The shared decision-making continuum. *JAMA.* 2010;304:903-904.

54. Munson D. Withdrawal of mechanical ventilation in pediatric and neonatal intensive care units. *Pediatr Clin North Am.* 2007;54:773-785, xii.

55. Truog RD, Cist AF, Brackett SE, et al. Recommendations for end-of-life care in the intensive care unit: the Ethics Committee of the Society of Critical Care Medicine. *Crit Care Med.* 2001;29:2332-2348.

56. American Academy of Pediatrics Committee on Bioethics. Guidelines on foregoing life-sustaining medical treatment. *Pediatrics.* 1994;93:532-536.

57. Ragsdale L, Zhong W, Morrison W, et al. Pediatric exposure to opioid and sedation medications during terminal hospitalizations in the United States, 2007-2011. *J Pediatr.* 2015;166:587-593.

58. Friedrichsdorf SJ, Kang TI. The management of pain in children with life-limiting illnesses. *Pediatr Clin North Am.* 2007;54:645-672.

59. Zernikow B, Michel E, Craig F, et al. Pediatric palliative care: use of opioids for the management of pain. *Paediatr Drugs.* 2009;11:129-151.

60. Nalamachu SR. Opioid rotation in clinical practice. *Adv Ther.* 2012;29:849-863.

61. Williams DG, Patel A, Howard RF. Pharmacogenetics of codeine metabolism in an urban population of children and its implications for analgesic reliability. *Br J Anaesth.* 2002;89:839-845.

62. Thrane S. Effectiveness of integrative modalities for pain and anxiety in children and adolescents with cancer: a systematic review. *J Pediatr Oncol Nurs.* 2013;30:320-332.

63. Ullrich CK, Mayer OH. Assessment and management of fatigue and dyspnea in pediatric palliative care. *Pediatr Clin North Am.* 2007;54:735-756.

64. Boyden JY, Connor SR, Otolorin L, et al. Nebulized medications for the treatment of dyspnea: a literature review. *J Aerosol Med Pulm Drug Deliv.* 2015;28:1-19.

65. Wusthoff CJ, Shellhaas RA, Licht DJ. Management of common neurologic symptoms in pediatric palliative care: seizures, agitation, and spasticity. *Pediatr Clin North Am.* 2007;54:709-733.

66. Santucci G, Mack JW. Common gastrointestinal symptoms in pediatric palliative care: nausea, vomiting, constipation, anorexia, cachexia. *Pediatr Clin North Am.* 2007;54:673-689.

67. Currow DC, Quinn S, Agar M, et al. Double-blind, placebo-controlled, randomized trial of octreotide in malignant bowel obstruction. *J Pain Symptom Manage.* 2015;49:814-821.

68. Beller EM, van Driel ML, McGregor L, et al. Palliative pharmacological sedation for terminally ill adults. *Cochrane Database Syst Rev.* 2015;(1):Cd010206.

69. de Graeff A, Dean M. Palliative sedation therapy in the last weeks of life: a literature review and recommendations for standards. *J Palliat Med.* 2007;10:67-85.

70. Gurschick L, Mayer DK, Hanson LC. Palliative sedation: an analysis of international guidelines and position statements. *Am J Hosp Palliat Care.* electronically published 7 May 2014.

72. Contro N, Kreicbergs U, Reichard W, Sourkes B. Anticipatory grief and bereavement. In: Wolfe J, Hinds P, Sourkes B, eds. *Textbook of Interdisciplinary Pediatric Palliative Care.* Philadelphia, PA: Elsevier; 2011: 41-54.

74. Robins PM, Meltzer L, Zelikovsky N. The experience of secondary traumatic stress upon care providers working within a children's hospital. *J Pediatr Nurs.* 2009;24:270-279.

76. Macdonald ME, Liben S, Carnevale FA, et al. Parental perspectives on hospital staff members' acts of kindness and commemoration after a child's death. *Pediatrics.* 2005;116:884-890.

77. Meert KL, Eggly S, Berg RA, et al. Feasibility and perceived benefits of a framework for physician-parent follow-up meetings after a child's death in the PICU. *Crit Care Med.* 2014;42:148-157.

Process of Organ Donation and Pediatric Donor Management

Thomas A. Nakagawa

PEARLS

- Involvement of pediatric critical care specialists has improved the quality and number of organs recovered. Additionally, more organs from pediatric donors are being transplanted into children.
- Donor management is crucial to the successful recovery of organs for transplantation. Management of the potential pediatric organ donor requires knowledge of the physiologic derangements associated with this specific patient population.
- Timely involvement of the organ procurement organization coordinator allows medical professionals to dialogue and improve authorization rates while assisting families with end-of-life care issues.
- Determination of neurologic death in children is based on clinical criteria that are consistent across the age spectrum.
- Donation after the circulatory determination of death (DCD) allows donation to occur from patients with a catastrophic brain injury who do not progress to neurologic death. Success with organs transplanted from DCD donors continues to occur in many centers.
- The sustained practice of pediatric DCD donation continues to account for more than 10% of the total number of DCD donors nationally.
- Neonatal donation provides another valuable source of organs for transplantation.

Introduction

The demand for transplantable organs continues to increase at a rapid pace, far exceeding the number of organs available for transplantation. Approximately 1.5% of the patients on the national transplant wait list are children 18 years of age or younger.[1] Similar to adults, the majority of children waiting for a transplant have end-stage renal failure and are in need of a kidney, followed by children with hepatic disease who are waiting for a liver.[1] In contrast to the increasing number of adults on the wait list, the number of children added to the national transplantation wait list has remained relatively stable. Importantly, the number of children receiving organ transplants has increased, and pediatric donors are providing more organs for pediatric patients awaiting transplantation.[1,2]

Additionally, wait listed patients in need of a transplant who in the past died from their organ failure are now living longer lives due to improved pharmacologic and medical management. In fact, some of these patients improve and may not require transplantation at all, further reducing the number of children on the national wait list. Nonetheless, children continue to die waiting for a lifesaving transplant, with the highest death rate observed in children younger than 1 year of age.[1,2] Although the number of children who die while on the wait list for a needed organ has decreased, the number of children who are removed from the wait list and die because they become too sick to transplant has increased.[1] The need for more organs and improved therapies to preserve organ function for those waiting for a transplant is clear in this population of patients. The American Academy of Pediatrics recognizes this need and supports organ donation emphasizing education, the need to shape public policy, and a system in which organ procurement, distribution, and cost are fair and equitable for children and adults.[3]

Each state has laws or regulations for the determination of death, which have in most cases been modeled after the Uniform Determination of Death Act (UDDA).[4] The UDDA states that an individual who has sustained either (1) irreversible cessation of circulatory and respiratory functions or (2) irreversible cessation of all functions of the entire brain (including the brain stem) is dead (see also Chapter 15). A determination of death must be made in accordance with accepted medical standards. Organ donation can occur following neurologic death (donation after brain death [DBD]), circulatory death (donation after circulatory death [DCD]), or through living donation. Donor organs recovered for transplantation include heart, lungs, liver, kidneys, pancreas, and intestines. However, the type of donation affects the organs recovered. Most organ donation occurs following death established by neurologic criteria. In both children and adults, the number of donors following neurologic death has decreased since the early 2000s.[1,5] This decline in pediatric donors has occurred for many reasons, including improved medical and surgical treatments, vaccinations that have reduced deaths associated with childhood infectious diseases, safety restraints, education and awareness regarding health hazards affecting children, and pediatric critical care specialists who have reduced morbidity and mortality for critically ill or injured children.

Missed opportunities for organ donation occur in many medical institutions.[6-8] Frequently these lost opportunities occur when families decline the option of donation. The hospital experience, difficulty understanding death, and racial barriers may contribute to the lack of authorization for donation.[9] Donor families are more likely to understand neurologic death and have a positive hospital experience compared with families that chose to not authorize donation.[10] In some cases families are not even given the opportunity for donation because the medical team may not recognize an eligible donor. Organs available for transplantation may be lost because of caregivers' lack of familiarity with appropriate donor management, or opportunities for donation may be denied by medical examiners or coroners who fear losing evidence and the ability to successfully prosecute cases in situations where accidental or nonaccidental trauma has claimed the life of a child.

Unique issues exist with the process of organ donation and transplantation in children. Parents and guardians must act as surrogate decision makers without benefit of being guided by the donor's wishes, as is often possible with adults. Size and weight constraints can the limit acquisition and use of organs recovered from children. Technical challenges related to surgical procedures in smaller children and infants and age-related variation in the timing associated with the declaration of brain death can result in organ deterioration and affect the viability of organs for transplantation. Specialized care required for the management of critically ill children and pediatric organ donors may be lacking at institutions that have limited expertise and support for children. This includes expertise from nursing and critical care specialists, as well as support from pediatric neurologists, neurosurgeons, general surgeons, other pediatric specialists, and pediatric support staff, who understand the unique needs of children and their families.

The process of donation involves identification of a potential donor, determination of neurologic death in a timely manner, authorization for organ donation, management of the donor, and recovery of organs for transplantation. The process of donation begins when a critically ill or injured child is identified as a potential donor with a timely referral to the organ procurement organization (OPO). Early involvement and collaboration with the OPO allows coordination of the donation process and enhances the chances of successful authorization and recovery of viable organs for transplantation.[3,7,11] Medical management of the potential pediatric organ donor requires knowledge of the physiologic derangements associated with this patient population. Hemodynamic instability, alterations in oxygenation and ventilation, metabolic and endocrine abnormalities, and coagulation disturbances are common. Support and care of the family provided by a team of physicians, nurses, social workers, chaplains, family service providers and organ donation specialists, and other support staff trained in the unique aspects of pediatric medicine are integral to the care of these children and their families.[7] Each of these elements is essential to ensure the successful recovery of organs from this select group of patients.

Role of the Pediatric Intensivist and Critical Care Team in the Process of Organ Donation

Effective donor management is crucial to the successful recovery of organs for transplantation. The integral involvement of the pediatric intensivist and the critical care team in the management of critically ill and injured children has been a foundation of the clinical practice in many successful pediatric

centers. Caring for critically ill children and their families through all phases of illness including end-of-life issues should be a seamless transition. The continuum of care for the dying patient who progresses to death and becomes a donor requires the expertise of the pediatric intensivist and critical care team to not only manage and prevent deterioration of organ systems and loss of transplantable organs but to help the family deal with the death of their child. Preserving the option of organ donation allows families to make the decision about donation for their child.[7,8] Involvement of critical care specialists, especially in pediatrics where there is a limited and decreasing number of donors improves the quality and number of organs recovered.

It is federally mandated that the OPO be informed of any impending death. The OPO should be notified in a timely manner prior to the death of the patient. Suitability of the potential donor needs to be determined and issues regarding donation need to be discussed with the medical team and the OPO prior to approaching the family. Utilizing OPO coordinators and appropriately trained requestors to obtain authorization by families has been a successful practice in the adult arena; however, pediatric critical care practitioners have learned that children and their families are different. Collaboration between the OPO and the pediatric intensivist is essential to determine the best way to approach families about authorization for donation.[7,8,11,12] Parents seem to prefer discussions regarding donation with the pediatric intensivist or a member of the health care team they have come to trust, rather than the OPO coordinator.[7,13] Additionally, one study noted that timing of the first request relative to discussions of brain death did not influence the decision to donate organs, but authorization for donation was more likely when parents had sufficient time to discuss this issue.[13] These concepts are vastly different from the traditional approach of the OPO coordinator requesting donation and decoupling the death and authorization process. Improved communication between the health care team and the OPO is imperative. Many institutions have adopted a team approach when discussing donation with families. This best practice is encouraged by the United States Department of Health and Human Services Organ Donation Collaborative, which has led to increased donation rates.[14] Best practices promote coordinated efforts between OPO coordinators and medical professionals to improve authorization rates while assisting families with end-of-life care issues. Involvement of palliative care teams has also been identified as another resource to assist the ICU team and parents and families facing end-of-life issues with their child.[15-18] In addition to the benefits of organ donation to the transplant recipient, there are psychologic and social benefits for the potential donor and the family.[3,8,19,20]

Determination of Neurologic Death

The majority of donations occur following neurologic death.[1] The dead donor rule states that patients must be declared dead before removal of vital organs in order for transplantation to occur.[21] Therefore accurate determination of neurologic death is essential before efforts at organ recovery proceed. Determination of neurologic death must occur in a timely and efficient manner for several reasons: It allows the family to begin the grieving process as they prepare for the loss of a loved one; it allows the process of organ preservation and preparation for recovery to begin; and if donation is not planned, medical therapies can be stopped, allowing redistribution of scarce ICU resources to other critically ill and injured patients.

Good donor management is imperative for the recovery of viable organs for transplantation. Hemodynamic instability and organ dysfunction account for a loss of up to 25% of potential donors when donor management is not optimized.[22] Furthermore, institution of hormonal replacement therapy (HRT) early in the donation process may assist with stabilization of the donor, improve the quality of organs recovered, and enhance posttransplant graft function.[23-27]

Determination of neurologic death in children is a clinical process based on specific criteria, which are consistent across the age spectrum. No unique legal issues differentiating the declaration of neurologic death exist for children. However, determination of irreversible injury and neurologic death can be more difficult in younger patients, resulting in age-based recommendations and two separate neurologic examinations.[28,29] Criteria for the determination of neurologic death in infants and children were revised in 2011.[28,29] The updated guidelines provide criteria to determine neurologic death for infants greater than 37 weeks' estimated gestational age to 18 years of age.[28,29] The clinical history, cause of coma, and neurologic injury must be determined to ensure that an irreversible condition has occurred. Physical examination criteria rely on the coexistence of coma and apnea in a child who is neither hypothermic nor hypotensive for age and whose examination is not affected by sedatives or neuromuscular blocking agents. The neurologic criteria to determine death in infants and children are listed in Table 17.1. Absence of neurologic function is defined by the following features on physical exam: midposition or fully dilated nonreactive pupils, absence of spontaneous eye movements induced by oculocephalic (when feasible) or oculovestibular testing, absence of bulbar function, cough, corneal, gag, and rooting reflexes, and absent respiratory effort when challenged with elevated carbon dioxide levels that would otherwise induce respiratory effort in such a patient. Two neurologic examinations and apnea tests separated by an

observation period are required to establish the diagnosis of neurologic death in the United States.[28,29] The duration of observation between examinations is based on age. Ancillary studies are not mandatory to make a determination of neurologic death. The need for ancillary studies will be determined by the physician caring for the child based on history and the ability to complete the clinical examination and apnea testing.[28,29] If clinical examination and apnea testing cannot be safely completed, an ancillary study should be used to assist with the determination of death. The examination results must remain consistent with neurologic death throughout the observation and testing period.

Determination of neurologic death for any infant or child requires establishing and maintaining normal physiologic parameters. Before the neurologic examination or neurodiagnostic testing can be meaningful, correction of hypotension and hypothermia must occur. Targeted temperature management and hypothermia protocols are being used more frequently as a treatment following cardiac arrest and traumatic brain injury. Hypothermia can affect drug metabolism and the clinical examination to determine neurologic death of a critically ill patient. Adequate time following rewarming is crucial prior to initiating testing for neurologic death. Current North American adult and pediatric guidelines emphasize a minimum core body temperature of >35°C (95°F).[28-31] The current pediatric guidelines for neurologic death suggest waiting at least 24 hours following rewarming before instituting testing for neurologic death. A period greater than 24 hours may be required to ensure that diagnostic error following targeted temperature management does not occur.[32-34] Additionally, conditions that can interfere with the neurologic examination or factors capable of imitating brain death must be excluded. Conditions such as severe hepatic or renal dysfunction, inborn errors of metabolism, metabolic disturbances, or toxic ingestions may play a role in the clinical presentation of the comatose infant or child. These conditions should be considered and, if identified, appropriate treatment instituted to correct the derangements resulting in coma. There may be instances where these conditions cannot be corrected and additional ancillary testing may be required to confirm neurologic death. Testing for drug intoxications including barbiturates, opiates, and alcohol should be performed as indicated. The half-life of sedative agents must be considered when determining the appropriate timing of the clinical examination. Longer-acting or continuous infusion of sedative agents and recent administration of neuromuscular blocking agents can interfere with the neurologic examination. These agents should be discontinued for a reasonable amount of time to allow adequate clearance of the drug(s) prior to initiating electroencephalogram (EEG) testing and clinical examination for neurologic death. Delayed drug metabolism in hypothermic patients or patients with hepatic or renal dysfunction should also be considered prior to testing for neurologic death. Barbiturates reduce cerebral blood flow (CBF); however, there is no evidence that high-dose barbiturate therapy completely arrests CBF. A radionuclide CBF study or cerebral arteriography can be utilized in patients with high-dose barbiturate therapy to demonstrate the absence of CBF.[28,29,35,36] Clearance of neuromuscular blockers can be confirmed by use of a nerve stimulator.

The apnea test is a critical and essential component of the clinical examination to determine neurologic death. Testing

TABLE 17.1	**Neurologic Examination Criteria for Brain Death Determination in Infants and Children**[28,29]

1. Coma. Patient must lack all evidence of responsiveness. Noxious stimuli should not produce a motor response other than spinally mediated reflexes.
2. Apnea. The patient must have the complete absence of documented respiratory effort (if feasible) by formal apnea testing demonstrating a $PaCO_2$ ≥60 mm Hg *and* >20 mm Hg increase above baseline $PaCO_2$.
3. Loss of all brain stem reflexes including the following:
   - Midposition or fully dilated pupils that do not respond to light
   - Absence of movement of bulbar musculature including facial and oropharyngeal muscles
   - Absent gag, cough, sucking, and rooting reflexes
   - Absent corneal reflexes
   - Absent oculovestibular reflexes
4. Flaccid tone and absence of spontaneous or induced movements, excluding spinal cord events such as reflex withdrawal or spinal myoclonus.
5. Reversible conditions or conditions that can interfere with the neurologic examination must be excluded prior to brain death testing.

for apnea must allow adequate time for the partial pressure of carbon dioxide ($PaCO_2$) to increase to levels that would normally stimulate respiration. Apnea testing must be performed safely while maintaining normal oxygenation and stable hemodynamics. Patients should be preoxygenated with 100% oxygen to prevent hypoxia and enhance the chances of successfully completing the apnea test. Mechanical ventilatory support should be adjusted to eliminate ventilation, allowing the $PaCO_2$ to rise while observing the patient for spontaneous respiratory effort. False reports of spontaneous ventilation have been described while patients were maintained on continuous positive airway pressure (CPAP) for apnea testing despite having sensitivity of the mechanical ventilator reduced to minimum levels.[28,29,37] Attaching a self-inflating bag valve system, such as a Mapleson circuit, to the endotracheal tube (ETT) or tracheal insufflation of oxygen using a catheter inserted through the ETT has also been employed to provide supplemental oxygen. High gas flow rates with tracheal insufflation may promote CO_2 washout preventing adequate $PaCO_2$ rise during apnea testing. Additionally, adequate gas outflow must be ensured to prevent barotrauma. The $PaCO_2$ should be measured and allowed to rise to 60 mm Hg or greater and 20 mm Hg above the baseline $PaCO_2$ while the patient is continually observed for any spontaneous respiratory movements over a 5- to 10-minute period. These respiratory criteria account for infants and children with chronic respiratory disease or insufficiency who may only breathe in response to supranormal $PaCO_2$ levels. The apnea test is consistent with neurologic death if no respiratory effort is observed during the testing period. The patient is placed back on mechanical ventilator support following apnea testing until death is confirmed with a second clinical examination and second apnea test. If apnea testing cannot be completed because of hemodynamic instability, desaturation, or an inability to reach a $PaCO_2$ of 60 mm Hg and a greater than 20 mm Hg increase above the baseline $PaCO_2$, or if there is any concern regarding the validity of the apnea test, an ancillary study should be pursued to make the determination of neurologic death. If an ancillary study is utilized, a second clinical examination and apnea test must also performed. Any respiratory effort is inconsistent with neurologic death.

Recommended clinical observation periods between examinations in children differ from those of adults, with a greater duration suggested for younger children. The updated guidelines continue to emphasize that the younger the child, the more cautious one should be in determining neurologic death. Table 17.2 lists the recommended observation periods based on the age of the infant or child from the Updated Guidelines for Determination of Brain Death in Infants and Children.[28,29]

Ancillary studies can provide additional supportive information to assist in the determination of neurologic death. These studies are useful when the clinical examination or apnea testing cannot be safely completed due to the underlying medical condition of the patient, when there is uncertainty about the findings of the neurologic examination, or if a confounding medication effect may be present. Ancillary studies are not necessary if the determination of neurologic death can be made based on clinical examination criteria and apnea testing. Ancillary studies may be utilized to expedite the determination of neurologic death by reducing the clinical observation period, potentially increasing viability of transplant

TABLE 17.2	Recommended Observation Periods to Determine Brain Death in Infants and Children[28,29]
Term infants (37 weeks estimated gestational age) to 30 days of age	
• Two examinations and apnea tests separated by at least 24 hours[a]	
Greater than 30 days of age to 18 years of age	
• Two examinations and apnea tests separated by at least 12 hours[a]	

[a]The observation period may be decreased if an approved ancillary study is used. A second clinical examination and apnea test must be performed following the ancillary study to declare death.

tissue. However, in the circumstance that an ancillary study is equivocal, the observation period can actually be increased until another study or clinical examination and apnea test can be performed to confirm neurologic death. Ancillary studies can be helpful for social and medical reasons. These studies may allow family members to better comprehend that neurologic death has occurred and may be important in situations where death is the result of homicide. Ancillary studies are not a substitute for a complete physical examination.

Four-vessel cerebral angiography evaluating anterior and posterior cerebral circulation remains the gold standard to determine blood flow when testing for neurologic death; however, this test is difficult to perform in small children and requires technical expertise that may not be available in every facility. Furthermore, transporting a potentially unstable patient to the angiography suite carries additional risk that can complicate this process. For these reasons, cerebral angiography is rarely performed in infants and children. EEG documentation of electrocerebral silence (ECS) and absence of CBF using radionuclide CBF study remain the most widely available and useful ancillary studies to assist with the diagnosis of neurologic death in infants and children. These studies are more easily accomplished at the bedside, without the need for extraordinary technical expertise. Radionuclide CBF studies have been used extensively with good experience.[38] Use of the portable gamma camera for radionuclide angiography has made CBF studies more accessible, allowing for the study to be undertaken at the bedside.[38,39] This study is becoming a standard in many institutions replacing EEG as an ancillary study to assist with the determination of neurologic death in infants and children.[28,29,40] EEG and radionuclide CBF studies are both accepted ancillary studies used to assist the clinician in determining neurologic death in infants and children. EEG may be more specific although less sensitive than the radionuclide CBF study. EEG testing evaluates cortical and cellular function, whereas radionuclide CBF testing evaluates flow and uptake into brain tissue. Each of these tests requires the expertise of appropriately trained and qualified individuals who understand the limitations of these studies to avoid misinterpretation. Specific criteria for these studies must be met to determine neurologic death.[28,29] Transcranial Doppler sonography and brain stem audio evoked potentials have been utilized[41-43] but have not been studied extensively or validated in children.[28,29,44,45] These studies along with CT angiography, perfusion MRI, and magnetic resonance angiography-magnetic resonance imaging (MRA-MRI) cannot be relied on as dependable or validated ancillary studies at this time.[28,29,45]

Ancillary studies are least sensitive in the neonatal age group.[28,29,46] Limited experience with ancillary studies performed in the newborn younger than 30 days of age indicates that EEG is less sensitive than CBF in confirming a diagnosis of brain death. Sensitivity remains quite low, however, even with CBF for this age group.[28,29,46,47] The younger the child, the more cautious one should be in determining neurologic death. If there is any uncertainty about the examination, apnea testing, or the ancillary study, continued observation is warranted. Additional clinical evaluations and apnea testing or a repeat ancillary study followed by a second clinical examination and apnea test should be performed to make the determination of neurologic death.

Once death has been declared, appropriate documentation of the clinical examination, apnea test, and any ancillary study should be noted. The updated guidelines for the determination of neurologic death in infants and children encourage the use of the incorporated guidelines checklist to assist with standardizing the process and documentation of neurologic death in children.[28,29]

Technologic advances continue to affect our ability to determine circulatory and neurologic death. In certain circumstances, determination of neurologic death may be complicated by mechanical support such as extracorporeal membrane oxygenation (ECMO) or the use of advanced ventilation modes.[48,49] The updated brain death guidelines state that apnea testing should be performed safely. Apnea testing should be aborted if the patient becomes hemodynamically unstable or pulse oximetry oxygen saturations fall to less than 85%.[28,29] Performing apnea testing for a patient supported with ECMO has been safely accomplished.[50,51] The patient is placed on a flow-inflating bag valve system and hypercapnia can be induced by reducing the sweep gas or adding exogenous CO_2 to the circuit, thus allowing CO_2 to rise to an appropriate level to stimulate respiration. The rate of CO_2 rise will be variable depending how much the sweep gas is reduced.[50] Adding exogenous CO_2 theoretically may reduce the duration of the apnea test; however, this technique has not been reported. Patients supported on advanced modes of ventilation may not tolerate apnea testing. Additionally, apnea testing may be impaired by sedation and use of neuromuscular blockades that are commonly used with advanced modes of ventilation. The updated guidelines for the determination of neurologic death in infants and children make no provisions for patients with cyanotic heart disease. These patients are desaturated, not desaturating, and there are no standards to determine what level of oxygen saturation should be used before apnea testing is terminated. In these situations an ancillary study such as radionuclide CBF is recommended to assist with the determination of neurologic death.

Determining neurologic death has great implications with profound consequences. The clinical diagnosis of neurologic death is highly reliable when made by experienced examiners using established criteria.[28,29,52,53] There are no reports of children recovering neurologic function who met adult brain death criteria on neurologic examination.[28,29,47] Diagnosis must never be rushed or take priority over the needs of the patient or the family. Appropriate emotional support for the family should be provided, including adequate time to grieve with their child after death has occurred. Readers are encouraged to become familiar with guidelines in their respective institution.

Brain Death Physiology

Progression to neurologic death results in neuroendocrine dysfunction requiring specific interventions to preserve organ function. Efforts to control cerebral perfusion pressure, hemodynamic manifestations of herniation, and loss of central nervous system (CNS) function all contribute to the instability that routinely occurs during and after the progression to neurologic death. These physiologic changes clearly affect end-organ viability in the prospective organ donor. Understanding the physiologic changes and anticipating associated complications with neurologic death are therefore critical for organ function and recovery.

Loss of CNS function causes diffuse vascular regulatory and cellular metabolic injury.[54] Neurologic death resulting from cerebral ischemia increases circulating cytokines,[55] reduces cortisol production,[56] and precipitates massive catecholamine release. The combination of these factors results in physiologic deterioration and ultimately end-organ failure if left untreated.

Cerebral blood flow is approximately 50 mL/100 g per minute and consumes 15% of the cardiac output.[57] Without substrate consumption by the brain, glucose needs are reduced and the patient is prone to hyperglycemia. As neurologic death occurs, cerebral metabolism is further decreased and carbon dioxide production falls resulting in a reduction in $PaCO_2$. Hypothermia should be anticipated as a result of hypothalamic failure and loss of thermoregulation. Additionally, impaired adrenergic stimulation results in loss of vascular tone with systemic vasodilation and increased heat loss. Ischemia of the anterior and posterior pituitary occurs, leading to neuroendocrine dysfunction and pituitary hormone depletion. This results in inhibition or loss of hormonal stimulation from the hypothalamus with subsequent fluid and electrolyte disturbances and eventually cardiovascular collapse, if left untreated.

Hemodynamic deterioration that occurs with neurologic death is initiated by a massive release of catecholamines, commonly referred to as a sympathetic, catecholamine, or autonomic storm. This release of catecholamines is associated with cerebral ischemia and intracranial hypertension and manifests clinically as systemic hypertension and tachycardia.[54,58] During this autonomic storm, organs are exposed to extreme sympathetic stress from direct neural stimulation or from significant increases in endogenous catecholamines. The local effects of this sympathetic stimulation include increased vascular tone, effectively reducing blood flow and potentially causing ischemia to these organs.

This autonomic storm also has direct effects on the myocardium, as the surge of catecholamines increases systemic vascular resistance (SVR), myocardial work, and oxygen consumption.[59] Ischemic changes occur as a result of the imbalance between myocardial oxygen supply and demand resulting in subendocardial ischemia.[54,60] Myocardial ischemia impairs cardiac output leading to dysfunction of other organs. Left ventricular end-diastolic pressure rises, causing pulmonary edema. This condition may be exacerbated by displacement of systemic arterial blood into venous and pulmonary circulations due to catecholamine-mediated systemic vasoconstriction. Increased pulmonary vascular resistance and right heart volume overload may displace the ventricular septum into the left ventricle, further impairing cardiac output by impeding left ventricular filling.[61] Progression to neurologic death results in a cascade of inflammatory mediators being released, causing vasodilation as loss of sympathetic tone and catecholamine depletion occurs.[61-63] Additionally, a shift from aerobic to anaerobic metabolism occurs as a result of ischemia and the depletion of pituitary hormones affecting cardiac performance and end-organ function.

Following the determination of neurologic death and the decision to proceed with organ donation, efforts to reduce intracranial pressure are abandoned and care shifts toward providing adequate circulation and oxygen delivery to preserve vital organ function for transplantation. Subsequent care may differ from management before death. Decreased intravascular volume, caused by efforts to reduce CBF and control intracranial pressure (eg, volume restriction and diuretic agents), must be corrected. Correction of metabolic derangements such as hypernatremia from the use of hypertonic saline and hyperglycemia associated with catecholamine release and reduced cerebral metabolism is essential to optimize organ function prior to transplantation. Attention to volume loss from osmotic diuresis associated with hyperglycemia and diabetes insipidus (DI) following neurologic death must be anticipated and addressed to prevent cardiovascular collapse. Hemodynamic management goals are directed at maintaining normal peripheral perfusion and blood pressure for age. Additional donor management goals include the normalization of carbon dioxide tension (PCO_2), normalization of temperature, and correction of any other metabolic disturbances. Any existing infections should continue to be treated until organ procurement occurs. Even if no infectious disease concerns exist, antibiotics are commonly administered prior to organ recovery. Donor management goals are listed in Table 17.3. Progression from neurologic death to somatic death and loss of transplantable organs can result if appropriate care is not instituted.[8,22,61] Aggressive donor management optimizes organ function and affects the quality of organs recovered.[8,26,61] Aggressive donor management results in more transplantable organs and improved graft function,[23-27] potentially reducing hospital stay and decreasing morbidity and mortality for the transplant recipient.

Physiologic Considerations in the Management of the Pediatric Organ Donor

Management of the donor is a continuum of care extending from admission of a critically ill child to the recovery of organs for transplantation. The critical care team must effectively treat the potential donor and correct the physiologic derangements that follow neurologic death. The goal of therapy is to restore and maintain adequate oxygenation, ventilation, and perfusion to vital organs, thus preserving their function for successful transplantation.

Treatment of Hemodynamic Instability

Cardiac instability is the greatest limiting factor to successful organ recovery. Of all the physiologic abnormalities encountered in the prospective organ donor, the cardiovascular system is fraught with the greatest complexity and variation. The tremendous physiologic derangements associated with

TABLE 17.3	Pediatric Donor Management Goals		
Hemodynamic Support		**BLOOD PRESSURE**	
		Systolic (mm Hg)	Diastolic (mm Hg)
Normalization of blood pressure	Neonate	60-90	35-60
Systolic blood pressure appropriate for age	Infant (6 mo)	80-95	50-65
Note: Lower systolic blood pressures may be	Toddler (2 yr)	85-100	50-65
acceptable if biomarkers such as lactate and S_VO_2	School age (7 yr)	90-115	60-70
are normal. CVP <12 mm Hg (if measured) Dopamine <10 mcg/kg/min or Use of a single inotropic agent Normal serum lactate	Adolescent (15 yr)	110-130	65-80

Oxygenation and Ventilation	**Fluids and Electrolytes**	
Maintain PaO_2 >100 mm Hg FiO_2 0.40 Normalize $PaCO_2$ 35-45 mm Hg Arterial pH 7.30-7.45 Tidal volumes 8-10 mL/kg and PEEP of 5 cm H_2O or Tidal volumes 6-8 mL/kg and PEEP of 8-10 cm H_2O	Serum Na+ (mEq/L) Serum K+ (mEq/L) Serum glucose (mg/dL) Ionized Ca++ (mmol/L)	130-150 3-5 60-200 0.8-1.2

Thermal Regulation
Core body temperature 36-38°C

Modified from Nakagawa TA. North American Transplant Coordinators (NATCO) Updated Donor Management and Dosing Guidelines. Lenexa, KS: NATCO; 2008.

neuroendocrine dysfunction require specific interventions to restore normal physiology.

The sympathetic storm associated with cerebral ischemia and intracranial hypertension is a predictably transient phenomenon. Although end-organ ischemia can occur from intense hypertension, treatment with antihypertensive agents may not be warranted and indeed can create additional problems with perfusion when this phase of sympathetic outflow has passed. If hypertension is severe and treatment is felt to be indicated, a single IV dose or continuous infusion of a short-acting antihypertensive agent such as hydralazine, sodium nitroprusside, esmolol, or labetalol can be administered and titrated to effect. One must anticipate the profound vasodilation and hypotension that will occur following neurologic death and be prepared to appropriately resuscitate the patient to restore normal circulation and perfusion.

Once neurologic death occurs, sympathetic outflow ceases and catecholamine depletion occurs leading to a loss of sympathetic tone and vasodilation. This results in profound and abrupt hypotension with release of proinflammatory mediators initiating a cascade of molecular and cellular events with resultant ischemia and reperfusion injury to vital tissues.[62] Management goals during this phase of patient care are directed at aggressive restoration of circulating volume, optimizing cardiac output and oxygen delivery to the tissues, and maintaining normal blood pressure for age (see Table 17.3). Aggressive restoration of circulating volume and utilization of catecholamines to support blood pressure are mainstays of treatment.[63] Intravascular volume replacement can occur with isotonic crystalloid solutions such as normal saline or colloid solutions such as 5% albumin. Packed red blood cells can be used for the anemic patient or plasma for the patient with a coagulopathy. The use of artificial plasma expanders such as Hespan or dextran for volume resuscitation should be avoided because large volumes of these agents can promote coagulation disturbances and impair renal function.[8,64-66] Commonly used inotropic agents such as dopamine, dobutamine, and epinephrine can be titrated to effect. Catecholamines and dopamine appear to have immunomodulating effects that may help blunt the inflammatory response associated with brain death and improve kidney graft function.[67,68] Vasopressors such as norepinephrine, vasopressin, and phenylephrine can be used in situations where there is profound vasodilation and low systemic vascular resistance. Although sometimes necessary, the administration of high-dose vasoactive agents can be associated with reduced perfusion to donor organs, potentially jeopardizing their viability prior to recovery and transplantation. Many OPOs routinely use a combination of inotropic support, volume resuscitation, and HRT for donor management. The use of HRT with agents such as thyroid hormone, steroids, vasopressin, and insulin is common during donor management, especially in situations where significant inotropic support is required.[23-26,62,69] In addition to the impact of hypovolemia, acidosis, hypoxia, and hypercarbia, electrolyte disturbances can alter myocardial performance affecting suitability of organs for transplantation. These disturbances must be corrected to enhance the chances of successful organ recovery. Clinical characteristics, such as blood pressure and central venous pressure (CVP), and biomarkers, such as mixed venous oxygen saturation and serum lactate levels, serve as guides to adequate cardiac performance and tissue oxygen delivery. Echocardiography can provide useful information about filling pressures, wall motion abnormalities, and ventricular shortening or ejection fractions. Serial echocardiograms are routinely employed in donor management and performed to assess cardiac function as treatment of the donor progresses. In many instances, cardiac performance will improve with aggressive resuscitation and institution of HRT following neurologic death.[8]

Certain clinical indicators of end-organ perfusion may not be reliable once brain death has occurred. Urine output may not be a good clinical indicator of intravascular volume when DI is present. After death of the brain stem, heart rate may not be a reliable sign of intravascular volume status because there is a loss of beat-to-beat variation, lack of vagal tone, and fixed heart rate. Perfusion may also be affected as temperature instability, and hypothermia can result in delayed capillary refill time. Biomarkers such as mixed venous oxygen saturation and serum lactate levels may usefully guide cardiac management and manipulation of oxygen delivery to tissues. Elevations in serum lactate and the development of a metabolic acidosis provide evidence of tissue ischemia and should prompt immediate attention. Importantly, an elevated serum lactate may be present following CNS or multisystem trauma and may persist following neurologic death or with profound hepatic dysfunction.

Arrhythmias can occur during progression to, or following, neurologic death. The catecholamine storm triggered by adrenergic stimulation results in myocardial ischemia and can cause necrosis of the conduction system promoting rhythm disturbances. Tachydysrhythmias can be seen prior to neurologic death in response to the catecholamine storm. Bradyarrhythmias may not be responsive to atropine because of denervation of the heart following neurologic death. Epinephrine is the pharmacologic treatment of choice if bradyarrhythmias occur. Other factors that contribute to arrhythmias include hypoxemia, hypothermia, cardiac trauma, and the pro-arrhythmic properties of inotropes. Hypotension from hypovolemia and vasodilation causes poor cardiac output and metabolic acidosis. Electrolyte and metabolic disturbances, specifically hypomagnesemia, hypocalcemia, and hypokalemia that occur with DI, may also precipitate rhythm disturbances. Identification and correction of the underlying cause of the arrhythmia are essential to address and treat rhythm disturbances.

Hormonal Replacement Therapy

Significant volume resuscitation and inotropic support are commonly required to correct severe cardiovascular derangements following neurologic death. Anterior pituitary hormone deficits can result in thyroid and cortisol depletion and may contribute to the hemodynamic instability encountered in patients who have progressed to neurologic death.[56] HRT to restore aerobic metabolism and replace hormone deficiency from the hypothalamus and pituitary, augment blood volume, and reduce the use of inotropic support while optimizing cardiac output is commonly used to support this patient population. The use of HRT has allowed a management strategy where blood pressure and normovolemia are maintained using a minimum number of vasoactive agents.

Hormonal replacement therapy in adult donors is controversial with correlations of hormone use, cardiac function, and variable clinical outcomes noted.[23-26,69,70-73] In one adult series HRT was shown to reduce the need for vasoactive infusions in 100% of unstable donors and to abolish the need in 53% of such donors.[74] Decreased inotropic requirements have also been noted in children who received levothyroxine and vasopressin as part of donor management following neurologic death.[75] Although studies are limited, HRT seems to be a reasonable consideration in situations where the hemodynamic status of the child is refractory to conventional therapy with fluid and inotropic administration. HRT has been associated with an increased number of organs recovered from donors.[22-25,76] No published studies are available in children; however, one unpublished abstract retrospectively reviewed 1903 pediatric donors.[1] HRT was associated with significantly increased odds of having the liver and at least one kidney and lung transplanted. There was no significant increase in the odds of the heart being transplanted. The greatest benefit of HRT in donor management may in fact be improved graft function following transplantation.[23,76-78] Given these observations many OPOs have adopted the use of HRT as a routine part of donor management.[8] Commonly used agents and doses for HRT in pediatric donors are listed in Table 17.4.

TABLE 17.4 Pharmacologic Agents Used for Hormonal Resuscitation in Children

Drug	Dose	Route	Comments
Desmopressin (DDAVP)	0.5 mcg/hr	IV	Terminal half-life = 75 min (range 0.4-4 hr) Titrate to control urine output (2-4 mL/kg/h) May be beneficial in patients with an ongoing coagulopathy
Vasopressin (Pitressin)	0.5 milliunits/kg/hr	IV	Half-life = 10-35 min Titrate to control urine output (2-4 mL/kg/h) Hypertension can occur
Levothyroxine (Synthroid)	0.8-1.4 mcg/kg/hr Maximum 20 mcg/hr	IV	Titrate to effect Bolus dose 1-5 mcg/kg can be administered (maximum dose 20 mcg) Smaller infants and children require a higher bolus and infusion dose
Triiodothyronine (T3)	0.05-0.2 mcg/kg/hr	IV	Titrate to effect
Methylprednisolone	20-30 mg/kg Maximum dose 2 grams	IV	Dose may be repeated in 8-12 hours Fluid retention and glucose intolerance can occur
Hydrocortisone infusion	<25 kg 1 mg/kg/hr 26-35 kg 50 mg/hr 36-45 kg 75 mg/hr >45 kg 100 mg/hr	IV	Maximum dose should not exceed 100 mg/hr
Insulin	0.05-0.1 units/kg/hr	IV	Titrate to effect to control blood glucose levels Monitor for hypoglycemia

Modified from Nakagawa TA. North American Transplant Coordinators (NATCO) Updated Donor Management and Dosing Guidelines. Lenexa, KS: NATCO; 2008.

Impaired cardiac performance following neurologic death is due to myocardial injury associated with the catecholamine storm. Additionally, reduced free triiodothyronine (T3) levels may impair mitochondrial function and deplete energy stores. Animal studies have shown that diminished circulating levels of triiodothyronine and thyroxine[54] impair oxygen utilization. The effects of thyroid hormone on myocardial contractility are complex and can be immediate or delayed. The acute inotropic properties of T3 may occur as a result of beta-adrenoreceptor sensitization or may be completely independent of beta-adrenergic receptors.[78-81] Furthermore, T3 administration may play an important role in maintaining aerobic metabolism at the tissue level after neurologic death has occurred.[82] Beneficial hemodynamic effects in brain-dead patients receiving T3 administration have been variable.[78,79] Levothyroxine (Synthroid) and triiodothyronine (T3) are the two IV thyroid agents available for administration. Triiodothyronine is used in some centers for HRT; however, the cost of this medication may be prohibitive. Dosing of thyroid hormone for the pediatric organ donor is weight based and not well established. One retrospective study in which younger children received larger bolus and infusion doses than older children demonstrated enhanced weaning of inotropic support in children who progressed to brain death.[75]

Corticosteroids such as hydrocortisone are another pharmacologic agent routinely used by many centers for HRT to assist with hemodynamic support. There are few data demonstrating that hydrocortisone provides hemodynamic benefit in the potential pediatric organ donor.[62] However, treatment of the donor with high doses of corticosteroids to reduce inflammation associated with neurologic death and modulate immune function may improve donor organ quality and posttransplant graft function.[8] Additionally, the potential benefit of hydrocortisone and other steroids may lie in their ability to alter adrenergic receptors and regulate vascular tone by increasing sensitivity to catecholamines.[83,84] Steroids have also been shown to stabilize pulmonary function, reduce lung water accumulation, and increase lung recovery from donors.[85-89]

The combination of thyroid hormone and corticosteroids may be used to reduce vasoactive agent dose requirements in children. Additionally, vasopressin for the control of DI can reduce the need for inotropic support. HRT may provide the greatest benefit to the recipient of transplanted organs by improving donor organ quality.

Management of Pulmonary Issues for the Potential Pediatric Organ Donor

Increasing success with lung transplantation for the treatment of patients with end-stage lung and pulmonary vascular disease has placed a premium on the acquisition of lungs from the donor pool. Children waiting for a lung transplant constitute less than 5% of the national pediatric wait list.[1] However, the demand for lungs far exceeds availability because lungs are the organs most likely to be found unsuitable for transplantation. Recovery of lungs for transplantation accounts for 7% to 22% of the multiorgan donor pool.[69,90] The low percentage of lung recovery for transplantation reflects stringent donor selection criteria and a lack of suitable organs for transplantation. Every effort should be made to preserve lung function using protective lung strategies. Lung protective strategies have the potential to salvage marginal lungs for transplantation; however, in many instances these strategies are not implemented, resulting in the loss of potential lung donors.[90]

Many factors contribute to the limitations associated with the acquisition of lungs for transplantation. Neurogenic pulmonary edema may develop during the progression or upon completion of neurologic death resulting in high ventilator settings. Blunt trauma in children resulting in pulmonary contusion/hemorrhage accounts for a large portion of injuries to the thoracic cavity. Inhalational or thermal injury can damage the lungs and airway structures. Infectious etiologies can compound the effects of existing lung disease or injury. Often these injuries are the reason the patient has become an organ donor. Furthermore, the lungs are particularly vulnerable in the face of critical illness, leaving them susceptible to complications such as fat emboli, pulmonary emboli, aspiration pneumonia, ventilator-associated pneumonia, and atelectasis.[87] Each of these disorders is associated with lung injury and impaired ventilation and oxygenation that diminish the lung suitability for transplantation.

The physiologic aberrations that accompany neurologic death can also result in end-organ damage rendering lungs unsuitable for transplantation. Management of pulmonary physiology is often complicated by the development of pulmonary edema as neurologic injury progresses.[61] The sympathetic storm associated with neurologic death causes systemic and pulmonary vasoconstriction. Neurogenic pulmonary edema occurs as pulmonary venous pressure rises, causing pulmonary capillary wall disruption and the evolution of pulmonary edema.[91] This predictable deterioration of pulmonary function increases the lung's vulnerability to injury following neurologic death.[90,92] Massive brain injury may in fact act as a preconditioning factor that renders the graft more susceptible to subsequent lung damage and increases the risk of post-transplant graft failure.[92]

Lung protective management strategies have been developed as a result of the complex physiology and vulnerability of the lungs following brain death. Measures to protect donor lungs have resulted in improved recovery and successful transplantation of these organs.[93,94] Management strategies include measures such as diligent pulmonary toilet with frequent suctioning, patient turning, clearance of mucous plugs, and airway evaluation with flexible bronchoscopy.[87,95] Ventilator management with attention to recruitment maneuvers such as sustained inflations and positive end-expiratory pressure (PEEP) have been advocated to avoid the development of atelectasis and treat pulmonary edema associated with the catecholamine storm that occurs with neurologic death.[94,95] The benefit associated with the use of inflation maneuvers and PEEP must be balanced against the risk of barotrauma and effects on preload that can potentially embarrass cardiac output in the donor with myocardial dysfunction. Volume administration and inotropic support may be required if blood pressure is affected by this maneuver. These cardiovascular effects can be minimized if adequate preload is provided prior to escalation of PEEP. Colloid solutions have been recommended to minimize the accumulation of pulmonary edema.[95] Additionally, albuterol has been shown to enhance clearance of pulmonary edema in an animal model[70] and to improve mucociliary clearance.[87] Corticosteroids are frequently utilized in the donor and have been shown to reduce lung water accumulation and stabilize pulmonary function.[85-88] Another novel therapy involves the use of naloxone to improve gas exchange in donor lungs.[96] The exact mechanism of action of naloxone to enhance pulmonary function is unknown, but free radical scavenging has been suggested.

Ventilatory requirements may become minimal in the donor as neurologic death occurs. Respiratory alkalosis is common as metabolic production of carbon dioxide from the brain ceases and compliance of the chest wall changes. Restoring normocarbia with a goal of 35 to 40 mm Hg in the child who has progressed to neurologic death is ideal given the effects of pH on unloading characteristics of oxygen from hemoglobin. Avoiding overdistention of the lungs during mechanical and manual ventilation is crucial to reduce the risk of barotrauma or further pulmonary injury.[87,94] Donor management goals include achieving a PaO_2 of >100 mm Hg, oxygen saturation of >95% using the least amount of oxygen necessary. Adequate alveolar recruitment can be obtained using a tidal volume of 8 to 10 mL/kg and PEEP of 5 cm/H_2O or lower tidal volumes of 6 to 8 mL/kg and higher PEEP of 8 to 10 cm/H_2O. Elevation of the head of the bed and use of a cuffed endotracheal tube with high cuff pressures to reduce aspiration risk are also advocated.[87] Additionally, oral care using chlorhexidine may reduce the chances of a ventilator-associated infection. Frequent turning, pulmonary toilet, and chest physiotherapy when appropriate are essential to prevent atelectasis. Prone positioning may be beneficial to optimize ventilation perfusion matching. Serial chest radiographs are commonly obtained to identify correctable issues or evaluate pulmonary pathology. Donor Management Goals for oxygenation and ventilation are summarized in Table 17.3.

An oxygen challenge test is routinely performed to determine the suitability of the lungs for transplantation. Transplant surgeons prefer a PaO_2/FiO_2 ratio >300 on a FiO_2 of 1 and a relatively clear chest radiograph. Many OPOs advocate early flexible bronchoscopic evaluation of the lungs to address correctable issues and maximize ventilation strategies to improve lung function. Bronchoscopy can help to clear mucous plugs or blood clots that may contribute to impaired oxygenation.

Fluid and Electrolyte Disturbances

Fluid and electrolyte disturbances in the pediatric donor are the result of physiologic abnormalities following neurologic death, as well as consequences of earlier medical management. Commonly encountered derangements include dehydration, hyperglycemia, sodium, potassium, and calcium disturbances. Metabolic fluctuations associated with progression toward neurologic death require meticulous management of fluids and electrolytes. If left untreated, these abnormalities can adversely affect organ viability.

Intravascular volume depletion is frequently encountered in the child with traumatic brain injury who has progressed to neurologic death. Fluid restriction is commonly employed along with hypertonic solutions and osmotic diuretics in the management of cerebral edema. Another contributor to intravascular volume depletion is osmotic diuresis from hyperglycemia secondary to corticosteroid and catecholamine use and the increased availability of glucose from a loss of cerebral metabolism. Furthermore, DI compounds sodium and water imbalance if not aggressively treated. The potential donor must be adequately volume resuscitated, as guided by CVP, perfusion, serum electrolyte concentrations, and serial lactate measurements. Restoring intravascular volume is crucial to maintain organ viability.

Diabetes Insipidus

Diabetes insipidus occurs in many neurologically dead patients, and if left untreated it can have profound effects on the donor (see also Chapter 85). Ischemia and ultimate necrosis of the posterior pituitary lead to a loss of central antidiuretic hormone (ADH). The loss of ADH results in uncontrolled urine output with free water losses resulting in severe hypernatremia, severe dehydration and hypovolemic shock, and eventual cardiovascular collapse. Hypernatremia (serum sodium >155 mEq/L) can affect organ suitability for transplantation and has been associated with poorer graft outcome following liver transplantation.[8,97]

In addition to hourly maintenance of intravenous fluids, one-quarter or one-half normal saline can be used to replace urine output in excess of 3 to 4 mL/kg, until pharmacologic replacement therapy is implemented. Glucose should be avoided in renal replacement fluids to prevent further exacerbation of hyperglycemia and osmotic diuresis. Enteral free water supplementation administered through a nasogastric tube can be used to correct severe hypernatremia. Rapid osmolar shifts during correction of hypernatremia are inconsequential because neurologic death has already occurred. DI frequently requires pharmacologic treatment with ADH to reduce ongoing free water loss. Pharmacologic agents such as vasopressin or desmopressin (DDAVP) are routinely utilized in HRT protocols to control excessive urine output associated with DI. These pharmacologic agents have specific indications and side effects that must be considered when contemplating their use to treat DI.[98] Donor management goals for treating DI include maintaining a normal serum sodium level and reducing excessive urine output. With refractory DI, a combination of vasopressin and desmopressin may be indicated to control urine output. Pharmacologic treatment is intended to reduce and not completely stop urine output.

Vasopressin is a polypeptide hormone secreted by the hypothalamus and stored in the posterior pituitary. Vasopressin acts on V_1 and V_2 vasopressin receptors stimulating contraction of vascular smooth muscle with resultant vasoconstriction. It has a short half-life of 10 to 20 minutes, and unlike desmopressin it has no effect on platelets.[8,99] Vasopressin can be administered by bolus or continuous IV infusion. The most desirable features of this agent derive from its ease of titration to control urine output. When discontinued, its effects are short lived. Vasopressin is administered at doses of 0.5 milliunits/kg/hr and can be titrated to control urine output to 2 to 4 mL/kg/hr.[98,99] By titrating in this way one preserves renal function and avoids volume overload and metabolic abnormalities such as hyponatremia and hyperkalemia. Vasopressin acts synergistically with catecholamines and can reduce the need for additional catecholamine support in the neurologically dead donor.[24,75] This pharmacologic agent is ideal for the donor with DI and hemodynamic instability requiring inotropic support. Vasopressin infusions commonly require rapid titration to control excessive urine output. The infusion may need to be reduced after several hours to avoid complete loss of urine output.[100] High doses of vasopressin, especially when combined with other vasopressors with alpha stimulation, may potentially reduce splanchnic perfusion including hepatic and pancreatic blood flow. Additionally, vasoconstriction and increased smooth muscle contractility may affect coronary and pulmonary blood flow.[60] Excessive dosing of vasopressin should be avoided to preserve end-organ function.

Desmopressin acetate (DDAVP) is a more potent synthetic polypeptide structurally related to vasopressin. This agent lacks smooth muscle contractile properties and is more specific for the V_2 vasopressin receptor. Desmopressin enhances platelet aggregation and has a longer half-life of 6 to 20 hours

when administered as a single IV dose.[101,102] Desmopressin may be a preferred agent for the correction of hypernatremia in hemodynamically stable donors who require no inotropic or vasopressor support or the donor with ongoing bleeding issues. Desmopressin can be administered by continuous infusion at 0.5 mcg/hr and titrated to control urine output or as a single IV dose.[98,103] Intramuscular and intranasal administration can result in erratic absorption and should be avoided. The terminal half-life of desmopressin administered by continuous IV infusion is 75 minutes with a range of 0.4 to 4 hours.[103] The longer half-life of desmopressin may be less desirable compared to the shorter half-life of vasopressin in potential kidney donors. However, desmopressin therapy may be discontinued 3 to 4 hours prior to organ recovery.[98] Fluid replacement for excessive urine output can be administered as needed for the short period of time prior to organ recovery.

Oliguria

Oliguria can be seen with volume depletion, acute renal insufficiency or failure, and overly aggressive pharmacologic management of DI. If urine output falls to less than 1 mL/kg/hr and does not improve after decreasing or discontinuing vasopressin or desmopressin, intravascular volume status must be evaluated and appropriately treated. If urine output is not improved following volume expansion, the initiation of inotropic or vasopressor support may improve urine output. Furosemide (Lasix) or mannitol can be utilized to stimulate urine output in the patient with adequate intravascular volume status. A selective dopamine agonist such as fenoldopam can be used to enhance urine output and may provide renal protection in the normotensive or hypertensive patient.[104]

Glucose, Potassium, and Calcium Derangements

Neurologic death causes major hormonal alterations resulting in insulin resistance and gluconeogenesis. Hyperglycemia as a result of corticosteroid and catecholamine use and increased availability of glucose due to the loss of cerebral metabolism can lead to an osmotic diuresis, exacerbating an already depleted volume status in the donor. Hyperglycemia can be avoided by frequently assessing blood glucose concentration and making appropriate adjustments in the dextrose concentration in IV fluids. If these simple maneuvers are unsuccessful in controlling blood glucose levels, an insulin infusion should be instituted to maintain glucose levels within a reasonable range (60–200 mg/dL). Although target glucose levels for insulin therapy in the deceased donor continue to be debated, uncontrolled hyperglycemia should be treated.[8] Serum glucose levels should be closely followed to avoid hypoglycemia.

Potassium derangements can result from diuresis, renal insufficiency, steroid administration, and acid-base disturbances. Potassium can be supplemented if hypokalemia is significant. The adverse effects of hyperkalemia are clearly more hazardous than those of hypokalemia. The adverse effects of hypokalemia most likely to affect the potential donor are dysrhythmias.

Hypocalcemia occurs commonly secondary to large volume replacement with colloids such as albumin, massive blood transfusions that result in large amounts of citrate reducing free calcium concentrations, and sepsis. Ionized calcium levels should guide the use of calcium supplementation.

Coagulation Abnormalities and Thermoregulatory Instability

Coagulation abnormalities can arise secondary to the release of tissue thromboplastin and cerebral gangliosides from injured brain.[60] Additionally, the catecholamine surge associated with traumatic brain injury may contribute to coagulation disturbances.[105] Synthetic plasma expanders such as hespan or dextran can promote coagulation disturbances and are not recommended for volume replacement.[8,64,66] Thrombocytopenia and platelet dysfunction can be induced by common drugs such as heparin, antibiotics, beta-blockers, calcium channel blockers, histamine H_2 receptor antagonists, tromethamine, and hespan.[106] Patients with liver disease have reduced synthesis of vitamin K–dependent clotting factors. A dilutional coagulopathy can occur from massive transfusions if coagulation factors are not replenished. Coagulation abnormalities can also be exacerbated by hypothermia. Coagulopathy can be corrected using fresh frozen plasma, platelets, cryoprecipitate, and restoring and maintaining normothermia. The goal of blood product replacement for coagulopathy should be tailored accordingly based on the abnormalities encountered. Coagulation abnormalities should be addressed prior to transport of the donor to the operating suite for organ recovery. A minimum platelet count of 75,000/uL should be obtained prior to recovery of organs in the operating suite. The use of aminocaproic acid (Amicar), an antifibrinolytic agent, and other similar hemostatic agents are not recommended for treatment of bleeding because microvascular thrombosis may be induced in donor organs.[60]

Hypothermia commonly occurs following neurologic death due to loss of hypothalamic-pituitary function controlling temperature response. Vasodilation with an inability to compensate for heat loss by shivering or vasoconstriction is a common cause of thermoregulatory instability in this patient population. Additionally, infusion of large volumes of room temperature IV fluids to treat DI and volume depletion contributes to hypothermia. Hypothermia can promote cardiac dysfunction, arrhythmias, coagulopathy, a cold-induced diuresis secondary to decreased renal tubular concentration gradient, and a leftward shift of the oxyhemoglobin dissociation curve resulting in decreased oxygen delivery to the tissues.[107] Radiant warmers, warm blankets, thermal mattresses, warm IV fluids or a blood warmer for infusion of blood products, and environmental warming will help maintain body temperature. Additionally, heating-inspired gases can assist in controlling body temperature. Prevention of hypothermia is essential to prevent deterioration of the potential organ donor.

Medical Examiner/Coroner Issues and Organ Donation for Children

Many children who die from head injuries are victims of trauma. When a child's death is ruled a homicide, great sensitivity is required to preserve the integrity of the criminal investigation. Successful recovery of organs from these patients, and prosecution of the perpetrator, can still occur in most cases with close cooperation between forensic investigators, treating physicians, the transplant team, and the OPO.[3,8,108-114] In fact, there is no reported case law where organ donation has resulted in loss of evidence and inability to prosecute a perpetrator involved with the death of a child. Early involvement of the medical examiner or coroner and protocols to facilitate organ recovery in homicide cases can decrease denials for organ donation.[110-113] Involvement of the district attorney during protocol development should also be a consideration. Efforts to reduce the number of medical examiner denials for donation continue to occur at a national level and are supported by the National Association of Medical Examiners.[114] Despite these national efforts many transplantable organs from potential pediatric donors continue to be lost because of medical examiner/coroner denials.[6]

Donation After Circulatory Death

Although the majority of recovered organs are from donors following neurologic death, donation after circulatory death (DCD) provides another source of valuable organs for transplantation. Formerly known as the non–heart-beating organ donor or donation after cardiac death, DCD is not a new way to recover organs for transplantation. Prior to guidelines to determine neurologic death, cadaveric organs were routinely recovered after death was declared following loss of circulation.

DCD allows recovery of organs from patients with catastrophic brain injury who do not progress to neurologic death. The discussions and decision to donate organs can only occur after the decision to withdraw life-sustaining medical therapies has been made. This avoids the perceived ethical conflict that the patient is being allowed to die primarily to recover organs. Routine end-of-life care, including comfort measures, is provided for these patients just as would be the case for any patient where withdrawal of medical therapies occurs. Specific criteria must be met for organs to be recovered by this method. Circulatory arrest must usually occur within 60 minutes of withdrawing medical therapies. The time constraint is important because longer periods to achieve circulatory arrest will result in organ ischemia rendering potential transplant tissue useless. Following loss of pulse pressure (mechanical asystole), the patient is observed for 2 to 5 minutes before recovery of organs can occur. This 2- to 5-minute observation period is crucial to ensure that auto resuscitation of the heart with restoration of circulation does not occur. If mechanical asystole is consistent with circulatory death following the observation period, organs are recovered for transplantation. Importantly, loss of circulatory function and not electrical activity (electrical asystole) is required to determine death. Determination of when a patient will develop loss of circulation can be difficult to predict. Scoring tools have been developed in an effort to determine if death will occur within the specified time period for donation to occur.[115-117] These tools should be used in conjunction with the physical examination, discussion with the critical care team and OPO to determine donor suitability, and likelihood of progressing to death in the allotted time period. If circulatory cessation does not occur within 60 minutes, the patient is returned to the ICU, procurement of organs is aborted, and continued comfort measures are provided for the patient. Families must be prepared for the possibility that death may not occur within the specified time period. If this situation occurs, continued comfort measures for the patient and ongoing family support should continue. DCD donation requires close collaboration among the critical care team, the operating room staff, and the OPO to ensure the successful recovery of organs.

The reevaluation of this method of donation was prompted by the increasing need to meet the demands of a growing national transplant wait list.[118,119] There have been significant increases in the number of DCD donors since the early 2000s.[2] This sustained practice of organ recovery in children accounts for more than 10% of all DCD donors during this time period.[1] DCD has the potential to increase organ donation in children.[2,120-124] Individual numbers of DCD donors may be small at any one pediatric center, but the collective impact from all pediatric centers actively recovering organs from this type of donor has significantly increased the number of organs available for transplantation.[2,118,121-124]

DCD focuses on recovery of the two most commonly needed organs for children: the liver and the kidney. Success with transplantation of DCD organs, primarily the kidney and the liver, is occurring in many centers. Rates of graft survival for some of these organs appear to be similar to that for organs recovered from donors following neurologic death.[125-130] Results from pediatric DCD renal transplants have been acceptable.[118] However, concern has emerged about DCD liver transplantation and an increased risk of biliary stenosis, hepatic infections, postoperative complications, and higher repeat transplantation rates.[8,118,131]

The neonatal donor population is being explored in more detail as another source of valuable organs for transplantation.[132-134] Recovery of neonatal kidneys has the potential to increase the number of kidneys available for transplantation.[8,118,135,136] En bloc renal transplant from neonatal and pediatric DCD donors is also occurring with good success, even in donors as small as 1.9 kg.[136-138] Experience is increasing with lung transplants from DCD donors; however, no children have received lungs from a DCD donor.[139-141] Additionally, the successful transplantation of three hearts recovered from neonatal DCD donors, under an established research protocol, has occurred.[142]

Some controversy exists over this mode of donation. The ethical concerns center primarily on when death occurs and if the potential donor meets criteria for death at the time of organ recovery.[143-147] Although an ethical discussion on DCD donation is beyond the scope of this chapter, many national organizations have reviewed DCD and concluded that this form of donation is ethically acceptable when performed within specific guidelines. The Society of Critical Care Medicine, Institute of Medicine, American Medical Association, American Academy of Pediatrics (AAP), and other medical societies support DCD as an acceptable means to recover organs for transplantation.[3,148-152] The AAP recognizes ethical concerns and encourages but does not mandate physician participation with this type of donation.[153] The AAP does state that institutions should provide access to DCD donation. Education regarding this mode of donation is crucial for all health care personnel to successfully identify and recover organs from this population of children.[7,154,155]

Contraindications to Organ Donation

There are relatively few medical contraindications to organ donation. The transplant surgeon and the medical director of the OPO ultimately determine whether an organ is acceptable for transplantation. This decision is based on the patient's history, laboratory studies, and inspection of organs at the time of recovery. Overwhelming sepsis is usually a contraindication to donation. In many of these cases, most organs will suffer from inadequate perfusion rendering the organ unacceptable for transplantation. However, patients with meningitis or bacteremia can donate organs if they have been appropriately treated with antibiotics for 24 hours.[8] Other CNS infections such as encephalitis or disseminated viral infections may pose too great a risk to the recipient, limiting the donation potential in these patients. Patients with hepatitis B and C can donate organs to patients who are infected with the same virus. Patients with HIV were once considered ineligible to become donors; however, the HIV Organ Policy Equity Act (HOPE) bill was passed and allows transplantation of HIV-positive organs from a donor with the same serotype. Active malignancies are a contraindication to donation. However, patients who have had cancer and are in remission may be candidates for donation depending on how long they have been in remission. Patients with central nervous system tumors that have not metastasized may be eligible to donate organs. Surgical intervention for these tumors including shunt placement or craniotomy may limit eligibility for donation. Concerns regarding donation potential should be discussed with the OPO medical director before a decision regarding donation eligibility can be established.

Evolving Areas of Transplantation

Improved donor management, operative techniques, postoperative care, and immunosuppressive therapy have advanced transplantation allowing for recovery of more organs and better graft function to meet the growing needs of those waiting for a lifesaving transplant. Uses of organs once considered less than optimal are now being considered for transplantation as technologies develop that can enhance donor organ function. Ex vivo perfusion of donor organs using specially designed organ support systems are being tested to improve the quality of organs prior to transplantation.[156-158] These organ preservation systems specifically designed for the kidney, heart, liver, and lungs may help overcome limitations and effects of cold ischemic preservation that can affect graft performance following transplantation. Ex vivo perfusion can maintain organs in a near physiologic state allowing for longer preservation time for procured organs prior to transplantation.

Infants waiting for a transplant continue to have the highest death rate on the waiting list.[2] Many infants waiting for a heart transplant may die because an organ never becomes available. ABO incompatible heart transplantation and recovery of hearts from neonatal DCD donors may provide needed organs to decrease infant deaths on the national wait list[133,141,159-161] (see also Chapter 39). The use of mechanical support devices can also provide a bridge to heart transplantation. Livers recovered from neonatal donors can undergo special processing for liver cell transfusion under an investigational study.[162] These hepatocytes are being infused into infants with urea cycle defects as a bridge to transplantation.[162,163] Advancement in vascularized composite allograft (VCA) transplantation continues to grow as more experience with face and extremity transplants occurs.[164-166] Vascularized composite allografts have been added under the definition of *organ* in the Organ Procurement Transplantation Network Final Rule.[167]

Summary

The process of organ donation begins when a critically ill or injured child is identified as a potential donor with a timely referral to the OPO. Identifying and caring for the pediatric organ donor requires a skilled team of specialists who deal not only with the deceased child but also with the family. Early involvement of the OPO allows coordination with physicians, social workers, chaplains, and family support services, enhancing the chance for the family to understand and authorize organ donation. Timely and accurate determination of neurologic death allows the focus of medical management to transition toward care and preservation of organs for transplantation once authorization has been obtained. Management of the pediatric organ donor is a natural extension of care for a critically ill or injured child. Meticulous care of the potential donor results in more transplantable organs with improved graft function. Increased numbers of organs recovered from pediatric donors are being transplanted into more children, although adults continue to receive the majority of these organs. The option for organ donation should be made available to every family. Preserving the option of donation provides an opportunity for every family to make decisions about donation when their child has died. Families should be emotionally supported and approached about donation opportunities in a professional, compassionate manner that allows for open discussion during the most difficult, agonizing time in their lives. The positive benefits of donation extend beyond the transplant recipient. Donation helps families heal as they deal with the loss of their child. Collaboration between pediatric critical care specialists, the critical care team, and other dedicated professionals providing specialized donor management can affect the lives of not only the donor family but also the many potential recipients and their families through the effects of a lifesaving and life-changing transplant.

For more information and additional resources about pediatric organ donation, readers are referred to the Organ Donation Toolbox at http://organdonationalliance.org/organ-donation-toolbox.

Key References

1. Data. OPTN. Organ Procurement and Transplantation Network. Available at: <http://optn.transplant.hrsa.gov/converge/data/>; Accessed 02.06.15.
2. Workman JK, Myrick CW, Meyers RL, et al. Pediatric organ donation and transplantation. Pediatrics. 2013;131:e1723-e1730.
3. Committee on Hospital Care, Section on Surgery, and Section on Critical Care. Policy statement—pediatric organ donation and transplantation. Pediatrics. 2010;125:822-828.
4. President's Commission for the Study of Ethical Problems in Medicine and Biomedical and Behavioral Research. Defining Death: A Report on the Medical, Legal and Ethical Issues in the Determination of Death. Washington, DC: U.S. Government Printing Office; 1981 Available at: <https://scholarworks.iupui.edu/bitstream/handle/1805/707/Definining%20death%20-%201981.pdf?sequence=1&isAllowed=y>; Accessed 02.06.15.
6. Webster PA, Markham L. Pediatric organ donation: a national survey examining consent rates and characteristics of donor hospitals. Pediatr Crit Care Med. 2009;10:500-504.
8. Kotloff RM, Blosser S, Fulda GJ, et al. Management of the potential organ donor in the ICU: Society of Critical Care Medicine/American College of Chest Physicians/Association of Organ Procurement Organizations Consensus Statement. Crit Care Med. 2015;43:1291-1325.
16. de Vos MA, Bos AP, Plötz FB, et al. Talking with parents about end-of-life decisions for their children. Pediatrics. 2015;135:e465-e476.
17. Boss R, Nelson J, Weissman D, et al. Integrating palliative care into the PICU: a report from the Improving Palliative Care in the ICU Advisory Board. Pediatr Crit Care Med. 2014;15:762-767.
18. Owens DA. The role of palliative care in organ donation. J Hosp Palliat Nurs. 2006;8:75-76.
21. The President's Council on Bioethics. Controversies in the determination of death: a white paper by the President's Council on Bioethics. Washington, DC: 2008 Available at: <https://bioethicsarchive.georgetown.edu/pcbe/reports/death/>; Accessed 02.06.15.
28. Nakagawa TA, Ashwal S, Mathur M, et al. Guidelines for the determination of brain death in infants and children: an update of the 1987 Task Force recommendations. Crit Care Med. 2011;39:2139-2155.
32. Mulder M, Gibbs HG, Smith SW, et al. Awakening and withdrawal of life-sustaining treatment in cardiac arrest survivors treated with therapeutic hypothermia. Crit Care Med. 2014;42:2493-2499.
44. Farrell MM, Levin DL. Brain death in the pediatric patient: historical, sociological, medical, religious, cultural, legal, and ethical considerations. Crit Care Med. 1993;21:1951-1965.
50. Jarrah RJ, Ajizian SJ, Agarwal S, et al. Developing a standard method for apnea testing in the determination of brain death for patients on venoarterial extracorporeal membrane oxygenation: a pediatric case series. Pediatr Crit Care Med. 2014;15:e38-e43.
51. Shah V, Lazaridis C. Apnea testing on extracorporeal membrane oxygenation: case report and literature review. J Crit Care. 2015;30:784-786.
59. Pérez López S, Otero Hernández J, Vázquez Moreno N, et al. Brain death effects on catecholamine levels and subsequent cardiac damage assessed in organ donors. J Heart Lung Transplant. 2009;28:815-820.
61. Lutz-Dettinger N, de Jaeger A, Kerremans I. Care of the potential pediatric organ donor. Pediatr Clin North Am. 2001;48:715-749.
70. Wood KE, Becker BN, McCartney JG, et al. Care of the potential organ donor. N Engl J Med. 2004;351:2730-2739.
73. Venkateswaran RV, Dronavalli V, Lambert PA, et al. The proinflammatory environment in potential heart and lung donors: prevalence and impact of donor management and hormonal therapy. Transplantation. 2009;88:582-588.
75. Zuppa AF, Nadkarni V, Davis L, et al. The effect of a thyroid hormone infusion on vasopressor support in critically ill children with cessation of neurologic function. Crit Care Med. 2004;32:2318-2322.
80. Cooper DK, Novitzky D, Wicomb WN, et al. A review of studies relating to thyroid hormone therapy in brain-dead organ donors. Front Biosci (Landmark Ed). 2009;14:3750-3770.
87. Mallory GB Jr, Schecter MG, Elidemir O. Management of the pediatric organ donor to optimize lung donation. Pediatr Pulmonol. 2009;44:536-546.
88. Venkateswaran RV, Patchell VB, Wilson IC, et al. Early donor management increases the retrieval rate of lungs for transplantation. Ann Thorac Surg. 2008;85:278-286.
93. Angel LF, Levine DJ, Restrepo MI, et al. Impact of a lung transplantation donor-management protocol on lung donation and recipient outcomes. Am J Respir Crit Care Med. 2006;174:710-716.
95. Rosengard BR, Feng S, Alfrey EJ, et al. Report of the Crystal City meeting to maximize the use of organs recovered from the cadaver donor. Am J Transplant. 2002;2:701-711.
98. Nakagawa TA, Mou SS. Management of the pediatric organ donor. In: LaPointe D, Ohler L, Rudow T, et al., eds. The Clinician's Guide to Donation and Transplantation. Lenexa, KS: North American Transplant Coordinators Organization (NATCO); 2006:839-835.
112. Shafer TJ, Schkade LL, Evans RW, et al. Vital role of medical examiners and coroners in organ transplantation. Am J Transplant. 2004;4:160-168.
114. Pinckard JK, Wetli CV, Graham MA, et al. National Association of Medical Examiners position paper on the medical examiner release of organs and tissues for transplantation. Am J Forensic Med Pathol. 2007;28:202-207.
115. Shore PM, Huang R, Roy L, et al. Development of a bedside tool to predict time to death after withdrawal of life-sustaining therapies in infants and children. Pediatr Crit Care Med. 2012;13:415-422.
116. Rabinstein AA, Yee AH, Mandrekar J, et al. Prediction of potential for organ donation after cardiac death in patients in neurocritical state: a prospective observational study. Lancet Neurol. 2012;11:414-419.
119. Kolovos NS, Webster P, Bratton SL. Donation after cardiac death in pediatric critical care. Pediatr Crit Care Med. 2007;8:47-49.
120. Morrissey PE, Monaco AP. Donation after circulatory death: current practices, ongoing challenges, and potential improvements. Transplantation. 2014;97:258-264.

124. Naim MY, Hoehn KS, Hasz RD, et al. The Children's Hospital of Philadelphia's experience with donation after cardiac death. *Crit Care Med*. 2008;36:1729-1733.

134. Stiers J, Aguayo C, Siatta A, et al. Potential and actual neonatal organ and tissue donation after circulatory determination of death. *JAMA Pediatr*. 2015;169:639-645.

136. Perez R, Santhanakrishnan C, Demattos A, et al. The neonatal intensive care unit (NICU) as a source of deceased donor kidneys for transplantation: initial experience with 20 cases (abstract #2289). *Am J Transplant*. 2014;14(suppl 3):134.

138. Lau KK, Berg GM, Schjoneman YG, et al. Pediatric en bloc kidney transplantation into pediatric recipients. *Pediatr Transplant*. 2010;14:100-104.

141. Krutsinger D, Reed RM, Blevins A, et al. Lung transplantation from donation after cardiocirculatory death: a systematic review and meta-analysis. *J Heart Lung Transplant*. 2015;34:675-684.

142. Boucek MM, Mashburn C, Dunn SM, et al. Pediatric heart transplantation after declaration of cardiocirculatory death. *N Engl J Med*. 2008; 359:709-714.

143. Bernat JL, Capron AM, Bleck TP, et al. The circulatory-respiratory determination of death in organ donation. *Crit Care Med*. 2010;38:963-970.

144. Joffe AR, Carcillo J, Anton N, et al. Donation after cardiocirculatory death: a call for a moratorium pending full public disclosure and fully informed consent. *Philos Ethics Humanit Med*. 2011;6:17.

149. Institute of Medicine. *Non-heart-beating organ transplantation: practice and protocols*. Washington, DC: National Academy Press; 2000. Available at: <http://www.iom.edu/reports/2000/non-heart-beating-organ-transplantation-practice-and-protocols.aspx>; Accessed 02.06.15.

150. American Medical Association. Opinion 2.157 - Organ Donation After Cardiac Death. Available at: <http://www.ama-assn.org/ama/pub/physician-resources/medical-ethics/code-medical-ethics/opinion2157.page?>; Accessed 02.06.15.

152. Gries CJ, White DB, Truog RD, et al. An official American Thoracic Society/International Society for Heart and Lung Transplantation/Society of Critical Care Medicine/Association of Organ and Procurement Organizations/United Network of Organ Sharing Statement: ethical and policy considerations in organ donation after circulatory determination of death. *Am J Respir Crit Care Med*. 2013;188:103-109.

153. Committee on Bioethics. Ethical controversies in organ donation after circulatory death. *Pediatrics*. 2013;131:1021-1026.

154. Curley MA, Harrison CH, Craig N, et al. Pediatric staff perspectives on organ donation after cardiac death in children. *Pediatr Crit Care Med*. 2007;8:212-219.

155. Mathur M, Taylor S, Tiras K, et al. Pediatric critical care nurses' perceptions, knowledge, and attitudes regarding organ donation after cardiac death. *Pediatr Crit Care Med*. 2008;9:261-269.

156. Andreasson AS, Dark JH, Fisher AJ. Ex vivo lung perfusion in clinical lung transplantation–state of the art. *Eur J Cardiothorac Surg*. 2014;46:779-788.

157. Ardehali A, Esmailian F, Deng M, et al. Ex-vivo perfusion of donor hearts for human heart transplantation (PROCEED II): a prospective, open-label, multicentre, randomised non-inferiority trial. *Lancet*. 2015;385:2577-2584.

161. Henderson HT, Canter CE, Mahle WT, et al. ABO-incompatible heart transplantation: analysis of the Pediatric Heart Transplant Study (PHTS) database. *J Heart Lung Transplant*. 2012;31:173-179.

165. Shores JT, Brandacher G, Lee WP. Hand and upper extremity transplantation: an update of outcomes in the worldwide experience. *Plast Reconstr Surg*. 2015;135:351e-360e.

166. Westvik TS, Dermietzel A, Pomahac B. Facial restoration by transplantation: the Brigham and Women's face transplant experience. *Ann Plast Surg*. 2015;74(suppl 1):S2-S8.

Pediatric Transport: Shifting the Paradigm to Improve Patient Outcome

Kate Felmet, Richard A. Orr, Yong Y. Han, and Kimberly R. Roth

PEARLS

- The goal of interfaculty transport is to bring critical care to the patient, providing aggressive stabilization and anticipating the evolution of respiratory failure and cardiovascular instability in a high-risk environment.
- Pathophysiology of acute respiratory and hemodynamic embarrassment in children differs from that in adults in ways that may impact care during transport and make it challenging for multidisciplinary teams to provide excellent care for pediatric patients.
- For most disease processes, speed of transport should not take precedence over providing quality resuscitation.
- Transfer by specialized pediatric transport teams may improve patient outcomes.
- Necessary components of a retrieval system include a communication center, appropriately trained team members, reliable equipment, continuing education, and safety monitoring.
- Although the legal responsibility for safety of interfacility transport rests mostly with the referring facility, the pediatric intensivist who acts as receiving or command physician can play an important role in recommending additional interventions and anticipating the deterioration of pediatric patients en route to tertiary care.

As pediatric emergency and critical care centers have become more regionalized, the need for quality interfacility transport increases. Eighty-nine percent of pediatric emergency department (ED) visits occur in nonpediatric EDs, where the extent of illness or injury is assessed and initial stabilization is provided.[1] Most community hospitals do not have the personnel, space, or facilities to provide critical care to infants or children beyond the period of initial stabilization, necessitating transfer. In transport, children are subjected to a high-risk environment with limited resources and monitoring capabilities. The goal during transport should be to minimize the risk of deterioration or secondary injury during transport while continuing and, in many cases, advancing the care initiated at the receiving facility.

For most pediatric critical illness, definitive care does not involve miracle drugs or technologies but rather the early, aggressive administration of simple therapies: Timely initiation of resuscitation fluids, inotropes administered via peripheral intravenous line, and antibiotic therapy can improve outcomes.[2,3] If appropriate resuscitation waits until the child arrives in the pediatric intensive care unit (PICU), the benefits of early action may be lost. Goal-directed therapy must begin before and continue during transport for the benefits noted in these studies to occur. Significant barriers to realizing this ideal state exist. A tension exists between the need to transfer patients as rapidly as possible and the desire to make transfers as safe as possible.

This chapter summarizes the physiology relevant to pediatric transport, particularly air transport, with attention to the differences between pediatric and adult patients. It is emphasized that a well-run interfaculty transport team that is focused on the specific needs of children can make a significant difference in patient outcomes. Information about appropriate vehicles, medication, and equipment for transport is best summarized in the American Academy of Pediatrics (AAP) Guidelines for Air and Ground Transport of Neonatal and Pediatric Patients.[4]

Adult-Oriented Medical Systems Frequently Fail Children

In many regions of the United States, medical transport teams that mostly focus on adults, like emergency medical services (EMS) or regional flight teams, are scattered throughout the community, close to referring hospitals, whereas pediatric retrieval teams are located at the sponsoring tertiary care facility. Because they are so accessible to referring hospitals, EMS and regional flight teams transport the majority of critically ill children. Training and protocols of these teams are primarily focused on the major causes of mortality in the adult population, like myocardial infarction, stroke, and trauma, disease processes for which rapid transfer definitive care is an important determinant of outcome.[5] Pediatric intensivists coordinating interfacility transfers need to be aware of the concerns that lead referring physicians to prefer rapid transport by a nonspecialized team over transfer by a team originating at the accepting facility. These concerns are summarized

BOX 18.1   Arguments Against and for Use of Specialized Pediatric Transport Teams

1. Specialized teams take too long to get to the patient.

   Concern for bed flow in small referring emergency departments is real, but when we bring goal-directed ICU care to the patient, the time to initiating time sensitive may be shortened.

2. Specialized teams spend too much time on the scene.

   Scene time is necessary for stabilization, but the need for additional measures may be underappreciated by the referring hospital.

3. Time to definitive care is longer with specialized teams.

   When interventions only available at the accepting facility are the most important determination of outcome, this may be true, but in general, with specialized team, total transport time has not been shown to correlate with negative outcomes.

4. Adult teams have Pediatric Advanced Life Support (PALS) training and can do the same thing.

   Nonspecialized teams lack experience with children, are less skilled in assessment of children, and have difficulty maintaining learned skills.

5. Specialized teams are expensive and resource-intensive.

   Resource use may be justified by improved outcomes.

in Box 18.1 and will be discuss in detail throughout the chapter.

Two independent studies reported that as recently as 2003, only 6% of emergency rooms were completely equipped to care for children.[6] In an assessment of the compliance by emergency departments with nationally recognized guidelines on the care of children in EDs, improvements since 2003 were noted, although deficits in equipment and safety procedures remain common.[7] Limited pediatric training coupled with limited exposure to pediatric patients may hamper the ability of ED and EMS providers to respond appropriately to pediatric emergencies. Fewer than 10% of all EMS runs nationwide involve infants and children, and a small percentage of these involve advanced life support (ALS) or critical care.[8,9] Babl and colleagues[10] demonstrated that in a program with 50 active ALS providers, each provider is expected to have one pediatric bag-valve-mask (BVM) case every 1.7 years, one pediatric intubation every 3.3 years, and one intraosseous cannulation every 6.7 years. Without repeated reinforcement, providers' knowledge and skills deteriorate over time.[11,12]

Underutilization of these skills may drive an aversion to performing procedures in children. With any given scenario in the EMS setting, adult patients are more likely to receive an appropriate intervention compared with a child having the same problem.[13-15] Multiple investigators have documented a disconcertingly low percentage of successful intubations in children compared with adult patients.[16-20] Historically, children have been twice as likely to die of trauma in the field compared with adults.[5,21,22] In a retrospective study comparing prehospital intervention of pediatric and adult patients with head injury, paramedics had difficulty with intubation in 69% of children compared with 21% of adults, and they were

unable to establish IV access in 34% of children versus 14% of adults.[13]

Referring hospitals that lack pediatric expertise may create suboptimal situations prior to transport. Esposito and colleagues found frequent errors occur in ED management of pediatric trauma, leading to preventable mortality of approximately 9%.[23] They reported a 64% error rate in the management of children, including gross violations of basic trauma care.[23] Han and associates[24] found that resuscitation practice in a community ED was consistent with American College of Critical Care Medicine-Pediatric Advanced Life Support (ACCM-PALS) guidelines in only 30% of children who presented with septic shock. Athey and coworkers[25] found that nearly 10% of all US hospitals without pediatric intensive care facilities admit critically ill and injured children, and that 7% of these hospitals routinely admit these children to adult intensive care units even though most of these lacked appropriate-sized equipment to care for children.[25]

Medical teams that mostly focus on adults often lack the training and the interventional skill to provide excellent initial stabilization. They may also lack an understanding of the physiologic differences between adults and children that impact the changes seen in the first few hours after presentation, the time window in which most patients are transported. An awareness of these differences will help emergency personnel to anticipate deterioration during transport and choose appropriate interventions before transport.

Critical Pediatric Physiology Relevant to Transport Medicine

Differences between the respiratory mechanics and cardiovascular physiology in adults and children mandate a need for earlier, more aggressive intervention in children with common pediatric problems. Failure to understand these differences can lead to a potentially injurious delay in advanced airway/pulmonary management and shock resuscitation.

Peripheral airway resistance in children younger than 5 years is approximately four times higher than in adults or older children, in whom the upper airway is the major contributor to airflow resistance.[24] For this reason, young children are more likely to have lower airway obstructive disease and are less likely to respond to airway positioning, an intervention that paramedics commonly use to defer intubation in adults.

Infants and small children are at higher risk for respiratory decompensation en route compared with older children adults. Infants and small children have more compliant chest walls with low elastic recoil, increasing the risk of lung collapse.[26] Muscular effort is required to stabilize the chest wall, and a portion of the force of contraction of the diaphragm is wasted in distorting the rib cage.[27] This mechanical disadvantage leads to increased energy expenditure and increases the likelihood that infants with lung disease may fatigue and stop breathing.[28-29] Functional residual capacity is only slightly higher than critical closing volume in infants and small children, leading to alveolar collapse much earlier in the course of respiratory failure. Lung growth appears to involve both an increase in the number of alveoli and an increase in the size of alveolar spaces,[30] which may also predispose the infant lung, with its smaller alveoli, to collapse. In addition, the adult lung contains anatomic channels that allow ventilation distal to an obstructed airway, also known as collateral ventilation; the absence of these pathways in young children further increases the risk for atelectasis.[31] The diffusing capacity across the alveolar-capillary membrane in a child is only about one-third that of an adult, making gas exchange less efficient.[32]

In general, positive pressure breathing applied early in the disease process can stop the progression of atelectasis and respiratory failure. Airway interventions should be planned carefully and performed early in the course of respiratory failure to avoid dealing with a respiratory crisis while en route. Gastric distention can further decrease the efficiency of the diaphragm in children and should be prevented or treated with a nasogastric tube.

Differences in cardiovascular physiology may hamper the ability of providers to recognize shock in children, which may delay the delivery of goal-directed therapy. Infants and children have a greater capacity to increase systemic vascular resistance in shock states and tend to preserve blood pressure until very late in the evolution of shock.[33] Pediatric shock resuscitation protocols developed by the consensus of experts in the field call for treatment of shock using clinical signs, including age-specific targets for heart rate and blood pressure, and relatively subtle indicators of perfusion as therapeutic endpoints.[34] These subtle signs may be difficult for adult-oriented providers to appreciate. Because children maintain diastolic blood pressure with vasoconstriction and tend to have normal coronary arteries, death from overwhelming shock and myocardial failure is uncommon. This creates the erroneous perception by emergency practitioners that goal-directed therapy is less critical in children and may lead to under-resuscitation.

Stresses of the Transport Environment

The physical stresses of the transport environment do not differ markedly between adults and children but deserve mention here. The transport environment is always risky. Movement of vehicles and ambient noise make examination difficult and monitor function less reliable. Each transfer of the stretcher or isolette from hospital to vehicle or between ambulance and aircraft adds potential for disruption of necessary tubes or devices. Fear and anxiety produced by the transport environment can worsen some conditions; at times it is advantageous to allow a parent to travel with the child. The transport team has to cope with these challenges, relying on only themselves, a limited number of medications, and the equipment they can carry. Depletion of medications and oxygen while en route can be catastrophic.

All of these physical stressors are magnified in air transport. Temperature drops significantly with increasing altitude. Helicopters are not climate controlled. The noise and vibration produced by rotorcraft make auscultation and simple procedures nearly impossible. Flight crews must rely on monitoring that does not depend on audible sounds, such as noninvasive blood pressure monitoring, capnometry, and pulse oximetry to monitor patients in flight. Although transport time in a helicopter may be short, physiologic changes are often missed, and new interventions are rarely initiated. For this reason, patients should be well stabilized prior to transport. In particular, the threshold for intubation in pediatric patients undergoing helicopter transport should be lower than in those undergoing ground transport.

Barometric pressure changes associated with increasing cabin altitude lower alveolar oxygen tension and increase the volume of gas entrapped in the bowel, sinuses, pleural space,

and so on. At the altitudes used by rotorcraft (generally less than 2000 feet above ground level), changes in oxygen tension are insignificant, and pressure changes have only a minor impact on the volume of air-filled spaces.[35] However, the relatively small volume of air in the tracheal tube cuff may be subject to clinically significant pressure changes at that altitude. A prospective study found that 98% of patients had tracheal tube cuff pressures >30 mm Hg and 72% had intra-cuff pressures >50 mm Hg during helicopter transport at a mean of 2260 feet.[36] Tracheal tube cuff pressures should be measured and adjusted during flight. Air removed at altitude will need to be replaced during descent.

The United States Federal Aviation Administration regulations mandate cabin altitude less than 8000 feet in fixed wing flight. Most medical flights maintain a cabin pressure equivalent to 6000 to 8000 feet.[37] Atmospheric pressure drops from 760 at sea level to 565 mm Hg O_2 at 8000 feet with a corresponding drop in the partial pressure of oxygen. Predicting PaO_2 at altitude is an inexact science; all that can be said conclusively is that patients with a marginal PaO_2 at ground level will be worse at cruising altitude. In practice, the impact of a cabin pressure in this range can usually be overcome with supplemental oxygen.[37] Oxygen should be used prophylactically in patients who are sensitive to alveolar hypoxia, like those with reactive pulmonary hypertension.

Ventilators are calibrated for performance at sea level, and those that compensate for changes in barometric pressure do exist but are not in common use. Tidal volumes delivered by the LTV 1000 (Pulmonetic Systems Inc. Minneapolis, MN), a commonly used transport ventilator, may vary from 5% to 12% at a simulated altitude of 4000 and 8000 in volume control mode. At 15,000 feet, LTV delivered tidal volumes may be 30% to 37% greater than set tidal volumes.[38] Similar findings have been reported with the Drager Oxylog ventilator.[38]

Acceleration and deceleration forces during takeoff and landing can cause clinically significant fluid shifts.[37] In most aircraft, the stretcher must be positioned head forward. This position will cause blood to pool in the legs during acceleration or takeoff and in the head during deceleration of landing.[37] In a patient with shock, raising the feet can minimize the decrease in cardiac output due to decreased venous return associated with takeoff. In a patient with increased intracranial pressure, the head should be raised during landing to minimize the increase in intracranial pressure associated with landing in this position.

Rapid Transfer, Goal-Directed Therapy, and the Golden Hour

Adult-focused EMS and regional flight teams operate under the assumption that the time between the moment of injury and arrival at a center capable of delivering definitive care is among the most important determinants of survival. This *golden hour* has been a driving force for clinical decision making since the concept was used to promote helicopter transports for trauma patients in the 1970s, an era when pretransport stabilization rarely went beyond supplemental oxygen[40] (Fig. 18.1). *Scoop and run* remains the prevailing philosophy in the world of adult interfacility transport.

There are a few disease processes in children in which rapid transport to a center that can provide definitive care is the most pressing issue. Aneurysms requiring neurosurgical intervention or complete transposition of the great arteries

TRADITIONAL MODEL

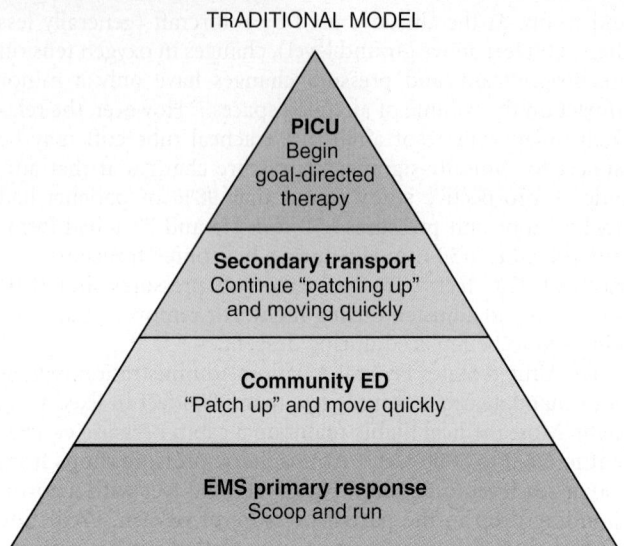

Fig. 18.1. Traditional model of emergency care based on the concept of the "golden hour." *ED,* emergency department; *EMS,* emergency medical services; *PICU,* pediatric intensive care unit.

requiring urgent atrial septostomy are examples and are thankfully rare. Respiratory insufficiency and shock are common reasons for referral of pediatric patients. One study identified shock in 37% of children transferred to tertiary centers *regardless of the reason for referral.*[41] It is increasingly recognized that rapid resuscitation is critical to the management of pediatric shock.[34] In adults and children, protocolized, aggressive, early resuscitation of septic shock has proved vastly more effective than any pharmacologic intervention.[2,24,41,42] Aggressive fluid resuscitation and the initiation of inotropes and antibiotics should be accomplished within the first hour after presentation. In adults with septic shock, a delay in antibiotic therapy is associated with worse survival, with mortality increasing by 7% for every 30 minutes that passes without delivery of appropriate antibiotic therapy.[3]

The American College of Critical Care Medicine (ACCM) clinical practice parameters for hemodynamic support of pediatric and neonatal septic shock prescribe simple interventions to be accomplished within the first hour after presentation. Definitive shock resuscitation can be initiated in community EDs and continued and refined in transport, provided that the treating physician and transferring team appreciate the urgent need and are sensitive to the subtle signs of shock in children. Han and colleagues reported that when community physicians aggressively resuscitated and successfully reversed shock before a transport team arrived, patients had a ninefold increase in their odds of survival.[24] These studies defy the popular notion that out-of-hospital stabilization wastes time and delays definitive therapy that should be rendered at the receiving facility. Bringing skilled transport personnel to the child rather than transporting the child with inadequately skilled personnel may markedly decrease the time to effective treatment.

Specialized Teams Improve Outcome

In 1978, Chance and associates[43] demonstrated reduced mortality and more stable physiology in neonates weighing less than 1.5 kg who were transported by a specialized team. Since that time several investigators have reported a decrease in the

number of preventable insults in children transported by a pediatric intensive care team compared with a multispecialty team.[44-47] In a study of children transported with head injury, Macnab and colleagues[48] determined that $135,952 in additional costs of care resulted from secondary adverse events occurring during transport by nonspecialized teams. In a prospective cohort study in which allocation of teams depended on team availability, not severity of illness, Orr and colleagues[49] showed that use of a specialized team resulted in decreased severity-adjusted mortality (9% versus 23%) compared with use of a nonspecialized team. Similarly, a large retrospective study of unplanned PICU admissions demonstrated that transfer by a specialty team was associated with improved survival in a multivariable analysis controlling for severity of illness with an odds ratio 0.58 (95% confidence interval [CI] 0.39–0.87).[50]

Pediatric specialized teams often perform additional stabilization maneuvers at the referring facility, prior to transport. In a prospective observational study, pediatric teams initiated sedation 23% of the time, inotropes 44% of the time, and osmolar therapies for intracranial hypertension nearly 50% of the time when the referring facility had failed to do so.[51] Retrieval teams also imitated mechanical ventilation, acquired central venous access, and placed or adjusted tracheal tubes (Fig. 18.2).[49] Time at the bedside for specialized retrieval teams can be relatively long due to these interventions (in this study, 97 minutes for neonates and 50 minutes for pediatric patients), but scene time has not been associated with mortality.[47]

Meaningful stabilization may also continue en route. In a before-and-after intervention trial, introduction of a goal-directed resuscitation protocol (Fig. 18.3) decreased the number of interventions required in the ICU and decreased the hospital length of stay for pediatric patients transported with systemic inflammatory response syndrome (SIRS).[52] In a prospective randomized controlled trial, enhanced monitoring of blood pressure during pediatric interfacility transport resulted in more aggressive resuscitation during transfer, shorter ICU stay, and less organ dysfunction.[53]

Components of a Specialized Interfacility Transport Team

Pediatric transport is part of a critical care continuum that includes EMS, the referring ED, secondary transfer, and the receiving critical care facility (Fig. 18.4). The continuum is often fragmented, resulting in poor communication, lack of continuity of care, and inadequate quality assessment. An ideal system would provide excellent communication between the referring and receiving hospitals, give clear advice to support the referring staff's care, bring high-level critical care to the patient at the referring institution, and continue optimal care through transport and into the PICU. Ideally, physicians and other caregivers from emergency medicine, neonatology, surgery, and intensive care all take an active role in designing each segment of the continuum and maintaining quality assurance. The critically ill child ultimately will be the responsibility of the pediatric intensivist, so it behooves him or her to have significant input into system design and protocols.

The retrieval system has a responsibility to the referral community to make tertiary care accessible. Differences in topography, weather patterns, and the distribution of hospitals and population centers mean that the ideal transport system will

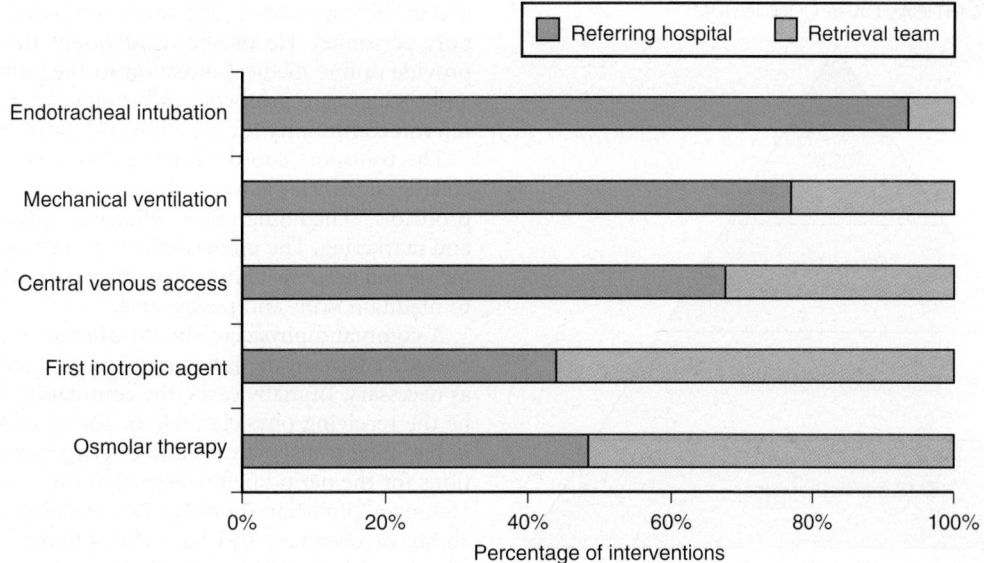

Fig. 18.2. Proportion of interventions performed by referring hospitals and intensive care retrieval teams during stabilization of critically ill children. (From Lampariello S, et al. Stabilisation of critically ill children at the district general hospital prior to intensive care retrieval: a snapshot of current practice. Arch Dis Child. 2010;95:681-685.)

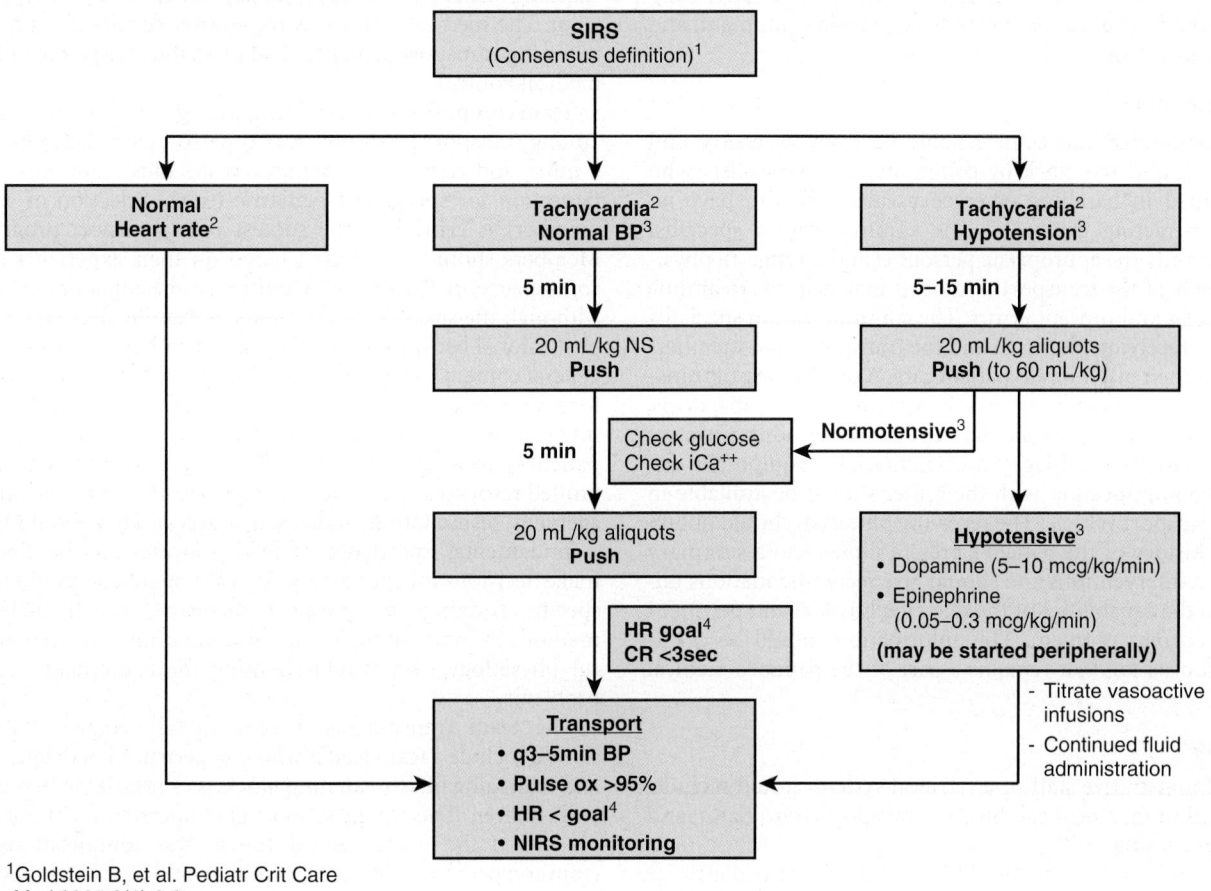

[1]Goldstein B, et al. Pediatr Crit Care Med 2005;6(1);2-8.
[2]See table for heart rate criteria.
[3]See table for age adjusted norms.
[4]See table for age adjusted HR goals.

Fig. 18.3. Transport goal-directed therapy protocol used by the Angel One Transport team at Arkansas Children's Hospital. *BP*, blood pressure; *CR*, cap refill time; *HR*, heart rate; *NIRS*, near-infrared spectroscopy; *NS*, normal saline; *SIRS*, systemic inflammatory response syndrome. (From Stroud et al. Goal-directed resuscitative interventions during pediatric interfacility transport. Crit Care Med. 2015;43:1692-1698.)

CRITICAL CARE CONTINUUM

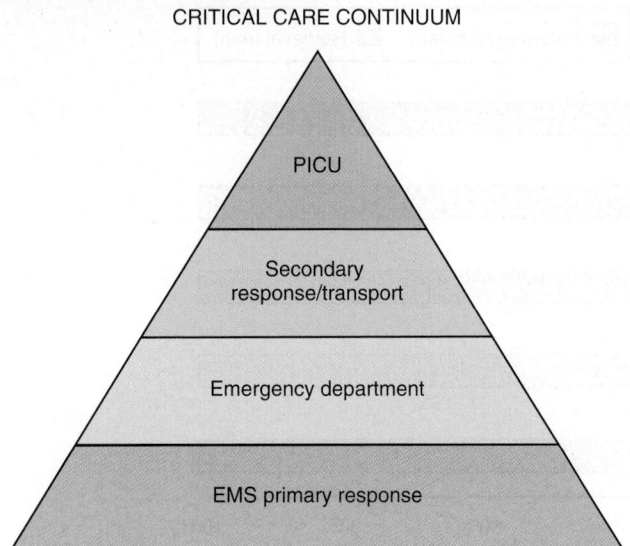

Fig.18.4. Pediatric transport as part of the critical care continuum. *EMS,* emergency medical services; *PICU,* pediatric intensive care unit.

differ from region to region. Regardless, a retrieval system should include a communications center, administrative staff, appropriately trained team members, reliable equipment, and a safety program.

Communications

The communications center should be easily accessible and staffed around the clock by communication specialists who are trained in handling emergency calls and who have no other distracting duties.[54-55] The communication specialist should notify the appropriate personnel and arrange all physical aspects of the transport. Protocols may help to streamline the process and prevent errors. The communication specialist frees the receiving physician and the transport team members to direct their attention to patient care. A detailed log of transport requests, including times, demographic data, diagnosis, and vehicle issues, should be kept for both administrative review and medical-legal documentation. Equipment for direct communication with the center should be available in every transport vehicle. The receiving physician should obtain a brief history of the patient's present illness and a summary of initial interventions and should give recommendations tailored to the capabilities of the referring hospital and pertinent to the current problem. This information should be documented on a log that remains a part of the patient's medical record.

Staffing

The administrative staff of a retrieval system should include, at a minimum, a medical director, transport coordinator, and medical command.[54-55]

The medical director should be a specialist in pediatric or neonatal critical care or emergency medicine. This individual should be experienced in both air and ground transport (as appropriate to his or her specific system) and should understand patient care capabilities and limitations in the transport environment.

The medical director must be actively involved in quality management, administrative decisions affecting medical care,

and the hiring, training, and continuing education of all transport personnel. He or she must orient the physicians who provide online medical direction to the policies, procedures, and patient care protocols and should act as a liaison to the referral community for teaching and outreach.[54-55]

The transport coordinator, usually a nurse or paramedic, collaborates with the medical director with regard to training, protocols, scheduling, data collection, quality management, and marketing. The medical director and transport coordinator should participate in patient transport, whenever possible, to maintain skills and perspective.

A command physician should oversee every transport and provide advice to the referring physician and transport team as necessary. In many cases, the command physician will also be the receiving physician. He or she should be experienced in handling transport calls and offering management suggestions for the period before arrival of the transport team. The command physician should be knowledgeable about the availability of resources and have the authority to accept transferred patients without further consultation, to perform triage, and to activate backup systems when necessary.

Medical control may be online, with direct real-time voice communication between the medical control physician and the transport team, or offline, through written protocols or standing orders for patient management by the transport team. The medical director is responsible for developing and renewing transport protocols and procedures used for offline medical control.

Team composition and training strategies vary considerably among transport programs. A two-person team composed of a nurse and respiratory therapist is the most common configuration for specialized pediatric teams. Selection of team members is critical to the success of a transport program. Members should be selected based on their experience and competence in the care of children in the inpatient setting. Although the specific requirements of training depend on the professional background of the team members, the goals and general content of training are the same for the nurse, respiratory therapist, physician, and paramedic. Transport crew members should be experienced in the care of critically ill patients and be able to deal with complex environments and limited resources. They must be highly skilled in airway management, resuscitation, and vascular access. They should have a fundamental knowledge of field priorities and be able to make decisions independently. All team members should have specific training in transport medicine, which includes methods of functioning in a moving environment, aeromedical physiology, and troubleshooting for equipment-related problems.

The team transporting a critically ill pediatric patient should include a team leader who is experienced in diagnosing and managing life-threatening illnesses or injuries in neonates and children. This caregiver must (1) understand pathophysiology and the usual clinical course and complications of common pediatric illnesses, (2) understand how to use appropriate laboratory and radiographic tests as diagnostic aids, and (3) have experience in managing neonates and children who require intensive pharmacologic intervention. In order to function independently, the team should be capable of performing, with high level of expertise, all standard emergency procedures required in the care of critically ill neonates and children.

Either an experienced nurse or physician commonly fills the team leader role. Many dedicated pediatric transport teams include a physician, although little objective evidence indicates this configuration improves outcome compared with nonphysician teams. Physician attendance is particularly controversial when the role is filled by physicians in training, as all but the most advanced trainees lack the knowledge and experience needed in the transport environment.

A transport program should define the cognitive knowledge and technical skills required for each professional group and should include a method to document the acquisition and maintenance of these skills. Instruction typically includes didactic sessions designed to assist personnel to acquire cognitive knowledge, a skill development and maintenance program, and a supervised orientation period. Simulation has been shown to improve adherence to protocols in the training of crisis-response teams and may be a useful adjunct to team member training.[56] The supervised orientation period should end only when the training program director and the trainee are confident in the trainee's abilities. A continuing education program must follow and include transport case conferences and review and ongoing competency-based training.

Equipment

For a thorough discussion of transport equipment and options, see the AAP Guidelines for Air and Ground Transport of Neonatal and Pediatric Patients.[4] Equipment taken on transport should be complete and adequate to provide continuing intensive care throughout the trip. Oxygen reserve should be calculated for each patient transported and should be at least twice the amount needed for the expected duration of the trip, in case of delays or equipment malfunction. Portable, compartmentalized equipment packs must be designed for easy access and must be able to withstand the stress of the transport environment. For air medical transport, weight and space restrictions must be considered when selecting equipment and range of medications. Transport monitors should have battery power that will last beyond the expected duration of transport, because of the possibility of unexpected delays or vehicle breakdowns, and should be free of movement artifact. Most important, the transport team should be self-sufficient and not dependent on the referring hospital for supplies. All equipment should be routinely checked and maintained after each transport by a team member dedicated to that task.

Safety

Safety should be a high priority in any transport program. Emergency vehicle operation carries substantial risks, not only to the crew and the patient but also to others in its vicinity. The medical director is responsible for thoroughly researching vendors of air or ground transport services in the areas of maintenance, safety records, experience of drivers and pilots, and reliability of equipment. Written contracts between the institution and the vendor should include specific insurance details. Ambulance drivers should be discouraged from exceeding the speed limit because no evidence indicates that use of lights and sirens has any positive effect on patient outcome.

Aeromedical transport involves a unique set of safety issues. Pilots who are under pressure to fly or who are sensitive to competition among aeromedical services within a region may fail to observe minimal weather standards, contributing to accidents. Pilots should be isolated from patient care issues to give them the freedom to make sound decisions based on the flight conditions. When aeromedical services compete, they should act jointly to establish regional safety guidelines, minimum weather standards, and a quality assurance program that examines compliance.

The transport team should be adept at survival techniques for their region and should always be prepared to deal with an off-airport landing. Regular sessions to review safety and emergency procedures for each transport mode should be provided for the transport team members.

Referring Hospital Responsibilities

Transfer of patients from one institution to another in the United States is regulated by federal statute. The current legal standard was established by the Consolidated Omnibus Budget Reconciliation Act (COBRA) of 1986 and its amendment in 1989, which created requirements for patient stabilization and transfer, guaranteeing equal access to emergency treatment to all regardless of ability to pay.[57,58] Violations can result in a number of penalties, including termination of Medicare privileges for the physician and hospital. The Emergency Medical Treatment and Labor Act (EMTALA) established by the COBRA legislation further delineates rules for interfacility transfer. Appropriate transfers must meet the following criteria: (1) the transferring hospital must provide care and stabilization within its ability; (2) the referring physician certifies that the medical benefits expected from the transfer outweigh the risks; (3) the patient consents to transfer after being informed of the risks of transfer; (4) the receiving facility must have available space and qualified personnel and agree to accept the transfer; (5) copies of medical records and imaging studies should accompany the patient; and (6) the interfacility transport must be made by qualified personnel with the necessary equipment.

Interfacility transport can be performed by a transport team from the referring facility, by the receiving facility, or by a third party. Under COBRA the referring hospital bears primary responsibility for the safety of interfacility transfer. Ideally, the decision about choice of team and mode of transport would be made jointly between the referring and receiving physicians. Physician-to-physician communication should include the following: (1) identification of the patient and medical history, (2) interventions performed during initial stabilization and patient's response, (3) pertinent physical examination findings, (4) ongoing therapy, and (5) potential complications that may occur during transport.

Summary

The limited pediatric training and exposure of EMS personnel, coupled with the differences in size, anatomy, physiology, and psychosocial aspects unique to children, will continually challenge the EMS provider. The approach that prioritizes rapidity of transport over stabilization and initiation of care, a pattern that is commonly accepted for adult patients, will not result in the best outcomes for most children. The need for pediatric-specific intensive care begins long before the patient arrives in the tertiary care center. Children transported by nonspecialized teams are at higher risk of transport-related adverse events and mortality. The primary goals in the majority of pediatric transports should be anticipatory management of respiratory insufficiency and early and attentive application of the principles of goal-directed shock resuscitation. Most pediatric patients with septic shock survive their acute illnesses, and emergency providers rarely witness the development of organ dysfunction in the first few hours of the shock state. The unique perspective of the pediatric intensivist is valuable and can help to change practice in the referring community.

References

1. Gausche-Hill M, Schmitz C, Lewis RJ. Pediatric preparedness of US emergency departments: a 2003 survey. *Pediatrics.* 2007;120:1229-1237.
2. de Oliveira CF, de Oliveira DS, Gottschald AF, et al. ACCM/PALS haemodynamic support guidelines for paediatric septic shock: an outcomes comparison with and without monitoring central venous oxygen saturation. *Intensive Care Med.* 2008;34:1065.
3. Kumar A, Roberts D, Wood KE, et al. Duration of hypotension prior to initiation of effective antimicrobial therapy is the critical determinant of survival in human septic shock. *Crit Care Med.* 2006;34:1589.
4. *American Academy of Pediatrics section on transport medicine: guidelines for air and ground transport of neonatal and pediatric patients.* 3rd ed. Elk Grove Village, IL: American Academy of Pediatrics; 2015.
5. Seidel JS, Hornbein M, Yoshiyama K, et al. Emergency medical services and the pediatric patient: are the needs being met? *Pediatrics.* 1984;73:769-772.
6. American College of Surgeons Committee on Trauma; American College of Emergency Physicians; National Association of EMS Physicians; Pediatric Equipment Guidelines Committee-Emergency Medical Services for Children (EMSC) Partnership for Children Stakeholder Group; American Academy of Pediatrics. Policy statement—Equipment for ambulances. *Pediatrics.* 2009;124:e166-e171.
7. Gausche-Hill M, Ely M, Schmuhl P, et al. A national assessment of pediatric readiness of emergency departments. *JAMA Pediatr.* 2015;169:527-534.
8. Glaeser PW, Linzer J, Tunik MG, et al. Survey of nationally registered emergency medical services providers: pediatric education. *Ann Emerg Med.* 2000;36:33-38.
9. Drayna PC, Browne LR, Guse CE, et al. Prehospital pediatric care: opportunities for training, treatment, and research. *Prehosp Emerg Care.* 2015;19:441-447.
10. Babl FE, Vinci RJ, Bauchner H, et al. Pediatric prehospital advanced life support care in an urban setting. *Pediatr Emerg Care.* 2001;17:36-37.
11. Su E, Schmidt TA, Mann NC, et al. A randomized controlled trial to assess decay in acquired knowledge among paramedics completing a pediatric resuscitation course. *Acad Emerg Med.* 2000;7:779-786.
12. Youngquist ST, Henderson DP, Gausche-Hill M, et al. Paramedic self-efficacy and skill retention in pediatric airway management. *Acad Emerg Med.* 2008;15:1295-1303.
13. Bankole S, Asuncion A, Ross S, et al. First responder performance in pediatric trauma: a comparison with an adult cohort. *Pediatr Crit Care Med.* 2011;12:e166-e170.
14. Scribano PV, Baker MD, Holmes J, et al. Use of out-of-hospital interventions for the pediatric patient in an urban emergency medical services system. *Acad Emerg Med.* 2000;7:745-750.
15. Gausche M, Tadeo RE, Zane MC, et al. Out-of-hospital intravenous access: unnecessary procedures and excessive cost. *Acad Emerg Med.* 1998;5:878-882.
16. Aijian P, Tsai A, Knopp R, et al. Endotracheal intubation of pediatric patients by paramedics. *Ann Emerg Med.* 1989;18:489-494.
17. Losek JD, Bonadio WA, Walsh-Kelly C, et al. Prehospital endotracheal intubation performance review. *Pediatr Emerg Care.* 1989;5:1.
18. Mishark KJ, Vukov LF, Gudgell SF. Airway management and air medical transport. *J Air Med Transport.* 1992;11:7-9.
19. Boswell WC, McElveen N, Sharp M, et al. Analysis of prehospital pediatric and adult intubation. *Air Med J.* 1995;14:125-127.
20. Doran JV, Tortella BJ, Drivet WJ, et al. Factors influencing successful intubation in the prehospital setting. *Prehosp Disaster Med.* 1995;10:259-264.
21. Ramenofsky ML, Luterman A, Quindlen E, et al. Maximum survival in pediatric trauma: the ideal system. *J Trauma.* 1984;24:818.
22. Seidel JS. Emergency medical services and the pediatric patient: are the needs being met? I. Training and equipping emergency medical services providers for pediatric emergencies. *Pediatrics.* 1986;78:808-812.
23. Esposito TJ, Sanddal ND, Dean JM, et al. Analysis of preventable pediatric trauma deaths and inappropriate trauma. *J Trauma.* 1999;47:243-251.
24. Han YY, Carcillo JA, Dragotta MA, et al. Early reversal of pediatric-neonatal septic shock by community physicians is associated with improved outcome. *Pediatrics.* 2003;12:793-799.
25. Athey J, Dean JM, Ball J, et al. Ability of hospitals to care for pediatric emergency patients. *Pediatr Emerg Care.* 2001;17:170-174.
26. Hogg JC, Williams J, Richardson JB, et al. Age as factor in the distribution of lower airway conductance and in the pathologic anatomy of obstructive lung disease. *N Engl J Med.* 1970;282:1283-1287.
27. Agostini E. Volume-pressure relationships of the thorax and lung in the newborn. *J Appl Physiol.* 1959;14:909-913.
28. Guslits BG, Gaston SE, Bryan MH, et al. Diaphragmatic work of breathing in premature human infants. *J Appl Physiol.* 1987;62:1410-1415.
29. Muller N, Volgyesi G, Bryan MH, et al. The consequences of diaphragmatic muscle fatigue in the newborn infant. *J Pediatr.* 1979;95:793-797.
30. Dunnill MS. The problem of lung growth. *Thorax.* 1982;37:561-563.
31. Macklem PT. Airway obstruction and collateral ventilation. *Physiol Rev.* 1971;51:368-436.
32. Bucci G, Cook C, Barrie H. Studies of respiratory physiology in children. *J Pediatr.* 1961;58:820.
33. *Pediatric Advanced Life Support Provider Manual.* Dallas: American Heart Association; 2012.
34. Brierley J, Carcillo JA, Choong K, et al. Clinical practice parameters for hemodynamic support of pediatric and neonatal septic shock: 2007 update from the American College of Critical Care Medicine. *Crit Care Med.* 2009;37:666-688.
35. Blumen IJ, Abernethy MK, Dunne MJ. Flight physiology. Clinical considerations. *Crit Care Clin.* 1992;8:597-618.
36. Bassi M, Zuercher M, Erne JJ, Ummenhofer W. Endotracheal tube intra-cuff pressure during helicopter transport. *Ann Emerg Med.* 2010;56:89-93.
37. Martin T, Glanfield M. The physiological effects of altitude. In: Martin T, ed. *Aeromedical Transportation: A Clinical Guide.* 2nd ed. Aldershot, Hampshire, England: Ashgate Publishing; 2006:39-54.
38. Rodriquez D Jr, Branson RD, Dorlac W, et al. Effects of simulated altitude on ventilator performance. *J Trauma.* 2009;66(4 suppl):S172-S177.
39. Flynn JG, Singh B. The performance of Dräger Oxylog ventilators at simulated altitude. *Anaesth Intensive Car.* 2008;36:549-552.
40. Cowley RA, Hudson F, Scanlan E, et al. An economical and proved helicopter program for transporting the emergency critically ill and injured patient in Maryland. *J Trauma Injury Infect Crit Care.* 1973;13:1029-1038.
41. Carcillo JA, Kuch BA, Han YY, et al. Mortality and functional morbidity after use of PALS/APLS by community physicians. *Pediatrics.* 2009;124:500-508.
42. Rivers E, Nguyen B, Havstad S, et al. Early goal-directed therapy in the treatment of severe sepsis and septic shock. *N Engl J Med.* 2001;345:1368-1377.
43. Chance GW, Matthew JD, Gash J, et al. Neonatal transport: a controlled study of skilled assistance. *J Pediatr.* 1978;93:662-666.
44. Bellingan G, Olivier T, Batson S, et al. Comparison of a specialist retrieval team with current United Kingdom practice for the transport of critically ill patients. *Intensive Care Med.* 2000;26:740-744.
45. Macnab AJ. Optimal escort for interhospital transport of pediatric emergencies. *J Trauma.* 1991;31:205-209.
46. Edge WE, Kanter RK, Weigle CG, et al. Reduction of morbidity in interhospital transport by specialized pediatric staff. *Crit Care Med.* 1994;22:1186-1191.
47. Orr R, Venkataraman S, Seidberg N, et al. Pediatric specialty care teams are associated with reduced morbidity during pediatric interfacility transport. *Crit Care Med.* 1999;27:A30.
48. Macnab AJ, Wensley DF, Sun C. Cost-benefit of trained transport teams: estimates for head-injured children. *Prehosp Emerg Care.* 2001;5:1-5.
49. Orr RA, Felmet KA, Han Y, et al. Pediatric specialized transport teams are associated with improved outcomes. *Pediatrics.* 2009;124:40-48.
50. Ramnarayan P, Thiru K, Parslow R, et al. Effect of specialist retrieval teams on outcomes in children admitted to paediatric intensive care units in England and Wales: a retrospective cohort study. *The Lancet.* 2010;376:698-704.

51. Lampariello S, Clement M, Aralihond AP, et al. Stabilisation of critically ill children at the district general hospital prior to intensive care retrieval: a snapshot of current practice. *Arch Dis Child.* 2010;95:681-685.

52. Stroud MH, Sanders RC Jr, Moss MM, et al. Goal-directed resuscitative interventions during pediatric interfacility transport. *Crit Care Med.* 2015;43:1692-1698.

53. Stroud MH, Prodhan P, Moss M, et al. Enhanced monitoring improves pediatric transport outcomes: a randomized controlled trial. *Pediatrics.* 2011;127:42-48.

54. Ehrenwerth J, Hackel A. Air-to-ground communication: a valuable aid in the transport of critically ill patients. *Crit Care Med.* 1986;14:543-547.

55. *Accreditation standards of the Commission on Accreditation of Air Medical Services.* 5th ed. Anderson, SC: Commission on Accreditation of Air Medical Services; 2001.

56. DeVita MA, Schaefer J, Lutz J, et al. Improving medical emergency team (MET) performance using a novel curriculum and a computerized human patient simulator. *Qual Saf Health Care.* 2005;14:326-331.

57. Fell MJ. The Emergency Medical Treatment and Active Labor Act of 1986: providing protection from discrimination in access to emergency medical care. *Spec Law Dig Health Care Law.* 1996;9-42.

58. Omnibus Budget Reconciliation Act of 1989, sec. 6018 42 USC 1395cc (West Supp 1990).

Chapter 19

Pediatric Vascular Access and Centeses

Sanjiv Pasala, Elizabeth A. Storm, Michael H. Stroud, Punkaj Gupta, Nahed El-Hassan, Thomas J. Lee, Olivia K. Irby, Xiomara Garcia-Casal, and Stephen M. Schexnayder

PEARLS

- Intraosseous infusion is a convenient means of emergency vascular access with new mechanical devices available. Vigilant observation of the needle insertion site is necessary to recognize extravasation and prevent serious complications.
- Pericardiocentesis may be required for both diagnostic and therapeutic purposes. Ultrasound imaging improves success and reduces complications, and it should be employed in all cases except with life-threatening tamponade.
- Umbilical arterial and venous access may be useful in neonates up to 2 weeks of age.

Intraosseous Infusion

Venous access in critically ill infants and children can be one of the most challenging aspects of their care. Peripheral veins in infants can be difficult to cannulate, particularly in the event of shock with shunting of blood away from the periphery and collapse of small veins. Because of these challenges, intraosseous (IO) infusion has become widely accepted as a quick, reliable means to establish short-term emergency venous access.[1,2]

IO infusion was first described in 1922 and became widely used in the 1930s and 1940s.[3] With the development of disposable needles and catheters, use of IO infusion fell out of favor. It was not commonly used again until the mid-1980s, when a series of publications demonstrated the utility of the technique for rapid venous access in critically ill children.[4,5]

The marrow space provides a noncollapsible access point to the vascular system. Marrow sinusoids drain into medullary venous channels that empty into the systemic circulatory system. Because of the noncollapsible nature of the marrow space and the direct connection to the venous circulation, fluids and medications infused into the marrow space are distributed rapidly through the venous circulation.

Indications

IO infusion is indicated in situations requiring the rapid acquisition of intravenous (IV) access in which the establishment of conventional peripheral access is difficult or impossible. The situations in which it is most often used include cardiopulmonary arrest, shock, burns, and status epilepticus. In these situations, limited attempts at standard peripheral access are usually made prior to placing an IO needle. In addition to its use in the hospital, IO access has been used successfully in the prehospital setting as well as in critical care transport.[6-8]

The success rate with the technique is high, greater than 95% with experienced practitioners.[9] Equal success using the newer mechanical intraosseous devices has also been demonstrated with equivalent pharmacokinetics.[10,11] Most fluids and medications that can be given through a conventional IV line can be given via an IO infusion with comparable results. In the event of cardiac arrest or severe shock, IO access is at least as effective as peripheral venous access in providing fluids and medications to the central circulation. Studies have shown that commonly used resuscitation, antiepileptic, and antibiotic drugs can be given effectively through an IO line. Three antibiotics produce subtherapeutic levels when given via an intraosseous line at standard IV doses: chloramphenicol, vancomycin, and tobramycin.[12]

In addition to the administration of fluids and medications, IO access can be used for certain clinical laboratory studies. No significant differences were found when comparing electrolytes, chemistries, pH, PCO_2, or hemoglobin from IO marrow specimens with either arterial or venous blood samples.[13] A marrow specimen can be cultured in lieu of a blood culture.[14] Finally, the marrow can be used for blood type and cross-matching.

Contraindications

IO infusion has few absolute contraindications. A fractured or previously punctured bone should not be used because infused fluid will extravasate and possibly cause compartment syndrome. Alternate sites in other bones can be used in such situations. Bone diseases such as osteogenesis imperfecta and osteopetrosis have been suggested as contraindications to intraosseous infusion.[15] Placing the needle into an area of cellulitis or burn could cause osteomyelitis or other infectious complications and is a relative contraindication, although if limited sites are available, placing the IO needle through burned skin is acceptable.

Supplies and Equipment

Bone marrow space is accessed with the use of one of several different types of needles. Conventional bone marrow needles (eg, Jamshidi needle, CareFusion, San Diego, California) work well. Needles made specifically for IO infusion use are available, including a straight needle or a needle with a threaded screw device (eg, Sur-Fast, Cook Medical, Bloomington, Indiana). Usually a 15- or 18-gauge needle is chosen. The smaller 18-gauge should be used in infants. Studies have shown no significant differences in time required to insert the needle, success rate, or extravasation rates between standard and threaded IO needles.[16,17] If bone marrow or IO needles are not available, standard lumbar puncture needles can be used,[9,18] although they are prone to bend. In neonates, even a 19- or 21-gauge butterfly needle can be used.[18] Needles with a stylet are preferred to prevent clogging of the needle by bone.

Two mechanical devices appropriate for the pediatric population have been introduced: the Bone Injection Gun (B.I.G., Waismed Ltd., Herzliya, Israel) and the EZ-IO (Vidacare Corporation, San Antonio, Texas; Figs. 19.1 and 19.2). The B.I.G. is a spring-loaded device, whereas the EZ-IO is a small battery-powered drill; both penetrate the bone marrow more quickly as compared to the manual method and are used more frequently than manual IO placement in many settings, including prehospital.[19] In addition, FAST1 (Chinook Medical Gear), a sternal injection gun, is used in the adult population but will not be discussed here.

Other equipment required for IO placement includes a towel or sandbag, syringes with saline or heparinized saline flush solution, IV fluid and tubing, a T-connector or stopcock, and antiseptic prep solution (iodine). Optional supplies include a pressure bag and materials for local anesthesia (syringe with 25-gauge needle and 1% lidocaine).

Technique

The IO needle can be placed into the bone marrow at one of several sites, including the proximal tibia, distal femur, distal tibia, iliac crest, and sternum. The proximal tibia is the site most commonly chosen. The sternum has been used in adults but should be avoided in children because of the possibility of perforating the smaller chest cavity. In addition, placing the needle in the sternum can interfere with airway and circulatory resuscitative efforts. When the needle is placed in the proximal tibia, the insertion site is located by palpation on the flat anterior tibial surface 1 to 3 cm (two fingers breadth) distal to the tibial tuberosity (Fig. 19.3). This site is chosen to avoid the proximal growth plate. The midshaft should not be used because of increased risk for fracture. Placing a towel or sandbag under the child's leg helps stabilize the leg and makes insertion easier. The skin overlying the area should be prepped with antiseptic solution. Local anesthesia by infiltration with 1% lidocaine should be performed if the patient is awake. If a needle with a plastic sheath is being used, adjust the sheath so that an adequate length of needle protrudes beyond the sheath. Some authors have suggested inserting the needle at a 60- to 75-degree angle away from the tibial growth plate, but others recommend using a perpendicular or 90-degree angle. The perpendicular angle helps prevent the needle from sliding along the bone. The needle is advanced using firm pressure and a twisting or rotary motion until a "give" or loss of resistance is felt, indicating entry into the marrow space. The force needed to penetrate the bony cortex is considerable; the twisting motion helps significantly in needle insertion. One disadvantage of using a threaded needle is that the "give" or loss of resistance that occurs when the needle enters the marrow space may not be felt; however, the needle may be more secure in the bone once the needle is placed.[20]

The stylet is removed and a syringe is attached to the needle to attempt to aspirate marrow. Correct placement of the

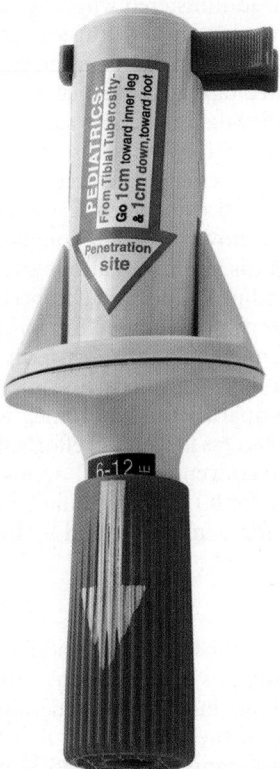

Fig. 19.1. Bone injection gun. (Courtesy Persys Medial and Waismed USA.)

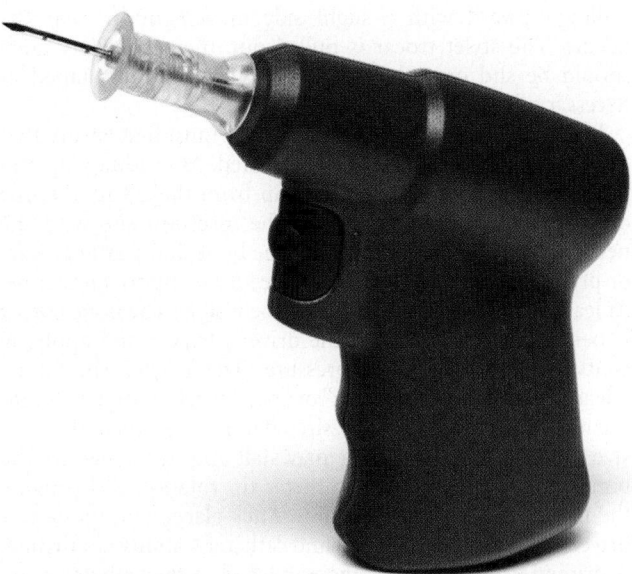

Fig. 19.2. EZ-IO. (Courtesy Vidacare Corporation.)

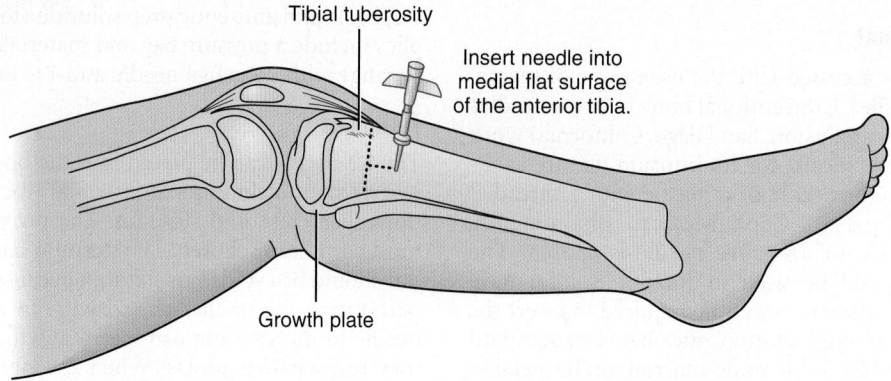

Fig. 19.3. Insertion of the intraosseous needle into the anterior tibia.

needle should be confirmed to avoid extravasation. Aspiration of bloody fluid into the syringe confirms that the needle is correctly placed. Additional evidence of correct needle placement includes the observation that the needle stands upright in the bone without support and lack of resistance when flush solution is infused into the needle with the syringe. Sometimes marrow cannot be aspirated even if the needle is correctly placed. If the "give" is felt on insertion and the needle stands alone in the bone but marrow cannot be aspirated, infusion of a small amount of fluid with the syringe can be attempted. Fluid should infuse easily with little pressure and without noticeable swelling of the soft tissues or extravasation of fluid.

Placement of IO needles with the newer mechanical devices has success rates equal to or higher than traditional manual methods, with the added benefit of ease of use and less risk to the user.[7,10] However, the high cost of this equipment may be a major limitation for use, especially in small facilities or resource-limited settings. In children, prehospital providers preferred the IO drill to the spring-loaded injection gun.[20,21]

When using the spring-loaded injection gun, after choosing the desired needle depth of penetration by dialing to the patient's age, the B.I.G. is positioned over the desired site with one hand while the other hand squeezes and pulls out the safety latch. The free hand is then used to activate the device at a 90-degree angle to the surface. The device is removed by pulling upward with a slight side movement to clear the needle. The stylet trocar is pulled out, then the safety latch should be slid over the needle and the apparatus taped as necessary for stabilization.

When using the IO drill, the operator must first ensure that driver and needle set are securely seated. After removing and discarding the needle set safety cap from the IO needle, the operator positions the driver at the insertion site with the needle set at a 90-degree angle to the bone and gently powers or presses the needle set until the needle set tip touches bone. At least 5 mm of the catheter must be visible. The bone cortex is penetrated by squeezing the driver's trigger and applying gentle, steady downward pressure. The trigger should be released when a sudden "give" or "pop" is felt upon entry into the medullary space and a desired depth is obtained. If excessive force is used, the driver may stall and not penetrate the bone. Gentle pressure and catheter tip rotation will provide the necessary penetrating action. After placement, the power driver and stylet are removed and catheter stability confirmed. A primed extension set is then attached to the catheter hub's Luer-Lok and the apparatus is flushed. The manufacturer does not recommend attaching a syringe directly to the IO needle hub, to reduce the risk of needle dislocation.

The possible insertion sites are the same whether using the manual or mechanical needles. When the needle is placed in the distal femur, it should be positioned approximately 2 to 3 cm proximal to the patella in the midline. In the distal tibia, the needle is placed 1 cm proximal to the medial malleolus midway between the anterior and posterior surfaces, posterior to the saphenous vein. The proximal tibia is usually selected in children younger than 4 years, but the distal tibia has been recommended in older children in whom the proximal tibial cortex is thicker. The proximal humerus can also be used, with the insertion site 1 to 2 cm proximal to the surgical neck of the humerus.

Maintenance

Once correct placement of the needle is confirmed, fluids and medication can be administered with a syringe via a stopcock or T-connector, or a standard IV infusion set can be connected to the needle. The needle is secured using gauze pads and tape. Some have suggested taping a clear plastic cup over the needle to help prevent dislodgment.[9] The site should be observed visually and by palpation for signs of extravasation, both immediately after placement and frequently (every 5 to 10 minutes) during use. If evidence of extravasation is seen, the needle should be removed to avoid compartment syndrome. If needle placement is attempted at one site and the cortex is penetrated but the line cannot be used because of extravasation, another bone must be chosen for subsequent attempts.

IO access is intended only for short-term use in emergency resuscitative situations; long-term use increases the risk of extravasation, compartment syndrome, and infection.[22,23] Therefore once IO access is secured, efforts should be directed toward obtaining conventional IV access. Once alternate access is obtained, the IO needle should be removed, manual pressure applied for 5 minutes, and a dressing applied to the site.

Complications

Significant complications of IO infusion are rare. The most common complication is extravasation of fluid. The causes of extravasation include incomplete penetration of the bony cortex, movement of the needle such that the hole is larger than the needle, dislodgment of the needle, penetration of the posterior cortex, and leakage of fluid through another hole in the bone, such as a previous IO site or fracture. Extravasation of a small amount of fluid is usually not problematic, but compartment syndrome may result after extravasation of larger volumes of fluid. Use of the IO line for prolonged periods and use of the IO line with pressure infusion appear to be risk factors for compartment syndrome. Compartment syndrome associated with IO infusion can result in the need for fasciotomy and amputation. Careful frequent observation of the IO site is necessary to detect extravasation and to prevent compartment syndrome. If extravasation occurs, the needle should be removed and the extremity observed for signs of compartment syndrome. Initial experience suggests the complications of the new mechanical devices are similar to that for the traditional IO needle.

Other rare complications include infection and bone fracture. Osteomyelitis, cellulitis, and sepsis have been reported in conjunction with IO infusion.[24] Risk for infection is increased when IO access is used in a bacteremic patient and when the line is used for a prolonged period. The risk of osteomyelitis is low. Although IO access is usually obtained in emergency situations, precautions to prevent infection should be taken, including use of sterile gloves and equipment and preparation of the skin with antiseptic solution (iodine or alcohol). Fracture of the bone has been reported.[25]

Summary

IO infusion is a valuable means of obtaining temporary, emergency vascular access in the critically ill infant or child. It has a high success rate and is associated with rare complications. Using appropriate technique and vigilantly monitoring the site for extravasation can usually prevent complications.

Arterial Catheter Placement

Frequent access to arterial blood is essential for a complete and thorough assessment of acid-base status, oxygenation, and ventilation in the critically ill patient. The dynamic, often rapidly evolving nature of critical illness in children, including the potential for rapidly changing hemodynamic status, routinely requires continuous measurement of blood pressure as an invaluable tool in planning timely interventions aimed at improving systemic oxygen delivery. Since the 1970s, arterial catheter placement in critically ill children has allowed continuous measurement of systolic, diastolic, and mean blood pressure, and it provides a visible pressure waveform that may contribute additional diagnostic information (see also Chapters 28 and 29). It also provides direct access to arterial blood for frequent, painless sampling. Hence the ability to place an arterial catheter is a fundamental skill in pediatric critical care medicine.

Indications

Indications for an arterial catheter include the following:
1. Need for frequent measurement of blood pressure to assess the patient's hemodynamic status and to allow for timely assessment of interventions aimed at improving hemodynamic status, such as fluid administration and titration of vasoactive infusions.
2. Need for frequent sampling of arterial blood for laboratory analysis. Access to arterial blood through an indwelling catheter increases the ease of painlessly obtaining blood samples for analysis. Obtaining arterial samples through a catheter also eliminates skewing of results by physiologic changes related to the stress of arterial puncture or venipuncture, such as increased respirations with crying, localized poor perfusion, or tourniquet use. Most notably, an indwelling arterial catheter allows for frequent assessment of arterial blood gas measurements, thereby providing the most accurate information on a patient's acid-base status, as well as measurement of PaO_2.
3. Need for continuous monitoring of cerebral perfusion pressure (CPP) in patients with traumatic brain injury or other causes of increased intracranial pressure (ICP) (see also Chapter 62).
4. Need for arterial access to facilitate therapeutic procedures, such as exchange transfusions and continuous arteriovenous hemodiafiltration.

Contraindications

Few absolute contraindications for placement of an arterial catheter exist. The skin at the site of arterial access must be intact prior to insertion of a catheter. Evidence of infection of the skin or underlying structures is a contraindication to catheter placement at this site. Other disruptions in skin integrity, such as burns, are a relative contraindication. Severe coagulopathy and systemic anticoagulation increase the risk of hemorrhage from unsuccessful arterial punctures associated with attempted arterial catheter placement, as well as the risks of bleeding at the site of arterial catheter insertion. These risks must be weighed against the potential benefits of improved monitoring when deciding to place an arterial catheter in a coagulopathic or anticoagulated patient.

A catheter should not be placed in an extremity with compromised perfusion. Evidence of adequate collateral circulation is desirable prior to placement of an arterial catheter. The traditional means of assessing collateral circulation to the hand is the Allen test. The radial and ulnar arteries are compressed until the distal extremity is blanched. Pressure over one artery then is released and capillary refill should return to the distal extremity in less than 5 seconds. The test is repeated releasing pressure over the other contributing artery. However, a normal Allen test does not guarantee adequate collateral circulation, nor does an abnormal test necessarily indicate possible complications.[26] The Allen test is considered less reliable for patients in shock. Additionally, an arterial catheter is often placed without assessing collateral circulation in emergent circumstances.

Procedure

Box 19.1 lists the supplies and equipment required for arterial catheterization.

Technique

The initial step in placing an arterial catheter is site selection. The radial, posterior tibial, and dorsalis pedis arteries are optimal sites, due to easy accessibility and typically good collateral circulation. Placement of the catheter in distal arteries of the extremities also allows for ease of site observation and hemorrhage control with direct pressure. Preductal placement in the right radial artery is preferred in infants with ductal-dependent heart lesions.

Catheters also can be placed in the axillary or femoral arteries if no peripheral sites are suitable. Insertion of a catheter into the axillary artery is technically more difficult than the other sites mentioned and is associated with a risk of

BOX 19.1   Supplies and Equipment for Arterial Catheterization

1. Appropriate size catheter (24 gauge for infants, 22 gauge for toddlers and older)
2. Sterile gloves
3. 10% povidone-iodine or chlorhexidine solution
4. Sterile towels
5. Syringe with 1% lidocaine and 25-gauge needle for local infiltration
6. Topical anesthetic cream
7. Luer-Lok connector with heparinized flush
8. 3-0 silk suture
9. Instrument tray with needle holder and scissors
10. Cloth tape
11. Plastic, nonocclusive dressing
12. Connecting tubing
13. Transducer
14. Fluids containing heparin (1 unit/mL) and papaverine

brachial plexus injury due to hematoma compressing the neurovascular bundle.[27] Traditionally, many physicians have been reluctant to place arterial catheters for long-term use into the femoral artery, particularly in infants and young children, for fear of complications, most notably severe ischemia of the limb. A retrospective study of 234 pediatric burn patients who underwent 745 femoral artery catheterizations revealed a 1.1% rate of loss of distal pulse. In this retrospective study, limb ischemia was associated with younger age, smaller patient size, and increased severity of the burn injury. Patients who suffered limb ischemia were managed with immediate catheter removal and systemic heparinization. Three underwent thrombectomy, with one requiring amputation of a digit.[28] Traditional teaching has held that the brachial arteries should not be used for arterial catheters because of the lack of collateral blood flow and risk of distal extremity ischemia. In a review of arterial catheter placements performed at a pediatric cardiac surgical center, 386 brachial artery catheters were placed in infants weighing 20 kg or less with no report of permanent ischemic damage and only three with temporary perfusion loss.[29] Despite these results, the complete lack of collateral circulation at the brachial artery requires careful consideration of risks and benefits before placement of a brachial artery catheter. Additionally, the superficial temporal arteries should not be used due to poor collateral flow and the possibility of retrograde flow resulting in showering of emboli into the cerebral circulation.

The selected site must be properly immobilized prior to placement of the indwelling catheter. If placing a radial artery catheter, the wrist is hyperextended 30 degrees to develop a straighter course and more superficial position of the radial artery. Typically, the radial pulse is best palpated in a position just proximal to the proximal wrist crease. The technique for radial arterial catheter placement has been expertly summarized in the "Videos in Clinical Medicine" series in the *New England Journal of Medicine*.[30]

Arterial catheter placement at any site is performed by initially preparing the site with a chlorhexidine solution and draping it with sterile towels. Lidocaine (1% without epinephrine) is infiltrated locally. Alternatively, lidocaine/prilocaine (EMLA) cream can be used as a local anesthetic. Systemic narcotics or anxiolytics may be administered, although cautiously in patients not receiving mechanically ventilation. Percutaneous placement of the catheter can be accomplished using one of several techniques. In the over-the-needle

technique, similar to placement of a peripheral IV catheter, the needle is inserted through the skin at a 30-degree angle (bevel up or down). When a flashback of blood is obtained in the hub, the catheter is advanced another 1 to 2 mm. While the needle is held stable, the catheter is advanced over the needle into the lumen of the vessel. Blood should be flowing continuously into the catheter hub prior to attempting to advance the catheter. Once the catheter is inserted through the skin to the hub, pressure is applied over the artery proximal to the catheter and a flushed Luer-Lok connector is attached to the hub. Correct placement of the catheter is verified by easily aspirating arterial blood into a syringe. The catheter is then flushed and securely sutured or taped into position. A transparent dressing is placed over the catheter as a protective barrier, usually after placement of a chlorhexidine-impregnated patch at the site of catheter insertion to decrease catheter-associated bloodstream infections.[31]

Transfixation, the second percutaneous technique, involves using the over-the-needle technique; however, when a flashback of blood is seen in the hub, the needle and catheter are further advanced through the posterior wall of the artery and this wall is transfixed to the underlying structures. The needle is pulled out, leaving the catheter in place. The catheter is then slowly withdrawn until the tip is again intraluminal, with blood flowing back into the hub. The catheter is then advanced into the artery up to the hub. Catheter advancement can be facilitated by attaching a syringe filled with flush to a connecter and gently flushing as the catheter is advanced. The position of the catheter is confirmed, and the catheter is secured as described earlier.

The final and most successful percutaneous method for catheter placement in critically ill patients involves use of the Seldinger technique.[32] A needle is used to pierce the anterior wall of the artery, and when return of arterial blood is seen, a guidewire is placed through the introducer needle and advanced into the lumen of the artery. The needle is then removed, and a catheter is advanced over the guidewire into the lumen of the vessel. This method also can be used with the over-the-needle technique. A study in pediatric patients showed improved success rates and time to insertion when arterial catheters are placed using a wire guide compared to no wire guide.[33] However, an adult study found no difference between wire guide versus no wire guide success rate or insertion times.[34] When placing a catheter into larger vessels such as the femoral artery, using the Seldinger technique, a longer catheter (eg, 5-8 cm) should be used.

Interest continues to grow in ultrasound-assisted placement of arterial catheters (see also Chapter 20). Studies have demonstrated decreased time to insertion and decreased number of attempts at catheter placement using ultrasound-guided compared to pulse palpation techniques.[35-37] However, a large randomized trial of pediatric patients receiving radial arterial catheter placement via ultrasound-guided versus traditional techniques by pediatric subspecialty trainees or anesthesiologists with minimal ultrasound experience found no difference in success rate.[38] A cutdown approach serves as an alternative if percutaneous attempts are unsuccessful. A superficial incision of the skin is made perpendicular to the artery. The subcutaneous tissues are bluntly dissected parallel to the vessel using hemostats. When the artery is identified, the posterior wall is gently dissected away from the adjacent structures. Two loops are placed around the vessel: one proximal and one distal. These loops are used to elevate the artery during cannulations; they should never be used to tie off the vessel. The artery is then cannulated under direct visualization using the over-the-needle technique. The catheter is secured with a suture through the skin, and the wound is closed with interrupted stitches. If excessive bleeding persists, gentle traction can be applied to the proximal loop in an attempt to control the hemorrhage.

Maintenance of an Arterial Catheter

To prolong patency of an arterial catheter, heparinized fluid is most commonly infused through the catheter. A common practice is to infuse 0.9% sodium chloride containing heparin 1 unit/mL at 3 mL/hr, although slower infusion rates may occasionally be used in small infants with a need for fluid restriction. There is conflicting literature supporting the use of heparin to positively impact patency and the risk of clot formation in peripheral arterial catheters.[39,40] However, more recent adult studies call into question the benefit of heparin and the need for more rigorous clinical investigation.[41,42] These studies do not take into account the smaller vessel size and prolonged monitoring common in critically ill children. A randomized, controlled trial of the addition of papaverine (60 mg/500 mL) to routine arterial catheter fluids demonstrated a significantly lower rate of catheter failure and longer catheter life in the papaverine group.[43] This study recommended avoiding the use of papaverine in neonates due to a perceived increased risk of intraventricular hemorrhage (IVH); however, a more recent study of neonates 25 to 36 weeks gestational age showed no increased risk of IVH.[44] Despite these results, many institutions routinely avoid the use of papaverine in arterial catheter fluids in preterm neonates and in patients with traumatic brain injury or some other preexisting intracranial hemorrhage.

The arterial catheter should always be visible so any bleeding around the catheter site or an inadvertent disconnection of the tubing from the catheter can be immediately observed to avoid significant hemorrhage. Securing the catheter with suture and the use of Luer-Lok connectors decreases the possibility of accidental detachment. The site of catheter insertion should be closely monitored for signs of infection or compromised perfusion. Mottling of the skin proximal or distal to the catheter may be indicative of intraarterial thrombus formation, and discoloration of fingers or toes distal to a catheter may result from emboli. The catheter must be removed if any of these complications are observed. Children with femoral artery catheters are at a higher risk of thrombus formation, and those of newborn age, lower body weight, low cardiac output, and elevated hematocrit have an even higher risk of femoral artery thrombosis.[45]

Arterial catheter transduction is performed with the transducer located as close as possible to the level of the right atrium and zeroed to atmospheric pressure for accurate measurements.[46] Studies in animal models have demonstrated that positioning the transducer level with the aortic root results in accurate measurement of mean arterial pressure regardless of patient position or catheter site, whereas placement of the transducer level with the catheter tip resulted in significant error in mean arterial pressure measurement.[47] Currently, changing arterial line fluids and tubing is recommended to occur every 96 hours.[48] The overlying dressing also is changed on a scheduled basis.

Inability to draw blood from a catheter or flattening of the waveform on the monitor is suggestive of either a kinked catheter or thrombus formation at the end of the catheter. If no evidence of compromised perfusion is present distal to the catheter, changing the catheter over a guidewire may be considered. However, strong consideration should be given to removing the existing catheter and placing another arterial catheter in a new position, as changing a catheter over a guidewire has been associated with an increased risk of catheter-associated bloodstream infection (CABSI), at least in central venous catheters.[49]

Complications

Complications related to arterial catheters include hemorrhage, thrombus formation, emboli, distal ischemia, and infection. Permanent ischemic complications related to radial artery catheters in adult patients are rare events.[27] A multiinstitutional diagnostic code database study demonstrated 10.3% of patients with arterial catheters also had a code associated with infection or inflammation and 7.5% had a thrombotic or embolic associated complication code. These complications were more common in younger children and those with longer hospitalizations.[50] In addition to bleeding, infection, and distal limb ischemia, an uncommon but well-recognized complication of arterial catheter placement is growth arrest due to physeal injury from extravasation, aneurysm formation, or ischemia.[51]

Catheter-related infections can be local or the focus for systemic sepsis. The risk of catheter-related infection has previously been thought to be lower for arterial catheters than for central venous catheters; however, a meta-analysis indicated arterial catheters are an underrecognized source of CABSI.[52] The risk of arterial catheter infection has been related to the duration of catheter use and to placement of a catheter in the femoral artery.[53-55] Presence of an arterial catheter has been noted to be a risk for CABSI, but it has been suggested that it is more likely that a positive culture is a surrogate marker for greater illness severity.[56] Regardless, the arterial catheter should be considered a possible source of sepsis, and strong consideration should be given to removing an arterial catheter when it is no longer necessary for optimal care.

Summary

Arterial catheterization is a necessary skill for the pediatric intensivist for the routine monitoring of many critically ill children. The potential risks and benefits of arterial catheter placement should be carefully weighed prior to the procedure. Rigorous studies investigating the complications associated with arterial catheterization are lacking for critically ill children, and further study is needed.[50]

Pericardiocentesis

Pericardiocentesis is the aspiration of fluid or air from the pericardial space. Pericardiocentesis can be performed emergently without imaging guidance techniques; however, this should only be undertaken in dire circumstances because of the risk of the procedure and the higher failure rate when no guidance is used.

Indications

Drainage of a pericardial effusion of any cause is absolutely indicated when cardiac tamponade is present. Often drainage is recommended if the effusion is large, even in the absence of tamponade, for diagnosis and fluid removal.[57] For small effusions, pericardiocentesis may be indicated for diagnosis alone. In pediatric patients, pericardial effusions most commonly occur with postviral or idiopathic pericarditis, but they are also seen with postpericardiotomy syndrome, collagen vascular disease, oncologic disease, and, rarely, uremia.[57] Purulent pericarditis resulting from *Staphylococcus aureus* or *Streptococcus pneumoniae* infection can be seen in cases of concomitant pneumonia with empyema. Although rare in developed countries, tuberculous pericarditis can occur. Drainage of purulent pericarditis is indicated for relief of tamponade, prevention of constrictive pericarditis, diagnosis, and drainage of infection. With purulent pericarditis, open drainage may be more effective because of the difficulty in draining thick pus.[58] If using a tube for pericardiocentesis and drainage, instillation of a fibrinolytic agent such as alteplase (recombinant tissue plasminogen factor) may be considered with purulent effusions. Traumatic pericardial effusions secondary to penetrating trauma often require surgical drainage of the blood, because tamponade is common. Pneumopericardium secondary to pulmonary air leaks in mechanically ventilated patients is usually well tolerated hemodynamically but may require drainage, especially in small infants, because of the development of tamponade.

Contraindications

There is no absolute contraindication to pericardiocentesis in an emergency situation. The presence of aortic dissection or myocardial rupture is considered a major contraindication. The presence of a bleeding diathesis or coagulopathy is another contraindication. Open drainage is preferred to closed drainage when the patient has traumatic tamponade and is in cardiac arrest. When the effusion is loculated in a location not easily reached using the subxiphoid approach, needle pericardiocentesis is contraindicated because the risk of complications increases and the possibility of successful drainage is low.

Procedure

Drainage of a pericardial effusion can be performed either by simple needle aspiration or by insertion of a drainage catheter. If the procedure is for diagnosis only and the effusion is small, then needle drainage is adequate. However, if tamponade is present, the effusion is sizable, or effusion likely will continue, insertion of a catheter for continuous drainage is indicated.

Equipment

1. *Needles for drainage* range in size from 14 to 20 gauge, depending on the type of fluid and the size of the patient. For thicker fluids, such as pus or blood, a larger-bore needle is used. A steel needle, such as a vascular introducer needle or a spinal needle, can be used, but often an IV catheter is more effective because once the fluid is reached, the steel inner needle can be removed from the IV catheter, leaving the softer, needleless catheter in place while the fluid is aspirated. This process decreases the risk of cardiac puncture.
2. *Syringes, three-way stopcock, and short extension tubing* are assembled for aspiration. A 5- or 10-mL slip-tip syringe is used when accessing the pericardium for easier manipulation. A larger 20- to 30-mL syringe may be needed for fluid drainage, depending on the predicted volume. The

stopcock and short tubing are useful when draining large amounts of fluid.
3. *Equipment for insertion* includes 2% chlorhexidine solution, sterile gloves and drapes, and 1% lidocaine for local anesthesia.
4. Appropriate *sterile sample tubes* should be available for collection of fluid for chemical, cellular, and microbiologic analysis.
5. A *cardiac monitor* is essential for determining arrhythmias during the procedure.
6. *Catheter, dilator, and flexible J-wire* are necessary when the catheter will be left in place. Placement in the pericardial sac of a 5- to 8-Fr pigtail catheter with multiple side holes is recommended. The size of the patient and the viscosity of the fluid determine the size of the catheter. If the fluid is fibrinous in appearance by echocardiography, then a larger-bore catheter should be placed. Several pigtail catheters are manufactured specifically for fluid drainage, often available as kits that also contain an appropriate-size dilator and J-wire guide. If a kit is not available, then a venous dilator of appropriate size with a separate J-wire can be used. A J-wire is used to prevent another puncture of the pericardium or heart using a straight wire. Before the needle is inserted, the wire, dilator, and catheter must be checked to ensure their sizes are compatible.

Monitoring for Pericardiocentesis

Monitor all critically ill patients continuously with both pulse oximetry and electrocardiograph (ECG) monitoring. Before pericardiocentesis, provide airway and respiratory support as clinically indicated. Procedures such as rapid sequence intubation or positive pressure ventilation can precipitate a sudden decrease in preload leading to acute events such as cardiac arrest. Monitoring the ECG tracing while advancing the pericardiocentesis needle enables the clinician to detect needle contact with the epicardium, which helps prevent cardiac puncture.

Echocardiographic guidance is recommended for most pericardiocentesis because it can be done at the bedside and is logistically less complex.[59] Echocardiographic scanning is indicated prior to needle drainage or catheter insertion for any reason except tamponade with cardiac arrest. The echocardiogram can show the size of the effusion, its distribution around the heart including any loculations, the presence of fibrin or clots, and evidence of tamponade. Tamponade can be diagnosed using two-dimensional imaging when the right atrium collapses during late diastole.

Technique

Needle aspiration can be performed blindly in the event of a true emergency such as traumatic tamponade; however, the technique has higher complication and failure rates. Among the potential chest sites for pericardiocentesis in infants and children, the subxiphoid approach is the safest and most common approach, although other approaches have been described. The approach is extrapleural and, in patients with normal anatomy, avoids major vessels such as the internal mammary, coronary, and pericardial arteries.[57] The subxiphoid and lower costal margin are prepared with 2% chlorhexidine. The area is draped in a sterile fashion. Lidocaine local anesthesia is infiltrated at the junction of the xiphoid and the left costal margin. The needle is inserted at a 30- to 45-degree angle and directed toward the left clavicle (Fig. 19.4). The slip-tip syringe is attached and is aspirated continually while the needle is inserted (Fig. 19.5). Needle advancement is halted when air or fluid is aspirated. During insertion the needle is guided using two-dimensional echocardiography. The echocardiographic probe is placed on the chest where the fluid is best seen. The needle tip is identified by ultrasound and followed as the needle is advanced.[60] Another technique involves mounting the needle on the echocardiographic probe, which has been placed in a sterile sleeve. The needle is advanced while the operator also handles the probe. This technique allows the use of locations other than the subxiphoid approach for insertion of the introducer needle, with the potential for better fluid visualization.[61] After the fluid has been echocardiographically evaluated, the patient is placed supine with the head elevated approximately 30 degrees.

If blood is obtained, analysis is necessary to determine whether the blood is of pericardial or intracardiac origin. Several techniques are helpful for this determination. The hematocrit of pericardial fluid will be lower than that of intracardiac blood, which will be equal to the patient's hematocrit. Dropping a few milliliters of the fluid on gauze sponges determines whether the fluid will clot. Fluid that does not clot is pericardial; fluid that does clot is most likely intracardiac blood. Another technique involves injection of small amounts of saline microbubble contrast (saline in a syringe that has been agitated) through the introducer needle while imaging with echocardiography. If contrast bubbles are seen in the heart, then the tip of the needle is intracardiac or intravascu-lar. If bubbles appear in the pericardial sac, then the needle is appropriately placed in the pericardium.

Once the needle is determined to be well positioned in the pericardial sac, if a catheter is to be inserted, then the J-wire can be passed through the needle as with standard Seldinger technique. The needle is removed, and the dilator is passed over the wire to open the tissues outside the pericardium and enlarge the puncture in the pericardium. The dilator is removed, taking care to leave the J-wire in good position. The catheter is passed over the wire into the pericardial sac. Its position can be confirmed echocardiographically. The wire is removed. The connecting tubing and three-way stopcock are connected and the fluid is aspirated. The tubing can be connected to a drainage bag for removal of fluid that continues to accumulate. A sterile sample of the aspirated fluid should be sent to the laboratory for appropriate analysis. The catheter is secured with suture and covered with an occlusive dressing. A chest radiogram should be taken at the end of the procedure and daily to confirm the catheter position.

Maintenance

The catheter is simple to maintain. The dressing should be changed according to the ICU protocol for central venous lines. The fluid in the drainage bag should be measured and the amount recorded on a regular schedule. If fluid is no

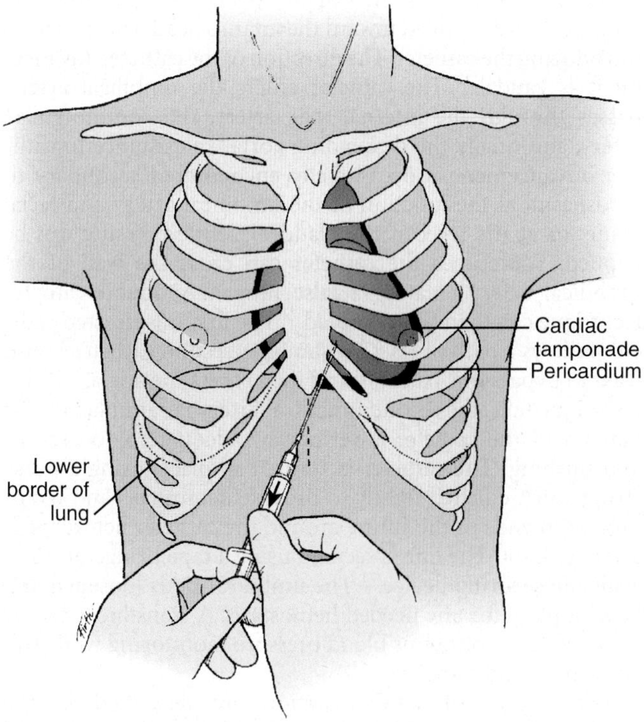

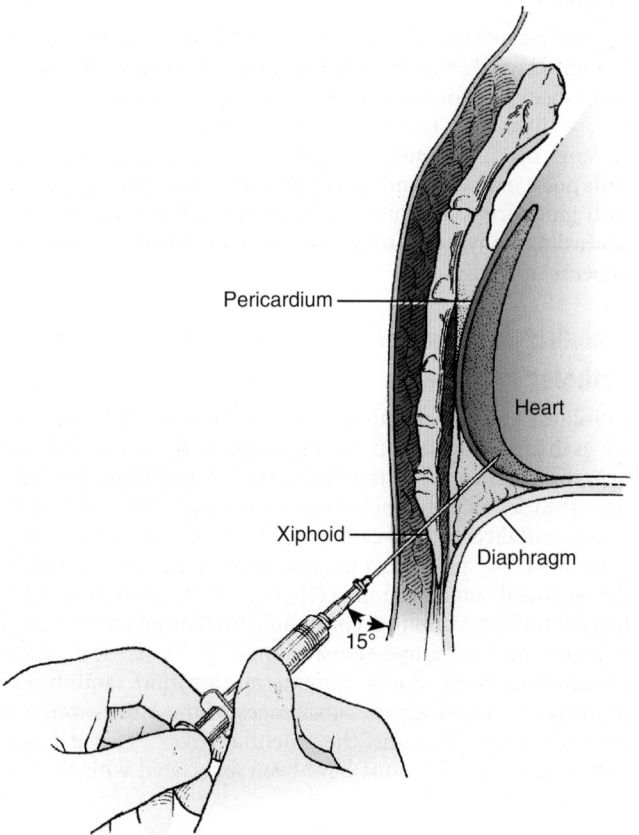

Fig. 19.4. Insertion of needle for pericardiocentesis at the junction of the xiphoid and the left costal margin, aiming toward the left shoulder. (From Brundage SI, Scott BG, Karmy-Jones R et al. Pericardiocentesis and pericardial window. In Shoemaker WC, Velmahos GC, Demetriades D, eds. Procedures and Monitoring for the Critically III. Philadelphia: Saunders Elsevier; 2002.)

Fig. 19.5. In pericardiocentesis, the needle is inserted slowly, under continuous aspiration, toward the heart at a 15-degree angle to the skin. (From Brundage SI, Scott BG, Karmy-Jones R et al. Pericardiocentesis and pericardial window. In Shoemaker WC, Velmahos GC, Demetriades D, eds. Procedures and Monitoring for the Critically III. Philadelphia: Saunders Elsevier; 2002.)

longer draining, then a small amount (1 to 2 mL) of heparinized saline can be infused into the pericardium through the stopcock after preparation with antiseptic solution. This process can release any fibrinous material occluding the catheter. If no fluid is forthcoming, then echocardiography can be performed to determine if residual pericardial fluid remains. If more fluid is present, flush the catheter again in an attempt to open up the catheter. If the fluid had originally been purulent, then instillation of a fibrinolytic agent may allow better drainage. If no fluid remains, the catheter can be removed, depending on the patient's condition and the underlying cause of fluid development.

Complications

The most serious and immediate mechanical complications of pericardiocentesis are myocardial puncture or laceration, vascular injury (coronary, intercostal, internal mammary, or intraabdominal), pneumothorax, air embolism, and arrhythmia (ventricular and supraventricular). Coronary laceration occurs rarely, resulting in acute myocardial ischemia. Transperitoneal needle passage can traverse intraabdominal organs. The liver is most commonly involved but is associated with low risk of significant hemorrhage. Perforation of a hollow viscus is theoretically possible but rarely reported. Infection of the indwelling catheter can occur but is rare because the catheter is not in place for more than 3 to 4 days.

Summary

Pericardiocentesis, with or without catheter placement, is a straightforward procedure that is indicated for relief of cardiac tamponade and for a diagnosis of certain pericardial effusions. It is a lifesaving technique for patients with tamponade. Patients needing emergency pericardiocentesis are checked with pulse oximetry and ECG monitors. Used in conjunction with guidance techniques such as echocardiography or electrocardiography, pericardiocentesis can be performed safely in patients of all ages.

Umbilical Arterial Catheter and Umbilical Venous Catheter Placement

Umbilical vein cannulation was first described in 1947 for an exchange transfusion in an infant with severe indirect hyperbilirubinemia.[62] Umbilical artery cannulation was later described in 1959 for blood gas sampling.[62] Since the early 2000s, umbilical arterial catheter (UAC) and umbilical venous catheter (UVC) placement have become routine procedures in the neonatal intensive unit (NICU).[63] UAC is indicated for frequent blood sampling, continuous measurement of blood pressure, and exchange transfusion.[63,64] UVC is needed for administration of fluids, parenteral nutrition, and blood products.[63,64] However, the advantages of these lines must be carefully balanced against the potential risks.[65,66] Several life-threatening complications have been associated with the use of these catheters.[65,66]

Supplies and Equipment

Prepackaged umbilical catheter insertion trays are commercially available and contain different sizes of catheters. The 3.5F and 5F are the most frequently used catheters.[63,64] Umbilical catheters are typically made of polyvinylchloride and have a single end hole, as side hole catheters have been linked with

higher incidence of thrombosis.[67,68] Umbilical catheters are available as single or multiple lumens. A single lumen can be used in either vessel, whereas a double- or triple-lumen catheter is used exclusively in the umbilical vein.[69] More than one lumen allows the administration of incompatible fluids. A 3.5F catheter is utilized for infants weighing <1500 g, and a 5F catheter is used for larger infants.[63,64]

Technique

The infant is kept in a supine position by using soft restraints of the arms and legs or via a swaddling technique. A catheter is prepared for insertion by connecting to a Luer-Lok stopcock and flushing with saline, with or without heparin. The umbilical stump and surrounding skin are thoroughly cleansed with 2% chlorhexidine or providone-iodine.[63,70] The antiseptic agent is allowed to dry and is then removed with sterile saline. The area is draped, sparing the head and chest to allow for appropriate patient monitoring. A cord tie is applied around the umbilical stump. Using a scalpel, the cord is horizontally cut 1 to 2 cm above the umbilical ring.[70] The larger, single thin-walled umbilical vein is typically located at 12 o'clock, whereas the two thick-walled generally constricted umbilical arteries are identified at 5 and 7 o'clock.[70] A single umbilical artery is sometimes isolated and can be a normal variation.[63,70]

I. Umbilical Arterial Cannulation

Once the umbilical artery is identified, the iris forceps is used to gently dilate the arterial lumen by first inserting the forceps in the closed position and subsequently allowing both prongs to spring open and dilate the lumen.[63,64] The catheter is introduced 0.5 cm in the lumen of the vessel.[63,64] Thereafter, the umbilical cord is pulled toward the infant's head before further introducing the catheter. The direction of the catheter advancement is caudal.[71] The catheter enters the umbilical artery, passes through the internal iliac artery, the common iliac artery, and finally the descending aorta.[71] Resistance to catheter advancement is occasionally encountered secondary to vasospasm, at the junction of the umbilical artery and facial plane, or at the level of the bladder. Gentle pressure can be applied. Sometimes the catheter can cross the wall of the umbilical artery creating a false lumen. A double-catheter technique can then be attempted.[72] The first misdirected catheter follows a path of least resistance. A second catheter is also used to bypass this pathway and then enters the aorta.[72] If this technique fails, the second umbilical artery is cannulated. The patency of the catheter is verified by adequate blood return and flushing. The catheter is sutured in place, using a purse string stitch cinched tightly to provide hemostasis and wrapping both ends of the suture around the catheter before tying a square knot. The line is secured using a tape bridge or other available securing device.[73] The umbilical tie is loosened and kept in place for any needed hemostasis. A transducer can be attached for continuous blood pressure monitoring while still allowing blood sampling.[74]

Two depths of UAC insertion are described in the literature.[75-77] Low or high placement of the catheter is based on the vertebral level at which the catheter resides in the aorta.[71,75-77] Low placement is defined as the catheter tip caudal to the origins of the renal arteries, whereas a high placement is described as the catheter tip in the descending aorta above the diaphragm and below the left subclavian artery.[71,75-77] A

Cochrane review evaluated the effects of the position of UACs and concluded that high-placed catheters led to fewer clinical vascular complications.[78] Although reference charts based on patient morphometric are available, there are simple formulas that predict the depth of insertion of arterial catheter.[75-77] Shukla's regression equation based on birth weight (BW) predicts UAC insertion length (cm) as $(3 \times BW (kg) + 9)$ for infants weighing ≥ 1500 g, whereas Wright's formula $(4 \times BW (kg) + 7)$ results in more accurate UAC placement (cm) for infants weighing <1500 g.[76,77]

II. Umbilical Venous Cannulation

Once the umbilical vein is identified, a catheter is introduced carefully in the lumen.[63,64,70] The umbilical vein does not always require routine dilation prior to the introduction of the catheter.[63,64,70] The umbilical cord is gently pulled toward the feet during placement to straighten the course of the vein. The direction of the catheter advancement is cephalad.[63,64,70] A properly placed UVC enters the inferior vena cava and the right atrium through the umbilical vein and the ductus venosus.[79] Sometimes, the catheter is misdirected into the portal, the splenic, or the mesenteric vein.[79] If there is resistance to insertion or poor blood return, inappropriate position of the catheter should be suspected. The double-catheter technique, described in the UAC section, can also be used in UVC placement.[79] The patency of the catheter is then verified by adequate blood return and flushing. The line is secured using the same technique described in the UAC paragraph.[63,64,70]

The length of catheter insertion is determined by the size of the infant and the indication for placement.[63,76,79] In emergency situations, the catheter is advanced to a depth where rapid blood return is achieved (2 to 4 cm in most infants).[63,75,76] A long-term UVC resides at the junction of the inferior vena cava and right atrium.[63,75,76] The two most commonly used methods to predict accurate depth of UVC are nomograms based on the measurement of the shoulder-umbilicus length and regressions equations based on BW.[75,76] Shukla's formula, $([3 \times BW (kg) + 9]/2) + 1$, is widely used to estimate the length of UVC insertion (cm).[76] Verheij suggested that Shukla's formula leads to over insertion of catheters and recommended a revised formula, $[3 \times BW (kg) + 9]/2$.[80]

Proper Placement of Umbilical Arterial and Venous Catheters

Anteroposterior and lateral views of a thoracoabdominal radiograph are required to confirm proper placement of the catheters.[81] Low UAC placement correlates with the third and fourth lumbar vertebrae on chest film, whereas a high placement correlates with the sixth and tenth thoracic vertebrae.[81] UVC tip should be positioned at or just above the diaphragm or between the eighth to tenth vertebrae.[81] Several studies have questioned the optimal diagnostic approach to determine the correct position of the umbilical catheters.[81] Questions were raised on the difficulty of relating anatomic structures to the projection of vertebral bodies on x-ray secondary to the variability of these structures in relation to bony landmarks. Bedside ultrasonography is suggested as a better modality for verifying the position of the umbilical catheters.[81] However, the disadvantage of this technique is the constant need for qualified personnel to perform the study at the time of the

catheter's placement.[81] Due to this limitation, most centers still rely on radiography to assess the catheter's position.

Maintenance

Infants are typically placed in the supine position or on their sides.[63,64,70] A dressing should not be applied to the umbilicus so that the catheter insertion site can be easily inspected.[63,64,70] The UVC is maintained as part of a closed system to prevent air embolism. A continuous infusion is needed to keep the lumen of the UAC clear, and the catheter is flushed after blood draws to minimize clot formation. Continuous fluid infusion containing heparin is needed in the arterial line.[82] The composition of the heparin-containing fluid varies by institution and is influenced by gestational age and electrolyte status. A typical infusion includes 38 to 77 mEq/L sodium chloride or sodium acetate or an isotonic amino acid solution with heparin 1 unit/mL.[82,83]

Removal

Umbilical line catheters are removed one at a time. Each catheter is pulled to approximately 5 cm, then the catheter is slowly withdrawn in increments of 1 cm/min.[84] This process is especially important during the removal of UACs because it allows the artery to spasm and provide hemostasis. If bleeding occurs, pressure is applied by elevating and pinching the skin just above the cord for venous bleeding or below the cord for arterial bleeding.[84] A hemostat can also be used to pinch the lumen of the vessel for persistent bleeding.[63,84]

Complications

Umbilical venous and arterial cannulations are associated with potential complications. These complications are related to placement and malposition of the catheters or prolonged catheter placement in the umbilical vessel.

Umbilical Arterial Cannulation

Several complications are linked to UAC placement and catheter tip position. Trauma to the vessel leading to hemorrhage can occur during placement.[85,86] Vasospasm of the umbilical artery with resulting blanching or cyanosis of the toes, feet, or buttocks has been described.[85,86] Warming of the unaffected limb may improve perfusion of the other extremity. Otherwise, catheter removal is warranted to prevent ischemic complication.[85,86] Other complications are peritoneal perforation, bladder injury, breaks of catheters, intravascular knots of catheters, or catheterization of the urachus resulting in urinary ascites.[64,85,86]

Additional complications can develop with prolonged indwelling of the UAC. McAdams and colleagues investigated the effects of UAC placement in an animal model and concluded that thrombus formation was detected in 80% of aortic sections.[87] In addition, the incidence of developing aortic thrombus increases proportionally to the duration of UAC placement and has been reported as 16% within 1 day, 32% within 7 days, and 80% within 21 days of UAC placement.[87] The presentation of emboli ranges from asymptomatic to limb-threatening ischemia or mesenteric artery occlusion with necrotizing enterocolitis or renal artery occlusion with renal failure and hypertension.[64,85-87] Furthermore, once the intima of the vessel has been traumatized, the vessel becomes susceptible to infection. In most instances, the microorganisms are coagulase negative staphylococci. These pathogens produce a biofilm that preferentially adheres to irregular catheter surfaces.[88] Catheter-related infection may also cause aortic aneurysm.[66] The Centers for Disease Control and Prevention (CDC) reaffirmed in 2011 that UACs should be removed as soon as possible and ideally should not be kept longer than 5 days.[88] It further states that UACs should be removed if signs of vascular insufficiency occur.[88]

Umbilical Venous Cannulation

A common complication of UVC placement is catheter tip malposition. A low positioned UVC within the confluence of the portal circulation may precipitate hepatic injury.[65] Clinical features of liver complications vary and can be asymptomatic or present as abdominal distension with hepatomegaly, hypotension, worsening respiratory status, or portal thrombosis with chronic portal hypertension.[65] A catheter tip in the right atrium can also result in pericardial effusion and tamponade.[89]

Complications related to UVCs indwelling over time include sepsis and thrombosis.[90] Both risks increase when the catheter is left in place for prolonged periods of time. Multiple interventions are recommended to prevent central line–associated bloodstream infection and include limiting central line access for injecting medications, enforcing *scrub the hub* before accessing the central line, and replacing UVCs as soon as possible with peripherally inserted central catheters (PICCs).[88] In 2011, the CDC recommended "removal of UVCs as soon as possible when no longer needed but UVCs can be used up to 14 days if managed aseptically."[88] Interestingly, Butler-O'Hara and colleagues completed a randomized controlled trial that showed similar infection rates with UVCs left in place up to 28 days compared to UVCs replaced by PICCs after 7 to 10 days.[91] However, the same authors later published a quality improvement project revealing a greater risk of infection with long-term compared to short-term UVC followed by PICC placement.[92] The authors hypothesized that the substantial decrease in PICC infection rates in their unit altered the risk-benefit ratios between the two strategies (short and long term) of UVC use.[92]

Summary

Umbilical lines are commonly used in the care of severely ill neonates. The use of UACs for blood collection and blood pressure monitoring and the use of UVCs for nutrition or medications have become commonplace in NICUs and can also be used in the pediatric intensive care unit (PICU). Although there are several benefits to their use, umbilical catheters are associated with potential problems. An awareness of the possible complications is important to minimize serious consequences and provide timely interventions.

Central Venous Line Placement

Central venous line (CVL) placement and use are frequently required in caring for critically ill patients. The need for central access should be anticipated so that circumstances surrounding the procedure, such as sterile technique and the patient's safety and comfort, can be optimized.

Indications and Contraindications

Indications for CVLs include the following:
- The need for reliable and durable venous access
- A lack of or inadequate peripheral venous access
- Administration of vasoactive infusions, total parenteral nutrition, and medications that require central venous delivery

- Frequent blood sampling
- Monitoring of central venous pressure and central venous oxygen saturation
- The need to provide access for extracorporeal support modalities such as continuous renal replacement therapy and apheresis

Contraindications to central access are not absolute and are primarily related to catheter placement at specific sites. In the presence of increased bleeding risk, sites where bleeding may be difficult to control, such as the subclavian, should be avoided if possible. In patients with significant intraabdominal or pelvic trauma, femoral catheters may pose increased risk. Bacteremia present at the time of catheter placement likely will colonize to central venous catheters. Catheters should not be inserted through obviously infected skin. The relative risk and benefit of catheter placement should be carefully considered before each procedure.[93]

Technique

Critically ill pediatric patients vary greatly in size, and the pediatric intensivist should have an awareness regarding the dimensions of the vein that is being accessed and the proximity and anatomic relation of the respective artery to the vein. The diameters of the central veins vary across the pediatric age groups (Table 19.1).

Appropriate-sized catheters for CVL placement in pediatric patients should be readily available. These catheters are

TABLE 19.1	Approximate Mean Femoral and Internal Jugular Vein Diameter Across the Pediatric Age Period	
Age	Mean IJV Diameter (mm)	Mean FV Diameter (mm)
25-27 weeks PCA[a]	2.1	1.5
31-33 weeks PCA[a]	3.3	1.9
37-39 weeks PCA[a]	4.2	2.3
1 month	5.5[b]	4.5[c]
1 year	6.2[b]	5.4[c]
2 years[d]	6.7	6.3
4 years[d]	7.8	7
6 years[d]	8.9	7.7
8 years[d]	10	8.5
10 years[d]	11.1	9.2
13 years[d]	12.8	10.4
16 years[d]	14.5	11.5
19 years[d]	16.2	12.6

[a]Tailounie M, McAdams LA, Frost KC, et al. Dimension and overlap of femoral and neck blood vessels in neonates. Pediatr Crit Care Med. 2012;13: 312-317.
[b]Alderson PJ, Burrows FA, Stemp LI, Holtby HM. Use of ultrasound to evaluate internal jugular vein anatomy and to facilitate central venous cannulation in paediatric patients. Br J Anaesth. 1993;70:145-148.
[c]Warkentine FH, Clyde Pierce M, Lorenz D, Kim IK. The anatomic relationship of femoral vein to femoral artery in euvolemic pediatric patients by ultrasonography: implications for pediatric femoral central venous access. Acad Emerg Med. 2008;15:426-430.
[d]Steinberg C, Weinstock DJ, Gold JP, et al. Measurements of central blood vessels in infants and children: normal values. Cathet Cardiovase Diagn. 1992;27:197-201.
FV, femoral vein; IJV, internal jugular vein; PCA, postconception age.

commonly plastic polymer and available in a variety of diameters, lumen numbers, and lengths. They can be packaged with appropriate-sized introducer needles, guidewires, and tissue dilators, along with other necessary equipment such as local anesthetic, skin cleanser, drapes, and suture for securing the catheter.

Adequate sedation and analgesia plus local anesthesia should be used not only to provide patient comfort during the procedure but also to make the procedure easier and safer with less patient movement.

Full barrier precautions should be used whenever a CVL is placed in the PICU and should include hair cover, mask, careful handwashing, sterile gown and gloves, a large area of skin prepped with antiseptic solution, and a draped sterile field large enough to eliminate the possibility of inadvertent contamination of equipment and sterile surfaces. Chlorhexidine is superior to povidone-iodine for skin disinfection.[94]

The majority of CVLs employed in the PICU are placed using the Seldinger technique. The technique is essentially the same regardless of the site used. The clinician places an introducer needle into the desired vein while aspirating with a syringe. When the lumen of the needle is fully within the lumen of the vein, blood flows freely into the syringe. The needle should be held in place with one hand while the syringe is disconnected with the other hand. The rate at which blood passively flows from the open needle hub depends on the gauge of the needle and the venous pressure; however, it should not be obviously pulsatile. A J-tipped guidewire is inserted into the open hub of the needle and advanced into the vein (Fig. 19.6A). The wire should meet little or no resistance as it is advanced. If resistance is met, attempts to advance the wire should cease. The position of the needle should be adjusted by either advancing or withdrawing slightly or changing the angle of entry. The wire can be carefully withdrawn and the syringe reattached to the needle in order to reidentify the lumen of the vein. If resistance is met while withdrawing the wire, the needle and wire should be withdrawn as a unit rather than risk breaking or cutting the wire. Once the guidewire is well within the lumen of the vein, a small incision is made adjacent to the needle to enlarge the puncture site to more easily accommodate the dilator and catheter. Next, the introducer needle is carefully withdrawn along the wire, holding the wire completely stationary. A dilator of appropriate size is advanced along the wire into the puncture far enough to dilate all tissue planes into the lumen of the vein. The dilator is withdrawn, and the desired catheter is advanced into position along the wire (Fig. 19.6B). The guidewire is removed, leaving the catheter in place. Blood should be easily aspirated from all lumens. Each lumen should be filled with sterile saline or heparinized saline to prevent thrombosis.

Several systems for securing catheters are commercially available. The most common technique uses silk suture. A large loop of suture should be placed in the skin, attached through the wings of the catheter hub, and tied tightly enough to prevent catheter movement but not so tightly as to cause necrosis of the skin within the loop of suture material (Fig. 19.6C).

Internal Jugular Vein Cannulation

Multiple approaches can be used to cannulate the internal jugular vein. For each of these approaches, the patient is supine in slight Trendelenburg position, with a roll of bed

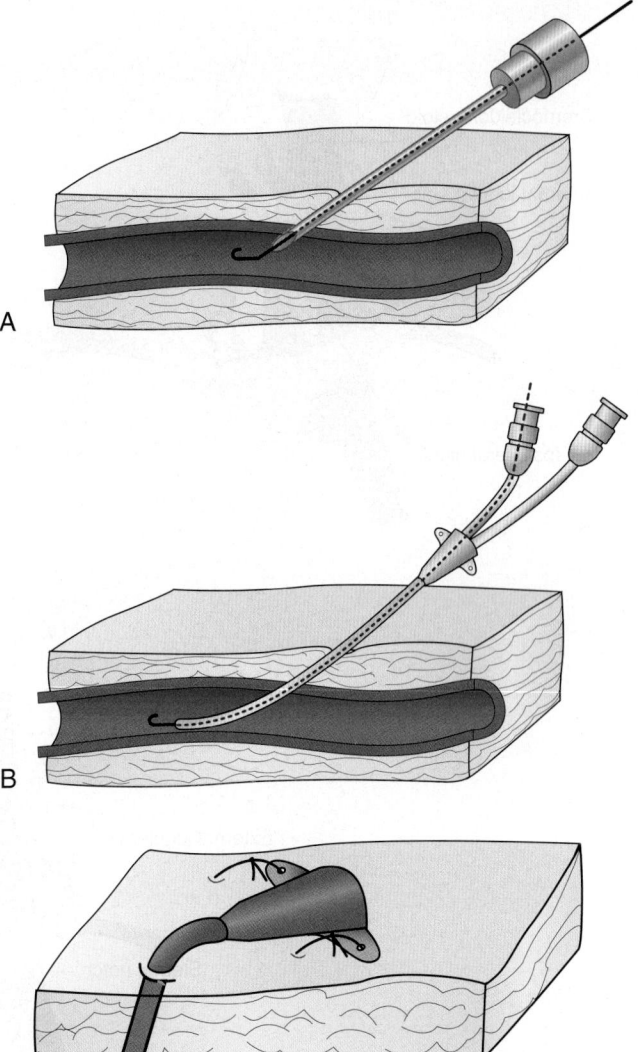

Fig. 19.6. (A) Guidewire is placed through the introducer needle into the lumen of the vein. (B) Catheter is advanced into the vein lumen along the guidewire. (C) Hub of the catheter is secured to the skin with suture.

linen under the shoulders to extend the neck and with the face turned to the contralateral side. The middle or low approach is most commonly used (Fig. 19.7A). The introducer needle enters the skin at the apex of the triangle formed by the clavicle and the heads of the sternocleidomastoid muscle at a 30-degree angle to the skin directed toward the ipsilateral nipple. For the anterior approach, the introducer needle enters the skin along the anterior margin of the sternocleidomastoid halfway between the mastoid process and the sternum and is directed at the ipsilateral nipple (Fig. 19.7B). Using the posterior approach, the needle enters the skin along the posterior border of the sternocleidomastoid halfway between the mastoid process and the clavicle and is directed toward the suprasternal notch (Fig. 19.7C).[95]

Subclavian Vein Cannulation

The patient is positioned supine in a slight Trendelenburg position. A narrow roll of bed linen is placed beneath the patient, between his or her shoulders. The introducer needle enters the skin inferior to the junction of the middle and

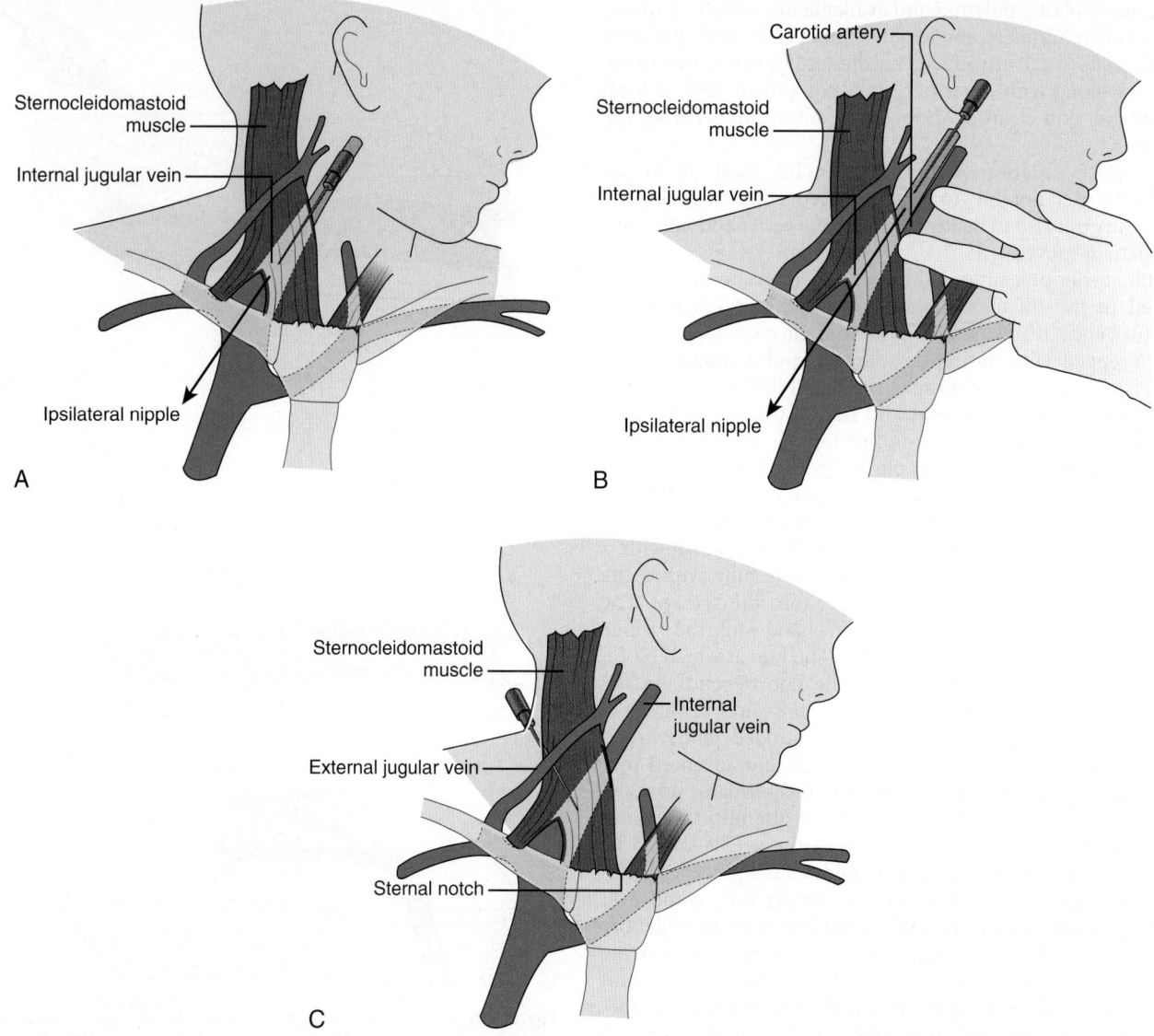

Fig. 19.7. Approaches to the internal jugular vein. The patient is supine, in slight Trendelenburg position, with the neck extended over a shoulder roll and the head rotated away from the side of the approach. (A) Middle approach. The introducer needle enters at the apex of the triangle formed by the heads of the sternocleidomastoid muscle and the clavicle and is directed toward the ipsilateral nipple at an angle of approximately 30 degrees with the skin. (B) Anterior approach. The carotid pulse is palpated and may be slightly retracted medially. The introducer needle enters along the anterior margin of the sternocleidomastoid about halfway between the sternal notch and the mastoid process and is directed toward the ipsilateral nipple. (C) Posterior approach. The introducer needle enters at the point where the external jugular vein crosses the posterior margin of the sterno-cleidomastoid and is directed under its heads toward the sternal notch.

lateral third of the clavicle and is directed toward the suprasternal notch. The needle passes slightly inferior to the clavicle and enters the subclavian vein (Fig. 19.8).[95]

Femoral Vein Cannulation

The patient is placed in a supine position either flat or in a slight reverse Trendelenburg position. A pad of bed linen is placed under the hips to slightly raise them off the bed surface. The leg on the side of catheter placement is slightly abducted and externally rotated. The femoral artery pulse is palpated just distal to the inguinal ligament about halfway between the anterior iliac crest and the pubic symphysis. The femoral vein is approximately 5 mm medial to the femoral artery in infants and toddlers and approximately 10 mm in adolescents and adults. The introducer needle enters the skin 1 to 2 cm distal

to the inguinal ligament at an approximately 30-degree angle with the skin surface and in line with the course of the vein, approximately parallel to the axis of the thigh (Fig. 19.9).[95]

Use of Ultrasound for Central Venous Line Placement

Ultrasonography is used increasingly to facilitate the placement of CVLs in the PICU. A number of studies demonstrate that the use of ultrasound reduces insertion-related complications in pediatric patients.[96-99] CVL placement success rates are improved with the use of ultrasound.[100] As familiarity with real-time ultrasound guidance is improving, novel techniques, including subclavian access, are successfully being implemented in pediatric patients.[101] Routine use of real-time ultrasound guidance for CVL placement is recommended (see also Chapter 20).

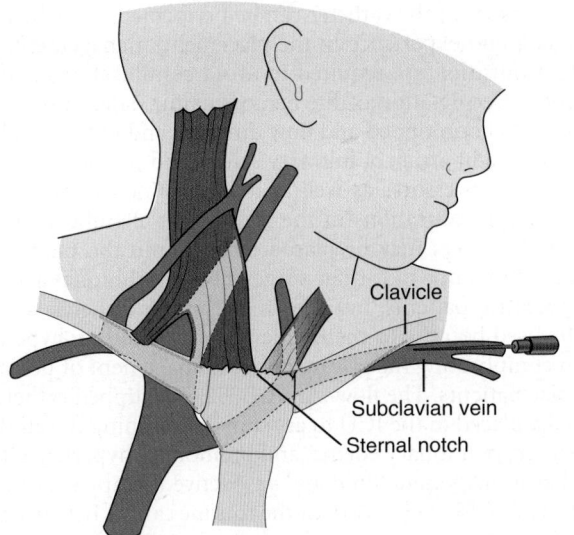

Fig. 19.8. Approach to the subclavian vein. The patient is supine, in slight Trendelenburg position, with a small roll along the spine between the shoulders. The needle enters the skin at the junction of the lateral and middle thirds of the clavicle and is directed toward the sternal notch in the horizontal plane.

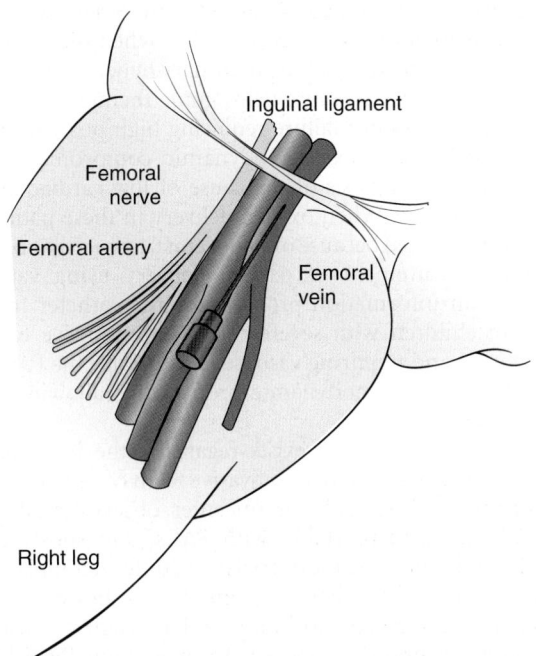

Fig. 19.9. Approach to the femoral vein. The patient is flat and supine, with the thigh slightly abducted and externally rotated. The introducer needle enters the skin 2 to 3 cm distal to the inguinal ligament and 0.5 to 1 cm medial to the pulse of the femoral artery.

Complications

Catheter-related bloodstream infection is the most common complication (see also Chapters 11 and 110). In children, the insertion site is not related to infection risk.[102] The risk of infection is decreased by use of a bundle of practices during insertion and ongoing maintenance of the CVL. The insertion bundle includes strict full barrier precautions and sterile technique. Dressing changes with chlorhexidine skin prep,

minimizing entry into the catheter, and daily assessment of the need of the catheter are all recommended during the maintenance of the catheter.[103] Currently available antibiotic impregnated catheters may decrease the risk of catheter-related infection.[104]

Pneumothorax may result if the lung is punctured during internal jugular or subclavian placement. This complication is less likely with careful patient positioning, attention to anatomic landmarks, and real-time use of ultrasonography as the introducer needle is advanced. Chest radiography should be performed after an internal jugular or subclavian catheter is attempted to document absence of pneumothorax. Thrombosis may occur in the vessel surrounding the catheter and is associated with malignancies and diabetic ketoacidosis.[105,106]

Bleeding at the time of placement can be serious and potentially life threatening. Bleeding at the skin puncture site from an inadvertent arterial puncture is easily controlled by direct pressure. However, bleeding caused by injury to a deeper vascular structure may result in difficult-to-control hemorrhage. Veins and arteries may be perforated or lacerated distant from the intended puncture site by the introducer needle, guidewire, vessel dilator, or the catheter itself. Injury to the femoral or iliac vessels may result in pelvic or retroperitoneal bleeding. Lacerations of the internal jugular, subclavian, or innominate veins or the superior vena cava may communicate with the thoracic cavity and result in hemothorax. Bleeding complications are more severe in the presence of a coagulopathy or thrombocytopenia, and these should be treated, if possible, before central access is attempted.[107,108]

A central venous catheter positioned such that it applies pressure to the wall of the vessel or to the wall of the heart increases the risk of perforation. This situation may result in acute blood loss or tamponade. Undesirable positioning of a CVL can be detected radiographically and should be corrected as soon as possible.[107,108]

Venous Cutdown

With the widespread use of central venous access and the use of intraosseous access during emergencies, venous cutdown is rarely performed. Venous cutdown is indicated when percutaneous access is not achievable and the need for IV access warrants the more invasive procedure. Materials needed depend on the technique of vein cannulation used. The skin should be prepped and draped, and sterile technique should be used. A skin incision is made perpendicular with respect to the vein. The tissue surrounding the vein is bluntly dissected to completely expose the vein. Ligatures are passed around the vein distal and proximal to the intended site of cannulation. A small venotomy is created and, using the ligatures to control the vein, a catheter is directly passed into the lumen of the vein. The distal ligature can be tightened to control bleeding and the proximal ligature to help secure the catheter (Fig. 19.10). Alternatively, an over-the-needle IV catheter can be directly introduced into the exposed vein without creating the venotomy or using ligatures. An introducer needle and then a guidewire can be inserted into the lumen of the vein using Seldinger technique placement. The latter approach is particularly useful for femoral venous cutdown. After the catheter is in place, it is secured with suture material and the wound is closed around the catheter.

The complications of venous cutdown are similar to the complications of other venous access techniques. The risk of

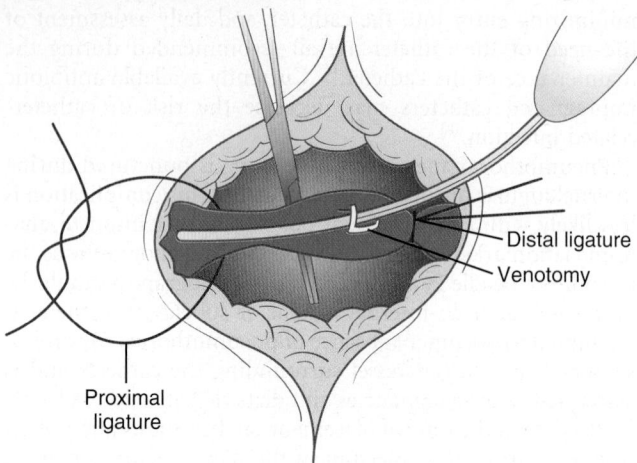

Fig. 19.10. Venous cutdown.

bleeding from the open wound should be considered, especially in patients with increased risk for bleeding (anticoagulation or other coagulopathy). The open wound also increases the risk of infection. Injury to adjacent structures, such as arteries and nerves, during incision and blunt dissection is a risk with cutdown.[95,109,110]

Peripherally Inserted Central Venous Catheters

PICCs are frequently used in PICU patients. For infants and smaller children, often only a single-lumen catheter can be placed. Multilumen catheters may be placed in older children. Although PICC lines can often be placed by visible location or palpation of veins in the antecubital fossae, ultrasound is frequently used to place these catheters proximal to the antecubital fossa. Success is more frequent when the catheters are inserted in the basilic vein.[111]

PICC lines are most often constructed of soft silicone or plastic polymer. The catheter length is measured prior to catheter insertion, and the catheter trimmed to the appropriate length. Placement of PICC lines is most commonly performed using a modification of the Seldinger technique. A needle or catheter is inserted into the vein, then a guidewire is placed, followed by a dilator. A soft peel-away introducer is often inserted next, with the catheter inserted through the introducer sheath; the sheath is peeled away after the catheter is in place. Outside of interventional radiology suites, chest radiography remains the primary method for documenting the location of the catheter tip.

Although PICC lines are associated with a lower risk of placement-related complications, they are subject to the same complications as percutaneous central venous catheters, including catheter-associated infection, thrombosis, perforation, embolization, and fracture.[112-115]

Pulmonary Artery Catheterization

Pulmonary artery catheter (PAC) monitoring was introduced into practice in 1970 by Swan and Ganz (see also Chapter 28). However, because of the invasiveness of the procedure and the lack of a proven survival benefit for patient management, other less invasive surrogate techniques have significantly decreased the use of the PAC.[116-119]

Placement of the catheter can be performed at the bedside, but skill and experience in the placement, management, and data acquisition are required to avoid complications and for proper interpretation of the hemodynamic data. Most catheters are balloon tipped and flow directed, and they are able to measure right atrial, pulmonary artery, and pulmonary capillary wedge pressures as well as to determine cardiac output and oxygen saturations in the right heart chambers. Single-lumen catheters may be placed directly into the pulmonary artery at the time of cardiac surgery. Both techniques are used in pediatric patients, but the single-lumen catheter is especially used because of the frequency of pulmonary hypertension complicating the postoperative management of pediatric cardiac patients. The flow-directed, balloon-tipped catheter is usually placed in the ICU to assist in determining the etiology of shock, pulmonary edema, and pulmonary hypertension, as well as to help guide fluid and vasoactive therapy over time.

PAC should not be used for the routine care of ICU patients, but it might be recommended in heart failure patients with persistent symptoms despite standard measures and also in patients undergoing heart transplant evaluation and patients with pulmonary hypertension.[118,119] Pulmonary hypertension may either be primary or secondary, the latter including pulmonary hypertension in postoperative congenital cardiac patients. These patients are prone to wide swings in pulmonary artery (PA) pressures associated with variations in oxygenation, ventilation, and even sedation. When nitric oxide is used to manage postoperative pulmonary hypertension, direct measurement of PA pressure helps guide therapy. In patients with severe respiratory failure requiring high positive airway pressure with associated hemodynamic compromise, PACs may aid in the diagnosis of the cause of low cardiac output and direct therapy. When oxygen delivery in these patients is significantly limited because of hypoxemia, low cardiac output, or both, measurement of oxygen delivery using variables derived from information provided by the catheter may be useful. In children with severe shock unresponsive to fluid resuscitation and requiring vasoactive infusions, the PAC may better define the hemodynamic profile, thus allowing more specific therapy.

Significant controversy exists regarding the benefits and potential harms caused by this invasive form of hemodynamic monitoring.[118-120] An older multicenter observational study reported increased mortality with PACs, and subsequently several randomized clinical trials failed to demonstrate a benefit to PAC-guided therapy. Some studies showed an association with increased morbidity and mortality,[117] whereas others did not find differences with or without PACs.[120] No studies in pediatric patients have demonstrated better outcomes with the use of the PAC.

Multiple barriers exist to PAC use, including patient risk with placement, the ability to measure similar variables via less invasive measures, increased cost, inaccurate measurement leading to misuse of PAC-derived variables, and incorrect interpretation and clinical application. Additionally, with the decreased use of this technology, the skill required to maintain competency in placement and interpretation of the data provided presents a significant challenge to many institutions.

Contraindications

There are no specific contraindications to placement of a PAC, but there are several relative contraindications, including bleeding diathesis increasing the risk for percutaneous access, as well as severe tricuspid or pulmonary insufficiency, which can make bedside catheter placement prohibitively difficult. Unstable cardiac arrhythmias that are easily triggered by catheter manipulation are also a relative contraindication. Catheter placement for measurement of cardiac output using the thermodilution technique is contraindicated in the presence of intracardiac shunts, tricuspid insufficiency, or pulmonary insufficiency, as the thermodilution measurement will be inaccurate.

Procedure and Equipment

Choosing the most appropriate size and type of catheter is often difficult because a variety of balloon-tipped, flow-directed catheters are available on the market. Catheters are available with two diameters, 5 Fr and 7 Fr. The 5-Fr diameter catheter is most appropriate for patients weighing less than 15 kg, and the 7-Fr diameter catheter is best for patients weighing more than 15 kg. Some PACs employ fiberoptic spectrophotometry for continuous measurement of mixed venous oxygen saturation. Single-lumen PACs are most commonly placed in the operating room at the time of heart surgery.

The standard PAC is 1 m long. The PAC is equipped with proximal and distal ports facilitating measurement of intravascular pressures, infusion of vasoactive agents, fluids, and blood sampling. The distance between the proximal and distal lumen ports varies depending on the catheter: Standards are 10, 15, 20, and 30 cm. Using the correct distance is crucial in order to monitor the appropriate pressure. At the tip are a thermistor used to calculate cardiac output and a balloon that may be inflated and deflated as necessary. Some catheters have an additional right ventricular port for temporary pacemaker insertion, and some have the fiberoptic oxygen saturation sensor for continuous measurement of mixed venous oxygen saturation. Other necessary equipment includes a monitor with cardiac output capability or a computer to determine cardiac output using thermodilution, as well as compatible pressure transducers. Carbon dioxide is used in some centers to inflate the balloon so as to minimize the risk of air embolization, although room air is most common. The catheters are placed through a percutaneous introducer sheath, which is placed with the same technique as described for central venous catheters.

Before placement, the catheter should be flushed and filled with fluid through which intravascular pressures are transmitted to a transducer. The equipment is then zeroed to atmospheric pressure at the level of the patient's left atrium (midaxillary line, fourth intercostal space) and calibrated. If all air bubbles are not removed from the tubing, they may result in *damping* of the waveform tracing and, consequently, erroneously low systolic pressure. Thrombus at the tip of the catheter may also alter the waveform.

The insertion site is prepared in sterile fashion with chlorhexidine solution and draped with sterile towels. It is important to drape a wide area with sterile sheets (full field barrier drape) in order to avoid exposure of the catheter, because of the length of the PAC. The PAC is inserted through the introducer sheath. A sterile sleeve is placed on the end of the sheath, and the catheter is passed through the sleeve, then through the introducer diaphragm and into the sheath.

Anatomically, the preferred sites of insertion are the right internal jugular, left subclavian, right subclavian, and left

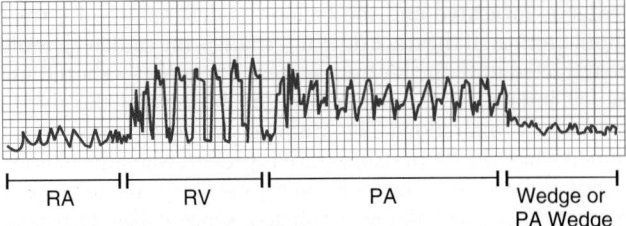

Fig. 19.11. Pressure tracing during placement of a pulmonary arterial catheter showing pressures from the right atrium (RA), right ventricle (RV), and pulmonary artery (PA), then pulmonary capillary wedge pressure. (From Adatia I, Cos P. Invasive and noninvasive monitoring. In Chang AC, ed. Pediatric Cardiac Intensive Care. Baltimore, MD: Lippincott Williams & Wilkins; 1998.)

internal jugular veins. Usually, the placement of the catheter is guided by pressure waveform monitoring (Fig. 19.11), but fluoroscopic visualization will occasionally be needed, particularly if the PAC is placed from a femoral site. Once the catheter tip enters the venous circulation, the balloon is inflated with air. From this point, the catheter should be advanced with the balloon inflated so as to prevent damage to the myocardium, cardiac valves, or pulmonary artery branches. If the catheter is withdrawn, the balloon must first be deflated to avoid valvular injury.

The catheter is advanced to the right atrium (RA), then across the tricuspid valve into the right ventricle (RV), and across the pulmonary valve into the PA. As the catheter continues to float with the balloon inflated, it will wedge in a branch PA, occluding the blood flow. The pulmonary artery occlusion pressure (PAOP), or wedge pressure (PAWP), will be recorded from the distal lumen. If the balloon is deflated, a PA pressure tracing will be recorded. If the waveforms are not obtained, the balloon should be deflated and the catheter pulled back to the RA before attempting placement again.

After insertion, a chest radiograph is obtained to ensure proper catheter placement and rule out pneumothorax. The catheter tip should be visualized ideally within West zone III of the lung (see also Chapter 28).

The pressure waveforms are characteristic; when the catheter is advanced to the RA, the atrial trace has a respiratory variation that helps to confirm the catheter is in the thorax. Once in the atrium the balloon is inflated and advanced to the RV, where the trace is characterized by a rapid upstroke in early systole with an equally rapid downstroke at the end of systole and diastolic pressure near zero. Turning the catheter with a clockwise motion usually helps in passing the PAC. The catheter is advanced to the PA. The PA trace has the same peak systolic pressure of the RV, but as systole ends, the trace shows a slower fall that continues through diastole, because the diastolic pressure in the PA is higher than the RV diastolic pressure. Once in the PA, the catheter is advanced slightly until a pulmonary wedge trace is seen. This trace is similar to the RA trace, although usually with a higher pressure. PAWP is obtained when the balloon is inflated and the catheter floats into the wedge position (see Fig. 19.11). Because the catheter floats to an area of greatest blood flow in the lung, it most likely will be in an area consistent with West zone III, where arterial pressure is higher than both venous and alveolar pressures.

Measurement of PAWP is best done at end-expiration to minimize the effect of changes in pleural pressure. Once the wedge is measured and the balloon is deflated, the PA trace should return. If the trace does not change, the catheter should be retracted until the PA trace is seen. The catheter should not be left inflated in the wedge position because of the risk of pulmonary infarction. The catheter is appropriately positioned when the PA pressure trace is present when the balloon is not inflated and the pulmonary capillary wedge trace is present when the balloon is inflated. Once it has been confirmed that the PAC is in good position by pressure trace and radiography, the catheter should be secured in the sleeve and taped to the patient.

Information Acquisition

Much hemodynamic and oxygen delivery information can be obtained from the Swan-Ganz–type PAC. Multiple hemodynamic pressures can be obtained, including RA, RV PA, and PA wedge pressures. Right atrial pressure is useful for determining preload of the right ventricle. Pulmonary artery pressure is useful for determining the presence of pulmonary hypertension both at baseline and with manipulation of oxygenation, ventilation, ventilator pressures, nitric oxide, and other procedures. PAWP reflects left ventricular preload. In most patients with normal cardiac function and anatomy, right atrial or central venous pressure adequately reflects LV preload as well. However, in the presence of certain congenital heart defects, with significant ventricular dysfunction, or with high mechanical ventilatory pressures, a significant discrepancy may exist between right and left ventricular preload. In such circumstances, measurement of PAWP may be useful for guiding fluid and inotropic therapy.

Mixed venous oxygen saturation ($S_{mv}O_2$) can be determined directly and continuously with a catheter containing the fiberoptic oximeter. In the absence of the oximeter, intermittent blood sampling from the distal port when in place in the pulmonary artery allows for $S_{mv}O_2$ measurement.

The thermistor at the tip of the catheter allows for measurement of cardiac output, using the thermodilution method. This method uses the Fick principle, based on the law of conservation of thermal energy. A specific amount of known temperature fluid is injected in the proximal port (upstream), and the temperature change downstream (at the thermistor) is recorded. The change in temperature over time allows for measurement of blood flow, in this case cardiac output. According to Jansen, this measure of cardiac output is accurate if the following conditions are met: (1) no loss of cold occurs between the injection site and the thermistor, (2) mixing of the cold injectate (indicator using Fick terms) and the blood is complete, and (3) the temperature change caused by the injection of cold fluid is sufficient to be detected by the thermistor.

To perform thermodilution cardiac output measurements, the catheter must be connected to the thermodilution computer, which is either freestanding or part of the cardiac monitor. A specific volume of injectate, either room temperature or iced, is injected rapidly into the proximal port of the catheter. The temperature difference over time that is detected at the thermistor is recorded as a curve. The computer then integrates the area under the curve, which is inversely proportional to the cardiac output. The cardiac output is calculated and projected. For pediatric patients, this number should be divided by their body surface area in square meters, deriving the cardiac index. The injectate can be either iced or room temperature. The disadvantages to iced injectate include risk of hypothermia in pediatric patients requiring frequent cardiac output measurements, the poor accuracy of the first injection because of warmer fluid in the catheter, and a greater signal-to-noise ratio. Room-temperature injectate prevents these problems and yet is accurate when cardiac output is stable. However, in conditions of high or low cardiac output, less variance occurs with iced injectate compared with room-temperature injectate. However, for convenience and the safety of pediatric patients, room-temperature injectate is recommended.

Usually three to five injections yield adequate results. Some error can be introduced by faulty technique. Injecting variable volumes or injecting with variable rates can result in inaccurate measures. Multiple injections and averaging of the results can overcome these problems. The presence of tricuspid or pulmonary insufficiency can lead to an overestimation of cardiac output. Echocardiography may be necessary to rule out the presence of valvular insufficiency. Intracardiac shunts, such as a ventricular septal defect, result in false values for cardiac output. Mechanical ventilation has been shown to alter stroke volume, which can result in a variability of cardiac output measurements. Therefore one should perform the injection at the same time in the ventilator cycle to standardize the cardiac output measurements.

Maintenance

Care of the PAC is similar to that for any central venous line. The catheter and sheath should be dressed sterilely at all times and the dressing changed according to protocol. The catheter is housed in a sterile sleeve that allows for aseptic technique if further manipulation is necessary. Pressure transduction of the distal (PA) and proximal (RA) ports and continuous ECG monitoring are mandatory. This setup continually confirms proper placement of the catheter. Whenever the balloon is inflated to determine PAWP, the balloon is allowed to deflate passively by opening the balloon port and removing the syringe. This step helps prevent balloon rupture. Balloon rupture should be suspected if blood is obtained when aspirating the balloon port. In this situation, remove and then replace the catheter if it is still clinically indicated. As noted earlier, arrhythmias can occur, particularly if the catheter becomes dislodged. A chest radiogram should be assessed daily for catheter position.

Interpretation

The hemodynamic data obtained or calculated with the PAC should be interpreted to make therapeutic decisions. There are not isolated "good" or "bad" cardiac output (CO) values, but appropriate cardiac output is that which permits an adequate oxygen delivery (DO_2). As a global index of adequacy between consumption (VO_2) and DO_2, $S_{mv}O_2$ is the target of choice for therapeutic decisions. $S_{mv}O_2$ should be kept above a threshold value between 65% and 70%, and all other PAC parameters should be used to choose how to maintain $S_{mv}O_2$ above this value. This $S_{mv}O_2$ goal can be achieved by fluid administration, blood transfusion, increasing or decreasing inotropic support, or vasopressors.[116,121]

Complications

PA catheterization is a significantly invasive procedure. Complications can occur during the Seldinger procedure to access the vein, during the passage of the PAC (across two heart valves), or during catheter use. Bleeding, infection, and pneumothorax may occur during venous access. Arrhythmias can be seen during placement of the PAC or due to dislodgment of the catheter. Their spectrum includes supraventricular tachycardia while the PAC tip is in the RA to premature ventricular beats or even ventricular tachycardia while the PAC tip is in the RV. Usually, the arrhythmias cease when the catheter tip reaches the pulmonary artery. Occasionally lidocaine, amiodarone, and defibrillation may be needed, so they should be readily available. Once the catheter is in place, pulmonary infarction or hemorrhage is a risk. Rupture of the distal pulmonary artery, endothelial damage, and valvular damage have been reported, as well as knotting of the catheter requiring fluoroscopic retrieval. The PAC should be removed as soon as possible to minimize the risk of complications.

Summary

Since the introduction of the PAC, controversy has surrounded the technology regarding the benefits and potential harms caused by this invasive form of hemodynamic monitoring. In adult clinical trials, the usefulness of the PAC has been challenged because no benefit in patient outcome has been observed, and some retrospective studies have described worse outcomes. Accurate acquisition and interpretation of PAC data are paramount for making appropriate therapeutic decisions.

Thoracentesis and Tube Thoracostomy

Thoracentesis

Thoracentesis is a procedure to remove fluid or air from the pleural space. In pediatric patients, thoracentesis is most frequently used as a diagnostic procedure. Pleural effusions in children are most commonly the result of an infectious process (50% to 70% parapneumonic effusions), with congestive heart failure (5% to 15%) and malignancy being less common causes.[122] Many other conditions may, rarely, cause pleural effusions in children (Box 19.2).

Indications

Thoracentesis may be used diagnostically or therapeutically to relieve respiratory distress resulting from large accumulations of fluid or air. If ongoing evacuation is required, tube thoracostomy should be considered (discussed later). Ultrasound is useful to identify fluid accumulations when there is complete opacification of the hemithorax on chest radiograph and to help characterize fluid consistency (complicated versus simple effusions). Ultrasound may also help to identify optimal locations for successful aspiration.[123]

Contraindications

Thoracentesis has no absolute contraindications. Positive pressure ventilation may increase the risk of pneumothorax. Uncorrected coagulopathy and thrombocytopenia predispose to bleeding complications; however, thoracentesis can generally be accomplished in this setting utilizing a small needle and careful technique. An uncooperative patient can lead to damage to the underlying vascular structures and lung parenchyma. This can be avoided by generous use of sedation and analgesia.

BOX 19.2   Causes of Pleural Effusion

Infection (exudates)
- Bacterial
- Viral
- Fungal
- Mycobacterial
- Mycoplasma

Cardiovascular
- Congestive heart failure
- Constrictive pericarditis
- Superior vena cava obstruction

Pulmonary
- Pulmonary infarction
- Atelectasis
- Asbestos exposure
- Drug-induced pleuritis

Intraabdominal disease
- Abdominal surgery
- Pancreatitis
- Hepatitis
- Peritonitis
- Subdiaphragmatic abscess
- Intrahepatic abscess
- Meigs syndrome
- Cirrhosis with ascites

Iatrogenic
- Extravascular central venous catheter placement

Collagen vascular disease
- Rheumatoid arthritis
- Systemic lupus erythematosus
- Sjögren syndrome
- Wegener granulomatosis

Neoplastic
- Lymphoma/leukemia
- Mesothelioma
- Chest wall tumors
- Metastatic carcinoma
- Bronchogenic carcinoma

Renal
- Uremia
- Urinary tract obstruction
- Nephrotic syndrome
- Peritoneal dialysis

Miscellaneous
- Esophageal rupture
- Hemothorax
- Chylothorax
- Lymphedema
- Hypoalbuminemia
- Myxedema
- Sarcoidosis
- Radiation therapy
- Immunoblastic lymphadenopathy
- Familial Mediterranean fever

Preparation

Sedation and analgesia are frequently required to safely perform thoracentesis in pediatric patients. Topical local anesthetic agents may reduce the discomfort associated with infiltration of local anesthetics and should be placed at the insertion site at least 15 to 30 minutes prior to the procedure (depending on agent).

Procedure

Box 19.3 lists the supplies and equipment required for thoracentesis.

Technique

If thoracentesis is being performed for evacuation of a pneumothorax, the patient should be placed in the supine position.

BOX 19.3   Supplies and Equipment for Thoracentesis

- Pillows or towels for positioning patient
- Sterile gloves
- Povidone-iodine or chlorhexidine solution
- Commercial thoracentesis tray (for older children and adolescents)
- Or assemble the following items:
  - Sterile gauze sponges
  - Sterile towels or drapes
  - 3- to 5-mL syringe for local anesthetic; 27- to 30-gauge needle for skin infiltration
  - 1% lidocaine; consider sodium bicarbonate to buffer lidocaine
  - Over-the-needle catheter: 14- to 20-gauge depending on the size of the patient
  - 10- or 20-mL syringes for fluid collection
  - Three-way stopcock or tubing extension set with clamp
  - Sterile dressing
  - Tape to secure dressing

BOX 19.4   Interpretation of Pleural Fluid

Characteristics of exudative effusions:
- Pleural to serum protein ratio >0.5
- Pleural to serum lactate dehydrogenase (LDH) ratio >0.6
- Pleural fluid LDH more than twice the upper limit of the normal serum value

---

Aspiration is performed at the second or third intercostal space in the midclavicular line. For removal of pleural fluid, the patient should be placed in the upright, seated position. Infants and young children may be held in the burping position by an assistant. The normal site for fluid aspiration is the seventh intercostal space in the posterior axillary line (near the tip of the scapula).

The site should be prepped with chlorhexidine and draped with sterile towels. The skin entry site is then generously infiltrated with a local anesthetic using a 27- to 30-gauge needle. The needle is then advanced perpendicular to the skin to infiltrate the underlying subcutaneous tissues, superior portion of the rib, and periosteum. A longer 22- to 25-gauge needle may be needed to accomplish this goal. The needle is then advanced over the superior border of the rib while gentle pressure is applied on the syringe plunger until the pleural space is reached. The depth of the needle where fluid aspiration occurs should be noted. An over-the-needle catheter of sufficient length is then used for aspiration of fluid with a syringe. If infection and exudate effusion are suspected, a larger catheter (16- to 18-gauge) may be needed.

Aspiration is continued until a sufficient quantity of fluid for diagnostic studies is obtained. A three-way stopcock with attached tubing may be placed on the catheter to facilitate this process. If fluid is being removed for the release of respiratory distress, aspiration is continued until fluid flow ceases. The catheter is subsequently removed and a sterile dressing is applied over the entry site.

Complications

The most common complication of thoracentesis is pneumothorax.[123] All patients undergoing thoracentesis should have a follow-up chest radiograph. Hemothorax may occur in patients with abnormal coagulation or thrombocytopenia. A platelet count of greater than 50,000/uL and normal coagulation studies are ideal, but the procedure can be safely performed with careful technique and avoidance of the neurovascular bundle found on the inferior border of the rib. In more urgent settings, platelets and clotting factors may be administered during the procedure. Soft tissue infections can be avoided with use of proper sterile technique. Reexpansion pulmonary edema has been reported in adult patients with removal of large fluid volumes and usually occurs in the first

hour following thoracentesis.[124,125] This complication has not been reported in children.

Interpretation

Analysis of pleural fluid is separated into two basic categories: exudates and transudates. The criteria used to distinguish between the two are largely dependent on adult data.[126] Box 19.4 lists the Light criteria for differentiating between transudative versus exudative fluid. Elevated triglyceride levels (greater than 110% of serum value) and lymphocyte predominance suggest chylothorax. Elevated amylase suggests pancreatitis or esophageal rupture.[127] Advances in polymerase chain reaction (PCR) technology allow for rapid and accurate diagnosis of *Staphylococcus aureus*, *Streptococcus pneumoniae*, and *Mycoplasma* in pleural fluid.[128]

Summary

Thoracentesis is a useful diagnostic procedure for pediatric pleural effusions. It can also be a useful technique resolving respiratory distress with significant fluid accumulations or pneumothoraces. Thoracentesis is a simple technique that can be performed with high yield and a minimal complication rate.

Tube Thoracostomy

Tube thoracostomy placement is a common procedure in the pediatric critical care setting. Many options, including less invasive techniques, are now available and are discussed here. Tube thoracostomy is required for a variety of reasons in critically ill pediatric patients. Pneumothoraces can develop spontaneously or as a result of acute lung injury. Large parapneumonic effusions and empyemas resulting from infectious pulmonary processes often require chest tube placement. Hemothoraces or hemopneumothoraces resulting from trauma frequently require drainage. Finally, chylothoraces in postoperative cardiac patients frequently require tube placement and continuous drainage. The technique utilized for placement depends on the nature (thick, thin, transudative, exudative) of the material to be removed.

Contraindications

As with thoracentesis, tube thoracostomy has no absolute contraindications. Attempts should be made to correct coagulopathy to prevent bleeding complications. However, when emergent or urgent intervention is required, tube thoracostomy should not be delayed.

Supplies and Equipment

Many institutions have specially designed chest tube trays with sterile instruments. Typical requirements include sterile gauze sponges, sterile towels for draping, syringes and needles for local anesthesia, a scalpel and blade, curved Kelly clamps of various sizes, needle driver, suture, and suture scissors. Other materials required are an appropriately sized chest tube, chlorhexidine solution, sterile gloves, a drainage apparatus (such as Pleur-Evac), local anesthetic, and tape.

Technique

Patients should receive sedation and analgesia for tube thoracostomy, along with generous local anesthesia. The technique for placement depends on the type of material expected to be removed from the chest. Thin, transudative fluid and pneumothoraces can often be evacuated with placement of a small-caliber tube (5 Fr to 9 Fr) via a modified Seldinger technique.[129]

After proper sedation and analgesia, the overlying skin is prepped with chlorhexidine and draped in sterile fashion. A needle attached to a syringe (5 or 10 mL) is inserted in the fourth or fifth intercostal space in the midaxillary line. Continuous suction is applied and the needle is advanced until fluid or air is obtained. A guidewire is then placed into the pleural space. A small skin incision is made and the overlying skin and subcutaneous tissues are dilated with a skin dilator. A small catheter with multiple side holes is then placed over the wire and advanced into the pleural space. The guidewire is removed and the catheter is attached to a standard chest tube suction device. The tube is anchored to the skin with a suture or a commercially available sutureless skin-anchoring device. Placement of pigtail catheters tends to be less painful than traditional tube thoracostomy (described later); however, the viscous fluids encountered with hemothoraces and empyemas generally do not drain well via this technique. Successful treatment of empyema with placement of pigtail catheters and use of fibrinolytic agents (alteplase and streptokinase) has been described.[130]

A variation of this technique allows for placement of larger caliber tubes. After placement of the guidewire as above, progressive skin dilators are used, allowing placement of a more standard-sized chest tube. Kits for placement of these over-the-wire devices are commercially available. Caution should be used with placement of these devices in diseases with poor pulmonary compliance or pulmonary hyperinflation, as these conditions may predispose to intraparenchymal tube placement and the development of bronchopleural fistulas.[131]

Traditional techniques for tube thoracostomy may be required for drainage of viscous fluids, including cases of empyema and hemothorax. Tube thoracostomy is a painful procedure and requires generous use of sedation and analgesia. Following administration of sedation and analgesia, the patient is placed in the supine position. The skin is prepped with chlorhexidine and draped in sterile fashion. The proper position for placement is the fourth or fifth intercostal space in the midaxillary line. The skin, subcutaneous tissues, intercostal muscles, underlying rib, and periosteum should be generously infiltrated with local anesthetic as described above.

A skin incision in the fourth or fifth intercostal space, large enough to allow placement of the chosen tube, is made parallel to the axis of the rib in the midaxillary line. A curved Kelly clamp is used to bluntly dissect the underlying subcutaneous tissue until the superior border of the upper rib is reached. The clamp is then used to push through and dilate the intercostal muscle and pleura insertion above the superior border of the rib. In a larger child, the index finger can be used to further dilate the subcutaneous tissues and intercostal muscles. Any intrapleural adhesions can also be manually broken up.

The end of the tube is then attached to a clamp and inserted into the pleural space. The clamp is opened and the tube advanced to the proper depth, ensuring all side holes are in the chest cavity. If possible, the tube should be advanced anteriorly for pneumothoraces and posteriorly for effusions. The tube is then attached to a pleural drainage system.

Many techniques are available for suturing the chest tube in place. The most important aspect of the choice of anchoring method is that the operator removing the tube knows how the tube was secured. Some operators prefer a horizontal mattress suture on both sides of the tube; others prefer to place a *pursestring suture* that can be pulled together after the tube is removed. If the latter technique is used, no knot is placed at the skin level, but extra suture is wrapped around the body of the tube and then tied to the tube itself. Upon removal, the extra suture serves as skin suture for the wound. Rarely, a suture is inadvertently placed through the tube while the device is anchored. In this event, a technique for cutting the suture using endoscopic scissors has been described.[132] Needleless anchoring devices for anchoring tubes without suture (eg, StatLock Multipurpose, Venetec International, San Diego, California) are commercially available.

Maintenance

Following successful chest tube placement, a chest radiograph should be obtained to verify proper position and to evaluate for resolution of pleural fluid or pneumothorax. Tubes should be evaluated for continued air leak by checking for air bubbles in the leak chamber of the suction apparatus. Persistent air leak with no evidence of pneumothorax by chest radiograph suggests the development of a bronchopleural fistula or airway injury. Some authorities suggest intermittent external negative pressure to "strip" the tube in order to maintain patency, although little evidence supports this practice.[133] Alteplase may also restore patency of tubes clogged by proteinaceous material.[130] Some advocate prophylactic antibiotic use, but little evidence supports this practice.[134]

Timing of tube removal depends on the indication for placement. Tubes placed for pneumothoraces may be removed following resolution of the air leak. The authors' practice is to place these tubes to water seal for at least several hours and obtain a chest radiograph prior to removal. This practice of placing tubes to water seal and evaluating with a chest radiograph is supported in the adult literature.[135] Tubes placed for drainage of pleural fluid may be safely removed once fluid drainage has decreased to 2 to 3 mL/kg/24 hours. Removal of large tubes may be painful and require analgesia or sedation, especially in small children. Tubes may be safely removed during either the inspiratory or expiratory phase.[136]

Complications

Several potential complications exist with placement of chest tubes. Any structure within the thorax may be inadvertently penetrated with use of undue force. For this reason, trocar chest tubes are not recommended for use in children, even in emergent situations. Placement in the lung parenchyma is relatively common, potentially leading to bronchopleural fistulas.[137] Vascular injury may occur with high placement, and subclavian artery obstruction has been reported as well.[138] Left-sided placement can lead to thoracic duct injury and development of chylothorax. Deep placement may lead to mediastinal perforation.[139] Computed tomography may be used to evaluate the exact placement of chest tubes in cases where inadvertent misplacement or complications are suspected.

Summary

Tube thoracostomy is a common procedure in pediatric critical care. With attention to detail, this procedure may be accomplished safely and with minimal risk. New techniques and smaller caliber tubes may be utilized in select cases. Fibrinolytic agents such as alteplase may be used to restore the patency of clogged tubes and may be of therapeutic benefit in cases of empyema.

Paracentesis

Paracentesis is the percutaneous sampling of peritoneal fluid by needle aspiration through the abdominal wall and is considered a relatively safe procedure. Analysis of ascitic fluid, combined with history and physical examination, will frequently confirm the cause of ascites.

Indications

Diagnostic paracentesis is indicated in any patient with new-onset ascites, when the cause of ascites is unknown, or cases of suspected bacterial peritonitis.[140,141] Paracentesis may also be used for the relief of respiratory distress or the end-organ effects of abdominal compartment syndrome secondary to massive ascites.[142]

Contraindications

Paracentesis in patients with ascites has no absolute contraindications, except when overt disseminated intravascular coagulation is present.[140,141,143,144] Severe renal dysfunction has the highest association with bleeding complications after paracentesis.[140,141,145] Due to the very low risk of bleeding complications and lack of data to support their use, the routine use of prophylactic fresh frozen plasma or platelets is not currently recommended.[140,141]

Procedure

When present, the physical examination findings of flank dullness, shifting dullness, and fluid waves support the presence of ascites and can guide selection of the needle insertion site.[140,141,143] Ultrasound guidance may improve the success rate of paracentesis.[146,147] Additionally, when physical exam findings are insufficient or difficult due to obesity, ultrasonography can detect smaller amounts of fluid, differentiate free from loculated fluid, and may be more sensitive than physical examination in diagnosing ascites.[140,141,148]

Supplies

Box 19.5 lists the supplies required for diagnostic paracentesis.

Technique

The patient is positioned in semirecumbent position. The bladder should be emptied by voiding or catheterization. The site of needle insertion is selected by physical examination or ultrasound. Outside of the neonatal period, preferred sites are midline along the avascular linea alba below both the umbilicus and the upper edge of dullness but above the bladder (usually midpoint between umbilicus and pubic symphysis suffices) or the left lower quadrant two finger breadths

---

BOX 19.5   Supplies for Diagnostic Paracentesis

- Antiseptic solution
- Alcohol preps
- Sterile gauze
- Sterile drapes
- Sterile gloves
- 1% lidocaine with or without epinephrine
- 3- to 10-mL syringe with small-gauge needle for local anesthesia
- 22- to 16-gauge spinal needle or intravenous catheter (22- to 20-gauge needle for small children, 16- to 20-gauge needle for larger children)
- 20-mL (or larger) syringe
- Specimen vials

(2–3 cm) in both the medial and cephalad directions from the anterior superior iliac spine. The right lower quadrant may also be used. Surgical scars should be avoided due to the risk of underlying bowel adhesions.[140,141,143] The inferior epigastric arteries running cephalad midway between the pubic symphysis and anterior iliac spine in the rectus sheath should be avoided. In patients with portal hypertension, the midline may become vascularized and should be avoided, as well as any visible collateral vessels, to reduce the chance of hemorrhagic complications.[140,141,143,149]

The entry site is disinfected with antiseptic solution, such as chlorhexidine or povidone iodine, and draped in sterile fashion. The skin and subcutaneous tissue down to the peritoneum are infiltrated with lidocaine using a small-gauge needle. Prior to needle insertion, the skin at the insertion site should be pulled downward approximately 2 cm, to create a nonlinear Z tract, and while holding negative pressure with the attached syringe, the clinician inserts the needle. The needle is advanced slowly until free flow of fluid into the syringe is noted, but it is removed immediately if frank blood is aspirated. If an IV catheter is utilized, the catheter should be advanced and needle removed at this time, with reattachment of the syringe to the catheter. Approximately 20 to 40 mL of fluid is collected for diagnostic evaluation, but much larger volumes, 1 to 5 liters depending on age, may be removed for tense ascites.[140-143] If fluid return stops or is sluggish, changing the patient's position may be helpful. Once fluid collection is complete, the needle or catheter is removed, direct pressure with gauze is applied, and then a sterile pressure dressing placed. When ongoing drainage is needed, a pigtail catheter can be placed using the Seldinger technique.

Complications

Potential complications of paracentesis occur in approximately 1%, most commonly abdominal wall hematoma or bleeding.[143] Additional, but rare (<0.1%), complications include persistent leakage of ascitic fluid, bladder perforation, intestinal perforation with and without resulting peritonitis, and scrotal edema.[141,143,150,151] In patients with bleeding complications, renal dysfunction was present in 70%, coagulopathy 59%, and thrombocytopenia 8%.[145] Appropriate selection of the needle insertion site minimizes the risk of hematoma or bleeding. The risk of intestinal perforation is increased in patients with previous abdominal surgical procedures with adhesions and can be minimized by avoiding abdominal surgical scars at the needle insertion site.[140,141,152,153] Additionally,

TABLE 19.2	Characteristics of Ascitic Fluid in Various Conditions	
Condition	**Clinical Characteristics**	**Laboratory Findings**
Portal hypertension	Straw colored, sterile	SAAG ≥1.1 g/dL Total protein <2.5-3 g/dL WBC <250-500/uL, <1/3 neutrophils
Spontaneous bacterial peritonitis	Cloudy or turbid Gram stain positive <10%, cultures may be negative, single organism[a]	Neutrophils ≥250/uL Total protein <1 g/dL LDH and glucose similar to serum
Secondary bacterial peritonitis	Multiple organisms	Neutrophils ≥250/uL Total protein >1 g/dL LDH elevated Glucose <50 mg/dL
Chylous ascites	Milky with recent fat ingestion	WBC 1000-5000/uL, predominately lymphocytes Triglycerides >200 mg/dL, cholesterol >48 mg/dL[b]
Pancreatic ascites	Turbid, brown or bloody	WBC and total protein increased Amylase and lipase levels >serum Amylase levels may be falsely low in young infants[c]
Urinary ascites		Protein <1 g/dL; urea and creatinine >serum[d]
Malignant ascites	Bloody	Protein and LDH elevated
Nephrotic syndrome	Straw colored	Total protein <2.5 g/dL[c]
Tuberculous ascites	Yellow or bloody, may have fibrin clots	Total protein >2.5 g/dL WBC >1000/uL, primarily lymphocytes PCR useful[¶]

[a]Kandel G, Diamant NE. A clinical view of recent advances in ascites. J Clin Gastroenterol. 1986;8:85-99.
[b]McGibbon A, et al. An evidence-based manual for abdominal paracentesis. Dig Dis Sci. 2007;52:3307-3315.
[c]Glauser JM. Paracentesis. In Roberts JR, Hedges JR, eds. Clinical Procedures in Emergency Medicine. Philadelphia: WB Saunders; 1991.
[d]Runyon BA. Care of patients with ascites. N Engl J Med. 1994;330:337-342.
[¶]Uzunkoy A, Harma M. Diagnosis of abdominal tuberculosis: experience from 11 cases and review of the literature. World J Gastroenterol. 2004;10: 3647-3649.
LDH, lactate dehydrogenase; *PCR,* polymerase chain reaction; *SAAG,* serum-ascites albumin gradient; *WBC,* white blood cells.

intestinal perforation has been reported with marked bowel distension, and, though rare, decompression should be considered prior to paracentesis.[151] Persistent leakage of ascitic fluid can be minimized by using the Z-tract method for needle insertion and a smaller bore needle. Ongoing fluid leaks can be managed by closing the defect with a suture or applying cyanoacrylate skin adhesive.[154] Bladder emptying decreases the risk of bladder perforation. Strict adherence to sterile technique and avoidance of areas of skin or soft tissue infection decrease the risk of infection.

Interpretation

Analysis of ascitic fluid may not yield a definitive diagnosis, but it is useful in the evaluation of ascites. Clinical assessment identifies the most likely diagnosis, helps determine which tests should be ordered, and influences the interpretation of results.[140,141,155,156]

Fluid studies that should be obtained include total protein, albumin, and white blood cell count with differential. Optional studies to consider are Gram stain, aerobic and anaerobic cultures (inoculated into culture bottles at the bedside), glucose, lactate dehydrogenase, and amylase. Rarely needed studies to consider are acid-fast bacilli (AFB) smear and culture, cytology, triglyceride, and bilirubin. Studies considered unhelpful are pH, lactate, cholesterol, fibronectin, and glycosamioglycans.[140,141] Corresponding serum chemistries should be obtained for comparison.

Analysis of the serum-ascites albumin gradient (SAAG) is useful for differentiating between ascites caused by portal hypertension and ascites resulting from other causes. A SAAG of 1.1 g/dL or higher correlates with portal hypertension with 97% accuracy.[141,155]

The characteristics of ascitic fluid in various conditions are summarized in Table 19.2.

Summary

Needle aspiration of ascitic fluid is a relatively safe procedure when performed with appropriate precautionary measures. Analysis of ascitic fluid obtained by paracentesis is useful in the evaluation of patients with new-onset ascites, unknown cause of ascites, or suspected bacterial peritonitis. Ongoing drainage through a catheter placed at the time of paracentesis may improve ventilation or reduce complications secondary to abdominal compartment syndrome in patients with massive ascites.

Key References

1. de Caen AR, et al. Part 10: Paediatric basic and advanced life support: 2010 International Consensus on Cardiopulmonary Resuscitation and Emergency Cardiovascular Care Science with Treatment Recommendations. *Resuscitation.* 2010;81(suppl 1):e213-e259.
2. Voigt J, Waltzman M, Lottenberg L. Intraosseous vascular access for in-hospital emergency use: a systematic clinical review of the literature and analysis. *Pediatr Emerg Care.* 2012;28:185-199.
14. Orlowski JP, et al. The bone marrow as a source of laboratory studies. *Ann Emerg Med.* 1989;18:1348-1351.
26. Brzezinski M, Luisetti T, London MJ. Radial artery cannulation: a comprehensive review of recent anatomic and physiologic investigations. *Anesth Analg.* 2009;109:1763-1781.
34. Ohara Y, et al. Use of a wire-guided cannula for radial arterial cannulation. *J Anesth.* 2007;21:83-85.
47. McCann UG 2nd, et al. Invasive arterial BP monitoring in trauma and critical care: effect of variable transducer level, catheter access, and patient position. *Chest.* 2001;120:1322-1326.
50. King MA, et al. Complications associated with arterial catheterization in children. *Pediatr Crit Care Med.* 2008;9:367-371.
56. Smith MJ. Catheter-related bloodstream infections in children. *Am J Infect Control.* 2008;36:S173.e1-S173.e3.
57. Maisch B, et al. Guidelines on the diagnosis and management of pericardial diseases executive summary; the task force on the diagnosis and management of pericardial diseases of the European society of cardiology. *Eur Heart J.* 2004;25:587-610.
59. Vayre F, et al. Subxiphoid pericardiocentesis guided by contrast two-dimensional echocardiography in cardiac tamponade: experience of 110 consecutive patients. *Eur J Echocardiogr.* 2000;1:66-71.
63. Green C, Yohannan MD. Umbilical arterial and venous catheters: placement, use, and complications. *Neonatal Netw.* 1998;17:23-28.
65. Grizelj R, et al. Severe liver injury while using umbilical venous catheter: case series and literature review. *Am J Perinatol.* 2014;31: 965-974.

66. Mendeloff J, et al. Aortic aneurysm resulting from umbilical artery catheterization: case report, literature review, and management algorithm. *J Vasc Surg.* 2001;33:419-424.

70. Lewis GC, Crapo SA, Williams JG. Critical skills and procedures in emergency medicine: vascular access skills and procedures. *Emerg Med Clin North Am.* 2013;31:59-86.

76. Shukla H, Ferrara A. Rapid estimation of insertional length of umbilical catheters in newborns. *Am J Dis Child.* 1986;140:786-788.

88. O'Grady NP, et al. Guidelines for the Prevention of Intravascular Catheter-Related Infections. 2011. Available from: <http://www.cdc.gov/hicpac/pdf/guidelines/bsi-guidelines-2011.pdf>. Accessed 14.07.15.

93. Olson ME, et al. Evaluation of strategies for central venous catheter replacement. *Crit Care Med.* 1992;20:797-804.

97. Froehlich CD, et al. Ultrasound-guided central venous catheter placement decreases complications and decreases placement attempts compared with the landmark technique in patients in a pediatric intensive care unit. *Crit Care Med.* 2009;37:1090-1096.

101. Rhondali O, et al. Ultrasound-guided subclavian vein cannulation in infants: supraclavicular approach. *Paediatr Anaesth.* 2011;21:1136-1141.

103. Miller MR, et al. Reducing PICU central line-associated bloodstream infections: 3-year results. *Pediatrics.* 2011;128:e1077-e1083.

117. Chatterjee K. The Swan-Ganz catheters: past, present, and future. A viewpoint. *Circulation.* 2009;119:147-152.

118. Shah MR, et al. Impact of the pulmonary artery catheter in critically ill patients: meta-analysis of randomized clinical trials. *JAMA.* 2005; 294:1664-1670.

128. Utine GE, et al. Pleural fluid PCR method for detection of *Staphylococcus aureus, Streptococcus pneumoniae* and *Haemophilus influenzae* in pediatric parapneumonic effusions. *Respiration.* 2008;75:437-442.

129. Aziz F, Penupolu S, Flores D. Efficacy of percutaneous pigtail catheters for thoracostomy at bedside. *J Thorac Dis.* 2012;4:292-295.

130. Thommi G, et al. Efficacy and safety of intrapleural instillation of alteplase in the management of complicated pleural effusion or empyema. *Am J Ther.* 2007;14:341-345.

140. Giefer MJ, Murray KF, Colletti RB. Pathophysiology, diagnosis, and management of pediatric ascites. *J Pediatr Gastroenterol Nutr.* 2011;52:503-513.

143. Runyon BA. Paracentesis of ascitic fluid. A safe procedure. *Arch Intern Med.* 1986;146:2259-2261.

145. Sharzehi K, et al. Hemorrhagic complications of paracentesis: a systematic review of the literature. *Gastroenterol Res Pract.* 2014;985141.

Emerging Role of Ultrasonography in the Pediatric Intensive Care Unit

Erik Su, Akira Nishisaki, and Thomas Conlon

PEARLS

- Intensivist-operated ultrasound is an important adjunct for vascular procedures at the pediatric intensive care unit bedside, and it is considered standard of care for percutaneous internal jugular vein central access. Evidence also suggests its utility in vascular access in other central vessels, peripheral veins, and arteries as well.
- Accuracy of intensivist-operated ultrasound examining the heart, lungs, abdomen, and cerebral circulation has also been explored. Cardiac ultrasound examinations by intensivists demonstrate sensitivity for pathology similar to studies performed by imaging specialists.
- Practice and familiarity with ultrasound's capabilities, advantages, and disadvantages contribute to responsible and effective practice.
- An image archival system is a core asset in the development of a program for documentation, quality improvement, education, and research purposes.

More than a technologic advancement in critical care medicine, ultrasound has been a positive innovation in the pediatric ICU, providing a means of facilitating procedure guidance and basic patient assessment. Since the 1980s, technologic advancements in imaging quality and digital storage have resulted in bedside ultrasound equipment that is both portable and powerful. Its use in the ICU results from recognition of its value for procedure guidance, interaction with cardiac intensivists in specialty ICUs, and shared interest from other clinical specialties such as emergency medicine. Ultrasound is emerging as standard of care for some ICU procedures and is increasingly recognized as a valuable diagnostic tool. Nonprocedural bedside ultrasound applications performed by intensivists contrasts with traditional diagnostic imaging in that it is often interpreted at the bedside, occurs synchronously with management decisions, and is readily used by the bedside clinician for serial assessment. In this sense, a clinician-operated exam is more focused on assisting the direct and immediate delivery of care, whereas diagnostic imaging by radiologists and cardiologists emphasizes optimizing study detail and longitudinal assessment.

Ultrasound Physics and Basics of Image Optimization

The physical principles that make ultrasound possible are well described. Ultrasound energy is transmitted in sound waves through substances at a frequency >20 kHz, beyond the range of human hearing. Probes used for bedside ultrasound typically use energies in the range of 1 to 20 MHz or more. Ultrasound impulses are transmitted in a coordinated manner from an array of piezoelectric elements in a transducer aimed at a target of interest. Reflected sound from tissue and interfaces between substances of differing density is received by the same piezoelectric array. Based on known speeds of ultrasound in tissue as well as image processing by the ultrasound device, a two-dimensional image is generated and cycled over time to compose a continuous video or cine. Variability in tissue sound velocity and attenuation properties including refraction, reflection, absorption, or scattering of returning ultrasound energy may introduce artifact in images (Fig. 20.1).[1]

A portion of image quality is naturally machine dependent, and a variety of parameters are adjustable for image optimization to reduce diagnostic error. Image size modification tools include depth, zoom, and scan area. Though a wide and deep scan area permits capture of a large field of view, short depth or high zoom factor facilitates imaging of small or superficial structures (Fig. 20.2).

Gain is also an important setting for image optimization and can be adjusted in several ways. Gain affects the sensitivity of the machine to returning ultrasound energy. Returning ultrasound energy is attenuated as it passes through tissue. Time to return of reflected ultrasound energy determines depth of visualized structures rendered on the screen, and time-gain compensation settings can be adjusted to emphasize gain at different depths based on when the return signal reaches the transducer. On various machines these may appear as sliding controls or knobs that control near and far gain. At the bedside, gain is adjusted relative to ambient room lighting so that relevant pathology can be visualized (Fig. 20.3).

Frequency is an adjustable control that also affects image quality. Higher ultrasound frequencies allow for higher resolution imaging as a function of improved spatial discrimination of structures. Higher frequencies also result in poorer imaging of deep structures due to signal attenuation; conversely, lower frequency imaging can identify deeper structures at the expense of image resolution (Fig. 20.4). Some devices permit use of harmonic frequencies that can improve

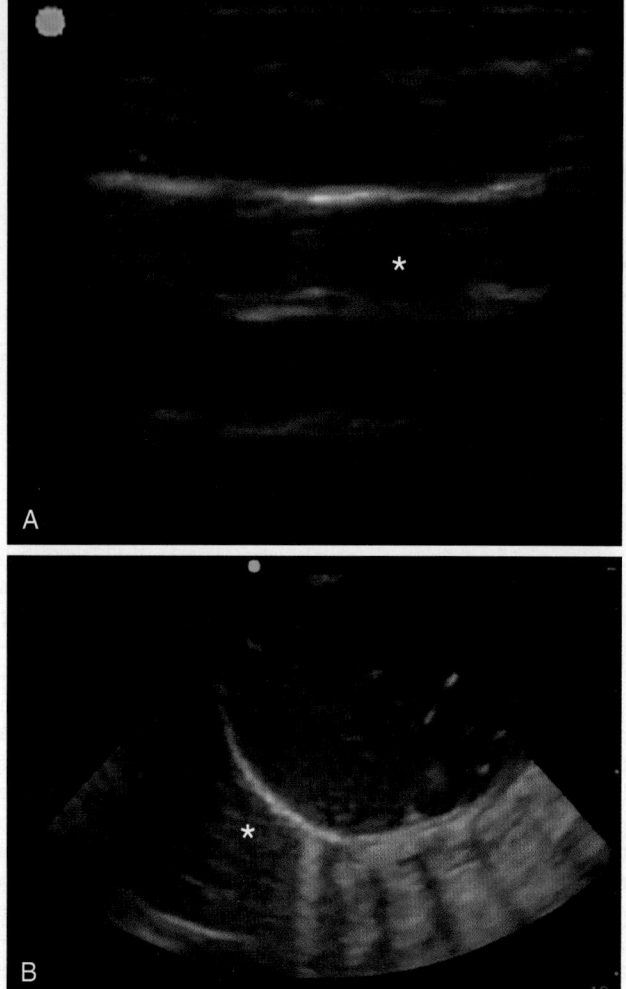

Fig. 20.1. Ultrasound artifacts. (A) Reflection artifact across the pleural line (*). (B) Mirror artifact across a diaphragm (*).

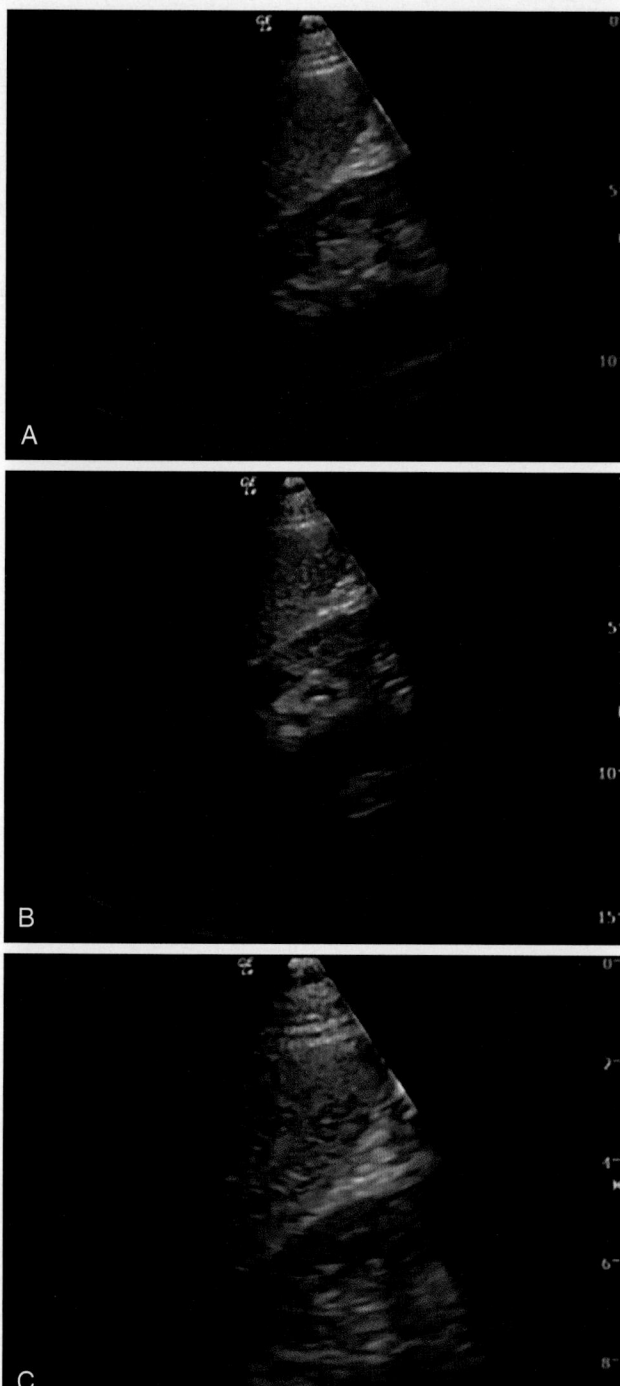

Fig. 20.2. Effects of depth on ultrasound image with B demonstrating same image as A at greater depth and C at shallower depth than A.

image quality of deep structures. In this mode, the machine only interprets frequencies of reflected sound that arrive at multiples of the fundamental transmitted frequency.

Doppler ultrasound is used in a variety of procedural and diagnostic applications to derive the speed of moving structures in the body, blood flow being a common target. Using color flow Doppler in vascular imaging, ultrasound machines color code areas on the two-dimensional image where tissue and fluid are moving: Returning reflected ultrasound frequency is either Doppler shifted higher (movement toward the transducer) or lower (movement away from the transducer). In the human body this can correspond not only to blood but also to the motion of fluid in the bladder and other potential spaces. Pulsed wave Doppler samples a small area of the screen for Doppler data that are then plotted along a velocity/time scale (Fig. 20.5). Doppler is most useful when the direction of blood flow is parallel to the ultrasound beam. In instances where the flow is not parallel, the angle is corrected by multiplying the velocity sampled in the area of interest by the cosine of the angle of the incident ultrasound beam to fluid flow. This correction only evaluates the angle within the plane of the ultrasound beam. If the flow travels out of plane of the ultrasound beam, accurate measurements cannot

be rectified with the correction function. For these reasons, use of angle correction is typically limited to approximately 30 to 45 degrees. By convention, in echocardiography angle correction is not used because of the difficulty in matching beam angles to nonlaminar flows in the heart.

Power Doppler displays amplitude of echoes from moving cells and is less angle dependent than traditional Doppler, thereby permitting improved visualization of vessel branching. For this reason, power Doppler can be a useful modality

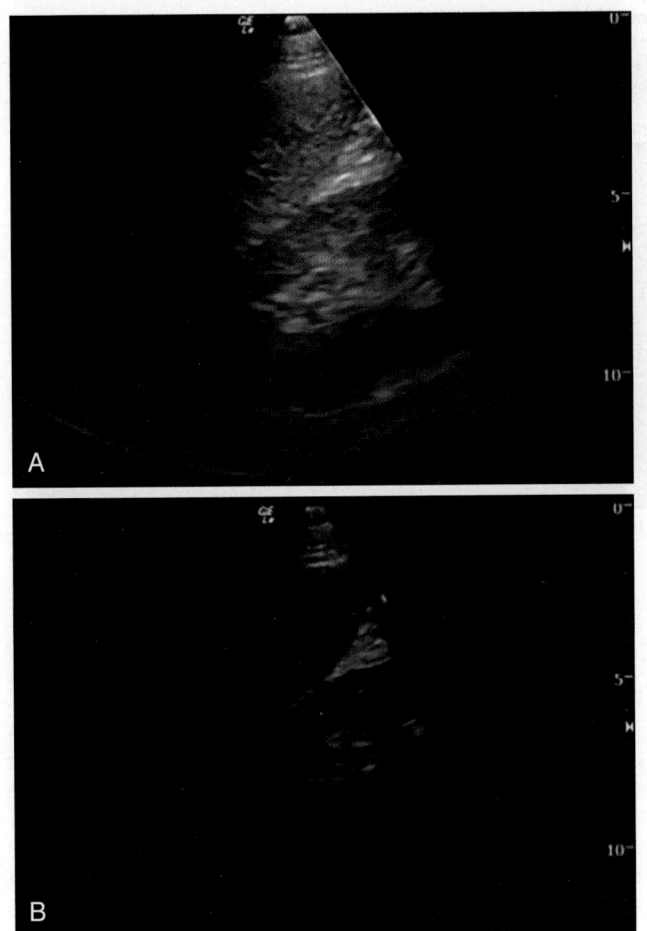

Fig. 20.3. Effects of gain on ultrasound image with B demonstrating same image as A at lower gain.

for vessel identification in procedure guidance. Power Doppler is typically displayed without directionality as seen in color flow Doppler; however, some machines permit superimposed directional color flow data.

M-mode ultrasound graphs the received ultrasound signal along a one-dimensional beam over time. This is useful for tracking objects in motion to quantify and characterize their movement (Fig. 20.6). Examples of M-mode applications include assessing respiratory variation of the inferior vena cava (IVC), calculating a left ventricular shortening fraction, and evaluating diaphragmatic excursion. When using M-mode, it is important that the operator's scanning hand be motionless because operator movement will be captured on the M-mode tracing as well.

Sweep speed is an important machine setting for M-mode and pulsed wave Doppler where data are plotted against time. Sweep speed is defined as the speed at which the data tracing is graphed on the screen. In some instances a faster sweep speed is necessary to reduce the amount of time displayed on the screen, thereby "stretching" the tracing so that finer details of movement are captured. This is helpful in echocardiography with a tachycardic heart so that cardiac motion is more easily discerned. Conversely, slowing sweep speed may be helpful in compressing more data into the screen (Fig. 20.7). Slowing sweep speed might be necessary for visualizing

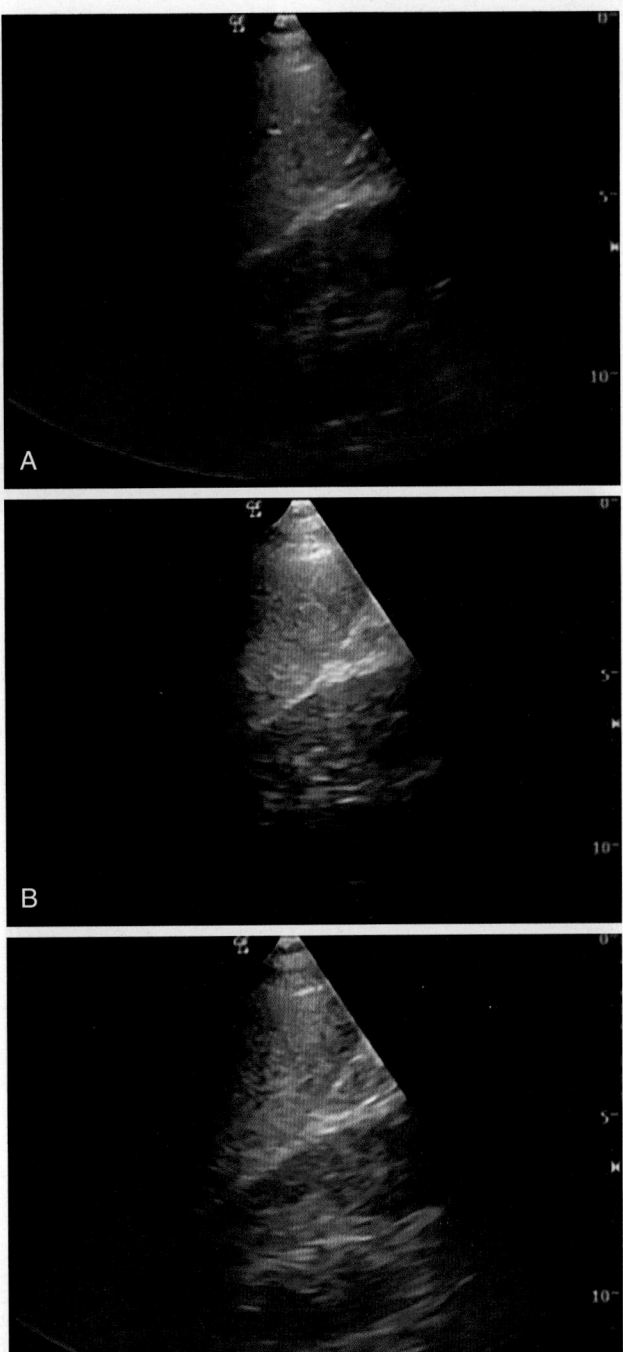

Fig. 20.4. Effects of frequency on ultrasound image with B demonstrating same image as A at higher frequency and C at lower frequency than A.

changes in cardiac ejection or inflow velocities over a respiratory cycle.

Transducers

Ultrasound transducers appear in a multitude of configurations that serve different specialized functions. They are largely divided into higher frequency linear array probes and lower frequency sector type probes, with occasional exceptions.

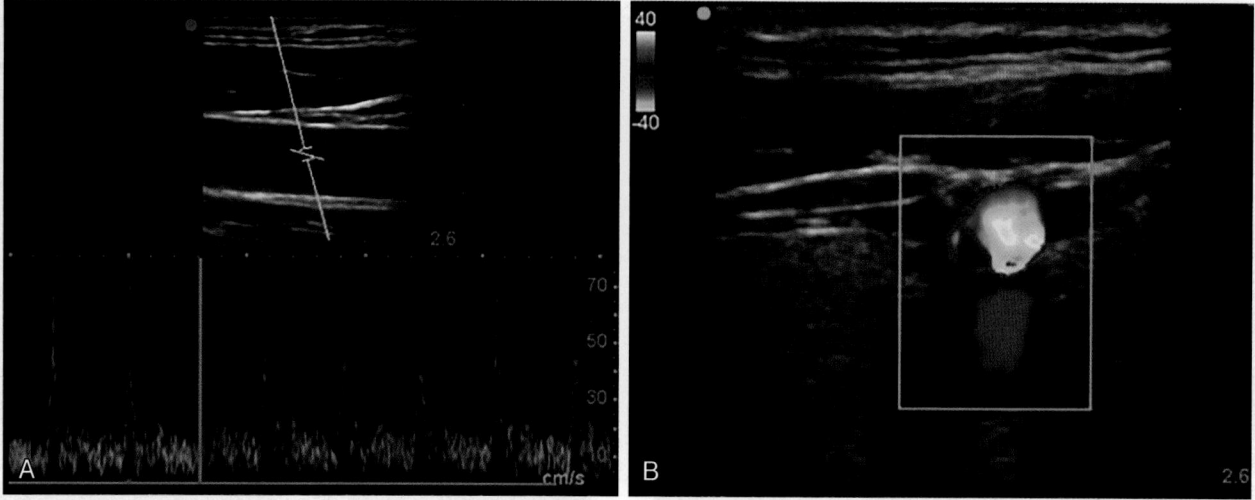

Fig. 20.5. Doppler modalities in ultrasound; (A) pulsed wave and (B) color flow Doppler.

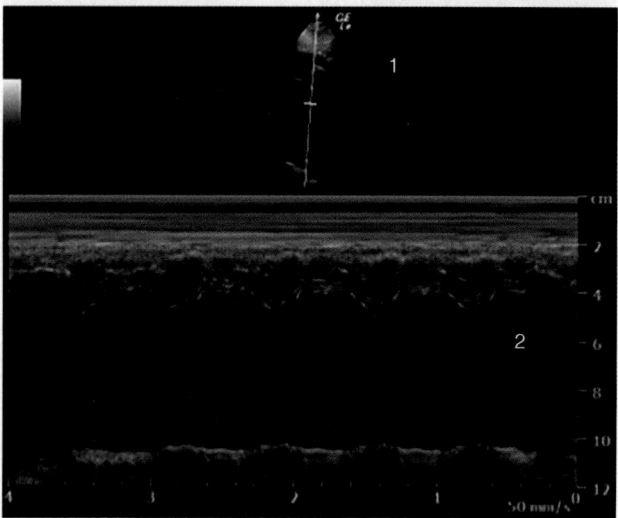

Fig. 20.6. M-mode imaging in ultrasound. (1) Two-dimensional image for cursor targeting. (2) M-mode tracing.

Linear array transducers are a mainstay of procedural guidance for intensivists and other clinical interventionalists using ultrasound (Fig. 20.8). They are configured with an array of parallel-oriented piezoelectric elements designed to image a field of tissue below the probe at close proximity to the skin. These probes also tend to emit higher frequencies (7 MHz or above) to visualize the region of interest at high resolution, with some small structure probes operating above 20 MHz. Linear array transducers are optimal for procedural guidance because needle localization is easier with their wide, shallow, and high-resolution field of view. Linear array transducers are also well suited to diagnostic imaging at shallow depths where higher resolution is preferred. Examples include thoracic imaging and vascular imaging. Linear arrays range in size and shape. In addition to conventional arrays in which the transducer face forms the end of the handpiece, linear transducers also include "hockey-stick"–shaped vascular probes, originally designed with improved ergonomics for carotid imaging but also useful for peripheral vascular procedures in children.

Sector-type transducers encompass phased array transducers and curvilinear transducers. The sector term refers to the image generated by the concave array appearing as a wedge-shaped sector on the ultrasound screen. Phased array transducers are low-frequency devices and have a small footprint on the skin, designed for deeper wide field imaging at depth (Fig. 20.9). Because these probes are largely used in cardiac imaging, the ultrasound hardware is optimized for fast frame-rate video at the expense of image resolution. Because of the small footprint and low frequency, these probes are also optimally suited for transcranial imaging for Doppler flow measurements of the cerebral arteries. This type of imaging requires a low fundamental frequency of approximately 1 MHz, with most probes ranging between 1 and 6 MHz. These probes can also be used for diagnostic imaging in the abdomen, particularly in infants and young children.

Curvilinear transducers operate at the same to slightly higher frequency (1-12 MHz) than phased array transducers and are engineered for improved image resolution at the expense of a slower frame rate. For this reason they excel at looking at relatively nonmobile structures such as the abdomen and its vasculature. Large curvilinear probes are often too large for children and therefore smaller radius microconvex curvilinear probes are preferred. These probes are also used for cranial ultrasound in infants due to their higher frequency and small footprint. Within the ICU, their higher resolution and footprint that is slightly wider than that of a phased array transducer also make them useful for procedure guidance, particularly for vascular access and regional anesthesia. In addition, they may facilitate visualizing the lung and thoracic structures.

Procedural Guidance

Long before entering the ICU, ultrasound became a mainstay for procedural guidance in the operating theater and interventional radiology suite. In the hands of intensivists, ultrasound has proved to be a useful adjunct in vascular access, increasing first-pass success and reducing adverse events during central venous catheter (CVC) insertion in a number of large series.[1-4] Though the majority of ultrasound trials for vascular access

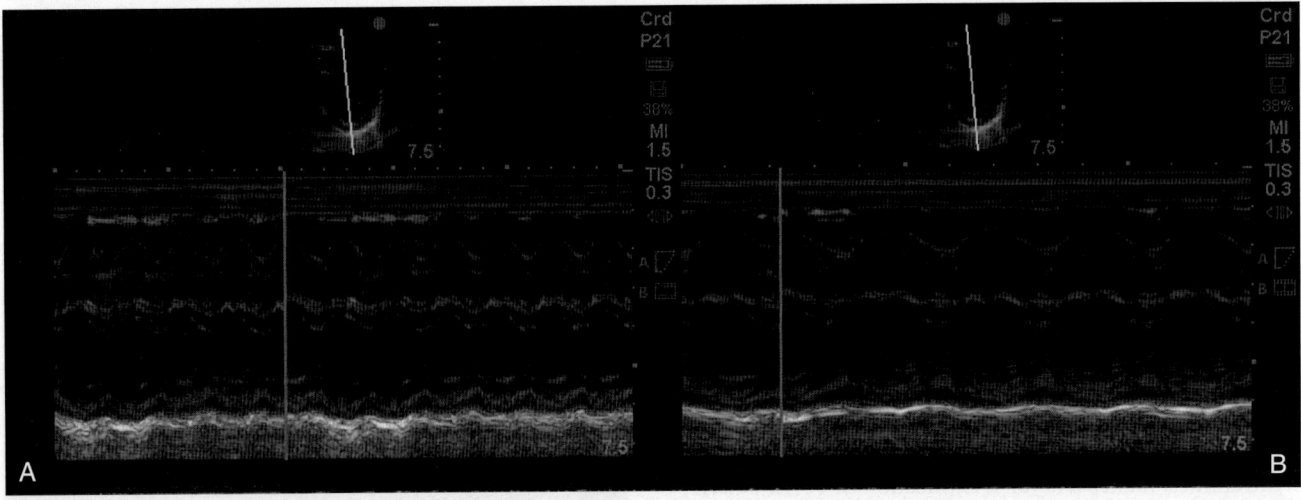

Fig. 20.7. Effect of sweep speed on time-based modalities. In this example of M-mode imaging, the image in A is running at a slower sweep speed than the image in B.

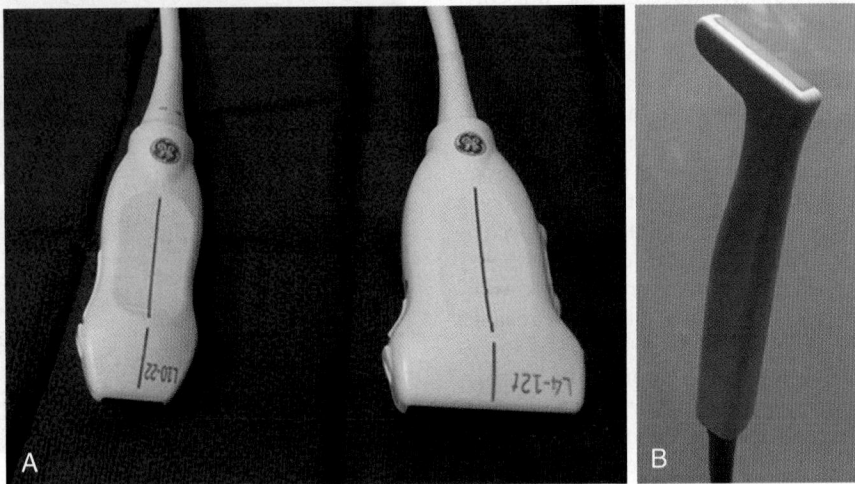

Fig. 20.8. Examples of linear array transducers. (A) Conventional linear array probes. (B) Carotid vascular or "hockey-stick" probe.

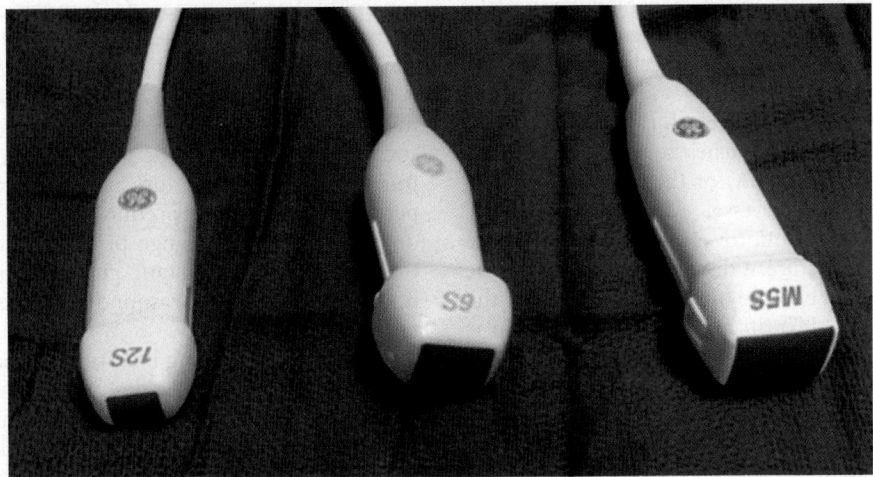

Fig. 20.9. Examples of phased array transducers.

have been conducted with trainees likely less familiar with landmark methods for CVC insertion, the preponderance of the primarily adult evidence supporting ultrasound guidance for internal jugular vein CVC cannulation has changed the procedure such that most practice environments would not have sufficient equipoise to have a landmark-only arm for a randomized trial. Although it appears that ultrasound guidance does improve safe vascular access, its use is a skill that requires training and practice. Novice providers should practice procedures with skilled operators before attempting them independently.

Before attempting procedural cannulation of a venous structure, it is important to identify surrounding arterial structures and demonstrate venous patency. Veins should be compressible and without distinct arterial pulsatility.

Similarly to techniques used during vascular examination of extremities, maneuvers for identification of vessel patency are helpful for targeting veins for cannulation. The primary and most reliable method is observing for compressibility of the venous structure and absence of pulsatility. Methods used in the vascular laboratory that can help identify a vessel include use of Doppler ultrasound to identify vessel flow and augmentation of vascular flow by squeezing the muscular extremity distal to the area being examined with ultrasound (eg, the calf when examining the common femoral vein). It is important to recognize, however, that in the setting of pulmonary hypertension, pulsatile venous flow can confound differentiation between vein and artery, as it can cause pulsatile distention as well as reversal of blood flow in the vein. Though this finding is most pronounced in patients who carry a known diagnosis of severe idiopathic pulmonary hypertension, it can also be seen in patients with acquired pulmonary hypertension from increased intrathoracic pressure or cardiogenic shock. Augmentation of flow is also not entirely reliable; this technique will show vascular flow in the setting of partial vessel obstruction as well, if flow can get around the obstruction. Additionally, a color Doppler signal may not match vessel dimensions because the signal may "bloom" or contract depending on the machine's Doppler gain setting.

In the event that these maneuvers do not demonstrate patency, a vessel may no longer be continuous due to sclerosis or thrombosis. Thrombi may or may not appear echogenic and may or may not obstruct venous flow. When identified they occupy space in the vessel lumen and are observed to obstruct venous flow and resist compression. Doppler modalities for identifying vessel occlusion are well described but have limited utility when thrombi are partially occlusive or in shock states when flow is very low.

Varying approaches to central vessel cannulation using ultrasound exist. Dynamic approaches to the central veins include the transverse (Fig. 20.10A) or the longitudinal (Fig. 20.10B) planes relative to the vessel. An advantage of the transverse approach is that it improves lateral steering of the needle to avoid arterial puncture. A disadvantage is that needle tip identification is harder, because only a cross section of the needle shaft is visualized. Identification of the needle tip is crucial for successful access and prevention of inadvertent injury, and it is performed by sliding the probe and staying over the needle tip throughout the procedure. This technique will avoid inadvertent puncture of deeper structures (ie, the pleura or carotid artery in internal jugular venous cannulation). The longitudinal approach has reciprocal advantages

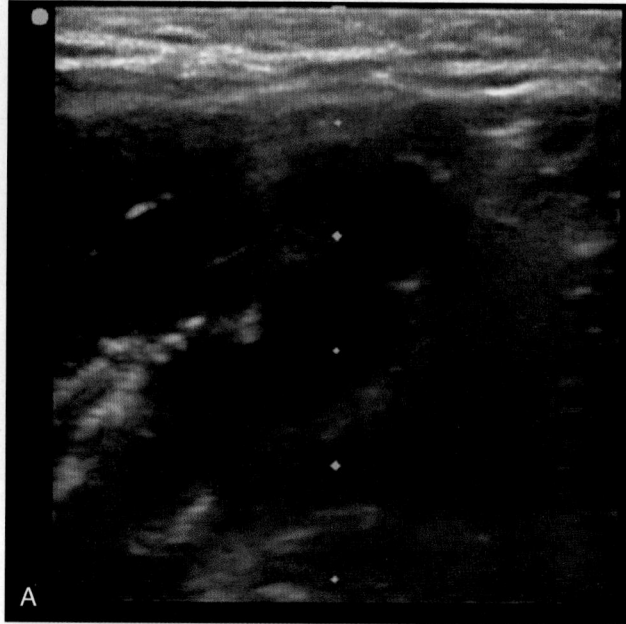

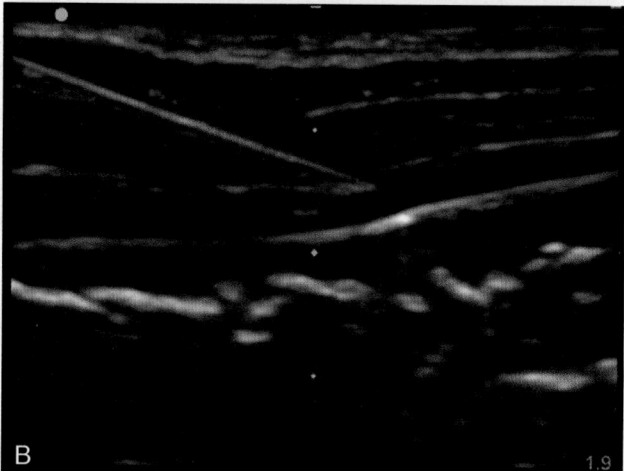

Fig. 20.10. Sonographic approaches to vascular access. (A) Transverse plane. (B) Longitudinal plane.

and disadvantages, facilitating observation of the advancing needle tip without moving the probe but losing lateral aiming capability. For these reasons, transverse visualization of the vessels is often more intuitive and most frequently taught to novice practitioners. *Static* ultrasound-guided central venous access uses the transducer to identify the vessel followed by marking of the site for needle puncture without direct ultrasound visualization of the needle during the attempted cannulation. This permits use of both hands for the technical performance of the procedure; however, patient positioning or physiology may change prior to venipuncture, rendering the mark inaccurate. Static guidance has been shown to be inferior to the active ultrasound guidance or so-called dynamic technique.[5]

Though most existing literature focuses on internal jugular venous access, experience describing other vessel access using ultrasound guidance has been published. There is limited adult patient experience reported on the placement of CVCs in the subclavian vein.[6,7] Ultrasound guidance for subclavian access may be stymied by relative probe to patient size issues in pediatric patients. In the longitudinal orientation, the transducer occupies the majority of the skin in the infraclavicular space and limits the area for target insertion. A number of authors have described a supraclavicular approach to the subclavian or brachiocephalic vein.[8-12] This is also approached using a longitudinal transducer orientation to the vessel and can be difficult in children for whom the length of the transducer displaces the needle insertion rather distal to the clavicle. In addition, the technique's dependence on the longitudinal approach makes it less accessible to novice learners. Use of a microconvex array to place a subclavian CVC is promising as a future adjunct for the procedure.[13]

Ultrasound guidance for femoral vein CVC placement remains contentious as the existing literature is limited methodologically and includes only small series or series that include femoral cannulation mixed with other catheterization sites.[14-16] Studies that compare different ultrasound approaches or ultrasound- versus landmark-guided approaches to femoral vein cannulation by pediatric intensivists are lacking and seem indicated, given different characteristics of the femoral vein in children compared to adults.[17-19]

The literature includes few descriptions of central axillary vein CVCs, but this site can be useful for patients with limited options for central access. When inserted in the axillary vein at a position in or distal to the axilla, the catheter takes a similar course to subclavian CVCs. A longer catheter length is necessary so that it reaches from the axilla to the turn of the brachiocephalic vein into the superior vena cava (SVC). In contrast to other CVCs, the redundancy of axillary tissues complicates venipuncture, and ultrasound guidance seems especially beneficial.

Outside of central veins, ultrasound has also been useful for peripheral IV access and arterial access. For patients with difficult peripheral access, ultrasound facilitates targeting and site selection leading to successful IV placement.[20] Ultrasound can identify sites difficult to detect from the surface, particularly collateral vessels that may become engorged due to obstruction of previously cannulated veins. An important consideration is vessel depth, because deep infiltrates are not as readily recognized as shallow ones, resulting in soft tissue injury and potential serious safety events.[21] Intravenous catheters exceeding an inch in length are useful to access deeper vessels and to increase maximize length of catheter within the vascular lumen. Their insertion benefits from placement in veins with sufficiently long straight courses. Deeper vessels require a steeper angle of insertion, and this increases the risk of penetrating the back wall of the vessel. Following the threading of the IV catheter into the vein under ultrasound visualization may help ameliorate this effect, as the operator can keep the device off of the back wall of the vessel. For these reasons, IVs deeper than a centimeter from the skin surface are poor candidate vessels.

A number of series have been published on ultrasound guidance for peripheral arterial access. Though historically the arterial pulse has been relied on for arterial catheterization, both adult[22] and pediatric studies[23] demonstrate that ultrasound guidance using methods similar to venous procedures facilitates arterial access.

Ultrasound can also help identify catheter position after CVC placement. Direct visualization of other CVCs in the IVC in addition to umbilical catheters is possible in patients.[24-26] However, identifying upper extremity CVCs is difficult because views of the superior cavoatrial junction are obstructed by lung artifact in older children and adults.[27-29] Another technique that has been demonstrated to verify central venous catheter position is use of agitated saline.[30,31] Agitated saline is produced by rapidly flushing approximately 0.5 to 1 mL of air and 9 to 9.5 mL of saline between two 10-mL syringes attached to a stopcock connected to the CVC until the distribution of small bubbles in the saline appears as homogenous as possible. At this time the saline is steadily, quickly, and carefully flushed into the patient such that the contrast is delivered promptly, though large bubbles are not injected. Agitated saline opacifies vascular structures and indicates continuity of the catheter within the proximal vessel or heart. Failure of the bubbles to appear in the venous space suggests that the catheter is not in the correct vessel. Pitfalls in this technique include slow injection, where bubbles may not reach the heart, and the presence of shunting, which could also diminish return of bubbles to the area being examined with ultrasound. Agitated saline techniques should be used with acceptance that the bubbles might travel into the systemic circulation, where there is a small risk that they could obstruct distal organ perfusion. These methods may ultimately decrease the need for radiography.

Umbilical access can also be facilitated by ultrasound in neonatal patients who may be in the pediatric ICU for specialized therapies such as advanced cardiac care or extracorporeal membrane oxygenation (ECMO).[24,25] Umbilical catheters can be placed using sagittal positioning of a small curvilinear or phased array transducer over the inferior vena cava as it enters the right atrium. Confirmation of tip position at the IVC–right ventricular (RA) junction is possible using this method because catheters are echogenic. This technique can be employed in umbilical arterial catheter placement by identifying the catheter in the descending aorta at the level of the diaphragm.

Drainage Procedures

Ultrasound is a useful adjunct to thoracentesis and thoracostomy. Pleural fluid collections are highly amenable to ultrasound interrogation. Simple effusions appear as an enclosed dark anechoic space sharply differentiated from surrounding tissues and often with underlying consolidated lung appearing to float within the fluid. Ultrasound is useful for characterizing effusion complexity: Proteinaceous septations and debris appear echogenic within the effusion.

Effusions can be visualized from several locations. During a pleural exam, using a linear array, effusions are recognizable as a dark anechoic space below the parietal pleura. Effusion can also be seen on echocardiographic views, particularly those capturing the dependent areas of the lower thorax such as subcostal or apical views (Fig. 20.11A). Additionally pleural effusion can be seen in abdominal exams of the right and left upper quadrant if the view captures the posterior aspects of the diaphragm. In these cases the effusion appears as an anechoic space cephalad to the diaphragm. An advantage of imaging an effusion using a phased array or curvilinear probe is that a large portion of the effusion tends to be visible in the far field of the sonographic sector, allowing identification of a deep effusion pocket, its extent, and its complexity (Fig. 20.11B). Color Doppler ultrasound may assist with effusion identification because its motion within the potential space will be detectable.

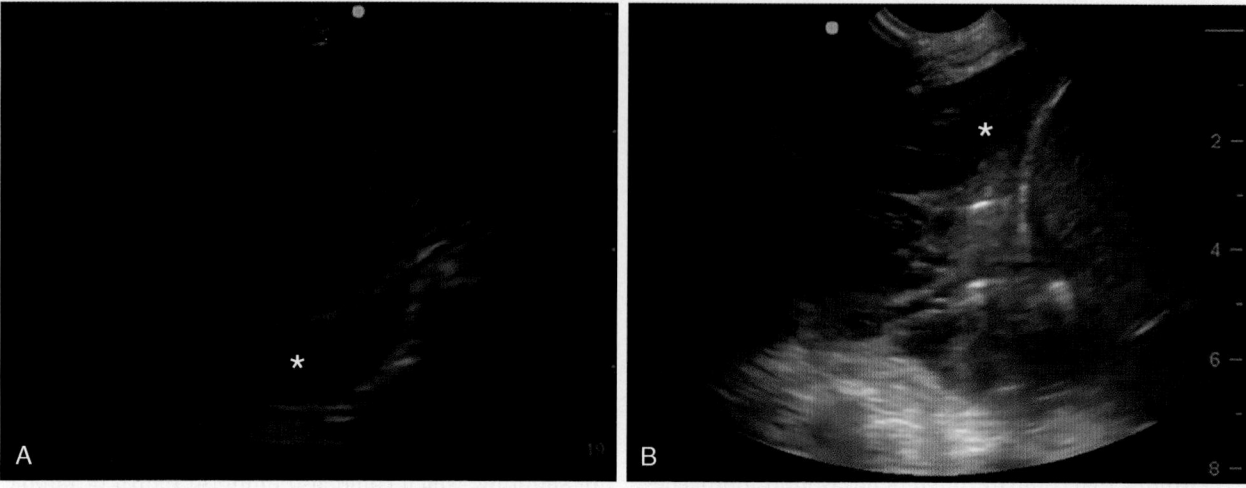

Fig. 20.11. Examples of pleural effusions seen with a phased array probe. (A) Simple effusion (*). (B) complex effusion (*).

Pleural fluid collections can be easily targeted for drainage using ultrasound to ensure safe needle insertion above the diaphragm. Though dynamic ultrasound guidance can be used during the drainage of an effusion, the *static* technique (ie, marking the location for needle insertion) simplifies the procedure without exposing the patient to increased procedural risk. There is presently no evidence to suggest clear superiority of one technique over another.

Thoracostomy tubes can also be identified in the effusion space, but they are less visible once fluid is drained. Prior to attachment of a thoracostomy tube to suction, visualization of the effusion space and position of the chest tube within can sometimes help determining whether the tube travels anterior or posterior to the lung.

Abdominal fluid collections are also characterized as simple or complex, and drainage of the peritoneal space is possible using ultrasound guidance. An important consideration in performing paracentesis is locating (and avoiding) the inferior epigastric arteries traveling from the iliac arteries cephalad along the inside of the anterior abdominal wall at the lateral edge of the rectus abdominis muscle. These vessels are identifiable on ultrasound and the machine can assist in planning a safe needle insertion.

With ultrasound, paracentesis is most easily performed from the lateral approach. After appropriately preparing the patient and identifying fluid for drainage, the arteries are identified. Rather than performing a traditional z track entry, the needle can be introduced obliquely into the peritoneal cavity with the probe oriented longitudinally over the needle for dynamic guidance (Fig. 20.12). The oblique track helps reduce the chance of leakage, is easier under ultrasound than the z track, and allows direct visualization of needle entry into the peritoneum to avoid underlying solid and hollow organ puncture. A temporary catheter can then be placed using the Seldinger technique for either one-time or ongoing drainage of ascites fluid.

Lumbar Puncture

Ultrasound-guided lumbar puncture provides limited advantage over landmark-based techniques in children as demonstrated in the literature,[32,33] though some hypothesize

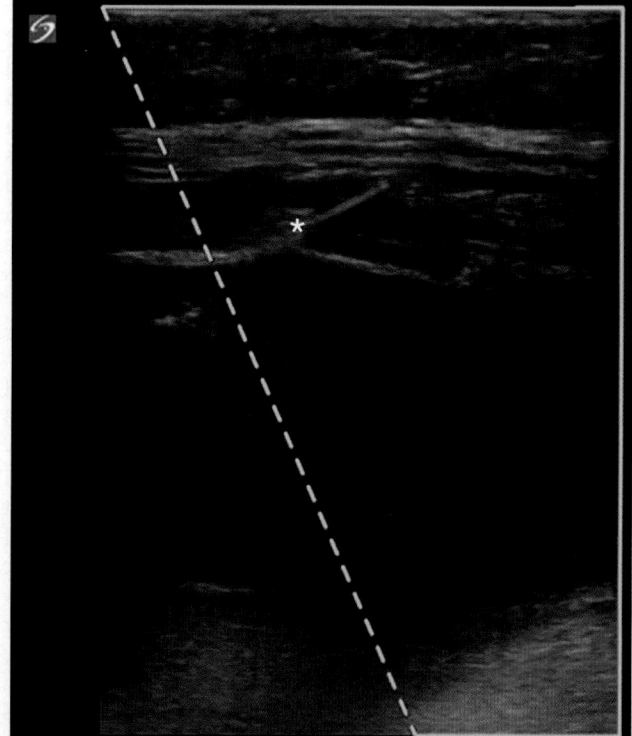

Fig. 20.12. Ultrasound-guided paracentesis. An asterisk (*) identifies the needle.

it is beneficial in patients who have difficult landmarks, such as older and obese patients[34] and perhaps children with spine abnormalities. Such patients can benefit from ultrasound-guided lumbar puncture due to difficulty in determining surface landmarks and insertion depth secondary to lumbar muscularity or adipose tissue. The technique can be performed under ultrasound visualization, but due to the near-perpendicular angle of needle insertion into the skin, the procedure is easier under static guidance using insertion markings (Fig. 20.13). This process involves visualizing the spine in two planes, both sagittally along the spine to identify

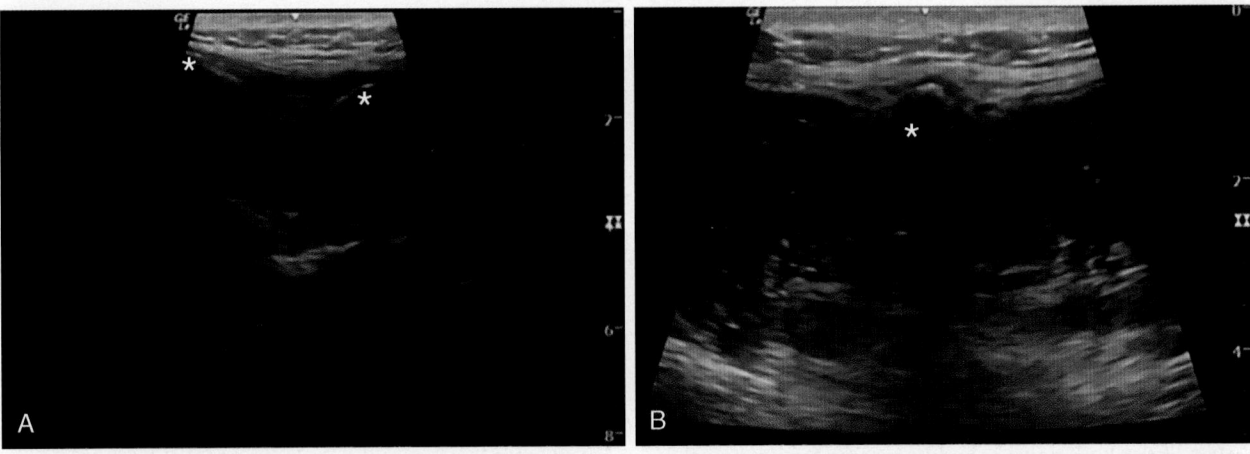

Fig. 20.13. Views of the lumbar spine. (A) Longitudinal view. (B) Transverse view. Spinous processes are indicated by *asterisks*.

the appropriate entry level and axially across it to center insertion in the midline. Additionally views of the spine can be used for measuring angle and depth of needle insertion to reach the dural space so that an appropriate needle can be selected.

Diagnostic Modalities

Pulmonary Ultrasound

Historically, pulmonary ultrasound has been considered impractical due to air-filled structures impeding ultrasound transmission.[35] Yet ultrasound images are produced within the thoracic cavity by the complex interaction of the ultrasound beam with interfaces between air- and water-filled structures. Seminal work done by intensivists examining the lungs of critically ill adults and children led to descriptions of pulmonary artifact patterns that reflect lung pathology.[36]

In the child, the patient's age can affect visualization of the thoracic cavity. Infants have excellent windows for thoracic visualization because of shallow imaging depths to reach the pleural space, higher body water content, and limited thoracic cage ossification. As children age, their imaging windows may become more difficult as a result of development, including increasing ossification and decreasing body water content, though imaging windows remain largely obtainable. If areas of the pleura are difficult to visualize due to ribs, rotating the probe parallel to the ribs within the intercostal space can improve the view. Lung motion is still appreciated as artifacts across the pleural plane. Alternatively a microconvex or phased array transducer can be used to see the pleural line, though these lower frequency probes often perform better in evaluating deep structures.

Thoracic ultrasound of the pleural space identifies overlying skin and soft tissue nearest to the probe, followed by deeper rib and intercostal structures, and then the pleural space. The visceral pleura slides against the parietal pleura through a thin and often invisible layer of normal pleural fluid.

Though the exact physiologic mechanisms underlying ultrasound lung artifacts is not definitively known, their similarity to artifactual findings associated with pathology in other organ systems and associations with pathology suggest their origins. Reverberation artifacts that replicate the pleural line

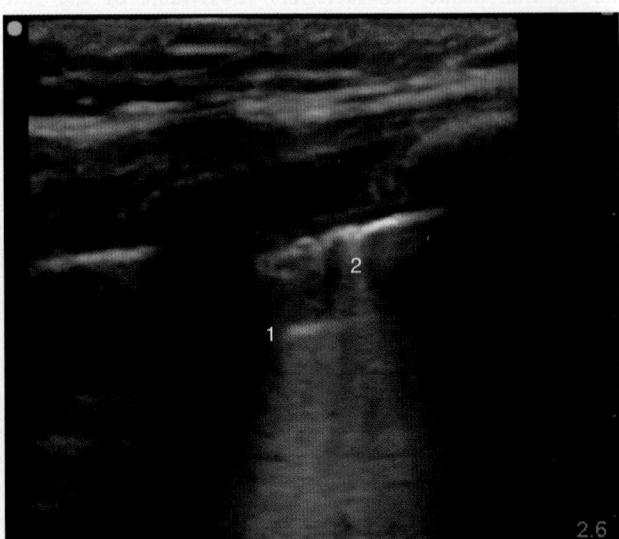

Fig. 20.14. Ultrasound of the thorax using a linear probe. (1) A-line. (2) B-line.

at regular intervals from proximal to distal field are called A-lines and often appear in the center of the ultrasound beam. These can appear regardless of pathology or whether tissue or air is underlying the parietal pleura, and therefore they need only be recognized as artifacts in the image. B-lines and Z-lines are generated radially from interfaces near the pleural line and appear to pierce through the lung parenchyma. B-lines reach the end of the viewable sector and obliterate A-lines, whereas Z-lines are limited reverberatory extensions from the pleural line (Fig. 20.14).

A pattern of increased B-lines suggests increased interstitial lung water. In the adult population this is consistent with pulmonary edema,[37] and it is reasonable to infer that it would bear similar implication in children. However, studies also suggest that B-lines indicate the presence of bronchiolitis in children in the emergency room setting.[38] Further elucidation of the significance of B-line patterns in critically ill children is lacking.

B-lines in children may also represent lung consolidation. Consolidated lung appears increasingly granular with the appearance of liver-like parenchyma, commonly referred to as *hepatization* due to the augmented visibility of consolidated lung parenchyma and vascular architecture appearing similar to hepatic structures. In the case of infectious pneumonias, diffuse geographic areas of consolidation, air, and necrosis may develop, resulting in what some authors term the *shred sign*. The diagnostic value of these lung consolidation patterns in critically ill children has not been well quantified to date.

Identification of pneumothorax with ultrasound has been described[37] as a dissociation of the visceral from parietal pleura by ultrasound-obstructing air, such that the parietal pleura is no longer visible (Fig. 20.15). Loss of pleural sliding is indicative of pneumothorax, and identification of the limit of a pneumothorax as the point where pleural sliding abuts an area where it is absent is described as the lung point. Identification of the lung point is highly specific for pneumothorax.[39] M-mode ultrasound is also useful for identification of pneumothorax. Placement of the M-mode cursor through the pleural surface characterizes movement of the lung parenchyma as a "granular" textured echogenic area distal to the pleural line. When contrasted with the more horizontal linear pattern of the proximal chest wall, this assumes a seashore-like appearance (Fig. 20.15B). When the M-mode cursor overlays pneumothorax, no lung parenchyma movement is seen, and the entire M-mode tracing over time appears to be a pattern of horizontal lines, otherwise described as a *barcode* or *stratosphere* sign (Fig. 20.15D).

Ultrasound views of the diaphragm can confirm tracheal placement of an endotracheal tube during intubation, though distance from the carina cannot be reliably determined in the older child. This is potentially useful in the management of a ventilated patient requiring rapid confirmation of tracheal placement such as in the case of a difficult airway patient for whom removal of the tube and reintubation could be dangerous. In this instance, subcostal views of the diaphragm capturing motion of each leaflet while the patient receives positive pressure breaths can be performed (Fig. 20.16). Confirmation that at least one leaflet moves with large positive pressure

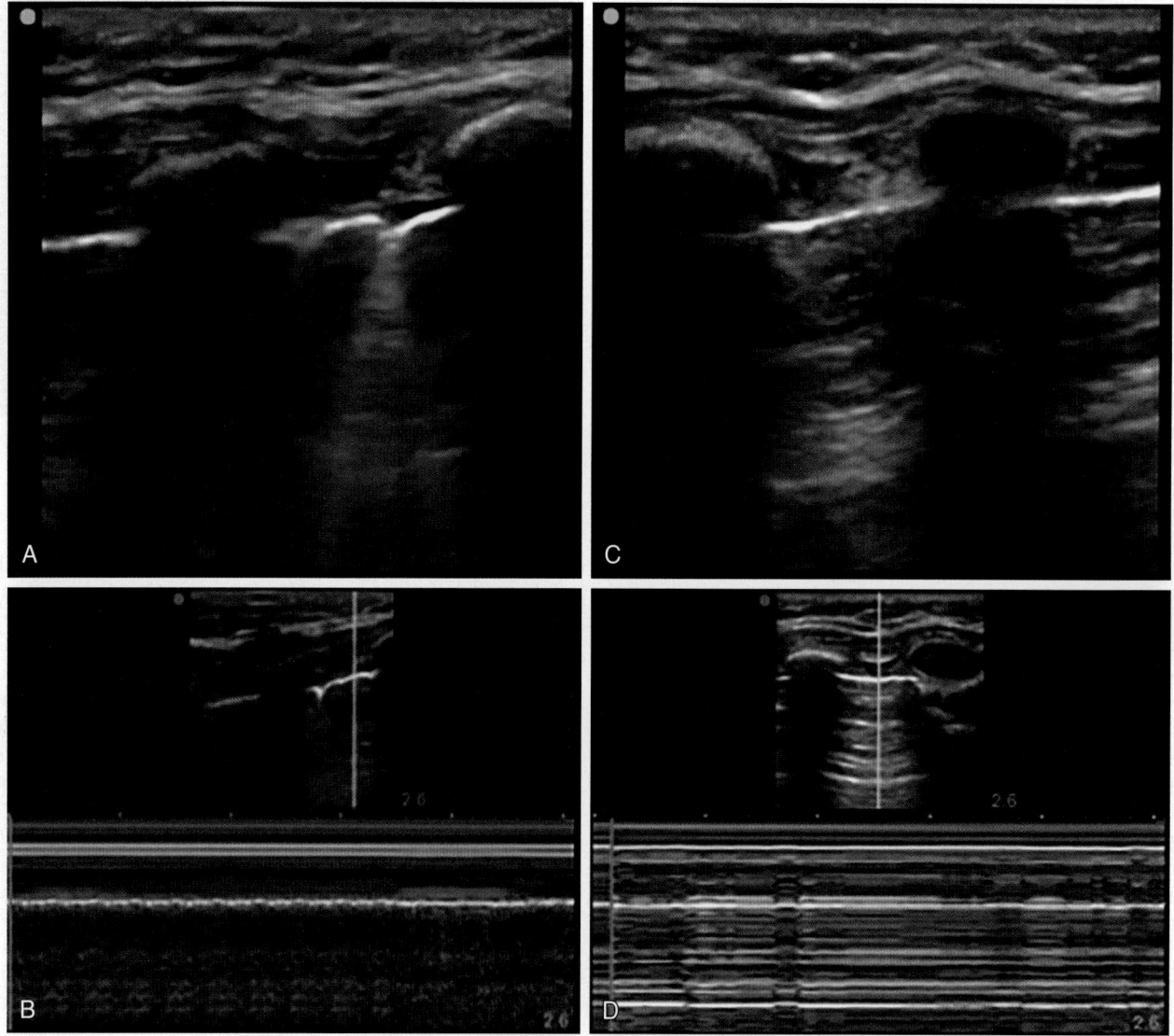

Fig. 20.15. Identification of pneumothorax via ultrasound. (A) Normal 2D lung ultrasound image. (B) Corresponding M-mode image. (C) Note lack of B-lines in pneumothorax in 2D image. (D) Corresponding pneumothorax M-mode image.

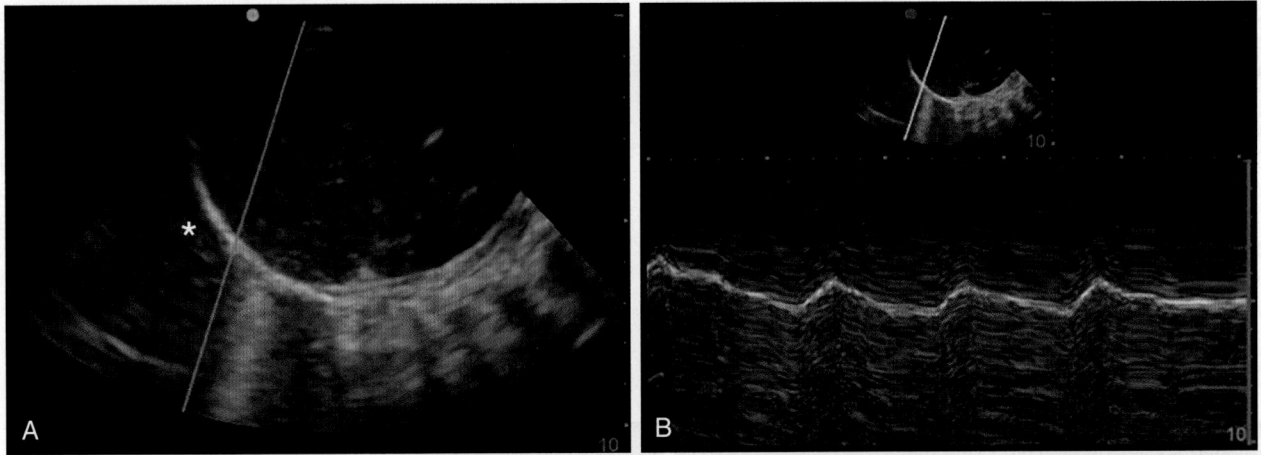

Fig. 20.16. Subcostal image of the diaphragm. (A) An asterisk indicates the diaphragm that is identifiable on M-mode imaging (B).

breaths will help verify that the tube is in the airway. Lack of excursion on one side might suggest main stem bronchus occlusion from secretions or inadvertent main stem bronchial intubation of the contralateral lung. This technique has been used to confirm tube placement in the operating theater[40] as well as in the pediatric emergency department,[41] though the distance between endotracheal tube (ETT) tip and carina cannot be accurately measured. In the neonatal population, the tube is visualizable in the sagittal plane from the parasternal view typically used for evaluation of the aortic arch and pulmonary arteries. Dennington and colleagues were able to accurately gauge depth of ETT position in neonates with high accuracy.[42] In larger infants and older children, this technique has not been successful due to thoracic growth and ossification.

Use of diaphragm windows to assess diaphragm paresis has also been described.[43-46] In multiple series, assessment of spontaneous diaphragm excursion using ultrasound in the oblique coronal (described previously) or sagittal planes accurately demonstrates diaphragm paresis. One would expect it to be similarly useful for patients with diaphragm paralysis from a variety of causes including protracted neuromuscular blockade or intrinsic neuromuscular dysfunction.

Abdomen

Assessment of abdominal pathology is frequently confounded by nonspecific complaints, particularly in sedated patients. Ultrasound as a noninvasive technology has potential for evaluating abdominal pathology without the radiation exposure of CT. However, as is the case with pulmonary pathology, air within the abdominal cavity creates challenging obstacles to ultrasound interrogation (Fig. 20.17). When air causes artifacts, determining whether the air is within the peritoneum or in the bowel is difficult and is a limitation of abdominal ultrasonography. Air localized within the liver vasculature, as well as bowel wall hypervascularity, has been associated with necrotizing enterocolitis in the at-risk neonate.[47-49]

Similarly, fluid in the abdomen can appear within or outside the intestinal lumen. The normal appearance of air artifact and stool is absent in fluid-filled ileus resulting in ultrasound visualization of distended, anechoic bowel loops. Peritoneal fluid as a result of ascites, hemorrhage, or peritoneal dialysis fluid is commonly seen in acute care settings.

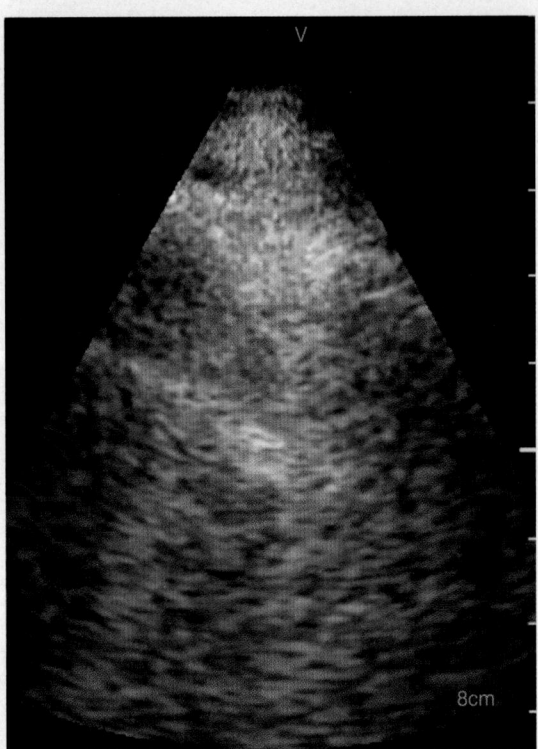

Fig. 20.17. Abdominal ultrasound with air interference obstructing view of abdominal contents.

A focused assessment with sonography in trauma (FAST) is performed in four abdominal windows where dependent fluid could appear from a traumatic injury. The probe is usually a curvilinear or phased array transducer. The FAST exam is widely used in adult trauma resuscitation for identification of intraperitoneal fluid, likely either from hemorrhage or ruptured viscus.[50-52] Though some adult literature supports the FAST exam as a replacement for computed tomography of the abdomen and diagnostic peritoneal lavage, successful performance of the application depends on operator expertise and time from the event. In children, the sensitivity of the test is as poor as 52% in some series,[53] likely because solid organ injury in children may result in smaller areas of bleeding. Despite its poor sensitivity, it has demonstrated good specificity in pediatric trauma,[53-59] and the finding of unexpected fluid in a pediatric trauma patient is likely a sign of an intraperitoneal injury.

Right Upper Quadrant (Fig. 20.18A)

The hepatorenal recess (Morison's Pouch) is the most dependent part of the peritoneum in the supine patient. Fluid can be seen between the retroperitoneal kidney and the intraperitoneal liver or above the liver as well. The transducer is placed near or below the lower ribs of the thorax in the posterior axillary line to visualize the right kidney with the indicator directed toward the patient's head. Fluid in the Morison's Pouch, inferior pole of the kidney, or the perihepatic space suggests intraperitoneal injury. The diaphragm is also seen in this view, and pleural effusion or intrathoracic hemorrhage in the trauma setting can also be identified or suspected when a classic mirror artifact of liver due to diaphragm is not visualized. The probe is usually oriented coronally but can be oriented axially with respect to the patient, and the entire organ should be scanned. If views from the posterior axillary line are difficult, the right kidney can be visualized in the anterior sagittal plane by placing the transducer at the lower edge of

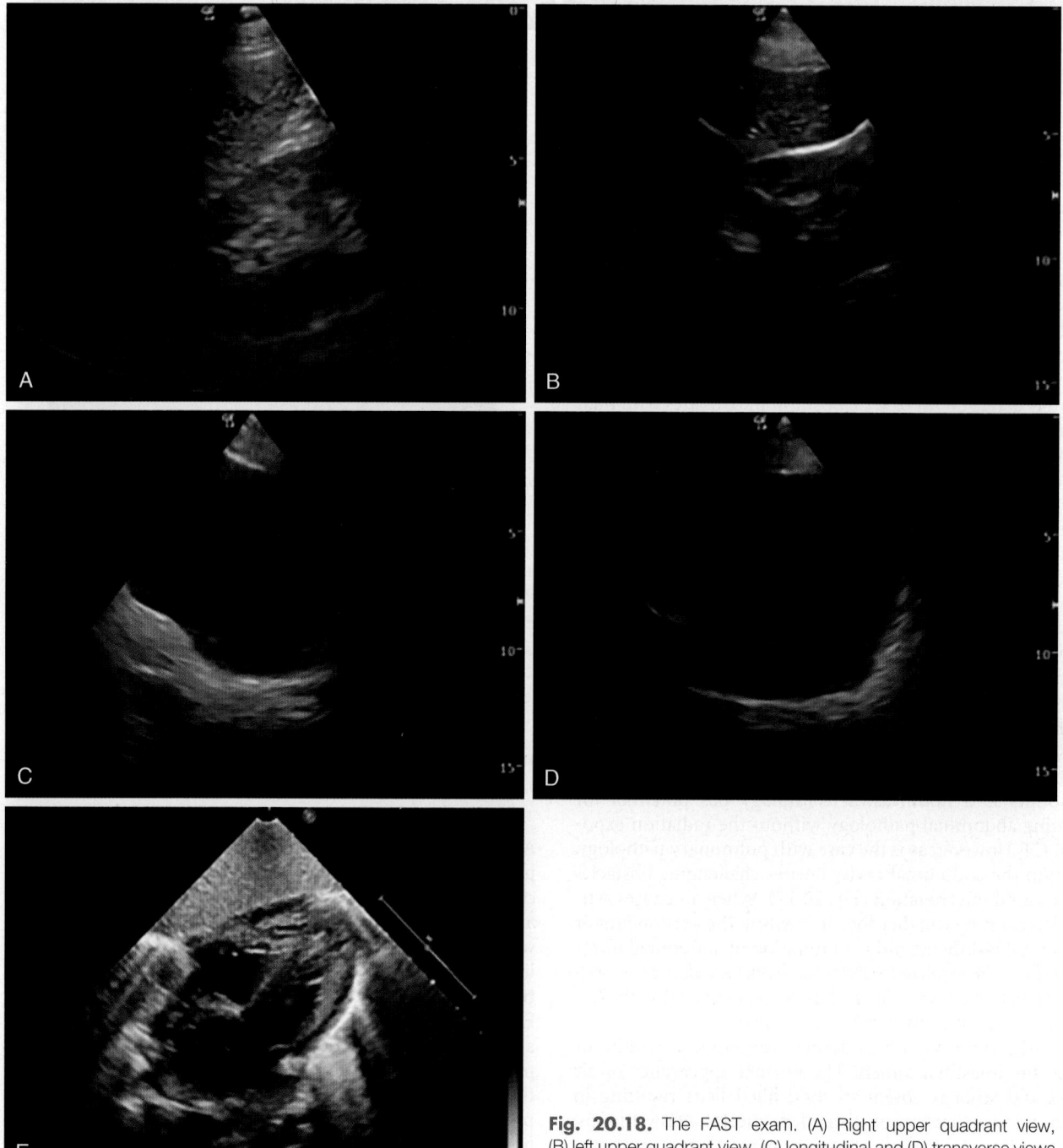

Fig. 20.18. The FAST exam. (A) Right upper quadrant view, (B) left upper quadrant view, (C) longitudinal and (D) transverse views of the bladder, and (E) subcostal cardiac view.

the costal margin just lateral to the midclavicular line with the indicator pointed toward the patient's head. In this view the Morison's Pouch can be visualized through the liver.

Left Upper Quadrant (Fig. 20.18B)

The splenorenal recess can be visualized from the left flank at the level of the posterior axillary line as well. It is visualized similarly to the view in the right with the probe indicator positioned toward the head for a coronal view of the kidney and surrounding spaces. Anterior windows are usually not feasible because of stomach contents. The left kidney is more cephalad in the abdomen than the right, and views from above the costal margin may be necessary. In this view pleural effusions can also be visualized.

Pelvis (Figs. 20.18C and D)

Particularly if a patient has been upright or inclined after trauma, fluid can accumulate in the pelvis in a manner not seen in the upper quadrants. As with visualization of the kidneys, the bladder can serve as an easily identifiable landmark from which to reference regional anatomy and discern pathology. The bladder is imaged in both the axial and sagittal planes. Fluid posterior to the bladder in the male or posterior to the bladder or uterus in the female patient suggests pathology.

Subcostal Cardiac (Fig. 20.18E)

The heart is visualized in the FAST scan from the subcostal margin below the xiphoid process, with the probe aimed toward the patient's left shoulder, and the indicator oriented toward the right flank if the machine remains set in a radiology convention setting with the screen indicator to the operator's left. The heart is imaged for pericardial effusion in this view, where dark fluid would appear adjacent to the heart.

Using FAST bladder views, verification of the presence of a urinary catheter can also be performed by visualizing the catheter itself or the water-filled balloon of the Foley catheter. A large volume in the bladder in an anuric patient indicates obstruction or malplacement of the urinary catheter. Though several authors have defined methods for calculating bladder volume, its variable geometry precludes easy approximation of volume. However, a practitioner can judge whether there is urine in the bladder despite efforts at diuresis or catheterization.

Solid echogenic structures in the distended abdomen suggest the abdomen is filled with a foreign mass (tumor), enlarged or swollen viscera, or a collection of a solidifying substance such as exudative ascites or clotting blood. Such findings should discourage needle drainage of a space in the evaluation of abdominal distention or intraabdominal hypertension, unless there is also a large volume of free fluid.

In shock management, some attention has been given to evaluation of renal perfusion as a surrogate for shock severity. A marked difference between systolic and diastolic renal arterial flow may suggest hypoperfusion.[60,61] However, to date examining this phenomenon has not consistently shown efficacy in evaluating shock states.[62-68] Whether this assessment will prove useful in children remains to be determined.

Cardiac Imaging

Imaging specialists often have a wide selection of phased array transducers for imaging the heart. Large adult-sized transducers, with more sophisticated technology and lower frequency transmission for adequate penetration, suit adolescents and young adults well. Smaller transducers allow use of slightly higher frequencies for imaging infants and young children, and their smaller faces permit better skin contact when the probe is held at shallow angles to the skin. It is therefore important that adequate equipment be available for accurate bedside ultrasound cardiac evaluation of critically ill patients.

Imaging of the heart is performed using locations, or "windows," on the body where acoustic transmission to the heart is adequate and less encumbered by effects of body position and tissue interference. These include the subcostal window immediately below the xiphoid process, the parasternal window to the left of the patient's sternum, and the apical window near the patient's point of maximal cardiac impulse, typically below the left pectoralis major muscle. These windows form standard echocardiography views (Fig. 20.19).

Of note, different groups (ie, cardiology, emergency medicine, critical care medicine) may use different screen indicator orientations during cardiac ultrasound evaluation. Within the scope of this text, the screen indicator is at the top right of the screen for all cardiac views. Subcostal windows can be used to visualize the base of the heart either longitudinally, such that all four chambers are seen (Fig. 20.19A), or in cross section, such that only the atria or ventricles are seen. The probe is placed in the subxiphoid region and beam aimed toward the patient's left shoulder. For a longitudinal view, the probe indicator is directed toward the patient's left flank, or approximately the 2 to 3 o'clock position with the top of the "clock" oriented toward the patient's head. For a transverse view, the probe indicator is directed at the patient's head and the view aligned across the chambers of interest. From the transverse view, the probe can also be directed directly posteriorly through the inferior vena cava (Fig. 20.19B) as it passes into the right atrium to assess its size variation through the respiratory cycle or through the aorta for evaluation of flow. Any view of the heart should be more than a single image, and fanning the transducer beam through the organ can provide the most complete impression of the heart. Septal defects are most easily visualized from the subcostal position using Doppler sonography because flow across them is most parallel to the ultrasound beam. In addition, the window is closest to the base of the heart and provides excellent imaging of effusion, particularly if the patient is slightly inclined head up. This window also has an advantage in small children with multiple dressings or monitoring devices on the chest because the subcostal window may be the only area not obscured.

Subcostal views are also important during active resuscitation from cardiac arrest when chest compressions must have priority. Ultrasound may reveal important information regarding the etiology of arrest including pericardial effusion, pulmonary embolism, and hypovolemia. Though subcostal windows benefit from not having intervening lung tissue obscure the heart, they can be hindered by interference from a gas-filled stomach and or bowel. In the case of internal interference from air-filled viscera, insonating the base of the heart from a position slightly overlying the right lobe of the liver can sometimes improve the view. Subcostal views may also be difficult in patients with substernal chest tubes or ventricular assist devices.

Views from the parasternal windows are commonly acquired from the third and fourth intercostal interspaces near the

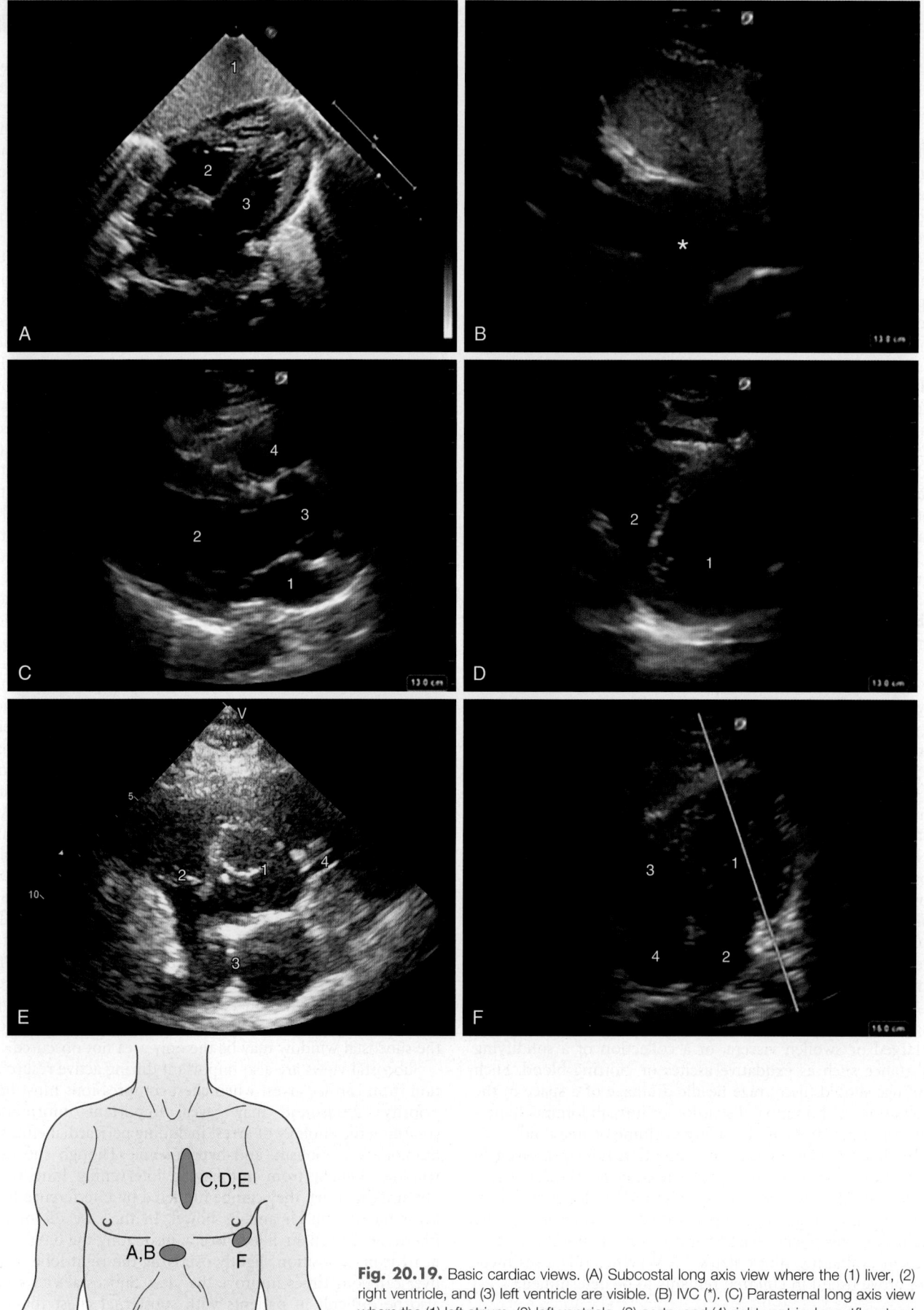

Fig. 20.19. Basic cardiac views. (A) Subcostal long axis view where the (1) liver, (2) right ventricle, and (3) left ventricle are visible. (B) IVC (*). (C) Parasternal long axis view where the (1) left atrium, (2) left ventricle, (3) aorta, and (4) right ventricular outflow tract are visible. (D) Parasternal short axis view at the midpapillary level where the (1) left ventricle and (2) right ventricle are visible. (E) Parasternal short axis at the aortic valve level where the (1) aortic valve, (2) tricuspid valve, (3) atrial septum, and (4) left coronary artery are visible. (F) Apical four-chamber view visualizing the (1) left ventricle, (2) left atrium, (3) right ventricle, and (4) right atrium.

sternum on the patient's left chest. To acquire the parasternal long axis view (Fig. 20.19C), the transducer indicator is toward the patient's right shoulder and aligned along the major axis of the left heart. From this view the left atrium, mitral valve, the left ventricular chamber, and left ventricular outflow tract (LVOT) are readily visible in continuity with the right ventricular outflow tract that appears anterior to the LVOT. This view can be modified to image the right ventricular inflow view by fanning the transducer anteriorly through the right heart. The right atrium and IVC are usually visible and the tricuspid valve opens into the right ventricle anterior and caudad to the right atrium. The SVC may be visualized in infants though it is frequently obscured by the lung in an older patient.

The parasternal window can also be used for visualizing the heart in a plane perpendicular to its major axis, or the short axis view (Fig. 20.19D). Short axis views are performed with the transducer indicator aligned toward the patient's left shoulder. There are several short axis views that span the length of the heart from atrium to apex. Imaging the ventricle at the midchamber level is useful for the pediatric intensivist to assess qualitative left ventricular function, as this location is where radial contractility is most pronounced. In this view the beam transects the ventricle such that the papillary muscles are the primary intraventricular structures visible, with the inferoseptal papillary muscle appearing in the lower left and the anterolateral papillary muscle appearing in the lower right of the image. A short axis view of the heart can also be performed at the aortic valve level. In this view the aortic leaflets are visible and roughly form a lambda sign in the middle of the appropriately centered image (Fig. 20.19E). With careful targeting the left or right coronary root is sometimes visible in this view. On the screen, the left atrium is directly posterior to the aortic valve (6 o'clock) and moving clockwise is the right atrium (8 o'clock), tricuspid valve (9 o'clock), right ventricle (12 o'clock), and pulmonary valve (2 o'clock) with the pulmonary artery and its bifurcation sometimes visualized at the 4 o'clock position.

Apical views (Fig. 20.19F) are very dependent on thoracic and abdominal structures. Increased intrathoracic pressure, as in asthma or high airway pressure ventilation, can cause the apex of the heart to move caudad and medially. Hyperinflated lung may obscure the apex. Conversely, high intraabdominal pressure can push the diaphragm cephalad and displace the heart cephalad and laterally. Apical views are insonated near the point of maximal impulse at the caudad aspect of the left pectoralis major muscle. The axis of the probe should be aligned with the major axis of the heart and point toward the center of the mediastinum. For the apical four-chamber view, the indicator is oriented toward the left flank, usually between the 2 and 3 o'clock positions. From this view the four chambers and both atrioventricular valves of the heart should be visible. In addition to the four chambers, this view allows visualization of both atrioventricular valves and their movement. The left heart appears on the right of the screen, and atria appear at the bottom when the probe face appears at the top of the screen. From the four-chamber view, the transducer can be fanned anteriorly so that the beam intercepts the LVOT for interrogation of outflow velocity. This is called the *apical five-chamber view*. From the four-chamber view, the probe can be rotated 60 degrees counterclockwise to obtain a two-chamber view of the left heart (left ventricle and atrium) for assessment of function.

Cardiac ultrasound can provide assistance in titrating fluid, inotropes, and vasopressors for persistent shock in children.[69,70] Initial pediatric experience has demonstrated that its use is feasible and associated with good outcome, complementing available adult data describing the utility of intensivist-driven cardiac ultrasound for hemodynamic assessment. It is reasonable to surmise that the value of focused cardiac ultrasound noted in adults[71] might be similar or better in children, as views of the heart may be better given pediatric body habitus.

Most literature related to cardiac ultrasound for hemodynamic assessment in children has focused on volume status assessment. Adult echocardiographers and pediatric nephrologists have used the collapsibility and distensibility of the compliant inferior vena cava as a noninvasive surrogate for volume status and estimation of dry weight for dialysis patients, respectively.[72,73] Beyond volume, IVC morphologic changes may also represent variable upstream pressures, and estimates of central venous pressure based on IVC imaging data have been published for adults.[74]

The diameter of the IVC is usually assessed in the sagittal view about 2 to 3 cm caudad to the inferior cavoatrial junction in adults. At this point the vessel diameter can be measured using M-mode or two-dimensional (2D) methods. Available evidence regarding IVC assessment for volume status is largely related to two physiologic conditions: (1) the patient who is pharmacologically paralyzed and intubated receiving a set tidal volume at near normal airway pressure and (2) the spontaneously breathing patient. IVC respiratory variation exceeding 12% to 18% in the neuromuscularly blocked adult patient[75,76] has been described as a threshold for volume responsiveness. Current convention in the adult is the use of maximum diameter observing for changes greater than 12%. Similar criteria have not yet been established in children. The degree to which airway pressure decreases respiratory variation and masks hypovolemia by increasing intrathoracic pressure is also not well delineated. Increasingly evidence, specifically in children, indicates that IVC behavior is not equivalent in the two respiratory conditions. In the pediatric operating room, titration of positive pressure ventilation as well as initiation of inhalational anesthesia changes the collapsibility of the IVC.[77] Increasingly evidence indicates that IVC behavior is not equivalent between patients receiving sedation and positive pressure ventilation compared to those spontaneously breathing.

Using a ratio of the size of the inferior vena cava to aorta diameter IVC:Ao in a transverse view may provide a useful assessment of volume status in children and avoids the challenge that results from the range of sizes in children. An IVC:Ao ratio of 0.8 or less appears to suggest clinically significant dehydration, whereas a ratio greater than 1.2:1 suggests hypervolemia.[72] Fluid responsiveness was not described, however; this study targeted diagnosis rather than evaluation of physiologic response to therapy. However, in critically ill children, limited data suggest that IVC:Ao and IVC collapsibility are poor surrogates for central venous pressure.[78] In addition, despite its use in septic shock algorithms as a surrogate marker for intravascular volume depletion, central venous pressure (CVP) measurements have come under considerable scrutiny given their poor accuracy.[79] Intensivists are only beginning to understand the complex interactions between pressure, volume, and compliance on IVC morphology in

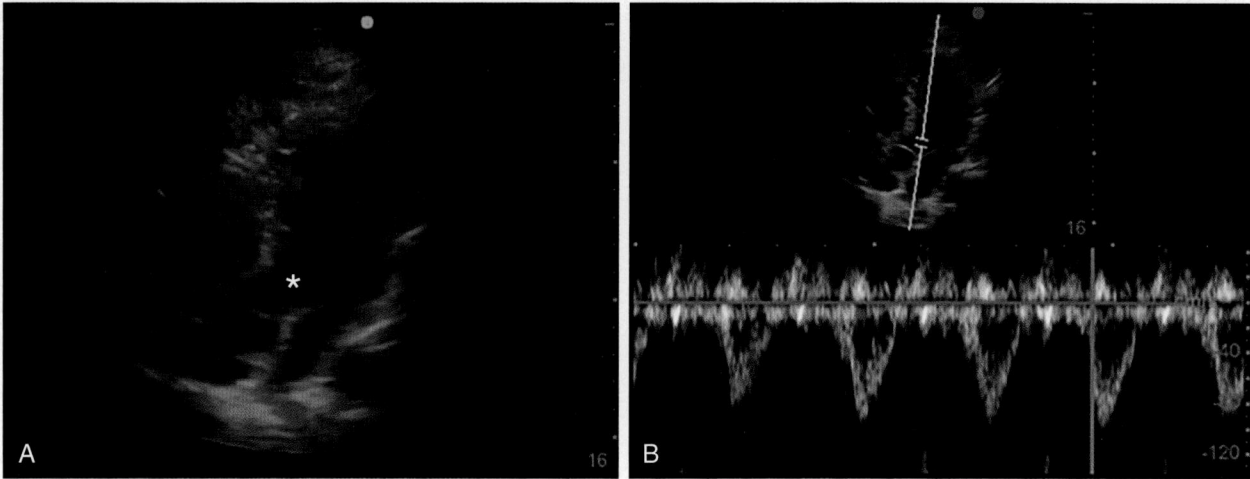

Fig. 20.20. Doppler interrogation of the left ventricular outflow tract. (A) Apical five-chamber view with (*) LVOT identified. (B) Pulsed wave Doppler of the LVOT.

individual patients undergoing life-sustaining therapies in states of critical illness.

Assessment of left heart performance as a surrogate for volume status has also been an area of interest in adults and children. Velocity of blood flow across LVOT has been used as a surrogate of stroke volume and indicator of intravascular volume status. Assessment of the left ventricular outflow tract using Doppler ultrasound is performed from the apical five-chamber view observing velocity of left ventricular ejection (Fig. 20.20). Stroke volume can be approximated by obtaining the Doppler velocity tracing of flow across the LVOT over time, calculating its integral (VTi), and multiplying this by the measured cross-sectional area of the LVOT. The cross section of the LVOT is usually measured from the parasternal long axis view using the diameter measured between the aortic valve leaflets in midsystole.

Using the estimated stroke volume and multiplying by the heart rate allows approximation of cardiac output. The LVOT Doppler tracing can also provide a beat-to-beat assessment of changes in stroke volume through the respiratory cycle. Respiratory changes in peak LVOT velocity exceeding 14% appear to identify volume responsiveness in intubated pediatric intensive care unit (PICU) patients.[80,81] In assessing variability in the Doppler flow tracing it is advisable to slow the sweep speed of the machine so multiple systolic ejection events are observed through the respiratory cycle. Variability of 14% is thought to indicate volume responsiveness. Pitfalls of this technique include limited apical views due to lung inflation and patient habitus. Further concerns particular to pediatric patients include the need for a smaller phased array transducer to maintain skin contact and small LVOT for appropriate placement of the Doppler cursor, made more challenging in the dehydrated child with a hyperkinetic heart.

Effusion in the pericardial space appears similar to pleural effusion as a largely dark and anechoic space separating the heart from the reflective pericardium (Fig. 20.21). Effusion may not be concentric and instead collect in dependent areas; therefore subcostal windows are often ideal for visualizing them. Effusions can also be complex as a result of accumulated protein in an empyema, solidification of hemorrhage, or presence of tumor.

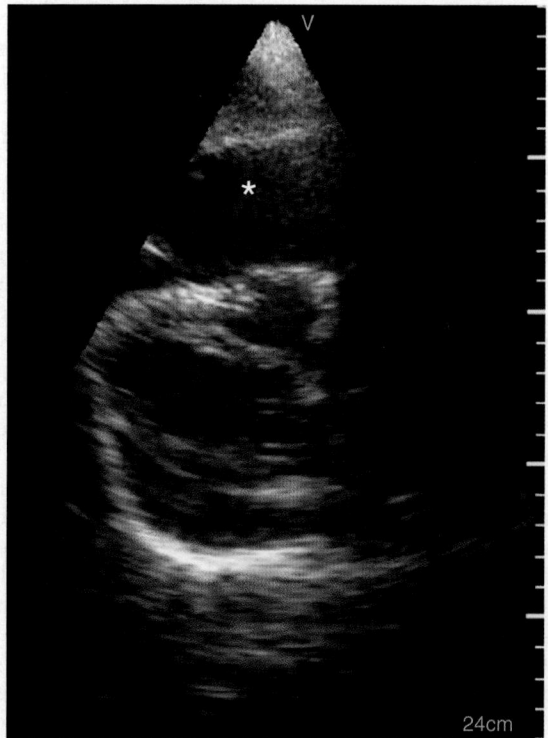

Fig. 20.21. Pericardial effusion. *Asterisk* indicates effusion.

Tamponade is a clinical diagnosis; however, the presence of an effusion and subsequent changes to cardiac morphology and function suggestive of tamponade physiology are detectable using ultrasound. The most specific indicator of tamponade is IVC engorgement secondary to impeded venous return to the heart. Other ultrasound findings consistent with tamponade may include collapse of the low-pressure right heart chambers during filling periods in the cardiac cycle, namely late diastole/early systole in the right atrium and early diastole in the right ventricle.[82] Respiratory variation in the left ventricular inflow is also associated with tamponade physiology as demonstrated by noticeably reduced mitral inflow during inspiration. Conversely, inflow across the tricuspid valve may increase during inspiration.

Pericardiocentesis

Concomitant imaging often facilitates pericardial effusion drainage. Use of a phased array probe in the apical position may not allow visualization of the needle but permits monitoring effective drainage of the effusion and wire placement for drain placement. Injecting a small quantity of agitated saline into the pericardiocentesis needle for sonographic contrast can help confirm that a needle is in the pericardial space rather than a vascular space, particularly if an effusion is bloody.[83] A dynamic visualization technique described for pericardiocentesis in adults uses a linear array transducer placed in the left parasternal area with the indicator pointed cephalad.[84] This technique allows visualization of an effusion anterior to the heart and an insertion site identified that avoids the internal mammary artery. A needle can then be inserted under long axis guidance, avoiding the artery from the caudad side of the probe toward the head, and drainage performed under direct needle guidance. Whether this has broad applicability in the pediatric setting remains undetermined.

Left Ventricular Cardiac Function

Although the best metric for characterizing cardiac contractility remains elusive, acute care practitioners can estimate cardiac function using qualitative and quantitative markers with reasonable accuracy when compared to echocardiography specialists.[85,86] The motion of the left ventricle (LV) assessed through the cardiac cycle is useful for this assessment. Visualizing the LV across the center of the chamber in multiple views, a sonographer can visually approximate or directly measure the excursion of the ventricular walls. These values are then compared to known standards (eg, a normal left ventricular fractional shortening [FS] measures between 25% to 45% of the LV end-diastolic diameter). This measurement is optimally performed quantitatively in the parasternal short axis view at the midpapillary level.

Area-based measurements of LV systolic function are also useful. These include changes in the cross section of the LV seen in the short axis or apical views (ejection fraction [EF]) by Simpson's method of discs. Area-based calculations are advantageous to single dimension assessments such as FS because they reduce the effects of regional wall motion abnormalities on accuracy of EF measurement. These calculations are prone to error from inaccurate inclusion of intracavitary structures such as the papillary muscles and trabeculae, as well as various artifacts. Apical views are also challenging in a child without appropriately sized transducers or if the lungs are hyperinflated, and this can compromise accurate assessment of the left ventricle EF. Substantial mentored practice is strongly recommended for skill development and accurate results.

M-mode modalities such as E-point septal separation (EPSS) and mitral valve annulus plane of systolic excursion (MAPSE) can also approximate systolic function. EPSS assesses the relative motion of the mitral valve anterior leaflet during diastole (Fig. 20.22). In the parasternal long axis view, at early diastole the leaflet is readily visualized as being more proximal to the probe and moving toward the septum both in the early passive phase of ventricular filling and late phase with atrial contraction. In the failing heart, end-systolic volume increases and diminishes the gradient across the mitral valve for flow into the LV during diastole. The excursion of the anterior mitral valve leaflet is therefore less pronounced and does not come as close to the septum. The distance between the leaflet and the septum is measured in the parasternal long axis view by placing the M-mode cursor across the mitral valve (MV) tips of the leaflets. In the adult, a normal EPSS is less than 6 mm and an abnormal one exceeds 10 mm. Normal values have been published in pediatric populations.[87,88]

MAPSE is assessed from the apical view of the MV by placing the M-mode cursor across the lateral end of the MV annulus (Fig. 20.23). In M-mode the vertical excursion of the MV apparatus is quantified as an approximation of the longitudinal contraction of the heart. The septal end of the MV can also be measured, though this tends to be a better indicator of biventricular function. Normal values have been published for pediatric populations.[89]

Right Ventricular Cardiac Function

In the PICU, assessment of the right ventricle (RV) can provide valuable information about the effects of pulmonary vascular resistance changes and mechanical ventilation on cardiac

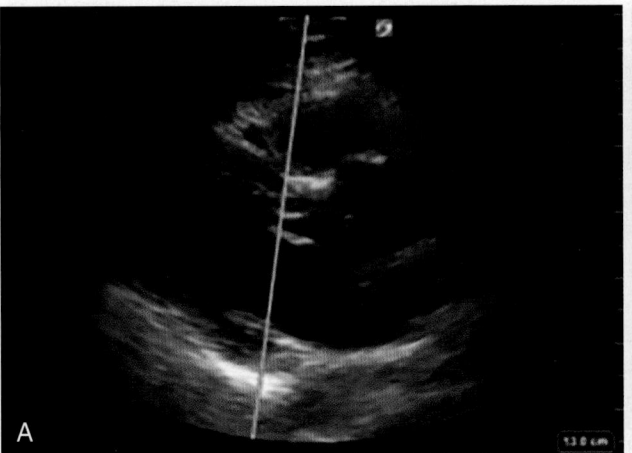
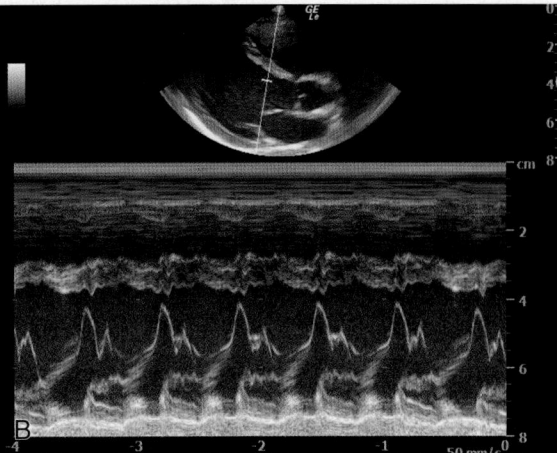

Fig. 20.22. E-point septal separation (EPSS). (A) Cursor alignment in 2D imaging for (B) M-mode measurement of EPSS.

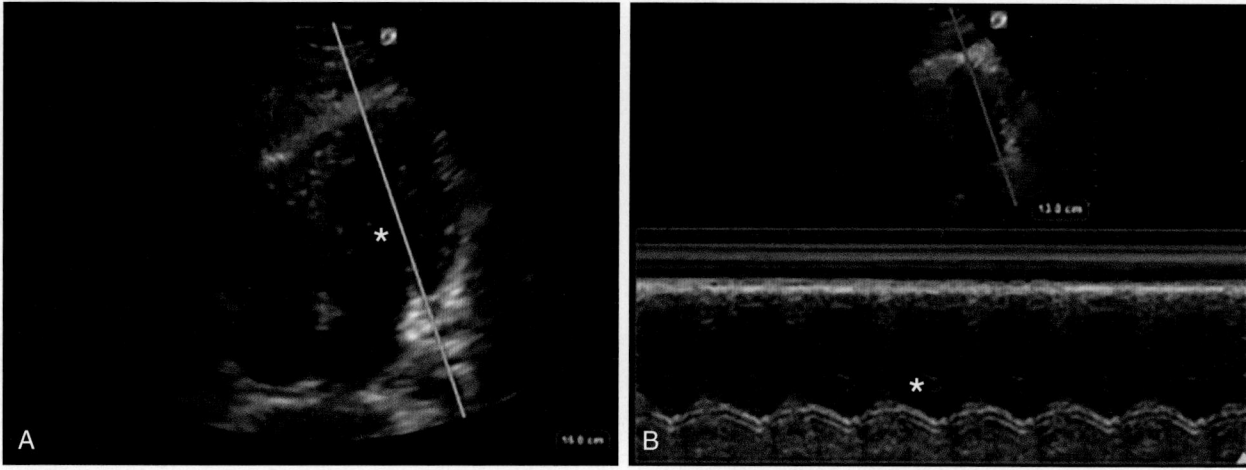

Fig. 20.23. Mitral annulus plane of systolic excursion (MAPSE). (A) Cursor alignment in 2D imaging for (B) M-mode measurement of MAPSE. Vertical excursion of the lateral side of the mitral valve annulus *(asterisk)* is measured to determine MAPSE.

performance. Assessment of the RV can, however, be difficult because of its position closer to the sternum and its triangular shape straddling the left ventricle and making characterization of its movement through the cardiac cycle difficult. Subtle signs of RV dysfunction can be seen with dilation and pulsatility in the inferior vena cava, although some pulsatility can be normal in both the IVC and subclavian veins. From the apical position or parasternal right ventricular inflow or parasternal short axis view at the aortic valve level, identification of a tricuspid valve regurgitant jet can potentially be used to evaluate RV systolic pressures. Quantification of jet peak velocity permits derivation of the pressure gradient between the right ventricle and atrium using the modified Bernoulli equation, where $\Delta P = 4(v_2\text{-}v_1)^2$ with v_1 representing velocity of blood flow distal to the tricuspid valve and v_2 representing velocity of flow in the jet. This simplifies to $\Delta P = 4v_2^2$ given v_1 approximates zero in systole. Body habitus and pulmonary inflation may make identification of a tricuspid regurgitation (TR) jet difficult in ICU patients,[90] and less severe RV dysfunction may not generate a jet.

Other clues to RV dysfunction include leftward interventricular septal deviation. Septal deviation can be visualized in multiple views; however, it is most prominent and appropriately evaluated in the parasternal short axis view at the mid-papillary level. Septal position can reveal right ventricular volume overload from pressure overload as a cause of RV dysfunction (Fig. 20.24). Volume overload is typically characterized by septal deviation occurring in diastole but not systole, resulting in the left ventricle assuming a predominantly circular conformation during systole. In the progression of RV failure to pressure overload of the ventricle, septal deviation is seen through the entire cardiac cycle.

Cardiac Arrest

During cardiac arrest, ultrasound may help immediately identify reversible causes of arrest, including critical hypovolemia and pericardial effusion with tamponade physiology.[38] In the modern PICU, ultrasound machines are easily deployed to the arresting patient's bedside for patient management. However, their use in cardiac arrest requires particular attention to patient and provider. Ultrasound gel conducts electricity and must be wiped from the skin between ultrasound views in the

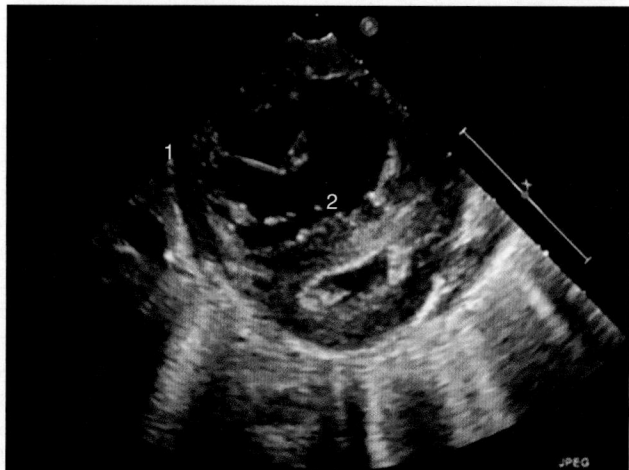

Fig. 20.24. Chronic severe right ventricular failure. Note thickened (1) right ventricular wall and (2) interventricular septum that bows into the left ventricle.

event defibrillation is necessary. The gel makes contact surfaces slippery for clinicians providing compressions and may dislodge pads and monitoring. Timing is also critical, and coordination of a sonographer's view of the heart should be performed briefly during pulse checks to minimize interference with chest compressions. The sonographer should not be the code team leader, so that sonography does not interfere with efficient CPR. Absent cardiac contractility, termed *cardiac standstill,* has been described as highly indicative of unlikely return of spontaneous circulation[91-93] in adults. In the pediatric setting, recovery of cardiac function after standstill has been described.[94] Placing the transducer in the subcostal position minimizes interference with compressors and defibrillator pads on the chest. Apical windows may also be possible but are often more difficult to acquire than subcostal windows, thereby consuming time in assessing for reversible causes of arrest.

Neurosonology

Distention of the optic nerve sheath demonstrated via direct ophthalmic ultrasound can potentially provide evidence of increased intracranial pressure.[95] The eye is imaged from the front over the closed eyelid to visualize the sheath approximately 3 mm behind the vitreous humor and retina. Careful measurement of the maximum sheath diameter is important to decrease the risk of underestimating pressure. Copious gel, preferably made for ophthalmic use, is advised to reduce eye irritation. There are limited data about normal or abnormal values for children of different ages or different intracranial disorders. A similar view surveying the posterior retinal space has also been described in examining retinal pathology for retinal hemorrhages in child abuse and has also been employed in examining traumatic and infectious pathologies involving the eye.[96] The diagnostic utility of this application remains under investigation.

Use of transcranial Doppler for assessing cerebral blood flow has become common for monitoring vasospasm in patients with subarachnoid hemorrhage and other disorders encountered in the adult neurocritical care unit. There is considerable interest in its application in pediatric neurocritical care as a noninvasive assessment tool for cerebral perfusion. Insonating the middle cerebral artery from the temporal window lateral to either eye requires a low-frequency transducer that can operate near 1 MHz. It is also possible to insonate the anterior cerebral artery in patients with an open anterior fontanelle, and the vertebrobasilar system can be insonated from the foramen magnum with some occipital support and care not to disrupt a critical airway or cervical spine. Color Doppler is used to image the cranial vessels, and pulsed wave Doppler can subsequently be employed to identify velocities in the vessel of interest. From the peak systolic (SBF) and diastolic flow (DBF), the resistive index can be calculated as RI = (SBF-DBF)/SBF or the pulsatility index as PI = (SBF-DBF)/(time-averaged mean velocity). An increasing RI or PI is suggestive of vascular constriction and a greater difference between systolic and diastolic flow.

Conclusion

Ultrasound technology is increasingly common in critical care medicine for procedural guidance and timely clinical assessment at the bedside. Optimal use requires an infrastructure to assure adequate training, but the dividends may have a powerful impact, including increased procedural safety, improved understanding of patient physiology, decreased time to diagnosis, and improved patient outcomes. More research is needed to determine ultrasound's role in the ICU, but with its ongoing incorporation into daily workflow new indications for its use are likely.

Key References

2. Brass P, Hellmich M, Kolodziej L, et al. Ultrasound guidance versus anatomical landmarks for internal jugular vein catheterization. *Cochrane Database Syst Rev.* 2015;(1):CD006962.
3. Brass P, Hellmich M, Kolodziej L, et al. Ultrasound guidance versus anatomical landmarks for subclavian or femoral vein catheterization. *Cochrane Database Syst Rev.* 2015;(1):CD011447.
9. Rhondali O, Attof R, Combet S, et al. Ultrasound-guided subclavian vein cannulation in infants: supraclavicular approach. *Paediatr Anaesth.* 2011;21:1136-1141.
10. Czarnik T, Gawda R, Perkowski T, et al. Supraclavicular approach is an easy and safe method of subclavian vein catheterization even in mechanically ventilated patients: analysis of 370 attempts. *Anesthesiology.* 2009;111:334-339.
13. Lanspa MJ, Fair J, Hirshberg EL, et al. Ultrasound-guided subclavian vein cannulation using a micro-convex ultrasound probe. *Ann Am Thorac Soc.* 2014;11:583-586.
14. Aouad MT, Kanazi GE, Abdallah FW, et al. Femoral vein cannulation performed by residents: a comparison between ultrasound-guided and landmark technique in infants and children undergoing cardiac surgery. *Anesth Analg.* 2010;111:724-728.
16. Froehlich CD, Rigby MR, Rosenberg ES, et al. Ultrasound-guided central venous catheter placement decreases complications and decreases placement attempts compared with the landmark technique in patients in a pediatric intensive care unit. *Crit Care Med.* 2009;37:1090-1096.
17. Hopkins JW, Warkentine F, Gracely E, et al. The anatomic relationship between the common femoral artery and common femoral vein in frog leg position versus straight leg position in pediatric patients. *Acad Emerg Med.* 2009;16:579-584.
19. Warkentine FH, Clyde Pierce M, Lorenz D, et al. The anatomic relationship of femoral vein to femoral artery in euvolemic pediatric patients by ultrasonography: implications for pediatric femoral central venous access. *Acad Emerg Med.* 2008;15:426-430.
20. Panebianco NL, Fredette JM, Szyld D, et al. What you see (sonographically) is what you get: vein and patient characteristics associated with successful ultrasound-guided peripheral intravenous placement in patients with difficult access. *Acad Emerg Med.* 2009;16:1298-1303.
21. Fields JM, Dean AJ, Todman RW, et al. The effect of vessel depth, diameter, and location on ultrasound-guided peripheral intravenous catheter longevity. *Am J Emerg Med.* 2011.
22. Shiloh AL, Savel RH, Paulin LM, et al. Ultrasound-guided catheterization of the radial artery: a systematic review and meta-analysis of randomized controlled trials. *Chest.* 2011;139:524-529.
23. Nakayama Y, Nakajima Y, Sessler DI, et al. A novel method for ultrasound-guided radial arterial catheterization in pediatric patients. *Anesth Analg.* 2014;118:1019-1026.
27. Matsushima K, Frankel HL. Bedside ultrasound can safely eliminate the need for chest radiographs after central venous catheter placement: CVC sono in the surgical ICU (SICU). *J Surg Res.* 2010;163:155-161.
30. Horowitz R, Gossett JG, Bailitz J, et al. The FLUSH study—flush the line and ultrasound the heart: ultrasonographic confirmation of central femoral venous line placement. *Ann Emerg Med.* 2014;63:678-683.
32. Hayes J, Borges B, Armstrong D, et al. Accuracy of manual palpation vs ultrasound for identifying the L3-L4 intervertebral space level in children. *Paediatr Anaesth.* 2014;24:510-515.
33. Neal JT, Woodford AL, Kaplan SL, et al. The effect of bedside ultrasound assistance on the proportion of successful infant lumbar punctures in a pediatric emergency department: a randomized controlled trial. *Acad Emerg Med.* 2015;22:S73.
36. Lichtenstein DA, Mauriat P. Lung ultrasound in the critically ill neonate. *Curr Pediatr Rev.* 2012;8:217-223.
37. Lichtenstein DA. Ultrasound examination of the lungs in the intensive care unit. *Pediatr Crit Care Med.* 2009;10:693-698.
38. Tsung JW, Blaivas M. Feasibility of correlating the pulse check with focused point-of-care echocardiography during pediatric cardiac arrest: a case series. *Resuscitation.* 2008;77:264-269.
41. Galicinao J, Bush AJ, Godambe SA. Use of bedside ultrasonography for endotracheal tube placement in pediatric patients: a feasibility study. *Pediatrics.* 2007;120:1297-1303.
42. Dennington D, Vali P, Finer NN, et al. Ultrasound confirmation of endotracheal tube position in neonates. *Neonatology.* 2012;102:185-189.
44. Miller SG, Brook MM, Tacy TA. Reliability of two-dimensional echocardiography in the assessment of clinically significant abnormal hemidiaphragm motion in pediatric cardiothoracic patients: comparison with fluoroscopy. *Pediatr Crit Care Med.* 2006;7:441-444.
46. Epelman M, Navarro OM, Daneman A, et al. M-mode sonography of diaphragmatic motion: description of technique and experience in 278 pediatric patients. *Pediatr Radiol.* 2005;35:661-667.
47. Faingold R, Daneman A, Tomlinson G, et al. Necrotizing enterocolitis: assessment of bowel viability with color Doppler US1. *Radiology.* 2005;235:587-594.
48. Kim W-Y, Kim WS, Kim I-O, et al. Sonographic evaluation of neonates with early-stage necrotizing enterocolitis. *Pediatr Radiol.* 2005;35:1056-1061.
49. Kim H-Y, Kim I-O, Kim WS, et al. Bowel sonography in sepsis with pathological correlation: an experimental study. *Pediatr Radiol.* 2010;41:237-243.
53. Fox JC, Boysen M, Gharahbaghian L, et al. Test characteristics of focused assessment of sonography for trauma for clinically significant abdominal

free fluid in pediatric blunt abdominal trauma. *Acad Emerg Med.* 2011;18:477-482.

54. Coley BD, Mutabagani KH, Martin LC, et al. Focused abdominal sonography for trauma (FAST) in children with blunt abdominal trauma. *J Trauma.* 2000;48:902-906.

55. Emery KH, McAneney CM, Racadio JM, et al. Absent peritoneal fluid on screening trauma ultrasonography in children: a prospective comparison with computed tomography. *J Pediatr Surg.* 2001;36:565-569.

59. Thourani VH, Pettitt BJ, Schmidt JA, et al. Validation of surgeon-performed emergency abdominal ultrasonography in pediatric trauma patients. *J Pediatr Surg.* 1998;33:322-328.

62. Dewitte A, Coquin J, Meyssignac B, et al. Doppler resistive index to reflect regulation of renal vascular tone during sepsis and acute kidney injury. *Crit Care.* 2012;16:R165.

69. Kutty S, Attebery JE, Yeager EM, et al. Transthoracic echocardiography in pediatric intensive care. *Pediatr Crit Care Med.* 2014;15:329-335.

70. Ranjit S, Aram G, Kissoon N, et al. Multimodal monitoring for hemodynamic categorization and management of pediatric septic shock. *Pediatr Crit Care Med.* 2014;15:e17-e26.

71. Bouferrache K, Amiel J-B, Chimot L, et al. Initial resuscitation guided by the Surviving Sepsis Campaign recommendations and early echocardiographic assessment of hemodynamics in intensive care unit septic patients. *Crit Care Med.* 2012;40:2821-2827.

72. Kosiak W, Swieton D, Piskunowicz M. Sonographic inferior vena cava/aorta diameter index, a new approach to the body fluid status assessment in children and young adults in emergency ultrasound—preliminary study. *Am J Emerg Med.* 2008;26:320-325.

74. Gunst M, Ghaemmaghami V, Sperry J, et al. Accuracy of cardiac function and volume status estimates using the bedside echocardiographic assessment in trauma/critical care. *J Trauma.* 2008;65:509-516.

75. Barbier C, Loubi res Y, Schmit C, et al. Respiratory changes in inferior vena cava diameter are helpful in predicting fluid responsiveness in ventilated septic patients. *Intensive Care Med.* 2004;30.

76. Feissel M, Michard FDR, Faller J-P, et al. The respiratory variation in inferior vena cava diameter as a guide to fluid therapy. *Intensive Care Med.* 2004;30.

78. Ng L, Khine H, Taragin BH, et al. Does bedside sonographic measurement of the inferior vena cava diameter correlate with central venous pressure in the assessment of intravascular volume in children? *Pediatr Emerg Care.* 2013;29:337-341.

80. Byon HJ, Lim CW, Lee J-H, et al. Prediction of fluid responsiveness in mechanically ventilated children undergoing neurosurgery. *Br J Anaesth.* 2013;110:586-591.

81. Durand P, Chevret L, Essouri S, et al. Respiratory variations in aortic blood flow predict fluid responsiveness in ventilated children. *Intensive Care Med.* 2008;34:888-894.

85. Pershad J, Myers S, Plouman C, et al. Bedside limited echocardiography by the emergency physician is accurate during evaluation of the critically ill patient. *Pediatrics.* 2004;114:e667-e671.

86. Spurney CF, Sable CA, Berger JT, et al. Use of a hand-carried ultrasound device by critical care physicians for the diagnosis of pericardial effusions, decreased cardiac function, and left ventricular enlargement in pediatric patients. *J Am Soc Echocardiogr.* 2005;18:313-319.

87. Engle SJ, DiSessa TG, Perloff JK, et al. Mitral valve E point to ventricular septal separation in infants and children. *Am J Cardiol.* 1983;52:1084-1087.

91. Breitkreutz R, Price S, Steiger HV, et al. Focused echocardiographic evaluation in life support and peri-resuscitation of emergency patients: a prospective trial. *Resuscitation.* 2010;81:1527-1533.

92. Blyth L, Atkinson P, Gadd K, et al. Bedside focused echocardiography as predictor of survival in cardiac arrest patients: a systematic review. *Acad Emerg Med.* 2012;19:1119-1126.

94. Steffen K, Thompson WR, Pustavoitau A, et al. Return of viable cardiac function following sonographic cardiac standstill in pediatric cardiac arrest. *Pediatr Emerg Care.* 2016.

95. Le A, Hoehn ME, Smith ME, et al. Bedside sonographic measurement of optic nerve sheath diameter as a predictor of increased intracranial pressure in children. *Ann Emerg Med.* 2009;53:785-791.

96. Riggs BJ, Trimboli-Heidler C, Spaeder MC, et al. The use of ophthalmic ultrasonography to identify retinal injuries associated with abusive head trauma. *Ann Emerg Med.* 2016;67:620-624.

Pediatric Critical Care in Resource-Poor Settings

Amélie von Saint André-von Arnim and Niranjan (Tex) Kissoon

PEARLS

- Global child mortality is declining due to decreasing poverty and increasing quality and access to basic medical care.
- Given the large burden and high mortality of critical illness and availability of low-cost therapies, there is ample rationale for expanding critical care services in least-developed countries.
- Basic critical care interventions can be successfully provided in resource-poor settings without an ICU.
- Publicly funded ICU care remains limited in low-income countries, and its introduction requires careful resource allocation.
- Health care systems improvements for the critically ill should involve a graded approach of strengthening capacity to provide health maintenance, basic critical care, and then publicly funded intensive care services as overall health indices improve.
- Critical care research from low-income countries is sorely needed to guide effective and efficient care and advocate for resources.

Life-threatening illnesses are a global phenomenon with markedly disparate outcomes depending on available resources. The term "resource-poor setting" defines a locale in developing or underdeveloped countries where mortality is high, and the capability to provide critical care for life-threatening illness is limited. In rich, industrialized countries, caring for critically ill patients involves a coordinated system of triage, transport networks, and emergency and intensive care provided in well-resourced units. This cohesive service is resource intensive and hence not affordable for many low-income countries where care is fragmented. Indeed, the burden of critical illness remains inordinately high in low-income countries,[1] despite an overall recent decrease in global childhood mortality. Thus care of the critically ill with sudden, serious reversible disease should be a universal goal. While the systems available in resource-rich areas cannot and should not be the near-term goal, a graded approach that involves strengthening capacity to provide health maintenance and implementing basic critical care followed by publicly funded intensive care services as overall health indices improve is a reasonable solution.

Child Mortality Rates

Current Trends and Health Maintenance

Globally, the under-5 mortality rate has decreased by nearly half (49%) since 1990, decreasing from 90 to 46 deaths per 1000 live births in 2013. This translates into 17,000 fewer children dying every day now compared with 1990 and a decrease in the contribution of deaths and disability of children younger than 5 years of age to the global disability-adjusted life years (adult and pediatric) from 41% to 25% between 1990 and 2010.[2] These gains may be partly attributed to attention to the Millennium Development Goals (MDGs), especially MDG numbers 4 and 5, which related to decreasing under-5 mortality by two-thirds and "improving maternal health" by reducing maternal mortality by three-quarters by 2015 from 1990 baseline.[3] These successes are due to decreasing poverty, increasing vaccination rates, access to medical care, improving quality of care, and other factors.

The under-5 mortality is currently falling faster than at any other time during the past 2 decades, but about 17,000 children younger than the age of 5 still die every day, with 6.3 million deaths annually.[4] In addition, gains have been patchy and the region with the world's highest under-5-mortality rates remains sub-Saharan Africa with roughly half (49.6%, 3.113 million) of those deaths. On average, 1 out of every 11 children born in sub-Saharan Africa dies before age 5. This is nearly 15 times the average rate in high-income countries.[4] The world's "bottom billion" living in poverty remains high even in rapidly emerging economies, such as India and China[5]: The five countries with the highest number of under-5 deaths in 2013 were India, China, Pakistan, Nigeria, and the Democratic Republic of the Congo.[6] Even if present trends in mortality continue, 4.4 million children younger than 5 years will die in 2030.[6] Thus despite substantial gains there are still great and burgeoning needs for critical care for children globally (Fig. 21.1).

Justification for Critical Care

Of the 6.3 million children who died in their first 5 years of life in 2013, 52% died of infectious causes.[6] Pneumonia, diarrheal diseases, and malaria were the leading infectious causes: pneumonia caused 0.935 million, diarrhea 0.578 million, and malaria 0.456 million deaths.[6] While substantial gains have been made in under-5 mortality, gains in neonates have been small with neonatal deaths contributing 44% of under-5

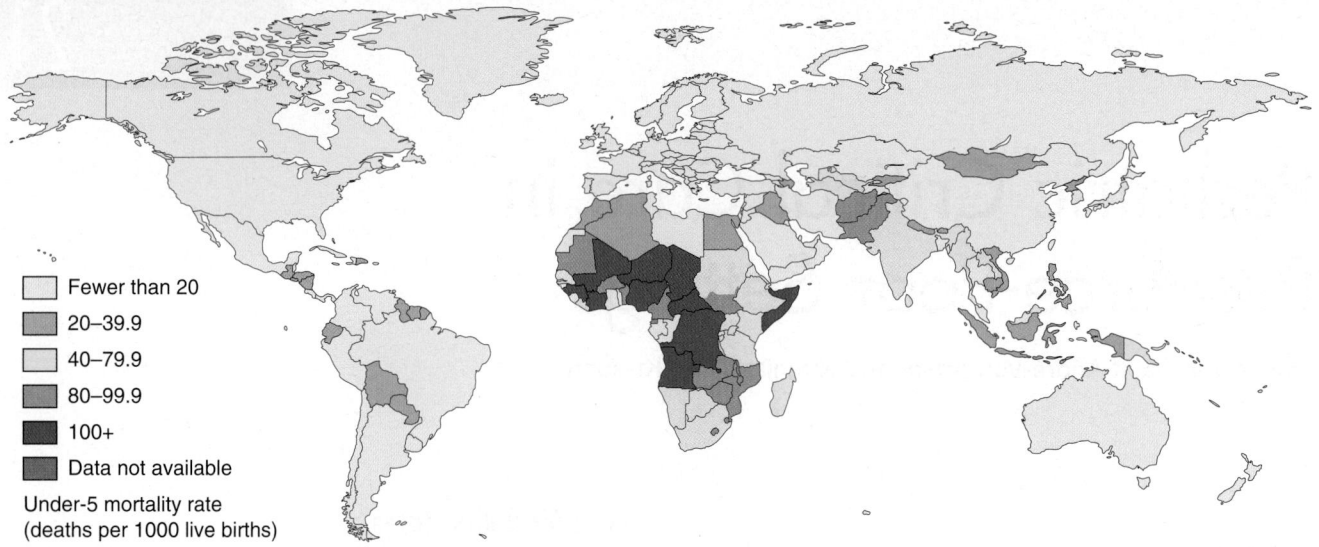

Fig. 21.1. Distribution of Global Under-5 Mortality Rates. United Nations Inter-agency Group for Child Mortality Estimation (IGME). (From UNICEF: Committing to child survival: A promise renewed progress report 2014, UNICEF, New York 2014. Available at: http://data.unicef.org/child-mortality/under-five#sthash.SSSCDvl3.dpuf.)

Legend (Under-5 mortality rate, deaths per 1000 live births):
- Fewer than 20
- 20–39.9
- 40–79.9
- 80–99.9
- 100+
- Data not available

deaths. Other important causes were injury, which contributed to 0.324 million deaths,[6] with overall 90% of global trauma deaths occurring in low- or middle-income countries.[7] Thus infectious diseases remain the leading cause for child mortality. Half of the infectious disease–related under-5 deaths are associated with malnutrition, mainly among the poor in low-income countries (Fig. 21.2).[3]

The number of deaths is clearly an underestimate because methods of measuring health outcomes are limited in middle- and low-income countries. For instance, in sub-Saharan Africa, only South Africa captures more than 50% of deaths in a vital registration system. The lack of death registries renders it difficult to estimate the burden of critical illness and hence limits the ability to hold governments accountable for their organization of health systems.[8,9]

The three general approaches that have been suggested to try to estimate global burden of critical illness have significant limitations.[10] These include the following: (1) counting patients admitted to ICUs around the world; (2) extrapolating from resource-rich countries' epidemiology; and (3) using the assumption that all deaths occurring in a region had a critical illness at some stage before their demise. The first two approaches will likely lead to an underestimation, and the third will lead to an overestimation of the burden of critical illness in resource-poor settings. However, by all indications the burden is enormous and likely to rise with increasing urbanization and epidemics.[1,11-13] Access to medical care may improve outcome but will increase the demand for critical care.

Given the high burden of critical illness in least-developed countries with a collective population of greater than 366 million children and adolescents,[14] the associated high mortality, and availability of low-cost strategies for the management of many critical illnesses, there is ample rationale for expanding critical care services in these regions of the world.

Critical Care in Resource-Poor Settings

Critical care can be defined by the severity of illness, complexity of the care that is offered, and training of the professionals who provide that care.[15] For the purposes of this chapter, however, we define pediatric *critical care* as the care of children who suffer a life-threatening illness or injury regardless of the location where care is provided. As an example, critical care includes treatment for severe pneumonia, malaria, or diarrheal diseases at district clinics and health centers, as well as tertiary-care hospitals. Thus critical care can be provided from the time of first presentation to the point of discharge home.[16] In contrast, we define *intensive care* as care provided for the critically ill or injured or those who have undergone major surgical procedures in an ICU. These units vary in resources (personnel, equipment, and supplies) and hence the level of care that can be provided but share the common characteristic of being a designated area in a hospital. Thus delivery of critical care services is not specific to a site and could be provided in the prehospital setting, emergency department, hospital wards, or intensive care unit.

In high-income countries, critical care services usually involve "a coordinated system of triage, emergency management, and ICUs" providing contemporary standards of care to the population.[17] Some urban university and private hospitals in sub-Saharan Africa, India, and China may offer critical and intensive care services close to high-income countries, but in many low- to middle-income countries (LMICs), health care systems are poorly organized, human and material resources are scant, and intensive care services are few or nonexistent, especially at the hubs of medical care, the district-level hospitals.[18-23] In sub-Saharan Africa, inadequate delivery of evidence-based, essential interventions continues to be a major obstacle.[24,25] Even quality of care for common childhood illnesses such as pneumonia and diarrheal diseases is poor in these settings.[20,26] Logistic and financial limitations, poorly resourced supporting disciplines (eg, laboratories, radiology, nursing), poor general health status of patients, underlying malnutrition, delayed presentation of severely sick children, and suboptimal care contribute to comparatively high mortality. As an example, a recent survey of Kenyan government hospitals revealed a median availability of

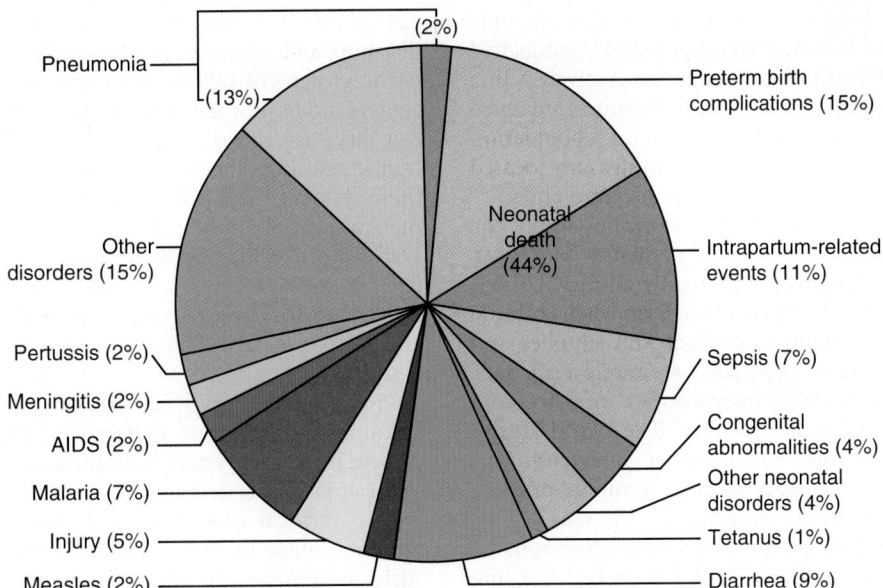

Fig. 21.2. Estimated number of deaths by cause in 2013. (From Liu L, et al. Global, regional, and national causes of child mortality in 2000-13, with projections to inform post-2015 priorities: an updated systematic analysis. Lancet. 2015;385:430-440.)

essential antibiotics in only 36% of the 22 surveyed facilities, with a wide range of essential resource availability from 49% to 93%.[27]

Intensive Care in Resource-Poor Settings

Where ICUs are available, the most common reasons for admission are for postsurgical and trauma care, infectious diseases, and peripartum maternal or neonatal complications.[28] These conditions are major contributors to the global burden of disease. Hence, building critical care capacity around the relevant disciplines (eg, surgery, obstetrics, pediatrics, internal medicine) where they already exist is a reasonable method to increase capacity. Increasing capacity may also entail providing more personnel, equipment, and supplies. For instance, an ICU in a public hospital often provides pressurized air or oxygen, but mechanical ventilation or renal replacement therapy is limited.[18] What may be found in a district-level hospital in sub-Saharan Africa is a four- to eight-bed ICU with one or two nurses. Fifty percent of the patients may have an empty IV drip and no patient monitors, mechanical ventilators, necessary disposable materials, or electricity. Oxygen is an expensive resource and not always available because of difficulties in refilling cylinders, and reliable electricity to power oxygen concentrators generally does not exist.[18]

Basic Critical Care in Resource-Poor Settings

Critically ill children in LMICs may benefit from timely care even without an ICU. Innovative and successful basic critical care interventions in these settings are increasingly evident. These include the training of villagers in basic first aid and resuscitation[29]; provision of low-cost simplified antimicrobial regimens and rapid diagnostic tests to rural health care workers, day clinics, and homes[30-32,33]; quality improvement of district hospital services[34,35]; reorganization of emergency services at referral hospitals[36,37]; provision of oxygen therapy for hypoxemic children with pneumonia in district clinics; and

medical treatment given by village workers or parents,[38,39] which all have proven to be effective and beneficial to critically ill children. Great gains have been made in treating pneumonia by the introduction of oxygen concentrators, oximetry monitoring, and supplemental oxygen administration in Papua New Guinea. These interventions decreased pediatric pneumonia case fatality by 35% at very low cost.[40] Noninvasive respiratory support such as Bubble-CPAP has been successfully and cost-effectively introduced for support of neonates and infants with respiratory compromise in limited-resource settings.[41-46] Use of simple nurse-initiated CPAP protocols for children up to 5 years of age has been successfully and safely introduced to some rural hospitals in Ghana.[47] Devices delivering CPAP or BiPAP can reduce the work of breathing and improve functional residual capacity, potentially avoiding intubation and preventing harm and high costs related to invasive mechanical ventilation.[48,49]

Cost of Intensive Care

Intensive care involving ICUs and mechanical ventilation is expensive, as opposed to the much lower-cost basic critical care interventions described earlier. The cost of intensive care includes expenditures for increased personnel, equipment, consumables, and expenses associated with potential long-term morbidity of survivors. The high fixed costs of ICU care contribute significantly to the limitations of an ICU infrastructure in low-resource settings.[9] Differing health insurance schemes and socioeconomic divisions can introduce significant variations in how patients are treated, both in terms of likelihood of admission to the ICU and care in the ICU.[50] The evidence indicates that universal health care coverage schemes in LMICs improve access and utilization of basic medical services,[51] which may positively affect ICU care going forward.

Defining the capacity to deliver intensive care in LMICs is challenging given the absence of uniform definitions of an ICU bed.[52,53] More than 50% of low-income countries lack any published data on ICU capacity.[53] In a recent review, the only countries with national ICU bed data, Nepal and Uganda, had 16.7 and 1.0 ICU beds per million people, respectively.[53] In a national survey in Zambia, only 7% of 68 hospitals surveyed offered ICU care, translating to 29 ICU beds for a population of 11.7 million.[54] Most ICUs in these settings are located in referral centers or university hospitals of large cities.[53,54] However, the presence of an ICU bed does not imply the ability to effectively care for critically ill patients.[55] Moreover, the data presented represent predominantly adult ICU beds that may accept a child on rare occasions. Even when children are admitted, age-appropriate equipment and supplies and care providers with pediatric experience are rarely available.

So one may ask, "Is increased intensive care infrastructure in limited-resource settings worthwhile?" The World Health Organization defines a "very cost-effective" intervention as one that costs less than the value of gross domestic product (GDP) per capita per disability-adjusted life year.[56] This includes many primary care and preventative interventions[57,58] and some surgical interventions.[59-62] ICUs in high-income countries function in large part by admitting and caring for complex patients with often incurable diseases,[63] whereas in many resource-limited settings, the ICU provides basic rescue interventions for children and young adults who are ill with curable diseases. Although provision of intensive care services may not seem rational or cost-effective in low-income countries, a short duration of critical care that is cost-effective and treats acute life-threatening illnesses affecting millions of young people worldwide may have a large impact on mortality from curable disease and reduce preventable deaths.[63] It is suggested that publicly funded expensive intensive care is justified in countries with under-5 mortality rates of less than 20 to 30 per 1000 live births. However, in settings where under-5 mortality rates are greater than 30 per live births, focus on basic critical care interventions specified earlier is more appropriate.[15,64] Research into cost-effective interventions in the setting of curable diseases is needed to further understand which critical care interventions are appropriate and sustainable, as well as how best to allocate resources.

Ethics of Intensive Care in Resource-Poor Settings

Development of publicly funded intensive care services in resource-poor settings raises many challenges. According to the global justice argument, health care services are a fundamental and universal human right available to everyone.[10] The *just* distribution of health care services across all human populations remains a serious challenge. Global justice would imply that those in resource-rich regions have a responsibility to combat critical illness and strengthen health care infrastructure for those in resource-poor settings.[65] In countries with per-capita health care investments less than $100 per person per year, the cost of intensive care renders its provision for everyone impractical. To attempt to provide access to ICUs at the standard of care accepted generally in the developed world will lead to serious distortion of health care budgets and have detrimental effects on overall health of the nation. Alternatively, access to different standards of care or differences in quality and breadth of critical care will develop or already has developed in LMICs. In such an inegalitarian health care policy, which is common in many developing nations, "centers of excellence can be maintained where

critical care technologies can be nurtured so that as a country develops and increases its standards of care, it will have its home-grown critical care resources on which to draw."[66] Such centers can harbor the skilled personnel within a country who can serve as catalysts in expanding high-quality care as economic resources increase and mortality gains are realized. In these systems, the key lies in extreme efficiency measures and meticulous attention to balancing the needs of individuals versus those of the population. Lessons learned from innovative methods in delivering critical care in less than ideal conditions and with fewer resources can lead to reverse innovations and be beneficial to both resource-rich and resource-poor worlds.

Providing ICU-level care also requires respecting family, cultural, and religious preferences. Different practices are present in different countries with respect to whom is accepted as the appropriate decision maker on initiation or discontinuance of critical care services. In particular, such decisions are often made by the family rather than patient.[66] In many African countries the idea of advanced directives and code status have yet to be discussed at the national judicial and medical community level.[67]

Resource allocation of intensive care services in deprived areas of the world is challenging and should be defined for each institution. As an example, the Red Cross War Memorial Hospital in South Africa published explicit patient exclusion criteria for offering critical care, in an attempt to provide a reasonable process for fair and equitable utilization of scarce resources.[68] Some of these exclusion criteria are futile care for children declared brain dead or status post cardiac arrest without establishment of normal respiratory pattern; children with underlying lethal conditions, such as children with burns on more than 60% of their body surface area with limited ability to provide timely surgical debridement; children with chronic renal failure with no ability to commit to long-term dialysis; children with severe/lethal chromosomal anomalies; and children with malignancies nonresponsive to therapy or inoperable cardiac lesions. Although this is a reasonable approach, implementation should be undertaken with great sensitivity to both the family and staff or it is likely to lead to failure, anger, and cynicism. In addition, careful decisions regarding the extent of ICU support need to be made in the context of potential impoverishment of the entire extended family, especially if the end result is a child's death or long-term morbidity.

Suggested ways to address ethical dilemmas of resource allocation in resource-poor settings include the following: obtaining data on disease prognosis with and without ICU care to inform clinical decision making; development of procedures for addressing level-of-care decisions openly and honestly; and articulating hospital policies on the use of critical care services, including policies regarding appropriate ICU admissions, cardiopulmonary resuscitation, and ventilator candidates.[67]

Strengthening Critical Care Infrastructure
Health Care Systems

There is no one blueprint for an ideal health care system, nor is there a remedy that will automatically elicit improved performance.[69] Building critical care services in LMICs requires a tiered approach, starting by improving delivery of evidence-based, basic, essential health care interventions, especially for countries with under-5 mortality rates greater than 30 per live births.[64,70,71] This requires broad strengthening of national health systems because a multitude of factors may influence how services are actually delivered, including financing, human resources, governance, and information systems, in addition to more traditional concerns over knowledge, skills, and availability of technologies.[72,73] A focus on district-level hospitals seems ideal because they are typically linked to a network of primary care and community-based health services and are more accessible to the local community.[10] In Africa, they consume approximately 50% of financial and human resources and, as the training ground for most health workers, have a major influence on increasing capacity building within health systems. Here, both basic and slightly more complex cost-effective interventions are provided in a multiprofessional setting that concentrates skills and resources.[19,24] However, care has been suboptimal in many areas. Recent efforts to identify indicators of quality hospital care for critically ill children and newborns suitable for use in low-income settings have suggested availability of intravenous fluids, epinephrine for injection, presence of a triage system, and prioritization and grouping of severely ill children for increased observation as valuable indicators.[74]

Introduction of publicly funded ICU care should be targeted in countries with under-5 mortality rates less than 30 per live births. Building regional centers of excellence to grow publicly funded intensive care resources and capacity over time may be a reasonable first step. However, there is no approach to improve health care systems that is suitable for all countries, and not all approaches are congruent with local values and ideologies or acceptable to all governments or their constituencies. Thus health care strengthening must be seen as a long-term process that involves complex systems and requires carefully orchestrated action on a number of fronts.[75] In order to avoid development of distrust in health care systems by local communities, focus on quality of care and its measurement are key for enhancing critical and intensive care services in resource-limited settings. The quality of care approach should include safety, effectiveness, and care delivery in ways that respect the dignity of individuals in the context of their own "local moral worlds."[76]

In recent years, the funding landscape has changed dramatically, and there is extensive private participation in the health care systems of LMICs, especially in service delivery. The private sector ranges from a limited number of formal not-for-profit and for-profit providers to numerous informal providers. There has been an increase in the number of private providers, driven by both rising incomes and the failure of public services to meet expectations.[69] The engagement of the private sector is a topic of considerable controversy, seen by some as inviting the privatization of health care and making it a commodity.[77] However, when the capacity of the public sector is limited and there is a concentration of human resources in the private sector, seeking a mix of public and private provision of services can be seen as a pragmatic response and may spur overall increases in services and care delivery.[78]

Capacity Building via Education

Most deaths among seriously ill children who come into contact with referral level health services occur within the first 48 hours of presentation.[79] Therefore, early recognition of critical illness and good quality immediate and effective care provided by skilled health professionals would likely reduce these deaths.[21,80] However, severe shortages of primary care providers, specialists, nurses, and prehospital-care providers remain a major challenge in LMICs. This crisis is exacerbated by the brain-drain of medical providers from resource-poor to resource-rich countries. To improve health workers' capacity to provide effective care for seriously ill newborns and children in low-income countries, various in-service life support training courses, based mainly on models of high-income countries, have been introduced in LMICs. These courses include (1) neonatal life support courses (eg, Newborn Life Support [NLS], Neonatal Resuscitation Program [NRP]); (2) pediatric life support courses (eg, Pediatric Advanced Life Support [PALS], Pediatric Life Support [PLS]); (3) advanced short courses in pediatric critical and trauma care (eg, Pediatric BASIC Course, Pediatric Fundamental Critical Care Support [PFCCS], and Advanced Trauma Life Support [ATLS]); (4) life support/emergency care elements within the Integrated Management of Pregnancy and Childbirth program (eg, Essential Newborn Care [ENC]); and (5) components of other in-service child health training courses that deal with the care of children with serious illness (eg, Emergency Triage, Assessment and Treatment [ETAT], Control of Diarrheal Diseases [CDD], and Acute Respiratory Infection [ARI] case management programs; training components of the Integrated Management of Childhood Illness [IMCI] strategy).

A recent Cochrane review assessed the effects of in-service emergency care training on health professionals' treatment of severely ill newborns and children in low-income countries.[81] It included only two neonatal resuscitation studies, both of which suggested a beneficial effect on health provider outcomes (resuscitation practices, assessment of breathing, resuscitation preparedness) in the short term. However, the effects on neonatal mortality outcomes were inconclusive, and improvement in health provider practices after training was not generalizable. The review authors concluded that decisions to scale up life support courses in low-income countries "must be based on consideration of costs and logistics associated with their implementation, including the need for adequate numbers of skilled instructors, appropriate locally adapted training materials and the availability of basic resuscitation equipment."[81]

ETAT was developed by the World Health Organization, specifically aimed at low-income countries, and is intended to improve prompt identification and institution of lifesaving emergency treatment for very ill children. This course was adapted to the East African context as "Emergency Triage Assessment and Treatment Plus admission care" (ETAT+).[82-84] Despite some positive results of ETAT+ implementation and further dissemination of these guidelines and training, reports indicated significant variation in uptake of best practices.[20-22,35,85] In Kenya, health workers at the hospital level were unable to provide appropriate care for severely ill newborns or children with inadequacies in key tasks such as prescription of antibiotics and feeds even when resources were available.[26] In attempting to rectify these deficiencies in care, the level of engagement of senior and particularly midlevel clinical managers was important.[86] The simple availability of authoritative WHO and national guidelines alone therefore does not improve hospital care for children as hoped. Broader, more system-oriented interventions addressing the many important influences on provider or user behavior are necessary.[73] A recent multifaceted approach addressing deficiencies in knowledge, skills, motivation, and organization of care utilizing face-to-face feedback of performance, supportive supervision, and provision of a local facilitator resulted in more sustained improvements of pediatric care in Kenya.[35]

The global community can help by supporting country-led processes of reform and capacity building in education and by helping to create a stronger evidence base that contributes to cross-country learning.

Critical Illness During Disease Outbreaks

As the recent H1N1 influenza, severe acute respiratory syndrome (SARS), and Ebola outbreaks have clearly illustrated, critical care resources are vital. With increasing global urbanization, the potential risks of emerging and reemerging infections grow, increasing critical care needs for large numbers of seriously ill patients.[87] Mass critical care preparedness in resource-limited settings has been largely ignored, despite the large densely crowded populations who are prone to suffer disproportionately from natural disasters.[88] A recent international consensus statement emphasizes the need to develop resilient health care systems. To prepare for disaster and mass critical care preparedness in resource-poor settings,[28] it recommends strengthening the primary care, basic emergency care, and public health systems and building critical care capacity in the fields with the highest burden of disease such as surgery, obstetrics, internal medicine, and pediatrics. To improve capacity building and quality of care at district hospitals, performance improvement activities should be instituted. District and regional level health centers should develop at least a minimal level of critical care. Prehospital care and transport of the critically ill could be improved through community-level education of medical and nonmedical laypersons.

How to Develop an ICU in Low- to Middle-Income Countries

Development of an ICU in LMICs should start with a needs assessment to build the care according to the local patient population needs, medical practices and culture, and available physical, equipment, and staffing resources.[89] For publicly funded ICUs, there should be early and close engagement with policy makers and administration to ensure long-term sustainability. Bed space sizes according to US standards[90] are likely not feasible in LMICs. However, because communicable diseases are highly prevalent in LMICs, adequate distance between bed spaces or a facility with separate isolation rooms needs to be taken into consideration.[91] Both adequate water and electricity supply are vital for an ICU. Backup power generators and equipment with prolonged battery life can help overcome temporary electricity shortages. Selection of ICU equipment (ventilators, monitors, blood gas machine, infusion pumps) for use in LMICs requires careful consideration of not only the initial cost but also the availability of ongoing maintenance and biomedical support from the supplier, cost of consumables (and their potential reusability), equipment durability, and ease of use.

Given the lack of trained critical care staff in LMICs, education of ICU nurses, physicians, pharmacists, and potentially respiratory therapists in basic critical and intensive care should be performed before opening ICU doors. Visiting content experts from high-income countries can play an important role in initial and ongoing capacity building. However, these trainers need to be well versed in the cultural context and should be educated on cultural sensitivity, the community, and medical problems of the host nation for the whole process to be effective.[89,92] Nursing staff turnover can be a challenge, leading to a significant burden of staff retraining.[67,89] In addition to ICU content, team work and organizational skills required for efficient ICU care need to be taught and maintained.

Given the limited ICU resources, their cost, and the principle of fee for service in many LMICs, an ethical framework including ICU patient inclusion and exclusion criteria should be set before ICU operation. Other important systems required for establishment of an ICU include infection control, reliable availability of medication and consumables (including their easy accessibility and restocking on code or procedure carts), radiology, laboratory medicine, and medical record systems that allow easy measurement of ICU patient outcomes.

Importance of Critical Care Research in Limited Resource Settings

Published data on critical care research from low-income countries remains limited yet is much needed.[9,67] Reasons for this gap in evidence may include lack of funding, lack of local critical care providers and researchers, lack of academic mentorship and infrastructure to do research, or barriers to turning available data into publishable research. The limited evidence in this field hinders effective and efficient care and advocacy for resources.

The research agenda should include increasing evidence regarding basic critical illness epidemiology and its outcomes in these settings. A more accurate estimate of the potential lives saved through critical care would serve to prove its role in health care systems in resource-poor settings.[10] Efficacy must be measured and validated for critical care interventions, with limited resources targeted to those practices that save lives, time, and resources. Dissemination of evidence and experience from successes and failures could help accelerate the pace of critical care infrastructure improvements. Data on critical care capacity and access to both critical care resources and health care professionals are essential for health system planning but generally lacking.

While recognizing that uptake of new recommendations can be slow in LMICs,[93] efforts should be made to adjust critical care guidelines from high-income countries to limited-resource settings including sepsis management guidelines.[18] Cost-effectiveness analyses of current and proposed critical care practices need to be emphasized.[67] Patient triage and clinical research would benefit from severity of illness scoring systems, adapted and validated for resource-poor settings. Low-cost critical care technology, such as low-cost mechanical ventilators[94,95] and noninvasive positive pressure ventilation, is much needed to support critical care in limited-resource settings. Locally available, ubiquitous technology such as cell phones should be used to enable better health care seeking and delivery and solve clinical challenges. Production of equipment within low-income countries or LMICs, rather than expensive import from the United States and Europe, may help drive down the cost of critical care interventions in these settings.[96] Technology development must be tightly woven into solving implementation challenges that result from not only technology cost and availability but also complexity of the political, social, and professional systems in LMICs.[93]

Key References

1. Dunser MW, Baelani I, Ganbold L. A review and analysis of intensive care medicine in the least developed countries. *Crit Care Med.* 2006;34: 1234-1242.
3. United Nations. *The Millennium Development Goals Report 2014.* New York, NY: United Nations; 2014.
4. UN Inter-agency Group for Child Mortality Estimation (UN IGME), T.I.-a.G.f.C.M.E.U. Levels and trends in child mortality. Report 2014. 2014.
6. Liu L, et al. Global, regional, and national causes of child mortality in 2000-13, with projections to inform post-2015 priorities: an updated systematic analysis. *Lancet.* 2015;385:430-440.
8. Children A.C.f.H.o.W.a. *Accountability for Women's and Children's Health.* Geneva, Switzerland: The World Health Organization; 2014.
9. Adhikari NK, et al. Critical care and the global burden of critical illness in adults. *Lancet.* 2010;376:1339-1346.
11. Murray CJ, Lopez AD. Measuring the global burden of disease. *N Engl J Med.* 2013;369:448-457.
16. Kissoon N, et al. World Federation of Pediatric Intensive and Critical Care Societies—its global agenda. *Pediatr Crit Care Med.* 2009;10:597-600.
18. Dunser MW, et al. Recommendations for sepsis management in resource-limited settings. *Intensive Care Med.* 2012;38:557-574.
19. English M, Lanata CF, Ngugi I, Smith PC. The district hospital. In: *Disease Control Priorities in Developing Countries.* Washington, DC: World Bank; 2006:1211-1228.
20. Reyburn H, et al. Clinical assessment and treatment in paediatric wards in the north-east of the United Republic of Tanzania. *Bull World Health Organ.* 2008;86:132-139.
24. Friberg IK, et al. Sub-Saharan Africa's mothers, newborns, and children: how many lives could be saved with targeted health interventions? *PLoS Med.* 2010;7:e1000295.
27. Gathara D, et al. Moving towards routine evaluation of quality of inpatient pediatric care in Kenya. *PLoS ONE.* 2015;10:e0117048.
28. Geiling J, et al. Resource-poor settings: infrastructure and capacity building: care of the critically ill and injured during pandemics and disasters: CHEST consensus statement. *Chest.* 2014;146(suppl 4):e156S-167S.
30. African Neonatal Sepsis Trial, et al. Simplified antibiotic regimens compared with injectable procaine benzylpenicillin plus gentamicin for treatment of neonates and young infants with clinical signs of possible serious bacterial infection when referral is not possible: a randomised, open-label, equivalence trial. *Lancet.* 2015;385:1767-1776.
31. Bhutta ZA, et al. Management of newborn infections in primary care settings: a review of the evidence and implications for policy? *Pediatr Infect Dis J.* 2009;28(suppl 1):S22-S30.
32. Baqui AH, et al. Effectiveness of home-based management of newborn infections by community health workers in rural Bangladesh. *Pediatr Infect Dis J.* 2009;28:304-310.
33. Yeboah-Antwi K, et al. Community case management of fever due to malaria and pneumonia in children under five in Zambia: a cluster randomized controlled trial. *PLoS Med.* 2010;7:e1000340.
34. English M, et al. An intervention to improve paediatric and newborn care in Kenyan district hospitals: understanding the context. *Implement Sci.* 2009;4:42.
35. Ayieko P, et al. A multifaceted intervention to implement guidelines and improve admission paediatric care in Kenyan district hospitals: a cluster randomised trial. *PLoS Med.* 2011;8:e1001018.
36. Molyneux E, Ahmad S, Robertson A. Improved triage and emergency care for children reduces inpatient mortality in a resource-constrained setting. *Bull World Health Organ.* 2006;84:314-319.
37. Molyneux E. Emergency care for children in resource-constrained countries. *Trans R Soc Trop Med Hyg.* 2009;103:11-15.
38. Ashraf H, et al. Randomized controlled trial of day care versus hospital care of severe pneumonia in Bangladesh. *Pediatrics.* 2010;126:e807-e815.
39. Addo-Yobo E, et al. Outpatient treatment of children with severe pneumonia with oral amoxicillin in four countries: the MASS study. *Trop Med Int Health.* 2011;16:995-1006.
40. Duke T, et al. Improved oxygen systems for childhood pneumonia: a multihospital effectiveness study in Papua New Guinea. *Lancet.* 2008; 372:1328-1333.
47. Wilson PT, et al. A randomized clinical trial evaluating nasal continuous positive airway pressure for acute respiratory distress in a developing country. *J Pediatr.* 2013;162:988-992.
53. Murthy S, Leligdowicz A, Adhikari NK. Intensive care unit capacity in low-income countries: a systematic review. *PLoS ONE.* 2015;10:e0116949.
63. Firth P, Ttendo S. Intensive care in low-income countries–a critical need. *N Engl J Med.* 2012;367:1974-1976.
64. Shann F. Role of intensive care in countries with a high child mortality rate. *Pediatr Crit Care Med.* 2011;12:114-115.
65. Caney S. *Justice Beyond Borders.* Oxford, England: Oxford University Press; 2005.
67. Riviello ED, et al. Critical care in resource-poor settings: lessons learned and future directions. *Crit Care Med.* 2011;39:860-867.
68. Argent AC, et al. Pediatric intensive care in South Africa: an account of making optimum use of limited resources at the Red Cross War Memorial Children's Hospital. *Pediatr Crit Care Med.* 2014;15:7-14.
74. Ntoburi S, et al. Development of paediatric quality of inpatient care indicators for low-income countries—a Delphi study. *BMC Pediatr.* 2010;10:90.
78. Balabanova D, et al. Good health at low cost 25 years on: lessons for the future of health systems strengthening. *Lancet.* 2013;381:2118-2133.
81. Opiyo N, English M. In-service training for health professionals to improve care of seriously ill newborns and children in low-income countries. *Cochrane Database Syst Rev.* 2015;(5):CD007071.
83. Irimu G, et al. Developing and introducing evidence based clinical practice guidelines for serious illness in Kenya. *Arch Dis Child.* 2008;93: 799-804.
84. Tuyisenge L, et al. Knowledge and skills retention following Emergency Triage, Assessment and Treatment plus Admission course for final year medical students in Rwanda: a longitudinal cohort study. *Arch Dis Child.* 2014;99:993-997.
86. English M, et al. Explaining the effects of a multifaceted intervention to improve inpatient care in rural Kenyan hospitals–interpretation based on retrospective examination of data from participant observation, quantitative and qualitative studies. *Implement Sci.* 2011;6:124.
88. Geiling J, et al. Resource-poor settings: response, recovery, and research: care of the critically ill and injured during pandemics and disasters: CHEST consensus statement. *Chest.* 2014;146(suppl 4):e168S-177S.
89. Basnet S, Adhikari N, Koirala J. Challenges in setting up pediatric and neonatal intensive care units in a resource-limited country. *Pediatrics.* 2011;128:e986-e992.
93. English M, et al. Adoption of recommended practices and basic technologies in a low-income setting. *Arch Dis Child.* 2014;99:452-456.
94. Williams D, et al. A low oxygen consumption pneumatic ventilator for emergency construction during a respiratory failure pandemic. *Anaesthesia.* 2010;65:235-242.
95. Beringer RM, Eltringham RJ. The Glostavent: evolution of an anaesthetic machine for developing countries. *Anaesth Intensive Care.* 2008;36:442-448.

Educating the Intensivist

Mary W. Lieh-Lai, Denise M. Goodman, David A. Turner, and Katherine Cashen

PEARLS

- Effective teaching should relate clearly to learners' current experience and knowledge.
- Adults learn best by active participation and practice; therefore educational efforts should emphasize these concepts and include bedside teaching, debriefing, simulation, case-based, and experiential learning.
- Skill acquisition in medicine is similar to the continuum of human developmental stages with learning that progresses from novice, advanced beginner, competent, proficient, expert, and, finally, master.
- The mature clinician is one who reflects on his or her daily medical experiences to place him or her in a larger context of previous encounters and critically evaluates his or her own performance, acknowledging both effective and ineffective aspects of patient care.

Pediatric critical care medicine is a discipline dedicated to the care of the critically ill child. The specialty focuses on the sick child as a whole and takes into account the impact of disease on all organ systems, addressing the physical, mental, and emotional needs of the child and those of his or her family. The education of pediatric intensivists is focused on patient care principles that include resuscitation, advanced life support, management of traumatic injury, postoperative care, application of mechanical ventilation, renal replacement therapy, cardiovascular support, and hemodynamic and neurologic monitoring. Knowledge of toxicology, pulmonology, hematology/oncology, and metabolic disorders; pharmacologic principles; transplantation; procedural sedation; and infectious diseases is also important. The complex needs of the critically ill child also require that intensivists be prepared to assume a leadership role in the coordination of care among team members from multiple disciplines (see Chapter 3). In addition, the pediatric intensivist must develop an understanding of the ethics of critical care medicine and be able to balance complex and high-technology care with humanistic principles and respect for the patient as a human being (see Chapters 14–16). The intensivist must be knowledgeable in patient safety and quality improvement methodology but should also lead these efforts in the intensive care unit environment (see Chapter 11). Skills for evaluating medical literature, clinical and/or basic science research, and the ability to teach learners of different levels effectively are all invaluable.

Adult Learning

Stuart and Hubert Dreyfus developed a model of skill acquisition on the basis of their studies of fighter pilots.[1] The Dreyfus model proposes that skill acquisition is not different from the continuum of human development, with stages of skill acquisition designated as novice, advanced beginner, competent, proficient, expert, and, finally, master. The learner needs to acquire certain skills and learn certain concepts at each level; therefore teaching methods have to match the level of development (Table 22.1).[2]

In addition to this developmental approach, principles of adult learning are crucial in the development of a curriculum that creates understanding and utilization of the competency domains by trainees and practitioners. Adult learning is fundamentally different from childhood learning because of the greater depth and breadth of experiences and knowledge on which adults build with new experiences.[3,4] In order to assimilate new information, adults must be able to integrate new ideas with what they already know, and information that conflicts with this knowledge may not be quickly integrated.[5] Adults have varied experiences and knowledge and do not all learn in the same way. They learn best when they are active participants in the learning process and are allowed to practice newly acquired skills and concepts,[4,6] and a multimodal approach to teaching with multiple exposures to content is more effective than any single approach or exposure method.

Adults are also self-directed and autonomous. As a consequence, education is typically most effective when programs facilitate self-learning with specific goals of acquiring practical information. Motivation for learning is both intrinsic (personal need for new knowledge or skill set) and extrinsic (professional expectations from colleagues or authority figures). Adults benefit from an appropriately challenging learning environment.[4,5] Finally, adult learners require and often seek out feedback, and they therefore learn more effectively when given timely feedback that reinforces newly acquired information.

ACGME Core Competencies

In 1999, the Accreditation Council for Graduate Medical Education (ACGME) initiated an outcome project to design a conceptual framework for education and training according to six general domains of competency.[7] The objective of the outcome project was to "ensure and improve the quality of graduate medical education (GME)."[8] The ACGME recommends that trainees demonstrate (1) *Patient care* that is compassionate, appropriate, and effective for the treatment of health problems and the promotion of health; (2) *medical knowledge* regarding established, as well as evolving,

TABLE 22.1	Dreyfus and Dreyfus Model of Skill Development Applied to the Development of a Competence in the Subspecialty of Critical Care Medicine	
Level of Learning and Characteristics	**Examples of Learner Level in Critical Care Medicine**	**Teaching Implications**
Novice: Rule driven Uses analytic reasoning and rules to link cause and effect Synthesis of information is based on knowledge acquired during residency training Big picture elusive	FIRST-YEAR FELLOW: Interviews patient and performs a physical exam that is focused on the critical illness May not be able to focus the information on the basis of a differential diagnosis Does not see the big picture	Teach basic critical care concepts Point out subtle but meaningful diagnostic information in the history and physical examination Eliminate irrelevant information Highlight discriminating features and their importance to the diagnosis Encourage reading about 2 diagnostic hypotheses at the same time
Advanced beginner: Sorts through rules and information to decide what is relevant on the basis of past experience Uses analytic reasoning and pattern recognition to solve problems Able to abstract from concrete and specific information to more general aspects of a problem	SECOND-YEAR FELLOW: Can generate more specific differential diagnosis while obtaining history and physical examination Capable of filtering relevant information to formulate a unified summary of the case Can abstract pertinent positives and negatives from the review of systems and incorporate them into the history of present illness	Expose learner to clinical cases proceeding from common to uncommon Emphasize the use of semantic qualifiers Encourage formulation and verbalization of differential diagnosis and treatment plan Good coaching: help learner become attentive to the meaningful pieces
Competent: Emotional buy-in allows learner to feel appropriate level of responsibility More expansive experience tips the balance on clinical reasoning from methodical and analytic to identifiable pattern recognition of common clinical problems Sees the big picture Complex/uncommon problems still require reliance on analytic reasoning	THIRD YEAR: Recognizes common patterns of illness based on previous encounters Sees consequences of clinical decisions, which leads to emotional buy-in to learning Will methodically attempt to reason through complex or uncommon problems Responsible for decision-making process	Balance supervision with autonomy in decision making Hold learners accountable for their decisions Do not tell them what to do; ask what they want to do Critical for learner to see a breadth and depth of patient encounters to construct and store in memory a large repertoire of illness scripts Tip the balance from clinical reasoning to pattern recognition
Proficient: Breadth of past experience allows reliance on pattern recognition of illness Problem-solving intuitive Still needs to fall back to methodical and analytic reasoning for managing problems because an exhaustive number of permutations and responses to management have provided less experience in this regard than in illness recognition Is comfortable with evolving situations, able to extrapolate from a known situation to an unknown situation Can live with ambiguity	CLINICAL INSTRUCTOR: Starts to match findings with those encountered in past experience Data gathering more effective and efficient Sees patient through different lens than the student Engages in process of clinical reasoning to find the best intervention	Needs to work alongside and be mentored by an expert Must develop capacity to know ones' limitations and step back and call on additional resources when stretched beyond one's capabilities
Expert: Thought, feeling, and action align into intuitive problem recognition and intuitive situational responses and management Open to notice the unexpected Clever Discriminates features that do not fit a recognizable pattern	ASSOCIATE PROFESSOR: Broad repertoire of illness scripts, based on clinical experience that allows immediate action for majority of clinical encounters Likes to deal with diagnostic dilemmas When presented with diagnostic dilemma, will slow down and look it up	Keep up the challenge Needs ongoing experience and ongoing exposure to interesting and complex cases to avoid complacency and to help transcend beyond this level Should be apprenticed to a master who models the skills of the reflective practitioner and a commitment to lifelong learning
Master: Exercises practical wisdom Goes beyond the big picture to that of culture and context of each situation Deep level of commitment to the work Great concern for right and wrong decisions that fosters emotional engagement Intensely motivated by emotional engagement to pursue ongoing learning and improvement Reflects in, on, and for action	ASSOCIATE PROFESSOR/ PROFESSOR: The clinician that everyone goes to with problem cases Recognizes subtle features of a current case reminiscent of cases seen over the years Painstakingly revisits past cases or identifies common thread that will help treat the current clinical problem Vision extends beyond individual practice Contributes to bigger context to improvements in the field Intense internal drive to learn and improve Practical wisdom	Self-motivated to engage in lifelong learning and practice improvement

Adapted from Carracccio CL, Benson BJ, Nixon LJ, Derstine PL. From the educational bench to the clinical bedside: translating the Dreyfus Developmental Model to the Learning of Clinical Skills. Acad Med. 2008;83:761-767.

biomedical, clinical, and cognitive sciences with the ability to apply these concepts to patient care; (3) *practice-based learning and improvement* involving self-evaluation with regard to patient care, appraisal, and utilization of scientific evidence; (4) *interpersonal and communication skills* that result in effective information exchange and partnership with patients, their families, and other health professionals; (5) *professionalism* manifested through a commitment to professional responsibilities, adherence to ethical principles, and sensitivity to a diverse patient population; and (6) an awareness of and responsiveness to the health care system and the ability to utilize system resources to provide optimal care in a *systems-based practice.*[7] These core domains of competency should be used to guide and coordinate evaluation of all residents or fellows in their development.[9]

Methods of Teaching

The quality of education in training programs is critical to fellow development. The importance of program quality was demonstrated in a study by Asch et al., which included almost 5 million deliveries performed by 4124 obstetricians from 107 residency programs in the United States.[10] The ranking (in five quintiles) for residency training programs was generated for the risk-adjusted maternal complications outcomes. In order to ensure that there was no residency selection bias, a secondary analysis was performed on data from medical licensure test scores obtained from the National Board of Medical Examiners and the Federation of State Medical Boards. The authors found that women treated by obstetricians who trained in programs in the bottom quintile had major maternal complication rates one third higher than those obstetricians who trained in programs in the top quintile.

Given the complexity of the intensive care unit (ICU) environment and the wide range of learners and educators, those in charge of education should consider the importance of the quality of teaching methods. The faculty members responsible for supervision in the ICU are the content experts and are also expected to be the facilitators/educators for all learners. To be an effective educator, there must be a clear understanding that a gap often exists between educators and learners regarding perceptions of adequate teaching and optimal teaching techniques.[11] One must overcome recognized barriers to education, which include lack of dedicated teaching time, high clinical workload, and lack of continuity between faculty and learners.[11-17] These factors are increasingly challenging in the current era of GME.[18]

Education in the ICU consists of teaching basic principles but should also include an ongoing, dynamic integration of new medical knowledge and technologic advances. In 2004, the Society for Critical Care Medicine released *Guidelines for Critical Care Medicine Training and Continuing Medical Education,* which addressed the needs of physician education in critical care medicine on a continuum from the resident to the intensivist. Table 22.2 demonstrates the broad scope of educational objectives for critical care medicine fellows and intensivists and includes two broad areas of learning: clinical and administrative.

Teaching tools should be designed and selected to optimize improvement of both physician performance and health care outcomes, and curricular development should focus on development of effective programs that include sequenced and multifaceted activities.[6] A review that evaluated 37 studies of

TABLE 22.2	Methods Used in the Education of Physicians
Teaching Method	**%**
Bedside, case-based teaching	94.4
Lecture series	79.0
Morbidity and mortality conference	72.6
Syllabus of articles	63.7
Journal club	62.9
Multidisciplinary rounds	60.5
Rounding sheets	58.1
Web-based articles	29.0
Psychomotor skills laboratories	24.0
Full-body simulator	15.3
Cadaver/animal laboratories	8.1
Computer simulation	4.8
Palm pilot algorithms	3.2
Standardized patients	3.2

Adapted from Chudgar SM, Cox CE, Que LG, et al. Current teaching and evaluation methods in critical care medicine: has the Accreditation Council for Graduate Medical Education affected how we practice and teach in the intensive care unit? Crit Care Med. 2009;37:49-60.

continuing medical education activities demonstrated that the use of multiple media, a variety of instructional techniques, and exposures to content to meet instructional objectives are all needed to improve clinical outcomes.[19] A recent review of techniques in critical care demonstrates the importance and benefit of multiple interactive strategies[20] that apply principles of adult learning. A survey of critical care medicine program directors across several specialties (pediatrics, surgery, internal medicine, and anesthesia) was conducted to determine current teaching methods, and these are summarized in Table 22.3.[21] In this survey, the most common teaching technique in the ICU was bedside, case-based teaching, with 80% of programs spending at least 2 hours a day on this activity. Eleven program directors planned on implementing computer or human patient simulation (45%), and 50% would also incorporate web-based learning modules, which also have been shown to be effective.[22] Debriefing is another teaching strategy that is commonly integrated into simulation-based education and is increasingly being used within the context of clinical care in the ICU to teach important principles. A debrief is a review of a situation led by an experienced facilitator to allow learners to explore steps that went well and identify opportunities for improvement and learning.[23] Another survey of PCCM program directors demonstrated that faculty role modeling is the most common technique used in pediatric critical care programs to teach the competencies of professionalism and communication.[24]

Some methods of teaching are particularly important in the ICU. These include case-based learning and experiential learning, both of which are based on principles of adult learning. Case-based learning uses scenarios or cases to address a particular curricular element and can be applied individually or in small group discussions. A faculty member who has the expertise to stimulate participants to think about the

TABLE 22.3   Essential Clinical and Administrative Learning Points

Clinical	Administrative
Identify and teach others to identify the need for/provide care for all critically ill patients.	Evaluate ICU policies and suggest improvements.
Provide and teach others resuscitation for any patient sustaining a life-threatening event.	Triage critically ill patients to optimize care delivery within the institution.
Initiate, manage, and wean patients from mechanical ventilation and teach others new methods and devices for management of respiratory failure.	Improve resource utilization and maintain patient care quality by facilitating triage of patients to limited institutional critical care beds and caregivers.
Initiate critical care to stabilize and manage patients who require transport.	Develop programs and change unit practice to improve care of critically ill patients.
Instruct other qualified caregivers and the lay public in the theory and techniques of CPR.	Develop programs for patient safety monitoring and error reduction.
Treat cardiogenic, traumatic, hypovolemic, and distributive shock with conventional and state-of-the-art approaches.	Actively participate in quality assurance processes, including morbidity and mortality conferences, process improvement teams, and the Joint Commission preparation.
Recognize potential for multiple organ failure and institute measures to avoid or reverse this syndrome.	Support the process of assessing patient and family satisfaction and participate in tool development and implementation.
Identify life-threatening electrolyte/acid-base disturbances and provide treatment/monitor outcome.	Encourage and enhance good relationships with other health care providers.
Identify and initiate discussions involving ethical issues and parent/patients' wishes in making treatment decisions, using advance directives, and other methods.	Understand advanced concepts important for compensation of critical care services and contractual issues related to providing critical care services and performing the business of medicine.
Diagnose and treat common and uncommon poisonings.	Develop skills for teaching critical care.
Teach appropriate use and monitoring of procedural sedation and use advanced pain management strategies.	Develop and evaluate curriculum changes for ICU caregivers, fellows, and residents.
Diagnose malnutrition and use/monitor advanced nutrition support methodologies.	Evaluate, modify, and approve ICU hospital policies.
Provide invasive and noninvasive monitoring for titrating therapy. Prioritize complex data to support action plan.	Improve resource utilization and maintain patient care quality by planning for future needs for institutional and regional critical care resources.
Use and teach medication safe practice guidelines and determine cost-effectiveness of therapeutic interventions.	Develop programs and change unit, institution, and regional practice to improve care of critically ill patients.
Develop skills of ICU nurses and ancillary personnel in caring for critically ill patients and provide in-service education.	Use existing tool sets to assess patient and family satisfaction and direct the development of new tools when appropriate.
Use, teach, and help enforce methods of infection control.	Develop programs and document improvement in patient safety monitoring and error reduction.
Communicate effectively with patients, families, and other involved members of the health care team about all treatment decisions and patient prognosis.	Develop high-quality relationships with other health care providers.
Continue to augment knowledge by assimilating peer-reviewed published medical literature through self-directed learning and CME activities.	Teach the business of medicine.
Diagnose and treat a sufficient number of patients with critical illness using conventional and state-of-the-art approaches to maintain clinical proficiencies.	Develop collaborative and productive relationships with other specialist physicians and model joint clinical planning in managing complex ICU problems.

Adapted from Dorman T, Angood PB, Angus DC, et al. Guidelines for critical care medicine training and continuing medical education. Crit Care Med. 2004;32:263-272.

knowledge and skills necessary to "solve" the case and eventually apply that to future practice generally leads the discussion.

Experiential learning is thought to be one of the most important ways by which medical students, residents, and fellows acquire clinical knowledge and skills. Kolb[25] and Atherton[26] described experiential learning as a cycle composed of four stages that include concrete experience, reflection, abstract conceptualization, and active experimentation. Concrete experience or knowledge by acquaintance is where the

learner is directly exposed to something and then reflects on what the experience means to him. Subsequently, the learner can apply theories that he or she has learned and use this information to modify his or her approach to future clinical encounters.

Teaching at the Patient's Bedside

In 1968, Reichman et al. demonstrated a 75% "incidence" of teaching at the bedside during attending rounds.[27] That number had declined to 16% in 1978[28] and may be lower today. Almost 20 years ago, LaCombe[29] expressed concerns about bedside teaching that remain today. "Profound advances in technology, in imaging, and laboratory testing and our fascination for these aspects of patient care, account for part of this decline, but faculty must also assume responsibility for the present lack of bedside teaching. If we are to reverse this trend, we will need to realize the barriers to bedside teaching, both real and imagined, and overcome them. And if we are to become effective bedside teachers, as were our mentors, we will need to sharpen our own physical diagnostic skills. We will need to learn how to be gentle with students and house staff, how to better communicate with patients, and how to teach ethics and professionalism with the patient at hand."

Very few data exist on the frequency of bedside teaching in the ICU in the modern era of medical education. Experiential learning and case-based learning at the bedside are traditionally thought to be the most effective means of educating clinicians in the understanding of disease processes and evaluation and management of critically ill patients. The impact of experiential learning at the bedside caring for a patient with fulminant meningococcemia and purpura fulminans is extremely valuable and difficult to quantify. Less dramatic but potentially equally effective are instances when one palpates a thrill, hears a gallop, feels an enlarged liver or spleen, listens to wheezing or stridor, or performs a detailed neurologic examination in a patient who has experienced a stroke or a spinal cord injury. Medical technology can be leveraged to enhance bedside teaching, as when flow-volume loops in a child with asthma are used to teach the principles of mechanical ventilation in the setting of bronchospasm or the waveforms on bedside monitors allow a demonstration of the impact of ventilation on hemodynamics. Showing learners extracorporeal membrane oxygenation circuits, continuous venovenous hemodialysis and ultrafiltration machines, high-frequency ventilators, and ventricular assist devices while they are being used in patient care reinforces prior learning and may provide the "aha" moment that is difficult to recreate in didactic lectures.

In addition, when trainees present the historical data and physical findings of their patients to the attending physician and the team during bedside rounds, they can be taught to describe the information relating to their patients in a succinct manner and discriminate between important and less important information, develop a list of differential diagnoses, and formulate a treatment plan. Bedside and experiential learning teach the important skill of "thinking on their feet," which will assist in their drawing correct conclusions regarding diagnosis and making management decisions. Bedside teaching and rounds are also important for the demonstration and role-modeling of professionalism (see also Chapter 2).

In the current era of limited duty hours and excessive time required for electronic medical recordkeeping, the focus on teaching and care of the patient at the bedside is sometimes lost.[30,31] However, it is important to remember that patients are often our best teachers, and developing into an outstanding practitioner hinges on exposure to a large and varied number of clinical situations to develop all of the domains of competency.

Procedural Training

Procedural expertise is crucial in the care of critically ill children. Specific skills that must be acquired during fellowship include peripheral arterial and venous catheterization, central venous catheterization, endotracheal intubation, thoracostomy tube placement, and procedural sedation (see Chapters 19 and 20).[32] In addition, knowledge of the indications, techniques, limitations, and complications of other procedures including cricothyroidotomy, tracheostomy, pericardiocentesis, and abdominal paracentesis is recommended.[33,34] Wide-ranging approaches to teaching procedures include didactics, video- and web-based training, and simulation. Regardless of the specific techniques implemented, initial performance under direct supervision is paramount, with progressive development of autonomy through the course of fellowship training.

Simulation Training

Simulation training is an interactive technique used to replicate real-world situations and experiences.[35] Historically, medical skills were developed by practicing on animals and cadavers, and sometimes this "practice" even occurred on actual patients. However, concerns regarding patient safety, quality of care, and ethics, along with advances in simulation technology, have led to a substantial increase in the use of simulation in medical education.[36-38] Modern medical simulation originated in the early 1960s with simple resuscitation manikins that were used in the field of anesthesiology, and this technique has both expanded and evolved substantially over time. Technologic advances in computer programming and manikin development, as well as increased affordability, have contributed to increasing use of this educational modality.[39]

Medical simulation can be generally divided into five different categories: role play, standardized patients, partial task trainers, computerized patients, and electronic patients. The most comprehensive form of simulation training is the electronic patient or high-fidelity, instructor-driven manikin.[35] These manikins are programmed to display normal and abnormal physical examination findings. The training session is divided into three sections: prebriefing, scenario exercise, and debriefing. Debriefing plays an important role in the educational process and allows the instructor to reemphasize the objectives of the exercise and address knowledge gaps that may have been unmasked during the scenario, and it allows the trainees to reflect on performance and discuss areas for improvement.[40-43]

Simulation training in medical education has gained widespread acceptance as a result of the ease of simulating critical events, safety of the learning environment, and reproducibility of the clinical scenarios.[44] Learners practice and develop skills without the consequences of negative patient outcomes. For procedures that are performed infrequently, simulation allows repeated opportunities to practice. Scenarios can be created to simulate a range of complications that the learner might otherwise not witness or experience. Recent evidence demonstrates that learners enjoy participation in medical simulation, and individual and team member performance are enhanced. In addition, self-confidence, knowledge, and operational performance improves with simulation training.[45-48] Some centers have implemented intense simulation-based orientation training for first-year pediatric critical care medicine fellows.

Other novel approaches for procedural training include senior pediatric resident–led mock code curricula use of "action-linked phrases" and real-time feedback during simulation.[49-51] Simulation-based medical education with deliberate practice to attain constant skill improvement is superior to traditional clinical education for acquisition of a wide range of medical skills.[52]

In-Situ Simulation

The ICU is a highly dynamic setting with complex patients and frequent high-risk situations and invasive procedures that need a well-functioning multidisciplinary team. In-situ portable simulation provides the added advantage of replicating the true working environment of the ICU. The learners are placed in the patient care setting and have the opportunity to use the actual equipment within the environment in which they work. In-situ simulation has been used to identify safety threats and reinforce resource location and teamwork behaviors.[53] It allows multidisciplinary team training in the setting of their clinical work.[54]

From the traditional code team to the performance of high-risk procedures, personnel must work together to accomplish many tasks. Training in teamwork and communication, known as Crew (or Crisis) Resource Management (CRM), was developed and implemented in the aviation industry to reduce or eliminate the contribution of human errors to catastrophic events. These principles have been adapted for use in anesthesia crisis management protocols and focus on competent team management, dynamic decision making, interpersonal behavior, situational awareness, effective use of resources, and stress management.[55] CRM training improves team functioning and dynamics in pediatric intensive care settings.[56-58] Clinical skills acquired during medical simulation have been shown to directly improve patient care practices and may improve patient outcomes.[44]

The effects of simulation on patient outcomes are more difficult to quantify due to multiple confounding factors. However, refresher training and practice for central venous catheter maintenance care on manikins and patients were associated with fewer central line–associated bloodstream infections in one pediatric intensive care unit (PICU).[59] The introduction of a pediatric medical emergency team with concurrent simulation team training was associated with improvements in patient outcomes related to more rapid recognition and timely management of patients with clinical deterioration.[60] A simulation-based mock code curriculum for pediatric residents has been associated with subsequently improved survival rates in children who required cardiopulmonary resuscitation.[61]

Additional studies are needed to identify the optimal modality, frequency of exposure, quality of assessment tools, and impact of simulation education on patient care. A multicenter pediatric network (International Network for Simulation-based Innovation, Research, and Education [INSPIRE]) has been formed to measure the impact of simulation on clinical outcomes. Despite some limitations, simulation training remains an important adjunct to traditional medical education in the ICU.

Web-Based Education

In recent years, online and web-based approaches to education have continued to become more prominent and are especially important for the current generation of learners.[62,63] Numerous resources that use technology for both content and process are available for learners. Information is now readily available and can be accessed from computers, tablets, and smart phones[64] including traditional textbooks and materials and a wide range of specifically developed online tools such as "podcasts," online modules, and complete online courses. Web-based distance education programs have been created, an example of which is OPENPediatrics, which is focused on bringing pediatric critical care education to the global community.[64] The "flipped" classroom approach to education wherein the learner engages in self-study before a classroom session to apply and consolidate learning is becoming more prominent as it often better meets the complex scheduling needs of learners in medicine.[62,63,65]

Teaching Professionalism

Professionalism is one of the competency domains used by ACGME and American Board of Pediatrics (ABP) and is arguably one of the most highly valued attributes of the accomplished clinician (see also Chapter 2). The first challenge is to arrive at a common definition, taking into account the complex culture of the PICU with its diverse interprofessional teams, encompassing different disciplines (nurse, intensivist, surgeon, pharmacist, etc.), hierarchies, and generations (baby boomers, Gen X, Millennials), as well as personal characteristics of the many individuals (individual personalities, experiences, and culture).

Professionalism incorporates mutual trust, as the patient must trust the clinician, the clinician trust the patient, clinicians trust each other, and all trust the system in which they practice. Moreover, professionalism requires self-insight as one is continually required to assess personal responses to the challenges of critical care practice and reflect on the interrelatedness of experiences at work and in one's personal life. Most importantly, professionalism is a continuum, for just as our understanding of character and integrity develops throughout our lifespan, the application of these attributes to professional practice also matures over time. The ACGME definition of professionalism incorporates the attributes of altruism, compassion, honesty, and integrity. Ethics, accountability, and respect are also counted among the core values of professionalism. Taken together, professionalism is a social contract wherein the professional pledges a duty to service over self-interest.[66-78]

Can professionalism be taught? The answer is an emphatic yes, and not only can it be taught, it must be taught. In the absence of a formal curriculum, these principles will be taught by the so-called hidden curriculum, which is a well-described phenomenon composed of the unwritten rules and assumptions, behaviors and attitudes, and accepted norms that are transmitted through informal interactions and hallway conversations. This hidden curriculum may be a powerful force for acculturation and exert a subtext even in the presence of a rigorous curriculum. That subtext may support or undermine the formal curriculum. For example, the principle that all patients should be treated with respect may be negated if derogatory comments about certain groups are common. To successfully teach professionalism, there must be explicitly articulated goals and expectations, as well as specific experiences through which to explore and apply key values, with sufficient guided reflection to integrate the concepts. A number of surveys and assessments have demonstrated that role modeling is one of the principal methods by which professionalism is taught, but this approach more likely reflects a reliance on ad hoc experiential learning. In fact, the identification of a role model rests with the learner, who recognizes someone as an exemplar whose behavior should be emulated.

More commonly, the resident or fellow is expected to learn professionalism by watching the behaviors of his or her faculty, but this is inadequate if done without intentionality and a mindful reflection of a given clinical encounter. At a minimum, faculty should take trainees aside after a variety of clinical encounters to reflect on what went well and what could improve. It is also important to note that a wide range of approaches including interactive seminars, standardized patients, reflective writing, and others can be successfully applied to teaching professionalism.

Professionalism can also be evaluated, and a variety of outcomes can be used to assess the impact of a specific curriculum. Some of these outcomes reflect everyday mundane activities but provide a sense of responsibility and accountability, such as timeliness of completing requests or replying to queries. Others are more difficult to quantify, but multisource feedback from interprofessional team members and families is helpful.

The concept of professionalism has evolved with time, societal changes, and changes in health care delivery, and this evolution will continue. Limitations on trainee duty hours have led to concerns regarding the balance between trainee self-care and limited patient contact time, potentially undermining trusting relationships. External events and forces, such as the proper role for social media, will also require continual consideration of appropriate professional behavior. Notwithstanding these challenges, medicine has moved beyond an implied assumption that professionalism is a given and now recognizes that it must be a focus of education and development throughout one's career.

Education in Research, Scholarship, and Leadership

Education in research and scholarship is an integral component of becoming a pediatric intensivist, as evidenced by the requirement for meaningful scholarly activity for board certification by the ABP and emphasis on faculty scholarly activity as a key component for fellowship program accreditation by the ACGME. Research in pediatric critical care is discussed in detail in Chapter 7, but education in this area should include a breadth of experiences. In addition to teaching basic techniques for laboratory and clinical investigation, research curricula should include conducting an efficient literature review, understanding evidence-based medicine techniques, presenting scientific findings, and medical writing. Trainees should not only learn these important skills but also begin developing techniques and approaches to teaching them.

In addition to research and scholarship, the pediatric intensivist has a central role in the education of his or her peers and team members while also managing ICUs and coordinating teams who provide multidisciplinary care to critically ill patients (see also Chapters 3 and 5). Leadership skills are crucial for every intensivist in both informal experiences (rounds, daily management of the ICU, crisis management) and formal administrative roles (committee chairs, medical director) (see also Chapter 2). In spite of these common leadership roles of intensivists in the ICU and hospital environment, specific curricula within training programs are often lacking.[79] A recent survey of multidisciplinary PICU team members demonstrated significant variation in the perceived importance of various leadership qualities for a pediatric intensivist. The field of leadership science is well developed outside of medicine, and education in this area represents an

opportunity for research to determine how the myriad leadership theories and models apply to the ICU environment and the pediatric intensivist.

Education in Safety and Quality for Learning and Patient Care

While medical errors have been attributed to the fatigue of residents,[80] this is only one of many contributing factors. Others include lack of supervision, deficiencies in transitions in care, lack of education related to quality improvement, and issues related to the lack of professionalism. A survey conducted by the American Hospital Association[81] found that there is a significant deficiency in communication, systems-based practice, and interprofessional teamwork in recent graduates of training programs. The Institute of Medicine report "To Err is Human" stated that errors are more commonly caused by system-related factors that led to either mistakes or the failure to prevent them. It is therefore imperative that the educational curricula of residents and fellows include an integrated approach to address the six focus areas recently outlined by the ACGME Clinical Learning Environment Review process (Table 22.4). When residents and fellows learn the principles in safety and quality and integrate them into their work during training, it is highly likely that they will include these principles in their everyday practice long after the completion of training (see also Chapter 11).

Evaluation and Assessment of Competency

Epstein and Hundert[82] define competence as the "habitual and judicious use of communication, knowledge, technical skills, clinical reasoning, emotions, values, and reflection in daily practice for the benefit of the individual and community being served." They further state that "competence builds on a foundation of basic clinical skills, scientific knowledge and moral development" and propose that competence is made up of

TABLE 22.4	Patient Safety and Quality Improvement Focus Areas
Focus Area	**Opportunities for Education**
Patient safety	Reporting errors, unsafe conditions, and near-misses; participation in interprofessional teams to promote and enhance safe care
Health care quality	Involvement in institutional efforts to improve systems of care, reduce health care disparities, and improve patient outcomes
Transitions in care	Effective standardization and oversight of transitions of care
Supervision	Appropriate-level specific supervision
Fatigue management and mitigation	Oversight of duty hours, fatigue management, and mitigation and effect education with regard to fatigue recognition and mitigation
Professionalism	Behavior of residents, fellows, and faculty members in fulfilling educational and other responsibilities; truthfulness in scholarly activities; ethical and respectful treatment of patients

From Clinical Learning Environment Review. Available at: http://www.acgme.org/acgmeweb/Portals/0/PDFs/CLER/CLER_Brochure.pdf.

several dimensions, each with a separate set of skills. Over time, a range of assessments has been utilized, including subjective assessment by supervisors, multiple choice examinations to evaluate factual knowledge and abstract problem-solving, and standardized patient assessments of physical examination and technical and communication skills. More recently, there is an increasing use of simulation-based assessment of competency. However, the evaluation of the ability to apply knowledge to patient care, the capability of working as a team member, and the development of physician-patient relationships can only be assessed by direct observation of real-life patient interactions. Pangaro[83] summarizes the issue of assessing competence very well: "The assessment of competence requires a whole series of performances that, in each moment of interaction with a patient, the competent physician must bring many qualities to bear, and what they will require varies from patient to patient."

Milestones

In order to fulfill the promise of the Outcome Project[84] to use educational outcome data in accreditation, milestones assessments in each specialty were developed by the ACGME in close collaboration with the members of the Review Committees, American Board of Medical Specialties (ABMS) certifying boards, medical specialty organizations, program director associations, and residents. Milestones describe the performance levels residents and fellows are expected to demonstrate for skills, knowledge, and behaviors in the six competency domains. They provide a framework of observable behaviors and attributes associated with the development of residents and fellows as physicians (Table 22.5, sample milestones template). The use of milestones assessment has a number of benefits for residents and fellows, and these include increased transparency of performance requirements by more explicit expectations, better feedback, and enhanced opportunities for early identification of underperformers.

Mentorship

And so it's been for me these long years. I've carried my mentor everywhere. If I get sloppy, I wonder "What would he think of me now?" And if I'm in a tight spot clinically, he prods me back to the literature. When I'm impatient with patients, I remember his patience with me. When I'm asked to teach, I do so willingly because that is what he did. When I begin to doubt myself, I remember his belief in me. And if I am ready to quit, I can see him standing there before me in his long white coat, with stern look and stethoscope, and I go on. What has he been for me, this mentor of mine? He's been like a father to me, but more than a father. He has been my companion in medicine, to help me through the loneliness that medicine can bring and to share with me the joy that medicine can be. My mentor has, through me and those of my students, cared decently and compassionately for countless patients. When I have cured a patient or two, why, so has he.

Michael A. LaCombe, MD, FACP
William Morgan Teaching Symposium,
University of Rochester, July 20, 1989

Mentorship is defined as a "dynamic, reciprocal relationship in a work environment between an advanced career incumbent (mentor) and a beginner (protégé), aimed at promoting the development of both."[85] Mentorship is at the core of the training of medical students, residents, and fellows in patient care, research, and education. While the benefits to the mentee are often emphasized, it is clear that mentors benefit as well[86,87] as they tend to have greater satisfaction in their careers. Mentorship takes place at many levels. It may begin during medical school where a mentor guides and even inspires a student to choose a certain career path. During fellowship, a mentor can be a major contributor to the development of the trainee's clinical knowledge and patient care skills. In addition, if the fellow decides to pursue a career that includes research, the

---

TABLE 22.5   Sample Template for Milestones Reporting

GATHERS AND SYNTHESIZES ESSENTIAL AND ACCURATE INFORMATION TO DEFINE EACH PATIENT'S CLINICAL PROBLEM(S). (PC1)

Critical Deficiencies			Ready for Unsupervised Practice	Aspirational
Does not collect accurate historical data. Does not use physical examination to confirm history. Relies exclusively on documentation of others to generate own database or differential diagnosis. Fails to recognize patient's central clinical problems. Fails to recognize potentially life-threatening problems.	Inconsistently able to acquire accurate historical information in an organized fashion. Does not perform an appropriately thorough physical examination or misses key physical examination findings. Does not seek or is overly reliant on secondary data. Inconsistently recognizes patients' central clinical problem or develops limited differential diagnoses.	Consistently acquires accurate and relevant histories from patients. Seeks and obtains data from secondary sources when needed. Consistently performs accurate and appropriately thorough physical examinations. Uses collected data to define a patient's central clinical problem(s).	Acquires accurate histories from patients in an efficient, prioritized, and hypothesis-driven fashion. Performs accurate physical examinations that are targeted to the patient's complaints. Synthesizes data to generate a prioritized differential diagnosis and problem list. Effectively uses history and physical examination skills to minimize the need for further diagnostic testing.	Obtains relevant historical subtleties, including sensitive information that informs the differential diagnosis. Identifies subtle or unusual physical examination findings. Efficiently uses all sources of secondary data to inform differential diagnosis. Models and teaches the effective use of history and physical examination skills to minimize the need for further diagnostic testing.

PC1: Patient Care Competency 1
Available at: http://www.acgme.org/acgmeweb/tabid/430/ProgramandInstitutionalAccreditation/NextAccreditationSystem/Milestones.aspx.

mentor can help identify a research focus and provide guidance in the entire process. For junior faculty members, mentorship provides opportunities to fine-tune clinical skills and diagnostic and therapeutic acumen. Research productivity is further enhanced by guidance in conducting basic science experiments and clinical trials, presenting findings, writing manuscripts, and obtaining extramural grant support. The mentor can help academic development of junior faculty members by sponsoring them for local, state, and national presentations or committee memberships and enlisting them as coauthors for book chapters and review articles. Mentorship in teaching is important as well. The mentor can help fellows and junior faculty members develop teaching skills by serving as an example and providing critique of teaching methods.

Although the importance of mentorship in academic development is clear, the process of finding the right mentor and developing the mentor-mentee relationship is altogether much more difficult. First, the mentee must decide his or her current and best sense of future goals before searching for his or her mentor. Junior faculty members should be provided with resources such as lists of senior faculty members who have successfully provided mentorships and what their areas of interest are. They should meet with many members of the department to determine who might be the best match. If no one in the department seems to fit that role, the mentee may need to look beyond his or her home institution. Perseverance is essential. Sometimes more than one mentor is necessary: One might serve as a clinical mentor and another for research activities. A forum should be available to junior faculty members to discuss their academic needs and concerns. Occasionally, when the mentoring relationship does not work out, the mentee should be allowed to seek out other mentors without being made to feel that it is wrong to do so. Academic departments should also foster mentorship by providing support for mentors including faculty development courses and recognition for their efforts.

Requirements

American Board of Pediatrics

The required elements for the education and training of pediatric intensivists in patient care have been defined over time and continue to evolve (see Chapter 1 for the history of the specialty). The ABP and sub-board of the Pediatric Critical Care Medicine have developed a list of content specifications for the subspecialty examination. This list is not intended to serve as a curriculum, but the pediatric intensivist sitting for the examination is expected to be familiar with more than 2000 items categorized into subsections and updated as the specialty evolves (https://www.abp.org/sites/abp/files/pdf/crit2010.pdf). To qualify for the ABP subspecialty examination, applicants are required to have a valid unrestricted allopathic and/or osteopathic license to practice, initial certification in general pediatrics, and successful completion of critical care medicine training in a program accredited by the ACGME. The applicant must also provide evidence of meaningful research during training.

Following initial certification, the Maintenance of Certification (MOC) program ensures that the intensivist invests in ongoing knowledge and skills necessary for the delivery of quality care. MOC is based on six competency domains that are evaluated during fellowship training and includes four parts: Part I—professional standing (medical license); Part II—lifelong learning and self-assessment; Part III—passing an examination; and Part IV—performance in practice with participation in ABP-approved quality improvement activities in patient care. Lifelong learning and MOC are detailed in Chapter 23).

Accreditation Council for Graduate Medical Education

Pediatric Critical Care Medicine is one of the subspecialties accredited by the ACGME. Accreditation and oversight for the training programs are provided by the ACGME Pediatric Review Committee. Program accreditation centers on the six competency domains noted earlier in this chapter, which were developed by the ACGME and the ABMS. These domains of competence are designed to provide a framework for education and training of fellows. In addition, meaningful scholarship by faculty members and fellows, requisite faculty credentials, and appropriate faculty-to-fellow ratio are components of accreditation. Program faculty must have an active role in the training program and research productivity. Fellowship training requirements include but are not limited to defined patient variety and numbers, with an adequate opportunity to develop procedural competence, a didactic curriculum that is comprehensive and regularly implemented, formal education related to developing teaching skills, and evaluation of competency.

Maintaining Competency After Training

In reviewing ratings of performance, Williams and colleagues[88] quote the work of Kane, defining clinical competence as embodying aspects of knowledge, skills, and judgment referable to the situation under observation but also generalizable to similar clinical situations. From this perspective, the six competency domains form a useful framework by which the practicing clinician may structure self-directed education and a program to integrate reflective practice into all aspects of professional development.

Medical knowledge and patient care encompass foundational knowledge, technical facility, and professional judgment. The conventional means to assess knowledge is through a certification examination. Technical competence may be assessed indirectly, such as through chart reviews, resource utilization, or case logs, or directly, including videos of patient encounters, standardized patients, and skills labs. The latter, while often used for trainees, is not practical for practicing physicians. Another approach is the establishment of a minimum number of procedures to be completed, but the number is usually set by consensus expert opinion and rarely validated. Arbitrary numeric standards disregard the variability in rates of acquisition and maintenance of skills between individuals. With any method, the data used to assess competence must meet several standards: The information must be accurate; observers and interpreters must agree on the implications of the findings; the observations must apply to a range of situations; and the tools must be feasible to use.[88] Once a skill is acquired, several factors influence maintenance of competency, including repetition, exposure to the procedure in different clinical situations, overall technical facility, and clinical judgment. Clinical judgment skills embody tangible and intangible qualities, including knowing when to perform or defer a procedure and recognizing when conditions deviate from the expected.[88]

Medical judgment in actual practice requires the application of knowledge to complex clinical situations, which rarely reflect the idealized descriptions of textbook medicine. Research in medical decision making shows that two major modes enter into these decisions.[89,90] Croskerry describes two phenotypes,[89,90] one of which is "intuitive, automatic, fast, frugal, and effortless." An example might be pattern recognition that a patient is following an expected trajectory of illness. A second approach described by the same author is "analytical, deliberate, slower, costly, and effortful,[90] for example, the classic diagnostic dilemma, where critical pieces of data are not concordant with our assumptions regarding the disease process. Unfortunately, it is human nature to undervalue information that differs from our preordained conclusions and to overvalue confirmatory information. The experienced clinician is ever vigilant for misapplying System 1 style when more cautious analysis is warranted, or vice versa.[89,90] Encouraging fellows to develop this habit of vigilance is challenging but essential.

The competency domains of practice-based learning and systems-based practice serve as a framework to reflect on one's clinical experiences and refine both thought patterns. The most common forum for this approach is morbidity and mortality conference where the context in which decisions were made is an essential part of the review.[91-94] However, many other opportunities exist, including, among others, daily rounds and case-based education sessions.

Communication is often cited as the most important factor in both good and bad outcomes. While good communication is sometimes believed to be an innate personality characteristic, communication skills can be taught, and one's life experiences can lead to more active, empathetic listening and responses (see also Chapter 4).[92,95]

The end of formal training as a fellow represents the beginning of a lifelong process of obtaining and refining one's knowledge and judgment, constituting the essence of professional development and maintenance of competency. While the medical profession and society at large have historically assumed physician proficiency by virtue of their continued practice, it is dangerous to assume that longevity is tantamount to expertise. Instead, the mature clinician is one who reflects upon his or her daily medical experiences to place him or her in a larger context of previous encounters; critically evaluates his or her own performance, acknowledging both effective and ineffective aspects of patient care; and seeks to fill in gaps in knowledge or performance.[43,47]

Critical care is practiced in an atmosphere of innate uncertainty. In this environment the practicing intensivist must be able to adapt "on the fly" and also, once a situation is resolved, to step back and pursue generalizable knowledge for the next encounter.

Another aspect of lifelong learning is the role teaching plays in ongoing self-directed learning. By reviewing and synthesizing contemporary literature, whether for a didactic lecture or for family and patient information, the seasoned intensivist creates an opportunity to address all aspects of professional development.

The ABP has incorporated this template of professional development into its Maintenance of Certification program. Over time the framework of the six competency domains will become an integral part of ongoing professional development. Rather than viewing these as administrative hurdles, the wise clinician may view them as reminders of the many facets of professionalism and learning that medical practice requires (see also Chapter 23).

Acknowledgment

We gratefully acknowledge the contribution of Drs. Melinda Fiedor Hamilton and Kevin M. Valentine, who coauthored this chapter in previous editions.

Key References

1. Dreyfus SE, Dreyfus HL. *A five stage model of the mental activities involved in direct skill acquisition (Air Force Office of Scientific Research under contract F49620-79-C-0063)*. Berkeley, CA: University of California; 1980 <http://oai.dtic.mil/oai?verb=getRecord&metadataPrefix=htm&identifier=ADA084551>. Accessed 21.11.09.
2. Carraccio CL, Benson BJ, Nixon LJ, Derstine PL. From the educational bench to the clinical bedside: translating the Dreyfus Developmental Model to the learning of clinical skills. *Acad Med*. 2008;83:761-767.
3. O'Brien G. What are the principles of adult learning? Available at: <www.southernhealth.org.au/meu/articles/adult-learning.htm>. Accessed 29.09.09.
4. Collins J. Education techniques for lifelong learning principles of adult learning. *Radiographics*. 2004;24:1483-1489.
10. Asch DA, Nicholson S, Srinivas S, et al. Evaluating obstetrical residency programs using patient outcomes. *JAMA*. 2009;302:1277-1283.
13. Wilkerson L, Irby DM. Strategies for improving teaching practices: a comprehensive approach to faculty development. *Acad Med*. 1998;73: 387-396.
14. Srinivasan M, Li ST, Meyers FJ, et al. "Teaching as competency": competencies for medical educators. *Acad Med*. 2011;86:1211-1220.
15. Turner DA, Narayan AP, Whicker SA, et al. Do pediatric residents prefer interactive learning? Educational challenges in the duty hours era. *Med Teach*. 2011;33:494-496.
17. Vaughn L, Baker R. Do different pairings of teaching styles and learning styles make a difference? Preceptor and resident perceptions. *Teach Learn Med*. 2008;20:239-247.
20. Tainter CR, Wong NL, Bittner EA. Innovative strategies in critical care education. 2015; doi: <http://dx.doi.org/10.1016/j.jcrc.2015.02.001>.
21. Chudgar SM, Cox CE, Que LG, et al. Current teaching and evaluation methods in critical care medicine: has the accreditation council for graduate medical education affected how we practice and teach in the intensive care unit? *Crit Care Med*. 2009;37:49-60.
23. Clay A, Que L, Petrusa E, et al. Debriefing in the intensive care unit: a feedback tool to facilitate bedside teaching. *Crit Care Med*. 2007;35: 738-754.
24. Turner DA, Mink RB, Lee KJ, et al. Are pediatric critical care medicine fellowships teaching and evaluating communication and professionalism? *Pediatr Crit Care Med*. 2013;14:454-461.
25. Kolb DA. Experiential learning: experience as the source of learning and development. Available at: <http://www.learningfromexperience.com/images/uploads/process-of-experiential-learning.pdf> (local filename: kolb84 Kolb Experiential learning. Pdf).
30. Block L, Habicht R, Wu AW, et al. In the wake of the 2003 duty hours regulations, how do internal medicine interns spend their time? *J Gen Intern Med*. 2013;28:1042-1047.
31. Fletcher KE, Visotcky AM, Slagle JM, et al. The composition of intern work while on call. *J Gen Intern Med*. 2012;27:1432-1437.
34. American College of Critical Care Medicine of the Society of Critical Care Medicine. Guidelines for advanced training for physicians in critical care. *Crit Care Med*. 1997;25:1601-1607.
37. Mileder LP. Addressing patient safety through dedicated simulation-based training. *Am J Med*. 2014;127:e25.
38. Institute of Medicine Committee on Quality of Health Care in America. In: Kohn LT, Corrigan JM, Donaldson MS, eds. *To Err Is Human: Building a Safer Health System*. Washington, DC: National Academies Press (US); 1999.
40. Rudolph JW, Simon R, Raemer DB, Eppich WJ. Debriefing as formative assessment: closing performance gaps in medical education. *Acad Emerg Med*. 2008;15:1010-1016.

42. Savoldelli GL, Naik VN, Park J, et al. Value of debriefing during simulated crisis management: oral versus video-assisted oral feedback. *Anesthesiology*. 2006;105:279-285.

43. Cheng A, Hunt EA, Donoghue A, et al. Examining pediatric resuscitation education using simulation and scripted debriefing: a multicenter randomized trial. *JAMA Pediatr*. 2013;167:528-536.

44. Cook DA, Hatala R, Brydges R, et al. Technology-enhanced simulation for health professions education: a systematic review and meta-analysis. *JAMA*. 2011;306:978-988.

45. Ottestad E, Boulet JR, Lighthall GK. Evaluating the management of septic shock using patient simulation. *Crit Care Med*. 2007;35:769-775.

46. Kim J, Neilipovitz D, Cardinal P, et al. A pilot study using high-fidelity simulation to formally evaluate performance in the resuscitation of critically ill patients: The University of Ottawa Critical Care Medicine, High-Fidelity Simulation, and Crisis Resource Management I Study. *Crit Care Med*. 2006;34:2167-2174.

47. Blackwood J, Duff JP, Nettel-Aguirre A, et al. Does teaching crisis resource management skills improve resuscitation performance in pediatric residents? *Pediatr Crit Care Med*. 2014;15:e168-e174.

48. van Schaik SM, Von Kohorn I, O'Sullivan P. Pediatric resident confidence in resuscitation skills relates to mock code experience. *Clin Pediatr (Phila)*. 2008;47:777-783.

52. McGaghie WC, Issenberg SB, Cohen ER, et al. Does simulation-based medical education with deliberate practice yield better results than traditional clinical education? A meta-analytic comparative review of the evidence. *Acad Med*. 2011;86:706-711.

53. Wheeler DS, Geis G, Mack EH, et al. High-reliability emergency response teams in the hospital: improving quality and safety using in situ simulation training. *BMJ Qual Saf*. 2013;22:507-514.

55. Howard SK, Gaba DM, Fish KJ, et al. Anesthesia crisis resource management training: teaching anesthesiologists to handle critical incidents. *Aviat Space Environ Med*. 1992;63:763-770.

56. Thomas EJ, Williams AL, Reichman EF, et al. Team training in the neonatal resuscitation program for interns: teamwork and quality of resuscitations. *Pediatrics*. 2010;125:539-546.

59. Hebbar KB, Cunningham C, McCracken C, et al. Simulation-based paediatric intensive care unit central venous line maintenance bundle training. *Intensive Crit Care Nurs*. 2015;31:44-50.

61. Andreatta P, Saxton E, Thompson M, Annich G. Simulation-based mock codes significantly correlate with improved pediatric patient cardiopulmonary arrest survival rates. *Pediatr Crit Care Med*. 2011;12:33-38.

63. Tainter CR, Wong NL, Bittner EA. Innovative strategies in critical care education. *J Crit Care*. 2015;pii:S0883-9441(15):00061-00061.

64. Wolbrink TA, Kissoon N, Burns JP. The development of an Internet-based knowledge exchange platform for pediatric critical care clinicians worldwide. *Pediatr Crit Care Med*. 2014;15:197-205.

66. van Mook WN, Gorter SL, de Grave WS, et al. Professionalism beyond medical school: an educational continuum? *Eur J Intern Med*. 2009;20:e148-e152.

67. Van Mook WN, de Grave WS, Wass V, et al. Professionalism: evolution of the concept. *Eur J Intern Med*. 2009;20:e81-e84.

71. Hochberg MS, Kalet A, Zabar S, et al. Can professionalism be taught? Encouraging evidence. *Am J Surg*. 2010;199:86-93.

74. Kesselheim JC, Atlas M, Adams D, et al. Humanism and professionalism education for pediatric hematology-oncology fellows: a model for pediatric subspecialty training. *Pediatr Blood Cancer*. 2015;62:335-340.

78. Stern DT, Papadakis M. The developing physician—becoming a professional. *N Engl J Med*. 2006;355:1794-1799.

79. Stockwell DC, Pollack MM, Turenne WM, Slonim AD. Leadership and management training of pediatric intensivists: how do we gain our skills? *Pediatr Crit Care Med*. 2005;6:665-670.

82. Epstein RM, Hundert EM. Defining and assessing professional competence. *JAMA*. 2002;287:226-235.

83. Pangaro LN. Investing in descriptive evaluation: a vision for the future of assessment. *Med Teach*. 2000;22:478-481.

84. Nasca TJ, Philibert I, Brigham T, Flynn TC. The next graduate medical education accreditation system—rationale and benefits. *N Engl J Med*. 2012;366:1051-1056.

85. Healy CC, Welchert AJ. Mentoring relations: a definition to advance research and education. *Educ Res*. 1998;19:17-21.

87. Palepu A, Friedman RH, Barnett RC, et al. Medical faculty with mentors are more satisfied. *J Gen Intern Med*. 1996;11(suppl 4):107.

89. Croskerry P. A universal model of diagnostic reasoning. *Acad Med*. 2009;84:1022-1028.

90. Croskerry P. Context is everything or how could I have been that stupid? *Healthc Q*. 2009;12 (special edition):e171-e177.

92. Epstein RM. Mindful practice. *JAMA*. 1999;282:833-839.

Lifelong Learning

Carrie A. Phillipi and Laura Marie Ibsen

PEARLS

- Adult learners are internally motivated to learn and have different styles and processes by which they learn.
- Active learning can occur in a variety of formats, including team-based, problem-based, simulation, and didactic teaching.
- Competency-based assessment is prominent in educational reform.
- Entrustable professional activities describe an *ability* to perform a task or responsibility without direct supervision once sufficient competency is attained.
- Milestones provide behavioral descriptors that indicate developmental progression along competencies.
- Educators and certification/accreditation bodies are piloting competency-based versus time-based progression in medical education and new assessment methods for physicians and trainees.
- Continuing medical education and maintenance of certification programs are working together to incorporate adult learning principles.

Lifelong Learning

The phrase *lifelong learner* implies the described individual has a voluntary interest in self-development and learning for pure enjoyment. It is assumed this attribute can be molded and influenced, even developed and promoted. These themes are prevalent in early childhood education. Montessori educational philosophy assumes a child is thirsty for knowledge and capable of initiating learning within a supportive learning environment.[1] Waldorf schools take a developmental approach to the child, taking advantage of natural tendencies in children to explore the natural world, arts, and sciences.[2] Adult learning principles build on these tenets.

Adult Learning Theory

Adult learning theory was theorized and modeled by Malcom Knowles in the 1970s.[3] He identified six principles of adult learning:
- Adults are internally motivated and self-directed.
- Adults bring life experiences and knowledge of learning experiences.
- Adults are goal oriented.
- Adults are relevancy oriented.
- Adults are practical.
- Adult learners like to be respected.

Given these general principles, Knowles drew on the work of Kolb,[4] where adult learning theory does not mean there is a one-size-fits-all approach to learning. For example, imagine two individuals who purchase a new electronic device. Whereas one may take the device out of the box, immediately turn it on, and begin experimenting with its features, the other purchaser may not even remove it from the box before reading the entire instruction manual. Adult learning theory celebrates the differences in learning approach, while making them overt and explicit. In designing and implementing curricula and assessments, medical educators may design curricula and evaluations attentive to these concepts (Fig. 23.1). Kolb described effective learning as a progression through a cycle of stages—having a concrete experience, reflection on that experience leading to information synthesis and future testable hypotheses. For those familiar with quality improvement principles, it is not unlike Plan-Do-Study-Act,[5] where small tests of change are implemented, observed, and the necessary modifications determined.

KOLB'S EXPERIENTIAL LEARNING THEORY

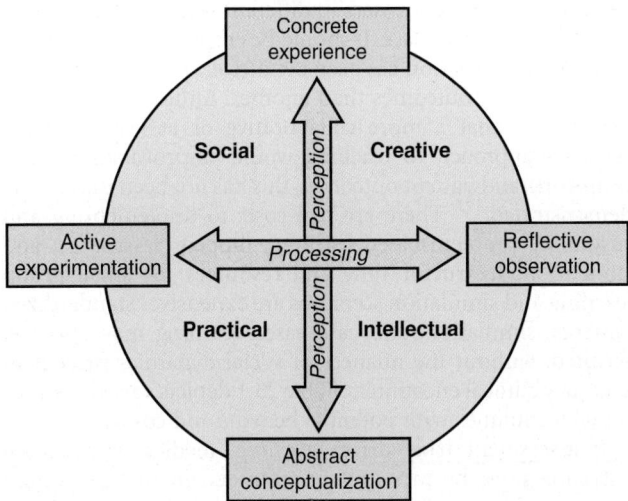

Fig. 23.1. Learning styles defined by Kolb's experiential learning theory. (Adapted from Kolb DA. Experiential Learning: Experience as the Source of Learning and Development. Upper Saddle River, NJ: Prentice-Hall; 1984:141.URL: http://www.learningfromexperience.com/images/uploads/process-of-experiential-learning.pdf. By Schaller DT, et al. One size does not fit all: earning style, play, and on-line interactives. In: Trant J, Bearman D, eds. Museums and the Web 2007: Proceedings. Toronto: Archives & Museum Informatics, published March 31, 2007, at http://www.archimuse.com/mw2007/papers/schaller/schaller.html.)

TABLE 23.1	Instructional Techniques According to Potential Costs and Benefits			
			Potential Benefits	**Potential Costs**
Didactic learning	Traditional Lecture	Teacher led	Easy to organize Inexpensive (both in teacher time and facility cost) Allows for independent learning	Noninteractive Noncollaborative
Problem-based learning	Small group cases	Student led Teacher facilitated	Active learning Motivation for learning Allows for complex thought Collaborative and interprofessional	Facilitator skill required High faculty, time, and space costs Students may have different styles and learning needs that are incompatible
Team-based learning	Out-of-class preparation followed by in-class application	Student led Teacher facilitated	Active learning Motivation for learning Allows for complex thought Collaborative and interprofessional Multiple assessments	Facilitator skill required High faculty, time, and space costs Advance student preparation required Students may have different styles and learning needs that are incompatible
Simulation	Practice of scenarios in simulated environments	Teacher led Students active	Hands-on skills practiced Literature from other industries (airlines) supports utility Collaborative and interprofessional	Resource and time expensive Can seem contrived/unrealistic

Applying Adult Learning Theory to Medical Education (Learner Assessment Drives Teaching Methods)

Learner assessment drives teaching methods in medical education and is increasingly incorporating adult learning theory. Adult learning theory places an emphasis on problem-based, collaborative learning, as opposed to didactic learning, and equality between teacher and student. Efforts to be inclusive of curricular methods that support adult learning principles are occurring in undergraduate, graduate, and continuing medical education. Problem-based and small group learning, flipped classrooms, and simulation exercises allow us many venues for reaching learners in different ways. Didactic learning is also firmly in place. It should be emphasized that no one method of instruction has been definitively proved to produce better learning outcomes than another. Although one would hypothesize that a more collaborative or at least student-centered approach to teaching would improve knowledge, teamwork, and patient outcomes, this has not been universally demonstrated.[6,7,8] There are real costs to implementing and sustaining problem-based learning, flipped classrooms, and simulation. Instructor time and resources for small group learning and simulation scenarios are expensive. Standardized patients, simulation, and case-based learning may also feel scripted, without the nuances of social dynamics present in everyday clinical encounters. Table 23.1 depicts varied instructional techniques with potential benefits and costs.

If assessment truly drives learning, medical educational curricula must be increasingly grounded in the assessment of knowledge and skills acquisition, now defined as abilities (or entrustable professional activities), and composed of individual competencies. Consider a teenager first learning to drive a car. The teen must be competent in many individual areas, such as knowledge of the laws of the road, and the skills of braking, using turn signals, mirrors, and seatbelts before embarking on this activity. Like supervising a learner performing a technical procedure on a critically ill child, the trust a parent affords a child in independent driving is fluid.

The teen may initially receive parental permission for driving around the neighborhood. As the adolescent demonstrates responsible and safe driving conduct, she may gain her parent's trust to drive on the freeway or with friends. Likewise, the graduated ownership a supervising intensivist will allow pediatric learners in performing central line placement will vary according to perceived knowledge and skills, but it is also highly contextual. Allowing an early driver or critical care fellow to navigate new territory is also inexorably tied to how individual parents (or faculty) inherently trust.

We describe evolving methods of assessment and their potential impact on learning in undergraduate, graduate, and continuing medical education within an historical context.

Undergraduate Medical Education

The traditional model of undergraduate medical education experienced in the 20th century and up until this day was largely born out of the Flexner Report.[9] In the early 1900s, 135 unregulated schools without universal requirements for entry or curriculum were functioning, largely as for-profit entities. Abraham Flexner, a prominent American educator, surveyed the scope of medical education; his scathing report led to the closure of all but 31 medical schools. Mergers and university affiliations resulted. The scientific method and the physician as a "social instrument" were championed in Flexner's report.[10] The two-by-two model of basic science (classroom) instruction followed by clinical training was adopted nearly universally, and as a result medical school education remains largely similar across the United States.

The two-by-two model has been questioned.[11] To better prepare physicians for projected needs (increased care coordination, interprofessional collaboration, quality/value-based care), medical schools around the United States are embarking on reform. Additionally, residency program leaders tell us that incoming interns are not residency ready.[12-14] It is unclear if a real decrease in intern readiness exists or if this represents simply anecdotal perception. Nevertheless, the myriad fourth-year medical student and intern "boot camps" common at

TABLE 23.2	Accreditation Council for Continuing Medical Education (ACGME) Core Competencies

Patient Care

Residents must be able to provide patient care that is compassionate, appropriate, and effective for the treatment of health problems and the promotion of health.

Medical Knowledge

Residents must be able to demonstrate knowledge about established and evolving biomedical, clinical, and cognate (eg, epidemiologic and social-behavioral) sciences and the application of this knowledge to patient care.

Practice-Based Learning and Improvement

Residents must be able to investigate and evaluate their patient care practices, appraise and assimilate scientific evidence, and improve their patient care practices.

Interpersonal and Communication Skills

Residents must be able to demonstrate interpersonal and communication skills that result in effective information exchange and teaming with patients, patients' families, and professional associates.

Professionalism

Residents must be able to demonstrate a commitment to carrying out professional responsibilities, adherence to ethical principles, and sensitivity to a diverse patient population.

Systems-Based Practice

Residents must be able to demonstrate an awareness of and responsiveness to the larger context and system of health care and the ability to effectively call on system resources to provide care that is of optimal value.

From ACGME Common Program Requirements. ACGME approved focused revision effective June 2013, pp. 7-10; https://www.acgme.org/acgmeweb/Portals/0/PFAssets/ProgramRequirements/CPRs2013.pdf.

TABLE 23.3	Core Entrustable Professional Activities for Entering Residency

EPA 1: Gather a history and perform a physical examination

EPA 2: Prioritize a differential diagnosis following a clinical encounter

EPA 3: Recommend and interpret common diagnostic and screening tests

EPA 4: Enter and discuss orders and prescriptions

EPA 5: Document a clinical encounter in the patient record

EPA 6: Provide an oral presentation of a clinical encounter

EPA 7: Form clinical questions and retrieve evidence to advance patient care

EPA 8: Give or receive a patient handover to transition care responsibility

EPA 9: Collaborate as a member of an interprofessional team

EPA 10: Recognize a patient requiring urgent or emergent care and initiate evaluation and management

EPA 11: Obtain informed consent for tests and/or procedures

EPA 12: Perform general procedures of a physician

EPA 13: Identify system failures and contribute to a culture of safety and improvement

From Core Entrustable Professional Activities for Entering Residency. Curriculum Developers' Guide. 2014. p 1. ©2014 Association of American Medical Colleges. May not be reproduced or distributed without prior permission. To request permission, please visit: www.aamc.org/91514/reproductions.html. https://members.aamc.org/eweb/upload/Core%20EPA%20Curriculum%20Dev%20Guide.pdf.

most institutions at least corroborate these worries. Critical physician workforce concerns as well as mounting student loan burdens compel us to act. Unanticipated challenges such as duty hour restrictions, coding and billing requirements, and the incorporation of the electronic health record into patient care have changed the duties students previously performed, and educators have been slow to adapt.

A desire to evaluate medical student skills (competencies) is a natural path forward. Undergraduate medical education has followed the lead from graduate medical education, adopting the six core competencies for teaching and assessment (Table 23.2). Two ongoing pilots sponsored by the American Association of Medical Colleges (AAMC) address competency-based assessment and progression.

Exploration of Medical School Progression According to Competency by the American Association of Medical Colleges With the Education in Pediatrics Across the Continuum and Entrustable Professional Activities Pilots

Education in Pediatrics Across the Continuum

In response to adult learning principles and with attention to the costs and rigidity of the traditional undergraduate medical education (UME) time-based model, an AAMC initiative is testing the feasibility of competency-based medical education with Education in Pediatrics Across the Continuum (EPAC).[15] A pilot group of medical students may advance through medical school as they master skill sets; progression is based on a demonstration of defined outcomes instead of time. In 2013, participating schools began to identify pediatric-leaning medical students to join the cohort. This pilot is currently ongoing, and outcomes are eagerly anticipated.

Entrustable Professional Activities

Residency program directors have been increasingly vocal about their perceptions that medical students are not *residency ready*. *Boot camps*, which are commonly held as capstone courses during the fourth year of medical school or early in internship, support this concern. The Core Entrustable Professional Activities for Entering Residency give a narrative voice for the progression of medical students to abilities required of a day-one, residency-ready intern. Thirteen entrustable professional activities (EPAs) have been defined with mapped competencies (Table 23.3). Writing orders, formulating a differential diagnosis, collaborating within an interprofessional team, and providing informed consent are examples. The AAMC seeks to determine how EPAs will be taught and assessed. Ten medical schools are currently participating in a pilot to study EPAs in undergraduate medical education.[16] It remains to be seen how program directors will use this information in their decision making when selecting medical students for their training programs.

Graduate Medical Education

Like undergraduate medical education, today's system of graduate medical education is a 20th-century phenomenon.[17] In the early 1900s, hospitals were primarily a place where one, especially if indigent, went to die. With the advent of technology, procedures, and aseptic technique, hospitals became a place of cures, leading to around-the-clock staffing needs. Specialization ensued and newly graduated MDs desired training in top-notch programs such as those offered by children's hospitals. By the end of World War I, with the advent of accreditation bodies, training programs as we know them today had largely replaced the apprenticeship (or "house pupil") models of the early 20th century. After World War II, increasing numbers of women and racial minorities, who were previously denied entry into the system, were included. The pace of specialization/subspecialization, combined later with federal funding, led to an explosion in the number of graduate medical education (GME) trainees. The passage of Medicare and Medicaid in 1965 allowed for hospitals to bill professional fees for faculty who oversaw the instruction and training of house officers, creating funding mechanisms to pay resident salaries. The resident as "employee" versus "student" remains a critical question today.

The long residency duty hours, historically born at least partially out of staffing needs, have been restricted. This has undeniably changed the landscape of learning. The need to transfer or hand over care has prompted educational reform with programs such as I-PASS.[18] Despite their universal acceptance and requirements for compliance monitoring, it is unclear whether duty hour changes have led to improved educational or patient care outcomes.[19,20]

Graduate Medical Education: Evaluation by Milestones

Building on the competencies, the Pediatric Milestone Project, a partnership between the Accreditation Council for Continuing Medical Education (ACGME) and American Board of Pediatrics, was designed for the evaluation of resident physicians participating in ACGME-accredited residency or fellowship training programs. Milestones are intended to provide a developmental framework for learner assessment. Fig. 23.2 provides an example of one milestone evaluation. Although they are not intended to address all competencies, milestones are anchored contextually in the development of the physician

1. Gathers and synthesizes essential and accurate information to define each patient's clinical problem(s). (PC1)				
Critical deficiencies			Ready for unsupervised practice	Aspirational
Does not collect accurate historical data	Inconsistently able to acquire accurate historical information in an organized fashion	Consistently acquires accurate and relevant histories from patients	Acquires accurate histories from patients in an efficient, prioritized, and hypothesis-driven fashion	Obtains relevant historical subtleties, including sensitive information that informs the differential diagnosis
Does not use physical exam to confirm history	Does not perform an appropriately thorough physical exam or misses key physical exam findings	Seeks and obtains data from secondary sources when needed	Performs accurate physical exams that are targeted to the patient's complaints	Identifies subtle or unusual physical exam findings
Relies exclusively on documentation of others [?] to generate own database or differential diagnosis	Does not seek or is overly reliant on secondary data	Consistently performs accurate and appropriately thorough physical exams	Synthesizes data to generate a prioritized differential diagnosis and problem list	Efficiently utilizes all sources of secondary data to inform differential diagnosis
Fails to recognize patient's central clinical problems	Inconsistently recognizes patients' central clinical problem or develops limited differential diagnoses	Uses collected data to define a patient's central clinical problem(s)	Effectively uses history and physical examination skills to minimize the need for further diagnostic testing	Role models and teaches the effective use of history and physical examination skills to minimize the need for further diagnostic testing
Fails to recognize potentially life threatening problems				
☐ ☐ ☐ ☐ ☐ ☐ ☐ ☐ ☐				
Comments:				

Fig. 23.2. Pediatric milestone used for evaluation. (From http://acgme.org/acgmeweb/Portals/0/PDFs/Milestones/PediatricsMilestones.pdf. The Pediatrics Milestone Project. A Joint Initiative of The Accreditation Council for Graduate Medical Education and The American Board of Pediatrics. January 2013, p. 1. Copyright © 2012 Accreditation Council for Graduate Medical Education and American Board of Pediatrics. All rights reserved. The copyright owners grant third parties the right to use the Pediatrics Milestones on a nonexclusive basis for educational purposes.)

in key elements of the competencies. Milestones are now routinely used in GME evaluations; UME evaluations will likely follow suit.

Beyond Undergraduate Medical Education and Graduate Medical Education
Continuing Medical Education, Board Certification, and Maintenance of Certification

The speed of medical and technical advance makes it difficult to argue against physicians practicing continuous learning. Continuing medical education is designed to promote the knowledge, skills, and performance of physicians and is managed by the ACGME.[21] Further, continuing medical education requirements are determined and monitored by state licensing boards. In Oregon, for example, the Oregon Medical Board, out of the office of the secretary of state, sets standards and monitors by audit the 30 hours/year of continuing medical education (CME) required by all practicing physicians.[22] Individual institutions, private agencies, and the American Academy of Pediatrics offer CME activities to fulfill these requirements. Additionally, states may require additional education; in Oregon, physicians are required to complete additional pain management education. Traditionally, methods of delivering CME for physicians involve didactic experiences such as grand rounds or other lecture series. It is reasonable to question whether these experiences are sufficient to drive outcomes, either in physician knowledge, practice, and, most important, patient-centered outcomes. Furthermore, evidence suggests physicians, like all learners, are unreliable self-assessors,[23] highlighting the need for external review to produce and ensure learning outcomes.

Board certification and maintenance of certification complements GME and CME in certifying practitioners in standards of excellence, *which are intended to lead to high-quality health outcomes for their patients.* Accreditation boards such as the American Board of Pediatrics[24] have a duty to the public, ensuring physicians participate in recertification through retesting and maintenance of certification activities. The requirements for pediatric board certification include graduation from medical school, completion of a 3-year ACGME-approved training program, a valid, unrestricted license, and a passing score on the American Board of Pediatrics Certification Examination. Introduced in 2010, the maintenance of certification (MOC) process for pediatricians is a points-based system with four components: part 1, professional standing; part 2, lifelong learning and self-assessment; part 3, cognitive expertise—secure examination; and part 4, performance in practice.

Although medical knowledge may be assessed through standardized testing, it is unclear whether this or other activities for certification truly lead to improved patient outcomes. How can this goal be achieved? Institutions and organizations that create CME programs are actively making connections with MOC requirements.[25] A physician can participate in practice-based improvement activities and receive both CME and MOC credit. To be effective, these experiences must incorporate adult learning principles, with high relevance to the learner, and require active participation. Additionally, they must be authentic on a local level, addressing local problems and opportunities. Organizations can actively incorporate CME/MOC activities into daily workflow for flexible, real-time learning and assessment.

New Methods of Assessment

Educators and those responsible for certification at all levels are currently actively engaged in discussion of new methods and concepts of assessment. There is a growing appreciation for the value in multiple low stakes assessments that include rich narrative feedback[26] and the integration of these assessments into a composite whole. Formative and summative assessment occurs along a spectrum instead of at discrete points in time. Innovations in higher stakes testing assessment are occurring in all phases of the test development cycle, including design and implementation of items and tests (assessment engineering, automated item generation), items and tasks used within the test (game-based assessment, computer-based simulations, use of Internet or key online resources during a test, and alternative text item types such as drag and drop or multiple correct answers), item selection during the test (computer adaptive testing), and delivery of the test (online proctoring versus test center proctoring versus no proctoring). The rapid development of computer and Internet technology makes innovation inevitable, and the resulting change needs to be managed carefully, with an eye to testing validity and reliability as well as test taker approval.

Assessment engineering is a comprehensive model-based view of test development, administration, and scoring. Components include a construct map, which represents the visual organization of knowledge about a particular problem; task models, which represent the building blocks of the construct map and are specific proficiencies; and templates, which include the information necessary for generating test items. Creation of a test using assessment engineering principles requires significant resources initially to develop the components (construct map, etc.) but decreased time and cost in the long term.[27] Automated item generation (AIG) is a related test development process in which models are developed, variables defined, and test items automatically generated. The Medical Council of Canada has used AIG and found that it reduced the cost to develop items. In addition, AIG items were more difficult and discriminating.[28]

The National Board of Medical Examiners in the Computer Case Simulation portion of the United States Medical Licensing Exam (USMLE), Step 3, has used computer-based simulations for many years. Case simulations can be realistic and are thought to help evaluate competencies that cannot be evaluated by multiple-choice items. Content experts develop the cases, and multiple experts' judgments about various actions are used to develop scoring tools. Although the potential for simulation to allow for assessment of clinical competency exists, it is less reliable (reproducible) than multiple-choice testing. The items are expensive and time consuming to develop, and test security is difficult.[29]

Game-based assessment is newer and has not yet been implemented in large-scale medical assessments, but it shows promise as the technology evolves. Games are developed based on construct maps and provide a means to evaluate students based on their responses to simulated clinical situations. They may offer another way to determine learner proficiency in more complex tasks.[30] As with computer case simulations as used by the USMLE, game-based assessments will require considerable commitment of resources for initial development.

There is considerable interest on the part of test takers to have open Internet or other online resources available during testing (so-called open-book testing). Although open-book testing may be more realistic and it is thought that it allows testing of higher cognitive skills, the data do not show that it drives deeper learning than closed-book tests.[31] Use of the Internet during testing (open-book testing) can help assess how efficiently and effectively the examinee uses the resource as well as the taker's knowledge. Barriers include security, connectivity, and out-of-date reference material.

Online proctoring refers to proctors monitoring an examinee over the Internet using a webcam and includes authentication of the examinee and monitoring of his or her behavior during the examination. Online proctoring became commercially available in 2006, and there are now several companies that provide the service. Benefits include greater convenience, lower cost, and the potential for greater security. Disadvantages include computer technical challenges, inability to deliver some types of testing over the Internet, and the potential perception of lower security.[32] No proctoring with candidate authentication is also an option but is not yet utilized for high-stakes examinations.

Current Controversies, Future Challenges
Time-Based Versus Competency-Based Progression

Individualized curricula and accelerated progress are highly en vogue. Reform is occurring across the country and brings up a debate not unlike what is held between liberal arts universities and vocational training programs around the country. Is a liberal arts education with its broad base necessary for the adaptability students will need when encountering and navigating an unpredictable workplace? Is the hands-on training that readies students more directly with real-world experiences more applicable and practical?[33] Or is there room to ensure transfer of skill (competence) with both?

Medical education reform must address this same conundrum head-on. Brian Hodges describes this conflict comparing "a tea-steeping versus an iDOC model for medical education."[34] The tea-steeping (or time-based) model has been in place and largely unchanged since the Flexner report. Although we encounter learners of varied strengths and weaknesses, the majority of medical students become physicians when they have completed 4 years of education; residency and fellowship programs likewise graduate trainees when their time is up. Consider instead an outcomes-based educational process by which the trainee is produced or manufactured. Can we produce quality physicians more cheaply and effectively by tailoring experiences toward the end product—for example, can we more efficiently manufacture an intensivist? In the end, Hodges argues for a marriage of time-based and outcomes-based training and highlights entrustable professional activities (abilities that translate competency into clinical practice) as a potential way forward.

Although beyond the scope of the chapter, we would be remiss to not mention factors such as the advent of the electronic health record, compensation and billing requirements, and faculty-driven care, which have undeniably affected the learning environment. Students and residents have different opportunities to learn from those available in the past. More opportunities for hands-on care by faculty and closer supervision of learners at all levels most likely are better for individual patients, but they may not provide some of the most powerful learning experiences of past eras. Even documentation experience may be limited: In some settings, students are not permitted to document patient information in the electronic health record, raising questions about their opportunities to write notes and, more important, organize their thoughts into coherent patient assessments and plans. Intensivists and physicians in general must be attuned to environmental and technologic advances, which change practices and the ways they teach, practice, and learn.

Continuing Medical Education and Maintenance of Board Certification

Some practicing physicians believe medical organizations have distinctly misstepped in pursuits to regulate learning activities. Internists have been particularly vocal in their complaints. In a letter to the Internal Medicine Community on February 3, 2015, the American Board of Internal Medicine admitted "they got it wrong" by establishing and requiring impractical and expensive programs physicians found unmeaningful.[35] Some feel the American Board of Pediatrics is similarly out of touch.[36] As recently as May of 2015, the American Board of Pediatrics initiated steps to simplify and expand options for MOC requirements[37] after criticism that its programs were time consuming, confusing, and expensive. This distress highlights the need for accrediting bodies to return to adult learning principles—if learners do not *care* about the material (relevance), it will not translate into meaningful outcomes, nor will it find acceptability within a discerning group of learners.

Conclusions

Reform is under way in medical education. New methods to encourage competency-based evaluation and active learning are readily visible. Resource utilization, especially faculty time and energy, is a finite and precious commodity. Reform should not be undertaken for the sake of reform, without clearly defined problems that can be addressed and studied for impact. Practitioners must also remember the less tangible aspects of inspiring future physicians to cultivate genuine passion for self-improvement and a thirst for knowledge in the absence of regulation.[38] How can adult learners capitalize on the natural tendencies for playful inquisitiveness so prevalent in early childhood education? How can medical educators empower physicians in training and in practice to best utilize adult learning principles? Medical education involves a group of individuals for whom society compels the practice of lifelong learning. Students and teachers must be equally compelled to get this right.

Key References

3. Knowles M. *Self-Directed Learning*. Chicago: Follet; 1975.
4. Kolb DA. *Experiential Learning: Experience as the Source of Learning and Development*. Upper Saddle River, NJ: Prentice-Hall; 1984.
9. Flexner A. *Medical Education in the United States and Canada*. Washington, DC: Science and Health Publications; 1910.
10. Duffy TP. The Flexner Report—100 years later. *Yale J Biol Med*. 2011; 84:269-276.

15. Education in Pediatrics Across the Continuum (The EPAC Project). American Association of Medical Colleges; <https://www.aamc.org/initiatives/epac/>. Accessed 05.15.

16. The Core Entrustable Professional Activities for Entering Residency. American Association of Medical Colleges; <https://www.aamc.org/initiatives/coreepas/>. Accessed 05.15.

23. Davis DA, Mazmanian PE, Fordis M, et al. Accuracy of physician self-assessment compared with observed measures of competence: a systematic review. *JAMA*. 2006;296:1094-1102.

25. Holmboe ES, et al. Continuing medical education and maintenance of certification: essential links. *Perm J*. 2007;11:71-75.

34. Hodges BD. A tea-steeping or i-Doc model for medical education? *Acad Med*. 2010;85(9 suppl):S34-S44.

38. Ludmerer KM. *Let Me Heal: The Opportunity to Preserve Excellence in American Medicine*. Oxford: Oxford University Press; 2014.

Public Health Emergencies and Emergency Mass Critical Care

Robert K. Kanter,[†] Carl O. Eriksson, and Mary A. King

"Keep your eye on the ball."

**Bob Kanter, trailblazer for children
in the world of disaster medicine**

PEARLS

- Public health emergencies (PHEs) can range from limited events that have no effect on critical care needs to catastrophic events that create demand for critical care beyond standard capacity.
- Pediatric intensivists must be engaged with hospital and regional PHE planning and preparedness efforts for all types of PHEs, whether limited in scope or catastrophic.
- The surge capacity continuum that spans *conventional* to *contingency* to *crisis* capacity should be employed during a PHE that requires an increase in critical care capacity.
- Emergency mass critical care (EMCC) is limited, essential critical care during disasters when critical care demand surpasses traditional resources.
- EMCC delivery can improve patient outcomes and lives saved by conserving, optimizing, and better matching critical care resources to critical care demand.

During a public health emergency like a natural disaster or influenza pandemic, a large number of children may need critical care in order to survive. Because pediatric critical care is so highly specialized, and because so few nonpediatric providers are comfortable caring for the sickest children, the pediatric ICU (PICU) represents an essential part of the response to a PHE. During such an event, the hospital incident command system (ICS) provides a leadership framework within and among organizations responding to an emergency, emphasizing flexibility and scalability, with clear lines of authority and consistent communications. Within this system the PICU will be a critical role.

Planning and preparedness for PHEs can save lives. Unfortunately, critical care providers receive little training in disaster medicine and response and are often underinvolved in hospital disaster preparedness efforts. Recent public health emergencies have exposed a lack of PHE awareness, training, and

preparation by critical care providers. The goal of this chapter is to educate the PICU provider in the principles and tools of PHE preparedness and emergency mass critical care (EMCC). Given the disproportionate scarcity of pediatric critical care resources, PICU providers must help to prepare their unit, hospital, and region for the next pediatric PHE. Preparing for pediatric critical care during small, limited, and routine PHEs can also help intensivists better prepare for any future catastrophic PHEs that necessitate EMCC.

PHEs in North America have included terrorist attacks on the New York World Trade Center and the 2013 Boston Marathon, Hurricanes Katrina and Sandy with subsequent flooding of New Orleans and New York City, a catastrophic tornado in Missouri, a major nightclub fire in Rhode Island, an influenza pandemic, and outbreaks of severe acute respiratory syndrome and Ebola. Whether we remember them as disasters or near misses, these emergencies provided important lessons. All-hazard and incident-specific planning and preparedness make a difference. When carried out, public health preparations (including evacuation, shelter, and aggressive infection control) limited major health effects. When critical care was necessary, existing resources were generally adequate to provide standard critical care when needed. However, small differences in circumstances in any of these recent emergencies might have resulted in much larger numbers of adults and children admitted to adult ICUs or PICUs. It is easy to imagine disasters that would overwhelm existing ICU resources, unless intensive care providers prepare to provide critical care in larger PHEs.

Basic Concepts

National Response Framework and Incident Command System

Responses to major public health emergencies are organized within a National Response Framework, as outlined by the federal US Department of Homeland Security.[1] Emergency responses are always coordinated at the most local jurisdictional level possible, usually at the city or county level. Responses to larger disasters need support from adjacent counties, the state, and sometimes the federal level. The hospital ICS[2] provides a leadership framework within and among organizations responding to an emergency. ICS emphasizes flexibility for any type of event, scalability to the size of the event, clear lines of authority, and consistent communications.

[†]Deceased

TABLE 24.1	Spectrum of Surge Capacity		
Magnitude of Surge	**Minor**	**Moderate**	**Major**
% Increase in capacity	20%	100%	200%
Response	Conventional	Contingency	Crisis
Response strategies	Conserve Substitute	Conserve Substitute Adapt Reuse	Conserve Substitute Adapt Reuse Reallocate

Data from Christian MD, Devereaux A, Dichter JR, et al. Introduction and executive summary: care of the critically ill and injured during pandemics and disasters: CHEST consensus statement. Chest. 2014;146(suppl 4):8S-34S.

Disaster plans at every hospital incorporate ICS principles, and PICU preparedness plans must align with these principles in order to most effectively use limited resources and communicate with the hospital and larger community.

Emergency Surge Capacity

Critical care responses to PHEs are scaled according to the size and severity of the emergency (Table 24.1).[3-5] Emergency surges are categorized as (1) minor, (2) moderate, and (3) major. For a sudden-impact event involving minor (up to 20%) increases above usual peak hospital capacity at one or more local hospitals, conventional surge methods would suffice to provide normal standards of critical care to all those who need it. Conventional critical care surge needs are met by canceling elective admissions, quickly discharging all patients who can safely leave the ICU, mobilizing staff, and adding beds, as feasible. Most hospitals have occasional experience with conventional critical care surge responses.

Moderate emergency surges result in an increased patient population of between approximately 20% and 100% of usual capacity and require an increased response to most effectively use limited resources. Contingency surge methods include all elements of the conventional response but include additional strategies. Non-PICU patient care areas may be repurposed for ICU-level care. Staff will need to be leveraged, either by changing provider-to-patient ratios or by using non-ICU staff (often in a tiered approach where bedside care is provided by non-ICU providers, who in turn are supervised by ICU providers). Supplies and equipment must be conserved when possible, and some substitutions, adaptations, and reuse may be necessary when safe. The goal of the contingency surge response is to significantly increase capacity while minimally affecting patient care practices, and thorough planning will increase the likelihood that a contingency surge response will adequately meet patient needs after a PHE.

Emergency Mass Critical Care

Emergency mass critical care (EMCC) approaches are required when a large PHE threatens to overwhelm critical care resources, as well as when conventional and contingency surge responses are inadequate to meet the critical care needs of the population. It is recommended that hospitals with a PICU be able to care for up to three times the usual number of critically ill patients for up to 10 days without outside help.[6] In these circumstances, population-based goals will attempt to maximize the number of survivors by providing immediate life-saving interventions to all persons who are likely to benefit from them, while delaying or forgoing other interventions. This represents a change from usual standards of care to crisis standards of care and should only be implemented if other approaches are inadequate.

Sudden impact events that stress the resources of a community may require the implementation of temporary reactive mass critical care such as has been orchestrated after events like a major fire.[7] A sustained PHE that exceeds resources in a large geographic area may require the sustained implementation of mass critical care. No historical precedents exist for sustained mass critical care. PHE powers are defined on a state-by-state basis,[8] and ICU leaders must be familiar with their own state and hospital incident command process for authorizing EMCC.

EMCC, whether temporary or sustained, should guarantee the following lifesaving interventions that can be performed immediately: (1) mechanical ventilation, (2) fluid resuscitation, (3) vasopressors, (4) antidotes and antibiotics, and (5) analgesia and sedation. Lifesaving EMCC interventions can be extended to much larger than usual numbers of patients by the following approaches (as depicted in Table 24.1): (1) conservation of resources; (2) substitution of equivalent available interventions for scarce or unavailable treatments; (3) adapting nearly equivalent available interventions instead of other scarce or unavailable treatments; (4) reuse of some single-use items; and (5) reallocation of multiuse resources (eg, a mechanical ventilator) from patients not expected to survive in spite of EMCC to patients with a higher likelihood of survival. The degree of deviation from usual practices must be proportional to the gap between patient needs and existing resources, and EMCC should be implemented in an organized way by each hospital's ICS.

Pediatric Critical Care Needs and Resources in a Public Health Emergency

If a PHE affected persons of all ages equally, children aged 0 to 14 years would account for 20% of all patients and those 0 to 19 years old would account for 28%.[9] Younger patients may be more vulnerable to infections, dehydration, toxins, and trauma and are less able to protect themselves in a dangerous environment. Thus children may be overrepresented in a patient population during a PHE.[3] Accidents involving a child-specific activity or violence intentionally targeting children may result in a patient population predominantly made up of children.

Survival rates from high-risk pediatric conditions tend to be better when children receive care at pediatric hospitals.[10-13] The younger the patient, the more age-specific are the treatment requirements. A national survey estimated a PICU peak capacity of 54 beds per million pediatric population.[14] Because normal PICU occupancy exceeds 50%, fewer than 30 vacant PICU beds per million age-specific population are generally available in a region. Because each region may only be served by a single or a few pediatric hospitals, events that disable a pediatric hospital may disproportionately degrade regional pediatric care.

Quantitative models indicate that survival in a PHE would be improved if a pediatric patient surge is distributed to pediatric beds throughout a region, rather than overloading facilities near the scene of an emergency.[15] Appropriate utilization of pediatric hospitals would be promoted by clear identification of pediatric hospitals, although every hospital must be prepared to stabilize and provide initial care for pediatric patients.[16,17] Unfortunately, control of patient distribution may be impossible in a PHE.[18] As a result, all hospitals must be prepared to care for some children.[19] Even if pediatric regional resources are used optimally, hospital vacancies to accommodate pediatric surges are much more limited than for adult patients.[20,21] Whether or not patients are distributed optimally to hospitals, outcomes from a hypothetical large PHE are likely to improve with EMCC approaches.[15,22] Additionally, using telemedicine for specialized and potentially unreachable resources such as pediatric critical care may significantly extend the reach of pediatric EMCC during a PHE.

Pediatric Disaster Timeline

When the PICU Is Notified of a Sudden-Impact Public Health Emergency

When a sudden-impact PHE is announced, PICU clinical leaders must immediately focus attention on safety of patients and staff. The hospital's ICS is activated. Normal operations continue until other instructions are received. Staff who are already in the hospital report to their normal assigned work area, notifying their supervisor of their arrival. PICU clinical leaders review the hospital disaster plan, including job action sheets, and discuss expectations with the staff. Hospitals and PICUs with robust emergency surge plans will be able to provide more practical and specific guidance to the on-site PICU clinical leadership, highlighting the need for planning before an event occurs. When possible, PICU clinical leaders will be informed about type, number, and arrival time of anticipated patients. However, such information is often unavailable and inaccurate. Patients in the PICU are evaluated for transfer to a lower level of care or discharge home, and scheduled admissions are reviewed for potential cancellation.

Based on the initial assessment, ICU leaders must determine the number of additional patients who could be accommodated with available staff, equipment, supplies, and space while providing the usual standard of care. Additional needs for staff, equipment, and supplies should be communicated through appropriate channels in the ICS. The ICS will direct the response to ensure adequate staff (including assigning and sometimes reassigning staff, as well as asking clinical leaders to call in additional staff when needed), supplies, equipment, and clinical space. As information about the event becomes available, PICU physician and nurse leaders provide incident-specific just-in-time teaching to staff when warranted. Just-in-time teaching is especially important when less experienced supplemental providers are assigned to the PICU.

At all times, clinical leaders must maintain awareness of the environment, operational problems, disaster-related communications, and reactions of staff, patients, and families.

Emergency Department Phase

To provide continuity of patient care and situational awareness, the PICU team must interact closely with the emergency department (ED). Rapidly accommodating patients from the ED or operating room will be essential to allow those areas to continue receiving new patients. In some cases, PICU staff may be temporarily reassigned to work in the ED, and the critical care team should be familiar with the ED perspective on disaster responses.

Triage

Triage sorts patients to match their needs with available resources. Triage is an evolving process relative to shifting needs and resources. Prehospital field triage and care are beyond the scope of this chapter, but when they are effective, patients who will benefit from ED care are selected. Some mild patients not requiring ED care may have been mistriaged to receive care, and others may arrive at the ED without prehospital assessment. The "worried well" may constitute a large proportion of patients arriving at an ED. Severely ill or injured patients may arrive later than those with less serious conditions in a sudden impact emergency. Triage categories are assigned in the ED by an experienced clinician whose sole role is to act as triage officer. Elements of the triage process may have to be repeated later according to evolving imbalances of patient needs and resources.

Triage in the ED is performed according to the nature of the PHE. When potential contamination of victims by toxins is involved, initial triage outside the hospital first identifies those needing immediate decontamination to protect the patient, staff, and entire hospital facility. Likewise, when a highly transmissible virulent infection is involved, triage prior to entering the ED identifies and isolates potentially infectious patients at the earliest time to avoid exposing staff and other patients. Failures of triage at the early stages of decontamination and infection control may place staff at risk and may have contributed to the infection of two nurses with Ebola virus in a US hospital during the 2014 Ebola outbreak.[23]

Physiologic triage identifies patients needing immediate lifesaving interventions. Physiologic triage tools identify patients in five categories: (1) those needing immediate lifesaving interventions; (2) those who need significant intervention that can be delayed; (3) those needing little or no treatment; (4) those who are so severely ill or injured that survival is unlikely despite major interventions; and (5) those who have already died. Care of patients triaged to group 4, those who are so severely ill or injured that survival is unlikely, must deviate most significantly from usual approaches to intensive care. Because of overall demands on the system, scarce resources must be allocated to other patients who are more likely to survive. Group 4 patients are sometimes referred to as "expectant." Expectant patients are defined by current resource constraints and physiologic observations. Palliative care is always provided to expectant patients. Also see the discussion of rationing at the end of this chapter.

No single triage tool is always rapid, completely accurate, appropriate for all ages and disorders, and already familiar to all providers.[24] Staff should be familiar with the physiologic triage tool in use locally. Pediatric experts can partner with regional health care coalitions to provide standardized pediatric health care education, such as pediatric triage, among other specialized pediatric topics.[25]

Decontamination

When indicated, decontamination reduces toxic effects for the victim and avoids contamination of staff and the hospital facility. The airway is monitored and maintained during decontamination. Antidotes are given after cleaning the site of administration. Age-specific issues include hypothermia in infants and behavioral limitations. Warm water may prevent hypothermia. Young children need assistance undressing, while some older children resist undressing and require encouragement and some privacy.[26-28]

Infection Control

For a public health emergency involving a highly virulent transmissible infection, infection control must begin outside the ED entrance and continue without interruption in the hospital while the patient is infectious. Infection control guidelines have been published[29,30] and should be readily available under hospital policies and procedures.

Some emerging infectious agents such as Ebola virus require specific infection control practices, and meticulous attention to infection control is required in order to limit secondary cases. In some cases, this may result in changes to the care made available (eg, for patients with severe Ebola virus disease, emergency cardiopulmonary resuscitation may present an unacceptably high risk of infecting staff members, and institutions may therefore not be able to offer patients these therapies).[31]

Keeping Families Together, Identifying and Tracking Children, Child Safety

Hospital care of children is more efficient, more effective, and less stressful when children are accompanied by a family member or familiar caregiver. This need must be balanced against other triage considerations. Unaccompanied children must be properly identified, tracked, and reunited with their families, requiring proper identification of adult caregivers before releasing children to them. Pediatric safe areas in hospitals with appropriate staff supervision are necessary. Sample child identification and tracking documents have been designed.[19]

Intensive Care Unit Phase

For a sudden impact event in which the ED phase lasts a few hours, the ICU phase may last weeks. On admission to the PICU, a "tertiary survey" is performed to detect injuries and disorders that were overlooked in the rapid primary and secondary survey. For standard interventions, template orders and an abbreviated hospital record may extend the capacity of an overloaded workforce. Every effort must be made to guarantee the essential critical care interventions: mechanical ventilation, fluid resuscitation, vasopressors, antibiotics and antidotes, and sedation and analgesia.

In order to provide essential interventions, some resource-intensive interventions that are ordinarily considered standard in an ICU may have to be delayed or foregone in a mass critical care situation, because standard care would reduce the population who could receive lifesaving care. Interventions that may have to be delayed include invasive hemodynamic monitoring, intracranial pressure monitoring, renal replacement therapy, extracorporeal life support, parenteral nutrition, and frequent recording of fluid balance and vital signs.[3,32] Clinical decision making may have to be based more often on clinical judgment and less often on laboratory and imaging studies.

PICU Operations in a Gradual-Onset and Sustained Public Health Emergency

Many of the same considerations pertain to sudden-impact and gradual-onset PHEs. However, a gradual onset allows event-specific preparation. Resources can be augmented, and procedures can be developed and practiced. Staff can be trained. Experience in the early phase of the emergency will provide evidence to refine event-specific recommendations. Rapid publication of such experience has provided rapid evolution of management recommendations in recent PHEs such as outbreaks of severe acute respiratory syndrome, H1N1 influenza, and Ebola virus disease.

Space

Patient care space may be adapted by converting single patient spaces to be used by two or three patients. After exhausting PICU space, additional space for EMCC may also be adapted by using intermediate care units, postanesthesia care units, EDs, procedure suites, or non-ICU hospital rooms. Overflow of critically ill adolescents or young adults may be shared between PICUs and adult ICUs. Overflow of young infants or term newborns may be shared by PICUs and neonatal ICUs. Nonhospital facilities should only be used for EMCC if hospitals become unusable.

Personnel

Supplemental providers may include physicians, nurse practitioners, physician assistants, nurses, respiratory therapists, pharmacists, and emergency medical technicians who have skills in non-ICU pediatrics or nonpediatric critical care. Rapid credentialing procedures, just-in-time education, and close supervision by experienced PICU clinicians will promote the role of supplemental providers. Hospitals should expect and plan for a need for significant psychosocial support for patients and providers during and after a PHE.[33]

Mechanical Ventilation

Most hospitals have only a small supply of standard ventilators and circuits in excess of usual ICU capacity. It may be necessary to consider temporary use of transport and anesthesia ventilators and bilevel positive pressure breathing devices. Some pediatric hospitals use a single type of ventilator for patients of all sizes, with appropriate circuits and software algorithms. In other hospitals, ventilators usually used for adults that have high compliance circuits and adult algorithms may have to be adapted for use in infants or small children. When local supplies have been exhausted in a major PHE, adult-focused pediatric-adaptable ventilators and supplies may be accessed through the Strategic National Stockpile.[34] Some difficulties may be encountered. The inspiratory flow or pressure sensor may not be sensitive to an infant's small inspiratory effort. Thus triggering of inspiration may fail for synchronized intermittent mandatory ventilation, assist control, or pressure support. Likewise, ventilator algorithms to terminate inspiration pressure support may fail in the presence of air leaks around endotracheal tubes. A substantial air leak around an uncuffed endotracheal tube may result in frequent ventilator alarms indicating low pressure or low exhaled tidal volume.

In a volume-controlled mode, adult ventilators may be unable to provide small tidal volumes and inspiratory flow appropriate for a small infant. Pressure-dependent losses of tidal volume in compressible spaces of adult ventilator circuits exaggerate breath-to-breath variation in delivered tidal volume if peak inspiratory pressure varies with patient effort or changing respiratory mechanics. Difficulties in providing small tidal volumes, as well as variation in ventilation due to leaks around uncuffed endotracheal tubes, may be alleviated by using a time-cycled, pressure-limited mode of ventilation. Supplemental providers need considerable assistance in caring for an infant on a ventilator. Maintaining endotracheal tube patency, stabilization, and proper cuff inflation and evaluating episodes of hypoxemia are challenges even for experienced PICU clinicians.

Manual Ventilation

Few hospitals stockpile enough mechanical ventilators to support three times the usual number of ICU patients. The temporary use of manual ventilation with a self-inflatable bag may be considered to meet mass critical care goals; however, this strategy is not without risk. Manual ventilation has been used successfully via tracheostomy tubes for days in a polio epidemic,[35] temporarily for hours via endotracheal tubes in a power failure,[36] and during weather emergencies.[37-39] It provides similar gas exchange compared with mechanical ventilation.[40-42] However, manual ventilation is labor intensive, is tiring to operators, may expose staff to infection risks as a result of close and prolonged bedside contact, and may lead to unnecessary patient risk of inappropriate gas exchange and barotrauma.

Equipment and Supplies

Mass critical care can only be provided if essential equipment and supplies are available on site. Resupply and rental deliveries may be impossible during a PHE. Thus hospitals must balance the benefits of an adequate stockpile against costs of keeping items on site that may never be used. The Task Force on Mass Critical Care[3] has recommended that a hospital first should target a mass critical care capacity of three times the usual maximum ICU capacity for 10 days.

Nonpediatric hospitals must also consider stockpiling for critically ill pediatric patients as transport and/or open pediatric ICU bed spaces may be unavailable. Although it may be possible to carry out many interventions by adapting nearly equivalent equipment and supplies, some adult equipment cannot be adapted to infants and small children. It is essential to stock adequate numbers of resuscitation masks, endotracheal tubes, suction catheters, chest tubes, intravenous catheters, and gastric tubes in pediatric sizes. If cuffed endotracheal tubes are used, it may be possible to cover all pediatric needs with 3.0-, 4.0-, 5.0-, and 6.0-mm cuffed tubes, reducing the need to stock uncuffed tubes in all other sizes. Guidelines for EMCC ventilators have been provided.[3,43]

Medications

In order to extend medication stockpiles in mass critical care, rules should be formulated ahead of time regarding appropriate substitutions, dose and frequency reductions, converting parenteral to enteral administration, restrictive indications, and shelf-life extension.[3] Experience in recent PHEs indicates that large quantities of analgesics and sedatives are essential.[7,44] Weight-based dosing may be simplified to improve efficiency by specifying a limited number of weight range categories.

When time constraints make it difficult to weigh patients, length-based estimates of weight may suffice.[45]

Evacuation

ICU providers must be aware of processes to ensure a safe and timely ICU evacuation. Hurricane Sandy demonstrated a lack of ICU evacuation knowledge, processes, and tools.[46] Pediatric patients are especially vulnerable during ICU evacuation as few hospitals can serve as recipient hospitals and few transport agencies are familiar with pediatric critical care transport for hospitalized pediatric patients. Thus PICU evacuation is critically dependent on regional coordination of PICU resources.[47] ICU-evacuation best practices were reviewed in the most recent Mass Critical Care Taskforce and include tools such as ICU evacuation checklists and job action sheets.[48]

Critical Care in Specific Types of Public Health Emergencies

While all-hazard planning prepares for PICU operations across all types of PHEs, some responses must be event specific. These responses are detailed extensively in standard references.[29,49] In addition to general critical care support, event-specific hospital responses and treatments are briefly outlined in Table 24.2. For any type of emergency, clinical interventions also will be necessary for illnesses and injuries that are indirectly related or unrelated to the primary event. These illnesses and injuries include patients hospitalized before the onset of the PHE.

Rationing

If a PHE overwhelms resources despite EMCC approaches, rationing of resources may be considered. Rationing might occur on a first-come, first-served basis or by selecting patients most likely to survive as a result of brief lifesaving interventions. Such criteria have been suggested for selecting patients for EMCC when needs exceed resources.[3,50] Proposed eligibility criteria include absence of severe chronic conditions, predicted mortality not exceeding an arbitrary upper limit, and improving clinical status on periodic reevaluations. EMCC exclusion criteria have been proposed that apply to both children and adults.[51] These criteria identify patients with low probability of survival and short life expectancy. In pediatrics, however, there is little consensus about, or data to support, which score to use, especially in light of typical PICU mortality of less than 5%.[6] Triage of resources, or rationing, should only occur using a formal hospital system triage policy and/or protocol and should be performed by trained triage officers with critical care training. At present, neither evidence nor consensus of opinion supports rationing, much less a particular rationing strategy.[52,53] For PHE rationing to be a feasible option, public and professional consensus is a necessary foundation. Only then could states create a legal basis and liability protections.[54]

As recently as during Hurricane Sandy, however, critical care leaders were asked by hospitals to formulate rationing plans during PHEs.[55] At Bellevue Hospital, there was imminent threat of losing all but six power outlets in the entire ICU on the 13th floor. A multidisciplinary clinical committee prioritized patients for those six electrical outlets using the Ontario Guidelines.[56] Fortunately, the generator power was maintained via the now famous "bucket brigade" that shuttled

TABLE 24.2   Specific Types of Public Health Emergencies and Event-Specific Management

Type of Event	Infrastructure	Decontamination	Infection Control	Disorders/Event-Specific Interventions
Emerging infectious illness (influenza, SARS) outbreak	Need for negative pressure isolation		Depending on organism, usually a combination of standard, droplet, airborne precautions	Pneumonia, sepsis Antibiotics/antiviral according to organism Antibiotics for bacterial coinfection
Major earthquake	Extensive damage Mass evacuation likely		Standard precautions	Multiple trauma including crush injuries requiring renal replacement therapy
Hurricane	Extensive damage Mass evacuation likely		Standard precautions	Multiple trauma
Nuclear detonation (terrorism)[57,59]	Extensive damage Mass evacuation likely	Radiation Contamination of body orifices, wounds, skin Treatment of life-threatening injuries is the priority	Standard precautions	Multiple trauma, burns, radiation (bone marrow, immunosuppression, gastrointestinal)
Radioactive dispersal bomb (terrorism)[58,59]	Local damage and contamination	Radiation Contamination of body orifices, wounds, skin Treatment of life-threatening injuries is the priority	Standard precautions	Multiple trauma, burns, radiation (bone marrow, immunosuppression, gastrointestinal)
Chemical attack Nerve agent (terrorism)		Essential, must be rapid	Standard precautions	Antidotes (atropine, pralidoxime) Anticonvulsants Bronchodilators
Chemical attack Vesicants/blister agent (terrorism)		Essential, must be rapid	Standard precautions	Chemical burns, potential airway injury
Chemical attack Pulmonary agent such as chlorine, phosgene (terrorism)		Move to fresh air Irrigate eyes, mucous membranes, skin	Standard precautions	Airway and pulmonary edema
Biological attack Anthrax (terrorism)		If known, direct exposure to spores	Standard precautions	Ciprofloxacin Doxycycline
Biological attack Pneumonic plague (terrorism)			Droplet precautions	Streptomycin Gentamycin
Biological attack Smallpox (terrorism)			Standard, contact, and airborne precautions	Vaccination

Adapted from Siegel JD, Rhinehart E, Jackson M, et al. Guideline for isolation precautions: preventing transmission of infectious agents in healthcare settings. Available at: <http://www.cdc.gov/hicpac/pdf/isolation/Isolation2007.pdf>. Accessed 07.15; and Foltin GL, Schonfeld DJ, Shannon MW, eds. Pediatric terrorism and disaster preparedness: a resource for pediatricians (AHRQ publication No. 06-0056-EF). Rockville, MD: Agency for Healthcare Research and Quality; 2006.

generator fuel up 13 flights of stairs until ICU evacuation could be achieved. Although these critical care triage plans were not implemented, their use was imminent. It is essential that critical care providers are knowledgeable about hospital and regional EMCC triage protocols and prepared for future events despite the lack of current consensus and data.

References

1. US Department of Homeland Security. *National response framework*. Washington, DC: Department of Homeland Security; 2014. Available at: <https://www.fema.gov/media-library/assets/documents/32230?id=7371>; Accessed 27.07.15.
2. Federal Emergency Management Agency, Emergency Management Institute. Introduction to the Incident Command System for healthcare/hospitals. 2013; Available at: <https://training.fema.gov/is/courseoverview.aspx?code=is-100.hcb>; Accessed 10.07.15.
3. Christian MD, Devereaux AV, Dichter JR, et al. Introduction and executive summary: care of the critically ill and injured during pandemics and disasters: CHEST consensus statement. *Chest*. 2014;146(suppl 4):8S-34S.
4. Phillips SJ, Knebel A. *Mass medical care with scarce resources: a community planning guide*. Rockville, MD: Agency for Healthcare Research and Quality (AHRQ Publication No. 07-0001); 2007.
5. Kanter RK, Cooper A. Mass critical care: pediatric considerations in extending and rationing care in public health emergencies. *Disaster Med Public Health Prep*. 2009;3:S166-S171.
6. Kissoon N, et al. Deliberations and recommendations of the Pediatric Emergency Mass Critical Care Task Force: executive summary. *Pediatr Crit Care Med*. 2011;12(suppl 6):S103-S108.
7. Mahoney EJ, Harrington DT, Biffl WL, et al. Lessons learned from a nightclub fire: institutional disaster preparedness. *J Trauma*. 2005;58:487-491.
8. Gostin LO, Sapsin JW, Teret SP, et al. The Model State Emergency Health Powers Act. *JAMA*. 2002;288:622-628.
9. US Census Bureau. *Age and sex, table S0101, American community survey*. Washington, DC: US Census Bureau; 2006.

10. Tilford JM, Simpson PM, Green JW, et al. Volume outcome relationships in pediatric intensive care units. *Pediatrics*. 2000;106:289-294.

11. Pollack MM, Alexander SR, Clarke N, et al. Improved outcomes from tertiary center pediatric intensive care: a statewide comparison of tertiary and nontertiary care facilities. *Crit Care Med*. 1991;19:150-159.

12. Osler TM, Vane DW, Tepas JJ, et al. Do pediatric trauma centers have better survival rates than adult trauma centers? An examination of the National Pediatric Trauma Registry. *J Trauma*. 2001;50:96-101.

13. Densmore JC, Lim HJ, Oldham KT, et al. Outcomes and delivery of care in pediatric injury. *J Pediatr Surg*. 2006;41:92-98.

14. Randolph AG, Gonzales CA, Cortellini L, et al. Growth of pediatric ICUs in the US from 1995 to 2001. *J Pediatr*. 2004;144:792-798.

15. Kanter RK. Strategies to improve pediatric disaster surge response: potential mortality reduction and tradeoffs. *Crit Care Med*. 2007;35:2837-2842.

16. American Academy of Pediatrics: American College of Critical Care Medicine. Consensus report for regionalization of services for critically ill or injured children. *Pediatrics*. 2000;105:152-155.

17. EMSC National Resource Center. Checklist of essential pediatric domains and considerations for every hospital's disaster preparedness policies. 2014.

18. EMSC National Resource Center. Available at: <http://www.emscnrc.org/EMSC_Resources/Publications.aspx>; Accessed 29.07.15.

19. Auf der Heide E. The importance of evidence-based disaster planning. *Ann Emerg Med*. 2006;47:34-49.

20. New York State Department of Health. Pediatric and obstetrical emergency preparedness toolkit: a guide for pediatric and obstetrical emergency planning. Available at: <www.health.state.ny.us/facilities/hospital/emergency_preparedness/guideline_for_hospitals/index.htm>; Accessed 29.07.15.

21. Kanter RK, Moran JR. Hospital emergency surge capacity: an empiric New York statewide study. *Ann Emerg Med*. 2007;50:314-319.

22. King MA, Koelemay K, Zimmerman J, et al. Geographical maldistribution of pediatric medical resources in Seattle-King County. *Prehosp Disaster Med*. 2010;25(4):326-332.

23. Kanter RK, Moran JR. Pediatric hospital and intensive care unit capacity in regional disasters. *Pediatrics*. 2007;119:94-100.

24. Chevalier MS, Chung W, Smith J, et al. Ebola virus disease cluster in the United States–Dallas County, Texas, 2014. *MMWR Morb Mortal Wkly Rep*. 2014; Available at: <http://www.cdc.gov/mmwr/preview/mmwrhtml/mm63e1114a5.htm>; Accessed 27.07.15.

25. Lerner EB, Schwartz RB, Coule PL, et al. Mass casualty triage: an evaluation of the data and development of a proposed national guidance. *Disaster Med Public Health Prep*. 2008;2:S25-S34.

26. Kenningham K, Koelemay K, King MA. Pediatric disaster triage education and skills assessment: a coalition approach. *J Emerg Manag*. 2014;12:141-151.

27. Fertel BS, Kohlhoff SA, Roblin PM. Lessons from the "Clean Baby 2007" pediatric decontamination drill. *Am J Disaster Med*. 2009;4:77-85.

28. Freyberg CW, Arquilla B, Fertel BS, et al. Disaster preparedness: hospital decontamination and the pediatric patient—guidelines for hospitals and emergency planners. *Prehosp Disaster Med*. 2008;23:166-173.

29. US Department of Homeland Security. Patient decontamination in a mass chemical exposure incident: national planning guidance for communities. 2014; Available at: <http://www.dhs.gov/sites/default/files/publications/Patient%20Decon%20National%20Planning%20Guidance_Final_December%202014.pdf>; Accessed 27.07.15.

30. Siegel JD, Rhinehart E, Jackson M, et al. Guideline for isolation precautions: preventing transmission of infectious agents in healthcare settings. 2009; Available at: <http://www.cdc.gov/hicpac/pdf/isolation/Isolation2007.pdf>; Accessed 27.07.15.

31. Centers for Disease Control and Prevention. Ebola virus disease. Infection prevention and control recommendations for hospitalized patients under investigation for Ebola virus disease in US hospitals. 2015; Available at: <http://www.cdc.gov/vhf/ebola/healthcare-us/hospitals/infection-control.html>; Accessed 27.07.15.

32. Eriksson CO, Uyeki TM, Christian MD, et al. Care of the child with Ebola virus disease. *Pediatr Crit Care Med*. 2015;16:97-103.

33. Kanter RK, Andrake JS, Boeing NM, et al. A method for developing consensus on appropriate standards of disaster care. *Disaster Med Public Health Prep*. 2009;3:27-32.

34. Young R, Hobson J. Before marathon bombings, Aurora helped Boston prepare. *Here & Now, WBUR, Boston National Public Radio*. Available at: <http://hereandnow.wbur.org/2013/08/27/aurora-boston-er>; Accessed 27.07.15.

35. Rubinson L, Vaughn F, Nelson S, et al. Mechanical ventilators in US acute care hospitals. *Disaster Med Public Health Prep*. 2010;4(3):199-206.

36. West JB. The physiological challenges of the 1952 Copenhagen poliomyelitis epidemic and a renaissance in clinical respiratory physiology. *J Appl Physiol*. 2005;99:424-432.

37. O'Hara JF, Higgins TL. Total electrical power failure in a cardiothoracic intensive care unit. *Crit Care Med*. 1992;20:840-845.

38. Norcross ED, Elliott BM, Adams DB, et al. Impact of a major hurricane on surgical services in a university hospital. *Am Surg*. 1993;59:28-33.

39. Nates JL. Combined external and internal hospital disaster: impact and response in a Houston trauma center intensive care unit. *Crit Care Med*. 2004;32:686-690.

40. Barkmeyer BM. Practicing neonatology in a blackout: the University Hospital NICU in the midst of Hurricane Katrina: caring for children without power or water. *Pediatrics*. 2006;117:S369-S374.

41. Gervais HW, Eberle B, Konietzky D, et al. Comparison of blood gases of ventilated patients during transport. *Crit Care Med*. 1987;15:761-763.

42. Hurst JM, Davis K, Branson RD, et al. Comparison of blood gases during transport using two methods of ventilatory support. *J Trauma*. 1989;29:1637-1640.

43. Johannigman JA, Branson RD, Johnson DJ, et al. Out-of-hospital ventilation: bag valve device vs transport ventilator. *Acad Emerg Med*. 1995;2:719-724.

44. Branson RD, Johannigman JA, Daugherty EL, et al. Surge capacity mechanical ventilation. *Respir Care*. 2008;53:78-90.

45. Kumar A, Zarychanski R, Pinto R, et al. Critically ill patients with 2009 Influenza A (H1N1) infection in Canada. *JAMA*. 2009;302:1872-1879.

46. Luten R, Zaritsky A. The sophistication of simplicity: optimizing emergency dosing. *Acad Emerg Med*. 2008;15:461-465.

47. Espiritu M, Patil U, Cruz H, et al. Evacuation of a neonatal intensive care unit in a disaster: lessons from Hurricane Sandy. *Pediatrics*. 2014;134(6):e1662-e1669.

48. Kanter RK. Regional variation in critical care evacuation needs for children after a mass casualty incident. *Disaster Med Public Health Prep*. 2012;6(2):146-149.

49. King MA, Niven AS, Beninati W, et al. Evacuation of the ICU: care of the critically ill and injured during pandemics and disasters: CHEST consensus statement. *Chest*. 2014;146(suppl 4):e44S-460S.

50. Foltin GL, Schonfeld DJ, Shannon MW. *Pediatric terrorism and disaster preparedness: a resource for pediatricians*. Rockville, MD: Agency for Healthcare Research and Quality (AHRQ publication No. 06-0056-EF); 2006.

51. Powell T, Christ KC, Birkhead GS. Allocation of ventilators in a public health disaster. *Disaster Med Public Health Prep*. 2008;2:20-26.

52. Christian MD, Sprung CL, King MA, et al. Triage: care of the critically ill and injured during pandemics and disasters: chest consensus statement. *Chest*. 2014;146(suppl 4):e61S-e74S.

53. Kanter RK. Would triage predictors perform better than first-come, first-served in pandemic ventilator allocation? *Chest*. 2015;147(1):102-108.

54. Johnson EM, Diekema DS, Lewis-Newby M, et al. Pediatric triage and allocation of critical care resources during disaster: northwest provider opinion. *Prehosp Disaster Med*. 2014;29(5):455-460.

55. Hoffman S, Goodman RA, Stier DD. Law, liability, and public health emergencies. *Disaster Med Public Health Prep*. 2009;3:117-125.

56. Uppal A, Evans L, Chitkara N, et al. In search of the silver lining, the impact of Superstorm Sandy on Bellevue Hospital. *Ann Am Thorac Soc*. 2013;10:135-142.

57. Christian MD, Hawryluck L, Wax RS, et al. Development of a triage protocol for critical care during an influenza pandemic. *CMAJ*. 2006;175:1377-1381.

58. Homeland Security Council Interagency Policy Coordination Subcommittee for Preparedness & Response to Radiological and Nuclear Threats. Planning guidance for response to a nuclear detonation. Available at: <http://www.remm.nlm.gov/planning-guidance.pdf>; Accessed 28.07.15.

59. Department of Health and Human Services. Radiation event medical management: guidance on diagnosis & treatment for health care providers. Available at: <http://www.remm.nlm.gov/index.html>; Accessed 28.07.15.

Cardiovascular System

Cardiovascular System

Structure and Function of the Heart

V. Ben Sivarajan and Steven M. Schwartz

PEARLS

- The basic form of the human heart and great vessels is complete 8 weeks after conception, after which the structures grow and mature. Recent data show some limited capacity for hyperplasia that persists even into adulthood.
- The parietal pericardium is a stiff membrane that surrounds the heart loosely, separated from the heart by a small amount of lubricating pericardial fluid.
- Immediately after birth, there is a large increase in total body oxygen consumption and cardiac output to approximately twice its later values.
- Although large arteries are regarded as conduits and capillaries as vessels allowing transport of substances to and from the tissues, many substances can move across arterial walls.
- Standard echocardiographic assessments (ejection and shortening fraction) reflect myocardial performance (load-dependent measure) as opposed to true contractility. Assessments of adequacy of ventricular-vascular coupling (adequacy of contractile status with a given preload given the afterload conditions) can be assessed by noninvasive or invasive methods.

Anatomic Development and Structure
Gross Anatomy

The basic form of the human heart and great vessels is complete 8 weeks after conception, after which the structures grow and mature. The ventricular mass enlarges by cellular hyperplasia and hypertrophy; hyperplasia previously assumed to cease after birth has recently been shown by carbon-14 dating to occur at an annual turnover rate of 1% at age 25 years, decreasing to half that value by age 75 years.[1] Increase of ventricular volumes is believed to depend on the increasing flow through each ventricle; diverting flow from a ventricle causes hypoplasia of that ventricle and its associated great artery. Before birth, left and right ventricles have equal wall thickness. After birth and clamping of the umbilical cord, there is a rise in systemic vascular resistance and a decrease in pulmonary vascular resistance; as a result, the left ventricle becomes thicker than the right ventricle. Left ventricular wall thickness is proportional to the logarithm of age from conception.[2] The ventricular septum is flat in the fetus. After birth, it bulges into the right ventricle and functions like part of the left ventricle.

In the embryo, coronary arteries form in the embryonic epicardial tissue[3] and join the aorta to supply flow to the thickening heart muscle, which can no longer get enough blood from sinusoids from the ventricular cavity.

Muscle fibers in the ventricles form a complex helical array. Fibers in the left ventricular midwall are circumferential, parallel to the atrioventricular groove. From this position the fibers twist gradually as they move toward each surface so that at the epicardial surface they are 75 degrees and at the endocardial surface 60 degrees from the circumferential fibers.[4] Some investigators believe that the muscle fiber layers form one continuous sheet that is wrapped around itself like a turban.[5] When the ventricle is dilated, the fiber angles change and become less effective in ejecting blood.[6]

Microscopic Anatomy

The myocardium is a syncytium made of branching fibers, each consisting of bundles of myocytes in series. The myocytes are joined to adjacent myocytes by the intercalated disk, a set of mechanical junctions: adherens junctions with N-cadherin, catenins, and vinculin; desmosomes with desmin, desmoplakin, desmocollin, and desmoglein; and gap junctions with connexins and N-cadherin.[7-9] The gap junctions transmit the electrical impulse from one cell to the next.

Myocyte

The major components of the myocyte are the sarcomeres, which contain the myofibrillar contractile apparatus; the mitochondria, which contain enzymes for energy production; the sarcolemma, which contains the cell envelope and its extensions into the cytoplasm; the sarcoplasmic reticulum; and the cytosol. The numerous proteins in these structures not only play a role in normal function but, if abnormal for genetic or extraneous reasons, contribute to myocardial dysfunction.[10]

Contractile Apparatus

The functional unit is the sarcomere, defined as the structure between two transverse Z lines,[11-13] representing disks that contain proteins such as α-actinin and filamin, which connect the actin and titin filaments of adjacent myocytes. On each side of the Z line is a light zone, the I (isotropic) band, and in the center of the sarcomere are two dark zones, the A (anisotropic) bands, separated by a light H band in the middle of which is a dark thin M band (Fig. 25.1). The I bands contain paired thin filaments of actin coiled in a helix and attached to the Z lines. In humans, cardiac α-actin makes up 80% of the actin in fetuses and neonates, while skeletal α-actin makes up 60% of the total in adults.[14] Two long tropomyosin filaments lie in the grooves between each pair of actin filaments

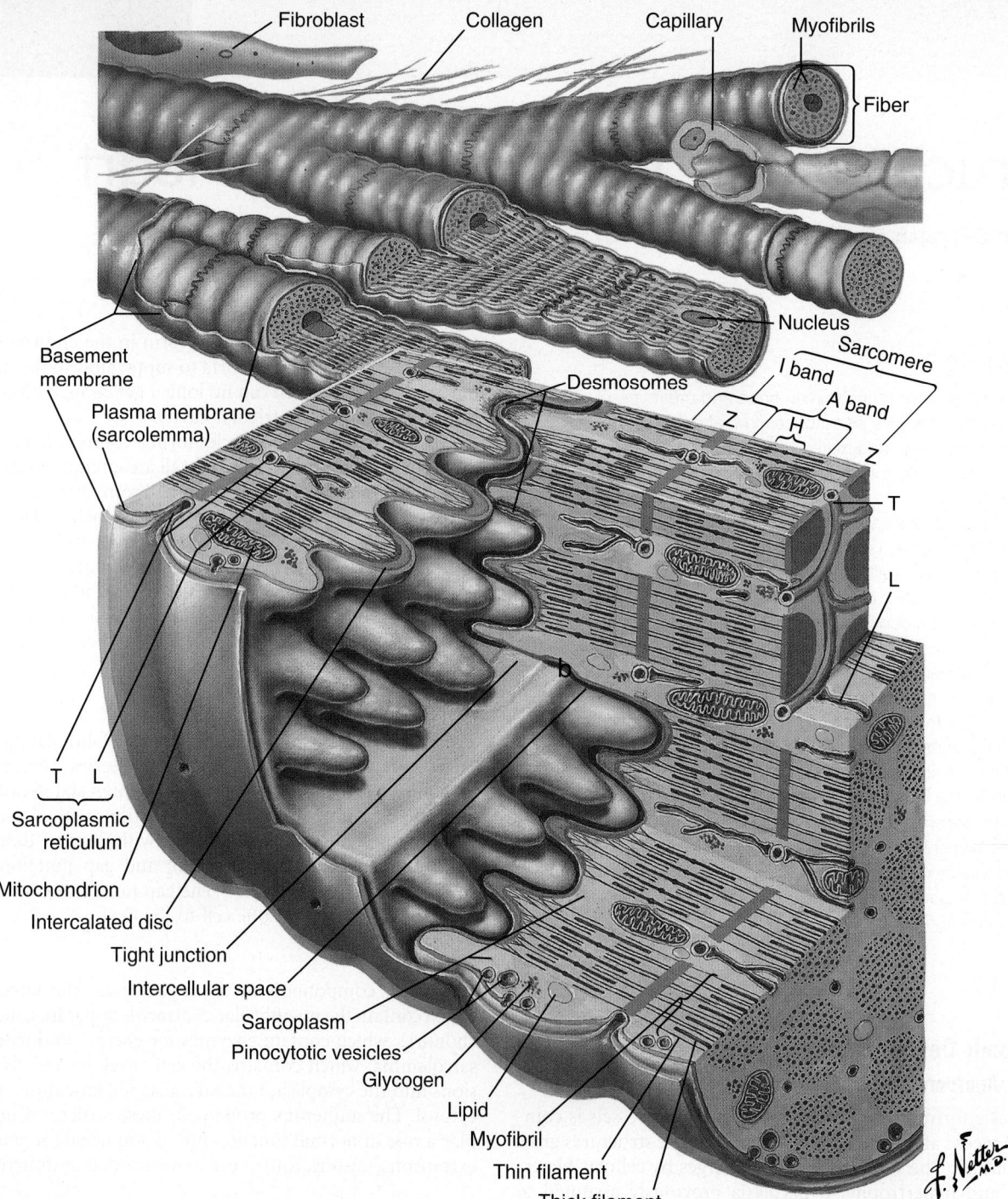

Fig. 25.1. Diagram of cardiac muscle unit showing organization of structural and contractile elements. (Netter illustration from www.netterimages.com. Elsevier Inc. All rights reserved.)

(Fig. 25.2).[15] Every 400 Å, near the crossover points of two actin filaments, is a troponin complex with the following three distinct troponins: (1) troponin T, which binds troponin to tropomyosin; (2) troponin I, which inhibits actin-myosin interaction; and (3) troponin C, which is a high-affinity calcium receptor. The thin actin filaments overlap with thick myosin filaments at the A bands. These myosin filaments are composed of light and heavy chains. The light chains coil around each other to form the long core of the myosin

molecule. The heavy chains form globular myosin heads that project from the sides of the thick filament toward the actin molecules (see Fig. 25.2). A collar of cardiac myosin-binding protein C encircles the thick filaments. Mutations of this protein are a common cause of hypertrophic cardiomyopathy.[16] Between two A bands there is usually a thin, lighter band, the H band, which has myosin but no actin filaments.[13,15]

Titin, the largest known molecule (molecular weight 3–3.6 MDa, 1-mm long), is the third most abundant fibrillar

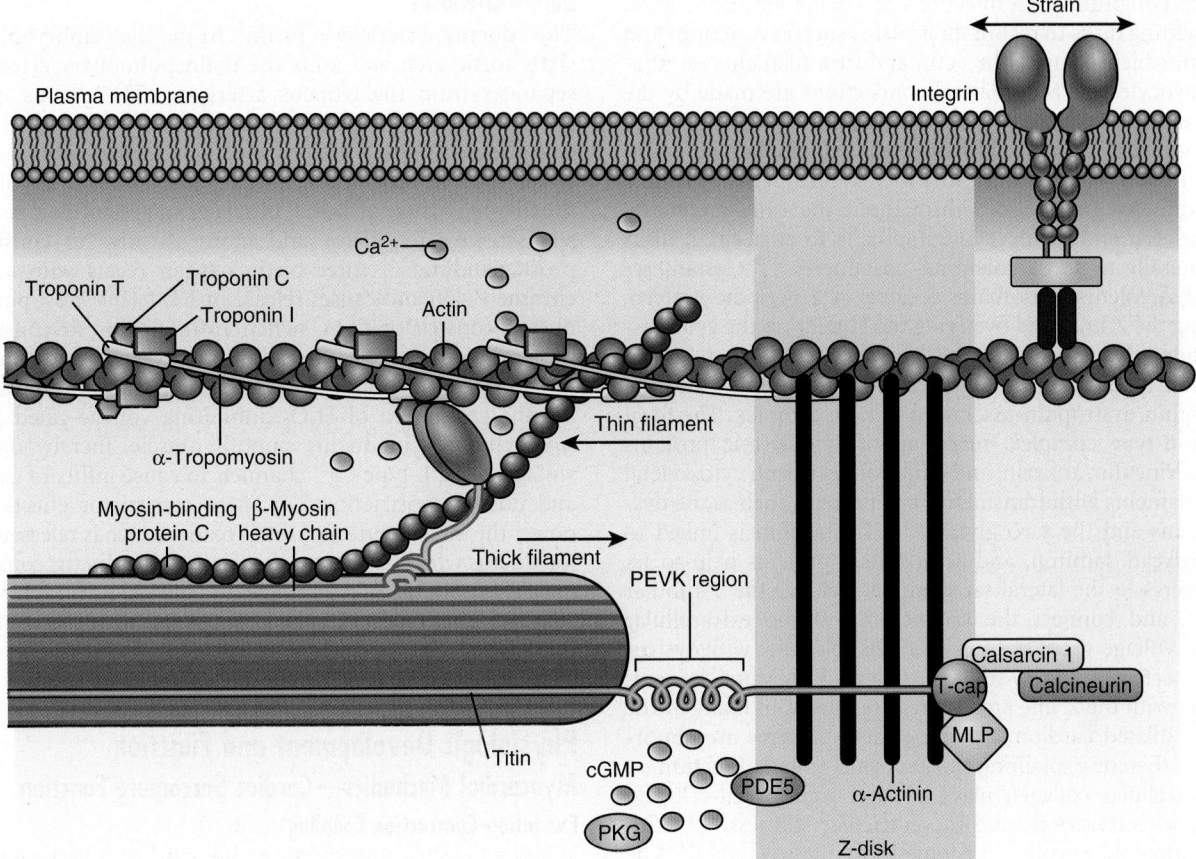

Fig. 25.2. Diagram showing the integration of myofibril contraction (actin-myosin complex formation) to attachments to the Z lines and cytoskeleton via various ultrastructural proteins. (Modified from Mudd JO, Kass DA. Tackling heart failure in the twenty-first century. Nature. 2008;451:919-928.)

protein. It extends from the Z band to the M band, has two isoforms, and is the main protein responsible for the elastic behavior of the myocyte.[17] It is essential for sarcomere assembly and for sensing sarcomere length[18] and, with myomesin (not shown in figure), supports the actomyosin filaments (see Fig. 25.2).

Myocytes have fewer myofibrils and more water and cytoplasm before birth than after birth, and the myofibrils do not have the uniformly parallel arrays that they will have after birth.[19]

Sarcolemma and Sarcoplasmic Reticulum
The cell membrane contains receptors, ion channels, pumps, and exchangers. It has indentations overlying the Z bands, and from these indentations small tubules termed *T (for transverse) tubules* penetrate the cell. Abutting against the T tubules are dilated expansions of the sarcoplasmic reticulum (junctional reticulum or cisternae), which join the free sarcoplasmic reticulum, a network of longitudinal tubules inside the cell that surround the thick (myosin) filaments. These tubular systems modulate the entry of calcium to, or its exclusion from, the cytoplasm.[11,19]

The cisternae contain the calcium-binding protein calsequestrin, whereas the longitudinal tubules contain phospholamban and the adenosine triphosphate (ATP)-dependent calcium pump.[19,20] Phospholamban inhibits the affinity of the sarcoplasmic reticulum Ca^{2+}-ATPase (SERCA) pump for calcium, and phospholamban phosphorylation relieves the

inhibition and increases calcium entry with a resulting increase in inotropy.[21-24] In heart failure, phospholamban phosphorylation is decreased by an increase in unphosphorylated calcineurin,[25] leading to decreased SERCA activity.[26,27] A similar decrease in SERCA has been found in sepsis[28] and in some forms of dilated cardiomyopathy.[29] Cisternae store and release activator calcium, whereas longitudinal tubules remove calcium from the cytosol. Calcium release is primarily via the calcium-activated calcium release channel termed the *ryanodine receptor*. Both T tubules and sarcoplasmic reticulum are sparse, undifferentiated, and disorganized early in gestation but increase and differentiate markedly late in gestation and after birth in mammals. Therefore the immature heart depends mainly on extracellular sources for activator calcium,[15,19] partly explaining its marked calcium sensitivity.

Cytoplasm
During development, the proportion of mitochondria in the myocyte increases, particularly at the time of birth, and mitochondria become larger and develop more complex cristae.[19] In the adult, approximately 30% to 40% of the muscle mass is made up of mitochondria. The cytosol contains other calcium-binding proteins[19,30] and other major proteins such as tubulin and desmin.

Cytoskeleton and Extracellular Matrix
For contractile proteins to shorten the whole myocyte, they must be linked to both the cell membrane and extracellular

matrix. Longitudinal connections are made via the Z lines, representing disks that contain proteins such as α-actinin and filamin, which connect the actin and titin filaments of adjacent myocytes.[31,32] More lateral connections are made by the extrasarcomeric skeleton. There is an intermyofibrillar cytoskeleton with intermediate filaments, microfilaments, and microtubules.[31,33-35] Desmin intermediate filaments provide a three-dimensional scaffold throughout the extrasarcomeric cytoskeleton and connect longitudinally to adjacent Z disks and laterally to subsarcolemmal costameres.[33,35] Costameres are subsarcolemmal domains located in a periodic pattern, flanking the Z lines and overlying the I bands on the cytoplasmic side of the sarcolemma.[36-40] They contain the focal adhesion-type complex, the spectrin-based complex, and the dystrophin/dystrophin-associated protein complex. The focal adhesion-type complex, made up of cytoplasmic proteins such as vinculin, ankyrin, and talin, connects with cytoskeletal actin filaments with transmembrane proteins such as the dystroglycans and the sarcoglycans.[41-43] Dystrophin is linked to dystroglycan, laminin, and actin. These proteins help to fix sarcomeres to the lateral sarcolemma, stabilize the T-tubular system, and connect the sarcolemma to the extracellular matrix. Voltage-gated sodium channels colocalize with dystrophin, spectrin, ankyrin, and syntrophins. Potassium channels interact with the Z line and intercalated disks. In many of the genetic dilated cardiomyopathies, these proteins are abnormal,[44-46] thereby explaining the abnormal muscle function.

Extracellular collagen plays a major role in cell-cell and cell-vessel interactions and in ventricular stiffness.[47-50] With maturation, more collagen is type III and less is type I.[51] The relationship between sarcomeres and cytoskeleton changes with maturation, perhaps accounting for maturational differences in the resting sarcomere's mean length in myocytes.[52] In addition, cell adhesion proteins stimulated by growth factors from the myocyte are present in greatest amount in the neonate, decrease with postnatal age, but increase again during hypertrophy.[53,54] Other elements in the extracellular matrix (eg, laminin, fibronectin, and tenascin) play a major role during morphogenesis and during contraction[55] and are important mediators in hypertrophy.

Nerves and Receptors

Adrenergic, muscarinic, and other receptors appear early and are functional even before innervation. Parasympathetic innervation precedes sympathetic innervation in all species.[19,56,57] Innervation is present in the earliest viable human premature infants but may not be fully mature. Innervation is most advanced in species that are most independent immediately after birth.

Cardiac sympathetic nerve fibers come from cervical sympathetic and stellate ganglia. Right sympathetic nerves innervate the right and anterior surfaces of the heart. Left sympathetic nerves innervate the left and posterior surfaces. Vagal nerve fibers descending from medullary centers supply both atria and ventricles and the proximal portion of the bundle of His; the distal part of the bundle of His has only sympathetic nerve supply. Sympathetic and vagal afferents leave the heart and carry information from baroreceptors that respond to high pressures in the ventricles and to lower pressures in the atria, cavae, and pulmonary veins, as well as from chemoreceptors that respond to locally produced substances such as bradykinin and prostaglandin.[58]

Ductus Arteriosus

The ductus arteriosus forms from the embryonic left sixth aortic arch and joins the main pulmonary artery that separates from the truncus arteriosus. The ductus is kept open by a balance between prostaglandin E2 (PGE2) and endothelin-1 (ET-1), both of which are formed in its wall and circulate from other sites. Initially, the ductus is sensitive to the dilating action of PGE2, but, later in gestation, it becomes less sensitive to dilator and more sensitive to constrictor prostaglandins.[59-61] After birth, oxygen reacts with a cytochrome P-450 and causes release of ET-1 (the most powerful ductus constrictor).[62] A switch from dilator to constrictor prostaglandins occurs. In addition, oxygen modulates the function of mitochondrial electron chain transport by increasing the generation of H_2O_2, inhibiting voltage-gated potassium channels in ductus smooth muscle, thereby opening voltage-gated L-type Ca^{2+} channels to cause influx of calcium and ductus constriction.[63-65] These constrictor effects overpower the dilating effect of nitric oxide, which is released from the ductus when oxygen tension rises.[66] The ductus constricts, usually within the first 24 hours and almost invariably within 3 weeks. The lumen then becomes permanently occluded by fibrosis.[61,67]

Physiologic Development and Function
Myocardial Mechanics—Cardiac Sarcomere Function
Excitation-Contraction Coupling

When an electrical impulse reaches cardiac muscle, myocyte membranes depolarize. Extracellular calcium in high concentration at the sarcolemmal membrane and the T tubules enters the cell rapidly. Spread of electrical excitation into the myocyte via the T tubules also causes release of intracellular calcium from the sarcoplasmic reticulum.[11,68,69]

Cytosolic calcium increases from a concentration of 10^{-7} M in diastole to 10^{-5} M in systole. When the calcium that entered the cytosol binds to troponin C, the inhibitory effect of troponin I is antagonized, and a conformational change of troponin and tropomyosin exposes the actin-myosin binding sites.[11,15,68,69] These sites interact with the myosin heads to form the cross-bridges (Fig. 25.3). The myosin heads rotate, generate force, and move the actin filaments, just as oars move a boat through the water. Interaction between actin and myosin pulls the two Z lines toward each other, shortening the muscle and generating force. Increasing intracellular calcium results in greater cross-bridge formation and a greater generated force. Isoforms of the troponins and tropomyosin change during development, but the functional effects of these changes are unknown.[19,70] Troponin I is less sensitive to a fall in pH in the fetus than in the adult, which could be protective in perinatal acidosis.

The myosin head contains an ATPase that liberates energy from ATP. The activity of the ATPase determines the velocity of shortening of unloaded muscle by affecting the rate of attachment and detachment of the cross-bridges.[19,71] In most mammalian species, fetal myocardium contains V_3 myosin isoform (having two β heavy chains) with a high ATPase activity rate. In humans and most of the larger mammals, however, almost all ventricular myocardial myosin is V_3 isoform at any age, although human atria contain V_1 myosin isoform.[19]

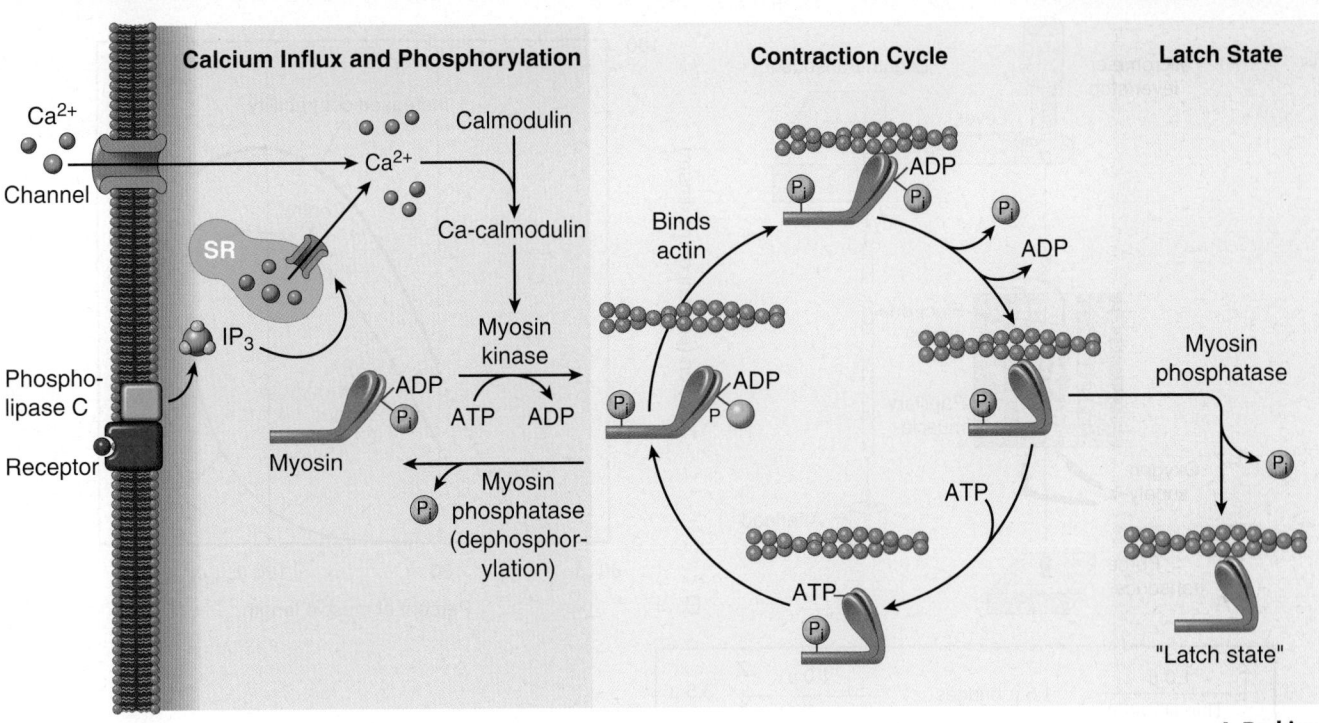

Calcium Influx and Phosphorylation **Contraction Cycle** **Latch State**

J. Perkins
MS, MFA

Fig. 25.3. Diagram of cardiomyocyte calcium cycling and adenosine-triphosphate (ATP) utilization during actin-myosin complex formation. (Netter illustration from www.netterimages.com. Elsevier Inc. All rights reserved.)

Sarcomere Length-Tension Relationships

Sarcomere length-tension relationships have been investigated in isolated cardiac muscle strips, usually papillary muscle with its nearly parallel fibers. The muscle strip is placed in a water bath. One end is tied to a lever and the other to a force transducer (Fig. 25.4A). Weights attached to the other end of the lever extend the muscle to any desired length before contraction (preload); excessive stretching is prevented by a stop. Other weights added to the lever after initial length is set affect the muscle only after contraction has started and so are termed the *afterload*. The muscle can be stimulated to contract by an electrical impulse. Instruments for measuring muscle length, sarcomere length by laser diffraction, calcium entry by various fluorescence methods, and a host of other specialized functions can be added.[69,72,73]

Stretching relaxed muscle produces an exponential-like increase in passive tension (Fig. 25.4B). This elasticity results mainly from titin.[17,73-75] At very low sarcomere lengths, the actin filaments from each Z line overlap each other. As the sarcomere lengthens, the Z lines move farther apart and a gap appears between the two sets of actin filaments. When the sarcomere reaches a length of approximately 2.2 μm, there is a maximal overlap between actin and myosin filaments[13,69,71] (Fig. 25.4C). At longer muscle and sarcomere lengths, actin and myosin filaments overlap less. The maximal sarcomere length is 3.0 μm. Further elongation of the muscle occurs by slippage of fibers and not by further sarcomere lengthening.[13,69,71]

Active contraction is studied in two ways[72] (Fig. 25.4D). First, muscle is stimulated to contract at different initial muscle lengths but is not allowed to shorten (isometric contraction). At the shortest lengths no force is generated; the

muscle remains slack. As sarcomere lengths increase, force is generated and increases to reach a maximum at sarcomere lengths of approximately 2.2 μm. At longer sarcomere lengths, there may even be a decrease in force.[71]

If, at any length, passive tension is subtracted from the tension generated during isometric contraction, the resulting curve demonstrates active tension as a function of length (see Fig. 25.4B).

Second, if afterload is small, the contracting muscle generates an appropriate force and then shortens while force remains constant (isotonic contraction). The rate of shortening is fastest at the onset of shortening, and from it, the velocity of shortening is measured (see Fig. 25.4D). The shortening velocity ranges from zero when the load is so heavy that it prevents shortening to a maximum when the external load is zero[69]; however, true zero loading is impossible because of internal viscosity and elastic forces.[19,71] Increases in cytosolic calcium increase the force generated during contraction but have little influence on the maximal velocity of shortening.

In fetal lambs, the passive tension of muscle strips is abnormally high. Active tension per mm² cross-sectional myocyte area at any given afterload is below adult values but is proportional to the reduced number of myofibrils.[19,30,57] Contractile material accounts for approximately 60% of cardiac muscle in adults but only 30% in fetuses. The extent and velocity of shortening are reduced in fetal heart muscle, but correcting for the amount of contractile machinery suggests the intrinsic performance of fetal and adult actin-myosin filaments is similar.[19] The change from fetal to adult performance seems to occur fairly soon after birth, when the myofibrillar array becomes regular and when the T tubules and the sarcoplasmic reticulum develop into their adult form.[19] For this reason,

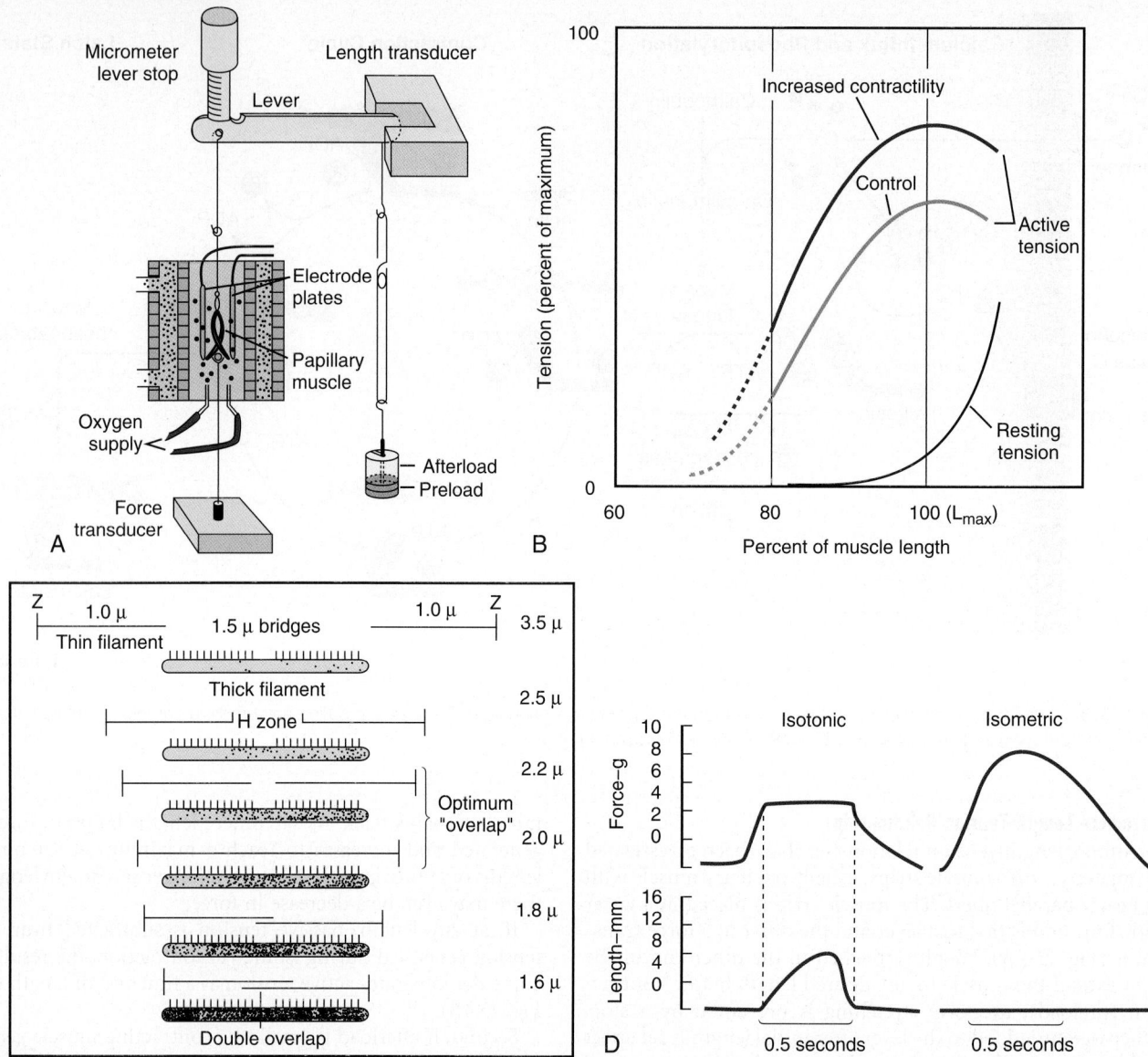

Fig. 25.4. A, Diagram of isolated muscle strip in a water bath and attached to transducers for measuring force and length. Preload is set by the lever stop. (From Parmley WW, Tyberg JV. Determinants of myocardial oxygen consumption. In: Yu PN, Goodwin JF, ed. Progress in Cardiology. Philadelphia: Lea & Febiger; 1976.) B, Relationship between muscle length and resting tension or active tension at three different contractile levels. (Original drawing by Albert Miller. Redrawn from Sonnenblick EH. Myocardial ultrastructure in the normal and failing heart. In: Braunwald E, ed. The Myocardium: Failure and Infarction. New York: HP Publishing; 1974.) C, Diagram showing relationships of sarcomere length, positions of the actin and myosin filaments, and contractile force. (Original drawing by Albert Miller. Redrawn from Sonnenblick EH. Myocardial ultrastructure in the normal and failing heart. In: Braunwald E, ed. The Myocardium: Failure and Infarction. New York: HP Publishing; 1974.) D, Typical length tracings for isotonic *(left)* and isometric *(right)* contractions. The *dashed vertical lines* in the left tracing indicate the portion of contraction in which the muscle shortens against a constant force. (Adapted from Parmley WW, Tyberg JV. Determinants of myocardial oxygen consumption. In: Yu PN, Goodwin JF, eds. Progress in Cardiology. Philadelphia: Lea & Febiger; 1976.)

prematurely born infants (and, to a lesser extent, full-term infants) have a much-reduced ability to tolerate an increase in afterload and are exquisitely sensitive to reductions in serum calcium concentrations.

Myocardial Mechanics — Myocardial Receptors and Responses to Drugs

α_1-Adrenoceptors appear early in gestation and in many species reach their highest density in the neonate.[19,56,76] These developmental changes may be associated with the normal cell hypertrophy that occurs during development. By contrast,

β-adrenoreceptors increase progressively with age. Both β_1 and β_2 are present on myocytes.[77,78] In addition, histamine H_2, vasoactive intestinal polypeptide (VIP), adenosine A_1, acetylcholine M_2, and somatostatin receptors have been identified. They act on the myocyte's contractile apparatus through one of two main pathways.

The major pathway involves the membrane-bound receptor–G protein–adenylate cyclase complexes. G proteins include the G_s (stimulatory) and G_i (inhibitory) proteins.[79] In their inactive state, these G proteins include α, β, and γ subunits and guanine diphosphate (GDP). When agonists stimulate β-adrenergic, histamine, or VIP receptors, the G proteins undergo a conformational change. The changes induce the Gs protein to exchange its GDP for guanine triphosphate (GTP) and release the β and γ subunits. The Gs-α-GTP complex interacts with adenylate cyclase to convert ATP to cyclic adenine monophosphate (cAMP), which activates a variety of protein kinases to phosphorylate proteins including voltage-dependent calcium channels, phospholamban, and troponin I. Consequently, calcium entry during depolarization and during uptake of calcium into the sarcoplasmic reticulum storage pool is increased, thus increasing contractility. The Gs-α-GTP complex has intrinsic GTPase activity that converts GTP to GDP. The β and γ subunits rejoin the complex, which now is available for further activation by the receptor. In this way, as long as receptors are occupied by the agonist, the Gs cycle produces increasingly more cAMP, thereby amplifying the stimulatory signal. The Gi protein complex undergoes a similar cycle when adenosine, acetylcholine, or somatostatin receptors are stimulated; however, activating Gi protein reduces cAMP formation and decreases contractility. β2 Adrenergic receptors also couple to Gi in addition to Gs.[80] Gi in this context is thought to oppose the effects of Gs to some degree, including limitation of the acute positive inotropic response to adrenergic stimulation and offering some protection from apoptosis.[81-83]

Another signal-transducing system in the human heart is the phospholipase C-diacylglycerol-inositol triphosphate pathway, activated by α1-adrenergic and M2-muscarinic receptors.[84-86] Occupation of the receptors activates phospholipase C, which cleaves phosphatidylinositol triphosphate in the cell membrane to produce diacylglycerol and inositol triphosphate. The former activates protein C kinase in the membrane, which may hinder the effects of cAMP. The latter facilitates calcium release from the sarcoplasmic reticulum. This pathway is important in smooth muscle contraction but is of less importance in heart muscle.

In heart failure, the number of β1-adrenergic and VIP receptors are down-regulated, and β2-adrenergic receptors are uncoupled from G proteins.[21,77,78,87,88] These changes make the myocardium less responsive to circulating or locally released catecholamines or VIP and play a role in the reduced contractility observed in heart failure. Treating heart failure with β-adrenergic blocking agents has been shown to reverse the receptor changes but has also been associated with improved function of muscle strips in adult patients.[89-92]

Coupling of β-adrenoreceptors is incomplete at birth. Milrinone is an agent that stimulates contractility by inhibiting phosphodiesterases; it bypasses the adenylate cyclase system. Although previously thought to be ineffective in the newborn,[93] a multicenter randomized trial[94] and subsequent widespread use has confirmed its efficacy in the neonatal population.[95,96] Because contractile mechanisms are almost fully developed at birth, the majority of mechanisms controlling contractility (except for changes in the source of calcium) are in place at birth.

Myocardial Mechanics — Integrated Muscle Function

Relationship Between Muscle Strips and Intact Ventricles

Preload stretching a muscle strip is equivalent to end-diastolic fiber length of the intact ventricle. This length can be measured by various devices in animals, but in the intact human ventricle it is best related to end-diastolic diameter or volume.

Frequently, end-diastolic pressure has been used interchangeably with end-diastolic volume as an index of preload, but this usage can be misleading if the distensibility of the ventricle changes or if pressure outside the heart (pericardial or intrathoracic) rises.[97-100]

Afterload is more complicated in the intact ventricle. Commonly, aortic systolic pressure is equated with afterload. However, in the muscle strip, afterload represents the force exerted by the muscle during contraction, and pressure and force are not the same.[75,101,102] It is preferable to calculate circumferential wall stress, which at the midwall is a function of ventricular pressure, diameter, and wall thickness. Both peak systolic and end-systolic wall stress can be used to assess ventricular function.

Calculations of wall stress are based on the Laplace relationship:

$$\text{Wall Stress} = \frac{Pr}{2h}$$

where P is pressure, r is radius of curvature, and h is wall thickness. Because the left ventricle is not a regular sphere, particularly in systole, the Laplace formula is an oversimplification.[103] A fairly simple and accurate formula was developed by Grossman and colleagues[104]:

$$\text{Wall stress} = \frac{Pr}{2h}\left[1+\frac{h}{2r}\right]$$

that is, as the Laplace equation modified by the expression in parentheses. Note that if the left ventricle dilates acutely, wall stress rises markedly because r gets bigger and h gets smaller.

The major findings from studies of muscle strips have been confirmed in intact ventricles. Increasing preload increases the pressure generated by an isolated ventricle that is not allowed to eject, as observed in the past century by Otto Frank. If the ventricle is allowed to eject, then increased preload allows the heart to eject the same stroke volume against an increased afterload or else to eject a greater stroke volume against a constant afterload. This is the Starling component of the Frank-Starling law.[105,106] The mechanism of this response is twofold: (1) lengthening the sarcomere narrows it and places the myosin and actin fibrils closer together for stronger interaction, and (2) increased calcium sensitivity is mediated in some way by titin stretching.[18] If an inotropic drug is given, then contractility increases and, from a given fiber length, greater force of contraction is achieved. This is a phenomenon seen every day in the ICU.

The force-frequency relationship can be determined in intact hearts[107,108] by examining the response of the maximal rate of change of pressure (dP/dt max) in the ventricles after premature beats. The results in intact ventricles and muscle strips are similar. Subsequently, Seed and colleagues[109] applied this technique to humans with normal or abnormal left ventricular function and found an optimal R-R interval of 800 ms. They also examined dP/dt max for two beats given at optimum intervals after the premature stimulus. As expected, the first normal beat after the premature beat was potentiated because the extra calcium introduced into the cytosol by the premature beat was available to potentiate the first beat after the premature stimulus. The second postpremature beat also was potentiated but less so. They used the ratio of the potentiation of these two beats to calculate the fraction of calcium recirculating from one beat to the next. This amount was constant in any one patient but was much less in those with left ventricular dysfunction.

Pressure-Volume Loops

If left ventricular pressure and volume are measured simultaneously, the resulting pressure-volume loop gives information about ventricular function and can be used to assess myocardial contractility in the intact heart.

The modern approach to analyzing these loops is based on the elastance concept of Suga and Sagawa.[110-112] Elastance is the ratio of pressure change to volume change. Consider an isolated ventricle containing a balloon that can be inflated to different volumes. At each volume the ventricle is stimulated to contract and generates a peak systolic pressure (Fig. 25.5A). As volumes increase, so do the peak systolic pressures generated, and the relationship is linear (Frank's law). The line joining the peak pressures intercepts the volume axis at a positive value, termed V_0, that indicates the unstressed volume of the ventricle. The equation for this line is as follows:

$$P_{es} = E_{es}(V - V_0)$$

where P_{es} is end-systolic pressure, E_{es} is slope of the line, V is the volume of interest and V_0 is unstressed volume. If contractility increases (more calcium enters the cells), the ventricle can generate greater pressures at any given volume, thereby generating a steeper pressure-volume line (higher value of E_{es}; purple line I in Fig. 25-5A). If contractility decreases, the ventricle generates lower pressures at any given volume, and the pressure-volume line is less steep (lower value of E_{es}; blue line D in Fig. 25-5A). E_{es} is also termed E_{max}.

If the ventricle is allowed to eject, the typical pressure-volume loop shown in Fig. 25.5B is seen. During diastolic filling, volume increases and diastolic pressure rises slightly because of the increase in passive tension. At the end of diastole, isovolumic systole occurs and ventricular pressure rises with no change in volume. When ventricular pressure exceeds aortic pressure, the aortic valve opens, blood is ejected, and ventricular volume decreases. Ejection ends, and pressure falls to diastolic levels as isovolumic relaxation occurs. The pressure and volume reached at the end of systole are those that would have been attained by the isolated ventricle at that same end-systolic volume. In other words, at a given volume, no higher pressure can be generated (loop 1; see Fig. 25.5B). The decrease in volume during ejection is the stroke volume, which, divided by the end-diastolic volume, gives the ejection fraction; normally, ejection fraction is greater than 65%.

If afterload is suddenly increased by raising aortic pressure, the normal heart responds as shown in Fig. 25.5B. In the first beat after the increase, the ventricle has to generate a higher pressure before the aortic valve opens (loop 2). It then ejects but cannot eject a normal stroke volume because that would require higher pressure from the same end-diastolic length (preload). In fact, the end-systolic volume is that which is appropriate for the higher pressure (compare Fig. 25.5A and B). If different afterloads are used, the end-systolic pressure-volume points define a sloping line that is the same as the line obtained in the isolated heart at those same volumes; this is the maximal ventricular elastance (E_{es}) or end-systolic elastance (E_{es}) line. If ventricular contractility increases, then the

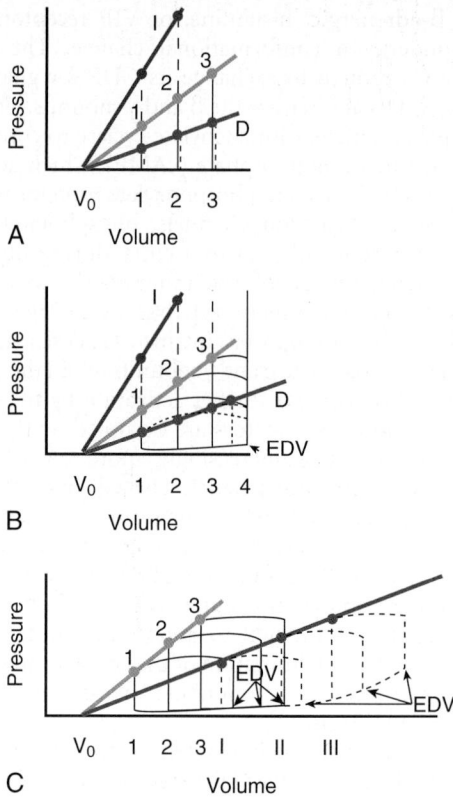

Fig. 25.5. Diagrams illustrating the concept of ventricular elastance. A, Isolated ventricle contracting at volumes 1, 2, and 3, generating corresponding pressures. *Purple line I* indicates results at increased contractility. *Blue line D* indicates results at decreased contractility. V_0, resting (unstressed) volume. B, Ventricular pressure-volume loops achieving end-systolic pressures of 1, 2, and 3 at corresponding volumes. *Purple line I* indicates results at increased contractility, with greater end-systolic pressures at each volume. *Blue line D* indicates results at decreased contractility. From a given end-diastolic volume, either the same ejection fraction is delivered at a lower end-systolic pressure *(dotted line 1)* or the same end-systolic pressure is achieved but at a much smaller stroke volume and ejection fraction *(line 4)*. C, When the ventricular end-diastolic volumes *(EDV)* increase as afterload increases, as is normal, then stroke volume can be maintained, even though ejection fraction decreases. If contractility is decreased *(blue line)*, then stroke volume can be maintained only with increasing end-diastolic pressures. 1, 2, 3, end-systolic volumes and pressures at normal contractility. I, II, III, end-systolic volumes at decreased contractility.

ventricle can attain higher ejection pressures at any given volume, and the end-systolic pressure-volume points lie on a steeper line that lies above and to the left of the normal line (purple line I in Fig. 25-5B). If ventricular contractility decreases, then the ventricle cannot generate normal pressures at any given end-diastolic volume and the end-systolic pressure-volume line lies below and to the right of the normal line (blue line in Fig. 25.5B). Note from Fig. 25.5B, that, from a given end-diastolic volume, the ventricle with impaired contractility can either eject a normal stroke volume at much reduced pressures or eject at a normal pressure only by reducing its stroke volume drastically (loop 4).

In beats that follow a sudden increase in afterload, the ventricles adjust. Because of the reduced stroke volume in the first beat, the end-systolic volume is larger than normal. During diastole, however, a normal stroke volume enters the ventricle so that end-diastolic volume increases (loop 2 in Fig. 25.5C). In normal ventricles, the increased end-diastolic fiber length causes little increase in diastolic pressure. The pressures during ejection and the end-systolic pressure-volume point are unchanged, but stroke volume and ejection fraction increase. After a few more cycles, a new equilibrium is established (loop 3) in which the ventricle ejects a normal stroke volume at the higher afterload. The ejection fraction, however, is subnormal because although the stroke volume is normal, the end-diastolic volume is increased. The ventricle has adapted to the higher afterload by increasing end-diastolic fiber length, a phenomenon described by Starling and discussed by Ross[101,102] under the term *preload reserve*. If the ventricle has decreased contractility (dashed loops), the same pattern of response occurs but with some important differences. With decreased contractility, the ventricle cannot eject a normal stroke volume from a normal end-diastolic volume. Compensation results in a larger than normal increase in end-diastolic volume, even at normal afterloads. Any increase in afterload causes a further increase in end-diastolic volume, and this increase causes diastolic pressures to rise to high values that cause pulmonary congestion. The normal preload reserve has been used up in the attempt to eject a reasonable stroke volume against a modestly increased afterload. In more depressed hearts, even normal afterloads cannot be handled by the ventricle without a pathologically raised diastolic pressure in the ventricles or a drastic decrease in stroke volume. Note that in these hearts, because of the relatively flat slope of the maximal ventricular elastance line, a slight reduction of afterload produces a relatively large increase in stroke volume and a relatively large decrease in ventricular end-diastolic volume and pressure. This is one of the mechanisms for cardiac improvement with afterload reduction.

The normal right ventricular (RV) pressure-volume curve is triangular in shape, unlike the more rectangular left ventricular (LV) pressure-volume curve.[113] This difference is accounted for by a relative lack of isovolumic contraction and relaxation times in the RV. The normally low afterload of the RV and the high compliance of the outflow portion of the ventricle allow ejection to begin almost instantaneously after the onset of contraction and proceed through pressure decline so that there is near complete emptying of the ventricle by the end of systole and the ejection time of the RV thus spans the entire period of systole. An important consequence of this relationship is that even small increases in RV afterload begin to make the RV pressure-volume curve begin to resemble the normal LV pressure-volume curve, with isovolumic contraction and relaxation times becoming more prominent.[114] Ejection fraction is reduced, although stroke volume may be maintained due to RV dilation,[115] and the thin-walled RV may handle this new physiology quite poorly.

Assessing Myocardial Contractility

An index of contractility must reflect the ability of the ventricle to perform work independent of changes in preload and afterload. Contractility can perhaps best be defined as the alterations in cardiac function that occur secondary to changes in cytosolic calcium availability or sarcomere sensitivity to calcium. Thus β-adrenergic agonists or phosphodiesterase inhibitors, which increase cytosolic calcium, and thyroxine,

which alters myosin ATPase sensitivity to calcium in some species by altering the dominant isoform, are positive inotropic agents. However, quantifying contractility in the intact heart or assessing contractile effects of an intervention is difficult[72] because all indices of contractility are indices of overall performance and are not independent of the other determinants of performance. For example, cardiac output is an excellent index of the systolic performance of the intact ventricle, but it is not a useful index of contractility because of its high sensitivity to preload, afterload, and heart rate. It is convenient to divide methods of assessing contractility into those based on early events in the cardiac cycle (isovolumic phase indices) and those that occur later (ejection phase indices).

Isovolumic Phase Indices

The concept of maximal velocity of contraction against zero load (V_{max}) once was popular, but the complexity of the mechanics of cardiac muscle made it difficult to assess what would have been the true index, namely, V_{max} of the contractile element alone.[116] In practice, too, it is not possible to abolish internal loading of the muscle fiber. Applying this concept to the intact heart was even more difficult.[117]

As a substitute for V_{max}, investigators used dP/dt max (maximal rate of change of ventricular pressure) or dP/dt at a developed ventricular pressure of 40 mm Hg. These values usually are achieved before the aortic valve opens and are relatively unaffected by changes in preload. The index is, however, affected markedly by changes in afterload and so must be used with care when afterloads are very different. This method is more useful for measuring acute changes in contractility than for assessing absolute contractility.

Ejection Phase Indices

The index of contractility most commonly used today is the maximal (end-systolic) ventricular elastance of Suga and Sagawa, which is independent of changes in preload (see previous text). Several different afterloads must be obtained, and either ventricular volumes must be measured or echocardiographic dimensions must be used as substitutes for volumes. The most clear-cut results have been obtained when reflex changes in contractility are prevented, which may explain why the relationship is less well established in conscious than in anesthetized animals.[75,118] Several studies have shown that the maximal elastance line often is alinear and gives a negative intercept on the pressure axis, that is, a negative resting volume.[119,120] To deal with this simply, some investigators use the values of E_{max} in the midrange of pressures.[120]

Ejection fraction and velocity of shortening also provide information about ventricular function. Because these two variables depend on afterload (see Fig. 25.5), it is necessary to adjust for changes in afterload. This adjustment has been made in adults and children[121-126] by providing normal data for the relationship between end-systolic wall stress and either velocity of shortening or ejection fraction (Fig. 25.6). However, the relationship is not linear,[127] so single-point determinations are of little use.

Ventricular Function Curves

Sarnoff and Mitchell[128] introduced the ventricular function curve. They measured LV diastolic pressure and stroke work, then infused fluids and examined the relationship between the two variables (Fig. 25.7A). If contractility increased, the curve shifted up and to the left; at any end-diastolic pressure, a greater stroke work was achieved. If contractility decreased, the curve shifted down and to the right. One problem with this technique, recognized by Sarnoff, was that curvilinearity of the diastolic length-pressure relationship produced an S-shaped curve when relating stroke work to end-diastolic pressure and that techniques for measuring fiber length or ventricular volume were inadequate. In addition, using pressure instead of fiber length or volume may lead to misinterpretations if pericardial or pleural pressures change substantially. Several groups of investigators adapted this function curve to examine the stroke volume to end-diastolic pressure relationship, but this is even less satisfactory because stroke volume is affected by the resulting increases of afterload.

More recently, the relationship of stroke work to end-diastolic fiber length or ventricular volume has been examined in conscious dogs with autonomic blockade.[105] This relationship, termed *preload recruitable stroke work*, was linear and independent of changes in afterload (Fig. 25.7B). The line intercepted the length or volume axis at values close to the unstressed length or volume, that is, at the length or volume

that the ventricle has at zero transmural pressure. Calcium infusion increased the slope of the line without changing the intercept on the length axis. Subsequently, the same group extended this analysis to ischemic ventricles.[129] Depression of ventricular function shifted the stroke work to end-diastolic segment length relationship to the right (increased intercept) and decreased the slope. This concept and the ventricular elastance concept have much in common. Both require measurements of wall force, stroke work, ventricular volume, or minor axis diameter and changing them over a range so that the lines or areas defining these indexes can be obtained.

Pericardial Function

The parietal pericardium is a stiff membrane that surrounds the heart loosely, separated from it by a small amount of lubricating pericardial fluid. Intrapericardial pressure is negative, reflecting the negative intrapleural pressure. On the other hand, the pericardium exerts a surface pressure on the heart that would exist even if all fluid were removed. If the pericardium had holes in it, fluid would leak out and there would be

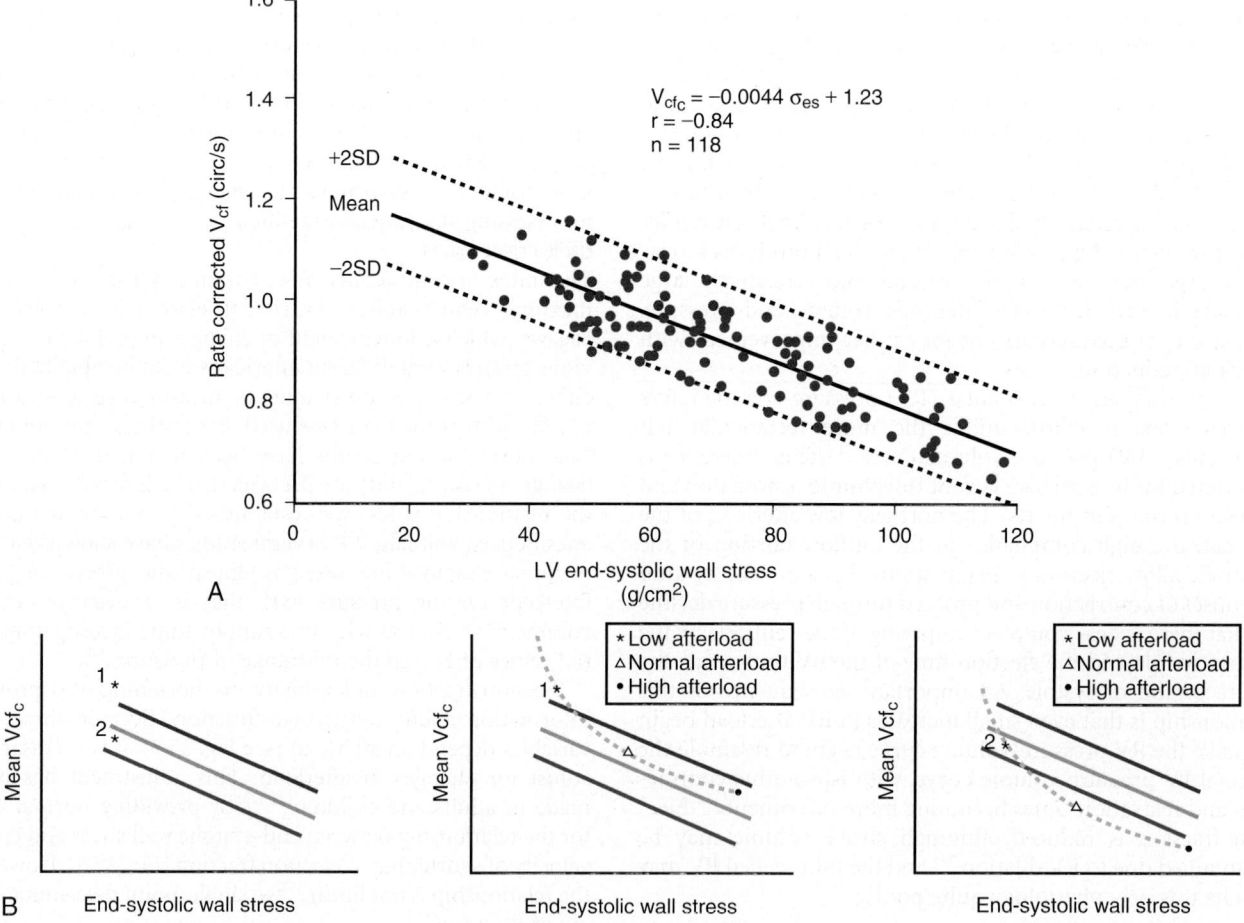

Fig. 25.6. A, Relationship between rate-corrected mean velocity of fiber shortening *(V_cf)* and left ventricular *(LV)* end-systolic wall stress. (From Colan SD, Borow KM, Neumann A. Left ventricular end-systolic wall stress-velocity of fiber shortening relation: a load-independent index of myocardial contractility. J Am Coll Cardiol. 1984;4:715.) B, Possibility of misinterpreting the relationship between mean velocity of fiber shortening and end-systolic wall stress. *Left,* Data point 1 is more than two standard deviations *(SD)* above normal relation (taken from left panel), suggesting increased contractility. Data point 2 is within the normal range, suggesting normal contractility. *Middle,* Alternative explanation for point 1 is that contractile state is normal, but points obtained at very low afterloads follow a hyperbolic, not a linear, relationship. *Right,* Alternative explanation for point 2 is that contractility is decreased, but because of the hyperbolic relationship and the low afterload it appears within the "normal" linear range. (Adapted from Banerjee A, et al. Nonlinearity of the left ventricular end-systolic wall stress-velocity of fiber shortening relation in young pigs: a potential pitfall in its use as a single-beat index of contractility. J Am Coll Cardiol. 1994;23:514.)

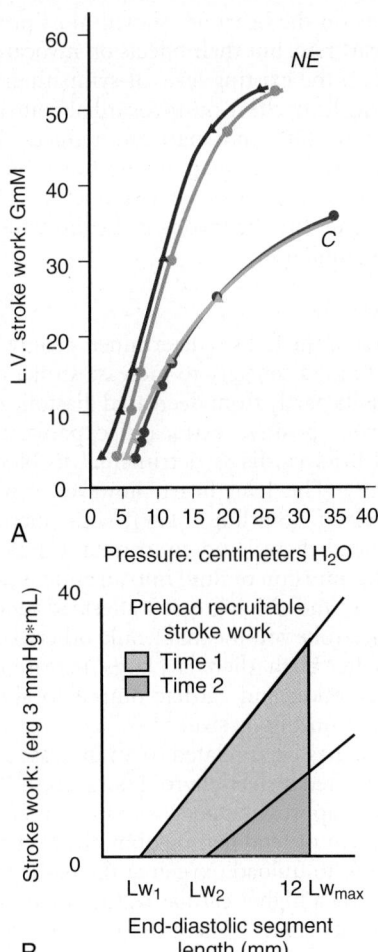

A

B

Fig. 25.7. Ventricular function curves. A, Typical function curve relating left ventricular diastolic pressure to left ventricular (external) stroke work. *C,* control state; *NE,* increased contractility resulting from norepinephrine infusion. *Pairs of lines* indicate repeatability of the measurement. (Redrawn from Sarnoff SJ, Mitchell JH. The control of the function of the heart. In: Hamilton WF, Dow P, eds. Handbook of Physiology, Section 2: Circulation, vol 1. Washington, DC: American Physiological Society; 1962.) B, Preload recruitable stroke work area, in which the area under the curve relating end-diastolic segment length to stroke work is indicated for two different contractile states of the ventricle. *Lw₁,* *Lw₂,* intercepts on the x-axis; *Lwmax,* maximal value of *Lw* for the whole experiment. For details, see reference. (Adapted from Glower DD, et al. Quantification of regional myocardial dysfunction after acute ischemic injury. Am J Physiol. 1988;255:H85.)

no fluid pressure, but the heart still could be compressed. This surface pressure varies in different regions but, in general, is similar to right atrial pressure.[99,130] As a result, in the usual situation transmural diastolic pressure across the wall of the left ventricle is not the same as left ventricular diastolic ventricular pressure. It can be estimated by subtracting right atrial pressure from LV pressure. The pericardium can restrict dilatation of the LV if there is a tense pericardial effusion (tamponade)[131] or if the ventricles dilate acutely. Thus if the ventricles enlarge because of sudden volume load or sudden myocardial depression, the pericardium becomes tense and restrains further enlargement of the ventricles.[99,100]

In some patients with acute myocardial ischemia, left ventricular diastolic pressure can be greatly increased without much change in ventricular volume because of tension in the pericardium. This mechanism makes it difficult to interpret changes in diastolic pressure-volume relations only in terms of myocardial stiffness.[97,98,130,132,133]

Ventricular Interaction

A closely related mechanism is ventricular interaction.[132] For example, if right ventricular output decreases, a series interaction reduces left ventricular filling and, therefore, LV output. Second, a direct interaction occurs because the left and right ventricles share the ventricular septum and are contained within the same relatively rigid pericardium. Consequently, RV distension, as in acute pulmonary embolism or congestive heart failure, pushes the septum to the left, thereby decreasing LV volume and preload. The resulting decrease in cardiac output should not be taken to indicate LV dysfunction.[99,134,135] Additionally, the LV generates a substantial portion of RV contractility[136] and the decrease in cardiac output that occurs with acute RV failure with an intact pericardium is at least partially attributable to a decrease in LV performance.[137] Cardiac output can be improved in this situation by opening the pericardium.

The effects of pericardial restraint and ventricular interaction come into play during positive pressure ventilation.[138] With a normal circulation, an increase in intrathoracic pressure will decrease transmural pressures, end-diastolic volumes, and stroke work of both ventricles. However, in the context of the normal circulation, these changes have no observable clinical effects. In congestive heart failure, however, where pericardial restraint regulates total cardiac volume, increased intrathoracic pressure decreases RV transmural pressure, filling, and volume, resulting in increased LV transmural pressure, end-diastolic volume, and stroke work via the Frank-Starling relationship. The ultimate effect of increased intrathoracic pressure in congestive heart failure (from a common intervention such as positive pressure ventilation) is highly dependent on intravascular volume status. In volume-depleted patients, the effects on the right heart will predominate, resulting in further reductions in cardiac output. Adequate volume status, however, will allow the beneficial effects of increased intrathoracic pressure on the LV to dominate, resulting in an increase in cardiac output.

Diastolic Ventricular Function

Diastolic function concerns the rate and extent of ventricular relaxation.[98,139] Many forms of heart disease manifest abnormalities of both systolic and diastolic function, but one or the other form of dysfunction may predominate and determine the type of therapy needed.

Diastolic dysfunction is manifested mainly by increased ventricular diastolic pressure at normal or even low ventricular volume.[139] This can result from increased passive stiffness of the ventricles because of chronic infiltrates (eg, amyloid), myocardial scars, constrictive pericarditis, or diffuse myocardial fibrosis. It also can result from impaired relaxation. Normally, relaxation of ventricular muscle in diastole is rapid and associated with rapid release of calcium bound to troponin and its subsequent uptake by the sarcoplasmic reticulum. Removal of calcium allows actin-myosin cross-bridges to dissociate and the sarcomeres to lengthen, thereby permitting the ventricle to dilate. Any decrease in calcium removal because of abnormalities in major contractile proteins or transport processes decreases the rate and extent of relaxation.[73,140,141]

Ischemia is one major factor that impairs calcium metabolism and diastolic ventricular function, but many other forms of heart disease have similar effects.[26,29,108,142] Clinically, diastolic function is assessed by relating end-diastolic pressure and volume, by observing the rate of ventricular filling by angiography or by Doppler studies of the mitral valve inflow, by measuring the peak rate of fall of ventricular pressure (−dP/dt max), or by calculating the time constant of the fall in ventricular pressure.

Neural Control of the Heart

The heart can function without any cardiac nerves, for example, after cardiac transplantation. However, the response to exercise in these denervated hearts is slow and due to increases in circulating catecholamines and the rise in body temperature. In intact animals and humans, β-adrenoreceptor blockade blunts the heart rate increase with exercise and abolishes inotropic response, as judged by the increase in dP/dt max.[143]

Studies of the neural control of the heart must consider the basal level of sympathetic and parasympathetic tone.[143] In conscious animals, resting sympathetic tone is low and resting parasympathetic tone is high. Therefore sympathetic blockade has little effect on heart rate and myocardial contractility, but parasympathetic blockade causes marked tachycardia. On the other hand, many anesthetics depress the sympathetic nervous system, leading to impaired contractility and bradycardia. Postoperatively, patients often have high circulating catecholamine concentrations, and the effects on myocardial function depend on the balance of catecholamine concentrations, stimulation of the sympathetic nervous system by pain, and extent of myocardial depression caused by the drugs used for sedation.

The carotid and aortic baroreceptors respond to changes in arterial blood pressure. If basal sympathetic tone is low, as is normal, then inhibiting sympathetic tone by raising aortic pressure has little effect on myocardial contractility. On the other hand, lowering arterial pressure causes a reflex increase in sympathetic tone, with increases in heart rate and contractility. Baroreceptor sensitivity increases throughout gestation in fetal lambs[144] but may decrease after birth.[145] Also in fetal lambs, denervating the baroreceptors did not alter mean arterial blood pressure or heart rate but did increase the variability of pressure and heart rate. Similar increased variability of pressures but not of heart rate occurred in adult sheep.[146] Denervation in the fetuses in the same study also decreased peripheral resistance.

Carotid and aortic chemoreceptors are stimulated by low P_{O_2}, high P_{CO_2}, and low pH, but the changes have to be marked, and even then the increase in myocardial contractility is modest. The fetus seems to be less sensitive than the adult to chemoreceptor stimulation.[147] The bradycardia that accompanies severe hypoxemia results from vagal stimulation. During exercise or hemorrhage, plasma catecholamines increase markedly, but the inotropic responses are different. With exercise, dP/dt max increases by as much as fourfold, the peripheral vascular bed is dilated, and cardiac output increases, whereas with hemorrhage, dP/dt max increases by only 30% to 50%, cardiac output falls, and most vascular beds vasoconstrict. Thus the pattern of sympathetic neural stimulation rather than the circulating catecholamine concentrations determines how the heart responds to these stimuli.

Vagal effects on the heart are shown most prominently by changes in heart rate, but their effects on myocardial contractility depend on the existing level of sympathetic tone. Vagal stimulation has little effect on myocardial contractility given little sympathetic tone but markedly reduces the inotropic effects of increases in circulating catecholamines or sympathetic nerve stimulation. Conversely, blockade of muscarinic receptors can intensify the myocardial contractile response to sympathetic stimulation.

Cardiac Output

Cardiac output in the fetus is determined mainly by heart rate because of a limited capacity to increase stroke volume. This limitation results partly from decreased diastolic distensibility and partly from positive extracardiac pressures.[148] Consequently, fetal bradycardia is detrimental to blood flow and oxygen delivery. The fetal heart, however, can respond to increased preload (Starling's law) with increased stroke volume, provided there is no concomitant increase in afterload.[149] Usually, infusion of fluid into an animal causes arterial pressure to rise, and the increased afterload tends to inhibit the increase in stroke volume that would otherwise occur.[149-151] Immediately after birth, there is a large increase in total body oxygen consumption and cardiac output to about twice its later values (per unit body size).[152]

This increase has been related to an increase in adrenergic receptors stimulated by fetal thyroid hormones.[153] In addition, because at birth approximately 80% of the infant's hemoglobin is in the form of fetal hemoglobin, the reduced ability of this hemoglobin to unload oxygen at the tissue level compels the infant to have a higher cardiac output than the infant will have 4 to 6 weeks later.[152] Therefore the neonate has limited cardiac output reserve and the heart has near-maximal contractility.[154,155] These features make the neonate unusually susceptible to diseases that impair cardiac function. The Frank-Starling mechanism, however, is intact at this time.[156] Evidence indicates β-adrenoreceptor stimulation helps the neonatal ventricle adapt to volume loads.[157] Thus β-adrenoreceptor blockade might be expected to be much more harmful in the neonate than in the older person with minimal sympathetic tone.

Myocardial Metabolism: Normal Myocardial Energy Metabolism

Basic Metabolic Processes

Basal metabolic processes can be studied by measuring oxygen uptake, production of heat, or utilization of high-energy phosphates. In isolated papillary muscle, most of the oxygen consumed is used in generating force (internal work), approximately 15% is used in shortening (external work), approximately 20% is used for basal metabolic processes (protein synthesis, sarcolemmal Na-K transport), and approximately 10% is used for the activity of Na/K-ATPase and Ca-ATPase.[158-160] Similar conclusions can be drawn from studies of whole hearts.[161]

The myocardium has a brisk rate of metabolism, consuming approximately 8 to 10 mL oxygen/100 g muscle/min under basal conditions. Potassium-induced cardioplegia can reduce myocardial oxygen consumption, but "resting" cardiac muscle still consumes more than five times as much oxygen as does resting skeletal muscle. During maximal exercise, the myocardium may consume as much as 60 to 80 mL oxygen/100 g muscle/min.[162]

Cardiac energy is generated by oxidizing substrates to carbon dioxide and water. During this process, energy is both used and stored, and most of the stored energy is in the form of ATP. When needed, ATP breaks down to adenosine diphosphate (ADP) or adenosine monophosphate (AMP) and releases energy for contractile or transport processes.[163] The substrates for energy production can be glucose, lactate, or fatty acids.[164] In a mixture, the fatty acids are preferred over the others, and an increase in plasma fatty acid concentrations, as in fasting or sympathetic stimulation, suppresses oxidation of carbohydrates by the heart.[55,164] Therefore lactate consumption or extraction cannot be used as an accurate guide to cardiac metabolism unless the concentration of the fatty acids is evaluated at the same time.[165] ATP is usually generated by oxidative phosphorylation. Various transport systems move the substrates into the mitochondria for oxidation by the tricarboxylic cycle. Other transport systems move the ATP out of mitochondria into the cytosol, where they can break down and supply energy. The ATP is replenished by transfer of a high-energy phosphate moiety from creatine phosphate to ADP, mediated by the enzyme creatine kinase.[163,166] When oxygen supply is restricted, ATP can be generated by anaerobic glycolysis, an inefficient but useful temporary pathway. Furthermore, products of glycolysis, if they accumulate, inhibit key enzymes and interfere with further ATP production. Therefore the myocardium is unable to build an oxygen debt without further depressing energy production and, hence, contractility. Oxidative metabolism is so important to the heart that more than 30% of the mass of the myocardium is mitochondria.[158]

Fetal lamb ventricles have the same oxygen consumption per unit mass as the adult left ventricle. Because fetal oxygen content is lower than that in the adult, however, myocardial blood flow per unit mass is about twice as high in the fetus as in the adult.[167,168] Oxidative capacity is relatively lower, and glycogen stores and glycolytic flux are relatively higher in the fetal heart. This condition may explain why the immature heart is more resistant to hypoxemia than is the adult heart, provided an adequate supply of glucose is available for glycolysis. The main substrates used by the fetal heart are glucose, lactate, and pyruvate, although ketones, amino acids, and short- and medium-chain fatty acids also can provide energy.[169] After birth, long-chain fatty acids become the predominant substrates. For these reasons, prolonged severe hypoglycemia can seriously depress cardiac function in the neonate but is unlikely to do so in the older person.

L-Carnitine is essential for fatty acid transport across the mitochondrial membrane. Most of the body's carnitine is produced endogenously when protein degradation releases trimethyl-lysine, which is transformed into carnitine. Carnitine is present in red meats and dairy products (including breast milk), but only small amounts are present in vegetable products. It can be absorbed by the intestine, is not broken down in the body, and is excreted by the kidney.

In all except young infants, the preferential source of energy for myocardial function comes from the β-oxidation of long-chain fatty acids. After fatty acids enter the cell, they are activated to fatty acid (or acyl) coenzyme A (CoA) compounds by palmitoyl-CoA synthetase, then linked by carnitine palmitoyl transferase I to carnitine to form acylcarnitines, thus releasing CoA. The acylcarnitines cross the mitochondrial membrane, and at the inner surface of the membrane another enzyme, carnitine palmitoyl transferase II, transfers the fatty acids back to CoA. The fatty acids can now undergo β-oxidation with the production of ATP. These enzymes also help transport acylcarnitine esters of CoA out of the mitochondria. These esters are toxic in high concentrations. Fetuses and neonates have decreased activity of carnitine palmitoyl transferase and palmitoyl-CoA synthetase, so glucose, lactate, and short-chain fatty acids are the preferred myocardial energy substrates at this age.[19,170]

Endogenous carnitine production is usually sufficient for growth, but plasma (and tissue) carnitine concentrations may decrease after 1 month of parenteral nutrition without carnitine supplements. Energy demands increase when renal excretion of carnitine increases in conditions of burns, sepsis, starvation, or after surgery; with excess excretion in Fanconi syndrome; with drugs such as valproic acid, pivampicillin, and pivmecillinam, which bind to carnitine and are excreted; with decreased production during chronic hemodialysis; and with cirrhosis of the liver.[171,172] Carnitine concentrations may be low in very premature infants.[173] Ischemia of heart or skeletal muscle depletes carnitine in the affected tissues, as does chronic congestive heart failure.[174,175] Most cases of severe carnitine deficiency in children, however, result from inherited defects in intermediary metabolism.[176]

Carnitine deficiency may produce acute or chronic syndromes, including a Reye syndrome–like encephalopathy, hypoglycemia, myopathy, cardiomyopathy, and failure to thrive. Once the diagnosis is established, treatment is with a diet high in carbohydrates and short-chain fatty acids, plus carnitine supplements by mouth (25–300 mg/kg/day) or even intravenously if needed. Patients with congestive heart failure who do not show overt evidence of carnitine deficiency may improve after taking carnitine supplements.[175]

Determinants of Myocardial Oxygen Consumption

In 1958, Sarnoff and Mitchell[128] reported that pressure work by the heart consumed more oxygen than did volume work and found a good correlation between the area under the LV pressure curve in systole (termed the tension-time index) and left ventricular oxygen consumption. Subsequently, others found that peak wall tension (or stress) was a better predictor of left ventricular oxygen consumption.[177-180] It is important to take account of wall thickness and ventricular dimensions in estimating myocardial oxygen consumption, which is why the tension-time index, which ignores wall stress, is not a good predictor. Increases of contractility or heart rate also increase myocardial oxygen consumption, but because they decrease ventricular size and thus wall stress, increased oxygen consumption is not as great as would be expected from studies in muscle strips.[181]

Stroke volume is an added predictor of myocardial oxygen consumption.[12,182-185] The approaches used include examining the area within the pressure-flow loop. This approach has been extended by Suga and colleagues,[112,186-191] who concluded that the best predictor of LV oxygen consumption was the area in the pressure-volume loop plus the area representing end-systolic pressure energy (Fig. 25.8). By subtracting the contributions of basal myocardial metabolism, they were able to show that the oxygen consumption–pressure-volume area (PVA) relationship was independent of contractile state. Further studies by these investigators showed that

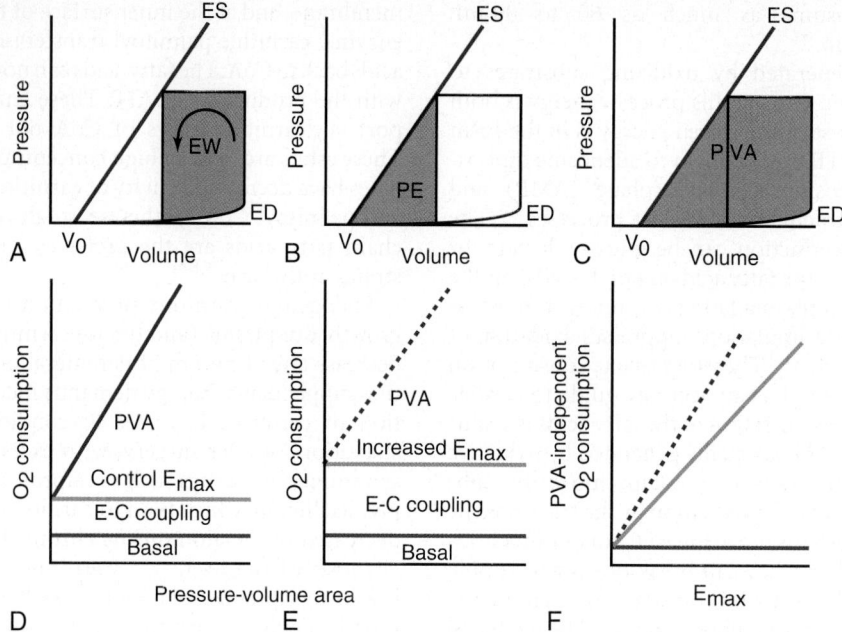

Fig. 25.8. Relationship of myocardial oxygen consumption to the pressure volume area (PVA). A, Ventricular pressure-volume loop with pressure plotted on the ordinate and volume on the abscissa. *Arrow* shows the direction of inscription of the loop. *ED,* end-diastolic pressure-volume line; *ES,* line of end-systolic pressure-volume points (end-systolic elastance); *EW,* area representing external mechanical work; V_0, unstressed ventricular volume. B, *Shaded area* to the left of the pressure-volume loop in the pressure-volume diagram represents potential energy (PE). C, Total area (PVA) is the sum of the external mechanical work area (EW) and the potential energy area (PE). D, PVA is linearly proportional to oxygen consumption, but some oxygen consumption is independent of PVA. The PVA-independent oxygen consumption shown below the *upper horizontal line* results from excitation-contraction (E-C) coupling and basal oxygen consumption. E, When contractility is increased, as indicated by the increased value for E_{max}, the relationship between PVA and oxygen consumption is unchanged, but PVA-independent oxygen consumption increases. F, Relationship between E_{max} and PVA-independent oxygen consumption is linear. With myocardial depression, the slope of this relationship is steeper *(dashed line).* Thus for any value of E_{max}, PVA-independent oxygen consumption is increased so that myocardial efficiency is reduced. (Data from references 61, 62, 125-127.)

PVA-independent oxygen consumption was a function of contractility, defined by E_{max}. Certain interventions, for example, acidosis, made the slope of this relation between PVA-independent VO_2 to E_{max} steeper, that is, they decreased the efficiency of the system.

Because oxidizing fats uses up more oxygen than does oxidizing carbohydrates, theoretically more oxygen should be used per unit of work when burning fatty acids. Though not consistently demonstrated, there are a few good studies of this phenomenon.[166]

Myocardial Oxygen Demand-Supply Relationship

One way of assessing myocardial oxygen demand is to note that it is roughly proportional to the ventricular systolic pressure generated and the duration of systole, that is, to the area under the real-time pressure curve of the ventricle in systole: the systolic pressure-time index (SPTI).[192,193] SPTI is dramatically influenced by cardiac afterload; for instance, aortic stenosis raises SPTI (at constant stroke volume). The correlation between SPTI and myocardial oxygen demand is imperfect because it does not take into account wall stress, which involves radius and wall thickness, or contractility.[194]

Because left ventricular myocardial perfusion is restricted to diastole (see Chapter 26), myocardial oxygen supply is proportional to both duration of diastole and myocardial perfusion pressure in diastole. In general, diastolic myocardial perfusion pressure can be represented graphically as the difference between superimposed aortic and left ventricular

pressure curves. The area between these curves, from the instant of aortic valve closure in diastole to reopening of the aortic valve in systole, has been termed the *diastolic pressure-time index* (DPTI) and is proportional to subendocardial blood flow. When multiplied by arterial oxygen content, this index correlates with subendocardial oxygen supply.[195]

The ratio DPTI × Arterial oxygen content/SPTI (Fig. 25.9) is a fair indicator of myocardial oxygen balance. At critical levels, subendocardial ischemia occurs.[192,193] This ratio is worsened by tachycardia, which shortens diastole and the duration of myocardial perfusion; by elevation of end-diastolic pressures in the ventricles; or by elevation of coronary sinus pressure. It is adversely affected by low aortic diastolic pressure (as in shock, aortic valve insufficiency, or other large diastolic runoff lesions) and by elevated ventricular systolic pressure (as in aortic stenosis, systemic hypertension, or pulmonary hypertension). The ratio is favorably affected by balloon aortic counterpulsation, which elevates aortic diastolic pressure and reduces systolic afterload. Given the imperfect nature of this ratio, too much emphasis should not be placed on any given value, but two points are clear: (1) A fall in the ratio in any patient moves that patient toward a supply-to-demand imbalance and (2) any ratio less than the 8.9 that typifies normal subjects likely indicates myocardial ischemia.[196]

Effects of Myocardial Ischemia on Cardiac Function and Metabolism

Ischemia indicates a flow that is inadequate to supply the demand for oxygen by an organ or tissue; it also implies

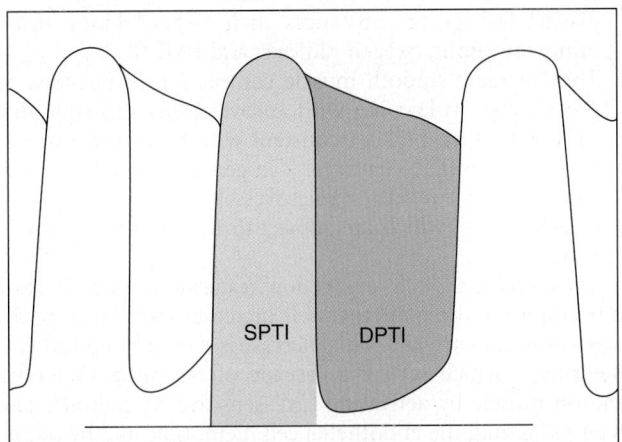

Fig. 25.9. Systolic pressure time index (SPTI) reflects myocardial work and oxygen demand. Diastolic pressure time index (DPTI) reflects myocardial blood flow. (Adapted from Fuhrman BP. Regional circulation. In: Fuhrman BP, Shoemaker WC, eds. Critical Care: State of the Art, vol 10. Fullerton, CA: Society of Critical Care Medicine; 1989.)

reduced clearance of metabolites.[197,198] The second part of the definition is what distinguishes ischemia from hypoxemia, in which there is a normal flow with a decreased oxygen delivery. Because the heart cannot sustain an oxygen debt, inadequate oxygen supply rapidly decreases the energy supply to the muscle cells, which cease to contract normally. If a branch of the left coronary artery is severely narrowed or occluded acutely, within 5 to 15 seconds the myocardium supplied by that branch stops contracting, turns blue, and bulges and thins during each systole. If the acute ischemia is global, that is, all coronary arteries have similar reductions in oxygen supply, then the subendocardial muscle becomes ischemic first because this muscle has the lowest coronary flow reserve. Subendocardial function is selectively decreased.[199-201] Global cardiac contractility decreases. Cardiac pump function is impaired, but survival is possible. More extensive global ischemia leads to death. Chronic imbalance of oxygen supply and demand leads to death of the affected muscle cells, producing either a localized infarct or diffuse, perhaps patchy, subendocardial fibrosis as occurs commonly with severe aortic stenosis, cyanotic heart disease, or dilated cardiomyopathy.

Temporary imbalance of supply and demand leads to two patterns of response, depending on the duration of the ischemia. If a branch coronary artery is occluded for 15 to 30 minutes and then the occlusion is removed, flow returns to normal rapidly, but the muscle may not contract normally for many hours. Some biochemical changes that occurred take many hours to reverse. This phenomenon is known as *reperfusion injury* or *stunning*.[202-205] It should be distinguished from the "no reflow" phenomenon in which, after a longer occlusion, release of the occlusion is followed by incomplete restoration of flow because of myocardial edema, cell swelling, plugging by neutrophils, and endothelial damage. Stunning may occur after prolonged cardiopulmonary bypass surgery and may account for some of the cardiac depression that often is observed in the early recovery period.[206,207]

Chronic ischemia of moderate severity causes myocardial hibernation, an adaptive response that leads to metabolic down-regulation and reduction of flow without extensive cell

death.[208-211] Regional function is reduced, but restoration of flow leads to functional recovery. This phenomenon is best known from studies of coronary artery disease but can be present in some children with normal coronary arteries and subendocardial ischemia.

Many biochemical changes occur when the heart becomes ischemic and which are the primary causes of the dysfunction is not always clear. As soon as oxygen supply is cut off, all components of the mitochondrial electron chain become reduced because of the absence of the final electron acceptor. Nicotinamide adenine dinucleotide (NAD) is reduced to NADH within 2 seconds after the onset of sudden ischemia.[212] Glycogenolysis increases rapidly, thereby helping to supply ATP, but then is progressively inhibited by increasing concentrations of hydrogen ion, NADH, and lactate. (This inhibition is less marked with pure hypoxemia because the associated high flows help to wash out these inhibitory metabolites.) The stores of high-energy phosphates become depleted. First creatine phosphate decreases and then ATP concentrations fall. For example, after sudden arterial occlusion, creatine phosphate is almost completely depleted within 3 minutes, and ATP is reduced to 35% of control concentration within 15 minutes. ATP is degraded to ADP and AMP, which then is deaminated to adenosine. Adenosine in turn is rapidly broken down to inosine and hypoxanthine. Because of these changes, the nucleotide pool of cardiac muscle is depleted so that even after flow is restored, a long time is required before normal high-energy stores are replenished. Furthermore, during ischemia, xanthine dehydrogenase in the tissues is converted to xanthine oxidase, which catalyzes the conversion of hypoxanthine to xanthine and superoxide radicals. These in turn can be converted by superoxide dismutase into hydrogen peroxide, which can be converted by catalase to produce highly reactive hydroxyl radicals. These free radicals can react with lipids in the cell membranes and cause lipid peroxidation, which produces several toxic and arrhythmogenic substances and impairs the functions of the cell membrane.[212] Oxygen-derived free radicals can be introduced by activation of neutrophils by the damaged endothelium and by the formation of peroxynitriles from nitric oxide.

Accompanying these changes are accumulations of hydrogen ions, lactate, and many other catabolites. These entities create an osmotic load within the cells, with resultant swelling of the cells and the mitochondria. The cell and mitochondrial membranes become impaired, and myoglobin and enzymes such as creatine kinase leak out of the cell, as do essential ions such as magnesium and potassium. Free calcium may accumulate in the cytosol (because of loss of chelating agents) and the mitochondria, particularly during reperfusion, and this calcium load may be highly detrimental to cell function. Finally, ischemia is associated with decreased myocardial carnitine concentrations, defective transport of long-chain fatty acids into the mitochondria, and accumulation of toxic acylcarnitine esters of CoA. These changes further delay the recovery of energy production and muscle contraction.

Systemic Vasculature

General Anatomy

The large arteries are elastic. Their media contain concentric lamellae of perforated elastic tubes cross-linked by transverse collagen (type III) and smooth muscle.[47,213] When smooth muscle contracts, the wall becomes stiffer. Smaller arteries have fewer lamellae. The media are bounded by the external and internal elastic laminae, beyond which are the adventitia with nerves and vasa vasorum and the intima with sparse fibrous tissue and a metabolically active endothelium, respectively. Arterioles have no lamellae and only a thin media with circular or spiral smooth muscle; the only elastic tissue is in the inner and outer elastic laminae. Capillaries are thin walled and nonmuscular, ideal for transport of materials into and from the tissues; however, they contain pericytes that have myosin, actin, and tropomyosin and so might have some contractile function. Veins have medial muscle but thinner walls relative to lumen diameter than do arteries. Their endothelium may have different properties. The numerous extracellular matrix components are reviewed by Buga and Ignarro.[214] The developmental aspects of blood vessels are reviewed by Stenmark and Weisen.[215]

Physiologic Mechanisms
General Features
Although large arteries are regarded as conduits and capillaries as vessels allowing transport of substances to and from the tissues, many substances can move across arterial walls. Oxygen and carbon dioxide can diffuse across arteriolar walls, and lipoproteins can penetrate the walls of large arteries. Whether atheromatous deposits form in arteries depends on the balance of the amount of lipoprotein that enters and leaves the arterial wall. This balance depends on the concentration and chemical nature of lipoproteins and the action of components of the wall, such as glycosaminoglycans, in binding altered lipoprotein molecules and preventing their transit through the wall.

Arteriolar tone controls peripheral resistance and, with cardiac output, determines blood pressure and regional flow. Regions of the circulation may differ markedly in their patterns of vascular regulation. A potent stimulus for increased vascular resistance in one region of the circulation may have a different effect in another. For example, during hemorrhagic shock, flow is maintained to heart and brain but is reduced to muscle, kidneys, and gut. Venous and venular tone, together with diuretic and antidiuretic factors, determine blood volume and venous pressure.

The two active components of the systemic circulation are the medial smooth muscle and the endothelium. They both have receptors for innumerable agonists and antagonists that diffuse from autonomic nerve endings, circulate from remote regions, or are produced locally. The smooth muscle is responsible for vasoconstriction or vasodilatation. The vascular endothelium is one of the metabolic powerhouses of the body and has several major functions:

1. Endothelial cells play important roles in the response to injury by causing leukocyte adhesion and extravasation, mediated by cell adhesion molecules such as selectins, cadherins, and integrins.[215,216]
2. They are intimately bound up with coagulation[215,217] by virtue of the production of procoagulant (eg, platelet-activating factor [PAF], von Willebrand factor, fibronectin, and factors V and X) and anticoagulant factors (eg, heparan, dermatan sulfate, thrombomodulin, ectonucleotidase) and by the production of nitric oxide and PGI_2, which inhibit platelet aggregation and degranulation.
3. They regulate capillary permeability by producing ET-1 (increase) or PGE1 (decrease) and respond with increased plasma leakage to substances such as bradykinin, histamine, thrombin, oxygen radicals, and PAF.[218]
4. They regulate smooth muscle contraction in response to shear stress, in keeping with an overriding principle that shear rate must be kept constant within narrow limits to prevent endothelial damage.[219] In general, most of the vascular resistance resides in microvessels smaller than 150 μm in diameter,[220] which are subject to the controls discussed here.

Any increase in local organ flow resulting from a decrease in resistance in these microvessels increases shear stress in the larger upstream arteries. This increase is sensed by endothelial integrins,[221] which set off a cascade of responses that relax smooth muscle by activating Ca^{2+}-sensitive K^+ channels and hyperpolarizing the endothelial cell membrane and by releasing acetylcholine, nitric oxide, PGI_2, ATP, and substance P.[215,222] A chronic increase in shear stress activates the nuclear factor-κB transcription complex and induces a number of early response genes.[215,222]

Control of Vascular Tone
In general, regional circulations regulate their flow so that they obtain required amounts of oxygen and nutrients. Any or all of the mechanisms discussed may be invoked. Vasomotor tone is strongly influenced by several mechanisms: (1) innervation and neural processes, (2) circulating endocrine and neuroendocrine mediators, (3) blood gas composition, (4) local metabolic products, (5) endothelial-derived factors, and (6) myogenic processes.

Receptors responsive to neural products (norepinephrine, acetylcholine, neuropeptides) are found throughout the circulation. Nevertheless, innervation and receptor distributions are organ specific, which allows rapid, patterned, coordinated redistribution of blood flow and an orchestrated response to hypoxia, changes in posture, and hemorrhage. Although these receptors respond to circulating agonists (including angiotensin II and adrenal epinephrine) and to those liberated locally, they are generally associated with innervation by autonomic nerves. In general, presynaptic α-adrenergic stimulation causes norepinephrine release and vasocontriction. β-Adrenergic stimulation generally causes vasodilatation. Cholinergic stimulation (whether sympathetic or parasympathetic) generally causes vasodilatation.

In all organs, sensory and efferent nerve endings contain nonadrenergic, noncholinergic (NANC) peptides, for example, neuropeptide Y, VIP, calcitonin gene-related peptide (CGRP), and substance P.[116,223-234] Neuropeptide Y is colocalized and released with norepinephrine,[235] and VIP is colocalized with acetylcholine and released upon stimulation of vagal nerve endings. Most of these peptides except neuropeptide Y are vasodilatory, and they help modulate blood pressure and regional flows. Substance P and CGRP are released when sensory nerves are stimulated by capsaicin, thus accounting for the flushing that accompanies the eating of hot peppers. (Many neuropeptides also occur throughout the central nervous system, where they may play roles in cardiovascular regulation.)

Humoral regulators of vascular tone and blood volume include angiotensin, adrenomedullin, aldosterone, arginine vasopressin (AVP), bradykinin, histamine, serotonin, thyroxine, natriuretic peptides, and various reproductive hormones. Most of these regulators have both direct effects and secondary effects, which tend to be organ specific or regional. They tend to have altered concentrations in hypertension, congestive heart failure, or shock, and their antagonists are used in therapy. Some agents, such as histamine, serotonin, and thyroxine, probably affect peripheral resistance only in abnormal states and are not physiologic regulators.

Angiotensin plays a special role in the homeostasis of blood pressure. Its concentration increases in hemorrhagic or hypovolemic shock, following increased renal production of renin that produces angiotensin I from angiotensinogen. Angiotensin I is converted to active angiotensin II by angiotensin-converting enzyme (ACE) in the endothelium, especially in the pulmonary vessels. However, angiotensin II is also produced locally in the heart and vessel walls by renin that enters from the blood and perhaps by other local proteases.[236,237] It causes generalized vasoconstriction in both systemic and pulmonary circulations, but locally it stimulates the release of vasodilating prostaglandins in the lung and kidney. Angiotensin II, via angiotensin I receptors, plays a role in cardiac and smooth muscle cell hypertrophy. In excess, it results in cardiac inflammation, fibrosis, and apoptosis.[238-241]

Adrenomedullin, originally found in pheochromocytomas, is produced in many normal cell types including endothelium. Among its many actions are long-lasting vasodilatation and diuresis.[242,243] It shares homologous sequences with CGRP, calcitonin, and amylin.[244] Its release may be stimulated by ET-1. It may play a role in treating heart failure.[245]

Aldosterone, known primarily for its effect on sodium excretion and potassium retention, has indirect central effects on blood pressure.[246-248] Its concentration increases when renin release is stimulated. In patients with congestive heart failure, its decreased breakdown in the liver accounts for high blood concentrations, which are harmful to the heart and blood vessels. Inhibition of aldosterone by spironolactone may have great clinical value.[247,249,250]

AVP, which is released from the axonal terminals of magnocellular neurons in the hypothalamus, causes vasoconstriction by stimulating VP_1 receptors. However, at low concentrations, AVP dilates coronary, cerebral, and pulmonary vessels. It is an antidiuretic hormone that acts on VP_2 receptors in the renal collecting ducts.[251] Its concentration is low in septic shock,[119] with ventricular arrhythmias, and after cardiac surgery[252] but is increased in myocardial and hemorrhagic shock, congestive heart failure, and cirrhosis of the liver.[106,251,253] Selective AVP antagonists promote free water excretion without concomitant electrolyte excretion[253-256] and are useful in treating fluid overload in patients with congestive heart failure, cirrhosis of the liver, and the syndrome of inappropriate antidiuretic hormone secretion without causing electrolyte imbalance.

Bradykinin is a potent pulmonary and systemic vasodilator released locally by the action of proteolytic enzymes on kallikrein after tissue injury.[257-260] Bradykinin is metabolized by kininase II, which is the same as ACE, so ACE inhibitors not only reduce angiotensin II production but also increase bradykinin concentrations. Bradykinin also causes endothelial cell release of tissue-type plasminogen activator.[261]

Histamine, released by mast cells in response to injury, is a potent vasodilator in most regions of the circulation but causes vasoconstriction in the lung. It also increases endothelial permeability.[262] No evidence indicates histamine plays a part in normal vasoregulation.

The natriuretic peptides are released from the heart when it is distended in congestive heart failure. They cause vasodilatation and increased diuresis. A-natriopeptide (mainly from atria) and B-natriopeptide (from ventricles) are released from myocardial cells, and C-natriopeptide is released from cardiac endothelium.[262-266] A recombinant B-natriopeptide (nesiritide) was initially shown to be safe and potentially more effective than dobutamine in treating acute severe congestive heart failure.[263-266] This is currently being tested in a large multinational randomized controlled trial (ASCEND-HF).[267] These natriopeptides and the kinins are broken down by neutral endopeptidase. Inhibition of this breakdown combined with inhibition of ACE by vasopeptidase inhibitors (eg, omapatrilat) greatly augments vasodilatation.[268-273]

Serotonin probably acts mainly in the central nervous system, but peripherally it can act on S_1 receptors to produce vasodilatation and on S_2 receptors to cause vasoconstriction. It also augments the action of other vasoconstrictors.[271,272]

Tissue levels of oxygen and carbon dioxide reflect adequacy of perfusion and oxygen delivery. These blood gases are potent determinants of regional blood flow and have effects that differ among regions of the circulation. They also have a more general effect mediated by carotid chemoreceptors.

Local metabolic regulation of vasomotor tone provides an ideal homeostatic mechanism whereby metabolic demand can directly influence perfusion. For instance, adenosine, which accumulates locally when tissue metabolism is high and tissue oxygenation is marginal, causes pronounced vasodilatation in the coronary, striated muscle, splanchnic, and cerebral circulations. Cerebral autoregulation has been suggested to take advantage of local metabolite production as an indicator of adequacy of blood flow. According to the argument, when perfusion pressure falls, cerebral blood flow might decline but for local accumulation of vasodilating metabolites. The perivascular concentration of these metabolites is restored to normal as flow rises, washing out the metabolites. Potassium is released from muscle in response to increased work, ischemia, and hypoxia.[273] Hypokalemia causes vasoconstriction.[274,275] Hyperkalemia, within the physiologic range, causes vasodilatation by stimulating K_{ir} channels.[276-278] Many of the agents previously discussed are produced locally and are effective as circulating hormones. At least four different types of potassium channels are present on arterial smooth muscle cells[278]: voltage-activated channels (K_v), calcium-activated channels (BK_{Ca}), inward rectifiers (K_{ir}), and ATP-dependent channels (K_{ATP}). These channels are activated by vasodilators. As a result, the cells hyperpolarize, voltage-dependent calcium channels close, intracellular calcium concentrations decrease, and vasodilatation results.[278] Pharmacologic vasodilators, such as cromakalim, pinacidil, and diazoxide, directly activate K_{ATP} channels, as do endogenous vasodilators such as CGRP, VIP, prostacyclin, and adenosine.[278] Inhibitors of K_{ATP} channels, such as glibenclamide, cause vasoconstriction.

The endothelial lining of blood vessels plays a prominent role in the regulation of vascular tone.[279] In addition to its roles in the elaboration of vasoactive eicosanoids[280] and in the metabolism of angiotensin, the endothelium secretes several other categories of vasoactive substances, including adrenomedullin (discussed previously), nitric oxide, endothelial cell hyperpolarizing factor, and endothelins.

Endothelium-derived relaxing factor (EDRF) has been identified as nitric oxide.[281] Nitric oxide is a potent vasodilator released from endothelium after stimulation and accounts for some or all of the activity generally ascribed to other agonists. For instance, acetylcholine causes constriction of vessels stripped of their intima and causes dilatation only in the presence of the vascular endothelium.[282] Adenosine, prostacyclin, and epinephrine dilate vessels stripped of their endothelium. Bradykinin, substance P, thrombin, and potassium cause only endothelium-dependent relaxation. Nitric oxide is also released from endothelium when flow increases, an example of positive feedback. Nitric oxide increases smooth muscle soluble guanylate cyclase activity, raises muscle cyclic GMP, and thereby relaxes vascular smooth muscle. In addition to EDRF, endothelial-derived hyperpolarizing factors, which are probably epoxyeicosatrienoic acids and hydrogen peroxide, are now thought to play major roles. The hydrogen peroxide is produced by the action of superoxide dismutase on superoxide anions that are generated by the metabolism of ATP.[282]

The vascular endothelium elaborates the endothelins (ET-1, ET-2, ET-3), a family of compounds that is vasoactive, structurally related peptides. ET-1 is the most potent vasoconstrictor known. It also promotes mitogenesis and stimulates the renin-angiotensin-aldosterone system and the release of vasopressin and atrial natriuretic peptide.[247,283-286] These peptides act on one of two receptor subtypes: ET_A and ET_B. ET_A is located mainly on vascular smooth muscle cells and is responsible for mediating vasoconstriction and cell proliferation. ET_B is present predominantly on endothelial cells and mediates vasorelaxation, as well as ET-1 clearance. Endothelins cause local vasoconstriction or vasodilatation, depending on dose and location in the circulation.[287] Individual endothelins occur in low levels in the plasma, generally below their vasoactive thresholds. This finding suggests they are primarily effective at the local site of release. Even at these levels, however, they may potentiate the effects of other vasoconstrictors such as norepinephrine and serotonin.[288] Endothelin antagonists, such as bosentan, now are being used, specifically in the setting of pulmonary arterial hypertension.[289,290]

Myogenic responses of vessels are changes in smooth muscle tone in response to stretch or increased transmural pressure. An increase in inflow pressure causes a rise in vessel wall tension and transmural pressure[291] that causes localized vasoconstriction. The reverse occurs when inflow pressure falls. The mechanisms of this response are complex. There is probably initial sensing by surface integrins,[292] followed by activation of cation channels with calcium entry.[293] In some way, protein kinase C, MAP kinases, and Rho kinase are also involved.[294-296]

As expected, a complex interplay exists among myogenic, flow-mediated, and metabolic regulation of vessel tone.[297] The relative importance of these mechanisms likely varies in different vascular beds.

Autoregulation

In all organs, when inflow pressure is suddenly raised or lowered while oxygen consumption remains constant, flow rises or falls transiently but then returns to the earlier value. The phenomenon is termed *autoregulation*. Myogenic tonic response is partly responsible for this phenomenon, but it is not the only mechanism. Some investigators believe tissues have oxygen sensors that respond to transient increases or decreases in oxygen supply.[298-300] Others believe the process is mediated by greater or lesser release of nitric oxide carried to

the tissues by hemoglobin in the form of S-nitrosohemoglobin or by ATP release by the red blood cell.[300-305] Carbon monoxide produced by the action of hemoxygenase in endothelium and smooth muscle may play a regulatory role.[306-313]

Acknowledgment

We gratefully acknowledge the contribution of Dr. Julien I. E. Hoffman, who authored this chapter in previous editions.

Key References

1. Bergmann O, et al. Evidence for cardiomyocyte renewal in humans. *Science.* 2009;324:98.
2. Huhta JC, et al. Left ventricular wall thickness in complete transposition of the great arteries. *J Thorac Cardiovasc Surg.* 1982;84:97.
3. Reese DE, et al. Development of the coronary vessel system. *Circ Res.* 2002;91:761.
4. Streeter DD Jr, Hanna WT. Engineering mechanics for successive states in canine left ventricular myocardium. 11. Fiber angle and sarcomere length. *Circ Res.* 1973;33:656.
5. Torrent-Guasp F, et al. The structure and function of the helical heart and its buttress wrapping. I. The normal macroscopic structure of the heart. *Semin Thorac Cardiovasc Surg.* 2001;13:301.
8. van Veen AA, et al. Cardiac gap junction channels: modulation of expression and channel properties. *Cardiovasc Res.* 2001;51:217.
11. Chidsey CA. Calcium metabolism in the normal and failing heart. In: Braunwald E, ed. *The Myocardium: Failure and Infarction.* New York: HP Publishing; 1974.
15. Katz AM. Contractile proteins in normal and failing myocardium. In: Braunwald E, ed. *The Myocardium: Failure and Infarction.* New York: HP Publishing; 1974.
19. Anderson PAW. Immature myocardium. In: Moller JH, Neal WA, eds. *Fetal, Neonatal, and Infant Cardiac Disease.* Norwalk, CT: Appleton & Lange; 1992.
21. Bristow M. Of phospholamban, mice, and humans with heart failure. *Circulation.* 2001;103:787.
22. Chu G, Kranias EG. Functional interplay between dual site phospholamban phosphorylation: insights from genetically altered mouse models. *Basic Res Cardiol.* 2002;97(suppl 1):143.
23. Frank K, Kranias EG. Phospholamban and cardiac contractility. *Ann Med.* 2000;32:572.
24. Schmidt AG, et al. Phospholamban: a promising therapeutic target in heart failure? *Cardiovasc Drugs Ther.* 2001;15:387.
25. Munch G, et al. Evidence for calcineurin-mediated regulation of SERCA 2a activity in human myocardium. *J Mol Cell Cardiol.* 2002;34:321.
26. Frank KF, et al. Modulation of SERCA: implications for the failing human heart. *Basic Res Cardiol.* 2002;97(suppl 1):172.
27. Pieske B, et al. Sarcoplasmic reticulum Ca2+ load in human heart failure. *Basic Res Cardiol.* 2002;97(suppl 1):963.
28. Wu LL, et al. Altered phospholamban-calcium ATPase interaction in cardiac sarcoplasmic reticulum during the progression of sepsis. *Shock.* 2002;17:389.
29. Lennon NJ, Ohlendieck K. Impaired Ca2+-sequestration in dilated cardiomyopathy (review). *Int J Mol Med.* 2001;7:131.
44. Towbin JA. The role of cytoskeletal proteins in cardiomyopathies. *Curr Opin Cell Biol.* 1998;10:131.
45. Towbin JA, Bowles NE. Molecular genetics of left ventricular dysfunction. *Curr Mol Med.* 2001;1:81.
55. Bristow JD. Cardiac and myocardial structure and myocardial cellular and molecular function. In: Gluckman PD, Heymann MA, eds. *Pediatrics and Perinatology. The Scientific Basis.* London: Edward Arnold; 1996.
59. Clyman RI. Developmental physiology of the ductus arteriosus. In: Polin Long WA, ed. *Fetal and Neonatal Cardiology.* New York: WB Saunders; 1989.
63. Michelakis ED, et al. O2 sensing in the human ductus arteriosus: regulation of voltage-gated K+ channels in smooth muscle cells by a mitochondrial redox sensor. *Circ Res.* 2002;91:478.
70. Mahony L. Development of myocardial structure and function. In: Emmanouilides GC, et al., eds. *Heart Disease in Infants, Children, and Adolescents, Including the Fetus and Young Adult.* Baltimore, MD: Williams & Wilkins; 1998.

73. Smith V-E, Zile MR. Relaxation and diastolic properties of the heart. In: Fozzard HA, et al., eds. *The Heart and Cardiovascular System: Scientific Foundations.* New York: Raven Press; 1991.

75. Strobeck JE, Sonnenblick EH. Myocardial contractile properties and ventricular performance. In: Fozzard HA, et al., eds. *The Heart and Cardiovascular System: Scientific Foundations.* New York: Raven Press; 1991.

76. McCormack J, et al. In vivo demonstration of maturational changes of the chronotropic response to alpha-adrenergic stimulation. *Pediatr Res.* 1988;24:50.

77. Bristow MR, et al. Beta 1- and beta 2-adrenergic-receptor subpopulations in nonfailing and failing human ventricular myocardium: coupling of both receptor subtypes to muscle contraction and selective beta 1-receptor down-regulation in heart failure. *Circ Res.* 1986;59:297.

83. Zaugg M, et al. Beta-adrenergic receptor subtypes differentially affect apoptosis in adult rat ventricular myocytes. *Circulation.* 2000;102:344-350.

87. Bristow MR. Mechanistic and clinical rationales for using beta-blockers in heart failure. *J Card Fail.* 2000;6:8.

92. Packer M, et al. Effect of carvedilol on the morbidity of patients with severe chronic heart failure: results of the carvedilol prospective randomized cumulative survival (COPERNICUS) study. *Circulation.* 2002;106:2194.

93. Artman M, et al. Inotropic responses change during postnatal maturation in rabbit. *Am J Physiol Heart Circ Physiol.* 1988;255:H335.

94. Hoffman TM, et al. Efficacy and safety of milrinone in preventing low cardiac output syndrome in infants and children after corrective surgery for congenital heart disease. *Circulation.* 2003;107:996-1002.

102. Ross J Jr. Mechanisms of cardiac contraction. What roles for preload, afterload and inotropic state in heart failure? *Eur Heart J.* 1983;4(suppl A):19.

107. Anderson PA, et al. Evaluation of the force-frequency relationship as a descriptor of the inotropic state of canine left ventricular myocardium. *Circ Res.* 1976;39:832.

111. Sagawa K. The end-systolic pressure-volume relation of the ventricle: definition, modifications and clinical use. *Circulation.* 1981;63:1223.

112. Suga H. Ventricular energetics. *Physiol Rev.* 1990;70:247.

114. Redington AN, et al. Changes in the pressure-volume relation of the right ventricle when its loading conditions are modified. *Br Heart J.* 1990;63:1.

123. Colan SD, et al. Use of the indirect axillary pulse tracing for noninvasive determination of ejection time, upstroke time, and left ventricular wall stress throughout ejection in infants and young children. *Am J Cardiol.* 1984;53:1154.

124. Colan SD, et al. Left ventricular end-systolic wall stress-velocity of fiber shortening relation: a load-independent index of myocardial contractility. *J Am Coll Cardiol.* 1984;4:715.

135. Belenkie I, et al. Ventricular interaction: from bench to bedside. *Ann Med.* 2001;33:236.

138. Tyberg JV, et al. Effects of positive intrathoracic pressure on pulmonary and systemic hemodynamics. *Respir Physiol.* 2000;119:171.

179. Strauer B-E. Myocardial oxygen consumption in chronic heart disease: role of wall stress, hypertrophy and coronary reserve. *Am J Cardiol.* 1979;44:730-740.

193. Hoffman JI, Buckberg GD. The myocardial supply:demand ratio—a critical review. *Am J Cardiol.* 1978;41:327.

214. Buga GM, Ignarro LJ. Vascular endothelium and smooth muscle function. In: Gluckman PD, Heymann MA, eds. *Pediatrics and Perinatology. The Scientific Basis.* London: Edward Arnold; 1996.

237. Muller DN, Luft FC. The renin-angiotensin system in the vessel wall. *Basic Res Cardiol.* 1998;93:7.

238. Burlew BS, Weber KT. Connective tissue and the heart. Functional significance and regulatory mechanisms. *Cardiol Clin.* 2000;18:435.

251. Holmes CL, et al. Physiology of vasopressin relevant to management of septic shock. *Chest.* 2001;120:989.

252. Zimmerman MA, et al. Vasopressin in cardiovascular patients: therapeutic implications. *Expert Opin Pharmacother.* 2002;3:505.

276. Murray PA, et al. The role of potassium in the metabolic control of coronary vascular resistance of the dog. *Circ Res.* 1979;44:767.

280. Sparks HV. Effect of local metabolic factors on vascular smooth muscle. In: Bohr DF, et al., eds. *Handbook of Physiology. The Cardiovascular System.* Vol 2. Bethesda, MD: American Physiological Society; 1980.

299. Budinger GR, et al. Hibernation during hypoxia in cardiomyocytes. Role of mitochondria as the O2 sensor. *J Biol Chem.* 1998;273:3320.

Regional Peripheral Circulation

Peter Oishi, Julien I. Hoffman, Bradley P. Fuhrman, and Jeffrey R. Fineman

PEARLS

- When delivering critical care, one must understand the specific properties that characterize the various regional circulations because therapies that benefit one region may be detrimental to another.
- Vascular tone is influenced by (1) innervation and neural processes, (2) circulating endocrine and neuroendocrine mediators, (3) local metabolic products, (4) blood gas composition, (5) endothelial-derived factors, and (6) myogenic processes.
- The transition from the fetal pulmonary circulation to the postnatal pulmonary circulation is marked by a dramatic fall in pulmonary vascular resistance and rise in pulmonary blood flow. The failure to successfully make this transition is integral to a number of neonatal and infant diseases.
- An important feature unique to the cerebral circulation is the presence of a blood-brain barrier. As a result, the cerebral vasculature responds differently from other vascular beds to humoral stimuli.
- Regulation of myocardial perfusion is tailored to match regional myocardial oxygen supply to demand over the widest possible range of cardiac workload. Increases in myocardial oxygen demand must be met by increases in myocardial blood flow.
- Critically ill patients are at risk for impaired splanchnic blood flow that can impair the two chief functions of the gastrointestinal system: (1) digestion and absorption of nutrients and (2) maintenance of a barrier to the translocation of enteric antigens. Splanchnic ischemia is associated with increased morbidity and mortality in critically ill patients.
- Although renal blood flow remains constant over a wide range of renal artery perfusion pressures, urinary flow rate varies as a function of renal perfusion pressure.

General Features
General Anatomy

Blood vessels comprise several distinct layers. Moving from the innermost layer outward are the metabolically active endothelium, intima (with nerves and vasa vasorum), media, and adventitia. Some vessels have fewer layers, depending on the position and function of the vessel within the circulation.

The large arteries are elastic. Their media contain concentric lamellae of perforated elastic tubes cross-linked by transverse collagen and smooth muscle. When smooth muscle contracts, the wall becomes stiffer. Smaller arteries have fewer lamellae. The media are bounded by the internal and external elastic laminae. Arterioles are less elastic, have no lamellae, and have a thin media with circular or spiral smooth muscle and inner and outer elastic laminae. Capillaries are thin walled and nonmuscular, ideal for transport of materials to and from the tissues. Veins have medial muscle but thinner walls relative to lumen diameter compared with arteries. The vascular endothelium has important metabolic characteristics, which may differ between vessel types (ie, arteries vs. veins) and different regions.[1,2]

Basic Physiology

Blood flow to a regional vascular bed is determined primarily by inflow pressure, vascular resistance, and outflow pressure. Inflow pressure is usually systemic arterial pressure. Outflow pressure approximates venous pressure but may at times exceed venous pressure if vascular tone is great enough to close the circulation above venous pressure or if external pressure impinges on the vasculature.

In a model to explain the relation of arterial pressure to flow, the circulation is represented by two capacitance vessels separated by a resistance. A standpipe full of blood is allowed to discharge its contents into the arterial vasculature (the proximal capacitance). Blood flows across the resistance site (the arterioles), traverses the venous vasculature (the distal capacitance), and drains to a reservoir at some outflow pressure (Po) (Fig. 26.1).

The pressure head of the system (Pi) is generated by the weight of the column of blood in the standpipe and is proportional to its height (Pi = blood column height in cm H_2O). As the standpipe discharges, the height decreases and Pi decreases. This in turn decreases the rate of flow (Q) through the vasculature. Q decreases almost linearly with Pi until the column is quite low. Ultimately, flow will cease while there is still pressure in the standpipe. The pressure at which flow ceases is the critical closing pressure of the circulation (Pc).[3] Pi below Pc is insufficient to maintain vessel patency and permit continued flow (Fig. 26.2).

Incremental resistance to flow is generally defined as the change in pressure per unit change in flow (dPi/dQ). At pressures well above critical closing pressure, this is nearly identical to the vascular resistance (R) defined clinically as:

$$R = (Pi - Po)/Q$$

When Pi does not greatly exceed Pc but Pc does greatly exceed Po, however, incremental resistance can differ substantially

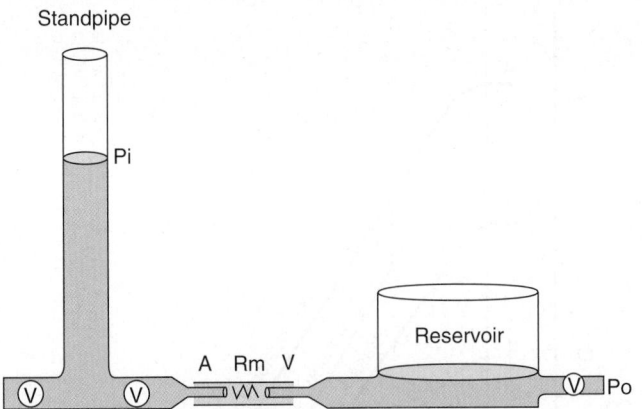

Fig. 26.1. Model for facilitating interpretation of vascular pressure-flow relations. When valves *(V)* are properly positioned, fluid filling the standpipe to height Pi discharges across the circulation to the reservoir at outflow pressure Po. *A,* artery; *Rm,* microvascular resistance; *V,* vein.

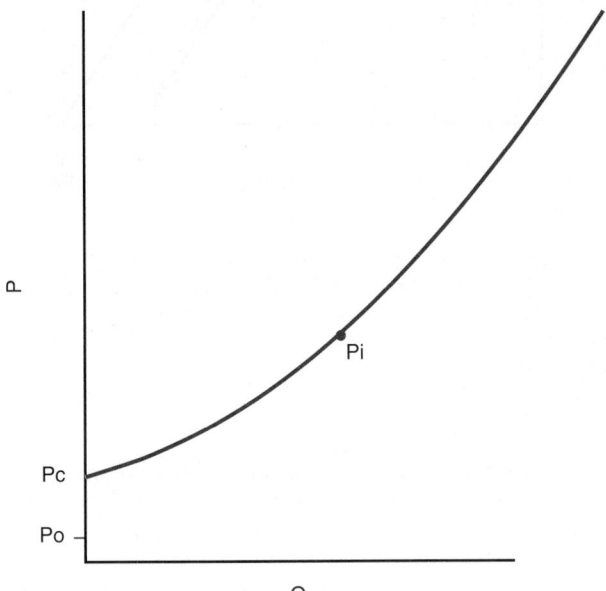

Fig. 26.2. As the standpipe in Fig. 26.1 discharges, Pi falls. Flow consequently slows and ultimately stops when Pi = Pc, the critical closing pressure of the circulation. Pi only reaches outflow pressure Po if Po ≥ Pc.

from this clinical estimate. Thus an increase in Pc can be confused with a true increase in incremental resistance. For example, a diagnosis of intrinsic pulmonary vascular disease (eg, pulmonary arterial hypertension) based on measured pulmonary artery pressures in a patient receiving mechanical ventilation with high airway pressures (that raise Pc) may be spurious.

Venous Return and Cardiac Output

A second model illustrates the relationship of cardiac output to intrinsic mechanical properties of the systemic vasculature. In this model, the heart acts as a roller pump, creating a circulation much like that achieved during venoarterial extracorporeal support (Fig. 26.3).

The roller pump displaces blood from the veins to the arteries and then across the resistance imposed by the arterioles.

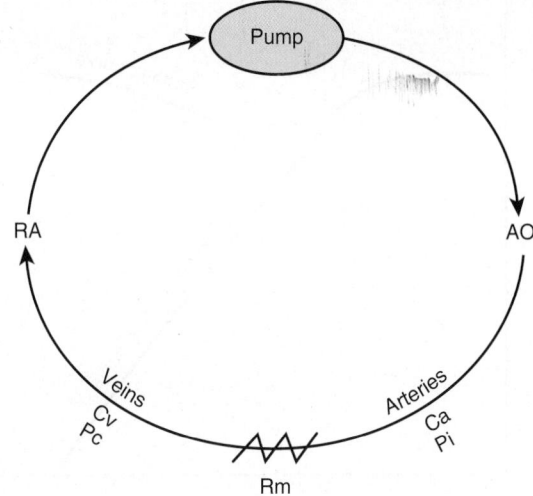

Fig. 26.3. Model for facilitating interpretation of the relation of venous return to right atrial pressure. The heart is replaced by a mechanical roller pump. The right atrium *(RA)* is drained by the pump, and blood is infused into the aorta *(AO)*. Blood then traverses the arteries, which have a capacitance *(Ca)* at an inflow pressure *(Pi)* determined by flow rate and microvascular resistance *(Rm)*. Blood then returns through veins having capacitance *(Cv)* and critical closing pressure *(Pc)* to the right atrium.

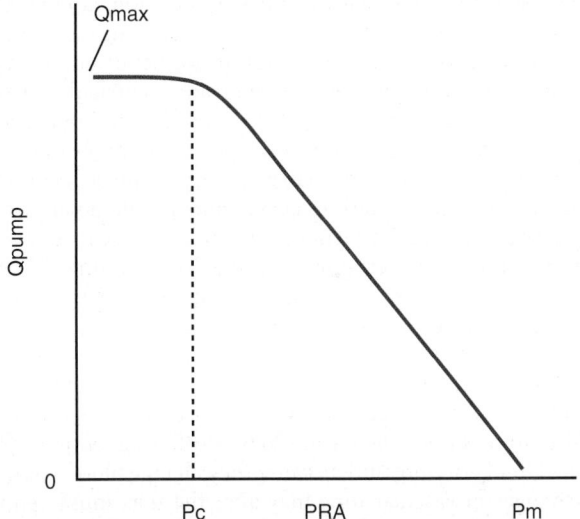

Fig. 26.4. Venous return curve. As pump flow *(Qpump)* varies, right atrial pressure *(Pra)* is altered by redistribution of blood between arteries and veins. Qpump cannot be increased above Qmax because Pra would fall below critical closing pressure *(Pc)* of the venous circulation. *Pm,* mean circulatory pressure of the vasculature at no flow.

As Q increases, more blood resides in the arteries and less in the veins. This partitioning of blood depends on arterial capacitance (Ca), venous capacitance (Cv), and resistance to flow. At maximal Q, Pi and arterial blood volume are high and venous pressure (Pv) is low. When Pv reaches Pc, the roller pump cannot be increased further because the veins will collapse when Pv is less than Pc.

As Q is reduced, by turning down the roller pump, arterial pressure (Pi) and volume fall and Pv increases. As Q approaches zero, venous pressure approaches the mean circulatory pressure (Pm) (Fig. 26.4). The importance of this model is that it

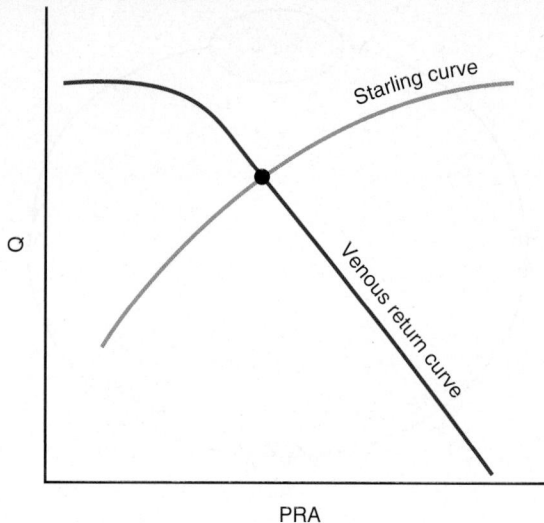

Fig. 26.5. Theoretical superimposition of venous return and Starling curves. For any state of the heart and vasculature, these curves intersect at a point that characterizes right atrial pressure *(Pra)* and cardiac output *(Q)*.

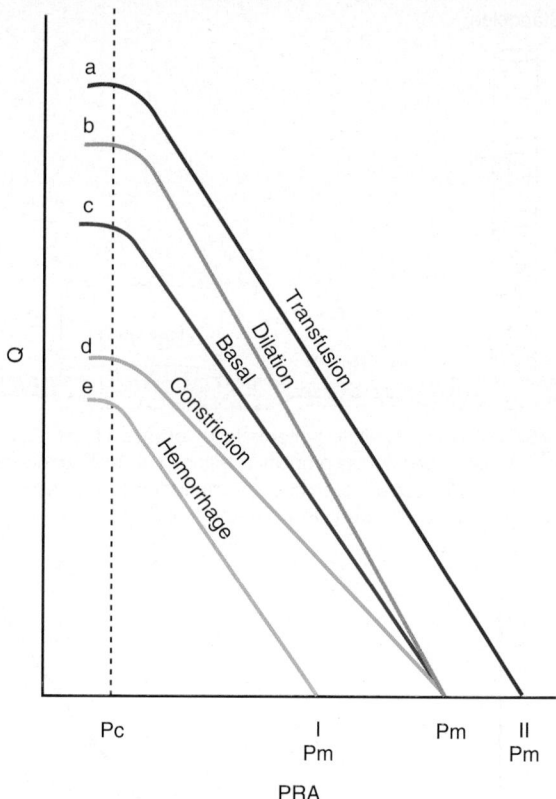

Fig. 26.6. Effects of changing blood volume and microvascular resistance on the venous return curve. Curves *a, c,* and *e* are parallel but have different mean circulatory pressure *(Pm)* at zero flow. Curves *b, c,* and *d* are nonparallel but have the same Pm. *Pc,* critical closing pressure; *Pra,* right atrial pressure.

can be used to illustrate the role of venous return as an independent determinant of cardiac output.

The Starling curve that describes the relationship between preload and contractility (and hence cardiac output) is illustrated in Fig. 26.5. Over the steep portion of the curve, optimization of myocardial preload increases ventricular stroke volume. This curve (see Chapter 25) can be superimposed on the venous return curve. Cardiac output occurs at the theoretical intersection of these two curves, representing a given state of cardiac function (Starling curve) and simultaneous set of vascular characteristics (venous return curve) (see Fig. 26.5).

It is important to recognize that the venous return curve is influenced by changes in blood volume and vascular tone. Transfusion elevates the maximal venous return and thus cardiac output that can be achieved before the system reaches Pc. Hemorrhage has the opposite effect. Because neither transfusion nor hemorrhage directly alters vascular tone, the slope of the curve is not altered (Fig. 26.6). Both interventions alter mean circulatory pressure because they change blood volume.

Changes in vascular tone may alter the maximum venous return (and thus cardiac output) attainable before venous collapse (Pc), at any given intravascular volume. At zero flow, the mean pressure in the system would relate most directly to the volume of blood within the vessels. Thus changes in vascular tone change the slope of the venous return curve (see Fig. 26.6).

In clinical practice, it is unusual for any of these changes in vascular mechanics to occur in isolation. For instance, arteriolar dilation and dilation of other capacitance vessels often occur together. Arteriolar dilation and dilation of capacitance vessels have opposite effects on the venous return curve and, consequently, different effects on cardiac output. It is for this reason that vascular volume expansion is often required in combination with nitroprusside or milrinone infusions in order to ensure adequacy of cardiac output despite a reduction in afterload.

In patients with sepsis, toxic vasodilation may cause either high or low cardiac output, depending on associated changes

in venous capacitance. Adequacy of vascular volume expansion, venous capacitance, vascular resistance, and the inotropic state of the heart can all profoundly influence cardiac output in patients with sepsis. Patients in septic shock are warm only if the circulation is adequately filled, cardiac function is sufficient, and incremental resistance is low.

Critical Closing Pressure

In many organs as inflow pressure is lowered, Q decreases and ceases at a pressure—the critical closing pressure (Pc)—that is higher than venous pressure. The probable mechanism is the vascular waterfall or Starling resistor. In 1910 Jerusalem and Starling[2] described a device designed to control afterload to the left ventricle and that made possible the study of cardiac contractility.[4] The device consisted of a collapsible rubber tube traversing a pressurized glass chamber (Fig. 26.7). When pressure surrounding the rubber tube exceeded the outflow pressure set by the reservoir, surrounding pressure opposed the flow of blood and became the true outflow pressure of the device. The physiologic counterpart of this occurs in small vessels surrounded by tissue pressure. In the heart, for example, a Starling resistor effect occurs in extramyocardial coronary veins, although there is also evidence for critical closure of small arterioles. No one has yet demonstrated vessel closure directly, but this might not be necessary because as small vessels narrow when they are compressed, the wall becomes convoluted and blood cells might become obstructed by the

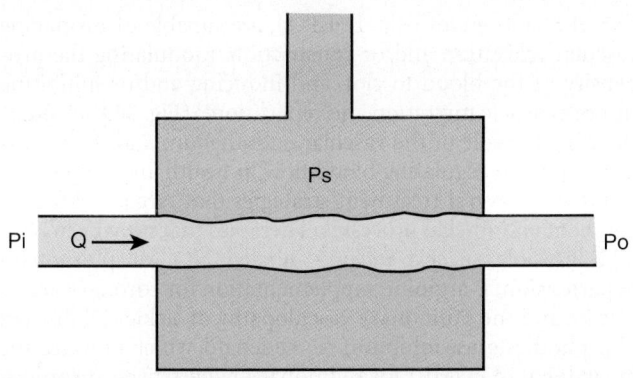

Fig. 26.7. Starling resistor is a compressible conduit exposed to surrounding pressure *(Ps)*. When Ps is less than outflow pressure *(Po)*, Ps does not oppose blood flow. When Ps is between inflow *(Pi)* and outflow pressures, it opposes blood flow. No flow is possible when Ps exceeds Pi.

folds even when externally the vessel does not appear to be closed.

Autoregulation

In all organs, when inflow pressure is suddenly raised or lowered while oxygen consumption remains constant, flow rises or falls transiently but then returns to its former value; the phenomenon is termed *autoregulation*. Several mechanisms, particularly related to oxygen sensing, have been implicated in this response, but the precise mechanisms are likely complex and multifactorial. For example, studies have described a role for nitric oxide (NO) carried to the tissues by hemoglobin in the form of S-nitrosohemoglobin.[5-7] Other locally produced gases such as hydrogen sulfide[8] and carbon monoxide[9,10] may also play a role. Importantly, some autoregulatory mechanisms are specific to individual microcirculations (eg, macula densa signaling in the renal circulation).

Distensibility and Compliance

The distensibility of a vessel is defined as the change in volume as a proportion of the initial volume for a given change in pressure:

$$\text{Distensibility} = \frac{\Delta V}{\Delta P} \times \frac{1}{V},$$

where V is volume and P is pressure. Veins are much thinner than arteries and are about eight times more distensible. Multiplying distensibility by volume yields DV/DP, which is the definition of compliance. Because venous volume is usually more than three times arterial volume, venous compliance is about 20- to 30-fold greater than arterial compliance. As a result, whenever fluids are infused, the veins accommodate the bulk of the fluid volume.

Vascular Resistance

Under normal circumstances, vascular resistance is the major control of organ flow and can be understood by considering the resistance of a Newtonian liquid passing through a rigid tube as defined by the Hagen-Poiseuille equation:

$$R = \left(\frac{8}{\pi}\right)\left(\frac{l}{r^4}\right)\eta$$

where R is resistance, l is tube length, r is the internal radius of the tube, and η is the fluid viscosity. Blood is not a Newtonian fluid, but this fact does not affect the accuracy of calculated vascular resistance much. However, vascular beds do contain many "tubes" in parallel. Thus for vascular systems, a factor k is added that represents the number of vessels. The equation thus becomes:

$$R = \left(\frac{8}{\pi}\right)\left(\frac{l}{kr^4}\right)\eta$$

Because the length and number of vessels and blood viscosity are relatively constant at any one time, change in vessel radius is the major factor responsible for a dynamic change in vascular resistance; because of the fourth power factor, small changes in radius cause large changes in resistance. Vessel radius is influenced by vascular elasticity and transmural pressure but is mainly regulated by changes in vessel wall smooth muscle tone.

Vascular Impedance

Resistance is strictly a steady state concept. In a pulsatile system the factors affecting the relationship of pressure dissipation to flow are resistance due to friction and viscosity, fluid inertia, and vessel wall compliance, which combine to produce an *impedance* to flow that varies with frequency. At zero frequency, steady state resistance is approximated by the change in mean pressure over flow, but there are substantial contributions made by the first three harmonics that are ignored by this calculation.

Local Regulatory Mechanisms

Regions of the circulation may differ markedly in their patterns of vascular regulation. A regulatory stimulus can have multiple effects that differ from one location to another. An agent that potently regulates vascular resistance in one region of the circulation may have no effect in another. For example, during hemorrhagic shock, flow is maintained to heart and brain but reduced to muscle, kidneys, and gut.

Vascular tone is strongly influenced by several mechanisms: (1) innervation and neural processes, (2) circulating endocrine and neuroendocrine mediators, (3) local metabolic products, (4) blood gas composition, (5) endothelial-derived factors, and (6) myogenic processes.

Innervation and Neural Processes

Receptors responsive to neural products (eg, norepinephrine and acetylcholine) are found throughout the circulation. Nevertheless, innervation and receptor distribution are organ specific, allowing rapid, patterned, coordinated redistribution of blood flow and an orchestrated response to events, such as hypoxia, changes in posture, and hemorrhage. Although these receptors respond to circulating agonists (including adrenal epinephrine), as well as to those liberated locally, they are generally associated with innervation by autonomic nerves. In general, presynaptic α-adrenergic stimulation causes norepinephrine reuptake, whereas postsynaptic α-adrenergic stimulation causes norepinephrine release and vasoconstriction. β-Adrenergic stimulation generally causes vasodilation. Cholinergic stimulation (whether sympathetic or parasympathetic) generally causes vasodilation (see Chapters 33 and 125).

Circulating Endocrine and Neuroendocrine Mediators

Humoral regulators of vascular tone include angiotensin, arginine vasopressin, bradykinin, histamine, and serotonin. Of less certain significance are aldosterone, thyroxine, antinatriuretic peptide, and various reproductive hormones. Most of these have both direct effects and secondary effects, which tend to be organ specific or regional in nature. Angiotensin plays a special role in the homeostasis of blood pressure and is produced in hemorrhagic or hypovolemic shock. It causes generalized vasoconstriction in both systemic and pulmonary circulations, but locally it stimulates the release of vasodilating prostaglandins in lung and kidney. Bradykinin is a potent pulmonary and systemic vasodilator released locally by the action of proteolytic enzymes on kallikrein after tissue injury. Histamine is released by mast cells in response to injury and is also a potent vasodilator in most regions of the circulation, but it causes vasoconstriction in the lung.

Local Metabolic Products

Local metabolic regulation of vasomotor tone provides an ideal homeostatic mechanism whereby metabolic demand can directly influence perfusion. The precise mechanisms underlying the coupling of blood flow with metabolic activity remain unclear. One theory holds that as the metabolic rate increases, so too does the formation of some vasodilating substance. Thus the regional vasculature relaxes, allowing more oxygen to be delivered in support of this work. As flow rises, the metabolites are washed out, restoring their concentration to normal. Adenosine, for instance, which accumulates locally when tissue metabolism is high and tissue oxygenation is marginal, causes pronounced vasodilation in the coronary, striated muscle, splanchnic, and cerebral circulations. Another example is potassium, which is released from muscle in response to increased work, ischemia, and hypoxia. Hypokalemia causes vasoconstriction, and hyperkalemia, within the physiologic range, causes vasodilation.

An increasing amount of data demonstrates the importance of the local redox state on the regulation of blood flow through the microcirculation. Reactive oxygen species, such as superoxide, hydrogen peroxide, and peroxynitrite, have been shown to influence normal regulatory processes and participate in the pathophysiology of a wide array of cardiovascular disorders. For example, the rapid reaction of NO with the superoxide anion results in the formation of peroxynitrite, a potent oxidant. Although peroxynitrite is known to have cytotoxic properties, under normal conditions peroxynitrite inhibits leukocyte adherence and platelet aggregation without evidence of cellular injury.[11] In disease states, however, peroxynitrite can lead to protein nitration and DNA damage. In addition, elevated levels of superoxide may decrease the bioavailability of NO leading to abnormal vasomotion.[12]

Blood Gas Composition

Tissue levels of oxygen and carbon dioxide have been shown to reflect adequacy of perfusion and oxygen delivery.[13] These blood gases are potent determinants of regional blood flow and have effects that differ from one region of the circulation to another. They also have a more general effect mediated by carotid chemoreceptors.

Endothelial-Derived Factors

The vascular endothelial cells are capable of producing a variety of vasoactive substances, which participate in the regulation of normal vascular tone. These substances, such as NO, CO, H_2S, and endothelin-1 (ET-1), are capable of producing vascular relaxation and/or constriction, modulating the propensity of the blood to clot, and inducing and/or inhibiting smooth muscle migration and replication[14] (Fig. 26.8). Understanding the role of the vascular endothelium and the factors it produces in regulating blood flow in health and disease has resulted in several treatment strategies that target, mimic, or augment endothelial processes. Therapies that have been used with variable success include inhaled NO for pulmonary hypertension; L-arginine supplementation for coronary artery disease and the pulmonary vasculopathy of sickle cell disease; phosphodiesterase inhibitors (ie, sildenafil, which prevents the breakdown of cGMP) for pulmonary hypertensive disorders; endothelin receptor antagonists for pulmonary hypertensive disorders and vasospasm following subarachnoid hemorrhage; and NO inhibitors for refractory hypotension secondary to sepsis.[15-20] Indeed, many older therapies used to promote vascular relaxation, such as nitrovasodilators, affect endothelial function, a fact not appreciated until relatively recently.

NO is a labile humoral factor produced by NO synthase from L-arginine in the vascular endothelial cell. NO diffuses into the smooth muscle cell and produces vascular relaxation by increasing concentrations of guanosine 3'5'-monophosphate (cGMP), via the activation of soluble guanylate cyclase. NO is released in response to a variety of factors including shear stress (flow) and the binding of certain endothelium-dependent vasodilators (such as acetylcholine, ATP, and bradykinin) to receptors on the endothelial cell. Basal NO release is an important mediator of both resting pulmonary and systemic vascular tone in the fetus, newborn, and adult, as well as a mediator of the fall in pulmonary vascular resistance normally occurring at the time of birth.[21] Dynamic changes in NO release are fundamental to the regulation of all vascular beds.

CO is a labile humoral factor produced by the action of hemoxygenase on heme in many tissues, including endothelial cells. Hemoxygenase-1 is constitutive and hemoxygenase-2 is inducible. CO interacts with NO, is an independent stimulator of cGMP, relaxes smooth muscle, inhibits its replication, and has powerful antithrombotic and antiinflammatory effects. It is beginning to enter the field of clinical medicine.[10,22]

Hydrogen sulfide (H2S) is produced in most tissues by a variety of mechanisms and may be the ultimate sensor that is stimulated by oxygen deficit or excess.[8]

ET-1 is a 21 amino acid polypeptide also produced by vascular endothelial cells.[23] The vasoactive properties of ET-1 are complex, and studies have shown varying hemodynamic effects on different vascular beds. However, its most striking property is its sustained hypertensive action. In fact, ET-1 is the most potent vasoconstricting agent discovered, with a potency 10 times that of angiotensin II. The hemodynamic effects of ET-1 are mediated by at least two distinctive receptor populations, ETA and ETB. The ETA receptors are located on vascular smooth muscle cells and mediate vasoconstriction, whereas the ETB receptors may be located on endothelial cells and mediate both vasodilation and vasoconstriction. Individual endothelins occur in low levels in the plasma, generally below their vasoactive thresholds. This suggests that they are primarily effective at the local site of release. Even at these levels, they may potentiate the effects of other vasoconstrictors such as norepinephrine and serotonin.[24] The role of endogenous ET-1 in the regulation of normal vascular tone is presently unclear. Nevertheless, alterations in endothelin-1 have

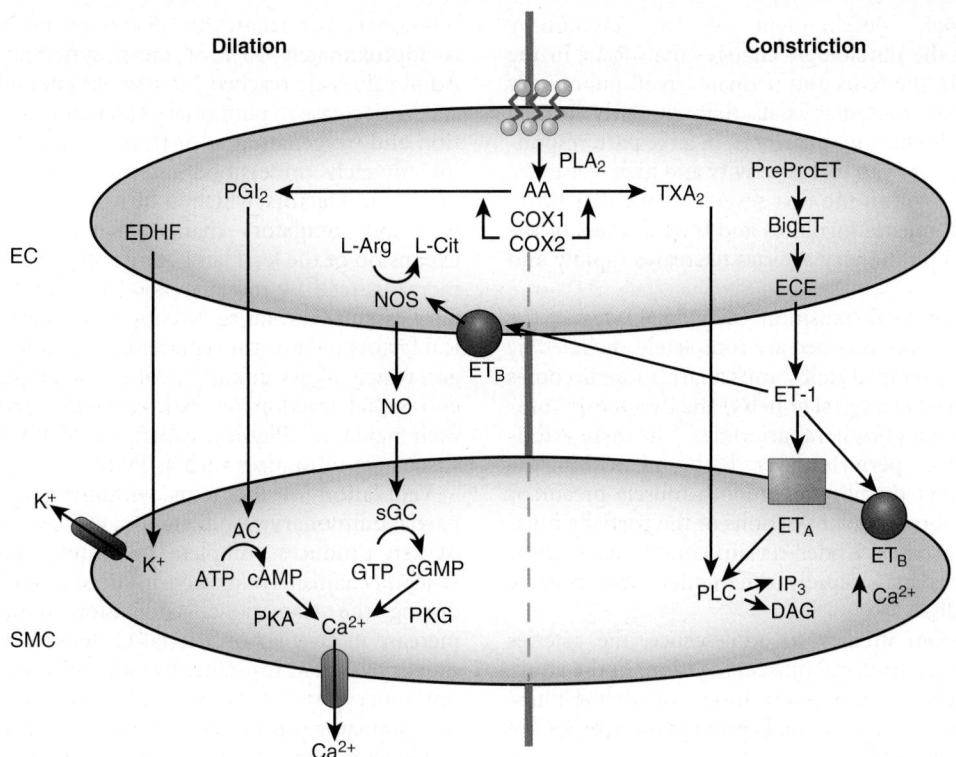

Fig. 26.8. Schematic of some endogenous vasoactive agents produced by the vascular endothelium. *AA,* arachidonic acid; *AC,* adenylate cyclase; *ATP,* adenosine triphosphate; *cAMP,* cyclic adenosine monophosphate; *cGMP,* cyclic guanosine monophosphate; *COX,* cyclooxygenase; *DAG,* diacylglycerol; *EC,* endothelial cell; *ECE,* endothelin-converting enzyme; *EDHF,* endothelial-derived hyperpolarizing factor; *ET-1,* endothelin-1; *GTP,* guanosine triphosphate; *IP3,* inositol 1,4,5, triphosphate; *L-arg,* L-arginine; *L-cit,* L-citrulline; *NO,* nitric oxide; *NOS,* nitric oxide synthase; *PGI2,* prostacyclin; *PKA,* protein kinase A; *PKC,* protein kinase C; *PLA,* phospholipase A2; *sGC,* soluble guanylate cyclase; *SMC,* smooth muscle cell; *TXA2,* thromboxane A2.

been implicated in the pathophysiology of a number of disease states.[25]

Endothelial-derived hyperpolarizing factor (EDHF), a diffusible substance that causes vascular relaxation by hyperpolarizing the smooth muscle cell, is another important endothelial factor. EDHF has not yet been identified, but current evidence suggests that the action of EDHF is dependent on K+ channels (Fig. 26.8). Activation of potassium channels in the vascular smooth muscle results in cell membrane hyperpolarization, closure of voltage-dependent calcium channels, and ultimately vasodilation. Potassium channels are also present in endothelial cells. Activation within the endothelium results in changes in calcium flux and may be important in the release of NO, prostacyclin, and EDHF. Potassium channel subtypes include ATP-sensitive K+ channels, Ca2+-dependent K+ channels, voltage-dependent K+ channels, and inward-rectifier K+ channels.

The breakdown of phospholipids within vascular endothelial cells results in the production of the important byproducts of arachidonic acid, including prostacyclin (PGI2) and thromboxane (TXA2). PGI2 activates adenylate cyclase, resulting in increased cAMP production and subsequent vasodilation, whereas TXA2 results in vasoconstriction via phospholipase C signaling (see Fig. 26.8). Other prostaglandins and leukotrienes also have potent vasoactive properties.

Myogenic Processes

In 1902 Bayliss described an intrinsic increase in vascular tone in response to elevated intravascular pressure.[26] This myogenic response results in alterations in vascular tone following changes in transmural pressure or stretch. This response is especially important at the arteriolar level and is thought to participate in regional autoregulation. Increases in intravascular pressure and/or stretch result in an increase in arteriolar smooth muscle tone, while decreasing pressures have the reverse effect. The precise mechanisms mediating this response are unclear, but a role for dynamic changes in intracellular Ca2+ and myosin light chain phosphorylation has been documented.[27] More recent work has focused on the role of tyrosine phosphorylation pathways, ENaC, transient receptor potential (TRP) channels, potassium channels, and alterations in Ca2+ sensitivity in this response.[28-32] Moreover, the myogenic response varies between the regional circulations and between vessels within a given circulation.

Regional Circulations
Pulmonary Circulation

Maldevelopment and/or maladaptation of the pulmonary vascular bed are important components of several neonatal and infant disease states (ie, chronic lung disease, persistent pulmonary hypertension of the newborn, and congenital heart disease). In addition, strategies aimed at altering postnatal pulmonary vascular resistance are commonly used in the management of these patients. Therefore an understanding of the regulation of postnatal pulmonary vascular tone is important.

The morphologic development of the pulmonary circulation affects the physiologic changes that occur in the perinatal period. In the fetus and neonate, small pulmonary arteries have thicker muscular coats than similarly located arteries in the adult. This muscularity is, in large part, responsible for the pulmonary vascular reactivity and high resistance found in the fetus. Within the first several weeks after birth, the medial smooth muscle involutes and the thickness of the media of the small pulmonary arteries decreases rapidly and progressively.[33]

Following this perinatal transition, the medial layers of the proximal pulmonary vascular bed are completely encircled by smooth muscle. Moving distally, muscularization becomes incomplete (arranged in a spiral or helix) and disappears completely from the most peripheral arterioles.[34] In these arterioles, an incomplete pericyte layer is found within the endothelial basement membrane. Smooth muscle precursor cells reside in the nonmuscular portions of the partially muscular pulmonary arteries. Under certain conditions, such as hypoxia, these cells may rapidly differentiate into mature smooth muscle cells.

Subsequently, from infancy to adolescence, the arteries undergo progressive peripheral muscularization. In the adult, complete circumferential muscularization extends peripherally such that the majority of small pulmonary arteries are completely muscularized.

Normal Fetal Circulation

In the fetus, normal gas exchange occurs in the placenta and pulmonary blood flow is low, supplying only nutritional requirements for lung growth and performing some metabolic functions. Pulmonary blood flow in near-term lambs is between 8% and 10% of total output of the heart.[35] Pulmonary blood flow is low despite the dominance of the right ventricle, which in the fetus ejects about two-thirds of total cardiac output. Most of the right ventricular output is diverted away from the lungs through the widely patent ductus arteriosus to the descending thoracic aorta, from which a large proportion reaches the placenta through the umbilical circulation for oxygenation. Fetal pulmonary arterial pressure increases with advancing gestation. At term, mean pulmonary arterial pressure is about 50 mm Hg, generally exceeding mean descending aortic pressure by 1 to 2 mm Hg.[36] Pulmonary vascular resistance early in gestation is extremely high relative to that in the infant and adult, probably due to the low number of small arteries. Pulmonary vascular resistance falls progressively during the last half of gestation, new arteries develop, and cross-sectional area increases; however, baseline pulmonary vascular resistance is still much higher than after birth.[36,37]

Changes in the Pulmonary Circulation at Birth

After birth, with initiation of ventilation by the lungs and the subsequent increase in pulmonary and systemic arterial blood O_2 tensions, pulmonary vascular resistance decreases and pulmonary blood flow increases by 8- to 10-fold to match systemic blood flow. This large increase in pulmonary blood flow increases pulmonary venous return to the left atrium, increasing left atrial pressure. Then the valve of the foramen ovale closes, preventing any significant atrial right-to-left shunting of blood. In addition, the ductus arteriosus constricts and closes functionally within several hours after birth, effectively separating the pulmonary and systemic circulations. Mean pulmonary arterial pressure decreases and, by 24 hours of age, is approximately 50% of mean systemic arterial pressure. Adult values are reached 2 to 6 weeks after birth[38,39] (Fig. 26.9).

The decrease in pulmonary vascular resistance with ventilation and oxygenation at birth is regulated by a complex and incompletely understood interplay between metabolic and mechanical factors, which in turn are triggered by the ventilatory and circulatory changes that occur at birth. Physical expansion of the fetal lamb lung without changing O_2 tension increases fetal pulmonary blood flow and decreases pulmonary vascular resistance, but not to newborn values.[40] Mechanical factors include the replacement of fluid in the alveoli with gas, which allows unkinking of the small pulmonary arteries, and radial traction on extra-alveolar vessels that maintain their patency.[41] Physical expansion of the lung also releases vasoactive substances such as PGI2.

Ventilation of the fetus without oxygenation produces partial pulmonary vasodilatation, while ventilation with air or oxygen produces complete pulmonary vasodilatation. The exact mechanisms of oxygen-induced pulmonary vasodilation during the transitional circulation remain unclear. The increase in alveolar or arterial O_2 tension may decrease pulmonary vascular resistance by either directly dilating the small pulmonary arteries or indirectly stimulating the production of vasodilator substances such as PGI2 or NO.

Therefore there are at least two components to the decrease in pulmonary vascular resistance with the initiation of ventilation and oxygenation. Both components are necessary for the successful transition to extrauterine life. Control of the

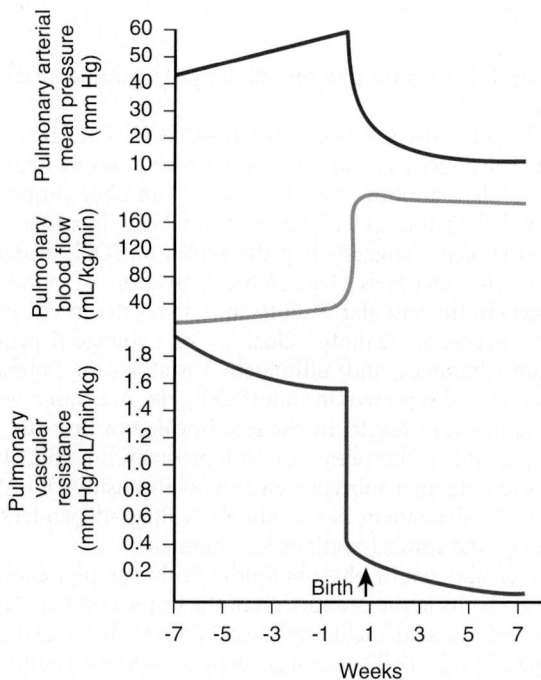

Fig. 26.9. Changes in mean pulmonary arterial pressure, pulmonary blood flow, and pulmonary vascular resistance at birth. (Data from Morin FC III, Egan E. Pulmonary hemodynamics in fetal lambs during development at normal and increased oxygen tension. J Appl Physiol. 1993;73:213-218; Soifer SJ, Morin FC III, Kaslow DC, et al. The developmental effects of prostaglandin D2 on the pulmonary and systemic circulations in the newborn lamb. J Dev Physiol. 1983;5:237-250.)

perinatal pulmonary circulation reflects a balance between factors producing pulmonary vasoconstriction (low O_2, leukotrienes, and other vasoconstricting substances) and those producing pulmonary vasodilatation (high O_2, PGI2, NO, and other vasodilating substances). The dramatic increase in pulmonary blood flow with the initiation of ventilation and oxygenation at birth reflects a shift from active pulmonary vasoconstriction in the fetus to active pulmonary vasodilatation in the newborn.

Failure of the pulmonary circulation to undergo this normal fall in pulmonary vascular resistance at birth (persistent pulmonary hypertension of the newborn) is associated with a variety of conditions including aspiration syndromes, sepsis, in-utero stress events, and certain congenital heart defects (eg, obstruction of pulmonary venous drainage, single ventricle with restrictive atrial septum).

Regulation of Postnatal Pulmonary Vascular Resistance

After the immediate postnatal state, the pulmonary circulation is maintained in a dilated, low-resistance state. Because the inflow pressure of the pulmonary circulation is quite low, there is a vertical gradation to the distribution of blood flow in the lung. Hydrostatic pressure must be adjusted for vertical height above the left atrium, both at the inflow and outflow of every alveolar capillary unit. For example, given a pulmonary artery mean pressure of 20 cm H_2O (zeroed at the level of the left atrium), an alveolar-capillary unit 12 cm above the left atrium will face an inflow pressure of only 8 cm H_2O. A left atrial pressure of 5 cm H_2O would generate no opposing outflow pressure to alveolar capillary units more than 5 cm above the left atrium. Critical closing pressure of postcapillary vessels would therefore set outflow pressure for a unit 10 cm above the left atrium. Were intrinsic vascular resistance identical throughout the lung, flow at any vertical height would be determined by hydrostatic driving pressure (inflow-outflow) and would be greatest at the base and least at the apex of the lung. West, Dollery, and Naimark reported that this phenomenon partitions the lung into three vertical regions (Fig. 26.10).[42] Zone I vessels are higher above the left atrium than pulmonary artery pressure (expressed in cm H_2O) and are not perfused by the pulmonary artery. Zone II vessels lie above the height defined by the hydrostatic left atrial pressure but below the height of pulmonary artery pressure. These units are perfused in proportion to the driving pressure across them, which is approximately pulmonary artery pressure less vertical height (or critical closing pressure, whichever is higher). Zone III vessels lie at a vertical height less than outflow pressure expressed in cm H_2O. Driving pressure across these units is independent of height because inflow and outflow pressures are comparably influenced by gravity. Of note, in a supine neonate, there is likely no Zone I.

Small pulmonary arteries course along with the branching airways, and small pulmonary vessels are intimately related with alveoli. Therefore airway pressure can directly modulate pulmonary blood flow.[43] Alveolar pressure can be loosely translated into surrounding pressure for alveolar vessels. Positive airway pressure applied to the lung can impinge on alveolar vessels whenever alveolar pressure exceeds the other determinants of outflow pressure. During positive pressure ventilation, outflow pressure of the pulmonary circulation may be determined predominantly by the mechanics of ventilation. The lung is partitioned into zones, but the distri-

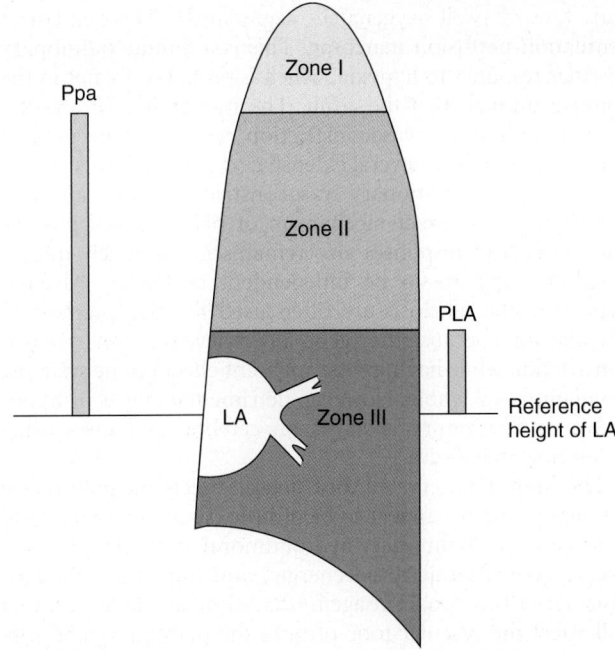

Fig. 26.10. The lung is divided vertically into three regions. Zone I alveolar capillary units are unperfused because they see no functional inflow pressure. Zone II units are perfused in proportion to their height above the left atrium (LA). Zone III vasculature is more uniformly perfused because gravity has comparable effects on inflow and outflow pressures. (Redrawn from Fuhrman BP. Regional circulation. In: Fuhrman BP, Shoemaker WC, eds. Critical Care: State of the Art, vol 10. Fullerton, CA: Society of Critical Care Medicine; 1989.)

bution of flow becomes a complex function of alveolar pressure, as well as left atrial and critical closing pressures.

To further complicate this view of the pulmonary circulation, lung volume and alveolar pressure both change during positive pressure ventilation. During inspiration, extra-alveolar vessels are dilated by radial traction, reducing their resistance to flow, whereas alveolar vessels narrow and elongate.[44] During lung inflation, alveolar surface tension rises, diminishing the transmission of alveolar pressure to alveolar vessels. There is also evidence that, in the infant lamb, lung stretch may directly augment pulmonary vascular tone in a manner that is dependent on calcium flux and subject to calcium channel blockade using verapamil. In fact, it is clear that mechanical ventilation can have profound direct effects on the intact pulmonary circulation that depends on the waveform of airway pressure applied, not on mean airway pressure alone.

In heterogeneous lung disease, the application of positive airway pressure can modulate and redistribute blood flow away from ventilated and toward unventilated regions of the lung by directly increasing the pulmonary vascular resistance of lung segments exposed to elevated airway pressure, that is, segments not protected by consolidation or airway obstruction.[44]

Two of the most important factors affecting pulmonary vascular resistance in the postnatal period are oxygen concentration and pH. Decreasing oxygen tension or pH elicit pulmonary vasoconstriction of the resting pulmonary circulation.[45] Alveolar hypoxia constricts pulmonary arterioles, diverting blood flow away from hypoxic lung segments and toward well-oxygenated segments.[46] This enhances ventilation-perfusion matching. This is a unique pulmonary vascular response to hypoxia, which is probably greater in the younger animal than the adult. The mechanism of alveolar hypoxic pulmonary vasoconstriction remains to be defined and is the subject of several extensive reviews. Acidosis potentiates hypoxic pulmonary vasoconstriction, and alkalosis reduces it.[45] The exact mechanism of pH-mediated pulmonary vasoactive responses also remains incompletely understood but appears to be independent of $PaCO_2$. Alveolar hyperoxia and alkalosis are often used to relax pulmonary vascular tone because they generally relieve pulmonary vasoconstriction while having little apparent effect on the systemic circulation as a whole. However, detrimental effects of hypocarbia or respiratory alkalosis on cerebral and myocardial blood flow may occur.

The lung is innervated, but neural effects on pulmonary vascular resistance appear to be of little consequence on basal tone. However, pulmonary neurohumoral receptors are sensitive to α-adrenergic, β-adrenergic, and dopaminergic agonists. Therefore vasoactive agents that stimulate these receptors will affect the vascular tone of both the pulmonary and systemic circulations. The degree of pulmonary to systemic alterations induced by these agents is variable and often dictated by the relative tone of each vascular bed. Therefore the response of these agents is difficult to predict in an individual critically ill patient.

A selective pulmonary vasodilator was long sought for treatment of pulmonary hypertension because, with the exception of oxygen, the response of the pulmonary circulation to humoral vasoactive agents is generally similar to that of the systemic circulation. To date, inhaled NO is the most commonly used agent for selective pulmonary vascular dilation. It is noteworthy that its selectivity is not based on a differential effect in the pulmonary and systemic circulations. Rather, when delivered as an inhaled gas, NO is rapidly bound to hemoglobin and inactivated, thus limiting its effects to the pulmonary circulation. Inhaled prostacyclin is another agent that offers relative pulmonary vascular selectivity due to its rapid metabolism.[47]

Cerebral Circulation

The brain makes up 2% of body mass, receiving approximately 14% of the cardiac output while accounting for close to 20% of the body's O_2 consumption in adults, up to 30% of cardiac output, 50% or more of total oxygen usage, and up to 98% usage of produced hepatic glucose in neonates. Other organ systems receive a larger percentage of the total cardiac output (eg, the lung) and use greater amounts of oxygen (eg, skeletal muscle), but the brain is unique in its intolerance for diminished blood flow. In fact, although some favorable outcomes have been reported, severe, if not irreversible, damage occurs often after just minutes of circulatory arrest under normal conditions.[48]

The cranium has three compartments: tissue, cerebral spinal fluid (CSF), and blood. The Monro-Kellie doctrine states that these compartments occupy a relatively fixed space and that an increase in one compartment can only occur at the expense of another. For example, with brain swelling, CSF and cerebral venous blood must be displaced if intracranial pressure (ICP) is to remain unchanged. As the limits of CSF and blood evacuation are approached, ICP rises. Raised ICP

and/or venous obstruction can impede cerebral blood flow (CBF). Cerebral perfusion pressure (CPP), defined as the difference between the mean arterial pressure and the ICP, is thus a more accurate descriptor of cerebral inflow pressure. CBF will decline when the CPP falls below the lower limit of the autoregulatory curve. In the setting of raised ICP this will occur even in the face of elevated systemic arterial pressures.

At rest, cerebral oxygen consumption is surprisingly high. Glucose is the primary energy substrate, although ketones can be used during periods of starvation. The brain has no functional capacity to store energy and thus is completely dependent on a steady supply of O_2 as up to 92% of its ATP production results from the oxidative metabolism of glucose.[48]

An important feature unique to the cerebral circulation is the presence of a blood-brain barrier (BBB). The vascular endothelium of brain capillaries forms a continuous sheet, with adjacent cells joined by tight junctions. Unlike the endothelium of non-neural capillaries, there are no intercellular clefts through which water-soluble particles can traverse and there is markedly diminished pinocytosis. Lipid-soluble substances, CO_2, and O_2, however, can freely diffuse across the endothelium. Metabolically important components, such as glucose, lactate, and amino acids, depend on specific carrier proteins to facilitate their diffusion into the brain. Furthermore, the BBB has a biochemical component, with high levels of degradative enzymes that protect the vascular smooth muscle and extracellular fluid from the effects of circulating vasoactive substances, such as catecholamines. Thus as a result of the BBB, the cerebral vasculature responds differently from other vascular beds to humoral stimuli. However, humoral stimuli can significantly alter the vascular tone of large cerebral arteries and can affect blood flow to parts of the brain that lack a complete BBB, such as the choroid plexus, median eminence, and area postrema.[49]

It has been recognized for nearly 80 years that CBF remains constant over a wide range of mean systemic arterial pressures (Fig. 26.11).[50] Constant CBF is maintained in the face of increasing inflow pressures by compensatory vasoconstriction. Conversely, in the setting of low systemic arterial pressures (ie, low inflow pressures) the cerebral vasculature dilates in order to maintain steady CBF. At systemic arterial pressures outside the autoregulatory range, further dilation or constriction can no longer maintain blood flow. At high pressures, disruption of the BBB ensues with subsequent edema and even hemorrhage from ruptured cerebral vessels. At low pressures, CBF begins to fall with continued decreases leading to ischemia and ultimately brain death.[51] Importantly, normal cerebral autoregulation can be impaired in the setting of disease. Traumatic brain injury, subarachnoid hemorrhage, and stroke, for example, can all abolish or impair the normal autoregulatory response.[52,53]

The brain's ability to autoregulate flow is well established, but the mechanisms underlying it are not completely understood. A myogenic response appears to be especially important in the setting of raised CPP. Large- and medium-sized cerebral arteries, including the ICA, have been shown to constrict both in vitro and in vivo in response to elevated transmural pressures. Although small arteries and arterioles primarily modulate cerebral resistance during normotension, at higher pressures the large cranial vessels dominate. Thus at high perfusion pressures, smaller, more delicate vessels are protected by changes in upstream resistance.

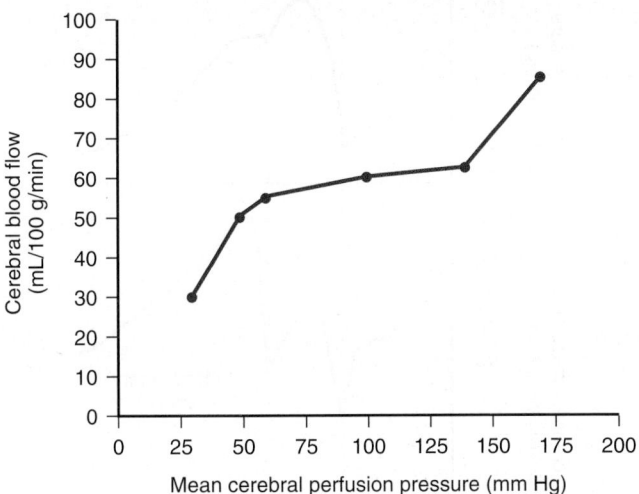

AUTOREGULATION OF CEREBRAL BLOOD FLOW

Fig. 26.11. Cerebral blood flow (CBF) autoregulates at perfusion pressures between 50 and 160 mm Hg. Below 50 mm Hg, CBF falls. Above 160 mm Hg, CBF rises. (Redrawn from Fuhrman BP. Regional circulation. In: Fuhrman BP, Shoemaker WC, eds. Critical Care: State of the Art, vol 10. Fullerton, CA: Society of Critical Care Medicine; 1989.)

In marked contrast to other vascular beds, neural stimuli have relatively little effect on basal CBF. Cerebral vessels display extensive perivascular innervation, especially by the sympathetic nerves arising from the superior cervical sympathetic ganglia, but the brain is well protected from circulating catecholamines by the BBB. Thus many of the vasoactive agents used in the critical care setting (α- and β-adrenergic agonists) have minimal effects of resting cerebral vascular tone. Mild to moderate electrical stimulation, as well as surgical resection of both the sympathetic and parasympathetic nervous systems, does not alter cerebral vascular tone under resting conditions. However, vigorous sympathetic stimulation, as would occur with strenuous exercise or hypertension, does result in vasoconstriction of large- and medium-sized cerebral vessels. Thus while a neurogenic mechanism may not mediate cerebral vascular resistance under normal conditions, it does provide protection during times of stress.[54] Indeed, patients with chronic hypertension have been shown to have a rightward shift of the autoregulatory curve.

As in other vascular beds, it appears that CBF is coupled to changes in metabolism.[55] For example, hypothermia decreases the cerebral metabolic rate of oxygen ($CMRO_2$), and therefore CBF, in both animal and human studies.[56-58] Seizure activity and fever both increase the $CMRO_2$ and CBF, which explains the deleterious consequences of both conditions for patients with raised ICP.[59] The mechanisms underlying this coupling of blood flow and metabolism are still unclear. A number of substances have been shown to affect cerebrovascular tone. These include carbon dioxide, oxygen, hydrogen ions, lactic acid, histamine, potassium ions, prostaglandin, ET-1, NO, and adenosine.

Carbon dioxide plays a critical role in the regulation of CBF. In fact, a linear increase in CBF is seen with increasing $PaCO_2$, making CO_2 one of the most potent known cerebral vasodilators.[60] Carbon dioxide exerts its effect via a reduction of the perivascular pH. Whereas arterial H+ cannot cross the BBB,

CO_2 can easily diffuse into the brain. Carbonic anhydrase facilitates the reaction between CO_2 and H_2O forming carbonic acid with subsequent dissociation producing H+ ions. Perivascular acidosis dilates the cerebral vasculature, while alkalosis leads to vasoconstriction.[61] In this way the cerebral vasculature is distinct in that respiratory acidosis and alkalosis will alter tone and CBF, while metabolic acidosis and alkalosis will not.[60,62] Interestingly, abnormal CO_2 reactivity has been associated with several disease processes, including traumatic brain injury, subarachnoid hemorrhage, stroke, carotid stenosis, and congestive heart failure.[52,53] Indeed, abnormal CO_2 vasoreactivity has been used as a means to prognosticate in some disease states.[53] Several studies have demonstrated that the cerebral vasculature adapts in the setting of chronically elevated $PaCO_2$ with changes in the pH of the brain extracellular fluid. This has obvious implications for the clinician attempting to treat raised ICP with chronic hyperventilation.

Arterial oxygen tension (PaO_2) also participates in the regulation of CBF. Arterial hypoxia dilates cerebral vessels at PaO_2 below 40 to 50 mm Hg. The relation between cerebral blood flow and arterial oxygen content is almost linear, and cerebral oxygen delivery can be maintained unless arterial oxygen content falls below 4 vol%. Hyperoxia does not appear to be a potent stimulus for vasoconstriction, however. The mechanisms of hypoxic vasodilation are not completely understood, but it is known that adenosine and both Ca2+-activated and ATP-activated potassium channels are particularly important. Adenosine, which leads to vasodilation through an increase in cAMP, has been found to increase by more than fivefold with hypoxia.[63]

A large body of evidence, both in animals and humans, implicates NO in a number of important processes within the cerebral circulation.[64-66] Vasodilation in response to acetylcholine, oxytocin, substance P, histamine, ET-1, ADP, ATP, and prostaglandin has all been shown to be NO dependent. Clinically, it is noteworthy that nitroprusside and other NO-donor compounds can dilate cerebral vessels.[67] This greatly complicates the management of hypertension in patients with increased intracranial pressure. In that setting, nitroprusside, for example, may reduce arterial pressure but raise both cerebral blood flow and blood volume, thereby causing herniation to occur. In addition, impaired NO signaling is important in the pathophysiology of subarachnoid hemorrhage where endothelial dysfunction has been well documented, leading to the important clinical problem of vasospasm.

ET-1 also mediates cerebrovascular tone.[68] Both ETA and ETB receptors have been identified in the cerebral vasculature. When given in high concentrations, ET-1 constricts cerebral vessels, probably via ETA receptor activation. In low concentrations, however, ET-1 relaxes cerebral vessels via endothelial cell ETB receptor activation, a response that is NO dependent. Sarafotoxin 6c (a selective ETB agonist) causes cerebral vasodilation. However, ETA and combined receptor antagonists do not alter basal cerebrovascular tone. Recently, ET-1 has been identified as an important mediator of vasospasm following subarachnoid hemorrhage. ET-1 levels are increased following subarachnoid hemorrhage. Associated with this increase, ETA receptor levels, smooth muscle cell ETB receptor levels (which mediate vasoconstriction), and endothelin-converting enzyme activity are increased. The potential clinical use of ET receptor antagonists following subarachnoid hemorrhage is under investigation, with promising preliminary results.[16]

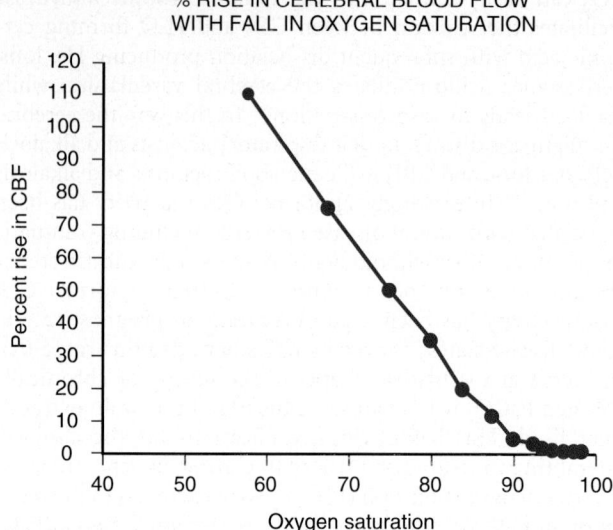

Fig. 26.12. Arterial hypoxia dilates cerebral vessels and maintains cerebral oxygen delivery. *CBF,* cerebral blood flow. (Redrawn from Fuhrman BP. Regional circulation. In: Fuhrman BP, Shoemaker WC, eds. Critical Care: State of the Art, vol 10. Fullerton, CA: Society of Critical Care Medicine; 1989.)

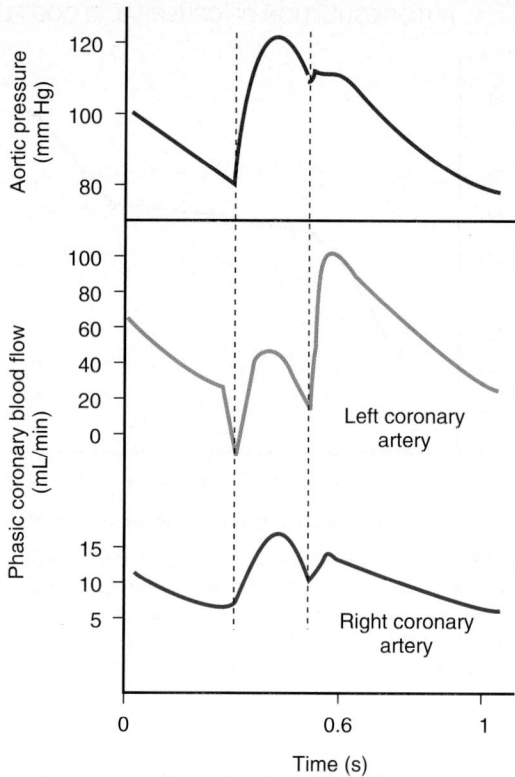

Fig. 26.13. Myocardial blood flow is modulated by ventricular wall tension. Most of the perfusion of the left ventricular myocardium occurs in diastole. (Adapted from Berne RM, Levy MN. Cardiovascular Physiology. 7th ed. St. Louis: Mosby; 1997.)

Coronary Circulation

Right and left coronary arteries arise from sinuses of Valsalva and course over the surface of the heart. Nutrient branches penetrate the myocardium to supply both superficial (epicardial) and deep (subendocardial) layers of the muscle. Venous blood drains primarily to the coronary sinus, although some returns by way of anterior coronary veins to the right atrium or via sinusoids directly to the ventricles.

Myocardial workload (which sets myocardial oxygen demand) is determined by not only the needs of the heart but also the demands of the body. Furthermore, the heart is required to generate its own perfusion pressure. Regulation of myocardial perfusion is, accordingly, tailored to match regional myocardial oxygen supply to demand over the widest possible range of cardiac workload and under conditions fashioned not so much for maximal cardiac efficiency but rather for benefit of the body.

Myocardial perfusion over a cardiac cycle is approximately the same per gram of tissue in the outer (subepicardial), mid, and inner (subendocardial) layers of the left ventricle, but the dynamics during the cardiac cycle are complicated. At the end of diastole, when the ventricle is relaxed and tissue pressures are generally under 10 mm Hg in any layer of the left ventricle, pressures in the intramural arteries are similar to each other and to aortic pressure. At the beginning of systole, tissue pressure rises to equal intracavitary pressure in the subendocardium but then falls off linearly across the wall to about 10 mm Hg in the subepicardium. These pressures are for an instant added to those inside the vessels because the vessels walls are not rigid. As a result, intravascular pressures in subendocardial arteries exceed aortic pressures, but aortic pressures are higher than pressures in subepicardial arteries. These pressure gradients and the greater shortening of subendocardial than subepicardial muscle fibers during systole compress the subendocardial vessels and squeeze blood out of them both forward into the coronary sinus and backward toward

the epicardium. In fact, narrowing of the subendocardial vessels facilitates thickening and shortening of the myocytes.[69] This backflow enters the subepicardial arteries to supply their systolic flow. In systole, there is indeed some forward flow into the orifices of the coronary arteries, but this does not perfuse the myocardium; it merely fills the extramyocardial arteries.[70] In fact, there is often reverse flow in the epicardial coronary arteries. In early diastole, blood flows first into the subepicardial vessels that have not been compressed but takes longer to refill the narrowed subendocardial vessels. Given enough time and perfusing pressure, all the myocardium will be perfused, but if diastole is too short or perfusion pressure too low, subendocardial ischemia occurs. Right ventricular myocardium, on the other hand, is normally perfused in both systole and diastole (Fig. 26.13) because of lower tissue pressures. We would expect perfusion of the hypertrophied right ventricle of severe pulmonic stenosis or tetralogy of Fallot to resemble that of the left ventricle.[71]

Myocardial Oxygen Demand-Supply Relationship

The left ventricle extracts most of the oxygen from the blood passing through the myocardium; coronary sinus oxygen saturation is normally about 30%. Therefore increases in myocardial oxygen demand have to be met by increases in myocardial blood flow. At rest, left ventricular myocardial blood flow is about 80 to 100 mL/100 g/min, and with maximal exertion, left ventricular oxygen consumption increases about fourfold, as does left ventricular blood flow in normal people and animals.[72] If coronary perfusion pressure does not change during exertion, the increased flow has to be achieved by a decrease in coronary vascular resistance; the response is termed *metabolic regulation*.

Coronary vascular resistance has three components: a basal low resistance in the arrested heart with maximally dilated vessels, an added resistance when vessels have tone, and a phasic resistance added whenever the ventricle contracts.[73] In the beating heart with vessels maximally dilated by a pharmacologic dilator, the second of these resistances is absent. Perfusion of the left ventricular myocardium then produces a steep pressure-flow relation that is linear at higher flows but usually curvilinear at low pressures and flows (Fig. 26.14A). Because the vessels are maximally dilated, flow is uncoupled from metabolism and depends only on driving pressure and resistance. If heart rate is increased, maximal flow at any perfusion pressure decreases because the heart is in a relaxed state for a smaller proportion of each minute.

If tone is allowed to return to the coronary vessels, then the pressure-flow relationship can be assessed at different perfusion pressures after cannulating the left coronary artery. It is necessary to do this because when cardiac metabolism and blood flow are coupled, increasing aortic blood pressure will increase coronary flow not only by increasing perfusion pressure but also by increasing myocardial oxygen demand. Under normal conditions coronary blood flow is autoregulated, such that if perfusion pressure is raised or lowered from its normal value, there is a range over which there is almost no change in flow; a rise in pressure has caused vasoconstriction, and a fall in pressure has caused vasodilatation. At perfusion pressures above some upper limit, flow increases, probably because the pressure overcomes the constriction. More importantly, at pressures below about 40 mm Hg (but varying, as discussed later) flow decreases predominantly in the deep subendocardial muscle (see Fig. 26.14A), indicating that some vessels have reached maximal vasodilatation and can no longer decrease resistance to compensate for the decreased perfusion pressure. In these vessels, flow and pressure are directly related. If this

pressure dependency occurs, then further decrease in perfusion pressure decreases local blood flow below its required amount, or if myocardial oxygen demands increase at the same low perfusion pressure (as will occur if the ventricle becomes dilated), the requisite increase in flow will not occur. These two conditions cause subendocardial ischemia.

At any given pressure, the difference between autoregulated and maximal flows is termed *coronary flow reserve*.[74-76] Coronary flow reserve can be measured in units of mL/min but can also be assessed by a dimensionless flow reserve ratio derived by dividing maximal flow by resting flow. Flow reserve depends on perfusion pressure because of the steepness of the pressure-flow relation in maximally dilated vessels. Coronary flow reserve indicates how much extra flow the myocardium can get at a given pressure to meet increased demands for oxygen; if reserve is much reduced, then flow cannot increase sufficiently to meet demands and myocardial ischemia will occur. What the figure does not show is that coronary flow reserve is normally lower in the subendocardium than in the subepicardium and that decreases in coronary flow reserve are always more profound in the subendocardium than in the subepicardium.

If autoregulated flow is normal but maximal flow is decreased, as indicated by the decreased slope of the pressure-flow relation during maximal dilatation (Fig. 26.14B), then coronary flow reserve will be reduced. Such a change can occur with marked tachycardia; a decrease in the number of coronary vessels due to small vessel disease, as in some collagen vascular diseases, especially systemic lupus erythematosus; increased resistance to flow in one or more large coronary vessels because of embolism, thrombosis, atheroma, or spasm; impaired myocardial relaxation due to ischemia; myocardial edema; a marked increase in left ventricular diastolic pressure; marked increase in left ventricular systolic pressure if coronary perfusion pressure is not also increased, as in aortic stenosis or incompetence; and an increase in blood viscosity, most commonly seen with hematocrits over 65%.

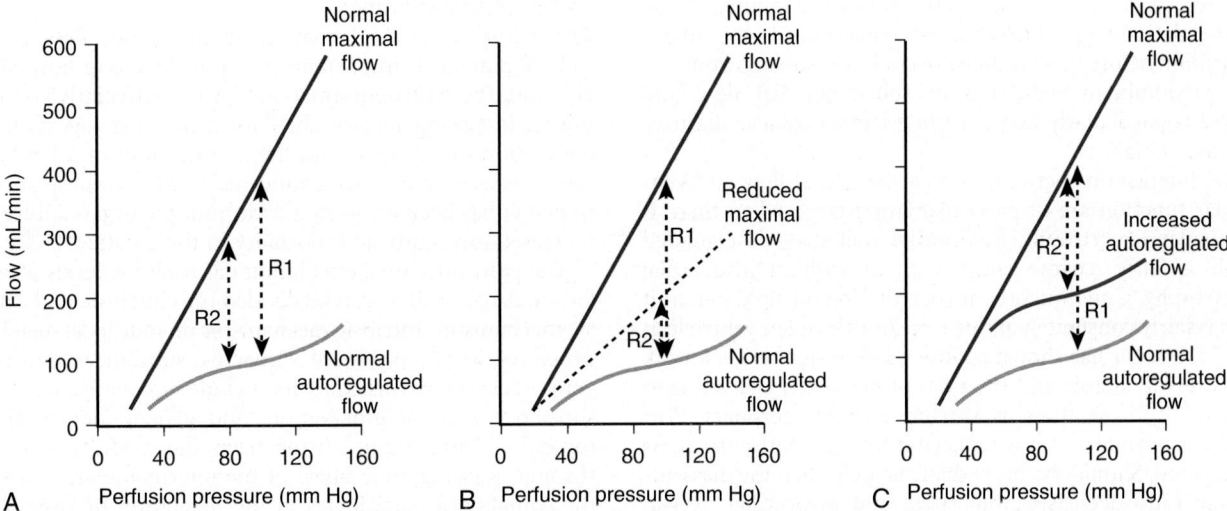

Fig. 26.14. (A) Normal pressure-flow relations in the left coronary artery during normal autoregulated flow and during maximal vasodilation. Values are appropriate for a left ventricle weighing approximately 100 g. R1, R2, coronary flow reserve measurements at two different coronary perfusing pressures. (B) Effect on coronary flow reserve of a reduced maximal flow. At the same coronary perfusing pressure, flow reserve is reduced from the normal R1 to R2. (C) Effect on coronary flow reserve of an increased autoregulated flow. Reserve is reduced from R1 to R2.

Coronary flow reserve can also be reduced if maximal flows are normal but autoregulated flows increase (Fig. 26.14C). Increased myocardial flows above normal values can occur with exercise, tachycardia, anemia, carbon monoxide poisoning, leftward shift of the hemoglobin oxygen dissociation curve (as in infants with a high proportion of fetal hemoglobin), hypoxemia, thyrotoxicosis, acute ventricular dilatation (because of increased wall stress), inotropic stimulation by catecholamines, and acquired ventricular hypertrophy. When hypertrophy occurs a few months after birth, ventricular muscle mass increases without a concomitant increase in conducting coronary blood vessels. Ventricular hypertrophy returns wall stress to normal, and myocardial flow per minute per gram of muscle is approximately normal. Therefore total left ventricular flow is increased in proportion to ventricular mass, but because maximal flow per ventricle is usually unchanged, the coronary flow reserve is diminished. Often autoregulated flow is increased and maximal flows are reduced at the same time (eg, with severe tachycardia or cyanotic heart disease with hypoxemia, ventricular hypertrophy, and polycythemia). Under these circumstances, coronary flow reserve can be drastically reduced. A third mechanism that reduces coronary flow reserve is a shift to the right of the pressure-flow line. If with maximally dilated vessels, diastolic coronary flow is measured at different mean diastolic perfusion pressures, a pressure-flow line is obtained that is linear at higher pressures but curved in the low pressure-flow region.[77,78] Zero flow occurs at a pressure of about 8 to 12 mm Hg; this is the critical closing pressure that is above right atrial pressure.[79,80] The whole pressure-flow line can be shifted to the right by several factors, most important of which are pericardial tamponade, a rise in right or left ventricular diastolic pressures, and α-adrenergic stimulation. Such a rightward shift decreases flow reserve (Fig. 26.14D). It is important to note that because the line of maximal pressure-flow relations slopes up and to the right, any decrease in that slope (Fig. 26.14B), any increase in autoregulated flow (Fig. 26.14C), or any rightward shift of the slope (Fig. 26.14D) raises the pressure at which autoregulation fails to compensate for decreased perfusing pressure. It is also important to reemphasize that any decrease in coronary flow reserve affects the subendocardium predominantly, so autoregulation will fail first and ischemia occur in the subendocardium before these changes occur in the subepicardium.[81] The predominant reduction in subendocardial flow and reserve is particularly marked when left ventricular diastolic pressure is high.

The interactions between myocardial blood flow and ventricular function are of particular importance when there is ventricular hypertrophy. Myocardial wall stress is regulated within a fairly narrow range, with or without myocardial hypertrophy. Consequently, myocardial blood flow per unit mass is fairly constant at about 1 mL/min/g of left ventricle at rest.[82-87] Strauer has shown a close relationship between peak wall stress in systole and the ratio of left ventricular mass to volume.[83,85,88,89] If there is no hypertrophy, coronary flow reserve is normal, but it is reduced if the left ventricular mass is increased. Should the heart dilate acutely, then the mass-to-volume ratio decreases, wall stress and myocardial oxygen consumption increase, and coronary flow reserve falls. If ventricular dilatation is marked, there can be subendocardial ischemia. Decreasing ventricular dilatation by afterload and preload reduction reverses these unfavorable events and is

another reason for the resulting improvement in ventricular function.

Right ventricular myocardial blood flow follows the general principles regarding coronary blood flow, but there are differences related to the low right ventricular systolic pressure and to the fact that alterations in aortic pressure change coronary perfusing pressure without altering right ventricular pressure work. If the normal right ventricle is acutely distended, for example, by pulmonary embolism, there will eventually be right ventricular failure; the increased wall stress increases its oxygen consumption, but the raised systolic pressure reduces the coronary flow, so when supply cannot match demand there will be right ventricular myocardial ischemia.[90] Raising aortic perfusing pressure mechanically or with α-adrenergic agonists increases right ventricular myocardial blood flow, relieves ischemia, and restores right ventricular function to normal. Improved coronary flow is not the only mechanism of this improvement; the increased left ventricular afterload moves the ventricular septum toward the right ventricle and improves left ventricular performance.[91] If right ventricular pressure is chronically elevated so that there is right ventricular hypertrophy, as in pulmonic stenosis, many forms of cyanotic congenital heart disease, and some chronic lung diseases, then right ventricular myocardial blood flow behaves in the same way as left ventricular blood flow, with one exception.[92-94] If aortic pressure is lowered, left ventricular pressure also decreases, as do left ventricular work and oxygen consumption. In the right ventricle, however, the workload may not be reduced (if there is no ventricular septal defect), so an imbalance between myocardial oxygen supply and demand may occur. The worst imbalance occurs when aortic systolic pressure is maintained but coronary perfusing pressure decreases, and this can occur in a child with tetralogy of Fallot who has too large an aortopulmonary anastomosis. The high aortic and left ventricular systolic pressures mandate an equally high right ventricular systolic pressure, but the low diastolic aortic pressure reduces coronary perfusion pressure in diastole and can cause both left and right ventricular ischemia and failure.[95]

Gastrointestinal Circulation

The maintenance of adequate splanchnic blood flow in critically ill patients is important. In a globally compromised circulation, the gastrointestinal system is particularly prone to injury, impairing its two chief functions: the digestion and absorption of nutrients and the maintenance of a barrier to the translocation of enteric antigens.[96-98] Moreover, splanchnic ischemia has been associated with multiple organ failure and increased morbidity and mortality in these patients.[99,100]

The gastrointestinal circulation has multiple levels of regulation. Broadly, these can be divided into intrinsic and extrinsic mechanisms. Intrinsic mechanisms include local metabolic processes, locally produced vasoactive substances, and myogenic reflexes. Extrinsic factors include circulating vasoactive substances, neural innervation, and general hemodynamic forces.[102] Neural input arising from the medulla oblongata through preganglionic fibers of the intermediolateral area of the spinal cord participates in the regulation of large blood vessels (>50 μm), largely through sympathetic α-adrenergic control. Blood flow to the intestinal circulation, like other vascular beds, is autoregulated such that oxygen delivery remains fairly constant with inflow pressures varying from 30 to 120 mm Hg.[102] Oxygen, carbon dioxide, H+ ions, and adenosine are important local metabolic mediators of this process. Other important vasoactive mediators of intestinal blood flow include serotonin, histamine, bradykinin, and prostaglandin, although their role in autoregulation is unclear.[103,104] Finally, various gastrointestinal hormones and peptides released from the intestinal mucosa and intestinal glands including gastrin, vasoactive intestinal polypeptide, cholecystokinin, secretin, glucagon, enkephalins, somatostatin, and kallidin are known to have vasoactive properties.[101]

A phenomenon unique to the gastrointestinal circulation is the increase in flow following the consumption of nutrients. This postprandial intestinal hyperemia appears to involve multiple factors. However, the composition of the chyme is particularly important. In fact, luminal distention, mechanical stimulation, and extrinsic neural stimulation are not necessary for the response to occur.[101] Lipids in combination with bile salts are the most potent triggers for postprandial hyperemia. Glucose is the most potent single stimulus for this response. Blood flow to skin and skeletal muscle decreases and cardiac output increases during postprandial hyperemia. Furthermore, nutrients that induce the largest increase in blood flow elicit the largest oxygen debt within the intestinal villi.

Interestingly, this postprandial hyperemia may be protective in some instances of low blood flow to the intestinal mucosa. Glucose has been shown to ameliorate mucosal ischemia in models of septic and hemorrhagic shock, and early enteral feeding has been advocated in human studies as well.[105] Conversely, enteral feeding has also been associated with bowel ischemia and injury in some patients, such as premature infants, thus complicating decisions around enteral feeding during or following low-flow states.[106]

Increasing data demonstrate a large role for NO in the regulation of gastrointestinal blood flow. NO, at least in part, mediates basal mesenteric and hepatic blood flow. Indeed, a number of studies implicate endothelial dysfunction, and aberrations in NO signaling in particular, in portal hypertension and cirrhosis.[107-109] NO also participates in the maintenance of the mucosal barrier function and is further protective by virtue of its inhibitory effect on platelet and leukocyte adhesion.[110] Furthermore, postprandial hyperemia has been shown to involve adenosine-mediated NO release.[111] Finally, neuronal NO synthase (nNOS) and inducible NO synthase (iNOS) are important in both normal and abnormal gastrointestinal motility and gastrointestinal inflammatory disorders, respectively.[112-114]

ET-1 is another important mediator of intestinal blood flow. The intestinal vasculature displays increased vasoconstriction in response to ET-1 compared with other vascular beds. This has particular importance for gastrointestinal blood flow in critically ill patients as ET-1 levels have been found to be elevated following surgery and in association with a number of disease states, including hypoxia, pancreatitis, and sepsis. ET receptor antagonism ameliorates ischemic injury to the bowel in several models of low-flow states.[115,116]

Finally, it should be remembered that drugs used to augment systolic blood pressure and/or to enhance cardiac output could have various effects on the gastrointestinal circulation. Fenoldopam, a dopamine-1 receptor agonist, has been shown to improve intestinal perfusion during hemorrhage.[117] Findings on more common agents such as norepinephrine, dopamine, and vasopressin, however, have had mixed results depending on the doses used and the models or clinical situations studied.[118-120] Thus investigations continue to target the determination of an optimum strategy to improve overall cardiac output and oxygen delivery without compromising flow to specific organs, such as the bowel.

Renal Circulation

Blood flow to the kidneys greatly exceeds the metabolic needs of the organs themselves. In a 70-kg adult, combined renal blood flow is approximately 1200 mL/min, accounting for just over 20% of total cardiac output supplying organs that represent under 0.5% of total body weight.[121] This high renal blood flow is necessary in order to support glomerular filtration, such that solute and fluid homeostasis can be maintained.

Blood is supplied to the kidneys by the renal arteries, which branch to form the interlobar, arcuate, and interlobular arteries. Interlobular arteries progress to form the afferent arterioles, which lead to the glomerular capillaries within the glomerulus, the site of fluid and solute filtration. The distal glomerular capillaries reform into the efferent arterioles, which then lead to a second capillary system, the peritubular capillaries. An elevated hydrostatic pressure within the glomerular capillaries supports filtration, whereas a much lower pressure within the peritubular capillary system supports absorption.[121] Alterations in the resistance of the afferent and efferent arterioles regulate these pressures and allow for dynamic changes in renal function in response to overall fluid and solute needs.

Renal blood flow is determined by the difference between renal artery pressure (which is generally equivalent to systemic arterial pressure) and renal vein pressure, over the renal vascular resistance. In general, three vascular segments limit renal vascular resistance: the interlobular arteries, afferent arterioles, and efferent arterioles. Regulation of renal vascular resistance can be broadly divided into extrinsic mechanisms and intrinsic mechanisms. Extrinsic mechanisms, which include the sympathoadrenal system, atrial natriuretic system, and renin-angiotensin-aldosterone axis, modulate renal blood flow by alterations in intrarenal vascular tone, mesangial tone, intravascular volume, and systemic vascular resistance.[121] Intrinsic mechanisms, which primarily alter afferent arteriolar resistance, are responsible for the autoregulation of renal blood flow in response to changes in renal perfusion pressure.

The juxtaglomerular apparatus, which includes the afferent and efferent arterioles, macula densa, and glomerular mesangium, is an important site in the regulation of renal perfusion and glomerular filtration. Glomerular filtration is largely a function of glomerular filtration pressure, which in turn is dependent on renal perfusion pressure and, importantly, the balance between afferent arteriolar and efferent arteriolar tone. Increased efferent arteriolar tone increases glomerular filtration by increasing glomerular pressure, whereas increased afferent arteriolar tone has the opposite effect.

Endogenous epinephrine and norepinephrine derived from sympathetic neural input have various effects on renal perfusion and glomerular filtration. Mild sympathetic output preferentially constricts the efferent arterioles, thereby increasing glomerular pressure and filtration.[122] However, intense sympathetic discharge results in afferent arteriolar constriction, which decreases glomerular filtration. Furthermore, sympathetic stimulation of afferent arterioles results in renin release, which leads to increased sodium reabsorption and fluid retention. Sympathetic stimulation can affect renal blood flow more generally by alterations in systemic arterial pressure. Indeed, clinically norepinephrine has been shown to increase renal perfusion and renal function (measured by changes in creatinine clearance) in patients with septic shock.

Angiotensin II, produced by cleavage of angiotensin I by the enzyme angiotensin-converting enzyme (ACE), also has important effects on renal perfusion. Like catecholamine stimulation, the effects of angiotensin II are dose related. At low levels, angiotensin II results in efferent arteriolar constriction, whereas at high levels both the afferent and efferent arterioles are constricted.[122] Angiotensin II alters renal blood flow further by alterations in intravascular volume through aldosterone and arginine vasopressin and by increasing systemic vascular resistance.

Arginine vasopressin (AVP) is synthesized in the anterior hypothalamus and released from the posterior pituitary gland. It plays a critical role in maintaining serum osmolality within a narrow range. Both V1 and V2 receptors have been identified. V2 receptors are located on the renal collecting ducts, and stimulation results in increased reabsorption of water. Activation of V1 receptors on systemic vessels results in vasoconstriction. Interestingly, V1 receptor activation in the pulmonary vasculature results in vasodilation, at least in part via NO production. Triggers for AVP release include changes in serum osmolality, hypovolemia, and hypotension. Patients with septic shock have been shown to have decreased levels of AVP, which has led to the use of AVP supplementation clinically. Unlike catecholamines and angiotensin II, high levels of AVP appear to preferentially constrict efferent arterioles, which preserves glomerular filtration.

ET-1 has diverse effects on the kidney.[123] In general, endothelin results in vasoconstriction, decreased renal perfusion, and decreased glomerular filtration. ET-1 constricts both the afferent and efferent arterioles. ET-1 has also been shown to stimulate cell proliferation within the kidney. Conversely, ET-1 may also promote natriuresis through ETB-receptor activation. Furthermore, alterations in ET-1 signaling have been implicated in a host of renal diseases including acute and chronic renal failure, essential hypertension, glomerulonephritis, renal fibrosis, and renal transplant rejection.[123]

Important vasodilators within the renal circulation include prostaglandins and atrial natriuretic peptide (ANP). The vasodilating prostaglandins (D2, E2, and I2) are synthesized from arachidonic acid by the enzyme phospholipase A2. Most of the important vasoconstricting factors, such as catecholamines, angiotensin II, and AVP, stimulate the release of prostaglandins, promoting increased renal perfusion and glomerular filtration. ANP is produced within the atrial myocytes and is released in response to increased atrial stretch. Through cGMP signaling, ANP results in afferent arteriolar dilation and increased renal perfusion and glomerular filtration. ANP also antagonizes the actions of endogenous catecholamines, angiotensin II, and AVP.

Like other organ systems, renal blood flow is autoregulated via mechanisms intrinsic to the renal vasculature.[121] Early studies demonstrate that renal blood flow and glomerular filtration remain constant at renal artery perfusion pressures of between 80 and 180 mm Hg.[124] Importantly, urinary flow rate is not constant within the autoregulatory range but rather changes as a function of renal perfusion pressure. The precise

mechanisms underpinning this autoregulation are unclear. However, recent evidence indicates that the mechanisms are likely complex involving interactions between tubuloglomerular feedback and myogenic processes that protect the kidney from damage in the setting of hypertension and also regulate renal function.[125-127]

A number of disease states that affect critically ill patients result in the loss of renal autoregulation. Acute tubular necrosis, septic shock, hepatic failure, and cardiopulmonary bypass have all been associated with renal dysfunction and a loss of renal autoregulation.

Conflicting Needs of Regional Circulations

The regional circulations maintain homeostasis independently and in concert. This is natural because individual organs have their own needs. Yet each region also has a responsibility to the body as a whole. There are times when individual need and responsibility conflict. Life-threatening illness accentuates these "conflicts of interest." An example follows:

The pulmonary and cerebral circulations respond differently to acute respiratory alkalosis. Alkalosis lowers pulmonary vascular resistance, but hypocarbia promotes vasoconstriction of the cerebral vasculature. The diametric behavior of these two circulations presents a challenge to clinicians managing patients following caval-pulmonary anastomosis for palliation of single ventricle congenital heart disease. With this anatomy, pulmonary blood flow is dependent on passive venous return (without a subpulmonary ventricle) from the superior vena cava (SVC). Pulmonary blood flow can be impaired if pulmonary vascular resistance increases. However, hyperventilation to decrease pulmonary vascular resistance actually decreases pulmonary blood flow if the resultant hypocarbia diminishes cerebral blood flow (due to cerebral vascular vasoconstriction) and SVC blood flow. This may result in a net decrease in pulmonary blood flow and desaturation.

It is possible that unsuccessful arbitration among regional circulations contributes to the genesis of the syndrome of multiple organ system failure (see Chapter 112). An increasing understanding of the mechanisms that regulate regional, microcirculatory blood flow will lead to new and improved treatments that optimize blood flow and allow the intensivist to successfully arbitrate the regional blood flow "conflict of interests" that will best serve the short- and long-term interests of the critically ill children.

Key References

1. Aird WC. Phenotypic heterogeneity of the endothelium: II. Representative vascular beds. *Circ Res*. 2007;100:174-190.
2. Aird WC. Phenotypic heterogeneity of the endothelium: I. Structure, function, and mechanisms. *Circ Res*. 2007;100:158-173.
3. Sylvester JT, Gilbert RD, Traystman RJ, Permutt S. Effects of hypoxia on the closing pressure of the canine systemic arterial circulation. *Circ Res*. 1981;49:980-987.
5. Stamler JS, Jia L, Eu JP, et al. Blood flow regulation by S-nitrosohemoglobin in the physiological oxygen gradient. *Science*. 1997;276:2034-2037.
7. Cannon RO 3rd, Schechter AN, Panza JA, et al. Effects of inhaled nitric oxide on regional blood flow are consistent with intravascular nitric oxide delivery. *J Clin Invest*. 2001;108:279-287.
8. Olson KR. Hydrogen sulfide and oxygen sensing in the cardiovascular system. *Antioxid Redox Signal*. 2009;12:1219-1234.

9. Chin BY, Otterbein LE. Carbon monoxide is a poison … to microbes! CO as a bactericidal molecule. *Curr Opin Pharmacol.* 2009;9:490-500.

10. Ryter SW, Alam J, Choi AM. Heme oxygenase-1/carbon monoxide: from basic science to therapeutic applications. *Physiol Rev.* 2006;86:583-650.

12. Cai H, Harrison DG. Endothelial dysfunction in cardiovascular diseases: the role of oxidant stress. *Circ Res.* 2000;87:840-844.

14. Moncada S, Higgs A. The L-arginine-nitric oxide pathway. *N Engl J Med.* 1993;329:2002-2012.

15. Humpl T, Reyes JT, Holtby H, et al. Beneficial effect of oral sildenafil therapy on childhood pulmonary arterial hypertension: twelve-month clinical trial of a single-drug, open-label, pilot study. *Circulation.* 2005;111:3274-3280.

16. MacDonald RL, Kassell NF, Mayer S, et al. Clazosentan to overcome neurological ischemia and infarction occurring after subarachnoid hemorrhage (CONSCIOUS-1): randomized, double-blind, placebo-controlled phase 2 dose-finding trial. *Stroke.* 2008;39:3015-3021.

17. Morris CR, Morris SM Jr, Hagar W, et al. Arginine therapy: a new treatment for pulmonary hypertension in sickle cell disease? *Am J Respir Crit Care Med.* 2003;168:63-69.

18. Rubin LJ, Badesch DB, Barst RJ, et al. Bosentan therapy for pulmonary arterial hypertension. *N Engl J Med.* 2002;346:896-903.

20. Roberts JD Jr, Fineman JR, Morin FC 3rd, et al. Inhaled nitric oxide and persistent pulmonary hypertension of the newborn. The Inhaled Nitric Oxide Study Group. *N Engl J Med.* 1997;336:605-610.

22. Otterbein LE. The evolution of carbon monoxide into medicine. *Respir Care.* 2009;54:925-932.

25. Vane JR, Anggard EE, Botting RM. Regulatory functions of the vascular endothelium. *N Engl J Med.* 1990;323:27-36.

27. Davis MJ, Hill MA. Signaling mechanisms underlying the vascular myogenic response. *Physiol Rev.* 1999;79:387-423.

30. Drummond HA, Grifoni SC, Jernigan NL. A new trick for an old dogma: ENaC proteins as mechanotransducers in vascular smooth muscle. *Physiology (Bethesda).* 2008;23:23-31.

31. Schubert R, Lidington D, Bolz SS. The emerging role of Ca2+ sensitivity regulation in promoting myogenic vasoconstriction. *Cardiovasc Res.* 2008;77:8-18.

36. Rudolph AM. Fetal and neonatal pulmonary circulation. *Annu Rev Physiol.* 1979;41:383-395.

42. West JB, Dollery CT, Naimark A. Distribution of blood flow in isolated lung; relation to vascular and alveolar pressures. *J Appl Physiol.* 1964;19:713-724.

43. Lopez-Muniz R, Stephens NL, Bromberger-Barnea B, et al. Critical closure of pulmonary vessels analyzed in terms of Starling resistor model. *J Appl Physiol.* 1968;24:625-635.

45. Rudolph AM, Yuan S. Response of the pulmonary vasculature to hypoxia and H+ ion concentration changes. *J Clin Invest.* 1966;45:399-411.

48. Vavilala MS, Lee LA, Lam AM. Cerebral blood flow and vascular physiology. *Anesthesiol Clin North America.* 2002;20:247-264.

49. Paulson OB. Blood-brain barrier, brain metabolism and cerebral blood flow. *Eur Neuropsychopharmacol.* 2002;12:495-501.

51. Panerai RB, Dawson SL, Eames PJ, Potter JF. Cerebral blood flow velocity response to induced and spontaneous sudden changes in arterial blood pressure. *Am J Physiol Heart Circ Physiol.* 2001;280:H2162-H2174.

55. Mintun MA, Lundstrom BN, Snyder AZ, et al. Blood flow and oxygen delivery to human brain during functional activity: theoretical modeling and experimental data. *Proc Natl Acad Sci U S A.* 2001;98:6859-6864.

56. Ehrlich MP, McCullough JN, Zhang N, et al. Effect of hypothermia on cerebral blood flow and metabolism in the pig. *Ann Thorac Surg.* 2002;73:191-197.

63. DiGeronimo RJ, Gegg CA, Zuckerman SL. Adenosine depletion alters postictal hypoxic cerebral vasodilation in the newborn pig. *Am J Physiol.* 1998;274:H1495-H1501.

65. Lavi S, Egbarya R, Lavi R, Jacob G. Role of nitric oxide in the regulation of cerebral blood flow in humans: chemoregulation versus mechano-regulation. *Circulation.* 2003;107:1901-1905.

69. Willemsen MJ, Duncker DJ, Krams R, et al. Decrease in coronary vascular volume in systole augments cardiac contraction. *Am J Physiol Heart Circ Physiol.* 2001;281:H731-H737.

74. Hoffman JIE. Maximal coronary flow and the concept of coronary vascular reserve. *Circulation.* 1984;70:153-159.

75. Hoffman JIE. A critical view of coronary reserve. *Circulation.* 1987;75(suppl I):6-11.

76. Hoffman JI. Problems of coronary flow reserve. *Ann Biomed Eng.* 2000;28:884-896.

78. Hoffman JIE, Spaan JAE. Pressure-flow relations in coronary circulation. *Physiol Rev.* 1990;70:331-390.

102. Matheson PJ, Wilson MA, Garrison RN. Regulation of intestinal blood flow. *J Surg Res.* 2000;93:182-196.

105. Revelly JP, Tappy L, Berger MM, et al. Early metabolic and splanchnic responses to enteral nutrition in postoperative cardiac surgery patients with circulatory compromise. *Intensive Care Med.* 2001;27:540-547.

107. Cahill P, Redmond E, Sitzmann JV. Endothelial dysfunction in cirrhosis and portal hypertension. *Pharmacol Ther.* 2001;89:273-293.

108. Pannen BH, Bauer M, Noldge-Schomburg GF, et al. Regulation of hepatic blood flow during resuscitation from hemorrhagic shock: role of NO and endothelins. *Am J Physiol.* 1997;272:H2736-H2745.

109. Clemens MG. Nitric oxide in liver injury. *Hepatology.* 1999;30:1-5.

117. Guzman JA, Rosado AE, Kruse JA. Dopamine-1 receptor stimulation attenuates the vasoconstrictive response to gut ischemia. *J Appl Physiol.* 2001;91:596-602.

118. Jakob SM, Ruokonen E, Takala J. Effects of dopamine on systemic and regional blood flow and metabolism in septic and cardiac surgery patients. *Shock.* 2002;18:8-13.

120. LeDoux D, Astiz ME, Carpati CM, Rackow EC. Effects of perfusion pressure on tissue perfusion in septic shock. *Crit Care Med.* 2000;28:2729-2732.

121. Dworkin LD, Sun AM, Brenner BM. The renal circulations. In: Brenner BM, ed. *The Kidney.* 6th ed. Philadelphia: WB Saunders Company; 2000:277-318.

123. Naicker S, Bhoola KD. Endothelins: vasoactive modulators of renal function in health and disease. *Pharmacol Ther.* 2001;90:61-88.

125. Bidani AK, Griffin KA, Williamson G, et al. Protective importance of the myogenic response in the renal circulation. *Hypertension.* 2009;54:393-398.

126. Cupples WA. Interactions contributing to kidney blood flow autoregulation. *Curr Opin Nephrol Hypertens.* 2007;16:39-45.

127. Loutzenhiser R, Griffin K, Williamson G, Bidani A. Renal autoregulation: new perspectives regarding the protective and regulatory roles of the underlying mechanisms. *Am J Physiol Regul Integr Comp Physiol.* 2006;290:R1153-R1167.

Endothelium and Endotheliopathy

Yves Ouellette

PEARLS

- Because of their location, endothelial cells have the ability to interact with blood components, such as flow, soluble factors, and other cells. Endothelial cells integrate these signals into a cohesive regulation of vascular responses.
- The endothelium controls the vascular tone of the underlying smooth muscle cells through the production of vasodilator and vasoconstrictor mediators.
- Endothelial cell activation in response to inflammation changes endothelial cellular physiology and alters vascular function.
- A large number of endothelial cell–active molecules are potential biomarkers for the early diagnosis of sepsis.

Until recently, scientists and clinicians considered the endothelium, the cell layer that lines the blood vessels, as an inert barrier separating the various components of blood and the surrounding tissues. The vascular endothelium is now recognized as a highly specialized and metabolically active organ performing a number of critical physiologic, immunologic, and synthetic functions. These functions include regulation of vascular permeability, fluid and solute exchange between the blood and interstitial space, vascular tone, cell adhesion, homeostasis, and vasculogenesis.[1]

The normal vascular endothelium is only one cell layer thick, separating the blood and vascular smooth muscle. The endothelium responds to physical and biochemical stimuli by releasing regulatory substances affecting vascular tone and growth, thrombosis and thrombolysis, and platelet and leukocyte interactions with the endothelium. Normal endothelial functions include control over thrombosis and thrombolysis, platelet and leukocyte interactions with the vessel wall, and regulation of vascular tone and growth. Of particular interest to intensivists is the fact that the endothelium secretes both powerful vasorelaxing (eg, nitric oxide [NO]) and vasoconstricting substances (eg, endothelin-1 [ET-1]). Because normal endothelial function plays a central role in vascular homeostasis, it is logical to conclude that endothelial dysfunction contributes to disease states characterized by vasomotor dysfunction, abnormal thrombosis, or abnormal vascular proliferation.

The endothelium lies between the lumen and the vascular smooth muscle, where it is uniquely positioned to "sense" changes in hemodynamic forces or blood-borne signals by membrane receptor mechanisms. The endothelial cells can respond to physical and chemical stimuli by synthesis or release of a variety of vasoactive and thromboregulatory molecules and growth factors.

The vascular endothelium possesses numerous enzymes, receptors, and transduction molecules, and it interacts with other vessel wall constituents and circulating blood cells. In addition to these universal functions, the endothelium may have organ-specific roles that are differentiated for various parts of the body, such as gas exchange in the lungs, control of myocardial function in the heart, or phagocytosis in the liver and spleen.

Normal Endothelial Function
Endothelial Cell Heterogeneity

Many vascular diseases appear to be restricted to specific vascular beds. For example, thrombotic events are often localized to single vessels. It is also common for certain vasculitides to specifically affect certain arteries, veins, or capillaries or to affect certain organs. Tumor cells often metastasize more commonly within particular vascular beds. The basis for this variability in vascular disease is poorly understood but may be explained by the heterogeneity of endothelial cells. There has been a greater understanding of how endothelial cell heterogeneity may contribute both to the maintenance of organ-specific function and to the development of disorders restricted to specific vascular beds.[1-3]

The morphologic appearance of capillary endothelium from different vascular beds may explain differences in tissue function. For example, the brain microcirculation is lined by endothelial cells connected by tight junctions that maintain the blood-brain barrier. By contrast, sinusoids found in the liver, spleen, and bone marrow are lined by endothelial cells that allow transcellular trafficking between intercellular gaps. Similarly, fenestrated endothelial cells found in the intestinal villi, endocrine glands, and kidneys facilitate selective permeability, which is required for efficient absorption, secretion, and filtering.[4]

Another example of endothelial cell heterogeneity lies in the expression of cell surface receptors involved in cell-to-cell signaling and cell trafficking. For example, in the mouse, lung-specific endothelial cell adhesion molecules are exclusively expressed by pulmonary postcapillary endothelial cells and some splenic venules. Similarly, specific mucosal cell adhesion molecules are expressed primarily on endothelial venules in the Peyer patches of the small intestine.[5,6] Tumor cells may show clear preferential adhesion to the endothelium of specific organs paralleling their in vivo metastatic propensities.[7] Distinct subsets of endothelial cells often exist within a single organ. During in situ studies, two distinct sinusoidal endothelial cell phenotypes can be recognized in the adult human liver: Hepatic periportal vessels express specific cell surface molecules such as PECAM-1 and CD34, whereas sinusoidal intrahepatic endothelial cells do not.

Endothelial Progenitor Cells

A significant amount of literature has shown that maintenance and repair of vasculature in ischemic diseases may be at least partially mediated through recruitment of endothelial progenitor cells (EPCs) from the bone marrow to areas of vascular injury.

An EPC is a specific subtype of hematopoietic stem cell that has been isolated from circulating mononuclear cells, bone marrow, and cord blood. EPCs migrate from the bone marrow to the peripheral circulation, where they contribute to vascular repair.[8,9] When injected into animal models of ischemia, EPCs are incorporated into sites of neovascularization[8,10,11] and have contributed to improved outcomes in patients with ischemic vascular disorders.[12] In addition, there has been accumulating evidence for the function of EPCs in critical illnesses such as sepsis.

Recruitment of EPCs to areas of endothelial and vascular damage may have prognostic implications and be associated with clinical outcome. The pathophysiologic changes associated with critical illness, notably sepsis and sepsis-related organ dysfunction, may lead to apoptosis and necrosis of endothelial cells from the vasculature and recruitment of EPCs from the bone marrow.

In various models of vascular injury and organ dysfunction, only a few studies have emerged regarding EPCs in particular as a therapeutic strategy. Transplanted EPCs have been shown to improve survival of mice following liver injury.[13] Infusion of EPCs also restored blood flow in a mouse model of hind limb ischemia.[9] A prospective randomized trial compared the effects of EPC transplantation in patients with idiopathic pulmonary arterial hypertension versus conventional therapy and showed that after 12 weeks, patients who had received EPCs had a significant improvement in their 6-minute walk test, mean pulmonary artery pressure, pulmonary vascular resistance, and cardiac output.[14]

Coagulation and Fibrinolysis

A normal physiologic function of the endothelium is to provide an antithrombotic surface inhibiting platelet adhesion and clotting, thus facilitating normal blood flow. Under pathophysiologic conditions, the endothelium transforms into a prothrombotic surface. A dynamic equilibrium exists between both states that permits a rapid response to an insult and a rapid recovery.[15]

Anticoagulant Mechanisms

The endothelium has anticoagulant, antiplatelet, and fibrinolytic properties.[16] Endothelial cells are the major sites for anticoagulant reactions involving thrombin. Thrombin plays a key role in coagulation, including the activation of platelets, activation of several coagulation enzymes and cofactors, and stimulation of procoagulation pathways on the endothelial cell surface. In the normal state, there is little thrombin enzyme activity. The surrounding endothelial cell matrix contains heparin sulfate and related glycosaminoglycans that activate antithrombin III. In addition, the subendothelial cell matrix

contains dermatan sulfate, which promotes the antithrombin activity of heparin cofactor II. Furthermore, microvascular endothelial cells release a tissue factor pathway inhibitor that inhibits the factor VIIa/tissue factor complex and further contributes to anticoagulation (Fig. 27.1).

Thrombin activity is also modulated by endothelial cell synthesis of thrombomodulin.[17,18] The binding of thrombin to thrombomodulin facilitates the enzyme's activation of the anticoagulant protein C. Activated protein C (APC) activity is enhanced by cofactor C, also called protein S, which is synthesized by endothelial cells as well as by other cells (see Fig. 27.1). APC inhibits factor Va and factor VIIIa. Thrombomodulin (TM) also inhibits prothrombinase activity indirectly by binding factor Xa (Fig. 27.2). Protein C has a special receptor on the endothelial cells: endothelial protein C receptor (EPCR). EPCR augments protein C activation approximately 20-fold in vivo by binding protein C and presenting it to the thrombin-TM activation complex. Both EPCR and TM can be found in plasma as soluble proteins. Activated protein C retains its ability to bind EPCR, and this complex appears to be involved in some of the cellular signaling mechanisms that down-regulate inflammatory cytokine formation (tumor necrosis factor, interleukin-6). In addition, platelet adhesion to endothelial cells is markedly inhibited by endothelium-derived prostacyclin.[19] The same stimuli that activate platelets, such as thrombin and adenosine diphosphate and adenosine triphosphate (ATP), also act to release prostacyclin from the endothelium, which allows the endothelium to limit the extent of platelet plug formation. The interactions between platelets and endothelium regulate platelet function, coagulation cascades, and local vascular tone.

Microvascular endothelial cells may secrete tissue-type plasminogen activator (t-PA), the powerful thrombolytic agent in frequent clinical use for treatment of coronary throm-

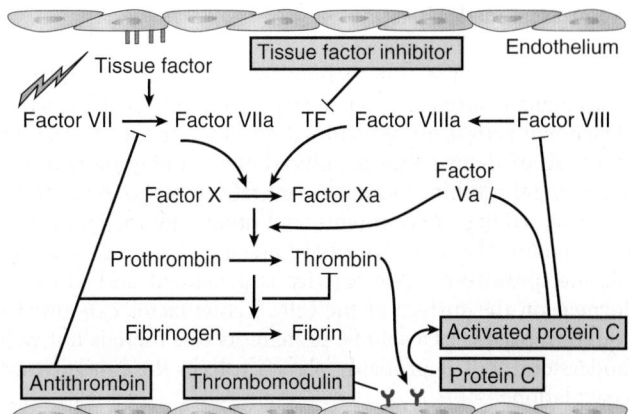

Fig. 27.1. Endothelium control of the coagulation cascade. An inflammatory stimulus up-regulates the interaction of tissue factor (TF) with factor VII, which generates activated factor VII (factor VIIa). The TF–factor VIIa complex then leads to the conversion of factor X to factor Xa. The interaction of factors Xa and Va results in the conversion of prothrombin to thrombin and the conversion of fibrinogen to fibrin. Three key anticoagulant pathways can inhibit this process. Protein C is activated through its interaction with cell-surface thrombomodulin and inhibits the activities of factors Va and VIIIa. Antithrombin blocks the activation of multiple factors including factor X and thrombin. Tissue factor pathway inhibitor interferes directly with the tissue factor–factor VIIa complex.

PROTEIN C PATHWAY

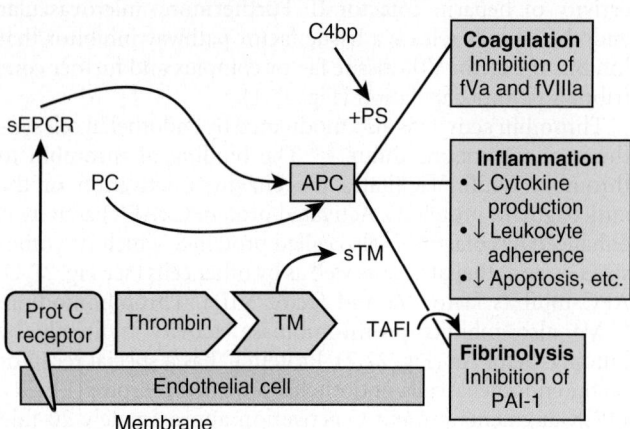

Fig. 27.2. The interaction of the protein C system with the endothelium: Thrombin bound to thrombomodulin (TM) modifies protein C bound to the endothelial protein C receptor on the cell surface to generate activated protein C (APC). APC acts as a natural anticoagulant by inactivating activated factors V (fVa) and VIII (fVIIIa), modulating inflammation by down-regulating the synthesis of proinflammatory cytokines, leukocyte adherence, and apoptosis and enhancing fibrinolysis by inhibiting thrombin-activatable fibrinolysis inhibitor (TAFI) and plasminogen activator inhibitor type-1 (PAI-1). *C4Bbp,* C4b binding protein (binds protein S); *+PS,* in the presence of protein S; *sEPCR,* soluble endothelial cell protein C receptor; *sTM,* soluble thrombomodulin. (Modified from Hazelzet J. Pathophysiology of pediatric sepsis. In: Nadel S. Infectious Diseases in the Pediatric Intensive Care Unit. London: Springer; 2008.)

botic occlusion.[20] t-PA release is stimulated in vivo by norepinephrine, vasopressin, or stasis within the vessel lumen. Thrombin may also stimulate t-PA release, providing a further endothelium-mediated safeguard against uncontrolled coagulation.

Procoagulant Mechanisms

The expression and release of tissue factor is the pivotal step in transforming the endothelium from an anticoagulant to a procoagulant surface.[21,22] Tissue factor accelerates factor VIIa-dependent activation of factors X and IX (see Fig. 27.1). The synthesis of tissue factor is induced by a number of agonists, including thrombin, endotoxin, several cytokines, shear stress, hypoxia, oxidized lipoproteins, and other endothelial insults. Once endothelial cells expressing tissue factor are exposed to plasma, prothrombinase activity is generated and fibrin is formed on the surface of the cells. Tissue factor can also be found in plasma as a soluble protein. Its role there is not well understood, but it probably plays a role in the initiation of coagulation.

Endothelium-Derived Vasodilators

The important role that the endothelium plays in controlling vascular tone has only recently been appreciated. Clinicians and researchers have come to appreciate that the endothelium controls underlying smooth muscle tone in response to certain pharmacologic and physiologic stimuli. This response involves a number of luminal membrane receptors and complex intracellular pathways and the synthesis and release of a variety of relaxing and constricting substances, described in the following sections.

Nitric Oxide

Furchgott and Zawadzki first postulated the existence of an endothelial-derived relaxing factor (EDRF) in 1980, when they noticed that the presence of endothelium was essential for rabbit aortic rings to relax in response to acetylcholine.[21] Later it was determined that the biological effects of EDRF are mediated by NO.[23]

NO is generated from the conversion of L-arginine to NO and L-citrulline by the enzyme nitric oxide synthase (NOS).[24] There are two general forms of NOS: constitutive and inducible. In the unstimulated state, NO is continuously produced by constitutive NO synthase (cNOS). The activity of cNOS is modulated by calcium that is released from endoplasmic stores in response to the activation of certain receptors. Substances such as acetylcholine, bradykinin, histamine, insulin, and substance P stimulate NO production through this mechanism. Similarly, shearing forces acting on the endothelium are another important mechanism regulating the release of NO. The inducible form of NOS (iNOS) is not calcium dependent but instead is stimulated by the actions of cytokines (eg, tumor necrosis factor-α [TNFα], interleukins) or bacterial endotoxins (eg, lipopolysaccharide). Induction of iNOS occurs over several hours and results in NO production that may be more than a thousandfold greater than that produced by cNOS. This is an important mechanism in the pathogenesis of inflammation (see Fig. 27.2). Inhibition of NOS using competitive analogs of L-arginine drastically reduces endothelium-dependent relaxation in vitro, particularly in large conduit arteries, thereby evoking vasoconstriction. Chronic treatment of animals with NOS inhibitors or suppression of the cNOS gene is reported to induce hypertension.[25-27]

Once NO is formed by an endothelial cell, it readily diffuses out of the cell and into adjacent smooth muscle cells where it binds and activates the soluble form of guanylyl cyclase, resulting in the production of cyclic guanosine-monophosphate (cGMP) from guanosine-triphosphate.[28] cGMP in turn activates a number of cGMP-modulated enzymes (Fig. 27.3). Increased cGMP activates a kinase that subsequently leads to the inhibition of calcium influx into the smooth muscle cell and decreased calcium-calmodulin stimulation of myosin light chain kinase. This, in turn, decreases the phosphorylation of myosin light chains, thereby decreasing smooth muscle tension development and causing vasodilation. There is also some evidence that increases in cGMP can lead to myosin light chain dephosphorylation by activating the phosphatase. In addition, cGMP-dependent protein kinase phosphorylates K$^+$ channels to induce hyperpolarization and thereby inhibits vasoconstriction.[29,30] Interestingly, NO inhibition of platelet aggregation is also related to the increase in cGMP. Drugs that inhibit the breakdown of cGMP such as inhibitors of cGMP-dependent phosphodiesterase (eg, sildenafil) potentiate the effects of NO-mediated actions on the target cell.

NO therefore contributes to the balance between vasodilator and vasoconstrictor influences that determine vascular tone.[31]

Prostacyclin

Another major endothelium-derived vasodilator is the prostaglandin prostacyclin (PGI$_2$), a derivative of arachidonic acid synthesized through the action of the enzyme cyclooxygenase. Endothelium cells are capable of producing a variety of

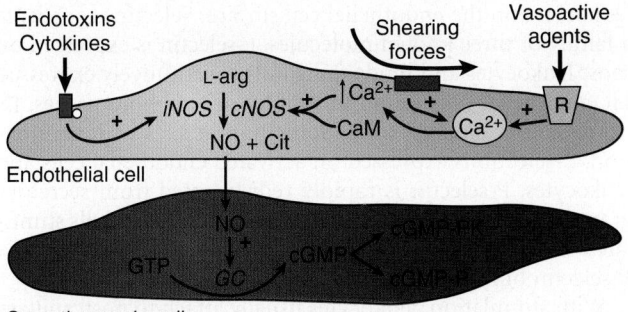

Fig. 27.3. Nitric oxide (NO) is generated from L-arginine (L-arg) by the action of nitric oxide synthase (NOS). In the resting state, constitutive NOS (cNOS) is modulated by intracellular Ca^{2+} and calmodulin (CaM). Stored Ca^{2+} is released in response to vasoactive agents (acetylcholine and bradykinin, for example) and other external stimuli such as shearing forces. Activation of endothelial cells by cytokines and endotoxins increases expression of inducible NOS (iNOS). Citrulline (Cit) is a byproduct of NO production. NO has a half-life of only a few seconds in vivo and quickly diffuses to surrounding cells such as smooth muscle cells. NO stimulates the production of the intracellular mediator cyclic GMP (cGMP). Increased cGMP activates a series of cGMP-dependent protein kinases (cGMP-PKs) and cGMP-dependent phosphatases (cGMP-Ps).

vasoactive substances that are products of arachidonic acid metabolism. Among these are prostaglandins, PGI₂, leukotrienes, and thromboxanes. These substances act as either vasodilators or vasoconstrictors, among their other biological activities. PGI₂ is a potent vasodilator and is active in both the pulmonary and systemic circulations. In addition to its vasodilatory effects, prostacyclin also has antithrombotic and antiplatelet activity. Its release may be stimulated by bradykinin and adenine nucleotides. Like NO, it is chemically unstable with a short half-life.[32] However, unlike NO, PGI₂ activity in arterial beds depends on its ability to bind to specific receptors in vascular smooth muscle. Its vasodilator activity is therefore determined by the expression of such receptors. PGI₂ receptors are coupled to adenylate cyclase to elevate cyclic AMP levels in vascular smooth muscle.[33] The increase in cAMP results in (1) stimulation of ATP-sensitive K^+ channels resulting in hyperpolarization of the cell membrane and inhibition of the development of contraction and (2) increased efflux of Ca^{2+} from the smooth muscle cell and inhibition of the contractile machinery.

In addition, PGI₂ facilitates the release of NO by endothelial cells, and NO potentiates the action of PGI₂ in vascular smooth muscle. Interestingly, NO may also potentiate the effects of prostacyclin. The NO-mediated increase in cGMP in smooth muscle cells inhibits a phosphodiesterase that breaks down cAMP and therefore indirectly prolongs the half-life of the second messenger of PGI₂.[34]

Endothelium-Derived Hyperpolarizing Factor

Endothelium stimulation by acetylcholine also produces hyperpolarization of the underlying smooth muscle and thereby induces vasorelaxation. This process is not mediated by NO but is instead mediated by another endothelium-derived factor. This factor increases K^+-channel conductance in smooth muscle cells, resulting in smooth muscle cell relaxation. The resulting vasodilation is not inhibited by L-NMMA,

the specific antagonist of NO, but is inhibited by ouabain, a Na^+/K^+-ATPase inhibitor. In addition, in most medium- to resistance-sized arteries, electrophysiologic studies have established that endothelium-dependent hyperpolarization of vascular smooth muscle is resistant to the combined inhibition of both NOs and cyclooxygenases. Accordingly, a component of the endothelium-dependent relaxation in these arteries is mediated by a substance different from NO and PGI₂. This component of endothelium-dependent vasodilatation has been attributed to a yet unidentified diffusible endothelium-derived hyperpolarizing factor (EDHF).[35]

Of significant clinical importance is the fact that EDHF-mediated effect increases as the arterial diameter decreases, such as in resistance arteries. EDHF likely plays a significant role in the regulation of peripheral vascular resistance and local hemodynamics. Unfortunately, in the absence of selective inhibitors of the EDHF pathway, it is not possible to evaluate the relevance of EDHF in vivo.[35]

Endothelium-Derived Vasoconstrictors

Endothelins (Endothelium-Derived Contracting Factors)

Endothelin is a 21-amino-acid peptide and is one of the most potent vasoconstrictors yet identified. Endothelial cells synthesize the prohormone big endothelin and express endothelin-converting enzymes to generate endothelin. There are three isoforms of endothelin, but only one (ET-1) has been shown to be released from human endothelial cells. ET-1 is synthesized in the endothelial cells and its release is mediated by a variety of stimuli. ET-1 release is stimulated by angiotensin II, antidiuretic hormone, thrombin, cytokines, reactive oxygen species, and shearing forces acting on the vascular endothelium. ET-1 release is inhibited by nitric oxide as well as by PGI₂ and atrial natriuretic peptide.[36,37]

ET-1 has a short half-life, suggesting that similarly to NO, ET-1 is mainly a locally active vasoregulator. Once released by endothelial cells, ET-1 binds to a membrane receptor (ET_A) found on adjacent vascular smooth muscle cells. This binding leads to calcium mobilization and smooth muscle contraction. The ET_A receptor is coupled with a G-protein linked to phospholipase-C, resulting in the formation of IP₃. Interestingly, ET-1 can also bind to an ET_B receptor located on the vascular endothelium, which stimulates the formation of NO by the endothelium. This release of NO appears to modulate the ET_A receptor-mediated contraction of the vascular smooth muscle. Its physiologic role includes maintenance of basal vascular resistance, and it is present in healthy subjects in low concentrations.

Reactive Oxygen Species

Endothelial cells secrete oxygen-derived free radicals and hydrogen peroxide in response to shear stress and endothelial agonists like bradykinin. Such reactive oxygen species are reported to inactivate NO, resulting in vasoconstriction. Reactive oxygen species may also facilitate the mobilization of cytosolic Ca^{2+} in vascular smooth muscle cells and promote Ca^{2+} sensitization of the contractile elements. Under conditions of hyperoxia, endothelium-derived superoxide anion may combine with NO with diffusion-limited kinetics to generate peroxynitrite, negating NO-mediated vasodilation, an effect inhibited by superoxide dismutase, which metabolizes superoxide anion to hydrogen peroxide.[38]

Vasoconstrictor Prostaglandins

The metabolism of arachidonic acid by cyclooxygenase in endothelial cells may lead to the secretion of precursors of thromboxanes and leukotrienes. These prostaglandins act on receptors in vascular smooth muscle to induce vasoconstriction. PGI_2, however, is the major endothelial metabolite of arachidonic acid that is generated through the cyclooxygenase pathway. Thus under normal circumstances, the influence of the small amounts of vasoconstrictor prostanoids released by endothelial cells is masked by the production of PGI_2, NO, and EDHF.[39,40]

Endothelium and Blood Cell Interactions

In addition to the interactions of the endothelium with blood coagulation factors, endothelial cells also express cell-surface molecules that orchestrate the trafficking of circulating blood cells. These cell-associated molecules help direct the migration of leukocytes into specific organs under physiologic conditions and accelerate migration toward sites of inflammation. They have also been implicated in the adhesion of platelets and erythrocytes in several common disorders associated with homeostasis.

Interactions of Leukocytes With the Vessel Wall

It is now well established that flowing leukocytes may adhere to specific regions of the endothelium in response to tissue injury or infection. These multicellular interactions are essential precursors of physiologic inflammation. Leukocytes interact with vessel surfaces through a multistep process that includes (1) initial formation of usually reversible attachments; (2) activation of the attached cells; (3) development of stronger, shear-resistant adhesion; and (4) spreading, emigration, and other sequelae[36] (Fig. 27.4).

Selectins are key molecules in the interaction of leukocytes and endothelial cells. They are transmembrane glycoproteins that recognize cell-surface carbohydrate ligands found on leukocytes and initiate and mediate tethering and rolling of

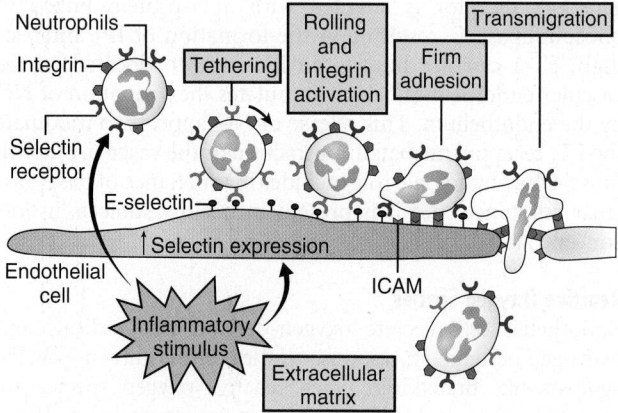

Fig. 27.4. Leukocyte recruitment process and transmigration. The multistep model for leukocyte recruitment at sites of inflammation begins with the activation of neutrophils and endothelial cells. Once activated, endothelial cells express selectins, whose binding to neutrophils initiates rolling and adhesion of neutrophils to the endothelium. Activated integrins on the surface of neutrophils bind to endothelial cell ICAMs, facilitating a firm adhesion. Transmigration through the endothelium further involves interactions with other molecules such as PECAMs and cadherins on the surface of endothelial cells.

leukocytes on the endothelial cell surface. Selectins constitute a family of three known molecules. L-selectin is expressed on most leukocytes and binds to ligands constitutively expressed on endothelial cells found in venules of lymphoid tissues. Its expression is induced on endothelium at sites of inflammation. E-selectin is expressed on activated endothelial cells and leukocytes. P-selectin is rapidly redistributed from secretory granules to the surface of platelets and endothelial cells stimulated with thrombin. Both endothelial cell E-selectin and P-selectin bind to ligands on leukocytes.[37]

With stimulation, leukocytes usually attach to postcapillary venule endothelial cells, where shear stresses are lowest. Leukocytes adherent to the endothelium can make contact with flowing leukocytes through the L-selectin molecule, resulting in amplification of leukocyte recruitment to sites of inflammation. It is generally understood that selectins initiate inflammatory, immune, and hemostatic responses by promoting transient multicellular interactions.[41]

Proinflammatory molecules presented on the surface of the endothelium proceed to activate a second family of adhesion molecules, the integrins, and cause cells to firmly adhere. After the initial tethering of leukocytes to endothelial cells, leukocytes then must roll prior to transmigrating through the endothelium. Inhibition of leukocyte adhesion does not reduce leukocyte rolling, suggesting that rolling and adhesion are distinct molecular events. In addition, inhibiting rolling reduces adhesion, suggesting that rolling is a prerequisite of leukocyte adhesion/recruitment and ultimately the inflammatory response.

Leukocytes subsequently migrate between endothelial cells into tissues by mechanisms that are not completely understood but that we know are affected by gradients of chemokines, integrins activation states, and interactions with PECAM-1, an Ig-like receptor. This migration requires disruption of endothelial-cell-to-endothelial-cell interaction of cadherins at tight junctions. Leukocyte recruitment to lymphoid tissues or inflammatory sites requires the coordinated expression of specific combinations of adhesion and signaling molecules. Diversity at each step of the cascade ensures that the appropriate leukocytes accumulate for a restricted period in response to a specific challenge.[4,41]

Platelet Adhesion

Endothelial cells and circulating platelets normally do not interact with each other due to the release of PGI_2, the release of NO, and the expression of CD39 on the surface of endothelial cells.[42] During vascular injury and inflammation, platelets adhere to exposed subendothelial components and are rapidly activated. Circulating platelets interact with the adherent platelets, producing a hemostatic plug that promotes thrombin generation and development of a stable fibrin clot. High shear stress, as seen in arteries, increases platelet adherence to the subendothelium where unactivated platelets attach to the subendothelium through interactions of platelet glycoproteins with immobilized von Willebrand Factor (vWF), a large, multimeric protein with binding sites for several other molecules, including subendothelial collagen. Flowing platelets attach transiently to vWF, resulting in continuous movement of the cells along the surface. Under the lower shear stresses found in veins, unactivated platelets interact with integrins to attach to and immediately arrest on immobilized fibrinogen.[43]

Once platelets adhere to either vWF or fibrinogen, they are activated by secreted products such as adenosine diphosphate or epinephrine or by surface molecules such as collagen that cross-link the integrins and other platelet receptors. The activated platelets spread and adhere more avidly to the subendothelial surface, which recruits additional platelets into aggregates. Shear-resistant adhesion may be further enhanced by interactions of other integrins or receptors with laminin, fibronectin, and thrombospondin. As thrombin is generated, converting bound fibrinogen to fibrin, the aggregated platelets contract to strengthen the clot.[43]

Endothelial Permeability

Transport across the endothelium can occur via two different pathways: through the endothelial cell (transcellular) or between adjacent cells (paracellular), through interendothelial junctions (Fig. 27.5). The endothelial cell is able to dynamically regulate its paracellular and transcellular pathways for transport of plasma proteins, solutes, and liquid. The semipermeable characteristic of the endothelium (which distinguishes it from the epithelium) is crucial for establishing the transendothelial protein gradient (the colloid osmotic gradient) required for tissue fluid homeostasis. The transcellular pathway, also known as transcytosis, is defined as vesicle-mediated transport of macromolecules, such as plasma proteins, across the endothelial barrier in a caveolae-dependent manner. The paracellular pathway is formed by the minute intercellular space between contacting cells. Its primary function is to restrict free passage of macromolecules in the range of 3 nm and above through interendothelial junctions (IEJs), while allowing the convective and diffusive transport of molecules of less than 3 nm in diameter. Permeability of the IEJs is determined by the adhesive properties of the proteins that comprise the tight junctions and adherens junctions. However, the junctional barrier is a dynamic structure. It responds to permeability-increasing agonists and migrating leukocytes with disassembly of IEJs and to barrier-stabilizing mediators by increasing the surface expression and adhesiveness of junctional proteins in order to strengthen IEJs.[44-46]

Endothelial Cell Dysfunction
Ischemia-Reperfusion Injury

Reperfusion of previously ischemic tissues can place the organs at risk for further cellular injury, thereby limiting the recovery of function. The microvasculature, particularly the endothelial cells, is vulnerable to the deleterious consequences of ischemia and reperfusion (I/R). I/R is now recognized as a potentially serious problem encountered during a variety of standard medical and surgical procedures, such as thrombolytic therapy, organ transplantation, and cardiopulmonary bypass.[47]

Hypoxia and inflammation are intimately linked on many levels and have functional roles in many human diseases. Indeed, a wide range of clinical conditions are characterized by hypoxia- or ischemia-driven inflammation or by inflammation-associated hypoxia. The molecular and

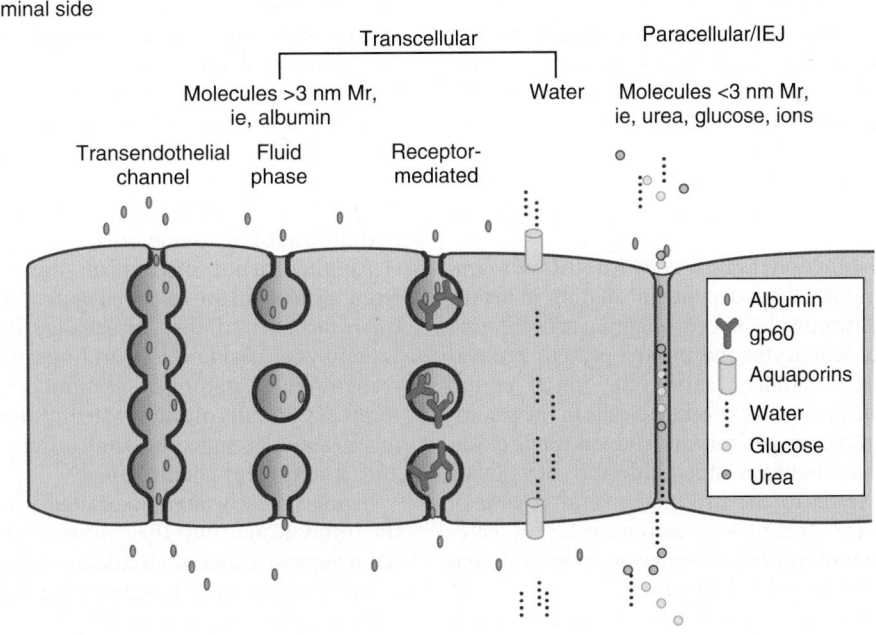

Fig. 27.5. Schematic of transport pathways in continuous endothelium. Under basal conditions, the transcellular pathway can mediate the transport of plasma proteins (>3 nm Mr) such as albumin by caveolae via an absorptive (receptor-mediated) or fluid-phase pathway. Transcellular channels can also form transiently in endothelial cells by fusion of multiple caveolae and allow albumin transport. Aquaporins form channels across the lipid bilayer that are highly selective for water molecules and allow their movement across the luminal or abluminal endothelial membrane, thus creating a transendothelial pathway for water. Small molecules including urea and glucose (<3 nm Mr) are transported around individual endothelial cells via the paracellular (ie, interendothelial junction [IEJ] pathway). *Mr,* molecular radius. (Modified from Mehta D, Malik AB. Signaling mechanisms regulating endothelial permeability. Physiol Rev. 2006;86:279-367.)

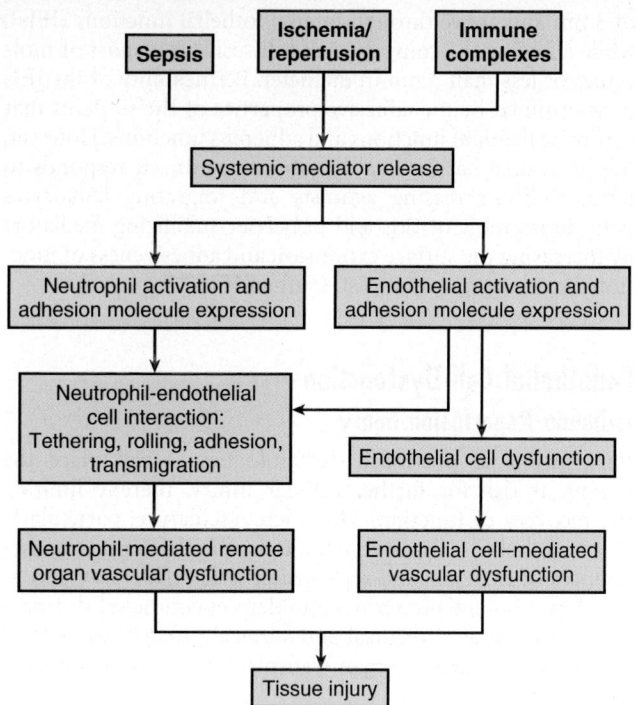

Fig. 27.6. Mechanisms that underlie the development of local and remote organ injury following an initial inflammatory event. The activation of endothelial cells and circulating neutrophils leads to the expression and activation of adhesion molecules that facilitate neutrophil invasion of vascular beds, resulting in local and remote organ dysfunction.

biochemical changes in the vascular wall during I/R are characteristic of an acute inflammatory response (Fig. 27.6). The intensity of this inflammatory response can be so severe that the injury response to reperfusion is also manifested in susceptible organs such as in the lungs and cardiovascular system. The resulting systemic inflammatory response syndrome (SIRS) and multiple organ dysfunction syndrome (MODS) are both associated with significant increases in mortality and morbidity.[48]

Microvascular dysfunction associated with I/R is manifested as impaired endothelium-dependent dilation in arterioles, enhanced fluid filtration, leukocyte plugging in capillaries, and the trafficking of leukocytes and plasma protein extravasation in postcapillary venules. During the initial period following reperfusion, activated endothelial cells in the microcirculation produce more oxygen radicals and less nitric oxide. The resulting imbalance between superoxide and nitric oxide in endothelial cells leads to the production and release of inflammatory mediators (eg, platelet-activating factor, TNF-α) and enhances the biosynthesis of adhesion molecules that mediate leukocyte-endothelial cell adhesion.[48]

Since its discovery in the early 1990s, hypoxia-inducible factor 1 (HIF-1) has been increasingly recognized for its key role in transcriptional control of more than a hundred genes that regulate a wide spectrum of cellular functional events, including angiogenesis, vasomotor control, glucose and energy metabolism, erythropoiesis, iron homeostasis, pH regulation, cell proliferation, and viability. Animal studies have provided compelling data to demonstrate a pivotal role for the HIF pathway in the pathogenesis of ischemic injury. For example,

HIF-1α has been shown to play a role in mediating cardioprotection.[49]

The inflammatory mediators released as a consequence of reperfusion also appear to activate endothelial cells in remote organs that are not exposed to the initial ischemic insult. Oxidants and activated leukocytes have been implicated as mediators of remote organ injury in I/R. This distant response to I/R can result in leukocyte-dependent microvascular injury that is characteristic of SIRS and MODS. The pulmonary damage associated with MODS can range from mild dysfunction to severe failure, as in acute respiratory distress syndrome (ARDS). The pulmonary injuries associated with ARDS include increased pulmonary microvascular permeability and the accumulation of neutrophil-rich alveolar fluid. Respiratory failure often is associated with cardiovascular, hepatic, gastrointestinal, and renal dysfunction as well as central nervous system involvement. MODS is associated with dysfunction of the coagulation cascade and the immune system, resulting in thrombosis, disseminated intravascular coagulation, and immunocompromise. The initiation of MODS may also lead to further tissue ischemia, resulting in additional insult.[50]

Sepsis

Although the pathophysiologic process of multiple organ dysfunction during sepsis is multifactorial, one common feature is the dysfunction of the microcirculation, including the resistance arteries, capillaries, and postcapillary venules. The microcirculation cannot be considered a simple passive conduit. Rather it is a functionally active system of interactions among the vascular wall; circulating and tissue-associated cells such as leukocytes, platelets, and mast cells; and extracellular mediators that contribute to the regulation of local, downstream, and upstream vascular tone. Sepsis is particularly associated with microvascular endothelial cell dysfunction leading to (1) the breakdown of endothelial barrier function, leading to tissue edema and uncontrolled inflammatory cell infiltration; (2) vasomotor dysfunction, leading to the formation of arteriovenous shunts in association with loss of peripheral resistance; and (3) disturbance of oxygen transport and utilization by tissue cells.[51]

Another major mechanism during sepsis is the change from anticoagulant to procoagulant and the contribution of microthrombi to the disturbance of the microcirculation. Lipopolysaccharide (LPS), an important pathogen product, is recognized by pathogen recognition receptors like toll-like receptors on cells of the innate immune system. This will lead to intracellular signaling and to the production of cytokines and other potent chemokines.

Septic shock is often associated with the loss of fluid from the intravascular into the extravascular space with the potential progressive loss of circulating blood, eventually leading to a depression of cardiac output. Similarly, loss of fluid into the extravascular space can lead to life-threatening edema in the lungs, kidney, and brain of septic patients. The loss of fluid is not believed to be associated with changes in hydrostatic or osmotic pressures within the vascular compartment but rather to the breakdown of endothelial barrier function. The permeability of the vascular barrier can be modified in response to specific stimuli acting on endothelial cells. Many inflammatory agonists mediate endothelial hyperpermeability via a calcium-dependent mechanism. Multiple cascades of intracellular signaling reactions are initiated when an inflammatory agonist binds to its respective receptor expressed on the endothelial surface (eg, thrombin binds the protease-activated receptor-1, histamine binds its receptor H1, and vascular endothelial growth factor binds its receptor vascular endothelial growth factor 2 (VEGFR-2). This breakdown allows migration of water and macromolecules, including proteins, into the extravascular space. The pathophysiologic mechanisms proposed include the separation of tight junctions between endothelial cells, as well as cytoskeleton contraction, rather than destructive changes of endothelial cells leading to defects in the endothelium.[44,52] Studies on the microcirculation of the gut have shown the development of a gap between microvascular and venous oxygen tension, suggesting enhanced shunting of the microcirculation. Defects in distributing blood to regional vascular beds or the microcirculation could be responsible for tissue hypoxia and limited oxygen extraction. Clinical evidence of decreased microvessel density in the sublingual microcirculation of fluid-resuscitated septic patients is consistent with findings of decreased functional capillary flow in the gut, liver, and skeletal muscle microcirculation in animal models of sepsis. This clinical finding raises the possibility that abnormal microvascular O_2 transport develops in multiple organs despite fluid resuscitation, leading to heterogeneous microvascular dysfunction and local tissue hypoxia in severe cases of sepsis.

Hemolytic-Uremic Syndrome

Thrombotic thrombocytopenic purpura (TTP) and the hemolytic-uremic syndrome (HUS) are related disorders characterized clinically by microangiopathic hemolytic anemia and thrombocytopenia. Pathologically, both conditions include the development of platelet microthrombi that occlude small arterioles and capillaries. Endothelial dysfunction plays a prominent role in the pathogenesis of both disorders. HUS commonly occurs in early childhood (approximately 90% of cases). It often follows an episode of bloody diarrhea caused by enteropathic strains of *Escherichia coli* that release an exotoxin, verotoxin-1 (VT-1) (see also Chapter 75). VT-1 binds with high affinity to receptors expressed in high density on renal glomerular endothelial cells. VT-1 is directly cytotoxic to endothelial cells where it promotes neutrophil-mediated endothelial cell injury. VT-1 induces the production of TNF-α by monocytes and cells within the kidney. In turn, TNF-α, in synergy with interleukin-1, increases VT-1 receptor expression and exacerbates the sensitivity of the endothelium to toxin-mediated and antibody-mediated cytotoxicity. It also promotes vWF release and impairs fibrinolytic activity.[53]

There is considerable evidence to suggest that endothelial cell injury plays a role in the pathogenesis of TTP. Platelet microthrombi in TTP contain abundant vWF but little fibrinogen, in contrast to those seen in disseminated intravascular coagulopathy. A subgroup of patients has been identified who suffer from chronic, relapsing TTP and whose plasma continues to contain elevated levels of unusually large vWF multimers (ULvWF) between relapses. ULvWFs may exacerbate microvascular thrombosis through their ability to aggregate platelets at high levels of shear stress. The secretion of ULvWF by cultured endothelial cells is stimulated by many agonists, including Shiga toxin. However, elevated levels of vWF occur in other thrombotic microangiopathies, and their exact role in TTP/HUS requires further study. Endothelial damage plays a pivotal role in the pathogenesis of the disease. The events that initiate TTP remain unknown. More recently, plasma from patients with TTP and HUS has been reported to induce apoptosis in microvascular endothelial cells. Interestingly, cells from dermal, renal, and cerebral origin were most susceptible, whereas pulmonary and coronary arterial cells were less susceptible.[54]

Vasculitic Disorders

Vasculitis is a disease that targets all levels of the arterial tree from aorta to capillaries and also affects venules, with leukocyte infiltration and necrosis. Different forms of vasculitis attack different vessels and are classified accordingly. The inflammatory process may target vessels of any type throughout the vascular system, although distinct clinicopathologic entities preferentially involve vessels of particular sizes and locations. Small vessels anywhere in the body may be affected by focal necrotizing lesions where extravasation of leukocytes drives the inflammatory responses, resulting in vasculitis. Leukocyte adhesion molecules participating in the interactions with endothelial cells belong to three major families: selectins, sialomucins, and integrins. Interestingly, it is recognized that these interactions participate in tissue specificity in various vasculitic conditions. For instance, specific selectin interactions mediate cutaneous tropism in several inflammatory disorders, including graft-versus-host disease and dermatomyositis.[55]

Biomarkers of Endothelial Activation

There is a strong rationale for targeting markers of endothelial cell activation as clinically informative biomarkers to improve diagnosis, prognostic evaluation, or risk-stratification of critically ill patients. During sepsis, a large number of endothelial cell-active molecules are potential biomarkers for the early diagnosis. These include regulators of endothelial activation, such as vascular endothelial growth factor (VEGF), the angiopoietin pathway (Ang-1/2), adhesion molecules (ICAM, VCAM, and E-selectin), mediators of permeability and vasomotor tone (ET- 1), and mediators of coagulation (eg, vWF).[56] Elevated endothelin levels have been found in systemic and pulmonary hypertension, coronary artery disease, and heart failure, although the role of ET-1 in the pathophysiology of these conditions has been postulated but not proved.[57,58]

Cellular markers such as EPC and endothelial microparticles (EMP) are also gaining interest as biomarkers. There is a positive correlation between EPC number and survival in sepsis.[59] In addition, there is a functional impairment of EPC with decreased proliferative and migratory capacities of EPC. These findings have led to therapeutic strategies (eg, statins) that focus on improving EPC number and function during sepsis.[60] In contrast, an elevation of EMP is considered a marker of endothelial dysfunction in cardiovascular disease. However, the number of EMP is positively related to survival and inversely correlated with the Sequential Organ Failure Assessment (SOFA) score in patients with sepsis. Because it is becoming increasingly clear that microparticles are more than simple markers of endothelial damage or activation, their interpretation as markers of endothelial dysfunction is less ambiguous.[61] Interestingly, EPCs show a biphasic response after traumatic brain injury; after an initial decrease, they peak 7 days after the insult. Furthermore they have been associated with an improved outcome after traumatic brain injury.[62]

However, the clinical utility of these biomarkers is limited by a lack of assay standardization, unknown receiver operating characteristics, and lack of validation. It remains speculative whether the use of endothelial cell biomarkers will guide therapy during critical care illness in the near future.

Conclusions

The endothelium can no longer be viewed as a static physical barrier that simply separates the blood from tissue. Rather, the endothelium coordinates key functions of different tissues in normal and pathophysiologic conditions. This is accomplished by the interaction of endothelial cells with circulating factors and cells and its ability to transmit biochemical and biophysical signals to surrounding tissues. A greater understanding of endothelial physiology will lead to novel therapeutic approaches in complex clinical conditions.

Key References

1. Rubanyi GM. The role of endothelium in cardiovascular homeostasis and diseases. *J Cardiovasc Pharmacol.* 1993;22(suppl 4):S1-S14.
2. Aird WC. Endothelial cell heterogeneity. *Crit Care Med.* 2003;31(4 suppl):S221-S230.
3. Kumar S, West DC, Ager A. Heterogeneity in endothelial cells from large vessels and microvessels. *Differentiation.* 1987;36:57-70.
4. Dejana E. Endothelial adherens junctions: implications in the control of vascular permeability and angiogenesis. *J Clin Invest.* 1996;98:1949-1953.
7. McCarthy SA, et al. Heterogeneity of the endothelial cell and its role in organ preference of tumour metastasis. *Trends Pharmacol Sci.* 1991;12:462-467.
8. Asahara T, et al. Isolation of putative progenitor endothelial cells for angiogenesis. *Science.* 1997;275:964-967.
9. Kalka C, et al. Transplantation of ex vivo expanded endothelial progenitor cells for therapeutic neovascularization. *Proc Natl Acad Sci USA.* 2000;97:3422-3427.
10. Asahara T, et al. Bone marrow origin of endothelial progenitor cells responsible for postnatal vasculogenesis in physiological and pathological neovascularization. *Circ Res.* 1999;85:221-228.
12. Schachinger V, et al. Intracoronary bone marrow-derived progenitor cells in acute myocardial infarction. *N Engl J Med.* 2006;355:1210-1221.
13. Taniguchi E, et al. Endothelial progenitor cell transplantation improves the survival following liver injury in mice. *Gastroenterology.* 2006; 130:521-531.
14. Wang XX, et al. Transplantation of autologous endothelial progenitor cells may be beneficial in patients with idiopathic pulmonary arterial hypertension: a pilot randomized controlled trial. *J Am Coll Cardiol.* 2007;49:1566-1571.
15. Bombeli T, Mueller M, Haeberli A. Anticoagulant properties of the vascular endothelium. *Thromb Haemost.* 1997;77:408-423.
16. Rosenberg RD, Rosenberg JS. Natural anticoagulant mechanisms. *J Clin Invest.* 1984;74:1-6.
18. Esmon NL. Thrombomodulin. *Semin Thromb Hemost.* 1987;13:454-463.
19. Majerus PW. Arachidonate metabolism in vascular disorders. *J Clin Invest.* 1983;72:1521-1525.
20. Levin EG, Santell L, Osborn KG. The expression of endothelial tissue plasminogen activator in vivo: a function defined by vessel size and anatomic location. *J Cell Sci.* 1997;110(Pt 2):139-148.
21. Furchgott RF, Zawadzki JV. The obligatory role of endothelial cells in the relaxation of arterial smooth muscle by acetylcholine. *Nature.* 1980;288:373-376.
23. Garland CJ, et al. Endothelium-dependent hyperpolarization: a role in the control of vascular tone. *Trends Pharmacol Sci.* 1995;16:23-30.
24. Stamler JS, Singel DJ, Loscalzo J. Biochemistry of nitric oxide and its redox-activated forms. *Science.* 1992;258:1898-1902.
25. Forstermann U. Biochemistry and molecular biology of nitric oxide synthases. *Arzneimittelforschung.* 1994;44:402-407.

28. Rapoport RM, Murad F. Agonist-induced endothelium-dependent relaxation in rat thoracic aorta may be mediated through cGMP. *Circ Res.* 1983;52:352-357.
29. Bolotina VM, et al. Nitric oxide directly activates calcium-dependent potassium channels in vascular smooth muscle. *Nature.* 1994;368: 850-853.
31. Stamler JS, et al. Nitric oxide regulates basal systemic and pulmonary vascular resistance in healthy humans. *Circulation.* 1994;89:2035-2040.
32. Moncada S, Vane JR. The role of prostacyclin in vascular tissue. *Fed Proc.* 1979;38:66-71.
35. Feletou M, Vanhoutte PM. Endothelium-derived hyperpolarizing factor. *Clin Exp Pharmacol Physiol.* 1996;23:1082-1090.
36. Kubes P, Kerfoot SM. Leukocyte recruitment in the microcirculation: the rolling paradigm revisited. *News Physiol Sci.* 2001;16:76-80.
37. McEver RP, Moore KL, Cummings RD. Leukocyte trafficking mediated by selectin-carbohydrate interactions. *J Biol Chem.* 1995;270:11025-11028.
38. Rubanyi GM, Vanhoutte PM. Superoxide anions and hyperoxia inactivate endothelium-derived relaxing factor. *Am J Physiol.* 1986;250(5 Pt 2):H822-H827.
39. Coleman RA, Smith WL, Narumiya S. International Union of Pharmacology classification of prostanoid receptors: properties, distribution, and structure of the receptors and their subtypes. *Pharmacol Rev.* 1994; 46:205-229.
40. Halushka PV, et al. Thromboxane, prostaglandin and leukotriene receptors. *Annu Rev Pharmacol Toxicol.* 1989;29:213-239.
41. Springer TA. Traffic signals on endothelium for lymphocyte recirculation and leukocyte emigration. *Annu Rev Physiol.* 1995;57:827-872.
42. Schafer AI. Vascular endothelium: in defense of blood fluidity. *J Clin Invest.* 1997;99:1143-1144.
43. Roth GJ. Platelets and blood vessels: the adhesion event. *Immunol Today.* 1992;13:100-105.
44. Kumar P, et al. Molecular mechanisms of endothelial hyperpermeability: implications in inflammation. *Expert Rev Mol Med.* 2009;11:e19.
45. Mehta D, Malik AB. Signaling mechanisms regulating endothelial permeability. *Physiol Rev.* 2006;86:279-367.
46. Vandenbroucke E, et al. Regulation of endothelial junctional permeability. *Ann N Y Acad Sci.* 2008;1123:134-145.
47. Grace PA, Mathie RT. *Ischemia-Reperfusion Injury.* London: Blackwell Science; 1999.
48. Neary P, Redmond HP. Ischemia-reperfusion injury and the systemic inflammatory response syndrome. In: Grace PA, Mathie RT, eds. *Ischemia-Reperfusion Injury.* London: Blackwell Science; 1999:123-136.
49. Orfanos SE, et al. Pulmonary endothelium in acute lung injury: from basic science to the critically ill. *Intensive Care Med.* 2004;30:1702-1714.
50. Lehr HA, Arfors KE. Mechanisms of tissue damage by leukocytes. *Curr Opin Hematol.* 1994;1:92-99.
52. Li H, Forstermann U. Nitric oxide in the pathogenesis of vascular disease. *J Pathol.* 2000;190:244-254.
53. Moake JL. Haemolytic-uraemic syndrome: basic science. *Lancet.* 1994;343:393-397.
54. Mitra D, et al. Thrombotic thrombocytopenic purpura and sporadic hemolytic-uremic syndrome plasmas induce apoptosis in restricted lineages of human microvascular endothelial cells. *Blood.* 1997;89: 1224-1234.
56. Xing K, et al. Clinical utility of biomarkers of endothelial activation in sepsis-a systematic review. *Crit Care.* 2012;16:R7.
57. Masaki T. The discovery, the present state, and the future prospects of endothelin. *J Cardiovasc Pharmacol.* 1989;13(suppl 5):S1-S4.
58. Yanagisawa M, et al. A novel peptide vasoconstrictor, endothelin, is produced by vascular endothelium and modulates smooth muscle Ca2+ channels. *J Hypertens Suppl.* 1988;6:S188-S191.
59. Rafat N, et al. Increased circulating endothelial progenitor cells in septic patients: correlation with survival. *Crit Care Med.* 2007;35:1677-1684.
60. Darwish NI, Liles WC. Emerging therapeutic strategies to prevent infection-related microvascular endothelial activation and dysfunction. *Virulence.* 2013;4:572-582.
61. Soriano AO, et al. Levels of endothelial and platelet microparticles and their interactions with leukocytes negatively correlate with organ dysfunction and predict mortality in severe sepsis. *Crit Care Med.* 2005; 33:2540-2546.
62. Liu L, et al. Endothelial progenitor cells correlate with clinical outcome of traumatic brain injury. *Crit Care Med.* 2011;39:1760-1765.

Principles of Invasive Monitoring

Molly V. Dorfman and Kenneth A. Schenkman

PEARLS

- Hemodynamic monitoring refers to measurement of the functional characteristics of the heart and circulatory system that affect the perfusion of tissues with oxygenated blood.
- Hemodynamic monitoring can be performed invasively or noninvasively and can be used for diagnosis, surveillance, or titration of therapy.
- The central venous waveform is composed of three waves (a, c, and v) and two wave descents (x and y).
- The arterial waveform has three components: rapid upstroke, dicrotic notch, and runoff.
- Cardiac output can be calculated using the Fick method or measured directly via thermodilution.
- Continuous SvO₂ monitors can guide goal-directed therapy in patients who are in septic shock.
- A pulmonary artery catheter can be used to measure cardiac output and indices of oxygen delivery and extraction.
- Newer minimally invasive modalities complement historically invasive devices for assessing hemodynamics.

Role of Invasive Hemodynamic Monitoring

Since William Harvey's observation in the early 1600s that the heart pumps blood in a continuous circuit, the function of the circulatory system has been the subject of intense scrutiny. Hemodynamic monitoring refers to measurement of the functional characteristics of the heart and the circulatory system that affect the perfusion of tissues with oxygenated blood in order to maintain homeostasis and to remove byproducts of metabolism. Several different types of invasive hemodynamic monitoring can be used concurrently to guide management. The goal of hemodynamic monitoring is to provide accurate diagnoses and to guide additional interventions to deliver improved care to the critically ill patient.

In his 1733 report "Statical essays: containing haemastaticks; or, an account of some hydraulick and hydrostatical experiments made on the blood and blood-vessels of animals," Hales[1] described early experiments in horses in which he used tubular devices inserted directly into arteries to measure intravascular pressures. Fig. 28.1 depicts Hales and an assistant in the process of these early experiments. This figure also illustrates a simple method for inferring arterial versus venous placement of a vascular catheter, which can also give a quick bedside estimate of central venous pressure.

Clinical hemodynamic assessment at the bedside begins with noninvasive measurements such as heart rate (HR), blood pressure, urine output, and peripheral perfusion. Other noninvasive studies that may contribute to assessment of hemodynamic status include electrocardiograms, chest radiographs, ultrasound, and echocardiography. Frequently, in the pediatric intensive care unit (PICU) these measurements are supplemented by invasive hemodynamic measures that require entrance into the intravascular space. Such invasive hemodynamic measurements include placement of central venous catheters to assess right atrial filling pressures and to measure mixed venous oxygen saturation, arterial catheters to assess arterial blood pressure, and pulmonary artery catheters (PACs) to assess left-sided pressures, cardiac output (CO), and vascular resistance. Although invasive hemodynamic monitoring can provide the skilled intensivist with a plethora of valuable information, it is not meant to take the place of, or minimize, the extensive amount of information that can be gained by less invasive techniques. Successful use of invasive hemodynamic measurements necessitates skills to obtain these measures safely with utmost attention to the multiple potential risks imposed upon the patient. Furthermore, for invasive hemodynamic measurements to be useful, the clinician must be able to successfully interpret the information provided by the measurements. Finally, as with any technology, the use of invasive hemodynamic monitoring is in evolution, and it is incumbent upon the clinician to be familiar with developments as they arise.

This chapter aims to be a practical guide to the use of hemodynamic monitoring in the PICU. The chapter reviews general principles of measurement and then discusses the three main types of invasive hemodynamic monitoring: central venous catheter, arterial catheter, and PAC. It addresses the indications and controversies, sites of insertion, interpretation of waveforms, and potential complications. It also reviews CO monitoring and calculation of oxygen consumption and delivery. New techniques coupling invasive monitoring with noninvasive devices are also discussed. Chapter 19 details the specific techniques for gaining access in order to make these measurements.

Indications for Invasive Hemodynamic Measurements

The three main indications for invasive hemodynamic monitoring are diagnosis, surveillance, and titration of therapy. Diagnosis may include the differentiation of septic shock (through assessment of factors such as diminished right heart filling pressures or preload and decreased systemic vascular

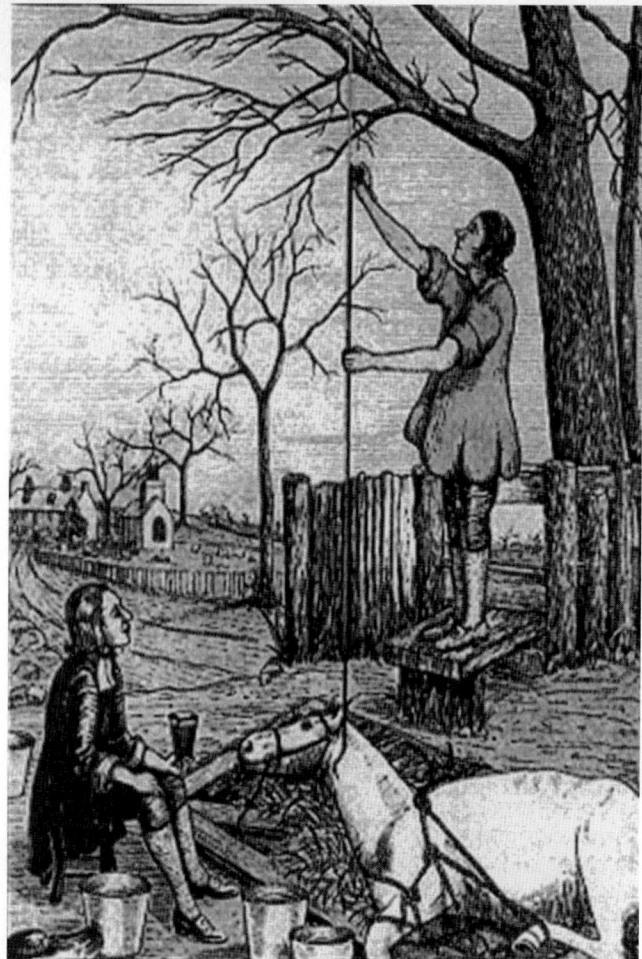

Fig. 28.1. Clinician and an assistant measuring the blood pressure of a horse. (From Pickering G. Systemic arterial hypertension. In: Fishman AP, Dickinson WR, eds. Circulation of the Blood: Men and Ideas. New York: Oxford University Press; 1964.)

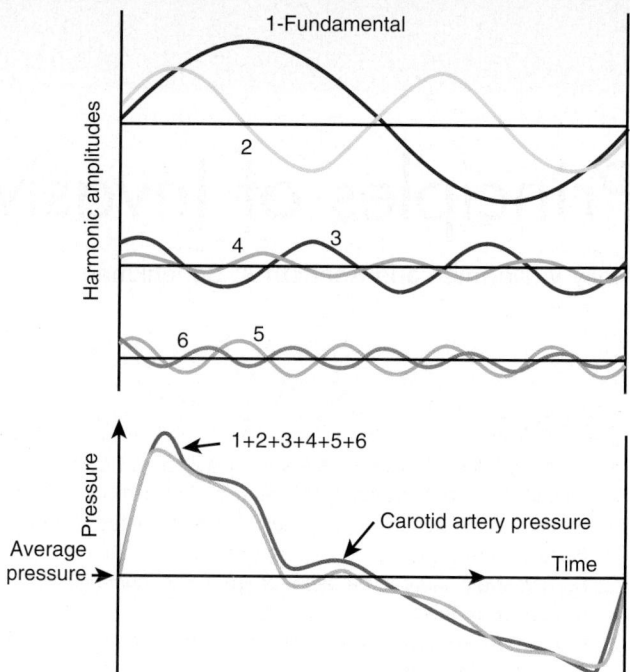

Fig. 28.2. Fourier series representation of an arterial pressure tracing. Bottom, High-fidelity carotid artery pressure tracing and the sum of the first six harmonics of its Fourier series representation. Despite the few terms used in the synthesis, the close fit of the two curves is evident. Top, Individual harmonic components labeled with their harmonic number. (Redrawn from RSC. Transducers for Biomedical Measurements: Principles and Applications. New York: John Wiley & Sons; 1974, from Hansen AT. Acta Physiol Scand. 1949;19[suppl 68]:1 and Perloff WH: Invasive measurements in the PICU. In: Fuhrman BP, Zimmerman JJ, eds. Pediatric Critical Care. 2nd ed. St. Louis: Mosby; 1998.)

resistance) from cardiogenic shock (characterized by elevated left heart pressures and afterload). Surveillance implies observation over time. The purpose of surveillance may be to assess the stability of a patient at risk for adverse changes or to determine the response to therapy. Invasive measurements performed for diagnostic purposes often are continued for surveillance. Titration of therapy is often based on information gleaned from invasive measurements.

Principles of Measurement

Intensive care clinicians rely on a wide variety of measurement systems to assess patient clinical status and response to therapy. However, not all clinicians have a good understanding of how physiologic variables are measured and, consequently, may not be able to troubleshoot monitoring systems or recognize when information obtained is inaccurate. A detailed discussion of monitoring is beyond the scope of this chapter, but a basic understanding of the principles of measurement is helpful in deciding which measurements to trust and how to assess a monitoring system for accuracy. Detailed descriptions of monitoring systems are provided elsewhere.[2-4]

Signal Analysis

Measurements generally are made directly by comparison with known standards or indirectly by use of a calibration system. Determination of length or weight usually is made by direct comparison with a standard ruler or standard mass. Most invasive measurements in the ICU are made indirectly, therefore requiring use of a calibration system. Thus understanding the basis for calibration of a system is important to determine the validity of the measurement.

Measurement systems detect and transform signals so that they can be presented in an interpretable way to the user. Signals can be characterized as static or dynamic. Slowly changing signals, such as body temperature, can be thought of as static. Hemodynamic measurements change from moment to moment and thus are dynamic. Physiologic signals may be periodic; for example, arterial pressure is periodic because it varies with the cardiac cycle.

Complex periodic signals, such as an arterial pressure waveform, can be described mathematically as the sum of a series of simpler waveforms called a Fourier series. Alternatively, the arterial tracing can be thought of as a sum of simpler waveforms, sine waves, and cosine waves. Fig. 28.2 depicts an arterial pressure waveform as the sum of the first six terms in the Fourier series. The sum of the first six terms in the series forms a waveform similar to the original tracing. Adding terms from the Fourier series, or higher harmonics, results in an increasingly better representation of the actual waveform. In general, to reproduce a pressure tracing without loss of significant characteristics for clinical use, the measurement system must have an accurate frequency response to approximately 10 times the fundamental frequency (first 10 harmonics).

The sampling rate of a measurement system determines how often a physiologic value is measured. For body temperature, sampling every few minutes might be sufficient, but for arterial pressure measurement, a higher rate is necessary. This principle may seem obvious, but as an example of the importance of sampling rate, consider the number of points needed to define a circle. If we place three equidistant points on a circle, we describe a triangle, not a circle. Similarly, four points describe a square. If we increase the number of points (sampling rate), we describe the circle more completely. For a sine wave, the minimum frequency of sampling needed to preserve the waveform is twice the frequency. This mathematical minimum is known as the Nyquist frequency.[4] For complex waveforms such as arterial pressure tracings, the sampling rate must be at least twice the highest frequency component in the waveform.

Measurement Systems

Hemodynamic monitoring in the clinical setting usually uses a fluid-coupled system where changes in pressure are transmitted via a column of (incompressible) fluid in a (ideally incompressible) tube to a mechanical transducer. The mechanical transducer, usually a displaceable screen diaphragm, converts a change in pressure to an electrical signal, which can be processed and displayed. In laboratory settings, vascular pressures can be measured by a transducer at the point of interest rather than remotely, as in the clinical setting. Measuring pressure at the point of interest—directly in the aorta, for example—decreases loss of signal integrity because of the measurement system. Most clinical pressure measuring systems have sufficient fidelity for clinical purposes. However, compliance, resistance, or impedance in the pressure tubing can result in damping or alteration of the recorded signal. The presence of bubbles in the fluid can further damp the recorded signal.

Errors in Measurement

The ideal measurement system determines the actual or "true" value for the measured variable. However, determination of a true value may be difficult. Every measurement system is subject to various errors. Errors in measurement can be classified as either systematic or random. Systematic errors occur in a predictable manner and are reproduced with repeated measures. Bias in a measurement system—for example, a baseline offset—results in a systematic error. Random errors are unpredictable and do not recur predictably with repeated measures.

Accuracy of a measurement is defined by the difference between the measured and true values, divided by the true value. Precision is defined by the reproducibility of the measurement; thus a more precise system yields more similar values for repeated measures under the same conditions than does a less precise system. Imprecision can be thought of as a representation of random errors, whereas bias can be thought of as a representation of systematic errors.

Calibration

Many measurement systems are linear, that is, based on an assumption that the relationship between the inputs and outputs from a measurement device can be fitted to a straight line. This assumption allows a system to be calibrated under two conditions, with the rest of the values falling on the line defined by those two points. Actual nonlinearity of the system adversely affects the measurements.

Calibration is a process in which the reading, or output of a device, is adjusted to match a known input value. For example, an electronic pressure transducer may be calibrated against a mercury manometer. If the input to the device is zero, the output should be adjusted so that the reading also is set to zero. This "zeroing" reduces any baseline offset, thus reducing systematic errors in subsequent readings. The system then is calibrated to a nonzero value, for example, 100 mm Hg pressure, and the system gain is adjusted to read this value as well.

Frequency Response

The ability of a measurement system to accurately measure an oscillating signal, such as arterial blood pressure, is dependent upon the system's frequency response. The system can either overestimate or underestimate the true amplitude of a signal. If the system is overdamped, the value reported underestimates the amplitude, and waveform characteristics may be lost. Resonance in the system may result in overestimation of the amplitude. Measurement of arterial systolic pressure—the amplitude of the arterial waveform—may be inaccurate because of overdamping, and important waveform characteristics may be lost if the frequency response of the measurement system is poor. Fig. 28.3 illustrates the effects of damping on measurement of blood pressure.

Impedance

Impedance is the ratio of the change in blood flow along a vessel to the change in the pressure in the vessel. Impedance has both resistive and reactive components. In a pulsatile system such as the cardiovascular system, resistance alone does not fully describe the impediment or impedance to forward flow of blood. The caliber, length, and arrangement of the blood vessels and the mechanical properties of the blood determine resistance in the blood vessels. Reactance includes compliance of the vessels and inertia of the blood and thus is a dynamic component of impedance. This is important because the pulsatile nature of the cardiovascular system is dynamic.

When blood is propelled through a vessel at a branch point, a reflected pressure wave back toward the heart increases the impedance of the system. The major sites of wave reflection from vessel branching are from vessels approximately 1 mm in diameter.[2] Thus these small vessels contribute significantly to overall impedance. Fig. 28.4 shows the relationships between pressure and flow velocity with distance along the length of the aorta. Because blood pressure increases with distance from the heart and flow velocity decreases with distance, the impedance increases toward the peripheral vasculature. Hemodynamic measuring systems are essentially physical extensions of the vascular system; thus the configuration and characteristics of the tubing and transducer system can alter the overall effect of impedance.

Invasive Techniques
Central Venous Pressure Catheters
Indications

Indications for CVP catheter placement in pediatric patients include assessment of right heart filling pressure (CVP),

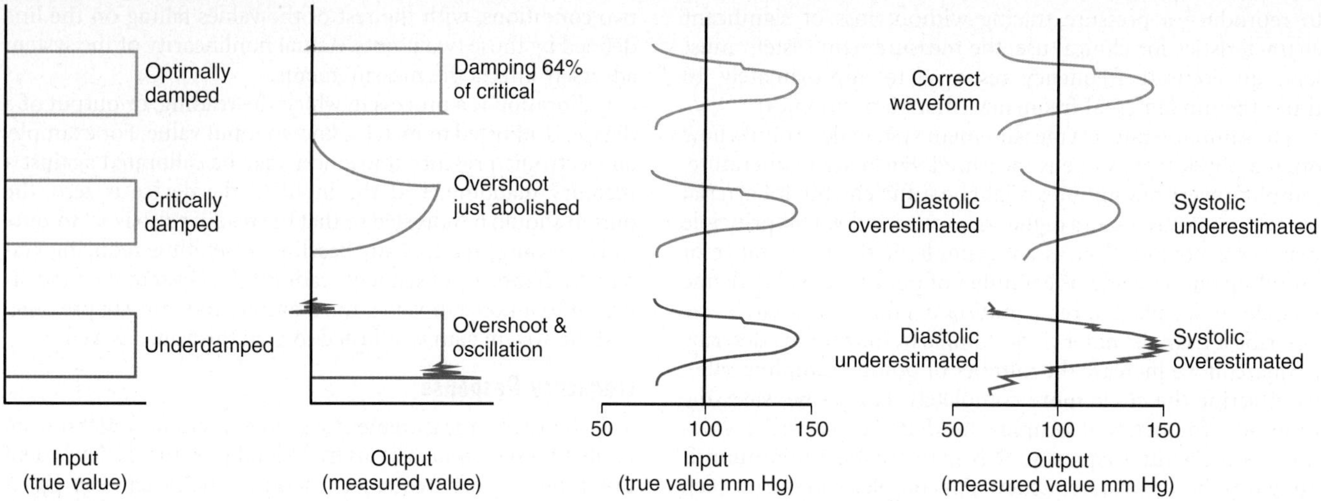

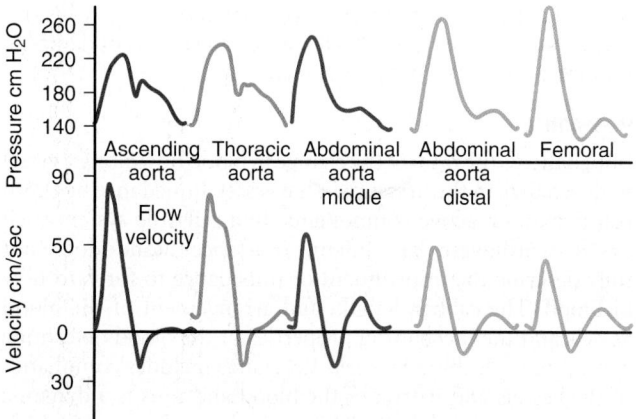

Fig. 28.3. Effects of damping on blood pressure measurement. Upper two graphs depict the response to a square-wave input from three different blood pressure transducers with different damping. Lower two graphs show the effect of damping on blood pressure measurement. (From Chatburn RL. Principles of measurement. In: Tobin MJ, ed. Principles and Practice of Intensive Care Monitoring. New York: McGraw-Hill; 1998.)

Fig. 28.4. Pressure pulses and flow velocity at various points in the systemic arterial circulation. Data were obtained from dogs and are similar to measurements made in humans. The data indicate that both peak and pulse pressure increase with distance from the heart, whereas oscillation in flow velocity shows a progressive decrease. Consequently impedance (discussed in the text) must increase toward the periphery. (From Perloff WH. Invasive measurements in the PICU. In: Fuhrman BP, Zimmerman JJ, eds. Pediatric Critical Care. 2nd ed. St. Louis: Mosby; 1998.)

monitoring of large fluid shifts between the intravascular and the extravascular space, infusion of vasoactive substances, monitoring mixed venous oxygen saturation, and infusion of hyperosmolar fluids and/or irritants.[5-7]

Interpretation of Waveforms

CVP is a measure of right atrial pressure, although it may be measured in the inferior or superior vena cava (SVC). It is a measure of preload—the force or load on the right ventricle during relaxation or filling. CVP is measured at the end of diastole, just prior to ejection. Final filling of the right

ventricle occurs at the end of atrial contraction. When the tricuspid valve is open during diastole, the right atrium and right ventricle form a continuous column; therefore right atrial pressure reflects right ventricular end-diastolic pressure. CVP is used to measure filling pressure or preload and is an indicator of volume status. It is commonly used in patients with hypovolemic or septic shock in whom volume resuscitation is desirable prior to institution of vasopressor therapy. In patients with decreased right ventricular function or pulmonary hypertension, an increased CVP well beyond normal limits may be observed and further fluid resuscitation may promote the development of congestive heart failure. Increases in the positive end-expiratory pressure can decrease preload despite a paradoxically increased CVP. Finally, increases in extrathoracic pressure, such as that caused by increased abdominal distension, can increase CVP.

The CVP waveform is divided into three components: a, c, and v waves (Fig. 28.5). Each component can be correlated with a specific portion of the electrocardiogram (ECG) tracing. The a wave occurs with atrial contraction and is seen after the P wave of the electrocardiogram during the PR interval. Thus the mean value of the a wave approximates right ventricular end-diastolic pressure. Cannon a waves (Fig. 28.6), which are enlarged a waves seen when the right atrium is ejecting against a closed tricuspid valve, may be seen when atrioventricular discordance occurs (ie, during junctional ectopic tachycardia, ventricular tachycardia, or heart block). The c wave occurs in early systole with closure of the tricuspid valve and is seen at the end of the QRS complex in the RST junction. The v wave occurs during filling of the right atrium in late systole before opening of the tricuspid valve and is seen between the T and P waves of the ECG. The v wave is increased in the setting of tricuspid regurgitation. The x descent is the decrease in pressure after the a wave, reflecting atrial relaxation. The y descent is the decrease in pressure that occurs after the v wave as the tricuspid valve opens and passive filling of the right ventricle occurs.

Continuous Mixed Venous Oxygen Saturation

Mixed venous oxygen saturation (SvO_2) can be measured continuously by using a specially designed central venous catheter. These catheters have two to three lumens and have the same capabilities of standard central venous line catheters, with the additional potential for spectrophotometric monitoring. The SvO_2 catheters use reflection spectrophotometry and are able to read hemoglobin oxygen saturation continuously. The reflected light is dependent on the oxygenated and deoxygenated hemoglobin concentration in the circulating blood.[8]

SvO_2 is another parameter used to monitor the relationship between oxygen delivery and demand and is often used as a surrogate for cardiac index. Rivers et al.[9] showed that when continuous SvO_2 monitoring was used to guide resuscitation and hemodynamic support in patients with severe sepsis and septic shock, survival rates improved. Guidelines set forth by the American College of Critical Care Medicine/Pediatric Advanced Life Support have recommended goal-directed therapy with a target SvO_2 of ≥70% in children and adolescents who are in septic shock.[7] A randomized controlled trial conducted by Oliveira and colleagues[10] supported the use of these guidelines in children and adolescents with severe sepsis or fluid-refractory septic shock. Most recently, there has been lacking evidence[11-13] to support continuous SvO_2 monitoring for early goal-directed therapy in severe sepsis and septic shock, so the role of these catheters, in light of complication risks with invasive monitoring, is still evolving.

Ideally, the catheter should be placed in the right internal jugular vein, with the tip taking measurements in the SVC. SvO_2 measurements obtained from the inferior vena cava exhibit greater variability because of fluctuations in splanchnic oxygen utilization and thus are less reliable. SvO_2 measurements from the right atrium contain coronary sinus blood and are more desaturated because of the high oxygen extraction rate of the myocardium. Studies in critically ill children have evaluated SvO_2 measurements obtained in the pulmonary artery and the SVC. Concordance analysis showed appropriate agreement in the measurements between these two sampling sites.[14] This finding has clinical importance because the use of PACs has declined, while central venous line use has increased.[15] Continuous SvO_2 monitoring can alert the intensivist to early changes in hemodynamic status, thus allowing for less frequent blood sampling through the central line and less risk of infection. Percutaneously placed SvO_2 central lines have even been used to monitor patients undergoing complex cardiac surgery, thus avoiding the risks associated with transthoracic lines following surgery.[16]

Arterial Pressure Catheters

Indications

The transition to direct monitoring of arterial blood pressure dates back to the mid-1950s when two separate studies compared invasive arterial measurements and noninvasive or cuff measurements in healthy adults.[17,18] Van Bergen and colleagues[18] noted a frequent difference between direct and indirect measurements, with indirect measurements increasingly lower than direct measurements as the systemic blood pressure increased. The greatest disparity was found in young hypertensive patients. Similarly, Cohn and Luria[19] observed that invasive arterial pressures were significantly greater than cuff pressures and emphasized the importance of direct measurements of systemic arterial pressure when caring for patients with hypotension and shock. Continuous direct monitoring of arterial blood pressure should be considered when

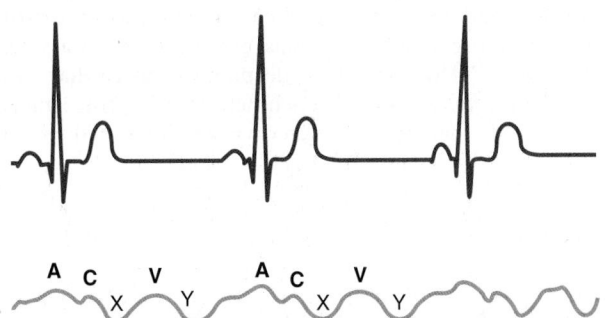

Fig. 28.5. Central venous pressure *(A)* tracing with corresponding electrocardiogram (ECG). The *a* wave is produced by atrial contraction and occurs after the P wave of the ECG during the PR interval. The *c* wave *(C)* is produced by closure of the tricuspid valve and takes place early in systole at the end of the QRS complex in the RST junction. The *v* wave *(V)* is caused by rapid filling of the right atrium late in systole before opening of the tricuspid valve and is seen between the T and P waves of the ECG. The x descent *(X)* reflects the decrease in pressure in the right atrium after the *a* wave as the tricuspid valve is pulled away from the right atrium by the right ventricle as it contracts during systole. The y descent *(Y)* is the decrease in right atrial pressure that occurs after the *v* wave as the tricuspid valve opens and blood moves from the right atrium into the right ventricle.

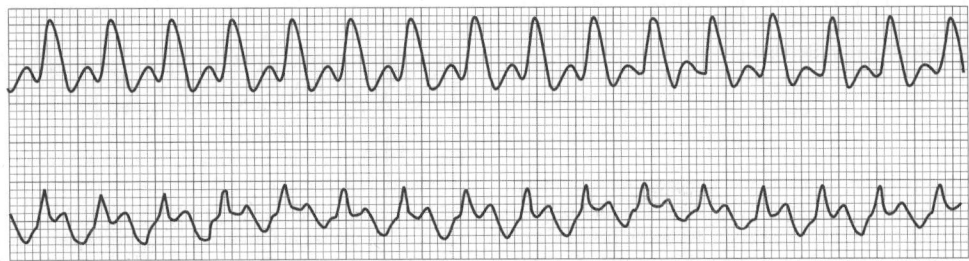

Fig. 28.6. Cannon *a* waves are enlarged *a* waves seen when the right atrium is ejecting against a closed tricuspid valve. These waves are typically seen when atrioventricular discordance occurs, such as during junctional ectopic or ventricular tachycardia or heart block.

treating patients who require more than minimal vasopressor therapy.

Indications for arterial catheterization include continuous monitoring of systemic arterial blood pressure, frequent blood sampling, and withdrawal of blood during exchange transfusions.[20] In addition to the value of the measurements themselves, these measurements provide components of derived measures of CO and oxygen delivery.

Interpretation of Waveforms

Systolic blood pressure (SBP) in children varies greatly with age and gender. As with the CVP waveform, the arterial waveform can be correlated with specific parts of the cardiac cycle. The arterial waveform has three main components (Fig. 28.7): (1) a rapid upstroke and downslope that correlates with systolic ejection, (2) a dicrotic notch that correlates with closure of the aortic valve, and (3) a smooth runoff that correlates with diastole. The dicrotic notch or incisura is decreased in situations of hyperdynamic CO in which left ventricular output and stroke volume (SV) are increased, pulse pressure is widened, and diastolic blood pressure (DBP) is increased (eg, surgical systemic-to-pulmonary shunts, patent ductus arteriosus, aortic regurgitation, anemia, fever, sepsis, hypovolemia, exercise). Conversely, cardiac tamponade and severe aortic stenosis can narrow the pulse pressure and are associated with a deflection (anacrotic notch) on the ascending limb of the waveform.[21]

Systolic pressures measured in the periphery typically are greater than those measured more centrally because of pulse amplification of pressure waves reflected back from arterial branch points[21,22] (see Fig. 28.4). More peripheral sites, such as the radial artery, have greater SBP and lower DBP than more central sites and thus taller and narrower waveforms with greater pulse pressures (difference between SBP and DBP). Important to note is that the mean arterial pressure (MAP in Eq. 28.1) represents the area under the waveform curve, and the overall magnitude of the reading remains the same regardless of the location of the tracing.

$$MAP = DBP + (SBP - DBP)/3 \qquad \text{Eq. 28.1}$$

The appearance of the arterial waveform also provides clinical information to the observer. Pulsus alternans (Fig. 28.8) is observed when regular variations occur in the amplitude of the peak systolic pressure during sinus rhythm. This phenomenon can be seen in patients with severe left ventricular failure. Pulsus paradoxus (Fig. 28.9) demonstrates an exaggerated decrease in the systolic pressure (>10 mm Hg) during the inspiratory phase of the respiratory cycle. This phenomenon can be observed in patients with pericarditis, pulmonary hyperinflation, and decreased intravascular volume.

Pulmonary Artery Catheters

History and Controversy

In 1847, Claude Bernard described a method for measuring intracardiac pressures in animals by inserting a glass tube in the heart.[23] However, the true pioneers of cardiac catheterization were two other Frenchmen: Jean Baptiste Auguste Chaveau, at that time a veterinarian interested in the

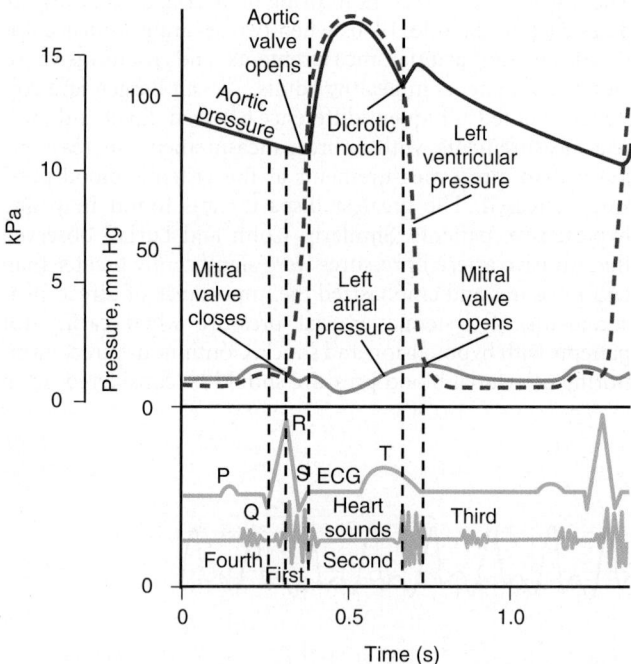

Fig. 28.7. Aortic, left ventricular, and left atrial pressure waveforms as they correspond to the electrocardiogram (ECG), opening and closing of the aortic and mitral valves, and heart sounds. Note the presence of the dicrotic notch on the descending limb of the aortic waveform. (From Peura RA. Blood pressure and sound. In: Webster JG, ed. Medical Instrumentation: Application and Design. Boston: Houghton Mifflin; 1978.)

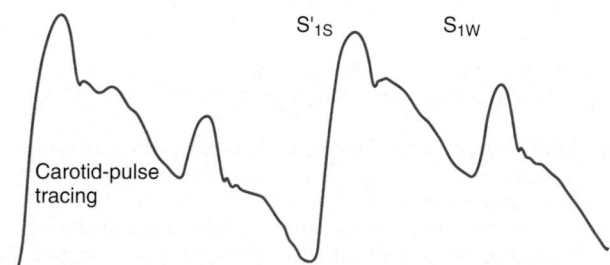

Fig. 28.8. Pulsus alternans occurs with left ventricular failure and is characterized by regular variations in the peak amplitude of systolic pressure during sinus rhythm. (Adapted from Cha K, Falk RH. Images in medicine: pulsus alternans. N Engl J Med. 1996;334:834.)

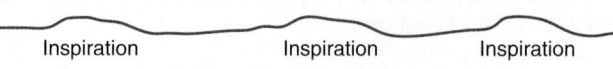

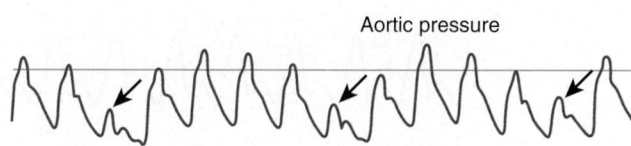

Fig. 28.9. Pulsus paradoxus is characterized by an exaggerated decrease in the systolic blood pressure during inhalation. It is commonly seen in conditions marked by great swings in intrathoracic pressure, such as in status asthmaticus, or when there are changes in cardiac function as in pericarditis. In severe hypovolemia, pulsus paradoxus also can be observed as a result of a decrease in preload. (Adapted from Wu LA, Nishimura RA. Images in clinical medicine: pulsus paradoxus. N Engl J Med. 2003;349:7.)

relationship between the dynamic motion of the heart and heart sounds, and Etienne-Jules Marey, a physician interested in the physiology of the circulation. In the early 1860s, using techniques adapted from Bernard's work, Chaveau and Marey inserted a double-lumen catheter into the right atrium of a horse to record phasic changes in intracardiac pressures as they simultaneously recorded the apical impulse.[23-26]

Right heart catheterization was not considered a safe practice in humans until the early 20th century. In 1929, Werner Forssman, a German surgeon, secretly performed a right heart catheterization on himself. In direct contradiction to his supervisor's instructions, Forssman inserted a urinary catheter into his own left antecubital vein, and then the remainder of the way to his right atrium under fluoroscopic guidance with the aid of a mirror. Forssman performed right heart catheterizations on himself a total of nine additional times without adverse consequences and expanded his findings by demonstrating the feasibility of injecting contrast dye during the procedure.[27,28]

In the early 1940s, Andres Cournand and Dickinson Richards, working at Bellevue Hospital in New York City, continued Forssman's work. They performed right heart catheterization in healthy humans and in those with cardiac failure.[28-31] In 1956, Forssman, Cournand, and Richards won the Nobel Prize in Physiology or Medicine for their discoveries relating to heart catheterization and pathologic changes in the circulatory system. They were the first investigators to measure pulmonary capillary wedge pressures using cardiac catheterization.[32,33]

In 1953, Lategola and Rahn,[34] performed experiments in dogs in which they were the first to use a self-guiding balloon-tipped catheter to measure pressures in the pulmonary circulation. Seventeen years later, Swan et al.[35] at the University of California, Los Angeles, used this technique to assess right heart pressures in humans and in doing so brought this methodology to the bedside, where it is still used today.

During the past 3 decades, much debate has occurred regarding the safety and efficacy of PACs in critically ill adults,[36-45] with multiple calls for a moratorium on PAC usage.[46,47] One randomized, controlled clinical trial underscored the lack of evidence supporting a benefit to therapy directed by PACs compared with standard care,[41] while another showed no significant effect on morbidity and mortality when PACs were used early in patients with sepsis, acute respiratory distress syndrome, or both.[42] An evidence-based review of PAC use reported no added benefit to its routine use, unless it is associated with a defined clinical protocol.[43] Shah and colleagues[44] performed a meta-analysis of 13 randomized clinical trials of the impact of PAC use in critically ill patients and found that it conferred no added benefit, nor did it cause an increase in mortality or hospital days. They concluded that use of evidence-based protocols in combination with PACs may prove to be beneficial. Studies have revealed a significant lack of knowledge and expertise on the part of physicians using PACs, suggesting the tool itself may not be the cause of the problems often associated with the PAC.[48,49] Notably, Friese and colleagues[45] reviewed more than 53,000 patients from the National Trauma Data Bank and found that PACs were used in the management of more severely injured trauma patients. They found that patients who arrived in severe shock and those aged 60 years or older had an associated survival benefit when a PAC was used.[45]

With regard to pediatric patients, the Pulmonary Artery Catheter Consensus Conference, based on a consensus of expert opinions, concluded that the PAC was useful for clarifying cardiopulmonary physiology in critically ill infants and children with pulmonary hypertension, shock refractory to fluid resuscitation and/or low-to-moderate doses of vasoactive medications, severe respiratory failure requiring high mean airway pressures, and on rare occasions, multiple organ failure. They found no data indicating that PAC use increases mortality in children; however, they also failed to find any controlled trials that proved a benefit of PAC use. The panel recommended PAC use for selected patients and called for randomized, controlled trials; a registry of PAC use; and studies to assess the impact of PAC use on cost and duration of ICU/hospital stay.[50] A further review of current studies[51] demonstrated level B and C evidence for most indications.

Indications
Although still controversial, current indications for PAC use in children include septic shock unresponsive to fluid resuscitation and vasopressor support,[52-54] refractory shock following severe burn injuries,[55] congenital heart disease (CHD),[54] multiple organ failure,[56] and respiratory failure requiring high mean airway pressures.[54,57]

Capabilities of PACs include determination of CVP, pulmonary artery pressure (PAP), and pulmonary artery occlusion pressure (PAOP), also referred to as pulmonary capillary wedge pressure (Pw). PAOP is a measurement of left atrial pressure and left ventricular end-diastolic pressure (when the mitral valve is open). PACs are also used to assess CO, SvO_2, oxygen delivery (DO_2) and consumption (VO_2), and pulmonary vascular resistance (PVR) and systemic vascular resistance (SVR). A fundamental application of the PAC is to examine the function of the right and left ventricles separately. PACs are used to establish diagnoses, guide response to therapy, and assess the determinants of oxygen delivery. PACs are especially helpful in cases of discordant ventricular function and can provide pacing.

One of the most common uses of the PAC in infants and children is monitoring pulmonary pressures during and after repair of CHD. In addition to flow-directed balloon-tipped PACs, transthoracic left atrial catheters are often used in these patients.[58] Use of PACs has altered the management of children with CHD by identifying residual anatomic defects and diagnosing pulmonary hypertensive crisis.[59,60] The ability to monitor PAP provides the means to titrate response to inhaled nitric oxide and other pulmonary vasodilators.[61,62] The lack of response to inhaled nitric oxide may suggest a residual structural anomaly in postoperative patients and indicate the need for repeat cardiac catheterization and/or repair.[62] In addition to monitoring for pulmonary hypertensive crisis, PACs can be used to assess the effects of changes in concentration of inspired CO_2 on mean pulmonary artery pressure (MPAP), pulmonary vascular resistance index (PVRI), and cardiac index (CI).[63]

Monitoring Techniques with the Pulmonary Artery Catheter

The functional features of the PAC are several. Its use as a method of indicator thermodilution, measurement of cardiac output, monitoring, and blood sampling is well documented.

Fig. 28.10 demonstrates the expected waveforms as the catheter passes through the cardiovascular system. Technical concepts are important for understanding the calculations needed for optimum use. Refer to Table 28.1 for a summary of the hemodynamic parameters that can be derived from a PAC.

Catheter Placement

PACs typically contain the following ports (Fig. 28.10). The proximal port is located 15 cm from the tip in 5-French catheters and 30 cm from the tip in larger catheters. It opens into or near the right atrium. The proximal port provides access for infusion of fluid or drugs, injection of cold saline solution as indicator (thermodilution method), CVP monitoring, and blood sampling. In infants or small children, PAC placement via the internal jugular or subclavian vein may result in the improper location of the proximal port before the right atrium such that the port lies inside the sheath or outside the body. Therefore it is essential to verify not only the placement of the distal tip in the pulmonary artery but also the location of the proximal port.

The distal port opens at the tip of the catheter. It is used for monitoring PAP and PAOP, blood sampling of mixed venous blood gases, and infusion of fluids. By monitoring pressure continuously through this port during catheter placement, the location of the tip can be determined from the characteristic pressure tracings shown in Fig. 28.10. After placement, PAP should be monitored continuously in order to identify inadvertent migration into the pulmonary capillary bed or "wedged" position. It is important to allow the catheter tip to "float" into the wedged position only when actively measuring PAOP in order to minimize risk of pulmonary artery infarct or rupture.

The balloon inflation port inflates the balloon, which is located 1 cm proximal to the catheter tip. The balloon is inflated for flow-directed catheter placement and PAOP monitoring.

The thermistor is located just proximal to the balloon and connects to a bedside computer to measure changes in the temperature of pulmonary artery blood.

The oximeter uses a fiberoptic-based sensor to continuously measure the $S\bar{v}O_2$.

Larger catheters also may have cardiac pacing ports. An adult-sized catheter is available for "continuous" CO determination when coupled with an appropriate bedside computer.

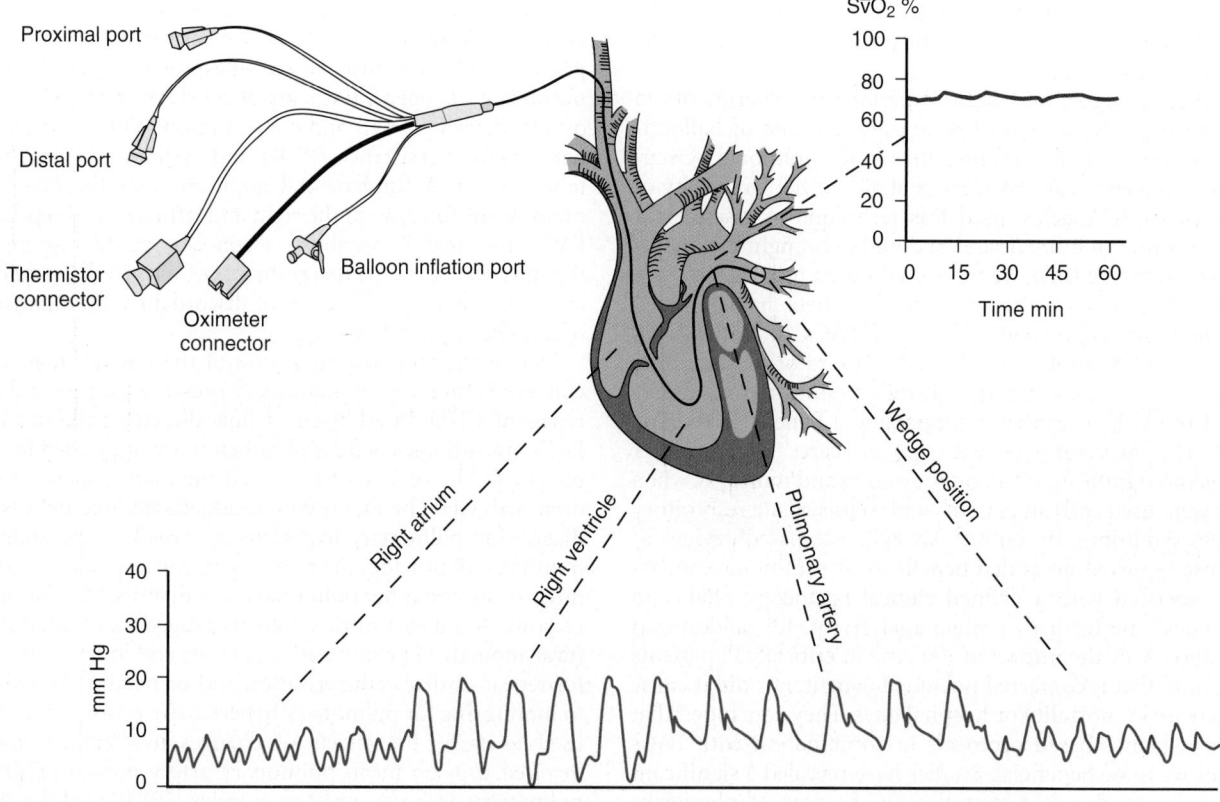

Fig. 28.10. Components and functional features of a thermodilution flow-directed pulmonary artery catheter. The flexible multilumen catheter with the balloon at the distal tip inflated is in the wedge position. The proximal ends of the five lumens are labeled. The distal port is connected to a pressure measurement system for catheter insertion and subsequent monitoring. When the distal tip is within the central venous circulation, the balloon is inflated to enhance flow direction of the tip through the right atrium into the right ventricle and then to the pulmonary artery. Recorded pressures *(lower panel)* correspond to these locations, confirming the course of the catheter. The *last tracing on the right* corresponds to the "wedge" position, commonly reflecting pressure transmitted from the left atrium via the pulmonary veins and capillaries. *Upper right panel* shows an example of a continuous $S\bar{v}O_2$ (venous oxygen saturation) tracing from the fiberoptic monitor available on adult-size catheters. (Modified from Daily EK, Tilkian AG. Hemodynamic monitoring. In: Tilkian AG, Daily EK, eds. Cardiovascular Procedures, Diagnostic Techniques and Therapeutic Procedures. St. Louis: Mosby; 1986.)

TABLE 28.1	Hemodynamic Parameters		
Parameter	**Formula**	**Normal Range**	**Units**
Cardiac index	$CI = CO/BSA$	3.5–5.5	$L/min/m^2$
Stroke index	$SI = CI/heart\ rate \times 1000$	30–60	mL/m^2
Arterial-mixed venous O_2 content difference	$avDO_2 = CaO_2 - CvO_2$	30–55	mL/L
O_2 delivery	$DO_2 = CI \times O_2$	620 ± 50	$mL/min/m^2$
O_2 consumption	$VO_2 = CI \times avDO_2$	120–200	$mL/min/m^2$
O_2 extraction ratio	$ERO_2 = avDO_2/CaO_2$	0.26 ± 0.02	
Arterial oxygen content	$(1.34 \times Hb \times SaO_2) + (PaO_2 \times 0.003)$		mL/L
Venous oxygen content	$(1.34 \times Hb \times SvO_2) + (PvO_2 \times 0.003)$		mL/L
Fick principle	$VO_2 = CO \times (CaO_2 - CvO_2)$		
Systemic vascular resistance index	$SVRI = 80 \times (MAP - CVP)/CI$	800–1600	$dyne{-}sec/cm^5/m^2$
Pulmonary vascular resistance index	$PVRI = 80 \times (MPAP - PAOP)/CI$	80–200	$dyne{-}sec/cm^5/m^2$
LV stroke work index	$LVSWI = SI \times MAP \times 0.0136$	56 ± 6	$gm{-}m/m^2$
RV stroke work index	$RVSWI = SI \times MPAP \times 0.0136$	0.5 ± 0.06	$gm{-}m/m^2$

avDO₂, arterial-mixed venous content difference; *BSA*, body surface area in m²; *CaO₂*, O₂ content of systemic arterial blood in mL/L; *CI*, cardiac index; *CO*, cardiac output; *CvO₂*, O₂ content of mixed venous blood in ml/L; *CVP*, central venous pressure in mm Hg; *DO₂*, oxygen delivery; *ERO₂*, O₂ extraction ratio; *Hb*, hemoglobin; *LVSWI*, left ventricular stroke index; *MAP*, mean systemic arterial pressure in mm Hg; 80 is the conversion factor used for the units in the table; *MPAP*, mean pulmonary arterial pressure in mm Hg; *PAWP*, pulmonary artery wedge pressure in mm Hg, which is approximately equal to the left atrial pressure under many circumstances; *PvO₂*, partial oxygen pressure in mixed venous blood; *PVRI*, pulmonary vascular resistance index; *RVSWI*, right ventricular stroke work index; *SI*, stroke index; *SvO₂*, venous oxygen saturation; *SVRI*, systemic vascular resistance index; *VO₂*, oxygen consumption. (Modified from Katz RW, Pollack MM, Weibley RE. Pulmonary artery catheterization in pediatric intensive care. In Advances in Pediatrics. Chicago: Year Book Medical Publishers; 1984.)

Indirectly Measured Variables

Measurements from PACs include directly and indirectly measured or derived variables. Directly measured variables include CVP, MAP, MPAP, PAOP, CO, SaO₂, and SvO₂. Derived parameters include CI, PVR, SVR, PVRI, and SVRI, as well as SV (in mL/beat) and stroke volume index (SVI; in mL/beat/m²). Stroke index (SI), or SVI, normally is 30 to 60 mL/m².[64,65]

$$SV = CO/HR \qquad \text{Eq. 28.2}$$

$$SVI = SV/BSA \qquad \text{Eq. 28.3}$$

Left ventricular stroke work index (LVSWI) and right ventricular stroke work index (RVSWI) normally are 56 ± 6 and 0.5 ± 0.06 gm-m/m², respectively.[64,65] Note that all values are for pediatric patients unless otherwise indicated.

$$LVSWI = SI \times MAP \times 0.0136 \qquad \text{Eq. 28.4}$$

$$RVSWI = SI \times MPAP \times 0.0136 \qquad \text{Eq. 28.5}$$

Measurement of Cardiac Output

CO is the volume of blood pumped by the heart each minute, or SV multiplied by the number of ejections per minute or HR (CO = HR × SV) and often is expressed as CI, which is CO divided by the body surface area (BSA) in m². The normal range for infants and children is approximately 3.3 to 6 L/min/m².[64,65] Two methods for calculating CO are discussed here: the Fick method and thermodilution.

Fick Method

In 1870, Adolph Fick was the first to study the relationship between blood flow and gas exchange in the lungs using a mathematic model.[66] Fick hypothesized that the amount of oxygen extracted by the body from the blood must equal the amount of oxygen taken up by the lungs during breathing. Fick also reasoned that the flow of blood through the lungs must equal the CO to the remainder of the body in the absence of a shunt. If the amount of oxygen consumed by the body and the amount of oxygen extracted by the body from the blood can be determined, then the CO can be determined. In Fick's time, oxygen consumption was measured using a basal metabolism spirometer, and the oxygen content in arterial and venous blood was measured using a rudimentary method.[66] Although Fick's method remains the gold standard, it is rarely used in the ICU because it is less practical than the more commonly used thermodilution method described in the next section. However, Fick's method is commonly used in the cardiac catheterization laboratory because the required data are readily available in this setting, although oxygen consumption, typically, is estimated.

As noted previously, Fick's equation is based on the assumption that the amount of oxygen extracted by the body from the blood equals the amount of oxygen taken up from the lungs during breathing.

The amount of oxygen extracted by the body from the blood equals the difference in oxygen content of arterial (CaO₂) and venous blood (CvO₂) in mL/L, also referred to as *arterial-mixed venous oxygen content difference* (avDO₂), multiplied by the total amount of blood pumped through the lungs or body (CO).

The oxygen content of the blood is a function of the hemoglobin (Hb) concentration of blood in g/dL, the arterial or venous oxygen saturation (SaO₂ or SvO₂) expressed in decimal form, and the arterial or venous partial pressure of arterial oxygen (PaO_2 or PvO_2) in mm Hg. The oxygen-carrying capacity of adult Hb is 1.34 mL O_2 per gram Hb, and the Bunsen solubility coefficient of O_2 in plasma at 37°C equals 0.003. A true SvO_2 is measured in the pulmonary artery; however, in the presence of an intracardiac shunt, SvO_2 should be measured in the SVC.

$$CaO_2 = 10 \times [(1.34 \times Hb \times SaO_2) + (PaO_2 \times 0.003)] \quad \text{Eq. 28.6}$$

$$CvO_2 = 10 \times [(1.34 \times Hb \times SvO_2) + (PvO_2 \times 0.003)] \quad \text{Eq. 28.7}$$

Note that the units for oxygen content in this chapter are milliliters of oxygen per liter of blood rather than milliliters of oxygen per deciliter of blood, as is in many other sources. (Thus the values for CaO_2 and CvO_2 must be converted to mL/L by multiplying in a correction factor of 10 dL/L.) Expressing oxygen content in these units allows for easy computation of CO, which is expressed as liters per minute.

The $avDO_2$ is the difference between CaO_2 and CvO_2 and normally ranges from 20 to 78 mL/L.[65]

$$avDO_2 = CaO_2 - CvO_2 \quad \text{Eq. 28.8}$$

As noted earlier, the amount of oxygen extracted (consumed) by the body from the blood equals $avDO_2$ multiplied by the amount of blood that flows through the lungs (Q_P). Assuming Q_P equals the flow of blood through the systemic circulation (Q_S), then Q_P is a measure of CO. (Note that pulmonary and systemic blood flows cannot be assumed to be identical in children with CHD with single-ventricle physiology or with shunts.)

$$O_2 \text{extraction} = (CaO_2 - CvO_2) \times CO \quad \text{Eq. 28.9}$$

The amount of oxygen taken up by the lungs equals the amount of oxygen consumed by the body. According to Fick, the amount of oxygen extracted by the body from the blood (Eq. 28.10) equals oxygen consumption (VO_2).

$$(CaO_2 - CvO_2) \times CO = VO_2 \quad \text{Eq. 28.10}$$

$$CO = VO_2 / (CaO_2 - CvO_2) \quad \text{Eq. 28.11}$$

As noted in Eqs. 28.6 and 28.7, the amount of dissolved oxygen in blood (PaO_2 or PvO_2) contributes an almost negligible amount to the oxygen content and can be left out for ease of computation. By rearranging Eq. 28.11, a rough estimate of CO can be calculated rather easily at the bedside without use of a PAC:

$$CO = VO_2 / (1.34 \times Hb \times (SaO_2 - SvO_2) \times 10) \quad \text{Eq. 28.12}$$

Oxygen consumption can be measured using the metabolic cart or taken from standardized tables.[14] Hb concentration can be measured directly. SaO_2 can be taken from the pulse oximeter. SvO_2 can be measured by the oximeter at the distal end of the PAC or determined from a venous blood gas sample from a catheter in the internal jugular or subclavian vein.

These data also can be used to calculate the intrapulmonary shunt fraction, which is the fraction of blood that passes through unventilated areas of lung:

$$Qs/Qt = (CpvO_2 - CaO_2) / (CpvO_2 - CvO_2) \quad \text{Eq. 28.13}$$

where CaO_2 is systemic arterial oxygen content and CvO_2 is mixed venous oxygen content.

$CpvO_2$ is the theoretical oxygen content in a normal pulmonary vein and can be calculated using the alveolar gas equation:

$$CpvO_2 = 10 \times [1.34 \times Hb \times SpvO_2 + PpvO_2 \times 0.003] \quad \text{Eq. 28.14}$$

where $SpvO_2$ is pulmonary vein O_2 saturation and $PpvO_2$ is pulmonary vein pO_2.

For the normal lung, $PpvO_2$ can be estimated from the alveolar air equation, and $SpvO_2$ is presumed to be 1.0:

$$PpvO_2 = PaO_2 = (PiO_2 - P_{wp}) - PaCO_2 / R \quad \text{Eq. 28.15}$$

where PaO_2 is alveolar partial pressure of oxygen, PiO_2 is inspiratory pO_2, P_{wp} is vapor pressure of water (47 mm Hg at 37°C), $PaCO_2$ is arterial CO_2, and R is respiratory quotient, which is normally assumed to be 0.8.

The normal shunt fraction is 3% to 7%.

Thermodilution Method

In 1921, Stewart[67] first described an indicator-dilution method for measuring CO. Flow was calculated by measuring the change in concentration of an indicator over time. The "ideal" indicator is "stable, nontoxic, uniformly distributed, and [does] not leave the system between sites of injection and detection. However, it should be rapidly cleared in a single circulation time to prevent recirculation interfering with measurement."[68]

In 1953, Fegler[69,70] demonstrated that a change in the heat content of blood could be used as an indicator for CO measurement. A bolus of cold liquid of a known temperature is injected into or proximal to the right atrium. A thermistor near the PAC tip in the pulmonary artery or a pulmonary artery branch measures a change in the temperature of the blood as the bolus passes by the end of the catheter. A computer calculates the flow by integrating the change in temperature at the thermistor.

The first law of thermodynamics, the conservation of heat, is the fundamental principle underlying thermodilution. Thermodilution makes several assumptions: physiologic conditions must remain constant during the period of observation, all heat exchange occurs between the indicator and the blood without heat loss to the surrounding tissues, mixing of the injectate and blood is complete upstream of the temperature measurement, and the temperature sensor is sufficiently sensitive, accurate, and rapidly responsive to depict accurately the change in temperature over time.

Measurement of CO using the thermodilution method can be understood by examining a modified version of the Stewart-Hamilton equation.[68] V_1 is injectate volume (in mL); Tb is temperature of the pulmonary artery at baseline (in degrees Celsius); Ti is temperature of the injectate (in degrees Celsius); K^1 is the density factor that equals the specific heat of the injectate multiplied by the specific gravity of the injectate, divided by the product of the specific heat and specific gravity of blood; and K^2 is a constant that figures in the dead space of the catheter and the loss of heat from the injectate as it moves through the catheter. The denominator of the equation is the integral of the change in the temperature of the blood (Tb) over time (t):

$$CO = V_1 (Tb - Ti) K^1 K^2 / \int \Delta Tb(t) dt \quad \text{Eq. 28.16}$$

The computer generates a CO curve with the area under the curve inversely related to the magnitude of the CO. In settings of low CO, less warm blood flows with the injectate and the injectate stays cooler. The difference between the injectate temperature and that of the blood remains large, and the CO curve has a high domed shape, with a slow return to baseline temperature. In situations of high CO, more pulmonary artery blood flows with the injectate and the temperature of the injectate approaches or equals that of the blood more rapidly. In these situations, because the difference between the final temperature of the injectate and that of the blood is small, the CO curve rapidly returns to baseline following a sharp spike from the cold injectate. In extreme low-flow states, the change in temperature of the injectate resulting from handling alone, before the injectate even enters the catheter from the proximal port, may be greater than the change caused by warming of the injectate by the flow of blood.

A correction factor is added to the equation to account for warming of the injectate because of handling alone; however, the correction factor may be inaccurate if the injection is too slow or the syringe is held in the injector's hands or too long. Therefore CO readings should be made as quickly as possible and should be repeated until three successive readings are within 15% of each other. Other sources of error include a falsely elevated CO because of inadvertent warming of the thermistor when it is up against the wall of the pulmonary artery. The thermodilution method generally should not be used in patients with an intracardiac shunt; however, if the shunt fraction is less than 10%, the error likely is negligible.[21]

Calculation of Oxygen Delivery and Consumption

Metabolic derangements, such as fever, sepsis, and shock, interfere with oxygen delivery (DO_2) to and consumption by (VO_2) the tissues. The SvO_2 is a measure of the oxygenation of blood returning to the heart. SvO_2 can be measured continuously by a fiberoptic oximeter (see description of PAC ports in the catheter ports section) and normally ranges from 65% to 75%. The oxygen extraction ratio (ERO_2) is $avDO_2$ (see Eq. 28.8) divided by CaO_2 (Eq. 28.11) and usually is approximately 25%[64,65]:

$$ERO_2 = avDO_2/CaO_2 \qquad \text{Eq. 28.17}$$

DO_2 also can be expressed as the product of CI and CaO_2 and VO_2 as the product of CI and $avDO_2$. The normal value for DO_2 is 620 ± 50 mL/min/m², whereas VO_2 typically ranges from 120 to 200 mL/min/m².[64,65]

$$DO_2 = CI \times CaO_2 \qquad \text{Eq. 28.18}$$

$$VO_2 = CI \times avDO_2 \qquad \text{Eq. 28.19}$$

Interpretation of Waveforms

The waveforms corresponding to the right atrium and the systemic arterial blood pressure were discussed in previous sections. The pressure in the right atrium ranges from approximately 3 to 12 mm Hg. As the PAC passes into the right ventricle, the diastolic pressure drops to 0 to 10 mm Hg and the systolic pressure increases to 13 to 42 mm Hg. As the catheter enters the pulmonary artery, the diastolic pressure increases to 3 to 21 mm Hg while the systolic pressure remains relatively similar to that of the right ventricle, 11 to 36 mm Hg. Once the catheter tip advances into the pulmonary capillary bed and the pulmonary artery is occluded by the inflated balloon, the measured pressure decreases to 2 to 14 mm Hg.[21]

By recognizing the changes in the various tracings, the movement of the catheter tip can be followed through the chambers of the right heart and into the pulmonary circulation, without simultaneous imaging.

The waveforms are affected by the components of the respiratory cycle. As expected, the effects of respiration differ during unsupported breathing (negative pressure) versus mechanical ventilation (positive pressure). During normal unsupported ventilation, PAPs decrease during inhalation and increase during exhalation. In contrast, during mechanical ventilation, PAP increases during inhalation and decreases during exhalation. The cyclical changes induced by the respiratory cycle cause the tracings to take on a sinusoidal pattern once the tip of the catheter enters the thorax. The effects of respiration on PAC determinations can be minimized by measuring pressures at the end of expiration, when pleural pressures are closest to zero.

Because CVP is a measure of preload or filling of the right ventricle, it reflects changes in volume status, right ventricular function, and pulmonary vascular tone. Similarly, PAOP measures filling pressures of the left atrium and ventricle. When the pulmonary artery is occluded, the pressure from the left atrium is transmitted back to the catheter tip. During diastole, when the mitral valve is open and the aortic valve is closed, a continuous fluid-filled column is formed from the catheter tip to the left ventricle and PAOP is equivalent to the left ventricular end-diastolic pressure. In patients with cardiogenic shock, an elevated PAOP may reflect decreased function of the left ventricle. In this situation, rather than providing further fluid resuscitation or preload, increasing contractility or decreasing afterload may be preferable. Afterload is the load that the heart must eject blood against and is inversely related to SV (volume of blood ejected by the heart with each beat) and CO. It is determined by the impedance of the vasculature, ejection pressure, preload, and ventricular wall stress.

According to Laplace's law, ventricular wall stress (T) is proportional to ventricular transluminal pressure (P) (Intraluminal pressure – Extraluminal pressure) and radius (r) and is inversely related to twice the wall thickness (t):

$$T = P \times r/2t \qquad \text{Eq. 28.20}$$

For a given pressure, wall stress is increased by an increase in radius (ventricular dilation); therefore volume administration may increase ventricular diameter and consequently wall stress. Thus afterload is preload dependent. Similarly, during spontaneous breathing the transluminal pressure and consequently the wall stress increase, whereas during mechanical ventilation (positive pressure) the transluminal pressure and wall stress both decrease. Ventricular hypertrophy increases wall thickness and therefore decreases wall stress.

Resistance

To understand resistance, returning to Ohm's law is helpful: voltage (V) varies directly with resistance (R) and current (I):

$$V = IR \qquad \text{Eq. 28.21}$$

Rearranging Eq. 28.21 by substituting pressure for voltage and flow for current gives Eq. 28.22:

$$R = (Pin - Pout)/Q \qquad \text{Eq. 28.22}$$

where R is resistance, *Pin* is pressure going into a vessel, *Pout* is pressure exiting the vessel, and Q is flow. According to

Poiseuille's law, the resistance of flow through a tube varies directly with the viscosity of the fluid and the length of the tube and is inversely proportional to the radius to the fourth power multiplied by pi (π):

$$R = 8\eta l/\pi r^4 \qquad \text{Eq. 28.23}$$

where η is viscosity, l is length, and r is radius. Unfortunately, Poiseuille's law assumes uniform viscosity, length, and radius, none of which holds true in the case of the pulmonary or systemic circulation; however, the principles behind the law are valuable in understanding the major determinants of resistance.

By substituting the appropriate values into Eq. 28.20, the formulas for SVR and PVR can be derived. CO is substituted for Qs and Qp in the absence of a right-to-left or left-to-right shunt or single-ventricle physiology. In the case of the equation for PVR (Eq. 28.25), PAOP is substituted for pulmonary vein pressure in determining Pout:

$$SVR = (MAP - CVP)/CO \qquad \text{Eq. 28.24}$$

$$PVR = (MPAP - PAOP)/CO \qquad \text{Eq. 28.25}$$

SVR and PVR are measured in mm Hg $\times$ minute $\times$ L^{-1} (or mm Hg/L per min). These units also are referred to as hybrid resistance units or Wood units after the cardiologist Paul Wood.[18] By multiplying by 80, hybrid resistance units or Wood units can be converted to the centimeter-gram-seconds (cgs) system, where resistance is measured as dynes sec/cm^5, also known as absolute resistance units.

PVR and SVR often are indexed for BSA (in square meters). The systemic vascular resistance index (SVRI) and pulmonary vascular resistance index (PVRI) are measured as dynes sec/cm^5/m^2:

$$SVRI = 80 \times (MAP - CVP)/CI \qquad \text{Eq. 28.26}$$

$$PVRI = 80 \times (MPAP - PAOP)/CI \qquad \text{Eq. 28.27}$$

SVRI usually is 800 to 1600 dynes sec/cm^5/m^2 in children[65,66] and 2180 $\pm$ 210 in adults.[71]

Calculation of Intracardiac Shunt

If the oxygen saturations throughout the cardiopulmonary circulation are known, derivation of the values for the ratio of pulmonary to systemic blood flow or intracardiac shunt (Qp/Qs) is possible:

$$Qp = VO_2/(1.34 \times 10 \times Hb (SpvO_2 - SpaO_2)) \qquad \text{Eq. 28.28}$$

$$Qs = VO_2/(1.34 \times 10 \times Hb (SaO_2 - SvO_2)) \qquad \text{Eq. 28.29}$$

$$Qp/Qs = (SaO_2 - SvO_2)/(SpvO_2 - SpaO_2) \qquad \text{Eq. 28.30}$$

where $SpvO_2$ is oxygen saturation in the pulmonary vein and $SpaO_2$ is oxygen saturation in the pulmonary artery. In the absence of severe intrapulmonary shunt, $SpvO_2$ approaches 98% to 100%. In a complete mixing lesion, $SpaO_2$ and SaO_2 should be equal by definition, enabling SaO_2 to be substituted for $SpaO_2$.

Novel Monitoring Devices

Recent application of novel devices has started bridging invasive and noninvasive monitoring of cardiac output. Modalities such as pulse wave analysis,[72] Doppler ultrasound,[73] bioimpedance,[74,75] and electrical velocimetry[76,77] have been validated to varying degrees and introduced into limited pediatric intensive care practice. These methods are noninvasive or relatively noninvasive in nature and often use algorithms that do not require frequent calibration. Their use may be limited by an understanding of the appropriateness of the data that they provide. Although the long-term utilization of such devices is not yet established, their relative ease of use or in placement, often using in-situ central venous catheters and arterial lines, in comparison with the PAC, as well as independence of influence from mechanical ventilation and additional monitoring capabilities, make them attractive to practitioners.

Conclusions

Invasive hemodynamic monitoring provides the intensivist with valuable information regarding the condition of critically ill children. Correct interpretation of this information is necessary to optimally aid in the management of these patients whose condition is often complex. New noninvasive monitoring modalities are emerging that may eventually supplant the need for these invasive measurements, but thus far invasive monitoring remains a cornerstone of pediatric critical care medicine.

Key References

1. Hales S. *Statical Essays: Containing Haemastaticks; or, an Account of Some Hydraulick and Hydrostatical Experiments Made on the Blood and Blood-Vessels of Animals.* London: Innis, Manby, and Woodward; 1733.
2. Tobin M. *Principles and Practice of Intensive Care Monitoring.* New York: McGraw-Hill; 1998.
3. Webster J. *Medical Instrumentation.* Boston: Houghton Mifflin Company; 1978.
4. Bronzino J. *The Biomedical Engineering Handbook.* Boca Raton, FL: CRC Press; 1995.
5. Lowrie L, Difiore J, Martin R. Monitoring in the pediatric and neonatal intensive care units. In: Tobin JMM, ed. *Principles and Practice of Intensive Care Monitoring.* San Francisco, CA: McGraw-Hill; 1998.
6. Heitmiller EWR. Hemodynamic monitoring considerations in pediatric critical care. In: Rogers M, ed. *Textbook Pediatric Intensive Care.* Baltimore: William & Wilkins; 1996.
7. Carcillo JA, Fields AI. Clinical practice parameters for hemodynamic support of pediatric and neonatal patients in septic shock. *Crit Care Med.* 2002;30:1365-1378.
9. Rivers E, Nguyen B, Havstad S, et al. Early goal-directed therapy in the treatment of severe sepsis and septic shock. *N Engl J Med.* 2001;345:1368-1377.
10. De Oliveira CF, de Oliveira DS, Gottschald AF, et al. ACCM/PALS haemodynamic support guidelines for paediatric septic shock: an outcomes comparison with and without monitoring central venous oxygen saturation. *Intensive Care Med.* 2008;34:1065-1075.
11. Yealy DM, Kellum JA, Huang DT, et al. A randomized trial of protocol-based care for early septic shock. *N Engl J Med.* 2014;370:1683-1693.
12. Peake SL, Delaney A, Bailey M, et al. Goal-directed resuscitation for patients with early septic shock. *N Engl J Med.* 2014;371:141001063014008.
13. Mouncey PR, Osborn TM, Power GS, et al. Trial of early, goal-directed resuscitation for septic shock. *N Engl J Med.* 2015;372:1301-1311.
14. Perez AC, Eulmesekian PG, Minces PG, Schnitzler EJ. Adequate agreement between venous oxygen saturation in right atrium and pulmonary artery in critically ill children. *Pediatr Crit Care Med.* 2009;10:76-79.
16. Muller M, Lohr T, Scholz S, et al. Continuous SvO$_2$ measurement in infants undergoing congenital heart surgery—first clinical experiences with a new fiberoptic probe. *Paediatr Anaesth.* 2007;17:51-55.
17. Roberts LN, Smiley JR, Manning GW. A comparison of direct and indirect blood-pressure determinations. *Circulation.* 1953;8:232-242.

18. Van Bergen FH, Weatherhead DS, Treloar AE, et al. Comparison of indirect and direct methods of measuring arterial blood pressure. *Circulation.* 1954;10:481-490.

19. Cohn JN, Luria MH. Studies in clinical shock and hypotension; the value of bedside hemodynamic observations. *JAMA.* 1964;190:891-896.

20. Kaye W. Invasive monitoring techniques: arterial cannulation, bedside pulmonary artery catheterization, and arterial puncture. *Heart Lung.* 1983;12:395-427.

21. Vargo T. Cardiac catheterization: hemodynamic measurements. In: Garson A, Fisher D, Neish S, eds. *Science and Practice of Pediatric Cardiology.* Baltimore, MD: Williams & Wilkins; 1998.

22. Murgo JP, Westerhof N, Giolma JP, Altobelli SA. Aortic input impedance in normal man: relationship to pressure wave forms. *Circulation.* 1980; 62:105-116.

35. Swan HJ, Ganz W, Forrester J, et al. Catheterization of the heart in man with use of a flow-directed balloon-tipped catheter. *N Engl J Med.* 1970; 283:447-451.

47. Dalen JE, Bone RC. Is it time to pull the pulmonary artery catheter? *JAMA.* 1996;276:916-918.

48. Iberti TJ, Fischer EP, Leibowitz AB, et al. A multicenter study of physicians' knowledge of the pulmonary artery catheter. Pulmonary Artery Catheter Study Group. *JAMA.* 1990;264:2928-2932.

49. Gnaegi A, Feihl F, Perret C. Intensive care physicians' insufficient knowledge of right-heart catheterization at the bedside: time to act? *Crit Care Med.* 1997;25:213-220.

50. Taylor R, Ahrens T, Yaakov B, PACCCP. Pulmonary Artery Catheter Consensus Conference: Consensus Statement. *Crit Care Med.* 1997;25:910.

51. Perkin RM, Anas N. Pulmonary artery catheters. *Pediatr Crit Care Med.* 2011;12:S12-S20.

52. Carcillo JA, Davis AL, Zaritsky A. Role of early fluid resuscitation in pediatric septic shock. *JAMA.* 1991;266:1242-1245.

53. Mercier JC, Beaufils F, Hartmann JF, Azema D. Hemodynamic patterns of meningococcal shock in children. *Crit Care Med.* 1988;16:27-33.

54. Pollack MM, Reed TP, Holbrook PR, Fields AI. Bedside pulmonary artery catheterization in pediatrics. *J Pediatr.* 1980;96:274-276.

55. Reynolds EM, Ryan DP, Sheridan RL, Doody DP. Left ventricular failure complicating severe pediatric burn injuries. *J Pediatr Surg.* 1995;30:264-269, discussion 269-270.

56. Thompson AE. Pulmonary artery catheterization in children. *New Horiz.* 1997;5:244-250.

57. DeBruin W, Notterman DA, Magid M, et al. Acute hypoxemic respiratory failure in infants and children: clinical and pathologic characteristics. *Crit Care Med.* 1992;20:1223-1234.

58. Wheedon D, Shore DF, Lincoln C. Continuous monitoring of pulmonary artery pressure after cardiac surgery in infants and children. *J Cardiovasc Surg (Torino).* 1981;22:307-311.

59. Damen J, Wever JE. The use of balloon-tipped pulmonary artery catheters in children undergoing cardiac surgery. *Intensive Care Med.* 1987;13:266-272.

60. Hopkins RA, Bull C, Haworth SG, et al. Pulmonary hypertensive crises following surgery for congenital heart defects in young children. *Eur J Cardiothorac Surg.* 1991;5:628-634.

61. Atz AM, Adatia I, Jonas RA, Wessel DL. Inhaled nitric oxide in children with pulmonary hypertension and congenital mitral stenosis. *Am J Cardiol.* 1996;77:316-319.

62. Adatia I, Atz AM, Jonas RA, Wessel DL. Diagnostic use of inhaled nitric oxide after neonatal cardiac operations. *J Thorac Cardiovasc Surg.* 1996; 112:1403-1405.

63. Morray JP, Lynn AM, Mansfield PB. Effect of pH and PCO_2 on pulmonary and systemic hemodynamics after surgery in children with congenital heart disease and pulmonary hypertension. *J Pediatr.* 1988;113:474-479.

64. Cayler GG, Rudolph AM, Nadas AS. Systemic blood flow in infants and children with and without heart disease. *Pediatrics.* 1963;32:186-201.

65. Krovetz LJ, McLoughlin TG, Mitchell MB, Schiebler GL. Hemodynamic findings in normal children. *Pediatr Res.* 1967;1:122-130.

66. Gottschall CA. The greatest medical discovery of the millennium (Fundamental steps to the understanding of cardiac performance). *Arq Bras Cardiol.* 1999;73:320-330.

68. Moise SF, Sinclair CJ, Scott DH. Pulmonary artery blood temperature and the measurement of cardiac output by thermodilution. *Anaesthesia.* 2002;57:562-566.

70. Fegler G. Measurement of cardiac output in anesthetized animals by a thermodilution method. *Q J Exp Physiol.* 1954;39:153-164.

71. Shoemaker W, Chang P, Bland R, Al E. Cardiorespiratory monitoring in postoperative patients: Pulmonary Artery Catheter Consensus Conference: consensus statement. *Crit Care Med.* 1979;7:243-249.

72. Kim JJ, Dreyer WJ, Chang AC, et al. Arterial pulse wave analysis: an accurate means of determining cardiac output in children. *Pediatr Crit Care Med.* 2006;7:532-535.

73. Tibby SM, Hatherill M, Murdoch IA. Use of transesophageal Doppler ultrasonography in ventilated pediatric patients: derivation of cardiac output. *Crit Care Med.* 2000;28:2045-2050.

74. Tibballs J. A comparative study of cardiac output in neonates supported by mechanical ventilation: measurement with thoracic electrical bioimpedance and pulsed Doppler ultrasound. *J Pediatr.* 1989;3476(89): 80710-80713.

75. Belik J, Pelech A. Thoracic electric bioimpedance measurement of cardiac output in the newborn infant. *J Pediatr.* 1988;113:890-895.

76. Blohm ME, Obrecht D, Hartwich J, et al. Impedance cardiography (electrical velocimetry) and transthoracic echocardiography for non-invasive cardiac output monitoring in pediatric intensive care patients: a prospective single-center observational study. n.d.

77. Norozi K, Beck C, Osthaus WA, et al. Electrical velocimetry for measuring cardiac output in children with congenital heart disease. *Br J Anaesth.* 2008;100(1):88-94.

Assessment of Cardiovascular Function

Melvin C. Almodovar, Thomas J. Kulik, and John R. Charpie

PEARLS

- Cardiovascular assessment and monitoring in the pediatric intensive care unit require careful integration of physical findings, laboratory studies, and electronic data to make appropriate therapeutic decisions.
- Noninvasive monitoring includes physical examination, chest radiography, echocardiography, blood pressure monitoring, and pulse oximetry. Invasive monitoring includes intravascular and intracardiac monitoring, cardiac output measurements (thermodilution or Fick method), and laboratory studies.
- Appreciating the quantity of therapy required to achieve and sustain adequate systemic oxygen delivery and perfusion pressure is useful for the clinician to understand the patient's overall condition, discern the patient's trajectory, and anticipate associated consequences of current management choices.
- Management of patients with single-ventricle physiology (such as the neonate with hypoplastic left heart syndrome) poses several unique challenges to the cardiac intensivist, including optimization of pulmonary-to-systemic blood flow ratios for best systemic oxygen delivery.

Pediatric patients undergoing surgical treatment for congenital heart disease (CHD) or those with severe systemic illnesses such as sepsis and other causes of multiple organ system failure commonly have impaired cardiovascular function.[1,2] In addition to treating the primary disease process, the pediatric intensivist should use strategies to reliably assess and monitor cardiovascular function, which specifically involve assessing adequacy of oxygen delivery (DO_2) and systemic perfusion pressure, the primary determinants of tissue oxygenation.

Cardiovascular Function

The function of the heart and vasculature is to deliver oxygen (O_2) and other nutrients to various tissues in order to meet the metabolic demands of the organism. Mild to moderate depression of DO_2 is normally compensated by augmented O_2 extraction at the tissue level, thereby maintaining a stable level of oxygen consumption (VO_2). When DO_2 falls below some critical level, this compensatory mechanism fails and a state of O_2 supply dependency exists[3] such that any further drop in DO_2 leads to a parallel fall in VO_2.[4-6] Under a state of supply-dependent O_2 consumption, affected tissues and organs attempt to maintain homeostasis partly through anaerobic metabolism. Several studies suggest the initial metabolic response to hypoxemia or decreased DO_2 differs between the newborn and older ages and varies among different vascular beds. In adults at rest, DO_2 is in great excess of VO_2. This "O_2 surplus" means moderate reductions of O_2 transport are generally well tolerated without compromise of VO_2. In contrast to the adult, the metabolism of the newborn may be particularly susceptible to modest alterations in O_2 transport because of the high resting demands for O_2, the ease with which these demands can be increased by small environmental changes, and the apparently limited reserve for augmenting cardiac output (CO) or O_2 extraction acutely.[7,8] Thus it is crucial that cardiovascular assessment and monitoring in the pediatric intensive care unit (PICU) involve continuous and reliable evaluation of the adequacy of systemic perfusion and DO_2 in order to select appropriate hemodynamic support strategies.

Quantity of Therapy

If one considers hemodynamic monitoring not only in terms of DO_2 and perfusion pressure but also in terms of what therapy is required to produce a given level of tissue oxygenation, one gains a much better understanding of the overall "condition" of the patient. It is therefore important to monitor not only DO_2 and perfusion pressure but also the "quantity of therapy" (QOT) needed to procure and maintain adequate tissue oxygenation. Consider two hypothetical 6-month-old infants, Destiny and Dakota, 2 hours after repair of tetralogy of Fallot. They have identical (and adequate) DO_2 and perfusion pressure, but Destiny has a left atrial (LA) pressure of 6 mm Hg and a right atrial (RA) pressure of 8 mm Hg, whereas Dakota has received volume infusion to achieve an LA pressure of 6 mm Hg and an RA pressure of 15 mm Hg. Assuming that the levels of intravascular volume provided are exactly those needed to achieve the (identical) DO_2 values and perfusion pressures, it is clear that the physiologies of these two patients are different. The clinician who has learned what to expect relative to the QOT in any given set of circumstances will find Dakota's sufficient tissue oxygenation only mildly reassuring and asks: Is there substantial residual right ventricular (RV) outflow tract obstruction or another problem or problems that I need to know about? Will Dakota have sufficient DO_2 in 10 hours when post–bypass myocardial depression is at its worst? Might additional therapy secure adequate DO_2 at a lower filling pressure, thereby minimizing adverse effects of systemic venous hypertension? As this example illustrates, the QOT concept is useful for three reasons:

1. The QOT is, in part, a function of the patient's overall "condition" and can reflect anatomic or physiologic problems that require further exploration.

2. Physiologic trajectory is key, especially early in the course of certain illnesses or after cardiopulmonary bypass, when DO_2 predictably declines over the first 12 hours.[2] Taking into account the QOT relative to tissue oxygenation at any point in time helps one better estimate the likelihood of the need for augmented support (eg, mechanical support of the circulation) as time passes.

3. Some therapies (eg, fluid infusion to obtain high filling pressure, or high airway pressure), while helpful at a point in time, can be pernicious over the longer run: High venous pressure, especially in infants, causes third spacing of fluid, and the effect of ventilator-associated lung injury on lung function can be devastating. By using high central venous or airway pressures, the intensivist is, in effect, incurring a debt to secure short-term perfusion that will have to be repaid later. Experienced clinicians always take the QOT into account in their work, thus influencing their level of concern about a patient and guiding subsequent timing and choice in adjusting therapy.

Almost any form of therapy might be included in the QOT concept, but in this chapter we focus on medical therapies that have the most important effect on hemodynamics, including DO_2 and perfusion pressure. These therapies include inotropic/vasoactive agents, volume infusion, and airway pressures used during mechanical ventilation. The amount of inotropic and vasoactive drugs administered, assuming that they are used appropriately, seems to be a crude indicator of patient illness.[2] Volume infusion to achieve adequate filling pressure is required even for the normal heart, but the QOT concept applies when higher than normal filling pressure is needed to maintain adequate CO. The consequences of high filling pressures are body edema (especially in infants), pleural and other cavity space effusions, and pulmonary edema. If high venous pressure is coupled with systemic hypotension (eg, with a "failing" Fontan circulation), there may be critically reduced transtissue perfusion pressure with a potentially negative impact on cerebral and splanchnic perfusion.

With respect to mechanical ventilation, the need for high mean airway pressure (P_{aw}) is most commonly a reflection of lung disease, but pulmonary edema on a hydrodynamic basis may occasion the use of high P_{aw} for optimal lung recruitment. High P_{aw} can reduce venous return to the heart, increase pulmonary vascular resistance (PVR), and contribute to ventilator-associated lung injury.

Variables That Determine Tissue Oxygenation

Tissue oxygenation is directly related to both DO_2 and systemic arterial blood pressure (SAP). DO_2, the quantity of O_2 delivered to the tissues per minute, is the product of systemic blood flow (SBF), which equals CO except in patients with certain cardiac malformations, and arterial O_2 content:

$$DO_2 \, (mL/min) = 10 \times CO \, (L/min) \times CaO_2$$
$$(mL/100 \, mL \, blood),$$

where *CO* is cardiac output or SBF in L/min or $L/min/m^2$ and CaO_2 is quantity of O_2 bound to hemoglobin plus the quantity of O_2 dissolved in the plasma in arterial blood. The O_2 content of arterial blood (mL O_2/dL blood) equals:

$$CaO_2 = (SaO_2 \times Hgb \times 1.36) + (PaO_2 \times 0.003)$$

where SaO_2 is arterial O_2 saturation, *Hgb* is hemoglobin concentration (g/dL), *1.36* (constant) is the amount of O_2 bound per gram of hemoglobin (mL) at 1 atm of pressure, PaO_2 is arterial partial pressure of O_2, and *0.003* (constant) multiplied by the PaO_2 equals amount of O_2 dissolved in plasma at 1 atm. The quantity of dissolved O_2 is generally considered to be negligible in the normal range of PaO_2. Hypoxia, because of poor gas exchange within the lungs (ie, intrapulmonary shunt), or in the setting of CHD with right-to-left shunting, is an important determinant of blood O_2 content.

CO is the product of stroke volume (quantity of blood ejected per beat) and heart rate, and SAP is determined by CO and systemic vascular resistance (SVR). The four primary determinants of cardiac function are preload (which determines the precontractile lengths of the myofibrils); end-systolic wall stress (function of systemic blood pressure and physical characteristics of the arterial system, ventricular wall thickness, and chamber dimension); myocardial contractility; and heart rate. These determinants of ventricular function can be altered by many factors in the intensive care setting. Preload, or end-diastolic volume, is affected by ventricular compliance (rate and extent of cardiomyocyte relaxation and cardiac connective tissue), intravascular volume, and intrathoracic pressure. Expansion of the heart resulting from transmural filling pressure, rather than the LA pressure per se, determines the force of contraction. Therefore intrathoracic (or intrapericardial) pressure is a key determinant of preload. Ventricular hypertrophy, vasodilator and diuretic therapies, and positive pressure mechanical ventilation all adversely affect preload. Similarly, cardiac function is inversely related to afterload, or end-systolic wall stress. Anatomic obstructions and systemic or pulmonary hypertension may negatively affect ventricular systolic and diastolic function. Excessively fast or slow heart rates and inappropriately timed atrial contraction (relative to ventricular systole) may negatively affect ventricular function. Finally, myocardial contractility is often negatively affected by the following factors: hypoxemia, acidosis, hypomagnesemia, hypocalcemia, hypoglycemia, hyperkalemia, cardiac surgery, sepsis, and cardiomyopathies.

Monitoring Tissue Oxygenation

CO can be assessed qualitatively by physical examination and other modalities and quantitatively by a variety of techniques using invasive and noninvasive devices, laboratory data, and other clinical indicators. DO_2 is easily derived if systemic blood flow can be measured, but it is only indirectly inferred if this information is lacking.

Qualitative Assessment of Cardiac Output
Physical Examination
The physical examination is often the initial and the most common technique used to assess and monitor cardiovascular function. Significantly diminished CO may manifest as diminished peripheral pulses, cool or mottled extremities, and delayed capillary refill. However, certain clinical signs of low

CO may be unreliable depending on the particular diagnosis. For example, in the context of cardiac lesions associated with a large arterial pulse pressure (eg, severe aortic insufficiency and aortopulmonary shunts), peripheral pulses may be increased despite low CO and reduced systemic DO_2. Patients in septic shock are often peripherally vasodilated and warm despite hypotension and reduced tissue DO_2. Impaired oxygenation may present as cyanosis of the skin, lips, and/or nail beds. Central cyanosis from either cardiac or respiratory causes results from arterial O_2 desaturation. In contrast, peripheral cyanosis results from vasoconstriction and low blood flow at the microcirculatory level. In some patients, cyanosis is a relatively subtle physical finding, particularly if the patient is anemic or has a dark complexion. Hydration status can be assessed by skin turgor, dryness of mucous membranes, and fullness of the anterior fontanel (in infants), but these manifestations of hydration status relate mostly to interstitial fluid and may poorly reflect intravascular volume, which must be directly measured.

Cardiac auscultation for abnormal heart sounds, including valve clicks, rubs, gallops, and murmurs, may provide the first indication of a significant functional or structural cardiac abnormality, although these sounds do not directly reflect DO_2. Unfortunately, the lack of a heart murmur, especially in low CO states, does not necessarily rule out a significant residual cardiac lesion. The presence of crackles on pulmonary auscultation, particularly in the older pediatric patient, may signify pulmonary edema. However, crackles are nonspecific and may be caused by lung disease or fluid overload, in addition to disorders of cardiac structure or function. Finally, jugular venous distension and hepatomegaly are indicative of high right-sided filling pressures often associated with RV dysfunction.

Chest Radiography

Although the chest radiograph is of little value in assessing a patient's hemodynamic profile per se, it may be helpful for assessing certain aspects related to cardiovascular status. Provided the chest radiograph is technically adequate, the clinician can assess heart size, contour and configuration, pulmonary vascularity, pleural effusions, lung parenchyma, and abdominal situs. Some of these findings, when abnormal, may help determine the etiology of cardiovascular dysfunction. Increased pulmonary arterial vasculature may be indicated by enlarged pulmonary arteries in the hila that radiate toward the periphery of the lung. Conditions that increase pulmonary blood flow (PBF, or Q_p) at least twice normal also increase the size of the pulmonary arteries. Increased pulmonary capillary pressure may be inferred by the presence of pulmonary edema. The edema may present as a "fluffy" hilum but may have a more diffuse granular appearance in neonates. Pleural effusions may accompany pulmonary edema, particularly in conditions associated with poorly compensated congestive heart failure. Increased pulmonary venous markings are indicative of elevated pulmonary venous pressures of any cause, although usually from decreased left ventricular compliance or obstruction in the pulmonary veins or left atrium.

In the early postoperative period, the most important information obtained from the chest radiograph is (1) the positions of the endotracheal tube, chest tubes, and intracardiac lines; (2) the presence of extrapulmonary fluid or air; and (3) the presence of pulmonary edema. The cardiothoracic ratio gives a quantitative estimate of cardiac size, which is obtained by dividing the transverse measurement of the cardiac shadow in the posteroanterior view by the width of the thoracic cavity. Cardiomegaly is present if this value is greater than 0.5 in adults and 0.6 in infants. Although useful for assessing left ventricular (LV) enlargement, the cardiothoracic ratio is not as sensitive to RV enlargement. RV enlargement results in lateral and upward displacement of the cardiac apex on the posteroanterior view and filling of the retrosternal space on the lateral view. It is perhaps more important to know what the chest radiograph may not reveal; significant cardiac problems, such as constrictive pericarditis, acute fulminant myocarditis, and even acute pericardial tamponade are often associated with a normal-sized heart on a chest radiograph.

Quantitative Assessment of Cardiac Output

Quantitative measures of CO in the ICU can be obtained by a variety of techniques, including the Fick method, thermodilution, dye dilution techniques, and Doppler echocardiography. Each of the first three methods applies a similar principle of dilution of an indicator: O_2, cold, or indocyanine green dye, respectively. The change in concentration of a substance is proportional to the volume of blood in which it is being diluted. In general, thermodilution is the method most widely used in the intensive care setting. However, for conditions of low CO, the Fick method is more reliable than the thermodilution or dye dilution techniques. Conversely, the Fick method is less accurate in conditions of high systemic blood flow because of difficulty in measuring narrow arteriovenous O_2 differences in the blood.

Thermodilution Technique

The thermodilution technique requires use of a specialized pulmonary artery (PA) catheter. CO is calculated by injecting a known volume of iced water or saline solution into the right atrium (proximal catheter port) and measuring the temperature change at the catheter tip in the PA. CO is calculated by the following equation:

$$CO = 1.08 \times V_i(T_b - T_i)/e_0 T_b(t)dt$$

where V_i is injectate volume (mL), T_b is temperature of blood, T_i is injectate temperature, and $T_b(t)dt$ is area under the curve. In general, thermodilution CO measures are performed using a completely automated system, and the calculations are performed by a computer. This method (as with any indicator dilution method) requires complete mixing and thus is most accurate in situations where a mixing chamber is located proximal to the thermistor. It is generally used only in patients who do not have intracardiac or great vessel–level shunts or an insufficient valve between the injection site and the sampling site. The injection must be made rapidly because a slow injection will give a falsely elevated CO. Possible sources of error with this method include inaccurate measurement of the volume of injectate or temperature of the blood or injectate, close approximation of the thermistor to a vessel wall, and inadequate mixing, as is sometimes seen in venous systems with low flow.

Fick Method

According to the Fick principle, CO equals O_2 consumption divided by the arteriovenous O_2 content difference:

$$CO = VO_2/(CaO_2 - CvO_2)$$

where VO_2 is O_2 consumption (mL/min) and CaO_2 and CvO_2 are arterial and venous O_2 content (mL O_2/100 mL blood), respectively. Care must be taken to select the appropriate sampling site for a true mixed venous blood sample. With a normal heart, the best site to obtain a mixed venous sample is within the PA. If a left-to-right shunt is present, however, the mixed venous site should be the cardiac chamber proximal to the site of the shunt. When a site other than the PA is used for the mixed venous site, the resultant value for arteriovenous O_2 difference is a less reliable reflection of the absolute CO, but it can be used for serial observations and for monitoring response to therapy over time.

Because measuring VO_2 in the intensive care setting requires special equipment and is somewhat cumbersome, the arteriovenous O_2 difference is often used as an indirect measure of CO. A wide arteriovenous O_2 difference generally reflects a low CO and indicates a large O_2 extraction by the tissues, whereas a narrow arteriovenous O_2 difference usually reflects a high CO. Unfortunately, studies suggest VO_2 is quite variable for any individual patient in an intensive care setting.[9] Furthermore, mixed venous O_2 saturation (and, hence, arteriovenous O_2 difference) may be misleading in patients with decreased tissue O_2 extraction.[10,11]

Doppler Echocardiography

Doppler techniques can be used to measure CO using the mean velocity of systolic flow, heart rate at the time of measurement, and cross-sectional area of the artery in which measurements are being made (usually the ascending aorta):

$$CO = A \times V \times HR$$

where A is the area of the orifice, V is integrated flow velocity, and HR is heart rate. To determine the integrated flow velocity, the area under the Doppler curve must be measured. The area of the aortic orifice is commonly obtained by measuring the aortic diameter from the two-dimensional image, where A = 0.785 ∞ d2. This technique requires special care for accurate Doppler interrogation of blood flow and is seldom used in the critical care unit.

Pulse Oximetry

Pulse oximetry measures the quantity of hemoglobin saturated with O_2 in peripheral arterial blood. It depends on two principles: (1) Oxygenated and reduced hemoglobin have different absorption spectra, and (2) at constant light intensity and hemoglobin concentration, O_2 saturation of hemoglobin is a logarithmic function of the intensity of transmitted light (Beer-Lambert law). Two wavelengths of light that have different absorption spectra for reduced hemoglobin and oxyhemoglobin are transmitted from the light-emitting diodes through the arterial bed. Light absorption at the two wavelengths is compared, yielding the ratio of oxyhemoglobin to reduced hemoglobin, or the O_2 saturation. Pulse oximeters have a high potential for error at saturations below 80%.[12] Furthermore, the O_2 dissociation curve flattens out at the high range so that at saturations greater than 95%, large changes in PaO_2 accompany small changes in saturation. This phenomenon should be kept in mind when monitoring premature infants, for whom it is important to avoid hyperoxia.

Other Measures of DO_2

Acid-Base Status

When tissue hypoxia occurs and affected tissues and organs resort, in part, to anaerobic metabolism, increased production of lactate, CO_2, and hydrogen ions occurs. The anion gap, the difference in unmeasured serum anions and unmeasured serum cations, can yield information regarding the cause of metabolic acidosis. If the anion gap is normal (8 to 16 mEq/L), loss of bicarbonate has occurred, usually via the kidneys or gastrointestinal tract, or rapid dilution of the extracellular fluid has occurred.

Blood Lactate

Blood lactate concentration is a laboratory measure that indirectly reflects perfusion.[13,14] Blood lactate measurements are extensively used for monitoring and evaluating response to therapy. We observed that initial absolute blood lactate levels were less important than the temporal trend in lactate concentrations for predicting mortality in postoperative cardiac patients.[15] Unfortunately, the specificity of blood lactate is imperfect and may lack sensitivity for detecting supply-dependent O_2 consumption, particularly if it is only regional. In addition, blood lactate depends on hepatic metabolism and the rate of production and clearance.

Gastric Tonometry

Gastric tonometry, a technique available for clinical use in adult and some pediatric ICUs, allows indirect assessment of perfusion by measuring gut intramucosal pH or partial pressure of carbon dioxide.[16,17] It may have an advantage over blood lactate concentration in that it can uncover regional hypoxia and hypoperfusion involving the gut and can be adapted for continuous online measurement.[17] Nonetheless, this technique assumes that a critical reduction in O_2 transport manifests in the splanchnic circulation before it can be detected systemically (probably a reasonable assumption), and tonometric methods are not entirely noninvasive.

Urine Output

Urine output generally reflects CO, but oliguria may occur in the first 24 hours after open heart surgery, especially in neonates, even in the context of good CO and blood pressure. It is therefore important to consider urine output in the context of other indicators of organ perfusion and not as an isolated variable. It should also be noted that the kidneys are quite sensitive to perfusion pressure and that good systemic blood flow coupled with low systemic arterial pressure (due to low SVR) may adversely affect urine output more than other measures of tissue perfusion.

Near-Infrared Spectroscopy

Near-infrared spectroscopy (NIRS), a noninvasive technique that has been applied to assess systemic and regional oxygen transport in several clinical and laboratory studies,[18-26] is gaining acceptance, particularly in patients with CHD, as a means of trending regional DO_2 or as a surrogate for mixed venous O_2 saturation or systemic DO_2.[27] Abdominal site NIRS has been shown to correlate with simultaneous intramucosal pH measurements by gastric tonometry in neonates and infants with CHD undergoing catheter-based or surgical intervention.[28] In an experimental setting in which DO_2 is controlled, NIRS has been used to correlate cytochrome *aa3* (the terminal link in the electron transport chain responsible for mitochondrial respiration), VO_2, and lactate flux.[23] Thus NIRS has the potential to identify a critical regional reduction in O_2 transport at the cellular level.

Systemic Arterial Blood Pressure

Invasive Blood Pressure Monitoring

Intravascular pressure monitoring is often essential in the management of critically ill neonates and infants in the ICU. Typically, an end-hole catheter is inserted into a vessel (or cardiac chamber) and connected to a pressure transducer by a coupling system composed of fluid-filled extension tubing, a stopcock for withdrawing blood and balancing the transducer to atmospheric pressure, and a continuous infusion device to flush out blood and air. The transducer translates pressure into an electrical signal that can be processed through a preamplifier into a waveform and numerical display on a monitor. The pressure transducer must be properly calibrated, dampened, and positioned (at mid-chest level). Inaccurate measurements can occur for a variety of reasons.

In the pediatric population, blood pressure is age dependent and is a relatively insensitive marker of CO and DO_2. Because blood pressure is the product of CO and SVR, hypotension may result from diminished CO and/or decreased SVR.[29] Because the treatment options are different, distinguishing low CO from low SVR is important.

Noninvasive Blood Pressure Monitoring

The auscultatory method of blood pressure measurement with a cuff and pressure gauge is difficult if access to the patient is limited, if the patient is small or uncooperative, and when frequent recordings are required. Therefore two techniques, Doppler and oscillometric measurements, have been developed. The Doppler technique uses a Doppler ultrasound probe that is applied to the radial or brachial artery. A cuff wrapped around the upper arm is inflated until the audible Doppler signal is obliterated and then deflated until the signal first becomes audible again (systolic blood pressure). This method has been validated in low-flow states and in small children.[30] The oscillometric method has the advantage of being readily automated. The device for indirect noninvasive mean arterial pressure (Dinamap) is based on the principle that blood flow through a vessel produces oscillation of the arterial wall that may be transmitted to an inflatable cuff encircling the extremity. As cuff pressure decreases, a characteristic change occurs in the magnitude of oscillation at the levels at which systolic, diastolic, and mean pressures are registered. Accuracy of Dinamap blood pressures has been validated in children, and it correlates well with direct intravascular radial artery pressures.[31] The accuracy of these two techniques relates to the cuff size. If the cuff is too narrow, the pressure recorded may be erroneously high; if the cuff is too wide, the pressure recorded may be too low. Both techniques are unreliable and inadequate in patients with low CO, hypotension, dysrhythmias, significant edema, or systemic vasoconstriction.

Central Venous or Intracardiac Pressure Monitoring

Pressures can also be measured in the cardiac chambers or in the pulmonary vasculature. However, the necessity for intravascular or intracardiac lines should always be carefully considered, and they should be removed as soon as the clinical condition permits. The placement of relatively large catheters in small vessels for prolonged periods carries a risk of thrombosis and systemic thromboembolism.

Central venous access affords the opportunity to measure central venous pressure (CVP), deliver drugs or high osmolarity nutritional solutions, and repeatedly sample blood to monitor venous O_2 saturations and for other laboratory studies. Intraarterial lines offer the opportunity to continuously monitor arterial pressure and for intermittent blood gas analysis.

Intravascular pressures provide information about ventricular preload and afterload. RV preload is assessed by the CVP. The CVP is determined by a variety of factors, including patient age, preoperative status (ie, a patient with RV hypertrophy and increased RA pressure), cardiac performance, intrathoracic pressure, blood volume, vasopressor therapy, and status of the pericardium. The CVP *a wave* reflects atrial contraction, and the *v wave* reflects atrial filling. Serial measurements of CVP are frequently used to evaluate the response to fluid administration. RV afterload can be assessed using a PA catheter. This catheter is particularly important for monitoring pulmonary artery pressure and therapeutic response to vasodilators in patients with elevated PVR. The PA wedge pressure reflects LA pressure (in the absence of pulmonary vein stenosis). In the postoperative cardiac patient, a direct LA line can be placed to directly assess LV preload. LV afterload is assessed by measurement of SAP, provided no LV outflow tract obstruction is present.

Assessing Variables That Affect the Quantity of Therapy

If it is important to take into account the QOT needed to secure adequate tissue perfusion, it follows that one would like to assess the variables that affect the QOT. Table 29.1 summarizes the effect of abnormalities of cardiovascular and pulmonary function on QOT. What follows is a brief description of how these cardiovascular variables may be assessed in the critical care unit.

Ventricular Systolic Function

Precise measurement of ventricular systolic function is difficult,[32] especially in the critical care setting. A commonly used surrogate is the echocardiographic demonstration of ventricular wall excursion/shortening. LV shortening and ejection fractions can be measured using echocardiography with reasonable accuracy, but these variables are influenced by preload and afterload and by inotropic conditions. RV morphology makes echocardiographic measurement of systolic function even more problematic, despite a variety of described techniques to assess this variable.[33] For either ventricle, most often one resorts to a qualitative assessment of ventricular wall excursion as a crude estimate of systolic function. Although cardiac magnetic resonance angiography/magnetic resonance imaging can accurately measure LV and RV ejection fraction, it is often of limited practical utility in the critically ill pediatric patient.

Ventricular Diastolic Function

Ventricular diastolic function is also difficult to measure precisely. In the critical care unit, diastolic dysfunction is usually manifested as a need for increased filling pressures for a given

TABLE 29.1	Cardiovascular Function and Quantity of Therapy (QOT)
Cardiac System Variable	**Impact on QOT**
Cardiac Function	
↓ Ventricular systolic function	↑ Filling pressure, ↑ inotropic/pressor support
↓ Ventricular diastolic function	↑ Filling pressure, ↑ pressor support
Abnormal rhythm	↑ Filling pressure, ↑ inotropic/pressor support
Intracardiac structural lesions (↓ efficiency)	↑ Filling pressure, ↑ inotropic/pressor support
Single ventricle with A-P shunt (↓ efficiency)	↑ Filling pressure, ↑ inotropic/pressor support
Peripheral Vasculature	
↑ SVR	↑ Ventricular work → ↑ filling pressure, ↑ inotropic/pressor support
↓ SVR	↑ Filling pressure, ↑ inotropic/pressor support
↑ PVR 2 ventricles	↑ Ventricular work → ↑ filling pressure, ↑ inotropic/pressor support
Aortopulmonary shunt	↓ PBF → ↓ O_2 → ↑ filling pressure, ↑ inotropic/pressor support
Bidirectional Glenn	↑ SVC pressure
Fontan	↑ filling pressure, ↑ inotropic/pressor support
Vascular Function	
"Leaky" vascular bed → edema → volume infusion → edema	↑ Filling pressure, ↑ inotropic/pressor support
Pulmonary Function	
↓ Lung compliance, ↓ gas exchange	↑ Airway pressure → ↓ venous return → ↑ systemic venous pressure, barotrauma

magnitude of ventricular output. Echocardiography sometimes will demonstrate an apparently underfilled ventricle despite adequate or high filling pressures, but most often a lack of compliance is inferred from high filling pressures alone. Echocardiographic measures of ventricular compliance exist, but many clinicians have found them to be of limited practical value. It is important to emphasize that *transmural filling pressure,* not atrial pressure per se, is what determines diastolic filling; elevated pericardial or intrathoracic pressure will reduce ventricular filling for any given atrial pressure.[34]

Rhythm Disturbance

A variety of abnormal rhythms can decrease systemic perfusion and therefore lead to increased QOT. A surface electrocardiogram may be sufficient to delineate the type and mechanism of an arrhythmia; however, especially with tachycardia, all too often one cannot clearly discriminate P waves from the T and QRS deflections. The use of atrial leads in conjunction with limb leads can be exceedingly helpful for both diagnosing and treating arrhythmias in postoperative patients. Alternatively, esophageal electrodes sometimes can be helpful, although they are somewhat cumbersome to use

(and cannot always effect atrial capture). It is important to frequently and carefully reassess the rhythm because significant changes (eg, from sinus rhythm to junctional ectopic tachycardia) may escape casual detection.

Abnormal Systemic Vascular Resistance

Abnormal systemic vascular resistance is determined by the following equation:

$$SVR = (SAP - CVP)/CO$$

where *SAP* is mean systemic arterial pressure (mm Hg), *CVP* is mean central venous pressure (mm Hg), and *CO* is cardiac output, usually indexed to surface area (L/min/m^2).

Increased SVR can be useful when CO is insufficient for adequate systemic perfusion pressure with normal SVR. On the other hand, SVR increased beyond that needed for adequate SAP increases systemic ventricular afterload and may therefore negatively affect CO.[35] For reasons discussed in the following section on single-ventricle physiology, increased SVR may also result in excess PBF in patients with an aortopulmonary shunt. Finally, increased SAP in a newly postoperative patient may contribute to excessive bleeding. In contrast, low SVR can cause systemic hypotension despite adequate or supranormal CO. Anecdotal observations and some published information indicate that low SVR may occur after cardiac surgery, as well as with other systemic illnesses (eg, sepsis).

As previously noted, because CO is infrequently measured in PICUs, SVR is most commonly inferred from observation of cutaneous perfusion and SAP. Indeed, it is important to evaluate systemic hypotension in the context of cutaneous perfusion (brisk capillary refill suggests low SVR) because rational therapy for decreased SVR with adequate CO (vasopressor support) is quite different from that useful for hypotension due to inadequate CO.

Increased Pulmonary Vascular Resistance

The clinical consequences of increased PVR are directly related to the specific cardiac anatomy and physiology. With two separate ventricles, high PVR can reduce systolic and diastolic function of the pulmonary ventricle and limit its output. In patients with a physiologically large aortopulmonary shunt, increased PVR, up to a point, can be useful because it reduces what would otherwise be excessive PBF. On the other hand, if PVR is too high, or in the setting of an excessively restrictive aortopulmonary shunt, inadequate PBF results. With a bidirectional Glenn circulation, elevated PVR may result in upper body congestion and hypoxemia. With a Fontan circulation, high systemic venous pressure, low CO, and hypoxemia (if a fenestration is present) may occur.

In patients with a structurally normal cardiovascular system, measuring PVR is analogous to measurement of SVR and is subject to the same practical difficulties. Echocardiographic estimation of RV pressure is a useful surrogate, using a tricuspid regurgitant jet, pulmonary regurgitant jet, or interventricular septal position. Unfortunately, in the absence of significant tricuspid regurgitation (or another defect that allows a pressure gradient to be measured between the right ventricle and a chamber of known pressure), echocardiographic estimation of RV pressure is crude.

For patients with an aortopulmonary shunt, PVR is rarely measured in the ICU; determining PBF requires measuring

VO_2 (an assumed VO_2 is questionable because it is so variable[9]), pulmonary arterial O_2 saturation, and pulmonary venous O_2 saturation. Because pulmonary venous catheters are rarely used, pulmonary venous O_2 saturations are usually assumed; however, this is a potential source of significant error because these saturations are variable and unpredictable.[36] Most important, pulmonary artery pressure is essentially never measured in the critical care unit in patients with shunts. For these patients, even estimating PVR is problematic because many variables (eg, PVR, systemic blood pressure, PBF and CO, hematocrit, and VO_2) influence the most obvious manifestation of increased PVR, low systemic arterial O_2 saturation. Circumstantial data may be used to infer that PVR is not elevated in hypoxemic patients with an aortopulmonary shunt; for example, echocardiographic demonstration of narrowing of the shunt suggests that increased PVR is likely not the cause of the hypoxemia. Alternatively, an increase in systemic arterial O_2 saturation with inhaled nitric oxide would also suggest that baseline PVR is increased.

Measuring PBF in patients with a cavopulmonary palliation (eg, bidirectional Glenn, hemi-Fontan, and Fontan) can also be done using the Fick method (thermodilution cannot be used to measure PBF because of inadequate mixing of the cold indicator in the systemic venous pathway). From a practical standpoint, increased PVR in this setting is often inferred from high systemic venous pathway pressures (superior vena caval pressures in a bidirectional Glenn patient), taking into consideration possible anatomic obstruction in the superior vena cava, pulmonary arteries, or pulmonary veins or increased systemic ventricular end-diastolic pressures.

Inefficient Circulation

The most important fundamental ways that structural defects can result in an inefficient circulation in patients with cardiac structural lesions are (1) increased ventricular afterload (eg, RV or LV outflow tract obstruction), (2) increased ventricular volume load (eg, ventricular septal defect and atrioventricular valve regurgitation), (3) impaired ventricular filling (eg, atrioventricular valve stenosis), (4) reduced PBF with shunting into the systemic circulation, (5) mixing of pulmonary and systemic venous blood, and (6) D-transposition of the great arteries physiology (ie, PVR predominantly directed to the PA and SVR predominantly directed to the aorta). Impaired coronary perfusion resulting in ventricular ischemia is perhaps not, conceptually, a problem of efficiency but a structural lesion that needs to be considered. Many patients have some combination of these lesions. It is beyond the scope of this chapter to discuss the evaluation of cardiac patients relative to structural lesions and their impact on DO_2, systemic perfusion pressure, and QOT. Suffice it to say that it is exceedingly important that the anatomy and associated physiology of patients with cardiac malformations be well defined. Echocardiography is the single most useful modality for delineating cardiac structure (and often even physiology) in the critical care unit. Cardiac catheterization and angiography remain important diagnostic and therapeutic tools, and MRI and CT are sometimes helpful.

Vascular Integrity

By vascular integrity we refer to the ability of the vascular (mostly microvascular) bed to keep fluid in the intravascular space. Leaky blood vessels result in organ, chest wall, and

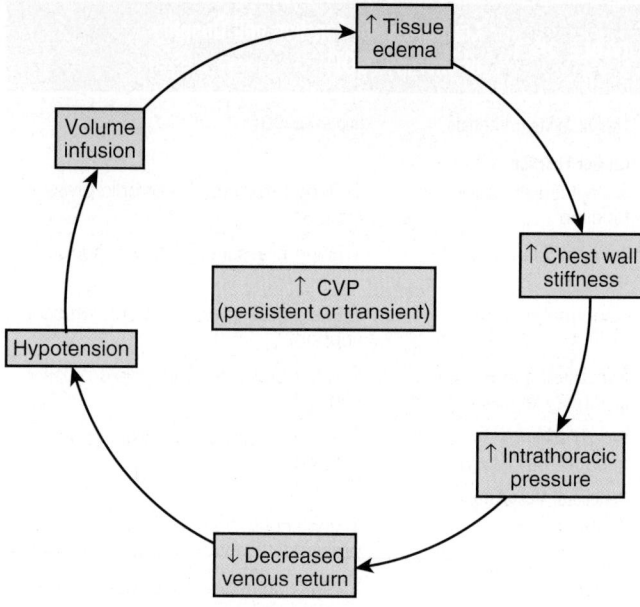

Fig. 29.1. Flow diagram.

peripheral edema, as well as fluid accumulation in the thoracic and abdominal cavities. This situation is exacerbated by high CVP, particularly when ventricular diastolic dysfunction exists, and tends to be self-perpetuating, especially in infants (Fig. 29.1).

It is important to assess third spacing, particularly in infants, where opening the chest may help minimize the hemodynamic effects of chest wall edema in post–cardiac surgical patients. Similarly, assessment for abdominal compartment syndrome due to ascites may allow surgical or catheter-based evacuation with improved pulmonary mechanics and urine output. Also, because progressive edema, even if relatively benign early on, is likely to eventually become a significant problem, this finding should figure prominently in the clinician's overall assessment of the patient's condition.

Pulmonary Function

Pulmonary dysfunction due to edema or acute or chronic lung injury can be a major physiologic liability for the obvious reasons related to impaired gas exchange. In addition, insofar as increased P_{aw} is required for adequate gas exchange, venous return to the heart may be impaired. This can be especially important in special circumstances, such as the patient after cavopulmonary palliation. Williams and colleagues[37] nicely showed the unfavorable impact of small increments of positive end-expiratory pressure in patients after Fontan palliation, which, as careful inspection of their data reveals, was mostly due to decreased venous return. Increased P_{aw}, especially if it causes overinflation of the lungs, also can increase PVR. Finally, increased P_{aw}, if applied for sufficient duration, can take a long-term toll by chronic reduction in lung function.

It is beyond the scope of this chapter to describe all available techniques for evaluating lung function. However, high P_{aw} is an important component of QOT and should lead the intensivist to consider alternatives (eg, permissive hypercapnia or extracorporeal life support).

Physiology of the Patient with a Single Ventricle

Patients with single-ventricle physiology differ from children with two functioning ventricles in many ways. They pose several unique challenges to the pediatric intensivist. For many patients with a single ventricle, initial palliation in infancy may involve placement of an aortopulmonary (eg, modified Blalock-Taussig) or right ventricle to PA ("Sano") connection as a source of PBF. The total output of the single-ventricle circulation is thus the sum of the pulmonary (Q_p) and systemic (Q_s) blood flows. The relative percentage of blood flow to the pulmonary and systemic circulations depends, in part, on the resistance in each vascular bed. Because PVR is usually substantially lower than SVR soon after birth, the size (diameter, length, and vessel of origin) of the aortopulmonary shunt is also a major contributor to total resistance to flow in the pulmonary circuit and hence an important determinant of Q_p/Q_s. SVR is often the single most important variable influencing Q_p[38] and the one most amenable to manipulation in the ICU. In patients with a single ventricle who have complete admixture of systemic and pulmonary venous blood, arterial O_2 saturation is influenced by not only lung function (eg, pulmonary venous O_2 saturation) but also Q_p and myocardial function (which influences Q_s and, hence, mixed venous O_2 saturation) (Figs. 29.2 and 29.3).

Computer modeling of shunt-dependent single-ventricle physiology[31] suggests that a Q_p/Q_s ~ 1.0 is ideal for optimizing systemic O_2 availability for a given pulmonary venous O_2 saturation, CO, and VO_2. The arterial O_2 saturation, considered in isolation, is a poor indicator of Q_p/Q_s because a low mixed venous O_2 saturation will depress arterial O_2 saturation, even in patients with a high Q_p/Q_s. Accurately measuring Q_p/Q_s, which equals systemic arterial O_2 saturation minus systemic venous O_2 saturation divided by pulmonary venous O_2 saturation minus pulmonary arterial O_2 saturation, requires determining O_2 saturation in blood in the proximal superior vena cava (SVC), as distinct from RA or inferior vena cava, and is subject to the previously noted variability and unpredictability of pulmonary venous O_2 saturations. That said, estimating Q_p/Q_s using the SVC O_2 saturation (as mixed venous) and the arterial O_2 saturation (which is also the PAO_2 saturation) and assuming the pulmonary venous O_2 saturation is helpful in estimating whether a patient with a single ventricle and an aortopulmonary shunt has appropriate (ie, associated with optimal systemic DO_2), increased, or decreased Q_p/Q_s. However, it is important to note that Q_p/Q_s is merely a number when considered in isolation. It must be placed into the context of the patient's overall status, considering the parameters previously outlined for assessing systemic DO_2. In particular, in patients following single-ventricle palliation, a progressive decline in the serum lactate concentration (regardless of the initial postoperative concentration) is a fairly sensitive and specific marker for early survival. In contrast, rising lactate levels are generally a robust predictor of early postoperative cardiovascular collapse or need for mechanical support unless therapy can improve the hemodynamic picture.[15]

$$DO_2 = CaO_2 \times SBF$$

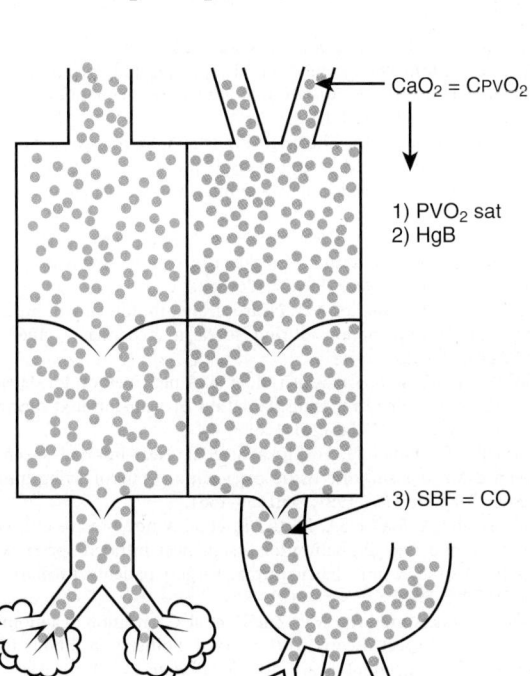

Fig. 29.2. Cartoon depicting the variables that determine systemic oxygen delivery (DO_2) with a normal heart. Blue dots depict desaturated (systemic venous) blood, and red dots depict fully saturated (pulmonary venous) blood. *CaO_2*, systemic arterial blood O_2 content; *CO*, cardiac output; *CpVO_2*, pulmonary venous blood O_2 content; *HgB*, blood hemoglobin concentration; *PvO_2 sat*, pulmonary venous O_2 saturation; *SBF*, systemic blood flow. Dissolved O_2 in the blood is ignored.

$$DO_2 = CaO_2 \times SBF$$

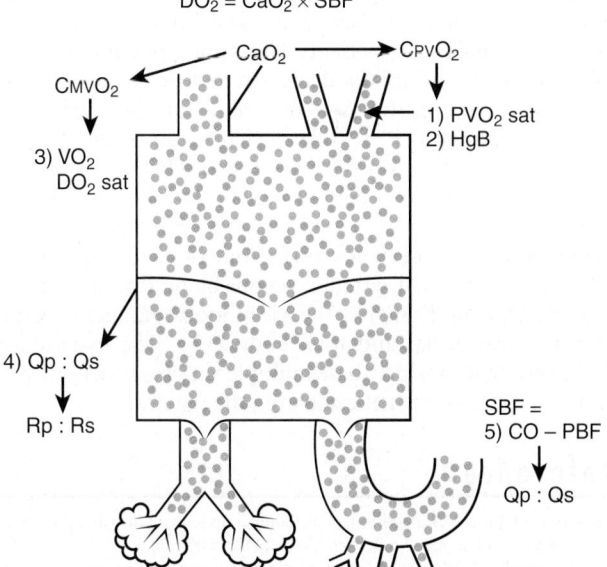

Fig. 29.3. Cartoon depicting the variables that determine systemic oxygen delivery (DO_2) with a cardiac malformation resulting in complete mixing of systemic and pulmonary venous blood. Blue dots depict desaturated (systemic venous) blood, and red dots depict fully saturated (pulmonary venous) blood. *CaO_2*, systemic arterial blood O_2 content; *CMvO_2*, systemic venous O_2 content; *CO*, cardiac output; *CpVO_2*, pulmonary venous blood O_2 content; *HgB*, blood hemoglobin concentration; *PvO_2 sat*, pulmonary venous O_2 saturation; *PBF*, pulmonary blood flow; *Qp:Qs*, ratio of pulmonary to systemic blood flow; *Rp:Rs*, ratio of pulmonary to systemic vascular resistance; *SBF*, systemic blood flow; *VO_2*, total body O_2 consumption. Dissolved O_2 in the blood is ignored.

It should be noted that the physiology is somewhat different in patients with two ventricles and an aortopulmonary shunt (eg, tetralogy of Fallot with severe RV outflow tract obstruction and a modified Blalock-Taussig shunt). Because PBF is usually made up of both systemic arterial blood and systemic venous blood, arterial O_2 saturation is higher for a given amount of PBF and cannot be calculated using systemic arterial O_2 saturation as the PAO_2 saturation.

Although the cardiopulmonary physiology of patients with bidirectional Glenn palliation differs somewhat from that of others (eg, the apparent paradoxical relationship between alveolar ventilation and arterial O_2 saturation[39,40]), cardiovascular assessment is much the same as for other patients. Two things are worth noting, however. First, because arterial O_2 saturations often increase significantly during the first several postoperative hours after Glenn palliation, lower than desired but acceptable O_2 saturations early on do not necessarily imply inadequate palliation. Second, although some degree of upper body edema and duskiness is not unusual soon after an operation, marked upper body congestion suggests the possibility of obstruction of the SVC to PA pathway, which requires prompt evaluation. Echocardiography may be sufficient to interrogate this pathway, although angiography may be required.

Evaluation of postoperative Fontan patients is also much the same as for other postoperative cardiac patients, but because Fontan patients are particularly sensitive to factors that impede transit of blood across the lungs and into the ventricle, it is important to identify any such factors, especially remediable ones, early on in the struggling patient. Anatomic abnormalities that might have little clinical importance in other circumstances (eg, partial obstruction of one or more pulmonary veins) can have a marked impact on the early postoperative Fontan patient. The same goes for modestly increased PVR and mildly decreased ventricular compliance. Catheters in the central systemic veins and left atrium are useful for estimating PVR and ventricular compliance, and the previously noted measures of systemic perfusion are helpful. The sick postoperative Fontan patient may pose the perfect storm of marginal SAP, acutely elevated CVP (relative to preoperative CVP), and hypoxemia (from right-to-left shunting of highly desaturated systemic venous blood through a fenestration), all complicated by the use of inotropic agents (which increase myocardial and total body VO_2). The experienced intensivist will consider these multiple variables, including the QOT, in aggregate when evaluating the patient.

References

1. Court O, Kumar A, Parrillo J, et al. Clinical review: myocardial depression in sepsis and septic shock. *Crit Care*. 2002;6:500-508.
2. Wernovsky G, Wypij D, Jonas RA, et al. Postoperative course and hemodynamic profile after the arterial switch operation in neonates and infants: a comparison of low-flow cardiopulmonary bypass and circulatory arrest. *Circulation*. 1995;92:2226-2235.
3. Schlictig R. Oxygen delivery and consumption in critical illness. In: Civetta J, Taylor R, Kirby RR, eds. *Critical Care*. 2nd ed. Philadelphia: Lippincott-Raven; 1997.
4. Adams RP, Dieleman LA, Cain SM. A critical value for O_2 transport in the rat. *J Appl Physiol Respir Environ Exerc Physiol*. 1982;53:660-664.
5. Cain SM. Oxygen delivery and uptake in dogs during anemic and hypoxic hypoxia. *J Appl Physiol Respir Environ Exerc Physiol*. 1977;42:228-234.
6. Schwartz S, Frantz RA, Shoemaker WC. Sequential hemodynamic and oxygen transport responses in hypovolemia, anemia, and hypoxia. *Am J Physiol*. 1981;241:H864-H871.
7. Lister G, Walter TK, Versmold HT, et al. Oxygen delivery in lambs: cardiovascular and hematologic development. *Am J Physiol*. 1979;237:H668-H675.
8. Klopfenstein HS, Rudolph AM. Postnatal changes in the circulation and responses to volume loading in sheep. *Circ Res*. 1978;42:839-845.
9. Jain A, Shroff SG, Janicki JS, et al. Relation between mixed venous oxygen saturation and cardiac index: nonlinearity and normalization for oxygen uptake and hemoglobin. *Chest*. 1991;99:1403-1409.
10. Scheinman MM, Brown MA, Rapaport E. Critical assessment of use of central venous oxygen saturation as a mirror of mixed venous oxygen in severely ill cardiac patients. *Circulation*. 1969;40:165-172.
11. Chang AC, Kulik TJ, Hickey PR, et al. Real-time gas-exchange measurement of oxygen consumption in neonates and infants after cardiac surgery. *Crit Care Med*. 1993;21:1369-1375.
12. Webb RK, Ralston AC, Runciman WB. Potential errors in pulse oximetry. II. Effects of changes in saturation and signal quality. *Anaesthesia*. 1991;46:207-212.
13. Kruse JA. Blood lactate and oxygen transport. *Intensive Care World*. 1987;4:121-125.
14. Kruse JA, Haupt MT, Puri VK, et al. Lactate levels as predictors of the relationship between oxygen delivery and consumption in ARDS. *Chest*. 1990;98:959-962.
15. Charpie JR, Dekeon MK, Goldberg CS, et al. Serial blood lactate measurements predict early outcome after neonatal repair or palliation for complex congenital heart disease. *J Thorac Cardiovasc Surg*. 2000;120:73-80.
16. Guzman JA, Lacoma FJ, Kruse JA. Relationship between systemic oxygen supply dependency and gastric intramucosal PCO_2 during progressive hemorrhage. *J Trauma*. 1998;44:696-700.
17. Guzman JA, Kruse JA. Development and validation of a technique for continuous monitoring of gastric intramucosal pH. *Am J Respir Crit Care Med*. 1996;153:694-700.
18. Slavin KV, Dujovny M, Ausman JI, et al. Clinical experience with transcranial cerebral oximetry. *Surg Neurol*. 1994;42:531.
19. Wyatt JS, Cope M, Delpy DT, et al. Quantitation of cerebral blood volume in human infants by near-infrared spectroscopy. *J Appl Physiol*. 1990;68:1086-1091.
20. Edwards AD, Wyatt JS, Richardson C, et al. Cotside measurement of cerebral blood flow in ill newborn infants by near infrared spectroscopy. *Lancet*. 1988;2:770-771.
21. Tateishi A, Maekawa T, Soejima Y, et al. Qualitative comparison of carbon dioxide-induced change in cerebral near-infrared spectroscopy versus jugular venous oxygen saturation in adults with acute brain disease. *Crit Care Med*. 1995;23:1734-1738.
22. Lewis SB, Myburgh JA, Thornton EL, et al. Cerebral oxygenation monitoring by near-infrared spectroscopy is not clinically useful in patients with severe closed-head injury: a comparison with jugular venous bulb oximetry. *Crit Care Med*. 1996;24:1334-1338.
23. Guery BP, Mangalaboyi J, Menager P, et al. Redox status of cytochrome a, a3: a noninvasive indicator of dysoxia in regional hypoxic or ischemic hypoxia. *Crit Care Med*. 1999;27:576-582.
24. Hampson NB, Piantadosi CA. Near infrared monitoring of human skeletal muscle oxygenation during forearm ischemia. *J Appl Physiol*. 1988;64:2449-2457.
25. Tashiro H, Suzuki S, Kanashiro M, et al. A new method for determining graft function after liver transplantation by near-infrared spectroscopy. *Transplantation*. 1993;56:1261-1263.
26. Noriyuki T, Ohdan H, Yoshioka S, et al. Near-infrared spectroscopic method for assessing the tissue oxygenation state of living lung. *Am J Respir Crit Care Med*. 1997;156:1656-1661.
27. Tortoriello TA, Stayer SA, Mott AR, et al. A noninvasive estimation of mixed venous oxygen saturation using near-infrared spectroscopy by cerebral oximetry in pediatric cardiac surgery patients. *Paediatr Anaesth*. 2005;15:495-503.
28. Kaufman JM, Almodovar MC, Zuk JP, et al. Correlation of abdominal site near-infrared spectroscopy with gastric tonometry in infants following surgery for congenital heart disease. *Pediatr Crit Care Med*. 2008;9:62-68.
29. Argenziano M, Chen JM, Choudhri AF, et al. Management of vasodilatory shock after cardiac surgery: identification of predisposing factors and use of a novel pressor agent. *J Thorac Cardiovasc Surg*. 1998;116:973-980.
30. Waltemath CL, Preuss DD. Determination of blood pressure in low-flow states by the Doppler technique. *Anesthesiology*. 1971;34:77-79.
31. Park MK, Menard SM. Accuracy of blood pressure measurement by the Dinamap monitor in infants and children. *Pediatrics*. 1987;79:907-914.

32. Susa H. Paul Dudley White Memorial Lecture: cardiac performance viewed through the pressure-volume window. *Jpn Heart J*. 1994;35:263.

33. Cacciapuoti F. Echocardiographic evaluation of right heart function and pulmonary vascular bed. *Int J Cardiovasc Imaging*. 2009;25:689-697.

34. Daughters GT, Frist WH, Alderman EL, et al. Effects of the pericardium on left ventricular diastolic filling and systolic performance early after cardiac operations. *J Thorac Cardiovasc Surg*. 1992;104:1084-1091.

35. Appelbaum A, Blackstone EH, Kouchoukos NT, et al. Afterload reduction and cardiac output in infants early after intracardiac surgery. *Am J Cardiol*. 1977;39:445-451.

36. Taeed R, Schwartz SM, Pearl JM, et al. Unrecognized pulmonary venous desaturation early after Norwood palliation confounds Gp:Gs assessment and compromises oxygen delivery. *Circulation*. 2001;103:2699-2704.

37. Williams DB, Kiernan PD, Metke MP, et al. Hemodynamic response to positive end-expiratory pressure following right atrium-pulmonary artery bypass (Fontan procedure). *J Thorac Cardiovasc Surg*. 1984;87:856-861.

38. Migliavacca F, Pennati G, Dubini G, et al. Modeling of the Norwood circulation: effects of shunt size, vascular resistances, and heart rate. *Am J Physiol Heart Circ Physiol*. 2001;280:H2076-H2086.

39. Bradley SM, Simsic JM, Mulvihill DM. Hyperventilation impairs oxygenation after bidirectional superior cavopulmonary connection. *Circulation*. 1998;98(suppl 19):II372.

40. Bradley SM, Simsic JM, Mulvihill DM. Hypoventilation improves oxygenation after bidirectional superior cavopulmonary connection. *J Thorac Cardiovasc Surg*. 2003;126:1033-1039.

Myocardial Dysfunction, Extracorporeal Life Support, and Ventricular Assist Devices

Ana Lía Graciano, Umesh Joashi, and Keith C. Kocis

PEARLS

- Advances in medical management, surgical techniques, and mechanical circulatory support for pediatric patients with congestive heart failure continue to improve patient outcomes.
- Indications for use of mechanical circulatory support continue to evolve.
- Patient size, expected duration of support, and goals of support (ie, bridge to recovery versus bridge to transplant) must be considered in the choice of a mechanical circulatory support device.
- Mechanical circulatory support is a lifesaving therapeutic option for patients with advanced heart failure. Device options in children are expanding but remain limited due to their size constraints.
- In children, most short-term mechanical circulatory support continues to be achieved with extracorporeal life support.
- Small patients (<6 kg), renal failure, and the need for biventricular support greatly increase the risk of death during support.
- A multidisciplinary team approach to the selection of the appropriate mechanical circulatory device is critical to a successful outcome.

Introduction

Mechanical circulatory support (MCS) is an invaluable tool in the care of children with severe refractory cardiac or respiratory failure. Two forms of mechanical support are currently available to infants and small children; these include extracorporeal life support (ECLS) and ventricular assist devices (VADs). Patient selection, timing of intervention, and device choice continue to pose a challenge in the treatment of pediatric patients.

This chapter reviews the basics of myocardial dysfunction in children with an emphasis on low cardiac output syndrome and its treatment with regard to mechanical circulatory support. Finally, we outline indications for MCS, salient technical details of specific devices, patient management, present

research, and future directions of these technologies for use in pediatric patients.

Pediatric Heart Failure

Heart failure (HF) is the final pathway of many pathophysiologic states affecting cardiovascular performance leading to inadequate cardiac output and decreased end-organ perfusion with diminished oxygen delivery to the vital organs. These include states of altered preload, afterload, contractility, and abnormal heart rate or rhythm. The etiology of the different types of heart failure in children is listed in Table 30.1,[1] with the largest disease burden being due to congenital malformations and cardiomyopathies.[2,3]

The primary goal in the management of myocardial dysfunction is to ensure adequate tissue oxygen delivery, as an imbalance between delivery and consumption results in organ dysfunction and failure. Initial therapies to treat decompensated heart failure target providing respiratory support; decreasing metabolic demands (ie, work of breathing); optimizing preload, afterload, and contractility; and optimizing heart rate and rhythm. Despite advances in pharmacologic therapies (eg, nesiritide, levosimendan, milrinone, amiodarone) a group of patients will continue to deteriorate or require excessive cardiopulmonary support. This group should be evaluated early for MCS before additional end-organ dysfunction or irreversible damage occurs. Several innovative types of MCS are being created and brought into clinical care while extended indications, management strategies, and outcomes are currently being developed. Simultaneously, ECLS continues to improve and remain the most commonly deployed form of MCS for infants and children.[4,5]

Low Cardiac Output Syndrome

Low cardiac output syndrome (LCOS) describes a clinical state with specific biochemical markers where there is inadequate systemic oxygen delivery (DO_2) to meet the metabolic demand (VO_2) of the patient. The condition has been recognized since the 1960s, and multiple studies have documented the predicted changes in physiologic parameters. LCOS has been an active area of research, and multiple reviews of current therapies are available to guide the intensivist.[6] LCOS is frequently seen in severe sepsis, myocarditis, cardiomyopathies,

TABLE 30.1 Etiology of Heart Failure in Children

Congenital Cardiac Malformations
Volume Overload
Left-to-Right Shunting
Ventricular septal defect

Patent ductus arteriosus

Atrioventricular or Semilunar Valve Insufficiency
Aortic regurgitation in bicommissural aortic valve

Pulmonary regurgitation after repair of tetralogy of Fallot

Pressure Overload
Left-Sided Obstruction
Severe aortic stenosis

Aortic coarctation

Right-Sided Obstruction
Severe pulmonary stenosis

Complex Congenital Heart Disease
Single Ventricle
Hypoplastic left heart syndrome

Unbalanced atrioventricular septal defect

Systemic Right Ventricle
L-transposition ("corrected transposition") of the great arteries

Structurally Normal Heart
Primary Cardiomyopathy
Dilated

Hypertrophic

Restrictive

Secondary
Arrhythmogenic

Ischemic

Toxic

Infiltrative

Infectious

Hsu DT, Pearson GD. Heart failure in children: part I: history, etiology, and pathophysiology. Circ Heart Fail. 2009;2:63-70.

and after pediatric cardiac surgery. Postoperative physiologic changes secondary to cardiopulmonary bypass, myocardial ischemia during aortic cross clamping, cardioplegia, residual lesions, ventriculotomy, changes in the loading conditions to the myocardium, and dysrhythmias may all contribute to the development of LCOS. A variety of proinflammatory triggers are activated during cardiopulmonary bypass as a result of blood contact with foreign surfaces, ischemia, reperfusion, tissue trauma, and temperature changes. This complex inflammatory response includes complement activation, cytokine release, leukocyte and platelet activation, and the expression of adhesion molecules. LCOS has been reported to affect up to 25% of infants and children, typically occurs between 6 and 18 hours after cardiac surgery, and results in a longer intensive care stay and increased mortality. It is associated with elevated systemic and pulmonary vascular resistances, impaired myocardial function, and dysrhythmias. When unrecognized or inadequately treated, LCOS can result in irreversible end-organ failure, cardiac arrest, and death. Prevention, early recognition, and optimal treatment are essential to ameliorate or reverse its course.[7]

Definitions

Achieving a balance between O_2 supply and demand is essential and can be accomplished by decreasing oxygen consumption (VO_2) or increasing oxygen delivery (DO_2). VO_2 is determined by tissue metabolism and is increased during periods of increased muscular activity (ie, seizures, exercise), infection, fever, or with increased levels of circulating catecholamines. Normally the ratio between DO_2 and VO_2 is 5:1 and when VO_2 increases according to increased metabolic demands, DO_2 adjusts accordingly. When the rate of oxygen consumption exceeds DO_2, anaerobic metabolism begins. Systemic oxygen delivery (DO_2) is defined as the amount of O_2 delivered to peripheral tissues each minute and is determined by cardiac output and the oxygen content of arterial blood as shown by the Fick equation that follows, where DO_2 refers to oxygen delivery and CO refers to cardiac output. Arterial oxygen content (CaO_2) is determined by hemoglobin (Hb) concentration, the arterial oxygen saturation (SaO_2), and the partial pressure of oxygen in the arterial blood (PaO_2). Cardiac output (CO) is defined as the product of heart rate (HR) × stroke volume (SV):

$$VO_2 = CO(CaO_2 - CvO_2)$$

$$DO_2 = CO \times CaO_2$$

$$CaO_2 = (Hb \times 1.36 \times SaO_2) + (PaO_2 \times 0.003)$$

$$CO = HR \times SV$$

Predictable changes in cardiac output have been demonstrated in newborns following the arterial switch operation for transposition of the great vessels. The median maximal decrease in cardiac index (32%) occurred approximately 6 to 12 hours after separation from cardiopulmonary bypass and nearly a quarter of these newborns reached a nadir of cardiac index that was <2 $L/min/m^2$.[8] The fall in cardiac index was coupled with a rise in the calculated systemic and pulmonary vascular resistance. Intraoperative perfusion strategy with either low-flow bypass or circulatory arrest was not associated with postoperative hemodynamic status or other postoperative events other than neurologic adverse events, which were higher with the use of deep hypothermic circulatory arrest (DHCA).[8]

Assessment

Although a complete assessment of oxygen delivery and consumption in critically ill infants and children is extremely challenging, numerous hemodynamic and biochemical parameters can be readily obtained to help guide the bedside clinician. Mixed venous oxygen saturation (SvO_2) or central venous oxygen saturation ($ScvO_2$), arterial lactate, and near-infrared spectroscopy (NIRS) are important biomarkers that can be serially measured in patients at risk for LCOS. SvO_2 and $ScvO_2$ are a reflection of the total body DO_2/VO_2 ratio and can be important metrics to follow in critically ill patients.[9,10] An elevated lactate level on admission (>4.5 mmol/L) and rising at 0.9 mmol/L/hr postoperatively is associated with major adverse events including death in infants after cardiac surgery.[11] Furthermore, lower SvO_2 may increase the predictive power of elevated arterial lactate levels for mortality after pediatric cardiac surgery.[6,12]

It is not uncommon to observe a disparity between direct measurements of DO_2 and cardiac output and estimates based on physical examination and interpretation of conventional laboratory and hemodynamic parameters.[7,13,14] Compensatory increases in systemic vascular resistance maintain arterial blood pressure as cardiac output decreases and central venous pressures may not correlate well with ventricular filling.[8,15] Femoral venous catheters are routinely placed in neonates and children, including an additional factor (intraabdominal pressure) in the accurate interpretation of these continuous variables. The effects of positive pressure ventilation on these measurements are well described.[16] Hemodynamic stability in the early postoperative period after the Norwood palliation depends on an adequate cardiac output and a balanced pulmonary-to-systemic blood flow ratio (Qp:Qs). The systemic oxygen saturation (SaO$_2$) alone is a poor predictor of Qp:Qs because of variability in systemic venous oxygen saturation (SvO$_2$) and pulmonary vein saturation (SpVO$_2$) after the Norwood operation. Monitoring and optimizing SvO$_2$ have been shown to improve outcomes in pediatric patients at risk for developing shock, including hypoplastic left heart syndrome.[9,17,18] Intermittent SvO$_2$ monitoring can be obtained to assess oxygen transport balance, but the presence of intracardiac shunts near the site of sampling and the need for repeated blood sampling limits its universal use. It has been reported that when SvO$_2$ monitoring is used in the postoperative care of critically ill neonates, significantly fewer adverse events are encountered, particularly with SvO$_2$ greater than 50%. Significant decreases in SvO$_2$ can occur without appreciable changes in arterial oxygen saturation, blood pressure, or heart rate. When low SvO$_2$ is recognized, increased inodilator support and measures that decrease metabolic demands (ie, sedation, neuromuscular blockade) often successfully return this metric to the normal range. In contrast, ventilator and inspired gas adjustments have less effect on SvO$_2$. The critical oxygen extraction ratio is defined by the onset of shock and ranges from 50% to 60%.[11,19,20] The critical DO$_2$ changes in parallel with changes in oxygen consumption even though the critical oxygen extraction ratio remains constant. When the critical oxygen extraction ratio is exceeded, SvO$_2$ decreases. This is an important consideration postoperatively when oxygen demand changes over time and with therapy.

Cerebral NIRS noninvasively assesses cerebral tissue oxygenation and relies on the relative lucency of biological tissue to near-infrared light where oxy- and deoxyhemoglobin have distinct absorption spectra,[18,21,22] and the oximeter monitors the nonpulsatile signal reflecting the microcirculation where 75% to 85% of the blood volume is venous. Thus the NIRS-derived oxygen saturation is an indicator of oxygen extraction for the region of brain beneath the optode. There is a good correlation between cerebral oxygen saturations, jugular bulb, and superior vena cava (SVC) saturations.[23,24] Cerebral oxygen saturations are closely and negatively correlated with the oxygen extraction ratio in neonates following the Norwood procedure. Strategies measuring regional venous weighted oxygen saturation in both cerebral and somatic regions provide better estimates of SvO$_2$ and a stronger relationship to outcome.

The pulse contour cardiac output (PiCCO) measurement system allows continuous hemodynamic monitoring using a large (femoral, brachial, or axillary) artery catheter and a central venous catheter. This technology uses intermittent transpulmonary thermodilution and pulse contour analysis. With the use of specific algorithms, various parameters such as cardiac output, extravascular lung water (EVLW), global end-diastolic volume (GEDV), pulse pressure variation (PPV), and stroke volume variation (SVV) can be obtained. PiCCO can assist in preload assessment in a volumetric manner. In patients with septic shock, GEDV calculated by PiCCO was found to be a better index of cardiac preload when compared with CVP in a prospective clinical study. The PiCCO may give inaccurate measurements in patients with arrhythmias, rapid temperature changes, intra/extracardiac shunts, aortic aneurysm, aortic stenosis, pneumonectomy, pulmonary embolism, and extracorporeal circulation.[19,25] The USCOM ultrasonic cardiac output monitor (USCOM Pty Ltd, Coffs Harbour, NSW, Australia) is a noninvasive device that determines cardiac output by continuous-wave Doppler ultrasound but pediatric data are limited.[26,27]

Specific Treatments to Improve Cardiac Function

In contrast to adult patients, tremendous heterogeneity exists between the etiology and pathophysiology of heart failure in pediatric patients. Despite these differences, treatment strategies for pediatric patients have followed the recommendations from large, randomized, multicenter trials in adult patients or "consensus" opinions based on single "best" institution clinical practices due to a lack of randomized, multicenter, pediatric clinical trials. With the expanded authority and mandates of the Food and Drug Administration (FDA) Pediatric Advisory Committee and the origins of the National Institutes of Health (NIH) Collaborative Pediatric Critical Care Research Network (CPCCRN) and the new Pediatric Cardiac Critical Care Consortium (PC4), the future is brighter for high-quality clinical trials in children.[28]

Outpatient management of chronic congestive heart failure with digitalis formed the basis of early therapy (~1970s) despite its narrow therapeutic index for safety. Loop or thiazide diuretics with the addition of the potassium-sparing antimineralocorticoid, spironolactone, were also commonly used, although drug compounding for children and potassium monitoring was problematic. Angiotensin-converting enzyme inhibitors (ACE-I) exert favorable effects on cardiac remodeling and survival in adults with congestive heart failure although their role in children is less clear, as a randomized, placebo-controlled trial in children evaluating the effect of ACE-I in single ventricle patients failed to demonstrate a beneficial effect.[29,30]

The nonselective β-blocker, propranolol, has been commonly used in pediatric cardiology for the treatment of dysrhythmias despite the need for frequent dosing. Selective β-blockers, like metoprolol, are a mainstay in adult cardiac patients with some use in children.[31,32] The nonselective β-blocker/α$_1$-blocker, carvedilol, has increased use in pediatric heart failure treatment. Most pediatric uses of these drugs have been extrapolated from the positive effects seen in adult trials that demonstrated a reduction in mortality and risk of hospitalization. Single-center trials have demonstrated both improved ejection fraction with the use of carvedilol in children awaiting heart transplantation with dilated cardiomyopathy and a delayed time to transplantation or death.[33] However, the most recent and largest multicenter, randomized, double-blind, placebo-controlled controlled trial of carvedilol in children and teenagers with symptomatic systolic heart failure did not demonstrate an improved survival benefit.[34]

For hospitalized children, LCOS has been traditionally managed using continuous infusions of catecholamines or their analogs (ie, dopamine, epinephrine, and dobutamine) to increase cardiac contractility (β_1) while avoiding tachycardia (β_1) and increases in systemic (SVR) or pulmonary vascular resistance (PVR) (α_1). Norepinephrine with its potent α_1 effects and lack of β_2 (vasodilatory) effects is generally not utilized unless a low SVR state is present (ie, septic shock). However, these agents when used in high doses can be deleterious on global and myocardial VO_2, induce myocardial cell apoptosis, and lead to increased mortality.

Milrinone, a phospodiesterase-3 inhibitor, has emerged as an important *inodilating* agent, which is now widely used in children after open-heart surgery after a landmark study showed that the prophylactic use of milrinone was associated with a decreased likelihood of LCOS in children after open-heart surgery in a dose-dependent fashion.[35] This benefit is thought to result from both improved myocardial contractility as well as pulmonary and systemic vasodilatory effects. Milrinone reduces right and left ventricular afterload through systemic and pulmonary vasodilatation and improves diastolic relaxation (lusitropy) of the myocardium through its enhanced cAMP-dependent diastolic reuptake of calcium.[36]

Sildenafil, an IV or oral drug that inhibits cGMP-specific phosphodiesterase type 5 (PDE5) causing smooth muscle relaxation, has proved to be beneficial in neonates with severe pulmonary hypertension and as an adjunct in weaning these patients from inhaled nitric oxide.[37,38]

Levosimendan, a relatively new drug, is a calcium sensitizer that enhances the contractility of the ventricle by binding to cardiac troponin C. In addition, the drug acts as a vasodilator by opening ATP-sensitive potassium channels in the vascular smooth muscle resulting in decreases in SVR and PVR. The improvement in myocardial performance is accomplished without an increase in intracellular calcium, thus providing a cardioprotective effect. Finally, an active metabolite with a half-life of ~3 days prolongs the duration of action for this continuously infused medication.[39]

Broad Treatment Strategies

Supportive care for decompensated heart failure begins with strategies aimed at improving the specific components of DO_2 and VO_2 listed previously (Fig. 30.1). This includes standard critical care therapies primarily focused on noncardiac support, such as intubation and mechanical support for respiratory insufficiency; temperature control, red cell transfusion for significant anemia; and control of pain and agitation with analgesia and anxiolysis. Mechanical respiratory support decreases metabolic demands by decreasing the work of breathing, reduces left ventricular afterload (wall stress), and can improve arterial oxygen saturation (SaO_2) by the administration of oxygen and PEEP, thus increasing CaO_2. However, endotracheal intubation can be risky in decompensated patients with HF, as the induction agents, laryngoscopy, and conversion to positive pressure ventilation can induce cardiac arrest. The benefits of noninvasive positive pressure

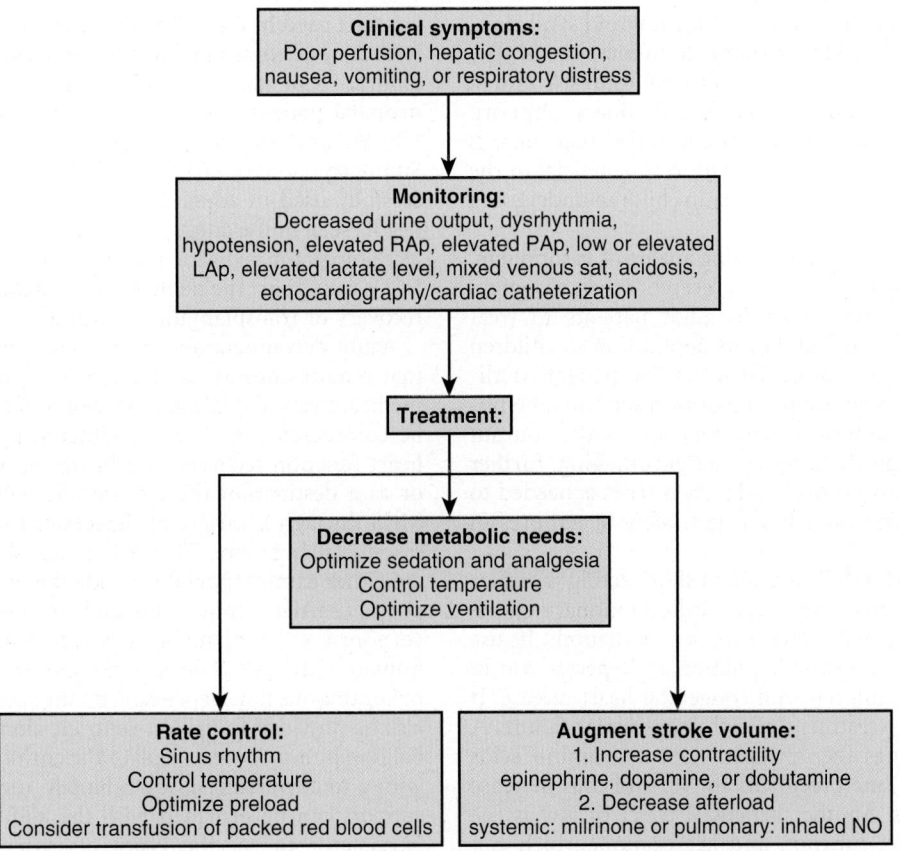

Fig. 30.1. Algorithm for treatment of ventricular dysfunction. *NO*, nitric oxide.

ventilation (facial BiPAP) have not been proved and the risks remain significant, particularly with regard to delay in timing for intubation and the need for additional sedation in children.

CaO_2 can also be increased by transfusing packed red blood cells (PRBCs) to increase hemoglobin concentrations in significant anemia. Research has not demonstrated a negative impact on patient outcomes when a restrictive transfusion practice was embraced, though the study did not examine complex or high-risk congenital cardiac patients or those with unrepaired or palliated cyanotic cardiac defects where a relative polycythemia is normally maintained to compensate for the decrease in SaO_2. Clearly, numerous, significant, deleterious effects on the recipient occur after allogenic blood transfusion, and the risk of donor-directed blood can be greater. In patients who are euvolemic, avoidance of hypervolemia with worsening pulmonary edema must be prevented when the decision to transfuse red cells is made.

Cardiopulmonary bypass results in numerous significant neurohormonal perturbations in the neonate after cardiac surgery. In particular, critical illness-related corticosteroid insufficiency and disruption of normal thyroid axis function can occur. Several studies have demonstrated acute salutary effects of postoperative therapy with both hydrocortisone and triiodothyronine without significant adverse effects,[40] although better clinical outcomes beyond the immediate hemodynamic improvements have yet to be shown. Adult patients who undergo open-heart surgery and receive triiodothyronine (T3) supplementation have demonstrated a dose-dependent increase in cardiac output, which has been associated with an improved clinical outcome. In multiple small studies in neonates and children after cardiopulmonary bypass, the serum thyroid panel identifies a pattern of sick euthyroid syndrome. Supplementation with T3 has variably led to increases in specific hemodynamic parameters, improved diuresis, and a decreased need for additional cardiopulmonary support. Regardless, a 2007 systematic review concluded that there is lack of evidence that T3 supplementation is beneficial in the prevention of morbidity and mortality in children undergoing cardiac surgery.[41]

Terlipressin is a synthetic long-acting analog of vasopressin, with a higher affinity for vascular V_1 receptors than vasopressin. Terlipressin has been used in adult patients to treat extremely low cardiac output, but its application in children is limited. In postoperative pediatric cardiac patients, terlipressin demonstrated an improvement in respiratory, hemodynamic, and renal indices in refractory low cardiac output syndrome.[42] Although these results are encouraging, further investigation with prospective randomized trials is needed to provide data regarding the efficacy and safety of terlipressin in infants and children.

Inhaled nitric oxide (iNO) is a potent short-acting vasodilator resulting in numerous beneficial cardiopulmonary effects on the pulmonary, systemic, and coronary circulations. Its use is standard for severe, reversible pulmonary hypertension in the neonate and in children with congenital heart disease. It is also useful in the treatment of right ventricular failure. A variety of other drugs (eg, nitroprusside) and amino acids (arginine, citrulline) are precursors to NO and thus increase its circulating levels. Another beneficial effect of NO is the inhibition of platelet function and aggregation, which can complicate a variety of cardiovascular diseases in children.[43]

Fenoldopam, a selective dopamine-1 receptor partial agonist, causes systemic vasodilatation and increased renal blood flow with improved renal function in adults. Two meta-analyses have concluded that fenoldopam use in critically ill adult patients at risk of acute kidney injury decreases the development of acute tubular necrosis, requirement for renal replacement therapy, length of ICU stay, and overall patient mortality. One study also demonstrated a reduction in the time on mechanical ventilation.[44] Data on the use of fenoldopam in pediatric patients are sparse, with one retrospective study demonstrating a significant improvement in diuresis in neonates after cardiopulmonary bypass with the addition of fenoldopam to conventional diuretic therapy, whereas another prospective trial failed to demonstrate a beneficial effect.[45]

Mechanical Circulatory Support in Pediatric Patients
Brief Historical Perspective

Since 1953 when John Gibbon first utilized extracorporeal perfusion in the operating room, the indications and utilization of MCS have continued to expand. Technologic advances have afforded support for thousands of patients per year with a variety of respiratory or cardiac indications. Early trials of extracorporeal membrane oxygenation (ECMO) were marked by mixed results. In 1985 Bartlett and colleagues reported the first successful use of ECMO in a newborn.[46] Since then, neonates with diagnoses of meconium aspiration syndrome, persistent pulmonary hypertension, and congenital diaphragmatic hernia have been treated for severe respiratory failure unresponsive to conventional therapies. ECMO for cardiac support was first used in the 1970s, but it was not until the 1990s that it became a common therapeutic technique for myocardial failure. As of January 2015, a total of 65,171 pediatric and neonatal patients were registered within the Extracorporeal Life Support Registry (ECLS Registry Report International Summary January 2015) (Table 30.2). VADs have been successfully used in adults since the early 1970s. The favorable results seen in the adult prompted the adaptation of the adult technology for pediatric patients. Worldwide experience with VADs to support the neonates and infants as a bridge to either recovery or transplantation continues to grow.

Acute decompensated heart failure is a critical condition that requires prompt and aggressive intervention and, when medical treatment is maximized or ineffective, patients should be considered for MCS for either temporary support until heart function recovers, as a bridge to heart transplantation, or as a destination therapy (ie, life with permanent MCS). MCS through a variety of devices can support right, left, or biventricular failure. This is accomplished with devices that are either extracorporeal (outside the human body), paracorporeal (partial within and outside the human body), or intracorporeal or implantable (residing completely within the human body). MCS devices can provide either pulsatile flow or continuous flow depending on the specific design. MCS can also be provided to the left ventricle alone with an intraaortic balloon pump or it can replace the entire function of the heart with a totally artificial heart. Finally, cardiac and pulmonary support can be provided with the addition of a membrane oxygenator to specific types of extracorporeal circulatory devices (ECLS). Venoarterial ECLS provides cardiopulmonary support, whereas venovenous ECLS provides only pulmonary support for severe respiratory failure.

Despite improvements in operative techniques, management of cardiopulmonary bypass, and myocardial protection, myocardial dysfunction and failure can occur after surgery for congenital heart disease with involvement of the left or right ventricles. Approximately 5% of children undergoing cardiac surgery require MCS. The patient's underlying pathophysiology, size, and expected length of support dictate which technique is most suitable. In children, most mechanical circulatory support continues to be achieved with ECLS. Since ECLS and VADs have advantages and disadvantages, determining the most appropriate modality for the individual patient requires significant expertise.

Extracorporeal Life Support

ECLS is the most utilized form of short-term MCS support for pediatric patients with decompensated heart failure unresponsive to medical therapy. Adaptations and simplification of the traditional cardiopulmonary bypass circuit have resulted in the standard venoarterial ECLS circuit (Fig. 30.2) through either extrathoracic (ie, carotid artery/jugular vein or femoral vessels) or transthoracic (right atrium/ascending aorta) placement after median sternotomy. The venous cannula allows for passive drainage of blood from the patient into a bladder, which then passes through a servo-regulated roller-head or centrifugal pump that propels blood through the remainder of the system at high pressure. Gas exchange (O_2 addition and CO_2 removal) occurs next through an artificial lung (oxygenator, comprising a silicone membrane or hollow fibers) where countercurrent sweep gas passes external to the blood phase. Blood temperature is controlled by a heat exchanger. Finally, blood is returned to the body into a major artery. Additional components include ports on the venous side (preoxygenator) for infusion of medications, pressure and flow monitors, oxygen saturation or blood gas analyzers for both the venous and arterial blood, bubble detectors, placement of a hemofilter for fluid control or dialysis (venovenous or arteriovenous), and, frequently, a bridge connecting the venous and arterial

TABLE 30.2	Extracorporeal Life Support Organization Registry Outcomes as of July 2015		
Category	Total	Survived Extracorporeal Life Support	Survived to DC or Transfer
Neonatal			
Respiratory	27,728	23,358 84%	20,592 74%
Cardiac	5,810	3,600 62%	2,389 41%
ECPR	1,112	712 64%	449 40%
Pediatric			
Respiratory	6,569	4,327 66%	3,760 57%
Cardiac	7,314	4,825 66%	3,679 50%
ECPR	2,370	1,313 55%	976 41%
Adult			
Respiratory	7,008	4,587 65%	4,026 57%
Cardiac	5,603	3,219 56%	2,294 41%
ECPR	1,657	639 39%	471 28%
Total	65,171	46,490 71%	38,636 59%

ECPR, extracorporeal cardiopulmonary resuscitation.

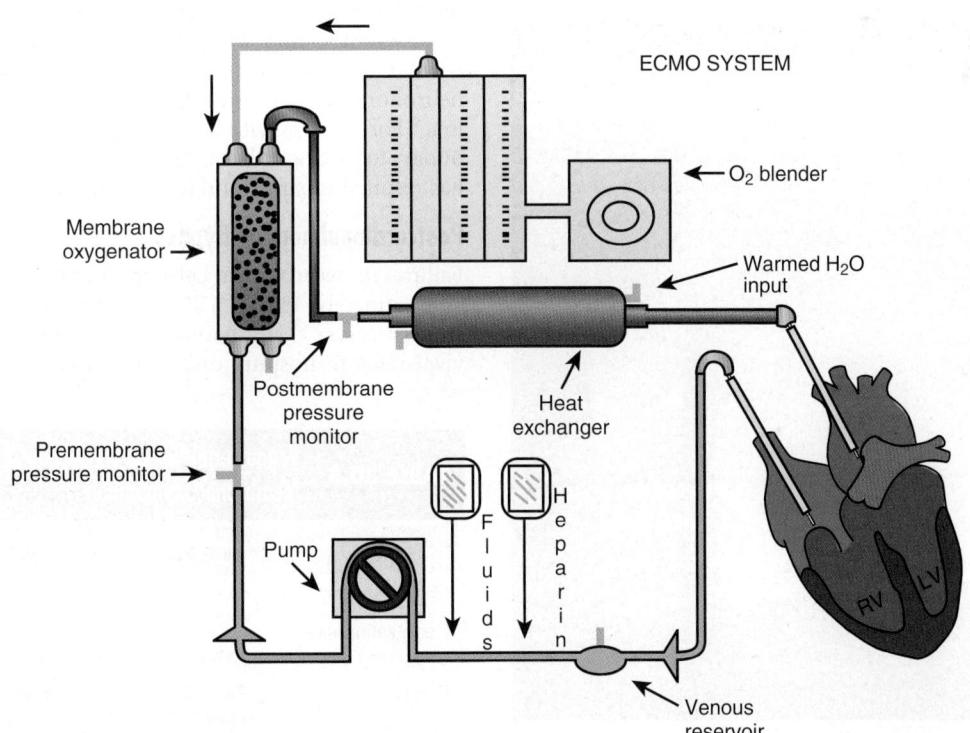

Fig. 30.2. Extracorporeal membrane oxygenation circuit.

sides of the circuit for use during trials off ECLS or in case of a circuit emergency.[47]

Venoarterial (V-A) ECLS provides biventricular and pulmonary support. It is important to note that complete cardiac bypass cannot be provided by V-A ECLS due to incomplete capture of the venous return by the venous cannula. Routine cannulation for V-A ECLS occurs via one of three vascular access points: The transcervical approach places the venous cannula in the right atrium (RA) via the right internal jugular vein and the arterial cannula in the transverse aortic arch via the right carotid artery; the transthoracic approach results in direct cannulation of the RA and ascending aorta through a median sternotomy for patients who either cannot be weaned from cardiopulmonary bypass or require MCS in the immediate postoperative period; and the femoral artery and vein cannulation for adolescents and adults, which utilizes longer cannulae to reach the RA and descending aorta. A combination of these approaches with more than one venous cannulation site can be employed when very high flows are required. The transcervical and transthoracic approaches are the preferred methods for small children. Fig. 30.3 demonstrates a chest radiograph obtained for evaluation of cannula placement in a patient supported by V-A ECLS. Venovenous (V-V) ECLS provides pulmonary support without cardiac support. In V-V ECLS a single double-lumen cannula is placed in the RA through a transcervical approach. This cannula provides both inflow and outflow for the circuit. V-V ECLS can improve right ventricular (RV) function as a result of oxygenated, pH-balanced blood flowing to the lungs, thus decreasing pulmonary vascular resistance (PVR) and right heart afterload.

Although some patients experience improvement in overall cardiac function with V-V ECLS, this might not be sufficient or sustained. Therefore when ECLS is necessary for significant myocardial dysfunction, V-A ECLS is the preferred modality. See Table 30.3 for comparison of V-A versus V-V ECLS.

Prior to pediatric VAD technology, the *No Membrane Oxygenator Ventricular Assist Device (NOMO-VAD)* was an adaptation of traditional ECLS whereby the oxygenator was omitted and the circuit shortened. This technique allows for MCS without the pulmonary support of ECLS, thus limiting some of the harmful inflammatory effects from exposure to the oxygenator and reducing the need for anticoagulation. It has been utilized successfully in neonates following first-stage palliation of hypoplastic left heart syndrome.[48,49]

Extracorporeal Membrane Oxygenation Indications and Contraindications

It is widely accepted that all patients considered for MCS should have either a reversible physiologic process or be a candidate for bridge to transplant or destination therapy. The time frame in which recovery is expected and the severity of cardiac or other organ failure are used to guide optimal device selection. Several studies emphasize that the importance of early institution of ECLS before a prolonged period of low cardiac output results in multiorgan dysfunction. Appropriate patient selection is vital to maximize survival.[50-52]

Myocarditis

The clinical course of myocarditis is variable with some patients presenting with subclinical disease and others with an indolent course progressing to a dilated cardiomyopathy, whereas a distinct subset presents with fulminant disease. Without MCS, these patients with rapidly progressive disease had expected survival rates of only 25% to 50%. With aggressive utilization of ECLS as bridge to transplantation or recovery, survival rates for patients are now reported as high as 90%.[53,54] It has been shown that the institution of MCS can normalize ventricular geometry, cellular composition, metabolism, and ultimately function, a phenomenon referred to as reverse remodeling. This process is thought to improve ventricular dysfunction because of favorable influences on the neurohormonal cardiovascular milieu and ventricular unloading.[55] For patients with end-stage dilated cardiomyopathy secondary to myocarditis, the use of MCS without transplantation has resulted in survival rates as high as 67% to 80%.

Postcardiopulmonary Bypass

Failure to wean from cardiopulmonary bypass occurs in approximately 1% to 3.2% of pediatric congenital cardiac surgery cases.[56,57] Individual institutions have reported survival rates to hospital discharge between 32% and 54% for

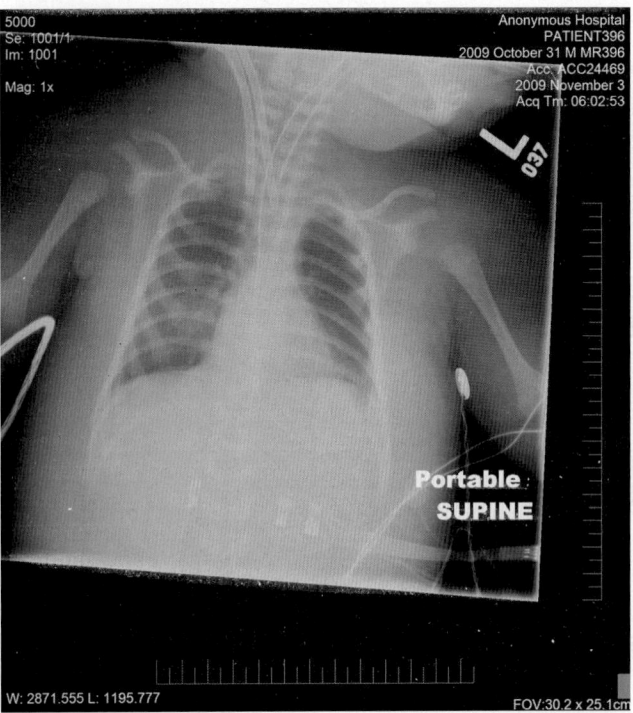

Fig. 30.3. Chest radiograph showing extracorporeal membrane oxygenation cannulas.

TABLE 30.3	Venoarterial Versus Venovenous Extracorporeal Membrane Oxygenation	
	VV ECMO	**VA ECMO**
Organ support	Pulmonary	Pulmonary and cardiac
Cannulation site	Transcervical or femoral	Transcervical, transthoracic, or femoral
Pump	Roller or centrifugal	Roller or centrifugal
Length of support	Days to weeks	Days to weeks

pediatric patients who require MCS after cardiac surgery. One small series has reported a survival rate as high as 80%.[58] However, the July 2015 Extracorporeal Life Support Organization (ELSO) registry report for postoperative cardiac surgery patients younger than 16 years of age noted an overall survival rate of only 47%. The use of MCS is currently widely accepted to support vital organs while allowing for myocardial recovery. It is imperative that these patients be evaluated for the presence of residual cardiac defects that may be causing or worsening cardiovascular collapse. Intraoperative transesophageal echocardiography (TEE), transthoracic echocardiography (TTE), and diagnostic cardiac catheterization may identify the need for reoperation or interventional cardiac catheterization to improve the patient's hemodynamic status.[59] Balloon valvuloplasty, angioplasty of aortic arch obstructions, device closure of residual septal defects, coil occlusion of aortopulmonary collateral vessels, or atrial septostomy all may be crucial interventions to improve the patient's hemodynamic state and allow for separation from MCS. Untreated and significant residual cardiac defects have been shown to be almost universally fatal for patients requiring MCS. The use of MCS for postcardiotomy support in neonates and infants with single ventricle physiology is technically more complex with worse outcomes, and thus it is considered a relative contraindication to MCS at some centers.[60] The 2015 ELSO report lists a 33% survival rate for ECLS use in patients following the stage I Norwood procedure, lower than for other postcardiotomy patients and falling to 19% if hemodialysis is required (Extracorporeal Life Support Organization: ECLS Registry Report. International Summary. Ann Arbor, MI, Extracorporeal Life Support Organization, 2015).

Extracorporeal Cardiopulmonary Resuscitation

In-hospital cardiac arrest in children continues to be associated with dismal outcomes despite advances in cardiopulmonary resuscitation (CPR). A prospective multicenter observational study from the National Registry of Cardiopulmonary Resuscitation reported a survival rate to hospital discharge of 27%, although a good neurologic outcome for 73% of survivors was seen.[61,62] A multicenter observational study from the Pediatric Emergency Care Applied Research Network (PECARN) reviewed in-hospital cardiac arrests that occurred during an 18-month period between 2003 and 2004 in which extracorporeal cardiopulmonary resuscitation (ECPR) was available. In this cohort, 49% survived to hospital discharge with the utilization of ECPR with a good neurologic outcome for 76% of survivors. Both studies excluded out-of-hospital, do-not-resuscitate, or neonatal intensive care unit patients. However, although neurocognitive outcome has improved for survivors of cardiac arrest, the duration of CPR remains inversely proportional to survival. One center demonstrated that a witnessed in-hospital cardiac arrest of >30 minutes in duration was universally fatal without the utilization of ECPR.[63] This result has led to an emerging interest in the use of ECPR for patients who failed to quickly reestablish a perfusing rhythm and adequate circulation with conventional CPR. The American Heart Association guidelines for in-hospital pediatric cardiac arrest now recommend consideration of MCS during cardiopulmonary resuscitation if the conditions leading to the arrest are likely to be reversible or amenable to heart transplantation. However, wide variability in patient selection and the ability to institute MCS in a timely fashion (ideally <60 minutes) has led to variable success with survival rates ranging from 0% to 100%.[64,65] Thus some large centers have created systems for rapid deployment ECLS utilizing a team that is immediately available to cannulate with a preprimed circuit. The 2015 ELSO Registry for neonatal and pediatric patients supported with ECLS following cardiac arrest reported a survival to hospital discharge of 38%.

Bridge to Transplantation

Although heart transplantation is the treatment of choice for end-stage myocardial failure, many children die every year waiting for a suitable organ to become available. As a result, MCS is now increasingly utilized as a bridge to heart transplantation. The most common indications for MCS as a bridge to transplant include cardiac failure due to congenital heart disease, cardiomyopathy, and graft rejection after heart transplantation.[66,67] Children with myocardial failure secondary to myocarditis also demonstrate increased short-term survival when treated with MCS and transplantation.[68]

Complications associated with ECLS generally limit the duration of support to approximately 2 weeks, but as long as complications precluding transplant have not developed, no arbitrary cutoff for duration of ECLS should be determined. A review of the United Network for Organ Sharing (UNOS) database from 1995 to 2005 evaluated both clinical status at transplantation and risk factors for the short- and long-term mortality of patients supported with various MCS devices. This study revealed that 30-day survival was significantly decreased for patients bridged to transplant with ECLS versus VAD, although long-term (10-year) survival was not affected. Not surprisingly, preoperative severity of illness predicted early survival following transplantation. The overall 10-year survival was 56.8% in patients supported with MCS prior to transplantation.[69]

Malignant Dysrhythmias

MCS can be lifesaving for pediatric patients with malignant dysrhythmias unresponsive to pharmacotherapy. A subset of patients with acute fulminant myocarditis will present with refractory LCOS and ventricular tachycardia or high degree heart block that further compromises end-organ perfusion. In this scenario, MCS may be used to bridge patients to recovery or transplantation. Several potentially lethal arrhythmias such as supraventricular tachycardia, junctional ectopic tachycardia, ventricular tachycardia, or torsades de pointes can occur congenitally, become acquired in the perioperative period, or manifest as a result of the ingestion of toxic substances or medications.[62,70] Again, ECLS can allow time for resolution of dysrhythmia with aggressive medical treatment and the subsequent recovery of cardiac function.

Refractory Respiratory Failure

Respiratory failure refractory to maximal medical therapy is the most common indication for ECLS in neonates. Causes include meconium aspiration syndrome, congenital diaphragmatic hernia, persistent pulmonary hypertension of the newborn, sepsis, or other congenital lung abnormalities. The first to perform a systematic comparison of neonatal ECLS practice patterns and respiratory failure deaths between countries demonstrated distinct differences between the United States (US) and the United Kingdom (UK). It concluded that US clinicians seem more willing to utilize ECLS for persistent pulmonary hypertension of the newborn and congenital diaphragmatic hernia. This difference in practice pattern was correlated with a decrease in the US neonatal death rate from congenital diaphragmatic hernia in comparison to the UK.

The most common diagnosis in the pediatric respiratory ECLS group of patients is acute respiratory distress syndrome (ARDS). Overall survival for this group of patients remains at 56%. The duration of ECLS is often longer for respiratory failure than cardiac failure. ECLS for respiratory failure is discussed in detail in Chapter 59.

Other Indications

Since the 1990s, successful treatment of pediatric patients with ECLS has increasingly being described in individuals that would have been excluded in the past, such as patients with trauma, immunosuppression, bleeding diatheses, sickle cell disease, status asthmaticus, septic shock, pulmonary embolism, established multiple organ system failure, among others.

Contraindications

Although individual institutions may have variations to this list, there are only a few absolute contraindications to ECLS, including irreversible cardiac failure without the option for transplantation, irreversible lung failure, severe neurologic dysfunction, grade III/IV intracranial hemorrhage, uncontrolled bleeding, and congenital anomalies/genetic syndromes with short expected life spans. Relative contraindications include prematurity (<34 weeks), weight <2 kg, grade II intraventricular hemorrhage, and recent bleeding.[71] Cardiac arrest is not a contraindication if rapid effective CPR was initiated, the underlying etiology is deemed reversible, and time for cannulation is <60 minutes. The challenge remains determining what is *irreversible, shortened life span, poor prognosis,* or *severe,* as these definitions have changed over time and with differing expectations for quality of life if survival is attained. Technical limitations are an inability to obtain vascular access secondary to thrombosis, abnormal anatomy, or prior surgery.

Critical Care Management During Extracorporeal Life Support

Patients who require MCS are by definition critically ill, often with multiple end-organ dysfunction, and thus it is not surprising that complications occur with a greater frequency for this group of patients than for other critically ill patients. The basic management principles are discussed in this section. Table 30.4 summarizes the most common reported complications for pediatric patients supported by ECLS.

Cardiac Output

When assessing the hemodynamic state of a patient, one must consider to what degree conventional support (ie, mechanical ventilation and vasoactive agents) is contributing to cardiac and pulmonary function versus the ECLS system. The amount of flow provided by the ECLS system is measured through ultrasonic flow probes on the high-pressure side of the circuit beyond where any shunts (ie, high-pressure to low-pressure connection through a hemofilter) may occur. An approximation of flow generated by the pump can be calculated from the product of the revolutions per minute (RPMs) and circuit tubing diameter. For most cardiac ECLS patients, flow is initiated at 120 to 150 mL/kg/min. However, it is important to note that flow should be adjusted to fit the physiologic needs of each

TABLE 30.4	Complications of Extracorporeal Membrane Oxygenation, Extracorporeal Life Support Organization Registry, July 2015				
% Reported	Respiratory Runs: Neonatal N = 23,495	Respiratory Runs: Pediatric N = 4263	Cardiac Runs: 0 to 30 Days N = 3980	Cardiac Runs: 31 Days to 1 Year N = 2,527	Cardiac Runs: 1-16 Years N = 2131
Raceway rupture	0.3%	0.7%	0.3%	0.7%	0.8%
Oxygenator failure	5.9%	13.3%	7.5%	8.4%	9.2%
Pump malfunction	1.7%	2.8%	1.6%	2.1%	2.3%
Seizures	9.9%	6.2%	7.8%	9.6%	5.2%
CNS infarct	7.8%	3.8%	3.6%	3.9%	4.1%
CNS hemorrhage	6.7%	5.7%	11.3%	5.2%	3.2%
Brain death	1%	5.7%	1.2%	3.9%	7.9%
Hypertension	12.6%	15.3%	8.2%	11.5%	10.8%
CPR	2.3%	5.8%	3.4%	3.1%	4.3%
Cardiac stun	5.1%	1.6%	6.9%	5%	5.5%
Tamponade	0.6%	2.2%	6.4%	5.7%	5.6%
Cannulation site bleeding	6.9%	14.4%	9.8%	10.6%	16.1%
Surgical site bleeding	6.2%	14.7%	32%	34.5%	30%
Gastrointestinal hemorrhage	1.7%	4.2%	1%	2%	2.9%
Infection	6.1%	18.9%	7.8%	12.6%	11.4%
Hemofiltration	14.3%	20.1%	25.6%	21.1%	18.8%
Continuous arteriovenous hemodialysis	1.4%	6.2%	5.6%	4.5%	6.1%
Dialysis	3.3%	14.5%	11%	12.5%	13.3%

patient. Patients with septic shock may require higher flows approaching 200 mL/kg/min to support their metabolic needs, assuming venous drainage is sufficient to yield such flows. A precise measurement of the patient's intrinsic cardiac output (ie, the amount of blood that is not bypassed through the ECLS circuit) is often unobtainable. However, indirect evaluation of the patient's cardiac output is possible through an assessment of arterial systolic blood pressure, pulse pressure, heart rate, organ perfusion, mixed venous oxygen saturation, and lactic acid levels on a given flow rate. Comparisons of these variables over time allow the clinician to make decisions regarding the adequacy of circulatory support or the readiness to wean from support. An echocardiogram can also provide valuable information about cardiac filling and function and guide therapy, particularly when weaning from ECLS or during a trial off ECLS. Mixed venous oxygen saturation (SvO_2) is measured in the venous return portion of the circuit, with a goal of 65% to 80%. However, if a left-to-right shunt exists such as a left atrial vent, the mixed venous saturation will be falsely elevated, particularly if the patient is receiving high FiO_2 and PEEP. Serial lactate measurements are often helpful to aid in the assessment of global end-organ perfusion. Elevated lactate levels may occur in patients with ongoing hepatic dysfunction, sepsis, low cardiac output, and end-organ hypoperfusion. A rough approximation of the relative contributions of the patient and circuit pulmonary parameters is possible by analyzing serial patient and circuit blood gas assays (pH, $paCO_2$, paO_2, SaO_2) while taking into consideration the mechanical ventilation settings (including FiO_2 and PEEP), circuit flow rate, gas sweep rate, and circuit oxygen concentration. Finally, *shunts* within the patient or the circuit must be taken into consideration. An example of a right-to-left patient shunt includes a patient with a patent ductus arteriosus, atrial septal defect, or ventricular septal defect in the setting of severe pulmonary artery hypertension. Circuit left-to-right shunts are generally limited to a left atrial *vent, open bridge,* the A-V hemodialysis filter, and in vivo continuous arterial blood gas device. Total blood flow for the patient on MCS requires the addition of ECLS circuit flow with the patient's native cardiac output minus any *shunt* within the system as a whole.

Troubleshooting

Hemodynamic compromise often continues despite MCS, and low-dose inotropes or inodilators can aid cardiac contractility to augment native cardiac output and reduce afterload to both the right and left ventricles. The most commonly utilized agents are dopamine (3–5 µg/kg/min), epinephrine (0.03–0.05 µg/kg/min), dobutamine (5 µg/kg/min), or milrinone (0.25–0.75 µg/kg/min). The use of catecholamines in high doses is detrimental to cardiac recovery and should be avoided by increasing circuit flow to provide adequate circulation. Tachydysrhythmias and pulseless electrical activity requiring cardiopulmonary resuscitation occurs in 3% of neonatal and pediatric ECMO runs (see Table 30.4). Chemical/electrical cardioversion of any dysrhythmia should be attempted quickly to promote recovery of cardiac function. Cardiac pacing can be utilized to optimize cardiac output.

Hypovolemia

Hypovolemia is a common occurrence during MCS for a variety of reasons. Inadequate venous drainage secondary to cannula malposition, cardiac tamponade, tension pneumothorax, or hemothorax may occur and generally results in hypotension requiring immediate correction (see Table 30.4). Ongoing evaporative losses from the oxygenator and bleeding secondary to coagulopathy can contribute to hypovolemia. Initiation of ECLS activates a host of inflammatory mediators resulting in capillary leak and hypovolemia.[72] Finally, attempts at mobilizing the large amount of *third spaced* fluid with either diuretics, hemofiltration, or through drains in pleural/peritoneal cavities can quickly cause either inadequate cardiac output from the patient or inadequate venous drainage to the ECLS circuit.

Hypertension

Hypertension secondary to neurohormonal dysregulation is one of the most common and unavoidable cardiovascular complications of ECLS (see Table 30.4). Although hypertension has not been demonstrated to negatively impact patient survival, its presence can worsen bleeding or further impair cardiac function and thus should be promptly addressed.[73]

Cardiac Stun

Cardiac stun, a term that describes reversible global dyskinesia of the ventricle, was coined by Braunwauld and Kloner in 1982.[74,75] Reversible cardiac dysfunction that results in the lack of antegrade left ventricular ejection during systole resembles electromechanical dissociation, which has been observed frequently in patients following the initiation of V-A ECLS. Excluding conditions of physiologic tamponade from thoracic tissues, blood, or air, an infant on ECLS should have sufficient cardiac function to generate a minimal pulse pressure of 10 mm Hg. Evaluations of patients who experience cardiac stun upon initiation of ECLS defined this condition as the absence of aortic valve opening during systole, equalizing of the patient preductal and postmembrane circuit PaO_2, and absence of pulse pressure in the aorta. The etiology of cardiac stun is multifactorial and hypothesized to be the sequelae of acute ischemia followed by reperfusion or severe electrolyte disturbances. The incidence of stun on ECLS is 5% to 12% in neonates and, when present and prolonged (>24 hours), results in a significant increase in mortality for these patients (see Table 30.4). Stun typically occurs during the initiation of bypass in patients who were more hypoxic, hypercarbic, acidotic, and suffered a cardiac arrest prior to ECLS. Important factors in trying to minimize cardiac stun upon the initiation of ECLS include correcting the pH and ionized calcium levels in the circuit and infusing calcium chloride to the patient upon commencing ECLS, followed by close monitoring of arterial blood gases and electrolytes with rapid correction of abnormalities.

Echocardiography and Cardiac Catheterization

Initial diagnostic and hemodynamic assessment should be attempted by transthoracic echocardiography, but imaging windows may be severely limited resulting in insufficient information. Transesophageal echocardiography (TEE) may improve diagnostic accuracy but may not be possible secondary to bleeding risks or patient size. Even if adequate imaging is obtained, the specific hemodynamic state of the patient on ECLS must be taken into account when interpreting these studies. Invariably, the loading conditions of the heart are markedly altered during ECLS. The echocardiographer should actively interface with the ECLS team (to potentially modify flows, add volume, increase mechanical ventilator support, etc.) in order to obtain the most comprehensive assessment of cardiac function to inform clinical decisions regarding the continuation or removal of further ECLS support. Cardiac catheterization can be a useful tool for select patients who fail to wean from ECLS. The specific loading conditions of the heart must be considered in the context of the acquired data in order to make sound clinical decisions. Therapeutic interventions that might be performed in the catheterization lab include balloon or blade atrial septostomy to alleviate left atrial hypertension, balloon valvuloplasty or angioplasty of vascular obstructions, device closure of residual atrial or ventricular shunts, and coil embolization of aortopulmonary shunts.[76] Correction of these types of residual defects in the catheterization laboratory or surgical correction in the operating room may be required to allow for separation from MCS. In a review of 216 courses of ECLS for pediatric patients, 50 of 60 catheterizations performed led to an intervention either during or after the catheterization procedure.[77] Complications of the catheterization included myocardial perforation in two infants, each weighing less than 3.5 kg. Both were treated for the complication and survived the procedure.[77] For patients with significant left ventricular failure, it may be necessary to decompress the left heart to prevent or reverse pulmonary edema or hemorrhage, decrease mitral regurgitation, and, importantly, improve coronary perfusion to increase the chances of myocardial recovery. In this scenario, *venting* of the left ventricle occurs through placement of a cannula in the left atrial appendage connected to the venous drainage to the ECLS circuit. This is accomplished in the operating room during transthoracic ECLS cannulation or in the catheterization laboratory through creation of an interatrial connection via balloon or blade septostomy. This procedure can markedly improve left ventricular function and increase the chances of survival.[78,79]

Single Ventricle

Lower survival rates are universally found in this subset of patients, which may be attributed to an imbalance of the systemic and pulmonary circulations, volume burden to the single ventricle after complex palliative surgery, compromised single ventricle function (particularly with right ventricular morphology), and impaired coronary perfusion to the systemic ventricle when a systemic-to-pulmonary artery connection (eg, modified Blalock-Taussig [BT] shunt) results in diastolic runoff from the aorta. Despite the challenges presented, larger centers continue to report improved outcomes with the accumulation of experience and application of innovative strategies. For example, initial efforts to balance the systemic and pulmonary circulations on ECLS included either completely or partially occluding the aortopulmonary shunt, which has now been demonstrated to increase mortality. The use of smaller size BT shunts or the use of the Sano modification (RV to PA nonvalved conduit for stage one hypoplastic left heart palliation) has contributed to decreasing the recirculation that would otherwise occur. Of note, higher ECLS with flows approaching 200 mL/kg/min may be required to provide adequate systemic and pulmonary support when the shunt is left open.[80,81]

Anticoagulation Strategies

ECLS requires meticulous management of hemostasis to limit patient morbidities. Hemorrhagic and thrombotic complications are a major concern for patients during ECLS,

particularly after cardiac surgery. Bleeding can manifest at surgical sites (arterial/venous cannulation sites, surgical repair sites (atriotomy, ventriculotomy, aortotomy sites, sternal incision, indwelling catheter sites, etc.) or masked in areas such as the thorax, intracranial vault, or the gastrointestinal tract (see Table 30.4). Prevention strategies that target reduction of hematologic complications focus on maintenance of the hemostatic regulatory mechanisms as close to normal as possible.[82-85] Apart from single-center experience, no well-defined consensus or protocol is available for pediatric and neonatal ECLS. The patient's age, diagnosis, clinical status in conjunction with the specific details of the ECLS device, and, finally, the flow through the circuit will dictate which anticoagulation strategy should be employed. The most commonly utilized agent for anticoagulation on ECLS is continuously infused unfractionated heparin. Most centers measure platelet counts, hematocrit, prothrombin time (PT), partial thromboplastin time (PTT), fibrinogen, specific factor levels (ie, anti-Factor Xa, antithrombin III), quantitative heparin levels, and activated clotting time (ACT). The ACT is the most commonly measured test for coagulation, as it can be performed quickly at the bedside, though other coagulation tests are available as point-of-care tests (ie, PTT).[86,87] Despite this advantage, ACT results vary markedly based on the technique used, and it is a nonspecific measure of coagulation because it measures the total time for a clot to form after ex vivo activation. The ACT is a global composite of the different individual components of coagulation, and thus more specific tests (listed above) must be used in concert to ascertain which specific component in the coagulation cascade is affected. Thus no single test is currently used to guide the anticoagulation regimen, but rather a panel of tests must be obtained and analyzed in concert. Several centers have reported on the effective use of thromboelastography (TEG) in determining patient coagulation status.[88] When "adequately anticoagulated on a continuous unfractionated heparin infusion," the goal ACT should be between 180 and 220 seconds when the ECLS pump is flowing at full flow (ie, >150 cc/kg/min). This goal can be decreased to 160 seconds on full flow if significant bleeding is present, particularly in the immediate postoperative period. Unfractionated heparin is metabolized via two mechanisms: at low doses, via a saturable mechanism representing clearance by the reticuloendothelial system and endothelial cells to which heparin binds with high affinity, and at high doses, via a nonsaturable mechanism represented by renal excretion. Thus close monitoring during ECLS must be followed when a patient's urinary output is oscillating between oliguria and polyuria.

Newer treatment strategies include the use of additional agents such as antithrombin III (ATIII) in either bolus or infusion form to correct abnormalities in the clotting cascade. ATIII is an alpha2-glycoprotein serine protease inhibitor that inactivates a number of enzymes from the coagulation system including the activated forms of factors II, VII, IX, X, XI, and XII. Replacement of ATIII is indicated when its level is low (<30%) and heparin infusion rates are increasing without a concomitant increase in ACT or PTT.[40,89,90] Anticoagulation with Coumadin, clopidogrel, low-molecular-weight heparin, and aspirin individually or in combination can be considered with certain MCS devices other than ECLS.[91]

Heparin-induced thrombocytopenia (HIT) is a relatively rare but serious complication of heparin administration caused by antibodies binding to a complex of heparin and platelet factor 4 (PF4) that leads to large vessel thrombosis and increased mortality. A drop in platelet count by more than 50% of the highest previous value should raise suspicion of HIT and trigger investigation. Treatment includes discontinuing heparin administration and initiating direct thrombin inhibitor therapy (ie, argatroban) if continued anticoagulation is needed.[82]

The lysine analogs tranexamic acid and epsilon aminocaproic acid are antifibrinolytic agents that have been shown to reduce bleeding in ECLS patients undergoing surgical procedures. However, prophylactic administration failed to reduce the incidence of intracranial hemorrhage in neonates.[86]

Profound abnormalities in many components of the coagulation cascade commonly occur in postoperative cardiac patients on ECLS. With this in mind, an attempt to normalize components of coagulation not impacted by heparin is important. Platelets are consumed at surgical bleeding sites, sequestered by the membrane oxygenator, so transfusions are required to maintain counts greater than 100,000/mm³. Administration of fresh frozen plasma to broadly increase multiple factor activities is also common. When hypofibrinogenemia occurs, cryoprecipitate infusion can be utilized due to the high concentrations of fibrinogen in the low volume of the cryoprecipitate unit. The availability of plasma protein concentrate (PPC) allows administration of highly concentrated factors in a substantially reduced volume, thus reducing the volume burden associated with conventional therapy. Although rare, the application of heparin-free ECLS has been reported in polytrauma patients.[92]

Ventilation Strategies
Ventilator management during ECLS remains controversial. Although data exist to guide clinicians regarding prevention of barotrauma, volutrauma, and oxygen toxicity for mechanically ventilated patients with acute respiratory distress syndrome in general, consensus lacks for patients on ECLS. Lung collapse strategies used for respiratory support on ECLS are not utilized by most cardiac centers. Goals continue to target the prevention of atelectasis with utilization of appropriate PEEP in order to maximize oxygenation of non-bypassed blood returning to the left atrium, which then is ejected by the left ventricle to perfuse the coronary arteries. In addition, providing modest levels of ventilator support can be achieved with either a pressure- or volume-limited mode of ventilation targeting a delivered tidal volume of 6 to 8 mL/kg. Respiratory rates between 10 and 25 are set depending on the age and *rest* strategy being employed and the degree that the patient's lungs are required for gas exchange. Optimizing PaO_2 to the patient and circuit by blending FiO_2 to keep the FiO_2 <0.6 reduces free radical formation and oxygen toxicity, providing adequate oxygenation to decrease pulmonary hypertension and optimize myocardial O_2 delivery. Chest radiographs are routinely performed to assess and guide strategies to optimize lung volume so that volutrauma and barotrauma are avoided.

Fluid, Nutrition, and Renal
Fluid overload and electrolyte disturbances such as high or low serum levels of potassium, calcium, magnesium, and phosphorous are common and need correction. Most cardiac patients on ECLS receive total parenteral nutrition due to the increased risk of gastrointestinal complications in patients

with cardiac defects, umbilical artery catheters, poor perfusion, or other bowel abnormalities. A select subset may tolerate trophic enteral feedings. Diuretics, commonly furosemide, are often employed to provide optimal fluid balance in patients with significant capillary leak and fluid retention (see Table 30.4). Optimization of fluid status is essential to weaning and eventual separation from ECLS support. For anuric or oliguric patients, early placement of an in-line hemofilter into the ECLS circuit with or without countercurrent dialysate is recommended. However, the management decisions that balance the use and timing of diuretics versus hemofiltration are center specific. The indications for initiation of dialysis are the same as for other critically ill patients with renal failure. Multiple retrospective reviews of patients supported by ECLS have found renal replacement therapy to be a risk factor for increased mortality. No causal relationship has been identified, and further investigation in this area is warranted.[93,94]

Analgesia and Sedation
Adequate analgesia and sedation are essential for both safety and comfort and to decrease metabolic demands in patients with circulatory compromise in the early postoperative recovery period. Typically, an opiate and a benzodiazepine class drug are utilized. Infusions may be utilized with cautious monitoring, as toxicity from propylene glycol and other solvents have been reported with benzodiazepine use.[95] Neuromuscular blockade should largely be avoided to limit critical care myopathy, allow for regular evaluation of the central nervous system, and limit soft tissue fluid accumulation. Central nervous system infarcts, hemorrhage, or seizures are all known complications of ECLS (see Table 30.4). For infants with an open fontanel, a daily head ultrasound should be performed regularly early in the course of treatment and with any change in clinical neurologic status. For older patients, a significant change in their neurologic status has a high likelihood of heralding major intracranial pathology, which needs to be promptly diagnosed by computed tomography in order to guide treatment and determine patient viability.

Several centers have reported a new approach in which patients are supported without the need of continuous analgesia and sedation and without the need of mechanical ventilation. This *awake ECLS* modality has been used as bridge to recovery, bridge to VAD, or bridge to transplantation.[96]

Infection
It is not surprising that patients on ECLS are at a high risk of developing nosocomial bloodstream infections (BSI). Identified risk factors include the duration of ECLS[97] open versus closed chest cannulation, the presence of central venous lines, and undergoing a major procedure prior to or while on ECLS. It appears that older patients on ECLS for respiratory failure may be at higher risk of health care–associated infection than neonates or cardiac patients (see Table 30.4). Bloodstream infections during ECLS for both pediatric cardiac patients postcardiopulmonary bypass and neonates with cardiac or respiratory failure have been associated with a poor outcome. The diagnosis of sepsis is difficult in patients supported with ECLS. Although variable degrees of leukopenia have been documented for neonates supported with ECLS, an increase in phagocytosis and intracellular killing by neutrophils also occurs. Temperature is controlled by the circuit's heat exchanger, so infection is generally not manifested by fever in

these patients. Hypotension or thrombocytopenia may occur for a variety of reasons. In view of this observation, the standard of care in many ECLS centers has been to perform routine surveillance cultures and provide prophylactic antibiotics. However, management strategies to limit infectious risks continue to evolve. Due to lack of a proved benefit and concerns regarding the long-term impact of broad-spectrum antibiotics on local bacterial resistance profiles, an increasing number of centers now perform daily blood cultures without the routine use of prophylactic antibiotics.[98] Additional retrospective data may suggest that routine surveillance cultures may not be warranted.[99] Further investigation is needed to determine the impact of prophylactic antibiotic use on the incidence of BSI, local antimicrobial flora, length of stay, survival, and cost.

Intrahospital Transport

Crucial situations exist for patients supported with ECLS that require intrahospital transport. This can include mobilization from the intensive care unit to a variety of locations such as the catheterization laboratory, radiology, or the operating suite. Reluctance to perform diagnostic or therapeutic interventions is often driven by fear of potentially disastrous complications during transport. These fears are largely unfounded. Guidelines designed to promote the establishment of an organized, efficient transport process supported by appropriate equipment and personnel have been recognized and are increasingly utilized in hospitals. Intrahospital transport for patients on ECLS is a labor-intensive process that should be approached in a coordinated effort with specific focus on the preparatory phase, the transfer phase, and the posttransport phase. However, with careful attention to these aspects, centers have demonstrated that intrahospital transport for patients on ECLS can be carried out safely and without major complications.[100]

Ventricular Assist Devices

The two main types of VADs are pulsatile pumps and continuous flow pumps. Continuous flow pumps have been preferred worldwide because of their smaller size and high performance. Based on the pump-patient interface, devices can be classified as intracorporeal, extracorporeal, or paracorporeal. Most VADS share similar basic principles. Cannulation depends on the type of support required. The right atrium (venous drainage) and pulmonary artery (arterial return) are cannulated for right ventricular assist device (RVAD), and the left atrium (venous drainage) and aorta (arterial return) are cannulated for left ventricular assist device (LVAD). A combination of both right and left ventricular assist devices is termed biventricular assist device (BiVAD). The pump is connected to a controller and power supply. Pumps have differences in modes of operation, size, and placement. A comparison of ECLS and VAD support is listed in Table 30.5.

Pulsatile VADs are devices that function on the principle of "positive displacement" by trapping a fixed amount of blood then forcing (displacing) that trapped volume into an exit cannula. Since the early report of pneumatically driven, pulsatile, paracorporeal VADs in children, the pediatric experience with pulsatile devices has continued to grow.[101,102] Advantages of these devices include the ability to provide long-term (weeks to months) biventricular support without an oxygenator, patient mobility out of the intensive care setting, need for low-level anticoagulation (heparin or warfarin with antiplatelet therapy), and, lastly, the pulsatile nature of flow. Disadvantages include a propensity for thromboembolic complications, high cost when compared to centrifugal VADs, and the need for exteriorization of the cannulae. Infection is also a serious complication, though immobilization of the cannulas close to the exit site can decrease its incidence. Only the paracorporeal Berlin Heart Excor and the Medos HIA (MEDOS Medizintechnik AG, Stolberg, Germany) pulsatile systems have been successfully deployed in children of all ages and as small as 2 kg. These devices have a special silicone system that connects the blood pump to the body. The cannulas are anastomosed to the right atrium and pulmonary artery for right ventricular assist (RVAD), to the apex of the left ventricle (or more rarely to the left atrium) and the ascending aorta for left ventricular assist (LVAD), or both (BiVAD).[103,104] Most times, LVAD insertion may be sufficient for bridging patients to heart transplantation, even in the presence of significant preoperative right ventricular dysfunction. Adequate unloading of the left ventricle reduces the left ventricular end-diastolic pressure and, in turn, reduces right ventricular afterload, which may improve RV systolic function.

The Berlin Heart EXCOR (Berlin Heart AG, Berlin, Germany) is the only labeled VAD available for long-term

---

TABLE 30.5 Extracorporeal Life Support Versus Ventricular Assist Devices

	ECLS	Centrifugal VAD	Pulsatile VAD
Oxygenator	Yes	No but can be added	No
Anticoagulation	ACT 180-200	ACT 160-180	Aspirin/warfarin/LMWH
Support	Cardiac + respiratory	Cardiac + respiratory	Cardiac
Type of ventricular support	Biventricular	Uni or biventricular	Uni or biventricular
Ventricular decompression	May need LA "venting"	Via direct drainage cannula in LA or LV apex	Via direct drainage cannula in LV apex
Risk of air embolus	Low	Yes (especially with LVAD)	Yes (especially with LVAD)
Length of support	Short term	Short term	Long term
Cannulation site	Transthoracic or transcervical	Transthoracic	Transthoracic

ACT, activated clotting time; *LA*, left atrial; *LMWH*, low-molecular-weight heparin; *LV*, left ventricular; *LVAD*, left ventricular assist device.

support of neonates and infants. This is a second-generation, paracorporeal pulsatile pneumatic pump with polyurethane valves and a transparent chamber through which the adequacy of filling and emptying can be assessed and evaluated for thrombus formation. This pump can be used to support left, right, or both ventricles. The blood-contacting surfaces of the pump are heparin coated, reducing anticoagulation requirements. Because it is available in a wide range of sizes, the Berlin Heart EXCOR VAD provides circulatory support options for pediatric patients ranging from 2.5 kg to adolescents. The Berlin Heart EXCOR was specially designed and developed for pediatric patients. The pump sizes vary between 10 mL and 80 mL. The 10-mL pumps are suitable for neonates and infants with body weight of up to 9 kg (body surface area of 0.2 m^2); the 25-mL and 30-mL pumps can be used in children up to the age of 7 years (weight 30 kg and body surface area of about 0.95 m^2); adult size pumps (50, 60 mL) can be implanted in older children. All Berlin Heart EXCOR cannulas exit the body through the upper abdominal wall (Fig. 30.4 device and cannulas). Survival with the Berlin EXCOR and the MEDOS VADs has been reported at 36% in children from 2 weeks up to age 16 years, including an infant with body surface area less than 0.3 m^2. Diagnosis included fulminant myocarditis, dilated cardiomyopathy, endocardial fibroelastosis, Ebstein anomaly, and status post redo aortic valve replacement. Neurologic complications vary between 25% and 30%.[105,106]

The Abiomed BVS 5000 VAD (Abiomed, Inc., Danvers, Massachusetts) was the first assist device approved by the FDA to be used in postcardiotomy patients. It is a pneumatically driven, pulsatile, extracorporeal pump used in adults for short-term uni- or biventricular support. The BVS 5000 can produce a stroke volume of 80 mL and flows up to 6 L/minute. It has been used in patients with a body surface area (BSA) ≥1.2 m^2, generally as a bridge to recovery in patients who have exhausted all other medical options.

The Thoratec Ventricular Assist System (Thoratec Corp., Berkeley, California) is a pneumatically driven, polyurethane sac enclosed in a plastic housing designed for intermediate and long-term use (weeks to years). The Thoratec VAD has a stroke volume of 65 mL and can be operated at rates up to 100 beats per minutes providing blood flow rates of almost 7 liters/minute. Patients require systemic anticoagulation for the duration of the VAD support. There are two Thoratec VAD systems, one paracorporeal (PVAD) and one implantable (IVAD). The Thoratec Paracorporeal Pneumatic VAD (PVAD) is indicated as a bridge to transplantation or bridge to recovery system. It can provide acute or intermediate uni- or biventricular support. The external position of the pump allows device exchange in cases of malfunction, thrombus, or infection. Furthermore, it can be used in smaller patients who are poor candidates for implantable devices with the smallest reported patient weighing 17 kg (BSA 0.73m^2). In a

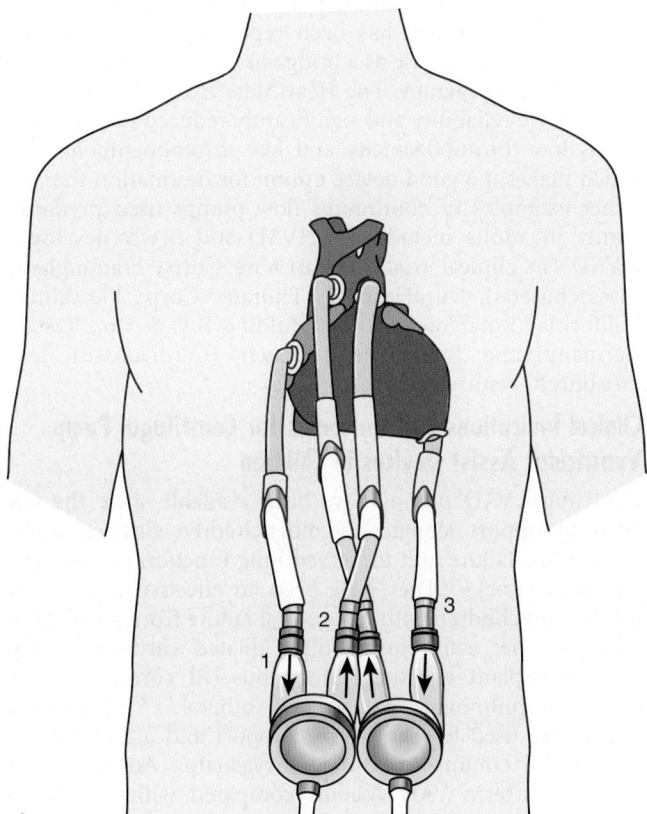

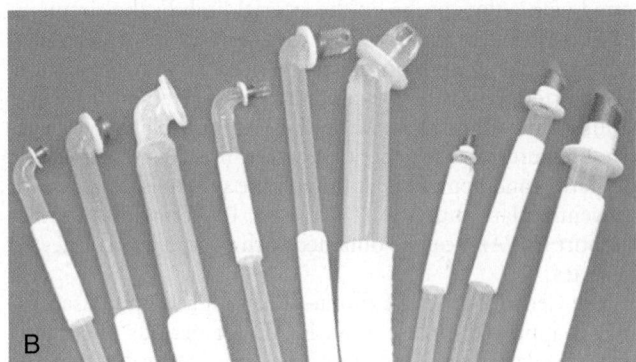

Fig. 30.4. (A) Schematic diagram of the Berlin Heart biventricular assist device showing apical cannulation, which allows better left ventricular unloading and decreased afterload to the right ventricle. 1, Deoxygenated blood flows from the body into the right atrium. Because the right ventricle is unable to pump blood into the lungs, the blood goes into the device. 2, The blood is pumped out from the device into the pulmonary artery. 3, Once the blood is oxygenated in the lungs, it flows into the left atrium. Because the left ventricle is unable to pump, the blood goes into the device. 4, The Berlin Heart pumps blood into the aorta and systemic circulation. (B) Set of cannulas available for the Berlin Heart assist device. The cannulas are available in different diameters, lengths, and tip configurations. (Courtesy Berlin Heart AG, Berlin, Germany.)

multicenter study (US and Germany), the Thoratec PVAD was used in 19 children with a mean BSA of 1.09 m^2, (range, 0.73–1.29), a mean age of 10 years (range, 7–14), and a mean weight of 31 kg (range, 17–41).[107] Indications for support were end-stage cardiomyopathy in eight patients, myocarditis in three, end-stage congenital heart disease in seven, and transplant graft failure in one patient. Mean duration of support was 43 days (range, 0–120). Survival through hospital discharge occurred in 8 of 11 (72%) patients with cardiomyopathy or myocarditis; however, only 1 of 7 patients with congenital heart disease survived. Neurologic complications were significant and predominant in the congenital heart disease group. Neurologic complications in these pediatric patients seem to be higher when cannulation is performed in the left atrium versus the left ventricle.[107] The Thoratec IVAD is a smaller, intracorporeal device with the same features as the Thoratec PVAD, except that it is used when longer support is anticipated. The device has been FDA approved since 2004 for circulatory assistance as a bridge to transplant or bridge to recovery. For adults, the pulsatile, axial flow pump, HeartAssist 5 (Reliant Heart, Houston, Texas) is a small LVAD implanted in the pericardial space, which is in clinical trials in the United States.

Continuous Flow VADs

The centrifugal pump that has been most available for use in pediatrics is the BioMedicus centrifugal pump (Medtronic, Eden Prairie, Minnesota) (Fig. 30.5). The BioMedicus centrifugal pump can be utilized for cardiopulmonary bypass, ECLS, or ventricular assistance depending on how the complete circuit is configured. The pump consists of a polycarbonate cone built around several rotator cones. It is magnetically coupled to a driver that controls the revolutions per minute (RPMs). The pump spins at an adjustable rate, generating a vortex continuous flow. This creates negative pressure that forces blood to drain (suctioned) from the venous cannula into the pump and redirects it out the top of the vortex (a tornado effect). The BP-80 and BP-50 models have cone volumes of 80 and 50 mL, respectively, with maximal flows of 10 L/minute. The centrifugal pump output (flow) is proportional to the rotational speed of the pump (RPM), preload to the pump (patient's intravascular volume), and pump afterload (impedance to outflow). Actual flow is measured with a flow probe on the arterial limb of the circuit, as RPM may not correlate accurately with flow. Heparin-bonded tubing can be used to minimize the need for anticoagulation. Mean arterial pressure is maintained by varying intravascular volume and adjusting RPM on the VAD console. Large negative pressures can be generated, which if excessive can create cavitation and hemolysis. Although the system is designed for univentricular support (LVAD or RVAD), biventricular support (BiVAD) can be obtained with two pumps connected in series.

The CentriMag VAD (Thoratec Corp., Pleasanton, California) is approved for use as an RVAD for periods of support up to 30 days for patients in cardiogenic shock due to acute right ventricular failure. It belongs to a new class of magnetically levitated devices operating in a bearing-less rotor that floats with a rotating magnetic field. Because of its contact-free environment and absence of seals or valves, this device minimizes blood trauma, thrombus formation, and hemolysis. It is capable of operating over a range of speeds up

to 5500 RPM generating flows up to 10 L/minute. The Thoratec PediMag blood pump, a miniaturized version of the CentriMag, is an extracorporeal circulatory support device providing hemodynamics stabilization for small patients (<10 kg) in need of cardiopulmonary assistance. It is cleared for clinical use up to 6 hours, so it can be used as a short-term solution to support the circulation while longer-term options are considered. It is a magnetically levitated pump and simple to implant. These devices are generally used for short- or intermediate-term support for recovery, conversion to a long-term VAD, or as a bridge to transplant.[108,109]

The HeartMate II (Thoratec Corp., Berkeley, California) is an axial flow rotary pump utilizing blood-immersed mechanical bearings with textured blood-contacting surfaces. The transcutaneous version is totally implantable. The HeartMate II is smaller than the first-generation devices, principally due to the elimination of the sac or reservoir necessary in pulsatile pumps. This device has two cannulas (inflow and outflow) without valves. It has smooth surfaces in the outlet and inlet stators but still requires anticoagulation. Clinical experience shows that the HeartMate II LVAD provides excellent support, with significant improvement in functional capacity. In a multicenter, prospective study, 42% of 133 adult heart transplant candidates supported with HeartMate II underwent transplantation within the 6 months of support, with an overall 6-month survival of 75% and 1-year survival of 68%.[110] More recently, an improved 6-month survival of 86.9% and 3% incidence of device malfunction with a mean duration of support of 6 months has been reported.[111] The FDA has already approved its use as a bridge to transplant therapy and for destination therapy. The HeartMate II has demonstrated great device reliability and significantly reduced device noise. It has low thrombogenicity and low thromboembolic risk, which makes it a good device option for destination therapy. Other examples of continuous flow pumps used predominantly in adults include the HVAD and newly developed mVAD (in clinical trials) (HeartWare Corp., Framingham, Massachusetts), DuraHeart II (Thoratec Corp., Pleasanton, California) RotaFlow (Maquet Holding B.V. & Co., Rastatt, Germany) and TandemHeart System (CardiacAssist, Inc., Pittsburgh, Pennsylvania).

Clinical Indications and Outcomes for Centrifugal Pump Ventricular Assist Devices in Children

Centrifugal VAD pumps have been available since the late 1970s to support neonates and older children with postoperative cardiac failure and preserved lung function (ie, no need for oxygenator).[112] They have been an effective support for infants and children with myocardial failure from a variety of etiologies (ie, acute myocarditis, dilated cardiomyopathy, acute transplant rejection, anomalous left coronary artery from the pulmonary artery, and others).[7,113] Centrifugal pumps are used for short-term support and are in essence mini ECLS circuits without an oxygenator. Advantages of these short-term VAD systems compared with traditional ECLS include lower priming volumes, adequate left (or systemic) ventricular decompression, lower heparin requirements, less hemolysis, ease of transport, and relatively low costs.[114] Centrifugal LVADs require a functional RV to supply preload to the left ventricle drained by the pump. Complications of the centrifugal VAD system include thrombus formation in the circuit, hemolysis, bleeding (including acquired

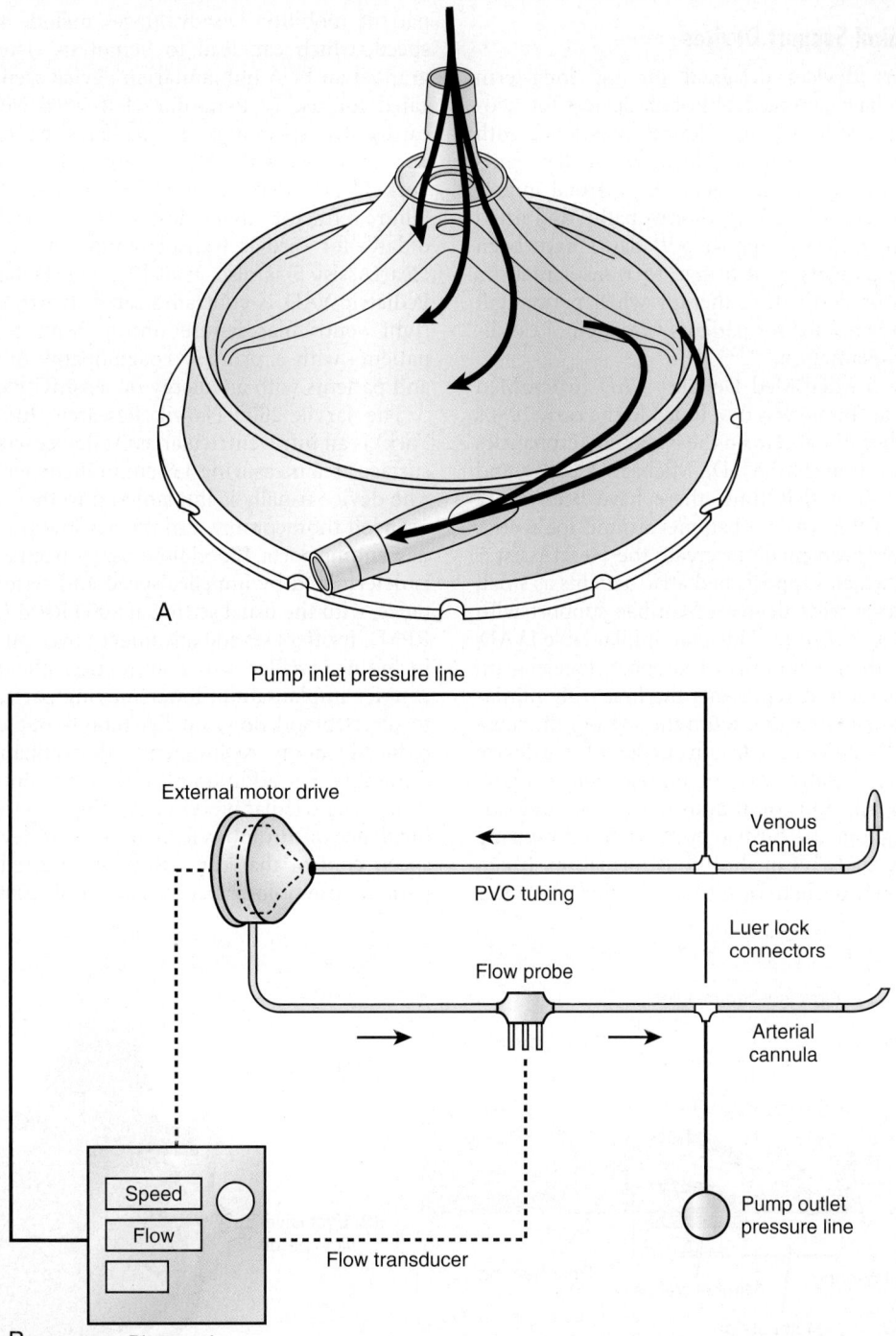

Fig. 30.5. (A) Schematic diagram of the BioMedicus centrifugal pump (Medtronic). Blood enters the cones via the apex of the cone, and the kinetic energy of the spinning cones is transferred to the blood leaving the side port. (B) Centrifugal pump setup. (From Karl TR, Horton SB. Centrifugal pump ventricular assist device in pediatric cardiac surgery. In: Duncan BW, ed. Mechanical Support for Cardiac and Respiratory Failure in Pediatric Patients. New York: Marcel Dekker; 2001.)

Von Willebrand disease),[115] and infection.[116] Duncan and colleagues reported the outcomes of 29 pediatric patients supported with the BioMedicus LVAD with a survival of 71% among patients with anomalous origin of the left coronary artery from the pulmonary artery or with cardiomyopathy. In those who underwent heart transplantation after LVAD support, survival was 50% and fewer instances of neurologic complications and hemolysis were seen than in the ECLS group reported in the same study.[48,117] Successful use of the centrifugal LVAD as a bridge to implantable VAD and then to heart transplantation in a patient with single ventricle physiology has been reported.[48,118] Single-center studies have shown little difference in survival rates of patients supported with either a centrifugal or a pulsatile pump.[118,119]

Long-Term Mechanical Support Devices

Mechanical support devices designed for the long-term support of patients have emerged, although devices for neonates and infants are still lacking. Clinical experience with these devices in adults is extensive and includes use in patients with postcardiotomy heart failure, acute myocardial infarction, cardiogenic shock, ischemic cardiomyopathy, and myocarditis. Long-term devices (support >30 days) have been placed in pediatric patients as a bridge to transplantation, bridge to recovery, or destination therapy when permanent circulatory support is needed for patients who are not candidates for heart transplantation.[120-122]

The Heart Assist 5 MicroMed DeBakey VAD (MicroMed Technology, Houston, Texas) was developed in the early 1990s as a result of a collaboration between the National Aeronautics and Space Administration (NASA), Dr. Michael DeBakey, and Dr. George Noon. Since that time, there have been more than 500 implants of this VAD in patients around the world. Design changes have been made to create the HeartAssist 5 (Fig. 30.6A and B), which supports pediatric patients as small as 18 kg. It provides a wide degree of cardiac support with blood flows from 1 to 10 L/min. This is an implantable LVAD, intended for more than 3 months of support, focusing on bridge to transplantation. It represents the first truly miniaturized device, approximately one-tenth the size of other currently marketed pulsatile VADs. The advantages of this device include its small size, relative ease of implant and explant, decreased infection risk, and continuous flow, which unloads the ventricle throughout the cardiac cycle while minimizing stasis and the associated risk of thrombus formation. It can operate up to 8 hours on batteries, thus allowing for better

patient mobility. Disadvantages include the rapid impeller speed, which can lead to hemolysis. This device has been granted an FDA humanitarian device exemption and is indicated for use as temporary left-sided MCS as a bridge to cardiac transplantation for pediatric patients between 5 and 16 years of age with BSA >0.7 m² and <1.5 m² who are in New York Heart Association (NYHA) class IV end-stage heart failure refractory to medical therapy and who are (listed) candidates for cardiac transplantation. An adult version of the HeartAssist 5 is also available. The DeBakey HeartAssist 5 Pediatric VAD is contraindicated in patients suffering from right ventricular failure unresponsive to medical therapy, patients with a primary coagulopathy or platelet disorders, and patients with an allergy or sensitivity to heparin.

The Jarvik 2000 (Jarvik Research, Inc., New York, New York) is an intraventricular assist device with a relatively small surface area measuring 1.8 cm in diameter by 5 cm in length. The device usually is implanted into the left ventricular apex via a left thoracotomy, and the outflow graft is placed into the descending aorta. Blood flow ranges from 2 to 7 L/minute and is determined by impeller speed and systemic vascular resistance, with the usual setting at 9000 RPM (range 8000-12,000 RPM). It offers several advantages over pulsatile flow pumps, including smaller size that reduces the risk of infections, simpler implantation, fewer moving parts, absence of valves to direct blood flow, smaller blood-contacting surfaces, and reduced energy requirements that enhance simplicity and durability. The addition of sintered titanium microspheres on its intraventricular blood-contacting surface has decreased the incidence of thrombus formation. This device has an external speed control that can easily be adjusted according to the patient's physiologic needs. The Jarvik 2000 is FDA approved

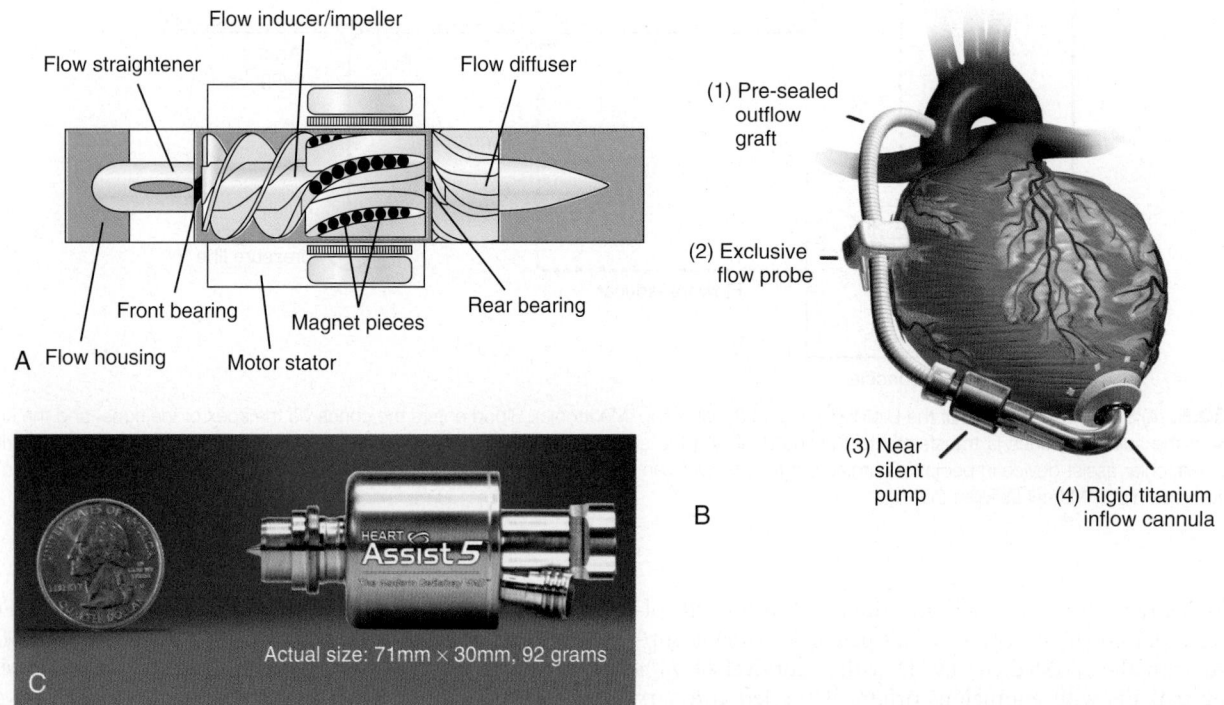

Fig. 30.6. HeartAssist 5 pediatric ventricular assist device (modern DeBakey ventricular assist device). (A) DeBakey ventricular assist device in a cutaway view. (B) HeartAssist 5 with its position in the heart. (C) HeartAssist 5 shown with a US quarter for size comparison. (Courtesy MicroMed Technology, Houston, Texas.)

as an investigational device to be used for bridge to transplantation. In Europe, the Jarvik 2000 is certified to be used both as a bridge to transplantation and destination therapy. A pediatric Jarvik 2000 is under investigation.[123]

Total Artificial Heart

Total artificial heart (TAH) devices completely replace the patient's native ventricles and all four cardiac valves and are used as destination therapy. Due to their large size, these devices have limited use in children.[124] CardioWest (SynCardia Systems, Inc.) is the modern version of the Jarvik 7 implanted in 1982. The CardioWest temporary TAH is the only artificial heart in the world. The CardioWest TAH is used as a bridge to heart transplant for eligible patients with severe end-stage biventricular failure. The 70-mL CardioWest TAH is suitable for patients with BSA ≥ 1.7 m^2; a 50-mL version of the device is under research investigation. The AbioCor Replacement Heart is a new mechanical device that replaces the pumping function of the diseased heart. It is used as destination therapy in patients who are ineligible for heart transplant and have no other suitable treatment options. The AbioCor has been granted FDA approval for the humanitarian device exemption.

Next Generation–Levitated Devices

New generations of devices include centrifugal continuous-flow pumps with an impeller or rotor suspended in the blood flow path using a noncontact bearing design, which uses either magnetic or hydrodynamic levitation. The levitation systems suspend the moving impeller within the blood field without any mechanical contact, thus eliminating frictional wear and reducing heat generation. This feature hopes to promise longer durability and higher reliability with a low incidence of device failure and need for replacement. Usually, magnetic levitation devices are larger owing to the need for complex position sensing and control system. Examples of third-generation devices are the VentrAssist (Ventracor Ltd., Sydney, Australia), Levitronix CentriMag (Thoratec Corporation), DuraHeart (Terumo, Inc., Ann Arbor, Michigan), HVAD (HeartWare Corp., Florida), and EVAHEART LVAS (Sun Medical Technology Research Corporation, Nagano, Japan).[125]

Device Selection

Three factors drive device selection: type of support (cardiopulmonary or cardiac), planned duration of support, and body surface area. Short-term support (less than 14 days) is used for acute myocarditis, graft dysfunction after cardiac transplant, and patients with unknown diagnoses or unknown neurologic status. It is also described for failure to wean from cardiopulmonary bypass. Long-term support (greater than 14 days) is often used in patients with known cardiomyopathy and failure to improve and in some with refractory heart failure and congenital heart disease. Venoarterial extracorporeal membrane oxygenation (ECMO/ECLS) has been successfully used since the mid-1970s and is the most widely available form of short-term biventricular cardiopulmonary support. It is most commonly employed for failure to wean from cardiopulmonary bypass, emergent support after cardiac arrest with failure of medical resuscitation, and early graft failure after cardiac transplantation. Biventricular support with ECMO requires either an opening in the atrial septum or an additional cannula placed in the left heart (pulmonary vein, left atrial appendage, or left atrium). It is important to note that after approximately 2 weeks, the risk of bleeding, thromboembolism, stocking and glove ischemia, and other major complications are common. Another device popular in Europe (FDA approval pending) and used for similar indications as ECLS is the Deltastream DP3 (Medos Medizintechnik AG, Stolberg, Germany).[126] This pump combines the effects of centrifugal and axial pumps. It requires a very small priming volume. These are very short-term devices until one of the following outcomes occur: Pulmonary (not cardiac) recovery leads to the insertion of longer-term cardiac support, cardiopulmonary recovery results in decannulation, or no recovery of either organ system leads to withdrawal of support.

A suggested algorithm for device selection is shown in Fig. 30.7.[127]

Patient Selection and Management

In general, the use of MCS in pediatric patients with acute or chronic end-stage heart failure is indicated when conventional medical therapy has failed. Despite listing for heart transplantation, the scarcity of organs usually necessitates consideration of mechanical support. Pediatric VADs are used almost exclusively as either bridge to transplant or bridge to recovery. Unlike in the adult population, the use of MCS as destination therapy is not a primary option in the pediatric population, but it has been reported in patients with Duchenne muscular dystrophy.[128]

Contraindications to the use of VADs in pediatric patients include irreversible end-organ dysfunction and active infection. Also, extreme prematurity, very low birth weight, and certain chromosomal defects are considered contraindications. It is important and often challenging to avoid initiating mechanical support too late. Moderate end-organ dysfunction often improves with MCS, especially renal and hepatic dysfunction.[129] Other considerations include thickness of the ventricular wall, semilunar valve regurgitation, and intracardiac shunts. Thick ventricles (such as those in hypertrophic cardiomyopathy) can prevent proper filling of the VAD, and these patients should be considered on a case-by-case basis.[130] Significant aortic insufficiency (or pulmonary insufficiency) will not permit adequate emptying of the ventricle and often necessitates closure of the aortic valve at the time of VAD implantation. Closure of intracardiac defects will prevent embolization of thrombus or air.[131]

Basic Management of the Ventricular Assist Device Patients

Patients assisted with VADs are not anticoagulated for the first 24 to 48 hours to decrease risk of bleeding. Intravenous unfractionated heparin is then started at 25 units/kg/hour and continued during the time of MCS, keeping anti-Xa levels between 0.35 and 0.7 units/mL. Once postoperative bleeding stops, antiplatelet therapy is started. Achieving optimal anticoagulation levels in children on VAD support remains a significant challenge. Children with ongoing VAD support often have issues with gastrointestinal function, such as feeding intolerance secondary to right heart failure, resulting in erratic absorption of enteral medications. The Edmonton protocol[85] involves a three-drug regimen, namely aspirin, dipyridamole, and either warfarin or enoxaparin depending on patient age.

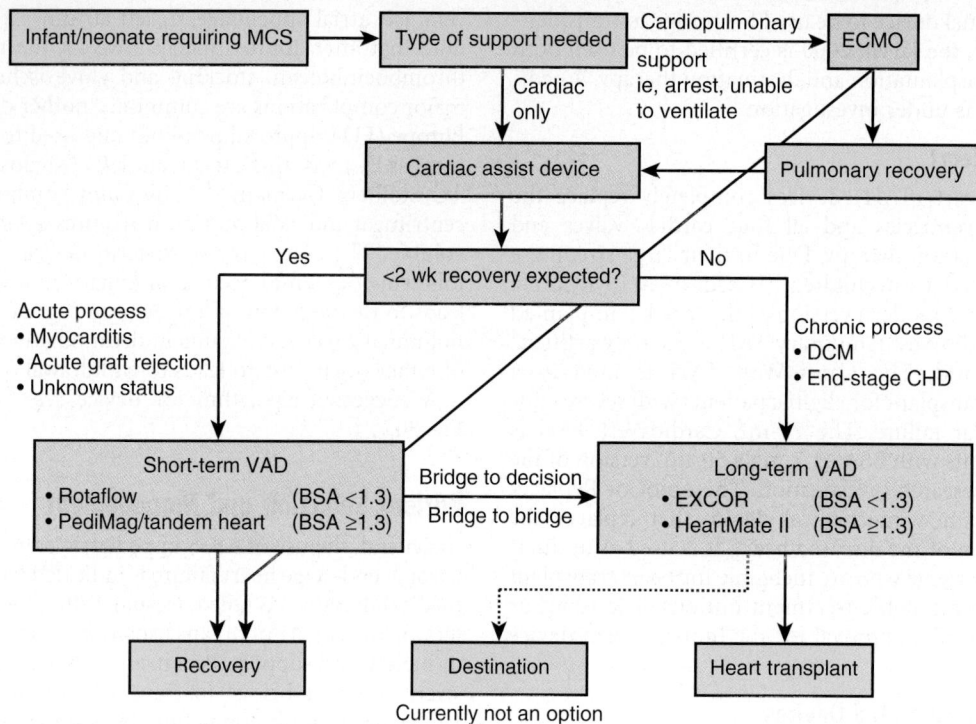

Fig. 30.7. Protocol for device selection; name of the devices used in the figure are authors' preference for each device type. (From Wilmot I, Lorts A, Morales D. Pediatric mechanical circulatory support. Korean J Thorac Cardiovasc Surg. 2013;46:391-401; with permission.)

This protocol was used as a guideline in the Berlin EXCOR Investigational Device Exemption (IDE) prospective trial.[106] Despite the guideline, the prevalence of major bleeding was significant: 42% in patients with BSA <0.7m² and 50% in patients with BSA 0.7-1.5 m². Unfortunately, there was also a significant prevalence of thrombosis, the most concerning of these events being stroke (29% in both cohorts). The occurrence of hemorrhagic and thrombotic complications appeared to be higher than those in the German trial.[104] Further randomized trials are warranted to further evaluate anticoagulation protocols in this patient population. At present, however, the EXCOR device remains the only pediatric VAD that can be used in all age groups. The prevalence of bleeding and stroke is of great concern and exhibits the same challenges that have plagued the use of all extracorporeal technology in critically ill children.

Infection prophylaxis using broad-spectrum antibiotics as well as antifungal drugs is continued for 48 hours after the implantation. Wound care consists of daily dressings using sterile saline. Once the drains are removed, the wound and cannula dressings are changed twice a week and surveillance cultures of the wound and cannula are obtained once a week.

Single-center studies have reported readmission rates after LVAD implantation of between 1.5 and 2.5 per patient-year of support, with an increased rate in the first 6 months after the implant. The leading cause of readmission was bleeding (primarily gastrointestinal), followed by heart failure/arrhythmia and infection.[132,133]

Mechanical Circulatory Support and Single Ventricle

Two general categories of patients with single ventricle physiology may require MCS support: those with prior palliative surgery but without complete separation of the systemic and pulmonary circulation and patients who are post-Fontan. In the first group, inflow is provided from the single ventricle with outflow to the ascending aorta. Pulmonary blood flow is maintained via a systemic-to-pulmonary artery shunt or a bidirectional Glenn shunt. In patients with a failing Fontan, cardiac failure may result from primary ventricular dysfunction producing high Fontan pressures or from failing Fontan physiology (preserved ventricular function but moderate to severe elevation of pulmonary vascular resistance) yielding chronic elevation of pressures in the Fontan pathway and sequelae of heart failure. In primary ventricular dysfunction and normal PVR, standard ventricle-to-aorta support may be sufficient. However, in the setting of failing Fontan physiology, cannulation choices are more challenging. If elevated pulmonary vascular resistance leads to systemic venous hypertension, then a second VAD may be required to support flow through the pulmonary circulation. In this situation, separation of the two circulations is performed by taking down the Fontan pathway.[134,135]

Some authors do not offer VADs to patients with single ventricle congenital heart disease and opt to support these children with ECLS. Nevertheless, there are several case reports describing the use of VAD support for single ventricle heart failure. The Edmonton group[136] reported the use of VAD support for a 3-year-old with early heart failure following a Fontan operation. The patient's anatomy was revised back to a bidirectional cavopulmonary connection, with initiation of ECMO. Support was later converted to a Berlin Heart EXCOR pediatric device, which was implanted with systemic right ventricular and aortic cannulation. This patient underwent successful heart transplantation after being supported with the EXCOR for 6 months. As the authors state: "the paucity of published reports on VAD support in single ventricle patients precludes firm recommendations regarding surgical management strategy."

Outcomes

The Berlin Heart EXCOR pediatric VAD multicenter trial results were published in 2012.[67] Although data from the trial suggest that 90% of children can be bridged to transplantation with the EXCOR, with a stroke risk of 29%, the primary cohort captured only one-fourth of all US children implanted with the EXCOR during the 3-year study period and did not include patients in whom the device was implanted as compassionate use. In a later publication, Almond and coworkers examined EXCOR outcomes in all 204 children implanted during the study period.[106] Overall survival in this unselected cohort was lower at 75%, and the risk of neurologic dysfunction was similar at 29%. Children were more likely to die on EXCOR support if they had significant renal or hepatic impairment at implantation or right ventricular failure requiring biventricular assist device support. In addition, children weighing <5 kg did significantly worse. These findings demonstrate that EXCOR survival varies considerably and depends heavily on patient characteristics at implantation, underscoring the need for careful patient selection. Specifically, excessive delay in implanting a device until renal, hepatic, or right ventricular function has significantly deteriorated increases the risk of death on EXCOR support, whereas implanting too early may also escalate mortality by unnecessarily exposing children to the risks of support (eg, stroke, death). Most of the neurologic events are secondary to left atrial cannulation; hence many centers favor ventricular apical cannulation. It is encouraging to note that even within the short 3-year time frame of this study, pediatric centers that have refined their patient characteristics over time are observing significantly lower patient mortality.[137,138]

Between 2003 and 2014, 15,745 patients who received a US FDA-approved MCS device were entered into the National Heart, Lung and Blood Institute Interagency Registry for Mechanically Assisted Circulatory Support (NHLBI INTERMACS) database. Of the 12,030 patients who received a continuous flow device, >90% received an LVAD. PediMACS, the pediatric component of INTERMACS, began collecting all pediatric data (patients <19 years of age) in September 2012. By April 2015, 36 centers had enrolled 251 devices in 216 patients (Fig. 30.8). The durable and temporary mechanical circulatory devices that have been entered into the registry are included in Table 30.6. Among patients up to 5 years of age, pulsatile LVADs (Berlin Heart EXCOR; Berlin Heart Steglitz, Berlin, Germany) accounted for nearly 50% of implants. Among patients between 6 and 10 years of age, continuous flow LVADs began to predominate, with an overall actuarial survival at 6 months of 90% and 66% of patients undergoing cardiac transplantation by 12 months.[139,139a] In 2016 the Pediatric Interagency Registry for Mechanical Circulatory Support (PediMACS) reported the outcome of children implanted with VADs in the United States. Between September 2012 and June 2015, 200 patients underwent 222 durable VAD implants. Ninety-one patients were supported with a pulsatile-flow device and 109 (55%) with a continuous flow (CF) device.

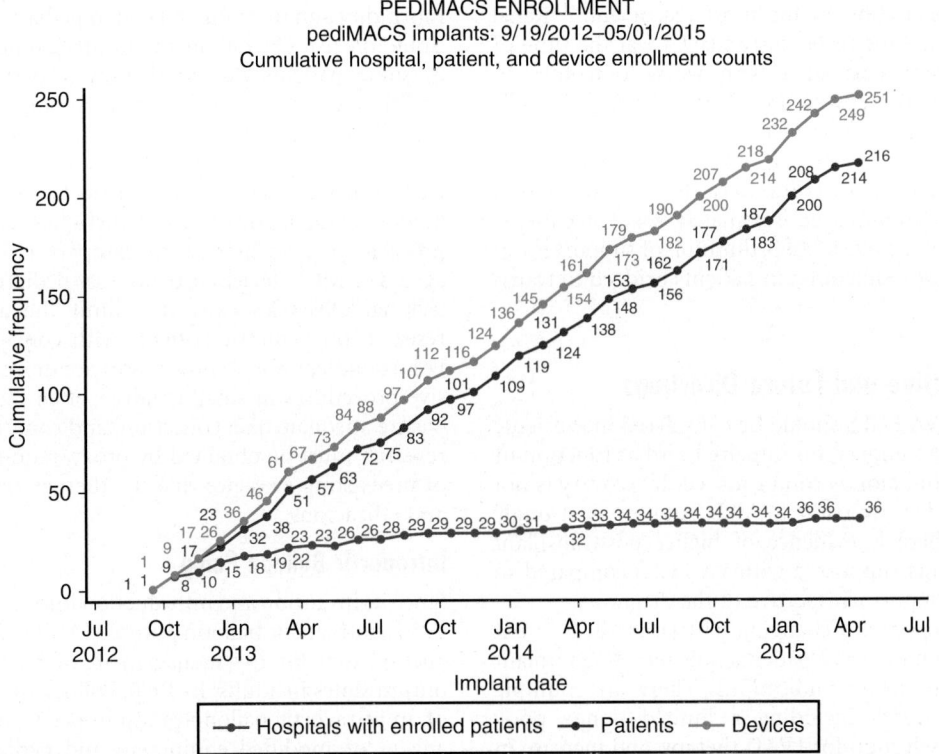

Fig. 30.8. Cumulative depiction of hospitals with enrolled patients, devices, and patients enrolled in the PediMACS Registry, September 19, 2012, to May 1, 2015. (From Kirklin JK, Naftel DC, Pagani FD, et al. Seventh INTERMACS annual report: 15,000 patients and counting. J Heart Lung Transplant. 2015;34:1495-1504; with permission.)

TABLE 30.6	Food and Drug Administration Approved Devices: Pediatrics (<19 Years of Age)
Type	**Device**
Durable Devices	
	Thoratec HeartMate II
Continuous flow	HeartWare HVAD
	MicroMed DeBakey Child VAD
Pulsatile extracorporeal	Thoratec PVAD
	HeartMate IP
Pulsatile intracorporeal	HeartMate VE HeartMate XVE Thoratec IVAD NovaCor PC NovaCor PCq
Total artificial heart	SynCardia CardioWest

VAD, ventricular assist device.
Kirklin JK, Naftel DC, Pagani FD, et al. Seventh INTERMACS annual report: 15,000 patients and counting. J Heart Lung Transplant. 2015;34:1495-1504.

There were 28 deaths. Reported serious adverse events included infection (n = 78), bleeding (n = 68), device malfunction (n = 79), and neurologic dysfunction (n = 52).

Diagnoses leading to pediatric heart transplantation are age specific and have also changed over time. Congenital heart disease remains the most common cause of heart failure leading to heart transplantation in infants but has significantly decreased over time, whereas cardiomyopathy is increasing. Unfortunately, infants have the highest waiting period due to lack of available organs and have the highest wait-list mortality.[138,140] Analysis of the Pediatric Heart Transplant Study (PHTS) registry demonstrated an overall survival of 83% at 5 years after transplantation in the most recent era.[141] Renal failure, ECLS at the time of listing, and ECLS at the time of transplantation were correlated with worse outcomes. A review of the United Network for Organ Sharing (UNOS) database[69] demonstrated improved survival when patients are supported with VADs. The use of ECLS as a primary means of mechanical support and a bridge to cardiac transplantation in the current era is minimal, approximately 4% of all patients listed for transplant. Unlike ECMO, duration of support is not a risk factor for worse outcomes in patients bridged to transplant with VADs.

Current Perspective and Future Directions

As a general rule, VA ECLS should be considered in the acute setting, after cardiac surgery, for impaired cardiac function or when respiratory function is compromised. If recovery is not promptly achieved, conversion to VAD support is strongly recommended. There is evidence of higher posttransplant mortality in patients supported with VA ECLS compared to those with VAD support irrespective of the diagnosis.

INTERMACS reported a changing pattern in MCS intent with an increasing number of patients now receiving implant under destination therapy indications. There are multiple reasons for this trend, including a limited donor pool, improved patient selection for LVAD therapy, and increase in the number of VAD implant centers. The growing population of patients supported by durable MCS devices has had an important effect on the infrastructure required to manage patients outside of the implanting hospital and on costs to the health care system.

With more effective devices available for pediatric patients, particularly the Berlin Heart EXCOR, the percentage of patients undergoing cardiac transplantation while supported on VADs has increased from under 5% before 2002 to greater than 20% since 2009. The superiority of VAD support compared with traditional ECLS among patients awaiting transplantation is evident from a study by the Pediatric Heart Transplant Study Group.[142] Despite the tremendous improvement in pediatric MCS since the Berlin Heart EXCOR became available in the United States in 2000 and received FDA approval in 2012, patients remain at risk for significant morbidity. Neurologic complications are high and continue to be the leading cause of mortality. Thromboembolic strokes are twice as frequent as intracranial hemorrhagic events.[143]

Options for circulatory support of pediatric patients under the age of 5 years are still limited to short-term extracorporeal devices. The need for devices suitable for small patients has been addressed by the National Heart, Lung, and Blood Institute (NHLBI), which has funded research for the development of mechanical support devices in children from 2 to 25 kg with congenital or acquired cardiovascular disease. The Pumps for Kids, Infants, and Neonates (PumpKIN) Trial launched by the NHLBI funded five novel pediatric circulatory support devices. Two investigational devices remain funded: the Jarvik (Jarvik Heart Inc., New York, New York) VAD, which is being randomized versus the Berlin Heart, and the Levitronix PediPL (Levitronix LLC, Waltham, Massachusetts) versus conventional ECMO.

Although advances in medical management, surgical techniques, and MCS for pediatric patients with cardiomyopathy or congenital heart defects continue to improve outcomes, morbidity and mortality related to pediatric heart failure continue to exist. Overall quality of life can be adversely affected in some patients due to therapy-related complications. In addition, caregivers of these patients may experience significant burden due to posttraumatic stress disorder, anxiety, depression, or poor physical health. Even though the randomized controlled trial remains the most powerful tool for unambiguous comparison of various therapies, it is a well-recognized problem that such trials to compare either pharmacologic agents or MCS devices used to treat pediatric heart failure are lacking. Obstacles exist that limit the ability to perform research on pediatric patients with congestive heart failure. For example, invasive procedures are more difficult, noninvasive procedures in small children often require anesthesia to ensure adequate data collection, and consent to participate in research must be obtained by proxy, requiring a greater level of preexisting evidence that the therapy being studied is safe and efficacious.

Intraaortic Balloon Pump

Since its invention and introduction into clinical practice in the 1960s, intraaortic balloon pumps (IABPs) have become a therapeutic tool for the management of refractory low cardiac output states in adults. In 1980, Pollock first described the use of an intraaortic balloon pump in pediatric patients with the advent of modified equipment and pediatric-sized balloon catheters. The IABP is a polyethylene balloon mounted on a catheter, which is usually inserted into the aorta via the femoral artery. The balloon is guided into the descending thoracic aorta approximately 2 cm from the subclavian artery. The balloon pump works by inflating during diastole (after aortic valve closure) for improved retrograde coronary flow augmentation; the balloon then deflates before systole to decrease left ventricular afterload. Cardiac output may be augmented by as much as 40%, decreasing left ventricular stroke work and myocardial oxygen requirements. The pump is available in a wide range of sizes (2.5-50 mL) and is driven by an external console. The use of an intraaortic balloon pump to support 24 postoperative cardiac patients with ages between 7 days and 17.5 years with low cardiac output syndrome despite optimal repair and maximal medical support resulted in successful separation from IABP in 18 out of 24 patients (75%) and 15 (62%) long-term survivors.[144] Major complications associated with increased mortality included two patients with limb ischemia and one patient with both limb and mesenteric ischemia, which resulted in a fatal outcome.[144] Additional complications included bleeding that necessitated reexploration of the chest and sepsis. A similar review of 29 patients supported with IABP for medical, postoperative surgical, and bridge-to-transplant indications demonstrated survival to hospital discharge of 18 of 29 patients (62%). Advantages of IABP include its relative ease of use and its placement without surgical dissection. Disadvantages include infrequency of use, limitations of an isolated left ventricular support modality, contraindication with certain anatomy/physiology (eg, patent ductus arteriosus or aortic insufficiency), and serious complications that include mesenteric ischemia and arterial injury. In children, failure to augment cardiac output can occur due to a highly elastic aorta. Pediatric IABP catheters differ from adult catheters in a variety of ways. The catheter shafts are smaller (4 or 5 French) with balloon sizes of 0.75 to 10 mL. Early failed reports of the use of IABP in children were primarily due to the use of inappropriately sized balloons and failure to gate to the ECG at fast heart rates. Adequate timing of the balloon inflation and deflation is essential; radial artery tracings were used in the past to aid timing of balloon inflation, but rapid heart rates led to significant timing errors. The use of M-mode echocardiography to aid in timing of the balloon inflation and deflation with aortic valve opening and closing has significantly improved the efficiency of intraaortic balloon pumping therapy. As a result of these difficulties, the use of intraaortic balloon pumping therapy in the pediatric population has remained limited to a small number of patients in a few institutions.[145]

Conclusions

Principles of MCS require an individualized approach. Indications include a variety of disease processes leading to LCOS such as myocarditis, septic shock, and surgery to repair congenital heart defects. Short-term experience with mechanical devices had been limited to ECLS, but pediatric experience with VADs is growing. Early institution of ECLS and transition to a VAD are necessary to avoid irreversible organ failure.

Pediatric MCS has demonstrated a number of significant advances; however, the limited options for mechanical support of the failing circulation in small children continue to be a challenge. Despite positive outcomes, several significant side effects remain, including bleeding, stroke, and infection. Patient selection, timing of support, device selection, and perioperative care continue to be critical components in a successful outcome for these patients.

Key References

3. Kantor PF, Lougheed J, Dancea A, et al. Presentation, diagnosis, and medical management of heart failure in children. Canadian Cardiovascular Society guidelines. *Can J Cardiol.* 2013;29:1535-1552.

7. Vogt W, Läer S. Prevention for pediatric low cardiac output syndrome: results from the European survey EuLoCOS-Paed. *Paediatr Anaesth.* 2011;21:1176-1184.

8. Wernovsky G, Wypij D, Jonas RA, et al. Postoperative course and hemodynamic profile after the arterial switch operation in neonates and infants: a comparison of low-flow cardiopulmonary bypass and circulatory arrest. *Circulation.* 1995;92:2226-2235.

10. Gasparovic H, Gabelica R, Ostojic Z, et al. Diagnostic accuracy of central venous saturation in estimating mixed venous saturation is proportional to cardiac performance among cardiac surgical patients. *J Crit Care.* 2014;29:828-834.

14. Osman D, Ridel C, Ray P, et al. Cardiac filling pressures are not appropriate to predict hemodynamic response to volume challenge. *Crit Care Med.* 2007;35:64-68.

16. Marik PE, Cavallazzi R, Vasu T, Hirani A. Dynamic changes in arterial waveform derived variables and fluid responsiveness in mechanically ventilated patients: a systematic review of the literature. *Crit Care Med.* 2009;37:2642-2647.

18. Murkin JM, Arango M. Near-infrared spectroscopy as an index of brain and tissue oxygenation. *Br J Anaesth.* 2009;103(suppl 1):i3-i13.

19. Proulx F, Lemson J, Choker G, Tibby SM. Hemodynamic monitoring by transpulmonary thermodilution and pulse contour analysis in critically ill children. *Pediatr Crit Care Med.* 2011;12:459-466.

21. Maldonado Y, Singh S, Taylor MA. Cerebral near-infrared spectroscopy in perioperative management of left ventricular assist device and extracorporeal membrane oxygenation patients. *Curr Opin Anaesthesiol.* 2014;27:81-88.

25. Fakler U, Pauli C, Balling G, et al. Cardiac index monitoring by pulse contour analysis and thermodilution after pediatric cardiac surgery. *J Thorac Cardiovasc Surg.* 2007;133:224-228.

29. Hsu DT, Zak V, Mahony L, et al. Enalapril in infants with single ventricle: results of a multicenter randomized trial. *Circulation.* 2010;122:333-340.

32. Margossian R. Contemporary management of pediatric heart failure. *Expert Rev Cardiovasc Ther.* 2008;6:187-197.

33. Huang M, Zhang X, Chen S, et al. The effect of carvedilol treatment on chronic heart failure in pediatric patients with dilated cardiomyopathy: a prospective, randomized-controlled study. *Pediatr Cardiol.* 2013;34:680-685.

35. Chang AC, Atz AM, Wernovsky G, et al. Milrinone: systemic and pulmonary hemodynamic effects in neonates after cardiac surgery. *Crit Care Med.* 1995;23:1907-1914.

36. Hoffman TM. Efficacy and safety of milrinone in preventing low cardiac output syndrome in infants and children after corrective surgery for congenital heart disease. *Circulation.* 2003;107:996-1002.

38. Hill KD, Sampson MR, Li JS, et al. Pharmacokinetics of intravenous sildenafil in children with palliated single ventricle heart defects: effect of elevated hepatic pressures. *Cardiol Young.* 2016;26:354-362.

39. Lechner E, Hofer A, Leitner-Peneder G, et al. Levosimendan versus milrinone in neonates and infants after corrective open-heart surgery: a pilot study. *Pediatr Crit Care Med.* 2012;13:542-548.

43. Ramakrishna H, Thunberg CA, Morozowich ST. Inhaled therapy for the management of perioperative pulmonary hypertension. *Ann Card Anaesth.* 2015;18:394.

44. Landoni G, Biondi-Zoccai GGL, Marino G, et al. Fenoldopam reduces the need for renal replacement therapy and in-hospital death in cardiovascular surgery: a meta-analysis. *J Cardiothorac Vasc Anesth.* 2008;22:27-33.

49. Jaggers JJ, Forbess JM, Shah AS, et al. Extracorporeal membrane oxygenation for infant postcardiotomy support: significance of shunt management. *Ann Thorac Surg.* 2000;69:1476-1483.

51. Kumar TKS, Zurakowski D, Dalton H, et al. Extracorporeal membrane oxygenation in postcardiotomy patients: factors influencing outcome. *J Thorac Cardiovasc Surg.* 2010;140:330-332.

54. Asaumi Y, Yasuda S, Morii I, et al. Favourable clinical outcome in patients with cardiogenic shock due to fulminant myocarditis supported by percutaneous extracorporeal membrane oxygenation. *Eur Heart J.* 2005;26:2185-2192.

57. Dyamenahalli U, Tuzcu V, Fontenot E, et al. Extracorporeal membrane oxygenation support for intractable primary arrhythmias and complete

congenital heart block in newborns and infants: short-term and medium-term outcomes. *Pediatr Crit Care Med*. 2012;13:47-52.

59. Allan CK, Thiagarajan RR, Armsby LR, et al. Emergent use of extracorporeal membrane oxygenation during pediatric cardiac catheterization. *Pediatr Crit Care Med*. 2006;7:212-219.

61. Nadkarni VM, Larkin GL, Peberdy MA, et al. First documented rhythm and clinical outcome from in-hospital cardiac arrest among children and adults. *JAMA*. 2006;295:50-57.

63. Morris MC, Wernovsky G, Nadkarni VM. Survival outcomes after extracorporeal cardiopulmonary resuscitation instituted during active chest compressions following refractory in-hospital pediatric cardiac arrest. *Pediatr Crit Care Med*. 2004;5:440-446.

64. Huang S-C, Wu E-T, Chen Y-S, et al. Extracorporeal membrane oxygenation rescue for cardiopulmonary resuscitation in pediatric patients. *Crit Care Med*. 2008;36:1607-1613.

67. Fraser CD, Jaquiss RDB, Rosenthal DN, et al. Prospective trial of a pediatric ventricular assist device. *N Engl J Med*. 2012;367:532-541.

69. Zafar F, Castleberry C, Khan MS, et al. Pediatric heart transplant waiting list mortality in the era of ventricular assist devices. *J Heart Lung Transplant*. 2015;34:82-88.

71. Chapman RL, Peterec SM, Bizzarro MJ, Mercurio MR. Patient selection for neonatal extracorporeal membrane oxygenation: beyond severity of illness. *J Perinatol*. 2009;29:606-611.

73. Heggen JA, Fortenberry JD, Tanner AJ, et al. Systemic hypertension associated with venovenous extracorporeal membrane oxygenation for pediatric respiratory failure. *J Pediatr Surg*. 2004;39:1626-1631.

75. Braunwald E, Kloner RA. The stunned myocardium: prolonged, postischemic ventricular dysfunction. *Circulation*. 1982;66:1146-1149.

78. Aiyagari RM, Rocchini AP, Remenapp RT, Graziano JN. Decompression of the left atrium during extracorporeal membrane oxygenation using a transseptal cannula incorporated into the circuit. *Crit Care Med*. 2006;34:2603-2606.

80. Roeleveld PP, Wilde R, de Hazekamp M, et al. Extracorporeal membrane oxygenation in single ventricle lesions palliated via the hybrid approach. *World J Pediatr Congenit Heart Surg*. 2014;5:393-397.

81. Sherwin ED, Gauvreau K, Scheurer MA, et al. Extracorporeal membrane oxygenation after stage 1 palliation for hypoplastic left heart syndrome. *J Thorac Cardiovasc Surg*. 2012;144:1337-1343.

85. Annich G, Adachi I. Anticoagulation for pediatric mechanical circulatory support. *Pediatr Crit Care Med*. 2013;14(5 suppl 1):S37-S42.

87. Maul TM, Wolff EL, Kuch BA, et al. Activated partial thromboplastin time is a better trending tool in pediatric extracorporeal membrane oxygenation. *Pediatr Crit Care Med*. 2012;13:e363-e371.

93. Smith AH, Hardison DC, Worden CR, et al. Acute renal failure during extracorporeal support in the pediatric cardiac patient. *ASAIO J*. 2009; 55:412-416.

96. Schmidt F, Jack T, Sasse M, et al. Awake veno-arterial extracorporeal membrane oxygenation. In pediatric cardiogenic shock: a single-center experience. *Pediatr Cardiol*. 2015;36:1647-1656.

98. Glater-Welt LB, Schneider JB, Zinger MM, et al. Nosocomial bloodstream infections in patients receiving extracorporeal life support: variability in prevention practices: a survey of the extracorporeal life support organization members. *J Intensive Care Med*. 2015;[Epub ahead of print].

104. Hetzer R, Potapov EV, Alexi-Meskishvili V, et al. Single-center experience with treatment of cardiogenic shock in children by pediatric ventricular assist devices. *J Thorac Cardiovasc Surg*. 2011;141:616-623, 623.e1.

105. Stein ML, Dao DT, Doan LN, et al. Ventricular assist devices in a contemporary pediatric cohort: morbidity, functional recovery, and survival. *J Heart Lung Transplant*. 2016;35:92-98.

106. Almond CS, Morales DL, Blackstone EH, et al. Berlin Heart EXCOR pediatric ventricular assist device for bridge to heart transplantation in US children. *Circulation*. 2013;127:1702-1711.

129. Miller LW, Guglin M. Patient selection for ventricular assist devices: a moving target. *J Am Coll Cardiol*. 2013;61:1209-1221.

134. Horne D, Conway J, Rebeyka IM, Buchholz H. Mechanical circulatory support in univentricular hearts: current management. Seminars in thoracic and cardiovascular surgery. *Semin Thorac Cardiovasc Surg Pediatr Card Surg Annu*. 2015;18:17-24.

136. VanderPluym CJ, Rebeyka IM, Ross DB, Buchholz H. The use of ventricular assist devices in pediatric patients with univentricular hearts. *J Thorac Cardiovasc Surg*. 2011;141:588-590.

139. Kirklin JK, Naftel DC, Pagani FD, et al. Seventh INTERMACS annual report: 15,000 patients and counting. *J Heart Lung Transplant*. 2015; 34:1495-1504.

142. Dipchand AI, Kirk R, Edwards LB, et al. The Registry of the International Society for Heart and Lung Transplantation: Sixteenth Official Pediatric Heart Transplantation Report—2013; focus theme: age. *J Heart Lung Transplant*. 2013;32:979-988.

143. Jordan LC, Ichord RN, Reinhartz O, et al. Neurological complications and outcomes in the Berlin Heart EXCOR® pediatric investigational device exemption trial. *J Am Heart Assoc*. 2015;4:e001429.

Echocardiographic Imaging: Noninvasive Cardiac Diagnostics

John L. Bass and Charles W. Shepard

PEARLS

- Echocardiography is a multipurpose imaging modality that is readily available and useful in a variety of intensive care settings.
- Echocardiography is employed in both noninvasive (transthoracic) and invasive methods (transesophageal and intracardiac).
- Echocardiography is the modality of choice in the evaluation of structural defects of the heart, ventricular function, volume status, valve function, degree of pulmonary hypertension, pericardial effusion, vascular abnormalities, cardiovascular communications, and cardiac function during extracorporeal membrane oxygenation/ventricular assist device placement or weaning.
- Echocardiography may be used for intraoperative or postoperative assessment, to guide intracardiac procedures, or for vascular access.
- Echocardiographic evaluations of cardiovascular communications provide valuable physiologic information about the connecting chambers/structures.

Introduction

Echocardiography is a relatively noninvasive technique that facilitates examination of the anatomy and flow in the heart and great vessels. The technique was first reported in the mid-1970s, initially as M-mode images with a single crystal transducer that demonstrated distance of structures from the chest wall and motion over time. This was rapidly expanded to two-dimensional (2D) imaging by moving the transducer mechanically through a sector, or forming a transducer with multiple crystals and electronically steering the echo beam. In the 1980s the signal and processing were further modified to detect the direction and velocity of blood using Doppler. Multigated pulsed Doppler was used to map flow throughout a sector and paint over the 2D image to provide an image of flow combined with anatomy. This combination of anatomy and flow has made echocardiography the primary diagnostic tool for congenital heart disease, supplanting cardiac catheterization. Further miniaturization allowed transducers to be placed at the end of endoscopes (transesophageal echocardiography [TEE]) and on small transducers for intravaginal imaging of the fetus, even on the end of catheters for intracardiac

echocardiography (ICE). Increasing computer processing power and speed provides the ability to generate real-time three-dimensional images. Echocardiography is limited by the ability to obtain images ("acoustic windows"), and patient cooperation is often necessary. Conditions that interfere with the ability of ultrasound to reach the cardiovascular structures from the chest wall, such as pneumothorax, pulmonary disease, or surgical resection of the thymus at cardiovascular operations, may also limit the ability to get good information. In these instances, TEE, a technique that images the heart from behind, may bypass these impediments and provide a different set of "windows" from which the heart can be imaged. The majority of patients, however, have adequate windows for ultrasound penetration so that echocardiography provides a primary diagnostic tool for evaluation of patients in the pediatric intensive care unit. Unlike Schroedinger's cat, the act of observation does not alter the state of the patient. The patient usually does not require additional sedation, does not have to be transported to a catheterization laboratory or radiology suite, and no contrast medium is necessary. Because of portability and the rapidity with which information can be acquired, echocardiography is ideally suited to serial observations and assessing the effects of therapy.

Diagnosis of Structural Defects

The full spectrum of congenital heart disease can be diagnosed using echocardiography. The connections, morphology of the atria and ventricles, anatomy, and defects of the semilunar and atrioventricular valves are easily defined. The relationships of vessels, valves, and defects of the atrial and ventricular septum are outlined in tomographic analysis. One disadvantage of echocardiography is that it is a tomographic technique, and the images of structures can be obtained from multiple windows with differing appearances. This led to a new generation of surgeons and interventional cardiologists who are able to recognize the different structures from these slices of anatomy and even perform interventional catheterization procedures while watching the ultrasound image alone without fluoroscopy. A full description of the diagnosis of congenital heart disease is beyond a single chapter on the uses of echocardiography in the ICU. Instead, we focus on how echocardiography helps in the evaluation of clinical problems that arise in patients admitted to the ICU for illness or those recovering from cardiovascular surgical or interventional procedures. Specifically, we discuss using echocardiography to assess ventricular function, volume status, valve function, pulmonary hypertension, pericardial effusion, vascular problems, catheter manipulation, transcatheter cardiac devices, ventricular assist device, and physiology derived from cardiovascular communications.

Ventricular Function

Diminished ventricular systolic function can account for hypotension or low cardiac output. This is measured traditionally for the left ventricle by looking at the percentage of decrease in an M-mode–derived internal diameter (diastolic left ventricular [LV] dimension-systolic LV dimension/diastolic LV dimension) or shortening fraction (Fig. 31.1). Normally this ratio is above 28%, and lower values indicate decreased LV systolic function. A more familiar calculation of systolic function is the LV ejection fraction. This calculation is the percentage of volume ejected by the left ventricle in systole using 2D measurements (diastolic volume-systolic volume/diastolic volume) and normally is 55% or above (Fig. 31.2). Mild dysfunction is in the range of 45% to 50%, and ejection fractions below 45% indicate significant systolic dysfunction. Calculations of ejection fraction usually are derived from an assumption of LV geometry (spinning the left ventricle around its long axis yields a true representation of its actual volume). When the left ventricle enlarges, it may assume a more spherical shape and these formulas become less accurate. Abnormalities of the ventricular septum motion can interfere with this calculation, as seen with ischemia, conduction abnormalities, and pressure or volume load of the right ventricle. Damage to the myocardium in select areas may produce regional wall motion abnormalities, particularly with abnormal perfusion or selective damage with global disease. Ejection fractions calculated in this circumstance are also less

accurate. Accuracy also depends on good definition of the endocardium so that the LV chamber can be traced. In larger patients, injecting protein or lipid microspheres that are small enough to cross the pulmonary capillary bed and opacify the left ventricle can yield a clearer delineation of the LV endocardial border. However, these agents are not approved for use in children and contraindicated in the presence of intracardiac right-to-left shunts. Calculation of right ventricular systolic function is more difficult as the right ventricle has a more

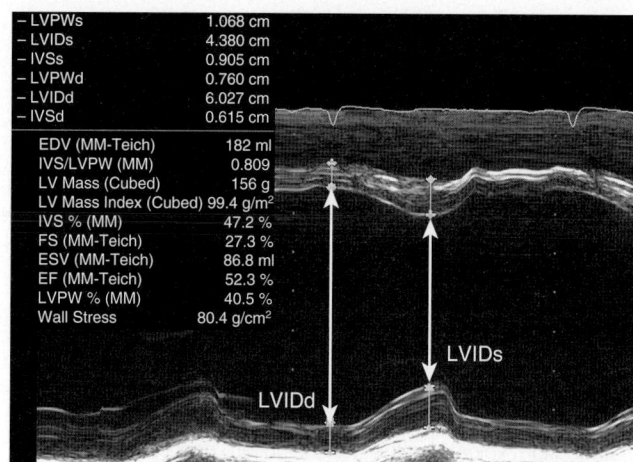

– LVPWs	1.068 cm
– LVIDs	4.380 cm
– IVSs	0.905 cm
– LVPWd	0.760 cm
– LVIDd	6.027 cm
– IVSd	0.615 cm
EDV (MM-Teich)	182 ml
IVS/LVPW (MM)	0.809
LV Mass (Cubed)	156 g
LV Mass Index (Cubed)	99.4 g/m²
IVS % (MM)	47.2 %
FS (MM-Teich)	27.3 %
ESV (MM-Teich)	86.8 ml
EF (MM-Teich)	52.3 %
LVPW % (MM)	40.5 %
Wall Stress	80.4 g/cm²

Fig. 31.1. Left ventricular (LV) function measured from an M-mode echocardiogram. The ultrasound beam passes through the left ventricle, and the motion relative to the chest wall and changes in thickness and diameter are represented on the vertical axis. Time is on the horizontal axis. Shortening fraction *(FS)*, a measure of LV systolic function, is calculated as the difference in LV diastolic *(LVIDd)* and systolic *(LVIDs)* dimensions, divided by the diastolic dimension.

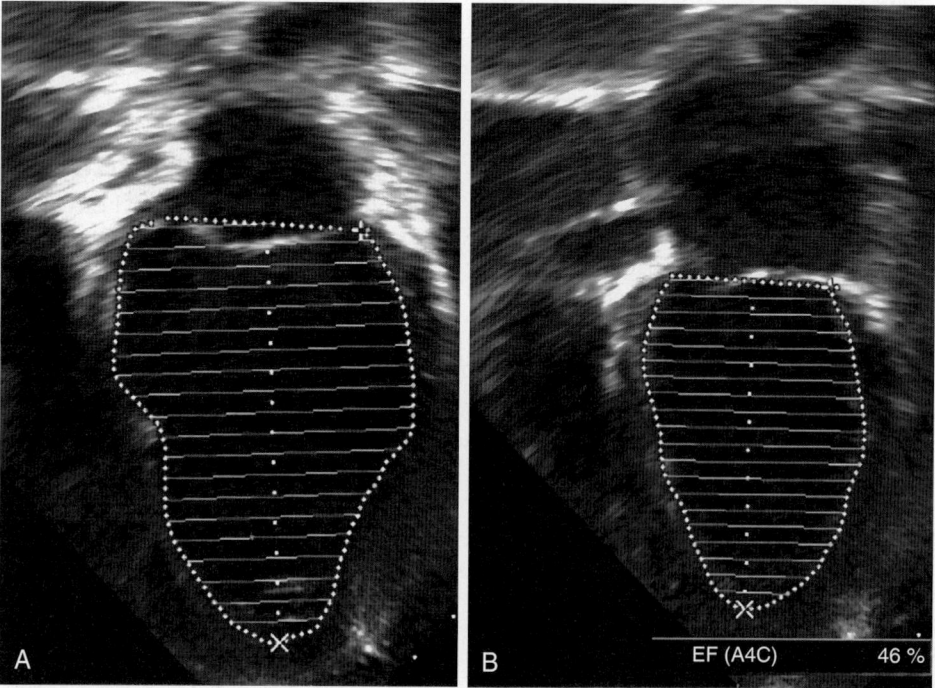

Fig. 31.2. Left ventricular ejection fraction. The ejection fraction (EF) is calculated from the difference in the diastolic volume (A), and the systolic volume (B) is divided by the diastolic volume. Normally the ejection fraction is 55% or above, with low normal 48% to 54%, mildly depressed 40% to 48%, moderately depressed 35% to 40%, and severely depressed less than 35%.

complex shape with different inflow and outflow geometries. This can be approximated from a four-chamber view and an inflow/outflow view from subcostal windows. But the most accurate method is careful reconstruction of the right ventricle from multiple slices or three-dimensional imaging.

Assessing Volume Status

The diastolic size of the ventricles is dependent on the preload and compliance. In a patient with normal myocardium, dehydration can produce small diastolic dimensions that increase with rehydration. This principle is useful in patients who have undergone acute large fluid shifts as seen after cardiopulmonary bypass. A small RV or LV size in the presence of hypotension, particularly with low central venous pressures, is an indicator of insufficient preload to fill the ventricular chamber. When compliance is decreased, the ventricular chambers may be small despite what would normally be considered adequate filling pressure. Postoperative tetralogy of Fallot patients have decreased right ventricular compliance due to RV hypertrophy and require a higher CVP to expand the RV and generate adequate cardiac output.

A corollary is conservation of mass when a larger ventricular cavity suddenly has a lower diastolic volume. This can occur with acute control of hypertension in an infant. Decrease in markedly elevated afterload with LV failure causes a sudden decrease in the diastolic volume. As the ventricular muscle is less stretched with a smaller chamber size, the ventricular walls become thicker (conservation of mass). This can also occur after cardiac transplantation. The large cavity left by the recipient heart allows implant of a larger donor organ. The new ventricle accommodates to the lower diastolic filling in a smaller person by decreasing diastolic volume. Again, LV mass is conserved by increasing the wall thickness. Over time, the "inappropriate" hypertrophy regresses.

Measuring Valve Function

Although 2D imaging of valves provides the anatomy of abnormalities, valve function is better assessed using Doppler. A combination of spectral and color flow Doppler yields measurements of timing and pressure differences, while color flow Doppler shows the relationship of abnormal flow to anatomic structures. For ease of discussion, we divide this into stenosis and regurgitation of semilunar and atrioventricular valves.

Semilunar valves are discrete in location, and the simplification of the Bernoulli equation (pressure difference = 4 × [peak velocity]^2) works well to calculate a systolic gradient. For the pulmonary valve, the peak instantaneous pressure gradient correlates best with the peak-to-peak gradient measured in the cardiac catheterization laboratory. For the aortic valve, however, the mean Doppler derived systolic pressure gradient seems to correlate best with the peak-to-peak gradient measured in the cardiac catheterization laboratory. Regurgitation is assessed directly by observing the size and distribution of the regurgitant jet on color flow Doppler and by evaluating chamber sizes affected by the regurgitant flow.[1] The length of the regurgitant jet is affected by the velocity difference across the valve. Pulmonary insufficiency usually reflects a lower diastolic pressure than aortic insufficiency, and significant regurgitation may produce a shorter regurgitant jet than an equivalent degree of aortic insufficiency. The regurgitant flow

comes from connected vascular systems for both pulmonary and aortic valves. Significant pulmonary or aortic insufficiency produces retrograde diastolic flow from the main pulmonary artery or abdominal aorta, supplementing assessment of the size of the regurgitant jet.

Atrioventricular valve stenosis and regurgitation can also be measured by spectral and color flow Doppler. The peak instantaneous gradient of tricuspid or mitral stenosis is less meaningful than the mean gradient derived from spectral Doppler. Obstruction may be reflected by enlargement of the connected atrial chamber in both instances. Atrioventricular valve regurgitation is more difficult to quantify. The jet length is greater with higher velocities independent of the amount of leakage. The regurgitant jet may move during systole or entrain along an atrial wall.[2,3] The proximal isovelocity surface area (PISA) has been used in adult patients to overcome this, measuring the area of a hemispheric shell of increasing velocity and velocity at which aliasing occurs.[1] This has less accuracy in pediatric patients because of multiple jets of regurgitation and the location of the regurgitant orifice. Systolic reversal of flow in the vessels connected to the chamber receiving the regurgitant flow (inferior vena cava or pulmonary veins) occurs when significant regurgitation is present.

Postoperative/procedural evaluation of valve competency or stenosis often is needed in the ICU, particularly because TEE in the operating room performed immediately postoperatively may not be accurate. The valve can be assessed for residual obstruction or regurgitation after balloon dilation of critical stenosis of the pulmonary or aortic valve. Difficulty weaning from ventilator support after atrioventricular septal defect repair may result from significant mitral valve regurgitation from dehiscence of the repair.

Evaluating Pulmonary Hypertension

Physiologic insufficiency of the tricuspid and pulmonary valves is common even in normal individuals and can be used to assess right ventricular and pulmonary arterial pressures. The peak velocity of tricuspid insufficiency reflects the peak systolic pressure difference between the right ventricle and right atrium. This normally ranges between 1.8 and 2.9 M/s. In this range of velocities, with normal right atrial pressure, pulmonary artery systolic pressure is normal. Higher velocities indicate elevated pulmonary artery systolic pressure[4] that may result from elevated pulmonary vascular resistance, right ventricular outflow obstruction, or transmission of systemic pressure from a ventricular septal defect (VSD) or patent ductus arteriosus (PDA). The end-diastolic velocity of pulmonary insufficiency can be used to calculate pulmonary artery diastolic pressure, as this reflects the difference in end-diastolic pressure between the pulmonary artery and right ventricle. This normally ranges between 0.5 and 1.5 M/s. With higher velocities, assuming a normal right ventricular diastolic pressure, pulmonary artery diastolic pressure can be estimated (Fig. 31.3). These calculations are especially useful with elevated pulmonary vascular resistance or indirect elevation in pulmonary artery pressure with elevated left atrial or pulmonary venous pressures.

The regurgitant velocities measured by Doppler across the pulmonary and tricuspid valves increase with increasing pulmonary artery pressure. At very high velocities, these estimates may be less accurate (any error in velocity is squared).

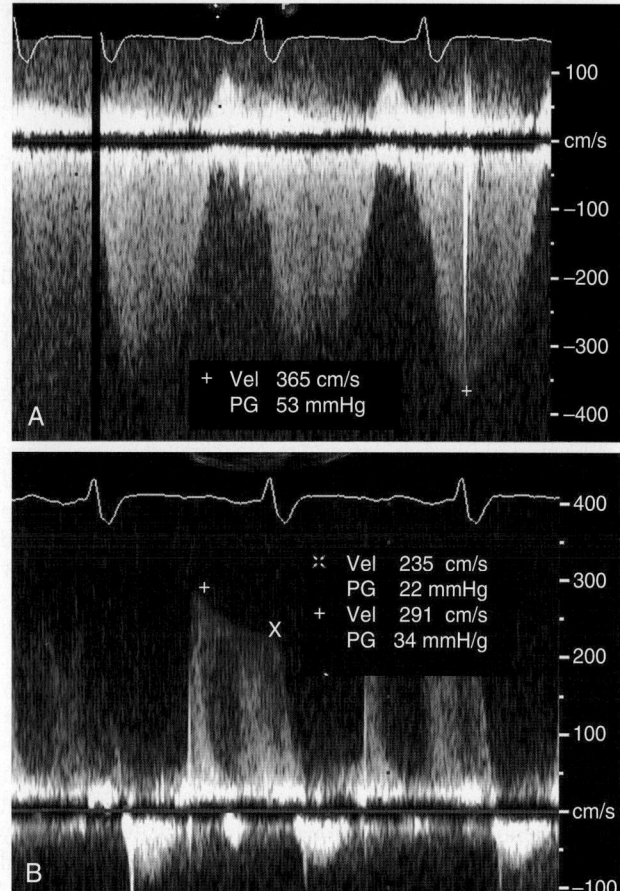

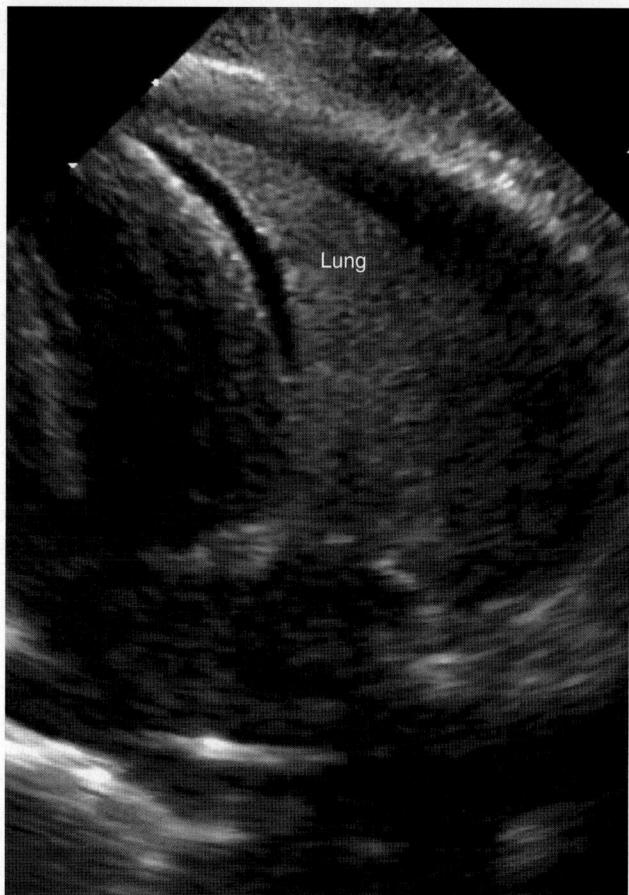

Fig. 31.3. Spectral Doppler tracings from pulmonary and tricuspid regurgitation in a patient with pulmonary hypertension. High-velocity tricuspid regurgitation (A) yields a calculated right ventricular systolic pressure 53 mm Hg above right atrial pressure (often assumed to equal central venous pressure). The pulmonary insufficiency signal (B) confirms that pulmonary artery pressure is elevated (end-diastolic velocity yields a calculated pulmonary artery diastolic pressure 22 mm Hg above right ventricular diastolic pressure). The velocity at the start of diastole may be an indicator of the mean pulmonary artery pressure.

Fig. 31.4. Two-dimensional echocardiogram performed from a left subcostal window. The apical left lung *(Lung)* is atelectatic, allowing reflection of ultrasound typical of tissue. There is small associated pleural effusion.

Hypertrophy of the right ventricle and the systolic contour of the ventricular septum (flattened or displaced toward the left ventricle) have also been used to evaluate systemic or higher right ventricular systolic pressure. In addition to the velocities of right-sided regurgitant flow, the velocity and direction of intracardiac shunts are useful in this assessment (in the absence of restriction or obstruction). Effectiveness of therapy directed to lower pulmonary artery resistance can be monitored noninvasively with a combination of these methods.

Assessing Pericardial Effusion

Pericardial effusion can occur in a number of circumstances: from primary pericardial infections (eg, bacterial [including tuberculosis], viral), a "sympathetic" collection in pulmonary infection, diffuse inflammatory processes (eg, uremia, post–bone marrow transplant, postpericardiotomy syndrome), or with mechanical trauma (eg, erosion of an atrial septal defect device, perforation by an umbilical venous catheter). The presence of an abnormal amount of pericardial fluid is easily

recognized by echocardiography with a separation between the visceral and parietal pericardium that has decreased acoustic density. This must be distinguished from fluid in the pleural space, or ascites. The heart is connected to pulmonary and systemic veins, as well as the great arteries, and pericardial effusions usually do not extend behind the left atrium or in front of the great arteries. Pleural effusions can occupy these areas and may extend around the lower lobes of the lungs. This fluid may accompany atelectasis that can be penetrated by the ultrasound beam (Fig. 31.4).

Excess pericardial fluid may interfere with filling of the heart by compromising expansion of the ventricular chambers. The amount of fluid that compromises filling depends on the speed with which the fluid accumulates. Fluid that accumulates rapidly (over minutes or hours) does not allow the pericardium to stretch so that a small volume may limit ventricular filling. Fluid accumulation over days or weeks allows the pericardium to stretch, and larger volumes of fluid may accumulate without causing compromise. The absolute amount of pericardial fluid may not indicate the degree of embarrassment.

Clinically, patients with compromised filling of the ventricles have tachycardia, tachypnea, and hypotension. True tamponade also has a pulsus paradoxus, an exaggerated respiratory variation of the systemic systolic blood pressure. This observation requires obtaining the blood pressure with a stethoscope as it is not recognizable with oscillometric blood pressure recorders. This is accompanied by late diastolic inversion of the right atrium[5] and/or early diastolic collapse of the right ventricle[6] (Fig. 31.5) and an inspiratory decrease of the velocity of blood ejected from the left ventricle.[7] The change in velocity must be considered carefully as the heart can "swing" in large effusions, changing the angle of incidence between flow and the echo beam. These signs indicate the need for emergent decompression of the pericardial space. Even in the absence of signs diagnostic of tamponade, a decrease in heart rate with improvement of blood pressure may be observed with removal of pericardial fluid, suggesting a lesser but real degree of compromise.

Removing fluid from the pericardium is easily and safely accomplished under echocardiographic guidance. The location of a safe entrance to the pericardium can be determined by finding a window where the pericardial space is a short distance from the skin, and there is no intervening lung. Traditionally this has been from a subxiphoid position. However, reaching the pericardial space through this approach could be challenging due to interposition of the liver, and the largest accumulation of fluid may not be reached through this approach. An easier approach may be from apical, parasternal, or even anterior/superior locations. Depending on adiposity, the fluid may be only a centimeter away from the skin. Lung that expands to cover the pericardial window with inspiration increases the risk of perforation of lung tissue and pneumothorax during the procedure.

Once a safe and close location to access a large accumulation of pericardial fluid has been selected, the passage of the pericardiocentesis needle into the pericardial space can be observed by echocardiography. This significantly reduces the chance of perforating the heart or coronary arteries. Visualizing that the needle is within the pericardial space is reassuring when the effusion is bloody. Once pericardial fluid is obtained, a guidewire is introduced into the posterior pericardium, followed by a dilator and placement of a pericardiocentesis catheter. As the fluid is evacuated, the decrease in effusion size can also be observed by echocardiography (Fig. 31.6). This procedure can be safely performed at the bedside without moving the patient to the cardiac catheterization laboratory or bringing C-arm fluoroscopy to the patient. Whether or not to leave the pericardiocentesis catheter in place at the end of drainage is a clinical decision. The procedure is sterile, and contamination of the pericardial space is unlikely.

Vascular

Echocardiography provides a clear picture of catheters in veins and arteries. In addition to location, the presence of thrombus associated with the catheter can be identified. In some instances, echocardiography can be used to position catheters and manipulate them through channels or intracardiac connections.[8] Indications to evaluate a catheter include persistent pleural effusions or facial edema in a postoperative patient, evaluation for access in a patient with previous indwelling catheters, arrhythmias in a patient with a central venous line that could fall through the tricuspid valve into the right ventricle, any infant with an umbilical venous line who is getting an echocardiogram for another reason, or direction of a balloon atrial septostomy catheter in a newborn infant with dextro-transposition of the great arteries.

Thrombi associated with venous catheters can vary from a fibrin cast left behind when the catheter is removed, to thrombi within the vessel where a catheter resides, to a thrombus

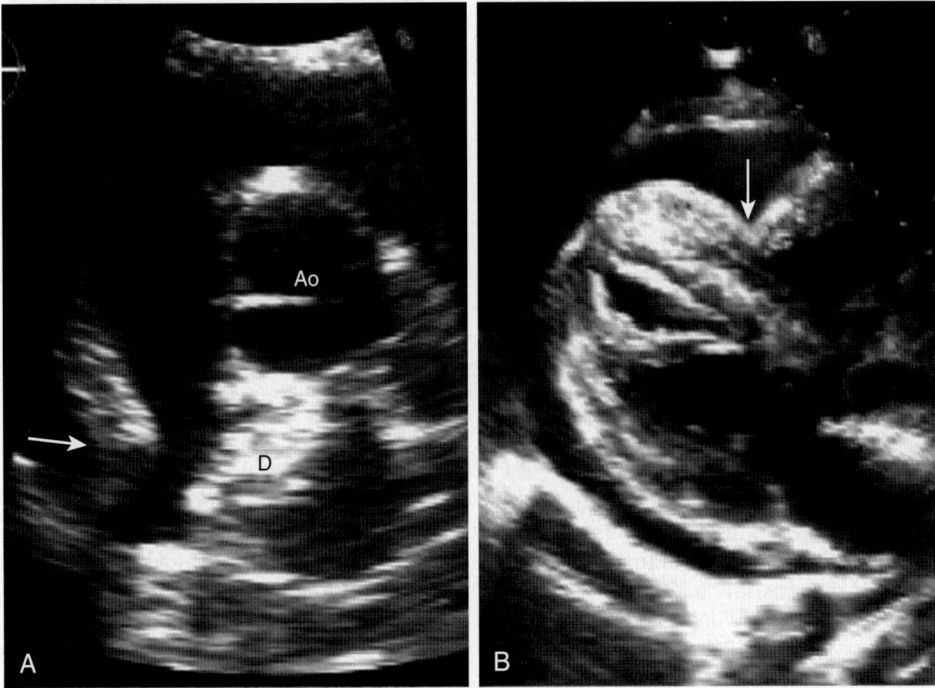

Fig. 31.5. Pericardial effusion in a patient with erosion of an Amplatzer Septal Occluder device *(D)* in contact with the aorta *(Ao)*. Tamponade is indicated by diastolic collapse of the right atrium *(arrow, Panel A)* and right ventricle *(arrow, Panel B)*. Erosion of the device is suggested by syncope, chest pain, or increasing exercise intolerance after implantation.

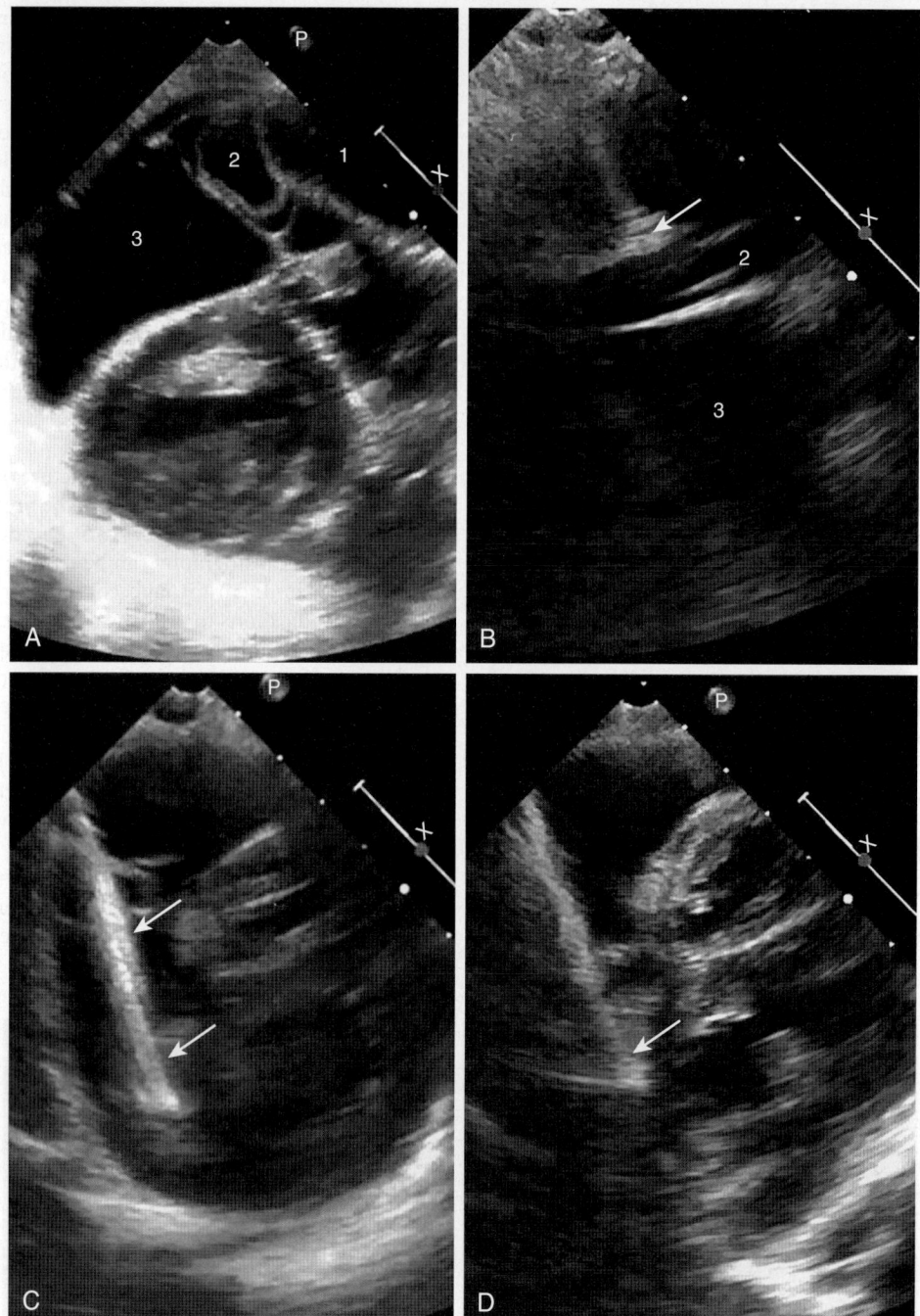

Fig. 31.6. Drainage of a complex pericardial effusion under echocardiographic guidance. In A, three separate chambers of a loculated effusion are present. In B, a needle is sequentially advanced through each chamber (*arrow* at limit of chamber 1). In C a guidewire (*arrows*) has been advanced to chamber 3. In D, chambers 2 and 3 have been evacuated by withdrawing a pigtail catheter (*arrow*) sequentially. The effusion was completely drained.

located where the tip of the catheter comes in contact with cardiac structures (Fig. 31.7). When the left innominate vein is occluded with thrombus, this may affect drainage from the thoracic duct. Early work suggests this may lead to chylous pleural effusions, or in the setting of Glenn/Fontan patients, protein-losing enteropathy or plastic bronchitis. Thrombi seem to be less common with umbilical venous catheters but can form across the foramen ovale when the catheter extends from the ductus venosus into the left atrium despite an apparently good position on a chest roentgenogram (Fig. 31.8). This

raises the possibility of air being instilled into the systemic circulation. Even when the catheter does not extend into the left atrium, the tip of the catheter is aimed at the foramen ovale, and injected fluid streams toward the left atrium. Also of concern is the possibility of erosion of the catheter through the atrial wall. This may be more likely when the catheter extends across the atrial septum (Fig. 31.9).

Vascular access has been significantly improved by direct ultrasonographic visualization of the vessel during puncture. The needle trajectory can be followed as it enters the vessel, and care can be taken to direct the entry point to "12 o'clock" position (Fig. 31.10) so that passage through the vascular lumen is ensured and the number of punctures to obtain access is reduced. This might lower the incidence of vascular thrombosis associated with acute vascular access and should

replace the classic approach of penetrating a vessel for access using landmarks and touch that becomes repeatable only with experience. The limitations of this technique are that landmarks (eg, the inguinal ligament) may be hidden by the ultrasound transducer, and care must be taken not to penetrate the sterile probe cover with the needle.

Caval anatomy can be important in care of children in the ICU. Although persistence of a left superior vena cava occurs with some frequency, the vessel usually connects to the coronary sinus and upper left systemic venous return reaches the right atrium. Rarely this can be associated with fenestrations of the coronary sinus that allow systemic venous blood to enter the left atrium or pulmonary venous blood to enter the coronary sinus (the equivalent of an atrial septal defect—a

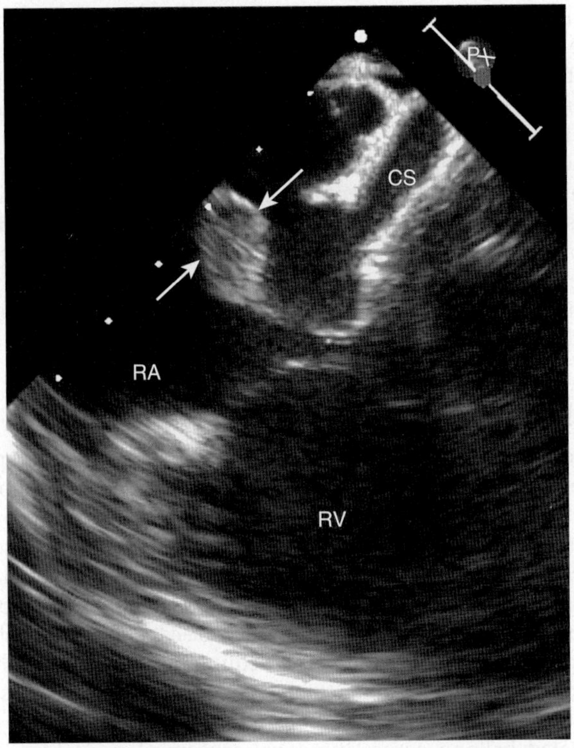

Fig. 31.7. A thrombus *(arrows)* is present attached to the right atrial *(RA)* wall. The thrombus formed at the tip of a central venous catheter. *CS,* coronary sinus; *RV,* right ventricle.

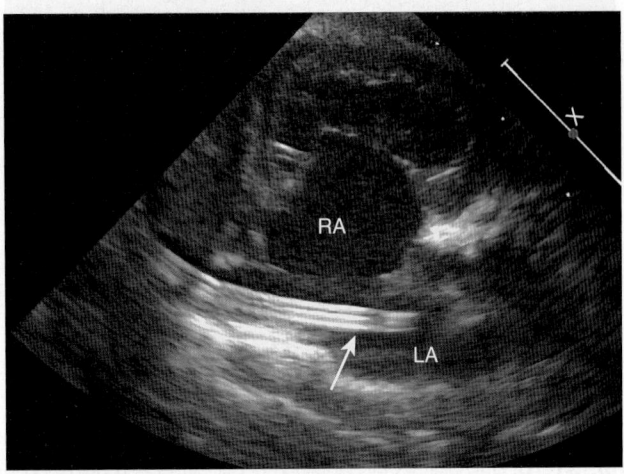

Fig. 31.9. An umbilical venous catheter *(arrow)* extending from the right atrium *(RA)* across the foramen ovale in the left atrium *(LA).*

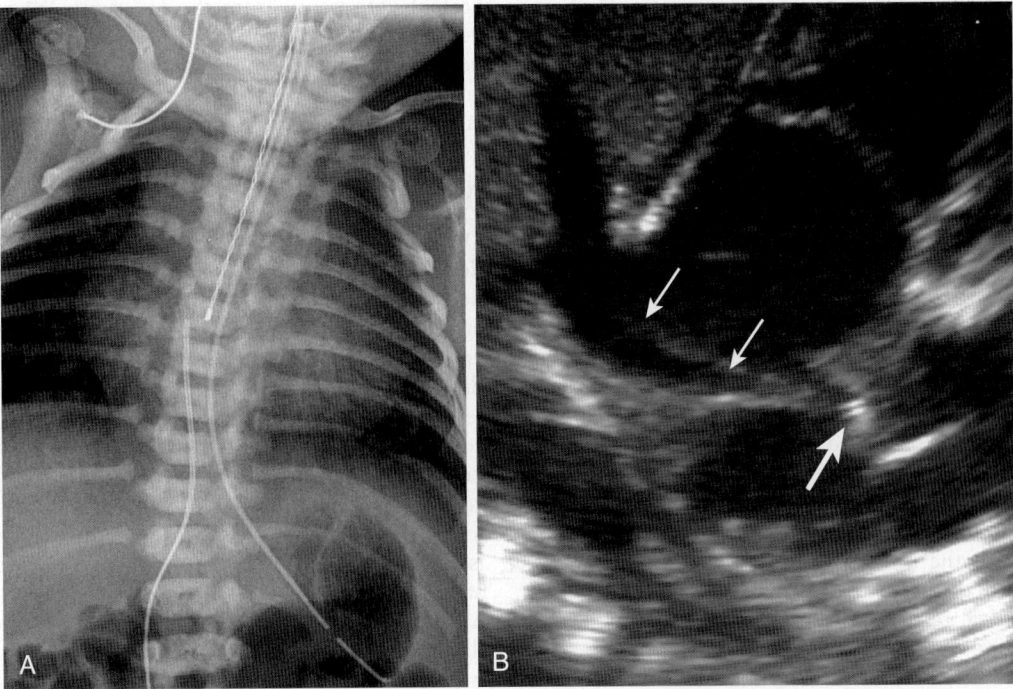

Fig. 31.8. Fibrin sheath from an umbilical venous catheter. On chest roentgenogram (A) the catheter tip appears to be in the mid right atrium. After removal of the catheter, echocardiography (B) reveals a fibrin sheath remaining *(small arrows),* and the tip of the thrombus extends across the foramen ovale *(larger arrow).*

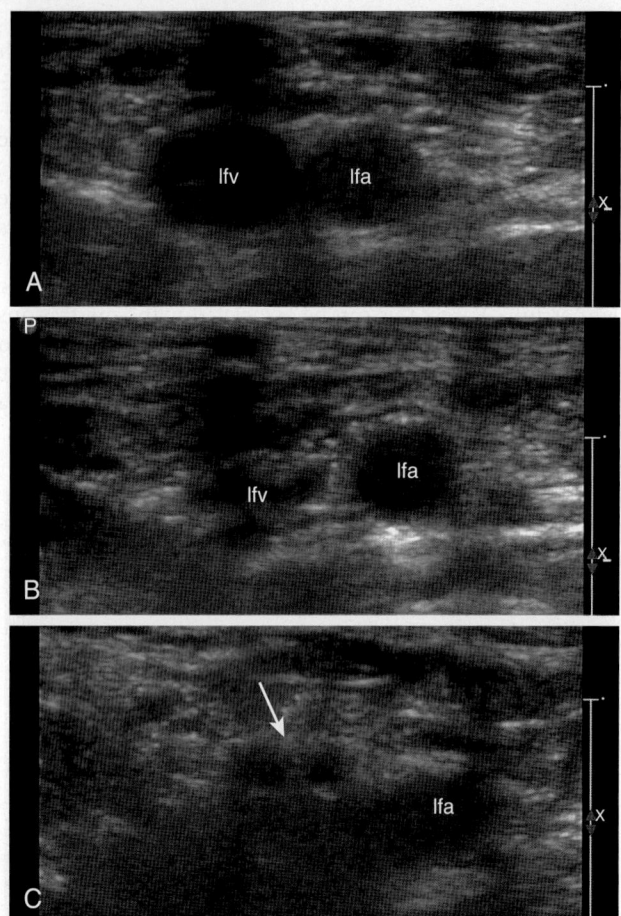

Fig. 31.10. Vascular access obtained under ultrasound guidance. In A the left femoral artery *(lfa)* and vein *(lfv)* are imaged. In B increased pressure on the transducer causes compression of the vein. The needle entering the vein can be seen at 12 o'clock *(arrow)* in C.

"coronary sinus atrial septal defect"). Another possible cause of cyanosis associated with a persistent left superior vena cava is direct attachment of the vein to the left atrium instead of the coronary sinus (Fig. 31.11). In this instance, the entirety of the left upper systemic venous return enters the left atrium directly, a cause of persistent cyanosis from birth that is not caused by pulmonary disease. This is easily resolved by transcatheter occlusion of the connection. After some surgical repairs (eg, cardiac transplantation) the anastomosis of the superior vena cava may be compromised and stenotic yielding higher velocity flow (Fig. 31.12), particularly when there has been a previous Glenn anastomosis. This may be manifested by edema of the face or upper body. Caval stenosis can be treated by stenting the narrowed segment.

Interruption of the inferior vena cava with azygous continuation leaves the hepatic venous return directly to the floor of the right atrium. This is not a cause of cyanosis. However, the connection of the inferior vena cava can be altered by surgical repair. Redirection of inferior vena caval flow may occur with surgical repair of an atrial septal defect, but the cyanosis is obvious at the time of surgery. Orientation of a surgical patch so that inferior caval flow is directed through a residual atrial communication may be less obvious. Subtle Doppler flow patterns may be difficult to elucidate, but an echo contrast study from the lower half of the body is

diagnostic. Fluid rapidly injected through a small bore needle or catheter reduces pressure where it enters the circulation, causing tiny gas bubbles to form transiently in the vessel or chamber. These persist for a short period of time before collapsing back into solution and are large enough that the pulmonary capillaries filter them out. These microbubbles reflect ultrasound providing a dense and graphic demonstration of the course of the blood in which they are produced and do not enter the systemic circulation from systemic venous injection unless there is an abnormal communication with a right-to-left shunt[9] (Fig. 31.13). Cryptogenic stroke may be associated with a transient right-to-left shunt (paradoxical embolus) through a patent foramen ovale (PFO). This is diagnosed with an echo contrast study during a Valsalva maneuver (transiently increasing systemic venous return and right atrial pressure) in patients who can cooperate. When there is no other cause of a stroke, the PFO may be closed with a transcatheter device.

Catheter Manipulation

The first catheter manipulation guided by echocardiography was probably balloon atrial septostomy. Patients with complete transposition of the great arteries often require improved mixing between the pulmonary and systemic circulations. In these cases, enlarging a small atrial communication can be lifesaving. Balloon atrial septostomy was traditionally performed under fluoroscopy in the cardiac catheterization laboratory. However, the entire procedure can be accomplished under ultrasound guidance at the bedside,[10] from access to crossing the atrial septal communication and pulling the inflated balloon across the atrial septum (Fig. 31.14). This avoids the need to move a fragile cyanotic newborn infant from the ICU to the cardiac catheterization laboratory. Visualization of the cardiac structures and balloon prevents inadvertent withdrawal from the LV cavity. When the umbilical vein is selected as the route of approach, but an umbilical venous catheter cannot be advanced into the inferior vena cava, direction of a catheter through the ductus venosus under echocardiographic guidance is possible (Fig. 31.15).

Devices

Over the past 15 to 20 years transcatheter devices have been developed that allow closure of simpler congenital heart defects, such as patent ductus arteriosus, atrial, and ventricular septal communications. Placement of these devices is enhanced by cardiac ultrasound—transesophageal, intracardiac, and epicardial. Surgically placed sutures may inadvertently impinge on adjacent cardiac structures (eg, the conduction system), and transcatheter devices have the same potential. An atrial septal defect occlusion device requires contact with the atrial septum throughout its entire circumference for stability. If this contact is not present or the device is undersized, it can become dislodged into the left or right atrial chamber (Fig. 31.16). The first indication that this has happened may be atrial or ventricular ectopy. Usually the device can be recaptured and repositioned or a larger device implanted. A rarer occurrence with an atrial septal occluder device is erosion of the edge of the device through the wall of the heart, resulting in an acute hemopericardium.[10] This usually occurs anteriorly and superiorly where the device is in

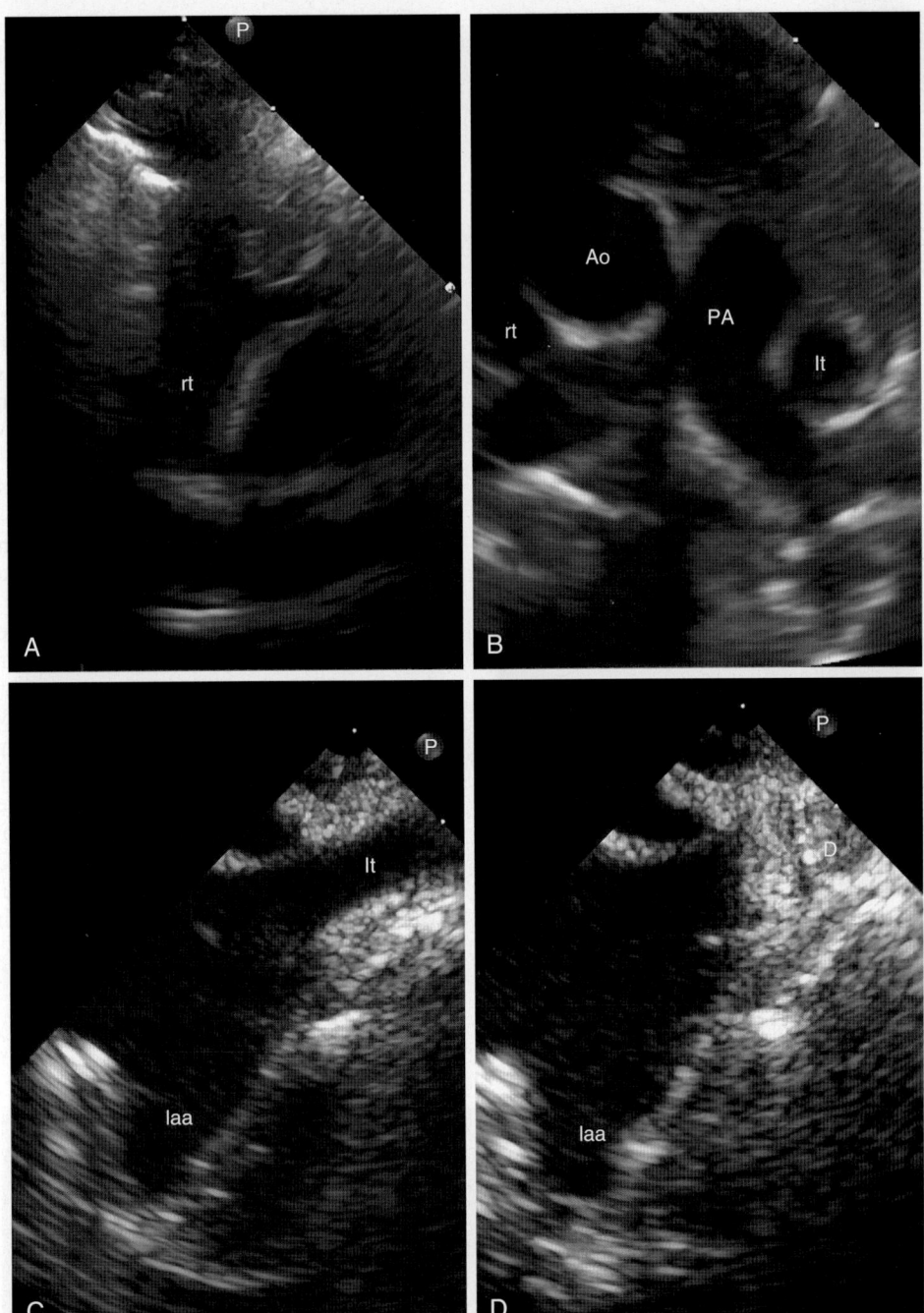

Fig. 31.11. Left superior vena cava *(SVC)* connecting directly to the left atrium. The normal right SVC *(rt)* is seen in A from a suprasternal notch view. A short axis view (B) shows the right SVC and left SVC *(lt)* in cross section to the right and left of the aorta *(Ao)* and pulmonary artery *(PA)*. Transesophageal imaging (C) shows the left SVC connecting directly to the left atrium. In D, a device (D) has been placed occluding the entrance of systemic venous blood to the systemic arterial circulation. *laa,* left atrial appendage.

contact with the atrial wall and aorta.[11] Symptoms are chest pain or syncope. When these occur, immediate echocardiography and pericardiocentesis when pericardial fluid is present are mandatory (Fig. 31.5). Early pericardiocentesis may prevent low cardiac output from tamponade.

Extracorporeal Membrane Oxygenation and Ventricular Assist Devices

Improved technology and miniaturization have led to increased utilization of ventricular assist devices (VADs) in

children. Echocardiography provides a noninvasive method of measuring effectiveness, changes in ventricular and valve function, and complications.[12] TTE usually provides adequate images in children, but TEE may be necessary in some. Both pulsatile and continuous-flow pumps are available, including venoarterial and venovenous extracorporeal membrane oxygenation (ECMO). Cannula position is readily ascertained with 2D imaging. Effective VAD support unloads the left ventricle, which translates into decreased LV dimensions. With pulsatile VADs, device ejection is not timed to the patient's

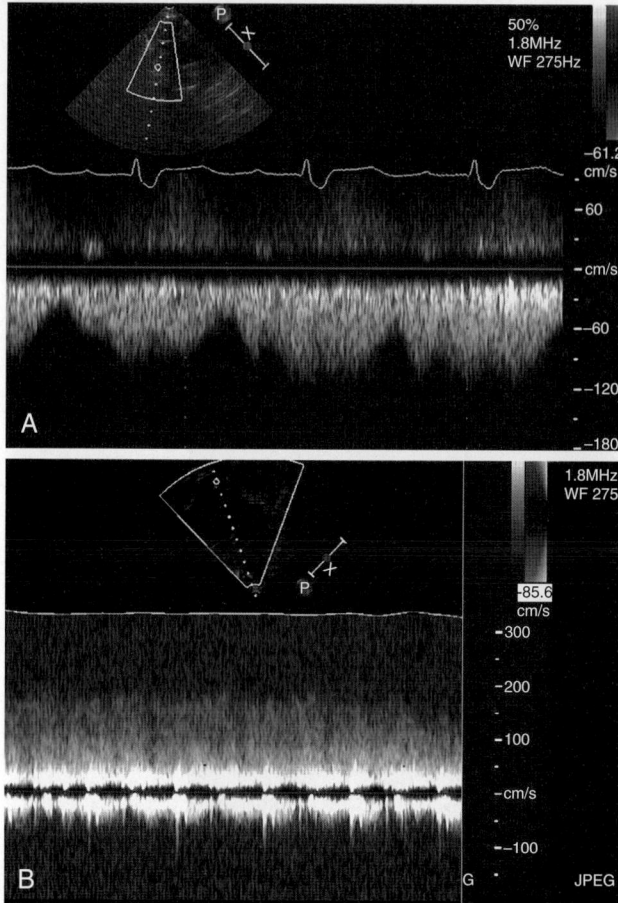

Fig. 31.12. Doppler recordings of superior vena caval *(SVC)* flow. The signal in A has a normal low-velocity signal and phasic variation with respirations and the cardiac cycle. The recording is made from the suprasternal notch, producing a negative signal. The signal in B is high velocity and continuous without variation, a result of SVC obstruction. The recording is made from a subcostal widow, producing a positive signal.

cardiac systole and maximum left ventricle end-diastolic dimension may not be synchronized with the ECG because of varying preload and afterload. The presence of a cannula in the ventricular apex may shadow this portion of the wall, and the EF may be calculated assuming an akinetic apex. The left ventricular assist device (LVAD) should decrease LV filling pressure with a consequent decrease in pulmonary artery pressure. This should affect RV size and function, TR velocity, and IVC size. Direct calculation of RV output can be made from the RVOT time-velocity integral and diameter in most patients. Significant mitral regurgitation (MR) can indicate inadequate decompression of the left ventricle. The aortic valve usually opens intermittently with pulsatile pumps. With continuous-flow VADs, aortic valve opening depends on the patient's LV function and the pump flow. Aortic insufficiency may worsen or become continuous (Fig. 31.17). Complete aortic valve closure may lead to thrombus formation in the cardiac apex or aorta (Fig. 31.18). Cannula obstruction may occur with cannula displacement or from thrombus. Expected velocities of Doppler evaluation of cannulas in children have not been confirmed.[13]

Atrial communications may be large enough to permit right-to-left shunting and systemic desaturation and may be closed at LVAD placement or by transcatheter approach. Pericardial effusions or hematomas may occur without symptoms on LVAD support but may affect the ability to wean support. Testing a patient's ability to be weaned from LVAD support is usually accomplished by stopping or lowering VAD output while observing LV size (LVEDd) and contractility (LVEF) along with calculated LV output (from LVOT, measured time velocity integral (TVI), and diameter). These supplement the usual measurements of aortic pressure and mixed venous saturation.

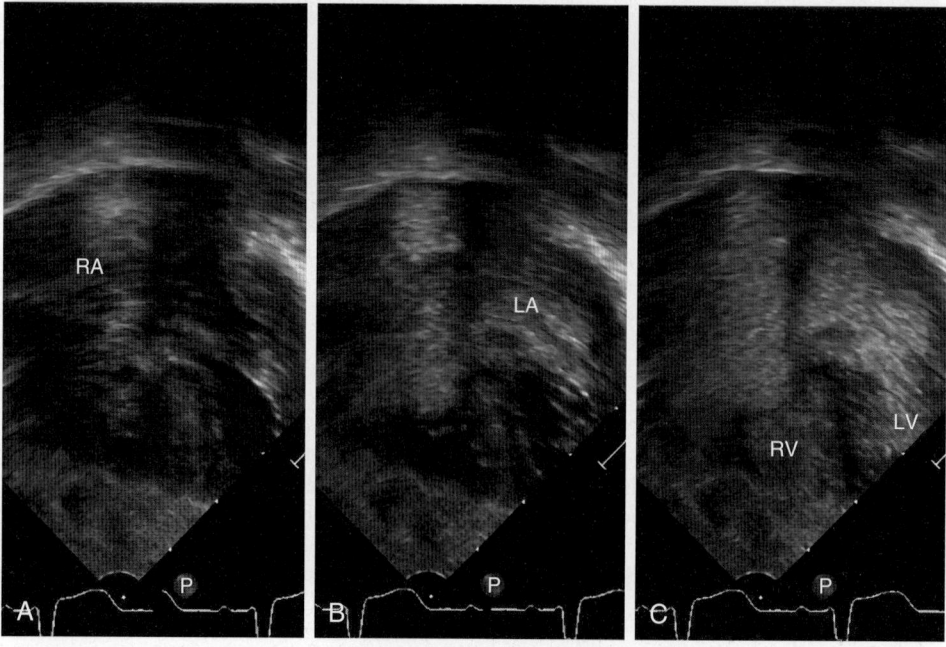

Fig. 31.13. An echo contrast study is performed injecting from the lower half of the body after repair of a complete atrioventricular septal defect. The right atrium (RA) is opacified first in A. In B the contrast effect has passed across an atrial septal communication to the left atrium (LA), and in C right *(RV)* and left *(LV)* ventricles are opacified. This documents a significant residual right-to-left shunt at atrial level.

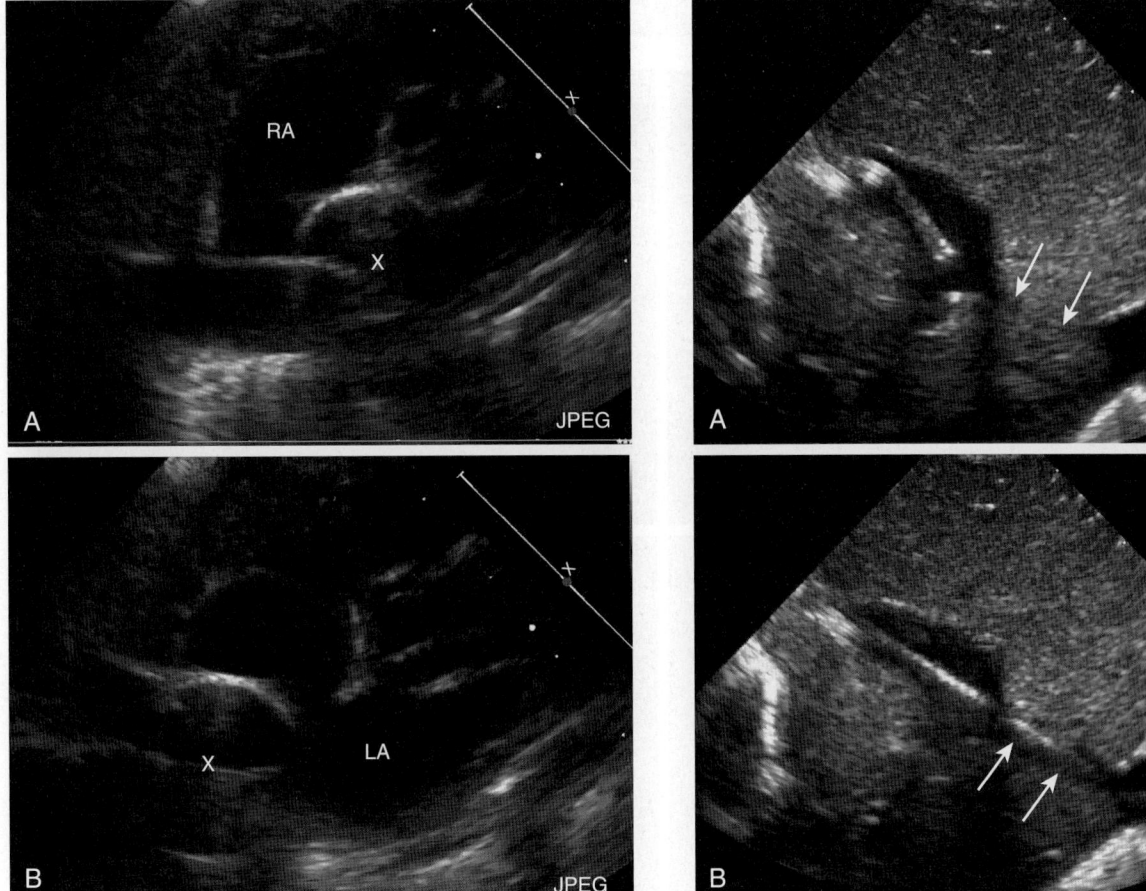

Fig. 31.14. Echocardiographic guidance of a balloon atrial septostomy. The inflated balloon *(X)* fills the left atrium (panel A). The balloon was sharply withdrawn across the atrial septum stopping at the inferior vena cava, leaving the left atrium *(LA)* empty with a hole in the atrial septum (panel B).

Fig. 31.15. Catheterization of the ductus venosus under echocardiographic guidance. Imaging is parallel to the long axis of the body with the head to image right and feet to image left. *Arrows* in A indicate the ductus venosus channel, while an angled glide catheter is seen proximally in the liver. In B, the catheter is rotated clockwise and advanced across the ductus venosus into the right atrium *(RA)*.

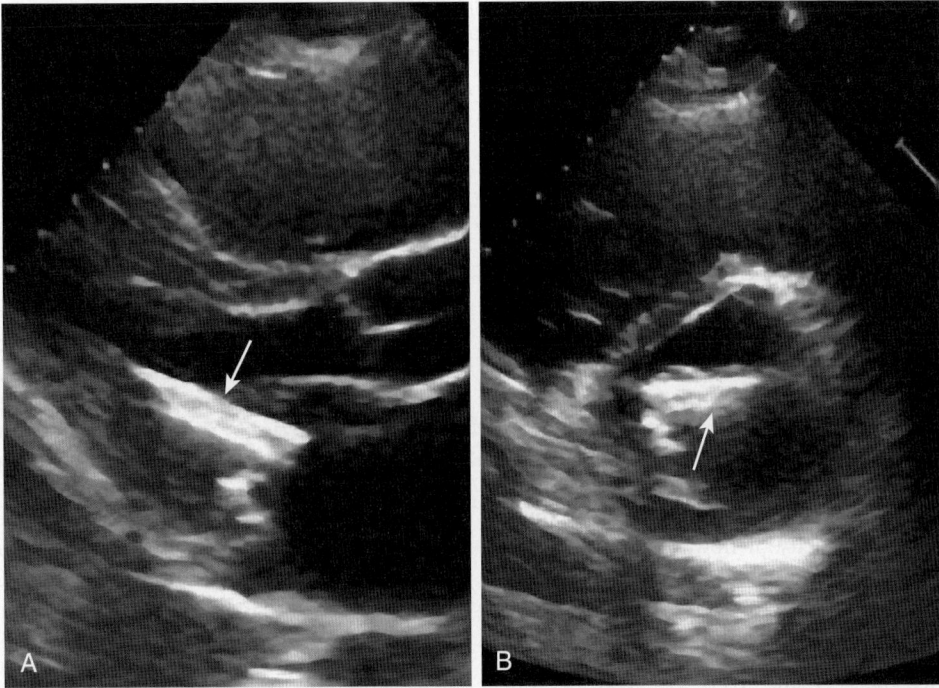

Fig. 31.16. An Amplatzer Septal Occluder device has embolized from its position in the atrial septum into the left atrium and across the mitral valve. In long axis (A) the device *(arrow)* is seen through the mitral orifice into the left ventricle. In short axis (B) the device *(arrow)* is seen sideways through the mitral orifice. Embolization of the device may be indicated by atrial and ventricular ectopy. Left in this position, the device could cause damage to the mitral valve.

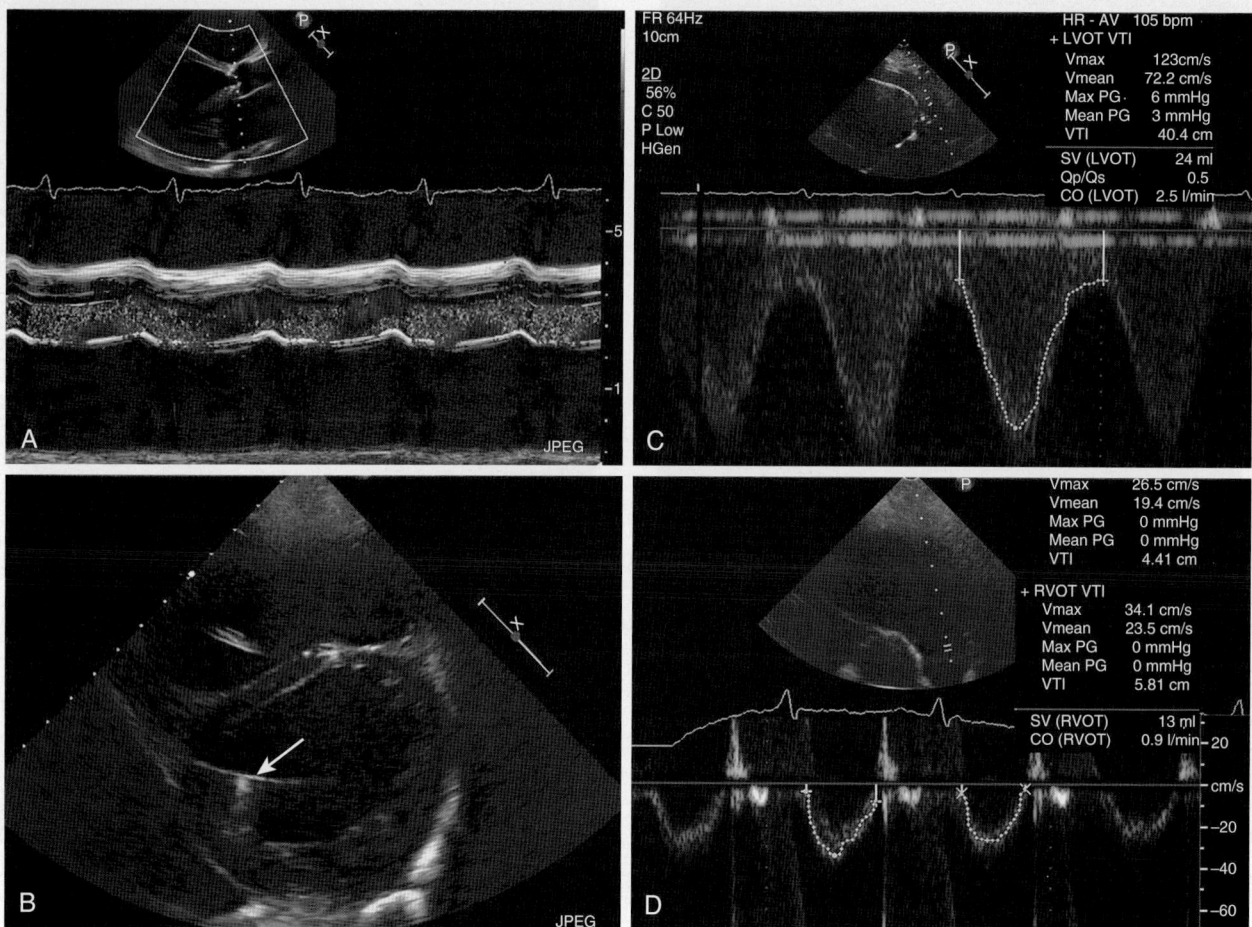

Fig. 31.17. Echocardiographic recordings in a patient on a continuous pump left ventricular assist device (LVAD). There is continuous aortic insufficiency (A) through an aortic valve that never opens. A cannula is seen entering the left ventricle (arrow) in B. An estimated output through the aortic cannula is made from the time velocity integral (TVI) and cannula diameter of 2.5 L/min (C). Right ventricular output is calculated from the right ventricular TVI and diameter of the right ventricular outflow tract (D) at 0.9 L/min. While calculation of LVAD output by Doppler may not be accurate with the long cannula and accelerated flow, the calculation was close to the flow from the device in this instance. It is clear that LVAD output does not equal cardiac output as aortic insufficiency is taken up by the pump and leaks back into the left ventricle, a circular shunt.

Cardiovascular Communications and Physiology

The patent ductus arteriosus (PDA) and PFO are normal cardiovascular communications that may persist for variable times after birth. Echocardiography is called on particularly when the patent ductus arteriosus is implicated in slow improvement of respiratory dysfunction in premature infants. The patency of a ductus arteriosus is confirmed by Doppler detectable flow. However, the significance of its contribution to respiratory function is defined by more than the simple demonstration of patency. The PDA provides a window on the relative pulmonary and systemic pressures and resistances. This is manifested by the velocity of flow, direction of flow, and effect on distal flows.[14] When the flow velocity is less than 1.5 M/sec, the pressures in the systemic and pulmonary circulations are equal. This is not an indication of the significance of the PDA. When pulmonary resistance is similar to systemic, the flow velocity will be low regardless of the size of the ductus. On the other hand, if the PDA is large enough, pressure will be equalized regardless of resistances. The significance of ductal shunting is reflected first by the direction of flow.

Typically we think of a PDA as shunting left to right throughout the cardiac cycle. However, elevation in pulmonary vascular resistance can result in systolic right-to-left flow, with left-to-right flow only in diastole (Fig. 31.19). As pulmonary resistance falls, the systolic flow becomes more left to right. The amount of diastolic left-to-right flow through the PDA is reflected in abdominal aortic flow (Fig. 31.20). Diastolic flow reversal results from "runoff" of blood from the aorta into the pulmonary arteries. A significant PDA can then be characterized as large enough to transmit high pressure to the pulmonary arteries (≥2- to 2.5-mm diameter) and shunting left to right and thus increasing pulmonary blood flow sufficiently to produce runoff from the abdominal aorta. It is less clear that a smaller pressure restrictive PDA without enough shunt to cause abdominal aortic runoff can still negatively impact respiratory disease. Bidirectional low-velocity PDA shunting with runoff from the abdominal aorta may have a negative impact on the pulmonary circulation, but removing the pop-off by closing the PDA may also lead to suprasystemic pulmonary arterial systolic pressures. Although pulmonary resistance equal to or greater than systemic causes PDA flow

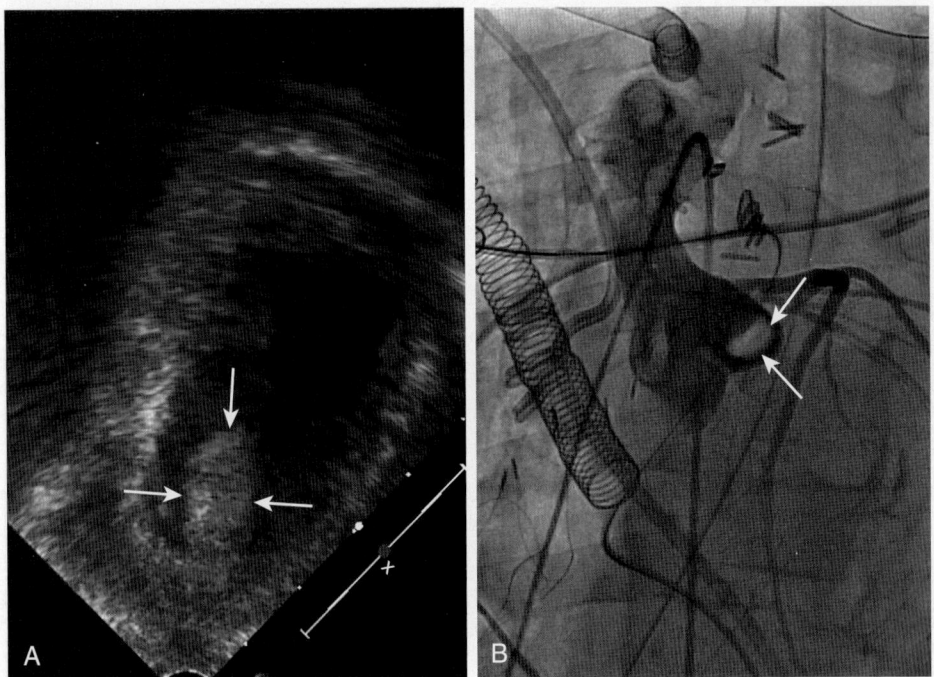

Fig. 31.18. With left ventricular (LV) dysfunction and an aortic valve that does not open on LV assist device support, thrombus may form in the left ventricular apex (A, *arrows*) or the noncoronary cusp of the aortic valve (B, *arrows*). The aortic thrombus could have been recognized on echocardiogram before cardiac catheterization.

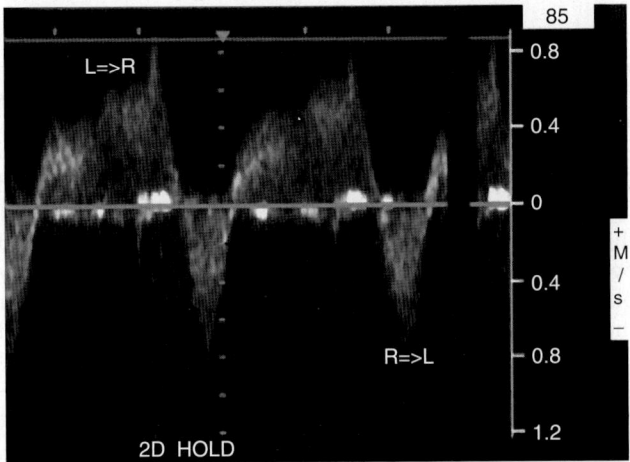

Fig. 31.19. Bidirectional flow through a patent ductus arteriosus due to elevated pulmonary vascular resistance. Systolic flow is right to left (R = >L) while diastolic flow is left to right (L = >R).

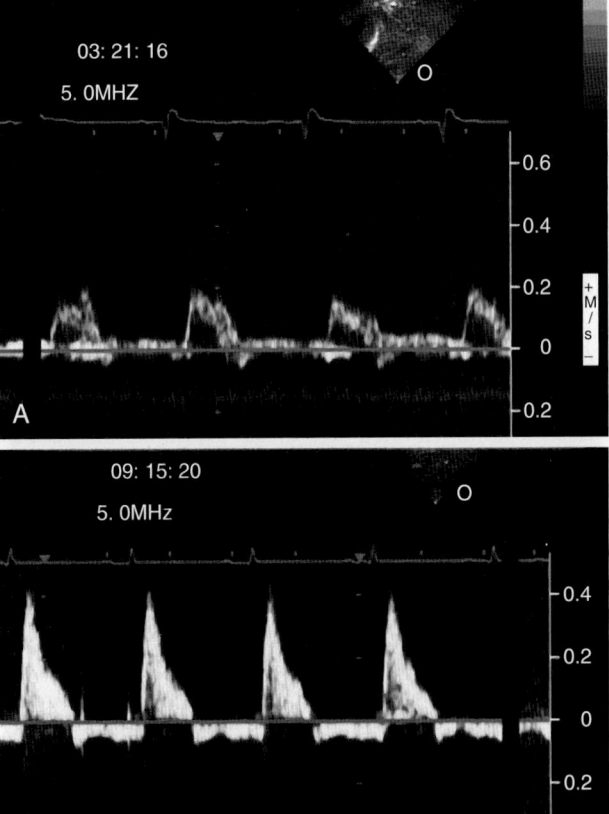

Fig. 31.20. Normal abdominal aortic flow is antegrade throughout the cardiac cycle except for an early diastolic reversal (A). When there is a patent ductus arteriosus and subsystemic pulmonary resistance, there is diastolic reversal of flow (B) as blood runs into the pulmonary circulation in diastole.

to go right to left, this pattern of flow may also occur when systemic vascular resistance is less than pulmonary.

This is further illustrated in the presence of an arteriovenous malformation in an infant (great vein of Galen or hepatic). In this circumstance, pulmonary resistance exceeds systemic resistance because of the low-resistance arteriovenous malformation. Ductal flow is right to left throughout the cardiac cycle, while there is "runoff" from the abdominal aorta also toward the malformation (Fig. 31.21).

Finally, left-sided obstructive lesions such as hypoplastic left heart, critical aortic stenosis, or preductal coarctation of the aorta may also produce systolic right-to-left flow through a PDA, even if pulmonary resistance is subsystemic. Nature

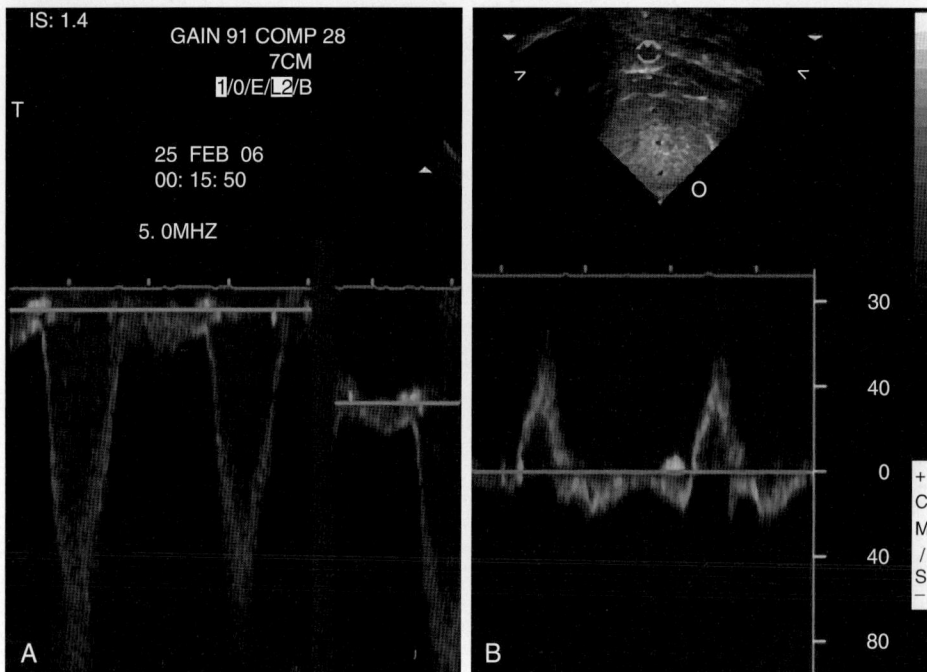

Fig. 31.21. Ductal (A) and abdominal aortic flow (B) with a cerebral arteriovenous malformation. Because systemic resistance is low, flow is continuously right to left through the ductus. But diastolic aortic flow runs toward the cerebral arteriovenous malformation in diastole. Were aortic runoff due to subsystemic pulmonary resistance, ductal flow would be left to right in diastole.

abhors a vacuum, and with inadequate blood flow to the systemic circulation, blood will flow right to left across the PDA to fill the void.

The PFO provides a similar window on the relative pressures and compliances of the right and left atria. There is often Doppler-detectable left-to-right flow in the valve component of the PFO until the communication seals, and the velocity allows determination of the pressure difference between right and left atria using the simplified Bernoulli equation ($P = 4 \times V^2$) (Fig. 31.22). Under normal conditions the pressure differences are small, and the velocity of the left-to-right shunt is less than 1.5 M/sec. LV diastolic dysfunction and mitral valve disease lead to elevated left atrial pressures, and a peak and mean pressure gradient between the atria can be calculated. Assuming a normal right atrial pressure, or when the right atrial pressure is directly measured in the ICU, absolute left atrial pressure can also be calculated. This supplements the assessment of mitral regurgitation by color flow Doppler and mitral stenosis from the diastolic velocity measured across the mitral valve. When right atrial pressure is elevated, with poor right ventricular compliance (due to myocardial issues or absolute volume, significant tricuspid regurgitation, or stenosis), a right-to-left shunt can be observed. With tricuspid or mitral atresia, the velocity of flow across the atrial septum adds to imaging in assessing the adequacy of the communication.

A VSD can also give information about relative ventricular pressures and outflow resistances. Low-velocity systolic left-to-right shunt confirms systemic right ventricular and pulmonary artery systolic pressures when there is no right ventricular outflow obstruction. When the defect is tiny and pulmonary resistance low, the left-to-right shunt is high velocity. A

moderate-sized VSD that is pressure restrictive but allows a "large" left-to-right shunt that produces left heart enlargement may show a high-velocity systolic shunt but also a pandiastolic left-to-right shunt because of LV volume overload (Fig. 31.23). An artificial but clinically useful application of this is the acute change in ventricular shunting demonstrated by Doppler during placement or adjustment of a surgically placed pulmonary arterial band. Not only are the diameter of the band from 2D imaging and the gradient across the band from Doppler seen but also the change in flow pattern across the VSD, which can become bidirectional. This can be evaluated in the operating room with TEE or once the patient returns to the ICU.

Summary

Echocardiography is often thought of as a diagnostic technique that reveals the anatomy and function of the heart and, occasionally, the presence of a pericardial effusion. However, there are many other occasions where it can provide assistance to the pediatric or neonatal intensivist, cardiologist, and cardiovascular surgeon in day-to-day management of ICU patients through evaluation of therapy or defining changing hemodynamics and physiology to assess medical therapy. Surveillance evaluation may detect changes before they become clinically apparent. It may be better to remove the occasional normal appendix—get an echocardiogram when no new information is obtained—than to overlook an unexpected alteration in condition that precedes clinical change. The noninvasive nature that does not impact the patient by transport or alter the clinical condition being observed makes echocardiography a primary management tool for the ICU patient.

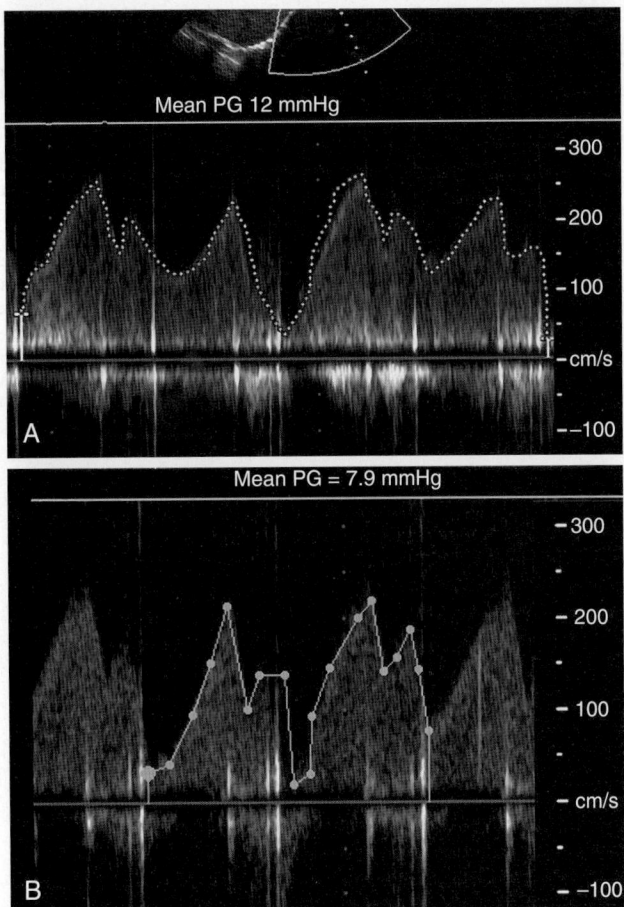

Fig. 31.22. Recordings of flow across an atrial communication in a patient with left ventricular hypoplasia and a "left ventricular growth" operation. There is significant diastolic restriction to flow. In A, a 12-mm Hg gradient between the right and left atria is calculated from the left-to-right atrial flow. After diuresis in B, the calculated pressure difference falls to 7.9 mm Hg, although the peak velocities are similar. Noninvasive measurement of atrial flow allows calculation of changes in hemodynamic state.

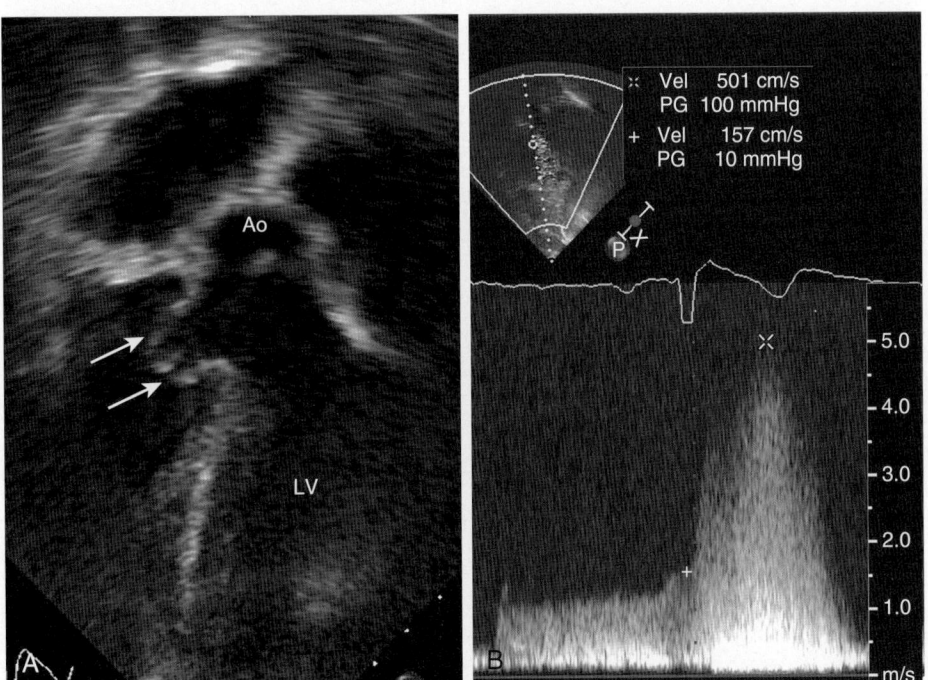

Fig. 31.23. Echocardiographic recordings from a patient with a moderate-sized perimembranous ventricular septal defect. *Arrows* point to the aneurysm of the atrial septum between the left ventricle *(LV)* and aorta *(Ao)* in Panel A from an apical five-chamber view. Doppler recorded from the left-to-right shunt in B shows a large systolic pressure difference between right and left ventricles. There is continuous diastolic left-to-right flow with velocities suggesting a 5- to 10-mm Hg pressure difference, presumably from a "large" left-to-right shunt with left ventricular enlargement and increased left ventricular diastolic pressures.

References

1. Zoghbi WA, Enriquez-Sarano M, Foster E, et al. Recommendations for evaluation of the severity of native valvular regurgitation with two-dimensional and Doppler echocardiography. *J Am Soc Echocardiogr.* 2013;16:777-802.
2. Enriquez-Sarano M, Tajik AJ, Bailey KR, et al. Color flow imaging compared with quantitative Doppler assessment of severity of mitral regurgitation: influence or eccentricity of jet and mechanism of regurgitation. *J Am Coll Cardiol.* 1993;21:1211-1219.
3. Chao K, Moises VA, Shandas R, et al. Influence of the Coanda effect on color Doppler jet area and color encoding. In vitro studies using color Doppler flow mapping. *Circulation.* 1992;85:333-341.
4. Berger M, Haimowitz A, Van Tosh A, et al. Quantitative assessment of pulmonary hypertension in patients with tricuspid regurgitation using continuous wave Doppler ultrasound. *J Am Coll Cardiol.* 1985;6:359-365.
5. Gillam LD, Guyer DE, Gibson TC, et al. Hydrodynamic compression of the right tirum: a new echocardiographic sign of cardiac tamponade. *Circulation.* 1983;68:294-301.
6. Armstrong WF, Schilt BF, Helper DJ, et al. Diastolic collapse of the right ventricle with cardiac tamponade: an echocardiographic study. *Circulation.* 1982;65:1491-1496.
7. Sharp JT, Bunnell IL, Holland JF, et al. Hemodynamics during induced cardiac tamponade in man. *Am J Med.* 1960;29:640-646.
8. Silvestry FE, Kerber RE, Brook MM, et al. Echocardiography-guided interventions. *J Am Soc Echocardiogr.* 2009;22:213-231.
9. Butler BD, Hills BA. The lung as a filter for microbubbles. *J Appl Physiol Respir Environ Exerc Physiol.* 1979;47:537-543.
10. Zellers TM, Dixon K, Moake L, et al. Bedside balloon atrial septostomy is safe, efficacious, and cost-effective compared with septostomy performed in the cardiac catheterization laboratory. *Am J Cardiol.* 2002;89:613-615.
11. Amin Z, Hijazi ZM, Bass JL, et al. Erosion of Amplatzer septal occluder device after closure of secundum atrial septal defects: review of registry of complications and recommendations to minimize future risk. *Catheter Cardiovasc Interv.* 2004;63:496-502.
12. Estep JD, Stainback RG, Little SH, et al. The role of echocardiography and other imaging modalities in patients with left ventricular assist devices. *J Am Coll Cardiol.* 2010;3:1049-1064.
13. Sachdeva R, Frazier EA, Jaquiss RDB, et al. Echocardiographic evaluation of ventricular assist devices in pediatric patients. *J Am Soc Echocardiogr.* 2013;26:41-49.
14. Musewe NN, Poppe D, Smallhorn JF, et al. Doppler echocardiographic measurement of pulmonary artery pressure from ductal Doppler velocities in the newborn. *J Am Coll Cardiol.* 1990;15:446-456.

Diagnostic and Therapeutic Cardiac Catheterization

Alan W. Nugent

PEARLS

- The cardiac catheterization laboratory plays important diagnostic and therapeutic roles in the management of children in the pediatric intensive care unit.
- For patients with cardiac disease whose critical care course is not progressing as expected, early exploration for diagnosis of unsuspected or residual defects by cardiac catheterization often improves outcomes.
- To maximize the utility of catheterization, effective communication between the intensive care physician and the interventional cardiologist is essential.

The cardiac catheterization laboratory plays an important diagnostic and therapeutic role in the management of children in the critical care environment. Obtaining comprehensive hemodynamic data and angiography in the catheterization laboratory helps formulate and tailor management strategies. In the postoperative cardiac patient, the diagnosis of unsuspected or residual anatomic defects may enable therapeutic surgical or catheter-directed interventions to improve a patient's outcome. Numerous interventions can be performed during cardiac catheterization. The pediatric critical team must be aware of the possible benefits and limitations of catheterization procedures, and effective communication between the intensive care physician and the physician performing the procedure is crucial.

Catheterization Laboratory Environment

Cardiac catheterization laboratories are remote from the ICU and rarely are configured to accommodate critical care personnel and equipment. Relative to patient size, the biplane fluoroscopic equipment used for imaging is in close proximity to the patient's head and neck, limiting access to the airway. A mechanical ventilator and monitors around the patient further confine space and limit access to the patient during a procedure. In addition, the environment is darkened to facilitate viewing of images, and full monitoring, either invasive or noninvasive, must be established before the procedure begins. Because of limited access to the patient and airway, end-tidal capnography and pulse oximetry are mandatory to ensure adequate ventilation and oxygenation during the procedure and to provide immediate detection of disconnection or dislodgment of the endotracheal tube that could inadvertently occur underneath sterile drapes. The environment is cooler because of computer and x-ray equipment, and without focus and monitoring of temperature, children may become hypothermic from conductive and convective heat loss; this is a particular problem in neonates and infants. In addition, frequent flushing of the catheters and sheaths contributes to hypothermia. Unnecessary exposure of the child must be prevented and convective warming blankets used where possible. Care must be taken when positioning a patient on the catheterization table because of the risk to pressure areas and of nerve traction injury. In particular, brachial plexus injury may occur when the patient's arms are positioned above the head for prolonged periods to enable better exposure for the lateral camera. To facilitate femoral vein and arterial access, the pelvis is commonly elevated from the catheterization table. This position may displace abdominal contents cephalad, restricting diaphragm excursion and increasing the risk for respiratory depression in a sedated patient.

Safe transportation of a critically ill child from the ICU to the catheterization laboratory can be a significant challenge but should not be a deciding factor as to whether or not the procedure should be performed. Safe transport requires planning and multidisciplinary coordination. This process includes physician and nursing staff accompanying the patient with complete monitoring and resuscitation equipment, respiratory therapy staff to assist with ventilation and establishing mechanical ventilation in the catheterization laboratory if indicated, coordinating timing with the laboratory staff to prevent needless delays, assistance with establishing adequate space for equipment and patient access in the laboratory, and correct positioning on the catheterization table to enable access for both the cardiologist and intensive care staff, as needed.

Adequate sedation and anesthesia during cardiac catheterization are essential to facilitate acquisition of meaningful hemodynamic data and to facilitate interventional procedures. For the most part, hemodynamic or diagnostic catheterization procedures can be performed with the patient under sedation.[1] For many interventional procedures, sedation may be appropriate; however, for procedures that are associated with significant hemodynamic compromise or are prolonged, general anesthesia is preferable. Whatever technique is used, hemodynamic data must be attained in conditions as close to normal as possible. For accurate calculation of the intracardiac shunt, reducing the inspired oxygen concentration to room air may be necessary, although this step may be inadvisable in patients with significant pulmonary vein desaturation and lung injury.

Hemodynamic and Oxygen Saturation Data

Hemodynamic cardiac catheterization is often unnecessary when echocardiographic analysis with Doppler measurements and color flow mapping is complete and unambiguous. However, in patients with complex cardiac anatomy, severe low cardiac output state, pulmonary hypertension, severe lung injury of uncertain etiology, or with concerns for important residual anatomic lesions after cardiac surgery, physiologic data from catheterization may provide important information.[2] Catheterization allows description of the direction, magnitude, and approximate location of intracardiac and intrapulmonary shunts. Intracardiac and intravascular pressures are measured to determine the presence of obstructions and whether shunt orifices are restrictive or nonrestrictive. Pressure gradients across sites of obstruction must be considered in light of estimated cardiac output, as a small pressure gradient measured at a time of low cardiac output is misleading.

Normally, no significant change in oxygen saturation from venae cavae to pulmonary artery is observed. In the child with congenital heart disease, the superior vena cava provides the simplest mixed venous oxygen saturation. A greater than 5% to 10% increase in oxygen saturation from the superior vena cava through to the pulmonary artery suggests the presence of a left-to-right shunt at the level of the right atrium with an atrial septal defect (ASD), in the right ventricle (RV) with a ventricular septal defect (VSD), and in the pulmonary artery with a patent ductus arteriosus (PDA) or aorto-pulmonary artery collateral vessels.[3] The magnitude of the left-to-right shunt can be calculated by applying the Fick equation to the pulmonary and systemic vascular beds separately:

$$Qp = VO_2/(SpvO_2 - SpaO_2)(Hb)(1.36)(10) \qquad \text{Eq. 32.1}$$

$$Qs = VO_2/(SaO_2 - SsvcO_2)(Hb)(1.36)(10) \qquad \text{Eq. 32.2}$$

where Qp is pulmonary blood flow, Qs is systemic blood flow, VO_2 is oxygen consumption, $SpvO_2$ is pulmonary vein saturation, $SpaO_2$ is pulmonary artery saturation, SaO_2 is arterial oxygen saturation, $SsvcO_2$ is superior vena cava oxygen saturation, and Hb is hemoglobin. (Note that saturation data in the equations is expressed as a decimal number and not as a percentage, eg, 98% saturation = 0.98.)

In pediatric patients, the pulmonary and systemic flows usually are indexed to body surface area:

$$CI = Qs/BSA \qquad \text{Eq. 32.3}$$

where CI is cardiac index and BSA is body surface area.

Thermodilution can be used to calculate the cardiac output in pediatric patients, although it is confounded by the presence of intracardiac or extracardiac shunts.[4] Measurement of oxygen consumption is preferable[5] because assumed values are unreliable in patients with critical illness and in those requiring substantial hemodynamic support. The practical reality is that many catheterization laboratories assume oxygen consumption,[6] especially in neonates and infants. Thus with the numerator assumed, the inherent error of all calculations should always be considered, particularly with respect to flow

and resistance calculations. A common error is to be unaware that the oxygen consumption tables commonly used are already indexed to BSA, and indexing a second time is a mistake.

The pulmonary to systemic blood flow ratio (Qp/Qs) can be derived simply from the measured oxygen saturation values because all other variables cancel out (from Equations 32.1 and 32.2):

$$Qp/Qs = (SaO_2 - SsvcO_2)/(SpvO_2 - SpaO_2) \qquad \text{Eq. 32.4}$$

The patient whose aortic blood is fully saturated can be assumed to have no significant right-to-left intracardiac shunt. However, when a right-to-left shunt is present, oxygen saturations also should be obtained from the pulmonary veins, left atrium, and left ventricle to determine the source of desaturated blood. Pulmonary venous desaturation implies a primary pulmonary source of venous admixture (eg, pneumonia, atelectasis, or other pulmonary disease).

Vascular resistance is calculated by the change in pressure divided by the flow (Dp/Q):

$$\text{Pulmonary vascular resistance (PVR)}$$
$$= (MeanPAP - MeanLAP)/Qp \qquad \text{Eq. 32.5}$$

$$\text{Systemic vascular resistance (SVR)}$$
$$= (MeanAoP - MeanSVCP)/Qs \qquad \text{Eq. 32.6}$$

where *PAP* is pulmonary artery pressure, *LAP* is left atrial pressure, *AoP* is aortic pressure, *SVCP* is superior vena cava pressure, *Qp* is pulmonary blood flow, and *Qs* is systemic blood flow.

Once again for pediatric patients, the vascular resistance is usually indexed to body surface area and expressed as Wood units.m[2]:

$$PVR = (MeanPAP - MeanLAP)(BSA)/Qp \qquad \text{Eq. 32.7}$$

$$SVR = (MeanAoP - MeanSVCP)(BSA)/Qs \qquad \text{Eq. 32.8}$$

Assessment of Critical Illness

The cardiac catheterization laboratory can be useful in a number of situations during the management of critically ill infants and children who have structurally normal hearts (Table 32.1) or congenital heart disease. Fluoroscopy can be used to assist with placing difficult central venous or pulmonary artery lines, performing pericardiocentesis and pleurocentesis, and assessing diaphragm function.

Patients with pulmonary hypertension can benefit from catheterization to diagnose or rule out structural disease involving the pulmonary arteries or pulmonary veins, as in cases of multiple thromboembolic disease or undiagnosed pulmonary vein stenosis. Acute vasoreactivity testing is important for evaluation of the response of pulmonary vasculature to vasodilator treatment, for example, with increased FiO$_2$ or inhaled nitric oxide.[7] Such evaluation and measurement of a specific response is important for prognostication and longer-term management strategies of patients with pulmonary hypertension. In the presence of structural heart disease with a left-to-right shunt and elevated PVR, pressure and saturation measurements are often repeated with pulmonary vasodilators to assess both the reactivity of the pulmonary vascular

TABLE 32.1	Indications for Cardiac Catheterization or Management in the Catheterization Laboratory of Pediatric Intensive Care Patients with Noncongenital Heart Disease
Diagnostic	Hemodynamic evaluation of intracardiac and intravascular pressures and oxygen saturations Evaluation of persistent hypoxemia: 　Pulmonary vein desaturation 　Decreased pulmonary blood flow 　Intracardiac right-to-left shunt Cardiac output measurement Pulmonary hypertension assessment and reactivity Fluoroscopy: 　Central venous catheter position 　Diaphragm movement 　Myocardial biopsy
Therapeutic	Pericardiocentesis Pleurocentesis Radiofrequency catheter ablation of an arrhythmogenic focus

bed and any contribution of ventilation/perfusion abnormalities to hypoxemia. If breathing 100% oxygen and inhaled nitric oxide increases pulmonary blood flow and dramatically increases Qp/Qs (with a fall in PVR), potentially reversible processes such as hypoxic pulmonary vasoconstriction may be contributing to the elevated PVR. The patient with a high, unresponsive PVR and a small left-to-right shunt may have extensive pulmonary vascular damage from the underlying lung injury or irreversible obstructive pulmonary vascular disease.

The reactivity of the pulmonary vascular bed and change in PVR are important components to the assessment of patients potentially listed for cardiac transplantation. An elevated PVR or pulmonary artery pressure is a risk factor for cardiac transplantation.[8] In patients with heart failure, left atrial hypertension can be a potent cause of elevated PVR. However, if PVR decreases with 100% FiO_2/inhaled nitric oxide during pretransplant catheterization, they still may be suitable candidates for cardiac transplantation.

Patients who present with severe cardiac failure because of myocarditis, idiopathic dilated cardiomyopathy, or intractable dysrhythmias often require cardiac catheterization, not only for hemodynamic assessment but also for endomyocardial biopsy. Biopsies in these circumstances can be associated with significant morbidity, and treatment of the baseline condition should not be delayed until catheterization is performed.[9] The risk of myocardial perforation is particularly increased in infants with thin-walled ventricles, and biopsies are generally contraindicated in infants with a very dilated and poorly functioning left ventricle. Patients who have a low cardiac output state associated with fulminant myocarditis are at risk for dysrhythmias during catheterization, and resuscitation resources must be immediately available, including mechanical support. The goal of biopsy is to firmly establish a diagnosis (thus management plan and prognosis). Although important, biopsy must not take priority over efforts to support the circulation and maintain cardiac output.

Transcatheter Radiofrequency Ablation

Pediatric patients undergoing radiofrequency catheter ablation (RFCA) vary in age and diagnosis.[10] Ablation may be indicated in newborns or infants with persistent reentrant tachycardia or ectopic atrial tachycardia[11,12] and in older children with ectopic foci but otherwise structurally normal hearts that are refractory to or poorly controlled by conventional antiarrhythmic drugs. If an incessant dysrhythmia, particularly a supraventricular tachycardia such as ectopic atrial tachycardia or permanent junctional reciprocating tachycardia, is the primary cause of a dilated poorly contracting heart at the time of presentation, electrophysiologic study and mapping of the dysrhythmia focus may be important diagnostic steps performed in the catheterization laboratory. Elective mechanical support of the circulation with extracorporeal membrane oxygenation (ECMO) may be indicated in order to preserve hemodynamic stability during ablation.[13] Successful RFCA in this circumstance may enable recovery of ventricular function.[14]

An increasing population of patients undergoing ablation consists of those with previous surgical repair of congenital heart defects. Patients with persistent volume or pressure load on the right atrium and those who required an extensive incision and suture lines within the right atrium, such as following a Mustard, Senning, or Fontan procedure, may be at increased risk for supraventricular tachyarrhythmias such as atrial flutter and fibrillation.[15,16] Ventricular tachyarrhythmias may develop late after repair of certain congenital heart defects, such as right ventricular outflow tract reconstruction for tetralogy of Fallot.[17]

RFCA procedures can be lengthy. Because children find it difficult to lie still for prolonged procedures, endotracheal general anesthesia is usually preferred. In addition, patients must remain immobile to prevent catheter movement at the time of ablation, because sudden patient movement may result in creation of a radiofrequency lesion at an incorrect site. For instance, if the focus is close to the atrioventricular (AV) node, inadvertent movement might displace the catheter and cause permanent AV conduction blockade.

On occasion, holding ventilation in either inspiration or expiration may be necessary to eliminate all movement and ensure adequate contact of the ablation catheter with the arrhythmic focus. For the most part, RFCA procedures are well tolerated hemodynamically and blood loss is minimal. During mapping, the focus is stimulated and the tachyarrhythmia induced. This situation may result in hypotension but usually is short-lived and can be readily converted via intracardiac pacing. If hypotension is prolonged and intracardiac conversion is unsuccessful, transthoracic cardioversion may be necessary; therefore a defibrillator should be immediately available.

Congenital Heart Disease

Although most congenital heart defects can be evaluated noninvasively by echocardiography, computed topography, or magnetic resonance imaging, further preoperative evaluation by angiography is essential in selected instances to assist with surgical planning.

Patients with pulmonary atresia and intact ventricular septum (PA/IVS) require careful examination of the coronary anatomy before decompressing the RV, either surgically or with catheterization techniques, because of the possible presence of RV-dependent coronary circulation (RVDCC).[18] RV to coronary artery fistulas can be seen on echocardiography, but selective right ventricular angiography, aortography, or selective coronary angiography is important to determine any associated coronary stenoses or atresia to diagnose RVDCC. If coronary perfusion is dependent on the high-pressure RV, myocardial ischemia will occur if the right ventricle is decompressed. Besides coronary artery lesions, a catheterization may be necessary to selectively image aortopulmonary collaterals in tetralogy of Fallot and pulmonary atresia with diminutive native pulmonary arteries. Angiography can delineate the exact location and anatomy of these collaterals and may be followed by coil occlusion if there is dual supply to the native pulmonary arteries. It is important to know the extent of collateral vessels before surgery and cardiopulmonary bypass because of the risk for impaired systemic perfusion from excessive runoff to the pulmonary circulation.

Patients with hypoplastic left heart syndrome with mitral stenosis and aortic atresia (MS/AA) may also be at higher risk for early mortality after stage 1 palliation with the Norwood procedure.[19] Analogous to the PA/IVS patient population, patients with MS/AA may have left ventricle–subepicardial coronary artery fistulae and be at risk for inadequate myocardial protection during cardiopulmonary bypass and ischemia following stage 1 palliation. Preoperative coronary angiography may also be warranted in this subgroup before surgical palliation.[20] Finally, preoperative angiography may be useful in patients with obstructed total anomalous pulmonary venous connection (TAPVC). Although pulmonary venous anatomy can often be determined by noninvasive methods, palliative transcatheter approaches to relief of pulmonary venous obstruction may be lifesaving in the critically ill neonate[21] and permit surgical repair when the patient is in much better overall condition.

Therapeutic Interventions in the Newborn

Interventional cardiac catheterization continues to evolve. Many specific anatomic defects can be treated in the catheterization laboratory to alleviate the need for surgical intervention.

Atrial Communication Procedures

The first therapeutic procedure performed in the catheterization laboratory for congenital heart disease was balloon atrial septostomy (BAS) in newborns diagnosed with transposition of the great arteries (TGAs) with intact ventricular septum.[22] A BAS is usually necessary in newborns with TGAs to facilitate mixing of systemic and pulmonary venous return at the atrial level before the arterial switch operation. This procedure can be performed with echocardiographic guidance[23] (Fig. 32.1) or in the cardiac catheterization laboratory if additional diagnostic information is required or there are potential vascular access problems. Via either the femoral or umbilical vein, a balloon catheter is advanced across the atrial defect from right atrium to left atrium and rapidly jerked back to the right atrium to tear the septum primum. It is always preferable to facilitate mixing at the atrial level and reduce left atrial pressure and risk for pulmonary hypertension before the arterial switch procedure. Although it has been reported that BAS may be associated with an increased risk for embolic neurologic

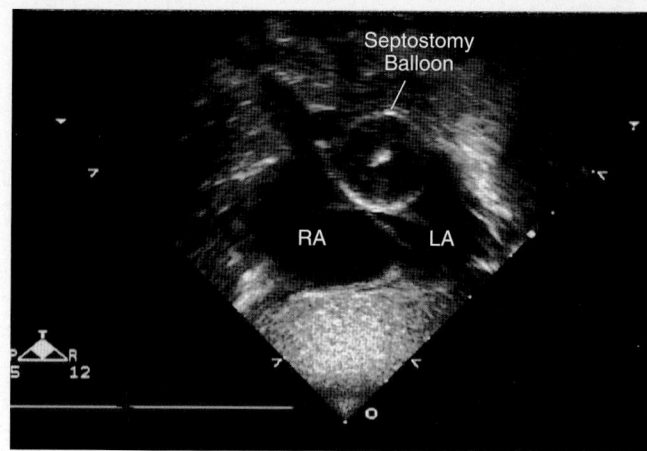

Fig. 32.1. Echocardiography-guided balloon atrial septostomy. From the subcostal view, the septostomy balloon is easily seen as it inflates in the left atrium (LA). *RA,* Right atrium.

injury,[24] this has not been the experience at the majority of institutions.[25,26] Whatever the mode of imaging, once access is obtained, anticoagulation with heparin can be administered theoretically to reduce the risk of thromboembolism.

In some patients with a single-ventricle lesion (such as mitral atresia or hypoplastic left heart syndrome) and a restrictive or near intact atrial septum, the left atrial pressure may be high at birth, causing pulmonary edema and pulmonary artery hypertension. The physiology in this circumstance is identical to that of patients with obstructed TAPVC. Patients are usually cyanotic and acidotic with a low cardiac output state. Survival is not possible without urgent left atrial decompression.[27] It is important to appreciate that the atrial septum is often thickened in these patients, which is quite different from the thin-walled restrictive foramen ovale of patients with TGA. Because of its thickness, disruption of the septum using a balloon atrial septostomy technique is not usually possible. In addition to the thickened atrial septum, the atrial cavity size usually is too small to even accommodate a septostomy balloon. Instead, decompression of the pulmonary atrium can be achieved with a Brockenbrough transseptal puncture (Fig. 32.2A) or radiofrequency perforation, followed by an atrial septoplasty involving balloon dilation and often stent placement across the thickened atrial septum (Fig. 32.2B). These infants are critically ill even with uncomplicated procedures. Because of the degree of cyanosis and the low cardiac output state, concurrent resuscitation with volume replacement, inotropic support, and mechanical ventilation are usually necessary during this procedure until adequate mixing is established and pulmonary veins are decompressed. In high-risk, single-ventricle neonates a more recent strategy has been the surgical use of bilateral PA bands to protect the pulmonary vascular bed and promote systemic output.[28] The same philosophy has been applied to optimize the preoperative status of hypoplastic left heart syndrome with intact atrial septum after successful left atrial decompression in the catheterization laboratory.[29]

Pulmonary Balloon Valvotomy

Congenital pulmonary valve stenosis may present as a murmur heard in the newborn period. If the obstruction is mild,

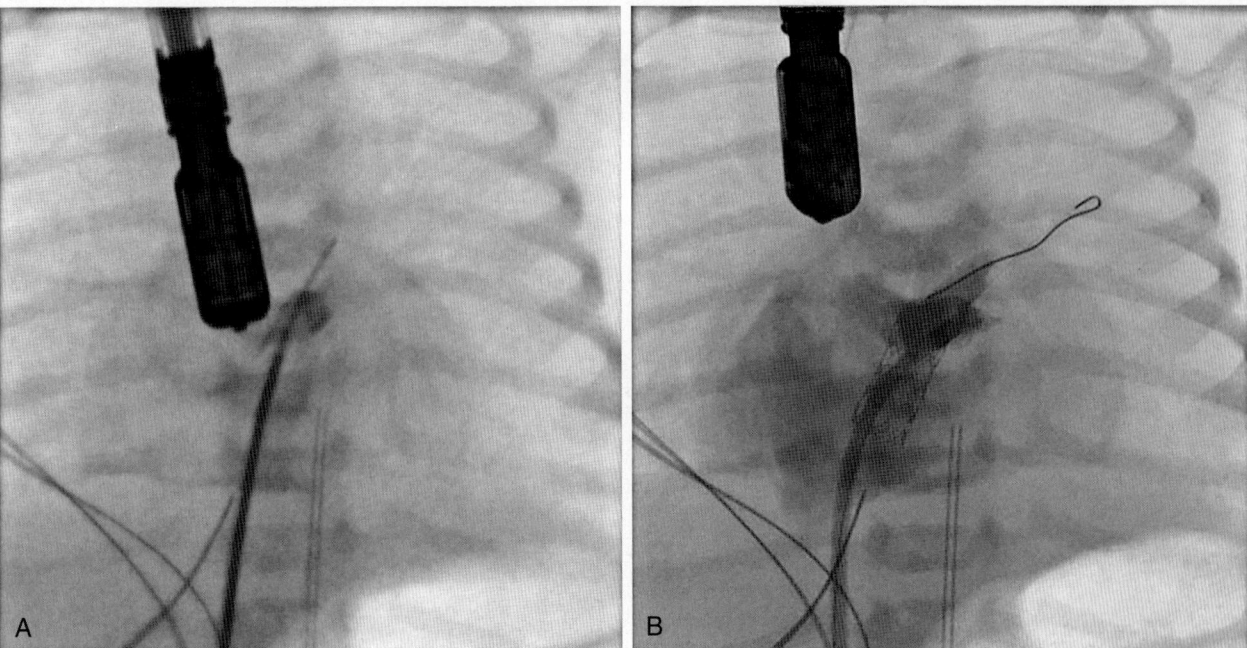

Fig. 32.2. Atrial septoplasty in a newborn with restrictive atrial septum and hypoplastic left heart syndrome. Note the severe pulmonary edema. (A) View of a Brockenbrough transseptal needle introduced across a stained thickened atrial septum. (B) Anteroposterior view following stent placement across the thickened atrial septum. Contrast is seen equally in both the hypoplastic left atrium and the right atrium.

intervention with balloon dilation can be deferred. Newborns with critical pulmonary valve stenosis or pulmonary valve atresia have severe restriction or absence of antegrade flow across the right ventricular outflow and, as a result, have ductus arteriosus-dependent pulmonary blood flow. Balloon dilation in the catheterization laboratory is the therapeutic procedure of choice (Fig. 32.3).[30] A balloon catheter is passed over a guidewire antegrade across the pulmonary valve, and balloon dilation, usually to approximately 120% size of the pulmonary valve annulus, is performed. Heart block and ventricular ectopy may occur with wire manipulation in the RV but are usually transient. Antegrade flow across the pulmonary valve may not increase significantly after balloon dilation until right ventricular compliance improves, and continuation of prostaglandin E1 (PGE1) infusion to maintain patency of the ductus arteriosus for several days following balloon dilation may be necessary. For some patients longer-term supplemental pulmonary blood flow is necessary, and this can be achieved with a PDA stent or surgical shunt. Perforation of the relatively thin right ventricular outflow tract with the guidewire is a potential complication, particularly in low-birth-weight and premature newborns.

Aortic Balloon Valvotomy

The newborn with critical valvar aortic stenosis who develops hypotension and acidosis as the ductus arteriosus closes (ductal dependent systemic blood flow) requires resuscitation with PGE1 to restore aortic flow, plus mechanical ventilation and inotropic support to achieve stabilization before an intervention is performed. Balloon dilation of the stenotic aortic valve during cardiac catheterization is the preferred intervention (Fig. 32.4),[31] although surgical valvotomy under direct vision using cardiopulmonary bypass (CPB) is the surgical alternative.[32] At catheterization, a guidewire is passed either retrograde (via femoral/carotid artery) or antegrade (via

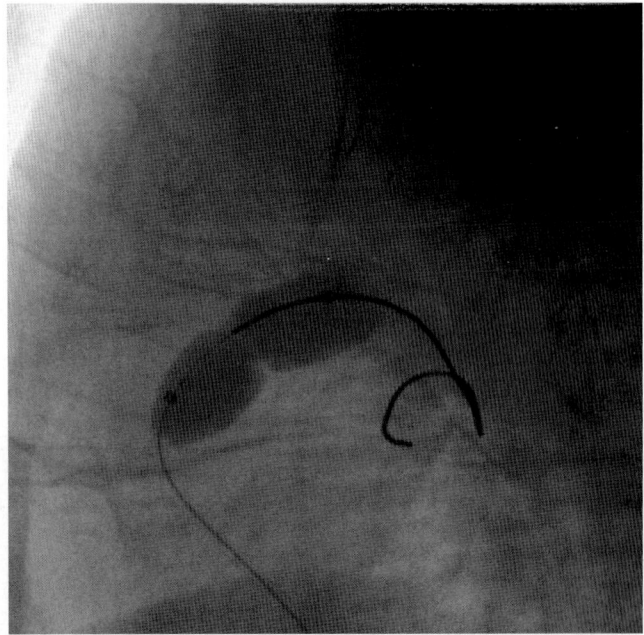

Fig. 32.3. Pulmonary valvuloplasty in a newborn with severe pulmonary valve stenosis. Lateral view with balloon catheter centered across a stenotic pulmonary valve. As the balloon is inflated, a "waist" representing the stenotic valve is seen.

femoral or umbilical vein) across the aortic valve. A balloon catheter is passed over the wire, and serial dilations are performed up to 90% to 100% size of the aortic valve annulus. The pressure gradient across the aortic valve is remeasured after each dilation, and an ascending aortogram is obtained to evaluate aortic valve regurgitation. Because of the initial minimal flow across the valve, balloon dilation of critical

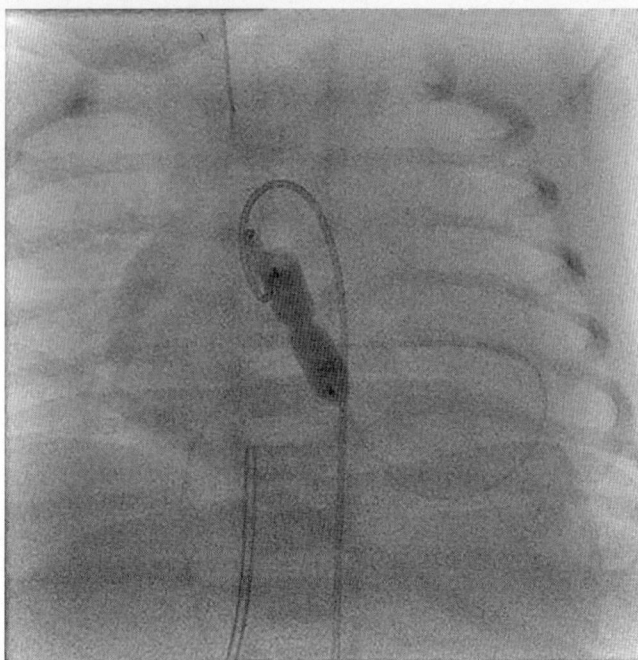

Fig. 32.4. Aortic valvuloplasty in a newborn with critical aortic stenosis. Anteroposterior view with antegrade catheter course from the femoral vein. The balloon, also with the "waist" apparent, is seen being inflated across the aortic valve.

neonatal aortic stenosis is usually well tolerated. Despite the successful relief of obstruction, antegrade flow across the valve may not increase significantly until left ventricular compliance and function improve; therefore continuation of PGE1 infusion, mechanical ventilation, and vasoactive drugs following dilation for some days may be necessary. Until flow across the valve increases, the residual gradient across the aortic valve will be underestimated by echocardiography, and serial studies usually are necessary to track the evolving gradient as left ventricular function improves. Other complications include possible mitral valve damage from either an antegrade or retrograde approach, ventricular fibrillation, and an acute low cardiac output state secondary to coronary ischemia in patients with a hypertrophied ventricle.

Perioperative Interventional Procedures

A thorough understanding of the anatomy and morphology of complex congenital heart defects is essential for successful management of patients with complex congenital heart disease. This is particularly critical when establishing a diagnosis and planning surgical intervention. Important for the successful perioperative management in the ICU is a thorough understanding of the pathophysiology of various defects. This understanding includes not only the preoperative pathophysiology associated with defects but also the potential alteration in pathophysiology related to surgical repair and/or development of complications in the postoperative period. As a general guide, if patients are not progressing as expected and low cardiac output persists, early cardiac catheterization should be performed to investigate and exclude the possibility of undiagnosed or residual structural defects. Despite biases to the contrary, early postoperative catheterization can be performed with no significant increased risk of adverse events.[33]

Scheduled Interventional Procedures

Transcatheter treatment of congenital cardiac defects continues to evolve and expand and, in some circumstances, is effectively replacing the need for conventional intraoperative surgical procedures.[34] For example, several centers are routinely palliating hypoplastic left heart syndrome with a hybrid approach including transcatheter-based ductal stent, along with bilateral pulmonary artery bands and balloon atrial septostomy, with favorable early results.[35] Transcatheter pulmonary valves have been successfully inserted in patients with right ventricular outflow tract conduit dysfunction.[36] Ductal dependent pulmonary blood flow lesions can now be treated with a PDA stent, in place of a Blalock-Taussig (BT) shunt. The impetus for the increasing numbers of PDA stent procedures is partly related to surgical morbidity but importantly due to technical advances in coronary artery stents, enabling low profile and ease of delivery in newborns.[37] Additional interventions now routinely performed in the catheterization laboratory include angioplasty, often combined with transcatheter placement of endovascular stents, for treatment of systemic and pulmonary arterial and venous stenoses, and device occlusion or embolization of systemic-to-pulmonary arterial communications, venous channels, fistulas, muscular VSDs, ASDs, and PDAs.

Risks and Complications

Placement of catheters in and through the heart increases the risk for dysrhythmias, perforation of the myocardium, damage to valve leaflets and chordae, cerebral vascular accidents, and air embolism. Use of radiopaque contrast material may cause an acute allergic reaction (rare in children with the use of nonionic contrast media), pulmonary hypertension, acute kidney injury, and myocardial depression. Blood loss may be sudden and unexpected when large-bore catheters are used or vessels are ruptured. More insidious blood loss may occur over several hours in heparinized small children or neonates because of bleeding around the catheter site or multiple aspirations and flushes of catheters. Transfusion requirements and appropriate vascular access should be continually assessed.

Arrhythmias, albeit transient, may be recurrent and even fatal if not promptly treated. Arrhythmias include catheter-induced supraventricular tachycardias, ventricular tachycardia, ventricular fibrillation, and occasionally complete heart block requiring temporary transvenous pacing. On most occasions, removing the wire or catheter resolves the arrhythmia, but full resuscitation and cardioversion equipment must be available in case the arrhythmia does not resolve.

The complications of various interventional procedures are related in part to the type of procedure, but all share the risks associated with percutaneous vascular access with large catheters that course through the heart and vessels.[38] Table 32.2 lists the specific problems that can occur during various transcatheter procedures. The pediatric catheterization community has matured in respect to quality improvement initiatives. There are now multiple prospective registries that shed more light on modern catheterization and the associated risks. This includes the IMPACT Registry with large participation.[39] And a smaller but more complex multicenter group has reported overall adverse event (AE) rates in the range of 5% to 18%, with higher AE rates reported in interventional (20%) versus

TABLE 32.2   Potential Complications in the Catheterization Laboratory

Procedure	Representative Lesion	Complications
Hemodynamic evaluation	Congenital heart disease Pulmonary hypertension Postoperative course; progress not as expected, persistent low cardiac output state, inability to wean from mechanical ventilation, persistent chylous effusions; evaluate residual intracardiac shunt or outflow tract obstruction	Blood loss requiring transfusion Air embolism Vascular access; trauma, dissection, occlusion, perforation Myocardial perforation and tamponade Arrhythmias; ventricular and supraventricular tachycardia, ventricular fibrillation, complete heart block
Coil embolization	Aortopulmonary collaterals Systemic-pulmonary shunts	Fevers Excessive hypoxemia Systemic embolization
Transcatheter device closure	Patent ductus arteriosus Atrial septal defect Ventricular septal defect Baffle leak	Air or device embolization Blood loss Interference with atrioventricular value function Arrhythmias; ventricular arrhythmias, complete heart block
Balloon and stent dilations	Pulmonary artery stenosis	Pulmonary artery tear and hemorrhage Pulmonary edema: high flow False aneurysm Right ventricle ischemia
	Pulmonary valve stenosis	As above Pulmonary valve regurgitation
	Mitral valve stenosis	Mitral insufficiency Pulmonary hypertension
	Coarctation of the aorta	Aortic dissection Hypertension
	Right ventricular conduit/Percutaneous pulmonary valve	Conduit disruption False aneurysms Stent embolization Pulmonary hemorrhage from distal wire injury
Atrial septostomy	Transposition of the great arteries, mitral stenosis (atresia) with restrictive atrial septum, hybrid procedure	Perforation of the heart and tamponade Atrial arrhythmia Mitral valve injury

noninterventional (10%) catheterization procedures.[40] This group has been able to develop a risk adjustment model that should allow comparisons of adverse events among other centers.[41] Many complications are potentially life-threatening, and successful treatment of complications depends on prompt action by critical care physicians and/or anesthesiologists cooperating closely with the interventional cardiologists who are manipulating the catheters.

Balloon Dilation of Pulmonary Arteries

Pulmonary artery balloon dilation and stent placement to relieve stenosis is a common procedure performed in the catheterization laboratory.[42] Pulmonary artery stenoses may be congenital or acquired lesions. They may be discrete, involving the main or branch pulmonary arteries, or multiple, involving distal segmental vessels. The increase in pulmonary artery pressure and fixed resistance to antegrade pulmonary blood flow may have related and deleterious consequences, which include the following:

1. An increase in the afterload on the RV, which in turn causes right ventricular hypertrophy. The RV can cope with a significant pressure load for some time. However, as right ventricular end-diastolic pressure increases and tricuspid regurgitation possibly develops, right atrial pressure increases and manifests as hepatomegaly, ascites, and persistent or recurrent pleural effusions.
2. Reduced antegrade flow across the pulmonary outflow, which in turn reduces preload to the left ventricle and

contributes to a low cardiac output state. Further, the hypertrophy of the ventricular septum reduces the compliance of the left ventricle and increases left ventricular end-diastolic pressure.
3. An increase in right ventricular pressure and ventricular hypertrophy may compromise coronary blood flow. Hypotension or tachycardia with altered coronary filling time may cause myocardial ischemia, with the subendocardium being at particular risk.
4. If the pulmonary valve is incompetent, for example, following right ventricular outflow reconstruction for repair of tetralogy of Fallot with or without pulmonary atresia, a considerable amount of pulmonary regurgitation may occur that causes an additional volume load on the RV, leading to right ventricular dilation and systolic failure. In addition, the increased pulsatility to the branch pulmonary arteries may cause extrinsic compression of the main stem bronchi.

Patients with persistent signs of right ventricular failure, such as low cardiac output state, hepatomegaly, ascites, recurrent pleural effusions (particularly if chylous in nature), and inability to wean from mechanical ventilation, should be considered for catheterization. Although echocardiography may help determine a specific problem, catheterization provides quantitative data that can direct vasoactive support and enable interventions such as pulmonary artery dilation, coiling of collateral vessels, and creation of an atrial communication that allows an atrial-level right-to-left shunt.

The function of the right ventricle is critical and often the cause of complications related to pulmonary artery dilation. At the time of balloon dilation, cardiac output may decrease significantly, causing hypotension, bradycardia, arterial oxygen desaturation, and a fall in end-tidal CO_2. Because the balloon is inflated for only a few seconds and provided preload is maintained, the procedure is usually well tolerated and the circulation usually recovers spontaneously. Patients who have a hypertrophied, poorly compliant RV with intraventricular pressures at systemic or suprasystemic levels may not tolerate the sudden increase in afterload associated with balloon dilation, even for a short period. In particular, myocardial ischemia and arrhythmias may occur, causing severe acute right ventricular failure and loss of cardiac output. General anesthesia and controlled ventilation are recommended before intervention in this at-risk group of patients.

Pulmonary artery disruption is signaled by local extravasation of contrast in the lung parenchyma, sudden hemodynamic deterioration from cardiac tamponade or acute hemothorax, or sudden onset of hemoptysis.[43] The tear in the pulmonary artery may be confined (Fig. 32.5A) and therefore controlled, or unconfined, resulting in hemodynamic collapse and the possible need for immediate surgical intervention. The potential for pulmonary artery disruption is increased because of the high pressure used to inflate the balloon and maintain tension on the vessel wall to tear the intima and media. The risk for pulmonary artery disruption may be increased in early postcardiac surgery patients if the dilation is performed across a recent pulmonary artery anastomosis; in the past waiting 6 weeks before dilatation was advocated. However, if there is a continuous suture, and using a stent to avoid recoil, interventions can be safely performed even in the early postoperative period.[33] Thus in the immediate postoperative period, particularly if the patient has severe right ventricular failure, low cardiac output state, or inability to wean from mechanical ventilation, pulmonary artery dilation should be performed. Cutting balloons have increased options available for achieving successful balloon dilation in resistant lesions with improved efficacy and similar safety profile to high-pressure dilation.[44] A high index of suspicion should be maintained in patients with peripheral pulmonary artery stenosis treated with high-pressure angioplasty or a cutting balloon. In the presence of substantial hemoptysis, immediate endotracheal intubation is indicated for airway control and ventilation. Hypertension and further airway stimulation should be avoided, the addition of positive end-expiratory pressure may be useful, and instillation of 1 mL of 1:100,000 epinephrine via the endotracheal tube may help reduce immediate bleeding by causing vasoconstriction of mucosal vessels. An immediate intervention by the catheterizer to tamponade the disrupted branch pulmonary artery with a balloon catheter may be lifesaving. Permanent occlusion of the vessel with a coil (Fig. 32.5B) or covered stent may be necessary to prevent further hemorrhage.

Transient unilateral or unilobar pulmonary edema is also seen in the setting of pulmonary artery dilation. This finding is related to sudden large increases in pulmonary blood flow and distal pulmonary artery pressure after dilation in a previously underperfused pulmonary vascular bed. Pulmonary edema after dilation usually occurs immediately following balloon dilation but can be delayed for up to 24 hours. Pulmonary edema and disruption of a pulmonary artery can occur abruptly, in isolation, or together, during pulmonary artery dilation procedures. Both can cause the appearance in the airway of frank blood or blood-tinged edema fluid in substantial quantities.

Patients who have a dilated RV secondary to a long-standing volume load, such as chronic pulmonary regurgitation, are at risk for arrhythmias and low output during catheter manipulations and interventions. As noted earlier, on most occasions the changes in rhythm are short-lived and settle once the catheters are withdrawn. Nevertheless, anesthesia and airway control are recommended if the circulation is compromised, and a defibrillator and transvenous pacing must be immediately available.

Potential movement at the time of critical balloon dilation or stent placement must be prevented. Dilation of pulmonary arteries is painful and often causes patients to waken from sedation and move. In addition, dilation of the pulmonary arteries may induce coughing. The coughing is usually not a problem for isolated pulmonary artery dilation, but if the patient moves during stent placement, stent malposition or

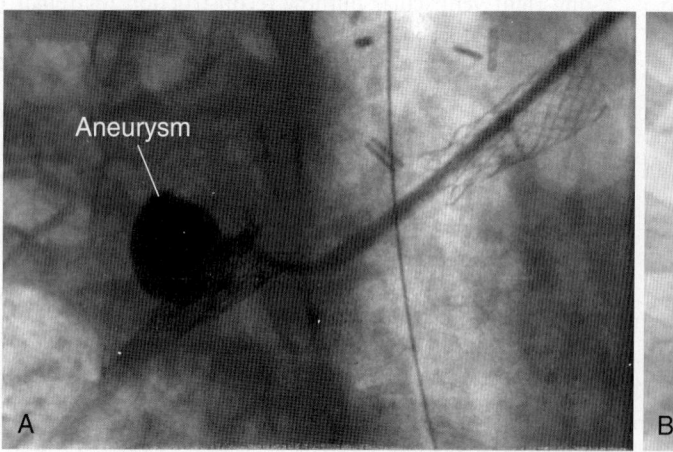
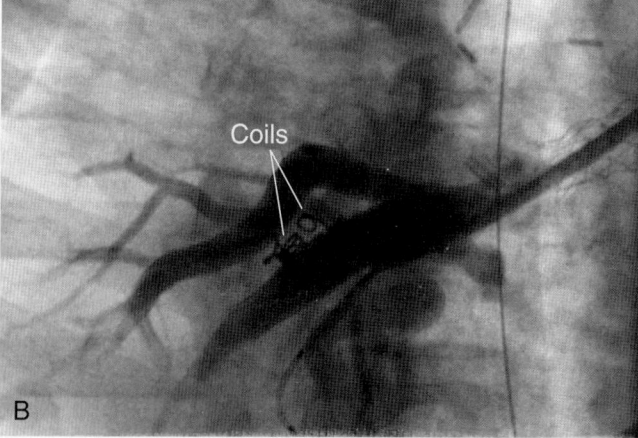

Fig. 32.5. Pulmonary artery trauma in a patient with multiple peripheral pulmonary artery stenoses. (A) Pulmonary artery aneurysm following balloon dilation. Note that a stent has been placed but the aneurysm is still present. (B) Resolution after coils are placed in the neck of the aneurysm.

embolization can occur. Therefore the patient must be immobile, and additional sedation should be considered immediately before stent placement.

Occlusion Device Insertion

Although device closures of PDA and ASD are commonly performed interventions in the catheterization laboratory, they are relatively uncommon procedures in pediatric intensive care patients. A persistent left-to-right shunt at the atrial level contributing to right ventricular volume overload, increased pulmonary blood flow, and inability to wean from mechanical ventilation may be one indication for occlusion, although often the ASD must be of considerable size to cause these symptoms and may be too large for safe deployment of the device. Conversely, a large right-to-left shunt across an ASD may result in significant cyanosis and increase the risk for paradoxical embolism and cerebral vascular accident. A similar circumstance exists in patients who have undergone a fenestrated Fontan operation. Placement of a PDA[45] or ASD[46] device is usually associated with minimal hemodynamic disturbance. Although placement can be performed in most patients using sedation techniques, endotracheal tube placement for airway protection may be necessary if transesophageal echocardiography is used to guide device placement.

Indications for VSD device placement include closure of a residual or recurrent septal defect, preoperative closure of defects that may be difficult to reach surgically while on CPB, and closure of acquired defects such as those due to myocardial infarction or trauma. A residual VSD may cause considerable volume load to the ventricles and result in a low cardiac output state and congestive heart failure requiring prolonged mechanical ventilation and inotropic or vasoactive support.

In contrast to closure of PDAs or ASDs, transcatheter VSD device closures are prolonged procedures that are often associated with profound hemodynamic instability and blood loss.[47] Although the technique has not changed over time, the devices available now have much smaller delivery systems that result in reduced sheath size and less hemodynamic compromise (Fig. 32.6).[48] However, all patients should be considered susceptible. Factors contributing to hemodynamic instability include blood loss, arrhythmias from catheter manipulation in the ventricles and across the septum, heart block from trauma to conduction system, atrioventricular or aortic valve regurgitation from stenting open of valve leaflets by stiff wire/catheters, and device-related factors such as malposition or dislodgment from the ventricular septum.

In all device closures, the long delivery sheath represents a potential space for air accumulation and risk for air embolism. In patients with intracardiac shunts, air embolization may be life-threatening and can be diagnosed by fluoroscopy. Extreme inspiratory efforts may introduce air into the sheath and the heart. Air in the right atrium may be shunted across an ASD even in the presence of nominal left-to-right shunting. Left heart air embolization produces ST-segment elevation and, often, hemodynamic changes as it passes into the aorta. The resultant ST-segment changes, hypotension, arterial desaturation, and bradycardia generally respond to aspiration and then sealing of the entry port, along with administration of atropine and inotropic and pressor support to maintain coronary perfusion. Meticulous purging of air from the catheter system and sealing of open ports help minimize the incidence of air embolism. Use of positive pressure ventilation through an endotracheal tube in an anesthetized, paralyzed patient also may decrease the potential for transcatheter air embolus.

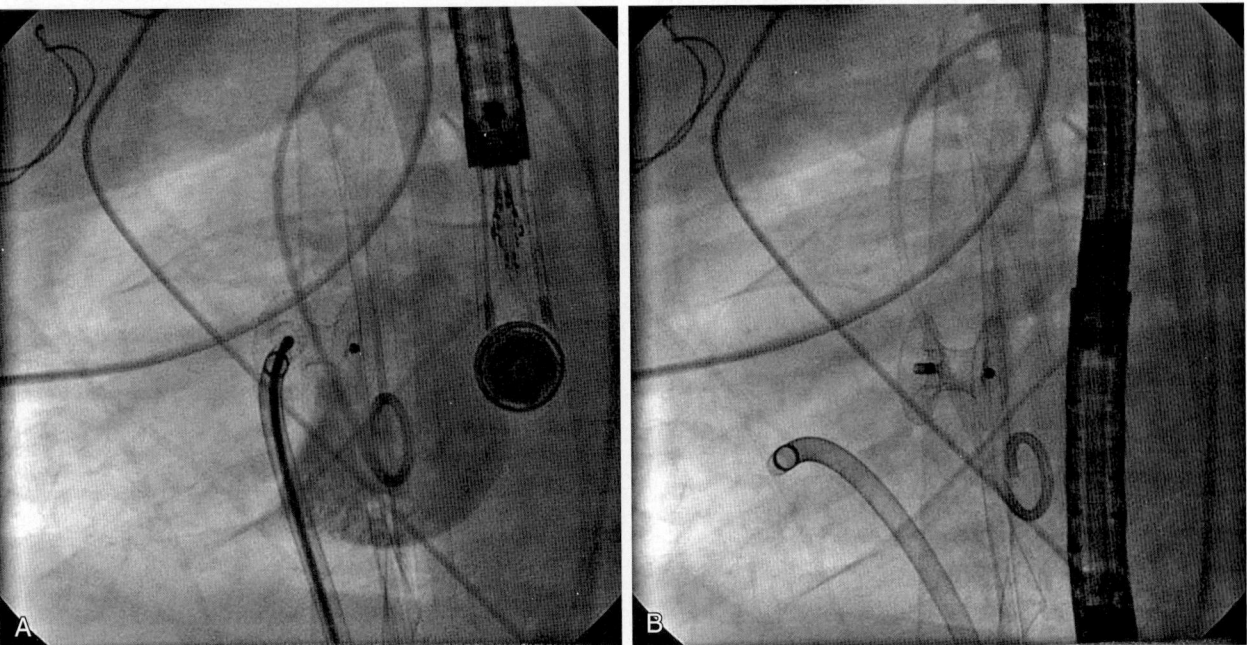

Fig. 32.6. Ventricular septal defect closure using the Amplatzer muscular VSD device. (A) Left ventricular angiogram during device delivery from the venous side. (B) Device after release. The pigtail catheter is in the left ventricle. The long sheath that delivered the device is in the right ventricle.

Cardiac Catheterization and Extracorporeal Membrane Oxygenation

Cardiac catheterization may be necessary in patients supported with ECMO for either diagnostic or therapeutic procedures, often to facilitate subsequent weaning and decannulation.[49] Reversible respiratory failure and pulmonary hypertension remain common indications for ECMO, but mechanical support of the failing circulation using ECMO has been increasingly used. Indications include refractory low cardiac output state, unexpected cardiac arrest, failure to wean from CPB, severe cyanosis, and refractory arrhythmias.[13,50] ECMO has also been used as a highly successful tool in the resuscitation of patients following hemodynamic deterioration due to catheter-induced complications, low output, or hypoxemia.[51]

A number of published series have described the feasibility and utility of cardiac catheterization of patients supported by ECMO.[52-54] Indications for catheterization have included assessment of surgical repair and interventions to treat residual defects, left heart decompression via a percutaneous transatrial vent in order to prevent overdistension of the left ventricle, hemodynamic assessment and myocardial biopsy in patients with fulminant myocarditis/cardiomyopathy, and catheter-based interventions such as arrhythmia ablation.

As already discussed in patients not following an expected clinical course, it is important to have a high index of suspicion for residual lesions in postoperative cardiac surgery patients who cannot be weaned from ECMO within 72 hours of expected myocardial recovery. Early catheterization and subsequent interventions may facilitate recovery of myocardial function, reduce ECMO duration, and lessen the potential for ECMO-related complications.

The use of percutaneously inserted mechanical circulatory support is a rapidly expanding field in adult cardiology,[55] and some of these technologies are applicable to pediatric patients.[56] An awareness of newer percutaneous means for providing short-term hemodynamic support is important for critical care physicians to be aware of, as well as an area likely to rapidly evolve.

Acknowledgment

I gratefully acknowledge the contribution of Peter Laussen, who authored this chapter in previous editions.

References

1. Javorski JJ, Hansen DD, Laussen PC, et al. Anesthesia for pediatric cardiac catheterization: innovations. *Can J Anaesth.* 1995;42:310-329.
2. Wilkinson JL. Haemodynamic calculations in the catheter laboratory. *Heart.* 2001;85:113-120.
3. Freed MD, Miettinen OS, Nadas AS. Oximetric detection of intracardiac left to right shunts. *Br Heart J.* 1979;42:690-694.
4. Freed MD, Keane JF. Cardiac output measured by thermodilution in infants and children. *J Pediatr.* 1978;92:39-42.
5. Lundell BPW, Casas ML, Wallgren CG. Oxygen consumption in infants and children during heart catheterization. *Pediatr Cardiol.* 1996;17:207-213.
6. LaFarge CG, Miettinen OS. The estimation of oxygen consumption. *Cardiovasc Res.* 1970;4:23-30.
7. McLaughlin VM, Archer SA, Badesch DB, et al. ACCF/AHA 2009 expert consensus document on pulmonary hypertension. *J Am Coll Cardiol.* 2009;53:1573-1619.
8. Davies RR, Russo MJ, Mital S, et al. Predicting survival among high-risk pediatric cardiac transplant recipients: an analysis of the United Network for Organ Sharing database. *J Thorac Cardiovasc Surg.* 2008;135:147-155.
9. Pophel SG, Sigfussen G, Booth KL, et al. Complications of endomyocardial biopsy in children. *J Am Coll Cardiol.* 1999;34:2105-2110.
10. Tanel RE, Walsh EP, Triedman JK, et al. Five-year experience with radiofrequency catheter ablation: implications for management of arrhythmias in pediatric and young adult patients. *J Pediatr.* 1997;131:878-887.
11. Blaufox AD, Felix GL, Saul JP. Pediatric Catheter Ablation Registry. Radiofrequency catheter ablation in infants ≤18 months old: when is it done and how do they fare? Short-term data from the pediatric ablation registry. *Circulation.* 2001;104:2803-2808.
12. Chiu SN, Lu CW, Chang CW, et al. Radiofrequency catheter ablation of supraventricular tachycardia in infants and toddlers. *Circ J.* 2009;73:1717-1721.
13. Carmichael TB, Walsh EP, Roth SJ. Anticipatory use of venoarterial extracorporeal membrane oxygenation for a high risk interventional cardiac procedure. *Respir Care.* 2002;47:1002-1006.
14. De Giovanni JV, Dindar A, Griffith MJ, et al. Recovery pattern of left ventricular dysfunction following radiofrequency ablation of incessant supraventricular tachycardia in infants and children. *Heart.* 1998;79:588-592.
15. Gelatt M, Hamilton RM, McCrindle BW, et al. Arrhythmia and mortality after the Mustard procedure: a 30-year single center experience. *J Am Coll Cardiol.* 1997;29:194-201.
16. Fishberger SB, Wernovsky G, Gentles TL, et al. Factors that influence the development of atrial flutter after the Fontan operation. *J Thorac Cardiovasc Surg.* 1997;113:80-86.
17. Deanfield JE, McKenna WJ, Presbitero P, et al. Ventricular arrhythmia in unrepaired and repaired tetralogy of Fallot. Relation to age, timing of repair and hemodynamic status. *Br Heart J.* 1984;52:77-81.
18. Guleserian KJ, Armsby LB, Thiagarajan RR, et al. Natural history of pulmonary atresia with intact ventricular septum and right-ventricle-dependent coronary circulation managed by the single-ventricle approach. *Ann Thorac Surg.* 2006;81:2250-2258.
19. Glatz JA, Fedderly RT, Ghanayem NS, Tweddell JS. Impact of mitral stenosis and aortic atresia on survival in hypoplastic left heart syndrome. *Ann Thorac Surg.* 2008;85:2057-2062.
20. Vida VL, Bacha EA, Larrazabal A, et al. Surgical outcome for patients with the mitral stenosis-aortic atresia variant of hypoplastic left heart syndrome. *J Thorac Cardiovasc Surg.* 2008;135:339-346.
21. Kyser JP, Bengur AR, Siwik ES. Preoperative palliation of newborn obstructed total anomalous pulmonary venous connection by endovascular stent placement. *Catheter Cardiovasc Interv.* 2006;67:473-476.
22. Rashkind WJ, Miller WW. Creation of an atrial septal defect without thoracotomy. A palliative approach to complete transposition of the great arteries. *JAMA.* 1966;196:991-992.
23. Steeg CN, Bierman FZ, Hordof AJ, et al. "Bedside" balloon septostomy in infants with transposition of the great arteries: new concepts using two-dimensional echocardiographic techniques. *J Pediatr.* 1985;107:944-946.
24. McQuillen PS, Hamrick SE, Perez MJ, et al. Balloon atrial septostomy is associated with preoperative stroke in neonates with transposition of the great arteries. *Circulation.* 2006;113:280-285.
25. Beca J, Gunn J, Coleman L, et al. Preoperative brain injury in newborn infants with transposition of the great arteries occurs at rates similar to other complex congenital heart disease and is not related to balloon atrial septostomy. *J Am Coll Cardiol.* 2009;53:1807-1811.
26. Petit CJ, Rome JJ, Wernovsky G, et al. Preoperative brain injury in transposition of the great arteries is associated with oxygenation and time to surgery, not balloon atrial septostomy. *Circulation.* 2009;119:709-716.
27. Vlahos A, Lock JE, McElhinney DB, et al. Hypoplastic left heart syndrome with intact or highly restrictive atrial septum. Outcome after neonatal transcatheter atrial septostomy. *Circulation.* 2004;109:2326-2330.
28. Guleserian KJ, Barker GM, Sharma MS, et al. Bilateral pulmonary artery banding for resuscitation in high-risk, single-ventricle neonates and infants: a single-center experience. *J Thorac Cardiovasc Surg.* 2013;145:206-214.
29. Barker GM, Forbess JM, Guleserian KJ, Nugent AW. Optimization of preoperative status in hypoplastic left heart syndrome with intact atrial septum but left atrial decompression and bilateral pulmonary artery bands. *Pediatr Cardiol.* 2014;35:479-484.
30. Colli AM, Perry SB, Lock JE, Keane JF. Balloon dilation of critical valvar pulmonary stenosis in the first month of life. *Cathet Cardiovasc Diagn.* 1995;34:23-28.

31. McElhinney DB, Lock JE, Keane JF, et al. Left heart growth, function, and reintervention after balloon aortic valvuloplasty for neonatal aortic stenosis. *Circulation*. 2005;111:451-458.

32. Siddiqui J, Brizard CP, Galati JC, et al. Surgical valvotomy and repair for neonatal and infant congenital aortic stenosis achieves better results than interventional catheterization. *J Am Coll Cardiol*. 2013;62:2134-2140.

33. Nicholson GT, Kim DW, Vincent RN, et al. Cardiac catheterization in the early post-operative period after congenital cardiac surgery. *JACC Cardiovasc Interv*. 2014;7:1437-1443.

34. Lock JE, Keane JF, Perry SB. *Diagnostic and Interventional Catheterization in Congenital Heart Disease*. Norwell, MA: Kluwer Academic Publishers; 1999.

35. Galantowicz M, Cheatham JP, Phillips A, et al. Hybrid approach for hypoplastic left heart syndrome: intermediate results after the learning curve. *Ann Thorac Surg*. 2008;85:2063-2071.

36. Armstrong AK, Balzer DT, Cabalka AK, et al. One-year follow-up of the Melody transcatheter pulmonary valve multicenter post-approval study. *JACC Cardiovasc Interv*. 2014;7:1254-1262.

37. Santoro G, Gaio G, Palladino MT, et al. Stenting of the arterial duct in newborns with duct-dependent pulmonary circulation. *Heart*. 2008;94:925-929.

38. Vitiello R, McCrindle BW, Nykanen D, et al. Complications associated with pediatric cardiac catheterization. *J Am Coll Cardiol*. 1998;32:1433-1440.

39. Martin GR, Beekman RH, Ing FF, et al. The IMPACT registry: improving pediatric and adult congenital treatments. *Semin Thorac Cardiovasc Surg Pediatr Card Surg Annu*. 2010;13:20-25.

40. Bergersen L, Marshall A, Gauvreau K, et al. Adverse event rates in congenital cardiac catheterization: a multi-center experience. *Catheter Cardiovasc Interv*. 2010;75:389-400.

41. Bergersen L, Gauvreau K, Foerster SR, et al. Catheterization for congenital heart disease adjustment for risk method (CHARM). *JACC Cardiovasc Interv*. 2011;4:1037-1046.

42. O'Laughlin MP. Catheterization treatment of stenosis and hypoplasia of pulmonary arteries. *Pediatr Cardiol*. 1998;19:48-56.

43. Baker CM, McGowan FX Jr, Keane JF, Lock JE. Pulmonary artery trauma due to balloon dilation: recognition, avoidance and management. *J Am Coll Cardiol*. 2000;36:1684-1690.

44. Bergersen L, Gauvreau K, Justino H, et al. Randomized trial of cutting balloon compared with high-pressure angioplasty for the treatment of resistant pulmonary artery stenosis. *Circulation*. 2011;124:2388-2396.

45. Pass RH, Hijazi Z, Hsu DT, et al. Multicenter USA Amplatzer patent ductus arteriosus occlusion device trial. Initial and one-year results. *J Am Coll Cardiol*. 2004;44:513-519.

46. Du ZD, Hijazi ZM, Kleinman CS, et al. Comparison between transcatheter and surgical closure of secundum atrial septal defect in children and adults. Results of a multicenter nonrandomized trial. *J Am Coll Cardiol*. 2002;39:1836-1844.

47. Laussen PC, Hansen DD, Fox LM, et al. Hemodynamic instability associated with VSD device closure: anesthetic implications. *Anesth Analg*. 1995;80:1076-1082.

48. Holzer R, Balzer D, Cao QL, et al. Device closure of muscular ventricular septal defects using the Amplatzer muscular ventricular septal defect occlude. Immediate and mid-term results of a U.S. registry. *J Am Coll Cardiol*. 2004;43:1257-1263.

49. Booth KL, Roth SJ, Perry SP, et al. Cardiac catheterization of patients supported by extracorporeal membrane oxygenation. *J Am Coll Cardiol*. 2002;40:1681-1686.

50. Duncan BW, Hraska V, Jonas RA, et al. Mechanical circulatory support in children with cardiac disease. *J Thorac Cardiovasc Surg*. 1999;117:529-542.

51. Allan CK, Thiagarajan RR, Armsby LR, et al. Emergent use of extracorporeal membrane oxygenation during pediatric cardiac catheterization. *Pediatr Crit Care Med*. 2006;7:212-219.

52. Ettedgui JA, Fricker FJ, Park SC, et al. Cardiac catheterization in children on extracorporeal membrane oxygenation. *Cardiol Young*. 1996;6:59-61.

53. DesJardins SE, Crowley DC, Beekman RH, Lloyd TR. Utility of cardiac catheterization in pediatric cardiac patients on ECMO. *Catheter Cardiovasc Interv*. 1999;46:62-67.

54. Haines NM, Rycus PT, Zwischenberger JB, et al. Extracorporeal life support registry report 2008: neonatal and pediatric cardiac cases. *ASAIO J*. 2009;55:111-116.

55. Rihal CS, Naidu SS, Givertz MM, et al. 2015 SCAI/ACC/HFSA/STS clinical expert consensus statement on the use of percutaneous mechanical circulatory support devices in cardiovascular care. *Catheter Cardiovasc Interv*. 2015;85:E175-E196.

56. Dimas VV, Murthy R, Guleserian KJ. Utilization of the Impella 2.5 microaxial pump in children for acute circulatory support. *Catheter Cardiovasc Interv*. 2014;83:261-262.

Pharmacology of the Cardiovascular System

Naomi B. Bishop, Bruce M. Greenwald, and Daniel A. Notterman

PEARLS

- Clinical acumen is necessary to distinguish between the need for an inotropic agent, which is used to increase cardiac contractility, and the need for a vasopressor agent, which is used to increase vascular tone.
- The failing myocardium may need to be supported with an agent that increases contractility and reduces afterload, such as milrinone or dobutamine.
- Multiple polymorphisms have been discovered in receptors relevant to the intensivist. Although the clinical importance of these polymorphisms has yet to be determined, physicians need to stay abreast of changes in this rapidly expanding area.

In many pediatric critical care units, disorders of the cardiovascular and respiratory systems are the most frequent reasons for admission. Children with these disorders constitute a large group who may require pharmacologic support to maintain adequate end-organ perfusion and oxygenation. The catecholamines are the class of drug most often used for this support, and they remain a mainstay of therapy for the pediatric critical care physician, although the role of other agents has expanded. Milrinone, a bipyridine, has been used to support patients with hemodynamic compromise of varying etiologies. In addition, the role of vasopressin and terlipressin in the management of patients with vasodilatory shock or after cardiopulmonary bypass continues to grow. This chapter examines the clinical pharmacology of the five clinically useful catecholamines, as well as newer agents and the venerable cardiac glycosides.

Mechanisms of Response

Pharmacologic manipulation of the cardiovascular system often entails increasing the inotropic state of the myocardium or altering the tone of the systemic vascular tree so as to improve perfusion. The final common mediator for both processes is the concentration of calcium in the cytosol. The pathway by which pharmacologic agents affect this parameter is a function of their specific cell surface receptors.

Adrenergic Receptors

Catecholamines modify cellular physiology through their interaction with specific adrenergic receptors. The classic

paradigm of α and β classes of adrenergic receptors remains unchanged, although new subtypes and sub-subtypes continue to be identified. Currently three subtypes of α_1 receptors (A, B, D), three subtypes of α_2 receptors (A, B, C), and three subtypes of β receptors (β_1, β_2, β_3) are recognized.[1] Advances in the biology of the adrenergic receptor have led to a greater understanding of role of the α receptor in the heart, adrenergic receptor regulation of cardiac myocyte apoptosis, and the coupling of the β_2 receptor to more than one G protein. The discovery of various genetic polymorphisms for the adrenergic receptors has added even more complexity, but the clinical relevance of many of these polymorphisms and their role in the pathogenesis of disease are only beginning to be elucidated. Despite this increase in our understanding of the adrenergic receptor, the clinical classification of the catecholamines into α and β agents remains functionally unchanged (Table 33.1).

Signal Transduction

Adrenergic receptors mediate their effects through G proteins and as such are classified as G protein–coupled receptors. The adrenergic receptor itself contains seven membrane-spanning α-helical domains, an extracellular N-terminal segment, and a cytosolic C-terminal segment (Fig. 33.1). G proteins are heterotrimeric proteins consisting of α, β, and γ subunits, each of which has multiple subfamilies.[2] There are at least twenty α subunits, five β subunits, and six γ subunits. The action mediated by a ligand binding to a particular adrenergic receptor is a function of the specific subunits comprising the G protein receptor complex.

Adrenergic receptors typically are coupled to one of three types of G proteins: G_s, G_i, or G_q. G_s proteins produce an increase in adenylate cyclase activity, while G_i proteins inhibit adenylate cyclase activity. G_q protein receptors stimulate phospholipase C to generate diacylglycerol and inositol 1,4,5-triphosphate. The nature of the G protein is usually a function of the type of α subunit (α_s, α_i, α_q, and $\alpha_{12/13}$).[2-4] Events involving interaction of G proteins, the receptor protein, and adenylate cyclase are summarized in Fig. 33.2. In the example of the G_s protein, ligand binding to the coupled receptor causes a conformational change in the G protein, resulting in guanosine diphosphate (GDP) disassociating from the Gsα subunit and guanosine triphosphate (GTP) binding to the α subunit. This GTP-Gα complex then disassociates from the Gβ subunit and binds to adenylate cyclase, leading to an increase in activity of this enzyme. Adenylate

TABLE 33.1   Adrenergic Receptors: Physiologic Responses, Agonist Potency, and Representative Antagonists

Receptor	G Protein	Physiologic Response	Agonist	Antagonist
α_1	G_q	Increase InsP$_3$, 1,2-DG, and intracellular Ca^{+2}; muscle contraction; vasoconstriction; inhibit insulin secretion	E > NE > D	Prazosin
α_2	G_i	Decrease cAMP; inhibit NE release; vasodilation; negative chronotropy	E > NE	Yohimbine
β_1	G_s	Increase cAMP; inotropy, chronotropy; enhance renin secretion	I > E ≥ D ≥ NE	Propranolol, metoprolol
β_2	G_s	Increase cAMP; smooth muscle relaxation; vasodilation; bronchodilation; enhance glucagon secretion; hypokalemia	I ≥ E > D > NE	Propranolol
D_1	G_s	Increase cAMP; smooth muscle relaxation	D	Haloperidol, metoclopramide
D_2	G_i	Decrease cAMP; inhibit prolactin and β-endorphin	D	Domperidone

cAMP, cyclic adenosine monophosphate; *D*, dopamine; *1,2-DG*, 1,2 diacylglycerol; *E*, epinephrine; *I*, isoproterenol; *InsP3*, Inositol 1,4,5-triphosphate; *NE*, norepinephrine.
Modified from Notterman DA. Pharmacologic support of the failing circulation: an approach for infants and children. Prob Anesth. 1989;3:288.

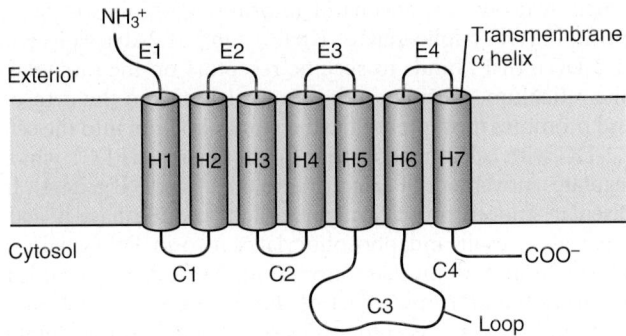

Fig. 33.1. Schematic representation of typical G protein–coupled receptor with seven membrane spanning regions (H1–H7), cytoplasmic (C1–C4), and extracellular (E1–E4) loops. (From Lodish H, et al. Molecular Cell Biology. 4th ed. New York, NY: WH Freeman; 1999.)

cyclase catalyzes the conversion of adenosine triphosphate (ATP) to cyclic adenosine monophosphate (cAMP), thus increasing cellular levels of cAMP. G$_i$ proteins have a different α subunit; when the G$_i$α GTP complex binds to adenylate cyclase, the enzyme is inactivated. By inhibiting this enzyme, G$_i$-coupled receptor agonists produce a decrease in the cellular concentration of cAMP. The specific cellular response that follows an alteration in the concentration of cAMP depends on the specialized function of the target cell.[2] Typically, an increase in concentration of cAMP leads to activation of a cAMP-dependent protein kinase. These kinases then phosphorylate and activate other structures and enzymes. Many compounds other than adrenergic agents also increase intracellular levels of cAMP. The question of how various agents produce specific responses through the expression of common second messengers continues to be investigated. One proposed mechanism involves anchoring proteins, such as A kinase anchoring proteins. These proteins localize protein kinase A (PKA) to particular cellular locales and also may offer binding sites for other regulatory proteins.[4] Similarly, anchoring proteins for both the active and inactive forms of protein kinase C have been described.[5] Different subtypes of anchoring proteins may serve to create another level of specificity in the effector response for a particular ligand by confining the response to a particular area of the cell.

β-Adrenergic Receptors

Myocardial β$_1$-adrenergic receptors are associated with G$_s$. When this receptor type is engaged by an agonist agent, the result is enhanced activity of adenylate cyclase and a rise in the concentration of cAMP. This process activates PKA. PKA in turn phosphorylates voltage-dependent calcium channels, increasing the fraction of channels that can be opened and the probability that these channels are open, producing an increase in intracellular calcium concentration (Fig. 33.3).[6] Calcium then binds to troponin C, allowing for actin-myosin cross-bridge formation and sarcomere contraction. In addition, PKA phosphorylates phospholamban, relieving the disinhibitory effect of the unphosphorylated form on calcium channels in the sarcoplasmic reticulum. The accumulation of calcium by the sarcoplasmic reticulum is thus enhanced, increasing the rate of sarcomere relaxation (lusitropy) and subsequently increasing the amount of calcium available for the next contraction. This process leads to both enhanced contractility and active diastolic relaxation.

Both β$_1$ and β$_2$ receptors are present in vascular smooth muscle, although β$_2$ receptors predominate.[1] The β$_2$ receptor is coupled to G$_s$; therefore activation of β$_2$ receptors promotes formation of cAMP. The activation of cAMP-dependent protein kinase in vascular smooth muscle, however, stimulates pumps that remove calcium from the cytosol and also promotes calcium uptake by the sarcoplasmic reticulum. As cytosolic calcium concentration decreases, smooth muscle relaxes and the blood vessel dilates.

α Receptors

Vascular smooth muscle contraction is mediated via α$_1$-adrenergic receptors, of which there are three subtypes: 1A, 1B, and 1D. The individual contributions of each of these subtypes to the control of vascular tone is an active area of investigation. Each subtype may be expressed in all of the vascular beds, but it is thought that one type predominates in any particular bed.[7] A mouse knockout model of the α$_{1D}$ receptor showed that α$_1$ binding in the aorta was lost but preserved in the heart. The knockout model also had lower blood pressures and a decreased response to norepinephrine.[8] α$_{1A}$ and α$_{1B}$ receptors are thought to be involved in both the heart and vasculature.[9,10] A knockout model of α$_{1A}$ demonstrated both decreased blood pressure and a decreased response

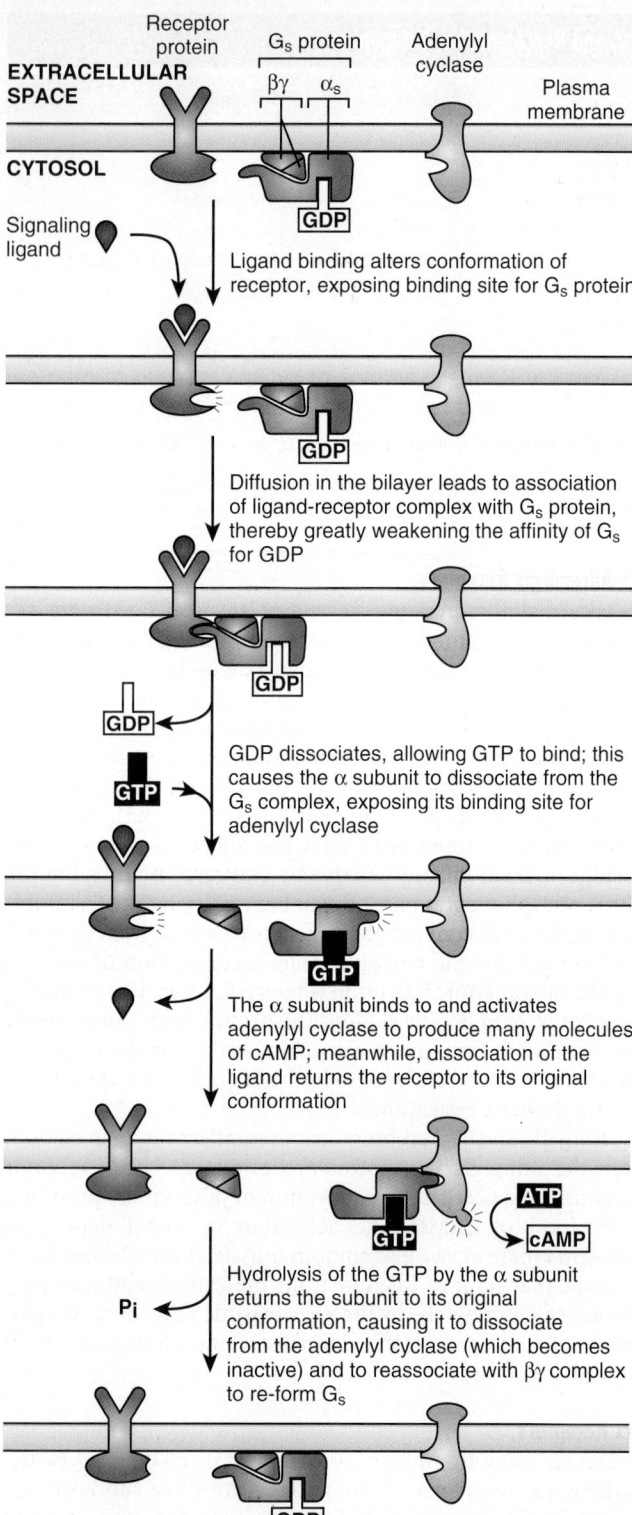

Receptor protein — G$_s$ protein — Adenylyl cyclase

EXTRACELLULAR SPACE βγ α$_s$ Plasma membrane

CYTOSOL

Signaling ligand

Ligand binding alters conformation of receptor, exposing binding site for G$_s$ protein

Diffusion in the bilayer leads to association of ligand-receptor complex with G$_s$ protein, thereby greatly weakening the affinity of G$_s$ for GDP

GDP dissociates, allowing GTP to bind; this causes the α subunit to dissociate from the G$_s$ complex, exposing its binding site for adenylyl cyclase

The α subunit binds to and activates adenylyl cyclase to produce many molecules of cAMP; meanwhile, dissociation of the ligand returns the receptor to its original conformation

Hydrolysis of the GTP by the α subunit returns the subunit to its original conformation, causing it to dissociate from the adenylyl cyclase (which becomes inactive) and to reassociate with βγ complex to re-form G$_s$

ATP → cAMP

P$_i$

Fig. 33.2. Adrenergic receptor complex. When the receptor is engaged by an appropriate ligand (eg, isoproterenol for a β$_1$ receptor), the receptor associates with the α$_s$ polypeptide of the G$_s$ protein. This causes the α$_s$ to extrude GDP and incorporate GTP; α$_s$ then associates with and activates the adenylate cyclase. The process is terminated when GTP is hydrolyzed to GDP and α$_s$ dissociates. (From Alberts B, et al. Molecular Biology of the Cell. 3rd ed. New York, NY: Garland Science; 1994. Reproduced by permission of Garland Science/Taylor Francis, LLC.)

to phenylephrine.[7] An animal model of overexpression of the α$_{1A}$ receptor was associated with marked increase in cardiac contractility without a change in blood pressure or heart rate.[11] In a knockout model of α$_{1B}$ receptors in mice, chronic exposure to norepinephrine did not lead to cardiac hypertrophy or vascular remodeling.[12] Overexpression of a mutant α$_{1B}$ receptor led to increased expression of mitogen-activated protein kinases and decreased responsiveness to isoproterenol in isolated cardiac preparations.[13] Thus while α receptors may have less inotropic effect than β-adrenergic receptors, they do have significant effects in the myocardium. Interestingly, in patients with heart failure, downregulation of β receptors has been noted while α receptors are preserved.[14] In fact, recent evidence suggests that α$_1$ receptors may display cardioprotective effects including activation of adaptive hypertrophy, increased contractility, and prevention of myocyte death.[15] The α$_1$ receptor is coupled to the family of G$_{q/11}$ proteins, which act independently of cAMP. Signal transduction across this receptor is initiated by the activation of phospholipase C, which hydrolyzes phosphatidylinositol 4,5-biphosphate to inositol 1,4,5-triphosphate (InsP$_3$) and 1,2-diacylglycerol (1,2-DG). InsP$_3$ binds to specific receptors on the sarcoplasmic reticulum, causing a release of calcium into the cytosol, and promotes movement of extracellular calcium into the cell. 1,2-DG with calcium activates protein kinase C (PKC), which regulates movement of calcium into the cytosol (Fig. 33.4). In vascular smooth muscle, medium light chain kinase is activated as a result and phosphorylates myosin light chain 2, leading to smooth muscle contraction.[16] A similar mechanism underlies the inotropic effect of the α$_1$ receptor in the myocardium.[17] The α$_{1A}$ receptor appears to be the most efficiently coupled of the different subtypes.[18] The α$_1$ receptors also activate calcium influx through voltage-dependent and voltage-independent calcium channels.[19] The α receptors also promote the activation of the mitogen-activated kinase family, which are key regulators of cell growth.

Receptor Downregulation

The mechanisms described provide numerous sites at which activity of the system can be modified, thereby affecting the sensitivity of target cells to both exogenous and endogenous catecholamines. Some of these receptor modifications are clinically important to the critical care physician. The best-documented type of modification involves agonist-mediated receptor desensitization. Exposure of receptors to agonists markedly reduces the sensitivity of the target cell to the agonist. Within seconds to minutes after agonist binding, the receptor may be uncoupled as a result of receptor phosphorylation. The receptor may be phosphorylated by PKA or PKC or by a member of the family of G receptor kinases (GRKSs). These kinases, which include β-adrenergic receptor kinases 1 and 2, phosphorylate only receptors that have agonist bound. Compared with PKA and PKC, phosphorylation by GRKS enhances the ability of β arrestin, a cytosolic protein, or clathrin to bind to the receptor and disrupt further signaling. The role of GRKS has been established for β$_1$, β$_2$, and α$_2$ receptors.[20,21] Sequestration of receptors within the target cell and degradation of sequestered receptors are other mechanisms by which receptors are downregulated. The desensitization of α$_1$ receptors has been extensively reviewed.[22] Homologous desensitization is mediated by GRKSs, which are activated by soluble Gβγ subunits and phosphatidylinositol biphosphate. As with

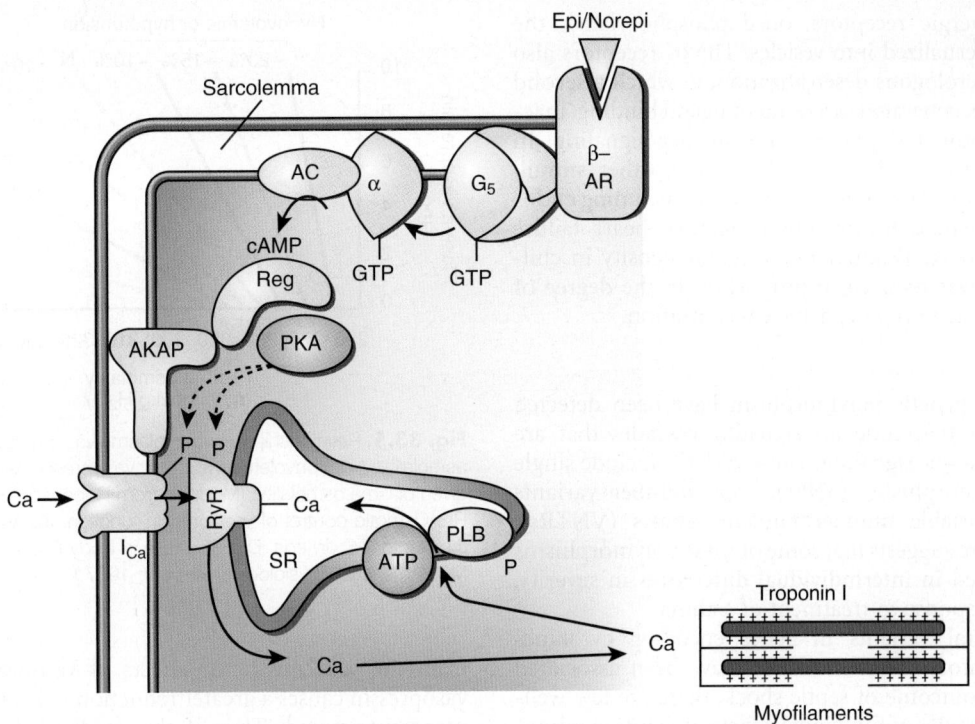

Fig. 33.3. β₁-Adrenergic receptor signaling cascade. Agonist (epinephrine/norepinephrine [Epi/Norepi]) to β-adrenergic receptor (β-AR) results in the α subunit binding to GTP, which activates adenylate cyclase (AC). AC then converts adenosine triphosphate (ATP) to cyclic adenosine monophosphate (cAMP), which binds to regulatory unit (Reg) on protein kinase A (PKA). PKA then promotes an increase in the intracellular concentration of calcium (Ca) by acting on voltage-gated channels (I_{Ca}) and on the sarcoplasmic reticulum (SR). Cardiac excitation-contact coupling then promotes sarcomere contraction. *AKAP,* A kinase anchoring protein; *PLB,* phospholamban; *RyR,* ryanodine receptor. (From Bers DM. Cardiac excitation-contact coupling. Nature. 2003;415:198.)

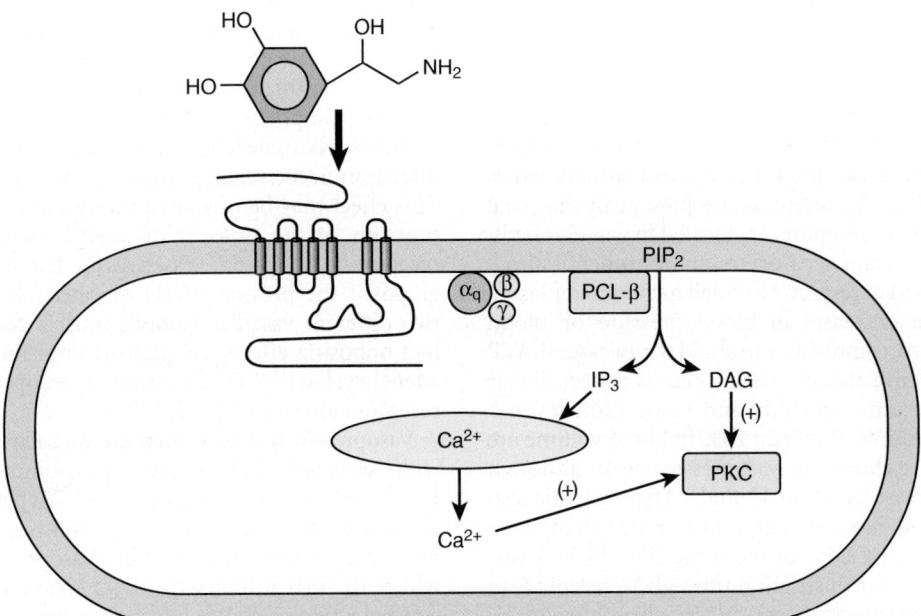

Fig. 33.4. α₁-Adrenergic receptor signaling cascade. Binding of an agonist such as norepinephrine to a G protein–coupled receptor activates the $G_{q/11}$ protein, leading to disassociation of the α and β subunits. Phospholipase C (PLC-β) is activated in turn and cleaves phosphatidylinositol 4,5-biphospate (PIP₂) to inositol 1,4,5-triphosphate (IP₃) and diacylglycerol (DAG). IP₃ and DAG promote an increase in intracellular calcium through the sarcoplasmic reticulum and protein kinase C (PKC). (From Zhong H, Minneman KP. α-1 adrenoreceptor subtypes. Eur J Pharm. 1999;375:26.)

the other adrenergic receptors, once phosphorylated, the receptors are internalized into vesicles. The α_1 receptors also demonstrate heterologous desensitization, in which a second messenger kinase, generated as a result of ligand binding, inactivates the receptor and prevents any further signaling. In addition to agonist-mediated desensitization, other stimuli also have been implicated in downregulation, including endotoxin, tumor necrosis factor, and congestive heart failure (CHF).[23] Lymphocyte β-adrenergic receptor density in children with CHF was reduced in proportion to the degree of elevation in plasma norepinephrine concentration.[24]

Polymorphisms

Several types of genetic polymorphism have been detected within the genes that code for signaling cascades that are involved in adrenergic signaling. These variants include single nucleotide polymorphisms (SNPs), copy number variants (CNVs), and variable number tandem repeats (VNTRs). Growing literature suggests that some of these polymorphisms may be implicated in interindividual differences in severity, periodicity, or response to treatment of asthma.[25]

Whereas several variants in genes encoding cytokines and other mediators of inflammation have been associated with severity or outcome of septic shock, there are few well-documented examples of functional genetic variants in adrenergic signaling that affect critical illness in children. In one study of adults with septic shock, an SNP in the β_2 receptor was associated with greater organ dysfunction and mortality.[26] Other polymorphisms have been associated with the β_1 receptor. Although these variants affect some properties of receptor function, clinical links are still being explored.[27-29] Recently, the Arg 389 β_1 variant has been shown to moderate the effect of β blockers on various cardiovascular measures, suggesting that it may become appropriate to test for this variant when considering therapy with an agent of this class. Interestingly, the Arg 389 β_1 variant has also been associated with increased cAMP generation, poorer prognosis in heart failure, and an increase in the predisposition to hypertension.[30]

Vasopressin Receptors

Arginine vasopressin is a nonpeptide hormone synthesized in the supraoptic and paraventricular nuclei of the hypothalamus. Three subtypes of vasopressin receptors exist, known as V_1, V_2, and V_3 (or V_{1b}). V_2 receptors are present in the renal collecting duct, while V_1 receptors are located in vascular beds, kidney, bladder, spleen, and hepatocytes, among other tissues.[31] Vasopressin is released in response to small increases in plasma osmolality or large decreases in blood pressure or blood volume.[32] The plasma osmolality threshold for release of AVP is 280 mOsm/kg; above this threshold there is a steep linear relation between serum osmolality and vasopressin levels.[32] Changes in blood volume of at least 20% in blood volume are necessary to effect a change in vasopressin levels, although levels may then increase by 20- to 30-fold.[32] Hypovolemia also shifts the vasopressin response curve to osmolar changes to the left and increases the slope of the curve (Fig. 33.5). Vasopressin can produce vasoconstriction through V_1 receptors in the vascular bed (discussed later), but it also activates V_1 receptors in the central nervous system (CNS), including receptors in the area postrema.[33] This region is responsible for the reflex bradycardia seen with vasopressin infusion, which attenuates the increase in blood pressure that would result

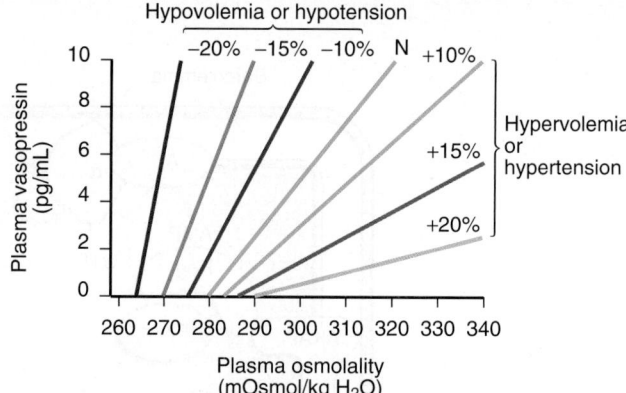

Fig. 33.5. Relationship between plasma vasopressin levels and plasma osmolality. As hypovolemia worsens, vasopressin levels increase for any given plasma osmolality. (Modified from Robertson GL, Athar S, Shelton RL. Osmotic control of vasopressin function. In: Androli TE, Grantham JJ, Rector FC Jr, eds. Disturbances in body fluid osmolality. Bethesda, MD: American Physiological Society; 1977.)

from the vasoconstrictor effects of vasopressin.[34,35] In fact, vasopressin causes a greater reduction in heart rate than other vasoconstrictors.[31] Thus if this feedback loop is abolished, vasopressin induces a greater vasopressor response than other agents.[33]

V₁ Receptors

Vasopressin receptors belong to the family of G protein–coupled receptors. V_1 receptors are coupled to G_q, and V_2 receptors are coupled to G_s.[32] When vasopressin binds to the V_1 receptor, phospholipase C is activated with the eventual production of $InsP_3$ and 1,2-DG. These molecules serve to increase the release of calcium from the endoplasmic reticulum, as well as increase the entry of calcium through gated channels (Fig. 33.6).[36] The increase in intracellular calcium leads to an increase in the activity of myosin light chain kinase. This kinase acts upon myosin to increase the number of actin-myosin cross-bridges, enhancing contraction of the myocyte. Of note, vasopressin has been shown to produce vasoconstriction in the skin, skeletal muscle, and fat while producing vasodilatation in the renal, pulmonary, and cerebral vasculature.[37] This effect may be mediated though nitric oxide or may be a function of the isoform of adenyl cyclase with which the receptor is coupled.[38] Vasopressin has also been shown to augment the pressor effects of catecholamines, although in two different vascular smooth muscle cell lines, vasopressin had opposing effects on isoproterenol-induced activation of adenyl cyclase.[39-41] Other effects of vasopressin binding to V_1 receptors are shown in Fig. 33.6.

Vasopressin may also increase vascular tone by interacting with so-called ATP-sensitive potassium channels termed K_{ATP}.[42] Activation of K_{ATP} channels hyperpolarizes the cell, closes calcium channels, and prevents contraction.[43,44] The result may be to protect the cell.[27] Vasopressin can induce PKC, which in turn inhibits the K_{ATP} channel when the cellular concentration of ATP is low,[28] allowing for cell depolarization and calcium entry, resulting in vasoconstriction (Fig. 33.7).[45] V_1 receptors have been demonstrated to have a weakly positive inotropic effect in the heart, although the clinical significance of this effect has not been established.[29]

V₁ RECEPTOR-EFFECTOR COUPLING

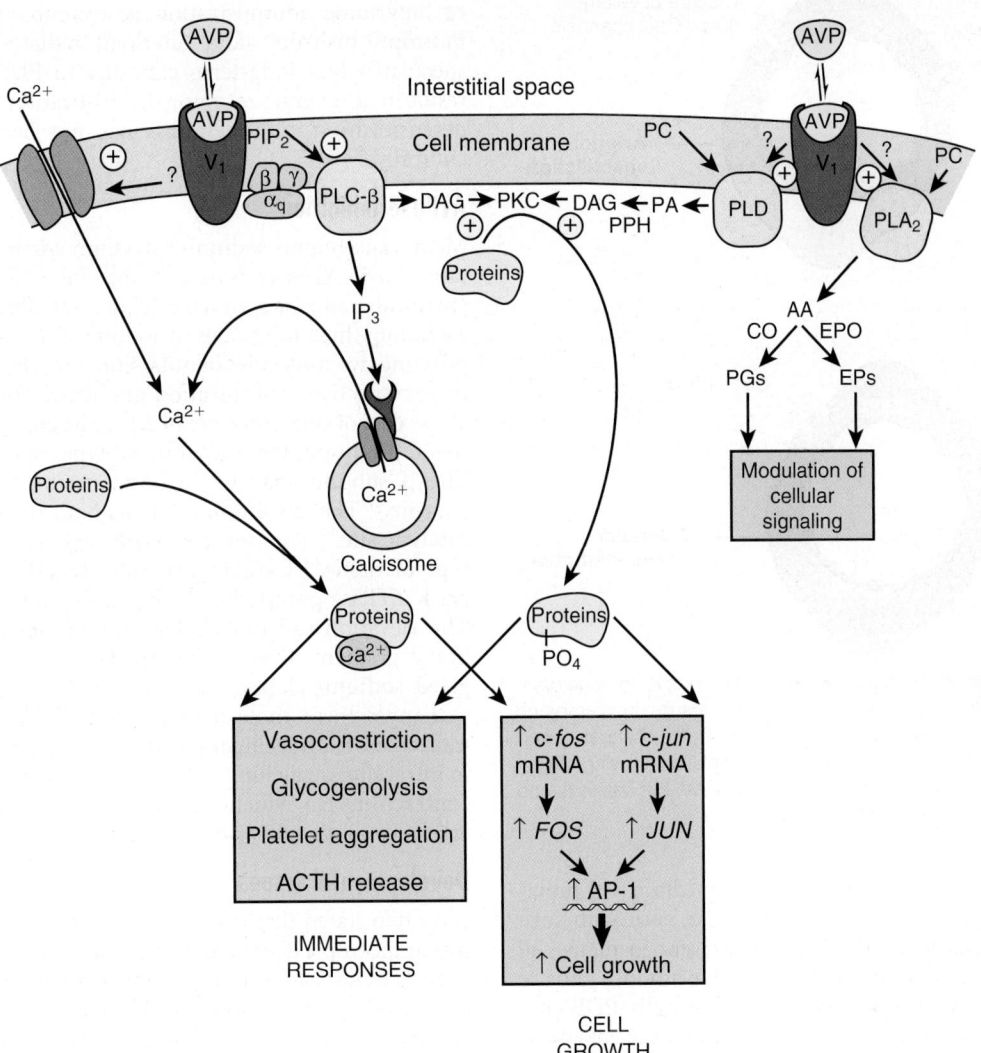

Fig. 33.6. V_1 receptor signaling cascade. Binding of arginine vasopressin (AVP) to the V_1 vasopressin receptor (V_1) leads to activation of phospholipase C (PLC-β) via the Gq protein with the production of inositol 1,4,5-triphosphate (IP_3). IP_3 promotes an increase in intracellular calcium, resulting in figure. *AA*, arachidonic acid; *ACTH*, adrenocorticotropic hormone; *AP-1*, transcription factor consisting of heterodimer of FOS and JUN; *CO*, cyclooxygenase; *DAG*, diacylglycerol; *EPO*, epoxygense; *EPs*, epoxyeicosatrienoic acids; *PA*, phosphatidic acid; *PC*, phosphatidylcholine; *PGs*, prostaglandins; *PIP₂*, phosphatidylinositol 4,5-biphosphate; *PKC*, protein kinase C; *PLA₂*, phospholipase A₂; *PLD*, phospholipase D; *PPH*, phosphatidate phosphohydrolase. "?" indicates the mechanism of coupling is unclear. (From Jackson EK. Vasopressin and other agents affecting the renal conservation of water. In: Hardman JG, Limbird LE, eds. Goodman and Gilman's the Pharmacologic Basis of Therapeutics. 10th ed. New York, NY: McGraw Hill; 2001.)

Receptor Downregulation

As with adrenergic receptors, vasopressin receptors undergo downregulation. Vasopressin promotes the phosphorylation of it own receptor immediately after binding. The receptor is removed from the cell surface within 3 minutes after binding.[46] As with adrenergic receptors, GRKSs catalyze the phosphorylation of the receptor. PKC also mediates this reaction and may serve as the means by which other agents downregulate the vasopressin receptor in a heterologous manner.[46]

Polymorphisms

Although numerous mutations in the V_2 receptor exist, some of which result in nephrogenic diabetes insipidus, much less is known about the V_1 receptor. One study established two polymorphisms in the V_1 receptor gene but failed to establish

a linkage with hypertension.[47] Another study involving 33 subjects, designed to evaluate a possible linkage to differences in platelet aggregation in response to vasopressin, identified four single nucleotide polymorphisms in the promoter region of the V1a receptor.[48] No difference in response was observed in subjects with and without the variant alleles. Still, the molecular basis for individual genetic variation remains an active area of investigation since discoveries in this area may inform risk stratification, prognostic accuracy, and individual response to therapy.

Phosphodiesterase Regulation of cAMP

Phosphodiesterases are a class of enzyme that catalyzes the hydrolysis of cAMP and cGMP into AMP and GMP, respectively. Therefore these enzymes can downregulate the signals

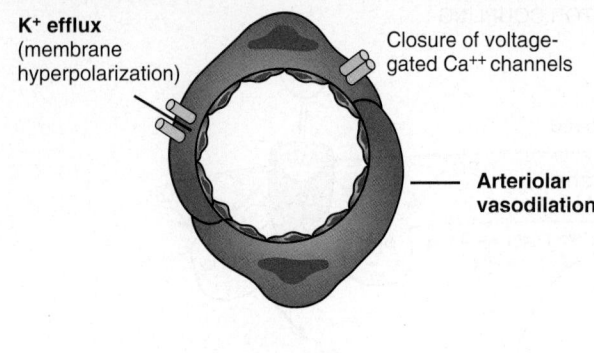

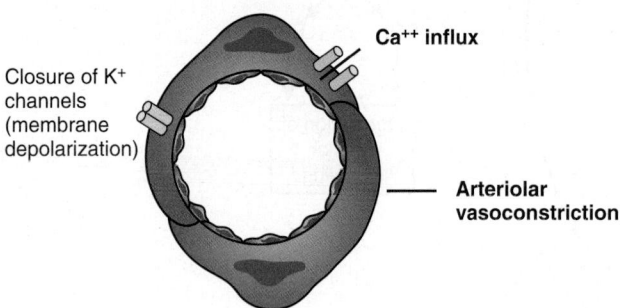

Fig. 33.7. K⁺ channels and vascular tone. Diffusion of K⁺ through open K_{ATP} channels in vascular smooth muscle cell results in membrane hyperpolarization, closure of voltage-gated Ca^{2+} channels, and decreased intracellular calcium, resulting in vasodilation. Closing of K_{ATP} channels has the opposite effects. (From Jackson W. Ion channels and vascular tone. Hypertension. 2000;35:173-178.)

transduced by cAMP, such as PKA activity (discussed previously). Several families of this enzyme exist, each with subtypes. Phosphodiesterase III (PDE3) is present in many cell types, including cardiac myocytes, vascular smooth muscle cells, adipocytes, platelets, and pancreatic islet cells. PDE3 has a much higher Vmax (ie, rate of reaction when the enzyme is saturated with substrate) for cAMP than it does for cGMP and therefore is functionally a cAMP esterase.[49] Different isoforms of PDE3 are present in cardiac (PDE3A1) and vascular smooth muscle cells (PDE3A2) and are localized to different cellular compartments. Thus they are able to regulate the function of their target enzymes in response to specific cellular signals.[50] The C-terminus of the enzyme codes for the central catalytic core that is the active binding site, and the N-terminus coding region (may) determine cellular targeting.[51] The bipyridines, such as milrinone, are competitive inhibitors of PDE3; that is, they bind to PDE3, preventing the enzyme from binding to cAMP.[52,53] They appear to bind near the binding site for cAMP, although different PDE3 inhibitors may have different binding sites.[54] Inhibition of PDE3 produces an increase in cAMP, resulting in a positive inotropic effect in the myocardium and vasodilatation in the systemic and pulmonary vasculature.[55] In contrast, methylxanthines such as theophylline, which inhibit all phosphodiesterases, cause levels of both cGMP (thought to decrease contractility) and cAMP to increase. This dual increase attenuates the overall inotropic effect. Bipyridines may also enhance contractility by increasing the sensitivity of myofilaments to cytosolic calcium.[56] Milrinone has been shown to enhance the sarcomere uptake of calcium and thereby augment left ventricular (LV) relaxation (lusitropy).[57] In the peripheral vasculature, PD3 inhibitors produce

vasodilatation via a cGMP mechanism.[58] The clinical effect of bipyridine administration is a combination of positive inotropy, lusitropy, and afterload reduction. It has been speculated that long-term exposure to PDE inhibitors may result in adrenergic receptor desensitization via heterologous desensitization, although this has not been demonstrated clinically.[59]

ATPase Inhibition

Membrane-bound sodium-potassium adenosine triphosphatase (Na-K ATPase) is responsible for maintaining electrochemical gradients across the cellular membrane. It does so by extruding three molecules of sodium from the cell and incorporating two molecules of potassium into the cell, both against their respective concentration gradients. This process occurs at the cost of one molecule of ATP. The enzyme consists of an α and β subunit; there are four subtypes of α and three of β.[60] The β subunit may be involved in the trafficking of the enzyme.[61] The α subunit contains both the binding site and catalytic site.[60] The isoforms expressed are dependent on the type of tissue.[62] Cardiac glycosides (eg, digoxin) inhibit the Na-K ATPase pump, thereby increasing intracellular sodium. The elevation in intracellular sodium alters the transmembrane gradient, thus inhibiting the activity of the voltage-gated sodium/calcium exchange (NCX) pump. This pump exchanges three molecules of extracellular sodium for one molecule of intracellular calcium.[63,64] The net result is a rise in intracellular calcium and, in the cardiac myocyte, enhanced contractility. No evidence exists to suggest the development of tolerance to digoxin with long-term use.[65]

Developmental Issues

It is often stated that the immature myocardium is less sensitive to inotropic agents than the adult heart. The exact nature of the mechanism responsible for these differences represents an area of active investigation. The majority of studies involve animal models or isolated human tissue. Because there are inherent differences between intact healthy animal models and the ill child, as well as pharmacokinetic differences between the infant and adult patient, caution must be exercised when extrapolating laboratory data to the bedside.[66] Nonetheless, a brief review of developmental differences is appropriate.

Age-related differences exist in the response of the developing myocardium to inotropic agents, receptor regulation, and calcium handling. However, the extent of these differences depends on the species studied and the model of illness to which the animals are exposed.[67-72]

Developmental differences also may exist in the expression of phosphodiesterase (PDE) isoforms. In a model of rabbit ventricular myocytes, administration of IBMX (a nonselective PDE inhibitor) and rolipram (a PDE type IV inhibitor) increased intracellular calcium currents in neonatal cells both at baseline and in response to isoproterenol but not in adult cells. In contrast, milrinone (a PDE type III inhibitor) increased intracellular calcium currents at baseline and in response to isoproterenol only in the adult cells.[73] Thus it would appear that in the neonatal myocardium, PDE type IV may be the dominant isoenzyme that regulates intracellular calcium currents.

Structural and ultrastructural differences also exist between immature and mature hearts. These differences include reduced ventricular compliance, greater ventricular interdependence, and a reduced ratio of myocardial contractile to noncontractile protein in the immature heart. The net effect is that the immature myocardium neither responds to nor tolerates volume loading as well as the adult heart. In addition to this diminished "preload reserve," the baseline heart rate of infants and children is quite high, which limits the extent to which tachycardia can augment cardiac output before diastolic filling is compromised.

The combination of impaired preload reserve, limited chronotropic reserve, and reduced sensitivity of the heart and peripheral vasculature to adrenergic agents implies that the response of the immature organism to inotropic and vasopressor agents may differ from the pattern noted in adults.[74,75] Indeed, a recent meta-review of the use of dobutamine in pediatrics concluded that although there is evidence to support the conclusion that this drug improves cardiac output in neonates, the underlying preclinical foundation of animal research was still inadequate to define the age-related effects of dobutamine on various physiologic measures or organ systems.[76] This limitation is likely to be present in the case of the other agents employed in pediatric critical care for the treatment of shock. Coupled with the wide variation in cardiac structure due to congenital heart disease, this means that individual differences in response to infusion of cardiovascular drugs may be difficult to predict and, to date, to explain. Meticulous observation to response must be the mainstay of safely administering these drugs to children.

Sympathomimetic Amines

Virtually all sympathomimetics currently used to treat hemodynamic problems are catecholamines. This class includes the endogenous compounds epinephrine, norepinephrine, and dopamine and the synthetic products isoproterenol and dobutamine. Catecholamines have a β-phenylethylamine core with hydroxyl (OH) substituents at the 3 and 4 aromatic ring positions (Fig. 33.8). Minor differences in molecular substitution about the N-terminus or the α or β carbons produce marked differences in activity. Structure-activity relationships are complex for the catecholamines and have been reviewed; it is possible to generalize by noting that increasing size of the substituent on the amino group enhances β-adrenergic activity, whereas decreasing size is associated with α-adrenergic selectivity.[77] Tyrosine serves as the base compound for the synthesis of catecholamines. Tyrosine hydroxylase catalyzes the conversion of tyrosine to dopa, which undergoes decarboxylation, producing dopamine. Dopamine β-hydroxylase converts dopamine to norepinephrine. In the adrenal medulla, norepinephrine is converted to epinephrine by N-methyl transferase (Fig. 33.9).

Catecholamines are subject to several different elimination processes.[78] Infused dopamine provides an example in which elimination occurs through a variety of processes. A small proportion is excreted unchanged in the urine. It is likely that a proportion undergoes neuronal reuptake. The principal means of elimination appears to be O-methylation by catechol O-methyltransferase (COMT) to form metanephrines, followed by either sulfoconjugation (by phenol sulfotransferase) or by deamination (by monoamine oxidase [MAO]) to homovanillic acid.[79] Substitution at the α carbon determines the rate of deamination by MAO.[80] The contribution of these pathways to total body clearance of catecholamines varies with

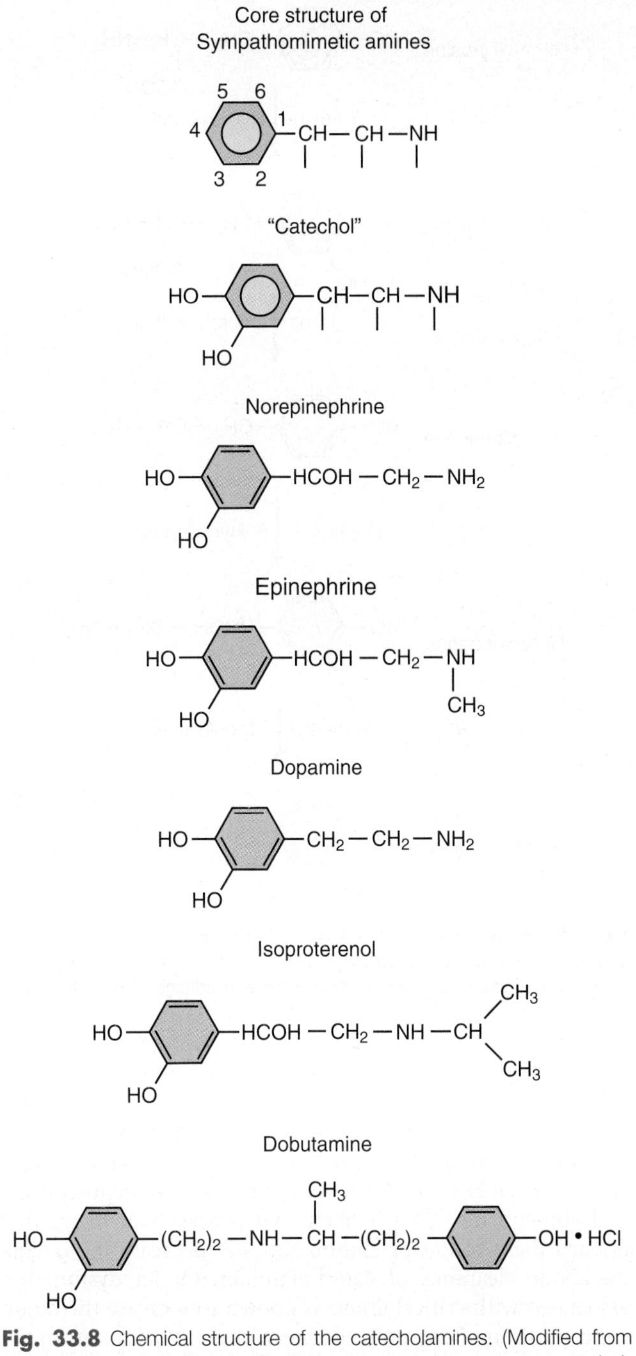

Fig. 33.8 Chemical structure of the catecholamines. (Modified from Chernow B, Rainey T, Lake R. Endogenous and exogenous catecholamines in critical care medicine. Crit Care Med. 1982;10:409.)

age and the particular circulatory bed. In newborn lambs, the lungs accounted for 35% of the total body clearance of norepinephrine and 15% of the clearance of epinephrine. Inhibition of MAO by desipramine decreased pulmonary clearance to near zero and decreased total body clearance of norepinephrine and epinephrine by 51% and 30%, respectively.[81] In adult rabbits, inhibition of COMT and MAO simultaneously decreased pulmonary clearance of norepinephrine, epinephrine, and dopamine but had only minor effects on total body clearance.[82] Inhibition of COMT did not change extracellular levels of catecholamines in the CNS.[83] Furthermore, individual

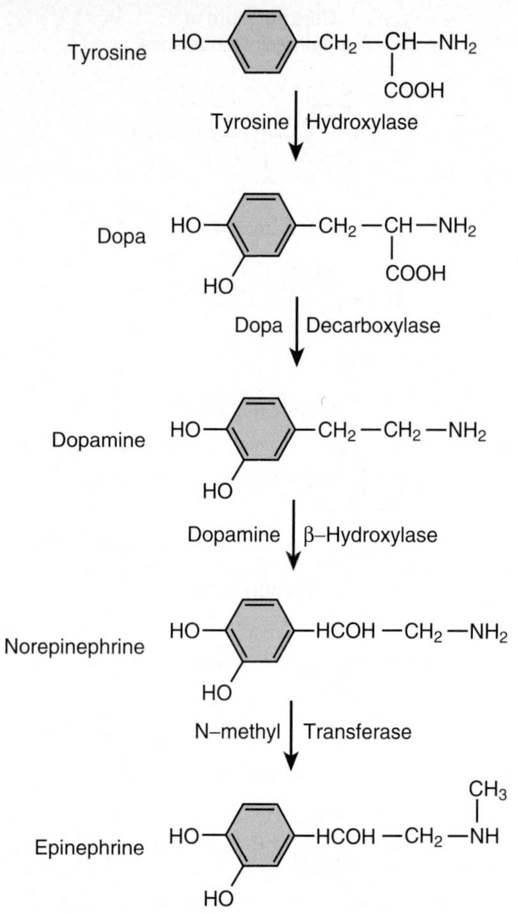

Fig. 33.9 Biosynthetic pathways of the endogenous catecholamines. (Modified from Chernow B, Rainey T, Lake R. Endogenous and exogenous catecholamines in critical care medicine. Crit Care Med. 1982;10:409.)

differences in COMT activity are not well correlated with dopamine clearance.[84] The liver and gut have been shown to clear between 30% and 52% of the circulating norepinephrine and epinephrine.[85,86] It is likely that processes or drugs that disturb these routes of elimination will decrease the overall metabolic clearance of catecholamines. Organ dysfunction associated with critical illness is known to increase the blood concentration of dopamine during a given infusion rate of the compound. For example, with liver dysfunction the clearance of dopamine is reduced.[87]

It is practical to divide the properties of catecholamines into their inotropic and vasopressor effects. An inotropic agent increases stroke work at a given preload and afterload. Typically, these agents engage receptors of the β_1-adrenergic class. Agents that stimulate β_1-adrenergic receptors also tend to increase heart rate modestly, unless other properties of the drug prevent this increase. Some inotropic agents also activate β_2 receptors, promoting peripheral vasodilatation and reflex tachycardia. In addition, the improvement in cardiac output that these agents provide may permit a reflex relaxation of vascular tone and systemic vascular resistance.

A vasopressor agent increases peripheral vascular tone, elevating systemic vascular resistance and blood pressure. Typically, vasopressors engage α_1-adrenergic receptors,

causing contraction of vascular smooth muscle. In principle, the physician will use a vasopressor agent to treat peripheral vasoplegia and an inotropic agent when the major problem is impaired cardiac contractility. In practice, most available agents display a blend of inotropic, chronotropic, and vasopressor activity that is often dose dependent. Norepinephrine has both inotropic and vasopressor effects, although it is most commonly used as a vasopressor agent. Phenylephrine (a noncatecholamine) has considerable specificity for the α-adrenergic receptor, so it is almost a pure vasopressor. Isoproterenol and dobutamine have little α-adrenergic agonist activity but considerable activity at the β receptor; they are mostly used as inotropes. Epinephrine and dopamine have both inotropic and vasopressor activity. At relatively low infusion rates, they enhance myocardial function and increase heart rate (β_1 and β_2). At higher rates, vasopressor activity (α_1) becomes manifest.

Dopamine

Basic Pharmacology

In the enzymatic pathway leading from tyrosine to epinephrine (Fig. 33.9), decarboxylation transforms L-dopa to dopamine. Dopamine is a central neurotransmitter and is also found in sympathetic nerve terminals and in the adrenal medulla, where it is the immediate precursor of norepinephrine.

Clinical Pharmacology

Dopamine stimulates dopamine (D_1 and D_2) receptors located in the brain and in vascular beds in the kidney, mesentery, and coronary arteries (Table 33.2).[88] It also stimulates α and β receptors, although the compound's affinity for these receptors is lower. D_1 receptors are coupled to G_s and thus enhance adenylate cyclase and produce a rise in cAMP, which evokes vasodilatation. This increases blood flow to these organs and enhances renal solute and water excretion by the kidney. Dopamine modulates release of aldosterone and prolactin (via D_2 receptors), which also may affect renal solute clearance.[89] The physiologic role of dopamine has been extensively reviewed.[67,90]

Low infusion rates of dopamine augment renal sodium excretion; intermediate rates (5–10 µg/kg/min) produce chronotropic and inotropic effects, and still higher infusion rates increase vascular resistance.[91] Renal blood flow, glomerular filtration rate, and sodium excretion are maintained or even increase during dopamine infusion in patients with poor cardiac output.

Research into the dose-physiologic response relationships in patients treated with dopamine has yielded inconsistent results,[92-95] suggesting that a patient's response to a given dose depends on multiple factors, including underlying condition, hemodynamics, and adrenergic receptor status and highlighting the importance of titration to individual response when using catecholamines in the management of critically ill patients. Despite these observed variations in dose response, there is now consensus that the augmentation in urine output seen in critically ill patients with poor cardiac output who are started on low-dose, "renal" dopamine results from improved renal blood flow rather than a direct, receptor-mediated diuretic effect on the kidney. Regardless, the use of low-dose dopamine in pediatric and neonatal ICUs to augment renal function continues despite the lack of evidence to suggest a beneficial effect.[96]

TABLE 33.2   Major Hemodynamic Effects of Adrenergic Receptor Activation by Catecholamines

Agent	RECEPTOR			
	α_1	β_1	β_2	D_1
Dopamine[a]	Vasoconstriction; ↑ SVR, PVR	Inotropy; chronotropy	Vasodilation	Vasodilation (renal)
Norepinephrine	Vasoconstriction; ↑ SVR, PVR	Inotropy (minor)	—	—
Epinephrine[b]	Vasoconstriction; ↑ SVR, PVR	Inotropy; chronotropy	Vasodilation	—
Isoproterenol	—	Inotropy	Vasodilation	—
Dobutamine	See text	Inotropy	—	—
Milrinone	Nonreceptor-mediated inotropy and vasodilation			

[a]Dose related. At low infusion rates, D1 receptor effects predominate; at intermediate rates, β1 and β2 receptor effects predominate; and at high rates, α receptor effects predominate.
[b]Dose related. At low infusion rates, β receptor effects predominate; at high rates, α receptor effects predominate.
D1, dopamine receptor; *PVR,* pulmonary vascular resistance; *SVR,* systemic vascular resistance.
Modified from Notterman DA. Pharmacologic support of the failing circulation: an approach for infants and children. Prob Anesth. 1989;3:288.

Both the receptor-mediated activity and clinical effects of dopamine depend in part on developmental factors such as age and, in the case of newborns, the degree of prematurity.[97] However, as reported in adults, trials in newborns have also yielded conflicting results. Nevertheless, dopamine remains one of the most widely used vasoactive medications in the neonatal ICU amid ongoing controversies concerning the indications for pharmacologic intervention and specific therapeutic goals (ie, optimal blood pressure vs. adequate organ perfusion) in this unique population. Additionally, uncertainty persists regarding the long-term effects of dopamine on neurologic development in premature infants.[98]

While there is limited evidence to support the observation that the inotropic and peripheral vasoconstrictor effects of dopamine predominate in the neonatal period,[68] controversies remain regarding the vasodilator effects on the renal, coronary, and cerebral vascular beds.[69] In addition, the view that infants display reduced sensitivity to dopamine is not very well supported. In support of reduced sensitivity, Perez and associates[70] found that in critically ill neonates, infusion rates greater than 20 μg/kg/min were necessary to achieve cardiovascular stability, but unlike in adults, reductions in urine output or peripheral perfusion were not observed. Much of the experimental evidence for diminished sensitivity to dopamine in infants emerged from studies in immature animals, and questions remain as to whether the results can be directly applied to humans. A contrary observation was made by Padbury and coworkers,[99] who found that dopamine at doses as low as 0.5 to 1 μg/kg/min increased cardiac output and stroke volume before heart rate, while increases in systemic vascular resistance did not occur until infusion rates exceeded 8 μg/kg/min. Seri and colleagues[97] attributed the increase in blood pressure they observed in critically ill premature infants at doses of 2.5 to 7.5 μg/kg/min to the enhanced α-adrenergic sensitivity of the immature myocardium, but reduced clearance of dopamine in this age group has also been proposed.[68]

Dopamine crosses the blood-brain barrier in preterm neonates, and in one recent study, Wong and associates[100] demonstrated improved cerebral venous saturations and coupling of cerebral blood flow to cerebral metabolic rate of oxygen consumption in 10 infants treated with dopamine when compared with 16 controls. Dopamine also inhibits the release of prolactin, thyrotropin, growth hormone, and the gonadotropins, but the clinical significance of these effects is unclear.[97,101,102]

Pharmacokinetics

Plasma dopamine clearance ranges from 60 to 80 mL/kg/min in normal adults and is lower in patients with renal or hepatic disease.[87,103] In subjects with normal renal function, the elimination half-life of infused dopamine is approximately 2 minutes.[104] Among critically ill children, the elimination half-life is 26 ± 14 minutes, and in neonates the elimination half-life is 5 to 11 minutes.[71,72] Wide interindividual variations in the rate of dopamine clearance have been reported in critically ill children and healthy adults.[105,106] Age has a striking effect on clearance of dopamine, and clearance in children younger than 2 years of age is approximately twice as rapid as it is in older children (82 vs. 46 mL/kg/min).[87] Allen and colleagues[84] demonstrated that clearance of infused dopamine decreased by almost 50% during the first 20 months of life, while an additional 50% decrease occurs between the ages of 1 and 12 years. Of note, another study did not show a correlation between advancing age and dopamine clearance, although the patients in this study had a mean age of 37 months.[105] Dopamine clearance may also decrease after 24 hours of continuous infusion.[4] Banner and colleagues[107] studied the pharmacokinetics of dopamine in 15 patients ranging in age from 3 days to 8 years and noted nonlinear behavior, and the authors questioned the utility of evaluating total body clearance in this age group. Differences in the rate of sulfoconjugation as a route of elimination may also contribute to the wide variations in the clearance of dopamine in critically ill children.[84,87,105] The possible role of concomitantly administered dobutamine on the clearance of dopamine has been suggested by some authors, but an in vitro study showed that although dopamine and dobutamine are competitors for both COMT and MAO, the concentrations achieved under clinical situations are unlikely to produce clinically significant levels of inhibition.[72,108] Pharmacokinetic differences between children and infants, rather than a difference in vascular or myocardial receptor sensitivity, may account for the observation that infants require and tolerate higher infusion rates. For a more detailed discussion on the pharmacokinetics of dopamine and other cardiovascular drugs, the reader is directed to one of many comprehensive reviews.[109]

Clinical Role

Dopamine has been shown to be an effective inotropic and vasopressor agent in neonates and infants with a variety of conditions associated with circulatory failure, including hyaline membrane disease, asphyxia, sepsis syndrome, and cyanotic congenital heart disease.[110,111] Fewer data evaluating the efficacy of dopamine in older children are available. However, it remains a mainstay of pharmacologic support for the child with inadequate perfusion. Dopamine may be used in children with fluid refractory septic shock or distributive shock,[112-114] but this topic is debated, and many practitioners favor the use of norepinephrine or epinephrine. Dopamine may also be appropriate for children with mild impairment of myocardial function and hypotension after resuscitation from cardiac arrest.[115,116] Severe impairment of vascular tone or of cardiac contractility suggests the need for other agents. Children with primary myocardial disease not complicated by frank hypotension will benefit from a more selective inotropic agent such as milrinone or dobutamine. Infusion rates of dopamine needed to improve signs of severe myocardial dysfunction may be associated with tachycardia, dysrhythmia, and increased myocardial oxygen consumption, and these adverse effects may outweigh any improvement in myocardial perfusion.

Adverse Effects

The clinical signs of dopamine toxicity are mainly cardiovascular: tachycardia, hypertension, and dysrhythmia. However, dopamine is less likely to produce severe tachycardia or dysrhythmias than either epinephrine or isoproterenol.[117] With the possible exception of the bipyridines, all inotropes increase myocardial oxygen consumption because they increase myocardial work. If the resulting increase in oxygen consumption is balanced by improved coronary blood flow, the net effect on oxygen balance is beneficial. The effect of dopamine on myocardial oxygen balance is better than that of isoproterenol, but not as good as dobutamine, and milrinone.[118] In the setting of cardiogenic shock, the improvement in myocardial contractility with the addition of an inotrope may reduce preload and afterload, improve coronary perfusion pressure, increase myocardial oxygen supply, and prolong diastolic coronary perfusion by reducing heart rate. If the same drug is administered to a patient with normal myocardial contractility, the result may be an increase in cardiac oxygen consumption without an increase in oxygen delivery to the myocardium. Tachycardia, due to both increasing oxygen consumption and shortening diastole, is a particular burden.

Dopamine depresses the ventilatory response to hypoxemia and hypercarbia by as much as 60%.[119] Dopamine (and other β agonists) decrease PaO_2 by interfering with hypoxic vasoconstriction.[120] In one study, dopamine increased intrapulmonary shunting in patients with acute respiratory distress syndrome (ARDS) from 27% to 40%.[121] The effect of dopamine on perfusion to the splanchnic bed is widely debated. Evidence suggests that in patients with sepsis dopamine may increase splanchnic blood flow and gastric pH and lead to less lactate production than epinephrine.[122-125] Dopamine may also increase oxygen delivery and reduce oxygen consumption in septic patients.[126,127] On the other hand, experiments in

animals suggest that dopamine is capable of modulating cellular immune functions in sepsis and may decrease survival. In a murine model, survival in dopamine-treated septic animals decreased by nearly 40%.[128] An increase in splenocyte apoptosis and decrease in splenocyte proliferation and IL-2 release, both of which indicate attenuated immune system function, were also observed.

In infants and children who have undergone cardiac surgery, dopamine may have several endocrinologic effects including decreases in prolactin and thyrotropin levels, as well as a reduction in the pulsatility of growth hormone.[89]

In patients with shock, dopamine can cause or worsen limb ischemia, gangrene of distal parts and entire extremities, and extensive loss of skin.[129] This is due to release of norepinephrine from synaptic terminals and in vivo conversion to norepinephrine. Hence, it is more often associated with limb ischemia than other adrenergic compounds. Extravasations of dopamine should be treated immediately by local infiltration with a solution of phentolamine (5–10 mg in 10 mL of normal saline solution) administered with a fine hypodermic needle.[130]

Preparation and Administration

Dopamine hydrochloride is available as premixed solutions in 5% dextrose or normal saline for infusion.[71] The use of standard concentrations and electronic "drip calculators"[131] is encouraged to prevent dosing errors. Dopamine is administered by central vein to avoid the risk of skin injury from extravasation, although it can be given safely through a peripheral intravenous catheter while central access is being secured. Dopamine may also be administered via the intraosseous route.[132] Table 33.3 provides information regarding compatibility.[133,134] Dopamine is not compatible with some of the 3-in-1 solutions used for parenteral nutrition or with sodium bicarbonate.[135] Dopamine is stable in solution for 24 to 84 hours.[136,137]

Interactions

Dopamine is metabolized by MAO, and concurrent use of an MAO inhibitor potentiates its effect.[77] In this rare circumstance, the initial dosage of dopamine should be reduced to one-tenth the usual dosage.[138] Both α-adrenergic blockers and β-adrenergic blockers antagonize the effects of dopamine. Other dopamine antagonists such as metoclopramide or haloperidol also may attenuate its effects. An increase in the infusion rate will often overcome the receptor blockade.

Summary

Dopamine is used to treat mild to moderate cardiogenic or distributive (septic, hypoxic-ischemic) shock associated with moderate degrees of hypotension. In the absence of hypotension, acute severe cardiac failure is treated with dobutamine or milrinone. When septic or cardiogenic shock is complicated by severe hypotension, epinephrine or norepinephrine is preferred, depending on hemodynamics and myocardial function (Table 33.4).

Norepinephrine

Basic Pharmacology

Dopamine is hydroxylated at the β carbon to produce norepinephrine, the principal neurotransmitter of the sympathetic nervous system (Figs. 33.8 and 33.9). Because there is no substituent on the N (amino)-terminus, norepinephrine has little

TABLE 33.3 Compatibility of Vasoactive Drugs With Commonly Used Continuous Infusions

PEDIATRIC INTENSIVE CARE UNIT CONTINUOUS INFUSION COMPATABILITIES

	Aminophylline	Cisatracurium	Dexmedetomidine	Dobutamine	Dopamine	Epinephrine	Fentanyl NYLI	Furosemide	Heparin	Isoproterenol	Lidocaine	Lorazepam	Midazolam	Milrinone	Norepinephrine[a]	Vasopressin	Vecuronium
Aminophylline	■	C/I	C	I	C	I	C	C	C	I	C	C	I	C	I	C	C
Cisatracurium	C/I	■	C	C	C	C	C	I	C/I	C	C	C	C	C	C	C	NT
Dexmedetomidine	C	C	■	C	C	C	C	C	C	C	C	C	C	C	C	C	C
Dobutamine	I	C	C	■	C	C	C	I	C	C	C/I	C	C/I	C	C	C	C
Dopamine	C	C	C	C	■	C	C	C/I	C	C	C	C	C/I	C	C	C	C
Epinephrine	I	C	C	C	C	■	C	C	C	C	C/I	C	C	C	C	C	C
Fentanyl	C	C	C	C	C	C	■	C	C	C	C/I	C	C	C	C	C	C
Furosemide	C	I	C	I	C/I	C	C	■	C	C/I	C	C	I	I	C	C	I
Heparin	C	C/I	C	C	C	C	C	C	■	C	C	C	C	C	C	C	C
Isoproterenol	I	C	C	C	C	C	C	C/I	C	■	C/I	C	C	C	NT	C	C
Lidocaine	C	C	C	C/I	C	C/I	C/I	C	C	C/I	■	C	C	I	C/I	C	C
Lorazepam	C	C	C	C	C	C	C	C	C	C	C	■	C	C	C	C	C
Midazolam	I	C	C	C/I	C/I	C	C	I	C	C	C	C	■	C	C	NT	C
Milrinone	C	C	C	C	C	C	C	I	C	C	I	C	C	■	C	C	C
Norepinephrine[a]	I	C	C	C	C	C	C	C	C	NT	C/I	C	C	C	■	C	C
Vasopressin	C	C	C	C	C	C	C	C	C	C	C	C	NT	C	C	■	C
Vecuronium	C	NT	C	C	C	C	C	I	C	C	C	C	C	C	C	C	■

[a]Norepinephrine = More stable in D5W at higher concentrations because of its high level of acidity (pH 3).
C, compatible; C/I, may be unstable at higher concentrations of additives; C/NS, this combination is more stable in normal saline solution (NS) than in D5W because of an exothermic reaction; I, incompatible.
From Trissel LA. Handbook on Injectable Drugs. 15th ed. Bethesda, MD: American Society of Health-System Pharmacists; 2009.

TABLE 33.4   Selecting Inotropic and Vasopressor Agents for Specific Hemodynamic Disturbances in Children

Hemodynamic Pattern	BLOOD PRESSURE OR SVR		
	Normal	Decreased	Elevated
Septic Shock			
Stroke index ↑ or ↔		Norepinephrine	
Stroke index ↓	Dobutamine or dopamine	Dopamine or epinephrine (or dobutamine and norepinephrine)	Dobutamine plus vasodilator and/or PDIII inhibitor
Cardiogenic shock	Dobutamine or dopamine or PDIII inhibitor	Dopamine or epinephrine	Dobutamine plus vasodilator and/or PDIII inhibitor
Myocardial dysfunction[a] (complicating critical illness)	Dobutamine or dopamine or PDIII inhibitor	Dopamine or epinephrine	Dobutamine plus vasodilator and/or PDIII inhibitor
Congestive heart failure	Dobutamine or dopamine or PDIII inhibitor		Dobutamine plus vasodilator and/or PDIII inhibitor
Bradycardia		Isoproterenol	

[a]For example, acute respiratory distress syndrome or anthracycline therapy.
PDIII inhibitor, milrinone; *SVR,* systemic vascular resistance.
Modified from Notterman DA. Pharmacologic support of the failing circulation: an approach for infants and children. Prob Anesth. 3:288.

β_2 activity and is considerably less potent at that receptor than epinephrine.[77] It is a moderately potent α and β_1 agonist.

Clinical Pharmacology

In normal subjects, norepinephrine elevates systemic vascular resistance (SVR) because α-adrenergic stimulation is not opposed by β_2 stimulation.[77] Reflex vagal activity reduces the rate of sinus node discharge, thereby blunting the expected β_1 chronotropic effect. In normal subjects renal, splanchnic, and hepatic blood flows decrease. The increase in afterload may augment coronary blood flow. This effect may be enhanced by α-adrenergic receptors located in the coronary arteries, although in coronary arteries from explanted human hearts, the vasodilatation in response to norepinephrine was mediated via β_2 receptors.[139] Norepinephrine does have inotropic effects on the heart, mediated via α_1 and β_1 receptors. The proportion of inotropic response related to α_1 stimulation may be affected by the pressure load on the right ventricle.[140] In the failing heart, the relative contribution from each type of adrenergic receptor appears to be equal.[141] In the isolated rat heart, the inotropic effects of norepinephrine are diminished in the presence of a nitric oxide synthetase inhibitor but restored when a nitric oxide donor is present.[142] In healthy volunteers norepinephrine produces a decrease in creatinine clearance because of the effect on renal blood flow; however, in patients with hypotension, the improvement in global perfusion produces an increase in urine output.[143]

The acute hemodynamic effects of norepinephrine are compared with those of epinephrine and isoproterenol in Fig. 33.10. Experience in critically ill children indicates that the hemodynamic responses are not different from those observed in adults. Use of norepinephrine in 18 neonates with persistent pulmonary hypertension–associated heart dysfunction produced significant increases in systemic blood pressure (33 ± 4 to 49 ± 4 mm Hg; $P <.05$) and LV output (172 ± 79 to 209 ± 90 mL/kg/min; $P <.05$), along with improvement in postductal transcutaneous oxygen saturation ($89\% \pm 1\%$ to $95\% \pm 4\%$; $P <.05$), pulmonary-to-systemic blood pressure ratio (0.98 ± 0.1 to 0.87 ± 0.1; $P <.05$),

and a 20% increase in the velocity of pulmonary artery blood flow ($P <.05$).[144] In a separate study in 22 neonates with septic shock refractory to fluid support and dopamine or dobutamine, norepinephrine (mean infusion rate 0.5 ± 0.4 µg/kg/min) significantly increased mean arterial blood pressure (36 ± 5 to 51 ± 7 mm Hg; $P <.001$) and urine output (1 ± 0.5 to 1.7 ± 0.4 mL/kg/hr; $P <.05$) while decreasing blood lactic acid concentrations (4.8 ± 2.3 to 3.3 ± 1.8 mmol/L; $P <.01$).[145]

Pharmacokinetics

Basal plasma levels of norepinephrine are much higher than basal plasma levels of epinephrine (250–500 vs. 20–60 pg/mL). The minimum concentration at which norepinephrine produces detectable hemodynamic activity is at least 1500 to 2000 pg/mL, suggesting that endogenous plasma norepinephrine simply represents "spillover" from sympathetic activity and that norepinephrine is not a true hormone.[146] The clearance of norepinephrine in healthy adults is 24 to 40 mL/kg/min, with the half-life averaging 2 to 2.5 minutes.[147] The clinical effect of norepinephrine ceases within 2 minutes of the infusion being stopped.[147] Little pharmacokinetic information in children is available. Norepinephrine is inactivated by reuptake into nerve terminals, with some elimination occurring by enzymatic degradation in the liver, adrenal glands, and kidney, either by methylation to normetanephrine (by COMT) or by oxidative deamination.[148] Most of the metabolites formed by either MAO or COMT are then reduced or oxidized further. 3-Methoxy-4-hydroxymandelic acid is the major metabolite in the urine.[77]

Clinical Role

Norepinephrine improves perfusion in children with low blood pressure and a normal or elevated cardiac index. Distributive or septic shock is the usual context in which norepinephrine is beneficial. Norepinephrine is administered in conjunction with repletion of intravascular volume and is best guided by estimates of cardiac output and SVR. The experience in adult patients provides a rationale for using this agent to

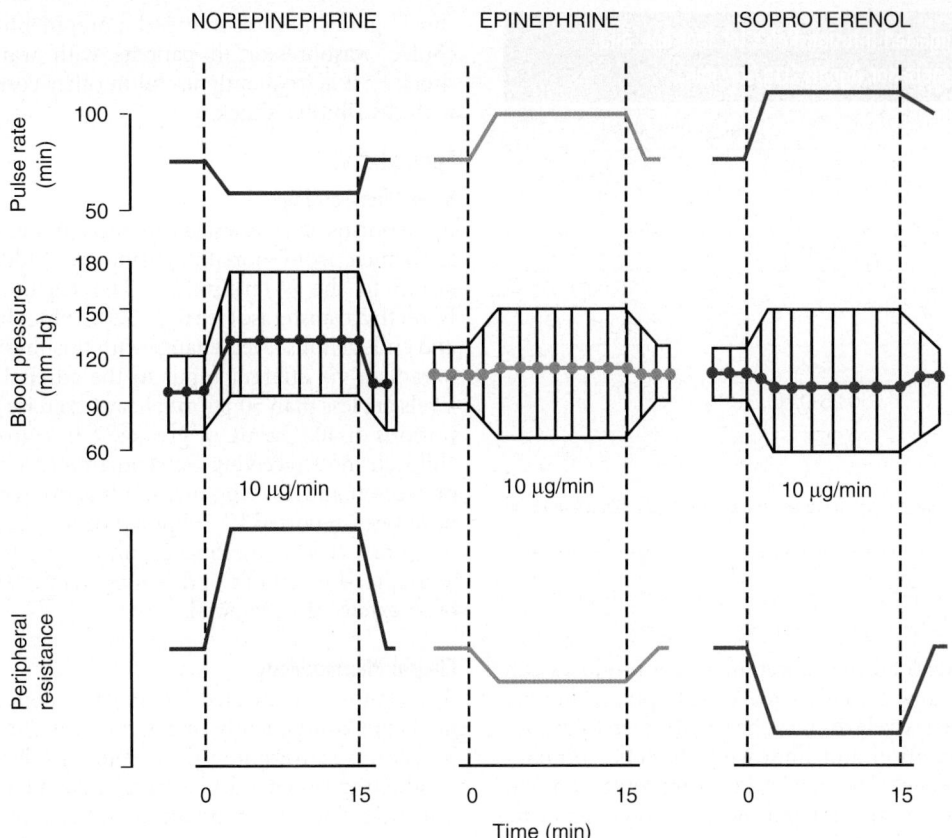

Fig. 33.10 Effects of intravenous infusion of norepinephrine, epinephrine, and isoproterenol in adult humans. (Modified from Allwood MJ, Cobbold AF, Ginsberg J. Peripheral vascular effects of noradrenaline, isopropylnoradrenaline and dopamine. Br Med Bull. 1963;19:132.)

treat hypotension that is unresponsive to volume reple-tion,[149-152] and norepinephrine is now a recommended agent for warm shock refractory to fluid loading in children as well.[114,153] A prospective, unblinded randomized study (in adults) indicates that high-dose norepinephrine is superior to high-dose dopamine for treating hypotension and other hemodynamic abnormalities associated with hyperdynamic septic shock.[154] Others have reported that lower average dosages (0.4 μg/kg/min) were effective in adults with sepsis.[155] Coronary and renal blood flow increased in lambs at a dose of 0.4 μg/kg/min while mesenteric blood flow decreased.[156] Thus titration is important and may entail fairly rapid escalation of dosage. One of several studies in children with septic shock treated with norepinephrine suggested that higher doses might be necessary in this population to restore adequate blood pressures and perfusion. A single-center retrospective review of 144 children with septic shock treated with norepinephrine between 2000 and 2010[157] reported a decrease in mortality from 82% to 17% over the study period and an associated increase in norepinephrine use. Mean doses ranged from 0.5 mcg/kg/min to 2.5 mcg/kg/min. The only complications observed were arrhythmias (not requiring treatment) in two patients and hypertension, which resolved with lowering of the norepinephrine dose. Notably, the authors reported no complications in 27 patients receiving the drug through a peripheral intravenous catheter for periods as long as 3 hours. Though the findings from this study suggest that norepinephrine is safe and effective for reversal of hypotension and hypoperfusion in

the context of septic shock, the authors caution that prospective studies are necessary to determine when and how norepinephrine should be used in this patient population.

Norepinephrine produces increases in SVR, arterial blood pressure, and urine flow. It is most valuable in the context of tachycardia because unlike dopamine at doses required to induce a vasopressor effect, norepinephrine does not produce significant elevation and may even lower heart rate through reflex mechanisms. In a study of adults with abdominal sepsis, norepinephrine infusion was associated with increases in systemic blood pressure and SVR. Stroke volume increased as heart rate declined. Cardiac index did not change, although creatinine clearance increased substantially.[155] Norepinephrine has also been shown to improve right ventricular (RV) performance in adults with hyperdynamic septic shock.[154]

The usual starting dosage for an infusion is 0.1 μg/kg/min (Table 33.5), with a goal of elevating perfusion pressure so that the flow to vital organs is above the threshold needed to meet metabolic requirements.[158] Arbitrary values of SVR or blood pressure are not appropriate end points for therapy, and the lowest infusion rate that improves perfusion as judged by clinical indices such as skin color and temperature, mental status, urine flow, and reduction in plasma lactate level should be used.[159]

Other causes of distributive shock (eg, vasodilator ingestion, intoxication with CNS depressants) also respond to norepinephrine when the predominant hemodynamic problem is low SVR and blood pressure.

TABLE 33.5 Suggested Infusion Rates for Inotropic and Vasopressor Agents (μg/kg/min)

Agent	CLINICAL INDICATION	
	Inotropic	Pressor
Dopamine	2-15	>12
Epinephrine	0.05-0.5	0.10-1
Norepinephrine		0.05-1
Vasopressin		0.0005-0.002[a]
Dobutamine	2.5-20	
Milrinone[b]	0.25-0.75	
Isoproterenol	0.05-1	

[a]Units/kg/min.
[b]The optimal dosage and infusion rates have not been established in children.

Adverse Effects

The increase in afterload that norepinephrine produces can potentially increase myocardial oxygen consumption, but norepinephrine may reflexively decrease heart rate, thereby reducing oxygen consumption and improving diastolic coronary perfusion.[77] Norepinephrine may lead to compromised organ blood flow in the setting of hypovolemia. Norepinephrine infusion may elevate blood pressure yet not improve clinical indices of perfusion. Poor clinical response is usually associated with a low cardiac index, stroke volume, LV stroke work index, and an elevated pulmonary artery occlusion pressure.[149,150] Employing excessive dosages or using norepinephrine to elevate blood pressure without improving perfusion may result in multiple organ system failure.

Preparation and Administration

See Table 33.3 for information regarding compatibility. Norepinephrine bitartrate is available in 4-mL ampules at a concentration of 1 mg/mL.[147] Norepinephrine should be diluted in 5% dextrose or 5% dextrose in 0.9% sodium chloride for preparation of infusions. Norepinephrine is administered only by central venous catheter, except in extreme emergency. Extravasation of norepinephrine should be treated immediately by local infiltration with a solution of phentolamine (5–10 mg in 10 mL of normal saline solution) administered with a fine hypodermic needle.[130,147] As with dopamine, norepinephrine should be administered by a syringe pump or other device that permits controlled and precise titration.

Interactions

Tricyclic antidepressants potentiate the action of norepinephrine by reducing neuronal uptake of the compound.[147] MAO inhibitors do not appear to enhance the activity of infused norepinephrine. α-Adrenergic blocking agents reduce efficacy of norepinephrine.

Summary

Norepinephrine is the agent of choice when the principal hemodynamic disturbance involves hypotension with an abnormally low SVR and a normal or high cardiac output after fluid resuscitation (Table 33.4). The most recent septic shock guidelines recommend norepinephrine as the "first choice" vasopressor in patients with warm (vasodilatory) shock.[114] It is frequently useful in other conditions associated with distributive shock.

Epinephrine

Basic Pharmacology

Epinephrine is synthesized in the adrenal medulla where it is formed from norepinephrine by addition of a methyl group to the N-terminus.[117] The reaction is catalyzed by N-methyl transferase (see Fig. 33.9). Epinephrine is a hormone, and endogenous levels change with the physiologic state of the organism via afferent input to the adrenal medulla. Resting levels are less than 50 pg/mL; heavy exercise produces concentrations of 400 pg/mL or greater.[146] In a group of critically ill children not receiving catecholamines, epinephrine levels between 0 and 1378 pg/mL at admission (mean, 508 pg/mL) have been reported.[160,161] Epinephrine activates α, β$_1$, and β$_2$ receptors. It is a principal hormone of stress and produces widespread metabolic and hemodynamic effects, which have been extensively reviewed.[117]

Clinical Pharmacology

β$_1$ receptors are affected by very low concentrations of epinephrine; consequently, one of the early effects of epinephrine infusion is activation of β$_1$ receptors in the myocardium and conducting systems, which accelerates phase 4 of the action potential. The rate of sinoatrial node discharge and heart rate increase, and systolic time intervals are shortened. The inotropic state of the myocardium is also enhanced, producing an increase in force of contraction and rate of rise of pressure. Evidence indicates that myocardial oxygen consumption is out of proportion to the increase in force of contraction, decreasing myocardial efficiency.[117] High concentrations of epinephrine or exposure to the compound when the myocardium is sensitive because of infarction, operation, or myocarditis may produce serious atrial and ventricular dysrhythmias.[117]

At low plasma concentrations, stimulation of peripheral β$_2$ receptors promotes relaxation of resistance arterioles; SVR decreases and diastolic blood pressure falls (Fig. 33.10). The decrease in SVR enhances the direct chronotropic effect of epinephrine. Higher concentrations are associated with activation of vascular α receptors, and SVR increases. The effect of epinephrine on the pulmonary vasculature may also vary as a result of the dosage used.[162] Higher doses are also associated with an increase in pulmonary vascular resistance (PVR), both from a direct effect and as a result of increased venous return to the right side of the heart.[117] During infusion of epinephrine, hepatic and splanchnic blood flow increase, while renal blood flow may be reduced.[117]

The thresholds for producing these effects in healthy adults have been examined.[146] Normal basal levels are around 40 pg/mL. Heart rate accelerates between 50 and 100 pg/mL; changes in blood pressure (systolic blood pressure increases, diastolic blood pressure decreases) occur between 75 and 100 pg/mL. Various metabolic effects (hyperglycemia, cytogenesis, and glycolysis) occur between 150 and 200 pg/mL. Concentrations of this magnitude are achieved during therapeutic infusion of the drug. Other metabolic effects include hypophosphatemia and hypokalemia. Desensitization to elevated levels of epinephrine occurs rapidly and may be present before administration of exogenous catecholamines in the ICU.

Pharmacokinetics

In healthy male volunteers the plasma clearance of epinephrine is 35 to 89 mL/kg/min.[163,164] The elimination half-life is approximately 1 minute.[104] Epinephrine is methylated by COMT to metanephrine in the liver and kidneys or deaminated via the action of MAO.[72] It also may be metabolized by extraneuronal uptake.[148] The resulting catabolites are then conjugated to sulfate or glucuronide and excreted in the urine. A wide interindividual variation in clearance is observed in healthy adults. In critically ill children receiving epinephrine at doses from 0.03 to 0.2 µg/kg/min, plasma concentrations at steady state ranged from 0.67 to 9.4 ng/mL and were linearly related to dose.[161] In this study, clearance ranged from 15 mL/kg/min to 79 mL/kg/min, demonstrating wide interindividual variation similar to dopamine. Variability between the ordered and the measured dose of catecholamines has also been observed.[165] Combined with the interindividual variation in clearance, there may be significant differences in plasma concentrations between patients receiving the "same" dose of epinephrine or dopamine.

Clinical Role

Epinephrine is employed to treat shock associated with myocardial dysfunction. Thus it is appropriate for treatment of cardiogenic shock or for inotropic support following cardiac surgery.[140] In a model of RV injury, epinephrine increased pulmonary artery blood flow and RV power with greater efficiency than did dopamine or dobutamine.[162] It can also be used to increase pulmonary flow across left-to-right shunts.[89] The patient with sepsis who continues to manifest cool extremities after intravascular volume repletion may benefit from an infusion of epinephrine. Epinephrine is most likely to be useful when hypotension exists in the context of a low cardiac index and stroke index ("cold shock").[112] At modest infusion rates (0.05–0.1 µg/kg/min), SVR decreases slightly; heart rate, cardiac output, and systolic blood pressure increase. At intermediate infusion rates, α_1-adrenergic activation becomes important but is balanced by the improved cardiac output and activation of vascular β_2 receptors. Even though epinephrine constricts renal and cutaneous arterioles, renal function and skin perfusion may improve. Very high infusion rates (more than 1–2 µg/kg/min) are associated with significant α_1-adrenergic–mediated vasoconstriction; blood flow to individual organs will be compromised, and the associated increase in afterload may further impair myocardial function. The effects of epinephrine on splanchnic blood flow continue to be investigated. Studies have shown decreased splanchnic blood flow, decreased oxygen uptake, and increased lactate with epinephrine compared with norepinephrine despite similar increases in global oxygen delivery.[166] Dopamine led to a decrease in lactate and an increase in arterial pH, whereas epinephrine was associated with increases in lactate and metabolic acidosis despite similar increases in cardiac index and oxygen delivery.[122] At a dose of 3.2 µg/kg/min in newborn piglets, epinephrine increased SVR and PVR, with a decrease in hepatic blood flow and oxygen delivery and an increase in lactate.[167] These effects were likely the result of the high dosages used and impaired hepatic utilization of lactate. Seguin and colleagues[168] demonstrated increased gastric blood flow with epinephrine compared with the combination of norepinephrine and dobutamine. They note that the doses of norepinephrine they used were higher than in previous studies. Other studies have shown that the degree of shock also may influence splanchnic blood flow.[169] In a study involving adult patients with septic shock, stepwise infusion of epinephrine was associated with linear increases in cardiac rate, mean arterial pressure, cardiac index, LV stroke work index, oxygen consumption, and oxygen delivery. In that study, neither pulmonary nor systemic vascular resistance was affected by epinephrine infusion.[79] Epinephrine is first-line treatment for severe anaphylaxis in both the prehospital and hospital settings. Although controlled studies cannot ethically be conducted, the case-fatality rate from food-related anaphylaxis has declined since the introduction of the epinephrine autoinjector.[170]

Epinephrine has been evaluated in very low-birth-weight infants with hypotension that did not respond to dopamine at doses as high as 15 µ/kg/min.[171] Blood pressure and heart rate increased while urine output was maintained. In fact, urine output increased among infants who had been oliguric.

Epinephrine is the most frequently used medication during pediatric cardiopulmonary resuscitation. Bolus injections of epinephrine are used to treat hemodynamically significant bradycardia, asystole, and pulseless arrest. Earlier studies in animals[172,173] demonstrated improved survival after primary cardiac arrest in subjects treated with epinephrine. This was attributed to higher rates of return of spontaneous circulation associated with improved coronary (and therefore myocardial) perfusion from an increase in aortic diastolic pressure. A study in adults following cardiopulmonary arrest attributed to ventricular fibrillation showed that early use of epinephrine was associated with improved survival to hospital discharge, while later initiation of the drug was not.[174,175] The recommended initial dosage is 0.01 mg/kg (10 µg/kg or 0.1 mL/kg of the 1:10,000 solution).[176] High-dose epinephrine (1:1000 concentration) is no longer recommended after clinical trials in adults and children comparing high-dose with standard-dose epinephrine showed no benefit in return of spontaneous circulation and possible decrease in 24-hour survival associated with the higher dose.[177-179]

Epinephrine may be given by endotracheal tube; the dosage is 100 µg/kg. Intraosseous administration is appropriate for both bolus and continuous administration of epinephrine. The dosage is the same as for IV injection. Epinephrine by infusion is also the agent of choice for hypotension or shock following successful treatment of cardiac arrest. Shock following an episode of hypoxemia or ischemia is usually cardiogenic and often responds to epinephrine.

Preparation and Administration

Epinephrine for injection at a concentration of 1:10,000 injection may be administered undiluted. The 1:1000 injection must be diluted with 0.9% sodium chloride for injection before administration. For continuous infusion, epinephrine should be diluted to a standard concentration, often 4 µg/mL.[176] Epinephrine should be infused by a pump capable of precise titration (eg, syringe pump) into a central vein, although low-dose infusions may be administered safely via peripheral intravenous catheters if central venous access is not available. Consult Table 33.3 for compatibility information.

Adverse Effects

Epinephrine produces CNS excitation manifested as anxiety, dread, nausea, and dyspnea.[118] Enhanced automaticity and increased oxygen consumption are the main serious cardiac toxicities.[117] Extreme tachycardia carries a substantial oxygen penalty, as does hypertension. A severe imbalance of myocardial oxygen delivery and oxygen consumption produces characteristic electrocardiogram changes of ischemia. A subischemic but persistently unfavorable ratio of oxygen delivery to consumption may also be harmful to the myocardium. This has not been adequately examined in critically ill children. Epinephrine may be arrhythmogenic. Increases in infusion rate lead to successively more serious events, including atrial and ventricular extrasystoles, atrial and ventricular tachycardia, and, ultimately, ventricular fibrillation. Ventricular dysrhythmias in the pediatric age group are not common but may occur in the presence of myocarditis, hypokalemia, or hypoxemia. Hypokalemia is produced by the infusion of epinephrine through stimulation of β_2-adrenergic receptors, which are linked to sodium-potassium-ATPase located in skeletal muscle.[180] Infusion of 0.1 μg/kg/min lowered serum potassium by 0.8 mEq/L. Hyperglycemia results from β-adrenergic–mediated suppression of insulin release. Increases in blood lactate levels have also been observed.[181] Epinephrine is an α_1-adrenergic agonist, and infiltration into local tissues or intraarterial injection can produce severe vasospasm and tissue injury.[117] Concurrent activation of β_2 receptors by epinephrine limits vasospasm, and local injury to tissue is less frequent than with norepinephrine, dopamine, or vasopressin.

Epinephrine overdose is serious. Several neonates died when inadvertently subjected to oral administration of huge amounts of epinephrine.[182] The syndrome mimicked an epidemic of neonatal sepsis with shock and metabolic acidosis. Intraaortic injection in infants (per umbilical artery) produces tachycardia, hypertension, and renal failure. IV overdose of epinephrine is immediately life threatening. Manifestations include myocardial infarction, ventricular tachycardia, extreme hypertension (up to 400/300 mm Hg), cerebral hemorrhage, seizures, renal failure, and pulmonary edema. Bradycardia also has been observed. Manifestations of acute overdose are treated symptomatically. β-receptor antagonists such as propranolol are contraindicated (see later). Hypertension is treated with short-acting antihypertensives (eg, nitroprusside).

Interactions

Tricyclic antidepressants and antihistamines such as diphenhydramine may potentiate the effects of epinephrine; use of fluorinated anesthetic agents such as halothane may increase the frequency of ventricular dysrhythmia.[117,183–185] Administration of epinephrine with a β-adrenergic antagonist such as propranolol may be dangerous because of residual unopposed α_1 activity; the result can be severe hypertension and bradycardia terminating in asystole. The concomitant use of α- or β-adrenergic antagonists also may antagonize the therapeutic effects of epinephrine.

Summary

Epinephrine is useful in treating shock associated with myocardial dysfunction and hypotension. In pediatric critical care, the most frequent indications for epinephrine infusion are resuscitation from cardiogenic shock, septic shock associated with hypotension and reduced stroke volume, and shock following severe hypoxemia-ischemia (Table 33.4).

Isoproterenol

Basic Pharmacology

Isoproterenol is the synthetic N-isopropyl derivative of norepinephrine (see Fig. 33.8). The bulky N-terminal substituent confers β_1- and β_2-receptor specificity; the compound does not affect the α-adrenergic receptor. Thus the principal cardiovascular activities of isoproterenol relate to its inotropic, chronotropic, and peripheral vasodilator effects.[117]

Clinical Pharmacology

Isoproterenol enhances cardiac contractility and heart rate.[117] Peripheral vasodilatation produces a fall in SVR, augmenting the direct chronotropic action of the drug. Significant tachycardia ensues. Systolic blood pressure increases while mean and diastolic pressures fall (see Fig. 33.10). If they were normal before infusion of isoproterenol, mesenteric and renal perfusions fall; however, if the subject was in shock, then the increase in cardiac output associated with isoproterenol administration may result in an increase in blood flow to these tissues.[117] Isoproterenol increases myocardial demand for oxygen and decreases supply by reducing diastolic coronary filling. In patients whose intravascular volume is not replete, hypotension may complicate initiation of isoproterenol infusion.

Pulmonary bronchial and vascular bed β_2-adrenergic receptors produce bronchodilation and pulmonary vasodilatation, respectively.[186] For this reason isoproterenol by continuous IV infusion was employed as adjunctive therapy in children with refractory or rapidly worsening status asthmaticus.[49] Continuously nebulized albuterol and IV infusion of terbutaline have supplanted isoproterenol for this indication.

Isoproterenol has few important metabolic effects. Hyperglycemia is not usually observed, although the drug does promote release of free fatty acids. Isoproterenol infusion causes sympathetic neurons to release norepinephrine, producing an increase in plasma levels; however, this effect relative to the hemodynamic response to isoproterenol has not been studied.[148]

Pharmacokinetics

Isoproterenol is metabolized by COMT.[117] The plasma elimination half-life of isoproterenol is 1.5 to 4.2 minutes.[187,188] Information about therapeutic isoproterenol concentrations in critically ill patients is not available. In healthy volunteers, tachycardia and increases in stroke volume were observed at 50 pg/mL.[148]

Clinical Role

In the past, isoproterenol was used for a variety of indications, including septic shock and cardiogenic shock associated with myocardial infarction; however, the tachycardia and increased myocardial oxygen consumption associated with its use, as well as a more sophisticated understanding of the pathophysiology of shock, have limited the use of this compound to very few specific indications.

Isoproterenol may be used to treat hemodynamically significant bradycardia.[189] However, epinephrine is probably preferable.[158] When bradycardia results from heart block, placement of a pacemaker is definitive treatment, but isoproterenol may be used in the acute setting as a bridge to pacemaker placement. Bradycardia due to anoxia will respond to oxygen and improving gas exchange.

Preparation and Administration

Before administration, isoproterenol should be diluted with 0.9% sodium chloride or D5W to a standard concentration, often 4 µg/mL.

Adverse Effects

Adverse effects associated with isoproterenol include fear, anxiety, restlessness, insomnia, and blurred vision.[190] Other effects may include headache, dizziness, tinnitus, sweating, flushing, pallor, tremor, nausea, vomiting, and asthenia. Cardiovascular effects may include ventricular tachycardia and other ventricular dysrhythmias that may be life threatening. Isoproterenol may cause hypertension and also can cause severe hypotension.

Interactions

The concomitant administration of a halogenated general anesthetic such as halothane or an IV methylxanthine such as aminophylline may potentiate the adverse cardiovascular effects of isoproterenol.[190] Propranolol given before an operation to repair tetralogy of Fallot attenuates the response to isoproterenol postoperatively.[191] Although it is no longer used regularly in the treatment of asthma, isoproterenol decreases serum theophylline concentrations, and it may be necessary to increase theophylline dosage when isoproterenol therapy is initiated and reduce theophylline dosage when isoproterenol is discontinued.[192]

Summary

Isoproterenol is rarely used to treat children or adults. More selective β_2 agonists are safer to use and are preferred. In the acute setting, it may play a role in the treatment of symptomatic bradycardia.

Dobutamine

Basic Pharmacology

The structure of dobutamine, a synthetic catecholamine, resembles dopamine in that the β carbon is not hydroxylated. Unlike other catecholamines, there is a large aromatic substituent on the N-terminus. Like isoproterenol, dobutamine is administered as a racemate; (+) dobutamine is a strong β agonist and an α antagonist, and (−) dobutamine is an α agonist and a weak β agonist.[193] This blend of receptor activities allows dobutamine to deliver significant inotropic and usually trivial chronotropic and vasopressor activity.

Clinical Pharmacology

In adults with CHF, dobutamine increased cardiac index from 2.4 to 2.9 L/min/m, decreased LV end-diastolic volume, and increased the LV dP/dt.[194] Although renal function and urine output may improve as the increase in cardiac output fosters relaxation of sympathetic tone and improved perfusion, dobutamine did not improve indices of renal function compared with dopamine in critically ill patients.[195] Dobutamine improved RV systolic function and decreased PVR in piglets with RV injury.[162] In healthy children, dobutamine increased LV systolic function and relaxation.[196] In the newborn piglet, dobutamine increased superior mesenteric and renal artery blood flow after 60 minutes, increased cardiac index, and decreased SVR.[197] A threshold model with a log-linear dose-response relationship above the threshold has been demonstrated in critically ill term and preterm neonates and in

children between 2 months and 14 years of age.[105,198] In one small study, dobutamine infusion (10 µg/kg/min) was associated with increases in cardiac output (30%), blood pressure (17%), and heart rate (7%). The plasma concentration thresholds for these increases were 13, 23, and 65 ng/mL, respectively, demonstrating that dobutamine is a relatively selective inotrope with little effect on heart rate at customary infusion rates.[199] Somewhat greater thresholds for improved cardiac output were observed in a second group of children and in infants, but in all studies, dobutamine improved cardiac contractility without substantially altering heart rate unless high infusion rates were employed.[198,200] In a Cochrane analysis that compared dobutamine with dopamine in premature neonates with low systemic blood flow on the first day of life,[201] dobutamine produced a significantly greater increase in superior vena cava flow, whereas dopamine produced a significantly greater increase in mean blood pressure. In addition, dobutamine has been shown to increase cerebral blood flow velocity but not cerebral oxygen consumption in patients with septic shock.[202]

Pharmacokinetics

The plasma elimination half-life of dobutamine in adults is approximately 2 minutes.[104] CHF increases the volume of distribution. In adults with CHF the terminal elimination half-life ($t_{1/2}\beta$) of dobutamine has been reported to be 2.37 minutes, with an apparent volume of distribution of 0.2 L/kg and total body clearance of 2.33 L/min/m².[203] Reported clearance values in children have ranged from 32 to 625 mL/kg/min in one study and from 40 to 130 mL/min/kg in another.[107,199] Infusions in the range used clinically yield plasma dobutamine concentrations from approximately 50 to 190 ng/mL in children and adults.[199] The principal route of elimination is methylation by COMT, followed by hepatic glucuronidation and excretion into urine and bile.[117] 3-O-methyldobutamine also represents a major route of elimination for dobutamine, with up to 33% of the infused drug being eliminated as the sulfoconjugated compound.[204] Dobutamine is also cleared from the plasma by nonneuronal uptake. Some investigators have reported nonlinear elimination kinetics, but other data suggest that dobutamine's kinetics can be adequately described by a simple first-order (linear) model.[105,107,109,199]

Clinical Role

In adults dobutamine produces improvement in a variety of conditions associated with poor myocardial performance, such as cardiomyopathy, atherosclerotic heart disease, and acute myocardial infarction. Dobutamine has been used following surgery for myocardial revascularization, cardiac transplantation, and other procedures associated with postoperative myocardial dysfunction, although undesirable chronotropic effects have been recorded when it has been used after cardiac surgery.[205] It is not clear that septic shock is an appropriate context in which to use dobutamine, unless the primary disturbance is complicated by myocardial dysfunction. Although impaired myocardial performance can be demonstrated early in patients with septic shock, the main problem relates to regulation of vascular tone, and preferred agents are those that increase systemic vascular resistance. When ventricular dysfunction complicates clinical management, dobutamine may be a useful adjunct. In this context, dobutamine alone or in combination with dopamine has produced an increase in cardiac output, LV stroke work, and blood pressure.[65] As indicated in Table 33.4, dobutamine also can be combined with norepinephrine in treating the patient with myocardial dysfunction that is associated with hyperdynamic shock (eg, a child who has received a cardiotoxic agent to treat cancer and in whom septic shock subsequently has developed).

Several studies in infants and children demonstrate that dobutamine improves myocardial function in a variety of settings.[105,198,199] Stroke volume and cardiac index improve without a substantial increase in cardiac rate. SVR and PVR may decrease toward normal.[203] Dobutamine has been evaluated in children following cardiac surgery with cardiopulmonary bypass. In a study by Bohn and colleagues,[66] dobutamine enhanced cardiac output by increasing heart rate; indeed, tachycardia prompted discontinuation of the infusion in several patients. The expected fall in SVR was not observed in children who received the drug after cardiopulmonary bypass. The authors found no benefit compared with isoproterenol or dopamine. These differences between adults and children may be due to the fact that myocardial dysfunction and CHF are not characteristic of the circulatory status of many children undergoing repair of congenital heart disease. Unlike in adults, the indication for surgery involves abnormalities in cardiac architecture or circulatory anatomy. Berner and associates[206] found that children undergoing operations for mitral valve disease responded to dobutamine with an increase in stroke volume, whereas children with tetralogy of Fallot repair did not, and their cardiac output increased only through a higher heart rate. A more recent report by the same group indicated that following repair of tetralogy of Fallot, dobutamine did enhance cardiac output when it was combined with atrial pacing to increase heart rate. Isoproterenol without pacing provided a higher cardiac output than either dobutamine alone or dobutamine in combination with pacing.[207] Booker and colleagues[208] found that dobutamine and dopamine had equivalent inotropic effects in children following cardiac surgery. Specific indications for dobutamine in the pediatric age group include low output CHF and a normal to moderately decreased blood pressure (see Table 33.4). Typical examples include viral myocarditis; cardiomyopathy associated with use of anthracyclines, cyclophosphamide, or hemochromatosis (related to hypertransfusion therapy); or myocardial infarction (Kawasaki disease).

Dobutamine is *not* a first-line agent to treat low output states that are caused by intracardiac shunt or abnormal cardiac chamber structure. Although dobutamine is used following corrective or palliative cardiovascular surgery in the child, in the context of demonstrated or suspected myocardial dysfunction, milrinone is now considered by many to be the preferred agent for providing inotropy and afterload reduction, despite insufficient evidence of superior effectiveness in a recent meta-analysis.[209] Dobutamine may be of adjunctive value in treating myocardial dysfunction that complicates a primary condition such as ARDS or septic shock. Dobutamine is rarely used as the sole agent to treat compromised hemodynamics associated with sepsis, ARDS, or shock following a severe hypoxic-ischemic event.

Adverse Effects

Dobutamine usually increases myocardial oxygen demand. In subjects with myocardial dysfunction, coronary blood flow and oxygen supply improve with the increase in demand. However, if dobutamine is used when myocardial contractility is normal, oxygen balance will be adversely affected.[210] Tachycardia greatly increases oxygen use by the heart and should prompt a reduction in the dosage of dobutamine (or use of an alternate agent).

Although dobutamine is less likely than other catecholamines to induce serious atrial and ventricular dysrhythmias, these may occur, particularly in the context of myocarditis, electrolyte imbalance, or high infusion rates.[211] Dobutamine and other inotropes should be administered cautiously to patients with dynamic LV outflow obstruction (hypertrophic aortic stenosis). Prolonged infusion of dobutamine inhibits the second wave of adenosine diphosphate–induced platelet aggregation; in a few adult patients petechial bleeding attributed to dobutamine has developed.[212]

Preparation and Administration

Dobutamine is available as a premixed solution in a variety of concentrations. For information regarding compatibility, refer to Table 33.3. Therapeutic dosing ranges between 2.5 and 20 µg/kg/min. Consideration should be given to selecting an alternative agent (epinephrine) if the desired clinical effect cannot be achieved at a dose of 20 µg/kg/min.

Adverse Effects

Adverse cardiovascular effects may include hypertension, tachycardia, and ectopic heart beats. Dobutamine may also cause headache, nausea, vomiting, paresthesia, and dyspnea. Dobutamine may also decrease serum potassium concentrations.

Interactions

The concomitant use of a β-adrenergic antagonist such as propranolol may antagonize the cardiovascular actions of dobutamine.[213] Halogenated anesthetic agents such as halothane may potentiate the adverse cardiovascular effects of dobutamine. Dobutamine may increase the insulin requirement of diabetic patients.

Summary

Dobutamine is a positive inotropic agent that should be reserved to treat poor myocardial contractility. Following cardiac surgery, dobutamine may be used when contractility is abnormal. For septic shock and other acute hemodynamic disturbances, dobutamine is an adjunct when the primary problem is complicated by poor myocardial function (see Table 33.4). In this context, concomitant use of a vasopressor such as norepinephrine may be appropriate.

Vasopressin

Basic Pharmacology

Vasopressin is a highly conserved hormone, and vasopressin-like peptides are present in numerous species. Its main function is to preserve fluid balance in the organism. In humans, it is released in response to two main stimuli: increases in plasma osmolality and decreases in effective circulating volume or blood pressure. Although vasopressin has long been used for the treatment of diabetes insipidus, its name derives from its vasopressor effect. Vasopressin has a number of effects beyond volume regulation. It acts as a neurotransmitter in the CNS, has a role regulating adrenocorticotropin hormone release, and is involved in thermoregulation, platelet aggregation, and smooth muscle contraction in the uterus and gastrointestinal tract.[31,32]

Clinical Pharmacology

As noted previously, the response patterns are different for the two stimuli for vasopressin release. An increase in plasma osmolality above 280 mOsm/kg leads to a dramatic increase in the release of vasopressin from the posterior pituitary, and the hormone exerts its effect by increasing water reabsorption in the renal collecting duct. The dose/response curve is so steep that when osmolality is 290 mOsm/kg, vasopressin levels exceed those that produce maximal urinary concentration. In contrast, the threshold for release in response to hypovolemia or hypotension is much higher, with decreases of greater than 20% required. However, once the threshold is reached, plasma levels rise 20- to 30-fold (far exceeding levels seen with hyperosmolality).[32] Vasopressin exerts its hemodynamic effects via the V_{1a} receptor, which is coupled to G_q. In the peripheral vasculature, intracellular calcium is increased, enhancing contraction and restoring systemic vascular tone. Vasopressin also inhibits potassium channels, further increasing intracellular calcium.[44,214] Baroreceptors in the left atrium, left ventricle, and pulmonary veins sense changes in volume while baroreceptors in the carotid sinus and aorta sense changes in arterial pressure.[32] Decreased pressure leads to a reduced rate of firing and release of the tonic inhibition of vasopressin release.[31]

Vasopressin is a potent vasoconstrictor when present in the plasma at high concentrations. At the lower concentrations associated with the vasopressin response to hyperosmolarity, it actually induces vasodilation in the pulmonary, renal, and cerebral circulation via the V_2 receptor or oxytocin-mediated nitric oxide release.[215] It does not elevate blood pressure because an associated decrease in heart rate offsets the increase in systemic vascular resistance. For this reason, vasopressin was not originally considered to be a clinically useful agent to treat hypotension.[216] Landry and colleagues[217] measured plasma vasopressin levels in 19 patients with septic shock and 12 patients with cardiogenic shock (all receiving catecholamine support). Surprisingly, plasma levels of vasopressin were not elevated in patients with septic shock (mean 3.1 pg/mL; normal <5 pg/mL). Patients with cardiogenic shock had an expected mean level of 22.7 pg/mL. Vasopressin infusion (0.04 units/min intravenously) in 10 patients with septic shock who were receiving catecholamines produced an increase in systemic vascular resistance and mean arterial pressure, which was associated with a decrease in cardiac index. The resulting plasma level of vasopressin was 30 pg/mL, an appropriate concentration considering the level of hypotension. Therefore vasopressin plasma levels are inappropriately low in patients with vasodilatory septic shock, possibly because of impaired baroreflex-mediated secretion. The authors hypothesized that this phenomenon contributes to the hypotension of vasodilatory septic shock.

It appears that in the early stages of septic shock, vasopressin levels are higher than normal but decrease to either low levels or levels that represent a relative deficiency (normal level in the setting of hypotension) as shock continues.[218] This pattern has also been demonstrated in a model of hemorrhagic shock.[219] In this study, neurohypophysis stores of vasopressin were depleted. In three patients with septic shock and low levels of vasopressin, the high intensity signal from the posterior pituitary on T1-weighted magnetic resonance imaging was lost, suggesting depletion of vasopressin.[218] Hence vasopressin deficiency may occur early in vasodilatory shock and contribute to its pathogenesis.

Pharmacokinetics

Vasopressin circulates as a free peptide and does not exhibit any protein binding.[37] It is degraded rapidly in the kidneys and liver, with 5% to 15% of an IV dose eliminated unchanged in the urine.[138] Renal failure or hepatic insufficiency can prolong the elimination half-life.[220,221] The normal elimination half-life is 10 to 20 minutes.[138]

Clinical Role

The original report by Landry and colleagues[217] generated intense investigation into the clinical applications of vasopressin in the setting of vasodilatory shock. The same group prospectively evaluated vasopressin in patients with vasodilatory shock after placement of an LV assist device.[222] At a dose of 0.1 units/min, vasopressin increased mean arterial pressure and SVR but not cardiac index. Among patients with a high level of endogenous vasopressin, the increase in blood pressure tended to be less. A rapid response to vasopressin was noted in all patients, allowing for the dose to be decreased to as low as 0.01 units/min. This group also published experience with vasopressin in patients with septic shock and children after cardiac surgery.[223,224] In five patients with septic shock, vasopressin was given at doses ranging from 0.03 to 0.05 units/min. Again, blood pressure and SVR increased, allowing for discontinuation of catecholamine support in four patients. Vasopressin was used to treat 11 children with hypotension, on epinephrine infusions following cardiac surgery. At vasopressin doses ranging from 0.0003 to 0.002 units/kg/min, blood pressure increased within 1 hour, and the epinephrine infusion could be decreased in five of eight patients. Two patients who had echocardiographic evidence of poor function died. The remaining nine patients with vasodilatory shock survived and were discharged from the ICU. The authors cautioned against the use of vasopressin in patients with cardiogenic shock, in view of the potential effect on cardiac index. Vasopressin levels were measured in three patients, two of whom had an absolute deficiency and one had a relative deficiency. In adults, vasopressin deficiency (relative or absolute) was associated with shock following cardiopulmonary bypass. Hemodynamic function improved with vasopressin, and the need for other vasopressors decreased.[225] In a small double-blind randomized study, prophylactic vasopressin (0.03 units/minute) decreased the need for norepinephrine and decreased ICU length of stay in patients receiving angiotensin-converting enzyme inhibitors who underwent cardiopulmonary bypass.[226] In another small study ($n = 10$), patients admitted to a trauma unit with the diagnosis of septic shock were randomly assigned to placebo or vasopressin at 0.04 units/min if they remained in shock with catecholamine support.[227] In the treatment group ($n = 5$), systolic blood pressure and SVR increased. Other vasopressors were discontinued within 24 hours in patients receiving vasopressin; in only one patient in the placebo group was other vasopressor support discontinued. In a larger, prospective, randomized study, the combination of vasopressin and norepinephrine was evaluated versus norepinephrine alone in patients with catecholamine-resistant vasodilatory shock.[228] Vasopressin was given at a dose of 0.06 units/min. The patients in the vasopressin-norepinephrine arm had a lower heart rate and higher blood pressure, SVR, and cardiac index. They also had reduced requirements for norepinephrine; additionally, the norepinephrine group had a higher rate of new-onset dysrhythmias. Gastric perfusion was also better preserved in the vasopressin group.

In summary, in several studies of patients with vasodilatory shock, vasopressin has been shown to improve blood pressure, increase SVR, lessen the need for catecholamines, improve markers of myocardial ischemia, and improve urine output.[71,229-231] Published experience in pediatric patients with septic shock is still limited. Liedel and colleagues[232] published their experience with five patients, ranging in age from 2 weeks (a 23-week premature infant) to 14 years. Doses used were between 0.0006 units/kg/min and 0.008 units/kg/min (one patient was given 0.06 units/min). In four patients, blood pressure increased and catecholamine support could be decreased. In three patients, urine output improved. Few formal randomized trials of vasopressin in pediatric patients with septic shock or following cardiac surgery have been published to date. In a multicenter, randomized trial involving 69 pediatric patients with vasodilatory shock,[233] vasopressin (0.0005–0.002 units/kg/min) or placebo was added to open-label vasoactive agents. There was no difference in the primary end point of time to vasoactive-free hemodynamic stability (49.7 vs. 47.1 hours) or in any of the secondary outcomes, which included mortality, ventilator-free days, length of critical care unit stay, and adverse events. Ten deaths occurred in the vasopressin group and five in the placebo group (no statistical significance). It was concluded that low-dose vasopressin did not demonstrate any beneficial effects. Vasopressin also has been used as a vasopressor in children undergoing evaluation for brain death.[234] At a dose of 0.04 units/kg/h, blood pressure increased and α agonist support was decreased. No deleterious effect on organ function was noted.

Prior to the most recent (2015) guidelines, vasopressin was part of the Advanced Cardiac Life Support protocol for ventricular fibrillation in adults.[115] For children who experience cardiac arrest, the guidelines state that based on inconsistent results in adult patients, there is insufficient evidence to make a recommendation either for or against the use of vasopressin.[235] Mann and colleagues[236] published their experience with vasopressin during cardiopulmonary resuscitation in pediatric patients in a retrospective case series. In six events involving four patients, vasopressin was given at a dose of 0.4 units/kg after conventional therapy had failed to achieve restoration of spontaneous circulation (ROSC). In all six events, pulseless electrical activity was the initial rhythm, while at the time vasopressin was given, events were asystole, pulseless ventricular tachycardia, and ventricular fibrillation. In four cases, ROSC was achieved for more than 60 minutes. One patient survived to discharge and was in a condition close to her neurologic baseline. A review of the American Heart Association National Registry of Cardiopulmonary Resuscitation in children suggested a lower rate of ROSC and longer arrest duration in patients to whom vasopressin was administered during in-hospital resuscitation.[237] The authors emphasize that this result should be interpreted with caution, however, because vasopressin was only administered in 64 (5%) of the 1293 cases reviewed, and all of these patients had longer arrest times and were also pretreated with epinephrine.

Dosing and Administration

No standards for pediatric dosing currently exist. The American Heart Association guidelines for pediatric advanced life support[235] suggest a bolus dose of 0.5 units/kg. Standard dosing

for vasopressin in vasodilatory shock has not been determined, but the dose used in a recent pediatric study ranged from 0.0005 units to 0.002 units/kg/min.[233] Current guidelines for management of severe sepsis and septic shock in adults suggest vasopressin (0.03 units/min) may be added to norepinephrine to raise mean arterial pressure to target or decrease norepinephrine dose, but that it should not be used as the initial vasopressor.[114]

Adverse Effects

Few adverse events have been reported with the use of vasopressin in the setting of vasodilatory shock. Elevation of liver enzymes and total bilirubin with a decrease in platelet count has been noted, and one series in adults noted six cardiac arrests among 50 patients receiving vasopressin for hemodynamic support.[230,238] All six patients had "severe refractory shock," and five were receiving a vasopressin dose greater than 0.05 units/min. In 30% of patients receiving vasopressin, ischemic skin lesions of the distal limbs, trunk, or tongue were noted. Preexisting peripheral arterial occlusive disease and the presence of septic shock were identified as risk factors.[238] Extravasation of vasopressin from a peripheral IV catheter was associated with skin necrosis.[239] Treatment with vasopressin at doses used to augment blood pressures and improve hemodynamics may cause hyponatremia, which, in most cases, resolves with discontinuation of the drug.[213] Yet in a case series involving 10 neonates with severe persistent pulmonary hypertension of the newborn who were treated with vasopressin, 0.0002 units/kg/minute, in addition to nitric oxide, no significant decrease in serum sodium was observed.[240] The effect on sodium levels may be a function of patient selection, dose, and duration of treatment.

Interactions

The antidiuretic effect of vasopressin may be antagonized with concomitant administration of epinephrine, heparin, lithium, or demeclocycline.[138] Tricyclic agents, chlorpropamide, carbamazepine, clofibrate, phenformin, and fludrocortisone may exert additive antidiuretic effects when used in combination with vasopressin. Concomitant use of vasopressin with a ganglionic blocking agent can enhance the vasopressor effect of vasopressin.

Summary

Vasopressin has been added to the pediatric ICU practitioner's armamentarium for the treatment of decreased systemic vascular resistance. Its use may elevate blood pressure and urine output in patients with catecholamine refractory vasodilatory shock. Vasopressin should not be used in settings where impaired myocardial function is the principal problem. The optimal dose has yet to be determined, and the pharmacokinetics of the drug in conditions such as septic shock or after cardiopulmonary bypass need to be further investigated. It may have a more defined role in the future in pediatric advanced life support, but thus far, there is insufficient evidence to make a recommendation for or against the routine use of vasopressin during cardiopulmonary resuscitation from cardiac arrest.

Terlipressin

Basic Pharmacology

Terlipressin (N-α-triglycyl-8-lysine vasopressin) is a synthetic analogue of mammalian lysine vasopressin, while arginine vasopressin is endogenous to humans.[241] Following IV administration, the three glycyl groups on terlipressin are enzymatically cleaved by endopeptidases, resulting in prolonged release of the active lysine vasopressin moiety. This allows for a longer duration of vasoconstrictive action (4–6 hours) than that of arginine vasopressin (6–20 minutes)[241,242] and obviates the need for administration as a continuous infusion. The vasoactive effects of terlipressin are due in part to direct effects of the parent drug and are not solely a function of the liberated lysine vasopressin moiety.[243,244]

Clinical Pharmacology and Adverse Effects

Clinical trials in adults with refractory septic shock have demonstrated terlipressin to be a potent vasoconstrictor when administered as an IV bolus, with significant increases in SVR, mean arterial pressure, PVR, and urine output, along with reductions in catecholamine requirements and blood lactate levels.[242,245-247] However, adverse effects on myocardial function, including significant reductions in cardiac index, heart rate, oxygen delivery, and oxygen consumption have been observed, raising concerns about the drug's safety profile.

A limited number of trials in children with refractory septic shock suggest a similar pharmacodynamic profile as that observed in adults.[248-251] One retrospective study involving 14 children with septic shock refractory to fluids and vasopressors evaluated the addition of terlipressin IV boluses at an initial dose of 7 μg/kg twice daily, titrated up every 6 hours to a maximum dose of 20 μg/kg, based on blood pressure response.[249] Terlipressin was associated with significant increases in MAP (54 ± 3 to 72 ± 5 mm Hg; $P = .001$) at 10 minutes, and urine output (1.6 ± 0.5 to 4.3 ± 1.2 mL/kg/h; $P = .011$) at 1 hour after administration. A significant reduction in heart rate (153 ± 6.5 to 138 ± 7.5 beats/min; $P = .003$) at 12 hours was also noted. Terlipressin has also been used as a rescue medication in the setting of prolonged pediatric cardiopulmonary resuscitation.[252] In a study of eight episodes of cardiac arrest, terlipressin was administered to 7 infants and children aged 2 months to 6 years, with asystole, who failed to respond to conventional resuscitative measures. Return of spontaneous circulation was achieved in six of the eight episodes, with four patients surviving to discharge from the hospital.

Terlipressin is not currently licensed for use in the United States, and as of this writing, approval is not imminent.

Bipyridines

Inamrinone (formerly known as amrinone), milrinone, enoximone, and piroximone are nonsympathomimetic inotropic agents. The structure of milrinone, a noncatecholamine inotrope, is shown in Fig. 33.11. Inamrinone, the earliest formulation to be introduced, was associated with an increased risk of thrombocytopenia in both adults and children[253,254] and potentially fatal hypotension,[255] and it is no longer available in the United States. Neither of these complications has been observed with milrinone, which has become the bipyridine of choice.

The pharmacologic effects of the bipyridines result from selective inhibition of phosphodiesterase III and not from interaction with adrenergic receptors or inhibition of sodium-potassium ATPase.[53] These agents produce positive inotropic and lusitropic effects on isolated ventricular tissue, as well as relaxation of vascular smooth muscle. They are often used to

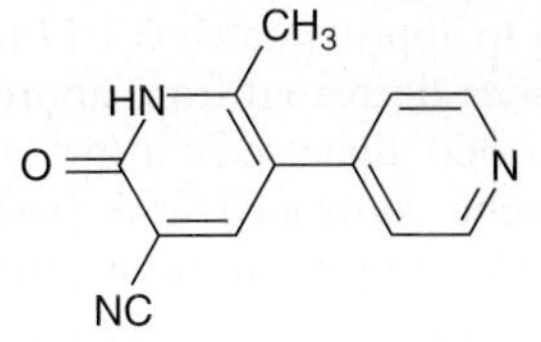

Fig. 33.11 Structure of milrinone.

improve myocardial contractility and decrease ventricular afterload.

Milrinone

Clinical Pharmacology

A derivative of inamrinone, milrinone shares the same mechanism of action and pharmacodynamic profile. In both adults and children, milrinone acts as an inotrope and vasodilator, producing a direct reduction in preload and afterload.[53,256] Administration to subjects with CHF results in increased cardiac index and reduced systemic vascular resistance, central venous pressure, and pulmonary capillary occlusion pressure,[257] while heart rate is not affected. Systemic hypertension is also reduced.[55,258,259] Patients experience a greater reduction in left and right heart filling pressures and SVR with milrinone than with dobutamine, even at equivalent contractility dosing.[260] Improvement in global hemodynamic function is associated with a more favorable ratio of myocardial oxygen delivery to consumption.[261] Blood pressure is usually maintained, even in the face of reduced SVR, because of the associated improvement in contractility and stroke volume. Increasing doses of milrinone have been shown to correlate with increasing mixed venous oxygen saturation (SvO_2).[262] Milrinone may improve contractility in patients who fail to respond to catecholamines and may further augment cardiac index in patients being treated with dobutamine. Caution is advised when administering milrinone to patients who are intravascularly volume depleted or in whom improvement in cardiac output does not occur, as hypotension may result.[263]

Animal models suggest that phosphodiesterase inhibitors are direct pulmonary vasodilators, even at doses lower than those that increase cardiac output.[264] Milrinone reduces PVR in children with intracardiac left-to-right shunts and elevated PVR, while in children with normal pulmonary pressure, a decrease in systemic but not pulmonary vascular resistance is observed.[265] PDE III inhibitors provide effective adjunctive therapy in the child with elevated pulmonary vascular resistance and reduced pulmonary blood flow. Milrinone has been used extensively following cardiac surgery in adults. When given perioperatively, milrinone attenuated decreases in gastric mucosal pH in patients undergoing coronary artery bypass grafting.[266] Splanchnic oxygenation improved and systemic levels of endotoxin and IL-6 were decreased. Although a cell culture study showed a possible increase rather than a decrease in proinflammatory markers in response to milrinone, serum levels of IL-1β and IL-6 in human subjects were decreased following cardiopulmonary bypass.[186,267] The decrease in IL-6 correlated inversely with levels of cAMP.

Several studies have evaluated milrinone in children following surgery for congenital heart disease. In one study, a loading dose of 50 μg/kg followed by a continuous infusion of 0.5 μg/kg/min was associated with mild tachycardia and a slight decrease in systemic blood pressure.[268] Cardiac index, however, increased from 2.1 to approximately 3.1 $L/min/m^2$, while SVR index and PVR index decreased from approximately 2100 to 1300 and 488 to 360 dyne-sec/cm^5/m^2, respectively. In a double-blind, placebo-controlled trial, high-dose milrinone (75 μg/kg bolus followed by continuous infusion at 0.75 μg/kg/min) was associated with a decreased incidence of low cardiac output syndrome.[90] Length of hospital stay was similar among the treatment groups, but prolonged stay (>15 days) was more common in the placebo arm. Milrinone has been shown to increase cardiac index and decrease systemic vascular resistance after the Fontan procedure.[90]

Milrinone also has been evaluated in children with nonhyperdynamic septic shock (ie, normal to low cardiac index and normal to elevated SVR). In a double-blind crossover study, milrinone increased cardiac index, stroke volume index, and oxygen delivery while decreasing SVR.[269] No differences in blood pressure or PVR were seen when milrinone was given at a dose of 0.5 μg/kg/min as a continuous infusion after a bolus dose of 50 μg/kg.

Pharmacokinetics

Milrinone is approximately 70% bound to plasma proteins, with approximately 85% renal elimination.[270] Hepatic glucuronidation accounts for a minor elimination pathway. In healthy adults, milrinone has an apparent volume of distribution of 0.32 ± 0.08 L/kg, clearance of 6.1 ± 1.3 mL/kg/min, and an elimination half-life of 0.8 ± 0.22 hours.[270] Both renal dysfunction and congestive heart failure affect the elimination profile of milrinone, extending the elimination half-life to approximately 2 hours.[271] In infants and young children undergoing cardiac surgery, the weight-adjusted clearance of milrinone was shown to increase with age, ranging from 2.6 mL/kg/min at age 3 months to 5.6 mL/kg/min at age 22 months.[272] In a separate study in infants and children (ages 1–13 years) following open heart surgery, milrinone clearance was significantly lower in infants than in children (3.8 ± 1 vs. 5.9 ± 2 mL/kg/min, respectively).[273] Importantly, the milrinone clearance values for both infants and children were significantly higher than those reported in adults following cardiac surgery (2 ± 0.7 mL/kg/min).[274] In the pediatric study just described, the plasma concentration versus time data fit a two-compartment model.[273] The apparent volume of distribution by area (Vβ), which reflects the volume of distribution during the terminal elimination phase, was not significantly different between infants and children (0.9 ± 0.4 vs. 0.7 ± 0.2 L/kg). However, the value reported for infants differed significantly from the value reported in adults following cardiac surgery (0.3 ± 0.1 L/kg).[274] In children with septic shock, the median half-life of milrinone was 1.5 hours.[275] Plasma levels did not correlate with changes in cardiac index or SVR. Milrinone clearance is significantly reduced in patients with acute renal dysfunction. A patient with acute renal failure may have as much as an eightfold increase in the serum level of milrinone when exposed to the same dosing regimen as patients with normal renal function.

Clinical Role

Milrinone augments cardiac contractility following cardiac surgery and improves perfusion in patients with "cold shock." Patients who respond with excessive vasodilation, as compared with inotropic effect, may be started on a low-dose catecholamine infusion to maintain target blood pressures. Milrinone's properties as a pulmonary vasodilator have made it a useful adjunct in the treatment of pulmonary hypertension.[276]

Preparation and Administration

Milrinone lactate is available in single-dose vials and as premixed solutions in 5% dextrose.[277,278] Loading doses may be drawn from a single-dose vial and administered undiluted over 15 minutes. A loading dose of 50 μg/kg is generally used in children.[268,272] For maintenance infusions, milrinone should be diluted with 0.45% or 0.9% sodium chloride or 5% dextrose to a final concentration of ≤200 μg/mL. Maintenance infusion rates are generally initiated at 0.5 μg/kg/min, titrated to clinical response. On the basis of the higher clearance and volume of distribution values previously discussed, Ramamoorthy and colleagues[273] suggested a loading dose of 104 μg/kg and initial maintenance infusion rate and 0.49 μg/kg/min, in infants, and 67 μg/kg and 0.61 μg/kg/min, respectively, in children. In patients not given a loading dose of milrinone, changes in cardiac index and plasma levels of milrinone after 3 hours were similar to those seen in patients who received a loading dose.[279] Milrinone is not compatible with furosemide but is compatible with a large number of drugs used in the pediatric ICU, including dopamine, epinephrine, fentanyl, and vecuronium.[280,281]

Adverse Effects

In a large pediatric study, serial measurements showed no difference in platelet count over time (baseline, 36 hours, 72 hours, and discharge) by treatment arm, and there was no difference in the incidence of thrombocytopenia (platelet count <50,000) during the study infusion (7.4% placebo, 8.8% low dose, and 2.6% high dose).[90] As previously stated, milrinone may cause hypotension in patients whose intravascular volume is not replete and in patients with renal dysfunction in whom drug clearance is reduced. Milrinone has been cited as a risk factor for early postoperative tachyarrhythmias in patients following congenital cardiac surgery. In one single-center prospective observational study of 603 patients following surgery for congenital heart disease, the incidence of early postoperative tachyarrhythmias was 50%.[282] Identified risk factors included age, cardiopulmonary bypass, aortic cross clamp time, and the use of milrinone at the time of admission to the cardiac ICU.

Summary

The bipyridines offer an attractive combination of positive inotropy with decreased systemic vascular resistance. They are useful in the short-term management of the infant and child with myocardial disease. Milrinone has an established role in the management of impaired cardiac contractility following cardiopulmonary bypass; its role in other settings has not been conclusively established by randomized trials.

Levosimendan

Basic Pharmacology

Levosimendan is a novel parenteral agent with inotropic and vasodilator properties that is classified as a calcium sensitizer.[283] Originally developed and marketed for inpatient management of acute decompensated heart failure in adults, it is now used in adults and children in the perioperative cardiac surgery setting, and case reports cite several additional applications. It is the R- (-) enantiomer of simendan and is a

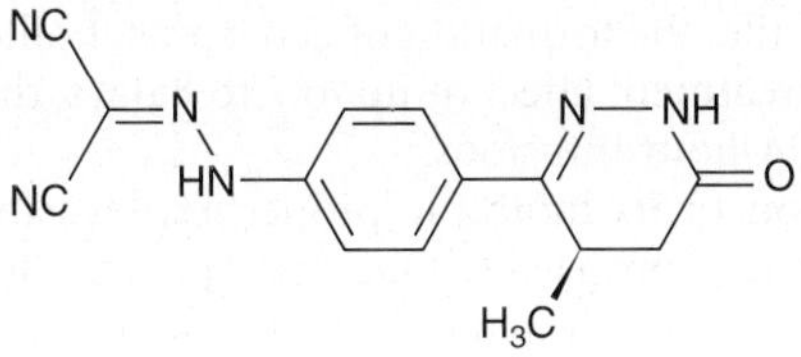

Fig. 33.12 Chemical structure of levosimendan.

pyridazole dinitrate derivative. The chemical structure (-)-(R)-([4-(1,4,5,6-tetrahydro-4-methyl-6-oxo-3-pyridazinyl)phenyl]-hydrazono) of propanedinitrile is shown in Fig. 33.12. The half-life of the parent compound is short, but the therapeutic effect is sustained for 7 to 9 days due to the formation of an active metabolite, OR-1896.[283-285] This allows levosimendan to be dosed weekly. No age or gender differences in efficacy or metabolism have been observed, and tolerance to the drug does not occur.[283,286]

Clinical Pharmacology

Classified as a cardioprotective inodilator, levosimendan displays three main clinical features: inotropy, vasodilation, and cardioprotection. It shares many of the functional properties of milrinone. As an inotrope, it acts by binding to calcium-saturated troponin C, stabilizing the calcium-bound conformation of troponin, thereby prolonging the actin-myosin interaction without altering cross-bridge cycling.[287-289] Unlike many inotropes, levosimendan does not increase intracellular calcium and therefore does not substantially increase the risk of arrhythmias or myocardial oxygen demand.[290,291] As with milrinone, phosphodiesterase III inhibition occurs, but at therapeutic doses, it is not the predominant mechanism via which levosimendan exerts its inotropic effects.[286,289]

As a vasodilator, levosimendan works by opening potassium-ATP channels on the sarcolemma of smooth muscle cells.[292,293] Hyperpolarization inhibits calcium channels and promotes sustained vasodilation, thus improving perfusion, in cardiac vessels, lungs, gastric mucosa, and the renal medulla.[294] Levosimendan also increases coronary blood flow by decreasing coronary vascular resistance[293,295] and through this mechanism may increase myocardial oxygen supply. Finally, levosimendan provides cardioprotection by opening mitochondrial potassium channels on cardiomyocytes.[287] These channels are said to be important mediators of ischemic preconditioning.[287,296] Although this theory has not yet been formally studied, this proposed cardioprotective property has led to the use of levosimendan preoperatively in patients at risk for myocardial ischemia during cardiac surgery on cardiopulmonary bypass.[297,298]

Levosimendan may also act as an antiinflammatory and antiapoptotic agent by decreasing proinflammatory cytokine production and downregulating NF-κ β-dependent transcription.[284,299]

Pharmacokinetics

The pharmacokinetics of levosimendan are linear at therapeutic dosages (0.05–0.2 μ/kg/min).[285] The relatively short half-life of the parent drug (approximately 1 hour) enables rapid onset of action, while the long elimination half-life of 70 to 80 hours of the active metabolite, OR-1896, in patients with heart failure allows for sustained activity.[285] Following IV administration, the majority of levosimendan is reduced via

glutathione to inactive metabolites and excreted in the urine as cysteineglycine and cysteine conjugates.[283,285] N-acetylated cysteineglycine conjugates are excreted in feces. Small amounts of levosimendan and its metabolites, OR-1855 and OR-1896, are eliminated unchanged in the urine. Approximately 6% of the drug is excreted into the small intestine and reduced by intestinal bacteria to an amino phenolpyridazinone metabolite (OR-1855) and then further metabolized by acetylation to the N-acetylated conjugate (OR-1896).[283] The maximal concentration of these two metabolites is observed approximately 48 hours after completing a 24-hour infusion. Small studies in children suggest the pharmacokinetics of levosimendan are similar to those in adults.[300,301] Pharmacokinetics are influenced by albumin levels and intestinal (bacterial) flora, as well as hepatic, renal, and gastrointestinal function.[283]

In patients with renal failure, the half-life of the active metabolites is prolonged 1.5-fold (to 94 to 97 hours) and the peak concentration and area under the concentration curve (AUC) are nearly twice that of patients with normal renal function.[284,302] Therefore caution is advised when treating patients with mild to moderate renal and hepatic dysfunction. Levosimendan is not recommended in patients with severe renal or hepatic failure.[294]

Clinical Role

Levosimendan was developed primarily as a parenteral inodilator for use in hospitalized adults with acute decompensated heart failure. In patients with severely elevated plasma brain natriuretic peptide (BNP), NT-proBNP (the promolecule), and endothelin 1 levels, treatment with levosimendan resulted in significant reductions in all three indicators.[303,304]

Use of levosimendan as a cardioprotective agent in adults and children undergoing cardiac surgery on cardiopulmonary bypass and in adults with heart failure undergoing noncardiac surgery is becoming more commonplace.[298,305,306] In adults with heart failure, when initiated before coronary artery bypass grafting, levosimendan was shown to prevent myocardial stunning and attenuate postoperative myocardial dysfunction.[298] Results from six phase IIb and phase III trials in Europe, comprising more than 3500 patients, comparing levosimendan with dobutamine in adults with acute decompensated heart failure, have been mixed. In one randomized trial[307] levosimendan demonstrated a significant mortality benefit at 28 days and at 6 months over dobutamine (8% vs. 17%), while results from another trial[308] failed to demonstrate reduced all-cause mortality at 180 days when levosimendan was compared with dobutamine. However, in this trial, levosimendan was superior to dobutamine when comparing morbidity in hospitalized patients. A 2012 meta-analysis by Landoni and colleagues[309] involving 45 studies and more than 5000 adult patients demonstrated a decrease in mortality and length of hospitalization when levosimendan was compared with dobutamine and placebo.

Case reports suggest levosimendan may improve myocardial function in sepsis and septic shock where cardiogenic shock is a major feature.[287,310] In postoperative and heart failure patients with renal dysfunction, levosimendan preserves renal function by improving renal blood flow and glomerular filtration rate through "preglomerular vasodilation."[294,311] The evidence for indications for levosimendan other than heart failure or perioperative cardiac and renal protection is anecdotal and limited to case reports and small, observational studies; large, randomized controlled studies have not been published.[312-314]

Although widely available in Europe for more than a decade, licensing of levosimendan in the United States was denied when the initial application was filed with the FDA in 1998, pending additional safety and efficacy data. Fast-track approval status was recently awarded to levosimendan for use in cardiac surgery patients at risk for low cardiac output syndrome pending results of a large industry-sponsored phase III trial.[298]

Currently, there are no official indications for levosimendan in patients younger than 18 years old, but published reports suggest it has been used as a rescue medication in more than 600 pediatric patients in the operating room and the PICU.[315,316] In one single-center study of 293 pediatric patients with cardiomyopathy or severe cardiac dysfunction following cardiac surgery, levosimendan as compared with milrinone was shown to delay the need for mechanical cardiac support.[316] In a second clinical trial, neonates undergoing cardiac surgery experienced an increase in cardiac index, while the group receiving milrinone demonstrated no change. Patients in the levosimendan group also had higher pH, lower blood glucose, and lower inotrope scores as compared with those on milrinone.[317]

Preparation and Administration

Levosimendan is marketed as a 2.5 mg/mL concentrated solution for IV infusion. The concentrate must be diluted with 5% dextrose solution to yield a final concentration of 0.025–0.05 mg/mL and should be used within 24 hours of preparation.[284] A loading dose of 6–12 µg/kg may be administered over 10 minutes before starting the continuous infusion if immediate effects are needed.[285] The lower bolus dosing should be used for patients who are receiving concurrent inotropic agents. Recommended dosing of the infusion ranges from 0.05–0.2 µg/kg/minute and is limited by the appearance of adverse effects.[307,318] Maximum infusion duration should not exceed 24 hours.[284,287] Caution should be taken in patients with renal and hepatic disease.

Adverse Effects

The most common adverse effects are hypotension, headache, palpitations, dizziness, tachycardia, atrial fibrillation, and hypokalemia.[311,319] Headache and hypotension are the direct result of vasodilation.[290] A clinically insignificant decrease in hemoglobin and erythrocyte counts has also been observed.[319] In adults with systolic blood pressures less than 100 mm Hg and/or diastolic pressures less than 60 mm Hg, use of levosimendan may increase mortality risk.[304]

Interactions

No significant drug interactions have been observed, but caution is advised when using levosimendan with agents that lower blood pressure. Unlike dobutamine (and other agents that employ β-adrenergic pathways), the effects of levosimendan are not attenuated by the coadministration of β-blocking agents.[307,320]

Summary

Levosimendan is a calcium-sensitizing agent with inotropic, vasodilator, and cardioprotective properties indicated for the short-term treatment of decompensated congestive heart failure in hospitalized patients. Although the parent drug has a short half-life, the formation of active metabolites confers a prolonged treatment effect of up to 7 to 8 days, thus allowing for weekly 24-hour infusions.

In addition to its inotropic properties, levosimendan has cardioprotective properties that have proven useful in the perioperative setting in patients at risk for ischemia and low cardiac output syndrome. Heart failure patients undergoing noncardiac surgery have also been pretreated with levosimendan with promising results.[306]

Although used extensively in adults and children in Europe for over a decade, the drug is not yet approved in the United States. There are no official indications for levosimendan in patients younger than 18 years of age.

Nesiritide

This once promising parenteral agent for the management of acute decompensated congestive heart failure is rarely used, due in part to cost, which approaches 40 times that of conventional therapies,[321] but more importantly because of concern over adverse effects. Studies comparing nesiritide with conventional therapy for decompensated heart failure did not find it to be superior, and a large meta-analysis[322,323] suggested a possible increased risk of renal dysfunction and mortality. As a result, the use of nesiritide rapidly declined,[324] and it is now indicated as a rescue medication in patients with life-threatening heart failure who do not respond to conventional therapy (eg, nitroglycerin, nitroprusside, milrinone, diuretics) or those in whom inotropic or chronotropic agents cannot be used due to the presence of arrhythmias.

Digitalis Glycosides

The role of digoxin in the acute care of critically ill children has always been limited by a narrow therapeutic index, slow onset of action, and the potential for life-threatening adverse effects. With the advent of new therapies for both the acute and chronic management of CHF and myocardial dysfunction, its role has further decreased. The practitioner in the pediatric ICU may still encounter patients receiving the drug, particularly for control of dysrhythmias. As is true for the catecholamines and other drugs discussed in this chapter, digoxin exerts its inotropic effects by increasing intracellular calcium.

Basic Pharmacology

Cardiac glycosides consist of a steroid moiety with one to four sugar molecules attached.[325] The number and composition of the associated sugar molecules affect the pharmacokinetics of the specific glycoside; all digitalis glycosides have similar pharmacodynamic properties. Glycosides bind to and inhibit sodium-potassium ATPase. Binding of digoxin to ATPase is affected by serum potassium. Hyperkalemia depresses digoxin binding, whereas hypokalemia has the opposite effect, accounting in part for potentiation of digoxin-induced dysrhythmias during hypokalemia.[326] As described earlier in this chapter, inhibition of ATPase produces an increase in intracellular calcium and enhances the inotropic state of the myocardium.

Clinical Pharmacology

In patients with CHF, the positive inotropic action of digoxin leads to increased cardiac output and reductions in filling pressures, edema, and sinus node rate. In a study of 10 adult patients with acute myocardial failure, a single dose of 10 μg/kg of digoxin produced a 69% increase in LV stroke work index, a 25% reduction in pulmonary capillary occlusion pressure, a 16% to 28% increase in cardiac index, and a 25% increase in stroke index within 2 hours of infusion.[327] Many of these changes were present within 60 minutes. In infants, digoxin is known to produce changes in echocardiographic measurements that are associated with an improved inotropic state, although detailed invasive hemodynamic measurements have not been made in infants or children.[10,200,327,328] When CHF is due to obstructive lesions or left-to-right shunts, it is more difficult to demonstrate benefit than when CHF is due to myocardial failure.

In patients with CHF who have a sinus rhythm, administration of digoxin produces a decrease in heart rate, likely because of improvement of the inotropic state and withdrawal of compensatory sympathetic activity. In addition, digoxin enhances vagal tone by increasing baroceptor sensitivity and directly stimulating central vagal centers,[326] which leads to direct slowing of heart rate, augmenting that produced by improved function. Another effect of digoxin-mediated enhanced vagal tone is slowed conduction of atrial impulses through the atrioventricular node to the ventricle. This property is exploited in use of digoxin to control or treat supraventricular tachycardia and atrial flutter or fibrillation. This aspect of digitalis pharmacology is reviewed in Chapter 35.

Use of digoxin in the pediatric ICU is further complicated by the large number of pharmacokinetic and pharmacodynamic interactions between digoxin and other pharmacologic agents used in critical care.[329] For example, carvedilol (a β-blocker) has been shown to decrease the elimination of digoxin in children, necessitating a reduction in digoxin dosage.[330] Toxicity is a major limiting factor in administering digitalis glycosides to critically ill patients. The most frequent side effects are gastrointestinal; the most serious are disturbances in cardiac rhythm.[10,325] Digitalis toxicity is reviewed in several of the references.[331,332] In adults and older children the dominant manifestations of digoxin toxicity are tachydysrhythmias such as ventricular premature contractions, ventricular tachycardia, and ventricular fibrillation. Atrial tachycardia and junctional tachycardia may also occur. Bradycardia and A-V conduction block are seen with acute, profound intoxication and in infants with enhanced vagal tone and diminished sympathetic activity, where the dominant findings are A-V conduction block and sinus bradycardia.

The risk of digitalis toxicity increases with factors that increase myocardial irritability, such as myocarditis, ischemia, hypoxemia, or catecholamine support. Hypokalemia and alkalosis also potentiate digoxin-induced dysrhythmias. Treatment of digoxin toxicity involves supportive treatment and correction of electrolyte disturbances.[333] Specific pharmacologic support (eg, with atropine, lidocaine, phenytoin, or magnesium sulfate) may be necessary (although frequently unsuccessful), and in life-threatening circumstances, treatment with digoxin-specific Fab antibody fragments is indicated.[334]

Pharmacokinetics

The dosage of digoxin prescribed for young children and infants is much higher than that applied to older children and adults. In the past, this disparity was ascribed to the incorrect belief that developmental immaturity was associated with decreased myocardial sensitivity to digitalis. It is now understood that neonates are not less sensitive to digoxin but eliminate digoxin more rapidly.[10] Clearance is dependent on age, although there is wide interindividual variation during the first year of life.[329] Thus infants may require higher loading ("digitalizing") and maintenance dosages to achieve therapeutically effective plasma concentrations of 1–2 ng/mL. Distribution of digoxin is relatively slow; therefore plasma levels will be misleadingly elevated if determined sooner than 6 hours following administration of a dose. At distribution equilibrium, the concentration of digoxin in the heart is 15 to 30 times greater than that in the plasma. In the nonacutely ill child, the half-life of digoxin is 36 hours with a clearance of 8.6 L/h.[40] Digoxin is eliminated through glomerular filtration and renal tubular secretion mechanisms, including the efflux pump, P-glycoprotein (P-gp). A polymorphism that decreases the activity of this enzyme was associated with increased serum digoxin levels.[335] Elimination is also strongly affected by renal dysfunction, complicating use of the agent in the critically ill child.

Clinical Role

The role of digoxin in the care of the pediatric patient continues to be refined and narrowed. Its role as an inotropic agent in the acute setting has been supplanted by other drugs (eg, milrinone) with a more favorable pharmacodynamic profile. Use of digoxin to improve cardiac function in children with systemic to pulmonary shunts has also decreased greatly, and it is used primarily now to control dysrhythmias and improve systolic function in children without structural lesions.[332] Because digoxin does not produce β-adrenergic receptor desensitization and has beneficial effects by virtue of decreased sympathetic activity, it continues to have a clinical role in the outpatient management of pediatric congestive heart failure.

Preparation and Administration

Digoxin is available in both parenteral and oral formulations. It may be administered undiluted, or it may be diluted with sterile water for injection, D5W, or 0.9% sodium chloride for injection. The injectable form must be diluted at least fourfold to avoid precipitation.

Adverse Effects

Cardiovascular adverse effects may include sinus bradycardia, atrioventricular block, ventricular tachycardia, and other dysrrhythmias.[329] Gastrointestinal adverse effects of digoxin include nausea, vomiting, anorexia, diarrhea, constipation, abdominal pain, and abdominal distension. Other effects may include visual disturbances, photophobia, headache, muscle weakness, fatigue, drowsiness, dizziness, vertigo, seizures, and neuropsychiatric abnormalities.

Interactions

The adverse cardiovascular effects of digoxin may be potentiated by agents that lower serum potassium or magnesium concentrations, such as thiazide diuretics, loop diuretics, ethacrynic acid, amphotericin B, corticosteroids, polystyrene sodium sulfonate, and glucagon.[329] The concomitant administration of digoxin with IV calcium results in additive or synergistic inotropic and adverse cardiovascular effects. β-adrenergic antagonists can cause complete heart block when administered with digoxin. Using digoxin with succinylcholine or sympathomimetics increases the risk of dysrhythmias.

Digoxin has a narrow therapeutic index; serum digoxin concentrations are increased with concomitant administration of amiodarone, flecainide, quinidine, propafenone, verapamil, captopril, itraconazole, and indomethacin.

Summary

Digitalis glycosides are inotropic agents that have the added benefit of slowing rather than accelerating heart rate. Given its narrow therapeutic window, long half-life, and with the emergence of newer medications, there is rarely a role for digoxin in the acute setting.

Conclusion

Significant advances have been made in our understanding of the mechanisms underlying adrenergic receptor signaling, the control of vascular tone, and the influence of genetic polymorphisms on the pathways involved in these processes. Despite this broader fund of knowledge, the therapeutic options for supporting the patient with impaired end-organ perfusion remain essentially unchanged. The catecholamines comprise the mainstay of therapy for patients in need of inotropic or vasopressor support. Although dopamine is still used, epinephrine and norepinephrine are increasingly becoming the mainstay of therapy for patients with poor cardiac performance or decreased systemic vascular tone, respectively.

Milrinone, levosimendan, or dobutamine can be used to increase myocardial contractility in the absence of hypotension. Milrinone is particularly useful for hemodynamic support after surgery for congenital heart disease. Vasopressin has emerged as an option for vasodilatory shock that is resistant to catecholamine therapy. Often the clinical picture is mixed, and the patient may require both inotropic and vasopressor support. Careful attention to hemodynamics and end-organ perfusion, as well as a thorough understanding of cardiovascular pharmacology, is necessary in order to select the agent(s) that will provide the optimal results in critically ill patients.

Acknowledgments

We gratefully acknowledge the contributions of Marc G. Sturgill and Michael Kelly, who coauthored this chapter in previous editions.

Key References

15. Connell TDO, Jensen BC, Baker AJ, et al. Cardiac alpha 1-adrenergic receptors: novel aspects of expression, signaling mechanisms, physiologic function, and clinical importance. *Pharmacological reviews.* 2014;8:308-333.

23. Singh M, Notterman DA, Metakis L. Tumor necrosis factor produces homologous desensitization of lymphocyte beta 2-adrenergic responses. *Circ Shock.* 1993;39:275-278.

25. Ortega VE, Meyers DA, Bleecker ER. Asthma pharmacogenetics and the development of genetic profiles for personalized medicine. *Pharmgenomics Pers Med.* 2015;8:9-22.

26. Nakada T-A, Russell J, Boyd JH, et al. Beta$_2$-adrenergic receptor gene polymorphism is associated with mortality in septic shock. *Am J Respir Crit Care Med.* 2010;181:143-149.

44. Landry DW, Oliver J. The pathogenesis of vasodilatory shock. *N Engl J Med.* 2001;345:588-595.

51. Omori K, Kotera J. Overview of PDEs and their regulation. *Circ Res.* 2007;100:309-327.

54. Zhang W, Ke H, Colman RW. Identification of interaction sites of cyclic nucleotide phosphodiesterase type 3A with milrinone and cilostazol using molecular modeling and site-directed mutagenesis. *Mol Pharmacol.* 2002;62:514-520.

57. Yano M, Kohno M, Ohkusa T, et al. Effect of milrinone on left ventricular relaxation and Ca(2+) uptake function of cardiac sarcoplasmic reticulum. *Am J Physiol Heart Circ Physiol.* 2000;279:H1898-H1905.

59. Booker PD. Pharmacological support for children with myocardial dysfunction. *Science.* 2002;12:5-25.

68. Gupta S, Donn SM. Neonatal hypotension: dopamine or dobutamine? *Semin Fetal Neonatal Med.* 2014;19:54-59.

76. Mielgo V, Valls I, Soler A, Rey-Santano C. Dobutamine in paediatric population: a systematic review in juvenile animal models. *PLoS ONE.* 2014;9:e95644.

79. Moran JL, O'Fathartaigh MS, Peisach AR, et al. Epinephrine as an inotropic agent in septic shock: a dose-profile analysis. *Crit Care Med.* 1993; 21:70-77.

87. Notterman DA, Greenwald BM, Moran F, et al. Dopamine clearance in critically ill infants and children: effect of age and organ system dysfunction. *Clin Pharmacol Ther.* 1990;48:138-147.

90. Hoffman TM, Wernovsky G, Atz AM, et al. Efficacy and safety of milrinone in preventing low cardiac output syndrome in infants and children after corrective surgery for congenital heart disease. *Circulation.* 2003; 107:996-1002.

96. Prins I, Plötz FB, Uiterwaal CS, et al. Low-dose dopamine in neonatal and pediatric intensive care: a systematic review. *Intensive Care Med.* 2001;27:206-210.

109. Steinberg C, Notterman DA. Pharmacokinetics of cardiovascular drugs in children. Inotropes and vasopressors. *Clin Pharmacokinet.* 1994;27: 345-367.

112. Carcillo JA, Fields AI. Clinical practice parameters for hemodynamic support of pediatric and neonatal patients in septic shock. *Crit Care Med.* 2002;30:1365-1378.

114. Dellinger RP, Levy MM, Rhodes A, et al. Surviving sepsis campaign. *Crit Care Med.* 2013;41:580-637.

116. ECC Committee, Subcommittees and Task Forces of the American Heart Association. 2005 American Heart Association Guidelines for Cardiopulmonary Resuscitation and Emergency Cardiovascular Care. *Circulation.* 2005;112:IV1-IV203.

128. Oberbeck R, Schmitz D, Wilsenack K, et al. Dopamine affects cellular immune functions during polymicrobial sepsis. *Intensive Care Med.* 2006;32:731-739.

131. Pon S. Integrated dosing calculator for emergency medications & medicated infusion tables. Available at: <http://www-users.med.cornell.edu/~spon/picu/calc/druginp5.htm>; 2013 Accessed 01.01.15.

141. Skomedal T, Borthne K, Aass H, et al. Comparison between alpha-1 adrenoceptor-mediated and beta adrenoceptor-mediated inotropic components elicited by norepinephrine in failing human ventricular muscle. *J Pharmacol Exp Ther.* 1997;280:721-729.

144. Tourneux P, Rakza T, Bouissou A, et al. Pulmonary circulatory effects of norepinephrine in newborn infants with persistent pulmonary hypertension. *J Pediatr.* 2008;153:345-349.

153. Brierley J, Carcillo JA, Choong K, et al. Clinical practice parameters for hemodynamic support of pediatric and neonatal septic shock: 2007 update from the American College of Critical Care Medicine. *Crit Care Med.* 2009;37:666-688.

157. Lampin ME, Rousseaux J, Botte A, Sadik A, et al. Noradrenaline use for septic shock in children: doses, routes of administration and complications. *Acta Paediatr Int J Paediatr.* 2012;101:e426-e430.

160. Notterman DA, DaBruin WM, Metakis L. Plasma catecholamine concentrations in critically ill children: evidence of early β-adrenergic receptor desensitization. *Pediatr Res.* 1989;25:42A.

169. De Backer D, Creteur J, Silva E, et al. Effects of dopamine, norepinephrine, and epinephrine on the splanchnic circulation in septic shock: which is best? *Crit Care Med.* 2003;31:1659-1667.

173. Zuercher M, Kern KB, Indik JH, et al. Epinephrine improves 24-hour survival in a swine model of prolonged ventricular fibrillation demonstrating that early intraosseous is superior to delayed intravenous administration. *Anesth Analg.* 2011;112:884-890.

179. Perondi MBM, Reis AG, Paiva EF, et al. A comparison of high-dose and standard-dose epinephrine in children with cardiac arrest. *N Engl J Med.* 2004;350:1722-1730.

181. Levy B. Bench-to-bedside review: is there a place for epinephrine in septic shock? *Crit Care.* 2005;9:561-565.

198. Martinez AM, Padbury JF, Thio S. Dobutamine pharmacokinetics and cardiovascular responses in critically ill neonates. *Pediatrics.* 1992;89:47-51.
209. Burkhardt B, Rücker G, Stiller B. Prophylactic milrinone for the prevention of low cardiac output syndrome and mortality in children undergoing surgery for congenital heart disease (protocol). *Cochrane Database Syst Rev.* 2015;(3):CD009515.
214. Robin JK, Oliver JA, Landry DW. Vasopressin deficiency in the syndrome of irreversible shock. *J Trauma.* 2003;54(suppl 5):S149-S154.
224. Rosenzweig EB, Starc TJ, Chen JM, et al. Intravenous arginine-vasopressin in children with vasodilatory shock after cardiac surgery. *Circulation.* 1999;100(suppl 19):II182-I186.
230. Holmes CL, Walley KR, Chittock DR, et al. The effects of vasopressin on hemodynamics and renal function in severe septic shock: a case series. *Intensive Care Med.* 2001;27:1416-1421.
233. Choong K, Bohn D, Fraser DD, et al. Vasopressin in pediatric vasodilatory shock: a multicenter randomized controlled trial. *Am J Respir Crit Care Med.* 2009;180:632-639.
236. Mann K, Berg RA, Nadkarni V. Beneficial effects of vasopressin in prolonged pediatric cardiac arrest: a case series. *Resuscitation.* 2002;52:149-156.
240. Mohamed A, Nasef N, Shah V, et al. Vasopressin as a rescue therapy for refractory pulmonary hypertension in neonates: case series. *Pediatr Crit Care Med.* 2014;15:148-154.
241. Westphal M, Rehberg S, Ertmer C, et al. Terlipressin—more than just a prodrug of lysine vasopressin? *Crit Care Med.* 2009;37:1135-1136.
245. Albanèse J, Leone M, Delmas A, et al. Terlipressin or norepinephrine in hyperdynamic septic shock: a prospective, randomized study. *Crit Care Med.* 2005;33:1897-1902.
248. Meyer S. Comment: terlipressin for children with extremely low cardiac output after open heart surgery. *Ann Pharmacother.* 2009;43:1375-1376, author reply 1376.
268. Chang AC, Atz AM, Wernovsky G, et al. Milrinone: systemic and pulmonary hemodynamic effects in neonates after cardiac surgery. *Crit Care Med.* 1995;23:1907-1914.
286. Kivikko M, Lehtonen L. Levosimendan: a new inodilatory drug for the treatment of decompensated heart failure. *Curr Pharm Des.* 2005;11:435-455.
289. Pierrakos C, Velissaris D, Franchi F, et al. Levosimendan in critical illness: a literature review. *J Clin Med Res.* 2014;6:75-85.
297. Parissis JT, Andreadou I, Bistola V, et al. Novel biologic mechanisms of levosimendan and its effect on the failing heart. *Expert Opin Investig Drugs.* 2008;17:1143-1150.
311. Nieminen MS, Fruhwald S, Heunks LM, et al. Levosimendan: current data, clinical use and future development. *Hear Lung Vessel.* 2013;5:227-245.
315. Hoffman TM. Newer inotropes in pediatric heart failure. *J Cardiovasc Pharmacol.* 2011;58:121-125.
323. Sackner-Bernstein JD, Skopicki HA, Aaronson KD. Risk of worsening renal function with nesiritide in patients with acutely decompensated heart failure. *Circulation.* 2005;111:1487-1491.
332. Hougen TJ. Digitalis use in children: an uncertain future. *Prog Pediatr Cardiol.* 2000;12:37-43.
335. Hoffmeyer S, Burk O, von Richter O, et al. Functional polymorphisms of the human multidrug-resistance gene: multiple sequence variations and correlation of one allele with P-glycoprotein expression and activity in vivo. *Proc Natl Acad Sci USA.* 2000;97:3473-3478.

Cardiopulmonary Interactions

Bradley P. Fuhrman and Ronald A. Bronicki

PEARLS

- Positive pressure ventilation (PPV) alters ventricular loading conditions and compliance.
- In patients who are hypovolemic, the effects of positive airway pressure on the right heart predominate, whereas in patients who have systemic ventricular systolic dysfunction, the effects of PPV on left ventricular afterload predominate.
- Large changes in arterial pulse pressure over the respiratory cycle help to identify mechanically ventilated patients who will have a favorable response to the administration of fluid or who may not tolerate high levels of positive end-expiratory pressure without fluid administration.
- PPV raises juxtacardiac pressure, thereby reducing left ventricular afterload.
- Respiratory effort imposes critical loads on the heart, and respiratory muscle failure from inadequate oxygen delivery is a final common pathway to death from shock.

Both spontaneous breathing and positive pressure ventilation (PPV) affect the circulation in predictable ways. The cardiovascular system also has important effects on respiration, ventilation, and gas exchange.

Effects of Ventilation on Circulation

As shown by Cournand[1] in his sentinel paper, PPV can have important effects on the circulation. The magnitude of these effects may be accentuated by factors that compromise cardiovascular homeostatic responsiveness, such as hypovolemia, cardiac dysfunction, or disordered vascular tone.

PPV alters ventricular loading conditions and compliance. These interactions may occur simultaneously and yet not act in the same direction on cardiac output. The net effect on cardiac output depends on which interactions predominate over the course of the respiratory cycle and on underlying cardiopulmonary function. For this reason, it is often easier to rationalize an interaction than to predict it.

For clarity of discussion, wherever the terms *positive pressure* or *mechanical ventilation* are used in this chapter, the patient is presumed to respond passively, as though subjected to neuromuscular blockade. In general, the term *preload dependence* is used in this chapter to connote patients in whom the dominant cardiovascular effect of positive pressure breathing is to reduce right heart filling with resultant fall in stroke volume. *Afterload dependence* is the term applied to

identify patients whose dominant effect is afterload reduction and consequent increase in stroke volume.

Right Ventricular Filling and Stroke Volume

The effects of PPV on filling of the right heart are the best understood of the various heart-lung interactions, are generally the preponderant effects on the circulation, and are mediated by changes in intrathoracic pressure and venous return over the respiratory cycle. Spontaneous breathing and PPV have opposite effects on intrathoracic pressure, which largely explains their different effects on cardiac output.

Venous Return

The mean systemic pressure of the circulation (P_{ms}) is thought to be the inflow pressure driving blood toward the right atrium.[2] This driving pressure is not measurable in the intact patient, but it can be thought of as the static mean pressure that might exist throughout the circulation if there were instantaneously no blood flow.[3] P_{ms} approximates the weighted average of pressures in venous reservoirs throughout the body during the circulation of blood.[4] The back pressure that opposes systemic venous return is the right atrial pressure (P_{ra}). The impact of these pressures on the return of venous blood to the heart is described by the venous return curve (Fig. 34.1A), which is drawn in such a way that the independent variable (Qpump) appears on the y-axis. Picture the systemic circulation as composed of noncompliant arteries functioning largely as conductive vessels and venous reservoirs functioning as capacitive vessels, which are separated by high-resistance arterioles and a pump that receives venous return and propels it into the systemic arterial circulation (Fig. 34.1B). The faster the pump circulates the blood, the more blood piles up before the arterioles and the higher the arterial pressure will be, and the faster the pump moves blood from venous to arterial system, the less blood resides on the venous side of the circuit and the lower the right atrial pressure will be (x-axis). As the pump is slowed down, venous pressure rises until flow reaches zero, at which point vascular pressures equilibrate throughout the circulation at P_{ms}. Resistance to venous return (R_{vr}) is the reciprocal of the slope of the linear part of the venous return curve.

$$\text{Simply stated: Venous Return} = (P_{ms} - P_{ra})/R_{vr} \quad \text{Eq. 34.1}$$

P_{ms} is a function of intravascular volume and compliance, the vast majority of which reside within and with the venous reservoirs. The P_{ms} can be altered by changes in venous tone and intravascular volume. P_{ms} is an extrathoracic measurement and is less sensitive than P_{ra} to changes in intrathoracic

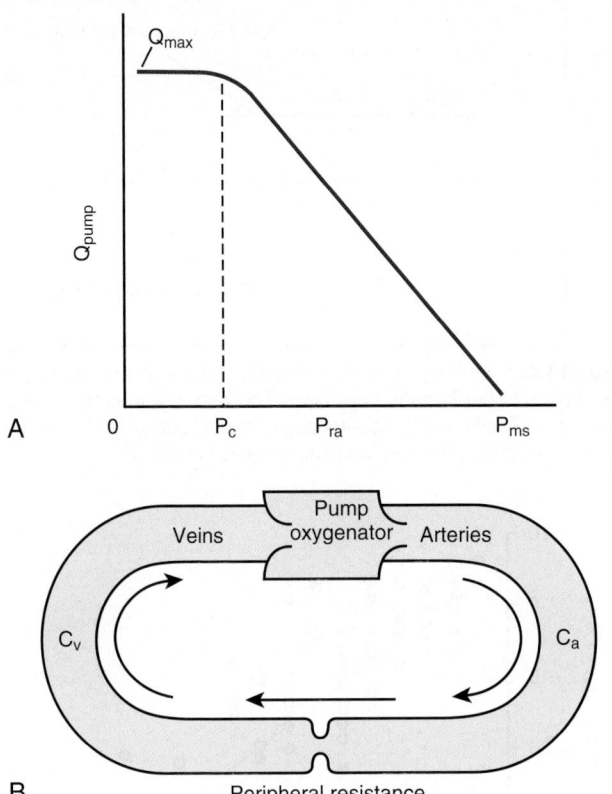

Fig. 34.1. (A) Systemic venous return curve. Flow (Q_{pump}) is plotted on the ordinate but is treated as the independent variable. Right atrial pressure (P_{ra}), the dependent variable, is plotted on the abscissa. (B) Circulation is treated as though a pump transferred blood from veins to arteries, generating arterial pressure sufficient to overcome peripheral arterial resistance. Arterial compliance (C_a) and venous compliance (C_v) determine the volume of blood distending arteries and veins at any Q_{pump}. When there is no flow, pressure equilibrates throughout the circulation at the mean systemic pressure of the circulation P_{ms}. As pump flow is progressively increased, venous pressure falls and arterial pressure rises because of the net transfer of blood from veins to arteries by the pump and because of the accumulation of blood before the peripheral resistance. When venous pressure falls to P_c, the critical closing pressure of the venous system, no further increase in pump flow is possible. (Modified from Guyton AC. Determination of cardiac output by equating venous return curves with cardiac response curves. Physiol Rev. 1955; 35:123.)

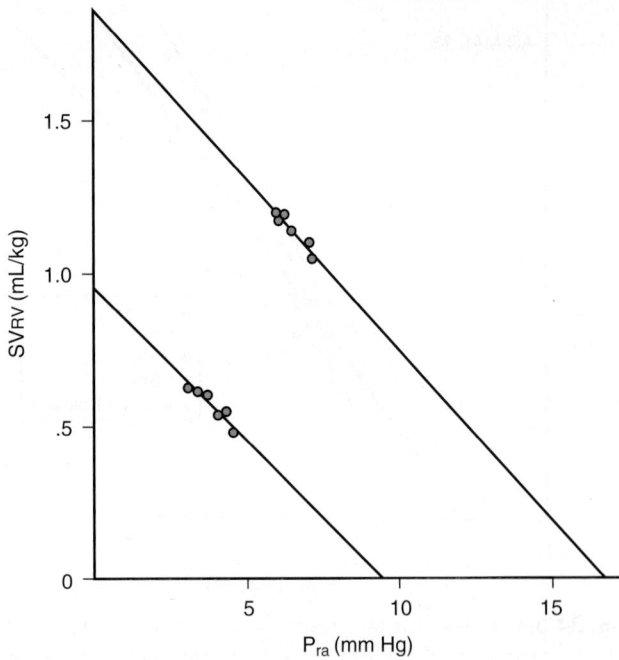

Fig. 34.2. During spontaneous inspiration, right atrial pressure (P_{ra}) falls, but this decline is associated with an increase in right ventricular stroke volume (SV_{RV}). Shown at two different mean P_{ra}. (From Pinsky MR. Instantaneous venous return curves in an intact canine preparation. J Appl Physiol. 1984;56:765.)

pressure.[5] P_{ra}, in contrast, is quite sensitive to changes in intrathoracic pressure.

At functional residual capacity (FRC), the thorax exerts recoil force, tending to spring outward, whereas the lung exerts recoil force (mostly as a result of alveolar surface tension), tending to collapse inward. These forces result in subambient pleural pressure. The cardiac fossa, or juxtacardiac space, which surrounds the pericardium and heart, shares in this balance of forces and has slightly negative pressure at apneic FRC. At any right atrial volume, P_{ra} is influenced by juxtacardiac pressure because these two forces act together to oppose the right atrium's balloon-like tendency to recoil inward. Therefore it is not surprising that all of these pressures (pleural, juxtacardiac, and right atrial) are influenced by the respiratory cycle.[6-8]

During spontaneous breathing, lung volume rises from FRC to end-inspiratory volume by expansion of the rib cage and descent of the diaphragm. This reshaping of the thorax stretches the lung, increasing its recoil tension, so pleural pressure and juxtacardiac pressure both become more negative (subambient). At any right atrial volume, spontaneous inspiration reduces P_{ra}. By the mathematic relationship in Eq. 1, this augments venous return.[9] Over the course of passive spontaneous expiration, all three pressures return toward their values at FRC. It follows that intrathoracic pressure, during relaxed spontaneous breathing, is always most negative at end-inspiration and becomes progressively less negative throughout the rest of the respiratory cycle.

Right Ventricular Preload and Stroke Volume

Transmural pressure is the pressure difference across (inside to outside) a hollow structure. This pressure difference and the wall tension of the structure determine its resting radius, or, at disequilibrium, its internal pressure. P_{ra} normally approximates the pressure within the right ventricle during cardiac filling, when the tricuspid valve is open. Juxtacardiac pressure approximates the pressure surrounding the ventricle. During spontaneous inspiration, systemic venous return to the right atrium and ventricle are augmented (Eq. 1), end-diastolic right ventricular (RV) volume rises, and right ventricular stroke volume increases by the Frank-Starling mechanism. Despite the falling P_{ra}, transmural pressure is increased by spontaneous inspiration and right ventricular stroke volume increases; hence there is a seemingly paradoxical inverse relationship between P_{ra} and right ventricular stroke volume over the spontaneous respiratory cycle (Fig. 34.2).[10] However, if *transmural* P_{ra} is plotted against right ventricular stroke volume during various respiratory maneuvers and with expansion of intravascular volume, the expected

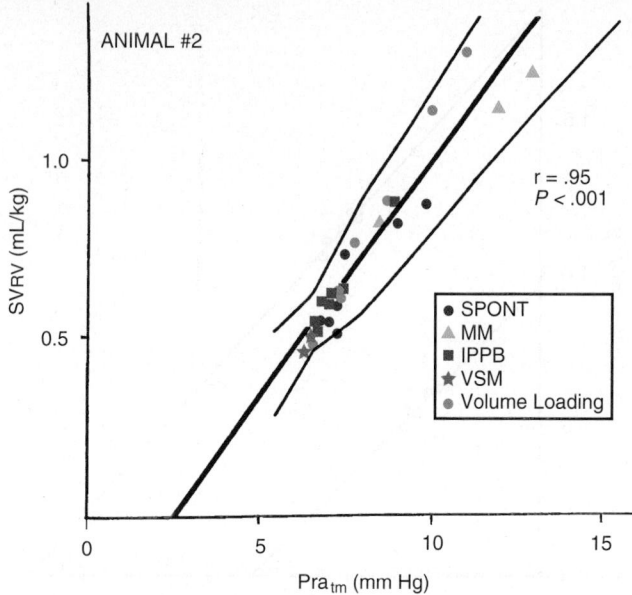

Fig. 34.3. Over a wide range of respiratory maneuvers, right ventricular stroke volume (SVRV) varies directly with transmural right atrial pressure (Pra_{tm}). IPPB, intermittent positive pressure breathing; MM, Müller maneuver; SPONT, spontaneous breathing; VSM, Valsalva maneuver. (From Pinsky MR. Determinants of pulmonary arterial flow variation during respiration. J Appl Physiol. 1984;56:1237.)

positive relation of RV filling pressure to stroke volume is revealed (Fig. 34.3).[11]

Positive Pressure Mechanical Ventilation and Right Ventricular Preload

The effects of PPV on pleural, juxtacardiac, and right atrial pressure are opposite those of spontaneous breathing. A common goal in the application of positive end-expiratory pressure (PEEP) is restoration of normal end-expiratory lung volume (normal FRC). All other things being equal, pleural pressure, which opposes thoracic recoil, should be the same at end-expiration whether breathing is spontaneous or mechanical. Pleural pressure is, after all, determined by thoracic volume during passive expiration.

During spontaneous inspiration, active reshaping of the thorax by the respiratory muscles and diaphragm inflates the lungs by reducing pleural pressure. In contrast, throughout positive pressure mechanical inspiration, pleural pressure rises because the passive thorax is pushed outward (from FRC to end-inspiratory volume) by the expanding lungs. Passive expiration restores pleural pressure to that of FRC. Averaged over the entire respiratory cycle, pleural pressure is higher during positive pressure breathing than it would be during spontaneous breathing (Fig. 34.4). (This elevation of pleural pressure during positive pressure mechanical ventilation may be thought of as transmission of airway pressure to the pleural space.) PPV, therefore, reverses the effects of spontaneous breathing on venous return[12] and RV transmural pressure.[13] RV stroke volume declines during positive pressure inspiration as P_{ra} rises. Averaged over the entire respiratory cycle, P_{ra} is raised and RV stroke volume is reduced by positive airway pressure relative to their expected values during spontaneous breathing (Fig. 34.5). It is easy to argue from these observations that PPV will invariably decrease venous return to the

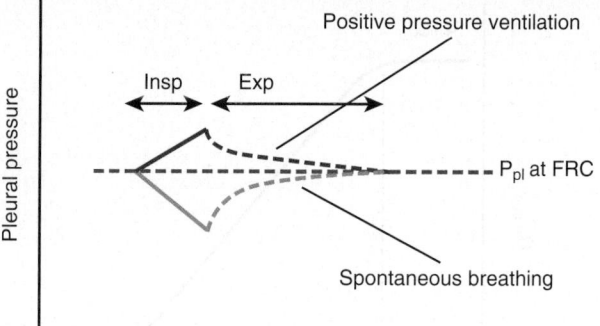

Fig. 34.4. Over the course of the respiratory cycle, if spontaneous and positive pressure breaths both begin and end at the same functional residual capacity (FRC), spontaneous breathing takes place at lower pleural pressure than does positive pressure ventilation.

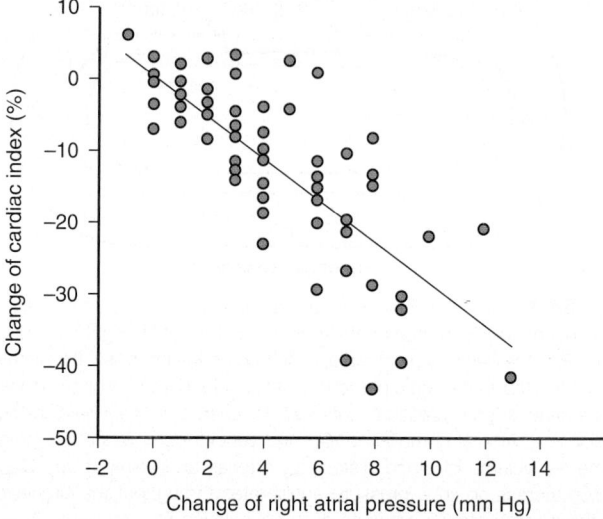

Fig. 34.5. Relationship between the percentage change in cardiac index and the percentage change in right atrial pressure that was produced by the application of graded levels of positive airway pressure in adults. (From Jellinek H, Krafft P, Fitzgerald RD, et al. Right atrial pressure predicts hemodynamic response to apneic positive airway pressure. Crit Care Med. 2000;28:672.)

right heart, but this is not always the case. In addition to the extent to which airway pressure is transmitted to the right atrium, discussed further later, the adequacy of circulatory reflexes to maintain an adequate albeit elevated P_{ms}, as well as underlying cardiac function, determines the extent to which cardiac output is adversely impacted by PPV. Venoconstriction and retention of intravascular volume act to elevate the P_{ms} and maintain an adequate pressure gradient for systemic venous return. During PPV, descent of the diaphragm may displace blood from the abdominal viscera[14,15] and positive airway pressure may displace blood from the pulmonary circulation, both of which raise P_{ms}.

Critical Illness and the Effects of Positive Pressure Breathing on the Right Heart

Among the effects of critical illness are capillary leak, chest wall edema, pulmonary edema, surfactant dysfunction, abnormal blood volume, and abdominal distension. Each of these modifies the effects of positive pressure breathing on the right

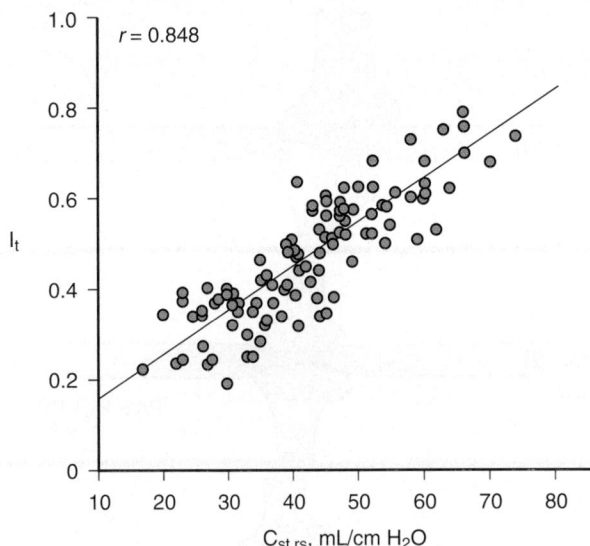

Fig. 34.6. Relationship between the static compliance of the respiratory system ($C_{st,rs}$) and the index of transmission (I_t, decimal fraction) of a change in static airway pressure to the pulmonary circulation in adults. I_t values for pleural and juxtacardiac spaces are presumed to be comparable. (From Teboul JL, Pinsky MR, Mercat A, et al. Estimating cardiac filling pressure in mechanically vented patients with hyperinflation. Crit Care Med. 2000;28:3631.)

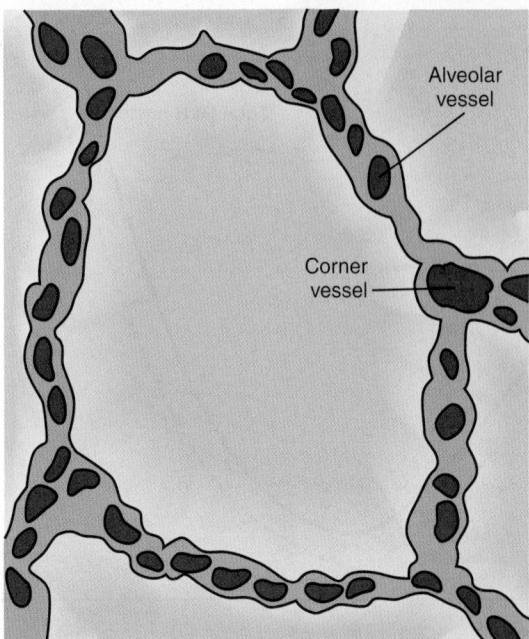

Fig. 34.7. Alveolus is encased in a network of capillaries. Alveolar vessels are those that lie between adjacent alveoli. Corner vessels are those that lie at the intersection of alveolar septa.

heart. Capillary leak alters the compliance of the atrial and ventricular chambers, modifying the responsiveness of the heart to changes in preload. Sepsis and inflammation decrease cardiac contractility, directly altering the way the heart responds to changes in preload. Chest wall edema, pulmonary edema, surfactant dysfunction, and abdominal distension alter thoracic and pulmonary compliances, which in turn alter pleural and juxtacardiac pressures.

Reduced respiratory system compliance diminishes the transmission of alveolar pressure to the juxtacardiac space.[16] The change in intrathoracic pressure that occurs with a change in static airway pressure is essentially the same as the change observed in pulmonary artery wedge pressure,[17] which is readily measured. Recognizing this relationship in adults has made it possible to estimate percent transmission of airway pressure to the juxtacardiac space by measurement of respiratory system compliance (Fig. 34.6).

Both abnormal blood volume and abnormal vascular compliance can change P_{ms} and thereby alter venous return. Vascular hypovolemia can exaggerate the adverse effects of PPV on preload, and hypervolemia can blunt that effect.

Pulmonary Circulation

By modifying pulmonary vascular resistance (PVR), the effects of breathing on pulmonary circulation modify RV afterload. The effects of breathing also can change the distribution of pulmonary blood flow within the lung. Both effects are significant.

Lung Volume
The alveolar septae are highly vascular (Fig. 34.7). More than 90% of the alveolar surface makes contact with alveolar capillaries. These vessels can be separated into two categories according to their location or response to lung inflation. Most

alveolar vessels are capillaries and lie in septa, which separate adjacent alveoli. Other alveolar vessels are termed *corner vessels* because they are located at the intersection of alveolar septae. These corner vessels are generally larger and most likely will divide later in their course to become alveolar capillaries located in septa between adjacent alveoli. When the lung is stretched by either spontaneous inspiration or positive pressure distension, corner vessels are pulled open by radial traction and their resistance to blood flow is reduced. When alveolar septae are stretched, alveolar capillaries are stretched, become thinner, and restrict flow. Moreover, lung distension by positive airway pressure compresses alveolar capillaries. The net effect of these factors is a U-shaped relation of PVR to lung volume (Fig. 34.8)[18-21]; PVR is least at FRC and rises with either atelectasis or overdistension.

Alveolar Pressure
When alveolar pressure is greater than ambient, as it is during PPV, the vessels that course through alveolar septae between adjacent alveoli can be compressed.[22,23] This behavior is akin to that of a Starling resistor, a collapsible tube traversing a rigid housing (Fig. 34.9). Flow (Q) is propelled through the tube by inflow pressure (P_i) and is opposed by outflow pressure (P_o). The tubing has some intrinsic resistance (R). If the housing is pressurized to a surrounding pressure (P_s), flow through the tube is determined as follows:

$$\text{for } P_s < P_o < P_i, Q = (P_i - P_o)/R \qquad \text{Eq. 34.2}$$

$$\text{for } P_o < P_s < P_i, Q = (P_i - P_s)/R \qquad \text{Eq. 34.3}$$

$$\text{for } P_o < P_i < P_s, Q = 0 \qquad \text{Eq. 34.4}$$

Except when $P_s < P_o$, alveolar pressure appears to modulate local pulmonary blood flow as though it surrounds the pulmonary capillary (Fig. 34.10).

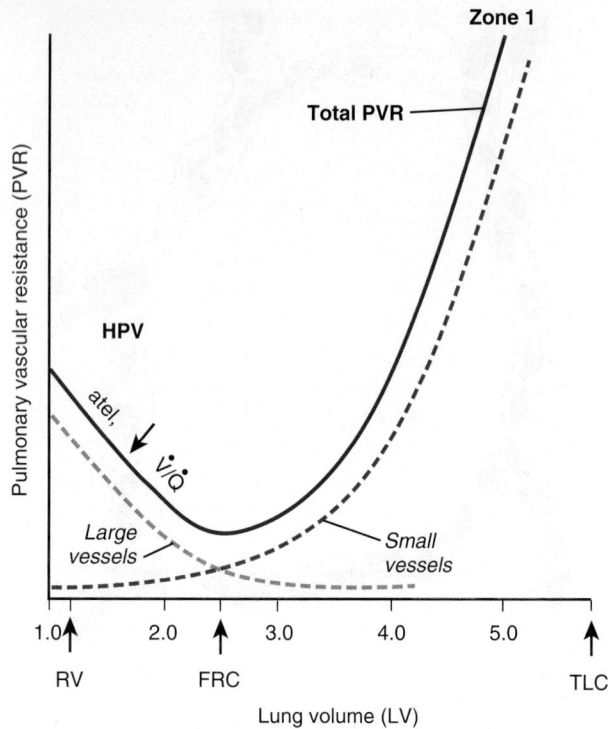

Fig. 34.8. Effects of lung volume on pulmonary vascular resistance *(PVR)*. As whole lung is distended from functional residual capacity *(FRC)* toward total lung capacity *(TLC)*, PVR rises, predominantly by increasing resistance to flow through the small alveolar vessels that course between adjacent alveoli (alveolar vessels). As whole lung is collapsed from FRC toward residual volume, PVR rises, predominantly by effects on corner vessel that traverse the intersection of alveolar septa. (Modified from Cassidy SS, Schwiep F. Cardiovascular effects of positive end-expiratory pressure. In: Scharf SM, Cassidy SS, eds. Heart Lung Interactions in Health and Disease, vol 42, Lung Biology in Health and Disease. New York: Dekker; 1989.)

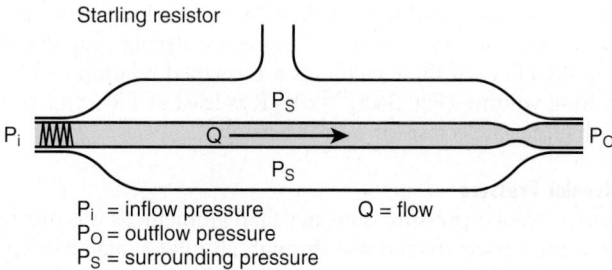

Fig. 34.9. Starling resistor is a compressible conduit traversing a rigid housing, which is pressurized to a surrounding pressure (P_s). Flow *(Q)* traverses the conduit, propelled by inflow pressure (P_i) and opposed by outflow pressure (P_o) such that driving pressure is $(P_i - P_o)$ for $P_s < P_o$. As P_s is increased, it begins to influence flow, but only after it exceeds P_o. At $P_s > P_o$, the driving force for flow becomes $(P_i - P_s)$. (Modified from Knowlton FP, Starling EH. The influence of variations in temperature and blood pressure on performance of the isolated mammalian heart. J Physiol. 1912;44:206-219.)

From this discussion, the degree to which P_s affects pulmonary blood flow is influenced by the magnitude of inflow pressure, which, for the pulmonary capillary, must be adjusted for vertical height. Alveolar pressure causes a greater reduction in flow at low inflow pressure, as seen in hypovolemia, than it

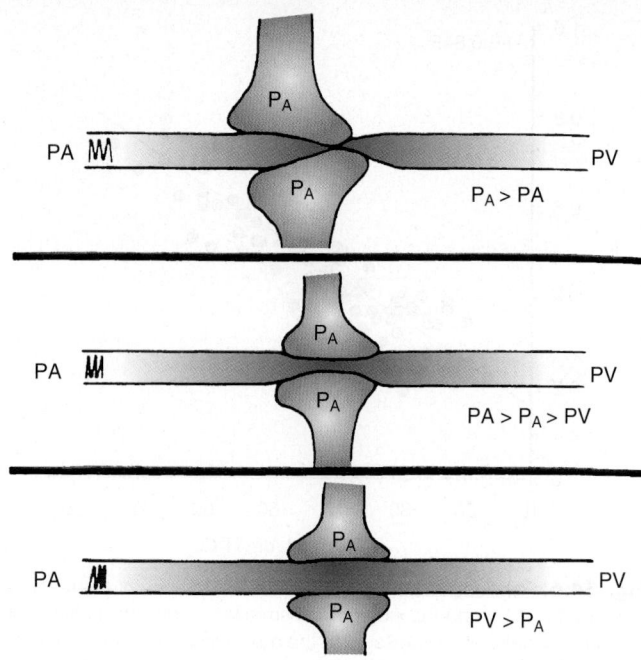

Fig. 34.10. Pulmonary capillaries are, in essence, surrounded by gas-filled alveoli. The influence of alveolar pressure (P_A) on regional lung blood flow is similar to the influence of surrounding pressure on flow through a Starling resistor. At ambient values of P_A, pulmonary vein pressure *(PV)* opposes inflow. As P_A rises, it begins to oppose inflow only after $P_A > PV$. It modulates inflow until P_A reaches hydrostatic inflow pressure *(PA)*, at which point flow ceases.

does at high inflow pressure, as seen with pulmonary venous hypertension and left heart failure.

Hydrostatic pressure in the lung is a function of vertical height (see Chapter 26).[24] To estimate the hydrostatic inflow pressure of a pulmonary capillary, a pressure equivalent to that exerted by a water column extending from the left atrium to the capillary must be subtracted from the pressure within the main pulmonary artery. The greater the vertical height of the pulmonary capillary, the lower is its inflow pressure and the greater is the attenuation of flow by alveolar pressure. This can produce areas of no flow, especially at peak inspiration, high in the supine lung. Regions of lung with high ventilation/perfusion ratios (V/Q) waste ventilation and can cause hypercapnia (see Chapter 47). Vertical height (h) of the capillary also alters the back pressure to flow. At a left atrial pressure of 10 cm H_2O (7 mm Hg), for example, there is $(10 - h)$ cm H_2O opposing flow up to a vertical height 10 cm above the heart. Above that, there is no back pressure and P_i and P_s alone determine flow through the capillary. Compression of pulmonary capillaries is a local phenomenon. It can divert pulmonary blood flow away from normal lung segments toward consolidated or atelectatic lung segments whose airways do not effectively transmit airway pressure to the alveolus.[25] The application of high PEEP in the presence of lobar pneumonia may increase blood flow through unventilated lung and worsen hypoxemia by this mechanism (Fig. 34.11). From a more positive perspective, PEEP may relieve atelectasis and improve ventilation, thereby relieving alveolar hypoxic vasoconstriction. Whether PEEP benefits or impairs pulmonary blood flow may depend on the balance of its effect on atelectasis and its effect on alveolar capillaries. It should also be

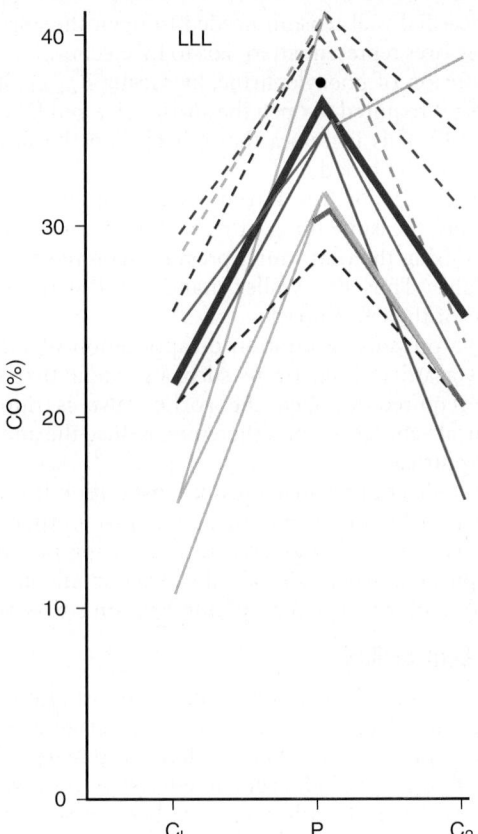

Fig. 34.11. Blood flow to the left lower lobes *(LLL)* of dogs with LLL pneumonia, measured at zero positive end-expiratory pressure *(PEEP)* (C_1), 6–12 cm H_2O PEEP *(P)*, and on cessation of applied PEEP (C_2). PEEP diverted blood flow away from more normal lung toward the consolidated LLL. (From Mink SN, Light RB, Cooligan T, et al. Effect of PEEP on gas exchange and pulmonary perfusion in canine lobar pneumonia. J Appl Physiol. 1981;50:517.)

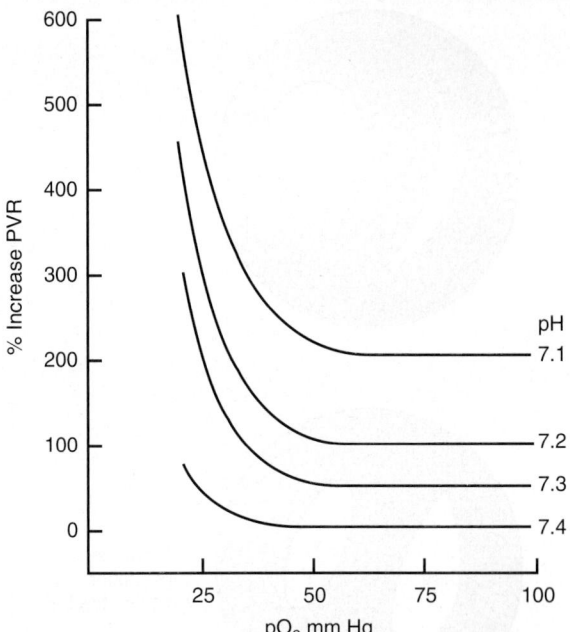

Fig. 34.12. Pulmonary vascular resistance *(PVR)* is a function of both pH and arterial pO_2. (From Rudolph AM, Yuan S. Response of the pulmonary vasculature to hypoxia and H^+ ion concentration changes. J Clin Invest. 1966;45:399.)

appreciated that while a manipulation of ventilator settings may improve oxygenation and arterial oxygen content, it may also cause cardiac output to decrease resulting in a net reduction in systemic oxygen delivery.

Regulation of Pulmonary Vascular Resistance

The resistance to flow through a vessel is described by the following:

$$R = 8\eta l/\pi r^4 \qquad \text{Eq. 34.5}$$

where η is viscosity, l is length, and r is radius. It follows that PVR can be effectively controlled by active changes in vessel radius. Mechanical ventilation may alter blood pH and alveolar oxygen tension (pO_2), both of which influence vessel tone and radius (Fig. 34.12).[26,27]

Hypoxic pulmonary vasoconstriction is a powerful mechanism for sustaining systemic oxygenation in the face of lung disease.[28-31] Relief of atelectasis and restoration of segmental ventilation not only increases the fraction of the lung that is ventilated but also restores blood flow to those segments by several mechanisms. Segmental alveolar hypoxia is relieved. Segmental volume is restored, which returns segmental vascular resistance toward its volume-dependent nadir. Gas exchange is also improved, favorably altering pH, pCO_2, and pO_2, and thereby reducing global PVR.

Direct Effects of Airway Pressure on Pulmonary Vascular Tone

Pulmonary vessels are stretched by lung inflation. The lung of infant lambs responds to abrupt changes in airway pressure with changes in vascular tone. Abrupt distension of one lung of the intact infant lamb increases the PVR of that lung alone.[32] The resistance change is sensitive to the waveform of the lung distension[33] and persists for some time after relief of distending pressure and return of lung volume to baseline.[34] This effect is calcium channel dependent[35] and resembles a myogenic reflex whereby direct vessel stretch causes constriction.

Left Ventricular Preload

Positive airway pressure can reduce left ventricular (LV) filling via several mechanisms as described earlier. In addition to the potential for limiting systemic venous return, increasing RV afterload, and decreasing RV ejection, positive airway pressure can compromise LV compliance and preload as a result of ventricular interdependence.

Ventricular Interdependence

The right and left ventricles share a common muscle mass and pericardial space. It follows that compliance of either ventricle will be influenced by volume of the other chamber (Fig. 34.13). Increased venous return to the right heart, as occurs during spontaneous inspiration and especially during execution of a Müller maneuver, shifts the interventricular septum to the left, reducing compliance of the left ventricle.[36,37] Similarly, excessive compression of the pulmonary circulation by positive airway pressure may impede RV ejection, causing the right ventricle to dilate and encroach on the left. Reduced LV compliance tends to diminish stroke volume by diminishing LV muscle stretch and ejection force (by the Frank-Starling mechanism).

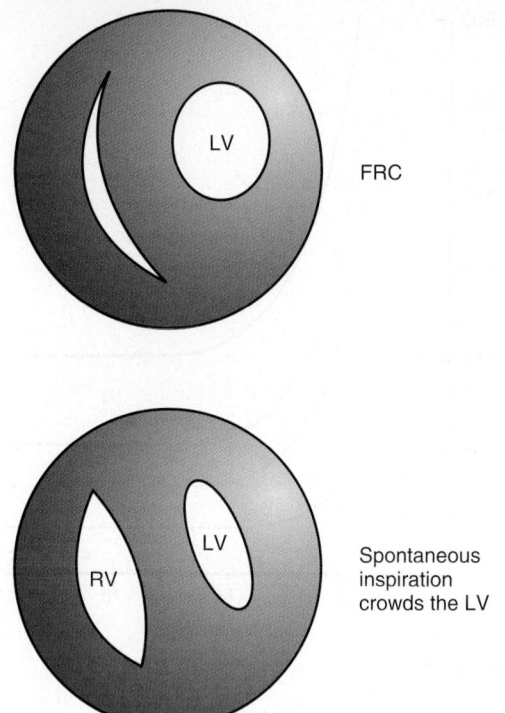

Fig. 34.13. Increasing the diastolic volume of the right ventricle *(RV)* reduces compliance of the left ventricle *(LV)*. *FRC,* functional residual capacity.

Cardiac Crowding

Overinflation of the lungs may crowd the cardiac fossa in which the heart resides. To the extent that this creates a mechanical barrier to cardiac filling, it may reduce LV compliance, end-diastolic volume, and force of contraction.

Left Ventricular Afterload

The left ventricle ejects blood from within the thorax to the extrathoracic arterial system. Most of the resistance to this forward flow resides in the arterioles. From a practical point of view, the pressure in the extrathoracic arteries can be described by the following equations:

$$(P_{artery} - P_{ms}) = Q \times R_{arteriole} \qquad \text{Eq. 34.6}$$

$$\text{or } P_{artery} = Q \times R_{arteriole} + P_{ms} \qquad \text{Eq. 34.7}$$

where Q is cardiac output, P_{artery} is inflow pressure before the arteriole, and P_{ms} is outflow pressure after the arteriole as defined for the venous return curve.

When the left ventricle contracts, it creates internal pressure against the closed aortic valve by generating tension in the myocardium that encircles the ventricular chamber. This "wall tension" causes ventricular pressure to rise until it reaches aortic diastolic pressure, opening the aortic valve and ejecting the stroke volume. Creation of wall tension and subsequent shortening of myocardial fibers perform the external mechanical work of the heart (see Chapter 25).

When the heart squeezes, it creates a pressure difference between the ventricle and the juxtacardiac space. In effect, the myocardium creates a transmural pressure to produce a ventricular pressure sufficient to open the aortic valve. Aortic diastolic pressure and external (juxtacardiac) pressure determine the myocardial wall tension needed to open the aortic valve. Both pressures represent afterloads to LV ejection.[38,39]

An infusion of phenylephrine, by raising $R_{arteriole}$, increases the pressure required to open the aortic valve and LV afterload (Fig. 34.14). This increases the wall tension the heart must generate to eject blood.

The Müller maneuver, forced inspiration against a closed glottis, does the same thing. It reduces juxtacardiac pressure, thereby raising the transmural pressure required to open the aortic valve. Thus the Müller maneuver also increases the afterload of the left ventricle.

Positive pressure inspiration or application of PEEP may raise juxtacardiac pressure to such an extent that the wall tension required to open the aortic valve is diminished. Mechanical ventilation may, therefore, reduce the afterload of the left ventricle.

The net effect of positive pressure inspiration is often augmentation of LV stroke volume and cardiac output. Arterial pressure is commonly observed to rise during positive pressure inspiration, whereas it falls during spontaneous inspiration. These are largely effects of afterload on stroke volume.

Cardiac Contractility

Studies of the effects of positive airway pressure on LV contractility have yielded conflicting results. Certainly ventilator changes in preload and afterload have secondary effects on stroke volume, but independent effects of positive airway pressure on LV contractility have not been consistently demonstrated. Negative inotropic effects modulated by reflexes, mediators, or alterations in coronary blood flow have been described,[40-45] but most animal and human studies fail to show that positive airway pressure has any primary effect on myocardial contractility.[46-49]

It has been suggested that high levels of PEEP may compress coronary vessels, cause myocardial ischemia, and thereby impair ventricular function.[50-52] LV myocardium is perfused predominantly in diastole. To the extent that juxtacardiac pressure exceeds diastolic pressure in the coronary sinus, such an effect is plausible. This assertion appears more compelling for patients in shock and for those with intrinsic coronary blood flow limitations than for otherwise normal individuals.

Preload Dependence Versus Afterload Dependence

The expected effects of a rise in airway pressure are as follows:
1. Decreased filling of the right ventricle acts to decrease RV stroke volume.
2. Pulmonary vascular compression increases RV afterload and acts to decrease RV stroke volume.
3. These effects may either increase or decrease RV size, depending on which effect predominates; if RV volume increases, ventricular interdependence adversely impacts LV function.
4. Both diastolic displacement of the interventricular septum toward the left ventricle (with resultant crowding of the left ventricle) and crowding of the juxtacardiac space by the expanding lungs reduce LV compliance. Both factors act to decrease LV filling and stroke volume.
5. The fall in LV afterload that results from increased juxtacardiac pressure acts to increase LV stroke volume.

These effects of positive airway pressure may have conflicting effects on stroke volume, so their aggregate effect on cardiac output is not entirely predictable.

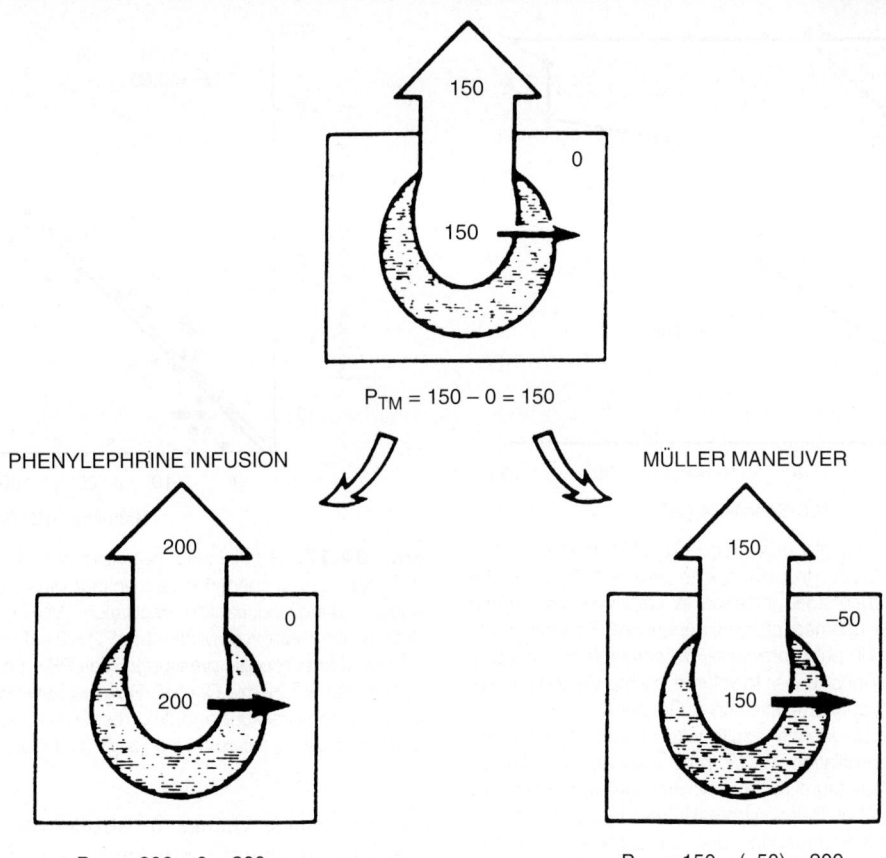

Fig. 34.14. Negative pressure in the juxtacardiac space (Müller maneuver) increases the wall tension required to eject blood into the aorta. This respiratory maneuver acts like a phenylephrine infusion to increase left ventricular afterload. (From Buda AJ, Pinsky MR, Ingels NB Jr, et al. Effect of intrathoracic pressure on left ventricular performance. N Engl J Med. 1979;301:453.)

In general, positive airway pressure has its most pronounced effect on the right heart; therefore positive airway pressure reduces cardiac output in most patients. This effect is greatest in patients who are hypovolemic because the driving pressure for systemic venous return ($P_{ms} - P_{ra}$) is more sensitive to change in P_{ra} when P_{ms} is low. In addition, pulmonary venous pressure is low and PPV increases the proportion of lung units where P_s (alveolar) $> P_i$, increasing RV afterload and decreasing RV ejection. In adults, the P_{ra} threshold (at zero PEEP) below which increasing airway pressure reduces cardiac output is approximately 12 mm Hg.[53] Another definition of preload dependence is responsiveness to vascular volume infusion. By this definition, when the dominant effect of positive airway pressure is to impede right heart filling, vascular volume infusion raises cardiac output. Four measurable parameters (Fig. 34.15) predict responsiveness to vascular volume infusion: (1) variation of pulse pressure over the respiratory cycle (Maximum – Minimum), (2) arterial systolic pressure, (3) P_{ra}, and (4) pulmonary artery wedge pressure.[54] Of these parameters, the inspiratory increase in arterial pulse pressure is the most sensitive and specific predictor of "preload dependence" (by receptor operating characteristic curve) (Fig. 34.16). Greater than 15% inspiratory rise in pulse pressure appears to identify adults with preload dependence during positive pressure ventilation.[55]

One might expect the converse also to apply. Reduced magnitude of the effects of PPV on RV filling or augmented effects on LV ejection may make the patient "afterload dependent."

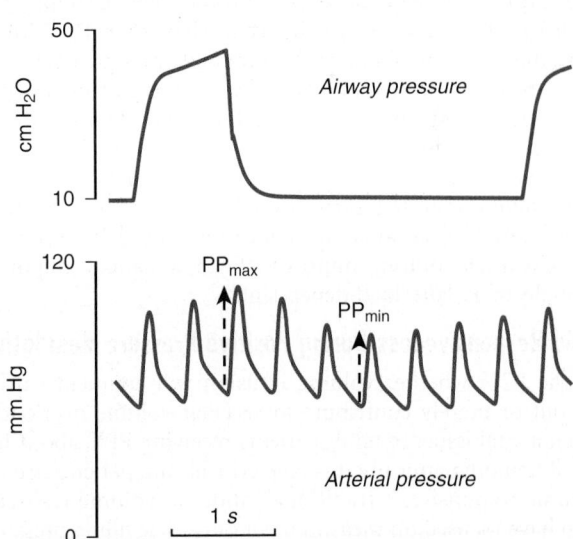

Fig. 34.15. Positive pressure inspiration generally raises aortic pulse pressure *(PP)*, systolic pressure *(SP)*, and diastolic pressure *(DP)*, as well as right atrial pressure and pulmonary artery wedge pressure. (From Michard F, Chemla D, Richard C, et al. Clinical use of respiratory changes in arterial pulse pressure to monitor the hemodynamic effects of PEEP. Am J Respir Crit Care Med. 1999;159:935.)

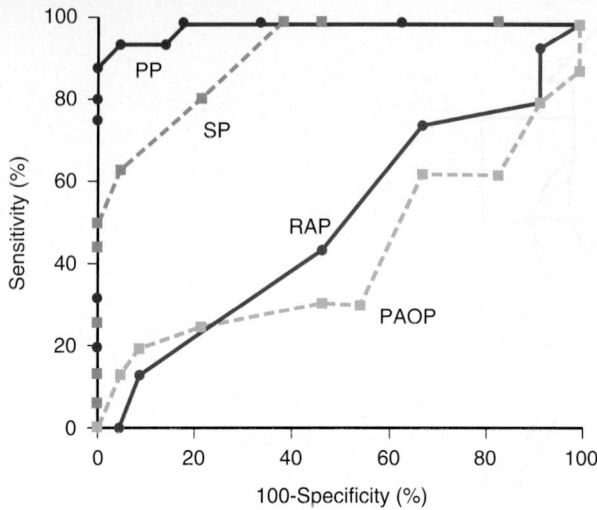

Fig. 34.16. Septic patients on positive end-expiratory pressure were challenged by volume infusion. In response to volume loading, some patients had a greater than 15% increase in cardiac index. These responsive patients were deemed preload dependent. The sensitivity and specificity of variation in pulse pressure *(PP)* across the respiratory cycle as a predictor of responsiveness to volume loading yielded a near-perfect receiver operating characteristic curve. Greater than 15% inspiratory rise in PP appears to identify adults with preload dependence during positive pressure ventilation. *PAOP,* pulmonary artery occlusion pressure; *RAP,* right atrial pressure; *SP,* systolic pressure. (From Michard F, Boussat S, Chemla D, et al. Relation between respiratory changes in arterial pulse pressure and fluid responsiveness in septic patients with acute circulatory failure. Am J Respir Crit Care Med. 2000;162:134.)

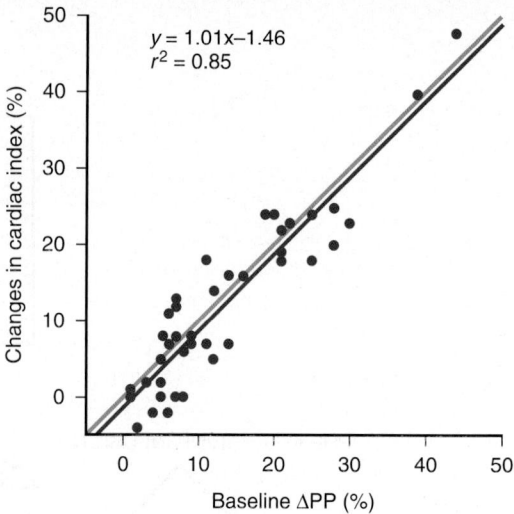

Fig. 34.17. Relationship between ΔPP before volume expansion (baseline) and % change in cardiac index in 40 adult patients with septic shock during mechanical ventilation. Volume expansion comprised 500 mL 6% hydroxyethyl starch. ΔPP = 2 × (Peak arterial pulse pressure − Lowest arterial pulse pressure)/(Peak PP + Lowest PP). (From Michard F, Boussat S, Chemla D, et al. Relation between respiratory changes in arterial pulse pressure and fluid responsiveness in septic patients with acute circulatory failure. Am J Respir Crit Care Med. 2000;162:134.)

Patients who have high blood volume, such as those in congestive cardiac failure or those with chronic anemia, should have high P_{ms} and decreased sensitivity to changes in P_{ra}.[56] Moreover, the patient with poor LV contractility may greatly benefit from the afterload reduction of PPV.[57] If positive airway pressure enhances the ejection of blood into the systemic circulation, this may directly reduce left atrial pressure. From these considerations, improved cardiac output reduces P_{ra} enhancing systemic venous return (see Fig. 34.1B). When favorable effects on LV ejection act to reduce right and left atrial pressures, cardiac output improves. Such a patient might be thought of as "afterload dependent."

Fluid Responsiveness During Positive Pressure Ventilation

In the ICU, whether volume infusion will augment cardiac output or merely contribute to vascular volume overload is often a vital issue. In adult patients receiving PPV, about half of all hemodynamically unstable critical care patients are not volume responsive.[58] Traditional guides to volume resuscitation have focused on measurement of cardiac filling pressures and responses to fluid challenges. In critically ill patients and in normal subjects, the stroke volume response to vascular volume infusion is poorly predicted by measurement of either right atrial or pulmonary artery occlusion pressure.[59] Much recent interest has focused on minimally invasive estimation of likelihood of responding to fluid infusion.

The cardiopulmonary interactions described previously can be used to predict response to fluid challenge. The change in stroke volume over the course of the positive pressure respiratory cycle strongly predicts fluid responsiveness; the greater the percentage change in stroke volume, the greater the response to volume infusion.[60] Similar relations have been shown between fluid responsiveness and respiratory variation in aortic blood flow velocity[61] and arterial pulse pressure.[53] Inspiratory collapsibility of the inferior[62] and superior[63] vena cavae has also been shown to predict volume responsiveness. The strong linear relationship of increase in cardiac index after fluid resuscitation to preinfusion pulse pressure variability over the respiratory cycle (ΔPP) is shown in Fig. 34.17, which depicts data from 40 mechanically ventilated adults with acute circulatory failure related to sepsis.

This same parameter, change in arterial pulse pressure over the respiratory cycle, can be used to estimate the effect of PEEP on cardiac index. The strong linear relationship of ΔPP to PEEP-induced change in cardiac index is shown in Fig. 34.18.

Changes in cardiac index induced by either fluid resuscitation or by application of PEEP appear to be predicted by measurement of ΔPP.[54] In general, in these patients, the greater the ΔPP, the more preload dependent the patient is to PEEP and the more responsive to fluid resuscitation.

Elevated Work of Breathing and the Circulation

During quiet respiration, the heart has no difficulty satisfying the demand of the respiratory muscles for perfusion and oxygen delivery. In respiratory failure, however, respiratory muscle perfusion may not be adequate. The diaphragm and accessory muscles of respiration are taxed to the limit by respiratory distress. Unlike cardiac muscle, respiratory muscles can accumulate a limited oxygen debt, and persistent hypoperfusion may interfere with their ability to perform the requisite work of breathing. In addition, in a low cardiac output state a competition among viscera for blood flow is created. The brain, myocardium, and respiratory pump lack adrenergic receptors and, under intense neurohormonal activation, do

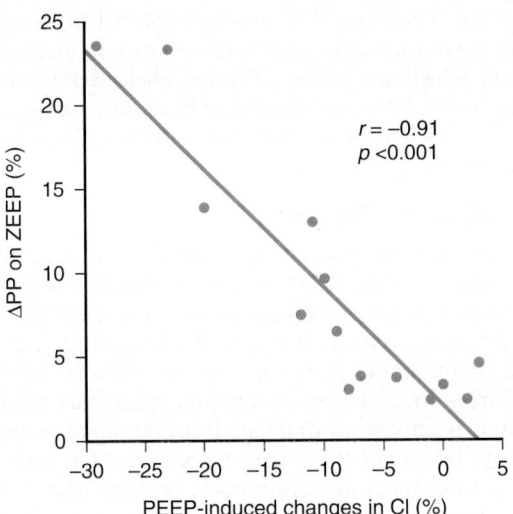

Fig. 34.18. Relationship between ΔPP on zero PEEP and % decrease in cardiac index on application of 10 cm H_2O PEEP. ΔPP = 2 × (Peak arterial pulse pressure – Lowest arterial pulse pressure)/(Peak PP + Lowest PP). (From Michard F, Chemla D, Richard C, et al. Clinical use of respiratory changes in arterial pulse pressure to monitor the hemodynamic effects of PEEP. Am J Respir Crit Care Med. 1999;159:935.)

not experience an increase in resistance to flow and thus compete for a limited cardiac output. Roussos and colleagues[64-66] demonstrated in animal models of cardiogenic and septic shock that mechanical ventilation and the unloading of the respiratory pump lead to a significant redistribution of blood flow from muscles of respiration to other vital organs, including the brain. Because it unloads the respiratory pump and decreases LV afterload, mechanical ventilation should be considered an essential tool in the armamentarium for treating heart failure and shock.

Pulsus Paradoxus in Respiratory Distress

Arterial pressure normally falls during spontaneous inspiration, which is best explained as a result of increasing LV afterload at a time in the respiratory cycle when ventricular interdependence restricts LV filling. It is well known that pericardial tamponade causes accentuation of the normal inspiratory decrease in systemic blood pressure, a phenomenon known as *pulsus paradoxus*. This phenomenon has been attributed to accentuation of normal ventricular interdependence, in the face of restricted biventricular diastolic volume of the heart. During loaded spontaneous inspiration, as in the Müller maneuver or in the presence of inspiratory airway obstruction (eg, croup), the inspiratory fall in juxtacardiac pressure is exaggerated and LV afterload is accentuated. Again, the result is pulsus paradoxus, an accentuated drop in blood pressure during inspiration.

The increase in blood pressure that occurs during positive pressure inspiration has been termed *reverse pulsus paradoxus*. This finding has been attributed to LV afterload reduction by the rise in juxtacardiac pressure that occurs during positive pressure inspiration.[67] Reverse pulsus paradoxus is a normal finding during positive pressure ventilation but may be accentuated in afterload-dependent states (eg, LV systolic dysfunction) as discussed earlier in the "Preload Dependence Versus Afterload Dependence" section).

Effects of Breathing on Measurement of Hemodynamic Parameters

Because hemodynamic measurements vary with respiration, mechanical ventilation may complicate assessment of cardiac function. Yet it may not be advisable to discontinue PEEP or mechanical ventilation to assess hemodynamics. Measuring vascular pressures at a consistent time in the respiratory cycle is usually sufficient. End-expiratory measurements are generally used because airway pressures are least at that time and hemodynamic measurements most closely approximate those at FRC.

It should be understood that the effects of mechanical ventilation on circulation are not merely artifactual. They are real. There is no greater accuracy of measurements made off the ventilator. Measurements performed after ventilator disconnect are subject to the effects of respiratory dysfunction and instability. Besides, the values of the hemodynamic parameters that are of interest are those that exist during stable mechanical ventilation.

A special circumstance can occur when a balloon flotation catheter with its tip in zone I lung is used to measure pulmonary artery pressure and when such a catheter with its tip in zone I or II lung is used to measure pulmonary artery wedge pressure.[68] Under such circumstances, airway pressures that exceed vascular pressures may be erroneously reported as vascular pressures.

Effects of Cardiovascular Function on Respiration
Shock States and Respiratory Function

Shock of any cause diminishes perfusion of respiratory muscles and can lead to respiratory failure and respiratory arrest. It also causes metabolic acidosis, which constricts pulmonary vessels and opposes lung blood flow.[69,70] Acidosis is a potent stimulus of respiratory effort and contributes to tachypnea and respiratory distress, which in turn worsen the demand on the heart. Shock is injurious to both heart and lung, and one final common pathway to recovery is the initiation of mechanical ventilation, which benefits both organ systems.

Hypovolemic shock can create extreme preload dependency.[71] In hypovolemic shock, diastolic blood pressure may fall during positive pressure inspiration, impairing coronary perfusion. This may cause myocardial ischemia and worsen cardiac function.

Cardiogenic shock, by reducing oxygen delivery to tissues, elevates percent tissue oxygen extraction from the blood. The resultant decline in venous oxygen tension has a paradoxical effect. It increases the efficiency of pulmonary blood flow by allowing greater oxygen uptake per unit of pulmonary blood flow. That is, the more desaturated the blood that enters the pulmonary circulation, the more new oxygen it can upload. This process requires that alveolar pO_2 not limit the amount of oxygen available for uptake and is one reason to administer oxygen to patients suffering cardiorespiratory failure.

Congestive Heart Failure

All that has been said about shock is equally true of congestive heart failure (CHF). In fact, there is a continuum from CHF to cardiogenic shock. CHF elicits physiologic responses that attempt to restore and maintain an adequate cardiac output. As these homeostatic responses are exhausted, cardiac output becomes inadequate and the patient develops obvious manifestations of cardiogenic shock and respiratory failure.

In addition to the impact of shock on respiratory function and reserve, CHF generally causes fluid retention and pulmonary edema. Treatment of cardiogenic shock by vascular volume expansion may, by augmenting cardiac filling pressures, improve cardiac output at the expense of pulmonary edema, which leads to elevated airway resistance, atelectasis, intrapulmonary shunt, and impaired oxygenation. Impaired respiratory mechanics leads to exaggerated negative pressure breathing and increased LV afterload while increasing circulatory demands by increasing respiratory muscle oxygen demand. Further, as the work of breathing increases, neurohormonal pathways are stimulated, which contribute importantly to increases in LV afterload, as described earlier.

PPV with PEEP improves lung function and oxygenation, eliminates exaggerated negative swings in intrathoracic pressure, and reduces sympathetic nervous system activation. In contrast to hypovolemic shock, cardiogenic shock generally causes elevated atrial pressures. When this is the case, pulmonary blood flow may be insensitive to airway pressures during positive pressure ventilation as a disproportionate number of lung units have $P_v > P_s$ (alveolar pressure). The patient is then usually afterload dependent and responds favorably to the afterload reducing effects of PPV. When treating the patient with CHF during PPV, there is a risk of worsening pulmonary edema during fluid resuscitation. It is wise to assess pulse pressure, as well as systolic and diastolic pressures, to predict volume responsiveness before administering volume.[72] These parameters may also prove useful in assessing the impact of changes in intrathoracic pressure on cardiac index.[54]

Cardiomyopathies and Congenital Heart Disease

Hypertrophic cardiomyopathy is characterized by intact LV systolic function but has varying degrees of diastolic dysfunction that may compromise output due to inadequate ventricular filling.[73] Thus the impact of increases in intrathoracic pressure on systemic venous return may not be tolerated. If pulmonary venous pressure is elevated secondary to impaired LV compliance, the impact of PPV and lung volumes on pulmonary vascular resistance will be mitigated as the proportion of lung units with $P_v > P_s$ increases. Hypertrophic cardiomyopathy may also obstruct LV outflow, either at rest or with exertion. PPV may not be tolerated as a decrease in preload and afterload leads to a decrease in ventricular operating volumes, exacerbating the obstruction.[74] Restrictive cardiomyopathies invariably have severe abnormalities of ventricular diastolic dysfunction. One would also expect these patients to not tolerate PPV due to its impact on systemic venous return.

The impact of intrathoracic pressure on ventricular diastolic disease is exemplified in some patients following repair of tetralogy of Fallot where varying degrees of RV diastolic dysfunction are common. In a subgroup of these patients, the degree of impairment is severe and has been termed *restrictive physiology*. In these patients, atrial systole causes RV diastolic pressure to rise above pulmonary arterial diastolic pressure generating pulmonary arterial flow during ventricular diastole. LV systolic function is, in most cases, normal; thus the primary impact of changes in intrathoracic pressure is on the right heart. Further, pulmonary venous pressure should not

be elevated. Therefore PPV may be expected to increase the proportion of lung units with P_s (alveolar) $> P_i$, increasing RV afterload, which may not be tolerated. Shekerdemian and colleagues[75] demonstrated a significant increase in cardiac output when patients were converted from PPV to negative pressure ventilation using a cuirass.

Glenn and Fontan Procedures

Hearts that cannot support two separate circulations after repair (univentricular hearts and hearts having one hypoplastic ventricle) are often palliated and then repaired by routing systemic venous return directly to the lung without an intervening subpulmonic pumping chamber (Glenn and Fontan procedures). In the Glenn circulation, pulmonary blood flow is derived from venous drainage from the upper extremities and brain by way of the superior vena cava flow and is thus sensitive to changes in intrathoracic pressure and its impact on the superior vena cava–pulmonary artery confluence, as well as lung volume and its impact on pulmonary vascular resistance. One would expect pulmonary blood flow and oxygenation to improve during spontaneous respiration. In the Glenn circulation the inferior vena cava drains directly to the single ventricle, and while systemic venous return is adversely affected by increases in intrathoracic pressure, it is not impacted by the lack of a subpulmonic pumping chamber and thus systemic output is generally well maintained following the Glenn procedure.

In the Fontan circulation, venous return from the lower body is diverted directly to the pulmonary arteries and thus all systemic venous return must traverse the pulmonary circulation without a subpulmonic pumping chamber to maintain adequate ventricular filling. The P_{ms} drives systemic venous return from the venous reservoirs to the central venous structures as in a normal circulation but is also responsible for driving systemic venous return across the pulmonary circulation to the single ventricle.[76]

Decreases in the common atrial pressure during the cardiac cycle contribute to the pressure gradient driving pulmonary venous return.[77] Because the pulmonary circulation and single ventricle reside entirely within the chest, changes in intrathoracic pressure do not contribute to driving pulmonary blood flow other than by altering the pressure gradient for systemic venous return to the vena cava–pulmonary artery confluence, as well as by altering the effective compliance of the ventricle as in the normal circulation. Shekerdemian and colleagues[78] demonstrated the importance of intrathoracic pressure in the Fontan circulation. Immediately following the Fontan procedure, negative pressure ventilation using a cuirass significantly improved cardiac output compared with PPV. Williams and colleagues[79] demonstrated the sensitivity of the Fontan circulation to PPV by exposing the inverse relationship between pulmonary vascular resistance and cardiac output with progressive increases in PEEP.

Key References

1. Cournand A, Motley HL, Werko L, et al. Physiologic studies of the effects of intermittent positive pressure breathing on cardiac output in man. *Am J Physiol*. 1948;152:162-174.
2. Brengelmann GL. A critical analysis of the view that right atrial pressure determines venous return. *J Appl Physiol*. 2003;94:849-859.
3. Guyton AC. Determination of cardiac output by equating venous return curves with cardiac output curves. *Physiol Rev*. 1955;35:123-129.

4. Guyton AC, Lindsey AW, Kaufmann BN, Richardson T. Venous return at various right atrial pressure and the normal venous return curve. *Am J Physiol*. 1957;189:609-615.

5. Fessler HE, Brower RG, Wise RA, Permutt S. Effects of positive end-expiratory pressure on the canine venous return curve. *Am Rev Respir Dis*. 1992;146:4-10.

6. Cassidy SS, Robertson CH Jr, Pierce AK, et al. Cardiovascular effects of positive end-expiratory pressure in dogs. *J Appl Physiol*. 1978;44:743-750.

8. Marini JJ, O'Quin R, Culver BH, et al. Estimation of transmural cardiac pressure during ventilation with PEEP. *J Appl Physiol*. 1982;53:384-391.

9. Brecher GA, Hubay CA. Pulmonary blood flow and venous return during spontaneous respiration. *Circ Res*. 1955;3:210-214.

10. Pinsky MR. Instantaneous venous return curves in an intact canine preparation. *J Appl Physiol*. 1984;56:765-771.

11. Pinsky MR. Determinants of pulmonary arterial flow variation during respiration. *J Appl Physiol*. 1984;56:1237-1245.

14. Takata M, Wise RA, Robotham JL. Effects of abdominal pressure on venous return: abdominal vascular zone conditions. *J Appl Physiol*. 1990;69:1961-1972.

15. Takata M, Robotham JL. Effects of inspiratory diaphragmatic descent on inferior vena caval venous return. *J Appl Physiol*. 1992;72:597-607.

16. Teboul JL, Pinsky MR, Mercat A, et al. Estimating cardiac filling pressure in mechanically ventilated patients with hyperinflation. *Crit Care Med*. 2000;28:3631-3636.

17. Pinsky MR. Recent advances in the clinical application of heart-lung interactions. *Curr Opin Crit Care*. 2002;8:26-31.

18. Burton AC, Patel DJ. Effect on pulmonary vascular resistance of inflation of the rabbit lungs. *J Appl Physiol*. 1958;12:239-246.

20. Benumof JL. Mechanism of decreased blood flow to atelectatic lung. *J Appl Physiol*. 1979;46:1047-1048.

22. Lopez-Muniz R, Stephens NC, Bromberger-Barnea B, et al. Critical closure of pulmonary vessels analyzed in terms of Starling resistor model. *J Appl Physiol*. 1968;24:625-635.

23. West JB, Dollery CT, Naimark A. Distribution of blood flow in isolated lung: relation to vascular and alveolar pressures. *J Appl Physiol*. 1964;19:713-724.

24. West JB, Dollery CT. Distribution of blood flow and the pressure flow relations of the whole lung. *J Appl Physiol*. 1965;20:175-183.

25. Mink SN, Light RB, Cooligan T, et al. Effect of PEEP on gas exchange and pulmonary perfusion in canine lobar pneumonia. *J Appl Physiol*. 1981;50:517-523.

28. Fishman AP. Vasomotor regulation of the pulmonary circulation. *Ann Rev Physiol*. 1980;42:211-220.

30. Wagner WW. Pulmonary circulation: control through hypoxic vasoconstriction. *Semin Respir Med*. 1985;7:124-135.

32. Fuhrman BP, Everitt J, Lock JE. Cardiopulmonary effects of unilateral airway pressure changes in intact infant lambs. *J Appl Physiol*. 1984;56:1439-1448.

33. Fuhrman BP, Smith-Wright DL, Kulik TJ, et al. Effects of static and fluctuating airway pressure on intact pulmonary circulation. *J Appl Physiol*. 1986;60:114-122.

34. Fuhrman BP, Smith-Wright DL, Venkataraman S, Howland DF. Pulmonary vascular resistance after cessation of positive end-expiratory pressure. *J Appl Physiol*. 1989;66:660-668.

35. Venkataraman ST, Fuhrman BP, Howland DF. PEEP-induced calcium channel-mediated rise in PVR in neonatal lambs. *Crit Care Med*. 1993;21:1066-1076.

36. Taylor RR, Covell JW, Sonnenblick EH, et al. Dependence of ventricular distensibility on filling of the opposite ventricle. *Am J Physiol*. 1967;213:711-718.

37. Mitchell JR, Whitelaw WA, Sas R. RV filling modulates LV function by direct ventricular interaction during mechanical ventilation. *Am J Physiol Heart Circ Physiol*. 2005;289:H549-H557.

38. Buda AJ, Pinsky MR, Ingels NB Jr, et al. Effect of intrathoracic pressure on left ventricular performance. *N Engl J Med*. 1979;301:453-459.

39. Pinsky MR, Summer WR, Wise RA, et al. Augmentation of cardiac function by elevation of intrathoracic pressure. *J Appl Physiol*. 1983;54:950-955.

48. Johnston WE, Vinten-Johansen I, Santamore WP, et al. Mechanism of reduced cardiac output during positive end-expiratory pressure in the dog. *Am Rev Respir Dis*. 1989;140:1257-1264.

51. Schulman DS, Biondi JW, Zohgbi S, et al. Coronary flow limits right ventricular performance during positive end-expiratory pressure. *Am Rev Respir Dis*. 1990;141:1531-1537.

52. Fessler HE, Brower RG, Wise R, et al. Positive pleural pressure decreases coronary perfusion. *Am J Physiol*. 1990;258:H814-H820.

53. Jellinek H, Krafft P, Fitzgerald RD, et al. Right atrial pressure predicts hemodynamic response to apneic positive airway pressure. *Crit Care Med*. 2000;28:672-678.

54. Michard F, Chemla D, Richard C, et al. Clinical use of respiratory changes in arterial pulse pressure to monitor the hemodynamic effects of PEEP in patients with acute lung injury. *Am J Respir Crit Care Med*. 1999;159:935-939.

55. Michard F, Boussat S, Chemla D, et al. Relation between respiratory changes in arterial pulse pressure and fluid responsiveness in septic patients with acute circulatory failure. *Am J Respir Crit Care Med*. 2000;162:134-138.

56. Van Den Berg P, Jansen JR, Pinsky MR. Effect of positive pressure on venous return in volume-loaded cardiac surgical patients. *J Appl Physiol*. 2002;92:1223-1231.

57. Pinsky MR, Matuschak GM, Klain M. Determinants of cardiac augmentation by increase in intrathoracic pressure. *J Appl Physiol*. 1985;58:1189-1198.

58. Michard F, Teboul JL. Predicting fluid responsiveness in ICU patients: a critical analysis of the evidence. *Chest*. 2002;121:2000-2008.

59. Kumar A, Anel R, Bunnell E. Pulmonary artery occlusion pressure and central venous pressure fail to predict ventricular filling volume, cardiac performance or the response to volume infusion in normal subjects. *Crit Care Med*. 2004;32:691-699.

60. Reuter DA, Kirchner A, Felbinger TW. Usefulness of left ventricular stroke volume variation to assess fluid responsiveness in patients with reduced cardiac function. *Crit Care Med*. 2003;31:1399-1404.

61. Slama M, Masson H, Teboul JL. Monitoring of respiratory variations of aortic blood flow velocity using esophageal Doppler. *Intensive Care Med*. 2004;30:1182-1187.

62. Feissel M, Michard F, Faller JP, Teboul JL. The respiratory variation in inferior vena cava diameter as a guide to fluid therapy. *Intensive Care Med*. 2004;30:1834-1837.

64. Aubier M, Trippenbach T, Roussos C. Respiratory muscle fatigue during cardiogenic shock. *Appl Physiol*. 1981;51:499-508.

66. Viires N, Aubier SM, Rassidakis A, et al. Regional blood flow distribution in dog during induced hypotension and low cardiac output. *J Clin Invest*. 1983;72:935-947.

71. Pepe PE, Lurie KG, Wigginton JG, et al. Detrimental hemodynamic effects of assisted ventilation in hemorrhagic states. *Crit Care Med*. 2004;32(suppl):S414-S420.

72. Pinsky MR. Using ventilation-induced aortic pressure and flow variation to diagnose preload responsiveness. *Intensive Care Med*. 2004;30:1008-1010.

76. Mace L, Dervanian P, Bourriez A, et al. Changes in venous return parameters associated with univentricular Fontan circulations. *Am J Physiol Heart Circ Physiol*. 2000;279:H2335-H2343.

78. Shekerdemian LS, Bush A, Shore DF, et al. Cardiopulmonary interactions after the Fontan operation. Augmentation of cardiac output using negative pressure ventilation. *Circulation*. 1997;96:3934-3942.

79. Williams DB, Kiernan PD, Metke MP, et al. Hemodynamic response to positive end-expiratory pressure following right atrium-pulmonary artery bypass (Fontan procedure). *J Thorac Cardiovasc Surg*. 1984;87:856-861.

Disorders of Cardiac Rhythm

Frank A. Fish and Prince J. Kannankeril

PEARLS

- Arrhythmias may result from ongoing therapies; ask, "What's the DEAL?"
  - *Drugs and drips*
  - *Electrolytes*
  - *Airway and acid base*
  - *Lines*
- Appropriate diagnosis is key. Always attempt to document arrhythmia in multiple leads before instituting therapy.
- For ventricular fibrillation or pulseless ventricular tachycardia, begin cardiopulmonary resuscitation and defibrillate immediately.
- Involve a cardiologist before initiating (chronic) antiarrhythmic drug therapy.
- Whenever possible, use available means to document atrial rate to discern correct ventricular-atrial relationship.
- "Supraventricular tachycardia" is a nonspecific electrocardiographic pattern. Multiple types of supraventricular tachycardia exist, and appropriate therapy depends on appropriate diagnosis.
- Whenever possible, opt for therapies that maintain atrioventricular synchrony.

Cardiac arrhythmias are frequently encountered in the intensive care setting. This chapter reviews diagnosis and management of arrhythmias representing a primary disease process and those that occur secondary to other conditions or therapies (Table 35.1).[1,2] Prompt restoration of hemodynamic stability concurrent with appropriate identification of the arrhythmia mechanism and predisposing factors is emphasized while providing a broader overview of arrhythmia mechanisms and their associated presentations in pediatric patients.

Classification of Arrhythmias

Arrhythmias can be classified according to rate, electrocardiographic findings, and, when possible, the underlying electrophysiologic mechanisms. Electrocardiographically, arrhythmias can be characterized as bradycardias, extrasystoles, or tachycardias. Bradycardias are further subdivided by the level of dysfunction (eg, sinus node dysfunction vs. atrioventricular [AV] block) and by the ensuing rhythm (sinus, junctional, or idioventricular). Extrasystoles and tachycardias are categorized as atrial, junctional, or ventricular in origin. Tachycardias are initially characterized by the level of origin

(supraventricular vs. ventricular), by electrocardiographic pattern, and functional mechanism: reentry, automaticity, or triggered activity. Whereas most treatment algorithms assume a reentrant mechanism, abnormal triggering and automaticity may be particularly important in the critically ill. Although differentiating between these mechanisms is sometimes difficult, it may be essential in guiding appropriate therapy, especially if initial therapies prove ineffective.

Bradycardias

Appropriate Versus Normal Heart Rate

Since normal heart rate ranges vary tremendously during childhood as a function of age and autonomic tone, "appropriate" heart rate is a more useful concept than "normal" heart rate. Thus any inappropriately fast or slow rates for a given circumstance warrant evaluation for factors affecting the sinus rate such as pain, agitation, respiratory insufficiency, oversedation, anemia, or acidosis, as well as the potential for a nonsinus arrhythmia.

Sinus Bradycardia and Sinus Pauses

Sinus bradycardia may result from high vagal tone, hypothermia, acidosis, increased intracranial pressure, drug toxicities, or direct surgical trauma to the sinoatrial (SA) node. Primary sinus node dysfunction in childhood is rare but has been described.[3] Transiently profound sinus bradycardia or prolonged sinus pauses of several seconds duration may be caused by intense vagal episodes, such as those occurring during neurocardiogenic syncope, apnea, or endotracheal suctioning. When clearly correlated with a vagal stimulus, pacing can usually be deferred. However, the hemodynamically tenuous patient with persistent or recurring bradycardias may warrant vagolytic, sympathomimetic, or pacing therapies.

It is important to recognize pauses due to blocked premature atrial depolarizations (PACs) where premature P waves may be obscured in the preceding T wave. Similarly, blocked PACs occurring in a bigeminal pattern may mimic sinus bradycardia. In cardiac patients, sinus node dysfunction may be the result of surgical injury or heterotaxy syndromes. Sinus bradycardia can also be a manifestation of long QT syndrome in infancy and of channelopathies.[4]

Atrioventricular Block

AV block is characterized as first-degree, second-degree, and third-degree, according to whether there is conduction delay, intermittent block, or complete loss of conduction between atria and ventricles. As with sinus bradycardia, AV conduction delay may be the result of intense vagal tone, metabolic derangements, drug toxicity, or direct injury to the AV node.

TABLE 35.1   Classification of Arrhythmias by Type and Basis

Arrhythmia	Primary	Secondary
Ventricular premature beats and supraventricular premature beats	+++	+++
Sinus bradycardia, sick sinus syndrome	++	++
Incomplete AV block		
Mobitz I	++	+++
Mobitz II		++
Congenital third-degree AV block	+++	++
Acquired third-degree AV Block		++
Paroxysmal SVT (AV reentrant tachycardia, AV nodal reentrant tachycardia)	+++	
Ectopic atrial tachycardia	++	
Atrial flutter and intraatrial reentry	++	+++
Atrial fibrillation	+	+++
Chaotic atrial tachycardia		++
Junctional ectopic tachycardia	+	+++
Monomorphic ventricular tachycardia	++	++
Torsades des pointes	+	+
Ventricular fibrillation	+	++
Bidirectional ventricular tachycardia	++	+

AV, atrioventricular; *SVT,* supraventricular tachycardia; +++, typical; ++, occasional; +, rare.

Second-degree block can be further characterized as Mobitz type I or Mobitz type II. In Mobitz I (Wenckebach conduction) there is progressive prolongation of the PR before block. It may be best recognized by comparing the last PR interval before block with the next conducted PR. Mobitz I usually represents block in the AV node and is less likely to progress suddenly to high-grade block. In some settings, such as in well-conditioned athletes, Mobitz I block may be benign.

Mobitz type II AV block is characterized by abrupt failure to conduct without prior lengthening of the PR interval. It is usually attributed to block within the His bundle and may portend a greater potential for sudden progression to complete AV block. Type II block may be more ominous and may require more aggressive and preemptive intervention with pacing.

Higher grades of second-degree AV block are best characterized by the ratio of atrial to ventricular depolarizations (2:1, 3:1, 4:1, etc.). Unless the onset is displayed, it cannot be characterized as Mobitz I or Mobitz II and the level of block cannot be inferred. High-grade AV block during sinus rhythm is usually pathologic but can occur as a normal response to rapid atrial tachyarrhythmias such as atrial flutter. Likewise, vagally mediated AV block may result in transient high-grade block (although the sinus rate usually slows concurrently).

Complete or third-degree AV block represents complete loss of AV conduction, usually with a junctional or idioventricular escape rhythm that is regular but may be quite slow. Changes in the RR interval usually indicate intermittent conduction during second-degree block (Fig. 35.1) or a junctional

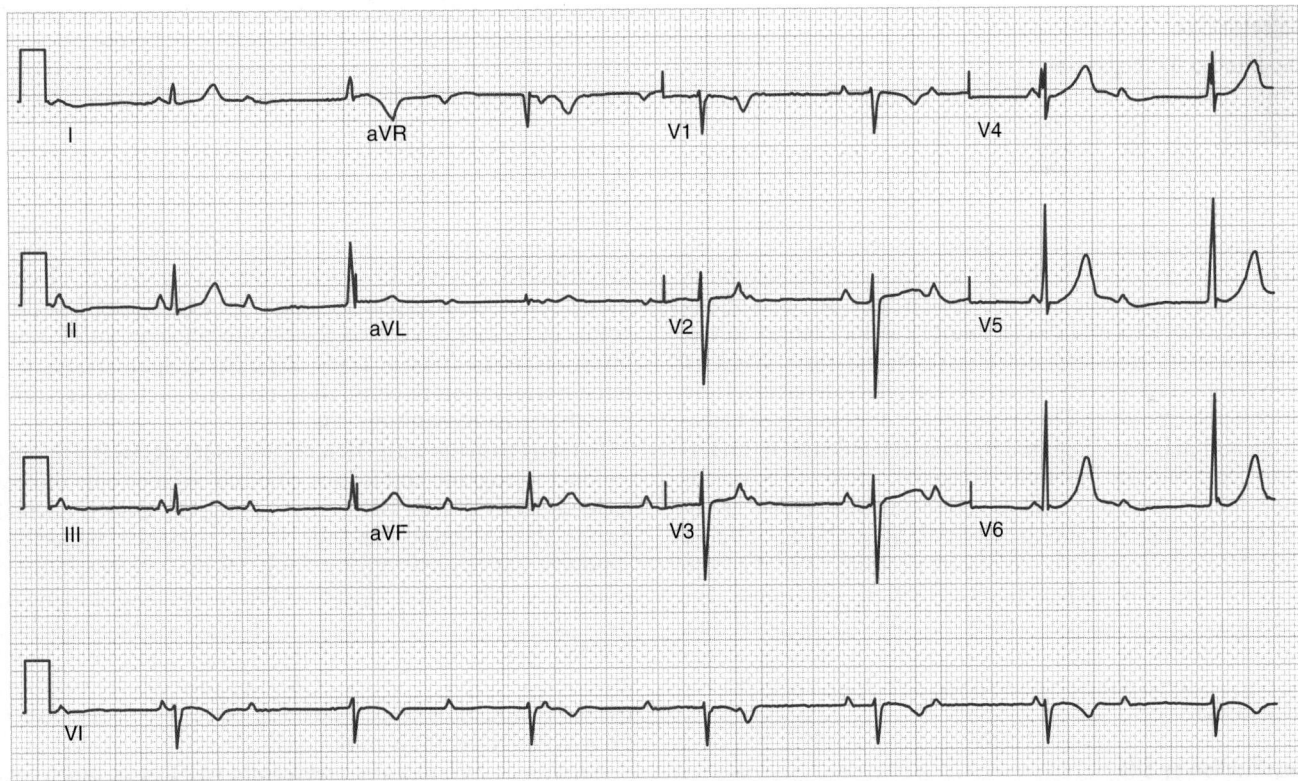

Fig. 35.1. Complete atrioventricular (AV) block, presumably congenital, in an asymptomatic 9-year-old with slow resting heart rate. Note the regular RR interval, which confirms complete rather than incomplete (second-degree) AV block.

rhythm with slower atrial rate and intermittent AV conduction (sinus capture complexes).

Bundle branch block patterns occur when impaired conduction in the specialized intraventricular conduction system results in delayed right or left ventricular depolarization, resulting in an aberrant widened QRS complex. Bundle branch block and AV block sometimes represent normal physiologic responses to abrupt shortening of the cycle length (as with premature atrial systoles or tachycardia initiation) or may result from drug effects, surgical injury, or primary disease within the specialized conduction tissue.

Escape Rhythms and Accelerated Rhythms

In the presence of sinus bradycardia or AV block, slower subsidiary rhythms typically emerge from the atrium, AV node, His-Purkinje system, or ventricular myocardium. When slower than the appropriate sinus rate, they are referred to as escape rhythms (atrial, junctional, or idioventricular). Similar rhythms may emerge and compete with an appropriate sinus rhythm, in which case they are referred to as an *accelerated rhythm*. Such rhythms can result from increased adrenergic tone, intrinsic mechanisms, or drug infusions. It is important to distinguish these accelerated subsidiary rhythms from escape rhythms resulting from AV block. Only rarely does an accelerated junctional or ventricular rhythm result in significant symptoms in a healthy child.[5] However, in the critically ill patient, atrial pacing at a slightly faster rate may be warranted to reestablish AV synchrony if cardiac output is compromised. The distinction between these accelerated junctional or ventricular rhythms and pathologic tachycardia can sometimes be arbitrary but is usually determined by the similarity in rates and gradual transitions between the accelerated rhythm with the normal sinus rhythm.

Tachycardias

Classification by Mechanism

While sinus tachycardia is the most common tachycardia of ill patients, pathologic tachycardias can occur due to three basic mechanisms: reentry, automaticity, or triggered. *Reentry* accounts for most forms of SVT, including atrial flutter and most sustained ventricular tachycardias (VTs). Reentrant tachycardias display an abrupt onset and termination, usually maintaining a relatively fixed rate. In contrast, *automatic* tachycardias arise from ectopic foci within the atrium, AV node, or ventricles and display more gradual changes in rate with "warm up" and "cool down" at onset and offset. *Triggered* tachycardias result from abnormal secondary depolarizations (afterdepolarizations). They typically occur as bursts of tachycardia and may be recognized by their dependence on underlying heart rate for initiation. Triggered activity is especially important in several specific situations such as cardiac glycoside toxicity (delayed afterdepolarizations) and drug-induced long QT syndromes (early afterdepolarizations), and they also are important in many hereditary arrhythmia syndromes. The dependence of triggered activity on underlying heart rate can sometimes be exploited therapeutically because either raising or lowering the underlying rate may suppress the tachycardia.

Classification by Site

Tachycardias usually are first characterized as either supraventricular or ventricular. However, both supraventricular and VTs include a diverse group of arrhythmias with varying substrates, mechanisms, and electrocardiographic features that become increasingly important when simple treatment algorithms fail or when arrhythmias become recurrent and require repeated or ongoing therapies.

Supraventricular Tachycardias

"Supraventricular tachycardia" (SVT), "paroxysmal atrial tachycardia," and "paroxysmal supraventricular tachycardia" (PSVT) are descriptive but nonspecific terms commonly used to describe any regular tachycardia (usually in excess of 200–220 beats/min) with normal QRS morphology and P waves that are either indiscernible or immediately follow the QRS complex. In otherwise healthy neonates and children this pattern usually represents a "reciprocating" tachycardia due to AV nodal reentry or AV reentry using an accessory connection (see next section). However, these same electrocardiographic features can be produced by a more diverse array of tachycardia mechanisms.[6] Furthermore, the most common SVTs can sometimes display variable patterns, including a "normal" PR interval, intermittent 2:1 conduction (in the case of AV node reentry), or a widened QRS, either because of rate-related bundle branch block or antegrade conduction through an accessory connection. Therefore it is most useful to adopt a broad and inclusive definition of SVT, which allows inclusion of nonreciprocating mechanisms such as atrial tachycardia, atrial flutter and fibrillation, junctional tachycardias, and wide QRS SVTs.

Atrioventricular Reciprocating Tachycardias (AV Reentry)

AV reciprocating tachycardias use one or more accessory AV connections in a reentrant circuit between the atria and ventricles. By definition, they display a fixed 1:1 AV relationship. In the most common pediatric mechanism of SVT, referred to as *orthodromic reciprocating tachycardia* (ORT), the AV node serves as the antegrade limb and retrograde conduction is over the accessory pathway,[6,7] with retrograde P waves immediately following each QRS complex.

Permanent junctional reciprocating tachycardia (PJRT) is a variant of ORT in which the accessory pathway displays slow, decremental ("AV node-like") conduction.[8] The result is typically a slower, more incessant tachycardia displaying a short or normal PR interval. In a single-lead rhythm strip, PJRT may mimic sinus tachycardia, although a 12-lead electrocardiogram (ECG) reveals atypical P wave morphology with P-wave inversion in the inferior leads. Repetitively spontaneous termination and prompt reinitiation are common features aiding in tachycardia recognition (Fig. 35.2).

In many patients with ORT, the accessory pathway can only conduct retrograde and is thus clinically evident only during tachycardia or during ventricular pacing; the QRS is normal during sinus rhythm. However, if the accessory connection conducts antegradely during sinus rhythm, "preexcitation" results in a delta wave: shortened PR interval and slurring of the QRS upstroke, the hallmark of Wolff-Parkinson-White (WPW) syndrome. Many patients with congenital heart disease may display a slurred QRS upstroke due to intraventricular conduction delay, which can be readily distinguished from WPW if the PR is prolonged.

Antidromic reciprocating tachycardia (ART) is a much less common form of AV reentry in which the circuit is reversed: Antegrade conduction from atrium to ventricle is over the

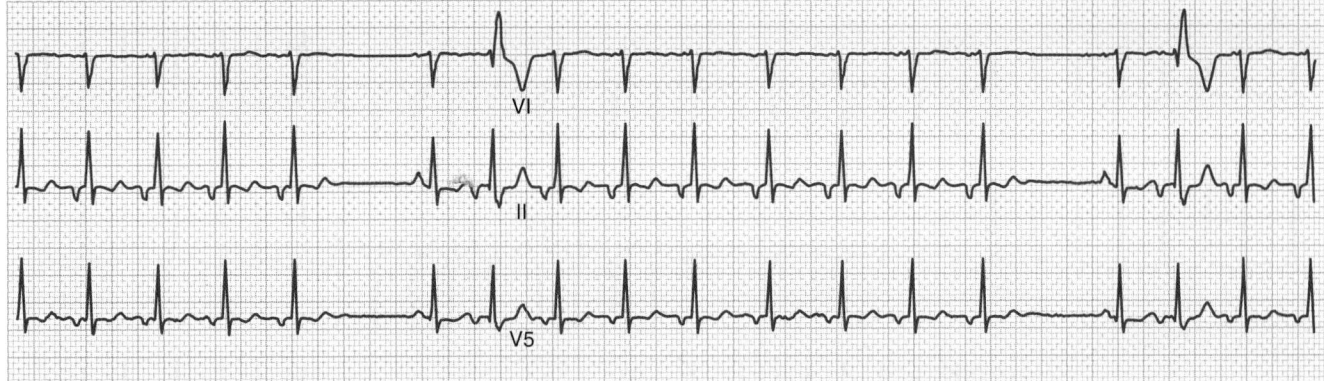

Fig. 35.2. Supraventricular tachycardia resulting from the permanent form of junctional reciprocating tachycardia. Note the slow rate, long RP and short PR interval, and inverted P waves in electrocardiogram leads II and III. At rest, this rhythm often shows incessantly repetitive termination (with retrograde block), followed by immediate reinitiation (after single, isolated sinus complexes). With exercise, this rhythm is often faster and sustained, rendering it electrocardiographically indistinguishable from the atypical form of nodal reentry.

accessory connection, resulting in a very wide ("maximally preexcited") QRS. ART can be difficult to distinguish from VT. Because it is a potentially more dangerous rhythm than ORT, it is most appropriately managed as VT in the acute setting. However, by definition, patients experiencing ART will display the WPW pattern after sinus rhythm is restored.

A specific form of antidromic AV reentry uses a Mahaim fiber. In the current era, this usually refers to a connection traversing the right AV ring, which displays decremental or AV nodelike conduction (atriofascicular connection). It results in wide QRS tachycardia resembling a left bundle branch block pattern and is particularly common in patients with Ebstein anomaly. Though usually responsive acutely to maneuvers interrupting AV node conduction, electrophysiologic study is required to confirm the diagnosis and distinguish it from VT or other forms of SVT with aberrancy.

Atrioventricular Nodal Reentrant Tachycardia

AV nodal reentrant tachycardia (AVNRT) is the second most common cause of SVT in older children and young adults without WPW syndrome or structural heart disease. It is seen less commonly in infants.[6,7] This tachycardia is attributed to so-called "dual AV nodal physiology" in which two or more separate inputs into the AV node (slow and fast pathways) conduct into and out of the AV node, providing the substrate for reentry.

Classically, two electrocardiographically distinct forms of AVNRT may occur. In "typical" AV node reentry, antegrade and retrograde conduction occurs over the slow and fast AV node inputs, respectively; retrograde P waves are obscured by the preceding QRS complex. In the "atypical" form of AV node reentry, the circuit is reversed, resulting in a long RP and short PR with an inverted P wave. Thus typical AVNRT resembles ORT and atypical AVNRT resembles PJRT (see previous section). Like PJRT, atypical AVNRT can also be mistaken for sinus tachycardia, as well as other atrial tachycardias (see next section). AVNRT with 2:1 conduction and other complex variations can be defined only with an intracardiac electrophysiologic study.

Primary Atrial Tachycardias

Atrial tachycardias present with diverse electrocardiographic patterns, including discrete and regular P waves (ectopic atrial

tachycardia, intraarterial reentry), sawtooth flutter waves (atrial flutter), or disorganized atrial activity (atrial fibrillation, chaotic atrial tachycardia).[9] Conduction to the ventricles can be variable, and the ventricular rate primarily determines the severity of symptoms, though loss of AV synchrony can also be important. When 1:1 conduction is present, adenosine or vagal maneuvers producing transient AV block will reveal the faster, ongoing atrial rate. Direct recordings of atrial activity (via esophageal, epicardial, or intraarterial recordings) are also useful, particularly in revealing 2:1 AV conduction. Despite the potential electrocardiographic similarities of the various primary atrial tachycardias, the varying mechanisms confer important differences in clinical behavior and management.

Most atrial tachycardias encountered in the pediatric intensive care setting are due to atrial reentry and are commonly referred to as "atrial flutter" regardless of whether the classic saw-toothed pattern (as in neonatal atrial flutter) is observed. In older patients with congenital heart disease (CHD), the term *intraatrial reentrant tachycardia* (IART) is often used to describe the slower, scar-dependent atrial reentry, which can result in normal-appearing P waves (rather than classic "flutter" waves). Because of the slower atrial rate, 1:1 AV conduction may be especially common, further confounding the diagnosis. Likewise, administration of an AV node–blocking agent may result in 2:1 AV conduction, leading to the erroneous conclusion that the tachycardia has been converted to sinus rhythm with first-degree AV block. Thus this arrhythmia should be suspected in any patient with postoperative CHD presenting with a monotonous and inappropriate tachycardia, otherwise suggestive of sinus tachycardia on ECG.

Atrial fibrillation, a common arrhythmia among the elderly, is far less common in pediatric patients. It may occur as the result of atrial myocarditis,[10] secondary to an underlying reentrant SVT[11] or mechanical stimulation by central venous catheters (Fig. 35.3). In patients with WPW syndrome, rapid conduction over the accessory pathway during atrial fibrillation can be life-threatening. When atrial fibrillation occurs in a young patient, the underlying basis should be sought because the long-term implications and treatment measures are much different than in adult patients.

Ectopic atrial tachycardia (EAT) is an automatic arrhythmia that typically presents as an incessant and chronically elevated

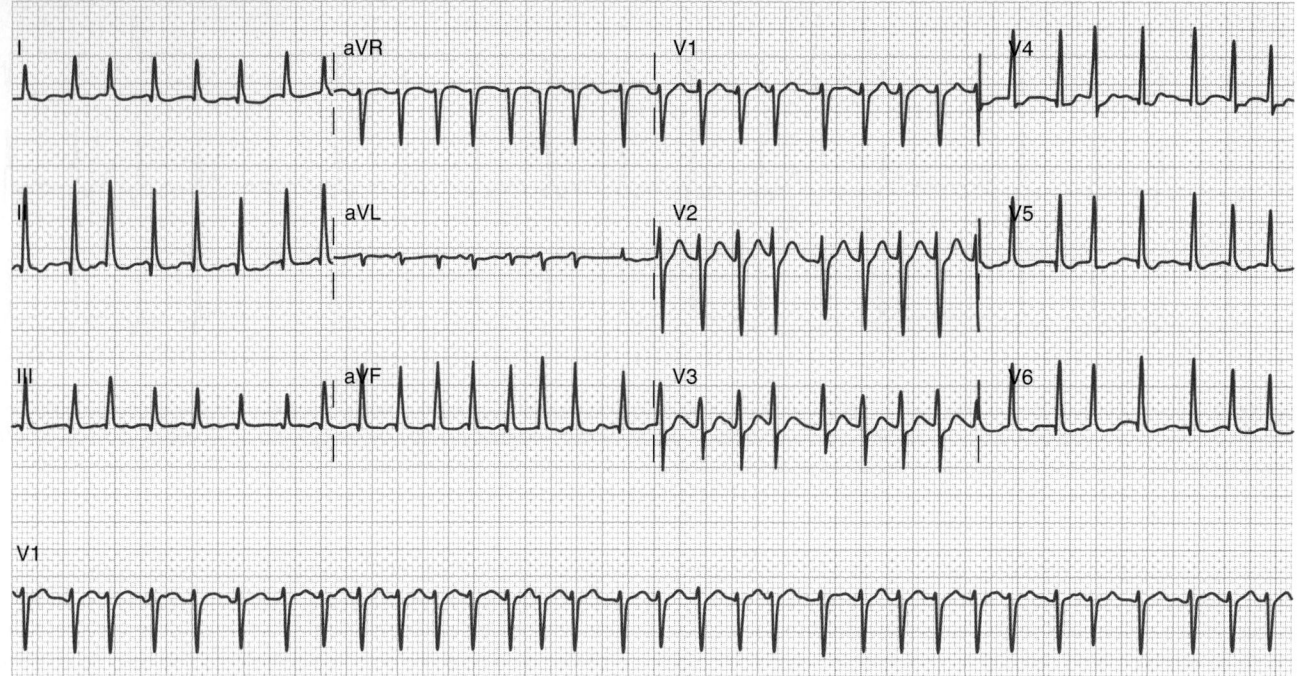

Fig. 35.3. Sustained atrial fibrillation in a previously healthy 17-year-old placed on extracorporeal membrane oxygenation for pneumonia and acute respiratory distress syndrome. Review of stored telemetry revealed atrial ectopy soon after cannulation, eventually initiating atrial fibrillation. Following direct current cardioversion to sinus rhythm, frequent ectopy persisted until the venous cannula was repositioned. Several months later, the patient remained free of further arrhythmias.

atrial rhythm that may be mistaken for sinus tachycardia, especially when the automatic focus is in the right atrium. First-degree AV block may be seen as a physiologic response to the inappropriately accelerated rate. Patients with EAT usually experience no overt palpitations but present instead with ventricular dysfunction and sometimes frank congestive heart failure (CHF). Because adenosine may transiently inhibit the automatic focus, termination with adenosine is nondiagnostic in distinguishing EAT from sinus tachycardia.

Instead, careful scrutiny of the P wave morphology, especially with transitions between the EAT and sinus, is necessary to establish the diagnosis.

Chaotic atrial tachycardia is an uncommon arrhythmia that is usually observed in infants and toddlers, often in association with a viral respiratory illness.[12] The hallmark features are a rapid and irregular atrial rate, often exceeding 300 bpm, and presence of multiple P-wave morphologies. The resulting ventricular response is irregularly irregular, simulating atrial fibrillation. However, this rhythm is probably the result of multiple triggered foci within the atria, and thus acute termination measures (ie, direct current cardioversion, adenosine, or pacing) are of little benefit. Usually this arrhythmia resolves within weeks or months of presentation. Treatment is based on the severity of symptoms.

Junctional Ectopic Tachycardia

Junctional ectopic tachycardia (JET) probably arises from an abnormal automatic focus or a protected microreentrant circuit in the region of the AV node or proximal His bundle. Antegrade conduction is usually over the normal His-Purkinje system with a narrow QRS. Retrograde (ventriculoatrial [VA]) block with complete VA dissociation and "sinus

capture" complexes aid in the recognition of this mechanism. Sometimes AV block coexists with JET. Variants include the common transient postsurgical JET, a congenital chronic JET, and paroxysmal JET described primarily in adults.[13,14] As in postoperative atrial tachycardias, direct atrial recordings aid the diagnosis. In some cases, JET is associated with 1:1 VA conduction, in which case additional pacing or pharmacologic maneuvers are necessary to distinguish it from other mechanisms of SVT.

Ventricular Tachycardias

VTs arise exclusively within the ventricle(s), and, by definition, the QRS duration is always aberrant and prolonged for a given age and heart rate. The QRS morphology may be either uniform or changing (bidirectional, polymorphic). Classically, VTs are associated with VA dissociation (atrial rhythm at a slower rate). Thus VA dissociation, when present, is helpful, but when it is absent (or uncertain) it does not exclude VT as the underlying mechanism. The presence of periodic fusion complexes (QRS morphology intermediate between tachycardia morphology and sinus morphology) is diagnostic. However, in infants and young children, ventricular tachycardia may be mistaken as SVT due to the relatively narrower QRS complexes and 1:1 VA conduction. JET with aberrancy is characterized by sinus capture complexes (or sustained AV conduction during atrial pacing) without change in QRS.

Like SVTs, VTs are diverse in pattern, mechanism, and severity, and they may result from each of the tachycardia mechanisms (reentry, automaticity, and triggered activity) with important therapeutic implications. The clinical setting, electrocardiographic pattern, and severity of symptoms dictate acute treatment approaches.

Approach to Diagnosis

Monitoring and General Assessment

In the intensive care setting, there may be a tradeoff between precision of diagnosis and urgency of therapy. Even so, appropriate diagnosis remains key to establishing appropriate ongoing therapy. When an arrhythmia develops, factors such as level of consciousness, ventilation, tissue perfusion, and acid-base status (including mixed venous saturation and lactate) govern what diagnostic measures can be employed before acute therapy. Minimal initial diagnostic evaluation should always include permanently recorded ECG rhythm strips, along with a rapid review of drugs being administered, potential toxic exposures, respiratory and acid-base status, and known associated illnesses that might be arrhythmogenic. Electrolytes, including calcium and magnesium, should be obtained along with drug screening in the patient presenting with altered mental status. The history of surgical procedures for CHD and trauma (chest and cranial) should be quickly reviewed. Indwelling catheter position should be noted on radiographs for potential intracardiac location. Concurrent with this brief survey, a differential diagnosis of the rhythm disturbance should be established quickly, followed by the most appropriate emergency therapy. If the patient is sufficiently stable, therapy may be deferred until a 12-lead ECG is obtained and other diagnostic measures taken for more precisely characterization.

Surface Electrocardiogram

The surface ECG remains the cornerstone of arrhythmia diagnosis. Certainly in patients with known cardiac abnormalities, and arguably in all patients admitted to the ICU, a baseline ECG should be obtained at admission. This ECG may provide a valuable baseline for later comparison in the event of a new arrhythmia. Because these arrhythmias occur in a monitored environment, a strip should be available to assess the rate, regularity, QRS morphology and duration, and AV relationship (Table 35.2), which should provide an initial differential diagnosis (Fig. 35.4). Ideally, multiple leads should be inspected. For sustained tachycardias, a full 12-lead ECG should be obtained whenever possible because diagnostic details, such as QRS aberrancy, atrial rate, and P-wave morphology, or hidden features, such as "flutter waves," may be evident only in selected leads (Fig. 35.5). Rate trends should be reviewed for abruptness of onset to help discriminate between sinus and nonsinus tachycardias in the critical patient.

While the surface ECG usually is sufficient to characterize bradycardias, additional diagnostic maneuvers, sometimes coupled with direct recording of atrial activity, may be required to accurately characterize tachycardias. Changes in ventricular rate and regularity, QRS duration and morphology, and atrial-to-ventricular relationship must be actively sought. When available, temporary atrial pacing wires or an esophageal ECG can facilitate the diagnosis (Fig. 35.6). Likewise, observing the response of an arrhythmia following perturbations such as PACs or PVCs may be informative. Repetitive patterns in ventricular activation referred to as "grouped beating" always provide important clues to the diagnosis.

Bradycardias

Perhaps the most important diagnostic issues in bradycardias are determination of AV conduction and the status of

TABLE 35.2	Electrocardiographic Patterns
Pattern	**Description**
AV Block	
Mobitz I	Shortened PR of first conducted beat after block
Mobitz II	No change in PR before/after block Periods of high-grade block
Third-degree	Fixed, rather than variable, RR interval
Supraventricular Tachycardias	
AV reentrant supraventricular tachycardia	P waves obscured or buried in ST segment
AV nodal reentrant supraventricular tachycardia	P waves obscured by terminal QRS "Pseudo" R′ in lead V_1 during tachycardia, not sinus
Junctional ectopic tachycardia	Narrow QRS tachycardia, VA dissociation RR periodically shortened because of sinus capture complexes[a]
Atrial ectopic tachycardia	Monotonous rate, inappropriately fast Abnormal P-wave morphology (may be subtle)
Intraatrial reentrant tachycardia	Inappropriately fast rate, discrete P waves, variable AV conduction in postoperative patient with congenital heart disease
Atrial flutter	Variable RR interval Rapid, sawtooth flutter waves (>280 beats/min)
Atrial fibrillation	Irregular ventricular rate Coarse baseline with no discernible P waves
Chaotic atrial tachycardia	≥3 P-wave morphologies, irregular atrial rate, variable AV conduction (periods or atrial flutter or fibrillation common)
Ventricular Tachycardias	
Monomorphic	Wide QRS for age, different from baseline Slurred upstroke of QRS Variable VA conduction[b] Sinus capture complexes[b]
Idiopathic types	Left bundle branch block, inferior axis (right ventricular outflow tract origin) Right bundle branch block, left superior axis (left ventricular septal origin)
Bidirectional	Alternating QRS axis (beat-to-beat)
Torsades des pointes	Initiation with "short-long-short" sequence QT-interval prolongation before onset "Twisting" of QRS axis

[a]Junctional ectopic tachycardia may be associated with third-degree AV block.
[b]Helpful when seen; absent if 1 : 1 VA relationship.
AV, atrioventricular; *VA*, ventriculoatrial.

underlying intrinsic escape rhythms. This should usually be straightforward when the atrial rate exceeds the ventricular rate during second-degree or third-degree AV block. In complete AV block, the resultant escape rhythm is usually regular; in second-degree AV block, the ventricular intervals vary (see Fig. 35.1). This is helpful when sinus node disease and AV block coexist where variation of the RR interval implies some

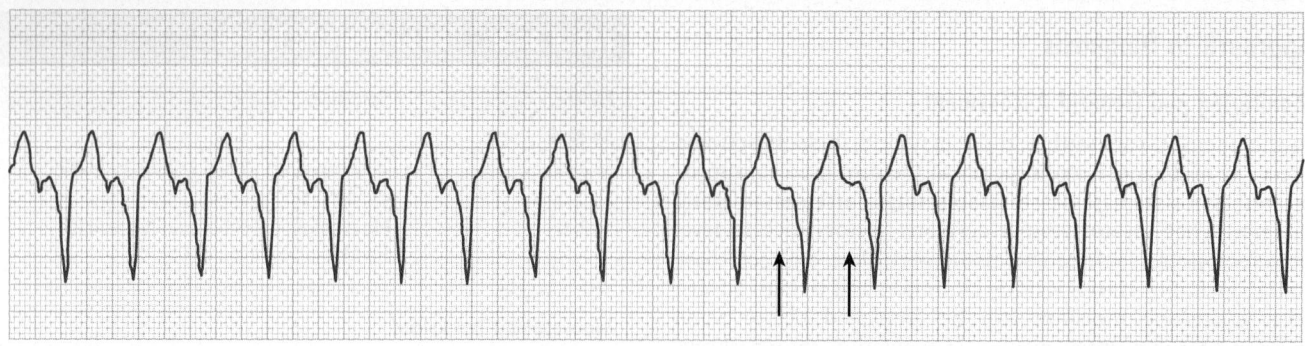

Fig. 35.4. Ventricular tachycardia in an 8-year-old with previous muscular ventricular septal defect repair. Note transient ventriculoatrial block *(arrows)*, excluding a supraventricular mechanism with aberrant conduction.

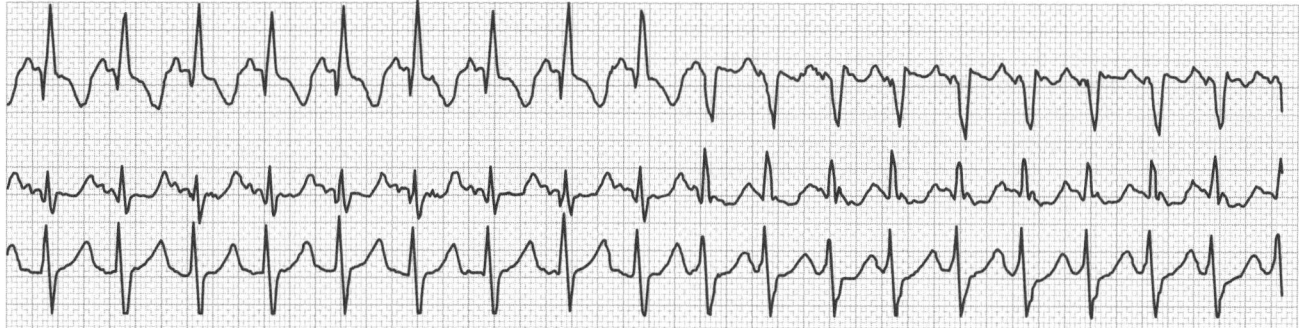

Fig. 35.5. Ventricular tachycardia following cardiac surgery. Note similarity between QRS complexes during sinus rhythm and ventricular tachycardia in two of three recorded leads.

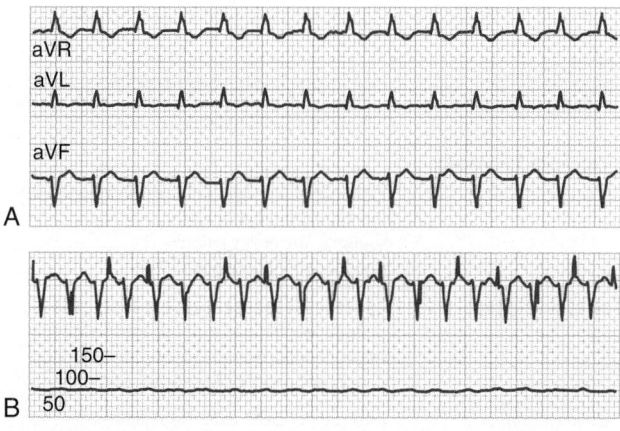

Fig. 35.6. (A) Narrow QRS tachycardia in an infant following a stage I Norwood operation. Possible atrioventricular (AV) dissociation is suggested, but P waves are not easily discerned on the surface electrocardiogram. (B) Atrial recording from the same patient (after rate increased) using an epicardial atrial pacing wire. AV dissociation with faster junctional rate is demonstrated, typical of junctional ectopic tachycardia. Absence of clearly shortened RR intervals because of sinus capture might indicate associated AV block.

degree of AV conduction. When atrial pacing is feasible (as in patients with recent cardiac surgery), AV conduction can be more directly characterized.

The distinction between bradycardia resulting from AV block and sinus nodal dysfunction may have important therapeutic implications. If AV nodal conduction is intact, it is usually most appropriate to pace the atrium only (see AAI

mode) rather than perform dual-chamber pacing. In contrast, isolated AV block is best managed by sensing and tracking the intrinsic atrial rate (see DDD mode).

Extrasystoles

Extrasystoles, or premature beats, are defined as supraventricular (supraventricular premature beats or premature atrial complexes) or ventricular (premature ventricular complexes, ventricular premature beats [VPBs]) in origin. True junctional extrasystoles are uncommon. When the extrasystole results in an early QRS with normal morphology and duration, a supraventricular extrasystole may be presumed. Usually, an early P wave can be discerned, but it may be obscured by the preceding T wave in certain leads. The ensuing sinus beat is usually advanced by the atrial extrasystole, but entrance block can result in a "full compensatory pause," often attributed to a ventricular extrasystole.

Isolated premature QRS complexes with prolonged QRS duration may represent either ventricular extrasystoles or aberrantly conducted atrial extrasystoles. Distinguishing the two may be difficult from a single rhythm strip. Premature P waves often may be obscured in a particular lead, or the ventricular extrasystole morphology may appear similar to the sinus QRS in one lead (but totally dissimilar in another). The ECG features favoring ventricular extrasystoles over aberrantly conducted atrial extrasystoles include (1) wide QRS morphology, (2) a full compensatory pause, (3) presence of fusion beats, and (4) absence of a discernible premature P wave. In the setting of ventricular preexcitation, variable fusion can occur as a result of exaggerated preexcitation with premature atrial depolarizations. As noted earlier, ventricular extrasystoles usually are followed by a full compensatory pause because the sinus node is not reset by the ventricular depolarization. However, an atrial extrasystole may also sometimes fail to reset the sinus node (because of entrance block) or a ventricular extrasystole may occasionally reset the sinus node because of retrograde (VA) conduction to the atrium.

The distinction between atrial and ventricular extrasystoles may be somewhat academic in otherwise asymptomatic individuals because neither generally warrants therapy. However, either might be a harbinger for myocardial irritability and should prompt a search for underlying causes. Occasionally, measures to suppress ectopy may appear to improve cardiac output by "regularizing" filling time in an otherwise tenuous patient. The relative advantages and risks of any such measure, whether achieved with medications or temporary pacing, need to be considered individually.

Tachycardias With Normal QRS

In otherwise healthy infants, children, and adolescents, SVT usually represents AV reentrant tachycardia or AVNRT (Fig. 35.7). Further distinction between these two mechanisms has little impact on acute management. However, in the ICU setting, primary atrial tachycardias (including sinus tachycardia) and junctional tachycardias are more prevalent (particularly following cardiac surgery). The finding of abnormal P-wave morphology (determined by 12-lead ECG), a PR interval greater than 50% of the RR interval, or completely obscured P waves favors a nonsinus mechanism. Finally, ensuring normal QRS duration for age, rather than simply relying on adult standards, is essential in discriminating from VTs.

Distinguishing sinus tachycardia from various types of SVT may be difficult. In young patients, intraarterial reentry, atrial flutter, and atrial fibrillation are usually seen following surgical treatment for congenital heart defects involving the atrium (atrial septal defects, atrial repair of transposition of the great arteries, or the Fontan operation).[15] The term *intraarterial reentrant tachycardia* (IART) is often used in this setting when discrete P waves are present rather the usual sawtooth "flutter waves." Because the atrial rate is often relatively slow in comparison with "typical" atrial flutter, a high index of suspicion is essential in recognizing this rhythm from sinus rhythm or sinus tachycardia, especially when fixed 1:1 conduction or 2:1 conduction (with blocked P waves obscured by the QRS or T wave). Again, direct atrial recordings using transesophageal electrocardiography or temporary epicardial atrial pacing wires usually facilitate the diagnosis and characterize the AV relationship (see Fig. 35.6B), as can vagal maneuvers or administration of adenosine to temporally interrupt AV conduction.

Tachycardias With Prolonged QRS

Generally, tachycardias with prolonged QRS should be presumed to be VTs until or unless evidence of an alternative diagnosis is clearly demonstrated. VA dissociation, the hallmark ECG feature of VT, may not be seen in childhood because of rapid retrograde conduction over the AV node (see Fig. 35.4). The distinction between VT and SVT with aberrant conduction can be difficult and may ultimately require invasive electrophysiologic study. Prolonged attempts to differentiate SVT from VT by noninvasive means may simply delay

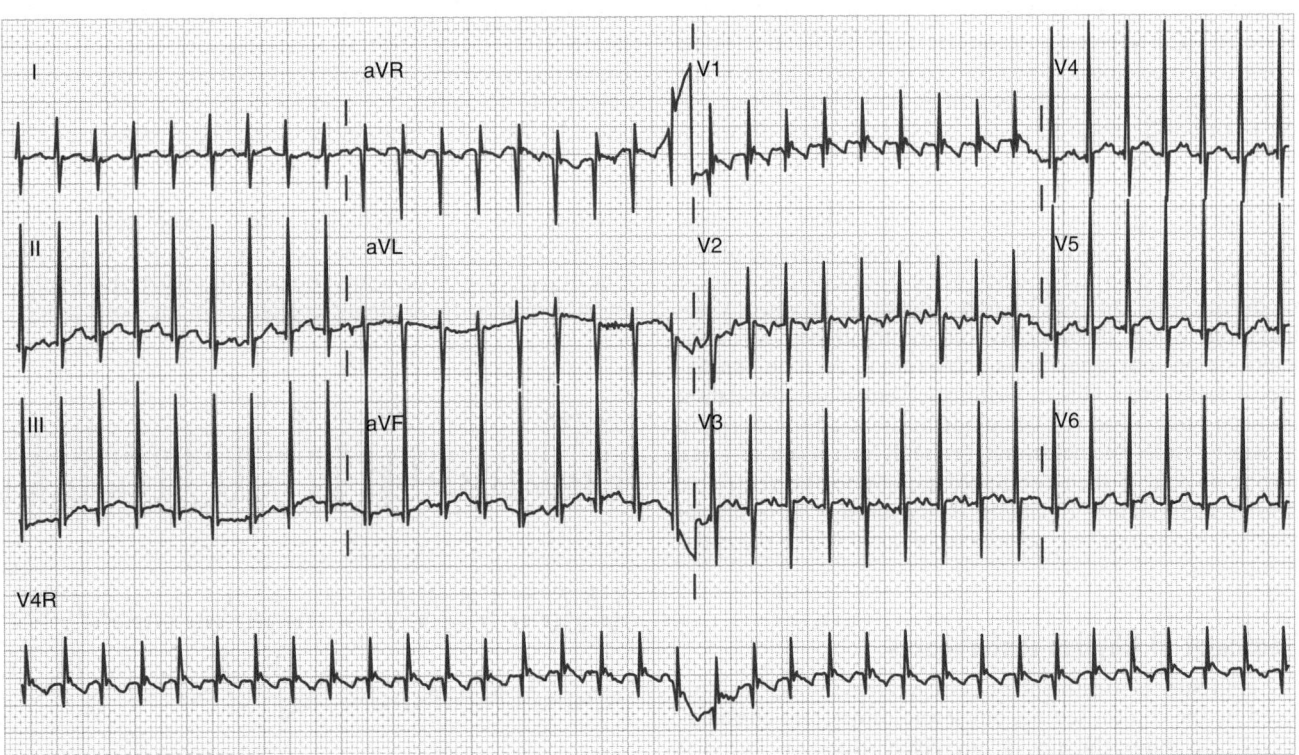

Fig. 35.7. Supraventricular tachycardia resulting from atrioventricular nodal reentry in an infant. Although considerably less common than orthodromic reciprocating tachycardia in this age group, the P wave on the terminal portion of the QRS complex results in a "pseudo rSr' pattern." During sinus rhythm, this terminal deflection on the QRS was absent, and the transesophageal recording confirmed the mechanism.

treatment, and the wrong conclusion may prove disastrous: acute treatment based on a presumed diagnosis of VT is rarely deleterious, even when the mechanism subsequently proves to be supraventricular. However, an erroneous presumption of "SVT with aberrant conduction" may result in rapid clinical deterioration. When feasible, a full 12-lead ECG may aid in the diagnosis, particularly when a baseline ECG in normal rhythm is available for comparison. Apparent hemodynamic stability should not be mistaken as evidence of SVT over VT, whether in an otherwise healthy child or in a patient with known cardiac disease.

Monitoring of Atrial Depolarization

When the AV relationship during a tachycardia is unclear, sometimes it can be inferred indirectly by other available monitoring. Invasive arterial and venous pressure waveforms can help define atrial contractile action in some situations. For example, cannon A waves are commonly noted in patients with atrial flutter or JET.

Direct recording of atrial activity is necessary when the AV relationship cannot be determined from the surface ECG or otherwise inferred by the means described. Patients recovering from cardiac surgery may have temporary atrial epicardial pacing wires that can be used to record atrial electrograms directly while simultaneously recording the surface ECG (see Fig. 35.6B). Attachment of the atrial wires to a unipolar precordial lead ("V lead") on the monitor is an easy way to observe atrial activation. Otherwise, atrial activity can be readily recorded with a bipolar esophageal catheter inserted in the esophagus behind the left atrium.

Diagnostic Uses of Adenosine

Although most widely used as an acute therapy for terminating SVT that involves the AV node, adenosine administration also may yield important diagnostic clues to the underlying arrhythmia mechanism.[16] By producing transient block in the AV node during tachycardia, it is often possible to distinguish AV reentrant tachycardias and AVNRTs (either of which should terminate) from atrial tachycardias and VTs. However, adenosine's effects are not confined to the AV node. Ectopic (automatic) atrial and junctional tachycardias, intraatrial reentry, and certain VTs may also terminate with adenosine. Extreme caution should be taken when administering adenosine during wide QRS tachycardia. Adenosine produces vasodilatation, which theoretically can result in hemodynamic deterioration and tachycardia acceleration, or even fibrillation, if tachycardia fails to terminate. Ventricular fibrillation has been rarely observed when adenosine is administered in the setting of WPW syndrome, probably as a result of atrial fibrillation that is then conducted rapidly to the ventricles. *Cardiac defibrillation capability should always be readily at hand when administering adenosine for diagnostic or therapeutic purposes.*

Treatment of Rhythm Disturbances

The approach to treatment of cardiac arrhythmias is influenced by the clinical setting, but several important considerations help guide therapy in any given situation. The first and most important concern is the degree of hemodynamic compromise associated with a particular arrhythmia. At one extreme, minor rhythm disturbances may be more readily recognized in the intensive care setting than in other situations simply because of the level of monitoring and may prompt undue attention and unnecessary treatment. At the other extreme, otherwise life-threatening arrhythmias ordinarily requiring acute therapy may be of little acute consequence in the setting of extracorporeal life support (ECLS) or mechanical ventricular assist devices. Indeed, ECLS may serve as adjunctive therapy for refractory arrhythmias. Even ventricular fibrillation in a patient with an LVAD rarely results in immediate decompensation. In contrast, arrhythmias that might ordinarily be well tolerated may be acutely destabilizing in an already critically ill patient and require immediate intervention.

A second important consideration in critically ill patients, particularly those after cardiac surgery, is to favor therapies that maintain appropriate AV synchrony, whenever feasible. In the setting of marginal hemodynamics, the practice of medically slowing the ventricular rate during arrhythmias such as atrial tachycardias and fibrillation, junctional tachycardia, or AV block may be inadequate to preserve cardiac output (see Fig. 35.8).

A third consideration in the management of arrhythmias in the ICU is the recognition that many arrhythmias in this setting are iatrogenic. Even minor arrhythmias may herald more serious issues, such as electrolyte disturbances, acidosis, subendocardial ischemia, excessive catecholamine infusions, or increased intracranial pressure. It is important to identify and correct any such underlying causes because therapies directed at the rhythm itself may not protect from more serious rhythm decompensation.

Finally, whenever feasible, acute and short-term measures with limited potential to impair hemodynamics generally should be favored over chronic therapies. Thus nonpharmacologic therapies, such as pacing or cardioversion, or ultrashort-acting drugs, such as adenosine and esmolol, may be preferable to chronic antiarrhythmic therapy. Whether chronic therapy is warranted for a given arrhythmia is determined more by its underlying mechanism, clinical setting, and frequency than by the severity of the arrhythmias encountered in the intensive care setting. Before beginning chronic antiarrhythmic therapy, consultation with a cardiologist versed in the spectrum of arrhythmias seen in childhood is advisable. The impact of acute measures on chronic arrhythmia management becomes increasingly crucial with the emergence of

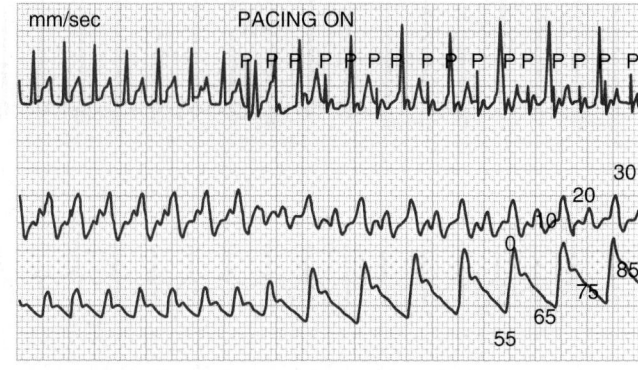

Fig. 35.8. Junctional ectopic tachycardia with hypotension immediately improved with faster atrial pacing (in this case, resulting in 2:1 atrioventricular [AV] block and AV synchrony).

amiodarone use in the ICU and the increasing availability of nonpharmacologic therapies such as radiofrequency catheter ablation and implantable defibrillators for a broader spectrum of arrhythmias and patient populations.[17-19]

Bradycardia Therapies

Whenever treatment is instituted for a rhythm disturbance, an underlying cause should be sought and corrected. This is especially important for bradycardias that occur in the intensive care setting, where airway compromise and respiratory insufficiency probably are the most common causes of acute bradycardias. Increased intracranial pressure, hypothermia, or iatrogenic causes also may produce bradycardias that require specific interventions beyond those outlined here. Emergency interventions for AV nodal and sinus nodal dysfunction are essentially identical. Chest compressions should be administered if there is no effective underlying rhythm.

Pharmacologic Treatment of Bradycardias

After appropriate confirmation or restoration of airway integrity and ventilatory function, initial treatment of symptomatic bradycardias is usually pharmacologic, whether the cause is sinus node slowing or AV nodal block. Atropine (0.01–0.04 mg/kg IV or, if necessary, IM or via endotracheal tube) may transiently ameliorate bradycardia caused by hypoxia (or other vagal stimulants), digoxin, intracranial hypertension, or AV block as a result of Lyme disease. Atropine is less likely to reverse bradycardic effects of β-blocking agents or other antiarrhythmic drugs, particularly in the setting of underlying sinus node disease. Epinephrine (0.1 μg/kg) can be administered by various routes to accelerate the heart rate. Continuous infusions of epinephrine (0.05–0.5 μg/kg/min) or isoproterenol (0.02–0.2 μg/kg/min) may be instituted. In general, high-dose epinephrine or isoproterenol infusions should be replaced by temporary pacing as soon as feasible. Even if lower doses of these agents prove adequate, temporary pacing should be available as a backup. Occasionally, methylxanthines are useful as an alternative to pacing for nonlethal bradycardias. Glycopyrrolate and ketamine may help augment rates in bradycardic patients, requiring sedation or anesthesia.

Temporary and Permanent Pacing for Bradycardias

Pacing is an essential adjunct to medical management of arrhythmias in the ICU. Several reviews of pacing in children are available.[20,21] Pacing can be accomplished using permanently implanted pacemaker and lead systems, temporary epicardial leads attached to the heart at the time of cardiac surgery, transvenous placement of a pacing lead, or transcutaneous patches. Most pacing is performed for bradyarrhythmias, although temporary pacing may be used to terminate reentrant tachyarrhythmias.

Principles of Pacing

All pacing requires a complete circuit with at least one lead on or near each chamber that is to be paced. Often, two leads are placed on each chamber (bipolar leads), although sometimes only the cathode is attached to the heart (unipolar leads), with a subcutaneous electrode acting as the anode. The metal can of a permanent pacemaker can also serve as the anode. The intensity of the pacing stimulus is related to the stimulus duration (pulse width) and its amplitude, which can be expressed as either current (mA) or voltage (V). Energy is proportional to the pulse width and the square of the amplitude. Most temporary pacemakers provide a fixed pulse width, with an adjustable current output (mA). Permanent pacemakers generally have both an adjustable pulse width and amplitude.

Sensing intrinsic activity of the chamber being paced is important to prevent asynchronous pacing that can induce inadvertent tachycardias. The sensitivity of permanent and temporary pacemakers is adjustable. The sensitivity setting (mV) actually refers to a sensing threshold for detection of spontaneous cardiac activity. The spontaneous activity must exceed that threshold to be detected. Thus a lower numeric sensitivity setting makes the pacemaker more sensitive to both spontaneous activity of the atrium or ventricle (appropriate sensing) and other electrical signals (oversensing).

The programmed mode and timing circuits of the pacemaker determine when the pacemaker fires and its response to sensed events. A simplified pacing code uses three letters to describe pacing modes.[22] The first two letters refer to the chamber(s) paced and chamber(s) sensed, respectively (A, atrium; V, ventricle; D, dual). The third letter refers to the response to sensed events (I, inhibit; T, trigger; D, dual). Thus a single-chamber atrial or ventricular pacing demand mode is AAI or VVI mode, whereas dual-chamber pacing is generally DDD mode. Corresponding asynchronous modes are AOO, VOO, or DOO and may be important to prevent inadvertent inhibition of pacing due to electrical interference, such as with electrocautery. Other pacing modes may be employed with permanent pacing systems, and recognizing the peculiarities of these modes is important when distinguishing observed pacing behaviors as appropriate or dysfunctional. Timing intervals most readily adjusted include low rate, AV delay, upper tracking rate (UTR), and postventricular atrial refractory period (PVARP). The sum of the AV delay and the PVARP in milliseconds determines the minimum atrial cycle length (60,000 divided by heart rate) and thus the maximum rate, which can be tracked and paced in the ventricle (UTR).

Temporary Pacing

In the pediatric ICU, temporary pacing is most commonly used in patients after surgical treatment of CHD. Temporary epicardial pacing wires are usually placed on the atria and ventricles, allowing pacing of either chamber. As previously noted, direct atrial recording (by attaching the wire to an ECG lead) may also aid in the diagnosis of tachyarrhythmias. Atrial burst pacing can be used to terminate reentrant supraventricular arrhythmias such as IART, AVNRT, and ORT. Pace termination of ORT is shown in Fig. 35.9. Although JET generally cannot be terminated with burst pacing, atrial pacing at a rate faster than the JET rate often improves hemodynamics

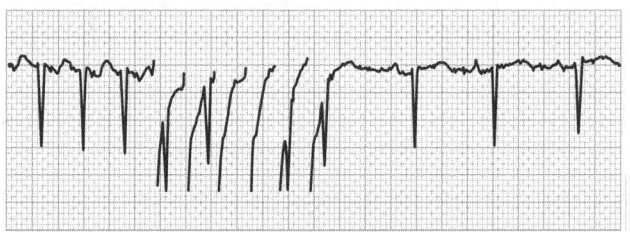

Fig. 35.9. Pace termination of orthodromic reciprocating tachycardia with a burst of atrial pacing.

by allowing AV synchrony until the JET resolves or is pharmacologically controlled (see Fig. 35.8).

In bradycardic patients who do not have temporary epicardial pacing wires, transcutaneous pacing can be performed acutely. It is important that electrodes and output are appropriate for the patient size, and positioning may be critical to maintaining capture. In general, transcutaneous pacing is used only for a short time while a temporary transvenous pacing lead is placed. At the bedside, placement of a balloon-tipped temporary transvenous lead is best accomplished via the internal jugular or subclavian vein because the catheter often can be directed to the ventricle "blindly." When fluoroscopy is available, a temporary active fixation may be preferred, allowing more secure positioning and the choice of pacing the atrium, ventricle, or both (in dual-chamber mode).

Setting Temporary Pacing Parameters

For AAI or VVI demand pacing, the pacemaker is usually initially set at a rate higher than the patient's intrinsic atrial or ventricular rate. The pacing threshold (lowest output that captures the chamber being paced) should be determined by decreasing the pacing current (mA) just until capture is lost and then setting output to twice threshold. Similarly, sensing threshold is determined by first lowering to a rate below the intrinsic rate of the chamber being paced, then adjusting the sensitivity to a higher numeric settings (less sensitive) until the pacemaker stops sensing the intrinsic activity as indicated by blinking markers on the device and/or inappropriate pacing on the monitor. The sensitivity is then reduced to a lower numeric value (more sensitive) to determine the highest numeric value at which the pacemaker senses appropriately (sensing threshold). Ideally, the sensitivity is programmed to one-half the sensing threshold, but this is not always possible, especially for temporary atrial leads. Failure to sense can result in inappropriate pacing, which can induce tachyarrhythmias. Fig. 35.10 shows a single inappropriate atrial stimulus initiating sustained ORT.

Dual-chamber pacing is more complex. The atrial and ventricular sensitivity and output are set using basically the same process described for single-chamber pacing. The other timing parameters discussed earlier must also be set, including the upper tracking rate (UTR), the AV delay, and (PVARP). Atrial

events occurring during the PVARP will be ignored by the pacemaker and will not result in a ventricular paced event. The pacemaker is also refractory to spontaneous atrial events during the AV interval. Thus the total atrial refractory period (TARP) includes both the AV interval and the PVARP and limits the upper tracking rate (UTR cannot exceed the TARP). Thus increasing the UTR often requires shortening the AV interval and/or the PVARP, thus decreasing the TARP.

The TARP also determines high-rate behavior when atrial rates exceed the UTR. If the spontaneous atrial cycle length (60,000 ms/min divided by the spontaneous atrial rate in bpm) is less than the TARP, only half of the spontaneous atrial beats will result in pacing. The point at which this occurs is known as the "2:1 block rate." In contrast, if the intrinsic atrial cycle length is greater than the sum of the AV delay and PVARP, atrial events exceeding the UTR will still be noted by the pacemaker. The resulting pattern of ventricular pacing resembles Wenckebach AV conduction and is referred to as "pacemaker Wenckebach." Thus it is desirable to program the AV delay and PVARP such that the resulting sum (TARP) is less than the upper tracking limit in milliseconds (60,000 divided by upper programmed rate) to favor pacemaker Wenckebach behavior and avoid acute drop in pacing rate by 50% when the UTR is reached. However, it is also important to distinguish appropriate pacemaker Wenckebach from failure to sense the atrium or failure to pace the ventricle. Fig. 35.11 shows 1:1 conduction, 2:1 block, and pacemaker Wenckebach at different pacemaker settings in a patient with a dual-chamber pacemaker for high-grade AV block.

When initiating dual-chamber pacing, it is important to be sure that the atrial lead senses appropriately and that the rates, intervals, and refractory periods are set appropriately to allow the pacemaker to track the spontaneous atrial rate. If the intrinsic atrial activity is not appropriately sensed and the dual-chamber temporary pacemaker's low rate is lower than the patient's intrinsic atrial rate, you may falsely assume that dual-chamber pacing is occurring when it is not. The presence of cannon A waves on the central venous pressure tracing may provide a clue that AV synchrony is not occurring. Reversing the atrial leads, lowering the numeric atrial sensitivity, or adjusting the AV interval, UTR, or PVARP may remedy this situation. If the atrium still cannot be sensed appropriately,

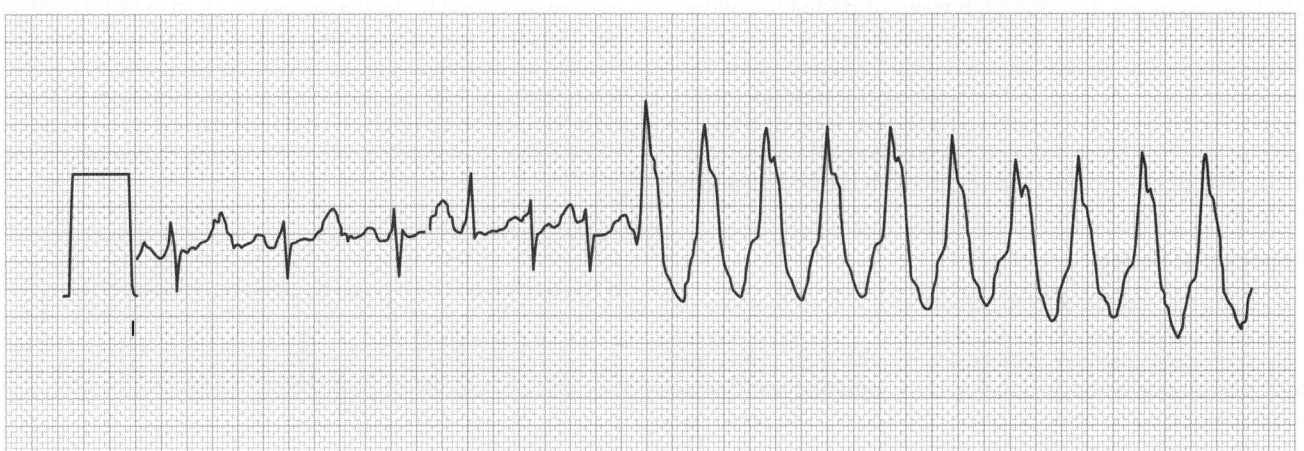

Fig. 35.10. Initiation of orthodromic reciprocating tachycardia with a single atrial paced beat that falls at a vulnerable time. After several narrow-complex beats, bundle branch block in tachycardia results in a wide-complex rhythm.

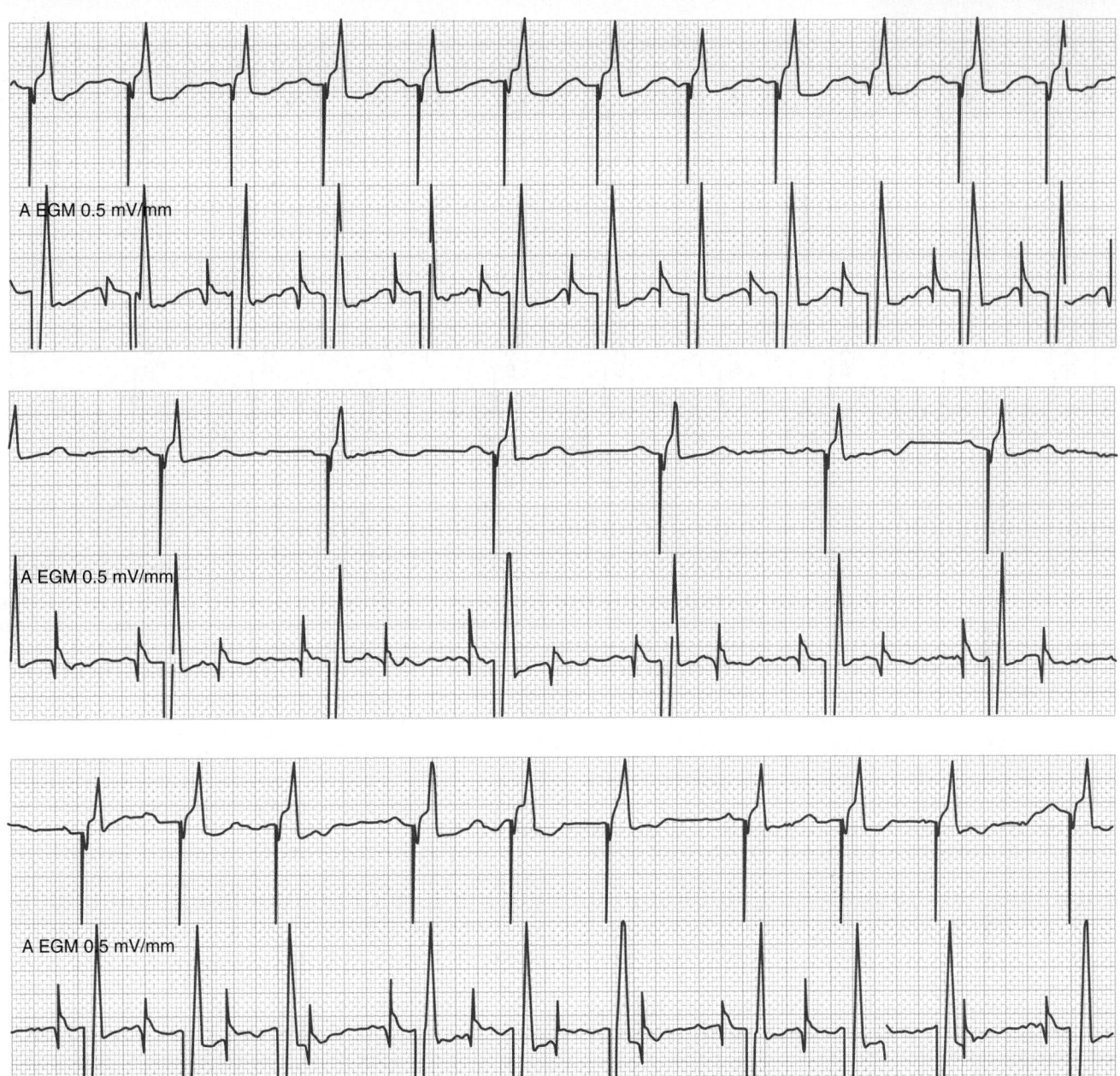

Fig. 35.11. Examples of pacemaker high-rate behavior. Each panel shows a surface electrocardiogram with the simultaneous atrial electrogram below. *Top,* 1:1 Atrioventricular conduction. Each sensed atrial event falls outside the total atrial refractory period, resulting in a corresponding paced ventricular event. *Middle,* 2:1 Block occurs when the total atrial refractory period exceeds the spontaneous atrial cycle length. Every other atrial beat falls within the refractory period and fails to trigger a ventricular pacing stimulus. *Bottom,* "Pacemaker Wenckebach" operation occurs when the atrial rate reaches the upper tracking rate. Gradual lengthening of the atrioventricular delay ensures that the ventricular pacing does not occur above the upper tracking rate. Eventually, an atrial sensed event falls within the refractory period so that a ventricular pacing stimulus is not triggered. All three recordings were obtained in the same patient over a short period by adjusting the programmable pacemaker parameters. (From Sliz NB Jr, Johns JA. Cardiac pacing in infants and children. Cardiol Rev. 2000;8:223-239.)

setting the pacemaker's low rate higher than the patient's own atrial rate will allow AV synchrony. In effect, this is pacing in DVI mode: pacing atrium and ventricle, sensing the ventricle, and inhibiting pacemaker output when spontaneous ventricular beats occur, avoiding asynchronous pacing by maintaining a higher atrial-paced rate.

Occasionally, a reentrant arrhythmia known as *pacemaker-mediated tachycardia* (PMT) may be seen, in which a DDD pacemaker (temporary or permanent) senses the atrium and

paces the ventricle, with the patient's own AV node conducting the impulse up from the ventricle to the atrium and the cycle repeating again. Thus the pacemaker acts as the antegrade limb of the reentrant circuit, while the patient's own AV node acts as the retrograde limb. Usually, PMT can be avoided with careful adjustment of the pacemaker's AV interval and PVARP. In a permanent pacing system, PMT can usually be terminated acutely by placing a magnet over the pacemaker; the resultant asynchronous pacing effectively interrupts the antegrade limb

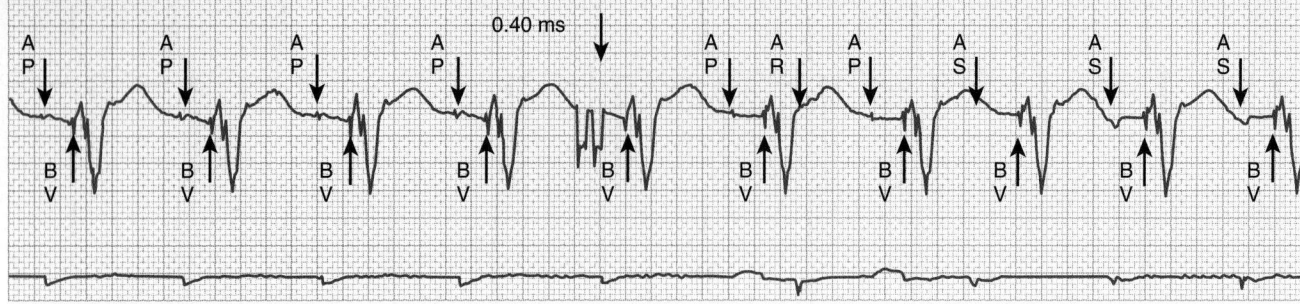

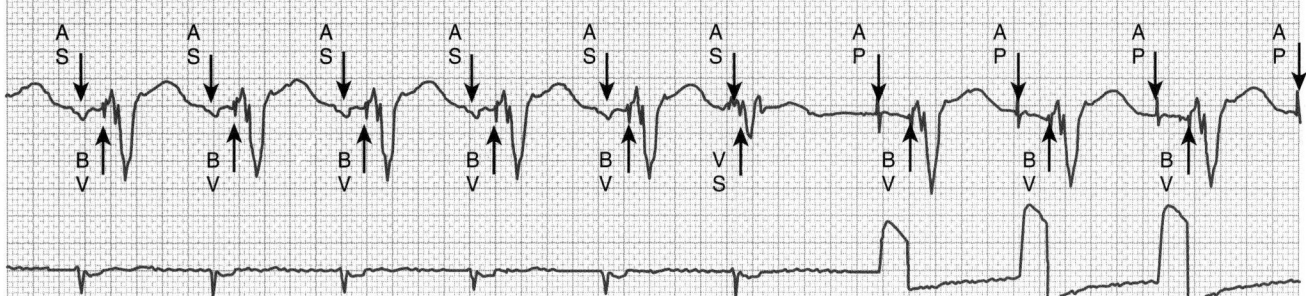

Fig. 35.12. Initiation and termination of pacemaker-mediated tachycardia. *Top,* Two atrial pacing stimuli fail to capture, followed by ventriculoatrial conduction of a ventricular paced beat. The resulting atrial beat *(AS)* is sensed and triggers another ventricular beat, and the process repeats. Had the retrograde atrial beat occurred during the postventricular atrial refractory period, it would not have triggered a ventricular paced beat. *Bottom,* Spontaneous ventricular beat inhibits the ventricular pacing, terminating the process. Atrial electrogram tracings are shown at the bottom of each panel. *AP,* atrial pace; *AR,* atrial refractory; *BV,* biventricular pace; *VS,* ventricular sense.

of the reentrant circuit. Fig. 35.12 shows initiation of PMT by loss of atrial capture with termination of the tachycardia by a spontaneous ventricular beat.

The selection of optimal temporary pacing mode and rate must be individualized for each patient. Usually atrial pacing (AAI) is preferred over dual-chamber pacing when AV conduction is intact. However, marked first-degree AV block may unfavorably affect ventricular filling such that dual-chamber pacing provides better hemodynamics. Periodic reassessment of pacing and sensing thresholds, as well as underlying rhythm, should be performed at least twice daily, and hemodynamic responses to changes in mode or timing parameters should be performed as needed with changes in clinical status.

Permanent Pacing

The two most common indications for permanent pacing are high-grade AV block and sinus node dysfunction. AV block may be congenital or acquired, with surgical damage to the conduction system the most common cause of acquired AV block. In patients with surgical AV block, there may be recovery of normal conduction with resolution of edema. In general, permanent pacing is not recommended unless there has been no recovery for 7 to 14 days.[23] Occasionally, if the surgeon is confident that the conduction system has been permanently damaged or if temporary pacing is not reliable, permanent pacemakers may be implanted before 7 days after the initial injury. Elective pacing for congenital AV block in the first decade of life is usually prompted by symptoms, low ventricular rates, or ventricular ectopy. Elective pacing is commonly recommended in the second decade of life even for asymptomatic patients with congenital heart block on the basis of studies showing that the first symptom in teenagers and adults may be catastrophic.[24] Pacing for sinus node dysfunction is

most commonly performed in patients with structural heart disease, usually following extensive atrial surgery such as Fontan operation or atrial repair of transposition of the great arteries.

In older children and adults, transvenous pacing is preferred to lower morbidity of implantation, optimize lead placement, and lower susceptibility to lead fractures as compared with epicardial leads, unless intracardiac shunting is present. In younger children, however, concern about venous occlusion in a patient who will require many decades of pacing often favors placement of epicardial pacemaker leads. The development of epicardial leads that elute a small amount of dexamethasone appears to improve epicardial lead performance,[25] although epicardial lead fractures remain a problem that is cause for concern. In patients requiring a lifetime of pacing, various approaches to allow atrial and ventricular pacing are commonly needed (Fig. 35.13). The recent development of "leadless" pacemakers represents an exciting prospect for future pacing options, but in their current design, they are not suitable for younger patients.[26]

Newer Indications for Pacing

Considerable data have shown that a prolonged QRS duration (either due to conduction delay or chronic pacing) results in mechanical dyssynchrony, which further impairs ventricular function. Biventricular pacing, with independent stimulation of the right and left ventricles, can reverse this dyssynchrony and improve ventricular function in some patients. Limited large-scale data are available in the pediatric population on this approach to heart failure treatment (often referred to as cardiac resynchronization therapy), but small studies suggest benefit.[27] Certainly, if pacing is otherwise required in a patient with impaired ventricular function, a biventricular pacing

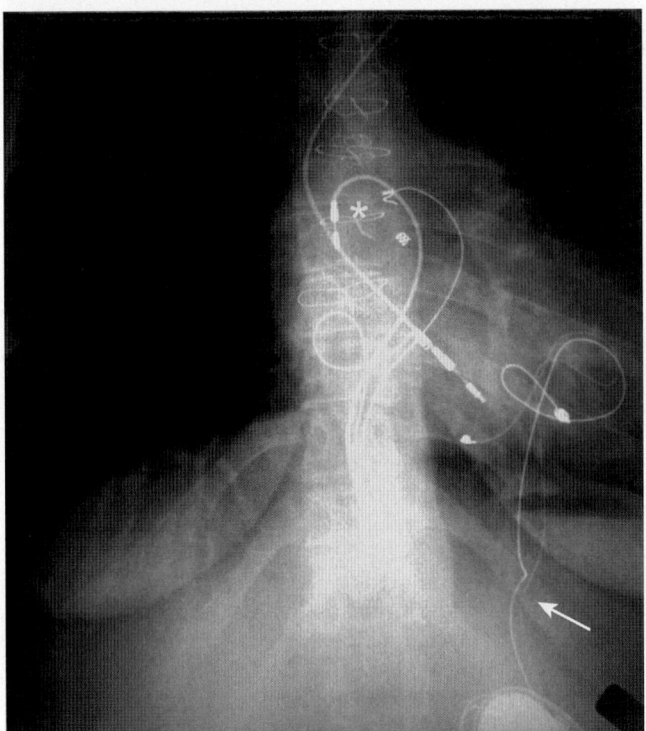

Fig. 35.13. Chest x-ray film of a patient with many abandoned pacing leads. There is a bipolar transvenous lead with the tip in the right ventricle. Another bipolar transvenous lead has been used as an epicardial atrial lead *(asterisk)*. There are two screw-in epicardial leads, one atrial and one ventricular. The atrial lead has a fractured electrode. Two other types of epicardial leads are more toward the apex, one of which is fractured *(arrow),* and the other of which is kinked. Only the kinked lead is functional. (From Sliz NB Jr, Johns JA. Cardiac pacing in infants and children. Cardiol Rev. 2000;8:223-239.)

system should be considered. Alternatively, with epicardial pacing, placement of the ventricular lead on the LV apex rather than RV may achieve similar benefit. However, identifying patients most likely to benefit from this modality and the best technique for optimizing the timing of activation between the ventricles remains unresolved. Ventricular pacing to intentionally introduce mechanical dyssynchrony has also been employed in patients with hypertrophic cardiomyopathy, though long-term benefit is probably limited.[28]

Tachycardia Therapies

Vagal Maneuvers

"Vagal maneuvers" were once the most commonly used intervention for terminating SVTs. They occasionally terminate VTs as well. Mechanical maneuvers such as the Valsalva maneuver or carotid sinus massage usually produce effective vagal stimulation beyond infancy. In infants, a similar reflex vagal response can sometimes be elicited by applying firm, steady abdominal pressure or by applying an ice pack to the face. These maneuvers should be attempted for 15 to 30 seconds. Endotracheal suctioning may also terminate tachycardias by this mechanism.

Acute Pharmacologic Therapies

Adenosine

An endogenous nucleoside with profound effects on SA node and AV node conduction, adenosine has become a mainstay in the acute treatment of SVT with normal QRS duration.[16] Administered as a rapid bolus, it produces transient but profound depression of AV nodal conduction and should reliably terminate reciprocating tachycardias (AV nodal reentry, AV reentry). Given the prevalence of AV reentry and AV nodal reentry among otherwise healthy young patients, adenosine is often advocated for wide QRS tachycardias as a therapeutic and/or diagnostic maneuver. It usually causes transient AV block without terminating most primary atrial tachycardias but may transiently suppress atrial automatic tachycardias (ectopic atrial or junctional) and occasionally may terminate atrial reentrant tachycardias. Certain VTs may be adenosine sensitive, particularly those originating because of abnormal triggering in the right ventricular outflow tract.

Adenosine (100–300 µg/kg) must be administered rapidly because of rapid metabolism by erythrocytes. If tachycardia is not terminated, determination must be made regarding whether a larger dose is warranted, the dose was given too slowly, or VA or AV conduction was altered without terminating tachycardia (see discussion on diagnosis). Therefore it is important to record an ECG strip during adenosine administration so that important diagnostic or therapeutic clues are not missed. Because of its brief effect (a half-life of 8–10 seconds), tachycardias sometimes immediately reinitiate following successful termination. If they reinitiate, readministration of the same dose should be attempted rather than increasing the dose further.

In addition to effects on the AV node, adenosine can produce sinus arrest, which may be prolonged in the setting of intrinsic SA nodal dysfunction after heart transplant; in the presence of drugs that interfere with its metabolism, such as dipyridamole and diazepam; or with drugs that may exaggerate its effects, such as class I, II, or III antiarrhythmic drugs. High doses should not be used indiscriminately in these situations. The use of adenosine in patients with reactive airway disease may be problematic because adenosine occasionally triggers severe bronchospasm. Conversely, its effects may be antagonized by aminophylline and other methylxanthines the patient may be receiving.

Adenosine produces dramatic but transient chest pain, along with systemic vasodilatation, both of which tend to increase sympathetic tone. As a result, adenosine may paradoxically accelerate tachycardias if termination is unsuccessful or, in the case of primary atrial tachycardias (atrial flutter or fibrillation), may produce more rapid conduction over the AV node (after initially slowing the ventricular rate). Various secondary arrhythmias may occur following administration of adenosine, particularly ventricular ectopy, atrial fibrillation, or, rarely, ventricular fibrillation. Although these effects are usually transient, *emergency external cardioversion should always be available whenever adenosine is administered.* The appropriateness of adenosine has been questioned in patients with known ventricular preexcitation syndromes (WPW syndrome) or suspected VTs. Nevertheless, its thoughtful and careful use remains invaluable for both diagnosis and treatment of many tachycardias.

Antiarrhythmic Agents

The addition of pharmacologic agents following adenosine administration should be guided by the clinical situation, known or suspected tachycardia mechanism, and response to adenosine administration. In some cases (such as in patients with wide QRS tachycardia or in hemodynamically compromised patients), it may be most appropriate to proceed directly to pacing termination or cardioversion if adenosine is unsuccessful in restoring sinus rhythm. In other instances, acute antiarrhythmic drug therapy may be warranted.[29]

The Vaughan Williams classification divides drugs according to their surface ECG effects, which often correlate closely with their cellular electrophysiologic effects: those that block cardiac sodium channels (class I); block β-adrenoreceptors (class II); prolong repolarization (class III); and block calcium channels (class IV). Digoxin and adenosine, which are not included in this classification scheme, exert their primary antiarrhythmic effects on the AV node. Magnesium also has depressant effects on the AV node and suppresses early and late afterdepolarizations (triggered activity). Many of the available drugs manifest properties of more than one class, which contribute collectively to their antiarrhythmic action.[30]

In general, class I drugs (particularly IA and IC) slow conduction in atrial, ventricular, or accessory pathway tissue and class III drugs prolong refractoriness in these same tissues. Class IA drugs usually accomplish both effects. β-Adrenergic antagonists, calcium channel antagonists, digoxin, and adenosine act primarily by slowing AV nodal conduction or inhibiting abnormal automaticity. Thus the latter group of drugs is primarily used for reciprocating tachycardias using the AV node (ART, ORT, AVNRT) or to induce second-degree AV block during a primary atrial tachycardia. In contrast, class IA, IC, and III drugs may be more effective in terminating or directly suppressing primary atrial tachycardias and also may be effective for reciprocating tachycardias.[6,29]

Despite the various antiarrhythmic agents available for chronic therapy, relatively few are suitable for acute administration to the critically ill patient either because the drugs are not available in intravenous formulation or they have significant negative inotropic effects when administered intravenously (Table 35.3). This discussion is limited to agents suitable for acute and short-term parenteral administration.

All antiarrhythmic agents have the potential for producing bradycardia, particularly when administered acutely, and most have negative inotropic and/or hypotensive effects. Careful observation is required during initial administration and subsequent infusion of all IV antiarrhythmic agents. Although many are contraindicated in cases of heart failure or hypotension, therapy may be necessary if the arrhythmia is contributing significantly to the patient's hemodynamic compromise.

Procainamide

Procainamide is useful for various SVTs and VTs in the intensive care setting. Its broad electrophysiologic effects include both conduction slowing and increased refractoriness in atrial tissue, ventricular tissue, and accessory AV connections. Unlike quinidine, procainamide can be administered intravenously. Effective plasma concentrations (6–10 µg/dL) can be readily achieved with a total loading dose of 15 mg/kg over 15 minutes (or in small-bolus increments at a similar rate). Careful and repeated blood pressure monitoring is required because of potential negative inotropic and direct vasodilator effects. If hypotension complicates infusion, administration should be momentarily interrupted until blood pressure returns to normal. In primary atrial tachycardias, a vagolytic effect may increase the ventricular response over the AV node. Occasionally, atrial tachycardia that is conducting 2:1 to the ventricle slows sufficiently to allow 1:1 conduction, converting a hemodynamically stable rhythm to an unstable rhythm. Thus one should always be prepared to use cardioversion if necessary.

Procainamide, like other class IA and class III drugs, is contraindicated in patients with the congenital or acquired long QT syndromes. Regular monitoring of plasma concentration every 6 to 12 hours is necessary during IV administration to maintain levels between 5 and 10 µg/dL. The active metabolite N-acetylprocainamide contributes to the antiarrhythmic action; higher levels of the parent drug may be necessary in patients lacking the enzyme to produce this metabolite.

Lidocaine

Intravenously administered lidocaine is useful for suppressing and sometimes terminating VTs in children. Although somewhat less likely to acutely terminate VTs than procainamide or amiodarone, lidocaine's lack of significant negative inotropic effect makes it attractive for this indication. The usual loading dose is 1–2 mg/kg acutely or 3 mg/kg over 20 to 30 minutes, followed by a 20–50 µg/kg/min infusion. Lidocaine levels should be monitored to prevent central nervous system (CNS) toxicity. With chronic use (4–7 days), accumulation of the metabolite glycine xylide may impair drug efficacy by interfering with the parent drug effect at the sodium channel. Despite traditional recommendations for its use in ventricular fibrillation, lidocaine actually increases defibrillation energy requirements.

β-Blocking Agents

A limited number of β-blocking agents are useful for intravenous treatment of tachycardias. Acutely, their role is generally limited to incessant tachycardias, which seem to be dependent on sympathetic tone, and VTs related to myocarditis, ischemia/reperfusion injury, or congenital long QT syndromes. In hemodynamically unstable patients, β-blocking agents should be used cautiously because of hypotension and potential sinus bradycardia once tachycardia terminates. All may produce bronchospasm, hypotension, or bradycardia or may depress ventricular function.

Esmolol, a short-acting, nonselective β-blocker with a half-life of 2 to 5 minutes, can be administered as a continuous infusion. A loading dose of 500 µg/kg is followed by an infusion of 50–100 µg/kg/min. The infusion can be titrated upward by doubling every 3 to 5 minutes up to 500 µg/kg/min. Repeat loading doses may be useful as the infusion is increased. Its very short half-life is excellent for short-term use, but extended efficacy is limited by tachyphylaxis. For longer-term intravenous administration, metoprolol (0.05–0.10 mg/kg) is administered by slow intravenous infusion every 4 to 6 hours, carefully observing for hypotension (or bradycardia).

Amiodarone

Amiodarone is arguably the single-most potent antiarrhythmic drug available, both in the acute, IV setting and when administered chronically. At sufficient doses, it is often effective in controlling various tachycardias refractory to other antiarrhythmic agents.[31] Although typically regarded as a class III agent, its effects are considerably more diverse. It not only prolongs repolarization (by blocking potassium channels), but to varying degrees it blocks some sodium channel (class I effect), calcium channel (class IV effect), and β receptors (class II effect).

Amiodarone is administered as a total loading dose of 5 mg/kg divided into 1-mg/kg aliquots given at 5- to 10-minute

TABLE 35.3   Treatment of Bradycardias, Supraventricular Tachycardias, and Ventricular Tachycardias

	Primary Therapies	Secondary Therapies	Long-Term Therapies
Bradycardias			
Sinus bradycardia	Atropine 0.01 mg/kg Epinephrine 0.1 mg/kg Transcutaneous pacemaker	Temporary pacemaker Isoproterenol infusion	Permanent pacemaker (AAIR, DDDR)
AV block (high-grade)	Transcutaneous pacemaker	Temporary pacemaker	Permanent pacemaker (DDDR)
Supraventricular Tachycardias			
Sinus tachycardia	Identify cause(s)	Sedation, pain control Adjust catecholamines Respiratory support	β-Blockers, if chronic Consider nonsinus mechanism
Paroxysmal supraventricular tachycardia, AV nodal reentrant tachycardia	Vagal maneuvers Adenosine Transesophageal termination Procainamide	Esmolol Verapamil Procainamide (IV) Amiodarone (IV) Class I, class III	β-Blockers, class I, class III Amiodarone Radiofrequency ablation Radiofrequency ablation
AET and other incessant supraventricular tachycardia	Amiodarone Esmolol Avoid cardioversion	β-blockers Amiodarone	
Atrial flutter <24 h	Rate-control (diltiazem IV) Procainamide Pace termination with pacemaker DC cardioversion Ibutilide (transesophageal echocardiography if duration unknown of >24 h to rule out thrombus)	Pace termination (transesophageal, intracardiac)	Radiofrequency ablation Antitachycardia pacemaker
Atrial fibrillation <24 h	Same as above, except pace termination not feasible)		
Chaotic atrial tachycardia	Procainamide, amiodarone	β-Blocker (rate control)	Propafenone, amiodarone
Ventricular Tachycardias			
Monomorphic (conscious, stable)	Procainamide/lidocaine DC cardioversion Pace termination if PM, ICD	Procainamide/lidocaine Amiodarone	Defined by substrate
Known heart disease	Same	Amiodarone	ICD, Radiofrequency ablation Amiodarone
Known idiopathic	Consider IV verapamil Avoid cardioversion	β-Blocker	Ca-channel blocker β-Blocker Radiofrequency ablation
Pulseless (monomorphic, polymorphic)	DC cardioversion β-Blocker Amiodarone	Amiodarone (unless long QT) β-blocker Magnesium	ICD
Ventricular fibrillation	Defibrillation	Epinephrine Vasopressin	ICD

AET, atrial ectopic tachycardia; *AV,* atrioventricular; *ICD,* implantable cardioverter-defibrillator; *PM,* pacemaker.

intervals. The loading can be truncated if arrhythmia control is achieved. If hypotension ensues, volume expansion or calcium chloride (10–30 mg/kg) should be administered. If arrhythmia control is not achieved, a second loading dose can be administered 30 to 60 minutes later. A continuous infusion of 10 mg/kg over 24 hours can be administered if ongoing therapy is desired.

Calcium Channel–Blocking Agents

Verapamil and diltiazem have proved useful for terminating SVT involving the AV node (AV reentry, AV nodal reentry). However, their acute efficacy is no greater than that of adenosine, and both may cause hypotension or cardiovascular collapse in young infants or patients with poor ventricular function.[32] Either drug can be useful as an alternative to adenosine when tachycardias have repeatedly reinitiated following termination with adenosine.

Both agents may help slow the ventricular response over the AV node during atrial flutter or fibrillation. Verapamil is administered as a bolus of 0.15 mg/kg. Diltiazem can be administered as a bolus of 0.15–0.35 mg/kg and can be infused continuously at 0.05–0.2 mg/kg/hr if ongoing effect is necessary. In addition to vasodilatation and negative inotropic effects, both can accelerate antegrade conduction over accessory pathways in patients with WPW syndrome. Therefore they are contraindicated for preexcited atrial fibrillation, and generally they should not be administered during uncharacterized wide QRS tachycardias. Likewise, oral calcium channel blockers generally should not be used as maintenance therapy for patients with WPW syndrome. If hemodynamic compromise develops, IV calcium gluconate should be administered immediately.

Magnesium Sulfate

Magnesium (administered as 25–50 mg/kg magnesium sulfate) has proved useful in the treatment of certain ventricular and supraventricular arrhythmias. Its actions appear to be mediated through depression of early and late afterdepolarizations; depressant effects on AV nodal conduction; and, at high doses, indirect inhibition of sodium-potassium adenosine triphosphatase. It is most effective in the acute treatment of torsades de pointes and as a temporizing measure in the treatment of arrhythmias associated with digoxin toxicity.[33] Therapeutic efficacy is not restricted to situations where hypomagnesemia is present. Although magnesium has efficacy comparable with that of adenosine in the acute termination of SVT resulting from AV reentry and AV nodal reentry, it has more severe and lasting adverse effects. It has little demonstrable effect in the acute treatment of monomorphic VTs or polymorphic VTs not associated with QT prolongation.

Digoxin

Digoxin has been used for various supraventricular arrhythmias, including AV reentry, AV nodal reentry, and primary atrial tachycardias. In a randomized controlled trial of infants younger than 4 months of age with SVT, recurrence rates were similar between digoxin and propranolol.[34] Digoxin may increase the risk of rapid antegrade conduction during atrial fibrillation in older patients and possibly infants with preexcitation. Like calcium channel–blocking agents, it should be avoided altogether in the treatment of patients with ventricular preexcitation (WPW syndrome). Its use is further confounded by potentially dangerous interactions with other medications including quinidine, verapamil, amiodarone, flecainide, phenytoin, and warfarin. At toxic dosages, its direct cellular effects may predispose to dangerous tachycardias and bradycardias.

Dexmedetomidine

Dexmedetomidine is a selective α2-adrenergic receptor agonist that provides sedation, anxiolysis, and analgesia with minimal to no respiratory depression. As a result it has become widely used in a variety of settings, including the pediatric ICU. Dexmedetomidine acts as a peripheral parasympathomimetic and a central sympatholytic, with electrophysiologic effects including sinus and atrioventricular node depression.[35] Studies have suggested that dexmedetomidine is effective for acute termination of SVT in children, with fewer side effects compared with adenosine.[36] Serious adverse events including sudden pauses, asystole, and loss of pacemaker capture have also been reported with dexmedetomidine infusion.[37,38]

Cardioversion and Defibrillation

Cardiovascular collapse or failure of mechanical and pharmacologic interventions for tachycardias may warrant cardioversion. For tachycardias with discrete QRS complexes, synchronization with the QRS should be confirmed (the default mode for most defibrillators is nonsynchronized, and most revert to nonsynchronized shocks after each shock is delivered). Proper synchronization may require changing the ECG lead configuration to achieve an upright QRS complex.

Several factors may determine the success of cardioversion and defibrillation. Energy requirements may vary from 0.25 to 1 J/kg for SVTs to greater than 2 J/kg for VTs. Newer defibrillators with a "biphasic" rather than "monophasic" waveform have reduced defibrillation energy requirements. Electrode (paddle) location is an important variable. If conversion is not achieved with low or moderate energy levels, consideration should be given to changing electrode position before using higher energy levels. Automatic tachycardias are characteristically refractory to cardioversion and may account for treatment failure. Finally, some antiarrhythmic drugs, particularly sodium channel–blocking drugs (see later discussion), increase defibrillation energy requirements and pacing thresholds, whereas other drugs (QT-prolonging drugs) appear to have a favorable effect.[39]

Approach to Therapy

Extrasystoles

In general, isolated extrasystoles do not require treatment unless they are sufficiently frequent to impair hemodynamics or they serve as frequent initiating events for tachycardias. In otherwise healthy children and adolescents, extrasystoles are a benign finding. In other settings, "complex" ventricular extrasystoles may identify patients at increased risk for cardiac arrest. Even in such situations, prophylaxis may not decrease and may actually increase the risk. Effort should instead be directed at identifying possible causes and correcting any predisposing factors, which include ischemia, electrolyte disorders, acidosis, pericarditis, or direct trauma from recent cardiac surgery, blunt or penetrating chest trauma, and intracardiac catheter-induced irritation. Numerous drugs, including digoxin, catecholamines, or drugs associated with the acquired long QT syndrome, may produce extrasystoles.

Sustained Tachycardias

Most sustained tachycardias observed in the intensive care setting warrant immediate attention and intervention. Sinus tachycardia may indicate the need for additional sedation and analgesia or may reflect hemodynamic compromise as a consequence of anemia, hypovolemia, or impaired myocardial function. Sinus tachycardia as a consequence of hyperthermia may be poorly tolerated in children already critically ill, especially following cardiac surgery. Sinus tachycardia may reflect an underlying neuroendocrine process such as hyperthyroidism or pheochromocytoma requiring acute medical intervention (β-blocker) while instituting therapy for the underlying disorder.

Nonsinus tachycardias in patients with primary rhythm disturbances may warrant therapy to prevent life-threatening events, prevent the development of myocardial dysfunction as a consequence of chronic (incessant) tachycardia, or simply alleviate acute tachycardia-related symptoms. The acuity of the situation dictates the approach to therapy. Tachycardias occurring secondary to other abnormalities (structural heart disease, metabolic derangements, drug toxicity) should always be regarded as high risk for serious hemodynamic deterioration.

Unstable Patients

The approach to patients with tachycardia is determined largely by the degree of hemodynamic compromise (see Table 35.3). Patients who are hemodynamically unstable or in cardiovascular collapse resulting from sustained tachycardia almost always warrant prompt cardioversion or defibrillation. Antiarrhythmic medications (and other supportive measures) should only replace cardioversion in the unstable patient when tachycardia is known to be incessant or is unresponsive to cardioversion (eg, JET, atrial ectopic tachycardia, chaotic tachycardia, and PJRT).

Cardiopulmonary resuscitation should always be instituted in the absence of a pulse or blood pressure, as is typically the case for polymorphic VT and ventricular fibrillation. Although hemodynamic and ventilatory support should be initiated immediately and maintained following tachycardia termination as needed, cardioversion (with bag and mask ventilation initially) should take precedence over other interventions.[40] Underlying factors contributing to the tachycardia should be sought, including hypoxia, infection (cardiac or systemic), drug toxicities (see later), and electrolyte derangements.

Once tachycardia is terminated, acute therapies may focus on either suppressing recurrences or terminating them when they recur. Although antiarrhythmic medications eventually may be necessary to suppress recurrences, most have negative inotropic or vasodilating effects, particularly when administered intravenously. Often it is preferable to delay specific therapy after initial termination until ventricular function improves. Most recurrences of SVTs can be safely treated with temporary pacing or adenosine rather than with repeated cardioversions. In the event of frequent recurrences, a transesophageal catheter may be left in place for this purpose, or a transvenous atrial pacing catheter may be warranted in selected patients. Similarly, temporary ventricular pacing may be useful in some circumstances for recurrent VT. Although adenosine can be administered repeatedly because of its short half-life, the resulting vasodilatation may be poorly tolerated in patients with tachycardia mechanisms unresponsive to adenosine.

Treatment Failure

When seemingly appropriate electrical and pharmacologic interventions fail to terminate tachycardias, three possibilities should be considered: erroneous diagnosis, unrecognized tachycardia reinitiation, or a technical error in the termination technique.

Errors in Diagnosis

As noted previously, automatic atrial tachycardias, JET, and occasionally chaotic atrial tachycardia might be mistaken for tachycardias with reentrant mechanism (ORT, AVNRT, and primary atrial reentry). Each of these conditions is usually refractory to electrical termination (either pace termination or cardioversion), yet the diagnosis may be subtle if atrial activity is obscured.

Confusion between VTs and SVTs with prolonged QRS probably remains the most frequent diagnostic error. Occasionally the presumption of VT may lead to ineffective treatments. For example, following cardiac surgery, incessant, monomorphic wide QRS tachycardia that is refractory to cardioversion may actually be JET with postsurgical bundle branch block. Brief atrial pacing at a faster rate may be necessary to confirm the diagnosis.

Certain tachycardias such as torsades de pointes related to long QT syndromes (congenital or drug-induced) or bidirectional VT resulting from digoxin toxicity must be recognized to provide more appropriate and specific therapies to prevent recurrences following cardioversion.

Unrecognized Reinitiation

Unrecognized reinitiation may occur following medical termination, pace termination, or cardioversion. In some tachycardias (as in PJRT or other incessant forms of SVT), reinitiation is expected, but it also may occur inadvertently as the result of continued pacing beyond the point of termination or may be facilitated by sinus pauses, junctional beats, or ectopic beats following adenosine or cardioversion. Again, measures to decrease the factors favoring reinitiation (eg, shorter pacing bursts, antibradycardia pacing, and coadministration of an antiarrhythmic drug) should be used rather than further increases in energy or dose of the terminating therapy. With frequent terminations and reinitiation of tachycardia, multiple repeated cardioversions are likely ineffective and may cause myocardial injury.

Improper Technique

Appropriate administration of adenosine is accomplished through an IV catheter (peripheral or central) by rapid push followed immediately with ample flush. Because of rapid metabolism by erythrocytes, arterial administration may be ineffective in terminating tachycardia (yet still produce vasodilatation). Errors in cardioversion or pacing technique are generally attributable to insufficient energy or improper electrode (or paddle) placement. For pace termination, the stimulator must be capable of sufficient output for the pacing modality being used (see section on temporary pacing). Intensive care personnel should be familiar with the defibrillation devices available in the ICU, including adjustment of electrocardiographic gain and lead selection to allow synchronous cardioversion when appropriate. However, in ventricular fibrillation or polymorphic tachycardia, asynchronous countershock is necessary. Use of excessive energy may damage the myocardium and, when repeated, may lead to preterminal bradycardias, which are refractory to all pacing modalities and progress to complete electromechanical dissociation if hypoxia and acidosis are not corrected.

Specific Arrhythmias

Primary Arrhythmias

Some arrhythmias require unique therapeutic approaches or are seen with sufficient frequency to warrant a brief review (Box 35.1).

Orthodromic Reciprocating Tachycardia in Infancy

Infants with ORT can present with tachycardia in utero, at birth, or within the first weeks to months of life. Postnatally, tachycardia sustained beyond a few hours may result in CHF that may progress to shock, acidosis, and complete cardiovascular collapse.[41] In the latter situation, ORT may be terminated

BOX 35.1 Rhythm Disturbances

Primary Rhythm Disturbances

Paroxysmal supraventricular tachycardias (atrioventricular nodal reentrant tachycardia, AVNRT)
Congenital AV block
Congenital long QT syndrome, Brugada syndrome
Other genetic arrhythmias
Ventricular tachycardias resulting from Purkinje hamartoma
Verapamil-sensitive ventricular tachycardias
Accelerated ventricular rhythm

Secondary Rhythm Disturbances

Early Postoperative Arrhythmias

JET
Postsurgical AV block
Early primary atrial tachycardia

Late Postoperative Arrhythmias

Ventricular arrhythmias (postoperative tetralogy of Fallot)
Sick sinus syndrome

Metabolic Derangements

Electrolyte disturbances
Endocrine derangements (thyroid)
CNS injury
Hypothermia, hyperthermia
Acute hypoxia (newborns)
Acute myocardial infarction

Drug Toxicity, Proarrhythmia

Digoxin
Cocaine
Tricyclic antidepressants
Antiarrhythmic drugs
Quinidine/sotalol
Flecainide/encainide
Organophosphates

Infectious

Lyme disease
Myocarditis, endocarditis

CNS, central nervous system; *JET*, junctional ectopic tachycardia.

during resuscitation efforts such that its causative role remains unrecognized. Thus SVT should be considered in the differential diagnosis of neonatal shock, along with other conditions such as sepsis, aortic coarctation, and congenital adrenal hyperplasia in which sinus tachycardia associated with cardiovascular collapse would be expected.

Tachycardia-Induced Cardiac Dysfunction

Although most SVTs are paroxysmal or episodic, chronic SVTs pose a unique problem. Many are minimally symptomatic and are recognized only by the inappropriately fast rate. However, with time, varying degrees of CHF become evident and ventricular dysfunction may be severe. Even then, the diagnosis may not be immediately evident. As a consequence, chronic tachycardia must be considered in any patient presenting with gradually progressive CHF. In one series, chronic atrial tachycardia was present in 37% of patients initially diagnosed with "idiopathic" cardiomyopathy and listed for heart transplant.[42]

In patients with structurally normal hearts, the most common incessant SVTs are PJRT and ectopic atrial tachycardia. These conditions may occur throughout infancy, childhood, and adolescence. The rates (often <200 beats/min) and

normal PR interval during tachycardia may lead to an erroneous diagnosis of sinus tachycardia secondary to the hemodynamic compromise (see "Approach to Diagnosis" section earlier). An abnormal P-wave axis on 12-lead ECG and Holter monitoring to look for interruptions in the tachycardia with changes in P-wave morphology are helpful. Electrophysiologic study may still be necessary to establish the diagnosis. In infants, incessant VTs and the rare congenital form of JET also are seen.

In each of these entities, it is important first to recognize the primary role of the tachycardia in producing secondary congestive symptoms and to recognize the futility of acute therapies such as adenosine, pace termination, and cardioversion. Most are catecholamine dependent so that inotropic agents may aggravate the situation and compromise the efficacy of antiarrhythmic regimens, whereas β-blocking agents may be useful despite the presence of heart failure. Once the diagnosis is established, chronic antiarrhythmic therapy is instituted to control or limit the tachycardia. Uncontrolled, severe cardiac symptoms may result, but ventricular dysfunction improves once tachycardia is suppressed medically or treated by catheter ablation.[43] Despite the severity of heart failure, antiarrhythmic medications that depress ventricular function are usually well tolerated.

Chaotic Atrial Tachycardia

Chaotic atrial tachycardia is a primary atrial tachycardia characterized by three or more different P-wave morphologies and irregular, rapid atrial rates (Fig. 35.14). Although atrial flutter may be associated with it, episodes are usually self-limited and cardioversion is neither indicated nor effective. Asymptomatic patients with slow or intermittent tachycardia may require no treatment. Occasionally digoxin is used to limit AV conduction when atrial rates are excessive or to enhance contractility in the setting of tachycardia-induced cardiomyopathy.[44] An association with respiratory syncytial virus has been described in some patients.[12] Various agents have been used in symptomatic cases; amiodarone and propafenone are the most effective.[44,45]

Long QT Syndromes

The long QT syndromes are a diverse group of disorders, both congenital and acquired, in which individuals are at risk for torsades de pointes and sudden death because of abnormalities in ventricular repolarization. In both congenital and acquired forms, the rate-corrected QT intervals usually exceed 0.46 second and, more typically, are greater than 0.48 to 0.50 second. Associated anomalies of T-wave morphology, including T-wave alternans, "bifid" T waves, and prominent U waves, are common. It may be difficult to establish the diagnosis of congenital long QT syndrome because QT prolongation may not be severe, and affected individuals sometimes have a normal QTc.[46] Congenital long QT syndrome should be considered in all patients with QT prolongation and a history of syncope, cardiac arrest, or seizures or a family history of unexplained sudden death. The diagnosis should be strongly considered in any child presenting with syncope or sudden death in whom polymorphic VT or multiform ventricular premature beats are documented. Incidental QT prolongation in an asymptomatic child (with a negative family history) may warrant further scrutiny. Finally, all infants presenting with second-degree or third-degree AV block should be evaluated for the possibility of long QT syndrome (Fig. 35.15).[4]

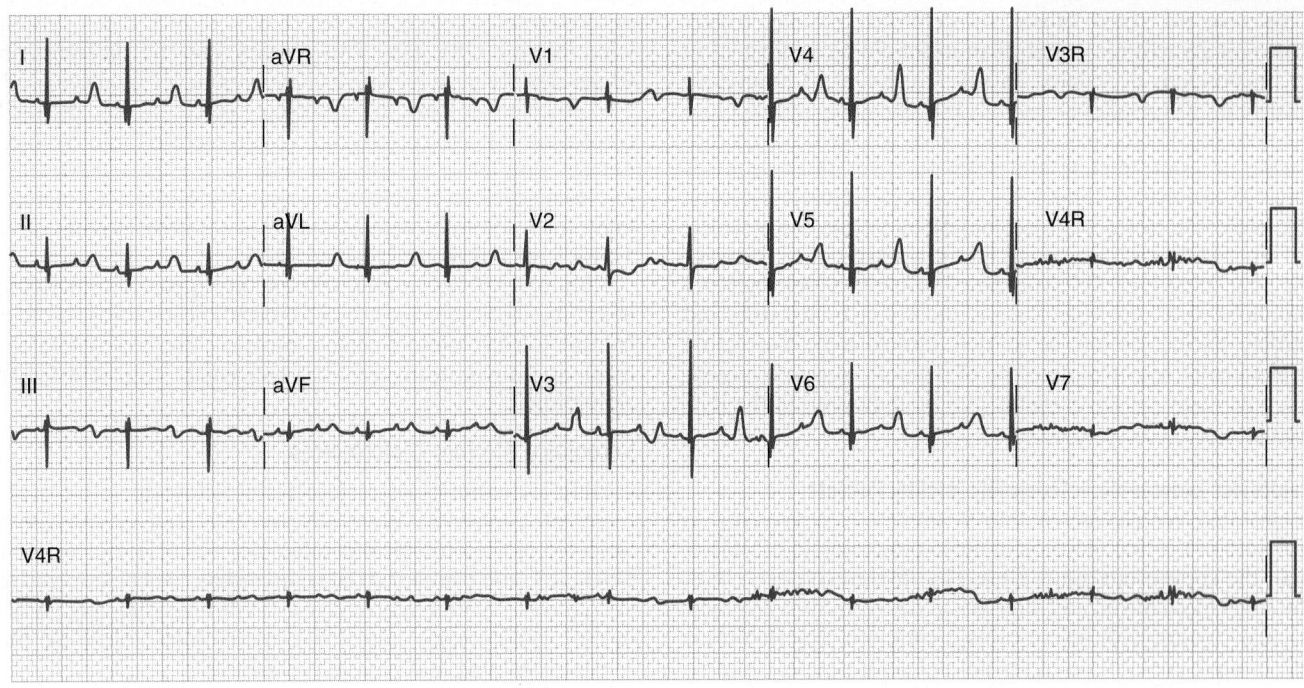

Fig. 35.14. Chaotic atrial tachycardia. Note two discrete P-wave morphologies before conversion to sinus rhythm.

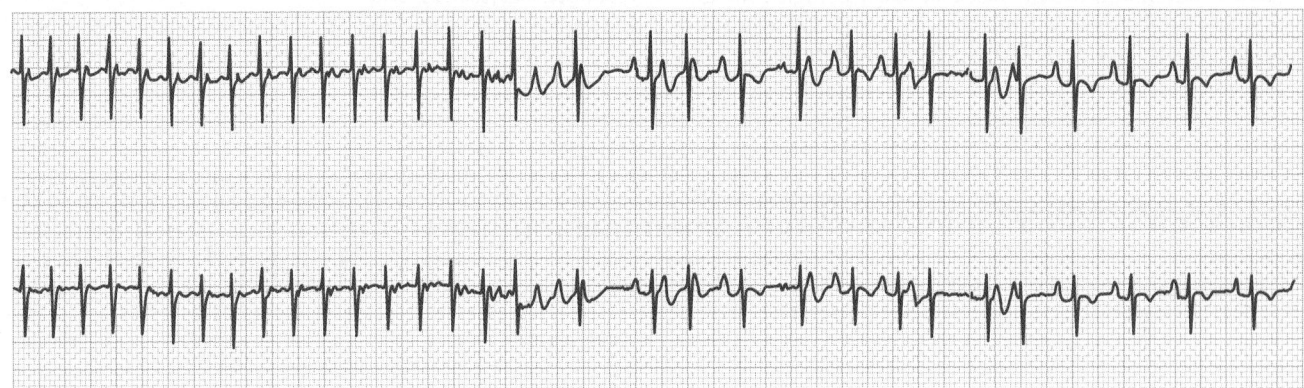

Fig. 35.15. Congenital long QT syndrome presenting with 2:1 atrioventricular block. The corrected QT interval is greater than 560 ms, resulting in "functional" block of every other sinus beat in the His-Purkinje system.

Patients with symptoms or arrhythmias associated with QT prolongation require careful evaluation for secondary causes, which include CNS injury, hypocalcemia, hypokalemia, and drugs that prolong the QT interval. The list of drugs that prolong the QT interval is extensive and includes antiarrhythmic and noncardiac drugs, most of which block I_{Kr}, the rapid component of the delayed rectifier potassium current.[47] Updated lists of these drugs are available at www.crediblemeds.org.

Torsade de pointes is the specific arrhythmia associated with long QT syndromes and is responsible for the symptoms (Fig. 35.16). This characteristic arrhythmia is recognized by progressive undulation in the QRS axis, resulting in a "twisting" appearance, and is usually associated with a specific initiation with a VPB following a pause (often following a previous VPB). Many episodes are not sustained, and even prolonged episodes may terminate spontaneously. Torsades de pointes that degenerates to ventricular fibrillation requires defibrillation.

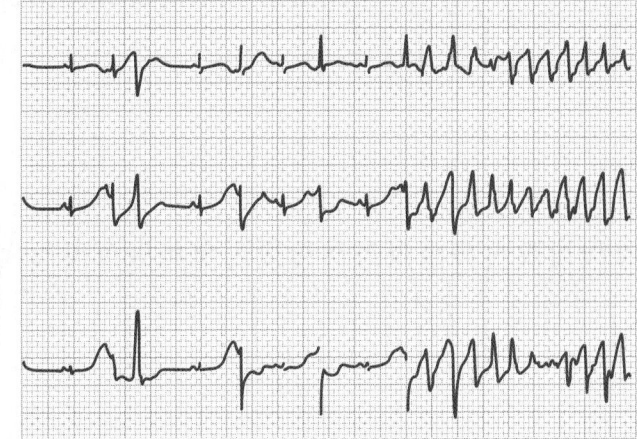

Fig. 35.16. Torsades des pointes in a teenage patient with long QT syndrome. This arrhythmia is associated with no pulse and results in syncope. It often terminates spontaneously but otherwise rapidly degenerates to ventricular fibrillation.

Because the stress caused by defibrillation may trigger recurrent arrhythmias, defibrillation should be performed in an unconscious or sedated patient. Treatment of immediate recurrence of torsades de pointes is challenging and includes magnesium sulfate, increasing the heart rate with temporary pacing or isoproterenol, and sedation.[48] For most acquired long QT syndromes (and some congenital forms), increasing the heart rate using isoproterenol or by pacing shortens the QT interval, but isoproterenol may exacerbate some forms of the congenital long QT syndrome.[49] Therefore isoproterenol should be used only when there is underlying bradycardia and cardiac pacing cannot be started immediately. Correcting hypokalemia, hypomagnesemia, or hypocalcemia and removing potentially causative agents may be important in the ICU setting.

Ventricular Tachycardia in Ostensibly Healthy Patients

Accelerated ventricular rhythm is observed occasionally in neonates in the first few days of life at rates only slightly faster than the appropriate sinus rates. The rhythm competes with the sinus mechanism, and alternation between sinus and ventricular rhythm with fusion beats is common. The rhythm is self-limited, does not usually result in hemodynamic compromise, and carries a good prognosis. No specific therapy is necessary unless rates are excessive.[50] A similar rhythm is seen in older children and usually has a similarly benign course.[51] Two other characteristic VTs may be seen in otherwise healthy children and adolescents. One arises from the right ventricular outflow tract, resulting in a left bundle branch block pattern with inferior QRS axis. This pattern may be incessant, in which case the term *repetitive monomorphic VT* has been used. The other arises from the posterior fascicle of the left-sided conduction system, producing a right bundle branch block pattern with leftward QRS axis (Fig. 35.17). This tachycardia has been called fascicular, or verapamil-sensitive VT. Interestingly, the response to verapamil may result in misclassification as "SVT with aberrant conduction."

Although VT can be seen without any apparent underlying heart disease, a rigorous search for occult heart disease is often fruitful. Cardiac tumors (rhabdomyomas, fibromas, hamartomas) and myocarditis can be associated with ventricular arrhythmias.[52]

Secondary Rhythm Disturbances

Certain arrhythmias characteristically follow operative treatment of congenital heart disease (CHD). Among those observed in the early postoperative period are complete heart block, JET, and primary atrial tachycardias. Late postoperative arrhythmias include ventricular arrhythmias following tetralogy of Fallot repair and atrial arrhythmias following the Mustard/Senning and Fontan procedures.

Postoperative Arrhythmias
Postsurgical Atrioventricular Block
Inadvertent damage to the AV conduction system may occur with cardiac surgery, especially after closure of ventricular

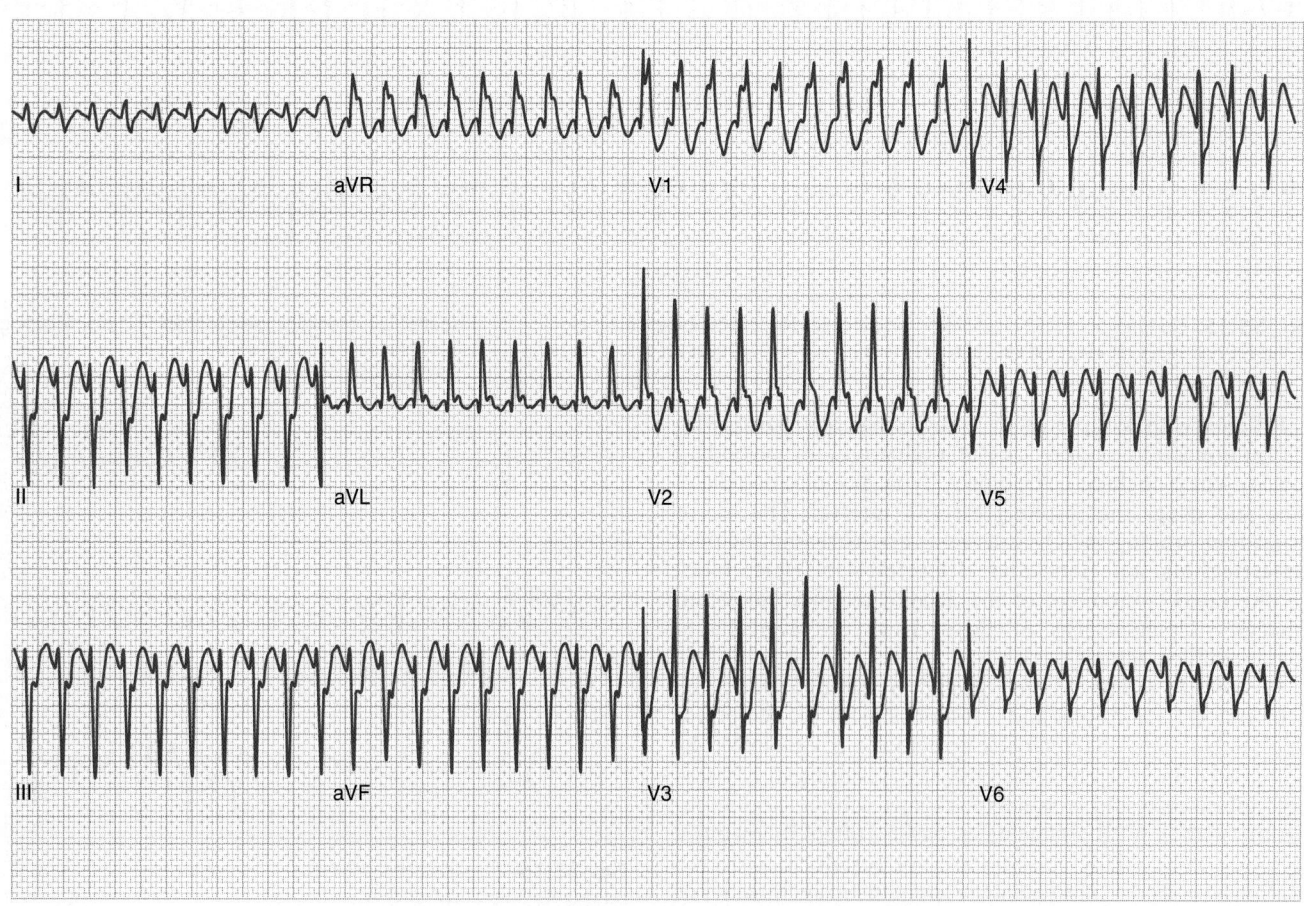

Fig. 35.17. Idiopathic ventricular tachycardia in an otherwise healthy 12-year-old. Note right bundle branch block pattern with superior axis, typical of origin within the left posterior fascicle region of the left ventricular septum.

septal defects (particularly associated with l-loop ventricles), during resection of septal tissue, or after insertion of prosthetic valves in the tricuspid, aortic, or mitral position. Bradycardia from AV block can be initially managed using isoproterenol to accelerate the ventricular rate or with epicardial temporary pacing wires placed at surgery. Although temporary pacing frequently is necessary for rate support, permanent pacemaker implantation should usually be delayed 7 to 14 days to allow for potential recovery of AV conduction. Most patients who recover AV conduction do so within 9 days of surgery.[53]

Junctional Ectopic Tachycardia

JET immediately following cardiac surgery may be mistaken for third-degree AV block, but on rewarming ventricular rates approach or exceed 200 bpm. Atrial wires or esophageal electrography confirms the key diagnostic features: AV dissociation with normal QRS and the regular ventricular rate faster than the atrial rate. Appropriately timed atrial systoles conducted to the ventricle result in "advancement" of the tachycardia cycle (without a change in QRS morphology or subsequent pause). If the QRS is normal but the RR interval does not shorten with appropriately timed atrial systoles, JET with retrograde (VA) conduction or third-degree AV block with JET as the escape rhythm should be suspected.

Infants with JET usually are often severely ill, and β-adrenergic agonists, fever, and endogenous catecholamines accelerate the tachycardia. Initial treatment of postoperative JET includes sedation and analgesia, withdrawal of adrenergic stimulants (to the extent possible), and cooling. The tachycardia may be suppressed by temporary overdrive (atrial) pacing, by pacing at a rate sufficient to produce 2:1 AV block, or by AVT mode pacing to provide AV synchrony.[54] IV amiodarone has been used with perhaps the greatest efficacy.[55] Although emergency radiofrequency ablation has been performed in rare instances, aggressive temporizing measures, including extracorporeal membrane oxygenation, appear warranted given the transient nature of this arrhythmia.

Late Postoperative Arrhythmias

Atrial tachycardia and bradycardia are common late sequelae following the Senning and Mustard operations for D-transposition of the great arteries, atrial septal defect closure, and the Fontan procedure for tricuspid atresia and single ventricle.[15] Patients with these arrhythmias appear to be at increased risk for sudden death, although whether death is the result of atrial tachycardia itself, associated bradycardia, degeneration to VT, or even nondysrhythmic events remains unclear.

Likewise, in patients with repaired or palliated CHD, ventricular arrhythmias that are associated with risk for sudden death may develop. There seems to be little justification for empirical drug therapy to suppress asymptomatic ventricular arrhythmias in these patients. Earlier repair is believed to decrease the incidence of serious problems. Still, the relative contributions of postoperative hemodynamic abnormalities, the natural history of the unrepaired lesions, and surgical technique to the development of late arrhythmias remain uncertain. Similarly, the roles of pacemaker/defibrillator therapy, prospective electrophysiologic study, and antiarrhythmic drug testing are not well established. Because both bradycardias and tachycardias develop in many patients, the correlation of symptoms with electrophysiologic abnormality is important in guiding therapy.

Metabolic Derangements

Electrolyte Disturbances

Hyperkalemia causes characteristically tall ("peaked" or "tente") T waves with a narrow base with progressive changes at higher concentrations, including decreased P-wave amplitude, QRS prolongation, SA nodal and AV nodal block, and ultimately ventricular fibrillation. Mild to moderate hypokalemia may cause prominent U waves, diminished T-wave amplitude, T-wave inversion, and fusion of the T wave and U wave, along with increased spontaneous ventricular ectopy and inducible ventricular arrhythmias. Arrhythmias caused by hypokalemia are potentiated by catecholamines, and hypokalemia itself potentiates the toxic effects of digoxin and the proarrhythmic effects of drugs associated with drug-induced long QT syndrome.[56] Severe hypokalemia is associated with ventricular fibrillation.

Hypercalcemia produces T-wave inversion and shortens the QT interval. Hypocalcemia prolongs the time to the peak of the T wave but not the QT interval itself. Isolated calcium abnormalities are uncommon, and arrhythmias caused by such abnormalities are rare, although hypercalcemia may aggravate digitalis toxicity.[2]

Endocrine Disorders (Thyroid)

Hyperthyroidism exerts both sympathetic-like and direct cardiovascular actions that produce sinus tachycardia and atrial fibrillation, but ventricular arrhythmias are uncommon. These arrhythmias respond to β-blockers and resolve when the euthyroid state is restored. Combination treatment with digoxin potentiates AV nodal block while minimizing negative inotropic effects. Hypothyroidism causes sinus bradycardia and AV conduction disturbances; QT interval prolongation is common but rarely associated with torsades de pointes.[57]

Central Nervous System Injury

The most common ECG change associated with CNS trauma and increased intracranial pressure is sinus bradycardia, usually with associated hypertension. These bradycardias appear to be vagally mediated and usually respond to atropine. However, potentially serious arrhythmias may occur within 24 hours following blunt trauma to the head, subdural hematoma, and subarachnoid hemorrhage. QT-interval prolongation is common and, in combination with bradycardia and hypokalemia, may provoke torsades de pointes.

Hypothermia and Hyperthermia

Mild hypothermia can cause a range of reversible ECG changes, including sinus bradycardia; prolongation of the PR, QRS, and QT intervals; and a characteristic secondary deflection on the terminal portion of the QRS (Osborn wave).[58] Severe hypothermia may cause more significant bradycardias, including AV block and asystole or VTs and ventricular fibrillation. Therapeutic hypothermia is associated with QT prolongation, and torsades de pointes has been reported.[59] In contrast, hyperthermia causes sinus tachycardia and may enhance other tachycardias such as PSVT, ectopic atrial arrhythmias, and especially JET in susceptible patients.

Acute Myocardial Infarction

Acute myocardial infarction is uncommon in young patients but may occur in cases of anomalous origin of the left coronary artery, when there is perinatal stress, following Kawasaki disease, with blunt chest wall trauma, and following cardiac transplantation and the arterial switch procedure. It can occur after air embolism in cyanotic CHD or after open-heart operations. The diagnosis may be overlooked in infants and children because of the inconsistency of symptoms and relatively poor (60%) clinical recognition by electrocardiography.[60] Nevertheless, acute infarction may result in various rhythm disturbances, including sinus bradycardia (as a result of the Bezold-Jarisch reflex), AV conduction disturbances, intraventricular block, and asystole.

Arrhythmias Resulting From Drug Toxicity
Digoxin

Digoxin toxicity may cause various arrhythmias and should be suspected in any patient in whom a new arrhythmia develops during digoxin therapy. Likewise, digoxin ingestion should be considered in patients with acute arrhythmias, particularly those associated with CNS and gastrointestinal symptoms. Accelerated junctional rhythm may be the first arrhythmia seen. Progressive AV block is common. Sinus bradycardia resulting from either SA node exit block or sinus arrest may occur, as can atrial fibrillation (but usually not atrial flutter). Ectopic atrial arrhythmias may occur. Nearly any ventricular arrhythmia may occur, including multiform ventricular extrasystoles, bigeminy, VT (particularly "bidirectional" VT, otherwise only seen in rare genetic arrhythmia syndromes; Fig. 35.18), and ventricular fibrillation.[61]

In general, digoxin concentrations less than 2 ng/mL are considered nontoxic. Neonates usually tolerate levels as high as 3.5 ng/mL. Nevertheless, neonates and other intensive care patients may be more susceptible to digoxin toxicity because of renal dysfunction, electrolyte imbalances, and hypoxia. Hypokalemia, excessive calcium infusions, and rapid sinus rates exacerbate digitalis-related arrhythmias.

Purified digoxin-specific Fab antibody fragment, which binds the drug and is eliminated in the urine, is used to treat digoxin toxicity. Prophylactic treatment with this preparation should be gauged according to the quantity ingested, the time since ingestion, and the serum digoxin level. Magnesium sulfate is a useful temporizing treatment while specific antibody treatment is being implemented. Cardioversion should be reserved for life-threatening tachycardias or those unresponsive to these therapies.

Cocaine

Life-threatening ventricular arrhythmias, cardiac arrest, and myocardial infarction can occur in healthy individuals with normal coronary arteries following cocaine ingestion and in prenatally exposed neonates.[62,63] Cocaine produces myocardial ischemia and infarction by inducing severe local coronary vasoconstriction, increasing myocardial-metabolic demand

through its potent chronotropic effects, and increasing afterload. In infarct models, cocaine directly potentiates arrhythmias induced by catecholamines.[64] These factors favor the use of β-adrenergic antagonists as first-line treatment for cocaine-related arrhythmias. Additionally, cocaine blocks fast inward sodium channels, similar to class I antiarrhythmic agents.[65] QT prolongation and torsades de pointes have been observed.

Tricyclic Antidepressants and Phenothiazine

Phenothiazines and tricyclic antidepressants produce electrophysiologic (and potentially antiarrhythmic) effects similar to quinidine and procainamide. They slow conduction velocity in atrial and ventricular tissue, prolong repolarization, and exert anticholinergic effects accounting for the observed ECG changes of conduction disturbances, prolonged QT intervals and QRS duration, and various tachycardias and bradycardias.[66] Sinus tachycardia, atrial and VTs, and AV conduction disturbances distal to the AV node occur occasionally during normal therapeutic administration and may reflect individual susceptibility to QT-prolonging agents.

Arrhythmias commonly follow intentional overdose, resulting in hypotension (due to α-blocking effects), severe anticholinergic effects (neuromuscular and mucosal), seizures, and coma. Quinidine and procainamide are contraindicated for tachycardias because of these agents. In patients manifesting early cardiotoxicity, arrhythmias may develop 3 to 7 days following ingestion, apparently because of release of tissue stores. Therefore ECG monitoring should be continued for at least 24 to 48 hours after apparent ECG and rhythm normalization and longer if severe arrhythmias are observed.

Infections

Myocarditis may cause atrial and VTs or acquired heart block. Lyme disease may produce high-grade acute AV block. Although AV conduction usually normalizes with appropriate antibiotic therapy, temporary pacing may be required.[67] Antibiotic treatment should be instituted on the basis of the history and electrocardiographic findings alone while awaiting confirmatory serology. Bacterial endocarditis can cause AV conduction disturbances, particularly when the aortic valve is involved. Unstable or persisting conduction abnormalities (longer than 7 days) carry a high risk of mortality (43%–80%) and are indications for early valve replacement.[68]

Myocarditis may be responsible for some cases of VT in otherwise healthy individuals and may range from chronic ventricular ectopy or tachycardia to fulminant and refractory arrhythmias leading to electromechanical dissociation. Chaotic atrial tachycardia may occur in the setting of infection with respiratory syncytial virus, although the cause of this association is unclear. Finally, paroxysmal tachycardias of any etiology may be exacerbated by acute infections that cause fever, dehydration, and increased sympathetic tone. Short-term modifications of chronic therapy may be necessary, particularly when oral administration becomes impractical.

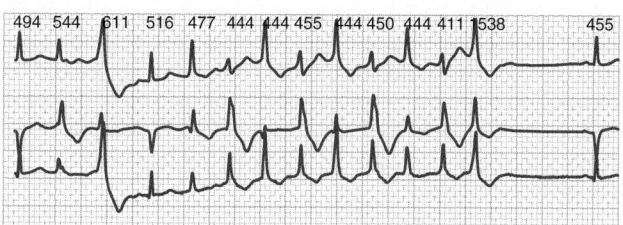

494 544 611 516 477 444 444 455 444 450 444 411 538   455

Fig. 35.18. Bidirectional ventricular tachycardia. This unusual arrhythmia is only seen in patients with digoxin toxicity and two rare genetic arrhythmia syndromes: Andersen-Tawil syndrome (periodic paralysis and ventricular arrhythmias) and catecholaminergic polymorphic ventricular tachycardia. The patient is asymptomatic during this arrhythmia, but patients appear to be at risk for ventricular fibrillation.

References

1. Valsangiacomo E, Schmid ER, Schupbach RW, et al. Early postoperative arrhythmias after cardiac operation in children. *Ann Thorac Surg.* 2002; 4:792-796.
2. Ramaswamy K, Hamdan MH. Ischemia, metabolic disturbances, and arrhythmogenesis: mechanisms and management. *Crit Care Med.* 2000; 28:N151-N157.

3. Benson DW, Wand DW, Dyment M, et al. Congenital sick sinus syndrome caused by recessive mutation in the cardiac sodium channel gene (SCN5A). *J Clin Invest.* 2003;12:1019-1028.

4. Lupoglazoff JM, Denjoy I, Villain E, et al. Long QT syndrome in neonates: conduction disorders associated with HERG mutations and sinus bradycardia with KCNQ1 mutations. *J Am Coll Cardiol.* 2004;43:826-830.

5. Pfammatter JP, Bauersfeld U. Idiopathic ventricular tachycardias in infants and children. *Card Electrophysiol Rev.* 2002;6:88-92.

6. Paul T, Bertram H, Bokenkamp R. Supraventricular tachycardia in infants, children and adolescents: diagnosis, and pharmacological and interventional therapy. *Paediatr Drugs.* 2000;2:171-181.

7. Anand RG, Rosenthal GL, Van Hare GF, et al. Is the mechanism of supraventricular tachycardia in pediatrics influenced by age, gender or ethnicity? *Congenit Heart Dis.* 2009;4:464-468.

8. Kang KT, Potts JE, Radbill AE, et al. Permanent junctional reciprocating tachycardia in children: a multicenter experience. *Heart Rhythm.* 2014;11:1426-1432.

9. Benditt DG, Benson DW Jr, Dunnigan A, et al. Atrial flutter, atrial fibrillation, and other primary atrial tachycardias. *Med Clin North Am.* 1984;68:895-918.

10. Frustaci A, Chimenti C, Bellocci F, et al. Histological substrate of atrial biopsies in patients with lone atrial fibrillation. *Circulation.* 1997;96:1180-1184.

11. Harahsheh A, Du W, Singh H, et al. Risk factors for atrioventricular tachycardia degenerating to atrial flutter/fibrillation in the young with Wolff-Parkinson-White. *Pacing Clin Electrophysiol.* 2008;31:1307-1312.

12. Donnerstein RL, Berg RA, Shehab Z, et al. Complex atrial tachycardias and respiratory syncytial virus infections in infants. *J Pediatr.* 1994;125:23-28.

13. Collins KK, Van Hare GF, Kertesz NJ, et al. Pediatric nonpost-operative junctional ectopic tachycardia medical management and interventional therapies. *J Am Coll Cardiol.* 2009;53:690-697.

14. Lan Y-T, Lee JCR, Wetzel G. Postoperative arrhythmia. *Curr Opin Cardiol.* 2003;18:73-78.

15. Khairy P, Van Hare GF, Balaji S, et al. PACES/HRS expert consensus statement on the recognition and management of arrhythmias in adult congenital heart disease. *Heart Rhythm.* 2014;11:e102-e165.

16. Pinter A, Dorian P. Intravenous antiarrhythmic agents. *Curr Opin Cardiol.* 2001;16:17-22.

17. McKee MR. Amiodarone: an "old" drug with new recommendations. *Curr Opin Pediatr.* 2003;15:193-199.

18. Campbell RM, Strieper MJ, Frias PA. The role of radiofrequency ablation for pediatric supraventricular tachycardia. *Minerva Pediatr.* 2004;56:63-72.

19. Walsh EP, Cecchin F. Recent advances in pacemaker and implantable defibrillator therapy for young patients. *Curr Opin Cardiol.* 2004;19:91-96.

20. Cohen MI, Bush DM, Vetter VL, et al. Permanent epicardial pacing in pediatric patients: seventeen years of experience and 1200 outpatient visits. *Circulation.* 2001;103:2585-2590.

21. Sliz NB Jr, Johns JA. Cardiac pacing in infants and children. *Cardiol Rev.* 2000;8:223-239.

22. Bernstein AD, Daubert JC, Fletcher RD, et al. The revised NASPE/BPEG generic code for antibradycardia, adaptive-rate, and multisite pacing. North American Society of Pacing and Electrophysiology/British Pacing and Electrophysiology Group. *Pacing Clin Electrophysiol.* 2002;25:260-264.

23. Gregoratos G, Abrams J, Epstein AE, et al. Guideline update for implantation of cardiac pacemakers and antiarrhythmia devices—summary article: a report of the American College of Cardiology/American Heart Association Task Force on Practice Guidelines (ACC/AHA/NASPE Committee to Update the 1998 Pacemaker Guidelines). *J Am Coll Cardiol.* 2002;40:1703-1719.

24. Michaelsson M, Riesenfeld T, Jonzon A. Natural history of congenital complete atrioventricular block. *Pacing Clin Electrophysiol.* 1997;20:2098-2101.

25. Horenstein MS, Walters H III, Karpawich PP. Chronic performance of steroid-eluting epicardial leads in a growing pediatric population: a 10-year comparison. *Pacing Clin Electrophysiol.* 2003;26:1467-1471.

26. Reddy VY, Knops RE, Sperzel J, et al. Permanent leadless cardiac pacing: results of the LEADLESS trial. *Circulation.* 2014;129:1466-1471.

27. Mah DY, Alexander ME, Banka P, et al. The role of cardiac resynchronization therapy for arterial switch operations complicated by complete heart block. *Ann Thorac Surg.* 2013;96:904-909.

28. Qintar M, Morad A, Alhawasli H, et al. Pacing for drug-refractory or drug-intolerant hypertrophic cardiomyopathy. *Cochrane Database Syst Rev.* 2012;(5):CD008523.

29. Bink-Boelkens MT. Pharmacologic management of arrhythmias. *Pediatr Cardiol.* 2000;21:508-515.

30. Roden DM. Antiarrhythmic drugs: from mechanisms to clinical practice. *Br Heart J.* 2000;84:339-346.

31. Vassallo P, Trohman RG. Prescribing amiodarone: an evidence-based review of clinical indications. *JAMA.* 2000;298:1312-1322.

32. Weindling SN, Saul JP, Walsh EP. Efficacy and risks of medical therapy for supraventricular tachycardia in neonates and infants. *Am Heart J.* 1996;131:66-72.

33. Redman J, Worthley LI. Antiarrhythmic and haemodynamic effects of the commonly used intravenous electrolytes. *Crit Care Resusc.* 2001;3:22-34.

34. Sanatani S, Potts JE, Reed JH, et al. The study of antiarrhythmic medications in infancy (SAMIS): a multicenter, randomized controlled trial comparing the efficacy and safety of digoxin versus propranolol for prophylaxis of supraventricular tachycardia in infants. *Circ Arrhythm Electrophysiol.* 2012;5:984-991.

35. Hammer GB, Drover DR, Cao H, et al. The effects of dexmedetomidine on cardiac electrophysiology in children. *Anesth Analg.* 2008;106:79-83.

36. Chrysostomou C, Morell VO, Wearden P, et al. Dexmedetomidine: therapeutic use for the termination of reentrant supraventricular tachycardia. *Congenit Heart Dis.* 2013;8:48-56.

37. Shepard SM, Tejman-Yarden S, Khanna S, et al. Dexmedetomidine-related atrial standstill and loss of capture in a pediatric patient after congenital heart surgery. *Crit Care Med.* 2011;39:187-189.

38. Webb CA, Weyker PD, Flynn BC. Asystole after orthotopic lung transplantation: examining the interaction of cardiac denervation and dexmedetomidine. *Case Rep Anesthesiol.* 2012;2012:203240.

39. Fish FA. Ventricular fibrillation: basic concepts. *Pediatr Clin North Am.* 2004;51:1211-1221.

40. The American Heart Association in collaboration with the International Liaison Committee on Resuscitation. Guidelines 2000 for cardiopulmonary resuscitation and emergency cardiovascular care. Part 10: pediatric advanced life support. *Circulation.* 2000;102:I-291-I-342.

41. Gikonyo BM, Dunnigan A, Benson DW Jr. Cardiovascular collapse in infants: association with paroxysmal atrial tachycardia. *Pediatrics.* 1985;76:922-926.

42. Zimmerman FJ, Pahl E, Rocchini A. High incidence of incessant supraventricular tachycardia in pediatric patients referred for cardiac transplantation. *Pacing Clin Electrophysiol.* 1996;19:663.

43. Moore JP, Patel PA, Shannon KM. Predictors of myocardial recovery in pediatric tachycardia-induced cardiomyopathy. *Heart Rhythm.* 2014;11:1163-1169.

44. Bradley DJ, Fischbach PS, Law IH, et al. The clinical course of multifocal atrial tachycardia in infants and children. *J Am Coll Cardiol.* 2001;38:401-408.

45. Fish FA, Mehta AV, Johns J. Characteristics and management of chaotic atrial tachycardia of infancy. *Am J Cardiol.* 1996;78:1052-1055.

46. Priori SG, Napolitano C, Schwartz P. Low penetrance in the long-QT syndrome: clinical impact. *Circulation.* 1999;99:529-533.

47. Yang T, Snyders D, Roden D. Drug block of I(kr): model systems and relevance to human arrhythmias. *J Cardiovasc Pharmacol.* 2001;38:737-744.

48. Khan IA, Gowda RM. Novel therapeutics for treatment of long-QT syndrome and torsades de pointes. *Int J Cardiol.* 2004;95:1-6.

49. Roden DM, Lazzara R, Rosen M, et al. Multiple mechanisms in the long-QT syndrome. Current knowledge, gaps, and future directions. The SADS Foundation Task Force on LQTS. *Circulation.* 1996;94:1996-2012.

50. Rehsia SS, Pepelassis D, Buffo-Sequeira I. Accelerated ventricular rhythm in healthy neonates. *Paediatr Child Health.* 2007;12:777-779.

51. Reynolds JL, Pickoff AS. Accelerated ventricular rhythm in children: a review and report of a case with congenital heart disease. *Pediatr Cardiol.* 2001;22:23-28.

52. Stratemann S, Dzurik Y, Fish F, et al. Left ventricular cardiac fibroma in a child presenting with ventricular tachycardia. *Pediatr Cardiol.* 2008;29:223-226.

53. Weindling SN, Saul JP, Gamble WJ, et al. Duration of complete atrioventricular block after congenital heart disease surgery. *Am J Cardiol.* 1998;82:525-527.

54. Janousek J, Vojtovic P, Gebauer RA. Use of a modified, commercially available temporary pacemaker for R wave synchronized atrial pacing in postoperative junctional ectopic tachycardia. *Pacing Clin Electrophysiol.* 2003;26:579-586.

55. Laird WP, Snyder CS, Kertesz NJ, et al. Use of intravenous amiodarone for postoperative junctional ectopic tachycardia in children. *Pediatr Cardiol.* 2003;24:133-137.

56. Yang T, Roden DM. Extracellular potassium modulation of drug block of IKr. Implications for torsades de pointes and reverse use-dependence. *Circulation.* 1996;93:407-411.

57. Klein I, Ojamaa K. Thyroid hormone and the cardiovascular system. *N Engl J Med.* 2001;344:501-509.

58. Mattu A, Brady WJ, Perron AD. Electrocardiographic manifestations of hypothermia. *Am J Emerg Med.* 2002;20:314-326.

59. Huang CH, Tsai MS, Hsu CY, et al. Images in cardiovascular medicine. Therapeutic hypothermia-related torsades de pointes. *Circulation.* 2006; 114:e521-e522.

60. Towbin JA, Bricker JT, Garson A Jr. Electrocardiographic criteria for diagnosis of acute myocardial infarction in childhood. *Am J Cardiol.* 1992; 69:1545-1548.

61. Hastreiter AR, van der Horst RL, Chow-Tung E. Digitalis toxicity in infants and children. *Pediatr Cardiol.* 1984;5:131-148.

62. Kloner RA, Rezkalla SH. Cocaine and the heart. *N Engl J Med.* 2003;348: 487-488.

63. Frassica JJ, Orav EJ, Walsh EP, et al. Arrhythmias in children prenatally exposed to cocaine. *Arch Pediatr Adolesc Med.* 1994;148:1163-1169.

64. Inoue H, Zipes DP. Cocaine-induced supersensitivity and arrhythmogenesis. *J Am Coll Cardiol.* 1988;11:867-874.

65. Chakko S. Arrhythmias associated with cocaine abuse. *Card Electrophysiol Rev.* 2002;6:168-169.

66. Witchel HJ, Hancox JC, Nutt DJ. Psychotropic drugs, cardiac arrhythmia, and sudden death. *J Clin Psychopharmacol.* 2003;23:58-77.

67. Pinto DS. Cardiac manifestations of Lyme disease. *Med Clin North Am.* 2002;86:285-296.

68. DiNubile MJ, Calderwood SB, Steinhaus DM, et al. Cardiac conduction abnormalities complicating native valve active infective endocarditis. *Am J Cardiol.* 1986;58:1213-1217.

Shock States

Lincoln S. Smith, Srinivasarao Badugu, and Lynn J. Hernan

PEARLS

- Shock is recognized by the features of tachycardia, tachypnea, and abnormalities of perfusion, as evidenced by skin perfusion, quality of pulses, mental status, and dysfunction of other organ systems.
- Pediatric patients with shock often present with myocardial dysfunction ("cold" shock), although older children and adolescents may present with the adult picture of vascular dysfunction ("warm" shock).
- Neonates in shock must be treated for both septic shock and cardiogenic shock resulting from ductal-dependent congenital heart disease until an echocardiogram can confirm the cardiac anatomy. These conditions cannot be ruled out by physical examination. Therefore all neonates with shock should be given prostaglandin infusion as part of their resuscitation. Pulmonary hypertension, hypocalcemia, and hypoglycemia frequently complicate shock in neonates.
- Pediatric patients in shock generally have absolute or relative hypovolemia, and the first line of resuscitation should be a fluid bolus of 20 mL/kg. Administration of more fluid should be based on rapid assessment of hemodynamic status.
- Early endotracheal intubation allows advantageous redistribution of the compromised cardiac output and reduces left ventricular afterload.
- Timely recognition and early aggressive goal-directed therapy reduce mortality in septic shock.

The clinical syndrome of shock is one of the most dramatic, dynamic, and life-threatening problems faced by the physician in the critical care setting. Although untreated shock is universally lethal, mortality may be considerably reduced with rapid, proper recognition; diagnosis; monitoring; and treatment.

Definition and Physiology

Shock is an acute, complex state of circulatory dysfunction that results in failure to deliver or use sufficient amounts of oxygen and other nutrients to meet tissue metabolic demands. If prolonged, it leads to multiple organ failure and death. Therefore shock can be viewed as a state of acute cellular energy deficiency. Shock can be caused by any serious disease or injury, but whatever the causative factors, it is always a problem of inadequate cellular sustenance. It is the final common pathway to death.

Delivery of oxygen (DO_2) is a direct function of cardiac output (CO) and arterial oxygen content (CaO_2):

Delivery of oxygen:

$$DO_2 = CO \times CaO_2 \qquad \text{Eq. 36.1}$$

Cardiac output:

$$CO = \text{Heart rate (HR)} \times \text{Stroke volume (SV)} \qquad \text{Eq. 36.2}$$

Oxygen content:

$$CaO_2 = (Hgb \times 1.34 \times SaO_2) + (0.003 \times PaO_2) \qquad \text{Eq. 36.3}$$

Stroke volume is a function of preload, afterload, contractility, and diastolic relaxation. Therefore optimizing heart rate, contractility, diastolic relaxation, preload, and afterload improves cardiac output. Oxygen-carrying capacity can be increased by raising hemoglobin and optimizing its saturation with oxygen. Oxygen delivery can be improved by manipulation of all these factors.

Calculation of global oxygen delivery may not reflect regional hypoperfusion and localized ischemia. Inadequate oxygen delivery can result from either limitation or maldistribution of blood flow. Reduced oxygen content (anemia, low arterial oxygen saturation) necessitates higher cardiac output to maintain oxygen delivery. In certain situations (fever, sepsis, trauma), metabolic demands may exceed normal oxygen delivery. Impairment of the extraction or utilization of oxygen by cells and mitochondria creates a functional arteriovenous shunt and may be the harbinger of multiorgan dysfunction syndrome.[1,2]

Recognition and Assessment of the Shock State

The early diagnosis of shock requires a high index of suspicion and knowledge of conditions that predispose children to shock. Interviews of the parents, physicians, nurses, and emergency medical services personnel caring for the child provide valuable information. A rapid and focused physical examination of a patient in shock is essential (Box 36.1).

Shock states have been divided into three phases: compensated, uncompensated, and irreversible (Box 36.2). In compensated shock, vital organ function is maintained primarily by intrinsic regulatory mechanisms. The ability to compensate for shock states varies with age and depends on developmental aspects of the autonomic nervous, circulatory, respiratory, renal, and immunologic systems, as well as the presence of other medical conditions. Previously healthy children can compensate for and maintain normal blood pressure during

BOX 36.1 Physical Assessment in Shock

State of consciousness: restless, anxious, agitated, comatose
Skin: temperature, perfusion, moistness, color, turgor, rash
Mucous membranes: color, moistness
Nail beds: color, capillary refill
Central capillary refill
Peripheral veins: collapsed or distended
Pulse: rate, rhythm, quality
Blood pressure: orthostatic changes, pulse pressure
Respiration: rate, depth, effort, crackles, adequacy of aeration
Urine: concentration, hourly output

BOX 36.2 Shock States

Hypovolemia
Cardiogenic
Obstructive
Distributive
Septic
Endocrine

states of reduced delivery and/or increased oxygen demand. Diagnosing a patient as having compensated shock, rather than mere dehydration, may be the difference between a patient who is appropriately resuscitated in a timely manner and one for whom resuscitative efforts are delayed.

Early signs of compensated shock may be subtle. Activation of peripheral and central baroreceptors produces catecholamines, and the resulting tachycardia and peripheral vasoconstriction are initially adequate to support blood pressure. Tachypnea, mildly prolonged capillary refill, orthostatic hypotension, and mild alteration of mental status (eg, lethargy, irritability) are signs of compensated shock. In patients with sepsis, other signs of early compensated shock may be plethora, warm extremities, bounding pulses, and a widened pulse pressure.

As shock progresses, compensatory mechanisms are exceeded, and oxygen delivery is no longer sufficient. Patients become hypotensive, acidotic, lethargic or comatose, and oliguric or anuric. Cellular function deteriorates, affecting all organ systems. Systemic vasoconstriction and hypotension produce ischemia and hypoxia in the visceral and cutaneous circulations. Altered cellular metabolism and function result in damage to blood vessels, kidneys, liver, pancreas, and bowel.

Terminal or irreversible shock implies damage to key organs of such magnitude that death occurs even if therapy restores cardiovascular function to adequate levels.

The contribution of laboratory tests to the initial evaluation of patients in shock is limited. Blood gases and serum lactate levels may quantify the degree of hypoxemia and acidosis and are widely used as markers for the effectiveness of treatment. Serum lactate[3-7] and troponin I[8,9] may be useful markers of severity of illness and for prognosis. Systemic mixed venous oxygen saturation greater than 70% suggests adequate cardiac output, but this assumes normal oxygen extraction.[10] However, an increased understanding of microcirculatory aberrations and cellular hypoxia has raised awareness of the limitations of tests on pooled venous samples. This has stimulated a search for a minimally invasive means of sampling regional circulations.[11-13] Gastric tonometry,[14,15] near-infrared spectroscopy,[16,17] rectal tonometry,[18] sublingual capnometry,[19,20]

muscle oxygenation,[21] tissue microdialysis,[22,23] and orthogonal polarization spectral imaging[24,25] are investigational methods to evaluate regional circulation, but their clinical utility remains unproven at this time. Repeated evaluations and monitoring of the patient in shock by a competent observer, with appropriate, timely interventions, remain the most effective and sensitive physiologic monitor available.

Treatment of Shock
General Principles

In addition to treatment of the primary underlying process, therapeutic efforts involve optimizing and balancing oxygen delivery and oxygen consumption. Therapy begins with the assurance of adequate oxygenation and ventilation; oxygen should always be the first drug administered. Efforts to reduce oxygen requirements when oxygen delivery is compromised are important. Sedation, paralysis, and control of fever are ways to reduce oxygen consumption. Even routine nursing procedures can increase oxygen consumption by up to 20% to 30% in healthy adults.[26]

Intubation and Mechanical Ventilation

During shock states, there is often increased work of breathing related to capillary leak, acidosis, and hypoxemia. In landmark studies in dogs, spontaneous breathing during shock states was associated with preserved blood flow and oxygen consumption by the diaphragm and intubation, paralysis, and mechanical ventilation resulted in redistribution of cardiac output from the muscles of respiration to vital organs.[27,28] A subsequent study in humans showed that central venous hypoxemia significantly improved after intubation and mechanical ventilation.[29] Although these data suggest that mechanical ventilation can substantially improve oxygen delivery to vital organs, suboptimal patient-ventilator interactions may result in increased oxygen consumption.[30,31] Positive pressure ventilation decreases preload and increases afterload on the right ventricle (see Chapter 34). The reduction of preload can often be overcome by treating the patient with a rapid fluid bolus before or during intubation. Positive pressure ventilation also reduces afterload to the left ventricle, which may improve stroke volume.

Fluid Resuscitation

Regardless of the underlying insult, most patients in shock have an absolute or relative hypovolemia, causing a decrease in preload and subsequent decrement of stroke volume and cardiac output. Early fluid resuscitation is the cornerstone of immediate therapy. Landmark studies of septic pediatric and adult patients showed that early fluid resuscitation was associated with improved patient outcomes, and these principles are incorporated in current treatment guidelines.[32-34] However, excessive fluid resuscitation in patients with cardiogenic shock and some forms of obstructive shock (massive pulmonary embolism or severe pulmonary hypertension) may rapidly push the patient over the Frank-Starling curve into congestive heart failure. Multimodal monitoring uses multiple variables and their changes over time to assess hemodynamic status and prognosis: Heart rate variability,[35] shock index[36] (HR/SBP), and speckle tracking imaging[37] have shown promise. Evidence associating positive fluid balance with increased mortality in critically ill adult and pediatric patients[38-41] suggests a need for better predictors of fluid responsiveness and end points of fluid resuscitation.[42,43] Therefore careful attention must be paid to the physiologic responses to fluid resuscitation by a competent observer. When sufficient preload has been achieved through fluid resuscitation but the patient remains in shock, other supportive therapies are indicated.

Inotropic, Chronotropic, Lusitropic, and Vasoactive Infusions

Infusions to increase cardiac output and improve peripheral vascular tone are indicated when patients have been adequately fluid resuscitated but hemodynamics remain deranged. Infusions of catecholamines (dopamine, dobutamine, epinephrine, norepinephrine); phosphodiesterase inhibitors (milrinone); and vasopressin are most commonly used. The choice of vasoactive infusion is dependent on the physiologic derangement (Table 36.1). Catecholamines work through

stimulation of α_1, α_2, β_1, β_2, and dopaminergic receptors to increase intracellular cyclic guanosine monophosphate (cGMP) (Table 36.2). Phosphodiesterase inhibitors increase cGMP by preventing its degradation within the cell (see Chapter 33). Vasopressin causes vasoconstriction by direct stimulation of vascular smooth muscle cell V1 receptors. Vasopressin also potentiates systemic adrenergic effects. Vasopressin and terlipressin (a synthetic analog of vasopressin with a similar pharmacodynamic profile but with a significantly longer half-life) have also shown some utility in the treatment of catecholamine-resistant shock.[44-46] Fenoldopam has been used to augment diuresis and improve hemodynamics after cardiac surgery and in septic shock.[47,48] There is not conclusive generalized evidence that the choice of medication influences outcome in critically ill adults.[49] Therefore therapies should be tailored to the unique patient situation, and patients should be closely monitored for expected responses.[35]

Other Therapies

The finding of hypocalcemia in infants who present in shock should raise the suspicion of left ventricular dysfunction. Hypocalcemia causes left ventricular dysfunction and is reversible with calcium therapy. Of note, 30% of neonates with DiGeorge syndrome are hypocalcemic.

Neonates, who have low glycogen stores and increased metabolic requirements during shock, may quickly develop hypoglycemia. Patients with mitochondrial disorders may also be highly sensitive to reductions in energy substrates. All patients in shock should be monitored and treated with appropriate energy substrates.

Adrenal insufficiency should be suspected in patients with refractory shock resulting from trauma (head or abdominal), history of steroid use within past 6 months, sepsis, or treatment with etomidate. Direct damage to the hypothalamus, anterior pituitary, or adrenals may result in cortisol deficiency. In septic shock, adrenal hemorrhage has been the paradigm of adrenal insufficiency, but evidence of transient relative or functional adrenal insufficiency in septic shock remains unclear (see section on septic shock).

Extracorporeal life support (ECLS) has been used to support patients of all ages with shock. The Extracorporeal Life Support Organization (ELSO) maintains a database of patients treated with ECLS from member institutions around the

TABLE 36.1	Therapies for Hemodynamic Patterns in Shock States		
	BLOOD PRESSURE OR SYSTEMIC VASCULAR RESISTANCE		
Hemodynamic Pattern	**Normal**	**Decreased**	**Elevated**
Septic shock			
Stroke index ↑ ↔	None	α_1, V_1	None
Stroke index ↓	β_1	α_1 and β_1	$\beta_1 + \beta_2$, or PDE
Cardiogenic shock	β_1	α_1 and β_1	$\beta_1 + \beta_2$, or PDE
Myocardial dysfunction (complicating critical illness)[a]	β_1 and/or β_2	α_1 and β_1	$\beta_1 + \beta_2$, or PDE
Congestive heart failure	β_1 and/or β_2	β_1	$\beta_1 + \beta_2$, or PDE
Bradycardia	None	β_1	None

[a]For example, acute respiratory distress syndrome or anthracycline therapy.
PDE, phosphodiesterase inhibitor.

TABLE 36.2	Vasoactive Medications				
	α_1	β_1	β_2	D_1	V_1
Dopamine[a]	Vasoconstriction	Inotropy, chronotropy	Vasodilation	Renal vasodilation	
Norepinephrine	Vasoconstriction	Inotropy			
Epinephrine[b]	Vasoconstriction	Inotropy, chronotropy	Vasodilation		
Dobutamine		Inotropy	Vasodilation		
Vasopressin	Potentiates	Potentiates			Vasoconstriction
Inamrinone, milrinone	Non–receptor-mediated inotropy, lusitropy, and vasodilation				

[a]Dose related: at low infusion rates, D_1 receptor effects predominate; at intermediate rates, β_1 and β_2 receptor effects predominate; at high rates, α_1 effects predominate on peripheral vasculature.
[b]Dose related: at low infusion rates, β receptor effects predominate; at high rates, α effects predominate on peripheral vasculature.

world. The registry was searched for data on patients treated with ECLS (from 1985 through January 2010) with any mention of the diagnosis of shock. The registry revealed 1512 pediatric patients (age ≤21 years old) who were treated with ECLS for any diagnosis that included the descriptor shock. The overall mortality was 60%. Sixty-five percent of patients were 1 year of age or younger, and 44% were neonates. In patients aged 21 years or younger treated with ECLS, the etiology of shock was cardiogenic (46%), septic (22%), hypovolemic (11%), traumatic or surgical (1%), and other or unspecified (20%). The mortality across the groups ranged from 56% to 64%.

Multisystem Effects of Shock

Management of the multisystem deterioration that occurs in shock states is as important as treating the underlying condition. Respiratory, gastrointestinal, central nervous system, renal, and hematologic abnormalities must be anticipated. Multiple organ dysfunction syndrome (MODS) is the derangement of two or more organs after an insult.[50] The severity of MODS has been associated with increased mortality in PICU patients.[51-54]

Respiratory

Respiratory failure frequently accompanies shock states. It may result from failure of the ventilator pump (ie, respiratory muscle fatigue) and/or deterioration of lung function (ie, acute respiratory distress syndrome). Therefore providing supplemental oxygen is essential in all children with shock. Early tracheal intubation protects the airway, provides relief from respiratory muscle fatigue, facilitates provision of positive airway pressure, redistributes blood flow from the muscles of respiration to core organs, reduces the left ventricle afterload, and reduces oxygen demands of respiratory muscles. Patients should be ventilated with a lung protective strategy (see Chapter 52).

Renal

Renal failure may develop in association with any of the shock syndromes. Shock-related renal failure is a continuum of acute prerenal azotemia through classic acute tubular necrosis to cortical necrosis. Although low-dose dopamine (3–5 µg/kg/min) improves renal blood flow,[55,56] it also impairs renal oxygen kinetics, inhibits protective feedback loops with the kidney, may worsen tubular injury, and has failed to show benefit in preventing or altering the course of acute renal failure in adults.[57,58] Acute anuric renal failure may require treatment with peritoneal dialysis, ultrafiltration, continuous hemofiltration or hemodiafiltration, or hemodialysis (see Chapter 78). Populations for whom early renal replacement therapies result in decreased mortality have not been consistently identified, but there is evidence that fluid overload is associated with mortality in critically ill children with renal dysfunction.[59] If renal dysfunction exists, all medications and therapies should be adjusted for creatinine clearance. High-output renal failure may occur in shock states without previous oliguria. The polyuria associated with this condition may falsely suggest adequate renal perfusion and adequate vascular volume at a time when the patient's intravascular volume is, in fact, depleted. Restoration of renal perfusion pressure remains the standard of care.

Coagulation

Coagulation abnormalities (eg, disseminated intravascular coagulation) probably occur to some extent in all forms of shock. Monitoring of prothrombin time, partial thromboplastin time, and platelet count and observation for abnormal bleeding are essential. Replacement therapies of absent clotting factors seem to be the most advantageous treatments. Use of vitamin K, fresh-frozen plasma, cryoprecipitate, and platelet transfusions should correct most coagulopathies. If general replacement therapy is ineffective and the patient is at risk for complications, specific factor therapy may be indicated (see "Septic Shock" later).

Hepatic

The degree of hepatic dysfunction may determine a patient's ultimate outcome in severe shock states. Maintaining adequate circulation helps maintain liver function and prevents further hepatocellular damage. Liver function tests should be performed early and followed frequently. If dysfunction exists, drugs requiring hepatic metabolism must be carefully titrated.

Gastrointestinal

Acute nonocclusive mesenteric ischemia is a devastating condition characterized by intense, prolonged splanchnic vasoconstriction; intestinal mucosal hypoxia; and acidosis. Mesenteric ischemia eventually leads to transmural necrosis of the bowel, bacterial translocation, sepsis, and multisystem organ dysfunction.[60-62] Morbidity and mortality for this condition are high because the signs and symptoms are nonspecific. Prevention of gut ischemia through adequate oxygen delivery may prevent bacterial translocation. Some clinicians advocate the use of selective gut decontamination and early enteral nutrition.[63,64] Most children with shock will tolerate postpyloric enteral feeding, although gastrointestinal feeding complications are more common than in critically ill patients without shock.[65,66] Other gastrointestinal disturbances after hypoperfusion and stress include bleeding, ileus, and bacterial translocation. Ileus may result from electrolyte abnormalities, administration of narcotic medications, or shock itself. Abdominal distension from ileus or ascites may cause respiratory compromise, especially in infants. The substantial morbidity and mortality of upper gastrointestinal bleeding due to "stress-related mucosal damage" have led to widespread prophylactic use of medications to suppress gastric acid production, but the benefit of this practice remains unproven.[67,68]

Endocrine

Multiple endocrine problems involving fluid, electrolytes, and mineral balance may arise and complicate the management of children in shock. Severe abnormalities of calcium homeostasis can occur during the course of acute hemodynamic deterioration. Patients who have been administered corticosteroids within 6 months preceding the onset of shock should be considered for stress doses of glucocorticoids. Patients in shock because of head or abdominal trauma may have disruption of the hypothalamic-anterior pituitary-adrenal axis. Adrenal hemorrhage has been demonstrated as a manifestation of severe sepsis, but more commonly patients may develop a relative or functional adrenal insufficiency. Dopamine may also inhibit secretion of prolactin, growth hormone, and thyrotropin in critically ill children.[40]

Functional Classification and Common Underlying Etiologies

Shock states can be classified into six functional categories (Box 36.2). Such tidy classification implies a degree of precision that will be misleading when approaching an individual patient. Vicious cycles play a prominent role in most shock syndromes. Any given patient, over time, may display features of any functional category or features of multiple categories. Hemodynamic profiles of these categories are summarized in Table 36.1.

Hypovolemic Shock

Hypovolemia is the most common cause of shock in infants and children. Etiologies include hemorrhage, fluid and electrolyte loss, endocrine disease, and plasma loss (Box 36.3). Acute losses of 10% to 15% of the circulatory blood volume may be well tolerated in healthy children who have intact compensatory mechanisms. An acute loss of 25% or more of the circulating blood volume, however, frequently results in hypovolemic shock that requires immediate, aggressive management.

Once the airway is assured or established, measures to restore an effective circulating blood volume should begin immediately. Placement of an adequate intravenous or intraosseous catheter and rapid volume replacement are the most important therapeutic maneuvers to reestablish the circulation. The choice of fluid depends on the nature of the loss. Hemorrhagic shock should be treated with transfusions of blood components, including emergency transfusion of uncrossmatched blood.[69,70] The hematocrit may be a poor early indicator of the severity of hemorrhage. Concomitant with colloid resuscitation of hemorrhagic shock, early surgical intervention may be indicated to control the source of bleeding.[71]

BOX 36.3 Etiologies of Hypovolemic Shock

I. Whole blood loss
   A. Absolute loss: hemorrhage
      1. External bleeding
      2. Internal bleeding
         a. Gastrointestinal
         b. Intraabdominal (spleen, liver)
         c. Major vessel injury
         d. Intracranial (in infants)
         e. Fractures
   B. Relative loss
      1. Pharmacologic (barbiturates, vasodilators)
      2. Positive pressure ventilation
      3. Spinal cord injury
      4. Sepsis
      5. Anaphylaxis
II. Plasma loss
   A. Burns
   B. Capillary leak syndromes
      1. Inflammation, sepsis
      2. Anaphylaxis
   C. Protein-losing syndromes
III. Fluid and electrolyte loss
   A. Vomiting and diarrhea
   B. Excessive diuretic use
   C. Endocrine
      1. Adrenal insufficiency
      2. Diabetes insipidus
      3. Diabetes mellitus

Isotonic crystalloid solutions, which are readily available, safe, and the least expensive, should be used in initial volume resuscitation for all other patients with hypovolemic shock. The first fluid bolus (20 mL/kg) should be administered as rapidly as possible. The amount of fluid necessary to restore effective circulating blood volume depends on the amount lost (deficit) and the rate of ongoing loss. The total amount of fluid given often exceeds the total volume lost because of expanded capacitance of the vascular space and dysfunction of cellular membranes. Ongoing fluid losses from chest tubes, biliary drains, bowel, capillary leak, or other losses of bodily fluids may dictate the use of solutions other than crystalloid.

The end point of fluid resuscitation should be normalization of arterial blood pressure, pulse pressure, peripheral perfusion, and heart rate. Uncomplicated, promptly treated hypovolemic shock usually does not lead to a significant capillary injury and leak. However, severe, prolonged hypovolemic shock, traumatic shock with extensive soft tissue injury, burn shock, or sepsis complicating hypovolemic shock may seriously impair capillary integrity. Therefore once adequate hemodynamics have been restored, fluid administration may be reduced unless there are demonstrable ongoing fluid losses. Continued assessment of hemodynamic status and vascular volume is essential to guide further therapy.

If the patient does not show improvement after several isotonic fluid boluses, more aggressive monitoring and reevaluation of the diagnosis may be required. Causes of ongoing vascular depletion should be sought, as well as other causes of refractory shock including unrecognized pneumothorax or pericardial effusion, intestinal ischemia (volvulus, intussusception, necrotizing enterocolitis), sepsis, myocardial dysfunction, adrenocortical insufficiency, and pulmonary hypertension. Arterial blood gases, hematocrit, serum electrolytes, glucose, and calcium should be reevaluated. Correction of acidosis, hypoxemia, or metabolic derangements is essential. Blood and other appropriate sites must be cultured and broad-spectrum parenteral antibiotic coverage begun if sepsis is suspected.

Cardiogenic Shock or Congestive Heart Failure

Cardiogenic shock or congestive heart failure (CHF) during infancy and childhood is a diagnostic and therapeutic challenge because of its myriad etiologies (Box 36.4). The common denominator in all forms of cardiogenic shock is depressed cardiac output. In most instances the underlying mechanism is systolic dysfunction or "pump failure." Cardiogenic shock can also be caused by diastolic dysfunction, as seen in postoperative patients, ischemic heart disease (anomalous left coronary artery from pulmonary artery [ALCAPA]), or disorders associated with ventricular hypertrophy.[72,73] Lack of myocardial relaxation increases left ventricular end-diastolic pressure resulting in pulmonary edema. Elevated left ventricular end-diastolic pressure also decreases myocardial perfusion pressure and can lead to subendocardial ischemia. Abnormalities of the heart rate and rhythm can also cause cardiogenic shock. While bradyarrhythmias cause low cardiac output due to decreased heart rate, atrioventricular dyssynchrony and tachyarrhythmias cause low cardiac output due to inadequate diastolic filling. Tachyarrhythmias also increase the myocardial oxygen consumption and compromise myocardial perfusion. Finally, myocardial dysfunction is frequently a late manifestation of shock of any etiology. It is important to

BOX 36.4   Etiologies of Cardiogenic Shock

I. Heart rate abnormalities
   A. Supraventricular tachycardia
   B. Ventricular dysrhythmias
   C. Bradycardia
II. Congenital heart defects
   A. Lesions with ductal dependent systemic blood flow in neonates (CoA, Critical AS, IAA, HLHS)
   B. Left-to-right shunt lesions
   C. Single ventricle dysfunction
   D. Systemic ventricular dysfunction (L-TGA)
   E. Ischemic cardiomyopathies (ALCAPA)
III. Cardiomyopathy, carditis
   A. Hypoxic-ischemic events
     1. Cardiac events
     2. Prolonged shock
     3. Head injury
     4. Anomalous coronary artery
     5. Excessive catecholamine state
     6. Cardiopulmonary bypass
   B. Infectious
     1. Viral
     2. Bacterial
     3. Fungal
     4. Protozoal
     5. Rickettsial
     6. Sepsis
   C. Metabolic
     1. Hypothyroid, hyperthyroid
     2. Hypoglycemia

     3. Pheochromocytoma
     4. Glycogen storage disease
     5. Mucopolysaccharidoses
     6. Carnitine deficiency
     7. Disorders of fatty acid metabolism
     8. Acidosis
     9. Hypothermia
    10. Hypocalcemia
   D. Connective tissue disorders
     1. Systemic lupus erythematosus
     2. Juvenile rheumatoid arthritis
     3. Polyarteritis nodosa
     4. Kawasaki disease
     5. Acute rheumatic fever
   E. Neuromuscular disorders
     1. Duchenne muscular dystrophy
     2. Myotonic dystrophy
     3. Limb girdle (Erb)
     4. Spinal muscular dystrophy
     5. Friedreich ataxia
     6. Multiple lentiginosis
   F. Toxic reactions
     1. Sulfonamides
     2. Penicillins
     3. Anthracyclines
   G. Other
     1. Idiopathic dilated cardiomyopathy
     2. Familial dilated cardiomyopathy

ALCAPA, anomalous origin of the left coronary artery from the pulmonary artery; *AS,* aortic stenosis; *CoA,* coarctation of the aorta; *Erb,* limb girdle musculodystrophy or scapulohumeral limb-girdle muscular dystrophy; *HLHS,* hypoplastic left heart syndrome; *IAA,* interrupted aortic arch; *L-TGA,* levo-transposition of great arteries.

understand the underlying pathophysiology of cardiogenic shock as therapy designed to improve certain conditions may also adversely affect prognosis in other conditions.[73]

Evaluation

The appropriate management of heart failure is dependent upon the specific etiology; accurate and rapid diagnosis is of prime importance. Recognition begins with a careful history and physical examination (Box 36.5) and is supplemented by noninvasive tests such as chest radiography, electrocardiography, and echocardiography. Further diagnostic workup may include laboratory investigations, cardiac catheterization, and endomyocardial biopsy.

Electrocardiography may give diagnostic hints by demonstrating chamber enlargement, ischemic changes, and arrhythmias. Two-dimensional and Doppler echocardiography has become the cornerstone for evaluation and management of children with cardiogenic shock. It is useful in diagnosing structural abnormalities and gives valuable information about the left ventricular volume, stroke volume, wall thickness, and contractility. Doppler investigation of the diastolic mitral inflow pattern is useful in assessing diastolic dysfunction.[73]

Nonspecific markers of inflammation (white blood cell count, C-reactive protein, and erythrocyte sedimentation rate) are often elevated in congestive heart failure caused by myocarditis. B-type natriuretic peptide and N-terminal pro-B-type natriuretic peptide can be elevated in myocarditis, and elevated levels may aid in distinguishing a cardiac from a noncardiac reason for respiratory symptoms in children. Confirmation of myocardial inflammation by endomyocardial biopsy may be required for a definitive diagnosis of myocarditis.[74]

BOX 36.5   Recognition of Congestive Heart Failure in Infants

History	Excessive respiratory effort
	Prolonged feeding time
	Poor weight gain
	Excessive sweating
	Frequent respiratory tract infections
Physical examination	Tachycardia
	Tachypnea
	Gallop rhythm
	Cold extremities
	Weak peripheral pulses
	Wheezing, rales
	Dyspnea, cough
	Cyanosis
	Diaphoresis
	Hepatomegaly
	Neck vein distension
	Peripheral edema
	Hypotension
Chest radiograph	Cardiomegaly
	Pulmonary venous congestion
	Hyperinflation

Therapy

Box 36.6 lists the general supportive and pharmacologic measures used in the treatment of severe CHF or cardiogenic shock. The initial therapy for cardiogenic shock is to support the heart with supplemental oxygen and mechanical ventilation. Preload should be optimized to allow the patient to take advantage of Starling mechanisms. Correction of metabolic derangements (eg, pH, glucose, calcium, magnesium) may enhance cardiac function, and pharmacologic interventions are usually

BOX 36.6 General Principles in Management of Cardiogenic Shock or Severe Congestive Heart Failure

I. Minimize myocardial oxygenation demands
   1. Intubation and mechanical ventilation
   2. Maintain normal core temperature
   3. Provide sedation
   4. Improve oxygen-carrying capacity by correcting anemia
II. Maximize myocardial performance
   1. Correct dysrhythmias
   2. Prostaglandins if suspecting ductal-dependent lesions
   3. Optimize preload: fluid boluses; if congested, appropriate salt and water restriction and appropriate use of venodilators and/or diuretics
   4. Improve contractility: provide oxygen, mechanical ventilation, correct acidosis and other metabolic abnormalities, inotropic and lusitropic drugs
   5. Reduce afterload: provide sedation and pain relief, correct hypothermia, positive pressure ventilation for LV afterload reduction, appropriate use of vasodilators
III. Mechanical circulatory support
   1. ECMO
   2. Ventricular assist devices
IV. Heart transplantation

ALCAPA, anomalous origin of the left coronary artery from the pulmonary artery; *AS,* aortic stenosis; *CoA,* coarctation of the aorta; *Erb,* limb girdle musculodystrophy or scapulohumeral limb-girdle muscular dystrophy; *HLHS,* hypoplastic left heart syndrome; *IAA,* interrupted aortic arch; *L-TGA,* levo-transposition of great arteries.

---

necessary to improve cardiac function (see Tables 36.1 and 36.2). In addition to inotropic effects, catecholamines also possess chronotropic properties and have complex effects on vascular beds of the various organs of the body. Consequently, the choice of an agent may depend as much on the state of the circulation as it does on the myocardium.

In neonates presenting in shock within the first 4 weeks of life, a lesion with ductal-dependent systemic output should be suspected and prostaglandin E_1 (PGE_1) (0.05–0.1 µg/kg/min) should be infused emergently until an echocardiogram can be obtained. This is a lifesaving intervention; opening and maintaining ductal patency is the only medical intervention that can restore adequate systemic cardiac output.

Proper use of the various vasoactive drugs often requires the presence of indwelling arterial and central venous catheters. A pulmonary artery catheter may be helpful if the patient is not responding to therapy and shock is not resolving as expected but is rarely used these days due to the potential complications. Many devices are available to measure cardiac output and other hemodynamic variables. Use of these monitoring devices allows the generation of data that will characterize the hemodynamic state, direct appropriate therapy, and allow for evaluation of the response to therapy.[75]

The digitalis glycosides may augment myocardial contractility, but because of a narrow therapeutic-to-toxic ratio, long half-life, and dependence of clearance on renal (digoxin) or hepatic function, their use in patients with cardiogenic shock should be avoided. These compounds have the advantage of improving contractility without further increasing the heart rate. They can be used once the shock is resolved.

Inamrinone, milrinone, and enoximone[76] belong to a class of nonglycoside, nonsympathomimetic inotropic agents that act via potent and selective inhibition of phosphodiesterase.

Inamrinone and milrinone are particularly useful in the treatment of cardiogenic shock because they improve diastolic function (lusitropy), increase contractility, and reduce afterload by peripheral vasodilation without a consistent increase in heart rate or myocardial oxygen consumption. Both of these drugs have relatively long half-lives, and they should be used cautiously in the presence of hypovolemia and/or hypotension. Milrinone is preferred over inamrinone because of inamrinone's tendency to cause thrombocytopenia. The use of milrinone has been shown to be effective in decreasing the risk of low cardiac output syndrome in postoperative cardiac patients.[77]

Use of vasodilators in shock generally is limited to situations in which cardiac dysfunction is associated with elevated ventricular filling pressures, elevated systemic vascular resistance, and normal or near-normal systemic arterial blood pressure. Occasionally, the combination of vasodilator and inotropic therapy results in hemodynamic improvement not attainable with either approach alone. Vasodilators improve cardiac performance and lessen clinical symptoms via arterial and venous smooth muscle relaxation. Arterial relaxation should increase ejection fraction, increase stroke volume, and decrease end-systolic left ventricular volume. Some evidence suggests some vasodilator drugs increase left ventricular compliance, which should improve diastolic function.[73] Venous relaxation should shift blood into the periphery and reduce right and left ventricular diastolic volume, with attendant beneficial effects on pulmonary and systemic capillary pressure. This ought to be reflected in decreased edema, reduced myocardial wall stress, and improved diastolic perfusion of the myocardium.

For treatment of cardiogenic shock, intravenous vasodilators with rapid onsets of action and short half-lives are preferred. Selection of a vasodilator agent should depend on its principal hemodynamic effects and the specific hemodynamic abnormalities in individual patients. Factors that increase systemic resistance, such as hypothermia, acidosis, hypoxia, pain, and anxiety, should be treated before vasodilator drugs are considered.

Afterload reduction of the failing right ventricle plays a pivotal role in some of the most frequently encountered and important cardiopulmonary disorders in children, including congenital heart disease, acute respiratory distress syndrome, bronchopulmonary dysplasia, and other chronic pulmonary disorders. The ability of the right ventricle to respond to the increased pulmonary vascular resistance seen in these situations often determines outcome. Therefore measures to decrease pulmonary vascular resistance have become more common in the treatment of many seriously ill pediatric patients. Such measures include supplemental oxygen, hyperventilation, metabolic and respiratory alkalosis, inhaled nitric oxide, prostaglandin E_1, prostacyclin, analgesia, and sedation.[78-80]

After the initial stabilization of children with cardiogenic shock, long-term management needs to be planned. Neurohumoral compensatory mechanisms that initially compensate for a fall in output of the failing heart, in time, become a major part of the problem.[75] Use of vasodilators to oppose systemic vasoconstriction and angiotensin-converting enzyme inhibitors to block the renin-angiotensin system may be necessary to break the self-perpetuating cycle caused by these neurohumoral compensatory mechanisms. Angiotensin-converting enzyme inhibitors improve ventricular function and clinical outcome in adults. However, their usefulness is not yet established in certain forms of pediatric heart failure, especially the failing single ventricle.[81]

Surgical Intervention

A number of congenital cardiac defects may present in severe CHF and cardiogenic shock. Diagnosis of these defects is critical because surgery is the definitive therapy. Prostaglandin E_1 infusion may allow for resuscitation and stabilization until surgery can be accomplished in ductal-dependent obstruction to systemic blood flow (eg, hypoplastic left heart syndrome, interrupted aortic arch, coarctation of the aorta).

Cardiac function may be supported temporarily by mechanical means, including left ventricular assist device (VAD), and ECLS. Cardiac transplantation has become an important tool for treating patients with severe myocardial dysfunction who otherwise would die of their heart disease.

Specific Etiologies

Cardiomyopathy

Patients with dilated cardiomyopathy may present in shock. The etiologies of acute dilated cardiomyopathies are listed in Box 36.7. Myocarditis is one of the more common causes of dilated cardiomyopathy in previously healthy children. Tachycardia (in the absence of fever) and tachypnea are usual presenting symptoms. In acute myocarditis, the history of illness

BOX 36.7	Organ Dysfunction Criteria
Cardiovascular	After isotonic fluid bolus ≥40 mL/kg in 1 h: Hypotension: BP <5th percentile for age *or* systolic BP <2 SD below normal age *or* Need for vasoactive drug to keep BP in normal range *or* ≥2 of the following: 1. Unexplained metabolic acidosis: base deficit >5.0 mEq/L 2. Lactic acidosis more than twice the upper limit of normal 3. Oliguria: urine output <0.5 mL/kg/h 4. Prolonged capillary refill: >5 s 5. Core to peripheral temperature gap >3°C
Respiratory	PaO_2/FiO_2 <300 in absence of cyanotic congenital heart disease or preexisting lung disease *or* $PaCO_2$ >65 torr or 20 torr over baseline *or* FiO_2 = 0.50 to keep saturations ≥92% *or* Need for invasive or noninvasive mechanical ventilation
Neurologic	GCS score ≤11 *or* Acute mental status change: decrease in GCS ≥3 points from abnormal baseline
Hematologic	Platelet count <80,000/mm³ or 50% decline in platelet count (for hematology/oncology patients) *or* INR >2
Renal	Serum creatinine ≥twice the upper limit of normal for age or twofold increase in baseline creatinine
Hepatic	Total bilirubin ≥4 mg/dL (outside neonatal period) *or* ALT twice upper limit of normal

ALT, alanine transaminase; *BP,* blood pressure; *GCS,* Glasgow Coma Scale; *INR,* international normalized ratio; *SD,* standard deviation.

is short (hours to days). Life-threatening dysrhythmias in patients with acute myocarditis include ventricular tachycardia and supraventricular tachycardia. Initial resuscitation of the patient with myocarditis is the same as for other forms of cardiogenic shock; however, patients with myocarditis and other dilated cardiomyopathies may not require much fluid resuscitation or respond as well to traditional inotropic therapy.[82,83] In addition, catecholamine infusions may promote the development of dysrhythmias.

Acute myocarditis in children with progressive heart failure may need mechanical circulatory support. Use of ECLS has been lifesaving in patients with acute myocarditis whose shock does not reverse with conventional therapy or in whom arrhythmias are unremitting. A number of studies have reported discharge rates of approximately 80% with approximately 60% of the patients experiencing myocardial recovery.[74] VADs have been used as a bridge to heart transplant. The primary VAD used for support in children is the pulsatile Berlin Heart EXCOR, which comes in various sizes, allowing support for infants as small as 3.5 kg. In the Berlin EXCOR trial, the mortality in patients on the device was 8%, and 87.5% of patients placed on the device received transplantations.[84]

On the basis of multiple case reports and case series, intravenous immunoglobulin (IVIG) has become part of routine practice for treating adults and children with acute myocarditis at many centers.[74] A recent meta-analysis showed that only children beyond the neonatal period who have viral encephalitis with myocarditis may benefit from IVIG.[85] Until more data are available, IVIG for presumed viral myocarditis should not be provided as routine practice in any situation.[74]

Hypoxic-Ischemic Injury

Shock following a generalized hypoxic-ischemic episode (eg, drowning, sudden infant death syndrome) is encountered frequently in infants and children with no preexisting cardiovascular or pulmonary disease. Data have shown that shock following hypoxic-ischemic events is cardiogenic and is characterized by a low cardiac index, elevated right and left heart filling pressures, elevated systemic and pulmonary vascular resistances, decreased oxygen consumption, and elevated oxygen extraction index.[86] However, in many patients, the mean systemic arterial blood pressure is elevated, suggesting an increase in systemic vascular resistance. Studies have documented progressive systolic and diastolic myocardial dysfunction immediately after successful cardiac resuscitation.[87] All of these observations have important therapeutic implications because the increased vascular resistance and decreased cardiac output may combine to prevent adequate tissue perfusion following anoxic injury.

Perioperative management of the transplanted heart poses a unique set of challenges in addition to the regular hypoxic-ischemic injury. The determinants of cardiac output, namely heart rate and stroke volume, are significantly affected in these situations. Due to the autonomic system denervation, heart rate is mainly dependent on circulating catecholamines. Stroke volume is affected by the diastolic dysfunction caused by the "down time." Appropriate management of the donor heart, followed by immunosuppression and judicious use of inotropic, chronotropic, and lusitropic agents in the transplanted patient have improved outcomes. The most recent data from the International Society for Heart & Lung Transplantation, including patients from 1982 through June 2011, demonstrate a median survival of 19.7 years for infants, 16.8 years for children ages 1 to 5 years, 14.5 years for children ages 6 to 10 years, and 12.4 years for children 11 to 17 years of age at the time of transplantation.[88]

Cardiac Injury in Trauma

Blunt cardiac injury can cause myocardial contusion, myocardial concussion, aneurysm, septal defects, chamber rupture, valvular rupture, and bleeding into or damage to the pericardium. Each of these entities has separate presentations, although the lesions often are concurrent. Every pediatric trauma patient deserves a careful cardiac evaluation. Of note, both left and right ventricular function may be impaired significantly in children with isolated head injury. The myocardial injury seen in children with head injury appears to be related to high levels of catecholamines with resultant myocardial ischemia.[89]

Obstructive Shock

Obstructive shock is caused by the inability to produce adequate cardiac output despite normal intravascular volume and myocardial function. Causative factors may be located within the pulmonary or systemic circulation or associated with the heart itself. Examples of obstructive shock include acute pericardial tamponade, tension pneumothorax, pulmonary or systemic hypertension, and congenital or acquired outflow obstructions. Recognition of the characteristic features of these syndromes is essential because most of the causes can be treated provided the diagnosis is made early.

Cardiac tamponade is defined as hemodynamically significant cardiac compression resulting from accumulating pericardial contents that evoke and defeat compensatory mechanisms. The pericardial space may contain effusion fluid, purulent fluid, blood, or gas. Clinical manifestations of tamponade may be insidious, especially when it occurs in conditions such as malignancy, connective tissue disorders, renal failure, or pericarditis. As cardiac output becomes restricted, the overall picture resembles CHF; however, the lungs are usually clear. Findings on physical examination that suggest cardiac tamponade include pulsus paradoxus, narrowed pulse pressure, pericardial rub, and jugular venous distension. Echocardiography is of particular value in detecting the presence of pericardial effusion and can provide clues about the presence of tamponade physiology before a patient is symptomatic. The normal effects of respiration are accentuated in cardiac tamponade. Echocardiography is useful in demonstrating the exaggerated phasic variation in cardiac volumes and flows caused by tamponade. Respiratory variation in tricuspid and pulmonary flow is more dramatic than mitral and aortic flow: With inspiration, the right ventricular early diastolic filling is augmented (>25%), while left ventricular diastolic filling diminishes (>15%). The stroke volume in the pulmonary artery increases with inspiration, while the aortic stroke volume decreases (>10%). The free walls of the right atrium and/or right ventricle collapse in diastole due to compression of these relatively low-pressure chambers by the higher-pressure pericardial effusion, and this collapse is exaggerated during expiration when right heart filling is reduced.[90]

The definitive treatment of cardiac tamponade is removal of pericardial fluid or air by surgical drainage or pericardiocentesis. Removal of even a small volume of fluid can rapidly improve blood pressure and cardiac output. Surgical drainage by either thoracotomy or a subxiphoid limited surgical approach should be considered for traumatic tamponade. Pericardiocentesis is a blind procedure; introduction of the needle should be monitored by echocardiography whenever possible. The subxiphoid approach is generally preferable (see Chapter 19).

Medical management is not a substitute for drainage but may avert a catastrophe until pericardiocentesis or surgical drainage can be safely performed. The principles of medical management include blood volume expansion to maintain venoatrial gradients and inotropic agents. In addition, any anticoagulant or thrombolytic therapy should be withheld or discontinued if pericardiocentesis is anticipated. Diuretics, which reduce blood volume, and digoxin or other agents, which slow the heart rate, are contraindicated in tamponade.

Congenital Heart Diseases With Ductal Dependent Systemic Blood Flow

Infants with critical aortic stenosis, aortic arch interruption, or juxtaductal coarctation of the aorta depend on patency of the ductus arteriosus to provide adequate lower body perfusion. Many of the signs and symptoms of coarctation with shock are indistinguishable from shock of other etiologies.[91] A high index of suspicion must be maintained for infants who present in shock in the first month of life. In severely ill infants in whom the diagnosis of coarctation, hypoplasia, or interruption of the aorta is clinically suspected, it is appropriate and often lifesaving to start a continuous prostaglandin E_1 infusion before a more complete diagnostic evaluation is performed.

Distributive Shock

Distributive shock results from maldistribution of blood flow to the tissue and can be considered to be relative hypovolemia. Abnormalities in distribution of blood flow may result in profound inadequacies in tissue oxygenation, even in the face of a normal or high cardiac output. Such maldistribution of flow generally results from widespread abnormalities in vasomotor tone. Distributive shock may be seen with anaphylaxis, spinal or epidural anesthesia, disruption of the spinal cord, or inappropriate administration of vasodilatory medication.

Treatment generally includes reversal of the underlying etiology and vigorous fluid administration. In severe cases of distributive shock that is unresponsive to fluids, vasopressor infusions may be necessary.

Septic Shock

Septic shock is often a combination of multiple problems, including infection, relative or absolute hypovolemia, maldistribution of blood flow, myocardial depression, and various metabolic, endocrine, and hematologic problems.[92] The most common presentation (80%) in children is low cardiac index with or without abnormalities of vascular tone.[93] These children have tachycardia, mental status changes, diminished peripheral pulses, mottled cold extremities, and prolonged capillary refill (>2 seconds). In many pediatric patients with septic shock, oxygen consumption is dependent on oxygen delivery.[94] This is similar to the physiologic relationship seen in pediatric patients with cardiogenic shock, suggesting that these two groups could be resuscitated with the same physiologic principles. Adults and some children (20%) present in a hyperdynamic state characterized by an elevated (or normal) cardiac output and decreased systemic vascular resistance.[93,95] These patients appear plethoric with warm extremities. They have tachycardia, bounding (or collapsing) pulses, a widened pulse pressure, high fever, mental confusion, and hyperventilation. There may be a rapid progression from high to low cardiac output state. As tissue perfusion worsens, anaerobic metabolism ensues and lactic acid accumulates. The hemodynamic profile changes over time due to evolution of the shock state and response to therapies.[93]

All patients with septic shock present with an absolute or functional hypovolemia. Increased microvascular permeability, arteriolar and venular dilation with peripheral pooling of intravascular volume, inappropriate polyuria, and poor oral intake all combine to result in reduced effective blood volume. Volume loss secondary to fever, diarrhea, vomiting, or sequestered third space fluid also contributes to hypovolemia.

Progressive deterioration in oxygen consumption and oxygen extraction portends a poor prognosis. Before the onset of cellular hypoxia,[2,96,97] changes in glycolysis and gluconeogenesis are early metabolic manifestations of sepsis.[98] Insulin responsiveness,[99] intracellular calcium stores,[100] glucose distribution,[101] and adrenergic effects[102] have all been implicated.

Therapy

An evidence-based guideline for the management of resuscitation and support of children and neonates with septic shock was issued in 2009, and the Surviving Sepsis Campaign updated guidelines in 2013.[33,103] Evidence-based algorithms for resuscitation for children (Fig. 36.1) and neonates (Fig. 36.2) are easy to use and have been shown to improve outcomes across diverse patient populations.[103] The emphasis remains on the first hour of fluid resuscitation and use of vasoactive infusions directed to age-appropriate goals of HR, BP, perfusion pressure (MAP-CVP), and capillary refill time of 2 seconds or less. Severity of shock states has been categorized according to hemodynamic responses (Table 36.3).[103] When resuscitation is delayed or inadequate, cellular hypoxia

and multiple system organ failure ensue and are the final common pathway to death.

There continues to be debate regarding the use of crystalloid or colloid solutions for volume expansion in sepsis.[104] Packed red blood cells (pRBCs) may be used if the hematocrit is less than 30% because red blood cell transfusion increases oxygen delivery to the tissues. However, expansion of oxygen-carrying capacity may not improve oxygen consumption.[105] Transfusion of pRBCs as part of a strategy to increase mixed venous oxygen saturation (SVO_2) to greater than 70% resulted in improved outcome in pediatric septic shock.[10]

Removal or control of microorganisms by surgical debridement, drainage, and antibiotic therapy is a crucial component of treatment of septic shock. Whenever possible, blood, urine, and samples from other potential infected sites should be sent for culture and susceptibility testing before broad-spectrum antibiotic therapy is initiated, but obtaining these cultures should never delay appropriate empiric antimicrobial therapy. Choice of antibiotic therapy is determined by the clinical scenario, likely organisms, and local antibiotic sensitivities.

Intubation and mechanical ventilation are also important in the resuscitation from pediatric septic shock for reasons already mentioned in this chapter. Although it has a favorable hemodynamic profile, induction with etomidate should be avoided because of its adverse effects on the adrenocortical function.[106-108]

Septic patients develop protein/caloric malnutrition as a principal manifestation of their metabolic response to sepsis.[104] In patients who were previously malnourished or remained hypermetabolic, this rapidly developing malnutrition is believed to contribute to morbidity and mortality. However, the abnormalities in intermediary metabolism make the provision of an adequate level of metabolic support challenging. Parenteral or enteral nutrition should begin as soon as cardiovascular stability is achieved. Many clinicians advocate the early use of enteral feedings to prevent gut mucosal atrophy and bacterial translocation.[65,66,109]

Experimental/Unproved Therapies

ECLS has been used to support myocardial and/or pulmonary function during sepsis. We queried the ELSO registry (1976 through January 2010) for ECMO use in all (neonatal, pediatric, and adult) patients with sepsis or septic shock. A total of 2960 patients were identified: 2409 neonates (81%) and 551 patients older than 1 month (19%). Overall survival was 67%, but there was a significant difference in the survival of neonates versus other patients. Survival in the neonatal group was 74% versus 40% in all other patients.

Continuous renal replacement therapy (CRRT) can improve survival in critically ill (including septic) children with MODS and fluid overload.[59,110,111] Therapeutic plasma exchange has shown benefit for critically ill (some septic) children with MODS.[112-115] Exchange transfusion and plasmapheresis have potential as therapeutic interventions.[116-119] Multicenter, randomized controlled studies showing efficacy for these therapies are lacking.

The presence of adrenal insufficiency in septic shock and critical illness has been widely studied. Knowledge of the effects of inflammatory mediators on the hypothalamic-pituitary-adrenal axis has led to the concept of "functional" or "transient" adrenal insufficiency.[120-122] The effect of critical illness on adrenal function is probably more complex and

TABLE 36.3	ACCM Hemodynamic Definitions of Shock
Cold or warm shock	Hypoperfusion manifested by: ↓ Mental status or capillary refill >2 s (cold shock) or flash capillary refill (warm shock) or ↓ (cold shock) or ↑ (warm shock) peripheral pulses or mottled cool extremities (cold shock) or ↓ urine output <1 mL/kg/h
Fluid-refractory, dopamine-resistant shock	Persistent shock after: ≥60 mL/kg fluid resuscitation (when appropriate) and dopamine to 10 μg/kg/min
Catecholamine-resistant shock	Persistent shock after use of direct-acting catecholamines: epinephrine and norepinephrine
Refractory shock	Persistent shock despite goal-directed use of inotropes, vasopressors, vasodilators, and maintenance of metabolic (glucose, calcium) and hormonal (thyroid, hydrocortisone, insulin) homeostasis

From Brierly J, Carcillo JA, Choong K, et al. International pediatric sepsis consensus conference: definitions for sepsis and organ dysfunction in pediatrics. Crit Care Med. 2009;37:666-688.

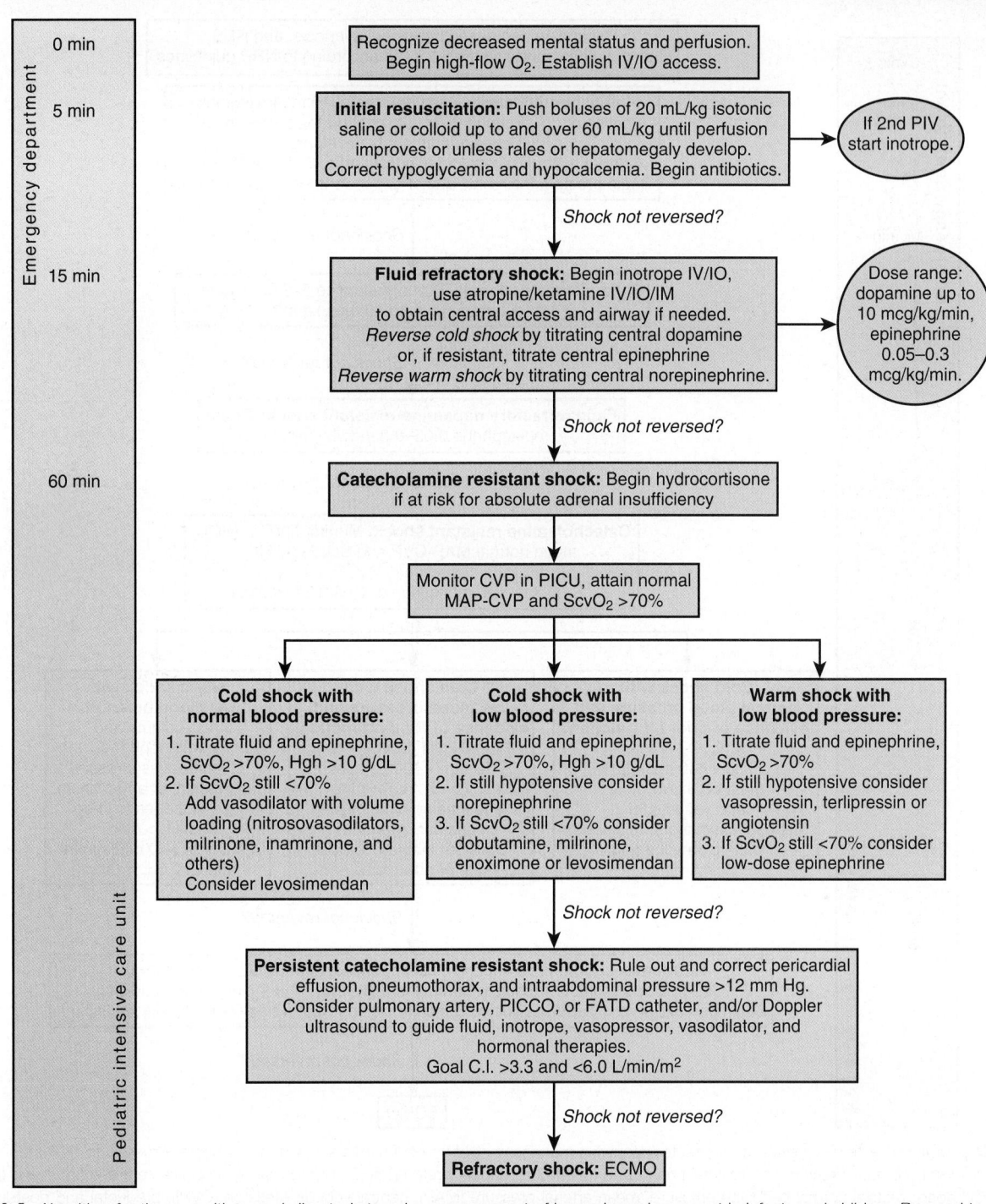

Fig. 36.1. Algorithm for time-sensitive, goal-directed stepwise management of hemodynamic support in infants and children. Proceed to next step if shock persists. (1) First-hour goals: restore and maintain heart rate thresholds, capillary refill ≤2 sec, and normal blood pressure in the first hour/ emergency department. Support oxygenation and ventilation as appropriate. (2) Subsequent ICU goals: if shock is not reversed, intervene to restore and maintain normal perfusion pressure (mean arterial pressure [MAP], central venous pressure [CVP]) for age, central venous O_2 saturation >70%, and CI >3.3, <6.0 L/min/m² in pediatric intensive care unit (PICU). *CI,* cardiac index; *CRRT,* continuous renal replacement therapy; *ECMO,* extracorporeal membrane oxygenation; *FATD,* femoral arterial thermodilution; *Hgb,* hemoglobin; *IO,* intraosseus; *IM,* intramuscular; *IV,* intravenous; *PICCO,* pulse contour cardiac output. (Modified from Brierley J, Carcillo JA, Choong K, et al. International pediatric sepsis consensus conference: definitions for sepsis and organ dysfunction in pediatrics. Crit Care Med. 2009;37:666-688.)

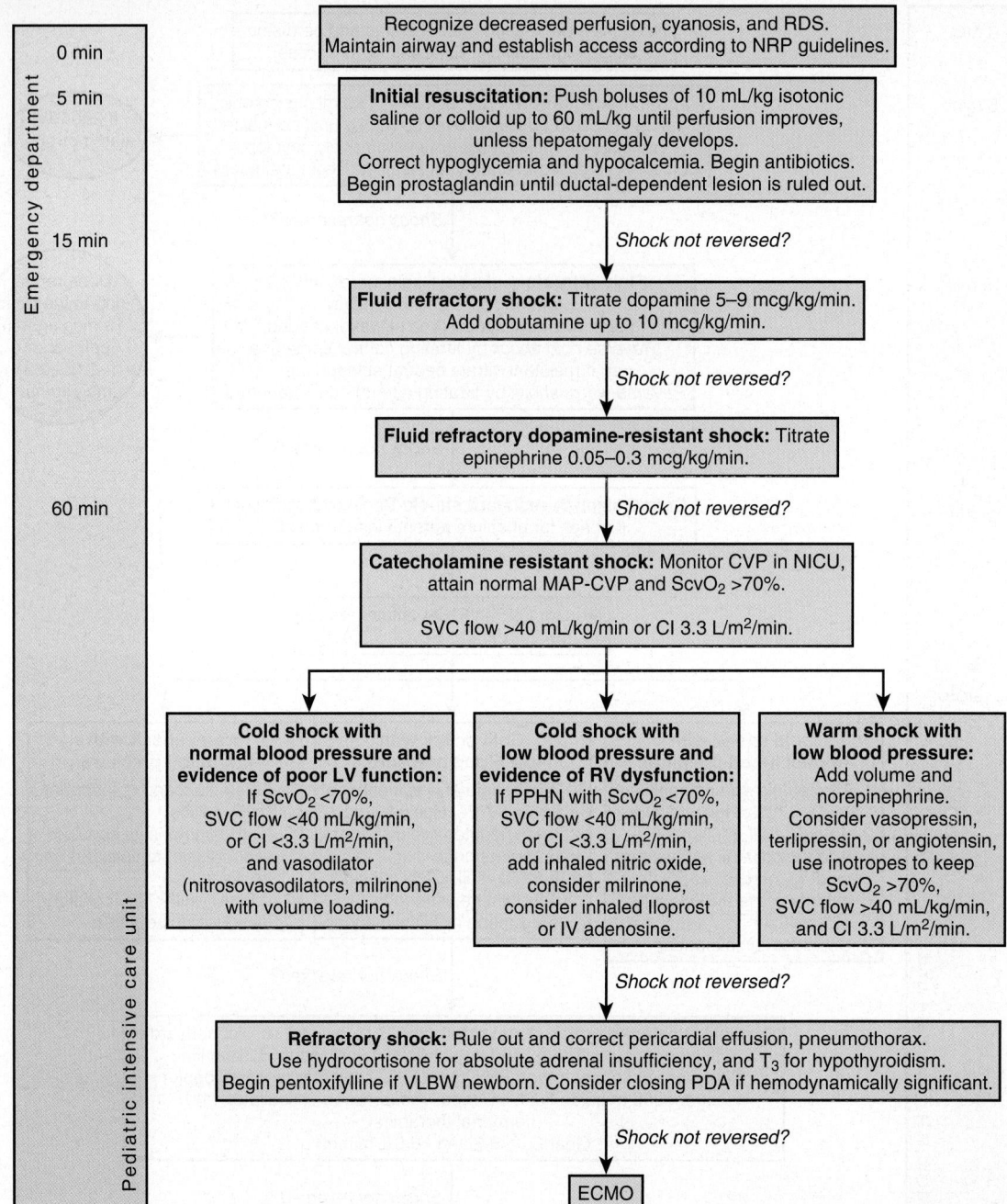

Fig. 36.2. Algorithm for time-sensitive, goal-directed stepwise management of hemodynamic support in newborns. Proceed to next step if shock persists. (1) First-hour goals: restore and maintain heart rate thresholds, capillary refill ≤2 sec, and normal blood pressure in the first hour. (2) Subsequent ICU goals: restore normal perfusion pressure (mean arterial pressure [MAP], central venous pressure [CVP]), preductal and postductal O_2 saturation difference <5%, and either central venous O_2 saturation (ScvO_2) >70%, superior vena cava (SVC) flow >40 mL/kg/min, or cardiac index (CI) >3.3 L/min/m² in the neonatal intensive care unit (NICU). *ECMO,* extracorporeal membrane oxygenation; *LV,* left ventricular; *NRP,* Neonatal Resuscitation Program; *PDA,* patent ductus arteriosus; *RDS,* respiratory distress syndrome; *RV,* right ventricular; *VLBW,* very-low-birthweight. (Modified from Brierley J, Carcillo JA, Choong K, et al. International pediatric sepsis consensus conference: definitions for sepsis and organ dysfunction in pediatrics. Crit Care Med. 2009;37:666-688.)

involves decreased glucocorticoid receptor protein expression and decreased clearance of cortisol.[123-125]

Adult studies have shown improved hemodynamics and antiinflammatory benefits of continuous low-dose hydrocortisone infusion in adult septic shock and survival benefit associated with increased vasopressor requirement and longer duration of shock.[126-128] Steroids should be given to patients with known adrenal insufficiency or who are at risk for adrenal insufficiency (chronic or recent steroid use; purpura fulminans; etomidate or ketoconazole administration; and hypothalamic, pituitary, or adrenal disease).[103,129] The safety and efficacy of stress-dose steroids administered to pediatric patients with "transient" adrenal insufficiency are unproven and pose potential risks to patients. Pediatric studies have not shown a consistent difference in mortality rates when steroids were used.[129,130]

Many pharmacologic agents and therapies have been evaluated as adjunctive treatments in sepsis and septic shock. Recombinant activated protein C was initially promising in adults with severe sepsis. Although the subsequent series of randomized controlled trials suggest it is not beneficial for pediatric or adult septic patients, a novel meta-analysis suggests there may be benefit.[131,132] Use of plasmapheresis, plasma exchange, and plasma filtration as therapy for treating sepsis-induced multiple organ system failure and improving outcome remains experimental.[133] Other therapies with potential therapeutic usefulness include inhibitors of arachidonic acid metabolism and inhibitors of thromboxane and leukotriene formation, white blood cell transfusions, passive immunotherapy, toxic oxygen scavengers, inhibitors of myocardial depressant factors, and fibronectin administration.[95,134] Therapies targeted at modulating inflammation, such as the administration of antagonists or antibodies to various cytokines (eg, tumor necrosis factor, IL-1), showed promise in early studies but subsequently showed no benefit.[134-138] Therapies designed to modulate the immune response,[139,140] inhibit neutrophil function, or inhibit synthesis of nitric oxide (endothelial-derived relaxing factor) have demonstrated no clinical benefit in septic shock.[137] Other areas being explored with regard to the pathophysiology and treatment of septic shock include factors that inhibit apoptosis and use of insulin to maintain tight glucose control and normoglycemia.[135,139,141] These therapies have shown some promise but remain unproven.

Summary

Shock is a life-threatening condition that has a myriad of causes. In order to survive shock, recognition and resuscitative efforts must be achieved early, the etiology elucidated, and ongoing monitoring and therapy instituted. The astute clinician who recognizes shock, institutes therapy, and continuously assesses response to therapy offers the child the best chance for a quality survival.

Key References

2. Fink MP. Bench-to-bedside review: cytopathic hypoxia. *Crit Care.* 2002;6: 491-499.
3. Wacharasint P, Nakada T-A, Boyd JH, et al. Normal-range blood lactate concentration in septic shock is prognostic and predictive. *Shock.* 2012; 38:4-10.
5. Scott HF, Donoghue AJ, Gaieski DF, et al. The utility of early lactate testing in undifferentiated pediatric systemic inflammatory response syndrome. *Acad Emerg Med.* 2012;19:1276-1280.
7. Kim YA, Ha E-J, Jhang WK, Park SJ. Early blood lactate area as a prognostic marker in pediatric septic shock. *Intensive Care Med.* 2013;39: 1818-1823.
10. de Oliveira CF, de Oliveira DSF, Gottschald AFC, et al. ACCM/PALS haemodynamic support guidelines for paediatric septic shock: an outcomes comparison with and without monitoring central venous oxygen saturation. *Intensive Care Med.* 2008;34:1065-1075.
11. Donati A, Tibboel D, Ince C. Towards integrative physiological monitoring of the critically ill: from cardiovascular to microcirculatory and cellular function monitoring at the bedside. *Crit Care.* 2013;17(suppl 1):S5.
29. Hernandez G, Peña H, Cornejo R, et al. Impact of emergency intubation on central venous oxygen saturation in critically ill patients: a multicenter observational study. *Crit Care.* 2009;13:R63.
32. Carcillo JA. Role of early fluid resuscitation in pediatric septic shock. *JAMA.* 1991;266:1242-1245.
33. Dellinger RP, Levy MM, Rhodes A, et al. Surviving sepsis campaign: international guidelines for management of severe sepsis and septic shock: 2012. *Crit Care Med.* 2013;41:580-637.
34. Rivers E, Nguyen B, Havstad S, et al. Early goal-directed therapy in the treatment of severe sepsis and septic shock. *NEJM.* 2001;345:1368-1377.
38. Acheampong A, Vincent J-L. A positive fluid balance is an independent prognostic factor in patients with sepsis. *Crit Care.* 2015;19:251.
39. Arikan AA, Zappitelli M, Goldstein SL, et al. Fluid overload is associated with impaired oxygenation and morbidity in critically ill children. *Pediatr Crit Care Med.* 2012;13:253-258.
40. Besen BAMP, Gobatto ALN, Melro LMG, et al. Fluid and electrolyte overload in critically ill patients: an overview. *World J Crit Care Med.* 2015;4: 116-129.
41. Flori HR, Church G, Liu KD, et al. Positive fluid balance is associated with higher mortality and prolonged mechanical ventilation in pediatric patients with acute lung injury. *Crit Care Res Pract.* 2011;2011:1-5.
43. Weber T, Wagner T, Neumann K, Deusch E. Low predictability of three different noninvasive methods to determine fluid responsiveness in critically ill children. *Pediatr Crit Care Med.* 2015;16:e89-e94.
49. Havel C, Arrich J, Losert H, et al. Vasopressors for hypotensive shock. *Cochrane Database Syst Rev.* 2011;CD003709.
51. Graciano AL, Balko JA, Rahn DS, et al. The Pediatric Multiple Organ Dysfunction Score (P-MODS): development and validation of an objective scale to measure the severity of multiple organ dysfunction in critically ill children. *Crit Care Med.* 2005;33:1484-1491.
52. Leclerc F, Leteurtre S, Duhamel A, et al. Cumulative influence of organ dysfunctions and septic state on mortality of critically ill children. *Am J Respir Crit Care Med.* 2005;171:348-353.
59. Sutherland SM, Zappitelli M, Alexander SR, et al. Fluid overload and mortality in children receiving continuous renal replacement therapy: the Prospective Pediatric Continuous Renal Replacement Therapy Registry. *Am J Kidney Dis.* 2010;55:316-325.
65. López-Herce J, Mencía S, Sánchez C, et al. Postpyloric enteral nutrition in the critically ill child with shock: a prospective observational study. *Nutr J.* 2008;7:6.
66. López-Herce J, Santiago MJ, Sánchez C, et al. Risk factors for gastrointestinal complications in critically ill children with transpyloric enteral nutrition. *Eur J Clin Nutr.* 2007;62:395-400.
68. Marik PE, Vasu T, Hirani A, Pachinburavan M. Stress ulcer prophylaxis in the new millennium: a systematic review and meta-analysis. *Crit Care Med.* 2010;38:2222-2228.
69. Spinella PC, Holcomb JB. Resuscitation and transfusion principles for traumatic hemorrhagic shock. *Blood Rev.* 2009;1-10.
71. Beekley AC. Damage control resuscitation: a sensible approach to the exsanguinating surgical patient. *Crit Care Med.* 2008;36:S267-S274.
73. Gaasch WH. Diagnosis and treatment of heart failure based on left ventricular systolic or diastolic dysfunction. *JAMA.* 1994;271:1276-1280.
74. Canter CE, Simpson KP. Diagnosis and treatment of myocarditis in children in the current era. *Circulation.* 2014;129:115-128.
75. Benedict CR. Neurohumoral aspects of heart failure. *Cardiol Clin.* 1994; 12:9-23.

Pediatric Cardiopulmonary Bypass

Richard M. Ginther, Jr., and Joseph M. Forbess

PEARLS

- Cardiopulmonary bypass (CPB), which originated in the mid-twentieth century, was designed to allow for the repair of congenital heart defects. Its history has since been characterized by perpetual technological advancements that have been instrumental in sustaining the momentum of clinical progress of this field.
- Because of the morbidity associated with the "time on-pump," many early surgeries were performed at profoundly hypothermic temperatures by utilizing circulatory arrest.
- The current philosophy underpinning the use of pediatric CPB is to meet the metabolic demands of the patient throughout the repair while minimizing the impact of associated nonphysiologic effects.
- All aspects of CPB have experienced major technological improvements. Circuits are miniaturized and cause less blood trauma, blood component therapy is highly directed, and on-pump patient monitoring techniques have advanced.
- The progress of pediatric CPB has played a major role in the steady reduction of morbidity and mortality associated with cardiac surgery in children. Pediatric mortality rates are now comparable to those in adult patients.

Background

History

Surgery for congenital heart disease has evolved into a relatively safe intervention considering its brief history and countless hurdles. This historical journey is of course filled with triumphs and tragic failures and tells a story of progressive intuition and challenges steadily surmounted. This has culminated in the generally successful model that is used today (Table 37.1). The early years of cardiac surgery spawned many novel techniques for operations that did not rely on cardiopulmonary bypass as used today. Surgeons initiated their efforts in cardiovascular surgery with attempts to repair extracardiac vascular anomalies such as patent ductus arteriosus and coarctation of the aorta. On August 26, 1938, at the Boston Children's Hospital, Dr. Robert Gross performed the world's first successful patent ductus arteriosus closure on a 7-year-old girl.[1] Soon, exposing the heart and attempting to correct life-threatening cardiac defects became a reality. In the early 1950s, surgeons began to explore several different approaches to repairing intracardiac defects. One technique, popularized by Dr. F. John Lewis, used total body hypothermia and vena cava inflow occlusion to achieve direct visualization of atrial septal defects.[2] Although this technique proved to be a fairly safe technique for simple atrial septal defects, failure was often the result when more complex defects were attempted.[3,4] Surgeons needed a way to safely perfuse the patient's circulatory system and extend the "safe" surgical time. In the late 1930s, Dr. John Gibbon and his wife Mary, a nurse and research assistant, began developing a heart-lung machine to do just this. By the early 1950s, Dr. Gibbon, in an interesting collaboration with International Business Machines Corporation (IBM), reported promising success in the laboratory using a heart-lung machine on cats and dogs.[5-7] After a previous fatal attempt to repair an atrial septal defect (ASD) in a 15-month-old child in February 1952, Dr. Gibbon successfully closed an ASD in an 18-year-old patient using his heart-lung machine on May 6, 1953.[8] Unfortunately, Dr. Gibbon was not able to repeat the same success with the heart-lung machine on subsequent cases, and his next four patients died. Other surgical teams devised their own versions of cardiopulmonary bypass but were unable to replicate laboratory successes, and no other human survivors were reported. It was theorized that perhaps these hearts were too sick to be repaired and that it was unrealistic to expect that these hearts could recover. Cardiopulmonary bypass became a widespread disappointment, and most investigators abandoned the technique. While others were reporting their attempts using the heart-lung machine, however,[9-12] Dr. C. Walton Lillehei and his colleagues at the University of Minnesota introduced a new approach for supporting patients during surgery: controlled cross circulation. During cross circulation, the patient's parent was used as the "heart-lung machine" and supported the patient during the operation (Fig. 37.1). Considering the potential for a 200% operative mortality, this was a highly controversial technique. However, using this method, Dr. Lillehei was able to effectively close an ASD on March 26, 1954.[13] Dr. Lillehei and his colleagues[14] continued a remarkable series of successes using cross circulation by performing 45 operations for anomalies including ventricular septal defect, atrioventricular canal, and tetralogy of Fallot, with an operative mortality of only 38%. This progress with more complex lesions prompted investigators to rethink their options for supporting, repairing, and recovering these patients. Two surgical camps ignited the resurgence of the artificial heart-lung machine: Dr. Lillehei and his colleagues at the University of Minnesota and Dr. John Kirklin and his colleagues at the nearby Mayo Clinic. Dr. Kirklin and colleagues[15] reported a 50% mortality among eight patients using a modification of the Gibbon-IBM pump oxygenator in the spring of

TABLE 37.1   Successful Congenital Cardiac Surgery Milestones

Year	Event	Surgeon
1938	Patent ductus arteriosus ligation	Gross
1944	Coarctation repair	Crafoord
1944	Blalock-Taussig shunt	Blalock, Taussig
1946	Potts shunt	Potts
1947	Closed pulmonary valvotomy	Sellors
1948	Atrial septectomy	Blalock, Hanlon
1951	Pulmonary artery band	Muller, Dammann
1952	Atrial septal defect closure using atrial well	Gross
1952	Atrial septal defect closure using hypothermia	Lewis
1953	Atrial septal defect closure using cardiopulmonary bypass	Gibbon
1954	Ventricular septal defect closure using cross circulation	Lillehei
1958	Superior cavopulmonary shunt (Glenn shunt)	Glenn
1958	Senning operation for transposition of great arteries	Senning
1963	Mustard operation for transposition of great arteries	Mustard
1968	Fontan procedure for tricuspid atresia	Fontan
1975	Arterial switch for transposition of great arteries	Jantene
1981	Norwood procedure for hypoplastic left heart syndrome	Norwood
1985	Neonatal heart transplantation	Bailey

1955. Months later, Lillehei and colleagues[16] reported a 29% mortality among seven patients using their own heart-lung machine and the groundbreaking DeWall Bubble Oxygenator. These two groups demonstrated that surgical repair of complex congenital defects could be performed in a more controlled environment than cross circulation or inflow occlusion, with promising results. What followed were many groups initiating open-heart programs primarily addressing congenital heart disease. Despite significant improvements in survival rates, congenital cardiac repairs remained a daunting undertaking with significant risk. Bypass circuits were enormous when compared with the patient blood volume, the systemic response was an extreme shock, and the understanding of the physiologic response to this "nonphysiologic" extracorporeal circulation was quite limited. Investigators sought to use cardiopulmonary bypass but limit the actual cumulative time that nonphysiologic blood flow is provided to the patient—with its attendant risk. The bypass circuit could be used to cool the patient down to profound hypothermia, after a lengthy period of topical cooling. The circulation of the patient could then be safely terminated for lengthy periods of time, allowing for complex cardiac repairs. At the conclusion of the repair, the heart-lung machine could be used to fully warm the patient. These hypothermic circulatory arrest techniques with limited periods of extracorporeal circulation were popularized in the early 1970s by Dr. Barratt-Boyes and proved to dramatically extend the "safe" period of support.[17] Surgeons began to perform increasingly complex congenital heart repairs. Pediatric cardiac surgical care was further refined over the subsequent several decades. The development of smaller, more efficient, and customizable heart-lung machine hardware and components, as well as improvements in myocardial protection, have allowed surgical teams to move away from the concept of limited cardiopulmonary bypass and toward a more "full-flow" philosophy wherein the metabolic demands of the body are continuously met while the patient is on the heart-lung machine. This chapter explores the concepts that form the basis of this philosophy and the techniques that surgical teams currently use to support pediatric patients during cardiovascular surgery.

Surgical Team

The surgical team consists of highly trained specialists, each of whom plays a vital role in the safety and success of the surgical procedure. This specialized team is led by the cardiac surgeon and typically includes an assistant surgeon or physician assistant, an anesthesiologist, a perfusionist, as well as several nurses, surgical scrub technologists, anesthesia assistants, and perioperative surgical assistants.

A perfusionist is a health care professional who specializes in all aspects of extracorporeal circulation. The primary focus of a perfusionist is to support the cardiac surgical patient during cardiopulmonary bypass. Because of this, the perfusionist's clinical expertise is a critical component of operative success. Perhaps the first perfusionist was Mary Gibbon, Dr. Gibbon's wife. In addition to helping design the Gibbon-IBM heart-lung machine, she assembled and operated it as well. The term *perfusionist* did not emerge until the early 1970s, and in the early days of cardiac surgery, surgical groups would typically use any locally available combination of physiologists, biochemists, cardiologists, or surgical residents to help operate the heart-lung machine. Now, cardiovascular perfusionists are highly trained, nationally certified (CCP; Certified Clinical Perfusionist), state-licensed allied health professionals. The common scope of practice for a perfusionist consists of cardiopulmonary bypass (CPB), extracorporeal membrane oxygenation (ECMO), isolated limb/organ chemoperfusion, ventricular assist device (VAD), autotransfusion, and intra-aortic balloon counterpulsation.

Equipment and Preparation for Cardiopulmonary Bypass
Heart-Lung Machine Console and Pumps

The cardiopulmonary bypass (CPB) machine, commonly referred to as the heart-lung machine, is the mechanical hardware that a perfusionist uses to support the patient during surgery. Until the late 1950s, the CPB hardware and circuitry were typically handmade, and many of the components had to be hand washed and sterilized for reuse. The hardware components were designed at that time with two objectives: to pump blood through the patient's cardiovascular system and to successfully perform respiratory gas exchange, hence the term "heart-lung machine." Unfortunately, this heart-lung

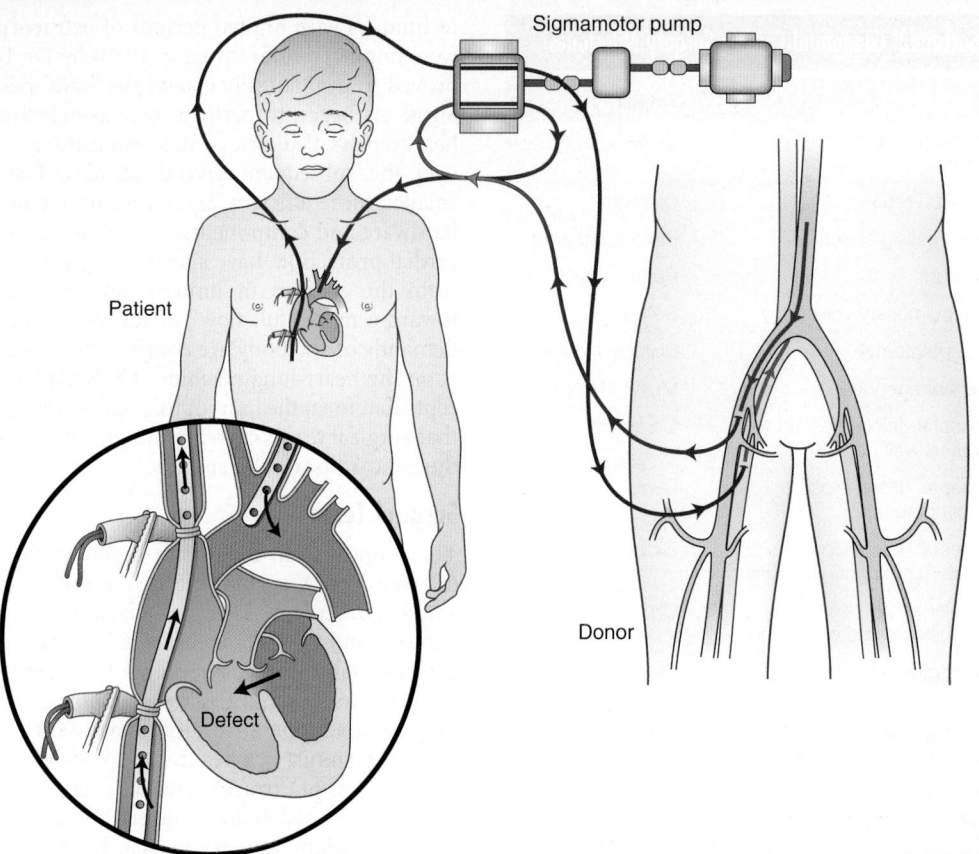

Fig. 37.1. Controlled cross circulation. (From Stoney WS. Evolution of cardiopulmonary bypass. Circulation. 2009;119:2844-2853.)

apparatus was large, difficult to move, had no safety features, and was not available to other institutions eager to operate. Surgeons interested in these handcrafted devices would often visit the surgical groups at the University of Minnesota and Mayo Clinic, but few could replicate their expensive and intricate systems. Eventually, industry developers began to commercially release heart-lung machines with hardware components consolidated onto a wheel-mounted console. Interestingly, although cardiac surgery began with the pediatric patient population, heart-lung machines were developed as "one-size-fits-all" units and were not customizable for smaller patients.

Modern heart-lung machine consoles are mobile, offer many pump configuration options, and are loaded with safety features. These design improvements allow for better configuration options for the pediatric surgical population. An ideal heart-lung machine for pediatric CPB is customizable for circuit miniaturization and offers safety devices and hardware that accommodate both smaller tubing sizes and circuitry. Customizations such as mast mounting pumps in various configurations and incorporating mini–roller pumps with shorter raceway lengths are two popular heart-lung machine configurations.[18,19]

Several different types of mechanical pumps have been used to substitute the function of the heart, and interestingly, the roller pump has remained a standard pump mechanism since the beginning of cardiopulmonary bypass. A roller pump functions by positive fluid displacement. Tubing is placed in a curved raceway, and as occlusive rollers rotate over the compressible tubing, blood is pushed forward

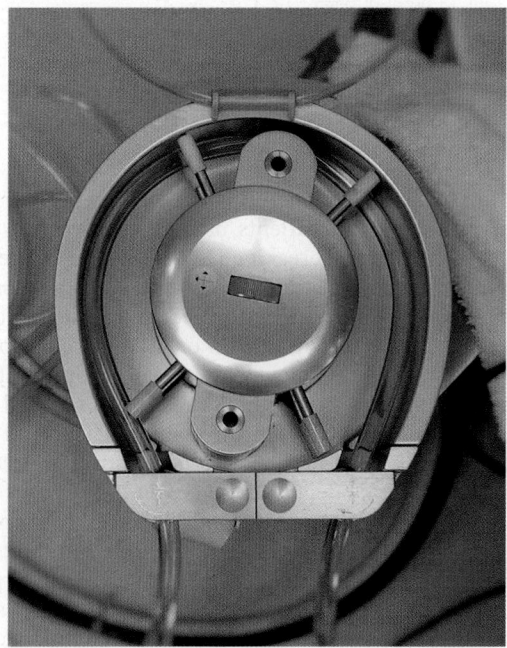

Fig. 37.2. Roller pump with ¼-inch tubing placed in the raceway.

creating a continuous nonpulsatile flow. The flow output is controlled by changing the revolution per minute (RPM) of the pump. Roller pumps are the most commonly used arterial (heart) pump in pediatrics (Fig. 37.2).[20] While roller pumps are used as the arterial pump, the heart-lung machine console also holds several other roller pumps used for cardiotomy field suction, venting the heart, and cardioplegia delivery.

The centrifugal pump is another type of arterial pump that has gained significant popularity since the mid-1970s. A centrifugal pump uses an impeller cone and rotational kinetic energy to propel the blood, and because it is nonocclusive, it is thought to be safer and cause less hemolysis than roller pumps. Centrifugal blood flow is controlled by the impeller cone RPMs and is also dependent on preload and sensitive to resistance distal to the pump. Because the pump is not occlusive, any resistance or occlusion will result in a reduction or cessation of flow. These pumps require the use of a flow probe to measure actual flow, and the nonocclusive property is considered a safety feature in the event of cannula obstruction or accidental arterial line occlusion. The use of centrifugal pumps during ECMO has become increasingly popular due to the suggested hemolytic and safety benefits; however, these benefits have often been refuted.[21-24] Roller pumps remain the main arterial pump type in pediatric CPB because they are simple, inexpensive, and, importantly, require a much smaller prime volume than centrifugal pumps.

Cardiopulmonary Bypass Circuit

The handmade circuits used on children in the mid-1950s were elaborate, and the large blood volume required to prime them was a burden on the blood bank. Perfusionists would have to spend the evening of surgery assembling the circuit and then tackle the tedious task of dismantling, rewashing, and sterilizing the same circuitry after surgery. Fortunately, manufacturers now offer a wide variety of disposable circuit components that are fairly simple to assemble. The modern CPB circuit is a series of components consisting of cannulas, tubing, venous reservoir, filters, oxygenator, heat exchanger, hemoconcentrator, suction, and cardioplegia delivery system.

Deoxygenated blood from the superior vena cava (SVC) and inferior vena cava (IVC) travels down a venous line, usually pulled by simple gravitational siphon effect, and into a venous reservoir. The deoxygenated blood in the reservoir is pumped through the oxygenator and then back to the patient's aorta (or other major artery) via the arterial line (Fig. 37.3). This blood pathway diverts blood away from the heart and lungs, creating a bloodless operative field. In the adult patient population, where the circuit prime volume is typically no

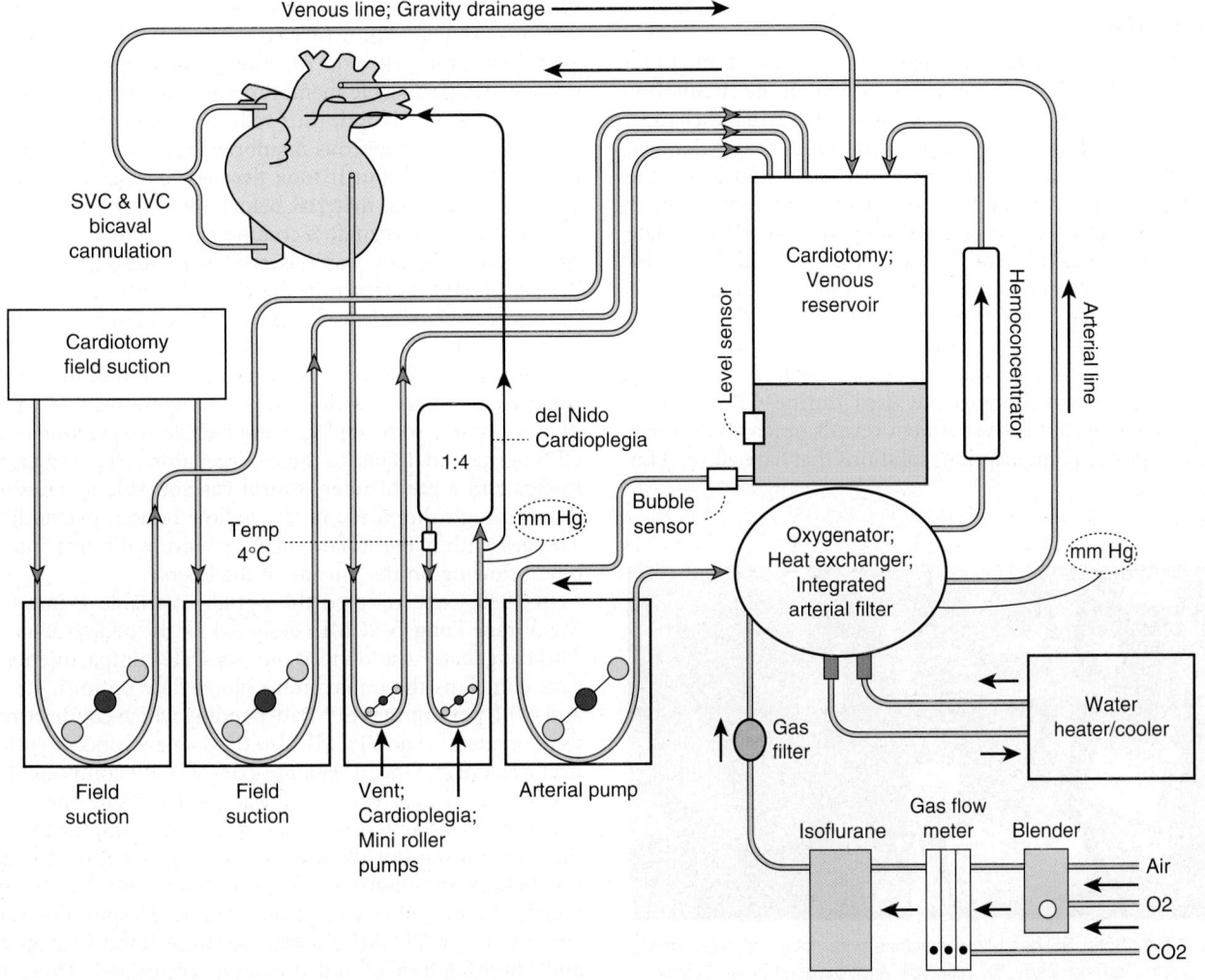

Fig. 37.3. Schematic of the cardiopulmonary bypass circuit at Children's Health Dallas.

greater than 25% of the patient's blood volume, a single circuit size can be used for almost all patient sizes. The small circuit prime-to-patient blood volume ratio helps to minimize patient hemodilution during CPB and ultimately reduces the likelihood of donor blood exposure. The same adult circuit, with a prime volume of about 1 L, would be approximately 500% of the circulating blood volume in a neonate. This discrepancy would seem outrageous considering current circuit options, but the prime-to-blood volume ratio was even higher before manufacturers began to release pediatric oxygenators in the mid-1980s. Since the oxygenator is one of the largest volume components of the CPB circuit, any significant reduction in size would result in large prime volume reductions. A circuit miniaturization movement began, and the new clinical challenge in pediatric CPB was to reduce both circuit prime volume and surface area. The goal of circuit prime and surface area reduction is to minimize hemodilution and the deleterious effects of foreign surface blood contact activation. Strategies such as using smaller diameter and shorter tubing lengths and incorporating neonatal and pediatric CPB components have allowed clinicians to reach this goal. At Children's Health Dallas, the perfusionists have made many circuit modifications to achieve a static prime volume of approximately 165 mL in our neonatal circuit. This prime volume lowers the circuit size to approximately 45% of the blood volume of a 3-kg patient (Fig. 37.4).

Oxygenators

An oxygenator, the artificial lung of the CPB circuit, might be considered the most important component of the circuit. It is responsible for oxygen and carbon dioxide (CO_2) gas exchange, as well as volatile anesthetic administration. A heat exchanger, used for cooling and warming the perfusate, and hence the patient, is housed inside the oxygenator, and certain newer models now integrate the arterial filter, to reduce particulate matter, into the oxygenator. A venous reservoir, which includes both venous line and cardiotomy suction filters and various ports for drug and fluid administration, is typically packaged with an oxygenator. Currently, hollow fiber membrane oxygenators, which fully separate the blood flow from gas flow by a thin polymer membrane, are used during CPB. A brief history of oxygenator development reveals much about some of the important "engineering" solutions that have allowed for

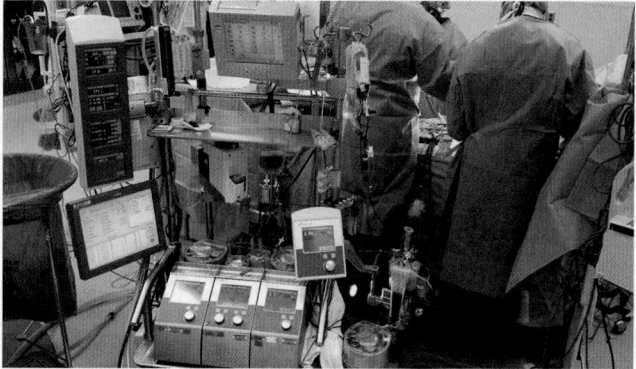

Fig. 37.4. Sorin S5 heart-lung machine with mast mounted arterial pump and Terumo Baby FX reservoir and oxygenator at Children's Health Dallas.

cardiac surgery to be performed more safely, in progressively smaller patients.

The first oxygenators used in the early days of cardiac surgery were hardware units that either used rotating discs or large mesh screens. These oxygenators worked by creating a large surface area film of blood, either over rotating discs in a pool of venous blood or trickling over large mesh screens, and exposing the film of blood to an oxygenated atmosphere.[25,26] Though these units were successful at oxygenating blood, they required extremely large priming volumes; were not disposable; were difficult to assemble, operate, and clean; and lost significant efficiency during hemodilution. In addition to these disadvantages, these oxygenators were not commercially available to clinicians looking to operate beyond the University of Minnesota and Mayo Clinic.

The University of Minnesota team dramatically changed this landscape in the late 1950s by releasing the simple, disposable, inexpensive, and commercially available DeWall-Lillehei bubble oxygenator.[27] Though the safety of actively adding bubbles to the blood was debated, the commercial availability of this device contributed to a rapid global expansion of cardiac surgery. The bubble oxygenator was a distinct improvement over the previous unwieldy direct blood contact oxygenators, yet it was still limited in that the direct blood air interface could produce significant blood trauma. This trauma accrues over time, so the safety margin for longer pump runs was diminished for longer, complex cases.

The next generation of oxygenators, membrane oxygenators, better mimicked the function of the lungs. These microporous, gas-permeable membranes eliminated direct contact between gas and blood, thus reducing blood trauma.[26] The concept of a microporous membrane separating the gas and blood was sound, but it took decades of research to find a suitable membrane material before these oxygenators could replace bubble oxygenators commercially. Initial success with silicone membranes was observed with long-term support during ECMO; however, in the operating room these membranes proved to be less efficient, prone to plasma leakage and thrombus formation.[26,28] The development and release of polypropylene microporous membranes allowed for efficient gas exchange over a wide range of temperatures and pump flow rates and soon replaced the bubble oxygenator during CPB in the mid-1980s. In these oxygenators, CO_2 and O_2 flow meters and a gas blender control gas and volatile anesthetic flow through the inside of the hollow polypropylene fibers. The gas within the hollow fibers passively diffuses into the blood flowing on the outside of the fibers.

In 1985 Cobe released the popular Variable Prime Cobe Membrane Lung (VPCML) designed for the pediatric market. This oxygenator was divided into separate compartments and gave clinicians three maximum blood flow options, 1.3, 2.6, and 4.0 L per minute (LPM), depending which compartments were opened.[29] The VPCML also tried a new concept with the heat exchanger. Once a separate external CPB component, the stainless steel heat exchanger was placed inside the venous reservoir. The stainless steel coil wrapped around the inside of the reservoir was not efficient unless a large amount of volume was held in the reservoir. This was counter to the efforts to reduce the overall circuit prime volume. Despite this shortcoming in the VPCML model, the move toward integration and consolidation of functionalities continued. These heat exchangers are now integrated within the oxygenator housing.

Considering that pediatric cardiac surgery is more likely than adult surgery to use moderate to deep hypothermia, these heat exchangers need to be extremely efficient with a small surface area.

As technology relentlessly improved, membrane hollow fibers were wrapped into tighter configurations. This eventually allowed for a priming volume low enough to release a dedicated neonatal oxygenator. In 2006, Dideco released the first neonatal oxygenator with a prime volume of 31 mL and max rated flow of 700 mL/min.[30] The new generation of neonatal and pediatric oxygenators achieves much higher maximum flow rates while keeping prime volumes appropriate for neonates. This has allowed clinical teams to achieve consistent physiologic outcomes after pump runs in neonates and small infants. A modern pediatric device like the Terumo Baby FX oxygenator with integrated arterial filter (Terumo Cardiovascular Group, Ann Arbor, Michigan, USA) offers a low total prime volume and a high maximum blood flow (Fig. 37.5). With arterial filter integration, this oxygenator has a total prime volume of 43 mL and a maximum rated blood flow of 1.5 LPM. This low prime oxygenator is suitable for neonates but also accommodates patients up to approximately 15 kg. This wide range of blood flow and low prime improves the likelihood of bloodless surgery—wherein an asanguineous prime is used—for the larger patients in range for this device. The Maquet Quadrox-i Neonatal oxygenator (Maquet Holding B.V. & Co. KG, Rastatt, Germany) is another oxygenator with an integrated arterial filter that has a 40-mL total prime volume and 1.5-LPM maximum flow. When considering the additional volume of an external arterial line filter, this high-efficiency oxygenator with an integrated filter offers the lowest total prime volume unit on the market today.[31] Current trends in oxygenator design and development include integration of the arterial line filter, biocompatible surface coatings for circuit tubing, decreasing flow resistance, and more efficient heat exchange.

Tubing

The tubing used to connect the various components of the CPB circuit to the patient is made of a medical-grade polyvinyl chloride (PVC). Tubing length and diameter are the two main factors to consider when designing a circuit. Shorter tubing with the smallest internal diameter will reduce prime volume, but the tubing must also be large enough to safely manage required blood flows and line pressures for a given patient. In the past, 1/4-, 3/8-, and 1/2-inch tubing were the only tubing options and thus made circuit miniaturization a difficult task. Currently, a wide range and selection of pediatric tubing and connector sizes are available, and tubing sizes such as 1/8, 3/16, and 1/4 inch have become the new standards in pediatrics. Changing the internal diameter of tubing affects blood flow resistance and must not impede venous drainage or arterial blood flow. At our institution, we select arterial-venous line sizes that accommodate gravity venous drainage and do not exceed an arterial line pressure of 350 mm Hg (Table 37.2). Large reductions in tubing length have been made possible by positioning the smaller new-generation pump consoles close to the patient and using mast mounted pumps to bring components closer together. The bioreactivity of blood coming into contact with artificial surfaces, such as tubing, is known to exacerbate the systemic inflammatory response and disrupt hemostasis. A major advancement has been the development of surface coatings that attempt to mimic the endothelial surface of blood vessels. These coatings have been shown to attenuate the increase of cytokines and inflammatory markers and preserve platelets.[32,33] When selecting tubing for the pediatric circuit, the goal is to safely achieve maximum blood flows, decrease prime volume, and attenuate blood trauma.

Hemoconcentrators

A hemoconcentrator is an ultrafiltration device that consists of semipermeable membrane fibers that remove plasma water

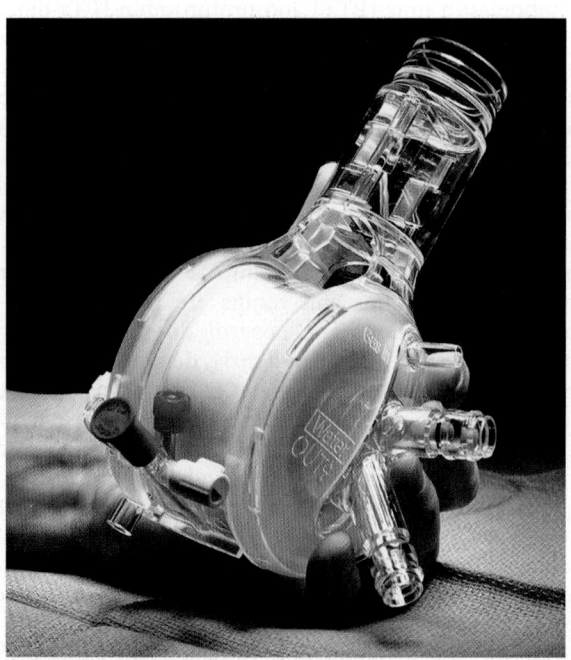

Fig. 37.5. Picture of the Terumo Baby FX05 pediatric oxygenator.

TABLE 37.2	Tubing Specifications and Maximum Blood Flow Ranges Tested at Children's Health Dallas				

TUBING SPECIFICATIONS			CHILDREN'S HEALTH DALLAS PROTOCOL	
Internal Diameter (inches)	mL/ft	mL/rev	Max Art Flow (mL/min)	Max Gravity Drainage (mL/min)
1/8	2.5	3.5	~450	
5/32	3.7	5	~750	
3/16	5	7	~1300	500-650
1/4	9.65	13	~3000	1300-1500
5/16	13.5	18	~5500	2000-2200
3/8	21.71	27	>5000	4000-4500
7/16	28.5	38		5000-5500
1/2	38.61	45		>5000
5/8	55.77	65		

and solutes. They function similarly to hemodialysis units but are simpler in that they do not require a dialysate solution. Blood flows through microporous membrane fibers, and since the hydrostatic pressure is higher inside the membrane fibers, effluent fluid permeates the membrane and can be removed. The membrane pore sizes are typically less than 55,000 daltons, which preserve plasma proteins such as albumin (65,000 daltons), and maintain the colloid oncotic pressure. The ultrafiltration rate of a hemoconcentrator is dependent on the hydrostatic pressure gradient across the membrane, blood flow rate through the membrane fibers, membrane pore size, and the hematocrit. Ultrafiltration is useful for increasing hematocrit, reducing high potassium levels after cardioplegia delivery, and removing harmful inflammatory mediators. Hemodilution during pediatric CPB is difficult to avoid, and a 2004 survey of pediatric cardiac surgery centers report that 98% of perfusionists routinely use a hemoconcentrator during the conduct of CPB.[20]

Circuit Prime

The CPB circuit is primed with a crystalloid replacement fluid. Common solutions include Plasma-Lyte A, lactated Ringer, and Normosol-R.[34] Lactated Ringer is a replacement fluid that contains 29 mEq/L of lactate but lacks magnesium. Plasma-Lyte A and Normosol-R both closely mimic human physiologic plasma electrolyte concentrations, osmolality, and pH. However, these two solutions do not contain calcium. At Children's Health Dallas, the perfusionists use Plasma-Lyte A because it does not contain lactate or calcium, thus allowing the perfusionists to lower CPB perfusate calcium levels, which is desirable, as is discussed later.

Once the CPB circuit is primed with a crystalloid solution and cleared of any air, the total prime volume of the circuit is estimated. The perfusionist must then choose between initiating CPB with or without adding heterologous blood. Unlike the adult patient population, blood products are often added to the neonatal and pediatric CPB circuits due to the small patient blood volume-to-circuit prime volume ratio. The dilutional effect of the crystalloid prime is determined by calculating the patient resultant hematocrit (HCTr). The HCTr formula, HCTr = (Patient blood volume × HCT)/(Patient blood volume + Circuit prime volume), is calculated once the patient hematocrit value is measured in the operating room before surgery. The institutional protocol at Children's Health Dallas is to maintain a CPB HCTr above 30%. If that value cannot be reached, then packed red blood cells (PRBCs) are added to the circuit. The institutional protocol also directs that a half unit of fresh frozen plasma, approximately 100 mL, will be added to the circuit prime for all patients less than 6 kg.

The pre-CPB circuit prime drug additives at our institution include heparin (1000 units/mL), 8.4% sodium bicarbonate, 20% mannitol, furosemide (10 mg/mL), methylprednisolone, tranexamic acid, and 25% albumin (Table 37.3). The ideal prime solution should be "physiologic" and also attempt to attenuate the adverse response to artificially supporting a patient with an extracorporeal circuit.

Anticoagulation

Due to the foreign surface contact and resultant intrinsic activation of the coagulation cascade, the patient must be anticoagulated before CPB. Heparin is the most widely used anticoagulant during CPB, and it acts by super-activating

TABLE 37.3 Cardiopulmonary Bypass Circuit Prime Drugs

Drug	Action	Prime Dose
Heparin	Anticoagulant	Calculated by Medtronic HMS and varies per patient
Sodium bicarbonate	Buffer	Achieve pH 7.40
Mannitol	Osmotic diuretic; oxygen radical scavenger	0.5 mg/kg; 12.5 g max dose
Furosemide	Loop diuretic	0.25 mg/kg; 20 mg max dose
Methylprednisolone	Corticosteroid	30 mg/kg; 1 g max dose
25% Albumin	Plasma protein	10% circuit prime volume
Tranexamic acid	Antifibrinolytic	20 mg/kg; 20 g max dose

antithrombin III (ATIII), which then inactivates thrombin and other proteases involved in coagulation. Heparin is used because it is fast-acting, and anticoagulation reversal can easily be achieved by administering protamine. Anticoagulation helps prevent circuit thrombus formation and avoid the devastating effects of potential arterial thromboembolism. Heparin was the anticoagulant used during Dr. Gibbon's first successful cardiac surgery in 1953, and its use during CPB has continued for more than 60 years. Before heparin administration and dosing protocols were available, anticoagulation methods were cumbersome and unsafe. The dosing was empiric, and the only methods for testing heparinization were lengthy laboratory heparin concentration tests. Fortunately, the activated clotting time (ACT) test was introduced in 1966 and this bedside whole blood test became the foundation of how heparinization is monitored in the cardiac operating room today.[35] Traditional laboratory tests such as partial thromboplastin time (PTT) and prothrombin (PT) time are sensitive to low doses of heparin and therefore are not useful during CPB. The ACT is a point-of-care test that measures the time (in seconds) needed for activated whole blood to form thrombin. In 1975, Bull et al.[36] reported a heparin management approach using the ACT test and the technique quickly became universally accepted. The report describes the heparin dose response curve technique and suggests an optimal ACT range of 480 seconds during CPB. In this technique, ACTs are run on various whole blood samples containing different heparin concentrations and results are plotted versus the heparin concentration. The heparin dose response curve, commonly referred to as the *Bull curve*, demonstrates the individualized ACT response to different levels of heparinization and is a useful tool in estimating the concentration of heparin necessary to achieve an ACT of 480 seconds (Fig. 37.6). Maintaining ACT results of at least 480 seconds during CPB remains the standard of care today. Though most clinicians will agree that 480 seconds is acceptable during CPB, there is debate whether or not that value should be universally applied, considering that not all ACT analyzers operate and activate blood in exactly the same manner.

Pediatric patients undergoing cardiac repair suffer disproportionate postoperative bleeding complications after CPB,

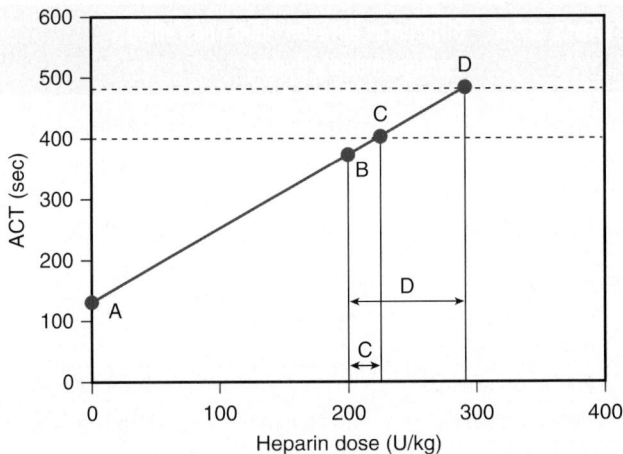

Fig. 37.6. An example of a heparin dose response curve wherein the patients baseline activated clotting time (ACT) is shown at point A. An initial heparin dose of 200 units per kilogram resulted in an ACT shown at point B. A linear extension of points A and B is drawn with an intersection at 400 (point C) and 480 seconds (point D), and these target intersects can be used to estimate further heparin doses to administer to the patient. (From Bull BS, Huse WM, Brauer FS, Korpman RA. Heparin therapy during extracorporeal circulation. II. The use of a dose-response curve to individualize heparin and protamine dosage. J Thorac Cardiovasc Surg. 1975;69:685-689.)

likely because of their size and immature coagulation system. Contributing factors to postoperative bleeding are dilution of coagulation factors during CPB, induction of the systemic inflammatory response, hematologic changes in cyanotic patients, hypothermia, and numerous coagulation factor deficiencies. All of these situations can inhibit adequate anticoagulation with heparin and ultimately lead to the generation of thrombin. It has been shown that prolonged ACT results of pediatric patients poorly correlate with the plasma levels of heparin during CPB.[37] Reports have shown that pediatric patients require higher plasma heparin concentrations than adults because they metabolize heparin faster, have a larger blood volume-to-body weight ratio, and have lower ATIII levels.[38,39] Weight-based heparin doses and ACT monitoring used with adult patients are therefore not recommended for use in pediatric patients.

The potential variability of a pediatric patient's response to heparin necessitates an individual dosing regimen and the use of different coagulation tests. A useful bedside hemostasis management tool in pediatric cardiac surgery is the Hepcon HMS PLUS (Medtronic Inc., Minneapolis, Minnesota, USA). The Hepcon HMS PLUS is fully automated and is used to run the following tests: ACT, heparin dose response (HDR) to identify individual heparin needs, and heparin-protamine titration (HPT) to verify heparin concentration. A baseline sample is collected from the arterial line before heparinization and is used to test the HDR. The HDR test determines the baseline ACT and patient response to increasing amounts of heparin. Results are used to identify heparin-resistant or heparin-sensitive patients and determine the patient heparin concentration needed to achieve appropriate anticoagulation. To test the blood heparin concentration with the HPT test, blood is added to tubes containing different mg/mL concentrations of protamine. Heparin and protamine bind in a 1:1 ratio, so the tube that produces a clot can be used to

determine the unit/mL heparin concentration. The HPT test is used frequently during CPB to maintain heparin concentrations suggested by the HDR and also run post CPB to verify proper heparin reversal after protamine administration. Without heparinization, hemodilution and the degree of hypothermia alone could extend the ACT beyond 480 seconds and this effect is amplified in the pediatric patient. Administering heparin to maintain a patient heparin concentration calculated by the HDR, despite an ACT above 480, will help to reduce consumptive coagulopathy, thrombin generation, fibrinolysis, neutrophil activation, and the need for transfusions.[40,41]

Once the patient is ready to be cannulated for CPB, a heparin bolus is administered to the patient by the anesthesiologist into an intravenous line or by the surgeon directly into the right atrium. In general, the patient receives a 400 U/kg dose of heparin minutes before arterial cannulation. Once the heparin has circulated within the patient for approximately 5 minutes, a blood sample from an arterial or intravenous line is used to run an ACT and HPT. If the ACT reaches 480 seconds or the HPT confirms an adequate heparin concentration, cardiotomy pump suction may be used and CPB may be initiated when the surgeon inserts the arterial and venous cannulas. ACT and HPT tests are run every 30 minutes during CPB, and heparin is administered if the ACT falls below 480 seconds or the heparin concentration falls below the maintenance value calculated by the HDR. If a parameter is low, the Hepcon HMS PLUS uses a formula based on the HDR, blood volume of the patient, and circuit prime volume to calculate the amount of heparin needed to adequately raise the ACT or HPT.

Cannulation

Cannulation refers to the process in which the surgeon attaches the venous limb of the CPB circuit to the systemic venous circulation of the patient, while attaching the arterial limb to the systemic arterial system of the patient. This is most commonly accomplished by placing an arterial cannula in the distal ascending aorta and venous cannulas in the SVC and IVC, respectively. The cannulas are inserted through appropriately sized purse-string sutures and secured with tourniquets. This bicaval configuration allows for the achievement of "total" CPB, and the vast majority of cardiac repairs can be accomplished using this technique. In pediatric cardiac programs, patients ranging in weight from approximately 1000 gm up to adulthood are placed on CPB. Therefore a wide range of cannula sizes must be kept in stock. Arterial cannulas range from as small as 8 French (Fr) (2.67 mm) in diameter up to over 20 Fr. Venous cannulas for CPB are available in straight and angled varieties and range down to as small as 10 Fr. Inserting these cannulas into the diminutive aorta and vena cavae of neonates is a taxing technical exercise that must be accomplished without complication in order to appropriately support the patient during the repair and leave the patient with undamaged vessels at the cannulation sites postoperatively.

Exceptions to standard bicaval cannulation are frequently seen in pediatric practice. First, patients can have anomalies of systemic venous return, such as bilateral superior vena cavae, ipsilateral hepatic veins, or interrupted inferior vena cava with azygous continuation to the SVC. All these anomalies have to be assessed, and an appropriate venous cannulation strategy must be devised. Occasionally, if these anomalies are prohibitive for selective cannulation, or the overall patient size is so small that the cavae are too small to cannulate, the right atrial appendage is cannulated in isolation, and periods of circulatory arrest, wherein venous return is not required, are used as to accomplish intracardiac portions of the repair.

Alternatives to standard ascending aortic cannulation are also used. In order to accomplish aortic arch reconstructions without resorting to circulatory arrest, a small prosthetic vascular tube graft is anastomosed to the innominate artery and the arterial cannula is inserted into this "chimney" graft. Alternatively, if the patient is large enough, the innominate artery can be cannulated directly. These innominate artery cannulation techniques allow the brain to be perfused up the right carotid artery while the aortic arch is being repaired.

Reoperations are common in congenital heart surgery. A number of these patients have pulmonary outflow conduits that are densely adherent to the sternum. Patients with transposition of the great arteries have an abnormally anteriorly located ascending aorta that can also be adherent to the chest wall in the midline. Peripheral cannulation via a femoral artery is sometimes necessary in these instances. Peripheral arterial cannulation in children should only be performed when absolutely necessary and converted to the ascending aorta as soon as possible. The obturation of the femoral artery by the cannula almost always causes hypoperfusion of the lower extremity. With longer cannulation times, the leg can be at significant risk for ischemic complications.

Cardiopulmonary Bypass
Pediatric Versus Adult Considerations

Although many of the management techniques governing pediatric and adult CPB are similar, several differences do exist (Table 37.4). The small size of the pediatric patient and nature of the surgical repair often expose these patients to moderate or deep hypothermic temperatures, wide ranges of perfusion flow rates, and hemodilution. These management techniques represent extreme shifts from normal physiologic parameters, and the harmful effects are potentially more pronounced in these small patients. Low-flow perfusion or circulatory arrest at deep hypothermia(15°C–20°C) is often required because of the complexity of the repair, significant aortopulmonary collateral blood flow returning to the operative field from the pulmonary veins, or simply because position of the perfusion cannulas interferes with access to the surgical site.

Compared with adults, hemodilution of the pediatric patient during CPB has a larger impact on the concentration of blood components, and the blood-to-foreign surface area exposure is much greater. This relatively greater exposure to nonendothelialized surfaces can lead to an increased inflammatory response and damage the formed elements of blood. Another important contrast between pediatric and adult support involves calcium management. The immature myocardium is susceptible to exacerbated postischemic injury due to overly rapid calcium "loading" at reperfusion.[42,43] Because of this, at Children's Health Dallas a perfusate that is relatively depleted of calcium is used until well after cross-clamp removal. Calcium is restored in a stepwise fashion before weaning from the circuit. The coagulation system of neonates

TABLE 37.4 Differences Between Adult and Pediatric Cardiopulmonary Bypass

Parameter	Adult	Pediatric
Hypothermic temperature	Rarely below 25°C-32°C	Commonly 15°C-20°C
Use of circulatory arrest	Rare	Common
Pump prime		
Dilution effects on blood volume	25%-33%	150%-300%
Additional additives		Blood, albumin
Perfusion pressures	50-80 mm Hg	25-50 mm Hg
Influence of α-stat versus pH-stat management strategy	Minimal at moderate hypothermia	Marked at deep hypothermia
Measured $PaCO_2$ differences	30-45 mm Hg	20-80 mm Hg
Glucose regulation		
Hypoglycemia	Rare—requires significant hepatic injury	Common—reduced hepatic glycogen stores
Hyperglycemia	Frequent—generally easily controlled with insulin	Less common—rebound hypoglycemia may occur

From Greely WJ, Cripe CC, Nathan AT. Anesthesia for pediatric cardiac surgery. In: Miller RD, Cohen NH, Eriksson LI, et al. Miller's Anesthesia. 8th ed. Philadelphia: Elsevier Saunders; 2015:2820.

and infants also differs from adults in that they have quantitative deficiencies of coagulation factors at baseline. These deficiencies of the immature coagulation system coupled with hemodilution discussed earlier result in significant postoperative coagulopathies and anemia that must be addressed with blood products much more commonly than in adult cases.

Initiation of Cardiopulmonary Bypass

Before starting a planned operation, the surgical team will discuss the procedure and form a detailed management plan for each team member. The perfusionist must understand the type and complexity of the surgery and discuss the proper cannula section, degree of hypothermia, myocardial protection technique, and any other unique patient variables that might affect perfusion management. The fundamental concepts of managing CPB for congenital patients are similar to adults, but anatomic variations and physiologic extremes complicate the approach. Once the surgical plan is established, the patient is prepped and draped for the skin incision and sternotomy. With the chest open, the surgeon exposes the heart and major vessels and then directs the anesthesiologist to administer heparin before cannulation. Alternatively, the surgeon can administer the heparin directly to the right atrium. Next, the arterial and venous cannulas are inserted, but before it is safe to initiate CPB, it is important to confirm an adequate anticoagulation level by obtaining an ACT and heparin concentration and that the arterial cannula is unobstructed. Congenital patients, especially cyanotic patients, often demonstrate variable dose responses to heparin. In addition, it cannot be assumed that the CPB dose of heparin is circulating in the patient, as intravenous line malfunction can occur. Initiating CPB on a pediatric patient with an obstructed aortic cannula could quickly exsanguinate the patient, as venous drainage commences without return of this blood to the patient, and cause severe hypotension. Once these two safety checks are complete, the patient is ready for CPB.

The venous line is unclamped to siphon deoxygenated blood from the patient, and the arterial flow is slowly increased as the heart begins to empty. Bicaval cannulation is often used in congenital surgery, but it is common to initiate CPB with only one cannula. This is done to verify adequate drainage from one cannula, as it would be difficult diagnose poor drainage from a single cannula if both were open. Once both cannulas are open, adequate venous drainage is confirmed when the central venous pressure (CVP) falls to zero and the SVC, IVC, and right atrium are collapsed. Total (also termed *full* or *complete*) CPB is achieved when all of the systemic venous blood is being diverted to the heart lung machine and full arterial flow can be achieved. When on total CPB, the mean arterial pressure (MAP) and CVP should confirm that the heart is empty by showing a flat tracing. However, the many anatomic variations of the congenital patient can lead to blood returning to the heart despite adequate drainage. Variations such as a patent ductus arteriosus, major aortopulmonary collateral arteries, an unrecognized left SVC draining to the coronary sinus, and aortic insufficiency can return blood to the heart and should be considered when evaluating venous drainage. Assessment of adequate venous drainage and perfusion flow rate is critical before proceeding to the surgical repair. A poorly positioned venous or arterial cannula can restrict optimal perfusion flow and addressing this issue during the aortic cross-clamp period would waste unnecessary myocardial ischemic time. Once cannula placement is deemed acceptable, full perfusion flow is achieved, and oxygenation from the oxygenator is confirmed, the anesthesiologist can turn off the ventilator.

Determining and Monitoring Effective Perfusion Flow Rate

The fundamental goals of bypass are to meet the metabolic demands of all tissues and to attenuate the deleterious pathophysiologic effects of artificially supporting a patient. Once the patient is transitioned to cardiopulmonary bypass, several management techniques are used to safely optimize the level of support. Perfusion flow rate, which represents the cardiac output during CPB, is altered to meet the oxygen consumption needs of the patient. Global adequacy of flow is estimated in real time by the display of oxygen saturation by a sensor in the venous return line. Assessing regional oxygen consumption to the brain, kidneys, or bowel, for instance, is a challenge. Additionally, due to age-related differences of body surface area (BSA)-to-blood volume ratios, flow rate indexes are higher in neonates than adults. The optimal effective flow rate or cardiac index for any size patient remains unclear; however, recommended flow ranges at normothermia are listed in Table 37.5. Considering that the perfusion flow rate is not fixed during the different phases of CPB, several variables are helpful in determining a safe minimal rate. Initial normothermic target rates are calculated for CPB initiation by weight and BSA. At Children's Health Dallas, in addition to the CPB initiation flow rates calculated by weight, the perfusionist calculates several cardiac indexes ranging from 2.4–3.0 L/min/

TABLE 37.5	Recommended Pump Flow Rates at Normothermia
Patient Weight (kg)	Pump Flow Rate (mL/kg/min)
<3	150-200
3-10	125-175
10-15	120-150
15-30	100-120
30-50	75-100
>50	50-75

From Jaggers J, Shearer IR, Ungerleider RM. Cardiopulmonary bypass in infants and children. In: Gravelee GP, Davis RF, Kuruz M, Utley JR. Cardiopulmonary Bypass Principles and Practice. 2nd ed. Philadelphia: Lippincott Williams and Wilkins; 2000:637.

m². Factors such as the degree of hypothermia, acid-base balance, depth of anesthesia and neuromuscular blockade, hematocrit, venous saturation, lactate level, urine output, and near infrared saturation trends are used to guide perfusion flow rates. Patient temperature is the greatest factor affecting perfusion flow, and rates as low as 40–50 mL/kg are routinely used at core temperatures in the 20°C range.

Arterial Pressure

The MAP will slowly lose its pulsatile trace and flatten out as the heart empties on CPB. Though the MAP is calculated by factoring the systolic and diastolic pressures, the value of the flat tracing is referred to as the MAP and perfusion pressure during CPB. The transition to CPB often leads to hypotension, and in contrast to adult cases, vasopressors (eg, phenylephrine) are not typically administered in the early phase of CPB in young patients. The goal in the early phase of CPB is to cool the patient and reduce the metabolic demands. Low perfusion pressure, 20–30 mm Hg, is accepted during the cooling phase, and vasodilators (eg, phentolamine) are actually used to reduce arterial tone and increase uniformity of perfusion and improve cooling. Vasodilation has been shown to improve temperature distribution and reduce lactate production in pediatric deep hypothermic CPB.[44] Hemodilution, hypocalcemia, and the inflammatory response are also factors that cause hypotension at the onset of CPB. Hemodilution will lower the perfusion pressure because of the viscosity reduction, and hemoconcentration performed by the perfusionist with the hemoconcentrator can easily increase perfusion pressure by raising the hematocrit. The systemic inflammatory response is triggered by the foreign surface contact of blood and bypass circuitry. This response releases many vasoactive mediators, which can quickly drop the perfusion pressure, and highlights the importance of minimizing circuit surface area for the pediatric patient. The decrease in pressure in an adult patient with coronary or carotid stenosis would likely be treated with a vasopressor, while increasing perfusion flow is the preferred method in young patients.

Arterial and Venous Oxygen Saturation

Most oxygen saturation monitoring techniques are noninvasive and inexpensive and can be used in real time. Changing perfusion flow rate and oxygen delivery will have immediate and direct effects on oxygen saturation levels. Pulse oximetry is a clinical mainstay and is used to monitor oxygen delivery to the extremities during the preoperative and postoperative periods. However, due to the nonpulsatile flow pattern generated during CPB, this technology is ineffective.

As mentioned earlier, a mainstay monitoring technique during CPB is to track the oxygen saturation of the venous line blood draining into the venous reservoir. As a general guideline, perfusion flow rate is adjusted to maintain this mixed venous saturation (SvO_2) greater than 70%. While this guideline is helpful during "normal" physiologic conditions, the many nonphysiologic variables of CPB cause shifts in the oxyhemoglobin dissociation curve (Fig. 37.7), and these venous oxygen saturations may fail to represent satisfactory oxygen delivery to the tissues. Leftward shifts in the curve prevent oxygen from being released from hemoglobin, which could deceivingly demonstrate an acceptable SvO_2 in the presence of tissue hypoxia. As the patient is cooled during CPB, regional deoxygenation has been shown to occur despite a normal or rising SvO_2 without increasing perfusion flow rate.[45] Hypothermia not only strengthens the hemoglobin oxygen affinity but also creates an alkaline blood pH and causes a further leftward oxyhemoglobin shift. In this situation, it is important to cool and warm patients methodically to minimize the temperature gradient between the blood and tissues and maintain perfusion flow so that the SvO_2 does not trend downward. As tissue temperature decreases, venous line SvO_2 can be used to help guide the reduction of perfusion flow rate.

It is especially critical to meet the metabolic needs of brain tissue, and global SvO_2 values may misrepresent regional oxygen consumption. It has been shown that considerable regional differences exist and SvO_2 can overestimate regional saturations from the brain.[46] The majority of venous blood analyzed by the venous line SvO_2 comes from IVC cannula, and IVC saturation is notoriously misleading as an estimate of oxygen consumption due to "contamination" by highly saturated renal venous blood. Though the SvO_2 does have its place in guiding perfusion flow rate, more specific, regional oxygenation assessment is currently recommended to ensure adequate perfusion flow distribution, particularly for the brain.

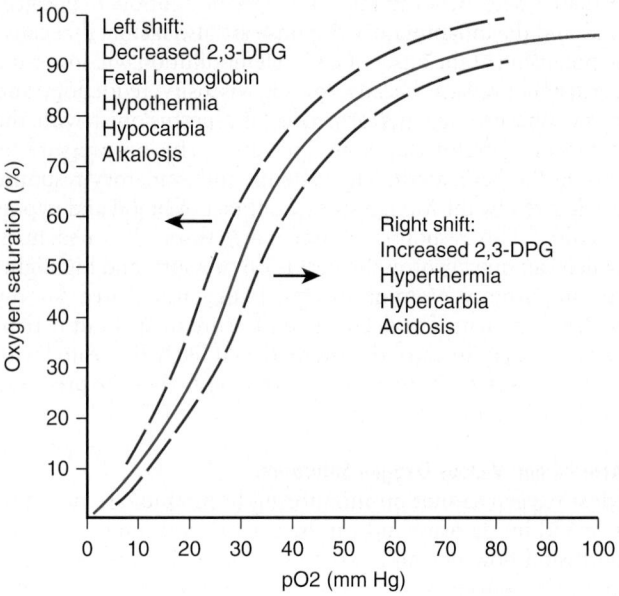

Fig. 37.7. The oxyhemoglobin dissociation curve.

Near-Infrared Spectroscopy

Near-infrared spectroscopy (NIRS) is a noninvasive optical sensor that can measure cerebral and somatic tissue oxygenation. NIRS monitoring is gaining considerable popularity because sensor pads may be placed over various regional tissue beds, particularly both cerebral hemispheres, and display real-time results. Somatic monitoring sites such as flank, abdominal, and muscle are suggested to help broaden the assessment of systemic hypoperfusion. The technology works by bouncing various wavelength arcs of near-infrared light from a sensor emitter and detector. These photodetectors allow for selective measurement of tissue oxygenation. This technology is widely used in the operating room and ICU, although interpreting the results has been a topic of debate. A validation study performed at Children's Health Dallas demonstrated that cerebral NIRS values accurately predicted the oxygen saturation in the SVC on CPB and that flank NIRS values were significantly associated with IVC saturation.[47] As increasing evidence validates tissue oximetry against invasive measurements, NIRS monitoring has shown its value in quickly detecting regional low flow.[48-51] At Children's Health Dallas, the perfusionists use NIRS trends and values to guide perfusion flow rate, hematocrit, blood gas strategy, temperature, and vasomotor tone (Box 37.1). It is important to note that NIRS helps to guide rather than dictate perfusion management. The upper limits and critical lower values reported by NIRS are poorly defined.

Considering the regional venous oxygen saturation variations of the neonatal and infant cardiac surgical patients, NIRS provides valuable information and early detection of poor perfusion in critical organs. NIRS has been particularly useful as a real-time monitor on patients with hypoplastic left heart syndrome, for example. Cerebral oxygen saturation measured after stage I palliation has been shown to strongly correlate with hemodynamic parameters and help to identify early postoperative complications.[49,52] Hoffman et al.[53] found that avoiding cerebral hypoxia with the use of NIRS monitoring was the most significant factor in improving childhood neurodevelopmental outcomes.

Methods to Optimize Physiologic Management
Target Hematocrit and Ultrafiltration

Despite the progress of reducing the pediatric circuit prime volume, hemodilution during CPB remains difficult to avoid.[54] Hemodilution can cause edema, coagulopathy, blood and colloid osmotic pressure reduction, and the need to transfuse blood products. Blood product transfusion is the most straightforward solution to address these complications; however, the risk-benefit assessment of blood transfusion must be considered. Transfusion-related complications include increased postoperative morbidity and mortality, prolonged mechanical ventilation and hospital stay, exacerbation

BOX 37.1	Methods to Improve Cerebral Near-Infrared Spectroscopy Values

Increase perfusion flow rate
Increase hematocrit
pH-stat blood gas strategy
Decrease temperature
Increase mean arterial pressure; vasopressor
Verify adequate superior vena cava drainage

of the inflammatory response, and infection.[55-58] Modern blood bank testing and donor screening have significantly reduced infectious complications, but noninfectious risk remains a major concern. In addition, smaller patients are exposed to a higher transfusion risk because the transfusion effects may be more pronounced than in adult patients. With a goal of minimizing hemodilution and donor blood exposure, the cardiac team must implement a transfusion algorithm and define a target hematocrit during CPB. Perioperative and developmental outcomes data reported from clinical trials at the Boston Children's Hospital demonstrate that, when compared with target CPB hematocrit values of 30%, hematocrit values at or below 20% are associated with adverse outcomes and that the benefits of hematocrit values higher than 25% should be further investigated.[59,60] The protocol at Children's Health Dallas is to maintain a hematocrit of at least 30% during cardiopulmonary bypass.

Reducing circuit prime volume and incorporating an ultrafiltration device can significantly reduce donor blood exposure. Originally, a hemoconcentrator added to the CPB circuit was used primarily to remove plasma water and raise the hematocrit. This process is referred to as "conventional ultrafiltration" (CUF) and its initial use was met with a few limitations. Perfusionists were accustomed to using diuretics to help increase the hematocrit; however, this strategy offered little control and required adequate kidney perfusion during CPB. When ultrafiltration emerged as a CPB technique in the mid-1980s, hemoconcentrators were viewed as an expensive option for removing excess circuit volume. Also, while fluid is removed from the circuit during CUF, the volume in the venous reservoir level diminishes and CUF must be stopped before the reservoir is emptied, which would have catastrophic consequences. Thus the amount of fluid removed during CUF is dependent on available volume in the venous reservoir, which limits the ability to effectively raise the hematocrit. In 1991 a report described a *modified ultrafiltration* (MUF) technique performed after weaning the patient from CPB and enabled the perfusionist to concentrate the entire circuit and return most of that volume back to the patient.[61] During this era, pediatric circuit prime volume was still rather high and various MUF techniques proved to be a valuable resource for reducing total body water post CPB. The popularity of MUF led investigators to explore the potential reduction of proinflammatory mediators during ultrafiltration. An additional ultrafiltration technique, *zero balance ultrafiltration* (ZBUF), emerged as alternate method to attenuate the inflammatory response. ZBUF is performed by removing the ultrafiltration effluent from the circuit during CPB while administering a replacement solution (eg, Plasma-Lyte A) to the venous reservoir in a 1:1 ratio. The high-volume filtration of fluid that is able to be exchanged allows the perfusionist to control electrolyte and glucose levels (eg, high potassium levels after delivering cardioplegia) and more effectively remove inflammatory mediators. The increasing acceptance of ultrafiltration during CPB led to developing many technique variations during the preoperative, perioperative, and postoperative phases and can thus be categorized into two groups: blood concentration and blood filtration.

In preparation for neonatal CPB at Children's Health Dallas, for example, the perfusionist adds approximately 300 mL of packed red blood cells to the venous reservoir after priming the circuit with Plasma-Lyte A. The circuit volume is

recirculated through the hemoconcentrator, and volume is removed until the reservoir is almost empty. The circuit prime is then "washed" by adding approximately 500 mL of Plasma-Lyte A and then removing that volume. This process is known as *prebypass ultrafiltration* (Pre-BUF), and in addition to concentrating the circuit, Pre-BUF has been shown to reduce high potassium, glucose, lactate, citrate, and bradykinin levels found in packed red blood cells. CUF is then performed during the early phase of CPB to remove any excess circuit volume and maintain a hematocrit of 30%. During the warming phase of CPB the perfusionist performs CUF and ZBUF. This combined ultrafiltration strategy, coupled with a miniaturized circuit, allows the perfusionist to filter the blood and exceed or meet baseline hematocrit values before weaning from CPB.

Hypothermia
DHCA versus SCP

The therapeutic potential of hypothermia has been known for centuries and has been routinely used in cardiac surgery since its inception. This concept relies on the fundamental physiologic relationship between oxygen consumption and temperature. In 1950, Bigelow and colleagues[62] compared the use of normothermia and topical cooling on dogs and reported superior ischemic tolerance by surface cooling after 15 minutes of circulatory arrest. The first clinical application in cardiac surgery was reported 1953 by Lewis and Taufic, who described the successful repair of an ASD in a 5-year-old girl using topical cooling and total body hypothermia.[2] To achieve this, patients were submerged in an ice bath to reduce their temperature to approximately 28°C, and then the defect was closed with the aid of inflow occlusion. In 1958, Sealy and colleagues[63] successfully reported the use of hypothermia in conjunction with CPB. The use of CPB with various degrees of hypothermia or deep hypothermic circulatory arrest (DHCA) dramatically increased the "safe" period of support, which enabled surgeons to repair increasingly complex anomalies, and allowed cardiac surgery to flourish.

Hypothermia suppresses metabolic activity, preserves high energy phosphate stores, and reduces the reaction rate of biochemical reactions. Several factors are used in determining the type and degree of hypothermia during CPB. The most significant factor is the degree of surgical difficulty and anticipated CPB support time. Complex surgical repairs requiring lengthy support times would benefit from more pronounced hypothermia. The degree of hypothermia varies greatly and is typically classified as mild, moderate, deep, and profound hypothermia (Table 37.6). Deep hypothermia might be seen as desirable when low flow (≤50 mL/kg/min) or DHCA is desired, as is the case in operations involving complete aortic arch reconstruction. Circulatory arrest is a process in which

TABLE 37.6   **Hypothermia Classifications in Cardiac Surgery**

Category	Core Temperature
Mild	32-34°C
Moderate	25-32°C
Deep	15-25°C
Profound	≤15°C

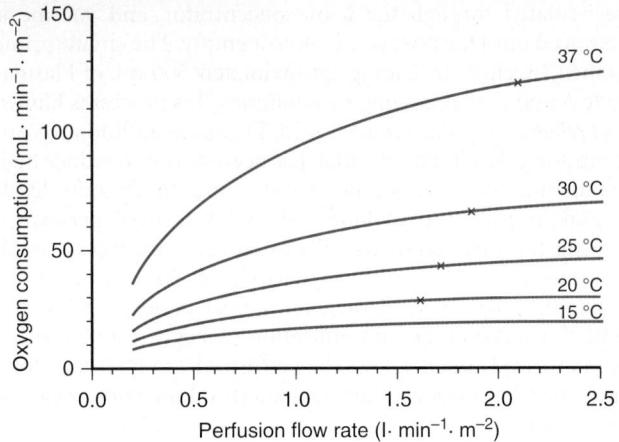

Fig. 37.8. Nomogram relating oxygen consumption (VO$_2$) to perfusion flow rate and temperature. (From Kirklin JW, Barratt-Boyes BG. Hypothermia, circulatory arrest, and cardiopulmonary bypass. In: Kirklin JW, Barratt-Boyes BG, eds. Cardiac Surgery. 2nd ed. New York, NY: Churchill-Livingstone; 1993:91.)

the perfusion flow is turned off and the patient's blood volume is allowed to drain into the venous reservoir. This dramatic application provides an asanguineous and completely motionless surgical field, facilitating complex repairs. In very small patients, the venous cannula may be obstructive and DHCA is required in order to remove the cannula and access the surgical site. Hypothermia also facilitates exposure of the surgical field by allowing decreased perfusion flow rates, which reduces the amount of collateral blood returning to the heart via the pulmonary veins (Fig. 37.8). Patients with pulmonary blood flow restrictions (eg, tetralogy of Fallot, pulmonary atresia) can develop major aortopulmonary collateral arteries, and these collaterals can flood the heart during the aortic cross-clamp period if CPB flow is maintained. This excessive blood return not only obscures the surgical site but may also warm the cold arrested myocardium or wash out cardioplegia from the coronary arteries. Hypothermia and perfusion flow rate reduction can attenuate this collateral flow while maintaining adequate oxygenation delivery to the patient.

The rate of cooling varies greatly between different tissue beds; thus multiple measurement sites are recommended to ensure uniform cooling distribution (Fig. 37.9). The optimal temperature measurement site is controversial, but choosing sites that closely reflect tissue temperatures of vital organs, particularly the brain, is widely accepted. At Children's Health Dallas, the patient's nasopharyngeal, rectal, and bladder temperatures are monitored during surgery. Nasopharyngeal closely correlates with brain temperature; however, it may underestimate the global core temperature considering the slower cooling rates of other tissue beds. For this reason, rectal and bladder temperature monitoring sites with slower rates of cooling are typically used to guide cooling end points.

The concept of a "safe" circulatory arrest time is controversial, and most guidelines are met with a degree of uncertainty. A nomogram focused on neurologic protection has been devised that estimates "safe" circulatory arrest times, but values should not be used as absolutes (Fig. 37.10). The historic incidence of perioperative cerebral injury during DHCA has led investigators to explore alternative techniques to protect the brain during complex repairs. Antegrade cerebral

perfusion (ACP, also known as selective cerebral perfusion) uses a cannulation technique that directs perfusion flow to only the brain with the theoretic advantage of protecting it from hypoxic ischemic injury. Though this technique has been adopted among many surgical centers, investigations comparing DHCA and ACP have failed to definitively demonstrate superiority of either technique[64-66] and not all of this work is focused only on neurologic issues. Recent literature has suggested that during ACP, the resultant partial perfusion from collateral vessels provides better protection to abdominal organs than DHCA.[67,68] In addition, the ideal temperature during ACP remains unknown. Recent reports, however, have demonstrated superior results using moderate to mild hypothermia, in the 25°C–30°C range, rather than deep levels of hypothermia.[69,70] Considering the coagulopathy, inflammatory response, as well as the vascular and organ dysfunction associated with deep hypothermia, a lesser degree of hypothermia may provide superior clinical outcomes.

pH and P$_a$CO$_2$ Strategy

CO$_2$ concentration and pH are primary determinants of cerebral blood flow. As body temperature decreases, the solubility of CO$_2$ increases, resulting in a decreased PaCO$_2$ and increased pH. Manipulating the acid-base management during hypothermic bypass can be classified by two mechanisms of control: alpha-stat or pH-stat. Both mechanisms have been studied intensely in reptiles (ectotherms) and hibernating mammals (endotherms), looking at their adaptive blood pH alterations that allow them to withstand extreme temperature fluctuations. pH-stat acid-base management is practiced by hibernating mammals and is accomplished by decreasing ventilatory rate and raising PaCO$_2$ while maintaining a constant pH during hypothermic conditions. Maintaining pH, while varying temperature during hibernation, is thought to preserve oxygen stores by decreasing metabolic activity. Alternatively, reptiles use alpha-stat and allow their pH to enter an alkaline state by reducing PaCO$_2$.

The perfusionist can maintain a pH-stat or "temperature-corrected" acid-base strategy during CPB by allowing CO$_2$ to passively rise or actually adding CO$_2$ to the CPB circuit. Cerebral blood flow has been shown to decrease during hypothermia using the alpha-stat strategy and demonstrates a linear relationship to the increased PaCO$_2$ when a pH-stat strategy is used.[71] In addition to preserving cerebral blood flow during hypothermia, a pH-stat strategy induces a rightward shift of the oxyhemoglobin dissociation curve (see Fig. 37.7) potentially allowing for increased oxygen "off-loading" from hemoglobin at the capillary level.

Whether pH-stat or alpha-stat acid-base management during hypothermic CPB demonstrates clear benefits on clinical outcomes has been difficult to demonstrate. However, it is suggested that a pH-stat strategy is optimal for pediatric patients and alpha-stat is the optimal strategy on adult patients.[72]

Myocardial Protection

Myocardial protection refers to the strategies and techniques employed to allow for the surgeon to work on the heart in a bloodless and motionless field yet recover the best possible postischemic myocardial function and cardiac output for the patient. Strategies for both adults and children attempt to reduce the cardiac workload and minimize the metabolic

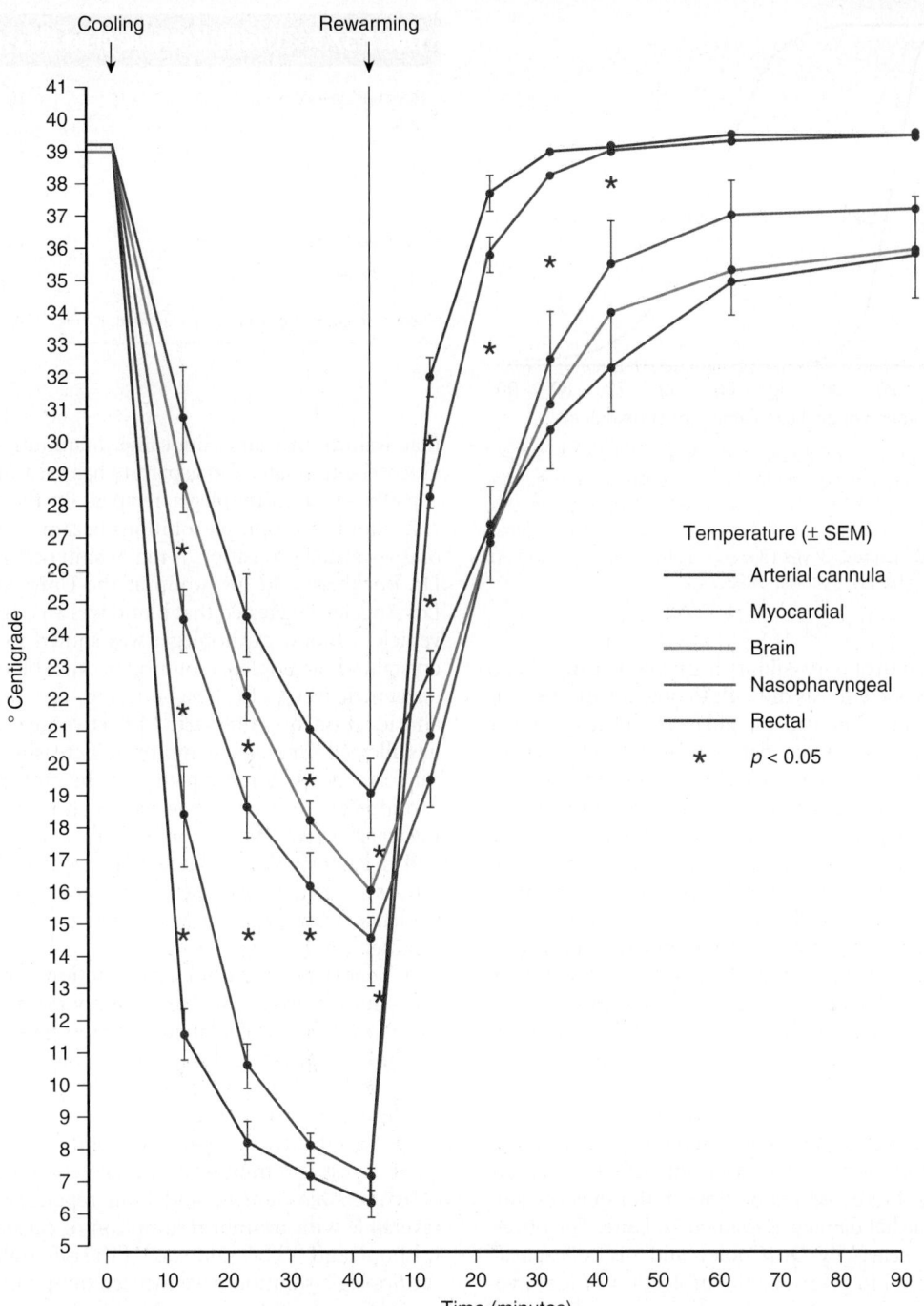

Fig. 37.9. Relationships of temperatures measured at various sites over time during cooling and warming from cardiopulmonary bypass. (From Stefaniszyn HJ, Novick RJ, Keith FM, et al. Is the brain adequately cooled during deep hypothermic cardiopulmonary bypass? Curr Surg 1983;40:294-297.)

demands and consequences of oxygen deprivation during ischemia. Reducing afterload and emptying the heart by initiating CPB is a myocardial protection technique during beating heart procedures (eg, palliative shunts, bidirectional Glenn procedure). When the heart needs to be stopped and opened for intracardiac repairs, the aorta is cross-clamped and cardioplegia is delivered to the coronary circulation to cause prolonged asystole. Cardioplegia is a myocardial arrest-producing solution that is formulated to prolong the myocardial tolerance to ischemia. There are many techniques to

protect the myocardium, but cardioplegia strategies are often the focus when discussing protection techniques. In North America, high potassium depolarizing solutions are the most common type of cardioplegia used.[34] Universal agreement on an optimal myocardial protective technique is widely debated, and most strategies are guided by surgeon or institutional preference.

After the first successful cardiac surgical correction using CPB in 1953, surgeons explored a variety of techniques to support the patient during the repair. It did not take long for

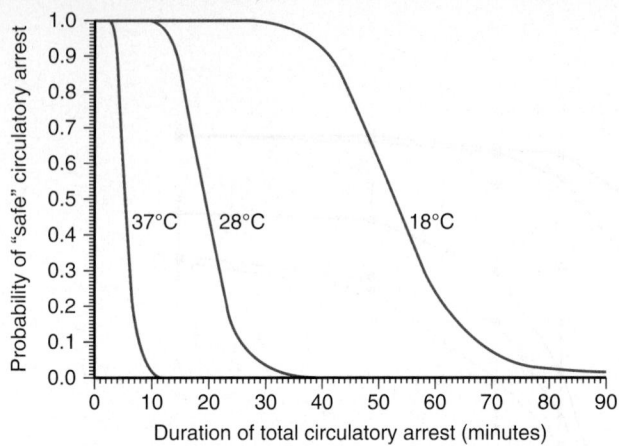

Fig. 37.10. Probability of a safe (absence of structural or functional damage) circulatory arrest according to duration. Estimate at nasopharyngeal temperatures of 37°C, 28°C, and 18°C. (From Kirklin JW, Barratt-Boyes BG. Hypothermia, circulatory arrest, and cardiopulmonary bypass. In: Kirklin JW, Barratt-Boyes BG, eds. Cardiac Surgery. 2nd ed. New York, NY: Churchill-Livingstone; 1993:74.)

TABLE 37.7	Crystalloid Formula of del Nido Solution
Plasma-Lyte A*	1000 mL
K-Cl	26 mEq
Na-HCO$_3$ 8.4%	13 mEq
Mannitol 25%	3.25 g
Lidocaine 2%	130 mg
Mg-SO$_4$ 50%	2 g

*Baxter Healthcare Corporation, Deerfield, Illinois, USA.

them to realize that the poor visibility in an open beating heart needed to be addressed. It was difficult to operate on a beating heart, and lethal air embolism (ie, air ejected out the aortic valve) claimed the lives of many patients. In 1955, Dr. Melrose and his colleagues[73] described a technique of stopping the heart to address these dangerous operative conditions. The report outlines how potassium citrate is used to achieve elective cardiac arrest. This sparked the interest of other investigators, and in 1958 Dr. Sealy and his colleagues at Duke reported an additive modification to the Melrose method and coined the term *cardioplegia*.[74] It is interesting to note that improving operative visibility, not protecting the heart, was the goal of arresting the heart. Further investigation began to show that these techniques caused damage to the myocardium and cardioplegia was abandoned. In the 1960s and early 1970s a number of investigators tried to find an alternative protection technique. Reports of using direct coronary perfusion with intermittent aortic occlusion, topical hypothermia, and normothermic ischemia with aortic occlusion failed to achieve consistent results, presented major time limitations for surgeons, and myocardial damage remained an issue. The observation of "stone heart" by Dr. Cooley and his colleagues[74] highlighted the need to prioritize the protection of the myocardium, and they proposed that depleting myocardium ATP stores would leave the heart frozen in systole. Fortunately, several European researchers continued to explore cardioplegia solutions throughout the 1960s. They discovered that the chelating action of the citrate ion of the potassium-citrate solution was responsible for myocardial damage because it interferes with cellular calcium and magnesium traffic. This finding resparked interest into pharmacologic cardiac arrest around the world, with a new focus of protecting the myocardium by membrane stabilization and managing calcium and other ion shifts. During the 1970s, a sequence of landmark reports hailed the worldwide return of cardioplegia and its use in protecting the myocardium. These publications identified potassium-chloride as a safe arresting agent and, moreover, showed that cold cardioplegia significantly extends the safe ischemic period. The use of cardioplegia additives such as

magnesium, procaine, lidocaine, mannitol, buffering agents, glucose, glutamate, and aspartate has led to much debate and a plethora of cardioplegia recipes. By the late 1970s, these crystalloid cardioplegia solutions became the dominant form of myocardial protection. A major shift occurred in 1978 when Dr. Buckberg and his group at the University of California, Los Angeles, suggested that blood was an optimal cardioplegia vehicle.[75] Blood cardioplegia was shown to be superior to a crystalloid cardioplegia solution because blood provides better oxygen delivery, effective buffering, free radical scavenging, and ideal oncotic pressure.[76] Effective myocardial protection has allowed surgeons to approach increasingly complex surgical corrections. A consequence of the motivation to optimize cardioplegia techniques has led to an incredible variation of myocardial protection techniques. Despite numerous advances and an extensive body of research, myocardial protection techniques continue to be largely program based because hard evidence, from prospective randomized trials, for instance, is lacking.[77]

A depolarizing cardioplegia solution uses a high dose of potassium, delivered to the coronary circulation in isolation, to decrease the cardiac membrane resting potential and arrest the heart in diastole. Delivering a cold dose of depolarizing cardioplegia does add a degree of protection, but simply arresting and cooling the heart does not offer optimal protection. An effective cardioplegia solution should (1) achieve quick arrest and minimize ATP depletion, (2) delay the onset of irreversible damage and limit reperfusion injury, (3) be reversible with prompt resumption of cardiac function upon washout, and (4) be nontoxic.[78] Efforts to optimize an effective cardioplegia solution have focused on myocyte calcium management and pH buffering. Modified depolarizing cardioplegia, a solution that combines a depolarizing agent with additional membrane stabilizing additives (eg, magnesium or lidocaine), has gained interest in attempting to optimize cardioplegia. A modified depolarizing solution that is gaining popularity in congenital surgery is del Nido cardioplegia (Compass; Baxter Healthcare Inc., Edison, New Jersey, USA) (Table 37.7).[79] Unlike most cardioplegia solutions that require frequent maintenance dosing to achieve effect protection, del Nido cardioplegia is known to provide excellent myocardial protection without the need to frequently redose.[80] This reported advantage allows the surgeon to operate uninterrupted while reducing the aortic cross-clamp time. Custodiol HTK (Essential Pharmaceuticals, LLC, Newton, Pennsylvania, USA) is an intracellular cardioplegia that achieves electrical and mechanical arrest by equilibrating the intracellular and extracellular ion concentrations. This solution is also gaining popularity in the congenital patient population because it does not require frequent maintenance doses.

At Children's Health Dallas, the surgical team uses del Nido cardioplegia with a customized pediatric cardioplegia circuit.[81] The cardioplegia is mixed at a 1:4 blood-to-crystalloid ratio, and upon aortic cross-clamp placement, a single, cold (4°C–6°C), 20 mL/kg antegrade dose is administered via the aortic root. Although there is no cardioplegia specifically designed for neonatal or congenital patients, several considerations are made to optimize protection. As previously discussed, tolerance of intracellular calcium shifts into the immature myocardium is impaired. The additives lidocaine and magnesium in del Nido cardioplegia both help to control intracellular calcium accumulation. Lidocaine prevents sodium shifts by blocking fast voltage sodium channels, which in turn limits calcium shifting into the myocyte. Magnesium, a calcium antagonist, inhibits calcium channel pumps and competes with calcium binding to troponin. These additives help the impaired immature myocardium to maintain effective electrical and mechanical arrest. Hypertrophic ventricles, as seen in tetralogy of Fallot, may not be adequately protected with standard cardioplegia doses and may require a higher cardioplegia dose and longer delivery time to properly cool and perfuse the hypertrophied myocardium. Cyanotic patients with inadequate pulmonary blood flow often have increased bronchial collateral flow. High collateral flow to the lungs ultimately returns to the heart via the pulmonary veins and is undesired while the aorta is cross-clamped. Collateral flow can fill the heart, warm the myocardium, and wash out the cardioplegia from the myocardium. Lowering the systemic temperature not only helps to offset myocardial warming but also allows the perfusionist to lower the perfusion flow and pressure, which in turn reduces this collateral flow. Also, adequate LV venting helps to minimize the effect of volume returning to the heart. High sensitivity to the inflammatory response in the immature myocardium can cause edema and reduce ventricular compliance. Mannitol is an additive in del Nido cardioplegia and helps reduce intracellular water accumulation. Care must be taken to not perfuse the myocardium at too high a pressure. This could injure fragile coronary vessels and create myocardial edema. A pressure of 30–50 mm Hg has shown to be adequate.[82]

Inflammatory Response to CPB

The systemic inflammatory response syndrome (SIRS) instigated by CPB is well documented, and limiting this response is associated with improved outcomes.[83-85] Multiple factors including blood exposure to nonendothelialized surfaces (eg, CPB circuit, air); surgical trauma (eg, intubation, sternotomy); ischemia-reperfusion; hypothermia; and allogenic transfusion have been linked to this inflammatory activation. This complex response includes cascade activations of complement, cytokine, coagulation-fibrinolytic, and various cellular activations. Perioperative and postoperative consequences include multiple organ failure (eg, myocardium, renal, pulmonary, neurologic, hepatic), coagulopathy, edema, elaboration of injurious oxygen-free radicals, and hypotension.[85]

The SIRS is more pronounced in neonates; the degree of hemodilution, the need for longer CPB and ischemic times, and the more prevalent use of profound hypothermia are all known to exacerbate SIRS and are contributors to the increased postoperative morbidity seen in neonates compared with older infants and children.[86-88]

A number of contemporary pharmacologic strategies and CPB techniques are designed to attenuate the inflammatory reactions and remove mediators during CPB. Corticosteroids have been used during CPB for many years and have been shown to mitigate many inflammatory processes such as increased capillary permeability, edema, and leukocyte migration. Various timing and dosing protocols have been suggested with conflicting results.[89,90] At Children's Health Dallas a 30-mg/kg (1-g maximum dose) perioperative dose of methylprednisolone is administered to the CPB circuit prime. Additionally, 10 mg/kg of methylprednisolone is administered 8–12 hours before the initiation of CPB in neonates. Despite the large variability of preoperative and perioperative corticosteroid administration in clinical use, the literature generally demonstrates the benefit of CPB-induced systemic inflammatory response attenuation.[91-93]

Common CPB-based techniques to attenuate SIRS include ultrafiltration, circuit miniaturization, and the use of biocompatible circuit coatings. Ultrafiltration during CPB has been shown to reduce inflammatory mediators, pulmonary injury and edema, postoperative mechanical ventilation support time, and the perioperative need for blood transfusion.[94-97] CPB circuit miniaturization and the use of biocompatible surface coatings provide two main benefits in attenuating the inflammatory response. First, the smaller surface area of a miniaturized circuit and biocompatible coating reduces the bioreactivity of blood coming into contact with foreign surfaces.[32,33] Second, smaller circuits reduce overall hemodilution and the need to transfuse donor blood, both of which have been shown to exacerbate the inflammatory response.[55,56] Although the inflammatory response to CPB cannot be avoided, a multimodal approach can significantly reduce CPB-related SIRS.

Termination of CPB

Once the surgeon has completed the cardiac repair, the entry sites into the heart are sutured closed. The venous return drainage is retarded, which fills the right heart. The anesthesiologist inflates the lungs, which facilitates the movement of this blood across the pulmonary vasculature and back to the left heart. Any active left heart venting is paused at this point, and the surgeon massages the filling heart to expel blood with any entrained air, out of a vent hole in the aortic root. Once there is no longer any air emanating from this site, the patient is placed into the Trendelenburg position and the cross clamp is removed from the aorta. The perfusionist then returns to full venous drainage, and the left heart vent can be placed to gentle suction again. The coronary circulation is now reperfused, washing out the cardioplegia. The heart is observed for any return of electrical activity. Temporary epicardial pacing wires are routinely placed, and pacing is initiated if the native rhythm does not promptly return. The left heart vent is removed before initiating ventilation to avoid entrainment air. Transesophageal echocardiography is then used to evaluate for the presence of air in the left heart as ventilation is restarted. If air is present, the vent site in the ascending aorta is kept open to evacuate it. Once the heart is confidently de-aired and the patient has returned to normothermia, the team agrees to wean from CPB. The perfusionist steadily reduces pump flow and venous return until the pump is fully off and the venous line is fully clamped. The patient's heart and lungs return to their native support roles at this point. Transesophageal, or in some cases epicardial, echocardiography is used to assess the adequacy of the repair. If the repair is deemed successful, a protamine dose, calculated by a heparin-protamine titration (discussed earlier in "Anticoagulation"), is administered. The cannulae are removed, and the purse strings are tied down. Adequate reversal of heparin is verified by measuring the ACT and heparin-protamine titration.

Key References

3. Lewis FJ, Varco RL, Taufic M. Repair of atrial septal defects in man under direct vision with the aid of hypothermia. *Surgery.* 1954;36:538-556.
4. Lewis FJ, Taufic M, Varco RL, Niazi S. The surgical anatomy of atrial septal defects: experiences with repair under direct vision. *Ann Surg.* 1955;142:401-415.
7. Miller BJ, Gibbon JH, Fineberg C. An improved mechanical heart and lung apparatus; its use during open cardiotomy in experimental animals. *Med Clin North Am.* 1953;1:1603-1624.
9. Dennis C, Spreng DS Jr, Nelson GE, et al. Development of a pump-oxygenator to replace the heart and lungs; an apparatus applicable to human patients, and application to one case. *Ann Surg.* 1951;134:709-721.
10. Dodrill FD, Hill E, Gerisch RA, Johnson A. Pulmonary valvuloplasty under direct vision using the mechanical heart for a complete by-pass of the right heart in a patient with congenital pulmonary stenosis. *J Thorac Surg.* 1953;26:584-594, discussion 195-197.
11. Helmsworth JA, Clark LC Jr, Kaplan S, Sherman RT. An oxygenator-pump for use in total by-pass of heart and lungs; laboratory evaluation and clinical use. *J Thorac Surg.* 1953;26:617-631, discussion 31-32.
12. Mustard WT. Heart pump and oxygenator. *Pediatrics.* 1957;19:1124-1128.
18. Kulat B, Zingle N. Optimizing circuit design using a remote-mounted perfusion system. *J Extra Corpor Technol.* 2009;41:28-31.
22. Barrett CS, Thiagarajan RR. Centrifugal pump circuits for neonatal extracorporeal membrane oxygenation. *Pediatr Crit Care Med.* 2012;13:492-493.
23. Lawson S, Ellis C, Butler K, et al. Neonatal extracorporeal membrane oxygenation devices, techniques and team roles: 2011 survey results of the United States' Extracorporeal Life Support Organization centers. *J Extra Corpor Technol.* 2011;43:236-244.
24. Meyer AD, Wiles AA, Rivera O, et al. Hemolytic and thrombocytopathic characteristics of extracorporeal membrane oxygenation systems at simulated flow rate for neonates. *Pediatr Crit Care Med.* 2012;13:e255-e261.
25. Hewitt RL, Creech O Jr. History of the pump oxygenator. *Arch Surg.* 1966;93:680-696.
28. Gaylor JD. Membrane oxygenators: current developments in design and application. *J Biomed Eng.* 1988;10:541-547.
29. Crockett J, Grey P. The Variable Prime Cobe Membrane Lung: first impressions. *Perfusion.* 1987;2:205-212.
30. Lawson DS, Smigla GR, McRobb CM, et al. A clinical evaluation of the Dideco Kids D100 neonatal oxygenator. *Perfusion.* 2008;23:39-42.
32. Albes JM, Stöhr IM, Kaluza M, et al. Physiological coagulation can be maintained in extracorporeal circulation by means of shed blood separation and coating. *J Thorac Cardiovasc Surg.* 2003;126:1504-1512.
37. Martindale SJ, Shayevitz JR, D'Errico C. The activated coagulation time: suitability for monitoring heparin effect and neutralization during pediatric cardiac surgery. *J Cardiothorac Vasc Anesth.* 1996;10:458-463.
38. D'Errico C, Shayevitz JR, Martindale SJ. Age-related differences in heparin sensitivity and heparin-protamine interactions in cardiac surgery patients. *J Cardiothorac Vasc Anesth.* 1996;10:451-457.
41. Koster A, Fischer T, Praus M, et al. Hemostatic activation and inflammatory response during cardiopulmonary bypass: impact of heparin management. *Anesthesiology.* 2002;97:837-841.
42. Bolling K, Kronon M, Allen BS, et al. Myocardial protection in normal and hypoxically stressed neonatal hearts: the superiority of hypocalcemic versus normocalcemic blood cardioplegia. *J Thorac Cardiovasc Surg.* 1996;112:1193-1200, discussion 200-201.

49. Mittnacht AJ. Near infrared spectroscopy in children at high risk of low perfusion. *Curr Opin Anaesthesiol.* 2010;23:342-347.
51. Yoshitani K, Ohnishi Y. The clinical validity of the absolute value of near infrared spectroscopy. *J Anesth.* 2008;22:502-504.
56. Kipps AK, Wypij D, Thiagarajan RR, et al. Blood transfusion is associated with prolonged duration of mechanical ventilation in infants undergoing reparative cardiac surgery. *Pediatr Crit Care Med.* 2011;12:52-56.
58. Whitney G, Daves S, Hughes A, et al. Implementation of a transfusion algorithm to reduce blood product utilization in pediatric cardiac surgery. *Paediatr Anaesth.* 2013;23:639-646.
59. Jonas RA, Wypij D, Roth SJ, et al. The influence of hemodilution on outcome after hypothermic cardiopulmonary bypass: results of a randomized trial in infants. *J Thorac Cardiovasc Surg.* 2003;126:1765-1774.
65. Algra SO, Kornmann VN, van der Tweel I, et al. Increasing duration of circulatory arrest, but not antegrade cerebral perfusion, prolongs postoperative recovery after neonatal cardiac surgery. *J Thorac Cardiovasc Surg.* 2012;143:375-382.
66. Misfeld M, Leontyev S, Borger MA, et al. What is the best strategy for brain protection in patients undergoing aortic arch surgery? A single center experience of 636 patients. *Ann Thorac Surg.* 2012;93:1502-1508.
67. Algra SO, Schouten AN, van Oeveren W, et al. Low-flow antegrade cerebral perfusion attenuates early renal and intestinal injury during neonatal aortic arch reconstruction. *J Thorac Cardiovasc Surg.* 2012;144:1323-1328, 8.e1-2.
70. Zierer A, El-Sayed Ahmad A, Papadopoulos N, et al. Selective antegrade cerebral perfusion and mild (28°C–30°C) systemic hypothermic circulatory arrest for aortic arch replacement: results from 1002 patients. *J Thorac Cardiovasc Surg.* 2012;144:1042-1049.
71. Murkin JM, Farrar JK, Tweed WA, et al. Cerebral autoregulation and flow/metabolism coupling during cardiopulmonary bypass: the influence of PaCO$_2$. *Anesth Analg.* 1987;66:825-832.
73. Melrose DG, Dreyer B, Bentall HH, Baker JB. Elective cardiac arrest. *Lancet.* 1955;269:21-22.
75. Follette DM, Mulder DG, Maloney JV, Buckberg GD. Advantages of blood cardioplegia over continuous coronary perfusion or intermittent ischemia. Experimental and clinical study. *J Thorac Cardiovasc Surg.* 1978;76:604-619.
76. Barner HB. Blood cardioplegia: a review and comparison with crystalloid cardioplegia. *Ann Thorac Surg.* 1991;52:1354-1367.
77. Bartels C, Gerdes A, Babin-Ebell J, et al. Cardiopulmonary bypass: evidence or experience based? *J Thorac Cardiovasc Surg.* 2002;124:20-27.
80. Matte GS, del Nido PJ. History and use of del Nido cardioplegia solution at Boston Children's Hospital. *J Extra Corpor Technol.* 2012;44:98-103.
82. Allen BS, Barth MJ, Ilbawi MN. Pediatric myocardial protection: an overview. *Semin Thorac Cardiovasc Surg.* 2001;13:56-72.
83. Butler J, Rocker GM, Westaby S. Inflammatory response to cardiopulmonary bypass. *Ann Thorac Surg.* 1993;55:552-559.
85. Wan S, LeClerc JL, Vincent JL. Inflammatory response to cardiopulmonary bypass: mechanisms involved and possible therapeutic strategies. *Chest.* 1997;112:676-692.
87. Hovels-Gurich HH, Vazquez-Jimenez JF, Silvestri A, et al. Production of proinflammatory cytokines and myocardial dysfunction after arterial switch operation in neonates with transposition of the great arteries. *J Thorac Cardiovasc Surg.* 2002;124:811-820.
88. Appachi E, Mossad E, Mee RB, Bokesch P. Perioperative serum interleukins in neonates with hypoplastic left-heart syndrome and transposition of the great arteries. *J Cardiothorac Vasc Anesth.* 2007;21:184-190.
89. Graham EM, Atz AM, McHugh KE, et al. Preoperative steroid treatment does not improve markers of inflammation after cardiac surgery in neonates: results from a randomized trial. *J Thorac Cardiovasc Surg.* 2014;147:902-908.
90. Scrascia G, Rotunno C, Guida P, et al. Perioperative steroids administration in pediatric cardiac surgery: a meta-analysis of randomized controlled trials*. *Pediatr Crit Care Med.* 2014;15:435-442.
91. Heying R, Wehage E, Schumacher K, et al. Dexamethasone pretreatment provides antiinflammatory and myocardial protection in neonatal arterial switch operation. *Ann Thorac Surg.* 2012;93:869-876.
92. Keski-Nisula J, Pesonen E, Olkkola KT, et al. Methylprednisolone in neonatal cardiac surgery: reduced inflammation without improved clinical outcome. *Ann Thorac Surg.* 2013;95:2126-2132.
94. Darling E, Searles B, Nasrallah F, et al. High-volume, zero balanced ultrafiltration improves pulmonary function in a model of post-pump syndrome. *J Extra Corpor Technol.* 2002;34:254-259.
96. Sever K, Tansel T, Basaran M, et al. The benefits of continuous ultrafiltration in pediatric cardiac surgery. *Scand Cardiovasc J.* 2004;38:307-311.
97. Song LO, Yinglong LI, Jinping LI. Effects of zero-balanced ultrafiltration on procalcitonin and respiratory function after cardiopulmonary bypass. *Perfusion.* 2007;22:339.

Critical Care After Surgery for Congenital Cardiac Disease

V. Ben Sivarajan and Alexandre T. Rotta

PEARLS

- The neonatal myocardium is less compliant than that of the older child, is less tolerant of increases in afterload, and is less responsive to increases in preload.
- Echocardiography is the preferred imaging modality for the assessment and delineation of intracardiac anatomic features before surgery in children. Accurate anatomic diagnosis is now routine, so most children can have surgery without preoperative cardiac catheterization.
- A predictable decrease in cardiac index typically occurs 6 to 12 hours after separation from cardiopulmonary bypass.
- Milrinone administered during the early postoperative period plays a significant role in decreasing the likelihood of low cardiac output syndrome.
- Patients with postoperative low cardiac output require an extensive evaluation for unanticipated residual lesions, as this is more likely to be the case than the classical low cardiac output syndrome.
- Patients with restrictive physiology from hypertrophy and diastolic dysfunction of the right ventricle, such as those after tetralogy of Fallot repair, require high right-sided filling pressures to achieve adequate cardiac output. Consequently, these patients are more prone to hepatic congestion, anasarca, pleural effusions, and ascites.
- Inhaled nitric oxide plays an important role in the management of postoperative pulmonary hypertension in the cardiac intensive care unit. It is particularly effective in the postoperative course of patients with venous hypertensive disorders, such as total anomalous pulmonary venous connection, once mechanical obstruction is relieved.
- Hyperglycemia is a frequent occurrence in the cardiac intensive care unit and has been associated with increased morbidity and mortality during the postoperative period. However, tight glycemic control has not been shown to improve outcomes in pediatric patients after cardiac surgery. In addition, the risks of significant hypoglycemia and its long-term attendant sequelae are greater in patients managed with a singular focus on tight glycemic control.
- Hypoxemia after bidirectional cavopulmonary anastomosis generally is a sign of decreased cardiac output, is poorly responsive to nitric oxide, and tends to improve with maneuvers that increase venous return through the superior vena cava, such as head elevation and controlled hypoventilation/mild hypercapnia.

- Liberation from positive pressure mechanical ventilation should be accomplished as soon as feasible in patients after a Fontan operation because spontaneous breathing improves pulmonary blood flow, arterial oxygen saturation, and ventricular preload.
- Ventricular ectopy and elevated atrial pressures after the arterial switch operation should raise suspicion of myocardial ischemia from insufficient coronary blood flow.
- Postoperative care of the patient with hypoplastic left heart syndrome after stage I palliation (Norwood procedure) requires adequate balancing of the pulmonary and systemic blood flows. A high arterial oxygen saturation denotes excessive pulmonary blood flow and is generally accompanied by decreased systemic blood flow, acidosis, and end-organ dysfunction.

Introduction

Congenital anomalies account for the largest diagnostic category among causes of infant mortality in the United States.[1] Structural heart disease leads the list of congenital malformations. Of the more than 4 million children born each year in the United States, nearly 40,000 have some form of congenital heart disease (CHD). Approximately half of these children appear for therapeutic intervention within the first year of life, and the majority of them require critical care expertise. Patients with congenital or acquired heart disease compose a major diagnostic category for admissions in large pediatric intensive care units (ICUs) across the country, representing 30% to 40% or more of ICU admissions in many centers.

Neonatal Considerations

Care of the critically ill neonate requires an appreciation of the special structural and functional features of immature organs, the interactions of the *transitional* neonatal circulation, and the secondary effects of the congenital heart lesion on other organ systems.[2-4] The neonate responds more quickly and profoundly to physiologically stressful circumstances, such as rapid changes in pH, lactic acid, blood glucose, and temperature. Neonates have diminished fat and carbohydrate reserves compared to older children. The higher metabolic rate and oxygen consumption of the neonate play a significant role in the rapid onset of hypoxemia when these patients become apneic. Immaturity of the liver and kidney may be associated with reduced protein synthesis and glomerular filtration such that drug metabolism is altered and hepatic synthetic function is reduced. These issues may be compounded by the normal increased total body water of the neonate compared with the older patient, along with the propensity for capillary leakage. This is especially prominent in the lung of the neonate in whom the pulmonary vascular bed is nearly fully recruited at rest and lymphatic recruitment required to handle increased mean capillary pressures associated with increases in pulmonary blood flow may be unavailable.[4] The neonatal myocardium is less compliant than that of the older child, is less tolerant of increases in afterload, and is less responsive to increases in preload. Younger age also predisposes the myocardium to the adverse effects of cardiopulmonary bypass (CPB) and hypothermic ischemia implicit in support techniques used during cardiac surgery. These factors do not preclude intervention in the neonate but simply dictate that extraordinary vigilance be applied to the care of these children and that intensive care management plans account for the immature physiology.

The observed benefits of neonatal reparative operations in patients with two ventricles are numerous (Box 38.1). They continue to dictate that care of the newborn with complex CHD after CPB be a central feature of cardiac intensive care. Elimination of cyanosis and congestive heart failure (CHF) early in life optimizes conditions for normal growth and development. Palliative procedures such as pulmonary artery banding and creation of systemic-to-pulmonary artery shunts do not fully address cyanosis or CHF and may introduce their own set of physiologic and anatomic complications. Examples of improved outcomes with a single reparative operation rather than staged palliation as a newborn are well known and evoke little controversy. Approaches that have been abandoned include banding the pulmonary arteries in truncus arteriosus,[5] staging repair of type B interrupted aortic arch (IAA),[6] and staging repair of transposition of the great arteries with IAA.[7] In other conditions (eg, severely cyanotic newborn with tetralogy of Fallot [TOF]), the risks and benefits of neonatal repair versus a palliative shunt are debatable.[8]

Whereas the neonate may be more labile than the older child, there is ample evidence that this age group is more resilient in its response to metabolic or ischemic injury. In fact, the neonate may be particularly capable of coping with some forms of stress. Tolerance of hypoxemia in the neonate is characteristic of many species,[9] and the plasticity of the neurologic system in the neonate is well known.[10] It is the rule

rather than the exception that neonates presenting with shock secondary to obstructive left heart lesions can be effectively resuscitated without persistent organ system impairment. The pliability and mobility of vascular structures in the neonate improve the technical aspects of surgery. Reparative operations in neonates take advantage of normal postnatal changes, allowing more normal growth and development in crucial areas such as myocardial muscle, pulmonary parenchyma, and coronary and pulmonary angiogenesis.

Postoperative pulmonary hypertensive events are more common in the infant who has been exposed to weeks or months of high pulmonary pressure and flow.[5] This is especially true for such lesions as truncus arteriosus, complete atrioventricular (AV) canal defects, and transposition of the great arteries (TGA) with ventricular septal defects (VSDs). Finally, cognitive and psychomotor abnormalities associated with months of hypoxemia or abnormal hemodynamics may be diminished or eliminated by early repair. However, if early reparative surgery results in more exposures to CPB (eg, repeated conduit changes) and associated adverse effects on cognitive or motor function, then the risk-to-benefit assessment must be modified accordingly.

Preoperative Care

Optimal preoperative care involves (1) initial stabilization, airway management, and establishment of adequate vascular access; (2) complete and thorough noninvasive delineation of the anatomic defect(s); (3) initiation/termination of prostaglandin therapy, as appropriate; (4) evaluation and treatment of secondary organ dysfunction, particularly the brain, kidneys, and liver; and (5) cardiac catheterization if necessary, typically for (a) physiologic assessment, (b) interventional procedures such as balloon atrial septostomy or valvotomy, or (c) anatomic definition not visible by echocardiography (eg, coronary artery distribution in pulmonary atresia with intact ventricular septum or delineation of aorticopulmonary collaterals in TOF with pulmonary atresia).

Physical Examination and Laboratory Data

Detailed history and physical examination are required, with focus on the extent of cardiopulmonary impairment, airway abnormalities, and associated extracardiac congenital anomalies.[11] Intrathoracic and extrathoracic airway problems in patients with Down syndrome, disorders of calcium homeostasis and immunologic deficiencies in patients with aortic arch abnormalities, and renal abnormalities in patients with esophageal atresia and CHD are a few of the associated conditions with which the anesthesiologist should be familiar. Intercurrent pulmonary infection is a common and significant finding in chronically overcirculated lungs. The presence, degree, and duration of hypoxemia are important details that, in the absence of iron deficiency, are reflected in the hematocrit. The nadir of physiologic anemia during infancy may contribute to left-to-right shunting by decreasing the relative pulmonary vascular resistance (PVR).[12]

Chest radiography can be used to assess heart size, pulmonary vascular congestion, airway compression, and areas of consolidation or atelectasis. The electrocardiogram (ECG) may reveal rhythm disturbances and demonstrate ventricular strain patterns (ST and T-wave changes) characteristic of unphysiologic pressure or volume burdens on the ventricles.

BOX 38.1 Advantage of Neonatal Repair

Early elimination of cyanosis
Early elimination of congestive heart failure
Optimal circulation for growth and development
Reduced anatomic distortion from palliative procedures
Reduced hospital admissions while awaiting repair
Reduced parental anxiety while awaiting repair

Electrolyte abnormalities caused by CHF and forced diuresis also must be evaluated preoperatively, as severe hypochloremic metabolic alkalosis may occur in some patients. It is important to discontinue digoxin preoperatively and to avoid hyperventilation and administration of calcium to these patients during induction of anesthesia, as the alkalotic hypokalemic, hypercalcemic, hypotensive, dilated, digoxin-bound myocardium fibrillates with ease.

Echocardiographic and Doppler Assessment

Advances in echocardiographic imaging have had an enormous impact on the diagnosis of CHD.[13] Accurate anatomic diagnosis now is routine in children without the need for cardiac catheterization. Echocardiography is the preferred imaging modality for the assessment of intracardiac anatomic features in young children. However, one should be aware of the current limitations of echocardiographic and Doppler techniques so that alternative diagnoses can be considered when intraoperative or postoperative findings are inconsistent with the working echocardiographic diagnosis.

Echocardiography can reliably determine atrioventricular and ventricular arterial alignment and the presence and location of intracardiac and great artery level shunts. Color Doppler is useful for estimating pressure gradients across discrete narrowings, such as septal defects and valves. It can also reliably estimate right ventricular systolic pressure, provided sufficient tricuspid regurgitation is present. Echocardiography is unreliable for imaging distal pulmonary artery stenosis and assessing gradients across long segments, such as a narrowed right ventricular to pulmonary artery conduit. Grading of AV valve regurgitation may be subjective and nonquantitative. Accuracy of transthoracic echocardiography can be limited by inadequate imaging windows in obese patients, older children, and some postoperative patients. The use of transesophageal or epicardial echocardiography in these patients can be helpful. In addition, selective use of three-dimensional echocardiography may improve diagnostic capabilities, such as defining the mechanism of valve regurgitation or visualization of complex anatomic features. As good as echocardiographic diagnosis of anatomic defects and Doppler measurements of pressure gradients and valve function have become, the standard for assessment of physiology when other clinical information is ambiguous or contradictory remains cardiac catheterization.

Cardiac Catheterization

When echocardiographic analysis with Doppler measurements and color flow mapping is complete and unambiguous, cardiac catheterization generally is not required in the preoperative assessment. Catheterization typically is not performed before infant or neonatal operations for VSDs, complete AV canal defects, TOF, TGA, IAA, hypoplastic left heart syndrome (HLHS), or coarctation of the aorta. However, in older patients with complex anatomy, such as a single ventricle, physiologic data from catheterization may be essential. This technique allows description of the direction, magnitude, and approximate location of intracardiac shunts. Intracardiac and intravascular pressures are measured to determine the presence of obstructions and whether shunt orifices are restrictive or nonrestrictive. Pressure gradients across sites of obstruction must be considered in light of simultaneous blood flow; a small pressure gradient measured at a time of low cardiac output is misleading.

Normal intracardiac pressure and saturation values in children are described in Chapter 32. In the normal heart, blood in the pulmonary artery (PA) represents complete mixing of the systemic venous return; thus sampling of PA blood yields the true mixed venous oxygen saturation. It is possible to have small step-ups in oxygen saturation sequentially from the superior vena cava (SVC) to the PA in the absence of significant left-to-right shunts due to sampling bias (streaming). In the child with CHD, the SVC gives the best indication of true mixed venous oxygen saturation; a 5% or greater step-up in saturation downstream suggests the presence of a left-to-right shunt.[14] It would occur at the level of the right atrium with an atrial septal defect (ASD), in the right ventricle with a VSD, and in the pulmonary artery with a patent ductus arteriosus (PDA). The magnitude of the left-to-right shunt can be calculated from the Fick equation. The frequently used term Qp/Qs (pulmonary-to-systemic blood flow ratio) can be derived simply from the measured oxygen saturation values.

The patient whose aortic blood is fully saturated can be safely assumed to have no significant intracardiac right-to-left shunting. However, when an intracardiac right-to-left shunt is present, aortic blood is hypoxemic. In this situation, blood samples should also be obtained from the pulmonary veins, left atrium, and left ventricle for oxygen saturation determination and ascertainment of the source of desaturated blood. Pulmonary venous desaturation implies a pulmonary source of venous admixture (eg, pneumonia, atelectasis, or other pulmonary disease). Intrapulmonary shunting may substantially alter the anesthetic plan and the postoperative ventilatory requirements of the patient.

In the presence of a left-to-right shunt and elevated PVR, pressure and saturation measurements often are repeated with the patient breathing 100% oxygen to assess both the reactivity of the pulmonary vascular bed and any contribution of ventilation-perfusion abnormalities to hypoxemia. If breathing 100% oxygen increases pulmonary blood flow and dramatically increases Qp/Qs (with a fall in PVR), potentially reversible processes such as hypoxic pulmonary vasoconstriction likely are contributing to the elevated PVR. The patient with a high, unresponsive PVR and a small left-to-right shunt despite a large shunt orifice may have extensive and irreversible obstructive pulmonary vascular disease. If so, surgical repair usually is contraindicated if the child is older than 1 year.[15]

During cardiac catheterization, anatomic abnormalities are identified angiographically. Special angled views provide specific information about the location and extent of congenital defects.[16] Ventricular function is assessed angiographically and physiologically (eg, by pressure measurements). The calculated size of a cardiac chamber may have important bearing on its ability to support the circulation of a child with a hypoplastic ventricle.

Magnetic Resonance Imaging and Angiography

Magnetic resonance imaging (MRI) and magnetic resonance angiography (MRA) have emerged as important diagnostic modalities in the evaluation of the cardiovascular system following the development of ECG-gated MRI. Image acquisition is synchronized to the patient's ECG to counter motion artifacts and to acquire cine sequences that allow detailed imaging of cardiac structures and visualization of blood flow throughout the cardiac cycle. In addition to providing excellent anatomic and three-dimensional images, particularly of the pulmonary veins and thoracic aorta, it also is possible with MRA to qualitatively assess valve and ventricular function and to quantify flow, ventricular volume, mass, and ejection fraction.[17,18] Whereas ferromagnetic implants near the region of interest might produce artifact, sternal wires and vascular clips produce relatively minor disturbances; therefore MRI generally can be performed in patients who have undergone previous cardiac surgery. Contraindications include patients with pacemakers, recently placed endovascular or intracardiac implants, and aneurysm clips on vessels that will be exposed directly to the magnetic field.

Assessment of Patient Status and Predominant Pathophysiology

Congenital heart defects can be complex and difficult to categorize or conceptualize. Rather than trying to determine the management for each individual anatomic defect, a physiologic approach can be taken. The following questions should be asked:

1. How does the systemic venous return reach the systemic arterial circulation to maintain cardiac output?
2. What, if any, intracardiac mixing, shunting, or outflow obstruction exists?
3. Is the circulation in series or parallel?
4. Are the defects amenable to a two-ventricle or single-ventricle repair?
5. Is pulmonary blood flow increased or decreased?
6. Is there a volume load or pressure load on the ventricles?

Appropriate organization of preoperative data, patient preparation, and decisions about monitoring, anesthetic agents, and postoperative care are best accomplished by focusing on a few major pathophysiologic problems, beginning with whether the patient is cyanotic, is in CHF, or both. Most pathophysiologic mechanisms that are pertinent to optimal patient preparation and to the perioperative plan focus on one of the following major problems: severe hypoxemia, excessive pulmonary blood flow, CHF, obstruction of blood flow from the left heart, and poor ventricular function. Although some patients with congenital heart disease present with only one of these problems, many have multiple interrelated issues.

Severe Hypoxemia

In the first few days of life, many of the cyanotic forms of CHD present with severe hypoxemia (PaO_2 <50 mm Hg) in the absence of respiratory distress. Infusion of prostaglandin E_1 (PGE_1) in patients with decreased pulmonary blood flow maintains or reestablishes pulmonary flow through the ductus arteriosus. This may also improve mixing of venous and arterial blood at the atrial level in patients with transposition of the great arteries.[19] Consequently, neonates rarely require surgery while they are severely hypoxemic. During preoperative stabilization with PGE_1, neurologic examination and blood chemistry analysis of renal, hepatic, and hematologic function are necessary to assess the effects of severe hypoxemia during or after birth on end-organ dysfunction.

PGE_1 dilates the ductus arteriosus of the neonate with life-threatening ductus-dependent cardiac lesions and improves the patient's condition before surgery. PGE_1 can reopen a functionally closed ductus arteriosus even several days after birth, or it can maintain patency of the ductus arteriosus for several months postnatally.[19,20] The common side effects of

PGE_1 infusion—apnea, hypotension, fever, central nervous system (CNS) excitation—are easily managed in the neonate when normal therapeutic doses of the drug (0.01–0.05 mcg/kg/min) are used.[21] However, PGE_1 is a potent vasodilator, so intravascular volume frequently requires augmentation. Patients with intermittent apnea resulting from administration of PGE_1 may require mechanical ventilation preoperatively; although apnea can resolve with the concomitant administration of aminophylline or caffeine.[22] PGE_1 usually improves the arterial oxygenation of hypoxemic neonates who have poor pulmonary perfusion as a result of obstructed pulmonary flow (critical pulmonic stenosis or pulmonary atresia) by providing pulmonary blood flow from the aorta via the ductus arteriosus. The improved oxygenation reverses the lactic acidosis that often develops during episodes of severe hypoxia. PGE_1 administration usually markedly improves the condition of a severely hypoxemic neonate with restricted pulmonary blood flow over minutes to hours.[23]

Excessive Pulmonary Blood Flow

Excessive pulmonary blood flow is frequently the primary problem of patients with CHD. The intensivist must carefully evaluate the hemodynamic and respiratory impact of left-to-right shunts and the extent to which it contributes to the perioperative course in the ICU. Children with left-to-right shunts may have chronic low-grade pulmonary infection and congestion that cannot be eliminated despite optimal preoperative preparation. If so, surgery should not be postponed further. Respiratory syncytial viral infections are particularly prevalent in this population, but advances in intensive care have markedly improved outcomes with this and other viral pneumonias.[24]

Aside from the respiratory impairment caused by increased pulmonary blood flow, the left heart must dilate to accept pulmonary venous return that might be several times normal. If the body requires more systemic blood flow, the heart responds inefficiently. Most of the increment in cardiac output is recirculated to the lungs. Eventually, symptoms of CHF appear. In the most severe cases, the evaluation reveals a severely malnourished child who is tachypneic, tachycardic, and dusky in room air. The child may have intercostal and substernal retractions and skin that is cool to the touch. Capillary refill may be prolonged. Expiratory wheezes usually are audible. Medical management with inotropes, systemic vasodilators, and diuretics may improve the patient's condition, but the diuretics may induce profound hypochloremic alkalosis and potassium depletion that often persist after surgery.

Obstruction of Left Heart Outflow

Patients who require surgery to relieve obstruction to outflow from the left heart are among the most critically ill children for whom the intensivist must care. These lesions include interruption of the aortic arch, coarctation of the aorta, aortic stenosis (AS), and mitral stenosis or atresia as part of the HLHS spectrum. These neonates present with inadequate systemic perfusion and profound metabolic acidosis. The initial pH may be below 7 despite a low $PaCO_2$. Systemic blood flow is largely or completely dependent on blood flow into the aorta from the ductus arteriosus.

Ductal closure in these neonates causes dramatic worsening of the patient's condition. The patient suddenly becomes critically ill and survival requires PGE_1 infusion to allow blood flow into the aorta from the pulmonary artery.[23,25] PGE$_1$ infusion improves perfusion and metabolism in neonates with acidosis, metabolic derangements, and renal failure because of inadequate systemic perfusion, so surgery generally can be deferred until stability is achieved. Ventilatory and inotropic support and correction of metabolic acidosis, along with calcium, glucose, and electrolyte abnormalities, should occur preoperatively. This stabilization period also allows assessment of the magnitude of end-organ dysfunction caused by the preceding period of inadequate systemic perfusion. Adequacy of stabilization, rather than severity of illness at presentation, appears to influence postoperative outcome the most.[26]

Ventricular Dysfunction

Ideally, the intensivist should participate in the preoperative care of all patients who are expected to recover in the ICU after surgery. Understanding the extent of ventricular dysfunction preoperatively provides considerable insight into intraoperative and postoperative events. Although patients with large shunts may have complete mixing but only mild-to-moderate hypoxemia as a result of their excessive pulmonary blood flow, the price paid for near-normal arterial oxygen saturation is chronic ventricular dilation and dysfunction and pulmonary vascular obstructive disease. Consequently, reducing the shunt fraction or using a staged approach to single-ventricle repair may be indicated. Older patients with CHD and poor ventricular function as a result of chronic ventricular volume overload (aortic or mitral valve regurgitation or long-standing pulmonary-to-systemic arterial shunts) present a different challenge, mitigated to some extent by afterload reduction. However, in all of these circumstances in hearts with chronic volume overload, there is a propensity for ventricular fibrillation during sedation, anesthesia, or intubation of the airway.

Assessment should include an estimation of the patient's functional limitation as an indicator of myocardial performance and reserve, quantification of the degree of hypoxia and amount of pulmonary blood flow, and evaluation of PVR. For patients with increased Qp/Qs, systemic blood flow should be optimized without further augmenting pulmonary flow during induction of anesthesia in the ICU or in the operating room. However, during maintenance and emergence from anesthesia, retraction of the lung, positional changes, and abdominal distension may increase the hypoxemia and compromise the function of a dilated, poorly contractile ventricle. If this sequence occurs during surgery, the management must be altered to improve pulmonary blood flow.

Postoperative Care

Assessment

When the clinical course of patients after cardiac surgery deviates from the usual expectation of uncomplicated recovery, our first responsibility is to verify the accuracy of the preoperative diagnosis and the adequacy of surgical repair. For example, a young infant who is acidotic, hypotensive, and cyanotic after surgical repair of TOF may tempt us to ascribe these findings to the vagaries of ischemia/reperfusion injury of CPB or transient, postoperative stiffness of the right ventricle. However, the real culprit may be an additional VSD undetected preoperatively and therefore not closed, a residual

---

BOX 38.2 | Ten Intensive Care Strategies to Diagnose and Support Low Cardiac Output States

1. Know in detail the cardiac anatomy and its physiologic consequences.
2. Understand the specialized considerations of the newborn and implications of reparative rather than palliative surgery.
3. Diversify personnel to include experts in neonatal and adult congenital heart disease.
4. Monitor, measure, and image the heart to rule out residual disease as a cause of postoperative hemodynamic instability or low cardiac output.
5. Maintain aortic perfusion and improve the contractile state.
6. Optimize preload (including atrial shunting).
7. Reduce afterload.
8. Control heart rate, rhythm, and synchrony.
9. Optimize heart lung interactions.
10. Provide mechanical support when needed.

VSD around the surgical patch, or residual right ventricle (RV) outflow obstruction. Getting the right postoperative assessment is imperative and treatment follows accordingly. Evaluation of the postoperative patient relies on examination, monitoring, interpretation of vital signs, and imaging. Only once the accuracy of the diagnosis and adequacy of the repair are established can a low cardiac output state be presumed and treatment optimized. Treating low cardiac output states and preventing cardiovascular collapse often are the central features of pediatric cardiac intensive care and are the focus of this chapter (Box 38.2). The details of the specific considerations for selected lesions are presented in their respective sections.

Optimizing preload involves more than just giving volume to a hypotensive patient. There are numerous considerations to fluid balance involving types of isotonic fluid, ultrafiltration in the operating room, optimal hematocrit, and the use of diuretics or vasopressors. Fluid itself can be detrimental if excess extravascular water results in interstitial edema and end-organ dysfunction of vital organs such as the heart, lungs, and brain. Occasionally, permitting a right-to-left shunt at the atrial level can optimize preload to the left ventricle in some conditions (discussed later). Maintaining aortic perfusion after CPB and improving the contractile state of the heart with higher doses of catecholamines are reasonable goals, but they may have particularly deleterious consequences in the newborn myocardium after hypothermic CPB. The benefits of afterload reduction are well known but, if excessive, may result in hypotension, coronary insufficiency, and cardiovascular collapse. Pacing the heart can stabilize the rhythm and hemodynamics, but it also may contribute to dyssynchronous, inefficient cardiac contraction or induce other arrhythmias. Although lifesaving in many instances, mechanical support of the failing myocardium in the form of extracorporeal life support (ECLS) or ventricular assist devices has its own set of limitations and morbidities. Almost every treatment approach has its own set of adverse effects. Supporting cardiac output in the postoperative patient is a balance between the promise and poison of therapy.

The initial assessment following cardiac surgery begins with review of the operative findings. This includes details of the operative repair and CPB, particularly total CPB or myocardial ischemic (aortic cross-clamp) times; concerns about myocardial protection; recovery of myocardial contractility; typical

<table>
<tr><td colspan="2">

BOX 38.3　Signs of Heart Failure or Low Cardiac Output States

</td></tr>
</table>

Signs
Cool extremities/poor perfusion
Oliguria and other end-organ failure
Tachycardia
Hypotension
Acidosis
Cardiomegaly
Pleural effusions

Monitor and Assess
Heart rate, blood pressure, intracardiac pressure
Extremity temperature, central temperature
Urine output
Mixed venous oxygen saturation
Arterial blood gas pH and lactate
Laboratory measures of end-organ function
Echocardiography

BOX 38.4　Common Causes of Elevated Left Atrial Pressure After Cardiopulmonary Bypass

1. Decreased ventricular systolic or diastolic function
2. Left atrioventricular valve disease
3. Large left-to-right intracardiac shunt
4. Chamber hypoplasia
5. Intravascular or ventricular volume overload
6. Cardiac tamponade
7. Arrhythmia

TABLE 38.1　Causes of Abnormal Right Atrial, Left Atrial, or Pulmonary Artery Oxygen Saturation

Location	Elevated	Reduced
RA	Atrial level left-to-right shunt	↑ Vo_2 (eg, low CO, fever)
	Anomalous pulmonary venous return	↓ Sao_2 saturation with a normal A-V O_2 difference
	Left ventricular-to-right atrial shunt	Anemia
	↑ Dissolved O_2 content ↓ O_2 extraction	Catheter tip position (eg, near CS)
	Catheter tip position (eg, near renal veins)	
LA	Does not occur	Atrial level right-to-left shunt
		↓ Pvo_2 (eg, parenchymal lung disease)
PA	Significant left-to-right shunt	↑ O_2 extraction (eg, low CO, fever)
	Small left-to-right shunt with incomplete mixing of blood	Sao_2 saturation with a normal A-V O_2 difference
	Catheter tip position (eg, PA "wedge")	Anemia

A-V, arteriovenous; *CO,* cardiac output; *CS,* coronary sinus; *LA,* left atrium; *PA,* pulmonary artery; *Pvo₂,* pulmonary vein oxygen tension; *RA,* right atrium; *Sao₂,* arterial oxygen saturation; *Vo₂,* oxygen consumption.

postoperative systemic arterial and central venous pressures; findings from intraoperative transesophageal echocardiography, if performed; and vasoactive medication requirements. This information guides subsequent examination, which should focus on the quality of the repair or palliation plus clinical assessment of cardiac output (Box 38.3). In addition to a complete cardiovascular examination, a routine set of laboratory tests should be obtained, including a chest radiograph, 12- or 15-lead ECG, blood gas analysis, serum electrolytes and glucose, ionized calcium and lactate measurements, complete blood count, and coagulation profile.

Monitoring

Monitoring central venous pressure is routine for many patients following cardiac surgery, except those who undergo the least complex procedures. For example, a central venous catheter is not routinely placed for patients undergoing thoracic procedures, such as repair of aortic coarctation, division of a vascular ring, PDA ligation, or in patients undergoing cardiotomy with a short period of mildly hypothermic CPB, such as an ASD repair. Intracardiac or transthoracic left atrial (LA) catheters are often used to monitor patients after complex reparative procedures. Pulmonary arterial (PA) catheters now are seldom used but may be particularly useful if the postoperative management anticipates a problem such as pulmonary hypertension, thereby allowing rapid detection of pressure changes and assessment of the response to interventions.

Left atrial catheters are especially helpful in the management of patients with ventricular dysfunction, coronary artery perfusion abnormalities, or mitral valve disease. The mean LA pressure typically is 1 to 2 mm Hg greater than mean right atrial (RA) pressure, which generally varies between 1 and 6 mm Hg in nonpostoperative pediatric patients undergoing cardiac catheterization. In postoperative patients, mean LA and RA pressures are often greater than 6 to 8 mm Hg. However, they generally should be less than 15 mm Hg. The compliance of the right atrium is greater than that of the left atrium except in the newborn, so pressure elevations in the right atrium of older patients with two ventricles typically are less pronounced.

Possible causes of abnormally elevated LA pressure are listed in Box 38.4. In addition to pressure data, intracardiac catheters in the right atrium (or a percutaneously placed central venous catheter), left atrium, and pulmonary artery

can be used to monitor the oxygen saturation of systemic or pulmonary venous blood and indicate the presence or absence of atrioventricular synchrony.

Table 38.1 lists the causes of abnormally high or low RA, LA, and PA oxygen saturations, which can be measured at the bedside in the ICU. Following reparative surgery, patients with no intracardiac shunts and adequate cardiac output may have a mild reduction in RA oxygen saturation to approximately 60%. Lower RA oxygen saturation does not necessarily indicate low cardiac output. If a patient has arterial desaturation (common mixing lessons, lung diseases, etc.), the arteriovenous oxygen saturation difference is normally <30%. Hence even a low RA saturation may be in keeping with appropriate oxygen delivery and extraction. Elevated RA oxygen saturation often is the result of left-to-right shunting at the atrial level (eg, from the left atrium, anomalous pulmonary vein, or left ventricular [LV]-to-RA shunt). Blood in the LA normally is fully saturated with oxygen (ie, approximately 100%). The two chief causes of reduced LA oxygen saturation are an atrial level right-to-left shunt and pulmonary venous desaturation from abnormal gas exchange.

In the absence of left-to-right shunts, PA oxygen saturation is the best representation of the "true" mixed venous oxygen saturation because all sources of systemic venous blood should be thoroughly combined as they are ejected from the right ventricle. When elevated, this saturation is useful in identifying residual significant left-to-right shunts following repair of a VSD. The absolute value of the PA oxygen saturation is a predictor of significant postoperative residual shunt. In patients following TOF or VSD repair, PA oxygen saturation greater than 80% within 48 hours of surgery with a fractional inspired oxygen concentration (FIO_2) <0.5 is a sensitive indicator of significant left-to-right shunt (Qp/Qs >1.5) 1 year after surgery.[27] Determination of PA oxygen saturation also can be useful in patients with systemic-to-pulmonary artery collaterals because flow from these vessels into the pulmonary arteries can increase oxygen saturation.

Low Cardiac Output Syndrome

Although low cardiac output after CPB is often attributable to residual or undiagnosed structural lesions, progressive low cardiac output states do occur. A number of factors have been implicated in the development of myocardial dysfunction following CPB including (1) the inflammatory response associated with CPB, (2) the effects of myocardial ischemia from aortic cross-clamping, (3) hypothermia, (4) reperfusion injury, (5) inadequate myocardial protection, and (6) ventriculotomy (when performed). The typical decrease in cardiac index has been well characterized in newborns following an arterial switch operation (ASO)[28] (Fig. 38.1). In a group of 122 newborns, the median maximal decrease in cardiac index that typically occurred 6 to 12 hours after separation from CPB was 32%.[28] One-fourth of these newborns reached a nadir of

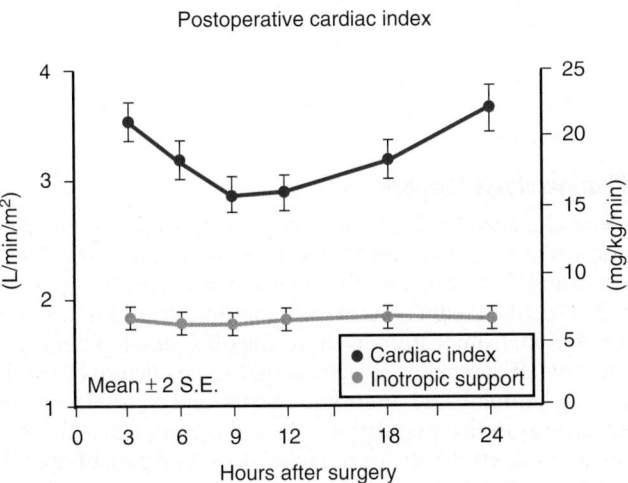

Fig. 38.1. Cardiac index (left axis) measured in infants following the arterial switch operation declined during the first 12 hours and was not the result of any reduction in inotropic support (right axis). One fourth of the patients reach a value less than 2 L/min/m². The median reduction in cardiac index the first night is 33%. (From Wernovsky G, et al. Postoperative course and hemodynamic profile after the arterial switch operation in neonates and infants: a comparison of low-flow cardiopulmonary bypass and circulatory arrest. Circulation. 1995;92: 2226-2235.)

the cardiac index that was less than 2 L/min/m².[28] Anticipation of this low cardiac output syndrome (LCOS) and appropriate intervention can do much to avert morbidity or the need for mechanical support. Mixed venous oxygen saturation, whole blood pH, and lactate are laboratory measures commonly used to evaluate the adequacy of tissue perfusion and, hence, cardiac output.

Volume Adjustments

After CPB, the factors that influence cardiac output, such as preload, afterload, myocardial contractility, heart rate, and rhythm, must be continuously assessed and manipulated as needed. Volume therapy (increased preload) is commonly necessary, followed by appropriate use of inotropic and afterload-reducing agents. Atrial pressure and the ventricular response to changes in atrial pressure must be evaluated. Ventricular response is judged by observing systemic arterial pressure and waveform, heart rate, skin color, peripheral extremity temperature, peripheral pulse magnitude, urine flow, core body temperature, and acid-base balance.

Preserving and Creating Right-to-Left Shunts

Selected children with low cardiac output may benefit from strategies that allow right-to-left shunting at the atrial level in the face of expected postoperative RV dysfunction. A typical example is early repair of TOF, when the hypertrophied and poorly compliant right ventricle may be further compromised by increased volume load from pulmonary regurgitation secondary to a transannular patch on the RV outflow tract. These children will benefit from leaving the foramen ovale patent to permit right-to-left shunting of blood, thus preserving cardiac output and oxygen delivery despite the attendant transient cyanosis. If the foramen ovale is not patent or is surgically closed, RV dysfunction can lead to reduced LV filling, low cardiac output, and ultimately LV dysfunction. In infants and neonates with repaired truncus arteriosus, the same concerns apply and may even be exaggerated if RV afterload is elevated because of pulmonary hypertension.

Other Strategies

Additional strategies to support low cardiac output associated with cardiac surgery in children include use of atrio-biventricular pacing for patients with complete heart block or prolonged interventricular conduction delays and asynchronous contraction.[29] Appreciation of the hemodynamic effects of positive and negative pressure ventilation may be used to assist cardiac output. Avoidance of hyperthermia and even induced hypothermia may provide end-organ protection during periods of low cardiac output and aid in the management of postoperative arrhythmias, such as junctional ectopic tachycardia. Antiinflammatory agents including monoclonal antibodies, competitive receptor blockers, inhibitors of compliment activation, and preoperative preparation with steroids are being actively investigated in an effort to protect major organs from ischemic injury imposed by CPB and the reperfusion injury associated with the recovery period.

Right Ventriculotomy and Restrictive Physiology

Right ventricular *restrictive* physiology has been demonstrated by echocardiography as persistent antegrade diastolic blood flow into the pulmonary circulation following reconstruction of the RV outflow in infants and children. This occurs in the setting of elevated RV end-diastolic pressure and RV hypertrophy, when the right ventricle demonstrates diastolic dysfunction with an inability to relax and fill during diastole. The poorly compliant RV usually is not dilated in this circumstance, and pulmonary valve regurgitation is limited because of the elevated RV diastolic pressure.[30,31]

The term *restrictive RV physiology* is also commonly used in the immediate postoperative period in patients who have a stiff, poorly compliant, and sometimes hypertrophied right ventricle. The elevated ventricular end-diastolic pressure restricts filling during diastole, causing an increase in right atrial filling pressure and, ultimately, systemic venous hypertension. Because of the phenomenon of ventricular interdependence, changes in RV diastolic function and septal position in turn affect LV compliance and function. Factors contributing to diastolic dysfunction include lung and myocardial edema following CPB, inadequate myocardial protection of the hypertrophied ventricle during aortic cross-clamp, coronary artery injury, residual outflow tract obstruction, volume load on the ventricle from a residual VSD or pulmonary regurgitation, and dysrhythmias. In many centers, a residual atrial communication is left to mitigate the perioperative sequelae associated with restrictive RV physiology, namely a low cardiac output state. In such a scenario, patients may be desaturated following surgery (typically 75% to 85% range) because of this right-to-left shunting, but they maintain systemic cardiac output while avoiding significant systemic venous hypertension. As RV compliance and function improve (usually within 2 to 3 postoperative days), the amount of shunt decreases and both antegrade pulmonary blood flow and SaO_2 increase.

If significant restrictive RV physiology develops in the absence of an unrestrictive atrial communication, a low cardiac output state with increased right-sided filling pressure (usually >10 mm Hg) ensues. Such patients often have cool extremities, are oliguric, and may have a metabolic acidosis. As a result of the elevated right atrial pressure, hepatic congestion, ascites, increased chest tube output, and pleural effusions may be evident. These patients may be tachycardic and hypotensive with a narrow pulse pressure. Preload must be maintained despite an already elevated RA pressure. Significant inotropic support often is required (typically dopamine 5 to 10 µg/kg/min or epinephrine 0.05–0.1 µg/kg/min). A phosphodiesterase inhibitor, such as milrinone, is potentially beneficial because of its lusitropic properties; however, one must be cautious in the use of these agents with renal impairment.[32] Sedation and paralysis often are necessary for the first 24 to 48 hours to minimize energy expenditure and associated myocardial work. Factors that further impair ventricular diastolic filling, such as loss of AV synchrony, accumulation of pleural fluid or ascites, and high tidal volume ventilation with air trapping, should be mitigated early in the postoperative course.

Mechanical ventilation may have a significant impact on RV afterload and the amount of pulmonary regurgitation. In addition, an increase in PVR because of hypothermia, acidosis, and either hypoinflation or hyperinflation of the lung also increases afterload on the right ventricle and pulmonary regurgitation. Synchronized intermittent positive pressure ventilation with the lowest possible mean airway pressure should be the aim, as discussed previously. This concept has been extended to older patients with single-ventricle

physiology. The Fontan circulation relies on passive flow of blood through the pulmonary circulation without benefit of a pulmonary ventricle. If a fenestration is left at the time of the Fontan procedure, the resulting right-to-left shunt helps to preserve cardiac output and results in fewer postoperative complications.[33,34] It is better to shunt blood right to left and accept some reduction in oxygen saturation (thus maintaining ventricular filling and cardiac output) than to have high oxygen saturation with a low cardiac output state.

Diastolic Dysfunction

Occasionally there is an alteration of ventricular relaxation, an active energy-dependent process, which reduces ventricular compliance. This is particularly problematic in patients with a hypertrophied ventricle undergoing surgical repair, such as TOF or Fontan surgery, and following CPB in some neonates when myocardial edema may significantly restrict diastolic function (ie, *restrictive physiology*).[30,31] The poorly compliant ventricle with impaired diastolic relaxation has a reduced end-diastolic volume and decreased stroke volume. β-Adrenergic antagonists and calcium channel blockers add little to the treatment of this condition. In fact, hypotension or myocardial depression produced by these agents often outweighs any gain from slowing the heart rate. Calcium channel blockers are relatively contraindicated in neonates and small infants because of their dependence on transsarcolemmal flux of calcium to both initiate and sustain contraction.

A gradual increase in intravascular volume to augment ventricular capacity, in addition to the use of low doses of inotropic agents, has proved to be of modest benefit in patients with diastolic dysfunction. Tachycardia must be avoided and AV synchrony maintained to optimize diastolic filling time and decrease myocardial oxygen demands. If low cardiac output continues despite treatment, therapy with vasodilators can be carefully attempted to alter systolic wall tension (afterload) and thus decrease the impediment to ventricular ejection. Because the capacity of the vascular bed increases after vasodilation, simultaneous volume replacement is often necessary. A noncatecholamine inodilator with vasodilating and lusitropic (improved diastolic state) properties, such as milrinone, is useful under these circumstances, in contrast with other inotropic agents.[35]

Pharmacologic Support

General principles of pharmacologic support in the neonatal and pediatric patient center on the recognition of the developmental limitations of the neonatal myocardium and the well-described reductions in cardiac output 6 to 12 hours after separation from CPB.[28] Despite ongoing development and maturity of adrenergic receptors and L-type calcium channels, catecholamine-based inotropic agents and vasodilators are efficacious in this population. These drugs have principles of use and side effects related to higher doses and patient-specific comorbidities. Other nonvasoactive agents serve as adjuncts to optimizing postoperative hemodynamics and fluid balance. The combination of a low-dose inotrope and an afterload reducing agent, or, more commonly, a phosphodiesterase inhibitor,[35] has been shown to decrease the occurrence of postoperative LCOS following CPB (Fig. 38.2).

It should be understood that the need for vasoactive and inotropic support varies greatly among patients recovering from cardiac surgery and even over time for an individual

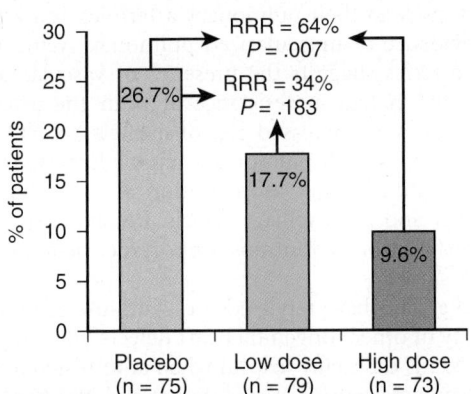

Fig. 38.2. Primary end point: development of low cardiac output syndrome (LCOS) or death in the first 36 hours. (From Hoffman, TM, et al. Efficacy and safety of milrinone in preventing low cardiac output syndrome in infants and children after corrective surgery for congenital heart disease. Circulation. 2003;107:996-1002.)

| **TABLE 38.2** | Critical Care Strategies for Postoperative Treatment of Pulmonary Hypertension |

Encourage	Avoid
Anatomic investigation	Residual anatomic disease
Opportunities for right-to-left shunt as *pop-off*	Intact atrial septum in right heart failure
Sedation/anesthesia	Agitation/pain
Moderate hyperventilation	Respiratory acidosis
Moderate alkalosis	Metabolic acidosis
Adequate inspired oxygen	Alveolar hypoxia
Normal lung volumes	Atelectasis or overdistension
Optimal hematocrit	Excessive hematocrit
Inotropic support	Low output and coronary perfusion
Vasodilators	Vasoconstrictors/increased afterload

patient progressing through the postoperative care continuum. The intensity of pharmacologic support employed must be constantly factored into the clinical assessment—the concept of intensity of therapy. One must not embrace a false sense of security when caring for a patient with adequate cardiac output when this requires disproportionate pharmacologic support. The current trend in cardiac critical care is to employ the lowest level of inotropic and vasoactive support necessary for adequate hemodynamic goals. Due to advances in preoperative stabilization, anesthetic strategies, surgical technique, myocardial protection, and CPB, it is not uncommon for a patient to return to the ICU requiring only modest doses of milrinone or epinephrine or no pharmacologic support at all. The specifics of cardiovascular pharmacology are discussed in Chapter 33.

Managing Acute Pulmonary Hypertension in the Intensive Care Unit

Children with many forms of CHD are prone to perioperative elevations in PVR.[36] This situation complicates the postoperative course, when transient myocardial dysfunction is further challenged by increased RV afterload.[37]

Although postoperative patients with pulmonary hypertension often are presumed to have active and reversible pulmonary vasoconstriction as the source of their pathophysiology, the intensivist is obligated to explore anatomic causes of mechanical obstruction that impose a barrier to pulmonary blood flow. Elevated LA pressure, pulmonary venous obstruction, branch pulmonary artery stenosis, or surgically induced loss of the vascular tree all raise RV pressure and impose an unnecessary burden on the right heart. Similarly, a residual or undiagnosed left-to-right shunt raises pulmonary artery pressure postoperatively and must be addressed surgically. Extended use of pulmonary vasodilator strategies only augments residual or undiagnosed shunts and increases the volume load on the heart.

Several factors peculiar to CPB may raise PVR: Pulmonary vascular endothelial dysfunction, microemboli, pulmonary leukostasis, excess thromboxane production, atelectasis, hypoxic pulmonary vasoconstriction, and adrenergic events all have been suggested to play a role in postoperative

pulmonary hypertension. Postoperative pulmonary vascular reactivity has been related not only to the presence of preoperative pulmonary hypertension and left-to-right shunts but also to the duration of total CPB. The threat of postoperative pulmonary hypertensive crises can be partially addressed by surgery at earlier ages, pharmacologic interventions, and other postoperative management strategies (Table 38.2).

Pulmonary Vasodilators

Many intravenous vasodilators have been used with variable success in patients with pulmonary hypertensive disorders requiring critical care. Older-style vasodilators such as tolazoline, phenoxybenzamine, nitroprusside, or isoproterenol have little biologic basis for selectivity or enhanced activity in the pulmonary vascular bed.[38] However, if myocardial contractility is depressed and the afterload reducing effect on the left ventricle is beneficial to myocardial function and cardiac output, then these drugs may be of some value. In addition to drug-specific side effects, they all have potential to produce profound systemic hypotension, critically lowering coronary perfusion pressure while simultaneously increasing intrapulmonary shunt.

In the setting of pulmonary hypertension where the right ventricular contractile function is affected but LV contractility is intact, one can utilize a systemic vasopressor (in addition to inotropic agents and RV vasodilators) to optimize the circulation. The increase in end-arterial elastance results in increased LV contractility to maintain the ventricle on the same end-systolic PV curve. The increased afterload shifts the interventricular septum resulting in improved LV diastolic filling. The increased systolic contractility of the LV results in improved systolic contractility of the RV through shared fibers in the interventricular septum (systolic ventricular interdependence). Finally, the high afterload induced by the vasopressor results in better RV coronary perfusion pressure.

Even with selective infusions of rapidly metabolized, intravenously administered vasoactive drugs into the pulmonary circulation, systemic drug concentrations and systemic hemodynamic effects can be appreciable. Prostacyclin appears to have somewhat more selectivity for the pulmonary circulation but at high doses can precipitate a hypotensive crisis in unstable postoperative patients with refractory pulmonary hypertension. It is best suited for chronic outpatient therapy in severe forms of primary pulmonary hypertension.[39-41] Agents that improve ventricular function in addition to reducing afterload (eg, type III phosphodiesterase inhibitors) are more appealing when cardiac output is low.

As an alternative approach to nonspecific vasodilators, it seems logical to target vasoconstrictors known to be associated with pathologic states or critical events. In this regard, endothelin, a potent vasoconstrictor, is elevated in persistent pulmonary hypertension of the newborn, in children with CHD, and in patients after CPB, and it seems a likely candidate for investigation of specific receptor blockers. Petrossian and colleagues[42] showed promising amelioration of postoperative pulmonary hypertension associated with CPB in animal models of increased pulmonary blood flow (from intracardiac shunts) when pretreated with endothelin-A receptor blockers. Undoubtedly, because the causes of pulmonary hypertension in the intensive care setting frequently are multifactorial, our "best" therapy will be multiply targeted. Adding phosphodiesterase V inhibitors to prostacyclin infusions, endothelin receptor blockers, thromboxane inhibitors, and inhaled nitric oxide (NO) all may have individual and combined merit with synergistic effects.

Nitric oxide is a selective pulmonary vasodilator formed by the endothelium from L-arginine and molecular oxygen in a reaction catalyzed by NO synthase. It then diffuses to the adjacent vascular smooth muscle cells where it induces vasodilation through a cyclic guanosine monophosphate-dependent pathway.[43,44] Because NO exists as a gas, it can be delivered by inhalation to the alveoli and then to the adjacent blood vessels. Once it diffuses across the wall of the pulmonary blood vessels, NO enters the vascular lumen where it is rapidly inactivated by hemoglobin, thus resulting in selective pulmonary vasodilation when pulmonary vasoconstriction exists. It has advantages over intravenously administered vasodilators that cause systemic hypotension and increase intrapulmonary shunting. Inhaled NO lowers pulmonary artery pressure in a number of diseases without the unwanted effect of systemic hypotension. This effect is especially dramatic in children with cardiovascular disorders and postoperative patients with pulmonary hypertensive crises.[37,45,46]

Therapeutic uses of inhaled NO in children with CHD abound in the ICU. For example, newborns with total anomalous pulmonary venous connection (TAPVC) frequently have obstruction of the pulmonary venous pathway as it connects anomalously to the systemic venous circulation. When pulmonary venous return is obstructed preoperatively, pulmonary hypertension is severe and demands urgent surgical relief. Increased neonatal pulmonary vasoreactivity, endothelial injury induced by CPB, and intrauterine anatomic changes in the pulmonary vascular bed in this disease contribute to postoperative pulmonary hypertension. In this postoperative setting, inhaled NO dramatically reduces pulmonary hypertension without adverse changes in heart rate, systemic blood pressure, or vascular resistance.

Patients with TAPVC, congenital mitral stenosis, and other pulmonary venous hypertensive disorders associated with low cardiac output are among the most responsive to NO. These infants are born with significantly increased amounts of smooth muscle in their pulmonary arterioles and veins. Histologic evidence of muscularized pulmonary veins and pulmonary arteries suggests the presence of vascular tone and capacity for change in resistance at both the arterial and venous sites. The increased responsiveness to NO seen in younger patients with pulmonary venous hypertension may result from pulmonary vasorelaxation at a combination of precapillary and postcapillary vessels. Resolving the primary venous obstruction is of utmost importance before using NO in these lesions.

Several groups have reported successful use of inhaled NO in a variety of other congenital heart defects following cardiac surgery. NO is especially helpful when administered during a pulmonary hypertensive crisis.[47] Successful NO use has been described after the Fontan procedure, following late VSD repair, and with a variety of other anatomic lesions where patients are at risk of developing postoperative pulmonary hypertensive crises.[46-48] Oxygen saturation in response to inhaled NO generally does not improve in very young infants who are excessively cyanotic after a bidirectional Glenn anastomosis.[49] For these, increasing cardiac output and cerebral blood flow will have a much greater impact on arterial oxygenation, because elevated pulmonary vascular tone is seldom the limiting factor in the hypoxemic patient after the bidirectional Glenn operation.[50]

Inhaled NO can be used diagnostically in neonates with RV hypertension after cardiac surgery to discern those with reversible vasoconstriction. In patients with Ebstein's anomaly, a clinical response to NO can accurately differentiate between functional and anatomic pulmonary atresia.[51] In addition, the use of NO in such patients can facilitate anterograde pulmonary blood flow and hemodynamic stabilization. Failure of the postoperative newborn to respond to NO should be regarded as strong evidence of anatomic and possibly surgically remediable obstruction.[51]

If NO must be discontinued before the pathologic process has been resolved, hemodynamic instability can be expected. The withdrawal response to inhaled NO can be attenuated by pretreatment with the type V phosphodiesterase inhibitor sildenafil.[52] Sildenafil inhibits the inactivation of cyclic guanosine monophosphate within the vascular smooth muscle cell and has the potential to augment the effects of endogenous or exogenously administered NO to effect vascular smooth muscle relaxation. Sildenafil can be administered in an oral or IV form and has a somewhat selective pulmonary vasodilating capacity while lowering LA pressure and providing a modest degree of afterload reduction in some postoperative children. Chronic oral administration of sildenafil to adults with primary pulmonary hypertension improves exercise capacity. This phenomenon has also been demonstrated in pediatric patients with a Fontan circulation, perhaps suggesting a broad therapeutic application in both early and more remote postoperative congenital heart disease.

Cardiac Tamponade

Chest closure is a time of particular instability after operations for CHD. The infant's crowded mediastinum makes compression of the heart and cardiac tamponade an ever-present possibility after chest closure, despite patent drainage tubes and surgical resection of the anterior pericardium. The warning signs of tamponade frequently are subtle in small children, even minutes before cardiovascular collapse. Any significant deterioration in hemodynamics after chest closure should first be attributed to tamponade if ventilation and cardiac rhythm are adequate. The signs of tamponade include tachycardia, hypotension, narrow pulse pressure, and high filling pressures on both the left and right sides of the heart.

Acute myocardial perforation with tamponade occasionally occurs during interventional cardiac catheterization procedures. Prompt support of the circulation with volume infusions and pressor support, along with immediate catheter drainage of the pericardial space, are essential in the event of this complication. Hemopericardium after ventricular puncture usually is self-limited, as the muscular ventricle seals the perforation after the responsible wire or catheter is removed. However, laceration of the thin-walled atrium may require suture repair under direct vision in the operating room.

Other causes of cardiac tamponade are seen in patients with CHD, and treatment frequently requires the assistance of an intensivist for either pericardiocentesis or sedation and monitoring for that definitive procedure. Postoperative tamponade from bleeding immediately after operation, as discussed earlier, is best handled by facilitation of chest tube drainage or reopening the sternotomy. Some children develop pericardial effusions during later phases of their illness because of hydrostatic influences (eg, patients with modified Fontan operations) or postpericardiotomy syndrome. Fluid in the pericardial space may accumulate under considerable pressure, and filling of the heart is impaired. If this problem is left unattended, the transmural pressure in the atria diminishes as intraatrial pressures rise, and diastolic collapse of the atria can be observed echocardiographically. Patients become symptomatic with a narrow pulse pressure, pulsus paradoxus, tachycardia, respiratory distress, decreased urine output, hyperkalemia, metabolic acidosis, and hypotension with tremendous endogenous catecholamine response.

In summary, aggressive identification and treatment of low cardiac output conditions after cardiac surgery are central to the critical care of children with CHD. Successful application of these strategies and thoughtful use of pharmacologic intervention undoubtedly have contributed to the remarkable decline in mortality associated with congenital heart surgery in the past two decades. However, despite these interventions, additional (mechanical) support is sometimes necessary as a bridge to recovery.

Diaphragmatic Dysfunction, Effusions, and Pulmonary Issues

Diaphragmatic paresis (reduced motion) or paralysis (paradoxical movement) may precipitate and promote respiratory failure, particularly in the neonate or young infant who relies on diaphragmatic function for breathing; older infants and children can recruit accessory and intercostal muscles if diaphragmatic function proves inadequate. Injury to the phrenic nerve, usually the left, may occur during operations that require dissection of the branch pulmonary arteries well out to the hilum (eg, TOF repair, ASO), arch reconstruction from the midline (eg, Norwood operation), manipulation of the SVC (Glenn shunt), takedown of a systemic-to-pulmonary shunt, or after attempted percutaneous central venous access. Phrenic nerve injury occurs more frequently at reoperation, when adhesions and scarring may obscure landmarks. Topical cooling with ice during deep hypothermia may also cause transient phrenic palsy. Increased work of breathing on low

ventilator settings, increased $PaCO_2$, and a chest radiograph revealing an elevated hemidiaphragm suggest diaphragmatic dysfunction. The chest radiograph may be misleading, however, if it is obtained at the end of inspiration when lung volume is at its highest. Ultrasonography or fluoroscopy is useful for identifying diaphragmatic motion or paradoxical excursion. Recovery of diaphragmatic contraction usually occurs; however, if a patient fails to tolerate repeated extubations despite optimizing cardiovascular and nutritional status and diaphragmatic dysfunction persists with volume loss in the affected lung, then surgical plication of the diaphragm may be required. Although only a temporary effect is gained, the prevention of collapse and volume loss in the affected lung often provides the critical advantage needed for liberation from positive pressure ventilation.

Pleural effusions and ascites may occur in patients after the Fontan operation or reparative procedures involving a right ventriculotomy (eg, TOF, truncus arteriosus) with transient RV dysfunction. Especially in young patients, pleural effusions and increased interstitial lung water may be a manifestation of right heart failure. This seems logically related to raised systemic venous pressure impeding lymphatic return to the venous circulation. The lymphatic circuit often is functioning at full capacity in these children. Pleural or peritoneal fluid and intestinal distension compete with intrapulmonary gas for thoracic space. Evacuation of the pleural space, drainage of ascites, and bowel decompression facilitate restoration of lung volume.

Pulmonary edema, pneumonia, and atelectasis are the most common causes of lower airway and alveolar abnormalities that interfere with gas exchange. If a bacterial pathogen is identified, antibiotics should be initiated promptly. If pulmonary edema is responsible for the gas exchange abnormality, therapy is aimed at lowering the LA pressure through diuresis and pharmacologic means to reduce afterload and improve the lusitropic state of the heart. For infants, fluid restriction frequently is incompatible with adequate nutrition; therefore an aggressive diuretic regimen is preferable to restriction of caloric intake. Adjustment of end-expiratory pressure and mechanical ventilation serve as supportive therapies until the alveoli and pulmonary interstitium are cleared of the fluid that interferes with gas exchange.

Separating From Mechanical Ventilation

Early tracheal extubation of children following congenital heart surgery is not a new concept but has received renewed attention with the evolution of fast-track management for cardiac surgical patients. Early extubation generally refers to tracheal extubation in the operating room or within a few hours (ie, 4-8 hours) after surgery, although in practice it means the avoidance of routine overnight mechanical ventilation. Factors to consider when planning early extubation are given in Table 38.3.

A number of published reports have described successful tracheal extubation in neonates and older children following congenital heart surgery, either in the operating room or soon after in the cardiac ICU.[53] This has been possible without adversely affecting patient care and with a low incidence of reintubation or hemodynamic instability. Such a process can reduce complications, like ventilator-associated events, and does not obviate meticulous attention to postoperative analgesia and sedation. The judicious use of this practice has

TABLE 38.3	Considerations for Planned Early Extubation After Congenital Heart Surgery
Patient factors	Limited cardiorespiratory reserve of the neonate and infant
	Pathophysiology of specific congenital heart defects
	Timing of surgery and preoperative management
Anesthetic factors	Premedication
	Hemodynamic stability and reserve
	Drug distribution and maintenance of anesthesia on bypass
	Postoperative analgesia
Surgical factors	Extent and complexity of surgery
	Residual defects
	Risks for bleeding and protection of suture lines
Conduct of bypass	Degree of hypothermia
	Level of hemodilution
	Myocardial protection
	Modulation of the inflammatory response and reperfusion injury
Postoperative management	Myocardial function
	Cardiorespiratory interactions
	Neurologic recovery
	Analgesia management

streamlined the care of children and highlights the advances in perioperative care of infants and older children after repair of congenital heart defects.[54]

Central Nervous System

The dramatic reduction in surgical mortality has been accompanied by a growing recognition of neurologic morbidity in some survivors. Central nervous system abnormalities may be a function of coexisting (preexisting) brain abnormalities or acquired events unrelated to surgical management (eg, embolism, brain infection, effects of chronic cyanosis), but CNS insults appear to occur most frequently during or immediately after surgery. In particular, support techniques used during neonatal and infant cardiac surgery (eg, CPB, profound hypothermia, circulatory arrest) have been implicated as important causes of brain injury.[55]

During hypothermic CPB, multiple perfusion variables may influence the risk of brain injury. These variables include (but are not limited to) (1) the total duration of CPB, (2) the duration and rate of core cooling, (3) pH management during core cooling, (4) duration of circulatory arrest, (5) type of oxygenator, (6) presence of arterial filtration, (7) position and function of cannulae, and (8) depth of hypothermia. Undoubtedly, there is interaction between these various elements, and CNS injury following CPB most likely is multifactorial. Early postoperative studies (in the ICU) revealed a higher incidence of neurologic morbidity in patients undergoing circulatory arrest, including a higher incidence of clinical and electroencephalographic (EEG) seizures, a longer recovery time to the first reappearance of EEG activity, and greater release of the brain isoenzyme of creatine kinase.[55]

Seizures are the most commonly observed neurologic complication of cardiac surgery with an incidence in older studies of 4% to 25%. Although the incidence of seizures in the cardiac ICU has dramatically declined, when seizures do occur they should be treated aggressively. In addition, the broad availability of continuous EEG monitoring has allowed timely detection of treatment of previously undetectable but relevant subclinical seizures. Importantly, one must limit practices that may have been associated with brain injury after CPB: rapid cooling on CPB and use of prolonged hypothermic circulatory arrest, extreme alpha-stat strategy of intraoperative pH management, extreme hemodilution to hematocrits less than 20, overheating infants upon arrival in the ICU, hypocapnic hyperventilation, and prolonged muscle relaxation (masking seizure observations). Elevated body temperature during critical illness is detrimental in the neurologic recovery of the critically ill and potentially brain-injured pediatric patient.

Intraventricular hemorrhage may occur as a consequence of perinatal events or circulatory collapse in the first few days of life and is commonly associated with prematurity. Although some centers routinely perform a head ultrasound on all newborns prior to cardiac surgery, data support limiting preoperative cranial ultrasound screening to those with existing risk factors.[56] Surgical intervention is delayed for several days if intraventricular bleeding is documented. The strategy of deferring operations in very premature newborns for several days after birth is associated with a low incidence of intraventricular hemorrhage in these high-risk patients despite use of CPB.[57]

Renal Function and Postoperative Fluid Management

Risk factors for postoperative renal failure include preoperative renal dysfunction, prolonged bypass time, low cardiac output, and cardiac arrest. In addition to relative ischemia and nonpulsatile blood flow on CPB, angiotensin II–mediated renal vasoconstriction and delayed healing of renal tubular epithelium have been proposed as mechanisms for renal failure. Postoperative sepsis and nephrotoxic drugs may further contribute to injury.

Because of the inflammatory response to bypass and significant increase in total body water, judicious fluid management in the immediate postoperative period is critical. Capillary leak and interstitial fluid accumulation may continue for the first 24 to 48 hours following surgery, necessitating ongoing intravascular volume replacement with colloid or blood products. A fall in cardiac output and increased antidiuretic hormone secretion contribute to delayed water clearance and potential prerenal dysfunction, which could progress to acute tubular necrosis and renal failure if a low cardiac output state persists.

During CPB, optimizing the circuit prime, hematocrit, and oncotic pressure; attenuating the inflammatory response with steroids; and use of modified ultrafiltration techniques have been recommended to limit interstitial fluid accumulation.[58] During the first 24 hours following surgery, maintenance fluids should be restricted to 50% to 66% of full maintenance and volume replacement titrated to appropriate filling pressures and hemodynamic response. Oliguria in the first 24 hours after complex surgery and CPB is common in neonates and infants until cardiac output recovers and neurohumoral mechanisms abate. Although diuretics are commonly prescribed in the immediate postoperative period, the neurohumoral influence on urine output is powerful. Time after

CPB and enhancement of cardiac output through volume and pharmacologic adjustments are the most important factors that will promote diuresis.

Peritoneal dialysis, hemodialysis, and continuous venovenous hemofiltration provide alternate renal support in patients with severe oliguria and acute kidney injury (AKI). Besides enabling water and solute clearance, maintenance fluids can be increased to ensure adequate nutrition. The indications for renal support vary but include pronounced uremia, life-threatening electrolyte imbalance such as severe hyperkalemia, ongoing metabolic acidosis, fluid restrictions limiting nutrition, and increased mechanical ventilation requirements secondary to persistent pulmonary edema or ascites.

A peritoneal dialysis catheter can be placed at the completion of surgery or as a bedside procedure later in the ICU. Indications include the need for renal support or for reducing intraabdominal pressure from ascites that may compromise mechanical ventilation and splanchnic perfusion. Drainage may be voluminous in the immediate postoperative period as third space fluid losses continue, and replacement with albumin or fresh-frozen plasma may be necessary to treat hypovolemia and hypoproteinemia.

Gastrointestinal Issues

Adequate nutrition is exceedingly important following cardiac surgery in neonates and children. These critically ill patients often have decreased caloric intake and increased energy demand after surgery; the neonate, in particular, has limited metabolic and fat reserves. Total parenteral nutrition can provide adequate nutrition in the hypercatabolic phase of the early postoperative period and generally is started on the first postoperative day if the prospect of meaningful enteral nutrition is unlikely.

Gastritis, ulcer formation, and upper gastrointestinal bleeding and may occur following the stress of cardiac surgery in children and adults. There are limited reports of the efficacy of proton pump inhibitors, histamine H_2 receptor blockers, sucralfate, or oral antacids in pediatric cardiac patients, although their use is common in most ICUs. Hepatic failure may occur after cardiac surgery, particularly after the Fontan operation, and typically is characterized by elevated liver enzymes and coagulopathy.

Necrotizing enterocolitis, although typically a disease of premature infants, is seen with increased frequency in neonates with CHD. Risk factors include (1) left-sided obstructive lesions, (2) umbilical or femoral arterial catheterization/angiography, (3) hypoxemia, and (4) lesions with wide pulse pressures (eg, systemic-to-pulmonary shunts and severe aortic regurgitation) producing diastolic runoff in the mesenteric vessels. Frequently, multiple risk factors exist in the same patient, making a specific etiology difficult to establish. Treatment includes continuous nasogastric suction, parenteral nutrition, and broad-spectrum antibiotics. Bowel exploration or resection may be necessary in severe cases.

Infection

Low-grade (<38.5°C) fever during the immediate postoperative period is common and may be present for up to 3 to 4 days, even without a demonstrable infectious etiology. However, one ought not to simply disregard the occurrence of fever in the days following surgery as it might signal an infection, especially in the multi-instrumented patient. CPB activates complement and other inflammatory mediators but also can lead to derangements of the immune system that increase the likelihood of infection.

Sepsis and nosocomial infection after cardiac surgery contribute substantially to overall morbidity. Despite the increased use of broad antibiotic coverage with third-generation cephalosporins, these agents do not seem to be more effective in decreasing postoperative infections. Meticulous catheter insertion and daily care routines, along with early removal of indwelling catheters in the postoperative patient, are important in reducing the incidence of sepsis.[59] Optimal head positioning, mouth care, sedation management, and consideration of an early-extubation strategy can reduce the rates of ventilator-associated events.

Mediastinitis occurs in up to 2% of patients undergoing cardiac surgery. Risk factors include delayed sternal closure, early reexploration for bleeding, or reoperation. Mediastinitis is characterized by persistent fever, purulent drainage from the sternotomy wound, instability of the sternum, and leukocytosis. Staphylococcus is the most common offending organism. Treatment usually involves debridement and irrigation with parenteral antibiotic therapy. Duration of therapy depends on the severity of the infection and is generally between 2 and 4 weeks.

Hyperglycemia

Hyperglycemia is a frequent occurrence in the pediatric cardiac intensive care unit.[60,61] As many as 97% and 78% of patients exhibit at least one blood glucose measurement above 125 mg/dl and 200 mg/dl, respectively, following surgical repair of congenital cardiac defects.[60,61] The duration of postoperative hyperglycemia in these patients has been strongly and independently associated with increased morbidity and mortality rates.[60,61]

Strict glycemic control with insulin administration has been shown to reduce morbidity and mortality rates significantly for adult patients admitted to a surgical intensive care unit.[62] The first glycemic control outcome trial conducted in children with a sample largely composed of postoperative cardiac patients showed decreased mortality, shorter ICU length of stay, and decreased markers of inflammation in patients treated with insulin to maintain fasting blood glucose levels.[63] Of significant concern in that trial, however, was the finding that 24.9% of children undergoing strict glycemic control had at least one episode of severe hypoglycemia (blood glucose <40 mg/dL [2.2 mmoL/L]).[63] The use of a more permissive glycemic range (90-140 mg/dL) has been postulated as an optimal target that would be associated with a lower incidence of hypoglycemia without incurring the negative effects of hyperglycemia, compared to an euglycemic range.[64] Subsequently, two large trials conducted in this population have decreased the enthusiasm for aggressive glucose control in the early postoperative period. The ChiP trial randomized 1369 pediatric patients in 13 centers to either conventional (blood glucose <216 mg/dL [12.0 mmoL/L]) or tight (glycemic control 72-126 mg/dL [4.0-7.0 mmoL/L]); 60% of trial participants had undergone cardiac surgery.[65] The primary end point of number of days alive and free from mechanical ventilation was comparable between the treatment groups (23.2 versus 23.6 days; mean difference [95% confidence interval] 0.36 [-0.42, 1.14]); no differences were noted in the cardiac subgroup.[65] The SPECS trial randomized 980 children in 2 centers after surgery with CPB to either tight-glycemic control (80-110 mg/dL [4.4-6.1 mmoL/L]) or standard care with no prespecified glucose target.[66] In this study, there was no difference in the primary outcome (rate of health care–associated infection) between the two study groups (8.9 versus 9.8 per 1000 patient-days, respectively; p = 0.67). With no clear benefit demonstrated with the use of a tight glycemic control strategy, there is now greater focus on the hypoglycemic complications associated with such practice. Both studies demonstrated a significantly increased risk of any (CHiP: 15.9% versus 3.7%; p <0.001, SPECS: 19% versus 9%, p <0.001) or severe hypoglycemia (CHiP: 7.3% versus 1.5%; p <0.001, SPECS: 3% versus 1%, p = 0.03) with tight glycemic control.[65,66]

Critical Care Management of Selected Specific Lesions

Single-Ventricle Anatomy and Physiology

For a variety of anatomic lesions, the pulmonary and systemic circulations are in parallel with complete mixing, with a single ventricle effectively supplying both systemic and pulmonary blood flow. The proportion of ventricular output to either the pulmonary or systemic vascular bed is determined by the relative resistance to flow in the two circuits. The pulmonary arterial and aortic oxygen saturations are equal. Assuming equal mixing, normal cardiac output, and full pulmonary venous saturation, SaO_2 of 80% to 85%, with MVO_2 of 60% to 65%, indicates Qp/Qs ≈1 and hence a balance between systemic and pulmonary flow. Although "balanced," the single ventricle still must receive and eject twice the normal amount of blood: one part to the pulmonary circulation and one part to the systemic circulation. A Qp/Qs >1 implies a volume burden on the heart that may have a clinical impact depending on the degree, duration, and myocardial reserve. Though lesion-specific considerations are important in the various types of single-ventricle physiology, common management principles to balance flow and augment systemic perfusion do apply.

Preoperative Management

Changes in PVR have a significant impact on systemic perfusion and circulatory stability, especially preoperatively when the ductus arteriosus is widely patent. In preparation for surgery, it is important that systemic and pulmonary blood flow be as well balanced as possible to prevent excessive volume overload and ventricular dysfunction that reduces systemic and end-organ perfusion. For example, a newborn with HLHS who has an arterial oxygen saturation greater than 90%, a wide pulse pressure, oliguria, cool extremities, hepatomegaly, and metabolic acidosis has severely limited systemic blood flow. Even though ventricular output is increased, the blood flow that is inefficiently partitioned back to the lungs is unavailable to the other vital organs. Immediate interventions are necessary to prevent imminent circulatory collapse and end-organ injury. In this "overcirculated" state, PVR is falling as it should in the normal postnatal state, and the ductus arteriosus is maintained widely patent to mitigate outflow obstruction from the RV to the systemic circulation. Blood flow manipulation by mechanical ventilation and inotropic support may temporarily stabilize the patient; this should accelerate the timeline for surgical intervention.

Similarly, in a patient with pulmonary atresia and an intact ventricular septum, LV-dependent pulmonary circulation occurs. Ductal patency is necessary for pulmonary blood flow. As PVR falls, pulmonary blood flow will be excessive and eventually will steal from the systemic circulation. Preoperative management should focus on an assessment of the balance between pulmonary (Qp) and systemic flow (Qs). This is best achieved by thorough and continuous reevaluation of the clinical examination for cardiac output state and perfusion; close monitoring of the oxygen saturation; evaluation of chest radiograph for cardiac size and pulmonary congestion; review of laboratory data for alterations in gas exchange, acid-base status, and end-organ function; and echocardiographic imaging to assess ventricular function and AV valve competence. A central venous line positioned in the proximal SVC may be useful to monitor volume status and sample central venous oxygen saturation as a surrogate of cardiac output and oxygen delivery. Central venous lines are not necessary in all circumstances; they may have significant complications in small newborns and do not substitute for clinical examination.

Initial resuscitation involves maintaining patency of the ductus arteriosus with a PGE_1 infusion at a rate of 0.01 to 0.05 µg/kg/min. Intubation and mechanical ventilation are not necessary in all patients. Patients usually are tachypneic, but provided the work of breathing is not excessive and systemic perfusion is maintained without a metabolic acidosis, spontaneous ventilation often is preferable to achieve an adequate systemic perfusion and balance of Qp and Qs. A mild metabolic acidosis and low bicarbonate level may be present but may not indicate poor perfusion and a lactic acidosis specifically. If the initial presentation involved circulatory collapse and end-organ dysfunction, then a period of days may be required to establish stability and allow return of vital organ function prior to surgery.

Patients may require intubation and mechanical ventilation because of apnea secondary to PGE_1, presence of a low cardiac output state, or for manipulation of gas exchange to assist balancing Qp/Qs. A SaO_2 greater than 90% indicates pulmonary overcirculation—that is, Qp/Qs >1. PVR can be increased with controlled mechanical hypoventilation to induce a respiratory acidosis, often necessitating sedation and neuromuscular blockade, and with a reduction of ambient FiO_2 to minimize hyperoxic pulmonary vasodilation. Ventilation in room air may suffice, but occasionally a hypoxic gas mixture is necessary. This is achieved by adding nitrogen to the inspired gas mixture, reducing the FiO_2 to around 0.17 to 0.19. Although these maneuvers often are successful in maintaining a relatively high PVR and reducing pulmonary blood flow, it is important to remember that these patients have a limited oxygen reserve and may desaturate suddenly and precipitously. Controlled hypoventilation reduces functional residual capacity (FRC) and therefore also decreases the oxygen reserve, which is further reduced by use of a hypoxic inspired gas mixture. An alternate strategy is to add carbon dioxide to the inspiratory limb of the breathing circuit, which also increases PVR, but because a hypoxic gas mixture is not used, systemic oxygen delivery is maintained.[67,68] Patients who have continued pulmonary overcirculation with high SaO_2 and reduced systemic perfusion despite these maneuvers require early surgical intervention to control pulmonary blood flow. At the time of surgery, a temporary snare can be placed around either branch of the pulmonary artery to effectively limit pulmonary blood flow. Alternatively, if there are important comorbidities that preclude a standard palliative operation (prematurity, intracranial hemorrhage), bilateral pulmonary arterial bands can be placed through a median sternotomy to effect optimization of systemic blood flow.

Decreased pulmonary blood flow in preoperative patients with a parallel circulation is reflected by hypoxemia with SaO_2 less than 75%. This may result from restricted flow across a small ductus arteriosus, increased PVR secondary to parenchymal lung disease, or increased pulmonary venous pressure secondary to obstructed pulmonary venous drainage or a restrictive ASD. In patients with a later postnatal presentation, blood flow through a restrictive ductus may be augmented by the administration of high-dose PGE_1 (0.1-0.2 µg/kg/min). Patients at this level of prostaglandin delivery should have their airway secured and may benefit from vasopressor therapy to both offset the vasodilating effects of PGE_1 and increase the systemic vascular resistance (SVR) to augment pulmonary blood flow. Sedation, paralysis, and optimization of mechanical ventilation to maintain an alkalosis may be effective if PVR is elevated. NO may be also be useful in selected cases. Systemic oxygen delivery is maintained by improving cardiac output and maintaining hematocrit >40%. Among some newborns with HLHS, pulmonary blood flow may be insufficient because mitral valve hypoplasia in combination with a restrictive or nearly intact atrial septum severely restricts pulmonary venous return to the heart. The newborn is intensely cyanotic and has a pulmonary venous congestion pattern on chest radiograph. Urgent interventional cardiac catheterization with balloon septostomy or dilation (or stent placement) of a restrictive ASD may be necessary.[69,70] Immediate surgical intervention and palliation are preferred in some centers. Increasingly, these patients are being identified prenatally with an option of fetal catheter-based intervention. Despite such advances, survival in this subgroup is reduced (between 48% and 69%).[70-74]

Systemic perfusion is maintained with the use of volume and vasopressor agents. Inotropic support often is necessary because of ventricular dysfunction secondary to the increased volume load. Systemic afterload reduction with agents such as phosphodiesterase inhibitors may improve systemic perfusion, although they also may decrease PVR and thus not correct the imbalance of pulmonary and systemic flow. Oliguria and a rising serum creatinine level may reflect renal insufficiency from a low cardiac output. Necrotizing enterocolitis is a risk secondary to splanchnic hypoperfusion, and we prefer not to enterally feed newborns with a wide pulse width and low diastolic pressure (usually <30 mm Hg) prior to surgery. It is important to continuously evaluate end-organ perfusion and function.

Postoperative Management

The postoperative management of patients with single ventricle anatomy and physiology will be discussed later in this chapter, in the section detailing postoperative care of newborns with HLHS following stage I palliation.

Bidirectional Cavopulmonary Anastomosis

In this procedure, also known as a bidirectional Glenn (BDG) shunt, the SVC is transected and connected end-to-side to the right pulmonary artery, while the pulmonary arteries remain in continuity. Therefore flow from the SVC is bidirectional into both left and right pulmonary arteries. The SVC becomes the only source of pulmonary blood flow, and IVC blood returns to the common atrium. Performed between age 3 to 6 months, the BDG has proved to be an important early staging procedure in single-ventricle physiology for relieving volume and pressure overload, pulmonary artery distortion, and coronary hypoperfusion associated with an aortopulmonary shunt. However, BDG circulation is not a stable source of pulmonary blood flow in the first few months of life when pulmonary cross-sectional area is inadequate to accommodate sufficient passive pulmonary blood flow for tolerable oxygenation. The BDG usually is performed on CPB using mild hypothermia with a beating heart. Therefore the complications related to CPB and aortic cross-clamping are minimal, and patients can be weaned and extubated in the early postoperative period.[75] In selected cases, the BDG anastomosis can be accomplished without CPB.

Systemic hypertension is common following a BDG. The etiology remains to be determined, but possible factors include improved contractility and stroke volume after the volume load on the ventricle is reduced, and brain stem–mediated mechanisms secondary to the increased systemic and cerebral venous pressure. Treatment with vasodilators may be necessary during the early postoperative period.

Following the BDG anastomosis, arterial oxygen saturation should be in the 80% to 85% range; however, stabilization to this level can take a number of days. In addition, positive pressure ventilation in these patients reduces passive pulmonary blood, so oxygen saturation frequently improves after extubation. Persistent hypoxemia (SaO_2 <70%) can be secondary to a low cardiac output state (low SvO_2), low pulmonary blood flow, or lung disease (Table 38.4). Treatment is directed at improving contractility, reducing afterload, and ensuring the patient has a normal rhythm and hematocrit. Increased PVR is an uncommon cause, and inhaled NO is rarely beneficial in these patients.[49] This finding is not surprising because PA pressure and resistance and vascular tone are not high enough following this surgery to see a demonstrable benefit from NO. Persistent profound hypoxemia should be investigated in the catheterization laboratory to evaluate hemodynamics, look for residual anatomic defects limiting pulmonary flow, such as SVC or PA stenosis or a restrictive ASD, and coil any significant venous decompressing collaterals (eg, azygous vein), if present.

Fontan Procedure

Since the original description in 1971,[76] the Fontan procedure and its subsequent modifications have been successfully used to treat a wide range of single-ventricle congenital heart defects.[77] The surgical reconstruction is "physiologic" in that the systemic and pulmonary circulations are in series and cyanosis is corrected. However, given the current long-term outcome data, its is important to remember that the operation is still palliative rather than curative.[78,79] The mortality and morbidity associated with this surgery have declined substantially over the years, and many patients with stable single-ventricle physiology can lead reasonably normal lives.[80]

Considerations in managing a cavopulmonary connection are given in Table 38.5. Systemic venous pressure of 10 to 15 mm Hg and LA pressure of 5 to 10 mm Hg—that is, a

TABLE 38.4 Factors Contributing to a Lower Than Anticipated Oxygen Saturation in Patients With Common Mixing Lesions

Etiology	Considerations
Low FiO_2	Low delivered oxygen concentration Failure of oxygen delivery device

Pulmonary vein desaturation	1. Ventilation-perfusion defects
	   Alveolar process (eg, edema/infection/atelectasis)
	   Restrictive process (eg, effusion/bronchospasm)
	2. Intrapulmonary shunt
	   Severe RDS
	   Pulmonary AVM
	   PA-to-PV collateral vessel(s)

↓ Pulmonary blood flow	Anatomic RV outflow obstruction Anatomic pulmonary artery stenosis Increased PVR Atrial level right-to-left shunt Ventricular level right-to-left shunt

↓ Oxygen content	1. Low mixed venous oxygen level
	   Increased O_2 extraction: Hypermetabolic state
	   Decreased O_2 delivery: Low cardiac output state
	2. Anemia

AVM, arteriovenous malformation; *Fio₂,* fractional inspired concentration of oxygen; *PA,* pulmonary artery; *PV,* pulmonary vein; *PVR,* pulmonary vascular resistance; *RDS,* respiratory distress syndrome; *RV,* right ventricle.

TABLE 38.5 Management Considerations Following a Modified Fontan Procedure

	Aim	Management
Baffle (right side)		→ or ↑ Preload
Pressure 10-15 mm Hg	Unobstructed venous return	Low intrathoracic pressure
	PVR <2 Wood units m²	Avoid increases in PVR, such as from acidosis, hypoinflation and hyperinflation of the lung, hypothermia, and excess sympathetic stimulation
Pulmonary circulation	Mean Pap <15 mm Hg Unobstructed pulmonary vessels	Early resumption of spontaneous respiration
Left atrial	Sinus rhythm	Maintain sinus rhythm
Pressure 5-10 mm Hg	Competent AV valve	→ or ↑ Rate to increase CO
	Ventricle	→ or ↓ Afterload
	Normal diastolic function	→ or ↑ Contractility
	Normal systolic function	PDE inhibitors useful because of vasodilatory, inotropic, and lusitropic properties
	No outflow obstruction	

AV, atrioventricular; *CO,* cardiac output; *Pap,* pulmonary arterial pressure; *PDE,* phosphodiesterase; *PVR,* pulmonary vascular resistance.

transpulmonary gradient of 5 to 10 mm Hg—is ideal. Intravascular volume must be maintained and hypovolemia must be treated promptly. Venous capacitance is increased, and as patients rewarm and vasodilate following surgery, a significant volume requirement of approximately 30 to 40 ml/kg on the first postoperative night is not unusual.

Changes in mean intrathoracic pressure and PVR have a significant effect on pulmonary blood flow. Pulmonary blood flow has been shown to be biphasic following the Fontan procedure, and earlier resumption of spontaneous ventilation is recommended to offset the detrimental effects of positive pressure ventilation.[81,82] Using Doppler analysis, it has been demonstrated that pulmonary blood flow predominantly occurs during inspiration in a spontaneously breathing patient—that is, when the mean intrathoracic pressure is subatmospheric. Therefore the method of mechanical ventilation following a Fontan procedure requires close observation. A tidal volume of 8 to 10 ml/kg with the lowest possible mean airway pressure is optimal. If appropriate selection criteria are followed, patients undergoing a modified Fontan procedure will have a low PVR without labile pulmonary vascular resistance. Vigorous hyperventilation and induction of a respiratory or metabolic alkalosis are often of little benefit in this group of patients, and the related increase in mechanical ventilation requirements may lead to injury. A normal pH and $PaCO_2$ of 40 mm Hg should be the goal and, depending on the amount of right-to-left shunt across the fenestration, the arterial oxygen saturation usually is in the 80% to 90% range. However, PVR may increase following surgery, particularly secondary to an acidosis, hypothermia, atelectasis and hypoventilation, vasoactive drug infusions, and stress response. Any acidosis must be treated promptly. If the cause is respiratory, ventilation must be adjusted. A metabolic acidosis reflects poor cardiac output and treatment directed at the potential causes, including reduced preload to the systemic ventricle, poor contractility, increased afterload, and loss of sinus rhythm. The effects of transient increases in PVR can be mitigated by the standard use of a fenestration of the Fontan circuit. This functions similarly to a residual PFO after a TOF repair where systemic hypoxemia (SaO_2) from the right-to-left shunt is the price paid for maintenance of systemic cardiac output.

The use of PEEP requires thoughtful consideration based on patient-specific postoperative circumstances. The beneficial effects of a PEEP-related increase in FRC, maintenance of lung volume, and redistribution of lung water must be carefully balanced against the possible detrimental effect of an increase in mean intrathoracic pressure on passive pulmonary blood flow. A PEEP of 3 to 5 cm H_2O, however, rarely has either hemodynamic consequence or substantial effect on effective pulmonary blood flow.

Alternative methods of mechanical ventilation have been used in these patients. High-frequency ventilation has employed successfully in selected cases, although the potential hemodynamic consequences of the raised mean intrathoracic pressure must be continually evaluated. Airway pressure-release ventilation has been shown to be superior in preserving systemic cardiac output when compared with standard pressure/volume control ventilation in patients post-Fontan completion.[83] Negative pressure ventilation can be beneficial by augmenting pulmonary blood flow.[84] The development of new negative pressure ventilators, cuirasses, and jackets have increased the interest in this mode of ventilation for this group of patients, but the experience is relatively small and indications are not defined. Application is cumbersome in the patient with surgical site dressings and chest tubes typically present after a midline sternotomy. In many centers, patients after a standard risk Fontan completion are identified for early extubation (in the operating room or within 6 hours of ICU admission), thus mitigating some of the aforementioned concerns. With proper selection criteria, optimal CPB management, and early extubation, most patients have an uncomplicated course after Fontan completion and can be discharged from the ICU environment within 1 or 2 days.

Nonspecific pulmonary vasodilators, such as sodium nitroprusside, glycerol trinitrate, PGE_1, and prostacyclin, have been used to dilate the pulmonary vasculature in an effort to improve pulmonary blood flow after a Fontan procedure, but the results have been variable. Although PVR may fall, pulmonary blood flow also could increase as a result of reduced ventricular end-diastolic pressure following improved ventricular function secondary to the fall in systemic afterload. The response to inhaled NO also is variable, and the improvement may be related to changes in ventilation/perfusion matching rather than a direct fall in PVR.

Afterload stress is poorly tolerated after a modified Fontan procedure because of the increase in myocardial wall tension and end-diastolic pressure. A phosphodiesterase inhibitor like milrinone is particularly beneficial. Besides being a weak inotrope with pulmonary and systemic vasodilating properties, its lusitropic action assists by improving diastolic relaxation and lowering ventricular end-diastolic pressure, thereby improving effective pulmonary blood flow and cardiac output.

Complications After the Fontan Procedure
Pleuropericardial Effusions
The incidence of recurrent pleural effusions and ascites has decreased since the introduction of the fenestrated baffle technique. Nevertheless, for some patients they remain a major problem with associated respiratory compromise, hypovolemia, and possible hypoproteinemia. They usually occur secondary to persistent elevation of systemic venous pressure, and reevaluation with cardiac catheterization may be indicated.
Rhythm Disturbances
Junctional bradycardia after Fontan completion is commonly observed postoperatively and rarely affects cardiac output significantly; in the rare circumstance where that occurs, the use of AAI pacing rapidly addresses the situation. Atrial flutter or fibrillation, heart block, and, less commonly, ventricular dysrhythmia may have a significant impact on immediate recovery and on long-term outcome.[85] Sudden loss of sinus rhythm initially causes an increase in LA and ventricular end-diastolic pressure and a fall in cardiac output. The SVC or PA pressure must be increased, usually with volume replacement, to maintain the transpulmonary gradient. Prompt treatment with antiarrhythmic drugs, pacing, or cardioversion is necessary.
Premature Closure of the Fenestration
Not all patients require a fenestration for a successful, uncomplicated Fontan operation. Those with ideal preoperative hemodynamics often maintain adequate pulmonary blood flow and cardiac output without requiring a right-to-left shunt across the baffle. Similarly, not all Fontan patients who received a fenestration use it for a right-to-left shunt in the

immediate postoperative period. These patients are fully saturated following surgery and may have an elevated right-sided filling pressure but nevertheless maintain an adequate cardiac output. The challenge is predicting which patients are at risk for low cardiac output after a Fontan procedure and who will benefit from placement of a fenestration. Even patients with ideal preoperative hemodynamics may manifest a significant low output state after surgery. In a review of 2747 Fontan completions from 68 centers contributing to the Society of Thoracic Surgeons (STS) database, 65% received a surgical fenestration at the time of initial operation.[86] Premature closure of the fenestration may occur in the immediate postoperative period, leading to a low cardiac output state with progressive metabolic acidosis and large chest drain losses from systemic venous hypertension. Patients may respond to volume replacement, inotrope support, and vasodilation; however, if hypotension and acidosis persist, cardiac catheterization and removal of thrombus or dilation of the fenestration may be urgently needed.
Persistent Hypoxemia
Arterial O_2 saturation levels may vary substantially following a modified Fontan procedure. Common causes of persistent arterial O_2 desaturation less than 75% include a poor cardiac output with a low SvO_2, a large right-to-left shunt across the fenestration, and additional "leak" in the baffle pathway producing more shunting. Persistent hypoxemia can also be caused by an intrapulmonary shunt or venous admixture from decompressing vessels draining from the systemic venous baffle to the pulmonary venous system. Reevaluation with conventional or bubble contrast echocardiography and cardiac catheterization may be necessary.
Low Cardiac Output State
An elevated LA pressure after a modified Fontan procedure may reflect poor ventricular function from decreased contractility or increased afterload stress, atrioventricular valve regurgitation, or loss of sinus rhythm (Table 38.6). Treatment consists of maintaining the high right-sided filling pressures (to maintain the transpulmonary gradient) and initiating inotropes and vasodilators. If a severe low output state with acidosis persists, takedown of the Fontan operation and conversion to a BDG anastomosis or other palliative procedure might be lifesaving. Central venoarterial extracorporeal membrane oxygenation (VA ECMO) support in this instance may be an effective bridging strategy to urgent reoperation. Emergent cannulation to VA ECMO after BDG and Fontan is associated with high morbidity and mortality and is generally contraindicated.[87,88]

Patent Ductus Arteriosus
Pathophysiology
The ductus arteriosus is a fetal vascular communication between the main pulmonary artery at its bifurcation and the descending aorta below the origin of the left subclavian artery. When patent, it provides a simple shunt between the systemic and pulmonary arteries. The magnitude and direction of flow between the systemic and pulmonary vessels are determined by the relative resistances to flow in the two vascular beds and the resistance of the ductus itself. With a large, nonrestrictive ductus and low PVR, the pulmonary blood flow is excessive and the volume load of the left heart is large. Systolic and diastolic flow away from the aorta may steal blood from vital organs and compromise end-organ function at many sites.[89]

TABLE 38.6 Etiology and Treatment Strategies for Patients With Low Cardiac Output Immediately Following the Fontan Procedure

Low Cardiac Output	Etiology	Treatment
Increased TPG		
Baffle >20 mm Hg LAp <10 mm Hg ↑ TPG ≫10 mm Hg	Inadequate pulmonary blood flow and preload to left atrium Increased PVR Pulmonary artery stenosis	Volume replacement Reduce PVR Correct acidosis Inotropic support
Clinical State		
High SaO$_2$/low SvO$_2$ Hypotension/ tachycardia Core temperature high Poor peripheral perfusion SVC syndrome with pleural effusions and increased chest tube drainage Ascites/hepatomegaly Metabolic acidosis	Pulmonary vein stenosis Premature fenestration closure	Systemic vasodilation Catheter or surgical intervention
Normal TPG		
Baffle >20 mm Hg LAp >15 mm Hg TPG normal 5-10 mm Hg	Ventricular failure Systolic dysfunction Diastolic dysfunction AVV regurgitation or stenosis	Maintain preload Inotrope support Systemic vasodilation Establish sinus rhythm or atrioventricular synchrony
Clinical State		
Low SaO$_2$/low SvO$_2$ Hypotension/ tachycardia Poor peripheral perfusion Metabolic acidosis	Loss of sinus rhythm ↑ Afterload stress	Correct acidosis Mechanical support Surgical intervention, including takedown to BDG and transplantation

AVV, atrioventricular valve; *BDG*, bidirectional Glenn anastomosis; *LAp*, left atrial pressure; *PVR*, pulmonary vascular resistance; *Sao$_2$*, systemic arterial oxygen saturation; *SVC*, superior vena cava; *SvO$_2$*, SVC oxygen saturation; *TPG*, transpulmonary gradient.

In addition, overcirculated lungs and elevated LA pressure increase the work of breathing.[90,91]

Critical Care Management

Although the PDA of premature infants can often be closed medically with indomethacin, contraindications to use of this agent (eg, intracranial hemorrhage, renal dysfunction, and hyperbilirubinemia) may require surgical closure of the defect.[92] Thoracotomy and surgical ligation of the ductus arteriosus are standard in term and preterm infants who are medically unstable. Beyond the newborn period, most centers now occlude the ductus with a percutaneously inserted vascular umbrella or using coils for smaller PDAs. In stable patients who are not candidates for an interventional cardiology approach (by nature of the length of the PDA), video-assisted thoracoscopic surgery (VATS) can be utilized.[93] Advantages of VATS compared with open thoracotomy include decreased postoperative pain, shorter hospital stay, and decreased incidence of chest wall deformity.[94]

Healthy asymptomatic patients undergoing surgery can be extubated in the operating room, allowing many options for anesthetic management. However, the fragile premature infant with severe lung disease may require mechanical ventilation for protracted periods after ligation of the ductus arteriosus. Fentanyl, pancuronium, oxygen, and air constitute a common anesthetic regimen for this procedure.[95] Many centers will bring the operative room environment to this patient population, performing the surgical ligation in the neonatal intensive care unit. Management of the premature infant in the operating room requires special considerations of gas exchange, hemodynamic performance, temperature regulation, metabolism, and drug and oxygen toxicity. Thoracotomy and lung retraction usually decrease lung compliance and increase oxygen and ventilatory requirements. A transient rise in systemic blood pressure with ligation of the ductus arteriosus may increase LV afterload or elevate cerebral perfusion pressure to the detriment of a premature patient. Inadvertent ligation of the left pulmonary artery or descending aorta has occurred because the ductus arteriosus often is the same size as the descending aorta.

The ductus is located near the recurrent laryngeal nerve (RLN), which may be damaged during the procedure. In addition to the close relationship of the RLN to the PDA and descending aorta, the RLN has a variable course that may be difficult to identify during dissection. Prior reports of PDA ligation performed by open thoracotomy indicate that the incidence of RLN injury is 1.2% to 8.8%.[96,97] RLN paralysis causes hoarseness and is not detected until the endotracheal tube is removed. The incidence may be reduced by location of the RLN within the thorax prior to ligation or clip placement using direct intraoperative stimulation of the RLN and evoked electromyogram monitoring.[98]

Ligation of an isolated ductus arteriosus generally results in normal cardiovascular function and reserve several months postoperatively.[99]

Atrial Septal Defect

Pathophysiology

There are three anatomic varieties of ASD. The most common, ASD secundum, is a defect in the septum primum, which ordinarily covers the region of the foramen ovale. ASD primum is a defect of the inferior portion of the atrial septum (endocardial cushion) usually accompanied by a cleft in the anterior leaflet of the mitral valve. Sinus venous defects are located near the junction of the right atrium and the SVC or IVC. They frequently are associated with a partial anomalous pulmonary venous connection.

Left-to-right shunting (simple) occurs at the atrial level, causing right ventricular volume overload. The degree of atrial level shunting is a function of the difference between right and left ventricular compliance as opposed to atrial pressure differential. Pulmonary blood flow is increased, but generally not enough to make these patients symptomatic during early childhood. However, later in life, as the left ventricle becomes less compliant and the LA pressures increase, the left-to-right shunt and volume load increase and symptoms of CHF may occur. In rare patients the long-standing increase in pulmonary blood flow causes pulmonary vascular obstructive disease.[100] Other problems associated with long-standing volume load from an atrial septal defect include atrial fibrillation.

Critical Care Management

The defect can be closed primarily with sutures or, if it is sufficiently large, with a synthetic patch. Sinus venosus defects associated with partial anomalous pulmonary venous connection require a more extensive patch that also directs the partial anomalous pulmonary venous return into the left atrium. These patients are among the healthiest encountered in the cardiac intensive care unit. Their anesthesia can be managed in many ways, but early tracheal extubation is the norm. Atrial arrhythmias, including atrial flutter and atrial fibrillation, are rarely seen during the postoperative period. Mitral regurgitation may occur in patients who have undergone repair of an ASD primum. Although transient LV failure has been reported, these patients rarely require inotropic support. Residual ASDs are uncommon, but occasionally failure to recognize partial anomalous pulmonary venous return results in a residual left-to-right shunt. Most patients can be extubated during the immediate postoperative period or in the operating room. With the exceptions mentioned, these patients usually have nearly normal cardiovascular function and reserve after repair.

Ventricular Septal Defect

Pathophysiology

Defects in the ventricular septum occur at several locations in the muscular partition dividing the ventricles. Simple shunting occurs across the ventricular septum. The magnitude of pulmonary blood flow is determined by the size of the VSD and the PVR.[101] With a nonrestrictive defect, high LV flows and pressures are transmitted to the pulmonary artery. Therefore surgical repair is indicated within the first 2 years of life to prevent the progression of pulmonary vascular obstructive disease.[102] In patients with established pulmonary vascular disease, the pulmonary arteriolar changes may not recede when the defect is closed. In such cases, there may be progressive PVR elevation.[103,104] The growth and development of the pulmonary vascular bed are significant factors in the patient's ability to normalize pulmonary vascular hemodynamics after surgery.[104] When PVR approaches or exceeds systemic vascular resistance, right-to-left shunting occurs through the VSD and the patients develop progressive hypoxemia (Eisenmenger syndrome). Closing the VSD in this circumstance adds the risk for acute right heart failure to that of progressive increases in PVR.

Critical Care Management

Closure of a VSD necessitates CPB. The most common septal defect, the membranous defect, is often repaired through the TV from a right atriotomy. However, lesions in the inferior apical muscular septum or those high in the ventricular outflow tract may require a left or right ventriculotomy. If so, postoperative ventricular function may be impaired. Concomitant RV muscle bundle resection can further impair ventricular function.

Before repair, measures that decrease PVR may appreciably increase left-to-right shunting in patients with a nonrestrictive defect and may increase the degree of CHF. Postoperative RV or LV failure may be a manifestation of the preoperative status of the myocardium, a result of the ventriculotomy and CPB,

or both. Small infants who fail to thrive, who are malnourished, and who have significant CHF preoperatively may have excessive lung water and may require prolonged mechanical ventilation postoperatively.[105] Such infants may have limited intraoperative tolerance for anesthetics that depress the myocardium or for maneuvers that increase pulmonary blood flow.

Persistent CHF and an audible murmur postoperatively, evidence of low cardiac output, or the need for extensive inotropic support intraoperatively suggests that a residual or previously unrecognized additional VSD is continuing to place a volume and pressure load on the ventricles. When PVR is increased preoperatively, the increase in RV afterload caused by closure of the VSD may be poorly tolerated, leading to the need for inotropic support of the heart and measures to decrease PVR.

Rarely, ventricular outflow tract obstruction is caused by placement of the septal patch. Transesophageal echocardiography performed in the operating room is an important tool in diagnosing this problem so it can be addressed prior to complete separation from CPB. Aortic regurgitation caused by prolapse of one of the aortic valve cusps can develop in subaortic or subpulmonic VSDs. In addition, heart block may occur after patch closure of a VSD. Temporary pacing may be needed to maintain an adequate heart rate and cardiac output. Generally, a permanent pacemaker is indicated when there is evidence of pacemaker dependence beyond 7 to 10 days.[106]

Critical Care Management for Late Postoperative Care

In the absence of residual VSDs, outflow obstruction, or heart block, most of these patients regain relatively normal myocardial function, especially if the VSD is repaired early.[107] However, a small percentage of patients, especially those in whom a large defect was repaired late in childhood, continue to have some degree of ventricular dysfunction and some pulmonary hypertension.[108]

Atrioventricular Canal Defects

Pathophysiology

The endocardial cushion defect, or complete common AV canal, consists of defects in the atrial and ventricular septa and the AV valvular tissue. All four chambers communicate and share a single common AV valve. The atrial and ventricular shunts communicate volume and systemic pressures to the right ventricle and pulmonary artery. The ventricular shunt orifice usually is nonrestrictive (simple shunt); therefore PVR governs the degree of excess pulmonary blood flow. Left AV valve regurgitation and direct left-ventricular-to-right-atrial shunting may further contribute to atrial hypertension and total left-to-right shunting.

Critical Care Management

Surgical repair of this lesion consists of division of the common AV valve and closure of the ASD and VSD with either a single-patch or two-patch repair technique. In addition, the left AV valve (and sometimes the right AV valve) requires suture approximation and resuspension of the separated portions.

Prior to surgical repair, these patients have large left-to-right shunts. As a result of their high pulmonary blood flows, they have CHF and pulmonary hypertension. Myocardial depressants and therapies that decrease PVR while increasing shunt flow may be poorly tolerated before repair. Some patients, especially older children, may have obstructive pulmonary vascular disease. All of the potential complications of ASD and VSD closures are seen in these patients. In addition, the left AV valve may be severely regurgitant.[109] Inotropic support for the failing heart, afterload reduction for mitral regurgitation, and measures to decrease PVR may be required intraoperatively and postoperatively after repair.

Patients with trisomy 21 frequently have an associated complete AV canal. Measures to decrease PVR and the use of prolonged ventilatory support are often necessary because of their tendency toward upper airway obstruction and abnormal pulmonary vascular reactivity. The large tongue, hypotonia, upper airway obstruction, and difficult vascular access of these patients pose additional problems. The most frequent postoperative problems in patients with trisomy 21 are residual VSDs, left AV valve insufficiency, and pulmonary hypertension.[110]

Truncus Arteriosus Communis
Pathophysiology
With truncus arteriosus communis, the embryonic truncus fails to separate normally into the two great arteries. A single great artery leaves the heart and gives rise to the coronary, pulmonary, and systemic circulations. The truncus straddles a large VSD and receives blood from both ventricles.

Complete mixing of systemic and pulmonary venous blood in the single great artery causes mild hypoxemia. Both pulmonary arteries usually originate from the ascending truncus, but occasionally only a single PA originates from the common trunk; the pulmonary artery orifice is seldom restrictive. The resulting shunt (simple) produces excessive pulmonary blood flow early in life as the PVR decreases. This *pulmonary steal* may elevate the arterial oxygen saturation and decrease the systemic blood flow. In such a case, net systemic oxygen transport decreases and lactic acidosis develops. Children with truncus arteriosus are at risk for developing early pulmonary vascular obstructive disease.[111] Regurgitation of blood through the truncal valve may place an additional volume load on the ventricles.

Critical Care Management
Complete repair of this lesion should be performed early, even in the neonate, before the development of irreversible pulmonary vascular changes.[112] The VSD is closed with a synthetic patch, and the pulmonary arteries are detached from the truncus. Continuity is established between the right ventricle and the pulmonary arteries with a valved conduit.[113] The truncal valve may require valvuloplasty if a significant amount of blood regurgitates through it. The presence of a dysplastic and moderately regurgitant truncal valve poses additional challenges; most data suggest that these patients are best served long term by cardiac transplantation. Pulmonary arterial banding or valve replacement may be considered as an interim bridging strategy to this destination.

Critical care management centers on control of pulmonary blood flow and ventricular support. Pulmonary blood flow may increase further with anesthetic agents, hyperventilation, alkalosis, and oxygen administration, resulting in hypotension and acute ventricular failure. If measures for increasing PVR do not decrease pulmonary flow, temporary occlusion of one branch of the pulmonary artery with a tourniquet limits pulmonary flow and restores systemic perfusion pressure until

CPB can be instituted. Because these patients are often in high-output CHF, myocardial depressants should be used with caution.

Immediately after repair, the combination of persistent pulmonary arterial hypertension and RV failure can be fatal. Hence, aggressive measures should be taken to provide adequate myocardial function and lower PVR. A residual VSD adds volume and pressure load on the ventricles and may have a devastating impact on the patient's hemodynamics and oxygenation. A VSD should be suspected in patients who are not doing well postoperatively. Any residual VSD should be repaired if feasible. Truncal valve regurgitation or stenosis may induce LV failure early during the postoperative period.

Critical Care Management for Late Postoperative Care
Obstruction of the pulmonary conduit and the accompanying RV hypertension may occur early or late during the postoperative course. Usually the conduit is unable to support flow in the growing child after several postoperative years. Late development of truncal (aortic) valve regurgitation is possible. For patients who underwent repair later in childhood, residual persistent pulmonary hypertension may be a problem.

Total Anomalous Pulmonary Venous Connection
Pathophysiology
Patients with TAPVC are cyanotic because their pulmonary veins connect to a systemic vein (complete mixing) and they have various degrees of pulmonary venous obstruction. The venous connection may be supracardiac (eg, to the SVC, innominate, or azygos vein), cardiac (eg, to the coronary sinus), or infracardiac (eg, to the hepatic veins, portal vein, or ductus venosus). Patients with this anomaly must have a patent foramen ovale or an ASD that allows blood flow to the left side of the heart.

This anatomic arrangement provides complete mixing of all systemic and pulmonary venous blood in the right atrium. Unless there is significant stenosis of the pulmonary venous connection, most of this right atrial blood passes through the right ventricle into the pulmonary artery, which increases pulmonary blood flow. If pulmonary venous return is significantly diminished due to obstruction, there is increased pulmonary venous congestion and decreased pulmonary blood flow.

Critical Care Management
These patients may be very ill, with hypoxemia, severe pulmonary edema, and pulmonary artery hypertension. Resuscitation, including mechanical ventilation, positive end-expiratory pressure (PEEP), and inotropic support of the myocardium, is followed by early surgical intervention to relieve the pulmonary venous obstruction. Although patients are hypoxemic, their primary pathology is caused by obstructed venous return from the lungs. Therapy that increases pulmonary blood flow (eg, PGE_1 or NO) must be avoided. Surgical repair of TAPVC requires attachment or redirection of the pulmonary venous confluence to the left atrium.

Intraoperative and postoperative problems often are related to residual or recurrent stenosis of the pulmonary veins. In patients who have severe preoperative pulmonary venous obstruction, the pulmonary vascular bed is poorly reactive, reflected by highly pulmonary vascular resistance indices (PVRi). This elevation in PVRi results in high pulmonary artery pressures and poor RV function after bypass and during the early postoperative period. Critical care management of these patients after completion of the repair should emphasize inotropic support of the right ventricle, avoidance of myocardial depressant drugs, and minimization of PVR. Prolonged mechanical ventilation with gentle hyperventilation and other postoperative therapy to decrease PVR are required. Inhaled NO has been particularly useful in this population, provided there is no residual pulmonary vein obstruction.[50]

Critical Care Management for Late Postoperative Care

Other than the potential for late development of recurrent pulmonary venous obstruction, these patients generally do well and have good cardiovascular reserve once recovery from the surgery is complete.[114] The size of the pulmonary veins at birth may be a predictor of late complications with recurrent pulmonary vein stenosis.[115]

Transposition of the Great Arteries

Pathophysiology

With transposition of the great arteries, the right ventricle gives rise to the aorta. Almost 50% of patients with this anomaly have a VSD, and some of them have a variable degree of subpulmonic stenosis. Oxygenated pulmonary venous blood returns to the left atrium and is recirculated to the pulmonary artery without reaching the systemic circulation. Similarly, systemic venous blood returns to the right atrium and ventricle and is ejected into the aorta again. Obviously, this arrangement is compatible with life only for a few circulation times unless there is some mixing of pulmonary and systemic venous blood via a PDA or an opening in the atrial or ventricular septum at birth. The physiologic disturbance in these patients is one of inadequate mixing of pulmonary and systemic blood rather than one of inadequate pulmonary blood flow.

Mixing of blood at the atrial level can be improved by balloon atrial septostomy. If dangerous levels of hypoxemia persist after the septostomy and metabolic acidosis ensues, an infusion of PGE_1 can maintain the patency of ductus arteriosus, increase pulmonary blood flow (by increasing left-to-right shunting across the PDA), and thereby increase the volume of oxygenated blood entering the left atrium. The volume-overloaded left atrium is likely to shunt part of its contents into the right atrium and thereby improve the oxygen saturation of aortic blood. Unlike other lesions, increased left-to-right shunting of blood during anesthesia improves arterial oxygen saturation before correction of the transposition.

Depending on the particular anatomy and the presence of a VSD or pulmonary stenosis, one of three corrective procedures is used. The intraoperative and postoperative problems encountered differ with each type of procedure.

Atrial Switch Procedure (Mustard and Senning)

An atrial level partition is created with baffling to redirect pulmonary venous blood across the TV to the right ventricle and thus to the aorta.[116] Systemic venous (SVC and IVC) return is directed across the atrial septum to the mitral valve, into the left ventricle, and out the pulmonary artery. Although the pulmonary and systemic circuits are then connected serially instead of in parallel, this arrangement leaves the patient with a morphologic right ventricle and tricuspid valve in continuity with the aorta. Therefore this ventricle must work against systemic arterial pressure and resistance.

One problem with atrial baffles is that they can obstruct systemic and pulmonary venous return.[117] When this occurs, the patient manifests signs and symptoms of systemic venous obstruction, as evidenced by signs of systemic venous hypertension. Often an overt SVC syndrome is avoided as the surgical technique focuses on leaving the IVC baffle unobstructed. As a result an SVC obstruction can be decompressed via the azygous vein into the IVC. When the pulmonary venous pathway is obstructed, pulmonary venous hypertension may be manifested by respiratory failure, poor gas exchange, and pulmonary edema. Severe pulmonary venous obstruction is manifested in the operating room by the presence of copious amounts of bloody fluid in the endotracheal tube, low cardiac output, and frequently poor oxygenation. Residual interatrial shunts also may cause intraoperative or postoperative hypoxemia. Long-term rhythm disturbances and the limitations of ventricular and AV valve function have made this operation nearly obsolete.

Arterial Switch Operation (Jatene Procedure)

Because of the complications associated with atrial baffle procedures, Jatene and others explored whether anatomic correction of this lesion, by dividing both great arteries and reattaching them to the opposite anatomically correct ventricle, would improve survival.[118,119] This procedure requires excision and reimplantation of the coronary arteries to the neoaorta (formerly the proximal main pulmonary artery). The success of the arterial switch procedure depends on adequate preparation of the left ventricle and technical proficiency with the coronary transfer. Anatomic correction of transposition of the great vessels is done during the neonatal period when PVR (LV afterload) and LV pressure are high. Left ventricular mass decreases progressively after birth in this lesion with the physiologic drop in PVR. If the left ventricle's ability to tolerate the work required is misjudged, the child may develop severe LV failure postoperatively necessitating significant vasoactive or mechanical support to maintain cardiac output. Infants with transposition of the great arteries who are older than a few weeks of age with an intact ventricular septum may have decreased LV pressure and mass. In such cases, the left ventricle may not tolerate the work required to perfuse the systemic vessels. However, if the neonate has a nonrestrictive VSD, the left ventricle is accustomed to high systemic resistances and will tolerate the increased workload at any age. In older patients with an intact ventricular septum, banding the pulmonary artery can prepare the left ventricle to function as a systemic ventricle by increasing its afterload and muscle mass. If the left ventricle is "conditioned" by banding the pulmonary artery and augmenting pulmonary blood flow with a modified Blalock-Taussig shunt, then an arterial switch procedure usually can be accomplished 1 week later, after hypertrophy and hyperplasia have occurred.[120] However, during this interval, these patients are cyanotic, with a volume-loaded right ventricle and a pressure-loaded left ventricle, and they may require considerable pharmacologic support.[121]

In experienced centers, the incidence of mortality after neonatal repair of transposition of the great arteries now is less than 3% and may be less than 2% for most anatomic arrangements of coronary arteries if the aortic arch is normal.[122] Mid- and longer term outcomes for the ASO are excellent demonstrating a 25-year survival and freedom from reoperation rates of 96.7% and 75%, respectively.[123] Alternative operations are reserved almost exclusively for patients with particularly difficult coronary anatomy[124,125] or pulmonic (neoaortic) stenosis.

Myocardial ischemia or infarction may occur after mobilization and reimplantation of the coronary arteries, especially if they are stretched or twisted. Inotropic support, maintenance of coronary perfusion pressures, control of heart rate, and treatment with vasodilators may be particularly useful, as in adult patients with myocardial ischemia. Postoperative bleeding and tamponade occur more commonly with this operation because of the presence of multiple arterial anastomoses.

Ventricular Switch (Rastelli Procedure)

This procedure can be used in TGA with VSD or double-outlet right ventricle when there is an unrestrictive outlet VSD and when coexisting pulmonary valve stenosis precludes a standard arterial switch operation. The pulmonary valve is oversewn and the right ventricle is connected to the pulmonary artery with a conduit.[126]

Complications of the Rastelli procedure include obstruction of LV outflow as a result of narrowing of the subaortic region by the VSD patch. The conduit also may obstruct during or after the immediate postoperative period. A small but significant incidence of heart block in these patients can be a difficult postoperative problem.

Critical Care Management

Management of patients following an atrial switch procedure rests on optimizing systemic oxygen delivery, monitoring for signs of baffle obstruction, and control of atrial arrhythmias. Most patients post-ASO without a VSD usually have an unremarkable postoperative course. Persistent ventricular dysfunction heralded by left atrial hypertension, hemodynamic instability, ventricular arrhythmia, or evidence of ischemic changes should prompt an intensive evaluation of the adequacy of the coronary anastomosis. Any of these perioperative issues or the unanticipated need for extracorporeal support necessitates immediate coronary evaluation and revision. Patients with delayed intervention (either due to late presentation or comorbidities that preclude a standard ASO timing of 2-10 days) usually will need to have a careful assessment for possible LV insufficiency. An aggressive strategy of systemic afterload reduction, deep sedation, and muscle relaxation while expecting a more protracted ICU course is often the norm for such patients. Occasionally, these patients will benefit from the use of ECLS or temporary left ventricular assist device (LVAD) support for retraining of the LV in the postoperative course.

Late Complications

Patients who have both a pulmonary ventricle and a morphologic right ventricle remaining as the systemic ventricle (ie, post-atrial baffle) can be regarded as having a physiologic or functional two-ventricle repair. Actuarial survival rates at 15 years have been quoted up to 85%; however, significant long-term functional deterioration is likely with increasing risk for right heart failure, sudden death, and dysrhythmias.[127,128] This situation is evidenced by systemic (right) ventricular dysfunction and TV regurgitation long after the repair.[129] These patients also are prone to develop significant atrial dysrhythmias, including supraventricular tachyarrhythmias and sick sinus syndrome later in life.[130] The arrhythmias may be preceded by RV dysfunction but also may be an isolated finding

and are potentially the major cause of sudden death in these patients. A number of large follow-up series have reported that the probability of a patient remaining in sinus rhythm after an atrial level repair is 50% at 10 years and 40% at 20 years. Function of the sinus node may be seriously impaired by the atrial manipulations during surgery, and sick sinus syndrome (requiring pacemaker insertion) may occur late in the postoperative period. The atrial baffle provides a functional repair, although despite this result, many patients continue to maintain relatively active lives with few subjective symptoms. Objective exercise testing on intermediate and late follow-up may demonstrate limited RV reserve in as many as 50% of patients. Exercise duration, peak heart rate response, and peak minute oxygen consumption are reduced compared with age-matched controls.[131]

Virtually all coronary artery patterns are amenable to ASO. No particular pattern has been associated with late death. A report of coronary artery angiography in 366 patients following ASO (median age at follow-up 7.9 years) revealed coronary artery stenosis or occlusion in 3% of patients.[132] The long-term significance of these coronary artery abnormalities has not been determined. Despite the angiographic findings, evaluation with serial ECG, exercise testing, and wall-motion abnormalities on echocardiography rarely demonstrate evidence of ischemia.[133]

After repair, the *native* pulmonary valve becomes the *neoaortic* valve. A 30% incidence of trivial-to-mild aortic regurgitation has been reported on intermediate-term follow-up, without significant hemodynamic changes.[134] Severe regurgitation is unusual.

There appears to be a very low incidence of significant rhythm disturbances after ASO.[135] Supravalvar pulmonary artery stenosis was an early complication but now is less common with surgical techniques that extensively mobilize, augment, and reconstruct the pulmonary arteries. Supravalvar AS may develop but is rare.

Assessment of myocardial performance using echocardiography, cardiac catheterization, and exercise testing following ASO has demonstrated function identical to that in age-matched controls. Based on the currently available clinical, functional, and hemodynamic data, a patient who has undergone ASO with no evidence of subsequent problems should be treated as any patient with a structurally normal heart when presenting for noncardiac surgery.

Late complications of the Rastelli procedure include progressive conduit obstruction and RV hypertension, residual VSDs, and occasionally subaortic obstruction from diversion of LV outflow across the VSD to the aorta.

Tetralogy of Fallot

Pathophysiology

The four anatomic features of TOF are VSD, RV outflow tract obstruction, overriding of the aorta, and RV hypertrophy. In addition, there may be VSDs of the muscular region of the septum and right-sided obstruction of the pulmonary valve and the main and branch pulmonary arteries.

Resistance to RV outflow forces systemic venous return from right to left across the VSD and into the aorta, producing arterial desaturation. The amount of blood that shunts right to left through the VSD varies with the magnitude of the RV outflow tract obstruction and with SVR. Distal PVR is low and has minimal influence on shunting. Systemic vasodilation, in conjunction with increasing dynamic infundibular stenosis, intensifies right-to-left shunting and can lead to hypercyanotic *spells*. Such spells can occur at any time before surgical correction of the anomalies and can be life threatening. Because the morbidity associated with recurrent hypercyanotic spells is significant, many physicians consider recurrent episodes of hypercyanosis an indication for corrective surgery at any age.

Critical care management of TOF patients with hypercyanotic episodes should focus on minimizing oxygen consumption, acidosis, tachycardia, and PVR while augmenting preload and SVR. Hypercyanotic spells in nonanesthetized children should initially be managed with 100% oxygen by facemask, a knee-chest position or squat position (to increase SVR), and morphine sulfate. This regimen can usually stabilize the dynamic infundibular stenosis while keeping SVR elevated. Deeply cyanotic and lethargic patients are given rapid IV crystalloid infusions to augment circulating blood volume. Continued severe hypoxemia is treated with a vasopressor bolus (eg, phenylephrine 1–2 µg/kg) to increase SVR and sometimes with judicious use of IV propranolol or esmolol to slow the heart rate. The latter allows more filling time and relaxes the infundibulum. If a hypercyanotic spell persists despite treatment, immediate surgical correction of the anomaly is indicated. The child can be anesthetized with IV narcotics, and an inhalation agent such as halothane may be beneficial to reduce hyperdynamic outflow tract obstruction. Anesthetic agents that predominantly decrease SVR, such as isoflurane, should be used with caution. The pattern of mechanical ventilation is critical, as excessive intrathoracic pressure can further reduces antegrade flow across the RV outflow.

Critical Care Management for the Early Postoperative Course

The surgical approach to the patient with TOF who presents with recurrent early hypercyanotic spells is variable. The traditional approach is to defer a complete repair until the standard elective repair can be completed (3-6 months of age). Delayed repair also is often necessary when a coronary artery crosses the RV outflow tract precluding transannular patch repair. There are currently two palliative interventions to facilitate a delayed repair strategy. The first is the use of a systemic-to-pulmonary artery shunt. Excellent outcomes have been achieved with this approach, and the need for a transpulmonary valve annulus outflow patch (transannular patch) at the time of definitive surgery is reduced.[136] The risks of cyanosis and complications related to a systemic-to-pulmonary artery shunt argue for early complete repair of TOF. The alternative approach, developed more recently, is stenting the RV outflow tract in the cardiac catheterization laboratory.[137] This procedure has the additional benefit of improving pulmonary artery growth prior to the definitive repair. Dohlen and colleagues reported on a series of nine patients who were effectively palliated with this approach at median age of 3 weeks.[138]

Another approach for patients with TOF is to proceed with an early complete repair. For that method, a ventriculotomy is performed in the RV outflow tract and frequently is extended distally through the pulmonary valve annulus and beyond any associated pulmonary artery stenosis. The outflow tract is enlarged with pericardium or synthetic material, and obstructing muscle bundles are resected to relieve the outflow tract obstruction.[139] Because they are smaller and younger, these patients may be at increased risk for complications associated with CPB. Pulmonary regurgitation results after a

transannular incision that may compromise ventricular function in the postoperative period. In approximately 8% of patients, abnormalities in the origin and distribution of the coronary arteries preclude placement of the RV outflow patch, making it necessary to bypass the stenosis by placing an external conduit from the body of the right ventricle to the pulmonary artery.[140,141] An analysis of 3059 TOF repairs between 2002 and 2007 demonstrated that 83% (2534) had a complete repair as their initial index procedure (with 6%, 19%, 38%, and 24% undergoing operation at the ages of 0 to 1, 1 to 3, 3 to 6, and 6 to 12 months, respectively).[142] There were 217 (7%) patients who underwent complete repair following an initial palliation. Rates of ventriculotomy, transannular patch, and RV-PA conduit use were significantly higher in those requiring an initial palliation. Discharge mortality was higher in palliative patients versus initial complete repair (7.5% versus 1.3%). There was less disparity in discharge mortality between the two approaches among neonates (6.2% versus 7.8%).[142]

When weaning patients from CPB following TOF repair, the aim of therapy is to support RV function and minimize afterload on the right ventricle. This is particularly important following repair in neonates or small infants. Although systolic dysfunction of the right ventricle may occur following neonatal ventriculotomy, more commonly the clinical picture is one of a *restrictive physiology* reflecting reduced RV compliance or diastolic function.[30,31] Factors contributing to diastolic dysfunction include ventriculotomy, lung and myocardial edema following CPB, inadequate myocardial protection of the hypertrophied ventricle during aortic cross-clamp, coronary artery injury, residual outflow tract obstruction, volume load on the ventricle from a residual VSD or pulmonary regurgitation, and arrhythmias.

Patients usually separate from CPB with a satisfactory blood pressure and atrial filling pressures less than 10 mm Hg on modest inotropic support, such as milrinone of 0.5 µg/kg/min or dopamine 5 to 10 µg/kg/min. However, in neonates during the first 6 to 12 hours after surgery, a low cardiac output state with increased right-sided filling pressures from diastolic dysfunction is common following a right ventriculotomy, and continued sedation and paralysis usually are necessary for the first 24 to 48 hours to minimize the stress response and associated myocardial work. Preload must be maintained, despite elevation of RA pressure.

In addition to high right-sided filling pressures, pleural effusions or ascites may develop. Significant inotropic support is often required, and a phosphodiesterase inhibitor, such as milrinone, is beneficial because of the lusitropic properties. Because of the restrictive physiology, even a relatively small volume load from a residual VSD or pulmonary regurgitation is often poorly tolerated in the early postoperative period, and 2 to 3 days may be required before RV compliance improves and cardiac output increases. Although the patent foramen ovale or any ASD usually is closed at the time of surgery in older patients, it is beneficial to leave a small atrial communication following neonatal repair. In the face of diastolic dysfunction and increased RV end-diastolic pressure, a right-to-left atrial level shunt maintains preload to the left ventricle and therefore cardiac output. Patients may be desaturated initially following surgery because of this shunting. As RV compliance and function improve, the amount of shunt decreases and both antegrade pulmonary blood flow and systemic arterial oxygen saturation increase.

Arrhythmias following repair include heart block, ventricular ectopy, and junctional ectopic tachycardia. Maintaining sinus rhythm is important to optimize end-diastolic filling and minimize end-diastolic pressure. Atrioventricular pacing may be necessary for heart block. Complete right bundle branch block is typical on the postoperative ECG.

Most patients recover systolic ventricular function postoperatively. However, in a small group of patients, especially those repaired at older ages, significant ventricular dysfunction remains.[143,144] These patients can have left ventricular subendocardial ischemia that impairs LV myocardial mechanics.[145] Pulmonary valve insufficiency may contribute to residual ventricular systolic dysfunction.[146] The most common cause of systolic dysfunction immediately after repair of CHD is a residual or previously unrecognized VSD, which causes a volume load on the left ventricle and pressure load on an already stressed right ventricle, leading to RV failure and poor cardiac output.[27] A residual VSD combined with residual RV outflow obstruction is particularly deleterious.

In some patients, the distal pulmonary arteries may be so hypoplastic and stenotic that they cannot be satisfactorily corrected. Suprasystemic pressure develops in the right ventricle, which in some cases can be ameliorated by partially opening the VSD to allow an intracardiac right-to-left ventricular shunt. This shunt unloads the compromised right ventricle at the expense of decreased arterial oxygen saturation.

Critical Care Management for Late Postoperative Care
Reconstruction of the RV outflow tract may lead to significant problems that affect RV function and risk for arrhythmias over time. Although most of the long-term outcome data pertain to patients following TOF repair, similar complications and risks are likely for those who have undergone an extensive RV outflow reconstruction, such as placement of a conduit from the right ventricle to the pulmonary artery for correction of pulmonary atresia, truncus arteriosus, and the Rastelli procedure for transposition of the great arteries with pulmonary stenosis.

Complete surgical repair of TOF has been successfully performed for more than 40 years, with studies reporting a 30- to 35-year actuarial survival of approximately 85%.[147] Many patients report leading relatively normal lives, but RV dysfunction may progress after repair and may be evident only on exercise stress testing or echocardiography. A spectrum of problems may develop, ranging from a dilated right ventricle with systolic dysfunction to diastolic dysfunction from a poorly compliant right ventricle, and these problems must be thoroughly evaluated preoperatively. In addition, continued evaluation is necessary because of the increased risk for ventricular arrhythmias and late sudden death. Factors that may adversely affect long-term survival include older age at initial repair, initial palliative procedures, and residual chronic pressure or volume load as occurs from pulmonary insufficiency or stenosis.

Systolic dysfunction secondary to a residual volume load from pulmonary regurgitation after tetralogy repair is a predictor of late morbidity. It is reflected as cardiomegaly on chest radiograph, an increase in RV end-diastolic volume and regurgitant volume by echocardiography and cardiac MRI,[17] and a reduction in anaerobic threshold, maximal exercise performance, and endurance on exercise testing.[148] Patients who have significant pulmonary regurgitation, RV dilation, and

reduced RV function are at potential risk for a fall in cardiac output during anesthesia, particularly as positive pressure ventilation may increase the amount of regurgitation.

An important group to distinguish consists of those who have continued restrictive physiology or diastolic dysfunction secondary to reduced ventricular compliance. They usually do not have cardiomegaly, they demonstrate better exercise tolerance, and the risk for ventricular dysrhythmias is possibly decreased. Although the right ventricle is hypertrophied, function is generally well preserved on echocardiography, with minimal pulmonary regurgitation. The incidence of significant RV outflow obstruction developing over time is low. Residual obstruction contributes to early mortality within the first year after surgery but is well tolerated in the long term.

A wide variation in the incidence of ventricular ectopy has been reported in numerous follow-up studies, including up to 15% of patients on routine ECG and up to 75% of patients on Holter monitor. Multiple risk factors, including an older age at repair, extent of ventriculotomy, residual hemodynamic abnormalities, and duration of follow-up, have all been considered important. In common with these factors are probable myocardial injury and fibrosis from chronic pressure and volume overload, combined with cyanosis. Although ventricular ectopy is common in asymptomatic patients during ambulatory ECG, Holter monitoring, and exercise stress testing, it often is low grade and does not identify those patients at risk for sudden death. Electrophysiologic induction of sustained ventricular tachycardia (VT), especially when monomorphic, is suggestive of the presence of a reentrant arrhythmic pathway. Although dependent on the stimulation protocol used to induce VT, the presence of monomorphic VT in a symptomatic patient with syncope and palpitations is significant and indicates treatment with radiofrequency ablation, surgical cryoablation, antiarrhythmic drugs, or placement of an implantable cardioverter-defibrillator.[149] The risk for ventricular dysrhythmias during anesthesia and ICU care for subsequent hospitalizations is unknown. Although preoperative prophylaxis with antiarrhythmic drugs is not recommended, a means for external defibrillation and pacing must be readily available.

Pulmonary Atresia
Pathophysiology
Atresia of the pulmonary valve or main pulmonary artery forms a spectrum of cardiac defects, the management of which depends on the extent of atresia, size of the right ventricle and tricuspid valve (TV), presence of a VSD and collateral vessels, surface area of the pulmonary vascular bed, and coronary artery anatomy. The timing of developmental abnormality defines the associated lesions. Pulmonary atresia with intact ventricular septum (PAIVS) is primarily an abnormality of tricuspid valve development that subsequently affects the pulmonary valve through its effects on fetal RV growth. Because the impact on the pulmonary valve is late, the fetal truncus arteriosus has already divided and the mesenchymal distal pulmonary vasculature can connect to a main pulmonary artery pressure head appropriately. As a result, this lesion predictably has well-developed central pulmonary arteries and pulmonary artery arborization.

At one end of the spectrum of PAIVS, platelike pulmonary atresia overlaps with critical pulmonary stenosis where there is a mild or negligible degree of hypoplasia of the right ventricle and TV. In these lesions, a fixed obligatory right-to-left atrial level shunt of all systemic venous return exists. Some blood may flow into the right ventricle, but because there is no outlet, blood regurgitates back across the TV and eventually reaches the left atrium and left ventricle. Pulmonary blood flow is derived exclusively or predominantly from a PDA. As a rule, these patients do not have extensive aortopulmonary collateral blood flow; consequently, they often become cyanotic when the PDA closes after birth. Critical pulmonary valve stenosis can be effectively treated by balloon valvuloplasty in the catheterization laboratory. Antegrade flow across the RV outflow may not improve immediately but may gradually increase over days as RV compliance improves. In platelike pulmonary atresia, radiofrequency perforation precedes balloon valvuloplasty.

Most patients with pulmonary atresia with intact ventricular septum have an underdeveloped TV and right ventricle. Depending on the degree of RV hypoplasia (which is directly related to the TV annulus Z score), the patient may be unsuitable for a biventricular repair in the long term. In this situation, initial palliation with an aortopulmonary shunt is necessary. Reconstruction of the RV outflow with a pericardial patch or interventional catheter techniques also may be considered if the right ventricle is of a sufficient size that a two-ventricle repair could be considered (approach overlaps with platelike pulmonary atresia with some RV hypoplasia). A large conal branch or aberrant left coronary artery across the RV outflow tract may restrict the size of a ventriculotomy and placement of a patch or conduit. Patients with pulmonary atresia, a hypoplastic right ventricle, and intact ventricular septum may have numerous fistulous connections (sinusoids) between the small hypertensive RV cavity and the coronary circulation.[150] This is distinct from right ventricular dependent coronary circulation where these sinusoidal connections are additionally accompanied by proximal stenoses in the true coronary arteries. This is a distinct risk in patients with a TV annulus Z score <−3, but it has been documented in moderate RV hypoplasia.[151] If decompression of the RV outflow tract is being considered in this population, a coronary angiogram is highly desirable to exclude this phenomenon.

At the other end of the spectrum, severe pulmonary atresia may be associated with an extremely hypoplastic right ventricle that is not suitable for biventricular repair. A palliative procedure with a modified Blalock-Taussig or central shunt usually is necessary at first to improve pulmonary blood flow, followed by staged single-ventricle repair (see the "Fontan Procedure" section).

In contrast to PAIVS, PA/VSD and TOF with PA represent an early failure of proper conotruncal development. As a result, the mesenchymal segmental pulmonary arteries do not see the main pulmonary artery pressure head and instead form connections with the nearest alternative (aorta). This is the nature of the development of the aortopulmonary collaterals (APCs) associated with the lesion. If the collaterals are substantial, defining a large pulmonary arterial segment, they are referred to as major aortopulmonary collateral arteries or MAPCAs. As a rule, these patients have two good-sized ventricles (unless accompanied by other lesions, such as an unbalanced AV septal defect). This disease can exist in a spectrum with confluent central pulmonary arteries and a short-segment main PA atresia to discontinuous PAs without a true central PA.

In the former situation, the pulmonary artery arborization is often close to normal with few MAPCAs. When antegrade flow is established from the right ventricle into the main pulmonary artery by a reparative procedure, the left-to-right shunt via collateral flow will impose a diastolic load on the left ventricle. Preoperative occlusion of these collateral vessels can be accomplished by interventional techniques in the cardiac catheterization laboratory but may leave the child precariously cyanotic in the hours before operation. The alternative is to complete the surgical procedure in a hybrid suite. This lesion is completely repaired in the neonatal period.

As mentioned, MAPCAs may be present to varying degrees, supplying some or all segments of the lung. They can be associated with a large left-to-right shunt, contributing to volume overload and pulmonary hypertension. Larger collateral vessels supplying significant portions of the lung can be anastomosed or "unifocalized" to the native pulmonary arteries, with the ultimate aim being to establish full antegrade pulmonary blood flow. Smaller vessels to some segments of lung can be coiled in the cardiac catheterization laboratory, provided there is antegrade flow from the native pulmonary arteries to those lung segments (dual supply).

When the pulmonary arteries are diminutive, it is important to establish early antegrade flow from the RV to the PA, in an effort to promote growth and establish a pathway to the pulmonary arteries for subsequent balloon dilation. A modified Blalock-Taussig or Mee shunt may initially be necessary to provide sufficient pulmonary blood flow if the pulmonary arteries are exceedingly small. Initially, the VSD can be left open, and postoperative management of cyanosis or CHF will be determined by the size of and the resistance offered by the pulmonary circulation. The course in these patients can be dynamic and demanding for even the most experienced practitioners. When collaterals are unifocalized in the operating room and right ventricle to diminutive pulmonary artery continuity is established, cyanosis may ensue and therapy is aimed at lowering PVR or (re)establishing adequate pulmonary blood flow. On the other hand, if the child is fully saturated in the aorta with elevated pulmonary artery oxygen saturation and LA pressure, then a left-to-right shunt through the VSD may be developing, which will produce a volume load on the left ventricle and an unstable postoperative course, dictating VSD closure. When the patient is not fully saturated in the aorta but is suffering from a volume-loaded left ventricle with low cardiac output and high LA pressure postoperatively, excessive systemic-to-pulmonary collaterals may be the culprits, requiring catheterization laboratory investigation and occlusion or immediate reoperation.

Critical Care Management

Critical care management of patients with pulmonary atresia is similar to that for TOF, except that hypercyanotic spells do not occur. Maintaining the patency of the ductus for the perioperative treatment of neonates with pulmonary atresia and critical pulmonary stenosis is essential. If there is platelike PA and the main pulmonary artery is present, it may be possible to perform a pulmonary valvotomy (interventional or surgical) and provide adequate pulmonary blood flow without a supplemental systemic-to-pulmonary artery shunt. The goal of therapy is to improve oxygenation and decrease RV afterload. Because the LV may be more pressure and volume loaded in this lesion than in the normal fetus, the RV may be relatively noncompliant postoperatively. This may manifest as requirements for high filling pressures and consequent right-to-left shunting through a purposefully patent foramen ovale. With growth and improved compliance of the right ventricle, the right-to-left shunting diminishes and the infant's oxygenation improves substantially. If hypoxemia persists, a PGE_1 infusion can be initiated to temporize either until accommodation of the restrictive RV physiology or for a Blalock-Taussig (BT) shunt.

In patients with long-segment pulmonary atresia, the need for a conduit to bridge the gap between the right ventricle and the pulmonary artery complicates the repair. Again, RV failure may occur postoperatively, especially when there is a residual VSD or RV outflow obstruction. The conduit may obstruct acutely during chest closure, further elevating pressure in the right ventricle. The relationship of the conduit to either normal or variant coronary anatomy is vital, as impingement of these structures can present as sudden inexplicable deterioration related to sternal closure.

After the VSD is closed and blood flow is from the right ventricle to the pulmonary arteries, there may be excessive pulmonary blood flow (Qp/Qs >1) as a result of the combined flow into the pulmonary arteries from the right ventricle and from aortopulmonary collaterals. If this occurs, the patient develops CHF and requires intraoperative inotropic support and an extended period of postoperative mechanical ventilation. With large collateral flow, the pulse pressure is wide and diastolic pressure low. The patient may require surgery to ligate the collateral vessels or may require embolization.

Critical Care Management for Late Postoperative Care
Patients with TOF and pulmonary atresia are subject to the same late problems and complications as patients with TOF alone. In addition, they will require conduit revisions over their lifetime. Some patients have accelerated conduit obstruction after surgery, which is often related to the presence of a porcine valve.[152] Consequently, many experts now prefer bovine-valved conduits or homografts except in a certain situations, such as when the distal pulmonary vascular impedence is high resulting in central pulmonary artery hypertension. In these situations a valve-less conduit that permits pulmonary insufficiency (and thus relieves central PA hypertension) is preferred. In cases when pulmonary regurgitant volume load to the RV is undesirable, some favor the placement of a heterologous bovine jugular vein bioprosthesis with a trileaflet venous valve.[153] This has been the valved conduit of choice in patients younger than 18 years of age, whenever pulmonary regurgitant volume load to the RV is undesirable.[153] Small-caliber bovine jugular vein conduits may result in significantly improved freedom from dysfunction at 5 and 10 years follow-up compared to pulmonary homografts in patients who received the operation during the first 2 years of life.[154]

Tricuspid Atresia
Pathophysiology
In this condition, an imperforate TV and hypoplasia of the right ventricle are present, often accompanied by a VSD of variable size and by pulmonic stenosis. The most common form of tricuspid atresia has normally related great arteries; when associated with transposition of the great vessels, the clinical presentation is similar to hypoplastic left heart syndrome.

In the usual type of tricuspid atresia, an obligatory atrial-level shunt exists from the right atrium through the patent foramen ovale or ASD into the left atrium, where complete mixing takes place. The degree of hypoxemia depends on the amount of pulmonary blood flow, which is regulated by the severity of the pulmonic stenosis. This in turn is regulated by the size of the VSD; patients with an extremely small/restrictive VSD will have pulmonary atresia in addition to tricuspid atresia. The common presentation is characterized by significant hypoxemia caused by the decreased pulmonary blood flow.

Critical Care Management
The ultimate palliative surgical course for tricuspid atresia is a modified Fontan procedure, but an initial palliative procedure may be required to improve pulmonary blood flow (modified BT shunt). Neonatal hypoxemia prior to surgery can be effectively stabilized on a PGE_1 infusion. A pulmonary artery band may be needed if the pulmonary blood flow is increased, or a shunt may have to be created for the severely hypoxemic child with decreased pulmonary blood flow upon ductal closure. The critical care management and complications are those discussed in the sections on shunts, banding, and modified Fontan procedures. Complications of chronic hypoxemia and cyanosis are also present.

Left-Sided Obstructive Lesions
Pathophysiology
This category includes valvar, subvalvar, and supravalvar mitral and aortic stenosis (AS), aortic coarctation, IAA, and the HLHS. Although these lesions can occur as isolated defects, they often are accompanied by other congenital cardiac defects. Identification of additional structural defects is necessary for optimal preoperative, surgical, and postoperative treatment.

Patients with LV outflow tract obstruction tend to present as either neonates or young infants with significant LV dysfunction and CHF or later in childhood with subclinical LV hypertrophy. The dramatic presentation of a neonate with circulatory collapse typically occurs with lesions that obstruct systemic blood flow so severely that right-to-left shunting at the ductus arteriosus is required to perfuse the body. As the ductus significantly narrows or closes, the LV becomes acutely pressure overloaded and begins to fail, leading to pulmonary edema and respiratory distress. When systemic perfusion becomes inadequate, the patient develops hypotension, weak pulses, metabolic acidosis, and oliguria. Classic examples include severe (or "critical") valvar AS, coarctation of the aorta, and HLHS (see the earlier single-ventricle discussion).

If the obstruction is less severe, the child can make the transition through ductal closure without notable LV dysfunction and maintain an adequate cardiac output. Over time, however, the pressure overload on the LV stimulates generalized hypertrophy. If untreated and significant, long-term pressure overload can cause LV diastolic dysfunction (compliance falls and end-diastolic pressure rises, causing pulmonary edema), LV systolic dysfunction, and episodic myocardial ischemia. Clinical manifestations of these changes can include reduced exercise tolerance, exertional chest pain, ventricular dysrhythmias, syncope, and sudden death. Significant LV dilation or clinical signs of CHF are ominous findings associated with a poor prognosis and an increased surgical mortality rate.

Aortic Stenosis

Of the three anatomic subtypes of AS, valvar AS occurs more frequently than subvalvar or supravalvar AS. The newborn with critical valvar AS who develops hypotension and acidosis as the ductus arteriosus closes requires resuscitation with PGE_1 to restore aortic flow plus mechanical ventilation and inotropic support to achieve stabilization before an intervention is performed. Currently, balloon dilation of the stenotic aortic valve during cardiac catheterization is the preferred intervention at most centers. A surgical valvotomy under direct vision using CPB is the surgical alternative. Despite successful relief of obstruction, significant LV dysfunction and low cardiac output often persist for days after the procedure and require continued treatment with mechanical ventilation and vasoactive drugs. Until LV function recovers and can support the entire cardiac output, continuation of prostaglandin infusion may be necessary to maintain patency of the ductus arteriosus. Patients should be carefully evaluated after balloon aortic valvuloplasty for residual AS and aortic regurgitation, the chief potential complication of valve dilation, especially if cardiac output does not improve over several days.

Older infants, children, and adolescents with moderate (pressure gradient 50-70 mm Hg at catheterization) or severe (pressure gradient >70 mm Hg at catheterization) valvar AS also are generally good candidates for balloon aortic valvuloplasty. If more than mild aortic regurgitation coexists with AS, however, a surgical intervention is preferred to balloon valvuloplasty. The pathophysiology produced by all types of aortic outflow obstruction is similar—that is, the pressure-overloaded LV becomes progressively hypertrophied and develops reduced compliance and an abnormally elevated end-diastolic pressure.

Initial assessment of obstruction relief can occur when the patient is still in the catheterization laboratory or operating room by either direct pressure measurements or echocardiography. Nevertheless, reevaluation for residual obstruction by physical examination or echocardiography in the ICU as patients recover from anesthesia and baseline physiology returns is important because outflow gradients can change. A significant residual obstruction should be suspected in any patient with persistent low cardiac output following the intervention.

Poor recovery of LV function after surgery can occur secondary to inadequate myocardial protection with cardioplegia in hearts with significant ventricular hypertrophy. Patients with marked hypertrophy are also at greater risk for developing VT and ventricular fibrillation early after surgery.

In patients with preserved LV systolic function who undergo an uncomplicated procedure, such as aortic valvuloplasty or subvalvar membrane resection, myocardial recovery after CPB is typically rapid and inotropic support is usually not required. Systemic hypertension is more common following relief of LV outflow obstruction, especially during emergence from anesthesia and sedation.

Antihypertensive therapy in the initial 24 to 48 hours may be necessary to prevent an aortic suture line and reconstructed valve leaflet disruption from excessive stress and to allow adequate hemostasis. Both beta-blockers (eg, labetalol, propranolol, and esmolol) and vasodilators (eg, nitroprusside), alone or usually in combination, are effective for lowering blood pressure in these patients.

In addition to assessing aortic valve and LV function, an evaluation for complications specific to each procedure is required. For example, if a myectomy is performed as part of the resection of fibromuscular subvalvar AS, the possibility of a new VSD, mitral valve injury, and left bundle branch block should all be assessed. Following the Ross procedure, it is important to assess patients for RV outflow tract and LV outflow tract obstruction, because the RV outflow tract is also reconstructed with a valved conduit. This procedure involves reimplantation of the native coronary arteries into the new pulmonary autograft placed in the aortic position; signs of coronary ischemia, unexplained hemodynamic collapse, or ventricular arrhythmia should prompt aggressive reevaluation of coronary flow adequacy.

Coarctation of the Aorta

Coarctation of the aorta is a narrowing in the descending aorta located at the level of insertion of the ductus arteriosus (juxta- or contraductal coarctation). Narrowing of the aortic lumen is asymmetric, with the majority of the obstruction occurring because of posterior tissue infolding, leading to the common description of a posterior aortic shelf. Depending on the severity and rapidity of development of the narrowing, patients can present as neonates with severe obstruction (a *critical* coarctation of the aorta) upon ductal closure, as infants with CHF, or as children/adolescents with asymptomatic upper extremity hypertension (especially with exercise).

Neonates presenting with critical coarctation of the aorta can often be distinguished clinically from patients with critical AS by their clearly discrepant upper versus lower body pulses, perfusion, and blood pressures. Other features at presentation, including evidence of CHF and inadequate blood flow to tissues, are similar. Because ductal narrowing or closure is common after hospital discharge, these patients often become critically ill and suffer end-organ damage before the ductus arteriosus can be reopened and resuscitation complete. Intestinal and renal ischemia leading to necrotizing enterocolitis and renal failure, respectively, are well-known complications of critical coarctation of the aorta. Echocardiography often reveals additional left-sided defects such as bicuspid aortic valve, valvar AS, aortic arch hypoplasia, and VSD. Preoperative stabilization and management in this clinical scenario includes initiation of PGE_1, mechanical ventilation, inotropic agents, and diuretic agents, as needed. In addition, these patients require adequate time for end-organ recovery before performing an intervention. In rare situations, the afterload on both ventricles cannot be relieved, as the PGE_1 infusion is unable to open the ductal and periductal arch tissue. In such a situation there is no prospect of facilitating cardiac and end-organ recovery; the patient should be taken to the operating room urgently for coarctation repair.

Coarctation of the aorta also occurs in association with complex defects such as D-transposition of the great arteries, single ventricle, and complete AV canal defect. If the ductus arteriosus is patent during echocardiographic evaluation of a neonate with suspected CHD, it often is not possible to predict the severity of coarctation of the aorta with confidence. A patient can have an abnormally narrowed aorta just proximal to the site of ductal insertion (ie, the aortic isthmus) and a posterior shelf but still not develop a severe coarctation of the aorta following ductal closure. Therefore evaluation of the potential severity of coarctation of the aorta in the ICU often involves discontinuing the PGE$_1$ infusion to allow for the ductus to close, followed by close clinical and echocardiographic reassessment for clinical manifestations of coarctation. An intervention to reduce aortic arch obstruction is indicated in any neonate with clinical or echocardiographic evidence of reduced ventricular function or impaired cardiac output related to coarctation development. These indications are more important than the systolic blood pressure difference between upper and lower body per se, although differences greater than 30 mm Hg often are accompanied by diminished ventricular function.

The postoperative management of patients following surgical repair of coarctation of the aorta can vary depending on the age at intervention. However, the key issues for assessment in all patients are adequate relief of obstruction and preservation of spinal cord function. Upper and lower body blood pressures and pulses should be compared serially and the lower extremities monitored closely for the return of sensation and voluntary movement in the early postoperative period. Equal pulses and a reproducible systolic blood pressure difference less than 10 to 12 mm Hg between upper and lower extremities indicate an excellent repair. Neonates and young infants typically require 1 to 2 days of mechanical ventilation postoperatively. Older children and adolescents often can be extubated in the operating room and rarely require inotropic support. In fact, these patients repaired at an older age are increasingly likely to have significant hypertension,[155] which should be treated aggressively early after surgery to reduce the risk of aortic suture disruption and bleeding. Beta-blockers and vasodilators, along with adequate analgesia and sedation, are effective. Patients with long-standing coarctation of the aorta frequently have persistent systemic hypertension despite an adequate surgical repair; continued treatment with angiotensin-converting enzyme inhibitors is advocated to achieve normal blood pressures. Due to the challenges in managing this cohort of older patients after coarctation repair and the advent of interventional catheterization approaches including the use of covered stents, a surgical repair strategy is increasingly falling out of favor.

Four uncommon complications are associated with surgical repair of coarctation of the aorta. Postcoarctectomy syndrome manifests as abdominal pain or distension in older patients and is presumably caused by mesenteric ischemia from reflex vasoconstriction after restoration of pulsatile aortic flow. Recurrent laryngeal nerve and phrenic nerve trauma can cause vocal cord paralysis and hemidiaphragm paresis or paralysis, respectively, with neonates and infants at highest risk. Disruption of lymphatic vessels or thoracic duct trauma can produce a chylous effusion that may require treatment by drainage or dietary modification.

Catheter-directed balloon angioplasty is used to treat both native and residual coarctation of the aorta.[156] The results of native coarctation of the aorta dilation after early follow-up appear similar to published surgical results, but aortic aneurysm formation has been reported. Balloon angioplasty of recurrent coarctation of the aorta after surgery is effective and is generally preferred to reoperation.

Interrupted Aortic Arch

Patients with IAA typically present as neonates with either a loud systolic murmur or circulatory compromise as the ductus arteriosus closes. Therefore patient presentation can be similar to other severe left-sided obstructive lesions such as critical AS, critical coarctation of the aorta, and HLHS. Unlike either critical AS or coarctation of the aorta, however, severe pressure overload on the LV does not occur in the presence of an unrestrictive VSD, which functions as a "pop off" for LV outflow. The approach to resuscitation is similar to that described for the other ductal-dependent left-sided obstructive lesions, with attention to the possibility of pulmonary overcirculation as for HLHS.

Postoperative management issues specific to patients with IAA include assessment of possible residual left-sided obstruction, both in the aortic arch and in the subaortic region, shunting across a residual VSD, hypocalcemia (related to DiGeorge syndrome), dysrhythmias, and LV dysfunction with low cardiac output secondary to global effects of CPB and deep hypothermic circulatory arrest (DHCA). Left-lung hyperinflation on postoperative chest radiographs suggests compression of the left main stem bronchus. This complication tends to occur after difficult arch reconstructions when tension on the aorta causes it to press on the anterior surface of the bronchus, thus producing distal air trapping.

Hypoplastic Left Heart Syndrome
Pathophysiology
Among the congenital heart lesions, perhaps the most controversial has been management of HLHS. Left untreated, HLHS is a uniformly fatal disease; debate continues regarding the optimal management strategy (ie, staged palliation, neonatal transplantation, comfort care). In the current era, the 14-month transplant free survival ranges from 65% to 75%, making the comparative waitlist mortality for transplantation in these patients unacceptable. The results of surgical management vary among institutions and are clearly dependent upon expertise and experience,[157] the clinical condition of the neonate at presentation,[158] prematurity, multiple congenital anomalies, presence of an intact atrial septum, later age of presentation,[159] and degree of hypoplasia of left heart structures.[160,161]

This common example of single-ventricle physiology also represents the most severe form of obstructive left heart lesion. An anatomic spectrum of disease is implied for the lesion, but in its most severe and common presentation there is atresia or marked hypoplasia of the aortic and mitral valves with critical underdevelopment of the left atrium, left ventricle, and ascending aorta. A 1- or 2-mm ascending aorta gives rise to the coronary circulation and the head vessels before converging with the ductus arteriosus, where the aorta becomes larger and supplies the circulation to the lower body. Pulmonary venous return arrives in the diminutive left atrium and cannot cross the atretic mitral valve; therefore it is directed to the right atrium and right ventricle, where common mixing occurs with the systemic venous return and all blood is ejected into the pulmonary artery. Systemic blood flow is then supplied from the pulmonary artery, right-to-left, across the PDA. As the PDA constricts in the neonatal period, systemic blood flow decreases and all ventricular output is directed to the lungs. The Qp/Qs ratio approaches infinity as Qs nears zero. Therefore the paradoxical presentation of high PaO$_2$ (70-200 mm Hg) in the face of shock and profound metabolic acidosis is seen. When the ductus arteriosus is reopened with PGE$_1$, systemic perfusion is reestablished, the acidosis resolves, and the PaO_2 returns to the range of 40 to 60 mm Hg, representative of a Qp/Qs ratio between 1 and 2.

Critical Care Management

Adequate preoperative resuscitation with PGE_1 and correction of metabolic acidosis and end-organ dysfunction are crucial to the stabilization and management of patients with this lesion. Further facilitation of resuscitation can be enhanced by judicious use of inotropic agents, which can optimize cardiac output and end-organ perfusion. However, excessive delay in the timing of surgical intervention results in gradual reduction in PVR over days, with excessive pulmonary blood flow and inadequate systemic perfusion. The surgical reconstructive approach to this lesion now commonly entails three operations that ultimately aim to provide a 2- to 5-year-old child with a reconstructed aortic arch and a Fontan-type circulation for single-ventricle physiology.[162,163] In the first stage of the reconstruction (Norwood operation),[163] the pulmonary artery is transected at the bifurcation and an anastomosis is performed to the ascending aorta, which has been surgically incised so that the aortic and pulmonary arterial confluence arise together from the single right ventricle as the neoaorta, which is extended into the remaining native aorta using homograft material. Pulmonary blood flow is established with either a modified BT shunt (usually 3.5 mm in diameter) or a RV-PA (Sano) conduit. The atrial septum is excised to ensure free flow of pulmonary venous return over to the TV. In addition to HLHS, the Norwood operation is used to repair other complex single-ventricle defects with systemic outflow obstruction or hypoplasia.[164]

The critical care considerations are the same as those outlined for patients with single-ventricle physiology. Perioperative management requires optimization of combined ventricular output, minimization of systemic oxygen consumption, and careful manipulation of Qp:Qs.

Postoperative Management

Evolution of Treatment Strategies. Common teaching has held that postoperative mortality and hemodynamic lability are attributable to myocardial dysfunction and the physiologic burden imposed by a shunt-dependent pulmonary circulation in parallel with systemic blood flow. Treatment strategies have emphasized factors that may affect the balance between pulmonary and systemic blood flow. Immediately following a Norwood operation, PVR may be transiently elevated but soon decreases. Once PVR falls, treatment is aimed at raising resistance to blood flow through the lungs and redirecting cardiac output to the systemic circulation. High inspired concentration of oxygen, hyperventilation, alkalosis, systemic vasoconstriction, and anemia will cause further increase in pulmonary blood flow and should be avoided. Therapies designed to raise PVR and thereby direct aortic blood flow to the systemic circulation have focused on lowering the FiO_2 or allowing the $PaCO_2$ to rise with the pH falling toward 7.3. Further measures, such as ventilation with hypoxic gas mixtures or added carbon dioxide, have been advocated by some centers and have been intermittently embraced and abandoned by others. Validation of the effectiveness of these techniques to balance the pulmonary and systemic circulations has been difficult.[68,165]

The clinical focus on caring for the newborn following Norwood palliation for HLHS has evolved in stages since the 1990s. The early emphasis was on manipulating the PVR by optimizing mechanical ventilation (ie, mean airway pressure, tidal volume, rate and inspiratory time, FiO_2, and $PaCO_2$). It soon became apparent that the majority of this effort was aimed in the postoperative period to raise PVR and lower pulmonary blood flow while increasing systemic blood flow. Like any therapeutic strategy, manipulating gas exchange and inspired gases had its own set of adverse effects. High FiO_2 has well-defined pulmonary toxicity that may appear in a matter of days or even hours after exposure. Use of low FiO_2 (below room air concentrations) to raise PVR transiently and stabilize patients is both counterintuitive and a relatively uncommon therapy in clinical medicine. Whether iatrogenically induced or as part of a pathologic process, alveolar hypoxia can be life threatening when aggravated by unexpected hypoventilation. A mechanically ventilated and sedated patient on an FiO_2 less than 0.21 has little safety margin for dangerous hypoxemia even in the most intensively monitored environments. Excellent animal models of chronic pulmonary hypertension are produced by relatively brief exposure to hypoxic gas. A newborn breathing hypoxic gas mixtures in the preoperative period of stabilization may have a favorable response by raising PVR and diminishing pulmonary blood flow. However, if this treatment is prolonged during preparation for reconstructive or transplantation surgery, the caretakers may be frustrated by subsequent elevation in PVR that persists during and after weaning from CPB.

In centers where neonates are allowed to awaken and breathe spontaneously during the immediate postoperative period, pulmonary blood flow may become excessive and further stimulate hyperventilation and respiratory alkalosis. Adding carbon dioxide to the inspired gas may reverse this trend toward respiratory alkalosis and stabilize the relative balance of the pulmonary and systemic circulations if the forces that drive minute ventilation are suppressed with agents for sedation or analgesia.[68,165] However, the metabolic cost of carbon dioxide breathing in an awakening child given little analgesia may discourage widespread application of this technique until the physiologic advantage over conventional means of controlling alveolar ventilation and $PaCO_2$ has been demonstrated. This is especially true in unsedated, preoperative patients where factors controlling respiration during carbon dioxide breathing may permit minimal change of $PaCO_2$ but substantially increase the respiratory rate and work of breathing.

The introduction of a 3.5-mm systemic-to-pulmonary shunt (rather than a 4-mm shunt) and the appreciation of the surgical complexity of an appropriately placed shunt did as much to reduce excessive pulmonary blood flow in infants as did manipulation of the ventilator. Although the smaller shunts were associated with a rare but real incidence of shunt thrombosis, those involved in postoperative care found patient management with a small shunt substantially easier than struggling with the tendency for pulmonary overcirculation with a 4-mm shunt. By the late 1980s it was apparent that this palliated circulation was required for only 10 to 12 weeks to reach an adequate patient size for the newly applied second stage of the procedure (bidirectional Glenn) to be performed. Therefore a relative increase in cyanosis (from a smaller shunt) was believed to be a justifiable price for more stable early postoperative hemodynamics. However, mortality rates did not plummet with the recognition of the advantage of smaller shunts and manipulating PVR, although by then many more centers were undertaking a staged reconstructive approach to HLHS. In the early 1990s attention was redirected to the observation that arterial oxygen saturation was only one variable in the assessment of Qp/Qs and that a perfectly acceptable arterial oxygen saturation of 80% in this disease may represent severe pulmonary overcirculation if the mixed venous oxygen saturation was only 20%. Hence a renewed interest in measuring and monitoring arterial and mixed venous oxygen saturations emerged. Thus in overcirculated patients with a small (3.5-mm) fixed-diameter shunt off of the subclavian artery, there was less emphasis on micromanagement of PVR and more interest in pharmacologically supporting cardiac output while reducing the systemic afterload to diminish the driving pressure across the shunt. Some have advocated use of the alpha-blocker phenoxybenzamine for blunting systemic vascular reactivity and dilating the peripheral circulation,[166] but its potent, long-lasting effects and associated hypotension that is not ameliorated by the usual alpha-agonist vasoactive agents can be challenging. The phosphodiesterase inhibitors then enjoyed a new and extensive application in pediatric critical care: lowering SVR, increasing cardiac output, and lowering filling pressures. The new strategy was to monitor (arteriovenous) DO_2, support cardiac output, and reduce SVR.

Later in the decade, the observation of limited coronary reserve, low mixed venous oxygen saturation, rising lactate, and hemodynamic collapse in the first 48 hours helped emphasize the fundamental limitation of myocardial function and cardiac output in the early postoperative period. The morphologic RV and TV seem ill suited to support adequate systemic plus pulmonary blood flow. Several centers then embraced mechanical support of the circulation temporarily for the failing Norwood patient in the early postoperative period.

Specific Considerations for the Norwood Operation. Management of patients following a Norwood-type operation is complex. Intensive monitoring is essential because the patient's clinical status can change abruptly with rapid deterioration. Persistent or progressive metabolic acidosis is a bad prognostic sign and must be aggressively managed. Considerations in the assessment of the circulation following the Norwood operation are given in Table 38.7.

Ideally the pH should be 7.4, $PaCO_2$ 40 mm Hg, and PaO_2 40 mm Hg in room air, with a mixed venous O_2 saturation of 60% reflecting a well-balanced circulation. Higher saturations can be achieved if the systemic circulation is well dilated without compromising perfusion pressure. Frequent adjustments in mechanical ventilation settings and FiO_2 may be necessary in the first few hours after surgery. However, manipulations of FiO_2 in the face of a restrictive 3.5-mm shunt may have less impact on pulmonary blood flow than would systemic vasodilation.[162] Leaving the sternum open after surgery may facilitate lower filling pressures, a balanced circulation, and a stable ventilation pattern.

Deep sedation or even muscle paralysis and anesthesia often are continued after surgery to minimize the stress response until the patient has a stable circulation and gas exchange. Inotropic support with dopamine and occasionally low doses of epinephrine usually are required, titrated to systemic pressure and perfusion. Afterload reduction with milrinone as a second-line agent is beneficial to reduce myocardial work and improve systemic perfusion. Monitoring SVC O_2 saturations, as a measure of mixed venous O_2 saturation (SvO_2) and

TABLE 38.7 Management Considerations for Patients Following a Norwood Procedure

Scenario	Etiology	Management
SaO_2 ~80% SvO_2 ~60% Normotensive	Balanced flow ($Q_p = Q_s$)	No intervention
SaO_2 >90% Hypotension	**Overcirculated ($Q_p > Q_s$)** Low PVR Large BT shunt Residual arch obstruction	Raise PVR — Controlled hypoventilation — Low FiO_2 (0.17-0.19) — Add CO_2 (3%-5%) — Increase systemic perfusion — Afterload reduction, vasodilation — Inotropic support — Surgical shunt revision
SaO_2 <75% Hypertension	**Undercirculated ($Q_p < Q_s$)** High PVR Small, kinked, thrombosed BT shunt	Lower PVR — Controlled hyperventilation — Alkalosis — Sedation/paralysis Increase cardiac output — Inotropic support Hematocrit >40% Surgical intervention
SaO_2 <75% Hypotension Low SvO_2	Low cardiac output Ventricular failure Myocardial ischemia Residual arch obstruction Atrioventricular valve regurgitation	Minimize stress response Inotropic support Surgical revision Consider mechanical support Consider transplantation

BT, Blalock-Taussig; *FiO₂,* inspired oxygen concentration; *PVR,* pulmonary vascular resistance; *Q_p,* pulmonary blood flow; *Q_s,* systemic blood flow; *SaO₂,* arterial oxygen saturation; *SvO₂,* mixed venous oxygen saturation.

cardiac output, is useful in this assessment. Volume replacement to maintain preload is essential, aiming for a common atrial pressure approximating 8 to 10 mm Hg.

The type, diameter, length, and position of the shunt affect the balance of pulmonary and systemic flow. Generally, a 3.5-mm modified BT shunt from the distal innominate artery provides adequate pulmonary blood flow without excessive steal from the systemic circulation for most full-term neonates. Nevertheless, a shunt resulting in a low diastolic pressure (<30 mm Hg) in turn affects perfusion to other vascular beds, particularly the coronary, cerebral, renal, and splanchnic perfusion. This may contribute to a prolonged and difficult postoperative course.

Overcirculation in the immediate postoperative period with an SaO_2 greater than 90% may reflect a low PVR or increased flow across the shunt if the shunt size is too large or the perfusion pressure is increased from residual aortic arch obstruction distal to the shunt insertion site. The increased volume load on the systemic ventricle results in congestive cardiac failure and progressive systemic hypoperfusion with cool extremities, oliguria, and metabolic acidosis. Although manipulation of mechanical ventilation and inspired oxygen concentration may help limit pulmonary blood flow, surgical revision to reduce the shunt size may be necessary.

If there is significant diastolic runoff through a large shunt, coronary perfusion will be reduced and lead to ischemia, low output, arrhythmias, and cardiac arrest. Rhythm disturbances are uncommon in the immediate postoperative period following a Norwood operation, and a sudden loss of sinus rhythm, particularly heart block or ventricular fibrillation, should increase the suspicion of myocardial ischemia and impending circulatory collapse.

In the immediate postoperative period, mild hypoxemia with a SaO_2 of 70% to 75% and PaO_2 of 30 to 35 mm Hg is preferable to an overcirculated state with high systemic oxygen saturations and falling mixed venous oxygen saturation. Pulmonary blood flow often increases on the first postoperative day as ventricular function improves and PVR falls during recovery from CPB. Pulmonary venous desaturation from parenchymal lung disease such as atelectasis, pleural effusions, and pneumothorax requires aggressive management.

Persistent desaturation and hypotension reflects a low cardiac output from poor ventricular function, thereby decreasing the perfusion pressure across the shunt. SvO_2 is low (often <40%), and treatment is directed first at augmenting contractility with inotropic agents and subsequently reducing afterload with a vasodilator. This is a serious clinical problem with a high mortality after a Norwood operation. The related myocardial ischemia and acidosis further impair myocardial function and systemic perfusion, leading to circulatory collapse.

Atrioventricular valve regurgitation and residual aortic arch obstruction are important causes of persistent low cardiac output and inability to wean from mechanical ventilation. Echocardiography is useful for assessing valve and ventricular function but is less accurate for assessing the degree of residual arch obstruction. Cardiac catheterization is sometimes necessary and will enable fine-tuning of hemodynamic support or balloon dilation of a hypoplastic segment of narrowed aorta. Occasionally, surgical revision of the aortic arch or atrioventricular valve is necessary, although this is seen more commonly in the interval before the bidirectional cavopulmonary shunt.

The advocated Sano modification of the Norwood procedure involves placement of a conduit from the right ventricle to the PA confluence (RV-PA shunt).[167,168] The primary advantage of this procedure in the immediate postoperative period is improved diastolic perfusion without runoff across an aortopulmonary shunt. Ventricular function is less likely to be compromised after surgery because the volume load to the ventricle is reduced from a lower Qp/Qs, along with a reduced risk for myocardial ischemia because of improved coronary perfusion. Perfusion to cerebral, renal, and splanchnic circulations also is likely to be improved with the lack of diastolic runoff to the pulmonary circulation, which may enhance postoperative recovery. Because pulmonary blood flow occurs only during ventricular systole across the right ventricle to the pulmonary artery conduit, there may be a critical reduction in pulmonary blood flow and excessive hypoxemia, especially during periods of low cardiac output or if there is dynamic obstruction to flow at the ventricular insertion site. Efforts to overcome this limitation by creating a larger RV incision run the longer-term risk of ventricular dysfunction, arrhythmias, or aneurysm formation.

A multicenter, randomized, controlled trial involving 549 neonates with HLHS demonstrated a significantly improved transplantation-free survival for patients randomized to receive a RV-PA shunt compared to those palliated with a modified BT shunt (74% versus 64%, P = 0.01).[169] The major benefit of the RV-PA shunt seems to be an increased survival rate in the early period after the procedure. The short-term survival advantage of the Sano modification of the Norwood operation for centers where mortality rate after the Norwood operation already was below 15% will be hard to demonstrate. More recent long-term follow-up, however, demonstrates an elimination of this survival advantage at 3 years of age with the RV-PA shunt group.[170] In addition, this group had worse RV ejection fraction validating concerns regarding the impact of an incision in the systemic ventricle.[170]

Orthotopic heart transplantation has gained acceptance as an alternative treatment for HLHS.[171] Neonatal transplants appear to be well tolerated, and some centers have avoided maintenance steroid therapy while achieving excellent midterm results using transplantation as the sole therapeutic option for this disease.[172,173] Others have successfully advocated a combined approach using either transplantation or staged reconstruction, depending on the pathophysiologic state of the child and the availability of a donor heart. However, the critical shortage of donor organs places a marked limitation on correction of this common congenital heart lesion.

It is apparent that many children have derived benefit from a completed, staged reconstruction or heart transplantation for this previously fatal illness. They are often able to lead active, productive lives, and many do develop normally.[174,175] Both survival and developmental outcomes for this disease are improving worldwide. However, the long-term prognosis for this evolving therapy will not be known for several years.

Hybrid Approach. An innovative alternative to the stage I Norwood palliation that eliminates the insult associated with CPB in the fragile neonate with HLHS has been developed. This approach combines interventional cardiac catheterization techniques with less involving surgery and is referred to as the hybrid procedure.[176,177] The goal is to replicate the physiologic state of the Norwood procedure by the combination of three interventions: (1) placement of bilateral pulmonary artery bands to limit flow to the lungs, (2) placement of an endovascular stent to maintain the long-term patency of the ductus arteriosus, and (3) balloon atrial septostomy with or without stenting of the atrial communication to ensure adequate mixing and unrestricted left-to-right atrial flow.[176-179] This is accomplished through a standard medial sternotomy and does not require CPB.

The procedure requires superb coordination between the surgical and cardiac catheterization teams. It is generally performed in a hybrid suite consisting of a large modern cardiac catheterization laboratory with enough room to accommodate the surgeons and supporting operating room staff, in addition to the interventional cardiology team and anesthesiologists. Outcomes have been encouraging with early mortality comparable with that of standard protocols (about 15%-20%).[180,181] Direct comparison of the two methods is complicated because, in most centers, the hybrid procedure generally has been reserved for patients regarded as high risk for bypass surgery (eg, low birth weight, unstable hemodynamics, and poor ventricular function). Interstage mortality can be significant (15%-20%),[180] and case-matched studies have shown no benefit over conventional surgery.[179] One barrier to the widespread implementation of the hybrid procedure is that results of conventional surgery in the low-risk groups are now so good that many centers of excellence have been reluctant to undertake a new procedure with its attendant learning curve.

The hybrid procedure poses some unique technical challenges: The ductal stent position is crucial and, if patients have a diminutive ascending and transverse aorta, then the procedure does not address this impediment to coronary flow. If the transverse aorta is small, the stent itself might distort or interfere with retrograde flow into the arch, and for this reason most centers do not recommend the hybrid approach in the setting of a small transverse arch. Nevertheless, the hybrid approach undoubtedly has a role in the management of patients with HLHS and, with continued encouraging results[182] beyond the centers of excellence that developed and advanced this technique, it has found a niche among high-risk patients or as a bridge to transplantation.

Up to 50% of patients that survive the stage I hybrid procedure require catheter reintervention due to stent migration or restrictive flow across the atrial communication.[180] The stage II procedure becomes much more extensive than the conventional stage II because the aortic arch needs to be reconstructed (excising the ductal stent), the bands removed, and the pulmonary arteries repaired with a patch in addition to creating the cavopulmonary connection. Consequently, the stage II after the hybrid procedure carries higher operative mortality (10% to 15%), and this needs to be taken into account when comparing it with conventional techniques.[180,182] No absolute consensus exists on the future of the hybrid procedure. This innovative approach offers potential benefits that should be scrutinized through careful study and long-term follow-up.

Summary

The cardiac ICU has become the epicenter of activity in large cardiovascular programs. Nowhere are collaborative practices and multidisciplinary skills more valued or necessary. A curriculum in cardiac intensive care is now formally incorporated into cardiology training. Pediatric intensive care training programs have a mandate to include curricula and experience in the management of postoperative cardiac patients. Additional cardiac intensive care training is offered in selected centers to pediatric intensive care specialists wishing to pursue a career in the cardiac intensive care unit. Specialists in this field must have in-depth training in pediatric intensive care and cardiology as the scope of practice goes well beyond the cardiovascular system and requires expertise in complex respiratory physiology, diagnosis and management of multiorgan system dysfunction, and the various supportive techniques vital to the discipline of intensive care, to name a few. Increased complexity of disease, advances in technology and applied research, shortened lengths of stay, and improved survival in contemporary series (Table 38.8) all describe the fast-paced specialized environment that has accompanied the development of this new specialty of pediatric cardiac intensive care. Although the dramatic reduction in mortality has been gratifying in cardiac intensive care and is attributable to many factors, achieving 100% survival with minimal morbidity remains our elusive goal. It will challenge the next generation of practitioners.

TABLE 38.8	Contemporary Outcomes for Benchmark Operations (January 2011 to December 2014)	
Procedure (Diagnosis)	Number of Operations	Operative Mortality Rate
Coarctation (off bypass)	3947	1.0%
Ventricular septal defect (VSD)	6985	0.7%
Tetralogy of Fallot	4519	1.0%
Atrioventricular canal defect	3116	3.2%
Arterial switch	1851	2.7%
Arterial switch + VSD	798	5.3%
Glenn/hemi-Fontan	3946	2.1%
Fontan	4164	1.4%
Truncus arteriosus	614	9.6%
Norwood (stage I palliation)	2828	15.6%

From the Society of Thoracic Surgeons (STS) National Database, Duke Clinical Research Institute.

Acknowledgment

We gratefully acknowledge the contributions of Peter C. Laussen and David L. Wessel, who authored this chapter in previous editions.

Key References

3. Romero TE, Friedman WF. Limited left ventricular response to volume overload in the neonatal period: a comparative study with the adult animal. *Pediatr Res.* 1979;13:910-915.
5. Hanley FL, et al. Repair of truncus arteriosus in the neonate. *J Thorac Cardiovasc Surg.* 1993;105:1047-1056.
8. Gladman G, et al. The modified Blalock-Taussig shunt: clinical impact and morbidity in Fallot's tetralogy in the current era. *J Thorac Cardiovasc Surg.* 1997;114:25-30.
9. Fisher DJ, Heymann MA, Rudolph AM. Fetal myocardial oxygen and carbohydrate consumption during acutely induced hypoxemia. *Am J Physiol.* 1982;242:H657-H661.
11. Greenwood RD. Cardiovascular malformations associated with extracardiac anomalies and malformation syndromes: patterns for diagnosis. *Clin Pediatr (Phila).* 1984;23:145-151.
12. Lister G, et al. Physiologic effects of increasing hemoglobin concentration in left-to-right shunting in infants with ventricular septal defects. *N Engl J Med.* 1982;306:502-506.
14. Freed MD, Miettinen OS, Nadas AS. Oximetric detection of intracardiac left-to-right shunts. *Br Heart J.* 1979;42:690-694.
21. Lewis AB, et al. Side effects of therapy with prostaglandin E1 in infants with critical congenital heart disease. *Circulation.* 1981;64:893-898.
24. Moler FW, et al. Respiratory syncytial virus morbidity and mortality estimates in congenital heart disease patients: a recent experience. *Crit Care Med.* 1992;20:1406-1413.
26. Jonas RA, et al. Anatomic subtype and survival after reconstructive operation for hypoplastic left heart syndrome. *J Thorac Cardiovasc Surg.* 1994;107:1121-1127, discussion 1127-1128.
28. Wernovsky G, et al. Postoperative course and hemodynamic profile after the arterial switch operation in neonates and infants: a comparison of low-flow cardiopulmonary bypass and circulatory arrest. *Circulation.* 1995;92:2226-2235.
30. Cullen S, Shore D, Redington A. Characterization of right ventricular diastolic performance after complete repair of tetralogy of Fallot. Restrictive physiology predicts slow postoperative recovery. *Circulation.* 1995;91:1782-1789.
31. Redington AN, et al. Antegrade diastolic pulmonary arterial flow as a marker of right ventricular restriction after complete repair of pulmonary atresia with intact septum and critical pulmonary valvar stenosis. *Cardiol Young.* 1992;2:382-386.

33. Lemler MS, et al. Fenestration improves clinical outcome of the Fontan procedure: a prospective, randomized study. *Circulation*. 2002;105:207-212.

35. Hoffman TM, et al. Efficacy and safety of milrinone in preventing low cardiac output syndrome in infants and children after corrective surgery for congenital heart disease. *Circulation*. 2003;107:996-1002.

37. Wessel DL. Current and future strategies in the treatment of childhood pulmonary hypertension. *Prog Pediatr Cardiol*. 2001;12:289-318.

38. Drummond WH, et al. The independent effects of hyperventilation, tolazoline, and dopamine on infants with persistent pulmonary hypertension. *J Pediatr*. 1981;98:603-611.

42. Petrossian E, et al. Endothelin receptor blockade prevents the rise in pulmonary vascular resistance after cardiopulmonary bypass in lambs with increased pulmonary blood flow. *J Thorac Cardiovasc Surg*. 1999;117:314-323.

43. Ignarro LJ, et al. Endothelium-derived relaxing factor produced and released from artery and vein is nitric oxide. *Proc Natl Acad Sci USA*. 1987;84:9265-9269.

44. Frostell C, et al. Inhaled nitric oxide. A selective pulmonary vasodilator reversing hypoxic pulmonary vasoconstriction. *Circulation*. 1991;83:2038-2047.

46. Journois D, et al. Inhaled nitric oxide as a therapy for pulmonary hypertension after operations for congenital heart defects. *J Thorac Cardiovasc Surg*. 1994;107:1129-1135.

47. Miller OI, et al. Inhaled nitric oxide and prevention of pulmonary hypertension after congenital heart surgery: a randomised double-blind study. *Lancet*. 2000;356:1464-1469.

49. Adatia I, Atz AM, Wessel DL. Inhaled nitric oxide does not improve systemic oxygenation after bidirectional superior cavopulmonary anastomosis. *J Thorac Cardiovasc Surg*. 2005;129:217-219.

52. Atz AM, Wessel DL. Sildenafil ameliorates effects of inhaled nitric oxide withdrawal. *Anesthesiology*. 1999;91:307-310.

53. Mittnacht AJ, Hollinger I. Fast-tracking in pediatric cardiac surgery–the current standing. *Ann Card Anaesth*. 2010;13:92-101.

55. Newburger JW, et al. A comparison of the perioperative neurologic effects of hypothermic circulatory arrest versus low-flow cardiopulmonary bypass in infant heart surgery. *N Engl J Med*. 1993;329:1057-1064.

58. Elliott M. Modified ultrafiltration and open heart surgery in children. *Paediatr Anaesth*. 1999;9:1-5.

64. Ulate KP, et al. Strict glycemic targets need not be so strict: a more permissive glycemic range for critically ill children. *Pediatrics*. 2008;122:e898-e904.

66. Agus MS, et al. Tight glycemic control versus standard care after pediatric cardiac surgery. *N Engl J Med*. 2012;367:1208-1219.

67. Ramamoorthy C, et al. Effects of inspired hypoxic and hypercapnic gas mixtures on cerebral oxygen saturation in neonates with univentricular heart defects. *Anesthesiology*. 2002;96:283-288.

70. Vlahos AP, et al. Hypoplastic left heart syndrome with intact or highly restrictive atrial septum: outcome after neonatal transcatheter atrial septostomy. *Circulation*. 2004;109:2326-2330.

72. Kalish BT, et al. Technical challenges of atrial septal stent placement in fetuses with hypoplastic left heart syndrome and intact atrial septum. *Catheter Cardiovasc Interv*. 2014;84:77-85.

75. Chang AC, et al. Early bidirectional cavopulmonary shunt in young infants. Postoperative course and early results. *Circulation*. 1993;88(5 Pt 2):II149-II158.

80. d'Udekem Y, et al. Redefining expectations of long-term survival after the Fontan procedure: twenty-five years of follow-up from the entire population of Australia and New Zealand. *Circulation*. 2014;130(11 suppl 1):S32-S38.

84. Shekerdemian LS, et al. Cardiopulmonary interactions after Fontan operations: augmentation of cardiac output using negative pressure ventilation. *Circulation*. 1997;96:3934-3942.

88. Sivarajan VB, et al. Pediatric extracorporeal life support in specialized situations. *Pediatr Crit Care Med*. 2013;14(5 suppl 1):S51-S61.

112. Bove EL, et al. Results of a policy of primary repair of truncus arteriosus in the neonate. *J Thorac Cardiovasc Surg*. 1993;105:1057-1065, discussion 1065-1066.

119. Jatene AD, et al. Anatomic correction of transposition of the great arteries. *J Thorac Cardiovasc Surg*. 1982;83:20-26.

120. Di Donato RM, et al. Age-dependent ventricular response to pressure overload. Considerations for the arterial switch operation. *J Thorac Cardiovasc Surg*. 1992;104:713-722.

122. Wernovsky G, et al. Factors influencing early and late outcome of the arterial switch operation for transposition of the great arteries. *J Thorac Cardiovasc Surg*. 1995;109:289-301, discussion 301-302.

125. Wernovsky G, Sanders SP. Coronary artery anatomy and transposition of the great arteries. *Coron Artery Dis*. 1993;4:148-157.

142. Al Habib HF, et al. Contemporary patterns of management of tetralogy of Fallot: data from the Society of Thoracic Surgeons Database. *Ann Thorac Surg*. 2010;90:813-819, discussion 819-820.

153. Brown JW, et al. Valved bovine jugular vein conduits for right ventricular outflow tract reconstruction in children: an attractive alternative to pulmonary homograft. *Ann Thorac Surg*. 2006;82:909-916.

156. McCrindle BW, et al. Acute results of balloon angioplasty of native coarctation versus recurrent aortic obstruction are equivalent. Valvuloplasty and Angioplasty of Congenital Anomalies (VACA) Registry Investigators. *J Am Coll Cardiol*. 1996;28:1810-1817.

163. Norwood WI, Lang P, Hansen DD. Physiologic repair of aortic atresia-hypoplastic left heart syndrome. *N Engl J Med*. 1983;308:23-26.

166. Hoffman GM, et al. Alteration of the critical arteriovenous oxygen saturation relationship by sustained afterload reduction after the Norwood procedure. *J Thorac Cardiovasc Surg*. 2004;127:738-745.

167. Sano S, et al. Right ventricle-pulmonary artery shunt in first-stage palliation of hypoplastic left heart syndrome. *J Thorac Cardiovasc Surg*. 2003;126:504-509, discussion 509-510.

170. Newburger JW, et al. Transplantation-free survival and interventions at 3 years in the single ventricle reconstruction trial. *Circulation*. 2014;129:2013-2020.

176. Barron DJ, et al. Hypoplastic left heart syndrome. *Lancet*. 2009;374:551-564.

180. Galantowicz M, et al. Hybrid approach for hypoplastic left heart syndrome: intermediate results after the learning curve. *Ann Thorac Surg*. 2008;85:2063-2070, discussion 2070-2071.

Cardiac Transplantation

F. Jay Fricker

PEARLS

- Indications for transplantation are cardiomyopathy and complex palliated congenital heart disease with severe myopathic ventricular dysfunction.
- Pediatric patients on inotropic support or circulatory support and who have life-threatening arrhythmia receive priority for available pediatric donors.
- Selection of the agent to initiate inotropic support has evolved from sympathomimetic agents (dobutamine/ dopamine) to the phosphodiesterase inhibitor milrinone.
- Virtual cross-match is now used in sensitized patients to improve organ allocation.
- It is imperative that immune suppression be initiated immediately after heart transplantation.
- The high-risk period for acute allograft rejection is in the first month after transplantation.
- Complications of immune suppression are infection, acute renal failure, malignancy, and hyperglycemia.

It has now been a quarter of a century since the first successful pediatric heart transplant was performed at Stanford University.[1] The introduction of cyclosporine as the primary immune suppressant agent used in solid organ transplantation was a key discovery because it was the first selective immunosuppressive agent used in solid organ transplant recipients. It has spared corticosteroid use and has made heart transplantation a cost-effective procedure.[2] In the past 25 years, perioperative mortality has become negligible even in patients with the most complex congenital heart defects. Advances have occurred in our understanding of the immune system, and improvement in critical care management of both donor and recipient patients has resulted in an increased survival benefit. This chapter reviews critical care management of the pediatric patient with cardiopulmonary failure who is evaluated for orthotopic heart transplantation. Donor management, physiology of the transplanted heart, and preoperative and perioperative critical care all play important roles in the successful outcome of critically ill children with no option other than heart replacement surgery.

Indications for transplantation are cardiomyopathy and complex palliated congenital heart disease with severe myopathic ventricular dysfunction.[3] The Pediatric Heart Transplant Study Group reviewed the causes of death after heart transplantation from a prospective database initiated in 1993. Patients were entered into the database on an intention-to-treat basis.[4-6] Using parametric data analysis with competing outcomes, death while waiting for transplant has been analyzed for all age groups, pretransplant diagnosis, blood type, and urgency status. Early death after heart transplant has been categorized as primary heart allograft failure. This includes inadequate preservation from long ischemic time and primary right ventricular failure from high pulmonary vascular resistance (PVR). Acute allograft rejection is an exceedingly rare event immediately after implantation. Late death after transplant is the result of posttransplant coronary vasculopathy, malignancy, or nonadherence to immune suppression regimens.[7,8]

The technical complexities of heart transplantation in children with palliated congenital heart disease contributed to the early perioperative mortality, which exceeded 30%. In addition, difficulties in estimating PVR, variable pulmonary artery anatomy, and complications from multiple repeat thoracotomy and sternotomy all contributed to early morbidity and mortality.[9] Solid organ preservation, surgical experience, and recipient selection have all improved with experience, resulting in reduced perioperative mortality that is equivalent to transplantation of the primary cardiomyopathic patient who has not had a previous sternotomy.[9,10] Primary transplantation in the neonate with hypoplastic left heart syndrome (HLHS) has caused controversy because an acceptable surgical alternative is available and infant donor heart resources are limited.[11] In reviews from the Pediatric Heart Transplant Study Group Database, the mortality of infants waiting for donor heart availability exceeds 25%.[4] In recent years, deaths while waiting for transplantation have decreased, but this decrease reflects the smaller number of infants listed and those who have opted for the Norwood procedure and single-ventricle palliation. The Norwood procedure does not preclude the possibility of future transplantation.

Late death after heart transplantation is related to either accelerated allograft coronary artery disease or primary malignancy.[12,13] The major cause of death in the adolescent heart transplant recipient is now noncompliance with the medical regimen.[7] With the decrease in perioperative mortality, we now expect 5-year survival after heart transplantation to exceed 80%. From the newest survival data (International Society for Heart and Lung Transplantation 2009 Report), the transplant half-life (the time at which 50% of the recipients remain alive) is 11.3 years for teens and 15.8 years for infants.[14] Rehospitalization after the first year is rare, and quality of life has been excellent.[15]

Critical Care of the Pediatric Patient Waiting for Heart Transplantation

The number of good donor hearts available to satisfy the number of potential adult recipients is not adequate. Statistics

BOX 39.1

BOX 39.1 Heart Transplantation Justification: Pediatric Cardiology Status IA

- Requires assistance with a ventilator
- Requires assistance with a mechanical assist device (eg, extracorporeal membrane oxygenation, left ventricular assist device)
- Requires assistance with an intra-aortic balloon pump
- Patient younger than 6 months with congenital or acquired heart disease exhibiting reactive pulmonary hypertension >50% of systemic blood pressure levels
- Requires infusion of a single high-dose inotrope (eg, dobutamine ≥7.5 µg/kg/min or milrinone ≥0.5 µg/kg/min)
- Patient does not meet any of the criteria specified above but has a life expectancy without a heart transplant of <14 days (ie, refractory arrhythmia)

from the United Network for Organ Sharing (UNOS) demonstrate this discrepancy between the number of potential recipients for heart and lung transplants and the availability of potential donors.[16] Donor availability for the pediatric patient is not as critical. Pediatric patients usually receive an appropriate donor offer unless they are infants or are adolescents of a size such that they are competing with critically ill adult patients. Guidelines from UNOS regarding organ distribution have changed to ensure that pediatric adolescent donors are available first to potential adolescent and young adult pediatric recipients for both heart and lungs.

For potential heart transplant recipients, urgency criteria have been established for the most critically ill patients. Pediatric patients on inotropic support or circulatory support or who have life-threatening arrhythmia receive priority for available donors (Box 39.1).

Management of the Potential Heart Transplant Recipient

The pretransplant management of the critically ill patient with end-stage myocardial dysfunction can determine the outcome of that patient after thoracic transplant. The principles of inotropic support, preservation of end-organ function, and attention to issues of nutrition and infection are the same for all critically ill patients in the pediatric ICU.

Evaluation of the potential heart transplant recipient requires a careful pretransplant hemodynamic assessment. This information can guide the fluid and inotropic therapy by optimizing preload and afterload while waiting for organ availability. The critical hemodynamic information influencing the function of the donor heart is an assessment of pulmonary artery pressure and PVR in the recipient before implantation. High PVR is associated with an increased perioperative transplant mortality rate and adverse long-term outcome.[17,18] A transpulmonary gradient greater than 15 mm Hg (mean pulmonary arterial pressure minus mean left atrial pressure) is associated with a higher incidence of heart graft dysfunction.[18] Preoperative hemodynamic assessment should include measurement of both left and right heart pressures with interventions to manipulate the PVR if elevated. Remeasuring hemodynamics with FiO_2 of 1, nitric oxide, prostacyclin, and aggressive vasodilator therapy to decrease systemic vascular resistance (SVR) can help determine whether the patient is a heart transplant candidate or if he or she should be considered for lung or heart and lung transplantation.[19,20]

Inotropic Support

Critically ill children with myopathic ventricular dysfunction severe enough for them to be in the ICU are on inotropic support. These agents increase contractility through a common pathway of increasing intracellular levels of cyclic adenylate monophosphate (cAMP). Increased cytoplasmic levels of cAMP cause increased release of calcium from the sarcoplasmic reticulum and increase contractile force generation. Increases in cAMP occur either by β-adrenergic–mediated stimulation (increase in production) or phosphodiesterase III (PDE III) inhibition (decreased degradation). Milrinone has proven to be a well-tolerated agent. IV administration of milrinone increases cardiac output and reduces cardiac filling pressures, PVR, and SVR, with minimal effect on heart rate. Milrinone has been well studied in the pediatric population, and the benefit is primarily related to effect on SVR and PVR rather than inotropy.[21,22] Milrinone is initiated at doses of 0.25 µg/kg/min and increased to 1 µg/kg/min without adverse effects. Although atrial and ventricular ectopy are less common with milrinone than dobutamine, ventricular ectopy/ventricular tachycardia can occur with the initiation of milrinone therapy. Tachyphylaxis is unusual with this agent. Milrinone has a long half-life and should be used cautiously in patients with hypotension. This drug is primarily excreted in the urine, so concentrations can increase in the presence of renal failure. We have observed severe hypotension and renal dysfunction precipitated by use of an angiotensin-converting enzyme inhibitor in a patient already on milrinone infusion. The addition of low-dose dobutamine (5–10 µg/kg/min) or epinephrine (dose 0.01–0.05 µg/kg/min) can help stabilize the critically ill child who is not responding adequately to milrinone therapy alone.

Nesiritide, a recombinant B-type natriuretic peptide, is now approved for treatment of acutely decompensated heart failure. Endogenous B-type natriuretic peptide is a cardiac hormone produced by the failing heart, and nesiritide is identical to the naturally occurring peptide. Nesiritide reduces preload and afterload, leading to increases in cardiac output/index without reflex tachycardia or direct inotropic effect. In addition, this drug promotes natriuresis and diuresis and suppresses the renin-angiotensin axis and endogenous catecholamines. Although this drug has not been studied extensively in the pediatric age group, in our and others' experiences, it has been found to be a safe and effective adjunctive therapy.[23,24]

Mechanical Support

Most patients waiting for transplantation who are on inotropic support do not remain hemodynamically stable indefinitely. Progressive end-organ dysfunction ensues, requiring escalation of support that includes multiple inotropic agents, in addition to respiratory and circulatory support. Mechanical circulatory support has become an important addition to the treatment armamentarium for the infant or child with decompensated heart failure and low cardiac output unresponsive to pharmacologic maneuvers.[25] Options include extracorporeal membrane oxygenation (ECMO), intra-aortic balloon, and left and right ventricular assist devices. Experience with ECMO as a bridge to heart transplantation has been reported by several pediatric transplant centers.[26,27] ECMO support can be used for 2 to 3 weeks without major complications from bleeding or infection, extending the window for donor organ availability. Isolated ventricular support devices, such as the Thoratec, Berlin Heart,[28] and DeBakey centrifugal pump, are now available for children.[29,30] The Berlin Heart EXCOR has become the primary extracorporeal circulatory device in infants and children. The current data from Berlin Heart show there have been a total of 698 patients supported for more than 47,000 days with this pneumatic-driven device (personal communication, Berlin Heart). The longest time of support in an individual patient was 902 days, with an average of 68 days of support before transplantation, explant, or death. The pediatric demography is that this device is used for all pediatric age ranges, but the mean age of 5 years and the median age of 2 years reflect the benefit in small children because of the availability of a pump size that can deliver 10-mL stroke volume. Actuarial survival of patients at 1 year who have been bridged to heart transplant or explanted now exceeds 80% (personal communication, Berlin Heart). In the past, use of these devices had always been considered extraordinary and usually proposed in patients with severe end-organ dysfunction. Placement of a device in a patient with multisystem organ failure usually results in a poor outcome. We propose that these devices be placed early, before end-organ dysfunction; doing so will enable rehabilitation of the patient, who then becomes a more optimal candidate for organ transplantation.

Anticoagulation

All patients with severe myocardial dysfunction are at risk for complications of systemic and pulmonary embolus. In our experience, nearly all explanted hearts have mural thrombi in both the left and right ventricles. Pulmonary emboli lead to increased PVR and the potential for lung abscess. The most devastating result of systemic embolus is stroke. All patients waiting for transplantation should be managed with systemic anticoagulation. Heparin is preferred, but warfarin is acceptable in a stable patient on inotropic support. We add a word of caution regarding the use of low-molecular-weight heparin for prophylaxis. Enoxaparin cannot be easily reversed in a patient who must go to the operating room emergently because a donor heart has been identified. Cardiovascular surgeons prefer using heparin for prophylactic anticoagulation.

Management of the Potential Heart Donor

Many potential heart donors are lost because of suboptimal management after brain death has occurred. Associated with brain death is a catecholamine surge causing unnatural circulatory physiology that rapidly evolves, making management of the donor difficult. This intense sympathomimetic outflow initially causes vasoconstriction resulting in tachycardia, hypertension, and increased myocardial oxygen demand. The result can be a direct injury to the myocardium in the potentially transplantable heart. Myocardial structural damage is seen and includes myocytolysis, contraction band necrosis, subendocardial hemorrhage, edema formation, and interstitial mononuclear infiltration.[31] This initial sympathetic outflow is followed by a loss of sympathetic tone resulting in marked vasodilatation and hypotension. The hypotension and cardiovascular collapse are related to decreased SVR rather than primary myocardial dysfunction. Large fluid volumes and high-dose inotropic agents at α-adrenergic dosing range are administered, causing volume overload and vasoconstriction

that can injure all donor organs. Hearts that are supported on high-dose inotropic agents will likely exhibit myocardial injury. A risk factor that predicts donor heart failure is a history of use of high-dose dopamine, dobutamine greater than 20 μg/kg/min, and epinephrine greater than 0.1 μg/kg/min.

Hormonal changes occur with brain stem injury and death. Early depletion of antidiuretic hormone causes inappropriate diuresis. Depletion of free triiodothyronine (T_3) has been implicated in myocardial dysfunction. Falling insulin levels lead to decreased intracellular glucose levels. A significant decrease in cortisol levels contributes to cardiovascular instability.[32,33]

Our present understanding of the physiology of brain death has resulted in "protocol" development for management of the potential donor. The principles of support include the following:

- Invasive cardiovascular monitoring maintaining a mean arterial blood pressure greater than 60 mm Hg and central venous pressure of 6 to 10 mm Hg.
- Vasopressin is now the first-line blood pressure support medication because it treats diabetes insipidus in addition to supporting blood pressure. Infusion of less than 2.5 U/hour is usually sufficient to increase mean arterial blood pressure and not cause end-organ injury.
- Respiratory support to maximize oxygen delivery to transplantable organs. Recommended ventilatory strategies are aimed at optimizing oxygenation and preventing lung injury.
- Hormonal support including high-dose corticosteroids in the form of Solu-Medrol, insulin, and, possibly, infusions of the thyroid hormone T_3 or T_4. The benefits of thyroid hormone replacement in the brain-dead donor are debated, but there are studies supporting their use.[32] Resuscitation of the "marginal donor heart" is worth the effort, given the shortage of available donor organs. Administration of T_3 has been advocated for reversal of myocardial dysfunction induced by the catecholamine surge of brain death.[32]

Pediatric heart transplantation after declaration of cardiocirculatory death has received significant interest in the transplant community because of the shortage of donor organs. Protocols are controversial because donor care is provided under the direction of the pediatric intensivists. The donor is moved to the operating room, and femoral arterial and venous lines are inserted for access to perform organ resuscitation. The donor is given comfort care, extubation is accomplished, and the donor is monitored for circulatory death by auscultation of the heart and palpation of pulses. When circulatory death has occurred, the donor is observed for a period of 1.25 to 3 minutes before death is declared. If cardiocirculatory death occurs within 30 minutes after extubation, the donor is declared a candidate for organ donation. Cold cardioplegia is infused into the catheter that was positioned in the ascending aorta, sternotomy is performed, and topical cooling of the heart is initiated. The inferior vena cava is opened to prevent distension of the heart. The routine technique for cardiectomy is then performed.[34] Organ donation after circulatory death for kidney and liver transplantation is becoming more common, but because the heart is more vulnerable to ischemia, this practice has not become common. The practice of transplantation after cardiocirculatory death for any organ remains an ethically controversial practice for many pediatric critical care intensivists.[35]

Critical Care Management of the Orthotopic Heart Transplant Recipient

Intraoperative Considerations

Heart replacement can be accomplished in virtually any congenital heart anomaly because the aorta, pulmonary arteries, and left atrium are in a relatively constant position near the midline. Regardless of malposition or positional relationships of the great arteries, the aorta of the recipient can be mobilized to make anastomosis with the donor aorta possible. The left atrium is a midline structure, and even when anomalies of the pulmonary venous return exist, pulmonary veins usually approach the midline and can be incorporated into the repair.[36]

Techniques of implantation have not changed significantly since the original description.[1,37] The newest innovation is the bicaval anastomosis.[38,39] This technique has the advantage of preserving sinus node function.[40] Implantation techniques require that the pulmonary veins come to the midline. The pulmonary artery and aorta can be malpositioned, but this adds little to the technical difficulty of the procedure. Aortic root size mismatch can, however, cause technical difficulty. Implantation of recipients with complex congenital heart disease can usually be accomplished by harvesting additional donor pulmonary artery, aorta, and caval tissue to replace deficient recipient tissue or to correct malposition of the vena cava or great arteries.[36,41]

Donor heart function is related to proper management of the donor and the total ischemic time of the donor heart. The amount of time the aorta is cross-clamped on the donor until the aortic anastomosis is completed on the recipient (total ischemic time) is a major factor determining early postoperative donor heart function. Nevertheless, donor hearts have been exposed to more than 8 hours of ischemia and recovered function after transplantation.

Early Perioperative Management

The early perioperative management of the recipient is not significantly different from the management of any postcardiac surgical patient. The physiologic responses of the newly transplanted heart are altered because of denervation. The major changes related to autonomic denervation include diastolic dysfunction and exaggerated response to exogenously administered catecholamines. The transplanted heart must also adapt to a new environment related to recipient lung function and elevated PVR.

Autonomic system denervation results in a relatively fixed heart rate without respiratory variation. Heart rates are between 90 and 110 bpm but can be faster because of exogenous catecholamine administration. (The sinus node is transplanted with the donor heart.) Heart rates can be slower if the recipient has been exposed to amiodarone pretransplant or if there was injury to the blood supply of the donor sinus node at the time of donor heart removal.

Early blood pressure instability is common because of loss of baroreceptor regulation and dependence of the transplanted heart on endogenous or exogenous catecholamines. Hypertension occurs because of a fixed stroke volume into a systemic vascular bed that is abnormal because of long-standing increase in systemic vascular resistance from compensatory heart failure. Size mismatch between donor and recipient can also contribute to the hypertension because of a large stroke volume from the transplanted heart. The other concern about donor heart/recipient mismatch is "big heart," or hyperperfusion syndrome. A well-functioning large allograft generates a large stroke volume causing systemic hypertension and high cardiac output in a patient who previously had a low cardiac output state. This increase in cerebral blood flow has the potential to cause cerebral vasoconstriction and symptomatic seizures, headache, or changes in mental status.[42] These symptoms are limited to the first few days after transplantation. There is a gradual adaptation in allograft stroke volume to the needs of the recipient. This adaptation of oversized cardiac allografts in children is part of the "shrink and grow" phenomenon previously described.[42] The oversized donor heart eventually undergoes remodeling with regression of hypertrophy. Although this is a rare problem in children, symptomatic hypertension must be treated aggressively early in the perioperative period.

Early myocardial function of the transplanted heart is dependent on catecholamine support. Small infusions of β-adrenergic agents such as isoproterenol for several days are often necessary to maintain optimal heart allograft function.[43]

The hemodynamics of the transplanted heart reflect a significant shift to the left of the pressure/volume curve. Diastolic dysfunction can be demonstrated from the early transplant period. Why this hemodynamic abnormality is present early because of preservation injury is understandable, but diastolic dysfunction persists well into the recovery phase and beyond. Fluid administration of 10 mL/kg to a heart transplant recipient months remote from transplant will uncover an occult restrictive hemodynamic pattern. Pulmonary artery wedge pressure will increase by twofold, and right atrial pressure will increase more than expected.[44] In the normal heart, right atrial pressure will not change and left atrial pressure will increase by 1 to 2 mm Hg in response to a fluid challenge.

Diastolic dysfunction is a significant impairment to early allograft function, limiting cardiac output. Diastolic dysfunction emphasizes the importance of heart rate and early sinus node function. The capability for temporary pacing in the early perioperative period is mandatory.

Management of Early Heart Allograft Dysfunction

Early heart allograft dysfunction is related to primary failure of the heart allograft because of unsuspected injury to the heart prior to procurement or because of preservation injury. The other major cause of primary allograft failure is elevated PVR in the recipient. Allograft failure is rarely caused by acute antibody-mediated injury. Risk factors associated with donor heart dysfunction, if present, should be factored into the decision of accepting that particular heart for your patient. Obviously the condition of the recipient and the expected length of survival would mandate, at least, consideration for acceptance of a "marginal heart."

Risk factors for donor heart dysfunction include "down time of the donor" (length of initial resuscitation), evidence of myocardial injury with elevation of troponin I, and a history of high-dose inotropic support (dopamine/dobutamine >20 μg/kg/min or epinephrine/norepinephrine >0.1 μg/kg/min) in the donor. Objective assessment of donor heart function can be made by obtaining an echocardiogram and electrocardiogram. The echocardiogram assesses donor heart systolic function (shortening fraction or left ventricular ejection fraction) and will detect the presence of mitral valve regurgitation or wall-motion abnormalities. The presence of any of these abnormalities makes the donor heart "marginal" for transplantation. In assessing the donor heart function, serial echocardiograms are imperative before determining that the heart is not usable for transplantation. Abnormal heart function seen in the midst of the catecholamine storm of brain death can recover. Repeating the echocardiogram remote from the initial resuscitation period or after the reduction or discontinuation of inotropic support can increase one's confidence in accepting the donor heart.

The other major reason for primary donor heart dysfunction is right heart failure from high PVR. We have known since the early days of heart transplantation that the donor right ventricle will not function when exposed to an abnormal pulmonary circulation. High PVR in the recipient increases perioperative morbidity and mortality and can affect late survival. All potential heart recipients undergo cardiac catheterization before heart transplantation to document the anatomy of systemic and pulmonary venous connections, determine pulmonary artery size and distribution, and calculate PVR. The upper limit of PVR associated with successful orthotopic heart transplantation is not known. Criteria developed from the adult heart transplant experience indicate that a PVR greater than 6 Wood units or a transpulmonary gradient (pulmonary artery mean pressure minus left atrial mean pressure) greater than 15 mm Hg is associated with increased perioperative mortality. The transpulmonary gradient is the most useful number for estimating PVR because measurement of cardiac output in the catheterization laboratory can be flawed. In children, PVR index (PVRI), determined by dividing transpulmonary gradient by cardiac index, is more useful, because children come in all sizes. PVRI less than 6 index units is associated with low perioperative mortality. Orthotopic heart transplants have been successful with PVRI greater than 6 and as high as 10 index units, but with increased morbidity and mortality rates. The diagnosis of high PVR is evident as the patient is weaned from cardiopulmonary bypass. Intraoperative transesophageal echocardiography demonstrates dilatation of the right ventricle and a small, underfilled left heart. Acute management of high PVR and right heart dysfunction includes high FiO_2 and administration of nitric oxide at 20 to 40 ppm. The need for continuous pulmonary vasodilator medications in the immediate perioperative period is unusual, but prostacyclin and sildenafil have both proved effective in this situation.[45]

The sinus node artery from the donor heart is at risk at the time of procurement, and the incidence of sinus node dysfunction causing junctional rhythm or atrial flutter/fibrillation is 10% to 20%. Nearly 5% of children require pacemaker therapy after transplantation because of sinus node dysfunction.[46] All transplant recipients have temporary pacing wires, so bradyarrhythmias are not an issue. If the patient is in atrial flutter/fibrillation, then cardioversion should be performed. Persistent sinus node dysfunction with bradycardia can be problematic because of early diastolic dysfunction of the heart allograft. In the usual scenario, the patient returns from the operating room in an atrial paced rhythm. When the pacemaker is turned off, the underlying rhythm is a junctional rate between 100 and 120 beats/min. As inotropic support is discontinued, the junctional rate slows to an unacceptable rate in the 50 to 80 beats/min range. Usually an occasional atrial

contraction is conducted, but the sinus node has been injured. Initiating theophylline at a dose of 10 mg/kg/day is helpful. Permanent pacing is recommended if sinus or atrial conducted rhythm has not returned within 2 weeks.

Heart Allograft Rejection and Immune Suppression

It is imperative that immune suppression be initiated early after heart transplantation. Solid organ transplants transfer antigen-presenting cells (APCs) that are recognized by the recipient's human leukocyte antigen (HLA) immune system as foreign, which sets up a cascade of lymphocyte stimulation and proliferation. These lymphocytes then migrate to the heart allograft, where they can adhere to myocytes and endothelial receptors and cause tissue destruction. T-cell activation is the prime mover of allograft rejection. The initial signal is T-cell receptor binding of antigen on the surface of an APC. The APC is derived from the donor in the form of a monocyte, or a tissue macrophage. Interaction of the APC and T-cell receptor causes release of interleukin (IL)-1 from the APC, which causes activation of the T cell. Activated T cells secrete IL-2 and other lymphokines that induce proliferation of activated T cells, which migrate to the allograft causing tissue damage.

Initial immune suppression protocols include high-dose corticosteroids, induction with IL-2 receptor blockade, or antithymocyte globulin, followed by introduction of the calcineurin inhibitors cyclosporine or tacrolimus (Table 39.1).

Induction protocols with lympholytic agents OKT3 or antithymocyte globulin are effective in delaying the time until the first allograft rejection episode but do not have a long-term survival benefit.[47] The benefit of induction with IL-2 receptor blockade in preventing early heart allograft rejection is supported by recent studies.[48]

Corticosteroids have been part of standard protocols since the early days of solid organ transplantation. High-dose methylprednisolone (5–10 mg/kg) is administered at the time of aortic cross-clamp removal and continued in tapering doses over the first several days after surgery. Corticosteroids have immunosuppressive properties and benefit the allograft because of membrane-stabilizing and antioxidant effects on the graft.

More controversial is the timing of the introduction of calcineurin inhibitors cyclosporine and tacrolimus. A major complication in the early perioperative course after heart transplantation is renal dysfunction. In the past, calcineurin inhibitors cyclosporine and tacrolimus were major contributors. The APC and lymphocyte receptor interaction occurs within hours of the transplant; therefore early introduction of calcineurin inhibitors is important. Because bioavailability of these drugs is so variable, early, continuous IV administration of these drugs has been a standard protocol.[49] We continue to experience a group of recipients who develop acute renal failure with IV administration of these drugs and therefore avoid IV use of cyclosporine and tacrolimus. Current protocols are based on oral/nasogastric administration of a standard dose of tacrolimus beginning on the day of transplant. Target levels of this drug are reached 3 to 5 days after transplant if subsequent doses are based on the trough level obtained each morning (see Table 39.1).[50]

The high-risk period for acute cellular rejection (ACR) is the first month after transplantation. ACR is a phenomenon that rarely occurs in the first week after transplant. Hyperacute

TABLE 39.1   Immune Suppression in the Intensive Care Unit

Agent	Mechanism of Action	Dose	Monitoring	Major Side Effect(s)
Induction Immune Suppression				
Corticosteroids	Redistribution of peripheral lymphocytes, inhibition of lymphokine IL-2 production, impairment of macrophage response to lymphocyte signals	Induction Immune Suppression Corticosteroids Dose 10 mg/kg every 8 hours times 3 doses 5 mg/kg every 8 hours times 3 doses 1 mg/kg every 8 hours times three doses 1 mg/kg/day tapering to 0.5 mg/kg at Hospital Discharge	Glucose	Infection, cushingoid appearance, hypertension, hyperlipidemia, glucose intolerance
Basiliximab	Monoclonal antibody binds to IL-2 receptor	20 mg >35 kg 10 mg <35 kg, administer days 1 and 4	CBC	Anaphylaxis
Antithymocyte globulin	Nonspecific T-cell lysis	Antithymocyte Globulin Dose 1 mg–1.5 mg/kg/day for 3–5 days Note: We are trying to decrease the total dose of ATG	T-lymphocyte subsets	Thrombocytopenia, anaphylaxis, infection, PTLD, localized pain with RATG administration, serum sickness
Cyclosporine	Calcineurin inhibitor, inhibition of T-cell receptor lymphokine production and T-cell proliferation	2.5 mg/kg/24 h IV	Monoclonal whole blood assay 100–400 ng/mL, depending on time since transplantation	Nephrotoxicity, central nervous system seizures, decreased magnesium, hypertension, hirsutism, gingival hyperplasia
Tacrolimus	Calcineurin inhibitor, inhibition of T-cell receptor lymphokine production and T-cell proliferation	Pretransplant 1.0 mg (given 4–8 hours before going to OR for transplant) IV: 0.03–0.05 mg/kg/24 hours Note: We avoid the use of tacrolimus IV because of high risk of renal failure; therefore do not recommend using this drug intravenously early after transplant Oral: 0.5–1.0 mg (or 0.1–0.3 mg/kg) twice daily and increase the dose to therapeutic level 10–15 ng/mL after transplant	10–15 ng/mL, whole blood	Nephrotoxicity, anemia/neutropenia, headache, tremors, insomnia, glucose intolerance
Maintenance Immune Suppression				
Cyclosporine		5–20 mg/kg 2× or 3× daily		
Tacrolimus		0.3 mg/kg/day divided 2× daily		
Sirolimus	Inhibition of T-cell activation and proliferation by preventing translation of mRNA		Triglycerides, platelets 5–10 mg/mL	Nephrotoxicity, hyperlipidemia, thrombocytopenia, leukopenia, gastrointestinal intolerance
Azathioprine	Antimetabolite inhibits purine and DNA synthesis	1–2 mg/kg/day	WBC <4000 ANC >1500	Bone marrow suppression
Mycophenolate mofetil		Mycophenolate mofetil or mycophenolic acid 30–60 mg/kg/day or 600 mg/m²/day	WBC <4000 ANC >1500	Bone marrow suppression, gastrointestinal intolerance
Prednisone		1–3 mg/kg/day		
Acute Cellular Rejection				
Methylprednisolone				
Antithymocyte globulin		1.5 mg/kg/day for 7–14 days		Peripheral lymphocyte count, platelet count

ANC, absolute neutrophil count <1000; *CBC,* complete blood cell count; *PTLD,* posttransplant lymphoproliferative disease; *RATG,* rabbit antithymocyte globulin; *WBC,* whole blood cell count.

rejection is uncommon but can occur when a heart transplant recipient has preformed HLA antibody that reacts with a donor who has those specific HLA antigens. A positive cross-match will be reported, which means the recipient's serum causes lysis of donor T cells obtained from lymph nodes from the donor at the time of organ procurement. Heart transplant recipients at risk for hyperacute rejection are identified by measuring the presence of HLA antibody in their serum. Specificity and quantification of these HLA antibodies can be measured by Luminex beads, which enable a virtual cross-match to be done between potential donors and recipients. Children with palliated congenital heart disease are at particular risk for HLA sensitization because of exposure to blood products at the time of their previous surgical procedures. Rapid institution of plasmapheresis immediately after implantation and continuing through the first several days after the operation is the optimal way to clear the offending antibody causing heart allograft dysfunction.

The diagnosis of ACR is made by endomyocardial biopsy. Histopathology in cardiac tissue obtained by endomyocardial biopsy remains the gold standard for diagnosis of acute cardiac allograft rejection. The numbers of infiltrating lymphocytes and the presence of myocyte injury are used to grade rejection and to guide allograft rejection therapy. Surveillance endomyocardial biopsies are performed within the first 2 weeks after transplant and then at strategic times depending on the size of the child, available access, and technical difficulty of obtaining tissue.

Clinical recognition of acute allograft rejection can be subtle but is obviously important because tissue diagnosis is not always possible, and surveillance techniques using peripheral blood, electrocardiography, and echocardiography have limitations. Acute cellular rejection can be present in the allograft without any symptoms or clinical findings. When ACR has progressed to hemodynamically significant allograft dysfunction, then symptoms of abdominal pain and vomiting are prevalent, and findings of systemic venous congestion, liver enlargement, and low cardiac output dominate. Symptoms of pulmonary venous congestion/pulmonary edema are rare findings. When ACR is suspected, histologic confirmation is always desirable if it can be safely performed. The principles of management are to acutely augment immune suppression with methylprednisolone or a lympholytic agent depending on the histologic and clinical severity of the heart allograft dysfunction. Following acute treatment, increases in maintenance of immune suppression agents are prescribed and follow-up endomyocardial biopsy is scheduled.

Complications of Immune Suppression in Heart Transplant Recipients Occurring in the Pediatric Intensive Care Unit

Infection

Infections are a major cause of mortality and morbidity in the early period after heart transplantation.[51,52] Factors that predispose to infection can be divided into preexisting factors related to the donor and recipient and factors secondary to events in the intraoperative and postoperative periods. For example, the site of the organ transplanted provides a clue to the site of infection. Renal transplant recipients acquire urinary tract infections, whereas heart transplant recipients

are exposed to chest cavity infections. The type and severity of the underlying illness leading to organ failure can increase the risk for rejection. Children with cardiomyopathy can be severely malnourished, require prolonged mechanical respiratory or circulatory support, and have chronic indwelling venous catheters, all of which predispose to infection. The presence of a pretransplant pulmonary infarction is associated with lung abscess in the posttransplant recovery period.[53] Neonates may experience severe sepsis from coagulase-positive staphylococci more often than older children.

The herpes virus family plays a significant role in infections occurring after transplantation. The clinical expression of cytomegalovirus and Epstein-Barr virus infection in the young patient is more severe because it is often a primary exposure.[54] Clinical infections related to these viruses rarely present before 1 month following organ transplantation and are most common in the first 6 months after heart transplantation.

Antibiotic management of the heart transplant recipient in the ICU can be focused primarily on clinical suspicion, time of infection after transplant, and predisposing factors. Immune suppression is selective and targets T cells. Neutrophil function is normal except for the effect of high-dose corticosteroids. Neutropenia can occasionally be a problem because of bone marrow suppression caused by antimetabolites and tacrolimus. Prophylactic antibiotics, in the form of third-generation cephalosporins, are used for patients after sternotomy and continued until chest tubes and central lines are removed. The strategy against infection includes initial isolation, routine surveillance cultures, and regular replacement of indwelling catheters. In the early setting after transplantation, temperature elevation should indicate active infection and serious complication. If an infection is suspected, early and aggressive investigation are necessary and broad-spectrum antibiotics/antifungal agents should be initiated until the source of the fever is identified.

Renal Function

Acute renal failure is a major complication following orthotopic heart transplantation. Renal failure is multifactorial in etiology, and the premorbid risk factors of heart transplant recipients cannot necessarily be controlled. We can monitor and control use of calcineurin-inhibitor immune suppression agents. Therapeutic strategies include delayed initiation of cyclosporine and tacrolimus by using antithymocyte globulin or IL-2 receptor blockade for induction of immune suppression. The other option is to use a modified oral/nasogastric protocol for tacrolimus administration.[55] This protocol targets tacrolimus levels to below 6 ng/mL in the first 3 days after transplantation and then aggressively increases dosing and target level over the next 4 days. It is important to avoid early IV administration of these agents because they invariably lead to renal afferent arteriolar vasoconstriction and oliguria. If renal dysfunction is complicating the posttransplant course, it is still difficult to withdraw calcineurin inhibitors completely, but lowering the target level to less than 6 ng/L and substituting higher doses of mycophenolate mofetil and adding sirolimus are reasonable options.[56] The other means for reversing renal toxicity is to target mechanisms of calcineurin inhibitor toxicity. Renal arteriolar vasoconstriction is an imbalance between vasodilator prostaglandins and vasoconstrictor thromboxane A_2. Thus prostaglandin E1 (PGE1) has been used for promoting renal vasodilatation, with some success. Oral

PGE1 analogs have received mixed reviews. Calcium channel antagonists have also been used to prevent renal toxicity. Felodipine has been shown to cause a natriuresis and to prevent the decline in renal hemodynamics produced by angiotensin II. We have not had enough experience with this potentially useful drug in reversing cyclosporine/tacrolimus nephrotoxicity.[57]

Diabetes Mellitus

Hyperglycemia is common after heart transplantation with tacrolimus-based immune suppression. The combination of decreased insulin production from islet cells caused by tacrolimus and decreased peripheral utilization related to high-dose corticosteroids results in nonketotic hyperglycemia. Insulin is initially mandatory in management but often can be discontinued if the tacrolimus dose is reduced and the corticosteroid portion of maintenance immune suppression is discontinued.[58]

Future Management Strategies for Critical Care of Infants and Children With Cardiopulmonary Failure

Heart transplantation in children has gained wide acceptance as an important adjunct to treatment of children with end-stage cardiomyopathic function from cardiomyopathy and palliated congenital heart disease. Successful transplantation has produced longer and better-quality lives for many infants and children. Ten-year survival free of malignancy and coronary vasculopathy is the expected outcome.[59]

The future is moving toward fewer transplant procedures in children. Palliation techniques for complex congenital heart disease (ie, single-ventricle Fontan procedure) are improving, and most of these patients will survive well into adulthood before requiring transplantation. Complications of adolescents with transposition of the great arteries who have undergone a Senning procedure and now present with systemic or right ventricular dysfunction will begin to disappear because of success with the arterial switch.

The natural history of cardiomyopathy is changing because of our understanding of the cellular mechanisms of myocardial function. New treatment strategies using angiotensin receptor and β-adrenergic blockade therapy are delaying or replacing the need for heart transplantation.

Circulatory support is being miniaturized by the development of the Berlin Heart and the DeBakey centrifugal pump. These devices can cause reversed ventricular modeling, allowing discontinuation of support without heart replacement therapy. The other major benefit of circulatory support is that, if initiated early, it can rehabilitate the child, recover end-organ function, and reduce the risks of heart transplantation surgery.

Acute and Chronic Heart Failure

Meaghan Doherty, Alejandro Lopez-Magallon, and Ricardo Munoz

PEARLS

- Admissions for symptoms associated with heart failure in children are common and place a significant burden upon the health care system.
- The etiology for heart failure is diverse, and appropriate therapy is dependent on proper identification of the underlying pathology.
- A solid understanding of cardiac biomechanics and physiology, as well as heart-lung interactions, is vital to proper management of patients in the pediatric critical care setting.
- The value of a comprehensive physical examination in a patient with heart failure is critical, and it should not be underappreciated.
- Echocardiography should be readily available to assess cardiac function, as well as structural or functional abnormalities leading to heart failure.
- When additional diagnostic data are necessary, such as direct measurement of intracardiac hemodynamics, assessment of coronary artery perfusion, or pathologic specimen for histologic diagnosis, cardiac catheterization should not be delayed.
- Targeted therapies may include medical management, catheter-based techniques, or surgical interventions.
- Patients with poor response to conventional medical therapy should be considered candidates for mechanical circulatory support before development of irreversible organ dysfunction.

Heart Failure

There has been increasing awareness regarding the impact of heart failure in pediatric patients and the significant associated morbidity and mortality. Although small in comparison with the numbers found in the adult population, children with heart failure are nowadays overrepresented in hospitals, as they require frequent office visits and unplanned hospital admissions. A recent study from a nationwide inpatient database estimated 11,000 to 14,000 annual admissions for children with heart failure in the United States.[1] In order to address the clinical needs of these patients, a comprehensive understanding of the underlying pathology and physiology is required, as well as in-depth familiarity with the current treatment options.

Not uncommonly, the patient with heart failure looks relatively well "on the surface" despite significant compromise in ventricular function, and the heart failure cardiologist must observe close vigilance with careful adjustments of anticongestive treatment. When further decompensation occurs, these patients can present a particular challenge to the critical care clinician, who is usually comfortable treating patients with overt hemodynamic compromise with early and invasive interventions. Sometimes delaying highly invasive interventions in order to allow time for improvement or heart transplant under optimal clinical conditions may be indicated, and a careful balance must then be pursued between these two apparently opposing strategies.

Definition

The myocardium functions to pump blood throughout the body in order to deliver oxygen and vital nutrients to the organs, which are necessary to meet systemic demands and maintain homeostasis. Heart failure occurs when the heart can no longer meet the metabolic needs of the body. The underlying pathologies that lead to this clinical syndrome are quite diverse, related to a combination of circulatory, neurohormonal, and molecular abnormalities.[2]

Systolic failure is due to a problem with the heart's ability to generate force during ventricular contraction, whereas diastolic failure is due to inadequate cardiac filling.

The ejection of blood occurs during the contractile phase, or ventricular systole. Problems during this period due to inadequate contractility result in insufficient generation of a pressure differential to drive an adequate blood flow through the body. As there is a deficiency in oxygen delivery and substrate availability, systolic heart failure results.

With diastolic dysfunction, there is impairment in the heart's ability to relax and dilate. A heart with diastolic dysfunction becomes stiff, resulting in elevated filling pressures and therefore a decrease in stroke volume and subsequent decrease in cardiac output. In addition, high atrial pressures develop, leading to pulmonary and systemic venous congestion. In oncology patients, serial echocardiography examinations due to the risk of chemotherapy-induced cardiomyopathy have demonstrated that subtle signs of diastolic dysfunction are often apparent before a decline in systolic dysfunction is evident.[3] Therefore careful assessment of diastolic indices may identify patients who are at increased risk for development of fulminant heart failure.

Although, by convention, the term *heart failure* is most often used to describe conditions in which impaired cardiac output results from derangements in ventricular filling or ejection, conditions of relative cardiac dysfunction may occur when there is increased metabolic demands and the heart is unable to sustain these increased needs.

Causes of Heart Failure

Identification of a primary etiology has important prognostic implications and helps to guide management strategies. Unfortunately, despite a thorough investigation, it is not always possible to determine the exact cause of failure in every patient and broad therapeutic strategies may be employed.

The physiologic circumstances resulting in heart failure are often related to an increased demand on the heart or an abnormality of myocyte structure or cellular regulation. These conditions may be congenital or acquired and may occur in isolation or in combination with other factors. Increased cardiac demands may be categorized as either pressure or volume load.

In children, structural abnormalities related to congenital heart disease are a common feature in patients presenting with heart failure. These abnormalities can result in pressure overload, volume overload, or a combination of both. The variations of lesions that occur are numerous and not discussed at this time. It is important to note that milder lesions may have delayed presentation, and structural heart disease may be found in a previously undiagnosed older child or adult who presents with signs and symptoms of cardiac dysfunction.

Structural abnormalities may be acquired, particularly in the postoperative patient. Septal hypertrophy and ventricular outflow obstruction may occur over time and present in older patients, and valve dysfunction may be a progressive occurrence due to infectious, rheumatologic, toxic, or traumatic insults.

Intrinsic abnormalities of heart muscle structure or metabolism lead to alterations in tissue mechanics or excitation-contraction coupling. These can also occur due to altered physiologic conditions such as electrolyte abnormalities, acidosis, hypoglycemia, or sepsis.

Cardiac arrhythmias can precipitate worsening heart function. This occurs in the presence of atrial or ventricular arrhythmias or complete heart block or may lead to a gradual decline of function due to an initially well-tolerated but incessant rhythm disorder.

High-output cardiac failure results when extra physiologic demands are placed on the myocardium due to an increase in metabolic requirements. This may occur during periods of acute illness or from chronic medical problems such as liver failure. Vascular malformations, such as arteriovenous malformations (AVMs), may also lead to a high-output state.

The myocardium undergoes adaptive mechanisms to accommodate increased workload; however, if these demands persist, the heart may be unable to keep up with the increased demand and dysfunction will result.

Physiologic Consideration in the Patient With Heart Failure

A more extensive discussion on cardiovascular function can be found elsewhere in this book (Chapter 29). Cardiac output is the product of heart rate and stroke volume, which is determined by contractility, preload, and afterload.

Preload

Preload is the amount of blood in the ventricle at the end of diastole. Otto Frank first reported in the late 19th century that stretching the ventricular tissue in frog hearts

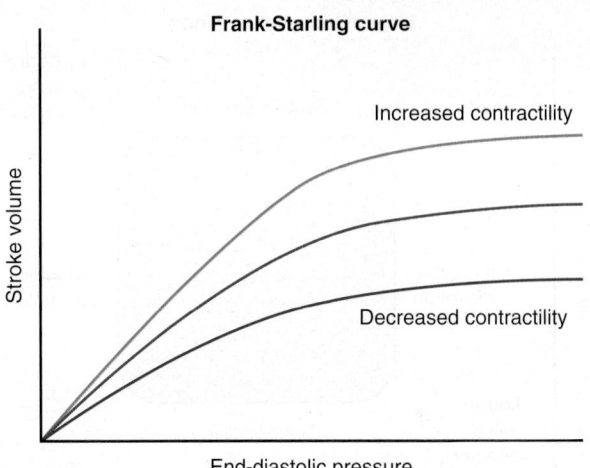

Fig. 40.1. The classic Frank-Starling curve with a graphic depiction of the relationship between preload and stroke volume under different inotropic conditions. For any given increase in preload (end-diastolic pressure), there will be a corresponding increase in stroke volume until a point of overstretching, beyond where there is a change in the slope with decreasing changes in stroke volume for any given increase in preload.

before contraction increased the strength generated by the myocardium. Later, Earnest Starling and his associates appreciated increased stroke volume in the setting of increasing venous return in dogs. We refer to the Frank-Starling curve as a graphic depiction of the myocardial fibers and ventricular chambers' ability to increase their contractility, and thus stroke volume, in response to changes in preload (Fig. 40.1).

This concept holds true until a certain point at which the myocardial fibers become overstretched and the length-tension relationship is no longer optimal for maximum contraction. At this point there is a change in slope of the curve to reflect a decrease in pressure generation at higher volumes. Clinically this represents the point where administration of additional fluid results in worsening symptoms of congestion. Another limitation of this graph is that it does not demonstrate the changes that occur in end-systolic volume with altered venous return. When afterload and contractility are kept stable, a pressure-volume loop can be used to demonstrate how changes in intraventricular volume affect pressure in the ventricle throughout the cardiac cycle (Fig. 40.2).[4]

If left ventricular pressure continues to rise at end diastole, several undesired effects occur. First, pulmonary congestion will develop with associated symptoms of cough, shortness of breath, and tachypnea. Worsening pulmonary edema may lead to poor gas exchange and decreased oxygenation. In addition, as stroke volume increases, so does wall tension and afterload. As the coronary arteries fill during diastole, coronary perfusion may become impaired by the increasing afterload and, combined with the increased oxygen consumption by the myocardium under these circumstances, may lead to tissue ischemia.

Afterload

Afterload can be thought of as the pressure or resistance against which the heart must pump in order to eject blood during systole. In the absence of left ventricular or aortic stenosis, the major determinant of the amount of force needed

LV pressure-volume loop

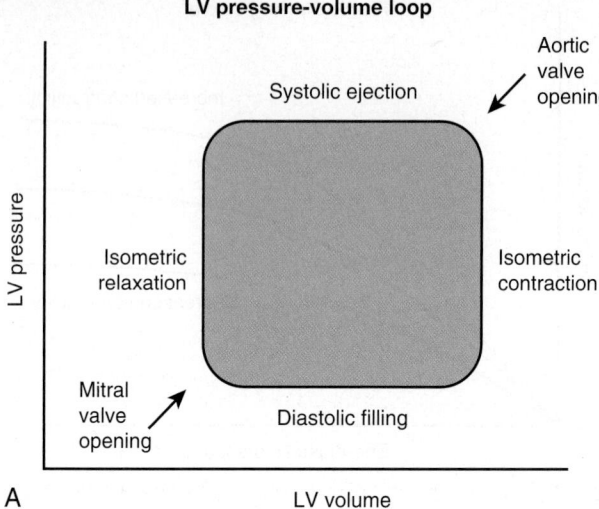

A

Preload and stroke volume with constant LV pressure

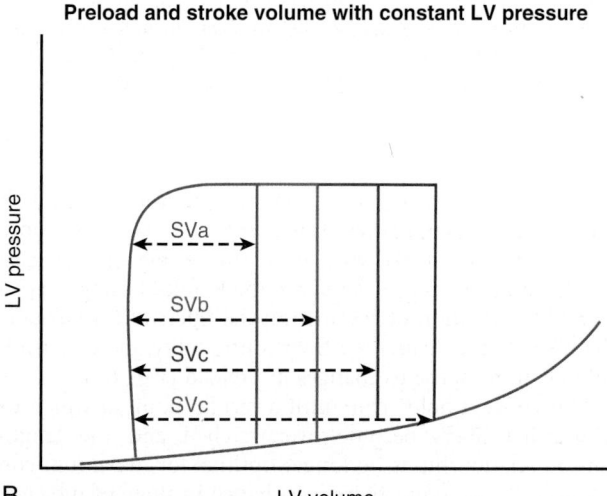

B

Fig. 40.2. Preload and stroke volume at constant left ventricular (LV) systolic pressure. (A) LV pressure-volume loop. Left ventricular pressure is plotted multiple times against chamber volume during the cardiac cycle. (B) Hemodynamic parameters like stroke volume, cardiac output, ejection fraction, and myocardial contractility can be determined from loop analysis.

is the systolic blood pressure. Although systolic blood pressure plays a major role in cardiac afterload, it is not the only variable at play. Afterload is better defined by the concept of wall stress, also called systolic wall tension (SWT), which accounts for intraventricular pressure, as well as both ventricular radius and ventricular wall thickness. As the ventricle dilates and its radius increases, there is an increase in wall stress. Conversely, when there is an increase in wall thickness, wall stress is reduced. This relationship is defined by the Law of LaPlace:

$$SWT = \frac{(transmural\ pressure \times ventricular\ radius)}{(wall\ thickness \times 2)}$$

Contractility

Contractility is the intrinsic ability of the heart muscle to generate force, and it occurs at the level of the sarcomere, where cross-bridge connections between actin and myosin

filaments are formed. In the resting state, calcium is stored in the sarcoplasmic reticulum and the adenosine triphosphate (ATP) binding sites of the myofilaments are covered. When calcium is released into the cytosol in response to cell membrane depolarization, it triggers a conformational change that results in exposure of ATP binding sites and allows binding between the thick and thin filaments.

Cardiac contractility is dependent on many factors including the structural integrity of myocardial fibers, proper electrolyte balance, adequate energy sources, and preload, as previously discussed. Alterations in cellular metabolism include a transition from fatty acid utilization to glucose metabolism. Mitochondrial dysfunction and free radical formation have a deleterious effect on excitation-contraction coupling and heart muscle mechanics.[5]

Oxygen Delivery

Oxygen delivery is the amount of oxygen delivered to the tissues each minute and is calculated by cardiac output multiplied by arterial oxygen content. The oxygen content of blood is determined by the hemoglobin concentration, hemoglobin saturation, and the amount of oxygen dissolved in the blood. This is another important concept to consider when managing a patient with poor cardiac output, as avoidance of anemia is a key treatment strategy.

Assessment of the Patient With Heart Failure

The development of low cardiac output syndrome (LCOS) can be assessed by both invasive and noninvasive means. Historic data including events preceding patient presentation and important features such as decreased urine output should be discussed. The clinical presentation will vary considerably with age, and these differences should be appreciated. Whereas infants may present with irritability or poor feeding, older children often complain of abdominal pain or discomfort.

Physical Examination in Patients With Heart Failure

A thorough physical examination is an essential part of the assessment of children with heart failure, perhaps more so than the typical patient in the critical care environment. The reliance on invasive monitoring alone may be insufficient to a complete understanding of a patient's status.

The physical examination begins with visual inspection of the patient and assessment of vital signs. Changes in heart rate or respiratory rate may be the earliest signs of a struggling myocardium; an altered heart rate may suggest underlying dysrhythmia. Changes in blood pressure may occur as a late manifestation of heart failure but are an important indicator of cardiac output. Respirophasic variation in pulse pressure should be noted, as this may suggest problems such as cardiac tamponade, and a wide pulse pressure may reflect a worsening aortic valve insufficiency. Oxygen saturation should be followed closely, as poor oxygenation may indicate worsening cardiac output or lung disease. In fact, this tool is often used to screen neonates for the presence of congenital heart disease. A pulse oximetry reading of less than 95% requires additional investigation.[6] In patients with mixed circulations, it is useful to estimate the amount of pulmonary blood flow.

During inspection, a patient's color, presence of dysmorphic features, level of alertness, and any visual signs of distress, such as increased work of breathing, should be noted. Patients in severe heart failure may have a pale or ashen discoloration. Overt cyanosis or digital clubbing will arise suspicion of pre-existent cyanotic heart disease or pulmonary hypertension with right-to-left shunting. Assessment of peripheral perfusion including pulses, temperature, and capillary refill is critical. Cool extremities with a warm core may be found in patients who are volume depleted or have a low cardiac output. Jugular venous distension may be difficult to identify in younger patients but is best assessed with the head of the bed at a 30-degree angle.

A careful respiratory examination is indicated in all patients. Changes in voice, cry, or audible stridor may suggest vocal cord dysfunction, whereas asymmetric chest movement is indicative of diaphragm paresis. Percussion and asymmetric breath sounds may help identify the presence of a pleural effusion. Rales during auscultation are suggestive of pulmonary edema, whereas wheezes or rhonchi suggest coexisting lung disease. Alternatively, wheezing can be appreciated in patients with airway compression due to vascular malformations or left atrial enlargement.

A focused cardiac examination begins with observation of the chest. Surgical scars offer a clue to preexisting pathology. Abnormal pulsations and displaced point of maximum impulse (PMI) should also be noted. The presence of a hyperdynamic precordium suggests a volume-overloaded heart, which can occur in the setting of increased intracardiac shunting or regurgitant valve function. A thrill may be appreciated due to high-velocity blood flow through a stenotic valve, vessel, or restrictive shunt. Pulses should be assessed in all extremities. Decreased pulsation in one extremity may suggest peripheral arterial thrombosis or may be due to a prior surgery such as a classic Blalock-Taussig shunt or subclavian flap repair of coarctation. Simultaneous palpation of upper and lower extremity pulses should be performed to assess for femoral delay secondary to a coarctation.

Auscultation of the heart should first focus on the rate and regularity of the heartbeat. The second heart sound should have variable splitting with respiration, although this may not be noted in the first day or two of life due to elevated pulmonary vascular resistance. A single heart sound is otherwise abnormal and may be due to valve atresia, pulmonary hypertension, or transposition of the great vessels. A second heart sound that is widely split is due to changes that delay closure of the pulmonary valve, such as right-sided volume overload or a right bundle branch block, whereas a narrow split S2 is found in conditions that result in early closure of the pulmonary valve or delayed closure of the aortic valve. Paradoxic splitting can occur with severe aortic stenosis.

Extra heart sounds can be either benign or pathologic. Although a third heart sound may be a normal finding in older children, a gallop rhythm with a third or fourth heart sound may reflect a stiff or volume overloaded ventricle, especially if accompanied with other signs and symptoms of heart failure. A fourth heart sound may be noted in late diastole and is nearly always abnormal, usually due to filling of a poorly compliant ventricle. Early systolic clicks suggest stenosis of a semilunar valve and are more easily appreciated when a patient leans forward. A midsystolic click suggests mitral valve prolapse, although this finding is uncommon in children. A pericardial friction rub is more easily appreciated over the apex and is common in the early postoperative period, although in the setting of recent-onset heart failure it may be due to acute myocarditis. A rub may not be appreciated in the presence of a large effusion.

Finally, careful assessment of organomegaly is required for a complete evaluation. Liver congestion and engorgement occurs due to high systemic filling pressures, and liver distension can be monitored over time to assess the patient response to anticongestive treatment. Care must be taken to distinguish true hepatomegaly from a downward displaced liver in the setting of pulmonary hyperinflation. This can often be distinguished by use of percussion.[7]

Diagnostic Studies in Patients With Heart Failure

A 12- or 15-lead electrocardiogram should be performed promptly in addition to continuous telemetry monitoring to assess for conduction abnormalities or other derangements in rhythm that can lead to rapid decompensation.

Biomarkers

Cardiac biomarkers are frequently used in the identification and surveillance of children with heart failure. The expanding field of metabolomics looks to identify metabolic differences in patients with early versus overt heart failure. The most commonly recognized and frequently utilized biomarkers are the natriuretic peptides (NPs), which are released from cardiac tissue in response to increased stress related to elevated pressure and/or volume load. Four NPs have been identified: A, B, C, and D. In clinical practice, brain natriuretic peptide (BNP), which is primarily secreted from the ventricle, is the most commonly measured peptide. NT-proBNP is a bioproduct of the BNP prohormone and can also be measured. These peptides function to decrease afterload by blocking endothelin release and promote diuresis and natriuresis by inhibiting the renin-angiotensin-aldosterone system. BNP has been found to have vasodilatory effects in the systemic, pulmonary, and renal blood vessels.[8]

In addition to being useful in the initial diagnosis of heart failure, these levels can be trended over time to monitor a patient's clinical status and response to therapy. Elevated BNP was found to be a risk factor for both readmission and death in a study of children with decompensated heart failure.[9]

The normal BNP level is appreciably elevated in the first few days of life, and normal values fall throughout the neonatal and childhood periods. These values also vary with patient size and gender and may be elevated in the setting of decreased clearance related to renal disease. It is important to remember that these levels may also be elevated in the setting of other diseases that cause increased demands on the heart, such as persistent pulmonary hypertension of the newborn or diaphragmatic hernia.

A study by Cheng et al.[5] evaluated plasma metabolite profiles using mass spectroscopy in control patients versus those with heart failure and those considered to be in recovery. A number of the metabolites investigated, particularly histidine, phenylalanine, spermidine, and phosphatidylcholine, were found to have independent prognostic significance similar to BNP, and analysis of these and other metabolites in combination was found to have improved prognostic value compared with BNP alone.

Echocardiography

Echocardiography is a vital tool in the evaluation of patients with cardiac dysfunction, offering a quick and comprehensive anatomic assessment, as well as determination of myocardial performance. Quick access to echocardiography is key to the assessment of a patient with changing hemodynamic circumstances, and identification of underlying etiology allows for timely initiation of targeted therapy. Measures of cardiac function include assessment of contractility, ejection fraction, and shortening fraction. Diastolic function can be investigated by tissue Doppler indices, and valve dysfunction can be demonstrated by color Doppler interrogation.

We focus specifically on measurements of global cardiac function. It is important to acknowledge that there are limitations to these tools, which do not assess for regional wall motion abnormalities or dyskinesis, which are particularly important when there is local injury suggestive of a coronary perfusion defect. In addition, these localized areas of dysfunction may not be properly accounted for in the calculations of global function and often add imprecision to the measurements. This is why a simple number is not sufficient to adequately describe overall cardiac performance, and these indices should be used together for an improved clinical picture.

Flow across the aortic valve can be quantified and used to estimate cardiac output. This is performed by obtaining a pulsed Doppler envelope at the level of the valve annulus in order to determine the velocity-time integral (VTI). This value is a correction for the change in velocity that occurs during the ejection time and is calculated by the computer. The VTI can then be multiplied by the cross-sectional area at the valve annulus to give an estimate of the stroke volume.[10] Once stroke volume is determined, it is multiplied by the patient's heart rate to determine cardiac output.

Determination of ejection fraction is based on the differences of ventricular chamber volume in diastole and systole, so errors associated with these volume measurements affect the estimated ejection fraction. The volume measurements are dependent on assumption of a normal ventricular shape, which is not necessarily true in hearts with significant dilation or hypertrophy. In addition, accurate measurement requires distinction between the cardiac wall and chamber interface, which is open to observer error, as well as issues related to image quality. Similar errors in these measurements are more dramatic in smaller patients. Left ventricle (LV) volume is calculated by 5/6 × LV length × cross-sectional area. LV ejection fraction is the percent change in ventricular volume between end diastole and end systole. The measurements are performed in the apical window using either the two- or four-chamber view. Normal estimated ejection fraction is between 54% and 75%.[10]

Right ventricle (RV) measurements are even more challenging due to its complicated geometry and the difficulty with two-dimensional (2D) imaging of this complex structure. Magnetic resonance imaging (MRI) is frequently used for more definitive analysis of RV size and function. Fractional area change (RV FAC) is a frequently used echocardiographic measurement to assess RV systolic function. It is measured as RVEDA-RVESA/RVEDA, where RVESA is RV end-systolic area and RVEDA is RV end-diastolic area. One important limitation to this calculation is that it does not account for the outflow portion of the RV, which is not visualized in the apical four-chamber view, where this measurement is performed. The use of three-dimensional echocardiography has been found to be more accurate compared with 2D echocardiography when compared with MRI measurements of RV size and function.[10] As the orientation of the muscle fibers in the RV

is aligned to contract in a more longitudinal plane, the degree of tricuspid valve systolic excursion during RV systole, known as TAPSE, correlates well with other measures of RV function. This is performed by obtaining an M-mode tracing through the lateral aspect of the tricuspid valve annulus in the apical view. Values can be interpreted as z scores on the basis of patient age and size.[11]

Shortening fraction (SF) is the percent change in the LV dimension from end diastole to end systole: LVEDD-LVESD/LVEDD × 100, where LVEDD is LV end-diastolic dimension and LVESD is LV end-systolic dimension. The normal value for LVSF is 28% to 38% and is highly dependent on ventricular loading conditions.[10]

Valve function should first be evaluated using 2D imaging. Valve size, leaflet excursion, and presence of infravalvar or supravalvar narrowing or dilation should be appreciated. Once the anatomy of the apparatus is established, color Doppler may be placed along the trajectory at an appropriate Nyquist limit, and turbulence of flow by color aliasing or presence of valvar insufficiency should be noted. Next spectral Doppler using both pulsed and continuous wave Doppler should be performed with the angle of interrogation parallel to the direction of blood flow. A pulsed Doppler signal will assess velocity at the specific level along the plane of interrogation, whereas a continuous wave Doppler will assess the velocities along the entire plane of interrogation. Thus it may be difficult to identify the precise level of obstruction using only continuous wave; however, the highest velocity along the trajectory will be determined. The velocities measured using spectral Doppler can be converted to pressure gradients using the Bernouli equation. Interpretation of these values must give consideration to the patient's hemodynamic state, as decreased contractility will result in lower valve velocities and potential underappreciation of valve stenosis, whereas hyperdynamic states may overestimate these gradients.

Additional Noninvasive Imaging Modalities

Although echocardiography is relatively quick, available, and inexpensive, there are many times when all of the desired information cannot be obtained from this modality alone and additional diagnostic tools should be considered. Other imaging modalities, such as MRI or CT scans, are frequently used to clarify a patient's anatomy when it is not clearly demonstrated by echocardiogram. This is the case when suboptimal images are obtained due to poor acoustics or when a question remains regarding coronary artery anatomy or anomalous venous drainage. Cardiac MRI is also useful for volume quantification and assessment of RV function,[12] which can be particularly challenging to assess by echocardiography. A myocardial perfusion scan to assess for delayed enhancement should be obtained when there is concern for regional ischemia related to impaired coronary blood flow.[13]

Cardiac Catheterization

Ready access to a cardiac catheterization laboratory with a skilled interventional cardiologist is necessary when direct measurement of intracardiac pressures is indicated, such as when a patient's course is not progressing as expected. Calculations of cardiac output, pulmonary vascular resistance, and Qp:Qs can be performed using data acquired in the cardiac catheterization laboratory to give a precise assessment of cardiac hemodynamics.

Cardiac catheterization is considered the gold standard for assessment of coronary perfusion and is also useful for assessing pulmonary venous desaturation secondary to pulmonary AVMs. Catheterization is also preferred over noninvasive studies when there is an indication for intervention, such as balloon atrial septostomy, angioplasty or valvotomy, or if a myocardial biopsy is required. Some patients may require emergent intervention, as may occur in a baby with transposition of the great arteries and acidosis secondary to a restrictive atrial septum. A more detailed analysis of catheter-based hemodynamic assessment and interventions is given in Chapter 32.

Management of Low Cardiac Output Syndrome

Medical management is used in acute heart failure to improve oxygen delivery capabilities to increase perfusion to vital organs.

Preload Management

Volume should not be withheld with the intention of preventing of edema in the setting of multiorgan dysfunction. Correction of the metabolic imbalances is of primary importance. Diuretics are indicated to limit the resulting pulmonary edema and require close monitoring of electrolyte imbalances and renal function. Acute kidney injury is a common and dose-related adverse effect from overaggressive diuresis. Most cases of acute kidney injury are reversible; however, particularly in patients with poor cardiac output and renal perfusion, irreversible renal damage may occur. Acute kidney injury is associated with increased risk of dialysis, prolonged intubation, infection, and prolonged ICU length of stay.[14]

Methods to Reduce Afterload

Systemic vascular resistance can be decreased by the use of vasodilators, as discussed in more detail later, thus decreasing ventricular workload. The use of mechanical ventilation is a powerful tool to reduce transmural pressure and therefore systolic wall tension and afterload in patients with decompensated heart failure (Fig. 40.3).

Methods of Optimizing Contractility

Inotropic agents are frequently used to enhance myocardial contractility. Factors to consider when choosing an inotrope include the resultant increase in myocardial oxygen consumption, its impact on the conduction tissue and propensity for arrhythmias, the effect on both systemic and pulmonary vascular resistance, and the specific type of heart disease being treated.

Oxygen Consumption

Oxygen consumption is the amount of oxygen consumed by the body. Because this value is equal to the amount of oxygen exchanged at the lungs, oxygen consumption can be measured via indirect calorimetry. In practice, the Fick principle is more commonly used to estimate oxygen consumption as the product of cardiac output and the difference in oxygen content between the arterial and venous systems. As increased cardiac output is necessary to compensate for relative anemia, maintenance of adequate hemoglobin is critically important in managing patients with heart failure.

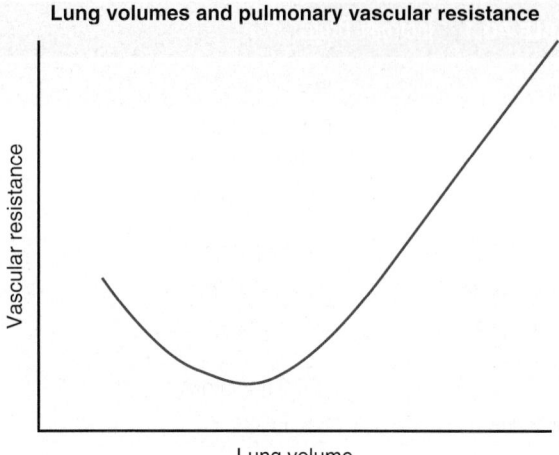

Lung volumes and pulmonary vascular resistance

Fig. 40.3. Lung volumes and pulmonary vascular resistance. At constant transmural pressure of the capillary bed, there is high resistance at low lung volumes due to stretching of extra-alveolar space. As lung volumes increase, the capillaries increase in diameter. Further increase in lung volumes will stretch the capillaries, resulting in narrowed vessel caliber.

Pharmacology of Heart Failure

Diuretics are used to manage systemic and pulmonary congestion. Although diuretics can provide marked symptomatic improvement, they do not affect contractility or afterload and are often used in conjunction with other agents. Loop diuretics are the most potent and rapid-acting diuretics and are therefore the drugs of choice in the ICU setting. See Table 40.1 for dosing guidelines.[15] They act by inhibiting the sodium-potassium-chloride cotransporter in the ascending limb of the Loop of Henle, resulting in decreased sodium and chloride resorption. Other classes of diuretics such as thiazide and aldosterone antagonists may be used as adjunctive therapy to augment diuresis.

Acute kidney injury is a serious and unfortunately common complication of diuretic use. Additional side effects of diuretics include electrolyte and acid-base imbalances. Hypokalemia, hypocalcemia, hypomagnesemia, and hypochloremic alkalosis may occur in a dose-dependent fashion. Hence close monitoring of renal function and electrolytes is indicated with use of these medications, with electrolyte repletion as indicated.

Vasoactives

Adequate calcium balance is necessary for proper cardiac muscle performance due to its role in excitation-contraction coupling. Avoidance of hypocalcemia, particularly in neonates who have a poorly developed sarcoplasmic reticulum, is crucial to optimize cardiac function and maintain proper vascular smooth muscle tone. Patients who have undergone cardiac bypass or have received large volumes of blood products are at particular risk for hypocalcemia. Monitoring ionized calcium levels is necessary to determine the need for supplemental calcium administration, as elevated intracellular calcium levels have been associated with increased cell injury and death during ischemia and reperfusion. Calcium infusion may lead to bradycardia, particularly if done rapidly. Calcium administration is not recommended in patients with

TABLE 40.1   Inotropic Drugs

Drug	Dose	Site of Action/Receptor	Effect
Calcium chloride	Bolus: 5-10 µg/kg Infusion: 10 mg/kg/hr	Cardiac myofilaments	↑ Contractility & SVR May ↑ PVR, ↓ HR
Epinephrine	0.01-0.05 µg/kg/min	β > α	↑ HR & contractility ↓ renalVR, may ↓ PVR & SVR
	>0.05 µg/kg/min[a]	α1 > β	↑ SVR
Norepinephrine	0.01-0.3 µg/kg/min[a]	α1 > β	↑ HR, contractility, SVR & PVR, ↓ renalVR
Dobutamine	2-10 µg/kg/min	β1 > β2, α1	↓ HR, contractility ↓ SVR & PVR
	10-20 µg/kg/min		
Dopamine	2-5 µg/kg/min	DA1, DA2	↓ renalVR
	5-10 µg/kg/min	β > α1	↑ HR, contractility, renalVR
	10-20 µg/kg/min[a]	α1 > β	↑ HR, contractility, SVR, PVR, renalVR
Isoproterenol	0.01-0.2 µg/kg/min	β1, β2	↑ HR, contractility ↓ SVR, PVR, renalVR
Milrinone	0.25-1 µg/kg/min Optional loading dose: 75-100 µg/kg	Phosphodiesterase III inhibitor	↑ HR, contractility ↓ SVR, PVR, renalVR
Levosimendan	Bolus: 6-12 µg/kg Infusion: 0.05-0.1 µg/kg/min	Troponin C, ATP-sensitive K+ channels	↑ contractility ↓ SVR, PVR, renalVR No effect on HR

[a]Higher doses may be used, but increase in cardiac afterload may be detrimental to myocardial performance.
HR, heart rate; SVR, systemic vascular resistance; PVR, pulmonary vascular resistance.
From Jones M, Klugman D, Fitzgerald R, et al. Pediatric Cardiac Intensive Care Handbook, Diuretics. Washington, DC: Pediatric Intensive Books, LCC; 2015 and Biaggioni I, Robertson D. Adrenoreceptor agonists and sympathomimetic drugs. In: Katzung BG, Masters SB, Trevor AJ, eds. Basic and Clinical Pharmacology. 11th ed. Stamford, CT: McGraw-Hill; 2009:127-148.

TABLE 40.2   Diuretics

Drug	Dosing	Oral		IV/IM	
Furosemide	Neonates & preterm	1-4 mg/kg/dose	Every 12-24 hours	1-2 mg/kg/dose	Every 12-24 hours
	Infants & children	0.5-6 mg/kg/day	Divided q 6-12 hours	0.5-4 mg/kg/day	Divided q 6-12 hours
	Adults	20-80 mg per dose	Every 6-8 hour	20-40 mg/dose; may increase by 20 mg	May repeat as needed
Bumetanide	Neonates	0.01-0.05 mg/kg/dose	Every 24-48 hours	0.01-0.05 mg/kg/dose	Every 24-48 hours
	Infants & children	0.015-0.1 mg/kg/dose	Every 6-24 hours; max: 10 mg/day	0.015-0.1 mg/kg/dose	Every 6-24 hours; max: 10 mg/day
	Adults	0.5-2 mg/dose	Every 12-24 hours; max: 10 mg/day	0.5-1 mg/dose	Every 6-24 hours; max: 10 mg/day

IM, intramuscular; IV, intravenous.
From Jones M, Klugman D, Fitzgerald R, et al. Pediatric Cardiac Intensive Care Handbook, Diuretics. Washington, DC: Pediatric Intensive Books, LCC; 2015.

preexisting bradycardia or asystole unless there is established hypocalcemia or hyperkalemia. In addition, caution must be used in patients on digoxin as calcium may enhance digitalis toxicity. See Table 40.2 for dosing guidelines and effects of the most commonly used vasoactive medications.[16,17]

Dopamine has a dose-dependent response on various tissues within the body. At low doses the dopaminergic-1 receptors are activated within the renal, mesenteric, and coronary vasculature. This so-called "renal dosing" of dopamine increases renal blood flow and glomerular filtration rate but is a controversial concept not universally accepted. At moderate doses there is activation of the B1 receptors in the heart, which has both inotropic and chronotropic effects. This results in increased cardiac output but minimal increase in blood pressure due to the peripheral vasodilatory effects of the dopaminergic receptors. As the medication is titrated to higher doses, there is activation of peripheral α1 receptors, as well as stimulation of endogenous norepinephrine release from nerve endings, both of which result in increased peripheral systemic vascular resistance (SVR) and cardiac afterload.[16] One concern with use of dopamine in infants is the potential pituitary gland suppression and alteration of thyroid function.[16,18]

Dobutamine acts primarily on β1 adrenergic receptors with less effect on α1 and β2 receptors. Therefore cardiac output is augmented by increased heart rate and contractility, with little to no increase in SVR, making this medication more appropriate for use in cases of cardiac dysfunction. However, increase in myocardial oxygen consumption may aggravate diastolic dysfunction in some patients.

Milrinone is a phosphodiesterase III inhibitor, which increases cAMP and results in increased calcium within the cardiac myocytes, improving both systolic and diastolic cardiac function. In addition to increased contractility, milrinone results in peripheral vasodilation by relaxing vascular smooth muscle cells. Therefore cardiac output and oxygen delivery are augmented without an increase in myocardial oxygen demand. Prophylactic milrinone therapy has been found to reduce the incidence of postoperative LCOS by up to 55% in neonates undergoing congenital heart surgery.[19] Milrinone may result in hypotension and reflex tachycardia. Slow-dose titration may be preferable to use of a loading dose to avoid an acute drop in blood pressure. Milrinone has a relatively long half-life, particularly in patients with renal dysfunction, and its effect persists for hours after its discontinuation.

Epinephrine has strong α and β effects, and its effect on different tissues within the body is also dose dependent. Low-dose epinephrine increases blood pressure primarily by increasing cardiac contractility by activation of the β1 receptor. There is also an effect on β2 receptors in skeletal muscle tissue that decreases vascular resistance and reduces cardiac afterload. As epinephrine dosing is titrated upwards, there is a greater effect on peripheral α receptors, resulting in increased blood pressure and cardiac afterload. There is an increase in renal vascular resistance at all doses, leading to risk of renal insufficiency due to diminished renal blood flow. Like most vasoactive medications, epinephrine can be proarrhythmic and continuous telemetry monitoring during infusion is required. The patient is at risk for both atrial and ventricular ectopy and reentrant tachycardias due to increased automaticity, as well as decrease in atrioventricular (AV) nodal refractory time. In addition, high-dose infusions of epinephrine can cause cardiac tissue necrosis in young infants and alternative methods of support should be considered should high doses be required.

Norepinephrine acts similarly to epinephrine; however, it is a more potent vasoconstrictor. There is little effect on peripheral β2 receptors, and therefore small doses of norepinephrine result in increased SVR and blood pressure, as opposed to low-dose epinephrine, which can decrease SVR. Norepinephrine also has a strong effect on β1 receptors within the heart to increase contractility, similarly to epinephrine. Norepinephrine is best indicated in cases of circulatory collapse and hypotension not responsive to other pressors. However, it is less commonly used in young children with cardiac dysfunction due to the significant increase in afterload.

Levosimendan works by altering the protein structure of troponin C and making it more sensitive to intracellular calcium, leading to increased inotropy without associated increase in myocardial oxygen consumption. It also results in vasodilation by increasing the activity of potassium-ATPase of the sarcolemma of smooth muscle tissue and provides a cardioprotective effect by acting on the same channel in the cardiac myocyte mitochondria. Its primary indication is in the treatment of acute-onset heart failure. Several ongoing prospective trials are looking at use of levosimendan in the immediate postoperative period with some encouraging results, and an experimental animal model comparing levosimendan with milrinone found similar and even advantageous effects of levosimendan in systemic and pulmonary vasodilation, as well as myocardial oxygen consumption profile.[20] The most common adverse effects include hypotension, tachycardia, atrial fibrillation, hypokalemia, and headache.

Isoproterenol is a nonselective β agonist with minimal α activity. Its physiologic effect is increased heart rate and contractility with decreased SVR. There is a greater chronotropic than inotropic effect, and isoproterenol is useful in patients with symptomatic bradycardia or heart block. Isoproterenol should be avoided in patients with ventricular outflow tract obstruction due to decreased preload. Significantly increased myocardial oxygen consumption may lead to demand ischemia, and high doses are associated with ventricular arrhythmias.

Mechanical Circulatory Support

Greater detail on the application, physiology, and technical issues of the various circulatory support devices are given elsewhere (Chapter 30). Unfortunately there are currently no established guidelines on the use of various methods of mechanical circulatory support in children and, therefore, the indications for and use of these devices vary widely across institutions. Overall, there seems to be a trend toward increased reliance on these devices as technology, surgical technique, and clinical outcomes have improved.[21]

The typical indication for mechanical circulatory support is when continued clinical decompensation is present despite highly aggressive medical management. Signs and symptoms that may be present under these circumstances include increased work of breathing, poor perfusion or other signs of LCOS, such as decreased mixed venous oxygenation, a rising base deficit or lactate levels, acidosis, and signs of multiorgan dysfunction such as decreased urine output or a change in neurologic status. When less invasive therapies are unable to correct these abnormalities, discussions regarding escalation of care among the multidisciplinary care teams should occur under semielective conditions and before further clinical deterioration that will lead to circulatory collapse and cardiac arrest.

The risk undertaken when deploying these devices can be substantial and must not be underappreciated. Infection is an obvious risk, and maintaining a low index of suspicion for sepsis with frequent surveillance cultures and judicial use of broad spectrum antibiotics is vital. Thrombosis is a common complication, and a strict anticoagulation protocol with full heparinization should be followed, unless medically contraindicated, in addition to close inspection of the visible portions of the circuit for thrombus formation or stranding.[22]

The successful management of a patient on mechanical circulatory support is best accomplished through the collaboration of a highly skilled interdisciplinary care team. Diligent bedside nursing combined with knowledgeable perfusionists, technically skilled surgeons, and an attentive intensive care team is necessary to provide the highest level of care to these most critically ill patients.

Extracorporeal Membrane Oxygenation

Extracorporeal membrane oxygenation (ECMO) requires surgically placed inflow and outflow cannulas in the major blood vessels or within the cardiac chambers. This can be done either centrally via a median sternotomy or by a vascular cutdown approach. Echocardiography is often used as an adjunct to confirm adequate cardiac decompression and cannulae position.

As many ECMO candidates may have congenital vascular anomalies or a history of previous vessel instrumentation in the cardiac catheterization laboratory or with central vascular access devices, knowledge of the anatomy, patency, and continuity of the vessels that may be chosen for ECMO cannulation is imperative before the procedure itself so as to avoid futile attempts and delays. ECMO can be rapidly instituted in patients with worsening cardiac dysfunction as a bridge to longer-term mechanical support using a ventricular assist device (VAD) or as a bridge to transplantation.

The use of VA ECMO has seen a dramatic increase. Once thought to be a last-effort salvage therapy for dying patients, ECMO is now used more routinely, particularly in larger centers. Because a patient's prognosis following ECMO is highly dependent on the patient's status before initiation of bypass, including organ dysfunction, residual cardiac lesions, or shunts and underlying disease pathology, it may be advantageous to consider initiation of ECMO sooner when the medical status of a patient is deteriorating, before development of multiorgan dysfunction, as these patients may have improved outcome following recovery of myocardial function or easier transition to longer-term therapies.[23]

ECMO allows time for ventricular recovery by decompressing the heart and lowering wall stress, improving coronary perfusion and supporting the circulation with adequate oxygenation. Of course, if the heart is not participating in cardiac output whatsoever, over time the heart muscle will atrophy, making the ability to wean from ECMO less likely. Just as early initiation and utilization of ECMO are key to prognosis, so too is an early exit strategy for weaning and ultimate decannulation in patients with recovery potential.

Managing Patients on ECMO

Immediately following successful cannulation and initiation of ECMO, systemic perfusion should be assessed and cannulae position should be confirmed. Mixed venous oxygenation, lactate levels, central venous pressure, blood pressure, and urine output are all critical components of an ongoing assessment and should be closely monitored with optimization of circuit flow rates and cardiac output, as indicated.

The patient should be monitored for signs of left atrial hypertension due to inadequate decompression as this may require placement of a left atrial vent to reduce wall stress and facilitate myocardial recovery. This can be evaluated on chest radiograph, echocardiogram, and by clinical examination findings suggestive of pulmonary edema.

As previously discussed, avoidance of anemia is necessary to optimize oxygen content and delivery. A higher flow rate needed to compensate for the presence of anemia leads to increased cell damage and hemolysis within the circuit. Hemoglobin of 14 to 15 gm/dL is considered optimal. A platelet count of at least 75,000 to 100,000 is considered adequate to minimize risk of bleeding.[24] As discussed earlier, a strict adherence to anticoagulation protocol to maintain optimal heparinization and minimize risk of thrombosis is critical.

Causes of decreased venous drainage may be related to hypovolemia in the setting of bleeding or fluid shifts, but sudden changes may signal compromised flow through the venous catheter, development of pericardial tamponade, or pneumothorax and mandate rapid investigation.

Echocardiography can be used to assess for cardiac distention and wall motion during attempts at weaning of ECMO flows and in observation of cardiac function during transient interruption of ECMO flows (clamping and bridging). Once underlying disease processes have been addressed and the patient is able to successfully wean flows and tolerate clamping, decannulation from ECMO should not be delayed.

Ventricular Assist Devices

VADs can be categorized as either continuous or pulsatile. Continuous flow ventricular assistance is provided by various types of centrifugal devices that are operated by a rotating magnet that drives a continuous roller pump. Cannulation for a centrifugal pump device is akin to that used for ECMO and can be used in most sizes of patients, including infants. The long-term risks of a centrifugal VAD are the same as a patient cannulated onto ECMO, and they are best used for short-term management as a bridge to recovery. However, due to the lack of an oxygenator and generally shorter tubing length, these devices have lower thrombotic risk compared with an ECMO circuit. Therefore the anticoagulation goals for a patient on a centrifugal pump can be less aggressive, which in turn may reduce the risk of bleeding. Patients are unable to ambulate with these devices, and like all mechanical support devices, shorter duration of support is associated with improved outcomes.[21]

Pulsatile VADs can be used for longer duration and are indicated in patients with persistent symptoms of low cardiac output or end-organ dysfunction on maximal support, often as a bridge to transplantation. This may include patients unable to wean from ECMO. Placement of a pulsatile device requires central cannulation through a midline sternotomy incision. Improved cardiac output and oxygen delivery result in improved end-organ perfusion. In addition, patients are able to ambulate and participate in higher levels of physical rehabilitation, which can improve pretransplant status. Unloading the heart with this type of device may allow for improved myocardial recovery. These devices are not currently approved as destination therapy in children, although they have been used for this indication in adults.

The external pulsatile VAD should be physically examined multiple times each day. The inlet and outlet valves of the bladder are a common location for thrombin stranding and clot formation, so careful inspection is critical. The membrane should be inspected for persistent wrinkling, which generally indicates inadequate bladder filling or ejection. Insufficient filling may reflect poor intravascular volume status, inadequate negative diastolic pressure, or development of cardiac tamponade. Inadequate bladder ejection suggests increased afterload, which may be related to clot formation, cannulae placement, patient agitation, or infection. Use of vasodilators or inotropic agents may be necessary to augment cardiac output under these circumstances.[21]

Heart Transplantation

Heart transplantation is the preferred treatment option in patients with advanced heart failure and inability to wean from higher levels of support, including continuous intravenous infusions or mechanical circulatory support.[25] Heart transplantation is best performed in a high-volume center with a dedicated multidisciplinary care team consisting of heart failure and transplant cardiologists, transplant nurse coordinators, social workers, pharmacists, nutritionists, and psychologists specially trained in the unique issues relative to this patient population.

The evaluation process for a potential transplant candidate is extensive and involves assessment of comorbid medical problems, infectious issues, alloimmunization status, as well as social and psychologic concerns. Any potential contraindications to transplantation must be explored carefully. Patient nutrition, rehabilitation status, and vaccinations should be optimized before transplantation, although live vaccines should be avoided due to immunosuppression at the time of transplantation.

When an organ becomes available, critical assessment of donor suitability is conducted, including cause of death, structure, function, rhythm abnormalities, and size of the donor relative to the recipient, as well as direct inspection of the organ at the time of procurement. An actual or virtual crossmatch for compatibility between the donor and recipient is also performed. Hyperacute rejection, which is due to preformed antibodies, is a rare but devastating complication. Acute humoral rejection often occurs days to weeks following transplantation but is much less common than acute cellular rejection. The most common cause of death in the early postoperative period is primary graft failure, which can be detected by lymphocyte infiltration on endomyocardial biopsy. Ischemia times of greater than 3 hours are associated with a higher risk of primary graft failure.[26]

Two techniques are commonly used for surgical anastomosis of the transplanted heart. The original technique used by Lower and Shumway involves anastomosis of the recipient atria with that of the donated heart. An alternative method involves venous anastomosis of the superior vena cava, inferior vena cava, and the right and left pulmonary veins. This approach may be better in patients who have undergone surgical palliation for congenital heart disease and results in less AV valve regurgitation and atrial arrhythmias; however, the procedure is more time consuming and has the added risk of acquired venous obstruction. A hybrid approach in which the left atrium is anastomosed as in the biatrial technique, together with complete resection of the recipient's right atrium and bicaval anastomosis as in the "total transplantation technique," has also been performed.[25] It is important to know which approach is used so that potential postoperative complications can be anticipated.

Intraoperative transesophageal echocardiogram is used to monitor cardiac function and potential complications, particularly right heart function and narrowing at the anastomosis sites. Poor cardiac function or rhythm abnormalities may require ECMO cannulation in some patients.

Postoperative management involves close attention to rhythm issues, fluid status, postoperative bleeding, and markers of hemodynamics including central venous pressures, mixed venous oxygen saturation, serum lactate, and urine output. Hypotension is common and may be due to LCOS or from systemic inflammatory process. Causes of LCOS include hypovolemia, cardiac tamponade, and poor ventricular function, as well as rhythm issues including bradycardia and atrial tachycardia. Temporary epicardial pacing or antiarrhythmics may be indicated. Echocardiography can also be useful in identifying primary cardiac causes. If corrective measures are not taken in a timely manner, secondary organ dysfunction will result. Care to avoid fluid overload in the early postoperative period is necessary to avoid exacerbation of right ventricular failure. Surgical reexploration or mechanical support may be indicated in some cases.

Immunotherapy

Use of induction of immunosuppression, which drastically reduces the likelihood of rejection in the early postoperative period, varies across different centers in terms of the patient selection and therapies used. Some centers use induction therapy on all patients, while others reserve this for those considered at higher risk of rejection. Use of induction allows delayed initiation of oral immunosuppression agents until renal and GI function have improved, yet it has been found to be associated with increased risk of later rejection.[26]

When used, induction should ideally begin within the first 12 hours, after postoperative bleeding is controlled. Steroid therapy is generally given in the operating room and continued throughout the postoperative period. Two commonly used induction agents are monomurab-CD3 (OKT3), which is a mouse monoclonal antibody, and antithymocyte globulin (RATG), which is a polyclonal rabbit antibody. Efficacy is similar between the two agents with different risk profiles. Risks include bacterial and viral infection and posttransplant lymphoproliferative disorder (PTLD).[25] Interleukin-2 receptor antibodies basiliximab and daclizumab, initially used in renal transplant patients, have also been employed after cardiac transplantation and seem to have a decreased risk of infection compared with older agents.[26] Maintenance immunosuppression with oral medications can be started following induction in so-called "sequential therapy." Some centers prefer to start these agents sooner, either in place of or at the time of induction therapy. Maintenance therapy generally consists of a calcineurin inhibitor, either cyclosporine or tacrolimus, which inhibits T-cell activation. Tacrolimus may be superior at preventing acute graft rejection when used in combination therapy. Calcineurin inhibitors are typically used in conjunction with an antiproliferative agent such as mycophenolate or azathioprine, which both interfere with purine synthesis. Mycophenolate has been associated with decreased mortality at 1 and 3 years relative to azathioprine.[25]

Conclusion

Management of patients with heart failure requires persistent ongoing assessment, with analysis of hemodynamic data and other contributing factors or underlying disorders. When a patient's clinical course is not as anticipated, rapid and sometimes highly invasive means are indicated to obtain additional diagnostic information to allow for specific targeted therapy. Maintenance of adequate cardiac output with avoidance of acidosis and multisystem organ dysfunction is the primary objective, and when this cannot be achieved with medical management alone, additional measures including use of mechanical circulatory support should be pursued. Although heart transplantation is a last-resort therapy, patients who require high levels of support without reasonable potential for recovery should be considered early, before development of irreversible organ damage or other risk factors that would worsen overall prognosis or deem them ineligible for organ listing.

References

1. Rossano J, Kim J, Decker J, et al. Morbidity and mortality of heart failure prevalence-related hospitalizations in children in the United States: a population-based study. *J Card Fail.* 2012;18:459-470.
2. Hsu D, Pearson G. Heart failure in children. *Circ Heart Fail.* 2009;2:63-70.
3. Bu'Lock F, Mott M, Oakhill A, et al. Left ventricle diastolic dysfunction after anthracycline chemotherapy in childhood: relation with systolic function, symptoms and pathophysiology. *Br Heart J.* 1995;73:340-350.
4. Patterson SW, Starling EH. On the mechanical factors which determine the output of the ventricles. *J Physiol.* 1914;48:357-379.
5. Cheng M, Wang C, Shiao M, et al. Metabolic disturbances identified in plasma are associated with outcomes in patients with heart failure. *J Am Coll Cardiol.* 2015;65:1509-1520.
6. Mahle W, Newburger J, Matherne GP, et al. Role of pulse oximetry in examining newborns for congenital heart disease: a scientific statement from the American Heart Association and American Academy of Pediatrics. *Circulation.* 2009;120:447-458.
7. Cassidy S, Allen H, Phillips J. History and physical examination. In: Allen HD, Driscoll DJ, Shaddy RE, Feltes TF, eds. *Moss and Adams' Heart Disease in Infants, Children and Adolescents.* 8th ed. Philadelphia: Lippincott, Williams & Wilkins; 2013.
8. Wong DT, George K, Wilson J, et al. Effectiveness of serial increases in amino-terminal pro-B type natriuretic peptide levels to indicate the need for mechanical circulatory support in children with acute decompensated heart failure. *Am J Cardiol.* 2011;107:573-578.
9. Rossano J, Shaddy R. Heart failure in children etiology and treatment. *J Pediatr.* 2014;165:228-233.
10. Lai W, Mertens L, Cohen M, et al. *Echocardiography in Pediatric and Congenital Heart Disease.* Oxford, UK: Whiley-Blackwell; 2013.
11. Koestenberger M, Ravekes W, Everett AD, et al. Right ventricular function in infants, children and adolescents: reference values of the tricuspid annular plane systolic excursion (TAPSE) in 640 healthy patients and calculation of z score values. *J Am Soc Echocardiogr.* 2009;22:715-719.
12. Helbing W, Ouhlous M. Cardiac magnetic resonance imaging in children. *Pediatr Radiol.* 2015;45:20-26.
13. Grant F, Treves ST. Nuclear medicine and molecular imaging of the pediatric chest: current practical imaging assessment. *Radiol Clin North Am.* 2011;49:1025-1051.
14. Toth R, Breuer T, Cserep Z, et al. Acute kidney injury is associated with higher morbidity and resource utilization in patients undergoing heart surgery. *Ann Thorac Surg.* 2012;93:1984-1991.
15. Jones M, Klugman D, Fitzgerald R, et al. *Pediatric Cardiac Intensive Care Handbook, Diuretics.* Washington, DC: Pediatric Intensive Books, LCC; 2015.
16. Munoz R, da Cruz E, Vetterly C. Handbook of pediatric cardiovascular drugs. In: Munoz R, da Cruz EM, Vetterly CG, Cooper DS, Berry D, eds. *Vasoactive Drugs in Acute Care.* 2nd ed. London: Springer-Verlag; 2014.
17. Biaggioni I, Robertson D. Adrenoreceptor agonists and sympathomimetic drugs. In: Katzung BG, Masters SB, Trevor AJ, eds. *Basic and Clinical Pharmacology.* 11th ed. Stamford, CT: McGraw-Hill; 2009:127-148.
18. Van den Berghe G, de Zegher F, Lauwers P. Dopamine suppresses pituitary function in infants and children. *Crit Care Med.* 1994;22:1747-1753.
19. Hoffman TM, Wernovsky G, Atz AM, et al. Efficacy and safety of milrinone in preventing low cardiac output syndrome in infants and children after corrective surgery for congenital heart disease. *Circulation.* 2003;107:996-1002.
20. Stocker C, Lara S, Shekerdemian L, et al. Mechanisms of a reduced cardiac output and the effects of milrinone and levosimendan in a model of infant cardiopulmonary bypass. *Crit Care Med.* 2007;35:252-259.
21. Annich G, Lynch W, MacLaren G, et al. *ECMO Extracorporeal Cardiopulmonary Support in Critical Care.* 4th ed. Ann Arbor, MI: Extracorporeal Life Support Organization; 2012.
22. Dalton H, Garcia-Filion P, Holubkov R, et al. Association of bleeding and thrombosis with outcome in extracorporeal life support. *Pediatr Crit Care Med.* 2015;16:167-174.
23. Chrysostomou C, Maul T, Callahan P, et al. Neurological outcomes after ECMO life support in children with cardiac disease. *Front Pediatr.* 2013;1:47.
24. Maul TM, Kamaneva MV, Wearden PD. Mechanical blood trauma in circulatory assist devices. In: Jahanmir S, Weiss W, Zapanta C, eds. *Mechanical Cardiovascular Assist Devices: Design and Performance Evaluation.* New York: ASME Press; in press.
25. Banner N, Hamour I, Lyster H, et al. *Postoperative Care of the Heart Transplant Patient, Surgical Intensive Care Medicine.* New York: Springer Science + Business Media; 2010.
26. Lindenfeld J, Miller G, Shakar S, et al. Drug therapy in the heart transplant recipient; Part 1: cardiac rejection and immunosuppressive drugs. *Circulation.* 2004;110:3734-3740.

Physiologic Foundations of Cardiopulmonary Resuscitation

Adnan M. Bakar, Kenneth E. Remy, and Charles L. Schleien

PEARLS

- Both the cardiac and thoracic pump mechanisms play a role in infants and children during cardiopulmonary resuscitation, so attention to excellent chest compression technique with an emphasis on "push hard, push fast" is critical to attaining sufficient cardiac output to maintain coronary and cerebral blood flow.
- Use of any vasoconstrictor (including vasopressin) should be sufficient to raise aortic diastolic pressure during cardiopulmonary resuscitation above the critical level for resuscitation success (>15–20 mm Hg).
- Amiodarone or lidocaine may be the most effective pharmacologic treatment for shock-resistant ventricular tachycardia or fibrillation.
- Use of the biphasic defibrillator is an important advance in the treatment of tachyarrhythmias and has advantages in its safety profile compared with monophasic defibrillators.
- Post–cardiac arrest resuscitative care is critical to survival and includes appropriate uses of inodilators and neuroprotective strategies, including avoidance of hyperthermia.

With the development of basic cardiopulmonary resuscitation (CPR) in the early 1960s, skilled resuscitation teams both in and out of the hospital were formed. The development of CPR saved lives; previously, every victim of cardiac arrest had died. Soon thereafter, successful resuscitation of patients by basic life support measures, defibrillation, and medications became common, even as long as 5 hours after commencement of CPR. Over the past decade, both survival and neurologic outcomes after in-hospital cardiac arrest have improved in adults and children.[1-3] Data show that the success of CPR depends on many factors. Rapid institution of basic life support measures (ie, bystander CPR for sudden out-of-hospital cardiac arrest and immediate electrical countershock for ventricular fibrillation [VF]) improve the chances of survival for patients experiencing sudden out-of-hospital cardiac arrest.[4] These measures led to the growing deployment of automatic external defibrillators (AEDs) in public places. Immediate defibrillation is currently the standard of care in witnessed VF arrests. However, evidence indicates that basic life support and other measures directed at restoring energy

substrates to the myocardium before countershock in patients with unwitnessed, out-of-hospital arrest may further improve outcome.[5-8]

Other preexisting factors that play a role in successful resuscitation include the patient's age, prior medical condition, presenting cardiac rhythm, and etiology of cardiac arrest. In 2008, a multi-institutional prospective study was published that examined these preexisting factors and further described in two additional studies the clinical characteristics, hospital course, and outcomes of a cohort of children after in-hospital or out-of-hospital arrest. Besides demonstrating differences in clinical characteristics, these studies offered future considerations for the care of children who had experienced cardiac arrest and post resuscitative care, including hypothermia.[9-11] The low resuscitation rate in children, even when the patient does not have preexisting disease, probably results from the high incidence of asystole as the presenting rhythm. Asystole is the most common presenting rhythm in both in-hospital and out-of-hospital arrests and is noted in 25% to 70% of victims.[12-16] Bradycardia and pulseless electrical activity (PEA) are other common rhythms. The high incidence of asystole in children who experience cardiac arrest can be explained by systemic disturbances such as hypoxia, acidosis, sepsis, and hypovolemia that commonly precede the arrest. Although ventricular arrhythmias are usually reported to be infrequent (range, 1.3%–3.8%), out-of-hospital series report VF in 10% to 19% of victims younger than 20 years.[17,18] These series, along with the observation that the frequency of witnessed arrest is much lower than in adults, suggests that ventricular rhythms may be more common than usually estimated and that delay in resuscitation results in progression of nonperfusing rhythms to asystole. Increasing availability of AEDs may be contributing to the increased recognition of ventricular arrhythmias in out-of-hospital pediatric cardiac arrest.[19] In specialized cardiac ICUs, ventricular arrhythmias account for as many as 30% of the arrests.[3,20,21]

In their original work on CPR, Kouwenhoven et al.[22] proposed that blood flow during closed-chest compressions resulted from squeezing of the heart between the sternum and vertebral column, now termed the *cardiac blood flow mechanism.* In fact, the precise mechanism by which forward circulatory flow is generated during closed-chest cardiac massage has major implications for current approaches to CPR. Other methods, such as vest CPR, simultaneous compression ventilation CPR (SCV-CPR), active compression-decompression CPR (ACD-CPR) both without and with an impedance threshold valve (ITV), and interposed abdominal compressions with CPR (IAC-CPR), take into account advances in our understanding of the mechanism of blood flow during resuscitation.

The pharmacology of resuscitation remains controversial, and these controversies have led to major changes in the guidelines for CPR. Use of sodium bicarbonate, calcium chloride, and glucose remains unresolved at this time. The role of high-dose epinephrine has been minimized because of concerns over postresuscitation deleterious effects on myocardial performance and poor outcomes. Evidence favoring a role for vasopressin, with a relatively pure vasoconstrictor effect, is accumulating. The role of lidocaine as the antiarrhythmic of choice for ventricular ectopy has been questioned as new data on the efficacy of amiodarone in persons in cardiac arrest have been generated.[3] Research is ongoing into alternative vasoconstrictors and the use of "pharmacologic cocktails" that may include β-blockers, antiarrhythmic agents, antioxidants, nitroglycerin, and a vasoconstrictor in attempts to improve the resuscitation outcome and postresuscitation cardiac function.[23-25]

Developments in the use of direct current countershock have occurred. Biphasic defibrillators are now widely in use and appear to improve the success of defibrillation at lower delivered energies and, it is hoped, decrease myocardial injury. As noted, the role of "shock first" is being reassessed because the success of electrical countershock in restoring spontaneous circulation declines rapidly after 3 to 4 minutes have elapsed.

Although postresuscitation cerebral preservation has become an important area of focus, therapeutic hypothermia has not been found to improve neurologic outcome after pediatric cardiac arrest.[11]

This chapter discusses the physiologic foundations of CPR. In the first section, the possible mechanisms of blood flow by the thoracic and cardiac pump mechanisms are discussed, including how the specific chest geometry of children and infants helps decide which of these mechanisms applies. Then newer CPR techniques, which take into account the physiologic mechanisms discussed in the first section, are discussed. Controversies and advances in pharmacologic management during CPR and current guidelines for use of drugs for resuscitation are addressed. New developments in the use of countershock, including the timing of shocks, the energy used, and the type of current delivery system used (biphasic or monophasic), are discussed. Finally, the role of therapeutic hypothermia is reviewed.

Mechanisms of Blood Flow
Cardiac Versus Thoracic Pump Mechanism

The cardiac pump hypothesis holds that blood flow is generated during closed-chest compressions when the heart is squeezed between the sternum and vertebral column. This mechanism of flow implies that ventricular compression causes closure of the atrioventricular valves and that ejection of blood reduces ventricular volume. During chest relaxation, ventricular pressure falls below atrial pressure, allowing the atrioventricular valves to open and the ventricles to fill. This sequence of events resembles the normal cardiac cycle and occurs during cardiac compression when open-chest CPR is used.

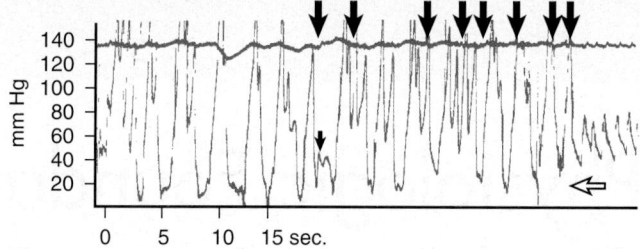

Fig. 41.1. Cough-cardiopulmonary resuscitation during prolonged ventricular asystole after coronary arteriographic injection. An 18-second period of asystole after right coronary arteriographic injection is depicted. During this period, the patient coughed every 2 seconds, generating peak aortic pressures greater than 140 mm Hg. *Large arrows* mark the intrinsic QRS complexes after the 18-second period of asystole. The *Small arrow* marks the resultant aortic pressure from the first intrinsic beat. The patient continued to cough until the cardiac rhythm stabilized 40 seconds later. (From Criley JM, Blaufuss AH, Kissel GL. Cough-induced cardiac compression. Self-administered form of cardiopulmonary resuscitation. JAMA. 1976;263:1246.)

Numerous clinical observations have conflicted with the cardiac pump hypothesis of blood flow. In 1964, Mackenzie et al.[26] found that closed-chest CPR produced similar elevations in arterial and venous intravascular pressures, the result of a generalized increase in intrathoracic pressure.[26] In 1976, Criley et al.[27] made the dramatic observation that several patients in whom VF developed during cardiac catheterization produced enough blood flow to maintain consciousness by repetitive coughing (Fig. 41.1). The production of blood flow by increasing thoracic pressure without direct cardiac compression describes the thoracic pump mechanism of blood flow during CPR.

During normal cardiac function, the lowest pressure in the vascular circuit occurs on the atrial side of the atrioventricular valves. This low pressure compartment is the downstream pressure for the systemic circulation, which allows venous return to the heart. Angiographic studies show that blood passes from the vena cava through the right heart into the pulmonary artery and from the pulmonary veins through the left heart into the aorta during a single chest compression.

Echocardiographic studies show that, unlike normal cardiac activity or during open-chest CPR, during closed-chest CPR in both dogs and humans, the atrioventricular valves are open during blood ejection and aortic diameter decreases rather than increases during blood ejection.[28,29] These findings during closed-chest CPR support the thoracic pump theory and argue that the heart is a passive conduit for blood flow (Fig. 41.2).[30]

Initial measurements of hemodynamic data during chest compression for CPR found the generation of almost equal pressures in the left ventricle, aorta, right atrium, pulmonary artery, and esophagus (Fig. 41.3).[31] The finding that all intrathoracic vascular pressures are equal implies that suprathoracic arterial pressures must be higher than suprathoracic venous pressures. The unequal transmission of intrathoracic pressure to the suprathoracic vasculature establishes the gradient necessary for blood flow. The transmission of intrathoracic pressure to the suprathoracic veins may be modulated by venous valves. The presence of these jugular venous valves has been demonstrated in animals and humans undergoing CPR.[32-34] An ultrasonography study of healthy children

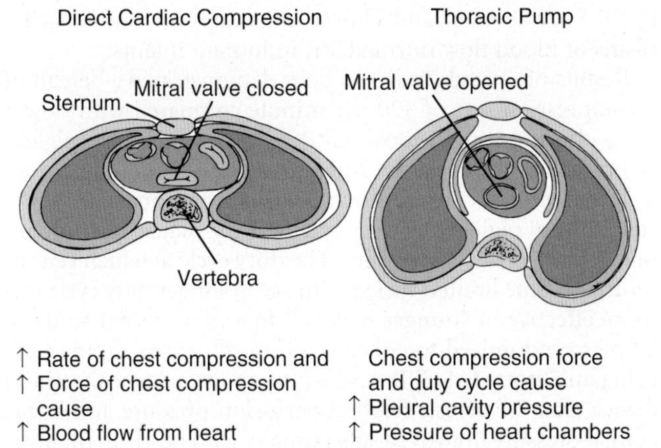

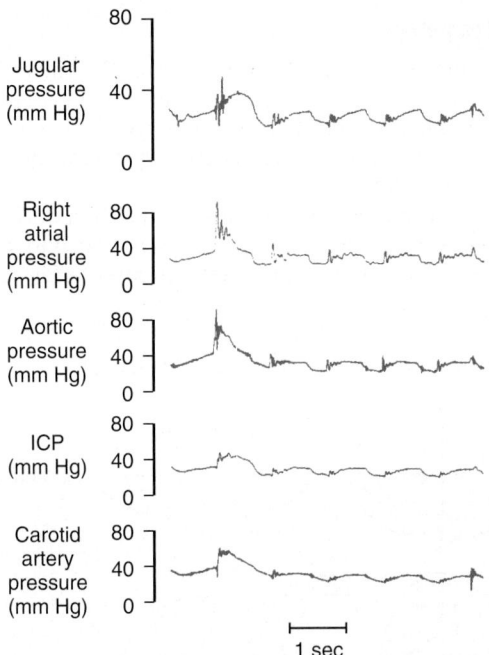

Direct Cardiac Compression

↑ Rate of chest compression and
↑ Force of chest compression cause
↑ Blood flow from heart

Thoracic Pump

Chest compression force and duty cycle cause
↑ Pleural cavity pressure
↑ Pressure of heart chambers

Fig. 41.2. Possible mechanisms for blood flow during cardiopulmonary resuscitation include direct cardiac compression *(left)* and the thoracic pump *(right)*. With direct cardiac compression, an increase in chest compression rate causes an increase in blood flow by squeezing the heart between the vertebral column and sternum. With the thoracic pump mechanism, factors that increase pleural pressure cause an increase in pressure within the heart chambers and ultimately an increase in blood flow. (From Schleien CL, et al. Controversial issues in cardiopulmonary resuscitation. Anesthesiology. 1989;71:135.)

Fig. 41.3. Original record during conventional cardiopulmonary resuscitation. The first compression for conventional cardiopulmonary resuscitation follows the lung inflation that occurred during the previous release phase. Note increase in pressure on this compression. *ICP,* intracranial pressure. (From Koehler RC, Chandra N, Guerci AD, et al. Augmentation of cerebral perfusion by simultaneous chest compression and lung inflation with abdominal binding after cardiac arrest in dogs. Circulation. 1983;67:266.)

confirmed the presence of these valves in 84% of 239 jugular veins studied. The valves were bilateral in 74% of children.[35] Transmission of intrathoracic pressure to the intracranial vault during CPR indicates that any such valve function is partial. Pathologic studies have also identified valves in the

subclavian vein in the large majority of cadavers studied (87%). The absence of these valves in some patients is postulated to lead to failure of closed-chest CPR.[36]

Subsequent hemodynamic and echocardiographic studies found different results. Deshmukh et al. demonstrated in a porcine model that mitral valve function persisted throughout resuscitation in 17 of 22 animals and that in successfully resuscitated animals, maximal aortic pressure exceeded that in the right atrium throughout the resuscitation.[32] In another porcine model of resuscitation, Hackl et al. manipulated the compressive force and depth of resuscitation by using a mechanical resuscitator.[37] The frequency of mitral valve closure during compressive systole was directly proportional to the force and depth of chest compression. When the depth of compression reached 25% of the anteroposterior diameter, valve closure occurred in 95% of cycles. They concluded that the mechanism of blood flow was dependent on the force and depth of compression. In a study of CPR using transesophageal Doppler echocardiography in adults, Porter et al. demonstrated mitral valve closure in compressive systole in the majority of patients (12 of 17) but not all patients.[38] Peak mitral flow occurred in diastole and was significantly higher in the group with mitral valve closure. Peak mitral flow occurred during compressive systole in those without valve closure. Left ventricular fractional shortening correlated with change in anteroposterior chest wall diameter and not mitral valve flow. These authors concluded that nonuniform increased intrathoracic pressure plays a role in determining whether valve closure occurs during chest compressions. As noted, a decrease in aortic dimension during CPR has been demonstrated by echocardiography and taken as evidence for the thoracic pump mechanism of blood flow. Hwang et al. readdressed this issue using transesophageal echocardiography.[39] They studied the aortic dimension of the proximal and distal thoracic aorta and noted a decrease in the aortic dimension in the distal aorta directly inferior to the zone of direct compression and an increase in the dimension of the proximal aorta. They also noted mitral valve closure in all subjects and a decrease in left ventricular (LV) volume of almost 50% at end compression. These findings were believed to be most consistent with the cardiac pump mechanism of blood flow.[40] Kim et al. also used transesophageal echocardiography to explore the role of the LV during nontraumatic arrests.[41] They noted that during the compression phase of CPR, there was anterograde flow from the ventricle to the aorta, as well as retrograde flow toward the mitral valve. The mitral valve remained closed during compression and opens during relaxation, while the aortic valve remained open during compression and closed during relaxation, which they concluded to be consistent with the cardiac pump mechanism.

The cardiac pump mechanism appears to predominate during closed-chest CPR in specific clinical situations. As noted, increasing the applied force during chest compressions increases the likelihood of direct cardiac compression. A smaller chest size may allow for more direct cardiac compression.[37,41] Adult dogs with small chests have better hemodynamics during closed-chest CPR than do dogs with large chests. Because the infant chest is smaller and more compliant than the adult chest, direct compression of the heart during CPR is more likely to occur. Blood flow during closed-chest CPR in a piglet model of cardiac arrest is higher than that achieved in adult models.[42] In contrast to adult animals, increasing intrathoracic pressure by SCV-CPR does not augment vascular pressure or regional organ blood flow during CPR in piglets.[43] The failure of SCV-CPR to increase blood flow in the infant implies that direct compression occurs with conventional CPR and that additional intrathoracic pressure is of no benefit. In a more recent study of 20 randomized swine to either a patient-centric blood pressure targeted approach with titration of compression depth to a systolic blood pressure of 100 mm Hg and vasopressors to a coronary perfusion pressure greater than 20 mm Hg or current usual practice, the blood pressure targeted group demonstrated improved 24-hour survival (8/10 vs. 0/10 survival, p = 0.001).[44] This study suggests that physiologic targets rather than absolute depths by age may in fact confer better outcomes.

Rate and Duty Cycle

In 2015 the American Heart Association (AHA) recommended a rate of chest compressions of at least 100 per minute.[45-49] At faster rates, blood flow is enhanced whether the thoracic pump mechanism or the cardiac pump mechanism is invoked. Duty cycle is defined as the ratio of the duration of the compression phase to the entire compression-relaxation cycle expressed as a percent. For example, at a rate of 30 compressions/min, a 1.2-second compression time produces a 60% duty cycle. If blood flow is generated by direct cardiac compression, then the stroke volume is determined primarily by the force of compression. Prolonging the compression (increasing the duty cycle) beyond the time necessary for full ventricular ejection should have no additional effect on stroke volume. Increasing the rate of compressions should increase cardiac output because a fixed, relatively small volume of blood is ejected with each cardiac compression. In contrast, if blood flow is produced by the thoracic pump mechanism, the volume of blood to be ejected comes from a large reservoir of blood contained within the capacitance vessels in the chest. With the thoracic pump mechanism, flow is enhanced by increasing either the force of compression or the duty cycle but is not affected by changes in compression rate over a wide range of rates.[33] Additionally, the "push hard, push fast" recommendation is based on the maintenance of a higher compression rate with a higher force of compression. Allowing total recoil of the chest allows for full blood return during the relaxation phase of the cycle.[50]

Mathematic models of the cardiovascular system confirm that blood flow is determined by both the applied force and the compression duration with the thoracic pump mechanism.[51] A mathematic model equating CPR to a circuit, constructed by Babbs, determined that while hemodynamics did not vary with compression rate, total flow and coronary flow were greatest when compression time equaled 30% of cycle time.[52]

It appears from experimental animal data that both the thoracic pump and cardiac pump mechanisms can effectively generate blood flow during closed-chest CPR. Differences between various studies may be attributed to differences in animal models or compression techniques. Important differences in animal models include chest wall geometry, compliance and elastic recoil, compliance of the diaphragm, and intraabdominal pressure. Differences in technique include the magnitude of sternal displacement, compression force, and momentum of chest compression, compression rate, and duty

cycle. Experimental and clinical data support both mechanisms of blood flow during CPR in human infants.

Results of several studies in dogs demonstrated a benefit of a compression rate of 120 per minute compared with slower rates during conventional CPR.[53-54] In studies of piglets, puppies, and humans, no differences were found comparing different rates of compression during conventional CPR.[34,55-57] In a study of piglet CPR, duty cycle was the major determinant of cerebral perfusion pressure. The duty cycle at which venous return became limited varied with age. A longer duty cycle was more effective in younger piglets.[57] In a more recent study of 22 pigs randomized to either head-up tilt versus supine CPR using an automated CPR device plus an impedance threshold device after VF arrest, cerebral perfusion pressure and intracranial pressure improved substantially with head-up tilt position.[58] This suggests that gravity has an effect on the venous circulation with high quality CPR and head tilted up positioning on cerebral perfusion. The discrepant importance of rate and duty cycle in various models (by different investigators) is confusing. However, increasing the rate of compressions during conventional CPR to 100 per minute satisfies both those who prefer the faster rates and those who support a longer duty cycle. This is true clinically because producing a longer duty cycle is easier when compressions are administered at a faster rate.

Chest Geometry

Chest geometry plays an important role in the ability of extrathoracic compressions to generate intrathoracic pressure. Shape, compliance, and deformability, which change greatly with age, are the chest characteristics that have the greatest impact during CPR.

The change in cross-sectional area of the chest during anterior to posterior delivered compressions is related to its shape (Fig. 41.4).[59] The ratio of the chest anteroposterior diameter

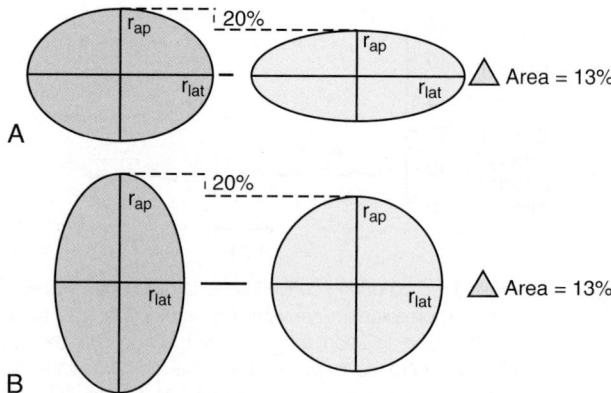

Fig. 41.4. Changes in area of ellipses with constant circumference. Each ellipse is labeled with the anteroposterior *(ap)* and lateral *(lat)* radii, and a 20% anteroposterior compression is applied. Indicated change in area equals relaxed area–compressed area. (A) Initial anteroposterior/lateral ratio = 0.7, and compression leads to positive ejection because relaxed area–compressed area is negative. (B) Initial anteroposterior/lateral ratio = 1.4, and compression toward a circular shape results in an increase in area. (From Dean JM, Koehler RC, Schleien CL, et al. Age-related changes in chest geometry during cardiopulmonary resuscitation. J Appl Physiol. 1987;62:2212.)

to the lateral diameter is referred to as the *thoracic index*. A keel-shaped chest, as seen in an adult dog, has a greater antero-posterior diameter and thus a thoracic index greater than 1. A flat chest, as in a thin human, has a greater lateral diameter and thus a thoracic index less than 1. A circular chest has a thoracic index equal to 1. A circle has a larger cross-sectional area than either of these elliptical chests. As an anteroposterior compression flattens a circle, the cross-sectional area decreases and compresses its contents. In contrast, as an anteroposterior compression is applied to the keel-shaped chest, the cross-sectional area increases as a circular shape is approached. The cross-sectional area of the keel-shaped chest does not decrease until the chest compression continues past the circular shape to flatten the chest. This implies a threshold past which the compression must proceed before intrathoracic contents are decreased and squeezed.[59] Thus the rounder, flatter chests of small dogs and pigs may require less chest displacement than the keel-shaped chests of adult dogs to generate thoracic ejection of blood. This dynamic has been demonstrated in small dogs having round chests compared with adult dogs having keel-shaped chests.[60]

As humans age, the cartilage of the rib cage calcifies and chest wall compliance decreases. Older patients may require greater compression force to generate the same sternal displacement. A 3-month-old piglet requires a much greater compression force for anteroposterior displacement than its 1-month-old counterpart.[59] Direct cardiac compression is more likely to occur in the more compliant chest of younger animals. Cerebral and myocardial blood flow during closed-chest CPR were much higher in infant piglets than in adults (Figs. 41.5 and 41.6).[61] This finding supports the cardiac pump mechanism of blood flow in infants because the level of organ blood flow achieved during closed-chest CPR in piglets approaches the level achieved during open-chest cardiac massage in adults.

Marked deformation of the chest can occur during prolonged CPR and may alter the effectiveness of CPR (Fig. 41.7).[61] Over time, the chest assumes a flatter shape, producing a larger percent decrease in cross-sectional area at the same absolute chest displacement. Progressive deformation may be beneficial if it leads to more direct cardiac compression. Unfortunately, too much deformation may decrease the recoil of the chest wall during the relaxation phase, leading to decreased cardiac filling. A progressive decrease in the effectiveness of chest compressions to produce blood flow is seen in piglets receiving conventional CPR.[61] Permanent deformation of the chest in this model approaches 30% of the original anteroposterior diameter. Attempting to limit deformation by increasing intrathoracic pressure from within during CPR with SCV-CPR was ineffective.[61] Using a thoracic vest to limit deformation when performing CPR greatly decreased the permanent chest deformation (3% vs. 30%) but did not attenuate the deterioration of vital organ blood flow with time.[63]

The characteristics of chest geometry of animals may relate to that in humans. Body weight, surface area, chest circumference, and diameter did not correlate with the magnitude of aortic pressure produced during CPR in a study of nine adults already declared dead.[62] A direct comparison of adult and pediatric human CPR has not been performed. The higher intravascular pressures and organ blood flow during CPR in infants compared with adults may result from more effective transmission of the force of chest compression because of the

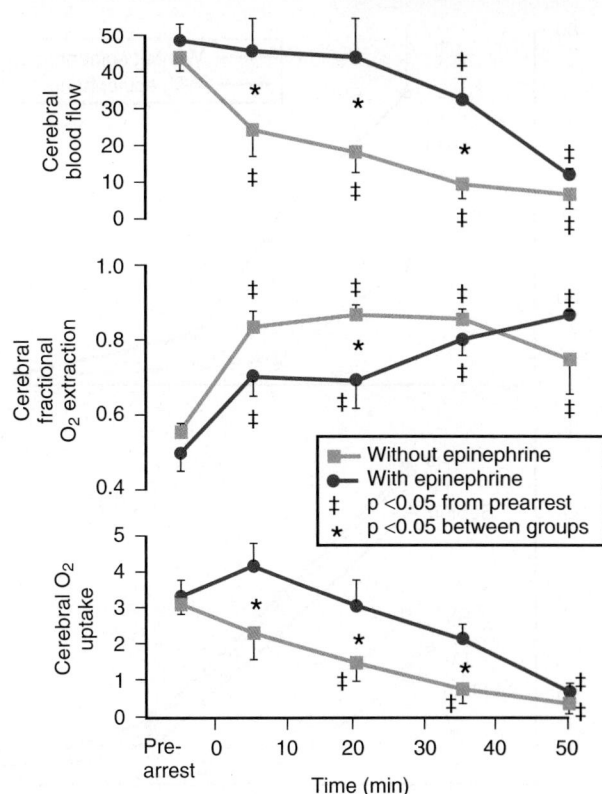

Fig. 41.5. Total cerebral blood flow, cerebral fractional O_2 extraction, and cerebral O_2 uptake before cardiac arrest and during 50 minutes of cardiopulmonary resuscitation in the groups with and without epinephrine.

higher compliance and greater deformability of the infant chest.

Effects of Cardiopulmonary Resuscitation on Intracranial Pressure

When chest compressions are applied, the increase in intrathoracic pressure is transmitted through the venous system of the head and neck to the intracranial vault, resulting in an increased intracranial pressure (ICP). Pressure is transmitted via the paravertebral veins and the cerebrospinal fluid during CPR in dogs.[64] Large swings in ICP corresponding to chest compressions occur in children undergoing CPR (Fig. 41.8).[65] This transmission of intrathoracic pressure to the intracranial contents accounts for the low cerebral perfusion pressure by increasing the downstream pressure and cerebral blood flow during closed-chest CPR. However, in a porcine model of CPR with an impedance threshold device, it was found that CPR done in a reverse Trendelenberg position (head up at 30°) reduced ICP and improved cerebral perfusion, likely because gravity improved venous drainage and thus reduced impedance to forward flow.[58]

The relationship of ICP to intrathoracic pressure during CPR is linear. In dogs receiving conventional CPR, ICP increased by one-third of the rise of intrathoracic pressure in a range from 10 to 90 mm Hg.[64] However, some modes of CPR change the intrathoracic to ICP relationship. In dogs, abdominal binding increases the transmission of pressure to the intracranial space to one half of the rise of intrathoracic pressure.[66] SCV-CPR, a mode of CPR designed to generate

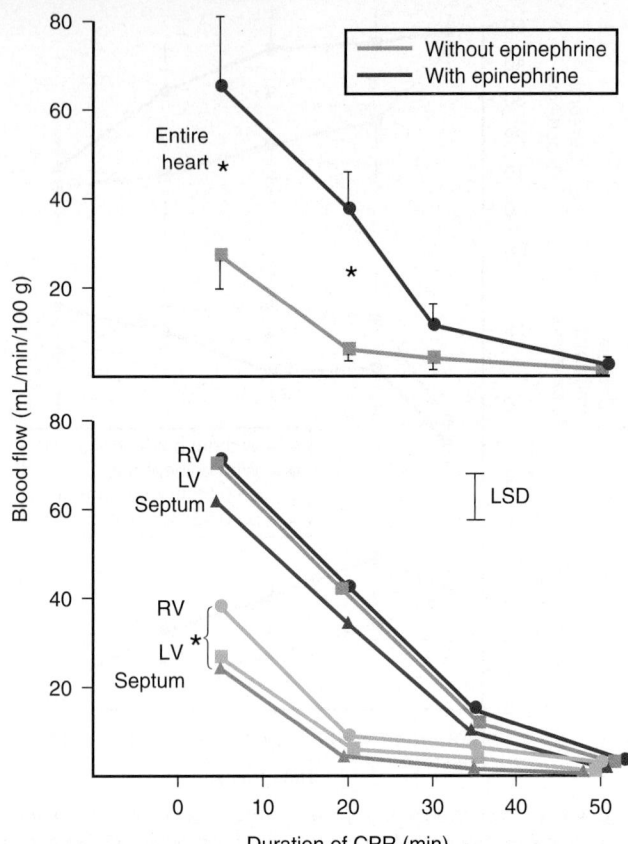

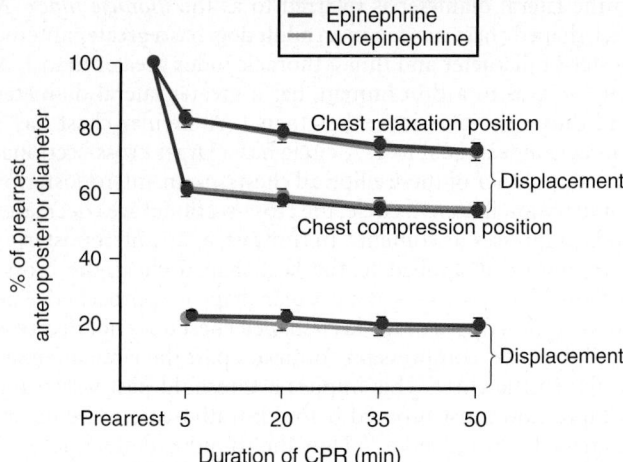

Fig. 41.7. Piston position during chest compression and relaxation phases of the cycle and net piston displacement expressed as a percent of prearrest anteroposterior chest diameter (12.0 ± 0.3 cm) in piglets. Note that displacement was essentially unchanged over the 50-minute duration, but marked deformation occurred during the relaxation phase by 5 minutes and continued to further deform over the 50-minute period in the groups with or without epinephrine. *CPR,* cardiopulmonary resuscitation. (From Schleien CL, Dean MJ, Koehler RC, et al. Effect of epinephrine on cerebral and myocardial perfusion in an infant animal preparation of cardiopulmonary resuscitation. Circulation. 1986;73:809.)

Fig. 41.6. *Top,* Total myocardial blood flow during cardiopulmonary resuscitation (CPR) in piglets with and without epinephrine. *Asterisk* indicates significant difference between groups at 5 and 20 minutes. *Bottom,* Blood flow to right ventricular free wall *(RV, circle),* left ventricular free wall *(LV, squares),* and interventricular septum *(triangles)* in the groups with and without epinephrine. Standard error bars are omitted for clarity, but the least significant difference bar *(LSD,* derived from Duncan multiple-range test) is shown for comparisons among heart regions within an animal group. (Means must differ by height of bar for $p < .05$.) LSD for comparing means between groups is twice that shown for within-group LSD. *Asterisk* indicates that RV blood flow was greater than LV and septal blood flows at 5 minutes in the group without epinephrine. Flows in all three regions in the group with epinephrine were greater than those in the respective regions in the group without epinephrine at 5 and 20 minutes. (From Schleien CL, Dean MJ, Koehler RC, et al. Effect of epinephrine on cerebral and myocardial perfusion in an infant animal preparation of cardiopulmonary resuscitation. Circulation. 1986;73:809.)

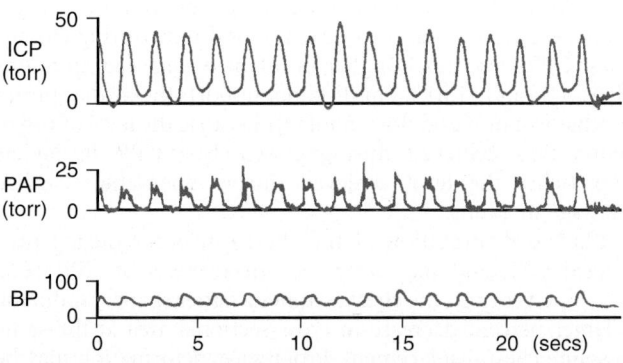

Fig. 41.8. Relationship of intracranial pressure *(ICP),* pulmonary artery pressure *(PAP),* and arterial blood pressure *(BP)* during closed-chest cardiac massage. Note that each chest compression is accompanied not only by a rise in arterial and pulmonary artery pressure but also by a sharp rise in intracranial pressure. (From Rogers MC, Nugent SK, Stidham GL. Effects of closed-chest cardiac massage on intracranial pressure. Crit Care Med. 1979;7:454.)

higher intrathoracic pressure, is similar to conventional CPR in its transmission of pressure to the cranium. Open-chest CPR decreases the transmission of pressure and improves cerebral perfusion pressure compared with conventional CPR. Thus increasing intrathoracic pressure may decrease cerebral blood flow because of the increase in downstream pressure, the ICP.

In this regard, ACD-CPR and ACD-ITV-CPR may have an advantage over conventional CPR. These techniques are designed to reduce intrathoracic pressure. Lindner et al. showed in a porcine model that cerebral perfusion is increased with ACD-ITV-CPR compared with standard CPR.[67] Using an adult porcine model of hypothermic VF arrest, the same group demonstrated by microdialysis techniques improved

lactate/pyruvate ratios and reduced glucose accumulation in the ACD-ITV group compared with standard CPR.[68] In a pediatric porcine model of resuscitation, Voelckel et al. found that ACD-CPR with ITV provided superior cerebral blood flow compared with standard CPR.[69]

Newer Cardiopulmonary Resuscitation Techniques
Simultaneous Compression Ventilation Cardiopulmonary Resuscitation

SCV-CPR is a technique designed to increase blood flow during conventional CPR by increasing the thoracic pump mechanism contribution to blood flow. Delivering a breath simultaneously with every compression, instead of after every fifth compression, increases intrathoracic pressure and augments blood flow produced by closed-chest CPR.

Experimental studies have shown that SCV-CPR increases carotid blood flow compared with conventional CPR alone.[70] Subsequent studies confirmed physiologic advantages of SCV-CPR in canine models.[31] However, in infant piglets and small dogs, SCV-CPR offered no advantage over conventional CPR.[60,62] In these small animals, the compliance and geometry of the chest may allow more direct cardiac compression. Thus higher intrathoracic pressure may be achieved with conventional CPR alone.[57,61] Coronary perfusion pressure (CPP) was either only minimally increased or even decreased in humans during SCV-CPR compared with conventional CPR. Survival was significantly worse in both animals and humans who received SCV-CPR compared with conventional CPR.[71,72] No study has shown an increased survival rate with this technique of CPR.

Interposed Abdominal Compression Cardiopulmonary Resuscitation

IAC-CPR is the delivery of an abdominal compression during the relaxation phase of chest compression. An extensive review by Babbs has been published.[73] IAC-CPR may augment conventional CPR in several ways. First, IAC-CPR may return venous blood to the chest during chest relaxation.[74,75] Second, IAC-CPR increases intrathoracic pressure and augments the duty cycle of chest compression.[74,76] Third, IAC-CPR may compress the aorta and return blood retrograde to the carotid or coronary arteries.[75] IAC-CPR is an attractive alternative to some of the newer techniques of CPR because it requires no additional equipment for implementation; however, it does require training and manpower.

In animal experiments, cardiac output and cerebral and coronary blood flow were improved when comparing IAC-CPR with conventional CPR but not in an infant model.[77,78] Additionally, in one animal experiment with newborn piglets examining chest compressions with manual sustained inflations of 30 cm H_2O versus current standard of care, ROSC was improved with better hemodynamic recovery in the group receiving sustained inflations.[79] Initial human studies also demonstrated an increase in aortic pressure and CPP during IAC-CPR compared with conventional CPR.[80] Four randomized controlled trials have compared IAC-CPR with standard CPR. The first trial reported in 1985 by Mateer et al. was the largest and included 291 patients.[81] IAC-CPR was applied in the field by paramedics until ambulance transport. No differences in mortality were found. The later trials involved a total of 279 hospitalized patients.[82-84] The results from these trials are more positive, and a meta-analysis of these studies found an increased likelihood of return of spontaneous circulation (ROSC) and intact survival to discharge with IAC-CPR versus standard CPR.[73,85] Although no intraabdominal trauma was detected in any of the 426 patients in these trials, one pediatric case report demonstrated direct pancreatic injury. Alternative techniques for abdominal hand position were studied in adult swine.[86,87] A stacked hand position similar to the usual position for chest compression over the abdominal aorta was compared with a diffuse hand position in which the hands were placed on the abdomen separately. This study demonstrated a significant increase in aortic diastolic pressure compared with standard CPR. However,

CPP was not augmented because the right atrial diastolic pressure was also elevated. Stacked hand position was found to produce a CPP equivalent to standard CPR. Diffuse hand position, however, was associated with decreased CPP, so if the technique is applied, this hand position should be avoided. Application of IAC-CPR is limited by the need for training and additional manpower. Although it has not been studied in a pediatric group, with skilled personnel available, IAC-CPR should be considered for use with inpatient arrests.

Active Compression-Decompression Cardiopulmonary Resuscitation and Impedance Threshold Valve Interposition

ACD-CPR uses a negative pressure "pull" on the thorax during the release phase of chest compression using a handheld suction device (Fig. 41.9).[88] This technique improves vascular pressures and minute ventilation during CPR in animals and humans.[67,88-90] The mechanism of benefit of this technique is attributed to enhancement of venous return by the negative intrathoracic pressure generated during the decompression phase; in addition, it reverses the chest wall deformation that accompanies standard CPR.[91] Preliminary results in adults were promising, and a large multi-institutional study of ACD-CPR completed in Europe found that ACD-CPR was superior to standard CPR.[90,92,93] In this study, a total of 750 patients were randomly assigned to receive standard CPR or ACD-CPR. In the experimental group, 5% survived to 1 year (12 patients with intact neurologic status) versus 2% (three patients with intact neurologic status) in the standard group.[94] However, a number of other trials have not shown a difference between standard CPR and ACD-CPR. A Cochrane Database Systematic Review concluded there was no consistent benefit from use of this technique.[95] The effectiveness of ACD-CPR appears to be relatively site specific. Explanations for this variability have focused on the effectiveness of training for providers and intersite variation of on-scene advanced life support techniques.[91] Use of ACD-CPR requires significantly more physical effort than conventional CPR, and this requirement may have influenced outcome.[96] No device is currently cleared for clinical use in the United States at this time.

Use of an inspiratory threshold valve has been evaluated in attempts to improve the outcome with ACD-CPR.[94,97] This technique involves the use of a valve placed between the ventilating bag and the airway, which is designed to close when the tracheal pressure falls below atmospheric pressure, enhancing the development of negative intrathoracic pressure during ACD-CPR (Figs. 41.10 and 41.11). Animal studies, including a young porcine model, showed improved organ perfusion, and brain microdialysis studies demonstrated decreased lactate accumulation and improved glucose utilization.[68,69,98,99] In a small series of patients, diastolic pressure was raised along with CPP and end-tidal CO_2 ($EtCO_2$) release.[100] These studies led to an inclusion of the technique as an acceptable alternative to standard CPR in the 2000 AHA guidelines and subsequent revised guidelines.[47,49] Plaisance et al. reported on a series of 400 patients randomly assigned to ACD-CPR with ITV or sham ITV. Survival at 24 hours was significantly improved in patients assigned to ACD-CPR.[94,100] There was a nonsignificant trend toward improved neurologic survival, with 6 of 10 discharged patients having intact survival compared with 1 of 8 discharged survivors in the sham ITV group. In two randomized control studies by Wolcke et al.[100a] and Plaisance et al. of 610 adults in cardiac arrest in

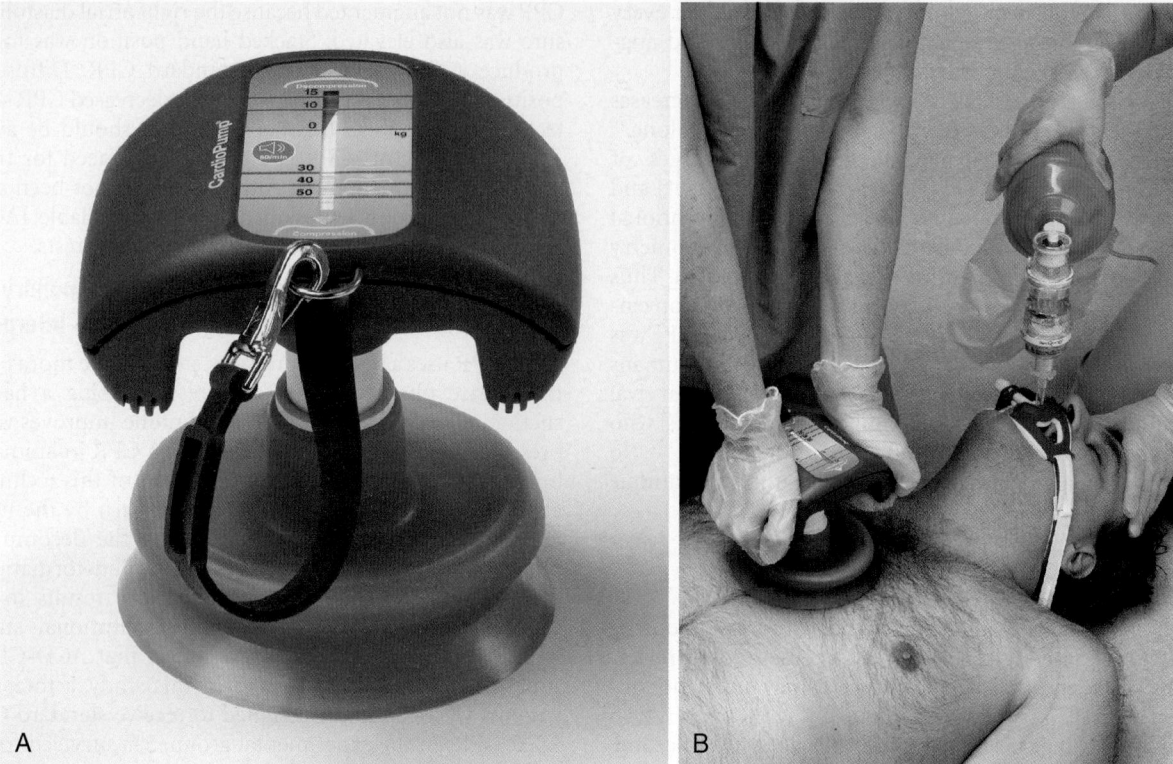

Fig. 41.9. (A) and (B) are properly placed. Device for performing active compression-decompression cardiopulmonary resuscitation. (B) The upper part is a handle and the lower part is a suction cup. (Courtesy AMBU Corporation. From Halperin H. New devices for generating blood flow during cardiopulmonary resuscitation. Curr Opin Crit Care. 2004;10:188-192.)

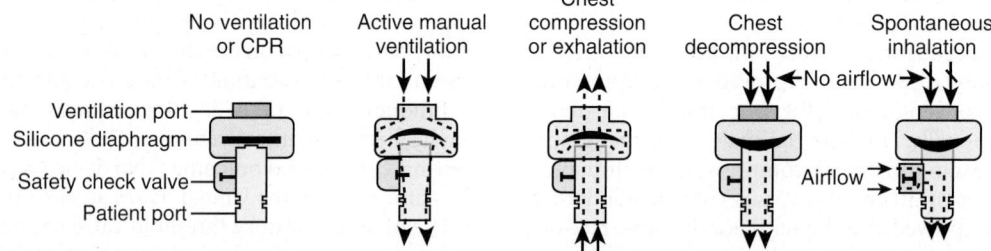

Fig. 41.10. Schematic diagram of impedance threshold valve. During a positive pressure ventilation the valve is open and gas flows. During chest compression or exhalation air moves freely through the valve. During chest decompression airflow is impeded by the valve decreasing intrathoracic pressure. During spontaneous ventilation the check valve opens allowing gas flow. *CPR,* cardiopulmonary resuscitation. (From Lurie KG, Barnes TA, Zielinski TM, et al. Evaluation of a prototypic inspiratory impedance valve designed to enhance the efficiency of cardiopulmonary resuscitation. Resp Care. 2003;48:52-57.)

the out-of-hospital setting, use of ACD-CPR plus the ITD was associated with improved ROSC and 24-hour survival rates when compared with CPR alone.[100] The addition of the ITD was associated with improved hemodynamics during standard CPR in one clinical study.[101] The ultimate role of this technique, which requires specialized equipment and significant resuscitator training, remains to be determined.[94,102]

Vest Cardiopulmonary Resuscitation

Vest CPR uses an inflatable bladder resembling a blood pressure cuff that is wrapped circumferentially around the chest with phased inflation to increase intrathoracic pressure. Because chest dimensions are changed minimally, direct cardiac compression is unlikely. In addition, the even distribution of the force of compression over the entire chest wall

decreases the likelihood of trauma to the skeletal chest wall and its thoracic contents.

Improvement of cerebral and myocardial blood flows and survival with vest CPR compared with conventional CPR was seen in dogs.[27,103-106] In piglets, a 3% permanent chest deformation was seen after 50 minutes of vest CPR, compared with an almost 30% deformation produced during an equivalent period of conventional CPR.[61,63] In a human study, vest CPR increased aortic systolic pressure but had little effect on aortic diastolic pressure compared with conventional CPR.[107] Despite its late application, vest CPR improved the hemodynamics and the rate of ROSC in adult patients in another study.[108] Evidence from a case control study of 162 adults documented improvement in survival to the emergency department when vest CPR was administered by adequately trained personnel

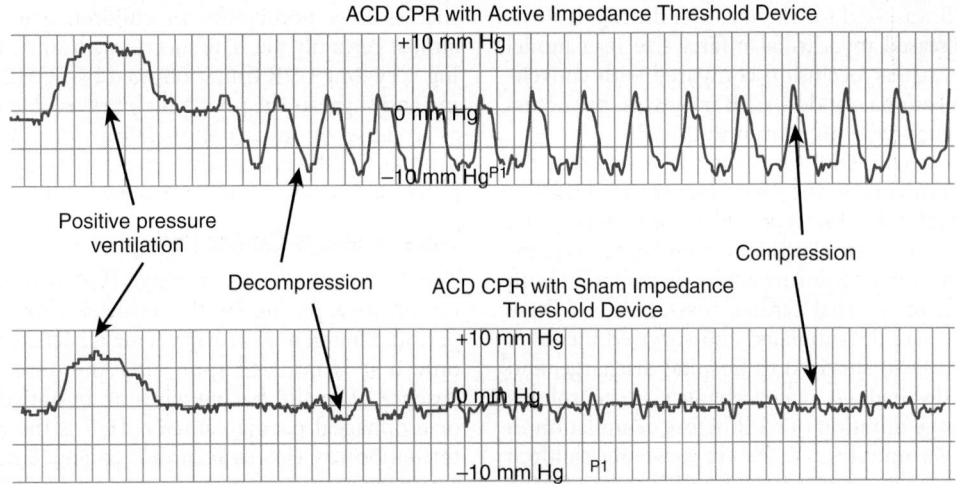

Fig. 41.11. Example of intratracheal pressures, a surrogate for intrathoracic pressures, in a patient undergoing cardiopulmonary resuscitation *(CPR)* with an automated compression device *(ACD)* with and without an impedance threshold device attached to a facemask. CPR was delivered at 100 compression/decompression cycles/min with a synchronized compression/ventilation ratio of 15:2. Note the absence of significant decreases in intratracheal pressures with a sham device. With the active impedance threshold device, wide fluctuations in intratracheal pressure are seen with each compression and decompression. (Courtesy M. Lurie, M.D., and Advanced Circulatory Systems, Inc.)

to patients in cardiac arrest in the out-of-hospital setting.[109] The lack of metallic parts has allowed vest CPR to be used experimentally during nuclear magnetic resonance spectroscopy to study brain intracellular pH.[110] The vest also has been used as an external cardiac assist device in nonarrested dogs with heart failure.[111] Clinically, the use of vest CPR depends on sophisticated equipment and remains experimental at this time.

Abdominal Binding

Abdominal binders and military antishock trousers have been used to augment closed-chest CPR. Both methods apply continuous compression circumferentially below the diaphragm. Three mechanisms have been proposed for augmentation of CPR by these binders. First, binding the abdomen decreases the compliance of the diaphragm and raises intrathoracic pressure. Second, blood may be moved out of the intrathoracic structures to increase circulating blood volume. Third, applying pressure to the subdiaphragmatic vasculature and increasing its resistance may increase suprathoracic blood flow. These effects increase aortic pressure and carotid blood flow in both animals and humans.[31,112] Unfortunately, as aortic pressure increases, the downstream component of CPP, namely, right atrial pressure, increases to an even greater extent, resulting in decreased CPP and myocardial blood flow.[28] These techniques also lower the cerebral perfusion pressure by enhanced transmission of intrathoracic pressure to the intracranial vault, which raises ICP (the downstream component of cerebral perfusion pressure). Clinical studies have failed to show an increased survival when an abdominal binder or military antishock trouser suit was used to augment CPR.

Open-Chest Cardiopulmonary Resuscitation

Use of open-chest cardiac massage has generally been replaced by closed-chest CPR. Compared with closed-chest CPR, open-chest CPR generates higher cardiac output and vital organ blood flow.[113] During open-chest CPR there is less elevation

of intrathoracic, right atrial, and intracranial pressure, resulting in higher coronary and cerebral perfusion pressure and higher myocardial and cerebral blood flow.[114]

Open-chest CPR is not a technique that can be applied by most health care personnel. It can be used in the operating room, ICU, or emergency department equipped with the necessary surgical and technical equipment and personnel. It is easily used in the operating room or ICU after cardiac surgery when the open chest can be easily accessed. Open-chest CPR is indicated for cardiac arrest resulting from cardiac tamponade, hypothermia, critical aortic stenosis, and ruptured aortic aneurysm. Other indications include cardiac arrest resulting from penetrating or crushed chest wall abnormalities that make closed-chest CPR impossible or ineffective.[115] Open-chest CPR is indicated for select patients when closed-chest CPR has failed, although exactly which patients should receive this method of resuscitation under this condition is controversial. When initiated early after failure of closed-chest CPR, open-chest CPR may improve outcome.[116] When performed after 15 minutes of closed-chest CPR, open-chest CPR significantly improves CPP and the rate of successful resuscitation.[117]

Cardiopulmonary Bypass

Because of the low rate of survival after prolonged CPR, more aggressive methods have been suggested to improve its success: cardiopulmonary bypass (CPB) and extracorporeal membrane oxygenation CPR (E-CPR).[118]

CPB is one of the most effective ways to restore circulation after cardiac arrest. Animal studies show that CPB increases survival at 72 hours, increases recovery of consciousness, and preserves the myocardium better than does conventional CPR.[119] In dogs, CPB resulted in better neurologic outcome than conventional CPR after a 4-minute ischemic period; however, neurologic outcome was dismal in both groups when the ischemic period lasted 12 minutes.[119] Some 90% of dogs survived 24 hours after 15 to 20 minutes of cardiac arrest, but only 10% survived when the arrest time was prolonged to 30 minutes when CPB was used for stabilization during defibrillation.[120] CPB decreased myocardial infarct size in a model involving coronary artery occlusion compared with conventional CPR.[121] In all animal models, CPB improves the success of resuscitation compared with conventional CPR.

Human experience with CPB for cardiac arrest outside the operating room is growing. In the first major series of pediatric patients undergoing E-CPR, reported by Morris et al., 64 children underwent 66 extracorporeal membrane oxygenation (ECMO) runs initiated during active resuscitation with chest compressions or internal cardiac massage.[122] Of these patients, 33 (50%) were decannulated and survived for more than 24 hours, 21 (33%) survived to hospital discharge, and 16 (26%) reportedly had no major changes in neurologic outcome. The average duration of CPR before cannulation in the survivors was 50 minutes. Of the six surviving children who required more than 60 minutes of CPR before ECMO, three had no apparent change in neurologic status. During the same period, 73 children underwent standard CPR; 10 received CPR for more than 30 minutes, with no survivors. Duncan et al. reported a series of 18 pediatric cardiac surgical patients at the Boston Children's Hospital who received ECMO during active chest compressions.[123] Of the first seven patients, only 29% survived. This led to the development of a rapid ECMO deployment strategy in which an ECMO pump is kept saline-primed in the ICU at all times, allowing initiation of extracorporeal support within 15 minutes. Precannulation support times dropped from an average of 90 minutes but still remained high at an average of 50 minutes. Of the remaining 11 patients, 10 were decannulated successfully, with 6 long-term survivors, 5 of whom were in New York Heart Association class I. This rapid deployment strategy likely will become more commonplace in large pediatric centers.

Many subsequent pediatric and adult studies have shown both the feasibility and varied success of E-CPR. Clear indications for its use include witnessed arrest in a biventricular circulation, and whereas contraindications include inability to provide effective CPR, there is uncertainty for the role of E-CPR in prolonged conventional resuscitation, because there are no guidelines on when to initiate it or which patient population it would be best suited for. This lack of criteria may explain the wide range of success of E-CPR, with survival ranging between 33% and 100%.[124]

Under the 2015 AHA guidelines, centers should consider ECMO CPR for in-hospital cardiac arrest refractory to standard resuscitation attempts if the condition leading to cardiac arrest is reversible or amenable to heart transplantation, if excellent conventional CPR has been performed after no more than several minutes of no-flow cardiac arrest, and if the institution is able to rapidly perform ECMO. Long-term survival has been reported even after more than 150 minutes of CPR in selected patients.[49]

Data are emerging involving the role of ECMO in persons with refractory ventricular fibrillation.[125] These data have solely been in the form of case reports but may represent a future direction for the care of patients with VF. In 2006, Samson et al. reported successful treatment of in-hospital VF in children with ECMO after cardiac arrest who had an initial rhythm of VF and immediate initiation of CPR.[126]

CPB and ECMO require a great deal of technical support and sophistication. In units with preprimed circuits on standby, CPB can be implemented quickly and with moderate success in a population of children who would otherwise almost certainly die. The success with some patients undergoing very long CPR times followed by ECMO use is encouraging and suggests the possibility of reversible myocardial injury as a cause of resuscitation failure in a subset of patients. Overall, ECMO is unlikely to have a major impact on pediatric outcome because of its limited availability.

Transcutaneous Cardiac Pacing

Transcutaneous cardiac pacing (TCP) is used as a method for noninvasive pacing of the ventricles for a relatively short period. Emergency cardiac pacing is successful in resuscitation only if it is initiated soon after the onset of arrest. In the absence of in situ pacing wires or an indwelling transvenous or esophageal pacing catheter, TCP is the preferred method for temporary electrical cardiac pacing. Since 1992, the AHA advanced cardiovascular life support (ACLS) guidelines have recommended the early use of an external pacemaker in patients with symptomatic bradycardia or asystole.[127]

Since Zoll established TCP in 1952 as a clinically useful method of pacing adult patients during ventricular standstill (Stokes-Adams attacks) and bradycardia-associated hypotension, numerous anecdotal reports have supported its use for bradycardic or asystolic arrests.[128] Zoll et al. reported successful in-hospital resuscitation of 12 of 16 patients with hypotensive bradycardia or asystole if TCP was initiated within 5 minutes of the arrest.[129] In contrast, if TCP was started between 5 and 30 minutes after the arrest, only 8 of 44 patients with either of these rhythms could be resuscitated.[129] In two controlled clinical trials of prehospital TCP, no differences in the survival rate or success of resuscitation were observed in paced and nonpaced patients who had asystole or PEA.[130,131] In patients with symptomatic bradycardia, TCP improved resuscitation and the survival rate.[132]

To date the efficacy of TCP in resuscitation of children has not been studied. Beland et al. showed that effective TCP could be achieved in hemodynamically stable children during induction of anesthesia for heart surgery.[133] They were successful in 53 of 56 pacing trials, and the patients experienced no complications.[131,133]

TCP is indicated for patients whose primary problem is impulse formation or conduction and who have preserved myocardial function. TCP is most effective in patients with sinus bradycardia or high-grade atrioventricular block with slow ventricular response who also have a stroke volume sufficient to generate a pulse. TCP is not indicated for patients in prolonged arrest because in this situation TCP usually results in electrical but not mechanical cardiac capture, and its use may delay or interfere with other resuscitative efforts.

To set up pacing, one electrode is placed anteriorly at the left sternal border and the other posteriorly just below the left scapula. Smaller electrodes are available for infants and children; adult-sized electrodes can be used in children weighing more than 15 kg.[133] Electrocardiographic leads should be connected to the pacemaker, the demand or asynchronous mode selected, and an age-appropriate heart rate used. The stimulus output should be set at zero when the pacemaker is turned on and then increased gradually until electrical capture is seen on the monitor. The output required for a hemodynamically unstable rhythm is higher than that for a stable rhythm in children in whom the mean stimulus required for capture was between 52 and 65 mA. After electrical capture is achieved, one must ascertain whether an effective arterial pulse is generated. If pulses are not adequate, other resuscitative efforts should be used.

The most serious complication of TCP is induction of a ventricular arrhythmia.[134] Fortunately, this complication is rare and may be prevented by pacing only in the demand mode. Mild transient erythema beneath the electrodes is common. Skeletal muscle contraction can be minimized by using large electrodes, a 40-ms pulse duration, and the smallest stimulus required for capture. Sedatives or analgesics may be necessary in the patient who is awake. If defibrillation or cardioversion is necessary, one must allow a distance of 2 to 3 cm between the electrode and paddles to prevent arcing of the current.

Pharmacology
Adrenergic Agonists

In 1963, only 3 years after the original description of closed-chest CPR, Pearson and Redding described the use of adrenergic agonists for resuscitation.[135] They subsequently showed that early administration of epinephrine in a canine model of cardiac arrest improved the success rate of CPR. They also demonstrated that the increase in aortic diastolic pressure by administration of α-adrenergic agonists was responsible for the improved success of resuscitation. They theorized that vasopressors such as epinephrine were of value because the drug increased peripheral vascular tone, not because of a direct effect on the heart.[136]

Yakaitis et al. investigated the relative importance of α- and β-adrenergic agonist actions during resuscitation.[137] Only 27% of dogs that received a pure β-adrenergic receptor agonist along with an α-adrenergic antagonist were resuscitated successfully, compared with all of the dogs that received a pure α-adrenergic agonist and a β-adrenergic antagonist (Fig. 41.12). Later studies reconfirmed this finding.[138] Michael et al. demonstrated that the α-adrenergic effects of epinephrine result in intense vasoconstriction of the resistance vessels of all organs of the body, except those supplying the heart and brain.[42] Because of the widespread vasoconstriction in nonvital organs, adequate perfusion pressure and thus blood flow to the heart and brain can be achieved despite the fact that cardiac output is very low during CPR (Fig. 41.13).[61]

The increase in aortic diastolic pressure associated with epinephrine administration during CPR is critical for maintaining coronary blood flow and enhancing the success of resuscitation. Even though the contractile state of the myocardium is increased by use of β-adrenergic agonists in the spontaneously beating heart, during CPR, β-adrenergic agonists actually may decrease myocardial blood flow by increasing intramyocardial wall pressure and vascular resistance. This decrease in myocardial blood flow could redistribute intramyocardial blood flow away from the subendocardium, increasing the likelihood of ischemic injury to this region.[139] Moreover, evidence indicates that left ventricular end-diastolic pressure (LVEDP) rises with epinephrine use, reducing the overall impact of the vasoconstrictor effects of epinephrine on CPP. Tang et al. showed elevated LVEDP and decreased measures of diastolic performance in epinephrine-resuscitated rats after induced VF compared with phenylephrine-resuscitated animals or epinephrine-resuscitated animals who

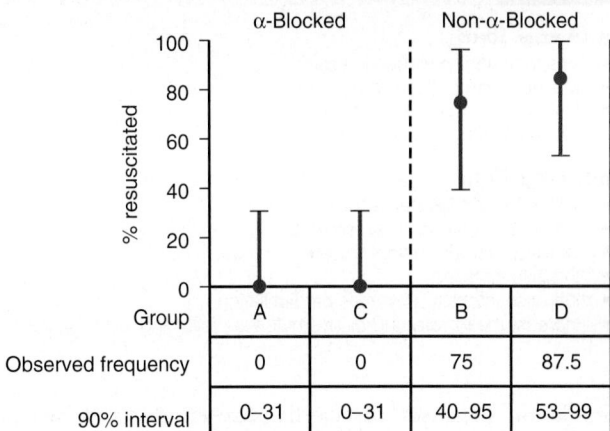

CARDIOPULMONARY RESUSCITATION

Fig. 41.12. Beneficial effect of α-adrenergic activity on resuscitation. Animals in group A received phenoxybenzamine; group B received propranolol; group C received phenoxybenzamine and propranolol; and group D received no drug. The 90% confidence intervals are reported for the sample size and observed resuscitation success. The lack of overlap between the α- and non–α-blocked groups indicates a significant benefit (p ≤.01) during resuscitation when α-adrenergic activity is intact. (From Yakaitis RW, Otto CW, Blitt CD. Relative importance of alpha and beta adrenergic receptors during resuscitation. Crit Care Med. 1979;7:293.)

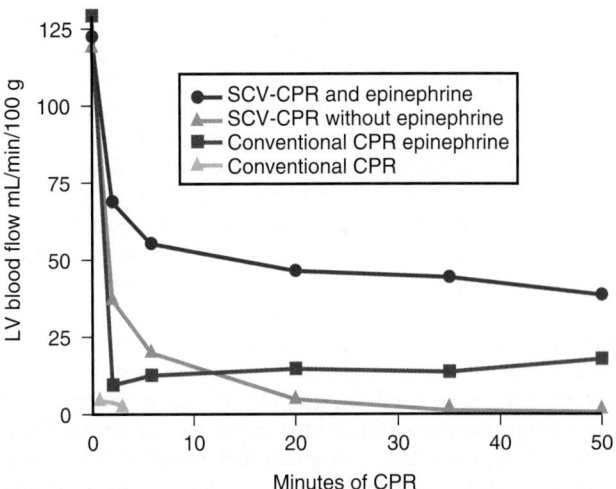

Fig. 41.13. Left ventricular (LV) blood flow before arrest and during four types of cardiopulmonary resuscitation (CPR). Note the rapid falloff of LV blood flow when epinephrine is not used. SCV-CPR, simultaneous compression ventilation CPR. (From Michael JR, Guerci AD, Koehler RC, et al. Mechanisms by which epinephrine augments cerebral and myocardial perfusion during cardiopulmonary resuscitation in dogs. Circulation. 1984;69:822.)

also received a β-blocker.[140] Similar data were found by McNamara, who used a rat pup model of asphyxial arrest.[141] LVEDP was increased and diastolic function indices decreased with epinephrine compared with either saline solution alone or epinephrine combined with verapamil. These data imply that excessive β-adrenergic effects prevent the intracellular calcium reuptake during diastole that is required for myocardial relaxation. By its inotropic and chronotropic effects, β-adrenergic

BOX 41.1 | α-Adrenergic vs. β-Adrenergic Agonist Effects

α-Adrenergic Effects
- Vasoconstrict peripheral vessels
- Maintain aortic diastolic pressure
- Improve coronary blood flow
- No metabolic stimulatory effect

β-Adrenergic Effects
- Vasodilate peripheral vessels
- Decrease aortic diastolic pressure
- Increase cellular metabolic rate
- Positive inotrope
- Increase intensity of ventricular fibrillation
- Increase heart rate and/or dysrhythmias following resuscitation

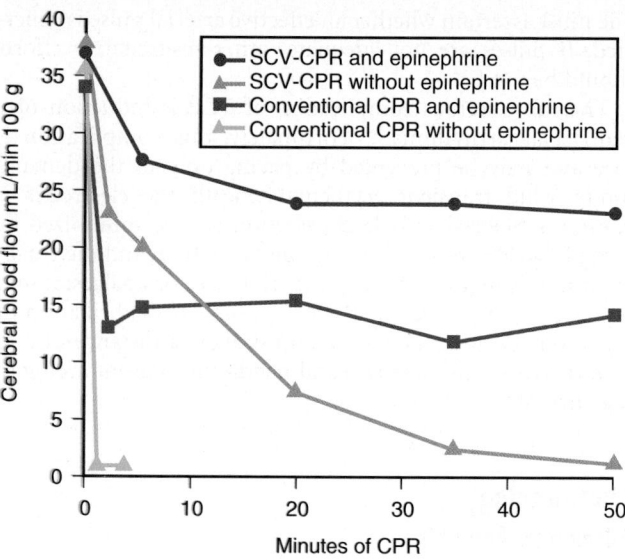

Fig. 41.14. Cerebral blood flow before arrest and during four types of 50 minutes of cardiopulmonary resuscitation (CPR). SCV-CPR, simultaneous compression ventilation CPR. (From Michael JR, Guerci AD, Koehler RC, et al. Mechanisms by which epinephrine augments cerebral and myocardial perfusion during cardiopulmonary resuscitation in dogs. Circulation. 1984;69:822.)

stimulation increases myocardial oxygen demand, which, when superimposed on low coronary blood flow, increases the risk of ischemic injury. This combination of increased oxygen demand by β-adrenergic agonists and decreased oxygen supply may damage an already ischemic heart, raising the question of whether a pure α-adrenergic agonist would be better than epinephrine, which has significant β-adrenergic effects (Box 41.1).[142] The effects on energy utilization and oxygen supply not only have implications for the success of the initial resuscitation but also for the postresuscitation function of the myocardium.

A number of studies have attempted to settle this controversy and actually have shown that pure α-adrenergic agonists can be used in place of epinephrine during CPR. Phenylephrine and methoxamine are two pure α-adrenergic agonists that have been used in animal models of CPR with success equal to that of epinephrine.[61,137,139] More recently, vasopressin has been studied as a noncatecholamine vasoconstrictor in the management of patients who experience cardiac arrest.[17] This agent is discussed in the section on vasopressin. These agents cause peripheral vasoconstriction and increase aortic diastolic pressure, resulting in improved myocardial and cerebral blood flow. This effect results in a higher oxygen supply/demand ratio in the ischemic heart and, at least, a theoretical advantage over the combined α- and β-adrenergic agonist effects of epinephrine. These agonists, as well as vasopressors such as vasopressin, have been used successfully for resuscitation.[17,136,143] These drugs maintain blood flow to the heart during CPR as well as epinephrine does. In an animal model of VF cardiac arrest, a resuscitation rate of 75% was reported for both epinephrine- and phenylephrine-treated groups. In this study, the ratio of endocardial to epicardial blood flow was lower in the group treated with epinephrine, suggesting the presence of subendocardial ischemia.[61] However, studies of this kind are difficult to interpret because of the inability to measure the degree of α-receptor activation by the different vasopressors. The higher subendocardial blood flow in the phenylephrine group may have been the result of less α-receptor activation.[144-146] Moreover, some investigators have questioned the merits of using a pure α-adrenergic agonist during CPR. Although the inotropic and chronotropic effects of β-adrenergic agonists may have deleterious hemodynamic effects during CPR administered for VF, increases in both heart rate and contractility increase cardiac output when spontaneous coordinated ventricular contractions are achieved.

Cerebral blood flow during CPR, like coronary blood flow, depends on peripheral vasoconstriction and is enhanced by

use of α-adrenergic agonists. This action produces selective vasoconstriction of noncerebral peripheral vessels to areas of the head and scalp without causing cerebral vasoconstriction.[61] As with myocardial blood flow, pure α-agonist agents are as effective as epinephrine in generating and sustaining cerebral blood flow during CPR in adult animal models and in infant models (Fig. 41.14).[61,143] No difference in neurologic deficits 24 hours after cardiac arrest was found between animals receiving either epinephrine or phenylephrine during CPR.[147]

Analogous to the heart, β-adrenergic agonists could increase cerebral oxygen uptake if a sufficient amount of drug crosses the blood-brain barrier during or after resuscitation. In addition, adrenergic agonists may vasoconstrict or dilate cerebral vessels, depending on the balance between α- and β-adrenergic receptors. Epinephrine and phenylephrine had similar effects on cerebral blood flow and metabolism, maintaining normal cerebral oxygen uptake for 20 minutes of CPR in dogs. This finding implies that cerebral blood flow was high enough to maintain adequate cerebral metabolism and that β-receptor stimulation did not increase cerebral oxygen uptake, despite the fact that the combined effects of brain ischemia and CPR can increase the permeability of the blood-brain barrier to drugs used during CPR or when enzymatic barriers to vasopressors (eg, by monoamine oxidase) are overwhelmed during tissue hypoxia. Mechanical disruption of the barrier could occur during chest compressions by large fluctuations in cerebral venous and arterial pressures or as a result of hyperemia, the large increase in cerebral blood flow that occurs during the early reperfusion period when the cerebral vascular bed is maximally dilated following resuscitation, particularly if systemic hypertension occurs.[148] No blood-brain barrier permeability changes during CPR immediately after resuscitation or 4 hours after resuscitation were found in adult dogs.[148] However, after 8 minutes of cardiac arrest and 6 minutes of

CPR in piglets, the blood-brain barrier was permeable to the small neutral amino acid α-aminoisobutyric acid 4 hours after cardiac arrest (Fig. 41.15).[149,150] The increase in permeability could be prevented by pre-arrest administration of conjugated superoxide dismutase and catalase, indicating a role of oxygen free radicals in the pathogenesis of this injury to the blood-brain barrier (Fig. 41.16).[151] These endothelial membrane changes frequently were associated with the presence of intravascular polymorphonuclear and monocytic leukocytes.[152] Whether leukocytes disrupt the blood-brain barrier by release of toxic substances, such as oxygen free radicals or proteases, or appear in the post-ischemic microvessels as an epiphenomenon of a more important derangement is unknown (Fig. 41.17).

Vasopressin

The role of vasopressin as a noncatecholamine vasoconstrictor in the management of patients who experience cardiac arrest has received a great deal of interest. Work by Lindner in Europe and Landry in the United States during the past 2 decades had established sufficient evidence of efficacy for its use to be included in the 2010 AHA Guidelines for Cardiopulmonary Resuscitation and Emergency Cardiovascular Care.[118,153] However, subsequent adult studies comparing standard dose epinephrine with vasopressin alone or in combination with standard dose epinephrine have showed that vasopressin offered no advantage in return of spontaneous circulation or survival to discharge,[154] and it has subsequently been removed from the 2015 AHA guidelines. However,

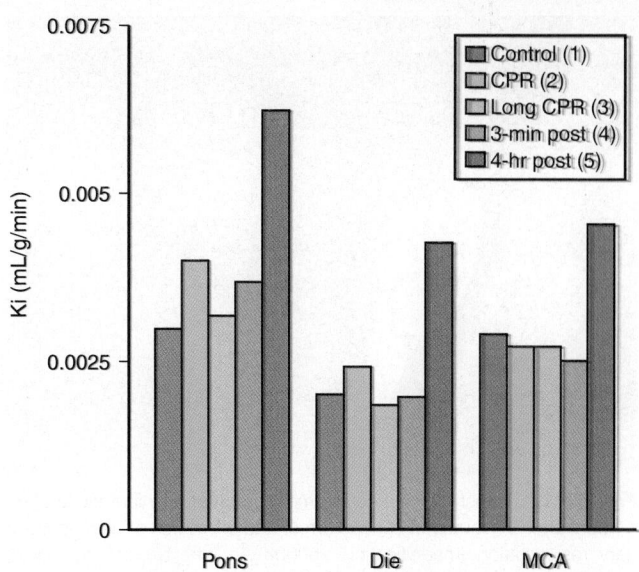

Fig. 41.15. Transfer coefficient *(Kᵢ)* of α-aminoisobutyric acid for pons, diencephalon *(DIE)*, and middle cerebral *(MCA)* artery regions. Control group; 8 minutes ischemia and 10 minutes cardiopulmonary resuscitation *(CPR)*; 8 minutes ischemia and 40 minutes cardiopulmonary resuscitation; 3 minutes after resuscitation; 4 hours after resuscitation. Group 5 in each region *p <.05, different from group 1 by one-way analysis of variance and Dunnett test for all three regions. (From Schleien CL, Koehler RC, Schaffner DH, et al. Blood-brain barrier disruption after cardiopulmonary resuscitation in immature swine. Stroke. 1991;22:477.)

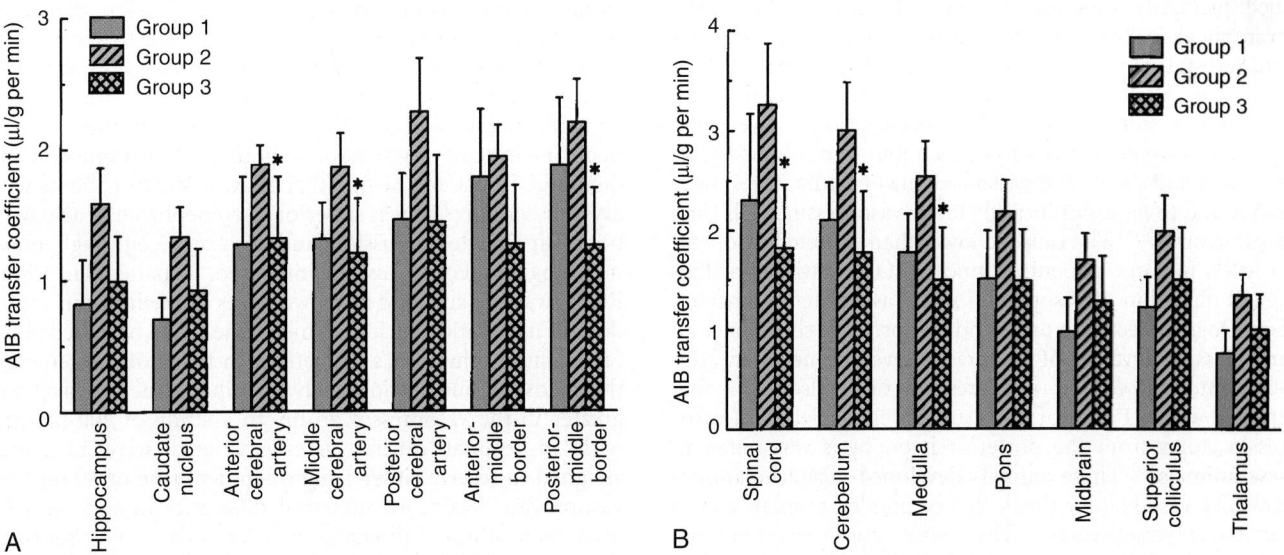

Fig. 41.16. (A) Bar graph showing transfer coefficient of α-aminoisobutyric acid *(AIB)* from plasma to brain in hippocampus, caudate nucleus, and primary supply and border regions of cerebral arteries in nonischemic time controls (group 1; *n* = 5), ischemia group treated with polyethylene glycol *(PEG)* (group 2; *n* = 8), and ischemia group treated with PEG-superoxide dismutase and PEG-catalase (group 3; *n* = 8). Error bars represent standard error of the mean *(SEM)*. *p <.05 between groups 2 and 3 by Mann-Whitney U test. (B) Transfer coefficient of AIB from plasma to brain in caudal brain regions in nonischemic time controls (group 1; *n* = 5), ischemia group treated with PEG (group 2; *n* = 8), and ischemia group treated with PEG-superoxide dismutase and PEG-catalase (group 3; *n* = 8). Error bars represent SEM. *p <.05 between groups 2 and 3 by Mann-Whitney U test. (From Schleien CL, Eberle B, Schaffner DH, et al. Reduced blood-brain barrier permeability after cardiac arrest by conjugated superoxide dismutase and catalase in piglets. Stroke. 1994;25:1830.)

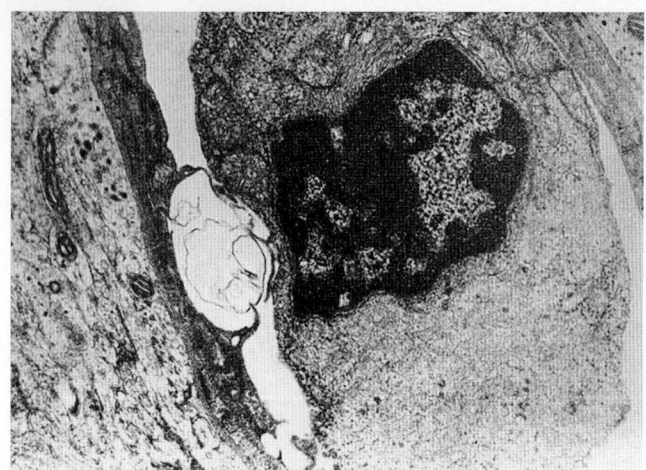

Fig. 41.17. Transmission electron micrograph of an infant piglet brain 4 hours after 8 minutes of cardiac arrest and 6 minutes of cardiopulmonary resuscitation (magnification ×5000). An intravascular leukocyte, which has the morphologic features of a monocyte, is adherent to the endothelial surface of a venule and appears to be occluding the lumen. The luminal surface of the endothelial cell contains membrane blebs and discontinuities. (From Caceres MJ, Schleien CL, Kuluz JW, et al. Early endothelial damage and leukocyte accumulation in piglet brains following cardiac arrest. Acta Neuropathol. 1995;90:582.)

increasing evidence indicates that vasopressin is a useful agent in the management of shock of multiple etiologies and therefore may have a role in postresuscitation management of the arrest victim.

Arginine vasopressin is a short peptide hormone secreted by the posterior pituitary gland in response to changes in tonicity and changes in effective intravascular volume, signaled primarily via baroreceptor unloading in the aorta. Severe shock is the most potent stimulus to vasopressin secretion. Serum levels 20- to 200-fold higher than normal may be found immediately after cardiac arrest, as well as in other severe shock states. Despite these observations, lower than expected vasopressin levels have been found in some patients with profound shock, and patients dying of cardiac arrest have been found to have significantly lower vasopressin levels than do survivors.[155-159] The cause of lower than expected vasopressin levels in some patients is unclear. Observations in dogs suggest depletion of vasopressin stores as a potential mechanism. Dogs subjected to profound hemorrhagic shock have an early massive elevation of vasopressin levels immediately after the event, followed by a depression of levels below that expected within 1 hour of the insult. Severe depletion of vasopressin stores from the posterior hypophysis was noted in these animals.[160] These animals developed a catecholamine-refractory vasodilatory shock that responded dramatically to low doses of vasopressin.[161] These observations have led to an exploration of the use of vasopressin in both cardiac arrest and shock states.

Vasopressin is an extremely potent vasoconstrictor. Its effects on vascular tone are primarily mediated through interaction with a specific G protein–coupled receptor referred to as the $V1_a$ receptor, which is distributed widely throughout vascular beds.[159] Of note, the $V1_a$ receptor is linked to the same second messenger system as the α-adrenergic receptor that mediates vasoconstriction through an alteration of intracellular calcium levels. However, in the pulmonary circulation, vasopressin activation of V1 receptors mediates the release of nitric oxide and causes pulmonary vasodilation. Vasopressin also interacts with its V_2 receptor, which regulates aquaporin expression on the renal collecting duct epithelium. Stimulation of the V_2 receptor occurs at substantially lower levels than those required to activate the $V1_a$ receptor.

Vasopressin use during resuscitation has been studied in animals and humans. In an adult porcine model of VF, vasopressin at a dose of 0.8 µg/kg was found to be superior to the maximally effective dose of epinephrine 200 µg/kg in restoring left ventricular myocardial blood flow, increasing diastolic CPP and total cerebral blood flow, as well as rates of ROSC.[141] Moreover, the duration of the effect was sustained for 4 minutes compared with 1.5 minutes for epinephrine.[17] Adverse effects noted in the postresuscitation phase included decreased renal and adrenal blood flow and reduced cardiac output.[162,163]

In a pediatric porcine model of cardiac arrest, vasopressin at a dose of 0.8 µg/kg was not as effective as epinephrine, 200 µg/kg, in restoring LV myocardial blood flow or achieving ROSC.[164] Only one of six animals achieved ROSC compared with six of six in the epinephrine group. A combination group that received both epinephrine, 45 µg/kg, and vasopressin, 0.8 µg/kg, fared better (ROSC in four of six animals). Possible explanations for the difference between adult and juvenile animals include different dose-response curves for the two drugs, failure of maturation of vasopressin receptors, a different distribution of vasopressin receptors than seen in adults, or the different experimental model.

In an initial small randomized clinical trial of vasopressin compared with epinephrine for refractory VF, the rate of achieving ROSC was higher in the vasopressin group.[165] These findings led to the inclusion of vasopressin in the adult guidelines. A large multicenter randomized trial of vasopressin for cardiac arrest in adults has been reported.[166] More than 1200 patients were randomly assigned in the field to receive two doses of either 40 international units (IU) of vasopressin or 1 mg of epinephrine followed by additional treatment with epinephrine, if necessary. Vasopressin was equivalent to epinephrine in achieving survival to both hospital admission and discharge in patients with either PEA or VF. In patients with asystole, vasopressin was superior to epinephrine in achieving both survival to admission and discharge, although intact neurologic outcome was not improved. In patients in whom ROSC was not achieved after two doses of medication, a third dose of medication such as epinephrine could be added at the resuscitating physician's discretion. In the group receiving a third dose of medication such as epinephrine, survival was greater in the vasopressin group. In a study of 200 patients with in-hospital cardiac arrest, patients were randomly assigned to receive either 1 mg of epinephrine or 40 units of vasopressin. Again, no statistical difference in survival to 1 hour or to hospital discharge was found between groups or subgroups.[167] The results of these studies led to the classification of evidence for vasopressin for use in adults as indeterminate in the 2010 AHA guidelines.[118] Subsequently, a meta-analysis of 10 randomized trials including a total of 6120 adult patients showed that the use of vasopressin was neither beneficial nor harmful in an unselected patient population in terms of ROSC, survival to hospital admission, survival to discharge, or favorable neurologic outcome. However, chance of ROSC was significantly higher in in-hospital cardiac arrest patients when vasopressin was used.[168] The published experience with vasopressin in children who experience cardiac arrest is limited. The first case series of vasopressin use in CPR reported the outcome of four children with six prolonged refractory cardiac arrests that were unresponsive to standard resuscitation efforts.[169] Each child received one or more bolus doses of vasopressin (0.4 µg/kg) as rescue therapy. In all children, the initial rhythm was a form of PEA that deteriorated to asystole in four of six events. Three children had ROSC for more than 60 minutes, including one child with asystole. Two children survived for more than 24 hours and one survived to hospital discharge. A second retrospective case series of pediatric cardiac arrests unresponsive to epinephrine found that ROSC was achieved in 6 of 8 episodes that were treated with terlipressin, a long-acting synthetic analog of vasopressin, at a dose of 15 to 20 µg/kg. Four of those patients survived without neurologic sequelae.[170] A review of a national registry of in-hospital CPR showed that patients who received vasopressin had a lower incidence of ROSC greater than 20 minutes (22 [34%] of 64) than patients who did not receive the medication (675 [55%] of 1229).[171] The association of poor outcome with vasopressin persisted even with multivariate analysis with logistic regression to attempt to control for other factors that might affect ROSC. The effect of vasopressin in pediatric arrest that was refractory to an initial epinephrine dose was evaluated in a pilot study. Patients were given vasopressin after an initial dose of epinephrine and were compared with a retrospective matched cohort of patients who experienced cardiopulmonary arrest that required greater than two doses of a vasopressor, not including vasopressin. Ten patients were enrolled, and although there was an increased 24-hour survival, there was no difference in ROSC, survival to hospital discharge, or favorable neurologic status at discharge.[172]

The current evidence only examines the use of vasopressin as a potential alternative when standard therapies, such as epinephrine, fail to cause ROSC. Unfortunately, variables such as dosing, timing of vasopressin infusion, or pediatric risk of mortality scores have not been controlled for in these studies. No double-blinded, randomized controlled studies have been performed, and thus no firm recommendations are available concerning the use of vasopressin for CPR in infants and children.

The current recommended dose of vasopressin for adults in cardiac arrest is 40 IU. No data comparing this dose to other doses are available, and concern exists regarding postresuscitation complications related to this dose. We have selected 0.5 µg/kg as the standard for cardiac arrest. Further data are necessary before more definitive dosing recommendations can be made.

Use of vasopressin in postresuscitation management may be considered. A relative vasopressin deficiency has been noted in a number of shock states, including hemorrhage, sepsis, and post-CPB, as well as in patients who have unsuccessful resuscitations. In these settings, shock may be refractory to catecholamines (norepinephrine doses of 2 to 4 µg/kg). These patients may respond to a vasopressin infusion, allowing the weaning of high-dose catecholamines. Although a role in the postresuscitation setting has not been demonstrated on the basis of the data related to refractory shock, consideration of the use of vasopressin for refractory hypotension may be appropriate.

Additionally, the additive effects of combination drug therapy for adults with cardiac arrest may be most beneficial. In a recent randomized, double-blind placebo control study investigating vasopressin plus epinephrine or saline placebo plus epinephrine with/without methylprednisolone, the group receiving combination therapy with vasopressin-epinephrine-methylprednisolone with CPR resulted in improved survival to hospital discharge with improved neurologic status.[173,174]

High-Dose Epinephrine

The physiologic responses of animals and humans to higher doses of epinephrine include higher cerebral blood flow, increased myocardial and submyocardial blood flow, improved oxygen delivery relative to oxygen consumption, and less depletion of myocardial adenosine triphosphate (ATP) stores with more rapid repletion of phosphocreatine.[145,175-179] Contrary results, with increased myocardial oxygen consumption and decreased myocardial blood flow, have been demonstrated during CPR following VF cardiac arrest.[40,43] In a piglet model, high-dose epinephrine (HDE) produced lower myocardial blood flow than achieved with standard-dose epinephrine (SDE).[171] In neonatal lambs following asphyxia-induced bradycardia, HDE resulted in higher heart rate but a lower stroke volume and cardiac output.[180]

Studies regarding survival of patients who were given HDE have been contradictory. In out-of-hospital patients who experienced cardiac arrest, HDE produced higher aortic diastolic pressure during CPR and increased the rate of ROSC compared with standard doses of epinephrine. Gonzalez et al. demonstrated a dose-dependent increase in aortic blood pressure by epinephrine in patients who failed to respond to prolonged resuscitative efforts.[181,182] Paradis et al.[183] showed that HDE increased aortic diastolic pressure and improved the rate of successful resuscitation in patients in whom ACLS protocols had failed. This group also reported on a series of 20 children treated with HDE and compared them with 20 historic control subjects consisting of children with cardiac arrest treated with SDE.[184] They reported that 14 of the children in the HDE group had ROSC, 8 survived to hospital discharge, and 3 were neurologically intact. There were no survivors in the SDE comparison group. Other centers have claimed that higher-than-standard doses of epinephrine during CPR in children improve the hemodynamics and increase the success of CPR; however, no one has provided any valid data that suggest that HDE improves survival beyond the immediate postresuscitation period.[94,183,185,186] On the basis of these studies, the 1992 AHA guidelines for pediatric advanced life support recommended HDE if an initial SDE failed to resuscitate the child.

Three large multicenter studies subsequently were published that dampened enthusiasm for the use of HDE. Stiell et al. studied 650 adult patients after cardiac arrests who were randomly assigned to receive either an SDE or HDE (7 mg) epinephrine protocol.[187] No differences were observed between the groups with regard to 1-hour survival (23% vs. 18%), rate of hospital discharge (5% vs. 3%), or neurologic outcome. Brown et al.[23] reported on 1280 adult patients who received either SDE (0.02 mg/kg) or HDE (0.2 mg/kg) after cardiac arrest. Again, no differences in ROSC, short-term survival, survival to hospital discharge, or neurologic outcome were observed between the two groups of patients. In a study of 816 adults, Callaham et al. reported a higher ROSC in the HDE group.[188] However, there were no differences in the rate of hospital discharge or ultimate survival of these patients. In addition to these studies, a specific pediatric animal study was published that failed to demonstrate a clear survival benefit for HDE, although the occurrence of ROSC appeared to be greater.[43] The 2000 AHA guidelines changed the recommendation for HDE to an option for second and subsequent doses of epinephrine.

More recently, a prospective, randomized, double-blind clinical trial of HDE in 68 pediatric inpatients was reported by Perondi et al.[14] ROSC for more than 20 minutes was achieved in 15 of 34 patients who received HDE but in only 8 of 34 patients who received SDE (p = .07). However, survival to 24 hours occurred in only two of the HDE group versus seven of the SDE group (p = .05). In the group that experienced an asphyxial arrest, none of 12 treated with HDE was alive at 24 hours, whereas 7 of 18 patients in the SDE group survived. Four survived to hospital discharge, and two patients were neurologically normal.[14] This trial reinforces concerns that HDE may account for some of the adverse effects that occur after resuscitation and is the basis of the 2015 AHA guidelines' recommendation against the use of HDE during CPR.[150,189,190] As discussed previously, epinephrine can worsen myocardial ischemic injury secondary to increased oxygen demand and result in tachyarrhythmias, hypertension, pulmonary edema, hypoxemia, and cardiac arrest.[150,191] Use of a β-adrenergic antagonist during or after ROSC has been suggested to attenuate the adverse effects of epinephrine.[76,105,192] Epinephrine causes hypoxemia and an increase in alveolar dead space ventilation by redistributing pulmonary blood flow.[193,194] In one study, HDE (>15 mg) given to adults during CPR resulted in a lower cardiac index, systemic oxygen consumption, and oxygen delivery immediately after resuscitation.[180] A meta-analysis of epinephrine use in adult cardiac arrest showed no difference in survival to discharge or neurologic outcome when using high dose over standard dose.[195] Prolonged peripheral vasoconstriction by excessive doses of epinephrine may delay or impair reperfusion of systemic organs, particularly the kidneys and gastrointestinal tract.

Atropine

Atropine, a parasympatholytic agent, acts by blocking cholinergic stimulation of the muscarinic receptors of the heart, which usually results in an increase in the sinus rate and shortening of the atrioventricular node conduction time. Atropine may activate latent ectopic pacemakers. Atropine has little effect on systemic vascular resistance, myocardial perfusion pressure, or contractility.[177]

Atropine is indicated for treatment of asystole, PEA, bradycardia associated with hypotension, second- and third-degree heart block, and slow idioventricular rhythms. In children who present in cardiac arrest, sinus bradycardia and asystole are the most common initial rhythms, which make atropine useful as a first-line drug. Atropine is particularly effective in clinical conditions associated with excessive parasympathetic tone.

The recommended dose of atropine is 0.02 mg/kg, with a minimum dose of 0.15 mg and a maximum dose of 2.0 mg. Smaller doses than 0.15 mg, even in small infants, may result paradoxically in bradycardia because of a central stimulatory effect on the medullary vagal nuclei by a dose that is too low to provide anticholinergic effects on the heart. Atropine may be given by any route, including IV, endotracheal, interosseous, IM, and subcutaneous. Its onset of action occurs within 30 seconds, and its peak effect occurs between 1 and 2 minutes after an IV dose. The recommended adult dose is 0.5 mg every 5 minutes until the desired heart rate is obtained up to a maximum of 2 mg. For asystole, 1 mg is given intravenously and repeated every 5 minutes if asystole persists. Full vagal blockade usually is obtained with a dose of 2 mg in adults.

Because of its parasympatholytic effects, atropine should not be used in patients in whom tachycardia is undesirable. In patients after myocardial infarction or ischemia with persistent bradycardia, atropine should be used in the lowest dose possible to increase heart rate. Using the lowest possible dose will limit tachycardia, a potent contributor to increased myocardial oxygen consumption, which could lead to VF. In addition, atropine should not be used in patients with pulmonary or systemic outflow tract obstruction or idiopathic hypertrophic subaortic stenosis because tachycardia decreases ventricular filling and lowers cardiac output in this setting.

Sodium Bicarbonate

The administration of sodium bicarbonate results in an acid-base reaction in which bicarbonate combines with hydrogen to form carbonic acid, which dissociates into water and carbon dioxide. Because of the generation of carbon dioxide, adequate alveolar ventilation must be present to achieve the normal buffering action of bicarbonate. Use of sodium bicarbonate during CPR remains controversial because of its potential adverse effects and the lack of evidence showing any benefit from its use during CPR.[196,197]

Sodium bicarbonate is indicated for correction of significant metabolic acidosis, especially when signs of cardiovascular compromise are present. Acidosis itself may have a number of negative effects on the circulation, including depression of myocardial function by prolonging diastolic depolarization, depressing spontaneous cardiac activity, decreasing the electrical threshold for VF, decreasing the inotropic state of the myocardium, and reducing the cardiac response to catecholamines. Acidosis also decreases systemic vascular resistance and attenuates the vasoconstrictive response of peripheral vessels to catecholamines. This effect is contrary to the desired effect during CPR. In addition, particularly in patients with a reactive pulmonary vascular bed, pulmonary vascular resistance is inversely related to pH. Rudolph and Yuan observed a twofold increase in pulmonary vascular resistance in calves when pH was lowered from 7.4 to 7.2 under normoxic conditions.[198] Therefore correction of even mild acidosis may be helpful in resuscitating patients who have the potential for increased right-to-left shunting through a cardiac septal defect, patent ductus arteriosus, or aortic-to-pulmonary shunt during periods of elevated pulmonary vascular resistance.

Multiple adverse effects of bicarbonate administration include metabolic alkalosis, hypercapnia, hypernatremia, and hyperosmolality. All of these adverse effects are associated with a high mortality rate. Alkalosis causes a leftward shift of the oxyhemoglobin dissociation curve, thus impairing release of oxygen from hemoglobin to tissues at a time when oxygen delivery already may be low. Alkalosis can result in hypokalemia, by enhancing potassium influx into cells, and ionic hypocalcemia, by increasing protein binding of ionized calcium. Hypernatremia and hyperosmolality may decrease tissue perfusion by increasing interstitial edema in microvascular beds.

The marked hypercapnic acidosis that occurs during CPR on the venous side of the circulation, including the coronary sinus, may be worsened by administration of bicarbonate.[199,200] Myocardial acidosis during cardiac arrest is associated with decreased myocardial contractility. The mean venoarterial P_{CO_2} difference was 24 ± 15 mm Hg in five patients during CPR and actually increased from 16 to 69 mm Hg in one patient after administration of bicarbonate.[201] Another group showed a mean difference of 42 mm Hg between partial pressure of carbon dioxide in mixed venous blood (Pv_{CO_2}) and Pa_{CO_2} during CPR. Paradoxical intracellular acidosis after bicarbonate administration is possible because of rapid entry of carbon dioxide into cells with a slow egress of hydrogen ion out of cells. Paradoxical intracellular acidosis in the central nervous system after bicarbonate administration has been proposed but not definitively shown. In neonatal rabbits recovering from hypoxic acidosis, bicarbonate administration increased both arterial pH and intracellular brain pH as measured by nuclear magnetic resonance spectroscopy.[202] In another study, intracellular brain ATP concentration in rats did not change during severe intracellular acidosis in the brain produced by extreme hypercapnia.[203] The rats who maintained ATP concentration even in the face of severe brain acidosis had no functional or histologic differences from normal control subjects. Using nuclear magnetic resonance spectroscopy of the brain in dogs during cardiac arrest and CPR, intracellular brain pH decreased to 6.29 with total depletion of brain ATP after 6 minutes of cardiac arrest. However, following effective CPR, ATP levels rose to 86% of pre-arrest levels and to normal by 35 minutes of CPR despite ongoing peripheral arterial acidosis (Fig. 41.18).[110] However, cerebral pH decreased in parallel with blood pH when CPR was started immediately after arrest. Bicarbonate administration ameliorated and did not worsen the cerebral acidosis, indicating that the blood-brain pH gradient is maintained during CPR.[204]

The 2015 AHA guidelines state that sodium bicarbonate has not been shown to improve outcome during CPR and only recommends its use in special situations, such as intoxications.[118] A Cochrane study looking at the use of empirical sodium bicarbonate administration versus placebo in out-of-hospital cardiac arrests in 874 adults found no difference in survival to the hospital.[205] Levy reviewed more than 30 animal studies evaluating the efficacy of sodium bicarbonate administration during CPR.[206] Among studies with survival as the primary outcome, four showed benefit and seven did not. When assessing myocardial performance, 12 studies concluded that sodium bicarbonate worsened performance, 2 studies showed no difference, and no study showed benefit. When reviewing 19 retrospective human adult studies examining mortality rates, 8 of these suggested a deleterious effect of sodium bicarbonate, 11 showed no difference in outcomes, and none showed benefit.[206]

In a large retrospective study of pediatric patients with in-hospital cardiac arrest, it was found that survivors were less likely to receive sodium bicarbonate than nonsurvivors. However, nonsurvivors were also observed to have a longer CPR duration, as well as more doses of calcium, vasopressin, and epinephrine.[9] A subsequent retrospective study by Raymond et al.[207] examined sodium bicarbonate use after the institution of the 2010 AHA guidelines. While they found that sodium bicarbonate use for in-hospital cardiac arrest had been decreasing, its use was still associated with decreased

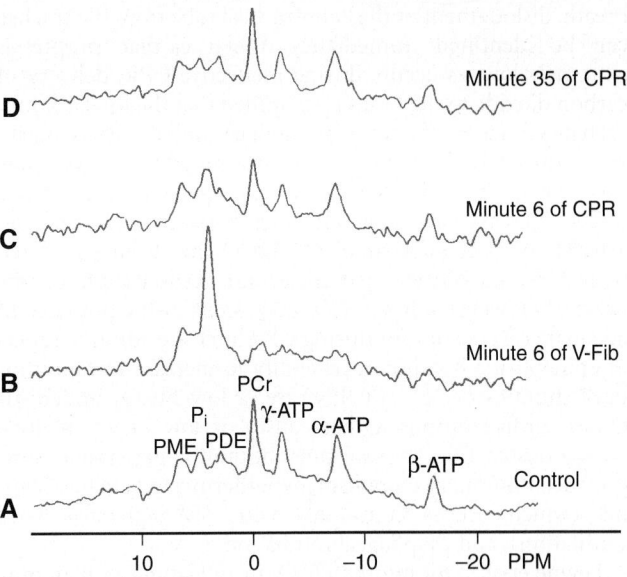

Fig. 41.18. [31]P magnetic resonance spectroscopy spectra from in situ dog brain during vest cardiopulmonary resuscitation *(CPR)* after a 6-minute delay in the onset of CPR from time of arrest. Each spectrum was acquired in 1 minute. The frequency of the inorganic phosphate *(P_i)* peak is pH dependent. Note complete absence of adenosine triphosphate *(ATP)* and phosphocreatine *(PCr)* and pH_i = 6.28 in *trace B* after 6 minutes of ventricular fibrillation *(v-fib)* without CPR. After 6 minutes of CPR *(trace C)*, ATP is more than 85% recovered, but pH is only 6.61. After 35 minutes of CPR *(trace D)*, pH_i has returned to 7. *PDE*, phosphodiesters; *PME*, phosphomonoesters; *PPM*, parts per million. (From Eleff SM, Schleien CL, Koehler RC, et al. Brain bioenergetics during cardiopulmonary resuscitation in dogs. Anesthesiology. 1992;76:77.)

survival at 24 hours and hospital discharge when given outside current pediatric advanced life support recommendations.[207]

When Pa_{CO_2} and pH are known, the dose of bicarbonate to correct the pH to 7.4 is calculated using the following equation:

$$\text{Sodium bicarbonate (mEq)} = 0.3 \times \text{weight (kg)} \times \text{Base deficit}$$

Eq. 41.1

(Because of its possible adverse effects and the large venous to arterial carbon dioxide gradient that develops during CPR, we recommend giving half the dose that would be given based on a volume of distribution of 0.6.) If blood gases are not available, the initial dose is 1 mEq/kg, followed by 0.5 mEq/kg every 10 minutes of ongoing arrest. Alveolar ventilation must be maintained because of the generation of carbon dioxide and can be assessed only by serial measurements of arterial blood gases and pH. Because of the potential adverse effects of bicarbonate, the indications for its use at this time are limited to cardiac arrest associated with hyperkalemia, patients with preexisting metabolic acidosis, and after approximately 10 minutes of CPR.

$EtCO_2$ monitoring is useful during CPR because it provides important information regarding both pulmonary and cardiac function. $EtCO_2$ is measured instantaneously in the exhaled gas of every breath. In the absence of lung disease, $EtCO_2$ correlates closely with Pa_{CO_2} provided pulmonary blood flow is at least 20% to 25% of normal. As a respiratory monitor, $EtCO_2$ analyzers accurately distinguish a tracheal ($EtCO_2$ >10) from an esophageal ($EtCO_2$ <5) intubation in infants and children.[208-213] Because measurements are made with every breath, dislodgment of the endotracheal tube from the trachea can be identified immediately. When cardiac output is extremely low, as occurs during ineffective CPR, delivery of carbon dioxide to the lungs is so limited that the total amount exchanged across the alveolar-capillary membrane is markedly reduced. In this situation, the measured $EtCO_2$ is very low even when $PaCO_2$ is elevated. As cardiac output increases, $EtCO_2$ increases and the difference between end-tidal and arterial CO_2 becomes smaller.[214] $EtCO_2$ has been correlated with CPP, the critical parameter for resuscitation of the heart.[214] However, a low $EtCO_2$ may occur in the presence of adequate cardiac output during CPR after the administration of epinephrine because of its ability to increase intrapulmonary shunting.[185,193,215] In this case, a low $EtCO_2$ underestimates cardiac output. Other causes of low $EtCO_2$ include airway obstruction, tension pneumothorax, pericardial tamponade, pulmonary embolism, hypothermia, severe hypocapnia (which occurs commonly with overaggressive hand ventilation), and esophageal intubation.

Levine et al.[211] monitored $EtCO_2$ in 150 adults with an out-of-hospital cardiac arrest who had electrical activity but no pulse.[216] They found that after 20 minutes of ACLS, an $EtCO_2$ level of 10 mm Hg or less successfully predicted survival to hospital admission with a sensitivity, specificity, and positive- and negative-predictive value of 100%. Grmec and Klemen prospectively studied the initial, average, maximal, minimal, and final $EtCO_2$ as a prognostic indicator for outcomes in adult resuscitation.[217] They found that using an initial, average, and final $EtCO_2$ level of 10 mm Hg identified 100% of patients who were successfully resuscitated, with specificity of 74%, 90%, and 81%, respectively.[217]

The 2015 AHA guidelines state that while use of $EtCO_2$ as an indicator of cardiac output may be useful in adults (evidence class IIb), currently no studies have evaluated the use of $EtCO_2$ in pediatric arrests.[118] There have been no human trials studying whether titrating resuscitation efforts to a specific number can affect clinical outcomes. In a piglet model of CPR, it was found that CPR guided by a target $EtCO_2$ was as effective as CPR guided by depth monitor, video monitor, and verbal feedback. Whereas no specific value has yet to be established, given the noninvasive nature of $EtCO_2$ monitoring and also extrapolating from adult data,[218] maintaining an $EtCO_2$ of greater than 10 to 15 mm Hg through the use of $EtCO_2$ monitoring is recommended during pediatric arrests.[153]

Other Alkalinizing Agents

A number of other alkalinizing agents have been used experimentally in animals and humans. However, none has demonstrated any real advantages over sodium bicarbonate. Carbicarb, a solution of equimolar amounts of sodium bicarbonate and sodium carbonate, corrects metabolic acidosis without many of the adverse effects of sodium bicarbonate.[74] The buffering action of sodium carbonate occurs by consumption of carbon dioxide with generation of bicarbonate ion, as illustrated in the following equation:

$$Na_2CO_3 + CO_2 + H_2O = 2\,HCO_3^- + 2Na^+ \qquad \text{Eq. 41.2}$$

During CPR, Carbicarb administration resulted in a greater increase in arterial pH and smaller increases in $PaCO_2$, lactate, and serum osmolality in animals.[74,219,220] However, Carbicarb was not superior to sodium bicarbonate when used for hypovolemic shock in rats.[221]

Dichloroacetate (DCA) increases the activity of pyruvate dehydrogenase, which facilitates the conversion of lactate to pyruvate.[222] When administered to patients with lactic acidosis, DCA decreased lactate concentration by half and increased bicarbonate concentration and pH.[223] In other studies, DCA improved cardiac output, possibly by increasing myocardial metabolism of lactate and carbohydrate.[224,225] In a multicenter trial of patients with lactic acidosis, DCA did not improve outcome when compared with sodium bicarbonate.[226]

Tromethamine (THAM; tris-hydroxymethyl-aminomethane) is an organic amine that combines with a hydrogen ion, causing CO_2 and H_2O to combine to form bicarbonate and a hydrogen ion. A dose of 3 mL/kg should raise the bicarbonate concentration by 3 mEq/L. Adverse effects of THAM include hyperkalemia, hypoglycemia, and acute hypocarbia resulting in apnea. In addition, peripheral vasodilation may occur after administration of THAM during CPR, which is an undesirable effect. THAM is contraindicated in patients with renal failure.

Calcium

Recommendations for use of calcium in CPR are restricted to a few specific situations, namely, hypocalcemia, hyperkalemia, hypermagnesemia, and calcium channel blocker overdose. These restrictions are based on the possibility that exogenously administered calcium may worsen ischemia/reperfusion injury. Intracellular calcium overload occurs during cerebral ischemia by the influx of calcium through voltage- and agonist-dependent (eg, N-methyl-D-aspartate) calcium channels. Calcium plays an important role in the process of cell death in many organs, possibly by activating intracellular enzymes such as nitric oxide synthase, phospholipase A and C, and others.[227,228] Calcium channel blockers improve blood flow and function after ischemia to the heart, kidney, and brain.[229-231] Calcium channel blockers also raise the threshold of the ischemic heart to VF.[232] For these reasons, it appears that the recommended restrictions for use of calcium during CPR are well founded. On the other hand, no studies have shown that elevation of plasma calcium concentration, which occurs after calcium administration, worsens outcome of cardiac arrest. Because the normal ratio of extracellular to intracellular calcium is on the order of 1000:1 to 10,000:1, it seems unlikely that the rate of influx of calcium into cells would be influenced by a relatively small increase in its extracellular concentration.

The calcium ion is essential in myocardial excitation-contraction coupling, in increasing ventricular contractility, and in enhancing ventricular automaticity during asystole. Ionized hypocalcemia is associated with decreased ventricular performance and peripheral blunting of the hemodynamic response to catecholamines.[233,234] In addition, severe ionized hypocalcemia has been documented in adults experiencing out-of-hospital cardiac arrest (mean Ca 0.67 mmol/L), during sepsis, and in animals during prolonged CPR.[234-236] Thus patients at risk for ionized hypocalcemia should be identified and treated as expeditiously as possible. Both total and ionized hypocalcemia may occur in patients with chronic or acute disease. Total body calcium depletion leading to total serum hypocalcemia occurs in patients with hypoparathyroidism, DiGeorge syndrome, renal failure, pancreatitis, and long-term use of loop diuretics. Ionized hypocalcemia occurs after massive or rapid transfusion of blood products, a result of citrate and other preservatives in stored blood products that bind calcium. The magnitude of hypocalcemia in this setting depends on the rate of blood administration, the total dose, and the hepatic and renal function of the patient. Administration of 2 mL/kg/min of citrated whole blood causes a significant decrease in ionized calcium concentration in anesthetized patients.

The pediatric dose of calcium chloride for resuscitation is 20 mg/kg. The adult dose is 200 mg (2 mL of the 10% solution). Calcium gluconate is as effective as calcium chloride in raising ionized calcium concentration during CPR. Calcium gluconate is given at a dose of 30 to 100 mg/kg, with a maximum dose of 2 g in pediatric patients. Calcium should be given slowly through a large-bore, free-flowing IV line, preferably a central venous line. Severe tissue necrosis occurs when calcium infiltrates into subcutaneous tissue. When administered too rapidly, calcium may cause bradycardia, heart block, or ventricular standstill.

Srinivasan et al. reviewed 1477 consecutive pediatric cardiopulmonary events submitted to the National Registry of Cardiopulmonary Resuscitation and reported on the prevalence of calcium administration.[237] Of the children in the registry, 659 were documented as receiving calcium. Calcium was more likely to be used in pediatric facilities, ICUs, and the settings of cardiac surgery, CPR performed for more than 15 minutes, asystole, and concurrently with other advanced life support medications. After controlling for confounding factors (demographics, immediate precipitating causes, arrest rhythm, concurrent ACLS medications, and duration of CPR), calcium administration during CPR was independently associated with poor survival to discharge and unfavorable neurologic outcomes. They found that 21% of patients survived to hospital discharge when calcium was used, compared with 44% who survived when calcium was not used. Only 15% of patients had a favorable neurologic outcome when calcium was used, compared with 35% with a favorable outcome when calcium was not administered.[237]

Glucose

Administration of glucose during CPR should be restricted to patients with documented hypoglycemia because of the possible detrimental effects of hyperglycemia on the brain during or following ischemia. Myers found that infant monkeys that received glucose before cardiac arrest were more likely to develop seizures, prolonged coma, and brain death with cerebral necrosis than were those that received saline solution.[238] Siemkowicz and Hansen confirmed this finding when they demonstrated that after 10 minutes of global brain ischemia, the neurologic recovery of hyperglycemic rats was worse than that of normoglycemic control subjects.[239] The mechanism by which hyperglycemia exacerbates ischemic neurologic injury may be increased production of lactic acid in the brain by anaerobic metabolism. During ischemia under normoglycemic conditions, brain lactate concentration reaches a plateau. In a hyperglycemic milieu, however, brain lactate concentration continues to rise for the duration of the ischemic period. The severity of intracellular acidosis during ischemia is directly proportional to the preischemic glucose concentration.[240] The negative effect of hyperglycemia during brain ischemia is predicated on the presence of at least a small amount of blood flow to brain tissue. In one study, collaterally perfused but not end-arterial brain tissue had greater neuronal damage during hyperglycemic focal ischemia (Fig. 41.19).[241]

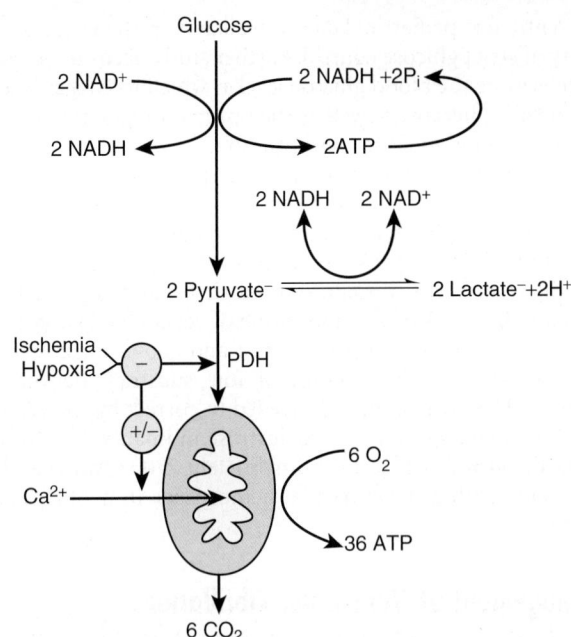

Fig. 41.19. Schematic diagram illustrating the aerobic/anaerobic metabolism of glucose. Oxidation of pyruvate to CO_2 (and H_2O) by pyruvate dehydrogenase and citric acid cycle enzymes is retarded to blocked by oxygen deficiency, causing a reduction of pyruvate to lactate. If the adenosine triphosphate *(ATP)* formed during glycolysis is hydrolyzed (ie, if the ATP concentration stays constant), one molecule of H^+ is released for each molecule of lactate formed. If the mitochondria retain a membrane potential, they will sequester excess calcium entering the cell; however, if they deenergized (with collapse of their membrane potential), they will release their calcium content. *ADP,* adenosine diphosphate; *NAD,* nicotinamide adenine dinucleotide; *NADH,* reduced nicotinamide adenine dinucleotide; P_i, intracellular phosphorus; *PDH,* pyruvate dehydrogenase.

Clinical studies show a direct correlation between the initial post–cardiac arrest serum glucose concentration and poor neurologic outcome.[230,242] However, a higher glucose concentration may just be an endogenous response to severe stress and thus a marker and not the cause of more severe brain injury.[75] In piglets, postischemic administration of glucose did not worsen neurologic outcome after global hypoxia-ischemia.[243] However, given the likelihood of additional ischemic and hypoxic events in the postresuscitation period, it seems prudent to maintain serum glucose in the normal range. Administration of insulin to hyperglycemic rats after global brain ischemia improved neurologic outcome.[244] The effect of insulin may be independent of its ability to lower blood glucose because these investigators later showed that normoglycemic insulin-treated rats had a better outcome than normoglycemic placebo-treated control subjects.[245]

Using intensive insulin therapy, Van den Bergh et al. strictly controlled the blood glucose levels of adults in a surgical ICU, maintaining levels between 80 and 110 mg/dL.[246,247] This control of blood glucose levels appeared to reduce mortality and protect the central and peripheral nervous systems. However, a subsequent study in a medical ICU showed no difference in mortality between the intensive insulin therapy and control groups.[248] Another study showed that the use of intensive insulin therapy to maintain normoglycemia was associated with increased episodes of hypoglycemia.[249]

Currently few pediatric data are available on the efficacy and safety of strict glucose control. Further study needs to be done to determine the blood glucose level at which to trigger intensive insulin therapy, as well as the optimal ranges at which to maintain blood glucose concentration.

Some groups of patients, including premature infants and debilitated patients with low endogenous glycogen stores, are more prone to the development of hypoglycemia during and after a physiologic stress (eg, surgery).[250] Hypoglycemia poses a higher risk in the immature pediatric brain compared with the adult brain. Bedside monitoring of serum glucose is critical during and after a cardiac arrest and allows for intervention before the critical point of low substrate delivery is reached. The dose of glucose needed to correct hypoglycemia is 0.5 to 1.0 g/kg given as 10% dextrose in infants. The osmolarity of 50% dextrose is approximately 2700 Osm/L and is associated with intraventricular hemorrhage in neonates and infants.

Management of Ventricular Fibrillation

The management of lethal ventricular arrhythmias traditionally has not played a major role in resuscitation teaching or management for children because of the low incidence of these arrhythmias. Newer evidence gathered in the environment of rapid access defibrillation suggests that up to 19% of the presenting rhythms in pediatric arrests is ventricular in origin, and this represents up to 5% to 15% of all pediatric victims of out-of-hospital cardiac arrest.[17,251] The incidence increases with age. Approximately 25% of children experiencing in-hospital cardiac arrest have ventricular tachycardia (VT) or fibrillation.[126] Moreover, the growing and aging population of children palliated for complex congenital heart disease in which the occurrence of ventricular arrhythmias may be much higher than in the general pediatric population requires greater attention to ventricular arrhythmias than in the past. Other potential causes of ventricular arrhythmias include familial and acquired prolonged QT syndrome, other arrhythmogenic ventricular conditions, cardiomyopathies, myocarditis, drug intoxications (such as illicit and accidental ingestion and therapeutic misadventures), electrolyte derangements (eg, magnesium, calcium, potassium, or glucose), and hypothermia.[252,253]

Advances have been made in the management of ventricular arrhythmias. Rapid access to defibrillation has been shown to reduce mortality in adults, and the development of public access defibrillation and AEDs has flowed from this knowledge. Initially AED devices had little utility for children, but the development of current-reducing electrodes and specific pediatric algorithms has made public access defibrillation a reality for children, and AEDs have been deployed in the many environments in which children would be the primary beneficiaries (eg, schools and public swimming pools). When automated external defibrillators are used within 3 minutes of adult-witnessed ventricular fibrillation in children, long-term survival can occur in more than 70% of cases.[254-256] The technique of current delivery has undergone change with the development and deployment of biphasic defibrillators, which may offer increased efficacy with reduced risk of myocardial injury. Finally, amiodarone has started to replace lidocaine as the drug of choice for refractory ventricular arrhythmias and atrial arrhythmias. The role of each of these factors in the resuscitation of pediatric arrest victims is discussed in the following section.

Defibrillation

VF is the chaotic electrical excitation of the ventricle, and the definitive treatment in accordance with the 2015 AHA guidelines is defibrillation.[47,189,257] The electrical mechanism is usually explained as a reentrant depolarization of the myocardium, initially in waves, which then take more circuitous routes and degenerate into smaller reentry circuits resulting in loss of the rhythmic contractile function of the ventricles.[258] This changing pattern of reentry circuits corresponds with the change from coarse to fine VF as the duration of fibrillation persists and may correlate with deterioration in energy stores associated with persistence of fibrillation.[5,259,260] Similarly, most cases of VT are attributable to reentrant mechanisms, although increased automaticity is the likely mechanism in persons with drug-induced torsades de pointes and electrolyte disturbances such as hypokalemia and hypomagnesemia.[261] Nonpulsatile VT with loss of effective contractile function of the heart rapidly deteriorates into VF. Loss of effective ventricular function with these arrhythmias requires emergent management.

The standard for management of VF and pulseless VT is immediate defibrillation and high-quality CPR. Although the lowest energy dose for effective defibrillation and the upper limit for safe defibrillation in infants and children are not known, energy doses greater than 4 J/kg (up to 9 J/kg) have effectively defibrillated children.[153] The standard voltage dose for pediatric defibrillation is 2 J/kg. If unsuccessful, successive doses of defibrillation are repeated at 4 J/kg or more, not to exceed 10 J/kg or the maximum adult dose.[115] This dosage is based on data reported by Gutgesell et al. in 1976.[262] They reported 71 defibrillation attempts in 27 children. Efficacy was 91% with 2 J/kg and 100% with 4 J/kg. After initial defibrillation, CPR is performed for 2 minutes, followed by a rhythm check and then repeat shock if required. This sequence may then be repeated, with consideration given to initiate vasopressor therapy. Rhythms that fail to respond to three rounds are defined as "shock resistant." In this setting, the standard as defined in the AHA guidelines is amiodarone, 5 mg/kg or lidocaine (or magnesium for torsades de pointes), followed by 2 minutes of CPR and continuation of the rhythm check-shock-CPR/vasopressor cycle (Fig. 41.21). Reversible causes of VT/VF should also be investigated. Success in resuscitation is incumbent on immediate defibrillation with immediate CPR in between delivery of shocks.

It is important to continue to deliver appropriate CPR while gathering defibrillation equipment.[263,264] Additional important considerations when delivering shocks include paddle size, position, contact pressure, and use of electrode paste. Large paddles reduce thoracic impedance, and infants older than 1 year or weighing more than 10 kg should be treated with adult paddles.[265] Adhesive patch electrodes are an acceptable alternative to paddles and can be used when available if their use does not cause a delay in therapy.[266-268] Paddles should be positioned to achieve current flow through the heart, and an anterior-apex or anterior-posterior placement is selected. Contact pressure has been demonstrated to reduce impedance. Firm pressure, which commonly is not properly applied, is required.[269] Proper electrode paste or gel is necessary. Care is required to avoid smearing paste across the chest wall because doing so can lead to arcing of the circuit and a resultant short circuit. Bare paddles, ultrasound gel, pads soaked in saline solution, and alcohol pads are not acceptable alternatives to electrode cream or paste.[189]

The role of immediate defibrillation has come under question. The efficacy of defibrillation declines rapidly as fibrillation persists. When an arrest is witnessed and a defibrillator is immediately available, defibrillation likely will be successful. With any delay in resuscitation, the success of initial defibrillation declines at a rate estimated at between 7% and 10% per minute of continued fibrillation.[154] A number of studies have demonstrated in both animals and adults that if more than 3 to 5 minutes of fibrillation have occurred before institution of defibrillation, use of CPR for 90 to 180 seconds to restore myocardial energy stores will improve the likelihood of conversion to a perfusing rhythm with defibrillation.[6,8,270,271] Given the frequency of unwitnessed arrest in children and the relatively low frequency of ventricular arrhythmias, CPR first may be the appropriate response in children.

Use of biphasic defibrillators is another important advance in the management of tachyarrhythmias. Studies suggest that defibrillation with a biphasic waveform can be achieved with lower energy and less myocardial injury than with a standard monophasic defibrillator current.[272,273] The first commercially available devices were approved by the US Food and Drug Administration in 1996. An evidence-based review was undertaken by the AHA and published in 1998.[45] The reviewers concluded that "low-energy, non-progressive biphasic waveform defibrillators may be used for both out-of-hospital and in-hospital VF arrest, including persistent or recurrent VF that does not respond to the initial low-energy shock." These conclusions were based on observational studies and case reports. Subsequently, Schneider et al. reported a randomized controlled trial of biphasic versus monophasic defibrillation for out-of-hospital cardiac arrest.[274] Of 338 arrests, 115 patients had VF and were shocked with an AED. Defibrillation in the initial shock series was successful in 98% of patients receiving biphasic shocks but in only 69% of those receiving monophasic shocks (p <.0001), providing further evidence that biphasic waveforms are more efficacious than monophasic waveforms (Fig. 41.20).

Biphasic shocks appear to be at least as effective as monophasic shocks and less harmful. Published data on children are limited to case reports.[275] Animal data are supportive of the use of biphasic defibrillators in infants and children. Clark et al. demonstrated in a piglet model that low-energy biphasic shocks were superior to monophasic shocks for converting

catheter-induced VF.[276] Both Tang et al. and Berg et al. studied the use of AEDs equipped with energy-reducing electrodes and found increased efficacy compared with monophasic waveforms.[5,277] Berg et al. also demonstrated improved LV function 5 hours after resuscitation.

According to the 2015 AHA recommendations, with a manual defibrillator, dosage recommendations for children remain 2 J/kg for the first attempt followed by 4 J/kg for subsequent attempts.[5,49,278] This dose was increased from the 2005 guidelines, which cited studies that demonstrated the ineffectiveness of 2 J/kg at achieving ROSC. Subsequent to the publication of the 2010 AHA recommendations, a review of the National Registry of Cardiopulmonary Resuscitation data compared the effect of 2 J/kg with historical controls and a 4 J/kg initial shock dose in VF and pulseless VT. The authors found that termination of the arrhythmia with an initial shock dose of 2 J/kg was significantly less effective than historical controls (56% vs. 91%). A higher initial dose of 4 J/kg was associated with less successful ROSC than the 2 J/kg dose. On the basis of these conflicting data, they concluded that the optimal initial shock dose has yet to be determined.

In the early 1990s, as part of an AHA campaign to improve the abysmal rates of resuscitation from out-of-hospital cardiac arrest in adults, the development and deployment of AEDs were initiated. Both fixed and escalating dose devices were developed; however, the initial dose usually was at least 150 J in adults. Because of the high fixed-energy doses, the devices were not recommended for use in children younger than 9 years. Moreover, use of these devices for young children was questioned because the arrhythmia detection algorithms used in these devices were developed for adults. Cecchin et al. used the Agilent Heartstream FR2 Patient Analysis System to analyze 696 five-second rhythms from 191 children younger than 12 years.[279] Analysis revealed 100% accuracy for nonshockable rhythms and 96% accuracy for VF. This is similar to the accuracy reported for adults. In a more recent study, Atkinson et al. tested the accuracy of the Lifepak 500 AED on 1561 fifteen-second rhythms from 203 children aged 1 day to 7 years.[261] The device correctly identified 99% of coarse VF as shockable and 99.1% of nonshockable rhythms. A number of manufacturers (Zoll and Agilent) have developed energy-reducing electrodes that should allow use of these devices in young children.[261]

Since the 2000 AHA guidelines, data have shown that AEDs can be safely and effectively used in children of all ages. Current guidelines recommend use of an AED in children between the ages of 1 and 8 years who have no signs of

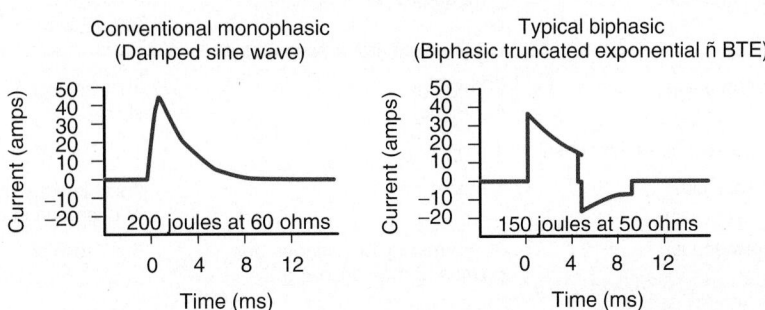

DEFIBRILLATION WAVEFORMS

Fig. 41.20. Schematic patterns of current flow for conventional monophasic and typical biphasic defibrillator waveforms.

circulation. The device should be adapted to deliver a pediatric dose with the use of a pediatric attenuator system that decreases the delivered energy to a dose suitable for children. When an attenuator system is not available, then the standard adult pads with corresponding dose should be delivered. In children younger than 1 year of age, a manual defibrillator is preferred; however, an AED with or without a pediatric attenuator may be used if necessary.[256]

Antiarrhythmics

Amiodarone is an effective antiarrhythmic agent for both atrial and ventricular arrhythmias. The role of amiodarone in cardiac arrest was established after a series of studies demonstrated efficacy and superiority of amiodarone over lidocaine in the management of refractory VF and pulseless VT in adults. Compared with lidocaine, amiodarone led to substantially higher rates of survival to hospital admission in patients with shock-resistant out-of-hospital VF.[280] These findings led to major changes in the AHA guidelines for management of ventricular arrhythmias (Table 41.1 and Figs. 41.21 and 41.22).

Early reports on use of oral amiodarone in children were favorable.[280-284] Data on amiodarone use in children are limited to case reports and descriptive case series.[285-289] Nevertheless, it is now used widely for serious pediatric arrhythmias. It appears to be effective and have an acceptable short-term safety profile. In 2008, we examined the practice patterns of amiodarone use during in-hospital cardiac arrest. In this retrospective cohort study, it was noted that there has been a significant increase in amiodarone use for VF/VT events during the past 5 years. It was also noted that the frequency of amiodarone use in adults correlated positively with the number of intensive care beds, suggesting that the emerging data and national guidelines affect resuscitation practice patterns.[84]

The growing pediatric experience among experts and inference from adult studies led to inclusion of amiodarone in the 2000 AHA pediatric advanced life support guidelines and continued in the 2015 AHA pediatric advanced life support guidelines as a drug of choice, alongside lidocaine, for pulseless

VT.[49] For hemodynamically stable VT, it is also a drug of choice, with the level of evidence classified as IIb. Procainamide remains an alternative drug choice. Amiodarone is commonly used for management of postoperative atrial and junctional ectopic tachycardia, especially in patients with ventricular pacing wires in place.

The wide range of effectiveness of amiodarone is demonstrated by the array of indications noted in the 2015 AHA guidelines for adults.[189] Its role in the management of atrial arrhythmias in adults includes the following: as an adjunct to electrical cardioversion of refractory paroxysmal supraventricular tachycardia and atrial tachycardia, for rate control when digoxin has been ineffective, for pharmacologic conversion of atrial flutter, and for control of rapid ventricular response in pre-excited atrial tachyarrhythmias. It is the drug of choice for junctional tachycardia with poor function. If function is preserved, amiodarone is an acceptable alternative to a β-blocker or calcium channel blocker. Its role in ventricular arrhythmias is outlined in Box 41.2.

The pharmacology of amiodarone is complex and may partially explain the wide range of efficacy. It is poorly absorbed orally and must be loaded intravenously in urgent situations. It is primarily classified as a Vaughn-Williams class III agent that blocks the ATP-sensitive outward potassium channels, causing prolongation of the action potential and refractory period. However, this effect requires intracellular accumulation. Upon IV loading, the antiarrhythmic effects primarily result from noncompetitive α- and β-adrenergic receptor blockade, calcium channel blockade, and effects on inward sodium current, causing a decrease in anterograde conduction across the atrioventricular node and an increase in the effective atrioventricular refractory period. The full antiarrhythmic impact requires a loading period for up to 1 to 3 weeks to achieve intracellular levels and full potassium channel blocking effects. Prolongation of the QT interval, an effect resulting from K-ATP channel blockade, is commonly described with amiodarone use; however, it does not manifest until several days into loading, underscoring its different effects during the acute period and after loading is accomplished. These effects

TABLE 41.1	**Drug Therapy for Pulseless Arrest**		
Drug	**Route of Administration**	**Dosage**	**How Applied**
Epinephrine	IV, intraosseous, endotracheal	10 µg/kg; max dose 1 mg IV/IO 100 µg/kg; max dose 2.5 mg ET	1:10,000 (0.1 mL/kg) 1:1000 should be used for ETT (0.1 mL/kg)
Atropine	IV, intraosseous, endotracheal, subcutaneous	0.02 IV/IO mg/kg; min dose 0.1 mg, max dose 0.5 mg, repeat once as needed, ET dose 0.04-0.06 mg/kg	
Sodium bicarbonate	IV, intraosseous	1 mEq/kg/dose or 0.3 × weight (kg) × base deficit	1 mEq/mL 0.5 mEq/mL
Calcium chloride	IV (intraosseous)	20 mg/kg 0.2 mL/kg	10% solution (100 mg/mL); administer slowly
Lidocaine	IV (intraosseous), endotracheal	1 mg/kg	1%, 2%, 4% solution
Amiodarone	IV (intraosseous)	5 mg/kg	If stable, load over 20-60 minutes IV push during cardiac arrest
Magnesium	IV (intraosseous)	25-50 mg/kg for torsades des pointes or max dose 2 g	50% solution

ETT, endotracheal tube; *IV,* intravenous.

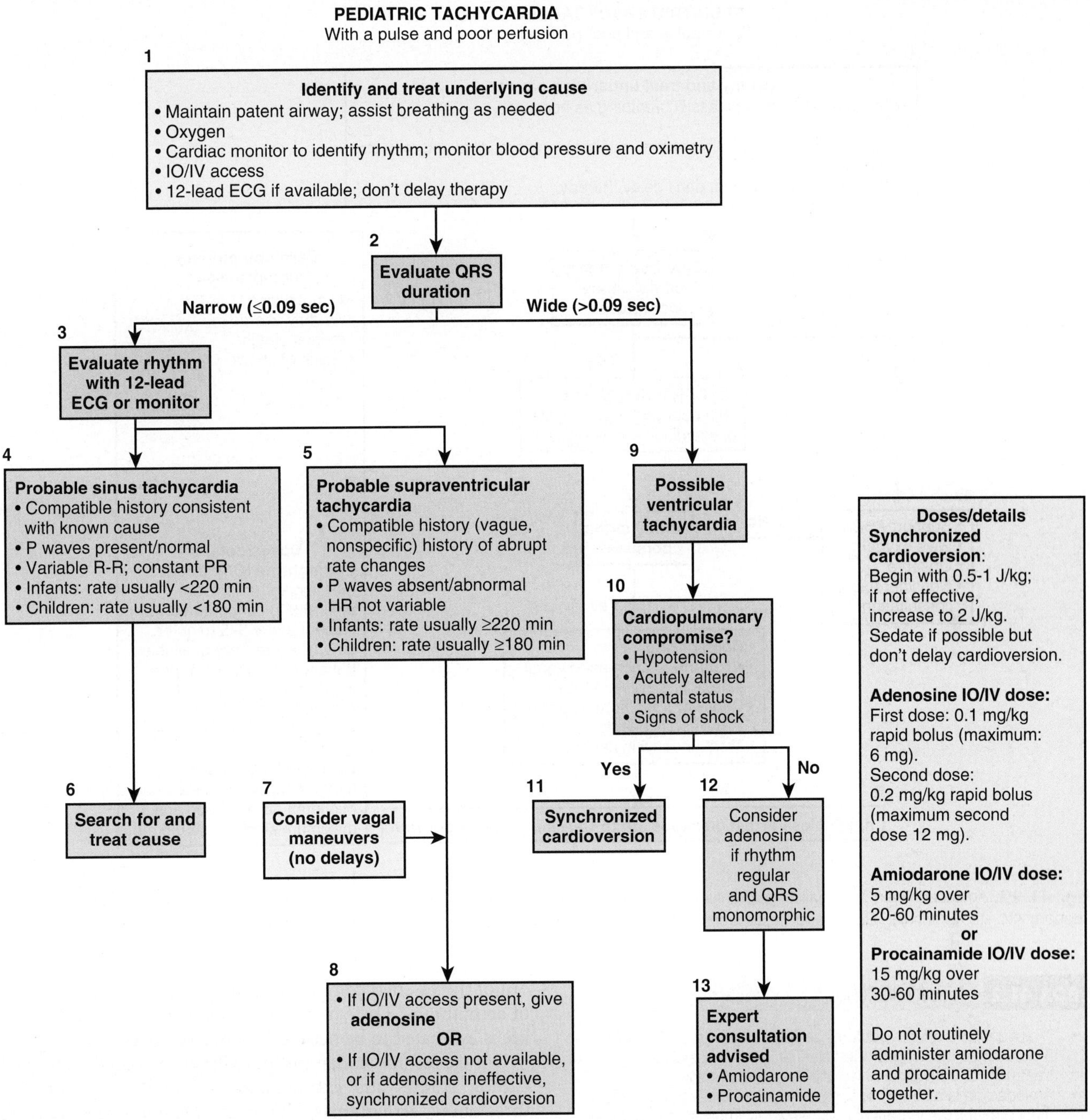

PEDIATRIC TACHYCARDIA
With a pulse and poor perfusion

1

Identify and treat underlying cause
• Maintain patent airway; assist breathing as needed
• Oxygen
• Cardiac monitor to identify rhythm; monitor blood pressure and oximetry
• IO/IV access
• 12-lead ECG if available; don't delay therapy

2

Evaluate QRS duration

Narrow (≤0.09 sec)   Wide (>0.09 sec)

3

Evaluate rhythm with 12-lead ECG or monitor

4

Probable sinus tachycardia
• Compatible history consistent with known cause
• P waves present/normal
• Variable R-R; constant PR
• Infants: rate usually <220 min
• Children: rate usually <180 min

5

Probable supraventricular tachycardia
• Compatible history (vague, nonspecific) history of abrupt rate changes
• P waves absent/abnormal
• HR not variable
• Infants: rate usually ≥220 min
• Children: rate usually ≥180 min

9

Possible ventricular tachycardia

10

Cardiopulmonary compromise?
• Hypotension
• Acutely altered mental status
• Signs of shock

Yes   No

6

Search for and treat cause

7

Consider vagal maneuvers (no delays)

11

Synchronized cardioversion

12

Consider adenosine if rhythm regular and QRS monomorphic

8

• If IO/IV access present, give **adenosine**
  OR
• If IO/IV access not available, or if adenosine ineffective, synchronized cardioversion

13

Expert consultation advised
• Amiodarone
• Procainamide

Doses/details
Synchronized cardioversion:
Begin with 0.5-1 J/kg; if not effective, increase to 2 J/kg. Sedate if possible but don't delay cardioversion.

Adenosine IO/IV dose:
First dose: 0.1 mg/kg rapid bolus (maximum: 6 mg).
Second dose: 0.2 mg/kg rapid bolus (maximum second dose 12 mg).

Amiodarone IO/IV dose:
5 mg/kg over 20-60 minutes
or
Procainamide IO/IV dose:
15 mg/kg over 30-60 minutes

Do not routinely administer amiodarone and procainamide together.

Fig. 41.21. American Heart Association guidelines for management of ventricular arrhythmias. *ABCs,* airway, breathing, and circulation; *BLS,* basic life support; *CPR,* cardiopulmonary resuscitation; *ECG,* electrocardiogram; *IO,* intraosseous; *IV,* intravenous; *PEA,* pulseless electrical activity; *TT,* tracheal tube; *VF,* ventricular fibrillation; *VT,* ventricular tachycardia.

are evident throughout all cardiac tissue, which may explain amiodarone's efficacy for so many arrhythmias, both atrial and ventricular. The α-adrenergic blockade leads to vasodilation, which may increase coronary blood flow.

Immediate hemodynamic effects of amiodarone are caused by the solubilizing agent Tween 80, which has both vasodilating and myocardial depressant effects.[290] Hypotension is commonly reported with IV administration and may limit the rate at which the drug can be given. The overall hemodynamic impact of intravenous administration depends on the balance

of its effect on rate control, myocardial performance, and vasodilation. Cardiac output is usually unchanged or increases despite the decreased contractility because of both rate control and vasodilation. The effect on systemic vascular resistance and the limited impact on contractility make amiodarone the drug of choice for use in patients with impaired cardiac function.

The drug is highly lipid soluble, giving it a large volume of distribution, which accounts for the need for loading over many days. Until all tissues are saturated, rapid redistribution

PEDIATRIC BRADYCARDIA
With a pulse and poor perfusion

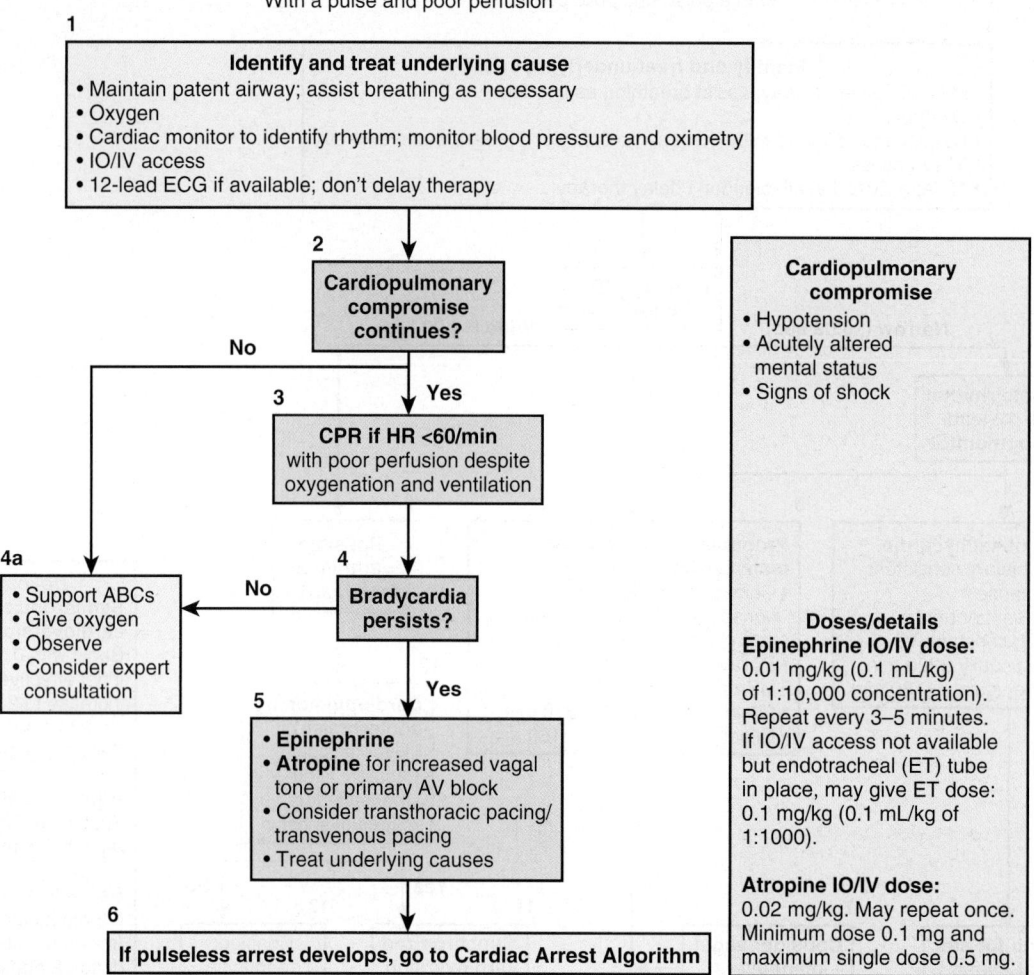

Fig. 41.22. American Heart Association guidelines for management of bradycardia. *ABCs,* airway, breathing, and circulation; *ALS,* advanced life support; *AV,* atrioventricular; *BLS,* basic life support; *CPR,* cardiopulmonary resuscitation; *IO,* intraosseous; *IV,* intravenous.

BOX 41.2 Amiodarone (IV)

- IV amiodarone affects sodium, calcium channels, and α- and β-adrenergic blocking properties. The drug is useful for treatment of both atrial and ventricular arrhythmias.
- Amiodarone is also helpful for ventricular rate control of rapid atrial arrhythmias in patients with severely impaired LV function when digitalis has proved ineffective. Amiodarone is recommended after defibrillation and epinephrine in cardiac arrest with persistent VT or VF.
- Amiodarone is effective for control of hemodynamically stable VT, polymorphic VT, and wide-complex tachycardia of uncertain origin.
- Amiodarone is an adjunct to electrical cardioversion of refractory PSVTs, atrial tachycardia, and pharmacologic cardioversion of AF.
- Amiodarone can control rapid ventricular rate due to accessory pathway conduction in preexcited atrial arrhythmias.

AF, atrial fibrillation; *LV,* left ventricular; *PSVT,* paroxysmal supraventricular tachycardia; *VF,* ventricular fibrillation; *VT,* ventricular tachycardia.

---

out of the vascular compartment may lead to early recurrence of arrhythmias. Once tissue saturation has occurred, the half-life is estimated to be between 13 and 103 days.

Dosage recommendations for children are based on limited clinical studies and extrapolation of adult data. For life-threatening arrhythmias, the usual recommended dose is 5 mg/kg administered intravenously. This dose can be repeated if necessary to control the arrhythmia. IV loading doses are followed by a continuous infusion of 10 to 20 mg/kg/day if there is a risk for arrhythmia recurrence. The ideal rate of bolus administration is unclear, but once diluted the drug is given by IV push in adults. The potential for profound vasodilation in children has led to concern by some pediatric intensivists and cardiologists, who recommend that amiodarone be given over 10 minutes as recommended in the package insert. This concern may not be valid in the pulseless arrest setting. Some delay always occurs with the current formulation of the IV drug because it must be diluted before it can be administered. Drug dilution should not delay administration of additional shocks. Averages of five shocks are delivered to adults with refractory VF before amiodarone is administered. An alternative dosing regimen for children is administration of 1 mg/kg pushes every 5 minutes up to 5 mg/kg. This dose can be repeated up to 10 mg/kg if the arrhythmia is not controlled. Use of the small-aliquot bolus technique may be particularly appropriate for infants younger than 6 to 12 months.

Amiodarone administered intravenously leaches plasticizers, particularly DEHP, from polyvinyl chloride. This effect is enhanced at low infusion rates and at higher drug concentrations and may be minimized by frequent intermittent boluses. Whether these plasticizers have any significant toxicity at these doses is unknown, although evidence indicates testicular vacuolization in rodents. Additional caution is warranted in neonates because the solution contains benzyl alcohol, which is associated with metabolic acidosis and death in premature infants (gasping syndrome). Identification of the potential for these adverse events has led the manufacturer to issue a statement to health care professionals stating that use of intravenously administered amiodarone in pediatrics is not recommended. The AHA has responded with a reiteration of the recommendation for IV amiodarone use in the 2015 guidelines for emergency cardiac care. In the recommendation it concludes that practitioners should obtain expert consultation because complications may include bradycardia, heart block, and torsades de pointes VT. Adverse reactions to amiodarone can be life-threatening. The drug prolongs the QT interval. In a series by Etheridge et al., 29 of 50 infants and children experienced mild-to-moderate prolongation of the QTc.[286] In the series by Burri et al., "most" infants experienced QTc prolongation.[285] Although none of the pediatric case series described the development of drug-induced arrhythmias in patients, amiodarone-induced torsades de pointes has been described in case reports, and, although less common than in adults, caution is warranted.[291] Use of amiodarone should be avoided in combination with other drugs that prolong the QT interval. In addition, caution should be exercised in the setting of hypomagnesemia and other electrolyte abnormalities that predispose to torsades de pointes. Severe bradycardia and heart block have been described, especially in the postoperative period, and ventricular pacing wires are recommended in this setting.

The manufacturer of the IV preparation (Pfizer, New York) reports in the product literature a series of 61 children receiving amiodarone, of whom 36% had hypotension, 20% had bradycardia, and 15% had atrioventricular block. These complications were severe or life-threatening in some cases. In the published case series of children, the incidence of adverse effects appears to be much lower. In a series reported by Etheridge et al., two of six patients who received intravenously administered amiodarone experienced hypotension.[286] In several other series, the incidence of hypotension ranged from 0 of 15 to 4 of 40.[285,287,289] All patients who were believed to require treatment responded to a saline solution infusion or calcium. One patient with symptomatic bradycardia responded to temporary pacing. Two other patients required a reduction in the rate of drug infusion for mild bradycardia.

Noncardiac adverse effects are often seen, especially with chronic dosing.[292] The most serious adverse effect is the development of interstitial pneumonitis, seen most often in patients with preexisting lung disease.[293] The incidence in children is unknown. Rarely an acute respiratory distress syndrome–like illness has been reported in both infants and adults at the initiation of treatment.[294,295] The lung disease may remit with early discontinuation of the drug. Thyroid disorders may

occur with chronic use. Desethylamidarone, the major metabolite of amiodarone, appears to have an antithyroid effect by noncompetitive binding to the nuclear receptors. Both hyperthyroidism with thyrotoxicosis and hypothyroidism have occurred. This may be of particular concern in the management of fetal tachycardias. Although amiodarone appears to be effective in controlling refractory life-threatening fetal tachycardias, evidence of fetal hypothyroidism was present in 19% of neonates based on cord blood thyroid-stimulating hormone.[296] Other forms of toxicity include hepatotoxicity that may progress to cirrhosis, photosensitivity and skin discoloration, and local inflammation and cellulitis at the infusion site. Injection site reactions occurred in 5 of 20 patients who received amiodarone through a peripheral IV line. Corneal opacities are a common finding with chronic therapy but apparently do not affect vision.

The published data on amiodarone use in pediatric cardiac arrest is sparse; its use is derived mostly from adult experiences and animal studies.[297,298] A case series of 40 pediatric patients with ventricular, atrial, or junctional tachyarrhythmias established the safety and efficacy of the drug in critically ill patients.[289] Subsequent to the publication of the 2015 AHA guidelines, Valdes et al. examined the use of amiodarone and lidocaine in in-hospital pediatric patients with pulseless VT or VF. They found that lidocaine was independently favorably associated with ROSC and 24-hour survival, but not survival to hospital discharge. However, amiodarone did not have any association with survival outcomes.[3] This led to the inclusion of lidocaine as a first line antiarrhythmic alongside amiodarone for pulseless VT and VF in the 2015 AHA guideines.[189]

Lidocaine is a Vaughn-Williams class Ib agent that inhibits fast inward sodium current, primarily affecting the ventricular myocardium, and produces a decrease in automaticity. Cells in the sinoatrial and atrioventricular node are minimally affected. It is highly selective for depressed myocardial tissue. Proarrhythmic effects are relatively uncommon, though high plasma concentrations are associated with depressed myocardial function especially in patients with underlying poor myocardial function. The half-life is 5 to 10 minutes, though hypokalemia can decrease its effect. The loading dose is 1 mg/kg, with an infusion rate of 20 to 50 mcg/kg/min. Since this agent does not increase the QTc interval, its use is preferable to amiodarone in patients with a prolonged QTc.

Procainamide is a Vaughn-Williams class Ia agent that slows the upstroke of the action potential by blocking sodium channels. This slows conduction in atrial and ventricular muscle cells and suppresses normal and abnormal automaticity. Procainamide increases the PR interval and the QRS duration and prolongs the QTc interval. Amiodarone and ranitidine increase procainamide levels. The IV bolus dose is 10 to 15 mg/kg, and a continuous infusion of 30 to 80 mcg/kg/min may be used. High doses have a negative inotropic effect and caution should be exercised in patients with a prolonged QT interval, left ventricular dysfunction, or sinus dysfunction. The risk of proarrhythmia, especially torsades de pointes, is moderate and not related to serum drug concentrations.

Postresuscitation Care

Hemodynamic instability is common after cardiac arrest. A persistently low cardiac index may lead to multiorgan failure and is associated with early death within the first 24 hours after arrest.[299,300] Systolic hypotension in the 6 hours after a

BOX 41.3 | Experimental Cerebroprotective Therapy

- Calcium channel blockers
- Glutamate receptor antagonists
- Opiate receptor antagonists
- Central α_2-receptor antagonists
- β-Receptor antagonists
- Oxygen radical scavengers
- Iron chelators
- Xanthine oxidase inhibitors
- Inhibitors of arachidonic acid metabolism
- Thrombolytic agents
- Lazeroids
- Cerebral vasodilators
- Metabolic activators/inhibitors
- Hypothermia
- Nitric oxide synthase inhibitors
- Adenosine agonists
- Antiplatelet agents
- Antineutrophil strategies
- Protease inhibitors
- Growth factors

pediatric cardiac arrest has also been found to be associated with in-hospital mortality and worse neurologic outcomes.[301] Therapies to address low cardiac output states have included the use of inodilators. Inodilators (inamrinone and milrinone) augment cardiac output with little effect on myocardial oxygen demand. An inodilator can be used to treat myocardial dysfunction with increased systemic or pulmonary vascular resistance.[302,303] Administration of fluids may be required because of the vasodilatory effects. Inodilators have a long half-life with a long delay in reaching a new steady-state hemodynamic effect after changing the infusion rate (18 hours with inamrinone and 4.5 hours with milrinone). In case of toxicity, adverse effects may persist for several hours after the infusion is discontinued.

Amelioration of neurologic injury after cardiac arrest has been a goal of many investigators over the past decades (Box 41.3). Two multicenter trials on mild hypothermia after cardiac arrest, one from Europe and the other from Australia, showed initial promise. In both studies, adult patients presenting with out-of-hospital VF who were resuscitated underwent rapid cooling to a target temperature between 32.8°C and 34.8°C. This temperature was maintained for 12 to 24 hours. Both neurologic outcome and mortality were improved compared with the control groups. The odds ratio for improved neurologic outcome was 1.4 in the European study, which included 275 patients, and 5.25 in the Australian study, which included 77 randomized patients. The hypothermia groups had lower mean blood pressure, required more frequent use of epinephrine, and had higher systemic vascular resistance.

Criticisms of these trials have included that they have a limited generalizability and that the control groups were not temperature controlled to avoid hyperthermia, which is known to worsen neurologic outcomes.[304,305] To that end, the Targeted Temperature Management trials sought to further investigate if mild hypothermia conferred any benefit over a controlled normothermia.[306] The trial compared temperature maintenance at 33°C versus 36°C in unconscious adult survivors of the entire out-of-hospital cardiac arrest patient population, regardless of the reason for arrest. The trial showed no difference in survival between the two groups,

nor in the secondary outcome of survival and neurologic outcome. Subsequent studies evaluating targeted temperature management did not find differences in the systemic inflammatory response or cognitive outcome at 6 months between the 33°C and 36°C groups.[307-309]

The Therapeutic Hypothermia after Pediatric Cardiac Arrest (THAPCA) trials sought to evaluate mild hypothermia versus controlled normothermia in unconscious children suffering from out-of-hospital cardiac arrest.[11] Eligible patients between the age of 48 hours and 18 years were randomized to mild hypothermia (target temperature of 33.0°C) or therapeutic normothermia (36.8°C). No difference between survival or functional outcome was found at 1 year. A trial of targeted temperature management in children after in-hospital cardiac arrest is currently being conducted.

Future Directions

Despite the aforementioned therapeutic advances, continued efforts to clarify their applicability to infants and children are vital. Clinical trials have been hampered by the federal regulation known as the "final rule" for resuscitation research.[310] In 1996, as part of a broad-ranging effort to protect patients' rights as human subjects, the standard of community consent for research that required immediate intervention was developed. Since that time, resuscitation research in both adults and children has been limited, with most trials conducted in Europe, Australia, and other countries, often with US collaborators. The feasibility of defining a community standard to perform a hypothetical trial of hypothermia after cardiac arrest in children was tested in 2004.[311] The relevant community was defined as hospital staff and the parents of ICU patients and parents of previously resuscitated children. They concluded that development of a study using an exemption from informed consent was feasible. However, in an accompanying editorial, Moler reiterates that, despite feasibility, practicality is very different as evidenced by the complete lack of pediatric resuscitation trials since 1996.[299,310] Whether revision of this rule will occur or techniques for acquiring community consent can be developed remains one of the major hurdles to future pediatric resuscitation research.

Key References

3. Valdes SO, et al. Outcomes associated with amiodarone and lidocaine in the treatment of in-hospital pediatric cardiac arrest with pulseless ventricular tachycardia or ventricular fibrillation. *Resuscitation*. 2014;85:381-386.
8. Wik L, et al. Delaying defibrillation to give basic cardiopulmonary resuscitation to patients with out-of-hospital ventricular fibrillation: a randomized trial. *JAMA*. 2003;289:1389-1395.
9. Meert KL, et al. Multicenter cohort study of in-hospital pediatric cardiac arrest. *Pediatr Crit Care Med*. 2009;10:544-553.
10. Moler FW, et al. In-hospital versus out-of-hospital pediatric cardiac arrest: a multicenter cohort study. *Crit Care Med*. 2009;37:2259-2267.
11. Moler FW, et al. Therapeutic hypothermia after out-of-hospital cardiac arrest in children. *N Engl J Med*. 2015;372:1898-1908.
14. Perondi MBM, et al. A comparison of high-dose and standard-dose epinephrine in children with cardiac arrest. *N Engl J Med*. 2004;350:1722-1730.
21. Meaney PA, et al. Effect of defibrillation energy dose during in-hospital pediatric cardiac arrest. *Pediatrics*. 2011;127:e16-e23.
22. Kouwenhoven WB. Closed-chest cardiac massage. *JAMA*. 1960;173:1064.
26. Mackenzie GJ, et al. Hæmodynamic effects of external cardiac compression. *Lancet*. 1964;283:1342-1345.

47. Brooks SC, et al. Part 6: alternative techniques and ancillary devices for cardiopulmonary resuscitation: 2015 American Heart Association guidelines update for cardiopulmonary resuscitation and emergency cardiovascular care. *Circulation.* 2015;132(18 suppl 2):S436-S443.

48. Atkins DL, et al. Part 11: pediatric basic life support and cardiopulmonary resuscitation quality: 2015 American Heart Association guidelines update for cardiopulmonary resuscitation and emergency cardiovascular care. *Circulation.* 2015;132(18 suppl 2):S519-S525.

49. de Caen AR, et al. Part 12: pediatric advanced life support: 2015 American Heart Association guidelines update for cardiopulmonary resuscitation and emergency cardiovascular care. *Circulation.* 2015;132(18 suppl 2):S526-S542.

50. Kleinman ME, et al. Part 5: adult basic life support and cardiopulmonary resuscitation quality: 2015 American Heart Association guidelines update for cardiopulmonary resuscitation and emergency cardiovascular care. *Circulation.* 2015;132(18 suppl 2):S414-S435.

56. Ornato JP, et al. Effect of cardiopulmonary resuscitation compression rate on end-tidal carbon dioxide concentration and arterial pressure in man. *Crit Care Med.* 1988;16:241-245.

68. Bahlmann L, et al. Brain metabolism during cardiopulmonary resuscitation assessed with microdialysis. *Resuscitation.* 2003;59:255-260.

85. Babbs CF. Interposed abdominal compression CPR: a comprehensive evidence based review. *Resuscitation.* 2003;59:71-82.

92. Cohen TJ, et al. A comparison of active compression-decompression cardiopulmonary resuscitation with standard cardiopulmonary resuscitation for cardiac arrests occurring in the hospital. *N Engl J Med.* 1993;329:1918-1921.

102. Pirrallo RG, et al. Effect of an inspiratory impedance threshold device on hemodynamics during conventional manual cardiopulmonary resuscitation. *Resuscitation.* 2005;66:13-20.

105. Ditchey RV, Rubio-Perez A, Slinker BK. Beta-adrenergic blockade reduces myocardial injury during experimental cardiopulmonary resuscitation. *J Am Coll Cardiol.* 1994;24:804-812.

122. Morris MC, Wernovsky G, Nadkarni VM. Survival outcomes after extracorporeal cardiopulmonary resuscitation instituted during active chest compressions following refractory in-hospital pediatric cardiac arrest. *Pediatr Crit Care Med.* 2004;5:440-446.

123. Duncan BW, et al. Use of rapid-deployment extracorporeal membrane oxygenation for the resuscitation of pediatric patients with heart disease after cardiac arrest. *J Thorac Cardiovasc Surg.* 1998;116:305-311.

126. Samson RA, et al. Outcomes of in-hospital ventricular fibrillation in children. *N Engl J Med.* 2006;354:2328-2339.

128. Zoll PM. Resuscitation of the heart in ventricular standstill by external electric stimulation. *N Engl J Med.* 1952;247:768-771.

154. Link MS, et al. Part 7: adult advanced cardiovascular life support: 2015 American Heart Association guidelines update for cardiopulmonary resuscitation and emergency cardiovascular care. *Circulation.* 2015;132(18 suppl 2):S444-S464.

159. Holmes CL, Landry DW, Granton JT. Science review: vasopressin and the cardiovascular system part 1—receptor physiology. *Crit Care.* 2003;7:427-434.

166. Wenzel V, et al. A comparison of vasopressin and epinephrine for out-of-hospital cardiopulmonary resuscitation. *N Engl J Med.* 2004;350:105-113.

171. Duncan JM, et al. Vasopressin for in-hospital pediatric cardiac arrest: results from the American Heart Association National Registry of Cardiopulmonary Resuscitation. *Pediatr Crit Care Med.* 2009;10:191-195.

174. Botnaru T, Altherwi T, Dankoff J. Improved neurologic outcomes after cardiac arrest with combined administration of vasopressin, steroids, and epinephrine compared to epinephrine alone. *CJEM.* 2015;17:202-205.

183. Paradis NA. Coronary perfusion pressure and the return of spontaneous circulation in human cardiopulmonary resuscitation. *JAMA.* 1990;263:1106-1113.

190. Rivers EP. The effect of the total cumulative epinephrine dose administered during human CPR on hemodynamic, oxygen transport, and utilization variables in the postresuscitation period. *Chest.* 1994;106:1499.

201. Falk JL, Rackow EC, Weil MH. End-tidal carbon dioxide concentration during cardiopulmonary resuscitation. *N Engl J Med.* 1988;318:607-611.

207. Raymond TT, et al. Sodium bicarbonate use during in-hospital pediatric pulseless cardiac arrest—a report from the American Heart Association Get With The Guidelines((R))-Resuscitation. *Resuscitation.* 2015;89:106-113.

209. O'Flaherty D, Adams AP. The end-tidal carbon dioxide detector. Assessment of a new method to distinguish oesophageal from tracheal intubation. *Anaesthesia.* 1990;45:653-655.

218. Sheak KR, et al. Quantitative relationship between end-tidal carbon dioxide and CPR quality during both in-hospital and out-of-hospital cardiac arrest. *Resuscitation.* 2015;89:149-154.

237. Srinivasan V, et al. Calcium use during in-hospital pediatric cardiopulmonary resuscitation: a report from the National Registry of Cardiopulmonary Resuscitation. *Pediatrics.* 2008;121:e1144-e1151.

242. Ashwal S, et al. Prognostic implications of hyperglycemia and reduced cerebral blood flow in childhood near-drowning. *Neurology.* 1990;40:820-823.

246. Van den Berghe G, et al. Intensive insulin therapy in critically ill patients. *N Engl J Med.* 2001;345:1359-1367.

256. Samson RA, Berg RA, Bingham R. Use of automated external defibrillators for children: an update—an advisory statement from the Pediatric Advanced Life Support Task Force, International Liaison Committee on Resuscitation. *Pediatrics.* 2003;112:163-168.

259. Kern KB, et al. Depletion of myocardial adenosine triphosphate during prolonged untreated ventricular fibrillation: effect on defibrillation success. *Resuscitation.* 1990;20:221-229.

261. Atkinson E, et al. Specificity and sensitivity of automated external defibrillator rhythm analysis in infants and children. *Ann Emerg Med.* 2003;42:185-196.

276. Clark CB, et al. Pediatric transthoracic defibrillation: biphasic versus monophasic waveforms in an experimental model. *Resuscitation.* 2001;51:159-163.

279. Cecchin F, et al. Is arrhythmia detection by automatic external defibrillator accurate for children? Sensitivity and specificity of an automatic external defibrillator algorithm in 696 pediatric arrhythmias. *Circulation.* 2001;103:2483-2488.

280. Dorian P, et al. Amiodarone as compared with lidocaine for shock-resistant ventricular fibrillation. *N Engl J Med.* 2002;346:884-890.

281. Coumel P, Fidelle J. Amiodarone in the treatment of cardiac arrhythmias in children: One hundred thirty-five cases. *Am Heart J.* 1980;100:1063-1069.

299. Laurent I, et al. Reversible myocardial dysfunction in survivors of out-of-hospital cardiac arrest. *J Am Coll Cardiol.* 2002;40:2110-2116.

Performance of Cardiopulmonary Resuscitation in Infants and Children

Robert M. Sutton, Robert A. Berg, and Vinay M. Nadkarni

PEARLS

- The four distinct phases of cardiac arrest and cardiopulmonary resuscitation (CPR) are as follows:
  1. Prearrest
  2. No flow (untreated cardiac arrest)
  3. Low flow (CPR)
  4. Postresuscitation
- The most common precipitating event for cardiac arrests in children is respiratory insufficiency; adequate ventilation and oxygenation are high priority.
- High-quality CPR (ie, push hard, push fast, allow full chest recoil, minimize interruptions, and do not overventilate) can improve cardiac arrest outcomes.
- Real-time monitoring and feedback combined with reflective debriefings of team performance can improve CPR quality and survival outcomes.
- Attention to meticulous postresuscitation care, specifically blood pressure and targeted temperature management, can improve survival outcomes.
- Strategically focused therapies to specific phases of cardiac arrest and resuscitation can lead to more successful resuscitation in children.

Pediatric cardiac arrest is not a rare event. Approximately 16,000 American children (8-20/100,000 children/year) experience cardiopulmonary arrest each year.[1-7] Approximately half of these cardiac arrests occur in the hospital and about half outside the hospital.[5,8] In times past, survival outcomes were not good and many children had severe neurologic injury after their arrest event. With advances in resuscitation science and implementation techniques, survival from pediatric cardiac arrest has improved substantially since the 1990s.[9,10] This chapter focuses on pediatric cardiac arrest, cardiopulmonary resuscitation (CPR), and other therapeutic interventions that have been specifically designed to improve outcomes from pediatric cardiac arrest.

Four Phases of Cardiac Arrest

The four distinct phases of cardiac arrest and CPR interventions are (1) prearrest, (2) no flow (untreated cardiac arrest), (3) low flow (CPR), and (4) postresuscitation. Interventions

to improve the outcome of pediatric cardiac arrest should optimize therapies targeted to the time and phase of CPR, as suggested in Table 42.1.[11-14]

Prearrest

The prearrest phase refers to relevant preexisting conditions of the child (eg, sepsis, pulmonary hypertension, neurologic, cardiac, respiratory, or metabolic problems) and precipitating events (eg, respiratory failure, hypotensive shock, pulmonary hypertension). It is known that pediatric patients who suffer an in-hospital cardiac arrest often have changes in their physiologic status in the hours leading up to their arrest event.[11-14] Therefore interventions during the prearrest phase focus on preventing the cardiac arrest, with special attention to early recognition and treatment of respiratory failure and shock. Rapid response teams or medical emergency teams (METs) are in-hospital emergency teams designed specifically for this purpose. These teams respond to patients on general inpatient units who are at high risk of clinical decompensation and transfer these children to more acute care areas, with the goal to prevent progression to full cardiac arrest. Implementation of pediatric METs has been moderately successful; decreased cardiac arrest frequency and mortality have been demonstrated.[13-18] Although METs cannot identify all children at risk for cardiac arrest, it seems reasonable to assume that transferring critically ill children to an intensive care unit (ICU) early in their disease process for better monitoring and more aggressive interventions can improve resuscitative care and clinical outcome.

No Flow/Low Flow

To improve outcomes from pediatric cardiac arrest, it is imperative to shorten the no-flow phase of untreated cardiac arrest. To that end, it is important to monitor high-risk patients to allow early recognition of the cardiac arrest and initiate basic and advanced life support. Effective CPR optimizes coronary perfusion pressure and cardiac output to critical organs to support vital organ viability during the low-flow phase. Important tenets of basic life support are push hard, push fast, allow full chest recoil between compressions, and minimize interruptions of chest compression. Achieving optimal coronary perfusion pressure, exhaled carbon dioxide concentration, and cardiac output during the low-flow phase of CPR is consistently associated with an improved chance for the return of spontaneous circulation (ROSC) and improved short- and long-term outcome in both animal and human

TABLE 42.1   Phases of Cardiac Arrest and Targeted Interventions

Phase	Interventions
Prearrest phase: *Protect*	Optimize community education regarding child safety Optimize patient monitoring Prioritize interventions to prevent progression to cardiac arrest Early recognition and activation of medical emergency response teams
Arrest (no-flow): *Preserve*	Minimize interval to BLS and ACLS phase Organized 911/code blue response system Preserve cardiac and cerebral substrate Minimize interval to defibrillation, when indicated
Low-flow (CPR): *Resuscitate*	Effective CPR to optimize myocardial blood flow and cardiac output Avoid overventilation Consider adjuncts to improve vital organ perfusion during CPR Match oxygen delivery to oxygen demand Consider extracorporeal CPR if standard CPR/ALS are not promptly successful
Postresuscitation: *Regenerate* Short term	Optimize cardiac output and cerebral perfusion Treat arrhythmias, if indicated Prevent hyper/hypoglycemia, hyperthermia Consider mild resuscitative systemic hypothermia
Long term	Early intervention with occupational and physical therapy Bioengineering and technology interface rehabilitation Possible future role for stem cell transplantation

ACLS, advanced cardiovascular life support; *ALS,* advanced life support; *BLS,* basic life support; *CPR,* cardiopulmonary resuscitation.

studies.[19–29] For ventricular fibrillation (VF) and pulseless ventricular tachycardia (VT), rapid detection and prompt defibrillation are vital for successful resuscitation. For cardiac arrests resulting from asphyxia or ischemia, provision of adequate myocardial perfusion and myocardial oxygen delivery are most important.

Postresuscitation

The postresuscitation phase includes management of the immediate postresuscitation stage, the next few hours to days, hospital course, and long-term rehabilitation and reintegration to the community. The immediate postresuscitation stage is a high-risk period for ventricular arrhythmias and critical organ (eg, heart, brain, kidney) reperfusion injuries. Interventions during the immediate postresuscitation stage and the next few days include delivering adequate tissue oxygen, treating postresuscitation myocardial dysfunction, and minimizing postresuscitation tissue injury (eg, preventing postresuscitation hyperthermia, targeting temperature management, targeting blood pressure management, avoiding hyperglycemia/hypoglycemia, recognizing and promptly treating seizures, and preventing secondary organ injury). This postarrest phase may have the greatest potential for innovative advances in the understanding of cell injury and death, inflammation, mitochondrial dysfunction and recovery, apoptosis, and

hibernation, ultimately leading to novel interventions. The rehabilitation stage concentrates on salvaging injured cells, recruiting hibernating cells, and reengineering reflex and voluntary communications of these cell and organ systems to improve functional outcome.

The specific phase of resuscitation dictates the focus of care. Interventions that improve outcome during one phase may be deleterious during another. For instance, intense vasoconstriction during the low-flow phase of cardiac arrest improves coronary perfusion pressure and the probability of ROSC. The same intense vasoconstriction during the postresuscitation phase increases left ventricular afterload and may worsen myocardial strain and dysfunction. Current understanding of the physiology of cardiac arrest and recovery allows us to only crudely manipulate blood pressure, oxygen delivery and consumption, body temperature, and other physiologic parameters in our attempts to optimize outcome. Future strategies likely will take advantage of increasing knowledge of cellular inflammation, thrombosis, reperfusion, mediator cascades, cellular markers of injury and recovery, and transplantation technology.

An overview of some of the pathophysiologic pathways perturbed by cardiac arrest and resuscitation, along with potential avenues for intervention, is shown in Fig. 42.1.

Epidemiology of Pediatric Cardiac Arrest

Cardiovascular disease remains the most common cause of disease-related death in the United States, resulting in approximately 1 million deaths per year.[30,31] It is estimated that more than 400,000 Americans will have a cardiac arrest each year, more than 50% in prehospital settings. Although data regarding the incidence of childhood cardiopulmonary arrest are less robust, the best data suggest that about 16,000 American children suffer a cardiac arrest each year (annual incidence: 8 to 20 per 100,000 children per year).[1–5,32–34] For in-hospital arrests specifically, it is estimated that approximately 1.4% of all children admitted to pediatric intensive care units[1,2,8,35] and 4% to 6% of children admitted to cardiac units will suffer a cardiac arrest.[36–40] In short, pediatric cardiac arrest is an important public health problem.

Outcomes from pediatric cardiac arrest have improved significantly since the 1990s. More than 70% of children who have an in-hospital cardiac arrest are successfully resuscitated initially (ie, attain sustained ROSC). Moreover, more than 35% of them will survive to hospital discharge, and many (nearly 75%) will have good neurologic function.[1–4,9,37–39,41–76] Factors that influence outcome from pediatric cardiac arrest include (1) the preexisting condition of the child, (2) the initial electrocardiographic (ECG) rhythm detected, (3) the duration of no-flow time (the time during an arrest when there is no spontaneous circulation or provision of CPR), and (4) the quality of the life-supporting therapies provided during the resuscitation. With this knowledge, it is no surprise then that out-of-hospital pediatric arrests have worse outcomes compared to in-hospital arrests.[3,32,35,44,49,52,55,59,61,77–83] As many of these out-of-hospital events are not witnessed and bystander CPR is not common (approximately 30% to 40% of children receive bystander CPR),[3,84] the duration of no-flow time can be prolonged. As a result, less than 10% of these children survive their initial event, and neurologic injury is common in those who do survive. These findings are

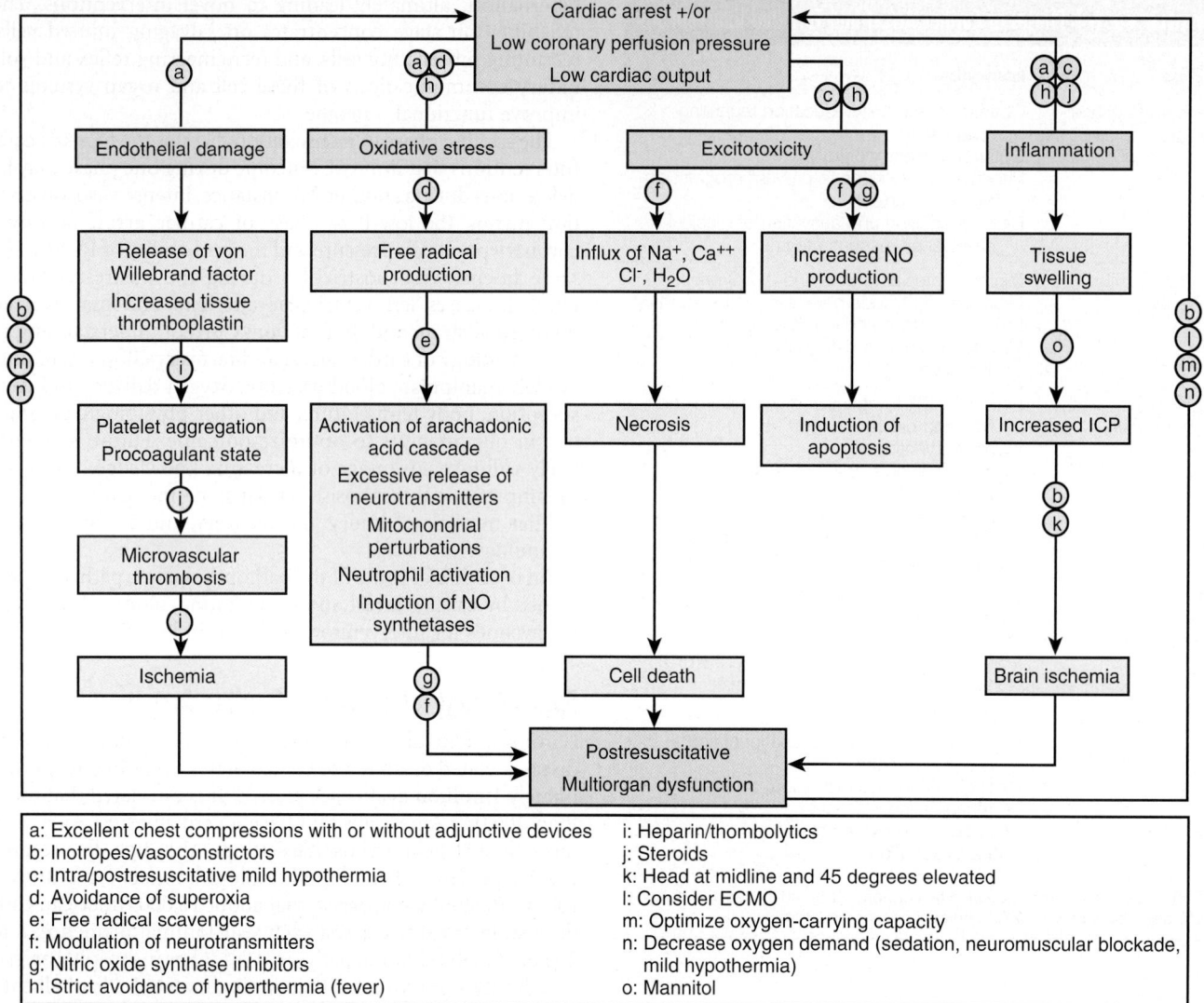

Fig. 42.1. Schematic of physiologic processes that result from cardiac arrest and initial resuscitation, with some promising interventions indicated by lowercase letters. Many complex interconnections and feedback loops among these processes are omitted from the schematic in order to generate an overview of the processes and potential interventions.

especially troublesome given that bystander CPR more than doubles patient survival rates.[85]

Compared to adults, superior survival rates are documented after pediatric cardiac arrest, specifically after in-hospital events; 27% of children survive to hospital discharge compared with only 17% of adults.[9] These findings may be due in part to differences in the initial ECG rhythm detected. Although pediatric arrests are less commonly caused by arrhythmias, such as ventricular tachycardia or ventricular fibrillation (10% of pediatric arrests versus 25% of adult arrests), the superior pediatric survival rate reflects a substantially higher survival rate among children with asystole or pulseless electrical activity compared with adults (24% versus 11%). Moreover, the higher survival rate seen in children is mostly attributable to a much better survival rate among infants and preschool-age children compared with older children.[86,87] Although this is speculative, the higher survival rates in children may be due to improved coronary and cerebral blood flow during CPR because of increased chest compliance in these younger arrest victims.[88,89]

Interventions During the Low-Flow Phase: Cardiopulmonary Resuscitation
Airway and Breathing

During the low-flow state of CPR, cardiac output and pulmonary blood flow are approximately 25% of that during normal sinus rhythm; therefore much less ventilation is necessary for adequate gas exchange from the blood traversing the pulmonary circulation. Moreover, animal and adult data indicate that a rapid rate of assisted ventilation (overventilation from exuberant rescue breathing) during CPR is common and can substantially compromise venous return and cardiac output by increasing intrathoracic pressure.[90–92] Moreover, these detrimental hemodynamic effects are compounded when one considers the effect of interruptions in CPR to provide airway management and rescue breathing.[93–98] Although overventilation is problematic, in light of the fact that most pediatric arrests are asphyxial in nature, provision of *adequate* ventilation is still important. The difference between arrhythmogenic and asphyxial arrests lies in the physiology.[27,28,99,100] In animal models of sudden VF cardiac arrest, acceptable PaO_2 and $PaCO_2$ persist for 4 to 8 minutes during chest compressions without rescue breathing.[101] This is in part because aortic oxygen and carbon dioxide concentrations at the onset of the arrest do not vary much from the prearrest state. As a result, the lungs act as a reservoir of oxygen during CPR, and adequate oxygenation and ventilation can continue without rescue breathing. However, during asphyxial arrest, blood continues to flow to tissues in the prearrest state, resulting in significant arterial and venous oxygen desaturation, elevated lactate levels, and depletion of the pulmonary oxygen reserve. Therefore at the onset of resuscitation, the arterial hypoxemia and acidemia are substantial. In this circumstance, rescue breathing with controlled ventilation can be lifesaving. In contrast, the adverse hemodynamic effects from overventilation during CPR combined with the interruptions in chest compressions to open the airway and deliver rescue breathing are lethal in certain circumstances such as VT/VF arrests. In short, the resuscitation technique should be titrated to the physiology of the patient to optimize patient outcome.

Circulation

Optimizing Blood Flow During Low-Flow Cardiopulmonary Resuscitation: Push Hard, Push Fast

When the heart arrests and no blood flows to the aorta, coronary blood flow ceases immediately.[102] At that point, the provision of high-quality CPR (push hard, push fast) is necessary to reestablish flow. The goal during CPR is to maximize the myocardial perfusion pressure (MPP), as related by the following equation:

$$MPP = \text{Aortic diastolic blood pressure (AoDP)} - \\ \text{Right atrial pressure (RAP)}$$

Myocardial blood flow improves as the gradient between AoDP and RAP increases. During the downward compression phase, aortic pressure rises at the same time as right atrial pressure with little change in the MPP. However, during the decompression phase of chest compressions, the right atrial pressure falls faster and lower than the aortic pressure, which generates a pressure gradient perfusing the heart with oxygenated blood during this artificial period of "diastole." Several animal and human studies have demonstrated in both VT/VF and asphyxial models the importance of establishing MPP as a predictor for short-term survival outcome (ROSC).[25,103–109]

Based on the preceding equation, MPP can be improved by strategies that increase the pressure gradient between the aorta and the right atrium. As an example, the inspiratory impedance threshold device (ITD) is a small, disposable valve that can be connected directly to the tracheal tube or facemask to augment negative intrathoracic pressure during the inspiratory phase of spontaneous breathing and the decompression phase of CPR by impeding airflow into the lungs. Application in animal and adult human trials of CPR has established the ability of the ITD to improve vital organ perfusion pressures and myocardial blood flow[93,110–113]; however, in a randomized trial during adult CPR, mortality benefit was limited to the subgroup of patients with pulseless electrical activity, and the quality of CPR was an important confounding factor.[114–117] Additional evidence that augmentation of negative intrathoracic pressure can improve perfusion pressures during CPR comes from the active compression-decompression device

(ACD). The ACD is a handheld device that is fixed to the anterior chest of the victim by means of suction—think household plunger—that can be used to apply active decompression forces during the release phase, thereby creating a vacuum within the thorax. By actively pulling during the decompression phase, blood is drawn back into the heart by the negative pressure.[118] Animal and adult studies have demonstrated that the combination of ACD with ITD acts in concert to further improve perfusion pressures during CPR compared to ACD alone.[111] In the end, although novel interventions such as the ITD and ACD are promising to improve blood flow during CPR, the basic tenants of "push hard, push fast, minimize interruptions, and do not overventilate" are still the dominant factors to improve blood flow during CPR and advance the chance of survival.

Chest Compression Depth

The pediatric chest compression depth recommendation of at least one-third anterior-posterior chest depth (approximately 4 cm in infants and 5 cm in children) is largely based on expert clinical consensus, using data extrapolated from animal, adult, and limited pediatric data. Maher and colleagues published data from a case series of infants postcardiac surgery associating arterial blood pressure with qualitative chest compression depths. In this small study of six infants, chest compressions targeted to one-half anterior-posterior chest depth improved systolic blood pressures compared to those at one-third anterior-posterior chest depth.[119] Though a small series with qualitatively estimated chest compression depths, this is the first study to collect actual data from children supporting the existing chest compression depth guidelines. On the contrary, two studies using computer-automated tomography[120,121] suggest that depth recommendations based on a relative (%) anterior-posterior chest compression depth are deeper than those recommended for adults, and that a one-half anterior-posterior chest depth is unattainable in most children. A report of 87 pediatric resuscitation events, most involving children >8 years, found that a compression depth >51 mm for more than 60% of the compressions during 30-second epochs within the first 5 minutes of cardiac arrest was associated with improved survival.[122] Thus the 2015 International Liaison Committee on Resuscitation (ILCOR) consensus on science and American Heart Association (AHA) guidelines recommend a compression depth of at least one-third the anterior-posterior diameter of the chest for children (birth to onset of puberty), which equates to approximately 1.5 inches (4 cm) in infants and 2 inches (5 cm) in children.[123,124] Once children reach puberty, a depth of at least 5 cm, but no more than 6 cm, is recommended. Future studies that collect data from actual children and that associate quantitatively measured chest compression depths with short- and long-term clinical outcomes (arterial blood pressure, end-tidal carbon dioxide, return of spontaneous circulation, survival) are needed.

Compression/Ventilation Ratios

The amount of ventilation provided during CPR should match, but not exceed, perfusion and should be titrated to the amount of circulation during the specific phase of resuscitation as well as the metabolic demand of the tissues. Therefore during the low-flow state of CPR when the amount of cardiac output is roughly 25% of normal, less ventilation is needed.[125]

However, the best ratio of compressions to ventilations in pediatric patients is largely unknown and depends on many factors including the compression rate, the tidal volume, the blood flow generated by compressions, and the time that compressions are interrupted to perform ventilations. Evidence has demonstrated that a compression/ventilation ratio of 15:2 delivers the same minute ventilation and increases the number of delivered chest compressions by 48% compared to CPR at a compression/ventilation ratio of 5:1 in a simulated pediatric arrest model.[126,127] This is important because when chest compressions cease, the aortic pressure rapidly decreases and coronary perfusion pressure falls rapidly.[102] Increasing the ratio of compressions to ventilations minimizes these interruptions, thus increasing coronary blood flow. These findings are in part the reason the 2015 AHA guidelines recommend a pediatric compression/ventilation ratio of 15:2.

Duty Cycle
In a model of human adult cardiac arrest, cardiac output and coronary blood flow are optimized when chest compressions last for 30% of the total cycle time (approximately 1:2 ratio of time in compression to time in relaxation).[128] As the duration of CPR increases, the optimal duty cycle may increase to 50%. In a juvenile swine model, a relaxation period of 250 to 300 milliseconds (duty cycle of 40% to 50% at a compression rate of 120/min) correlates with improved cerebral perfusion pressures compared with shorter duty cycles of 30%.[129]

Circumferential Versus Focal Sternal Compressions
In adult and animal models of cardiac arrest, circumferential (vest) CPR has been demonstrated to improve CPR hemodynamics dramatically.[130] In smaller infants, it is often possible to encircle the chest with both hands and depress the sternum with the thumbs while compressing the thorax circumferentially (thoracic squeeze). In an infant animal model of CPR, this two-thumb method of compression with thoracic squeeze resulted in higher systolic and diastolic blood pressures and a higher pulse pressure than traditional two-finger compression of the sternum.[131]

Open-Chest Cardiopulmonary Resuscitation
Excellent standard closed-chest CPR generates cerebral blood flow that is approximately 25% of normal. By contrast, open-chest CPR can generate cerebral blood flow that approaches normal. Whereas open-chest massage improves coronary perfusion pressure and increases the chance of successful defibrillation in animals and humans,[132–134] performing a thoracotomy to allow open-chest CPR is impractical in many situations. A retrospective review of 27 cases of CPR following pediatric blunt trauma (15 with open-chest CPR and 12 with closed-chest CPR) demonstrated that open-chest CPR increased hospital cost without altering rates of ROSC or survival to discharge. However, survival in both groups was 0%, indicating that the population may have been too severely injured or too late in the process to benefit from this aggressive therapy.[135] Earlier institution of open-chest CPR may warrant reconsideration in selected special resuscitation circumstances.

Medications Used to Treat Cardiac Arrest
Although animal studies have indicated that epinephrine can improve initial resuscitation success after both asphyxial and VF cardiac arrests, no single medication has been shown to improve survival outcome from pediatric cardiac arrest. A variety of medications are used during pediatric resuscitation attempts including vasopressors (epinephrine or vasopressin), antiarrhythmics (amiodarone or lidocaine), and other drugs such as calcium chloride and sodium bicarbonate. Each is discussed separately next.

Vasopressors
Epinephrine (adrenaline) is an endogenous catecholamine with potent α- and β-adrenergic stimulating properties. The α-adrenergic action (vasoconstriction) increases systemic and pulmonary vascular resistance. The resultant higher aortic diastolic blood pressure improves coronary perfusion pressure and myocardial blood flow even though it reduces global cardiac output during CPR. The adequacy of myocardial blood flow is a critical determinant of ROSC. Epinephrine also increases cerebral blood flow during CPR because peripheral vasoconstriction directs a greater proportion of flow to the cerebral circulation.[136–138] However, evidence suggests that epinephrine can decrease local cerebral microcirculatory blood flow at a time when global cerebral flow is increased.[139] The β-adrenergic effect increases myocardial contractility and heart rate and relaxes smooth muscle in the skeletal muscle vascular bed and bronchi; however, the β-adrenergic effects are not observed in the peripheral vascular beds secondary to the high dose used in cardiac arrest. Epinephrine also increases the vigor and intensity of VF, boosting the likelihood of successful defibrillation. One study showed that among children with in-hospital cardiac arrest with an initial nonshockable rhythm who received epinephrine, delay in the administration of epinephrine >5 minutes from time of cardiac arrest was associated with a decreased chance of survival to hospital discharge with a favorable neurologic outcome.[140]

High-dose epinephrine (0.05–0.2 mg/kg) improves myocardial and cerebral blood flow during CPR more than standard-dose epinephrine (0.01–0.02 mg/kg) in animal models of cardiac arrest and may increase the incidence of initial ROSC.[141,142] Administration of high-dose epinephrine, however, can worsen a patient's postresuscitation hemodynamic condition. Retrospective studies indicate that use of high-dose epinephrine in adults or children may be associated with a worse neurologic outcome.[143,144] A randomized, controlled trial of rescue high-dose epinephrine versus standard-dose epinephrine following failed initial standard-dose epinephrine in pediatric in-hospital cardiac arrest demonstrated a worse 24-hour survival in the high-dose epinephrine group (1/27 versus 6/23, p <.05).[145] Based on these clinical data, high-dose epinephrine cannot be recommended routinely for either initial or rescue therapy.[146]

Vasopressin is a long-acting endogenous hormone that acts on specific receptors to mediate systemic vasoconstriction (V_1 receptor) and reabsorption of water in the renal tubule (V_2 receptor). The vasoconstriction is most intense in the skeletal muscle and skin vascular beds. Unlike epinephrine, vasopressin is not a pulmonary vasoconstrictor. In experimental models of cardiac arrest, vasopressin increases blood flow to the heart and brain and improves long-term survival compared with epinephrine. However, vasopressin can decrease splanchnic blood flow during and following CPR and can increase afterload in the postresuscitation period.[147–151] Adult randomized controlled trials suggest that outcomes are similar after the use of vasopressin or epinephrine during CPR.[152,153] During pediatric arrest, a case series of four children who received vasopressin during six prolonged cardiac arrest events suggested that the use of bolus vasopressin may result in ROSC when standard medications have failed.[154] However, a more recent retrospective study of 1293 consecutive pediatric arrests from the National Registry of CPR (NRCPR) found that vasopressin use, though infrequent (administered in only 5% of events), was associated with a lower likelihood of ROSC. Therefore it is unlikely that vasopressin will replace epinephrine as a first-line agent in cases of pediatric cardiac arrest. However, the available data suggest that its use in conjunction with epinephrine may deserve further investigation.

Calcium

Calcium is used frequently in cases of cardiac arrest, despite the lack of evidence for efficacy when it is administered routinely during resuscitation attempts. In the absence of a documented clinical indication (ie, hypocalcemia, calcium channel blocker overdose, hypermagnesemia, or hyperkalemia), administration of calcium does not improve outcome from cardiac arrest.[51,155–163] To the contrary, three pediatric studies have suggested a potential for harm, as routine calcium administration was associated with decreased survival rates or worse neurologic outcomes.[51,155,156]

Buffer Solutions

There are no randomized controlled studies in children examining the use of sodium bicarbonate for management of pediatric cardiac arrest. Two randomized controlled studies have examined the value of sodium bicarbonate in the management of adult cardiac arrest[164] and in neonates with respiratory arrest in the delivery room.[165] Neither was associated with improved survival. One multicenter retrospective in-hospital pediatric study found that sodium bicarbonate administered during cardiac arrest was associated with decreased survival, even after controlling for age, gender, and first documented cardiac rhythm.[155] Therefore during pediatric cardiac arrest resuscitation, the routine use of sodium bicarbonate is *not* recommended.

Clinical trials involving critically ill adults with severe metabolic acidosis did not demonstrate a beneficial effect of sodium bicarbonate on hemodynamics despite correction of acidosis.[166,167] However, the presence of severe acidosis may depress the action of catecholamines, so the use of sodium bicarbonate may be considered in an acidemic child who is refractory to catecholamine administration.[168,169] Acidosis may increase the threshold for myocardial stimulation in a patient with an artificial cardiac pacemaker[170]; therefore administration of bicarbonate or another buffer is appropriate for management of severe documented acidosis in these children. Administration of sodium bicarbonate also is indicated in the patient with a tricyclic antidepressant overdose, hyperkalemia, hypermagnesemia, or sodium channel blocker poisoning. The buffering action of bicarbonate occurs when a hydrogen cation and a bicarbonate anion combine to form carbon dioxide and water. If carbon dioxide is not effectively cleared through ventilation, its buildup counterbalances the buffering effect of bicarbonate. Because carbon dioxide readily penetrates cell membranes, intracellular acidosis may increase without adequate ventilation. Therefore bicarbonate should not be used to manage respiratory acidosis.

Unlike sodium bicarbonate, tromethamine (THAM) buffers excess protons without generating carbon dioxide. Carbon dioxide is consumed following THAM administration. In a patient with limited ventilation, tromethamine may be preferable when buffering is necessary. Tromethamine undergoes renal elimination, and renal insufficiency may be a relative contraindication to its use. Carbicarb, an equimolar combination of sodium bicarbonate and sodium carbonate, is another buffering solution that generates less carbon dioxide than sodium bicarbonate. In a canine model of cardiac arrest comparing animals given normal saline, sodium bicarbonate, THAM, or Carbicarb, the animals given any buffer solution had a higher rate of ROSC than the animals given normal saline. In the animals given sodium bicarbonate or Carbicarb, the interval to ROSC was significantly shorter than in animals given normal saline. However, at the end of the 6-hour study period, all resuscitated animals were in a deep coma, so no inferences regarding meaningful survival can be drawn.[171] The AHA does not recommend either THAM or other alternatives over bicarbonate when a buffering agent is desired during CPR.[146]

Postresuscitation Interventions

Targeted Temperature Management

Hyperthermia following cardiac arrest is common in children, and fever following cardiac arrest is associated with poor neurologic outcome.[172,173] Two seminal articles addressing adult out-of-hospital VF cardiac arrest have established that mild induced hypothermia (32°C-34°C) is a clinically promising goal-directed postresuscitation therapy. In these randomized studies of comatose patients older than 18 years after VF cardiac arrest, outcomes were improved.[174,175] However, extrapolation of these findings to the pediatric arrest victim is difficult, as fever, trauma, stroke, and other ischemic conditions, common in pediatric cardiac arrest, are associated with poor neurologic outcome. Neonatal trials of selective brain cooling and systemic cooling show promise in neonatal hypoxic-ischemic encephalopathy, suggesting that induced hypothermia may improve outcomes.[176,177] Using an approach of *therapeutic normothermia* with scheduled administration of antipyretic medications and the use of external cooling devices may be necessary to prevent hyperthermia in this population.

A large multicenter, prospective, randomized study of children aged 2 days to 18 years who remained comatose after out-of-hospital cardiac arrest (OHCA) found a strong trend of 20% versus 12% survival with favorable neurologic outcome, but no significant difference in survival with good functional outcome at 1 year and no additional complications in comatose patients who were treated with therapeutic hypothermia (32°C-34°C), compared to those treated with normothermia (36°C-37.5°C). Additional observational data of children resuscitated from either in-hospital cardiac arrest (IHCA) or OHCA[178–180] have suggested that ICU duration of stay, neurologic outcomes, and mortality are not improved with therapeutic hypothermia. However, one small study of therapeutic hypothermia in survivors of pediatric asphyxia cardiac arrest[181] showed an improvement in survival to hospital discharge, but without a significant difference in neurologic outcome. At the time of publication, results are pending from a large multicenter randomized controlled trial of targeted temperature management for pediatric patients with IHCA (Therapeutic Hypothermia After Cardiac Arrest website: www.THAPCA.org). Thus the AHA states that for infants and children remaining comatose after OHCA, it is reasonable either to maintain 5 days of continuous normothermia (36°C-37.5°C) or to maintain 2 days of initial continuous hypothermia (32°C-34°C) followed by 3 days of continuous normothermia. Continuous measurement of temperature during this time period is recommended and fever (temperature 38°C or higher) should be aggressively treated.[182]

Glucose Control

Both hyperglycemia and hypoglycemia following cardiac arrest are associated with worse neurologic outcome.[183–186] Although it seems intuitive that hypoglycemia would be associated with worse neurologic outcome, whether hyperglycemia per se is harmful or is simply a marker of the severity of the stress hormone response from prolonged ischemia is not clear. In critically ill adult patients, tight glucose control using an insulin infusion was associated with improved survival.[187,188] However, subsequent studies of nonsurgical adult populations and neonatal/pediatric trials have demonstrated no survival benefit or the potential for harm when rates of inadvertent hypoglycemia were high during treatment.[186,189–196] Using the available data, there is insufficient evidence to formulate a strong recommendation on the management of hyperglycemia in children with ROSC following cardiac arrest. If hyperglycemia is treated following ROSC in pediatric patients, blood glucose concentrations should be carefully monitored to avoid hypoglycemia.

Blood Pressure Management

Compared with healthy volunteers, adults resuscitated from cardiac arrest have impaired autoregulation of cerebral blood flow.[197] Hence they may not maintain adequate cerebral blood flow in the context of low systemic pressure and, likewise, may not be able to protect the brain from excessive blood flow and microvascular perfusion pressure in the context of systemic hypertension. However, in animal models, briefly induced hypertension following resuscitation improves neurologic outcome compared with normotensive reperfusion.[198,199] Therefore a practical approach to blood pressure management following cardiac arrest is to attempt to minimize blood pressure variability in this high-risk period following resuscitation. Three small observational studies after pediatric IHCA and OHCA[200–202] demonstrated worse survival to hospital discharge when children exhibited hypotension after ROSC. One of these studies associated post-ROSC hypotension (defined as a systolic blood pressure less than the fifth percentile for age) after IHCA with a lower likelihood of survival to discharge with favorable neurologic outcome. In 2015, the AHA recommended that a systolic blood pressure >5 percentile for age be maintained. Continuous arterial blood pressure monitoring is recommended to rapidly identify and effectively treat hypotension.[202,203]

Postresuscitation Myocardial Dysfunction

Postarrest myocardial stunning and arterial hypotension occur commonly after successful resuscitation in both animals and humans.[174,175,204–211] Animal studies demonstrate that postarrest myocardial stunning is a global phenomenon with biventricular systolic and diastolic dysfunction. This postarrest myocardial stunning is pathophysiologically and physio-logically similar to sepsis-related myocardial dysfunction and post–cardiopulmonary bypass myocardial dysfunction, including increases in inflammatory mediators and nitric oxide production.[204,206,207,210] Because cardiac function is essential to reperfusion following cardiac arrest, management of postarrest myocardial dysfunction may be important to improving survival. The classes of agents used to maintain circulatory function (ie, inotropes, vasopressors, and vasodilators) must be carefully titrated during the postresuscitation phase to the patient's cardiovascular physiology. Trials in animal models have shown that various vasoactive medications can effectively ameliorate postarrest myocardial dysfunction (eg, dobutamine, milrinone, levosimendan).[212–216] Similarly, in human observational studies, fluid resuscitation and various vasoactive medications (ie, epinephrine, dobutamine, and dopamine) have been provided for myocardial dysfunction syndrome.[174,175,205–209,217,218] In the end, optimal use of these agents involves close goal-directed titration, and the use of invasive hemodynamic monitoring may be appropriate.

Other Considerations
Quality of Cardiopulmonary Resuscitation

The quality of health care provider CPR during adult resuscitations typically does not comply with American Heart Association clinical practice guidelines. Long CPR-free intervals, shallow chest compressions, incorrect chest compression rates, and overventilation are common.[219,220] The quality of CPR performed during the resuscitation attempt is directly related to patient outcome.[94,221,222] Studies have shown in adults and in children that patients with a witnessed cardiac arrest[4] and those who receive bystander CPR[223] have an increased chance of survival. Those who suffer their in-hospital cardiac arrest at night or during weekends (presumably when the quality of resuscitation is not as good as in the daytime or on weekdays) have higher mortality.[224] Furthermore, pediatric outcomes are improved in hospitals staffed with highly trained pediatric-specific providers.[32] Taken together, these findings establish that the quality of resuscitative care, specifically early high-quality CPR, is an important determinate of patient survival.

In an effort to improve CPR quality, CPR-monitoring defibrillators with audiovisual feedback have been used during adult resuscitation, and CPR quality and clinical outcomes have improved.[222,225] The combination of focused bedside training and automated feedback defibrillators improved CPR guideline compliance of in-hospital providers.[226] However, there were still significant portions of the resuscitation that suffered from substandard resuscitative care. The addition of environmental debriefings has been demonstrated to improve short- and long-term outcomes following cardiac arrest in the ICU.[227]

Extracorporeal Membrane Oxygenation Cardiopulmonary Resuscitation

Venoarterial extracorporeal membrane oxygenation (ECMO) has been increasingly used as a rescue therapy during CPR, especially for potentially reversible acute postoperative myocardial dysfunction or arrhythmias. Studies of extracorporeal CPR (E-CPR) have demonstrated favorable early survival outcomes in children with primary cardiac disease when E-CPR protocols were in place at the time of the arrest.[45,228–239] Interestingly, data have been mixed regarding the relationship between outcome and CPR duration before ECMO cannulation. CPR and ECMO are not curative treatments. They are simply cardiopulmonary supportive measures that restore tissue perfusion until the patient has recovered from the precipitating disease process. As such, they can be powerful tools. Thus E-CPR should be considered for children with cardiac arrest who have heart disease amenable to recovery or transplantation, if the arrest occurs in a highly supervised environment such as an intensive care unit with existing clinical protocols and available expertise and equipment to rapidly initiate extracorporeal life support (ECLS).

Ventricular Fibrillation and Ventricular Tachycardia in Children

Pediatric VF or VT has been an underappreciated pediatric problem. Reports indicate that VF and VT (ie, shockable rhythms) occur in 27% of in-hospital cardiac arrests at some time during the resuscitation.[42] In a population of pediatric cardiac intensive care unit patients, as many as 41% of arrests were associated with VF or VT.[36] According to the NRCPR database, during in-hospital arrest, 10% of children had an initial rhythm of VF/VT. In all, 27% of the children had VF/VT at some time during the resuscitation.[42] The incidence of VF varies by setting and age.[240] In special circumstances, such as tricyclic antidepressant overdose, cardiomyopathy, status post–cardiac surgery, and prolonged QT syndromes, VF and pulseless VT are more likely.

The treatment of choice for short-duration VF is prompt defibrillation. In general, the mortality rate increases by 7% to 10% per minute of delay to defibrillation. Because VF must be considered before defibrillation can be provided, early determination of the rhythm by electrocardiography is critical. An attitude that VF is rare in children can be a self-fulfilling prophecy with a uniformly fatal outcome. The recommended defibrillation dose is 2 J/kg, but the data supporting this recommendation are not optimal and are based on old monophasic defibrillators. In the mid-1970s, authoritative sources recommended starting doses of 60 to 200 J for all children. Because of concerns for myocardial damage and animal data suggesting that shock doses ranging from 0.5 to 1 J/kg were adequate for defibrillation in a variety of species, Gutgesell and colleagues evaluated the efficacy of their strategy to defibrillate with 2 J/kg monophasic shocks. Seventy-one transthoracic defibrillations in 27 children were evaluated. Shocks within 10 J of 2 J/kg resulted in successful defibrillation in 91% of defibrillation attempts. The major determinant of successful defibrillation other than VF duration is countershock current. This current depends on the defibrillator energy and transthoracic impedance. Studies in children indicate that the transthoracic impedance of infants and children greatly overlap. Although there is a statistically significant correlation between size and transthoracic impedance, the correlation is weak. These studies provide only weak support for the present dogma that the defibrillator energy dose should vary directly with weight. Although the limited data regarding pediatric defibrillation used monophasic waveform shocks, most modern defibrillators use biphasic waveform shocks. Defibrillation with these biphasic waveforms is theoretically safer and more effective than monophasic waveform defibrillation.

Therefore the use of 2 to 4 J/kg biphasic waveform shocks should be at least as effective as 2 to 4 J/kg monophasic shocks and possibly safer.

Antiarrhythmic Medications: Lidocaine and Amiodarone

The administration of antiarrhythmic medications should not delay the administration of shocks to a patient with VF. However, after an unsuccessful attempt at electrical defibrillation, medications to increase the effectiveness of defibrillation should be considered. Epinephrine is the current first-line medication for both pediatric and adult patients in VF. If epinephrine and a subsequent repeat attempt to defibrillate are unsuccessful, lidocaine or amiodarone should be considered.

Lidocaine traditionally has been recommended for shock-resistant VF in adults and children. In one study, amiodarone improved survival to hospital admission (but not hospital discharge) in the setting of adult shock-resistant VF compared with placebo.[241] In another study of shock-resistant out-of-hospital VF, patients receiving amiodarone had a higher rate of survival to hospital admission than patients receiving lidocaine.[242] A study of adult shock-resistant VF did not show benefit of either amiodarone or lidocaine compared with placebo, but the drugs were administered late in the course of resuscitation.[243] None of these studies included children. An observational analysis of the American Heart Association Get With the Guidelines-Resuscitation registry showed an association of improved ROSC and short-term survival with lidocaine, and not with amiodarone, for pediatric refractory VF in the in-hospital setting.[244] Because there is moderate experience with amiodarone use as an antiarrhythmic agent in children and because of the adult studies, it is rational to use amiodarone similarly in children with shock-resistant VF/VT. The recommended dosage is 5 mg/kg by rapid intravenous bolus. There are no published prospective or randomized comparisons of antiarrhythmic medications for pediatric refractory VF. Although extrapolation of adult data and electrophysiologic mechanistic information suggest that amiodarone may be preferable for pediatric shock-resistant VF, the optimal choice is not clear.

Pediatric Automated External Defibrillators

Automated external defibrillators (AEDs) have improved adult survival from VF.[245,246] AEDs are recommended for use in children 8 years or older with cardiac arrest.[247,248] The available data suggest that some AEDs can accurately diagnose VF in children of all ages, but many AEDs are limited because the defibrillation pads and energy dosage are configured for adults. Adapters having smaller defibrillation pads that dampen the amount of energy delivered have been developed as attachments to adult AEDs, allowing their use in children. However, it is important that the AED diagnostic algorithm is sensitive and specific for pediatric VF and VT. Four studies have been conducted demonstrating the accuracy of AEDs to recognize pediatric arrhythmias. Case reports suggest AEDs can be used in children, including infants. The algorithms used by AEDs have high sensitivity and specificity for pediatric arrhythmias and rarely recommended a shock inappropriately. The energy doses delivered by AEDs are high, but they are below the range demonstrated to cause harm in laboratory animal studies of shock toxicity. The diagnostic algorithms from several AED manufacturers have been tested for such sensitivity and specificity and therefore can be reasonably used in younger children.

Summary

Outcomes from pediatric cardiac arrest and CPR appear to be improving. Perhaps the evolving understanding of pathophysiologic events during and after pediatric cardiac arrest and the developing fields of pediatric critical care and pediatric emergency medicine have contributed to these apparent improvements. In addition, exciting breakthroughs in basic and applied science laboratories, such as E-CPR, are on the immediate horizon for study in specific subpopulations of cardiac arrest victims. By strategically focusing therapies to specific phases of cardiac arrest, there is great promise that critical care interventions will lead the way to more successful cardiopulmonary and cerebral resuscitation in children.

Key References

1. Slonim AD, Patel KM, Ruttimann UE, Pollack MM. Cardiopulmonary resuscitation in pediatric intensive care units. *Crit Care Med.* 1997;25: 1951-1955.
2. Suominen P, Olkkola KT, Voipio V. Utstein style reporting of in-hospital paediatric cardiopulmonary resuscitation. *Resuscitation.* 2000;45:17-25.
3. Young KD, Seidel JS. Pediatric cardiopulmonary resuscitation: a collective review. *Ann Emerg Med.* 1999;33:195-205.
4. Donoghue AJ, Nadkarni V, Berg RA, et al. Out-of-hospital pediatric cardiac arrest: an epidemiologic review and assessment of current knowledge. *Ann Emerg Med.* 2005;46:512-522.
5. Atkins DL, Everson-Stewart S, Sears GK, et al. Epidemiology and outcomes from out-of-hospital cardiac arrest in children. The resuscitation outcomes consortium epistry of cardiac arrest. *Circulation.* 2009;119: 1484-1491.
6. Atkins DL, Berger S. Improving outcomes from out-of-hospital cardiac arrest in young children and adolescents. *Pediatr Cardiol.* 2012;33: 474-483.
7. Rajan S, et al. Out-of-hospital cardiac arrests in children and adolescents: incidences, outcomes, and household socioeconomic status. *Resuscitation.* 2015;88:12-19.
8. Berg RA, Nadkarni VM, Clark AE, et al. Incidence and Outcome of CPR in PICUs. *Crit Care Med.* 2016;44(4):798-808.
9. Nadkarni VM, Larkin GL, Peberdy MA, et al. First documented rhythm and clinical outcome from in-hospital cardiac arrest among children and adults. *JAMA.* 2006;295:50-57.
10. IOM (Institute of Medicine). *Strategies to improve cardiac arrest survival: a time to act.* Washington, DC: The National Academies Press; 2015: 60-61.
11. Buist MD, Jarmolowski E, Burton PR. Recognising clinical instability in hospital patients before cardiac arrest or unplanned admission to intensive care. A pilot study in a tertiary-care hospital. *Med J Aust.* 1999;171: 22-25.
12. Chaplik S, Neafsey PJ. Pre-existing variables and outcome of cardiac arrest resuscitation in hospitalized patients. *Dimens Crit Care Nurs.* 1998; 17:200-207.
13. Brady PW, Zix J, Brilli R, et al. Developing and evaluating the success of a family activated medical emergency team: a quality improvement report. *BMJ Qual Saf.* 2015;24:203-211.
14. Bonafide CP, Localio AR, Song L, et al. Cost-benefit analysis of a medical emergency team in a children's hospital. *Pediatrics.* 2014;134:235-241.
15. Brilli RJ, Gibson R, Luria JW, et al. Implementation of a medical emergency team in a large pediatric teaching hospital prevents respiratory and cardiopulmonary arrests outside the intensive care unit. *Pediatr Crit Care Med.* 2007;8:236-246.
16. Sharek PJ, Parast LM, Leong K, et al. Effect of a rapid response team on hospital-wide mortality and code rates outside the ICU in a children's hospital. *JAMA.* 2007;298:2267-2274.
17. Tibballs J, Kinney S. Reduction of hospital mortality and of preventable cardiac arrest and death on introduction of a pediatric medical emergency team. *Pediatr Crit Care Med.* 2009;10:306-312.
18. Raymond TT, Bonafide CP, Praestgaard A, et al. American Heart Association Get With the Guidelines–Resuscitation Investigators. Pediatric medical emergency team events and outcomes: a report of 3647 events from the American Heart Association's Get With the Guidelines–Resuscitation Registry. *Hosp Pediatr.* 2016;6:57-64.
19. Kern KB, Carter AB, Showen RL, et al. Twenty-four hour survival in a canine model of cardiac arrest comparing three methods of manual cardiopulmonary resuscitation. *J Am Coll Cardiol.* 1986;7:859-867.
20. Kern KB, Ewy GA, Voorhees WD. Myocardial perfusion pressure: a predictor of 24-hour survival during prolonged cardiac arrest in dogs. *Resuscitation.* 1988;16:241-250.
21. Kern KB, Lancaster L, Goldman S, Ewy GA. The effect of coronary artery lesions on the relationship between coronary perfusion pressure and myocardial blood flow during cardiopulmonary resuscitation in pigs. *Am Heart J.* 1990;120:324-333.
22. Sanders AB, Ewy GA, Taft TV. Prognostic and therapeutic importance of the aortic diastolic pressure in resuscitation from cardiac arrest. *Crit Care Med.* 1984;12:871-873.
23. Sanders AB, Kern KB, Atlas M. Importance of the duration of inadequate coronary perfusion pressure on resuscitation from cardiac arrest. *J Am Coll Cardiol.* 1985;6:113-118.
24. Sanders AB, Kern KB, Otto CW. End-tidal carbon dioxide monitoring during cardiopulmonary resuscitation. A prognostic indicator for survival. *JAMA.* 1989;262:1347-1351.
25. Paradis NA, Martin GB, Rivers EP, et al. Coronary perfusion pressure and the return of spontaneous circulation in human cardiopulmonary resuscitation. *JAMA.* 1990;263:1106-1113.
26. Ornato JP, Levine RL, Young DS. The effect of applied chest compression force on systemic arterial pressure and end-tidal carbon dioxide concentration during CPR in human beings. *Ann Emerg Med.* 1989;18:732-737.
27. Friess SH, Sutton RM, French B, et al. Hemodynamic directed CPR improves cerebral perfusion pressure and brain tissue oxygenation. *Resuscitation.* 2014;85:1298-1303.
28. Sutton RM, Friess SH, Maltese MR, et al. Hemodynamic-directed cardiopulmonary resuscitation during in-hospital cardiac arrest. *Resuscitation.* 2014;85:983-986.
29. Sutton RM, French B, Nishisaki A, et al. American Heart Association cardiopulmonary resuscitation quality targets are associated with improved arterial blood pressure during pediatric cardiac arrest. *Resuscitation.* 2013;84:168-172.
30. Zheng ZJ, Croft JB, Giles WH, Mensah GA. Sudden cardiac death in the United States, 1989 to 1998. *Circulation.* 2001;104:2158-2163.
31. IOM (Institute of Medicine). *Strategies to improve cardiac arrest survival: a time to act.* Washington, DC: The National Academies Press; 2015.
32. Donoghue AJ, Nadkarni VM, Elliott M, Durbin D. American Heart Association National Registry of Cardiopulmonary Resuscitation Investigators. Effect of hospital characteristics on outcomes from pediatric cardiopulmonary resuscitation: a report from the national registry of cardiopulmonary resuscitation. *Pediatrics.* 2006;118:995-1001.
33. Atkins DL, Berger S. Improving outcomes from out-of-hospital cardiac arrest in young children and adolescents. *Pediatr Cardiol.* 2012;33: 474-483.
34. Rajan S, et al. Out-of-hospital cardiac arrests in children and adolescents: incidences, outcomes, and household socioeconomic status. *Resuscitation.* 2015;88:12-19.
35. Kuisma M, Suominen P, Korpela R. Paediatric out-of-hospital cardiac arrests: epidemiology and outcome. *Resuscitation.* 1995;30:141-150.
36. Rhodes JF, Blaufox AD, Seiden HS, et al. Cardiac arrest in infants after congenital heart surgery. *Circulation.* 1999;100(suppl 19):194-199.
37. Parra DA, Totapally BR, Zahn E, et al. Outcome of cardiopulmonary resuscitation in a pediatric cardiac intensive care unit. *Crit Care Med.* 2000;28:3296-3300.
38. Gupta P, Jacobs JP, Pasquali SK, et al. Epidemiology and outcomes after in-hospital cardiac arrest after pediatric cardiac surgery. *Ann Thorac Surg.* 2014;98:2138-2143, discussion 2144.
39. Lowry AW, Knudson JD, Cabrera AG, et al. Cardiopulmonary resuscitation in hospitalized children with cardiovascular disease: estimated prevalence and outcomes from the kids' inpatient database. *Pediatr Crit Care Med.* 2013;14:248-255.
40. Ortmann L, Prodhan P, Gossett J, et al. American Heart Association's Get With the Guidelines–Resuscitation Investigators. Outcomes after in-hospital cardiac arrest in children with cardiac disease: a report from Get With the Guidelines–Resuscitation. *Circulation.* 2011;124:2329-2337.

41. Reis AG, Nadkarni V, Perondi MB. A prospective investigation into the epidemiology of in-hospital pediatric cardiopulmonary resuscitation using the international Utstein reporting style. *Pediatrics.* 2002;109:200-209.

42. Samson RA, Nadkarni VM, Meaney PA, et al. Outcomes of in-hospital ventricular fibrillation in children. *N Engl J Med.* 2006;354:2328-2339.

43. Hintz SR, Benitz WE, Colby CE, et al. Utilization and outcomes of neonatal cardiac extracorporeal life support: 1996-2000. *Pediatr Crit Care Med.* 2005;6:33-38.

44. Lopez-Herce J, Garcia C, Dominguez P, et al. Outcome of out-of-hospital cardiorespiratory arrest in children. *Pediatr Emerg Care.* 2005;21:807-815.

45. Thiagarajan RR, Laussen PC, Rycus PT. Extracorporeal membrane oxygenation to aid cardiopulmonary resuscitation in infants and children. *Circulation.* 2007;116:1693-1700.

46. Tibballs J, Kinney S. A prospective study of outcome of in-patient paediatric cardiopulmonary arrest. *Resuscitation.* 2006;71:310-318.

47. Chamnanvanakij S, Perlman JM. Outcome following cardiopulmonary resuscitation in the neonate requiring ventilatory assistance. *Resuscitation.* 2000;45:173-180.

48. Torres A Jr, Pickert CB, Firestone J. Long-term functional outcome of inpatient pediatric cardiopulmonary resuscitation. *Pediatr Emerg Care.* 1997;13:369-373.

49. Tunstall-Pedoe H, Bailey L, Chamberlain DA. Survey of 3765 cardiopulmonary resuscitations in British hospitals (the BRESUS Study): methods and overall results. *BMJ.* 1992;304:1347-1351.

86. Meaney PA, Nadkarni VM, Cook EF, et al. Higher survival rates among younger patients after pediatric intensive care unit cardiac arrests. *Pediatrics.* 2006;118:2424-2433.

Respiratory System

Structure and Development of the Upper Respiratory System in Infants and Children

Robert H. Chun and Joan C. Arvedson

PEARLS

- The structures of the upper airway undergo extensive changes from infancy through young adulthood. An understanding of the numerous variations, congenital anomalies, and resulting special vulnerabilities of the developing airway and underlying illness should result in improved health outcomes and a lower morbidity rate in children with airway disease.
- The upper and lower respiratory tracts develop separately. Thus there are few coincident congenital anomalies between these two contiguous areas.
- An understanding of possible congenital anomalies of the airway will improve diagnosis and treatments.

The respiratory tract can be divided into the upper or conducting airways and the lower or gaseous exchange airways. For the purposes of this chapter, the trachea down to the carina is included as part of the "upper" or conducting airways. The upper airway shares its development with that of the upper digestive tract, and the lower airway shares its development with the cardiovascular system.

Developmental Anatomy of the Upper Airway

The embryologic development of the nasal cavity, mouth, nasopharynx, and hypopharynx occurs in a separate environment from that of the larynx, trachea, bronchi, and lung parenchyma. Because the upper airway and lower respiratory tract develop separately, there are few coincident congenital anomalies between these two contiguous but developmentally distinct areas.

The branchial arches derived from the neural crest cells begin to appear during the fourth week of embryogenesis. The branchial arches give rise to formation of the face, neck, nasal cavities, mouth, larynx, pharynx, and striated muscles in the head and neck that are involved in breathing and swallowing. The development of these structures is usually complete by week 14.

The respiratory system, including parts of the larynx, trachea, and lungs, also begins to appear during week 4, when the laryngotracheal groove develops into a diverticulum that subsequently separates from the pharynx. In the fourth and fifth weeks, the longitudinal tracheoesophageal folds fuse, forming the tracheoesophageal septum and dividing the foregut into ventral and dorsal portions. The ventral portion becomes the larynx, trachea, bronchi, and lungs, and the dorsal portion becomes the esophagus. Abnormalities in development of the esophagus and trachea can lead to tracheoesophageal fistula (TEF). A rare but significant tracheoesophageal fistula is the H type that could present with recurrent lower airway disease (Fig. 43.1).

The embryogenesis of the larynx is complex. The cartilages and muscles are derived from the fourth and sixth branchial arches. The epithelium is derived from the endoderm of the laryngotracheal tube. As this epithelium proliferates rapidly, the larynx is temporarily occluded until the 10th week, when recanalization occurs. Failure to recanalize can result in laryngeal webs, stenosis, or, rarely, atresia (Fig. 43.2). The epiglottis forms by mesenchymal proliferation of the third and fourth branchial arches (Fig. 43.3).

Another developmental abnormality is a laryngeal cleft that presents as a defect in the posterior arytenoid muscles and sometimes tracheal cartilage leading to aspiration. The cleft can vary from mild to severe depending on the extent of the defect that may extend from the top of the cricoid cartilage into the thoracic trachea (Fig. 43.4). Findings on videofluoroscopic swallow studies (VFSSs) are suspicious for laryngeal cleft when liquid is seen to move into the trachea posteriorly and lower than typically seen with simple delayed airway closure. Those findings typically lead to further workup to include operative endoscopy with palpation of the larynx, which is the definitive diagnostic procedure.

The tracheobronchial tree also has several embryonic origins. Its epithelium is derived from the laryngotracheal tube. The connective tissue, cartilages, and muscles are derived from the surrounding splanchnic mesenchyme. All cartilages of the trachea are C-shaped with a membranous posterior tracheal wall, giving the airway flexibility to expand, except for the cricoid cartilage immediately below the true vocal folds. The cricoid cartilage is anatomically considered part of the larynx. It is the only cartilage in the airway to form a complete

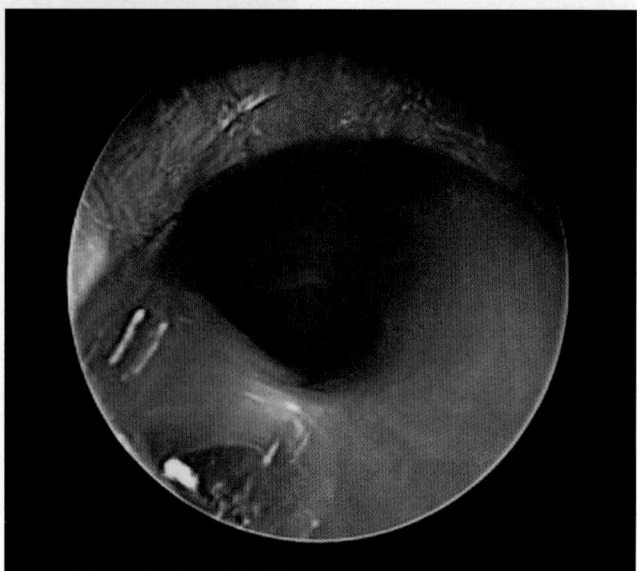

Fig. 43.1. Bronchoscopy with trachea above with tracheoesophageal fistula below.

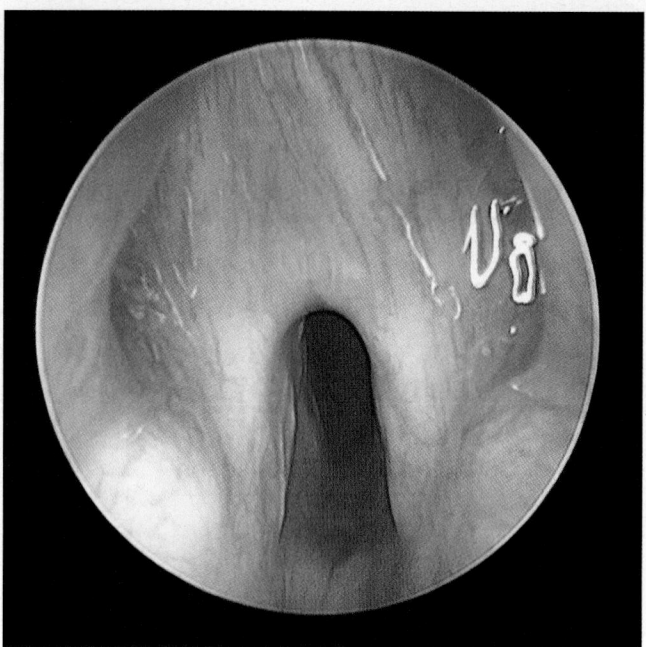

Fig. 43.2. Laryngeal web.

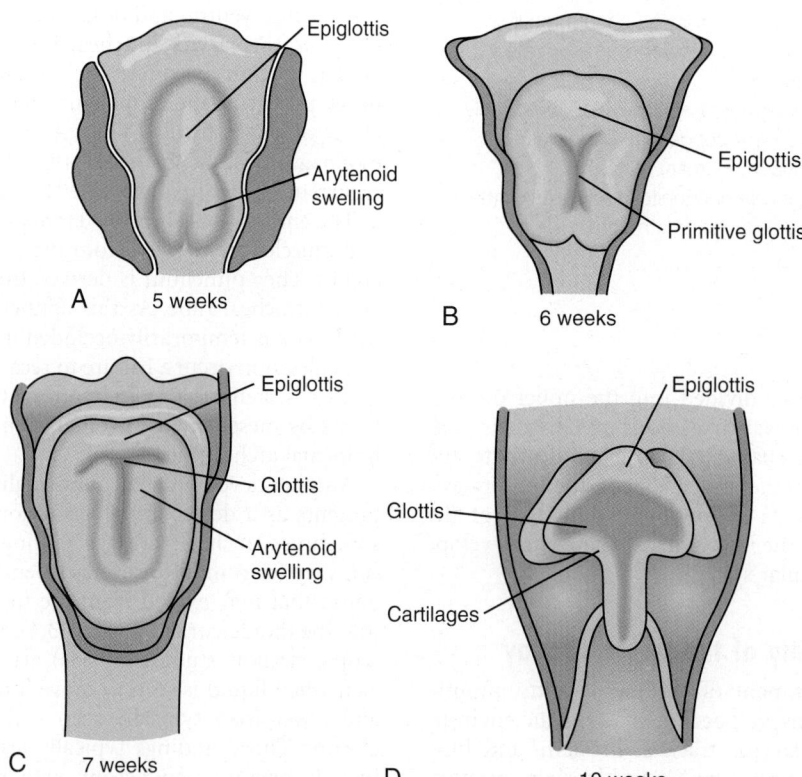

Fig. 43.3. (A–D) Embryologic development of the larynx. (Modified from Arvedson J, Brodsky L. Pediatric Swallowing and Feeding: Assessment and Management. 2nd ed. Boston: Thomson Learning [Cengage Learning]; 2002.)

ring. Because of its inflexibility, edema from intubation and inflammation can result in serious injury that should be avoidable in most cases.

Laryngeal web or subglottic stenosis can present with stridor, likely biphasic, and respiratory distress in a newborn infant (Fig. 43.5). While medical treatment such as steroids, racemic epinephrine, heliox, or intubation may manage these infants in the acute setting, many infants with congenital webs or stenosis will need surgical intervention. Laryngeal atresia that is not diagnosed prenatally will lead to often fatal respiratory distress at birth (Fig. 43.6). The infants' mothers will likely present with severe polyhydramnios and fetal

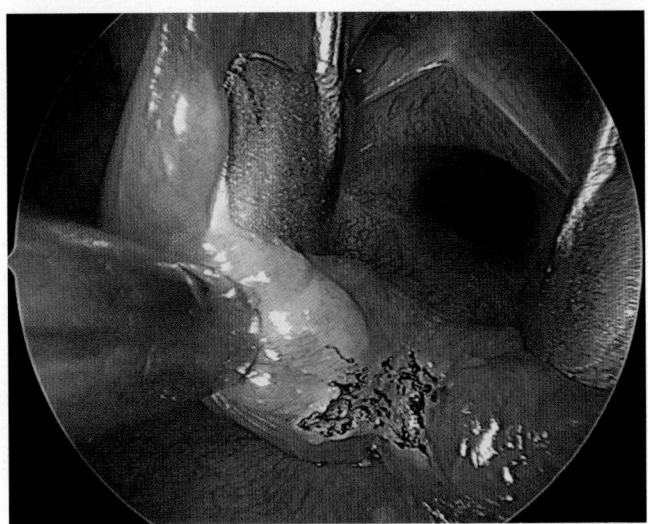

Fig. 43.4. Laryngeal cleft during repair.

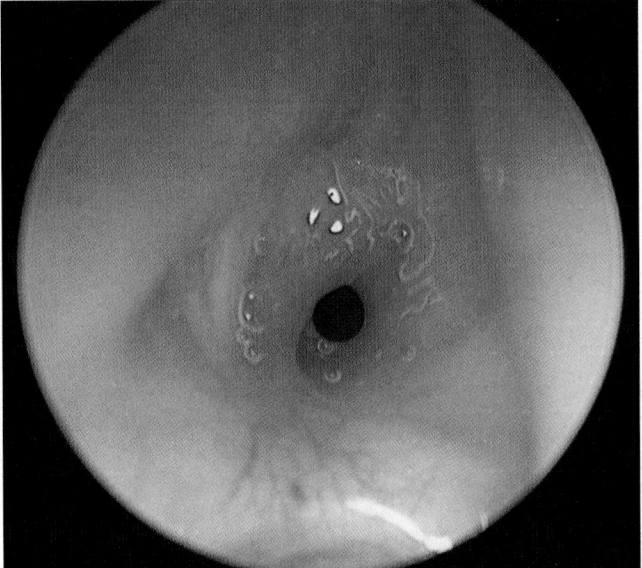

Fig. 43.5. Subglottic stenosis.

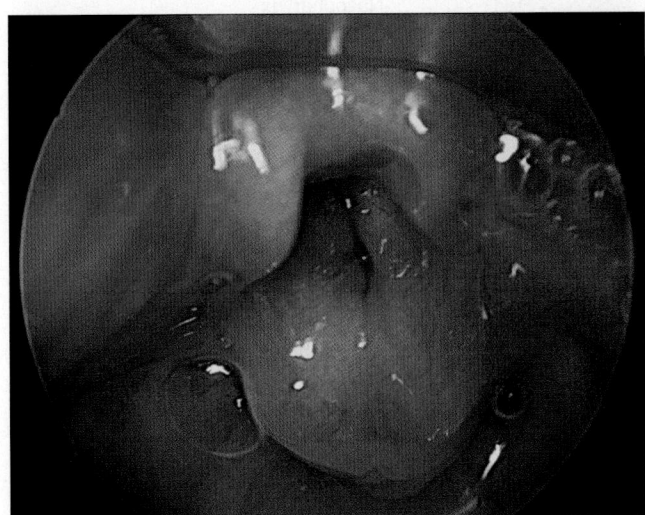

Fig. 43.6. Laryngeal atresia.

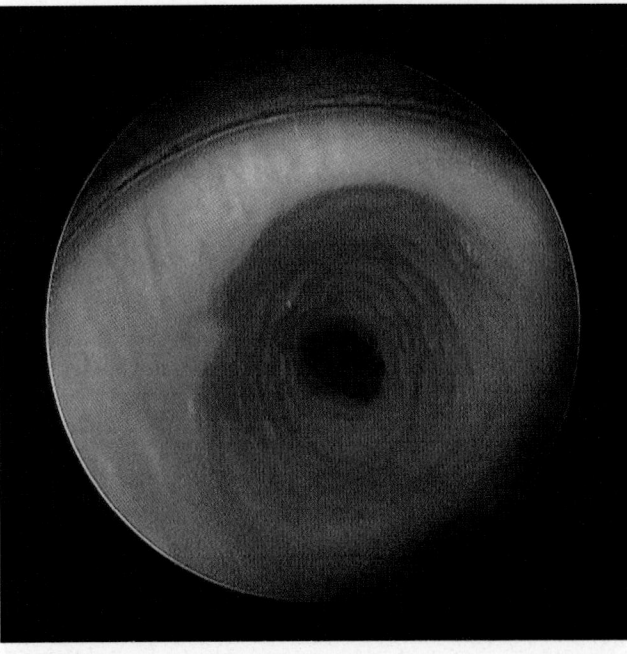

Fig. 43.7. Bronchoscopy demonstrating distal complete tracheal rings.

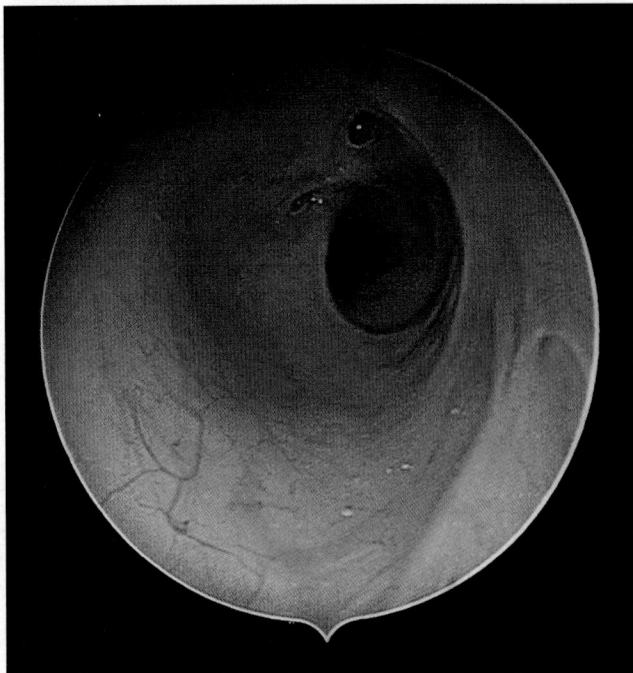

Fig. 43.8. Congenital tracheal stenosis.

hyperinflation of the lungs. Fetal MRI assists in the diagnosis. A tracheostomy in the newborn period is necessary in coordination with an ex utero intrapartum treatment for airway management.

Abnormalities of the lower airway can lead to critical airway distress. Although the only normal complete tracheal ring is the cricoid cartilage, complete tracheal rings or tracheal stenosis can lead to difficult intubations and respiratory distress. Depending on the severity of distress and tracheal stenosis, surgical management is needed in the majority of cases (Figs. 43.7 and 43.8). Children with Down syndrome can present with multilevel airway problems as a result of midface hypoplasia, a small nasopharynx, relatively large tongue, and a congenitally narrowed subglottic space. If a child with Down syndrome requires intubation, a smaller endotracheal that is one half size to one full size lower than a child with a normal airway should be used.

Anatomy and Physiology of the Upper Airway
Nasal Passages

The upper airway begins at the tip of the nose and the vermilion border of the lips. Both the nasal and oral passages allow air to stream from the environment through the larynx into the lungs, where oxygen and carbon dioxide are exchanged in alveolar-capillary units. Oral passages (oral cavity, oropharynx, and hypopharynx) are conduits for ingestion of the food and liquid needed to support growth and development.

The structures of the upper airways of the infant (Fig. 43.9) gradually change in the first few years of life to assume their adult configuration (Fig. 43.10). Preferential nasal breathing is present in typical term neonates and persists until 6 months of age because of the high position of the larynx in the neck with the soft palate and valleculae in close anatomic approximation. Nasal breathing is a necessary underpinning for nipple feeding at the breast or bottle in order for infants to coordinate sucking, swallowing, and breathing sequencing.

Infants with upper airway obstruction who require enteral feeds are served better with an orogastric (OG) tube than a nasogastric (NG) tube and oxygen delivered by mask rather than by nasal cannula to avoid obstruction and injury to this area. The nasal cavity courses posteriorly to reach the nasopharynx.

The adenoid pad is located in the nasopharynx and sits against the muscles covering the cervical spine at the base of the skull. During the first several years of life, the adenoid may enlarge. In most instances the adenoids involute between age 8 and puberty unless ongoing inflammation occurs as a result of allergy, infection, or gastrointestinal reflux.

In the newborn infant, abnormal development of the nasal cavity can lead to airway obstruction. Pyriform aperture stenosis is an overgrowth of the maxillary crest leading to anterior nasal obstruction. Choanal atresia is a failure of recanalization of the posterior nasopharynx leading to obstruction that may be unilateral or bilateral (Fig. 43.11). An oral airway or intubation can bypass these airway obstructions in an acute setting. Choanal atresia is associated with CHARGE syndrome. Pyriform aperture stenosis is associated with holoprosencephaly, pituitary abnormalities, and central mega incisor syndrome. Therefore comprehensive genetic and systemic evaluations are critical.

The nasal passage is divided by the nasal septum, which is cartilaginous anteriorly and bony posteriorly. Injury to the anterior nasal septum is not uncommon with the use of nasal tubes, nasal cannula, or nonhumidified oxygen because of the thin epithelium overlying the cartilage anteriorly. Bacterial colonization frequently occurs when the nasal passages become dry and stasis of secretions occurs. In the critically ill patient, injury to this anterior mucosa can lead to epistaxis. This can be treated with pressure, oxymetazoline, and packing if needed.

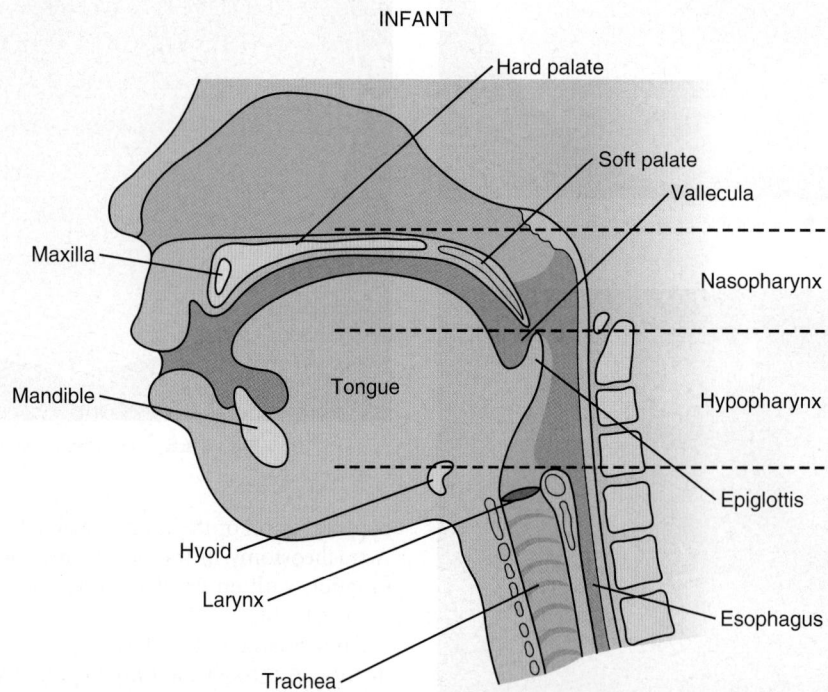

INFANT

Fig. 43.9. Lateral view of the infant's upper airway. The soft palate and valleculae form a tongue and groove relationship that effectively separates the oral cavity from the nasal cavity during the first 6 months of infancy when most children are primarily nasal breathers. This anatomic proximity effectively separates the oral route for ingestion from the nasal route for respiration. Anterior placement of the larynx has implications for intubation technique. (Modified from Arvedson J, Brodsky L. Pediatric Swallowing and Feeding: Assessment and Management. 2nd ed. Boston: Cengage Learning; 2002.)

OLDER CHILD

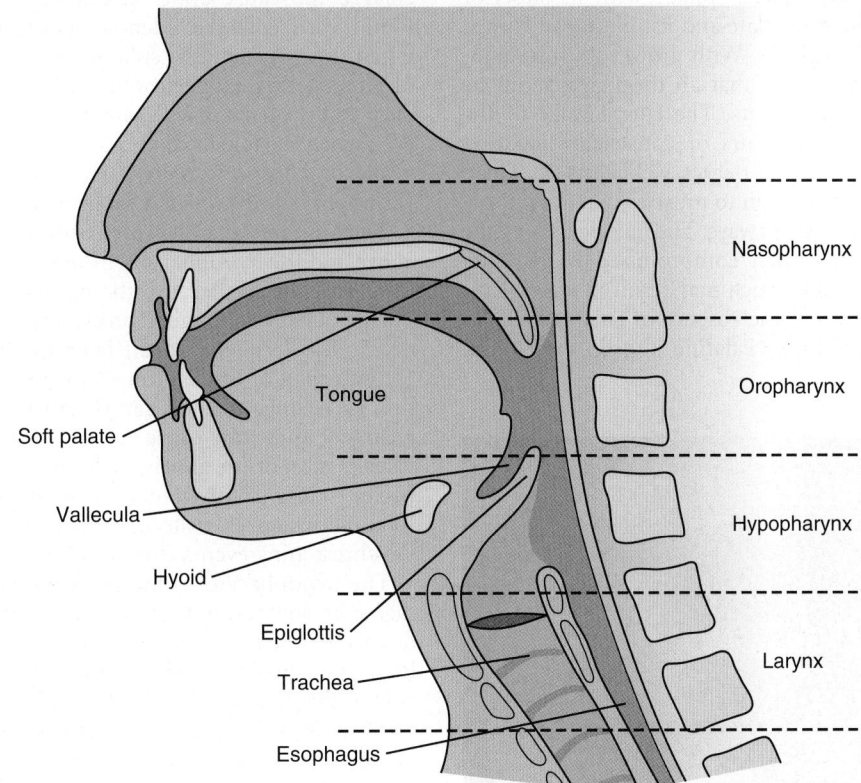

Nasopharynx

Oropharynx

Tongue

Soft palate

Hypopharynx

Vallecula

Hyoid

Epiglottis

Larynx

Trachea

Esophagus

Fig. 43.10. Lateral view of the older child's upper airway. Note the development of the oropharynx, a shared passage for eating and breathing. The tongue occupies less of the oral cavity. The larynx sits lower in the neck, which is unique to humans and has allowed for the development of human speech production. However, the shared passageway with the digestive system creates challenges in airway protection, particularly during intubation. (Modified from Arvedson J, Brodsky L. Pediatric Swallowing and Feeding: Assessment and Management. 2nd ed. Boston: Cengage Thomson Learning; 2002.)

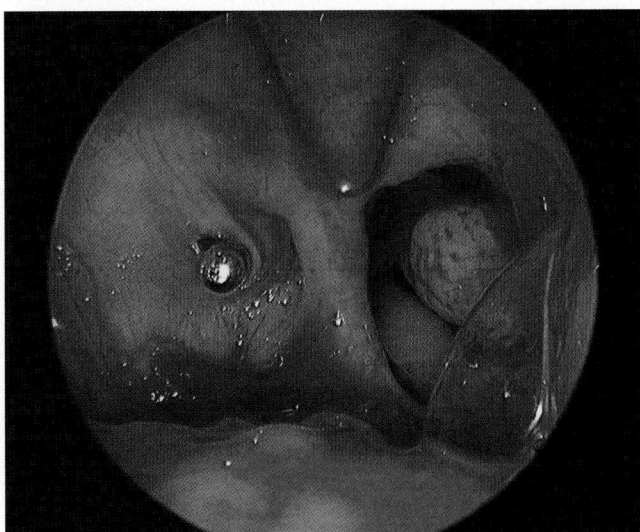

Fig. 43.11. Unilateral choanal atresia undergoing repair. Posterior view.

The ostia of the paranasal sinuses drain into the nasal cavity. Any obstruction secondary to tubes or inflammation can lead to poor mucus clearance, bacterial overgrowth, and sinusitis. In the critically ill and immunocompromised patient, invasive fungal sinusitis can be a rare but fatal source for fever of unknown origin. Nasal endoscopy and possible biopsy and debridement are needed for evaluation of this disease (Fig. 43.12).

Mouth (Oral Cavity) and Pharynx

The structures of the oral cavity include the lips, teeth, tongue, palate, and palatine tonsils. The anterior structures are primarily involved in speech and bolus preparation of food and liquid. The tongue in young infants fills the oral cavity. Children with Beckwith-Wiedemann syndrome have macroglossia. The tongue often protrudes out of the mouth. In some instances, tongue reduction may be necessary or the airway may need to be bypassed. Some craniofacial anomalies are characterized by micrognathia or retrognathia, when even a normal- or smaller-sized tongue may be posteriorly placed, causing upper airway obstruction. Glossoptosis can produce airway obstruction that prevents ventilation by natural or mechanical means. In the critical care setting, an endotracheal tube may be required to bypass the obstruction. Infants with Pierre Robin sequence (micrognathia, glossoptosis, posterior U-shaped cleft palate) may present with severe airway obstruction, especially in supine positioning. Nasal trumpets, oxygen, prone positioning, and intubation may be necessary in the critical setting for airway management. Intubation is difficult with usually a grade 3 to 4 (Cormack and Lehane) laryngeal view. Fiberoptic intubation may be helpful.

The oropharynx that is not seen in young infants begins posterior to the posterior tonsillar pillars with its superior border at the edge of the soft palate and its inferior border at the superior tip of the epiglottis. With growth and development, the pharynx elongates so that an oropharynx can be noted between ages 2 and 3 years. The lateral walls of the pharynx consist of the three pairs of constrictor muscles, which are innervated by cranial nerves V, IX, and X. These cranial nerves provide innervation to muscles that are important in protection of the lower airways. The muscle tone of the pharyngeal constrictors is often compromised in children with neurologic impairment, which may result in airway collapse and obstruction even in the absence of enlarged tonsils and adenoid or glossoptosis. Palatine tonsils are found laterally, and when chronically or severely inflamed, they may enlarge and cause upper airway obstruction similar to that found with enlarged adenoid at the nasopharyngeal level. Often, but not always, enlargement of tonsils and adenoid occurs together. Hypertrophied palatine tonsils can be noted deep in the pharynx with lateral view VFSS in some children even when the tonsils did not appear markedly enlarged upon visual oral inspection. Hypertrophied tonsils may interfere with bolus transit of solid foods in some children.

The oropharynx is the crossroads for the nasopharynx from above and the hypopharynx from below. Infants have no distinct oropharynx because the nasopharynx is contiguous to the hypopharynx. Lingual tonsil hypertrophy in older children occurs less frequently than hypertrophy of palatine tonsils. Hypertrophy of lingual tonsils may result in airway obstruction or feelings of food getting stuck in the pharynx. When enlarged, they can cause airway obstruction that prevents visualization of the glottis. Vallecular cysts may present in the newborn infant with dysphagia and upper airway obstruction. In some instances, vallecular cysts are associated with acute life-threatening events (Fig. 43.13).

The hypopharynx is the most inferior of the shared passageways for respiration and deglutition. Superiorly it is defined by the tip of the epiglottis, which in the adult is at the level of the hyoid bone in the neck, a relationship that is variable in the infant and child. The inferior border of the hypopharynx is at the level of the cricopharyngeus muscle, which is the primary muscle unit in the upper esophageal sphincter located directly posterior to the cricoid cartilage. Protection of the airway occurs in this area, particularly during deglutition. The anterior boundary of the hypopharynx is the larynx. Although immunization has nearly eradicated epiglottitis, toxic-appearing children with stertor, respiratory difficulty, and drooling should still have epiglottis or necrotizing epiglottis in the differential diagnosis (Fig. 43.14). The critical treatment is operative airway management with possibility of tracheotomy.

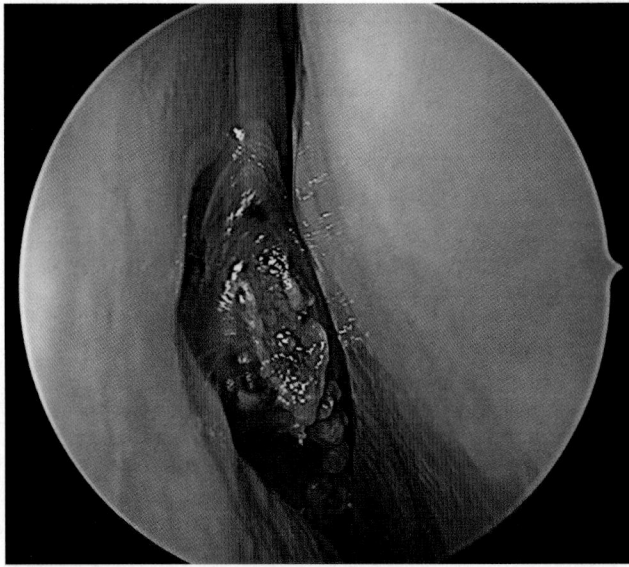

Fig. 43.12. Invasive fungal sinusitis of right necrotic middle turbinate.

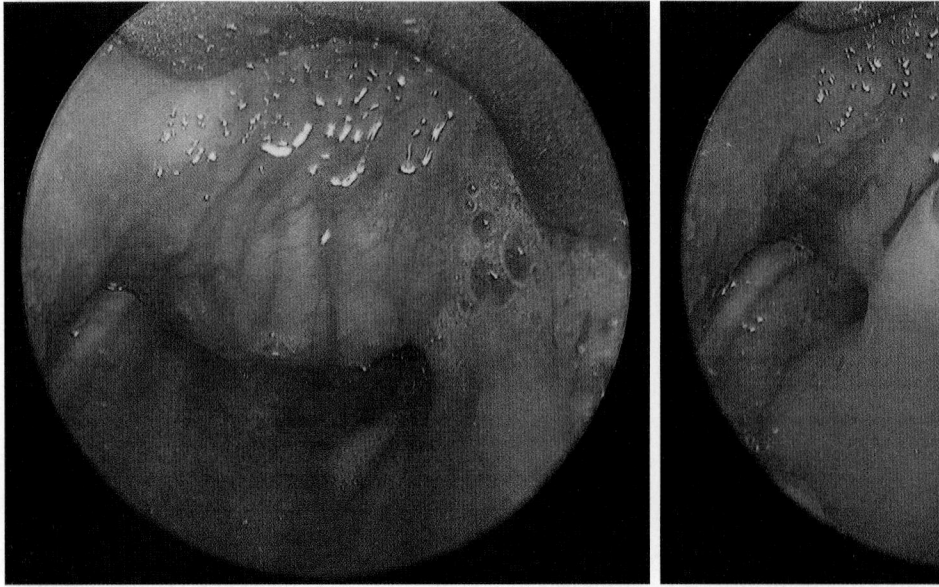
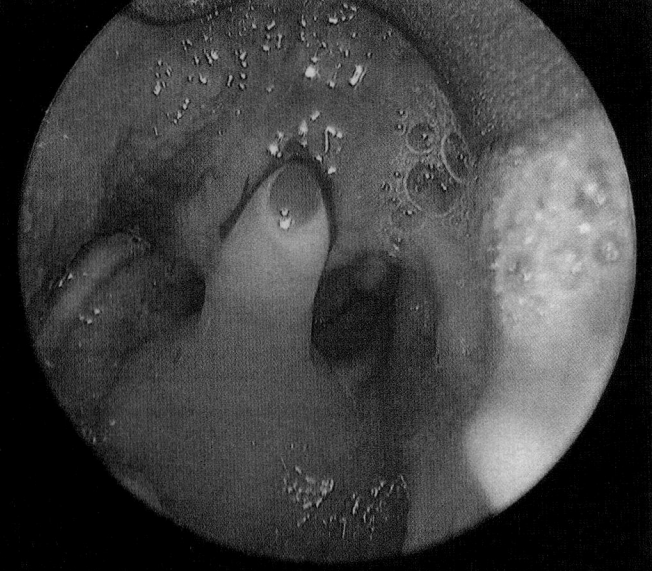

Fig. 43.13. Vallecular cyst at the base of tongue.

Larynx

The larynx is a complex structure of cartilage, ligaments, and muscles involved in respiration, protection of the lower airways, and phonation. The larynx begins at the level of the true vocal folds and extends to the inferior border of the cricoid cartilage.

Proper airflow requires that the larynx have functioning vocal folds so that during inspiration there is abduction of the true vocal folds, allowing the least restrictive inflow of air. During expiration, slight adduction occurs and the false vocal folds (also known as the ventricular folds) modulate the expiratory airflow.

Protection of the lower airways is key to survival. Prevention of aspiration of secretions or ingested food requires multilevel coordination of several sphincters. The most superior level is the epiglottis, which has a flattened lingual surface directing secretions laterally and posteriorly as it folds into the larynx during deglutition. The paired arytenoid cartilages sit at the posterior aspect of the larynx and provide the next level of protection. These cartilages, along with the coordination of the aryepiglottic folds, contract medially to close the glottis.

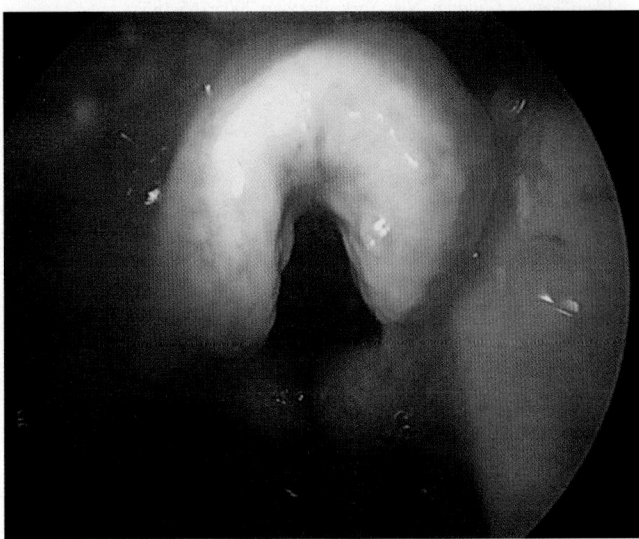

Fig. 43.14. Necrotizing epiglottitis.

Simultaneously, the larynx is elevated and pulled forward by hyolaryngeal excursion, which provides the airway with further protection during swallowing. Finally, the paired true and false vocal folds adduct and provide yet another level of protection. During quiet respiration, the highly innervated larynx repels unwanted secretions by the highly sensitive cough reflex, mediated primarily through cranial nerves IX and X. In the intubated, often sedated, or paralyzed child, these protective mechanisms are absent and the dangers of aspiration of secretions become of great concern. Frequent suctioning of oral cavity secretions may reduce this risk but is unlikely to eliminate aspiration completely.

Innervation of the larynx for its protective and respiratory functions is located centrally in the brain stem, making it reflexive. The sensory and motor innervations to this area are critical to proper function. Thus following prolonged intubation, immediate return of function is unrealistic. A cautionary approach to the reestablishment of oral feeds is prudent. Another issue to consider is that intubation may cause recurrent laryngeal nerve injury with vocal fold paralysis or paresis. The mechanism for this injury is believed to result from pressure on the cricoarytenoid joint close to where the nerve enters the larynx.

Children presenting with bilateral vocal fold paralysis should be evaluated for their airway obstruction, as well as for intracranial or thoracic causes of their obstruction, such as an Arnold-Chiari malformation. Unilateral vocal fold paralysis is a known complication following pediatric heart surgery, especially patent ductus arteriosus (PDA) ligation. Spontaneous recovery may occur in 25% to 45% of cases in 1 to 2 years of time. If feeding, voice, and breathing are appropriate, no intervention is required.

Laryngomalacia is a prolapsing of the posterior arytenoid mucosa and foreshortened aryepiglottic folds that cause a spectrum of airway obstruction. Laryngomalacia is characterized by inspiratory stridor, associated airway obstruction, and dysphagia. Most children (>80%) outgrow this condition, but children with sleep apnea, failure to thrive, and pectus excavatum many need further surgical management. Nearly 20% of these children will also have a synchronous airway lesion in the lower airway.

Anatomic differences between the upper aerodigestive tracts of infants and children are listed in Table 43.1.

TABLE 43.1	Anatomic Airway Differences Between Infants and Children	
Anatomic Location	**Infant**	**Older Child**
Oral cavity	Tongue fills mouth Edentulous Tongue rests between lips and sits against palate Relatively smaller mandible	Mouth is larger, tongue rests on the floor of the mouth Dentulous Tongue rests behind teeth and not against palate Mandibular-maxillary relationship relatively normal
Pharynx	No definite/distinct oropharynx Obtuse angle at skull base in nasopharynx	Elongation from nasopharynx through hypopharynx with distinct oropharynx 90-degree angle at skull base
Larynx/ tracheobronchial tree	One-third adult size Half of true vocal fold is cartilage Narrow, vertical epiglottis Subglottis size in a full-term newborn neonate fits a 3.5 uncuffed endotracheal tube Tracheal rings more compliant	Less than one-third of true vocal fold is cartilage Flat, wide epiglottis Subglottis enlarges with age

Modified from Arvedson J, Brodsky L. Pediatric Swallowing and Feeding: Assessment and Management. 2nd ed. Boston: Thomson Learning; 2002.

Trachea and Bronchi

Inferior to the larynx is the trachea. It conducts air to the bronchi, which branch to ever smaller lumen tubes that eventually become alveoli, the anatomic location of gas exchange. The trachea is made of cartilaginous rings that are essentially the same diameter until they reach the carina, where the trachea splits into left and right main stem bronchi.

The right main stem bronchus is shorter, wider, and takes off at a less acute angle than does the left main stem bronchus. Bronchial foreign body aspiration is seen more often in the right main stem bronchus than in the left main stem bronchus. Bronchial intubation is more often encountered on the right. The right main stem bronchus leads to the right upper, middle, and lower lobes of the lungs.

The left main stem bronchus is longer, narrower, and more acutely angled than the right main stem bronchus. Its bronchi lead to the left lower and upper lobes. As mentioned previously, these airways are lined by pseudostratified, ciliated columnar epithelium. This epithelium is readily injured through suctioning. Prolonged intubation, particularly after tracheotomy, results in diffuse squamous metaplasia. Without functioning cilia, airway secretions remain in the airway and can be the source of irritation, inflammation, and atelectasis, all complicating factors in the management of the upper airway during a critical illness.

Acknowledgment

The authors would like to dedicate the chapter to the memory of Dr. Linda Brodsky.

Key References

1. Brodsky L, Arvedson J. Anatomy, embryology, physiology, and normal development. In: Arvedson J, Brodsky L, eds. *Pediatric Swallowing and Feeding: Assessment and Management.* 2nd ed. Boston: Cengage Learning; 2002:13-80.
2. Laitman J, Reidenberg J. Specializations of the human upper respiratory and upper digestive systems as seen through comparative and developmental anatomy. *Dysphagia.* 1993;8:318-325.
3. Marcus C, Smith R, Mankarious L, et al. Developmental aspects of the upper airway: report for the NHLBI Workshop, March 5-6, 2009. *Proc Am Thorac Soc.* 2009;6:513-520.
4. Minocchieri S, Burren J, Bachmann M, et al. Development of the premature infant nose throat-model (PrINT-model)—an upper airway replica of a premature neonate for the study of aerosol delivery. *Pediatr Res.* 2008;64:141-146.
5. Randall D, et al. Development of the respiratory system and respiration. In: Chamley C, Carson P, Duncan R, eds. *Developmental Anatomy and Physiology of Children.* New York: Elsevier; 2005:165-185.

Structure and Development of the Lower Respiratory System in Infants and Children

John E. Baatz and Rita M. Ryan

PEARLS

- Lungs increase in volume from about 250 mL at birth to 6000 mL in the adult.
- Each lung lobe is subdivided into 19 bronchopulmonary segments, which receive a primary segmental bronchus and a tertiary pulmonary artery branch and are drained by pulmonary veins.
- The airway branching pattern in the lung undergoes multiple generations, yielding a total of 27 or 28 divisions when counting begins from the primary bronchus.
- The aggregate length of the airways in the adult lung spans approximately 1500 miles or 2400 km.
- The bronchial mucosa contains several epithelial cell types with the ciliated cell comprising more than 90% of the epithelial cell population in the conducting airways, but the proportion and number of cilia per cell decrease from the proximal to distal airways.
- The acinus, which is approximately spherical in shape and has a diameter of about 7 mm and a length of 0.5 to 1 cm, is the gas exchange portion of the lung.
- At the alveolar level, many changes occur in the postnatal period. Although there is disparity concerning the time alveolarization is completed, alveoli in a normal adult number from 300 to 500 million and have a diameter of 150 to 200 μm.
- The two epithelial cells of the alveolus are the gas-exchanging type I cell and type II cell, which are responsible for the production of pulmonary surfactant and have a central role in repair.
- The alveolar-capillary unit is composed of three major constituents: epithelial lining of the alveolus, capillary endothelial cells, and a mixture of cellular and extracellular interstitial components.
- Following birth the pulmonary vasculature undergoes extensive remodeling and, when fully matured, thickness of the pulmonary artery is only about 60% that of the aorta.
- The large pulmonary arteries traverse the lung with the cartilaginous airways and extend from the hilum nearly halfway down the bronchial tree.
- Smaller pulmonary arteries measure between 100 and 1000 μm in diameter, branch with the bronchial tree, and lie close to bronchi and bronchioles.
- Pulmonary veins do not course with the bronchial tree; instead, they are seen within the interlobular septae.

Lower Respiratory System

Overview of the Lungs

While the upper airway of the respiratory system is involved in uptake of air for delivery to the lungs and in the removal of large particulates from the air, the primary purpose of the lower respiratory tract is to efficiently deliver oxygen to the blood and remove expired carbon dioxide. The main components of the lower respiratory tract are the trachea, bronchial tubes, and lungs. The lungs are dense, spongy structures composed of smaller branches of the bronchi called bronchiolar tubes, which, after several branching generations, terminate at alveolar sacs, where oxygen and carbon dioxide are exchanged with the blood of alveolar sac–associated capillaries. The trachea, bronchial tubes, and bronchioles serve to provide rapid delivery of large volumes of air, whereas the alveolar sacs provide the large surface area required for sufficient gas diffusion.

Externally, the lungs are paired structures that, with the mediastinum, fill the thoracic cavity. Normally, the right lung is composed of three lobes and the left lung consists of two lobes and the lingula, arising from the left upper lobe. The lobes are separated by fissures and have hili that receive a primary lobar bronchus, pulmonary artery and veins, bronchial arteries and veins, lymphatics, and nerves (Fig. 44.1).[1,2] The lobes are further subdivided into 19 bronchopulmonary segments that receive primary segmental bronchi, a tertiary pulmonary artery branch and are drained by pulmonary veins. Pulmonary veins do not course with the airway and pulmonary artery; instead, they course midway between the dyads and can be readily identified in the intersegmental septa. The connective tissue septa that demarcate each bronchopulmonary segment define the smallest surgically resectable portions of the lung.

The lung bud develops in the first month of the embryonic period, after which extensive branching progresses (≈20 generations) forming the bronchial tree by mid-second trimester.[3] The most rapid period of human lung development occurs between 22 weeks' gestational age (wga) and term (≈40 wga). This is during the saccular period, when alveolarization is initiated and accelerates, yielding approximately 20,000,000 to 50,000,000 alveoli at birth—only 6% to 16% of that in the full-grown adult lung.[4] The beginning of the third trimester

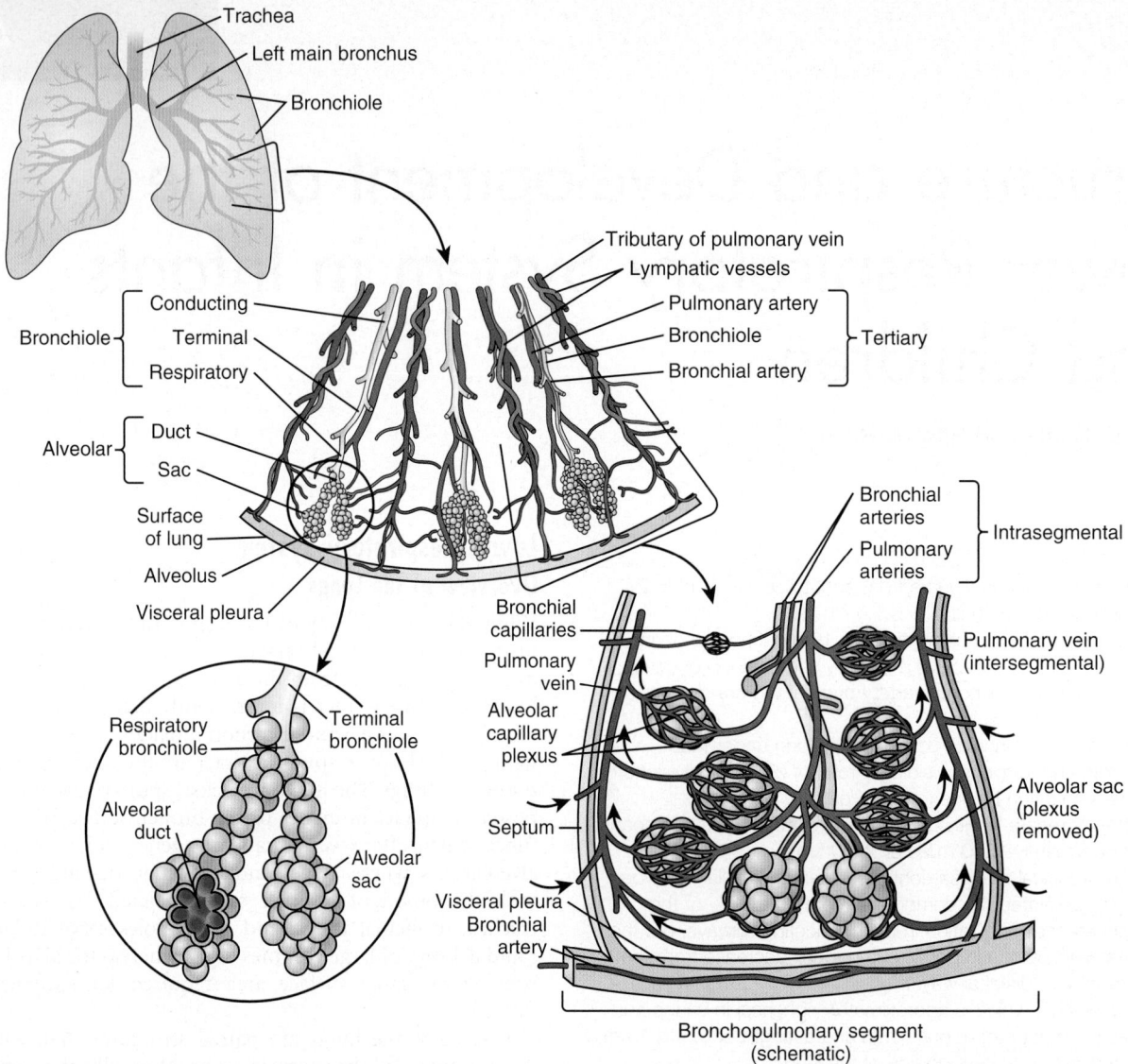

Fig. 44.1. Internal structure and organization of lungs. Within the lungs, the bronchi and pulmonary arteries are paired and branch in unison. Segmental (tertiary) branches supply the bronchopulmonary segments. Each intrasegmental pulmonary artery ends in a capillary plexus in the walls of the alveolar sacs and alveoli. The pulmonary veins arise from the pulmonary capillaries and drain toward and then course within the septa between adjacent segments. Bronchial arteries are distributed along and supply the bronchial tree. Their distal-most branches supply capillary beds drained by the pulmonary veins, such as those of the visceral pleura (even though this small amount of blood is poorly oxygenated). (Modified from Moore KL, Dalley AF. Clinically Oriented Anatomy. 5th ed. Philadelphia: Lippincott Williams & Wilkins; 2006.)

(22-27 wga) is not only critical with respect to premature births but also because early development of fetal human lungs primarily occurs in the presence of fetal hemoglobin ($\alpha_2\gamma_2$), while later stages (~27 wga-~38 wga) of human fetal lung development (which includes initiation of both pulmonary surfactant expression and accelerated alveolarization) occur during the main γ to β globin transition, ie, from fetal to adult hemoglobin ($\alpha_2\beta_2$).[5-7] Fetal hemoglobin binds oxygen more efficiently than adult hemoglobin, yielding higher oxygen tensions in lung tissue of developing human fetuses. Therefore treatment of premature infants with regard to oxygen delivery should consider potential risks associated with the oxygen-binding properties of the predominant hemoglobin form.

At birth, the lungs weigh about 40 g and double in weight by 6 months. Lung volume increases from about 250 mL at birth to 6000 mL in the adult.[8] Mature respiratory alveoli

appear at approximately 36 weeks of gestation and continue to develop until about 2 years of age, with an approximate total surface area of 2.8 m². By age 2 years, most of the alveolarization process is completed, but newly formed alveolar septa still contain a double capillary network rather than a single one observed in adult lungs. Therefore over the next several years, the capillary bed will reorganize well after alveolar formation. After 8 years of age, the lung enters the phase of natural growth.[9]

Airways

In the lung, the airway undergoes multiple generations of branching, yielding a total of 23 to 28 divisions when counting begins from the primary bronchus. The bronchi are the larger intrinsic cartilaginous airways and comprise 9 to 12 generations starting with the primary bronchus and terminating in bronchi, having a diameter of approximately 1 mm. Bronchioles, sometimes called *membranous bronchioles* or *distal noncartilaginous airways,* are conducting airways. They comprise an additional 12 generations before ending as terminal bronchioles, the last purely conducting structure in the lung. Horsfield and Cumming showed that the course from the trachea to the alveolar level may comprise as few as 8 or as many as 24 airway branch points.[10] The first 16 generations of branching are genetically determined, while more distal branching and alveolarization are more plastic and are much more likely to be influenced by maternal nutrition and other extrinsic factors.[11] For this reason, a particular airway diameter may be found at various points along the course of the airway. Determination of the total cross section of airways is important in understanding the distribution of airway resistance. Weibel[12] showed that as the peripheral generations of the airways are approached, the total cross-sectional area of the lung is markedly increased, suggesting that peripheral airways account for only a small proportion of total airway resistance. In the adult, an asymmetric dichotomous branching pattern is seen, each daughter branch having a cross-sectional area about 75% of its parent branch. This results in an increase of combined cross-sectional area of the two daughter branches. It is well known, however, that peripheral airway resistance in children's lungs is disproportionately high. The size of the conducting airways is related to stature, so the airways' cross-sectional area in children increases at a slow rate with growth and aging. Because the peripheral airways make up a significant portion of the total respiratory resistance in children, disease in the bronchioles can be serious.

The bronchi maintain the histologic appearance of the trachea in that mucosa, submucosa, muscularis, adventitia, and cartilaginous support are present. As the bronchi branch deeper into the lung parenchyma, the cartilage rings become plates and less regular, and the muscularis becomes continuous, being located between the submucosa and cartilage plates. Also contained within the bronchial submucosa are mucus-secreting submucosal glands, nerves, ganglia, and bronchial arterial branches (Fig. 44.2). As the bronchi decrease in diameter, the pseudostratified columnar epithelium becomes lower and the mucoserous glands become fewer in number. Although the glands wane in number in the more distal parts of the lung, mucous cells persist and can be found in very small bronchi and some membranous bronchioles.

The bronchial mucosa contains several epithelial cell types: ciliated, mucus producing (goblet cells), basal, brush, and neuroendocrine.[13,14] The ciliated cell constitutes more than 90% of the epithelial cell population in the conducting airways, but the proportion and number of cilia per cell decrease from the proximal to distal airways. The 9 + 2 microtubular structure within the cilia has been shown to be altered in the primary ciliary syndromes (Fig. 44.3). In addition to its ciliary beating movement, the ciliated columnar cells regulate the depth of the composition of the periciliary fluid and transport ions across the epithelium. The basal cell has a progenitor cell role and also functions to maintain adherence of columnar cells to the basement membrane. The brush cell, thought to have a role in fluid absorption and/or chemoreceptor function, is found rarely in the tracheobronchial and alveolar epithelia.

The mucociliary apparatus is the primary defense mechanism in the respiratory system. Although mucous goblet cells secrete mucin, it is the submucosal glands that produce more than 90% of the mucus needed for mucociliary function. The glandular unit of the bronchial submucosa comprises mucous, serous, myoepithelial cells, collecting duct cells, and occasionally neuroendocrine (Kulchitsky) cells.[14,15] The physical characteristics of the mucous layer reveal that the superficial layer is more viscous than the deeper layer. This difference in consistency of the mucous layer allows the cilia to function properly, allowing a power and recovery stroke mechanism. The secretions include lysozyme, antileukoprotease, lactoferrin, and IgA. The secretory component of IgA is synthesized in bronchial gland cells and expressed on their basolateral cell surfaces, to which IgA dimers synthesized by plasma cells bind. The complex is endocytosed by the glandular cell and then is secreted from its luminal surface. Neuroendocrine cells can be solitary near the basal lamina between columnar cells or in

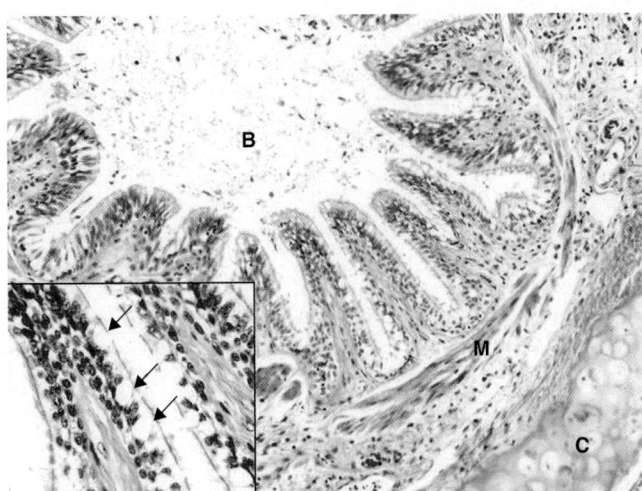

Fig. 44.2. Bronchus *(B)* with surrounding smooth muscle *(M)* and cartilage *(C).* The airway mucosa (inset) is composed of ciliated epithelial cells and vacuolated goblet cells *(arrowheads).* (Gomori trichrome; ×40 and ×400.)

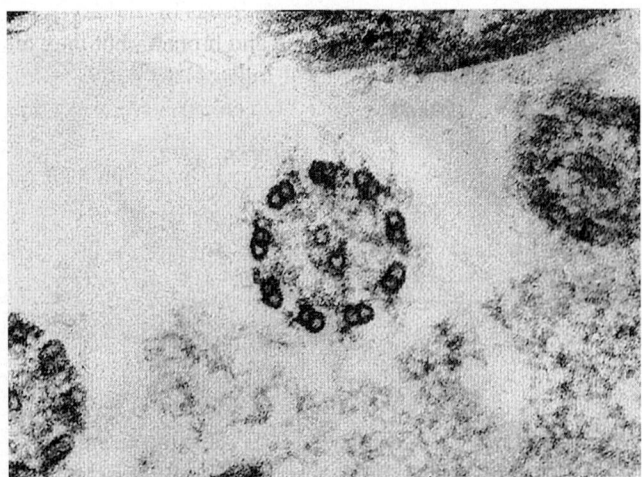

Fig. 44.3. Internal structure of a cilium (no cell membrane evident) in which two axial tubules and nine peripheral duplex tubules are seen. Dynein arms are attached to several of the peripheral duplex tubules (×13,500).

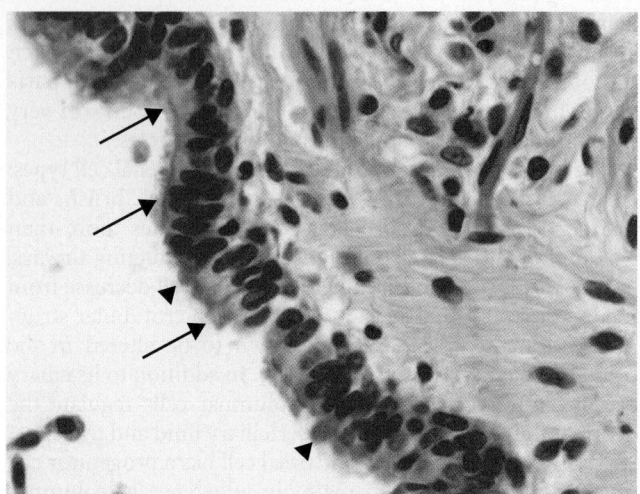

Fig. 44.4. Distal conducting airway mucosa composed of some ciliated epithelial cells showing a terminal bar *(arrows)* and a nonciliated Clara cell *(arrowheads)*. (Hematoxylin-eosin stain; ×400.)

collections called *neuroepithelial bodies* that occur near branch points of bronchi.[15] The neuroendocrine cells are more abundant in the fetus and likely have a role in lung growth or maturation.

Although originally defined as having a lumen diameter less than 2 mm, the term *small airway* usually refers to a bronchiole. Histologically, the bronchiole is characterized by a transition from pseudostratified tall columnar epithelium to a more cuboidal ciliated form. In addition, the mucous goblet cell is replaced by the nonciliated Clara cell (Figs. 44.4 and 44.5). In the bronchiolar epithelium, a ratio of about three ciliated cells to two nonciliated cells lines the lower airways. The Clara cell is identified as a dome- or tongue-shaped cell that protrudes into the bronchiolar lumen among the shorter ciliated cells. The Clara cell has varying features according to species but possesses an abundance of agranular reticulum and secretory granules. Clara cells synthesize and secrete Clara cell secretory protein (CC10, CC16), a unique 10-kDa protein similar to rabbit uteroglobin that has antiinflammatory and immunoregulatory functions.[16] In addition, Clara cells secrete

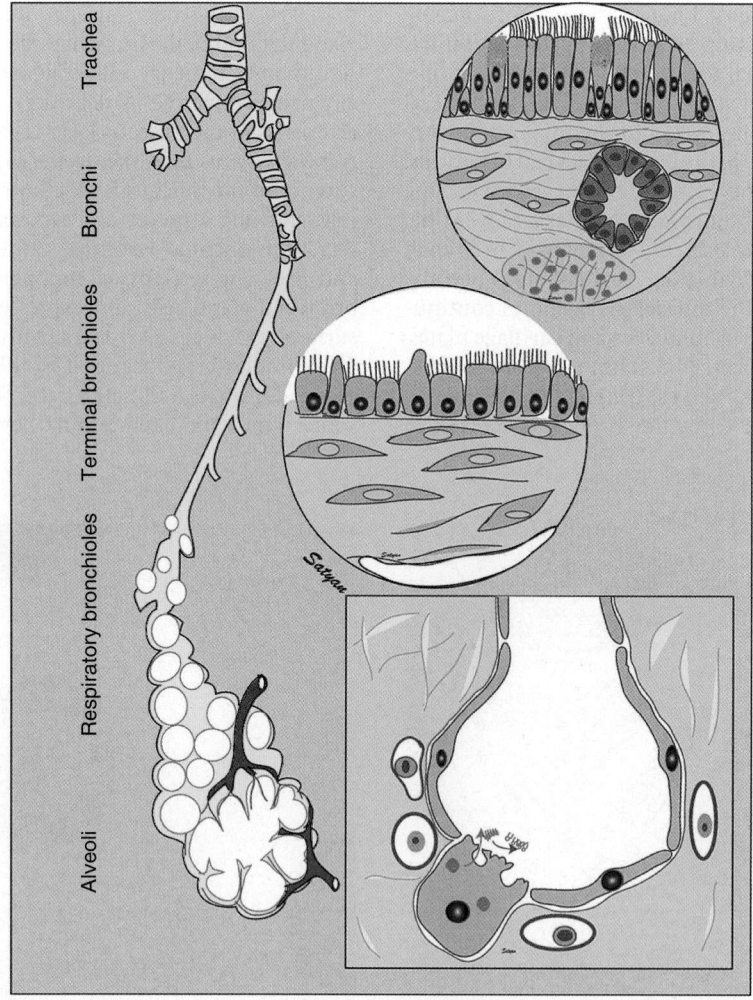

Fig. 44.5. Respiratory tract epithelia. There is a progression from pseudostratified columnar epithelium with ciliated, goblet, and basal cells in the large conducting airways (top circle) to a more cuboidal ciliated epithelium in the small conducting airways with nonciliated Clara cells (middle circle). In the alveolar epithelium, flattened type I pneumocytes and cuboidal type II pneumocytes are present and are associated with an extensive capillary network (box). (Copyright Satyan Lakshminrusimha.)

surfactant-associated proteins A, B, and D. Importantly, the Clara cell also functions as a progenitor cell that differentiates into ciliated cells following injury, and some investigators have shown that the Clara cell can differentiate into a type II epithelial cell.[17]

Within the wall of the bronchiole, the muscular layer becomes more prominent and submucosal glands and cartilage are absent. The bronchiole segment ends as a terminal bronchiole, which marks the terminus of the conducting portion of the airway. The terminal bronchiole branches into two generations of respiratory bronchioles, which through further divisions give rise to additional respiratory bronchioles that have more alveoli in their walls, so-called second- and third-order respiratory bronchioles. By definition, respiratory bronchioles are alveolated, and they branch into two to three generations of alveolar ducts. The alveolar ducts are defined as those channels from which a series of alveoli open and are histologically characterized by having small clublike ends that contain muscle sphincters and elastic fibers. The ducts open into a final generation of alveolus-lined spaces, the multiloculated cup-shaped alveolar sacs (Fig. 44.6).

Definitions of Special Lung Unit and Alveolar Formation

Each bronchopulmonary segment is further compartmentalized into smaller units termed *pulmonary lobules*. Each pulmonary lobule is supplied by a bronchiole that divides into a cluster of three to five terminal bronchioles and their associated respiratory tissue situated at the end of a bronchial pathway. The pulmonary lobule is roughly 1 to 2 cm in diameter and pyramidal in shape. It is bound by delicate connective tissue septa in which small proximal branches of pulmonary veins travel. The portion of the pulmonary lobule distal to the terminal bronchioles and consisting of several respiratory bronchioles, alveolar ducts, and ultimately alveoli is termed the *pulmonary acinus*. The acinus, which is approximately spherical in shape and has a diameter of about 7 mm and a length of 0.5 to 1 cm, is the gas exchange portion of the lung.

At the alveolar level, many changes occur in the postnatal period. Although there is disparity concerning the time alveolarization is completed, evidence links the postnatal development of alveoli with elastic tissue fiber deposition.[18] At birth, primitive alveoli called *saccules* are evident, but approximately 50 million alveoli are already formed.[19] The number of alveoli in a normal adult can vary from 300 to 500 million, and they have a diameter of 150 to 200 μm. The early work by Dunnell[20] suggesting that new alveolar formation ceased at about age 8 years has been challenged by Thurlbeck,[21] who has shown that alveolarization appears to be nearly complete at about age 2 years. Lung volume correlates with body size, but alveolar surface area correlates with metabolic activity; thus alveoli become more complex in shape during maturation and as increasing O_2 is required.

Alveolar-Capillary Unit

The alveolar-capillary unit is highly specialized to maximize diffusion between the blood and air gases (Fig. 44.7). The alveolar-capillary unit is composed of three major constituents: (1) the epithelial lining of the alveolus; (2) capillary endothelial cells; and (3) a mixture of cellular and extracellular interstitial components.[22] This alveolar-capillary bed is the most extensive in the body and is contained within the epithelium-lined walls of adjacent alveoli forming a gridlike network. The internal surface area of the adult lung is 70 to 80 m^2, of which 90% covers the pulmonary capillaries; thus the air-blood surface available for gas exchange is 60 to 70 m^2.[22] The endothelial cells, which constitute about 30% of the total lung cells, contain few intracellular organelles that are clustered together within the cytoplasm allowing the cell to maximize its surface area. A number of adenine nucleotides, vasoactive amines, prostaglandins, vasoactive peptides, and lipoproteins can be metabolized and taken up within the numerous pinocytotic vesicles characteristic of pulmonary endothelial cells.

In addition to gas exchange, endothelial cells synthesize and secrete various locally acting substances such as nitric oxide, endothelins, prostacyclin, tissue plasminogen activator, and thrombomodulin. Other functions include liquid and solid exchange and enzyme activity within the walls of the caveolae.

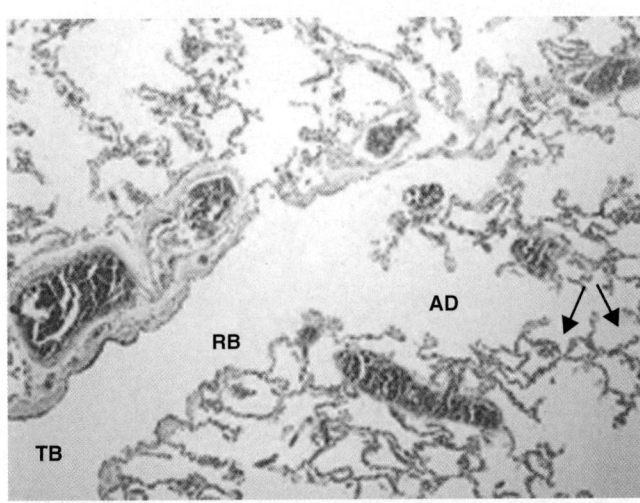

Fig. 44.6. Distal conducting airway with transition to respiratory airway. *AD*, alveolar duct; *RB*, respiratory bronchiole; *TB*, terminal bronchiole. Individual alveoli are indicated by *arrows*. (Hematoxylin-eosin stain; ×40.)

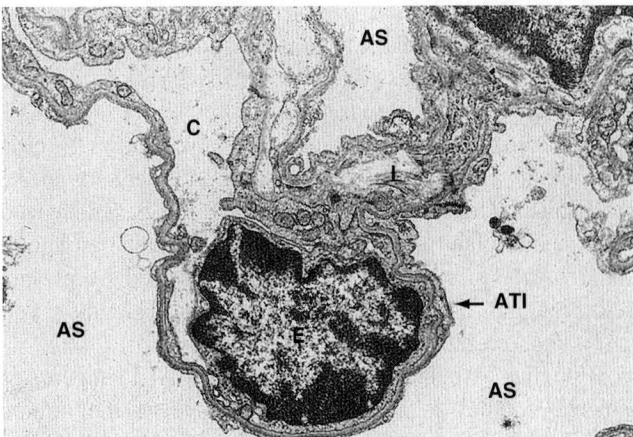

Fig. 44.7. Both surfaces of the alveolar wall that separates the alveolar spaces (*AS*) are covered by thin extensions of alveolar type I (*ATI*) epithelial cells. The capillary (*C*) is lined by endothelium (*E*). The epithelium and endothelium rest on a fused basement membrane on the thin portion of the alveolar wall and are separated by an interstitial space (*I*) in the thick portion of the alveolar wall (×5500).

At the ultrastructural level the blood-air barrier consists of a 0.1- to 0.2-μm thick septum composed of a capillary endothelial cell and the type I pneumocyte with their intervening fused basal laminae. Within thicker portions of the alveolar wall, the alveolar epithelium and capillary endothelium are separated by the interstitial space.

The connective tissue space, or interstitium of the lung at the alveolar level, does not have lymphatics, but it can accumulate fluid that can be absorbed into the lymphatic system, which usually ends at the respiratory bronchiolar level. The interstitial cell population includes resident and migratory cell populations. Normally, the interstitium contains macrophages, pericytes, myofibroblasts, mast cells, infrequent lymphocytes, and a few cells that are best termed *undifferentiated, mesenchymal,* or *pluripotent* because in disease they can differentiate into various cell types including fibroblasts, smooth muscle cells, and others. Greater than 25% of the interstitial cells cannot be identified definitively with the electron microscope, so it is understandable why most of the cells cannot be identified by light microscopy without special cell marker stains.

Two epithelial cell types line the alveoli. Type I cells have thin cytoplasmic extensions and a large surface area covering approximately 90% of the total alveolar surface (Fig. 44.8). Numerically, they form only about 40% of the epithelial cells, whereas the type II cell, which is cuboidal, constitutes 60% of the total number of epithelial cells but contributes less than 10% of the total alveolar surface area. Type I cells are exquisitely well adapted to allow for the rapid exchange of gases, and their micropinocytotic system likely plays a major role in the transport of solutes, such as albumin and immunoglobulin, in small quantities. They can be induced to ingest some particulates and can increase their number of pinocytotic vesicles, but they are not active in surfactant uptake.

The type II cell is the regenerative cell of the alveolar epithelium, serving as the stem cell following injury. It can repopulate the alveolar surface in about 5 days. It is cuboidal in shape and only numbers about one per alveolus. Ultrastructurally the type II cell has characteristic surface microvilli and cytoplasmic multilamellar inclusions, which are the intracellular cytoplasmic storage forms of pulmonary surfactant (Fig. 44.9). The inclusions evolve from multivesicular bodies or lysosomal granules, which progressively acquire the characteristic lamellae through fusion and condensation. In addition to its roles in the synthesis, secretion, and reuptake of surfactant, the type II cell synthesizes arachidonic acid metabolites, synthesizes and secretes connective tissue components of the basement membrane including fibronectin, synthesizes and secretes components of the complement system, expresses class II proteins of the major histocompatibility complex among others, and has been found to be a critical source of many different growth factors during injury and repair.[23]

Considerable data demonstrate clearly that there are several populations of macrophages: intraalveolar, septal (interstitial), pulmonary intravascular, and airway. Within the alveolar spaces, alveolar macrophages are abundant and form an

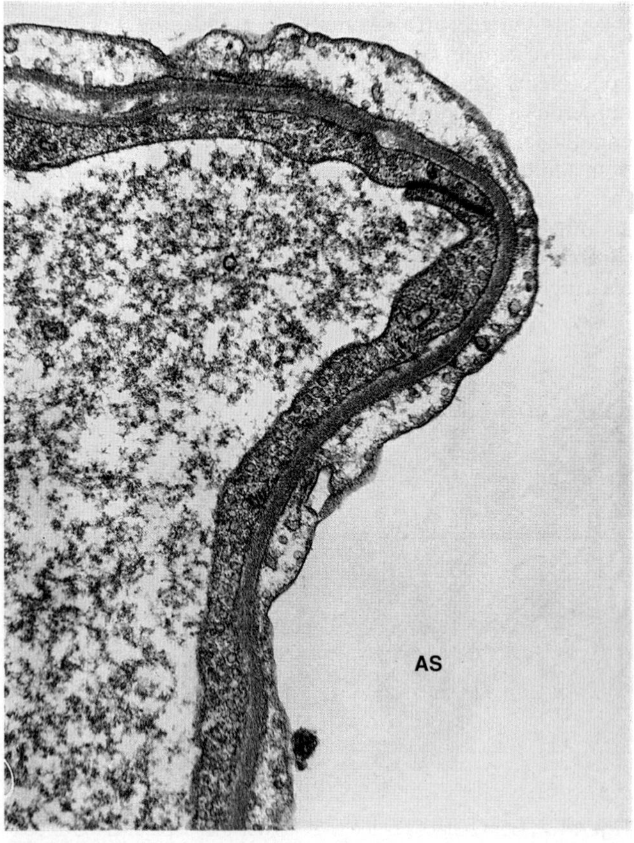

Fig. 44.8. Electron micrograph showing the thin side of the air-blood barrier. The thin cytoplasmic extension of the type I epithelium contains only a few vesicles and shares a fused basement membrane with the endothelium, which contains many caveolae (×18,000). *AS,* alveolar space; *C,* capillary.

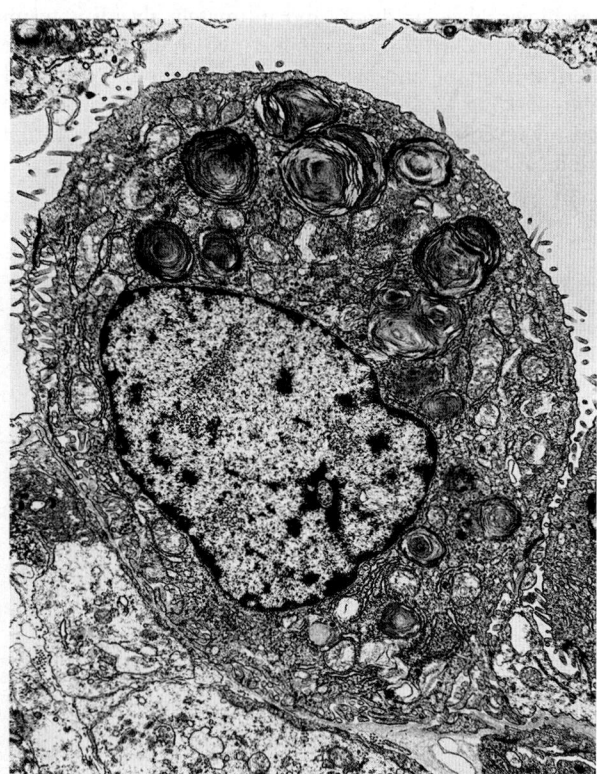

Fig. 44.9. Cytoplasm of the alveolar type II cell has abundant lamellar inclusion bodies and surface membrane microvilli (×7500).

important arm of the defense mechanism of the lung (Figs. 44.10 and 44.11). They number approximately 23×10^9 in the lung (10% of the total cells of the alveolar compartment), and 50 to 100 are estimated per alveolus. They derive from three sources: bone marrow via blood monocyte, the interstitial macrophage pool, and proliferation of macrophages in the alveolar space. They are actively phagocytic and scavenge the surface of the alveoli for respired particulates (macrophages as so-called "dust cells"). Although seen free-floating in alveolar spaces in light microscopic preparations, the alveolar macrophage crawls along the surface of epithelium, adhering with its filopodia. The macrophage has remarkable metabolic activities, has known immune functions, and is involved in lung injury and repair phenomena. Alveolar macrophages also play a role in surfactant uptake, removal, or catabolism. More than 100 macrophage-synthesized mediators have been identified, including many proinflammatory cytokines, and numerous ligands have been demonstrated. In normal bronchoalveolar lavage fluid, 90% of the cells are alveolar macrophages and 1% to 5% are lymphocytes (T-cell lymphocytes constituting 60% to 70% and B cells 5% to 10%).

Lung Circulation

Pulmonary Vascular System

The pulmonary circulation is furnished by the pulmonary and bronchial vascular systems.[24,25] During gestation, branches of the pulmonary arterial system are thick walled and contain a medial layer of smooth muscle. At birth, the pulmonary artery and aorta are comparable in medial thickness and configuration. Elastic fibers tend to be long, uniform, unbranched, and parallel with one another. Following birth the pulmonary vasculature undergoes extensive remodeling and by 2 years of age shows a media composed of short, branched, and loosely arranged elastic fibers. When fully matured the pulmonary artery and its thickness are only about 60% that of the aorta. Only a few muscular arteries are seen accompanying terminal bronchioles at birth. Following birth, when pulmonary arterial pressures fall to normal levels, the muscle fibers diminish. Initially new vessels without muscle are formed, along with new respiratory units during lung growth. Smooth muscle extends peripherally into small arteries slowly, reaching arterioles at the respiratory bronchiolar level at 4 months, alveolar duct level at 3 years, and some alveoli at age 10 years.[26]

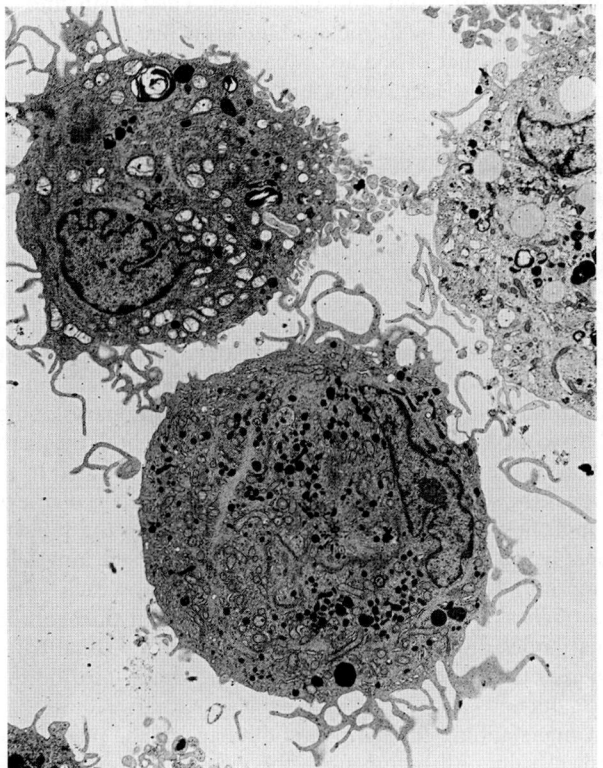

Fig. 44.10. Alveolar macrophages recovered from bronchoalveolar lavage fluid contain abundant lysosomes and other cytoplasmic contents, including lipid droplets and surfactant remnants (×5300).

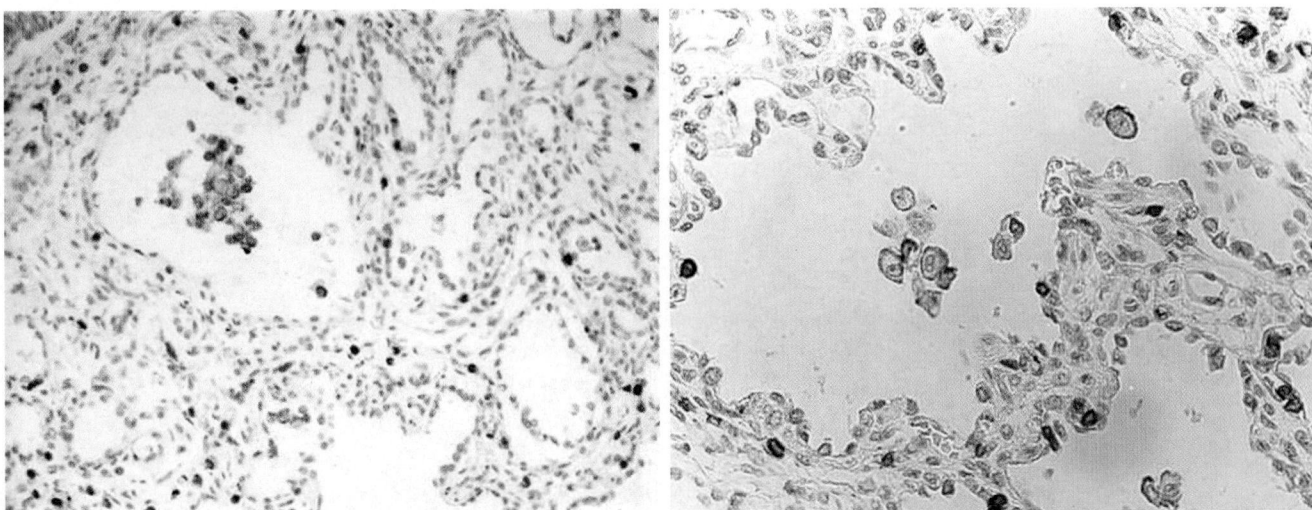

Fig. 44.11. Sections obtained from infants who died with bronchopulmonary dysplasia. Pulmonary macrophages present within air spaces were immunostained (brown stain) with anti-CD45, a general leukocyte marker. Leukocytes are also identified within the alveolar walls and capillaries. (hematoxylin counterstain; ×200 left, ×400 right.) (Original lung section courtesy Dr. Gloria Pryhuber.)

The criteria for recognizing various types of pulmonary vessels were put forth by Brenner in 1935.[27] The pulmonary arteries, which exceed 1000 μm in external diameter, are called elastic pulmonary arteries and traverse with the cartilaginous airways. They extend from the hilum to nearly halfway in the bronchial tree of the newborn, a pattern completed by week 16 of gestation and retained into adulthood. Pulmonary arteries measure between 100 and 1000 μm in diameter and have a distinct muscular media and internal and external limiting elastic membranes. The muscular arteries of the lung have thinner media than their counterparts in the systemic circulation. Muscular pulmonary arteries branch with the bronchial tree and lie close to bronchi and bronchioles (Fig. 44.12). Pulmonary arterioles are vessels that measure 100 μm in diameter and have only an endothelial lining and a single elastic lamina with little, if any, muscular media. These vessels usually are seen at the level of the alveolar ducts and in certain sites within the alveolar walls. Pulmonary capillaries are non-fenestrated, whereas bronchial capillaries are fenestrated. The appearance of pulmonary venules is identical to that of pulmonary arterioles, and serial sections are required to differentiate the two. In contrast with the pulmonary arteries, the larger branches of pulmonary veins do not course with the bronchial tree; instead, they are seen within the interlobular septa. The media of larger veins is composed of smooth muscle fibers, collagen, and elastin. Unlike their arterial counterpart, these veins show no clear internal and external elastic lamina (Fig. 44.13).

Bronchial Vascular System

Whereas the pulmonary circulation returns all venous blood to the lung and serves some nutritive function to peripheral capillaries, the bronchial circulation is the primary blood source for the lung. Although two major bronchial arteries for each lung is a common pattern, this is present less than 40% of the time. There usually are two bronchial arteries in the left lung and one in the right lung. Although variable, the left bronchial arteries usually arise from the upper portion of the descending aorta. The right bronchial artery arises from the descending aorta, one of the right intercostal branches, or

subclavian or internal thoracic arteries. The bronchial arteries traverse along the dorsal portion of each bronchus. They lose their distinctness along the respiratory bronchioles and drain with the alveolar capillaries into the peribronchiolar venous network. They form a capillary plexus in the bronchi that supplies the submucosa and muscle. The capillary plexus communicates with branches of the pulmonary artery that empty into pulmonary veins. Other bronchial arteries supply the interlobular tissue and the pleura. They drain into the bronchial veins. The diameter of the bronchial artery is much smaller than that of the accompanying pulmonary artery. It has an internal elastic lamina and media but no external elastic lamina.

Pulmonary Lymphatics and Bronchus-Associated Lymphoid Tissue

Pulmonary lymphatics[24] invariably have less elastic tissue in their walls than either arteries or veins.[24,25] They are lined by endothelium, and valves are present especially near and in the visceral pleura. There are two lymphatic systems in the human lung: a superficial network in the pleura and a deep network around the bronchi and pulmonary arteries and veins and in the connective tissue septa between the pulmonary lobules. The two separate systems have anastomoses, in both the pleura and near the hilum. Lymphatics can be demonstrated to the level of the septal walls but are not found at the alveolar level. Lymph flow from both lower lobes drains into the infratracheal lymph nodes. The remaining right and left lung lobes drain into the tracheobronchial lymph nodes on each side of the trachea, respectively. Lymph from the right tracheobronchial nodes drains into the right bronchomediastinal trunk, whereas the left tracheobronchial nodes drain into the thoracic duct.

Understanding the lymphatic drainage of the pleura is of clinical value. All lymph from the visceral pleura eventually reaches parabronchial and hilar lymph nodes by flowing on the surface or in lymphatic trunks that course through the lung. Lymphatic vessels in the parietal pleura are in communication with the pleural space via 2- to 6-mm stomas found on the mediastinal pleura or the intercostal surfaces of the

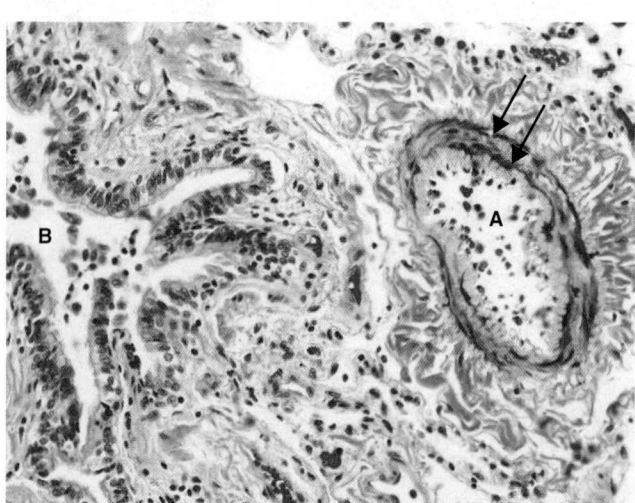

Fig. 44.12. Small muscular pulmonary artery *(A)* traveling with a bronchiole *(B)*. Two layers of smooth muscle cells are present in the vascular media *(arrows)*. (Gomori trichrome; ×200.)

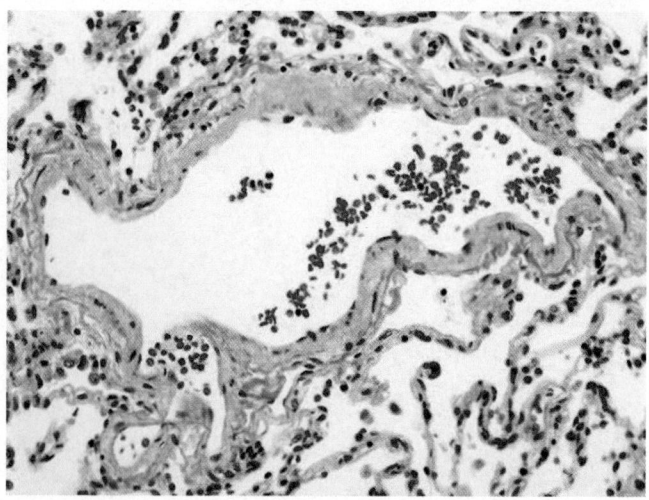

Fig. 44.13. Pulmonary vein. The media is composed of loose, pale, blue-staining collage fibers with scarce smooth muscle present. (Gomori tricrome, ×200.)

lower thorax.[28] The parasternal nodes in the second and third interspaces receive lymph from a significant portion of the parietal pleura, so biopsy of these nodes may reveal an etiology of the pleural effusion. The portion of lymph that drains caudally from the lower parietal pleural region into retroperitoneal nodes can explain metastases of tumor to adrenals and kidneys.

Bronchus-associated lymphoid tissue (BALT) appears as isolated nodules in the connective tissue of the lamina propria of the bronchial tree and produces primarily IgG and secretory IgA.[29] Collections of BALT cells tend to occur at airway bifurcations and are covered by a special epithelium that can pinocytose and transport solutes and particulate antigens. BALT is sparse at birth but starts accumulating thereafter. It is prominent in lungs of children and in diseased lungs of patients with bronchiectasis. Although more than 50% of the cells are B lymphocytes, T lymphocytes are also found (18%), along with follicular dendritic cells. Sometimes these nodules bulge into the bronchial lumen.[29] Additional lymphoid tissue in the lung is a rich supply of lymph nodes within the lung, at the carina, and along the trachea.

Diaphragm

Although the diaphragm is the principal muscle of respiration, it is not essential for breathing in the awake state. It becomes essential during deep anesthesia because other muscles of respiration become inactive. The diaphragm is a musculotendinous sheet that is the main source of inspiratory muscle force.[24,28] Anatomically it separates the thoracic from the abdominal cavity. It has two distinct muscular components: the sternocostal portion and the crural. These two portions have distinct embryologic origins and have separate segmental innervations and varying muscle fiber composition. There are changes in fiber composition following birth. The muscle fibers vary morphologically, physiologically, and cytochemically. The diaphragm has three openings near its central portion for the aorta, inferior vena cava, and esophagus. The vagus nerve passes through the esophageal hiatus, whereas the azygos vein and thoracic duct pass through the aortic hiatus. There are small paravertebral perforations for splanchnic nerves. Because of the way the fibers originate from the bones and traverse to the central tendon, triangular areas may result in spaces or clefts in the diaphragm. Anteriorly these are called Morgagni foramina, and posteriorly they are known as the *foramina of Bochdalek*. Both are potential sites for hernias. The phrenic nerve innervates the diaphragm.

During contraction in adults, the dome of the diaphragm descends and the lower ribs elevate. In infants, because of their compliant rib cage, descent opposes elevation of the lower ribs and results in the subcostal retractions.[28] Other muscles of respiration include the intercostals, the majority of which are arranged to enhance inspiration by elevating the lower ribs, and the abdominal muscles, which are powerful muscles of expiration but do not participate in expiration during quiet breathing. Scalenes act to elevate the first two ribs and are active even during quiet breathing. Although the sternocleidomastoid muscles usually are not active in quiet breathing, when inspiratory efforts are marked, they become the most important accessory muscles of inspiration. This is well seen in infants with respiratory distress who elevate the upper portion of their sterna.

Summary

The respiratory portion of the lung is a complex organ with more than 40 cell types. It undergoes remodeling over the first few years of life. Altered structure, whether due to congenital abnormalities or injury and repair, is a critical determinant of survival and quality of life. Understanding the structure of the lung is critical to the management and treatment of lung disease in critically ill children.

Acknowledgments

We gratefully acknowledge the contributions of Christopher A. D'Angelis and Jacqueline J. Coalson, who authored this chapter in a previous edition.

Physiology of the Respiratory System

Mark J. Heulitt and Katherine C. Clement

PEARLS

- During childhood, the most important chest diseases have obstructive pictures that are best measured using interrupter and oscillation techniques.
- Wheezing is a sound heard when there is flow limitation in a compliant tube. It is a sign of expiratory flow limitation. The wheezing is caused by "flutter" of the walls at the site of flow limitation secondary to the conservation of energy in the system.
- The respiratory system is not a linear system; resistance and compliance are not constants. They are dependent on volume, volume history, and flow.
- The equation of motion changes when a spontaneously breathing patient is placed on positive pressure mechanical ventilator support. The pressure applied to the airway (P_{APP}) equals the sum of pressure generated by the patient's muscles (P_{mus}) plus the ventilator pressure (P_{vent}). Thus:

$$P_{mus} + P_{vent} = \frac{1}{C}V + R\dot{V}$$

Physiology of the Respiratory System

Because of the increasing emphasis on molecular biology today, many physicians currently in training have received limited exposure to physiologic principles that form the basis of clinical medicine. However, a resurgence of interest in translational research has occurred recently with a reemphasis on molecular research and applied animal physiology before these principles are used in clinical research.[1] In a recent editorial in the *European Journal of Physiology*, Rossier[2] stated that research is refocusing itself to make a change from the past, where its mantra was "from function to the gene," to the future, where the focus must be on the "gene to function." That "structure determines function" relates to that first lecture in physiology when it was discussed that changes in the shape of a protein, cell, or organ will usually result in a change of function of that structure. This is never so true as in a discussion of the physiology of positive pressure mechanical ventilation in pediatric patients. The focus of this chapter is to expose the reader to the important basic principles of respiratory physiology and to serve as a primer to other chapters in this book that use these principles.

The main function of the lungs is (rapid) gas exchange. This process is accomplished by a well-coordinated interaction of the lungs with the central nervous system, the diaphragm and chest wall musculature, and the circulatory system.

Gas exchange occurs in the alveolus, where the thin laminar blood flow and inspired air are separated only by a thin tissue layer. Gas exchange takes 0.25 seconds or one-third of the total transit time of a red cell. The entire blood volume of the body passes through the lungs each minute in the resting state, approximately 5 L/min. The total surface area of the lung is about 80 meters square, equivalent to the size of a tennis court. The primary function of the lungs is to supply oxygen (O_2) and to remove carbon dioxide (CO_2) from the tissues of the body. For the lungs to do this, two interrelated processes must occur: ventilation, which is the movement of air between the outside body and the alveoli, and gas exchange, which is the transfer of O_2 and CO_2 between the alveolar gas and the mixed venous blood entering the lungs.

Approximately 10% of the lung is occupied by solid tissue, whereas the remainder is filled with air and blood. However, it should be noted that changes occur with development. A gram of lung from an infant probably represents more airway tissue and less parenchymal (alveolar and interstitial) tissue than the same amount of lung from an adult. Supporting structures of the lung must be delicate enough to allow gas exchange yet strong enough to maintain the architectural integrity needed to sustain alveolar structure. The functional structure of the lung can be divided into (1) the conducting airways (dead air space) and (2) the gas exchange portions. The two plumbing systems are airways for ventilation and the circulatory system for perfusion. Both systems are under low pressure.

Conducting Airways

The diameter of the lower airways is maintained by a balance of forces. Sympathetic impulses relax and parasympathetic impulses constrict the muscles. Airway dilatation may occur as a result of sympathomimetic agents (eg, epinephrine or adrenaline). Narrowing forces are bronchial smooth-muscle contraction, mediated by efferent autonomic nerve control. Constriction also can occur as a result of irritants (eg, dust, smoke, or cold); hyperventilation; and vasoactive agents (eg, acetylcholine, histamine, or bradykinin).

Additional narrowing occurs during forced expiration, when there is dynamic airway compression caused by pleural and peribronchial pressures. This narrowing is counteracted by intraluminal pressure and tethering action of the surrounding lung. The luminal diameter of a branch is related to the number of alveoli at the end of that branch (axial and lateral pathways). Because the longer airways with more branches and more alveoli usually have a wider lumen that allows greater airflow, newly inspired air reaches all of the alveoli throughout both lungs at the same time and in approximately the same amount, that is, an even distribution of inspired air throughout all lobes in a given period of time. There are approximately 23 airway divisions to the level of the alveoli. The divisions include main bronchi, lobar bronchi, segmental bronchi (to designated bronchopulmonary segments), and so on to the smallest bronchioles, which do not have alveoli and are lined completely by bronchial epithelium. These are the terminal bronchioles. Although the base airway diameter decreases with branching, the overall or total cross-sectional diameter increases tremendously so that peripheral airway resistance decreases.

Model of the Respiratory System

The respiratory system can be represented by a collection of physical components interacting with one another and with their environment. Although in vivo analysis demonstrates that the lungs do not function as a single compartment, analyzing the respiratory system in a linear model simplifies the presentation.

A single balloon on a pipe is the simplest model, although this model has its deficiencies because the airway is more complex than a simple pipe. Also, it now appears that the alveolus is not simply a single balloon or group of balloons similar to a cluster of grapes. It is now known that the alveoli are not physically independent structures but are actually interconnected.[3] An excellent review of the structure of the alveoli and the role of surfactant is offered by Gatto et al.[4] However, to lay the groundwork for our understanding of respiratory mechanics, we consider the simple model of a balloon on a pipe.

The relationship at any moment (t) between the pressure applied at the opening of the model (P[t]) and the volume in the model (V[t]) during emptying of this balloon can be described as a first-order model:

$$P(t) = E \cdot V(t) + R \cdot \dot{V}$$

where E is the elastance of the balloon, R is the resistance of the pipe, and $\dot{V}$ is the flow through the opening. Using regression analysis, E and R can be calculated from P(t), V(t), and V(t).

The values of R and E, as applied to the respiratory system, reflect the resistance of the airways and the elastance of the respiratory system, whereas V(t) is the volume increase from functional residual capacity (FRC) when the mouth pressure is zero.

The three important components of this linear model are the time constant (τ), compliance (C) or elastance (E), and resistance (R). The relationship of these is given by the equations:

$$\tau = C \times R \text{ or } \tau = R/E$$

Each of these components will be discussed separately.

Elastic Properties of the Respiratory System

The respiratory system is composed of a collection of elastic structures. The response to a force applied to the elastic struc-

ture of the respiratory system is to resist deformation by producing an opposing force, known as *elastic recoil*, to return the structure to its relaxed state.[5] In the respiratory system this opposing force produces a pressure known as the *elastic recoil pressure* (P_{EL}). The force required to stretch an elastic structure depends on the volume at which the outward recoil of the chest wall balances the inward recoil, known as the *elastic equilibrium volume*. The pressure of the elastic recoil or P_{EL} divided by the lung volume (V) gives a measure of the elastic properties of respiratory system and is called *elastance* (E):

$$E = P_{EL}/V$$

When lung volume is plotted on the ordinate and P_{EL} is plotted on the abscissa, the slope of the static pressure-volume curve is equivalent to the reciprocal of elastance, called *compliance*.

For ventilation of the lungs to occur, the forces necessary to overcome the elastic, flow-resistive, and inertial properties of the lungs and the chest wall must be produced to create motion of the respiratory system. In normal circumstances, respiratory muscles produce these forces.

Overcoming forces to move gas into the airway can be exemplified by moving a block of wood over a surface. The movement of the block is determined by the friction between the block of wood and the surface and how fast the wood is moving. It is irrelevant what the block's position is. Similarly, the pressure required to produce a flow of gas between the atmosphere and the alveoli must overcome the frictional resistance of the airways. This pressure is proportional to the rate at which volume is changing or flow $(\dot{V})$ as follows:

$$P_{mouth} - P_{alv} = P_{fr}\alpha\dot{V} \text{ or } P_{ao} - P_A = P_{fr}\alpha\dot{V}$$

where P_{ao} is pressure at the airway opening (usually atmospheric pressure), P_A is the alveolar pressure, and P_{fr} is the pressure required to overcome frictional resistance. The pressure required to produce a unit of flow is known as *flow resistance* (R):

$$R = P_{fr}/\dot{V}$$

If the respiratory system is modeled as a single compartment with a single constant elastance (E) and a single constant resistance (R), then the equation of motion describes the balance of forces acting on the system as follows:

$$P = EV + R\dot{V} + I\dot{V}$$

The inertia *(I)* is usually negligible and therefore ignored. Of the pressure produced during normal tidal respiration, most is required to overcome the elastic forces and a minimal amount is required to overcome the flow-resistant forces.

Traditionally it was thought that little energy was dissipated by the tissues of the respiratory system and that the majority of the force developed during breathing was required to move gas through the airways. The lung parenchyma is a complex system consisting of alveolar walls composed of collagen, elastin, and proteoglycan macromolecules; an air-liquid interface of surfactant; and cells that have the capacity to act in a contractile fashion, called *interstitial cells*. The viscoelastic behavior of the pulmonary parenchyma could potentially explain this behavior. In addition, this action is difficult to study because it is unclear where the boundary of the airways end and parenchyma begins. Airway smooth muscle exists in the terminal bronchioles and alveolar ducts, and the behavior of these structures may well influence parenchymal mechanics.

The energy expended moving the tissue is called the *tissue viscance* or resistance, although it is a non-Newtonian resistance. In other words, the viscosity depends on the force applied. When measured during inspiration, the tissue resistance increases with increasing lung volume, whereas airway resistance falls. Tissue resistance comprises approximately 65% of respiratory system resistance at FRC in mechanically ventilated animals and increases as much as 95% at higher lung volumes.[6] The contribution of tissue resistance to respiratory system resistance in humans under the same circumstances is unknown.

Resistance is expressed as changes in pressure divided by changes in flow:

$$R = \Delta P / \Delta \dot{V}$$

The other part of elastic recoil depends on the surface tension at the alveolar gas-liquid interface (surface forces). Surface tension is produced by the interface between air in the alveolus and the thin film of liquid that covers the alveolar surface. Surface tension in the alveolus is created by interacting water molecules that direct a force inward and could cause the alveoli to collapse. This action is described by La Place's equation where the pressure inside a bubble exceeds the pressure outside the bubble by twice the surface tension, divided by the radius. In other words, the smaller a bubble, the more the pressure inside exceeds the pressure on the outside. La Place's equation is defined as:

$$P = 2T/r$$

where *P* is the internal pressure, *T* is the tension in the wall of the structure, and *r* is the radius. When comparing two different alveoli with the same surface tension, the smaller the radius, the greater the pressure created by a given surface tension. Air will flow from high pressure (small alveoli) to lower pressure (larger alveoli). Thus smaller alveoli are more likely to collapse. The surface tension of the alveoli is affected by a substance produced in the alveoli called *surfactant.* Surfactant contains a mixture of lipids and proteins, is manufactured by alveolar type II cells, and exists as a monolayer on top of the alveolar subphase. Three surfactant-associated protein groups have been identified.[7] Surfactant acts to lower surface tension at the alveolar air-liquid interface and thereby decreases elastic recoil of the lungs.[8] Another action of surfactant is to reduce the development of pulmonary edema by diminishing one component of the pressure gradient driving transudation. In the lung there is a gradient between pulmonary capillary pressure and the interstitial pressure that surrounds the capillary. In most of the lung, the pulmonary capillary pressure is greater than the interstitial pressure; thus pulmonary edema would develop if not checked by the oncotic pressure of the plasma proteins. By reducing surface tension, the surfactant reduces the interstitial pressure and transcapillary gradient, but if there is a deficiency of surfactant and thus a rise in surface tension, pulmonary edema may develop.[9] Also, surfactant has been described as an antiwetting agent that helps to keep the lungs dry.[10] Currently there is agreement on the fact that surfactant plays an essential role in alveolar mechanics, but its mechanism is debated. The aforementioned description outlines the classic discussion on the role of surfactant, but diverse opinions exist on its true role. Scapelli[11] has described the role of the surfactant foam bubbles within the alveoli as "inner tubes." In contrast, Hills proposes that surfactant coats the alveolar walls as a "biologic wax."[12,13] The clinical implications of a deficiency of surfactant has been described in a famous editorial by Lachman entitled "Open Up the Lung and Keep the Lung Open."[14]

Compliance and Elastance

Compliance is how much a compartment will expand if the pressure in that compartment is changed. An elastic balloon has a high compliance because a small pressure increase inside the balloon will greatly expand the balloon. A rigid tube has a low compliance because a small pressure increase inside the rigid tube will not result in a significant increase in the volume of the rigid tube. Two major forces contribute to lung compliance: tissue elastic forces and surface tension forces. The compliance (C) is determined by the change in elastic recoil pressure (ΔP) produced by a change in volume (ΔV):

$$C = \Delta V / \Delta P$$

The compliance of the lungs (C_L), chest wall (C_{CW}), and respiratory system (C_{RS}) can be determined by measuring the change in distending pressure and the associated change in volume. The distending pressure represents the pressure change across the structure, where P_{ao}, P_{pl}, and P_{bs} represent the pressure measured at the airway opening, pleural pressure, and pressure at the body surface (atmospheric pressure), respectively:

$$C_L = \Delta V / \Delta (P_{ao} - P_{pl})$$
$$C_{CW} = \Delta V / \Delta (P_{pl} - P_{bs})$$
$$C_{RS} = \Delta V / \Delta (P_{ao} - P_{bs})$$

Lung volume and volume-pressure relationships (eg, compliance) reflect parenchymal (air space) development, whereas airflow and pressure-flow relationships (resistance and conductance) predominantly reflect airway development. The lungs become stiffer (compliance decreases) at higher lung volumes.

Pulmonary compliance changes with growth and maturation depending on the number of expanded air spaces, size and geometry of the air spaces, characteristics of the surface lining layer, and properties of the lung parenchyma. This shift is represented by changes in the shape of the volume-pressure curve. When these curves are corrected by expressing the volumes as a percentage of the maximal observed lung volume, they are more curved in infants than in older children (Fig. 45.1).[15] It is important to note that there may be boundaries for dynamic changes in alveolar size and shape during ventilation because of the tensile forces of the connective tissue and surface tension supporting the alveoli and alveolar ducts.

The developmental change in shape of the volume pressure curve represents the maturation of alveoli and hence differences in the elastin-collagen ratio with age.[15] The lung volume (as a percent of maximal lung volume) at which airway closure occurs is higher in children younger than 7 years[16] and is closer to their functional residual volume. Pressure-volume relationships are also more curvilinear in infants.[17] Chest wall compliance is 50% greater in infants.

Elastance is defined as the change in distending pressure divided by the associated change in volume:

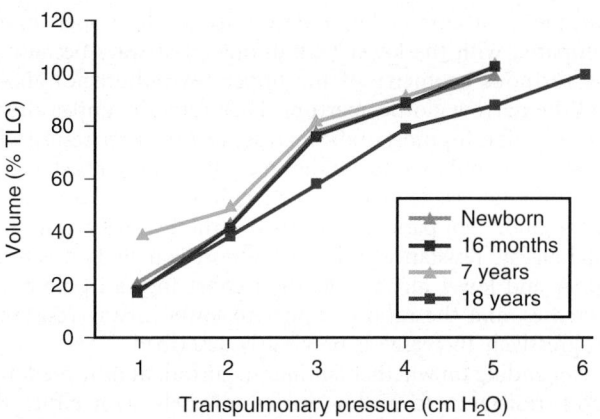

Fig. 45.1. Deflation volume-pressure curves of the lung at different ages (obtained from studies on excised lungs).[9] With increasing age up to young adulthood, the curves become straighter and, at a given lung volume, elastic recoil pressure is greater. The curve from elderly individuals resembles that from a 7-year-old respiratory system. *TLC,* total lung capacity.

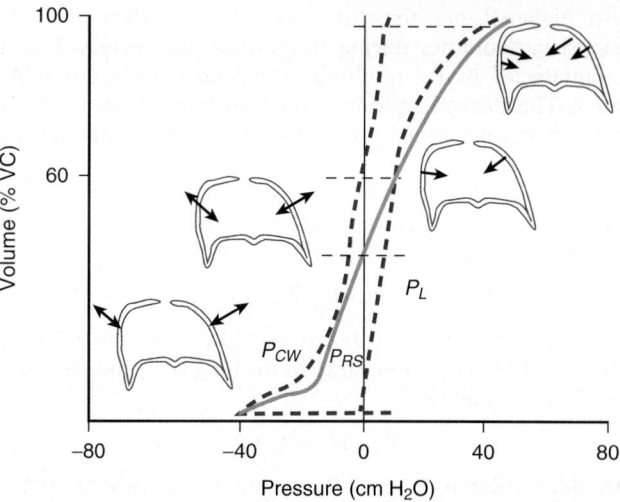

Fig. 45.2. Pressure-volume relationship of the lung (P_L), chest wall (P_{CW}), and entire respiratory system (P_{RS}). *Large arrows* represent the elastic recoil of the lungs and the chest wall. (Modified from Agostoni E, Mead J. Statics of the respiratory system. In: Fenn WO, Rahn H, eds. Handbook of Physiology, Respiration, vol 1. Washington, DC: American Physiological Society; 1964:392.)

$$E = \Delta P / \Delta V$$

Elastance is therefore the reciprocal of compliance; thus stiff lungs have a high elastance.

Elastic Recoil of the Respiratory System

In the intact thorax, the inward recoil of the lungs is opposed by the outward recoil of the chest wall (when it is below its resting volume). Both the lungs and chest wall recoil inward when chest volume exceeds its resting volume. These recoil forces act as though arranged in series.

The pressure required to balance the elastic recoil of the lungs, chest wall, and respiratory system (elastic recoil pressure) may be determined by having a subject exhale in increments from total lung capacity (TLC) to residual volume. At each volume, the subject relaxes against a fixed obstruction with glottis open, and the pressure difference across the lung, chest wall, and entire respiratory system is recorded. Pressure volume curves are derived in this way for the respiratory system, and its components are shown in Fig. 45.2.[18] The static pressure-volume curves of the respiratory system, lung, and chest wall are different during inspiration and expiration. Thus lung volume at a given transpulmonary pressure is higher during deflation than during inflation. This phenomenon is called *hysteresis*. Hysteresis is the failure of a system to follow identical paths of response on application and withdrawal of a forcing agent, as occurs during inspiration and expiration. Hysteresis in the respiratory system depends on viscoelasticity, such as stress adaptation (ie, rate-dependent phenomenon), and on plasticity (ie, a rate-independent phenomenon). In the lungs, hysteresis is due primarily to surface properties and alveolar recruitment-derecruitment. In comparison, the chest wall hysteresis is related to the action of both muscles and ligaments because both skeletal muscles and elastic fibers exhibit hysteresis. Hysteresis is negligible when volume changes are minimal, such as during quiet breathing. This phenomenon is important because the area of the hysteresis loop represents energy lost from the system.

The resting volume of the respiratory system, the FRC, is the volume at which the elastic recoil of the lungs and the chest wall exactly balances each other. Above and below this equilibrium point, progressively increasing pressure is required to change the volume of the respiratory system. The total pressure required at each volume is the sum of the pressures required to overcome the elastic recoil of the lungs and chest wall.

Flow Resistance of the Respiratory System

The response of the lung to movement is governed by its response to the physical impedance of the respiratory system. The impedance can be categorized into (1) elastic resistance between the alveolar gas/liquid interface and tissue and (2) frictional resistance to gas flow. Under static conditions, pressure is required only to oppose the elastic recoil of the respiratory system. However, when the lungs and chest wall are in motion and movement of air into and out of the lungs occurs, pressure also must be provided to overcome the frictional or viscous forces. The ratio of this additional pressure (P) and the rate of air flow that it produces $(\dot{V})$ is defined as the resistance:

$$R = P / \dot{V}$$

In other words, the flow $(\dot{V})$ measured at the mouth depends on the driving pressure (ie, the pressure difference between alveoli $[P_{alv}]$ and mouth $[P_{mo}]$) and the airway resistance (R_{aw}):

$$\dot{V} = (P_{mo} - P_{alv}) / R_{aw}$$

If the mouth pressure is zero (ie, atmospheric pressure), the driving pressure is the alveolar pressure.

Airways resistance (R_{aw}) is the sum of the peripheral airways resistance (peripheral intrathoracic airways <2 mm diameter; R_{awp}), the central airways resistance (large intrathoracic airways >2 mm diameter; R_{awc}), and the extrathoracic airways resistance (especially glottis; R_{ext}). In healthy people, R_{ext} accounts for 50% of the total R_{aw} and R_{awp} for about 15%. R_{awp} and R_{awc} are influenced by lung volume. Higher lung volumes give higher P_{el} and therefore increase airway diameter. With increasing volumes during inspiration, the increased P_{el} is counteracted by P_{pl}, resulting in increased radial distending force. This distending force is the transmural pressure and is the difference between pressure in (P_{in}) and pressure outside (P_{out}) the airway.

At zero airflow the pressure inside the airways (P_{in}) equals atmospheric pressure and transmural pressure (P_{tm}) equals the elastic recoil pressure (P_{el}):

$$P_{in} = P_{mo}, P_{tm} = P_{el}$$

The total respiratory resistance (R_{rs}) consists of the resistance of the airways (R_{aw}), resistance of the lung (R_L), and resistance of the chest wall (R_{cw}):

$$R_{rs} = R_{cw} + R_L + R_{aw}$$

In older children, R_{cw} and R_L represent only 10% to 20% of R_{rs},[19] but in newborns, R_L could be higher.[20]

Airway diameter of the intrathoracic airways approximates to a sigmoidal relationship with P_{tm}. This relationship results in volume dependency of R_{aw}. At higher lung volumes R_{awp} decreases. The specific relation between R_{awp} (or its reciprocal conductance G_{aw} [$=1/R_{aw}$]) and volume is mirrored by the specific R_{aw} (sR_{aw}) and specific G_{aw} (sG_{aw}):

$$sR_{aw} = R_{aw}/V$$

The resistance of the airways (R_{aw}), lungs (airway and parenchyma) (R_L), chest wall (R_{cw}), and entire respiratory system (R_{RS}) can be calculated by measuring the rate of airflow and the associated trans-structural pressure by subtracting from the total pressure the amount required to overcome elastic recoil:

$$R_{aw} = (P_{ao} - P_{alv})/\dot{V}$$
$$R_L = (P_{ao} - P_{pl})/\dot{V}$$
$$R_{cw} = (P_{pl} - P_{bs})/\dot{V}$$
$$R_{RS} = (P_{ao} - P_{bs})/\dot{V}$$

where P_{ao}, P_{alv}, P_{pl}, and P_{bs} represent the pressure at the airways opening, alveolar pressure, pleural pressure, and pressure at the body surface, respectively. The resistance of the lung parenchyma may be derived by subtracting airway from total lung resistance.

The relationship between the flow rate and the airway pressure gradient is nonlinear because of the relative contribution of the various components of the respiratory system to the total pressure required to overcome the viscous forces and its dependence on volume, volume history, and flow. The viscous forces increase disproportionately as the flow rate increases and as airway resistance increases. In contrast, the resistance of the chest wall and lung parenchyma remains constant over a wide range of flow rates.[21] During quiet breathing by mouth, airway resistance accounts for greater than 50% of the total respiratory system resistance.[22] However, as flow rate increases, the contribution of the airways to total resistance progressively increases.

Changing patterns of airflow result in the nonlinear flow-resistance characteristic of the airways. Subsequently, as the flow rate to the airway increases, airflow becomes progressively more turbulent. The more turbulent the flow, the greater the pressure required to overcome the viscous forces.

Turbulence occurs at lower flow rates in the upper airway compared with the lower (intrathoracic) airways because of the tortuous geometry of the upper (extrathoracic) airway and the narrow glottic aperture. Therefore, the upper airway is responsible for most of the increase in airway resistance with an increase in flow rate. Studies have shown the resistance of the lower airways to be nearly constant up to flow rates of 2 L per second.[21] For patients who are breathing quietly by mouth, total airway resistance is divided almost equally between the upper and lower airways. As their effort increases, flow rate increases, and the ratio of upper to lower airway resistance progressively increases as previously described.

Depending on whether laminar or turbulent flow predominates, resistance to airflow varies inversely with either the fourth or fifth power of airway radius.[23] Therefore major changes in airway resistance are caused by factors that affect airway diameter.[24] During spontaneous lung inflation, airway diameter increases as airway resistance decreases. This change is produced by two mechanisms. First, as lung volume increases, the increasing elastic recoil of the pulmonary parenchyma provides a tethering effect that dilates the intrapulmonary airways. Second, extrapulmonary and large intrapulmonary airways are surrounded by pleural pressure, which becomes increasingly negative during inspiration. This phenomenon leads to an increasing pressure gradient across the airway wall and therefore to an increasing diameter. The change in airway resistance with lung volume is curvilinear and is illustrated in Fig. 45.3.[24] When the reciprocal of airway resistance, airway conductance (G_{AW}), is plotted against lung volume, this relationship is nearly linear.

Dynamic Change in Airway Caliber During Respiration

Airway caliber is partially dependent on the transmural pressure. The transmural pressure is the difference between the interstitial pressure and atmospheric pressure. The external airway wall for the intrathoracic airways is subjected to the interstitial pressure, which is approximately equal to the pleural pressure. In contrast, the external walls of extrathoracic airways are subjected to atmospheric pressure. The

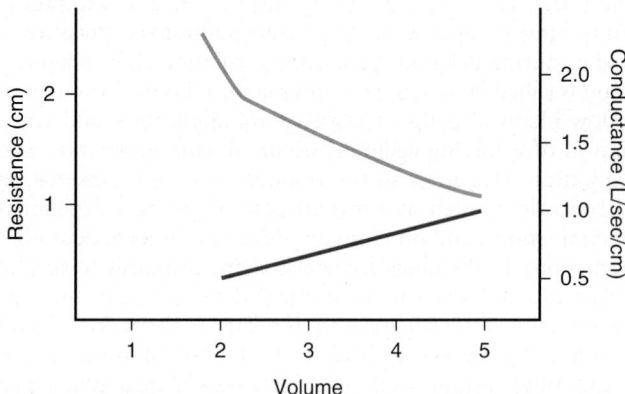

Fig. 45.3. Relationship between lung volume and airway resistance *(solid line)* and conductance *(dashed line)*. (Modified from Briscoe WA, Dubois AB. The relationship between airway resistance, airway conductance, and lung volume in subjects of different age and body size. J Clin Invest. 1958;37:1280.)

intraluminal pressure is dependent on the generation of the airway. During inspiration, pleural pressure is negative relative to atmospheric pressure. Alveolar pressure is approximately equal to pleural pressure, and pressure at the mouth is equal to atmospheric pressure. This pressure difference creates a gradient from the mouth to the alveoli. Extrathoracic airways tend to narrow during inspiration because the transmural pressure is positive. In contrast, the transmural pressure in the intrathoracic airways is negative, causing a tendency for these airways to dilate during inspiration. The degree of airway caliber change during inspiration depends on both the magnitude of the transmural pressure and airway wall compliance. At the end of inspiration there is a relaxation of the inspiratory muscles, and the elastic recoil of the respiratory system produces, relative to atmospheric pressure, a positive pleural and alveolar pressure. Because of the dynamic pressure changes previously described, there is a tendency for intrathoracic airways to narrow and extrathoracic airways to dilate during expiration.

Applied Forces

Ventilation of the lungs involves motion of the respiratory system, which is produced by the forces required to overcome the flow resistive, inertial, and elastic properties of the lungs and chest wall. Under normal circumstances, these forces are produced by the respiratory muscles.

If ventilation is to occur, opposing forces must be overcome by a pressure applied to the respiratory system to create motion. At each instant, the applied pressure (P_{APP}) must equal the sum of the pressure required to balance elastic recoil (P_{ER}) and the pressure lost to viscous (resistive) forces (P_R). The maximal pressures that can be generated by the respiratory muscles are determined by both lung volume and gas flow:

$$P_{APP} = P_{ER} + P_R$$

With use of the aforementioned equations, this may be converted to:

$$P_{APP} = (1/C)V + R\dot{V}$$

This equation is known as the *equation of motion of the respiratory system.*

Fig. 45.4 illustrates the pressure involved in respiration. Gradients must occur to allow for gas to flow into the lungs. The airway pressure gradient that drives airflow into the lungs is defined as:

$$P_M - P_{ALV}$$

where P_M is the pressure at the mouth, which is normally atmospheric, and P_{ALV} is the alveolar pressure. Transpulmonary pressure (P_{TP}) is defined as:

$$P_{TP} = P_{ALV} - P_{pl}$$

where P_{ALV} is the alveolar pressure and P_{pl} is the intrapleural pressure. P_{TP} is equal to elastic recoil of the lungs when there is no airflow. P_{TP} increases and decreases with lung volume. Transchest wall pressure (P_{TC}) is defined as:

$$P_{TC} = P_{pl} - P_{bs}$$

where P_{pl} is the intrapleural pressure and P_{bs} is the pressure at the body surface that is usually atmospheric. P_{TC} and P_{pl} are equal in magnitude to the elastic recoil of the chest when there

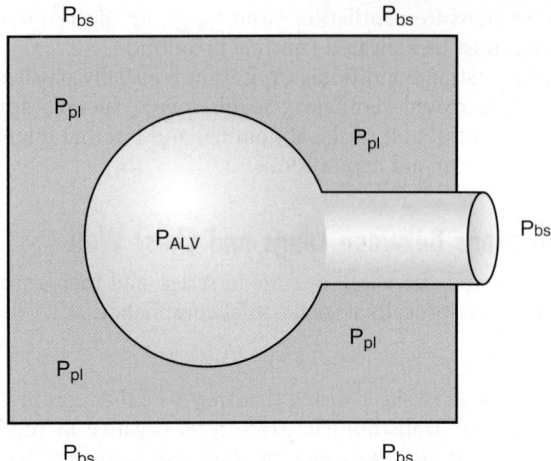

Fig. 45.4. Illustration of the pressure involved in respiration. Gradients must occur to allow for gas to flow into the lungs. P_{ALV}, alveolar pressure; P_{bs}, pressure at the body surface; P_{PL}, intrapleural pressure.

TABLE 45.1	Balance of Forces	
$P_{RS} + P_{MUS}$	=	$P_L + P_{CW}$
$P_{ALV} - P_{bs} + P_{MUS}$	=	$P_L + P_{CW}$
Inspiratory muscle contraction		Lung, chest wall elastic recoil
Outward acting forces when positive		Inward acting forces when positive

is no airflow and, like P_{TP}, they increase and decrease with lung volume.

The transmural pressure (P_{RS}) is defined as:

$$P_{RS} = P_{ALV} - P_{bs}$$

where P_{ALV} is the alveolar pressure and P_{bs} is the pressure at the body surface. P_{RS} represents the transmural pressure across the entire respiratory system, including the lungs and the chest wall, and is equal to the net passive elastic recoil pressure of the whole respiratory system when airflow is zero.

During inspiration the respiratory muscles provide the applied pressure that expands the chest wall and lungs, causing the alveolar and airway pressure to fall. The net result is that the alveolar pressure becomes less than atmospheric pressure. Once alveolar pressure is less than atmospheric pressure, air flows into the lungs along a pressure gradient and the lungs inflate, storing potential energy in the elastic structures for expiration. In order for gas flow to occur, there must be a balance of forces. Table 45.1 illustrates these forces (expressed as pressures).

Expiration is usually passive (excluding disease states where the patient actively tries to empty their lungs). That is, the energy stored in the elastic recoil of the lungs and the chest wall produces the positive alveolar and airway pressure needed to overcome flow resistance and air is forced from the lungs.

In order to inflate the lungs there must be an increase in alveolar pressure, which is usually done with positive pressure ventilation or a decrease in body surface pressure, such as in negative pressure ventilation (iron lung), or the respiratory muscles must be activated (normal breathing).

Under resting conditions, expiration is usually passive. At times of increased ventilatory requirements, such as during exercise, contraction of the abdominal and internal intercostals muscles can aid expiration.

Interactions Between Lungs and Chest Wall

The lungs and chest wall operate in series, and their compliance adds reciprocally to make total compliance:

$$1/C_T = 1/C_L + 1/C_{CW}$$

The chest wall is like a spring that may be either compressed or distended. Transthoracic pressure is negative at residual volume and at FRC, meaning the chest wall is smaller than its unstressed volume and its tendency is to spring out. Normal tidal breathing is entirely in the negative pressure range for transthoracic pressure. When examining the compliance curve of the chest wall (lung volume versus transthoracic pressure), pressure is 0 at about 65% of TLC. Thus the chest is at its unstressed volume and has no tendency to collapse or expand. Transthoracic pressure is positive at volumes above 65% TLC. The chest tends to collapse above its unstressed volume.

Volume-pressure loops observed during breathing are based on the flow resistance of gas and tissue. It had been previously suggested that the static volume-pressure relationship is represented by a single line, suggesting that the static pressures depend only on volume. However, the static pressure will vary depending on the volume history of the lung. Thus if the lung is fully expanded, at deep inspiration, static pressures will be lower. This concept is important because of the hysteresis of the lungs and tendency not to follow identical paths of response on the application and withdrawal of forces on the lung. Hysteresis applies to both the lung and chest wall.

Time Constant of Emptying

The time taken for volume in the respiratory system to be reduced by 63% when the respiratory system is allowed to empty passively and the volume-time profile is measured is known as the time constant (τ) of the respiratory system.[25] If we use a model of the respiratory system with a single compartment and a single, constant elastance and a single, constant resistance, then the following occurs:

$$\tau = R/E$$

In a single compartment model the volume-time profile can be represented by a single exponential decay.

In healthy adults the time constant of the passive respiratory system is short—approximately 0.5 seconds. Such a short time constant allows the lungs to empty to the end-expiratory volume (EEV) at the end of each expiration. Thus the FRC and EEV are equal. Since the respiratory system is relaxed at the end of expiration, inspiration can begin as soon as inspiratory muscle activity is initiated. The expiratory time constant is shorter in children, with values approximating 0.3 seconds reported in infants with normal lungs.[26] Infants with hyaline membrane disease have stiffer than normal lungs with expiratory time constants reported as low as 0.1 seconds. In the case of patients with obstructive airway diseases such as asthma, resistance is increased and the expiratory time constant is longer. Therefore, a longer time is required for the lungs to

empty and return the respiratory system to EEV. Patients with chronic airway obstruction frequently have carbon dioxide retention and an increased respiratory drive. This phenomenon results in an increased respiratory rate with a shorter respiratory cycle and less time available for expiration. In this situation the respiratory system frequently does not have time to return to EEV before the next inspiration starts; thus FRC occurs at a volume higher than EEV, not equal to EEV, which prevents relaxation of the respiratory system at the end of expiration. This lack of relaxation of the respiratory system at the end of expiration causes a positive recoil pressure. This pressure is called *intrinsic positive end expiratory pressure,* or PEEP$_i$. Before inspiratory flow can begin, the patient's inspiratory muscle must produce enough force to overcome the PEEP$_i$; thus this force is "lost" to produce inspiratory flow and represents a load that must be overcome by the inspiratory muscle. In patients with severe airway obstruction, this pressure can be as high as 15 to 20 cm H_2O.

Physiology of Positive Pressure Mechanical Ventilation

Up to this point our discussion has focused on patients breathing spontaneously without artificial support. To understand the respiratory physiology principles that apply to the critically ill pediatric patients, we must briefly examine the effects of positive pressure breathing on the pediatric respiratory system.

The respiratory system, like most biological systems, is closely associated with exponential functions. An exponential function is a mathematic expression that describes an event where the rate of change of one variable is proportional to its magnitude.

For example, in a passive breath, expiratory flow will be higher at the beginning of expiration than at the end, as the lung volume decreases toward FRC.

Among various forms of exponential functions, the two most important ones for the clinician in mechanical ventilation are the rising and decaying exponential functions.

Rising exponential function expresses an increase of one variable as a function of time—for example, flow, pressure, or volume versus time. A rising exponential function expresses the behavior of a physical system where the rate of change of one variable is proportional to its magnitude and a constant. In this relationship, the largest rate of change is always observed at the beginning of the event, and the smallest rate of change is always observed at the end of the event.

Decaying exponential function expresses a decrease of one variable as a function of time: flow, pressure, or volume versus time. An example of this relationship can be seen with the pressure decrease during lung deflation in a passive expiration. Flow returns to a baseline during a passive expiration, reflecting a negative decaying function. This expression of a physical system is expressed where the rate is proportional to its magnitude only. Therefore the rate of change will always have the largest value at the beginning of the event and the smallest value at the end of the event. The rate of decay is not constant over time.

As previously discussed, the respiratory system is governed by various laws of physics that describe the various dynamic forces involved in the movement of the system. In physiology, force is measured as Pressure = Force/Area, displacement is measured as Volume = Area × Displacement, and the relevant rate of change is measured as flow (eg, Average flow =

$\Delta V/\Delta$Time; Instantaneous flow = dv/dt [the derivative of volume with respect to time]). The pressure necessary to cause flow of gas into the airway and increase the volume of the gas in the lung is the key component in positive pressure mechanical ventilation. The volume of gas (ΔV) to any lung unit and the gas flow ($\dot{V}$) is related to the applied pressure (ΔP) by:

$$\Delta P = (\Delta V/C) + V \times R + K$$

where R is the airway resistance and C is the lung compliance. This equation is the same one previously described as Newton's equation of motion for the respiratory system. The applied pressure to the respiratory system measured at the inlet is the sum of the muscle pressures P_{mus} (pressure generated by the patient's spontaneous muscular forces) and the ventilator pressure $P_{applied}$ (pressure generated by ventilator). Muscle pressure is patient generated but cannot be directly measured. Muscle pressure represents the pressure generated by the patient to expand the thoracic cage and lungs. In contrast, ventilator pressure is the transrespiratory pressure generated by the ventilator during inspiration. Combinations of these pressures are generated when a patient is breathing on a positive pressure ventilator. In spontaneously breathing patients, the pressure measured at the patient's airway is a mix of the two pressures dependent on the mode of ventilator support used. For example, in continuous positive airway pressure, all pressure generated will be by the patient muscles, whereas in pressure support, the pressure generated will be a mix of the pressure generated by the patient's respiratory muscles and that generated by the ventilator. When respiratory muscles are at complete rest, the muscle pressure is zero; therefore the ventilator must generate all the pressure necessary to deliver the tidal volume and inspiratory flow. The reverse is also true, and there are degrees of support depending on the amount of force generated by the patient's respiratory muscles. The application of the equation of motion to the generation of gas flow is the next important step. Total pressure applied to the respiratory system (P_{RS}) of a patient undergoing ventilation is the sum of the pressure generated by the ventilator (measured at the airway) (P_{AO}) and the pressure generated by the respiratory muscles (P_{MUS}). Therefore:

$$P_{RS} = P_{Applied} + P_{MUS} = (V/C) + \dot{V} \times R + K$$

where P_{RS} is the respiratory system pressure, $P_{Applied}$ is the applied pressure by the ventilator, P_{MUS} is the pressure developed by the respiratory muscles, $\dot{V}$ is flow, R is airway resistance, V/C is respiratory system compliance, and K is the pressure. $P_{Applied}$ and $\dot{V}$ can be measured by the pressure and flow transducer in the ventilator. Volume is derived mathematically from the integration of the flow waveform.

To generate a volume displacement, the total forces have to overcome elastic and resistive elements of the lung and airway/chest wall represented by V/C and V × R, respectively. V/C depends on both the volume insufflated in excess of resting volume and the respiratory system compliance. To generate gas flow, the total forces must overcome the resistive forces of the airway and the endotracheal tube against the driving pressure gradients. At any moment during inspiration, there must be a balance of forces opposing lung and chest wall expansion measured as the airway pressure (P_{AO}). The opposing pressure can be summarized as the sum of elastic recoil pressure ($P_{elastic}$), flow-resistive pressure ($P_{resistive}$), and inertial pressure ($P_{resistance}$) of the respiratory system. Therefore:

$$P_{AO} = P_{elastic} + P_{resistive} + P_{inertance}$$

Inertial forces are usually negligible during conventional ventilation, which depends on bulk convective flow—unlike in high-frequency ventilation, where volumes are at the level of dead space. Therefore, for conventional ventilation, the forces exemplified in the equation of motion can expressed as:

$$P_{AO} = P_{elastic} + P_{resistive}$$

If elastic forces are recognized as the product of elastance and volume ($P_{elastic} = E \times V$) and the resistive forces as the product of flow and resistance (Resistive $\dot{V} \times R$), the formula can be written as:

$$P_{AO} = (Elastance \times Volume) + (Resistance \times Flow)$$

If compliance (the inverse of elastance) is substituted for elastance, the equation of motion, as described in the preceding text, becomes:

$$P_{AO} = Volume/Compliance + Resistance \times Flow$$

The quotient of volume displacement over compliance of the respiratory system represents the pressure necessary to overcome the elastic forces above the resting lung volume or FRC. It is essential to remember that the pressure to distend the alveoli is inversely related to the size of the alveoli. Thus, if the lung volume is below the resting volume, more pressure must be generated to distend those alveoli. This is reflected as La Place's law, and the resting lung represents the quantity of air remaining in the lungs at the end of a spontaneous expiration. Of course, just as in so many aspects of medicine, this is not as clear as it appears. The reader must remember that La Place's law is applied to spheres. Alveoli are thought to be prismatic or polygonal in shape (ie, their walls are flat), and Laplace's law considerations in their inflation apply only to the very small curved region in the fluid where these walls intersect. Even though it has been invoked as a mechanical model for the forces of alveolar inflation and as an explanation for the necessity of pulmonary surfactant in the alveolus, it still represents a reasonable model for alveolar behavior and consequences of lack of recruitment of the lung.

Pressure, flow, and volume are all measured relative to their baseline values. The pressure necessary to cause inspiration is measured as the change in airway pressure above PEEP. For example, in a patient breathing spontaneously on continuous positive airway pressure, the ventilator pressure is zero; the patient must use his or her respiratory muscles to generate all the work of breathing. The same can be applied to the volume during inspiration or the tidal volume, which is the change in volume above FRC. The pressure necessary to overcome the resistive forces of the respiratory system is the product of the maximum airway resistance (R_{MAX}) and inspiratory flow. Flow is measured relative to its end-expiratory value, which is usually zero, unless a $PEEP_i$ is present. The ultimate result of the gas movement or flow is to allow gas to reach and be exchanged at the alveolar unit.

Gas Exchange

The basic function of the respiratory system is to supply oxygen to the body and to remove excess carbon dioxide. The following are the essential steps involved in this process:

1. Ventilation, the exchange of gas between the atmosphere and alveoli

2. Diffusion across the alveolar-capillary membrane
3. Transport of gases in the blood
4. Diffusion of the gases from the capillaries of the systemic circulation to the cells of the body
5. Use of the oxygen and production of carbon dioxide within the cells as a byproduct of metabolism

During the process of ventilation, air is transported back and forth between the outside of the body and the terminal respiratory units of the lungs. In the alveoli, the air is exposed to a thin film of blood. O_2 diffuses across the alveolar-capillary membrane, enters the blood, and combines with hemoglobin. Simultaneously, CO_2 diffuses from the blood and enters the alveolar gas. In this way, the mixed venous blood entering the lungs is altered through the addition of O_2 and removal of CO_2. This is the process of gas exchange.

The partial pressure of O_2 (PaO_2) and CO_2 ($PaCO_2$) in the arterial blood, and therefore the adequacy of gas exchange, is dependent on a number of factors. These factors include the composition of the alveolar gas and the extent to which equilibrium is reached between the alveolar gas and pulmonary capillary blood. The alveolar gas composition is, in turn, dependent on the content of the inspired air and mixed venous blood, the quantity of air (ventilation) and blood (perfusion) reaching the alveoli, and the ratio of alveolar ventilation to perfusion ($\dot{V}_A/Q$). Of the factors determining the adequacy of gas exchange, the structure and function of the lungs primarily influence the ventilation-perfusion relationships, alveolar ventilation, and diffusion of O_2 and CO_2. Alveolar ventilation and oxygenation are related by the alveolar gas equation. The alveolar air equation for calculating P_AO_2 is essential to understanding any PaO_2 value and in assessing if the lungs are properly transferring oxygen into the blood. This is discussed further as follows in regard to its relation to ventilation and perfusion.

$$P_AO_2 = F_iO_2 * (P_B - P_{H2O}) - P_aCO_2/RQ$$

P_AO_2	The alveolar partial pressure of oxygen (pO_2)
F_iO_2	The fraction of inspired gas that is oxygen (expressed as a decimal)
P_B	Barometric pressure
P_{H2O}	The saturated vapor pressure of water at body temperature and the prevailing atmospheric pressure
P_aCO_2	The arterial partial pressure of carbon dioxide (pCO_2)

The respiratory quotient or respiratory coefficient (RQ) is the ratio of CO_2 produced to the O_2 consumed, and its value is typically 0.8.

Ventilation Perfusion Relationships

In the normal, upright lung, both alveolar ventilation and perfusion increase from the apex to the bases largely because of the effects of gravity. Blood flow increases more rapidly from apex to base than ventilation, and therefore $\dot{V}_A/Q$ ratios are high at the apex and decrease progressively toward the base of the lungs. The regional differences in perfusion are called *West's zones of perfusion*.[27-29] West's zone I occurs when mean pulmonary arterial pressure is less than or equal to alveolar pressure; thus no blood flow occurs. In zone I, the apices of the lung of an upright adult, there are unperfused yet ventilated alveoli, which is dead space ventilation. (Bronchial arterial flow nourishes the lung.) In zone II, which consists of the mid lung, pulmonary artery pressure is greater than alveolar

pressure. Conditions in this zone are governed by the fact that blood flow is not influenced by venous pressure but by the difference between arterial and alveolar pressures, which is a function of (hydrostatic) height. In zone III, the lower zone of the lung, pressure at the alveolus is exceeded by the pressures in both pulmonary artery and vein. Flow in this zone is a function of pulmonary artery and pulmonary venous pressures and is independent of height. At the base of the lung, because of higher perivascular pressures and reduced lung expansion, flow is again diminished.[30]

Any disorder affecting the airways or the parenchyma of the lung will result in an increased imbalance between ventilation and perfusion and therefore a greater than normal range of $\dot{V}_A/Q$ ratios. The presence of varying $\dot{V}_A/Q$ ratios, whether in the normal or the diseased lung, has several important effects on gas exchange. The PO_2 and the PCO_2 of an alveolus, and therefore of the capillary blood leaving it, is dependent on the ratio of ventilation to perfusion. As this ratio decreases, the PO_2 decreases and the PCO_2 increases. The opposite occurs as the $\dot{V}_A/Q$ ratio increases. Fig. 45.5 demonstrates the relationship between the ventilation/perfusion ratios P_AO_2 and P_ACO_2.

Lung units with low $\dot{V}_A/Q$ ratios therefore decrease arterial PO_2 and increase arterial PCO_2. In the extreme cases in which no ventilation reaches a lung unit, $\dot{V}_A/Q$ is zero and mixed venous blood is added unchanged to the arterial circulation. A right-to-left shunt occurs. The contribution of low $\dot{V}_A/Q$ units and shunts to arterial blood may be determined through the calculation of the venous admixture Q_S/Q_T:

$$Q_S/Q_T = (C_C - C_a)/(C_C - C\overline{V}),$$

where C_c, C_a, and $C\overline{V}$ are the O_2 contents of pulmonary end-capillary, arterial, and mixed venous blood, respectively. This contribution also may be assessed by calculating the difference between the alveolar and arterial PO_2 ($A - aDO_2$), which varies directly with the extent of venous admixture. Because of difficulties in accurately measuring it, the mean alveolar PO_2 (P_AO_2) is calculated from the alveolar air equation:

$$P_AO_2 = P_IO_2 - PCO_2/R,$$

where P_IO_2 represents the PO_2 of inspired air and R is the respiratory exchange quotient—the ratio of CO_2 production to O_2 consumption. In healthy young subjects, the $A - aDO_2$ averages 8 mm Hg.[31]

When ventilation to a lung unit exceeds its perfusion (that is, $\dot{V}_A/Q > 1$), the excess ventilation is considered to be "wasted" because it does not participate in gas exchange. The sum of the excess ventilation contributed by lung units with high $\dot{V}_A/Q$ ratios is referred to as *alveolar dead space*.

The effects of increasing ventilation/perfusion imbalance on gas exchange are that as the amount of inequality increases, both the ratio of physiologic dead space to tidal volume and venous admixture increases and arterial PO_2 falls. Arterial PCO_2 also progressively increases.

Alveolar Ventilation

The volume of air entering the lungs each minute that actually participates in gas exchange is called the *alveolar ventilation* ($\dot{V}_A$). It is therefore the difference between the total volume of air entering the lungs each minute (minute ventilation, $\dot{V}_E$) and the volume of air entering the lungs that does not participate in gas exchange (dead space: $\dot{V}_D$): $\dot{V}_A = \dot{V}_E - \dot{V}_D$.

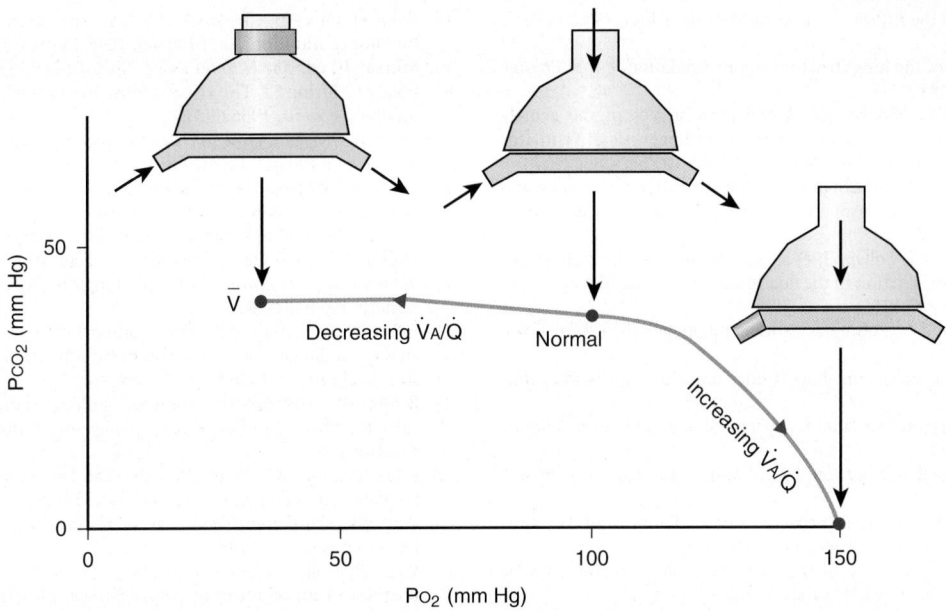

Fig. 45.5. Relationship between the ventilation/perfusion ratio $(\dot{V}_A/Q)$ of an alveolus and the P_{O_2} and P_{CO_2} of the alveolar gas and end-capillary blood. The P_{O_2} and P_{CO_2} vary from the mixed venous blood $(\dot{V})$ to inspired air (I) as $\dot{V}_A/Q$ changes from zero to infinity. (Modified from West JB. Ventilation blood flow and gas exchange. 3rd ed. Oxford, England: Blackwell Scientific; 1977:37.)

The type of dead space $(\dot{V}_D)$ depends on the location of the volume not exchanged, either in the anatomic airways or in the alveolus. The anatomic dead space is equal to the volume of airways proximal to the terminal respiratory units. Approximately 25% of each tidal volume is lost in these conducting airways. The ultimate volume is dependent on body size and equals approximately 1 mL/lb.[32] This volume is divided almost equally between the upper and lower airways. An alveolar dead space is produced by all alveoli that are overventilated relative to their perfusion. Thus, more gas is available than blood for diffusion. The physiologic dead space is usually expressed as a fraction of the tidal volume (V_D/V_T).

The alveolar ventilation is an important determinant of gas exchange because it, along with the rate at which tissue metabolism produces CO_2 $(\dot{V}_{CO_2})$, determines the P_{CO_2} of arterial blood:

$$P_{CO_2} = \dot{V}_{CO_2}/\dot{V}_A$$

When $\dot{V}_{CO_2}$ is constant, P_{CO_2} varies inversely with $\dot{V}_A$. It is evident that at given minute ventilation, the P_{CO_2} will vary directly with the amount of physiologic dead space. As dead space changes, the P_{CO_2} can be kept constant only by increasing or decreasing $\dot{V}_E$ by an identical amount.

The measurement of dead space has evolved from the original description by Bohr in 1891 when dead space was considered simply the gas from the conducting airways. One can calculate the physiologic dead space as:

$$V_D/V_T = (Pa_{CO_2} - P\bar{E}_{CO_2})/Pa_{CO_2}$$

where $P\bar{E}_{CO_2}$ is end-tidal P_{CO_2}.

Diffusion of Oxygen and Carbon Dioxide

Gas must travel through a number of barriers between the alveolus and blood. These barriers include the alveolar epithelial lining, basement membrane, capillary endothelial lining, plasma, and red blood cell. The amount of gas (Q) diffusing through a membrane is directly proportional to the surface area available for diffusion (S), the pressure difference for the gas on either side of the membrane (p1 − p2), and a constant (K) that depends on the solubility coefficient of the gas, membrane characteristics, and liquid used. This association is defined by the Fick principle of the diffusion state as follows:

$$Q/\min = K\lambda(p1 - p2)/d$$

where Q is inversely proportional to the distance it has to diffuse, whereas K is proportional to the solubility of the gas and inversely proportional to the square root of the molecular weight.

In healthy subjects at rest, equilibration of the P_{O_2} and P_{CO_2} of the alveolar gas and pulmonary capillary blood is achieved in approximately 0.75 seconds.[33] This is about one-third of the time spent by the blood in the capillary network. The rate of pulmonary blood flow can increase greatly, to the point that it prevents equilibration. For this reason, diffusion disequilibrium has been demonstrated in healthy persons, but only during strenuous exercise at high altitudes.

In the presence of parenchymal disease, diffusion impairment may occur solely as a result of thickening of the alveolar-capillary membrane. Much more commonly, however, diffusion disequilibrium is associated with destruction of the pulmonary capillary bed. This destruction results in a greatly increased blood flow velocity in the remaining capillaries, which may allow insufficient time for equilibration. Even when parenchymal disease is severe, however, diffusion disequilibrium usually occurs only when cardiac output, and therefore rate of flow, is markedly increased.

References

1. Hall JE. The promise of translational physiology. *Am J Physiol Lung Cell Mol Physiol.* 2002;283(2):L235-L236.

2. Rossier B. "Back to the future … " a word from the editor. *Pflugers Arch.* 2003;445:455.
3. Fung YC. A model of the lung structure and its validation. *J Appl Physiol.* 1988;64(5):2132-2141.
4. Gatto LA, Fluck RR, Nieman GF. Alveolar mechanics in the acutely injured lung: role of alveolar instability in the pathogenesis of ventilator induced lung injury. *Respir Care.* 2004;49(9):1045-1055.
5. Karlinsky JB, Snyder GL, Franzblaw C, et al. In vitro effects of elastase and collagenase on mechanical properties of hamster lungs. *Am Rev Respir Dis.* 1976;113:769-777.
6. Ludwig MS, Dreshaj I, Solway J, et al. Partitioning of the pulmonary resistance during constriction in the dog: effects of volume history. *J Appl Physiol.* 1987;62(2):807-815.
7. Wright JR, Hawgood S. Pulmonary surfactant metabolism. *Clin Chest Med.* 1989;10:83.
8. Bangham AD. Lung surfactant: how it does and does not work. *Lung.* 1987;165:17-25.
9. Hills BA. What forces keep the air spaces of the lung dry? *Thorax.* 1982;37(10):713-717.
10. Hills BA. Water repellency induced by pulmonary surfactants. *J Physiol.* 1982;325:175-186.
11. Scapelli EM. The alveoli surface network: a new anatomy and its physiologic significance. *Anat Rec.* 1998;251(4):491-527.
12. Hills BA. An alternative view of the roles surfactant and the alveolar model. *J Appl Physiol.* 1999;87(5):1567-1583.
13. Scapelli EM, Hills BA. Opposing views on the alveolar surface, alveolar models, and the role of surfactant. *J Appl Physiol.* 2000;89(2):408-412.
14. Lachmann B. Open up the lung and keep the lung open. *Intensive Care Med.* 1992;18(6):319-321.
15. Fagan DG. Post-mortem studies of the semistatic volume-pressure characteristics of infant's lungs. *Thorax.* 1976;31:534.
16. Mansell AL, Bryan C, Levison H. Airway closure in children. *J Appl Physiol.* 1988;319:1112.
17. Thorsteinsson A, Larsson A, Jonmarker C, et al. Pressure-volume relations of the respiratory system in healthy children. *Am J Respir Crit Care Med.* 1994;150:421.
18. Rahn H, Otis AB, Chadwick EL, et al. The pressure-volume diagram of the thorax and lung. *Am J Physiol.* 1946;146:161-178.
19. Murray JF, ed. *The Normal Lung.* Philadelphia: WB Saunders; 1986.
20. Polgar G, String ST. The viscous resistance of the lung tissues in newborn infants. *J Pediatr.* 1966;69:787.
21. Ferris BG, Mead J, Opie LH. Partitioning of respiratory flow resistance in man. *J Appl Physiol.* 1964;19:653-658.
22. Hogg JC, Williams J, Richardson JB, et al. Age as a factor in the distribution in the distribution of lower airway conductance and in the pathologic anatomy of obstructive lung disease. *N Engl J Med.* 1970;282:1283.
23. Dubois AB. Resistance to breathing. In: Fenn WO, Rahn H, eds. *Handbook of Physiology, Respiration.* Vol 1. Washington, DC: American Physiological Society; 1964:451-462.
24. Brisco WA, Dubois AB. The relationship between airway resistance, airway conductance and lung volume in subjects of different age and body size. *J Clin Invest.* 1958;37:1279-1285.
25. Brody AW. Mechanical compliance and resistance of the lung-thorax calculated from the flow during passive expiration. *Am J Physiol.* 1954;178:189-196.
26. Kano S, Lanteri CJ, Pemberton PJ, et al. Fast versus slow ventilation for neonates. *Am Rev Respir Dis.* 1993;148:578-584.
27. West JB. *Ventilation/Blood Flow and Gas Exchange.* 3rd ed. London: Blackwell Scientific; 1979.
28. West JB, Dollery CT. Distribution of blood flow and the pressure-flow relations of the whole lung. *J Appl Physiol.* 1964;19:713.
29. West JB, Dollery CT, Naimark A. Distribution of blood flow in isolated lung: relation to vascular and alveolar pressure. *J Appl Physiol.* 1964;19:713.
30. Hughes JMB, Glazier JB, Maloney JE, et al. Effect of lung volume on the distribution pulmonary blood flow in man. *Respir Physiol.* 1968;4:58.
31. Mellemgaard K. The alveolar-arterial oxygen difference: its size and components in normal man. *Acta Physiol Scand.* 1966;67:10-20.
32. Radford EP. Ventilation standards for use in artificial respiration. *J Appl Physiol.* 1955;61:1560.
33. Roughton FJ. Average time spent by blood in human lung capillary and its relation to the rates of CD uptake and elimination in man. *Am J Physiol.* 1945;143:621.

Noninvasive Respiratory Monitoring and Assessment of Gas Exchange

Beryl F. Yaghmai and Kenneth A. Schenkman

PEARLS

- Pulse oximetry is based on the principles that the pulsatile component of the optical absorbance detected from tissue is primarily from arterial blood and that oxyhemoglobin and reduced (deoxy-) hemoglobin have different optical absorption spectra.
- Limitations of pulse oximetry include motion artifact, effects of ambient light, presence of pigmentation or dyes, low perfusion states, and dyshemoglobinemia.
- Most pulse oximeters measure only oxyhemoglobin and deoxyhemoglobin; however, blood cooximeters and noninvasive cooximeters now account for other absorbing species such as methemoglobin and carboxyhemoglobin.
- Capnography can be a good global indicator of the patient's condition and can detect alveolar hypoventilation before changes detected by pulse oximetry.
- The accuracy of the capnogram depends on the sampling site. If the tidal volume is small and the sample flow rate is large, the gas sample may be diluted by entrained fresh gas.

Noninvasive monitoring in the form of vital signs (ie, heart rate, respiratory rate, noninvasive blood pressure, fluid intake and output, and temperature) has been used routinely for all patients receiving care in the ICU since the birth of the specialty. Guidelines for equipment and monitoring and for levels of care for pediatric ICUs (PICUs) were specified by the American College of Critical Care Medicine in 2004.[1] The majority of children admitted to the PICU present with cardiorespiratory disease or with an acute illness that may progress to involve the respiratory system, emphasizing the specific need for careful monitoring of respiratory parameters. Close respiratory examination and monitoring allow titration of therapies to minimize oxygen toxicity, ventilator-induced injury, optimize patient-ventilator interaction, and aid in weaning from the ventilator.[2] Pulse oximetry and capnometry have significantly affected the practice of critical care medicine and are now standards of care. New technologies currently under development to noninvasively monitor physiologic function may significantly decrease the need for more invasive monitoring and lessen the associated risks of such modalities.

Pulse Oximetry

Pulse oximetry is a significant technologic advance that has improved patient safety.[2-6] Its ease of application and accuracy have resulted in widespread use, and it is now a standard monitoring modality for many aspects of medical care. Indications for pulse oximetry monitoring in the pediatric population now include screening for neonatal congenital heart disease.[7-9] In the ICU, pulse oximetry is used to detect hypoxia and wean the oxygen concentration in patients undergoing mechanical ventilation.

Takuo Aoyagi, working for the Nihon Kohden Corporation in Japan, first proposed the theory for pulse oximetry in 1972. His idea was developed into a working oximeter, which subsequently was patented in Japan in 1974 and marketed as the world's first commercial pulse oximeter. In 1977 a fiberoptic-based pulse oximeter with improved accuracy was marketed by Minolta, and in 1982 Nellcor began marketing a pulse oximeter that ultimately became an industry standard.[10] Since then numerous companies have produced and marketed pulse oximeters, and improvements in technology continue to improve the accuracy and reliability of these devices. More recently, Masimo Corporation (Irvine, Calif.) introduced pulse oximeters with signal extraction technology[11] that minimizes motion artifact and interference from ambient light and is able to function in relatively low perfusion states. This approach has improved the accuracy of pulse oximetry readings and has decreased the frequency of false alarms in clinical settings.[12-16]

Standard pulse oximeters are not accurately calibrated for the low saturations seen with some congenital cardiac lesions. There is, however, a "blue" sensor that is particularly sensitive in patients with cyanotic congenital heart disease.[17] Accurate pulse oximetry is especially vital in the neonatal population, who benefit from tight control of oxygenation in order to minimize oxidative stress and to decrease the risk of retinopathy of prematurity.[18]

Principles of Pulse Oximetry

Pulse oximetry is based on the principles that (1) the pulsatile optical absorbance detected in biological tissue is primarily due to arterial blood and that (2) oxyhemoglobin and reduced (deoxygenated) hemoglobin have different optical absorption spectra.[3] The attenuation of light passing through blood-perfused tissue changes with pulsation of blood and the

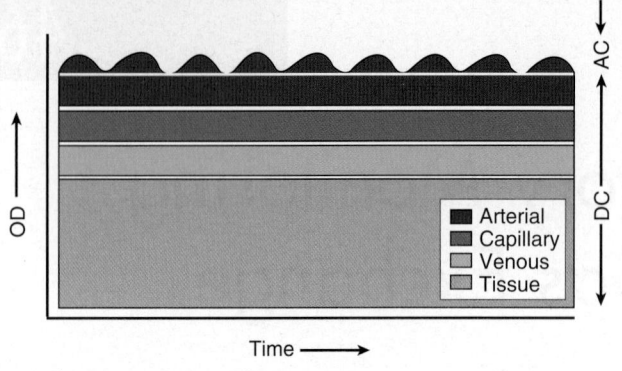

Fig. 46.1. Light passing through a pulsating tissue will be absorbed by multiple components of tissue and blood. The alternating component (AC) is composed of only arterial blood.

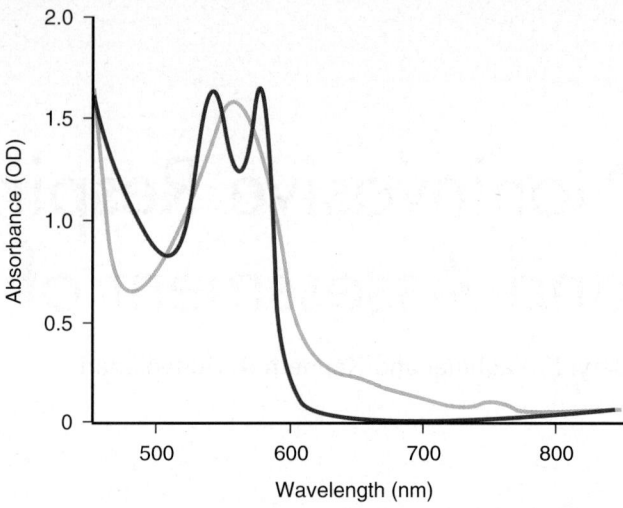

Fig. 46.2. Absorption spectra of hemoglobin in the visible and near-infrared spectral region. The deoxy form of hemoglobin (blue) has a single peak in the visible and near-infrared region. Oxyhemoglobin (red) has two peaks in the visible region but no significant peak in the near-infrared region.

alternating component of the light attenuation results from the composition of arterial blood.[19] Fig. 46.1 is a schematic diagram showing that the component of light attenuation as a result of pulsatility comes from arterial blood. This information can be analyzed to determine the hemoglobin saturation in the arterial blood. Absorption of light as a result of other tissue components and capillary and venous blood in the static (nonpulsatile) portion of the signal is ignored in the analysis.

Light passing through a turbid media such as tissue is attenuated by absorption and scattering. If light scattering in tissue is assumed to be fairly constant, then measured changes in the attenuation of the transmitted light can be assumed to result from changes in absorption. Beer's law describes the theoretic absorption of light as follows:

$$\text{Absorbance (OD)} = -\log_{10}(I/I_O) = \varepsilon bc \qquad \text{Eq. 46.1}$$

where I is light emerging from the sample, I_o is incident light illuminating the sample, ε is molar extinction coefficient of the specific absorbing species at a specific wavelength, b is path length (in centimeters) the light traverses, and c is molar concentration of the absorbing species. Thus changes in the concentration of an absorber, that is, oxyhemoglobin, result in changes in absorbance.

Hemoglobin has characteristic light-absorbing properties that change with oxygen binding. Fig. 46.2 shows absorption spectra of oxyhemoglobin and deoxyhemoglobin in the visible and near-infrared spectral region. At any given wavelength there is a difference in absorption between oxyhemoglobin and deoxyhemoglobin except where the spectra cross at wavelengths called *isosbestic wavelengths,* where the absorption is the same for each state. At nonisosbestic wavelengths, the difference in absorption can be used to determine the fraction of oxyhemoglobin. Saturation of hemoglobin is defined as follows:

$$\text{Hb}_{sat} = [\text{OxyHb}]/([\text{OxyHb}] + [\text{DeoxyHb}]) \qquad \text{Eq. 46.2}$$

where Hb_{sat} is fractional saturation of hemoglobin, [$OxyHb$] is concentration of oxyhemoglobin, and [$DeoxyHb$] is concentration of deoxyhemoglobin. Hemoglobin percent saturation, as commonly reported, is determined by multiplying Hb_{sat} by 100.

Pulse oximeters typically use red (660-nm) and infrared (940-nm) wavelengths of light to determine the ratio of

oxygenated to deoxygenated blood.[11] Deoxygenated blood absorbs more red light, whereas oxygenated blood absorbs more infrared light. The two wavelengths are passed through an arterial bed, and the ratio of infrared and red light transmitted to the photodetector is determined. The absorption around 940 nm is relatively low and fairly constant over the range of saturations; thus a change in absorbance at 660 nm can be referenced to the absorption at the 940-nm wavelength and is used to determine the saturation. The ratio is calibrated against measurements of arterial oxygen saturations from human volunteers and their absorbance ratios. Each pulse oximeter uses a complex algorithm to convert the change in absorbance at the two wavelengths to an absolute saturation value. More wavelengths can be used to improve the accuracy of the measurement.

In the presence of other forms of hemoglobin, primarily carboxyhemoglobin or methemoglobin, the saturation of hemoglobin is correctly determined by the more complex relationship:

$$\text{Hb}_{sat} = [\text{OxyHb}]/([\text{OxyHb}] + [\text{DeoxyHb}]$$
$$+ [\text{MetHb}] + [\text{CarboxyHb}]) \qquad \text{Eq. 46.3}$$

where [$MetHb$] is concentration of methemoglobin and [$CarboxyHb$] is concentration of carboxyhemoglobin. Most pulse oximeters cannot accurately account for the presence of these other forms of hemoglobin. Blood cooximeters, however, do account for these species, as do the newer Masimo pulse oximeters.

Validation

Numerous studies have been performed to validate existing pulse oximeters.[20,21] Pulse oximeters also must be subjected to extensive testing before obtaining US Food and Drug Administration (FDA) approval for marketing in the United States. Despite all of the current testing, difficulties in both calibration and validation remain. One of the most significant issues surrounding calibration is the development of an appropriate universal test that will accurately test the pulse oximeter for a wide range of potential clinical applications. Pulse oximeters must be accurate for a wide range of skin thickness and color and over a wide range of saturations. In general, pulse oximeters are most accurate at higher saturations, usually above 75%.[22-24]

Sources of Error

Although pulse oximetry is widely accepted as a valid clinical monitor and provides valuable minute-to-minute clinical data, pulse oximeters are subject to multiple potential sources of error. Pulse oximetry measures oxygen saturation (SaO_2). SaO_2 and PaO_2 are not linearly related; the oxyhemoglobin dissociation curve is sigmoid in shape (Fig. 46.3). Large changes in PaO_2 at high levels of oxygen, the upper flat portion of the oxyhemoglobin dissociation curve, occur with little change in saturation. Saturations measured by pulse oximetry on average overestimate SaO_2 in the range of 76% to 90%,[25] and the accuracy of pulse oximetry falls with arterial oxygen saturations less than 70%.[2,3] At arterial oxygen saturations below 70%, pulse oximetry may be more appropriate for showing trends.[3]

Pulse oximetry sensors may be unable to distinguish a true signal from background in low perfusion states that result in diminished pulsations (eg, vasoconstriction, low cardiac output, and hypothermia).[26] This situation is usually displayed as an inadequate pulse message.[2] Low peripheral perfusion and motion artifact are the most common causes of inaccurate pulse oximetry readings.[6,11,27] Newer designs of pulse oximeters with signal-progressing algorithms that detect and ignore motion and pulse rate interferences help overcome these limitations.[11,27]

Other sources of error include interfering dyes or other pigments in the blood and ambient light.[26] Intravenous dyes and certain colors of nail polish may falsely lower pulse oximetry readings. The extent of ambient light interference has been questioned for some of the pulse oximeters studied,[28] and shielding of the probe from ambient light is often used clinically to improve performance.

The presence of dyshemoglobinopathies is an infrequent clinical problem but can result in erroneous pulse oximetry readings.[26] Abnormal hemoglobin levels (carboxyhemoglobin, methemoglobin) that have similar absorbance spectra can lead to overestimation of the true SaO_2.[3] In methemoglobinemia, the iron in the heme groups in hemoglobin becomes oxidized from the ferrous (Fe^{2+}) state to the ferric (Fe^{3+}) state. The oxidized form of hemoglobin, called methemoglobin, cannot bind oxygen. Thus the presence of significant quantities of methemoglobin leads to tissue hypoxia because these molecules no longer participate in oxygen transport. However, light absorbance by methemoglobin more closely resembles oxyhemoglobin than deoxyhemoglobin at the measured wavelengths, erroneously leading the pulse oximeter to indicate a higher percentage of oxygen saturation than expected.[29,30] Similarly, the presence of carboxyhemoglobin may result in erroneous reading in pulse oximetry because carbon monoxide–bound hemoglobin also does not participate in oxygen transport.[31]

Masimo has developed a pulse oximeter, known as the Masimo Rainbow SET, that uses eight wavelengths of light

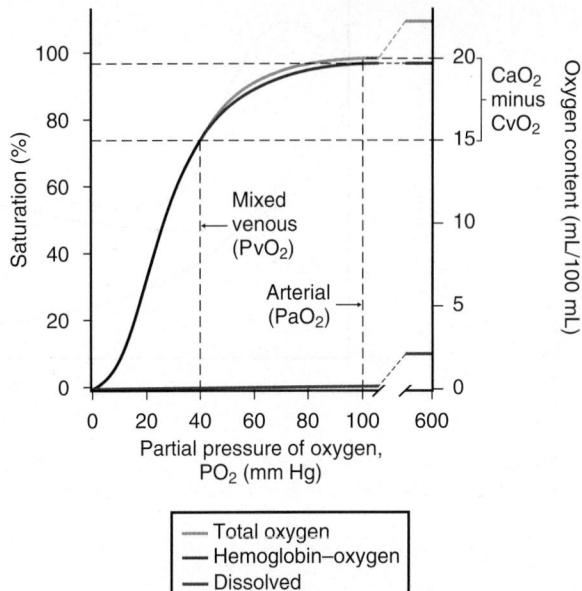

HEMOGLOBIN–OXYGEN DISSOCIATION CURVE

Fig. 46.3. Hemoglobin-oxygen (Hb-O_2) dissociation curve shows the percentage saturation of hemoglobin at each PO_2. When the hemoglobin concentration is known, the content of oxygen can be calculated. The total content includes the small additional content of oxygen in solution, which becomes significant at high levels of PO_2. The saturation scale on the left applies only to the Hb-O_2 line. The scale on the right shows content values for a normal hemoglobin level of 15 g/100 mL blood. (Modified from Hlastala MP. Blood gas transport. In: Culver BH, ed. The Respiratory System. Seattle: ASUW Publications; 1997. Redrawn in Albert RK, Spiro SG, Jett R, eds. Clinical Respiratory Medicine. 2nd ed., St. Louis: Mosby Elsevier; 2004.)

(Fig. 46.4) and thus is able to determine carboxyhemoglobin and methemoglobin levels in addition to oxygenated and deoxygenated hemoglobin.[32] Because these other species of hemoglobin are recognized, it is also possible to have a continuous readout of total hemoglobin. The Rainbow oximeter will be useful not only for monitoring patients with dyshemoglobinemias but also in situations where occult blood loss may be occurring because of its ability to report total hemoglobin. Because the technology is relatively new, confirmation with laboratory samples may still be necessary, but trends can then be followed with the oximeter, minimizing the need for blood sampling.[33]

Because cooximeters account for the presence of both carboxyhemoglobin and methemoglobin, blood gas samples sent for cooximetry should correctly measure hemoglobin saturation in cases where measurable levels of either methemoglobin or carboxyhemoglobin are present or suspected. Fetal hemoglobin has a sufficiently similar absorbance spectrum to adult hemoglobin, such that the presence of fetal hemoglobin does not significantly affect the determined saturation.[34] The presence of bilirubin also does not appear to significantly affect pulse oximetry readings.[35]

Probe Placement

Pulse oximetry probes typically are placed on fingers or toes, with the light-emitting diodes placed across the digit, opposite

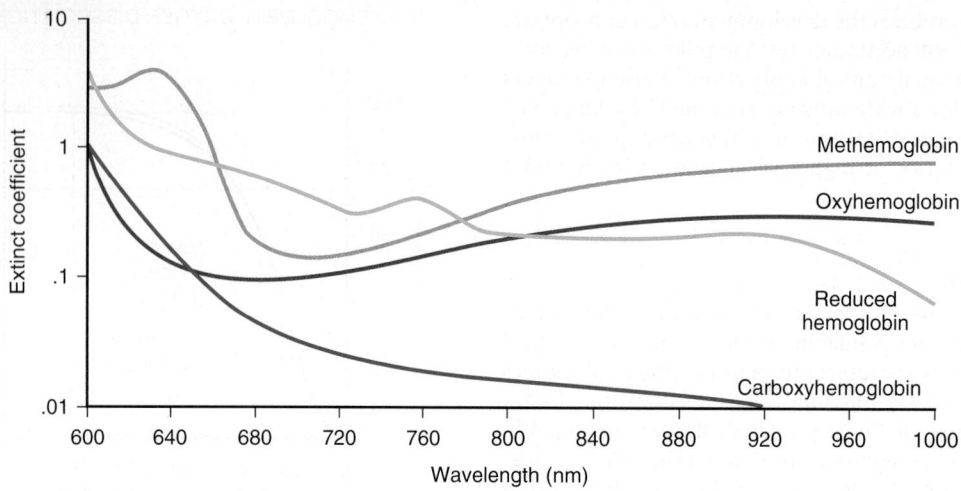

Fig. 46.4. Absorption spectra for carboxyhemoglobin, deoxyhemoglobin, oxyhemoglobin, and methemoglobin used in the Masimo SET Rainbow pulse oximeter. (Modified with permission from Masimo Corporation.)

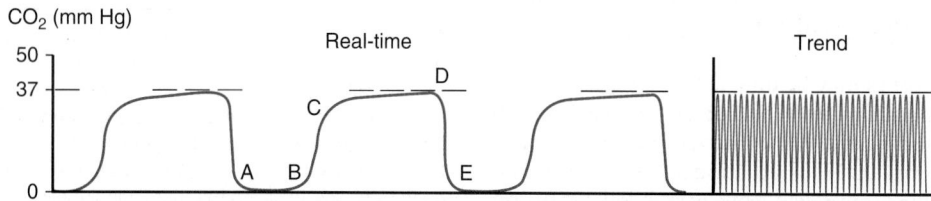

Fig. 46.5. Normal capnogram. (A-B) baseline during inspiration or dead space. (B-C) Expiratory upstroke (mix of dead space and alveolar gas). C-D: expiratory or alveolar plateau. D- end-tidal volume or $P_{ET}CO_2$. D-E: inspiratory downstroke. (Modified with permission from Zwerneman K. End-tidal carbon dioxide monitoring: a VITAL sign worth watching. Crit Care Nurs Clin N Am. 2006;18:217-225. Fig. 1.)

from the detector. For premature and small infants, the probe often is placed around the entire palm or foot with good results. In larger pediatric patients the nasal ala may also be used.[36] Because of scattering of light in tissue, pulse oximeter probes also can be used in a reflectance mode. In this manner, both light-emitting diodes and detectors are on the same surface and can be placed, for example, on the forehead.[37,38] Transesophageal probes have been designed and are used for care of operative or critically ill patients with potentially poor peripheral perfusion.[39-41] The complications of pulse oximetry are rare. They include skin burns and pressure necrosis in newborns.[2,3] Limited understanding of pulse oximetry by health care providers may be an underrecognized problem, along with time spent determining whether alarms are false.[6,42]

Capnometry and Capnography

Another monitoring technology routinely used in the critical care unit is the measurement of carbon dioxide (CO_2). Capnometry is the measurement of the partial pressure (or concentration) of CO_2 in the patient's airway during the entire ventilatory cycle. A capnometer provides a numeric measurement of inspired and expired, end-tidal CO_2 ($P_{ET}CO_2$). Capnography is the graphic display of the partial pressure or concentration of CO_2 as a waveform (capnogram), usually plotted as P_{CO_2} versus time. When the waveform display is calibrated, capnography includes capnometry.

Physiologic Basis

$P_{ET}CO_2$ monitoring is the noninvasive measurement of exhaled carbon dioxide at the plateau of the carbon dioxide waveform. $P_{ET}CO_2$ concentration reflects $PaCO_2$, cardiac output, percentage of dead space, and airway time constants. In healthy subjects, the $P_{ET}CO_2$ concentration is 1 to 5 mm Hg less than the $PaCO_2$.[43] $P_{ET}CO_2$ concentration represents the P_{CO_2} of all ventilated alveoli, whether or not they are perfused. Therefore any condition that reduces pulmonary perfusion of ventilated alveoli increases the difference between $PaCO_2$ and $P_{ET}CO_2$. When ventilation and perfusion are well matched throughout the lung, the arterial partial pressure of CO_2 ($PaCO_2$) and the partial pressure of $P_{ET}CO_2$ are nearly equal, normally 40 mm Hg. If a discrepancy between ventilation and perfusion exists, a difference between the $PaCO_2$ and $P_{ET}CO_2$, also known as $(a-et)\Delta P_{CO_2}$, occurs. Comparison between $P_{ET}CO_2$ concentration and $PaCO_2$ helps to differentiate between change in alveolar ventilation, CO_2 production, or pulmonary perfusion as a cause of the change in $P_{ET}CO_2$ concentration.

The capnogram displays the CO_2 concentration in the patient's airway over time (Fig. 46.5). The essentials of a normal capnogram are (1) zero baseline during early exhalation, which reflects gas exhaled from the anatomic dead space; (2) sharp upstroke during midexhalation, which reflects the transition to alveolar gas; (3) relatively horizontal alveolar plateau (the final peak is also known as $P_{ET}CO_2$ [or end-tidal CO_2] because it reflects the end of expiration; prolonged exhalation caused by obstructive lung disease causes a steeper plateau); and (4) sharp downstroke and return to a zero baseline at the start of inhalation. A capnogram without these normal attributes suggests an anomaly in the patient's cardiopulmonary system, a malfunction in the airway, a malfunction in the gas delivery system, or an error in the measurement system.[44]

Clinical Applications

The role of $PETCO_2$ monitoring has expanded in recent years to include prehospital and emergency department settings.[45-46] It can be used to verify tracheal intubation, detect complete airway obstruction, and monitor ventilation during sedation.[43,47-49] Capnometry and capnography are useful in verifying endotracheal tube position following intubation and serve as continuous monitors of endotracheal tube location. This is based on the observation that CO_2 is exhaled through the trachea and not from the esophagus, which allows differentiation between endotracheal and esophageal intubation.[50-51] Confirmation of endotracheal intubation with a calorimetric detector is highly accurate in pediatric patients and is more sensitive and specific when compared with pulse oximetry and auscultation on physical examination.[50] Capnography can also be employed during transport of patients for early detection of endotracheal tube dislodgement, allowing for faster correction and avoidance of life-threatening consequences related to hypoxic arrest.[52] This is particularly significant in the pediatric population where the distance between the vocal cords and carina is small.

$PETCO_2$ monitoring can also be helpful in monitoring the respiratory status of patients placed on noninvasive positive pressure ventilation or during procedural sedation where a nonintubated patient's respiratory efforts are difficult to visualize.[53-54] Capnography may detect alveolar hypoventilation, earlier than pulse oximetry in patients receiving moderate sedation.

Finally, $PETCO_2$ monitoring is becoming a routine monitoring parameter during cardiopulmonary resuscitation (CPR).[45,54] Of all prehospital vital signs, $PETCO_2$ has been found to be the most predictive and consistent for mortality.[55] Recent Advanced Cardiac Life Support (ACLS) guidelines recommend using capnography to monitor the effectiveness of chest compressions during CPR.[56] A sudden decrease in $PETCO_2$ is seen with loss of pulmonary blood flow in cardiac arrest. Increasing $PETCO_2$ values generated during CPR are associated with chest compression depth and ventilation rate,[57] and an acute rise in $PETCO_2$ exceeding 10 mm Hg is seen with return of spontaneous circulation.[58] Patients with ROSC after CPR have statistically higher levels of $PETCO_2$, suggesting better lung perfusion and cardiac output.[59] Current guidelines suggest achieving a threshold of 10 to 15 mm Hg to ensure adequate delivery of chest compressions, although an average $PETCO_2$ level of 25 mm Hg was found in patients with ROSC in a recent systematic review and meta-analysis.[59-61] Ongoing studies will further elucidate $PETCO_2$ goals and may be used to predict outcomes in the resuscitation setting.

Operating Principles of Capnometry

Sampling of exhaled CO_2 can be at the patient-ventilator interface (mainstream), diverted to a monitor (sidestream), or an intermediate connection.[49] In the most common sampling method, gas is diverted from the airway and aspirated through a tube (sidestream) to the CO_2 monitor. A low dead space sidestream CO_2 monitor is optimal for use in patients <10 kg in weight. An alternative to the diverting instrument is the nondiverting or "mainstream" capnometer in which a special flow-through adapter and CO_2 monitor are placed in the patient's airway. The exhaled gas sample is exposed to various wavelengths of infrared light. The relative amount of light absorbed by the exhaled sample is compared with the amount of light absorbed by a sample that does not contain CO_2. By comparing the difference in absorption between the two samples, the capnometer determines the amount of CO_2 in the sample gas, which it then displays as the CO_2 concentration. CO_2 also can be measured semiquantitatively using a pH-sensitive indicator that changes from purple to yellow when exposed to CO_2.[47] The Easy Cap $PETCO_2$ detector is placed between the endotracheal tube and resuscitation bag after intubation, and a color change from purple to yellow should be observed. Up to six breaths may be necessary to allow for washout of retained CO_2 in the event of esophageal intubation. A constant purple color indicates that the tube is not in the trachea or the presence of poor pulmonary perfusion while a tan color may indicate tracheal intubation with poor pulmonary perfusion or esophageal intubation with retained CO_2.

Clinical and Technical Issues

Both physiologic anomalies and technical factors can result in $PETCO_2$ values that do not approximate $PaCO_2$. For $PETCO_2$ to approximate $PaCO_2$, two assumptions must be met: (1) the lung units must empty synchronously with uniform time constants and (2) ventilation and perfusion must be well matched in the lung units. Additionally, technical variables can produce $PETCO_2$ values that do not approximate $PaCO_2$. These include the design of the gas sampling system, distance the gas must be transported, and instrument's calibration methods.

Gas Sampling Issues

The gas sampling method used by a capnometer affects the accuracy of the capnogram and $PETCO_2$ measurements. Relevant factors include the location of the ventilatory circuit from which the gas is sampled, the distance over which the gas is transported before analysis, and the sample flow rate of the instrument. With a nondiverting or mainstream device, the CO_2 monitor is placed on the airway, so there is no need to divert gas from the airway. This sampling configuration typically is available only in infrared capnometers because only infrared CO_2 monitors can be designed small enough to fit on the airway. A study comparing mainstream proximal end-tidal CO_2 to a novel method that sampled distal end-tidal CO_2 via a special double-lumen tube found that the distal end-tidal samples had the best correlation with $PaCO_2$ and remained reliable even when severe lung disease was present.[62] Another sampling configuration is seen in the proximal-diverting device. A lightweight, low-profile airway adapter is placed in the patient's airway, and gas is sampled from the airway and transported to the sensor, which is placed near the patient but not in the airway itself. A third sampling configuration is found in the distal-diverting device, the classic "sidestream" capnometer. In a distal-diverting system, gas is sampled from the airway and transported to the CO_2 monitor, which is located in the display unit distal to the patient.

The accuracy of the capnogram, $P_{ET}CO_2$ measurements, and displayed values depends on the sampling site (Fig. 46.6). In continuous gas flow circuits, sampling in or at the endotracheal tube results in the most accurate values because there is little contamination with fresh gas from the breathing circuit (point A). The Y-connector of the breathing circuit is the next best sampling site (point B). However, if the fresh gas flow is large compared with the expiratory flow rate of the patient (as may be the case in neonates and small children), the capnogram and $P_{ET}CO_2$ values may be distorted as a result of dilution with the fresh gas flowing through the Y-connector. If gas is sampled "downstream" from the patient, the waveform and $P_{ET}CO_2$ are increasingly diluted by fresh gas from the circuit (points C and D). If gas is sampled "upstream" from the patient in the fresh gas supply, none of the exhaled CO_2 is detected and the measured $P_{ET}CO_2$ is zero (point E). Therefore the best sampling site is within the patient's endotracheal tube or at the tube connector, as far as possible from the Y-connector of the breathing circuit.[63]

In breathing circuits with intermittent flow (demand-valve ventilators) and in larger children with large exhaled tidal volumes, the capnogram and $P_{ET}CO_2$ values are usually unaffected by minor changes in sampling location. If the tidal volume is small (eg, as in infants and children) and the sample flow rate is large (ie, >150 mL/min), the capnogram and $P_{ET}CO_2$ measurements may be significantly diluted by the entrainment of fresh gas. Using a capnometer system with a low sample flow rate, typically less than 75 mL/min, restores the waveform and $P_{ET}CO_2$ readings to more accurate values.

Dead Space Ventilation

Dead space is the volume of gas in the airways and lung that participates in tidal breathing but does not participate in gas exchange. Obvious examples are the volume of the endotracheal tube and ventilator circuit (apparatus dead space) and the volume of the tracheal lumen and central airways (anatomic dead space). A less obvious, but still important, source of error in critically ill patients is alveolar or physiologic dead space. This dead space is attributable to lung units in which ventilation greatly exceeds perfusion. Gas exchange in these overventilated, relatively underperfused lung units is less efficient than normal.

The fraction of the tidal volume that is delivered to all dead spaces taken together can be calculated using the Bohr equation. A sample of mixed expired air collected over numerous breaths is analyzed for mixed PCO_2 (P_ECO_2). The total fraction of dead space per tidal volume is given by:

$$V_D/V_T = (PaCO_2 - P_ECO_2)/PaCO_2 \qquad \text{Eq. 46.4}$$

Physiologic dead space (V_D/V_T) can be determined from a variant of the Bohr equation:

$$V_D/V_T = (PaCO_2 - P_{ET}CO_2)/PaCO_2 \qquad \text{Eq. 46.5}$$

or

$$V_D/V_T = 1 - (P_{ET}CO_2/PaCO_2) \qquad \text{Eq. 46.6}$$

where $P_{ET}CO_2$ is used in place of a sample of mixed expired air.

In many clinical situations, dead space ventilation is an appreciable fraction of tidal breathing, including severe respiratory dysfunction,[64] pulmonary hypoperfusion, pulmonary thromboembolism, and cardiac arrest (Box 46.1). In these conditions, the clinician using a capnometer may see a large arterial to end-tidal PCO_2 gradient (typically >10 mm Hg). This gradient can be used as an indicator of severity of disease, and $P_{ET}CO_2$ can be used to evaluate trends rather than as a specific measure of alveolar PCO_2.

Differential Diagnosis of Abnormal Capnograms

The capnogram probably is the single most reliable and effective monitor of pulmonary ventilation. The integrity and function of the patient's cardiopulmonary system and the breathing circuit both affect the capnogram, and malfunctions often can be detected by changes in the capnogram.[62,65]

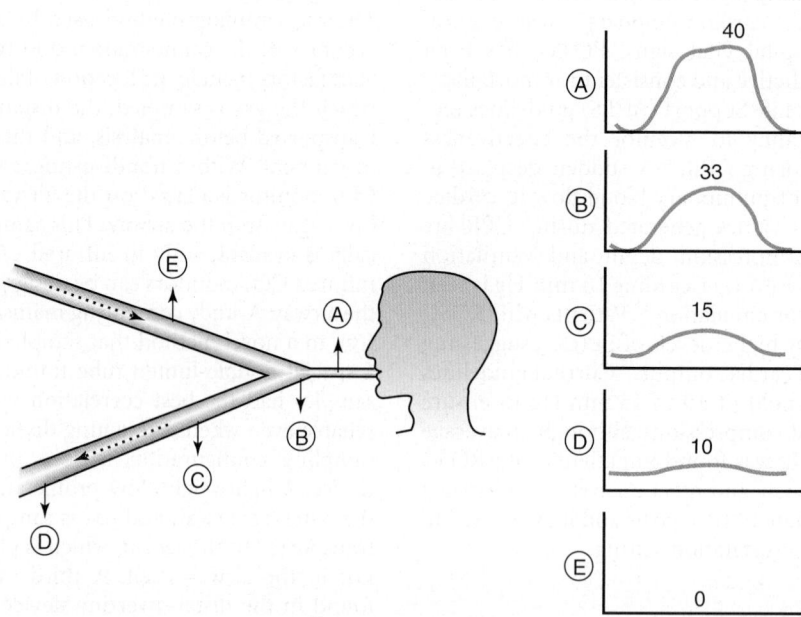

Fig. 46.6. Accuracy of end-tidal CO_2 measurements is highly dependent on obtaining good samples of expiratory gas from the patient. If sampled gas is contaminated with fresh gas from the breathing circuit, the measured values will not be accurate. The best samples are obtained from a site nearest to the source of CO_2, the patient (point A).

Gradually Decreasing End-Tidal CO₂ Concentration

When the capnogram retains its normal morphology but there is a slow, progressive drop in PETCO₂ (Fig. 46.7), the possible causes include falling body temperature, slowly decreasing systemic or pulmonary perfusion, and hyperventilation. Sedation and neuromuscular blockade attenuate the normal body mechanisms for generating heat to preserve body temperature. As body temperature falls, the patient's rate of metabolism and CO₂ production also fall. If ventilation is controlled and kept constant as body temperature decreases, alveolar CO₂ concentration and arterial PCO₂ decrease. This decrease is reflected in the capnogram as a slow decrease in

PETCO₂ over many minutes. Another cause of decreasing PETCO₂ is a fall in total body perfusion associated with blood loss or cardiovascular depression. As systemic and pulmonary perfusion decrease, alveolar dead space increases with a resultant fall in PETCO₂.

Sustained Low End-Tidal CO₂ Concentrations Without Plateaus

Occasionally, with no apparent malfunction in the breathing circuit or in the patient's cardiopulmonary status, the capnogram shows sustained low PETCO₂ values without a good alveolar plateau (Fig. 46.8). In this situation, PETCO₂ is not a good estimate of alveolar PCO₂. The absence of a good alveolar plateau suggests that either full exhalation is not occurring before the beginning of the next breath or the patient's tidal volume is being diluted with fresh gas because of a small tidal volume, high aspirating sample rate, or high fresh gas dilution from the circuit. Several maneuvers are available to distinguish between these possibilities.

Incomplete emptying of the lungs may be suggested by adventitial sounds such as wheezing or large airway rhonchi with compromise of small airway patency caused by bronchospasm or secretions. If rhonchi are present, tracheal suctioning often corrects the partial obstruction and restores full exhalation. Bronchospasm may be treated with a variety of bronchodilators. An endotracheal tube that is kinked or partially obstructed by secretions may prevent full exhalation. Passing a suction catheter down the endotracheal tube usually confirms or eliminates this possibility. Gently squeezing the child's chest to assist with a forced exhalation often produces a waveform in which the CO₂ concentration continues to rise toward an alveolar plateau. If the plateau is present, the "squeeze PETCO₂" value may be taken as a good estimate of alveolar CO₂ concentration.

When no signs of partial airway obstruction are present, another explanation for this type of capnographic waveform should be considered. In infants and other patients who have small tidal volumes, the aspirating sample rate may exceed the expiratory flow rate near the end of exhalation. When this occurs, the aspirating sample is diluted with fresh gas from the breathing circuit, resulting in a drop-off of the plateau

BOX 46.1	Clinical Conditions Associated with Abnormalities in PETCO₂

Increases in PETCO₂

Sudden
   Sudden increase in cardiac output
   Release of a tourniquet
   Injection of sodium bicarbonate

Gradual
   Hypoventilation
   Increased metabolism (carbon dioxide production)

Decreases in PETCO₂

Sudden
   Sudden hyperventilation
   Sudden decrease in cardiac output
   Massive pulmonary embolism
   Air embolism
   Ventilator disconnection
   Ventilator circuit leakage
   Obstruction of the endotracheal tube

Gradual
   Hyperventilation
   Decrease in metabolism (carbon dioxide production)
   Decreased pulmonary perfusion

Absent PETCO₂
   Esophageal intubation
   Accidental extubation

Modified from Tobin M. Respiratory monitoring. JAMA. 1990;264:244-251.

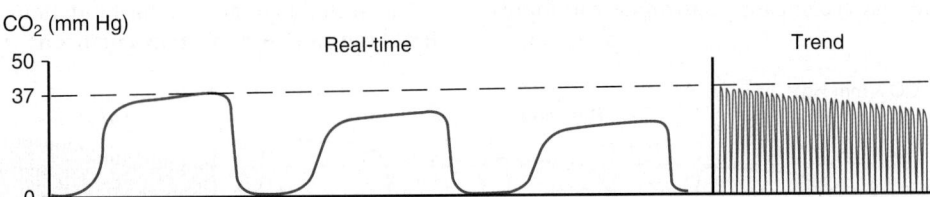

Fig. 46.7. Decreasing PETCO₂ level. (Modified with permission from Zwerneman K. End-tidal carbon dioxide monitoring: a VITAL sign worth watching. Crit Care Nurs Clin N Am. 2006;18:217-225. Fig. 6.)

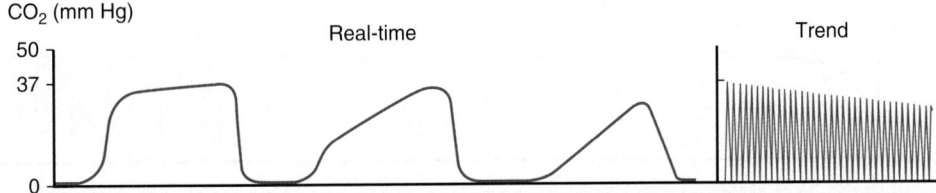

Fig. 46.8. Airway obstruction or obstruction in breathing circuit. (Modified with permission from Zwerneman K. End-tidal carbon dioxide monitoring: a VITAL sign worth watching. Crit Care Nurs Clin N Am. 2006;18:217-225. Fig. 7.)

and a fall in PETCO₂ as a result of dilution. Reducing the flow rate of fresh gas or moving the sampling site closer to the endotracheal tube connector usually corrects the problem. In very small newborns, a sample rate of 100 to 250 mL per minute may be too high to result in good plateaus despite instituting the preceding corrective measures. Then either a capnographic system having a very low sampling rate (50 mL/min) can be used or the capnogram can be used as a gross monitor of the integrity of the ventilatory circuit and trends in cardiopulmonary function rather than as an accurate estimate of alveolar ventilation.

Sustained Low End-Tidal CO₂ Concentration With Good Plateaus

In some circumstances, the capnogram demonstrates a low PETCO₂ with a widened (a-et) ΔPCO₂ and preservation of a good alveolar plateau. This discrepancy may indicate that the capnograph is malfunctioning or miscalibrated. The clinician can evaluate this possibility by sampling his or her own exhaled CO₂ and verifying that the PETCO₂ concentration is between 5% and 6% (equivalent to approximately 38 to 46 mm Hg). If the instrument is functioning properly and is well calibrated, a wide (a-et) ΔPCO₂ is an indication of excessive dead space ventilation in the patient.

Exponential Decrease in End-Tidal CO₂

An exponential drop in PETCO₂ that occurs within a short time (eg, a dozen or so breaths) almost always signals a sudden and probably catastrophic event in the patient's cardiopulmonary system (see Fig. 46.7). The basis for this capnogram is a sudden and dramatic increase in alveolar dead space ventilation. Possible causes include sudden hypovolemia, circulatory arrest with continued pulmonary ventilation, and pulmonary embolus with thrombus or air. Only after ruling out these catastrophic events and determining that the patient is hemodynamically stable should more mundane explanations for the exponential decay in PETCO₂ be considered. The most common noncatastrophic cause is an accidental increase in ventilation attributable to an incorrect ventilator adjustment, resulting in a gradual decrease in PETCO₂. However, it is important to note that even doubling the alveolar ventilation decreases the PETCO₂ to only half of the preadjustment value, not to the near-zero values that may accompany catastrophic cardiopulmonary events.

Gradual Increase in Both Baseline and End-Tidal CO₂

A gradual rise in both baseline and PETCO₂ value indicates that previously exhaled CO₂ is being rebreathed from the circuit (Fig. 46.9). In this situation, the inspiratory portion of the capnogram fails to reach the zero baseline, and there may actually be a premature rise in CO₂ concentration during the inspiratory phase of ventilation. PETCO₂ usually increases until a new equilibrium alveolar CO₂ concentration is reached, when excretion once again equals production.

Transcutaneous Monitoring

Transcutaneous measurements reflect both gas exchange and skin perfusion. The development of portable, miniaturized electrodes led to the use of this technology to continuously measure both oxygen and CO₂ tension transcutaneously. In this technique, a probe composed of a heater, an electrode, and a thermistor is applied to the patient's skin. The skin is warmed and softened to improve diffusion and permeability. This step also causes capillaries to dilate, resulting in better approximation of arterial oxygen values. This technology works under the assumption that transcutaneous values reflect those from the arterial circulation. Heating the skin allows more rapid diffusion of both oxygen and carbon dioxide from the subcutaneous tissues to the surface of the electrode. However, the heating affects both tissue and blood by decreasing oxygen solubility, shifting the oxyhemoglobin dissociation curve to the right, and dilating local arterioles. Temperatures of 44°C to 45°C increase diffusion and prevent vasoconstriction in the local area of the skin.[66]

Oxygen Monitoring

Transcutaneous Clarke electrodes measure oxygen tension in a local segment of the heated skin. Because skin is the organ most responsive to adrenomedullary induced vasoconstriction, local oxygen tension may not be the same in all skin segments or other tissues. In essence, transcutaneous oxygen tension (TcPO₂) is only an indirect reflection of arterial oxygen tension; it is more directly related to local tissue perfusion and oxygenation.

This technology has several limitations and disadvantages that limit the use of transcutaneous monitoring to the

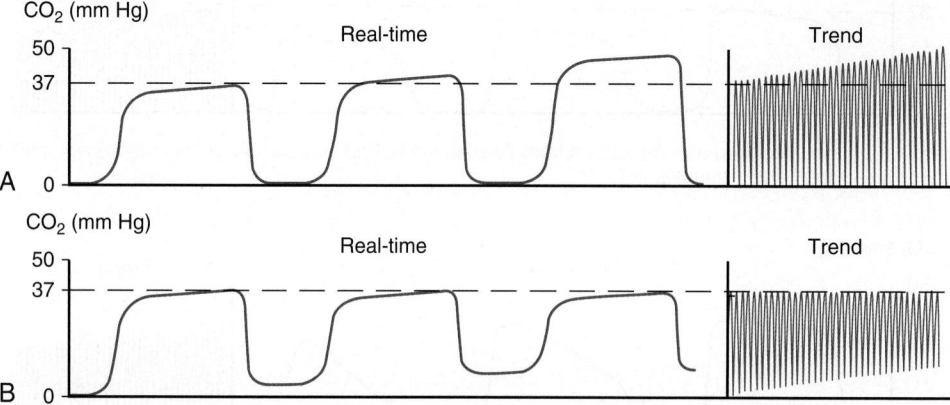

Fig. 46.9. (A) Increasing PETCO₂ level. (Modified with permission from Zwerneman K. End-tidal carbon dioxide monitoring: a VITAL sign worth watching. Crit Care Nurs Clin N Am. 2006;18:217-225. Fig. 3.) (B) Rising baseline. (Modified with permission from Zwerneman K. End-tidal carbon dioxide monitoring: a VITAL sign worth watching. Crit Care Nurs Clin N Am. 2006;18:217-225. Fig. 4.)

newborn population. Skin thickness increases with age, making transcutaneous measurements less predictable. Electrode placement must be changed every 4 to 6 hours to prevent thermal injury to the site of measurement or when readings become unstable. A thermal neutral environment to limit peripheral vasoconstriction increases the correlation between transcutaneous and arterial tensions. Finally, the electrode membranes must be calibrated before each use and each change of measurement site, and comparison with arterial blood gases is necessary. However, displaying $TcPO_2$ has been shown to result in less time spent hyperoxemic and less time spent hypoxemic than displaying the SpO_2, which may be particularly useful in infants.[67] Because of these limitations and the ease of application of pulse oximetry and $PETCO_2$ monitoring, transcutaneous oxygen monitoring has nearly been replaced by other monitoring methods.

Carbon Dioxide Monitoring

Transcutaneous CO_2 tension using a Stowe-Severinghaus electrode has been widely used in the neonatal population to approximate $PaCO_2$. Transcutaneous CO_2 values parallel but consistently overestimate $PaCO_2$ values in hemodynamically stable neonates and adults.[68] The difference in arterial and transcutaneous values reflects accumulation of CO_2 in the tissues as a result of inadequate perfusion. Transcutaneous monitoring of CO_2 more closely approximates arterial CO_2 tension in infants and children who are experiencing respiratory failure than does $PETCO_2$.[69-71] This technology is also useful in settings where nonconventional forms of ventilation (high-frequency ventilation) preclude the use of end-tidal monitoring.

Conclusion

Noninvasive monitors, such as pulse oximetry and capnometry, are standards of care in the pediatric critical care environment. It is therefore important to understand key clinical and technical issues that determine how these instruments can be used most effectively. These noninvasive technologies provide early warning of potential catastrophic events and facilitate early intervention, with potential for better outcomes. Concerns for complications related to invasive monitors will continue to drive the search for newer and better devices for noninvasive physiologic monitoring. Promising recent advances have been made in the technology of pulse oximeters, allowing measurements of all types of hemoglobin, including dyshemoglobins and total hemoglobin, with less artifact resulting from patient movement, which is a vital consideration in the PICU patient population. However, with all of the technologic advances, we must remember the importance of basic vital sign monitoring and clinical observation, such as heart rate, respiratory rate, temperature, and fluid balance.

References

1. Rosenberg DI, Moss MM. Guidelines and levels of care for pediatric intensive care units. *Crit Care Med.* 2004;32:2117-2127.
2. Jubran A. Pulse oximetry. *Intensive Care Med.* 2004;30:2017-2020.
3. Salyer JW. Neonatal and pediatric pulse oximetry. *Respir Care.* 2003; 48:386-396.
4. Miyasaka K. Pulse oximetry in the management of children in the PICU. *Anesth Analg.* 2002;94:S44-S46.
5. Cote CJ, Notterman DA, Karl HW, et al. Adverse sedation events in pediatrics: a critical incident analysis of contributing factors. *Pediatrics.* 2000;105:805-814.
6. Poets CF, Urschitz MS, Bohnhorst B. Pulse oximetry in the neonatal intensive care unit (NICU): detection of hyperoxemia and false alarm rates. *Anesth Analg.* 2002;94:S41-S46.
7. Zhao QM, Ma XJ, Ge XL, et al. Pulse oximetry with clinical assessment to screen for congenital heart disease in neonates in China: a prospective study. *Lancet.* 2014;384:747-754.
8. Ewer AK. Review of pulse oximetry screening for critical congenital heart defects in newborn infants. *Curr Opin Cardiol.* 2013;28:92-96.
9. Kemper AR, Mahle WT, Martin GR, et al. Strategies for implementing screening for critical congenital heart disease. *Pediatrics.* 2011;128: 1259-1267.
10. Aoyagi T, Miyasaka K. Pulse oximetry: its invention, contribution to medicine, and future tasks. *Anesth Analg.* 2002;94:S1-S3.
11. Goldman JM, Petterson MT, Kopotic RJ, et al. Masimo signal extraction pulse oximetry. *J Clin Monit Comput.* 2000;16:475-483.
12. Barker SJ. "Motion-resistant" pulse oximetry: a comparison of new and old models. *Anesth Analg.* 2002;95:967-972.
13. Malviya S, Reynolds PI, Voepel-Lewis T, et al. False alarms and sensitivity of conventional pulse oximetry versus the Masimo SET technology in the pediatric postanesthesia care unit. *Anesth Analg.* 2000; 90:1336-1340.
14. Hay WW, Rodden DJ, Collins SM, et al. Reliability of conventional and new pulse oximetry in neonatal patients. *J Perinatol.* 2002;22: 360-366.
15. Noblet T. Patient safety and staff satisfaction following conversion to Masimo SET pulse oximetry—experience in neonatal ICU. *Respir Care.* 2001;46:1140.
16. Workie FA, Rais-Bahrami K, Short BL. Clinical use of new-generation pulse oximeters in the neonatal intensive care unit. *Am J Perinatol.* 2005; 22:357-360.
17. Whitney GM, Tucker LR, Hall SR, et al. Clinical evaluation of the accuracy of Masimo SET and Nellcor N595 oximeters in children with cyanotic congenital heart disease. *Anesthesiology.* 2005;103:A1344.
18. Bohnhorst B, Peter CS, Poets CF. Detection of hyperoxaemia in neonates: data from three new pulse oximeters. *Arch Dis Child Fetal Neonat Ed.* 2002;87:F217-F219.
19. Alexander CM, Teller LE, Gross JB. Principles of pulse oximetry: theoretical and practical considerations. *Anesth Analg.* 1989;68:368-376.
20. Van de Louw A, Cracco C, Cerf C, et al. Accuracy of pulse oximetry in the intensive care unit. *Intensive Care Med.* 2001;27:1606-1613.
21. van Oostrom JH, Melker RJ. Comparative testing of pulse oximeter probes. *Anesth Analg.* 2004;98:1354-1358.
22. Bohnhorst B, Peter CS, Poets CF. Pulse oximeters' reliability in detecting hypoxemia and bradycardia: comparison between a conventional and two new generation oximeters. *Crit Care Med.* 2000;28:1565-1568.
23. Carter BG, Carlin JB, Tibballs J, et al. Accuracy of two pulse oximeters at low arterial hemoglobin-oxygen saturation. *Crit Care Med.* 1998;26: 1128-1133.
24. Fanconi S. Reliability of pulse oximetry in hypoxic infants. *J Pediatr.* 1988;112:424-427.
25. Ross PA, Newth CJ, Khemani RG. Accuracy of pulse oximetry in children. *Pediatrics.* 2014;133:22-29.
26. Trivedi NS, Ghouri AF, Shah NK, et al. Effects of motion, ambient light, and hypoperfusion on pulse oximeter function. *J Clin Anesth.* 1997;9: 179-183.
27. Robertson FA, Hoffman GM. Clinical evaluation of the effects of signal integrity and saturation on data availability and accuracy of Masimo SE and Nellcor N-395 oximeters in children. *Anesth Analg.* 2004;98: 617-622.
28. Fluck RR Jr, Schroeder C, Frani G, et al. Does ambient light affect the accuracy of pulse oximetry? *Respir Care.* 2003;48:677-680.
29. Reynolds KJ, Palayiwa E, Moyle JT, et al. The effect of dyshemoglobins on pulse oximetry: part I, theoretical approach and part II, experimental results using an in vitro test system. *J Clin Monit.* 1993;9:81-90.
30. Watcha MF, Connor MT, Hing AV. Pulse oximetry in methemoglobinemia. *Am J Dis Child.* 1989;143:845-847.
31. Hampson NB. Pulse oximetry in severe carbon monoxide poisoning. *Chest.* 1998;114:1036-1041.
32. Barker SJ, Curry J, Redford D, et al. Measurement of carboxyhemoglobin and methemoglobin by pulse oximetry: a human volunteer study. *Anesthesiology.* 2006;105:892-897.

33. Macknet MR, Kimball-Jones PL, Applegate RL, et al. Non-invasive measurement of continuous hemoglobin concentration via pulse co-oximetry. *Anesthesiology.* 2007;107:A1545.
34. Harris AP, Sendak MJ, Donham RT, et al. Absorption characteristics of human fetal hemoglobin at wavelengths used in pulse oximetry. *J Clin Monit.* 1988;4:175-177.
35. Ralston AC, Webb RK, Runciman WB. Potential errors in pulse oximetry. III: Effects of interferences, dyes, dyshaemoglobins and other pigments. *Anaesthesia.* 1991;46:291-295.
36. Morey TE, Rice MJ, Vasilopoulos T, et al. Feasibility and accuracy of nasal alar pulse oximetry. *Br J Anaesth.* 2014;112:1109-1114.
37. Cheng EY, Hopwood MB, Kay J. Forehead pulse oximetry compared with finger pulse oximetry and arterial blood gas measurement. *J Clin Monit.* 1998;4:223-226.
38. Dassel AC, Graaff R, Meijer A, et al. Reflectance pulse oximetry at the forehead of newborns: the influence of varying pressure on the probe. *J Clin Monit.* 1996;12:421-428.
39. Kyriacou PA, Powell S, Langford RM, et al. Esophageal pulse oximetry utilizing reflectance photoplethysmography. *IEEE Trans Biomed Eng.* 2002;49:1360-1368.
40. Ramirez FC, Padda S, Medlin S, et al. Reflectance spectrophotometry in the gastrointestinal tract: limitations and new applications. *Am J Gastroenterol.* 2002;97:2780-2784.
41. Vicenzi MN, Gombotz H, Krenn H, et al. Transesophageal versus surface pulse oximetry in intensive care unit patients. *Crit Care Med.* 2000;28:2268-2270.
42. Elliott M, Tate R, Page K. Do clinicians know how to use pulse oximetry? A literature review and clinical implications. *Aust Crit Care.* 2006;19:139-144.
43. Nagler J, Krauss B. Capnography: a valuable tool for airway management. *Emerg Med Clin North Am.* 2008;26:881-897.
44. Swedlow DB. Capnometry and capnography: the anesthesia disaster warning system. *Semin Anesth.* 1986;5:194.
45. Bhende MS, LaCovey DC. End-tidal carbon dioxide monitoring in the prehospital setting. *Prehosp Emerg Care.* 2001;5:208-213.
46. Nagler J, Krauss B. Capnography: a valuable tool for airway management. *Emerg Med Clin North Am.* 2008;26:881-897.
47. Bhende MS, Allen WD. Evaluation of a Capno-Flo resuscitator during transport of critically ill children. *Pediatr Emerg Care.* 2002;18:414-416.
48. Zwerneman K. End tidal carbon dioxide monitoring: a VITAL sign worth watching. *Crit Care Nurs Clin North Am.* 2006;18:217-225.
49. Lightdale JR, Goldmann DA, Feldman HA, et al. Microstream capnography improves patient monitoring during moderate sedation: a randomized controlled trial. *Pediatrics.* 2006;117:e1170-e1178.
50. Grmec S. Comparison of three different methods to confirm tracheal tube placement in emergency intubation. *Intensive Care Med.* 2002;28:701-704.
51. Wyllie J, Carlo WA. The role of carbon dioxide detectors for confirmation of endotracheal tube position. *Clin Perinatol.* 2006;33:111-119.
52. Langhan ML, Ching K, Northrup V, et al. A randomized controlled trial of capnography in the correction of simulated endotracheal tube dislodgement. *Acad Emerg Med.* 2011;18:590-596.
53. Tai CC, Lu FL, Chen PC, et al. Noninvasive capnometry for end-tidal carbon dioxide monitoring via nasal cannula in nonintubated neonates. *Pediatr Neonatol.* 2010;51:330-335.
54. Bhende MS. End-tidal carbon dioxide monitoring in pediatrics—clinical applications. *J Postgrad Med.* 2001;47:215-218.
55. Hunter CL, Silvestri S, Ralls G, et al. The sixth vital sign: prehospital end-tidal carbon dioxide predicts in-hospital mortality and metabolic disturbances. *Am J Emerg Med.* 2014;32:160-165.
56. Kodali BS, Urman RD. Capnography during cardiopulmonary resuscitation: current evidence and future directions. *J Emerg Trauma Shock.* 2014;7:332-340.
57. Sheak KR, Wiebe DJ, Leary M, et al. Quantitative relationship between end-tidal carbon dioxide and CPR quality during both in-hospital and out-of-hospital cardiac arrest. *Resuscitation.* 2015;89:149-154.
58. Pokorná M, Necas E, Kratochvíl J, et al. A sudden increase in partial pressure end-tidal carbon dioxide ($P_{ET}CO_2$) at the moment of return of spontaneous circulation. *J Emerg Med.* 2010;38:614-621.
59. Hartmann SM, Farris RW, Di Gennaro JL, et al. Systematic review and meta-analysis of end-tidal carbon dioxide values associated with return of spontaneous circulation during cardiopulmonary resuscitation. *J Intensive Care Med.* 2014;30:426-435.
60. Kolar M, Krizmaric M, Klemen P, et al. Partial pressure of end-tidal carbon dioxide successful predicts cardiopulmonary resuscitation in the field: a prospective observational study. *Crit Care.* 2008;12:R115.
61. Eckstein M, Hatch L, Malleck J, et al. End-tidal CO_2 as a predictor of survival in out-of-hospital cardiac arrest. *Prehosp Disaster Med.* 2011;26:148-150.
62. Kugelman A, Zeiger-Aginsky D, Bader D, et al. A novel method of distal end-tidal CO_2 capnography in intubated infants: comparison with arterial CO_2 and with proximal mainstream end-tidal CO_2. *Pediatrics.* 2008;122:e1219-e1224.
63. Gravenstein N, Lampotang S, Beneken J. Factors influencing capnography in the Bain circuit. *J Clin Monit.* 1985;1:6.
64. Yamanaka M, Sue D. Comparison of arterial-end-tidal P_{CO_2} difference and dead space/tidal volume ratio in respiratory failure. *Chest.* 1987;92:832.
65. St John RE. Exhaled gas analysis. Technical and clinical aspects of capnography and oxygen consumption. *Crit Care Nurs Clin North Am.* 1989;1:669.
66. Tremper KK, Waxman K, Shoemaker WC. Transcutaneous oxygen monitoring of critically ill adults with and without low flow shock. *Crit Care Med.* 1979;7:526-531.
67. Quine D, Stenson BJ. Does monitoring method influence stability of oxygenation in preterm infants? A randomised crossover study of saturation versus transcutaneous monitoring. *Arch Dis Chil Fetal Neonatal Ed.* 2008;93:F347-F350.
68. Tremper KK, Shoemaker WC, Shippy CR, et al. Transcutaneous P_{CO_2} monitoring in adults patients in the ICU and operating room. *Crit Care Med.* 1981;9:752-755.
69. Tobias JD, Meyer DJ. Noninvasive monitoring of carbon dioxide during respiratory failure in toddlers and infants: end-tidal versus transcutaneous carbon dioxide. *Anesth Analg.* 1997;85:55-58.
70. Urbano J, Cruzado V, Lopez-Herce J, et al. Accuracy of three transcutaneous carbon dioxide monitors in critically ill children. *Pediatr Pulmonol.* 2010;45:481-486.
71. Tobias JD. Transcutaneous carbon dioxide monitoring in infants and children. *Paediatr Anaesth.* 2009;19:434-444.

Overview of Breathing Failure

Katherine V. Biagas, Robert K. Kanter,[†] Navyn Naran, and Bradley P. Fuhrman

PEARLS

- Three pathways to breathing failure are (1) impaired neural control, (2) failure of the muscles of breathing, and (3) dysfunction of the mechanics of breathing.
- Though diverse stimuli drive respiratory cycling and effort, all must be processed by the brain to affect respiratory muscles. For this reason, brain death entails loss of all respiratory effort.
- Volitional control of breathing is supratentorial and may dominate automatic control in the awake state, but it may be lost in brain injury with or without loss of automatic control.
- Automatic control of breathing is integrated in the medulla and involves numerous separate brain stem regions, which are so widely dispersed that some evidence of respiratory drive may persist even after near-total loss of brain function.
- Muscles of breathing include the diaphragm, intercostals, and accessory muscles. The diaphragm works like a piston to expand the thorax and displace abdominal organs caudad. Intercostal muscles participate in both inspiration and expiration. The thoracic accessory muscles (scalenes, sternocleidomastoids, pectoralis minor, and erector spinae) all elevate the ribs and facilitate inspiration. The abdominal muscles (rectus abdominis, transverse abdominis, and the obliques) facilitate expiration.
- The respiratory muscles can fail from overwork (as might occur in asthma) or from inadequate supply of blood, oxygen, or nutrients (as might occur in shock or sepsis, even when there is no evidence of lung disease).
- Dysfunction of the mechanics of breathing can contribute significantly to respiratory muscle workload, predominantly through imposition of inefficiencies. Assisted ventilation can (1) prevent breathing failure from progressing to respiratory arrest, (2) improve gas exchange, and (3) reduce metabolic expenditure for muscle work in the patient with limited reserve.

Respiration involves movement of air (breathing), diffusion of gases between alveolus and pulmonary circulation, circulation of blood between tissue and lung, and tissue energy metabolism. This chapter provides an overview of spontaneous breathing and breathing gone awry and sets the stage for later chapters on respiratory disorders. The term "breathing failure" is used here to limit consideration to mechanical failure of the respiratory pump that drives air movement.

[†]Deceased

Breathing failure is arguably the most common cause of arrest in infants and children.

Physiology of Breathing

Diaphragm

The diaphragm arises from the embryologic pleuroperitoneal fold. Myoblasts migrate from cervical somites to the pleuroperitoneal fold, where they arrange themselves into a sheet on a mesenchymal substrate that separates the peritoneum from the abdomen. Once fully formed, the diaphragm originates from bilateral tendinous crura attached to the spinal column and inserts as a costal tendon attached to the chest wall between the sixth and twelfth ribs. The dome of the diaphragm remains largely tendinous. This configuration, a circular attachment to the thoracic wall, vertical muscle orientation adjacent to the thorax, and attachment to a flattened central tendinous dome (Fig. 47.1), works like a piston during breathing to enlarge the thorax and displace abdominal contents downward.

Approximately 50% of the diaphragm consists of type I fast-twitch muscle fibers, which have high endurance and are resistant to fatigue. The remainder of the diaphragm is made up of type IIA and type IIB fibers, which have different properties.[1] Type IIA fibers are important in achieving high levels of minute ventilation quickly, have good endurance, and can contract rapidly, but they are unable to sustain long-term power output. Type IIB fibers cannot sustain their force of contraction because they possess lower oxidative capacity and are more susceptible to fatigue. The greater the force of contraction required, the more motor units of the diaphragm are recruited. There appears to be little difference between the activity of costal muscles and crural muscles, either during normal breathing or in response to hypoxia and hypercapnia.

When a patient lies supine, the diaphragm rests against the inner surface of the rib cage. When the diaphragm contracts and its muscle fibers shorten, the whole diaphragm moves down, lowering pleural pressure and increasing intraabdominal pressure. The increase in intraabdominal pressure generated by descent of the diaphragm acts as a caval pump to enhance cardiac filling.[2] Because of its alignment against the lower ribs (zone of apposition), descent of the diaphragm also expands the caudal portion of the rib cage.

The muscle of the diaphragm extends from the costal insertion to the dome of the diaphragm. When the diaphragm is "high," it is loaded for greater force of contraction. When it is "low" or "flat," it is unloaded and mechanically disadvantaged.

The diaphragm is the major inspiratory muscle of the neonate. It increases in thickness with age (as its muscle mass increases). It also becomes appositional to a longer segment

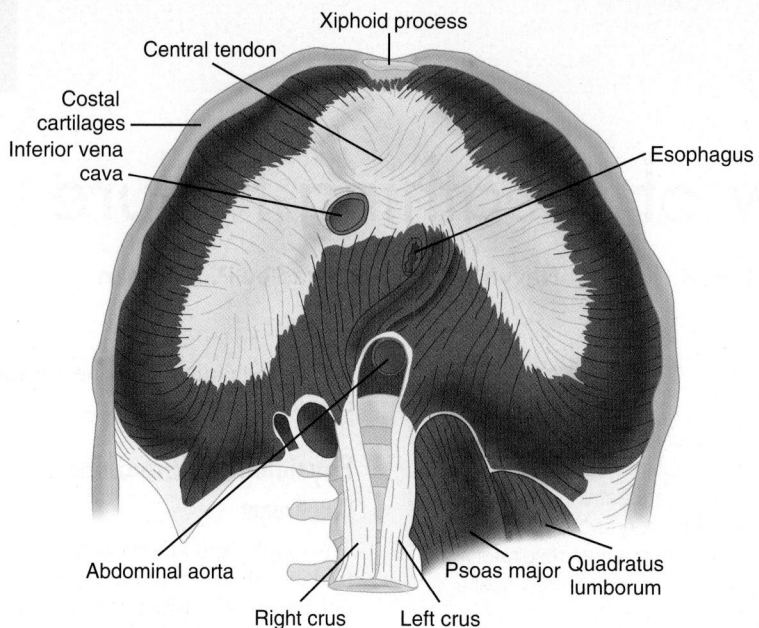

Fig. 47.1. The diaphragm is attached circumferentially to the thoracic wall. Its muscular portion extends onto the dome, where it is tendinous and flattened. When the muscle contracts, the dome descends like a piston, enlarging the thorax and displacing abdominal contents downward.

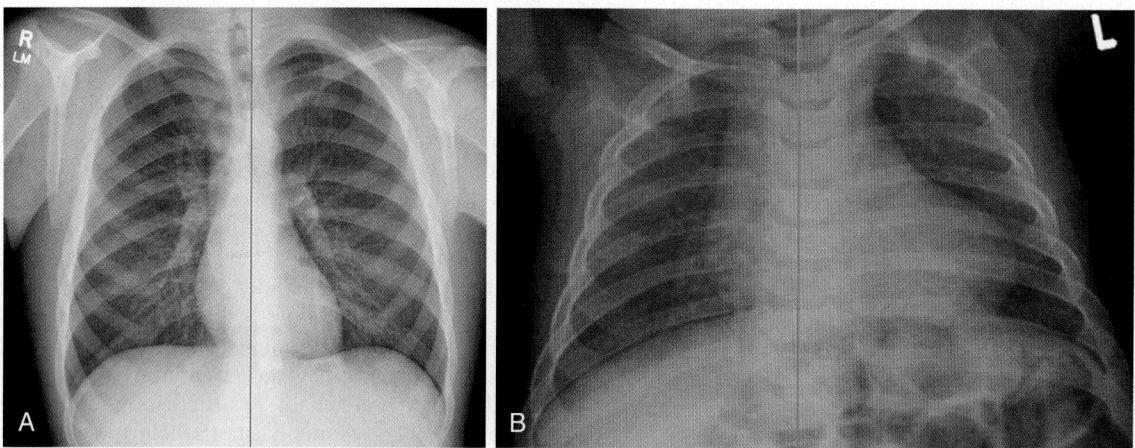

Fig. 47.2. The angle of the muscular diaphragm to the vertical is narrow in the older child (A) and adult than it is in the infant (B). This more horizontal traction on the dome may be disadvantageous when the muscle of the infant diaphragm contracts. (Courtesy Women & Children's Hospital of Buffalo, NY.)

of chest wall with growth, enhancing its effectiveness as an inspiratory piston.[3] In the neonate, the muscular diaphragm has a greater angle from the vertical than that of the adult, which reduces its effectiveness as an air pump (Fig. 47.2). This angle approaches zero with growth, increasing the diaphragm's effectiveness with advancing age. The importance of this angle as an impediment to diaphragmatic effectiveness becomes exaggerated at total lung capacity, with air trapping, and when the abdomen is distended, all of which flatten and unload the diaphragmatic muscle (Fig. 47.3).

Intercostal Muscles

The rib cage is fixed to the spine and sternum. The spine maintains a relatively fixed separation between adjacent ribs. Vertical mobility of the sternum allows lift and descent of the anterior rib cage. Thoracic volume is modified during breathing primarily by changing the angle of the anterior ribs

to the horizontal. At rest, the ribs slope caudad from their spinal attachments. The rib cage tilts upward during inspiration. The intercostal muscles form three functional sheets. The outermost (external) sheet and the parasternal sheet act to displace the ribs cephalad as they shorten. This increases both the anteroposterior and lateral dimensions of the thorax. There is also a deep (internal) layer of intercostal muscle at right angles to the external sheet that acts to displace the ribs caudad when it contracts. Thus the intercostal muscles play both inspiratory and expiratory roles in breathing by reshaping the thorax.

Accessory Muscles of Respiration

Though quiet expiration is largely passive, resulting mostly from inward elastic recoil of the lung, active expiration may be assisted by contraction of abdominal muscles (rectus abdominis, transverse abdominis, and the obliques). During

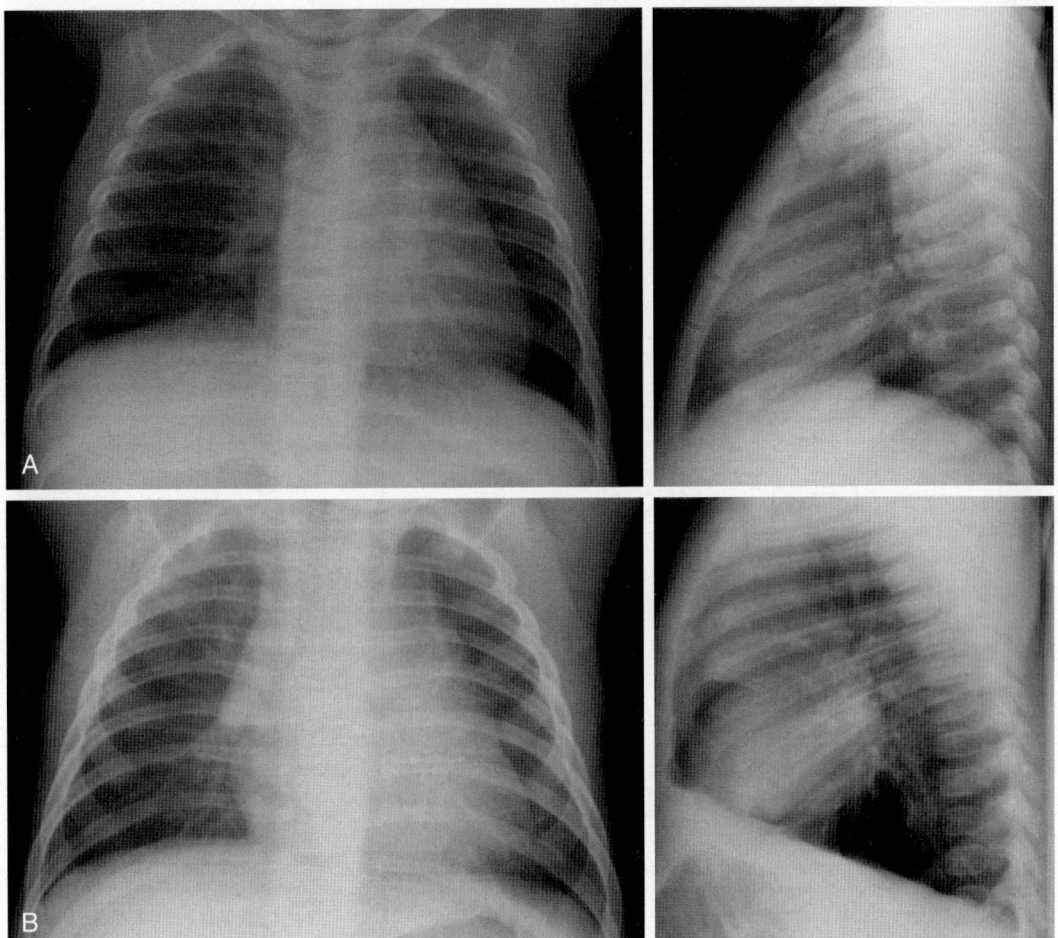

Fig. 47.3. The normal position of the diaphragm (A) allows it to stretch or "load" during expiration. In inspiration, its muscular attachment to the thorax pulls it vertically downward. Air trapping (B), abdominal distension, or other disorders that cause flattening of the diaphragm interfere with "loading" and with the direction of contraction. (Courtesy Women & Children's Hospital of Buffalo, NY.)

quiet breathing, abdominal muscle tone elevates the diaphragm during expiration, increasing the zone of apposition and loading the diaphragm for greater inspiratory contractile efficiency.

Accessory muscles of inspiration include the scalenes, sternocleidomastoids, pectoralis minor, and erector spinae, all of which elevate the ribs during contraction. During quiet breathing, accessory muscles play a minor role, but during respiratory exertion, they may play a major role and act to unload and unburden the diaphragm and intercostals. Even profoundly neurologically impaired children, who exhibit little volitional activity, can use accessory muscles of breathing when distressed. Children with dysfunction of the primary muscles of respiration may rely on their accessory muscles even at rest.

Controls of Breathing

Powerful neural regulation of breathing maintains a constant supply of oxygen to the tissues, despite wide variations of metabolic rate and respiratory system disorders, until an advanced stage of respiratory failure is reached. Sick or injured patients usually hyperventilate in compensation for stressful disorders. Stressed patients with irregular breathing or inappropriately comfortable effort to breathe probably have a severely depressed respiratory drive warranting ventilator support. Derangements of respiratory controls may be the primary cause of acute respiratory failure or one of multiple causes in a critically ill or injured patient. In other patients, disorders of respiratory regulation prolong dependence on mechanical ventilation. Disorders of respiratory controls may be difficult to distinguish from, and may combine with, muscle failure and altered respiratory mechanics.

Normal Regulation of Breathing

Rhythmic discharges whose timing corresponds to inspiratory and expiratory phases are generated in the pre-Bötzinger complex of the ventrolateral medulla oblongata.[4,5] During resting breathing, inspiratory efferent activity stimulates diaphragm flattening, as well as increased pharyngeal muscle tone and vocal cord abduction essential to keep the upper airway patent during inspiratory airflow. When inspiratory muscles relax, resting expiration is passive, driven by elastic recoil of the lung and chest wall.

The respiratory rate, inspiratory time, and motor intensity are modified by a variety of rostral neural, chemical, and mechanical stimuli (Fig. 47.4). With high-intensity stimulation, accessory muscles of breathing are activated, including intercostals and neck muscles. Nasal flaring occurs. Stimulated breathing also may include end-inspiratory vocal cord closure

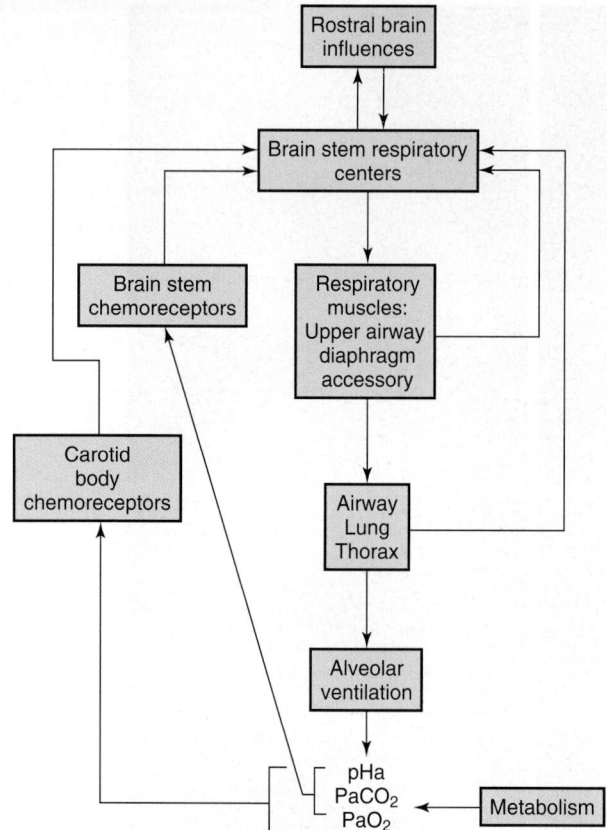

Fig. 47.4. Elements of the respiratory control system.

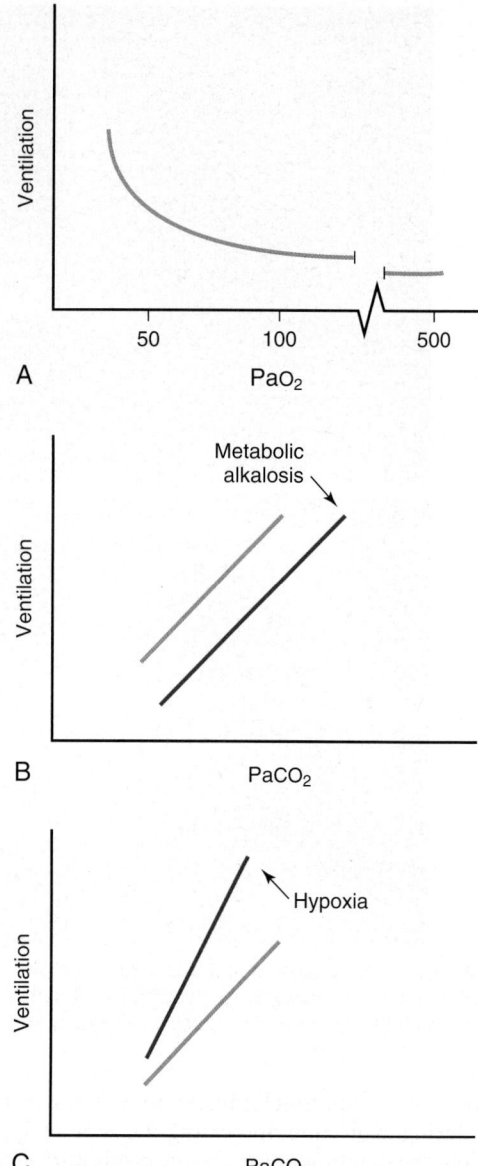

Fig. 47.5. Chemoreceptor activity, as measured by minute ventilation, varies as a function of PaO₂ (A), PaCO₂ (B) (superimposed metabolic alkalosis inhibits breathing), and PaCO₂ (C) (superimposed hypoxia further stimulates breathing).

that prolongs lung inflation with little energy expenditure, clinically evident as a grunting vocalization when the vocal cords open at the beginning of expiration. In highly stimulated breathing, abdominal muscles contract to force expiratory airflow. Other normal respiratory control behaviors include periodic deep inspirations, sneezing, and coughing to maintain expansion of basal lung areas and clear secretions from the respiratory tract. Breathing is normally coordinated with swallowing, vocalizing, and airway protective reflexes to prevent aspiration.[6] Pharyngeal muscle tone is also adjusted with neck flexion and extension to maintain airway patency.

Hypoxemia is a powerful stimulus to ventilation mediated by sensory input originating in the carotid body chemoreceptor. Peripheral chemoreceptor activity and ventilation increase slightly as Pao_2 falls below 500 mm Hg. Ventilation rises steeply as Pao_2 falls below 50 mm Hg (Fig. 47.5A). Low arterial oxygen tension, rather than low oxygen content, is the ventilatory stimulus. Little carotid body response results from profound anemia. Hydrogen ion concentration and carbon dioxide tension independently activate chemoreceptors in the carotid body and brain stem (Fig. 47.5B). The simultaneous presence of hypoxia augments the hypercapnic ventilatory response (Fig. 47.5C).

Mechanical loads on breathing influence respiratory efforts immediately, independent of chemical stimuli. Sensors for load-compensating reflexes are located in respiratory muscles and the chest wall. Reduction in lung volume is also detected by pulmonary stretch receptors. Afferent signals pertaining to loaded breathing travel via the spinal cord, vagus nerves, and perhaps the phrenic nerves. Both conscious and reflex responses are involved in compensatory increases of effort, including the recruitment of accessory muscles in response to increased respiratory resistance or to a decrease in compliance. Stimulation to breathe is further augmented by hypercapnia or hypoxemia when loaded breathing reduces ventilation. Respiratory compensation for mechanical loads accounts for the increased respiratory effort in patients who maintain normal blood gas tension or hypocapnia despite abnormal respiratory mechanics. Dyspnea and anxiety exacerbate the tendency to hyperventilate even without a chemical ventilatory stimulus.

Sleep modifies breathing, and compensation for respiratory illness is most likely to fail during sleep.[7] In some persons ventilatory responses to hypercapnia and hypoxia diminish during sleep. Sleep-induced reduction in upper airway tone and cough reflexes worsens the risk of obstruction and aspiration. In infants, whose thorax is compliant, awake lung volume is maintained by thoracic muscle tone and breathing at sufficiently high frequencies that expiration seldom reaches the passive resting lung volume. During sleep, inspiratory muscle tone diminishes and respiratory rate decreases, with resulting reduction in infants' expiratory lung volume. Infants' compensation for mechanical loads is compromised during the rapid eye movement stage of sleep more than during quiet sleep.

Breathing Failure

When challenged, muscle tension can be augmented by increasing either the frequency of firing or number of motor units being fired. At low muscle tension, the *number* of motor units participating in contraction may be increased before frequency is raised. Recruitment is used to increase work. To achieve an even greater increase in force, the *frequency* of firing of individual motor units may be raised, such that while the number of motor units is held constant the *work* of each motor unit is increased.

Working skeletal muscles rely on a continuous supply of oxygenated blood. Diaphragmatic function can be impaired if blood flow or oxygenation is reduced. Diaphragmatic muscle cannot operate at optimal length (force-length relationship) to generate the appropriate contraction (force-velocity relationship) if energy demand outstrips energy supply. The combination of suboptimal force-length and force velocity relationships causes rapid, shallow breathing, largely from dysfunction of type IIB fast-twitch glycolic fibers.

Respiratory muscle fatigue develops during exhaustive exercise. Prolonged malnutrition has also been shown to affect the diaphragm's muscle structure and impair its ability to generate force. On the other hand, it has been shown that respiratory muscle training can lessen the development of respiratory muscle fatigue.[8] Training of the diaphragm can increase capillary density, myoglobin content, mitochondrial enzyme concentration, and the concentration of glycogen, but persistent mechanical ventilation (particularly during deep sedation or paralysis) decreases muscle strength by allowing disuse muscle atrophy.

In acute illness, breathing fails if respiratory muscle demand for blood flow, metabolic substrate, and oxygen delivery outstrips supply, just as it does in exhaustive exercise.[9] The point at which this occurs is influenced by many factors, including the energy cost of breathing, duration of contraction per breath, velocity of contraction, operational length of muscle fibers, energy supply, efficiency of muscles, and state of muscle training.[10] Breathing failure, if untreated, may cause respiratory arrest and death.

Final Common Pathways to Breathing Failure

Several discrete mechanisms may cause breathing failure (Table 47.1). Each of these final common pathways may be triggered or compounded by other discrete adversities, and independent pathways of breathing failure may converge to cause respiratory arrest (or need for mechanical support of breathing).

Failure of Respiratory Controls

Disorders of respiratory controls may present with impaired respiratory cycle generation (central apnea), deficient

TABLE 47.1   Failure of Breathing

Mechanism	Examples
Failure of neural control	Uncal herniation, central hypoventilation
Failure of muscles of breathing	Insufficient muscle blood flow, hypoxemia
Failure of mechanics of breathing	Flail chest, diaphragmatic paralysis

responses to respiratory stimuli (hypoventilation during stress and failure to arouse from sleep hypoxia), or inadequate motor control of the vocal cords or pharynx (causing stridor or stertor). These patterns of regulatory dysfunction may occur individually or in combination. Pulmonary hypertension as a result of recurrent hypoxia, or aspiration pneumonia associated with impaired airway protective reflexes, may complicate the clinical situation.

Acute Failure

Patients with a critical illness or injury generally hyperventilate. When a stressed patient fails to hyperventilate, depressed respiratory controls and impending respiratory failure should be suspected.

Moderate brain injuries are typically associated with hyperventilation, whether the injury is traumatic, infectious, or hypoxic-ischemic. The hypermetabolic state, lung pathology, and loss of inhibitory cortical influences probably combine to augment ventilation. Even when the brain-injured patient does hyperventilate, airway protective reflexes are usually impaired, seizures may ensue, and subtle progression of the brain lesion may lead to hypoventilation. Resulting hypoxia exacerbates the brain injury.

Seizures impair breathing in various ways. Apnea or slowing of respiratory rate, impairment of upper airway protective reflexes, and poor inspiratory effort are common. The clinician must have a high index of suspicion to recognize occult seizures in infants. The seizure-induced respiratory depression may be difficult to distinguish from the brain pathology that caused the seizure, as well as the respiratory-depressing effects of anticonvulsant medications.

Respiratory depression by analgesic, sedative, anticonvulsant, and anesthetic agents is common. Relative effects on upper airway patency and hypoxic, hypercapnic, and loading responses may be dissociated. Concern regarding respiratory depression does not warrant withholding analgesia. Rather, monitoring should be appropriate. In fact, the patient suffering pain may breathe shallowly, exacerbating hypoxia. Sedatives and analgesics that are rapidly cleared after a single dose may have a more prolonged duration of action when given repeatedly or continuously. Clearance rates for medications may vary with systemic disease, immaturity, or genetic factors. Sedation and analgesic-induced respiratory depression may unnecessarily prolong the need for mechanical ventilation.

Opioid-induced respiratory depression can be reversed with naloxone. In patients with cardiovascular compromise (eg, those who have had cardiac surgery), naloxone should be avoided in the immediate postoperative period because the stress of abruptly eliminating opioid anesthesia is hazardous. In the patient with multiple chronic drug ingestions, naloxone may induce vomiting without improving airway protective reflexes, predisposing the patient to aspiration. The benzodiazepine antagonist flumazenil reduces the respiratory depression that results from taking benzodiazepines, but little pediatric experience with this agent has been reported. Flumazenil lowers the threshold for seizures and may cause a more hazardous condition than the initial respiratory depression. The duration of action of antagonists may be shorter than the agent that is depressing breathing. Close monitoring of the patient is essential, and repeated doses of antagonists may be necessary. In other cases of drug-induced respiratory depression, mechanical ventilation provides greater safety than do pharmacologic antagonists. This is the case with multifactorial central depression or in severely ill patients.

Other medications may depress breathing without alteration of consciousness. For example, prostaglandin E_1, which is given to maintain patency of the ductus arteriosus in infants with congenital heart disease, is frequently associated with respiratory depression. The respiratory inhibitory action of metabolic alkalosis may contribute to prolonged dependence on mechanical ventilation in children receiving chronic doses of diuretic agents. When metabolic alkalosis accompanies prolonged recovery from respiratory failure, correction of the alkalosis with potassium chloride and occasionally acetazolamide may promote ventilator weaning.

In the advanced stage of respiratory failure, the vigorous respiratory effort of the dyspneic patient may become counterproductive. Agitation increases oxygen consumption, and forced respiratory efforts may cause dynamic obstruction of airways. Dynamic airway obstruction in the dyspneic child may account for rapid progression of respiratory failure in some cases.

As the severely dyspneic patient decompensates, exhausted efforts may rapidly give way to periodic breathing and apnea. While this phenomenon is commonly observed in infants with lower respiratory infections[11] and pertussis,[12] observations in adults with near-fatal asthma reveal a similar tendency for respiratory arrest to precede cardiovascular collapse.[13] The mechanism of this terminal respiratory depression with severely loaded breathing is not well understood, but it appears to occur in some patients before the development of life-threatening hypoxia and hypercapnia.

Chronic Failure

Congenital or long-standing acquired disorders of the central nervous system may impair respiratory centers, leading to respiratory failure. Acute respiratory insufficiency may accompany progression of a central lesion. A static regulatory impairment may be revealed by failure to compensate for acute systemic illness.

Structural Brain Lesions. Recognition of structural brain lesions as the cause of impaired respiratory regulation is important because some of the lesions are correctable. Congenital structural neurologic malformations may manifest as apnea or profound hypoventilation at birth or may be recognized later. In particular, patients with Chiari malformations often have central and obstructive sleep apnea.[14] Surgical decompression may be associated with improvement even when performed in adults.[15] Acquired lesions such as posterior fossa tumors may interfere with respiratory regulation before or after surgical resection.

Nonstructural Congenital Disorders. Some genetic conditions are associated with derangements in regulation of breathing. Children with congenital central hypoventilation syndrome[16] have characteristic mutations in the *PHOX2B* gene. These patients may first come to medical attention because of growth failure, neurodevelopmental disabilities, or cor pulmonale. Abnormalities include autonomic dysfunction and cardiovascular instability, occasional association with Hirschsprung disease, tumors of neural crest origin, as well as impaired controls of breathing. The syndrome may be recognized in the newborn period, later in childhood, and rarely in adults. Sleep hypoventilation predominates in persons with congenital central hypoventilation syndrome, although some patients also experience respiratory insufficiency while awake. The disorder is often fatal without mechanical ventilation. Early mechanical ventilation may reduce the sequelae and improve long-term neurodevelopmental outcome.

Prader-Willi syndrome is a multigenic disorder initially presenting with hypotonia and then with progressive obesity, growth failure, neurodevelopmental disabilities, reduced ventilatory response to hypoxia and hypercapnia, sleep hypoventilation, and apnea.[17]

Rett syndrome is an X-linked disorder affecting development, behavior, autonomic and respiratory regulation, and seizures. Occurring only in girls, most cases involve spontaneous mutations, although occasionally other family members are affected. Abnormalities are often present in the *MECP2* gene, although some patients with characteristic clinical features have other genetic findings. Multiple phenotypes exist in regard to the respiratory control disorder, with hyperventilation, hypoventilation while awake or asleep, and apneustic breathing.[18]

Many other genetic syndromes with severe neurologic manifestations have impaired upper airway motor function, respiratory cycle timing, and respiratory effort nonspecifically associated with their brain disorder. Nongenetic congenital disorders may impair respiratory controls. For example, children with cerebral palsy occasionally have neurologic deficits of pharyngeal tone, although the central drive to breathe is usually intact.

Nonstructural Acquired Chronic Disorders. Some patients with severe chronic respiratory disease have blunted ventilatory responses to hypoxia, hypercapnia, or respiratory mechanical loads. A concern regarding supplemental oxygen is sometimes raised in the care of patients with acute exacerbations of chronic respiratory disease. It is sometimes argued that administration of supplemental oxygen causes respiratory failure in patients with chronic CO_2 insensitivity who might depend on hypoxic drive to breathe. However, the adverse effects of hypoxia are a greater concern. Because the hypoxic drive to breathe only increases substantially at oxygen tension below 50 mm Hg (Fig. 47.5A), it is virtually impossible to maintain stable respiratory stimulation with mild and "safe" hypoxia without risking episodic life-threatening hypoxia. If a patient is so poorly compensated that removal of hypoxic drive results in hypoventilation, then mechanical ventilation may be the safest management strategy, unless end-of-life plans specifically exclude mechanical ventilation.

Obesity causes hypoventilation by a complex interaction of factors including mechanical loads on the respiratory system, reduction of lung volume, upper airway obstruction, and impaired respiratory regulation. In obese patients, weight loss often improves hypoventilation.[19]

Apparently healthy preterm infants may have postanesthetic apnea until the age of 60 weeks' postconceptional age.[20,21] Apneic events occurred within 2 hours of surgery in 72% of patients, but in the remainder, respiratory irregularity began as late as 12 hours postoperatively. Both obstructive and central mechanisms of apnea were observed. Continuous monitoring for at least 12 hours after anesthesia is warranted when surgery is required for infants born prematurely who are still younger than 60 weeks' postconceptional age.

Sleep hypoventilation tends to occur in adults with hypothyroidism and diabetes mellitus.[22] Little information is available regarding the pediatric patient or the specific role of the endocrine disorder versus obesity.

Recognizing Depressed Respiratory Drive. Respiratory neural output is not routinely directly measured in the clinical setting. Interpreting ventilation as a measure of the intensity of drive to breathe is confounded by dependence of ventilation on the multiple factors of muscle strength, respiratory system mechanics, as well as respiratory neural motor output. Nevertheless, the stressed patient who appears inappropriately comfortable, with little accessory muscle activity, or with periodic breathing, should be presumed to have depressed controls of breathing warranting assisted ventilation.

Failure of Neural Control

The brain may fail to drive rhythmic breathing for a variety of reasons. The brain is susceptible to injury, ischemic stroke, central nervous system hemorrhage, suppression of brain function by cold, structural dysfunction, chemical suppression, signal disruption, and intrinsic disorders of respiratory control. Efferent neural pathways may be blocked by spinal cord lesions, spinal anesthesia, phrenic nerve injury, or neuromuscular disorders. Examples are cited in Table 47.2.

Note that volitional and automatic control of breathing may be separately and independently affected. In Ondine's curse (resulting from stroke involving the lateral medulla), automatic control is impaired, whereas volitional control may persist in the awake state. Supratentorial stroke may impair volitional control of breathing, though automatic control of breathing may be preserved. Central hypoventilation is abnormal respiratory control by the brain and results in hypercapnia. Patients with central hypoventilation may have otherwise normal neurologic functioning or concomitant neurologic injury. Unless mixed with peripheral neuromuscular disease, patients have normal muscle strength, but the essential feature is altered responses to respiratory acidosis.[23] Respiratory patterns may also be abnormal. Central hypoventilation is most apparent when patients are sleeping. Apnea of prematurity, which may persist beyond term, is still not well understood but is clearly aggravated by concomitant infection.

Peripheral (extracranial) neural disorders include spinal cord injury, myasthenia gravis, anticholinesterase poisoning, and Guillain Barré syndrome. The hallmark of these diseases is muscle paresis or paralysis. Hypercapnia is a common feature. Depending on the extent of weakness, patients will be unable to increase their work of breathing in the face of lung disease. Clinical signs such as tachypnea and accessory muscle usage cannot be relied on. Abnormal arterial blood gases may be the only indications of worsening breathing failure, especially in patients with altered sensorium. Patients with spinal cord lesions develop muscle weakness below the level of injury. For instance, patients with lower cervical cord injury may have preservation of suprasternal muscle action but have loss of other accessory muscle function, as well as diaphragmatic

TABLE 47.2	Causes of Failure of Neural Control of Breathing
Mechanism	**Example**
Brain injury	Closed head trauma Ischemic stroke
Severe supratentorial stroke	"Locked-in" syndrome (loss of volitional control of breathing)
Lateral medullary stroke	Ondine's curse (loss of automatic control)
Subarachnoid hemorrhage	Intracranial hypertension with uncal herniation
Brain suppression by cold	Cold-water drowning
Structural brain dysfunction	Brain stem glioma
Chemical suppression	Narcotic overdose
Signal disruption	Seizure
Intrinsic Disorders	
Idiopathic	Ondine's curse
Immaturity	Apnea of prematurity
Spinal cord lesion	Poliomyelitis, traumatic cord transection
Spinal anesthesia	Inadvertent spinal anesthesia
Phrenic nerve injury	Cardiac surgical phrenic nerve injury
Neuromuscular disorder	Curare poisoning, botulinum, and many snake venoms

TABLE 47.3	Causes of Muscle Failure
Mechanism	**Example**
Overwork	Lung dysfunction, airway obstruction
Inadequate substrate	Shock, hypoxemia
Muscle plegia	Hypokalemia
Muscle tetany	Tetanus, hypocalcemia

dysfunction or paresis. These patients will have vigorous suprasternal retractions that expand the lung apices but have little other movement.

Failure of Muscles of Breathing

Causes of breathing muscle failure are listed in Table 47.3, along with examples. They may be crudely divided into causes of muscle exhaustion, causes of muscle plegia or paralysis, and causes of muscle tetany.

In pediatric critical care, the most common cause of failure of the muscles of breathing is exhaustion. The respiratory muscles may become exhausted when responding to excessive workload. Airway obstruction (fixed or functional), lung stiffness, thoracic stiffness (eg, anasarca), abdominal distension, air trapping, and inefficient ventilation-perfusion matching (eg, high ventilation-perfusion mismatch, which functionally wastes ventilation) are examples. Respiratory muscles may also become exhausted if their effort is not supported by adequate nutrition, blood supply, and oxygen delivery. Respiratory distress can be likened to running a marathon. There can be a "wall" beyond which respiratory muscle metabolism is not able to sustain further respiratory effort. Without assistance, after these muscles reach their "wall," respiratory arrest occurs.

In both shock and hypoxemia, oxygen delivery to respiratory muscle may prove inadequate to meet demand on a minute-by-minute basis.[24] Skeletal muscle may sustain a transient oxygen debt by unloading oxygen from myoglobin, but such reserve is limited. Skeletal muscle can also perform anaerobic metabolism to generate adenosine triphosphate, but only until levels of reducing substances (diphosphopyridine nucleotide) build up to such a degree that they inhibit the activity of Kreb cycle enzymes. Over a range of oxygen delivery, metabolic use of oxygen is insensitive to rates of supply (delivery), but below some threshold, muscle aerobic metabolism must inevitably be reduced.[25]

Mitochondrial dysfunction may aggravate deficient muscle metabolism in sepsis. Impaired oxygen utilization may contribute to failure of breathing in other mitochondrial crises as well. One of the indications for intubation and mechanical ventilation in patients with septic shock is to avert respiratory arrest from failure of oxidative metabolism and exhaustion of the muscles of breathing.

There are a few conditions in which muscle contraction may be impaired by dysfunction of the myocyte. Tetrodotoxin (puffer fish) blocks the fast voltage-gated sodium channel of the muscle cell, thereby causing paralysis. Hypokalemia may impair muscle contraction, and hypokalemic periodic paralysis has similar effects. Tetanus and hypocalcemia are capable of causing tetanic contraction that can impair breathing.

Failure of Mechanics of Breathing

Mechanical factors may pose acute or chronic impediments to breathing. Some place such a burden on respiratory muscles that they become exhausted (eg, flail chest, severe thoracic dystrophy, chest deformity). Others cannot be overcome by any effort (eg, foreign body, pneumothorax). Chest and spinal deformities, diaphragmatic eventration, prune belly syndrome (in which abdominal musculature is virtually absent), and deformities that flatten the diaphragm may either cause chronic respiratory insufficiency or contribute to intolerance of intercurrent processes such as pneumonia.

Breathing Failure From Lung Disease

Acute lung disease may progress to breathing failure along one of several pathways. The primary mechanism is respiratory muscle exhaustion. Both excessive demand and impaired supply may come into play, and, in many children, poor thoracic mechanics and neurologic impairment contribute to breathing failure from acute lung disease.

Typically, lung disease increases the work of breathing. Hypoxia and hypercarbia drive the respiratory muscles toward exhaustion. Efficiency of the respiratory system is impaired by lung regions of high ventilation-perfusion ratio. Because these regions see scant blood flow, they actually waste ventilation and breathing effort. On the other hand, low ventilation-perfusion ratio segments cause hypoxemia, which impairs oxygen delivery to tissue and makes circulation inefficient. When oxygen delivery is too low, muscle oxygen utilization becomes delivery dependent, and muscle work capacity declines. Add to these factors others, such as the compliance of the infant chest (which wastes breathing effort),

the deformity of kyphoscoliosis (which makes breathing less efficient), the inefficiency of the infant diaphragm that operates at a wide angle to the chest wall, abdominal distension (which further widens that angle and opposes descent of the diaphragm), and the nutritional issues of chronic illness, and progression toward respiratory arrest is accelerated. Superimposed immaturity, neuromuscular dysfunction, or other comorbid conditions may also exacerbate breathing failure.

As breathing failure worsens, fatigue causes the patient's respiratory effort to deteriorate. Patients use accessory muscles less, they develop brief respiratory pauses, and they progress to apnea followed by respiratory arrest. Respiratory pauses are a subtle but helpful warning sign that should be interpreted as impending respiratory arrest. Pauses warn that respiratory support is indicated. Another helpful sign is grunting. Grunting is a low-pitched sound produced by partial or total closure of the glottis in expiration. Grunting is thought to augment expiratory lung volume (FRC) and increase arterial oxygen tension much like positive end-expiratory pressure (PEEP).[26] Grunting is also a warning of possible impending arrest in children and adults with respiratory failure,[27] though it also often occurs immediately after birth and may quickly resolve as the neonate successfully navigates transition. Patients may appear anxious and describe a feeling of air hunger. Mental status changes ranging from panic to obtundation may occur. Abrupt respiratory slowing and gasping are harbingers of respiratory arrest.

Ventilator-induced lung injury (VILI) and the acute respiratory distress syndrome are histologically inseparable. Two of the mechanisms of VILI are excessive tidal volume and repeated opening and closing of diseased lung units (see Chapter 51). The distress of breathing failure drives breathing. This exertion may overdistend some lung units while contributing to closure and reopening of others. The ausculatory finding of rales in patients with pneumonia supports the contention that closure and reopening of lung units are characteristic of parenchymal lung disease. Ventilation-perfusion mismatch suggests the presence of both overdistended and collapsed alveoli. One must ask: Can spontaneous breathing during respiratory failure promote an injury identical to VILI? Can spontaneous breathing of the patient with severe lung disease and breathing failure worsen lung mechanics and accelerate breathing failure?

After a patient has been intubated for breathing failure, tidal volume can be controlled, alveoli can be stinted open by PEEP, and the risk that superimposed secondary lung injury may worsen lung disease may actually be reduced (compared with the risk of an analogous injury by spontaneous breathing). Intubation also interrupts the progression from breathing failure to respiratory arrest.

Restrictive Versus Obstructive Respiratory Disease

Though restrictive and obstructive pulmonary processes act through the same final common pathways of breathing failure, their mechanics and clinical manifestations often differ. Restrictive diseases are those that limit lung expansion. These include processes that (1) fill alveoli with blood, infectious material, edema, or other debris; (2) involve expansion or swelling of the alveolar interstitium; (3) compress the lung, as with pneumothorax or effusion; or (4) impair excursion of the chest wall or thoracoabdominal region because of neuromuscular dysfunction, skeletal deformity, abdominal distension, ascites, or anasarca. These processes are characterized by a reduction in vital capacity, small resting lung volumes, but normal or near-normal airways resistance. The physical examination reflects these processes. Patients are tachypneic, taking rapid, shallow breaths. Auscultation of the chest may reveal fine inspiratory crepitations (crackles) or rales, evidence of parenchymal lung disease. Poor excursion of the chest wall is usually readily appreciated. Retractions (subcostal and intercostal) are common and indicate significant respiratory effort.

Obstructive diseases of the lung are common in childhood and are characterized by obstruction to flow in airways. Obstructive diseases may be classified as extrathoracic (above the thoracic inlet) or intrathoracic (below). Obstruction may be the result of occluding material or tissue in airways, reduction in lumen caliber from elevated tone of the smooth muscle of airway walls or swelling of tissue, weakness of the airway wall causing collapse and impeding gas flow, or extrinsic compression of airways. In some diseases, several of these processes occur simultaneously. Indeed, secondary obstruction is a common phenomenon. Obstruction in a proximal airway may cause turbulent gas flow downstream in distal airways. Turbulent gas flow causes the wall of the still developing airway to flutter, further weakening the wall's structure and exacerbating overall obstruction.

The hallmark of extrathoracic obstruction is inspiratory noise (stridor or stertor). The affected airway segment lies between the nose and proximal trachea. Inspiratory stridor is a vibratory sound heard because the reduction of intrathoracic pressure during inspiration narrows the extrathoracic (subglottic) airway, generating an inspiratory noise. Stertor is a snoring noise generated in the nasopharynx. Airways with severe obstruction flutter in both inspiration and exhalation, causing biphasic stridor or noise heard in both phases of the respiratory cycle. Other characteristic sounds may help to identify the obstructed airway segment (Table 47.4). In extreme obstruction, patients may position themselves to maximize airway caliber (remaining upright, leaning slightly forward, and holding the head in the "sniffing position" to enhance alignment of the pharynx and larynx). It should be noted that generation of noise requires airflow. With severe obstruction, there is little airflow and little noise is generated. Loss of noise, despite increased effort, is an ominous sign and is indicative of complete obstruction and impending respiratory arrest.

The hallmark of intrathoracic obstruction is an expiratory sound. In intrathoracic obstruction, forced expiration compresses soft airways, causing a musical wheeze. This obstruction may be largely relieved by inspiration, which tends to dilate intrathoracic airways. In severe intrathoracic obstruction, sounds may be heard during both phases of the respiratory cycle. The classic pediatric disease of intrathoracic obstruction is asthma. High-pitched wheezes on exhalation are heard early in the episode. As airway obstruction worsens, wheezes are heard in inspiration as well. With severe obstruction, wheezes diminish because there is little gas flow.

The character of the voice and ability to speak (in words, phrases, or sentences) may be helpful in the evaluation of airway obstruction. Observation of the respiratory rate can be revealing in obstructive disease. With mild obstruction, the respiratory rate is often slower than normal but may rise as ventilation perfusion inequality develops and increases respiratory drive. Physical examination will often reveal the use of accessory muscles of breathing.

Compensatory Mechanisms in Breathing Failure

A patient may try to compensate for the functional effects of lung disease. These compensatory mechanisms generally come into play before there is evidence of breathing failure. Many of the clinical signs of respiratory distress, discussed previously, are evidence of compensatory mechanisms. Understanding these mechanisms improves in the recognition of impending failure.

Compensatory Mechanisms in Restrictive Lung Disease

Tachypnea is the patient's primary compensation for the small lung volume of restrictive lung disease and is the earliest detectable clinical sign. Additional compensation is achieved by recruitment of accessory muscles. Patients with restrictive disease may take periodic sigh breaths, which are larger than tidal breaths, to recruit collapsing units. Compensatory mechanisms also operate to maximize gas exchange in diseased lungs. Hypoxic pulmonary vasoconstriction is an important mechanism to improve gas exchange in normal lungs. Hypoxic pulmonary vasoconstriction is a direct response of the vascular smooth muscle to low PaO_2 alveolar units. The precapillary arteriole of such units constricts in response to low O_2 tension in the adjacent postcapillary venule, thereby directing blood away from poorly functioning alveoli. In a lung with patchy disease, the overall effect of the hypoxic pulmonary vasoconstriction response is to shunt blood away from diseased segments and allow flow to healthier areas. This may, paradoxically, increase pulmonary vascular resistance and oppose right ventricular ejection. Inhaled nitric oxide (iNO) provides a putative exogenous means to improve ventilation perfusion matching (by preferentially dilating vessels to ventilated lung segments) without afterloading the right ventricle, although enduring benefits with iNO have not been demonstrated.[28]

Compensatory Mechanisms With Obstructive Lung Disease

The major compensations in obstructive disease focus on maximizing airflow. As previously stated, patients naturally position themselves to maximize opening of their airway. If this is the case, repositioning patients, especially to the supine position, may worsen airflow. For the infant, carefully

TABLE 47.4	Abnormal Sounds Indicative of Extrathoracic Airway Obstruction
Sound	**Condition**
Hoarseness	Unilateral vocal cord paralysis
Muffled voice	Supraglottic or infraglottic processes, including epiglottitis
"Hot potato" voice	Oral, retropharyngeal abscess Cellulitis or connective tissue infection of the floor of the mouth also known as Ludwig's angina
"Barking" cough	Laryngotracheobronchitis (croup)
Monotone, hurried sentences	Bilateral vocal cord paresis

monitored prone positioning may aid gas exchange and assist spontaneous breathing.[29,30] Control of respiratory rate provides another means of compensation. In mild obstructive disease, the respiratory rate is lower than normal. As resistance to airflow rises, total work of breathing also rises greatly. To maximize efficiency, the respiratory rate falls. Longer respiratory cycle times allow longer times for gas flow. Having said this, the clinician will recognize that many patients with obstructive lung disease present with tachypnea, not decreased respiratory rates. The causes of tachypnea are (1) ventilation/perfusion mismatching with hypoxemia, and sometimes hypercarbia, driving the respiratory rate and (2) development of atelectasis in unventilated lung segments resulting in the superimposition of a restrictive process on an obstructive one. Tachypnea in such patients is counterproductive, greatly increasing the work of breathing and further diminishing gas flow.

Special Conditions

Several conditions deserve special note. In these, physical findings may reflect specific aberrations that generate specific compensatory mechanisms.

Infancy

Young infants are at a mechanical disadvantage for efficient breathing. The configuration of the infant's chest wall differs from that of adults. Orientation of the ribs is more horizontal in infants than in adults, and they move less during breathing. The chest wall is more compliant and is composed of more cartilaginous tissues. Strength of intercostals muscles is less. In the absence of muscular action, FRC is determined by the elastic forces of the lung and the chest wall, which oppose each other. Accordingly, the infant's more compliant chest wall and weaker musculature results in lower FRC. Infants with lung disease use expiratory braking (grunting), which involves constriction of pharyngeal muscles and glottis, to increase end-expiratory lung volume. Although this promotes higher FRC, it imposes a disadvantageous increase in muscular work.

Infant respiratory muscle fibers differ from those of adults. The infant diaphragm contains a greater proportion of type II fibers, which are unable to sustain repeat strenuous activity.[31] Hence, the infant's diaphragm fatigues more quickly than that of the adult.[32] The infant's diaphragmatic anatomy is also disadvantageous. The reduced appositional area and greater diaphragmatic angle of the infant causes less lung volume expansion with diaphragmatic contraction. Because pulling the rib cage cephalad produces less outward chest displacement in the infant than in the adult, the infant's tidal volume is, in the aggregate, more dependent on diaphragmatic contraction than that of the adult.

Superimposition of breathing failure on infant respiratory function exacerbates these mechanical disadvantages. In normal respiration, the chest wall and abdomen move inward and outward in synchrony. With restrictive lung disease, the respiratory pattern may be out of phase, called *paradoxical breathing*. Contraction of the diaphragm pulls the compliant infant chest wall inward during inspiration and pushes abdominal contents outward. This respiratory pattern is greatly exaggerated by severe restrictive lung disease. With decreased lung compliance, the pleural pressure swing is exaggerated, pulling the chest wall farther inward. Prolonged respiration in this manner can cause inward deformation of the sternum, or acquired *pectus excavatum,* and is a clinical sign of prolonged respiratory insufficiency. In the infant with severe restrictive disease, recruitment of additional diaphragmatic and accessory muscles, use of compensatory braking and grunting maneuvers, and increases in respiratory rate may be insufficient to maintain a normal FRC. Fatigue comes quickly. Moreover, such work is extremely energy expensive. Infants with chronic respiratory insufficiency can use as much as 50% of their caloric intake for breathing, leaving few calories for growth and other functions and resulting in failure to thrive.

Infants are disadvantaged with respect to obstructive lung disease. In infants and young children, a greater percent of total airways resistance is apportioned to large airways than in adults. Infants are particularly susceptible to nasal obstruction, as occurs during upper respiratory infection, because the nose may comprise as much as 50% of total airway resistance. Moreover, resistance to airflow is proportional to the inverse of the airway radius to the fourth power:

$$R = 8\eta L/\pi r^4$$

where η is gas viscosity, L is airway length, and r is radius of the airways. Resistance is greater in infants and young children because of their intrinsically small airways. Further reduction in airways caliber with obstructive disease (eg, bronchiolitis) magnifies this problem.

The infant's airways are also less endowed with cartilage than are those of the adult and may be subject to flow limitation during active expiration. The trachea and bronchi may be pathologically compressed during expiration, causing severe obstruction that is worsened by expiratory effort. Such regions of severe and pathologic flow limitation (tracheomalacia and bronchomalacia) may be localized. Similarly, the larynx may be compressed (by atmosphere) during forced inspiration (laryngomalacia) if there is proximal (supraglottic) obstruction.

Thoracic Dysfunction

Neuromuscular disorders generally result in restrictive lung defects. Coexisting obstructive lung disease can be seen with some thoracic defects or with scoliosis. Persistent atelectasis and long-standing lung hypoplasia may lead to atrophy and may destroy supporting airway architecture resulting in air trapping. Deformities of the rib cage and spinal column result in restriction to lung expansion as occurs with isolated scoliosis.[33,34] The most severe of these are classified as "asphyxiating thoracic dystrophies" in which the chest fails to expand at all during breathing. As with the other forms of neuromuscular diseases, hypercapnia predominates. Muscle strength may be normal, but abnormal configuration of intrathoracic muscles and diaphragm may make muscle work inefficient.

With many of these disorders, patients live in a chronic state of increased work of breathing and muscle fatigue. Growth failure is common. They tend to have little ability to meet the added demands of acute respiratory processes, such as respiratory infections. Total breathing failure often ensues. They may have frequent and recurring need for positive pressure support. Yet the usual signs of impending breathing failure may be absent in patients who are weak, nonresponsive, or have chest wall distortions. In such cases, close monitoring and measurement of arterial blood gases are essential.

Altered Nutritional States: Malnutrition and Obesity

A major functional consequence of malnutrition is altered muscle function. Protein-calorie malnutrition results in decreased muscle energetics.[35] Protein deficiencies alone may have a similar effect. Catabolism of skeletal muscle to meet body protein needs results in decreased muscle mass. Malnourished states are easy to recognize when they are the result of long-standing inadequate caloric intake, as in marasmus, but this is rarely seen in developed countries. More common are subtler forms of insufficient nutrition in children who live in a chronically high metabolic state, such as chronic congestive heart failure. Such patients may be unable to consume enough calories for effective positive nitrogen balance. Catabolism is ongoing, sacrificing muscle mass and function. Chronic respiratory insufficiency results in a cycle of progressive breathing failure, increasing work of breathing, and worsening imbalance between calorie intake and expenditure. Recognition of this cycle is imperative; metabolic demands must be decreased by treating the underlying condition and caloric intake must be increased. In the young child, reversal of this cycle is signaled by resumption of somatic growth. The clinician should also note that in patients with malnutrition the superimposition of an acute respiratory process, such as an intercurrent respiratory infection, will result in more rapid progression to breathing failure. The patient has little or no reserve for the added metabolic demands and work of breathing.

At the other end of the nutritional spectrum, obesity has major respiratory consequences. As with obese adults, obese children are at risk from obstructive sleep apnea syndrome. Obstructive sleep apnea syndrome may cause frequent obstructive events. Hypercarbia and hypoxemia may occur. Obstructive sleep apnea syndrome is diagnosed by polysomnography. Treatment includes weight loss, removal of tonsils and adenoids, palatoplasty procedures in some patients, and nightly positive pressure support in others. Additionally, obesity alters lung volumes, especially when children are supine. With abdominal contents pushing up on the diaphragm, FRC and total lung capacity are reduced, representing another form of chronic restrictive disease. This effect is exaggerated in the supine (as opposed to upright) position.

Conclusion

Breathing failure occurs when neural, muscular, or mechanical challenges cannot be overcome by compensatory mechanisms. A common final pathway is muscle exhaustion, either from excessive demand on respiratory muscles or from inadequate supply to these muscles of blood flow, oxygen, or nutrients. Assisted ventilation is important to not only improve gas exchange but also prevent respiratory arrest from breathing failure. This is true in both lung disease and other conditions that impair neural, muscular, or mechanical breathing capacity.

References

1. Smith-Blair N. Mechanisms of diaphragm fatigue. *AACN Clin Issues.* 2002;13:307-319.
2. Takata M, Robotham JL. Effects of inspiratory diaphragmatic descent on inferior vena caval venous return. *J Appl Physiol.* 1992;72:597-607.
3. Rehan VK, McCool FD. Diaphragm dimensions of the healthy preterm infant. *Acta Paediatr.* 2003;92:1062-1067.
4. Smith JC, Ellenberger HH, Ballanyi K, et al. Pre-Bötzinger complex: a brainstem region that may generate respiratory rhythm in mammals. *Science.* 1991;254:726.
5. Ruangkittisakul A, Kottick A, Picardo MC, et al. Identification of the pre-Bötzinger complex inspiratory center in calibrated "sandwich" slices from newborn mice with fluorescent Dbx1 interneurons. *Physiol Rep.* 2014;19:2.
6. Moore JD, Kleinfeld D, Wang F. How the brainstem controls orofacial behaviors composed of rhythmic actions. *Trends Neurosci.* 2014;37:370-380.
7. Casey KR, Cantillo KO, Brown LK. Sleep-related hypoventilation/hypoxemic syndromes. *Chest.* 2007;131:1936-1948.
8. Verges S, Lenher O, Andrea C, et al. Increased fatigue resistance of respiratory muscles during exercise after respiratory muscle endurance training. *Am J Physiol Regul Integr Comp Physiol.* 2007;292:R1246-R1253.
9. Roussos C, Zakynthinos S. Fatigue of the respiratory muscles. *Intensive Care Med.* 1996;22:134-155.
10. Roussos C, Koutsoukou A. Respiratory failure. *Eur Respir J.* 2003;22(suppl 47):3s-14s.
11. Hill RV. Incidence of apnea in infants hospitalized with respiratory syncytial virus bronchiolitis: a systematic review. *J Pediatr.* 2009;155:728-733.
12. Surridge J, Segedin ER, Grant CC. Pertussis requiring intensive care. *Arch Dis Child.* 2007;92:970-975.
13. Molfino NA, Nannini LJ, Martelli AN, et al. Respiratory arrest in near-fatal asthma. *N Engl J Med.* 1991;324:285.
14. Khatwa U, Ramgopal S, Mylavarapu A, et al. MRI findings and sleep apnea in children with Chiari I malformation. *Pediatr Neurol.* 2013;48:299-307.
15. Botelho RV, Bittencourt LR, Rotta JM, et al. The effects of posterior fossa decompressive surgery in adult patients with Chiari malformation and sleep apnea. *J Neurosurg.* 2010;112:800-807.
16. Rand CM, Patwari PP, Carroll MS, et al. Congenital central hypoventilation syndrome and sudden infant death syndrome: disorders of autonomic control. *Semin Pediatr Neurol.* 2013;20:44-55.
17. Pavone M, Caldarelli V, Khirani S, et al. Sleep disordered breathing in patients with Prader-Willi syndrome: a multicenter study. *Pediatr Pulmonol.* 2015;50:1354-1359.
18. Ramirez JM, Ward CS, Neul JL. Breathing challenges in Rett syndrome: lessons learned from humans and animal models. *Respir Physiol Neurobiol.* 2013;189:280-287.
19. Piper AJ, Grundstein RR. Big breathing—the complex interaction of obesity, hypoventilation, weight loss and respiratory function. *J Appl Physiol.* 2010;108:199-205.
20. Kurth CD, Spitzer AR, Broennle AM, et al. Postoperative apnea in preterm infants. *Anesthesiology.* 1987;66:483.
21. Kurth CD, LeBard SE. Association of postoperative apnea, airway obstruction, and hypoxia in former premature infants. *Anesthesiology.* 1991;75:22.
22. Bottini P, Tantucci C. Sleep apnea in endocrine diseases. *Respiration.* 2003;70:320-327.
23. Panitch HB. The pathophysiology of respiratory impairment in pediatric neuromuscular diseases. *Pediatrics.* 2009;123(suppl 4):S215-S218.
24. Aubier M, Trippenbach T, Roussos C. Respiratory muscle fatigue during cardiogenic shock. *J Appl Physiol.* 1981;51:499.
25. Fahey JT, Lister G. Postnatal changes in critical cardiac output and O_2 transport in conscious lambs. *Am J Physiol.* 1987;253:H100.
26. Dinwiddie R, Russell G. Artificial grunting in respiratory distress syndrome. *Arch Dis Child.* 1972;47(255):837-838.
27. Young Infants Clinical Signs Study Group. Clinical signs that predict severe illness in children under age 2 months: a multicentre study. *Lancet.* 2008;371(9607):135-142.
28. Afshari A, Brok J, Møller AM, Wetterslev J. Inhaled nitric oxide for acute respiratory distress syndrome (ARDS) and acute lung injury in children and adults. *Cochrane Database Syst Rev.* 2010;(7):CD002787.
29. Gillies D, Wells D, Bhandari AP. Positioning for acute respiratory distress in hospitalised infants and children. *Cochrane Database Syst Rev.* 2012;(7):CD003645.
30. Wells DA, Gillies D, et al. Positioning for acute respiratory distress in hospitalised infants and children. *Cochrane Database Syst Rev.* (2):2005;CD003645.

31. Sieck GC, et al. Diaphragm muscle fatigue resistance during postnatal development. *J Appl Physiol.* 1991;71:458-464.

32. Greenspan JS, Miller TL, et al. The neonatal respiratory pump: a developmental challenge with physiologic limitations. *Neonatal Netw.* 2005;24:15-22.

33. Koumbourlis AC. Scoliosis and the respiratory system. *Paediatr Respir Rev.* 2006;7:152-160.

34. Hawes M. Impact of spine surgery on signs and symptoms of spinal deformity. *Pediatr Rehabil.* 2006;9:318-339.

35. van Waardenburg DA, et al. Critically ill infants benefit from early administration of protein and energy-enriched formula: a randomized controlled trial. *Clin Nutr.* 2009;28:249-255.

Ventilation/Perfusion Inequality

Thomas V. Brogan and David J. Vaughan

PEARLS

- Gravity affects the distribution of pulmonary blood flow and ventilation. Both perfusion and ventilation increase down the lung. Despite these changes, perfusion is tightly matched to ventilation.
- There is also significant heterogeneity of pulmonary blood flow and ventilation in isogravitational fields. The pattern of both perfusion and ventilation is fractal in nature.
- The primary ventilation/perfusion abnormality in acute respiratory distress syndrome (ARDS) is intrapulmonary shunt.
- In persons with asthma, ventilation/perfusion mismatch is responsible for hypoxemia, but no correlation exists between measurements of overall airway obstruction and V_A/Q mismatch.
- Although positive end-expiratory pressure decreases the proportion of shunt in ARDS, at high levels it also increases dead space.

The primary function of the lung is to exchange oxygen and carbon dioxide between inspired air and blood. Efficient gas exchange requires the close matching of regional ventilation and perfusion. The lung is influenced by external and internal factors that affect ventilation/perfusion (V_A/Q) relationships. Early studies supported the concept that vertical gradients of both ventilation and perfusion produced close V_A/Q matching. Newer studies demonstrated that perfusion and ventilation have much greater heterogeneity, even in isogravitational planes, which serves to match ventilation to perfusion.

Lung diseases commonly produce abnormalities in functional residual capacity (FRC) and closing capacity, which distort normal V_A/Q matching (Table 48.1). Lung units that are poorly ventilated in relation to blood flow (low V_A/Q) produce blood with low oxygen content (desaturated blood), but units with high V_A/Q ratios cannot compensate because the oxygen content of blood leaving these areas has oxygen content only slightly higher than that from normal V_A/Q regions due to the sigmoid shape of the hemoglobin oxygen dissociation curve (Fig. 48.1).

The alveolar gas equation helps to explain the pathophysiology of abnormal gas exchange by providing information on alveolar oxygen tension. According to the Fick equation, under steady state conditions, the quantity of O_2 taken up by the lungs equals the amount of O_2 removed from inhaled air:

$$O_2 = {}_A(FIO_2 - FAO_2) \qquad \text{Eq. 48.1}$$

where O_2 represents O_2 consumption, FIO_2 is the fraction of inspired O_2, A represents alveolar ventilation, and FAO_2 is the fraction of alveolar O_2. This equation can be rearranged to read:

$$FAO_2 = FIO_2 - O_2/_A \qquad \text{Eq. 48.2}$$

Then, by changing the fraction of gases to their partial pressures, the equation takes the following form:

$$PAO_2 = PIO_2 - (O_2/_A)(P_B - 47 \text{ mm Hg}) \qquad \text{Eq. 48.3}$$

where PIO_2 is the inspired PO_2 and P_B is barometric pressure.

The concept underlying this equation is that alveolar oxygen level (PAO_2) is the difference between inspired oxygen (PIO_2) and the amount taken up by the pulmonary capillaries [$(O_2/_A)$ $(P_B - 47 \text{ mm Hg})$]. The ratio $O_2/_A$ can be estimated from a surrogate for the ratio between O_2 and $_A$. By using PCO_2 in arterial blood as an estimate of alveolar CO_2, $CO_2/_A$ as an estimator of $FACO_2$, and the respiratory quotient $R = CO_2/O_2$, the second term of Eq. (3) can be estimated by $PACO_2/R$. The alveolar gas equation can then be derived as follows:

$$PAO_2 = FIO_2 \times (P_B - 47 \text{ mm Hg}) - (CO_2/R/_A) \times (P_B - 47 \text{ mm Hg}) \qquad \text{Eq. 48.4}$$

$$PAO_2 = FIO_2 \times (P_B - 47 \text{ mm Hg}) - (F_ACO_2/R) \times (PB - 47 \text{ mm Hg}) \qquad \text{Eq. 48.5}$$

$$PAO_2 = FIO_2 \times (P_B - 47 \text{ mm Hg}) - (PACO_2/R) \qquad \text{Eq. 48.6}$$

According to this equation, PAO_2 may be decreased by increases in the $PACO_2$ or by decreases in the atmospheric pressure and R.

Distribution of Ventilation

Regional lung ventilation is influenced by many factors, including gravity, posture, and experimental technique. Gravity has been considered paramount because it creates variation in pleural pressure from the lung apex to the base, imposing a globular shape on the lung. Pleural pressure is more negative at the apex of the lung compared with the base, increasing approximately 0.25-cm H_2O per centimeter of vertical distance toward the base, making transpulmonary pressure greater at the apex. Consequently, apical alveoli are large, at the upper end of the normal pressure volume curve, and distend less for a given pressure change (lower compliance). In the spontaneously breathing upright human, maximal gas distribution occurs at the base and progressively diminishes toward the lung apex.[1,2] This gradient also exists when

TABLE 48.1 Causes of Hypoxemia

Intrapulmonary Factors	Extrapulmonary Factors
PRIMARY	PRIMARY
Ventilation/perfusion mismatch	Decreased cardiac output
Shunt	
Alveolar-end capillary diffusion limitation	SECONDARY Decreased P50
Decreased minute ventilation	Decreased hemoglobin concentration
Decreased Fio$_2$	Alkalosis

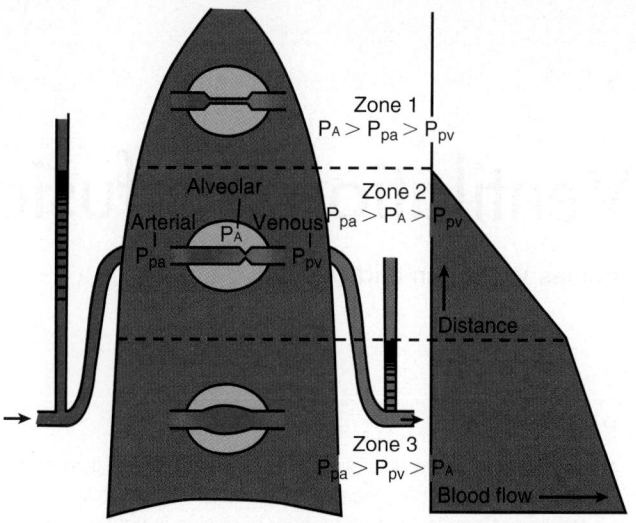

Fig. 48.2. Normal distribution of pulmonary blood flow: gravitational model. According to the model, the gravitational driving force for pulmonary blood flow increases down the lung. At the apex (zone 1), flow is absent as alveolar pressure (P_A) exceeds pulmonary artery (P_{PA}) and pulmonary venous (P_V) pressures. In *zone 2*, flow is determined by the driving pressure $(P_{PA} - P_A)$. Flow is constant and maximal in *zone 3* because both P_{PA} and P_V exceed P_A where the driving pressure is $P_{PA} - P_V$.

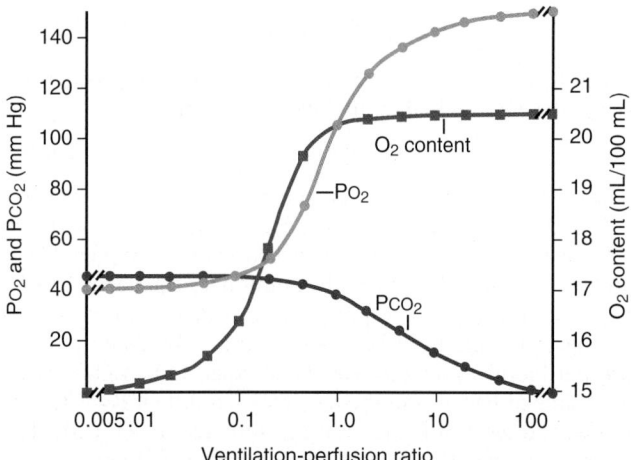

Fig. 48.1. Gas exchange in a single lung unit. Changes in Po$_2$, Pco$_2$, and end-capillary O$_2$ content in a lung unit as its ventilation/perfusion ratio is increased from shunt (V/Q = 0) to dead space (V/Q = ∞). Hemoglobin concentration is 14.8 g/dL.

inhalation occurs in the recumbent position, although to a lesser degree.

Ventilation heterogeneity does not depend solely on gravitational influences. The time constant (the product of resistance and compliance) is the time required for inflation to 63% of final lung volume. Therefore a given lung unit with a slow time constant fills more slowly than one with a fast time constant and empties more slowly. When time constants of different lung units vary, as frequently happens in lung disease, gas distribution will be determined in part by the rate, duration, and frequency of breathing.

Distribution of Perfusion

The pulmonary circulation is a low-pressure circuit with a mean pulmonary artery pressure (P_{PA}) of approximately 15 mm Hg, compared with mean systemic pressure on the order of 100 mm Hg. According to the classical model of lung perfusion, gravity affects PBF in a similar fashion to ventilation but to a greater extent. The P_{PA} decreases by 1 cm H$_2$O per centimeter of vertical distance up the lung, so the driving pressure rapidly drops with minimal blood flow to the apices.

In the erect human, pulmonary blood flow (PBF) progressively increases from apex to base.[3]

The three-zone model of PBF has been widely used to explain the heterogeneity of perfusion within the lung (Fig. 48.2).[3] Three variables comprise the components of this model: pulmonary arterial (P_{PA}), alveolar (P_A), and pulmonary venous (P_V) pressures. PBF within the lung zones depends on the relative magnitudes of these pressures within each zone. Zone 1 ($P_A > P_{PA} > P_V$) has negligible blood flow, as high alveolar pressure is believed to compress collapsible capillaries. This region is one of minimal gas exchange or "wasted" ventilation. Zone 1 conditions are rare except in cases of diminished PBF (eg, hypotension or cardiac failure) or increased P_A encountered during positive pressure ventilation.

Zone 2 consists of the midportions of the lungs in which $P_{PA} > P_A > P_V$, where PBF is determined by the difference between pulmonary arterial and alveolar pressures. Venous pressure does not influence the flow rate. Blood flow progressively increases with descent through this zone as P_{PA} increases, whereas P_A remains relatively constant.

In the lowest lung region, zone 3, $P_{PA} > P_V > P_A$; therefore the arteriovenous pressure gradient ($P_{PA} - P_V$) determines PBF.[3] A zone 4 region in the most dependent areas of the lung has also been described. In this region, transudated pulmonary interstitial fluid increases interstitial pressures, thereby reducing blood flow; this effect is exaggerated as lung volume diminishes from total lung capacity to residual volume.

PBF in immature animals differs in several important ways from that of adult animals. The immature pulmonary vascular bed appears to be fully recruited, with no contribution of Starling resistors in the pulmonary circulation during exposure to acute or chronic hypoxia.[4,5] Furthermore, neonatal piglets show a relative hypoxemia with an increased dispersion of PBF.

Fractal Model of Pulmonary Blood Flow and Ventilation

Studies employing increased resolution showed PBF to possess greater heterogeneity than described in the gravitational model.[6-8] Isogravitational PBF was shown to be nearly as heterogeneous as that of the entire lung (Fig. 48.3) rather than being random PBF correlated with that of neighboring regions.[8] High-flow regions bordered other high-flow regions while low-flow regions abutted other low-flow regions. The distribution of PBF was shown to be independent of the scale of measurement, suggesting a fractal nature of PBF.

A fractal structure or process has a characteristic form that remains constant over a magnitude of scales (Fig. 48.4).[8] This concept of self-similarity has been recognized within the bronchial and pulmonary vascular trees.[9] In animal models and in humans under conditions of microgravity, gravity's contribution to overall perfusion heterogeneity was of secondary importance. PBF had a hilar to peripheral gradient.[9-11] The asymmetry of flow at pulmonary artery branches accounts for the heterogeneity of flow within isogravitational planes. Thus regions that share a parent or grandparent branch have more similar flows than do branches that are separated by a greater distance. This fractal pattern extends to the subacinar level.[12]

Fractal Model of the Pulmonary Ventilation

The close correlation between regional ventilation and perfusion suggests that ventilation has spatial characteristics similar to perfusion.[13-16] The correlation of regional heterogeneities of ventilation and perfusion ensures a narrow distribution of V_A/Q normally. Fractals possess a large area-to-volume ratio,

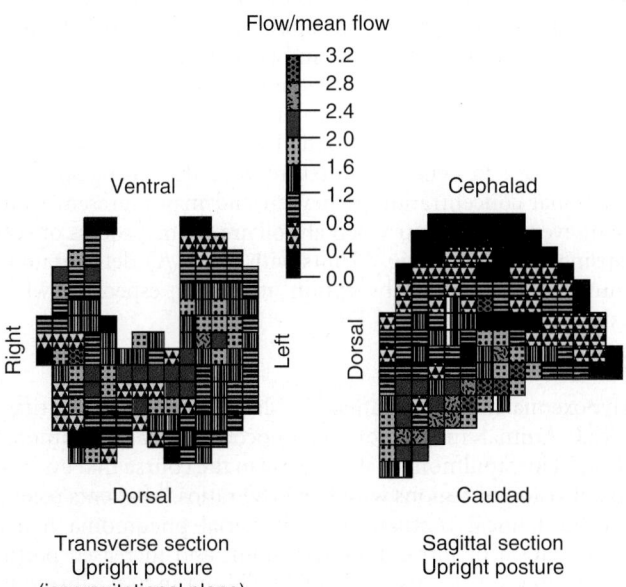

Fig. 48.3. Isogravitational heterogeneity of pulmonary blood flow. Reconstruction of transverse and sagittal plane from a single baboon animal during upright posture. Each *square* depicts location and relative blood flow to a piece of lung in a given plane. Heterogeneity of blood flow is present in isogravitational planes. Flow is not random; rather, neighboring pieces tend to have similar magnitudes of flow. Cephalad-caudad (gravitational) gradient is apparent in the sagittal section.

ensuring that all cells are serviced by capillaries and efficiently ensuring gas exchange and substrate irrespective of an organism's size. The correlation between regional ventilation and perfusion may be explained by the close association of the developing bronchial tree and pulmonary arterial tree during organogenesis.[17]

The innate structure of the lung itself appears to underlie the precision of V_A/Q matching.[18] Basal pulmonary vascular tone is minimal, suggesting that vasoregulation is of minor importance for maintaining close V_A/Q matching normally.[19-21] Passive matching of perfusion and ventilation by pulmonary structure suggests that lung perfusion is an optimally engineered system. That is, it requires no active feedback mechanism during normal function, which tends to sustain effective performance (Fig. 48.5).[22] Furthermore, a fractal system delivers substrate with a minimum of energy expended because the fractal structure minimizes the total hydrodynamic resistance of the system, as well as the amount of biological material to construct the vascular and bronchial trees while still filling the space occupied by the lung.[22] Finally, the fractal structure efficiently uses the amount of genetic code to construct the vascular and bronchial structure by using a recursive construction mechanism that requires only a handful of proteins. A much greater amount of genetic code would be needed if each branch in the system required unique genetic code.

V_A/Q Abnormalities in Pulmonary Disease
Hypoxemia

The primary causes of hypoxemia in children are intrapulmonary shunt and V_A/Q mismatch. Shunt differs from V_A/Q mismatch in that it does not respond to increases in inspired O_2. Oxygen content of arterial blood represents a weighted average of the O_2 content of shunted blood (Q_s/Q_t) and the remaining fraction ($1 - Q_s/Q_t$):

$$C_aO_2 = C_vO_2 \times Q_s/Q_t + C_cO_2 \times (1 - Q_s/Q_t) \qquad \text{Eq. 48.7}$$

Q_s and Q_t represent shunt and total lung blood flow, respectively, and C_aO_2, C_vO_2, and C_cO_2 are the arterial, venous, and pulmonary capillary oxygen contents, respectively. This equation can then be rearranged to solve for shunt fraction:

$$Q_s/Q_t = \frac{C_cO_2 - C_aO_2}{C_cO_2 - C_vO_2} \qquad \text{Eq. 48.8}$$

Regional alveolar hypoxia causes pulmonary vasoconstriction, restricting blood flow to the area.[23,24] (A similar though less robust response occurs with decreased mixed venous oxygenation [P_{VO_2}].) This compensatory response, hypoxic pulmonary vasoconstriction (HPV), is best when hypoxia is localized and when the P_AO_2 is in the 70 to 90 mm Hg range.[24] The degree of HPV varies across the lung and is affected by sepsis, vasodilators, anesthetics, and changes of inspired oxygen. Inspiration of 100% O_2 worsens V_A/Q mismatch substantially by opposing HPV.[25]

Alterations in inspired or arterial CO_2 tensions also have been shown to alter V_A/Q ratios. Inspired CO_2 (3%–5%) improves V_A/Q matching and perfusion heterogeneity in normal and injured lungs, while hypocapnia produces the opposite effect.[26-28] These changes in V_A/Q heterogeneity appear to be dependent on changes in pH.

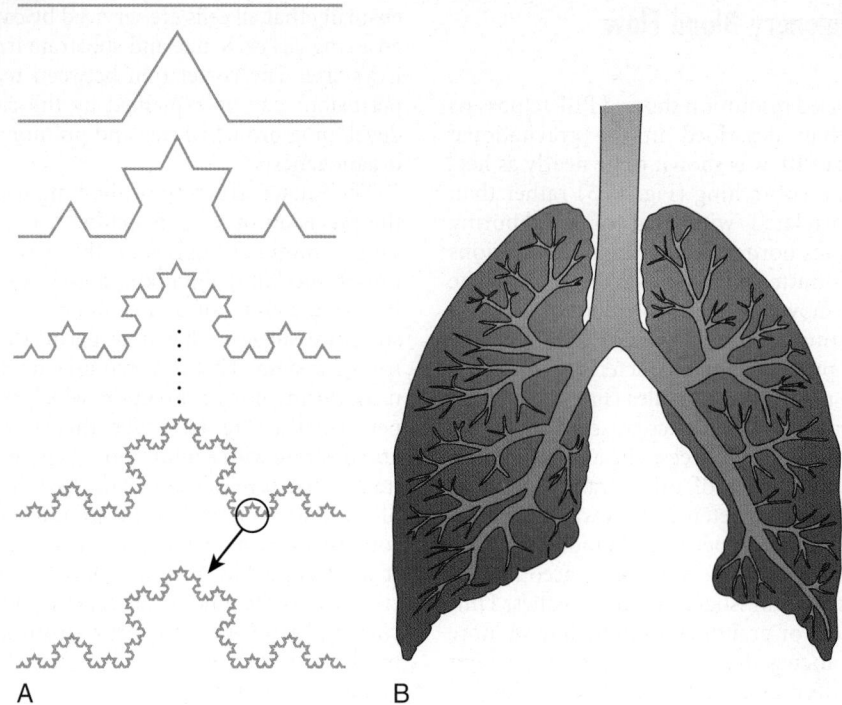

Fig. 48.4. Fractal structures. (A) This curve is produced by a simple iterative transformation beginning with a straight line. At each step the middle third of all lines is replaced with two segments, one-third length of the line, forming part of an equilateral triangle. An infinite number of iterations can be performed. Thus as increasing magnification reveals more detail, the overall appearance of the new segment remains similar to that of the previous segment. (B) The pulmonary vascular (and bronchial) tree is a repetitive pattern of dichotomous branches that become progressively smaller and fill a predetermined area.

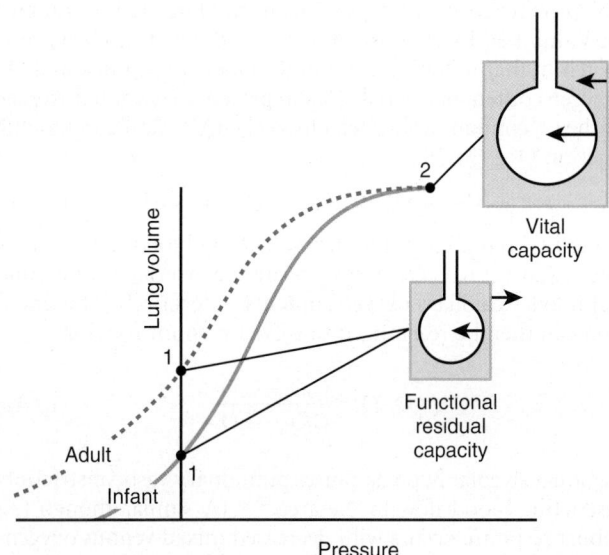

Fig. 48.5. Relative ventilation and perfusion maps. Regional ventilation and perfusion scaled to the measured minute ventilation and cardiac output in the pig. Both regional ventilation and perfusion show clustering in which adjacent units have similar flows. There is strong correlation in which areas of high ventilation receive high perfusion and areas of low ventilation receive low perfusion. (These pig lungs were examined in cubes of 1.5 to 2.0 cm³ volume.)

Acute Respiratory Distress Syndrome

Acute respiratory distress syndrome (ARDS) is marked by profound hypoxemia refractory to high FiO_2, suggesting shunt.[29] Hypoxemia in ARDS is due to shunt that is proportional to cardiac output.[29] Intrapulmonary shunt results from alveolar flooding, atelectasis, and right-to-left shunt through a patent foramen ovale. Some patients also have units with very low V_A/Q ratios as well as substantial ventilation to regions that are underperfused. The low V_A/Q units explain the increase in venous admixture with decreasing inspired fractional concentration of oxygen and may represent transient events that occur when alveoli are in the process of collapsing or reexpanding.[30] Units with low V_A/Q deteriorate to shunt as a result of absorption atelectasis, especially when exposed to high levels of FiO_2.

Pneumonia

Hypoxemia found in patients with pneumonia is multifactorial. Animal models of pneumococcal lobar pneumonia showed intrapulmonary shunt early in the course that evolved to perfusion of regions with low V_A/Q ratios.[31] Patients receiving mechanical ventilation for bacterial pneumonia had a combination of intrapulmonary shunt and increased perfusion to low V_A/Q units.[32] High F_IO_2 did not increase intrapulmonary shunt but did oppose HPV in pneumonia patients. Similar, less severe findings also were observed in spontaneously breathing patients with pneumonia.[33]

Asthma

Ventilation/perfusion abnormalities have been found across the spectrum of patients with asthma. Asthmatics usually have a bimodal distribution of blood flow with normal units and large areas of low V_A/Q with little intrapulmonary shunt.[34] No correlation exists between measurements of airway obstruction and inert gas exchange,[35] so maximum airflow rates and V_A/Q inequalities appear to be unrelated, suggesting that spirometric changes reflect bronchoconstriction in larger and medium-sized airways, whereas V_A/Q abnormalities are mainly related to edema and/or mucus formation occurring in the distal small airways.[35] High F_IO_2 may prevent HPV and place low V_A/Q regions at risk for absorption atelectasis. Bronchodilators may enhance the perfusion of low V_A/Q areas, exacerbating V_A/Q mismatch. However, the beneficial effects of bronchodilators on airway resistance generally outweigh the worsening in V_A/Q mismatch.

Pulmonary Embolism

Pulmonary emboli tend to travel to high-flow regions of the lung, producing a shift of PBF toward regions that previously had seen low flow, preferentially in nondependent areas, which have greater capacity for capillary recruitment.[21] Before embolization, regions with high blood flow had good V_A/Q matching. After embolization, regional ventilation changed little. The areas to which blood flow shifted now became low V_A/Q regions, resulting in hypoxemia. Nonperfused areas added to dead space, increasing P_ACO_2.

Primary Pulmonary Hypertension

V_A/Q inequalities tend to be moderate even in late stages of pulmonary hypertension.[36] Much of the cardiac output is distributed to lung units with almost normal V_A/Q ratios, whereas less than 10% of flow perfused underventilated or unventilated areas. When Q is reduced, hypoxemia often occurs because of low mixed venous PO_2. Oxygen, sodium nitroprusside, isoproterenol, and nifedipine worsen V_A/Q matching, but patients do not usually experience hypoxemia due to increased flow, resulting in an increase in SvO_2 that raises end-capillary PO_2.

Therapeutic Considerations
Positive End-Expiratory Pressure

Positive end-expiratory pressure (PEEP) decreases the proportion of shunt units by recruiting atelectatic units, thereby improving FRC, closing capacity and oxygenation. By decreasing cardiac output (Q), PEEP also decreases intrapulmonary shunt. However, even when Q is preserved, PEEP decreases shunt because of increased flow to recruited units.[30] With constant Q, PEEP decreases venous admixture and increases P_vO_2.

PEEP also affects dead space. Low levels of PEEP decrease dead space by reductions in shunt, but high levels of PEEP increase dead space. The increase in dead space with high PEEP results from overinflation of some lung units, leading to compression of capillaries and zone 1 conditions.

Prone Positioning

Studies have shown that prone positioning, especially when employed early in the course of ARDS, improves survival, although this benefit remains undemonstrated in children.[37-39] Prone positioning improves oxygenation by producing more evenly distributed ventilation and an increase in the matching of ventilation to perfusion.[40-42] In ARDS and other lung injury

models, nonaerated or poorly aerated portions of the lung are found mainly in the dependent areas. The majority of perfusion goes through dorsal lung regions, whether in the prone or supine position.[4] Positive pressure ventilation, especially PEEP, redistributes perfusion toward the dependent portion of the lungs by creating conditions of zones 2 and 1.[4,32] This redistribution may increase the vertical perfusion gradient in the supine position but may reduce it in the prone position.

Nitric Oxide

Nitric oxide (NO) improves gas exchange in persons with acute lung diseases by preferentially increasing blood flow to well-ventilated regions of the lung. NO reaches the well-ventilated units, producing vasodilation and reducing shunt fraction.[43] Beneficial effects appear over a wide range of doses. A randomized trial in children with ARDS showed a significantly greater extracorporeal membrane oxygenation-free survival in the inhaled NO group compared with controls.[44] NO does not appear to be beneficial in persons with chronic lung diseases, possibly because the structural damage precludes rapid vascular changes or because shunt usually is not found in such diseases.

References

1. West JB. Regional differences in gas exchange in the lung of erect man. *J Appl Physiol.* 1962;17:893-898.
2. Hughes JMB, Grant BJB, Greene RE, et al. Inspiratory flow rate and ventilation distribution in normal subjects and in patients with simple bronchitis. *Clin Sci.* 1972;43:583-595.
3. West JB, Dollery CT, Naimark A. Distributions of blood flow in isolated lung: relation to vascular and alveolar pressures. *J Appl Physiol.* 1964;19:713-724.
4. Gibson RL, Truog WE, Redding GJ. Hypoxic pulmonary vasoconstriction during and after infusion of group B *Streptococcus* in neonatal piglets: vascular pressure-flow analysis. *Am Rev Respir Dis.* 1988;137:774-778.
5. Redding GJ, Gibson RL, Standaert TA, et al. Regional pulmonary blood flow in piglets during group B streptococcal bacteremia. *Am Rev Respir Dis.* 1990;141:1209-1213.
6. Reed JH, Wood EH. Effect of body position on vertical distribution of pulmonary blood flow. *J Appl Physiol.* 1970;28:303-311.
7. Hakim TS, Dean GW, Lisbona R. Gravity independent inequality in pulmonary blood flow in humans. *J Appl Physiol.* 1987;63:1114-1121.
8. Glenny RW, Robertson HT. Fractal properties of pulmonary blood flow: characterization of spatial heterogeneity. *J Appl Physiol.* 1990;69:532-545.
9. Glenny RW, Bernard S, Robertson HT, et al. Gravity is an important but secondary determinant of regional pulmonary blood flow in upright primates. *J Appl Physiol.* 1999;86:623-632.
10. Glenny RW, Lamm WJ, Albert RK, et al. Gravity is a minor determinant of pulmonary blood flow distribution. *J Appl Physiol.* 1991;71:620-629.
11. Prisk GK, Guy HJ, Elliot AR, et al. Ventilatory inhomogeneity determined from multiple-breath washouts during sustained microgravity on Spacelab SLS-1. *J Appl Physiol.* 1995;78:597-607.
12. Glenny RW, Bernard S, Robertson HT. Pulmonary blood flow remains fractal down to the level of gas exchange. *J Appl Physiol.* 2000;89:742-748.
13. Altemeier WA, McKinney S, Glenny RW. Fractal nature of regional ventilation distribution. *J Appl Physiol.* 2000;88:1551-1557.
14. Harris RS, Schuster DP. Visualizing lung function with positron emission tomography. *J Appl Physiol.* 2007;102:448-458.
15. Hopkins SR, Levin DL, Emami K, et al. Advances in magnetic resonance imaging of lung physiology. *J Appl Physiol.* 2007;102:1244-1254.
16. Petersson J, Sanchez-Crespo A, Larsson SA, et al. Physiological imaging of the lung: single-photon-emission computed tomography (SPECT). *J Appl Physiol.* 2004;102:468-476.
17. Weibel ER. Fractal geometry: a design principle for living organisms. *Am J Physiol Lung Cell Mol Physiol.* 1991;261(6 Pt 1):L361-L369.

18. Melsom MN, Kramer-Johansen J, Flatebo T, et al. Distribution of pulmonary ventilation and perfusions measured simultaneously in awake goats. *Acta Physiol Scand.* 1997;159:199-208.

19. Celermajer DS, Dollery C, Burch M, et al. Role of the endothelium in the maintenance of low pulmonary vascular tone in normal children. *Circulation.* 1994;89:2041-2044.

20. Vaughan DJ, Brogan TV, Kerr ME, et al. Contributions of nitric oxide synthase isozymes to exhaled nitric oxide and hypoxic pulmonary vasoconstriction in rabbit lungs. *Am J Physiol Lung Cell Mol Physiol.* 2003;284: L834-L843.

21. Altemeier WA, Robertson HT, McKinney S, et al. Pulmonary embolization causes hypoxemia by redistribution regional blood flow without changing ventilation. *J Appl Physiol.* 1998;85:2337-2343.

22. West GB, Brown JH, Enquist BJ. A general model for the origin of allometric scaling laws in biology. *Science.* 1997;276:122-126.

23. Duke HN. The site of action of anoxia on the pulmonary blood vessels of the cat. *J Physiol (Lond).* 1954;125:373-382.

24. Grant BJB, Davies EE, Jones HA, et al. Local regulation of pulmonary blood flow and ventilation-perfusion ratios in the coatimundi. *J Appl Physiol.* 1976;40:216-228.

25. Dantzker DR, Wagner PD, West JB. Proceedings: instability of poorly ventilated lung units during oxygen breathing. *J Appl Physiol.* 1974;242: 72P.

26. Swenson ER, Robertson HT, Hlastala MP. Effects of inspired carbon dioxide on ventilation-perfusion matching in normoxia, hypoxia, and hyperoxia. *Am J Respir Crit Care Med.* 1994;149:1563-1569.

27. Domino KB, Swenson ER, Hlastala MP. Hypocapnia-induced ventilation/perfusion mismatch: a direct CO_2 or pH-mediated effect? *Am J Respir Crit Care Med.* 1995;152:1534-1539.

28. Keenan RJ, Todd TRJ, Wood W, et al. Effects of hypercarbia on arterial and alveolar oxygen tensions in a model of gram negative pneumonia. *J Appl Physiol (1985).* 1990;68:1820-1825.

29. Dantzker DR, Bower JS. Pulmonary vascular tone improves VA/Q matching in obliterative pulmonary hypertension. *J Appl Physiol Respir Environ Exerc Physiol.* 1981;51:607-613.

30. Walther SM, Domino KB, Glenny RW, et al. Positive end-expiratory pressure redistributes perfusion to dependent regions in supine but not prone lambs. *Crit Care Med.* 1999;27:37-45.

31. Wagner PD, Laravuso RB, Goldzimmer E, et al. Distribution of ventilation-perfusion in dogs with normal and abnormal lungs. *J Appl Physiol.* 1975;38:1099-1109.

32. Gea J, Roca J, Torres A, et al. Mechanism of abnormal gas exchange in patients with pneumonia. *Anesthesiology.* 1991;75:782-789.

33. Lampron N, Lemaire F, Teisseire B, et al. Mechanical ventilation with 100% oxygen does not increase intrapulmonary shunt in patients with severe bacterial pneumonia. *Am Rev Respir Dis.* 1985;131:409-413.

34. Wagner PD, Dantzker DR, Iacovoni VE, et al. Ventilation-perfusion inequality in asymptomatic asthma. *Am Rev Respir Dis.* 1978;118:605-612.

35. Roca J, Ramis L, Rodriguez-Roisin R, et al. Serial relationships between ventilation-perfusion inequality and spirometry in acute severe asthma requiring hospitalization. *Am Rev Respir Dis.* 1988;137:579-584.

36. Dantzker DR, Bower JS. Pulmonary vascular tone improves VA/Q matching in obliterative pulmonary hypertension. *J Appl Physiol Respir Environ Exerc Physiol.* 1981;51:607-613.

37. Guerin C, Reignier J, Richard J-C, et al. Prone positioning in severe acute respiratory distress syndrome. *N Engl J Med.* 2013;368:2159-2168.

38. Pelosi P, Brazzi L, Gattinoni L. Prone position in acute respiratory distress syndrome. *Eur Respir J.* 2002;20:1017-1028.

39. Curley MA, Hibbard PL, Fineman LD, et al. Effect of prone positioning on clinical outcomes in children with acute lung injury: a randomized controlled trial. *JAMA.* 2005;294:229-237.

40. Beck KC, Vetterman J, Rehder K. Gas exchange in dogs in the prone and supine positions. *J Appl Physiol (1985).* 1992;72:2292-2297.

41. Mure M, Domino KB, Lindahl SGE, et al. Regional ventilation-perfusion distribution is more uniform in the prone position. *J Appl Physiol (1985).* 2000;88:1076-1083.

42. Musch G, Layfield JD, Harris RS, et al. Topographical distribution of pulmonary perfusion and ventilation, assessed by PET in supine and prone humans. *J Appl Physiol (1985).* 2002;93:1841-1851.

43. Cooper CJ, Landzberg MJ, Anderson TJ, et al. Role of nitric oxide in local regulation of pulmonary vascular resistance in humans. *Circulation.* 1996;93:266-271.

44. Bronicki RA, Fortenberry J, Schreiber M, et al. Multicenter randomized trial of inhaled nitric oxide for pediatric acute respiratory distress syndrome. *J Pediatr.* 2015;166:365-369.

Mechanical Dysfunction of the Respiratory System

J. Julio Pérez Fontán

PEARLS

- Workload and efficiency define the demands that disease imposes on the respiratory muscles and therefore are the relevant variables in the analysis of the mechanical function of the respiratory system.
- The work done by the respiratory muscles and, by extension, the energy that must be supplied to these muscles are defined by the combined volume-pressure relationships of the lungs and chest wall.
- Volume changes within the respiratory system are dictated primarily by the body's need to take up oxygen and eliminate carbon dioxide and therefore are determined by factors such as physical activity or metabolic rate, which are relatively independent of the condition of the lungs and chest wall. Pressure changes, on the other hand, depend on physical processes that take place in the respiratory system's constituents.
- The efficiency of the respiratory pump is influenced by factors that the astute clinician must consider when assessing a child's ability to sustain an increased respiratory workload. These include the configuration of the diaphragm, presence of rib cage distortion, and nutritional state and conditioning of the respiratory muscles.
- It is a common clinical observation that different types of mechanical derangement result in distinctive patterns of breathing. These patterns generally agree with the principle of minimal power expenditure and can be useful to categorize the type of derangement the patient has during the initial evaluation.

From a mechanical perspective, the mammalian respiratory system functions like a reciprocating pump that aspirates fresh air into the pulmonary alveoli and exhausts spent alveolar gases into the atmosphere. The pump is powered by a specialized group of skeletal muscles (the respiratory muscles) that, through their insertions on the skeletal structures of the chest and abdomen, create movements that expand and sometimes compress the lungs. As often happens with systems that contain moving parts, the respiratory system is particularly vulnerable to mechanical dysfunction. The inefficiencies imposed by this dysfunction and the attempts that the organism makes to compensate for them are responsible for the

majority of the signs and symptoms of respiratory disease. Whether compensation occurs before the appearance of intolerable alterations in gas exchange and, if so, at what cost for the organism are the all-important questions that often define both the therapeutic course and ultimate outcome of respiratory disease at all ages. As we will see, both questions can be analyzed in the simple thermodynamic terms of a balance between the work that must be done and the energy that is available to do it.

This chapter provides a basic understanding of the mechanical function of the respiratory system in health and disease, focusing on factors that determine both respiratory work and energy expenditure. The first portion of the chapter discusses the forces responsible for the volume-pressure behavior of the lungs and chest wall and how this behavior relates to the work of breathing in both normal and disease conditions. The second portion analyzes the elements that influence the translation of the work of breathing into energy expenditure, with special attention to the factors that define the efficiency of the respiratory system. Throughout the chapter, the unique characteristics of the developing respiratory system and the mechanical features that are relevant for the diagnosis and management of respiratory disease are highlighted.

Work, Power, and Energy Expenditure in the Respiratory System

In simple intuitive terms, the variable that best sums up the function of a muscle-powered pump is the mechanical load that the contraction of the powering muscles must overcome with each pump cycle. Over time, mechanical load translates into power (the work divided by the time that it takes to carry it out) and energy expenditure. Accordingly, whether the respiratory muscles can carry a given mechanical load is ultimately determined by their ability to generate work from the limited amount of energy that they can mobilize from their blood supply. The first law of thermodynamics stipulates that when a certain amount of energy is added to a closed system by an external source (in this case the metabolism of fuels supplied by the circulation to the respiratory muscles), the resultant change in the system's internal energy may be either applied to perform external work (W) over a period of time (t) or dissipated as heat (Q). Implicit in this statement is the fact that only a portion of the energy that the respiratory muscles derive from metabolic substrates is transformed into respiratory work. This proportion varies depending on the system's efficiency (E), defined as:

$$E = \frac{W \cdot t}{W \cdot t + Q} \qquad \text{Eq. 49.1}$$

Thus workload and efficiency define the demands that the contractile machinery of the respiratory muscles must meet and therefore are the relevant variables in the analysis of the mechanical function of the respiratory system.

Determinants of Respiratory Work

Every high school physics student learns to calculate the external work done to move an object between two points as the product of the force needed to overcome all resistances to the movement by the distance between the points. Because the force may change along the way, the same student may learn at some point that it is more practical to break the movement into many elementary components and then add up all the work components by integration, as shown in Fig. 49-1A.

The calculation of the external work during breathing follows the same general principle, with one caveat: Allowances must be made for the fact that the lungs and chest wall move in all the dimensions of space. In other words, their displacements are measured in terms of volume, not distance, and determined by pressure, not force. The mathematic subtleties of this distinction may become a little clearer if we compare the breath to the action of a syringe, where, by pushing or pulling on the plunger, we create a pressure (P), positive or negative, that has the effect of changing the volume contained in the barrel (V). The work done in this process can be determined by integrating the product P · dV, as shown in Fig. 49.1B. The obvious corollary is that the work done by the respiratory muscles and, by extension, the energy that must be supplied to these muscles are both defined by the volume-pressure relationships of the lungs and the chest wall.

Volume-Pressure Relationships

Before analyzing the volume-pressure behavior of the various components of the respiratory system, it is helpful to clarify the terminology. Throughout this chapter, the term *thorax* is used in reference to all the moving components of the respiratory system, including the walls of the thoracic cavity (the skeletal rib cage and its soft tissues), abdomen, and lungs themselves. Similarly, the term *chest wall* is used to indicate all the structures that form the enclosure of the lungs, including the thoracic wall, diaphragm, abdominal wall, and abdominal organs.

The volume changes of the respiratory system can be easily measured with the help of devices such as spirometers (which measure gas flow) or plethysmographs (which measure volume displacement). For any breath, the thorax (defined by the suffix TH), lungs (L), and chest wall (W) all undergo the same change in volume, or:

$$\Delta V_{TH} = \Delta V_L = \Delta V_W \qquad \text{Eq. 49.2}$$

This identity results from the manner in which the lungs and chest wall are linked at the pleural interface, which prevents them from changing volume independently of each other.

The pressures needed to inflate the thorax, lungs, and chest wall are, in contrast, different from each other. Respiratory physiologists have traditionally approached the analysis of these pressures by taking an imaginary walk from the mouth down the airways to the alveolus, across the lung tissue and visceral pleura to the pleural space, and finally across the chest wall to the surface of the chest (Fig. 49.2). In this path, we would first encounter gas (from the mouth to the alveolus) and then successive barriers of tissue (alveolar wall, lung interstitium, pleura, and skeletal and soft tissues of the chest wall). If we were to measure the local pressure at strategic points along the way, then we could easily apportion how the pressure generated by the respiratory muscles is used to mobilize

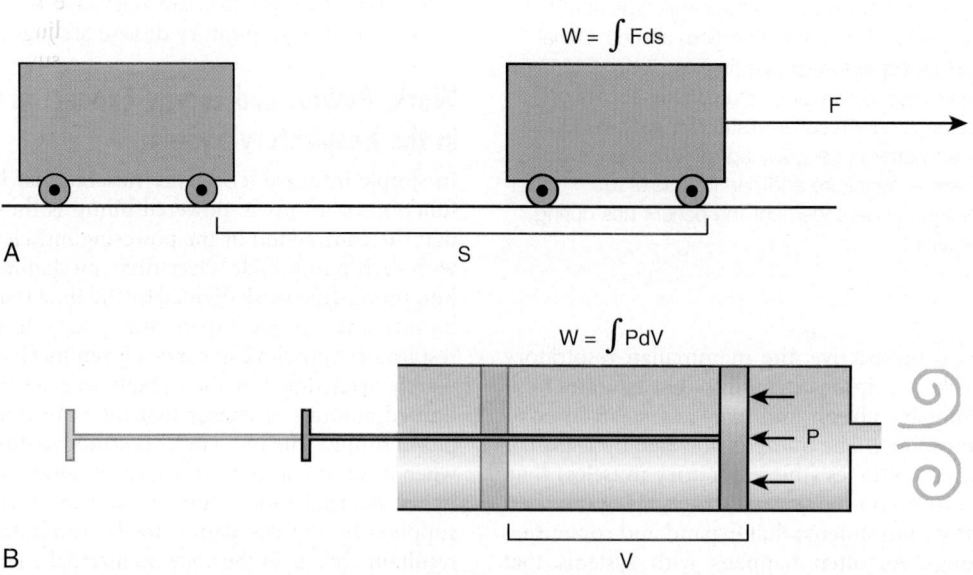

Fig. 49.1. (A) The amount of work that a force *(F)* must perform to move an object over a linear distance *s* is equivalent to the product *F* × *s*. If the force varies during the displacement, then it is more precise to integrate the product of F by the change in *s (ds)*. (B) By analogy, the work needed to produce a volume displacement *V* in a syringe, a better analogy for the respiratory pump, is determined as the integral of the product of the pressure inside the pump (the tridimensional analog of *F*) by *dV* (the tridimensional analog of *ds*).

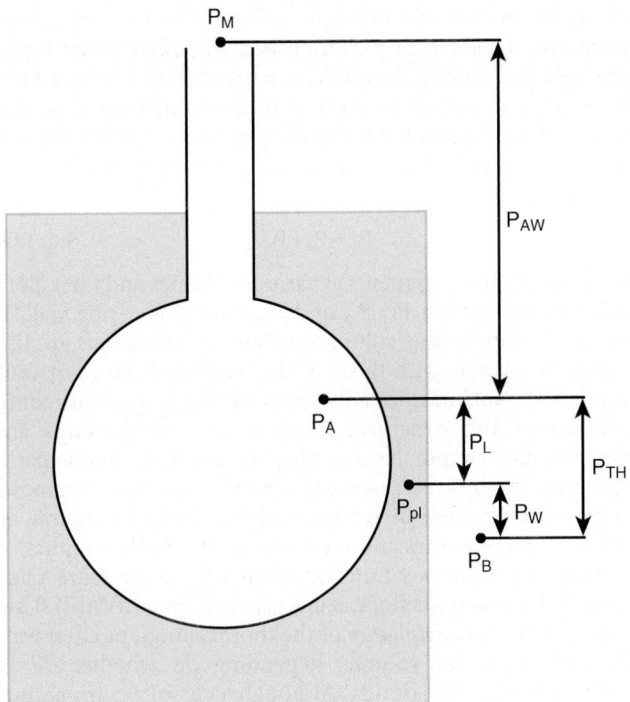

Fig. 49.2. Schematic representation of the thorax demonstrating the relevant pressure gradients generated during breathing. The difference (P_{AW}) between the pressure at the mouth (P_M) and the pressure at the alveoli (P_A) drives gas flow back and forth between the atmosphere and the alveolar spaces. The transpulmonary pressure (P_L) is the pressure that distends the lungs and is calculated as the difference between P_A and pleural pressure (P_{pl}). The transmural pressure of the chest wall (P_W) is the effective pressure distending the rib cage and abdomen and is defined as the difference between P_{pl} and atmospheric pressure (P_B).

the components of the respiratory system. This would be a useful exercise because it allows us to isolate the components that are performing poorly from a mechanical perspective and to quantify the extent of their dysfunction. For instance, the difference between the pressures measured at the mouth (P_M) and the alveolus (P_A) is the pressure needed to force air through the conducting airways (P_{AW}):

$$P_{AW} = P_M - P_A \qquad \text{Eq. 49.3}$$

An increase in this pressure above what is expected would alert us that there is undue resistance to the passage of air through the airways. Similarly, the difference between the pressures measured in the alveolus and the pleural space (P_{pl}) is the pressure required to overcome the forces that the muscles must overcome to inflate the lungs beyond their resting state and is known as the transpulmonary pressure (P_L).

$$P_L = P_A - P_{pl} \qquad \text{Eq. 49.4}$$

Finally, the difference between the pleural space and atmospheric pressure outside the chest wall $(P_B$, conventionally considered to be zero or reference) is a measure of the forces that the muscles have to surmount in order to force the chest wall (interestingly, including the muscles themselves) to increase or decrease its volume to accommodate the inflation and deflation of the lungs:

$$P_W = P_{pl} - P_B \qquad \text{Eq. 49.5}$$

For the sake of simplicity, we will consider first the particular situation in which the lungs undergo passive distention without participation of the respiratory muscles. This is what happens during positive airway pressure ventilation, when the pressure drive for inflation of the whole thorax is provided by the gradient $(P_M - P_B)$. By performing a series of substitutions in Eqs. 3 through 5 and assuming $P_B = 0$, we can easily arrive at the following equality:

$$P_M = P_{AW} + P_L + P_W \qquad \text{Eq. 49.6}$$

This formula informs us that, from a mechanical point of view, the airways, lungs, and chest wall are arranged *in series,* and thus the total pressure needed to generate a movement is the sum of the pressures generated by each of these three components. Respiratory physiologists have often borrowed from electrical theory, assuming, perhaps to the dismay of many readers, that the simplicity of electrical circuitry is less intimidating than the complexities of Newtonian mechanics. When speaking of electrical circuits, the term *series* indicates that every element in the circuit experiences the same current as the circuit as a whole, but the total voltage across the circuit is the sum of the voltages across the individual elements. Because current is the electrical analog of flow (volume per unit of time) and voltage is the analog of pressure, it is easy to see how Eqs. 2 and 6 justify the electrical analogy.

The mechanical behavior of the airways and lungs does not change substantially during muscle-powered breathing. The behavior of the chest wall, on the other hand, is greatly influenced by the contraction of the respiratory muscles. Because the muscles are part of the chest wall and change their mechanical characteristics as they contract, any attempt to define mathematically the behavior of the chest wall during a spontaneous breath is a futile exercise. For our purposes here, however, it may suffice to say that, during spontaneous breathing, Eq. 6 may be written as:

$$P_{mus} = P_{AW} + P_L + P_W \qquad \text{Eq. 49.7}$$

where P_{mus} represents the pressure generated by the muscles' contraction. Thus every time we take a breath, the neural output to the respiratory muscles is adjusted to overcome as precisely as possible the opposing pressures generated by the respiratory system.

Nature of the Mechanical Forces Acting on the Respiratory Pump

Volume changes within the respiratory system are dictated primarily by the body's need to take up oxygen and eliminate carbon dioxide and therefore are determined by factors such as physical activity or metabolic rate, which are relatively independent of the condition of the lungs and chest wall. Pressure changes, on the other hand, depend on the complex physical processes that take place in the respiratory system's constituents as they undergo motion. For instance, elastic pressures result primarily from the tendency of tissue components such as collagen and elastin fibers to recover their original shape after being stretched during lung inflation, but they also include pressures generated by surface tension at the alveolar gas-liquid interface. Airway resistive pressures relate to friction and overcome the adherence of the moving gas molecules to the airway walls (viscous pressures) and, to a lesser extent, compensate for the loss in gas kinetic energy at points where the movement and direction of the gas change rapidly.

Tissue-resistive pressures are applied primarily to produce molecular rearrangements in the tissue and at the gas/liquid alveolar interface as the lungs inflate and deflate. Finally, inertial pressures derive from the acceleration and deceleration of the gas and tissue contained in the thorax during breathing. (Inertial pressure losses are negligible in children during normal breathing and therefore deserve no more than a passing reference here.)

Disease alters these physical processes and therefore also influences the forces and pressures that result from them. To relate these alterations to the disease's clinical manifestations, it is helpful to classify both processes and pressures into nondissipative and dissipative, depending on whether the potential energy used by the respiratory muscles to produce movement stays in or leaves the system. For instance, elasticity is typically a nondissipative process because the energy needed to produce elastic deformation during inspiration is accumulated in the tissues and then used to empty the lungs during expiration; it never leaves the system. In contrast, all resistive processes are dissipative: The energy liberated by the friction of the gas against the airway walls or by the molecular interactions within the tissue is transformed into heat, which is then transported outside of the system (dissipated) by the blood or the expired gas.

Nondissipative Phenomena: Elastic Behavior of the Respiratory System

Elastic pressures result from the tendency of the components of the lungs and chest wall to recover their original shape after undergoing deformation. Because this tendency increases proportionally to the magnitude of the deformation, elastic pressures are volume dependent. Thus they are most easily studied when the volume of the thorax is kept constant, a situation in which the absence of movement renders all resistive pressures irrelevant. This can be accomplished by inflating the lungs passively to the desired level (as in a breath hold) or by asking the subject to inspire to a given volume and then close the glottis while relaxing the respiratory muscles (something that a trained individual can do). In such circumstances, $P_{AW} = 0$, and therefore:

$$P_A = P_L + P_W \qquad \text{Eq. 49.8}$$

By obtaining measurements at various volumes and then plotting volume against P_A, P_L, and P_W (remember our walk!), we can compare the volume-pressure relationships of the thorax as a whole with those of the lungs and the chest wall (Fig. 49.3). Not unexpectedly given the heterogeneous composition of the structures involved, the relationships are complex and cannot be described in a simple mathematic equation. In all three cases, the plotted curve has a sigmoid shape, with pressure increasing rapidly relative to volume at low and high volumes and more slowly at middle volumes.[1]

Being a continuous function, each volume-pressure relationship has a defined slope at any given volume (dV/dP). This slope defines the *compliance* of the thorax, lungs, or chest wall for that particular volume, depending on whether dP is replaced by dP_A, dP_L, or dP_W. Although a cursory examination of Fig. 49.3 reveals that both the lung and chest wall compliances defined in this manner vary markedly over the entire range of volumes, on closer inspection, the ratio dV/dP is relatively constant at normal breathing volumes. Thus for these volumes, it is safe to write:

$$\Delta P_{el} = \Delta V/C \qquad \text{Eq. 49.9}$$

where ΔP_{el} represents the change in elastic recoil pressure of the thorax (ΔP_A), lungs (ΔP_L), or chest wall (ΔP_W) for a lung volume excursion ΔV, and C is the compliance of the

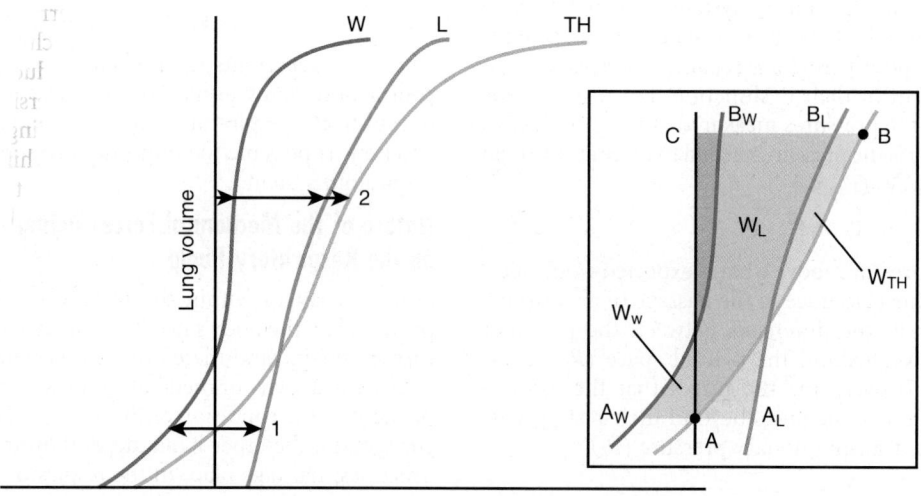

Fig. 49.3. Idealized representation of the static volume-pressure relationships of the thorax *(TH)*, lungs *(L)*, and chest wall *(W)*. Pressure, on the abscissa, represents the pressure across the thorax as a whole ($P_{TH} = P_A - P_B$), lungs ($P_L = P_A - P_L$), and chest wall ($P_W = P_{pl} - P_B$; see Fig. 49.2). The *arrows* indicate the magnitude and direction of the pressures acting on the thorax and its components at two volumes: (1) the relaxation volume of the thorax, where the recoils of the lung and the chest wall neutralize each other; and (2) an arbitrary volume where the recoils of the lungs and the chest wall act both in the direction of reducing thoracic volume. *Inset:* Detail of the same curves, indicating the elastic work done on the thorax as a whole and each of its components for a volume displacement starting at a volume A (the relaxation volume of the thorax) and ending at a volume C. The work done on the thorax as a whole is represented by the area A-B-C; the work done on the lungs by A-A_L-B_L-C; and the work done on the chest wall by A_W-A-B_W-C. A portion of the work done on the chest wall (the *triangular area in purple* between A_W and the ordinate axis) is contributed by the recoil of the chest wall, which between those points facilitates the action of the respiratory muscles.

corresponding component. As lung volume decreases or increases beyond this linear range, dV/dP starts to decrease in a volume-dependent manner and the respiratory muscles must generate progressively larger pressures to produce the same volume change. Disease frequently causes the lungs to operate on the fringes of the volume-pressure range, thereby increasing rapidly both the work of breathing and the energy needed to do it.

At any given volume, the lungs, chest wall, and thorax each generate a certain elastic pressure or recoil. This recoil can act to increase or decrease volume (as indicated by the direction of the *arrows* in Fig. 49.4). By definition, elastic recoil drives the thorax and its individual components to adopt a volume, known as the *relaxation volume,* at which recoil itself is extinguished. The relaxation volumes of the lungs and the chest wall are the volumes that each of these components would adopt if all the mechanical constraints imposed by their mutual attachments and interactions were removed. The relaxation volume of the thorax, in contrast, is defined by the mechanical interaction of the lungs and the chest wall. It coincides with the point at which the opposing elastic recoils of these two components neutralize each other (as shown by the equal magnitude but opposite pressure vectors at the points labeled 1 in Fig. 49.4).

In the adult, at relaxation volume, the gas contained in the lungs is less than the residual volume (the volume of gas contained in the lungs at the end of a forced expiration). The relaxation volume of the chest wall, by contrast, exceeds 50% of the volume at vital capacity (the maximal volume of gas that can be inhaled from residual volume). This discrepancy in the relaxation volumes of the lungs and chest wall has three

important consequences. First, it forces the relaxation volume of the thorax as a whole to occupy a position intermediate between the relaxation volumes of the lungs and the chest wall (at approximately 35% of vital capacity). Under most circumstances, this volume coincides with the functional residual capacity (FRC), which is the volume contained in the lungs at the end of a tidal expiration at steady state. Second, as the thorax starts to rise above its relaxation volume during inspiration, the outward recoil of the chest wall contributes to the expansion of the lungs, thereby reducing the work that the respiratory muscles need to perform during normal breathing (see Fig. 49.3, *inset,* where the work done by the chest wall at the beginning of a breath is labeled W_W). Finally, at normal breathing volumes, the opposing actions of the lungs and chest wall recoils create a negative pressure at the boundaries of the lung tissue with the chest wall and other intrathoracic structures. This negative pressure is an important contributor to the return of venous blood to the chest. The static volume-pressure relationships of the lungs and chest wall vary depending on their state of maturation and health (see Fig. 49.4). In the infant, the chest wall generates remarkably little outward recoil within the normal range of breathing volumes.[2-4] Because the inward recoil of the lungs varies little with respect to lung size and age during development,[5,6] the relaxation volume of the infant's thorax is proportionally smaller than that of the adult (as shown in Fig. 49.4 by the lower intercept of the volume-pressure relationship of the thorax and the ordinate axis). If, as occurs in the adult, the FRC coincided with this relaxation volume (15% of vital capacity compared with 35% in the adult), then the infant would be at a definite disadvantage in terms of alveolar stability and oxygenation. The newborns of most mammalian species, however, have developed physiologic strategies to maintain their FRC above the relaxation volume of the thorax.[7] These strategies, which may be even more important in the presence of respiratory illness,[8] are generally directed at interrupting expiratory flow before expiration is complete and include shortening of the expiratory time,[9] contraction of adductor muscles of the glottis to retard exhalation,[10] and persistence of the tonic activity of the inspiratory muscles during expiration.[11] Being so dependent on the pattern of breathing, the FRC of the newborn and small infant is vulnerable to changes in muscle coordination and tone. As an example, the decrease of tonic activity of the respiratory and laryngeal muscles associated with rapid eye movement sleep[11] may cause a substantial reduction in thoracic lung volume at these ages. Similarly, muscle weakness, anesthesia, deep sedation, and central nervous system depression in general tend to lower FRC below levels compatible with alveolar stability. Under such circumstances, alveoli close and both the shunt fraction and work of breathing increase.

In addition to its effects on the FRC, the reduced outward recoil of the chest wall in the infant reduces the chest wall's contribution to lung expansion. It also limits the amplitude of the pleural pressure variations as the lungs expand, an effect that helps to explain the surprising cardiovascular tolerance of many infants to the application of high levels of positive airway pressure.

Lungs/Chest Wall Interactions

Although, considered in isolation, the lungs and chest wall have different volume-pressure relationships, their mechanical

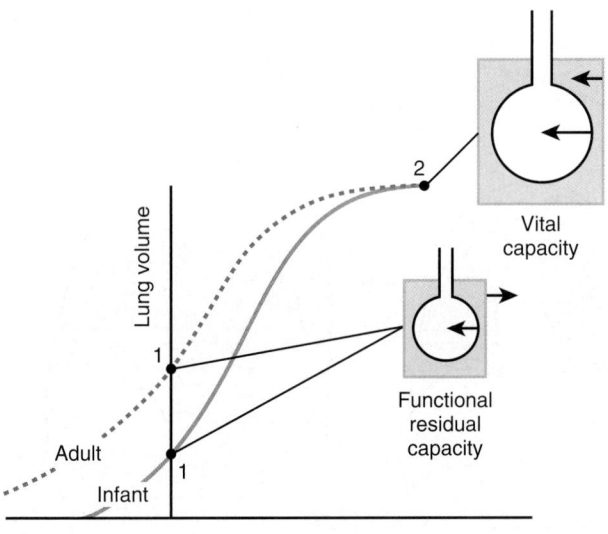

Fig. 49.4. Idealized volume-pressure relationships illustrating the differences in the elastic behaviors of the infant and adult thoraxes (normalized for vital capacity). The difference between the two points (labeled *1*) highlights the effect of maturation on the relaxation volume of the thorax. In the infant the chest wall is considerably more compliant than in the adult and, as a result, the opposite recoils of the lungs and the chest wall neutralize each other at a lower relaxation volume. Thus infants have a lower functional residual capacity *(FRC)* than do adults. At volumes higher than the relaxation volume of the chest wall, the recoils of the lungs and chest wall act in the same direction, opposing further increases in volume (as highlighted here at vital capacity, labeled *2*).

linkage at the pleural space prevents them from changing volume independently. By sharing a common boundary, the lungs and chest wall are also influenced simultaneously by variations in the pressure at this boundary. The resultant interplay is well illustrated by the effects of a pneumothorax, a complication that is quite familiar to readers who practice intensive care medicine. When a certain volume of gas enters the pleural space, the most immediate effect is an increase in pleural pressure (ΔP). This increase causes the effective transmural pressures of the lungs and chest wall to change by the same absolute amount but in opposite direction: transpulmonary pressure ($P_A - P_{pl}$) decreases by $-\Delta P$, whereas chest wall transmural pressure (P_{pl}) increases by ΔP. No longer held together by a rigid boundary, the lungs and chest wall respond to the change in transmural pressure by decreasing and increasing volume along their respective volume-pressure relationships (Fig. 49.5A). Consequently, one could say that the volume of air originally introduced in the pleural cavity is

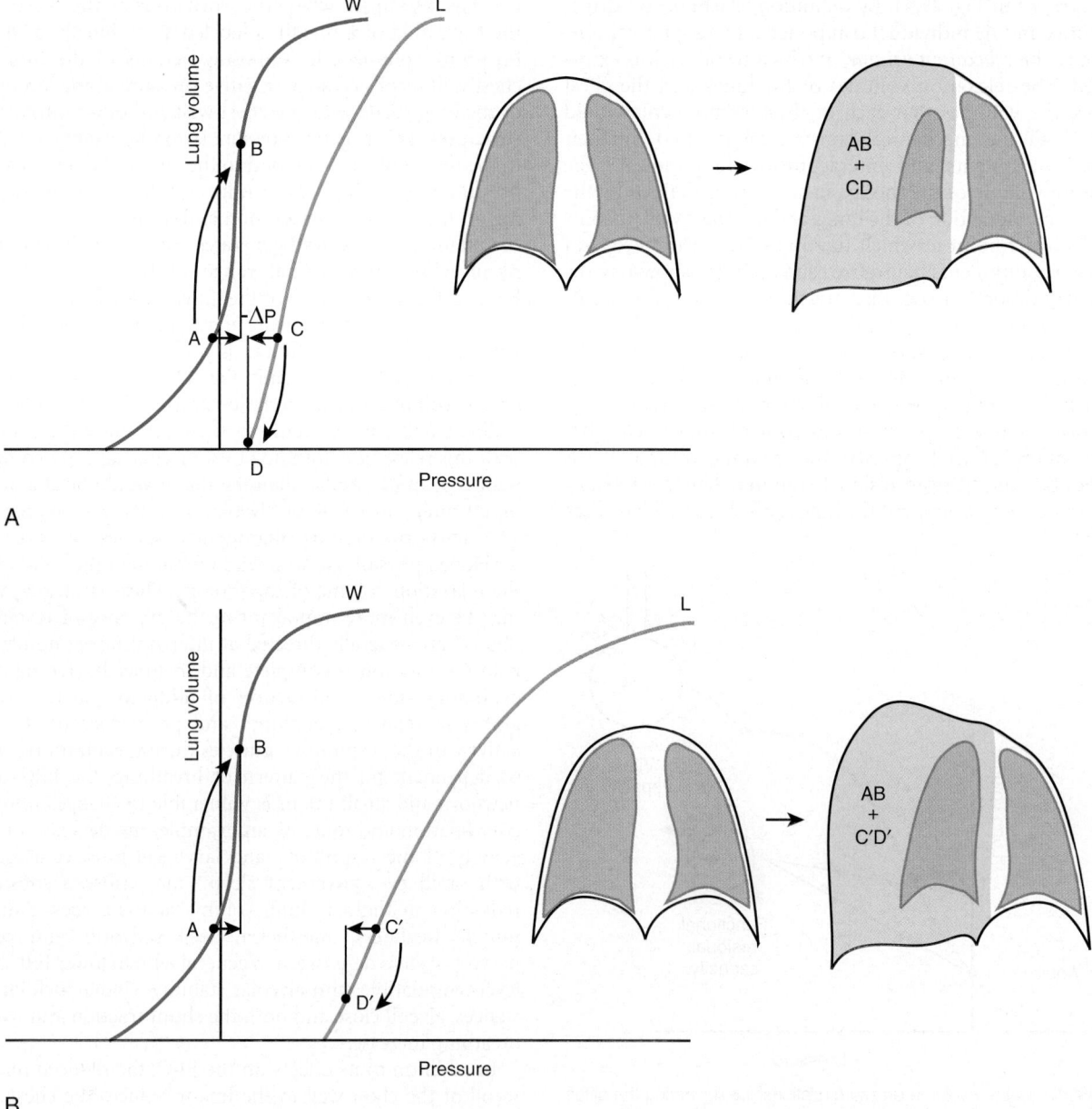

Fig. 49.5. (A) The effects of a pneumothorax are used here to illustrate the interactions between the elastic recoils of the lungs and the chest wall. Pressures, on the abscissa, represent the transmural pressures of the lungs (L, $P_A - P_{pl}$, see Figs. 49.2 and 49.3) and chest wall (W, $P_{pl} - P_B$). The introduction of a volume of gas into the pleural space raises pleural pressure by a magnitude ΔP, which changes both transmural pressures by the same absolute magnitude but in opposite directions. Lungs and chest wall respond to the change in transmural pressure by decreasing ($C{\rightarrow}D$) and increasing their volume ($A{\rightarrow}B$) along their respective volume-pressure relationships. The volume of the pneumothorax is thus partitioned between the lungs and the chest wall according to their relative compliances. (B) When lung compliance is decreased by disease, the volume-pressure relationship of the lungs is displaced to the right and has a lower slope (or compliance). Under these circumstances, the chest wall is forced to accommodate the majority of the volume change introduced by the pneumothorax ($AB \gg C'D'$), giving perhaps the wrong impression that the stiffness of the lungs prevents them from collapsing further.

partitioned into two components, one corresponding to the volume lost by the lungs as they collapse and the other corresponding to the volume gained by the chest wall as it expands. The relative extents to which the lungs collapse and the chest wall expands are dictated by the volume-pressure relationships of the lungs and chest wall. If the compliance of the chest wall exceeds the compliance of the lungs (as is usually the case in the infant), then the chest wall expands more than the lungs collapse. The difference is even greater when lung compliance is reduced by disease (Fig. 49.5B). Then the chest wall absorbs the majority of the volume change while the lungs barely decrease their volume. This simple analysis explains why noncompliant lungs show surprisingly little collapse when a pneumothorax develops, a finding that is often mistakenly attributed to the "stiffness" of the lung parenchyma. It also provides an opportunity to point out that the magnitude of the chest wall expansion, although frequently overlooked when a pneumothorax is diagnosed radiographically, relates more directly to the true malignancy of the process (the impediment of cardiac filling by the compression of the intrathoracic vessels) than does the usually more apparent collapse of the lungs.

One important idea to emerge from these considerations is that, respiratory muscle activity aside, the pressure inside the pleural space is really determined by the elastic recoil of the chest wall and volume of the thoracic contents. As long as lung volume is not forced above its normal range and chest wall compliance is unaltered by disease, pleural pressure (and thus the pressure around the major vessels and the heart) remains low, regardless of the airway pressures. Conversely, excessive lung distension (eg, in asthma or other conditions in which the lungs are overinflated) is always associated with a high pleural pressure and is, for that reason, less well tolerated from a cardiovascular point of view. The dependence of pleural pressure on chest wall compliance explains why premature infants and newborns, who have very large chest wall compliance, have limited changes in this pressure during positive pressure ventilation, even if physiologic lung volumes are exceeded. Disease-induced reductions in chest wall compliance, on the other hand, always increase pleural pressure and reduce venous return to the heart. This is one reason why patients with abdominal distension typically have low cardiac output and why relief of the distension (eg, by paracentesis in patients with ascites) reduces pleural pressure and increases cardiac output.

Dissipative Phenomena: Resistive Behavior of the Respiratory System
Dynamic Volume-Pressure Relationships

Analysis of the volume-pressure relationships of the thorax and its components becomes more complicated when we consider the pressure changes generated by gas flow and movement of the lung and chest wall tissue as the lungs inflate and deflate. These pressure changes result from molecular interactions between the gas and airway walls, within the gas stream itself, and among the components of the gas-liquid interface and tissue. The same interactions are responsible for well-known physical phenomena such as viscosity (the internal resistance of a fluid to flow), turbulence (the development of

chaotic, energy-consuming movements within a flowing fluid), or viscoelasticity (a property of tissues and fluids that causes their deformations to be time dependent; ketchup provides a good example when it hangs stubbornly to the bottle before being released after multiple taps).[12-14]

Regardless of their ultimate physical nature, all the phenomena that occupy our attention at this point have two characteristics in common. The first is that they always result in a net loss or dissipation of energy from the respiratory system. The lost energy can no longer be used to perform work, and consequently dissipative pressure losses cause the volume-pressure relationships of the respiratory system to follow a different trajectory depending on the direction of the volume change. This property, known as *hysteresis*, is responsible for the development of loops when the volume-pressure relationships are plotted continuously during a breath (Fig. 49.6). In this graphic representation, the dissipative pressures can be easily identified as the horizontal distance between the volume-pressure tracing and the corresponding point on the elastic volume-pressure relationship. The work done against these pressures can be quantified as the area enclosed by the loop.

The second common characteristic of dissipative pressures losses is that they occur only when there is volume change or flow in or out of the lungs (flow is the first derivative of volume with respect to time, dV/dt, and is usually represented with the engineering symbol $\dot{V}$. The relationship between resistive pressure loss (P_{res}) and $\dot{V}$ is, under most

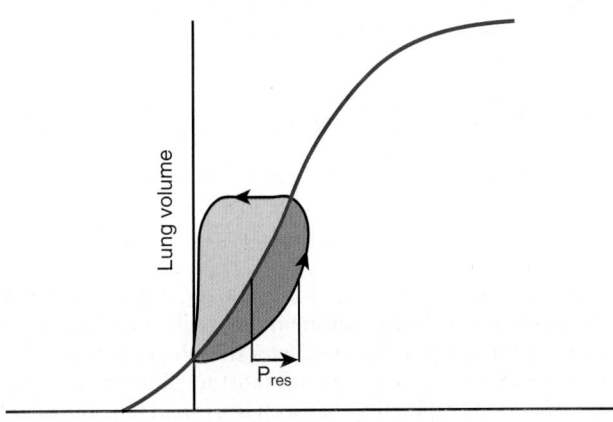

Fig. 49.6. Idealized representation of the dynamic or real-time volume-pressure relationship of the respiratory system during a single breath (the *arrows* indicate the direction of the movement). Because energy is dissipated as the lungs change volume, the relationship follows a different trajectory during inspiration and expiration, forming a loop (hysteresis). The horizontal distance between any point in the loop and the line describing the elastic volume-pressure relationship of the respiratory system *(black)* is the pressure needed to overcome the dissipative forces present at that point in the breath (P_{res}). The area enclosed by the loop *(shaded area)* is the amount of energy used in overcoming these forces. The inspiratory portion of this work *(darker shading* between the loop and the elastic volume-pressure relationship) must be performed by the respiratory muscles. The expiratory portion of the work *(lighter shading)* is normally done by the elastic recoil of the lungs and chest wall and requires no muscle effort or energy consumption. The resistance of the respiratory system is calculated by dividing P_{res} by the airway flow.

circumstances, simple enough to be summarized with a linear equation:

$$P_{res} = R \cdot \dot{V}$$ Eq. 49.10

where the coefficient R defines the flow resistance of the corresponding component (thorax, lungs, or chest wall). While the concept of resistance is useful as a pulmonary function assessment and reporting tool, the idea of assigning a fixed value to R involves a gross oversimplification. Indeed, resistive pressure losses are influenced by factors other than the absolute flow rate, including among others lung volume, flow direction (inspiratory or expiratory), and breathing pattern. An understanding of the role played by these factors during normal breathing provides valuable insights for the recognition and treatment of airway obstruction.

Effect of Flow Rate and Pattern on the Dynamics of the Gas Stream

The airway tree is a complex fractal-like structure. A particle traveling in the gas stream from the mouth to the alveolus would likely encounter obstacles and bifurcations and experience periods of acceleration and deceleration along the way. Thus in real life, the pressure losses, and thus the amount of work that needs to be done to sustain these losses, are a complex function of flow and geometry. In the simplest of circumstances, a tube with a uniform diameter, gas flow tends to adopt a *laminar* arrangement with a *parabolic velocity profile*, whereby the gas molecules in the middle move faster than the ones near the wall, which are slowed down by their viscous interaction with the wall (in fact, the molecules next to the wall may not move at all). Under these circumstances, energy dissipation is minimal and the pressure loss in the tube can be estimated with Pouiselle's law:

$$P_{res} = \frac{128 \cdot \mu \cdot L}{\pi \cdot d^4} \times \dot{V}$$ Eq. 49.11

where μ is the viscosity of the gas, L the length of the tube, and d its diameter. It is easy to see that the complex fraction on the right side of this equation corresponds to the coefficient R in Eq. 10.

Considerable theoretic and empiric evidence exists that although laminar flow is common, Pouiselle flow conditions are rare in the airways. The reason for this phenomenon is that airway segments are generally too short to allow the development of velocity differences between layers and thus the establishment of a parabolic profile. The resultant blunt velocity profile (ie, the molecules move at similar speed in the center lines as in the vicinity of the airway wall) results in greater friction and causes the relationship between P_{res} and $\dot{V}$ to become nonlinear. Or, put in a different way, the value of R becomes dependent on $\dot{V}$.

The dependence of R on $\dot{V}$ becomes even more pronounced when an obstacle disturbs the laminar organization of the flow stream. Under these circumstances, the velocity and direction of the gas molecules can vary vigorously and randomly and a turbulent flow pattern is created. When flow becomes turbulent, energy dissipation increases exponentially with flow rate and the density of the gas becomes more relevant than its viscosity in determining both pressure losses and work. This is the reason why helium, which has a much lower density than air, can decrease the work of breathing substantially in patients with some forms of airway obstruction (even though its viscosity is slightly greater than the viscosity of air).

Airway Dynamics

The airways provide a distribution network to transport gas to and from the gas-exchanging units of the lungs. Although often idealized as a system of passive pipes, the airway network is in reality a highly specialized organ. Each airway segment, from the nose to the alveoli, has evolved to not only serve specific functions such as humidification and phonation but also ensure maximal patency under the changing mechanical conditions present during breathing.

Indeed, the activity of the respiratory muscles exposes the airways to considerable transmural stresses (or pressures) during breathing (Fig. 49.7). The caliber and length of the airways change in response to these stresses in a manner that is only limited by the passive rigidity of its wall tissues and by the tone of the airway intrinsic muscle. Thus airway transmural pressure (the difference between the pressures measured on the inside and outside surfaces of the airway wall) and airway wall compliance (defined both as compressibility and distensibility) are the two determinants of airway caliber and, ultimately, also the determinants of airway resistance.

Airway transmural pressure varies during breathing. Its variations result from the fact that inspiration and expiration have very different effects on the pressures inside and outside the airways. The pressure inside all airways undergoes qualitatively similar changes during each phase of the breathing cycle. During inspiration, for instance, there is a gradient of increasingly negative pressures from the mouth, where pressure is atmospheric (or the zero reference), to the alveolar spaces, where the pressure must be negative (or subatmospheric) for gas to flow in. This negative pressure is of course driven by the actions of the respiratory muscles and transmitted to the lungs via the link between the chest wall and lungs at the pleural space. During expiration, alveolar pressure becomes positive and the gradient is inverted, with the pressures inside the airways being always positive but diminishing toward the mouth.

The pressure outside the airways is influenced in a different fashion by inspiration or expiration depending on whether the airways are extrathoracic or intrathoracic. Extrathoracic airways are included in the tissues of the neck, where the pressure can be considered to be atmospheric (at least in nonobese individuals, in whom tissue gravitational forces are neutralized by the skeletal support of the neck). Most of the intrathoracic airways are embedded in the lung tissue, where multiple tethering elements transmit the stresses (or pressures) generated by the tissue recoil to the airway wall (a phenomenon known as *pulmonary interdependence*[15]). Therefore the pressure outside the intrapulmonary airways approximates the pleural pressure and, as we have seen, relates to lung volume in a manner that depends on the pressure-volume characteristics of the chest wall (see the section on Lungs/Chest Wall Interactions).

Taking these considerations altogether, it follows that the effect of inspiration and expiration on airway caliber is very different depending on whether the airway is outside or inside the chest cavity. During inspiration, the extrathoracic airways (ie, the pharynx, larynx, and extrathoracic portion of the trachea) become narrower because the pressure inside their lumen decreases while the pressure immediately outside their

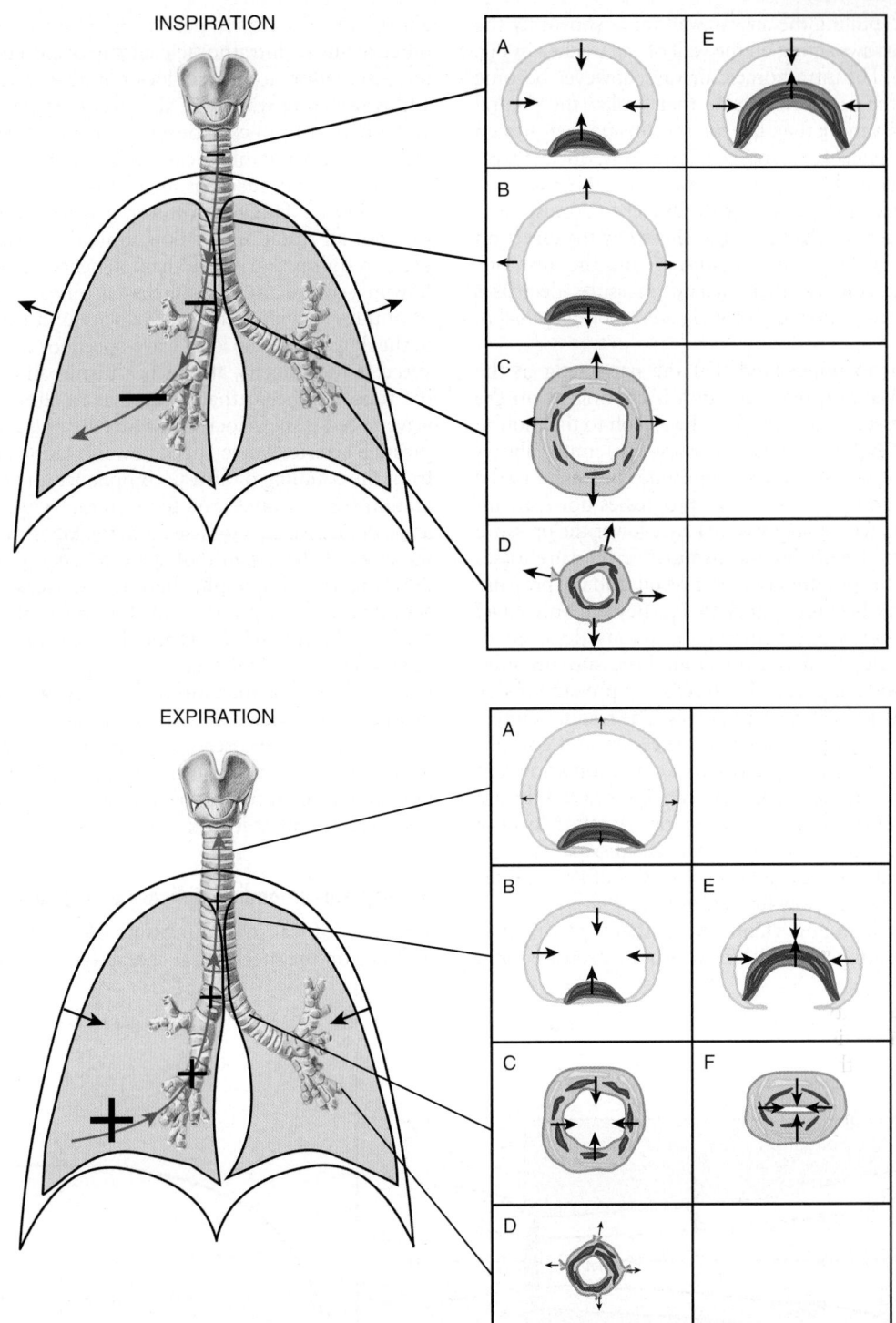

Fig. 49.7. Schematic representation of the differential effects of inspiration and expiration on the configuration of the extrathoracic and intrathoracic airways. During inspiration, the contraction of the respiratory muscles creates a negative pressure (relative to atmospheric) in the alveoli. This pressure drives inspiratory flow and, depending on the flow itself and the resistance of the airways, results in progressively less negative—but negative nonetheless—pressures in the direction of the mouth (as shown by the progressively smaller size of the negative signs in the picture). During expiration, the recoil of the thorax (and, at times, the contraction of the expiratory muscles) reverses the situation, and pressures are more positive in the alveoli than in the more proximal airways. The caliber of the airways is determined by the difference between airway pressure and the pressure acting on the outside surface of their walls (airway transmural pressure). The latter approximates atmospheric pressure (zero reference) for the extrathoracic airways and pleural pressure for the intrathoracic airways. Thus during inspiration, airway transmural pressure (which is represented in magnitude and direction by the *arrows*) acts to decrease the caliber of the extrathoracic airways (represented here by the extrathoracic portion of the trachea, *A*) and to increase the caliber of the intrathoracic trachea *(B),* large bronchi *(C),* and bronchioles *(D).* Note that, in the case of the bronchioles and other intrapulmonary airways, the relevant pressure outside the airways is transmitted to the airway wall by the tissue elements that tether them to the surrounding tissues in the lung. During expiration, the phenomenon is reversed, and, although the transmural pressure is positive in the distal portions of the airway tree, it decreases progressively and may eventually become negative (as shown in the example by the inward-directed *arrows* in *C*). Abnormalities in the tone of the airway muscle or the stiffness of the airway cartilage exaggerate these effects and promote collapse of the extrathoracic airways during inspiration (shown here for the trachea, *E*) and the intrathoracic airways during expiration (*E* and *F*).

walls is constant (pulling the airway wall in, as shown by the direction of the arrows acting on the wall of the trachea in Fig. 49.7, *top panel A*). The intrathoracic airways, however, become dilated because the pressure outside their walls (the pleural pressure) decreases more than the pressure inside their lumen (see Fig. 49.7, *top panel B, C, and D*). Conversely, during expiration the extrathoracic airways increase their caliber as their inside pressure becomes positive with respect to atmospheric pressure (pushing the wall out, as also shown by the direction of the arrows in Fig. 49.7, *bottom panel A*) and the intrathoracic airways narrow as their inside pressure decreases with respect to pleural pressure (see Fig. 49.7, *bottom panel B, C, and D*).

It is important to understand that the narrowing of the intrathoracic airways during expiration is contingent on the existence of a pressure gradient from the alveoli to the mouth. As predicted by Eq. 4, alveolar pressure (P_A) must always exceed pleural pressure (P_{pl}) by a magnitude equivalent to the elastic recoil of the lungs. As the gas progresses downstream during expiration, frictional pressure losses lower the pressure inside the airways. Eventually the cumulative pressure losses can be as large as the pulmonary elastic recoil, and the pressure inside the airways becomes equal to P_{pl}. Beyond this *equal pressure point* (somewhere between the points depicted in *bottom panels D and C*), airway transmural pressure becomes negative (ie, the pressure outside exceeds the pressure inside the airway) and acts to collapse the airway. The resultant interplay between the negative transmural pressure and compliance of the airway wall can give rise to a condition known as *flow limitation*,[16,17] whereby gas flow can no longer increase even if the subject makes a greater expiratory effort to raise alveolar pressure. Because the majority of the dissipative pressure losses are related to gas viscosity, this type of flow limitation is known as *viscous* flow limitation (Fig. 49.8).

Flow limitation is an important concept that is pertinent to many clinical situations in which flow is both decreased and effort independent. It occurs in subjects with asthma and other forms of intrathoracic airway obstruction[18,19] when the increased effort to exhale does not accelerate lung emptying and is therefore wasted. It also occurs in persons with croup and other forms of extrathoracic airway obstruction when the increased effort to inhale cannot increase inspiratory flow, and the attempt only succeeds in creating more stridor and respiratory muscle fatigue. However, it is important to point out that not all situations of flow limitation relate to dissipative pressure losses. For more than 30 years we have known that flow in a compliant tube, such as an airway, cannot exceed the minimum flow at which the velocity of a particle suspended in the flow equals the local wave-speed for the tube. The wave-speed is the velocity at which a disturbance travels through the tube, a concept that is familiar to clinicians because the wave-speed is the velocity at which the pulse waveform travels through arteries. Wave-speed flow limitation ultimately results from the coupling of airway compliance and convective acceleration (see Fig. 49.8). As the respiratory gas moves through areas of decreasing cross-section, the kinetic energy of the gas increases at the expense of the total energy contained in the flow stream. As a result, there is a decrease in the pressure acting on the inner surface of the airway (this decrease is the basis for the Venturi effect) and the transmural pressure of the airway decreases. Once again, if the airway is sufficiently compliant, there is a maximum flow beyond which the inside pressure would decrease faster than can be accommodated by the decrease in cross-sectional area and flow becomes limited. Regardless of its causal mechanism (viscous or wave-speed), flow limitation occurs at lower flows in the presence of airway obstruction and at low lung volumes, when airway diameter is minimal.

Airway Muscle and Compliance of the Airways

The effect of transmural pressure on the caliber of an airway depends on the mechanical characteristics of the airway itself

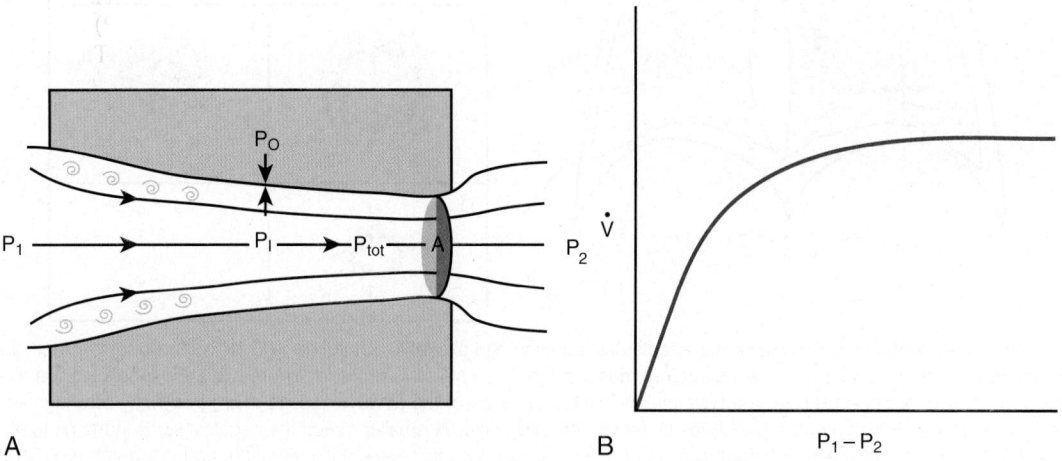

A

B

Fig. 49.8. (A) Flow limitation develops when the transmural pressure *(P_I – P_O)* of a collapsible tube (such as an airway) and the flow in the tube interact in such a manner that the cross-section of the tube (A) cannot support an increase in the flow rate, independent of the pressure driving the flow *(P₁ – P₂)*. Viscous flow limitation occurs when viscous friction (illustrated by the eddies at the edge of the flow stream) causes the pressure acting on the inner surface of the tube wall *(P_I)* to decrease faster than can be accommodated at any given flow. Wave-speed flow limitation takes place when the increase in the kinetic energy of the fluid or gas at a point of narrowing causes P_I to decrease relative to the head pressure *(P_{tot}* or the pressure that we would register with a probe facing the direction of flow) so that any further increase in flow cannot be supported by a further reduction in A. (B) Regardless of the mechanism, when flow is limited, any increase in the driving pressure (or, in the case of the airways, the effort of the respiratory muscles) cannot increase flow V̇.

or, more specifically, on its ability to undergo collapse or distension, a property that is often described as airway wall compliance. The structure of each segment of the airway tree has evolved to minimize luminal distortion in response to the varying stresses that act on the airway wall during breathing. The pharynx and larynx, for example, contain skeletal muscle, which stiffens their walls or dilates the pharyngeal lumen and the glottis during inspiration under the control of cranial nerves IX and X. Loss of pharyngeal or laryngeal tone during sleep or after pharmacologic inhibition or injury of the controlling neurons is the most important cause of upper airway obstruction during inspiration.

The smooth muscle of the trachea and bronchi has a similar function. For instance, the trachea is composed of a series of incomplete cartilaginous rings forming a relatively rigid arrangement that resists the collapsing effects of positive intrathoracic pressures during expiration. The rings leave a dorsal gap, where the wall of the trachea is soft. This weak point is bridged by the trachealis muscle, which, upon contracting, can approximate the edges of the cartilage rings and prevent the soft portion of the wall from bulging into the airway lumen (see Fig. 49.7). Like the smooth muscle in other airway segments, the trachealis muscle is innervated by local parasympathetic ganglia. The ganglia in turn receive inputs from parasympathetic preganglionic neurons located in the medulla via nerve fibers carried by the vagus nerves.[20,21] The medullary preganglionic neurons are anatomically and functionally integrated in the control of breathing. As a result, the traffic of impulses reaching the airway ganglia (and thus the tone of the muscle) varies with the phase of the breathing cycle and increases when the respiratory drive is increased, such as during exercise, hypercapnia, or hypoxemia.[22,23] Malformations or physical or pharmacologic interventions that disrupt the trachealis muscle or its nerve supply lead to tracheal obstruction when the intrathoracic pressure increases during expiration or when the child cries or exhales forcefully. This form of tracheal obstruction is often diagnosed as tracheomalacia, even though no true softening of the tracheal cartilage occurs.

The bronchial smooth muscle is also innervated by the parasympathetic system.[24] In cartilaginous bronchi, the stiffening effect of the muscle contraction is augmented by the cartilage and prevents the bronchial lumen from collapsing when the transmural pressure decreases during expiration, coughing, or crying. In bronchioles, which in humans lack cartilage, contraction of the smooth muscle stiffens the airway walls as well. However, in these smaller airways, smooth muscle contraction may have a more important function of preventing excessive airway distension during inspiration, when the stressed transmitted to the airway wall may disrupt the delicate bronchiolar structure.

Airway Obstruction

Airway obstruction causes an exaggeration of the reciprocating changes in airway caliber that we have just described during normal breathing. Thus the clinical manifestations of the obstruction depend on its location (extrathoracic or intrathoracic) and direction of flow (inspiratory or expiratory). When the obstruction is extrathoracic (eg, as occurs with croup, glossoptosis, and tonsil or adenoid hypertrophy), during inspiration the respiratory muscles must create a more negative pressure inside the airway segment downstream from

the obstruction to overcome the increased resistance. Therefore this segment of the airway tends to decrease its diameter even further, worsening the obstruction and producing a characteristic turbulent noise (inspiratory stridor) as gas accelerates through the narrowest point and induces vibrations in the airway mucosa. The obstruction is relieved during expiration because the pressure inside the airway segment becomes positive with respect to atmospheric pressure.

When the obstruction is intrathoracic (eg, as occurs with extrinsic compression of the trachea and bronchi, tracheobronchomalacia, and asthma), during inspiration the pressure inside the airways downstream from the obstruction becomes much lower than it would be under normal circumstances. However, no matter how low, the pressure inside the airways still must be less negative than the pleural pressure (Eqs. 3 and 4) because otherwise lung recoil ($P_A - P_{pl}$) would be negative, which is unimaginable. Thus during inspiration the transmural pressure of intrathoracic airways always remains positive. In contrast, during expiration the pressure inside the airway segment located between the obstruction and the thoracic outlet may become lower than pleural pressure at some point (see the section on Airway Dynamics). This situation, coupled with the Venturi effect created by the acceleration of flow at the obstructed segments, causes these airways to collapse and produce high-pitched vibrations (wheezing), expiratory delay, and dynamic hyperinflation (often referred to as *gas trapping*).

A Specific Case Study in Airway Mechanics: Mechanical Ventilation

The application of positive pressure in the airways changes the balance of pressures that determines airway caliber. When positive end-expiratory pressure (PEEP) is used, pressure inside the airways is offset in the positive direction (relative to atmospheric pressure) during the entire respiratory cycle. As a result, any portion of the extrathoracic airway that is not bypassed by an endotracheal tube (or the entire extrathoracic airway when mask ventilation is used) experiences a net increase in transmural pressure, which is the reason why continuous positive airway pressure (CPAP) is helpful in the management of extrathoracic obstruction. The pressure inside the intrathoracic airways also increases, but the increase is negated to some extent by the effects that PEEP has on lung inflation and therefore on elastic recoil and pleural pressure (remember the always important principle enunciated in Eq. 4). For this reason, the effects of PEEP in patients with intrathoracic airway obstruction and gas trapping are unpredictable.[25] Although PEEP is beneficial in some of these patients, in others, it increases lung volume,[26] interferes with cardiovascular function, and ultimately decreases oxygen delivery to the tissues.[27] These individual variations may simply reflect differences in the mechanisms of dynamic hyperinflation or simply heterogeneity of lung disease.[28,29] In patients who have gas trapping without expiratory flow limitation, proximal airway pressures (and thus also PEEP) are transmitted faithfully to the alveoli. As a result, their lung hyperinflation worsens. By contrast, in patients who have both gas trapping and expiratory flow limitation, PEEP may not influence the pressures upstream of the flow-limiting point; therefore, alveolar pressure and lung volume may not increase as much, but the increase in the transmural pressure at the choking segment may be sufficient to reset the maximum (limited flow rate) at a higher level. Although PEEP is not recommended in every patient, its judicious use may be considered, under careful monitoring, to improve the mechanical function of the lungs of some selected infants and children with severe obstructive airway disease.

Determinants of Regional Gas Flow Distribution in the Lungs

From a mechanical perspective, the lungs form a parallel arrangement of acinary or multialveolar units, each supported by a conducting airway. The development of inequalities in the mechanical and gas-exchanging functions of these units is a fundamental factor in the manifestations of lung disease. To understand how mechanical inequality affects the distribution of ventilation in the lungs, it is essential to realize that the potential filling volume of any alveolar unit is determined by the unit's compliance. However, the actual filling volume during a breath depends on the rate at which the unit can fill relative to other units.[30] This rate is a function of the unit's compliance and resistance in a manner that is best defined by

the product of these two variables, a constant with the dimension of time known as the time constant (represented by the Greek letter τ).

The mathematic formulations that describe the distribution of flow among units with different time constants can be complex. However, it is possible to make some basic predictions of how a certain flow pattern will influence the distribution of tidal volume among these units. Imagine a simplified lung composed of three units (Fig. 49.9), one with a normal compliance and resistance (normal τ), another with a low compliance and a normal resistance (short τ), and the third with a normal compliance and a high resistance (long τ). As long as the inspiratory time is sufficiently long to allow equilibration of alveolar pressures within the lungs, a decelerating inspiratory flow pattern (pressure-controlled ventilation) will inflate all three units proportionally to their compliances, thus favoring the two units with normal compliance. If the inspiratory time is shortened, however, gas is still flowing at the end of inspiration. This situation results in pressure and inflation inequalities among the units, with a disproportionate portion of the tidal volume being directed to units with a short time

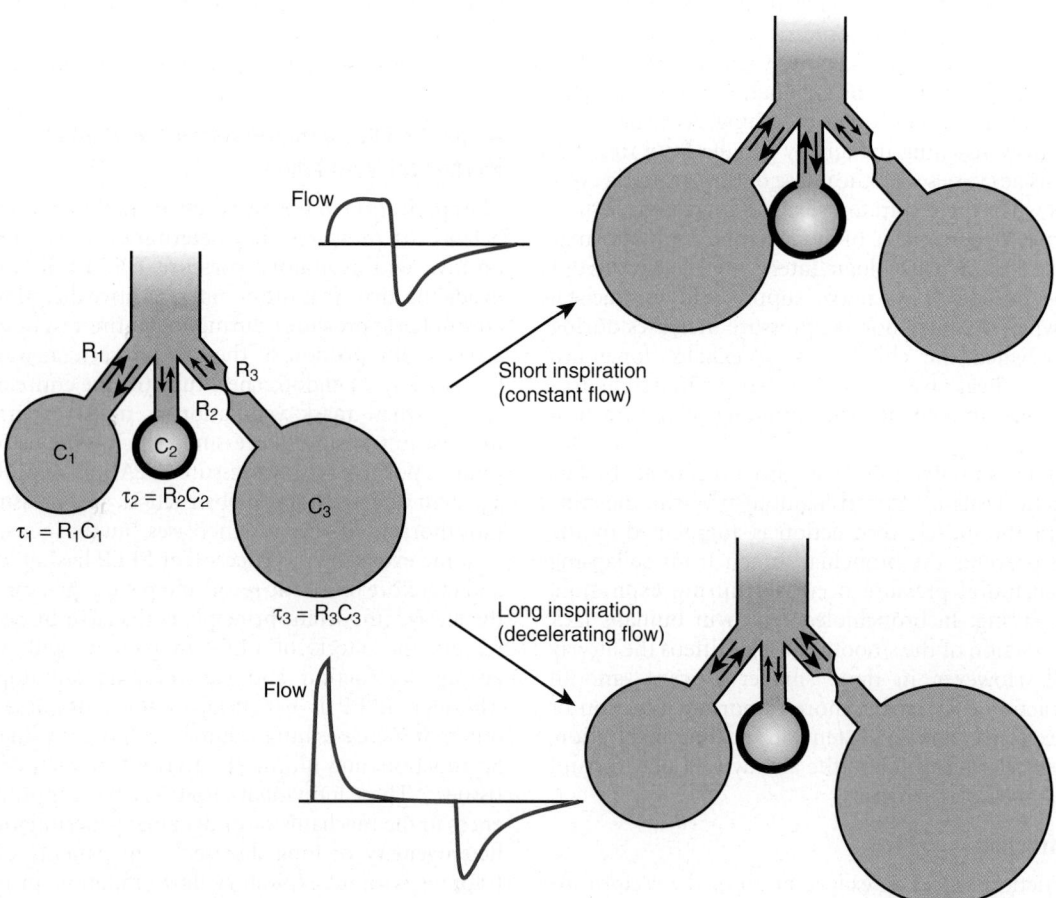

Fig. 49.9. Schematic representation of the lung showing the effects of ventilatory pattern on the distribution of inspiratory gas flow. The rate of inflation or deflation of an airway-alveolar unit can be characterized by a time constant (τ) equal to the product of its resistance (R) and compliance (C). Three types of units are represented in the scheme (each identified by the corresponding numerical subscript): (1) a normal unit with normal compliance and resistance (normal τ); (2) a restrictive unit with decreased compliance and normal resistance (short τ); and (3) an obstructed unit with normal compliance and increased resistance (long τ). Inflation with a decelerating pattern of flow (typical of modern pressure-controlled ventilator modes) favors units with normal compliance (1 and 3). Inflation with a short inspiratory time and a constant flow (more typical of volume-controlled modes) directs flow away from the unit with a long time constant (3), causing the tidal volume of the other units (1 and 2) to be disproportionately larger relative to their compliance.

constant (once again proportionally to their compliance) and away from the unit supplied by an obstructed airway. The effect of such redistribution on gas exchange depends on the blood supply received by each type of unit and is therefore difficult to predict in diseased lungs. However, the astute clinician may derive some insight into the mechanism of a given patient's gas exchange abnormalities by observing carefully the changes induced by variations in the flow rate and duration of inspiration during mechanical ventilation.

Restrictive and Obstructive Respiratory Disease

As seen, inertial pressure losses are relatively insignificant at normal breathing frequencies in children, and viscoelastic pressure losses are usually small and lumped together with other dissipative pressure losses. Therefore the pressure that the respiratory muscles must generate to produce a certain volume excursion of the thorax can simply be considered the sum of elastic and resistive pressures that need to be overcome in the process (see Eqs. 6 and 7). Because work is calculated by integrating these pressures relative to the same volume change, it immediately follows that the total work done by the respiratory muscles is the sum of the works done to overcome elastic and resistive pressures.

When applying these formulations, it is important to realize that elastic and resistive forces do not always act in the same direction. During inspiration, the respiratory muscles must generate the force to overcome both elasticity and flow resistance. Thus both elastic and resistive works have the same sign and their effect on total work is additive. During expiration, however, the elastic recoil of the lungs normally provides the force needed to overcome resistance. Elastic and resistive works are of similar magnitude and opposite sign, and the total work done by the muscles is zero. When there is intrathoracic airway obstruction, however, the absolute value of resistive work often exceeds that of elastic work. Under these circumstances the expiratory value of total work is no longer negligible and the expiratory muscles must do the balance of the expiratory work.

The term *restrictive respiratory disease* encompasses all conditions in which elastic or nondissipative work is primarily increased. One could also say that restrictive disease is caused by a decrease in thoracic compliance. Whether originating in the lungs or the chest wall, a decrease in thoracic compliance has two important mechanical consequences. First, the work of breathing increases, but only during inspiration; expiration continues to be passive and, in fact, takes place at a faster rate as elastic recoil increases. Second, the relaxation volume of the thorax and FRC decreases. The resultant decrease in lung volume, which may further reduce lung compliance, may be more pronounced in the infant, whose resting relaxation volume is already low. At low lung volumes, alveoli lack the support provided by the recoil of neighboring structures at higher volumes (mechanical interdependence[15]) and become inherently unstable, particularly if the surfactant system is affected by the disease and surface tension is increased. To prevent alveolar collapse, infants and small children with restrictive respiratory disease often close their glottis toward the end of expiration, causing each breath to end in a grunt. PEEP and continuous positive airway pressure are effective therapeutic modalities to achieve the same objective of preserving the end-expiratory inflation volume.[31,32] Deep lung inflations during positive pressure ventilation (often described as recruitment maneuvers) also may maintain unstable alveoli open for a period. This effect of volume history on alveolar volume decreases the work needed for spontaneous breaths following the inflation, adding to the more obvious benefits of intermittent mandatory ventilation in patients with restrictive lung disease.

Obstructive respiratory disease includes all conditions in which resistive or dissipative work is predominantly increased. The small caliber and high wall compliance of the developing airways render the infant and child more vulnerable to the development of airway obstruction.[33] Under normal breathing conditions, the small caliber of the airways represents no mechanical disadvantage because there is good correspondence between airway cross-sectional area and gas flow. When obstruction develops, however, airway resistance increases as an exponential function of the reduction in airway diameter (see Eq. 11). Because the same absolute decrease in caliber causes a much greater proportional reduction in airway diameter in a small than in a large airway, obstructive lesions tend to have more severe consequences in children than in adults.

Determinants of Respiratory Efficiency

The respiratory system has a notable ability to compensate for mechanical dysfunction. However, compensation does not come cheap. It raises the work of breathing in almost every instance, usually by combining increases in the force of contraction of the respiratory muscles with changes in ventilatory pattern. If the increase in work is sufficient to overcome the additional restrictive and obstructive loads applied on the respiratory system, minute alveolar ventilation and arterial PCO_2 are maintained within normal limits and respiratory failure is averted. In contrast, if the metabolic and contractile machinery of the respiratory muscles cannot meet the greater work demands, alveolar ventilation becomes insufficient to support gas exchange and respiratory failure ensues.

In the final analysis, the success or failure of the compensatory effort is a simple matter of balance between the energy resources available to the respiratory muscles and the energy demands imposed on these muscles. The energy resources are relatively well defined and limited by the blood supply of the muscles, their ability to metabolize substrates, and the internal efficiency of the muscle's metabolic apparatus. The energy demands on the respiratory muscles are more variable, however, and depend on the workload these muscles must perform per unit of time (ie, the power they must generate) and the overall efficiency with which the work is performed.

In thermodynamic terms, efficiency is defined as the proportion of the free energy available within a system that is transformed into external work (Eq. 1). In the case of the respiratory system, this notion can be reshaped to define efficiency as the quotient of respiratory muscle breathing power (W × t) divided by respiratory muscle energy consumption.

The breathing power is difficult to measure in spontaneously breathing subjects (remember that the respiratory muscles are themselves part of the chest wall) and has to be estimated from the volume-pressure relationships of the lungs. The energy consumption of the respiratory muscles is in turn estimated from their oxygen consumption,[34] which we can compute (also suboptimally) as the difference between the total body oxygen consumptions measured during spontaneous and supported ventilation. Some obvious sources of energy consumption, which are not included in the breathing power, reduce the respiratory system's efficiency. For example, the work of breathing does not account for isometric activity of the respiratory and postural muscles, which is not proper work in a physical sense (no volume change) but consumes energy. Other forms of volume-pressure work usually are not taken into account when calculating respiratory efficiency, so they also become sources of apparent inefficiency. The work performed to inflate the chest wall, as we just noticed again, cannot be determined during spontaneous breathing when contraction of the muscles changes the wall's passive properties. Similarly, the work done to deform the rib cage is difficult to measure and often is ignored. Thus it is not surprising that the published efficiencies tend to be artifactually low.[35,36]

As defined here, the poor overall efficiency of the respiratory system implies that, during each breathing cycle, a substantial amount of energy derived from metabolic substrates is dissipated as heat and cannot be converted into volume-pressure work. Respiratory disease can increase this energy dissipation by various mechanisms, leading to efficiency values as low as 1% to 3%.[35,37,38] Disease-induced alterations in chest wall configuration, for example, can limit force generation by the muscles, thus interfering with the transformation of chemical energy into mechanical energy.[39] Changes in the geometry of the chest wall also modify the spatial relationships of the muscles and can interfere with the transformation of mechanical energy into work. Finally, disease-related anomalies in the contractile state of the muscles produced by fatigue or poor nutrition further decrease muscle force and the work of breathing without decreasing muscle energy demands.[40,41]

Power of Breathing and Breathing Frequency

Unlike work, which is a function of the volume-pressure characteristics of the thorax, respiratory power (work/time) is influenced by the pattern of breathing. It has been held for some time that, at any given time, each subject has an optimal breathing frequency at which minimum power, and thus a minimum energy consumption, is necessary to attain a certain minute alveolar ventilation (Fig. 49.10).[36,42] Although this view has been challenged by those who believe that breathing frequency is adjusted to minimize average muscle force rather

than power (after all, there are no known energy or power receptors anywhere in the body),[43] it is a common clinical observation that different types of mechanical derangement result in distinctive patterns of breathing. These patterns generally agree with the principle of minimal power expenditure. For instance, patients with restrictive lung disease breathe rapidly and shallowly. In contrast, patients with airway obstruction breathe more slowly and prolong their inspiration or expiration, depending on whether the obstruction is extrathoracic or intrathoracic. By simply inspecting the effort and frequency of the breathing movements, the clinician can therefore assess not only the severity but also the specific nature of a patient's respiratory dysfunction.

Alterations in Chest Wall Configuration
Diaphragmatic Configuration
The amount of force developed by a muscle depends on its resting length. An optimal resting length for which maximal force is developed can be defined for each muscle. In the case of the diaphragm, the optimal length is attained at thoracic volumes close to the normal FRC. At these volumes, the muscle has the shape of a dome-capped cylinder, a configuration that has several advantages. First, diaphragmatic contraction shortens the cylinder in the axial direction, producing a pistonlike motion that displaces more volume than if the diaphragmatic dome simply became flatter (assuming the same degree of fiber shortening). Second, the descent of the diaphragmatic dome increases the surface of contact between the rib cage and the lungs. Therefore the increase in lung surface produced by lung inflation can be accommodated without changing the shape of the lung or the chest wall. Finally, at normal breathing volumes, the sides of the diaphragmatic cylinder are apposed to the internal surface of the rib cage. This area of apposition establishes a mechanical link between intraabdominal pressure and lung volume.[44] As the diaphragm contracts during inspiration, intraabdominal pressure increases, pushing the lower portion of the rib cage forward and laterally. Thus diaphragmatic contraction has an additional contribution to lung inflation at low energy cost and may help to stabilize the lower rib cage against inspiratory distortion.

The configuration of the chest in the infant and small child minimizes these advantages. At these ages, the lower portion of the infant's rib cage has relatively large anteroposterior and

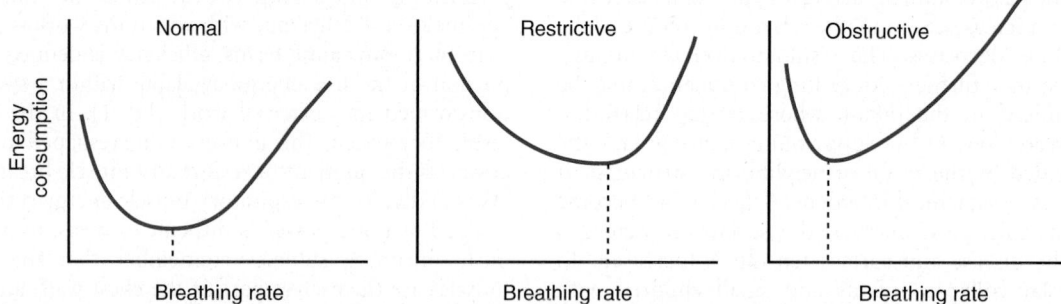

Fig. 49.10. Each combination of mechanical conditions is associated with an optimal breathing rate for which the power (work × time) and thus the energy consumption of breathing are minimal. Restrictive disease increases the optimal rate, while obstructive disease decreases it. Actual breathing rates adhere remarkably to predictions on the basis of minimal power. Consequently, it is safe to assume that, under most circumstances, the presence of tachypnea is indicative of a restrictive derangement and that a decrease in respiratory rate or, more precisely, a prolongation of inspiration or expiration indicates an obstructive derangement.

lateral diameters. As a result, the insertions of the diaphragm are spread out, thereby reducing the axial shortening range of the muscle. Moreover, the lack of a substantial area of apposition of the diaphragm and rib cage abolishes the inspiratory and stabilizing effects of intraabdominal pressure on the rib cage.

Thoracic hyperexpansion and abdominal distension exaggerate these limitations by widening the diameters of the lower portion, spreading out the diaphragmatic insertions. The length of the muscle fibers is diminished to a suboptimal length, and the force generated during inspiration is decreased. Abdominal distension has the additional disadvantage of raising intraabdominal pressure, which opposes diaphragmatic contraction and raises the work that the muscle has to do.

Rib Cage Distortion

Until now, we have assumed that the rib cage and abdomen have the same configuration during spontaneous breathing and passive inflation-deflation maneuvers. This assumption implies that all the various parts of the chest wall move with a single degree of freedom and that there are no volume shifts between parts. However, it has been known for quite some time that, under certain conditions, the rib cage and abdomen can change volume independently of one another and even in opposite directions.[45] In other words, the chest wall has multiple degrees of freedom and can undergo regional distortion.

Regional chest wall distortion results from the coupling of changes in pressure (pleural or intraabdominal) and the local compliances of the rib cage and abdominal wall. Rib cage distortion is more pronounced during inspiration, when pleural pressure decreases with respect to atmospheric pressure or the diaphragm pulls the rib cage by its costal insertions, forcing the thoracic wall inward in the expiratory direction. This inward movement of the rib cage causes visible retractions in areas where the chest wall has no bony support (intercostal, subcostal, or suprasternal spaces) or where the support has been abnormally weakened (eg, costal fractures). Abdominal distortion, in contrast, usually involves alterations in the contractile state of the diaphragm or abdominal wall muscles. When one hemidiaphragm becomes paralyzed, for example, the negative pleural pressure generated by other inspiratory muscles pulls the paralyzed muscle upward, into the rib cage, during inspiration. As a result, the abdominal wall of the affected side moves paradoxically in the inward direction, and the chest wall becomes distorted. As another example, contraction of the abdominal muscles stiffens the abdominal wall, raising intraabdominal pressure and shifting all volume changes to the rib cage during both inspiration and expiration.

The developing chest wall is particularly susceptible to distortion. As we have seen, the rib cage is compliant in the newborn.[2,4,46] Although this high compliance facilitates passage through the birth canal, it also promotes distortion of the rib cage during inspiration. In addition, the intercostal muscles, whose main contribution to breathing is to stabilize the rib cage by contracting simultaneously with the diaphragm, appear to have decreased tone at early ages, especially during rapid eye movement sleep and in preterm infants.[47] Finally, the lack of a substantial area of apposition between the diaphragm and rib cage removes the stabilizing effect of the intraabdominal pressure on the lower rib cage. Accordingly,

in infants chest wall retractions tend to develop in the presence of minimal mechanical lung dysfunction.

Chest wall distortion represents a pressure-induced change in volume, and therefore it constitutes a form of work. Distortional work is usually not computed as part of the work of breathing. However, it has a measurable energy cost, and therefore it needs to be viewed as a source of respiratory inefficiency. Both the distortional work and its energy cost can be better understood if we analyze the volume-pressure relationships of the thorax in the particular case of rib cage retractions during inspiration. Regardless of whether such retractions are present, at any point, the volume change of the lungs (ΔV_L) must be equivalent to the sum of the volume changes of the rib cage (ΔV_{rc}) and abdomen (ΔV_{ab}):

$$\Delta V_L = \Delta V_{rc} + \Delta V_{ab} \qquad \text{Eq. 49.12}$$

Consequently, if ΔV_L is to remain constant, decreases in ΔV_{rc} caused by rib cage retractions during inspiration must be accompanied by a proportional increase in ΔV_{ab} (Fig. 49.11). If, as often occurs, ΔV_{rc} is negative, then ΔV_{ab} becomes greater than ΔV_L. Because the volume displacement of the diaphragm approximates ΔV_{ab}, chest wall retractions inevitably result in an increase in the diaphragmatic excursion.

The amount of work done by the diaphragm is calculated by integrating the pressure developed by the muscle relative to the volume displacement produced by the diaphragmatic contraction. In practical terms, the pressure developed by the diaphragm or transdiaphragmatic pressure is defined as the difference between the intraabdominal pressure (P_{ab}, often estimated from measurements of gastric pressure) and the pleural pressure (P_{pl}, estimated from the esophageal pressure). The volume displaced by the diaphragm is estimated as ΔV_{ab} in Eq. 12. Thus diaphragmatic work (W_{di}) can be computed as:

$$W_{di} = \int (P_{ab} - P_{pl}) \cdot dV_{ab} \qquad \text{Eq. 49.13}$$

The work done on the airways and lungs to move gas in and out of the alveoli (see Eqs. 3 and 4) is:

$$W_L = \int (P_M - P_{pl}) \cdot dV_L \qquad \text{Eq. 49.14}$$

P_{ab} is generally greater than P_M (which is 0 in the absence of positive airway pressure), particularly in a recumbent subject. In the presence of rib cage retractions, dV_{ab} greatly exceeds dV_L and consequently W_{di} substantially exceeds W_L. The volume displacement of the diaphragm may be up to twice the tidal volume of the lungs in premature infants without apparent lung disease,[48] an increase that could be responsible for the poor weight gain and development of fatigue of infants recovering from the respiratory distress syndrome.

Alterations in Contractile State of the Respiratory Muscles

Respiratory efficiency is affected by the functional state of the respiratory muscles. Sustained increases in activity will likely eventually result in decreased contractile force and lower minute alveolar ventilation, a condition often classified as muscle fatigue. When muscle fatigue is present, the energy consumption of the muscle may be increased with respect to the actual work performed. Similar decreases in contractility without a decrease in energy consumption can be present in a variety of clinical situations. Some result from an imbalance between the energy demands of the muscle's contractile

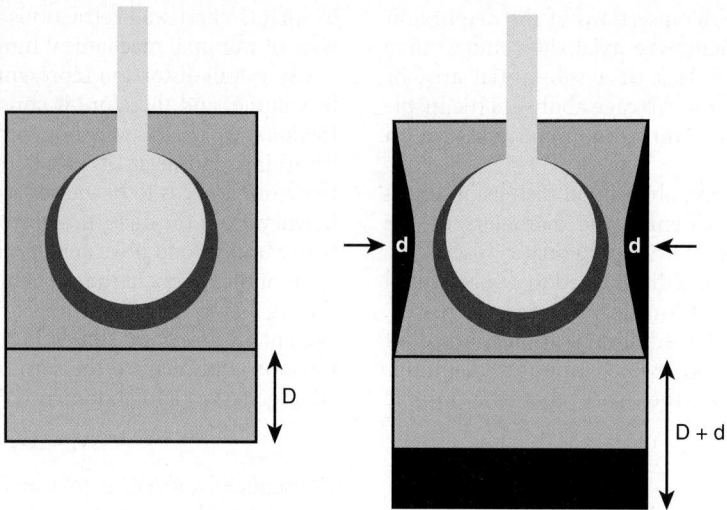

Fig. 49.11. Effect of inspiratory rib cage distortion on the volume displacement of the diaphragm. When the rib cage caves inward during inspiration, to generate the same tidal volume in the lungs (shown in *red*), the diaphragm must increase its volume excursion above the nondistorted value (*D*) by an amount equivalent to the volume of the inward movement of the rib cage (*d*). Rib cage distortion usually relates to the combination of an increased rib cage compliance and increased respiratory effort, which translates into more negative pleural pressures acting on the inner surface of the rib cage. However, it can occur without apparent increase in effort, especially in premature infants, or as a result of disease- or trauma-induced chest wall distortion (eg, rib fractures or unilateral phrenic palsy).

machinery and its substrate availability (eg, shock[49]). Others are simply the expression of the inadequate coupling of the excitation-contraction processes inside the muscle cell, changes in the recruitment of specific fiber populations within the muscle,[50] or chronic depletion of the muscle's energetic resources as a result of malnutrition.[40]

Conclusion

Although the developing respiratory system has obvious mechanical disadvantages, the reader should not be left with the idea that infants and children are constantly on the brink of respiratory failure. Quite the contrary, they have a remarkable capability to tolerate respiratory disease. This capability is in great part based on a proficient system of mechanical compensation. The information contained in this chapter is intended to provide an overview of the factors involved in both mechanical dysfunction and its compensation. Unfortunately, the physiologic principles underlying the basic concepts presented here are receiving less and less attention in our training programs. The reader is encouraged to visit and study the many classical references contained in the bibliography. Although many of them certainly show the signs of age, they provide the critical foundation for a more rational approach to the therapy of respiratory disease in the critically ill child.

References

1. Salazar E, Knowles JH. An analysis of pressure-volume characteristics of the lungs. *J Appl Physiol.* 1964;19:97-104.
2. Gerhardt T, Bancalari E. Chest wall compliance in full-term and premature infants. *Acta Paediatr Scand.* 1980;69:359-364.
3. Papastamelos C, Panitch HB, England SE, Allen JL. Developmental changes in chest wall compliance in infancy and early childhood. *J Appl Physiol.* 1995;78:179-184.
4. Richards CC, Bachman L. Lung and chest wall compliance of apneic paralyzed infants. *J Clin Invest.* 1961;40:273-278.
5. Fagan DG. Shape changes in static V-P loops from children's lungs related to growth. *Thorax.* 1977;32:198-202.
6. Stigol LC, Vawter GF, Mead J. Studies on elastic recoil of the lung in a pediatric population. *Am Rev Respir Dis.* 1972;105:552-563.
7. Mortola JP. Dynamics of breathing in newborn mammals. *Physiol Rev.* 1987;67:187-243.
8. Latzin P, Roth S, Thamrin C, et al. Lung volume, breathing pattern and ventilation inhomogeneity in preterm and term infants. *PLoS ONE.* 2009;4:e4635.
9. Olinsky A, Bryan MH, Bryan AC. Influence of lung inflation on respiratory control in neonates. *J Appl Physiol.* 1974;36:426-429.
10. Fisher JT, Mortola JP, Smith JB, et al. Respiration in newborns: development of the control of breathing. *Am Rev Respir Dis.* 1982;125:650-657.
11. Muller N, Volgyesi G, Becker L, et al. Diaphragmatic muscle tone. *J Appl Physiol.* 1979;47:279-284.
12. Bachofen H. Lung tissue resistance and pulmonary hysteresis. *J Appl Physiol.* 1968;24:296-301.
13. Perez Fontan JJ. Effect of lung lavage on the stress relaxation of the respiratory system. *J Appl Physiol.* 1993;75:1536-1544.
14. Perez Fontan JJ, Ray AO, Oxland TR. Stress relaxation of the respiratory system in developing piglets. *J Appl Physiol.* 1992;73:1297-1309.
15. Mead J, Takishima T, Leith D. Stress distribution in lungs: a model of pulmonary elasticity. *J Appl Physiol.* 1970;28:596-608.
16. Dawson S, Elliott EA. Wave-speed limitation on expiratory flow: a unifying concept. *J Appl Physiol.* 1977;43:498-515.
17. Wilson T, Rodarte J, Butler J. Wave-speed and viscous flow limitation. In: Macklem P, Mead J, eds. *Handbook of Physiology: Respiration.* 3rd ed. Bethesda, MD: American Physiological Society; 1986.
18. Fakhoury KF, Sellers C, Smith EO, et al. Serial measurements of lung function in a cohort of young children with bronchopulmonary dysplasia. *Pediatrics.* 2010;125:e1441-e1447.
19. Turner SW, Palmer LJ, Rye PJ, et al. Infants with flow limitation at 4 weeks: outcome at 6 and 11 years. *Am J Respir Crit Care Med.* 2002;165:1294-1298.
20. Perez Fontan JJ, Kinloch LP, Donnelly DF. Integration of bronchomotor and ventilatory responses to chemoreceptor stimulation in developing sheep. *Respir Physiol.* 1998;111:1-13.
21. Perez Fontan JJ, Velloff CR. Neuroanatomic organization of the parasympathetic bronchomotor system in developing sheep. *Am J Physiol.* 1997;273(1 Pt 2):R121-R133.
22. Pérez Fontán JJ, Kinloch LP, Donnelly DF. Integration of bronchomotor and ventilatory responses to chemoreceptor stimulation in developing sheep. *Respir Physiol.* 1998;111:1-13.

23. Richardson CA, Herbert DA, Mitchell RA. Modulation of pulmonary stretch receptors and airway resistance by parasympathetic efferents. *J Appl Physiol.* 1984;57:1842-1849.

24. Pérez Fontán JJ, Velloff CR. Neuroanatomical organization of the parasympathetic bronchomotor system in developing sheep. *Am J Physiol.* 1997;273:R121-R133.

25. Martin JG, Shore S, Engel LA. Effect of continuous positive airway pressure on respiratory mechanics and pattern of breathing in induced asthma. *Am Rev Respir Dis.* 1982;126:812-817.

26. Smith PG, el-Khatib MF, Carlo WA. PEEP does not improve pulmonary mechanics in infants with bronchiolitis. *Am Rev Respir Dis.* 1993;147: 1295-1298.

27. Tuxen DV. Detrimental effects of positive end-expiratory pressure during controlled mechanical ventilation of patients with severe airflow obstruction. *Am Rev Respir Dis.* 1989;140:5-9.

28. Marini JJ. Should PEEP be used in airflow obstruction? *Am Rev Respir Dis.* 1989;140:1-3.

29. Marini JJ. Does positive end-expiratory pressure improve CO_2 exchange in controlled ventilation of acute airflow obstruction? *Crit Care Med.* 2011;39:1841-1842.

30. Otis AB, McKerrow CB, Bartlett RA, et al. Mechanical factors in distribution of pulmonary ventilation. *J Appl Physiol.* 1956;8:427-443.

31. Kumar A, Falke KJ, Geffin B, et al. Continuous positive-pressure ventilation in acute respiratory failure. *N Engl J Med.* 1970;283:1430-1436.

32. Suter PM, Fairley B, Isenberg MD. Optimum end-expiratory airway pressure in patients with acute pulmonary failure. *N Engl J Med.* 1975;292:284-289.

33. Shaffer TH, Bhutani VK, Wolfson MR, et al. In vivo mechanical properties of the developing airway. *Pediatr Res.* 1989;25:143-146.

34. Campbell EJ, Westlake EK, Cherniack RM. The oxygen consumption and efficiency of the respiratory muscles of young male subjects. *Clin Sci (Lond).* 1959;18:55-64.

35. Cherniack RM. The oxygen consumption and efficiency of the respiratory muscles in health and emphysema. *J Clin Invest.* 1959;38:494-499.

36. Milic-Emili J, Petit J. Mechanical efficiency of breathing. *J Appl Physiol.* 1960;15:359-362.

37. Fritts HW Jr, Filler J, Fishman AP, Cournand A. The efficiency of ventilation during voluntary hyperpnea: studies in normal subjects and in dyspneic patients with either chronic pulmonary emphysema or obesity. *J Clin Invest.* 1959;38:1339-1348.

38. Thibeault DW, Clutario B, Awld PA. The oxygen cost of breathing in the premature infant. *Pediatrics.* 1966;37:954-959.

39. Finucane KE, Panizza JA, Singh B. Efficiency of the normal human diaphragm with hyperinflation. *J Appl Physiol.* 2005;99:1402-1411.

40. Donahoe M, Rogers RM, Wilson DO, Pennock BE. Oxygen consumption of the respiratory muscles in normal and in malnourished patients with chronic obstructive pulmonary disease. *Am Rev Respir Dis.* 1989;140: 385-391.

41. Larson DE, Hesslink RL, Hrovat MI, et al. Dietary effects on exercising muscle metabolism and performance by 31P-MRS. *J Appl Physiol.* 1994;77:1108-1115.

42. Crossfill M, Widdicombe J. Physical characteristics of the chest and lungs and the work of breathing in different mammalian species. *J Physiol (Lond).* 1961;158:1-14.

43. Mead J. Control of respiratory frequency. *J Appl Physiol.* 1960;15: 325-336.

44. Mead J. Functional significance of the area of apposition of diaphragm to rib cage [proceedings]. *Am Rev Respir Dis.* 1979;119(2 Pt 2):31-32.

45. Konno K, Mead J. Measurement of the separate volume changes of rib cage and abdomen during breathing. *J Appl Physiol.* 1967;22:407-422.

46. Heldt GP, McIlroy MB. Dynamics of chest wall in preterm infants. *J Appl Physiol.* 1987;62:170-174.

47. Henderson-Smart DJ, Read DJ. Reduced lung volume during behavioral active sleep in the newborn. *J Appl Physiol.* 1979;46:1081-1085.

48. Heldt GP, McIlroy MB. Distortion of chest wall and work of diaphragm in preterm infants. *J Appl Physiol.* 1987;62:164-169.

49. Aubier M, Trippenbach T, Roussos C. Respiratory muscle fatigue during cardiogenic shock. *J Appl Physiol.* 1981;51:499-508.

50. Coirault C, Riou B, Bard M, et al. Contraction, relaxation, and economy of force generation in isolated human diaphragm muscle. *Am J Respir Crit Care Med.* 1995;152(4 Pt 1):1275-1283.

Specific Diseases of the Respiratory System: Upper Airway

David Jardine, Andrew Inglis, Jr., and Agnes I. Hunyady

PEARLS

- Diseases leading to compromise of the airway are the most frequent causes of cardiac arrest in pediatric patients. A small reduction in the caliber of the child's airway may lead to a life-threatening reduction of airflow.
- Laryngomalacia is the most common congenital anomaly of the larynx. Infants tend to outgrow this problem during the first year of life; however, the condition may be of sufficient severity in some infants that activities such as feeding are compromised.
- The trachea may be compressed by the presence of an abnormal vascular structure. Children affected by this problem may have such diverse symptoms as stridor, wheezing, lobar atelectasis, or recurrent pulmonary infections.
- The practice of treating laryngotracheobronchitis with corticosteroids is a standard of care, especially for hospitalized patients. A meta-analysis in which the efficacy of corticosteroids was evaluated suggests that corticosteroids may reduce the need for endotracheal intubation and hasten improvement when given in the first 24 hours of illness.
- Epiglottitis, a bacterial infection of the supraglottic tissues historically caused by *Haemophilus influenzae* type B, is now most frequently caused by group A β-hemolytic streptococcus.
- Patients with bacterial tracheitis usually do not respond to inhaled racemic epinephrine, have a high fever, and appear very ill.

Diseases leading to compromise of the airway are the most frequent causes of cardiac arrest in pediatric patients. Various processes can lead to respiratory failure, including disorders of the respiratory tract causing obstruction, mechanical impairment of ventilation (pneumothorax, chest wall injury), neuromuscular failure (severe weakness, coma), and failure to deliver oxygen to the tissue (cardiac insufficiency, septic shock).[1] Prompt recognition of the general process causing respiratory failure quickly eliminates many diagnostic possibilities, permitting the clinician to focus on a smaller group of causes and a narrower range of therapeutic interventions. Specific diseases of the airway leading to obstruction are discussed here.

The small size of the infant's trachea makes airway obstruction more likely and particularly dangerous. The normal anteroposterior diameter of the infant's glottis is 4.5 mm. One millimeter of circumferential tracheal edema reduces the glottic lumen to 30% of its normal size. Poiseuille's law stipulates that laminar flow of gas through a tube is inversely proportional to the fourth power of the radius of the lumen:

$$R = \frac{8 l n}{\pi r^4}$$

where R is the resistance to gas flow, l is the length of the tube, n is the viscosity of the gas, and r is the radius. Unfortunately, airflow through a narrowed trachea is usually turbulent, which worsens the situation because resistance to turbulent flow of gas past an obstruction is inversely proportional to the fifth power of the radius of the lumen.[2,3] Gas exchange will be dramatically reduced by minor degrees of impingement on an infant's trachea. A child may not tolerate lesions that would not even produce symptoms in an adult. Rapid triage and expeditious treatment of upper airway obstruction in children are essential.

Initial Management

Once the diagnosis of upper airway obstruction is made, efforts should be undertaken to minimize disturbing the patient unless the respiratory embarrassment is severe enough to be life threatening. Airway obstruction often worsens when infants and children are alarmed during a diagnostic evaluation. Humidified oxygen should be administered through a nasal cannula or facemask. These devices may frighten younger children who may more readily accept oxygen delivered through flexible tubing held by the parent. If the child will tolerate placement of a pulse oximeter probe, this provides a noninvasive way of evaluating oxygenation. Because arterial oxygen saturation is easily determined noninvasively, arterial blood gas is should be reserved to determine which patients may be hypercapnic; however, this procedure will further upset the child. Using clinical judgment to assess the severity of airway obstruction is a standard practice.[4]

After upper airway obstruction has been diagnosed, a combination of physical and radiographic findings may help localize the lesion. Once the anatomic site of the lesion has been identified, the diagnostic possibilities narrow greatly. During the diagnostic evaluation, the child may sit in the parent's lap if this reduces anxiety. This position usually does not interfere with diagnostic evaluation, like lateral neck and chest radiography.

Gentle, nonthreatening examination of the patient's head and neck may reveal the cause of the illness. During the initial evaluation, an assessment should be made regarding the likely location of the obstruction. Extrathoracic airway obstruction usually results in stridor (the obstruction is most severe during inspiratory phase), whereas intrathoracic airway obstruction usually results in wheezing (the obstruction is most severe during expiratory phase). Localizing the obstruction in this manner helps to narrow the diagnostic possibilities. In the emergency room setting, it may be possible to use a small fiberoptic scope to identify supraglottic causes of airway obstruction. This should not be attempted unless individuals are present who are skilled in the fiberoptic evaluation of the pediatric airway and if such an examination does not worsen the patient's distress.

The initial evaluation should be accomplished expeditiously with the goals of making decisions about the management and further evaluation of the patient with upper airway compromise. In the case of severe respiratory compromise, it may be necessary to plan for invasive procedures (endotracheal intubation or operative intervention) while the diagnostic evaluation is being performed. Finally, it should not be forgotten that pulmonary edema might follow relief of severe upper airway obstruction.[5] Postobstructive pulmonary edema may be severe enough to require intensive therapy, including endotracheal intubation, mechanical ventilation, and positive end-expiratory pressure.

Congenital Malformations

A variety of congenital malformations can affect the pediatric airway. Many of these become evident in the delivery room. Some congenital malformations do not present until the child is older and somatic growth has made the airway impairment more evident.

Choanal Atresia

Choanal atresia is estimated to occur about once in every 5000 to 9000 live births.[6] Choanal atresia is seen commonly with other defects, especially CHARGE syndrome, which accounts for 25% of all patients with choanal stenosis.[7] Unilateral choanal atresia, the most common form, is often seen without accompanying congenital defects and may not be diagnosed at the time of delivery. Bilateral choanal atresia almost always occurs in the presence of other congenital defects.[7] For the first 5 months of life, many infants breathe only through their noses and do not open their mouths when the nasal passages are occluded; consequently, bilateral choanal atresia often results in respiratory distress shortly after birth. Bilateral choanal atresia (Fig. 50.1) is diagnosed through examination of the naris with the mouth closed. If no airflow is present, a presumptive diagnosis of choanal atresia is established. Some authorities advocate passing a thin, flexible catheter through the naris. This will confirm the diagnosis of choanal atresia; however, if the symptoms are resulting from choanal stenosis, edema formation following even minor trauma of the nasal mucosa after catheter placement may lead to complete occlusion of the nasal airway and worsening of respiratory distress. Surgery is indicated for the correction of bilateral choanal

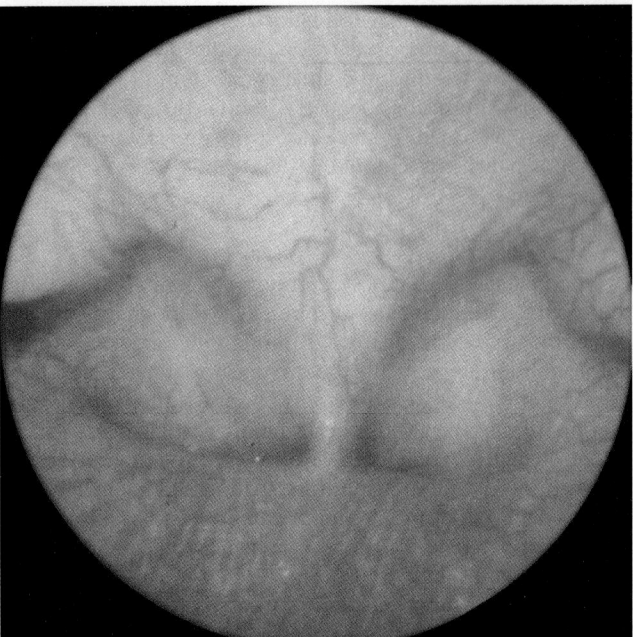

Fig. 50.1. Choanal atresia before repair. View of choanal atresia from posterior nasopharynx. There is complete absence of choanae. (Copyright Andrew F. Inglis, Jr.)

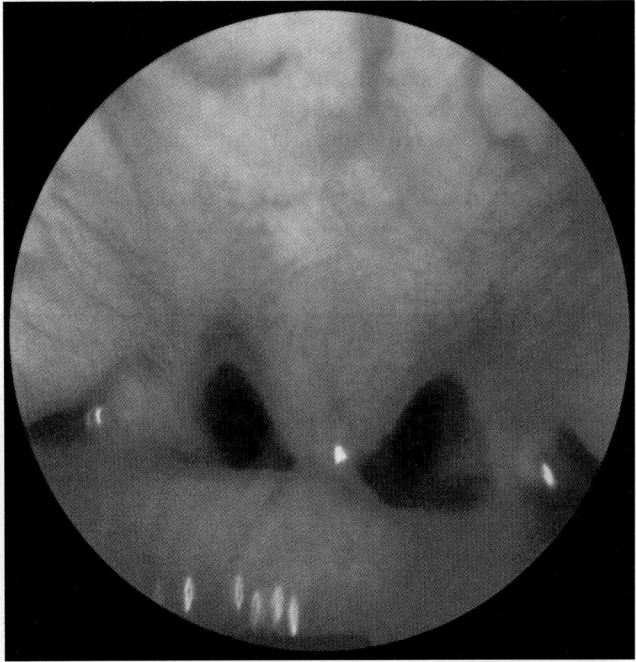

Fig. 50.2. Choanal atresia after repair. View from the posterior of the nasopharynx demonstrating patency of choanae following surgery. (Copyright Andrew F. Inglis, Jr.)

atresia if the infant has symptoms[8] (Fig. 50.2). Infants with bilateral choanal atresia generally have surgery within the first 3 months of life, whereas infants with unilateral choanal atresia typically have surgery after the second year of life.[9] Various surgical approaches and adjuncts have been reported; however, there is insufficient evidence to indicate which are the most successful.[10] Although choanal atresia is the most common cause of nasal airway obstruction, midline nasal masses such as meningoencephaloceles, gliomas, or dermoid tumors can also cause obstruction. Because these lesions may originate from within the cranial vault, computed tomography (CT) scanning or magnetic resonance imaging (MRI) should be performed before a biopsy or surgical correction of the abnormality is attempted.[11]

Laryngomalacia

Laryngomalacia is the most common congenital anomaly of the larynx. The infant has inspiratory stridor that is exacerbated by crying or distress. Although no gross anatomic abnormalities are present, the laryngeal cartilages lack their usual rigidity. When the larynx is observed during fiberoptic examination of the glottis, the arytenoid cartilages and supraglottic structures collapse inward (toward the glottis) during inspiration, leading to inspiratory stridor. During exhalation, the laryngeal structures are more patent but may still be narrowed compared to a normal infant larynx (Fig. 50.3). The negative intrathoracic pressure generated during inspiration contributes to a high incidence of gastroesophageal reflux[12] and pulmonary aspiration.[13,14]

In some patients with laryngomalacia, gastroesophageal reflux may be the primary cause of the airway compromise, whereas in others it may be a significant cofactor exacerbating preexisting neurologic or anatomic abnormality.[15] The respiratory embarrassment associated with this problem is usually minor and self-limited, although hypoxia and hypercapnia have been documented.[16] During infancy, laryngomalacia accompanies sleep apnea in 27% of patients.[17] Infants tend to outgrow this problem during the first year of life; however, the condition may be severe enough in some infants to compromise activities such as feeding. In the most severe cases, surgical intervention may be necessary.[18] The goal is to relieve airway obstruction by excision of tissue that collapses into the glottis during inspiration.

Laryngeal Webs, Stenosis, and Tumors

Laryngeal webs usually occur at the level of the glottis and are usually located anteriorly. These may be congenital or acquired and are generally thin membranes of soft tissue that partially occlude the tracheal opening, producing symptoms of feeble cry and dyspnea shortly after birth (Fig. 50.4).[19] Surgical lysis of these lesions corrects the problem. Laryngeal cysts and laryngoceles are soft tissue masses that protrude into the glottic lumen (Fig. 50.5). The resulting respiratory compromise is usually recognized as inspiratory stridor. Treatment is surgical excision of the lesion.[20]

Another lesion presenting as inspiratory stridor is congenital laryngotracheal (subglottic) stenosis. This is the second most frequent cause of stridor in infants.[21] The infant with this problem may have symptoms when newborn but often comes to medical attention later when the tracheal edema produced by a minor respiratory infection causes severe inspiratory stridor. This may be initially diagnosed as croup (laryngotracheobronchitis) but is noted to recur with each subsequent upper respiratory infection. Although the diagnosis of laryngotracheal stenosis may be made radiographically, it is usually established with bronchoscopy. If endotracheal intubation is necessary, a smaller than normal endotracheal tube should be used to reduce trauma and ischemia of the subglottic tissues. Depending on the severity of the lesion, surgical intervention may be necessary (see "Laryngotracheal (Subglottic) Stenosis" for details of the surgical procedures).

Soft tissue masses may reduce the caliber of the tracheal lumen, either by extrinsic compression, as happens with a cystic hygroma, or by growth into the tracheal lumen from the

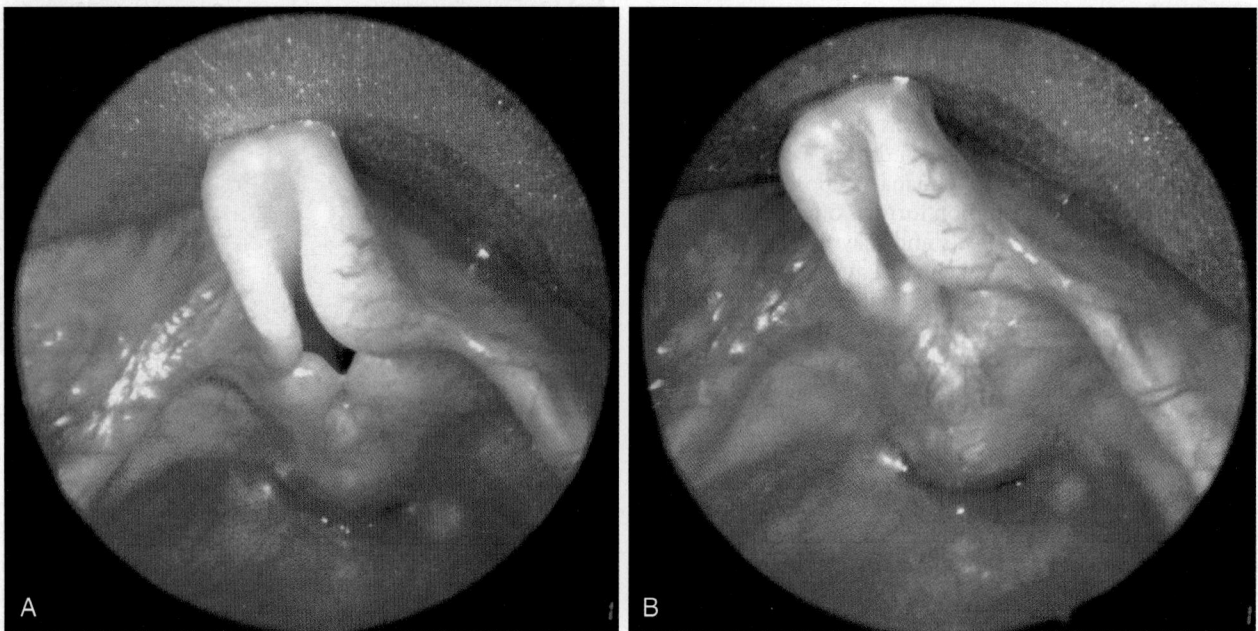

Fig. 50.3. Laryngomalacia demonstrates narrowing of the larynx in inspiration and expiration. During exhalation (A) note the tightly curled epiglottis and the slitlike opening to the laryngeal inlet caused by the medialization of the superior edges of the aryepiglottic folds. During inhalation (B) the aryepiglottic folds are drawn further inward, causing obstruction of the larynx. (Copyright Andrew F. Inglis, Jr.)

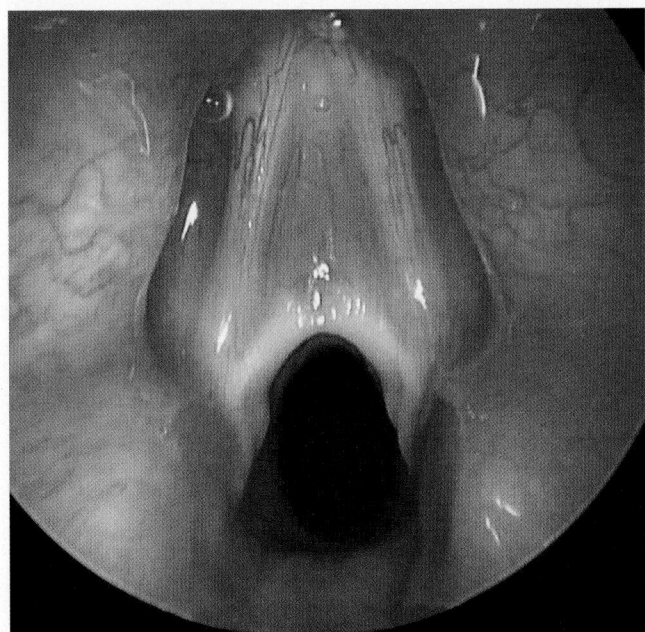

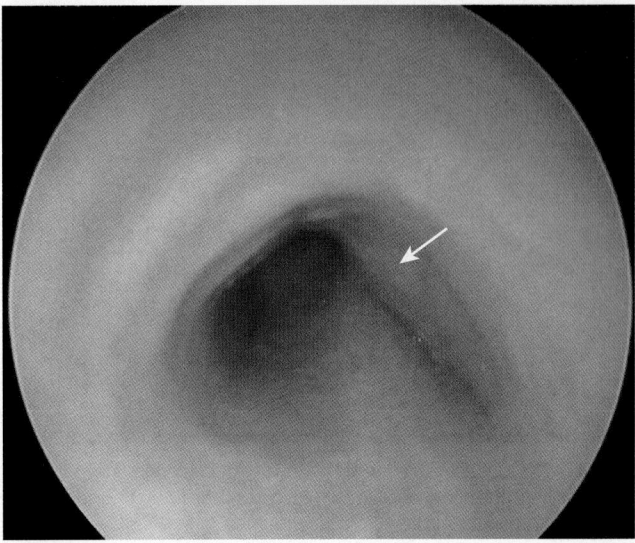

Fig. 50.6. The lateral portion of the tracheal lumen is severely compressed by the impingement of the vascular ring. (Copyright Andrew F. Inglis, Jr.)

Vascular Impingement on the Trachea

The trachea may be compressed by the presence of an abnormal vascular structure (Fig. 50.6).[24] The innominate artery is the most common vessel causing tracheal compression. Vascular rings and enlarged pulmonary arteries are also known to cause tracheal compression, as are a variety of other vascular abnormalities.[25] These lesions may present with physical findings such as stridor or wheezing. Alternatively, the patient may be symptom-free but may suffer respiratory problems such as recurrent lobar atelectasis or frequent pulmonary infections. For this reason, it is difficult to recognize a vascular ring as the underlying cause of illness.[26] Careful inspection of the chest radiograph may reveal indentation of the trachea, but often this sign is absent. Barium swallow has been the historic method of diagnosing vascular impingement of the trachea. CT scanning and MRI have become the diagnostic modalities of choice (Figs. 50.7 and 50.8). These noninvasive methods are effective at showing complex three-dimensional cardiovascular anatomy, especially the extracardiac morphology. Treatment involves surgical correction of the vascular anomaly, in severe cases.[27] Respiratory distress may persist postoperatively because prolonged compression of the trachea has made the affected segment softer and collapsible.

Bronchomalacia and Intrathoracic Tracheomalacia

During normal respiration, the upper airway is subject to cycles of positive and negative intraluminal pressure. The cartilaginous components of the upper airway are rigid ringlike structural elements that resist the tendency to collapse caused by the cycling of pressure within the airway lumen. When these structures lack their characteristic rigidity, the mechanics of breathing are altered.[28] The symptoms produced by these changes depend on the location of the damaged cartilages. Characteristically, intrathoracic cartilaginous lesions such as bronchomalacia or tracheomalacia impede exhalation. The diagnosis of airway malacia should be suspected in children who have recurrent lower airway infections or asthmatic

Fig. 50.4. A laryngeal web occludes most of the tracheal lumen in this patient. This web, which is a thin membrane of soft tissue at the level of the glottis, has many of the features typical of this class of lesions. (Copyright Andrew F. Inglis, Jr.)

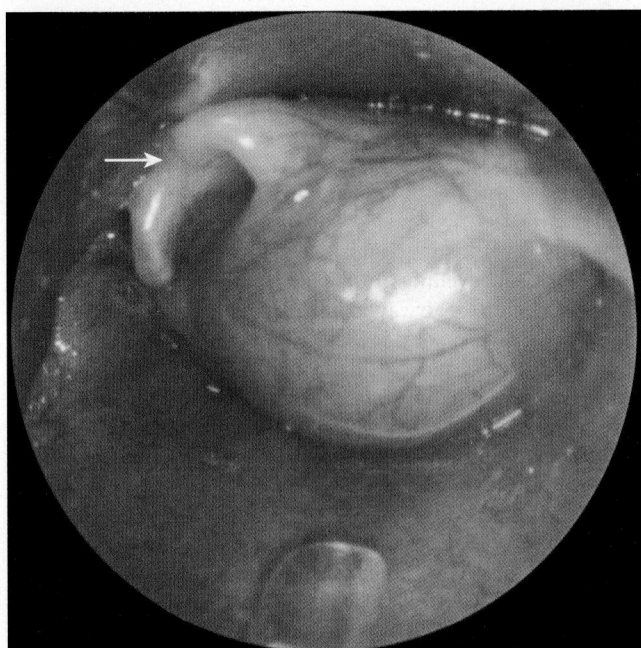

Fig. 50.5. A large laryngeal cyst protrudes from the lateral wall of the trachea, just below the level of the glottis. (Copyright Andrew F. Inglis, Jr.)

tracheal wall, as happens with a hemangioma. Although these lesions may be present at birth, they often do not produce symptoms for the first few months until the growing lesion further impinges on the trachea. Although surgery is frequently used for treatment of tracheal hemangiomas,[22] pioneering work by Judah Folkman was instrumental in demonstrating that some of these lesions respond to steroid therapy.[23]

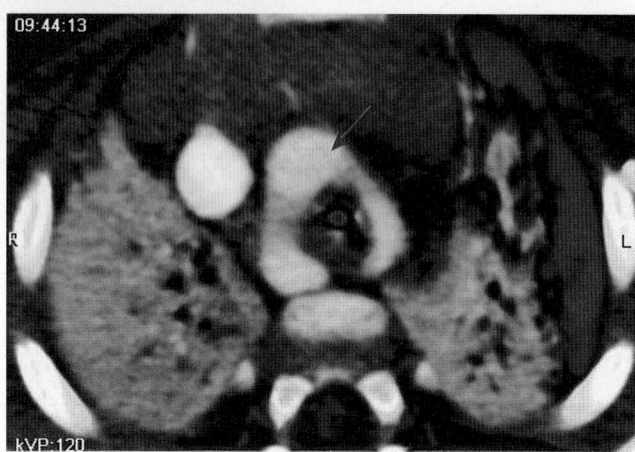

Fig. 50.7. Contrast CT scan showing the vascular ring encircling and compressing the trachea (*arrow* indicates vascular ring encircling trachea). (Copyright Andrew F. Inglis, Jr.)

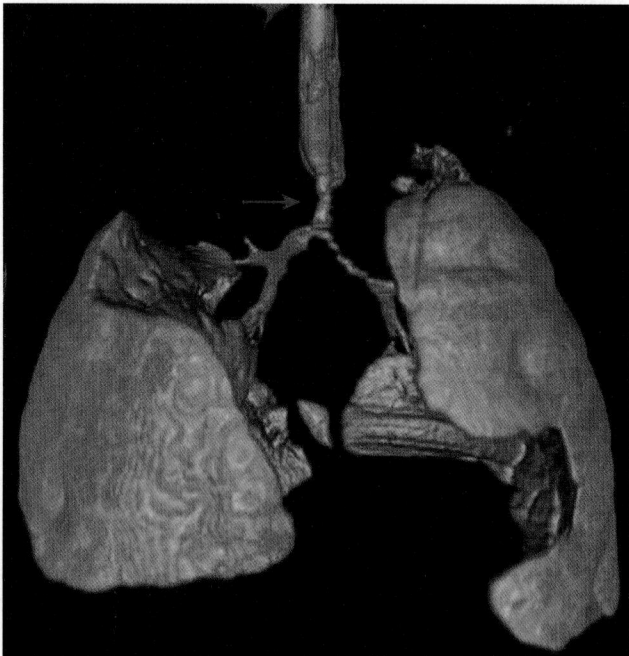

Fig. 50.8. High-resolution three-dimensional reconstruction of CT scans clearly shows severe tracheal compression caused by the vascular ring (*arrow* indicates tracheal narrowing caused by vascular ring). (Copyright Andrew F. Inglis, Jr.)

symptoms that do not respond to medical therapy.[29] Confirmation of this problem may be made through observation of collapse of the upper airways during active exhalation, such as occurs while crying. Collapse can be observed with several diagnostic modalities including fluoroscopy, flexible or rigid bronchoscopy, and ultrafast CT scanning.[30]

Although these lesions may be congenital, many of the cases of tracheomalacia and bronchomalacia seen in the pediatric intensive care unit (PICU) are the result of an infectious or mechanical insult to the trachea. Infants with bronchopulmonary dysplasia and persistent respiratory problems may be affected by bronchomalacia alone or in combination with

tracheomalacia.[31] Airway malacia is frequently associated with purulent bacterial airway infections that may require recurrent antibiotic therapy.[32] The obstructive symptoms produced by these lesions may be relieved by continuous positive airway pressure to maintain patency of the airway during exhalation.[33] The level of continuous positive airway pressure necessary to improve respiratory function may be assessed clinically (relief of obstructive symptoms), mechanically (measurement of flow-volume loops), or bronchoscopically (maintenance of airway patency throughout the respiratory cycle).[34] With sufficient time, many of these infants outgrow their respiratory difficulties. As an alternative to tracheostomy and positive airway pressure, some have advocated surgical intervention with pericardial flap aortopexy[35] or, in extreme situations, metallic airway stents.[36]

Infectious Processes

A variety of infectious processes may affect the pediatric airway. Poiseuille's law dictates that airway compromise from the swelling that accompanies an infectious process is greater in infants and young children than it is in adults. A small reduction in the caliber of the smaller child's airway may lead to a life-threatening reduction of airflow.

Laryngotracheobronchitis

Laryngotracheobronchitis (croup) is a common childhood infection, affecting approximately 3% of children each year.[37] Parainfluenza virus is the most common cause (approximately 75% of cases),[37] whereas coronavirus and rhinovirus constitute the remainder of infections.[38] This is a seasonal illness, occurring predominately during winter months and most commonly affecting children from age 6 months to 3 years. There is frequently a history of prodromal infection accompanied by an unusual cough (described as sounding like the bark of a seal). Swelling of the tracheal mucosa in the subglottic region causes airway compromise (Fig. 50.9). Medical attention is usually sought when the child develops inspiratory stridor and respiratory distress. Various scales have been devised to quantify the severity of the stridor to document the progression of the illness and the response to therapy. One of the most commonly employed scales is the Westley scale,[39] which has been validated (Table 50.1).[40]

When a chest radiograph is obtained during an episode of laryngotracheobronchitis, the trachea is seen to have a gradual progressive narrowing of its lumen, reaching the narrowest point just below the vocal cords (the "steeple sign") (Fig. 50.10). The upper glottis, as seen on a lateral neck radiograph, is normal.

Many care providers believe that exposing the child to cold or misty air often dramatically improves the symptoms, although evidence in support of this therapy is lacking.[37,41,42] When the illness is refractory to these measures, racemic epinephrine has been shown to produce measurable reduction of airway obstruction.[43] This probably is accomplished by stimulation of the α-adrenergic receptors, producing vasoconstriction and resulting in diminished tracheal edema. Rebound tracheal edema may occur several hours later as the effect of the racemic epinephrine dissipates. Because this problem is unpredictable, the child should be admitted to the hospital for observation after racemic epinephrine has been used.

TABLE 50.1 Westley Croup Score

	0	1	2	3	4	5
Chest wall retraction	None	Mild	Moderate	Severe		
Stridor	None	With agitation	At rest			
Cyanosis	None				With agitation	At rest
Level of consciousness	Normal					Disoriented
Air entry	Normal	Decreased	Markedly decreased			

Total score ranges from 0-17 points (severe croup).[37]
From Johnson DW. Croup. BMJ Clin Evid. 2014;2014.

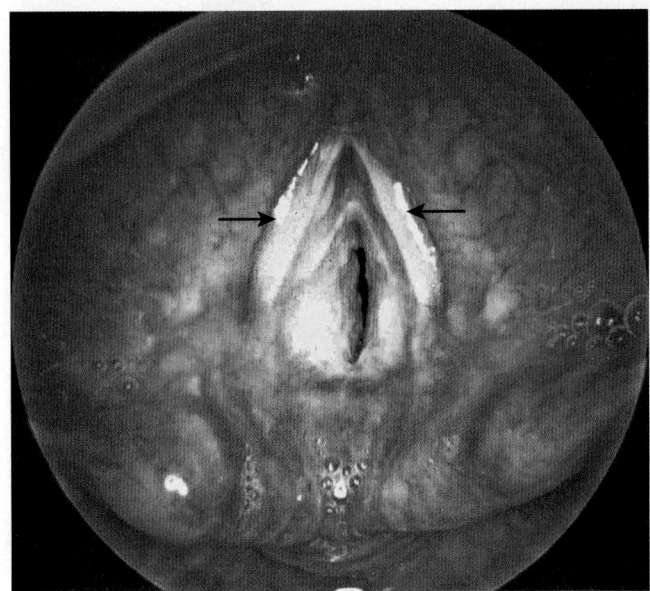

Fig. 50.9. Laryngotracheobronchitis: Below the level of the vocal cords the trachea appears swollen and the tracheal walls are covered with purulent material (vocal cords are indicated by *arrows*).

The practice of treating laryngotracheobronchitis with corticosteroids is widespread, especially for hospitalized patients.[44] Oral, intramuscular, and nebulized corticosteroids have been shown to be beneficial in randomized, blinded trials.[45,46] Meta-analyses in which the efficacy of corticosteroids was evaluated suggest that corticosteroids reduce the need for endotracheal intubation or inhaled epinephrine, hasten improvement in the first 24 hours of illness, shorten the duration of hospitalization, and reduce the frequency of readmission.[37] Mixtures of 70% helium and 30% oxygen (heliox) may be beneficial in more severe cases of laryngotracheobronchitis because the characteristics of this mixture permit greater gas flow past areas of airway narrowing.[47]

Endotracheal intubation is occasionally necessary when laryngotracheobronchitis proves refractory to medical intervention. Unless merited by special circumstances, such as severe subglottic stenosis in association with laryngotracheobronchitis, tracheostomy offers no advantages over endotracheal intubation. The endotracheal tube should be smaller than would normally be used to avoid additional injury to the swollen tracheal mucosa. If the tracheal edema is severe, even a small tube may fit tightly in the trachea.

Later, when an audible leak around the endotracheal tube is present, the trachea may be extubated with a high probability that reintubation will not be necessary.[48] If a leak does not become audible after 2 to 4 days, it is our practice to extubate the trachea, because prolonged intubation may increase the risk for subglottic injury. Racemic epinephrine is commonly needed to treat stridor after extubation. If a patient should have especially severe or recurrent laryngotracheobronchitis, an anatomic lesion causing tracheal narrowing should be suspected.

Recurrent croup is a frequently encountered problem. Physicians caring for these patients are often pressed to consider further evaluation to determine if an anatomic abnormality may be responsible for the problem. A review of the experience of rigid bronchoscopic evaluation of children with recurrent croup indicates that gastroesophageal reflux is common in these children (45%), whereas only 11% of the children had anatomic anomalies requiring surgical intervention.[49]

Epiglottitis

Epiglottitis caused by *Haemophilus influenzae* type B was once a common cause of serious respiratory illness in pediatric patients, but because of widespread use of the *H. influenzae* type B vaccine, this is now an uncommon illness in young children.[50] Patients who present with epiglottis are now older, with an average age of 11.6 years as opposed to an average age of 5.8 years before the advent of Hib vaccination.[51] Although cases of *H. influenzae* epiglottis continue to occur, even among vaccinated patients,[52] other causes of epiglottitis have assumed greater importance in the postvaccination era. Group A β-hemolytic *Streptococcus* is now identified as the cause of epiglottitis in many patients and is clinically indistinguishable from epiglottitis caused by *H. influenzae* type B.[53] Thermal injury to the epiglottis from ingesting hot liquids can also cause epiglottitis.[54] Several points serve to distinguish epiglottitis from laryngotracheobronchitis (Table 50.2).

Although infrequently seen, the management of epiglottitis in young children is a multidisciplinary undertaking, involving pediatric intensive care specialists, anesthesiologists, and otolaryngologists. When a child with presumed epiglottitis is admitted to the emergency department, this team should be notified in anticipation of taking the child to the operating room to secure his or her airway. As the team members are being notified, lateral radiographs of the neck may be obtained if tolerated by the patient. This may be done with the child sitting on the parent's lap to minimize the child's anxiety. In

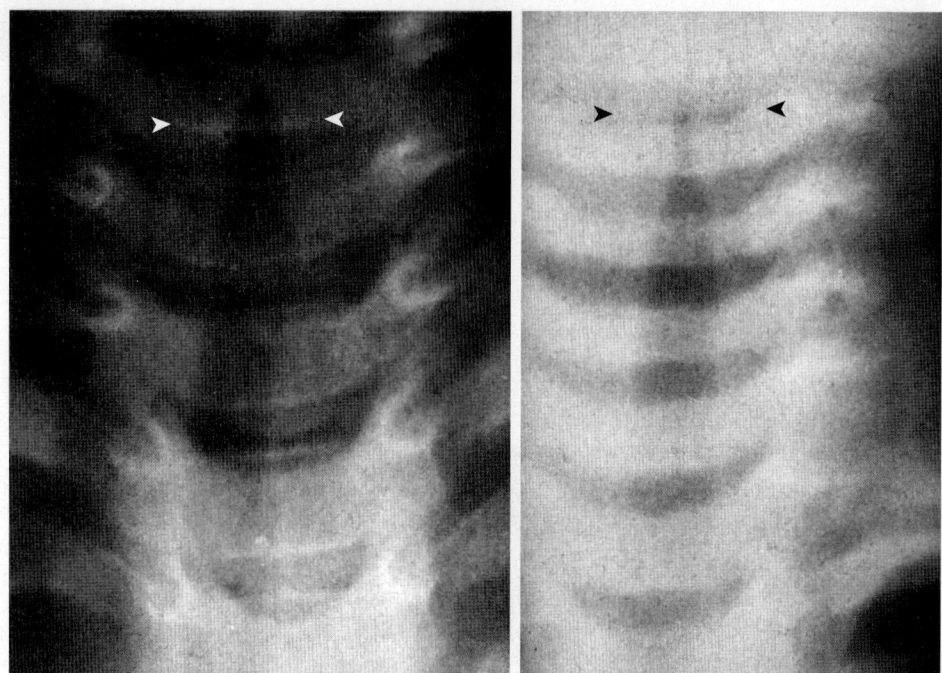

Fig. 50.10. Anteroposterior radiograph of the neck. *(Left)* A normal tracheal air column (between the *arrows*). *(Right)* Trachea narrowed by laryngotracheobronchitis.

TABLE 50.2	Characteristics of Laryngotracheobronchitis, Bacterial Tracheitis, and Epiglottitis		
	Laryngotracheobronchitis	**Bacterial Tracheitis**	**Epiglottitis**
Age	3 mo to 3 yr	6 mo to 12 yr	12 yr (average)
Onset	Gradual	Intermediate	<24 hr
Fever	Usually low	Usually high	High
Cough	Characteristic "barking"	Characteristic "barking"	None
Sore throat	None	Usually absent	Often severe
Drooling	No	No	Usually
Posture	Any position	Any position	Sitting forward, mouth open, drooling
Voice	Normal	Normal or hoarse	Muffled
Appearance	Nontoxic	Toxic	Toxic
Seasonal distribution	Usually winter, epidemic	Throughout the year	Throughout the year

epiglottitis, the anteroposterior view of the trachea appears normal, but a lateral neck radiograph shows a markedly swollen and edematous epiglottis (Fig. 50.11). The diagnostic evaluation of the patient should proceed expeditiously, while care is taken to disturb the patient as little as possible. For this reason, fiberoptic examination of the epiglottis in the awake patient is usually not advisable. Attempts to examine the oropharynx directly or to start an intravenous line should be discouraged. The apprehension caused by these events may lead to tracheal obstruction by the enlarged epiglottis. If the patient will tolerate it, humidified oxygen should be administered, preferably through a plastic hose held by the parent.

If the diagnosis of epiglottitis is strongly suspected or confirmed on the lateral neck x-ray film, the child should go to the operating room as quickly as possible. In the operating room, the patient is anesthetized with an inhaled anesthetic

(sevoflurane) and oxygen while the patient is spontaneously breathing. Once the patient has been anesthetized, an intravenous catheter is inserted. Laryngoscopy is then performed (Fig. 50.12). It may be exceedingly difficult to obtain a direct view of the glottis and trachea because of the large swollen epiglottis. Nevertheless, it is almost always possible to pass an endotracheal tube through the edematous tissues and into the trachea. Nasotracheal intubation is preferred to orotracheal intubation because the tube is more readily secured to the face, the patient cannot bite the tube, and salivation is decreased. An otolaryngologist should be in the operating room and ready to do an emergency tracheostomy if an airway cannot be secured by endotracheal intubation, although this is rarely necessary. As with laryngotracheobronchitis, endotracheal intubation is preferred to tracheostomy because it has been shown that complications are more common when a

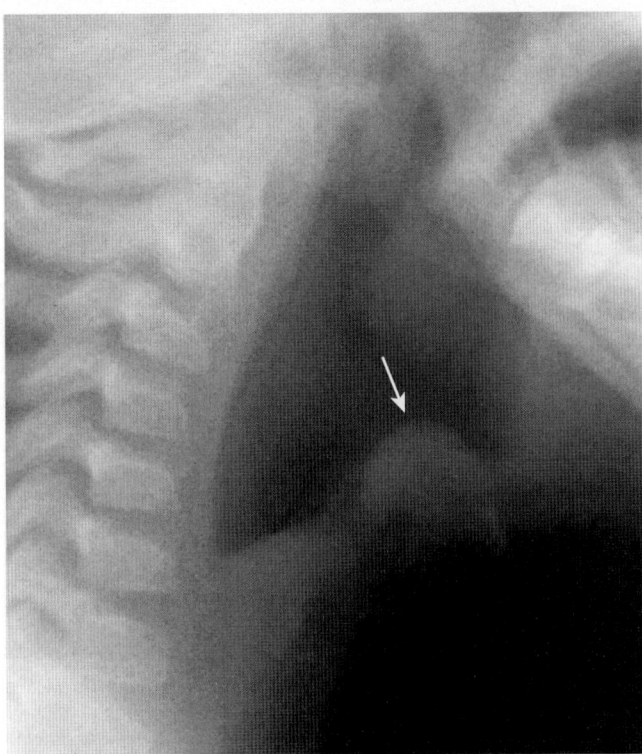

Fig. 50.11. Lateral radiograph of the neck of a patient with epiglottitis. Note the large, swollen epiglottis *(arrow)*.

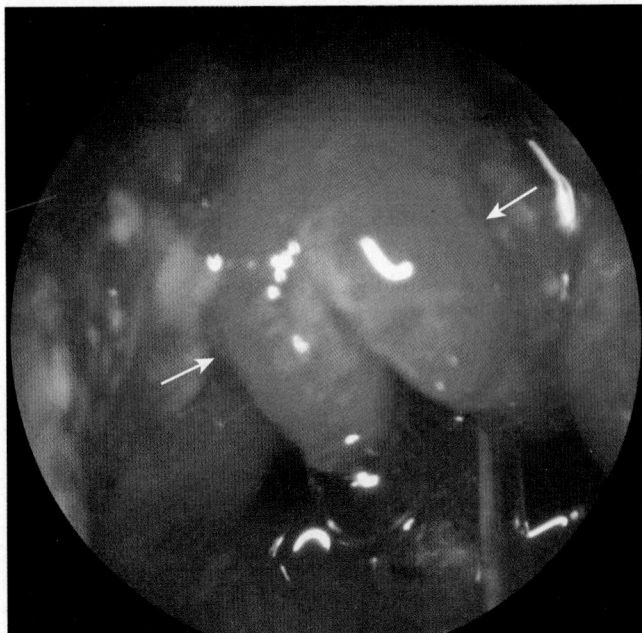

Figure 50.12. Epiglottitis causing a severely swollen epiglottis *(between the arrows)*. In the lower portion of the picture, the endotracheal tube can be seen. (Copyright Andrew F. Inglis, Jr.)

tracheostomy has been routinely used to treat epiglottitis. After the airway is secured, blood cultures and cultures of the epiglottis are obtained, and antibiotic therapy is initiated with a penicillinase-resistant antibiotic because of the high incidence of *H. influenzae* resistance to ampicillin.[55]

In the PICU, patients usually require endotracheal intubation for 24 to 72 hours while the swollen epiglottis returns to normal size. The patient may be allowed to breathe spontaneously through the endotracheal tube or may undergo mechanical ventilation. Variable amounts of sedation are usually necessary. Extraepiglottic sites of *H. influenzae* infection are common.

The management of epiglottitis depends on the patient's age. Adults and teenagers with epiglottitis usually present with severe pharyngitis but usually have mild or absent airway obstruction. In contrast to younger unsedated children, teenagers and adults are more likely to tolerate examination of the airway with a small fiberoptic bronchoscope. This procedure may have superior diagnostic sensitivity compared to lateral neck radiographs. Although the management of epiglottitis in young children is almost always accomplished with placement of an endotracheal tube, teenagers and adult patients may be admitted to the hospital for close observation and expectant airway management. Endotracheal intubation is reserved for patients who develop respiratory compromise.[56,57]

Peritonsillar Abscess

The initial presentation of peritonsillar abscess may resemble that of epiglottitis. The child usually has a severe sore throat and may have a muffled voice and drooling. Imaging studies such as CT scan or transcervical ultrasonography may be used to confirm the physical findings.[58] Approximately half of the children with peritonsillar abscess are managed medically and the other half require surgical intervention, either abscess drainage or tonsillectomy.[59] Although trismus may be of concern in evaluation of the patient for anesthesia, there is usually no anatomic restriction of jaw movement. Once the patient has been anesthetized, the mouth may be easily opened. Extubation can usually be performed immediately after the abscess has been drained, unless there is severe inflammation and swelling extending well beyond the tonsillar bed. Commonly encountered microorganisms include group A *Streptococcus*[60] and *Fusobacterium* species.[61]

Retropharyngeal Abscess

Over 80% of children with retropharyngeal abscess are younger than 6 years.[62] Patients may have fever, stiff neck, sore throat, and, in severe cases, respiratory distress. During examination of the oropharynx, the posterior pharyngeal wall may be observed to bulge, but most commonly the findings are unremarkable. Palpation of the posterior pharyngeal wall should be avoided because it may cause rupture of the abscess with possible spillage of the contents into the tracheobronchial tree. The presence of torticollis is seen much more frequently when an abscess is present.[62] An inspiratory radiograph of the lateral neck may show thickening of the prevertebral soft tissue, and occasionally an air-fluid level may be present (Fig. 50.13). A chest radiograph should be obtained to evaluate possible mediastinal extension of the infection. Contrast CT scanning is commonly employed to evaluate these infections; however, evidence of abscess on CT scan does not reliably predict the quantity of purulent material obtained at the time of surgical drainage.[63]

Depending on the severity of the abscess, a large proportion of patients treated with antibiotic therapy can be cured

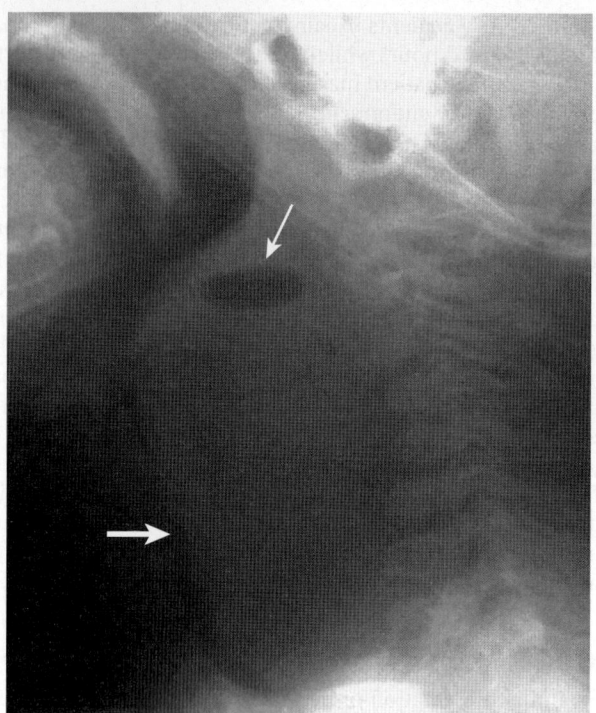

Fig. 50.13. Lateral radiograph of the neck of a patient with retropharyngeal abscess. Note the thickening of the prevertebral soft tissue and the radiolucent area caused by the presence of air in the tissue *(arrows)*. (Copyright Andrew F. Inglis, Jr.)

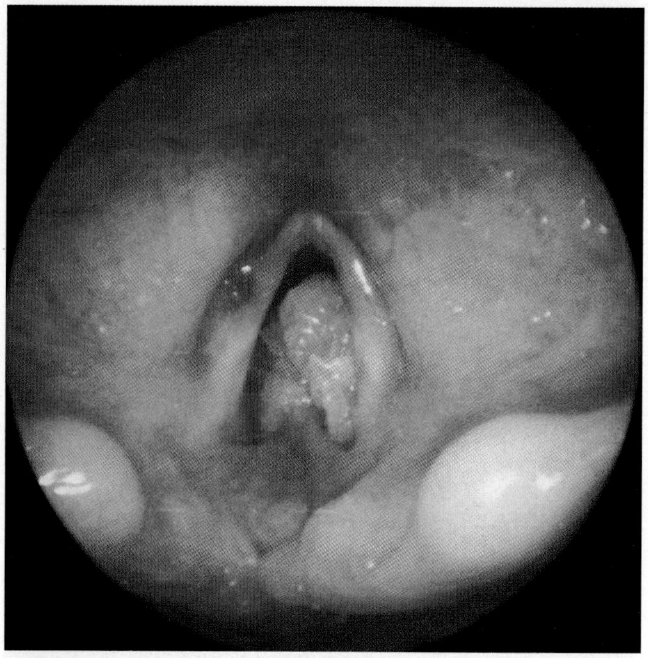

Fig. 50.14. Large, pedunculated papilloma is seen just below the vocal cords. These papillomas almost completely occluded the tracheal lumen and produced marked respiratory distress. (Copyright Andrew F. Inglis, Jr.)

without surgical intervention.[64-66] Surgical treatment of this lesion is drainage of the abscess, after the patient has been anesthetized and an endotracheal tube has been inserted to protect the patient from pulmonary aspiration of the purulent fluid.

Bacterial Tracheitis

The peak incidence of this infection occurs in the fall and winter and tends to affect children between 6 months and 8 years of age. Bacterial tracheitis is a secondary infection that begins during a viral upper respiratory infection.[67-69] Frequently, but not always, bacterial tracheitis will resemble viral laryngotracheobronchitis (croup); however, patients with bacterial tracheitis usually have a high fever and may appear very ill at the time of presentation (see Table 50.2). Unlike patients with croup, these patients show little or no response to nebulized racemic epinephrine. Bronchoscopy, which is the definitive diagnostic procedure, shows normal supraglottic structures and diffuse inflammation of the larynx, trachea, and bronchi,[70] with adherent or semiadherent purulent membranes in the trachea.[71] Endotracheal intubation is often necessary because of severe, progressive respiratory distress. Following endotracheal intubation, aggressive tracheobronchial toilet may be necessary because thick, tenacious purulent debris may rapidly occlude the endotracheal tube.

A variety of bacterial agents have been reported in association with this illness, including *Moraxella catarrhalis, Staphylococcus aureus, Haemophilus influenzae* type B, and *Pneumococcus*.[72,73] The injury to the respiratory epithelium caused by the virus may predispose the patients to bacterial superinfection. The most common complication of bacterial

tracheitis is pneumonia, which is observed in approximately 60% of patients with this illness. Antibiotics are an important aspect of therapy and should be directed by the results of bacterial cultures obtained during bronchoscopy or immediately after endotracheal intubation.

Laryngeal Papillomatosis

The laryngeal papilloma is the most common benign tumor of the larynx during childhood. The agent causing this disease is human papilloma virus, with types 6 and 11 causing the majority of cases.[74] Despite its nonmalignant structure, the propensity of this tumor to cause respiratory obstruction may result in injury to the patient or death. The onset of symptoms occurs between infancy and 4 years of age. New onset of infection is less frequent after age 5 years. The most common medical complaint in these children is voice change, which occurs in more than 90% of the patients. Airway obstruction is present in almost half of the patients, although it is mild in many of these. The presence of inspiratory stridor may misdirect the diagnostician to think that the child has laryngotracheobronchitis. The diagnosis is typically made with laryngoscopy (Fig. 50.14).

The treatment for this illness is surgical excision of the polyps.[75] Induction of anesthesia in the child with severe airway obstruction may be hazardous, because it may be difficult or impossible to ventilate the child's lungs after loss of consciousness. Although patients characteristically require multiple surgical resections of these lesions (an average of 11 resections over the course of the disease), the mortality with this illness is low. Carbon dioxide laser vaporization of the papillomata is widely used. During laser excision of lesions caused by a similar viral agent, anogenital condylomas, medical personnel have become infected with the virus, presumably from viable virus particles carried in the smoke plume.[76]

A variety of adjuvant therapies have been developed to reduce the frequency of relapse following surgical treatment.[77] These adjuvant therapies include interferon-α, acyclovir, valacyclovir, and cidofovir, among others. It has been suggested that the human papillomavirus (HPV) vaccine may reduce the incidence and recurrence of laryngeal papillomatosis.[78]

Vocal Cord Paralysis

The recurrent laryngeal nerves supply the bulk of the motor innervation to the larynx. These nerves originate in the nucleus ambiguous in the brain stem, travel to the chest with the vagus nerve, and then loop back up to the larynx in the tracheoesophageal groove. The left recurrent laryngeal nerve loops under the ductus arteriosus in the chest, and thus it is vulnerable to injury during ligation of this vessel and with other thoracic vascular procedures.[79] Symptoms associated with even complete unilateral vocal cord paralysis vary greatly in severity. In infants, they may range from a mildly diminished cry to a severely disabled larynx with significant stridor, feeding difficulties from aspiration, and loss of voice.[80] Bilateral vocal cord paralysis almost always produces significant stridor with varying degrees of airway distress.[81] Stridor in these instances is typically inspiratory and may be confused with laryngomalacia, a much more common entity. Over half of the patients have associated anomalies including concomitant airway diseases.[37,81] Diagnosis can usually be made at the bedside by fiberoptic laryngoscopy.[82]

Congenital vocal cord paralysis is usually idiopathic and often resolves spontaneously over several months. This is the most common cause of bilateral vocal cord paralysis in children.[83] Other neurologic causes, such as Arnold-Chiari malformation, are occasionally seen, and workup usually includes an MRI. The cause of acquired vocal cord paralysis is usually obvious, with most cases coming after thoracic or cervical surgery.[81,84]

The treatment of vocal cord paralysis in the critical care setting is primarily supportive. Airway support may include temporizing with high-flow nasal oxygen or continuous positive airway pressure/biphasic positive airway pressure (CPAP/BiPAP).[37] Over 60% of patients with bilateral and some with unilateral vocal cord paralysis require tracheostomy,[37,81] but procedures aimed at enlarging the glottic airway—vocal cordotomy, arytenoidectomy, vocal cord lateralization, and posterior cricoid split and cartilage grafting[82]—should be delayed, as spontaneous recovery is possible within the first 2 years.[85] If a specific lesion may be addressed medically or surgically (such as decompression of the brain stem in Arnold-Chiari malformation), such therapy should be undertaken.

Intrathoracic Mass Lesions Causing Respiratory Obstruction

The intrathoracic trachea may be compressed by a variety of anterior mediastinal masses. Because the symptoms produced by a malignant mass impinging on the trachea can worsen dramatically over several days, the child with respiratory compromise resulting from a mediastinal mass deserves rapid evaluation and aggressive medical therapy.

Before caring for a child with this problem, the parents should be asked if the child refuses to lie in certain positions. The child's reluctance to recline in a given position may be caused by airway compromise from the mass. Forcing the child to lie down may result in airway obstruction or even cardiac arrest.[86] Endotracheal intubation is indicated only if respiratory function becomes severely compromised. Unfortunately, this measure may be of little benefit, because the lesion may compress the bronchi distal to the tip of the endotracheal tube requiring advancing the endotracheal tube into the mainstem bronchi.[87] In addition, it may be impossible to ventilate the child's lungs after muscle relaxants have been administered to facilitate placement of the endotracheal tube. Mechanical support with extracorporeal membrane oxygenation (ECMO) has been used to assist patients with large mediastinal masses; however, the mass may distort the great vessels and pose unusual challenges for the ECMO team.[88] Obtaining tissue for a pathologic diagnosis can be a challenge, as these patients are at significant risk for anesthetic complications.[89,90] It is therefore recommended that the least invasive and lowest risk diagnostic intervention is employed first, when appropriate. When mediastinal biopsy under anesthesia is inevitable, preparations should be made to rapidly treat intraoperative complications by changing patient position, opening the intrathoracic airway with rigid bronchoscopy, performing emergency thoraco/sternotomy, or implementing ECMO cannulation via the femoral vessels.[91]

Trauma

Postextubation Stridor

After endotracheal intubation that lasts more than a few hours, postextubation stridor is a relatively common problem in small children and is most frequently caused by laryngeal edema. Estimates of the frequency of postextubation stridor in children vary widely. Most authors cite figures of less than 2% to 9%,[92,93] although the incidence may be as high as 37% in patients with trauma or burns.[94]

In addition to audible stridor, patients with this problem show decreased air movement, flaring of the alae nasi, and, in more severe cases, decreased arterial oxygen saturation and mental status changes. The severity of these signs reliably indicates the severity of airway obstruction.[95]

Several risks are associated with the development of postextubation stridor. Endotracheal tube size plays an important role, because too large an endotracheal tube may compress the tracheal mucosa, causing submucosal ischemia. When the endotracheal tube is removed, the injured tissue may swell and partially obstruct the larynx. Endotracheal tube movement within the trachea may produce trauma to the tracheal mucosa, resulting in tissue injury and swelling. Whether stridor occurs depends on the extent of the swelling and the diameter of the child's airway. Small patients are more likely to have postextubation stridor because a larger proportion of their airway is obstructed with a given degree of swelling and because of the unfavorable characteristics of turbulent flow through small passages. Lack of an audible leak of air around the endotracheal tube is frequently used as a predictor of postextubation stridor in children; however, one study suggests that this measure may be valid only in children ages 7 years and older.[96]

The presence of an endotracheal tube cuff was felt to contribute to the risk of postextubation stridor in children younger than 8 years of age, where the subglottic region is the narrowest portion of the airway. More recent data, however, show that with careful monitoring of cuff pressure,[97,98] the use of endotracheal tubes with low pressure–high volume cuff is not only safe in term neonates, infants, and children[92,93,99] but, given their numerous advantages, are preferable.[100,92,93,99,93]

Postextubation stridor has a greater risk of developing in children with trisomy 21; as many as one-third of these patients have stridor after extubation. There appear to be several causes for this problem, including hypotonia and facial abnormalities, such as a large tongue.

Although most cases of postextubation stridor are caused by laryngeal edema, when this problem persists, other causes should be sought. Anatomic airway anomalies, which may not be visible during endotracheal intubation (such as tracheal hemangioma), may cause persistent postextubation stridor. Vocal cord paralysis is one of the more common causes of persistent postextubation stridor and may be caused by increased intracranial pressure, brain stem compression,[101] trauma to the brain stem after neurosurgery, or recurrent laryngeal nerve during thoracic surgery.[102]

The therapy of postextubation stridor is aimed at reducing airway edema. Racemic epinephrine and dexamethasone are the most widely used therapeutic agents. Racemic epinephrine, delivered by aerosol nebulizer, probably works by stimulation of α-adrenergic receptors; this stimulation causes vasoconstriction, which, in turn, reduces tracheal edema. Racemic epinephrine works rapidly, so improvement, when it occurs, should be observed within a few minutes of completion of therapy. Mixtures of helium and oxygen have also proved helpful in the treatment of postextubation stridor.[103]

The practice of using dexamethasone to treat postextubation stridor is widespread,[104] although the efficacy of this therapy remains controversial. Although data from animal studies suggest that corticosteroid use at the time of extubation may reduce tracheal edema, inflammation, and capillary dilation, a meta-analysis of prior studies failed to show reduction of postextubation stridor after corticosteroid use.[105] Nevertheless, many practitioners think that dexamethasone (or an equivalent dose of another steroid) will ameliorate postextubation stridor, especially if the medication is administered several hours before extubation.

In most cases, postextubation stridor is self-limited, but occasionally, endotracheal intubation may be necessary. If the degree of airway obstruction before reintubation was severe, postobstructive pulmonary edema may be observed and should be treated with positive end-expiratory pressure. When reintubation is contemplated, the size of the previous endotracheal tube should be determined, and a smaller endotracheal tube should be selected in the hope of preventing additional tracheal injury. Ideally, the trachea should remain intubated until a leak around the endotracheal tube is observed, indicating resolution of the laryngeal edema.

Laryngotracheal (Subglottic) Stenosis

Laryngotracheal stenosis is most commonly seen as a complication of prolonged endotracheal intubation, and as such it is

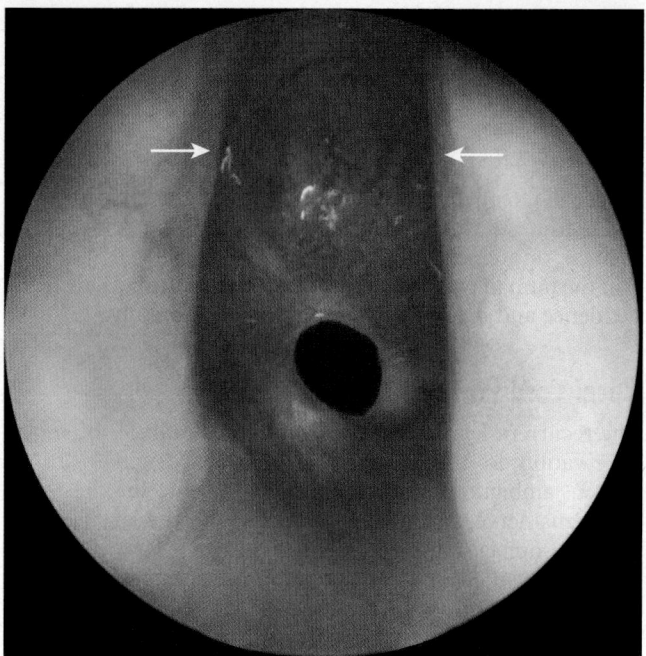

Fig. 50.15. A cicatricial ring *(between the arrows)* is demonstrated just below the glottis. This was caused by trauma from prolonged endotracheal intubation. (Copyright Andrew F. Inglis, Jr.)

of special interest to the critical care practitioner (Fig. 50.15). Injury most commonly occurs in the larynx at the level of the cricoid cartilage, just below the vocal cords, the only part of the airway below the nose that is surrounded by a complete circumferential ring of cartilage. This region cannot expand under pressure and is thus more susceptible to pressure necrosis and scarring (subglottic stenosis). Airway stenosis also can occur at the level of the vocal cords (glottic stenosis) when scarring occurs within the cricoarytenoid joints (cricoarytenoid ankylosis) or between the arytenoid cartilages (interarytenoid fibrosis). Glottic stenosis prevents vocal cord abduction and occasionally may be confused with bilateral vocal cord paralysis. Rarely, tracheal stenosis may be seen as a result of endotracheal tube (ETT) cuff injury, often in the setting of infection requiring high-pressure ventilation.

Laryngeal intubation injury appears to result from an interaction of several elements, including individual susceptibility, movement of the endotracheal tube, size of the ETT, presence of infection, and duration of intubation. Fortunately, the incidence of this complication in neonates appears to be decreasing.[106] The odds of prevention will be enhanced by choosing the smallest tube that allows adequate ventilation and pulmonary care; this reduces the risk of subglottic stenosis. It is also thought that nasotracheal intubation may reduce movement of the ETT within the airway and thus diminish trauma, although this benefit comes with an increased risk of sinusitis secondary to obstruction of drainage from the sinus cavities. Gastroesophageal reflux is frequently present and perhaps plays a significant role in the development of laryngotracheal stenosis.[106] The role of early intervention with a tracheotomy for the prevention of laryngeal stenosis is controversial.[107]

Chronic laryngeal stenosis can be managed a variety of ways.[108] The obstruction may be bypassed with a tracheotomy or may be managed with high-pressure balloon dilatation, endoscopic excision of scar, cricoid expansion via cricoid split and cartilage grafts, and excision of the stenotic segment and reanastomosis via partial cricotracheal resection.[109] Postoperative management of these patients is frequently complicated by the need to allow the larynx to heal for 5 to 14 days while maintaining a patent airway with an endotracheal tube. Management of the patient during this critical period is controversial. Some favor heavy sedation including the use of neuromuscular blocking agents to minimize the chance of movement of the ETT and accidental extubation. Others favor the opposite, actually allowing the patient to be alert and active with the ETT in place.[110,111]

Ideally, reconstruction will be performed at a young age (younger than 25 months) to minimize the time period the child is exposed to the hazards of being dependent on the tracheotomy airway and so that the child's speech and language development are not impaired.[112] Earlier laryngotracheal reconstruction may, however, be more prone to failure and require revision procedures.

Foreign Body Aspiration

Airway obstruction may be produced by aspiration of a variety of foreign bodies, with nuts, seeds, and legumes (peanuts) being the most frequent offenders in children.[113,114] Most of the patients aspirating foreign bodies are aged 1 to 3 years, with more than 95% being younger than 10 years. Fewer than 30% of patients aspirating foreign bodies receive medical attention within the first 24 hours, with many patients experiencing a significant delay before seeking medical attention.[115] Patients with an aspirated foreign body may initially be symptom-free or may have a cough, wheezing, and evidence of respiratory embarrassment. Patients without symptoms who do not seek medical attention may have a persistent cough and may develop pneumonia distal to the obstructed bronchus. Recurrent bouts of pneumonia may lead to bronchiectasis if the foreign body is not removed.

Foreign bodies may become lodged in the airway anywhere from the posterior pharynx to the bronchi. The symptoms produced by foreign body aspiration vary according to the site of the foreign body and the degree of obstruction it produces. Foreign bodies of the extrathoracic airway characteristically produce inspiratory stridor. Foreign bodies lodged in the intrathoracic trachea and bronchi tend to produce expiratory stridor and wheezing.

Radiographic evaluation should include inspiratory and expiratory radiographs because a single anteroposterior radiograph will be unremarkable in 18% of children with an aspirated foreign body (Fig. 50.16).[115] If the foreign body is producing ball-valve bronchial obstruction, hyperinflation of the involved lung will be seen during the expiratory radiogram. Many foreign bodies are not radiopaque,[116] so failure to see a foreign body on the chest radiograph cannot exclude this diagnosis. If a suspicion of an aspiration is high, a bronchoscopy is warranted (Fig. 50.17).

Foreign bodies are removed from the tracheobronchial tree with a rigid or, less commonly, with a flexible bronchoscope.[117] Occasionally this is impossible and tracheostomy or thoracotomy for bronchotomy or lobectomy is required.[118] Cardiopulmonary bypass has been successfully used to support a patient who had extensive foreign body aspiration.

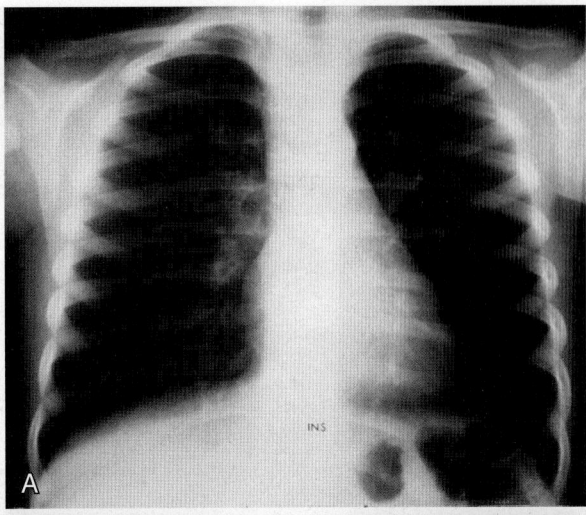
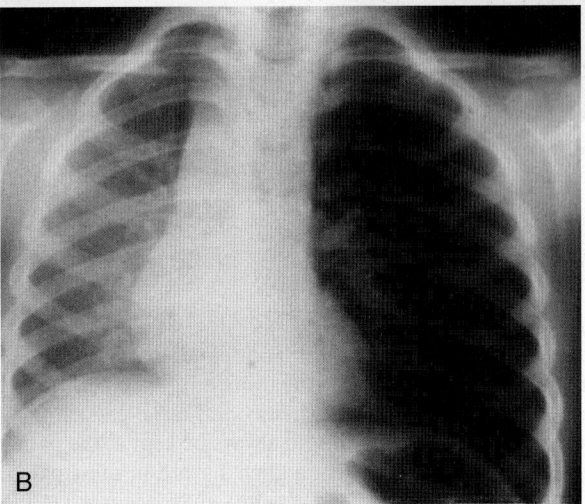

Fig. 50.16. Inspiratory chest radiograph with foreign body present in left mainstem bronchus. During inspiration (A), the left lung is slightly hyperinflated but could be considered normal. The expiratory radiograph (B) clearly demonstrates that the left lung is hyperinflated because of air trapping by the foreign body. (A and B, Courtesy Eric Effmann, MD.)

Traumatic Injury to the Airway

Traumatic injury to the upper airway may be divided into two broad categories: oral facial trauma and laryngeal/tracheal trauma. Patients with obvious oral facial trauma may be at risk for upper airway obstruction. Even if the patients have no sign of respiratory distress at the time of presentation, swelling of soft tissues and hemorrhaging to the airway may lead to airway compromise.

Patients who must undergo operative intervention to treat their traumatic injuries need careful evaluation of their airway, including radiographs and CT scan examination. Traumatic injuries may make intubations in the trachea difficult in these patients. For this reason, sedation is to be avoided and endotracheal intubation with the patient awake should be considered. This may be accomplished with direct laryngoscopy after local anesthesia has been applied to the patient's oropharynx. In more difficult cases, it may be necessary to use a fiberoptic bronchoscope to guide the ETT into the trachea.

Postoperatively, patients undergoing repair of facial trauma may have their jaw wired shut and the nasal/submental ETT

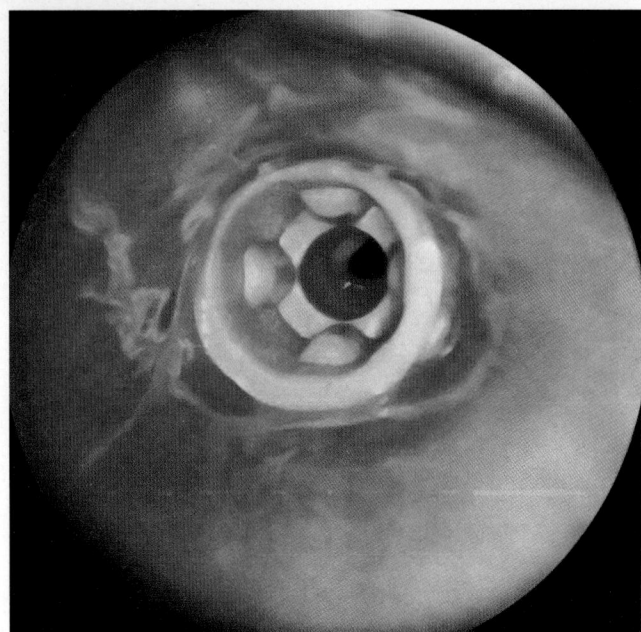

Fig. 50.17. Hollow plastic foreign body in patient's trachea. Because the object was not radiopaque, it could not be observed on a chest radiograph, and because the lumen of the foreign body was aligned with the tracheal lumen, severe respiratory embarrassment did not occur. (Copyright Andrew F. Inglis, Jr.)

sutured in place to prevent accidental extubation. These patients should undergo extubation only when fully awake and after resolution of their airway and facial edema. Instruments to open the wires should always be kept at the patient's bedside. Emesis may present a grave hazard in these patients.

Injury to the larynx and trachea may occur after blunt trauma such as automobile accidents, after penetrating trauma, clothesline injury, or with crush injuries such as hanging. Blunt trauma to the neck may lead to fracture of the cartilaginous rings supporting the trachea or to disruption of the tracheal mucosa. In the latter case, attempted endotracheal intubation may worsen a partial tracheal transection and create an airway emergency.[119] Signs of laryngeal injury include dyspnea, altered phonation, odynophagia, hoarseness, hemoptysis, swelling, and subcutaneous emphysema of the neck. The development of subcutaneous emphysema after blunt trauma to the neck suggests that a laryngeal fracture or tracheal tear has occurred. The quantity of air in the subcutaneous tissues does not correlate with the severity of the injury.[120] Establishment of an adequate airway is an essential consideration. Although the standard of care in management used to be surgical repair, often preceded by tracheostomy placement, conservative management with prolonged endotracheal intubation is now acceptable,[121] and tracheostomy is only necessary in about one-third of cases.[122]

Blunt thoracic trauma can cause tracheal or bronchial disruption. Most commonly, these are blowout injuries that result in tracheobronchial disruption. These injuries usually occur near the carina, and most involve mainstem bronchi.[123] Because children have flexible ribs, severe intrathoracic injuries can occur without rib fractures. The signs of tracheobronchial disruption include persistent air leak, failure to expand the lung with thoracostomy tube drainage, and massive atelectasis (from failure to conduct gas through an injured bronchus). Diagnosis of these injuries is usually made with bronchoscopy. Although small tracheobronchial disruptions may be managed conservatively, most of these lesions require surgical repair.[123]

Burn Injury to the Upper Airway

Thermal injury to the upper airway may complicate the management of a patient with burns. The presence of facial burns and singed nasal hairs, hoarseness, or inspiratory stridor should suggest the possibility of burn injury to the upper airway. Although respiratory compromise may not be present at the time of admission, it may develop later as swelling of the injured airway becomes more severe. Because of the efficient cooling capacity of the upper air passages, thermal injury to the airway below the vocal cords is uncommon, occurring in less than 5% of all hospitalized patients with burns.

Evidence of respiratory embarrassment in a patient with burns should be rapidly evaluated. Neck radiographs and fiberoptic examination of the larynx may show swelling of the soft tissues of the airway. If these findings are present, endotracheal intubation should be expeditiously performed to secure the airway before obstruction occurs. Because of the risk of infection, attempts are made to avoid tracheostomy placement in the patient with burns, and data suggest this is a safe practice.[107] Upper airway embarrassment is often accompanied by smoke inhalation injury to the lower airway, resulting in hypoxemia and hypercapnia. The products of combustion result in severe carbon monoxide intoxication or cyanide poisoning, both of which have nonspecific symptoms but require prompt medical therapy.[124]

Angioedema

Angioedema is a well-demarcated localized edema involving the deep layers of skin, including the subcutaneous tissue. Angioedema may occur in response to a variety of systemic disorders, including allergic reactions that are mediated with immunoglobulin E, anaphylactic and anaphylactoid reactions, and other illnesses. Angioedema may lead to swelling of the soft tissue of the face, particularly the eyes and lips. If this should involve the soft tissues of the upper respiratory tract, laryngeal obstruction may result. Administration of subcutaneous epinephrine may dramatically reduce swelling caused by this condition. Compared to adults, children often have a rapid response to antihistamines and steroids.[125] Occasionally, respiratory embarrassment caused by this condition is so severe that endotracheal intubation is warranted. The evaluation of patients with this disorder should be directed at (1) the identification of the causative agents so that the patients can avoid these in the future and (2) the anatomic site of presentation to allow stratification of airway risk and planning of appropriate triage for airway intervention.[126]

Tracheostomy

Indications for the placement of a tracheostomy fall into three broad, frequently overlapping categories: airway obstruction, assisted ventilation, and pulmonary toilet. Pediatric anatomic anomalies that may necessitate tracheostomy are most often manifested in the neonatal period or in infancy, although some may not appear until childhood. The most common abnormalities include vocal cord paralysis (congenital and postbirth injury), subglottic stenosis, tracheal stenosis, cystic hygroma, tracheal hemangioma, and laryngeal cyst. The accurate diagnosis of these problems is frequently made during bronchoscopic examination of the larynx and trachea while the patient is anesthetized. If the obstruction is of sufficient magnitude, consideration should be given to doing a tracheotomy at the time of bronchoscopy.

Infants may require a tracheostomy because of the need for prolonged periods of assisted ventilation. The advent of neonatal intensive care has enabled small preterm infants to survive despite severe respiratory illness. Many of these patients will need lengthy periods of mechanical ventilation to treat infant respiratory distress syndrome and bronchopulmonary dysplasia. Prolonged intubation may lead to subglottic stenosis.[127] For a reduction in the frequency of this complication, a tracheostomy may be performed. The optimal timing of tracheostomy for children who need long-term intubation is controversial. In many neonatal ICUs, infants needing mechanical ventilatory support for more than 30 to 45 days will undergo a tracheostomy. Placement of a tracheostomy is not a trivial matter, with several large studies showing a tracheostomy-related mortality rate of 0.5% to 0.7%.[128,129] One study provided evidence that long-term tracheostomy is associated with airway inflammation (number of cells, neutrophils), more frequent bacteria, and reduced concentration of surfactant protein-D.[130] The decline of polio in the United States during the decade following 1950 dramatically decreased the number of tracheostomies performed to facilitate mechanical ventilation and pulmonary toilet. Nevertheless, several pediatric diseases predictably lead to prolonged neuromuscular failure. Infants with infant botulism may have prolonged neuromuscular weakness and may undergo a tracheostomy to simplify management of mechanical ventilation. Similarly, older children with Guillain-Barré syndrome and respiratory failure may need a tracheostomy if a lengthy course of mechanical ventilation is expected. The use of tracheostomy has been advocated to promote pulmonary toilet and improve ventilation during the treatment of flail chest.

The timing of the tracheostomy will depend on several issues, including the patient's underlying illness and the severity of the condition that makes tracheostomy necessary. If possible, emergency tracheostomy under unfavorable conditions should be avoided because the complications are more common in this setting. Percutaneous placement of a tracheostomy has been widely used in the adult population; however, experience in children remains limited. One small retrospective series suggests that placement in the ICU can be done safely with adherence to sound techniques and prudent patient selection.[131]

Postoperative Nursing Care

Care from attentive, trained nurses is essential for the well-being of the patient with a tracheostomy. Until a tract of granulation tissue has formed in the stoma between the cervical and tracheal epithelium, precautions should be taken to prevent the accidental displacement of the tracheostomy tube. Although stay sutures simplify replacement of the tracheostomy tube, this procedure may be difficult, especially in an emergency situation with a struggling patient. A hastily replaced tube may be incorrectly located in the pretracheal soft tissue, resulting in asphyxiation. If positive pressure ventilation is attempted with the tube in this position, subcutaneous and mediastinal emphysema may be followed by a life-threatening tension pneumothorax. Because of these risks, patients routinely stay in the ICU for 5 to 7 days postoperatively. Smaller children have arm restraints placed to prevent them from pulling at the tracheostomy tube. If necessary, sedation is given until the child grows accustomed to the tracheostomy and the tract matures with the formation of granulation tissue. If accidental displacement of the tracheostomy tube does occur, replacement may be facilitated with a gentle insertion of a 0 Miller laryngoscope blade into the stoma and the identification of the tracheal lumen before the tube is passed.

Besides avoiding accidental displacement of the tracheostomy, the nurse must constantly monitor the patient for obstruction of the tracheostomy tube. The tube may be obstructed by dried tracheal mucus. Sometimes the patient's chin may obstruct the tube. Humidified gas may be administered to prevent drying and inspissation of secretions.

Complications

Any operation on the airway involves risk. The complication rate after tracheostomy has been reported to be 10% to 30%, with a death rate of 3%. Early postoperative complications include air leak, hemorrhage, and aspiration. Air leak is seen more often in children than in adults and may be life threatening. The risk of complications declines as the patient ages. Some life-threatening complications, such as accidental decannulation or tracheostomy tube obstruction, may occur anytime after the placement of a tracheostomy. The safety and well-being of patients with a tracheostomy require constant vigilance to prevent these mishaps.

Swallowing dysfunction after tracheostomy may lead to aspiration of saliva and food. This may be due in part to anchoring of the trachea to the skin of the neck, preventing the cephalad movement of the trachea during swallowing. Children who have a tracheostomy often have difficulty learning to eat. The high frequency of pneumonia observed after tracheostomy may be in part due to the problem of recurrent aspiration. Aerophagia, another form of swallowing dysfunction, occurs with modest frequency in pediatric patients after tracheostomy.

Late complications include granulation tissue formation, tracheal stenosis, infection of the stoma, pneumonia, fused vocal cords, and distal tracheomalacia. Although infection of the stoma and distal tracheomalacia may be evident before decannulation, granulation formation and fused vocal cords may not be apparent until decannulation is attempted. An uncommon but particularly dangerous late complication is erosion of the tracheostomy tube into the innominate artery.

Decannulation

Problems at the time of decannulation occur in up to 36% of children. These difficulties are most frequent in patients younger than 1 year. Structural abnormalities that result in decannulation problems include subglottic stenosis, tracheomalacia at the tracheostomy site, granuloma tissue obstructing the trachea, and fused vocal cords. If respiratory distress is encountered during decannulation, it should not be attributed to the patient's psychological dependence on the tracheostomy tube. Evaluation of the airway with bronchoscopy or a lateral neck radiograph is important. Psychological factors should not be considered until structural causes of respiratory embarrassment have been eliminated.

Key References

1. Hammer J. Acute respiratory failure in children. *Paediatr Respir Rev.* 2013;14:64-69.
2. Badgwell JM, McLeod ME, Friedberg J. Airway obstruction in infants and children. *Can J Anaesth.* 1987;34:90-98.
5. Galvis AG, Stool SE, Bluestone CD. Pulmonary edema following relief of acute upper airway obstruction. *Ann Otol Rhinol Laryngol.* 1980;89(2 Pt 1):124-128.
11. Coates H. Nasal obstruction in the neonate and infant. *Clin Pediatr (Phila).* 1992;31:25-29.
12. Dickson JM, Richter GT, Meinzen-Derr J, et al. Secondary airway lesions in infants with laryngomalacia. *Ann Otol Rhinol Laryngol.* 2009; 118:37-343.
14. Richter GT, Wootten CT, Rutter MJ, et al. Impact of supraglottoplasty on aspiration in severe laryngomalacia. *Ann Otol Rhinol Laryngol.* 2009;118:259-266.
17. Qubty WF, Mrelashvili A, Kotagal S, et al. Comorbidities in infants with obstructive sleep apnea. *J Clin Sleep Med.* 2014;10:1213-1216.
23. Folkman J. Toward a new understanding of vascular proliferative disease in children. *Pediatrics.* 1984;74:850-856.
24. Smith BM, Lu JC, Dorfman AL, et al. Rings and slings revisited. *Magn Reson Imaging Clin N Am.* 2015;23:127-135.
29. Boogaard R, Huijsmans SH, Pijnenburg MW, et al. Tracheomalacia and bronchomalacia in children: incidence and patient characteristics. *Chest.* 2005;128:3391-3397.
32. Kompare M, Weinberger M. Protracted bacterial bronchitis in young children: association with airway malacia. *J Pediatr.* 2012;160: 88-92.
37. Johnson DW. Croup. *BMJ Clin Evid.* 2014;2014.
39. Westley CR, Cotton EK, Brooks JG. Nebulized racemic epinephrine by IPPB for the treatment of croup: a double-blind study. *Am J Dis Child.* 1978;132:484-487.
42. Moore M, Little P. Humidified air inhalation for treating croup. *Cochrane Database Syst Rev.* 2006;(3):CD002870.
43. Bjornson C, Russell K, Vandermeer B, et al. Nebulized epinephrine for croup in children. *Cochrane Database Syst Rev.* 2013;(10):CD006619.
47. Moraa I, Sturman N, McGuire T, et al. Heliox for croup in children. *Cochrane Database Syst Rev.* 2013;(12):CD006822.
49. Duval M, Tarasidis G, Grimmer JF, et al. Role of operative airway evaluation in children with recurrent croup: a retrospective cohort study. *Clin Otolaryngol.* 2015;40:227-233.
51. Shah RK, Roberson DW, Jones DT. Epiglottitis in the Hemophilus influenzae type B vaccine era: changing trends. *Laryngoscope.* 2004;114: 557-560.
56. Cheung CS, Man SY, Graham CA, et al. Adult epiglottitis: 6 years experience in a university teaching hospital in Hong Kong. *Eur J Emerg Med.* 2009;16:221-226.
58. Fordham MT, Rock AN, Bandarkar A, et al. Transcervical ultrasonography in the diagnosis of pediatric peritonsillar abscess. *Laryngoscope.* 2015;125:2799-2804.
63. Malloy KM, Christenson T, Meyer JS, et al. Lack of association of CT findings and surgical drainage in pediatric neck abscesses. *Int J Pediatr Otorhinolaryngol.* 2008;72:235-239.
65. Novis SJ, Pritchett CV, Thorne MC, et al. Pediatric deep space neck infections in U.S. children, 2000-2009. *Int J Pediatr Otorhinolaryngol.* 2014;78:832-836.
70. Eckel HE, Widemann B, Damm M, et al. Airway endoscopy in the diagnosis and treatment of bacterial tracheitis in children. *Int J Pediatr Otorhinolaryngol.* 1993;27:147-157.
74. Goon P, Sonnex C, Jani P, et al. Recurrent respiratory papillomatosis: an overview of current thinking and treatment. *Eur Arch Otorhinolaryngol.* 2008;265:147-151.
77. Boltežar IH, Bahar MS, Žargi M, et al. Adjuvant therapy for laryngeal papillomatosis. *Acta Dermatovenerol Alp Pannonica Adriat.* 2011; 20:175-180.
81. Jabbour J, Martin T, Beste D, et al. Pediatric vocal fold immobility: natural history and the need for long-term follow-up. *JAMA Otolaryngol Head Neck Surg.* 2014;140:428-433.
85. Lesnik M, Thierry B, Blanchard M, et al. Idiopathic bilateral vocal cord paralysis in infants: case series and literature review. *Laryngoscope.* 2015;125(7):1724-1728.
89. Anghelescu DL, Burgoyne LL, Liu T, et al. Clinical and diagnostic imaging findings predict anesthetic complications in children presenting with malignant mediastinal masses. *Paediatr Anaesth.* 2007; 17:1090-1098.
91. Garey CL, Laituri CA, Valusek PA, et al. Management of anterior mediastinal masses in children. *Eur J Pediatr Surg.* 2011;21:310-313.
93. Weiss M, Dullenkopf A, Fischer JE, et al. Prospective randomized controlled multi-centre trial of cuffed or uncuffed endotracheal tubes in small children. *Br J Anaesth.* 2009;103:867-873.
94. Kemper KJ, Benson MS, Bishop MJ. Predictors of postextubation stridor in pediatric trauma patients. *Crit Care Med.* 1991;19:352-355.
96. Mhanna MJ, Zamel YB, Tichy CM, et al. The "air leak" test around the endotracheal tube, as a predictor of postextubation stridor, is age dependent in children. *Crit Care Med.* 2002;30:2639-2643.
97. Kako H, Goykhman A, Ramesh AS, et al. Changes in intracuff pressure of a cuffed endotracheal tube during prolonged surgical procedures. *Int J Pediatr Otorhinolaryngol.* 2015;79:76-79.
100. Litman RS, Maxwell LG. Cuffed versus uncuffed endotracheal tubes in pediatric anesthesia: the debate should finally end. *Anesthesiology.* 2013;118:500-501.
101. King EF, Blumin JH. Vocal cord paralysis in children. *Curr Opin Otolaryngol Head Neck Surg.* 2009;17:483-487.
105. Khemani RG, Randolph A, Markovitz B. Corticosteroids for the prevention and treatment of post-extubation stridor in neonates, children and adults. *Cochrane Database Syst Rev.* 2009;(3):CD001000.
107. Kadilak PR, Vanasse S, Sheridan RL. Favorable short- and long-term outcomes of prolonged translaryngeal intubation in critically ill children. *J Burn Care Rehabil.* 2004;25:262-265.
109. Sittel C. Pathologies of the larynx and trachea in childhood. *GMS Curr Top Otorhinolaryngol Head Neck Surg.* 2014;13:Doc09.
113. Sidell DR, Kim IA, Coker TR, et al. Food choking hazards in children. *Int J Pediatr Otorhinolaryngol.* 2013;77:1940-1946.
115. Wolach B, Raz A, Weinberg J, et al. Aspirated foreign bodies in the respiratory tract of children: eleven years experience with 127 patients. *Int J Pediatr Otorhinolaryngol.* 1994;30:1-10.
118. Singh H, Parakh A. Tracheobronchial foreign body aspiration in children. *Clin Pediatr (Phila).* 2014;53:415-419.
120. Shires CB, Preston T, Thompson J. Pediatric laryngeal trauma: a case series at a tertiary children's hospital. *Int J Pediatr Otorhinolaryngol.* 2011;75:401-408.
121. Wood JW, Thornton B, Brown CS, et al. Traumatic tracheal injury in children: a case series supporting conservative management. *Int J Pediatr Otorhinolaryngol.* 2015;79:716-720.
122. McCormick ME, Fissenden TM, Chun RH, et al. Resource utilization and national demographics of laryngotracheal trauma in children. *JAMA Otolaryngol Head Neck Surg.* 2014;140:829-832.
123. Heldenberg E, Vishne TH, Pley M, et al. Major bronchial trauma in the pediatric age group. *World J Surg.* 2005;29:149-153, discussion 53-54.
124. Fidkowski CW, Fuzaylov G, Sheridan RL, et al. Inhalation burn injury in children. *Paediatr Anaesth.* 2009;19(suppl 1):147-154.
125. Shah UK, Jacobs IN. Pediatric angioedema: ten years' experience. *Arch Otolaryngol Head Neck Surg.* 1999;125:791-795.
128. Carr MM, Poje CP, Kingston L, et al. Complications in pediatric tracheostomies. *Laryngoscope.* 2001;111(11 Pt 1):1925-1928.
130. Griese M, Felber J, Reiter K, et al. Airway inflammation in children with tracheostomy. *Pediatr Pulmonol.* 2004;37:356-361.
131. Klotz DA, Hengerer AS. Safety of pediatric bedside tracheostomy in the intensive care unit. *Arch Otolaryngol Head Neck Surg.* 2001;127: 950-955.

Pediatric Acute Respiratory Distress Syndrome

Lincoln S. Smith and Robinder G. Khemani

PEARLS

- The acute respiratory distress syndrome (ARDS) is a restrictive lung disease with clinical manifestations of hypoxemia, poor respiratory system compliance (high work of breathing), and new pulmonary infiltrates. Pathologically ARDS is characterized by diffuse alveolar damage, pulmonary edema and atelectasis, and the presence of alveolar neutrophils.
- Direct insults leading to ARDS include pneumonia, gastric content aspiration, lung contusion, hydrocarbon ingestion, smoke inhalation, and mechanical ventilation. Indirect insults include sepsis, severe trauma and burn, blood transfusions, pancreatitis, major surgery, and ischemia-reperfusion injury.
- Injury to the alveolar epithelium or endothelium results in loss of the alveolar epithelial-endothelial barrier function with resultant accumulation of proteinaceous fluid in the alveolar space and surfactant inactivation.
- Cellular and soluble mediators of inflammation, surfactant inactivation and loss, coagulation dysfunction, alveolar fluid clearance, and apoptosis are pathobiological mechanisms of lung injury.
- Ventilator management for children with ARDS should embrace limiting both tidal volume (V_T) and inspiratory pressure, allowing for permissive hypercarbia with sufficient levels of positive end-expiratory pressure to prevent alveolar derecruitment and limit high concentrations of inspired fraction of oxygen.
- There is not clear evidence to support the routine use of pulmonary or nonpulmonary ancillary therapies for children with PARDS, including surfactant and iNO, but data supporting prone positioning are growing.

Introduction

The terms *wet lung, Da Nang lung,* and *shock lung* were used from the 1940s through the 1960s to describe patients who died from severe hypoxia and had diffuse pulmonary edema.[1] In 1967 Ashbaugh and colleagues described a case series of patients with severe acute hypoxemic respiratory failure, poor lung compliance, and diffuse alveolar infiltrates on chest x-ray. Although there was an 11-year-old among the 12 patients in

the case series, they coined the term *acute respiratory distress syndrome in adults,* which they later called *adult respiratory distress syndrome.*[2,3] Acknowledgment that this disease process also occurred in children did not come until the 1994 American-European Consensus Conference, where it was renamed *acute respiratory distress syndrome (ARDS).*[4,5]

Clinical Features: Pathophysiology

ARDS is characterized by the rapid onset of respiratory failure in patients with severe pulmonary or systemic inflammation (Table 51.1). ARDS is a restrictive lung disease (reduced respiratory system compliance) due to pulmonary edema, atelectasis, pulmonary consolidation, surfactant dysfunction, and chest wall restriction (chest wall edema, ascites, peritonitis, etc.). Hypoxemia results from intrapulmonary shunt (V/Q = 0) and V/Q <1 due to heterogeneous pulmonary edema and endexpiratory lung volumes falling below functional residual capacity (FRC). Furthermore, increased physiologic dead space (V/Q >1) is also common in ARDS from endothelial injury and coagulation, impaired cardiac output or pulmonary perfusion, and regional overdistension.

Chest imaging shows patchy, asymmetric to diffuse infiltrates. In patients for whom the syndrome does not resolve, persistent hypoxemia and low lung compliance persists, but increased alveolar dead space worsens. In these patients, chest imaging begins to show linear opacities and formation of bullae, and pneumothoraces may develop.

Definition

The Berlin Definition of ARDS was published in 2012, and it addressed perceived limitations of the American European Consensus Conference (AECC) definition.[6,7] Validation of the Berlin definition in pediatrics was limited by differences in the epidemiology and management of children with ARDS as compared with adults.[8,9] The Pediatric Acute Lung Injury Consensus Conference was convened to develop a pediatric definition of ARDS (Fig. 51.1).[10-12] Major differences between the Berlin and the Pediatric Acute Lung Injury Consensus Conference (PALICC) definitions are as follows:
1. The PALICC definition does not require bilateral infiltrates on chest x-ray.
2. The PALICC definition allows substitution of SpO_2 when PaO_2 is not available to assess hypoxemia severity, providing $SpO_2 \leq 97\%$.

Age	Exclude patients with perinatalrelated lung disease
Timing	Within 7 days of known clinical insult
Origin of edema	Respiratory failure not fully explained by cardiac failure or fluid overload
Chest imaging	Chest imaging findings of new infiltrate(s) consistent with acute pulmonary parenchymal disease

Oxygenation	Noninvasive mechanical ventilation		Invasive mechanical ventilation		
	PARDS (no severity stratification)		Mild	Moderate	Severe
	Full face mask bilevel ventilation or CPAP ≥5 cm H$_2$0[2]		4≤ OI <8	8≤ OI <16	OI ≥16
	PF ratio ≤300 SF ratio ≤264[1]		5≤ OSI <7.5[1]	7.5≤ OSI <12.3[1]	OSI ≥12.3[1]

Special populations	
Cyanotic heart disease	Standard criteria above for age, timing, origin of edema, and chest imaging with an acute deterioration in oxygenation not explained by underlying cardiac disease.[3]
Chronic lung disease	Standard criteria above for age, timing, and origin of edema with chest imaging consistent with new infiltrate and acute deterioration in oxygenation from baseline that meet oxygenation criteria above.[3]
Left ventricular dysfunction	Standard criteria for age, timing, and origin of edema with chest imaging changes consistent with new infiltrate and acute deterioration in oxygenation that meet criteria above not explained by left ventricular dysfunction.

Fig. 51.1. Pediatric acute respiratory distress syndrome (PARDS) definition. [1]Use PaO2-based metric when available. If PaO2 is not available, wean FIO2 to maintain SpO2 ≤97% to calculate oxygen saturation index (OSI; [FIO2× mean airway pressure × 100]/SpO2) or SpO2:FIO2 (SF) ratio. [2]For nonintubated patients treated with supplemental oxygen or nasal modes of noninvasive ventilation, see Fig. 51.2 for at-risk criteria. [3]Acute respiratory distress syndrome severity groups stratified by oxygenation index (OI; [FIO2 × mean airway pressure × 100]/PaO2) or OSI should not be applied to children with chronic lung disease who normally receive invasive mechanical ventilation or children with cyanotic congenital heart disease. *CPAP,* continuous positive airway pressure; *PF,* PaO2:FIO2.

TABLE 51.1	Acute Respiratory Distress Syndrome Risk Factors
Direct	**Indirect**
Pulmonary infections	Sepsis
Inhalations	Multiple trauma
Pulmonary contusions	Blood transfusion
Aspiration	Severe burns
Mechanical ventilation	Pancreatitis
	Major surgery
	Ischemia-reperfusion injury

3. The PALICC definition introduces the use of oxygenation index (OI) or oxygenation-saturation index (OSI) to stratify severity groups.

The PALICC definition of pediatric ARDS (PARDS)[11,12] identifies an at-risk group and criteria to identify PARDS patients with chronic lung disease, cyanotic heart disease, or left ventricular dysfunction.

Pathobiology

The primary pathologic description of ARDS is disruption of alveolar epithelial-endothelial barrier resulting in noncardiogenic pulmonary edema. Disruption of surfactant and alveolar fluid clearance, dysregulated inflammation, and coagulopathy are pathobiologic mechanisms associated with worse lung injury (Fig. 51.2).[13] Etiologies associated with ARDS can be divided into direct (alveolar epithelial) and indirect (alveolar capillary) injuries (see Table 51.1). There are three conceptual phases of ARDS (acute, fibrosing, and resolution), which have substantial temporal overlap but different pathobiological mechanisms and pathology.[14]

Alveolar Epithelial-Endothelial Barrier

The large surface area and thin structure of the lung is efficient for gas exchange but makes it susceptible to injury. The integrity of the alveolar epithelial-endothelial barrier requires maintenance of a thin layer of alveolar wall liquid (AWL) coating the alveolar epithelium. The AWL is necessary for dispersion of surfactant, and it is dependent on regulated flow of water, proteins, and small solutes across postcapillary venules into the alveolar airspace.[15] Excess alveolar fluid is removed by sodium-dependent transport by type II alveolar epithelial cells.[16]

Direct injuries to the alveolar epithelium causing disruption of alveolar fluid clearance (AFC) lead to pulmonary edema. Indirect injuries that increase endothelial permeability can overwhelm intact AFC, again resulting in pulmonary edema. Accumulation of pulmonary edema fluid is a cause of reduced respiratory system compliance and impaired gas exchange (ventilation/perfusion mismatch and shunt). The rate of AFC has been associated with mortality in adult patients with ARDS.[17] Catecholamines, glucocorticoids, growth factors, thyroid hormone, and Fas/FasL affect AFC,[16,18] although therapies targeting AFC have not thus far improved outcomes in adults with ARDS.[19] Regulation of postnatal lung development may be a protective factor in children with ARDS, in part through preservation of AFC.[20]

Pulmonary Endothelial Injury

Mechanical, chemical, and cellular injuries to the pulmonary endothelium cause alveolar barrier dysfunction, activate inflammatory and coagulation cascades, change pulmonary

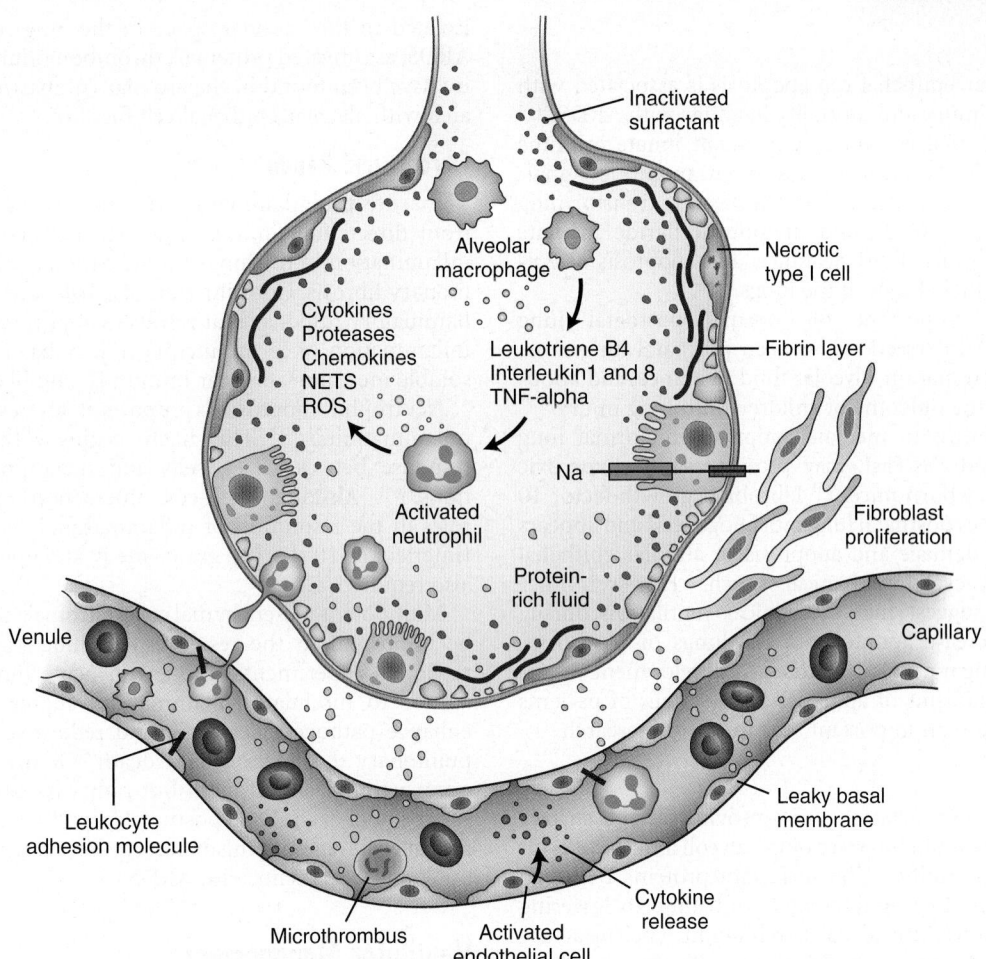

Fig. 51.2. Schematic of pathophysiology in acute respiratory distress syndrome. There is a loss of epithelial and endothelial barrier integrity and loss of function leading to increased permeability pulmonary edema. Solutes and large molecules such as albumin enter the alveolar space. In the presence of proinflammatory mediators and activated endothelium, leukocytes traffic into the pulmonary interstitium and alveoli. There is activation of coagulation and deposition of fibrin in capillaries and alveoli with increased concentrations of fibrinogen and fibrin-degradation products in the edema fluid. Surfactant depletion and degradation result in large increases in surface tension and loss of alveolar shape and integrity. Recovery is preceded by fibroblast proliferation. *NETs,* neutrophil extracellular traps; *ROS,* reactive oxygen species; *TNF,* tumor necrosis factor.

vascular resistance, and may lead to multiorgan dysfunction.[21,22] Elevated pulmonary vascular resistance and thrombosis of pulmonary capillary beds can increase alveolar dead space. Thrombomodulin is shed during endothelial injury, which has been associated with mortality in children and adults with ARDS.[23,24] Activation of the pulmonary endothelium results in increased permeability by both para- and transcellular pathways.[25] Studies of endothelial and platelet activation and coagulation in cardiovascular disease and sepsis led to a single-blinded randomized trial of recombinant human-activated protein C in adult patients with ARDS, but it did not change outcome.[26] Von Willebrand factor (vWF) has correlated with ARDS mortality in children and adults, but studies investigating other biomarkers of endothelial activation and coagulation have not consistently correlated with disease severity.[13,22] Neutrophil reactive oxygen species, supplemental oxygen, and altered endothelial nitric oxide signaling may contribute to elevated pulmonary vascular resistance. Pulmonary endothelial angiotensin-converting enzyme (ACE) and ACE2 genetic polymorphisms and activity correlate with mortality in children and adults with ARDS.[13,27] ACE and

ACE2 are other mechanisms by which pulmonary endothelial biology, pulmonary vascular resistance, inflammation, apoptosis, and coagulation may intersect in the pathobiology of ARDS.[28]

Leukocytes and Inflammation

Macrophages are the only resident leukocyte in the quiescent alveolar airspace. Leukocyte infiltration into the alveolar airspace is a pathologic hallmark of ARDS.[29] The alveolar epithelium, endothelium, and activated leukocytes contribute to local and systemic inflammation. The inflammatory response is crucial to the early response to direct injury to the lungs, but it contributes to reduced lung compliance and V/Q mismatch.

Severe systemic inflammation (high levels of circulating cytokines and chemokines) activates the alveolar endothelium and circulating leukocytes resulting in indirect lung injury. In addition to alveolar fluid accumulation, the cell surface adhesion molecules adherent to activated alveolar endothelium regulate neutrophil rolling, binding, activation, and migration into the alveolar space by both para and transcellular mechanisms.[13,30,31]

Apoptosis

Increased alveolar epithelial cell apoptosis is associated with severity of lung injury and mortality in adults with ARDS.[32,33] Nuclear factor kappa-B (NFκB)–dependent innate immune signaling via Toll-like receptors results in apoptotic signaling.[34,35] Studies also suggest that Fas ligand, transforming growth factor β (TGF-β), and lipopolysaccharide mediate inflammation, alveolar fluid clearance, and apoptosis of epithelial and endothelial cells in the lungs.[18,36-45]

Apoptosis is important for normal postnatal lung development.[46-48] Intersections between postnatal lung morphogenesis, inflammation, alveolar fluid clearance, and apoptosis may affect the outcome of children with lung injury.[20,49] Fas has been shown to mediate apoptosis in normal lung development, and Fas/FasL may protect against hyperoxic lung injury in newborn mice.[50,51] Fibroblast growth factor 10 (FGF-10) regulates postnatal lung morphogenesis and appears to reduce DNA damage and apoptosis of alveolar epithelial cells treated with cyclic mechanical stretch.[52] However, other animal studies suggest that mechanical ventilation during infancy may increase apoptosis in the lungs of newborns, thereby disrupting normal postnatal lung development.[53] Age-dependent mechanisms of apoptosis in the lungs of patients with ARDS remain an important area for future research.

Surfactant

Primary functions of surfactant are to provide variable surface tension at the air-liquid interface of the alveoli and to contribute to innate immunity.[54] The surfactant proteins B (SP-B) and C (SP-C) are hydrophobic and contribute to lowering the surface tension of the alveolar wall liquid. The surfactant proteins A (SP-A) and D (SP-D) are collectins and have important roles in innate immune responses to microbial pathogens. All four of the surfactant proteins have immuno-modulatory effects and affect pulmonary fibrosis and lung remodeling.[55,56]

Adults with ARDS have low levels of SP-A, B, and D in bronchoalveolar lavage (BAL) fluid, and increased serum levels of these proteins in children and adults are associated with severity of lung injury.[57-61] There are lower levels of phospholipids in BAL fluid, as well as changes in the overall composition of the phospholipids present in BAL fluid of patients with ARDS.[62] Reactive oxygen species from high concentrations of supplemental oxygen and activated neutrophils in the alveolar spaces of patients with ARDS may cause surfactant dysfunction.[63,64] Finally, patients with genetic polymorphisms within the surfactant protein B genes that result in lower levels of SP-B have a higher risk of developing ARDS or have more severe lung injury when they become ill.[65-67] Similar findings are also seen with SP-A and D with regard to the development of ARDS for adults with pneumonia.[68]

Coagulation

Endothelial function, inflammation, and coagulation are inextricably linked.[69,70] Activation or injury to the endothelium results in expression of tissue factor (TF) and von Willebrand factor (vWF) antigen, and vWF has been associated with mortality in pediatric and adult ARDS patients.[71,72] Plasminogen activator inhibitor-1 (PAI-1) has also been associated with severity of illness and mortality in adult and pediatric patients with ARDS.[13,73,74] Coagulopathy and fibrinolysis are not

isolated to the vascular space in the lungs of patients with ARDS, as activated protein C, thrombomodulin, and TF activity have been found in the alveolar compartment and associated with alveolar epithelial cell function.[13,73,75]

Fibrosis and Repair

The acute proinflammatory response is essential to recover from direct lung injury. However, unnecessarily prolonged inflammation in the lungs can be pathologic and lead to pulmonary fibrosis. Coordination of a balanced pro-and antiinflammatory response that results in appropriate resolution of inflammation once the inciting injury has resolved requires soluble mediators, cellular immunity, and likely stem cells.

Neutrophil apoptosis is important for resolution of lung inflammation.[33,76,77] This likely begins with a coordinated response between Treg cells and macrophage subpopulations.[78-81] Although cell-cell interactions play important roles in the resolution of inflammation,[82] soluble mediators (interleukin-10 [IL-10], granzyme B, and lipid mediators) are also required.[83-85]

Multipotent mesenchymal stem (stromal) cells (MSCs) may be important to the resolution of lung inflammation and repair. In experimental models of acute lung injury, MSCs appear to modulate inflammation, augment tissue repair, enhance pathogen clearance, and reduce severity of injury, pulmonary dysfunction, and death.[86] Many of these effects occur without engraftment but rather by paracrine effects.[87] A fixed pool of MSCs in postnatal lungs that are depleted with age may be a mechanism for age-dependent differences in outcomes of patients with ARDS.

Ventilator Management

Adult and animal data support ventilator strategies in ARDS that limit tidal stretch of the alveoli (avoiding volutrauma), limit inspiratory (driving) pressure (barotrauma), allow permissive hypoxemia and hypercapnia, and provide adequate positive end-expiratory pressure (PEEP) to maintain end expiratory lung volume to limit cyclic opening and closing of the alveoli (Chapter 52). Theoretic constructs of ventilator management in ARDS advocate ventilation in a safe zone characterized by location on the deflation limb of quasi-static pressure-volume curve, in the zone of optimal compliance. Adequate PEEP during conventional ventilation or mean airway pressure during high-frequency ventilation may prevent atelectrauma by limiting cyclic opening and closing of alveoli. Limiting tidal stretch (by limiting tidal volume or peak inspiratory pressure) prevents overdistention, particularly of relatively spared alveoli with longer inspiratory time constants.

Despite these theoretic constructs, there is limited high-level pediatric evidence regarding the optimal methods or targets to achieve these strategies.

Considerations for Ventilator Mode

There is limited evidence to support the belief that one mode of ventilation is superior to another for PARDS,[88,89] but volume control (constant flow pattern) used in the ARDS Network ARMA trial in adults is infrequently used in pediatrics in favor of a decelerating flow pattern of pressure-controlled or pressure-regulated volume control (PRVC).[90] This factor, among others, may limit the direct applicability of adult ARDS data to pediatrics. However, regardless of the mode of ventilation, the principles of lung protective ventilation are applicable and should be used for children with ARDS (Chapter 52).

Tidal Volume

Targeted tidal volume (V_T) of 6 mL/kg ideal body weight (IBW) is an evidence-based standard in adult ARDS, but pediatric data are not conclusive. Observational pediatric studies demonstrate lower mortality for patients treated with higher V_T = 6 to 10 mL/kg.[91] This is likely due to V_T commonly being the response versus the set variable in pediatric mechanical ventilation. Higher V_T for a set pressure represents better respiratory system compliance, implying the patient is less ill. Location of measurement of V_T (proximal airway versus at the ventilator without compensation for ventilator tubing compliance), IBW versus actual body weight, and correction for leak around endotracheal tubes are practice differences between adult and pediatric ICU providers that complicate extrapolation of adult V_T data to children.[92] Nevertheless, current recommendations are to use V_T in or below the physiologic range (5–8 mL/kg) IBW, with lower V_T targets in children with more compromised respiratory system compliance.[93]

Peak or Plateau Pressure

There are few data to support limit for peak or plateau pressure in pediatrics. These terms are commonly interchanged when pressure-controlled ventilation is used. There may be few differences between peak and plateau pressure for children with ARDS managed with the decelerating flow pattern of pressure-controlled ventilation, unless they concurrently have significant lower airway disease. Measuring plateau pressure requires a period of no flow during inspiration (an inspiratory hold). This maneuver may not be implemented routinely or consistently in pediatric critical care, and *plateau* pressure is often mislabeled. However, recommendations are to limit plateau pressure to 28 cm H_2O for children with normal chest wall compliance, allowing slightly higher pressures when chest wall compliance is reduced.[93] Ultimately, the shear stress induced by positive pressure ventilation is a function of transpulmonary pressure (alveolar pressure minus pleural pressure), affording the use of higher inspiratory pressure when pleural pressure is also increased (obesity). Tidal volume gets the most attention, but the ARDSNet lung protective 6 mL/kg strategy recommends decreasing V_T below 6 mL/kg if needed to limit plateau pressure to 30 cm H_2O (ARDSNet ARMA). High driving pressure (delta P), independent of both plateau pressure and V_T, is associated with higher mortality in adults with ARDS.[94]

Positive End-Expiratory Pressure

PEEP should be set to prevent lung collapse and recruitment-derecruitment injury during tidal ventilation. Unfortunately, given the inhomogeneity of lung disease in PARDS, it is difficult to use this principle to guide specific PEEP recommendations for individual patients. The optimal method to set PEEP for an individual patient remains a research question, and existing data do not support a single PEEP level (high or low) that improves outcome for adults or children with ARDS. Pediatric practice appears highly variable with respect to PEEP application, and PEEP is uncommonly increased to levels frequently used in adults with ARDS.[95,96] Adult studies that

protocolize PEEP and FiO_2 for oxygenation targets support higher levels of PEEP.[97,98] Evidence is lacking in children, but moderately elevated levels of PEEP (10–15 cm H_2O) titrated to oxygenation and hemodynamic responses are recommended for children with severe PARDS, with the potential for higher levels of PEEP in the most severe patients.[93] Importantly, plateau pressure should still be limited, and markers of oxygen delivery, respiratory system compliance, and hemodynamics should be closely monitored as PEEP is increased.

Unconventional Ventilation Strategies

Various forms of unconventional ventilation are considered for children with PARDS, particularly those with severe disease. The most common unconventional mode is high-frequency oscillatory ventilation (HFOV). Although many practitioners use HFOV in PARDS, there are no data supporting improved outcomes; albeit there are data suggesting improved gas exchange. As such, HFOV is frequently used as a rescue ventilator mode. The concept of HFOV is to ventilate with V_T approximating anatomic dead space, leading many to believe it is an optimal form of lung protective ventilation and should be considered earlier in the course of ARDS. However, adult and observational pediatric data do not support use of HFOV early in ARDS.[99-102] Current recommendations are to consider HFOV for patients with moderate to severe ARDS when adequate gas exchange cannot be maintained without exceeding suggested limits of plateau pressure (ie, lung protection is not maintained with conventional ventilation).[93]

Alternative modes of unconventional ventilation such as airway pressure release ventilation (APRV) and high-frequency jet ventilation (HFJV) have some theoretic advantages for patients with moderate to severe ARDS, but there are no controlled data demonstrating that these are superior to conventional modes of ventilation or HFOV for children with PARDS.

Pulmonary Ancillary Therapies
Exogenous Surfactant

The efficacy of exogenous surfactant for PARDS may depend on the concentration of individual surfactant proteins as well as other phospholipids.[103] Investigations have used exogenous surfactant preparations rich in either surfactant protein B or C, given their direct properties on alveolar surface tension.[104-106]

Preclinical or Adult Data

Lung injury studies in animals suggest exogenous surfactant improves oxygenation, pulmonary compliance, alveolar edema, total lung water, and alveolar protein concentrations and may have an effect on lung inflammation.[107-111]

Heterogeneous patient populations and study designs make interpreting adult data difficult. Exogenous surfactant appears to transiently improve oxygenation without affecting mortality, but some studies suggest harm related to adverse events such as hypoxemia (7%-50%), hypotension (9%-35%), transient airway obstruction, or rare events like bradycardia, leukopenia, air leak syndrome and pneumonia.[104,112-117] Posthoc analyses suggesting that treatment with recombinant protein-C surfactant benefited the subgroups of adults with ARDS direct injury were not confirmed in randomized trials.[104,118-120]

Pediatric Data

Early pediatric studies of exogenous surfactant for ARDS showed improvements in oxygenation and suggested reduced duration of ventilation and reduced mortality.[121] Unfortunately, subsequent multicenter, randomized, placebo-controlled, blinded trials of calfactant did not show improved mortality or ventilator-free days.[106,114]

A phase II placebo-controlled, double-blind, randomized controlled trial (RCT) of a synthetic surfactant preparation (lucinactant), which mimics the actions of surfactant protein B, was performed in 165 non-premature children with persistent hypoxemia.[105] The most common diagnoses were bronchiolitis and pneumonia, and only 37 children met the criteria for ARDS. Lucinactant was shown to be safe, it improved oxygenation without an effect on the duration of mechanical ventilation, and mortality was extremely low (<5%).

In summary, there is not evidence to suggest that exogenous surfactant reduces mortality for children or adults with ARDS. Exogenous surfactant can be safely administered in children, and oxygenation may transiently improve. The effects of surfactant seem to be confounded by the dosing regimen, drug delivery, drug concentration, surfactant formulation, degree of lung recruitment, lung disease severity, etiology of ARDS, comorbidities, and a multitude of other factors. Future research is warranted to identify whether subgroups of patients benefit from exogenous surfactant.

Nitric Oxide

Physiologic Rationale

Nitric oxide (NO) is normally synthesized in the vascular endothelium, causing vasodilation by relaxing smooth muscle via intracellular cyclic guanosine monophosphate (cGMP). Nitric oxide also affects inflammation by altering endothelial interactions with leucocytes and platelets.

Because inhaled NO (iNO) is theoretically delivered only to ventilated lung units, its major effect is improved V/Q balance by increasing blood flow to ventilated units, thereby reducing physiologic dead space and improving oxygenation.[122,123] iNO may also be important for lowering pulmonary vascular resistance and supporting the right ventricle in some ARDS patients with preexisting pulmonary hypertension.[124-129]

Preclinical and Adult Studies

In addition to effects on pulmonary vascular resistance, animal data suggest iNO may both aggravate and ameliorate lung injury. Some lung injury models suggest iNO reduces neutrophil migration and oxidative burst,[130] decreases lung inflammation,[131-133] decreases platelet aggregation,[134-136] and promotes lung repair.[137] iNO may improve pulmonary bacterial clearance through mechanisms related to endothelial permeability.[138,139] Other models suggest that iNO has no effect[140] or may potentiate lung injury through proinflammatory mechanisms.[141-143]

Meta-analyses of iNO for adults with ARDS suggest that iNO does not reduce mortality.[144,145] Most studies demonstrate transient improvements in oxygenation within the first 24 hours, but there may be an increased risk of renal impairment (RR 1.59, 95% CI 1.17-2.16) among adults treated with iNO as compared with controls. However, there appears to be persistent use of iNO as a rescue therapy.[146]

Pediatric Data

There have been a number of uncontrolled trials and small RCTs demonstrating improvements in oxygenation but not mortality or duration of ventilation with iNO administration for children with ARDS or hypoxemic respiratory failure.[129,144,145,147-151] A third small RCT on 32 children with ARDS examined the potential synergistic effects of prone positioning and iNO, demonstrating more sustained improvements in oxygenation with the combination of prone positioning and iNO over the first 24 hours of ventilation.[152] A multicenter trial has shown that iNO reduced the length of mechanical ventilation, mostly through lower use of ECMO.[153] Unlike the adult studies, there does not appear to be evidence of significant toxicity with iNO administration in pediatric ARDS.

Pediatric and adult evidence suggests iNO is probably best reserved for situations when refractory hypoxemia needs to be temporarily reversed (ie, as a bridge to extracorporeal support) or for patients with a true clinical indication such as documented pulmonary hypertension with right heart failure.[154]

Nonpulmonary Therapies

Prone Positioning

Physiologic Rationale

The best described and cited rationale for prone positioning of ARDS patients is that it improves regional V/Q matching due to a more uniform distribution of aerated lung, particularly in dorsal lung regions, thereby reducing physiologic dead space and improving oxygenation.[155,156] The effects of prone positioning on gas exchange are conventionally thought to be due to gravitational effects on the distribution of atelectasis and edema, as well as the effects of the weight of the heart and position of the dorsal diaphragm on the expansion of dorsal lung units.[157,158] Interestingly, prone positioning also appears to improve the cephalocaudal distribution of ventilation, because the heart, mediastinal structures, and abdominal contents rest on the sternum. The prone position reduces regional differences in pleural pressure near the diaphragm that are normally present when upright or supine (Fig. 51.3).[158-161]

Prone positioning may also reduce inequalities in regional time constants and promote more effective alveolar ventilation to "slower" compartments.[162,163] These effects ultimately may influence lung stress and reduce the development of ventilator-induced lung injury.[164,165] When used in conjunction with high PEEP strategies currently recommended for ARDS, prone positioning may also increase alveolar recruitment and prevent cyclic recruitment/derecruitment and atelectrauma.[166] Minimizing derecruitment may be a physiologic explanation of why additional recruitment strategies such as HFOV sustain temporary improvements obtained by prone positioning.[167]

Patients with more compliant chest walls may have more benefit from prone positioning due to the reduction in chest wall compliance caused by limiting expansion of the sternum. This reduction in chest wall compliance, in addition to decreasing compression of lungs by the heart and decreasing the vertical pleural pressure gradient in the lungs, theoretically allows preferential distribution of ventilation to dorsal regions of lungs.[158] However, there is contradictory evidence for this mechanism and the overall effect of chest wall properties on

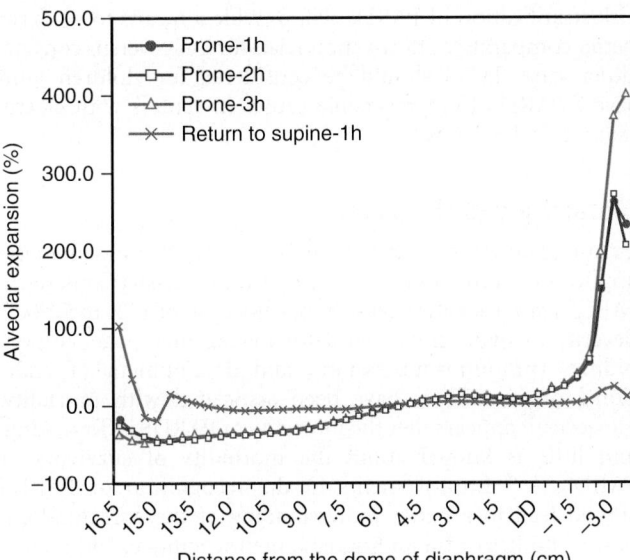

Fig. 51.3. Percentage of alveolar expansion along cephalocaudal axis. Zero line indicates cutoff between alveolar expansion and contraction. In prone group, alveolar expansion was observed in caudal regions and was most prominent in lung regions below diaphragmatic cupola. In upper lung, with 5 to 6 cm above the diaphragm as a turning point, alveolar contraction occurred. (Reproduced with permission Lee HJ, Im JG, Goo JM, et al. Acute lung injury: effects of prone positioning on cephalocaudal distribution of lung inflation—CT assessment in dogs. Radiology. 2005;234:151-161. Copyright © 2005 Radiological Society of North America.)

the oxygenation response in prone positioning of ARDS patients.[168] It is also important to note that none of these studies were performed in children.

Other potential mechanisms for the beneficial effects of prone positioning include promoting airway secretion clearance[158] and lowering pulmonary artery pressure via attenuation of hypoxic pulmonary vasoconstriction, although due to compromised preload, this effect may not directly translate into improvements in cardiac index.[169,170]

Preclinical or Adult Data

Animal models support the physiologic mechanisms detailed earlier. Adult data demonstrate that the gas exchange response to prone positioning is not universal and benefits only a subset of patients.[158,171,172] Moreover, the immediate improvement in oxygenation is inconsistently associated with a survival advantage in adults with ARDS.[173-175] However, prone positioning has been associated with improved survival in adults for whom dead space ventilation improved.[176,177]

There have been close to a dozen randomized controlled trials of prone positioning for ARDS in adults.[173,175,178-183] Two meta-analyses highlight significant heterogeneity in these trials, which may be due to duration of prone positioning, use of concurrent lung protective ventilation, tidal volume, hypoxemia severity, use of high frequency oscillatory ventilation, and duration of respiratory failure prior to prone positioning.[182,183] Nevertheless, both of these meta-analyses concluded that prone positioning affords a survival advantage for adults with ARDS, with the effect most pronounced in those who receive a longer duration of prone positioning, are managed with lung protective ventilation strategies with regard to PEEP

and tidal volume, and have more severe lung injury and hypoxemia. However, when pooling the adverse events, those in the prone positioning group had a higher incidence of pressure ulcers, airway problems, and endotracheal tube obstruction.[182]

The Proning Severe ARDS Patients (PROSEVA) trial in adults is a major driver of the conclusions with regard to survival advantage with prone positioning.[179] Prone positioning was maintained for a minimum of 16 consecutive hours, and ventilator management was standardized with a lung protective ventilation protocol. Mortality was 32.8% in the supine group and 16% in the prone group at 28 days (p <0.001). Unlike other studies, there were no increased adverse events in the prone group as compared with controls. The study suggests that prone positioning may benefit adults with severe ARDS when done by experienced providers, with a long consecutive duration of prone positioning and meticulous lung protective ventilation.

Pediatric Data

The results of the PROSEVA trial question existing data on prone positioning in children. Multiple uncontrolled trials and one randomized controlled trial on prone positioning have not demonstrated a survival advantage in children with ARDS.[184-188] The highest level of pediatric evidence comes from a multicenter randomized controlled trial in 2005,[189] which had detailed multidisciplinary protocols and guidelines for lung protective ventilation, sedation, extubation readiness, hemodynamic support, nutrition, and skin care.[190] This unblinded clinical trial was stopped early secondary to futility: There was no difference in the primary outcome of ventilator-free days or the secondary outcomes of mortality, time to recovery of lung injury, organ failure, cognitive impairment, and functional health. Most of the patients would now be considered to have moderate ARDS, and at the time study procedures began, nearly half of the children had PF ratios >150. Because of adult data supporting more benefit from prone positioning for those with severe hypoxemia and repeated findings that strategies for lung protective ventilation may be important confounders on the relationship between prone positioning and outcome, the high use of high-frequency oscillatory ventilation in pediatrics may further confound these results.

Finally, although theory supports that children may have more pronounced benefits from prone positioning due to chest wall compliance, this benefit may be counteracted by less substantial compression of the lungs by the heart when supine as compared with adults. Future studies may benefit from the inclusion of measurements of transpulmonary pressure gradients as well as chest wall versus static lung compliance changes with prone positioning.

Monitoring

Pediatric patients with or at risk of PARDS should receive at least clinical monitoring of respiratory frequency, heart rate, continuous pulse oximetry, and noninvasive blood pressure.[191] Exhaled V_T should be measured at the endotracheal tube, especially in the smallest patients, or corrected for tubing compliance if measured at the ventilator. Exhaled V_T should likely be normalized to ideal body weight, although spinal deformities and contractures complicate measurement of height for calculation of "ideal" body weight. Inspiratory pressure (peak pressure in pressure modes and plateau pressure in volume modes), flow, and volume should be measured continuously. Continuous monitoring of SpO_2 (with titration of FiO_2 titrated to keep SpO_2 <97%), PEEP, and mean airway pressure (MAP) are essential to diagnose PARDS and monitor disease progression. Continuous capnography is important to determine the adequacy of support provided and monitor physiologic dead space, which is associated with disease severity. Arterial blood sampling may be required when the accuracy of noninvasive monitoring is unclear, and placement of arterial catheters may be indicated for hemodynamic assessments. Standard plain film chest x-rays are intermittently indicated for diagnosis, determining appropriate position of equipment, and diagnosing complications (pneumothorax), but it is not clear whether routine daily chest x-rays add value to the care of mechanically ventilated patients.

Noninvasive Support

Despite the widespread increased use of noninvasive support for pediatric and adult patients with acute respiratory failure, there are scant data to determine the utility of these modes of respiratory support for ARDS patients. Noninvasive support of ARDS patients has theoretic benefits, including avoidance of complications of intubation, preservation of spontaneous breathing and airway clearance, and reduced need for sedation. Noninvasive respiratory support can be considered for children with mild PARDS in a setting where trained and experienced staff can closely monitor for response to therapy and rapidly identify and treat deterioration.[192] Immunocompromised patients may particularly benefit from noninvasive respiratory support by avoiding the infectious risks of artificial airways. Uncontrolled descriptive pediatric studies suggest that it is feasible, and adult data suggest that it is superior to medical therapy alone.

The severity of underlying disease and an early response to noninvasive support appear to be primary determinants of success. The presence of a second organ failure, requirement of >12 cm H_2O mean airway pressure, FiO_2 >0.6 or SF <190, high severity of illness scores (PELOD or PRISM), or moderate to severe ARDS suggest that noninvasive support will not be sufficient.[192-195] Once a patient is started on noninvasive support for respiratory failure, the patient must be closely monitored for evidence that she or he has responded. Failure to respond to noninvasive respiratory support within the first few hours has been associated with a need for intubation, higher complications rates at the time of intubation, and higher mortality in adults. Evidence that a patient has failed to respond to noninvasive respiratory support may include absence of a reduction in respiratory rate, ph <7.25 after 2 hour, increased oxygen requirement ($FiO2$ >80% after 1 hour), a decreased PaO_2/FiO_2 ratio or an SF <190, an increase of $PaCO_2$, or an altered level of consciousness.[192,195]

Extracorporeal Life Support

There are data from clinical trials of extracorporeal life support (ECLS) for neonates and adults with severe respiratory failure, but none in children. Data from the Extracorporeal Life Support Organization (ELSO) registry suggest that the average survival of >3500 children treated with ECLS for respiratory failure is 57% (51%–69%).[196] Improvements in diagnosis and

risk stratification of PARDS will provide a means to perform better comparative effectiveness trials for ECLS versus conventional care. ECLS should be considered for children with severe PARDS from reversible causes in centers with clearly defined ECLS teams.[196]

Morbidity and Outcomes

Existing knowledge of the outcomes of PARDS is based on the application of the American-European Consensus Conference (AECC) criteria and suggests mortality rates of 15% to 50%.[197] Severity of hypoxemia, ventilator management, age, comorbidities (immunosuppression), and development of additional organ failures have been associated with mortality. However, it appears that the mortality of PARDS is decreasing, and little is known about the morbidity of survivors of PARDS.[197,198] Improvements in the recognition of PARDS should lead to a better understanding of the epidemiology. Future studies of the pulmonary, neurocognitive, and neuromuscular morbidities are needed in survivors of PARDS.

Key References

6. Force ADT, et al. Acute respiratory distress syndrome: the Berlin definition. *JAMA*. 2012;307:2526-2533.
7. Ferguson ND, et al. The Berlin definition of ARDS: an expanded rationale, justification, and supplementary material. *Intensive Care Med*. 2012;38:10.
11. Pediatric Acute Lung Injury Consensus Conference Group. Pediatric acute respiratory distress syndrome: consensus recommendations from the Pediatric Acute Lung Injury Consensus Conference. *Pediatr Crit Care Med*. 2015;16:428-439.
12. Khemani RG, et al. Pediatric acute respiratory distress syndrome: definition, incidence, and epidemiology: proceedings from the Pediatric Acute Lung Injury Consensus Conference. *Pediatr Crit Care Med*. 2015;16(5 suppl):S23-S40.
13. Sapru A, et al. Pathobiology of acute respiratory distress syndrome. *Pediatr Crit Care Med*. 2015;16:S6-S22.
19. National Heart, Lung, and Blood Institute Acute Respiratory Distress Syndrome (ARDS) Clinical Trials Network, Matthay MA, Brower RG, et al. Randomized, placebo-controlled clinical trial of an aerosolized β_2-agonist for treatment of acute lung injury. *Am J Respir Crit Care Med*. 2011;184:561-568.
20. Smith LS, Zimmerman JJ, Martin TR. Mechanisms of acute respiratory distress syndrome in children and adults: a review and suggestions for future research. *Pediatr Crit Care Med*. 2013;14:631-643.
21. Maniatis NA, Orfanos SE. The endothelium in acute lung injury/acute respiratory distress syndrome. *Curr Opin Crit Care*. 2008;14:22-30.
24. Sapru A, et al. Plasma soluble thrombomodulin levels are associated with mortality in the acute respiratory distress syndrome. *Intensive Care Med*. 2015;41:470-478.
55. Whitsett JA, Wert SE, Weaver TE. Diseases of pulmonary surfactant homeostasis. *Annu Rev Pathol*. 2015;10:371-393.
58. Todd DA, et al. Surfactant phospholipids, surfactant proteins, and inflammatory markers during acute lung injury in children. *Pediatr Crit Care Med*. 2010;11:82-91.
59. LeVine AM, et al. Surfactant content in children with inflammatory lung disease. *Crit Care Med*. 1996;24:1062-1067.
71. Flori HR, et al. Early elevation of plasma von Willebrand factor antigen in pediatric acute lung injury is associated with an increased risk of death and prolonged mechanical ventilation. *Pediatr Crit Care Med*. 2007;8:96-101.
74. Sapru A, et al. Elevated PAI-1 is associated with poor clinical outcomes in pediatric patients with acute lung injury. *Intensive Care Med*. 2010;36:157-163.
93. Rimensberger PC, Cheifetz IM. Ventilatory support in children with pediatric acute respiratory distress syndrome. *Pediatr Crit Care Med*. 2015;16:S51-S60.
94. Amato MBP, et al. Driving pressure and survival in the acute respiratory distress syndrome. *N Engl J Med*. 2015;372:747-755.

95. Khemani RG, et al. Variability in usual care mechanical ventilation for pediatric acute lung injury: the potential benefit of a lung protective computer protocol. *Intensive Care Med.* 2011;37:1840-1848.

96. Santschi M, et al. Acute lung injury in children: therapeutic practice and feasibility of international clinical trials. *Pediatr Crit Care Med.* 2010;11:681-689.

97. Briel M, et al. higher vs lower positive end-expiratory pressure in patients with acute lung injury and acute respiratory distress syndrome: systematic review and meta-analysis. *JAMA.* 2010;303:865-873.

99. Ferguson ND, et al. High-frequency oscillation in early acute respiratory distress syndrome. *N Engl J Med.* 2013;368:795-805.

100. Young D, et al. High-frequency oscillation for acute respiratory distress syndrome. *N Engl J Med.* 2013;368:806-813.

101. Gupta P, et al. Comparison of high-frequency oscillatory ventilation and conventional mechanical ventilation in pediatric respiratory failure. *JAMA Pediatr.* 2014;168:243-249.

102. Bateman DST, et al. Early high frequency oscillatory ventilation in pediatric acute respiratory failure: a propensity score analysis. *Am J Respir Crit Care Med.* 2016;193:495-503.

105. Thomas NJ, et al. A pilot, randomized, controlled clinical trial of lucinactant, a peptide-containing synthetic surfactant, in infants with acute hypoxemic respiratory failure. *Pediatr Crit Care Med.* 2012;13:646-653.

106. Willson DF, et al. Pediatric calfactant in acute respiratory distress syndrome trial. *Pediatr Crit Care Med.* 2013;14:657-665.

114. Willson DF, et al. Effect of exogenous surfactant (calfactant) in pediatric acute lung injury: a randomized controlled trial.[Erratum appears in *JAMA.* 2005;294:900]. *JAMA.* 2005;293:470-476.

152. Ibrahim T, El-Mohamady H. Inhaled nitric oxide and prone position: how far they can improve oxygenation in pediatric patients with acute respiratory distress syndrome? *J Med Sci.* 2007;7:390-395.

153. Bronicki RA, et al. Multicenter randomized controlled trial of inhaled nitric oxide for pediatric acute respiratory distress syndrome. *J Pediatr.* 2015;166:365-369 e1.

154. Tamburro RF, Kneyber MCJ. Pulmonary specific ancillary treatment for pediatric acute respiratory distress syndrome. *Pediatr Crit Care Med.* 2015;16:S61-S72.

155. Richter T, et al. Effect of prone position on regional shunt, aeration, and perfusion in experimental acute lung injury. *Am J Respir Crit Care Med.* 2005;172:480-487.

156. Tang R, et al. Relationship between regional lung compliance and ventilation homogeneity in the supine and prone position. *Acta Anaesthesiol Scand.* 2012;56:1191-1199.

158. Lee DL, et al. Prone-position ventilation induces sustained improvement in oxygenation in patients with acute respiratory distress syndrome who have a large shunt. *Crit Care Med.* 2002;30:1446-1452.

179. Guerin C, et al. Prone positioning in severe acute respiratory distress syndrome. *N Engl J Med.* 2013;368:2159-2168.

189. Curley MA, et al. Effect of prone positioning on clinical outcomes in children with acute lung injury: a randomized controlled trial. *JAMA.* 2005;294:229-237.

190. Curley MA, et al. Clinical trial design–effect of prone positioning on clinical outcomes in infants and children with acute respiratory distress syndrome. *J Crit Care.* 2006;21:23-32, discussion 32-37.

191. Emeriaud G, Newth CJL. Monitoring of children with pediatric acute respiratory distress syndrome. *Pediatr Crit Care Med.* 2015;16:S86-S101.

192. Essouri S, Carroll C. Noninvasive support and ventilation for pediatric acute respiratory distress syndrome. *Pediatr Crit Care Med.* 2015;16:S102-S110.

193. Mayordomo-Colunga J, et al. Predicting non-invasive ventilation failure in children from the SpO2/FiO2 (SF) ratio. *Intensive Care Med.* 2013;39:1095-1103.

194. Essouri S, et al. Noninvasive positive pressure ventilation: five years of experience in a pediatric intensive care unit. *Pediatr Crit Care Med.* 2006;7:329-334.

195. Demaret P, et al. Non-invasive ventilation is useful in paediatric intensive care units if children are appropriately selected and carefully monitored. *Acta Paediatr.* 2015;104:861-871.

196. Dalton HJ, Macrae DJ. Extracorporeal support in children with pediatric acute respiratory distress syndrome. *Pediatr Crit Care Med.* 2015;16:S111-S117.

197. Quasney MW, et al. The outcomes of children with pediatric acute respiratory distress syndrome. *Pediatr Crit Care Med.* 2015;16:S118-S131.

198. Aspesberro F, Mangione-Smith R, Zimmerman JJ. Health-related quality of life following pediatric critical illness. *Intensive Care Med.* 2015; 41:1235-1246.

Ventilator-Induced Lung Injury

Jean-Damien Ricard, Nicolas de Prost, Alexandre T. Rotta, Georges Saumon, and Didier Dreyfuss

PEARLS

- Although essential to the support of patients with respiratory failure, mechanical ventilation can be associated with the development of pulmonary tissue injury, termed *ventilator-induced lung injury (VILI)*.
- The concept of VILI has been elegantly tested in the research laboratory in both normal and diseased lungs, where the individual contribution of various factors such as tidal volume, positive end-expiratory pressure, and overall state of lung distention can be determined. Lung volume at the end of inspiration (ie, the overall degree of lung distension) probably is the main determinant of VILI severity.
- One must take the magnitude of the loss of aerated lung volume and alterations in lung mechanics into account to assess the risk of VILI.
- Experimental and clinical data support the idea that reasoned tidal volume reduction designed to prevent volutrauma can be advantageous in the management of these patients.

Mechanical ventilation is essential to the life support of patients with respiratory failure. Several potential drawbacks to mechanical ventilation were identified early in its history.[1] More recent experimental studies have shown that certain ventilation modalities may produce subtle tissue damage similar to that seen in early acute respiratory distress syndrome (ARDS) and termed *ventilator-induced lung injury (VILI)*. This issue has received much attention in the clinical field.[2,3] This chapter describes the pathophysiologic events leading to VILI and places these observations into a clinical perspective of ventilatory management of patients with ARDS.

Evidence for Ventilator-Induced Lung Injury
Ventilation of Intact Lungs
High Lung Volume Ventilator-Induced Lung Injury

Webb and Tierney[4] found that pulmonary edema rapidly developed in rats subjected to 45 cm H_2O peak airway pressure ventilation. Edema severity and rate of development increased with peak airway pressure magnitude. It was later confirmed that such a ventilation modality produces endothelial and epithelial cell damage and lung capillary permeability changes that result in nonhydrostatic pulmonary edema.[5]

The respective roles of increased airway pressure and increased lung volume in this injury were clarified when mechanical ventilation at high and low tidal volume (V_T) were compared at identical (45 cm H_2O) peak airway pressures.[6] The injury was found only in rats subjected to high V_T and not in those undergoing ventilation at high airway pressure in which lung distention was limited by thoracoabdominal strapping (Fig. 52.1).[6] Furthermore, in animals undergoing ventilation at high V_T by negative external distending pressure, pulmonary edema still developed, confirming that excessive airway pressure is not the causal factor of this type of injury.[6] This VILI that depends mostly on end-inspiratory volume has been called volutrauma.[7,8] Several investigators reached the same conclusions in other species using different protocols,[9,10] confirming the fact that large tidal volumes are more critical than high intrathoracic pressures in the genesis of ventilator-induced lung edema in intact animals. The effects of gradual lung inflation on alveolar epithelial and pulmonary microvascular permeability to proteins were evaluated using a scintigraphic study in rats.[11] Two tracers were used, ^{99m}Tc-albumin (in the alveolar instillate) and ^{111}In-transferrin (in the blood), which allowed for measuring both alveolar epithelial permeability (estimated from the rate at which ^{99m}Tc-albumin left the lungs) and microvascular permeability (measured from the accumulation of ^{111}In-transferrin in the lungs). Increasing lung tissue stretch by ventilation at high airway pressure immediately increased microvascular and alveolar epithelial permeability to proteins. The same end-inspiratory pressure threshold (between 20 and 25 cm H_2O) was observed for epithelial and endothelial permeability changes (Fig. 52.2). The existence of a lung distention threshold above which lung edema would develop was further confirmed in healthy pigs by Gattinoni and colleagues using the stress/strain approach. Indeed, when a lung strain (ie, the ratio between volume change and lung resting volume[12]) greater than 1.5 to 2 was achieved, corresponding to tidal volumes larger than 20 mL/kg in healthy animals,[13] a dramatic lung edema developed. This strain approach also allowed for the development of a unifying rule in various mammal species relating the time course of VILI with the lung strain applied.[14] Obviously, the lower the denominator (ie, low lung resting volume, the so-called baby lung effect), the greater will be the strain for a given lung inflation. In most of the definitions of strain, the numerator (ie, lung volume change) includes tidal volume plus positive end-expiratory pressure (PEEP) volume. However, it was previously suggested that the contribution of tidal volume and PEEP volume on lung strain are not equivalent (ie, *dynamic* and *static* lung strain). Indeed, Protti and colleagues showed in a pig model of VILI that the development of lung edema depended not only on the global strain applied but also on its components, large dynamic strains (ie,

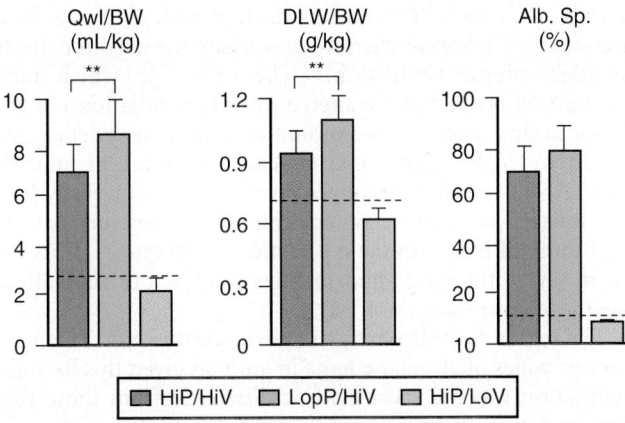

Fig. 52.1. Comparisons of the effects of high-pressure–high-volume ventilation *(HiP-HiV)* with those of negative inspiratory airway pressure high tidal volume ventilation (iron lung ventilation, *LoP-HiV)* and of high-pressure–low-volume ventilation (thoracoabdominal strapping, *HiP-LoV). Dotted lines* represent the upper 95% confidence limit for control values. See Fig. 53.4 for details on edema indices. Permeability edema occurred in both groups receiving high tidal volume ventilation. Animals undergoing ventilation with a high peak pressure and a normal tidal volume had no edema. *BW,* body weight; *DLW,* dry lung weight; *Qwl,* extravascular lung water. (From Dreyfuss D, Soler P, Basset G, et al. High inflation pressure pulmonary edema. Respective effects of high airway pressure, high tidal volume, and positive end-expiratory pressure. Am Rev Respir Dis. 1988;137:1159-1164.)

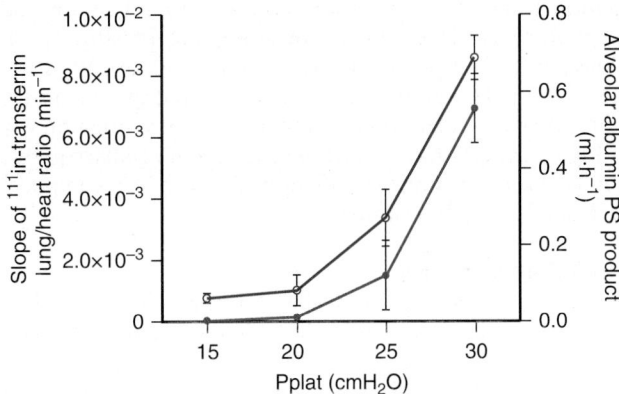

Fig. 52.2. Relationship between plateau pressure *(Pplat)* and ^{111}In-transferrin lung-to-heart ratio slope (an index of lung microvascular permeability; *left axis, open circles)* and alveolar ^{99m}Tc-albumin permeability-surface area product (an index of alveolar epithelium permeability; *right axis, full circles)* in mechanically ventilated rats. Both indexes dramatically increased for plateau pressures composed between 20 and 25 cm H_2O. (From de Prost N, Dreyfuss D, Saumon G. Evaluation of two-way protein fluxes across the alveolo-capillary membrane by scintigraphy in rats: effect of lung inflation. J Appl Physiol. 2007;102:794-802.)

large tidal excursions) being more harmful than large static strains (ie, high PEEP and small V_T).[15]

Pediatric experimental models of VILI showed consistent results from those obtained with older animals. For instance, lung injury developed in infant mice with healthy lungs when V_T's greater than 20 mL/kg were used[16] and, using a two-hit model of injurious mechanical ventilation and lipopolysaccharide (LPS) exposure, Roth-Kleiner and associates showed

that there was a synergistic response on cytokines production and histologic lesions in animals receiving both insults.[17] Several studies compared the effects of injurious mechanical ventilation strategies between pediatric and adult models of VILI and revealed that there was an age-related susceptibility to VILI, the former being less sensitive than the latter.[18] The factors accounting for these differences are not totally understood; the fact that the functional residual capacity-to-body weight ratio is greater in the immature than in the mature lung implies that for the same V_T applied in mL/kg of body weight, pediatric lungs would in fact experience a lower strain than adult lungs.[18] Nevertheless, even after adjusting V_T's for baseline total lung capacity, Kornecki and coworkers found greater susceptibility to an injurious mechanical ventilation strategy in adult than in pediatric rats,[19] suggesting less susceptibility of pediatric patients to VILI and making it difficult to directly extrapolate the results obtained from large randomized-controlled trials conducted in the adult population to the pediatric population.[18]

Low Lung Volume Ventilator-Induced Lung Injury

Unlike volutrauma, ventilation at low lung volumes does not seem to injure healthy lungs. Intact animals tolerate mechanical ventilation with physiologic V_T and low levels of PEEP for prolonged periods of time without any apparent damage. Taskar and colleagues[20] have shown that the repetitive collapse and reopening of terminal units during 1 hour of mechanical ventilation did not result in appreciable lung damage, although it did alter gas exchange and reduce compliance, as does spontaneous (low V_T) ventilation under deep anesthesia.

Ventilation of Damaged Lungs

High-Volume Lung Injury

Several investigators have evaluated the effect of overdistention on damaged lungs. These studies consistently demonstrated the increased susceptibility of diseased lungs to the detrimental effects of some modalities of mechanical ventilation.

Hernandez and colleagues[21] compared the effects of oleic acid alone, mechanical ventilation alone, and their combination on lung capillary filtration coefficient and wet-to-dry lung weight ratio in young rabbits. Filtration coefficient and wet-to-dry weight were not significantly affected by low doses of oleic acid or by mechanical ventilation at a peak inspiratory pressure of 25 cm H_2O for 15 minutes. However, the filtration coefficient as well as the wet-to-dry weight ratio increased significantly when oleic acid injury was followed by mechanical ventilation at these pressures, suggesting that ventilation at high volume and pressure might favor VILI in abnormal isolated lungs and that it might occur at lower airway pressure than in the normal lung. Whether this could also occur in lungs in situ was investigated by comparing the effects of different modalities of mechanical ventilation in rats with α-naphthylthiourea (ANTU)-injured lungs[22] (Fig. 52.3). ANTU infusion alone caused moderate permeability pulmonary edema. Mechanical ventilation alone resulted in a permeability edema of severity related to magnitude of V_T. Strikingly, lungs of animals injured by ANTU had more edema than predicted when they underwent ventilation with a high V_T (45 mL/kg body weight), indicating that the two insults acted in synergy. Even slight lung alterations, such as those produced by spontaneous ventilation during prolonged

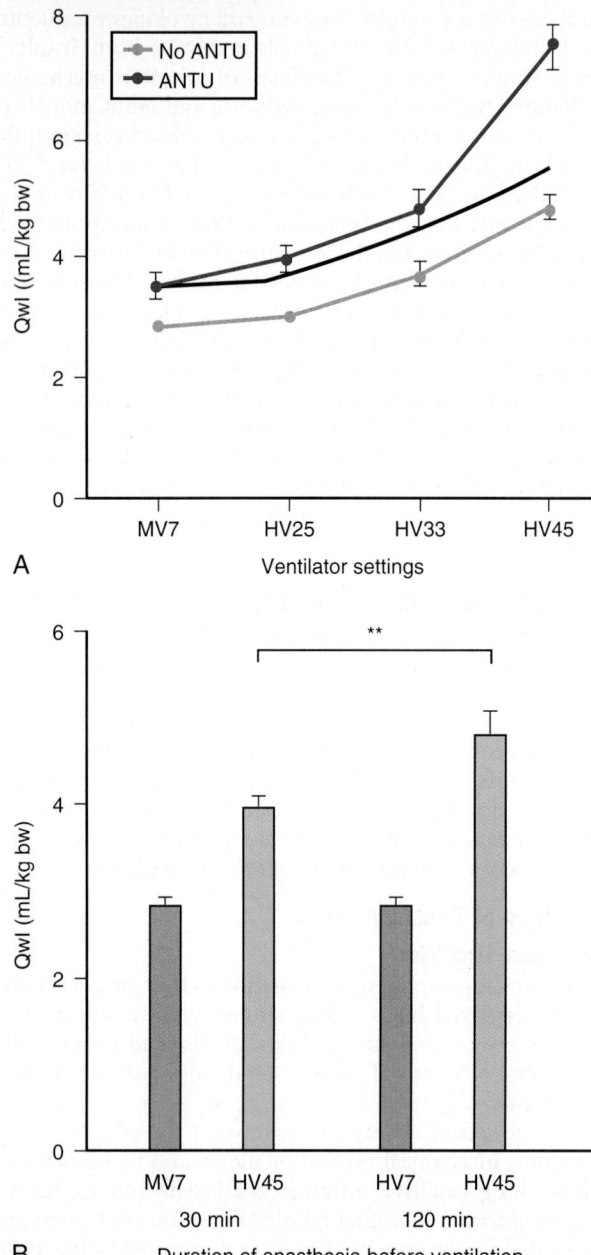

A

B   Duration of anesthesia before ventilation

Fig. 52.3. Interaction between previous lung alterations and mechanical ventilation on pulmonary edema. (A) Effect of previous toxic lung injury. Extravascular lung water *(Qwl)* after mechanical ventilation in normal rats *(orange circles)* and in rats with mild lung injury produced by α-naphthylthiourea (ANTU) *(purple circles)*. Tidal volume (V_T) varied from 7 to 45 mL/kg body weight *(bw)* *Black line* represents the Qwl value expected for the aggravating effect of ANTU on ventilation edema assuming additive. ANTU did not potentiate the effect of ventilation with V_T up to 33 mL/kg bw. In contrast, ventilation at 45 mL/kg bw V_T resulted in an increase in edema that greatly exceeded additivity, indicating synergy between the two insults. (B) Effect of lung functional alteration by prolonged anesthesia. Intact rats were anesthetized and breathed spontaneously for 30 or 120 minutes prior to mechanical ventilation with 7 mL/kg bw *(open bars)* or 45 mL/kg bw *(shaded bars)* V_T in intact rats. Qwl of animals that underwent ventilation with a high V_T was significantly higher than in those that underwent ventilation with a normal V_T. Qwl was not affected by the duration of anesthesia in animals that underwent ventilation with a normal V_T. In contrast, 120 minutes of anesthesia before high V_T ventilation resulted in a larger increase in Qwl than did 30 minutes of anesthesia. **p <.01. (From Dreyfuss D, Soler P, Saumon GL. Mechanical ventilation-induced pulmonary edema. Interaction with previous lung alterations. Am J Respir Crit Care Med. 1995;151:1568-1575.)

anesthesia (which inactivates surfactant and promotes focal atelectasis[23,24]), are sufficient to exacerbate the harmful effects of high-volume ventilation.[22] The extent to which lung mechanical properties are altered prior to ventilation is a key factor in this synergy. The amount of pulmonary edema produced by high-volume mechanical ventilation in animals given ANTU, or after prolonged anesthesia, was inversely proportional to respiratory system compliance measured at the beginning of high-volume mechanical ventilation.[22] Thus the more severe the lung abnormalities were before ventilation, the more severe was the VILI.

The reason for this synergy requires clarification. The presence of zones of alveolar edema in animals given this harmful ventilation was the most evident difference from those that underwent ventilation with lower, less harmful V_T.[22] Because alveolar flooding reduced the number of alveoli available for ventilation, they were more prone to overinflation, more vulnerable, and at greater risk of alveolar flooding. This in turn would further reduce aerated lung volume and result in positive feedback. Thus, uneven distribution of ventilation during acute lung injury[25] favors regional overinflation and injury. To substantiate this phenomenon, rats underwent ventilation with V_T of up to 33 mL/kg after alveolar flooding by instillation of saline solution into the trachea. Flooding with saline solution did not significantly affect microvascular permeability when V_T was low. As expected, capillary permeability alterations were more important in animals that experienced alveolar flooding than in intact animals that underwent ventilation at high V_T. Correlations also were found among end-inspiratory (plateau) airway pressure, the pressure at the "lower inflection point" on the pressure-volume (PV) curve, and the capillary permeability changes found in animals that experienced alveolar flooding and underwent ventilation with at high V_T (Fig. 52.4).[26] Thus the changes in capillary permeability caused by lung overinflation are more severe in poorly recruitable (and less compliant) lungs.

Low-Volume Lung Injury

An increase in trapped-gas volume during pulmonary edema and acute lung injury probably occurs because of airway

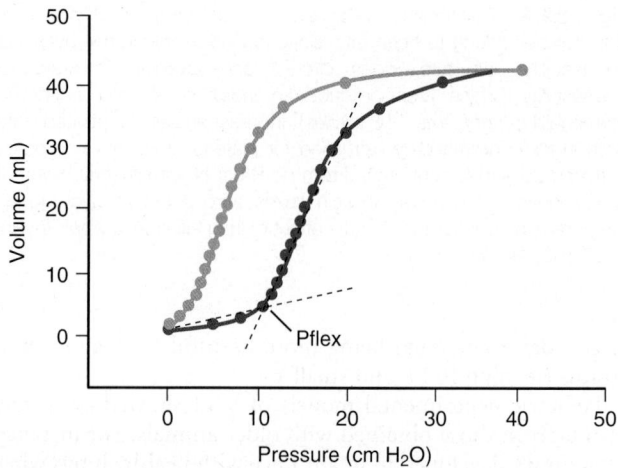

Fig. 52.4. Static volume-pressure relationship for the total respiratory system of a surfactant-depleted juvenile rabbit. *Pflex* indicates the lower inflexion point.

closure and is worsened by impaired surfactant function.[27] Under such conditions, the slope of the inspiratory limb of the respiratory system PV curve often displays a sharp increase at low lung volume. This change reflects the sudden and massive opening of units previously excluded from ventilation and has been termed the *lower inflection point.* This phenomenon often has a dramatic effect on arterial oxygenation, because setting PEEP above the pressure at this inflection point often decreases shunt and increases PaO_2.[28-31]

The possibility that pulmonary dysfunction may be aggravated if this inflection point lies within the V_T has been a focus of attention. Studies performed on surfactant-depleted lungs ventilated at various levels of PEEP suggest that repeated closure and reopening of terminal units can cause lung injury.[32-34] Indeed, during volume-controlled ventilation, lung compliance fell over time. However, when PEEP was adjusted to be either above or below the lower inflection point of the inspiratory limb of the PV curve, arterial PaO_2 was better preserved and less hyaline membrane formation occurred in the high-PEEP group.[32,33] Muscedere and colleagues[35] reported similar results in isolated, unperfused rabbit lungs lavaged with saline solution and ventilated with a low (5 to 6 mL/kg) V_T and with a PEEP set below or above the inflection point. However, Sohma and colleagues[34] did not find this injury in vivo in rabbits whose lungs had been injured with hydrochloric acid,[34] and Martynowicz and coworkers[36] have questioned the existence of the repetitive collapse-reexpansion phenomenon during tidal ventilation using the parenchymal marker technique for studying regional lung expansion in oleic acid–injured dog lungs. Their findings therefore did not support the hypothesis that a more important gravitational gradient during VILI produces atelectasis by compression of the dependent lung, cyclic recruitment and collapse, and ultimately shear stress injury.[36] They proposed that the displacement of air-liquid interfaces along the tracheobronchial tree would cause the lower inflection point on the PV curve and speculated that this would reflect the mechanics of partially fluid-filled alveoli with constant surface tension and not the abrupt opening of airways or atelectatic parenchyma.[37] It therefore remains unsettled whether injury caused by the repetitive reopening of collapsed terminal units and the protective effect of PEEP is restricted to the peculiar situation of surfactant depletion by bronchoalveolar lavage. In the clinical arena, the negative results of three randomized controlled trials comparing higher to lower PEEP levels[2,38,39] cast doubt on the clinical existence of repetitive opening and closing lung injury.

Roles of Tidal Volume, Positive End-Expiratory Pressure, and Overall Lung Distention

The influence of PEEP on acute lung injury (and more specifically on ventilator-induced pulmonary edema) must be studied in the context of the level of V_T. Indeed, PEEP increases functional residual capacity (FRC) and recruits the lung but also increases end-inspiratory volume when V_T is kept constant, thus possibly favoring overinflation. PEEP application also may depress hemodynamics and affect lung fluid balance. Therefore close analysis of the numerous studies that have been done to clarify the relationships between PEEP, oxygenation, and extravascular lung water accumulation during hydrostatic or permeability type edema must take into account

the experimental approach used, that is, intact animals or isolated lungs (for which lung water content will differ), and whether or not V_T is reduced (thus increasing or not increasing end-inspiratory lung volume).

Effects of Positive End-Expiratory Pressure When Tidal Volume Is Kept Constant

Application of PEEP may result in lung overinflation if it is followed by a significant change in FRC because of the increase in end-inspiratory volume. Overinflation will affect preferentially the more distensible areas that receive the bulk of ventilation, which may explain the lack of reduction or even the worsening of edema reported following PEEP application in most experiments.[40] PEEP does not affect the severity of hydrostatic[41] or permeability[41,42] edema in intact animals, although it improves oxygenation[41] because of the recruitment of flooded alveoli (Fig. 52.5). In isolated ventilated-perfused lungs, PEEP rather aggravates edema fluid accumulation[43] (Fig. 52.6). Thus when V_T is left unchanged, increasing FRC with PEEP affects edema differently in isolated lungs or in intact animals. In the latter, the lack of effect of PEEP depends on the balance between PEEP-induced increase in end-inspiratory lung volume, which decreases interstitial pressure and increases filtration pressure in extra-alveolar vessels, and the hemodynamic depression due to elevated intrathoracic pressure that, in the opposite, decreases filtration pressure. In contrast, preservation of perfusion rate in isolated-perfused lungs favors edema formation.[43]

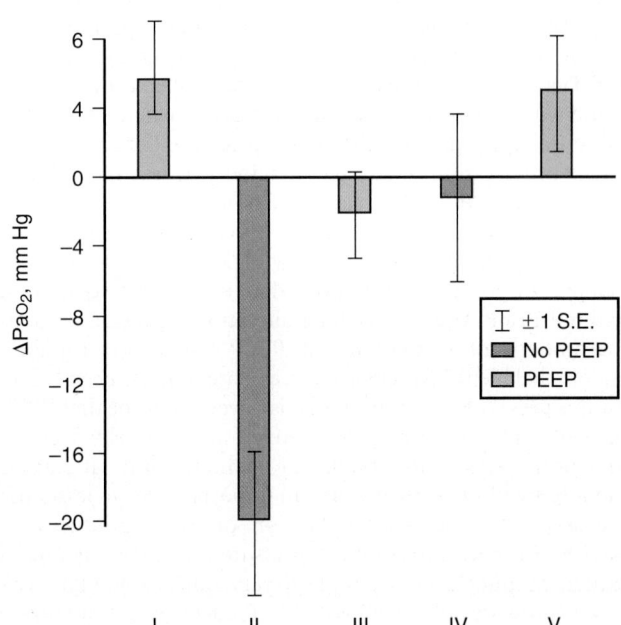

Fig. 52.5. Change in arterial oxygen tension (ΔPaO_2, mm Hg) during the 1-hour period between the initial and final measurements for groups I (control), II, and III (severe hydrostatic pulmonary edema, without and with positive end-expiratory pressure [PEEP], respectively) and IV and V (moderate pulmonary edema, without and with PEEP, respectively). The difference between ΔPaO_2 for groups II and III is significant (p <.01). (From Hopewell PC, Murray JF. Effects of continuous positive-pressure ventilation in experimental pulmonary edema. J Appl Physiol. 1976;40:568-574.)

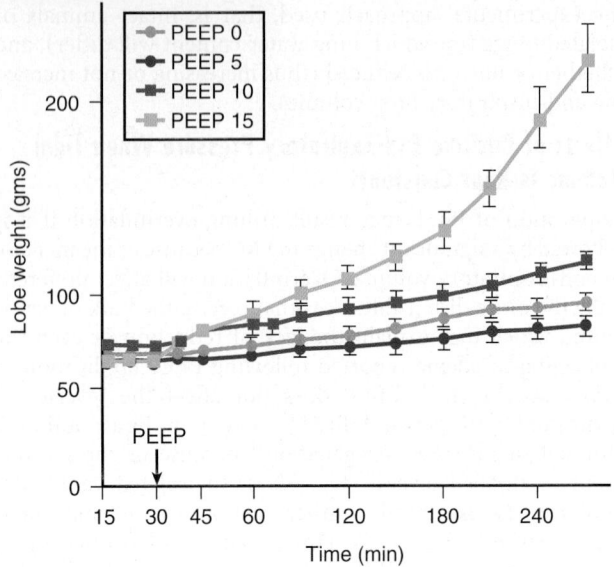

Fig. 52.6. Effect of three levels of positive end-expiratory pressure (PEEP) on water accumulation in hydrochloric acid–injured ventilated-perfused dog pulmonary lobes. The highest PEEP resulted in a further increase in pulmonary edema. (From Toung T, Saharia P, Permutt S, et al. Aspiration pneumonia: beneficial and harmful effects of positive end-expiratory pressure. Surgery. 1977;82:279-283.)

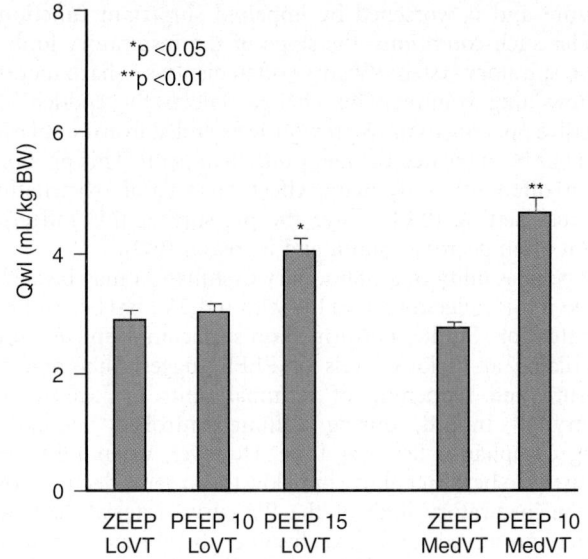

Fig. 52.7. Effect of increasing positive end-expiratory pressure (PEEP) from 0 to 15 cm H_2O during ventilation with two different tidal volume (V_T) values (7 mL/kg body weight [BW]: LoV$_T$ and 14 mL/kg BW: MedV$_T$). Pulmonary edema (as evaluated by increases in extravascular lung water [Qwl]) occurred when PEEP was increased. PEEP required to produce edema varied with V_T: 15 cm H_2O PEEP during ventilation with low V_T and 10 cm H_2O PEEP during ventilation with moderately increased V_T. *p <.05; **p <.01 versus zero end-expiratory pressure (ZEEP) and the same V_T. (From Dreyfuss D, Saumon G. Role of tidal volume, FRC, and end-inspiratory volume in the development of pulmonary edema following mechanical ventilation. Am Rev Respir Dis. 1993;148:1194-1203.)

Effects of Positive End-Expiratory Pressure When Tidal Volume Is Reduced

Edema is less severe during high-volume ventilation (even though FRC is increased by PEEP) when end-inspiratory lung volume is kept constant by decreasing V_T (Fig. 52.7). Webb and Tierney[4] showed that less edema developed during ventilation with 45 cm H_2O peak airway pressure when 10 cm H_2O PEEP was applied. The authors attributed this benefit of PEEP to the preservation of surfactant activity. It was later shown that, although PEEP decreased the amount of edema, it did not prevent alteration of capillary permeability.[6] However, animals undergoing ventilation with PEEP had no alveolar damage in contrast with those that underwent ventilation without PEEP. The only cellular alterations found in animals that underwent ventilation with PEEP consisted of capillary endothelial blebs.[6] No satisfactory explanation has been found for this preservation of the epithelial layer. It may be that PEEP prevented fluid movement in terminal units, thereby decreasing shear stress at this level. The hemodynamic alterations induced by PEEP probably play an important role in lessening the severity of edema. Application of PEEP produces an increase in mean intrathoracic pressure that adversely affects cardiac output.[44,45] For example, in rats subjected to high peak airway pressure and 10 cm H_2O PEEP, edema was more severe when the hemodynamic alterations induced by PEEP were corrected with dopamine infusion.[46] The amount of extravascular lung water was correlated with systemic blood pressure, suggesting that restoration of cardiac output increased filtration pressure and was responsible for aggravation of edema. The reduction of edema and of the severity of cellular damage by PEEP during ventilation-induced pulmonary edema may be linked to reduced tissue stress by decreasing volume-pressure excursion, movement of foam in distal airways, preservation of surfactant activity, and a decrease in capillary filtration.

Possible Mechanisms of Ventilator-Induced Lung Injury

It is now clear that ventilation-induced pulmonary edema is essentially the result of severe changes in the permeability of the alveolar-capillary barrier. Small increases in filtration pressure may combine with altered permeability to aggravate edema.

Ventilation may damage lungs by two different mechanisms, and the severity of damage depends on both intensity and duration of the insult. A rapidly occurring and severe permeability pulmonary edema may be produced in small animals as a consequence of acute lung stretch. This edema does not appear to require the involvement of inflammatory cells or secretion of mediators and can occur within a few minutes. Edema develops more slowly in larger animals for the same plateau pressure, rendering the situation more complex. A low lung volume injury may contribute its own effects to high end-inspiratory volume damage. Further, ventilation without PEEP may reduce aerated lung volume and gradually worsen mechanical nonuniformity. This lung inhomogeneity will in turn promote overinflation of the more compliant and probably healthier zones, leading to positive feedback aggravation. In addition, when lung lesions develop slowly, inflammatory pathways have enough time to be activated and may participate in tissue injury (Fig. 52.8).

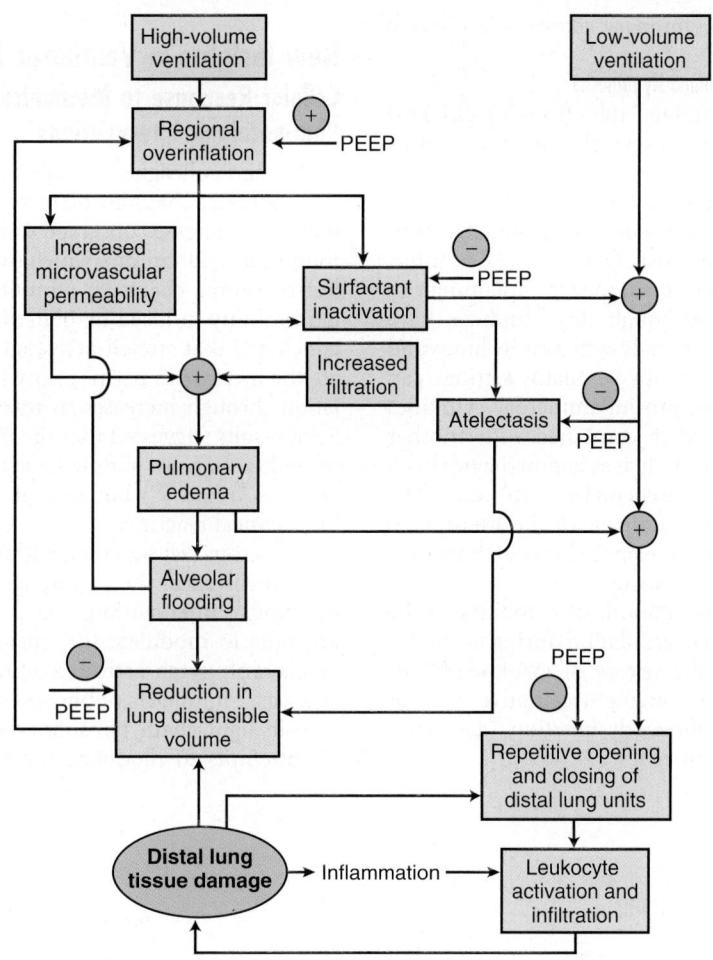

Fig. 52.8. Flow diagram summarizing the contributors to mechanical ventilation–induced lung injury. Positive end-expiratory pressure (PEEP) generally opposes injury or edema formation *(minus sign)* except when it contributes to overinflation *(plus sign)*. (From Dreyfuss D, Saumon G. Ventilator-induced lung injury: lessons from experimental studies. Am J Respir Crit Care Med. 1998;157:294-323.)

Mechanisms of Increased Vascular Transmural Pressure

Increased fluid filtration may occur at both extra-alveolar[47,48] and alveolar[49-51] sites during mechanical ventilation. Increased transmural pressure in extraalveolar vessels results from the increase in lung volume, and the decrease in perivascular interstitial pressure is the consequence of lung stretch.[45,52,53] Increased filtration across alveolar microvessels also may be promoted by the surfactant inactivation[4,49] that accompanies ventilation at high V_T or because of the presence of plasma proteins (such as fibrinogen and albumin) in airspaces.

Mechanisms of Altered Permeability

Although capillary permeability alterations are obvious and may be severe during ventilator-induced edema, the underlying mechanisms are not fully understood and may vary according to the extent and duration of lung overdistention.

Effects of Surfactant Inactivation

In addition to its effects on fluid filtration, surfactant inactivation and elevated alveolar surface tension may increase alveolar epithelial permeability to small solutes. Surfactant inactivation by detergent aerosolization increases diethylenetriaminepentaacetic acid (DTPA) clearance in rabbits[54] and dogs.[55] This effect has been ascribed to the ventilation

inhomogeneities and regional overexpansion that result from uneven inactivation of surfactant and maldistribution of lung mechanical properties rather than to the elimination of peculiar barrier properties of surfactant.[55] The effects of surfactant inactivation and large V_T ventilation on alveolocapillary permeability (as assessed by pulmonary DTPA clearance) are additive.[56] Endothelial permeability may be altered because the increased surface tension due to surfactant inactivation augments radial traction on pulmonary microvessels.[49]

Participation of Inflammatory Cells and Mediators
Role of Inflammatory Cells
The endothelial cell disruption observed during overinflation edema in small animals may allow direct contact between polymorphonuclear cells and the basement membrane. This contact may promote leukocyte sequestration. A striking feature of the VILI that occurs after several hours is the infiltration of inflammatory cells into the interstitial and alveolar spaces. In one of the earliest studies on this subject, Woo and Hedley-White[57] observed that overinflation produced edema in open-chest dogs and that leukocytes accumulated in the vasculature and macrophages in the alveoli. Further studies have confirmed these results[58] and have shown that high transpulmonary pressure increased the transit time of leukocytes in the lungs of rabbits.[59] Conversely, when animals are depleted

of neutrophils, high-volume pulmonary edema is less severe than in nondepleted animals.[60]

Role of Inflammatory Mediators (Biotrauma Hypothesis)

Tremblay and colleagues[61] examined the effects of different ventilatory strategies on the level of several cytokines in bronchoalveolar lavage fluid of isolated rat lungs ventilated with different end-expiratory pressures and V_T. High V_T ventilation (40 mL/kg) with zero end-expiratory pressure resulted in considerable increases in tumor necrosis factor (TNF)-α, interleukin (IL)-1β and IL-6, and macrophage inflammatory protein (MIP)-2 (Fig. 52.9). Although these findings have been inconstantly replicated in animals with healthy lungs and it remains unclear whether injurious ventilator settings can result in primary production of pro-inflammatory cytokines in the lungs,[62,63] it will do so when combined with another aggression (ie, the two-hit theory), such as hemorrhagic shock and resuscitation[64] or mesenteric ischemia-reperfusion.[65] The biotrauma hypothesis forms the rationale for the attempts to modulate pharmacologically the imbalance between lung pro- and antiinflammatory mediators during VILI.

In addition to increasing the amount of cytokines in the lung, it has been suspected that overinflation during mechanical ventilation may promote the release of cytokines[66,67] or bacteria[68,69] into the blood, thus giving a causative role for mechanical ventilation in multiorgan dysfunction.[70] However, this hypothesis remains to be proved.[71]

New Insights in Ventilator-Induced Lung Injury
Cellular Response to Mechanical Strain and Pharmacologic Interventions

Parker and colleagues[72] studied the different signal transduction pathways that may be involved in the microvascular permeability increases observed during experimental VILI. They found that gadolinium, which blocks stretch-activated nonselective cation channels, annulled the increases in vascular permeability induced by high airway pressure.[73] The authors concluded that stretch-activated cation channels might initiate the increase in permeability induced by mechanical ventilation through increases in intracellular Ca^{2+} concentration. Such results suggested that the increase in microvascular permeability may not simply be a passive physical phenomenon (a *stress failure*[74,75]) but may at least in part be the result of biochemical reactions.

Numerous cell signaling pathways have indeed been shown to be involved in the pathophysiology of VILI. Several pharmacologic interventions have been tested, including (1) attempts to modulate the microvascular permeability using blockers of stretch-activated cation channels,[73] beta-adrenergic agonists,[76] inhibitors of phosphotyrosine kinase,[77] or reducing myosin light chain phosphorylation with adrenomedullin[78]; (2) attempts to modulate the imbalance between pro- and

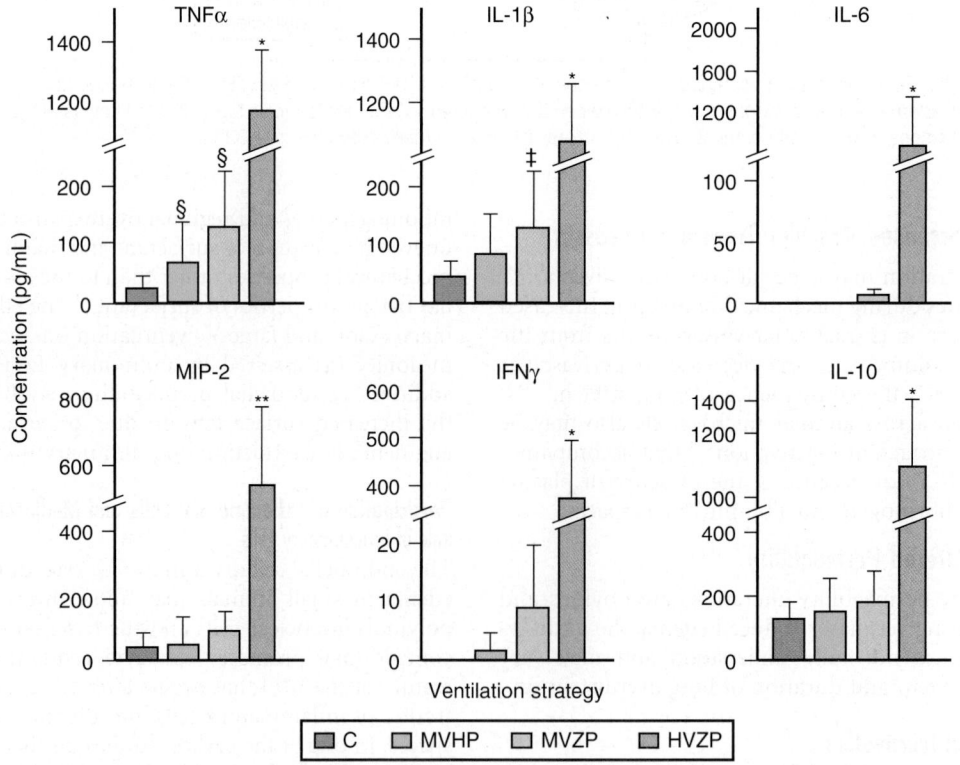

Fig. 52.9. Effect of different ventilatory strategies on cytokine concentrations in lung lavage of isolated unperfused rat lungs. Four ventilator settings were used: controls (*C*, normal tidal volume [V_T]), moderate V_T + high positive end-expiratory pressure (PEEP) (*MVHP*), moderate V_T + zero PEEP (*MVZP*), and high V_T + zero PEEP (*HVZP*) resulting in the same end-inspiratory distention as MVHP. Major increases in cytokine concentrations were observed with HVZP. *IFN*, interferon; *IL*, interleukin; *MIP*, macrophage inflammatory protein; *TNF*, tumor necrosis factor. (From Tremblay L, Valenza F, Ribeiro SP, et al. Injurious ventilatory strategies increase cytokines and c-fos m-RNA expression in an isolated rat lung model. J Clin Invest. 1997;99:944-952.)

antiinflammatory mediators in the lung (eg, administration of anti–TNF-α antibody[79-81] and inhibition of MIP-2 activity,[82,83] which reduced neutrophilic infiltration and lung injury); and (3) attempts to modulate hormonal and metabolic pathways. For instance, inhibition of the renin-angiotensin system[84,85] and pretreatment with atorvastatin or simvastatin[86,87] decreased alveolar-capillary barrier permeability and lung inflammation in experimental models of VILI. Nevertheless, none of those pharmacologic interventions has proved beneficial for the prevention and treatment of VILI in patients. Although it is probably illusory to believe that a single pharmacologic intervention might be beneficial in patients, the description of those pathways illustrates the complexity of the cellular mechanisms involved in VILI.

Influence of Carbon Dioxide Tension on Ventilator-Induced Lung Injury

Deleterious effects of hypocapnia have been extensively reviewed.[88] However, it is important to note that, in addition to detrimental effects of hypocapnia[89] and hypercapnia[90] on ischemia-reperfusion lung injury, experimental studies suggest that hypercapnia may protect from the acute increase in capillary permeability caused by overinflation[91] and from inflammation during VILI.[92]

Strategies to Reduce Ventilator-Induced Lung Injury: Use of the Pressure-Volume Curve and Analysis of the Mechanics of the Respiratory System

The ARDS network trial[93] has undisputedly shown that reducing V_T from 12 mL/kg to 6 mL/kg resulted in a 22% reduction in mortality rate (Fig. 52.10). By protocol, the same reduction of V_T was applied to all patients allocated to the low V_T group. However, it has repeatedly been shown that pressures and the volumes considered safe for some patients with ARDS may cause lung overdistention in others.[94-97] Conversely, arbitrary settings may result in an unnecessary reduction in V_T, which a meta-analysis has suggested as being potentially harmful.[98]

Taking the presence and value of a lower inflection point (LIP) on the pressure-volume curve into account when setting the level of PEEP may lessen VILI in some[32,33,35] but not all instances.[34] The concept on lung protection against VILI with the setting of a PEEP level above the LIP, however, relies on a putative stabilizing effect of PEEP that would reduce the repetitive opening and closing of distal lung units. As discussed earlier, serious criticisms have been raised against this opening and closing theory,[99] casting doubt on the usefulness of measuring LIP to prevent VILI.

The overall degree of lung distention resulting from the settings of both PEEP and tidal volume is a fundamental determinant of VILI. Although the exact physiologic significance of an upper inflection point (UIP) is debated, it may indicate lung overstretching. Ventilation that takes place above the UIP was found to be markedly deleterious.[100] Thus, determination of the volume at which the UIP is observed may help reduce the risk of VILI, because it indicates the maximum stretch that the lung can sustain without noticeable damage.[100] Analysis of the airway pressure-time curve during mechanical ventilation has also proved useful in determining the stress applied to lungs. Indeed, an upward concavity of the pressure-time curve suggests that compliance decreases as tidal volume is delivered, with resulting high-volume stress.[101] Such a ventilation pattern was associated with histologic lung injury in an isolated, nonperfused, lavage model of acute lung injury[101] and with overdistention, as attested by CT-scan analysis of the lungs of intact animals with saline lavage-induced lung injury.[102] The same group of authors demonstrated that in patients with ARDS, a ventilation strategy achieving a stress index greater than 1.05 (ie, the shape of the pressure-time curve demonstrating an upward concavity) had a negative predictive value of 0.86 for the presence of tidal hyperinflation, as assessed by chest CT scan.[103]

Amato and colleagues proposed using the driving pressure, which is the tidal volume normalized by the compliance of the respiratory system, to reconcile discrepant findings from clinical studies reporting conflicting responses from the manipulation of tidal volume, plateau pressure, and PEEP.[2,38,39,93,104,105] Reanalyzing the results of previously published clinical studies, using a mediation analysis of individual data from 3562 patients, they concluded that among the ventilator parameters studied, the driving pressure was most closely associated with mortality, with each 1 SD increment (7 cm H_2O) being associated with a relative risk of 1.41.[106] Although clinical evidence is still lacking to ascertain that ventilation strategies aiming at reducing the driving pressure would improve outcomes of patients with ARDS, this parameter might help explain the negative results of these studies comparing higher versus lower PEEP levels.[2,38,39]

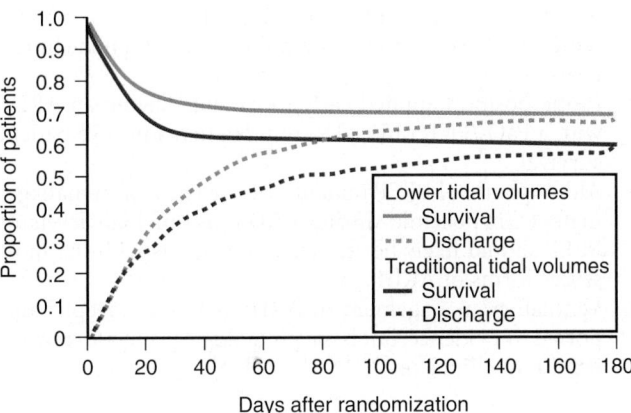

Fig. 52.10. Probability of survival and of being discharged home and breathing without assistance during the first 180 days after randomization in patients with acute lung injury and acute respiratory distress syndrome. (From The Acute Respiratory Distress Syndrome Network. Ventilation with lower tidal volumes as compared with traditional tidal volumes for acute lung injury and the acute respiratory distress syndrome. N Engl J Med. 2000;342:1301-1308.)

Strategies to Reduce Ventilator-Induced Lung Injury: Mechanical Measures

Prone position was shown to be lung protective in experimental models because it favors a more homogeneous distribution of transpulmonary pressure gradient,[107] it increases lung recruitment of collapsed areas, thereby lowering lung strain,[108,109] and it improves gas exchanges through regional perfusion alterations.[110] As compared to supine position, prone position homogenized the distribution of lung injury in dogs with normal lungs subjected to injurious ventilation[111] and lessened the histologic lesions in dogs with previously injured lungs and similar ventilator settings.[112] These benefits have led to the realization of clinical studies assessing the impact of prone position in ARDS patients. Three randomized controlled trials in ARDS showed no benefit to prone positioning on 28-day mortality and ventilator-free days in spite of significant improvement in oxygenation.[113-115] However, a randomized-controlled trial including 466 patients with ARDS and a PaO_2/FiO_2 ratio <150 mm Hg who were randomized to receive a conventional ventilation strategy alone or associated with early and protracted (ie, 16 hours a day) prone position showed a significant reduction in mortality at day 28 (16% versus 33%, p <0.001).[116] This dramatic reduction in mortality is ascribed to a reduction of VILI, and prone position is now believed to be a crucial aspect of management of patients with severe (ie, PaO_2/FiO_2 ratio <150 mm Hg) ARDS.

The effect of surfactant administration was assessed in experimental models of VILI demonstrating that (1) the preventive intratracheal administration of exogenous surfactant reduced impairment of lung mechanics, oxygenation, and alveolar permeability in rats subjected to an injurious ventilation strategy[117] and (2) that a pretreatment with surfactant altered the systemic spread of lung-borne TNF-α of LPS-exposed[118] but not of previously healthy rats.[119] Yet the results of the clinical trials that tested the effects of surfactant administration in ARDS patients were disappointing: Aerosolized[120] or tracheally instilled[121] surfactant had no effect on survival and lung mechanics in an adult population of ARDS patients in spite of an effect on oxygenation during the 24 hours following administration in one study.[121] These negative results might be attributed to both the types of surfactant used and administration modalities. As a matter of fact, in pediatric patients with acute lung injury (premature infants being excluded), and as compared to placebo, the intratracheal administration of a natural surfactant (calfactant) was associated with reduced mortality (19.5% versus 36%) and improved lung mechanics and oxygenation, but there were no differences in ventilator-free days.[122]

Perfluorocarbons have physical properties that allow for decreasing the mechanical heterogeneity of acutely injured lungs by the suppression of air-liquid interfaces and the reopening of collapsed or liquid-filled areas. Partial liquid ventilation (PLV)[123] with perfluorocarbons has thus been tested as an alternative to conventional gas ventilation for the treatment of acute respiratory failure. In experimental models of acute lung injury, PLV was shown not only to improve gas exchanges and lung mechanics dose-dependently[124] but also to decrease histologic lung lesions.[125] However, when both large perfluorocarbon and tidal volumes were used, PLV led to a high incidence of barotrauma.[126] The mechanical properties of rat lungs flooded with saline in order to reduce the aerated volume were studied after injurious mechanical ventilation with and without intratracheal perfluorocarbon instillation. The instillation of a low dose (3.3 ml/kg) of perfluorocarbon in these flooded lungs not only improved lung mechanics but also decreased permeability alterations.[26] The effect of perfluorocarbon dosing was further tested in rats ventilated with high tidal volumes having previously healthy[127] or preinjured[128] lungs: Lower doses (10 mL/kg) of perfluorocarbon were protective, whereas larger doses (13 and 16 mL/kg) aggravated lung edema. A clinical trial comparing conventional ventilation to PLV with low (10 mL/kg) and high (20 mL/kg) doses of perfluorocarbon yielded consistent results. Indeed, both PLV groups exhibited not only higher plateau pressures and poorer oxygenation than the conventional ventilation group but also fewer ventilator-free days and a trend toward greater mortality, as well as a higher incidence of pneumothoraces (17% versus 6%, p <0.05).[129] The failure of PLV when large perfluorocarbon volumes are used, and thus high plateau pressures generated, highlights the clinical relevance of VILI.

Conclusion and Clinical Applications

The experimental concept of VILI is undeniably relevant to clinical practice.[93] High-volume injury contributes to the mortality of patients with ARDS and may be reduced by decreasing V_T and plateau pressure. On the other hand, the concept of low lung volume injury that should benefit from high levels of PEEP has not received the same convincing clinical confirmation, given the negative survival data from three randomized controlled trials comparing two levels of PEEP,[2,38,39] but still, current guidelines, which mainly rely on a meta-analysis of these three trials,[130] recommend using high PEEP levels for the most severe ARDS patients.[131] Thus the ideal ventilatory strategy has yet to be determined. For the time being and until further evidence is obtained, one may put forward the following conclusions:

- Tidal volume reduction should likely apply to all mechanically ventilated patients, and a 6-mL/kg V_T with a plateau pressure <28 cm H_2O is typically used because of the lack of readily available tools that allow for measuring the aerated lung volume at bedside, thus limiting the possibility to titrate individually an ideal V_T. In the meantime, the analysis of the respiratory mechanics can provide meaningful tools, which can indicate that the ventilation strategy is likely to be safe.[103,106]
- Superprotective ventilation strategies relying on techniques such as extracorporeal CO_2 removal or extracorporeal membrane oxygenation (ECMO), rendering it possible to drastically reduce the V_T applied (ie, in the range of 3 and 6 mL/kg), have yet to be assessed by well-designed clinical trials.
- Prone position applied early to patients having an ARDS with a PaO_2/FiO_2 ratio <150 mm Hg may improve patient survival.
- Although use of PEEP remains the cornerstone of management of hypoxemia during ARDS, use of high levels of PEEP should likely be restricted to patients with the most severe forms of ARDS.
- Ventilatory management of ARDS is not yet deeply supported by evidence, but basic physiologic principles remain helpful to clinicians.[62,99,132,133]

Key References

2. Brower RG, et al. Higher versus lower positive end-expiratory pressures in patients with the acute respiratory distress syndrome. N Engl J Med. 2004;351:327-336.
4. Webb HH, Tierney DF. Experimental pulmonary edema due to intermittent positive pressure ventilation with high inflation pressures.

Protection by positive end-expiratory pressure. *Am Rev Respir Dis.* 1974;110:556-565.

5. Dreyfuss D, Basset G, Soler P, Saumon G. Intermittent positive-pressure hyperventilation with high inflation pressures produces pulmonary microvascular injury in rats. *Am Rev Respir Dis.* 1985;132:880-884.

6. Dreyfuss D, Soler P, Basset G, Saumon G. High inflation pressure pulmonary edema. Respective effects of high airway pressure, high tidal volume, and positive end-expiratory pressure. *Am Rev Respir Dis.* 1988;137:1159-1164.

8. Dreyfuss D, Soler P, Saumon G. Spontaneous resolution of pulmonary edema caused by short periods of cyclic overinflation. *J Appl Physiol.* 1992;72:2081-2089.

11. de Prost N, Dreyfuss D, Saumon G. Evaluation of two-way protein fluxes across the alveolo-capillary membrane by scintigraphy in rats: effect of lung inflation. *J Appl Physiol.* 2007;102:794-802.

12. Chiumello D, Carlesso E, Cadringher P, et al. Lung stress and strain during mechanical ventilation for acute respiratory distress syndrome. *Am J Respir Crit Care Med.* 2008;178:346-355.

13. Protti A, Cressoni M, Santini A, et al. Lung stress and strain during mechanical ventilation: any safe threshold? *Am J Respir Crit Care Med.* 2011;183:1354-1362.

14. Caironi P, Langer T, Carlesso E, et al. Time to generate ventilator-induced lung injury among mammals with healthy lungs: a unifying hypothesis. *Intensive Care Med.* 2011;37(12):1913-1920.

21. Hernandez LA, Coker PJ, May S, et al. Mechanical ventilation increases microvascular permeability in oleic injured lungs. *J Appl Physiol.* 1990;69:2057-2061.

22. Dreyfuss D, Soler P, Saumon G. Mechanical ventilation-induced pulmonary edema. Interactions with previous lung alterations. *Am J Respir Crit Care Med.* 1995;151:1568-1575.

26. Dreyfuss D, Martin-Lefevre L, Saumon G. Hyperinflation-induced lung injury during alveolar flooding in rats: effect of perfluorocarbon instillation. *Am J Respir Crit Care Med.* 1999;159:1752-1757.

29. Falke KJ, Pontoppidan H, Kumar A, et al. Ventilation with end-expiratory pressure in acute lung disease. *J Clin Invest.* 1972;51:2315-2323.

30. Matamis D, Lemaire F, Harf A, et al. Total respiratory pressure-volume curves in the adult respiratory distress syndrome. *Chest.* 1984;86:58-66.

31. Suter PM, Fairley B, Isenberg MD. Optimum end-expiratory airway pressure in patients with acute pulmonary failure. *N Engl J Med.* 1975;292:284-289.

32. Argiras EP, Blakeley CR, Dunnill MS, et al. High peep decreases hyaline membrane formation in surfactant deficient lungs. *Br J Anaesth.* 1987;59:1278-1285.

35. Muscedere JG, Mullen JBM, Gan K, et al. Tidal ventilation at low airway pressures can augment lung injury. *Am J Respir Crit Care Med.* 1994;149:1327-1334.

36. Martynowicz MA, Minor TA, Walters BJ, Hubmayr RD. Regional expansion of oleic acid-injured lungs. *Am J Respir Crit Care Med.* 1999;160:250-258.

38. Meade MO, Cook DJ, Guyatt GH, et al. Ventilation strategy using low tidal volumes, recruitment maneuvers, and high positive end-expiratory pressure for acute lung injury and acute respiratory distress syndrome: a randomized controlled trial. *JAMA.* 2008;299:637-645.

39. Mercat A, Richard JC, Vielle B, et al. Positive end-expiratory pressure setting in adults with acute lung injury and acute respiratory distress syndrome: a randomized controlled trial. *JAMA.* 2008;299:646-655.

46. Dreyfuss D, Saumon G. Role of tidal volume, FRC and end-inspiratory volume in the development of pulmonary edema following mechanical ventilation. *Am Rev Respir Dis.* 1993;148:1194-1203.

58. Tsuno K, Miura K, Takey M, et al. Histopathologic pulmonary changes from mechanical ventilation at high peak airway pressures. *Am Rev Respir Dis.* 1991;143:1115-1120.

60. Kawano T, Mori S, Cybulsky M, et al. Effect of granulocyte depletion in a ventilated surfactant-depleted lung. *J Appl Physiol.* 1987;62:27-33.

61. Tremblay L, Valenza F, Ribeiro SP, et al. Injurious ventilatory strategies increase cytokines and c-fos m-RNA expression in an isolated rat lung model. *J Clin Invest.* 1997;99:944-952.

63. Ricard JD, Dreyfuss D, Saumon G. Production of inflammatory cytokines in ventilator-induced lung injury: a reappraisal. *Am J Respir Crit Care Med.* 2001;163:1176-1180.

65. Bouadma L, Schortgen F, Ricard J, et al. Ventilation strategy affects cytokine release after mesenteric ischemia-reperfusion in rats. *Crit Care Med.* 2004;32:1563-1569.

66. Imai Y, Kawano T, Miyasaka K, et al. Inflammatory chemical mediators during conventional ventilation and during high frequency oscillatory ventilation. *Am J Respir Crit Care Med.* 1994;150:1550-1554.

68. Nahum A, Hoyt J, Schmitz L, et al. Effect of mechanical ventilation strategy on dissemination of intratracheally instilled Escherichia coli in dogs. *Crit Care Med.* 1997;25:1733-1743.

69. Verbrugge S, Sorm V, van 't Veen A, et al. Lung overinflation without positive end-expiratory pressure promotes bacteremia after experimental Klebsiella pneumoniae inoculation. *Intensive Care Med.* 1998;24:172-177.

72. Parker JC, Townsley MI, Rippe B, et al. Increased microvascular permeability in dog lungs due to high airway pressures. *J Appl Physiol.* 1984;57:1809-1816.

73. Parker JC, Ivey CL, Tucker JA. Gadolinium prevents high airway pressure-induced permeability increases in isolated rat lungs. *J Appl Physiol.* 1998;84:1113-1118.

77. Parker JC. Inhibitors of myosin light chain kinase and phosphodiesterase reduce ventilator-induced lung injury. *J Appl Physiol.* 2000;89:2241-2248.

93. Ventilation with lower tidal volumes as compared with traditional tidal volumes for acute lung injury and the acute respiratory distress syndrome. The Acute Respiratory Distress Syndrome Network [see comments]. *N Engl J Med.* 2000;342:1301-1308.

94. Gattinoni L, Pelosi P, Crotti S, Valenza F. Effects of positive end-expiratory pressure on regional distribution of tidal volume and recruitment in adult respiratory distress syndrome. *Am J Respir Crit Care Med.* 1995;151:1807-1814.

95. Gattinoni L, Pesanti A, Avalli L, et al. Pressure-volume curves of total respiratory system in acute respiratory failure. Computed tomographic scan study. *Am Rev Respir Dis.* 1987;136:730-736.

97. Roupie E, Dambrosio M, Servillo G, et al. Titration of tidal volume and induced hypercapnia in acute respiratory distress syndrome. *Am J Respir Crit Care Med.* 1995;152:121-128.

99. Hubmayr RD. Perspective on lung injury and recruitment: a skeptical look at the opening and collapse story. *Am J Respir Crit Care Med.* 2002;165:1647-1653.

101. Ranieri VM, Zhang H, Mascia L, et al. Pressure-time curve predicts minimally injurious ventilatory strategy in an isolated rat lung model. *Anesthesiology.* 2000;93:1320-1328.

102. Grasso S, Terragni P, Mascia L, et al. Airway pressure-time curve profile (stress index) detects tidal recruitment/hyperinflation in experimental acute lung injury. *Crit Care Med.* 2004;32:1018-1027.

103. Terragni PP, Filippini C, Slutsky AS, et al. Accuracy of plateau pressure and stress index to identify injurious ventilation in patients with acute respiratory distress syndrome. *Anesthesiology.* 2013;119:880-889.

104. Talmor D, Sarge T, Malhotra A, et al. Mechanical ventilation guided by esophageal pressure in acute lung injury. *N Engl J Med.* 2008;359:2095-2104.

105. Amato MBP, Barbas CSV, Medeiros DM, et al. Effect of a protective-ventilation strategy on mortality in the acute respiratory distress syndrome. *N Engl J Med.* 1998;338:347-354.

106. Amato MB, Meade MO, Slutsky AS, et al. Driving pressure and survival in the acute respiratory distress syndrome. *N Engl J Med.* 2015;372:747-755.

113. Guerin C, Gaillard S, Lemasson S, et al. Effects of systematic prone positioning in hypoxemic acute respiratory failure: a randomized controlled trial. *JAMA.* 2004;292:2379-2387.

114. Taccone P, Pesenti A, Latini R, et al. Prone positioning in patients with moderate and severe acute respiratory distress syndrome: a randomized controlled trial. *JAMA.* 2009;302:1977-1984.

116. Guerin C, Reignier J, Richard JC, et al. Prone positioning in severe acute respiratory distress syndrome. *N Engl J Med.* 2013;368:2159-2168.

121. Spragg RG, Lewis JF, Walmrath HD, et al. Effect of recombinant surfactant protein C-based surfactant on the acute respiratory distress syndrome. *N Engl J Med.* 2004;351:884-892.

127. Ricard JD, Dreyfuss D, Laissy JP, Saumon G. Dose-response effect of perfluorocarbon administration on lung microvascular permeability in rats. *Am J Respir Crit Care Med.* 2003;168:1378-1382.

129. Kacmarek RM, Wiedemann HP, Lavin PT, et al. Partial liquid ventilation in adult patients with the acute respiratory distress syndrome. *Am J Respir Crit Care Med.* 2006;173:882-889.

130. Briel M, Meade M, Mercat A, et al. Higher vs lower positive end-expiratory pressure in patients with acute lung injury and acute respiratory distress syndrome: systematic review and meta-analysis. *JAMA.* 2010;303:865-873.

Asthma

Steven L. Shein, Richard H. Speicher, Howard Eigen, and Alexandre T. Rotta

PEARLS

- Patients with severe acute asthma exacerbations should be promptly and aggressively managed in the emergency department with inhaled β-agonist agents, inhaled ipratropium bromide, oxygen, and a systemic corticosteroid. Patients who fail to improve or who further deteriorate should be admitted to the intensive care unit for escalation of therapy and a higher level of monitoring.
- Standard treatments include administration of intravenous fluids, oxygen, β-agonist agents by intermittent or continuous nebulization, ipratropium bromide, parenteral corticosteroids, and intravenous infusion of a β_2-agonist agent. Other therapies available in the intensive care unit include intravenous infusions of magnesium sulfate and methylxanthine agents, and breathing helium-oxygen mixtures.
- Failure to respond to treatment can lead to further deterioration and the development of respiratory failure, necessitating noninvasive ventilatory support or even intubation and mechanical ventilation. When needed, ventilation should be initiated with a strategy that avoids dynamic hyperinflation. Select patients may benefit from inhalational anesthetic agents for bronchodilatation, bronchoscopy to relieve airway obstruction or atelectasis resulting from mucous plugging, or extracorporeal life support.
- Aggressive medical treatment and a mechanical ventilation strategy that minimizes dynamic hyperinflation result in low morbidity and near-zero mortality rates in patients with critical or near-fatal asthma.

Asthma is a highly prevalent chronic disease that affects both children and adults. It is the most common medical emergency in the pediatric population. Despite adequate treatment and access to medical care, patients with asthma are at risk for episodic acute respiratory deterioration, commonly known as reactive airway disease exacerbations or asthma attacks. These episodes vary greatly in severity, ranging from those that are easily managed in the outpatient setting by increasing corticosteroid and bronchodilator therapy to severe episodes with intense airway obstruction that rapidly evolve to respiratory failure.

Several terms are used to denote severe asthma attacks, including *status asthmaticus, acute severe asthma, critical asthma,* and *near-fatal asthma.* Definitions vary among sources, and many consider *status asthmaticus* to be an outdated term.[1-5] For this text, *acute severe asthma* is defined as an asthma attack unresponsive to repeated doses of beta-agonists and requiring hospital admission,[1] *critical asthma* is defined as acute severe asthma necessitating ICU admission,[6,7] and *near-fatal asthma* is defined as critical asthma that requires endotracheal intubation and mechanical ventilation.[7]

Epidemiology and Risk Factors

Asthma is the most common chronic illness in childhood, affecting 9.5% of all children in the United States.[8] Overall global prevalence is approximately 11% to 13% and varies widely, from approximately 5% in some Asian and Eastern Europe countries to nearly 25% in parts of Central America, South America, Oceania, and the United Kingdom.[9] Asthma is a common reason for hospitalization, with approximately 150,000 pediatric asthma admissions occurring in the United States annually.[10] It is also a common comorbidity among children hospitalized for other reasons, present in 21.8% of all-cause pediatric hospitalizations.[11] In some countries, including the United States, asthma hospitalizations are becoming less frequent, but admissions are increasing in other developed countries.[10,12,13] Even in areas where the incidence of acute severe asthma is decreasing, admissions to the pediatric intensive care unit (PICU) are increasing. In New Jersey, the incidence of critical asthma increased from 0.09 to 0.31 per 1000 children between 1992 and 2006, and 35% of acute severe asthma admissions received ICU care during the most recent epoch.[14] In Ohio, ICU utilization averages approximately 25% among six children's hospitals, with greater than 40% of hospitalized children receiving ICU care at some centers.[15] Rates of positive pressure ventilation for asthma have increased in the United States and Spain.[10,12] Among critical asthma patients in the United States, 5% to 12% are treated with invasive mechanical ventilation, and 3% to 5% are treated with noninvasive ventilation.[14,16,17] Intubation prior to PICU admission is common and associated with shorter duration of mechanical ventilation.[16] Despite this increase in critical care utilization, mortality rates from acute severe asthma (<0.1%), critical asthma (~0.3%), and near-fatal asthma (~4%) are quite low. Many of the deaths from asthma occur in patients who suffered prehospital cardiac arrest.[7,12,14,16]

Risk factors for severe asthma exacerbations are of particular importance to the practicing intensivist (Box 53.1). Critical asthma is disproportionately more common in boys, Hispanic children, and African-American children.[16] Risk factors for near-fatal asthma include African-American race, older age, concurrent pneumonia, and the presence of comorbid conditions.[7,10,14]

BOX 53.1 Risk Factors for Near-Fatal Asthma

Medical Factors

Previous asthma attack with the following:
- Admission to intensive care unit
- Respiratory failure and mechanical ventilation
- Seizures or syncope
- Paco$_2$ >45 torr
- High consumption (>2 canisters per month) of β-agonist metered-dose inhalers
- Underuse of corticosteroid therapy

Psychosocial Factors
- Denial of or failure to perceive severity of illness
- Associated depression or other psychiatric disorder
- Noncompliance
- Dysfunctional family unit
- Inner-city residents

Ethnic Factors
- Nonwhite children (black, Hispanic, other)

The majority of patients with asthma who progress to near-fatal asthma or cardiac arrest do so prior to arrival at the emergency department or during the first stages of therapy.[7,18] Therefore early identification and close monitoring of patients at high risk for near-fatal asthma could be advantageous. High-risk patients often have a history of ICU admissions,[19] mechanical ventilation,[4,19] seizures or syncope during an attack,[20] PaCO$_2$ greater than 45 torr,[4,19] attacks precipitated by food,[19] or a history of rapidly progressive and sudden respiratory deterioration.[5] High-risk patients are likely to use more than two canisters of β-agonist metered-dose inhalers per month[21] and often are poorly compliant or are receiving insufficient steroid therapy.[22,23] Denial and failure to perceive the severity of an attack are factors frequently associated with near-fatal asthma.[24,25] Although unquestionably some patients at risk for near-fatal asthma simply ignore early warning signs and do not seek medical attention, a subgroup of patients actually lacks normal perception of disease severity. Some patients with near-fatal asthma exhibit reduced chemosensitivity to hypoxia and blunted perception of dyspnea.[26] Other patients have a decreased perceptual sensitivity of inspiratory muscle loads and display abnormal respiratory-related evoked potentials.[27]

Although many of these high-risk factors are commonly present in patients with near-fatal asthma, they fail to identify a significant number of cases. In one case series, 33% of patients who died of asthma were judged to have a history of trivial or mild asthma, whereas 32% had never been admitted to the hospital with an asthma exacerbation.[5] The Collaborative Pediatric Critical Care Research Network (CPCCRN) reported that 13% of 260 children with near-fatal asthma had no prior history of asthma and that only 37% of known asthmatics had required hospitalization in the 12 months preceding the episode of near-fatal asthma.[7] Some of these patients may in fact have what likely represents a distinct clinical entity known as sudden asphyxial asthma, a condition marked by acute onset of severe airway obstruction and hypoxia that rapidly leads to cardiorespiratory arrest in patients known to have only mild asthma or no asthma history at all.[28,29]

Pathophysiology

Asthma is primarily an inflammatory disease and, as such, it is marked by highly complex interactions among inflammatory cells, mediators, and the airway epithelium[30] (Fig. 53.1). Functionally, asthma is characterized by variable airflow obstruction and airway hyperresponsiveness associated with airway inflammation. Though various inflammatory phenotypes cause clinical asthma, asthmatic patients commonly have airway inflammation dominated by eosinophils, T$_H$2 cytokines, and IgE.[31] Pathologically, it is marked by mast cell degranulation, accumulation of eosinophils and CD4 lymphocytes, hypersecretion of mucus, thickening of the subepithelial collagen layer, and smooth muscle hypertrophy and hyperplasia.[32]

Mast cells, eosinophils, neutrophils, macrophages, and T lymphocytes are central to the derangements that occur during an acute attack (see Fig. 53.1). The usual cascade begins with the activation and degranulation of mast cells in response to allergens or topical insults. Mast cells release mediators including histamine, prostaglandins, and leukotrienes that cause acute bronchoconstriction. Additionally, the mast cells promote activation of T lymphocytes via allergen presentation. The inflammatory process is then amplified by T-lymphocyte release of cytokines and chemokines, predominantly T$_H$2 cytokines, such as interleukin (IL)-4, IL-5, IL-8, and IL-13.[33] The presence of these T$_H$2 cytokines leads to further augmentation of the inflammatory process through excessive production of immunoglobulin E (IgE) by B cells, stimulation of airway epithelial cells, and eosinophil chemotaxis. IgE stimulates mast cells to release leukotrienes, whereas interleukins (particularly IL-5) promote maturation and migration of activated eosinophils into the airway.[34] This highly inflammatory state results in stimulation of airway epithelial cells and continued augmentation of the inflammatory process by further release of leukotrienes, prostaglandins, nitric oxide, adhesion molecules, and platelet-activating factor. This process results in overproduction of mucus and in epithelial cell destruction, leading to airway plugging and denuding of the airway surface. Disruption of the epithelial surface exposes nerve endings, resulting in hyperirritable airways[35] that become more susceptible to spasm and obstruction when challenged by subsequent exposures to allergens and irritants.[36] Airway irritants that trigger acute asthma include cigarette smoke and inhaled particulates,[37] respiratory tract viruses,[38] psychologic stress,[39] and cold air.[40] The mucus secreted in the airways of asthmatics contains large amounts of cellular debris and is thicker than in normal persons.[42] Mucus hypersecretion may be a principal cause of respiratory failure in persons with severe asthma and has been underappreciated as a factor in respiratory failure.[41-43]

Inflammation-mediated airway edema, mucus hypersecretion, airway plugging, and bronchospasm lead to the severe airway obstruction seen in patients with severe asthma exacerbations. The resulting obstruction and increased airway resistance create an impediment for inspiratory and expiratory gas flow, which leads to deranged pulmonary mechanics and increased lung volumes.[41]

Airway plugging can result in ventilation/perfusion mismatching and an increased oxygen requirement. Hypoxemia is nearly universal in patients with a severe asthma attack, but generally it is easily corrected with supplemental oxygen[44] and

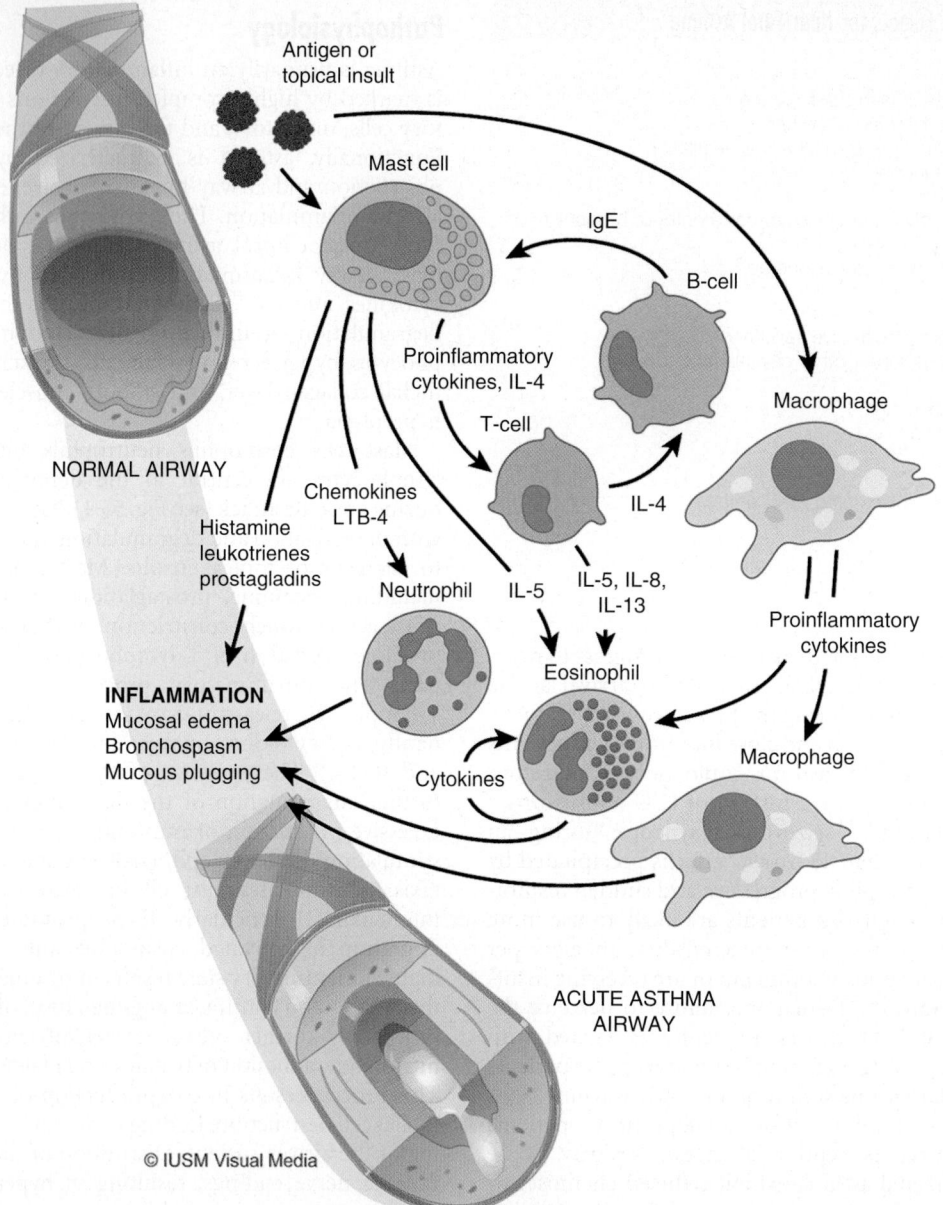

Fig. 53.1. Cellular and humoral mediators that lead to mucosal edema, bronchospasm, and mucous plugging in patients with acute asthma. *IL*, interleukin; *LTB-4*, leukotriene B-4.

is only weakly correlated with pulmonary function abnormalities.[45] More frequently, heterogeneous airway plugging and obstruction lead to regional alveolar hyperinflation associated with reduced perfusion, resulting in a significantly increased pulmonary dead space. Most patients with acute asthma exhibit an increased respiratory rate in attempt to achieve a higher minute volume and compensate for the ventilation abnormality. In asthmatics with acute exacerbations, airway obstruction results in significant prolongation of the expiratory time. The subsequent breath is initiated before the last one has emptied leading to dynamic hyperinflation. The small airways collapse and close at a higher than normal lung volume contributing further to dynamic hyperinflation and air trapping. At higher lung volume there is a higher alveolar driving pressure to empty the lung, which should serve as an adaptive mechanism. However, the net result in acute asthma

is high-energy use. Expiration becomes active with the use of the abdominal muscles. At high lung volumes the lung is less compliant and the inspiratory accessory muscles are engaged to help move an adequate tidal volume[46,47] (Fig. 53.2).

During a severe attack, inspiratory transpulmonary pressures in excess of 50 cm H_2O may be generated, compared with approximately 5 cm H_2O during normal breathing.[48] The increased muscle work is accompanied by an increase in blood flow to the diaphragm, but this flow often is insufficient to meet the much greater metabolic demands.[49] Failure to promptly relieve the airway obstruction and reduce the work of breathing eventually leads to respiratory muscle fatigue, inadequate ventilation, and respiratory failure.

States of advanced airway obstruction and dynamic hyperinflation typical of severe asthma attacks have a significant impact on the circulatory system. The highly negative

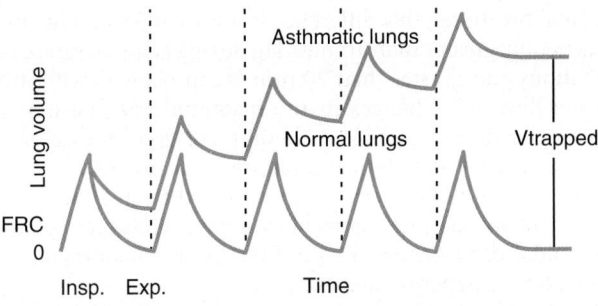

Fig. 53.2. Mechanics of dynamic pulmonary hyperinflation in the setting of severe airflow obstruction. The next inspiration begins before complete exhalation, leading to gas trapping and increased end-expiratory lung volume. *Exp.,* expiration; *FRC,* functional residual capacity; *Insp.,* inspiration; *Vtrapped,* volume of trapped gas above FRC. (From Levy BD, Kitch B, Fanta CH. Medical and ventilatory management of status asthmaticus. Intensive Care Med. 1998;24:105-117.)

TABLE 53.1   Clinical Asthma Evaluation Score*

	0	1	2
PaO$_2$ (torr) *or* Cyanosis	70-100 in 21% O$_2$ None	<70 in 21% O$_2$ In 21% O$_2$	<70 in 40% O$_2$ In 40% O$_2$
Inspiratory breath sounds	Normal	Unequal	Decreased to absent
Accessory muscles used	None	Moderate	Maximal
Expiratory wheezing	None	Moderate	Marked
Cerebral function	Normal	Depressed or agitated	Coma

*A score of 5 or more is thought to be indicative of impending respiratory failure. A score of 7 or more with PaCO$_2$ >65 torr indicates existing respiratory failure. Data from Wood DW, Downes JJ, Lecks HI. A clinical scoring system for the diagnosis of respiratory failure. Preliminary report on childhood status asthmaticus. Am J Dis Child. 1972;123:227-228.

intrapleural pressures generated by spontaneously breathing patients during inspiration favor transcapillary fluid movement into the interstitium and air spaces, promoting pulmonary edema.[47] They also cause a phasic increase in left ventricular afterload and a decrease in cardiac output[50] that is clinically manifested as pulsus paradoxus.[51] Right ventricular afterload may be increased during severe asthma as a result of pulmonary vasoconstriction related to hypoxia and acidosis. A state of increased pulmonary vascular resistance resulting from dynamic hyperinflation also can increase right ventricular afterload, further affecting cardiac output.[51-53]

Clinical Assessment

History

The child with an asthma exacerbation usually presents with complaints of difficulty breathing and shortness of breath. The presence of these complaints in a child known to have had previous asthma exacerbations is highly suggestive of the diagnosis. A significant percentage of children have a history of a coexisting viral upper respiratory infection, whereas some describe exposure to known allergic triggers. Circumstances permitting, time should be taken to inquire about the presence of high-risk factors (discussed earlier) for severe disease and the adequacy of maintenance therapy.

Physical Examination

Children with severe forms of acute asthma commonly present with tachypnea, diaphoresis, increased use of accessory muscles, and nasal flaring. Sick nonverbal children may appear anxious, agitated, or simply unable to be distracted from the task of breathing. Older children often assume a tripod sitting position and may voice a sensation of impending doom. Speech occurs in short phrases because of the rapid respiratory rate. The presence of intercostal, subcostal, and suprasternal retractions; nasal flaring; the inability to speak in sentences; and agitation are signs of impending respiratory failure. Evolution or persistence of these signs is followed by slower labored breathing, confusion or obtundation, and respiratory arrest.

Wheezing, which is a common clinical finding in patients with acute asthma exacerbations, is the audible manifestation of the transmitted turbulence to airflow in the intrathoracic intrapulmonary airways. Wheezing is usually expiratory as a result of the dynamic compression of conducting airways, but it can be inspiratory as well. Wheezing in persons with severe asthma usually is bilateral. Asymmetrical wheezing suggests regional mucous plugging, atelectasis, pneumothorax, or the presence of a foreign body. The degree of wheezing correlates poorly with disease severity,[54] because wheezes are heard only in the presence of sufficient airflow. A patient with severe airway obstruction and limited airflow may have a silent chest upon initial examination, but loud wheezes may develop after effective therapy is instituted. Likewise, in a patient with loud wheezes who continues to worsen, a reduction in wheezing may occur as a prelude to respiratory failure.

An objective assessment of disease severity is important in evaluating a patient's response to therapy. Several asthma severity scores are widely used in clinical practice, including the Clinical Asthma Score (CAS), the Pediatric Asthma Severity Score (PASS), and the Preschool Respiratory Assessment Measure (PRAM).[55-57] Wood and colleagues[58] developed a practical clinical asthma score specifically intended to identify near-fatal asthma. It is composed of five variables with three different grades that allows for semiquantitative assessment of disease severity (Table 53.1), and it correlates well with the need for prolonged bronchodilator therapy and hospitalization.[59] Increasing scores correlate with progressive hypercarbia, and scores >5 often indicate respiratory failure. However, although clinical asthma scores seem to be useful for assessing the severity of an attack, they are not as effective in prospectively identifying patients who require prolonged hospitalization or in whom complications and subsequent disability develop.[60,61] There is still a need for a single scoring system with sufficient validity, reliability, and utility for universal clinical application.[62]

A less frequently used but more objective method of assessing disease severity and progression in patients with severe asthma is measurement of the pulsus paradoxus. Originally described by Adolf Kussmaul[63] in a patient with constrictive pericarditis, pulsus paradoxus also is observed in conditions in which pleural pressure swings are exaggerated, such as

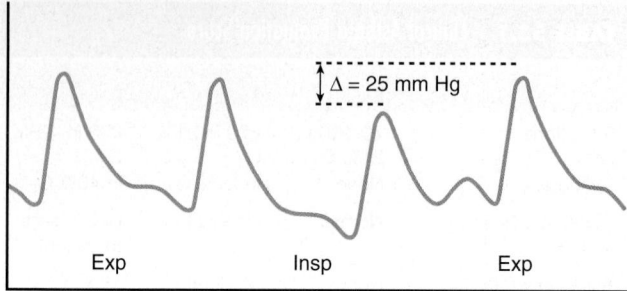

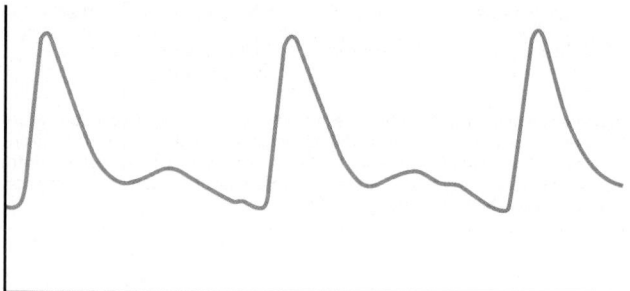

Fig. 53.3. Pressure recording from a radial artery catheter of a spontaneously breathing patient with airway obstruction. *Upper panel:* Abnormally high pulsus paradoxus of 25 mm Hg is measured as the difference (Δ) in systolic blood pressure between expiration (Exp) and inspiration (Insp). *Lower panel:* Normal slight physiologic variation of the systolic blood pressure as a function of the respiratory cycle 12 hours after the onset of treatment.

critical asthma. The simplest definition of pulsus paradoxus is an exaggeration of the physiologic inspiratory decrease in systolic blood pressure[64] (Fig. 53.3). Several mechanisms have been proposed for the occurrence of pulsus paradoxus in persons with asthma, and it is likely that various mechanisms contribute differently depending on the adequacy of intravascular volume, the magnitude of pleural pressure swings, the degree of pulmonary hyperinflation, and the state of cardiac contractility. These mechanisms include cyclic increases in left ventricular afterload and in venous return to the right heart[51] from highly negative intrapleural pressure during inspiration[65]; decreased left ventricular preload as a result of inspiratory blood pooling in the pulmonary vasculature[66]; impaired left ventricular diastolic filling caused by a leftward shift of the interventricular septum resulting from increased venous return to the right heart[67]; constraint of cardiac filling because of longitudinal inspiratory deformation of the pericardium[51]; and increased right ventricular afterload with decreased filling of the left ventricle as a result of hyperinflation, acidosis, and hypoxia.[68] The pulsus paradoxus can be measured easily in a patient who is spontaneously breathing by transducing pressure signals from an indwelling arterial catheter. Alternatively, it can be measured with a manual sphygmomanometer by inflating the cuff 20 mm Hg above the systolic pressure and then deflating it slowly until the first Korotkoff sounds are heard (systolic blood pressure). Initially, Korotkoff sounds are heard only during expiration. The cuff is then carefully deflated until the point where the sounds are appreciated during both inspiration and expiration and correspond to every heartbeat. The difference between the highest systolic pressure and the pressure at which all Korotkoff sounds are heard is the magnitude of the pulsus paradoxus. During

normal breathing, this difference is less than 5 mm Hg, but it is generally greater than 10 mm Hg during acute asthma exacerbations and greater than 20 mm Hg in patients with more severe disease.[69] Changes in the magnitude of pulsus paradoxus during the course of therapy are good indicators of disease severity and clinical response to treatment.[51,69]

In patients with severe asthma exacerbations, the liver is often palpable despite a normal liver span, a finding explained by caudal displacement of the liver by the diaphragm, flattened by the hyperinflated lungs.

Radiography

A chest radiograph is not routinely indicated in acute severe asthma[16] but may be useful in patients suspected of having a pneumothorax, pneumomediastinum, pneumonia, or clinically important atelectasis. In children presenting with a first episode of severe wheezing, a chest radiograph may help diagnose anatomic abnormalities (such as vascular rings or a right-sided aortic arch) or foreign bodies. We generally obtain a chest radiograph in patients who are sick enough to require monitoring and treatment in the ICU to exclude the possibility of unsuspected extrapulmonary or airspace disease.

Laboratory Data
Arterial Blood Gas Analysis

Arterial blood gas measurements provide objective information on the adequacy of ventilation and oxygenation of the patient with asthma. The typical blood gas abnormality in the early phase of acute asthma is hypoxemia with hypocapnia ($PaCO_2$ <35 torr), reflecting hyperventilation.[70] With worsening airway obstruction, $PaCO_2$ measurements return to the normal range of approximately 40 torr. However, this "normal" $PaCO_2$ should not be viewed as reassuring when taken in the context of prolonged expiratory time, tachypnea, and accessory muscle use.[71] In fact, $PaCO_2$ greater than 40 torr in a patient with a severe asthma exacerbation should be interpreted as a sign of evolving respiratory muscle fatigue and warrants close clinical observation. Sicker patients often exhibit a mixed respiratory and metabolic acidosis.[72] Lactic acidosis is frequently encountered in these patients and usually is secondary to excess sympathetic stimulation (type B lactic acidosis),[73] though it may also reflect tissue hypoxia and impending respiratory failure.[74] Measurement of the lactate: pyruvate ratio may help distinguish the etiology of lactic acidosis.

Abnormal arterial blood gas measurements alone should not be the basis for the decision of whether to intubate a child with asthma. This is dictated by the overall clinical status and may come before blood gas measurements reach the usual criteria for respiratory failure. In children requiring mechanical ventilation, frequent blood gas measurements are essential to monitor disease progression and the adequacy of ventilatory support. Additionally, blood gas analysis may be the only means to diagnose significant hypercarbia in critical asthma patients who have neurologic comorbidities or static encephalopathy.

Electrolytes and Complete Blood Cell Count

Routine blood chemistry analysis and blood cell counts generally are not helpful in patients with acute severe asthma.

Children who present with a protracted asthma attack may have evidence of dehydration with elevated blood urea nitrogen or decreased bicarbonate as a result of inadequate oral fluid intake and increased insensible water losses. Patients undergoing repeated treatments with nebulized or intravenous (IV) β-agonist agents might show evidence of hypokalemia from the potassium shift to the intracellular space. The white blood cell count usually is normal, although some atopic patients may exhibit elevated eosinophil counts. The presence of leukocytosis does not necessarily indicate infection and often is related to adaptive stress or the administration of exogenous corticosteroids.

Muscle Enzymes

Myoglobin, a heme protein present in skeletal and cardiac muscle, is often elevated in patients with near-fatal asthma.[75] At least one-third of patients with acute severe asthma exhibit an elevated plasma creatine kinase (CK).[75] Although such elevations seem to be more pronounced in patients with marked acidemia or with more severe respiratory insufficiency, a convincing correlation between disease severity and CK elevation has not been established.[75] Though the CK-myocardial bound (CK-MB) isoenzyme is increased in some patients, most elevations in CK are not secondary to cardiac disease.[75] However, patients with acute severe asthma do have risk factors for acute cardiac injury, including hypoxemia, acidosis, and high myocardial energy demand. Troponin may be elevated even in patients without known cardiac disease. In one study, 36% of critical asthma patients without known cardiac disease (n = 64) who had troponin measured as part of clinical care had elevated levels,[76] and all eight cases of troponin >0.5ng/mL (range: 1–12.6 ng/mL) were associated with sustained diastolic hypotension. Diastolic hypotension develops in many children treated with continuous β-agonist medications, potentially decreasing coronary perfusion,[76] and should be observed for.

Electrocardiography

Patients with significant airway obstruction and hyperinflation may exhibit a change in the mean frontal P-wave vector. A P-wave axis greater than 60 degrees has been associated with hyperinflation in both pediatric and adult patients with airway obstruction and is thought to represent positional atrial changes caused by inferior displacement of the diaphragm.[77]

Twelve-lead electrocardiography and continuous cardiac monitoring are valuable tools in the care of patients with critical asthma in the ICU. These patients usually receive high doses of β-agonist drugs and may show evidence of hypokalemia (low-voltage T waves) or cardiac arrhythmias.[78,79] The already increased myocardial energy demand resulting from airway obstruction is compounded by the chronotropic and vasodilatory effects of β-agonist drugs and may lead to myocardial ischemia, particularly in adult patients with restricted coronary perfusion. Pediatric patients may exhibit electrocardiographic (ECG) and enzymatic evidence of myocardial ischemia, particularly during treatment with intravenously administered isoproterenol.[80] However, despite the fact that a study reported that a high percentage (66%) of patients exhibited nonspecific ST segment changes or other criteria suggestive of ischemia, these changes were not well correlated with

initiation of terbutaline therapy or elevations in cardiac troponin T.[81]

Spirometry

Measurement of peak expiratory flow rates can be used to estimate the degree of airway obstruction and response to therapy in patients presenting to the emergency department with an acute asthma attack. This is less useful in the ICU because sick patients with severe respiratory distress may be unable to perform an adequate forced expiratory maneuver. Measurements also may not be reliable in younger patients who are incapable of coordinating a rapid forced expiratory effort.

Treatment

Initial Management in the Emergency Department

Pediatric patients with mild acute asthma exacerbations generally are treated in the emergency department with one or more doses of an inhaled β-agonist, such as albuterol (salbutamol). Most of these patients also should receive a systemic corticosteroid, such as prednisone, and then can be sent home to complete a 3- to 5-day course of therapy. Patients with mild disease often respond well to initial treatment and do not require the attention of a pediatric intensivist.

Patients with moderate or severe acute asthma attacks require aggressive treatment from the outset. Because most patients with moderate or severe attacks have enough intrapulmonary shunt to result in hypoxemia, supplemental oxygen therapy should be initiated at the earliest time possible. The inspired oxygen can be adjusted once SpO_2 is measured and can be kept above 92%. It should be obvious that use of supplemental oxygen will cause an increase in SpO_2 but will have no impact on ventilation. Therefore one must not assume that ventilation is adequate in a patient with normal SpO_2 during administration of supplemental oxygen therapy.

Nebulized β-agonist agents, such as albuterol (salbutamol), are the most commonly used first-line therapy in the emergency department. The usual albuterol dose ranges between 0.05 and 0.15 mg/kg, diluted with 1 or 2 mL of normal saline solution. However, from a practical standpoint, patients weighing 20 kg or more usually are administered 5-mg doses, whereas patients weighing less than 20 kg receive 2.5-mg doses. Albuterol doses are repeated every 20 minutes during the first hour, with the need for additional doses dictated by clinical response.

Patients with moderate or severe acute asthma also should receive a dose of systemic corticosteroid in the emergency department, which usually is administered prior to the second dose of albuterol. Prednisone (2 mg/kg) can be administered orally and generally is well tolerated. Oral prednisone is superior to inhaled fluticasone in children with severe asthma as evidenced by greater improvement in pulmonary function and lower hospitalization rates.[82] Alternatively, dexamethasone administered as a single intramuscular dose (0.3–1.7 mg/kg) or enterally (0.6 mg/kg daily for 2 days) has been shown to be equivalent to 5-day courses of prednisone with less emesis.[83] The role of corticosteroid drugs in reversing an acute asthma attack in the emergency department has been the subject of debate, considering that these drugs require at least

4 to 6 hours for peak effects to be manifested.[84] However, regardless of considerations about onset of action, acute suppression of inflammation is a cornerstone of acute asthma treatment, and there is evidence that early administration may reduce the rate of hospitalization.[85] Patients with more severe asthma exacerbations, those unable to tolerate oral medication because of respiratory distress or emesis, or those with a history of nausea during intensive β-agonist therapy should be given parenteral corticosteroid drugs such as methylprednisolone (2 mg/kg administered intravenously, followed by 0.5 to 1 mg/kg/dose administered intravenously every 6 hours).

Inhaled or nebulized anticholinergic agents such as ipratropium bromide are an important adjunct to the treatment of asthma exacerbations in the emergency department. In patients treated with one dose of a corticosteroid, use of ipratropium bromide (500 μg/2.5 mL) in conjunction with the second and third albuterol doses has been associated with greater clinical improvement[86] and reduced hospitalization rates compared with corticosteroid and albuterol alone.[87]

Magnesium sulfate administered as a single intravenous bolus (25–40 mg/kg over 20 minutes) has been shown to reduce hospitalization rates in children with moderate to severe asthma when administered in the emergency department.[88,89] In practice, magnesium sulfate is more commonly used as an adjunct in severe asthma to prevent respiratory failure and ICU admission.[90]

Admission Criteria

Most patients with an acute asthma exacerbation respond to treatment in the emergency department and are discharged home. Among patients whose symptoms persist despite initial treatment, most can safely be managed in the general pediatric inpatient ward. Indications for hospitalization after treatment in the emergency department are loosely defined but may include (1) an inadequate response to three or four aerosol treatments; (2) relapse within 1 hour of receiving treatment with aerosols and steroids; (3) persistent SpO$_2$ measurements of less than 91% in room air; (4) the need for oxygen therapy; (5) a significant reduction in peak expiratory flow rate, especially with a poor response to bronchodilators; (6) having unreliable family support or being unable to comply with outpatient treatment; and (7) multiple visits for the same episode.[91,92] Patients who require higher levels of monitoring, more invasive and aggressive treatment, or who deteriorate during hospitalization in the general pediatric ward should be admitted to the PICU.

Management in the Intensive Care Unit
General

Patients with critical asthma who are admitted to the ICU represent a heterogeneous group, thus requiring different levels of monitoring and treatment. However, all patients who are sick enough to warrant admission to the ICU should be monitored using continuous ECG tracing, continuous respiratory rate, noninvasive blood pressures, and SpO$_2$. Sicker patients who require frequent blood sampling will benefit from an indwelling arterial catheter. Patients in respiratory failure requiring mechanical ventilation should have reliable and adequate central venous access.

Oxygen

Patients with more severe asthma exacerbations universally exhibit hypoxemia as a result of intrapulmonary shunts caused by mucous plugging, atelectasis, and hyperinflation. Treatment with β-agonist agents also contributes to hypoxemia by abolishing regional pulmonary hypoxic vasoconstriction and increasing intrapulmonary shunt.[93,94] Patients may have hypoxemia despite a normal-appearing chest radiograph, as regional hyperinflation may result in the conversion of lung segments from West zone 2 to zone 1, increasing ventilation-perfusion mismatch. Therefore humidified oxygen should be used for nebulization and continuously between treatments.[95] Supplemental oxygen can safely be incorporated into the treatment algorithm, because, unlike in some adult patients with severe chronic obstructive pulmonary disease[96] or asthma,[97] no evidence exists to suggest that supplemental oxygen suppresses the respiratory drive in children with critical asthma.

Fluids

Patients with critical asthma usually present with decreased total body water because of decreased oral fluid intake and increased insensible water losses. Therefore most patients require some degree of volume expansion. This should be carefully balanced with the need to avoid overhydration because of the propensity for transcapillary fluid migration and alveolar flooding exhibited by some patients with large swings in intrathoracic pressures. The need for rapid fluid expansion often becomes obvious shortly after intubation of patients with low intravascular volumes who are receiving β-agonist agents. Patients should remain NPO and on isotonic intravenous fluids until an improvement in respiratory status allows for the safe initiation of enteral nutrition.

Corticosteroids

Corticosteroids play a central role in the treatment of patients with critical and near-fatal asthma, considering that these conditions are predominantly inflammatory in nature. Glucocorticosteroid agents modulate airway inflammation by a number of mechanisms, including direct interaction with cytosolic receptors and glucocorticosteroid response elements in gene promoters and indirect effects on binding of transcription factors, such as nuclear factor–κB, and on other cell signaling processes, such as posttranscriptional events.[98] Gene products suppressed by glucocorticosteroid agents include a wide range of cytokines (IL-1, IL-2, IL-3, IL-4, IL-5, IL-6, IL-7, IL-8, IL-11, IL-12, IL-13, tumor necrosis factor-α, and granulocyte-macrophage colony-stimulating factor), adhesion molecules (intracellular adhesion molecule-1 and vascular cell adhesion molecule-1), and inducible enzymes, including NO synthase and cyclooxygenase-2.[99] Transcription of other genes, such as lipocortin-1 and the β$_2$-adrenergic receptor, may be enhanced.[99] Glucocorticosteroid agents also decrease airway mucus production, reduce inflammatory cell infiltration and activation, and attenuate capillary permeability.[100-103]

In children with critical or near-fatal asthma, glucocorticosteroids should be administered by the IV route. The oral route may be used in selected cases, but inhaled glucocorticosteroids play no role in the treatment of the hospitalized patient.[30,82] The most common agent used in the United States is methylprednisolone because of its wide availability as an IV preparation and lack of mineralocorticoid effects. The usual dose of methylprednisolone is 0.5 to 1 mg/kg/dose, administered intravenously every 6 hours. Hydrocortisone, an agent with both glucocorticoid and mineralocorticoid activity, can be used as an alternative at doses of 2 to 4 mg/kg/dose, administered intravenously every 6 hours. Short courses of steroids usually are well tolerated without significant adverse effects.[102] However, hypertension, hyperglycemia, mood disorders, and serious viral infections, such as fatal varicella, have been reported in previously well patients with asthma who have received glucocorticosteroid drugs.[102,104,105] Duration of corticosteroid therapy is dictated by the severity of illness and clinical response, but airway inflammation continues long after the clinical symptoms improve. Once initiated, treatment with systemic corticosteroids is continued for 5 to 7 days and followed by long-term inhaled steroids. Longer treatment courses necessitate gradual weaning of the drug to decrease the chances of symptomatic adrenal insufficiency or relapse. Prophylaxis with an H_2 blocker or proton pump inhibitor should be considered because of the possibility of steroid-associated gastritis and gastric perforation.[106]

β-Agonists

The β-agonist properties of the sympathomimetic agents cause bronchial smooth muscle relaxation and, hence, bronchodilatation. These agents also can increase diaphragmatic contractility, enhance mucociliary clearance, and inhibit bronchospastic mediators from mast cells.[107] Therefore β-agonists, along with systemic corticosteroids, are the mainstay of pharmacotherapy in persons with critical and near-fatal asthma. $β_2$-receptor selectivity is desirable to avoid adverse effects of nonselective α- and $β_1$-adrenergic receptor stimulation. However, despite relative $β_2$ selectivity, cardiovascular adverse effects remain a dose-limiting factor. The relative potency of various agents for the $β_2$ receptor is as follows: isoproterenol > fenoterol > albuterol > terbutaline > isoetharine > metaproterenol.[108] Of these, only albuterol and terbutaline are widely used in clinical practice, with some centers still using isoproterenol in selected occasions.

Once bound to the β-adrenergic receptor, β-agonists activate adenyl cyclase, resulting in increased intracellular cyclic adenosine monophosphate (cAMP) levels, which leads to bronchial and vascular smooth muscle relaxation. Dose-response curves demonstrate that large dose increases fail to enhance bronchodilation significantly. However, as the degree of bronchial constriction increases, the bronchodilation dose-response curve shifts to the right, indicating the need for a higher dose to achieve the desired response.[108]

In persons with near-fatal asthma, parenteral and aerosol routes of administration are used exclusively. Traditional therapy for persons with critical asthma previously included subcutaneous doses of epinephrine, but epinephrine is no longer widely used because of the development of newer, more selective β-agonist agents with longer durations of action and fewer adverse effects.

The most frequent adverse effects of β-agonist agents are skeletal muscle tremor, nausea, and tachycardia. These adverse effects are common to nonselective and selective $β_2$-agonist drugs administered either by IV or inhalational routes. Other cardiovascular adverse effects include blood pressure instability (predominantly diastolic hypotension) and cardiac dysrhythmias.[109,110] Myocardial ischemia has been well documented as a serious complication of IV (and inhalational) isoproterenol administration to children with critical asthma.[80,111] However, continuous IV infusions of terbutaline generally are safe and are not associated with significant cardiotoxicity.[81] Prolongation of the QTc interval and hypokalemia have been observed during IV infusions of β-agonist drugs.[112] Hypokalemia occurs even with a relatively stable total body potassium and is the result of intracellular potassium shifting resultant, at least in part, from an increased number of sodium-potassium pumps and not from augmented potassium elimination.[113] Therefore supraphysiologic potassium supplementation is rarely necessary. A significant adverse effect of β-agonist agents is hypoxemia. This is related to drug-mediated pulmonary vasodilation overcoming local hypoxic vasoconstriction and increasing perfusion to poorly ventilated lung units and intrapulmonary shunt.[93,94]

Albuterol (Salbutamol)

Albuterol is the most $β_2$-specific aerosol agent available in the United States. It usually is administered every 20 minutes during the initial phase of treatment at a dose of 0.05 to 0.15 mg/kg. The optimal dose and frequency of albuterol are variable and affected by spontaneous tidal volume, breathing pattern, device, and technique. On average less than 1% of the nebulized drug is deposited in the lung.[114] After the initial series of three albuterol treatments, continuous albuterol nebulization should be started for patients who require nebulization treatments more frequently than every hour.

Continuous albuterol nebulization appears to be superior to repeated intermittent dosing and does not cause significant cardiotoxicity.[115-117] A small prospective randomized study in children with critical asthma and impending respiratory failure indicated that children treated with continuous albuterol nebulization had more rapid clinical improvement and shorter hospitalizations than children treated with intermittent albuterol doses.[116] Continuous administration of albuterol also was associated with more efficient allocation of respiratory therapists' time[116] and could offer the added advantage of more hours of uninterrupted sleep to patients who often are already exhausted.[118] The usual dose of continuously administered albuterol ranges between 0.15 and 0.45 mg/kg/h, with a maximum dose of 20 mg/h. Higher doses of albuterol have been used in patients who are unresponsive to standard treatment.[119] However, we do not support this practice, because the intensification of adverse effects usually outweighs any small incremental gain in bronchodilatation. It should be remembered that a major component of bronchial obstruction in severe asthma is from airway wall edema and mucus obstruction of the airways, neither of which is responsive to bronchodilators.

Albuterol is a 50:50 mixture of R-albuterol (levalbuterol), the active enantiomer that causes bronchodilation, and S-albuterol, which was thought to be inactive in humans. Levalbuterol, the pure R-isomer, is approved for use in the United States as a preservative-free nebulizer solution. The purported advantage levalbuterol over albuterol stems from the fact that S-albuterol may not be completely inert and has a longer elimination half-life than R-albuterol.[120,121] However, the notion that S-albuterol is not inert and that it is capable of clinically significant adverse effects is not universally accepted.[122-124] A large randomized controlled trial of levalbuterol versus racemic albuterol in children with asthma demonstrated a decreased rate of hospitalization in patients treated with levalbuterol.[125] However, this study had methodological problems, as the primary outcome variable (rate of hospital admission) was left to the discretion of the treating physicians and none of the secondary outcome variables were significantly different between treatment groups once the patients had been admitted to the hospital.[125] More recent randomized clinical studies in children with asthma failed to show that levalbuterol is superior to racemic albuterol.[126-128] Furthermore, although the cost of levalbuterol has decreased significantly, this drug continues to be more expensive than albuterol (M.L. Biros, PharmD, Rainbow Babies & Children's Hospital, personal communication, 2015). Considering the lower cost of albuterol and the paucity of clinical evidence supporting the superiority of levalbuterol, we favor albuterol as the routine bronchodilator of choice in children with critical and near-fatal asthma.

Intravenously administered albuterol is not available in the United States. However, the efficacy of albuterol infusions in patients with severe asthma has been well established in countries where the IV preparation is available.[129,130]

Terbutaline

Terbutaline is a relatively selective β_2-agonist with a mechanism of action similar to that of albuterol. It is the most commonly used parenteral β-agonist in the United States and is available for nebulization, subcutaneous injection, and IV use. Because of its lower β_1-receptor affinity, subcutaneous administration of terbutaline has largely supplanted the use of epinephrine in persons with severe acute asthma. Subcutaneous terbutaline is rarely used in the PICU; it is reserved for patients with acute worsening of the respiratory status who do not have vascular access and in whom access cannot be easily obtained. Subcutaneous terbutaline is more commonly used in the acute management of sick patients in the emergency department and before hospital contact. The usual subcutaneous terbutaline dose is 0.01 mg/kg/dose (maximum 0.25 mg) subcutaneously every 20 minutes for three doses, as necessary.

Terbutaline is more commonly used in the ICU by IV infusion. This therapy is indicated for patients with critical asthma who fail to improve or who show signs of deterioration during treatment with nebulized β_2-agonists, ipratropium bromide, and steroids. The usual range of IV terbutaline dosage is 0.1 to 10 µg/kg/min, as a continuous infusion prepared in 0.9% normal saline solution or D_5W.[109] In our clinical experience, however, most patients are started on a dose of 1 µg/kg/min and the dose is titrated to effect, with doses higher than 4 µg/kg/min rarely necessary. Patients starting therapy at doses lower than 1 µg/kg/min can be given a loading dose of 10 µg/kg over 10 minutes to accelerate the onset of action.

Anticholinergic Agents

Anticholinergic agents have become an important part of the treatment of children with severe acute asthma. The typical anticholinergic agent used in treating patients with asthma is ipratropium bromide, a quaternary ammonium compound formed by the introduction of an isopropyl group to the N atom of atropine. Unlike atropine (a tertiary ammonium compound), ipratropium bromide does not cross the blood-brain barrier and does not cause central anticholinergic adverse effects. Considering that bronchial smooth muscle

tone is influenced by the parasympathetic input, ipratropium bromide can produce bronchodilation by inhibition of cholinergic-mediated bronchospasm.[131] An important property of ipratropium bromide is the lack of negative effect on ciliary bronchial epithelium, unlike the marked inhibition of ciliary beating and mucociliary clearance produced by atropine.[131]

Nebulized ipratropium bromide (250- to 500-µg doses) can be used every 20 minutes during the first hour in the emergency department. The recommended dose for continuation therapy is 250 to 500 µg, given every 6 hours. After inhalation, peak responses usually develop over 30 to 90 minutes, and clinical effects may persist for more than 4 hours.[131] Systemic effects are minimal because less than 1% of an inhaled dose of ipratropium bromide is absorbed into the circulation. However, extrapulmonary effects such as mydriasis and blurred vision have been reported as a result of inadvertent topical ocular absorption of the drug.[132,133]

The addition of ipratropium bromide to nebulized albuterol in the treatment of bronchospasm makes pharmacologic sense, because albuterol causes bronchodilatation by increasing cAMP levels, whereas the effect of ipratropium bromide is mediated by a decrease in cyclic guanosine monophosphate. The combined use of ipratropium bromide and nebulized albuterol in treating children with asthma who present to the emergency department has proved to be cost effective and reduces the rate of admission to the hospital.[86,87] However, the routine addition of repeated doses of nebulized ipratropium bromide to a standard regimen of β_2-agonist agents and systemic steroid drugs in hospitalized children with asthma does not appear to confer a significant benefit.[134,135] Considering the high safety profile of inhaled ipratropium bromide treatments and the benefits of its use in the emergency department, we find it reasonable to administer ipratropium bromide along with standard therapy for critically ill patients with asthma despite the lack of robust data specific to the PICU population.

Magnesium Sulfate

Magnesium is a physiologic calcium antagonist that inhibits calcium uptake and relaxes bronchial smooth muscle. It has been known since the 1940s that magnesium causes bronchorelaxation in patients with asthma,[136] but its use as an adjunct in treating patients with severe asthma has occurred only recently. Numerous reports, case series, and randomized controlled trials have suggested clinical improvement when asthmatic patients receive IV magnesium sulfate infusions in the emergency department or ICU.[137,138] Although there is some evidence that magnesium is as effective as albuterol when delivered by nebulization[139] and has been used successfully as a liquid vehicle for albuterol nebulization,[140] a larger trial failed to show a significant benefit on hospital length of stay.[141]

The indication for IV magnesium sulfate in children with critical or near-fatal asthma is still unclear because of the paucity of randomized controlled trials. Some studies suggest that magnesium sulfate infusions are associated with significant improvements in short-term pulmonary function,[88,142,143] whereas another study failed to show improvement in disease severity or a reduction in hospitalization rates.[89] The usual dose of magnesium sulfate in children with critical or near-fatal asthma is 25 to 40 mg/kg/dose, infused intravenously, over 20 to 30 minutes.[144] The onset of clinical response is rapid (occurring in minutes) and generally is observed during the initial infusion. Patients should be carefully monitored for adverse effects during the infusion, which include hypotension, nausea, and flushing. Serious toxicity—such as cardiac arrhythmias, muscle weakness, areflexia, and respiratory depression—is not a significant concern with the use of magnesium sulfate in persons with acute asthma, when used as directed. The IV infusion of magnesium sulfate under controlled conditions appears to be safe, and a subset of patients with critical and near-fatal asthma clearly responds to this therapy, which may reduce need for mechanical ventilator support.[88,142-145] A systematic review of the published randomized controlled trials supports the use of magnesium sulfate in addition to β2-agonist agents and systemic steroid drugs in the treatment of persons with acute severe asthma.[146]

Methylxanthine Agents

Methylxanthine agents, as the name implies, are substances formed by the methylation of xanthine and include caffeine, theobromine, and theophylline. The water solubility of methylxanthine agents is very low but can be greatly enhanced by formation of complexes with a variety of compounds. Most notably, the combination of theophylline and ethylenediamine yields aminophylline, a water-soluble salt. A large number of methylxanthine derivatives have been developed, but only theophylline and aminophylline are relevant to the treatment of patients with asthma.

The exact molecular mechanism of theophylline-mediated bronchodilation is unclear but is thought to involve its action as a phosphodiesterase-4 inhibitor, reducing the degradation of cAMP, which in turn mediates cellular responses that result in bronchial smooth muscle relaxation.[147] Other mechanisms of action have been proposed, including inhibition of phosphoinositide 3-kinase activity,[148] adenosine receptor antagonism,[149] increasing histone deacetylase activity, stimulation of endogenous catecholamine release,[150] prostaglandin antagonism,[151] and alterations in intracellular calcium mobilization.[152] Theophylline is also known to cause inhibition of afferent neuronal activity,[153] thereby leading to inhibition of bronchospasm mediated by reflex activation of cholinergic pathways. Theophylline has antiinflammatory and immunomodulatory actions[154] and is known to augment diaphragmatic contractility and increase respiratory drive.[155]

In isolated human bronchial preparations in vitro theophylline concentrations greater than 70 μmol/L can induce a 50% reversal of bronchoconstriction.[156] Such high local concentrations presumably would be achieved with plasma levels greater than 10 to 20 μg/mL.[157] In clinical practice, however, this range poses a difficult problem because of the narrow window between therapeutic levels and toxicity, which often overlap. The half-life of theophylline ranges from 3 to 7 hours.[158] Therefore aminophylline, which is equivalent to 80% theophylline, generally is administered as a continuous IV infusion to avoid significant fluctuations in serum concentrations. When a decision is made to initiate therapy with theophylline or aminophylline, a loading dose is given to achieve serum levels between 10 and 20 μg/mL. Assuming a normal average volume of distribution, a 1-mg/kg dose of theophylline (1.25 mg/kg of aminophylline) raises the serum concentration by 2 μg/mL. The loading dose should be administered over 20 minutes and should be followed immediately by the continuous infusion of

the drug. Empiric doses of aminophylline can be started for patients with normal hepatic and cardiac function as follows: infants younger than 6 months: 0.5 mg/kg/h; infants aged 6 months to 1 year: 0.85 to 1 mg/kg/h; children aged 1 to 9 years: 1 mg/kg/h; and children older than 9 years: 0.75 mg/kg/h. Patients with compromised hepatic or cardiovascular function should be started at a dose of 0.25 mg/kg/h. Obese patients should have doses calculated on ideal body weight to prevent toxicity. Serum drug levels should be monitored 30 to 60 minutes after the loading dose and frequently during the continuous infusion, considering that steady-state concentrations are not achieved until approximately five half-lives, which corresponds to 24 to 36 hours of infusion.

A number of studies in adults and children with acute asthma indicate that therapy with theophylline or aminophylline is of no clinical benefit.[159-161] More recently, randomized, placebo-controlled trials tested the efficacy of aminophylline[18] and theophylline[162] in children with critical asthma. Aminophylline treatment resulted in significantly improved physiologic outcomes, such as oxygenation and pulmonary function testing, but did not decrease ICU length of stay and was associated with adverse effects such as nausea and vomiting.[18] Theophylline was associated with faster clinical improvement, but it had no effect on PICU length of stay and led to a significantly higher frequency of vomiting compared with control subjects.[162]

Considering the narrow therapeutic window (10 to 20 μg/mL), which often overlaps the toxicity (>15 μg/mL), the questionable evidence of clinical efficacy, and that methylxanthine agents have been associated with adverse effects ranging from nausea, vomiting, and fever to dyskinesias, seizures, and death, use of these agents has decreased significantly. In fact, methylxanthines were used in less than 6% of children with critical and near-fatal asthma admitted to pediatric ICUs in a multicenter study in the United States.[16] With these considerations in mind, we use methylxanthine agents only in occasional selected patients who fail to respond to maximal therapy with β-agonist agents, steroids, anticholinergic drugs, magnesium sulfate, and other adjuncts.

Helium-Oxygen Mixtures

Helium is a biologically inert gas that is less dense than any gas except hydrogen and is about one-seventh as dense as air. The medicinal application of helium and oxygen mixtures (heliox) in the treatment of asthma and extrathoracic airway obstruction has been known for nearly 8 decades.[163] Because of its low density, heliox reduces the Reynolds number. This effect is associated with a reduced likelihood of turbulent gas flow while facilitating laminar gas flow in the airways, thus decreasing the work of breathing in situations associated with high airway resistance.[164] Heliox provides a theoretic benefit in patients with obstructive lesions of the extrathoracic and intrathoracic airways. Several reports advocate the benefit of heliox in the management of children with extrathoracic airway obstruction.[164,165] The role of heliox in patients with asthma is less clear.

Research using heliox mixtures has demonstrated a greater percentage of lung particle retention and a greater delivery of albuterol from both metered-dose inhalers and nebulizers,[166,167] suggesting that one of the beneficial effects of heliox use in patients with asthma is improved deposition of aerosolized drugs. Although there is some evidence that 70%/30%

heliox-driven continuous nebulized albuterol treatments are associated with a greater degree of clinical improvement compared with oxygen-driven continuous nebulized albuterol in children with moderate to severe asthma exacerbations,[166] other studies have shown no significant improvement in hospital or ICU length of stay.[168] The higher the needed FIO2, the less effective the heliox mixture.

Heliox has been recommended by some investigators as a useful adjunct in adult patients with severe asthma, both during spontaneous breathing and during mechanical ventilation.[169-172] Anecdotal reports suggest that heliox is associated with improvement in pulmonary function in children with acute asthma.[173,174] However, a small randomized crossover trial of heliox in spontaneously breathing patients with severe asthma failed to show improvement in pulmonary function or dyspnea scores.[175] Additionally, a systematic review of seven prospective, controlled trials in children and adults did not support the use of heliox in patients with moderate or severe acute asthma.[176] The paucity of well-executed, randomized, controlled studies makes it impossible to assess the therapeutic effect of heliox in children with asthma. In addition, should heliox be beneficial in some patients, the duration of administration and optimal helium-oxygen mixture remain undetermined. Until more sound information emerges, heliox remains an unproved therapy for pediatric asthma, and its use should be restricted to individual attempts in selected patients with severe refractory critical or near-fatal asthma who do not respond to conventional treatment.[177] To get full benefit from the lower gas density, 80:20 or 70:30 helium-oxygen mixtures must be used, limiting the therapy to those with low inspired oxygen needs.

Ketamine

Ketamine hydrochloride is a dissociative anesthetic agent with bronchodilatory properties that is available in a solution for IV or intramuscular administration. After IV administration, a sensation of dissociation is generally experienced within 15 seconds, followed by unconsciousness after another 30 seconds. This reaction is followed by profound analgesia that lasts 40 to 60 minutes and amnesia that may persist for 2 hours. Some patients, particularly older children, may experience a postanesthesia emergence reaction with confusion, agitation, and hallucinations. Usual ketamine doses do not significantly affect hypoxic or hypercarbic respiratory drive. Pharyngeal and laryngeal reflexes are maintained, and although the cough reflex is somewhat depressed, airway obstruction does not normally occur. Aside from its anesthetic properties, ketamine causes sialorrhea and increases airway secretions, cardiac output, heart rate, blood pressure, metabolic rate, cerebral blood flow, and intracranial pressure.[178] Pulmonary vascular resistance is not altered, and hypoxic pulmonary vasoconstriction is preserved. Ketamine inhibits bronchospasm and lowers airway resistance, presumably through blockage of N-methyl-D-aspartate receptors in airway smooth muscle.[179] The bronchodilatory effect of ketamine makes it an attractive agent in patients with asthma who require sedation and anesthesia for intubation or mechanical ventilation.[180,181] However, the bronchodilatory effects of ketamine may be counteracted by the observed increase in airway secretions and sialorrhea.

Questions exist regarding the use of ketamine in nonintubated patients with critical asthma. In the emergency department, ketamine infusion added to standard therapy of nonintubated patients has not shown a clinical benefit.[182] However, limited evidence suggests that this therapy may be helpful in selected patients when trying to avoid the need for mechanical ventilation.[183] In our experience, the administration of ketamine to nonintubated children with critical asthma frequently precedes the need to intubate and is rarely associated with significant and noticeable clinical improvement. For this reason, attempts at administering ketamine to nonintubated children with severe critical asthma should always take place in the ICU under strictly monitored conditions and with personnel capable of rapidly establishing an airway for initiation of ventilatory support.

Ketamine usually is administered as an IV bolus of 2 mg/kg, followed by a continuous infusion of 1 to 2 mg/kg/h. The resulting sialorrhea and increased airway secretions can be attenuated by administration of glycopyrrolate or atropine. The concurrent use of benzodiazepines may attenuate the agitation and hallucinations in patients who experience emergence reactions following ketamine anesthesia.

Mechanical Ventilation
Indications

Only a small minority of patients with near-fatal asthma admitted to the PICU (10% to 12%) will require endotracheal intubation and mechanical ventilation.[16] The indications for intubation are not precisely defined, and the decision to proceed with intubation is largely based on clinical judgment. Absolute indications are obvious and include cardiac or respiratory arrest, profound hypoxemia refractory to supplemental oxygen administration, and respiratory failure. The decision to intubate should not be based solely on blood gas results. However, the presence of a mixed respiratory and metabolic acidosis, persistent hypoxemia, and agitation or obtundation, despite maximal therapeutic efforts, indicate impending respiratory arrest and signal the urgent need to proceed with intubation and mechanical ventilation.

Some patients may benefit from attempts to attenuate respiratory muscle fatigue with a trial of noninvasive ventilation.[184,185] However, the use of bilevel positive airway pressure requires patient cooperation and a well-sealed mask, which may prove difficult, if not impossible, to achieve in an anxious and agitated child with impending respiratory failure.

Intubation

The intubation of patients with near-fatal asthma is complicated by the fact that these patients are, by definition, fatigued, acidotic, and often also hypoxemic or agitated. Once the decision to intubate is reached, someone skilled and experienced in rapid sequence intubation should promptly perform the procedure. Intubation should be preceded by the administration of an anesthetic, such as an opiate, propofol, or ketamine; a benzodiazepine; and a neuromuscular blocker. Ketamine is the preferred anesthetic because of its properties as a bronchodilator. Our practice is to use ketamine with a benzodiazepine, such as midazolam or lorazepam, to ensure adequate sedation and reduce the risk of hallucinations during emergence from anesthesia. Propofol may cause bronchodilatation and could be used as an alternative to ketamine, although this drug currently is not approved in the United States for continued use for anesthesia in the PICU after induction. Among the opiates, fentanyl is a widely available choice; morphine should be avoided because it is associated with histamine release and could, at least in theory, contribute to the allergic and inflammatory process. A rapid-acting neuromuscular blocker such as succinylcholine can be used to induce chemical paralysis. More commonly, a nondepolarizing neuromuscular blocker such as vecuronium, rocuronium, or cisatracurium is used. The patient should be preoxygenated with 100% oxygen by facemask during spontaneous breathing. Assisted breathing with a bag-mask apparatus can be performed with care taken to avoid worsening of dynamic hyperinflation and gastric distension. Whenever possible, a nasogastric tube should be placed in advance to decompress the stomach.

A cuffed endotracheal tube should be introduced and its placement confirmed by a colorimetric method or capnography, auscultation, and chest radiograph. Special attention to the manual ventilation technique is needed to avoid fast rates that often are inadvertently applied immediately following intubation. Rapid respiratory rates applied to intubated children with severe airway obstruction lead to iatrogenic hyperinflation, hypoxemia, and hemodynamic instability (hypotension). These patients require slow respiratory rates with prolonged expiratory times to allow for adequate gas exchange and lung volumes. A helpful technique is to use a stethoscope to auscultate for the disappearance of expiratory wheezes, prior to starting the next inspiration. The occurrence of desaturation and hypotension following intubation should prompt an equipment check and confirmation of tube placement. A tension pneumothorax must be considered in patients with hypoxemia and hypotension who fail to improve rapidly after administration of fluids and optimization of ventilation (or brief endotracheal tube disconnection), particularly when unequal breath sounds are present.

Ventilator Settings

The goal of mechanical ventilation in patients with near-fatal asthma is to reverse hypoxemia (if present), relieve respiratory muscle fatigue, and maintain a level of alveolar ventilation compatible with an acceptable pH, while avoiding iatrogenic hyperinflation and levels of intrathoracic pressure that reduce cardiac output. Therefore the choice of mechanical ventilator settings must take into consideration the significant derangements of lung mechanics and function that are inherent in persons with severe acute asthma. Ill-advised attempts to achieve a normal $PaCO_2$ would require fast respiratory rates, high minute volumes, and very high airway pressures, which are associated with the development of air leak (pneumothorax and pneumomediastinum) and high mortality rates.[186-188]

A paradigm shift in the ventilatory management of patients with asthma occurred with the introduction of a strategy of controlled hypoventilation reported by Darioli and Perret.[187] Their strategy resulted in no mortality in 34 episodes of mechanical ventilation in 26 patients and significantly lower complication rates in comparison with historical controls.[187] This approach used tidal volumes between 8 and 12 mL/kg and targeted peak airway pressures up to 50 cm H_2O. Tidal volumes were reduced if the peak pressure limit could not be respected and higher $PaCO_2$ measurements were tolerated.[187] A similar approach using respiratory rates lower than 12 breaths/min, tidal volumes between 8 and 12 mL/kg, peak inspiratory

pressures of 40 to 45 cm H_2O, and permissive hypercapnia also resulted in few complications and no mortality or long-term morbidity in 19 mechanically ventilated children with near-fatal asthma.[186]

The modes of ventilatory support for patients with severe acute asthma can be divided between pressure and volume preset. No definitive evidence exists to suggest that one mode of ventilation is superior to the other. However, to safely ventilate a patient with asthma, the characteristics of each mode must be understood. Pressure control modes use a decelerating gas flow and have the advantage of ensuring that a particular inspiratory pressure limit is respected. The main disadvantage of pressure control modes is that tidal volumes can vary greatly with changes in airway resistance and pulmonary compliance. Volume control modes deliver a constant tidal volume, provided there is no significant air leak around the endotracheal tube. An added advantage of volume control is that it allows for comparison of peak inspiratory pressure and plateau pressure measurements (peak-to-plateau pressure), which can serve as a longitudinal indicator of airway resistance and response to therapy. For these measurements, the plateau pressure is obtained by performing an inspiratory hold (a feature available on most ventilators) and is then compared with the peak inspiratory pressure (Fig. 53.4). An increasing peak-to-plateau pressure indicates increasing airway resistance, whereas a decreasing peak-to-plateau pressure suggests response to therapy. A disadvantage of volume control ventilation is that very high lung volumes can develop if exhalation is incomplete, because tidal volumes remain constant breath to breath. The option of using pressure-regulated volume control, a mode available on several ventilators, offers some of the advantages of pressure control and of volume control, including optimal decelerating inspiratory gas flow, assured tidal volumes, and minimized airway pressures.

Use of positive end-expiratory pressure (PEEP) in intubated patients with asthma has been the focus of controversy. Externally applied PEEP may benefit patients with expiratory flow limitation resulting from dynamic compression of small airways by moving the equal pressure point further down the airway and enabling decompression of upstream alveoli.[189] The application of low levels of PEEP that are, by definition, lower than the level of auto-PEEP also may relieve dyspnea by

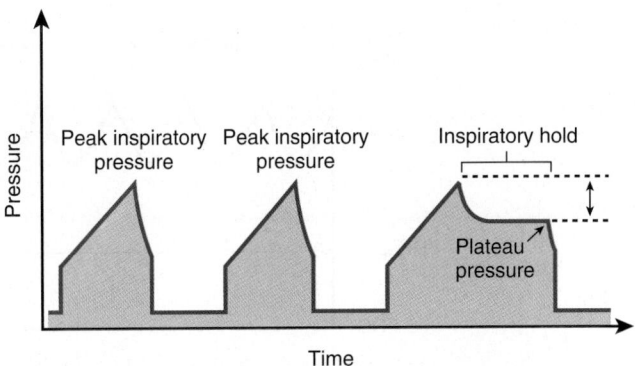

Fig. 53.4. Schematic representation of the airway pressure waveform over time during volume control ventilation. The peak-to-plateau pressure difference (*double-headed arrow*) is obtained after an inspiratory hold by comparing the peak pressure and the measured plateau pressure.

facilitating ventilator triggering and synchronization for intubated patients capable of drawing spontaneous breaths.[189,190] However, as elegantly demonstrated by Tuxen,[191] the use of PEEP in chemically paralyzed patients with severe airflow obstruction is uniformly associated with higher lung volumes, increased airway and intrathoracic pressures, and circulatory compromise (Fig. 53.5).

Our preference is to use the volume control synchronized mandatory ventilation mode or the pressure-regulated volume control mode, with tidal volumes of 8 to 12 mL/kg, which can be reduced as needed to generate peak inspiratory pressures of 45 cm H_2O or less and plateau pressures 30 cm H_2O or less. The initial tidal volume target of 8 to 12 mL/kg might seem high, particularly in the era of lung protective ventilation with reduced tidal volumes for patients with acute respiratory distress syndrome. However, it is important to note that the typical patient with near-fatal asthma does not have significant parenchymal lung injury or the heterogeneously decreased lung compliance characteristic of patients with acute respiratory distress syndrome. Furthermore, once clinical stability is achieved, tidal volumes can often be reduced to achieve conservative peak and plateau pressure goals, as previously discussed. Respiratory rate is initially set between 6 and 12 breaths/min, and inspiratory time is set between 1 and 1.5 seconds, allowing for expiratory times between 4 and 9 seconds. PEEP is set at zero for the patient under neuromuscular blockade. With intensification of therapy and clinical improvement, neuromuscular blockade is stopped and trigger sensitivity for spontaneous breaths is optimized. Once the patient no longer requires neuromuscular blockade, a low level of PEEP (lower than the measured auto-PEEP and generally not in excess of 8 cm H_2O) is applied to facilitate synchronization between the ventilator and the patient capable of triggering a breath. The resultant spontaneous breaths should be assisted by the application of pressure support. To be clear: The use of PEEP *should be avoided* in the patient with near-fatal asthma without significant parenchymal lung disease under neuromuscular blockade, as any applied expiratory pressure will translate into a proportional increase in hyperinflation. PEEP *should be applied* to the spontaneously breathing intubated patient, as it shifts the equal-pressure point distally, decreases inspiratory intrathoracic pressure swings, and facilitates ventilator trigger and synchrony.

Use of a ventilation strategy consisting of pressure support with PEEP has gained acceptance in the management of spontaneously breathing intubated patients with asthma, with the goal of reducing inspiratory work.[192] In fact, pressure support with PEEP was the most commonly used strategy (36% of patients) in a study of 261 patients with fatal and near-fatal asthma.[7] In this strategy, PEEP is used to facilitate ventilator triggering by narrowing the gap between proximal and distal airway pressures during a hyperinflated obstructed state. Pressure support is then applied to facilitate inspiration while reducing associated work of breathing. The patient initiates and terminates every breath and dictates the inspiratory time, respiratory rate, and depth of each breath, making this a comfortable mode for the patient with some degree of awareness.

Ventilatory Monitoring

Regardless of the chosen mode of ventilation, patients with near-fatal asthma undergoing mechanical ventilation require close monitoring. Frequent auscultation provides valuable information regarding symmetry of breath sounds (assessing for pneumothorax or mucous plugging) and optimal length of exhalation. Monitoring modules capable of analyzing and displaying permutations of important variables, such as pressure, volume, flow, and time, can provide important information that assists in the optimization of ventilator settings (Fig. 53.6). Monitoring the peak-to-plateau pressure difference allows for inferences regarding airway resistance and response to treatment. The shape of the capnography curve also may provide insights regarding adequacy of lung emptying (Fig. 53.7), whereas integrated volumetric capnography can track changes in alveolar dead space over time.

Analgesia, Sedation, and Muscle Relaxation

Patients with near-fatal asthma undergoing mechanical ventilation require adequate analgesia and sedation to avoid tachypnea, breath stacking, and ventilator dyssynchrony, particularly in the setting of hypercapnia. Ketamine is the anesthetic agent of choice because of its bronchodilatory properties. Its use with continuous infusions of midazolam or lorazepam can provide deep sedation while decreasing the chance of postanesthetic hallucinatory reactions. Despite its bronchodilatory effects, some practitioners do not favor the use of ketamine

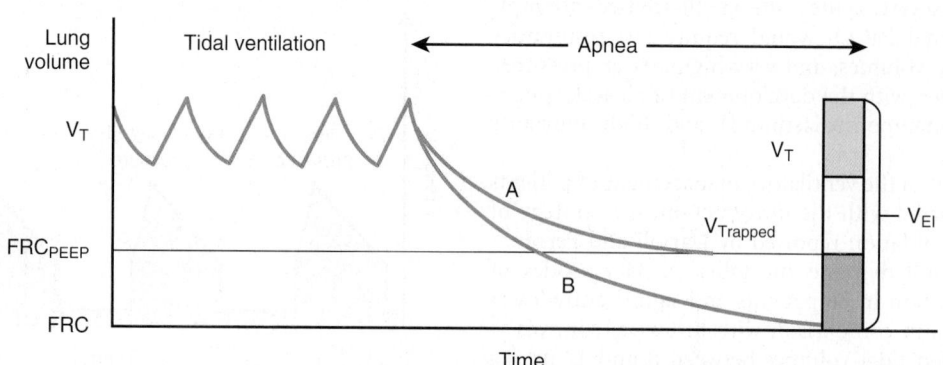

Fig. 53.5. Schematic representation of the measurement of V_{EI} both on and off PEEP by a period of apnea during steady-state ventilation. (A) V_{EI} measured with PEEP left on. (B) V_{EI} measured with PEEP turned off. *FRC,* functional residual capacity; *FRC_{PEEP},* functional residual capacity resulting from PEEP; *PEEP,* positive end-expiratory pressure; V_{EI}, end-inspiratory lung volume above FRC; V_T, tidal volume; $V_{Trapped}$, volume of trapped gas above FRC. (From Tuxen DV. Detrimental effects of positive end-expiratory pressure during controlled mechanical ventilation of patients with severe airflow obstruction. Am Rev Respir Dis. 1989;140:5-9.)

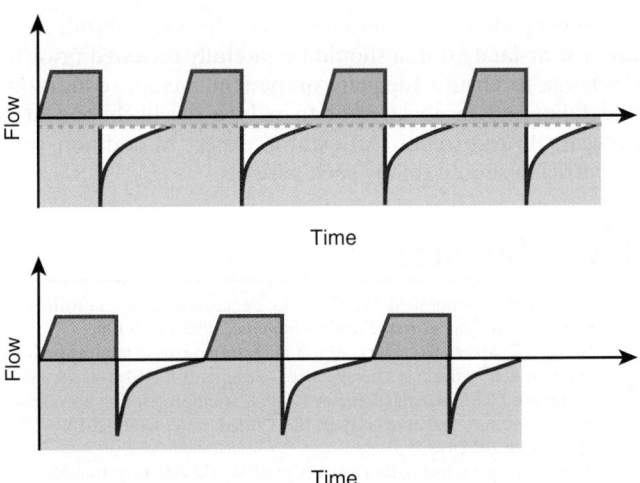

Fig. 53.6. Schematic representation of the airway flow tracing over time during volume control ventilation. *Upper panel:* Expiratory flow does not return to zero prior to the initiation of the following breath, resulting in auto-PEEP. *Lower panel:* Expiratory flow returns to baseline prior to the initiation of the following breath after optimization of ventilator settings (lower respiratory rate and longer expiratory time).

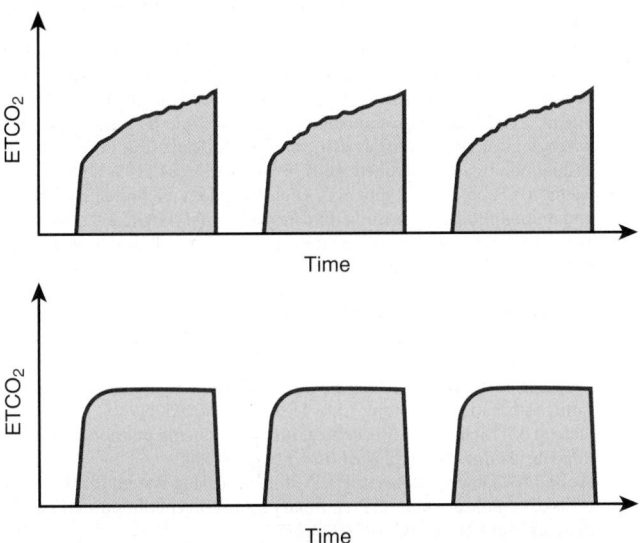

Fig. 53.7. Schematic representation of a capnogram in near-fatal asthma *(upper panel)* and under normal conditions *(lower panel)*. Severe airflow obstruction in persons with near-fatal asthma is manifested by sloping of the expiratory phase tracing and absence of a plateau, suggesting incomplete exhalation prior to the following inspiration. *ETCO₂*, end-tidal carbon dioxide.

because of concerns about the negative impact of increased secretions on an already hypersecretory and narrowed airway. When opiates are used instead, fentanyl is the preferred agent because morphine can cause histamine release and, theoretically, aggravate an acute attack.

Muscle relaxation with neuromuscular blockers should be maintained following initiation of mechanical ventilation until satisfactory gas exchange and clinical stability are achieved. Patients who exhibit significant hypercapnia during mechanical ventilation require continuation of neuromuscular blockers

to abolish spontaneous respiratory movements that could worsen dynamic hyperinflation. However, use of neuromuscular blockers should be discontinued as soon as feasible to reduce the likelihood of serious neurologic complications, such as prolonged muscle weakness or paralysis, from the interaction of these agents and corticosteroid drugs.[193,194] Reports of prolonged paralysis and myopathy after the concomitant use of corticosteroid drugs and aminosteroid-based neuromuscular blockers, such as vecuronium and pancuronium, led to the preferential use of benzylisoquinolinium compounds, such as cisatracurium, in patients with asthma. However, this combination may not be completely safe, because prolonged muscle weakness has also been observed after treatment with cisatracurium and corticosteroids.[195]

Inhalational Anesthetic Agents

Inhalational anesthetic agents have been used for their bronchodilatory effects in the treatment of mechanically ventilated patients with near-fatal asthma that is refractory to more conventional treatment modalities.[196] The exact mechanism responsible for bronchodilatation during inhalational anesthesia is unknown but may involve direct inhibition of vagal tone.[197] Various agents have been used successfully in both adult and pediatric patients with refractory near-fatal asthma, including halothane,[198] isoflurane,[199,200] enflurane,[201] and sevoflurane.[201,202] Sevoflurane compares favorably with halothane and appears to be less noxious to human airways than isoflurane or enflurane.[203]

Inhalational anesthetics can be delivered by means of an anesthesia machine that feeds into the low-pressure gas port of a conventional mechanical ventilator or via a dedicated anesthesia ventilator with its own vaporizer. It is important to ensure proper disposal of exhaled gases into a scavenger system to prevent release of the anesthetic agent into the environment. A monitor capable of continuously analyzing inspiratory and expiratory drug concentrations is helpful in ascertaining the actual amount delivered and signaling interruptions in therapy, such as those caused by an empty vaporizer reservoir or inadvertent failure to resume therapy after a refill. Usual doses of isoflurane range from 0.5% to 2% and should be titrated for effect. Clinical response usually can be observed within 30 minutes.

Therapy with an inhaled anesthetic agent for persons with refractory near-fatal asthma should be performed in a well-monitored ICU, under the direction of personnel experienced in the administration of these agents and knowledgeable in their adverse effects. Patients treated with halothane can experience significant hypotension as a result of myocardial depression and require rapid fluid expansion and inotropic support.[204,205] Halothane is associated with cardiac arrhythmias, particularly during concurrent administration of epinephrine,[206] which explains why many physicians prefer a nonarrhythmogenic alternative such as isoflurane. Isoflurane does not have negative inotropic effects but may still cause hypotension because of vasodilatation.[177] Considering that halothane and isoflurane result in equivalent bronchodilation, isoflurane is preferred for use in children because of its less significant adverse effects. The use of subanesthetic doses of inhalational anesthetic agents in an attempt to avoid mechanical ventilation in spontaneously breathing patients with severe asthma during maximal medical treatment is an intriguing strategy that warrants further study.[207]

Antibiotics

In children, acute asthma exacerbations frequently are triggered by a viral infection. Thus antibiotic agents are not indicated as part of standard treatment. A subset of school-aged children may present to the hospital with shortness of breath, accessory muscle use, hypoxemia, and expiratory wheezing caused by *Mycoplasma pneumoniae* pneumonia that simulates an acute asthma exacerbation. These patients usually have bilateral interstitial disease on a chest radiograph and should be treated with appropriate antibiotics, such as a macrolide.

Patients with near-fatal asthma who require intubation and prolonged mechanical ventilation should be monitored for the development of nosocomial infections. The presence of fever and abundant thick white or purulent tracheal secretions warrants obtaining a protected tracheal specimen for Gram stain and culture to guide appropriate antibiotic coverage.

Bronchoscopy

Increased bronchial secretions and mucous plugging play a major role in the continued deterioration observed in some patients.[41-43] Mucous plugging and casts can cause atelectasis of large segments and worsen the heterogeneity of ventilation and dynamic hyperinflation. Thus a small percentage of mechanically ventilated patients with severe near-fatal asthma may require selective suction of mucous plugs, casts, or thick secretions by bronchoscopy.[208] The combination of bronchial lavage with mucolytic agents such as *N*-acetylcysteine[209] or recombinant human deoxyribonuclease[210] and aggressive selective suction through a bronchoscope may be beneficial in patients with clinically significant mucous plugging who fail to respond to maximal therapy and traditional tracheal suction.

Extracorporeal Life Support

The use of extracorporeal life support (ECLS) has been reported in the management of the very few patients with near-fatal asthma who continue to exhibit a profound degree of clinical instability despite maximal therapy.[211,212] Such cases are extremely unusual and constitute less than 1% of patients in the Extracorporeal Life Support Organization registry (256 of 32,975 [0.78%] pediatric and adult ECLS runs).[213] Interestingly, the survival rate for persons with near-fatal asthma necessitating ECLS is approximately 83%,[213] which is remarkable considering that the majority of these patients were extraordinarily sick and had failed to respond to aggressive treatment.

Prognosis

The prognosis of patients with critical or near-fatal asthma who receive proper medical therapy is excellent. Better understanding of the pathophysiology of airway obstruction and dynamic hyperinflation, coupled with improved mechanical ventilation strategies and aggressive pharmacologic treatment, has reduced the ICU mortality rate to nearly zero in these patients.[7,214-216] Asthma fatalities still occur in patients with sudden onset of severe airway obstruction who do not come to medical attention prior to the development of respiratory failure or cardiorespiratory arrest.[217,218] The postdischarge

treatment plan for patients admitted to the hospital with critical or near-fatal asthma should be carefully reviewed prior to discharge to ensure adequate outpatient therapy, education, and follow-up in an attempt to reduce the likelihood of a preventable recurrence. An asthma expert in addition to a pediatrician should follow such patients.

Key References

5. Robertson CF, Rubinfeld AR, Bowes G. Pediatric asthma deaths in Victoria: the mild are at risk. *Pediatr Pulmonol.* 1992;13:95-100.
7. Newth CJ, Meert KL, Clark AE, et al. Fatal and near-fatal asthma in children: the critical care perspective. *J Pediatr.* 2012;161:214-221, e3.
8. Akinbami LJ, Moorman JE, Bailey C, et al. Trends in asthma prevalence, health care use, and mortality in the United States, 2001-2010. *NCHS Data Brief.* 2012;1-8.
9. Asher MI, Montefort S, Bjorksten B, et al. Worldwide time trends in the prevalence of symptoms of asthma, allergic rhinoconjunctivitis, and eczema in childhood: ISAAC Phases One and Three repeat multicountry cross-sectional surveys. *Lancet.* 2006;368:733-743.
10. Hasegawa K, Tsugawa Y, Brown DF, Camargo CA Jr. Childhood asthma hospitalizations in the United States, 2000-2009. *J Pediatr.* 2013;163:1127-1133, e3.
15. Biagini Myers JM, Simmons JM, Kercsmar CM, et al. Heterogeneity in asthma care in a statewide collaborative: the Ohio Pediatric Asthma Repository. *Pediatrics.* 2015;135:271-279.
16. Bratton SL, Newth CJ, Zuppa AF, et al. Critical care for pediatric asthma: wide care variability and challenges for study. *Pediatr Crit Care Med.* 2012;13:407-414.
17. Sheikh S, Khan N, Ryan-Wenger NA, McCoy KS. Demographics, clinical course, and outcomes of children with status asthmaticus treated in a pediatric intensive care unit: 8-year review. *J Asthma.* 2013;50:364-369.
20. Strunk RC, Mrazek DA, Fuhrmann GS, LaBrecque JF. Physiologic and psychological characteristics associated with deaths due to asthma in childhood. A case-controlled study. *JAMA.* 1985;254:1193-1198.
28. Saetta M, Fabbri LM, Danieli D, et al. Pathology of bronchial asthma and animal models of asthma. *Eur Respir J Suppl.* 1989;6:477s-482s.
31. Wenzel SE. Asthma phenotypes: the evolution from clinical to molecular approaches. *Nat Med.* 2012;18:716-725.
41. Kuyper LM, Pare PD, Hogg JC, et al. Characterization of airway plugging in fatal asthma. *Am J Med.* 2003;115:6-11.
43. Hays SR, Fahy JV. The role of mucus in fatal asthma. *Am J Med.* 2003;115:68-69.
46. Levy BD, Kitch B, Fanta CH. Medical and ventilatory management of status asthmaticus. *Intensive Care Med.* 1998;24:105-117.
47. Stalcup SA, Mellins RB. Mechanical forces producing pulmonary edema in acute asthma. *N Engl J Med.* 1977;297:592-596.
58. Wood DW, Downes JJ, Lecks HI. A clinical scoring system for the diagnosis of respiratory failure. Preliminary report on childhood status asthmaticus. *Am J Dis Child.* 1972;123:227-228.
69. Knowles GK, Clark TJ. Pulsus paradoxus as a valuable sign indicating severity of asthma. *Lancet.* 1973;2:1356-1359.
70. McFadden ER Jr, Lyons HA. Arterial-blood gas tension in asthma. *N Engl J Med.* 1968;278:1027-1032.
73. Meert KL, McCaulley L, Sarnaik AP. Mechanism of lactic acidosis in children with acute severe asthma. *Pediatr Crit Care Med.* 2012;13:28-31.
76. Sarnaik SM, Saladino RA, Manole M, et al. Diastolic hypotension is an unrecognized risk factor for beta-agonist-associated myocardial injury in children with asthma. *Pediatr Crit Care Med.* 2013;14:e273-e279.
82. Schuh S, Reisman J, Alshehri M, et al. A comparison of inhaled fluticasone and oral prednisone for children with severe acute asthma. *N Engl J Med.* 2000;343:689-694.
84. Rowe BH, Spooner C, Ducharme FM, et al. Early emergency department treatment of acute asthma with systemic corticosteroids. *Cochrane Database Syst Rev.* 2000;(2):CD002178.
86. Qureshi F, Zaritsky A, Lakkis H. Efficacy of nebulized ipratropium in severely asthmatic children. *Ann Emerg Med.* 1997;29:205-211.
87. Qureshi F, Pestian J, Davis P, Zaritsky A. Effect of nebulized ipratropium on the hospitalization rates of children with asthma. *N Engl J Med.* 1998;339:1030-1035.
91. Geelhoed GC, Landau LI, Le Souef PN. Evaluation of SaO2 as a predictor of outcome in 280 children presenting with acute asthma. *Ann Emerg Med.* 1994;23:1236-1241.

116. Papo MC, Frank J, Thompson AE. A prospective, randomized study of continuous versus intermittent nebulized albuterol for severe status asthmaticus in children. *Crit Care Med.* 1993;21:1479-1486.

119. Werner HA. Status asthmaticus in children: a review. *Chest.* 2001 119:1913-1929.

125. Carl JC, Myers TR, Kirchner HL, Kercsmar CM. Comparison of racemic albuterol and levalbuterol for treatment of acute asthma. *J Pediatr.* 2003;143:731-736.

128. Andrews T, McGintee E, Mittal MK, et al. High-dose continuous nebulized levalbuterol for pediatric status asthmaticus: a randomized trial. *J Pediatr.* 2009;155:205-210, e1.

134. Craven D, Kercsmar CM, Myers TR, et al. Ipratropium bromide plus nebulized albuterol for the treatment of hospitalized children with acute asthma. *J Pediatr.* 2001;138:51-58.

146. Cheuk DK, Chau TC, Lee SL. A meta-analysis on intravenous magnesium sulphate for treating acute asthma. *Arch Dis Child.* 2005;90:74-77.

159. Strauss RE, Wertheim DL, Bonagura VR, Valacer DJ. Aminophylline therapy does not improve outcome and increases adverse effects in children hospitalized with acute asthmatic exacerbations. *Pediatrics.* 1994;93:205-210.

162. Ream RS, Loftis LL, Albers GM, et al. Efficacy of IV theophylline in children with severe status asthmaticus. *Chest.* 2001;119:1480-1488.

166. Kim IK, Phrampus E, Venkataraman S, et al. Helium/oxygen-driven albuterol nebulization in the treatment of children with moderate to severe asthma exacerbations: a randomized, controlled trial. *Pediatrics.* 2005;116:1127-1133.

168. Bigham MT, Jacobs BR, Monaco MA, et al. Helium/oxygen-driven albuterol nebulization in the management of children with status asthmaticus: a randomized, placebo-controlled trial. *Pediatr Crit Care Med.* 2010;11:356-361.

177. Tobias JD, Garrett JS. Therapeutic options for severe, refractory status asthmaticus: inhalational anaesthetic agents, extracorporeal membrane oxygenation and helium/oxygen ventilation. *Paediatr Anaesth.* 1997;7:47-57.

181. Nehama J, Pass R, Bechtler-Karsch A, et al. Continuous ketamine infusion for the treatment of refractory asthma in a mechanically ventilated infant: case report and review of the pediatric literature. *Pediatr Emerg Care.* 1996;12:294-297.

182. Allen JY, Macias CG. The efficacy of ketamine in pediatric emergency department patients who present with acute severe asthma. *Ann Emerg Med.* 2005;46:43-50.

184. Akingbola OA, Simakajornboon N, Hadley EF Jr, Hopkins RL. Noninvasive positive-pressure ventilation in pediatric status asthmaticus. *Pediatr Crit Care Med.* 2002;3:181-184.

186. Cox RG, Barker GA, Bohn DJ. Efficacy, results, and complications of mechanical ventilation in children with status asthmaticus. *Pediatr Pulmonol.* 1991;11:120-126.

187. Darioli R, Perret C. Mechanical controlled hypoventilation in status asthmaticus. *Am Rev Respir Dis.* 1984;129:385-387.

191. Tuxen DV. Detrimental effects of positive end-expiratory pressure during controlled mechanical ventilation of patients with severe airflow obstruction. *Am Rev Respir Dis.* 1989;140:5-9.

192. Wetzel RC. Pressure-support ventilation in children with severe asthma. *Crit Care Med.* 1996;24:1603-1605.

196. Rooke GA, Choi JH, Bishop MJ. The effect of isoflurane, halothane, sevoflurane, and thiopental/nitrous oxide on respiratory system resistance after tracheal intubation. *Anesthesiology.* 1997;86:1294-1299.

199. Shankar V, Churchwell KB, Deshpande JK. Isoflurane therapy for severe refractory status asthmaticus in children. *Intensive Care Med.* 2006;32:927-933.

200. Turner DA, Heitz D, Cooper MK, et al. Isoflurane for life-threatening bronchospasm: a 15-year single-center experience. *Respir Care.* 2012;57:1857-1864.

212. Mikkelsen ME, Woo YJ, Sager JS, et al. Outcomes using extracorporeal life support for adult respiratory failure due to status asthmaticus. *ASAIO J.* 2009;55:47-52.

214. Bellomo R, McLaughlin P, Tai E, Parkin G. Asthma requiring mechanical ventilation. A low morbidity approach. *Chest.* 1994;105:891-896.

216. Rampa S, Allareddy V, Asad R, et al. Outcomes of invasive mechanical ventilation in children and adolescents hospitalized due to status asthmaticus in United States: a population based study. *J Asthma.* 2014;1-8.

217. Bohn D, Kissoon N. Acute asthma. *Pediatr Crit Care Med.* 2001;2:151-163.

Neonatal Respiratory Disease

Devaraj Sambalingam and Lewis P. Rubin

PEARLS

- Pulmonary or nonpulmonary disorders can lead to neonatal respiratory distress or failure.
- Increasingly, recognized variations in inherited risk and susceptibility to treatments in respiratory disorders relate to genetics, epigenetic change, intrauterine environment, race, ethnicity, and gender.
- The outcome of neonates with respiratory disorders greatly depends on early recognition of respiratory distress, the ability to distinguish respiratory disorders from the normal neonatal transition, and prompt intervention.
- The three most common reasons of respiratory distress are transient tachypnea of the newborn, respiratory distress syndrome, and persistent pulmonary hypertension of the newborn.
- Knowledge of cellular and molecular mechanisms of the pulmonary surfactant system has facilitated recognition of hereditary disorders previously described as idiopathic.
- In addition to respiratory distress syndrome, many other neonatal clinical respiratory disorders may be associated with *functional* surfactant deficiency.
- Noninvasive positive pressure ventilator techniques have dramatically reduced the need for endotracheal intubation.
- The term *congenital thoracic malformation* is recommended for all congenital lung and thoracic malformations; nomenclature and classification of these entities are evolving.
- In the neonate, significant congenital heart disease can present as (1) cyanosis with minimal or no respiratory distress or (2) cardiorespiratory failure.

Respiratory distress in the newborn is a frequent cause of admission to special care nurseries, second only to prematurity/low birth weight, and occurs in up to 7% of all newborn infants.[1] The rise in cesarean sections and the growing numbers of premature deliveries have increased the incidence of respiratory distress in the newborn.

Effective gas exchange within the lung requires both adequate ventilation and perfusion. Determinants include central respiratory drive, muscle strength, chest wall recoil, right ventricular output, and pulmonary vascular resistance. Consequently, a wide range of pulmonary and nonpulmonary derangements can lead to respiratory insufficiency.

Lung Maturation and Physiologic Changes at Birth

Branching morphogenesis is mediated by complex signaling and transcriptional programs. Thyroid transcription factor–1(TTF-1), SOX2 (larger airways), and SOX9 (smaller airways and epithelial cells) are required for branching and cell differentiation.[2-6] The developing human lung evolves through embryonic (<7 weeks), pseudoglandular (7-17 weeks), canalicular (16-26 weeks), saccular (26-37 weeks), and alveolar (36 weeks into childhood) stages. Surfactant production by type 2 epithelial cells accelerates from 36 weeks onward.

A critical adaptive change for newborns is intolerance to lower PaO_2 compared to fetal life the few minutes before birth. This complex and incompletely understood mitochondrial switch occurs in both term and preterm babies. Lung expansion, clearance of lung fluid, and cardiopulmonary changes following cord clamping lead to increased systemic vascular resistance and decreasing pulmonary vascular resistance with resultant decreased shunting across the ductus arteriosus and it eventual closes. In the first approximately 6 hours following birth, adequate functional residual capacity (FRC) is achieved, intrapulmonary shunting decreases, and a regular rhythmic, modulated respiratory pattern is established. Any disruption in this cardiopulmonary transition may manifest as respiratory distress in the form of tachypnea (>60 breaths/min), cyanosis, expiratory grunting, chest retractions, and nasal flaring.

Acute or Early-Onset Respiratory Disorders
Transient Tachypnea of the Newborn or Retained Fetal Lung Liquid Syndrome

The chloride-rich fetal lung fluid is actively secreted at a rate of 4 to 5 ml/kg/h (measured in fetal lambs),[7] maintaining a pressure in the presumptive airways of +2 cm H_2O, which is critical for lung growth.[8] Secreted lung mixes with amniotic and is swallowed by the fetus. The high resistance in the upper airway in the fetus relaxes during fetal lung excursions (breathing movements); the combination of swallowing and diaphragmatic contractions maintains pressure for continued respiratory tract expansion and growth. The mechanisms of fetal lung liquid production and reabsorption involve active ion transport and hormonal regulation[9] (Fig. 54.1).

Chloride ions enter the developing terminal air sac epithelium from the basolateral membrane via a Na/K/2CL cotransporter (the transporter on which furosemide acts). Transepithelial (reabsorptive) movement of lung fluid at the time of birth involves passive movement of sodium through epithelial sodium channels (ENaC),[10] which are inactive during fetal life and are activated during parturition by

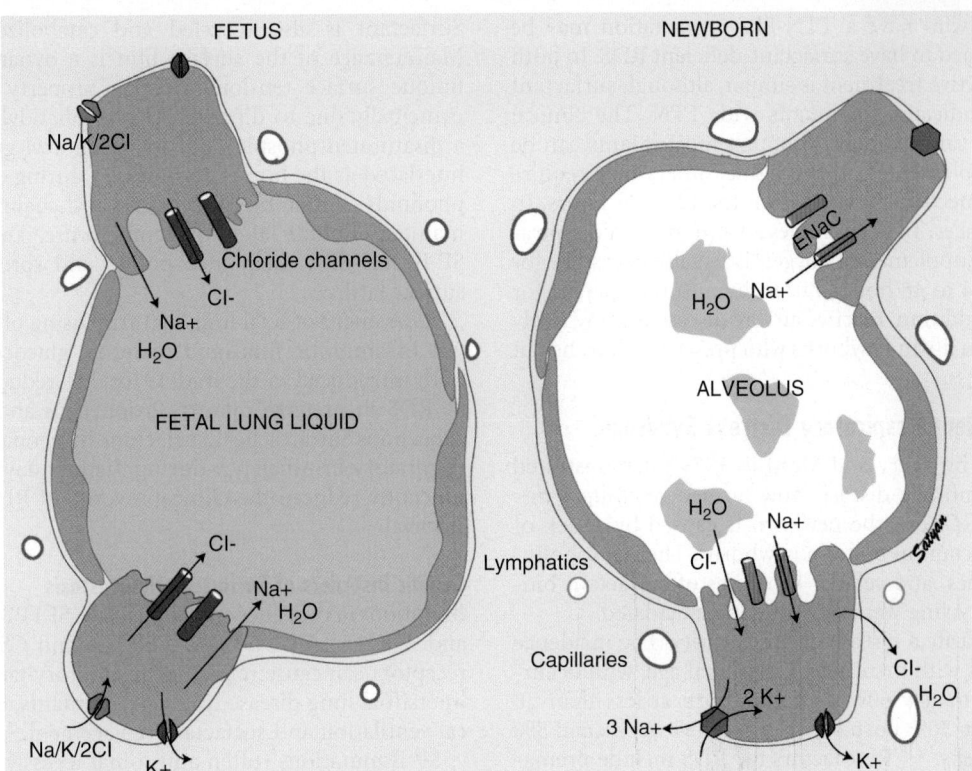

Fig. 54.1. Mechanism of fetal and neonatal lung fluid transport. (Modified from Guglani L, Lakshminrusimha S, Ryan RM. Transient tachypnea of the newborn. Pediatr Rev. 2008;29:e59-65. Copyright Satyan Lakshminrusimha.)

adrenergic stimulation. Although β-adrenergic agents such as terbutaline and epinephrine enhance Na ion trafficking and liquid reabsorption, in animal studies β-adrenergic blockade does not inhibit the reabsorption of lung liquid during spontaneous labor and delivery. Additional hormones of parturition, such as vasopressin, may contribute to this process.

The pulmonary circulation also plays a key role in fetal lung fluid clearance; interstitial liquid drains directly into the circulation, and the dramatic increase in pulmonary blood flow occurring after birth enhances reabsorption of liquid from fetal airspaces. It is estimated that lung fluid approximates to 20 to 30 mL/kg near term.[11] In the hours to days leading up to delivery, net lung fluid accumulation diminishes and, during labor, reabsorption predominates. As a result, extravascular lung liquid volume (ie, liquid within the airspaces and interstitium) decreases. Any excess fluid remaining within the airspaces at the time of delivery is further resorbed as air entry into the lungs displaces liquid from the airways into the interstitium. Residual interstitial liquid is then taken up into the circulation over the next several hours, partly due to the dilatation of lymphatic channels resulting from paracrine interactions. Excessive residual extravascular liquid can impair gas exchange as interstitial liquid pressure compresses small airways leading to atelectasis and gas trapping. Excess liquid remaining within airspaces will impair alveolar gas exchange.

The onset of breathing increases the surface area for liquid reabsorption and is associated with the opening of pores through which liquid can readily enter the interstitium. Drainage of interstitial liquid is generally complete by the end of initial neonatal transition (4 to 6 hours). Interstitial liquid appears to be directly absorbed into the microcirculation in a process governed by Starling forces; the contribution

of lymphatic drainage appears to be negligible. Retention of liquid in airspaces and interstitium leads to impaired gas exchange and respiratory distress with variable clinical presentations.

Excess liquid within the airspaces also reduces compliance and increases intrapulmonary shunting, which results in tachypnea and mild to moderate hypoxemia. The chest radiograph may show opaque areas similar in appearance to neonatal pneumonia or surfactant-deficient respiratory distress syndrome (RDS). This picture is sometimes described as "prolonged neonatal transition" or "delayed extrauterine adaptation." Excess interstitial liquid reduces compliance and compresses small airways, which leads to the clinical signs of tachypnea and air trapping. The chest radiograph may show streaky densities within the lung (wet lung), fluid collection within interlobar fissures, or even small pleural effusions; the lungs may also appear hyperinflated because of gas trapping. This clinical picture is often termed *retained fetal lung liquid* or *transient tachypnea of the newborn (TTN)*.

Delayed fetal lung liquid clearance represents the most common type of respiratory disorder in the neonate and occurs in an estimated 3.6 to 5.7 per 1000 term infants and in up to 10 per 1000 preterm infants. Infants who are born precipitously or by cesarean delivery, those who are male, and those born to mothers with diabetes are at highest risk for this disorder.[12-14] The differential diagnosis includes neonatal pneumonia and meconium aspiration syndrome. Definitive diagnosis is often retrospective, once the respiratory signs resolve, most often within 1 to 5 days and requiring minimal interventions.

Infants stressed in utero or whose mothers have received β-mimetic agents are less likely to have retained lung liquid.

Preterm infants who have a TTN-like presentation may be mistakenly assumed to have surfactant-deficient RDS. In both instances, supportive treatment is similar, although surfactant therapy is not indicated for infants with TTN. The clinical severity of TTN varies widely. Although most infants can be treated with supplemental oxygen alone, others may require intubation and mechanical ventilation for 12 to 24 hours. In these latter instances, TTN resembles an amniotic fluid aspiration syndrome. Supplemental oxygen is usually necessary for not more than 24 to 48 hours, but tachypnea may persist for several days. In addition, reactive airway disease is more likely to develop later in life in newborns who present with transient respiratory distress.

Surfactant-Deficient Respiratory Distress Syndrome

A seminal study by Avery and Mead in 1959[15] demonstrated that hyaline membrane disease, now termed *respiratory distress syndrome (RDS)* of the newborn is caused by a lack of pulmonary surfactant in preterm newborns. The phospholipids, proteins, genes, and cellular processes of surfactant biosynthesis and recycling were subsequently elucidated.

RDS is a primarily a disease of prematurity. The incidence of RDS decreases with increasing gestational age, with occurrence in approximately 60% of babies born at less than 28 weeks of gestation 30% born between 28 to 34 weeks, and 5% born after 34 weeks.[16-18] Risk factors for RDS include prematurity, male sex, maternal gestational diabetes, perinatal asphyxia, hypothermia, and multiple gestations.

Surfactant-deficient alveoli are more prone to collapse, leading to diffuse atelectasis and the classic ground glass appearance of chest radiographs. There is reduced ventilatory compliance, atelectasis, and intrapulmonary shunting. Infants with surfactant deficiency have stiff, noncompliant lungs and require significant distending pressure for lung expansion and adequate ventilation. Affected neonates exhibit tachypnea, respiratory muscle (diaphragmatic, subcostal, and intercostal) retractions, and expiratory grunting. Complications include pulmonary air leak, pulmonary hemorrhage, intracranial hemorrhage, and chronic lung disease. Infants who require prolonged intubation and mechanical ventilation also are at risk for subglottic injury including subglottic stenosis and tracheomalacia. Before the availability of exogenous surfactant therapy, the mortality rate from RDS exceeded 20%; currently, infants treated in neonatal intensive care units (NICUs) rarely succumb to RDS unless they are extremely preterm or suffer severe complications.

Pulmonary surfactant disperses at the air-liquid interface of alveoli, reduces surface tension at this interface, and prevents alveolar collapse at end expiration. Pulmonary surfactant consists of lipids 90% and proteins 10%. Phospholipids (including phosphatidylcholine [PC] and phosphatidylglycerol [PG]) are enriched surfactants produced by alveolar type 2 pneumocytes. The lipids are synthesized in the endoplasmic reticulum and transferred into lamellar bodies (LBs) via an ATP-binding cassette transporter A3 (ABCA3) pathway.[19-21] The hydrophobic surfactant apoproteins (SP-B and SP-C) are assembled into LBs and secreted into the alveolar space with lipids via G-protein coupled receptor (GPR 116)[22,23] at the epithelial surface. Under the influence of extracellular calcium ions, the LBs then unwind and interact with hydrophilic surfactant proteins (SP-D and SP-A) to form a tubular myelin mesh, which spreads into the surfactant film surface monolayer.

Surfactant is also recycled and catabolized or reutilized. Maintenance of the surface film is a dynamic process. The unique surface tension–lowering property of surfactant is principally due to dipalmitoyl phosphatidylcholine (DPPC), a disaturated phospholipid in which acyl groups are tightly interlaced as the film is compressed during exhalation. Phospholipids containing unsaturated acyl chains and cholesterol maintain fluidity at body temperature. During inhalation, SP-B and SP-C help incorporate and spread lipids in the surface lattice.

Assessment of fetal lung maturity using phospholipid analysis of amniotic fluid and maternal glucocorticoid therapy, both introduced in the mid-1970s, has reduced the incidence of RDS in preterm infants. Prophylaxis and treatment with exogenous intratracheal surfactant in neonates with signs of respiratory insufficiency during the first days of life have significantly reduced the clinical severity of RDS and improved survival.

Genetic Disorders of Surfactant Homeostasis

Mutations in the genes encoding SP-B (SFTPB), SP-C (SFTPC), and ABCA3 (ABCA3) and CSF2RA and CSF2RB (GM-CSF receptor) can cause refractory respiratory failure and chronic interstitial lung disease in full-term infants, despite mechanical ventilation and surfactant replacement.[24]

SP-B mutations (often autosomal recessive) can result in a complete loss of SP-B. Affected patients almost always present with respiratory failure in the neonatal period and usually die (without lung transplantation) in the first few months of life. SP-C mutations are inherited as an autosomal dominant disorder, can present in infancy or later childhood, and are variable in severity. ABCA3 and CSFR mutations are inherited as autosomal recessive disorders and can present as a neonatal form or much later in life as chronic childhood interstitial lung disease (chILD syndrome).[19] Histopathologic changes resulting from these gene mutations include pulmonary alveolar proteinosis in the more severe neonatal form and chronic interstitial pneumonitis in the later-onset, less severe forms.

Congenital alveolar proteinosis is a rare disease entity with histopathologic similarities to alveolar proteinosis occurring in older children and adults. However, the clinical course of congenital alveolar proteinosis is severe, with rapid progression to death within several hours to days.

Therapeutic bronchoalveolar lavage has been helpful in adults and some children with alveolar proteinosis, but it has not been systematically studied in infants with congenital disease. Extracorporeal support does not alter the long-term prognosis of infants who have this condition. To date, the only survivors are those who have undergone lung transplantation. Molecular genetic diagnosis can identify affected infants and help predict fatal outcome, permitting more individualized counseling for parents whose infants have this fatal disorder.

Pulmonary Air Leak Syndromes

Pulmonary air leak syndrome encompasses a spectrum of entities including pneumothorax, pneumomediastinum, pneumopericardium, and pulmonary interstitial emphysema (PIE). Subcutaneous emphysema and pneumoperitoneum are rarer forms.

As a group, pulmonary air leaks are more common during the neonatal period than at any other time of life. The two most common types of air leak, pneumothorax and pneumomediastinum, occur spontaneously in 1% to 2% of term neonates[25] and are apparently symptomatic only in an estimated 10% of these newborns. Preterm infants with surfactant-deficiency RDS historically had reported rates of air leaks in excess of 30%; these rates fell rapidly with the advent of surfactant therapy in the 1980s but still remain at about 5%.[26] Infants who have meconium aspiration or hypoplastic lungs have much higher air leak rates.

Air leak initiates as rupture of an overdistended alveolus. Overdistention may be due to generalized air trapping or uneven distribution of air. Alveoli most susceptible to this injury are those that border on arterioles and other structural elements of the lung, locations where more uniform protection by surrounding alveoli is lacking. After rupture of the alveolus or terminal airspace, air escapes into the lung interstitium and tracks along the perivascular connective tissue sheaths toward the hilum. If air leaks into the intrapleural space, pneumothorax results. If the leak is at the hilar pleural reflection, pneumomediastinum occurs; air leak at the pericardial reflection results in pneumopericardium. Rarely, air can dissect into the soft tissue planes of the neck, causing subcutaneous emphysema, or across the diaphragmatic apertures and into the peritoneal abdominal space, leading to a pneumoperitoneum.

In the past, pulmonary air leaks most commonly occurred as a result of excessive ventilatory pressures due to either overly aggressive mechanical ventilation (barotrauma) or air trapping caused by partial airway obstruction by meconium or other debris (ball valving). More recently, air leaks are more commonly seen during the recovery phase of acute respiratory disease, when lung compliance dramatically improves and pressure-limited ventilation leads to excessive tidal volumes (volutrauma). This phenomenon explains the clinical observations that air leaks tend to occur during the recovery phase of RDS and why the incidence of air leaks actually increased during early trials of surfactant therapy. Both observations underscore the need to closely monitor ventilatory volumes and wean pressure aggressively as compliance improves. Moreover, evidence indicates volume-limited ventilation may be a safer mode for neonatal mechanical ventilation, even during the recovery phase of acute neonatal respiratory disease.

Pneumomediastinum is one of the most common air leaks and, considering the pathways by which air will track, is often the harbinger of further air leaks. Infants with isolated pneumomediastinum generally display few or no signs other than chest x-ray low-density widening of the mediastinum. Distention of the mediastinum has the potential to compress the great vessels and compromise circulation. This situation rarely occurs in clinical practice because air will usually track into the soft tissues of the neck and scalp or rupture into the pleural spaces before pressure needed for circulatory compromise is attained. On an anteroposterior view of the chest x-ray, air may form a lucency around the heart, whereas on a lateral view, air lifts the lobes of the thymus away from the cardiac silhouette (spinnaker sail sign).

Pneumothorax is a clinically common and more worrisome form of pulmonary air leak. The initial signs of pneumothorax result from lung compression and diminished lung compliance. If compromise is minimal, the infant will maintain minute ventilation simply by increasing ventilatory rate (tachypnea); an additional sign may be increased use of accessory muscles (retractions) in an effort to improve tidal volume. If positive pressure within the pleural space builds to the point of vascular compromise (ie, tension pneumothorax), cardiac return will decrease, and the heart rate will rise to compensate for diminished stroke volume. Eventually, blood pressure may fall and, if oxygen delivery cannot be maintained, bradycardia and cardiopulmonary arrest may ensue.

Pneumopericardium is a rare but often life-threatening form of pulmonary air leak. The clinical signs closely resemble those of tension pneumothorax, with the addition that diminished heart sounds are invariably present. Mortality may be as high as 80%. Diagnosis is suspected if an infant experiences acute circulatory collapse; it is confirmed by lucency around the heart on x-ray or by return of air on pericardiocentesis using an angiocatheter and syringe.

Pneumoperitoneum occurs when air dissects from the chest through a foramen of the diaphragm. This condition is generally benign and causes little clinical difficulty. It can, however, be confused with perforation of a viscus. Pneumoperitoneum is often distinguishable from bowel perforation by a clinical history of a prior pneumomediastinum or pneumothorax, especially when there is an absence of gastrointestinal signs. Although pneumoperitoneum usually requires no treatment, it may occasionally compromise ventilation. In that case, aspiration of air from the pneumoperitoneum is both therapeutic and diagnostic; oxygen tension in ventilatory gas is markedly higher than that in bowel gas.

PIE is a more severe manifestation of the same pathophysiologic process that leads to other air leak syndromes. In this instance, air accumulates in the interstitial space rather than tracking toward the hilum. The chest x-ray may show a variable number of cystic or linear lucencies in the lung fields. Some lucencies may be elongated or sausage shaped; others appear as enlarged subpleural cysts ranging in size from a few millimeters to several centimeters in diameter.[27,28] This air accumulation produces compression of the airways and vasculature, making ventilation more difficult. This situation creates a need for higher airway pressures in order to maintain open airways, which, in turn, can increase the air leak and therefore the PIE. Avoiding this escalation of therapy is a primary principle in the treatment of PIE.

The approach to management of air leaks in infants is similar to that in older children. Pneumothorax, pneumopericardium, and occasionally pneumoperitoneum are acute, life-threatening emergencies because they can seriously impair cardiac output by decreasing venous return. There should be a high degree of suspicion for air leaks in a patient who has a sudden, unexpected cardiovascular deterioration. Transillumination of the relatively translucent neonatal chest wall using an intensely focused light source is a quick and useful tool for diagnosing a large pneumothorax. Immediate aspiration of the air, preferentially with a large bore angiocatheter, should be done even before radiographic confirmation if the infant is severely compromised. An unstable or recurrent pneumothorax may require a thoracotomy tube. However, tube thoracostomy can be associated with significant complications, including parenchymal lung injury, phrenic nerve paralysis, chylothorax, and hemorrhagic pericardial effusion. Penetration of the chest tube into the pulmonary parenchyma is a complication that often is not appreciated by chest radiographs. One study of autopsies of infants with pneumothorax reported a lung perforation rate of 25%.[29,30]

Cardiac tamponade resulting from a pneumopericardium may be suggested by distant heart tones and hypotensive shock with a normal-appearing electrocardiogram tracing *(electromechanical dissociation)*. Pneumomediastinum often is asymptomatic and rarely benefits from drainage, even in the presence of clinical signs. PIE occurs predominantly in preterm infants and often leads to a vicious cycle of increasing ventilator delivery pressures to open alveoli compressed by extrinsic air, which, in turn, leads to more extravasation of air and further collapse. Previously used treatment maneuvers for PIE, including positioning, selective main stem intubation, and steroids, have been unsatisfactory.

Both high-frequency oscillatory ventilation (HFOV) and high-frequency jet ventilation (HFJV) can provide adequate gas exchange using extremely low tidal volumes and a supraphysiologic rate in neonates with acute pulmonary dysfunction, and they may reduce the potential risk of air leak syndrome in neonates.[31] However, there is no conclusive evidence that HFOV or HFJV reduces the incidence of air leaks in neonates.[32,33]

Pulmonary Hemorrhage

Pulmonary hemorrhage (PH) in the newborn is a life-threatening condition that has an incidence of 1 to 12 per 1000 live births and 50 per 1000 high-risk infants.[34] Risk factors for PH include prematurity, intrauterine growth restriction, patent ductus arteriosus (PDA) with systemic steal, asphyxia, congenital heart disease, coagulopathy, RDS, surfactant therapy, hypothermia, multiple births, oxygen toxicity, male gender, urea cycle defects, meconium aspiration, and the need for positive pressure ventilation. Antenatal corticosteroids seem to be protective.

In most cases, what is called pulmonary hemorrhage is actually the most severe manifestation of pulmonary edema rather than anatomic vascular disruption. This conclusion is validated by determining measures of the hematocrit of hemorrhagic fluid suctioned from the airway. The hemorrhagic fluid hematocrit generally will be 15% to 20% lower than venous hematocrit in the same patient at the time. Finding whole blood in the airway is rare and usually results from trauma from mechanical injury.

The major forces involved in this process seem to be circumferential tension in the capillary wall secondary to capillary transmural pressure, surface tension of the alveoli that supports the bulging capillaries, and longitudinal tension in the alveoli as a result of lung inflation.[34-37] Factors that alter capillary transmural pressure are increased perfusion pressure (eg, left ventricular failure), increased pulmonary blood flow (eg, from a left-to-right shunt across a PDA), increased microvascular permeability (eg, associated with sepsis or oxygen toxicity), and decreased oncotic pressure (eg, protein malnutrition or water overload). Most infants with PH will have more than one risk factor. In the neonate, the factors most commonly associated with hemorrhagic pulmonary edema are those that increase pulmonary blood flow, such as a left-to-right shunt or treatment with surfactant. PH also has been associated with neurologic disorders, including seizures, stroke, subarachnoid hemorrhage, and massive intraventricular hemorrhage. Sudden improvement in lung compliance after surfactant therapy, with resultant decrease in pulmonary vascular resistance producing increased left-to-right shunting, may lead to PH. Hypothermia causes platelet aggregation that

can result in thrombocytopenia, a process that continues or accelerates upon warming.

The diagnosis is made when the appearance of bloody secretions within an endotracheal tube coincides with acute respiratory deterioration that requires increased oxygen and ventilator support. The chest radiograph is nonspecific and may show fluffy opacities, focal ground-glass opacities, or appear as a complete whiteout of the lung fields.

The goal of management is to stop hemorrhage while maintaining adequate gas exchange. Increasing positive end-expiratory pressure (PEEP) reduces alveolar flooding and can improve oxygenation and left ventricular function. Although the airway must be kept clear, frequent suctioning not only may be traumatic but also can aggravate the condition by reducing PEEP. High mean airway pressures, which can be safely achieved with high-frequency ventilation (HFV), can be effective in massive pulmonary hemorrhage yielding rapid improvement in oxygenation.

Administration of endotracheal or nebulized epinephrine or iced saline solution via the endotracheal tube has been advocated in the past but has questionable efficacy, and epinephrine may worsen the condition by elevating pulmonary vascular pressure. Aggressive volume resuscitation also should be avoided for the similar reasons. Antibiotics should be considered if sepsis is suspected, but the efficacy of prophylactic antibiotics to prevent bacterial contamination of the airways is unproved. If an underlying cause such as a PDA or coagulopathy is suspected, it should be treated.

Additional therapies that may be beneficial in specific instances include surfactant, recombinant activated factor VII (rFVlla), and hemocoagulase.[38-40] The rationale for surfactant therapy is that red blood cell products, including hemoglobin, proteins, and lipids, can inactivate the infant's pulmonary surfactant.[41] Recombinant FVlla is a vitamin K–dependent glycoprotein that activates the extrinsic pathway and binds to tissue factor promoting sealing of vascular injury sites and restoring hemostasis. Its effect may be augmented by concomitant transfusion of platelets. Hemocoagulase is a purified enzyme mixture that has a thromboplastin-like effect by converting prothrombin to thrombin and fibrinogen to fibrin.

Prevention also may be possible in some cases; in preterm infants at high risk for the development of hemodynamically significant PDA, indomethacin prophylaxis appears to reduce the incidence of severe hemorrhagic pulmonary edema.

Even with aggressive management, mortality from hemorrhagic pulmonary edema may exceed 25%. The Trial of Indomethacin Prophylaxis in Preterm infants (TIPP) study (post-hoc analysis) showed risks of death or survival with neurosensory impairment were doubled after serious PH. Approximately 60% of preterm infants who survive PH developed bronchopulmonary dysplasia. An increased incidence of cerebral palsy and cognitive delay (odds ratio 2.86 and 2.4, respectively)[42] has been reported. PH is also associated with an increased risk of seizures and periventricular leukomalacia in survivors at 18 months of age.[43]

Pneumonia

Neonatal pneumonia is a common cause of significant morbidity and mortality. In developed countries, term infants have an incidence of <1%, whereas the incidence in preterm and sick infants may approach 10%.[44] The World Health Organization (WHO) estimated approximately 800,000 infants die annually from neonatal respiratory infections, mostly pneumonia.[45] Neonatal pneumonia can be congenital (acquired before labor and rupture of amniotic membrane via hematogenous or ascending infection or by aspiration), intrapartum (acquired during labor via ascending or hematogenous infection), or postnatal (acquired after birth).

The lungs represent the most commonly affected organ in neonates with sepsis. Bacterial or viral infection in the neonate may begin in utero, by transplacental passage or, more commonly, by ascending infection from the maternal genital tract or by hematogenous spread. Prolonged rupture of membranes (>18 hours) increases the risk of an ascending infection, although some organisms may invade through intact membranes. Cervical bacterial colonization with group B streptococci (GBS) or primary herpes viral cervical infection during pregnancy increases the risk of transmitting those diseases. Nevertheless, routine cervical cultures taken during pregnancy often do not reliably predict bacterial flora present at the time of delivery. Also, infants born vaginally are invariably colonized with organisms from the vaginal canal and typically swallow organisms during vaginal passage. Cesarean delivery is not necessarily protective because fetuses may swallow contaminated amniotic fluid or aspirate organisms in utero. Infection occurring during the perinatal period may not present clinically for several days. Consequently, congenitally acquired infections may be indistinguishable from infections postnatally acquired (ie, nosocomial).

As a result, organisms that cause perinatal pneumonias are typically those found in the genital tract of the mother and include streptococci (groups A, B, and D), gram-negative rods (eg, *Escherichia coli* and *Klebsiella* species), *Listeria monocytogenes,* ureaplasma, genital hemophilus, and herpesvirus. Although the incidence of GBS pneumonia has decreased dramatically due to maternal screening and intrapartum treatment, GBS remains a common bacterial cause of neonatal pneumonia.

GBS expresses a pore-forming cytolysin (beta-hemolysin), which is inhibited by surfactant phospholipid. Consequently, in preterm babies, morbidity is higher. Less commonly, maternal viral infections (eg, adenovirus, enteroviruses, or varicella) can be vertically transmitted to the fetus. Although perinatal tuberculosis is rare compared with other causes of neonatal pneumonia, there is an increasing prevalence of this disease in women of child-bearing age. Perinatal infection with other organisms, most typically chlamydia, may not present for several weeks. *Citrobacter diversus* is associated with abscess formation in the brain and lungs.[46] *Bacillus cereus* is associated with a necrotizing form of pneumonia and has frequently been found in contaminated ventilator circuits.[47,48]

Pneumonia may develop as a nosocomial infection in neonates, particularly in those who require mechanical ventilation for other critical illnesses. Although reported rates vary widely, in part because of the lack of a diagnostic standard in this population, some authors have suggested that the incidence of ventilator-associated pneumonia (VAP) may be as high as 30% in selected NICU populations. In addition to the presence of an endotracheal tube, risk factors for VAP include low birth weight, prolonged mechanical ventilation, sedation with opiates, frequent endotracheal tube suctioning, and crowding that is typical in some units. If a VAP is suspected, typical nosocomial pathogens such as staphylococcus, Klebsiella and Pseudomonas species, and the pathogens previously listed for

congenital pneumonias should be considered as possible causes. *U. urealyticum* and *U. parvum* have frequently been recovered from endotracheal aspirates shortly after birth in very low-birth-weight infants and have been variably associated with various adverse pulmonary outcomes, including bronchopulmonary dysplasia.

Diagnosis of congenital pneumonia may be challenging because clinical and radiographic signs may be nonspecific. Although congenital infections are generally introduced through the respiratory tract, signs are rarely limited to those of pneumonia; the neonate is particularly prone to rapid dissemination of either bacterial or viral infections and typically has signs of sepsis or meningitis in addition to respiratory distress. The chest radiograph initially may appear normal, except for slight streakiness or hyperinflation, or the lung fields may be sufficiently opaque to be confused with surfactant-deficient RDS. Meconium aspiration with resultant severe chemical pneumonitis may be indistinguishable radiographically from bacterial pneumonia. Heart failure or obstructed anomalous pulmonary venous drainage also can present with a clinical and radiographic picture similar to pneumonia/sepsis.

Congenitally acquired pneumonia/sepsis can be a rapidly fatal disease, especially in the case of group B streptococcal or herpetic viral infections, for which mortality rates as high as 50% have been reported. A high degree of suspicion is therefore warranted. Antibiotics are routinely used in neonates with suspected pneumonia or sepsis and antiviral therapy should be considered if the infant has systemic signs such as shock or disseminated intravascular coagulation or is not responding to initial therapy.

Revised guidelines for antenatal screening and antepartum prophylaxis published by the Centers for Disease Control and Prevention in 2010[49] aim to improve the screening rate of pregnant women. The further guidelines from the Committee of the Fetus and Newborn of the American Academy of Pediatrics (COFN) in 2013 have helped to focus the management of infants born after maternal chorioamnionitis.[49] Also, because current microbiologic screening may not identify all GBS carriers, GBS continues to be an important cause of early-onset neonatal sepsis. Vaccination may be the most effective means for preventing neonatal GBS disease, and this issue is currently under review.

Meconium Aspiration Syndrome

Passage of meconium in utero is a sign of fetal distress (acute or chronic) and occurs because of relaxation of the fetal anal sphincter. Moderate distress occurring during labor results in passage of meconium in the final stages of delivery (terminal meconium), whereas more severe or chronic distress results in earlier passage, with resultant staining of the amniotic fluid and fetus. Meconium staining is a significant marker of fetal distress and occurs in 10% to 20% of all deliveries, but meconium aspiration syndrome (MAS) occurs in only 4% to 5% of these; MAS is most common in postmature infants.[50-52] Intrauterine meconium passage is a maturational phenomenon meconium; it is rarely observed in fetuses younger than 34 weeks' gestation. Maternal risk factors for MAS include preeclampsia, diabetes, chorioamnionitis, and illicit substance use.

Meconium is a lipid- and protein-rich substance containing desquamated cells from the gastrointestinal (GI) tract, skin, lanugo hair, bile salts, pancreatic enzymes, and mucopolysaccharides and is highly irritating to mucous membranes of the distal airways, resulting in a chemical pneumonitis. Dissolved meconium may travel down the respiratory tree and inactivate pulmonary surfactant. Meconium induces a potent inflammatory response, and MAS is associated with alterations in the pulmonary vasculature, including remodeling and thickening of the vessel muscle walls. This process results in pulmonary vascular hyperreactivity, vasoconstriction, and high resistance and pressure. Activation of the complement cascade leads to inflammation and constriction of pulmonary veins. As the proinflammatory cytokine profile improves, so does pulmonary function. More particulate meconium will remain trapped in small airways, and this can lead to a ball-valve type of gas trapping. In most cases, the meconium is gradually removed from the respiratory tract through phagocytosis, and normal pulmonary function returns in 5 to 7 days. In more severe cases, meconium aspiration syndrome may lead to respiratory failure, and even death, despite aggressive intervention.

Infants with meconium aspiration are typically postmature and exhibit elongated nails, peeling skin, and staining of the umbilical cord, skin, and nails. Respiratory distress develops shortly after birth. The infant's respirations initially may be depressed if meconium passage occurred in response to a recent intrauterine asphyxial episode. Gas trapping may lead to a barrel-shaped appearance of the chest, and respiratory distress may be severe. Chest radiographs often show characteristic patchy densities, hyperinflation, and areas of collapse. Air leaks are especially common. Aspiration of blood during delivery results in a similar clinical and radiographic picture. However, blood aspiration usually has a much milder course.

Routine airway suctioning on the perineum or routine endotracheal suctioning for all meconium-stained newborns is no longer recommended. The American Academy of Pediatrics and American Heart Association Neonatal Resuscitation Program currently recommends that visualization of the airway and suctioning should be limited to infants who are not vigorous at delivery. Because MAS results in a ventilation-perfusion mismatch, severe hypoxemia may occur and further elevate pulmonary vascular resistance.

Another antenatal intervention aimed at reducing disease from meconium aspiration is amnioinfusion, the process of instilling isotonic fluid into the amniotic space before delivery. The theoretic benefits of this approach include dilution of thick meconium and reducing cord compression by providing support to the umbilical cord. However, a large randomized clinical trial has questioned the efficacy of this practice.[53] Distressed fetuses may aspirate in utero, long before delivery. Severe complications such as persistent pulmonary hypertension of the newborn (PPHN) are more likely to be the result of the antecedent stress and are not due to meconium aspiration per se.

Supplemental oxygen to maintain arterial oxygen saturation, endotracheal suctioning to clear remaining meconium, and ventilatory strategies aimed to minimize gas trapping have been mainstays of management. HFV may help to prevent the development of air leaks. Antibiotics are commonly used because distinguishing the clinical and radiographic picture from sepsis is difficult and because damage to the airways may predispose to subsequent bacterial infection. A systematic review of four clinical trials in term and near-term infants concluded that surfactant administration significantly reduced the need for extracorporeal membrane oxygenation (ECMO), although overall mortality was not affected.[54,55] Nevertheless, surfactant replacement therapy is sometimes combined with other therapies including high-frequency ventilation and inhaled nitric oxide.

Despite the intense inflammatory nature of meconium aspiration, the efficacy of steroid administration remains uncertain. Although several small randomized trials have suggested clinical improvement, the mortality rate for MAS remains high.

Because intrauterine meconium passage and MAS are frequently associated with a hypoxic event, long-term neurologic outcome remains guarded. The overall mortality rate for MAS in the United States remains at 1% to 2%.[51] Moreover, mortality from MAS resulting from severe parenchymal pulmonary disease and pulmonary hypertension is as high as 20%, and air leak syndromes occur in 20% of affected infants. Recent data suggest meconium aspiration during the perinatal period may be associated with an increased risk of reactive airway disease in early childhood. Induction of labor at 41 weeks' gestation reduces the risk of MAS and perinatal death without increasing the risk of cesarean section.

Congenital Malformations of the Lung

In utero the organ of gas exchange is the placenta and fetal viability does not depend on a functioning lung. Not surprisingly, substantial abnormalities of the lung can exist antenatally with little or no clinical indication until delivery of the neonate, when the lung must assume the function of gas exchange.

Pulmonary Hypoplasia

Both static and dynamic expansions of the fetal lung are important determinants of normal fetal lung development. Static lung expansion occurs as a result of fetal lung liquid production. Epithelial cells within the lung actively secrete fluid into the lung lumen, distending the future airspaces.

Inadequate production or excessive drainage of fetal lung liquid leads to pulmonary hypoplasia. Dynamic lung expansion occurs during fetal breathing movements, which are rhythmic and occur with increasing frequency during the latter part of gestation. Absent or abnormal fetal breathing also results in pulmonary hypoplasia. Hypoplastic lungs are small in volume and DNA content relative to body size. They have reduced numbers of alveoli (mean alveolar count, MAC), bronchioles, and arterioles per unit mass. Although its pathophysiologic origins are not well understood, pulmonary hypoplasia can result from impairment of normal fetal lung expansion. It generally occurs in conjunction with one of the following conditions: (1) a space-occupying lesion within a hemithorax, such as a diaphragmatic hernia, or a massive pleural effusions associated with fetal hydrops can cause pulmonary hypoplasia; (2) an inadequate thoracic cage, as occurs in some types of osteochondrogenesis like asphyxiating thoracic dystrophy or achondrogenesis may cause hypoplasia; (3) a deficiency of amniotic fluid (oligohydramnios), due to leakage (preterm rupture of fetal membranes) or underproduction (renal dysplasia), may have similar consequences; (4) inadequate vascular supply to the developing lung, as may be seen with pulmonary artery atresia, hypoplastic right heart syndrome, or tetralogy of Fallot, may cause lung hypoplasia;

(5) it may be due to an absence of fetal breathing movements; or (6) pulmonary hypoplasia may occur with chromosomal anomalies such as trisomy 13 or 18. If the insult occurs before the pseudoglandular stage of lung development (7 to 17 weeks), the degree of hypoplasia is severe. Pulmonary hypoplasia may occur in the absence of any of these conditions, but such cases of primary isolated pulmonary hypoplasia are rare.

Infants with pulmonary hypoplasia generally show signs of respiratory failure in the immediate newborn period. Reduced lung volume impairs ventilation and leads to hypercarbia. Decreased surface area for gas exchange (due to a reduced number of alveoli) leads to hypoxemia. A decreased cross-sectional area of the vasculature makes these infants particularly susceptible to pulmonary hypertension, which further exacerbates the hypoxemia. The chest radiograph in infants with pulmonary hypoplasia shows low lung volumes but may be otherwise unremarkable. The severity of the respiratory distress depends on the degree of hypoplasia and the presence of associated conditions such as fetal hydrops or cyanotic heart disease. The most common association is renal dysplasia or agenesis; in these cases, infants have a history of moderate to severe oligohydramnios and have severe respiratory distress and compression deformities of the face and extremities (Potter sequence). An antenatal sonographic assessment of lung-to-head ratio can be a useful predictor of pulmonary hypoplasia.

Treatment of infants with pulmonary hypoplasia is supportive, and outcome depends on the severity of the hypoplasia and the presence of associated lethal anomalies such as renal agenesis or achondrogenesis. The lungs of infants with severe pulmonary hypoplasia may be extremely difficult to ventilate, and pneumothoraces are common because of the need for high distending pressures. HFV may be an effective means of ventilating these infants' lungs using a combination of high ventilatory rates with extremely low tidal volumes. Due to high impedence and delay in pulmonary vasculature development, the pulsatility indices are high, and peak systolic velocity is significantly lower than normal. Peak systolic velocity can be a marker of severity.

Survival depends on etiology or associated conditions. Survival rates due to congenital diaphragmatic hernia have improved and range from 60% to 70%. In certain forms of cystic adenomatoid malformation (CAM), the survival rates range between 25% and 30%.

Congenital Diaphragmatic Hernia

Congenital diaphragmatic hernia (CDH) occurs in approximately 1 in 2500 to 3000 live births and is the most common cause of pulmonary hypoplasia in the neonate.[56,57] At least 750 babies die of CDH in the United States annually, excluding a 15% prenatal termination rate. CDH can be associated with other anomalies as part of chromosomal defects, single gene defects (Denys-Drash syndrome, spondylocostal dysostosis, or neonatal Marfan syndrome), or multiple gene disorders. Most cases of CDH are nonsyndromic.

Failure of the pleuroperitoneal canal to close at 6 to 8 weeks' gestation results in a diaphragmatic defect that allows gastrointestinal structures to enter the thoracic cavity as the intestines return from outside the fetus into the abdominal cavity. The resulting mass effect in the chest impairs ipsilateral lung growth, characterized by a quantitative reduction in airways

and their associated preacinar arteries. The defect occurs on the left side in 80% to 85% of cases, because closure of the right pleuroperitoneal membrane normally precedes the left during development. Because herniation often occurs before the 10th week of gestation when normal gut rotation occurs, malrotation is common. Nongastrointestinal anomalies are found in approximately 25% of cases; the most common involve the cardiovascular system. A wide variety of those have been reported. Other associated anomalies include esophageal atresia, trisomies (13, 18, and 21), Turner syndrome, neural tube defects, and renal anomalies. It has been assumed the pulmonary hypoplasia seen with CDH is secondary to mechanical forces, but studies in newborn babies and in animals have suggested that CDH may also be associated with nutritional deficiencies. In the rat model of nitrofen-induced CDH, prenatal retinoic acid improves alveologenesis[58-60]; experimental data regarding vitamin E supplementation have yielded conflicting results.

The clinical presentation of CDH depends on the degree of pulmonary hypoplasia present. In addition, the abdomen is often scaphoid because of a paucity of abdominal contents. As the infant cries and swallows air, the degree of lung compression may worsen, and an infant who appears healthy at delivery may undergo respiratory decompensation within minutes. The chest radiograph will show a cystic lesion in the lower lung field, often extending upward along the lateral chest wall. Initially, when the intestines remain fluid filled, the radiograph may be similar to that seen with pulmonary sequestrations or fluid-filled cysts. As the infant swallows more air, the radiographic findings may be confused with congenital emphysema or even pneumothorax. Small or right-sided defects may not present for weeks or even months. Indeed, cases have occasionally been incidentally diagnosed during childhood when chest radiographs are obtained for other reasons. With the widespread use of antenatal sonography, most cases of CDH are diagnosed before birth, facilitating planned neonatal stabilization. In cases where sonographic findings are equivocal, prenatal magnetic resonance imaging may be particularly useful.

Initial management focuses on stabilization, including immediate endotracheal intubation and gastrointestinal decompression. Ventilation by bag and mask is avoided to prevent introducing more gas into the gastrointestinal tract. As with pulmonary hypoplasia, the clinical course may be complicated. CDH with persistent pulmonary hypertension may have a mortality of 80%. The introduction of neonatal ECMO has decreased early mortality, which nevertheless remains significant.[61,62] The contralateral non-hypoplastic lung in experimental CDH is functionally immature, implying potential benefit for surfactant therapy, but this maneuver has not been effective in a review of a large, national CDH registry.[63-65] In postmortem samples, concentration of SP-A has been dramatically reduced, more so in the affected lung than on the contralateral side.

Attempts at intrauterine intervention, either to close the defect or to encourage lung growth through temporary obstruction of fetal lung liquid egress at the trachea, have been disappointing. Fetal surgery for CDH has been associated with an unacceptably high incidence of complications, including recurrence of the defect, preterm delivery, and miscarriage.[66-68] Fetoscopic tracheal occlusion by clips or removable balloons[69] has also been attempted.

In infants with significant pulmonary hypoplasia who require ECMO, distending the lung with perfluorochemical in experimental protocols may promote lung growth.

Although early postnatal corrective surgery was advocated in the past, there has been a more recent shift toward delayed repair, in large measure because respiratory function often worsened in the immediate postoperative period. Consequently, early aggressive cardiorespiratory stabilization followed by delayed surgical plication is the recommended approach and is associated with improved outcome. An alternative to an initial period of attempted stabilization maybe an ex utero intrapartum therapy procedure (EXIT), in which the delivering fetus is orally intubated and placed on mechanical ventilation prior to umbilical cord ligation. In this approach, a brief trial of ventilation may be given; if oxygen saturation does not improve during the trial, the fetus is cannulated and ECMO (EXIT to ECMO) is initiated, followed by delivery of the infant. The validity of this approach remains unproved.

Surviving children with CDH may have brain injury, neurodevelopmental disability, hearing loss, feeding difficulties, gastroesophageal reflux, lung disease, scoliosis, and recurrence after repair.[70] In patients who required ECMO, 35% had brain abnormalities assessed by computed tomography (CT), and 35% to 45% needed a hearing aid.[71-73] Perhaps the most successful advance since the 1990s has been improvement in postnatal treatment to preserve and protect lung parenchyma using gentler ventilatory strategies.

Congenital Pulmonary Airway Malformation

Congenital pulmonary airway malformation (CPAM), previously known as congenital cystic adenomatoid malformation (CCAM), is a relatively infrequent lesion, estimated to occur in 1 in 10,000 pregnancies.[74,75] CPAM is a discrete nonfunctioning, intrapulmonary mass characterized by overgrowth of terminal respiratory bronchioles that form cysts ranging from <1 mm to >10 cm. These cysts suppress alveolar growth and can communicate with the tracheobronchial tree, evidenced by air trapping seen after postnatal resuscitation. Cysts may also communicate with each other. Histologically, the lesions are notable for a preponderance of elastic tissue and for an absence of cartilage. The cysts are usually multiple, and in more than 95% of cases the cystic malformations lie within a single lobe. No single lobar predilection exists. A contributory gene influencing CPAM development is HOXB5[76]; its expression is maintained at a level typical of early lung development. Other growth and maturational factors including FGF7, KGF, and FGF10 have been implicated.

CPAMs are often divided into three types, which vary in anatomic and clinical characteristics according to the Stocker classification scheme.[77] A revised classification has added two new types, type 0 and type 4. Type 0 is bronchial dysplasia, and type 4 is the peripheral form of CPAM.[78,79] Type 1 CPAM, which accounts for about half of cases, occurs as a few large (>2 cm) cysts, usually one to four in number, or as a single large cyst surrounded by much smaller *satellite* cysts. Type 2 CPAM, which accounts for about 40% to 45% of cases, consists of multiple, small (<2 cm), evenly spaced cysts scattered throughout the affected area. Compared with type 1 CPAM, type 2 cysts are associated with a much higher incidence (about 25%) of anomalies in other organs, particularly in the genitourinary tract (eg, renal dysgenesis). Type 3 CPAM, which accounts for fewer than 10% of cases, occurs as large

collections of tiny cysts; the affected area can be large, and this type often leads to early cardiovascular compromise, resulting in fetal hydrops or immediate postnatal complications. In the alveolo-acinar type of CPAM, small cysts are formed later in development, and in the bronchial epithelial type, larger cysts are formed early in the pseudoglandular phase of development.

Depending on the type, CPAM presents during the neonatal period in 50% to 85% of infants, but presentation may be delayed for up to several years. Cases are occasionally discovered incidentally. Lesions may be detected prenatally during routine sonography.

The most common presentation of CPAM is respiratory distress that results from obstruction, although infection of the cyst leading to recurrent lobar pneumonias can also occur. The elastic walls of the cyst allow easy expansion on inspiration, but the lack of cartilaginous support results in premature closure during exhalation and a ball-valve type of respiratory compromise.

Chest radiograph findings are variable and depend on the type of CPAM. In the neonate, a solid space-occupying mass will appear, becoming air filled over the next several hours or days. In types 1 and 2, multiple air-filled cysts may become evident. This appearance may be confused with diaphragmatic hernia. Placement of a nasogastric tube to determine the location of the stomach and intestines as well as the absence of a scaphoid abdomen helps distinguish between the two entities. The multiple small cysts of type 3 CPAM cannot be delineated on a chest radiograph. In this case, a CT scan of the chest can be helpful.

Treatment of symptomatic infants may require positive pressure ventilation. In some infants, PEEP may facilitate emptying of the cysts. Definitive treatment is surgical removal of the affected lobe, which can often be performed thoracoscopically. Even if an infant is asymptomatic, surgical resection is recommended by 3 to 6 months of age because of the high risk of expansion or infection if the cysts are left untreated.

Prognosis depends on the type and extent of the CPAM. The large type 3 lesions are more likely to cause immediate respiratory distress and have higher mortality, especially if associated with pulmonary hypoplasia or fetal hydrops. The prognosis in type 2 CPAM depends on the presence and nature of associated anomalies.[80,81] In addition, malignant transformation of CPAM (mucinous adenocarcinoma) has been reported.[82,83] Most cases of CPAM, however, have a good prognosis.

A CPAM volume ratio (CVR) may be measured prenatally by sonography. An index of length × width × height × 0.52 that exceeds 1.6 at initial diagnosis predicts an increased risk for fetal hydrops.[81] Maternal prenatal glucocorticoid treatment increases survival rates and favors the resolution of hydrops in some cases. Fetal lobectomy has been performed after failure of glucocorticoid therapy in large lesions; EXIT procedures with lobectomy (EXIT to resection) while on placental circulation have also been attempted.

Bronchogenic Cysts

Bronchogenic cysts are rare[84] and occur as a result of anomalous budding of the ventral or tracheal diverticulum of the foregut during the 6th week of gestation, with subsequent separation from the normally developing bronchi by the 16th week of gestation. If separation occurs early (<12 weeks), the bronchogenic cyst tends to be located in the mediastinum (the most common type); if separation occurs later, it is more likely to be located in the peripheral pulmonary parenchyma. The cyst walls are cartilaginous and receive either systemic or pulmonary blood supply, depending on location.[85] Bronchogenic cysts are more common in male infants, are usually singular, are more commonly right sided, and are generally under 10 cm in diameter. These lesions generally do not communicate with the airway and remain fluid filled, which differentiates them from pulmonary parenchymal cysts.

Bronchogenic cysts generally do not present in the neonatal period unless they are large, expand rapidly, or are located near major airways; in these instances, infants may show moderate to severe respiratory distress. More commonly, the young child will have recurring episodes of wheezing or infection. Occasionally, asymptomatic bronchogenic cysts are visualized on chest radiographs taken for other reasons. Chest radiographs can readily reveal most bronchogenic cysts. The cyst typically appears as a round or oval water density mass, commonly in the mediastinal or perihilar area. If the cyst has become infected, an air-fluid level may be present.

Mediastinal bronchogenic cysts usually appear immediately inferior to the carina and extend to the right. Pulmonary bronchogenic cysts are usually sharply circumscribed and are located near the periphery. Two-thirds of these cysts are located in the lower lobes and show no right or left predilection. About 25% of bronchogenic cysts may be difficult to visualize with a chest radiograph. In these cases, CT scan can delineate the lesion and determine associated anomalies, such as a pulmonary sequestration.

Treatment may require ventilatory support for infants with respiratory distress. In all cases, surgical resection is indicated.[86] The prognosis for infants who have a bronchogenic cyst, whether mediastinal or pulmonary, is good.[87]

Pulmonary Parenchymal Cysts

Pulmonary parenchymal cysts may represent a disorder of bronchial growth, although they may alternatively be acquired. Like adenomatoid malformations and bronchogenic cysts, congenital cysts arise early in fetal life. Pulmonary parenchymal cysts are thought to develop when completion of the terminal bronchioles and development of the alveoli occurs. Pulmonary cysts are typically thin walled, singular, multilocular, and located in the periphery. Unlike bronchogenic cysts, some communication usually exists between the pulmonary cyst and the tracheobronchial tree, so approximately 75% fill with air.

Like adenomatoid malformations, pulmonary cysts contain mostly elastic tissue and little or no cartilage. Although pulmonary cysts are generally small (1 to 2 cm in diameter), they can expand dramatically and are much more likely to cause respiratory insufficiency than are bronchogenic cysts. As in adenomatoid malformations, an absence of cartilaginous support leads to trapping of air. But unlike adenomatoid malformations, pulmonary cysts are rarely associated with other anomalies. Rupture of a peripheral cyst can result in a pneumothorax. Rarely, multiple cysts occur, and they may extensively involve both lungs. These cases are generally fatal within the perinatal period.

Chest radiographs typically reveal thin-walled, round cysts with an air density. Often, faint strands of lung tissue can be seen within the cysts. A large pulmonary cyst may be confused

with congenital lobar emphysema. In this circumstance, a CT scan can easily distinguish the cystic nature of the former condition. Bronchogenic cysts are identified prenatally in 70% of cases using high-resolution ultrasonography. Reports of spontaneous resolution of pulmonary cysts have been infrequent. As with other cystic lesions of the lung, surgical resection of the affected lobe is usually indicated.

Pulmonary Sequestrations

Like bronchogenic cysts, pulmonary sequestrations result from an abnormal budding of the foregut, which retains its embryonic systemic arterial connections. Thus a sequestration is a mass of nonfunctioning, ectopic pulmonary tissue that has its own (systemic) blood supply. Sequestrations do not communicate with the trachea-bronchial tree.[88]

There are two types of pulmonary sequestrations, which are histologically similar. Extralobar sequestrations are surrounded by a separate pleura, whereas intralobar sequestrations are surrounded by lung tissue and have no separate pleural covering. Extralobar sequestrations account for about 25% of cases, are more common (90%) on the left side, are more common in males (80%), and are usually located in a subpulmonic location. Extralobar sequestrations are commonly associated (50% to 60%) with other anomalies, including direct esophageal communication, bronchial atresia, colonic duplication, CPAM, pulmonary hypoplasia, and diaphragmatic hernia. Most cases of extralobar sequestration become apparent during infancy. Presentations range from fetal hydrops with massive pleural effusions or pulmonary hypoplasia to recurrent lower respiratory infections (particularly if a gastrointestinal communication is present).

Intralobar sequestrations are the more common type (75%). They are usually left sided (65% to 70%) and typically occur in the lower lobes. Unlike extralobar sequestrations, they are rarely associated with other anomalies. Most cases are asymptomatic and are discovered on chest radiographs obtained for other reasons. Symptomatic cases typically present in late childhood with recurrent infections. Distinguishing between extralobar and intralobar sequestrations on chest radiographs may be difficult. Both lesions can appear as either solid or cystic structures, although extralobar lesions are more often solid and intralobar lesions are more often cystic. Delineation of the vascular supply to the sequestration is important to differentiate extralobar sequestrations from CPAMs and to guide surgical management. Magnetic resonance imaging has replaced arteriography for obtaining this information. Some authors recommend a study of the GI tract, particularly if communication with the sequestration is suspected. As with other cystic lesions of the lung, surgical removal is indicated and may be done thoracoscopically. Whereas extralobar sequestrations can be removed en bloc because of their separate pleural covering, intralobar sequestrations require lobectomy. Partial success with a nonsurgical approach using transumbilical artery embolization during the newborn period has been reported.

Congenital Lobar Emphysema

Congenital lobar emphysema is an unusual disorder characterized by progressive lobar overdistention of the lung as a consequence of developmental disruptions.[77,89,90] Other terms include *congenital lobar overinflation* and *infantile lobar emphysema,* although the term *overinflation* may be a misnomer.

In fewer than 25% of cases, clinical and radiographic findings are typical of a ball-valve type of obstruction. More commonly, the cause for air trapping remains uncertain.[91] Intrinsic bronchial obstruction may result from a deficiency of cartilaginous support or an intraluminal mass such as a mucous plug. Extrinsic bronchial obstruction usually results from an underlying cardiovascular abnormality, such as a vascular sling or, rarely, a PDA. An intrathoracic mass, such as an enlarged lymph node or a bronchogenic cyst, also can cause extrinsic obstruction.

Congenital lobar emphysema is more common in male infants[90] and typically occurs in the upper lobes or the right middle lobe. Fewer than 1% of cases occur in the lower lobes. Up to 20% of the cases show bilateral involvement. Associated cardiovascular anomalies are common. Rib cage anomalies and aplasia/dysplasia of the kidneys have been reported in a small percentage of cases. In most infants with congenital lobar emphysema, the condition presents within the first month of life, and about one-third of infants exhibit respiratory signs within hours of birth. Respiratory compromise is directly related to the degree of overinflation. Typically, infants have mild to moderate tachypnea, asymmetric inflation of the chest, and cyanosis. A chest radiograph reveals the overinflated lobe with ipsilateral atelectasis and flattening of the hemidiaphragm; mediastinal shift away from the affected side may be observed. A CT scan may help to identify the cause of obstruction, if one is present. Lobectomy is the definitive treatment and may be performed thoracoscopically. Surgery is limited to symptomatic cases. Favorable outcomes are reported in asymptomatic or minimally symptomatic cases in which surgery was not performed.[92]

Pulmonary Agenesis and Aplasia

Pulmonary agenesis and aplasia are rare, highly lethal disorders with similar underlying causes that differ from causes of pulmonary hypoplasia. Pulmonary agenesis and aplasia result from an arrested development of the embryonic lung. The earlier in development arrest occurs, the more severe the defect. In pulmonary agenesis, the bronchial tree, pulmonary parenchyma, or pulmonary vasculature does not develop. In pulmonary aplasia there is a rudimentary bronchial pouch.

The resulting lesions may involve one lobe or the entire lung. Focal or bilateral defects are rare. Pulmonary agenesis or aplasia may be associated with other nonpulmonary anomalies including microphthalmia/anophthalmia, cleft palate, cardiac defects, congenital diaphragmatic hernia/eventration, and limb abnormalities. Abnormal blood flow in the dorsal aortic arch during the 4th week of gestation has been hypothesized to cause pulmonary agenesis. The contralateral lung may develop as many as twofold more alveoli in response to pulmonary aplasia/agenesis.

The clinical presentation is variable. If the defect is focal and isolated, the infant may have normal respirations, though mild respiratory distress may be present. A chest radiograph reveals unilateral lung or lobar collapse with a shift of mediastinal structures, which leads to a suspicion of bronchial or bronchiolar obstruction. Misdiagnosis may subject the infant to unnecessary risks of bronchoscopy despite CT being readily available for diagnosis. Associated anomalies of the cardiovascular, gastrointestinal, genitourinary, central nervous, and musculoskeletal systems have all been described. If the defect is isolated to a single lobe, surgical resection will reduce

respiratory signs and lower the risk for infection. If the defect is extensive but the fetus is potentially viable, an ex utero intrapartum procedure may be attempted.

Prognosis depends on the degree of pulmonary involvement, whether or not there have been recurrent pulmonary infections, and the presence of associated anomalies. Bilateral defects are invariably lethal. If the defect is focal, the remaining normal lung undergoes compensatory hypertrophy. Nevertheless, mortality exceeds 50%, generally because of the presence of associated malformations. Right-sided defects have a poorer prognosis than left-sided lesions, partly because of a higher association with other anomalies and partly because of an increased risk for disseminating infection. Right-sided lesions also may produce a more severe mediastinal shift, distorting the trachea and great vessels. Repeated lower respiratory infections can result in progressive pulmonary debilitation and increase the risk of death.

Special Treatment Considerations for Acute Respiratory Failure
Surfactant Replacement

Exogenous surfactant therapy has significantly decreased the incidence, severity, and morbidity of RDS and improved the survival of low-birth-weight infants. Exogenous surfactants in current clinical use are considered natural because they are derived from either bovine or porcine lungs. Newer synthetic forms of surfactant that incorporate recombinant human proteins are increasingly available. Both natural and synthetic surfactant extracts are effective in the prevention and treatment of respiratory distress syndrome. A meta-analysis showed natural surfactant demonstrates greater early improvement in the requirement for ventilator support, lower incidence of pneumothorax, and risk of mortality when compared to earlier generations of synthetic surfactant. Human surfactant, purified and concentrated from pooled amniotic fluid, has also been studied clinically and is effective, but it is not generally in use. The three commercial animal-derived surfactants are compositionally different from one other, even though two use the same animal species source. These differences are, in large part, due to the methods by which the surface-active components are extracted or supplemented in the different preparations. Although most compositional differences have little biophysical or clinical importance, differences in SP-B content appear to affect onset and duration of activity and resistance to inhibition.

Conditions such as meconium aspiration, persistent pulmonary hypertension, hemorrhagic pulmonary edema, congenital diaphragmatic hernia, pulmonary hypoplasia, acute respiratory distress syndrome (ARDS), pneumonia, bronchiolitis, and asthma are associated with surfactant dysfunction and inactivation so that persons with these conditions might also benefit from exogenous surfactant therapy.

High-Frequency Ventilation

Two types of high-frequency ventilation (HFV) are commonly available for use in neonates. One type (Bunnell Life Pulse) uses a highly pressurized, intermittent jet of gas delivered at rates of 120 to 600 Hz and is called high-frequency jet ventilation (HFJV). The other type (Sensormedics Oscillator) uses an oscillating diaphragm or piston to provide active instillation and withdrawal of gas and is called high-frequency oscillatory ventilation (HFOV).

Although the effects of ventilator settings have been well studied in HFV, the actual mechanics of gas exchange during HFV are less well understood. Similar to conventional rate ventilation, oxygenation is affected primarily by inspired oxygen concentration and mean airway pressure. Although ventilation is affected by both volume and frequency, the effect of volume is much more pronounced than during conventional rate ventilation, and the effect of frequency is contrary to what might be expected because the frequency inversely affects tidal volume. In practice, frequency is not a critical variable within the ranges afforded by high-frequency ventilators and is not a principal adjustment during HFV use. One key advantage to HFV use in the neonate is the capability for using high-end expiratory pressures without the need for high-inspiratory pressures in order to maintain normal tidal volumes. This feature permits the adjustment of mean airway pressure more or less independent of volume. This ability is particularly desirable when significant V/Q mismatch exists, such as in the neonate who has idiopathic persistent pulmonary hypertension and whose lungs may be easy to ventilate but who is marginally oxygenated with 100% oxygen. Another advantage of HFV is the ability to use low, usually subphysiologic tidal volumes. The use of low volumes prevents alveolar overdistention and rupture of more compliant alveoli, thereby reducing the risk of pneumothorax. Furthermore, HFV reduces airflow across existing air leaks, potentially promoting their closure and facilitating more effective ventilation in situations such as severe PIE or bronchopleural fistula. Nevertheless, a specific advantage of HFV over conventional volume-triggered or pressure ventilation in preterm infants with RDS, other than managing air leaks, has not been demonstrated.

Complications reported with HFV use include hypotension (more commonly with HFOV), pulmonary hypertension, tracheobronchitis, and, in preterm infants, intraventricular hemorrhage. Because use of excessive airway pressures may impede cardiac return and increase pulmonary vascular resistance, hyperinflation should be avoided. Necrotizing tracheobronchitis, which was seen in the early years of HFV, is now rare, in part due to attention to humidification and avoidance of excessive mean airway pressures. Although some studies have suggested very low-birth-weight (less than 1500 g) infants treated early with HFOV may have a lower incidence of chronic lung disease, others have suggested that HFOV increases the risk of intracranial hemorrhage in preterm infants, perhaps because of altered cerebral blood flow and drainage. Other clinical studies have found no such association. Animal studies have found significant effects of HFV compared to conventional rates ventilation on the cerebral circulation.

Extracorporeal Membrane Oxygenation

Extracorporeal membrane oxygenation (ECMO) evolved from cardiac bypass technology with the introduction of membrane oxygenators that operate for days without significantly disrupting blood cells and plasma proteins. However, when applied to premature neonates with RDS, ECMO initially was disappointing. ECMO did not reduce mortality rates in patients with ARDS and was associated with a high risk of intracranial hemorrhage in preterm infants. Nevertheless, subsequent use of ECMO in term infants with

cardiorespiratory failure, particularly those with persistent pulmonary hypertension and congenital diaphragmatic hernia for whom conventional therapies had failed, has led to its increasing neonatal application, despite the absence of controlled clinical trials. In neonates with respiratory failure, compared with other indications for ECMO, respiratory syncytial virus (RSV)/lower airway disease has a far higher survival rate (96%) and a very low rate of neurologic sequelae.

Most causes of neonatal respiratory failure in the newborn are self-limited, and ECMO allows time for lung recovery from the underlying disease process and for reversal of pulmonary hypertension, which frequently accompanies respiratory failure in the newborn.

Nitric Oxide Inhalation

In mammals, vascular smooth muscle relaxation is, in part, regulated by nitric oxide, which is released by adjacent endothelial cells in response to flow and shear stimuli and stimulates guanylate cyclase to produce the potent vasodilator, cyclic guanosine monophosphate. Inhaled nitric oxide causes significant pulmonary vasorelaxation without exerting significant systemic effects because it is rapidly scavenged by hemoglobin in the pulmonary microvascular circulation. Inhaled nitric oxide reaches and selectively vasodilates lung units that are better ventilated, thereby optimizing ventilation-perfusion matching. Inhaled nitric oxide is approved for use in term and near-term (≥34 weeks' gestation) infants who have persistent pulmonary hypertension. Although it does not alter the long-term outcome in patients with this condition, it significantly reduces the need for rescue treatment with ECMO.[93]

Although nitric oxide inhalation has received much interest in the management of term infants with persistent pulmonary hypertension, other applications remain under evaluation. Animal studies suggest nitric oxide may have a significant role in the successful perinatal transition to air breathing. Clinical studies suggest inhaled nitric oxide may be beneficial in infants with surfactant-deficient RDS, particularly those who do not respond to exogenous surfactant therapy. The basis for these applications is the observation that pulmonary hypertension also occurs in preterm infants with RDS. In preterm animal studies, nitric oxide production modulates basal pulmonary vascular tone.

Rare clinical complications of inhaled nitric oxide include methemoglobinemia (because of the high affinity for hemoglobin) and prolonged bleeding times. The toxicity of nitric oxide metabolites includes the potential for injury to the pulmonary epithelium and surfactant system.

Liquid Ventilation

Liquid ventilation with perfluorochemicals, in a complete departure from traditional ventilation with gases, is an alternative ventilatory strategy that has received interest especially in adult critical care. Specific advantages of liquid instead of gas expansion of the lungs were first demonstrated in the 1920s, but application to the clinical setting was hampered by the poor solubility of most liquids for oxygen and carbon dioxide and technical difficulties in achieving liquid tidal volume exchange. The introduction of perfluorochemicals, which have high solubility for respiratory gases, and development of specific liquid ventilators enabled researchers to study liquid ventilation in animals in the 1970s. The demonstration that complete tidal liquid movement was not necessary to capitalize on the advantages of liquid ventilation made liquid ventilation a clinical reality in the 1990s.

Partial liquid ventilation (PAGE, PFC (perfluorocarbon)-associated gas exchange) is the term applied to conventional gas tidal volume ventilation superimposed on liquid-filled alveoli (ie, alveoli filled to functional residual capacity). Although, in animal studies, gas exchange can be impaired by too rapid liquid ventilation in the healthy lung, it is improved in many injured lung models. Possible mechanisms for this improvement include reducing surface tension and maintaining alveolar stability, thereby eliminating the need for alveolar surfactant by filling the alveoli with liquid and removing the air-liquid interface normally present.

Perfluorochemicals also may produce a mechanical PEEP, holding the alveoli open because of the higher liquid density. Consequently, partial liquid ventilation may offer the potential to manage infants with respiratory distress resulting from surfactant deficiency or dysfunction, for whom exogenous surfactant replacement has failed or becomes impractical (eg, those with a heterogeneous lung disease such as ARDS). In animal models, perfluorochemicals also reduce neutrophil accumulation and the inflammatory response to lung injury, and they inhibit hydrogen peroxide and free radical production by macrophages. Studies in animals also show partial liquid ventilation leads to a marked improvement in respiratory mechanics compared with conventional ventilation strategies.

Large randomized human trials have been limited by the dose-dependent risk of hypoxia and barotrauma associated with perfluorocarbon.[94,95] No studies of perfluorochemical liquid ventilation have been conducted in term neonates with respiratory disease. Current information is limited to clinical trials and individual case reports.

Chronic Pulmonary Disease

Chronic Lung Disease (Bronchopulmonary Dysplasia)

The classical phenotype of bronchopulmonary dysplasia (BPD) of severe alveolar septal fibrosis and cavitation, first described by Northway and coworkers,[96] is less commonly seen in the postsurfactant era. A milder form of BPD *(new BPD)* is associated with disruption of lung development, specifically in extremely preterm infants, an arrest of alveolar septation, and vascular development in the distal part of the lung leading to impaired pulmonary function in later life. Microvascular disruption has marked angiogenesis proportionate to the growth of air-exchanging lung parenchyma. Prominent corner vessels with variable capillary density in adjacent alveoli or vessels most distant from the air surface are prominent features of this new BPD.[97-99] The reported incidence of BPD in infants born at less than 28 weeks' gestation varies between 15% and 50% and increases with earlier gestational age.[100]

The changing spectrum of BPD has led to multiple revisions in the definition. A National Institutes of Health consensus meeting in 2001 proposed new criteria based on supplemental oxygen requirement and severity (Table 54.1).

The pathogenesis of BPD involves prolonged injury and repair in the immature lung. Imbalance in the release of pro- and antiinflammatory cytokines results from volu/barotrauma,

TABLE 54.1	Diagnostic Criteria for Bronchopulmonary Dysplasia: National Institutes of Health, 2001		
	Mild Supplemental O₂ for 28 Days and	**Moderate** Supplemental O₂ for 28 Days and	**Severe** Supplemental O₂ for 28 Days and
<32 weeks GA at birth	RA at 36 weeks corrected GA or at discharge	<0.3 FiO₂ at 36 weeks corrected GA or at discharge	≥0.3 FiO₂ at 36 weeks corrected GA or at discharge
≥32 weeks GA at birth	RA by postnatal day 56 or at discharge	<0.3 FiO₂ by postnatal day 56 or at discharge	≥0.3 FiO₂ by postnatal day 56 or at discharge

GA, gestational age; *RA*, room air.

hyperoxia, pulmonary edema, and sometimes superimposed infection. The inflammatory and repair responses are modulated by genetic susceptibilities.

The association of mechanical ventilation and oxygen therapy with BPD has been demonstrated in multiple animal models. In preterm lambs, chronic ventilation with less than 30% oxygen can produce BPD-like pulmonary changes. These observations have led to the postulate that even room air might be hyperoxic to the very preterm human lung. The preterm human lung has low FRC and total lung capacity and may require airway pressures >20 cm H_2O to maximally recruit lung volume. The lung volume available between FRC and TLC for safe mechanical ventilation may be as low as 15 ml/kg (50 ml/kg for term infants). Injury can occur during neonatal resuscitation because of the physiologic difficulties of establishing an FRC while avoiding overdistention of the lung. During the urgent interventions to ventilate a distressed newborn, overly aggressive ventilation can promote excessive lung volumes.

Animal models have characterized ranges of fetal lung responses to inflammatory exposures. Mediators of epithelial lung injury include proinflammatory cytokines, including interleukin-1β (IL-1β), IL-6, IL-8, and tumor necrosis factor (TNF)-α,[101-103] and impaired signaling of growth factors such as vascular endothelial growth factor (VEGF).[104,105] Antenatal inflammation potentiates postnatal inflammatory pathways. Most extremely low-birth-weight (ELBW) infants are exposed to antenatal corticosteroids and many may be exposed to chorioamnionitis. Ureaplasma species are frequently associated with BPD. Additional risk factors include maternal infection, neonatal sepsis, and PDA.

Although better monitoring, improved ventilation strategies, and new technologies have helped to reduce the incidence and severity of BPD in more mature neonates, increased survival of ELBW infants has increased the overall prevalence of this condition in NICU graduates.

The clinical presentation of BPD depends on the severity and extent of the acute lung injury. In the most severe cases, infants may require a considerable ventilatory and oxygen support beyond the age of 1 week. These infants are slow to wean from mechanical ventilation, require supplemental oxygen for weeks to months, and have episodes of bronchospasm or desaturation. Infants with severe BPD can exhibit varying degrees of right ventricular failure or, in less severe cases, simply display fluid intolerance. In the less severe and more common instances, onset is more insidious. For the first 2 to 3 weeks of life, these ELBW infants may appear stable on minimal ventilatory and oxygen support, but the need for increased ventilatory and oxygen support slowly develops. These infants often have episodes of apnea, desaturation, or carbon dioxide retention. Increased secretions from the endotracheal tube may occur. The chest radiograph may show areas of atelectasis, but more commonly the lung fields appear clear in the early stages or show minimal, homogeneous increased lung field density. Depending on clinical signs, confounding conditions such as a PDA, pneumonia, or aspiration must be considered.

The goal of management is to promote lung growth while supporting respiratory needs and minimizing further lung injury by preventing oxygen toxicity (and ensuing pulmonary hypertension and complications) and ventilator-induced lung injury (VILI). Guides for pressure-cycled mechanical ventilation include short inspiratory times (0.24-0.4 sec), rapid rate (40-60/min), low PiP (14-20 cm H_2O), moderate PEEP (4-6 cm H_2O), and low tidal volume (3-6 ml/kg). Bronchodilators may be helpful, particularly during exacerbations, due to the large airway component in BPD. Fluid restriction or diuretics may be helpful in infants who have evidence of cor pulmonale or fluid intolerance. At initial presentation, infants often receive antibiotics until infection is ruled out. Infants with pulmonary insufficiency have increased energy needs, making nutritional support particularly important.

An approach aimed at reducing the inflammation and ongoing fibrotic injury has included the use of glucocorticoids. Dexamethasone has been shown to be effective in weaning off mechanical ventilation when used moderately early and delayed.[106-110] However, early use (<4 days) is associated with neurologic sequelae.[111] Postnatal steroid courses to improve BPD remain controversial. Infants who receive long courses of steroids for BPD usually show biochemical evidence of adrenal suppression, which may last for several months. Inhaled steroids offer no advantage over the intravenous route, aside from ease of administration.

New therapies to prevent or reduce the severity of BPD have been studied. Antioxidants like N-acetyl cysteine and recombinant superoxide dismutase (rSOD) have not shown decreases in BPD. Vitamin A has improved septation and alveolar capillary growth in animal studies and modestly decreased BPD rates in clinical studies.[112] Nitric oxide and high-frequency ventilation have protective effects in animal models but have not consistently shown benefit in several clinical trials. Antiproteases and thyrotropin-releasing hormone also have shown mild protective effects in animal models.[113-117]

Preconditioning is a concept in which antenatal exposures modulate postnatal experience.[118] When mice were exposed to intraamniotic lipopolysaccharide (LPS), a BPD-like phenotype was exhibited in newborn mice.[119] Postnatal exposure to >95% oxygen increases BPD-like abnormalities, but postnatal exposure to 65% oxygen has had the opposite effect of accelerated lung growth and attenuated pulmonary hypertension. In sum, antenatal inflammation can cause the BPD phenotype to be substantially modified.

Animal experiments have suggested promising lung protection and regeneration strategies using mesenchymal stem cells (MSCs) or progenitor cells from the endothelial lineage in experimental animal models. In a small phase 1 clinical trial involving nine infants between 23 and 29 weeks' gestation, a single intratracheal transplantation of MSCs derived from human umbilical cord cells was associated with a reduction in the severity of BPD and had no reported adverse effects.[120] Another mechanism contributing to the long-term efficacy of MSCs may be the transfer of mitochondria from MSCs to damaged lung cells.

The long-term outcome for infants with classic BPD has improved over the years, although these infants remain at risk for significant morbidity and mortality. VLBW infants with BPD have greater impairment of fine and gross motor skills and language and cognitive skills than infants without BPD.[121,122]

Infants who have BPD may require supplemental oxygen for the first several months of life, and some may require chronic diuretic and bronchodilator therapy. High-caloric formulas should be considered for infants who cannot tolerate fluid loading. Rehospitalizations may occur as a result of respiratory exacerbations, often brought on by infection, during the first 2 years of life.[123] These infants are also at risk for sudden death due to pulmonary hypertension or bronchospasm.

Mortality from BPD has markedly improved, but it remains high in infants with complicating conditions such as cardiovascular disease or in those who have intercurrent respiratory infections, particularly RSV or adenovirus. Passive immunization against RSV is recommended for high-risk premature neonates but it is not uniformly protective. Minimizing exposure to environmental hazards, whether infectious or irritant (eg, from kerosene burners or cigarette smoke), cannot be overemphasized.

Congenital Defects of the Lymphatics

Congenital chylothorax is thought to result from a failure of peripheral and central lymphatic channels to fuse or, perhaps, from a rupture of inadequately fused channels at birth. The congenital condition has a different course and prognosis from postoperatively acquired chylothorax. Most affected infants show respiratory signs within hours from birth and may require mechanical ventilation. Congenital chylothorax may be associated with chromosomal abnormalities or other malformations, as described in a case series of 11 newborns. Familial cases are especially common in babies with associated congenital pulmonary lymphangiectasis with bilateral chylothoraces.

Progressive respiratory compromise develops as fluid accumulates in the hemithorax. Pleural drainage is both diagnostic and therapeutic. Initially, the lymphocyte-rich fluid is clear, but it becomes opaque when milk feedings are introduced. Nutritional support is critical because of a loss of protein in the chylous drainage. Most cases spontaneously resolve in 2 to 3 weeks. Occasionally, a several-day course of a somatostatin analog, which reduces chyle flow, or surgical closure of the thoracic duct is indicated.[124] Whether congenital or postoperative, common chylothorax complications include nosocomial infection, hemodynamic disturbance, and protein loss.

In the congenital form, time to resolution is significantly affected by additional underlying problems. Pulmonary lymphangiectasia is a rare condition that can be a primary or due to secondary dilation of pulmonary lymphatics from obstructed pulmonary venous flow. Primary lymphangiectasia can be isolated, termed *congenital pulmonary lymphangiectasia,* or it can be part of a generalized condition that includes intestinal lymphangiectasia, in which pulmonary involvement is less severe. Congenital pulmonary lymphangiectasia may result from the failure of connective tissue elements to regress during fetal lung development. In some cases, a hereditary pattern has been suggested. Affected infants usually show respiratory signs soon after birth. However, some infants may remain symptom free for several weeks. Affected infants are usually born at term and may have a normal examination except for mild tachypnea, they may be more severely affected with cyanosis, or they may be frankly hydropic. Preterm infants may be mistaken as having surfactant-deficient RDS. Radiographs generally reveal streaky reticular densities as a result of engorged lymphatics, and occasionally a finer, ground-glass appearance may be confused with surfactant deficiency.

Pleural effusions have been reported but are unusual. The condition is progressive and untreatable. Most infants die within days, but occasional survivors beyond infancy have been reported.

Lymphatic dysplasias, formerly termed *cystic hygromas (CHs)*, are cystic lymphatic lesions that can affect many anatomic sites. These lesions usually occur in the head and neck (~75%), with a predilection for the posterior triangle on the left side. Less common sites include the axilla (20%), mediastinum, groin, and retroperitoneum.[125] Other terms, including *lymphangioma, cavernous lymphangioma, cystic lymphangioma,* and *lymphangioma circumscriptum,* have been abandoned due to confusion with and absence of risk for malignant transformation.

Nonpulmonary Conditions That Result in Respiratory Disease

Many nonpulmonary disorders may present with respiratory distress in the neonate (Table 54.2). Conditions that affect the control or mechanics of breathing, patency or integrity of the upper airway, perfusion to and from the lung, or acid-base balance can present with increased respiratory effort or signs of respiratory insufficiency (ie, respiratory acidosis or hypoxemia).

The clinical and radiographic picture may be consistent with an underlying pulmonary pathologic condition, but nonpulmonary causes should be considered, particularly if an infant is gravely ill or does not respond to conventional treatments. In many nonpulmonary conditions, a delay in diagnosis can lead to progressive injury and death.

Neonatal Apnea

Apnea is one of the most common respiratory problems encountered in the neonatal population. The incidence of apnea is inversely proportional to gestational age at birth, and more than 75% of infants born before 27 weeks will have apnea at some point during their hospital stay. For infants born at 30 to 31 weeks, the risk is approximately 50%, and for those born at 32 to 33 weeks, the risk is about 14%. The risk for those born at 34 to 35 weeks is 7%. Apnea can be broadly classified as physiologic (ie, apnea of prematurity) or pathologic (ie, resulting from an underlying disorder such as sepsis). The American Academy of Pediatrics has defined apnea as "an unexplained episode of cessation of breathing for 20 seconds or longer, or a shorter respiratory pause associated with bradycardia, cyanosis, pallor, or marked hypotonia."

Apnea can be classified into three main types. The first is central apnea, which results from decreased/altered central

TABLE 54.2 Nonpulmonary Conditions That Cause Respiratory Distress in the Newborn

Disorders of Respiratory Control
- Central hypoventilation disorder
- Apnea

Airway Obstruction/Patency
- Choanal stenosis/atresia
- Mandibular hypoplasia/micrognathia
- Laryngomalacia
- Laryngeal web/stenosis
- Vocal cord injury
- Airway vascular tumors/malformations
- Tracheobronchomalacia
- Tracheoesophageal fistula
- Vascular compression

Interference With Respiratory Mechanics
- Neuromuscular disorders
- Phrenic nerve injury
- Eventration of the diaphragm
- Pleural effusion
- Chest wall anomalies

Perfusion Abnormalities
- Persistent pulmonary hypertension of the newborn
- Hyperviscosity
- Congenital heart disease

Disorders of Acid-Base Balance
- Metabolic disorders (eg, organic acidemias)
- Intestinal bicarbonate wasting
- Renal bicarbonate wasting
- Sepsis
- Iatrogenic metabolic acidosis/alkalosis

responsiveness to respiratory stimuli, such as hypoxia and hypercarbia. Responsiveness improves as the infant matures and approaches term gestation. This type of apnea is characterized by cessation of respiratory effort, which usually occurs at the end of exhalation. The second type of apnea is obstructive apnea due to anatomic or physiologic restriction of the airway. Common examples include tracheomalacia and Pierre Robin sequence. The respiratory pattern of obstructive apnea demonstrates increasing respiratory effort with little to no air movement. Mixed apnea represents the third type of apnea. Initially, the infant may have a central apneic event, but when respiratory effort is made, an obstructive pattern is revealed.

The obstructive pattern is thought to result from gradual airway collapse during the initial central apneic portion of the episode. Most apneic episodes lasting longer than 20 seconds fall into this category.

Although apneic spells are a common cause of readmission following NICU discharge, apnea of prematurity remains a diagnosis of exclusion. Most infants who have apnea of prematurity achieve complete resolution of symptoms by 34 to 36 weeks, postconceptional age. Once apnea of prematurity has resolved, it does not return. Pathologic causes such as hypoglycemia, hypoxemia, hypothermia or hyperthermia, infection, left-to-right shunt, and intracranial hemorrhage should be ruled out. New-onset apnea in a previously symptom-free infant presents diagnostic concern. Apnea also increases in response to less stressful stimuli, such as immunizations or an ophthalmic examination. Apnea in a term or near-term infant is almost always pathologic. Isolated apnea may be treated with simple tactile stimulation in many cases. Infants who remain apneic after stimulation may require blow-by oxygen, nasal cannula therapy, nasal continuous positive airway pressure, nasal intermittent mechanical ventilation, or even reintubation and mechanical ventilation, depending on the severity, recurrence, and presence of underlying pathology.

Caffeine is the pharmacologic agent of choice to treat apnea because of its long plasma half-life and low toxicity. However, not every infant responds to caffeine therapy. One study identified genetic markers (adenosine receptor gene polymorphisms) that may predict an individual's response to caffeine. Studies show that 4% to 13% of sudden infant death syndrome (SIDS) cases have a history of apnea. However, multiple studies have failed to demonstrate a link between acute life-threatening events (ALTEs) and SIDS. More than 80% of SIDS cases occur between midnight and 6 am, whereas more than 80% of ALTEs occur between 8 am and 8 pm.

Choanal Atresia/Stenosis

Choanal obstruction resulting from a failure of bony or membranous regression is the most common supralaryngeal congenital defect. It occurs in approximately 1 in 4000 live births. Choanal atresia is often associated with defects in other organs or with syndromes that include other craniofacial anomalies, especially CHARGE syndrome (coloboma of the eye, heart anomaly, choanal atresia, retardation, and genital and ear anomalies). Choanal atresia is usually unilateral, typically on the right side; a 2:1 excess of choanal atresia has been reported in girls. Unilateral choanal atresia occurs more frequently in isolated cases, whereas bilateral choanal atresia should prompt further evaluation for other congenital anomalies. Associated findings include a high-arched palate, thickening of the vomer, and medial bowing of the lateral wall of the nose. Clinical presentation depends on the degree of obstruction. Bilateral choanal atresia or severe bilateral stenosis becomes evident in the newborn period, whereas unilateral cases or mild stenosis may not present for weeks, months, or years. Infants who have respiratory signs typically are distressed during times of sleep or feeding, when nasal breathing predominates. Clinical presentation in infants with unilateral obstruction or mild stenosis may occur only when the nares become obstructed, as during the passage of a nasogastric tube or inflammation in an upper respiratory infection. With occlusion of the patent nares, an infant may suddenly decompensate with signs of severe respiratory distress.

Infants in severe distress may require elective intubation if an oral airway proves insufficient or cannot be easily maintained. Direct visualization of the obstruction is best performed by an otolaryngologist using a fiberoptic scope. A cranial CT scan can determine the presence and thickness of the bony plate within the nasal cavity, which is an important surgical consideration. Definitive treatment generally involves drilling through the bony plate and stenting the nasal passage with tubes for 6 weeks to allow proper healing. A high degree of suspicion is key to diagnosing and properly treating this disorder, and if true bilateral choanal atresia is present, associated anomalies must be excluded.

Laryngomalacia

Laryngomalacia is the most common cause of stridor in the neonate. It is a dynamic lesion resulting in collapse of the supraglottic structures during inspiration, leading to airway obstruction. Infants have an omega-shaped epiglottis (curled onto itself). Similar to infants with mandibular hypoplasia, infants with laryngomalacia tend to have more respiratory insufficiency in the supine position because it allows the relatively unsupported anterior tissue to drop into hypopharynx, causing obstruction. Affected infants may be stridulous during periods of crying or distress. Rarely, the lesion may cause sufficient hypoxemia or hypoventilation to interfere with normal growth and development. Treatment includes prone positioning, and resolution is common by age 1 to 2 years.

Vocal Cord Paralysis

Vocal cord paralysis may be unilateral or bilateral. Unilateral cord paralysis usually presents with a weak or sometimes hoarse cry. Obstructive signs, such as stridor or retractions, are less severe and less common. The infant may also cough or choke while feeding because of an inability to prevent aspiration while swallowing. Common causes are stretch injury during delivery or recurrent laryngeal nerve injury during ductus ligation. Consequently, left-sided paralysis or paresis is most common. Respiratory signs from unilateral cord paralysis usually improve over several weeks or months without intervention but may take years to resolve.

Bilateral cord paralysis is a more serious problem and is often the result of an intracranial pathologic condition, such as Chiari malformation, intracranial hemorrhage, or hypoxic-ischemic encephalopathy. These infants may have near total airway obstruction and moderate to severe stridor. Many will require tracheostomy to maintain a stable and patent airway.

Airway Vascular Tumors/Malformations

Hemangiomas are the most common vascular tumors of the airway and occur in isolation or as part of a spectrum of posterior fossa malformation, arteriovenous malformations, cardiac/aortic defects, eye anomalies, and sternal defect (PHACES) syndrome. Congenital hemangiomas located just below the level of the vocal cords are another relatively uncommon cause of stridor in neonates, with or without expiratory wheeze. Hemangiomas often enlarge as the newborn grows and can threaten the airway. Positional changes tend to have little effect on the severity of respiratory signs. Superficial, capillary hemangiomas on the skin of the neck are often present, suggesting the diagnosis. For acute exacerbations, systemic and intralesional steroids are a mainstay of first-line therapy. For steroid unresponsive lesions, some evidence suggests antiangiogenic agents (IFN-α2a and IFN-α2b) may be effective. Anti-VEGF agents like bevacizumab are under evaluation. Nevertheless, symptomatic infants eventually may require surgical removal of the lesions. The availability of laser surgical ablation has markedly reduced the need for tracheostomy in children with subglottic hemangioma. Open excision has an estimated 90% success rate. Propranolol has had a beneficial role in the involution of hemangiomas.

Tracheobronchomalacia

Tracheobronchomalacia is characterized by an abnormally compliant airway cartilage, leading to intermittent airway collapse during normal respiration. Specific classification depends on the area(s) involved (eg, tracheomalacia, tracheobronchomalacia, and bronchomalacia). Infants may be mildly or severely affected, depending on the extent of involvement and the capacity of surrounding supporting tissues to maintain airway patency. Affected infants generally have respiratory signs in the newborn period, but presentation may be delayed for days or weeks if the defect is mild. In these milder cases, infants may remain free from respiratory distress until inter-current infection leads to increased airway secretions and increased work of breathing. Signs include expiratory wheez-ing and respiratory distress including tachypnea and retrac-tions, and the infant may receive a mistaken diagnosis of reactive airway disease. Paradoxically, the use of bronchodila-tors may actually worsen the condition. A chest radiograph may show hyperinflation.

Definitive diagnosis is made by direct visualization, typi-cally with flexible tracheobronchoscopy. Treatment is sup-portive as airway compromise generally lessens as the infant grows. However, more severe cases may require stenting with continuous positive airway pressure or even surgical plication. Tracheostomy alone may not be helpful if the affected area extends beyond the proximal trachea. A high association with other congenital anomalies, including vascular rings or tra-cheoesophageal fistula (discussed later in this chapter), also should be considered. A history of recurrent coughing or choking should prompt further investigation.

Tracheoesophageal Fistula

Esophageal atresia with tracheoesophageal fistula (TEF) occurs in approximately 1 in 4500 live births, making it one of the most common congenital malformations. Usually iso-lated, it can be associated with other anomalies including complex syndromes and malformation sequences such as VATER (vertebral defects, anal atresia, TEF, esophageal atresia, and renal anomalies), VACTERL (VATER plus cardiac and upper limb defects), and CHARGE (coloboma, heart defect, choanal atresia, mental retardation, genital hypoplasia, ear anomalies, and deafness). In the absence of a recognized syn-drome, TEF may also be associated with isolated cardiac defects, present in up to 50% of cases. Whether as part of a syndrome or an isolated anomaly, TEF usually is associated with esophageal atresia; in 5% to 7% of cases there is no asso-ciated esophageal atresia (H-type TEF).

TEF and associated esophageal atresia and TEF as part of a more general disorder invariably present in the immediate newborn period. Infants with an isolated H-type fistula may remain clinically silent for many weeks or even months.

Although relatively rare (approximately 1 in 100,000 live births), an H-type fistula must be suspected in any infant who coughs during feedings and has recurrent pneumonitis. In preterm infants it can present as apnea spells with no other signs. The diagnosis of an H-type fistula can be difficult but is best discovered by a cine esophagram. In cases in which this study is inconclusive, bronchoscopy may be necessary. Suc-cessful repair and preservation of pulmonary function depends on early diagnosis.

Vascular Compression

Vascular compression of the trachea or main stem bronchus can result from incomplete regression of the embryonic bran-chial arch arteries during fetal development. The most common anomaly is a vascular "ring" consisting of a double aortic arch in which the vessel completely encircles the trachea and esophagus. Other variants include an ectopic aortic arch

(passing behind the esophagus) or an aberrant origin of the right brachiocephalic artery.

Vascular rings cause inspiratory stridor and expiratory wheezing, neither of which change appreciably with the infant's position. Intermittent worsening of signs is sometimes seen during feeding as milk passing through the esophagus, further compressing the trachea. Additionally, feeding diffi-culty may occur because of esophageal compression.

When a previously undiagnosed infant first presents with these upper airway signs, she or he may be misdiagnosed as having tracheomalacia, bronchomalacia, or tracheobron-chomalacia, until further imaging confirms the vascular abnormality.

The presence of an abnormally shaped mediastinum on a chest film often provides a clue to diagnosis. Endoscopy may identify tracheal or esophageal compression. An echocardio-gram may define the vascular anomaly. Occasionally, cardiac catheterization may be indicated. Decisions regarding surgical correction of this defect depend on the relative compromise of the trachea and esophagus. As a caution, the degree of compression may worsen as the infant grows.

Phrenic Nerve Paralysis

Stretch injury to the cervical nerve roots C3 to C5 during delivery can lead to temporary paralysis of the hemidia-phragm, and avulsion of the nerve roots can lead to perma-nent injury without intervention. Phrenic nerve paralysis occurs more commonly on the right. Brachial plexus injury or Horner syndrome is present in 70% to 80% of cases, and clavicular fracture is common. Infants who are at highest risk are those with birth weights greater than 4 kg, shoulder dys-tocia, or difficult breech presentations. Diminished ventilation is present on the affected side and the infant may be tachy-pneic or even be cyanotic if severely compromised. The chest radiograph will show varying degrees of atelectasis, a raised hemidiaphragm on the affected side, and the heart and medi-astinum shifted toward the contralateral side. Fluoroscopy will demonstrate that the paralyzed diaphragm elevates during inspiration and descends on expiration (paradoxical move-ment). Treatment is supportive in most cases because function usually will spontaneously return in several weeks. When there is nerve avulsion or permanent dysfunction, surgical plication may be necessary.

Eventration of the Diaphragm

The diaphragm consists of three layers: a muscular layer sand-wiched between the pleural and peritoneal layers. Eventration of the diaphragm occurs when all or part of the diaphragmatic muscle is replaced by fibroelastic tissue. It is a rare disorder that results in a nonfunctioning diaphragm having highly elastic fibrous tissue. Partial defects are more common and usually occur on the right side. However, complete defects are more common on the left side and often are associated with other organ anomalies. Normal abdominal pressure permits the viscera easily to push the affected diaphragm upward into the hemithorax. In utero, this phenomenon may lead to pul-monary hypoplasia (although this is usually mild) whereas, occurring after birth, eventration can cause respiratory com-promise by affecting lung expansion. Radiographic and fluo-roscopic findings are similar to those of a paralyzed diaphragm, but a history of birth trauma or associated injuries is usually absent. With large defects, the appearance of bowel in the thoracic cavity on a chest radiograph may be mistaken for a diaphragmatic hernia. However, close inspection should reveal the thin, overlying diaphragmatic pleura. Treatment is supportive; defects that remain symptomatic beyond the neonatal period may require plication.

Pleural Effusion

Collection of fluid within the pleural cavity, if excessive, can result in significant respiratory embarrassment. Pleural effusions in the neonate may result from inflammation, fluid transudation, or frank leakage from disrupted vessels (either vascular or lymphatic). Small pleural effusions normally are present during the first hours of life as fetal lung liquid resorbs from the airspaces, but a large pleural effusion or persistence beyond the first day of life is abnormal. Large effusions can result in significant respiratory compromise. Although initial management is similar regardless of cause, successful long-term management depends on accurately identifying the source of the pleural effusion.

Congenital Anomalies of the Chest Wall

Thoracic cage abnormalities represent a group of uncommon but frequently overlooked causes of respiratory distress in the neonate. They may be structural or functional in nature. The structural abnormality may be limited to the sternum or it may involve the entire thoracic cage. Sternal deformities include pectus excavatum, which is a relatively common but usually benign condition, and complete separation of the sternum often accompanies ectopia cordis and usually is lethal. Generalized structural abnormalities invariably involve some degree of thoracic restriction and pulmonary hypoplasia. Many of these abnormalities are themselves lethal or are part of a more generalized lethal disorder. Some conditions, however, such as achondroplasia and Ellis-van Creveld syndrome, are compatible with normal life. Functional anomalies result from dysfunctional chest wall musculature. Like structural defects, they may be restricted to the thoracic cage but, more often, they are part of a systemic disorder, such as congenital muscular dystrophy, glycogen storage disease, or myasthenia gravis. Severe congenital kyphoscoliosis does not itself usually cause neonatal respiratory problems but it may augment mild respiratory illness from another cause.

Most infants with thoracic cage abnormalities are readily recognized in the immediate newborn period, although a relatively protuberant abdomen may distract the clinician from the primary problem. Infants with restrictive thoracic cages (either structural or functional) will have tachypnea and retractions. The radiograph shows a narrow, elongated thoracic cage with high clavicles and depressed hemidiaphragms. Treatment is supportive, and in the absence of severe pulmonary hypoplasia or an underlying lethal disorder, infants may do relatively well, despite requiring initial mechanical ventilation.

Persistent Pulmonary Hypertension of the Neonate

The organ of gas exchange for the fetus is the placenta, not the lung. Placental blood flow is high and pulmonary blood flow is minimal. To achieve intrauterine gas exchange, blood returning to the right side of the heart is directed to the systemic (and thereby placental) circulation. This blood flow path occurs via two fetal right-to-left shunts, namely the foramen ovale, which shunts blood from the right to left

atrium, and the ductus arteriosus, which shunts blood from the pulmonary artery to the descending aorta. Due to these shunts, less than 10% of the combined fetal ventricular output goes to the lungs.

At birth, dramatic lung changes must occur for the fetus to undergo a successful transition from placental to pulmonary gas exchange. Liquid is removed from the potential airspaces (see "Retained Fetal Lung Liquid Syndrome," presented earlier), and blood flow course is redirected. After inflation of the lungs with air and a dramatic increase in oxygen tension within the lungs, a marked increase in cyclic nucleotides occurs within pulmonary vascular smooth muscle, leading to vasodilatation. The resultant drop in pulmonary vascular resistance leads to a 10-fold increase in pulmonary blood flow, which causes left atrial pressure to exceed right atrial pressure, allowing the one-way flap across the foramen ovale to close. Flow across the ductus arteriosus reverses and, combined with increased blood oxygen tension, leads to gradual ductal closure over the first few hours of life.

In the syndrome of persistent pulmonary hypertension of the newborn (PPHN), this transition of the pulmonary circulation fails to occur normally (see section 3 of Chapter 56, Diseases of Pulmonary Circulation). Pulmonary vascular resistance and pulmonary arterial pressure remain high and blood flow continues largely to bypass the lungs as in fetal life. (This is why the term *persistent fetal circulation* has been used, although in a strict sense it is inaccurate because there is no longer a placental/umbilical circulation.) PPHN should be suspected if the degree of hypoxemia is out of proportion to pulmonary disease. PPHN is associated with many neonatal disorders, including RDS, meconium aspiration, air leak syndromes, perinatal asphyxia, congenital sepsis, and structural lung disorders such as pulmonary hypoplasia or alveolar-capillary dysplasia. PPHN can also be idiopathic. Infants with PPHN may be affected moderately or severely, depending on the extent of shunting. PPHN can be a self-limited disease, running a course over several days. In more severe cases, severe hypoxemia can lead to significant morbidity and mortality.

PPHN mortality previously has been as high as 50% to 60% but has improved significantly since the introduction of new treatment modalities including HFV, inhaled nitric oxide, and ECMO. Because nitric oxide increases cyclic guanosine monophosphate levels, selective phosphodiesterase inhibitors such as sildenafil are sometimes utilized in infants who have a prolonged course of PPHN or in whom pulmonary arterial hypertension develops after the newborn period, either idiopathic or as a result of underlying cardiorespiratory disease. The long-term benefits and risks of sildenafil are unknown.

Hyperviscosity Syndrome

Neonates with polycythemia (ie, a central hematocrit greater than 65%) are at risk for abnormally high blood viscosity, which interferes with regional tissue perfusion. Polycythemia may occur in several situations, including twin-twin transfusion, maternal-fetal transfusion, prolonged delayed cord clamping, home delivery, maternal diabetes, small-for-gestational-age infants, postmature infants, and infants with Down syndrome or Beckwith-Wiedemann syndrome. Signs generally relate to the degree of hyperviscosity and range from tachypnea to apnea, listlessness to irritability, hypoglycemia, and jitteriness to seizures.

Hyperviscosity syndrome presents during the first hours of life. The presentation may mimic congenital pneumonia, meconium aspiration, persistent pulmonary hypertension, or congenital heart disease. Affected infants are at risk for thrombotic injury unless the condition is reversed by partial blood volume exchange.

Congenital Heart Disease

In the neonate, significant congenital heart disease (CHD) typically presents as cyanosis with minimal or no respiratory distress or cardiorespiratory failure. Congenital heart disease in which pulmonary blood flow is either excessive or nonrestrictive often presents with respiratory distress.

Infants who have right ventricular outflow tract obstructive lesions, such as D-transposition of the great arteries with an intact ventricular septum or tetralogy of Fallot, may be visibly cyanotic but appear to be comfortable. Cyanotic heart disease should be suspected in these infants, even if a murmur is absent, particularly if the infant has persistent low oxygen saturation or is hypoxemic in 100% oxygen. Conditions with left ventricular outflow tract obstruction or a large ventricular septal defect (VSD) may present without cyanosis but have pallor, systemic hypotension, marked respiratory distress, and often a loud murmur. Chest radiographs may show cardiomegaly or pulmonary vascular congestion. Simple left-to-right shunt lesions including small VSD, atrial septal defect, atrioventricular septal defect, and PDA do not often present with severe pulmonary edema or distress during the neonatal period because a relatively high pulmonary vascular resistance can restrict pulmonary blood flow. In contrast, PDA in preterm infants can present with pulmonary edema and respiratory distress. In the mixed types of CHD, there is an overlap in presentation and infants may be cyanotic as well as display signs of respiratory conditions such as tachypnea and retractions. This type of presentation, common with hypoplastic left heart syndrome and obstructed total anomalous pulmonary venous return (TAPVR), may initially be confused with sepsis, pneumonia, meconium aspiration, or even RDS. TAPVR deserves particular mention because it is not detected in utero and sometimes may be missed postnatally, even on repeated echocardiograms.

In fact, TAPVR with pulmonary venous obstruction is a surgically correctable congenital heart lesion for which neonates may mistakenly be placed on ECMO. A high index of diagnostic suspicion is warranted in a term or near-term infant who has a clinical and radiographic picture similar to surfactant-deficient respiratory distress or group B streptococcal sepsis.

Metabolic Disorders

Several hundred human inborn errors of metabolism (IEM) have been identified. These are a heterogeneous group, have variable presentations, and are relatively rare. Consequently, the possibility of an IEM may be overlooked. Even in an era of expanded newborn screening in many US states and in several other countries, newborn screening results may be initially unavailable or require special expertise for interpretation. An infant with an IEM that causes metabolic acidosis or metabolic encephalopathy may have deep and labored respirations (Kussmaul breathing). In many cases, the condition will rapidly progress to respiratory failure and apnea. Other manifestations of IEM result either from accumulation of a toxic product or deficiency of an essential substrate. In many IEMs, there may not be dysmorphic features, seizures, or vomiting. Instead, a there may be a pattern of worsening but nonspecific signs of multiple organ dysfunction that may not respond to routine intervention. It is important to maintain a high index of suspicion for IEMs, especially when there are no identified risk factors for respiratory distress. A delay in diagnosis and treatment can be catastrophic.

Intestinal or Renal Bicarbonate Wasting

Low plasma bicarbonate represents a metabolic acidosis that may present as tachypnea and respiratory distress in the neonate, although it usually does not occur in isolation. Of note, metabolic acidosis with a normal anion gap may be a feature of neonatal diabetes or may indicate bicarbonate loss via the kidneys or intestines. Gastroenteritis, renal tubular acidosis, and mineralocorticoid insufficiency are common causes. Differentiating the source of the acidosis is important because bicarbonate therapy may be harmful depending on the underlying problem.

Key References

1. Kumar A, Bhat BV. Epidemiology of respiratory distress of newborns. *Indian J Pediatr.* 1996;63:93-98.
4. Warburton D, El-Hashash A, Carraro G, et al. Lung organogenesis. *Curr Top Dev Biol.* 2010;90:73-158.
6. Whitsett JA, Wert SE, Weaver TE. Diseases of pulmonary surfactant homeostasis. *Annu Rev Pathol.* 2015;10:371-393.
8. Vilos GA, Liggins GC. Intrathoracic pressures in fetal sheep. *J Dev Physiol.* 1982;4:247-256.
12. Clark RH. The epidemiology of respiratory failure in neonates born at an estimated gestational age of 34 weeks or more. *J Perinatol.* 2005; 25:251-257.
13. Edwards MO, Kotecha SJ, Kotecha S. Respiratory distress of the term newborn infant. *Paediatr Respir Rev.* 2013;14:29-36, quiz 36-37.
14. Yurdakok M. Transient tachypnea of the newborn: what is new? *J Matern Fetal Neonatal Med.* 2010;23(suppl 3):24-26.
15. Avery ME, Mead J. Surface properties in relation to atelectasis and hyaline membrane disease. *AMA J Dis Child.* 1959;97(5 Pt 1): 517-523.
16. Sweet DG, Carnielli V, Greisen G, et al. European consensus guidelines on the management of neonatal respiratory distress syndrome in preterm infants—2010 update. *Neonatology.* 2010;97:402-417.
19. Dishop MK. Paediatric interstitial lung disease: classification and definitions. *Paediatr Respir Rev.* 2011;12:230-237.
20. Kurland G, Deterding RR, Hagood JS, et al. An official American Thoracic Society clinical practice guideline: classification, evaluation, and management of childhood interstitial lung disease in infancy. *Am J Respir Crit Care Med.* 2013;188:376-394.
22. Bridges JP, Ludwig MG, Mueller M, et al. Orphan G protein-coupled receptor GPR116 regulates pulmonary surfactant pool size. *Am J Respir Cell Mol Biol.* 2013;49:348-357.
24. Whitsett JA. The molecular era of surfactant biology. *Neonatology.* 2014;105:337-343.
25. Davis C. Value of routine radiographic examinations of the newborn, based on a study of 702 consecutive babies. *Am J Obstet Gynecol.* 1930;20:73.
33. Rojas-Reyes MX, Orrego-Rojas PA. Rescue high-frequency jet ventilation versus conventional ventilation for severe pulmonary dysfunction in preterm infants. *Cochrane Database Syst Rev.* 2015;(10):CD000437.
43. Kluckow M, Evans N. Ductal shunting, high pulmonary blood flow, and pulmonary hemorrhage. *J Pediatr.* 2000;137:68-72.
44. Dennehy PH. Respiratory infections in the newborn. *Clin Perinatol.* 1987;14:667-682.
45. Garenne M, Ronsmans C, Campbell H. The magnitude of mortality from acute respiratory infections in children under 5 years in developing countries. *World Health Stat Q.* 1992;45:180-191.

49. Prevention of perinatal group B streptococcal disease: a public health perspective. Centers for Disease Control and Prevention. *MMWR Recomm Rep.* 1996;45(Rr–7):1-24.

51. Singh BS, Clark RH, Powers RJ, Spitzer AR. Meconium aspiration syndrome remains a significant problem in the NICU: outcomes and treatment patterns in term neonates admitted for intensive care during a ten-year period. *J Perinatol.* 2009;29:497-503.

54. Choi HJ, Hahn S, Lee J, et al. Surfactant lavage therapy for meconium aspiration syndrome: a systematic review and meta-analysis. *Neonatology.* 2012;101:183-191.

55. Hahn S, Choi HJ, Soll R, Dargaville PA. Lung lavage for meconium aspiration syndrome in newborn infants. *Cochrane Database Syst Rev.* 2013;(4):CD003486.

56. Deprest J, Brady P, Nicolaides K, et al. Prenatal management of the fetus with isolated congenital diaphragmatic hernia in the era of the TOTAL trial. *Semin Fetal Neonatal Med.* 2014;19:338-348.

57. McGivern MR, Best KE, Rankin J, et al. Epidemiology of congenital diaphragmatic hernia in Europe: a register-based study. *Arch Dis Child Fetal Neonatal Ed.* 2015;100:F137-F144.

58. Babiuk RP, Thebaud B, Greer JJ. Reductions in the incidence of nitrofen-induced diaphragmatic hernia by vitamin A and retinoic acid. *Am J Physiol Lung Cell Mol Physiol.* 2004;286:L970-L973.

59. Kutasy B, Friedmacher F, Pes L, et al. Antenatal retinoic acid administration increases trophoblastic retinol-binding protein dependent retinol transport in the nitrofen model of congenital diaphragmatic hernia. *Pediatr Res.* 2016;79:614-620.

60. Schmidt AF, Goncalves FL, Regis AC, et al. Prenatal retinoic acid improves lung vascularization and VEGF expression in CDH rat. *Am J Obstet Gynecol.* 2012;207:76.e25-76.e32.

63. Van Meurs K. Is surfactant therapy beneficial in the treatment of the term newborn infant with congenital diaphragmatic hernia? *J Pediatr.* 2004;145:312-316.

68. Deprest J, Jani J, Van Schoubroeck D, et al. Current consequences of prenatal diagnosis of congenital diaphragmatic hernia. *J Pediatr Surg.* 2006;41:423-430.

70. Ahmad A, Gangitano E, Odell RM, et al. Survival, intracranial lesions, and neurodevelopmental outcome in infants with congenital diaphragmatic hernia treated with extracorporeal membrane oxygenation. *J Perinatol.* 1999;19(6 Pt 1):436-440.

74. Priest JR, Williams GM, Hill DA, et al. Pulmonary cysts in early childhood and the risk of malignancy. *Pediatr Pulmonol.* 2009;44:14-30.

76. Wilson RD, Hedrick HL, Liechty KW, et al. Cystic adenomatoid malformation of the lung: review of genetics, prenatal diagnosis, and in utero treatment. *Am J Med Genet A.* 2006;140:151-155.

79. Stocker JT. Congenital pulmonary airway malformation: a new name for and an expanded classification of congenital cystic adenomatoid malformation of the lung. *Histopathology.* 2002;41:424-430.

83. Granata C, Gambini C, Balducci T, et al. Bronchioloalveolar carcinoma arising in congenital cystic adenomatoid malformation in a child: a case report and review on malignancies originating in congenital cystic adenomatoid malformation. *Pediatr Pulmonol.* 1998;25:62-66.

85. Correia-Pinto J, Gonzaga S, Huang Y, Rottier R. Congenital lung lesions—underlying molecular mechanisms. *Semin Pediatr Surg.* 2010;19:171-179.

86. Stefanova P, Ivanov B. Treatment of congenital lung cysts in childhood. *Khirurgiia.* 2014;75-79.

88. Corbett HJ, Humphrey GM. Pulmonary sequestration. *Paediatr Respir Rev.* 2004;5:59-68.

91. Congenital malformations of the lungs and airways. *Pediatr Respir Med.* 1999;1123.

93. Inhaled nitric oxide in full-term and nearly full-term infants with hypoxic respiratory failure. *N Engl J Med.* 1997;336:597-604.

95. Leach CL, Greenspan JS, Rubenstein SD, et al. Partial liquid ventilation with perflubron in premature infants with severe respiratory distress syndrome. The LiquiVent Study Group. *N Engl J Med.* 1996;335:761-767.

97. Coalson JJ. Pathology of new bronchopulmonary dysplasia. *Semin Neonatol.* 2003;8:73-81.

100. Ehrenkranz RA, et al. Validation of the National Institutes of Health consensus definition of the bronchopulmonary dysplasia. *Pediatrics.* 2005;116:1353-1360.

105. Thebaud B, Ladha F, Michelakis ED, et al. Vascular endothelial growth factor gene therapy increases survival, promotes lung angiogenesis, and prevents alveolar damage in hyperoxia-induced lung injury: evidence that angiogenesis participates in alveolarization. *Circulation.* 2005;112:2477-2486.

106. Doyle LW, Ehrenkranz RA, Halliday HL. Late (> 7 days) postnatal corticosteroids for chronic lung disease in preterm infants. *Cochrane Database Syst Rev.* 2014;(5):CD001145.

109. Halliday HL, Ehrenkranz RA, Doyle LW. Late (>7 days) postnatal corticosteroids for chronic lung disease in preterm infants. *Cochrane Database Syst Rev.* 2009;(1):CD001145.

110. Halliday HL, Ehrenkranz RA, Doyle LW. Early (< 8 days) postnatal corticosteroids for preventing chronic lung disease in preterm infants. *Cochrane Database Syst Rev.* 2010;(1):CD001146.

112. Tyson JE, Wright LL, Oh W, et al. Vitamin A supplementation for extremely-low-birth-weight infants. National Institute of Child Health and Human Development Neonatal Research Network. *N Engl J Med.* 1999;340:1962-1968.

113. Ballard RA, Ballard PL, Creasy RK, et al. Respiratory disease in very-low-birthweight infants after prenatal thyrotropin-releasing hormone and glucocorticoid. TRH Study Group. *Lancet.* 1992;339:510-515.

117. Stiskal JA, Dunn MS, Shennan AT, et al. alpha1-proteinase inhibitor therapy for the prevention of chronic lung disease of prematurity: a randomized, controlled trial. *Pediatrics.* 1998;101(1 Pt 1):89-94.

120. Chang YS, Ahn SY, Yoo HS, et al. Mesenchymal stem cells for bronchopulmonary dysplasia: phase 1 dose-escalation clinical trial. *J Pediatr.* 2014;164:966-972.e6.

Pneumonitis and Interstitial Disease

Daiva Parakininkas

PEARLS

- Most pediatric pulmonary parenchymal disease occurs as the result of an infectious agent.
- Clinical evaluation for parenchymal lung disease in the pediatric patient should include a search for symptoms and signs associated with pulmonary disease, such as difficulty with feeding, exercise intolerance, chest pain, cough, tachypnea, dyspnea, cyanosis, orthopnea, clubbing of the nail beds, weight loss, and lethargy.
- Factors predisposing a child to bacterial pneumonia include having numerous siblings, having parents who smoke, preterm delivery, living in an urban environment, poor socioeconomic status, presence of an airway foreign body, impaired immune response, congenital and anatomic lung defects, abnormalities of the tracheobronchial tree, cystic fibrosis, and congestive heart failure.
- Viral agents are the leading cause of lower respiratory tract infection in infants and children.
- Three major clinical syndromes are associated with lower respiratory tract viral illnesses: (1) bronchitis, (2) bronchiolitis, and (3) pneumonia.
- Fungal infections are important in the differential diagnosis of pulmonary infections, particularly in children whose immunity is compromised and in healthy children who are exposed to pathogens in a particular geographic or environmental setting.
- Three forms of disease patterns in pneumocystosis are (1) childhood/adult, (2) infantile, and (3) chronic fibrosing observed in some patients infected with the human immunodeficiency virus.
- Chemical pneumonitis and/or pneumonia may be acquired by (1) aspiration, (2) inhalation, (3) ingestion, or (4) injection.
- Pulmonary hemorrhage is a potentially life-threatening event that can occur at any age. Clinical presentation varies from massive fatal hemoptysis to silent bleeding with respiratory distress and anemia.

Pneumonitis, or inflammation of the lung parenchyma, is perhaps the most common cause of life-threatening lower respiratory tract disease in pediatric patients. Although pneumonitis may result from noninfectious processes (Box 55.1), most pediatric pulmonary parenchymal disease occurs as the result of an infectious agent. Pneumonitis may involve the pleura, interstitium, and airways; pneumonia by definition must include alveolar consolidation. Whereas early parenchymal lung injury is associated with increased cellularity with minimal fibrosis, advanced disease is characterized by extensive fibrosis and destruction of gas exchange units. Physiologic changes may include the following: low lung volumes, diminished lung compliance, impaired gas exchange, and airflow limitation. This chapter addresses the principal potential causes of pediatric pulmonary parenchymal disease, including alveolar and interstitial disorders.

Pathogenesis

Regardless of the cause, pneumonitis often follows a common pathogenesis. The initial parenchymal injury can result from mechanisms that directly damage the endothelium or epithelial cells. Other agents may injure the lung indirectly by one or more of the following processes:

1. Generation of toxic radicals
2. Recruitment of inflammatory cells (eg, neutrophils)
3. Activation of complement and/or release of chemotactic factors

If these processes go unchecked, alterations may occur in the lung parenchyma and connective tissues leading to end-stage fibrosis. This condition is characterized by severe destruction of gas exchange units and airways and the development of parenchymal cystic lesions.

Pathophysiology

Changes in lung volumes in pulmonary parenchymal disease depend primarily on the intensity of the alveolitis and stage of the disease process. Acute severe pneumonitis with intense alveolitis is characterized by moderate to severe reduction in both vital capacity (VC) and total lung capacity. It is also associated with a reduction in pulmonary compliance. In the early stages, patients with chronic interstitial diseases involving the lung parenchyma often have normal VC and total lung capacity. Subsequent reduction in lung volumes and pulmonary compliance occurs as the disease progresses and pulmonary fibrosis ensues.[1] Expiratory flow rates are usually preserved in persons with pneumonitis involving the lung parenchyma, and major obstructive defects, although reported, are rare. The carbon monoxide diffusing capacity, one of the earliest and most sensitive tests of parenchymal inflammation, is diminished in persons with interstitial lung disease (ILD). A reduction in the carbon monoxide diffusing capacity is not specific and may be found with other parenchymal disorders. Early in the course of parenchymal disease, resting arterial oxygen tension may be normal, but there is often mild alveolar hyperventilation with reduction in alveolar carbon dioxide tension and widening of the alveolar-arterial oxygen gradients

BOX 55.1	Etiology of Pediatric Interstitial Lung Disease

Infectious
- Bacteria
- Virus
- Mycoplasma
- Chlamydia
- Rickettsia
- Protozoa
- Fungus

Noninfectious
- Acute lung injury
- Chemical agents
- Physical agents
- Radiation
- Drugs
- Congenital lymphangiectasia
- Metabolic disorders
- Bronchopulmonary dysplasia
- Hypersensitivity pneumonitis
- Cardiovascular causes
- Collagen/vascular disorders
- Mixed connective tissue disorders
- Idiopathic pulmonary fibrosis
- Pulmonary hemorrhage syndromes
- Pulmonary hemosiderosis
- Pulmonary venoocclusive disease
- Desquamative interstitial pneumonia
- Lymphocytic infiltrative disorders
- Lymphocytic interstitial pneumonitis
- Familial erythrophagocytic lymphohistiocytosis
- Angioimmunoblastic lymphadenopathy
- Sarcoidosis
- Inherited diseases
- Malignancy
- Leukemia
- Hodgkin disease
- Non-Hodgkin lymphoma
- Histiocytosis X

($PAO_2 - PaO_2$). With exercise, hypoxemia and an increased $PAO_2 - PaO_2$ become exaggerated because of ventilation/ perfusion (V/Q) imbalance. V/Q mismatch is attributed to regional alterations of flow, altered parenchymal compliance, and increased obstruction to pulmonary airflow. Progressive alveolitis and subsequent derangement of gas exchange lead to deterioration of ventilatory efficiency and markedly increased work of breathing. Adequate oxygenation may become impossible even with the use of high-flow supplemental oxygen. Resting hypercapnia, pulmonary hypertension, and eventual right ventricular dysfunction with heart failure are common sequelae.[2-4]

Diagnosis

Diagnosing parenchymal lung disease in the pediatric patient may be quite challenging because of extreme variability in the presentation of disease. Clinical evaluation of the child should include a search for symptoms and signs associated with pulmonary disease, such as difficulty with feeding, exercise intolerance, chest pain, cough, tachypnea, dyspnea, cyanosis, orthopnea, clubbing of the nail beds, weight loss, and lethargy. In the child with diffuse alveolar disease, auscultative findings may be normal unless significant consolidation or small airway involvement is present. Fine crackles that may be heard throughout the chest late in inspiration are a characteristic

finding of small airway disease. These rales are produced by the opening of occluded small peripheral airways.

Laboratory Diagnosis

The chest radiograph is critical in the diagnosis and management of pulmonary parenchymal disease. In children with ILD the classic radiographic features that are present in adults may be absent. Computed tomography scanning,[5-7] gallium lung scanning, and bronchoalveolar lavage (BAL)[8-10] are useful techniques in the diagnosis and management of diseases involving the lung parenchyma. Pulmonary function testing is important and usually can be performed reliably in children who are older than 4 years.[1,11]

Bacterial Pneumonitis

Bacterial infections of the lower respiratory tract continue to account for a significant number of hospital admissions. The frequency of bacteria as etiologic agents of lower respiratory tract infection varies from 10% to 50%, depending on the study population and the methods of evaluation used.[12,13] In a large study of pediatric patients with lower respiratory tract infection, an etiologic agent was identified in nearly 50% of the patients. Bacteria accounted for 10% to 15% of the causative agents identified.

Factors predisposing to bacterial pneumonia include having numerous siblings, having parents who smoke, preterm delivery, living in an urban environment, and poor socioeconomic status. Hospitalization also increases the risk of contracting bacterial pneumonia because of the clustering of ill patients in confined areas, administration of immunosuppressive therapy, and various medical and surgical interventions that enhance the opportunity for colonization and infection. Additional factors that increase susceptibility to bacterial pneumonia include the presence of an airway foreign body,[14] impaired immune response,[15-19] congenital and anatomic lung defects, abnormalities of the tracheobronchial tree, cystic fibrosis,[20] and congestive heart failure.

Definition

Bacterial pneumonia is an inflammatory process of the lungs that may involve interstitial tissue and pleura in its evolution but always progresses to alveolar consolidation.

Pathophysiology

Pneumonia occurs when pulmonary defense mechanisms are disrupted and bacteria invade the respiratory system by aspiration or hematogenous spread. In most instances pneumonia appears to be a consequence of aspiration of a high inoculum of pathogenic bacteria. Viruses are often responsible for enhancing the susceptibility of the respiratory tract to bacterial infection. Less frequently, bacterial pneumonia may be the result of defects in host immunity because of young age, underlying immune dysfunction, or immunosuppressive therapy. Pneumonia may also occur when host defenses are mechanically disrupted because of tracheostomy or endotracheal intubation. The presence of respiratory pathogens in the terminal bronchioles and alveoli induces an outpouring of edema fluid and large numbers of leukocytes into the alveoli.[2,21] Macrophages subsequently remove cellular and bacterial debris. The infectious process may extend further within the lung segment or disseminate through infected bronchial fluid to other areas of the lung. The pulmonary lymphatic system enables bacteria to reach the bloodstream or visceral pleura.

With consolidation of lung tissue, VC and lung compliance markedly decrease and intrapulmonary right-to-left shunt and V/Q mismatch occur, resulting in hypoxia. Subsequently, pulmonary hypertension may occur because of significant oxygen desaturation and hypercapnia, often leading to cardiac overload.

Clinical Features

Signs and symptoms of bacterial pneumonia vary with the individual pathogen, the age and immunologic condition of the patient, and the severity of the illness. Clinical manifestations, especially in newborns and infants, may be absent. General or nonspecific complaints include fever, chills, headache, irritability, and restlessness. Individual patients may have gastrointestinal complaints including nausea, vomiting, diarrhea, abdominal distention, or pain. Specific pulmonary signs include nasal flaring, retractions, tachypnea, dyspnea, and occasionally apnea.

Tachypnea is the most sensitive index of disease severity. The sleeping respiratory rate is often a valuable guide to diagnosis. On auscultation, diminished breath sounds are frequently noted. Fine crackles that may be heard in children and older patients are commonly absent in infants. Because of the relatively small size of the child's thorax and the thin chest wall, broad transmission of the breath sounds occurs and the classic findings of consolidation are often obscured. Pleural inflammation may be accompanied by chest pain at the site of inflammation. This pleuritic pain may cause "splinting," which restricts chest wall movement during inspiration and reduces lung volume.

Extrapulmonary infections that may be present in some children include abscesses of the skin or soft tissue (*Staphylococcus aureus);* conjunctivitis, sinusitis, otitis media, and meningitis (*Streptococcus pneumoniae* or *Haemophilus influenzae*); and epiglottitis (*H. influenzae*).

Radiographic Features

Bacterial pneumonia is typically characterized by defined areas of consolidation with either segmental or lobar involvement. Lobar consolidation is the most characteristic, but multilobed disease is not unusual. The findings of pleural effusion, pneumatocele, or abscess are also strongly indicative of a bacterial infection. Staphylococcal pneumonia is suggested by rapid clinical and radiographic progression of disease, particularly in a young infant. Evidence of an abscess or pneumatocele further suggests a diagnosis of staphylococcal or gram-negative pneumonia such as *Klebsiella*. Group A streptococcal pneumonia may initially present with a diffuse interstitial pattern before the development of consolidation. Except for *Pseudomonas,* which may have a diffuse nodular appearance in the lower lobes, pneumonias caused by gram-negative organisms have no specific radiographic pattern. Anaerobic pulmonary infection is also associated with lung abscesses or air fluid levels.

Diagnosis

Bacterial pneumonia is suggested by fever, leukocytosis (>15,000 white blood cells), and increased band forms on the peripheral blood smear. Examination of the sputum may be helpful in establishing the diagnosis of bacterial pneumonia;

however, it is often difficult to obtain a satisfactory sputum sample in pediatric patients unless transtracheal aspiration or bronchoscopy is used. Transtracheal aspiration, although useful in adolescents and adults, is associated with significant complications in infants and young children. If a sputum sample is obtained (an adequate specimen must have >25 polymorphonuclear cells and <25 epithelial cells per high-power field), the Gram stain should be examined for a predominant bacterial pathogen and cultures should be performed with the appropriate antibiotic susceptibility studies. Counterimmune electrophoresis (CIE) performed on sputum specimens has proved helpful in establishing the diagnosis in both adults and children. Bacterial pneumonia is accompanied by bacteremia in a significant number of cases; hence blood cultures should be obtained before initiation of antibiotic therapy. Circulating antigens in *S. pneumoniae* and *H. influenzae* may be detected in the blood with CIE,[22] polymerase chain reaction (PCR),[23-25] or latex agglutination.[26,27]

If a significant pleural effusion is present, a diagnostic thoracentesis should be performed for the purposes of Gram stain and culture. Culturing pleural fluid has a relatively high yield in patients who have not received previous antibiotic therapy. If the Gram stain of pleural fluid is negative, CIE or latex agglutination should be performed because bacterial antigen may be detected in the fluid even after the initiation of antibiotics.

BAL should be considered in the management of a severely ill child in order to make a prompt diagnosis.[9,10] Making a prompt diagnosis is essential for the patient with progressive disease who has responded poorly to initial therapy or for the child with underlying immunodeficiency for whom empiric antibiotic treatment may be hazardous. In such instances, if the BAL is nondiagnostic, then lung aspiration or biopsy should be considered.[28] Material may be obtained through closed-needle biopsy, percutaneous needle aspiration, or an open lung biopsy. Positive results for such procedures in carefully selected cases identify an etiologic agent in 30% to 75% of cases, with open lung biopsy having the highest yield.[18,29]

Specific Pathogens

Group B Streptococci

Group B streptococci can cause infection in people of any age; however, these organisms are common pathogens in infants younger than 3 months.[30] Early-onset illness is often associated with maternal fever at the time of delivery, prolonged rupture of membranes, amnionitis, prematurity, and low birth weight.

Infected neonates usually manifest clinical symptoms within the first 6 to 12 hours of life. Symptoms include fever, respiratory distress, apnea, tachypnea, and hypoxemia. By 12 to 24 hours of age, signs of cardiovascular collapse are often apparent. Frequently, the syndrome of pulmonary hypertension of the newborn is present, and pulmonary or intracranial hemorrhage may become the terminal event.

Isolation of the organism establishes the diagnosis. Cultures from blood and cerebrospinal fluids must be obtained in all instances of suspected group B streptococcal pneumonia. Rapid diagnostic techniques have been helpful in providing early diagnoses. The radiographic findings in neonates with group B streptococcal pneumonia can be either a lobar (40%) or a diffuse reticulonodular pattern with bronchograms similar to findings of respiratory distress syndrome.

Aggressive cardiovascular and ventilatory support is usually required, particularly in the early stages of the disease. Antibiotic therapy should include a combination of ampicillin or penicillin and an aminoglycoside agent.

Although in the past the mortality rate of patients with group B streptococcal pneumonia could be as high as 50% to 60%, recent studies suggest improvement with prompt initiation of therapy and even better outcomes with maternal prophylaxis.[31] Some infants experience a second episode of infection 1 to 2 weeks after discontinuation of antibiotic therapy. Infants with group B streptococcal pneumonia and meningeal involvement (30%) may demonstrate significant neurologic deficits (20%-50%).

Streptococcus pneumoniae

S. pneumoniae is a gram-positive diplococcus with at least 84 sera types; however, 80% of the serious infections are caused by only 12 sera types. Streptococci are a major cause of pneumonia in the United States. Victims are usually infants younger than 2 years, with a peak age between 3 and 5 months. Patients with asplenia, functional hyposplenia, or malignancy or those receiving immunosuppressive drugs are at special risk of the development of invasive disease.[32]

The radiographic finding in infants is often a patchy bronchopneumonia. Lobar consolidation is not uncommon. Penicillin is the drug of choice in the treatment of persons with streptococcal pneumonia. However, organisms relatively resistant to penicillin occur in 3% to 40% of culture-positive patients recorded in studies from different parts of the United States.[33] In such instances, pneumonias have been effectively treated with vancomycin or high-dose β-lactam cephalosporin agents such as cefuroxime, ceftriaxone, or cefotaxime. Disease resulting from penicillin-resistant pneumococci should be considered in patients who received therapy with β-lactam antibiotics.[33-35]

The pneumococcal 13-valent conjugate vaccine is recommended for all children aged 5 and younger. It is also recommended for certain children aged 60 to 71 months with chronic medical conditions, immunosuppressive conditions, functional or anatomic asplenia, cerebrospinal fluid leaks, or cochlear implants. The pneumococcal polysaccharide vaccine, a 23-valent formulation, is recommended in children 2 years and older with an increased risk of invasive pneumococcal disease.[36]

Haemophilus influenzae

Haemophilus organisms are small, nonmotile, gram-negative rods that occur in both encapsulated and nonencapsulated forms. Approximately 90% to 95% of invasive disease is caused by the encapsulated sera type B. A pleural effusion or empyema is detected in nearly 40% of patients with H. influenzae pneumonia. There is an extremely high incidence of bacteremia in this disease. Serious complications such as epiglottitis, meningitis, and pericarditis can be diagnosed in 15% to 20% of patients. Cellulitis, anemia, and septic arthritis occur infrequently.

In a hospitalized patient, administration of the combination of ampicillin and chloramphenicol or a single cephalosporin such as cefuroxime, cefotaxime, or ceftriaxone generally is effective therapy.[33,37] The mortality rate in appropriately treated patients is generally considered less than 5% and often is related to associated meningitis, epiglottitis, or pericarditis

rather than the pneumonic process itself. Hib conjugate vaccine is an important measure in reducing the incidence of Haemophilus-related disease and should be administered to all children.[33,38,39]

Staphylococcal Pneumonia

Primary S. aureus pneumonia has decreased in frequency in recent years but still accounts for approximately 25% of cases in young infants. The incidence of secondary or metastatic dissemination has increased since 1972. Patients with primary pneumonia present with fever and respiratory symptoms, whereas those with metastatic disease often present with fever, generalized toxicity, and musculoskeletal symptoms. In patients presenting with primary staphylococcal pneumonia, the disease is often preceded by an upper respiratory tract infection.[40,41] Pleural effusion or empyema develops in nearly 80% of the patients with primary staphylococcal pneumonia and is extremely common in patients with metastatic disease. It is not unusual for patients with staphylococcal pneumonia to remain bacteremic long after the initiation of appropriate antibiotic therapy.

Radiographic findings of S. aureus pneumonia differ according to the stage of disease. They vary from minimal changes to consolidation (most common) and are associated with pleural effusion (50% to 60%) or pneumothorax (21%). Pneumatoceles usually appear during the convalescent stage and may persist for prolonged periods in asymptomatic patients. Antibiotic therapy should be administered intravenously and include a drug that is resistant to inactivation. Strong consideration should be given to providing antibiotic coverage for methicillin-resistant S. aureus, which can account for 1% to 30% of isolates, depending on the prevalence in the area.[40] The duration of therapy is usually lengthier in patients with staphylococcal disease than for patients with other bacterial pneumonias and consists of 21 days or more of treatment. The mortality rate of staphylococcal pneumonia varies from 23% to 33%. An increased incidence of mortality is usually associated with younger age, inappropriate initial antimicrobial therapy, or failure to drain an empyema appropriately.

Mycoplasma Pneumonia

Mycoplasma organisms are the smallest free-living microorganisms. They lack a cell wall and are pleomorphic. Mycoplasma is an uncommon cause of pneumonia in children younger than 5 years but is the leading cause of pneumonia in school-aged children and young adults. Illness can range from a mild upper respiratory tract infection to tracheobronchitis to pneumonia. Symptoms include malaise, low-grade fevers, and headache. In 10% of children a rash develops that usually is maculopapular. Cough, if it develops, usually occurs within a few days and may continue for 3 to 4 weeks. Initially the cough is nonproductive but then may become productive and is usually associated with widespread rales on physical examination. Roentgenographic abnormalities vary but are usually bilateral and diffuse.[33]

Isolation of Mycoplasma by culture is complicated by the requirement for special enriched broth or agar media, which are not widely available; it is successful in only 40% to 90% of cases and requires 7 to 21 days. A fourfold increase in antibody titer between acute and convalescent sera is diagnostic, but the time involved is lengthy, providing only a retrospective diagnosis. Complement fixation and immunofluorescent and several enzyme immunoassay antibody tests have been developed but are of limited diagnostic value.[33] Serum cold agglutinins with titers of 1:32 or greater are present in more than 50% of patients with pneumonia by the beginning of the second week of illness. PCR test has become an important means of diagnosing *M. pneumoniae* infections in clinical practice and allows for institution of therapy directed at the causative pathogen.[41] Treatment of upper respiratory tract infections or acute bronchitis is rarely indicated, but treatment with erythromycin or another macrolide such as azithromycin is indicated for persons with pneumonia or otitis media.

Gram-Negative Bacteria

Pneumonia caused by gram-negative enteric bacteria, especially *Pseudomonas,* is almost always found in patients with underlying pulmonary disease, compromised immune status, or those receiving prolonged respiratory therapy.[42,43] Gram-negative enteric bacteria are a frequent cause of nosocomial infection in critical care units. These organisms can produce a severe necrotizing pneumonia that is associated with an increase in morbidity.[44]

Legionella pneumophila

Pneumonia that occurs as a result of *Legionella pneumophila* has been reported infrequently in the pediatric age group.[45-48] The onset of this disease is characterized by high, unremitting fever; chills; and a nonproductive cough.[46] Extrapulmonary manifestations include gastrointestinal symptoms such as diarrhea, liver involvement, and confusion. Chest radiographs typically consist of peripheral nodular infiltrates and pleural effusions. Cavitation occurs only in immunosuppressed individuals. Death in the normal host is unusual if prompt therapy with azithromycin or erythromycin is initiated.

Anaerobic Bacteria

Pneumonia resulting from anaerobic upper respiratory flora is uncommon in healthy children. When it does occur, it is frequently associated with risk factors such as underlying pulmonary disease, a CNS disorder (including seizures), a postanesthetic state, and aspiration of a foreign body. Lung abscess and empyema are frequent complications in persons with anaerobic bacterial pneumonias.

Complications

The mortality rate in persons with uncomplicated bacterial pneumonia is less than 1%. Death is more common in children with complicated disease or an underlying disorder. The most frequent complications of bacterial pneumonia are pleural effusion and empyema (Table 55.1). Thoracentesis should always be performed if fluid is present to facilitate an etiologic diagnosis and establish the character of the fluid. Tube thoracostomy is indicated if a large amount of fluid is present and is producing respiratory compromise or if purulent fluid is obtained by thoracentesis. Empyema may extend locally to involve the pericardium, mediastinum, or chest wall. Evidence of empyema extension should be considered in the child who is unresponsive to antibiotic therapy.[28]

When tube thoracostomy/surgical drainage is required, it should be discontinued as soon as drainage has substantially decreased. For patients with staphylococcal empyema, streptococcal pneumonia, or *H. influenzae* empyema, 3 to 7 days of

TABLE 55.1	Major Sequelae/Life-Threatening Complications Associated With Bacterial Infections
Complication/Sequelae	**Organism**
Necrotizing pneumonia	Anaerobic, GNB
Respiratory failure	GBS
Shock	GBS, SP, H. flu, GNB
Apnea	GBS
Pneumothorax	H. flu
Pneumatoceles	H. flu, anaerobic, staph, SP, GAS
Abscess (lung)	Staph, SP, anaerobic
Pleural effusion	H. flu, GAS, SP, staph
Empyema	H. flu, staph, SP
Epiglottitis	H. flu, GAS
Meningitis	H. flu, GBS, SP
Encephalopathy	Legionella
Pericarditis	H. flu
Bone/joint	H. flu, staph
Kidneys	Staph

GAS, Group A streptococcus; GBS, group B streptococcus; GNB, gram-negative bacteria; *H. flu, Haemophilus influenzae;* SP, *Streptococcus pneumoniae;* Staph, *Staphylococcus aureus.*

drainage is usually sufficient. Patients with empyema require prolonged antimicrobial therapy and careful follow-up.

Pneumothorax and pneumatoceles can be seen with almost any bacterial pneumonia but are especially common with staphylococcal disease.[49] Such pneumatoceles require no special therapy and usually resolve. Lung abscess is an infrequent complication of *H. influenzae* and pneumococcal pneumonia and is most often encountered with staphylococcal disease or anaerobic bacteria.

Prognosis is usually excellent even in persons with severe bacterial pneumonia complicated by empyema. Long-term follow-up of children with empyema has demonstrated remarkably few, if any, residual pulmonary function abnormalities and remarkable clearing of chest roentgenograms. In contrast to adults with empyema, children seldom require surgical procedures such as decortication. However, follow-up chest radiographs should be obtained on all patients with bacterial pneumonia to document complete resolution. Such radiographic follow-up studies are probably not indicated until at least 6 to 8 weeks following the initiation of antibiotic therapy.

Therapy

Therapy for persons with bacterial pneumonia should include appropriate IV antibiotic treatment directed toward the specific pathogen, if it is known (Table 55.2). Localized or compartmental complications such as empyema, lung abscess, pericarditis, or septic joints require appropriate surgical drainage and antibiotic therapy. Prevention via immunization or chemoprophylaxis has changed the incidence and epidemiology of pneumonitides significantly. Options for

TABLE 55.2   Bacterial Pneumonia Therapy

Disease/Organism	Therapy
Undetermined Organisms	
Serious, life-threatening pneumonia, nonsuppressed host	Cefotaxime or ceftriaxone + azithromycin + vancomycin Bronchial lavage or needle aspiration of lung may be necessary to establish diagnosis
Suppressed neutropenic host	Imipenem/meropenem *or* piperacillin or ceftazidime + aminoglycoside ± clindamycin Vancomycin not included in initial therapy unless high suspicion or if patient has indwelling line. Ampho not used unless still febrile after 3 days/high suspicion. Bronchial lavage, needle/open biopsy may be necessary to establish diagnosis
Lung abscess	Clindamycin *or* ticarcillin/clavulanate *or* piperacillin/tazobactam
Specific Organisms Pneumonia With Empyema *Streptococcus pneumoniae,* group A strep	
Penicillin susceptible	Cefotaxime or ceftriaxone + chest tube drainage
Penicillin resistant	Vancomycin ± rifampin + chest tube drainage
Staphylococcus	
Methicillin sensitive	Nafcillin or oxacillin + chest tube drainage
Methicillin resistant	Vancomycin + chest tube drainage
Pneumonia Without Empyema *Haemophilus influenzae*	Ampicillin or cefotaxime or ceftriaxone + chloramphenicol
Klebsiella pneumonia	Meropenem
Escherichia coli, Enterobacter	Aminoglycoside or cephalosporin
Legionella	Azithromycin or erythromycin ± rifampin
Pseudomonas	Aminoglycoside + anti-*Pseudomonas* penicillin or aminoglycoside + ceftazidime
Mycoplasma pneumoniae	Erythromycin or azithromycin or clarithromycin

immunization, active or passive, and chemoprophylaxis for various etiologic agents are listed in Table 55.3.

Viral Pneumonitis

Infection is the most common cause of pulmonary interstitial disease in children, and viral agents are the leading cause of lower respiratory tract infection in infants and children. The viral agents listed in Table 55.4 account for the greatest percentage of pediatric pulmonary disease. Nearly 85% of all hospitalizations of children younger than 15 years occur during outbreaks of respiratory syncytial, parainfluenza, or influenza virus.

The diagnosis of viral pneumonia in children is frequently based on the clinical presentation, epidemiologic setting, and exclusion of bacterial pathogens by negative cultures. A specific agent is identified in only approximately 50% of cases of presumed viral pneumonia. Pediatric viral respiratory tract infections occur most commonly during the winter, with distinct peaks during midwinter and early spring in temperate climates. Closed population groups provide for greater spread of respiratory viruses and increased recognition of viral pneumonias.

Pathophysiology

The mechanism of infection for most respiratory viruses appears to be a progressive spread from the larger airways to the alveoli. The respiratory epithelial cell is the major target of cytopathic effect. The normal ciliated columnar epithelium may become markedly dysplastic with loss of the overlying cilia.[50,51] Areas of ulceration then occur as segments of the mucosal surface desquamate into the bronchial lumen. Impaired mucociliary clearance occurs, and altered stimulation of nerves mediating bronchial smooth muscle tone leads to increased airway resistance.[52] Enhanced mucus formation along with mucosal debris may lead to obstruction of the bronchioles, luminal narrowing, distal air trapping, and hyperinflation of various lung segments. In advanced disease with complete small airway obstruction, atelectasis results, causing hypoxemia as a result of intrapulmonary shunting and V/Q imbalance.

In persons with severe viral pneumonia, widespread parenchymal injury caused by a necrotizing alveolitis may occur. Alveolar round cell infiltrates occur often, with subsequent hyaline membrane formation and intraalveolar hemorrhage, which produces extensive parenchymal destruction and diminished lung compliance, decreased lung volumes, and intrapulmonary shunting.[53]

Diagnosis

Although the clinical presentations of illness by respiratory viruses overlap, presumptive diagnosis of the specific etiology is based on clinical presentation, setting, and, most importantly, epidemiologic information. In the past, virus isolation

TABLE 55.3 Preventive Measures

Organism	Immunization	Chemoprophylaxis
Cytomegalovirus	IVIG: prophylaxis in seronegative transplant recipients	Ganciclovir or valganciclovir
Haemophilus influenzae type b	Capsular polysaccharide vaccine *or* conjugate vaccine	Rifampin in the face of incomplete immunization and exposure
Influenza	Inactivated virus produced in chicken embryos	Oseltamivir (A or B) *or* amantadine/rimantadine (A)
Measles	Live virus vaccine *or* IVIG for immunocompromised patients	None
Streptococcus pneumonia	Purified capsular polysaccharide antigens of 23 pneumococcal serotypes vaccine *or* multivalent protein conjugate vaccine	Penicillin VK for functional or anatomic asplenia until age 5 yr
Pneumocystis carinii	None	Trimethoprim-sulfamethoxazole *or* pentamidine or dapsone or atovaquone
RSV	RSV-IVIG *or* palivizumab (monoclonal antibody)	None
Group B strep	None	Intrapartum antibiotics

IVIG, intravenous immunoglobulin; *RSV*, respiratory syncytial virus.

TABLE 55.4 Viral Agents Associated With Pediatric Interstitial Lung Disease

Agent	Frequency
Respiratory syncytial virus	+++++
Parainfluenza virus	++++
Adenovirus	+++
Influenza virus	+++
Cytomegalovirus	+
Enterovirus	+
Rhinovirus	+
Measles	+

or seroconversion was necessary for a definitive diagnosis. Today many respiratory viral infections can be diagnosed through the use of new techniques.[54]

Viral specimens should be obtained as early as possible during the period of greatest viral excretion. Cultures may be negative in up to 40% of patients during acute viral respiratory tract disease; failure to isolate a virus is not definitive evidence against the diagnosis of viral pneumonia. Serologic tests including complement fixation, hemagglutination inhibition, enzyme-linked solid-phase assays (enzyme-linked immunosorbent assays), and antibody assays have been used in the diagnosis of viral infection. Histologic evidence of infection in biopsy or postmortem specimens may be helpful, particularly when intranuclear inclusions are documented. Rapid diagnostic techniques focus on detection of the virus or its components in the sample. These new techniques include refinements in the use of immunofluorescence, enzyme immunoassay, time-resolved fluoroimmunoassay, latex agglutination assays, and use of nucleic acid hybridization methods, such as DNA probes and PCR.[55-58]

Three major clinical syndromes are associated with lower respiratory tract viral illness:
1. Bronchitis: Acute bronchitis is a febrile illness associated with a new productive cough. Symptoms of upper respiratory tract infection may be present. Acute bronchitis can adversely affect respiratory function, particularly in patients with chronic pulmonary impairment, leading to hospitalization of persons with marginal lung function.
2. Bronchiolitis: Symptoms result from airflow obstruction caused by localized inflammation of the terminal respiratory bronchioles. The development of cough; tachypnea with intercostal retractions; fine, moist, inspiratory crackles; and expiratory wheezes are characteristic. Hypoxemia and cyanosis are often present.[59]
3. Pneumonia: Primary viral pneumonia is frequently a mild illness characterized by a mild cough and one or more segmental infiltrates on chest radiograph. Although it is usually a self-limited process, in some persons the pneumonic process may progress with extensive parenchymal injury, diffuse interstitial alveolar infiltrates, and severe hypoxemia. Bacterial superinfection is heralded by increased temperature, change in sputum, and signs of localized consolidation several days after the initial onset of symptoms.

Radiographic Findings

Differentiation of bacteria from viral pneumonia cannot be made solely on the radiographic appearance. Children with presumed viral pneumonia, however, may have several radiographic findings, including the following:
1. Peribronchial thickening and perihilar linear densities
2. Partial lobar or patchy involvement in multiple areas of the lung
3. Shifting regional infiltrates
4. Areas of hyperinflation and atelectasis

Hilar adenopathy is usually absent. Diffuse bilateral infiltrates similar to those reported in acute respiratory distress syndrome (ARDS) have been found in persons with severe influenza, adenovirus, and respiratory syncytial virus (RSV) pneumonias.[60] Pleural effusions can occur in both adenovirus and parainfluenza pneumonias. Pulmonary calcifications/nodules have been described in the convalescent phase of varicella and measles.

Specific Pathogens

We review the most common viral pathogens that cause pneumonitis in children but have elected to exclude such viruses as Hantavirus that are beyond the scope of this chapter. There continue to be viruses that are identified as pathogens in viral pneumonitis but as of yet do not have effective chemoprophylaxis or therapy such as the human metapneumovirus or the bocavirus, but their inclusion would not add to our discussion. Please refer to more up-to-date journal articles for specific pathogens of interest.[25,61]

Respiratory Syncytial Virus

RSV is the most common cause of bronchiolitis and pneumonia in the United States in children between the ages of 6 months and 3 years. The disease produced by RSV varies from upper respiratory tract infection to severe bronchiolitis and pneumonia with wheezing and respiratory failure.[59] Higher mortality rates and greater severity with prolonged symptoms occur in infants and children younger than 6 weeks of age and in those who have a history of prematurity, chronic lung disease, cardiopulmonary disease, congenital heart disease, pulmonary hypertension, or neuromuscular impairment, as well as in those receiving chemotherapy or immunosuppressive therapy.[16,62-69] Signs of RSV pneumonia include wheezing, dyspnea, pulmonary infiltrates, and areas of atelectasis and hyperinflation on the chest radiograph. RSV infection may result in increased airway reactivity and airway resistance that persists for months. Significant respiratory tract shedding of virus continues for up to 21 days from the onset of illness. Nosocomial spread of RSV infection is common, and early diagnosis and appropriate isolation techniques are critical in hospitalized patients.

Methods for diagnosis of RSV include viral isolation in cell culture, immunofluorescence of exfoliated nasopharyngeal epithelial cells for detection of RSV antigens, and enzyme immunoassay for detection of RSV antigens in nasal secretions.[70,71] PCR technology is available for diagnosis of RSV illness.

All hospitalized patients with bronchiolitis and RSV pneumonia should be monitored for hypoxia, hypercarbia, and the need for ventilatory assistance. Supportive care includes the use of humidified oxygen, secretion clearance, and hydration.[72,73] Mechanical ventilation for respiratory failure is usually well tolerated. Extracorporeal membrane oxygenation has been used successfully in infants who do not respond to conventional ventilation.[74,75] The routine administration of bronchodilators and corticosteroids is not warranted; use should be individualized on the basis of clinical reponse.[75,76] Passive immunoprophylaxis has proved useful in high-risk populations in preventing RSV infection, as has palivizumab, a humanized mouse monoclonal antibody.[33,77-81] The incidence of bacterial superinfection in persons with RSV disease is low; therefore prophylactic antibiotics are not recommended for RSV disease.[62,82,83] It is not unusual for an infant with RSV to require hospitalization for 7 to 10 days following the onset of illness. Long-term complications of RSV infection may include persistent bronchial reactivity, with lower respiratory tract symptoms in more than 70% of infants in the year following hospitalization.[84] Whether moderately severe RSV infection predisposes a person to asthma later in life remains controversial.[85-89]

Parainfluenza Virus

Parainfluenza virus (types 1 and 2) is more often associated with laryngotracheobronchitis and croup than with pneumonia (usually type 3). Parainfluenza is second only to RSV as an etiology of lower respiratory tract disease responsible for the hospitalization of children.[90-96] The pneumonia associated with parainfluenza is typically mild; however, fatal cases with prolonged viral shedding have been reported in patients with severe combined immunodeficiency disease.[97-100] Conferred immunity following infection is low; repeat infection occurs in nearly 50% of patients by age 30 months, although they result in progressively milder illness. Parainfluenza virus, like RSV, has demonstrated ability to elicit an immunoglobulin IgE-specific antibody response.[93] Rapid identification of parainfluenza virus by either fluorescent or enzyme-linked immunologic techniques is possible, but results are variable depending on the viral type and antisera used. Viral culture may take up to a week. PCR methods are available for detection and differentiation, with high sensitivity and specificity. Treatment is supportive.

Adenovirus

Adenoviruses are responsible for approximately 3% of the pneumonias occurring in children. Clinical features are similar to other viral pneumonias except that the onset of illness is often gradual, occurring over several days. Of the 51 serotypes, types 3, 4, and 7 are the most common causes of lower respiratory tract disease in children. Adenovirus type 7 is most commonly associated with severe pneumonitis in infants and children and has a significant incidence of mortality and morbidity.[41,101-105] In 2007, a new strain of adenovirus 14 was isolated in previously healthy infants and young adults in the United States in whom fatal pneumonia developed.[106] A clinical presentation similar to that of bacterial pneumonia, with massive pleural effusion, rhabdomyolysis, and myoglobinuria, has been reported with adenovirus type 21.[107] In many infants with documented adenovirus respiratory tract infection, chronic pulmonary disease that manifests as persistent atelectasis, bronchiectasis, and recurrent pneumonitis with areas of hyperinflation and interstitial fibrosis develops. Bronchiectasis and restrictive lung disease have been documented in children following acute adenovirus infection. Adenovirus pneumonia is the most common cause of bronchiolitis obliterans in children, and unilateral hyperlucent lung syndrome has been reported.[108-112] Disseminated adenovirus occurs and is usually associated with infection by serotype 3, 7, or 21. It occurs most frequently in infants younger than 18 months and usually involves the heart, pericardium, liver, pancreas, kidneys, CNS, and skin.[113] Fatal cases of adenovirus and pneumonia can occur in previously healthy young individuals. Diagnosis is made by cell culture and antigen and DNA detection by PCR. Adenovirus typing is available from some reference and research laboratories. Treatment is mainly supportive in immunocompetent patients, but cidofovir and IV immunoglobulins have been used in some immunocompromised patients.[114]

Influenza

Three antigenically distinct influenza viruses exist—types A, B, and C. All three have hemagglutinin surface antigen, but only types A and B have neuraminidase surface antigen. Antigenic drift for types A and B produces minor changes in the surface antigens, resulting in endemic illness. Antigenic shift only occurs with influenza type A, resulting in a major change or new surface antigen, for which there may be low or no immunity in the population. Influenza type A is subtyped by its surface antigens, and currently three influenza strains are circulating worldwide, including influenza A/H1N1, H1N2, and H3N2.[33,115]

Clinical signs of uncomplicated influenza pneumonia include coryzal symptoms followed by dyspnea, fever, cyanosis, cough, and wheezing. Children with influenza typically have a more sudden onset of "toxic" signs than do those with other viral diseases. Infection is associated with myalgia, encephalopathy, and cardiac involvement. Pathologically, influenza virus infection is similar to RSV in that the virus destroys ciliated respiratory epithelial cells with subsequent edema and an acute inflammatory response. Influenza has been associated with Reye syndrome and with significant bacterial suprainfections.[116] In patients in whom bacterial infection develops, there often is a period of apparent improvement before a sudden worsening that is heralded by the production of purulent sputum, return of fever, and development of pulmonary consolidation.[117] Fatal outcomes have been reported in previously healthy children, as well as in high-risk groups.

Prevention of influenza disease is possible with either administration of multivalent influenza vaccine (influenza A/H1N1, A/H3N2, and B) or chemoprophylaxis with oseltamivir and zanamivir (influenza A, B, and A/H1N1) or amantadine hydrochloride and its closely related analog rimantadine (influenza A). One study showed efficacy of aerosolized ribavirin in the treatment of persons with influenza B.[118,119] Diagnosis of influenza pneumonia may be made by a culture of the virus from respiratory secretions or with serologic techniques. Rapid diagnosis by means of immunofluorescence of exfoliated nasopharyngeal cells may be helpful, as well as by PCR. Treatment includes supportive care, monitoring of respiratory status, and administration of antiviral medications.

Measles

Measles is a highly contagious disease that is preventable by vaccine; the incidence fell below the endemic threshold in the United States in 2000.[120] Endemic outbreaks continue in developing countries and when international travelers import measles to nonimmunized persons in the United States.[33,120] Typical disease manifests as high fever, cough, runny nose, and generalized rash. Respiratory symptoms are nearly universal in this illness, making the prevalence of measles pneumonia difficult to determine. Moist crackles develop in most children, and approximately 20% have expiratory wheezes and hypoxia. In cases in which radiographs have been obtained, a fine reticular infiltrate was present, compared with the nodular infiltrates in children with atypical measles. Although the clinical syndrome usually resolves over 1 to 2 weeks, both radiographic and pulmonary function abnormalities may persist for months. Severe life-threatening tracheitis may occur during the course of measles or bacterial suprainfection.[121-123] In fatal cases, severe respiratory and nervous system disease are manifested, and lung tissue

demonstrating interstitial pneumonitis with diffuse endothelial cells, pneumatocyte degeneration, and presence of multinucleated giant cells has been reported.[124]

Diagnosis is made by isolation of the virus, standard serology, or identification of viral ribonucleic acid by reverse transcription PCR. All suspected cases should be reported to local and state health departments. No antiviral agent is available; treatment is supportive. Two doses of vitamin A (200,000 International Units on consecutive days) have been shown to reduce pulmonary-specific and overall mortality rates in patients up to 2 years of age.[125] Administration of IV immunoglobulin may be of benefit to high-risk or immunosuppressed patients when it is started within 6 days of exposure.[33]

Human Immunodeficiency Virus

HIV infection in children most commonly presents with recurrent bacterial infections. The major morbidity and mortality in pediatric AIDS are associated with lung disease, ranging from opportunistic infections such as *Pneumocystis carinii* pneumonia to entities such as chronic interstitial pneumonitis.[126,127] Treatment for specific pulmonary pathogens is discussed throughout this chapter, but specific guidelines for HIV/AIDS treatment are lengthy, rapidly changing, and beyond the scope of this chapter. \More specific and current information regarding HIV/AIDS is available at www.aidsinfo.nih.gov/guidelines. This website provides the most current information regarding HIV/AIDS clinical research, HIV treatment and prevention, and medical practice guidelines. This information can also be obtained by phone at 1-800-HIV-0440 within the United States or 1-301-315-2816 outside the United States or by mail at AIDS Info, P.O. Box 4780, Rockville, MD 20849-6303.

Complications

The actual mechanisms by which viruses predispose the lung to secondary bacterial infection are not precisely understood. Viruses are capable of altering both cellular and noncellular defenses of the respiratory tract.[52,53,128] Viral infection of the epithelial cells appears to predispose the upper respiratory tract mucosa to bacterial colonization by allowing bacterial pathogens to adhere to injured cells.[51,52] Viral infection may cause significant impairment of both intracellular killing and ingestion of bacteria by the pulmonary macrophage. Significant defects in polymorphonuclear leukocyte chemotaxis and phagolysosome fusion occur during acute viral infection. The greatest impairment of macrophage function occurs 1 week after the onset of viral infection, which correlates with the peak incidence of bacterial suprainfection. Thus suprainfection during the course of viral lower respiratory tract disease appears to be the result of a combination of the cytopathic effects of the virus on the respiratory mucosa and various alterations in host immune response.

Significant life-threatening complications of viral lower respiratory tract disease are noted in Box 55.2. Respiratory failure with viral pneumonitis resembling ARDS is frequently seen in patients in the pediatric critical care unit. It is often associated with influenza or adenovirus but can occur with varicella, cytomegalovirus, and RSV.[60]

Diagnosis

A number of techniques are available for establishing a viral diagnosis. In the critical care setting, the decision to undertake these diagnostic measures should be guided by how awareness

<table>
<tr><td>BOX 55.2</td><td>Major Sequelae/Life-Threatening Complications Associated With Viral Pneumonitis</td></tr>
</table>

Subacute Sclerosing Panencephalitis: Measles
- Guillain-Barré syndrome: influenza, varicella
- Reye syndrome: influenza, VZV
- Encephalitis: adenovirus, measles, RSV, CMV
- Seizures: influenza
- Bacterial superinfection: influenza, VZV, Epstein-Barr virus, measles
- Asthma: RSV, parainfluenza, rhinovirus
- Apnea: RSV, influenza
- Bronchiolitis obliterans: influenza, adenovirus, measles
- Chronic obstructive pulmonary disease: RSV
- Fatal pneumonitis: influenza, measles, adenovirus, RSV, parainfluenza, CMV
- Tracheitis, life-threatening: measles, parainfluenza
- Appendicitis: adenovirus, measles
- Intussusception: adenovirus, CMV
- Hepatitis: adenovirus, influenza measles, CMV
- Nephritis: adenovirus, influenza, measles
- Myocarditis: adenovirus, influenza, measles
- Pericarditis: adenovirus, influenza, measles
- Arthritis: adenovirus
- Deafness: adenovirus
- Keratoconjunctivitis: adenovirus
- Myositis: influenza
- Stevens-Johnson syndrome: measles
- Coagulopathy: measles
- Thrombocytopenia: measles, CMV

CMV, cytomegalovirus; RSV, respiratory syncytial virus; VZV, Varicella zoster virus.

of the specific viral illness will affect the clinical management. Potential benefits include (1) a guide to selection of appropriate antiviral therapy and avoidance of unnecessary treatments with antibiotics and (2) initiation of appropriate infection control measures and use of vaccine or drug prophylaxis. Direct isolation of viruses is a sensitive method of diagnosis early in the course of disease when a large number of infectious particles are present in respiratory secretions. Nasopharyngeal washings are the preferred specimens for viral cultures because large quantities of secretions for culture are easily available. Unfortunately, viral isolation may require up to 2 weeks for positive culture results. Serologic testing or diagnosis depends on demonstration of a rising antibody titer between acute and convalescent sera. Although serologic data may provide a diagnosis, they are of little value in guiding therapeutic critical care interventions. The more commonly used methods for viral diagnosis involve detection of viral antigens present in the respiratory secretions. These antigen-detection techniques using radioimmune or enzyme-linked assays can detect all riboviruses and adenoviruses that commonly produce lower respiratory tract infections. Antibody detection has also been used successfully in the diagnosis of lower respiratory tract viral disease (cytomegalovirus pneumonia).[129] A major advantage of tests capable of detecting viral components is that these studies can be performed rapidly and the results made available to the critical care physician in hours, thus allowing timely management.

Prevention and Treatment

Guidelines for influenza chemoprophylaxis and treatment are lengthy and rapidly changing. Specific and current information regarding the use of antiviral drugs is available at www.aapredbook.org/flu or www.cdc.gov/flu/professionals/antivirals/index.htm.

Vaccination

Passive immunization is also available for some viruses that can be associated with pneumonitis, but recommendations are ever changing, so please check the Centers for Disease Control and Prevention (CDC) recommendations as well (see Table 55.3 for further details).

Chemoprophylaxis

Amantadine, rimantadine, oseltamivir, and zanamivir are approved for prophylaxis of viral respiratory tract infection caused by influenza. Amantadine and rimantadine have been shown to be effective prophylaxis for influenza type A; however, they are not active against influenza type A/H1N1 or influenza type B. Amantadine resistance has been reported in persons with influenza type A/H3N2. Oseltamivir and zanamivir have activity against influenza types A, B, and A/H1N1. Oseltamivir resistance has been reported among persons with influenza type A/H1N1 strains globally, but no significant resistance has been reported among persons with influenza type A/H1N1 strains circulating in the United States. All four drugs are recommended for persons at high risk for serious influenza infection who have not been vaccinated or who have received the vaccine within 2 weeks of the onset of an epidemic. They are also recommended for persons in whom appropriate immune response may not develop following vaccination and for persons who cannot receive the influenza vaccine because of allergic reactions.[33,130,131]

Therapy

A number of antiviral agents inhibit the replication of respiratory viruses in vitro, and some of these drugs have been used clinically in both experimental and naturally occurring respiratory infections (Table 55.5). Amantadine can be used to treat seasonal influenza A virus infections. Numerous studies have demonstrated that amantadine shortens the course of illness in uncomplicated influenza infections in otherwise healthy children if initiated within the first 48 hours of the disease. Amantadine is not effective against influenza type B or A/H1N1.[132] Currently circulating influenza A and H1N1 viruses are resistant to adamantanes, so these medications are not recommended for use currently. Most influenza A and B virus strains are susceptible to oseltamivir and zanamivir.[133] These neuraminidase inhibitors have been shown to reduce the severity and duration of illness.[134-137] Resistance to oseltamivir has been reported in persons with influenza type A/H1N1 strains but not A/H3N2 or B strains.[138-141] Zanamivir is effective against influenza type A, B, and A/H1N1, but it has not been approved for therapeutic use in children younger than 7 years.[33] Peramivir was approved to treat influenza infection in adults on December 19, 2014. Peramivir is the first neuraminidase inhibitor approved in the IV form. Peramivir is a neuraminidase inhibitor and should not be administered if the patient has a severe allergy to oseltamivir, zanamivir, or one of their metabolite components.[142] Resistance patterns are perpetually changing, and for the most up-to-date information regarding resistance patterns, see the CDC website at www.cdc.gov/flu/professionals/antivirals/.

Ribavirin is a synthetic nucleoside analog licensed for use in aerosol form for treatment of persons with severe RSV

TABLE 55.5 Antiviral Agents Used in Viral Pneumonia

Agent	Indication	Route	Side Effects
Acyclovir	HSV, varicella Prophylaxis/treatment	IV, PO	Phlebitis, seizures, leukopenia, renal dysfunction
Valacyclovir	HSV, varicella Prophylaxis/treatment	PO	Bone marrow suppression, renal failure
Ganciclovir	CMV in immunocompromised host Prophylaxis/treatment	IV, PO	Renal failure, bone marrow suppression, seizure
Valganciclovir	CMV prophylaxis	PO	Same as ganciclovir
Amantadine	Influenza A Prophylaxis/treatment	PO	Nausea, dizziness, ataxia, diarrhea
Rimantadine	Influenza A Prophylaxis	PO	Similar to amantadine
Zanamivir	Influenza A and B Treatment, prophylaxis under study	Diskhaler	Bronchospasm
Oseltamivir	Influenza A and B Prophylaxis/treatment	PO	Nausea, vomiting, vertigo
Peramivir	Influenza A and limited B treatment	IV	Stevens-Johnson syndrome, erythema multiforme, neuropsych events, and diarrhea
RSV-IVIG	RSV prophylaxis (high-risk population)	IV	Allergic, fluid overload, not approved for CCHD
Palivizumab	RSV prophylaxis	IM	Anaphylaxis
Ribavirin	RSV (parainfluenza, influenza A and B, measles)	Small-particle aerosol	Conjunctival edema
Foscarnet	CMV retinitis, HSV resistant to acyclovir	IV	Renal dysfunction, nausea, bone marrow suppression
Pieconaril (under investigation)	Enterovirus and rhinovirus Prophylaxis/treatment	PO	Under investigation

CCHD, cyanotic congenital heart disease; *CMV,* cytomegalovirus; *HSV,* herpes simplex virus; *IVIG,* intravenous immunoglobulin; *RSV,* respiratory syncytial virus.

infection. This therapy may shorten the course of the illness and improve oxygenation in high-risk patients. A few children with severe combined immune deficiency have been treated with ribavirin with resulting clinical improvement and decrease in viral shedding.[65,143-153] Ribavirin aerosol may be effective in shortening the course of both influenza type A and B in infections in college students, and it is possible that parainfluenza and the measles virus can be treated with ribavirin.[154] Various case reports of treatment in seriously ill adults with complicated viral infections suggest that ribavirin may be an effective treatment. Overall, the documented therapeutic benefit of antiviral agents has been inconclusive. Improvement is most apparent when the therapy was initiated early after the onset of infection. Future investigations are necessary to define the optimum dose/route of antiviral agents for each respiratory virus/pneumonia and to clarify the ability of antiviral therapy to modify serious lower respiratory tract infection in high-risk infants and children.

In persons with varicella or zoster, acyclovir reduces the period of viral shedding and the time needed to heal skin lesions, and it can prevent dissemination of localized zoster in immunocompromised children. Thus the use of acyclovir in immunosuppressed patients can be justified by the low toxicity of the drug and potential severity of the illness. Ganciclovir (DHPG) is an antiviral drug with significant activity against cytomegalovirus.[155] It has been used successfully in immunocompromised patients with disseminated cytomegalovirus and

pneumonia.[156] Symptomatic infection of the lower airway with herpes viruses is rare. When it occurs, it usually does so in an immunosuppressed child. Antiviral therapy for herpes viruses includes acyclovir, foscarnet, and adenine arabinoside.[157,158]

Fungal Pneumonitis

Fungal infections are becoming increasingly important in the differential diagnosis of pulmonary infections, particularly in immunocompromised hosts. The majority of pulmonary mycotic infections occur in two microbiologic and clinical groups (Box 55.3). In general, different patient groups are at risk for infection because of either opportunistic or pathogenic dimorphic pulmonary fungi. Primary pulmonary mycotic infections generally infect healthy children exposed to the pathogen in a particular geographic or environmental setting, whereas the opportunistic mycoses occur in children whose immunity is compromised.[159,160] The increase in opportunistic fungal infections can be attributed to numerous factors, including the following:

1. Selection of fungal organisms as flora by the use of broad-spectrum antibiotics
2. Leukopenia secondary to use of cytotoxic agents
3. Suppression of humoral and cell-mediated immunity by cytotoxic and suppressive therapy
4. Increased use of immunosuppressive drugs in patients with organ transplant or collagen vascular disease

BOX 55.3   Major Pulmonary Mycoses

Primary (Endemic; Pathogenic to Normal Children)
Dimorphic Soil
- Histoplasmosis
- Blastomycosis
- Coccidioidomycosis
- Paracoccidioidomycosis
- Sporotrichosis

Nondimorphic Soil
- Cryptococcosis

Opportunistic (Ubiquitous; Abnormal Host)
- Aspergillosis
- Mucormycosis
- Candidiasis

5. An increasing number of patients with AIDS
6. An increased number of invasive surgical procedures in hospitalized children, which create portals of entry for fungi[19]

Primary Pulmonary Fungi

Fungi that cause primary pulmonary infection in otherwise healthy hosts are generally endemic mycoses found in a particular geographic distribution. The four major mycoses in this group are histoplasmosis, blastomycosis, coccidiomycosis, and paracoccidiomycosis.[161] Chemiluminescent DNA probes are available for identification of blastomycosis, coccidioidomycosis, and histoplasmosis. We review these primary pulmonary mycoses in the following section but exclude paracoccidiomycosis because this infection occurs primarily in South America, Central America, and Mexico. For information regarding paracoccidiomycosis infections, please refer to up-to-date journal articles.

Pathogenesis

The dimorphic fungi cause infection following inhalation of spores (conidia) into the pulmonary system. In the lower respiratory tract the conidia transform into the yeast phase, which is susceptible to phagocytosis by the pulmonary macrophages. These yeast forms may persist in the nonimmune host. As the yeast-laden macrophages are transported via the lymphatics to the peribronchial and mediastinal lymph nodes, hematogenous dissemination may occur. However, with the primary pulmonary infection in the immunocompetent host, extrapulmonary infection is rare.

Progressive primary pulmonary infection in the absence of host defenses (such as in a patient who is immunocompromised or an infant) may lead to seeding of extrapulmonary sites, dissemination, and death if left untreated. Cellular immunity is the primary host defense against these deep mycoses, many of which are subclinical and require no therapy. However, children with severe life-threatening infections should be treated (Table 55.6).

Histoplasmosis

Histoplasmosis is caused by *Histoplasma capsulatum,* which is endemic in the east-central United States, particularly the Mississippi and Ohio River valleys. Primary pulmonary histoplasmosis is asymptomatic in more than 50% of patients.

Patients usually become ill 2 weeks following exposure, manifesting influenza-like illness with fever, chills, myalgia, headache, and a nonproductive cough. Occasionally children have a skin rash, arthritis, and erythema nodosum.

The chest radiograph may show patchy areas of pneumonitis and prominent hilar adenopathy. After exposure to an usually heavy inoculum, a more diffuse pulmonary involvement may occur with extensive nodular infiltrates. Children with this condition frequently have significant dyspnea and may progress to respiratory failure. The chest radiograph frequently returns to normal after a primary pulmonary infection; however, a number of residual abnormalities may be seen, including multiple nodules with a dense core of calcium (a target lesion), scattered calcifications within lymph nodes, and occasionally small "buckshot" calcifications scattered throughout both lung fields.[161]

Diagnosis

The skin test is of epidemiologic value but is useless in individual case diagnosis because a positive test only indicates prior exposure to this disease. Neither are direct smears of the sputum helpful for diagnosis. Most cases are recognized by serologic studies and include immunodiffusion (M and H bands) and complement fixation. Unfortunately, the immune diffusion test is relatively insensitive, and a response may be delayed following a primary infection. The complement fixation test is more sensitive but less specific.[162] A titer of 1:32 or higher against the yeast antigen is diagnostic if the clinical picture suggests histoplasmosis. Children with rapidly progressive pneumonia that is not responding to antibacterial antibiotic therapy or those in impending respiratory failure need urgent diagnosis, and invasive procedures such as BAL, diagnostic lung aspiration, or open lung biopsy are necessary to obtain the required information.

Complications

Disseminated histoplasmosis refers to progressive extrapulmonary infection that occurs most frequently in children younger than 2 years and in patients with altered cellular immunity.[17,163] The clinical features of disseminated disease include fever, weight loss, hepatosplenomegaly, cough, diarrhea, gastrointestinal ulcers, and skin lesions. Anemia, leukopenia, and thrombocytopenia may occur as a result of bone marrow involvement in young children and may lead to rapid death. Chronic disseminated disease, which is uncommon and insidious, may present as a nonspecific afebrile illness without cough or radiographic abnormalities. Occasionally, disseminated histoplasmosis presents as a localized infection involving the CNS. Chorioretinitis and pleural effusion, along with isolated gastrointestinal findings involving terminal ileum, can occur.

Treatment

The usual primary pulmonary infection requires no treatment. Amphotericin B should be used for persons with a severe infection, especially if it is life threatening or associated with respiratory failure. Upon clinical improvement, itraconazole should be given to complete the course of therapy. Chronic cavitary histoplasmosis can be treated with IV amphotericin B or a long-term course of oral itraconazole or ketoconazole. Pericarditis therapy should include antiinflammatory agents such as indomethacin or aspirin. Failure of

TABLE 55.6 Antifungal Therapy

Drug	Indications	Route	Side Effects
AmB	All life-threatening mycoses, empiric therapy in febrile granulocytopenic patients	IV	Fever, chills, nephrotoxicity, anemia, hypokalemia, thrombophlebitis
AmB lipid complex, AmB cholesteryl sulfate, AmB liposomal	Failure or intolerance to AmB, organ transplantation with renal insufficiency	IV	Same as AmB with decreased nephrotoxicity and infusion-related adverse events
Flucytosine (5-FC)	With AmB for life-threatening infections with *Cryptococcus, Candida* (central nervous system, ophthalmitis, disseminated, renal) or invasive disease refractory to AmB	PO	Neutropenia with elevated serum levels (if levels are not available, this agent should not be used)
Ketoconazole	Not indicated for acute treatment of severe invasive disease; alternative for mild blastomycosis, histoplasmosis, *Candida,* or coccidiomycosis	PO	Nausea, vomiting, hepatotoxicity, testosterone synthesis blockade
Miconazole	Deep infection: *Pseudallescheria* and *Scedosporium*	IV	Cardiac dysrhythmias, cardiovascular collapse with rapid infusion
Fluconazole	*Cryptococcus, Candida* (question in critically ill), coccidiomycosis	PO	Nausea, vomiting, dizziness
Itraconazole	Non–life-threatening blastomycosis, sporotrichosis, histoplasmosis, paracoccidioidomycosis	PO	Pediatric dosage not yet established; nausea, hypokalemia, edema, hypertension, adrenal insufficiency, epigastric pain
Voriconazole	*Aspergillus* and *Cryptococcus,* resistant *Candida* spp.	IV	Visual changes, fever, nausea, vomiting, elevated liver enzymes
Caspofungin	Treatment for resistant *Aspergillus* and possible combination therapy for *Candida* and endemic mycoses	IV	Fever, phlebitis, nausea, headache, elevated liver enzymes
Mycamine	*Candida*	IV	Fever, nausea, vomiting, hemolysis, elevated liver enzymes
Posaconazole	*Candida* *Aspergillus* *Zygomycetes*	PO	Fever, headache, prolonged QT, elevated liver enzymes, renal impairment, increased midazolam levels if used together

AmB, amphotericin B.

pericarditis to improve with nonsteroidal antiinflammatory medication should not prevent use of a brief course of steroids because steroid use does not appear to predispose to dissemination.[164-168]

Blastomycosis

Blastomycosis is endemic to the southeastern region of the United States but extends northward along the western shores of Lake Michigan across to northern Wisconsin and Minnesota and into Canada. An intimate exposure to an infected site is required for infection rather than the casual exposure often found with histoplasmosis and coccidioidomycosis.[169-171] Most pediatric cases of blastomycosis occur in older children and adolescents in rural areas.

The pathophysiology is similar to that of histoplasmosis. The clinical course of primary pulmonary blastomycosis is variable. The symptoms are similar to those of acute bacterial pneumonia and include high fever, cough with productive purulent sputum, occasional pleuritic chest pain, and myalgias. Such symptoms generally last 2 to 3 weeks.

The chest radiograph frequently demonstrates patchy areas of alveolar consolidation affecting one or both lower lobes. Pleural effusions and cavitation can occur but are unusual. A rather dense lobar infiltrate similar to pneumococcal pneumonia is uncommon but occurs more frequently in

pulmonary blastomycosis than with other pulmonary fungi. Clearing of the chest x-ray film may take 3 to 4 months.

Blastomycosis is not always self-limited, and progressive pulmonary infection can occur with acute dissemination to distant sites. In such instances the child remains febrile and toxic with rather rapid progression. Diffuse pulmonary involvement with acute miliary spread can lead to rapid respiratory failure and radiographic findings of ARDS.

Children may have asymptomatic primary pulmonary blastomycosis that is diagnosed only with reactivation blastomycosis involving the skin, bones, or other distant organ sites. Reactivation blastomycosis appears to be most common in the first 1 or 2 years immediately after the initial pulmonary infection and probably occurs in less than 5% of all infected patients. A chronic form of pulmonary blastomycosis may occur in patients who have no significant history of acute pneumonia but present with respiratory symptoms that have persisted for weeks or months. These persons have a chronic cough, productive sputum, nocturnal fevers, night sweats, weight loss, and dyspnea. Chest radiographs in persons with chronic blastomycosis may reveal a single large mass, often perihilar in location. A more common finding is a fibronodular infiltrate with small cavities and fibrosis radiating toward the hila. Such findings mimic tuberculosis.

Diagnosis

No reliable skin test exists for pulmonary blastomycosis. Sputum and material aspirated from BAL, lung aspiration, skin, or bone lesions may be examined directly after potassium hydroxide digestion, and the pathognomonic yeast forms are identified. Such positive direct smears provide a rapid, accurate, inexpensive test. Serologic tests include immunodiffusion using purified antigen. The complement fixation test is less sensitive and less specific than the immunodiffusion test.[172] Most acute cases are diagnosed by direct sputum smears or from BAL.

Complications

Patients whose illnesses are clinically similar to bacterial pneumonia frequently have a self-limited process. Life-threatening progressive respiratory failure similar to ARDS can occur. In such instances, diagnosis and therapy including mechanical ventilation must be initiated promptly. Dissemination occurs only in the most severe cases.[173,174] With dissemination, characteristic skin lesions (ie, raised and crusted) may occur on the face and upper extremities. In persons with disseminated disease, bone involvement often includes the spine, ribs, and skull.

Treatment

Acute pulmonary blastomycosis does not require treatment in all cases. Treatment with IV amphotericin should be given if the patient is severely ill or if progressive illness occurs. Oral itraconazole and ketoconazole have been used for treatment of chronic pulmonary blastomycosis (similar to tuberculosis) but should not be used for severe life-threatening infections.[175,176]

Coccidioidomycosis

Coccidioidomycosis is a relatively common infection that occurs primarily in the southwestern United States. Sixty percent of patients with primary pulmonary infection have no symptoms or minimal symptoms. Children 5 years or younger have a higher frequency of progressive disease than do older children and healthy adults. The clinical course of coccidioidomycosis is a flulike illness usually associated with fever, cough, and chest pain. There may be a transient maculopapular eruption similar to erythema nodosum in children. Radiographic abnormalities range from hilar adenopathy to patchy infiltrates with pleural effusion.

Diagnosis

Diagnostic studies include skin testing, which has some usefulness if the patient has compatible respiratory illness and a past negative skin test. Direct smears of potassium hydroxide–digested sputum are helpful if characteristic spherules are found. Antibody detection through complement fixation may be a useful measure of severity of disease.[174] In cases of suspected coccidioidal meningitis, complement fixation tests on cerebrospinal fluid should be obtained because many patients have a negative spinal fluid culture with positive complement fixation studies. Use of chemiluminescent DNA probes may aid in rapid diagnosis.

Complications

Complications include chronic progressive coccidioidal pneumonia, which is similar to tuberculosis but uncommon in pediatric patients. Disseminated coccidioidomycosis does occur and is often accompanied by persistent fever and rapid progression with development of meningitis, bony lesions, and skin and soft tissue disease. A fulminant primary miliary spread of disease with severe respiratory failure and diffuse lung involvement has been observed in patients with altered immune status. The disseminated disease frequently has an insidious onset, following the primary pulmonary infection by weeks. The meninges are the most worrisome site of extrapulmonary involvement because coccidioidal meningitis requires intrathecal amphotericin B therapy, and cure is unlikely.[177,178]

Treatment

If the infection causes prolonged fever, progressive pulmonary disease, significant mediastinal adenopathy, or disseminated lesions, antifungal therapy with amphotericin B should be initiated. Ketoconazole has been used in skeletal, cutaneous, and other localized infection but not for meningitis. Coccidiomeningitis is the most difficult complication of this disease to treat; it requires intrathecal and systemic therapy with amphotericin B.[179-181]

Opportunistic Pulmonary Mycoses
Pulmonary Aspergillosis

Invasive pulmonary aspergillosis occurs almost exclusively in immunocompromised patients.[15,182-185] Despite treatment, unless the underlying immune defect is ameliorated, invasive pulmonary aspergillosis is often fatal. Many cases are nosocomially acquired, usually in hospitals undergoing renovation or new construction.[171] Children with hematologic malignancies (eg, myelogenous and lymphocytic leukemia) or organ transplantation are at the highest risk for development of invasive disease, presumably because of the abnormal immune cells and the cyclic neutropenia induced by repeated doses of chemotherapy. Persons with heart and bone marrow transplants are at higher risk for aspergillosis infection than are persons with kidney transplants.

Neutropenia is an important risk factor for the development of aspergillosis because both the absolute neutrophil count and the duration of neutropenia have been related to the incidence of infection. Use of steroids and immunosuppressive drugs also appears to predispose to invasive aspergillosis.[186] Immune and myelosuppressed patients exposed to heavy aerosol concentrations of aspergillosis spores have an increased chance of the development of invasive pneumonia. Efforts should be made to eliminate the risk of airborne conidiospores in patient areas. If such elimination is not possible, then susceptible patients should be moved away from areas of excavation or construction.

Clinical signs of invasive aspergillosis are nonspecific. The usual presentation includes pulmonary infiltrates and fever that do not respond to empiric antibacterial therapy. Patients may exhibit dyspnea, a nonproductive cough, pleuritic chest pain, and pleural friction rubs. Symptoms are usually difficult to identify in small children, and auscultatory changes are typically found only with advanced disease. Hemoptysis is uncommon in children.

Diagnosis

Radiographs of the chest reveal virtually any infiltrative pattern, including patchy infiltrates, necrotizing pneumonitis, miliary nodules, and lung abscesses. Early findings may include a round, patchy pneumonia that progresses to a wedge-shaped density characteristic of pulmonary infarctions.[187] Definitive diagnosis of invasive pulmonary aspergillosis requires histopathologic identification of fungus in tissue specimens. Positive sputum cultures do not prove the presence of invasive disease even in compromised hosts, although isolation should be taken seriously and multiple positive cultures should be considered strong evidence of fungal infection in patients whose immunity is compromised. Serologic antibody tests have no value in the diagnosis of invasive aspergillosis. In severely ill children, fiberoptic bronchoscopy with bronchial lavage is the initial diagnostic test of choice in patients with suspected pneumonitis. If the results of fiberoptic bronchoscopy are nondiagnostic, a lung biopsy (open or needle) may be required, though not often done. Enzyme immunoassay detecting galactomannan antigen, a constituent of the *Aspergillus* cell wall, may aid in the diagnosis. Sensitivity and specificity of this test depends on many factors.[188] This assay may be run on blood or BAL specimens, and this along with cultures and CT findings may aid in the diagnosis of aspergillosis without requiring a biopsy specimen.

Complications

Untreated invasive pulmonary aspergillosis is usually fatal in immunocompromised patients. Fatality rates greater than 80% are reported; however, survival may improve if appropriate therapy is initiated early in the disease. Death usually results from progressive pneumonitis, pulmonary infarction, and massive hemoptysis. On rare occasions, endocarditis, osteomyelitis, meningitis, or infection of the eye or orbit occurs.

Treatment

Therapy with amphotericin B should be initiated early in the course of the disease. Surgical resection is usually not indicated in the treatment of critically ill patients with uncontrolled disease. However, it may be considered in patients who have only partial response to antifungal therapy or with relapsing disease in a well-defined lung segment or in those identified with massive hemoptysis. In critically ill patients who are unresponsive to therapy or in whom aspergillosis develops while they are receiving amphotericin B, the addition of flucytosine or rifampin may be helpful. Use of the lipid formulations of amphotericin is indicated in patients who are intolerant of or refractory to conventional amphotericin for reasons such as renal toxicity or persistent infusion-related adverse events. Itraconazole is an option for use after an initial course of amphotericin B. Change from amphotericin to the oral itraconazole must take into account the patient's status.[189-190] New antifungal agents such as voriconazole and micafungin have shown effectiveness in treating aspergillosis.[191-193]

Pulmonary Candidiasis

Of all the opportunistic pulmonary mycoses, candidiasis may be the most difficult to diagnosis and treat effectively because the *Candida* organism routinely colonizes the upper respiratory tract, resulting in positive cultures without significant disease. The prevalence of *Candida pneumonitis* has increased remarkably in the past 3 decades as a result of the increased use of broad-spectrum antibiotic therapy, immunosuppressive drugs, indwelling vascular lines, prosthetic devices, and organ transplantation.

Pathogenesis

Pulmonary candidiasis may occur by hematogenous seeding of the lung parenchyma from a distal infected site or through direct invasion of inhaled or aspirated organisms. *Candida* acquired through the hematogenous route demonstrates pulmonary lesions that are diffuse, bilateral, and miliary. The endobronchial form of infection does not have a significant interstitial component such as that seen with a hematogenous form. The endobronchial form radiographically demonstrates pulmonary lesions that are small, asymmetrical, patchy, and frequently found in the lower lobes.

Diagnosis

There are no pathognomonic signs and symptoms of pulmonary candidiasis. The diagnosis should be considered in an immunocompromised febrile patient with a pulmonary lesion, particularly if broad-spectrum antibiotics were used without a response. Oral pharyngeal involvement (thrush) indicates that the patient is harboring the organism in an invasive stage. Retinal lesions on ophthalmoscopic examination may help identify invasive *Candida*. A cutaneous lesion often seen in persons with invasive *Candida* is a discrete erythematous papule with an erythematous halo. The radiographic findings of *Candida* pneumonia are nonspecific. Early in the course of infection, patients have normal chest radiographs. The isolation of *Candida* in culture from an otherwise sterile body fluid or tissue and the identification of the organism in a biopsy specimen are diagnostic of invasive *Candida*. Serologic studies are of no diagnostic value. Proof of *Candida* pneumonia requires tissue examination or evaluation of alveolar lavage or protected brush samples from bronchoscopy as direct evidence of tissue invasion. If these studies fail to identify the disease process, the diagnosis of pulmonary candidiasis may be established with a lung biopsy.

Complications

As with other mycoses, pulmonary candidiasis may be complicated by systemic dissemination affecting other organs. Concomitant infection with other organisms, particularly bacteria, is not uncommon.

Treatment

Effective treatment includes correction of the patient's immunosuppression in addition to administration of amphotericin B. The concomitant and synergistic effect of flucytosine has been demonstrated with amphotericin B for most *Candida* species and is recommended for use in critically ill patients.

Pneumocystis carinii Pneumonia

Pneumocystis carinii, which is probably a protozoan, produces a unique infection. In the early stages of the infection with cysts, trophozoites are found distributed within the alveoli, most commonly adjacent to the alveolar septum. Usually in this phase, no clinical signs or symptoms are evident. With extension of infection, the number of organisms increases and bilateral diffuse distribution occurs throughout the lungs. Eventually desquamation of the alveolar septal cells occurs, with subsequent phagocytosis of the organisms by the alveolar macrophages. Minimal inflammation occurs in discrete areas of the alveolar septum at this stage of the disease, and a child may or may not be symptomatic. Ultimately the alveolar septum becomes thickened with inflammatory cells producing the clinical manifestations of childhood pneumocystosis.[194] In the infantile form there is extensive involvement of alveolar septa with plasma cell and lymphocyte infiltration. The normal septal thickness may be increased 5 to 20 times, which results in occupation of much of the alveolus by the distended septum.

Clinical Features

The three forms of disease patterns in pneumocystosis are the childhood/adult form, the infantile form, and a more chronic fibrosing form observed in some HIV-infected patients.[195] The typical child/adult type of pneumocystosis occurs in children beyond infancy who have congenital or acquired immunodeficiency disorders or malignancies and in organ transplant recipients.[196-198] Clinical symptoms of pneumonitis include fever, cough, tachypnea, cyanosis, flaring of the nasal ala, and retractions. Chest auscultation usually reveals no adventitious sounds until the terminal stage of infection, at which time bilateral crackles may be present. The chest roentgenogram initially may be normal, and changes may be seen only late in the course of the disease.[199]

In the infantile form of pneumocystosis, symptoms often begin insidiously and presentations include poor feeding, failure to thrive, and diarrhea. Increasing tachypnea may be detected, with respiratory rates frequently in the range of 80 to 120 breaths per minute. A dry, nonproductive cough with increased retractions and flaring of the nasal alae becomes prominent. Diffuse crackles may be heard bilaterally on auscultation of the chest, and most infants remain afebrile. The clinical course in neonates and infants may be quite rapid, with progressive cyanosis and death resulting from respiratory failure within days. More commonly, however, the course extends over a period of several weeks, with a mortality rate varying from 20% to 50% without treatment.[198,200]

The chronic fibrosing type of *Pneumocystis* pneumonia identified in patients with HIV is associated with the presence of long-standing symptoms, localized radiologic changes, and interstitial fibrosis.[195]

Diagnosis

A definitive diagnosis requires documentation of *P. carinii* in lung tissue. The standard surgical open lung biopsy provides histologic details; however, the necessity for general anesthesia presents additional risk, particularly in the critically ill child. Identification of the organism in sputum is sufficient for the diagnosis, but inducing and obtaining sputum in young children are often difficult; in such cases, bronchoscopy should be considered.[201] Fiberoptic bronchoscopy with BAL, although not achieving yields as high as open lung biopsy, offers a useful and safe alternative to open lung biopsy.[9,10,29] Transthoracic percutaneous needle aspirate and thoracoscopy have been used successfully and can be obtained without the use of a general anesthetic.[202,203] However, pneumothorax can be expected in up to 30% of children. Once a specimen is obtained, it can be stained with one of the array of preparations by which the organism can be confidently identified. PCR techniques amplifying *P. carinii* DNA have been shown to be sensitive, and specific detection methods can be applied to BAL samples, sputum, and nasopharyngeal aspirates with success.[204] Serum lactate dehydrogenase is usually elevated in patients with *P. carinii* pneumonia and appears to be related to the degree of lung injury.[205] The chest radiograph often may be normal early in the course of *P. carinii* pneumonia. However, as the disease progresses, the pattern demonstrates a diffuse bilateral alveolar disease process with hyperinflation and eventually development of air bronchograms. The bilateral densities are frequently more intense in the middle and lower lung fields. Only late in the course of disease do the upper lung fields become involved. Atypical lesions have been reported, including pneumonitis limited to lobar areas. Pneumatoceles and pleural effusions have been reported.[206]

Complications

P. carinii usually remains localized to the lungs, even with extensive disease. A disseminated form has been documented, with recovery of the organism from extrapulmonary sites including bone marrow, liver, and spleen. Life-threatening complications that can arise in patients with *P. carinii* pneumonitis include pneumothorax and pneumomediastinum. Pneumothorax, both spontaneous and iatrogenic, occurs frequently in patients with *P. carinii* pneumonitis. Some evidence indicates that upper lobe predominance of pneumothorax may be more frequent in those previously treated with inhaled pentamidine. Pneumomediastinum, with associated respiratory failure, may be noted in patients receiving assisted ventilation.

Treatment

Therapy for *P. carinii* should include specific anti-*Pneumocystis* chemotherapy, inhibition of the pulmonary inflammatory response, and enhancement of the immunologic status of the patient.[207-212] Several drugs have been used for treatment of pneumocystosis (Table 55.7).

Trimethoprim-sulfamethoxazole may be administered either orally or intravenously and is the drug of choice for treatment of this disease.[3,180] The second most widely used drug for treatment of *P. carinii* pneumonitis is pentamidine isethionate.[211,212] Its effectiveness has been well documented over several years, but it has an increased number of undesirable adverse effects and treatment failures compared with trimethoprim-sulfamethoxazole.[197] Secondary to the prevalence of sulfa allergy and therefore a need for an alternative

TABLE 55.7	*Pneumocystis Carinii* Pneumonitis Therapy		
Drug	**Route**	**Duration of Therapy (Days)**	**Comments**
TMP-SMX	IV/PO	21	DOC
Pentamidine isethionate	IV	21	DOC
TMP dapsone	PO	21	Alternative
Trimetrexate folinic acid	IV	21	Alternative
Clindamycin primaquine	PO	21	Alternative
Atovaquone	PO	21	Alternative
Prednisone	IV/PO	21	Adjunctive agent

DOC, drug of choice; *IV*, intravenous; *PO*, by mouth; *TMP-SMX*, trimethoprim-sulfamethoxazole.

therapy for *P. carinii*, pneumonitis studies continue to find new medication regimens and new medications that may be used as alternatives to trimethoprim-sulfamethoxazole. They all have their own side effect profile and their own risk benefit profile.[213-215] Administration of a corticosteroid such as prednisone should occur at the initiation of specific anti-*Pneumocystis* therapy to improve survival and attenuate or prevent the initial decline in oxygenation. In addition to the specific therapies, efforts should be made to reverse the immune dysfunction that allowed occurrence of *P. carinii* (ie, reduce or discontinue immunosuppressive medications).

Chemical Pneumonitis

A large number of chemical and physical agents may produce intense inflammation of the lower respiratory tract in children. Chemical pneumonitis and/or pneumonia may be acquired in several different ways, such as by aspiration, inhalation, ingestion, or injection.

Aspiration Pneumonia

Aspiration pneumonia is composed of a diverse group of disorders that have in common the soiling of the lower respiratory tract by foreign, nongaseous substances. For purposes of this chapter, neither the solid foreign body nor the infectious component of aspiration is discussed.

Gastroesophageal reflux (GER) has been defined as the retrograde passage of stomach contents into the esophagus. This condition may be asymptomatic or associated with significant regurgitation and vomiting, esophagitis, failure to thrive, and anemia.[216] Aspiration into the pulmonary tree can cause significant complications including apnea, pulmonary fibrosis, severe necrotizing pneumonias, recurrent bronchospasm, and death. Diminished lower esophageal sphincter pressure is often the result of physiologic immaturity; hence GER is more frequent in younger infants. This disorder also occurs in older children, especially those with central nervous and neuromuscular dysfunction. Other high-risk pediatric populations include patients with congenital abnormalities of the tracheal-bronchial tree and those with severe chronic pulmonary disease (Box 55.4).

Pathophysiology

The association of GER and lung disease has been well documented; however, the actual cause and effect of the relationship has not been firmly established. Massive aspiration of gastric fluid produces direct injury to the mucosal surface of the respiratory tract, resulting in diffuse alveolar damage, hemorrhage, and necrotizing bronchiolitis. This may be followed by a rapid interstitial reaction, resulting in an acute inflammatory polymorphonuclear cell infiltration involving the interalveolar septa. Bronchiolitis obliterans and fibrosis can occur. In severe instances the initial onset of disease closely resembles that of ARDS with similar outcomes. Repeated aspiration of small amounts of gastric contents may lead to recurrent pneumonia, airway hyperreactivity, bronchitis, and bronchiectasis with eventual fibrosis and involvement of the pulmonary interstitium.

Clinical Findings

Clinical symptoms of GER vary with age.[216,217] In older children, heartburn, acid/bitter taste, retrosternal pain, or

---

| **BOX 55.4** | Pulmonary Aspiration and Gastroesophageal Reflux: Associated Disorders |

Associated Disorders
- Bronchopulmonary dysplasia
- Asthma
- Cystic fibrosis
- Infantile apnea

Central Nervous System
- Convulsive disorders
- Anoxic encephalopathy
- Neurologic impairment
- Myopathies

Congenital Malformations
- Tracheoesophageal fistula
- Hiatal hernia

General
- Failure to thrive
- Achalasia
- Cardiopulmonary resuscitation
- Emergency surgery

---

abdominal pain may be reported. Infants may be irritable and exhibit stridor, poor sleeping patterns, or intermittent apnea. Esophagitis can lead to microcytic anemia because of repeated episodes of gastrointestinal blood loss. Chronic respiratory symptoms may include coughing, wheezing with choking episodes occasionally resulting in apnea, or life-threatening events similar to those seen in infants with sudden infant death syndrome. In the hospitalized pediatric patient, significant aspirations may occur during or after general anesthesia. Severe aspiration may be seen in patients receiving tube feedings as a result of displacement of the feeding catheter.

Findings on a chest radiograph may vary from slight hyperinflation to a pattern of diffuse interstitial and alveolar densities. In mild cases a picture of bilateral diffuse infiltrates compatible with ARDS may be seen. Although a barium esophagogram can help to evaluate esophageal motility and detect esophagitis, it reflects only a single point in time. Therefore a negative study does not rule out the presence of GER. Radionuclide scans permit observation of esophageal function following administration of a radioactive tracer. Thus the frequency and severity of reflux and information on esophageal and gastric dysmotility may be obtained. If delayed aspiration occurs, the radionuclide may be observed in the lung fields on a delayed scan.[217] Esophageal motility and intraluminal pressures may be measured by esophageal manometry. Intraesophageal pH measurement is helpful in that it allows long-term monitoring of acid reflux by detecting frequency, duration, and intensity of reflux.[218,219] Esophagoscopy is also useful for assessing the extent of mucosal injury by allowing direct visualization and obtaining a mucosal biopsy. Use of BAL for assessment of lipid-laden macrophages has been useful in establishing or corroborating the diagnosis of aspiration in complex patients.[218,219]

Treatment

Treatment of patients with GER frequently includes placing the patient in an upright prone position and using thickened feedings. Use of antacid preparations, omeprazole, cimetidine, ranitidine, and other inhibitors of H_2 gastroreceptors may be helpful in decreasing acid production and neutralizing its effects on the esophageal mucosa. Omeprazole has on rare occasions been associated with electrolyte disturbances. It has also been reported to possibly result in atrophic gastritis with prolonged use, but its use continues to increase despite these possible adverse effects.[220-224] Metoclopramide is used before meals to help improve lower esophageal function and aid gastric emptying. With the suspension of cisapride from the marketplace as an effective prokinetic agent because of potentially fatal toxicity, interest in erythromycin as a prokinetic agent has resurfaced, and many trials evaluating its dose and efficacy are under way.[225] Bronchodilators are used frequently to treat bronchospasm associated with GER. Because theophylline decreases the lower esophageal sphincter pressure, aerosolized β_2-agonists are preferred. In instances where medical therapy was attempted and failed or in life-threatening situations, antireflux surgery is indicated. In such instances a fundoplication, partial plication, or percutaneous gastrojejunostomy is the appropriate treatment of choice.[216] The most favorable outcome and lowest incidence of morbidity in such instances are achieved when surgery is delayed until the patient is adequately nourished and optimal pulmonary status has been obtained.

Inhalation Injury

Acute inhalation injuries are a leading cause of fatalities in pediatric patients. Smoke inhalation accounts for the largest number of pediatric lives lost to inhalation injury each year. A significant number of inhalation injuries as a result of irritant gases occur through industrial or household accidents.[226,227] Serious pulmonary inhalation injury may be manifested immediately or delayed in onset (Table 55.8).[228-230]

Pathogenesis

Direct injury to the mucosal surface is the most common mode of pulmonary injury. Inhalation of noxious substances may cause extensive physical damage to the lungs and seriously impair subsequent gas exchange. The epithelial cells of air passages may become necrotic and desquamate, causing marked airway obstruction. Bronchospasm caused by irritation from the inhaled gases or particles may lead to further airway obstruction. Severe damage to the basement membrane may occur and cause subsequent leakage of intravascular fluid and blood into the alveolar and interstitial spaces. Injury may occur at all levels of the respiratory tract, depending on the physical and chemical properties of the irritant, the agent concentration, duration of exposure, and breathing pattern of the person exposed.[228,231,232] The clinical course usually has three phases: (1) the acute phase, which occurs within minutes or hours of the insult, resulting in pulmonary edema, hypoxemia, and respiratory failure; (2) the delayed phase, which occurs within the first few days and may include continuing effects of the lung injury such as pulmonary edema, airway obstruction, and superinfection; and (3) the phase in which long-term sequelae may be noted because of the hypoxic or ischemic injury to other organ systems and recurrent pulmonary problems resulting from reactive airways disease or interstitial fibrosis.

Clinical Findings

Clinical manifestations are nonspecific for inhalation of various irritant gases and may differ, depending on the individual child. Injury of the airways may be manifested as upper airway obstruction resulting in laryngotracheitis, bronchitis, and upper airway edema. More peripheral airway obstruction may present with classic findings of asthma and airway edema with hypersecretion. In cases of massive exposure the presenting symptoms may be those associated with acute respiratory distress syndrome, manifested by profound V/Q mismatch, cyanosis, dyspnea, and respiratory failure. Severe nasopharyngeal and laryngeal edema with hypersecretion may present as stridor.[229,231] Chest radiograph findings are nonspecific, ranging from scattered areas of atelectasis and infiltrate to dense bilateral alveolar infiltrates.

Treatment

Prompt physical removal from the offending agent and maintenance of upper airway patency are imperative. Endotracheal intubation is a high-risk procedure, and meticulous attention must be directed toward maintaining proper pulmonary toilet and removal of upper airway secretions and debris from the artificial airway once it is secured.

Oxygenation should be monitored closely. High oxygen concentrations, mechanical ventilation, and use of positive end-expiratory pressure may be necessary in the event of acute respiratory failure because the diminished compliance and formation of pulmonary edema occur rapidly. Use of steroids may be justified in the treatment of patients who have been exposed to oxides of nitrogen; however, use after exposure to other irritant gases has not been validated.

Bronchoscopy may be indicated and useful in assessing the severity of airway injury and as an aid to endotracheal intubation and treatment of major areas of atelectasis. However, use of BAL is usually not indicated except in instances in which significant particulate or carbonaceous material is likely. Humidification of air and oxygen mixtures to thin secretions is necessary, and chest percussion/postural drainage may help to mechanically clear the airways.

Use of prophylactic antibiotics in persons with inhalation injuries is not recommended. If pulmonary infection is

TABLE 55.8	**Irritant Gases**
Agent	**Exposure/Environment**
Direct Mucosal Injury	
Acrolein	Plastic, rubber, textiles
Ammonia	Fertilizer, refrigerants, explosives
Chlorine	Bleaching, disinfectant
Formaldehyde	Disinfectant, paper, photography
Hydrogen chloride	Refining, dye making
Hydrogen fluoride	Etching, petroleum
Nitrogen dioxide	Welding, fertilizer, farming
Phosgene	Insecticide, dyes, chemicals
Sulfur dioxide	Bleaching, refrigeration
Asphyxiation Injury	
Carbon dioxide	Mining, foundry
Carbon monoxide	Smoke, foundry, mining
Natural gas	Mining, petroleum

suspected, prompt therapy with broad-spectrum antimicrobial agents should be started. Use of bronchodilators is advocated because of a high incidence of bronchospasm. No critical studies have evaluated this therapy in persons with an inhalation injury; however, the risk associated with its use is low, and administration to the child with obvious airflow obstruction is warranted. Use of aerosolized β_2-agonists is preferred. Special attention is required in the presence of smoke inhalation with regard to treatment of carbon monoxide poisoning. Hyperbaric oxygen, if available, or sustained administration of 100% oxygen is recommended in the initial treatment of patients with significant carbon monoxide intoxication. Development of upper or lower airway edema may necessitate intubation and mechanical ventilatory support.[228,232,233] Administration of artificial surfactant may be beneficial in patients in whom ARDS develops.[233] Use of prophylactic steroids and antibiotics for persons affected by smoke inhalation is not recommended, especially if burn injuries are present, because complications are more frequent.

Prognosis

The prognosis of children with acute pulmonary injury produced by inhalation of toxic gases is generally good. Restrictive and obstructive pulmonary function abnormalities have been observed following recovery. Residual defects such as bronchiolitis obliterans, bronchiectasis, and reactive airways disease have been observed following smoke inhalation.

Ingestion/Injection of Pharmacologic Agents

Several chemotherapeutic agents and other commonly used drugs have potentially serious pulmonary toxicity (Box 55.5).

BOX 55.5   Pharmacologic Agents Associated With Pulmonary Toxicity

Cytotoxic Agents
Antibiotics
- Bleomycin: IP/PF, H, PEFF
- Mitomycin C: IP/PF, PE, PEFF

Alkylating Agents
- Cyclophosphamide: IP/PF, PE, B
- Chlorambucil: IP/PF
- Melphalan: IP/PF

Antimetabolites
- Methotrexate: IP/PF, PE, H, PEFF
- Azathioprine: IP/PF
- G-mercaptopurine: IP/PF
- Cytosine arabinoside: IP/PF, PE
- Nitrosoureas
- Carmustine: PF

Noncytotoxic Agents
- Amiodarone: IP/PF
- Carbamazepine: H, B
- Gold salts: IP/PF, H
- Nitrofurantoin: AH, PEFF, H, B, IP/PF
- Diphenylhydantoin: H
- Sulfasalazine: H, FA, BO, B
- Penicillamine: DA, AH, H, BO

AH, alveolar hemorrhage; *B*, bronchospasm; *BO*, bronchiolitis obliterans; *DA*, diffuse alveolitis; *FA*, fibrosing alveolitis; *H*, hypersensitivity lung reaction; *IP*, interstitial pneumonitis; *PE*, pulmonary edema; *PEFF*, pleural effusion; *PF*, pulmonary fibrosis.

Pulmonary toxicity is thought to be a direct effect in most instances, but immunologic and hypersensitivity mechanisms may also be involved. Toxicity may occur during therapy or after discontinuation of the agent.[234] The development of blebs in the capillary endothelium is followed by an interstitial fibrinous edema and mononuclear cell response with eventual hyaline membrane formation. Some studies have shown a significant decrease in type 1 pneumocytes with evolution of type 2 pneumocytes, septal thickening, and a proliferation of fibrous tissue with a decrease in the number of alveolar septa. Pleural thickening may accompany the pneumonitis.

Diagnosis/Clinical Findings

Characteristic clinical features of drug-induced pulmonary disease include fever, malaise, dyspnea, and a nonproductive cough. Initial radiographic studies may be normal but usually demonstrate a diffuse alveolar and/or interstitial involvement. Pulmonary function studies may be of either an obstructive or restrictive pattern. Hypoxemia enhanced by exercise is an early and clinically important finding because interstitial pneumonitis and pulmonary fibrosis constitute a major portion of drug-induced pulmonary disease. Histologic examination of lung tissue is frequently indicated to confirm the clinical diagnosis and to rule out other potential causes of pneumonitis such as *Pneumocystis*, viral, or fungal infections that often occur in children treated with these agents.

Other complications such as hypersensitivity lung disease, noncardiogenic pulmonary edema, bronchiolitis obliterans, alveolar hemorrhage, and pleural effusion may occur in these patients. Persistent and fatal lung dysfunction may follow drug-induced pulmonary damage. Therapy should be directed at early recognition of the problem, discontinuation of the offending agent, and supportive therapy.

Idiopathic Interstitial Lung Disease

ILD of undetermined etiology is rare in adults but is even more uncommon in children. Histologic classification of the idiopathic type of ILD can be somewhat confusing, and in past years, pediatric classification mirrored the adult classification scheme. As research progressed, some overlap was noted, but it was found that pediatric interstitial lung diseases have features that are unique to pediatrics. Usual interstitial pneumonitis has never been identified in children as the diagnostic fibroblastic foci were not found in any of the cases that had initially been labeled UIP. Other interstitial pneumonias such as desquamative interstitial pneumonitis (DIP) and lymphocytic interstitial pneumonia (LIP) are seen in children but remain quite rare and have some features that are different from their adult counterparts. DIP in children is not associated with smoking, and the histologic picture is one of macrophage being the primary inflammatory cell that fills the alveolus, although histiocytes, lymphocytes, eosinophils, and plasma cells are also present. Hyaline membrane formation is not seen in DIP, and the structural integrity of the alveolar unit is usually maintained. DIP tends to be responsive to steroids.[233] LIP is seen mostly in patients with immune deficiencies and connective tissue disorders. LIP tends to be insidious in onset and appears as a result of infiltration of the interstitium by plasma cells, mature lymphocytes, and histiocytes. Nonspecific interstitial pneumonitis histologically is a mixture of inflammation and fibrosis. This entity has been identified in children. Cryptogenic organizing pneumonia has been identified in children as an isolated phenomenon or with infection, asthma, drug reactions, malignancies undergoing chemotherapy, bone marrow transplantation, and autoimmune disorders. Prognosis is usually excellent, and patients have an excellent response to corticosteroids. Acute interstitial pneumonia is a rapidly progressive disorder with a histologic appearance consistent with the organizing form of diffuse alveolar damage. This diagnosis generally has a poor prognosis. Some interstitial lung diseases that are unique to infancy most likely in the past had been labeled under the aforementioned interstitial lung diseases but truly belong in their own classification scheme. These syndromes are persistent tachypnea of infancy (neuroendocrine cell hyperplasia of infancy), follicular bronchitis, cellular interstitial pneumonitis (pulmonary interstitial glycogenosis), chronic pneumonitis of infancy, and genetic abnormalities of surfactant function.[235] Detailed discussions of these disorders of infancy or the other interstitial lung diseases and their management are beyond the scope of this chapter but can be found in various review articles.[236-241] Patients who do not respond to medical therapy should be considered candidates for lung transplantation.

Pediatric Pulmonary Hemorrhage

Pulmonary hemorrhage (PH) is a potentially life-threatening event that can occur at any age. The clinical presentation varies from massive fatal hemoptysis to silent bleeding with respiratory distress and anemia. Rapid determination of the etiology of the PH and institution of specific therapy are often difficult. This section examines the less common causes of PH. PH resulting from trauma and infection is not discussed.

Definition

PH is defined as extravasation of blood into airways and/or lung parenchyma. Massive PH in adults is defined as blood loss of 600 mL or more in 24 hours.[242-246] In infants, Esterly and Oppenheimer[245] characterized massive PH as the involvement of at least two pulmonary lobes by confluent foci of extravasated erythrocytes. Loss of 10% of a patient's circulating blood volume into the lungs regardless of age causes a significant alteration in cardiorespiratory function and should be considered massive. The diagnosis of PH following an episode of silent bleeding is established by pulmonary hemosiderosis, which is the abnormal accumulation of iron within lung parenchyma and alveolar macrophages.

Pathophysiology

Accumulation of blood in the airways following a significant episode of PH creates multiple problems. These problems include production of a diffusion barrier resulting in hypoxemia and reduction in the diameter of involved airways, which in turn increases airway resistance and may lead to airway obstruction.

Reduction in pulmonary compliance and impairment of ventilation may occur.[246-248] These changes in respiratory function increase both the ventilatory and myocardial work necessary to maintain a normal arterial oxygen tension. Interstitial fibrosis that develops following repeated episodes of PH results in reduced carbon monoxide diffusion and diminished static and dynamic lung compliance.

Etiology

Classification of the etiologies of PH provides a simple framework to proceed with diagnostic and therapeutic interventions (Box 55.6). Diffuse PH is usually associated with less total blood loss and can occur from either immune or nonimmune mechanisms. Diffuse, immune PH typically affects adolescents and, less commonly, school-aged children. Focal PH is commonly responsible for massive PH and carries a mortality rate greater than 50%.[247,249-250] Focal PH typically affects preschool-aged children but may occur in infancy.

Diffuse/Nonimmune Pulmonary Hemorrhage

PH in the neonate occurs in 0.7 to 4 per 1000 live births and is present in 6% to 26.3% of neonates at postmortem examination. Risk factors associated with PH in the neonate include asphyxia, infection/sepsis, CNS injury, weight less than 1500 g and/or small-for-gestational age, male sex, congenital heart disease, idiopathic respiratory distress syndrome, and coagulation disorders.[250,251] Intraalveolar hemorrhage appears to occur more commonly in neonates of older gestational age. Pulmonary hemorrhage in neonates as a primary occurrence is uncommon.[250] Pathogenesis of PH in the neonate is considered to result from the development of persistent pulmonary hypertension with right-to-left intracardiac shunting of blood, resulting from hypoxia and acidosis. Left ventricular failure ensues, causing an increase in pulmonary capillary pressure and subsequent disruption of pulmonary capillary and alveolar membranes. Severe CNS injury may indirectly affect cardiac function, causing increased left ventricular end-diastolic pressure.[252]

Severe hemoptysis and life-threatening PH are rare in the preadolescent child with congenital heart disease. However, a drastic increase in pulmonary capillary pressure in children with pulmonary atresia, unilateral pulmonary venous atresia, total anomalous pulmonary venous drainage, mitral stenosis,

---

BOX 55.6   Causes of Pulmonary Hemorrhage

Diffuse

Nonimmune
- Neonatal
- Congenital heart disease
- Hematologic

Immune
- Lower respiratory and renal
- Goodpasture syndrome
- Idiopathic rapid progressive glomerulonephritis
- Upper and lower respiratory and renal
- Wegener granulomatosis
- Multisystem organ involvement
- Systemic lupus erythematosus
- Polyarteritis nodosa
- Behçet syndrome
- Henoch-Schönlein syndrome
- Rheumatoid arthritis

Focal
- Foreign body aspiration and chronic retention
- Sequestration
- Arteriovenous fistula
- Bronchogenic and gastroenteric cysts
- Thrombus or embolus
- Neoplasms: angiomas, adenomas

cor triatriatum, or hypoplastic left heart syndrome may result in massive PH.[252,253]

Although the lungs are an infrequent site for early manifestations of primary bleeding disorders,[243,246] a coagulopathy should be ruled out during the management of any patient with PH. In patients with leukemia, PH occurs most frequently when the platelet count is lower than 10,000/mm.

Diffuse/Immune Pulmonary Hemorrhage

The classic clinical triad of hemoptysis, microcytic hypochromic anemia, and diffuse alveolar-filling opacities on a chest radiograph (Fig. 55.1) is found in most episodes of PH in this category. Although the lung may be the only organ affected, more frequently multiple organs are involved. In patients with PH, establishing which extrapulmonary organs are involved by the disease helps to narrow the differential diagnosis of which of the immune-mediated disorders is most likely present.

Diffuse parenchymal bleeding without evidence of extrapulmonary involvement occurs in patients with idiopathic pulmonary hemosiderosis, Heiner syndrome, and drug-induced PH. Idiopathic pulmonary hemosiderosis, a disease of childhood, is a diagnosis of exclusion. Clinically, episodes of PH recur, with 30% to 50% of patients eventually dying of exsanguination and/or respiratory failure.[254,255] Microscopic examination of the lungs is compatible with nonspecific injury rather than a specific cause such as vasculitis or immune deposits.[254] Heiner syndrome, which affects children between the ages of 6 months and 2 years, usually manifests as other symptoms, such as chronic rhinitis, recurrent otitis media, and growth retardation.[255] Tests for precipitating antibodies to milk proteins are positive. Symptoms resolve when milk and milk products are eliminated from the diet.

Although uncommon, exposure to or inhalation of D-penicillamine, lymphangiography dye, trimellitic anhydride, cocaine, and exogenous surfactant[256,257] has been associated with development of PH. Acute PH of an undetermined etiology occurring in infants has been reported.[258,259]

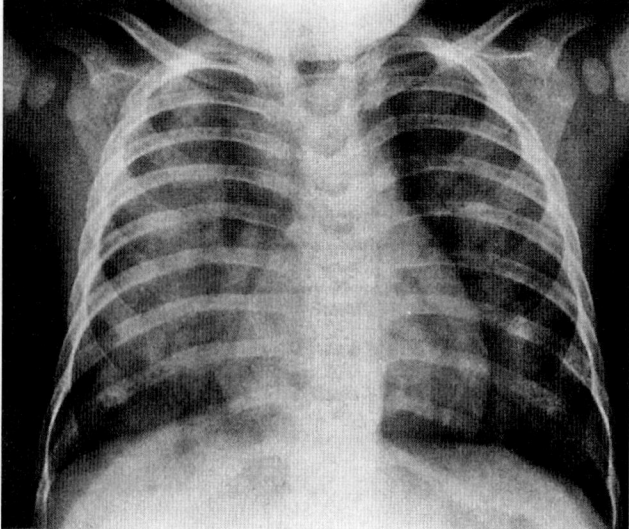

Fig. 55.1. Chest radiograph of a patient with diffuse immune pulmonary hemorrhage.

Idiopathic rapidly progressive glomerulonephritis is usually a disease of older adults (mean age, 55-60 years). In children with PH and either proteinuria, hematuria, or red cell casts, Goodpasture syndrome is the most likely etiology. The presence of a linear immunofluorescent staining of Ig and C3 along glomerular capillary walls and antibasement membrane antibody (ABMA) in the serum confirms the diagnosis of Goodpasture syndrome. Renal biopsy is the preferred primary method of confirming the diagnosis because an ABMA assay is not readily available at most institutions. ABMA is a cytotoxic plasma Ig that reacts immunologically with components of alveolar and glomerular basement membrane. Stress failure of pulmonary capillaries because of alteration of the alveolar and glomerular basement membrane may contribute to the likelihood of PH in these patients.[260] Fifty percent of patients with Goodpasture syndrome die of asphyxia as a result of massive PH. The presence of sinusitis and/or bilateral, multiple cavitary pulmonary nodules and evidence of glomerulonephritis in patients with PH help distinguish Wegener granulomatosis from the other vasculitides.[261] Serositis, arthritis, facial erythema, fever, and glomerulonephritis are present before the development of PH in patients with systemic lupus erythematosus (SLE).[262] Ten percent of all cases of immune-mediated PH are associated with SLE.[262] The onset of PH in patients with SLE is abrupt. Pulmonary histology may or may not reveal a small vessel vasculitis characterized by neutrophilic infiltration of vessel walls and necrosis of capillaries and alveolar septa. Renal histology shows a vasculitis represented by focal and segmental glomerulonephritis with absent or minimal immune deposits. The majority of patients who have SLE and PH die.[262] PH has been reported with most of the vasculitides, but the incidence is much lower than in the SLE population. Constitutional signs and symptoms, such as musculoskeletal involvement, blood dyscrasias, and dermatitis, are the predominant clinical features of polyarteritis nodosa, the second most likely vasculitis-associated disease to cause PH.[263,264] A segmental necrotizing (granular pattern) vasculitis is the characteristic lesion of polyarteritis nodosa, with PH a dominant feature.[265] Recurrent uveitis, mucocutaneous ulcerations, and genital ulcerations in a patient with PH suggests Behçet syndrome as the etiology. Other clinical features seen with Behçet syndrome include arthritis, gastrointestinal disease, cardiovascular involvement, and CNS disease.[266,267] A necrotizing vasculitis of small- to medium-sized arteries and veins and thromboses of the terminal vascular beds or vena cava confirm the diagnosis.

Although PH is an extremely rare complication of Henoch-Schönlein purpura or syndrome (when abdominal pain and arthritis precede the purpura), it should be treated aggressively because it may be fatal. In a few patients with rheumatoid arthritis, syndromes resembling idiopathic pulmonary hemosiderosis without evidence of vasculitis or renal disease have developed.

Focal Pulmonary Hemorrhage

Congenital malformations that may be responsible for PH during infancy include angiomas and bronchogenic and gastroenteric cysts.[249] Angiomas are located in the subglottic area and present with symptoms of airway obstruction by age 6 months in almost 90% of cases. Bronchogenic cysts arise from abnormal branching of the tracheobronchial tree, are lined with ciliated columnar epithelium, are filled with mucoid fluid, and if they are in communication with the airway, they may demonstrate an air-fluid level. They are prone to infection and may bleed if contiguous vessels erode. Gastroenteric cysts, which are enteric duplication cysts lined with gastric mucosa, produce acid peptic secretions that may erode through adjacent vessels to cause bleeding. Pulmonary sequestration, arteriovenous fistula, and bronchial adenomas are congenital malformations that may present in childhood or later life with PH. With its tendency to become recurrently infected, a sequestered lobe may suffer erosion into its systemic arterial supply, causing massive PH.[249] Pulmonary arteriovenous fistula with or without telangiectasia (isolated or familial) may produce massive PH during childhood, but this usually does not occur until adulthood.[265,266,268] Adenomas are highly vascular tumors that, with minor trauma or inflammation, can cause PH. Acquired causes of focal PH include aspiration of an organic foreign body and development of a pulmonary arterial thrombus or embolus.[247] A patient presenting with PH and wheezing should lead the clinician to suspect a diagnosis of foreign body aspiration. Prolonged retention of an organic foreign body leads to hyperplasia of tortuous bronchial vessels, varicosities, and bronchiectasis, any of which may cause PH. Thrombi or emboli may develop in postoperative immobile children with central venous or pulmonary catheters, in female adolescents using oral contraceptives, or in patients with homozygous deficiency of antithrombin III, protein S, and protein C. Focal PH may develop in children with cystic fibrosis as a result of bronchiectasis.

Treatment

General

The primary objectives in treatment of PH are twofold: (1) to rapidly control the bleeding to prevent tissue hypoxia and/or ischemia resulting from airway obstruction and exsanguination and (2) to stabilize hemodynamics to prevent further damage to the kidneys or other extrapulmonary organs by the underlying disorder.[244,267] Initial management of the patient with severe PH should occur in the setting of a critical care unit because of the potential lethality of this event (Box 55.7). General care measures include use of the Trendelenburg position as tolerated, oxygen supplementation, mechanical ventilation, and hemostasis therapy when indicated. The Trendelenburg position may help clots propagate superiorly and exit the airway. This position may not be well tolerated by patients with respiratory or cardiac embarrassment. Positive end-expiratory pressure during mechanical ventilation may become necessary to reverse hypoxemia and may provide a measure of tamponade to the site of hemorrhage.[244] Coagulation factors should be administered when indicated to lessen the severity of bleeding. Hemodynamic monitoring with a pulmonary arterial catheter may be beneficial in some instances because high pulmonary artery occlusion pressure may worsen PH of any etiology. Short-term control of bleeding may be obtained with insertion, under direct vision, of a balloon-tipped (Fogarty) catheter into the affected portion of the airway. Right upper lobe bleeding is best managed by intubating the left main stem bronchus with a cuffed endotracheal tube and inflating the cuff of the tube. Utilization of a "double-lumen" or Carlens-type endotracheal tube may also be helpful in isolating the bleeding segment. However, the diameter of these tubes precludes their use in smaller children, and proper positioning may prove difficult.[244,269]

BOX 55.7   Treatment of Pulmonary Hemorrhage

General
- Admission to pediatric ICU
- Positioning (intermittent Trendelenburg)
- Oxygen supplementation
- Mechanical ventilation (positive end-expiratory pressure)
- Hemodynamic monitoring
- Hemostasis replacement therapy
- Endobronchial tamponade (Fogarty catheter, cuffed endotracheal tube)

Specific

Immune
- Corticosteroids
- Other immunosuppressive agents (azathioprine, cyclophosphamide)
- Plasmapheresis (Goodpasture syndrome)
- Bilateral nephrectomy
- Deferoxamine, milk-free diet

Focal
- Surgical resection
- Selective embolization of bronchial vessels

Rigid bronchoscopy is the best means of identifying the source and type of bleeding, but it also has therapeutic applications.[269-271] The rigid scope readily establishes an adequate airway and can be used for large-volume isotonic saline solution lavage and for suctioning large volumes of blood. Fiberoptic bronchoscopy should be reserved for diagnostic purposes, including definitive identification of the bronchopulmonary segments involved and BAL. BAL provides useful information by permitting culture of the lavage for bacteria, fungi, mycobacteria, and viruses and quantitative assessment of the hemosiderin content of the alveolar lavage. Interpreting the presence or absence of hemosiderin-laden macrophages should be done cautiously because macrophages may not appear for up to 48 hours following an acute episode of bleeding and usually disappear by 2 weeks.

Specific

Despite the different etiologies in the category of immune-mediated PH, the response to corticosteroid therapy is swift (within 24-48 hours) as assessed by transfusion requirements, hemoglobin concentration, hemoptysis, and absence of new infiltrates.[255] Although controlled clinical trials have not been performed to validate this temporal relationship suggestive of therapeutic benefit, the risk of administering a short course of high-dose corticosteroids in this setting is low. Hence, the corticosteroids adrenocorticotropic hormone (10–25 units/day), methylprednisolone (2–4 mg/kg/day), or hydrocortisone (4 mg/kg/day) should be administered early in a patient with an acute, life-threatening episode of immune-mediated PH. Once remission is achieved, corticosteroids should be tapered until they are discontinued or symptoms recur. In cases of inadequate response to corticosteroids alone, other immunosuppressive agents (eg, azathioprine, cyclophosphamide, chlorambucil) have been administered with some success in persons with the immune-mediated PH syndromes.[272] Azathioprine (1.2–5 mg/kg/day) with prednisone (5–20 mg every 6 hours) is a typical treatment combination. Cyclophosphamide is the drug of choice for treatment of patients with Wegener granulomatosis.[273] Once a specific diagnosis is made for the various etiologies of immune-mediated PH, directed therapies are available, including immunosuppression and plasmapheresis. These therapies are beyond the scope of this chapter and are discussed in the literature.[273-275] Administration of IV vasopressin to a patient with massive hemoptysis may temporarily control the bleeding. Surgical resection of a bleeding focus remains the procedure of choice if feasible. Severe bleeding at the time of resection resulting in single lung ventilation increased the mortality rate from 12% to 25% in one series. Pulmonary embolectomy should be considered for patients with an acute large embolus, especially if fibrinolysis is contraindicated.[246,276,277] For focal PH resulting from increased bronchial circulation, selective embolization or occlusion of bronchial vessels with glass microspheres, small pledgets of absorbable gelatin sponge or polyvinyl alcohol sponge may provide temporary hemostasis. Embolization should be considered in the unstable or poor surgical candidate with focal PH. Complications of embolization include inadvertent CNS or coronary artery occlusion and transverse myelitis with resulting paraplegia.

Summary

PH that does not occur in the familiar setting of trauma or infection can be classified according to extent of pulmonary involvement (ie, diffuse or focal). PH occurs most commonly during the neonatal period as a result of diffuse nonimmune mechanisms. PH in the neonate is a preterminal complication of severe disorders of the cardiovascular and respiratory systems. The best initial approach to diagnosis and specific therapy in the older child is determining the extent of extrapulmonary organ involvement. Diseases that lead to focal hemorrhage are more likely to cause massive hemoptysis, typically affect younger children, and may be amenable to surgical resection. If the suspected cause of PH is a diffuse, immune-mediated process, a trial of corticosteroids should be administered early because of the rapid, dramatic response seen in patients with some disorders. A systematic approach to diagnosis in persons with PH will improve the odds of a favorable outcome for patients with this rare phenomenon.[246,270]

Key References

5. Fan L. Evaluation and therapy of chronic interstitial pneumonitis in children. *Curr Opin Pediatr.* 1994;6:248.
12. Khamprad T, Glezen W. Clinical and radiologic assessment of acute lower respiratory tract disease in infants and children. *Semin Respir Infect.* 1987;2:130.
15. Davies S, Sarosi G. Aspergillosis in the immunosuppressed patient. In: Al-Doory Y, Wagner G, eds. *Aspergillosis.* Springfield, IL: Charles C. Thomas; 1985.
19. Walsh T, Pizzo P. Fungal infections in granulocytopenic patients current approaches to classification, diagnosis and treatment. In: Holmgerg K, Meyer R, et al., eds. *Diagnosis and Therapy of Systemic Mycoses.* New York, NY: Raven Press; 1989.
25. Lee L, Henderson D. Emerging viral infections. *Curr Opin Infect Dis.* 2001;14:467-480.
30. Philip A. The changing face of neonatal infection: experience at a regional medical center. *Pediatr Infect Dis J.* 1994;13:1098.
33. Pickering L, et al. *Red Book: 2009 Report of the Committee on Infectious Diseases.* 28th ed. Elk Grove Village, IL: American Academy of Pediatrics; 2009.
36. Use of 13-valent pneumococcal conjugate vaccine and 23-valent pneumococcal polysaccharide vaccine among children aged 6-18 years with

immunocompromising condition: recommendations of the Advisory Committee on Immunization Practices (ACIP). *MMWR Morb Mortal Wkly Rep.* 2013;62:521-524.
37. Gilbert D, et al. *The Sanford Guide to Antimicrobial Therapy.* Hyde Park, NY: Sanford; 2002.
41. Principi N, Esposito S. *Mycoplasma pneumoniae* and *Chlamydia pneumoniae* cause lower respiratory tract disease in paediatric patients. *Curr Opin Infect Dis.* 2002;15:295-300.
44. Zhang F, et al. Risk factors for ventilator-associated pneumonia in the neonatal intensive care unit: a meta-analysis of observational studies. *Eur J Pediatr.* 2014;173:427-434.
50. Carson J, et al. Acquired ciliary defects in nasal epithelium of children with acute viral upper respiratory tract infections. *N Engl J Med.* 1985;312:463.
54. Dennehy P. Rapid diagnosis of viral infections. In: Hilman B, ed. *Pediatric Respiratory Disease.* Philadelphia: WB Saunders; 1993.
58. Henderson F, et al. The etiologic and epidemiologic spectrum of bronchiolitis in pediatric practice. *J Pediatr.* 1995;183:179.
61. Welliver RC. Review of epidemiology and clinical risk factors for severe respiratory syncytial virus (RSV) infection. *J Pediatr.* 2003;143(suppl 5):S112-S117.
72. Panitch H. Respiratory syncytial virus bronchiolitis: supportive care and therapies designed to overcome airway obstruction. *Pediatr Infect Dis J.* 2003;22:S83-S88.
76. Scarfone R. Controversies in the treatment of bronchiolitis. *Curr Opin Pediatr.* 2005;17:62-66.
78. The IMpact-RSV Study Group. Palivizumab, a humanized respiratory syncytial virus monoclonal antibody, reduces hospitalization from respiratory syncytial virus infection in high-risk infants. *Pediatrics.* 1998;102:531-537.
89. Mejias A, Chavez-Bueno S, Ramilo O. Respiratory syncytial virus pneumonia: mechanisms of inflammation and prolonged airway hyperresponsiveness. *Curr Opin Infect Dis.* 2005;18:199-204.
93. Welliver R, et al. Natural history of parainfluenza virus infection in childhood. *J Pediatr.* 1983;101:180.
107. Moro MR, et al. Clinical features, adenovirus types, and local production of inflammatory mediators in adenovirus infections. *Pediatr Infect Dis J.* 2009;28:376-380.
115. Glezen W. Influenza viruses. In: Feigin R, et al., eds. *Feigin & Cherry's Textbook of Pediatric Infectious Disease.* Philadelphia: Saunders Elsevier; 2009:2395-2414.
126. Rubinstein A, et al. Pulmonary disease in children with acquired immune deficiency syndrome and AIDS-related complex. *J Pediatr.* 1986;108:498-503.
134. Harper SA, et al. Seasonal influenza in adults and children—diagnosis, treatment, chemoprophylaxis and institutional outbreak management: clinical practice guidelines of the Infectious Disease Society of America. *Clin Infect Dis.* 2009;48:1003-1032.
143. Ventre K, Randolph AG. Ribavirin for respiratory syncytial virus infection of the lower respiratory tract in infants and young children (update of Cochrane Database Sys Rev 2004;(4):CD000181; PMID: 15494991). *Cochrane Database Sys Rev.* 2007;CD000181.
151. Shigeta S. Recent progress in antiviral chemotherapy for respiratory syncytial virus infections. *Expert Opin Investig Drugs.* 2000;9:221-235.
158. Bueno J, et al. Current management strategies for the prevention and treatment of cytomegalovirus infection in pediatric transplant recipients. *Paediatr Drugs.* 2002;4:279-290.
168. Wheat J, et al. Practice guidelines for the management of patients with histoplasmosis: Infectious Diseases Society of America. *Clin Infect Dis.* 2000;30:688-695.
170. Vyas KS. Pulmonary blastomycosis. *Semin Respir Crit Care Med.* 2011;32:745-753.
174. Wheat L, et al. State-of-the-art review of pulmonary fungal infections. *Semin Respir Infect.* 2002;17:158-181.
179. Feldman B, Snyder L. Primary pulmonary coccidioidomycosis. *Semin Respir Infect.* 2001;16:231-237.
185. Soubani A, Chandrasekar P. The clinical spectrum of pulmonary aspergillosis. *Chest.* 1988;121:1988-1999.
188. Leeflang MM, et al. Galactomannan detection for invasive aspergillosis in immunocompromised patients. *Cochrane Database Syst Rev.* 2008;CD007394.
189. Patterson KC, Strek ME. Diagnosis and treatment of pulmonary aspergillosis syndromes. *Chest.* 2014;146:1358-1368.
197. Neville K, et al. Pneumonia in the immunocompromised pediatric cancer patient. *Semin Respir Infect.* 2002;17:21-32.

209. Masur H, et al. Prevention and treatment of *Pneumocystis* pneumonia. *N Engl J Med*. 1992;327:1853.

216. Vandenplas Y, Hegar B. Diagnosis and treatment of gastro-oesophageal reflux disease in infants and children. *J Gastroenterol Hepatol*. 2000;15:593-603.

224. Wilde M, McTavish D. Omeprazole: an update of its pharmacology and therapeutic use in acid-related disorders. *Drugs*. 1994;48:91.

225. Curry J, et al. Review article: erythromycin as a prokinetic agent in infants and children. *Aliment Pharmacol Ther*. 2001;15:595-603.

227. Rorison D, McPherson S. Acute toxic inhalations. *Emerg Med Clin North Am*. 1992;10:409.

228. Ruddy R. Smoke inhalation injury. *Pediatr Clin North Am*. 1994;41:317.

230. Ainslie G. Inhalational injuries produced by smoke and nitrogen dioxide. *Respir Med*. 1993;87:169.

235. Fan L, et al. Pediatric interstitial lung disease revisited. *Pediatr Pulmonol*. 2004;38:369-378.

238. Deterding R, Fan L. Surfactant dysfunction mutations in children's interstitial lung disease and beyond. *Am J Respir Crit Care Med*. 2005;172:940-941.

243. Kumar S, et al. Pulmonary hemorrhage in a young infant. *Ann Allergy*. 1989;62:209.

244. Noseworthy T, Anderson B. Massive hemoptysis. *Can Med J Assoc*. 1986;135:1097.

246. Cahill B, Ingbar D. Massive hemoptysis: assessment and management (review). *Clin Chest Med*. 1994;15:147.

247. Donald K, et al. Alveolar capillary basement membrane lesions in Goodpasture's syndrome and idiopathic pulmonary hemosiderosis. *Am J Med*. 1975;59:642.

254. Susarla SC, Fan LL. Diffuse alveolar hemorrhage syndromes in children. *Curr Opin Pediatr*. 2007;19:314-320.

268. Pouwels H, et al. Systemic to pulmonary vascular malformation (review). *Eur Respir J*. 1992;5:1288.

275. Fox H, Swann D. Goodpasture syndrome: pathophysiology, diagnosis, and management. *Nephrol Nurs J*. 2001;28:305-310.

Diseases of Pulmonary Circulation

Satyan Lakshminrusimha and Vasanth H. Kumar

PEARLS

- A normal fetus is in a state of physiologic pulmonary hypertension and is dependent on the placenta for gas exchange.
- The onset of breathing and lung inflation at birth and the resultant increase in oxygen tension decrease pulmonary vascular resistance (PVR), which is essential for establishing a normal postnatal circulatory pattern.
- Elevated pulmonary vascular resistance relative to systemic vascular resistance, which may result from either vasoconstriction or structural remodeling of the pulmonary vasculature, characterizes persistent pulmonary hypertension of the newborn (PPHN).
- An increase in pulmonary vascular smooth muscle can occur in utero or after birth and result in peripheral extension of the smooth muscle onto vessels that do not normally have muscle layers. This process may contribute to the pathology of PPHN.
- The gold standard in defining PPHN rests on the echocardiographic findings of right-to-left shunting of blood at the foramen ovale and/or ductus arteriosus, as well as evidence of elevated pulmonary arterial pressure in the absence of structural heart disease.
- High-frequency oscillatory ventilation, surfactant therapy, and nitric oxide have decreased the need for extracorporeal membrane oxygenation in infants with PPHN.
- In children, it is important to establish an accurate diagnosis with respect to etiology because therapy may depend on the etiology of pulmonary hypertension.
- Echocardiography is a useful screening tool in children with suspected pulmonary arterial hypertension (PAH). Before committing to therapy specific to childhood PAH, diagnosis needs to be confirmed by catheterization.
- Calcium channel blockers are useful only for patients who respond to vasodilator testing during cardiac catheterization.
- Overall exercise capacity, symptoms as assessed by World Health Organization classification, and hemodynamic parameters of right ventricular function help not only in the management of these patients but also correlate well with survival.
- Recent advances in the medical management of PAH have widened the spectrum of therapeutic modalities available for children to include prostanoids, oral endothelin receptor antagonists, PDE5 inhibitors, and some forms of combination therapies.
- Aggressive medical therapy combined with prompt and meticulous follow-up will improve quality of life and survival of children with pulmonary hypertension. Early referral to expert centers is crucial to patient survival.

Etiology and Treatment of Pulmonary Hypertension

This chapter addresses the neonatal and pediatric aspects of pulmonary hypertension (PH). First, unique aspects of fetal and postnatal development of pulmonary vasculature, transitional circulation, and developmental regulation of pulmonary vascular tone are briefly discussed. This background helps in understanding the pathophysiology and treatment of pulmonary vascular disorders in newborns and children.

Developmental Pulmonary Vascular Anatomy

The vascular network of the developing endodermal pair of lung buds is derived from the surrounding mesenchyme of the splanchnic mesoderm beginning at 4 weeks of gestation. These vessels accompany the developing airways, differentiate into arteries, and join the larger pulmonary arteries that originate from the sixth aortic arch. The veins arise separately within the loose mesenchyme of the lung septa and subsequently connect to the developing left atrium.

In the normal fetal lung, fully muscularized thick-walled preacinar arteries extend to the level of terminal bronchioles, whereas the intraacinar arteries (ie, those accompanying respiratory bronchioles) are partially muscular (surrounded by a spiral of muscle) or nonmuscular. Arteries at alveolar ducts and alveolar walls are nonmuscular.[1] An increase in intrauterine vascular smooth muscle, resulting from peripheral extension of smooth muscle into vessels that do not normally contain muscle layers, may contribute to the pathophysiology of persistent pulmonary hypertension of the newborn (PPHN).[2] Increased muscularization of the pulmonary arteries has been described in infants with severe meconium aspiration syndrome (MAS) with PPHN.[3] Neonates who die of PPHN may have a striking distal extension of smooth muscle in the intraacinar region, thickening of the media and adventitia, and excessive accumulation of the matrix protein in the pulmonary vessels.[4] The increase in vascular smooth muscle and its peripheral extension can occur either prenatally or postnatally. In utero ductal ligation 1 to 2 weeks before delivery results in severe PPHN at birth associated with distal extension of vascular smooth muscle in newborn lambs[5] similar to the changes seen in human infants dying with severe PPHN.

Developmental Pulmonary Vascular Physiology

The normal fetus is in a state of physiologic pulmonary hypertension. Most of the right ventricular output crosses the ductus arteriosus to the aorta (≈8%-10% of combined ventricular output in an ovine fetus and 13%-21% in human fetuses).[6-8] The ratio of blood entering the pulmonary arteries to the ductus arteriosus is determined by the fetal pulmonary vascular resistance (PVR) and can vary with fetal oxygenation status and gestation.[9,10]

The lung increases in weight by 6-fold from midgestation to term and the number of pulmonary vessels increases more than 10-fold.[11,12] Thus the tremendous increase in cross-sectional area of pulmonary vasculature permits pulmonary blood flow (Q_p) to increase throughout gestation. However, Q_p remains relatively constant when corrected for wet lung weight with advancing gestation.[13] A gradual increase in pulmonary arterial pressure (PAP), accompanied by a relatively constant flow per unit lung tissue, results in increasing fetal pulmonary vascular resistance (PVR) with advancing gestation.[13] A major part of this increase comes from elevated pulmonary vascular tone associated with low PO_2 in the fetal lung.[14,15] Maintaining high PVR in utero is important because the function of gas exchange is performed by the placenta, not by the lungs.

Regulation of Pulmonary Vascular Tone in Utero

Low oxygen tension and various mediators play a crucial role in maintaining elevated fetal PVR.[16] Vasoconstriction in response to low oxygen tension contributes to high PVR in the fetal lamb as it approaches term.[13-15] Arachidonic acid metabolites such as prostaglandin $F_{2\alpha}$ ($PGF_{2\alpha}$) and thromboxane A_2 (TXA_2) are synthesized by the fetal lung via the cyclooxygenase pathway[17] and are pulmonary vasoconstrictors in the fetal and newborn lungs. Blocking prostaglandin or thromboxane synthesis does not decrease fetal PVR but prevents the decrease in PVR in response to rhythmic distention of the lung in fetal lambs.[18] Serotonin increases fetal PVR.[19,20] The use of selective serotonin reuptake inhibitors (SSRIs) during the last half of pregnancy has been associated with an increased incidence of PPHN in at least three human population studies.[21-24] While the mechanism by which SSRIs induce pulmonary hypertension in newborn is not known, it is speculated that higher drug-induced serotonin levels result in pulmonary vasoconstriction. However, recent studies have questioned the association between maternal SSRI intake and PPHN.[25,26] Furthermore, the severity of PPHN following fetal exposure to SSRI has not been well described and a recent report observed no differences in right pulmonary artery Doppler pulsatility index (PI) in fetuses of mothers exposed to SSRI antidepressants.[27]

Endothelins (ETs) are 21-residue peptides[28,29] whose role in regulating vascular tone and vasomotor responses has been studied intensively in the past decade. Three distinct ET isoforms have been described: endothelin-1 (ET-1), endothelin-2 (ET-2), and endothelin-3 (ET-3), cleaved from ET precursors big ET-1, big ET-2, and big ET-3, respectively, by an ET-converting enzyme. Endothelin-1 synthesized by vascular endothelial cells is a potent vasoconstrictor.[30] Infusion of big ET-1, the precursor of ET-1, into fetal lambs causes sustained pulmonary vasoconstriction.[31] Currently at least two receptor subtypes, ET_A and ET_B, are thought to mediate responses to ETs (Fig. 56.1). The ET_B receptor plays a role in vasodilation and ET_A receptor in vasoconstriction. Selective blockade of the ET_A receptor causes fetal pulmonary vasodilation.[32-34] Some investigators suggest a significant role for an endothelial ET_B receptor in vasodilation and a smooth muscle ET_B receptor and ET_A receptor in vasoconstriction.[35,36] Vasoconstriction

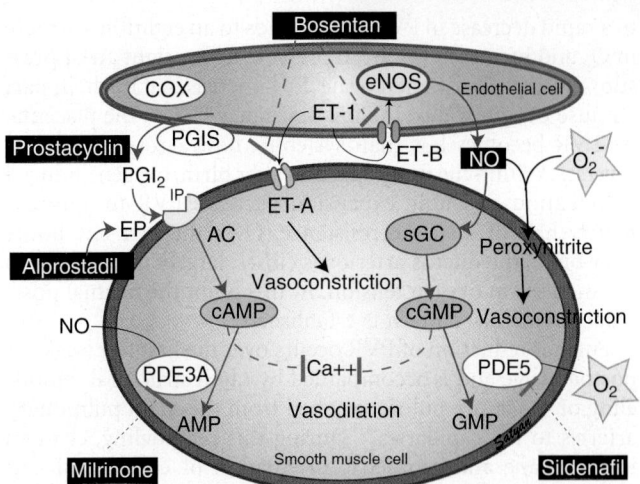

Fig. 56.1. Endothelium-derived vasodilators—prostacyclin (PGI_2), nitric oxide (NO), and vasoconstrictor (endothelin, ET-1). Cyclooxygenase (COX) and prostacyclin synthase (PGIS) are involved in the production of prostacyclin. Prostacyclin acts on its receptor (IP) in the smooth muscle cell and stimulates adenylate cyclase (AC) to produce cyclic adenosine monophosphate (cAMP). Cyclic AMP is broken down by phosphodiesterase 3A (PDE 3A, the enzyme most prevalent in vasculature) in the smooth muscle cell. Milrinone inhibits PDE 3A and increases cAMP levels in arterial smooth muscle cells and cardiac myocytes resulting in pulmonary (and systemic) vasodilation and inotropy. Nitric oxide (NO) stimulates PDE 3A.[362,363] Endothelin is a powerful vasoconstrictor and acts on ET-A receptors in the smooth muscle cell and increases ionic calcium concentration. A second endothelin receptor (ET-B) on the endothelial cell stimulates NO release and vasodilation. Endothelial nitric oxide synthase (eNOS) produces NO, which diffuses from the endothelium to the smooth muscle cell and stimulates soluble guanylate cyclase (sGC) enzyme to produce cyclic guanosine monophosphate (cGMP). Cyclic GMP is broken down by PDE5 enzyme in the smooth muscle cell. Sildenafil inhibits PDE5 and increases cGMP levels in pulmonary arterial smooth muscle cells. Natriuretic peptides stimulate particulate guanylate cyclase (pGC) to produce cGMP. Cyclic AMP and cGMP reduce cytosolic ionic calcium concentrations and induce smooth muscle cell relaxation and pulmonary vasodilation. Nitric oxide is a free radical and can avidly combine with superoxide anions to form a toxic vasoconstrictor, peroxynitrite. Hence the bioavailability of NO in a tissue is determined by the local concentration of superoxide anions. Hyperoxic ventilation with 100% oxygen can increase the risk of formation of superoxide anions in the pulmonary arterial smooth muscle cells and limit the bioavailability of NO and stimulate PDE5 activity.[138] Medications used in persistent pulmonary hypertension are shown in black boxes. (Copyright Satyan Lakshminrusimha.)

induced by ET-1 is mediated by calcium,[37] whereas the vasodilator properties are mediated by endothelium-derived nitric oxide (NO).[36,38] ET-1 may play a role in the change that occurs in the pulmonary vasculature at birth. It is possible that prenatally endogenous ET-1 primarily stimulates ET_A receptors to cause vasoconstriction and that ET_B receptors are less active in fetal life.[32] However, ET_B receptors mediate the vasodilator responses to ET-1 in the fetus, and there is a suggestion that abundance of ET_B receptors may be of physiologic importance in decreasing PVR at birth.[39]

Transitional Circulation

Successful transition is accomplished when the fluid-filled fetal lungs are distended with air during breathing[16] leading to a rapid decrease in PVR.[40] This leads to an eightfold increase in Q_p and increased left atrial pressure above right atrial pressure, closing the foramen ovale. SVR increases at birth, in part because of removal of the low resistance bed of the placenta. As PVR becomes less than systemic, flow across the ductus reverses. Within the first 5 minutes after birth, oxygen-induced vasodilation and lung expansion decrease PVR to approximately half of systemic resistance. Over the first few hours after birth, the ductus arteriosus closes, largely in response to the increase in oxygen tension. At this point the normal postnatal circulatory pattern is established.

Further reduction of PVR occurs over the first few weeks of postnatal age and is accompanied by rapid structural remodeling of the entire pulmonary bed from the main pulmonary arteries to the capillaries.[41] During this remodeling, changes in the shape and geometric orientation of endothelial and smooth muscle cells cause luminal enlargement. Maturation of smooth muscle function, thinning of endothelial cells, and more gradual changes in elastic and connective tissue occur over the next few weeks.

Factors Responsible for Decrease in Pulmonary Vascular Resistance at Birth

The onset of ventilation with rhythmic inflation of the lungs at birth with a resultant increase in oxygen tension in the lungs leads to a decrease in PVR. Each of these stimuli has been shown to decrease vascular resistance and increase blood flow in the lungs of fetal lambs.[13,16,40,42]

The drop in PVR soon after birth is accompanied by production of prostacyclin (PGI_2) and nitric oxide (NO). PGI_2 synthesized by endothelial cells appears to relax smooth muscle by producing cyclic adenosine monophosphate (cAMP). Even though blockade of prostaglandin synthesis, by either indomethacin[43,44] or meclofenamate,[18] blunts the decrease in PVR, it does not completely disrupt the transition to gas exchange. In addition cyclooxygenase through the PGE_2 pathway plays an important role in maintaining patency of the ductus arteriosus. PPHN has been observed in infants of mothers receiving aspirin or nonsteroidal antiinflammatory drugs that inhibit cyclooxygenase activity,[45] although this association has been recently called into question.[46]

Acetylcholine,[47] bradykinin,[48] and histamine[49] are fetal pulmonary vasodilators, which in many species act by an endothelium-dependent mechanism (Fig. 56.1). They stimulate the production of NO by vascular endothelium. NO activates soluble guanylate cyclase (sGC) to produce the second messenger cyclic guanosine monophosphate (cGMP). cGMP induces relaxation of vascular smooth muscle through activation of a cGMP-dependent protein kinase that produces a lowering of cytosolic ionic calcium, in part through activation of potassium channels.[50,51] There is strong evidence that NO is an important mediator of the decrease in PVR at birth.[52] The dilation of the fetal pulmonary circulation caused by an increase in oxygen tension is mediated in large part by endogenous synthesis of NO.[53] Prolonged administration of nitric oxide synthase (NOS) inhibitors in late-gestation lambs to block endogenous NO synthesis does not affect basal PVR but markedly blunts the decrease in PVR observed at birth.[54]

Evidence suggests that many other mediators can act as pulmonary vasodilators during fetal life and at birth. The purines adenosine triphosphate (ATP) and adenosine[10,55-58]; natriuretic peptides such as atrial natriuretic peptide (ANP),

B-type natriuretic peptide (BNP), and C-type natriuretic peptide (CNP)[59]; and arachidonic acid metabolites such as EETs, generated through the cytochrome P-450 pathway, are potent pulmonary vasodilators.[60] As pulmonary vasodilation at birth is a vital step in establishing postnatal life, it is logical that there would be sufficient redundant vasodilators to compensate for failure or inadequacy of any single pathway.[61]

Persistent Pulmonary Hypertension of the Newborn

PPHN is a serious clinical condition that can result from diverse etiologies and is characterized by failure of the pulmonary circulation to adapt to extrauterine life. Elevated pulmonary-to-systemic vascular-resistance ratio (PVR/SVR) resulting from either vasoconstriction, structural remodeling of the pulmonary vasculature, intravascular obstruction, or lung hypoplasia (Fig. 56.2) characterizes PPHN. This leads to right-to-left shunting of blood across the foramen ovale and ductus arteriosus, resulting in hypoxemia. Numerous disease states with diverse etiologies can result in a similar final pathophysiology. About 10% of cases with PPHN are idiopathic, with no associated pulmonary airspace pathology. However, PPHN is usually associated with other acute respiratory conditions, such as meconium aspiration syndrome (MAS), respiratory distress syndrome (RDS), pneumonia, or congenital diaphragmatic hernia (CDH) (Fig. 56.3). Hypoxemia in these conditions can be due to ventilation/perfusion (V/Q) mismatch and intrapulmonary, as well as extrapulmonary, right-to-left shunting of blood. In some newborns with hypoxic respiratory failure, a single mechanism predominates (eg, extrapulmonary right-to-left shunting in idiopathic PPHN). However, more commonly, several of these mechanisms contribute to hypoxemia. In MAS, obstruction of the airways by meconium results in decreasing V/Q ratios and increasing intrapulmonary right-to-left shunt. Other segments of the lungs may be overventilated relative to perfusion, causing increased physiologic dead space. The same patient may also have severe PPHN with extrapulmonary right-to-left shunting at the ductus arteriosus and foramen ovale. The PPHN in MAS may result from alveolar hypoxia, inflammatory mediators, or abnormal pulmonary vascular muscularization (Fig. 56.4).

Clinical Presentation

PPHN must be included in the differential diagnosis of hypoxic respiratory failure in term or preterm infants. Prenatal and perinatal history may provide clues to the etiology of PPHN. These include the presence of meconium, acidosis, and asphyxia at delivery and maternal risk factors for infection such as prolonged rupture of membranes, maternal fever, or positive group B *Streptococcus* status. Postmaturity also appears to be a risk factor.

Although PPHN is traditionally considered a disease of term and late-preterm infants, it is increasingly being diagnosed in extremely preterm infants.[62,63] Pulmonary hypertension in preterm infants has a bimodal postnatal age of presentation. Some preterm infants with RDS present with PPHN in the first few days of life[62] while preterm infants with bronchopulmonary dysplasia (BPD) may be diagnosed with pulmonary hypertension later in the hospital course[64] or after discharge from the neonatal ICU or during a subsequent admission to the pediatric ICU with an intercurrent illness.

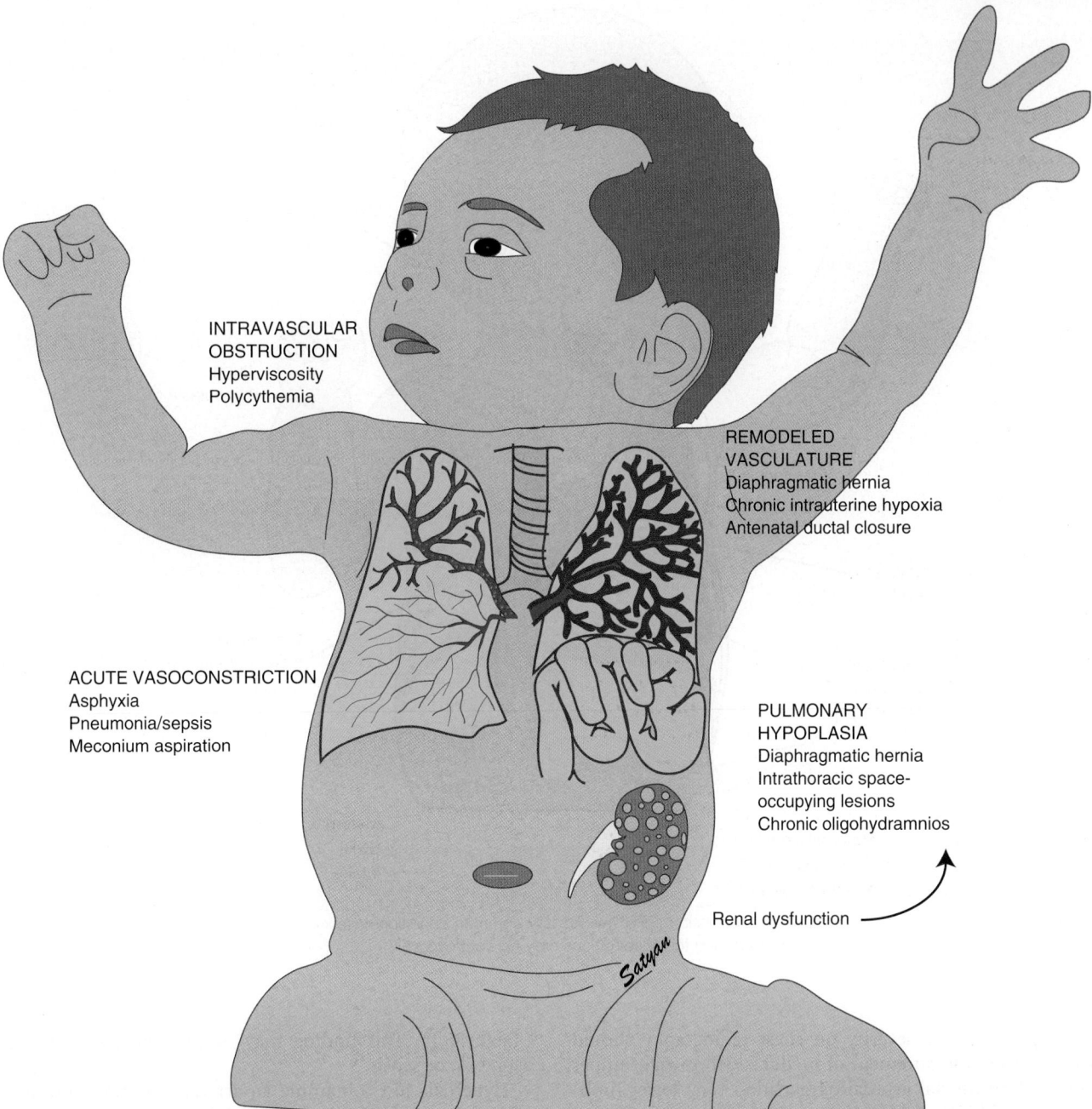

Fig. 56.2. Mechanisms of persistent pulmonary hypertension (PPHN)—Elevated pulmonary vascular resistance (PVR) is typically secondary to four mechanisms. Parenchymal lung disease (such as hyaline membrane disease [HMD]) resulting in acute alveolar hypoxia leads to pulmonary vasoconstriction. Intravascular obstruction secondary to hyperviscosity often due to polycythemia can lead to PPHN. Remodeled vasculature (maladaptation of pulmonary circulation) due to congenital diaphragmatic hernia, intrauterine closure of ductus arteriosus, and chronic intrauterine hypoxia leads to PPHN. Pulmonary hypoplasia secondary to intrathoracic space-occupying lesions such as congenital pulmonary malformations, diaphragmatic hernia, and oligohydramnios due to renal disease or chronic leakage leads to PPHN. Finally, infants born with malformations of alveolar and vascular development such as alveolar capillary dysplasia (ACD) with malalignment of pulmonary veins (MPV) have intractable and often lethal PPHN. (Copyright Satyan Lakshminrusimha.)

Preterm infants with fetal growth restriction and born after prolonged rupture of membranes are at higher risk for developing pulmonary hypertension.[65] Pulmonary vascular disease significantly increases morbidity and mortality in BPD.[66]

Labile hypoxemia is the hallmark of PPHN (Fig. 56.5). A newborn infant who is extremely labile, with frequent desaturation episodes and wide swings in arterial Po_2, without changes in ventilator settings, should suggest the possibility of PPHN. Lability can also occur in the face of significant parenchymal disease when V/Q mismatch is severe. Auscultation of the heart in babies with PPHN may reveal a single S_2, which can be loud, and a systolic murmur of tricuspid regurgitation. Chest x-ray findings may vary depending on the etiology of PPHN. Hypoxemia out of proportion to the degree of

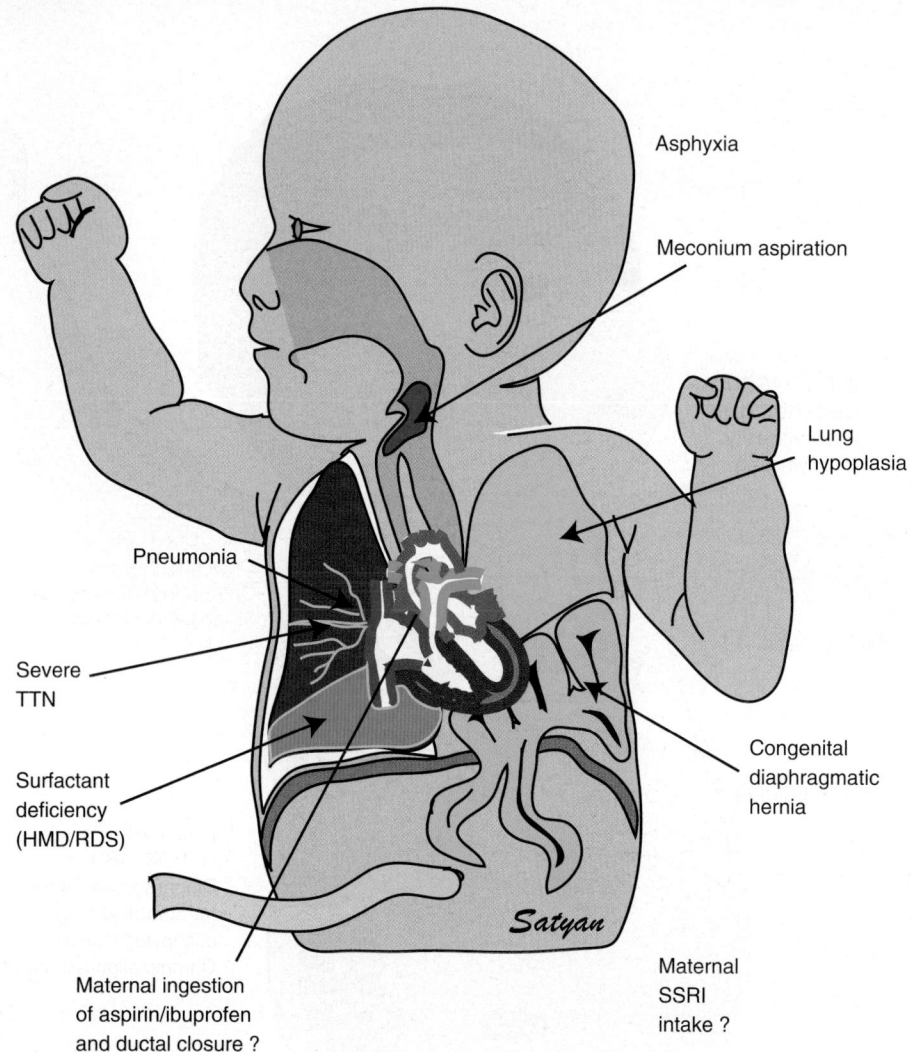

Fig. 56.3. Etiology of persistent pulmonary hypertension (PPHN)—clinically common conditions associated with PPHN (see text for details; the ? sign indicates that the association between PPHN and these conditions may be controversial).

parenchymal disease severity on chest radiography should suggest PPHN. Measurement of preductal (from right upper limb) and postductal arterial oxygenation (any lower limb) can confirm PPHN. A difference in arterial $Po_2 \geq 10$ to 20 mm Hg or oxygen saturation $\geq 5\%$ to 10% should be considered significant. Absence of a difference in oxygen tension does not exclude PPHN because shunting at the atrial level produces no ductal gradient and is probably the most common site of shunting. Thus in clinical practice, the gold standard in defining PPHN rests on the echocardiographic findings of right-to-left shunting of blood at the foramen ovale and/or the ductus arteriosus, as well as estimates of PAP. Doppler measurements of atrial and ductal level shunts provide essential information when managing a newborn with hypoxic respiratory failure. For example, left-to-right shunting at the foramen ovale and ductus arteriosus with marked hypoxemia suggests predominant intrapulmonary shunting, and interventions should be directed at optimizing lung inflation. Similarly, presence of right-to-left shunting at the ductal level and left-to-right shunting at the atrial level suggests PPHN with left ventricular dysfunction with some pulmonary venous hypertension

(Table 56.1). This finding may be associated with CDH,[67] asphyxia, or sepsis.[68]

Hyperoxia test (obtaining an arterial gas after 15 minutes of exposure to 100% oxygen) and/or hyperoxia-hyperventilation (hyperoxia and alkalosis to induce pulmonary vasodilation and improve PaO_2) is no longer widely practiced due to the known adverse effects of hyperoxia and alkalosis. PPHN can alternatively be confirmed by demonstrating elevated pulmonary pressures by an early echocardiogram, when available.

B-type natriuretic peptide (BNP) concentrations in plasma correspond well with echocardiographic findings of ventricular strain.[70] Reynolds et al.[71] suggested BNP as an early indicator of PPHN in the presence of respiratory illness in neonates without CHD. BNP has been proposed as a biomarker in PPHN, especially to assess efficacy of treatment and to predict rebound PPHN.[71,72] However, its value in the practical management of PPHN is presently unclear. Some centers obtain serial (monthly) echocardiograms with BNP levels to screen for pulmonary hypertension associated with BPD in preterm infants.

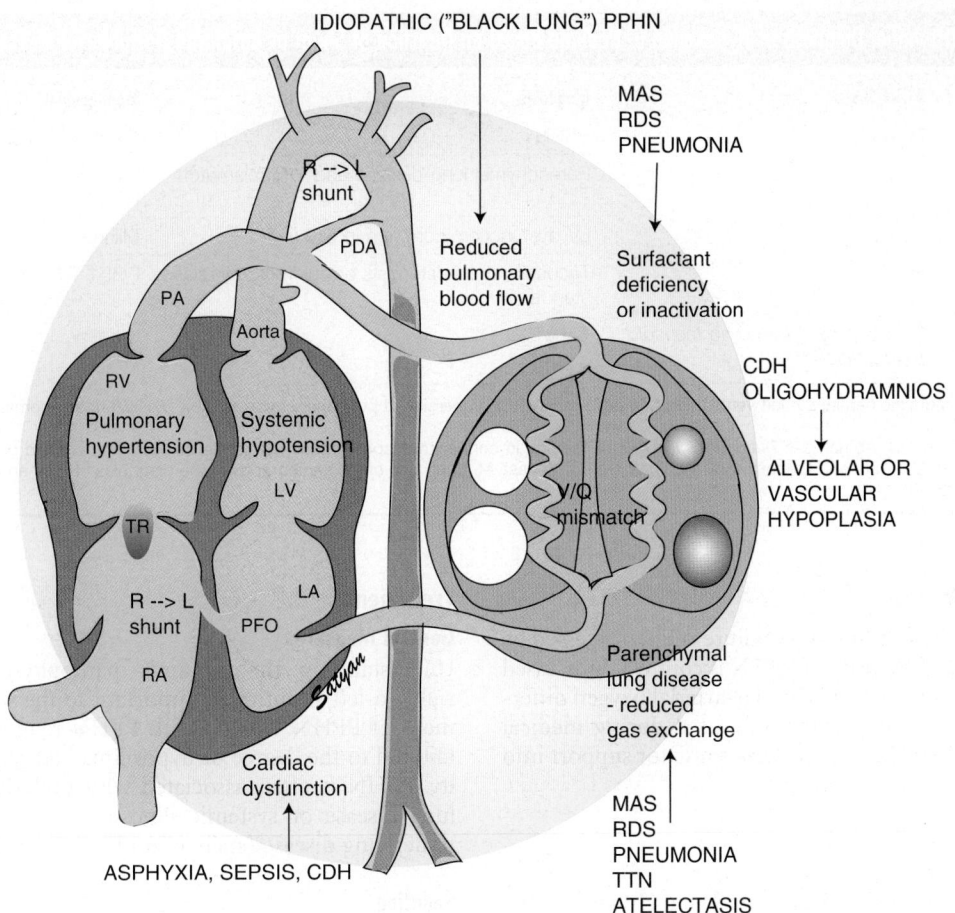

Fig. 56.4. Various etiologic factors causing persistent pulmonary hypertension (PPHN) and hemodynamic changes in PPHN/HRF. *CDH,* congenital diaphragmatic hernia; *HRF,* hypoxemic respiratory failure; *LA,* left atrium; *LV,* left ventricle; *MAS,* meconium aspiration syndrome; *PA,* pulmonary artery; *PDA,* patent ductus arteriosus; *PFO,* patent foramen ovale; *RA,* right atrium; *RDS,* respiratory distress syndrome; *RV,* right ventricle; *TTN,* transient tachypnea of the newborn; *TR,* tricuspid regurgitation. (Copyright Satyan Lakshminrusimha.)

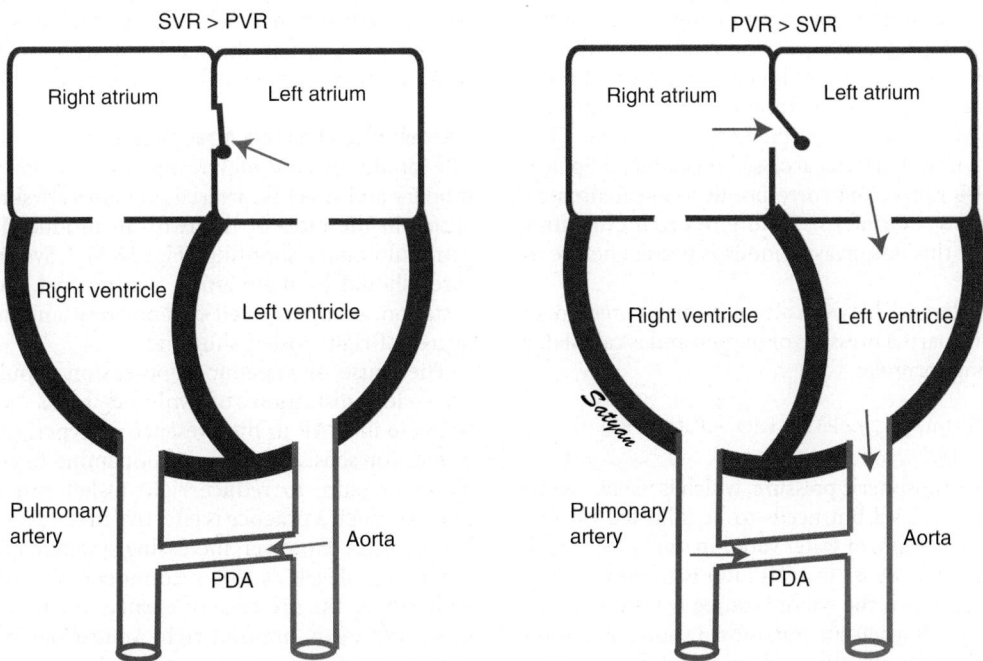

Fig. 56.5. Physiology of labile oxygenation in persistent pulmonary hypertension. When systemic vascular resistance (SVR) is higher than pulmonary vascular resistance (PVR), there is no right-to-left shunt. When PVR is close to or exceeds SVR, variable right-to-left shunt at foramen ovale and ductal levels results in labile hypoxemia. (Copyright Satyan Lakshminrusimha.)

TABLE 56.1   Differential Diagnosis of Hypoxemia in Neonate Based on Direction of Shunt at Atrial and Ductal Level on Echocardiography

Ductal Shunt	Atrial Shunt	Diagnosis	Management
R → L	R → L	PPHN	Oxygenation and inhaled NO
L → R	L → R	Parenchymal lung disease and V/Q mismatch	Lung recruitment, specific therapy NO may be beneficial
R → L	L → R	LV dysfunction (common in CDH)[67]	Milrinone
L → R	R → L	Tricuspid atresia/stenosis or pulmonic atresia/stenosis	PGE1 + Surgery
R → L (Large PA)	R → L (small LA and *no tricuspid regurgitation*)[69]	TAPVR	Surgery

CDH, congenital diaphragmatic hernia; *LV,* left ventricular; *NO,* nitric oxide; *PPHN,* persistent pulmonary hypertension; *TAPVR,* total anomalous pulmonary venous return.
Data from Kinsella JP, Ivy DD, Abman SH. Pulmonary vasodilator therapy in congenital diaphragmatic hernia: acute, late, and chronic pulmonary hypertension. Semin Perinatol. 2005;29:123-128; and Lakshminrusimha S, Wynn RJ, Youssfi M, et al. Use of CT angiography in the diagnosis of total anomalous venous return. J Perinatol. 2009;29:458-461.

Severity of PPHN

In the PICU, severity of respiratory failure is often assessed by P/F ratio (PaO_2/F_{IO2}). Severity of PPHN is commonly assessed by oxygenation index (OI) and alveolar-arterial oxygen difference ($AaDO_2$). OI is more commonly used during medical management of PPHN because it takes ventilator support into consideration and is calculated as:

$$OI = MAP \times F_{IO_2} \times 100/PaO_2$$

where *MAP* is the mean airway pressure in cm H_2O, F_{IO2} is the fraction of inspired oxygen, and PaO_2 is partial pressure of oxygen in arterial blood (in mm Hg). Hypoxemic respiratory failure can be classified into mild (OI ≤15), moderate (OI >15 to 25), severe (OI 25-40), and very severe (OI >40).[73] Disadvantages of OI include (1) it can be manipulated by changing F_{IO2} or MAP or based on the type of ventilator; (2) it requires arterial access; (3) the value may vary on the basis of the site of arterial access—right radial (preductal) versus umbilical or posterior tibial (postductal). More recently, oxygen saturation index (OSI = MAP × FiO_2 × 100/Preductal SpO_2) has been used in patients without arterial access.[74] If preductal SpO_2 is in the 70% to 99% range, OSI corresponds to approximately half of OI (OSI of 8 = OI of 16).[75] More research evaluating the clinical role for this noninvasive index is needed before its widespread use.

$AaDO_2$ is the difference between alveolar partial pressure of oxygen and arterial partial pressure of oxygen and is calculated using the following formula:

$$AaDO_2 = (Patm - P_{H_2O}) \times FiO_2 - PaO_2 - PaCO_2/RQ$$

where *Patm* is the atmospheric pressure, which is usually equal to 760 mm Hg at sea level but needs to be adjusted in high altitude. P_{H_2O} is the pressure of water vapor in one ATM, which is usually considered to be 47 mm Hg. RQ is the respiratory quotient and equal to 1 if the energy source is purely carbohydrate or equal to 0.8 when the nutritional source is a combination of carbohydrate, protein, and lipid. The disadvantage of $AaDO_2$ is that it does not take ventilator pressure into account but is useful in patients on noninvasive supplemental oxygen (eg, oxygen hood, mask, cannula).

Treatment

General Measures

Understanding the dynamic pathophysiology underlying right-to-left shunting is important to the successful management of PPHN. Infants with PPHN require supportive care tailored to the degree of hypoxemia and physiologic instability. PPHN is often associated with underlying parenchymal lung disease or systemic illness; therapy should target the underlying disease (such as antibiotics for sepsis).

Sedation

In PPHN, even mild stress can cause Po_2 to plummet within minutes. Accordingly, neonates and children with PPHN are often sensitive to activity and agitation. Minimal stimulation and sedation with narcotics such as fentanyl and morphine are commonly used to achieve this goal. Systemic hypotension due to excessive narcotic use should be avoided as it can worsen right-to-left shunts. Paralysis should be avoided, if possible, as it is associated with increased mortality.[76]

Systemic Blood Pressure Management

The lability in Pao_2 may result from the fact that when pulmonary and systemic arterial pressures are similar, small alterations in the ratio of the two can produce large changes in extrapulmonary shunting (Fig. 56.5).[77] Systemic blood pressures should be maintained at a normal range for age and gestation, as an increased systemic resistance may decrease the degree of right-to-left shunting.

The cause of systemic hypotension should be addressed first—administration of volume bolus in hypovolemia, decrease in MAP in the presence of hyperinflation, and antibiotics for sepsis. The use of dopamine to increase systemic blood pressure to reduce right-to-left shunt is a common practice. Such a practice is effective in the presence of systemic hypotension. However, increasing systemic pressure to supraphysiologic levels is not recommended.[68] In some patients with PPHN, the presence of a patent ductus arteriosus acts as a pop-off valve, limiting right ventricular preload and dysfunction. Increasing systemic blood pressure limits right-to-left shunt across the PDA and may add to right ventricular strain. In addition, the optimal therapy for reduced pulmonary blood flow is selective pulmonary vasodilation. If, instead, pulmonary blood flow is forced by elevating systemic pressure (and limiting right-to-left shunts) through the constricted pulmonary circuit, endothelial dysfunction due to increased shear stress[5] is likely to exacerbate PPHN. Dopamine (especially at >10 mcg/kg/min) is not selective to systemic vasculature and can increase pulmonary arterial pressure in PPHN.[9] Norepinephrine infusion is also effective in stabilizing systemic blood pressure and improving oxygenation in neonates with PPHN.[78] Vasopressin may be an effective therapeutic agent with some selectivity to systemic vasoconstriction.[79] Intractable catecholamine-resistant hypotension may require a dose of hydrocortisone to stabilize blood pressure in PPHN.

Temperature

Maintaining normothermia is an important supportive measure during management of PPHN. However, therapeutic hypothermia may be required in some patients with asphyxia, PPHN, and hypoxic-ischemic encephalopathy. Asphyxia is an important risk factor for PPHN, especially if associated with meconium aspiration syndrome.[80] The use of moderate hypothermia (33.5°C for 72 hours as recommended by AAP by either whole-body cooling or selective head cooling) does not result in a significant increase in the incidence of PPHN (25% vs. 22% with conventional management without hypothermia).[81] However, as compared with moderate hypothermia (33.5°C), deeper whole-body cooling to 32°C is associated with a tendency to increased PPHN (34% vs. 25%, $p = 0.06$), increased need for inhaled NO (34% vs. 24%, p-0.03), and ECMO (9 vs 4%, p-0.005)[82] and should be avoided. Case reports indicate that patients with hypoxemic respiratory disorders before the onset of cooling (especially those that need >50% inspired oxygen and/or iNO)[83] may experience exacerbation of PPHN with hypothermia and/or rewarming.[84] Mild therapeutic hypothermia by itself is not a cause for PPHN. However, infants predisposed to elevated PVR due to the presence of asphyxia and respiratory disease may not tolerate hypothermia-induced pulmonary vasoconstriction.[85] These findings emphasize the need for close monitoring of core temperature, systemic/pulmonary hemodynamics, and oxygenation during hypothermia and rewarming for asphyxia.

In many centers, confusion exists regarding optimal reporting of $PaCO_2$ during whole-body hypothermia. The laboratory may report $PaCO_2$ levels either at baby's temperature (known as the pH-stat method) or corrected to 37°C (alpha-stat method). Decreasing temperature increases the solubility of CO_2 in the blood and decreases $PaCO_2$ and may have implications for PPHN management with potential of overventilation or underventilation. We recommend the pH-stat method and reporting of $PaCO_2$ at actual (and not corrected) body temperature.[68]

Supportive Care

All patients with PPHN benefit from a core group of therapies that includes management of hypothermia, hypocalcemia, acidosis, hypoglycemia, and polycythemia. Surprisingly, there have been few prospective randomized trials of most of the supportive therapeutic modalities advocated for treatment of PPHN. Older therapies such as hyperventilation and alkalosis were introduced into clinical practice on the basis of animal studies or short-term studies that included very small numbers of patients and used physiologic response rather than patient

outcome as the end point. Only the newer therapies of inhaled nitric oxide (iNO) and extracorporeal membrane oxygenation (ECMO) have been rigorously evaluated in controlled clinical trials.

Optimal Pulmonary Hypertension During Acute PPHN Management

Animal studies documented the sensitivity of the pulmonary vasculature to both hypoxia and acidosis.[86] Short-term studies during cardiac catheterization showed reductions in PAP and elevation of oxygen tension following hyperventilation.[77,87] On the basis of these studies, hyperventilation became the mainstay of ventilation of term infants with hypoxic respiratory failure and PPHN. Subsequent observations have raised concern of impaired cerebral perfusion and neurosensory deafness at extremes of alkalosis.[88,89] Studies of infants with PPHN maintaining normal Pco_2 (40-60 mm Hg) indicate similar or better outcomes and with less chronic lung disease.[90,91] Many neonatologists have moved away from the practice of hyperventilation in neonates with PPHN. Animal studies have shown the beneficial effects of hyperventilation result from altered pH rather than from changes in Pco_2 or minute ventilation.[92,93] At one time alkali infusion to maintain alkaline pH to induce pulmonary vasodilation was a standard practice. In a National Institute of Child Health and Human Development observational study, the group treated with alkali had a greater chance of treatment with ECMO compared with those treated with hyperventilation and an increased rate of supplemental oxygen at 28 days.[76] Alkali infusion with bicarbonate increases CO_2 production, necessitating higher ventilator support. Lack of patient outcome data with both hyperventilation and alkali infusion and availability of better therapeutic options have led to less use of these outdated management strategies. We recommend maintaining pH >7.25, preferably 7.30 to 7.40 during the acute phase of PPHN.[68]

Oxygen

Oxygen is a specific and potent pulmonary vasodilator and increased oxygen tension is an important mediator of reduction in PVR at birth. Alveolar hypoxia and hypoxemia increase PVR and contribute to the pathophysiology of PPHN. However, exposure to hyperoxia may result in formation of oxygen free radicals and lead to lung injury. Recent evidence suggests that brief exposure to 100% oxygen in newborn lambs results in increased contractility of pulmonary arteries[94] and reduces response to inhaled NO.[95,96] The biological half-life of endogenous NO is related to the local concentration of superoxide anions.[97] Administration of intratracheal recombinant human superoxide dismutase (SOD, an antioxidant that breaks down superoxide anions) results in improved oxygenation in lambs with PPHN.[98,99] On the basis of these studies, it appears that avoiding hyperoxia is as important as avoiding hypoxia in the management of PPHN.

The optimal PaO_2 in the management of PPHN is not clear. Wung et al.[91] have suggested that gentle ventilation with avoidance of hyperoxia and hyperventilation results in good outcome in neonates with respiratory failure. Decreasing PaO_2 below 45 to 50 mm Hg results in increased PVR in newborn calves[86] and lambs.[96] In contrast, maintaining PaO_2 >70 to 80 mm Hg does not result in additional decrease in PVR in both control lambs and lambs with PPHN. In animal studies, hypoxemia results in pulmonary vasoconstriction. Normoxemia reduces PVR, but hyperoxemia does not result in additional pulmonary vasodilation. But to date, randomized studies comparing different PaO_2 targets have not been conducted in infants with PPHN. We recommend maintaining preductal oxygen saturations in the low to mid-90s with PaO_2 levels between 55 and 80 mm Hg during management of infants with PPHN.[68]

Surfactant

Exogenous surfactant therapy improved oxygenation and reduced the need for extracorporeal membrane oxygenation (ECMO) in neonates with PPHN secondary to parenchymal lung disease such as MAS.[100] A post-hoc analysis of the randomized trial of early nitric oxide use showed that early use of surfactant before randomization decreased the risk of death/ECMO, especially in infants with parenchymal lung disease.[101] Over the past decade, the use of surfactant in treating secondary PPHN and respiratory failure has increased and might have contributed to improved effectiveness of iNO with reduced need for ECMO. Surfactant inactivation and deficiency are observed in many neonatal respiratory disorders such as pneumonia, RDS, and MAS.

It is not clear if surfactant therapy is beneficial in infants with CDH. Animal studies show benefit,[102-104] but a review of the CDH registry did not support the use of surfactant.[105] We recommend administration of surfactant only in the presence of clinical, radiologic, or biochemical evidence of surfactant deficiency in CDH.

High-Frequency Ventilation

Many clinicians use high-frequency ventilation (HFV) to manage infants with PPHN. Considering the important role of parenchymal lung disease in specific disorders resulting in PPHN, adequate lung inflation and optimal ventilation are as essential as pharmacologic vasodilator therapy. In the case of inhaled vasodilators, optimal inflation and ventilation may be necessary for drug delivery.[106] Infants with PPHN from a variety of causes have been successfully treated with HFV.[107] High-frequency oscillatory ventilation (HFOV) decreases $Paco_2$ and increases oxygenation in infants with PPHN. HFOV may improve oxygenation through safer use of higher mean airway pressures to maintain lung volume and prevent atelectasis. Two studies have evaluated the effectiveness of HFV compared with conventional ventilation in rescuing infants with respiratory failure and PPHN from potential ECMO therapy.[108,109] Neither mode of ventilation was more effective in preventing ECMO in these infants. In clinical pilot studies using iNO, combination of HFOV and iNO resulted in the greatest improvement in oxygenation in some newborns who had severe PPHN complicated by diffuse parenchymal lung disease and underinflation.[110] A randomized controlled trial demonstrated that treatment with HFOV and iNO was often successful in patients who failed to respond to HFOV or iNO alone in severe PPHN, and the differences in responses were related to the specific disease associated with PPHN. Infants with RDS and MAS benefit most from a combination of HFOV and iNO therapy.[111,112] If a PIP of >28 cm H_2O or tidal volumes >6 mL/kg are required to maintain $PaCO_2$ <60 mm Hg on conventional ventilation, we recommend switching to high-frequency (jet or oscillator) ventilation.[68]

Nitric Oxide

The physiologic rationale for using iNO for treatment of PPHN[113,114] is based on its ability to achieve potent and selective pulmonary vasodilation without decreasing systemic vascular tone (Fig. 56.6). Once iNO enters the intravascular space, it combines with hemoglobin to form methemoglobin and does not exert a vasodilator effect on the systemic circulation. Inhaled NO also exerts a microselective effect and reduces V/Q mismatch. Being an inhaled vasodilator, NO enters only ventilated alveoli and redirects pulmonary blood by dilating adjacent pulmonary arterioles and reduces V/Q mismatch (see Fig. 56.6). Studies in newborn lambs have shown that prolonged administration of NO increased survival rates without

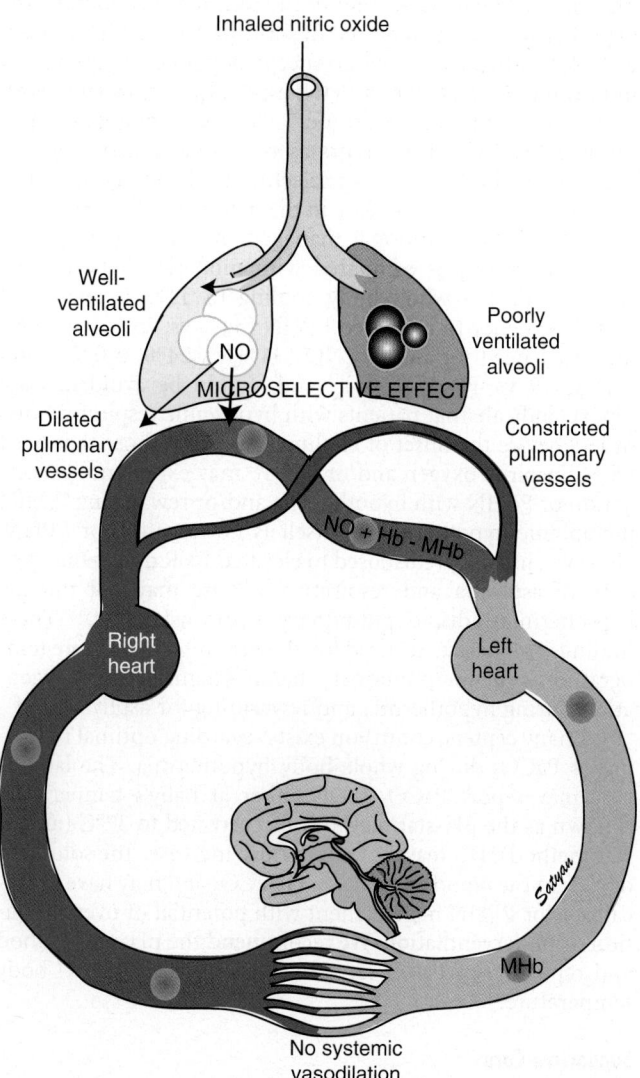

Fig. 56.6. Selective and microselective action of inhaled nitric oxide (NO). Inhaled NO is a selective dilator of the pulmonary circulation without any significant systemic vasodilation as it combines with hemoglobin to form methemoglobin (MHb). Because it is an inhaled vasodilator, it selectively goes to the well-ventilated alveoli. It improves blood flow to these alveoli and reduces V/Q mismatch (microselective effect). (Copyright Satyan Lakshminrusimha.)

increasing the incidence of acute lung injury in lambs with PPHN.[115]

Studies have shown that iNO therapy causes marked improvement in oxygenation in term newborns with PPHN.[116] Multicenter randomized clinical studies confirmed that iNO therapy reduces the need for ECMO in term neonates with hypoxemic respiratory failure.[117-119] Inhaled NO therapy is approved by the FDA for clinical use in term/near-term newborn infants (>34 weeks' gestation) with hypoxic respiratory failure and PPHN.

Initiation of iNO
There has been a debate regarding the timing of initiation and optimum starting dose of iNO in PPHN.[68] An OI of 25 is associated with a 50% risk of requiring ECMO or mortality[61] in the absence of specific pulmonary vasodilator therapy. Konduri et al. initially demonstrated that earlier initiation of iNO with an OI of 15 to 25 did not reduce the need for ECMO but may have a tendency to reduce the risk of progression to severe hypoxemic respiratory failure.[120,121] Post-hoc analysis of the same study suggested that the use of surfactant before randomization and enrollment (and use of iNO) at an OI of ≤20 was associated with reduced incidence of ECMO/death.[101] Such early initiation is associated with fewer hospital days, fewer days on ventilation, and fewer hours on ECMO.[122]

Dosing of iNO
Previous clinical trials suggested that the ideal starting dose for iNO is 20 parts per million (ppm) with the effective doses between 5 and 20 ppm.[120] Doses >20 ppm did not increase the efficacy and were associated with more adverse effects in these infants[118] such as elevated methemoglobin (>7%) and nitrogen dioxide (NO_2) (>3 ppm).[116] A dose of 5 ppm results in improved oxygenation in PPHN. A dose of 20 ppm results in improved oxygenation *and* results in the most optimal decrease in pulmonary to systemic arterial pressure ratio.[123] To summarize, we recommend initiation of iNO if OI is ~20 at a dose of **20** ppm. A complete response to iNO is defined as an increase in PaO_2/FiO_2 ratio of ≥**20** mm Hg. (20-20-20 rule for initiation of iNO, Fig. 56.7).[68] Methemoglobin levels are monitored at 2 hours and 8 hours after initiation of iNO and then once a day for the duration of iNO therapy. High inspired oxygen and high mean iNO dose are risk factors for elevated methemoglobin in term infants.[124]

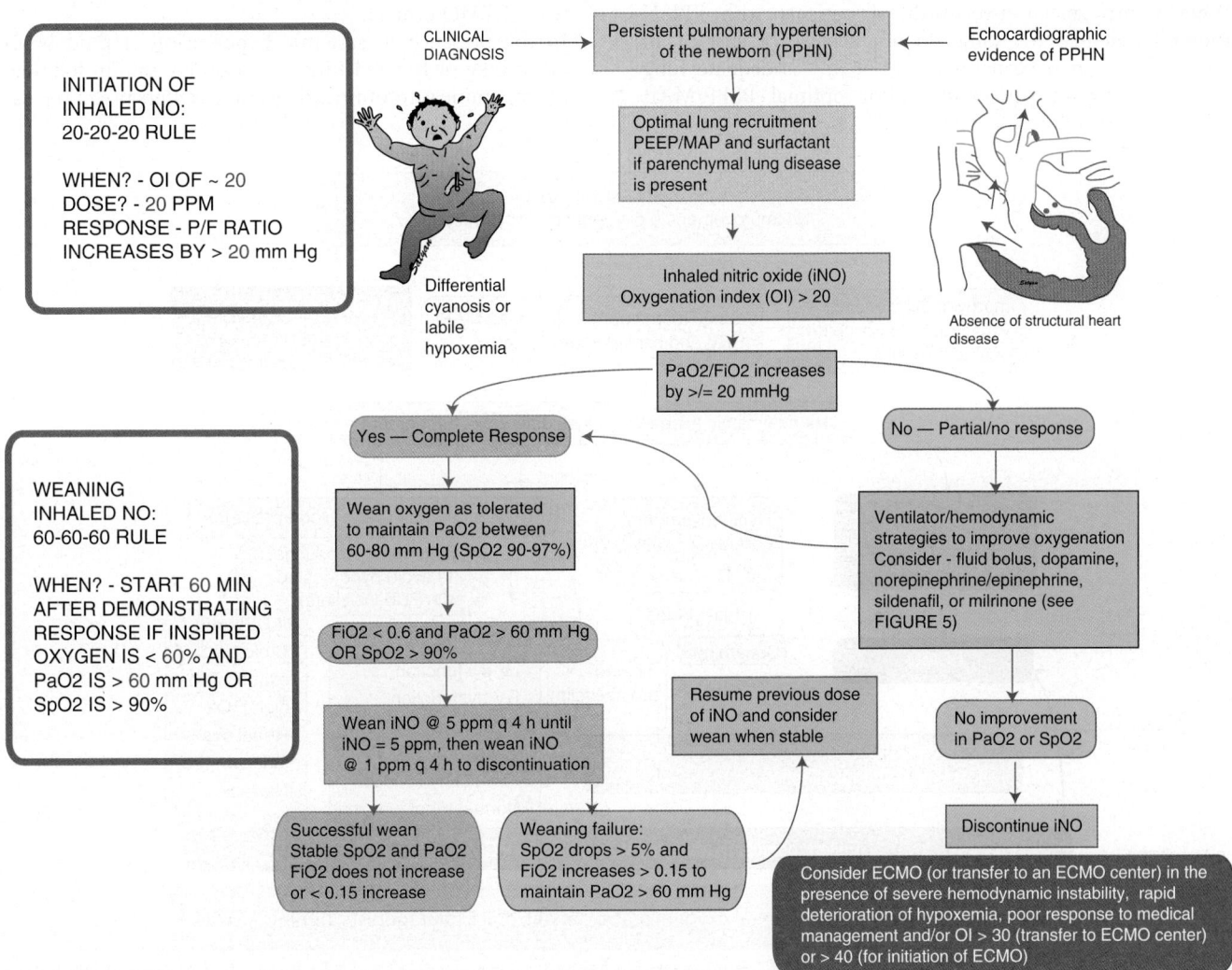

Fig. 56.7. Weaning protocol for inhaled nitric oxide in use at Women and Children's Hospital of Buffalo. (Copyright Satyan Lakshminrusimha.)

Weaning iNO

Due to rebound vasoconstriction and resultant pulmonary hypertension on abrupt withdrawal, iNO needs to be weaned gradually.[125] Weaning in steps from 20 ppm gradually over a period of time before its discontinuation has been shown to prevent the rebound effect.[126] If there is oxygenation response, inspired oxygen concentration is first weaned below **60**% and then iNO is weaned only if PaO_2 can be maintained $\geq$**60** mm Hg (or preductal SpO_2 $\geq$90%) for **60** minutes (60-60-60 rule of weaning iNO).[68] At our center, we wean iNO at a rate of 5 ppm every 4 hours. Once iNO dose is 5 ppm, gradual weaning by 1 ppm q 4 hours is performed (see Fig. 56.7). Continuing iNO in the absence of a response or not weaning iNO or extremely slow weaning can potentially lead to suppression of endogenous eNOS.[127,128]

Contraindications

Inhaled NO is contraindicated in the treatment of neonates known to be dependent on right-to-left shunting of blood (such as hypoplastic left heart syndrome). Also, patients with preexisting left ventricular dysfunction treated with iNO, even for short durations, have a high risk of pulmonary edema (package insert INOmax 2009).

Management of iNO-Resistant PPHN

While approximately two-thirds of patients with PPHN respond well to iNO, some do not achieve or sustain an improvement in oxygenation (Fig. 56.8).[118] Adequate lung recruitment (with surfactant and/or optimal PEEP/MAP,

preferably with high-frequency ventilation) is crucial to deliver iNO to its target site—the pulmonary vasculature.[9] A repeat echocardiogram to evaluate ventricular function and severity of PPHN (and to rule out cyanotic heart disease such as total anomalous pulmonary venous return [TAPVR] that may have been missed on the first echocardiogram[69]) is the next step. Management of systemic hypotension in PPHN is discussed previously. If lung recruitment and hemodynamic stability are achieved and iNO is still not effective, the patient should be managed in a tertiary center with access to ECMO. Our recommendations for management of iNO-resistant PPHN not responding to iNO in spite of lung recruitment with increased MAP and surfactant are outlined in Fig. 56.8 and summarized here.

a. Hemodynamic evaluation: A repeat echocardiogram should be performed to exclude structural heart disease, left ventricular dysfunction, and right ventricular dysfunction and to evaluate ventricular output. For example, if left ventricular dysfunction is associated with high left atrial pressures and a left-to-right shunt at the level of the oval foramen in the presence of a right-to-left shunt at the ductus arteriosus (Table 56.1), iNO is contraindicated and an inodilator such as milrinone should be initiated.

b. Rapid deterioration with hemodynamic instability should necessitate cannulation for ECMO (or immediate transfer to an ECMO center).

c. In the presence of systemic hypotension, a fluid bolus (10 mL/kg of lactated Ringer or isotonic saline) followed by dopamine is recommended. Some centers prefer the use

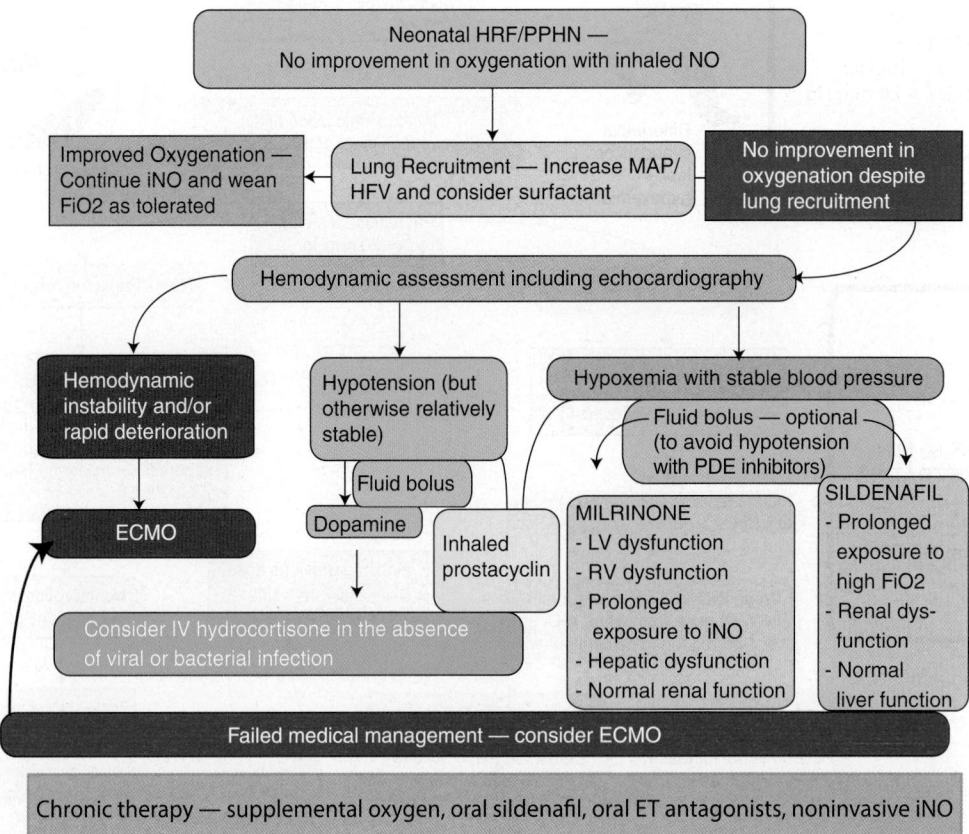

Fig. 56.8. Flowchart showing the author's suggested guidelines for management of iNO-resistant persistent pulmonary hypertension. (Copyright Satyan Lakshminrusimha.)

of norepinephrine or vasopressin. A cortisol level is drawn in these patients. If the levels are low relative to the infant's stress level and there is no evidence of infection (viral or bacterial), the authors recommend a stress dose of hydrocortisone.

d. If blood pressure is relatively stable but hypoxemia persists, consider the use of PDE inhibitors. Sildenafil is preferred if normal liver and ventricular function are present and may have added benefit in the context of prolonged hyperoxia. Ventricular dysfunction or hepatic compromise is an indication for milrinone rather than sildenafil as long as normal renal function is present. Chronic therapy (especially in the presence of CDH or BPD) involves PDE5 inhibitors followed by endothelin receptor antagonists and noninvasive iNO (Fig. 56.8).

Side Effects of iNO

Inhaled NO by itself is toxic at higher concentrations. Potential side effects include methemoglobinemia, pulmonary edema, and platelet dysfunction. NO reacts with superoxide anion to form peroxynitrite, which causes lipid peroxidation and other oxidative injury to cell membranes. NO_2 is even more toxic. Careful monitoring of both NO and NO_2 levels during administration is mandatory.

Long-Term Outcomes Following iNO in PPHN

Outcome of infants treated with iNO collectively supports both the efficacy and safety of this mode of treatment. Reports identify significant medical and neurodevelopmental sequelae of PPHN with or without iNO and point out the necessity for coordinated multidisciplinary follow-up for these infants. The overall rate of neurodevelopmental handicap in infants treated with NO was 46%, with 25% mildly affected and 21% severely affected at age 1 year in one study.[129] In another study, mild and severe neurodevelopmental handicaps were 14% and 12% at age 1 year and 9% and 12% at age 2 years.[130] In these studies sensorineural hearing loss was present in 6% to 19% of infants with PPHN treated with iNO. No difference was noted between control and treatment groups for these outcomes. Published reports on the use of iNO in ECMO centers have not substantiated early concerns that iNO would adversely affect outcome by delaying ECMO utilization. Inhaled NO treatment may play an important role in stabilizing patients before ECMO is initiated, thus improving the chances of ECMO cannulation without further clinical deterioration. The Committee on the Fetus and Newborn, American Academy of Pediatrics, has suggested that iNO use be limited to tertiary care centers where ECMO is available.[131] In non-ECMO centers, a system should be in place to continue iNO during transport even if a response occurs, as not all physiologic responders avoid ECMO. For the same reason, the combination of HFOV and iNO should be used cautiously in non-ECMO centers.

Prostaglandin E1 (PGE1)

Aerosolized prostaglandin E1 (Alprostadil) has been used to treat pulmonary hypertension in adults. In a small pilot phase I-II study, Sood et al.[132,133] suggested that inhaled PGE1 was a safe and selective pulmonary vasodilator in hypoxemic respiratory failure with or without use of iNO. PGE1 solution for aerosolization is prepared from Alprostadil (Prostin VR 500, Pfizer, New York, New York, USA) and administered as a continuous nebulization through a MiniHeart low-flow jet nebulizer (WestMed Inc., Tucson, Arizona, USA) at 150 to 300 ng/kg/min diluted in saline to provide 4 mL/hr.[133]

IV PGE1 has also been used in patients with CDH in combination with iNO to promote pulmonary vasodilation and to maintain ductal patency and reduce right ventricular afterload.[134]

Inhaled Prostacyclin

Prostacyclin administered intravenously is a common therapy in adults with pulmonary arterial hypertension. Inhaled PGI_2 has been used in PPHN resistant to iNO at a dose of 50 ng/kg/min.[135] The IV formulation Flolan (Glaxo-Wellcome, Middlesex, UK) is dissolved in 20 mL of manufacturer's diluent (a glycine buffer, pH = 10). Fresh solution is added to the nebulization chamber every 4 hours.[135] The effect of such alkaline pH on neonatal respiratory tract is not known.

Phosphodiesterase Inhibitors
Sildenafil (PDE5 Inhibitor)

Studies have shown that cGMP is decreased in response to exogenous NO in animal models of PPHN,[136] and increased clearance of cGMP by one or more phosphodiesterases has been proposed as one of the causes.[137] Sildenafil acts by inhibiting cGMP-specific phosphodiesterase type 5 (PDE5), an enzyme that promotes degradation of cGMP. The activity of this enzyme is significantly increased following hyperoxic ventilation in lambs with PPHN.[138,139] Studies have shown that oral sildenafil (dose range 1–2 mg/kg every 6 hours) improves oxygenation and reduces mortality in centers limited by nonavailability of iNO and ECMO.[140,141]

IV sildenafil was shown to be effective in improving oxygenation in patients with PPHN with and without prior exposure to iNO.[142] The use of IV sildenafil should be restricted to refractory cases at a center with ECMO backup due to the potential risk of systemic hypotension[143] and pulmonary hemorrhage, presumably due to sudden reversal of ductal shunt.[144] On the basis of pharmacokinetic data in neonates with PPHN, IV sildenafil is administered as a load of 0.42 mg/kg over 3 hours (0.14 mg/kg/hour) followed by 1.6 mg/kg/day as a continuous maintenance infusion (0.07 mg/kg/hour).

Milrinone (PDE3 Inhibitor)

Milrinone inhibits PDE3 and increases concentration of cAMP in pulmonary and systemic arterial smooth muscle and in cardiac muscle. Milrinone relaxes pulmonary arteries in the fetal lamb model of PPHN.[145] Infants with PPHN refractory to iNO therapy have responded to IV milrinone in three case series[146-148] and appears to be particularly useful in the presence of ventricular dysfunction.[149,150] A loading dose (50 mcg/kg over 30-60 minutes) followed by a maintenance dose (0.33 mcg/kg/min and escalated to 0.66 and then to 1 mcg/kg/min based on response) is commonly used. The loading dose is not recommended in the presence of systemic hypotension and in premature neonates.[149] As with any systemic vasodilator, hypotension is a clinical concern and blood pressure needs to be closely monitored. A fluid bolus (10 mL/kg of lactated Ringer solution) before loading dose may decrease the risk of hypotension. In addition, one case series described an increased incidence of intracranial hemorrhage with the use of milrinone in PPHN.[147] Milrinone may be the pulmonary vasodilator of choice in the presence of PPHN with left ventricular dysfunction (Fig. 56.5).

Bosentan (Endothelin-1 Receptor Blocker)

Endothelin receptor antagonists are beneficial and well tolerated in adult patients with pulmonary arterial hypertension.[151] Initial reports suggested that bosentan was an effective drug in the management of PPHN.[152] The results of a multicenter, randomized, double-blind, placebo-controlled exploratory trial of bosentan in PPHN were recently reported. Bosentan (2 mg/kg/dose twice daily) did not show any additive effect on the top of iNO in term neonates with PPHN.[153] However, endothelin receptor antagonists may have a role in the management of chronic pulmonary hypertension associated with BPD or CDH.

Steroids

Antenatal betamethasone attenuated oxidative stress and improved in vitro response to vasodilators in a fetal lamb model of pulmonary hypertension.[154] Glucocorticoids have been found to improve oxygenation and attenuate the pulmonary hypertensive response in animal models of meconium aspiration syndrome, which is a common cause of PPHN.[155] Steroids have been reported to decrease hospital stay and duration of oxygen use in infants with meconium aspiration.[156,157] It is proposed that hydrocortisone attenuates ROS production by induction of superoxide dismutase and normalization of PDE5 activity.[158] Looking at the evidence this far, we do not recommend routine use of steroids in patients with PPHN, especially if there is suspicion of viral or bacterial sepsis. Anecdotal use of stress dose hydrocortisone in iNO-resistant PPHN associated with systemic hypotension in our unit has resulted in stabilization of systemic blood pressure and improved oxygenation possibly secondary to hemodynamic stability and PDE5 inhibitory effects.[159,160]

Extracorporeal Membrane Oxygenation

Extracorporeal membrane oxygenation (ECMO) is a technique of modified cardiopulmonary bypass used over a prolonged period to support heart and lung function. If the heart and lungs cannot support the newborn, they can be bypassed with ECMO. Several randomized trials have indicated improved survival of infants supported with ECMO. In a large prospective trial conducted in the United Kingdom, 121 infants with severe respiratory failure were randomized to ECMO or conventional management.[161] Survival in the ECMO-treated patients was significantly greater than in the control group (68% vs. 41%). Neurologic outcome was similar among survivors of either treatment arm, indicating ECMO likely did not contribute to morbidity in this group of critically ill infants. ECMO has been shown to be both clinically[161] and economically[162] justifiable for mature newborn infants with severe respiratory failure. ECMO is not a specific treatment for any disease but rather a method of supportive treatment, in which the patient is kept alive while the lungs and their vasculature recover. As newer treatment modalities including HFOV, surfactant therapy, and NO have become available for treatment of hypoxemic respiratory failure, ECMO use in newborns has decreased considerably.[163,164] Because of serious inherent risks, such as systemic and intracranial hemorrhage, for infants with PPHN the procedure presently is reserved for newborn infants with reversible pulmonary disease in whom alternative therapies have failed. However, ECMO should be initiated before the infant is moribund. The technical details of ECMO including appropriate

indications for venovenous (VV) versus venoarterial (VA) in PPHN are provided in Chapter 59.

The use of neonatal ECMO has declined from a peak of 1516 cases per year in 1992 to 750 to 865 cases/year from 2008 to 2012. This decline is likely due to improvements in both perinatal care and availability of advanced therapies for neonatal hypoxemic respiratory failure including high-frequency ventilators, surfactant, and iNO.[165] In newborns with PPHN, mechanical ventilation with oxygen and iNO is the initial treatment, but prolongation of iNO with high oxygen levels may induce chronic lung disease and extend the length of stay in the NICU.[166] On the other hand, initiating ECMO too early may expose newborns to major vessel cannulation and systemic anticoagulation.[167] General accepted criteria to start ECMO is persistent hypoxemia (with an OI of >40 or AaDO$_2$ >600 in spite of aggressive medical management of PPHN with mechanical ventilation and iNO) and the presence of hemodynamic instability (Fig. 57.1).

Future Therapies

Newer experimental therapies such as antioxidants, Rho-kinase inhibitors, L-citrulline, and inhaled prostacyclin analogs are under investigation. While the need for ECMO for neonates with PPHN is decreasing, this syndrome continues to be associated with high mortality and morbidity emphasizing the need for novel treatment strategies to improve outcome in PPHN.

Pulmonary Arterial Hypertension in Children
Introduction

After the newborn period, pulmonary arterial hypertension (PAH) in children is an uncommon disease characterized by elevated PAP either at rest or during exercise. Progressive obliteration of the pulmonary vascular bed with increased PVR is the hallmark of PAH and is associated with substantial morbidity and mortality. The updated classification of pulmonary hypertension (PH) (Table 56.2) has identified five groups of disorders that cause PH.[168] The groups share similar pathologic and hemodynamic characteristics and therapeutic approaches in the management of PAH. This classification represents a comprehensive, common classification for both children and adults. Pulmonary arterial hypertension can be idiopathic (IPAH) or heritable (HPAH) or associated with many other conditions listed in Table 56.2. Group 3 encompasses developmental lung disorders, a large group of diseases unique to infants and children, who go on to develop significant lung disease, hypoxic respiratory failure, and pulmonary hypertension (see Table 56.2, section 3.7). With an estimated prevalence of 15 to 50 cases per 1 million adults, PAH is a rare disease. PAH is even less common in children, with an estimated prevalence of <10 cases per 1 million children. Five-year survival from diagnosis from a recent observational study in the United States was 74% ± 6%, with no significant difference between the idiopathic PAH/heritable PAH (n = 122, 75% ± 7%) and PAH associated with congenital heart disease (n = 77, 71% ± 13%) cohorts.[169]

In a global perspective study designed to collect information on etiologies and outcomes with confirmed PAH (defined as pulmonary arterial pressures of ≥25 mm Hg; pulmonary capillary wedge pressure of ≤12 mm Hg; and pulmonary vascular resistance index ≥3 WU/m^2) from 19 countries over 2 years, 57% (182/317) had idiopathic or familial

TABLE 56.2   Updated Classification of Pulmonary Hypertension[168]

1. Pulmonary arterial hypertension (PAH)
   - 1.1 Idiopathic PAH
   - 1.2 Heritable PAH (1.2.1-BMPR2; 1.2.2-ALK-1, ENG, SMAD9, CAV1, KCNK3; 1.2.3-Unknown)
   - 1.3 Drug and toxin induced
   - 1.4 Associated with connective tissue disease (1.4.1), HIV infection (1.4.2), portal hypertension (1.4.3), congenital heart diseases (1.4.4), and schistosomiasis (1.4.5)
   - 1'. Pulmonary venoocclusive disease and/or pulmonary capillary hemangiomatosis
   - 1". *Persistent pulmonary hypertension of the newborn (PPHN)*

2. Pulmonary hypertension due to left heart disease
   - 2.1 Left ventricular systolic dysfunction
   - 2.2 Left ventricular diastolic dysfunction
   - 2.3 Valvular disease
   - 2.4 Congenital/acquired left heart inflow/outflow tract obstruction and congenital cardiomyopathies

3. Pulmonary hypertension due to lung diseases and/or hypoxia
   - 3.1 Chronic obstructive pulmonary disease
   - 3.2 Interstitial lung disease
   - 3.3 Other pulmonary diseases with mixed restrictive and obstructive pattern
   - 3.4 Sleep-disordered breathing
   - 3.5 Alveolar hypoventilation disorders
   - 3.6 Chronic exposure to high altitude
   - 3.7 Developmental lung diseases [CDH, BPD, ACD, ACD with misalignment of pulmonary veins, lung hypoplasia, surfactant protein (SP) abnormalities—SPB deficiency, SPC deficiency, ATP-binding cassette A3 mutation, thyroid transcription factor 1/Nkx2.1 homeobox mutation, pulmonary interstitial glycogenosis, pulmonary alveolar proteinosis, pulmonary lymphangiectasia]

4. Chronic thromboembolic pulmonary hypertension

5. Pulmonary hypertension with unclear multifactorial mechanisms
   - 5.1 Hematologic disorders: chronic hemolytic anemia, myeloproliferative disorders, splenectomy
   - 5.2 Systemic disorders: sarcoidosis, pulmonary histiocytosis
   - 5.3 Metabolic disorders: glycogen storage disease, Gaucher disease, thyroid disorders
   - 5.4 Others: tumoral obstruction, fibrosing mediastinitis, chronic renal failure, segmental PH

ACD, alveolar capillary dysplasia; *BMPR2*, bone morphogenetic protein receptor type II; *BPD*, bronchopulmonary dysplasia; *CAV1*, caveolin-1; *CDH*, congenital diaphragmatic hernia; *ENG*, endoglin; *HIV*, human immunodeficiency virus; *PH*, pulmonary hypertensiion; *SPB*, surfactant protein B; *SPC*, surfactant protein C.
Simonneau G, Gatzoulis MA, Adatia I, et al. Updated clinical classification of pulmonary hypertension. J Am Coll Cardiol. 2013;62(suppl 25):D34-41.

PAH. Forty-three percent (145) had PAH associated with other disorders, of which 115 had congenital heart disease (CHD). Forty-two patients (12%) had PAH associated with respiratory disease or hypoxemia, with bronchopulmonary dysplasia (BPD) being the most frequent. Chromosomal anomalies, mainly trisomy 21, were reported in 47 (13% of) patients. Median age at diagnosis was 7 years (IQR 3-12) and 59% (268 of 456) were female. Despite severe pulmonary hypertension, 64% of these children had functional class of I or II, consistent with preserved right ventricular function.[170]

Molecular Mechanisms and Pathology of PAH

PAH is a syndrome resulting from restricted flow through the pulmonary arterial circulation, leading to pathologic increase in PVR and ultimately to right heart failure. The disease spectrum varies from mild to severe PAH, as infants and children present in various stages of PAH with symptoms related to decompensation of right ventricular function. However, the pathology appears to be restricted to the pulmonary vasculature itself. The typical pathology is mostly a progressive panvasculopathy predominantly affecting the small pulmonary arteries characterized by a variety of arterial abnormalities, including endothelial cell (EC) hyperplasia, medial hypertrophy, adventitial proliferation, thrombosis in situ, varying degree of inflammation, and plexiform arteriopathy, depending on the degree of progression of the vessel pathology. Pulmonary vascular remodeling involves structural changes in the normal architecture of the walls of PA, occurring as a primary response to injury, such as hypoxia or toxin, within the resistance PAs of the lung. The developmental phase of vascular maturation influences the degree and progression of vessel changes and also the symptomatology of PAH. A common feature of all forms of pulmonary hypertensive remodeling is the appearance of a layer of smooth muscle cells (SMC) in small, peripheral, normally nonmuscular arteries, especially the precapillary vessels, wherein the intermediate cells inside the internal elastic lamina proliferate and differentiate into SMCs. However, in vessels that lack elastic lamina (20- to 30-μ diameter), pericytes and surrounding interstitial fibroblasts contribute to the process of muscularization. In the presence of alveolar hypoxia, as in hypoxic lung disease or high altitudes, distal neomuscularization occurs, leading to formation of inner muscular tubes characteristic of hypoxia-induced PH in humans.[171,172] Increased muscularization of muscular arteries occurs in more proximal arteries, in response to endothelial damage or release of factors from endothelial cells. Activation of elastases disrupts the elastic lamina of the vessel and promotes proliferation of SMCs and deposition of extracellular matrix. Endothelial injury along with increased flow results in neointimal formation, a layer of cells between the endothelium and the internal lamina, contributing significantly to PVR. Neointimal formation is more common in congenital heart disease. It comprises cells such as myofibroblasts that lack the mature markers of SMC (such as myosin) and endothelial markers (such as CD31, CD34, or factor VIII). It has been postulated that these cells may be from the media or the adventitial fibroblasts migrating to the subendothelial space.[173] An overview of the pathologic processes occurring in the pulmonary vasculature is depicted in Fig. 56.9A.

The endothelial cell is central to the pathogenesis of PAH, translating the hemodynamic responses to histopathologic changes in the vessel wall, through a complex set of signaling mechanisms, which are still being studied. The initiating injury of the endothelial cell in PH may be hypoxia, increased flow (as in congenital heart disease), toxins, or drugs on the background of genetic susceptibility. Irrespective of the initiating process, secreted vasoactive factors direct the vascular remodeling through cell proliferation, thrombosis, and vasoconstriction. Pulmonary arterial endothelial cells from patients with IPAH produce decreased amounts of NO, a suppressor of SMC proliferation.[174] In the chronically hypoxic rat model of PH, the labeling index for endothelial cells increased threefold (measured by 3H-thymidine uptake in vivo) in main pulmonary arteries within 24 hours, and an increase in replicating endothelial cells was seen in small muscular arteries at 7 and 10 days.[175] Thus endothelial cell proliferation appears to contribute to intimal thickening, as do edema and thickening

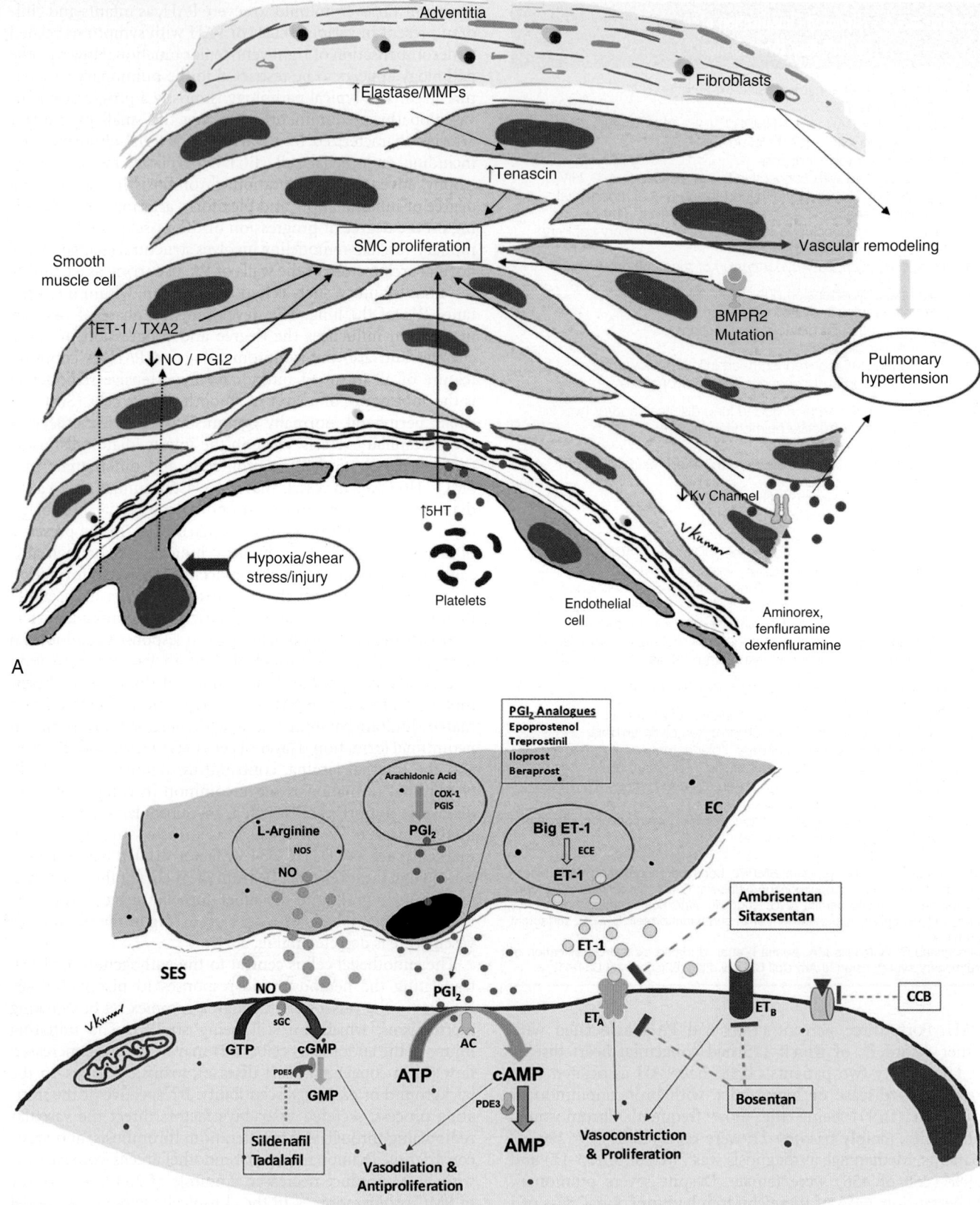

Fig. 56.9. (A) Schematic depicting the pathways involved in the pathogenesis of pulmonary arterial hypertension in children. (B) Schematic diagram of vascular mediators of the lung, their mechanism of action, interaction between the endothelial cell and the smooth muscle cell in the pulmonary vasculature and its relationship to drugs used in the management of pediatric pulmonary hypertension. The three predominant signaling pathways are shown—nitric oxide-GMP system, PGI2-cAMP system, and the endothelin-1 pathway. *AC,* adenylate cyclase; *BMPR2,* bone morphogenetic protein receptor type 2; *CCB,* calcium channel blocker; *cGMP,* cyclin GMP; *COX1,* cyclo-oxygenase type 1; *EC,* endothelial cell; *ECE,* endothelin converting enzyme; *ET-1,* endothelin-1; ET_A, endothelin receptor type A; ET_B, endothelin receptor type B; *5 HT,* 5 hydroxytryptamine; *Kv Channel,* voltage-gated potassium channel; *MMPs,* matrix metalloproteinases; *NO,* nitric oxide; *NOS,* nitric oxide synthase; *PDE3,* phosphodiesterase type 3; *PDE5,* phosphodiesterase type 5; *PGIS,* prostaglandin synthase; PGI_2, prostacyclin; *SES,* subendothelial space; *sGC,* soluble guanylyl cyclase; *SMC,* smooth muscle cell; *TXA2,* thromboxane A2. See text for details. (Copyright Vasanth H. S. Kumar.)

of the endothelial basement membrane.[176] In response to the stimuli (hypoxia, increased shear stress, injury), endothelial cells in the hypertensive pulmonary circulation produce more of factors such as ET-1, angiopoietin-2 (Ang-2), and thromboxane A_2 (TXA$_2$), which induce vasoconstriction and cell proliferation and less of mediators such as NO and prostacyclin (PGI$_2$), that are vasodilators and antiproliferative. The net effect of this imbalance in mediators is maintenance of the vessel wall in the remodeled hypertensive state. Hypertrophy of smooth muscle cells makes a greater contribution than hyperplasia in the larger-sized more proximal vessels, whereas hyperplasia is more prevalent than hypertrophy in the smaller resistance arteries.[176] Alterations in endothelial coagulation and fibrinolytic factors also contribute to the pathogenesis of idiopathic and thromboembolic pulmonary hypertension. In situ thrombosis in small pulmonary arteries is a feature of patients with idiopathic pulmonary hypertension. In addition, anticoagulant therapy with warfarin improves the survival of these patients. Thrombin disrupts the endothelial barrier, causing leak of proteins and interstitial edema, and promotes growth and differentiation of fibroblasts. Recent evidence supports an active role for the adventitial fibroblast in the remodeling of the pulmonary circulation during the development of pulmonary hypertension.[177]

Various stimuli can initiate vasoconstriction of the vessels of the lung in individuals with PH, predisposing these reactive vessels for subsequent development of characteristic vascular lesions.[172] The vascular endothelium is regarded as an important source of locally active mediators that contributes to the control of vasomotor tone. Thromboxane/PGI$_2$ and NO/ET-1 system are two of the important balances that control pulmonary vasomotor tone.

Endothelin-1 (ET-1) is a potent vasoconstrictor and stimulates pulmonary artery smooth muscle cell (PASMC) proliferation (Fig. 56.9B). Plasma levels of ET-1 are increased in PAH and correlate with severity of PAH and prognosis.[178] Of the two ET-1 receptors, ET$_A$ receptors, expressed mainly in the smooth muscle, mediate vasoconstriction and cell proliferation, whereas ET$_B$ receptors, expressed mainly in the endothelial cells, are important for clearance of ET-1 and release of NO and PGI$_2$.[28,179] In experimental studies of hypoxia-induced[180] and monocrotaline-induced PH,[181] chronic ET receptor blockade lowered PAP and the incidence of vascular and pulmonary injury and improved NO-mediated pulmonary vasodilation. Studies with L-ω-nitroarginine methyl ester [L-NAME]–induced PH suggest that ET-1 is linked to the dysfunction of the L-arginine/NO pathway[182] because ET$_A$ selective[183] but not combined ET blockade[184] improves endothelial function. Thus selective inhibition of ET$_A$ receptors improves the endothelial L-arginine/NO pathway, which agrees with observations in humans.[185] ET-1 expression in pulmonary arteries is increased in patients with primary and secondary PH.[186,187] ET-1 increases at high altitudes in mountaineers and correlates with pulmonary pressures and oxygen tension.[188] ET increases even more in mountaineers prone to high-altitude pulmonary edema.[189] Increased local production[187] and elevated circulating levels of endothelin[190] have been demonstrated in patients with Eisenmenger syndrome,[191] IPAH,[192] and in PAH associated with CHD.[193]

Prostacyclin (PGI$_2$) is a powerful vasodilator and an inhibitor of platelet aggregation, whereas thromboxane A_2 (TXA2) is a vasoconstrictor and induces platelet aggregation leading to microvascular thrombus formation and hence vascular injury. As thromboxane A_2 and PGI$_2$ have opposing effects on platelet aggregation and pulmonary vascular smooth muscle, an imbalance in their biosynthesis could contribute to the progressive increase in PVR seen in older untreated patients with pulmonary hypertension from congenital heart disease.[194] Decreased urinary excretion of 2, 3-dinor-6-keto prostaglandin $F_{1\alpha}$, a metabolite of PGI$_2$, occurs in patients with IPAH.[195] In PAH, the balance between these two molecules is shifted toward TXA2,[195] favoring thrombosis, proliferation, and vasoconstriction. A decrease in expression of the enzyme PGI$_2$ synthase (PGI$_2$-S) in the lung may be an important manifestation of pulmonary endothelial dysfunction in severe PH. Prostacyclin synthase is decreased in small- and medium-sized pulmonary arteries, and the loss of expression of PGI$_2$-S may represent one of the phenotypic alterations present in the pulmonary endothelial cells in severe PAH.[196] Pulmonary PGI$_2$-S overexpression in transgenic mice protects against development of hypoxic pulmonary hypertension.[197] PGI$_2$-S may play a major role in modifying the pulmonary vascular response to injury. Intratracheal transfer of human PGI$_2$-S gene has been shown to augment pulmonary prostacyclin synthesis, ameliorate MCT-induced pulmonary hypertension, and improve survival in MCT rats.[198]

Potassium (K$^+$) channels play an important part in smooth muscle cell electrophysiology, which has implications for the development of PAH. The inhibition of voltage-gated K$^+$ (Kv) channels results in an accumulation of K$^+$ ions within the cell, depolarizing the cell and activating the voltage-gated, L-type calcium channel.[199] Intracellular calcium initiates a number of signaling cascades in the cell, leading to vasoconstriction and possibly initiating cell proliferation. Expression array analysis has demonstrated a depletion of Kv1.5 channels in pulmonary tissue derived from PAH patients.[200] It is currently unknown if these Kv channels are congenital or acquired, yet a number of polymorphisms in the Kv1.5 channel gene have been described,[201] which may suggest a genetic predisposition to channel depletion. The use of anorexic agents like aminorex, fenfluramine, and dexfenfluramine is associated with the development of PAH,[202] and these agents are thought to act by blocking the Kv channel.[203] Kv2.1 is inhibited by dexfenfluramine, a weight-loss drug that is associated with the development of PAH.[203] Anorexigen-induced Kv channel inhibition and membrane depolarization can contribute to pulmonary vasoconstriction.[204,205] Fenfluramine reduces the Kv1.5 mRNA levels by 50% in PASMCs from normotensive patients,[206] suggesting that expression of Kv channels may play an important role in anorexigen-induced PAH. Inhibition of Kv currents in pulmonary SMCs may be regulated by serotonin, thromboxane, and nitric oxide.[176] Furthermore, BMP signaling can regulate Kv receptor expression,[207] suggesting Kv channels may represent a common pathway of regulation in pathogenesis of PAH.

An association between human immunodeficiency virus (HIV) infection and pulmonary hypertension has been noted, with a rate 6 to 12 times higher than the general population.[208] Mechanisms of disease include infection of the smooth muscle with dysregulation of proliferation, imbalance of vascular mitogens in response to systemic HIV infection, and endothelial cell injury precipitated by HIV-infected cells.[209] The direct actions of HIV-encoded proteins have also been implicated in PAH.[210] It has been thought that human herpes virus 8 (HHV-8), the causative agent for Kaposi sarcoma and an opportunistic pathogen associated with HIV, may play a role in the development of PAH, but the link has not been consistently validated.[211,212] Heightened circulating levels of cytokines and their receptors have been demonstrated in IPAH patients, including fractalkine, MCP-1, and GM-CSF.[213] Loss of BMPR2 induces IL-6, a cytokine that can cause severe PVD in rodents in association with SMC proliferation.[214] An increase in perivascular macrophages, an essential component of hypoxia-induced PAH that is seen in experimental animals, is observed in the lung tissue from patients with IPAH.[215] Matrix metalloproteinases (MMPs) and extracellular matrix are thought to be important in vascular remodeling and hence proliferation of SMCs. Endothelial abnormalities early in the course of PAH may permit extravasation of factors that stimulate SMC production of vascular serine elastase.[216,217] This results in the liberation of matrix-bound SMC mitogens, such as basic fibroblast growth factor, and enhances matrix degradation by activating other MMPs. Elevated serine elastase activity has been documented in rodent and murine models of PAH,[218] which has led to successful experimental use of elastase inhibitors to prevent the pulmonary vascular pathology. MMPs stimulate the production of mitogenic cofactor, tenascin, leading to phosphorylation of growth factor receptors and SMC proliferation. When MMPs are inhibited, tenascin levels fall, leading to apoptosis.[219] Direct inhibition of MMP-2 and serine elastases lead to complete regression of experimental PH in rats,[216] suggesting they regulate vascular tone. MMP-2 and MMP-9 can activate platelets,[220] and intravascular MMP-2 can enhance the formation of vasoconstrictors and inhibit the action of endogenous vasodilators.[220]

Genetics of PAH

More than half (70%) of patients with heritable PAH (HPAH) and 10% to 20% of patients with sporadic PAH are heterozygous for a mutation in bone morphogenetic protein (BMP) receptor type 2 (BMPR2). The penetrance of heritable PAH is low with 80% of family members carrying BMPR2 mutations not developing PAH,[221] but the functional link between BMPR2 and PAH is reinforced by the fact that IPAH patients have reduced BMPR2 protein expression, as do some patients with other conditions associated with PAH. In addition, mutations in the TGF-β superfamily of receptors have also been described in patients with PAH and IPAH.[222] For example, activin-like kinase type I (ALK1) and endoglin are mutated in patients with hereditary hemorrhagic telangiectasia and PAH.[223,224] BMPR2 is a receptor with serine/threonine kinase activity, activating a broad range of intracellular signaling pathways. It phosphorylates one of the smad family of proteins, followed by nuclear translocation, DNA binding, and gene transcription.[225] Alternatively, it can activate via the p38/MAP kinase/ERK/JNK pathways or c-Src pathways.[226] Under normal conditions, BMP ligands bind BMPR2 to suppress the growth of vascular smooth muscle cells.[227] Failure of the protective effects of BMP ligands on endothelium may trigger vascular proliferation and remodeling. Accordingly, the proliferation of vascular SMCs[228] is facilitated by the absence of apoptosis[229] in patients with familial PAH resulting from BMPR2 mutations. Furthermore, response of pulmonary SMCs to BMP signaling appears regulated by hypoxia, a known precipitant of pulmonary hypertension.[230] Thus dysregulation of BMP signaling pathway may be a common pathogenic finding in

multiple types of PAH due to genetic or exogenous stimuli.[176] The reduced expression of BMPR2 appears to be estrogen dependent as the female predisposition of IPAH is related to aberrant expression of a cytochrome, CYP1B1, which leads to a mitogenic estrogenic metabolite.[231]

Similar to BMP pathway, serotonin (5-hydroxytryptomine or 5-HT) signaling pathway has been implicated as a potential causative factor of PAH. Serotonin is both a vasoconstrictor and a mitogen that promotes SMC hyperplasia and hypertrophy.[232] It is primarily stored in the platelets and binds the G-protein–coupled serotonin receptors with intracellular action via the adenylyl-cyclase pathway. Serotonin transporter (5-HTT) transports extracellular serotonin into cytoplasm of the SMC, activating proliferation. Elevated serotonin and serotonin transport have been implicated in the pathology of experimental and clinical PAH. Serotonin exaggerates pulmonary vasoreactivity in fawn-hooded rats,[233] and there is attenuation of pulmonary vascular disease in mice lacking the serotonin transporter gene.[234] In contrast, mice overexpressing the serotonin transporter globally,[235] or specifically in SMCs,[236] develop worsened hypoxia-induced PAH. PDGF-mediated proliferation of SMCs can be compounded by increased activity of the serotonin transporter because this enhances PDGF receptor β–mediated signaling.[237]

Clinical Presentation

There is often no correlation among the time PAH is thought to have started, the age at which it is diagnosed, and the severity of symptoms. The disease seems to progress fairly rapidly, especially in children. Median age at diagnosis was 7 years (IQR 3-12 years) with 59% (268 of 456) female preponderance in the Tracking Outcomes & Practice in Pediatric Pulmonary Hypertension (TOPP) registry[170] and 4.3 ± 4.9 years (50% <2 years) from a Spanish registry.[238] Frequent tiredness, dyspnea, dizziness, and fainting spells are the typical early symptoms. Other symptoms include edema of legs, cyanosis, palpitations, and chest pain. Exertional dyspnea, chest pain, and syncope result from the inability to increase cardiac output in the presence of increased oxygen demand. Examination findings compatible with PH in children include jugular venous distention, systolic murmur of tricuspid regurgitation, loud second heart sound at the base of the heart, and a diastolic murmur of pulmonary regurgitation. In patients with PAH and right heart failure hepatomegaly, ascites and peripheral edema may be seen. Initially the right ventricle (RV) hypertrophies to maintain cardiac output at rest, although the ability to increase cardiac output during exercise may be impaired. As pulmonary vascular disease progresses, right ventricular dysfunction ensues, resulting in right heart failure. Although the left heart is not directly affected by pulmonary vascular disease, progressive right heart dilatation can impair left ventricular filling.[239] The New York Heart Association (NYHA), the classification widely used in adults, describes the functional impact of heart failure on the degree of physical limitation. The functional level of patients is graded from I to IV with higher grades representing severe disease and worse prognosis. The NYHA classification of dyspnea was published by the World Health Organization (WHO) in 1998 as a consensus document to assess functional class in adults. The NYHA classification was graded into four classes depending on the functional ability of the patient to perform work depending on the severity of the heart disease: Class I—ability to perform work without any limitation of physical activity; Class II—slight limitation of physical activity; Class III—marked limitation of physical activity, however comfortable at rest; Class IV—inability to carry out any physical activity without discomfort. A new functional classification of pulmonary hypertension in children has been proposed because age, physical growth, and maturation influence the way in which functional effects of the disease are expressed. The classification should allow the clinician to review progress with time as the child grows up, as consistently and as objectively as possible, and to monitor response to treatment over the years. A new pediatric functional classification has been proposed for different age groups of 0 to 0.5 years; 0.5 to 1 year; 1 to 2 years; 2 to 5 years; and 5 to 16 years.[240] The following table describes the functional class through development of the child with pulmonary hypertension based on the report of the pediatric taskforce (Table 56.3).[240]

Diagnostic Approach

The diagnosis of PAH is made on the basis of a clinical and a comprehensive diagnostic evaluation. Chest radiographs, pulmonary function tests (PFTs), and sleep study will help in ruling out pulmonary causes of PH. Chest radiographs may demonstrate enlarged central pulmonary arteries, right heart enlargement, or evidence of left-sided heart lesion. Etiologic clues of parenchymal lung disease or an airway lesion may be demonstrated. PFT and exercise testing are important for not only diagnosis but also monitoring progression of the disease. Other tests that may help in the diagnosis include autoantibody testing for collagen vascular disorders, HIV testing, and LFTs in cases of portopulmonary hypertension. Electrocardiographic abnormalities are common in pediatric PAH. Right axis deviation (RAD) and right ventricular hypertrophy (RVH) on electrocardiogram are commonly associated with worse hemodynamics, whereas their absence is suggestive of a lack of disease progression.[241] In catheterization-confirmed PAH patients ≤18 years of age, 93% had an electrocardiographic abnormality, with 78% demonstrating RVH and 52% had RAD for age.[241] If PH is suspected on the basis of history, risk factor assessment, and physical examination, an echocardiogram is the next appropriate study.

Doppler echocardiography may offer clues to the potential etiologies of PH, particularly left-sided heart lesions. However, tricuspid or pulmonary regurgitation velocity measurements with pulsed Doppler are more reliable in determining the presence of pulmonary hypertension.[242] Right ventricular systolic pressures >35 to 40 mm Hg in a patient with unexplained dyspnea may warrant further evaluation of PAH. A Doppler-derived ratio of tricuspid regurgitation velocity (TRV) to velocity time integral (VTI) of the right ventricular outflow tract (RVOT) [TRV/VTI$_{RVOT}$] is a simple, noninvasive method to estimate PVR and can be used to follow up patients post catheterization and to assess response to treatment.[243] Common echocardiographic findings of PAH include right atrial and right ventricular (RV) enlargement, reduced RV function, tricuspid regurgitation, flattening of intraventricular septum, and underfilling of the left ventricle. Despite limitations and interobserver variability, findings on echocardiography strengthen the diagnosis of PAH; however, right heart catheterization (RHC) will eventually be required for an accurate assessment of PVR and to confirm the diagnosis. Other noninvasive modalities such as CT and/or MRI should be explored

before subjecting the patient to a catheterization procedure. CT scanning may suggest an etiology of PAH such as a severe airway or parenchymal lung disease. Chronic thromboembolic pulmonary hypertension (CTEPH) is a form of PH and should be sought in all patients with clinically significant PH because it is curable with surgery. CT and V/Q scans help in the diagnosis of CTEPH. Presence of ground-glass opacities, particularly with a centrilobular distribution, septal lines, and adenopathy on CT scan, are suggestive of pulmonary veno-occlusive disease in a patient displaying symptoms of PH.[244] Pulmonary veno-occlusive disease is an unusual form of PH, characterized by elevated PAP with a normal pulmonary capillary wedge pressure and evidence of venous congestion on CXR. Cardiac MRI accurately assesses size and function of the RV with a high degree of reproducibility and hence is used a prognostication tool in the management of PAH.[245] Despite the previously mentioned noninvasive investigations, catheterization may be necessary to define the hemodynamic profile, confirm the diagnosis of PAH, perform vasoreactivity testing on confirmation of diagnosis, and, most importantly, begin a specific management plan for the treatment of PAH.

The current hemodynamic definition of PAH is a mean PAP ≥25 mm Hg, a pulmonary capillary wedge pressure (PCWP), left atrial pressure (LAP) or left ventricular end-diastolic pressure (LVEDP) of ≤15 mm Hg, and a pulmonary vascular resistance index (PVRI) of ≥3 Wood units/m.[2,246] Any patient with suspected PAH requires a careful invasive assessment of pulmonary hemodynamics, as elevated PA pressure is not always caused by pulmonary vascular disease. Pulmonary hypertension commonly occurs with high transpulmonary flow states such as exercise, anemia, pregnancy, sepsis, portopulmonary syndrome, or thyrotoxicosis. In these states, the pulmonary vascular bed is anatomically normal and the PH resolves when the cardiac output returns to normal. The consensus document on pulmonary hypertension requires elevated PVR as opposed to simply elevated mean PAP in the setting of normal left heart filling pressures. PVR is a more robust diagnostic criterion for PAH because it reflects the influence of transpulmonary gradient and cardiac output and is only elevated if the vascular obstruction occurs within the precapillary pulmonary circulation. PVR is a useful measure to apply to patients with increased mean PAP. PVR distinguishes passive PH (elevated mean PAP, normal PVR) from PAH caused by pulmonary vascular disease (elevated mean PAP, elevated PVR). By definition, PVR and PAP are both elevated in PAH.[247]

All patients suspected of having PAH after noninvasive evaluation should undergo right heart catheterization before initiation of therapy specific to PAH. Although RHC and pulmonary angiography are invasive, they can be performed safely by experienced operators even in patients with severe PH and right heart failure. In a recent review of 7218 RHC procedures collected retrospectively and prospectively, 76 (1.1%) serious events were reported. Most of them were related to venous access (hematoma, pneumothorax), followed by arrhythmias and hypotensive episodes related to vagal reactions or pulmonary vasoreactivity testing with an overall procedure related mortality of 0.05% (4/76).[248] In a recent review, the mean age of cardiac catheterization (CC) for PHVD was 4 years (0.3-17), with 75 patients undergoing 97 CC. Twenty-nine percent of the patients had heritable PAH, and 52% had CHD with 14% with lung

TABLE 56.3 Functional Classification for Assessment of Pulmonary Hypertension in Infants and Children Up to 16 Years of Age[240]

Age	Class I	Class II	Class IIIa	Class IIIb	Class IV
0-6 Months	Asymptomatic, growing and developing normally, no limitation of physical activity; has head control with normal body tone; rolls over & has no head lag. Sitting with support	Slight limitation of physical activity, unduly dyspneic and fatigued; falling behind physical developmental milestones; growing along centiles	Marked limitation of physical activity, unduly fatigued; comfortable at rest; regression of learned physical activities; quiet & needs frequent naps; less than ordinary activity causes undue fatigue, syncope, or presyncope; growth compromised; poor appetite; requires excessive medical attention	Growth severely compromised; poor appetite; supplemental feeding; less than ordinary activity causes undue fatigue or syncope + features of Class IIIa	Unable to carry out any physical activity without undue dyspnea, fatigue, or syncope; not interacting with family; syncope and/or right heart failure + features of Class III
6-12 Months	Mobile, sitting, grasping, starting to stand, crawling, playing	Delayed physical development; growing along centiles; comfortable at rest	Regression of learned physical activities; stops crawling; quiet and needs frequent naps; hesitant, cautious & unadventurous; growth compromised; poor appetite; comfortable at rest; less than ordinary activity causes undue fatigue or syncope; requires excessive medical attention	Growth severely compromised; poor appetite; supplemental feeding; less than ordinary activity causes undue fatigue or syncope + features of Class IIIa	Unable to carry out any physical activity without undue dyspnea, fatigue, or syncope; not interacting with family; syncope and/or right heart failure + features of Class III
1-2 Years	Standing, starting to walk/walking, climbing	Delayed physical development; unduly dyspneic & fatigued when playing; continues to grow along centiles	Regression of learned physical activities; reluctant to play; quiet & needs frequent naps; hesitant, cautious & unadventurous; growth compromised; poor appetite; less than ordinary activity causes undue fatigue or syncope; comfortable at rest	Growth severely compromised; poor appetite; supplemental feeding; less than ordinary activity causes undue fatigue or syncope + features of Class IIIa	Unable to carry out any physical activity without undue dyspnea, fatigue, or syncope; not interacting with family; syncope and/or right heart failure + features of Class III
2-5 Years	Asymptomatic, growing normally; attending nursery/school regularly, playing games with his/her peers	Unduly dyspneic & fatigued when playing with friends; nursery/school attendance—75%; no chest pain	Regression of learned physical activities; reluctant to play with friends; comfortable at rest; nursery/schooling compromised (<50% attendance); less than ordinary activity (dressing) causes undue dyspnea, fatigue, syncope, or chest pain	Unable to attend nursery/school, but mobile at home; wheelchair needed outside home; growth compromised; poor appetite; supplemental feeding; less than ordinary activity causes undue fatigue, syncope, or chest pain + features of Class IIIa	Unable to attend school, wheelchair dependent, not interacting with friends; syncope/chest pain and/or right heart failure + features of Class III
6-15 Years	Asymptomatic, growing along centiles; children attending school regularly, playing games with his/her peers	Unduly dyspneic & fatigued when playing with friends; school attendance 75% normal; no chest pain; comfortable at rest	No attempts at sports; comfortable at rest; schooling compromised (<50% attendance); less than ordinary activity causes undue dyspnea, fatigue, syncope, or chest pain	Unable to attend school but mobile at home and interacting with friends; wheelchair needed outside the home; growth compromised; poor appetite; supplemental feeding; less than ordinary activity (dressing) causes undue dyspnea, fatigue, syncope and/or presyncope, or chest pain + features of Class IIIa	Unable to attend school, wheelchair dependent, not interacting with friends; syncope/chest pain and/or right heart failure + features of Class III

Lammers AE, Adatia I, Cerro MJ, et al. Functional classification of pulmonary hypertension in children: report from the PVRI Pediatric Taskforce, Panama 2011. Pulm Circ. 2011;1:280-285.

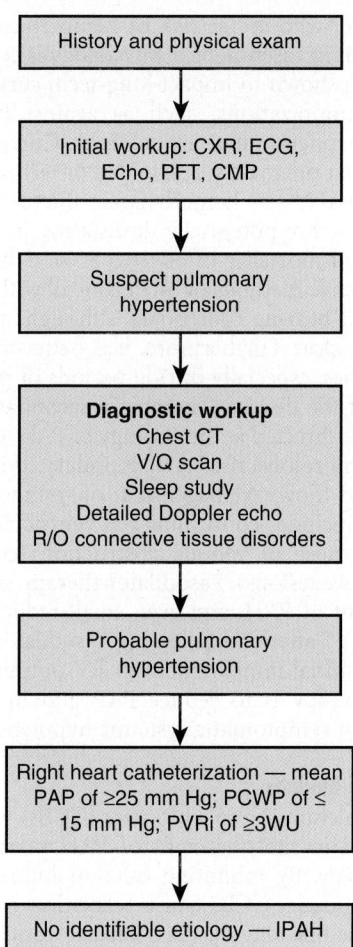

History and physical exam

↓

Initial workup: CXR, ECG, Echo, PFT, CMP

↓

Suspect pulmonary hypertension

↓

Diagnostic workup
Chest CT
V/Q scan
Sleep study
Detailed Doppler echo
R/O connective tissue disorders

↓

Probable pulmonary hypertension

↓

Right heart catheterization — mean PAP of ≥25 mm Hg; PCWP of ≤ 15 mm Hg; PVRi of ≥3WU

↓

No identifiable etiology — IPAH

Fig. 56.10. Algorithm for diagnostic workup for pulmonary hypertension in children. *CMP,* comprehensive metabolic panel; *CT,* computed tomography; *CXR,* chest radiograph; *ECG,* electrocardiogram; *Echo,* echocardiogram; *IPAH,* idiopathic pulmonary arterial hypertension; *PAP,* pulmonary artery pressure; *PCWP,* pulmonary capillary wedge pressure; *PFT,* pulmonary function tests; *PVRi,* pulmonary vascular resistance index; *V/Q,* ventilation-perfusion scan.

disease.[249] No deaths or serious arrhythmias were noted in any patients. Three percent of patients undergoing CC had adverse events, and 45% of patients from follow-up CC resulted in alteration of therapy. A simple but not an exhaustive workup of the child with suspected pulmonary hypertension is illustrated in Fig. 56.10.

Acute Vasodilator Testing

Vasodilator testing establishes the relative contribution of reversible vasoconstriction versus fixed stenosis in patients with PAH over a brief period of minutes to hours, and this can be used as a screen to identify patients who may benefit from long-term therapy with oral calcium channel blockers (CCBs). Responders seem have better prognosis than nonresponders.[250] Acute vasodilator testing (AVT) is usually performed during diagnostic catheterization using inhaled NO,[251] IV PGI$_2$,[252] or IV adenosine.[253] The decision to proceed with AVT has to be individualized; however, patients with idiopathic PAH or congenital heart disease often benefit the most from this testing. Patients with PAH secondary to connective

tissue disorders, NYHA functional class IV, and elevated left heart filling pressures or those on calcium channel blockers are not candidates for vasodilator testing.[254] Significant response to acute vasodilator has been complicated by a variety of definitions, such as a decrease in mPAP by at least 10 mm Hg to an absolute level of <40 mm Hg without a decrease in cardiac output[255]; a fall in PVR of ≥30%[256]; or a decrease of >20% in both mPAP and PVRI.[257] The percentage of positive tests depends on the criteria used and is about 10% to 15%.[258] Half of the patients with a positive test will benefit from long-term therapy with CCBs.[259]

Inhaled NO is the commonly used drug for AVT at doses of 10 to 80 ppm for 15 minutes,[257] but the vasodilator response to NO is not dependent on the concentration and most of the response is obtained at 10 ppm with 2 minutes of inhalation.[256] Acute vasodilator testing with inhaled treprostinil at a dose of 1.5 µg/kg (0.7–2.9 µg/k) has recently been shown to be well tolerated in children with PAH.[260] Other drugs such as inhaled iloprost at doses of 5 to 50 µg in 10 to 15 minutes have been tested with good results.[261] A positive test estimates the degree of vasoconstriction at a given time, but it does not predict the activity of the underlying disease process. It is possible that those patients who have a significant vasodilation but later fail chronic CCB therapy have a more aggressive form of the disease. In patients with IPAH and positive pulmonary vasoreactivity test, CCBs have a pulmonary vasodilator effect with reduction in mPAP and increase in quality of life and survival.[255] The current approach is to initiate CCBs if the patient has a positive vasodilator test, adequate systemic blood pressure, and stable dyspnea in NYHA class I to IV before initiation of therapy.[262]

Treatment

The prognosis of children with PAH has improved in the past decade owing to new therapeutic strategies and aggressive treatment strategies. Although management decisions were often extrapolated from adult studies, emerging literature from pediatric clinical trials helps in forming management decisions specific to children. The natural history of idiopathic PAH in children is worse than adults; however, with treatment, the outcome appears to be better in children. The ultimate goals of treatment should be improved survival and allowing for maximum activities of childhood without any limitations. Improvement in symptomatology (dyspnea, fatigue, and chest pain) and hemodynamic profile (lowered PAP) help in preventing the progression of the disease and improve survival.

Management of Acute Exacerbation of PAH

Clinically significant deteriorations of PAH such as progressive worsening of symptoms, syncope, right ventricular failure, or postoperative PAH need prompt diagnosis and management in order to decrease morbidity and mortality associated with acute PAH.

Oxygen

As hypoxemia is a potent pulmonary vasoconstrictor, it is recommended to start supplemental oxygen to maintain oxygen saturation ≥90%. O$_2$ supplementation is used to avoid acute/chronic hypoxemia and is considered in patients with severe right heart failure or hypoxemia following exercise and in nonhypoxic patients in exacerbation.[263] Some patients may benefit from chronic O$_2$ supplementation as home therapy along with maintenance therapy with medications to slow the progression of the disease.[264]

Nitric Oxide

Nitric oxide (NO) is currently the first-line drug in the acute management of PAH or in cases of postoperative PAH arising from CHD repair or other causes. Nitric oxide is produced endogenously in the vascular endothelium. It acts by increasing cGMP in the smooth muscle by stimulating guanylate cyclase, relaxing the smooth muscle, and contributing to reduced PAP and hence PVR. Inhaled NO (iNO) dilates the pulmonary circulation, deactivated by combining with hemoglobin while avoiding systemic vasodilation, and is extremely effective in the management of PH in critically ill patients in intensive care setting.[265] Inhaled NO, however, is expensive and requires a fairly sophisticated delivery and monitoring system. Inhaled nitric oxide has been used to assess the vasodilator capacity of the pulmonary vascular bed in children with CHD and elevated PVR.[266,267] Low-dose iNO (2–20 ppm) has been effective in the management of postoperative PH following corrective surgery in infants with CHD.[268]

The acute responsiveness to iNO seems to predict the subset of patients who might be responsive to oral calcium channel blockers and thus is a relatively safe and easy test to perform during cardiac catheterization.[269] NO at higher doses (20–80 ppm) produces selective pulmonary vasodilatation in children with CHD and PH.[270] In a randomized trial, high-risk infants undergoing congenital heart surgery, prophylactic use of NO at 10 ppm continuously until extubation had fewer pulmonary hypertensive crises compared with controls.[271] It can help discriminate anatomic obstruction to pulmonary blood flow from pulmonary vasoconstriction and may be used in the treatment or prevention of pulmonary hypertensive crisis after cardiopulmonary bypass in neonates.[272,273] A trial of iNO may diminish the need for ECMO in patients with cardiopulmonary failure following cardiac surgery.[274,275] Inhalation of low levels of NO appears to be safe. The major clinical toxicity is due to the formation of NO_2 and methemoglobinemia.

Maintenance Therapies of PAH in Children
Conventional Therapies

The therapeutic regimen must be tailored in a given child and adjusted according to the clinical and hemodynamic response to improve the quality of life in children with PAH. Most important are avoidance and treatment of chronic hypoxemia. As hypoxemia is a potent pulmonary vasoconstrictor, it is recommended to maintain oxygen saturation ≥90% during the chronic phase of the disease. Children are advised to avoid heavy physical exercise because this may evoke exertional syncope and to be on O_2 supplementation to avoid chronic hypoxemia following exercise. A sodium-restricted diet is advised and is particularly important to manage volume status in patients with RV failure. Diuretic therapy is often necessary in children with heart failure but should be initiated carefully. Children with PAH may be preload dependent to maintain adequate cardiac output. The use of diuretics remains essential in the management of patients with PH related to left ventricular dysfunction.[276] Although its role is not well studied in children, chronic anticoagulation may be beneficial in patients with low cardiac output states, central venous lines, or hypercoagulable states at risk for thrombosis in situ. Risks and benefits of anticoagulation should be weighed, particularly in

young children, who are at risk of hemorrhage. The use of anticoagulation in Eisenmenger physiology is controversial—it has not been shown to impact long-term survival.[277]

Routine immunizations, such as against influenza and pneumococcal pneumonia, are advised. Current guidelines recommend that pregnancy be avoided or terminated early in women with PAH,[255] as hemodynamic fluctuations of pregnancy and labor, are potentially devastating to PAH patients with a maternal mortality of 30% to 50%.[278] It is important to discuss effective methods of birth control with women with PAH of child-bearing potential, although the preferred method is not clear. Furthermore, it is better to avoid major elective surgeries, especially during periods of progression or bad control of the disease. Therapy in secondary pulmonary hypertension is directed at the etiology of PAH. Closure of the heart defect will resolve the PAH secondary to increased pulmonary blood flow. Management of pulmonary venous hypertension includes controlling left ventricular failure and relieving the cause of venous obstruction (commonly left heart obstructive lesions). Vasodilator therapy is the mainstay in management of PAH, and even small reductions in right ventricular (RV) afterload following vasodilator therapy will produce substantial improvement in RV output. The goal of vasodilator therapy is to reduce PAP and increase cardiac output without symptomatic systemic hypotension.

Calcium Channel Blockers

Historically, calcium channel blockers (CCBs) were the drugs primarily used in the treatment of PAH in the absence of alternate therapy. By inhibiting calcium influx into cardiac and smooth muscle, CCBs cause relaxation of the vascular smooth muscle but may decrease cardiac contractility. Acute response to the vasodilator drug during cardiac catheterization will help in determining the desirability of using chronic oral CCBs. The response to acute vasodilator testing is higher in children compared with adults (41% vs. 12% in adults).[279] The acute response in children is also age dependent. Patients who meet criteria for oral CCBs should be followed closely for both safety and efficacy of CCB therapy. CCBs should be avoided in patients with severe ventricular dysfunction, high right atrial pressures, and decrease in cardiac output and in patients <1 year of age. If the patient meets the definition of an acute response and does not improve to functional class I or II on CCB therapy, he or she should not be considered a chronic responder and alternative PAH therapy should be considered. Long-acting nifedipine, diltiazem, and amlodipine are the most commonly used calcium channel blockers. Verapamil should be avoided due to its potentially negative inotropic effects. Oral CCBs help in reducing PAP in about 40% of children with PAH.[280] In the remaining 60%, acute vasodilator testing with agents such as iNO or IV PGI_2 failed to demonstrate responsiveness and these children have not benefited from chronic oral CCB therapy.[280] Chronic CCB therapy improved survival and quality of life in children who acutely respond to vasodilator drug testing.[281] A 5-year survival rate for patients treated with chronic oral calcium channel blockade who respond acutely to vasodilator testing was 97% versus 35% for those who do not respond acutely.[280] Regular, noninvasive monitoring of PAP and cardiac function is as essential part of the management of patients on chronic CCBs, as they may deteriorate over time. Chronic use of calcium channel blockers in patients with fixed PVR and unfavorable hemodynamics may worsen right heart failure.

Prostacyclin Agonists

Prostacyclin (PGI_2) increases cAMP by stimulating the enzyme adenylate cyclase within the vascular smooth muscle, resulting in vasodilatation. Prostacyclin is reduced in patients with PAH and administering PGI_2 or its analogs has been the mainstay in the management of these patients. Currently commercially available prostanoids include epoprostenol, treprostinil, iloprost, and beraprost.

Epoprostenol

Prostacyclin (sodium epoprostenol) has been studied extensively over the past decade. Long-term, continuous IV PGI_2 has been shown to improve survival, quality of life, and exercise capacity and to significantly reduce PAP in children with PAH.[279,280,282,283] Until recently, chronic IV PGI_2 was the mainstay of PAH in children who were not considered responders to vasodilator testing. In both nonresponders and responders who fail to improve on CCBs, continuous IV infusion with PGI_2 improved survival.[280] Since the consistent availability of epoprostenol, the survival of children with idiopathic PAH at 1, 5, and 10 years was 97%, 97%, and 78% with a treatment success rate of 93%, 86%, and 60%, respectively.[284] Chronic PGI_2 therapy lowered mPAP, PVR, and quality of life in patients with PH and associated CHD who failed conventional therapy.[285] Children are on PGI_2 therapy for months to years, depending on the progression of the disease and patient needs. Some children who were previously believed to have fixed pulmonary vascular disease with irreversible obstruction may be reversible with long-term IV PGI_2, perhaps via remodeling of the pulmonary vascular bed.[280,286] However, epoprostenol has a short half-life (2-3 minutes), necessitates administration by continuous IV administration and placement of a central catheter, and is delivered by a portable infusion pump. Due to a complicated nature of delivery mechanism, epoprostenol therapy should be initiated at a specialist center, well versed in PGI_2 administration. Epoprostenol is initiated at a dose of 1 to 3 ng/kg/min and scaled up over days to weeks to a maintenance dose of 50 to 80 ng/kg/min. Side effects are dose dependent, occurring within hours of dose titration, and commonly include flushing, headache, jaw pain, diarrhea, and thrombocytopenia.[287,288] Despite its short half-life, it has a potential for systemic hypotension from high doses and significant desaturations from ventilation-perfusion mismatching in patients with significant lung disease.[276] Tolerance develops in some patients requiring dose escalation, resulting in additional adverse events and increased drug costs. More importantly, complications are associated with administration of PGI_2 such as risk of serious infections, catheter thrombosis, and rebound PAH due to pump failure with subsequent interruptions in therapy.[289,290] Given its considerable complexity, epoprostenol use should be limited to centers experienced with its administration and systematic follow-up of these patients. Although in the late 1980s and early 1990s, the aim of chronic PGI_2 therapy was to act as a bridge to lung or heart/lung transplantation,[291] currently continuous PGI_2 is being used as an alternative therapy to transplantation in selected children.[279]

Treprostinil

The propensity for serious catheter-related infections with epoprostenol administration led to the development of treprostinil, a stable prostacyclin analog for management of PAH. Its administration was initially approved for subcutaneous infusion followed subsequently by intravenous and inhaled routes. Treprostinil has a longer half-life (about 4 hours), stable at room temperatures with fewer side effects. Treprostinil delivered by subcutaneous route (40 ng/kg/min) demonstrated a significant improvement in functional class, hemodynamics, and 6-minute walk (6MW) distance, suggesting it has the potential for rescue therapy in children.[292] Bloodstream infection with PGI_2 is one of the reasons for switching to subcutaneous treprostinil. Although injection site pain due to subcutaneous infusion remains a major disadvantage, subcutaneous treprostinil may be tolerated in children.[292] In a recent study, children with PAH were successfully switched to IV treprostinil to decrease side effects from IV PGI_2.[293] Recently inhaled treprostinil has shown promising results.[294,295] Children with PAH received three to nine breaths (6 μg/breath) of inhaled treprostinil four times/day. Inhaled treprostinil was associated with improvement in exercise capacity and WHO functional class when added to background-targeted PAH therapy in children. Side effects include cough and sore throat, occasionally needing discontinuation of treatment.[294] In PAH patients who remained symptomatic on bosentan or sildenafil, inhaled treprostinil improved exercise capacity and quality of life and was safe and well tolerated.[295] Inhaled treprostinil is currently used as an add-on therapy for progressive PAH or with serious effects with another drug. IV or subcutaneous treprostinil is generally started at 1.25–2 ng/kg/min and gradually increased to 50–80 ng/kg/min on the basis of clinical status, hemodynamic profile, and side effects. Given the complexity of administration of both IV and subcutaneous treprostinil, administration should be limited to centers experienced with this agent. The Centers for Disease Control and Prevention report raised concern for an increased risk of bloodstream infections, particularly with gram-negative organisms, in patients receiving IV treprostinil.[296] Despite the concerns with treprostinil remaining the same as with IV epoprostenol, the availability of subcutaneous, IV, and inhaled preparation and fewer side effects allow for greater flexibility in the management of PAH in children.

Iloprost

Iloprost is a stable prostacyclin analog with a serum half-life of 20 to 25 minutes. Aerosolization of prostacyclin or its stable analog iloprost causes selective pulmonary vasodilatation, increases cardiac output, and improves venous and arterial oxygenation, probably by minimizing ventilation-perfusion mismatch in patients with severe PH.[297] Inhaled iloprost represents a significant advance from IV PGI_2 in the management of PAH, offering a new strategy for treatment of this disease. Long-term treatment with aerosolized iloprost has been shown to be safe and has sustained effects on exercise capacity and pulmonary hemodynamics in patients with PPH.[298] In a placebo-controlled trial, iloprost inhalation (2.5 μg or 5 μg per inhalation; median dose of 30 μg per day) improved pulmonary hemodynamics and quality of life in patients with severe PH.[299] Inhaled iloprost might be an alternative to iNO for early testing of vascular reactivity and postoperative treatment of acute PH in children with CHD.[300-303] Common side effects of inhaled iloprost include cough, headache and flushing, and jaw pain. Iloprost was approved by the FDA in 2004 for functional class III and IV PAH. Its short half-life and frequent inhalations (six to nine times daily) do not make it an ideal candidate for chronic treatment of PAH in children.

Beraprost

Beraprost is a prostacyclin analog for oral administration. It has been shown that beraprost reduces PVR in patients with PAH[304-306] and may also be effective in the treatment of secondary precapillary pulmonary hypertension.[307] Oral administration of beraprost sodium may also improve exercise capacity and ventilatory efficiency in patients with both primary and chronic thromboembolic pulmonary hypertension.[308] In a randomized study, beraprost (80 μg four times a day) improved exercise capacity and symptoms in NYHA functional class II and III patients with PAH and, in particular, in those with primary pulmonary hypertension.[309] Limited studies suggest the efficacy of oral beraprost in infants and children with PH secondary to congenital heart defects.[310]

Endothelin Receptor Antagonists

Endothelin-1 mediates vasoconstriction and smooth muscle cell proliferation contributing to the development of PAH. Its action is mediated mainly through the ET_A receptor. Both nonselective (ET_A and ET_B receptor) and selective (ET_A receptor) antagonists are being evaluated in animal and clinical studies.

Bosentan

Bosentan, a dual endothelin receptor antagonist and an oral antagonist of both ET_A and ET_B receptors, is the most widely studied endothelin receptor antagonist (ERA) in clinical trials. Several clinical studies in children have demonstrated the usefulness of bosentan therapy, including an improvement in exercise capacity, functional class, and long-term outcomes in idiopathic PAH and PAH associated with CHD.[311-314] In one of the first studies published in children, the risk of worsening was lower in patients in WHO functional class I/II than in patients in WHO class III/IV at bosentan initiation with Kaplan-Meier (K-M) for survival at 2 years of 91%[315] and the K-M estimate for disease progression of 54% at 4 years.[316] In another large observational study, bosentan was safe and effective in slowing the progression of the disease.[317] Bosentan, when administered over 3 years in patients with IPAH or associated with CHD, led to improvement in both functional class and 6MW distance up to 3 years. After 3 years, bosentan was continued as monotherapy in only 21% of children with IPAH but in 69% of repaired cases and 56% of those with Eisenmenger syndrome. K-M survival estimates for the 101 patients studied were 96%, 89%, 83%, and 60% at 1, 2, 3, and 5 years, respectively.[317]

The Bosentan Randomized Trial of Endothelin Antagonist Therapy-5 (BREATHE-5) was a 16-week, multicenter, randomized, double-blind study evaluating the effect of bosentan on systemic pulse oximetry and pulmonary vascular resistance in patients with WHO functional class III Eisenmenger syndrome.[318] Bosentan was used at a dose of 62.5 mg twice daily for 4 weeks followed by 125 mg twice daily for the duration of the study. In this first placebo-controlled trial in children with ES, bosentan was well tolerated and improved exercise capacity and hemodynamics without compromising peripheral oxygen saturation. The lack of changes in the SpO_2 was due to similar decreases in PVRi and SVRi, resulting in a limited impact on right-to-left shunt. The reductions in hemodynamic parameters such as PVR index (PVRi), SVR index (SVRi), mPAP, and SBP might have decreased the workload on the right and left ventricles and contributed to the delay in the progression of right ventricular failure.[318] Side effects in the bosentan-treated group were comparable with those reported in the literature and include edema, palpitations, headache, chest pain, and elevated liver enzymes.[318] Potentially serious hepatotoxicity and teratogenicity has been reported with bosentan, which requires close monitoring and cautious use. Due to the risk of hepatic toxicity, the FDA requires that liver function tests be performed at least monthly and hematocrit every 3 months on these patients. Experts are concerned that endothelin antagonists as a class may be capable of causing testicular atrophy and male infertility. Younger males who may consider conceiving should be counseled regarding this possibility before taking these drugs. In a pharmacokinetic assessment of bosentan in pediatric PAH (pediatric FormUlation of bosenTan in pUlmonary arterial hypeRtEnsion–FUTURE-1 study), plasma concentration of bosentan in children was lower than in adults despite doubling the dose from 2 mg/kg bid to 4 mg/kg bid, suggesting exposure plateau is reached at 2 mg/kg twice daily. This could be related to a smaller size of their intestinal surface area or other absorption characteristics resulting in lower absorption, given that elimination half-life was similar in both children and adults.[313] It is worth noting that after an oral administration, maximum concentrations are reached in 3 to 5 hours with elimination half-life of 5 hours. Bosentan is metabolized primarily by CYP2CP and 3A4 isoenzymes in the liver, and its metabolites are excreted in the bile. The new pediatric formulation is well tolerated with a sweet taste and has a favorable risk-benefit profile at 2 mg/kg/dose twice daily.[313]

Selective ET_A Receptor Antagonists

Sitaxsentan and ambrisentan are the two commercially available selective ETA receptor antagonists. In adult PAH patients with NYHA functional class II, III, or IV, sitaxsentan treatment improves WHO functional class and exercise capacity as assessed by a 6-mile walk (6MW) test.[319,320] In a double-blind study, ambrisentan was evaluated at four dosages (1, 2.5, 5, or 10 mg) once daily for 12 weeks followed by 12 weeks of open label ambrisentan.[321] Initial experience with ambrisentan in children suggests that treatment is safe with similar pharmacokinetics to those in adults.[322] In a study of pediatric patients with PAH, 15 of 38 patients were switched from bosentan to ambrisentan and the remaining 23 children were treated with ambrisentan as an add-on therapy due to disease progression. In both patients, mPAP significantly improved (transition patients -55 ± 18 vs. 45 ± 20 mm Hg, $n = 13$, $P = 0.04$, add-on -52 ± 17 vs. 45 ± 19 mm Hg, $n = 13$, $P = 0.03$) during follow-up. WHO functional class improved in 31% of patients. Ten patients (26%) had side effects associated with ambrisentan treatment, including nasal congestion, headache, and flushing. However, no patients had aminotransferase abnormalities and there were no deaths after initiation of ambrisentan during follow-up. In patients with Eisenmenger syndrome, ambrisentan was safe and associated with increased exercise capacity at short-term follow-up with patients maintaining functional class, SpO_2, and hemoglobin with no significant evidence of clinical deterioration at long-term follow-up.[323] Ambrisentan use in children is increasing due to once-daily dosing, lack of drug interaction with PDE5 therapy, and decreased risk of elevated liver enzymes. Pediatric dosing is not available due to insufficient clinical data, but pediatric patients can be started on ambrisentan at 2.5 mg (<20 kg) or 5 mg (≥20 kg) and the dose can be titrated to 5–10 mg depending on the clinical response and disease progression. Ambrisentan was FDA approved in 2007 for PAH patients with functional class II and III symptoms. As a class, endothelin receptor antagonists have a potential for liver injury and teratogenicity. Monthly monitoring of liver function tests, a monthly pregnancy test in women of child-bearing potential, and a periodic hemoglobin measurement are required. Precautions regarding contraception and testicular atrophy are similar to bosentan.

Phosphodiesterase Type 5 Inhibitors

Type 5 phosphodiesterase (PDE5) is primarily responsible for degradation of cGMP to inactive metabolite GMP. PDE5 appears to be particularly abundant in pulmonary vessels. One way of augmenting the concentration of cGMP in pulmonary vessels is by inhibiting the activity of PDE5. PDE5 inhibitors, such as sildenafil and tadalafil, have antiproliferative, proapoptotic, and vasodilating effects on the pulmonary vasculature by increasing cGMP.[324] PDE5 inhibitors are administered orally and are well tolerated. Side effects include headache, flushing, dyspepsia, epistaxis, and erections in males. Vision abnormalities are dose related and rarely occur with therapeutic dosing, yet visual and hearing assessments should be considered in premature infants on PDE5 therapy.

Sildenafil

The FDA approved sildenafil in 2005 for the treatment of adult PAH at doses of 20 mg three times daily. Two small studies have shown that oral sildenafil improves hemodynamics and exercise capacity (6MW test) for up to 12 months at doses of 0.25 to 1 mg/kg four times daily[325] and improved oxyhemoglobin saturations and exercise tolerance in children with PAH without any side effects.[326] STARTS-1 is a multicenter trial of children randomized to low (10 mg), medium (10–40 mg), or high (20–80 mg) doses of sildenafil (ages: 1-17 years) for 16 weeks with PAH.[327] The doses of sildenafil were adjusted on the basis of body weight and steady state maximum concentration of sildenafil. Although the primary outcome of percent change in peak oxygen consumption (PVO_2) for the three sildenafil groups was only marginally significant, the improvement in exercise capacity, functional class, and hemodynamic improvements with the medium and high doses suggests efficacy of sildenafil at these doses.[327] The most frequent adverse events included headache, pyrexia upper respiratory tract infection, and diarrhea. In STARTS-2, sildenafil-treated patients continued STARTS-1 dosing and placebo-treated patients were randomized to one of the three sildenafil dose groups ($n = 1234$).[328] All children received sildenafil for ≥3 years from STARTS-1 baseline; 37 deaths were reported (26 on study treatment). Most patients who died (28/37) had idiopathic PAH (76% vs. 33%) and baseline functional class III/IV disease (38% vs. 15%); patients who died had worse baseline hemodynamics. K-M estimated that 3-year survival rates from the start of sildenafil were 94%, 93%, and 88% for patients randomized to low-, medium-, and high-dose sildenafil, respectively; 87%, 89%, and 80% were known to be alive at 3 years. Hazard ratios for mortality were 3.95 (95% CI, 1.46–10.65) for high versus low and 1.92 (95% CI, 0.65–5.65) for medium versus low dose.[328] Although children randomized to higher compare with lower sildenafil doses had an unexplained increased mortality, all sildenafil dose groups displayed favorable survival for children with PAH. In 2012 the

FDA released a strong warning against the chronic use of sildenafil for pediatric (ages 1 through 17) with PAH, citing that children taking high doses of Revatio (sildenafil) had a higher risk of death than children taking a low dose and low doses of Revatio are not effective in improving exercise ability. A consensus statement of experts strongly recommended avoiding high doses of sildenafil and adjusting the dosage to 10 mg three times daily (8–20 kg body weight) or 20 mg three times a day (>20 kg).[329] The current FDA review is not relevant regarding the short-term use of sildenafil in the critical care setting. Sildenafil is also useful to treat rebound PH in the settings of withdrawal from nitric oxide therapy,[330,331] management of postoperative pulmonary hypertensive crisis,[332] and treating pulmonary hypertension resulting from bronchopulmonary dysplasia.[333,334] For children <8 kg body weight, the dose of 0.25–1 mg/kg three times a day is recommended,[335] but it has been dosed four times a day in some centers. As sildenafil is metabolized by hepatic CYP-450, coadministration of sildenafil with CYP3A inducers or inhibitors such as ketoconazole or rifampin should be avoided.[276]

Tadalafil

Tadalafil is a phosphodiesterase-5 (PDE5) inhibitor that was approved by the FDA in 2009 for the treatment of PAH. Tadalafil has a greater affinity (10,000-fold) for PDE5 compared with the other PDE inhibitors and is long-acting with a half-life of 17.5 hours. In a controlled clinical study in patients with PAH, patients receiving tadalafil in a total daily dose of 40 mg had significant improvements in their 6MW distance and time to clinical worsening.[336] In a recent study, oral tadalafil (1 mg/kg once a day) was administered easily and tolerated well, and it improved mean pulmonary artery pressure in children with PAH, suggesting oral tadalafil may be more effective and safer than sildenafil in the treatment of PAH.[337] Patients were switched from sildenafil to tadalafil with no significant side effects and were shown to improve functional capacity and oxygen capacity better than sildenafil with fewer daily doses, suggesting that tadalafil may be the better drug.[338]

Combination Therapy

The goal of combination therapy is to maximize efficacy and minimize toxicity. The safety and efficacy of combination therapy in PAH are subjects of active investigation. As noted earlier, agents that inhibit degradation of cGMP (PDE5 inhibitors) may act synergistically with iNO. Similarly, inhibiting PDE3, a principal metabolizer of cAMP, might be expected to augment the response to PGI_2. Inhaled milrinone, either alone or in combination with inhaled PGI_2, selectively dilates the pulmonary vasculature without systemic effects in cardiac surgical patients with PH.[339] Inhaled iloprost has been studied in patients who remained symptomatic (NYHA functional class III or IV) while on stable bosentan therapy for at least 3 months.[340] After 12 weeks, the primary efficacy measure, postinhalation 6MW test improved significantly in the iloprost group, along with improvements in mean PAP and functional class. Sildenafil in patients who remained symptomatic on a stable dose of epoprostenol for at least 3 months demonstrated an improvement in the 6MW test, mean PAP, and time to clinical worsening.[341] Oral bosentan and sildenafil in combination have been shown to be effective in the treatment of IPAH and PAH-CHD in children.[342] There is a mutual pharmacokinetic interaction between bosentan and sildenafil that may influence the dosage of each drug in a combination treatment. Bosentan decreases the maximum plasma concentration of sildenafil (C_{max}) by 55.4% on Day 16, whereas sildenafil increased bosentan C_{max} by 42.0%. Hence close monitoring is advisable with coadministration.[343] However, Bosentan and sildenafil in combination were well tolerated, with no serious adverse events reported. Side effects in pediatric PAH were more commonly reported in patients on combination therapy with an ERA and/or prostacyclin, likely due to a synergistic effect and commonly include flushing, diarrhea, dyspepsia, headache, and hyperactivity.[344]

Pulmonary Thromboendarterectomy

Patients with suspected PAH should undergo evaluation for chronic thromboembolic pulmonary hypertension. Chronic thromboembolic pulmonary hypertension (CTEPH) is a rare form of pulmonary hypertension that can lead to progressive right heart failure and death. CTEPH should be an important diagnostic consideration in symptomatic children with a known hypercoagulable state, a history of thromboembolism or venous catheter placement, and/or a diagnosis of pulmonary hypertension. The screening tool of choice is the perfusion scanning. If indicative of CTEPH, pulmonary angiography should be performed. Patients are considered to be candidates for surgery if they have surgically accessible disease and present an acceptable risk. Pulmonary thromboendarterectomy surgery in pediatric patients with CTEPH is well tolerated with improved postoperative hemodynamics, functional status, minimal postoperative complications, and low perioperative mortality, similar to that reported for adults with CTEPH, with the notable exception being a higher rate of rethrombosis in pediatric patients.[345] The surgery has to be performed at a center experienced in performing this procedure with excellent technical skills and support systems in place.

Atrial Septostomy

Despite advances in medical treatment for PAH, many patients experience progressive functional decline, largely from worsening right heart failure. Fortunately, it is uncommon to see patients in the pediatric age group in end-stage PAH compared with adults. In these patients, interventional and surgical options including atrial septostomy and lung or combined heart and lung transplantation should be considered. In patients with symptomatic cor-pulmonale secondary to pulmonary vascular disease, atrial septostomy can improve symptoms and may serve as a palliative bridge to heart and/or lung transplantation.[346,347] The procedure permits right-to-left shunting, decompresses the right heart, and increases left ventricular preload. Several case series have reported hemodynamic and clinical improvement following atrial septostomy.[346,347] Improved cardiac output appears to be the principal hemodynamic benefit. Improvements in NYHA functional class and 6MW test have also been reported.[348] The success rates for bridging patients to transplantation, with septostomy, ranges from 30% to 40%.[346,347] In a retrospective study in children with IPAH, 19 underwent atrial septostomy at a mean age of 8.4 years.[349] There were no deaths, with improvement in syncope, WHO functional class, and echocardiographic assessment of right ventricular function.[349] Procedural mortality rate and complications are high and hence

atrial septostomy has to be performed in experienced centers only. Currently, atrial septostomy is recommended for patients with severe PAH and intractable right heart failure despite maximal medical therapy, including optimized PAH specific agents and inotropes. The goals of the procedure are palliation and restoration and maintenance of clinical stability until a transplant can be performed.

Lung and Combined Heart/Lung Transplantation

Before PGI_2 became available as the long-term therapy, lung transplantation was the only option for survival for patients with severe pulmonary hypertension. Single-lung, double-lung, and heart-lung transplantation have all been advocated as the operation of choice in PAH. Transplantation is offered after maximal therapeutic effort with vasodilators and oxygen has been attempted and when the estimated 2-year survival is less than 50%.[350] Most centers now perform bilateral lung or heart-bilateral lung transplantation for PAH. IV PGI_2 has been used as a bridge to stabilize the patient until transplantation is accomplished. Extracorporeal membrane oxygenation (ECMO) is a safe and effective means of bridging well-selected patients with refractory respiratory failure to lung transplantation or return to their baseline condition, notwithstanding the considerable consumption of resources.[351] To date, more than 1800 lung transplants have been performed, most frequently in children >5 years of age.[352] Idiopathic PAH is the second most common indication for lung transplantation (LTx) in pediatric patients overall and the most common indication among children aged 1 to 5 years old. The 2013 IHSLT registry data of pediatric LTx performed between 1990 and 2011 reports a median survival of 4.9 years for pediatric patients. This observed survival is statistically similar to that of adult LTx recipients (4.9 years vs. 5.4 years). Like in adults, there has been a clear improvement in survival of 3.3 years among those transplanted between 1988 and 1999 versus median survival of 5.8 years in those transplanted in 2000 to 2011.[352] The most common causes of death following LTx include graft failure (first 30 days), non-CMV infection (1 month to 1 year), and bronchiolitis obliterans (after the first year). In a single-center study of LTx for IPAH, the median survival for those transplanted was 5.8 years, with 1- and 5-year survival rates of 95% and 61%, respectively. Compared with the transplanted group, children who died waiting had a significantly higher incidence of suprasystemic right heart pressures and hemoptysis.[353] As outcomes for infants listed for lung or heart/lung transplantation are similar to that of children, very young age should not be considered a contraindication to lung or heart/lung transplantation.[354] Earlier diagnosis and listing may decrease pretransplant mortality.[354] Even though the early outcome following lung transplantation has improved considerably, long-term complications, including infections, bronchiolitis obliterans, and complications of immunosuppression remain significant problems.[355] Aggressive medical therapy combined with early recognition of lung transplant candidates will improve quality of life and overall survival of these children.

Prognosis and Survival in PAH

Despite advances, vasodilators remain the mainstay in the management of PAH in children. Fig. 56.11 presents an overview of the complex management of PAH in children, with various options to choose at this time. The treatment

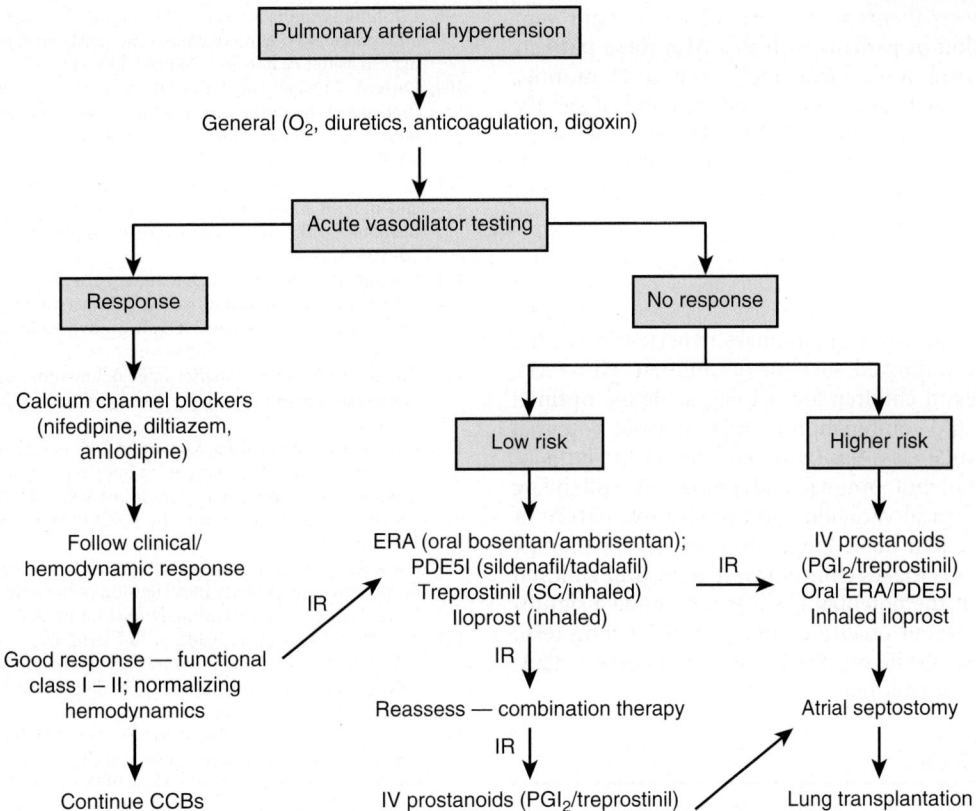

Fig. 56.11. Treatment algorithm for pulmonary arterial hypertension. See text for details. Diuretics are used in management of right heart failure. O_2 is recommended to maintain SpO_2 >90%. Calcium channel blockers (CCBs) are indicated for patients who have a positive acute vasodilator response. For patients who do not respond to acute vasodilator testing and are considered lower risk on the basis of clinical assessment, oral therapy with endothelial receptor antagonist (ERA) or phosphodiesterase 5 inhibitors (PDE5I), inhaled treprostinil, or iloprost would be the first line of therapy. For patients who are considered high risk on the basis of clinical assessment, continuous treatment with IV prostacyclin (PGI2) or treprostinil would be the first line of therapy recommended with or without oral ERA/PDE5I. Iloprost is a prostacyclin analog delivered as an aerosol. Combination therapy should be considered when patients are not responding adequately to initial monotherapy. Timing for lung transplantation and/or atrial septostomy is challenging and reserved for patients who progress despite optimal medical treatment. *IR,* incomplete response; *SC,* subcutaneous. (Modified from the Expert Consensus Document on Pulmonary Hypertension. McLaughlin VV, Archer SL, Badesch DB, et al. ACCF/AHA 2009 expert consensus document on pulmonary hypertension: a report of the American College of Cardiology Foundation Task Force on Expert Consensus Documents and the American Heart Association developed in collaboration with the American College of Chest Physicians; American Thoracic Society, Inc.; and the Pulmonary Hypertension Association. J Am Coll Cardiol. 2009;53:1573-1619.)

algorithm is a minor modification with emphasis on initial diagnosis and management of these patients from the expert consensus document for pulmonary hypertension.[247] The goal of therapy should be to improve the quality of life and survival of these children with PAH. While most of the studies have been focusing on short-time end points such as 12 weeks' duration or 6MW test and long-term follow-up data on these patients are lacking. Although the therapies are evolving rapidly in the management of PAH, long-term experience with epoprostenol has suggested the importance of early follow-up because patients who remain in functional class III or IV despite therapy have poor outcomes and should be considered for lung transplant.[287] Data from the REVEAL registry suggest that the median age at diagnosis was 7 years. At diagnosis the mPAP and PVRI were 56 mm Hg and 17 WU/ m^2, respectively, with a 5-year survival from diagnosis of 74% ± 6%. Increased survival from enrollment included the ability to respond to vasoreactivity testing and lower brain natriuretic peptide.[169] In a study comparing factors impacting survival at three major referral centers (NY, Denver, and Netherlands), diagnosis, WHO functional class, mPAP/mSAP, and PVRi

were identified as independent predictors of outcome among center cohorts. Moreover, the treatment of PAH-targeted combination therapy during the study period was independently associated with transplant-free survival.[356] In a recent single-center study of 65 children with PAH, the 5-, 10- and 15-year survival rates were 96%, 92%, and 65%, respectively, and there was no significant correlation between outcome and immediate response to the vasodilators.[357]

For clinical decision making in the treatment of these patients, it is important to be able to predict survival using prognostic factors.[358] In a systematic review and meta-analyses, WHO-functional class, (N-terminal pro-) brain natriuretic peptide, mean right atrial pressure, cardiac index, and acute vasodilator response were consistently reported prognostic factors for outcomes in pediatric PAH.[359] While echocardiography has been a pivotal screening test, the presence of any degree of pericardial effusion has been proven to be a consistent predictor of mortality.[360] More recently, tricuspid annular plane systolic excursion (TAPSE) on echocardiography has been shown to be a robust measure of RV function and a powerful predictor of patient survival in PH.[361] TAPSE of less than 1.8 identifies patients with more advanced right ventricular dysfunction in patients with PH. Also these patients had reduced survival over a median follow-up of 19 months. Cardiac MRI accurately assesses size and function of the RV with a high degree of reproducibility. RV function is an important prognostic indicator in PAH, and MRI of poor RV function was found to be an independent predictor of mortality and treatment failure.[245]

Conclusions

Advances in the treatment of pulmonary hypertension in the past decade have improved survival of children with PAH. New clinical trials in children are helping to define optimal dosing of mono and combination therapy to avoid potential toxicities. Functional class has been evolving on the basis of child development, but optimal end points are still being defined. The biological variability and progressive nature of the disease in children make longer observations to therapy problematic. All this makes clinical investigations in children more difficult, but the potential rewards for having a significant impact on overall quality of life, as well as long-term survival, far outweigh the hurdles in developing newer management options for children.

Key References

6. Dawes GS. Pulmonary circulation in the foetus and new-born. *Br Med Bull.* 1966;22:61-65.
9. Lakshminrusimha S. The pulmonary circulation in neonatal respiratory failure. *Clin Perinatol.* 2012;39:655-683.
21. Chambers CD, Hernandez-Diaz S, Van Marter LJ, et al. Selective serotonin-reuptake inhibitors and risk of persistent pulmonary hypertension of the newborn. *N Engl J Med.* 2006;354:579-587.
40. Teitel DF, Iwamoto HS, Rudolph AM. Changes in the pulmonary circulation during birth-related events. *Pediatric Res.* 1990;27:372-378.
41. Haworth SG. Normal structural and functional adaptation to extrauterine life. *J Pediatrics.* 1981;98:915-918.
52. Abman SH, Chatfield BA, Hall SL, et al. Role of endothelium-derived relaxing factor during transition of pulmonary circulation at birth. *Am J Physiol.* 1990;259:H1921-H1927.
53. Tiktinsky MH, Morin FC 3rd. Increasing oxygen tension dilates fetal pulmonary circulation via endothelium-derived relaxing factor. *Am J Physiol.* 1993;265:H376-H380.
54. Fineman JR, Wong J, Morin FC 3rd, et al. Chronic nitric oxide inhibition in utero produces persistent pulmonary hypertension in newborn lambs. *J Clin Investig.* 1994;93:2675-2683.
62. Kumar VH, Hutchison AA, Lakshminrusimha S, et al. Characteristics of pulmonary hypertension in preterm neonates. *J Perinatol.* 2007;27:214-219.
63. Van Meurs KP, Wright LL, Ehrenkranz RA, et al. Inhaled nitric oxide for premature infants with severe respiratory failure. *N Engl J Med.* 2005;353:13-22.
64. Mourani PM, Sontag MK, Younoszai A, et al. Early pulmonary vascular disease in preterm infants at risk for bronchopulmonary dysplasia. *Am J Respir Crit Care Med.* 2015;191:87-95.
76. Walsh-Sukys MC, Tyson JE, Wright LL, et al. Persistent pulmonary hypertension of the newborn in the era before nitric oxide: practice variation and outcomes. *Pediatrics.* 2000;105:14-20.
80. Lapointe A, Barrington KJ. Pulmonary hypertension and the asphyxiated newborn. *J Pediatrics.* 2011;158(suppl 2):e19-e24.
81. Shankaran S, Laptook AR, Ehrenkranz RA, et al. Whole-body hypothermia for neonates with hypoxic-ischemic encephalopathy. *N Engl J Med.* 2005;353:1574-1584.
88. Bifano EM, Pfannenstiel A. Duration of hyperventilation and outcome in infants with persistent pulmonary hypertension. *Pediatrics.* 1988;81:657-661.
89. Hendricks-Munoz KD, Walton JP. Hearing loss in infants with persistent fetal circulation. *Pediatrics.* 1988;81:650-656.
96. Lakshminrusimha S, Swartz DD, Gugino SF, et al. Oxygen concentration and pulmonary hemodynamics in newborn lambs with pulmonary hypertension. *Pediatr Res.* 2009;66:539-544.
100. Lotze A, Mitchell BR, Bulas DI, et al. Multicenter study of surfactant (beractant) use in the treatment of term infants with severe respiratory failure. Survanta in Term Infants Study Group. *J Pediatr.* 1998;132:40-47.
101. Konduri GG, Sokol GM, Van Meurs KP, et al. Impact of early surfactant and inhaled nitric oxide therapies on outcomes in term/late preterm neonates with moderate hypoxic respiratory failure. *J Perinatol.* 2013;33:944-949.
111. Kinsella JP, Abman SH. High-frequency oscillatory ventilation augments the response to inhaled nitric oxide in persistent pulmonary hypertension of the newborn: Nitric Oxide Study Group. *Chest.* 1998;114(suppl 1):100S.
113. Kinsella JP, Neish SR, Shaffer E, et al. Low-dose inhalation nitric oxide in persistent pulmonary hypertension of the newborn. *Lancet.* 1992;340:819-820.
116. Davidson D, Barefield ES, Kattwinkel J, et al. Inhaled nitric oxide for the early treatment of persistent pulmonary hypertension of the term newborn: a randomized, double-masked, placebo-controlled, dose-response, multicenter study. The I-NO/PPHN Study Group. *Pediatrics.* 1998;101:325-334.
117. Clark RH, Kueser TJ, Walker MW, et al. Low-dose nitric oxide therapy for persistent pulmonary hypertension of the newborn. Clinical Inhaled Nitric Oxide Research Group. *N Engl J Med.* 2000;342:469-474.
118. NINOS. Inhaled nitric oxide in full-term and nearly full-term infants with hypoxic respiratory failure. The Neonatal Inhaled Nitric Oxide Study Group. [Erratum appears in N Engl J Med 1997;337:434]. *N Engl J Med.* 1997;336:597-604.
119. Roberts JD Jr, Fineman JR, Morin FC 3rd, et al. Inhaled nitric oxide and persistent pulmonary hypertension of the newborn. The Inhaled Nitric Oxide Study Group. *N Engl J Med.* 1997;336:605-610.
120. Konduri GG, Solimano A, Sokol GM, et al. A randomized trial of early versus standard inhaled nitric oxide therapy in term and near-term newborn infants with hypoxic respiratory failure. *Pediatrics.* 2004;113:559-564.
131. AAP. American Academy of Pediatrics. Committee on Fetus and Newborn. Use of inhaled nitric oxide. *Pediatrics.* 2000;106:344-345.
140. Baquero H, Soliz A, Neira F, et al. Oral sildenafil in infants with persistent pulmonary hypertension of the newborn: a pilot randomized blinded study. *Pediatrics.* 2006;117:1077-1083.
151. Rubin LJ, Badesch DB, Barst RJ, et al. Bosentan therapy for pulmonary arterial hypertension. *N Engl J Med.* 2002;346:896-903.
161. UK collaborative randomised trial of neonatal extracorporeal membrane oxygenation. UK Collaborative ECMO Trail Group. *Lancet.* 1996;348:75-82.
168. Simonneau G, Gatzoulis MA, Adatia I, et al. Updated clinical classification of pulmonary hypertension. *J Am Coll Cardiol.* 2013;62(suppl 25):D34-D41.
169. Barst RJ, McGoon MD, Elliott CG, et al. Survival in childhood pulmonary arterial hypertension: insights from the registry to evaluate early and long-term pulmonary arterial hypertension disease management. *Circulation.* 2012;125:113-122.
174. Rabinovitch M. Molecular pathogenesis of pulmonary arterial hypertension. *J Clin Investig.* 2012;122:4306-4313.
185. Verhaar MC, Strachan FE, Newby DE, et al. Endothelin-A receptor antagonist-mediated vasodilatation is attenuated by inhibition of nitric oxide synthesis and by endothelin-B receptor blockade. *Circulation.* 1998;97:752-756.
205. Weir EK, Reeve HL, Johnson G, et al. A role for potassium channels in smooth muscle cells and platelets in the etiology of primary pulmonary hypertension. *Chest.* 1998;114(suppl 3):200S-204S.
247. McLaughlin VV, Archer SL, Badesch DB, et al. ACCF/AHA 2009 expert consensus document on pulmonary hypertension: a report of the American College of Cardiology Foundation Task Force on Expert Consensus Documents and the American Heart Association developed in collaboration with the American College of Chest Physicians; American Thoracic Society, Inc.; and the Pulmonary Hypertension Association. *J Am Coll Cardiol.* 2009;53:1573-1619.
252. Rubin LJ, Groves BM, Reeves JT, et al. Prostacyclin-induced acute pulmonary vasodilation in primary pulmonary hypertension. *Circulation.* 1982;66:334-338.
262. Barst RJ, Gibbs JS, Ghofrani HA, et al. Updated evidence-based treatment algorithm in pulmonary arterial hypertension. *J Am Coll Cardiol.* 2009;54(suppl 1):S78-S84.

270. Roberts JD Jr, Lang P, Bigatello LM, et al. Inhaled nitric oxide in congenital heart disease. *Circulation.* 1993;87:447-453.

280. Barst RJ, Maislin G, Fishman AP. Vasodilator therapy for primary pulmonary hypertension in children. *Circulation.* 1999;99:1197-1208.

295. McLaughlin VV, Benza RL, Rubin LJ, et al. Addition of inhaled treprostinil to oral therapy for pulmonary arterial hypertension: a randomized controlled clinical trial. *J Am Coll Cardiol.* 2010;55:1915-1922.

313. Beghetti M, Haworth SG, Bonnet D, et al. Pharmacokinetic and clinical profile of a novel formulation of bosentan in children with pulmonary arterial hypertension: the FUTURE-1 study. *Br J Clin Pharmacol.* 2009;68:948-955.

324. Archer SL, Michelakis ED. Phosphodiesterase type 5 inhibitors for pulmonary arterial hypertension. *N Engl J Med.* 2009;361:1864-1871.

327. Barst RJ, Ivy DD, Gaitan G, et al. A randomized, double-blind, placebo-controlled, dose-ranging study of oral sildenafil citrate in treatment-naive children with pulmonary arterial hypertension. *Circulation.* 2012;125:324-334.

328. Barst RJ, Beghetti M, Pulido T, et al. STARTS-2: long-term survival with oral sildenafil monotherapy in treatment-naive pediatric pulmonary arterial hypertension. *Circulation.* 2014;129:1914-1923.

Mechanical Ventilation and Respiratory Care

Shekhar T. Venkataraman

PEARLS
- Modern pediatric respiratory care requires a major institutional commitment in resource allocation for state-of the-art management of the patient requiring mechanical ventilation.
- A team approach in which the roles and responsibilities of each of the team members (physicians, respiratory therapists, bedside nurses, and the family) are clearly defined and respected is required.
- Every team member must be abreast of the technologic advances in the design and implementation of mechanical ventilation.

Introduction

This chapter reviews the applied physiology relevant to gas exchange and lung mechanics, design and function of ventilators including a modern classification of the modes, guidelines for the use of mechanical ventilation based on pathophysiology, philosophy and practice of weaning, respiratory care adjuncts to mechanical ventilation, high-frequency ventilation, adverse effects of mechanical ventilation, and home respiratory care. The topic of noninvasive mechanical ventilation including negative pressure ventilation is covered elsewhere (see Chapter 58).

Applied Respiratory Physiology

Lung Volumes and Capacities

Air gets in, air gets out; oxygen is taken up, carbon dioxide is eliminated; this is the essence of breathing. Tidal volume is the volume of gas that is moved in and out of the lungs per breath and is normally 6 to 8 mL/kg for a spontaneous breath, regardless of age. Total lung capacity (TLC) is the volume of gas present in the lung with maximal inflation (60–80 mL/kg). Vital capacity is the volume of gas that can be maximally expired from TLC (40–50 mL/kg). Functional residual capacity (FRC) is the volume of gas that is present in the lung at the end of a normal expiration. FRC results from the balance between forces that favor alveolar collapse and maintain alveolar inflation. The normal FRC is about 30 mL/kg. Residual volume is the volume of gas present in the lung at the end of

a maximal expiratory effort. Closing volume refers to the volume of gas present in the lung at which small conducting airways begin to collapse. When FRC exceeds closing volume, the small airways and the alveoli remain open. On the other hand, when closing volume exceeds FRC, the small airways and alveoli tend to collapse. In infants and children younger than 6 years, the closing volume exceeds FRC. This explains the propensity for atelectasis in infants and young children. With development, FRC exceeds closing volume in children older than 6 years.

Physiology of Inflation and Deflation

Impedance to Lung Inflation

Thoracic structures impede lung inflation, and a certain amount of force is required to overcome this impedance. Elasticity of the lung and chest wall is a major factor that impedes lung inflation. Elastance is defined as the change in pressure for a unit change in volume. Compliance is the reciprocal of elastance. Lung compliance is defined as the change in lung volume for a unit change in transalveolar pressure (alveolar pressure minus the pleural pressure). Chest compliance is the change in thoracic cage volume produced by a unit change in transthoracic pressure (ambient pressure minus the pleural pressure). Total respiratory system compliance is the total change in lung volume (lung and chest) for a unit change in transrespiratory pressure (alveolar pressure minus the ambient pressure). Disease processes that result in an abnormal lung or chest wall compliance are given in Table 57.1. Specific lung compliance refers to lung compliance that is normalized to the lung volume or body weight (similar in children and adults). The pressure required to overcome compliance is:

$$P_{Compliance} = Volume/Compliance \text{ or } Volume \times Elastance$$

Total respiratory system resistance is the second factor that impedes inflation and is defined as the change in transpulmonary pressure (proximal airway pressure minus the alveolar pressure) required to produce a unit flow of gas through the airways of the lung. Total resistance can be partitioned into airway resistance and frictional resistance to deformation of the lungs, chest wall, and abdominal contents.[1] In the infant, the airway resistance is equally distributed between the upper and lower airways. With increasing age, most of the airway resistance resides in the upper airways. Frictional resistance is also known as the *nonelastic viscous resistance*. In certain pathologic conditions, such as pulmonary edema, interstitial lung disease, and pulmonary fibrosis, frictional resistance may

TABLE 57.1	Factors Associated With Decreased Total Respiratory Compliance

Decreased Lung Compliance

Surfactant deficiency or alteration
Respiratory distress of the newborn
Adult respiratory distress syndrome
Interstitial inflammation
Diffuse pneumonitis
Fibrosis
Pulmonary edema
Alveolar edema
Interstitial edema
Hyperinflation
Airway obstruction—both upper and lower
Excessive CPAP/PEEP or auto-PEEP
Atelectasis

Decreased Chest Compliance

Restrictive pleural disease
Pleural collection of air or fluid
Fibrosis
Increased intercostal muscle tone
Upper motor neuron disease
Drugs
Restrictive chest diseases
Deformations—kyphosis, scoliosis, or both
Ankylosis
Restrictive bandages

Diaphragmatic Restriction

Abdominal distention
Abdominal binding
Increased abdominal pressure—peritoneal dialysis,
    postlaparotomy, etc.

CPAP, continuous positive airway pressure; *PEEP*, positive end-expiratory pressure.

be increased. The pressure required to overcome this total resistance can be written as:

$$P_{\text{Total Resistance}} = P_{\text{Resistance}} + P_{\text{Frictional resistance}}$$
$$= \text{Total Respiratory Resistance} \times \text{Flow}$$

Inertance of the respiratory gas is another factor that impedes inflation, and the pressure required to overcome inertial forces of the gas is normally low and can be omitted.[1] Then, the total pressure (P_{tp}) required to inflate the lung can be mathematically expressed as follows, termed the "Equation of Motion":

$$P_{tp} = P_{\text{Compliance}} + P_{\text{Total Resistance}}$$

Concept of Time Constant

With a constant inflation pressure, it takes a finite amount of time to inflate the lung with a given volume of gas. The rate of inflation and deflation of the lung is approximately mono-exponential and is directly proportional to the compliance and the resistance. Time constant is calculated as the product of compliance and resistance. It takes one, three, and five time constants to cause a 63%, 95%, and a 99% change in lung volume, respectively (Fig. 57.1).[1] Normal expiration is passive because of the elastic recoil of the lung, which is attributable to alveolar surface tension and tissue elasticity. Surface tension is greatest at high lung volumes and lowest at FRC. Elastic recoil of the lung provides most of the force required to expel the gas from the lungs. Inspiratory and expiratory time constants may be different because the inspiratory and expiratory resistances are different.

Work of Breathing

During normal breathing, the work of breathing is performed entirely by the inspiratory muscles (Fig. 57.2), and almost all

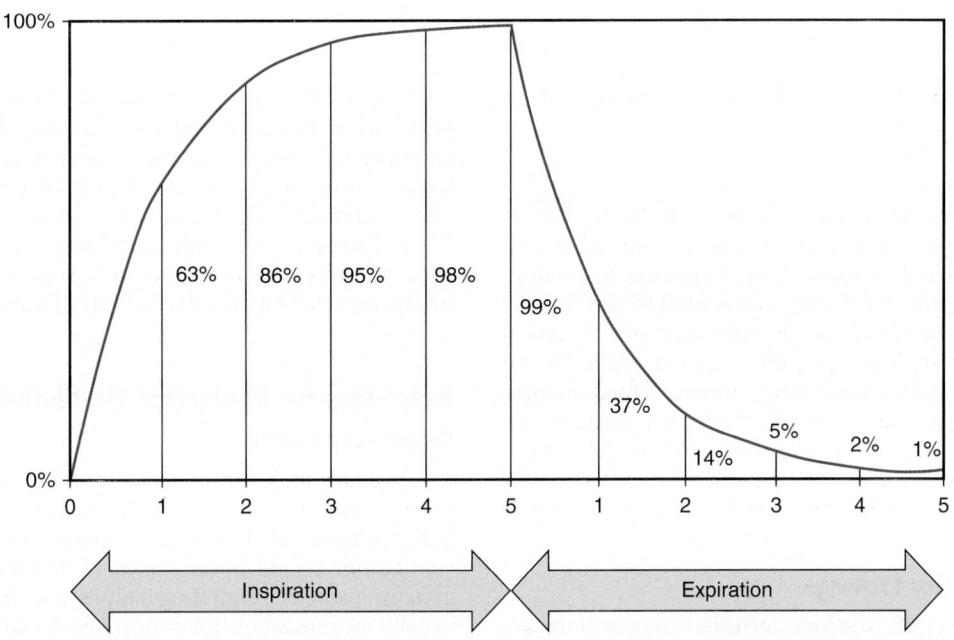

Fig. 57.1. Inspiratory and expiratory time constants. This graph shows the change in lung volume during inspiration and expiration by time constants. It takes 1, 2, 3, 4, and 5 time constants to cause a 63%, 86%, 95%, 98%, and 99% change in lung volume.

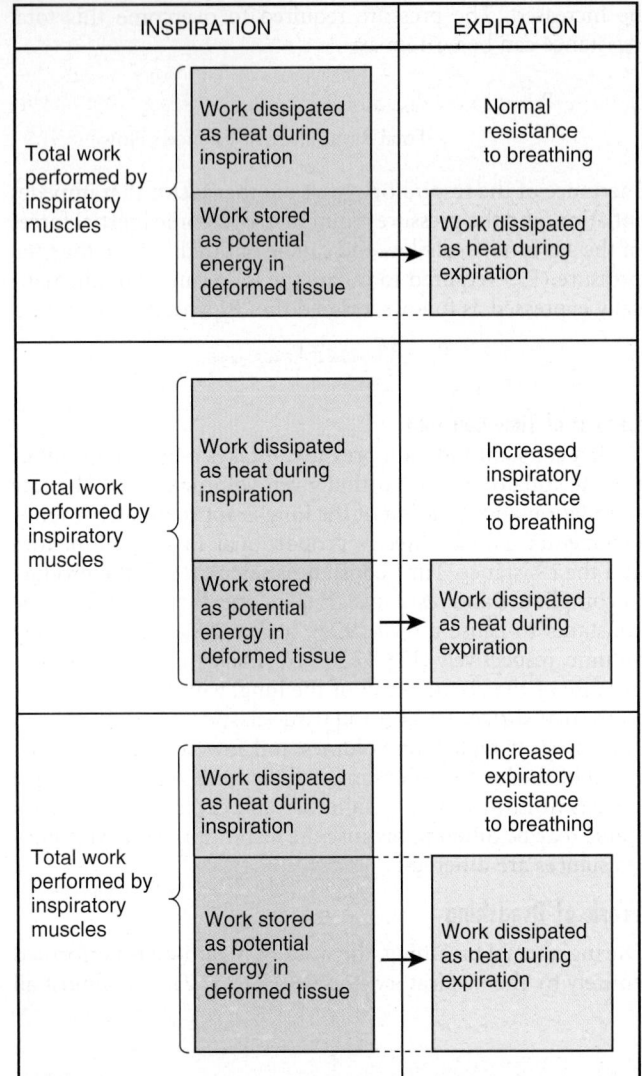

	INSPIRATION	EXPIRATION

Fig. 57.2. Work of breathing of respiratory muscles. The area in each box represents the amount of work performed. The left side shows the total amount of work performed with normal resistance and increased inspiratory and expiratory resistances to breathing. (Reproduced with permission from Nunn JF. Applied Respiratory Physiology. 3rd ed. London: Butterworths; 1987.)

of the work is performed during inspiration. Nearly half of the work of breathing during inspiration is dissipated as heat to overcome frictional resistance.[1] The remaining inspiratory work is stored as potential energy that is used to perform the expiratory work. Increased airway resistance and decreased chest and lung compliances would require a greater P_{tp} to inflate the lung to the same lung volume. These changes impose a greater workload on the respiratory muscles and increase the oxygen cost of breathing. When the oxygen supply-demand balance to the respiratory muscles is perturbed, respiratory failure may ensue because of muscle fatigue.

Determinants of Gas Exchange

The determinants of systemic arterial oxygenation are inspired oxygen concentration and tension, lung volume, cardiac output, ventilation-perfusion (V/Q) matching, and

TABLE 57.2   Causes of Ventilatory Pump Failure

Decreased Respiratory Muscle Capacity
Decreased respiratory center output (central nervous system disorders)
Phrenic nerve injury
Decreased muscle strength or endurance
Malnutrition
Prolonged neuromuscular blockade
Muscle fatigue
Electrolyte abnormalities

Increased Respiratory Muscle Load
Increased work of breathing
Hyperinflation
Lower airway obstruction
Decreased respiratory system compliance
Increased ventilatory requirements
Increased carbon dioxide production (eg, excessive carbohydrate intake)
Increased dead space
Hypercatabolic states (eg, sepsis)

the magnitude of venous admixture or intrapulmonary shunting. Lung volumes increase during inspiration and fall during expiration. During expiration, the presence of alveolar surfactant prevents alveolar collapse. A critical opening pressure is required to maintain both the patency of the terminal airways and alveolar volume. When the airway pressure is below the critical opening pressure, the terminal airway closes and the alveoli collapse because of continued absorption of gases into the bloodstream. Surfactant deficiency, loss, or alteration promotes alveolar collapse and increases the critical opening pressure. In parenchymal lung disease, which is characterized by an increased critical closing pressure, alveoli collapse during expiration if the airway pressures cannot be maintained above the critical opening pressure. Alveolar collapse leads to inadequate oxygenation due to increased intrapulmonary shunting resulting from (V/Q) mismatch.

The determinants of systemic arterial carbon dioxide ($PaCO_2$) include the tidal volume and the ventilator rate. $PaCO_2$ reflects the balance between metabolic production of CO_2 and its elimination. Decreased CO_2 elimination usually results from decreased central drive, lower airway obstruction, parenchymal disease, and muscle weakness. Inadequate ventilation causes CO_2 retention when it becomes insufficient to clear metabolic CO_2 production at a normal $PaCO_2$ (Table 57.2). Increased metabolic production of carbon dioxide usually results from hypermetabolic states or excessive caloric intake, especially high-carbohydrate alimentation.

Indications for Mechanical Ventilation
Respiratory Failure

The primary indication for institution of assisted ventilation is respiratory failure. Respiratory failure is generally defined as the presence of (1) inadequate oxygenation, (2) inadequate ventilation, or (3) both. Apnea or respiratory arrest is an extreme form of respiratory failure, and prolonged apnea is usually an indication for immediate mechanical ventilation. *Inadequate oxygenation*, objectively, is defined as partial pressure of arterial oxygen (PaO_2) less than 60 torr or an arterial hemoglobin oxygen saturation of less than 90% in room air. Oxygenation can also be expressed as the ratio of PaO_2 to fractional concentration of oxygen in inspired gas (FiO_2). *Inadequate oxygenation* can also be defined as a PaO_2-FiO_2 ratio of less than 300. Other indices include an alveolar-to-arterial oxygen gradient of more than 300 torr with a FiO_2 of 1.0. Inadequate oxygenation due to intrapulmonary shunting can be overcome with the addition of increased inspired oxygen concentration, provided the magnitude of the shunt is less than 15% (Fig. 57.3). Intrapulmonary shunt can be decreased by with the re-expansion of collapsed alveoli or with the decrease in the fraction of pulmonary blood flow going to the collapsed/consolidated alveolar segments. *Inadequate ventilation* is defined as a $PaCO_2$ greater than 45 torr with an arterial pH of less than 7.35 in the absence of chronic hypercapnia. Acute-on-chronic ventilatory failure is defined as a change in $PaCO_2$ of at least 20 torr with a corresponding decrease in arterial pH. Impending respiratory failure, characterized by rapidly rising $PaCO_2$, progressive respiratory distress, $PaCO_2$ out of proportion to the respiratory effort, or fatigue of respiratory muscles, is a relative indication for mechanical ventilation. Intubation and institution of mechanical ventilation in impending respiratory failure are likely to be more controlled than when full-blown respiratory failure develops. Therefore in critically ill children, establishing mechanical ventilation before respiratory failure develops is preferable. Chronic respiratory failure is defined as requirement for mechanical ventilation for more than 28 days. Children with chronic lung disease often fail to grow despite adequate caloric intake. In these patients, mechanical ventilation may decrease the work of breathing enough to allow the child to grow.

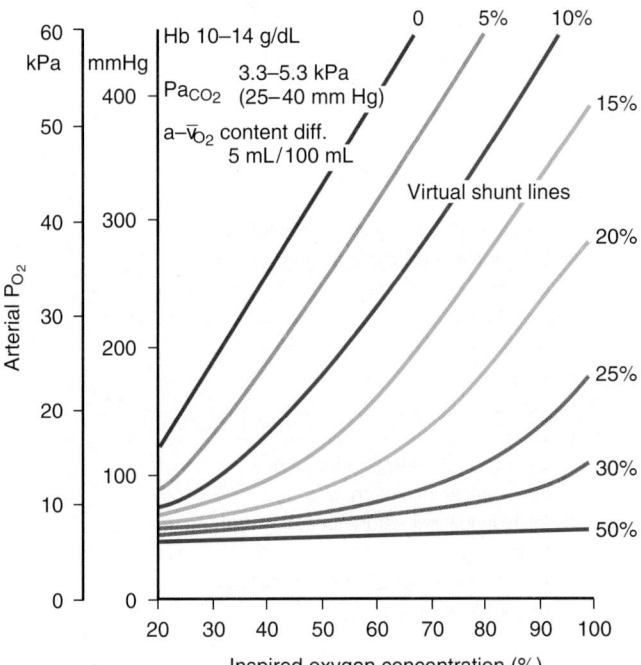

Fig. 57.3. Iso-shunt diagram. This shows the relationship among the magnitude of intrapulmonary shunt, the inspired oxygen concentration, and the arterial oxygen tension for a hypothetical patient. (Reproduced with permission from JF Nunn. Applied Respiratory Physiology. 3rd. London: Butterworths; 1987.)

Cardiovascular Dysfunction

Moderate to severe cardiovascular dysfunction is another major indication for mechanical ventilation. The cardiovascular and respiratory systems must act in concert to maintain adequate gas exchange and thereby meet the metabolic demands of the whole body. Therefore the two systems cannot be functionally divorced from each other. Cardiovascular dysfunction can result in a decrease in respiratory reserve and an increase in respiratory work and may ultimately result in respiratory failure. Positive pressure ventilation decreases lactic acid production by respiratory muscles during circulatory shock, and withdrawal of ventilatory support results in a marked increase in cardiac work with poor cardiac reserve.[2,3]

Neurologic and Neuromuscular Disorders

Acute neurologic disorders may require mechanical ventilation for many reasons. First, neurologic disorders may result in decreased ventilatory drive and therefore result in acute hypercapnia. Second, loss of airway protective reflexes may require an artificial airway for maintaining airway integrity and for providing an access for suctioning pooled secretions. Third, mechanical ventilation may be instituted to deliberately cause hyperventilation in disorders associated with intracranial hypertension to produce hypocapnia and respiratory alkalosis. Fourth, certain acute neuromuscular disorders such as Guillain-Barré syndrome, transverse myelitis, botulism, and drugs may result in decreased ventilatory effort because of muscle weakness and may result in hypoventilation and hypercarbia. Mechanical ventilation is usually instituted under these circumstances until the patient recovers from the primary disorder. Mechanical ventilation is also instituted for various chronic neuromuscular disorders such as muscular dystrophy and for permanent neurologic disorders such as spinal cord transection for prolonged home ventilator support.

Design and Functional Characteristics of Ventilators

A detailed review of the physical characteristics and functional design of ventilators is beyond the scope of this chapter, and the reader is referred to several excellent reviews on this subject.[4-16] In 1991, Chatburn proposed a new system for understanding the design of mechanical ventilators.[7] Since the initial publication in 1991, this classification has been subsequently updated and revised.[8-15] Most recently, Chatburn et al.[16] published fundamental maxims that describe the taxonomy of mechanical ventilation. The following is a summary that incorporates Chatburn's classification and taxonomy.[7-16]

Ventilator as a Machine

The concept is a simple one—a ventilator is simply a machine that performs external work.[6] This requires energy to be applied to the device, which is then altered, transmitted, and directed in a predetermined manner to perform the work of breathing. This work can either replace the patient's work of breathing completely or partially or augment a patient's breathing efforts. Therefore a ventilator is a mechanical device that is used to move gas into the lungs by increasing P_{tp}. Positive pressure ventilators create P_{tp} by raising the airway pressure (Paw) above the intrapleural pressure (P_{pl}), whereas negative pressure ventilators create P_{tp} by decreasing P_{pl} below Paw.

Classification of Ventilators

The scheme to classify mechanical ventilators is shown in Table 57.3. All ventilators include an input power, a drive system, a control system, a cycling mechanism, and a system to provide positive end-expiratory pressure (PEEP).[4-12] The accessories include a heated humidifier and an oxygen blender. The input power provides the energy to operate the ventilator and is usually electric or pneumatic. The drive system provides the force required to generate a gas flow. For gas flow to be provided, a pressure gradient needs to be created between the ventilator and the lungs. This is most commonly accomplished with compressed gases at high pressures from wall outlets or cylinders or a small compressor designed to be used with individual ventilators. In this scheme, the ventilator acts only to modulate the flow of gas and will not function if the external source of gas fails. Alternatively, some ventilators have a built-in compressor such as a piston and cylinder or a system of bellows, or a rotating vane. A ventilator that has an internal compressor does not need an external source of gas to inflate the lung.

The pressure generated within the ventilator can be thought of as the driving pressure that forces the gas into the lungs through the conducting system involving the ventilator circuit and the patient's airways. During mechanical ventilation, for a single breath, P_{tp} may be generated either by the ventilator or a spontaneous breath or a combination of both. Therefore the equation of motion can be reexpressed as:

$$P_{tp} = P_{mus} + P_{vent} = (Volume \times Elastance) + (Total\ Resistance \times Flow)$$

where P_{mus} is the pressure exerted by the respiratory muscles and P_{vent} is the pressure exerted by the ventilator.

Compliance and resistance are assumed to remain constant during lung inflation and are called *parameters*. Pressure, volume, and flow in the respiratory system change with time

---

TABLE 57.3   Outline of Ventilator Classification System

I. Input
   A. Electric
      1. AC
      2. DC (battery)
   B. Pneumatic
II. Power Conversion and Transmission (drive mechanism)
   A. Compressor
      1. External
      2. Internal
   B. Motor and linkage
      1. Electric motor/rotating crank and piston rod
      2. Electric motor/rack and pinion
      3. Electric motor/direct
      4. Compressed gas/direct
   C. Output control valves
      1. Electromagnetic poppet valve
      2. Pneumatic poppet valve
      3. Electromagnetic proportional valve
      4. Pneumatic diaphragm
III. Control Scheme
   A. Control circuit
      1. Mechanical
      2. Pneumatic
      3. Fluidic
      4. Electric
      5. Electronic
   B. Control variables and waveforms
      1. Pressure
      2. Volume
      3. Flow
      4. Time
   C. Phase variables
      1. Trigger variable
      2. Limit variable
      3. Cycle variable
      4. Baseline variable
   D. Modes of ventilation and conditional variables

IV. Output
   A. Pressure
      1. Rectangular
      2. Exponential
      3. Sinusoidal
      4. Oscillating
   B. Volume
      1. Ramp
      2. Sinusoidal
   C. Flow
      1. Rectangular
      2. Ramp: (a) ascending ramp, (b) descending ramp
      3. Sinusoidal
   D. Effects of the patient circuit
V. Alarm Systems
   A. Input power alarms
      1. Loss of electric power
      2. Loss of pneumatic power
   B. Control circuit alarms
      1. General systems failure (ventilator-inoperative)
      2. Incompatible ventilator settings
      3. Inverse I:E ratio
   C. Output alarms
      1. Pressure
      2. Volume
      3. Flow
      4. Time
         (a) high/low ventilatory frequency
         (b) high/low inspiratory time
         (c) high/low expiratory time
      5. Inspired gas
         a) high/low inspired gas temperature
         b) high/low FiO_2

Reproduced from Chatburn RL. Classification of Mechanical Ventilators, Respiratory Care Equipment. Philadelphia: JB Lippincott; 1995.
FiO_2, fractional concentration of oxygen in inspired gas; *I:E*, inspiratory-to-expiratory time ratio.

and are therefore referred to as *variables*. Fig. 57.4 shows the classification scheme that is based on the equation of motion.

A ventilator can also be viewed as a form of mechanical controller that "controls" either pressure (in a pressure generator) or flow (in a flow generator). A pressure generator is a ventilator that generates a fixed pattern of pressure within the ventilator and at the mouth, regardless of the lung conditions, whereas the flow waveform is free to vary.[4,5] This occurs when the generated pressure is low (generally between 20 and 50 cms H_2O), which results in a high initial flow rate that decays to zero as the alveolar pressure approaches the generated pressure.[4,5] The generated pressure can be constant, nonconstant, increasing, or decreasing. The Hand-E-Vent (Ohio Medical Products), Bird Asthmatik (Bird Corporation), Bennett PR-1, and Bennett PR-2 ventilators are examples of pressure generators. A flow generator is a ventilator that generates a high driving pressure (3–50 psig corresponding to 200–3500 cm H_2O) and controls the inspiratory flow of gas into the patient by interposing a high series resistance system between the generated pressure and the patient. The flow generated may be constant, nonconstant, increasing, or decreasing.[4,5]

Patterns of Gas Flow

The pattern of gas flow from the ventilator to the patient depends on the driving mechanism and the driving pressure in the ventilator. Four distinct flow patterns can be recognized: (1) a constant flow, (2) a decelerating flow, 3) an accelerating flow, and (4) a sinusoidal or sine-wave flow (Figs. 57.5–57.7). A constant inspiratory flow is generated when the driving pressure is high (eg, 50 psig) relative to the airway pressure. The drive mechanism is usually a high-pressure gas system (compressed air or oxygen at 10–50 psig). The driving force generally exceeds 1000 cm H_2O and is many times higher than the

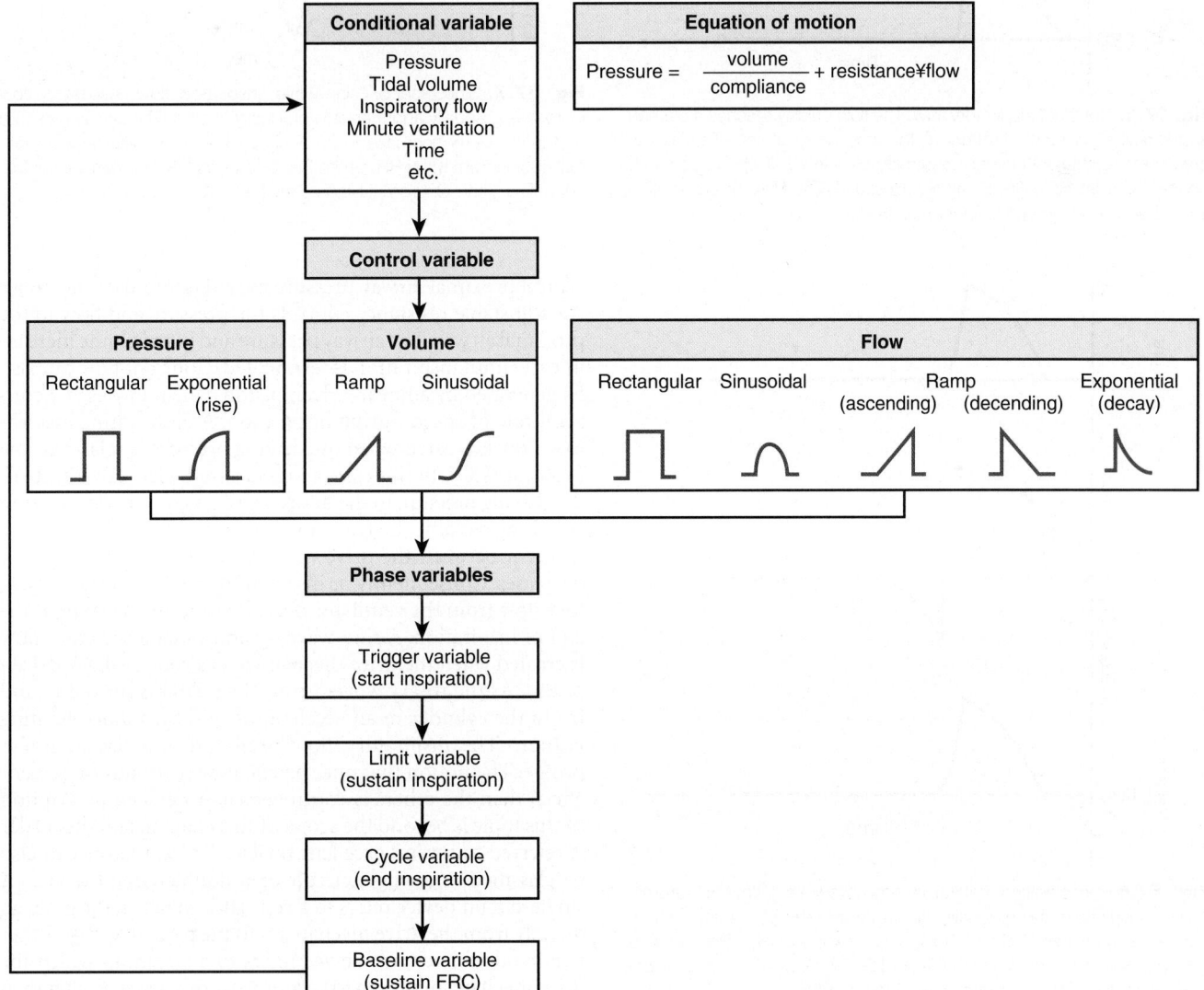

Fig. 57.4. Chatburn classification system based on a mathematic model known as the equation of motion for the respiratory system. This model indicates that during inspiration the ventilator is able to directly control one and only one variable at a time (eg, pressure, volume, or flow). Some common waveforms provided by current ventilators are shown for each control variable. Pressure, volume, flow, and time are also used as phase variables that determine the parameters of each ventilatory cycle (eg, trigger sensitivity, peak inspiratory flow rate or pressure, inspiratory time, baseline pressure). (Reproduced with permission from Chatburn RL. Classification of Mechanical Ventilators, Respiratory Care Equipment. Philadelphia: JB Lippincott; 1995.)

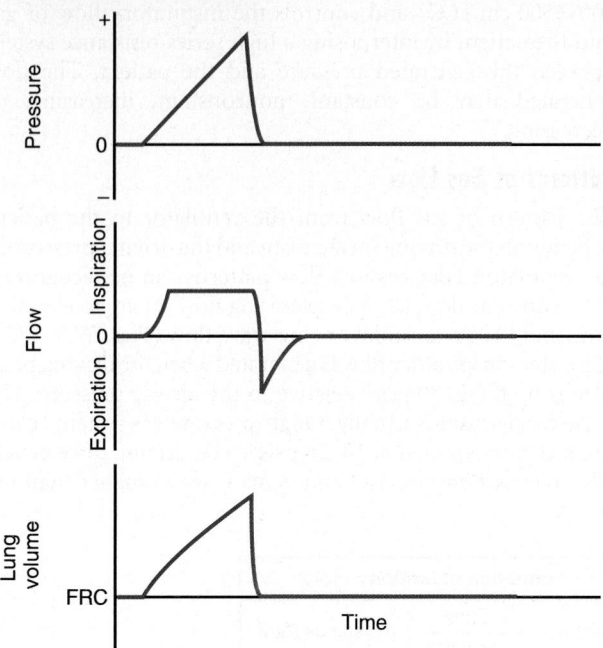

Fig. 57.5. Constant inspiratory flow. The flow quickly reaches a plateau and remains constant throughout the inspiratory phase. The airway pressure and lung volume increase relatively linearly. (Reproduced with permission from Kirby RR, Smith RA, Desautels DA. Mechanical Ventilation. New York: Churchill Livingstone; 1985.)

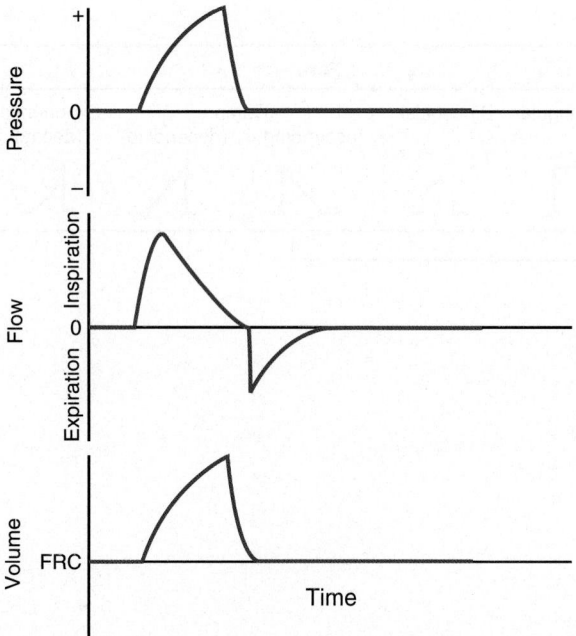

Fig. 57.6. Decelerating inspiratory flow. Inspiratory flow is maximal early in inspiration and gradually falls to zero at the end of inspiration. The airway pressure and lung volume rise exponentially. (Reproduced with permission from Kirby RR, Smith RA, Desautels DA. Mechanical Ventilation. New York: Churchill Livingstone; 1985.)

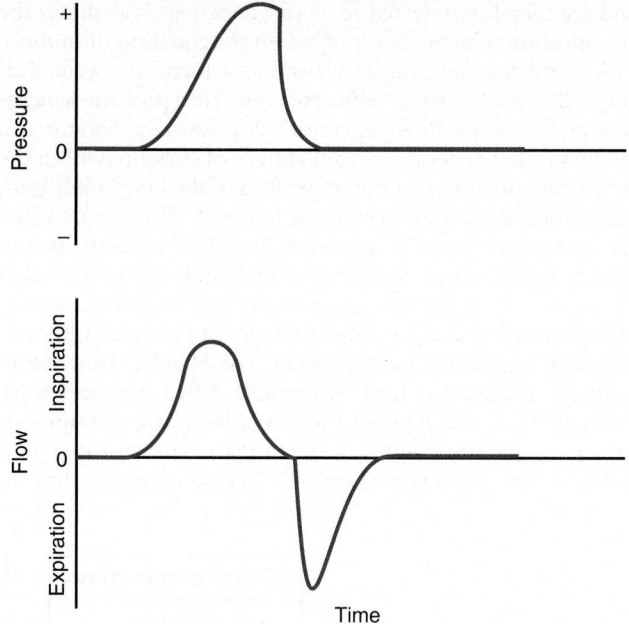

Fig. 57.7. Sinusoidal or "sine-wave" inspiratory flow. Inspiratory flow increases gradually and then falls gradually to zero. The airway pressure and lung volume increase in an S-shaped fashion. (Reproduced with permission from Kirby RR, Smith RA, Desautels DA. Mechanical Ventilation. New York: Churchill Livingstone; 1985.)

typical proximal airway pressure required to inflate the lungs. An adjustable resistance controls the pressure and flow to the proximal airway. The airway pressure and lung volume increase linearly until inspiration is terminated. Constant flow can also be generated by a linear-driven piston, which moves at a constant rate of speed during inspiration. A decelerating inspiratory flow is created when the driving pressure is relatively low (<60 cm H$_2$O). In this case, a pressure-reducing valve controls the driving pressure to the desired level. As the airway pressure and lung volume increase during inspiration, the pressure gradient between the drive mechanism and proximal airway decreases. Consequently, as inspiration progresses, the inspiratory flow from the ventilator decreases and finally stops at the end of inspiration. A sine-wave or sinusoidal inspiratory flow is created when the drive mechanism is a rotary wheel–driven piston. As the rotary wheel turns, the piston is moved to and fro in the cylinder in an accelerating and then a decelerating fashion. The inspiratory flow produced also has a similar profile. The notion that one specific flow pattern is more beneficial than the others is controversial. A detailed description of this topic is beyond the scope of this chapter, and the reader is referred to several excellent reviews.[4-12] Ventilators can also be classified as a single-circuit or a double-circuit device. A single-circuit device refers to a ventilator in which the gases go directly from the drive mechanism to the patient. On the other hand, a double-circuit device refers to a system in which the drive mechanism is used to compress another system that then delivers the tidal volume.[4-12]

Modes of Ventilation

The section below is a summary of several excellent articles.[7-16] A mode of ventilation can be defined by a predetermined pattern of patient-ventilator interaction that has three components. They are (1) the ventilator breath control variable, (2) the breath sequence, and (3) the targeting scheme.

Ventilator Breath Control Variable

A breath is defined as one cycle of positive flow (inspiration) and negative flow (expiration) defined in terms of the flow-time curve.[16] Inspiratory time is defined as the period from the start of positive flow to the start of negative flow. Expiratory time is defined as the period from the start of negative flow to the start of positive flow. Total cycle time is the sum of inspiratory and expiratory times and is equal to the inverse of breathing frequency. The inspiratory-expiratory (I:E) ratio is defined as the ratio of inspiratory time to expiratory time. Percent inspiratory time (also called the *duty cycle*) is defined as the ratio of inspiratory time to total cycle time. The tidal volume (VT) is the integral of flow with respect to time. For constant flow inspiration, this simply reduces to the product of flow and inspiratory time.[16]

An unassisted breath is defined as one in which the ventilator provides the flow rate required by the patient's efforts, and the transrespiratory system pressure stays nearly constant throughout the breath.[16] Breaths occurring during continuous positive airway pressure (CPAP) are an example of unassisted breaths. An assisted breath is defined as one in which the ventilator performs some or all of the work of breathing. A fully supported breath is one in which the ventilator performs all of the mechanical work of inspiration (eg, drug-induced neuromuscular blockade) when the respiratory muscles are inactive. In a fully supported breath, a ventilator assists breathing using either pressure control or volume control based on the equation of motion for the respiratory system.

It is important to understand that the term *volume control* means that the volume and inspiratory flow are predetermined. Only when both the parameters are preset can it be referred to as *volume control*. For example, if the tidal volume is preset but the ventilator is allowed to change the flow during inspiration, it would not be a volume-controlled breath. Similarly, if the inspiratory flow is preset but the volume delivered is dependent on the inspiratory pressure and/or the respiratory mechanics, then it cannot be referred to as volume control. It is important to understand that the term *volume control* is used as a standard term based on the taxonomy and does not refer to a manufacturer's mode.[16] Similarly, in pressure control, inspiratory pressure as a function of time is predetermined, which means presetting a particular pressure waveform or an inspiratory pressure proportional to the patient's effort (such as with neutrally adjusted ventilator assist [NAVA]). In pressure control, the flow and volume depend on the compliance and resistance of the respiratory system.[16] Again, pressure control does not refer to a specific manufacturer's mode. Time control is a category of ventilator modes in which the flow, volume, and pressure during inspiration depend on the mechanics of the respiratory system. High-frequency oscillatory ventilation (HFOV) and high-frequency percussive ventilation are examples of time control.[16]

Breath Sequence
Phases of a Breath

Trigger is a signal that starts inspiration. Time, pressure, flow, minimum minute ventilation, apnea interval, and electrical signals are used as inspiratory triggers. Cycling refers to the termination of inspiration and start of expiration. Inspiratory time, pressure, volume, flow, and electrical signals are used as cycling signals.[16] All ventilators are equipped with mechanisms to provide four basic functions: (1) inflate the lungs, (2) terminate lung inflation, (3) allow lungs to empty, and (4) start lung inflation.[7,8,10,11,16] The ventilator performs these functions through four phases: (1) the inspiratory phase, (2) the changeover from the inspiratory to the expiratory phase, (3) the expiratory phase, and (4) the changeover from the expiratory phase to the inspiratory phase.

Classification of Breaths

The criteria used to start (trigger) and stop (cycle) inspiration are used to classify breaths. Both triggering and cycling events can be initiated by either the ventilator or the patient. When inspiratory flow starts with a ventilator-generated signal, it is referred to as *ventilator triggering* and is independent of a patient-initiated signal. Similarly, when inspiration starts on a patient-generated signal, it is referred to as patient triggering and is independent of a ventilator-generated signal. Ventilator cycling refers to ending inspiration based on signals from the ventilator independent of signals based on patient factors. Time cycling is a common criterion and refers to the time that has elapsed from the start of inspiration and is breath-to-breath. Patient cycling occurs when a signal based on the patient's respiratory mechanics, which affects the equation of motion, reaches a threshold value. For example, in flow cycling, which is a form of patient cycling, the inspiratory flow decays to the threshold value dependent on the patient's respiratory mechanics.[16]

Spontaneous Versus Mandatory Breaths

When the start and end of a breath are determined by the patient, it is referred to as a *spontaneous breath*.[16] This means that a spontaneous breath is both patient triggered and patient cycled and is independent of any ventilator settings. A spontaneous breath may be unassisted or assisted. An unassisted spontaneous breath refers to a breath where the patient determines both the timing and size of the breath. Normal breathing is unassisted spontaneous breathing. T-piece breathing or breaths during CPAP are also examples of unassisted spontaneous breathing.[16] The size of the breath is determined solely by the effort of the patient with no additional help from the ventilator. An assisted spontaneous breath refers to a breath where the ventilator does some of the inspiratory work indicated by an increase in airway pressure above the baseline. For an assisted breath, the patient must initiate a breath, and then the ventilator is triggered to provide a positive pressure breath. The trigger can be either pressure or flow. With an assisted spontaneous breath, the ventilator contributes to the size of the breath but it is important to understand that the patient determines the timing of the breath. Pressure-supported breath is an example of an assisted spontaneous breath. A mandatory breath is one in which the start or end of inspiration (or both) is determined by the ventilator, independent of the patient. The inspiratory time is not under the control of the patient. A mandatory breath may occur during a spontaneous breath (eg, high-frequency jet ventilation).[16] A spontaneous breath may occur during a mandatory breath (eg, airway pressure release ventilation). The criteria for determining the phase variables during a mechanical breath are shown in Fig. 57.8.

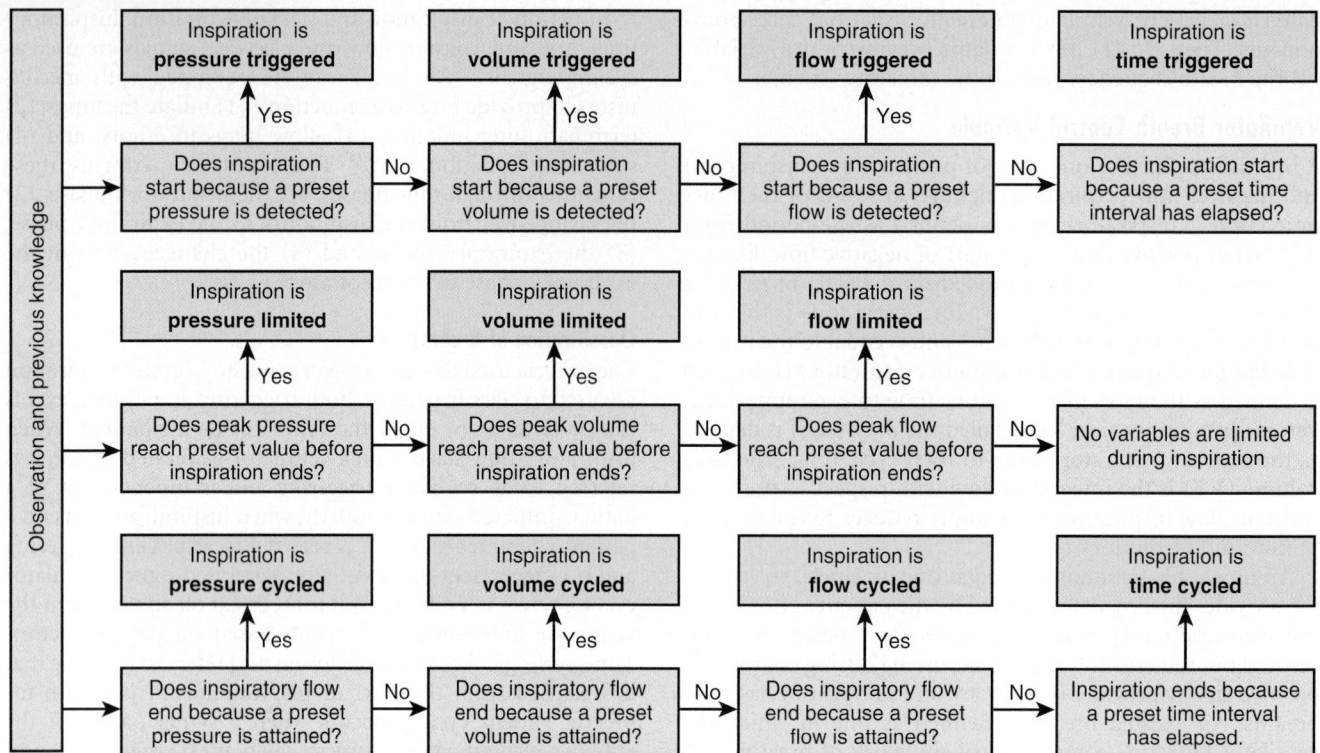

Fig. 57.8. Criteria for determining phase variables during a ventilator-assisted breath. (Reproduced from Chatburn RL. Classification of Mechanical Ventilators, Respiratory Care Equipment. Philadelphia: JB Lippincott; 1995.)

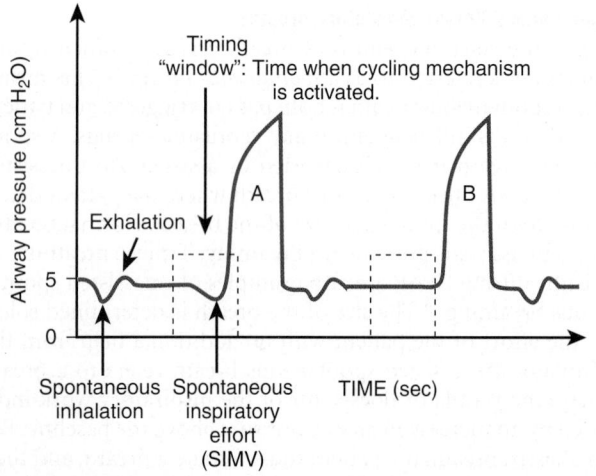

Fig. 57.9. Synchronized intermittent mandatory ventilation. At set intervals, the ventilator's timing circuit becomes activated and a timing "window" appears *(dotted line)*. If the patient initiates a breath in the timing window, then the ventilator will deliver a mandatory breath. If no spontaneous effort occurs, then the ventilator will deliver a mandatory breath a fixed time after the timing window. (Reproduced with permission from Kirby RR, Smith RA, Desautels DA. Mechanical Ventilation. New York: Churchill Livingstone; 1985.)

Breath Sequences

Ventilators deliver three basic breath sequences: (1) continuous mandatory ventilation (CMV), (2) intermittent mandatory ventilation (IMV), and (3) continuous spontaneous ventilation (CSV).[8,10,11,16] CMV refers to a breath sequence when all the breaths are mandatory. Even if there is a patient-triggered signal, it will result in a mandatory breath. During CMV, spontaneous breaths are not permitted or do not occur between mandatory breaths. If the patient is breathing spontaneously during CMV, each spontaneous breath may trigger a mandatory breath. Assist-control refers to a mode of ventilation when a patient receives a combination of ventilator-initiated and patient-initiated mandatory breaths. The total number of mechanical breaths will be the sum of the preset frequency of ventilator breaths and the number of patient-triggered breaths. When all minute ventilation is provided by the ventilator, it is referred to as *total ventilatory support*. Total ventilatory support is provided when the patient does not take any spontaneous efforts because of a primary disease process (eg, quadriplegia, muscle disease), pharmacologic therapy (eg, induced neuromuscular blockade), or suppression of spontaneous breathing efforts (eg, hyperventilation). Spontaneous efforts are used only for triggering (assist-control). Total ventilatory support is provided entirely by CMV (Fig. 57.9).

Intermittent Mandatory Ventilation

IMV refers to a breath sequence in which spontaneous breaths occur between mandatory breaths. The concept of IMV where spontaneous breathing occurred with a preset mechanical ventilator rate was first developed by Kirby et al.[17] in 1971 with the use of a continuous flow circuit in the management of respiratory distress syndrome of the neonate. The total ventilatory support time and duration of weaning were significantly reduced in infants using IMV compared with CMV.[18,19] IMV was later introduced as a mode by Downs et al.[20] in 1973 to describe a mode of ventilation that allowed the patient to

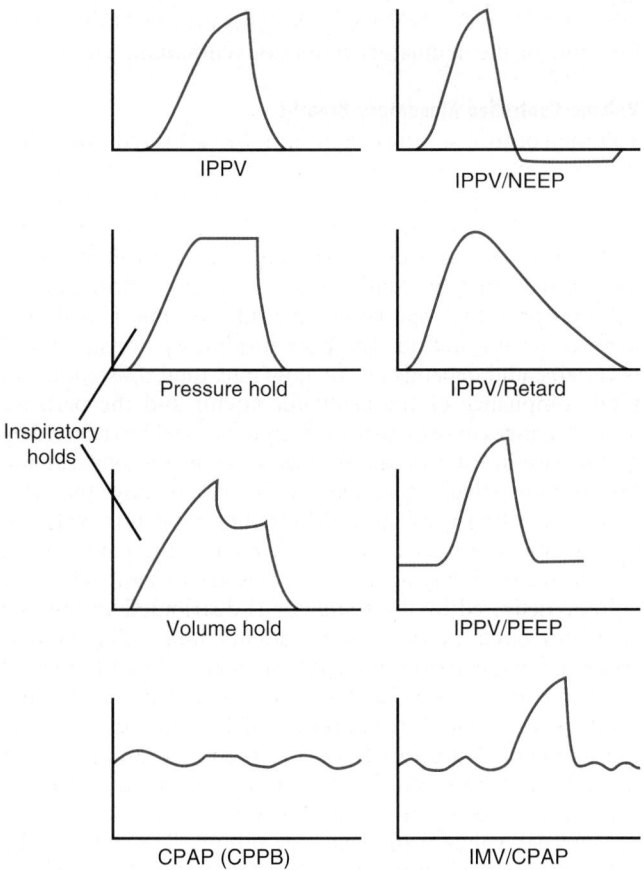

Fig. 57.10. Pressure-time curves of some of the mandatory modes of ventilation. (Reproduced with permission from Kirby RR, Smith RA, Desautels DA. Mechanical Ventilation. New York: Churchill Livingstone; 1985.)

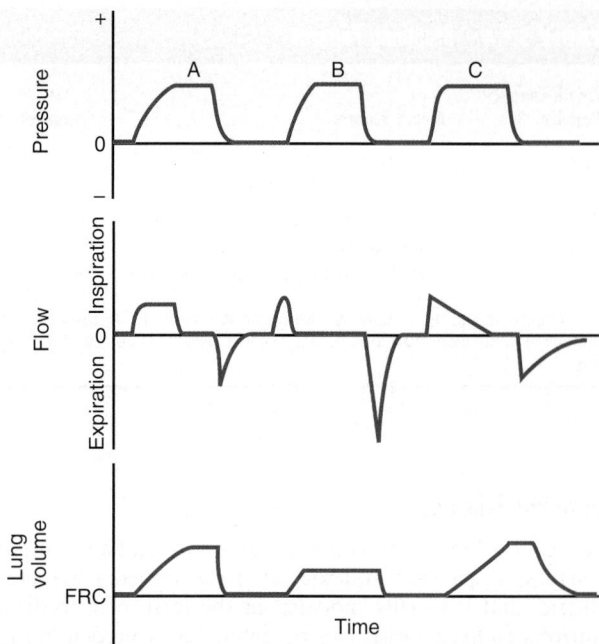

Fig. 57.11. Pressure-control ventilation. Inspiratory flow pattern is constant. Airway pressure and lung volume rise relatively linearly. The airway pressure reaches a preset pressure limit and does not change throughout inspiration. Lung volume follows the time course of the pressure curve with a slight lag. *(A)* Normal lung. *(B)* Lung with decreased compliance. *(C)* Lung with increased resistance. With decreased compliance the tidal volume delivered is decreased. With increased resistance, it takes longer to deliver the tidal volume. (Reproduced with permission from Kirby RR, Smith RA, Desautels DA. Mechanical Ventilation. New York: Churchill Livingstone; 1985.)

breathe spontaneously with a preset ventilator rate. The total minute ventilation is due to a combination of mandatory mechanical breaths and spontaneous breaths. There are three forms of IMV. In the first, mandatory breaths are always delivered at the set frequency. Two systems are currently available to deliver this form of IMV: One uses continuous flow, and the other uses a demand valve. These breaths may or may not be synchronized. When IMV is synchronized to the patient's inspiratory efforts, it is referred to as *synchronized IMV* (SIMV) (Fig. 57.11). The ventilator accomplishes this by creating a timing window just before the next mandatory breath is scheduled to be delivered. If the patient takes a spontaneous breath in this timing window and the ventilator senses this breath on the basis of the trigger sensitivity, then the mandatory breath is synchronized with the patient's effort. Each time a synchronized breath is delivered, the machine recomputes the time required to deliver the next mandatory breath. In SIMV, the total number of mandatory breaths will only be equal to the preset frequency of mandatory breaths. SIMV breaths can be either volume regulated or pressure limited. If a synchronization window is used, the ventilatory period of the previous mandatory breath may actually be shorter than the set period. In some ventilators, the next mandatory breath may be longer to maintain the set mandatory breathing frequency. In the second type of IMV, mandatory breaths are delivered only when the spontaneous breathing rate falls

below a threshold (set individually for each patient). If the spontaneous rate is above the threshold, then all the breaths are assisted spontaneous breaths. But when the spontaneous rate falls below the set frequency, the breath sequence becomes IMV. The IMV rate is often referred to as a "backup rate." In the third form of IMV, when the spontaneous minute ventilation drops below a threshold, mandatory breaths are delivered to maintain the minimum minute ventilation (Fig. 57.10).

Ventilatory Pattern

A ventilatory pattern is a sequence of breaths (CMV, IMV, or CSV) with a designated control variable (volume control [VC] or pressure control [PC]). Thus there are six theoretically possible ventilatory patterns based on three breath sequences and two control variables. These are VC-CMV, PC-CMV, VC-IMV, PC-IMV, VS-CSV, and PC-CSV.[16] The VC-CSV combination is not possible because volume control implies ventilator cycling (time or volume) and therefore, by definition, is a mandatory breath. Thus we are left with five ventilatory patterns (Table 57.4).[16] These five ventilatory patterns are what are available in what would be termed "conventional ventilators." Time can also be a control variable so that both CMV and IMV are possible time control ventilatory patterns such as in high-frequency oscillatory ventilation (HFOV) or high-frequency percussive ventilation. Only one ventilatory pattern can be present in a mode of ventilation. The ventilatory pattern can be used as a mode classification system.[16]

TABLE 57.4 Breathing Patterns

Breath-Control Variable	Breath Sequence	Acronym
Volume	Continuous mandatory ventilation	VC-CMV
	Intermittent mandatory ventilation	VC-IMV
Pressure	Continuous mandatory ventilation	PC-CMV
	Intermittent mandatory ventilation	PC-IMV
	Continuous spontaneous ventilation	PC-CSV

From Chatburn RL, El Khatib, M, Mireles-Cabodevila E. A taxonomy for mechanical ventilation: 10 fundamental maxims. Respir Care. 2014;59:1747-1763.

Targeting Schemes

The relationship between operator inputs to ventilator outputs to achieve a specific ventilator pattern is termed a "targeting scheme" and is usually modeled in the form of a feedback control system. A target can be defined as a predetermined goal of the ventilator output. Targets can be set either within breaths or between breaths. Within-breath targets or parameters relate to pressure, flow, and volume waveforms. Between-breath targets, mainly used within advanced targeting schemes, may be set to modify the within-breath targets and/or the overall ventilatory pattern (between-breath targets).[16]

There are currently seven basic targeting schemes: (1) set-point targeting, (2) dual targeting, (3) biovariable targeting, (4) servo targeting, (5) adaptive targeting, (6) optimal targeting, and (7) intelligent targeting. In set-point targeting, the operator sets all of the parameters of the waveform (pressure or volume/flow). Dual targeting refers to a scheme in which the ventilator is allowed to switch between pressure and volume control. When the ventilator randomly sets the inspiratory pressure or the tidal volume to mimic the variability seen with normal breathing, it is referred to as biovariable targeting. Servo targeting allows the ventilator output to be automatically adjusted to a varying input. In adaptive targeting, the ventilator automatically sets one target (pressure in a breath) to achieve another (average tidal volume over several breaths). When a performance characteristic (eg, work rate of breathing) is minimized or maximized, by automatically adjusting the ventilatory pattern, it is referred to as optimal targeting. In the recent article on the taxonomy, Chatburn et al.[16] have used the modern taxonomy to describe the several manufacturers' different modes. It is important to understand that many of the modern modes have not been tested in infants and children. Many of the modes are currently being investigated in adults. The following is a description of some of the most common modes used in infants and children, as well as some newer modes in more detail.

Commonly Used Mandatory Modes

The two most common forms of controlled mandatory mechanical ventilation modes that are used in infants and children are pressure-limited time-cycled and volume-controlled time-cycled modes of ventilation. Pressure-limited time-cycled ventilation would be classified as PC-CMV or PC-IMV according to the modern taxonomy. Similarly, volume-controlled time-cycled ventilation would be classified as VC-CMV or VC-IMV. Fig. 57.8 shows pressure-time curves for some of the mandatory modes of ventilation.

Volume-Controlled Mandatory Breaths

Volume-controlled ventilation can be delivered by either volume-cycled breath, where inspiration is terminated after a preset volume is delivered and inspiratory time is allowed to vary, or volume-controlled time-cycled breaths, where the cycling mechanism is preset time and the tidal volume delivered is regulated by adjusting the inspiratory flow rate. In volume-controlled ventilation, the tidal volume is delivered throughout inspiration. The peak inspiratory pressure (PIP) is variable and depends on the flow rate, total resistance, and total compliance of the ventilator circuit and the patient's lungs. Changes in resistance or compliance will be reflected by an increase in PIP, and the ventilator can be set to alarm at a pressure limit that is generally set 5 to 10 cm above the PIP.

Most modern ventilators deliver the preset tidal volumes reliably, but the tidal volumes delivered to the patient on a breath-to-breath basis may not always be constant. The tidal volume delivered by the ventilator is distributed among the ventilator circuit, airways, and patient's lungs. The compliances and resistances of the ventilator circuit, the endotracheal or tracheostomy tube, and the patient independently and together affect the distribution of tidal volume delivered by the ventilator. A decrease in the compliance or an increase in the resistance of the ventilator circuit will affect the actual tidal volume delivered to the patient. The ventilator circuit includes an internal volume and external tubing. The actual tidal volume or the effective tidal volume (VT_{eff}) delivered to the patient can be approximated by the following formula:

$$VT_{eff} = VT_{del} + VT_{circuit}$$

where VT_{del} is tidal volume delivered by the ventilator and $VT_{circuit}$ is the volume of gas that is distributed to the ventilator circuit.

VT_{del} is equal to the inspired tidal volume, when there is no leak in the total respiratory system. When there is a leak in the system, however, such as with the use of uncuffed endotracheal tubes, then VT_{del} is less than the inspired tidal volume. $VT_{circuit}$ can be estimated by the following formula:

$$VT_{circuit} = C_{vent} \times (PIP - PEEP)$$

where C_{vent} is the compliance of the ventilator circuit, PIP is the peak inspiratory pressure reached in the circuit during inspiration, and $PEEP$ is the level of positive end-expiratory pressure.

An increase in resistance or compliance of the ventilator circuit (including the endotracheal tube) or the patient's airways or lungs will increase the time constant to inflation. If the inspiratory time is less than five times the time constant of the whole respiratory system, which includes the ventilator circuit and the patient's airways, then the VT_{del} will be less than the preset tidal volume. During inspiration, after the tidal volume is delivered, an inspiratory hold will maintain inspiratory pressure and prolong the duration of inspiration (see Fig. 57.8). During exhalation, expiratory flow curves depend on the type of expiratory resistance or PEEP valve in the system.

Pressure-Limited Mandatory Breaths

Pressure-limited ventilation can be either pressure-cycled or pressure-limited time-cycled ventilation. In pressure-cycled ventilators, inspiration is terminated when a preset pressure limit is reached. In this mode of ventilation, the inspiratory time may vary depending on the changes in resistance and compliance of the total respiratory system. This mode of ventilation is not widely used these days except for intermittent positive pressure breathing treatments. Pressure-limited, time-cycled ventilation is most commonly used in the neonate with respiratory distress syndrome and in children with acute respiratory distress syndrome (ARDS). In this mode, inspiratory and expiratory times are constant and the PIP reaches a preset limit quickly early in inspiration and is then maintained at that level during the rest of the inspiratory phase. Usually a high flow rate is used (4–10 L/kg/min). The tidal volume delivered depends on the compliance and resistance of the ventilator circuit and the patient's lungs. Pressure-controlled ventilation results in higher mean airway pressure for the same amount of minute ventilation. Fig. 57.11 shows the time course of changes in airway pressure, inspiratory flow, and lung volume with normal lungs, lungs with decreased compliance, and lungs with increased resistance. As shown in Fig. 57.11, with PIP remaining the same, lung volume delivered is affected by changes in lung compliance and airway resistance. Factors that would increase mean airway pressure during pressure-controlled ventilation are shown in Fig. 57.12.

Continuous Flow Versus Demand Flow

Some ventilators that can provide pressure-limited ventilation have both inspiratory and expiratory valves. Once PIP is reached, both inspiratory and expiratory valves close and the lung is held in inflation until the end of inspiration. For use in infants, ventilators were modified to provide continuous flow throughout the respiratory cycle.[17] A continuous flow

device refers to a ventilator in which the flow of respiratory gas occurs throughout the respiratory cycle. Most infant ventilators are continuous flow devices (eg, Infant Star, Baby Bird). In most continuous flow infant ventilators, inspiratory valves are lacking and the cycling is controlled by the exhalation valve. Closure of the exhalation valve begins inspiration, and the flow of gas going through the circuit is diverted to the patient. If the inspiratory flow rate is low (1–3 L/kg) and if the PIP is not limited, the tidal volume delivered by the patient can be calculated from the inspiratory flow rate and inspiratory time. This would result in a time-cycled, volume-controlled breath. For pressure-control ventilation, the flow rates used are usually higher (4–10 L/kg). Once the preset PIP is reached, the excess flow is vented through a pressure relief valve and the lungs are maintained in inflation throughout the rest of inspiration. During exhalation there is continuous flow of gas, allowing the patient to breathe from the circuit rather than open a demand valve. A demand flow ventilator refers to a ventilator that allows inspiratory flow of gas to the patient between ventilator breaths through a demand valve that is opened by the patient's inspiratory efforts. Work of breathing is higher with a demand flow ventilator compared with a continuous flow device because of the effort required to open the demand valve.

CPAP/PEEP

CPAP refers to the maintenance of positive airway pressure throughout the respiratory cycle with no positive pressure breaths being delivered to the patient. PEEP refers to the maintenance of positive airway pressure above atmospheric pressure at the airway opening at end expiration.[21] CPAP/PEEP can be applied by a variety of devices. These include (1) an underwater column, (2) a water-weighted diaphragm, (3) a venturi valve, (4) a spring-loaded valve, (5) a pressurized exhalation valve, (6) a magnetic valve, and (7) a fixed or adjustable orifice. Devices that retard expiratory flows (eg, venturi valve, fixed, or adjustable orifice) tend to produce higher mean airway pressure than those that do not retard expiratory flow rates.

CPAP may be provided by several means:
1. Endotracheal CPAP[5,22]: This is the most reliable method of applying CPAP. The advantages of endotracheal CPAP are precise control of airway pressure and FiO$_2$; access to the airway for tracheobronchial toilet; maintenance of enteral feeding through a nasogastric tube; and, if necessary, immediate institution of mechanical ventilation. The disadvantages are those associated with those of endotracheal intubation and the long-term presence of an artificial airway.
2. Nasal CPAP: Specially designed nasal prongs,[23] a single cannula or a shortened uncuffed endotracheal tube inserted into the nasopharynx, and nasal masks[24] provide a means of applying CPAP. Because of the location in the nasopharynx, there will be a loss of pressure in the hypopharynx so that the actual CPAP delivered to the trachea may vary. This technique is easy to apply and can be instituted by less-skilled personnel. This technique is most useful in infants who are obligatory nose breathers. Mouth breathing reduces the efficiency of this technique considerably. Nasal prongs are more prone to obstruction with thick secretions and require proper humidification and frequent suctioning. Nasal prongs have also been reported to increase the work of breathing.[25]

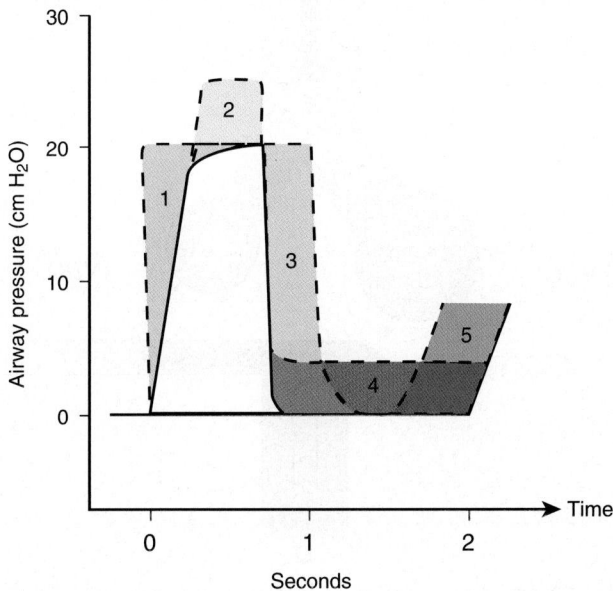

Fig. 57.12. Factors that increase mean airway pressure during pressure-controlled ventilation: *(1)* increased inspiratory flow rate, *(2)* increased preset pressure limit, *(3)* increased inspiratory time, *(4)* increased positive end-expiratory pressure, and *(5)* increased ventilator rate. Note that with each maneuver, the area under the curve increases. Area under the curve represents mean airway pressure. (Reproduced with permission from Goldsmith JP, Karotkin EH, eds. Assisted Ventilation of the Neonate. Philadelphia: WB Saunders; 1988.)

3. Facemask CPAP: A tight-fitting mask is placed on the face covering the nose and mouth. CPAP is provided with the application of positive airway pressure to the mask. This technique is only useful in patients who are alert and cooperative, without a tendency for nausea and vomiting. A tight-fitting mask may produce pressure lesions on the face if applied too tight. Gastric distention with vomiting and aspiration are potential problems.

The primary effect of CPAP/PEEP is an increase in end-expiratory lung volume due to the increased P_{tp}. In lung diseases characterized by increased closing volume and decreased FRC, alveoli are unstable and tend to collapse. Recruitment of collapsed alveoli requires a P_{tp} greater than that required to sustain inflation once the alveoli are open. An increase in FRC above the closing volume restores this balance, prevents alveolar collapse, and maintains alveolar stability (Fig. 57.13). This reduces the magnitude of V/Q mismatching because of improved distribution of alveolar ventilation.[26,27] Airway closure and alveolar collapse can be prevented if the level of CPAP/PEEP is above the critical opening pressure. In lung disease with nonuniform or heterogeneous parenchymal involvement, CPAP/PEEP may hyperinflate normal lung segments, and this hyperinflation results in redistribution of blood toward the diseased segments, increasing intrapulmonary shunt on one hand and increasing alveolar dead space on the other (Fig. 57.14).

Selection of Parameters for Mandatory Breaths
The first parameter is the tidal volume. A practical approach to determining an adequate tidal volume is to evaluate the desired degree of chest expansion during manual ventilation and reproduce that when the patient is connected to the ventilator. A desirable VT_{eff} for most patients is 8 to 10 mL/kg. Patients with normal lung compliance may require a preset tidal volume of 12 to 15 mL/kg to produce a VT_{eff} of 8 to 10 mL/kg. Ideally, the end-inspiratory alveolar pressure should be less than 30 cms of H_2O. The end-inspiratory alveolar pressure can be measured using an inspiratory hold maneuver. With an inspiratory hold, inspiratory flow is stopped, both inspiratory and expiratory valves are closed, and the proximal airway pressure equilibrates with the alveolar pressure. The end-inspiratory hold pressure is called the "pause pressure," "plateau pressure," or simply "end-inspiratory airway pressure." A large VT_{eff}, especially that which results in an end-inspiratory airway pressure greater than 40 cm of H_2O, should be avoided. During mechanical ventilation, end-inspiratory alveolar pressure can be estimated through the measurement of the end-inspiratory airway pressure with an end-inspiratory hold maneuver.

Ventilator rate is the next parameter to be selected. The initial rate selected depends on the age of the patient and ventilatory requirements of the patient and may subsequently be adjusted according to the $PaCO_2$. The initial ventilator rate for a newborn infant usually ranges from 25 to 30 breaths per minute; for a 1-year-old, between 20 and 25 breaths per minute; and for an adolescent, from 15 to 20 breaths per minute. The inspiratory time is selected to provide an inspiratory-to-expiratory time (I:E) ratio of at least 1:2 in most patients. Inspiratory time can be set as either a percentage of the total respiratory cycle or as a fixed time in seconds

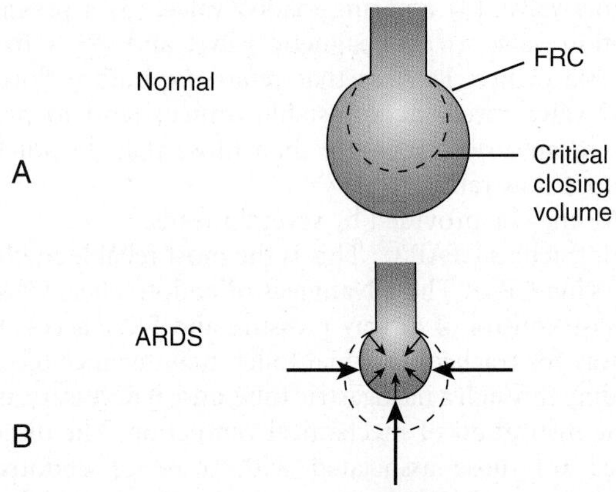

Fig. 57.13. Effect of continuous positive airway pressure (CPAP) on functional residual capacity (FRC). In normal lungs (A), FRC is greater than critical closing volume. In acute respiratory distress syndrome (ARDS) (B), FRC is less than critical closing volume. CPAP restores FRC to be greater than critical closing volume and prevents alveolar collapse (C). (Reproduced with permission from Kirby RR, Smith RA, Desautels DA. Mechanical Ventilation. New York: Churchill Livingstone; 1985.)

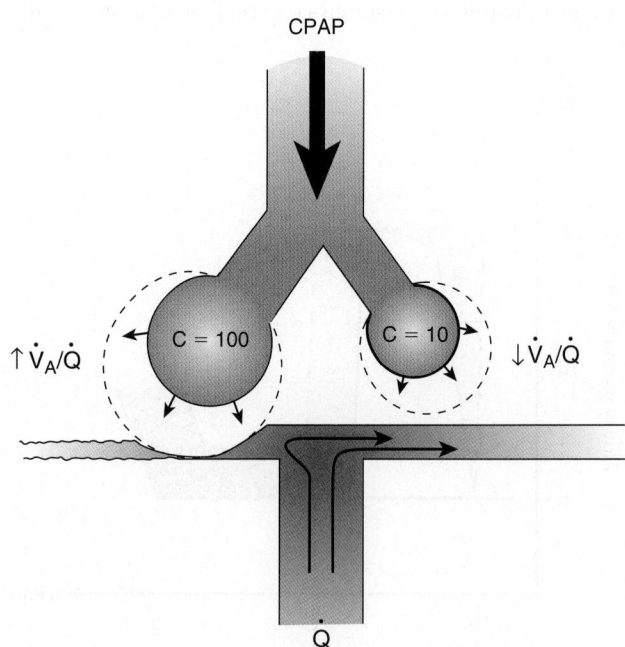

Fig. 57.14. Effect of continuous positive airway pressure (CPAP) on nonhomogenous lung disease. CPAP increases functional residual capacity (FRC) in the lung segment with decreased ventilation-perfusion ratio (V̇A/Q̇) and decreases shunt reaction. CPAP overdistends lung segments with high V̇A/Q̇ and redistributes blood toward the segments with low V̇A/Q̇, increasing the amount of shunt. The net effect depends on the balance between the two. (Reproduced with permission from Kirby RR, Smith RA, Desautels DA. Mechanical Ventilation. New York: Churchill Livingstone; 1985.)

depending on the ventilator. Inspiratory time must be selected to allow sufficient time for all lung segments to be inflated. In heterogenous lung disease with varying regional time constants, a short inspiratory time may not be sufficient to inflate all lung segments and may contribute to underventilation and underinflation. Similarly, sufficient expiratory time must be provided for all lung segments to empty. If inspiration starts before the lung has completely emptied, this will result in air trapping and inadvertent positive end-expiratory pressure. The I:E ratio can be adjusted according to the pathophysiologic cause of the lung disease. In infants with bronchiolitis and in children with asthma, the expiratory time may have to be lengthened to avoid air trapping.[28-30]

PEEP is the next parameter to be selected. The level of PEEP will depend on the clinical circumstance. PEEP increases mean Paw during both volume-controlled and pressure-controlled ventilation, which results in a higher mean lung volume. The goals of PEEP are (1) increasing end-expiratory lung volume above closing volume to prevent alveolar collapse, (2) maintaining stability of alveolar segments, (3) improving oxygenation, and (4) reducing work of breathing. The optimum PEEP is the level at which there is an acceptable balance between the desired goals and undesired adverse effects. The desired goals are (1) reduction in inspired oxygen concentration to "nontoxic" levels (usually $\leq 50\%$); (2) maintenance of PaO_2 or SaO_2 (arterial oxygen saturation) of more than 60 mm Hg or more than 90%, respectively; (3) improvement of lung compliance; and (4) maximal oxygen delivery.[28-30] Arbitrary limits cannot be placed on the level of PEEP or mean airway pressure that will be required to maintain adequate gas exchange. When the level of PEEP is high, peak inspiratory pressure may be limited to prevent it from reaching dangerous levels that contribute to air leaks and barotrauma.

FiO_2 is the next parameter to be selected. FiO_2 is adjusted to maintain an adequate PaO_2. High concentration of oxygen can produce lung injury and should be avoided. The exact threshold of inspired oxygen that increases the risk of lung injury is not clear. An FiO_2 less than 0.5 is generally considered safe. In patients with parenchymal lung disease with significant intrapulmonary shunting, the major determinant of oxygenation is lung volume, which is a function of the mean airway pressure. With a shunt fraction of more than 20%, oxygenation may not be substantially improved by higher concentrations of oxygen.

Other Modes Used in Infants and Children

Pressure-Support or Pressure-Support Ventilation

A pressure-supported breath is one that is patient triggered, pressure controlled, and flow cycled. It is an assisted spontaneous breath in which the ventilator assists the patient's own spontaneous effort with a mechanical breath with a preset pressure limit. Fig. 57.15 shows the important components of a pressure-support breath. As with any form of support that is designed to respond to the patient's effort, the inspiratory pressure assist of PSV requires a signal to trigger the demand valve to initiate flow.[42] Since this breath is patient triggered and patient cycled with pressure as the control variable, it would be classified as PC-CSV according to modern taxonomy.

The patient's spontaneous breath creates a negative pressure (pressure triggering) or a change in flow through the circuit (flow triggering), which triggers the ventilator to deliver a

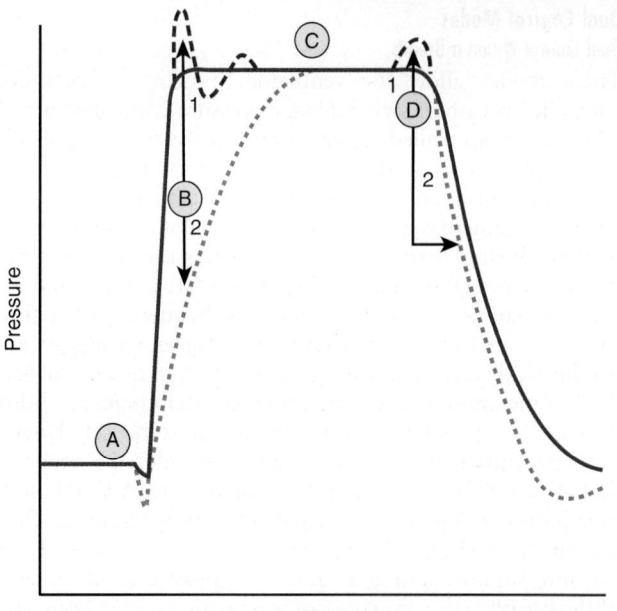

Fig. 57.15. Components of a pressure-support breath. *Point A* is the patient's effort indicated by a negative deflection. When the ventilator senses this trigger (change in pressure or flow), it will deliver flow to reach the desired pressure-support level *(Point B)* as rapidly as possible. Ventilator-delivered flow is then servo-adjusted to patient demand to maintain this pressure plateau *(Point C)*. Inspiration is terminated when a minimal flow criterion is reached *(Point D)* and airway pressure returns to baseline. (Reproduced from MacIntyre NR. Pressure support ventilation. Mechanical ventilation and assisted respiration. In Grenvik A, Downs J, Rasanen J, Smith R, eds. Contemporary Management in Critical Care. New York: Churchill Livingstone; 1991.)

breath. With initiation, the machine delivers high inspiratory flow to achieve a peak airway pressure level that is selected by the operator.[32-34] The pressure limit stays constant as long as the patient's inspiratory effort is maintained with a variable gas flow rate from the ventilator.[33,34] As inspiration continues, the inspiratory flow rate decreases. A threshold reduction in the flow rate is a signal for the termination of the inspiratory assist, with the opening of an expiratory valve, after which passive exhalation occurs.[32-34] The termination signal can be a predetermined percentage of the peak inspiratory flow (10% or 25%) or a fixed flow (usually 5 L/min).[35-37] Many ventilators also incorporate backup flow termination criteria, such as the duration of inspiration greater than 5 seconds or an increase in the airway pressure above the set pressure-support level (eg, when a patient attempts to cough). In summary, PSV is patient triggered, pressure limited, and flow cycled. PSV is entirely dependent on the patient's effort; if the patient becomes apneic, the ventilator will not provide any mechanical breath.

Martin et al. demonstrated in a bench study of a modified pediatric volume ventilator that work of breathing during pressure-support ventilation can be reduced by a high sensitivity and a low-volume displacement in the circuit.[38] The effectiveness of pressure-support ventilation in children was first demonstrated in six children (age 3–5 years) after cardiac surgery.[39] With increasing pressure-support levels, the tidal volume increased with a corresponding decrease in respiratory frequency.[39] Increasing pressure support also improved thoracoabdominal synchrony in infants.[40]

Dual Control Modes
Dual Control Within a Breath

These modes allow the ventilator to deliver a pressure-controlled breath or switch from a pressure-controlled breath to a volume-controlled breath within the breath. This is shown in Fig. 57.15. This mode is referred to as VAPS (Bird 8400ST and Tbird, Bird Corp., Palm Springs, California, USA) and pressure augmentation (PA) (Bear 1000). Both techniques can operate during mandatory breaths (pressure-limited time-cycled) or pressure-supported breaths. During VAPS and PA, the clinician must set the respiratory frequency, peak flow, PEEP, inspired oxygen concentration, trigger sensitivity, and minimum desired tidal volume. During VAPS or PA, the ventilator's inspiratory flow waveform is constant (square). Additionally, the pressure-support setting must be set. During pressure support, VAPS and PA can be considered a safety net that always supplies a minimum tidal volume. A VAPS or PA breath may be initiated by the patient or time triggered. Once the breath is triggered, the ventilator attempts to reach the pressure-support setting as quickly as possible. This portion of the breath is the pressure-control portion and is associated with a rapid variable flow, which may reduce the work of breathing. As this pressure level is reached, the ventilator's microprocessor determines the volume that has been delivered from the machine (NOTE: This is not exhaled tidal volume), compares this measurement with the desired tidal volume, and determines whether the minimum desired tidal volume will be reached. If the ventilator determines that the ultimate delivered tidal volume will be equivalent to the set tidal volume, the breath is delivered as a pressure-support breath. If the ventilator determines that the ultimate delivered tidal volume will be less than the set tidal volume, then the breath changes from a pressure-limited to a volume-limited breath. At that point inspiratory flow remains constant, and the ventilator increases the inspiratory time until the desired volume has been delivered. Inspiratory pressure will increase above the set pressure-support setting. Setting the high-pressure alarm remains important during VAPS. If pressure increases abruptly, the high-pressure alarm setting is reached and the breath is pressure cycled (Fig. 57.16). VAPS breath can allow the patient a tidal volume larger than the set volume.

Mandatory Dual-Control Breath-to-Breath Modes

Dual-control breath-to-breath mode with mandatory pressure-limited time-cycled breaths is referred to as pressure-regulated volume control (PRVC) (with Siemens 300), adaptive pressure ventilation (APV) (with Hamilton Galileo), autoflow (Evita 4), or variable pressure control (Venturi), depending on the manufacturer. In this form of pressure-limited, time-cycled ventilation, delivered tidal volume is used as a feedback control for continuously adjusting the pressure limit. All breaths in these modes are time or patient triggered, pressure limited, and time cycled. One difference between devices is that the Siemens 300 only allows PRVC in the CMV mode. The newer Servo-i ventilator and the other ventilators allow dual-control breath to breath with CMV or SIMV. During SIMV, the mandatory breaths are the dual-control breaths. PRVC is selected on the mode selector switch, and the desired tidal volume is set. A "test breath" is delivered, and total system compliance is calculated. The next three breaths are delivered at a pressure limit that is 75% of that necessary to achieve the desired tidal volume on the basis of the compliance calculation. The ensuing breaths increase or decrease the

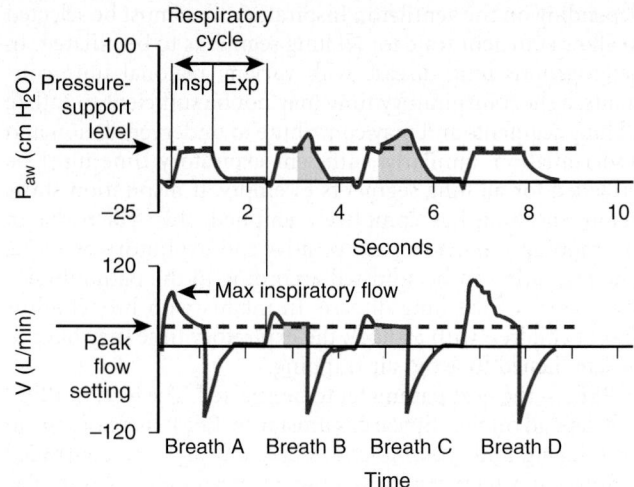

Fig. 57.16. Pressure and flow waveforms illustrating volume-assured pressure support. (Reproduced with permission from Branson RD, MacIntyre NR. Dual-control modes of mechanical ventilation. Respir Care. 1996;41:294-305.)

pressure limit at less than 3 cm H_2O per breath in an attempt to deliver the desired tidal volume. The pressure limit fluctuates between 0 cm H_2O above the PEEP level and 5 cm H_2O below the upper-pressure alarm setting. The ventilator sounds an alarm if the tidal volume and maximum pressure limit settings are incompatible. With changes in lung compliance and resistance, the delivered tidal volume may not be equivalent to the set tidal volume. If the delivered tidal volume is less than the set tidal volume, the pressure limit is increased to achieve the set tidal volume until the pressure limit is equal to a level 5 cm H_2O below the upper pressure limit alarm. The upper pressure-limit alarm must be adjusted with this in mind. It should be set to the maximum allowable pressure plus 5 cm of H_2O. When the delivered tidal volume is larger than the set tidal volume, then the ventilator will lower the pressure limit to achieve the set tidal volume. There is no lower limit for the reduction in the pressure-limit level. This mode of ventilation appears to be most beneficial when there are rapid changes in lung compliance (such as after surfactant administration[41-43]). Clinically controlled trials are required to evaluate the benefits of PRVC ventilation in acute lung disease, in ventilation of healthy lungs (ie, in patients undergoing neurosurgical procedures), and during weaning from the ventilator.

Assisted Dual-Control Breath-to-Breath Mode

Dual-control breath to breath in the pressure-support mode is simply closed-loop pressure-support ventilation, with tidal volume as the input variable. It is referred to as *volume support* (Siemens 300, Servo-i) and *variable pressure support* (Venturi). All breaths are patient triggered, pressure limited, and flow cycled. Volume support is selected with the mode selector switch, and the desired tidal volume is set. The ventilator initiates volume support by delivering a "test breath" with a peak pressure of 5 cm H_2O when a patient effort is sensed. The delivered tidal volume is measured, and total system compliance is calculated. The subsequent three breaths are delivered at a peak inspiratory pressure of 75% of the pressure calculated to deliver the minimum tidal volume. Each subsequent breath uses the previous calculation of system compliance to manipulate peak pressure to achieve the desired tidal volume.

From breath to breath, the maximum pressure change is less than 3 cm H_2O and can range from 0 cm H_2O above PEEP to 5 cm H_2O below the high-pressure alarm setting. The primary cycling mechanism is flow cycling of the pressure-supported breath. Similar to the PRVC mode previously described, the pressure-support level is adjusted to maintain the set tidal volume with changes in compliance and resistance. In addition to the volume-support settings, a mandatory ventilator frequency must be set. This frequency is set according to the age of the patient; the frequency for ages younger than 6 months is 16 to 20 breaths per minute; for 6 months to 2 years, 14 to 18 breaths per minutes; for 2 to 5 years, 12 to 16 breaths per minute; and for older than 5 years, 10 to 16 breaths per minute. A secondary cycling mechanism is activated if inspiratory time exceeds 80% of the set total cycle time. There is also a relationship between the set ventilator frequency and tidal volume. The minute ventilation calculated by the set tidal volume and the backup ventilator rate gives the minimum minute ventilation that needs to be achieved. If the patient is breathing at a frequency faster than the set ventilator rate, then the only adjustment that is made by the ventilator is to manipulate the pressure-support level to achieve the desired tidal volume. The total minute ventilation in this instance will be larger than the minimum level that needs to be achieved. When the patient's breathing rate is less than the set frequency, then the total minute ventilation will decrease to a level below the set minimum level. Next, the tidal volume target is automatically increased by raising the pressure-support level up to a maximum of 150% of the initial set value. If the tidal volume has to be increased beyond the 150% of the initial set value or the minute ventilation cannot be maintained at the set minimum level, then the ventilator will alarm and switch to the PRVC mode to ensure that at least the set minimum minute ventilation is delivered.

AutoMode

AutoMode combines mandatory and assisted dual-control breath-to-breath modes. The patient's effort or lack of breathing effort determines whether the breaths are flow cycled or time cycled. AutoMode is available on the Siemens 300A ventilator. Simplistically, AutoMode can be thought of as the combination of volume support and PRVC in a single mode. When the patient is breathing spontaneously, then the patient is in volume-support mode. If the patient becomes apneic or is paralyzed, the ventilator provides PRVC. The apneic threshold setting is 12 seconds for adults, 8 seconds for children, and 5 seconds for neonates. The change from PRVC to volume support or from volume support to PRVC is accomplished at equivalent peak pressures.

Automatic Tube Compensation

Automatic tube compensation (ATC) is a technique of overcoming the imposed work of breathing caused by artificial airways available in the Evita 4 ventilator. It accomplishes this by using the known resistive characteristics of the artificial airways. ATC is essentially pressure support in which the ventilator adjusts the pressure support to compensate for the imposed work of breathing by the artificial airways and the flow demand of the patient. The equation for calculating tracheal pressure (Ptrach) is:

$$Ptrach = Paw - (K \cdot V2)$$

where *Paw* is airway pressure, *V* is flow, and *K* is the tube coefficient describing the nonlinear pressure/flow curve of the ETT.

To select the level of ATC required, the operator needs to input type of tube, endotracheal or tracheostomy, and the percentage of compensation desired (10%-100%). Most of the interest in ATC revolves around eliminating the imposed work of breathing during inspiration. Under static in vitro conditions, pressure support can eliminate the endotracheal resistance, but in vivo, where the inspiratory flow demands of the patient are changing, a single level of pressure support is unlikely to be effective. Moreover, there are no in vivo measurements of the minimal pressure support needed to overcome the endotracheal tube resistance. During periods of tachypnea, the level of pressure support no longer eliminates work imposed by the endotracheal tube. Additionally, the resistance of the endotracheal tube creates a condition early in the breath in which ventilator flow is high, tracheal pressure remains low, and undercompensation for imposed work occurs.[44] Late in the breath, when pressure begins to equilibrate during the pressure plateau, pressure support tends to overcompensate, prolong inspiration, and exacerbate overinflation.[44] During expiration, however, there is also a flow-dependent pressure decrease across the tube. ATC also compensates for this flow-resistive component and may reduce expiratory resistance and unintentional hyperinflation. During expiration, the calculated tracheal pressure is greater than airway pressure.

Airway Pressure Release Ventilation

Airway pressure release ventilation (APRV) is a method of mechanical ventilation introduced by Stock and Downs.[45,46] It was based on the premise that most patients with ARDS required positive pressure support to maintain an adequate lung volume and required minimal, if any, ventilatory assistance.[45,46] These authors theorized that if a sufficiently high level of CPAP was provided with a high gas flow rate, it would maintain an adequate lung volume and oxygenation while ventilatory needs would be met entirely by spontaneous breathing. If additional ventilatory assistance were to be required, CPAP level could be abruptly reduced for a short period of time and this could be repeated several times in a minute to enhance ventilation. It is important to review the original design of an APRV circuit and contrast that with what is currently available in ventilators.

The original circuit included a CPAP device and a mechanism to release airway pressure periodically to some desired low pressure (Fig. 57.17). Gas was delivered from a high-pressure tank through a Venturi device at a flow rate of 90 to 100 L/min. The gas flowed through a T-piece circuit, which has a threshold-resistor expiratory valve to generate CPAP. Proximal to the threshold resistor, an automatic switch was placed to periodically allow gas to bypass the expiratory valve. This bypass could be set to either ambient pressure or another resistor valve, which would generate a pressure much lower than the CPAP pressure (Fig. 57.17). A timing device controlled the opening and closing of the switch. In the original description, the gas flow through the circuit was continuous and allowed unrestricted spontaneous breathing. In the original report, APRV was used in 10 dogs with normal lungs and abnormal lungs. With normal and injured lungs, APRV could maintain the same level of oxygenation for the same mean

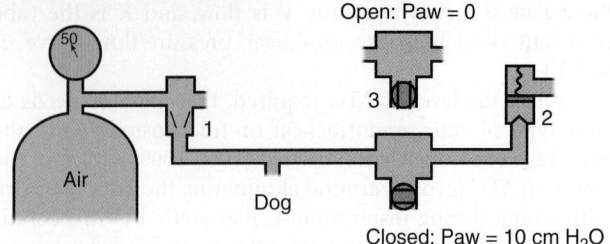

Fig. 57.17. Airway pressure release ventilation. Gas is delivered from a high-pressure source through the inspiratory limb of a T-piece circuit *(1)*. When the switch in the expiratory limb *(3)* is closed, continuous positive airway pressure is generated by the expiratory resistor valve *(2)*. When the switch is open, gas escapes through the bypass limb to a predetermined pressure.

airway pressure but with a lower peak inspiratory pressure. The I : E ratio used was about 1 : 0.7 with a rate of about 20/min. With lung injury, APRV could maintain the same oxygenation with a lower dead space.[45] Hemodynamic status was similar during both modes. Several studies with acute respiratory failure have shown that APRV results in improvement in gas exchange with much lower airway pressures.[45,47-49] Lower peak airway pressures are the consistent major advantage of ARPV. Because airway pressures are lower, APRV results in less adverse cardiovascular effects than IMV.[47,49]

In the accompanying editorial, the authors described how APRV would be used:[46]

"To provide APRV, continuous positive airway pressure (CPAP) is maintained so that the patient can breathe spontaneously without significant airway pressure (Paw) fluctuation. The appropriate level of CPAP may be determined by observing, measuring, and calculating a variety of physiologic responses to varying levels of CPAP. Changes in respiratory effort, respiratory rate, depth of respiration, PaO_2, calculated right-to-left shunting of blood, and lung-thorax compliance help the clinician to determine an appropriate Paw. Once a satisfactory level of CPAP is selected, if mechanically assisted ventilation is required, APRV may be initiated by cyclically releasing Paw to a lower level. This decreased Paw will allow gas to passively leave the lungs, eliminating CO_2. When the brief release period ends, Paw rapidly returns to the original CPAP level, thus increasing lung volume. The degree of ventilatory assistance provided by the APRV will be determined by the frequency of pressure release, the duration of pressure release, the CPAP level, the pressure release level, the patient's lung-thorax compliance, and flow resistance in the patient's airways and in the pressure release valve."

The authors also stated that:

"A continuous or intermittent flow of pressured gas and a variety of threshold resistor valves may be independently, or in combination, used to provide CPAP and to allow pressure release. Gas flow must at least equal the patient's peak inspiratory flow."[46]

With APRV, minute ventilation occurs with both spontaneous breaths and the periodic inflation and deflation that occur with the two levels of airway pressure. Gas exchange can occur throughout the respiratory cycle.

APRV is, by the modern taxonomy, PC-IMV usually using an inverse I : E ratio. Spontaneous breaths are also allowed during the mandatory breaths. The mandatory breaths applied by APRV are time-triggered, pressure-targeted, time-cycled breaths, which can be synchronized to a patient's breathing. Four major variables determine an APRV breath: Phigh, Plow, Thigh, and Tlow. Phigh is defined as the pressure of the triggered mandatory breath and Thigh is the duration that Phigh is maintained. Plow is the release pressure and Tlow is the time of the pressure release. Currently, some of the modern ventilators have incorporated features that allow spontaneous breathing through a demand-flow system during both the inspiratory and expiratory phases of a pressure-controlled time-cycled breath. These are called by different names such as *biphasic positive airway pressure* and *intermittent mandatory pressure-release ventilation*. These different modes have been classified under the acronym APRV. Some ventilators incorporate pressure support to be provided for the spontaneous breaths during these modes. It is clear that the patient-ventilator interactions are clearly different between the original APRV circuit and the modern "APRV" systems. Generally, demand-flow systems increase the trigger work of breathing and therefore are not necessarily unrestricted, especially in infants and children.

APRV use in children is relatively new and not well studied. Most of the articles published on the use of APRV are mostly case reports or case series.[50-64] It has been used mainly as a rescue therapy with refractory hypoxemia. Most of the studies showed improvement in oxygenation, but improvement was probably related to using a higher mean airway pressure with APRV.[50-64] None of the studies used the original approach as suggested by the original authors.[50-64] Habashi published a review of APRV with guidelines for optimal settings for adults and pediatric patients.[65] These guidelines have not been formally validated in any prospective study.

Proportional Assist Ventilation

Proportional assist ventilation (PAV) is a mode of mechanical ventilation based on the equation of motion. It accomplishes this by taking into account the instantaneous elasticity and flow resistance of the respiratory system. When PAV is initiated, the ventilator provides "test breaths" (controlled breaths with fixed flow and volume), which allows estimation of the respiratory system mechanics, minute ventilation, and the work of breathing (resistive and elastic ventilator muscle loads). These are repeated at regular intervals to recompute the load estimations. These estimations provide inputs for the PAV algorithm. The clinician can set the level of PAV (usually a percentage of the total work) to be provided breath-by-breath by the ventilator. The design of PAV allows the ventilator to change the pressure output (pressure control) to always perform work proportionally to patient effort.[66,67] In PAV, when the patient makes an inspiratory effort, the ventilator monitors the instantaneous rate and volume of gas flow.[66,67] The ventilator then amplifies the patient's effort during the breath by applying an additional pressure, which is based on the equation of motion. PAV can also be conceptualized as simply PSV, in which the level of pressure support is adjusted as a multiple of the sum of the volume and flow signals. The ventilator tries to maintain a constant percentage of work performed by the patient per breath irrespective of the volume of the breath or the inspiratory flow of the breath.

Unlike conventional breaths, where volume, flow, or pressure is predetermined, in PAV the ventilator applies the pressure in relation to the patient effort after the breath has started.[66,67] The tidal volume and minute ventilation are completely determined by the patient. In PAV, the ventilator unloads the patient's effort to a preset proportion of the patient's effort and the ventilating pressure is shared between the patient and ventilator. PAV is designed to improve patient-ventilator synchrony. Exhalation is generally flow cycled. Unlike conventional modes, in PAV, the pressure applied by the ventilator is directly proportional to the patient effort (ie, pressure applied by the ventilator increases as the patient effort increases to unload the respiratory muscles and decreases as the patient effort decreases).[66-68] There are few clinical studies in infants and children.[69-72] These studies show that PAV can maintain gas exchange with lower airway and transpulmonary pressure and improve thoracoabdominal synchrony.[69-72] Despite these studies, PAV is currently not recommended for patients less than 20 kg.

Neurally Adjusted Ventilatory Assist

In neurally adjusted ventilatory assist (NAVA), the ventilator assist is controlled by changes in electromyographic activity of the diaphragm.[73] NAVA is a mode of ventilation in which the ventilator assists a spontaneous breath with a pressure that is proportional to the integral of the electrical activity of the diaphragm (EAdi).[73] NAVA involves the transesophageal recording of EAdi using a specifically designed catheter. In order for NAVA to be effective, it is critical that the esophageal catheter measuring EAdi be positioned correctly.[74] The EAdi signal should reliably monitor and control the ventilatory assist.[75] The EAdi signal is used to both trigger and cycle-off the breath. With NAVA, the magnitude of the ventilator support will depend on a mathematic function that represents diaphragmatic electrical activity times a gain factor as shown by the equation:

$$Paw = NAVA\ level \times EAdi$$

where *Paw* is the instantaneous airway pressure (cms H_2O), *EAdi* is the instantaneous integral of the diaphragmatic electrical activity signal (μV), and the *NAVA* level (cms $H_2O/\mu V$ or per arbitrary unit) is a proportionality constant or gain factor. Similar to PAV, this allows the patient to control the tidal volume and flow within the breath. By coordinating the diaphragmatic activity and the ventilator support, the delivered pressure should be synchronous with EAdi and the level of assistance can be automatically adjusted depending on the changes in neural drive, respiratory mechanics, and inspiratory muscle function.[73] It is critical to understand that using EAdi to estimate respiratory center output requires that the phrenic nerve is intact and functioning and assumes that the diaphragm is the primary inspiratory muscle.

It is important to understand that pressure, flow, volume, or time during inspiration is not predetermined. In NAVA, the ventilator assists the spontaneous breath with a pressure applied per millivolt of diaphragmatic electrical activity and the ventilating pressure is shared between the patient and ventilator. NAVA is designed to improve patient-ventilator synchrony. Similar to PAV, when the patient effort increases, the pressure applied by the ventilator during the breath also increases to unload the patient effort in NAVA. Studies in infants and children demonstrate that NAVA is feasible and

may be of potential advantage over other modes of mechanical ventilation.[74-80] By allowing better patient-ventilator synchrony, it may be possible to reduce the amount of sedation that needs to be used in these children.

Mandatory Minute Volume Ventilation

Mandatory minute volume ventilation (MMV) was first introduced by Hewlett et al.[81] in 1977. In this mode, the patient is guaranteed a preset delivered minute ventilation. If the spontaneous minute ventilation exceeds the preset value, then the ventilator reduces the rate to zero and does not deliver a mechanical breath. If there is no spontaneous minute ventilation, then the ventilator will deliver sufficient breaths to match the preset minute ventilation. If the spontaneous minute ventilation is insufficient to match the preset value, then the ventilator will provide the remainder of the minute ventilation. Different mechanisms are used by manufacturers to achieve this goal. In the Ohmeda CPU1 ventilator, the preset minute ventilation is compared with the patient's total minute ventilation (spontaneous and mechanical) every 24 cycles and then adjusted. In the Engstrom Erica ventilator, it is done on a breath-by-breath basis. Currently there is not much experience with MMV in pediatric patients. The indications of MMV are in patients after abdominal surgery, especially with complications; patients who are recovering from respiratory muscle paralysis (eg, Guillain-Barré syndrome, myositis, myasthenia gravis); and patients who have widely fluctuating respiratory drive (encephalopathy).

Ventilation for Selected Underlying Pathophysiology
Primary Respiratory Muscle Failure ("Respiratory Pump Failure")

The primary difficulty in these disorders is inadequate ventilation due to weakness of the respiratory muscles (pump failure). Tidal volumes and ventilatory rates are set to provide normal minute ventilation to maintain normocarbia. Complete control of ventilation may result in disuse muscle atrophy and complicate weaning from mechanical ventilation. Therefore spontaneous breathing should be encouraged as much as possible. Assisted ventilation is a useful mode of ventilation in these disorders because the trigger sensitivity can be adjusted to encourage spontaneous breathing on the one hand and prevent muscle fatigue on the other. FiO_2 is usually kept to a minimum (≤ 0.3) because these disorders are not associated with inadequate oxygenation. In chronic hypoventilation, hypercarbia is often acceptable, provided the arterial pH is within the normal range. PEEP is usually set at a relatively low level (3–5 cm H_2O).

Disorders With Airway Obstruction

Provision of an artificial airway relieves respiratory distress due to upper airway obstruction (eg, epiglottitis, croup). Respiratory failure due to lower airway obstruction poses a special problem during mechanical ventilation. Depression of cardiac output and hypotension may occur during intubation because of the institution of positive airway pressure to already hyperinflated lungs. This causes further impedance to venous return and increased pulmonary vascular resistance. Volume-controlled ventilation is the preferred mode of ventilation. Inspiratory-expiratory ratio should be at least 1:2. The expiratory time required depends on the severity of the lower airway obstruction. If the expiratory time is inadequate to empty the lung, "auto-PEEP" or "inadvertent PEEP" will result. Inadvertent PEEP results in air trapping and hyperinflation with its attendant complications. The level of PEEP selected for patients with lower airway obstruction is controversial. There are two schools of thought: "low PEEP" and "high PEEP." Low PEEP advocates usually apply a PEEP of 3 to 5 cm H_2O because of the concern for pulmonary barotrauma from air trapping and alveolar hyperinflation. In lower airway disease, air trapping often results in an end-expiratory alveolar pressure that is higher than the proximal airway pressure because of incomplete emptying of the alveoli. This results in "auto-PEEP" or "inadvertent PEEP." End-expiratory lung volume and therefore the level of alveolar inflation will not be affected by the level of proximal set PEEP as long as it is less than the amount of auto-PEEP. In adults with severe asthma, high levels of PEEP, which is closer to the level of auto-PEEP, have been shown to decrease the magnitude of air trapping and work of breathing without significant complications.[82-85] In children with tracheomalacia or bronchomalacia, PEEP decreases the airway resistance by distending the airways and preventing dynamic compression during expiration. The use of low levels of PEEP compared with high levels has been described previously.

Parenchymal Lung Disease

ARDS, hyaline membrane disease of the newborn, and interstitial pneumonias are examples of parenchymal lung disorders that are characterized by a reduction in FRC, an increase in closing volume above FRC, and diffuse subsegmental atelectasis. These diseases are characterized primarily by inadequate oxygenation due to V/Q mismatching and intrapulmonary shunting. Therapy should be directed toward maintaining lung volumes above closing volume throughout the respiratory cycle, increasing FRC above closing volume, and reducing V/Q mismatching and intrapulmonary shunting. The most effective method of achieving these goals is with an increase of mean lung volume, which is usually obtained with an increase of the mean airway pressure. During spontaneous breathing without any ventilatory assistance, CPAP is the most reliable method to increase lung volume. CPAP is effective in improving oxygenation in hyaline membrane disease and ARDS.[85,86] During positive pressure breathing, the level of PEEP required to maintain adequate oxygenation primarily depends on the severity of the underlying lung disease. The degree of intrapulmonary shunting, ventilation-perfusion mismatching, alveolar edema, alveolar collapse, and decreased compliance is directly proportional to the severity of lung disease. As the severity of lung disease increases, the airway pressures required to maintain adequate gas exchange also increase. Therefore arbitrary limits cannot be placed on the level of PEEP or mean airway pressure that will be necessary to maintain adequate gas exchange. Tidal volumes should be limited to 6 to 8 mL/kg. Studies in adults, including the ARDS Network study, have demonstrated that using high tidal volumes of 12 mL/kg is detrimental to patient outcome.[87,88] When high levels of PEEP are used, PIP may reach levels that contribute to pulmonary air leak and barotrauma. Attempts to decrease PIP with the reduction of tidal volume will result in decreased mean airway pressure, mean lung volume, and decreased minute ventilation. With a high airway pressure

maintained throughout inspiration, pressure-control ventilation may provide higher mean airway pressure and maintain a higher mean lung volume compared with volume-control ventilation. A general rule of thumb is to consider switching to pressure-limited time-cycled ventilation when PEEP requirement is more than 10 cm H_2O. For hyperinflation to be avoided, the end-inspiratory pause pressure should not exceed 35 cm H_2O. Hypercapnia may be permitted under these circumstances provided arterial pH is adequate (permissive hypercapnia). It has been recommended that the optimal PEEP should be set above the critical closing or critical opening pressure of the airways. This can be deduced by the lower inflection point generated with static pressure-volume loops (Fig. 57.18). As the lung is inflated from zero end-expiratory pressure, in many lungs there is an abrupt change in compliance as denoted by the "lower inflection point." It is generally thought that this is the critical opening pressure of the airways above which the alveoli and airways remain open. As the lung is further inflated in increments, the pressure-volume slope increases and then abruptly changes direction as noted in Fig. 57.18 as the "upper inflection point." It is generally thought that the upper inflection point reflects overdistention of the alveoli. The general recommendation is to keep the PEEP level above the lower inflection point and the end-inspiratory pause pressure below the upper inflection point. Currently, bedside use of static pressure-volume loops to set PEEP is not a standard practice in infants and children. Therefore the level of PEEP should be set by titrating the level of PEEP and selecting the level by the maximal level of improvement in oxygenation compliance seen without affecting systemic hemodynamics. The repeated collapse and reopening of the lung units at low lung volume have been

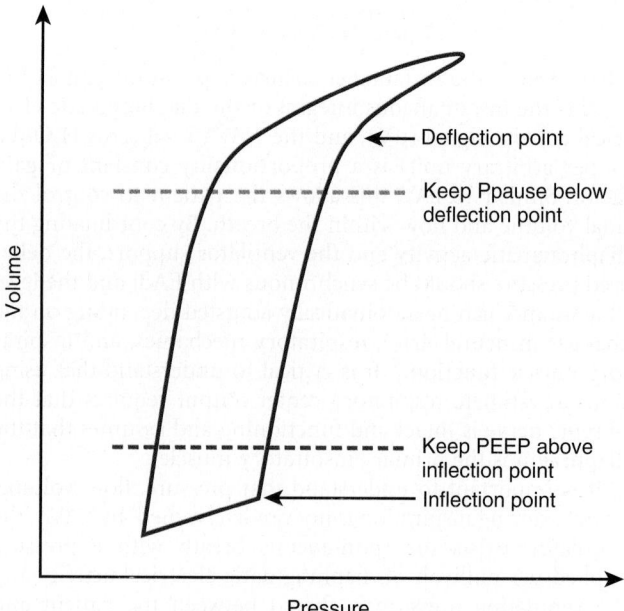

PRESSURE-VOLUME LOOP IN ACUTE LUNG INJURY

← Deflection point

Keep Ppause below deflection point

Keep PEEP above inflection point
Inflection point

Volume

Pressure

Fig. 57.18. Optimal positive end-expiratory pressure (PEEP) and peak alveolar pressure setting in acute lung injury/acute respiratory distress syndrome on the basis of static pressure-volume loop. The goal is to keep the PEEP level above the lower inflection point and to keep the end-inspiratory pause pressure below the upper inflection point.

shown to contribute to ventilation-induced lung injury.[89-92] A strategy combining recruitment maneuvers, low-tidal volume, and higher PEEP has been shown to decrease the incidence of barotrauma or volutrauma.[89-93]

Alveolar Recruitment and Derecruitment

Alveolar recruitment, by definition, means opening up of closed alveoli. In ARDS and other parenchymal lung diseases, atelectasis and consolidation are common pathologic features that result in intrapulmonary shunting. The goals of positive pressure support in ARDS are to recruit closed alveoli and present derecruitment of open alveoli. The benefits of optimal lung recruitment and prevention of derecruitment are (1) a reduction in the intrapulmonary shunt fraction and venous admixture resulting in an improvement in arterial oxygenation; (2) improvement in lung compliance; and (3) prevention of repeated alveolar collapse and reopening, which may ameliorate or prevent ventilator-induced lung injury. The primary determinants of alveolar recruitment and derecruitment are transpulmonary pressure and PEEP, both of which increase mean airway pressure. Mean lung volume depends on mean alveolar pressure. Mean airway pressure has been shown to be an excellent marker of mean alveolar pressure.[94] Increasing mean airway pressure will improve oxygenation if there is alveolar recruitment.

Currently several techniques of alveolar recruitment have been described in the literature. These include manual inflation to high airway pressures, the increase of PEEP in a stepwise manner, application of a sign maneuver, the use of pressure-limited time-cycled ventilation with a high peak inspiratory pressure, and the combination of titrated levels of PEEP with increased inflation pressures. Ventilatory sighs are effective in recruiting alveoli in ARDS.[95] They are effective, however, only from an optimal level of PEEP that does not result in derecruitment. At optimal PEEP, a sigh maneuver increases end-expiratory lung volume and improves oxygenation.[96] Gattinoni et al.[97,98] showed and quantified alveolar recruitment induced by PEEP and showed that the primary role of tidal volume inflation was to open the lung and the primary role of PEEP was to avoid derecruitment. Not all patients have recruitable lungs. In some patients, the lungs may be maximally recruited and any further increase in airway pressures may either cause no change in lung mechanics or gas exchange or result in a deterioration of lung mechanics and gas exchange due to overdistention.[99] The low tidal volume and moderate PEEP approach used in the ARDS Network study has been shown to result in derecruitment in many patients. Richard et al. showed that increasing PEEP or performing periodic recruitment techniques counteracted the derecruitment in these patients.[100] Periodic high levels of PEEP, high inflation plateau pressures, or both have shown to be beneficial in improving lung mechanics and oxygenation, through alveolar recruitment.[101-103]

Prone Positioning

Prone positioning has been proposed as a means to improve gas exchange in patients with ARDS with severe hypoxemia. Oxygenation improves in most adult patients with acute lung injury (ALI)/ARDS when they are placed prone.[104-107] A large, multicenter trial of prone positioning for almost 7 hours a day did not show improvement in mortality rates in patients with ALI/ARDS; however, a post hoc analysis suggested improvement in those patients with the most severe hypoxemia.[108] A recent multicenter trial of prone positioning for almost 20 hours a day also suggested improvement in this patient subgroup that did not reach statistical significance.[109] A recent Cochrane Review identified nine relevant RCTs that studied the effect of prone positioning for acute respiratory failure on outcomes.[110] While prone positioning resulted in a relative risk of less than 1, it was not statistically significant when all patients were included. Early implementation of PP, prolonged adoption of PP, and severe hypoxemia at study entry were three subgroups that showed a statistically significant mortality benefit.[111-117]

Bruno et al.[118] reported the short-term effects of 1 to 2 hours of prone positioning in children with respiratory failure. They found that only 28% of the patients had a significant improvement in oxygenation.[118] Curley et al.,[119] in a preliminary single-center study in children with ALI/ ARDS, showed that oxygenation improved with prone positioning in 84% of patients without any critical incident. Relvas et al.[120] also reported a retrospective study on the effects of prone positioning in children with ARDS and showed that the improvement in oxygenation was much more sustained if the duration of prone positioning was between 18 and 24 hours than when the duration of prone positioning was between 6 and 10 hours.[120] A recent multicenter study on prone positioning in children with ALI/ARDS showed that patient recruitment within 48 hours of meeting acute lung injury criteria and prone positioning for 20 hours a day for a maximum of 7 days did not show any differences in the number of ventilator-free days between the two groups.[121] There were no differences in the secondary end points, including proportion alive and ventilator free on day 28, mortality from all causes, the time to recovery of lung injury, organ failure–free days, and cognitive impairment or overall functional health at hospital discharge.[121]

Although the magnitude of the response varies widely from marginal to dramatic, there is no adequate model predicting where a particular patient with ARDS will fall in the spectrum. Furthermore, patients' response times vary from immediate to several hours. As a result, little is known about the optimal time period to maintain the prone position. Some patients respond to a return to a supine position after a trial of prone positioning by reverting to their original oxygenation, others have a reduction in oxygenation that is better than the original supine value, and some patients show an improvement. Prone positioning may have potentially life-threatening complications, including accidental dislodgement of the endotracheal tube and central venous catheters. Marcano et al.[122] reported that prone positioning resulted in cephalad movement of the endotracheal tube within the trachea in children with ARDS ranging from 10% to 57% of their thoracic tracheal length. Their study also suggested that if the tip of the endotracheal tube is not deeper than one-third of the thoracic tracheal length before prone positioning, it might slide into the cervical trachea as a result of prone positioning.[122]

Unilateral Lung Disease or Severely Differential Lung Disease

Unilateral or asymmetrical lung disease in infants and children poses special problems during mechanical ventilation. Some of these patients may have severe intrapulmonary shunts leading to hypoxemia requiring mechanical ventilation. Because of regional differences in compliance and resistance, the time constants for inflation and deflation may vary widely between lung segments. During conventional ventilation, tidal volume delivered tends to preferentially inflate the more compliant lung and underventilate the stiffer, more affected lung. This may result in overinflation of the relatively "normal" lung and cause redistribution of pulmonary blood flow away from the hyperinflated lung, thus exaggerating the ventilation-perfusion mismatching. Such overinflation may contribute to further barotrauma. In such circumstances, with unilateral or asymmetrical lung disease, simultaneous independent lung ventilation (SILV) may allow each lung to be ventilated according to its needs without affecting the opposite lung. Currently, SILV can be generally indicated in the treatment of unilateral lung disease, such as unilateral atelectasis or consolidation, emphysema, pneumonia, pneumothorax, and bronchopulmonary fistula. In postoperative care, ILV can be used for lung reexpansion after thoracic surgery, for correction of V/Q mismatch in the lung remaining dependent during surgery, and for the treatment of pulmonary complications arising during anesthesia and surgery (eg, pneumothorax or aspiration syndrome). A new possible indication for SILV can be the selective administration of drugs to one lung, such as antibiotics or surfactant. SILV requires a bilumen tube with one tube being the longer "bronchial" tube and the other shorter "tracheal" tube. Usually, the bronchial tube is advanced into the right main stem bronchus so that both lungs can be ventilated separately.

In adults, SILV has been shown to be useful in the treatment of unilateral lung disease.[123-126] In infants and children, SILV has been limited because of the lack of a suitable bilumen tube. Marraro[127] reviewed their experience with SILV in infants and children younger than 1 year with a bilumen tube developed in their department, but it is currently available through Portex Ltd. (Mythe, Kent, United Kingdom). The indications included bronchopneumonia with unilateral prevalence, unilateral pneumonia, lobar atelectasis, and diaphragmatic hernia. Nine of 41 patients treated with SILV had rapid improvement in lung disease, whereas the other 32 recovered more slowly. No major complications were attributed to SILV. In newborns and infants, it is possible to provide ILV with a double-lumen endotracheal tube manufactured by Portex as special equipment. In children older than 6 to 8 years, selective bronchial intubation is possible using a cuffed double-lumen tube similar to that used in adults (26- to 28-Fr Bronchocath Mallinckrodt, Bronchoport Rusch). The Marraro Paediatric Endobronchial Bilumen Tube, produced by SIMS-Portex, may be used in neonates and children age 2 to 3 years.[128] It is uncuffed to maximize the internal diameter of the tube and has no carinal hook; this minimizes tracheal trauma.[107-109] ILV requires two ventilators that permit the application of different modes of ventilation and different PEEP levels for each lung. Synchronization of the beginning of the inspiratory phase and the inspiratory time can avoid mediastinal shifts that impede venous return and reduce cardiac output.[127-129]

Heart Failure

The goals in respiratory management in congestive heart failure are prevention and relief of alveolar collapse from alveolar and interstitial edema due to pulmonary vascular congestion, as well as decreased oxygen demand on the heart with a reduction in the work of breathing. CPAP/PEEP will provide relief of atelectasis. Hyperinflation should be avoided because it may increase pulmonary vascular resistance and increase right ventricular afterload. The oxygen cost of breathing can be reduced with a decrease in the work of breathing. This can be provided by a judicious combination of controlled ventilation and sedation. By unloading the respiratory muscles, mechanical ventilation can also reduce the work of breathing. In extreme cases, muscle relaxation by neuromuscular blockers may provide additional reduction in oxygen cost of breathing. As a general principle, the greater the inotropic support a heart needs, the greater should be the respiratory support provided. Tidal volumes should be generally maintained on the lower range (8–10 mL/kg). In adults with congestive heart failure, positive intrathoracic pressure has been shown to improve cardiac output.[130,131] This effect has been attributed to decreased left ventricular afterload provided by positive airway pressure.

Postoperative Management After Repair of Congenital Heart Disease

After open heart surgery, many infants and children require mechanical ventilation during the postoperative period. The duration of requirement of mechanical ventilation depends on several factors such as age of the patient, complexity of the cardiac lesion, complexity of the operative procedure, duration of bypass, duration of circulatory arrest, and postoperative cardiopulmonary status. Prolonged intubation and mechanical ventilation are more likely in children younger than 1 year of age, with more complex heart lesions, prolonged bypass and prolonged circulatory arrest times, and postoperative respiratory failure and hemodynamic instability. In the immediate postoperative period, patients should be supported with controlled mechanical ventilation until hemodynamic functions improve. Adequate PEEP should be applied to prevent and relieve atelectasis. Initially, the ventilator rate should be appropriate for the age. As the hemodynamic function improves, the rate can be weaned, as dictated by the clinical status. The choice of ventilatory parameters depends on the goals for each patient. In patients with pulmonary hypertension or pulmonary vascular disease, hyperventilation to provide respiratory alkalosis will decrease pulmonary vascular resistance and right ventricular afterload. In patients with marginal cardiac output, high airway pressures are to be avoided. In patients who have undergone a Fontan procedure, early extubation is desirable, and if that is not possible, then spontaneous ventilation should be encouraged. Because these patients are totally dependent on venous return for their cardiac output, airway pressures must be kept at a minimum. High intrathoracic pressure may not only impede venous return but also decrease pulmonary blood flow from increased pulmonary vascular resistance.

Diseases With Abdominal Distention

The presence of abdominal distention poses a special problem. Positive intraabdominal pressure tends to elevate the diaphragm, decrease P_{tp} in the lung bases, and decrease alveolar lung volumes in the lung bases. For normal lung volumes to be maintained, a greater P_{tp} has to be generated. This increases the airway pressures during positive pressure ventilation and increases work of breathing during spontaneous breathing. During positive pressure ventilation, a higher P_{tp} may cause hyperinflation of the apical regions while restoring normal volumes in the bases. Therapy should be directed primarily toward reducing the intraabdominal pressure.

Neurologic and Neuromuscular Diseases

Hyperventilation with respiratory alkalosis is an effective method of reducing intracranial pressure. High intrathoracic pressure may impede venous return from the brain by increasing central venous pressures. Therefore high levels of PEEP are to be avoided. The goals of respiratory support in patients with acute neuromuscular diseases that are self-limiting are (1) provision of respiratory assistance to maintain adequate minute ventilation and (2) avoidance of disuse muscle atrophy from mechanical ventilation. Spontaneous breathing must be encouraged as much as possible. Neuromuscular blockade must be avoided.

Patient-Ventilator Asynchrony

One of the primary goals of mechanical ventilation is to reduce the patient's work of breathing. This can be achieved only if the patient's respiratory muscles and the ventilator act in a coordinated manner. The patient should not be attempting to inspire when the ventilator is in the expiratory phase and should not be attempting to exhale when the ventilator is attempting to deliver a breath. Patient-ventilator asynchrony is defined as a mismatch between the inspiratory times of the patient and the ventilator. Asynchrony can occur during intermittent mandatory ventilation, patient-triggered mandatory breaths, supported spontaneous breaths, and assist-control ventilation. It is important to recognize patient-ventilator asynchrony and take measures to either minimize or eliminate it.

A detailed description and analysis of patient-ventilator asynchrony is beyond the scope of this chapter, and the reader is referred elsewhere.[132-142] There are different types of asynchrony related to the different phases of breathing. The triggering phase is from onset of patient effort to onset of flow delivery.[138-142] The post-triggering inspiratory phase comprises the onset of flow delivery to the termination of machine inspiration. The cycling phase or expiratory triggering refers to the termination of machine inspiration and the onset of expiration. Brief summaries of the types of asynchrony in the different phases are described as follows.

Asynchrony Associated With Breath Triggering

It is important to first understand the different components of the trigger phase. Trigger threshold refers to the variable that determines the onset of a breath. The four common types of trigger mechanism available on commercial ventilators are time, pressure, volume, and flow. There is a fifth type called the shape-signal or "shadow" trigger that is available on the Respironics noninvasive ventilators.[141-143] For time triggering, the trigger threshold is a set interval of time from the previous breath; in pressure triggering, it is the minimum pressure decrease from PEEP; and in flow and volume triggering, it is the minimum change in flow or volume in the circuit that is sensed by the ventilator to initiate a breath. The inspiratory trigger time is the time elapsed between the initial patient effort and the point at which the airway pressure reaches the maximum baseline. Time to return trigger pressure to zero is the time taken after the ventilator is able to supply flow to returning the airway pressure to the pretrigger baseline. This is influenced by the rise time setting in the ventilator. Triggering time delay is the time from onset of triggering to the onset of flow delivery and is the sum of the inspiratory trigger time and the time to return trigger pressure to zero. Asynchrony associated with breath triggering can be classified into (1) missed triggering, (2) delayed triggering, (3) autotriggering, (4) double triggering, and (5) reversed triggering.

Missed triggering: Missed triggering refers to a spontaneous breath that is not accompanied by a synchronous assisted/supported mechanical breath. Missed triggering results in a patient's effort that fails to trigger a ventilator breath. This can be due to either poor patient effort or an insensitive threshold. Poor patient effort may result in a breath that is not strong enough to reach the trigger threshold. This may be due to muscle weakness that results in an effort that is below the trigger threshold. It may also be due to an increased load on the muscles at the start of inspiration such as induced by intrinsic PEEP, when the patient effort is insufficient to trigger the breath. It can also be due to the trigger threshold being set too high (insensitive trigger). Ineffective triggering can be detected as a pressure drop in the airway with a change in flow but not followed by a ventilator breath. Ineffective triggering can be resolved by setting the trigger sensitivity low enough to capture the patient's efforts but not result in autotriggering (see later). On the other hand, the threshold may be set too high or may not sense the effort that results in a wasted spontaneous breath. Delayed triggering is defined as a lag from sensing the trigger to delivering the mechanical breath. Delayed triggering refers to the delay in the start of the ventilator breath after the patient's effort has been detected. This is usually intrinsic to the trigger sensitivity and electronic response of the ventilator circuit.

Autotriggering: When a breath is delivered neither in response to a scheduled event nor triggered by a patient effort, it is referred to as autotriggering. It is best detected with esophageal monitoring where a breath is delivered in the absence of a diaphragmatic contraction. Ventilator factors that are associated with autotriggering are a low triggering threshold, circuit leak, and water in the circuit. Patient-related factors include cardiac oscillation and low respiratory drive. Autotriggering is the most common type of patient-ventilator asynchrony during noninvasive ventilation, usually due to leaks around the interface.[144]

Double triggering: When two consecutive inspirations occur within an interval of less than half of the mean inspiratory time, it is referred to as double triggering.[141,142] The usual reason for double triggering is a mismatch between a neural inspiratory signal that is longer than the machine's inspiratory time. This results in the second breath being triggered after the first breath has been delivered. Double triggering can also occur when a pressure-supported breath has a high termination criterion.[142] These breaths may occur on top of each other or soon after each other.[141,142] When the breaths are stacked, the peak inspiratory pressure may be increased by the second breath. While missed trigger events are due to the low patient effort relative to the trigger threshold, double triggering is usually due to excessive patient demand or effort. Double triggering may also occur with sighs or coughing.[141,142]

Asynchrony During Inspiration (Flow Asynchrony)

Once the breath is initiated, the flow of gas into the patient must match the needs of the patient. When the patient's demand is met by the ventilator, the profile of the pressure-volume and pressure-time curves is more "physiologic."[141] Most common form of flow asynchrony occurs when the patient's demand exceeds the delivered flow and is more likely to occur with acute respiratory failure from ARDS. The pressure-time curve in ventilator graphics display can be useful in assessing flow asynchrony. Less common is a delivered flow that is in excess of the patient's needs resulting in larger tidal volumes.

Asynchrony During Cycling

Cycling asynchrony occurs when the ventilator drive and cycling criteria are mismatched. Either the ventilatory drive is abnormal or the cycle criteria are set too long or too short. With a high respiratory drive, cycling may occur sooner as the ventilator breath ceases abruptly. When the ventilator cycling occurs later than the patient's intrinsic cycling, machine cycling is prolonged. Delayed cycling refers to the prolongation of the ventilatory inspiration breath beyond the start of the patient's expiration. This can occur during pressure-support ventilation and can induce adverse effects such as increasing hyperinflation and intrinsic PEEP due to a shortened expiratory time. Premature cycling refers to the ventilator terminating inspiration while the patient is still continuing to have inspiratory efforts. This most commonly occurs in the presence of a leak in the ventilator circuit or around the endotracheal tube.

Ideally, ventilator breaths should be synchronized with spontaneous breaths. Asynchrony between mechanical ventilation and spontaneous breathing is common, especially in small infants. The most common form of asynchrony is active exhalation during a ventilator-delivered inspiratory breath. This has several detrimental effects. These are increased expiratory work of breathing, decreased overall minute ventilation with hypercarbia, patient discomfort, and increased risk for air leak.[145,146] Patients exhibiting asynchrony during mechanical ventilation have shown improved oxygenation and ventilation after neuromuscular blockade.[147,148]

Patient-ventilator asynchrony has been recently studied in infants and children mainly in the context of comparing NAVA with conventional modes.[77-79,149,150] These show a high prevalence of asynchrony. NAVA did decrease the overall magnitude of asynchrony but did not completely eliminate it.[77-79,149,150] Two recent studies show that asynchrony events are frequent during pressure-support ventilation in children during both invasive and noninvasive ventilation.[151,152] Despite adjusting the cycling-off criteria, the asynchrony persisted. NAVA reduced the magnitude of asynchrony significantly in both forms of ventilation.

Use of Neuromuscular Blockade

Neuromuscular blockers are often used as adjunctive therapy to mechanical ventilation. Although spontaneous breathing is to be encouraged as much as possible, respiratory muscle paralysis becomes necessary at times as an aid to mechanical ventilation. The indications for the use of neuromuscular blocking agents during mechanical ventilation are (1) asynchrony between the patient and ventilator; (2) use in controlled ventilation; (3) a decrease in oxygen demand of skeletal muscles, especially in patients with hemodynamic instability; and (4) prevention of coughing, especially in patients with intracranial hypertension. Neuromuscular blockade is also

used in patients when ventilation is to be controlled so that the appropriate minute ventilation is delivered. Paralysis of respiratory muscles may also be required in patients after congenital heart surgery to reduce the oxygen demand on the heart. Prolonged neuromuscular blockade is to be avoided because it tends to promote muscle atrophy. This, in turn, will prolong weaning from mechanical ventilation.

High-Frequency Ventilation
Definitions

High-frequency ventilation (HFV) refers to diverse modes of ventilation characterized in general by supraphysiologic ventilatory frequencies (>60 cycles/min) and low tidal volumes (less than or equal to physiologic dead space during conventional ventilation). Four distinct methods of HFV are recognized: high-frequency positive pressure ventilation (HFPPV), high-frequency jet ventilation (HFJV), high-frequency oscillatory ventilation (HFOV), and high-frequency chest wall oscillation (HFCWO).

1. HFPPV: HFPPV was first described by Oberg and Sjostrand in 1969[153] and refers to ventilation at a frequency of 60 to 100 cycles per minute with a tidal volume of 3 to 4 mL/kg using a ventilator with a small internal dead space, low internal compliance, and minimal compression of gases within the ventilator. HFPPV was initially instituted by insufflation through a catheter positioned within the endotracheal tube, with expiration occurring through an expiratory valve connected to the outer orifice. Since 1973, a pneumatic valve, based on the Coanda or wall effect, was developed in which the gas mixture was intermittently delivered through a sidearm branching off the main channel of the pneumatic valve connector (Fig. 57.19).

   This main channel remains open for insertion of a bronchoscope or a laryngoscope.

2. HFJV: HFJV, which was first described by Sanders in 1967[154] to assist bronchoscopy, refers to delivery of inspiratory gases through a jet injector at a high velocity into the trachea at a rate of 100 to 400 cycles per minute (Fig. 57.20). Tidal volumes delivered are usually 3 to 5 mL/kg.

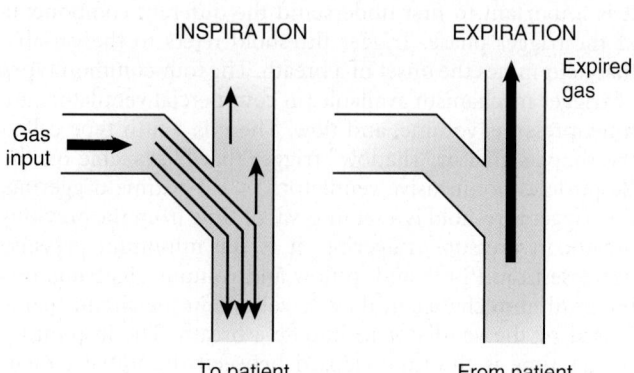

Fig. 57.19. High-frequency positive pressure ventilator. The inspiratory limb is angled so that the inspiratory gas can be directed to the patient. During inspiration, some gas escapes through the expiratory limb, preventing entrainment. During expiration, the gas flows out into the expiratory limb. (Reproduced with permission from Shoemaker WC, Ayres S, Grenvik A, et al., eds. The Textbook of Critical Care. Philadelphia: WB Saunders; 1989.)

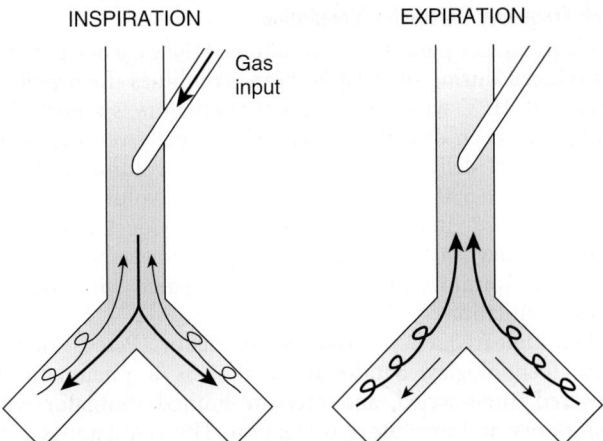

INSPIRATION   EXPIRATION

Gas input

Fig. 57.20. High-frequency jet ventilator. Gas is introduced into the trachea at a high pressure through a small catheter. *Arrows* represent coaxial and turbulent flow patterns. (Reproduced with permission from Shoemaker WC, Ayres S, Grenvik A, et al., eds. The Textbook of Critical Care. Philadelphia: WB Saunders; 1989.)

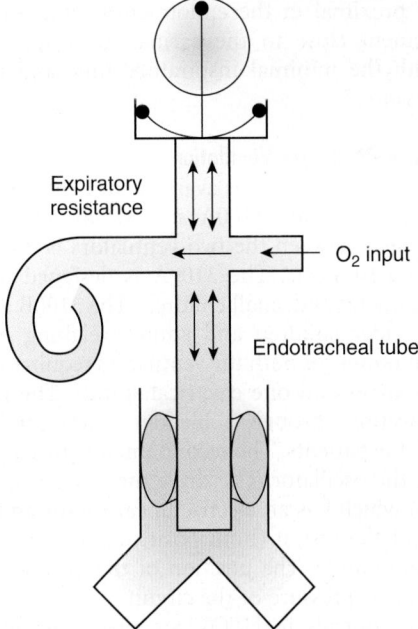

Expiratory resistance

O_2 input

Endotracheal tube

Fig. 57.21. High-frequency oscillation system. Uses a reciprocating pump *(top)* to oscillate a column of gas that is a mixture of inspired and expired gases. Excess gas is vented through the overflow side port *(left)*. (Reproduced with permission from Shoemaker WC, Ayres S, Grenvik A, et al., eds. The Textbook of Critical Care. Philadelphia: WB Saunders; 1989.)

3. HFOV: HFOV was first described by Lunkenheimer in 1972[155] and refers to ventilation at frequencies of 900 to 3600 cycles per minute, with an alternating positive and negative pressure in the airway. This oscillatory flow may be produced by a piston pump or a diaphragm with tidal volumes of 1 to 3 mL/kg (Fig. 57.21).
4. HFCWO: HFCWO was first described by Zidulka et al.[156] in 1983 and refers to a method of ventilation in which a rigid harness surrounds the chest and is oscillated at a frequency of 180 to 600 cycles per minute; minute ventilation is controlled with adjustment of the inflation pressure and frequency. A variant of HFCWO is high-frequency body surface oscillation (HFBSO), in which the body is encased in an air-tight tank.

Only HFPPV, HFJV, and HFOV have been extensively used clinically.

Mechanism of Gas Flow in High-Frequency Ventilation in the Normal Lung

The exact mechanism of gas transport in HFV is currently not clear. It is possible that each mode of ventilation may have differing mechanisms of gas flow from the proximal airway to the alveoli. If gas flow to the lungs is increased more than 200 times the minute volume of oxygen demand, the lung parenchyma can be made to oscillate.[157,158] At ventilatory frequencies less than 7 Hz, regional alveolar ventilation depends on segmental compliance and airway resistance. At a ventilatory frequency greater than 7 Hz, a frequency-dependent excitation of the lung parenchyma and airway conduits occurs,[159] and at frequencies greater than 10 Hz, ventilation becomes independent of regional compliance. When the gas in the airways is oscillated at high frequency, the airways begin to undergo spatial oscillation inside the chest. These oscillations are composed of periodic changes in length and width, movements of curved or angular bronchi, and wave motions in the bronchi. When the frequency of oscillation approaches the natural resonant frequency of the lung structures, the oscillations of the airways and lung parenchyma are amplified. These result in shaking and squeezing of the neighboring parenchyma,

resulting in intraparenchymal and interparenchymal gas mixing.[160] Other mechanisms involved in gas transport during HFV include accelerated axial dispersion, increased collateral flow through pores of Kohn, intersegmental gas mixing or Pendelluft phenomenon, Taylor dispersion, asymmetric gas flow profiles, and gas mixing within the airway due to the nonlinear pressure-diameter relationship of the bronchi.

Parameters to Be Selected
High-Frequency Jet Ventilation
The main controls in HFJV are the driving pressure, inspiratory time, and rate. The driving pressure is usually initiated at a desired mean airway pressure and adjusted according to the level of lung expansion and gas exchange. Inspiratory time is usually kept to a minimum at 20%. A higher inspiratory time may be used but may result in air trapping. The rate can be adjusted up to 600 breaths per minute depending on the jet ventilator used. PEEP is applied through a separate bias flow circuit with continuous flow. FiO_2 delivered to the patient is adjusted through regulation of the inspired oxygen concentration of the bias flow circuit. In certain circumstances, conventional ventilation can be combined with HFJV. Here, conventional ventilation provides "sigh breaths" of approximately 10 to 12 mL/kg to prevent atelectasis and maintain lung volumes during HFJV. The size of each breath increases with a higher driving pressure, increased inspiratory time, and a decreased frequency. Because there is entrainment of gas with HFJV, it is difficult to predict the effect of ventilator parameters on minute ventilation. Ventilation is most effective when the jet catheter is close to the carina. The main concerns with HFJV are airway injury and air trapping. Airway injury can be minimized with placement of the tip of the catheter

sufficiently proximal in the endotracheal tube and without close placement close to the carina. Air trapping can be avoided with the minimal inspiratory time and the lowest driving pressure.[161]

High-Frequency Oscillatory Ventilation

Currently, the HFOV systems available in North America are the Viasys Critical Care 3100A and 3100B ventilators. The main difference between the two ventilators is the age range each of them supports. The 3100A is designed to support HFOV in neonates and small children. The 3100B is designed to support older children and adults weighing more than 35 kg. Input power for both the ventilators requires two pneumatic gas sources and one electrical source. The first pneumatic connection through a blender determines the FiO_2 delivered to the patients. The second pneumatic connection is for cooling the oscillator. The drive mechanism is a square-wave driver, which has an electric linear motor and a piston. The stroke of the piston (both positive and negative) determines the amplitude. The position of the piston determines the mean airway pressure of the circuit.

The main controls in HFOV are mean airway pressure, oscillatory pressure amplitude, bias flow, frequency, and inspiratory time. With piston-driven oscillators, piston-centering is an additional control mechanism. Mean airway pressure determines the mean lung volume of the lung. Oscillatory amplitude is the total change in pressure around the mean airway pressure produced by forward and backward displacement of the piston. The pressures developed in the patients' airways are considerably dampened because of the impedance of the endotracheal tube. Similarly, the pressure profile is further dampened in the distal airways because of the impedance of the proximal airways. If the oscillatory frequency approaches the natural resonant frequency of the lung and airways, then there may be amplification of the pressure waves. The oscillatory amplitude determines the volume displacement with each stroke of the piston. If the volume of gas displaced is less than the dead space of the airways and lungs, then there is little chest displacement. If sufficient chest displacement is seen with each stroke, then the volume of gas displaced tends to be larger than the physiologic dead space and results in some direct alveolar ventilation. Frequency is the next parameter that can be controlled and is usually in the range of 5 to 10 Hz. For a given amplitude, a lower frequency will result in less attenuation of pressures along the airways and improve gas exchange. Inspiratory time is generally controlled at 33% of the total cycle time. In certain circumstances a lower inspiratory time may be used. Bias flow is a continuous flow of fresh humidified gas and allows replenishing oxygen and removing carbon dioxide from the circuit. Determinants of oxygenation during HFOV are mean airway pressure and FiO_2. Minute ventilation during HFOV is directly proportional to the frequency and the square of the tidal volume. Tidal volume is determined by the amplitude and the duration of each stroke. With increased frequency, the time for each stroke is reduced, decreasing the tidal volume. When the ventilatory frequency is decreased, this increases the time for each stroke and thereby increases the tidal volume. The primary determinant of ventilation is oscillatory amplitude. Decreasing the frequency to reduce attenuation and increasing the inspiratory time are less effective strategies to improve carbon dioxide elimination.

High-Frequency Percussive Ventilation

High-frequency percussive ventilation (HFPV), a newer mode introduced during the past 20 years, combines the beneficial effects of HFV with conventional ventilatory support.[162-164] HFPV has been described as an exceptionally versatile form of HFV that delivers subphysiologic tidal volumes at rapid rates (up to 500 breaths/min) using the volume-diffusive respirator.[162-164] It has been shown to provide the same or improved oxygenation and ventilation at lower peak, mean, and end-expiratory pressures when compared with conventional ventilation.[162-164]

The high-frequency percussive ventilator (Percussionaire, Bird Technologies, Sandpoint, Idaho) is a pneumatically powered, time-cycled, and pressure-limited ventilator with inspiratory and expiratory oscillation. The ventilator is connected to a high-pressure flow generator, fed by an air-oxygen blender. Two inspiratory circuits come off the ventilator—one a high-pressure and the other a low-pressure circuit. The low-pressure circuit is connected to the humidifier and a nebulizer system. The humidifier and nebulization system provide a gas mixture that is appropriately heated and fully humidified. The high-pressure circuit is a low-compliant tubing. Both the circuits attach to a system called the "Phasitron," which is a sliding Venturi that acts as both an inspiratory and expiratory valve. The Phasitron is driven by a high-pressure gas supply at a high-frequency rate of 200 to 900 beats/min superimposed on a conventional inspiratory/expiratory pressure-controlled cycle that is set at a desired rate. From the Phasitron, there are two branches: an inspiratory limb that attaches to the endotracheal tube and an expiratory limb. The Phasitron consists of a hollow cylinder in which there is a spring-controlled piston driven by the high-pressure circuit. Two safety valves, one inspiratory and one expiratory, regulate the pressure delivered to the airway. There are seven control variables: (1) peak inspiratory pressure, (2) positive end-expiratory pressure, (3) continuous positive airway pressure, (4) inspiratory time, (5) expiratory time, (6) percussive frequency, and (7) rate. The tidal volume delivery is a product of the peak inspiratory pressure (PIP) setting and subtidal volumes produced by the oscillatory function. During inspiration, lung volumes are progressively increased in a controlled, stepwise fashion by repetitively diminishing subtidal volume deliveries until an oscillatory plateau is entered and maintained. At the end of inspiration, the lung is allowed to empty passively until the preset expiratory baseline is reached. Gas exchange has been noted to be as good, if not better, than CV at lower airway pressures. The endotracheal tube cuff should be left partially deflated to allow for a continuous air leak through the trachea.

Clinical Uses of High-Frequency Ventilation

The principal theoretical advantage for the use of HFV lies in the ability to ventilate effectively at low airway pressures. The most common use of HFV is in the operating room for use in airway operations; in laryngoscopies; in bronchoscopies; and in emergency airway management, in which airway movement has to be reduced to a minimum.[161] HFV has been used to manage neonates with idiopathic respiratory distress syndrome with the goal of decreasing the incidence of pulmonary barotrauma. Initial studies showed improvement in gas exchange with lower airway pressures, provided periodic sigh maneuvers were performed.[165-168] HFV has also been shown to support adequate gas exchange with severe pulmonary interstitial emphysema (PIE) in neonates.[169,170] The initial enthusiasm for HFOV as a method for reducing pulmonary barotrauma in premature neonates with idiopathic respiratory distress syndrome requiring mechanical ventilation has been tempered by a recent multicenter trial in which HFOV did not prove to be superior to conventional mechanical ventilation.[171] One area of relatively proven benefit of HFV is in the management of bronchopleural fistulae. HFJV has proven useful in the management of bronchopleural fistula, with consistent improvement in arterial blood gas, when conventional ventilation had previously failed.[172] Recent studies have suggested a role for HFV in children after cardiac surgery and with ARDS.[173-178] HFJV has been shown to improve cardiac function after a Fontan procedure.[173] HFJV and HFOV have been shown to improve oxygenation and ventilation compared with conventional ventilation in children with respiratory failure.[175-178] Our results indicate that high-frequency oscillatory ventilation, utilizing an aggressive volume recruitment strategy, results in significant improvement in oxygenation compared with a conventional ventilatory strategy designed to limit increases in peak airway pressures. In a prospective study of HFOV compared with conventional ventilation, HFOV resulted in improved oxygenation, lower requirement for supplemental oxygen at 30 days, and improved outcome compared with conventional mechanical ventilation.[178]

The most common approach to HFOV in infants and children is as a rescue therapy when conventional mechanical ventilation proves to be insufficient to recruit the lungs and maintain adequate gas exchange. There are many reported strategies with the use of HFV: (1) "high lung volume strategy," which requires HFV to be provided at a mean airway pressure that is at least 3 to 5 cm higher than with conventional ventilation; (2) combined HFV and conventional ventilation (usually used with HFJV), in which conventional tidal breaths are interposed during HFV usually at a rate of 5 to 8 breaths per minute; or (3) application of HFV at the same mean airway pressure as conventional ventilation. The high lung volume strategy seems to be the most promising one at least for HFOV. When transitioning the patient to HFOV from conventional ventilation, the mean airway pressure on HFOV is set to 3 to 6 cm H_2O above the mean airway pressure on conventional ventilation. It is important to recruit the lung before placing the patient on HFOV. Amplitude is set by adjusting the power control while observing for adequacy of chest wall vibrations. The goal for oxygenation is to employ a mean airway pressure that will allow reduction of FiO_2 to at least 0.6 while maintaining an arterial oxygen saturation of at least 90%. This may require titrating the mean airway pressure from the initial setting. Adequacy of lung recruitment is usually verified by ensuring that both hemidiaphragms are displaced to the level of the ninth posterior rib on a chest radiograph. Once an appropriate degree of lung inflation and patency of the endotracheal tube are verified, ventilation needs to be addressed. Arterial $PaCO_2$ can be maintained at the desired level by changing the amplitude or frequency. Ventilation is increased by an increase in amplitude and a decrease in frequency. It is also important to deflate the cuff of the endotracheal tube, if a cuffed tube is used. Adjusting the bias flow can also aid in ventilation but is seldom done in routine clinical practice.

Case series in neonates with respiratory failure showed that HFPV can result in improvement in oxygenation and ventilation with a reduction in FiO_2 and PEEP requirements.[179-181] One other purported advantage to high-frequency percussive ventilation is the mobilization of secretions. This has generated much interest from the burn community, particularly for the treatment of children and adults with inhalation injury.[182-188] Two prospective, randomized trials of HFPV have been reported in the pediatric burn population. Compared with the conventional ventilation, high-frequency percussive ventilation resulted in similar ventilation and improved oxygenation at significantly lower peak inspiratory pressures. Pneumonia and mortality rates were lower in the high-frequency group.[183,184]

Adverse Effects of Mechanical Ventilation
Yin-Yang of Mechanical Ventilation

Mechanical ventilation has profound effects on various organ systems; some are beneficial and others have adverse effects. The beneficial and adverse effects can occur simultaneously; the net effect of mechanical ventilation results from the interaction of useful and deleterious effects. The beneficial effects in the lung are related to improvements in pulmonary mechanics and gas exchange. Adverse effects of positive pressure ventilation are related to (1) consequences of positive intrathoracic pressure and (2) injury to the airway. Some of the important adverse effects of mechanical ventilation are shown in Table 57.5.

Airway Injury

The presence of an endotracheal tube traversing the upper airway can be associated with significant airway injury. Oropharyngeal and nasopharyngeal injuries are rare. Ulceration of the ala nasi from pressure necrosis may occur following prolonged nasotracheal intubation, particularly if the skin perfusion of the ala nasi is compromised by tight taping. Similar ulceration may occur at the angles of the mouth from

TABLE 57.5	Adverse Effects of Mechanical Ventilation

Respiratory system
  Airways
    Mucosal swelling
    Ulceration
    Granuloma formation leading to airway obstruction
    Infection
  Lung
    Infection
    Adverse effects on gas exchange
    Effects on extravascular lung water
    Air leaks
Cardiovascular system
  Heart
    Decreased venous return
    Decreased left ventricular compliance
    Decreased left ventricular afterload
Pulmonary circulation
    Compression of alveolar vessels
    Increased pulmonary vascular resistance
Other systems
    Decreased renal blood flow
    Decreased hepatic blood flow
    Decreased cerebral venous drainage

tight taping of orotracheal tubes.[200,201] Palatal grooves and traumatic cleft palate can occur in infants.[202] Laryngeal injury may extend from minor swelling to ulceration of the mucosa of the vocal cords and aryepiglottic folds. Similarly, injuries in the subglottic region may extend from minor swelling to major ulceration. Healing of the severe injuries may lead to scarring or granuloma formation with airway obstruction, which may be partial or complete. The majority of the subglottic tracheal lesions is due to compression of the tracheal mucosa by the endotracheal tube. High-pressure cuffs, cardiovascular instability, upper respiratory tract infection, duration of intubation, and head-neck movement all increase the risk of tracheal injury. Airway injury can also result from suction catheters.[192] Necrotizing tracheobronchitis is a severe form of airway injury seen in patients on mechanical ventilation, which is characterized by extensive ulceration and mucosal damage. The sequelae of tracheal injuries include tracheal stenosis, tracheomalacia, tracheoesophageal fistula, and tracheoinnominate artery fistula.

Injury to the airway can be prevented by attention to several details. The endotracheal tube should be of the proper size, with a gas leak around it at less than 20 cm H_2O positive pressure. Excessive pressure on the skin should be avoided while taping of the endotracheal tube. Excessive patient movement should be prevented by adequate sedation and restraints. Endotracheal tube cuffs should be inflated with pressures less than 20 cm H_2O. Suctioning should be gentle, preferably with a catheter with multiple side holes. Suction catheters should not be routinely advanced beyond the tip of the endotracheal tube.

Effects on the Lung

Adverse effects of mechanical ventilation on the lung are due to the following factors: (1) high airway pressures, (2) overdistention of the alveoli, (3) altered mucociliary clearance, (4) lung water clearance, and (5) oxygen toxicity. The adverse effects of positive pressure ventilation may be manifested as (1) parenchymal injury, (2) altered ventilation-perfusion relationship leading to impaired gas exchange, and (3) increased risk for infection. Increased airway pressure may cause hyperinflation of the alveoli and predispose to alveolar rupture. Hyperinflation may increase alveolar dead space, impair cardiac filling, and compress alveolar vessels. "Pulmonary barotrauma" is a loose term that encompasses many entities of parenchymal injury. Alveolar rupture from overdistended alveoli is the most common manifestation of pulmonary barotrauma. Air leak may occur from the lung into the pleura (pneumothorax), interstitium (pulmonary interstitial emphysema, PIE), mediastinum (pneumomediastinum), pericardium (pneumopericardium), peritoneal cavity (pneumoperitoneum), and subcutaneous tissue (subcutaneous emphysema). Even though the term implies high airway pressures as the main mechanism of parenchymal injury, pulmonary barotrauma is often multifactorial.[193-196] The physiologic consequences of extra-alveolar air may range from no adverse effect to life-threatening cardiorespiratory compromise. A pneumothorax may be small and inconsequential or may be large and under tension. Tension pneumothorax would need immediate evacuation of the pleural air. PIE may decrease lung compliance and increase pulmonary vascular resistance.[197] Pneumomediastinum requires careful observation. The natural tendency of pneumomediastinum is to track along fascial planes either cephalad to produce subcutaneous emphysema or caudad to produce pneumoperitoneum or pneumoretroperitoneum. Pneumomediastinum rarely requires evacuation. Pneumopericardium can range from a minimal inconsequential amount of air to life-threatening cardiac tamponade. Cardiovascular compromise is an indication for immediate evacuation of pericardial air.

A special form of pulmonary air leak is a bronchopleural fistula, where a fistulous track develops between the bronchus and the pleural space. This results in an almost continuous flow of air from the airway into the pleural space. The fistula flow is wasted ventilation and may result in hypercarbia. Attempts to increase minute ventilation by increasing tidal volume will only serve to increase the fistula flow by increasing the pressure gradient across the fistula. If attempts to decrease airway pressures with conventional ventilation are not possible without compromising gas exchange, a trial of high-frequency ventilation may be tried.

Barotrauma can be minimized by avoiding factors that predispose to pulmonary air leakage. The principal factors that can be controlled are airway pressures and lung volumes. As long as acceptable gas exchange is maintained, every effort must be made to reduce airway pressures to a minimum. Hyperinflation must be avoided. When the lung disease is severe, deliberate hypercarbia may be tolerated provided the arterial pH is normal. Inspired oxygen concentration should be maintained at nontoxic levels (usually <50%).

Effects on Circulatory System

The cardiovascular effects of positive intrathoracic pressure are complex and depend on the underlying lung disease, uniformity of lung disease, transmission of airway pressure to the pleural space, lung volume, etc. Cournand's laboratory was one of the first to demonstrate that positive pressure ventilation decreased cardiac output.[198,199] Positive intrathoracic pressure impedes right ventricular filling by decreasing the pressure gradient to venous return.[198-201] Positive airway pressure also increases pulmonary vascular resistance, provided the airway pressure exceeds left atrial or critical closing pressure.[202] Positive intrathoracic pressure has also been shown to decrease left ventricular afterload. The net effect is a combination of all the effects mentioned earlier and the reflex cardiovascular adjustments that accompany these changes. Positive pressure breathing also decreases urine output, and decreases hepatic, portal venous, and mesenteric perfusion.[203-207] Many of these effects can be offset by volume loading.

Specialty Gases
Altering Inspired Oxygen and Carbon Dioxide Concentration

A low alveolar oxygen tension increases pulmonary vascular resistance (hypoxic pulmonary vasoconstriction), and a high alveolar oxygen tension decreases pulmonary vascular resistance.[208] With certain types of congenital heart disease such as hypoplastic left heart syndrome, it is critical to control pulmonary blood flow and prevent pulmonary overcirculation. One approach is to decrease the FiO_2 to less than 0.21 with a blending of room air with nitrogen. The exact FiO_2 delivered must be monitored to avoid administering excessively low inspired oxygen. Several studies have shown that hypoxic gas mixtures can be used both preoperatively and postoperatively to balance the pulmonary and systemic circulations.[209-211]

The other approach, especially in patients undergoing mechanical ventilation, both preoperatively and postoperatively, is to increase the inspired carbon dioxide concentration ($FiCO_2$). Increased $FiCO_2$ also increases pulmonary vascular resistance. During mechanical ventilation, increased $FiCO_2$ allows one to hyperventilate and prevent atelectasis without producing hypocarbia. One of the difficulties with a boost in $FiCO_2$ is increased spontaneous ventilatory drive due to an increased $PaCO_2$. This increases the work of breathing and with marginal cardiac reserve may impose undue strain on the heart. Therefore in spontaneously breathing patients, neuromuscular blockade and total ventilatory support may be necessary with increased $FiCO_2$ to avoid an increased workload on the heart. Morray et al.[212] were the first to report on this technique to increase PVR to prevent pulmonary overcirculation. This finding has been confirmed in both an experimental model[213] and in infants with hypoplastic left heart syndrome.[214]

Helium-Oxygen Mixture

Helium-oxygen mixture has much lower density compared with oxygen-nitrogen mixture and offers a reduced resistance to breathing.[214a] A detailed description of the properties of helium-oxygen mixture and its clinical applications is beyond the scope of this chapter, and the reader is referred to excellent reviews on this topic.[215-221] On the basis of the physics of airflow and the properties of heliox, the behavior can be predicted with its use. The predictions are (1) heliox will result in a higher flow when transairway pressures are held constant, (2) heliox will result in a lower airway pressure when the airflow is constant, (3) density-dependent flow meters will underestimate flow, (4) heliox can decrease the degree of air trapping and hyperinflation associated with lower airway obstruction, (5) heliox can decrease the work of breathing, and (6) heliox can result in better deposition of aerosols administered with it.[221] Helium is usually administered in at least 30% to 40% oxygen through a tight-fitting facemask. Use of an Oxyhood is not indicated because helium tends to separate and layer at the top of the Oxyhood with the patient breathing little helium.

Several studies have shown that heliox administration improves symptoms and relieves the respiratory distress associated with upper airway obstruction due to viral croup, subglottic narrowing, and postextubation stridor.[222-231] The use of heliox in asthma is increasing. It is being used as the carrier gas for bronchodilator aerosols, as well as continuously to relieve lower airway obstruction in status asthmaticus.[232-244] Most of the studies show improvement in clinical scores of respiratory distress, relief of wheezing, and faster resolution of symptoms.[232-244] It is important to remember that the quality of the breath sounds may be altered by heliox and may appear diminished due to the effect on airflow in the lungs. The patient may have relief of symptoms while having a "silent chest" during heliox administration, and this may not be an ominous sign. It is important to auscultate the chest by discontinuing the heliox to appreciate if the lower airway obstruction and wheezing are still present. Heliox has also been used in acute bronchiolitis with or without positive airway pressure.[245-253] Similar to the studies in asthma, there is improvement in the clinical score and work of breathing in these infants.[245-253] Recently, helium-oxygen mixture has been shown to improve gas exchange in neonates with respiratory distress syndrome.[254] Oxygenation should be monitored during administration of helium-oxygen mixture to avoid hypoxia, especially in neonates.[255]

Inhaled Nitric Oxide

Inhaled nitric oxide produces selective pulmonary vasodilation. Indications for inhaled nitric oxide include diaphragmatic hernia, pulmonary hypertension after repair of congenital heart disease, primary pulmonary hypertension, and isolated right heart failure. In babies with severe hypoxemia and pulmonary hypertension, inhaled nitric oxide rapidly increases arterial oxygen tension without causing systemic hypotension.[256-259] Randomized controlled studies showed that nitric oxide inhalation safely improves arterial oxygen levels and decreases the need for extracorporeal membrane oxygenation (ECMO) therapy.[256-259] Oxygenation improves in approximately 50% of infants receiving nitric oxide. In addition, Kinsella and Abman[260] showed that high-frequency ventilation seems to augment the response to inhaled nitric oxide probably by better recruitment of alveoli. In children with ALI/ARDS, Ream et al.[261] showed an improvement in oxygenation in more than two-thirds of the patients. Researchers of a randomized controlled trial of inhaled nitric oxide in children with acute hypoxemic respiratory failure have also reported an improvement in oxygenation.[262] Results from several adult studies, however, showed that several participants failed to show any improvement.[263-266] In these multicenter studies in children and adults, there were no differences in ventilator-free days and no effect on mortality between treatment groups. Not all patients respond to inhaled nitric oxide. It seems prudent to test whether a patient will respond to inhaled nitric oxide. At Children's Hospital of Pittsburgh, a 2-hour trial of inhaled nitric oxide with 20 to 40 ppm is administered to infants and children with ALI/ARDS with hypoxemic respiratory failure. A good response is defined as improvement in PaO_2/FiO_2 ratio of greater than 100%. A partial response is defined as an improvement in PaO_2/FiO_2 ratio between 50% and 100%. If the response is less than 50%, the patient is considered a nonresponder. Inhaled nitric oxide is then continued in only those patients who show a partial or good response. Nitric oxide binds to hemoglobin to produce methemoglobin. Therefore methemoglobin levels should be monitored during administration of nitric oxide. In addition, nitric oxide combines with oxygen to form nitrogen dioxide. Nitrogen dioxide is known to cause lung injury. Therefore the concentration of nitrogen dioxide should be monitored in the inspired gas to keep it below 1 to 2 ppm.

Respiratory Care During Mechanical Ventilation
Pulmonary Hygiene

The primary objectives of airway clearance therapy are (1) to prevent and treat atelectasis from mechanical obstruction of airways and (2) to remove toxic substances including infective materials, proteolytic enzymes, and other mediators of inflammation.[267] Various airway clearance techniques have been reviewed recently and describe the evidence underlying each one of the techniques in children with and without neuromuscular disease.[268,269] On the basis of all these studies, it appears that the most effective method of clearing secretions is a combination of changing body position and vigorous coughing by the patient.[270] When the patient is unable to cough effectively, it is common practice to resort to chest physiotherapy and active suctioning of the trachea. Suctioning the trachea usually requires disconnecting the patient from the ventilator, passage of a suction catheter into the endotracheal tube, and application of suction to the catheter while the catheter is withdrawn from the endotracheal tube. In patients with marginal oxygenation, suctioning may result in hypoxia; arrhythmias; hemodynamic instability; and, in rare instances, cardiac arrest.[271-273] This can be prevented by prior hyperoxygenation. Suctioning may also result in cardiac arrhythmias. Chest physiotherapy refers to a variety of respiratory maneuvers performed to aid in the clearance of airway secretions and promoting lung expansion. These are (1) postural drainage, (2) chest percussion and chest vibration, and (3) deep breathing exercises. The efficacy of chest physiotherapy in patients who have undergone intubation is unclear. In adults, some studies have shown a benefit when all the components of the chest physiotherapy regimen are performed.[274] In children with cystic fibrosis, no additional benefit was provided by chest physiotherapy maneuvers when compared with spontaneous coughing.[275] Recently, several devices have been proposed as an adjunct to the standard chest physiotherapy. They include an intrapulmonary percussive ventilator (IPV); a mechanical insufflator-exsufflator (CoughAssist); the FLUTTER mucus clearance device and Acapella devices; intermittent positive pressure breathing (IPPB); mechanical percussors; and the ABI Vest, formerly known as the ThAIRapy Vest. The IPV is used in mechanized chest physical therapy; the IPV device delivers high-flow jets of air to the airways by a pneumatic flow interrupter at a rate of 100 to 300 cycles per minute through a mouthpiece. The patient controls variables such as inspiratory time, peak pressure, and delivery rates. Initial studies showed that in children with cystic fibrosis, IPV was as effective as standard aerosol and chest physiotherapy.[276,277] IPV was recently reported to improve atelectasis in children, compared with conventional chest physiotherapy.[278] A more recent study suggests that IPV may be more beneficial in secretion clearance in children with cystic fibrosis.[279] The mechanical insufflator-exsufflator (CoughAssist) is a portable electric device that uses a blower and a valve to alternately apply a positive and then a negative pressure to a patient's airway to assist the patient in clearing retained bronchopulmonary secretions. This device attempts to simulate a cough. Air is delivered to and from the patient through a breathing circuit incorporating a flexible tube; a bacterial filter; and a facemask, a mouthpiece, or an adapter to a tracheostomy or endotracheal tube. Miske et al.[280] reported that in children with neuromuscular disease and impaired cough, the use of a mechanical insufflator-exsufflator was safe, well tolerated, and effective in preventing pulmonary complications. The FLUTTER mucus clearance device and Acapella device are small handheld devices that provide positive expiratory pressure (PEP.) Exhaling through the device creates oscillations, or "flutter," in pressures in the airway resulting in loosening of mucus. Other PEP devices are used with a small volume nebulizer and function in conjunction with medication delivery. A recent Cochrane Review concluded that there was no clear evidence that PEP was a more or less effective

intervention overall than other forms of physiotherapy, and there was limited evidence that PEP was preferred by participants compared with other techniques.[281] IPPB devices use pressure to passively fill the lungs when a breath is initiated. An incorporated manometer and mechanical valves serve to terminate the flow of inspired air when a predetermined pressure is reached on inhalation. IPPB breathing circuits are designed to nebulize inhaled medication. Most IPPB devices are powered by compressed air and are not suitable for home use. Mechanical percussors are typically electrical devices used in lieu of a caretaker's hands for chest percussion or vibration. Conventional chest physiotherapy is both labor intensive and time consuming. A high-frequency chest wall vibrating/oscillating device is currently available (The ABI Vest). Arens et al.[282] showed that in hospitalized patients with cystic fibrosis, high-frequency chest compression with the vest conventional chest physiotherapy was equally safe and effective when used during acute pulmonary exacerbations.

Humidification Systems

During spontaneous breathing, inspired air is warmed and almost completely humidified as it passes through the upper airways.[283] The use of an endotracheal or a tracheostomy tube bypasses the natural warming and humidifying functions of the upper airway. The mucosal surface below the artificial airway must then provide both humidification and heat to the inspired air. This may adversely affect mucociliary clearance.[283,284] If the inspired gases are not warmed to the body temperature, insensible water loss in the lung is increased. All gases used in respiratory therapy are dry with no moisture. Therefore these gases must have moisture added to them during delivery to the patients. When a gas is warmed, its relative humidity decreases.

Humidifiers can be classified into those that provide only humidity and those that provide both heat and humidity. There are several types of nonheated simple humidifiers. The simplest in design is the pass-over or blow-by humidifier. The second type is the bubble humidifier, probably the most common device used in respiratory therapy. In this device, the gas is directed below the surface of the water and allowed to bubble to the surface. A jet-humidifier produces an aerosol; humidity is provided by evaporation of the aerosol particles. An underwater jet humidifier uses a combination of jet and bubble humidification principles. In the clinical setting, the amount of humidity provided by the simple humidifiers is about the same. Although the more efficient humidifiers increase humidification, they also tend to cool the inspired air. Therefore the absolute humidity delivered tends to be similar among the simple humidifiers. Relative humidity of 100% at room temperature is less than 40% relative humidity at body temperature. When inspired gases are humidified with one of these devices, the balance of the moisture is provided by the airway mucosa. Therefore when the upper airway is bypassed by the presence of an artificial airway, then the inspired gases must be additionally heated to provide 100% humidity at body temperature. The factors that determine the efficiency of humidifying devices depend on (1) time of contact with the gas and water, (2) temperature of both the gas and water, and (3) the surface area of contact of the gas-water interface. The efficiency of humidification increases as the time of contact increases and as the surface area of contact increases. Increasing the temperature of the inspired gas before delivery decreases the humidity that needs to be provided by the airway mucosa and adds to patient comfort. Heated humidifiers use the same principle as the simple humidifiers and have in addition a heating element. The relative humidity with these systems can be as high as 100%. The heating system can be servo-controlled to adjust the heat according to the relative humidity.

Aerosol Therapy

Aerosolized drug administration is often used in the treatment of infants and children with respiratory diseases including reversible lower airway obstruction, pneumonias due to *Pneumocystis carinii* and respiratory syncytial virus, and hyaline membrane disease. Common drugs used as aerosol agents include beta-2 agonists, atropine, ipratropium bromide, cromolyn sodium, antiviral agents, corticosteroids, antibiotics, surfactant, pentamidine, and mucolytics. A drug aerosol increases the therapeutic index of the drug by delivering it directly to the site of action with minimal side effects. The factors that affect deposition of aerosol particles are gravity, viscosity of the gas, kinetic activity of the particles, particle inertia, physical nature of the particle, temperature and humidity of the aerosol, and the ventilatory pattern. Compared with that in adults, deposition of aerosolized particles in infants and children is poor because of factors such as a small airway caliber, greater airway resistance, high respiratory rate with a short inspiratory time, increased chest wall compliance, ineffective coordination effort, and inconsistent breath-holding maneuvers. Despite poor aerosol deposition, a clinical response to inhaled medications can often be seen. The dose and the delivery method should be individualized to each patient to ensure a good clinical response.

Nebulizers are devices that generate aerosols. Particle size has to be at least 1 to 5 microns for deposition in the distal airways. Currently, four types of delivery systems are available for clinical use that generate medication aerosols. These are the jet nebulizers (small-volume and large-volume nebulizers), ultrasonic nebulizers, metered-dose inhalers, and dry-powder inhalers. A jet nebulizer uses the Bernoulli principle to create an aerosol. The size of the particle depends on the jet flow rate and size of the capillary tube. Baffles placed in the path of the aerosols tend to remove larger particles, allowing delivery of smaller particles to the patient. A pneumatic nebulizer is a device that creates the aerosol using the same principle as the jet nebulizer, but the aerosol particles are carried to the patient by a main gas flow. A pneumatic nebulizer may be a mainstream nebulizer in which the aerosol is generated in the path of the main gas flow or a sidestream nebulizer in which the aerosol is generated in a separate chamber and carried passively into the path of the main gas flow. The ultrasonic nebulizer uses a piezoelectric crystal that produces a highly concentrated output of aerosol particles and has been used primarily for cough and sputum production or broncho-provocational challenges. Ultrasonic nebulizers have not been routinely used for drug delivery in infants and children. With the replacement of the saline solution with medication, however, the highly concentrated output from the ultrasonic nebulizer may perform better than a small-volume nebulizer in accomplishing greater deposition of medications in children. The metered-dose inhaler uses a pressurized canister that dispenses a single bolus of aerosolized medication. Such inhalers are convenient, cost effective, and versatile, and

generally have an effective deposition rate of 10% to 15%. The canister is activated into the spacer and the medication remains suspended in the chamber until the patient inhales. A dry-powder inhaler delivers a large bolus of medication during a single inspiration maneuver and produces therapeutic effects similar to a metered-dose inhaler and an aerosol nebulizer. The dry-powder medication, released from a capsule and deposited into a small canister, is delivered to the lungs during inspiration. The inspired flow rate causes a turbulent state within the canister, and the powder is directed toward the respiratory tract.

Aerosolized medications are often delivered through mechanical ventilators for the treatment of bronchospasm. Aerosol delivery is inefficient when delivered through a ventilator. The endotracheal tube is the most significant barrier to effective delivery. The smaller the inner diameter of the tube, the less efficient is aerosol delivery. The nebulizer is most effective when it is synchronized to fill the inspiratory limb of the circuit with aerosolized particles during the exhalation phase of ventilation, thereby improving the delivery of medication during the subsequent inspiration. The inspiratory portion of the circuit serves as a spacer chamber, similar to the spacer used for metered-dose inhalers. Some current ventilators offer a synchronized nebulization capability, in which a portion of the preset inspiratory gas is diverted to power the nebulizer. The effects of added volume delivered to the inspiratory limb should be taken into account and minimized with the addition of a pressure relief valve to the circuit. Metered-dose inhalers can be equally effective as nebulizers during mechanical ventilation.

Weaning From Mechanical Ventilation

Weaning from mechanical ventilation is defined as liberation from mechanical ventilation while spontaneous breathing is allowed to assume the responsibility for effective gas exchange. Weaning can be considered a success when a patient can maintain effective gas exchange, with complete spontaneous breathing and without any mechanical assistance. Weaning can be considered a failure when spontaneous efforts are incapable of sustaining effective gas exchange without mechanical ventilator support. Extubation is defined as the removal of an endotracheal tube. The timing of extubation should coincide with an assessment that the patient is capable of maintaining effective gas exchange without any mechanical ventilator support. Avoiding both premature extubation and unnecessary prolongation of mechanical ventilation is important.

When the indications that were met for provision of mechanical ventilation are no longer present, then the patient can be weaned from mechanical ventilation (Table 57.6). Weaning should start (1) when the underlying disease process is improving; (2) when gas exchange is adequate; (3) when no conditions exist that impose an undue burden on the respiratory muscles, such as cardiac insufficiency, severe hyperinflation, severe malnutrition, and multiple organ system failure; and (4) when the patient is capable of sustaining spontaneous ventilation as ventilator support is decreased without expending an excessive amount of energy. It is the patient who dictates the initiation of the weaning process and pace of the weaning process. Patients cannot be arbitrarily forced to wean. Improvement of the underlying disease process can be assessed with measurement of indices of gas exchange, pulmonary

TABLE 57.6   Criteria to Be Met Before Initiating Weaning

1. Alert mental status
2. Good cough and gag reflexes
3. Core temperature below 38.5°C
4. Spontaneous respiratory effort
5. pH 7.32-7.47
6. Partial pressure of arterial oxygen (PaO_2) >60 mm Hg or pulse oximetry reading <95%
7. Fractional inspired oxygen (FiO_2) ≤0.50
8. Positive end-expiratory pressure (PEEP) ≤7 cm H_2O
9. Partial pressure of carbon dioxide ($PaCO_2$) <50 mm Hg
10. No further need for vasoactive agents
11. No clinical need for increased ventilator support in the past 24 hours
12. No planned operative procedures requiring heavy sedation in the next 12 hours

TABLE 57.7   Criteria for Terminating a Spontaneous Breathing Trial

1. Inability to maintain gas exchange
   Pulse oximeter saturations <95% with 40% inspired oxygen
   Needing >50% inspired oxygen to maintain oxygen saturations >95%
2. Inability to maintain effective ventilation
   Measured exhaled tidal volume <5 mL/kg
   An increase in $PaCO_2$ >50 mm Hg or an increase of >10 mm Hg
   Respiratory acidosis with pH <7.3
3. Increased work of breathing
   Respiratory rate outside of the acceptable range for their age for age

<6 mo	20-60/min
6 mo-2 yr	15-45/min
2-5 yr	15-40/min
>5 yr	10-35/min

   Use of accessory respiratory muscles
   Intercostals/suprasternal/supraclavicular retractions
   A paradoxical breathing pattern
4. Other signs of distress
   Diaphoresis
   Anxiety
   Heart rate higher than the 90th percentile for a given age
   Change in mental status (agitation or somnolence)
   Systolic blood pressure lower than the third percentile for a given age

If a patient has any of these signs at any time during the breathing trial, the trial should be terminated and mechanical ventilation should be reinstituted. *PaCO₂,* partial pressure of carbon dioxide.

mechanics, ventilation-perfusion relationships, and x-ray findings. The patient's ability to take over the responsibility from the ventilator depends on several factors: (1) respiratory muscle strength, (2) stability of the cardiovascular system, (3) work of breathing, (4) general nutritional status of the patient, and (5) the presence or absence of an underlying hypercatabolic state (eg, sepsis). Weaning cannot be accomplished unless all of these factors are optimal. The pathophysiologic determinants of weaning outcome include the following: (1) adequacy of pulmonary gas exchange; (2) respiratory drive; (3) respiratory muscle performance and capacity; (4) respiratory muscle load; (5) amount of dead-space ventilation; and (6) work of breathing and ventilatory requirements. Table 57.7 shows the specific parameters to be met before initiating weaning. There are currently two approaches to weaning. One is the "traditional" method of slowly reducing the ventilator support, including inspired oxygen concentration, to a minimal acceptable level and then assessing the patient's readiness to extubate. The other is the "modern" concept of assessing the patient's readiness to extubate as soon as the patient meets criteria to initiate weaning.

Traditional Method of Weaning

In the traditional method, the exact sequence of the weaning process will be dictated by the clinical circumstance. At each step of weaning, the patient must demonstrate an ability to sustain effectiveness of breathing. Minute ventilation is reduced primarily with a decrease in the ventilator rate. Mean airway pressure is then reduced to a minimum with a decrease in CPAP/PEEP. Most children are currently weaned with SIMV or IMV alone, with SIMV and added pressure support, or with pressure support alone. Despite earlier indications that weaning with IMV was useful,[285,286] current studies do not advocate weaning with IMV in adults.[287,288] In infants, provision of a continuous flow device has been shown to decrease work of breathing and aid in weaning.[17] PSV has been advocated as a weaning mode because it can result in better synchrony between the patient and the ventilator than IMV, volume-assisted ventilation, or pressure-control ventilation.[289-292] Pressure support will allow ventilatory muscle loads to be returned gradually during the weaning process.[289-292] Because each breath is assisted, it alters the pressure-volume relationship of the respiratory muscles in such a way as to improve its efficiency.[289-292] The parameters

that can be manipulated to titrate the muscle loading are the magnitude of the trigger threshold and the preset pressure limit. PEEP is provided to maintain FRC and prevent alveolar collapse. The amount of pressure support to be provided depends on the clinical circumstance. PSVmax, or the maximum pressure support needed to reduce the respiratory work to zero, requires a pressure limit that delivers a VTeff of about 10 to 12 mL/kg. PSVmax is not necessary at the start of weaning. The level of pressure support that should be selected should allow for spontaneous respiration without undue exertion and still result in normal minute ventilation. No strict criteria can be established; they have to be applied and titrated on an individual basis. Weaning of PSV is accomplished with a decremental reduction of the pressure limit. Similar to that previously mentioned in the weaning guidelines, with each wean, the effect of weaning on muscle loading has to be evaluated clinically. An increase in respiratory rate is an early indication of increasing muscle load. Retractions and use of accessory muscles would indicate a more severe muscle load. If respiratory rate increases during the weaning process, the level of pressure support should be increased until there is reduction in the respiratory rate. A relative contraindication to the use of PSV is a high baseline spontaneous respiratory rate. There is a finite lag time involved from the initiation of a breath to the sensing of this effort and from the sensing to the delivery of a mechanical breath. In infants breathing at a relatively fast rate (>50 breaths per minute), this lag time may be too long, and this may result in asynchrony between the patient and the ventilator.

"Modern" Method of Weaning

The premise underlying the modern method is that not all patients require a prolonged weaning process. Esteban et al.[287] showed that 76.2% of patients successfully underwent a 2-hour trial of spontaneous breathing, and 89.4% of them immediately underwent extubation. In a recently completed randomized, controlled trial of weaning modes in children, 42% of the patients initially tested with a minimal pressure-support trial passed the test and underwent extubation.[293] These studies validate the modern method of weaning patients from mechanical ventilation. If patients meet the criteria for weaning as outlined in Table 57.8, they can be subjected to a Readiness to Extubate Trial (RET) to test their ability to breathe spontaneously and maintain gas exchange. If the RET is successful, then the patient is ready to be extubated. If the patient fails an RET, there are two choices, either continuation of invasive mechanical ventilation or extubation to noninvasive ventilation. If invasive mechanical ventilation is continued, then the RET can be repeated in 24 hours. The level of invasive mechanical ventilator support should keep the patient comfortable with no increased work of breathing. If the decision is to extubate to noninvasive positive pressure support, then it would be prudent to test the patient on a level of pressure support that is necessary to maintain gas exchange and decrease the work of breathing. The criteria for terminating an RET are shown in Table 57.8.

Readiness to Extubate Trial (RET)

Currently, there are three methods of RETs: (1) T-piece trials, (2) CPAP trials, and (3) minimal pressure-support trials.[287,288,293-296] In T-piece trials, the patient is removed from the ventilator but does not undergo extubation. Humidified supplemental oxygen is provided to the airway without any positive pressure support through a T-piece (Fig. 57.22).

In this system, a corrugated tubing from the nebulizer/humidifier attaches to one end of the T-piece, and an extension of corrugated tubing attaches to the other end of the T-piece. The flow rate should be adjusted to produce a constant mist coming from the extension piece on the T-tube during both inspiration and expiration so that the patient's minute ventilation is matched by the device. Roughly, this

TABLE 57.8	Threshold Values for Low- and High-Risk of Reintubation for Bedside Parameters of Respiratory Function		
Respiratory Parameter		**Low Risk (≤10%)**	**High Risk (≥25%)**
Spontaneous tidal volume (mL/kg)		>6.5	<3.5
FIO_2		<0.3	>0.4
Mean airway pressure (cm H_2O)		<5	>8.5
Peak inspiratory pressure (cm H_2O)		<25	>30
Dynamic compliance (mL/kg/cm H_2O)		>0.9	<0.4
Fraction of the total minute ventilation provided by the ventilator (%)		<20	>30
Mean inspiratory flow (mL/kg/sec)		>14	<8

Respiratory parameters were measured just before extubation. Risk of reintubation is percent of patients who were reintubated within 48 h of extubation.

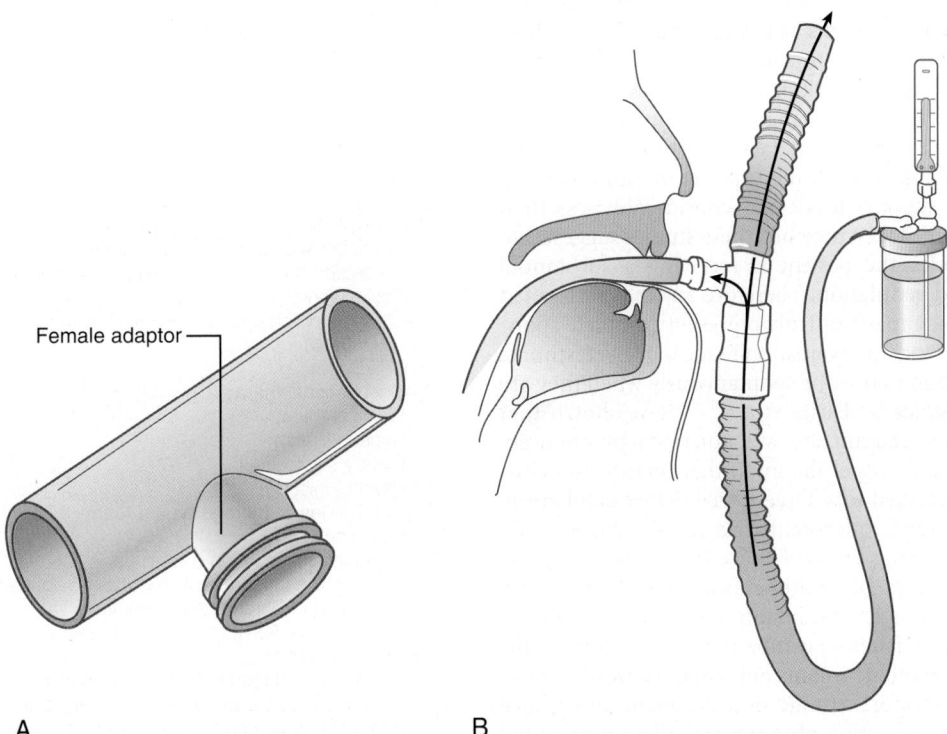

A   B

Fig. 57.22. (A and B) T-piece circuit. (Reproduced with permission from Kofke WA. Postoperative respiratory care techniques. Part III. Weaning from mechanical ventilation and oxygen therapy. Curr Rev RACN. 1992;13:161.)

Female adaptor

corresponds to at least about three times the minute ventilation of the patient.

The RET can also be conducted without removing the patient from the ventilator with a low level (eg, 5 cm H_2O) of CPAP or with a low level of PSV. Randolph et al.[293] described a minimal pressure-support technique in which the level of pressure support was adjusted for the endotracheal tube size (3–3.5 mm = pressure support of 10 cm H_2O; 4–4.5 mm = pressure support of 8 cm H_2O; >5 mm = pressure support of 6 cm H_2O). On the other hand, in a study comparing minimal pressure support with T-piece trials, Farias et al.[294-296] used a pressure support of 10 cm H_2O for all patients. The duration of the trial can range from 30 minutes to 2 hours. The proponents of a "minimal pressure-support" approach to the RET speculate that this overcomes the resistance to breathing through the artificial airway. Ishaaya et al.[297] showed that minimal pressure support based on in vitro studies overestimated the amount of support required to overcome the resistance of the endotracheal tube and ventilator circuitry. There are no measurements in vivo validating this concept in children. In one study of adults, the authors reported a similar resistance to breathing through the upper airway after extubation as that with the endotracheal tube in place.[298] Resistance through the artificial airway is affected by many factors, including the inspiratory flow of the patient, inner diameter of the tube, use of either an endotracheal or a tracheostomy tube, and presence of secretions in the tube. In children, Farias et al.[295] recently compared two methods of RET, one with pressure support of 10 cm H_2O and the other with a T-piece circuit. The extubation failure was not different between the two groups.[295]

Physicians are reluctant to subject infants and young children to a trial of complete spontaneous breathing with either CPAP or a T-piece circuit because of concern about the work of breathing imposed by the endotracheal tube and the breathing circuit. Proponents of this paradigm routinely extubate patients after a "minimal pressure-support" RET. Willis et al.[299] showed elegantly that the work of breathing associated with T-piece breathing was similar to that with complete spontaneous breathing after extubation. In fact, this study showed that the work of breathing with all the support modes including minimal pressure support mode was considerably less than that after extubation. Taken together, these studies suggest that with support modes the patient is receiving a substantial amount of assisted ventilation. Therefore an RET performed with a support mode may not truly represent complete spontaneous breathing, and any evaluation made may overestimate the ability of children to breathe spontaneously when they are extubated. The studies by Farias et al.[294-296] have shown that RETs with a T-piece circuit are well tolerated by children. These should serve to dispel the myth that infants and children cannot be subjected to a T-piece trial before extubation. Despite these theoretic concerns, Farias et al.[295] showed that patients extubated using either T-piece or pressure-support trials had similar rates of reintubation. There is currently another school of thought that infants and children need not be subjected to an RET before extubation. Proponents of this practice routinely extubate infants and children from a "low" level of ventilator support. Studies in children, however, have shown that when the fraction of minute ventilation provided by the ventilator is more than 30%, the risk of extubation failure is increased.[300,301] It is preferable that the ability to breathe effectively be determined with complete spontaneous breathing without ventilator support. An important dictum to remember is that "the test for extubation readiness is not extubation."[302]

Extubation

When RET is successful, the patient can undergo extubation and be liberated from mechanical ventilation. The patient must be awake, be alert, and have airway protective reflexes. The patient must be breathing effectively, without undue exertion. Adequate gas exchange with a relatively low FiO_2 must be established. A stable cardiovascular system must be established. Metabolic, nutritional, and electrolyte balance must be ensured. Airway pressures must be reduced to a minimum. Extubation failure can be predicted using simple measures of respiratory function such as inspiratory drive, lung mechanics, gas exchange, and level of ventilator support before extubation.[300,301] A low risk is defined as an extubation failure rate of less than 10%, and a high risk of failure is defined as an extubation failure rate of at least 25%.[300,301] Table 57.9 lists the

---

TABLE 57.9   Factors to Be Considered in Children for Home Care

Patient selection
    Medical assessment
    Cardiopulmonary stability
    Positive trend in weight gain and growth curve
    Freedom from frequent respiratory tract infections
Characteristics of the family and child
    Awareness
    Motivation
    Commitment
Home requirements
    Safe electrical, plumbing, and heating systems
    Telephone
    Space
Health care support personnel
    Nurses
    Aides
    Family and friends
Funding
    Third-party
    State
    Other
Multidisciplinary home care team from the discharging institution
    Physician specializing in technology-dependent patients
    Nurse specializing in technology-dependent patients
    Social worker
    Respiratory therapist specializing in technology-dependent patients
Other services
    Occupational therapy
    Physical therapy
    Speech therapy
    Dietary services
    Psychologist
Responsibilities of the home care team
    Coordinator
    Physician available on a 24-h basis
    Referral to a local durable medical equipment company
    Instruction of parents and caretakers
    Assistance of family in securing funding
Family preparation
    Training in cardiopulmonary resuscitation
    Instruction in all aspects of home care plan
    Instruction in use and maintenance of equipment
    Psychologic impact
    Techniques of instruction

threshold values for the respiratory parameters with identified low- and high-risk values.[300,301] Additional parameters that may be useful in determining eligibility for extubation are an intrapulmonary shunt fraction less than 15% (requires pulmonary artery catheterization), a physiologic dead space less than 40%,[303] a vital capacity of at least 15 mL/kg, and a maximum negative inspiratory force of at least 30 cm H_2O.

Weaning Problems

Farias et al.[294-296] distinguish between two types of failure: trial failure and extubation failure. Trial failure is defined as a failure to sustain effective gas exchange and breathing during a trial of spontaneous breathing while the patient is still intubated. Extubation failure is defined as the requirement for reintubation within 48 hours after extubation. Some patients take longer than others to wean. Factors that prolong the weaning process are (1) slow resolution of the underlying disease process, (2) ventilatory pump failure, and (3) psychologic factors. In many instances, weaning is delayed because of the slow resolution of the underlying disease process. Ventilatory pump failure can be due to increased respiratory work load, decreased respiratory muscle capacity, or a combination of both. Decreased ventilatory drive may result from respiratory center dysfunction caused by sedative agents; neurologic disease, particularly if it affects the brain stem; sleep deprivation; and metabolic alkalosis. Phrenic nerve injury usually results as a complication of birth trauma or operative procedures involving the heart and other thoracic structures.[304-306] This may result in either paresis or paralysis of one or both hemidiaphragms. When muscle weakness is present, weaning should generally be slow, allowing sufficient time for regaining muscle strength and endurance. Muscle training through an incremental increase in muscle work can be achieved by a gradual increase in the trigger threshold for assisted ventilation. Ventilatory requirements can be reduced with a decrease in carbon dioxide production with a reduction in excess caloric intake. Muscle loading may occur during IMV because of patient asynchrony. Asynchrony between the patient's breathing and the mechanical breaths may occur during both phases of the respiratory cycle. When the patient exhales while the ventilator delivers a mechanical breath, the airway pressures will be higher and the mechanical breath is wasted. This increases the work of breathing during exhalation. Prolonged asynchrony may result in muscle fatigue and may contribute to prolonged weaning. Considering nonrespiratory factors that may affect extubation failure is important. In a study by Khamiees et al.,[188] although all patients passed an RET, poor cough strength and endotracheal secretions were synergistic in predicting extubation failure. A recent article describes the current state of knowledge and evidence for many of the issues related to weaning and extubation.[307]

Tracheostomy and Weaning

Most airway resistance resides in the upper airways. Tracheostomy may aid in the weaning by several mechanisms. First, it reduces airway resistance by bypassing the upper airway. This reduces the work of breathing. Second, it increases patient comfort and allows better interaction between the patient and the caretakers, especially the parents. Third, it increases nursing comfort. Tracheostomy is not without risk. The procedure and complications of tracheostomy are described in detail elsewhere. Immediate complications are those related to

bleeding, those related to pulmonary air leak, and those associated with anesthesia. Long-term complications include infections of the trachea and lung, granuloma formation with subglottic stenosis from scarring, erosion of the trachea, and bleeding from erosion into a major thoracic vessel (eg, innominate artery).

Home Respiratory Care

Chronic respiratory failure is defined as the requirement for mechanical ventilation for longer than a month. Due to improved medical care and technology, the prevalence of children surviving with chronic respiratory failure is increasing. In 1984, the Ad Hoc Task Force on Home Care of Critically Ill Infants stated that "the goal of a home care program for infants, children, or adolescents with chronic conditions is the provision of comprehensive, cost-effective health care within a nurturing home environment that maximizes the capabilities of the individual and minimizes the effects of disabilities."[310] Respiratory care requirements in these children may range from supplemental oxygen to long-term mechanical ventilation. Long-term care in a tertiary care center is expensive and can alternatively be provided in a specialized chronic care rehabilitation center or at home. In 1986, the American College of Chest Physicians published guidelines for the management of ventilator-dependent patients in the home and at alternate community sites.[311] Since the late 1970s and early 1980s, home care has been shown to be as safe as hospital care for infants with tracheostomies and infants and children requiring long-term mechanical ventilation.[312-318] The diagnoses included neuromuscular disease, spinal cord trauma, and respiratory failure from chronic cardiorespiratory disease.[172-178] Home care is psychosocially more acceptable to the families, is less expensive, and may provide a better quality of life for respiratory technology-dependent children.[319,320]

Indications for Home Respiratory Care

The goals of long-term home respiratory care include (1) provision of comprehensive, cost-effective respiratory care, (2) enhancement of quality of life, (3) reduction of morbidity, and (4) wherever possible, extend life. The major indication for home respiratory care is chronic respiratory failure. This may occur in children with parenchymal or airway disease or in children with normal lungs. In children with normal lungs, respiratory failure is usually due to central or peripheral nervous system dysfunction, neuromuscular disorders, or chest wall abnormalities. Patients who require home respiratory care generally fall under the following categories: (1) patients whose underlying disease is most likely to recover and therefore would need respiratory care during the recovery phase such as infants with bronchopulmonary dysplasia and children recovering from adult respiratory distress syndrome, (2) patients whose underlying disease is irreversible but not progressive such as patients with spinal cord injury, and (3) patients whose underlying disease is irreversible and progressive such as patients with muscular dystrophy. The approach to home care planning will be different depending on the natural course of the underlying disease.

Logistics of Home Care

Home care requires a team approach with interaction among several health care personnel—primary physician, home care nurses, respiratory therapists, social workers, sometimes the State Health Agency, and the family and patient (Table 57.9). First, the patient must be ready for home care.[318,320,321] In some patients, a stable tracheostomy with a mature stoma is essential. Inspired oxygen requirement should not be greater than 35%. PaO_2 should be greater than 60 to 70 torr with a $PaCO_2$ less than 60 torr with a normal arterial pH at relatively low ventilator settings. The family must demonstrate not only a desire to provide home care but also a minimal ability to provide various aspects of home care. Health care personnel must be available in the local community to assist the family in providing care. The home must have adequate facilities to maintain and run all necessary equipment and supplies. Contingency plans must be made for emergencies. The location of the home has major implications for home care. The home must be easily accessible by standard transportation. A home care provider should be available on a 24-hour basis to respond to emergencies. The home must have adequate space to accommodate all the caretakers and the required equipment. Discharge planning must be thorough and take into account all the factors listed in Table 57.9. A detailed description of the various respiratory care equipment used for home care is beyond the scope of this chapter, and the reader is referred elsewhere.[322,323] A thorough knowledge of the limitations of various devices is essential for the respiratory care personnel coordinating home care. Parents who are motivated to providing home care for their children are willing to take on the cumbersome responsibility of carrying all the necessary equipment from place to place just to have the benefit of having the child at home.

Key References

1. Nunn JF. *Applied Respiratory Physiology*. 3rd ed. London: Butterworths & Co.; 1987.
7. Chatburn RL. A new system for understanding mechanical ventilators. *Respir Care.* 1991;36:1123-1155.
10. Chatburn RL, Primiano FP Jr. A new system for understanding modes of mechanical ventilation. *Respir Care.* 2001;46:604-621.
11. Chatburn RL. Classification of ventilator modes: update and proposal for implementation. *Respir Care.* 2007;52:301-323.
22. Gregory GA, Kitterman JA, Phibbs RH, et al. Treatment of idiopathic respiratory-distress syndrome with continuous positive airway pressure. *N Engl J Med.* 1971;284:1333-1340.
28. Suter PM, Fairley HB, Isenberg MD. Optimal end-expiratory airway pressure in patients with acute pulmonary failure. *N Engl J Med.* 1975;292:284.
45. Stock MC, Downs JB, Frolicher DA. Airway pressure release ventilation. *Crit Care Med.* 1987;15:462.
68. Sinderby C, Beck J. Proportional assist ventilation and neurally adjusted ventilatory assist—better approaches to patient ventilator synchrony? *Clin Chest Med.* 2008;29:329-342.
79. Alander M, Peltoniemi O, Pokka T, Kontiokari T. Comparison of pressure-flow, and NAVA-triggering in pediatric and neonatal ventilatory care. *Pediatr Pulmonol.* 2012;47:76-83.
81. Hewlett AM, Platt AS, Terry VG. Mandatory minute volume. A new concept in weaning from mechanical ventilation. *Anaesthesia.* 1977;32:163-169.
83. Martin JG, Shore S, Engel LA. Effect of continuous positive airway pressure on respiratory mechanics and pattern of breathing in induced asthma. *Am Rev Respir Dis.* 1982;126:812.
84. Qvist J, Anderson JB, Pemberton M, et al. High level PEEP in severe asthma. *N Engl J Med.* 1982;307:1347.
85. Tyler DC. Positive end-expiratory pressure. A review. *Crit Care Med.* 1983;11:300.
86. Weisman IM, Rinaldo JE, Roger RM. Positive end-expiratory pressure in adult respiratory failure. *N Engl J Med.* 1982;307:1381.
88. Acute Respiratory Distress Syndrome Network. Ventilation with lower tidal volumes as compared to traditional tidal volumes for acute lung injury and the acute respiratory distress syndrome. *N Engl J Med.* 2000;342:1301-1308.
93. Slutsky AS. Lung injury caused by mechanical ventilation. *Chest.* 1999;116(suppl):9S-15S.
103. Foti G, Cereda M, Sparacino ME, et al. Effects of periodic lung recruitment maneuvers on gas exchange and respiratory mechanics in mechanically ventilated acute respiratory distress syndrome (ARDS) patients. *Intensive Care Med.* 2000;26:501-507.
104. Lamm WJ, Albert RK. Mechanism by which prone position improves oxygenation in acute lung injury. *Am J Respir Crit Care Med.* 1994;150:184-193.
108. Gattinoni L, Tognoni G, Pesenti A, et al. Effect of prone positioning on the survival of patients with acute respiratory failure. *N Engl J Med.* 2001;345:568-573.
119. Curley MAQ, Thompson JE, Arnold JH. The effects of early and repeated prone positioning in pediatric patients with acute lung injury. *Chest.* 2000;118:156-163.
120. Relvas MS, Silver PC, Sagy M. Prone positioning of pediatric patients with ARDS results in improvement in oxygenation if maintained 12 h daily. *Chest.* 2003;124:269-274.
121. Curley MAQ, Hibberd PL, Fineman LD, et al. Effect of prone positioning onclinical outcomes in children with acute lung injury. a randomized controlled trial. *JAMA.* 2005;294:229-237.
127. Marraro G. Simultaneous independent lung ventilation in pediatric patients. *Crit Care Clin.* 1992;8:131.
130. Buda AJ, Pinsky MR, Ingels NB Jr, et al. Effect of intrathoracic pressure on left ventricular performance. *N Engl J Med.* 1979;301:453.
133. Kallet RH. Patient-ventilator interaction during acute lung injury, and the role of spontaneous breathing. Part 1: respiratory muscle function during critical illness. *Respir Care.* 2011;56:181-189.
134. de Wit M. Monitoring of patient-ventilator interaction at the bedside. *Respir Care.* 2011;56:61-72.
138. Branson RD. Patient-ventilator interaction: the last 40 years. *Respir Care.* 2011;56:15-24.
140. Tobin MJ, Jubran A, Laghi F. Patient-ventilator interaction. *Am J Respir Crit Care Med.* 2001;163:1059-1063.
171. HiFi Study Group. High frequency oscillatory ventilation compared with conventional mechanical ventilation in the treatment of respiratory failure in preterm infants: assessment of pulmonary function at 9 months of corrected age. *J Pediatr.* 1990;116:933.
178. Arnold JH, Hanson JH, Toro-Figuero LO, et al. Prospective, randomized comparison of high-frequency oscillatory ventilation and conventional mechanical ventilation in pediatric respiratory failure. *Crit Care Med.* 1994;22:1530-1539.
182. Cortiella J, Mlcak R, Herndon D. High frequency percussive ventilation in pediatric patients with inhalation injury. *J Burn Care Rehabil.* 1999;20:232-235.
200. Cassidy SS, et al. Cardiovascular effects of positive-pressure ventilation in normal subjects. *J Appl Physiol.* 1979;47:453.
215. Myers TR. Therapeutic gases for neonatal and pediatric respiratory care. *Respir Care.* 2003;48:399-422.
240. Kim IK, Phrampus E, Venkataraman S, et al. Helium/oxygen-driven albuterol nebulization in the treatment of children with moderate to severe asthma exacerbations: a randomized, controlled trial. *Pediatrics.* 2005;116:1127e1133.
246. Hollman G, Shen G, Zeng L, et al. Helium-oxygen improves Clinical Asthma Scores in children with acute bronchiolitis. *Crit Care Med.* 1998;26:1731-1736.
256. Inhaled nitric oxide and hypoxic respiratory failure in infants with congenital diaphragmatic hernia. The Neonatal Inhaled Nitric Oxide Study Group (NINOS). *Pediatrics.* 1997;99:838-845.
262. Dobyns EL, Cornfield DN, Anas NG, et al. Multicenter randomized controlled trial of the effects of inhaled nitric oxide therapy on gas exchange in children with acute hypoxemic respiratory failure. *J Pediatr.* 1999;134:406-412.
263. Dellinger RP, Zimmerman JL, Taylor RW, et al. Effects of inhaled nitric oxide in patients with acute respiratory distress syndrome: results of a randomized phase II trial. Inhaled Nitric Oxide in ARDS Study Group. *Crit Care Med.* 1998;26:15-23.
268. Schechter MS. Airway clearance applications in infants and children. *Respir Care.* 2007;52:1382-1390.
284. Egan DF. *Aerosol and Humidity Therapy in Fundamentals of Respiratory Therapy*. 3rd ed. St. Louis: CV Mosby; 1977.

287. Esteban A, Frutos F, Tobin MJ, et al. A comparison of four methods of weaning patients from mechanical ventilation. *N Engl J Med*. 1995;332:345-350.

288. Brochard L, Rauss A, Benito S, et al. Comparison of three methods of gradual withdrawal from ventilatory support during weaning from mechanical ventilation. *Am J Respir Crit Care Med*. 1994;150:896-903.

293. Randolph AG, Wypij D, Venkataraman ST, et al., Pediatric Acute Lung Injury and Sepsis Investigators (PALISI) Network. Effect of mechanical ventilator weaning protocols on respiratory outcomes in infants and children: a randomized controlled trial. *JAMA*. 2002;288:2561-2568.

296. Farias JA, Alia I, Retta A, et al. An evaluation of extubation failure predictors in mechanically ventilated infants and children. *Intensive Care Med*. 2002;28:752-757.

300. Khan N, Brown A, Venkataraman ST. Predictors of extubation success and failure in mechanically ventilated infants and children. *Crit Care Med*. 1996;24:1568-1579.

309. Deleted in review.

310. Ad Hoc Task Force on Home Care of Chronically Ill Infants. Guidelines for home care of infants, children and adolescents with chronic disease. *Pediatrics*. 1984;74:434.

311. O'Donohue WJ Jr, Giovanni RM, Keens TG, Plummer AL. Long-term mechanical ventilation. Guidelines for management in the home and at alternate community sites. Report of the Ad Hoc Committee, Respiratory Care Section, American College of Chest Physicians. *Chest*. 1986;90:1S.

Noninvasive Ventilation: Concepts and Practice

Shekhar T. Venkataraman

PEARLS

- Not all patients are suitable for noninvasive ventilation. Careful selection is important for success.
- Noninvasive ventilation can be used for both short-term and long-term indications.
- Technologic advances in interfaces and equipment have allowed noninvasive ventilation to be used both at home and in the hospital.
- A team approach is crucial.
- Family involvement is essential for success.

Introduction

Conventional mechanical ventilation provided through endotracheal intubation or a tracheostomy is a lifesaving technique in the management of patients with respiratory failure. Endotracheal intubation and tracheostomy are associated with complications including injury to the airway and nosocomial infections. In addition, mechanical ventilation of children with endotracheal intubation often requires use of sedatives with its attendant side effects and complications. Positive pressure noninvasive ventilation (NIV) is provided by an interface that increases the proximal airway pressure, whereas negative pressure NIV is provided by creating a negative pressure around the chest wall. In both instances, the transpulmonary pressure is raised, causing airflow into the lungs. Continuous positive airway pressure (CPAP) refers to application of a constant pressure to the airway in which the patient's breathing efforts are unassisted. Continuous negative expiratory pressure (CNEP) refers to application of a constant negative pressure around the chest in which the patient's breathing efforts are unassisted. Spontaneous breaths may also be assisted using positive pressure delivered through the facial interface. Mechanical ventilation may be provided using negative pressure ventilation. Noninvasive ventilation can be provided using either positive or negative pressure ventilators. This review describes the various noninvasive ventilatory techniques available, published reports on their efficacy, their advantages and disadvantages, and future directions. Throughout this chapter, NIV refers to assisted positive pressure noninvasive ventilation, CPAP is referred to separately, and negative pressure ventilation is described at the end of the chapter.

Historical Perspective

The first tank respirator was described in 1832 by John Dalziel of Scotland.[1] He designed an airtight box in which the patient was placed in a sitting position with the head and neck outside. Negative pressure was created inside the box using a system of bellows, a piston rod, and a one-way valve.[1] Dalziel, in 1832, reported the use of a bellows-operated box with a seal around the neck or shoulders to provide artificial respiration to a drowned seaman.[1] The first workable, manually operated, noninvasive negative pressure ventilator was designed by Woillez in 1867.[2] Doe, in 1889, described a box used for resuscitating newborns.[3] Since then there have been many designs of tank respirators in the late 19th and early 20th century. A detailed description is beyond the scope of this chapter, and the reader is referred to excellent reviews on this topic by Woollam.[4,5]

Drinker developed the first tank ventilator in 1928, but the first demonstration of prolonged use of this tank respirator was published in 1929 by Drinker and McKhann.[6]

Artificial respiration was maintained almost continuously for 122 hours in a girl, aged 8 years, suffering from acute anterior poliomyelitis, without discomfort or apparent harm to the patient. Administration of artificial respiration did not prohibit sleeping or the taking of nourishment. Though the patient died of pneumonia and cardiac failure, this report showed the feasibility of prolonged mechanical ventilation with a tank respirator. The description of the apparatus for use in adults, children, and infants was subsequently published in 1929.[7,8] The Drinker tank ventilator was subsequently used with great clinical value in patients with poliomyelitis.[9-15]

Negative pressure ventilation was introduced for use with neonates in the 1960s.[16,17] In 1953, Lassen reported that positive pressure ventilation administered using an endotracheal tube or a tracheostomy was more successful that negative pressure ventilation in treating patients with poliomyelitis.[18] Major technologic advances in the design of positive pressure ventilators led to the marked decrease in negative pressure ventilation. Noninvasive positive pressure ventilation by face mask was first employed by Barach et al.[19] for the treatment of hypoxemic respiratory failure secondary to acute pulmonary edema. Gregory et al.,[20] in 1971, reported that CPAP through nasal prongs was effective in improving oxygenation in neonates with hyaline membrane disease. Vidyasagar and Chernick[21] showed that constant negative pressure applied about the chest and abdomen was as effective as CPAP in improving oxygenation in neonates with hyaline membrane disease. Despite these early reports, noninvasive ventilation did not become popular until more recently. Ellis et al.[22] were the first to report the successful use of NIV through a nasal mask on a 6-year-old with severe alveolar hypoventilation. There is currently a renewed interest in noninvasive ventilation coinciding with technologic advances in the manufacture and design of noninvasive ventilators. NIV through a mask for neuromuscular disorders was pioneered in the 1980s by Rideau et al.[23] and subsequently by Bach et al.[24]

Indications

The indications for the use of NIV can be categorized into short-term and long-term NIV. Short-term NIV is indicated where positive pressure support is needed acutely in a hospital setting in acute care or critical care areas for conditions that are reversible within a few days. Long-term NIV is indicated in conditions where respiratory failure is likely to be chronic or progressive.

Short-Term Noninvasive Ventilation

The indications for use of NIV in acute care and critical care situations are given in Table 58.1. The selection guidelines are given in Table 58.2. Four questions must be answered before attempting short-term NIV. They are as follows:
1. Does the patient have an irreversible cause of respiratory failure?
2. Can the patient's gas exchange be maintained without positive pressure?
3. Does the patient require immediate intubation and invasive mechanical ventilation?
4. Does the patient have any contraindications to the use of NIV (see Table 58.2)?

If the answer to any of these question is in the affirmative, then the patient may not be a suitable candidate for short-term NIV. If the answers to all these questions are in the negative, then the patient can be considered a candidate for NIV. Additional questions that the clinician needs to consider are the following:

1. Does the patient only need increased positive airway pressure to recruit the lung to improve oxygenation? If the patient needs only increased airway pressure to recruit atelectatic lung and to maintain lung volumes, then the patient can be placed on noninvasive CPAP through an appropriate interface.
2. Does the patient need additional ventilatory assistance on the basis of clinical signs and symptoms or gas exchange derangements? If the patient needs ventilatory assistance, the patient is a candidate for NIV.

Fig. 58.1 shows the algorithm to be followed for initiation and weaning of NIV in acute respiratory failure. If NIV is used in acute situations, there should be a determination every hour for up to 2 to 3 hours whether the patient has improved (see Fig. 58.1). Signs of success and failure are given in Table 58.3. A good response to NIV is indicated by (1) decreased respiratory rate, (2) reduced work of breathing, (3) improvement of dyspnea, (4) an increase in pH, (5) better oxygenation, and (6) decreased arterial carbon dioxide ($PaCO_2$) levels. Additionally, there may be hemodynamic effects such as a reduction in heart rate, improved blood pressures, and perfusion. Generally, for short-term use, NIV is used continuously until the patient improves or fails NIV. The goals of short-term NIV are given in Table 58.4.

Adult Studies on the Short-Term Use of Noninvasive Ventilation

Acute Cardiogenic Pulmonary Edema

CPAP was described by Barach et al.[19] for the treatment of acute cardiogenic pulmonary edema. Several studies, including multiple randomized trials, have shown that the use of CPAP or NIV improves outcomes in cardiogenic pulmonary edema.[25-34] These studies show that the use of CPAP/NIV has the following favorable effects: (1) a rapid reduction in respiratory rate, dyspnea, and work of breathing; (2) a reduced rate of endotracheal intubation; and (3) a trend toward

TABLE 58.1	Indications for Short-Term Noninvasive Ventilation
Acute Hypoxemic Respiratory Failure	
Acute lung injury	
Acute cardiogenic pulmonary edema	
Pneumonia	
Acute Lower Airway Disease	
Acute asthma	
Avoiding Intubation	
Immunocompromised patients	
Restrictive chest diseases	
Neuromuscular disorders	
Postoperative respiratory failure	
Do not intubate patients	
Postextubation respiratory failure	
Facilitate Weaning and Extubation	

TABLE 58.2	Selection Guidelines for Short-Term Noninvasive Ventilation

A. Potentially reversible condition
B. Need for ventilatory assistance
  Moderate to severe increase in work of breathing
    Tachypnea
    Retractions
    Paradoxical breathing
    Accessory muscle use
  Gas exchange criteria
    Ventilatory failure ($PaCO_2$ >45 mm Hg with a pH <7.35)
    Oxygenation failure (PaO_2/FiO_2 ratio <200)
C. Contraindications to noninvasive ventilation
  Respiratory or cardiac arrest
  Unstable (hypotension, shock)
  Poor airway protective reflexes
  Recent upper airway and esophageal surgery
  Excessive secretions
  Uncooperative
  Agitation
  Untreated pneumothorax
  Inability for a good mask fit
  Rapidly progressive neuromuscular weakness (eg, Guillain-Barré syndrome)

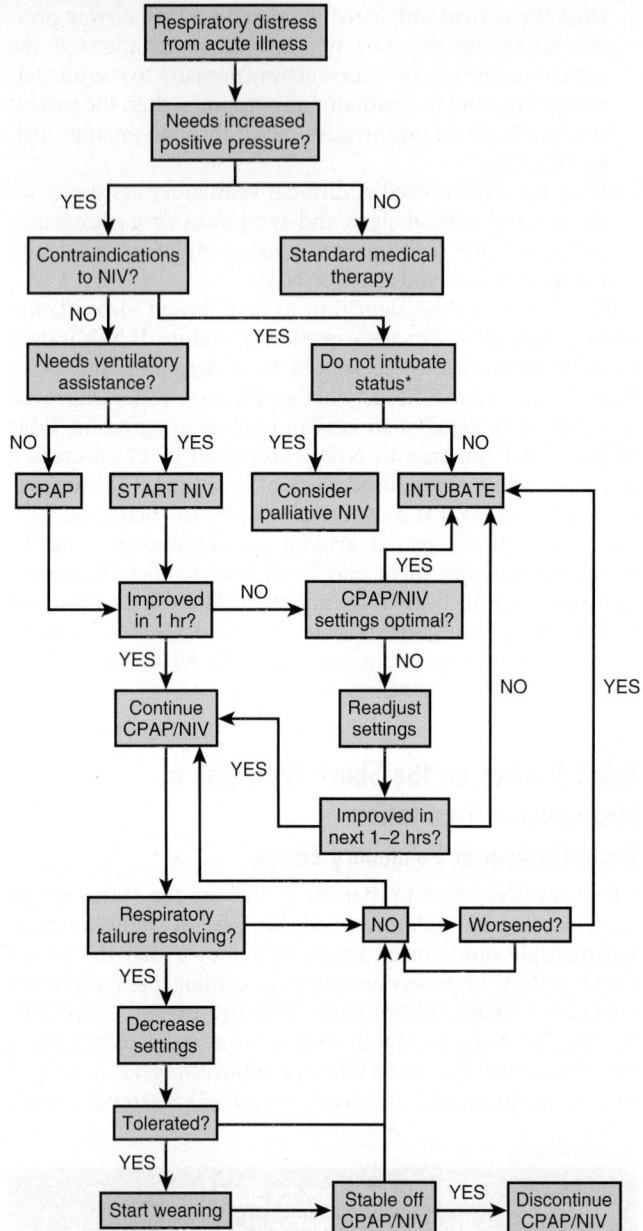

Fig. 58.1. Algorithm for initiation and weaning of short-term continuous positive airway pressure and noninvasive ventilation.

TABLE 58.3	Signs of Success and Failure Within 1 to 2 Hours of Application of Noninvasive Ventilation (NIV) for Short-Term NIV

Signs of success
  Reduction in respiratory rate to a range that is normal for age
  Absence of retractions
  Absence of paradoxical breathing
  Improvement in gas exchange
    Improved pH
    Improved PaO_2/FiO_2
    Reduction in $PaCO_2$
Signs of failure
  No change in signs of work of breathing
  No change in gas exchange
  Hemodynamic instability
  Signs of respiratory fatigue
  Change in mental status
  Increased agitation

TABLE 58.4	Goals of Noninvasive Ventilation (NIV)

Short-Term NIV
Relieve respiratory distress
Decrease work of breathing
Improve gas exchange
Avoid intubation
Long-Term NIV
Ameliorate symptoms
Improve gas exchange
Improve quality of life
Improve sleep duration and quality
Improve survival

reduced mortality.[25-34] Physiologic mechanisms underlying the improvement are likely due to an increase in functional residual capacity, increased lung compliance, reduced work of breathing, and an improved cardiac performance due to reduced preload and afterload.

Acute Respiratory Failure/Acute Respiratory Distress Syndrome/Pneumonia

Adult studies have shown that NIV can be used in hypoxemic respiratory failure with an arterial oxygen tension to fraction of inspired oxygen (PaO_2/FiO_2 ratio) of less than 300, with bilateral parenchymal disease to prevent endotracheal intubation. Ferrer et al.[35] showed that NIV reduced the intubation rate from 52% to 25% with a reduction in ICU mortality from 39% to 18%. But this finding must be tempered with studies

that show that NIV may not reduce the need for endotracheal intubation.[36,37] A recent systematic review showed that NIV for acute hypoxemic respiratory failure was associated with a significantly lower rate of endotracheal intubation than standard management with a risk reduction of about 25%.[37] Overall, there was a reduction in hospital mortality of about 10% to 17%.[38]

Chronic Obstructive Pulmonary Disease

In adults with acute exacerbations of chronic obstructive pulmonary disease (COPD), NIV has improved both short-term and long-term outcomes.[39-45] Compared with standard therapy, NIV decreased the need for endotracheal intubation, reduced hospital mortality, and reduced the length of stay in the hospital, especially for those who had hypercapnia with respiratory acidosis.[46-51] A recent review strongly recommended the use of NIV for an acute exacerbation of COPD.[46] It is reasonable to expect a similar response to acute asthma since many of the pathophysiologic features are similar. Uncontrolled studies showed improvement in patients with an acute asthmatic attack.[47,48] Three small RCTs have been published on using NIV with acute exacerbation of asthma.[49-51] Holley et al.[49] did not find any difference in outcomes with the use of NIV. Sorosky et al.[50] showed that there was a rapid improvement measure of lower airway obstruction and fewer patients were admitted to the hospital.[50] In a recent three-arm trial, there was a greater reduction in dyspnea and a greater increase in the forced expiratory volume in the first second with NIV.[51]

Immunocompromised and Oncology Patients

It is desirable to reduce the probability of nosocomial infections in immunocompromised patients. Therefore it is appealing to apply NIV to avoid endotracheal intubation in these patients. Adult studies have shown that NIV can reduce the rate of endotracheal intubation, make possible earlier hospital discharge, and reduce the incidence of serious complications.[52-55] Despite aggressive management, some end-stage oncology patients experience breathlessness and dyspnea due to respiratory failure. NIV may alleviate the symptoms and provide comfort.[56-58] Nava et al. showed that application of NIV to these patients reduced their breathlessness and reduced the total dose of morphine administration to suppress dyspnea.[59]

Perioperative Respiratory Failure

Adult studies have shown that respiratory insufficiency that develops postoperatively in patients can be successfully treated with NIV. NIV reduces the rate of intubation and is more effective than CPAP or chest physiotherapy.[60,61] In patients after lung resection surgery, NIV reduced the rate of intubation and mortality compared with conventional therapy.[62] Adults with restrictive chest diseases who develop respiratory failure after surgery such as spinal fusion are also good candidates for NIV if they develop postoperative respiratory failure provided they do not have any other contraindications.

Facilitation of Weaning and Extubation

Endotracheal intubation and invasive mechanical ventilation are associated with complications including ventilator-associated pneumonia, ventilator-induced lung injury, and airway trauma. To minimize these complications, it is desirable to extubate the patient as quickly as possible. Generally, extubation coincides with the end of weaning (ie, the patient is not placed on any form of positive pressure support post extubation). In patients who take a long time to wean but require fairly low ventilatory assistance, it is possible to extubate them to NIV. Theoretically, it would reduce the incidence of complications associated with endotracheal intubation and invasive mechanical ventilation. Udwadia et al.[63] were one of the first to test this paradigm in 22 adult patients who were successfully stabilized on NIV following extubation. Recent adult studies have demonstrated that the use of NIV resulted in a reduction in the duration of mechanical ventilation, a reduction in the incidence of nosocomial pneumonia, and a reduction in the duration of hospital stay.[64-67]

Weaning and Postextubation Failure

NIV has been successfully used in weaning patients who had acute-on-chronic respiratory failure.[68] Recently, some adult studies have examined the use of NIV for postextubation respiratory failure (ie, respiratory failure that develops after extubation on complete spontaneous breathing).[69,70] The rationale for the use of NIV in this circumstance is the avoidance of endotracheal intubation. In at least one study in the adults, this approach was shown to increase the time from respiratory failure to intubation with an increase in mortality rate.[69,70]

Pediatric and Neonatal Studies

In 1993, Akingbola et al.[71] published a case report describing effective NPPV therapy in two pediatric-age patients with acute respiratory distress. Padman et al.[72] published a preliminary report on 15 patients aged 4 to 21 years who had respiratory failure due to cystic fibrosis (4 patients) and neuromuscular disease (11 patients). In 14 patients, the placement of an artificial airway was avoided. They observed significant improvement in hospital days, respiratory rate, heart rate, serum bicarbonate, arterial carbon dioxide, dyspnea, activity tolerance, and quality of sleep. Since that time, NIV has been applied to pediatric patients with a variety of respiratory disorders. There has been a significant increase in the number of articles since 2004 showing the growing interest and expertise in the use of NIV in children.[73] The following is a summary of the studies of acute short-term NIV in infants and children.

Acute Short-Term Indications
Acute Respiratory Failure

Just as in adults, NIV has been used successfully in infants and children with acute respiratory failure due to parenchymal lung disease, acute respiratory distress syndrome (ARDS), bronchiolitis, pneumonia, and other lung infections.[74-76] In 1995, Fortenberry et al. reported a retrospective study on the efficacy and complications of NIV in 28 children with acute hypoxemic respiratory insufficiency.[76] NIV significantly decreased respiratory rate and improved both oxygenation and ventilation. The use of NIV decreased hospitalization rate and increased patient comfort. Only 3 of 28 patients required intubation or reintubation.[76] Padman et al.[77] conducted a prospective study in 34 patients with impending failure, all of whom required airway or oxygenation/ventilation support and required admission to the pediatric ICU. A decrease in respiratory rate, heart rate, and dyspnea score, as well as an improvement in oxygenation, was noted in more than 90% of patients studied. The frequency of intubation in these patients was only 8%.[77] In a study by Essouri et al.,[78] a total of 114 patients were treated with NIV, among whom 83 (77%) were successfully treated without intubation. NIV failure was associated with more severe illness and a diagnosis of ARDS.[78] Joshi and Tobias[79] reported on a 5-year experience with primary respiratory failure and postoperative respiratory failure. Application of NIV improved gas exchange, decreased inspired oxygen requirement, and decreased respiratory rate in 29 patients with primary respiratory failure.[79] Munoz-Benet et al.[80] reported on a 3-year prospective noncontrolled study in 26 children with acute respiratory failure (ARF). Pneumonia was observed in most of the children (46.8%). There was a significant improvement in the respiratory rate, heart rate, pH, carbon dioxide levels, and oxygen saturation at 2 to 4 hours, which was sustained for 24 hours. Only four patients required intubation. All patients survived.[80]

Cambonie et al.[81] were the first to demonstrate the efficacy of nasal CPAP in young infants with respiratory failure secondary to acute respiratory syncytial virus bronchiolitis. Nasal CPAP improved respiratory symptoms and signs as measured by a clinical score.[81] Inspiratory time to total time ratio decreased, and work of breathing assessed by esophageal manometry also decreased significantly.[81] The mechanism of improvement with CPAP is unloading of respiratory muscles.[81] Javouhey et al.[82] reported their experience using NIV as a primary means of support in infants with respiratory failure secondary to acute bronchiolitis. In the year before using NIV, there were 53 patients and 27 patients in the year when NIV was used as a primary mode of respiratory support.[82] Eighty-nine patients were intubated in the year before NIV was applied, but only 52% were intubated during the NIV period. Fewer patients required supplemental oxygen (10/27) for more than 8 days compared with 33/53 patients in the previous year.[82] NIV also reduced the incidence of ventilator-associated pneumonia.[82] Several moderately large retrospective studies have shown that CPAP or NIV decreased work of breathing, respiratory symptoms, and signs; improved gas exchange; and reduced the need for intubation.[83-86]

In 2008, Yanez et al.[87] reported on a prospective, randomized, controlled trial of NIV in children with acute respiratory failure. Compared with control patients, children treated with NIV had improvement in heart rate, respiratory rate, and gas exchange.[87] The NIV group had a significantly lower rate of endotracheal intubation than control patients (28% vs. 60%, respectively).[87] There have been two RCTs using CPAP with bronchiolitis.[88,89] Thia et al.,[88] in 2008, showed that infants with bronchiolitis randomized to receive CPAP for hypercarbia had improvement in capillary PCO_2 while the control infants had a slight increase in capillary PCO_2.[88] Chidini et al.[89] compared CPAP delivered by helmet or facial mask in infants with acute respiratory failure secondary to bronchiolitis due to respiratory syncytial virus.[89] CPAP by helmet had a lower rate of intolerance (17% vs. 54%) while the intubation rates were similar. In patients who tolerated CPAP, gas exchange and breathing pattern improved with both interfaces.[89] CPAP by mask had a greater incidence of cutaneous sores and leaks.[89]

Status Asthmaticus

Initial reports of the use of NIV with status asthmaticus were mainly case reports.[72,76,77] In one of the first reports of the use of NIV in children by Fortenberry et al.,[76] there were two patients with status asthmaticus. In the case series reported by Padman et al.,[77] there were two patients with reactive airway disease. Teague et al.[90] reported that NIV treatment acutely improved oxygenation and reduced cardiorespiratory distress in 19 out of 26 patients with status asthmaticus. This group of "NIV responders" had significantly shorter lengths of stay in both the ICU and hospital. However, the seven nonresponders required endotracheal intubation as respiratory distress progressed despite sedation. Akinbola et al.[91] reported the use of NIV in three children with status asthmaticus and showed an improvement in ventilatory parameters. Thill et al.,[92] in a randomized, crossover study in children with lower airway obstruction, showed that NIV decreased signs of work of breathing such as respiratory rate, accessory muscle use, and dyspnea as compared with standard therapy with no serious associated morbidity. Carroll et al.[93] reported the use of NIV in five children, four of whom were obese. Needleman et al.[94] was the first to demonstrate that application of NIV improved work of breathing, phase angles, and other respiratory parameters, and discontinuation of NIV was associated with worsening of the respiratory signs. Since then, there have been several large series on the use of NIV in status asthmatics.[95,96] In 2007, Beers et al.[95] reported a

retrospective study on the application of NIV in 83 children with status asthmaticus. There was an immediate improvement in symptoms in almost 80% of the patients.[95] Almost 90% of the patients tolerated NIV, and of those 22% did not require admission to the PICU.[95] In 2011, Mayordomo-Colunga et al.[96] prospectively enrolled 72 patients with status asthmaticus. Sixty-seven responded to NIV with improvement in clinical scores, respiratory rate, heart rate, and blood gas parameters.[96] Response was seen within an hour of placement of NIV and was sustained.[96] Only five patients failed and required intubation.[96]

Cardiac Patients

Chin et al.[97] reported on the successful use of NIV after congenital cardiac surgery in two infants younger than 1 year of age. Gupta et al.[98] reported a large, retrospective study on the use of NIV after cardiac surgery. NIV was used as either a "prophylactic" approach (58 events), where NIV was applied on extubation from invasive mechanical ventilation, or a "nonprophylactic" approach (163 events), where NIV was applied after extubation only when there were signs and symptoms of respiratory failure.[98] CPAP was used in 201 events with a success rate of 78%, and NIV was used in 20 events with 80% success rate.[98] Factors associated with response to NIV were a lower risk-adjusted classification for congenital heart surgery, presence of atelectasis, steroid therapy received within 24 hours after NIV, and normal heart rate and oxygen saturations demonstrated within 24 hours after initiation of NIV.[98] A similar but prospective study was reported by Kovacikova et al.[99] over a 3-year period. There were 107 episodes of NIV use in 82 patients. In almost 60% of the patients, NIV was used successfully without the need for tracheal intubation.[99]

Immunocompromised and Oncology Patients

Although oncology patients have been included in previous reports on the use of NIV in acute respiratory failure, Otonello et al.[100] were the first to report on the use of NIV of only oncology patients. Twenty patients with either hypoxemic or hypercapnic respiratory failure were treated with NIV. Fifteen out of 20 patients showed marked improvement in oxygenation and ventilation.[100] Pancera et al.[101] reported an 8-year experience of using NIV in children with oncologic disorders. NIV as the first-line therapy was compared with invasive mechanical ventilation.[101] This study included 120 patients who were treated with NIV and 119 who were intubated and mechanically ventilated as the first-line therapy.[101] The overall success rate of NIV was 74.2%. Seventy-five percent of the patients treated with NIV did not require endotracheal intubation, showing that NIV is a viable first-line therapy for respiratory failure in immunocompromised patients for preventing endotracheal intubation.[101] Cardiovascular dysfunction, severe illness score, and solid tumors were predictive of NIV failure in these patients. Piastra et al.[102] enrolled 23 consecutive immunocompromised children with ARDS who were treated with NIV using a helmet or face mask. For all the patients, NIV response rates were 82% and 74%, for early and sustained improvement, respectively.[102] NIV was successful in improving gas exchange and respiratory distress when there were both early and sustained responses.[102] Severe sepsis and septic shock were associated with NIV failure. All patients who were successfully managed by NIV survived.[102]

Other Indications

There are several small reports of the use of NIV for postextubation respiratory failure.[77,79,103-105] More recently, NIV has been suggested as an alternative to endotracheal intubation for the perioperative management of scoliosis correction in patients with muscular dystrophy.[106] NIV has also been used in children after liver transplantation to facilitate extubation and prevent reintubation.[107,108]

NIV has been used successfully to improve symptoms of obstructive sleep apnea.[109-112] Teague et al.[109] showed that NIV improves gas exchange in children with upper airway obstruction. Rosen et al.[110] also showed that CPAP and NIV were used successfully to manage the preoperative and/or postoperative upper airway obstruction in children with obstructive sleep apnea. Friedman et al.[111] reported using NIV on nine patients after adenotonsillectomy to treat postoperative obstructive symptoms. They showed that NIV is effective after adenotonsillectomy to avoid the risks of intubation and ventilator dependence.[111] Essouri et al.[112] published a prospective, randomized, controlled study comparing standard therapy with CPAP and NIV in upper airway obstruction in the postoperative period. During spontaneous breathing, patients were tachypneic with a high inspiratory time (Ti) to total respiratory time (Ttot) (Ti/Ttot). Esophageal pressure measurements and swings were elevated, reflecting an increased work of breathing, but could not maintain normal gas exchange.[112] Both CPAP and NIV resulted in a significant decrease in all indices of respiratory effort.[112] During NIV, there were significantly high ineffective inspiratory efforts due to ineffective or delayed triggering.[112]

Long-Term Noninvasive Ventilation

Long-term NIV is indicated in conditions that result in chronic respiratory failure. This can be either progressive or nonprogressive. Generally, long-term NIV is intermittent with periods of time off NIV. The most common form of long-term NIV is nocturnal NIV with off-periods during the daytime. The goals of long-term NIV are given in Table 58.4. The indications for long-term NIV are given in Table 58.5.

Physiologic Effects and Outcomes of Long-Term Noninvasive Ventilation
Neuromuscular Disorders

Patients with neuromuscular and chest wall disorders often have sleep-related disturbances.[113] In adults, intermittent

TABLE 58.5   Indications for Long-Term Noninvasive Ventilation

Restrictive thoracic diseases
    Chest wall deformity—kyphoscoliosis
Slowly progressive neurologic disorders
    Postpolio syndrome
    Muscular dystrophies
    Spinal muscular atrophy
Nonprogressive chronic respiratory failure
    High spinal cord injury
Chronic lung disease
    Cystic fibrosis

NIV consistently improves daytime gas exchange.[114,115] NIV ameliorates hypoventilation, intermittent sleep apneas, and other sleep-disordered breathing.[116] NIV, applied appropriately, improves the quality of life with restrictive thoracic disorders.[117]

In the 1970s and 1980s, intermittent positive pressure ventilation through a mouthpiece was used to treat respiratory failure late after poliomyelitis or Duchenne muscular dystrophy.[118-120] In 1993, Bach et al.[121] published the results of application of a clinical protocol to manage patients with Duchenne muscular dystrophy. The protocol consisted of using NIV and assisted coughing (both manually and mechanically operated) to maintain normal oxygen saturation monitored by a pulse oximeter, particularly during intercurrent upper respiratory tract infections.[121] They showed that strict adherence to the protocol was associated with decreased hospitalization and increased survival.[121,122] These studies show that noninvasive respiratory aids can prolong survival and permit extubation or decannulation of patients with Duchenne muscular dystrophy with no breathing tolerance.[121,122] Mellies et al.[123] showed that long-term noninvasive ventilation in children and adolescents with neuromuscular disorders (non-Duchenne muscular dystrophy) improved both nocturnal and diurnal gas exchange and sleep.

Initial reports on the use of NIV in children with infantile SMA showed that it was feasible, but survival was not prolonged.[124] In 2002, Bach et al.[125] reported comparing the outcomes of patients with SMA type 1 who developed respiratory failure before age 2 years and either had tracheostomy tubes or used NIV-assisted coughing. Tracheotomized patients were hospitalized less frequently until they were 3 years of age but had more after 5 years of age when compared with the patients who were treated with NIV and assisted coughing.[125] With respiratory support as outlined earlier, both groups survived between 8 and 12 years on average.[125] The use of NIV along with assisted coughing has increased survival in children with SMA type 1.[126-130] In children with neuromuscular disorder, symptoms of daytime sleepiness, headache, and sleep quality improve after initiation of NIV.[129] Hospitalization rates and health care costs decreased. Quality of life remained stable after NIV, despite disease progression.[129] Children with spinal muscular atrophy (types 1 and 2) often develop thoracoabdominal asynchrony, especially during sleep. NIV improved sleep breathing parameters and thoracoabdominal coordination during sleep in SMA types 1 and 2.[130]

Cystic Fibrosis

The role of NIV in patients with cystic fibrosis is emerging. Initially, NIV was used in end-stage lung disease as a bridge to transplantation.[72,131-133] These studies suggest that the waiting time can be extended while keeping the patient comfortable.[72,131-133] It is also being used to treat acute or chronic respiratory failure and sleep disturbance.[134-139]

In 1981, Sullivan et al.[140] first demonstrated that nasal CPAP was effective in reversing obstructive sleep apnea in four adults and one teenager. Guilleminault et al.,[141] in 1986, reported that nasal CPAP reversed or reduced obstructive sleep apnea in some children while there were problems related to poor cooperation from parents and difficulty in preventing leaks around the nasal mask. Since the first report, several studies have shown that nasal CPAP was effective in obstructive sleep apnea in infants and children.[142-146] In 1995, Guilleminault et al.[147] reported that nasal CPAP was successful in 70 out of 72 infants with sleep-disordered breathing. In many instances, it provided an interim solution while allowing the patient to grow and postponing surgery.

Interfaces

A properly fitting facial appliance is essential for the optimal application of NIV. There are currently several devices in use: (1) Adam's Circuit and nasal pillows, (2) nasal masks, (3) oral-nasal masks, (4) total face masks, and (5) helmet or head hood and six mouthpieces. A correctly sized interface minimizes leaks, improves effectiveness of positive pressure support, and improves comfort.

Adam's Circuit: This device uses a "nasal pillow," which attaches to a manifold that is placed over the top of the head (Fig. 58.2). Some patients prefer this to the nasal mask. "Nasal pillows" are available in various sizes (see Fig. 58.2).

Nasal masks: A nasal mask rests between the bridge of the nose and above the upper lip (Fig. 58.3). As a rule, the smaller the mask, the better the fit. In patients who are unable to keep their mouth closed, chin straps may be used to close the mouth.

Oral-nasal masks: This is the most common interface used to provide NIV (Fig. 58.4). The ideal face mask should (1) be made of a clear material to allow visual inspection, (2) conform to the contours of the patient's face, (3) be easily moldable from its factory shape, (4) be soft and not apply excess pressure on the skin of the face, and (5) maintain its deformed shape (has "memory") when it is removed. The mask should extend from the bridge of the nose to just below the lower lip. The mask is secured using an anchoring system that goes around the head.

Total face mask: This mask covers the whole face including the eyes (Fig. 58.5). The advantage of a total face mask is that it does not have to conform to the shape of the face and therefore does not have to be molded to fit every patient. The disadvantage is that it has an increased dead-space, and therefore there may be difficulty in eliminating CO_2.

Head hood: Also called a "helmet," it has been used successfully in a number of European ICUs (Fig. 58.6). It appears best suited for application of CPAP. Dead space is a major concern and therefore should be reserved for patients in the ICU.

Mouthpieces: These are simple devices to be pursed between the lips for domiciliary mechanical ventilation (Fig. 58.7).

Equipment

A detailed description of the devices available for NIV at home is beyond the scope of this chapter, and the reader is referred to several excellent reviews.[148,149] This discussion focuses on the characteristics of positive pressure ventilators that can be used for providing NIV. Negative pressure ventilators are discussed elsewhere in the chapter. The ventilators that are used for NIV can be classified into three categories: (1) conventional ICU ventilators with a double-limb circuit without leak compensation, (2) devices with a single-limb circuit with leak compensation, and (3) devices that combine the previous two

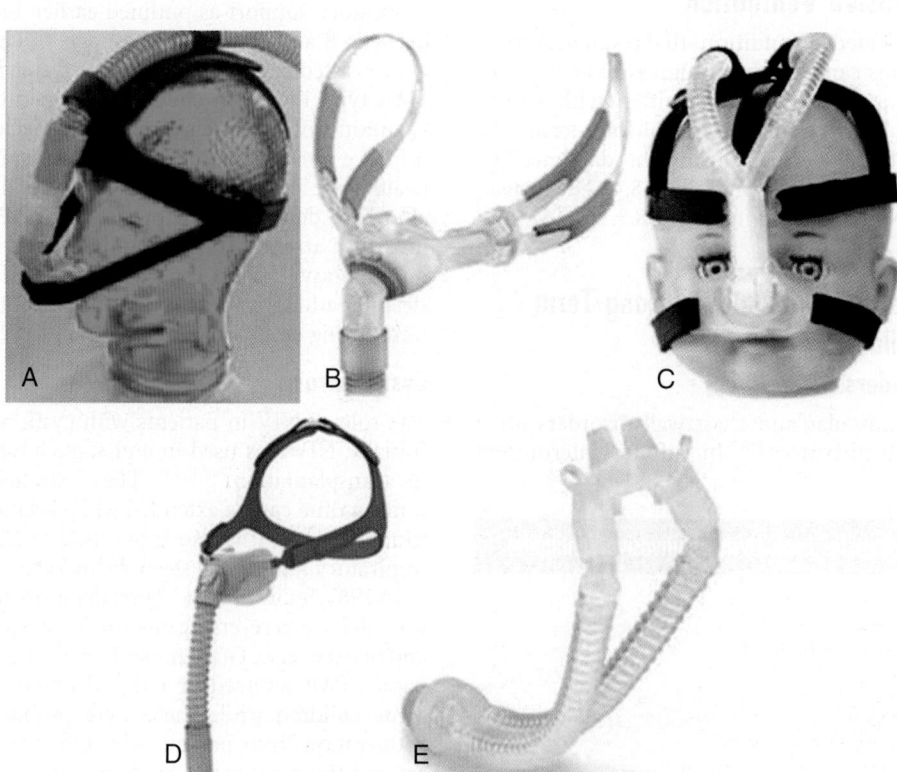

Fig. 58.2. Adam's Circuit and nasal pillows. Adam's Circuit (A), ResMed SwiftTM FX Bella (B), Medical Innovations PediFlow (C), Fisher and Paykal Pilairo Q (D), and Innomed Technologies Nasalaire II Petite (E). (Courtesy manufacturers.)

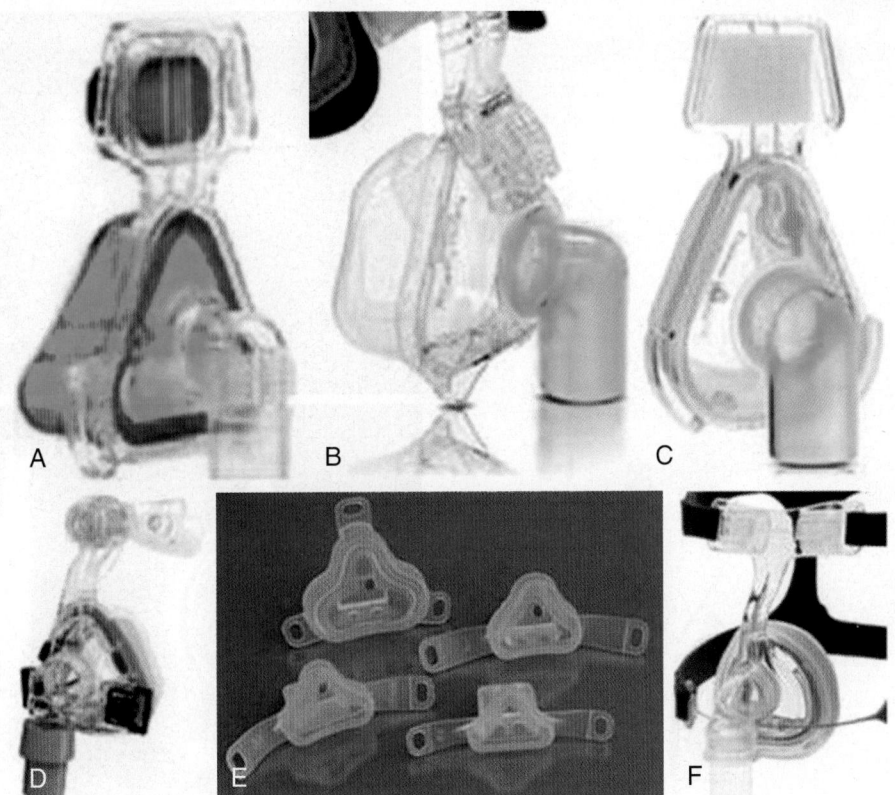

Fig. 58.3. Nasal masks. Respironics PN831 (A), Respironics PerformaTrak (B), Respironics Contour Deluxe (C), ResMed Mirage (D), Airon Nasal Masks (E), and Fisher and Paykal HC407 (F). (Courtesy manufacturers.)

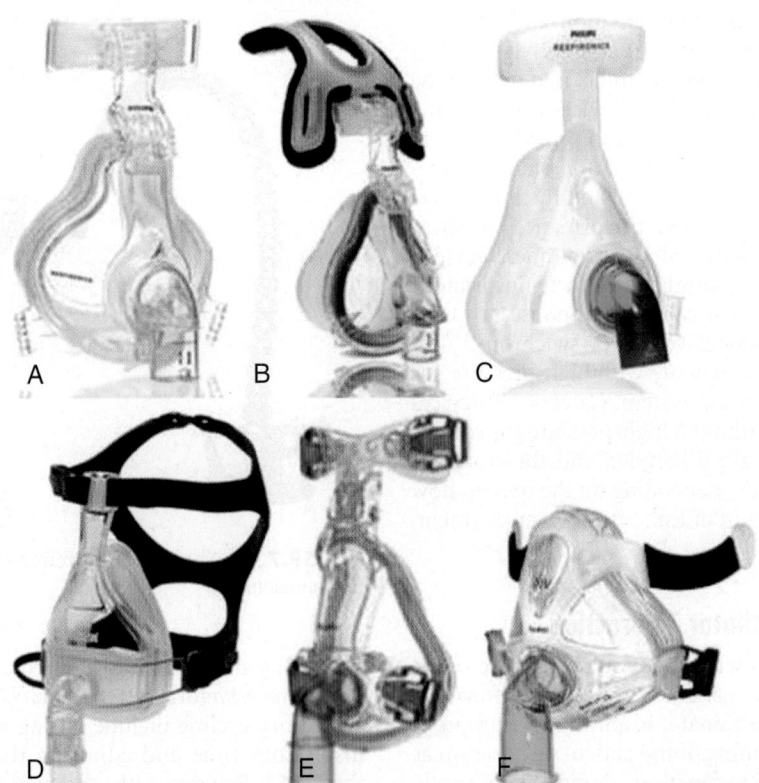

Fig. 58.4. Oronasal masks. Respironics AF531 (A), Respironics AF811 (B), Respironics AF421 (C), Fisher and Paykal HC431 (D), ResMed Ultra Mirage (E), and ResMed Quattro FX (F). (Courtesy manufacturers.)

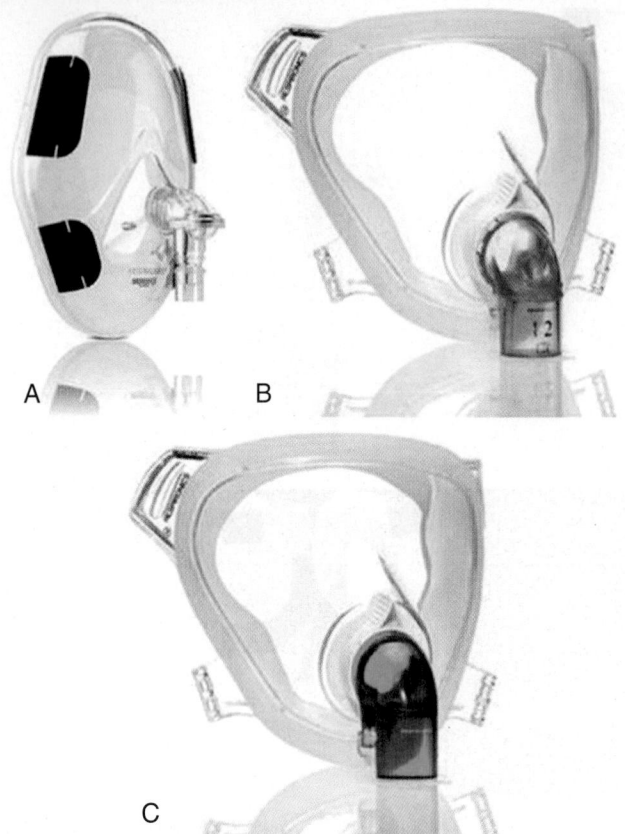

Fig. 58.5. Full-face masks. Respironics Total (A), Respironics Perfor-Max Single Use (B), Respironics PerforMax Multi-Use (C).

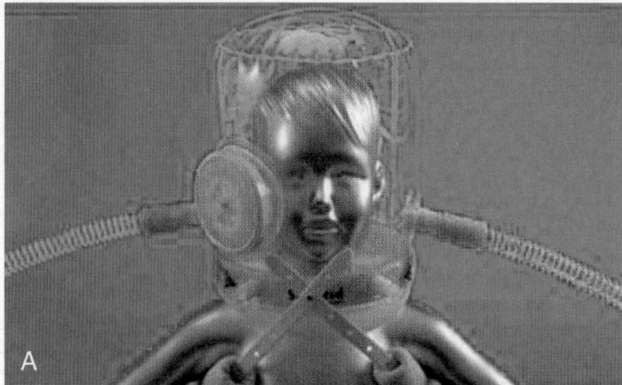

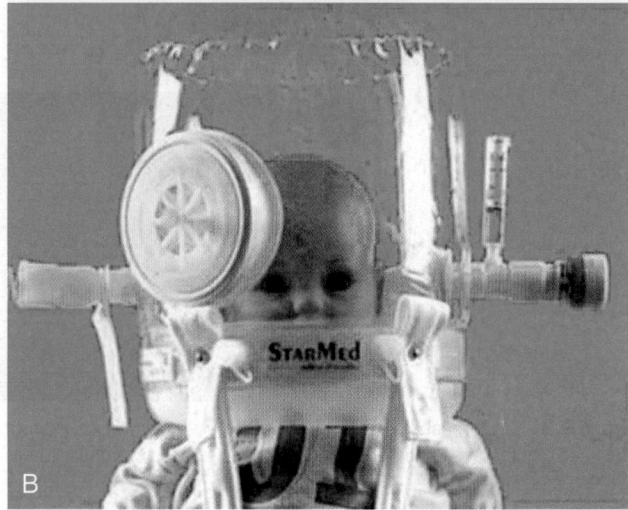

Fig. 58.6. Helmet or head hood. StarMed CaStar Ped (A) and StarMed CaStar Infant (B).

categories to include both leak compensation and having a double-limb circuit. Category 1 devices can only be used in the hospital. Category 2 and 3 devices can be used in both the hospital and at home. Examples of these devices would be any of the conventional ICU ventilators that can provide pressure support with positive end-expiratory pressure (PEEP) (Category 1), Respironics Bi-PAP (Category 2), and the Pulmonetics LTV ventilator (Category 3). The performances of these ventilators vary widely in delivered tidal volumes, air-leak compensation, response to simulated effort, inspiratory trigger, expiratory cycling, rebreathing, response to high ventilatory demands, and patient-ventilator synchrony.[150-150b] Category 1 or ICU ventilators operate with high-pressure gas sources with an oxygen blending system. Category 2 devices and 3 devices can operate without a high-pressure gas source. Bilevel ventilators do not have a blender, and therefore the delivered FiO_2 is unpredictable depending on the oxygen flow rate, ventilator settings, amount of leak, site of O_2 enrichment, and type of exhalation port.[151]

Optimizing Patient-Ventilator Interaction

Optimal patient-ventilator interaction requires that the ventilator be able to detect the patient's inspiratory efforts as quickly as possible and terminate inspiration (expiratory cycling) as close to the beginning of the patient's expiration as possible. Inspiratory trigger function differs significantly among the ventilators.[152-154] Factors affecting the inspiratory trigger function include trigger response to the inspiratory

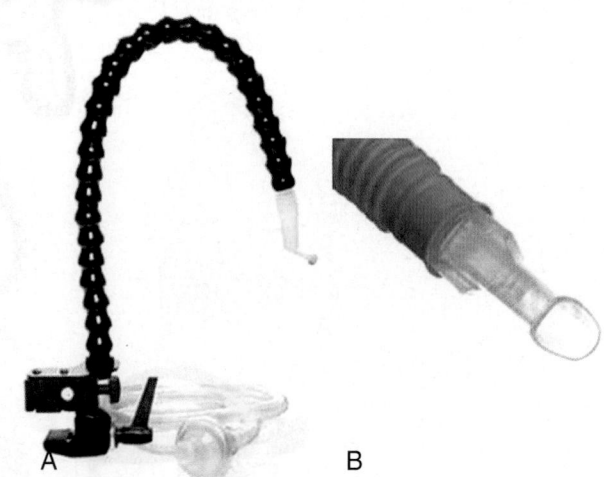

Fig. 58.7. Mouthpieces. Respironics (A) and Colorbox (B). (Courtesy of manufacturers).

flow, leak-induced autotriggering, and pressure-time and flow-time waveform heterogeneity.[152-154] Strategies to optimize expiratory cycling include setting a suitable threshold for the inspiratory time and adjusting the expiratory cycling flow-threshold. Patients with obstructive lung disease tend to do better with high inspiratory flow, whereas patients with neuromuscular disease seem to do better with low inspiratory flows.[155] An adjustable backup rate is available in most modern ventilators used for NIV. It is particularly useful when sedation is used to improve patient compliance with NIV. Leaks around the interface reduce its effectiveness. Some amount of leak around the interface is expected with NIV. Complete elimination of air leak is not desirable as it comes at the expense of a very tight-fitting mask, which may lead to patient discomfort and skin breakdown. Ventilators differ in their capacity to compensate for leaks. One of the drawbacks of a large air leak is autotriggering. Humidification is important to prevent mucosal drying. Humidification can be provided using a heated humidifier, heat and moisture exchanger, or a pass-over humidifier.

Ventilator Settings

With CPAP, the level of CPAP is selected on the basis of the clinical needs. There should be relief of symptoms within 1 to 2 hours of application of CPAP. With short-term NIV, two strategies have been employed. One approach is to start with a high inspiratory pressure (about 20–25 cms H_2O). The goal of such an approach is for rapid relief of symptoms. If intolerant, a lower level that is tolerated is then selected. This approach is called the *high-low approach*. The other approach starts with a lower inspiratory pressure (about 8–10 cms H_2O) and gradually increases to produce relief of symptoms. The aim of this approach is to maximize patient comfort and tolerance. This is called the *low-high approach*. Within the first 1 to 3 hours, subsequent adjustments may be necessary depending on the patient response. Expiratory pressure is used routinely during short-term NIV. Maximal fraction of inspired oxygen (FiO_2) with bilevel ventilators is usually about 45% to 50%. If a higher FiO_2 is required, and endotracheal intubation is not indicated, then an ICU-type ventilator may be used.

Complications and Concerns During Short-Term Noninvasive Ventilation

Aerophagia and gastric distention can occur with NIV. The higher the pressures used, the greater the chance of gastric distention. Regurgitation of gastric contents and aspiration into the lungs are major concerns with the use of an oronasal, total face masks, and a helmet. Close monitoring is necessary to prevent aspiration. A nasogastric tube to keep the stomach decompressed is necessary in these acutely ill patients. Pressure sores related to the masks are the other major concern. It should be possible to pass one or two fingers between the headgear and the face. Care should be taken to avoid fitting the interface too tightly. A spacer with soft padding can reduce the incidence of pressure sores on the face.

Circuit and CO_2 Rebreathing

Single-limb circuits that are employed with bilevel ventilators can result in significant CO_2 rebreathing. All single-limb circuits have an exhalation port that is placed close to the patient interface through which exhaled gas will escape. If the exhaled gas flow exceeds the rate of escape through the exhalation port, exhaled air is rebreathed with the next inspiration. This results in significant CO_2 rebreathing and can cause hypercarbia. Rebreathing also depends on the level of EPAP, location of the exhalation port, and design of the exhalation port.

Earlier devices had significant CO_2 rebreathing of the exhaled air, especially if the EPAP levels were set too low. In the newer designs, this problem has been largely minimized. The closer the exhalation port to the patient interface, the lower the rebreathing of CO_2. In fact, if the exhalation port is located in the mask itself, it results in the lowest amount of CO_2 rebreathing. Dual-limb circuits eliminate the risk of rebreathing.

Ventilator Settings

Similar to short-term NIV, the ventilator settings must relieve patient symptoms. The approach that is generally recommended for long-term NIV is the low-high approach with gradual increase in support. A backup rate sufficiently high to control breathing nocturnally can rest the respiratory muscles and prevent apnea, especially in patients with neuromuscular disease. NIV can be provided both intermittently and continuously. There has been an increase in the continuous use of NIV, especially in patients with neuromuscular disorders. This has resulted in prolonging survival in these patients.

Monitoring of Patients With Long-Term Noninvasive Ventilation

Monitoring patients who are on long-term NIV requires an assessment of their respiratory function. Pulse oximeters are useful in detecting hypoxemia especially during sleep. End-tidal CO_2 monitors are only used in the clinic or hospital. Treatment of sleep-disordered breathing improves the quality of life and may prolong survival. Polysomnography may be required to document sleep disorders but is more expensive than nocturnal pulse oximetry. If a patient has bulbar weakness or severe obesity, there may be obstruction of the upper airway or obstructive sleep apnea in addition to sleep hypoventilation. Both problems are treated with nocturnal ventilation.

Negative Pressure Ventilation
Design and Modes of Negative Pressure Ventilators

All negative pressure ventilators have a chamber in which subatmospheric pressure is generated and a pump that generates this pressure. The chamber may cover only the chest and the upper abdomen (cuirass, Fig. 58.8) or all the extracranial portions of the body (tank respirator [Fig. 58.9], isolette, or a body suit). The tank respirator has both the chamber and pump in one unit. In all other cases the two units are separate. The cuirass can be prefabricated or custom designed to fit the contours of the chest. Custom designed cuirasses are especially useful in patients with skeletal or spinal deformities. All body suits fit over a hard shell similar to the cuirass placed over the chest and upper abdomen. Most negative pressure pumps in use today are pressure cycled. Some volume-cycled pumps have been used, but their use has been limited because the pump cannot compensate for the variable amounts of air leak.

Tank/Whole Body Ventilator

Most of the modern tank ventilators are either made of aluminum or plastic and have separate rotary pumps. Older ventilators had bellows pumps either separately or incorporated into the unit.[7,8] There is a mattress inside the chamber on which the patient's body rests and a head and neck rest that are outside the chamber. Most models have windows and

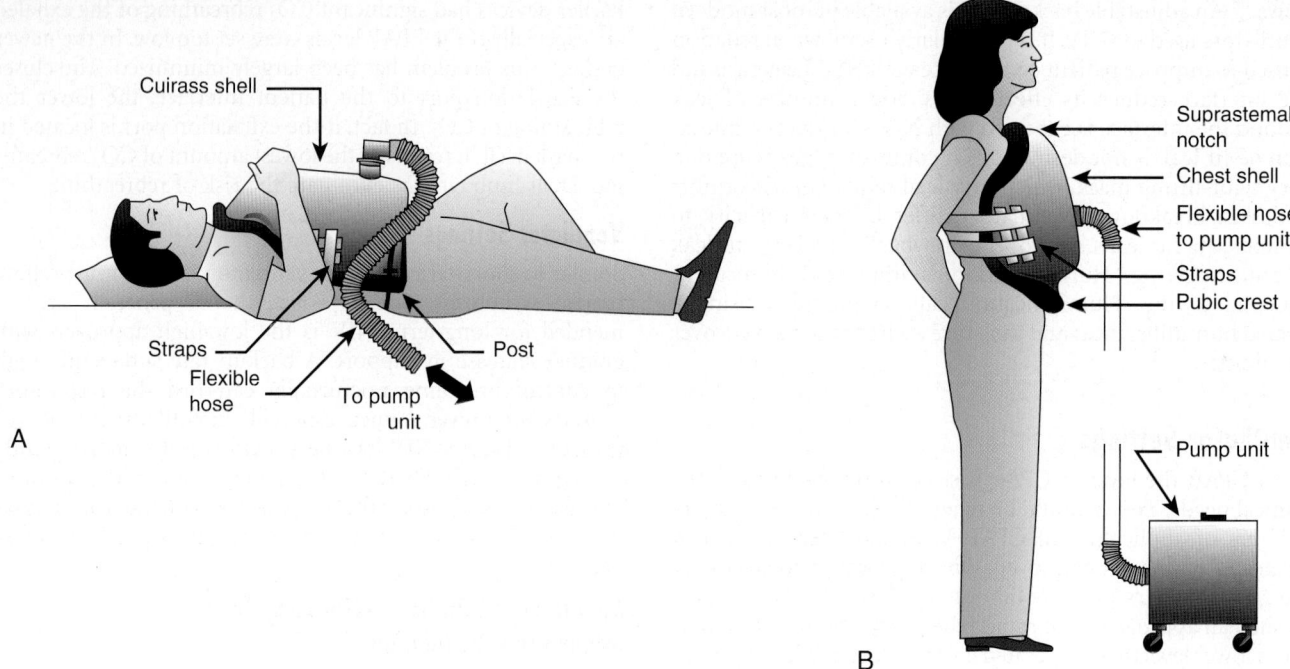

Fig. 58.8. Cuirass ventilator. During inspiration, a negative pressure is created in the cuirass shell using an external pump. Expiration (A) can be either passive or assisted with positive pressure (so-called biphasic ventilation). This can be applied in both the supine (A) and nonsupine (B) positions.

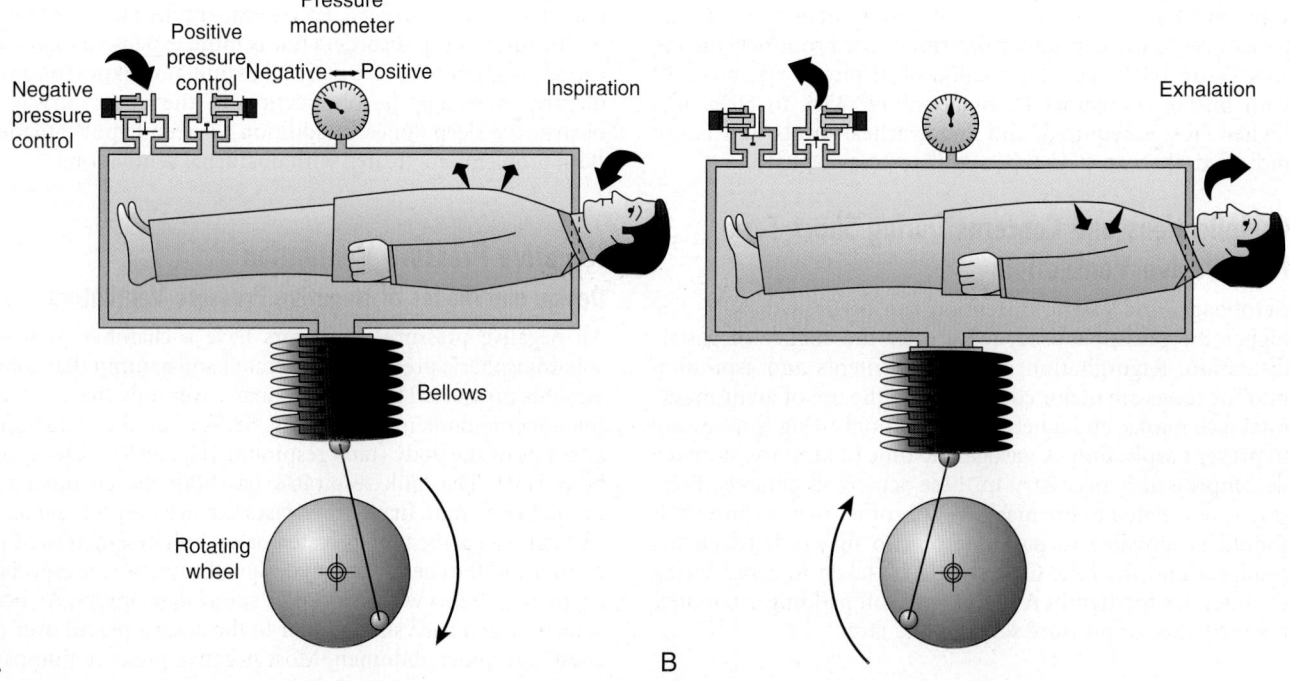

Fig. 58.9. Tank respirator. During inspiration (A), a negative pressure is created in the chamber using a bellows system (shown in figure) or a piston. Expiration (B) can be either passive or assisted with positive pressure (so-called biphasic ventilation).

portholes that allow observations of the patient and access to the patient as well. In some models, the head or feet can be raised, as well as tilting of the whole body. One advantage of the tank respirator is that it does not need to be designed to fit each patient. It requires only one effective seal at the level of the neck. The disadvantage is that it is difficult to access the patient. Aspiration of material from the pharynx into the

trachea and bronchi may occur, especially with swallowing dysfunction. The tidal volume is directly proportional to the peak negative pressure within the chamber.[156]

Isolette Ventilator
An isolette-type respirator is a negative pressure ventilator consisting of two Plexiglas chambers, one for the body and

one for the head.[157,158] The two chambers are connected by an opening equipped with a neck sleeve. The infant's body is placed on a mattress in the body chamber with the neck placed in the opening between the two chambers. The head rests on a head rest. When the neck sleeve is gently closed around the neck to obtain a relatively tight seal with all the openings in both chambers being closed, negative pressure ventilation can be instituted. The depth of ventilation is controlled by the peak inspiratory negative pressure. Ventilator rate and the inspiratory/expiratory ratio are selected by adjusting the appropriate controls.[157,158] Humidified oxygen is delivered by a face mask or into the head chamber. The infant's body temperature can be controlled using servo control regulation. In ventilators using synchronized modes, a self-triggering device that detects either inspiratory flow or breathing movements is usually attached to the patient.

Cuirass Ventilation

Theoretically, a cuirass that covers only the chest should be easier to use than the tank ventilator. Unfortunately, standard sizes may fit poorly and fail to provide an airtight seal around the chest. Therefore many of the cuirasses may have to be custom fit for use so that the cuirass should not only seal the chest without leaks but also enable the anterior abdominal wall to be free to expand during inspiration.[159,160] Customized cuirasses are usually constructed from a cast of the patient's chest.[159,160] The cuirass is made of a synthetic material (Vitrathene or fiberglass), which makes it light and can be made airtight by padding the edges and covering it with airtight material such as neoprene. Sometimes, a back strap may be necessary to maintain an airtight seal between the cuirass and patient. Development of pressure sores at the points of contact between the cuirass and the patient is a disadvantage that needs to be monitored. Similar to the tank ventilator, the tidal volume achieved with a cuirass is proportional to the peak negative pressure within it.

Hayek Cuirass Ventilator

The Hayek oscillator is currently the most versatile cuirass-type negative pressure ventilator (Fig. 58.10). The cuirass is a lightweight, flexible chest enclosure with large soft seals to fit around the chest and abdomen. It rests on either a backplate or flexible cushion forming an airtight enclosure around the

chest and abdomen. This is in contrast to previous cuirass designs, which were heavy, bulky, and nontransparent. There is a range of sizes for patients ranging from preterm infants to adults. The ventilator unit is attached to the cuirass and is capable of biphasic ventilation. The unit is capable of providing ventilation with frequencies ranging from 6 breaths/min to 20 Hz. This machine can behave as a conventional negative pressure ventilator at frequencies to 2 Hz. Tidal volume increases in proportion to the negative pressure span generated within the cuirass, and minute ventilation is related to

TABLE 58.6	Indications, Advantages, Disadvantages, and Contraindications of Negative Pressure Ventilation

Indications
1. Parenchymal lung disease
   Respiratory distress of the newborn
   Interstitial pneumonias
   Acute respiratory distress syndrome
   Acute pulmonary edema
2. Respiratory pump failure
   Poliomyelitis
   Neuromuscular diseases
   Skeletal deformities
   Persistent flail chest deformity
3. Cardiovascular disorders
   After Fontan-type operations
   Repair of total cavopulmonary connection
   Tetralogy of Fallot
   Phrenic nerve palsy after pediatric cardiac surgery

Advantages
1. Avoidance of intubation or tracheostomy
2. Preservation of physiologic functions such as speech, cough, swallowing, and feeding
3. Allows fiberoptic bronchoscopy to be performed without disconnection from the ventilator
4. Promotes venous return by creating negative intrathoracic pressure

Disadvantages
1. They are noisy
2. Access to patient is difficult
3. Tank ventilators produce abdominal pooling of blood resulting in hypotension (tank shock)
4. Regulation of inspiratory-expiratory ratio is difficult (more recent ventilators such as the Hayek negative pressure ventilator allow for regulation of inspiratory-expiratory ratio and application of negative end-expiratory pressure)
5. Difficult to sterilize
6. Lack of protection of the upper airway, especially in unconscious patients or those with bulbar dysfunction
7. Upper airway obstruction can be minimized with an oral airway
8. Difficulty in achieving an adequate seal
9. Discomfort

Contraindications
1. Gastrointestinal bleeding
2. Rib fracture
3. Recent abdominal surgery
4. Uncooperative patients
5. Sleep apnea syndrome
6. Neurologic disorders with bulbar syndrome
Clinical Side Effects
1. Tiredness
2. Musculoskeletal pain or tightness
3. Esophagitis
4. Rib fractures and pneumothorax
5. Impaired sleep quality
6. Poor compliance

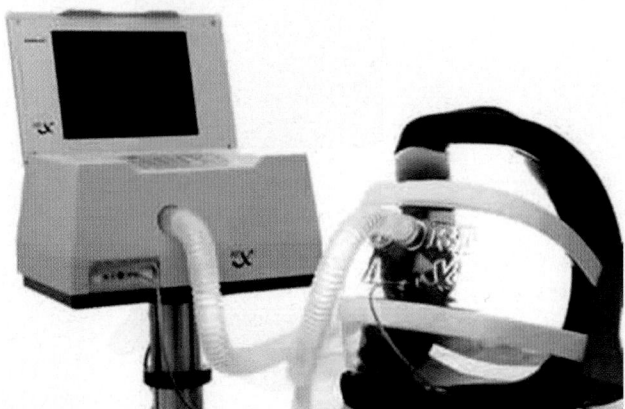

Fig. 58.10. Hayek cuirass ventilator. The chest cuirass is made of flexible plastic. This ventilator is capable of conventional negative pressure ventilation, as well as high-frequency chest wall oscillations.

the tidal volume and frequency. At a frequency above 2 Hz, however, the Hayek oscillator behaves more as a high-frequency oscillator and oxygenation is achieved largely by diffusion. Three frequencies of up to 15 Hz can be obtained with this machine, and frequency, inspiratory, and expiratory pressures and I:E ratio are dialed in for individual patients. Adjusting the expiratory pressure permits ventilation above, at, or below the patient's FRC.

Jacket Ventilation

The first effective jacket ventilator was the Tunnicliffe jacket, developed in the 1950s.[161] The design consists of an airtight synthetic garment with an inner framework made of metal or plastic. Most of the models cover the chest and abdomen and end at a level just below the hips (Fig. 58.11). Though several sizes are available, they are still too large for infants and children. They are also not quite effective in patients with skeletal abnormalities. A pump intermittently evacuates the air within the jacket similar to that used in a cuirass ventilator. The developed tidal volumes are usually smaller than that of a tank respirator. The most commonly used are the Tunnicliffe jacket, Lifecare PulmoWrap, and Lifecare Numo Garment.

Current Modes

At present, there are four modes of negative pressure application: (1) cyclical negative pressure, (2) negative/positive pressure, (3) CNEP, and (4) negative pressure/CNEP. Cyclical negative pressure ventilation refers to a mode where the ventilator generates the preset subatmospheric pressure during inspiration while expiration is passive. Negative/positive pressure ventilation refers to a mode that is a combination of negative pressure during inspiration with positive pressure during expiration. CNEP refers to a mode where a constant subatmospheric pressure is provided throughout the respiratory cycle and the patient breathes spontaneously. Negative pressure/CNEP refers to a mode where negative pressure inspiratory cycles are superimposed on CNEP. Additionally, some ventilators provide an inspiratory assist mode. Respiratory synchronized mode, available in the RTX Respirator, allows full synchronization using the patient's inspiratory and expiratory efforts.

Table 58.6 shows the indications, advantages, disadvantages, contraindications, and clinical side effects of negative pressure ventilation.

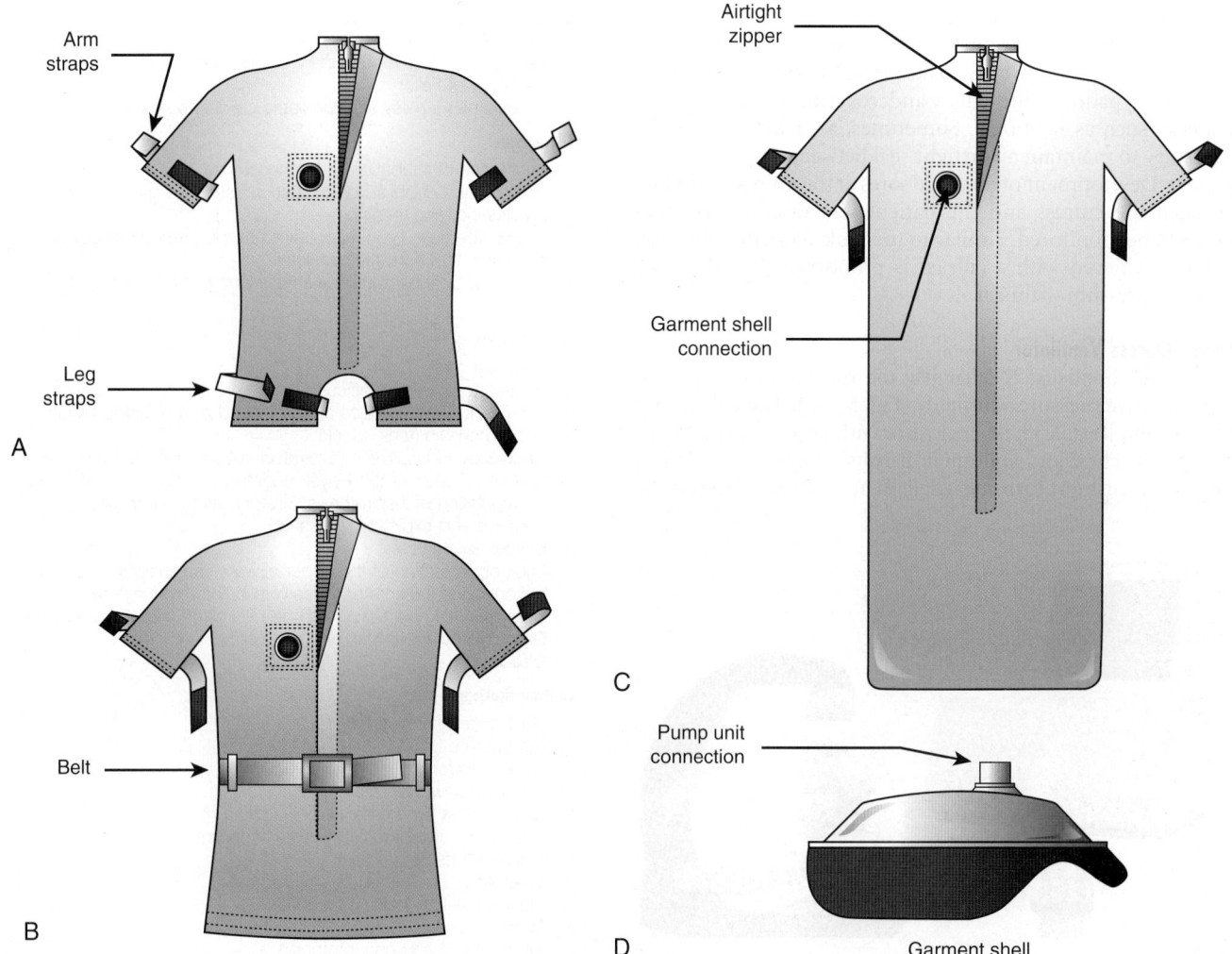

Fig. 58.11. Jacket ventilation. Jackets of different sizes are shown with an inlet port to connect the ventilator tubing. A, B, and C are jackets with seals at different locations. D is the garment shell with a pump connection.

Summary

NIV is a viable alternative to invasive mechanical ventilation in children. NIV can be used for both short-term and long-term needs to treat respiratory failure. Selection of patients is crucial to ensure success with NIV.

Key References

4. Woollam CHM. The development of apparatus for intermittent negative pressure respiration. (1) 1832-1918. *Anaesthesia.* 1976;31:537-547.
5. Woollam CHM. The development of apparatus for intermittent negative pressure respiration. (2) 1919-1976, with special reference to the development and uses of cuirass respirators. *Anaesthesia.* 1976; 31:666-685.
20. Gregory GA, Kitterman JA, Phibbs RH. Treatment of the idiopathic respiratory distress syndrome with continuous positive airway pressure. *N Engl J Med.* 1971;284:1333-1340.
27. Nava S, Carbone G, DiBattista N, et al. Noninvasive ventilation in cardiogenic pulmonary edema. A multicenter randomized trial. *Am J Respir Crit Care Med.* 2003;168:1432-1437.
29. Masip J, Roque M, Sanchez B, et al. Noninvasive ventilation in acute cardiogenic pulmonary edema: systematic review and meta-analysis. *JAMA.* 2005;294:3124-3130.
35. Ferrer M, Esquinas A, Leon M, et al. Noninvasive ventilation in severe hypoxemic respiratory failure: a randomized clinical trial. *Am J Respir Crit Care Med.* 2003;168:1438-1444.
40. Kramer N, Meyer TJ, Meharg J, et al. Randomized prospective trial of noninvasive positive pressure ventilation in acute respiratory failure. *Am J Respir Crit Care Med.* 1995;151:1799-1806.
47. Meduri GU, Cook TR, Turner RE, et al. Noninvasive positive pressure ventilation in status asthmaticus. *Chest.* 1996;110:767-774.
48. Fernandez MM, Villagra A, Blanch L, et al. Noninvasive mechanical ventilation in status asthmaticus. *Intensive Care Med.* 2001;27:486-492.
55. Hilbert G, Gruson D, Vargas F, et al. Noninvasive ventilation in immunosuppressed patients with pulmonary infiltrates, fever, and acute respiratory failure. *N Engl J Med.* 2001;344:481-487.
56. Curtis JR, Cook DJ, Sinuff T, et al. Noninvasive positive pressure ventilation in critical and palliative care settings: understanding the goals of therapy. *Crit Care Med.* 2007;35:932-993.
64. Nava S, Ambrosino N, Clini E, et al. Noninvasive mechanical ventilation in the weaning of patients with respiratory failure due to chronic obstructive pulmonary disease. A randomized, controlled trial. *Ann Intern Med.* 1998;128:721-728.
73. Najaf-Zadeh A, Leclerc F. Noninvasive positive pressure ventilation for acute respiratory failure in children: a concise review. *Ann Intensive Care.* 2011;1:15.
76. Fortenberry JD, Del Toro J, Jefferson LS, et al. Management of pediatric acute hypoxemic respiratory insufficiency with bi-level positive pressure (BiPAP) nasal mask ventilation. *Chest.* 1995;108:1059-1064.
77. Padman R, Lawless ST, Kettrick RG. Non-invasive ventilation via bi-level positive airway pressure support in pediatric practice. *Crit Care Med.* 1998;26:169-173.
78. Essouri S, Chevret L, Durand P, et al. Noninvasive positive pressure ventilation: five years of experience in a pediatric intensive care unit. *Pediatr Crit Care Med.* 2006;7:329-334.
79. Joshi G, Tobias JD. A five-year experience with the use of BiPAP in a pediatric intensive care unit population. *J Intensive Care Med.* 2007;22: 38-43.
80. Munoz-Bonet JI, Flor-Macian EM, Rosello PM, et al. Noninvasive ventilation in pediatric acute respiratory failure by means of a conventional volumetric ventilator. *World J Pediatr.* 2010;6:323-330.
82. Javouhey E, Barats A, Richard N, et al. Non-invasive ventilation as primary ventilator support for infants with severe bronchiolitis. *Intensive Care Med.* 2008;34:1608-1614.
83. Lazner MR, Basu AP, Klonin M. Non-invasive ventilation for severe bronchiolitis: analysis and evidence. *Pediatric Pulmonol.* 2012;47:909-916.
87. Yanez LJ, Yunge M, Emilfork M, et al. A prospective, randomized, controlled trial of noninvasive ventilation in pediatric acute respiratory failure. *Pediatr Crit Care Med.* 2008;9:484-489.

89. Chidini G, Piastra M, Marchesi T, et al. Continuous positive airway pressure with helmet versus mask in infants with bronchiolitis: an RCT. *Pediatrics.* 2015;135:e868-e875.
91. Akingbola OA, Simakajornboon N, Hadley EF Jr, Hopkins RL. Noninvasive positive pressure ventilation in pediatric status asthmaticus. *Pediatr Crit Care Med.* 2002;3:181-184.
93. Carroll CL, Schramm CM. Noninvasive positive pressure ventilation for the treatment of status asthmaticus in children. *Ann Allergy Asthma Immunol.* 2006;96:454-459.
95. Beers SL, Abramo TJ, Bracken A, Wiebe RA. Bilevel positive airway pressure in the treatment of status asthmaticus in pediatrics. *Am J Emerg Med.* 2007;25:6-9.
98. Gupta P, Kuperstock JE, Hashmi S, et al. Efficacy and predictors of success of noninvasive ventilation for prevention of extubation failure in critically ill children with heart disease. *Pediatr Cardiol.* 2013;34: 964-977.
101. Pancera CF, Hayashi M, Fregnani JH, et al. Noninvasive ventilation in immunocompromised pediatric patients: eight years of experience in a pediatric oncology intensive care unit. *J Pediatr Hematol Oncol.* 2008;30: 533-538.
102. Piastra M, De Luca D, Pietrini D, et al. Noninvasive pressure-support ventilation in immunocompromised children with ARDS: a feasibility study. *Intensive Care Med.* 2009;35:1420-1427.
103. Mayordomo-Colunga J, Medina A, Rey C, et al. Noninvasive ventilation after extubation in paediatric patients: a preliminary study. *BMC Pediatr.* 2010;10:29.
104. Lum LC, Abdel-Latif ME, de Bruyne JA, et al. Noninvasive ventilation in a tertiary pediatric intensive care unit in a middle-income country. *Pediatr Crit Care Med.* 2011;12:e7-e13.
105. Dohna-Schwake C, Stehling F, Tschiedel E, et al. Non-invasive ventilation on a pediatric intensive care unit: feasibility, efficacy, and predictors of success. *Pediatric Pulmonol.* 2011;46:1114-1120.
108. Murase K, Chihara Y, Takahashi K, et al. Use of noninvasive ventilation for pediatric patients after liver transplantation: decrease in the need for reintubation. *Liver Transpl.* 2012;18:1217-1225.
109. Teague WG, Kervin L, Dawadkar V, Scott P. Nasal bi-level positive airway pressure acutely improves ventilation and oxygen saturation in children with upper airway obstruction. *Am Rev Respir Dis.* 1991;143: 505.
114. Leger P, Jennequin J, Gerard M, Robert D. Home positive pressure ventilation via nasal masks in patients with neuromuscular weakness and restrictive lung or chest wall disease. *Respir Care.* 1989;34:73-79.
117. Nauffal D, Domenech R, Martinez Garcia MA, et al. Noninvasive positive pressure home ventilation in restrictive disorders. Outcome and impact on health-related quality of life. *Respir Med.* 2002;96:777-783.
121. Bach JR, Ishikawa Y, Kim H. Prevention of pulmonary morbidity for patients with Duchenne muscular dystrophy. *Chest.* 1997;112:1024-1028.
122. Gomez-Merino E, Bach JR. Duchenne muscular dystrophy: prolongation of life by noninvasive ventilation and mechanically assisted coughing. *Am J Phys Med Rehabil.* 2002;81:411-415.
125. Bach JR, Baird JS, Plosky D, et al. Spinal muscular atrophy type 1: management and outcomes. *Pediatr Pulmonol.* 2002;34:16-22.
126. Oskoui M, Levy G, Garland CJ, et al. The changing natural history of spinal muscular atrophy type 1. *Neurology.* 2007;69:1931-1936.
127. Lemoine TJ, Swoboda KJ, Bratton SL, et al. Spinal muscular atrophy type 1: are proactive respiratory interventions associated with longer survival? *Pediatr Crit Care Med.* 2012;13:e161-e165.
128. Gregoretti C1, Ottonello G, Chiarini Testa MB, et al. Survival of patients with spinal muscular atrophy type 1. *Pediatrics.* 2013;131:e1509-e1514.
129. Young HK, Lowe A, Fitzgerald DA, et al. Outcome of noninvasive ventilation in children with neuromuscular disease. *Neurology.* 2007;68: 198-201.
130. Petrone A, Pavone M, Chiarini Testa MB, et al. Noninvasive ventilation in children with spinal muscular atrophy types 1 and 2. *Am J Phys Med Rehabil.* 2007;86:216-221.
133. Caronia CG, Silver P, Nimkoff L, et al. Use of bilevel positive airway pressure (BiPAP) in end-stage patients with cystic fibrosis awaiting lung transplantation. *Clin Pediatr (Phila).* 1998;37:555-560.
136. Madden BP, Kariyawasam H, Siddiqi AJ, et al. Noninvasive ventilation in cystic fibrosis patients with acute or chronic respiratory failure. *Eur Respir J.* 2002;19:310-313.

139. Fauroux B, Le Roux E, Ravilly S, et al. Long-term noninvasive ventilation in patients with cystic fibrosis. *Respiration*. 2008;76:168-174.

140. Sullivan CE, Issa FG, Jones MB, Eves L. Reversal of obstructive sleep apnea by continuous positive airway pressure applied through the nares. *Lancet*. 1981;1:862-865.

142. Waters KA, Everett FM, Bruderer JW, Sullivan CE. Obstructive sleep apnea: the use of nasal CPAP in 80 children. *Am J Respir Crit Care Med*. 1995;152:780-785.

147. Guilleminault C, Pelayo R, Clerk A, et al. Home nasal continuous positive airway pressure in infants with sleep-disordered breathing. *J Pediatr*. 1995;127:905-912.

158. Samuels MP, Southall DP. Negative extrathoracic pressure in treatment of respiratory failure in infants and young children. *Br Med J*. 1989;299:1253-1257.

160. Kinnear W, Petch M, Taylor G, Shneerson JM. Assisted ventilation using cuirass respirators. *Eur Respir J*. 1988;1:198-203.

161. Spalding JMK, Opie L. Artificial respiration with the Tunnicliffe breathing-jacket. *Lancet*. 1958;i:613-615.

Extracorporeal Life Support

Heidi J. Dalton, Tom Preston, and Hanneke IJsselstijn

PEARLS

- Venovenous cannulation for extracorporeal membrane oxygenation (ECMO) is currently preferred for patients with adequate cardiac function and is used in over 50% of reported children.
- Venoarterial access for ECMO remains the most common cannulation technique for patients with cardiac dysfunction.
- In venoarterial ECMO, desaturated venous blood is drained from the body and reinfused into a large artery after being oxygenated in the ECMO circuit.
- Venovenous ECMO differs from venoarterial ECMO in that blood is both withdrawn and returned into the venous circulation of the patient.
- The use of ECMO in patients with neonatal respiratory failure has decreased as new methods of support, such as inhaled nitric oxide, surfactant, and high-frequency oscillation, have been developed.
- As experience with ECMO support in older patients has grown, expansion to clinical situations such as cancer, sepsis, burns, and trauma has occurred.
- One quickly expanding area of extracorporeal support is as a means of resuscitation in cardiac arrest (extracorporeal cardiopulmonary resuscitation).
- Improvements in extracorporeal pumps, cannulae, circuitry, and oxygenators are making ECMO easier to implement and potentially safer.

Aided by the discovery of heparin in 1916 and by advances in the technology of membrane oxygenators,[1] extracorporeal life support has changed dramatically since the early 1950s, when John Gibbon first used a machine of his own design to provide extracorporeal life support for a cat whose pulmonary artery was occluded with a clamp.[2] Early experiences with the use of cardiopulmonary bypass for operations on the heart were mixed, but as experience and technology have continued to advance, the field of cardiopulmonary bypass has expanded at a rapid rate.

As experience with bypass techniques in the operating suite grew, investigation of the use of extracorporeal support of patients with cardiopulmonary failure outside the operating room began.[3-6] Infants with severe respiratory disease or pulmonary hypertension were among the groups for whom use of a temporary cardiopulmonary bypass system seemed appropriate. This technique of modified cardiopulmonary bypass came to be known as "extracorporeal membrane oxygenation" (ECMO).[7-11] Although premature infants had an unacceptably high incidence of intracranial hemorrhage as a result of systemic heparinization, infants of more than 35 weeks' gestation with respiratory failure were successfully supported with ECMO. An abandoned infant with severe hypoxemia, named Esperanza (meaning "hope") by her caregivers, was among the first to be treated with ECMO by Bartlett in 1976. Today, Esperanza is a grown woman with children of her own.

Efforts to organize and collate data on patients treated with ECMO resulted in the formation of the Extracorporeal Life Support Organization (ELSO).[12] In 2014 ELSO celebrated its 25th anniversary. This largely volunteer network of physicians, surgeons, nurses, respiratory therapists, and all those with an interest in extracorporeal life support comprises more than 130 centers and contains data on more than 60,000 patients treated with extracorporeal life support throughout the world. The rise in new ECMO centers and support of older children and adults is exciting, but unfortunately many patients who receive ECMO are not reported to ELSO. This hampers efforts to obtain a fully accurate description of ECMO use and outcomes throughout the world.

As more patients have been treated and techniques have been refined, ECMO procedures and management of patients have evolved to the point that ECMO now can be offered to patient groups previously excluded from consideration.[13-19] The decision regarding when a patient should be treated with ECMO remains empirical and is often based on clinical judgment and case discussion with involved clinicians and family. Similarly, although there is little complete standardization of ECMO circuit design, cannulation technique, and patient management, the general principles are fairly constant. Guidelines for ECMO center training, equipment selection, and patient selection and management have been developed by expert consensus and are posted on the ELSO website (www.ELSO.org). Although the guidelines are fairly general, the expectation is that they will enable more standardization of practice in the future. The information in this chapter represents general practice, the authors' experience, and a review of the literature. For more detailed information regarding extracorporeal life support, the reader is directed to the excellent text regarding this subject published by the ELSO organization.

Materials and Methods
Cannulation Techniques

Several modes of ECMO, or extracorporeal life support (ECLS), as it is also known, have been developed that

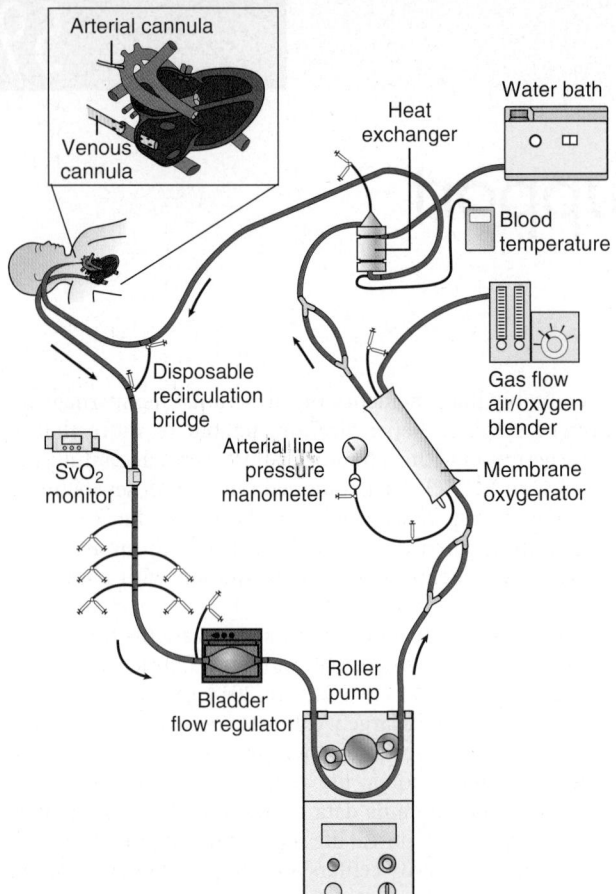

Fig. 59.1. Cervical venoarterial ECMO with roller pump/silicone lung.

Labels in figure: Arterial cannula; Venous cannula; Heat exchanger; Water bath; Blood temperature; Disposable recirculation bridge; Gas flow air/oxygen blender; Membrane oxygenator; SvO₂ monitor; Arterial line pressure manometer; Roller pump; Bladder flow regulator

differ according to cannulation site and minor physiologic principles.[20-31] However, the basic circuit is similar for all modes. Cannulation may be venoarterial or venovenous. Venoarterial access has been used most commonly in the past and will be discussed first.

Cannulation for Extracorporeal Membrane Oxygenation
Venous Access

In venoarterial ECMO, desaturated systemic venous blood is drained from the body and reinfused into a large artery after being oxygenated in the ECMO circuit (Fig. 59.1). The right atrium is the usual site accessed for ECMO cannulation. The internal jugular (IJ) vein is a large vessel with a fairly short, straight course to the right atrium and thus is preferred during cervical cannulation. To augment cerebral venous drainage in patients who undergo cannulation via the right IJ vein, some centers also place a smaller cannula retrograde in the vessel to the level of the jugular venous bulb at the base of the skull. This catheter can facilitate cerebral venous drainage and provide a means of monitoring jugular venous oxygen saturation. Some clinicians believe that monitoring jugular venous saturation provides information on the adequacy of oxygen delivery to the brain and that it is valuable during ECMO, although this practice is relatively controversial. Reports of an increase in venous drainage via the retrograde cannula of up to one-third have been noted, although the practice seems relatively infrequent in most centers.[21,22] The retrograde cath-

eter is connected by a Y adapter into the larger venous drainage line.

In older children and adults, the femoral vessels can be used for cannulation. Venous access is obtained from the femoral vein into the inferior vena cava (IVC), or the cannula can be advanced further up the IVC to the right atrial/IVC junction. Although femoral vein cannulation diverts less venous return to the pump than a catheter positioned in the right atrium, the amount of blood drained is often adequate to meet the needs of the patient. Femoral cannulation is generally restricted by age, vessel size, and to patients who are at least 15 kg. For patients with femoral venous access who exhibit venous stasis or obstruction of the extremity distal to the cannula, a similar catheter to that used for jugular venous drainage can be directed distally to facilitate decompression of the leg and augment venous return. This catheter is then connected by a Y adapter into the venous drainage line of the ECLS circuit. Compartment syndrome from venous stasis in femoral venous cannulation has been described, and thus careful monitoring of the extremity is mandatory.

In patients who undergo cannulation via the mediastinum, the venous cannula is often placed directly into the right atrial appendage. Other vessels, such as the subclavian or axillary vessels, have been associated with limb perfusion abnormalities or difficulties with adequate blood flow in the past. New cannulas with better flow dynamics or use of side grafts onto vessels that do not occlude distal blood flow may allow use of vessels that have been previously avoided.

Arterial Access

Access is obtained for cervical venoarterial ECMO by cannulating the right carotid artery and advancing the cannula to the arch of the aorta. Care must be taken not to position the end of the cannula close to the aortic valve, because this position may result in aortic insufficiency induced by the high-velocity blood flow returning from the ECMO circuit and being directed toward the aortic valve leaflets. Alternatively, if the arterial cannula is advanced too far down the aortic arch, it can occlude blood flow to the left carotid artery and the brain. Cervical venoarterial ECMO is associated with risk of emboli from the ECMO circuit into the brain and potential risk for neurologic abnormalities or stroke later in life. Sixty-four percent of patients <18 years of age reported to the ELSO registry from 2007–2008 received cervical cannulation, with 66% of these patients comprising neonates. Other sites included the femoral artery in 15% and the aorta in 32%. Neurologic injury occurred in 22% of patients and cervical cannulation independently increased odds of neurologic complications (odds ratio [OR] 1.4, 95% confidence interval [CI] 1.01–1.69). No interaction between age and cannulation site was noted.[23-26]

Use of the femoral artery for access during venoarterial ECMO requires careful monitoring of upper body oxygenation to avoid the *red lower body, blue upper body* syndrome. If a long femoral artery cannula that reaches the thorax is used, good oxygenation to the upper body is assured, but resistance to blood flow is high. Most often, a short femoral artery cannula is used (18 cm), which normally sits in the iliac vessels. The amount of arterial return reaching the upper body, heart, and brain in this mode of ECMO is dependent on antegrade flow out of the native left heart and the retrograde flow from the ECMO arterial return. In patients with severe cardiac dysfunction, arterial return from the ECMO circuit flows further up the aorta and may predominate. In patients with good cardiac function, the majority of upper body arterial flow may be from native left heart ejection. Arterial flow from low-lying ECMO cannulas with good native heart function may thus preferentially flow to the lower body. This arterial flow will mix with venous return from the lower body before the oxygenated blood flows through the cardiopulmonary circuit and out the aorta. In patients with impaired gas exchange, the amount of venous mixing prior to reaching the ascending aorta reduces the amount of oxygen that is delivered to the upper body (heart and brain). Thus the PaO_2 and arterial oxygen saturations in the upper body are lower than that obtained with cervical venoarterial ECMO. One study of various configurations of ECMO in an animal model of respiratory failure noted that venous saturations in the superior vena cava during femoral venous and arterial cannulation only reached 40%. Successful use of ECMO has been achieved, however, with this mode, and it is extremely common in adults, especially those placed on ECMO during arrest. Monitoring upper body oxygenation with a pulse oximeter, near infrared spectroscopy, or other measures is recommended to assess the amount of oxygenated flow getting to the head during this mode of ECMO. Echocardiography often can determine the extent of retrograde aortic flow versus native heart ejection.

One method to improve upper body oxygenation in the event of hypoxia with femoral arterial cannulation is to add another cannula in the right internal jugular vein and Y this into the return portion of the ECMO circuit. This will direct some oxygenated blood into the right heart and improve overall upper body saturation. This so-called hybrid model works well in many reports, although flow to both the femoral artery and the right IJ cannula must be monitored to ensure that adequate flow is directed to both sites and avoid thrombosis from stagnant blood flow.

Femoral arterial cannulation also can be associated with impaired flow to the distal limb and resultant ischemia.[27,28] A small *feeder* cannula can be directed distally down the leg artery and then connected by a Y adapter into the arterial cannula to improve perfusion. Additionally, placement of a 14-gauge catheter into the posterior tibial artery that is then connected by a Y adapter into the arterial side of the ECMO circuit has been reported. Ischemia and the need for amputation with femoral artery cannulation occur even with such precautions, therefore meticulous attention to limb perfusion is required to prevent this complication.[27,28] Establishing a graft onto the femoral artery through which the cannula is inserted or ultrasound-based sizing of the femoral vessels and use of a cannula that will not completely occlude the femoral artery have also been suggested to limit risk of ischemia. Side graft techniques have also been used successfully to allow ECMO support via subclavian or axillary vessels.[29]

In mediastinal cannulation, the arterial return cannula is usually placed into the aortic arch under direct vision. During mediastinal cannulation, patients with severe left ventricular dysfunction who cannot open the aortic valve to eject blood often have a left atrial venting catheter inserted to allow decompression of the left heart. This technique prevents pulmonary venous hypertension, which can lead to severe pulmonary edema or hemorrhage. This catheter can be connected by a Y adapter into the venous drainage of the ECLS circuit to provide adequate left heart decompression.[30,31]

Patients with intact sternums who require left atrial decompression often are taken to the cardiac catheterization suite for a blade atrial septostomy that then allows the left heart to decompress into the right atrium and the blood to be drained into the venous ECMO cannula.[31] Experience with use of an Impella device to provide left heart drainage or use of an intraaortic balloon pump (in larger patients) has also been successful.

The primary modality to verify proper cannula position has traditionally been chest radiography; however, use of echocardiography is known to be more accurate and should be considered the gold standard for evaluation of cannula placement.[32]

Venovenous Extracorporeal Membrane Oxygenation

Venovenous ECMO differs from venoarterial ECMO in that blood is both withdrawn and reinfused into the patient's venous circulation (Fig. 59.2). Cannulation can be introduced via either the cervical or femoral vessels.[33] Currently several types of multiple-lumen, single cannulas exist. One such cannula, manufactured by Origen Inc. (Austin, Texas), is available in sizes from 13 to 32 Fr and can support patients of all sizes. This cannula is placed into the right IJ vein and requires only one surgical site. The drainage and infusion lumens in this cannula are separated by a distance of a few centimeters. Reinforcement of the drainage lumen now prevents collapse of this lumen, which had limited its effectiveness with centrifugal pump systems in the past. Careful placement and orientation of the cannula can reduce recirculation of reinfused blood from the ECMO circuit, although some amount of recirculation (which will be discussed later in further detail) always occurs. Another cannula, especially popular with adults and larger children, is manufactured by Avalon Inc. (Maquet).

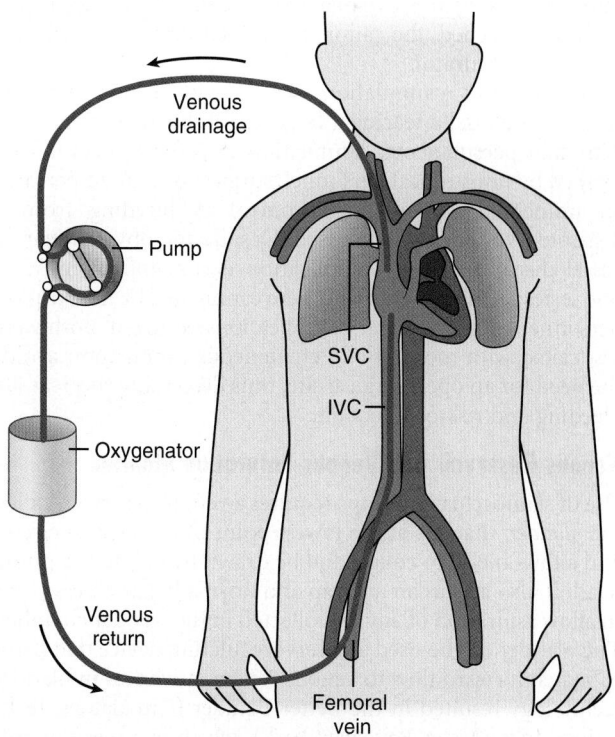

Fig. 59.2. Venovenous ECMO with two site cannulas.

It is also available in sizes from 15 to 31 Fr and is able to obtain flow rates to support even large adult patients. This cannula has two drainage lumens, one of which is positioned in the IVC and one in the superior vena cava. A reinfusion port that sits between the two lumens is directed at the tricuspid valve when placed properly—thus limiting recirculation of oxygenated blood. Placement of this cannula requires meticulous assessment with echocardiography or fluoroscopy for optimal performance. Although experience with the Avalon cannula has been good, especially among adolescents and adults, late cardiac perforation or difficulty in maintaining proper placement has been reported in children (especially infants). Reconfiguration of the distal IVC port in the 13-Fr cannula has been completed, but its effectiveness is not yet well documented. Time will tell if the advantages of this cannula outweigh its increased cost.

Venovenous ECMO also can be provided via two (or more) separate access sites. The right IJ and femoral vein provide access in the majority of patients. Patients with venovenous cannulation may have venous blood drained from the right atrium via the IJ vein or from the IVC via the femoral vein. Although more venous drainage usually can be obtained from a cervical cannula (which is usually shorter and larger than a cannula that can be placed into the femoral vein), the femoral site often may prove adequate and draining from the femoral vessel and reinfusing into the IJ results in less recirculation. Older children and adults also may undergo bilateral femoral cannulations, with one cannula placed into the high IVC and the other ending in the low IVC or iliac vessels (see Fig. 59.2).

Percutaneous Cannulation

Although the historical approach to vessel access has been via an open procedure with placement of cannulas under direct vision, kits for percutaneous placement now exist in many sizes. These kits use a modified Seldinger technique with obturators increasing in size to dilate the vessel. Once the appropriate size is reached, the cannula is passed into the vessel over the largest obturator.

Percutaneous cannulation carries with it the inherent risks of potentially tearing a large vessel during cannulation. Although percutaneous cannulation in some centers is performed by nonsurgical personnel, surgical backup to perform an immediate cutdown for control of bleeding from a disrupted vessel may be needed. Despite the obvious fear of vessel disruption, this complication occurs infrequently. In one series of 100 patients who were cannulated by nonsurgical personnel, only 2 vascular complications occurred. Both were associated with mortality.[34] Percutaneous cannulation avoids the need for an open surgical site, thus decreasing surgical site bleeding and risk of infection.

Venous Reservoir and Venous Saturation Monitor

Use of semiocclusive pumps requires a venous reservoir, called the *bladder,* that sits at the lowest point of the ECMO circuit and allows blood to collect and be drawn from it to the pump head. It also acts as an air trap and normally has access ports to allow aspiration of any air collected in the bladder chamber. The bladder can be used as a servoregulating device that helps to match forward flow to venous return. Advances in bladder technology resulted in the Better Bladder (Circulatory Technology Inc., Oyster Bay, New York), which is a piece of collapsible tubing encased in a hard shell. Changes in venous

return cause the tubing to contract. This device helps servoregulate flow and can be used with either semiocclusive or centrifugal pumps. Servoregulation by monitoring of direct negative and positive pressure within the ECMO circuit has eliminated the use of the bladder in some centers, although most still incorporate some sort of "bladder" within the circuit.[35,36]

Another important feature of the ECMO circuit is the venous saturation monitor that is placed along the venous drainage line. Most new pump systems incorporate this into their monitoring apparatus. Transonic flow probes can provide venous saturation monitoring and may be used to provide additional information. Monitoring venous saturation over time gives information regarding the balance of oxygen delivery and extraction. Use caution when interpreting venous saturation in the presence of left atrial drains or left-to-right intracardiac shunts (which allow oxygenated blood returning from the lungs to be directed into the venous drainage line), as observed venous saturation may not reflect tissue levels of venous saturation but be falsely elevated. Venous saturation should be monitored at a site proximal to entry of oxygenated blood into the circuit.[36,37]

Types of Pumps and Oxygenators

Roller-Head Pumps

The majority of ECMO prior to 2011 was performed using a roller-head semiocclusive pump.[38,39] Venous blood is siphoned via gravity to the roller heads, which are enclosed in a box (the pump housing). Compression of the raceway tubing advances blood forward at high pressure to the membrane lung (if gas exchange is required), from which it is returned to the patient. The gravity siphon, the need to reposition tubing within the raceway to avoid rupture, and the need for pressure monitoring with multiple access points within the circuit combine to require a large priming volume. This increases the exposure to blood products and the associated inflammatory response from contact with the artificial surface of the circuit. Hemolysis from red cell destruction within the raceway or other areas of turbulent flow in the circuit may also occur. Roller pumps generate high pressure in the circuit distal to the raceway/roller heads. Thus acute interruption to forward flow as may occur with kinking of the arterial cannula or elevated resistance to blood flow on the high-pressure side of the circuit can result in an immediate and potentially lethal circuit rupture. Monitoring of the high-pressure side of the ECMO circuit is universal, with critical high limits for arterial line pressure determined based on tubing size and pump flow. Pressures below 300 to 350 mm Hg are desired, and safety mechanisms will stop the ECMO pump if line pressure limits are exceeded. Many centers use filters in the ECMO circuit prior to blood return to the patient, which can help detect air bubbles or trap debris. While using a filter seems practical, in reality these devices may be so sensitive that they result in many episodes of stopping ECMO to check alarms or maintain the filters. A more complete description of roller-head ECMO support can be found in prior editions of this chapter.

Newer pumps may provide pulsatile flow. The nonpulsatile nature of venoarterial ECMO flow has been implicated in the renal dysfunction sometimes noted in patients treated with venoarterial ECMO. The pulsatile flow of the newer pumps has yet to be effectively linked to native heart ejection, although this remains a goal.[40,41]

Centrifugal Pumps

Many centers have transitioned to centrifugal pumps for ECMO support.[42] Although older models were plagued with hemolysis at the low flows that infants and children require, newer devices now employ small pump heads, which may be magnetically levitated or function via bearings that are low resistance, extremely durable, and create less heat, which may lessen risk of hemolysis. Although both roller and centrifugal pumps can create high negative pressure on the venous inflow side, centrifugal pumps only create forward flow if downstream pressure is lower than that in the pump head. Thus occlusion of the postcentrifugal pump circuit will not generate high pressures than can result in tubing rupture as can occur in semiocclusive, roller-head systems. Loss of venous return with continuous rotation of either roller-head or centrifugal pumps results in generation of high negative pressure in the ECMO tubing that can lead to hemolysis and cavitation as air is drawn out of solution. The collapse of the tubing and cannula that can be induced by high negative pressure also can lead to damage of the endothelium of the affected vessel or the right atrium. To protect the patient as venous return is lost and negative pressure develops, a signal is sent to the pump head that causes it to slow down or stop until adequate venous return is achieved. Older versions of the servoregulation system stop the pump whenever venous return diminishes and then restart it when venous return is adequate. This on/off action of servoregulation has been shown to result in acute changes in cerebral blood flow in patients who have undergone cannulation via the cervical route, which may be harmful. Centrifugal devices contain a magnetically controlled spinning head. Blood enters at the inner apex and is propelled tangentially to the outer wall of the pump head. There it is expelled into the circuit. In the past, hemolysis has limited the use of centrifugal pumps, especially in small children. The longer blood sits in the centrifugal head and the faster the head spins, the more hemolysis will be created. It is also postulated that as clots develop in the membrane oxygenator over time and increase outflow resistance, hemolysis worsens in the rotor head. Centrifugal pumps may also create microemboli, which can reach the patient if they are not trapped in the membrane lung. Newer pump designs have small heads that require little priming volume. Technical advances in "spinning" the head may also reduce hemolysis. New low-resistance hollow fiber membrane lungs allow easy propulsion of blood from the centrifugal device and are a major reason that centrifugal pumps have become so popular for patients of all ages.[45,46]

Blood flow to the centrifugal head is augmented by the suction effect of the spinning pump head and thus is not as dependent on gravity drainage as are roller-head pumps. Thus centrifugal pumps can be placed at any level as long as it is below the level of the patient's heart, which makes transporting the patient easier than with roller-head devices. Circuit length can also be reduced, which allows for smaller priming volumes and the potential for less exposure to blood products. The active suction effect of centrifugal heads can create levels of negative pressures as high as −200 to −700 within the venous inlet tubing. Monitoring of venous pressure with alarm limits to signal when excessive negative pressure is occurring is common in most centers. Setting an appropriate venous line or inlet pressure is an important part of circuit management but seems frequently misunderstood. Optimal servoregulation alarms or interventions require a number of factors that should be taken into consideration. The most important fact is that the total resistance on the venous side of the circuit is the sum of the resistances. The major contributor to this negative pressure is the pressure drop across the venous cannula. Most manufacturers provide pressure drop curves for each of their cannula across a range of flow rates (Fig. 59.3). Although these curves are created using water instead of blood, and thus do not represent the effect of viscosity of blood, they provide a suitable surrogate for the resistance induced by the cannula. Selecting a cannula that will provide the expected blood flow at a pressure drop of less than 100 mm Hg is recommended[47] (see Fig. 59.3). Pressure drops greater than 100 mm Hg will increase the risk of hemolysis. Another factor to consider is that exposure of the right atrium to pressures more negative than 20 mm Hg can damage the intima. Taking these two points into consideration, if the venous cannula chosen to provide the expected blood flow rate has a pressure drop of 40 mm Hg from inlet to outlet, the venous servo limit should be set at −60 mm Hg to protect the right atrium from damage and provide adequate blood flow. Thus the venous pressure limit to be set will vary from patient to patient. Clinicians also vary as to where best the venous pressure should be measured—at the junction of the catheter to the circuit tubing, which will reflect negative pressure closest to the heart, or at the pre–pump head site, which reflects the most negative pressure within the total circuit.

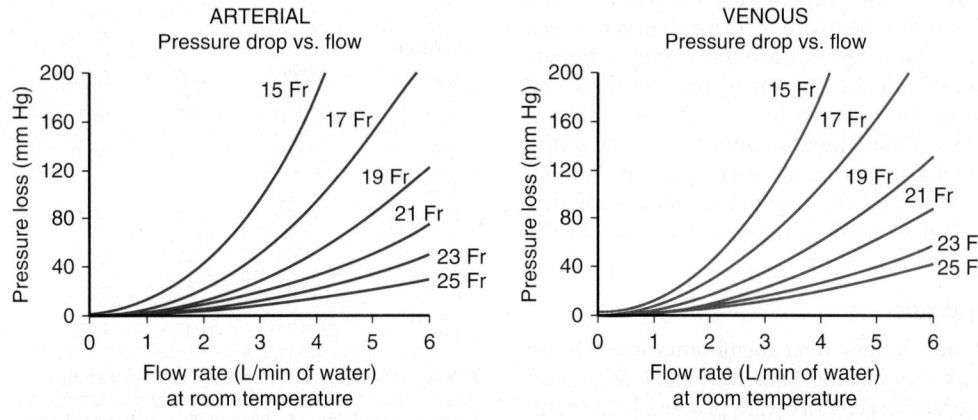

Fig. 59.3. Pressure drop across cannulas based on flow. (Reproduced from Medtronic, Inc., with permission.)

Monitoring venous return and understanding the function of centrifugal pumps are keys to safe and appropriate use of this form of support. Another advantage of centrifugal pumping devices is that air and debris are trapped within the vortex of the pump head and may be less likely to embolize than with roller-head circuits. This advantage is countered by some reports that centrifugal pumps generate more microbubbles than do roller-head devices. A publication examining causes of hemolysis noted that the direct interaction of blood with air and high negative pressure (such as occurs with cardiotomy suction during bypass surgery) resulted in the greatest amount of hemolysis. Centrifugal circuits contain a flow probe that displays how much blood is being returned to the patient. Servoregulation occurs by the same method as with roller pumps, in that venous and arterial pressure limits and goals are set and the pump (or the specialist) adjusts the revolutions per minute of the pump head or the desired flow to maintain set goals. Centrifugal pumps are easy to set up and have many potential benefits, but they are very sensitive to preload and afterload.[48] Understanding physiology to optimize centrifugal pump–driven ECMO is mandatory. Although the majority of centers have changed to centrifugal/hollow fiber ECMO systems, there is no evidence that they are superior to older roller-pump systems. A few reports note increased survival and need for fewer blood products with new systems.[49] Other reports have noted an increase in hemolysis and renal failure in patients receiving centrifugal pump ECMO, although this study included older devices.[50] Centrifugal pump/hollow fiber systems have allowed miniaturization of ECMO, which allows for easier patient transport and less exposure to blood products for priming, making patients more mobile with fewer safety concerns. Circuit tubing and components have a variety of surface coatings to minimize the inflammatory response that occurs when blood contacts a foreign surface, although none have eliminated need for anticoagulation during ECMO support.

Advances in ECLS will likely be drawn from continuing work with artificial heart or ventricular support devices. The advent of percutaneous mechanical support devices other than ECMO allows for newer forms of support for patients with cardiac failure. Investigation into both short- and long-term ventricular assist devices for infants and children is ongoing, and several devices now exist that are applicable to children (the Berlin Heart is the most common).[51]

Membrane Lung

Until recently, the predominant membrane oxygenator was a silicone membrane envelope (with a plastic spacer screen inside) wound in a spiral fashion around a polycarbonate spool.[5,52] Gas flows within the interior of the envelope, and blood flows between the turns in the membrane envelope. Blood flow to the membrane lung is controlled by the pump setting. It is extremely efficient in gas exchange, but the high resistance to blood flow and the development of clots within the device have led to a reference for newer versions of the membrane lung.

Hollow-Fiber Oxygenator

Almost overnight, new hollow-fiber membranes have almost completely replaced the silicone lung during ECMO use.[33] Early versions of these oxygenators were plagued by difficulties with plasma leakage that resulted in very short life spans

for the oxygenator and limited their use. The development of polymethylpentane membranes, which are extremely resistant to plasma leakage and have excellent gas exchange characteristics, make them the preferred device. These devices have a low resistance to blood flow and a lower priming volume than the traditional silicone membrane lung, which makes them faster and easier to prime. Newer versions maintain excellent gas exchange, have little hemolysis, and have durability for days to weeks without failure. In the United States, the Quadrox D device (Maquet INC) and the Medos oxygenators are currently available. Other countries use similar devices. An evaluation of pumps and oxygenators in more than 500 patients from 2012 to 2014 revealed that centrifugal pumps were used in 67% of patients and polymethylpentane devices in nearly 100%.[33]

Patient Populations Treated With Extracorporeal Life Support

The demographics of patients who have received ECMO support are shown in Table 59.1.[12,56]

Neonatal Cardiopulmonary Failure

The majority of ECMO patients reported to the ELSO registry are neonates with respiratory failure.[57-60] The advent of inhaled nitric oxide, surfactant, high-frequency ventilation, and improved pre- and postnatal care has decreased the frequency of ECMO use in these small patients. Nonetheless, an average of 800 infants receive ECMO each year. Although neonatal respiratory distress syndrome has virtually disappeared, patients with meconium aspiration syndrome, persistent pulmonary artery hypertension of the newborn (PPHN), and sepsis still require ECMO support. These infants experience a combination of pulmonary parenchymal and vascular dysfunction that impairs gas exchange. The diagnosis,

TABLE 59.1	Overall Extracorporeal Membrane Oxygenation Results				
	Total	Surv Extracorporeal Life Support		Surv to DC	
Neonatal					
Respiratory	27,728	23,358	84%	20,592	74%
Cardiac	5810	3600	62%	2389	41%
ECPR	1112	712	64%	449	40%
Pediatric					
Respiratory	6569	4327	66%	3760	57%
Cardiac	7314	4825	66%	3679	50%
ECPR	2370	1313	55%	976	41%
Adult					
Respiratory	7008	4587	65%	4026	57%
Cardiac	5603	3129	56%	2294	41%
ECPR	1657	639	39%	471	28%
Total	65,171	46,490	71%	38,636	59%

ECPR, extracorporeal cardiopulmonary resuscitation.
Adapted from the International Extracorporeal Life Support Organization (ELSO) Registry, Ann Arbor, MI, January 2015, with permission.

outcome, and mode of ECMO applied in neonatal patients are shown in Table 59.2.

ECMO provides adequate gas exchange and circulatory support without further exposure to high oxygen concentrations or high airway pressures, thus fostering healing of the damaged lungs. The circulatory changes that result from the initiation of ECMO also lower pulmonary vascular resistance. Draining right atrial blood reduces right atrial pressure and promotes closure of the foramen ovale. In addition, the reduced blood flow to the pulmonary vascular bed decreases pulmonary flow, reduces pulmonary artery pressure, and relieves right-to-left shunting through the patent ductus arteriosus. Well-oxygenated blood flowing left to right through the patent ductus arteriosus promotes its closure. By relieving hypoxia, hypercapnia, and acidosis, ECMO promotes relaxation of pulmonary vascular tone. The amount and extent of pulmonary arteriolar smooth muscle begin to regress. These changes allow the transition to a mature circulation. The infant continues to receive ECMO until parenchymal lung disease heals sufficiently to allow adequate gas exchange or fetal pulmonary artery flow converts to a mature state and adequate gas exchange occurs. However, pulmonary function tests indicate that commonly infants are weaned from ECMO with only moderate improvement in mechanical lung function. These observations support the impression that circulatory abnormalities contribute importantly to neonatal "respiratory" failure and may partially explain the difference in outcome between neonates and older patients treated with ECMO. Historically, neonates have had the best survival of all ECMO groups (>70%). As more complex patients with multiple organ failure have received ECMO, overall survival in neonates has shown some decline.

Infants with congenital diaphragmatic hernia constitute a special subgroup of patients treated with ECMO for severe pulmonary hypertension and respiratory failure. Severe pulmonary hypertension or lung hypoplasia leads to about 50% mortality even with ECMO support. Morphologic examination, better understanding of the pathophysiology of this lesion, and stabilization with ECMO as needed preoperatively or perioperatively have improved the survival rate in some centers in this challenging group of patients.

Pediatric and Adult Patients

Approximately 400 non-neonatal pediatric patients undergo ECMO each year for severe respiratory failure, with an overall survival rate of 53% (see Table 59.2). Most of these patients have severe hypoxia, hypercapnia, or intractable air leaks. Pulmonary dysfunction resulting from bacterial or viral pneumonia, aspiration syndromes, intrapulmonary hemorrhage, acute respiratory distress syndrome, and less well-defined disorders have also been treated successfully with ECMO.[61,62] The uncertainties accompanying the use of ECMO in neonates, who

TABLE 59.2	Common Diagnoses and Outcomes for Extracorporeal Membrane Oxygenation Patients				
NEONATAL RESPIRATORY RUNS BY DIAGNOSIS					
	Total Runs	**Average Run Time**	**Longest Run Time**	**Survived**	**Percentage Survived**
CDH	7228	254	2549	3691	51%
MAS	8684	133	1327	8128	94%
PPHN/PFC	4800	155	1176	3696	77%
RDS	1546	136	1093	1300	84%
Sepsis	2856	143	1200	2084	73%
Pneumonia	376	249	1002	218	58%
Air Leak Syndrome	133	171	979	98	74%
Other	2498	183	1843	1519	61%
PEDIATRIC RESPIRATORY RUNS BY DIAGNOSIS					
	Total Runs	**Average Run Time**	**Longest Run Time**	**Survived**	**Percentage Survived**
Viral Pneumonia	1450	317	2968	940	65%
Bacterial Pneumonia	686	284	1411	402	59%
Pneumocystis Pneumonia	35	373	1144	18	51%
Aspiration Pneumonia	304	249	2437	208	68%
ARDS, Postop/Trauma	185	248	935	115	62%
ARDS, Not Postop/Trauma	550	304	3086	297	54%
Acute Resp Failure, Non-ARDS	1186	255	2429	641	54%
Other	2306	219	2465	1195	52%

Run time in hours. Survived = survival to discharge or transfer based on number of runs.
ARDS, acute respiratory distress syndrome; *CDH,* congenital diaphragmatic hernia; *MAS,* meconium aspiration syndrome; *PFC,* persistent fetal circulation; *PPHN,* persistent pulmonary hypertension of the newborn; *RDS,* respiratory distress syndrome.
Adapted from the International Extracorporeal Life Support Organization (ELSO) Registry, Ann Arbor, MI, January 2015, with permission.

compose a homogeneous group relative to other age groups, are compounded in older children. The enormously heterogeneous older pediatric population spans nearly two decades of physiologic development, and cardiorespiratory failure develops as a result of a multitude of different disorders. Furthermore, many patients have varying degrees of multiple organ failure along with respiratory disease at the time ECMO is instituted. Both lung disease and secondary organ dysfunction must be resolved to achieve survival. These factors result in lower survival rates in older patients treated with ECMO than that achieved with the neonatal patient population.

One small subgroup of ECLS patients with excellent survival is made up of those with status asthmaticus.[59] One study of 64 asthmatic patients supported by ECLS noted the mean duration of ECMO was 94 hours, and 94% of the patients survived. Venovenous support was the cannulation mode in 86% of patients.[63]

One common theme in pediatric ECMO is the increasing complexity of patients. The multiple exclusion criteria used in the early days of ECMO have now been essentially eliminated, and each potential patient is generally considered on a case-by-case basis. Even patients with known bleeding disorders such as hemophilia have successfully received ECMO support.[64]

A review of the International Extracorporeal Life Support Registry (ELSO) found that patients with comorbidities prior to ECMO increased from 18% to 47% between 1993 and 2007 (Fig. 59.4).[65] Although such patients had decreased survival as compared to patients without comorbidities, overall 40% to 50% survived to hospital discharge. Patients with pertussis and fungal pneumonia continue to show increased mortality

when compared to other groups. The willingness of clinicians to apply ECMO to groups previously excluded is highlighted by the numbers of patients with trauma who receive ECMO support.[62] More than 550 patients with respiratory failure and trauma are reported with survival of 50%. Patients with underlying malignancy also form an increasingly large percentage of ECMO support, rising from 0.3% to 1% of pediatric ECMO cases in the most recent review. Of 171 patients analyzed from 2008 to 2012, 55% survived their ECLS run and 48% survived to hospital discharge. A questionnaire sent to 118 ECMO centers noted that 95% of responding sites would consider the use of ECMO in a patient with malignancy. This response demonstrates the change in attitude among many clinicians with regard to patients with cancer.[19,66]

One group that remains the most difficult is made up of patients with underlying bone marrow transplant. Although ECLS has been applied to such children, usually for refractory respiratory failure, none have been reported as survivors to discharge in the ELSO registry. Anecdotal reports, however, of sporadic survival, combined with pleas from oncologists that the rapid rise of stem cell transplants and today's conditioning and posttransplant regimens are less toxic and lead to rapid engraftment, make this a controversial area that is still being explored. Selected patients are still receiving ECLS on a case-by-case basis. Anecdotal reports have noted that patients with newly discovered malignancy have also received successful induction therapy while on ECMO support.[68,69]

Although it is desirable to initiate ECMO prior to the onset of multiple organ system failure, many patients present with established organ failure. ECMO may provide an optimal environment for organ recovery in such patients, not just providing respiratory or cardiac support. Further, the ability to add adjunctive devices such as hemofiltration or dialysis (Fig. 59.5) to augment renal function and allow use of plasmapheresis, plasma exchange, or hepatic support devices is another aspect of ECMO support that may facilitate patient care and organ recovery.[70] Implementation of ECMO during multiple organ systems failure now occurs under a variety of conditions, with resolution of organ dysfunction and often with good outcome. Furthermore, because it avoids the circulatory derangements that often result from extreme forms of

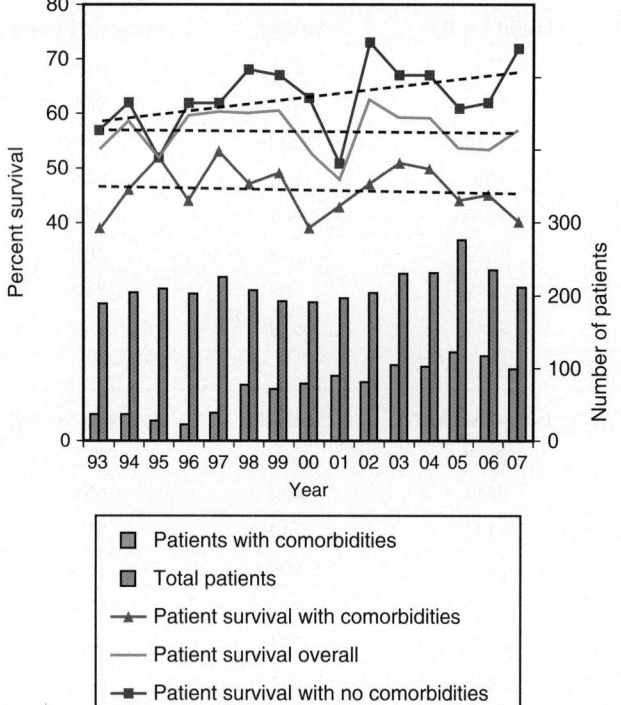

Fig. 59.4. Changes in pediatric ECMO for respiratory failure and outcome. *Dashed lines* depict linear trend. (Reproduced from Zabrocki L, Brogan T, Statler K, et al. Extracorporeal membrane oxygenation for pediatric respiratory failure: survival and predictors of mortality. Crit Care Med. 2011;39:364-370.)

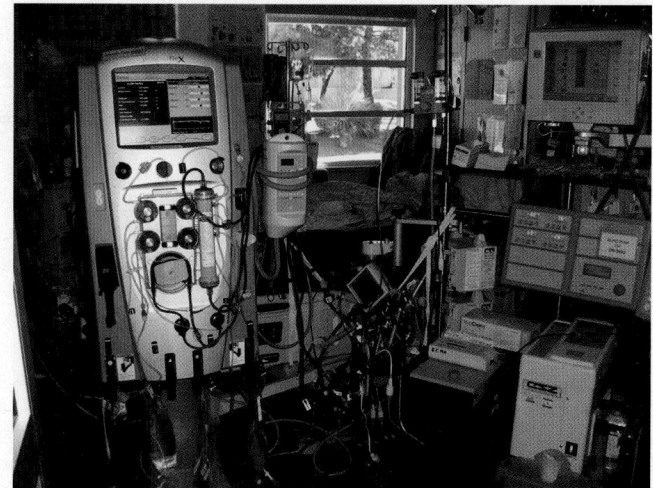

Fig. 59.5. Hemofiltration with a centrifugal pump/hollow fiber lung. (Courtesy of H.J. Dalton, MD, with permission.)

mechanical ventilation and provides systemic perfusion without the need for high-dose levels of inotropic agents, ECMO also may prevent damage to other systems.[62]

Extracorporeal Membrane Oxygenation in Adults

The most rapid rise in the use of ECMO is in adult patients. Since 2009, ECMO use has increased over 400% in this population, with overall survival similar to that of pediatric patients (Table 59.3).[72-74] Early randomized trials of ECMO use in adults that did not show benefit have been criticized for poor study design and had complication rates in both control and ECLS groups that are much higher than those noted today. The randomized trial of venovenous ECMO compared with conventional mechanical ventilation in adults with respiratory failure in the United Kingdom (the Conventional Ventilation or ECMO for Severe Adult Respiratory Failure [CESAR] study) found a benefit to patients referred to a single ECMO

center when outcome was examined at 6 months after discharge. A total of 180 patients were enrolled and randomly allocated to receive treatment (n = 90) at the single ECMO center in the United Kingdom or to receive conventional management ventilation (CMV) (n = 90) at a designated CMV center. Randomization criteria included a Murray score of >3 or severe respiratory acidosis with pH <7.20. Study results noted that 63% of patients allocated to "consideration for treatment by ECMO" survived to 6 months without disability compared with 47% of those allocated to conventional management (P = .03; risk ratio, 0.69; 95% confidence interval 0.05 to 0.97). Of note, 17 of 90 patients randomly assigned to "consideration for treatment by ECMO" who were treated within the ECMO center with a "gentle ventilation" (low tidal volume, limited pressure) strategy were not treated with ECMO and 14 survived.[75] Whether this finding represents the beneficial effects of increased expertise within centers that support patients with severe respiratory failure with ECMO availability or other factors is unknown. Early transfer of patients with potentially reversible respiratory failure who meet similar criteria to those in the CESAR study may be recommended. This study also found a cost-benefit ratio in terms of quality of life and economics that was favorable in the ECMO group. As with most randomized studies, critics questioned some aspects of the CESAR study design, most notably that there was no mandated protocol for ventilator management in the CMV arm, and this has led to another randomized trial of ECMO versus CMV in Europe, which is ongoing.

As with pediatric patients, use of ECMO in adults with trauma (even with recent head injury and intracranial hemorrhage), sepsis, HIV, and other disease processes that may have been excluded from ECMO consideration in the past is on the rise.

One special patient population is those patients awaiting lung transplant. With the advent of new equipment and patient management techniques that allow patients to be awake, mobile, and undergo active rehabilitation while on ECMO support, this area represents a new growth region where excellent results are being reported in both pre- and posttransplant care. This is especially the case in adults with chronic obstructive pulmonary disease (COPD) or similar diseases who require carbon dioxide removal more than oxygenation support. Such gas exchange is extremely efficient even with venovenous cannulation and requires only a fraction of circulating blood volume to be lifesaving.[76-79]

The new, large, percutaneous cannulas for venovenous ECMO support, along with small centrifugal pumps and less cumbersome total ECMO systems, are all advantageous to the adult population. Alternative support techniques such as pumpless extracorporeal support and the implantable artificial lung are additional clinical modalities for adult respiratory failure.[80]

Extracorporeal Membrane Oxygenation for Myocardial Dysfunction

The International ELSO Registry lists more than 9000 patients who have received ECMO for cardiac failure, predominantly following surgical repair of congenital heart defects (Table 59.4). Outcome of neonatal and pediatric patients notes that 60% are successfully weaned from ECMO and 43% survive to be discharged from the hospital. Adult cardiac patients have

TABLE 59.3	Proposal for and Relevance of Long-Term Follow-Up After (Neonatal) Extracorporeal Membrane Oxygenation Treatment	
	Specific Topics	**Relevance/Intervention**
Infancy	Growth	Hyperalimentation
	Hearing assessment	Early referral audiology
	Screening CKD	Early recognition and treatment
	Neurologic impairment	Early recognition, rehabilitation
	Mental and motor development	Referral physical therapist
Toddler	Growth (mainly in CDH)	Hyperalimentation
	Screening CKD	Early recognition and treatment
	Neurologic impairment	Rehabilitation
	Language development	Hearing assessment, speech-language pathologist
	Motor function development	Referral physical therapist
School age	Lung function assessment	Evaluate reversibility of airflow obstruction
	Exercise capacity	Exercise training, sports participation
	Growth (mainly in CDH)	Hyperalimentation
	Screening CKD	Early recognition and treatment
	Motor function development	Referral physical therapist
	Neuropsychologic assessment	Hearing assessment, early school support
	Self-esteem	Early intervention, support
Adolescence into adulthood	Exercise capacity	Exercise training, sports participation
	Screening CKD	Early recognition and treatment
	Growth (mainly in CDH)	Hyperalimentation
	Neuropsychologic assessment	School support, choice of profession/career
	Self-esteem	Support

Neuropsychologic assessment should include intelligence, attention, memory, executive functioning, visual-spatial processing, and behavior.
CDH, congenital diaphragmatic hernia; *CKD*, chronic kidney disease.
Courtesy of H. IJsselstijn, MD, PhD.

TABLE 59.4	Cardiac Extracorporeal Membrane Oxygenation Patients and Outcome (Under Age 16 Years)	
	Runs	**% Survived**
Congenital defect	9807	43
Cardiac arrest	309	38
Cardiogenic shock	286	46
Myocardiopathy	825	61
Myocarditis	431	67
Other	2056	50

Adapted from the International Extracorporeal Life Support Organization (ELSO) Registry, Ann Arbor, MI, January 2015, with permission.

slightly worse survival rates, with 48% weaned off ECMO and 34% discharged from the hospital.[81-85]

Although center-specific factors separating patients with myocardial dysfunction who will not survive from those who will recover adequate function without such invasive support have been put forth in the literature, none have proved to be universally accepted. Patients with evidence of low cardiac output and shock (including low urine output, poor perfusion, hypotension, elevated cardiac filling pressures, and low mixed venous oxygen saturation) despite maximal respiratory and pharmacologic support are candidates for ECMO rescue. The absence of clear criteria for using ECMO and the reluctance to initiate such invasive support often delay use until cardiac arrest has occurred. As a result, a significant number of patients treated with ECMO have recovered myocardial function only to die of hypoxic/ischemic encephalopathy that was experienced before ECMO was initiated. Such events have now led to a trend in cardiac patients to consider ECMO earlier in the course of dysfunction. Availability of ECMO is now a recommended part of pediatric cardiac surgical programs. As newer and smaller cardiac assist devices are developed for pediatric patients, the need for ECMO support in this population may wane, but at this time ECMO provides the most readily available support technique over a wide range of patient ages and sizes for cardiac failure.

Most patients requiring ECMO for circulatory support have undergone venoarterial ECMO because of its capacity to provide both respiratory and circulatory support. The majority of survivors recover myocardial function within 72 hours of ECMO support, although patients with myocarditis or cardiomyopathy can have good survival rates even after prolonged ECMO support. In most reports, patients whose myocardial function has not improved substantially within 24 to 72 hours of rest on ECMO are not likely to recover cardiac function sufficient to support life. Transplantation may be an option in these patients if their underlying cardiac anatomy and general clinical condition make them appropriate candidates. Patients who fail to improve often are evaluated by cardiac catheterization early during ECMO to identify residual lesions (if postoperative) or abnormalities that may be amenable to further surgical repair or catheterization laboratory interventions. Cardiac patients with good respiratory function may not routinely require ventilator support. Such patients may require only low levels of ventilator support or

can be extubated during ECMO, which may alleviate the need for heavy sedation to maintain endotracheal tube position.

Myocarditis and cardiomyopathy are two categories of nonsurgical cardiac failure that have increasingly received ECLS support.[83] Although it may be difficult acutely to differentiate unknown cardiomyopathy from viral myocarditis, both diseases may benefit from mechanical support with ECMO or ventricular assist devices that create a stable hemodynamic milieu where the heart can "rest" and recover. One review of the ELSO registry noted a 61% survival rate in 255 children with myocarditis. Seven patients received cardiac transplantation, with six surviving to discharge. The average duration of ECLS in nontransplant patients was 168 hours, with a range of 145 to 226 hours. Multivariate analysis showed that female gender, arrhythmia while undergoing ECMO, and renal failure requiring dialysis were associated with increased in-hospital mortality.

One analysis of a single institution's experience of ECLS following cardiac surgery in children spanning a 17-year period found that 38% of cardiac patients survived to discharge. One-third of the children had single ventricle cardiac pathology. Cannulation occurred in the operating room in 46% of patients, and 51% of cannulations took place in the ICU. Complications included reexploration for bleeding (56%), neurologic complications such as ischemic brain injury or intracranial hemorrhage (17%), renal dysfunction (10%), and pulmonary hemorrhage (5%). Factors associated with mortality were renal failure, neurologic complications, longer ECLS duration, and need for recurrent ECMO support. Mortality also may have been affected by the lack of a cardiac transplant program for patients not recovering myocardial function.[84]

In another review of 58 patients receiving ECMO following congenital heart defect repair (January 2003 through June 2008), 67% of patients were weaned off ECMO support and 41% survived to hospital discharge. Single ventricle repair was noted in 53% of patients. When analyzed for factors associated with outcome, ECMO duration longer than 10 days (OR, 6.1), urine output less than 2 mL/kg/h in the first 24 hours (OR, 15), renal failure (OR, 9.4), and pH less than 7.35 after 24 hours of ECMO (OR, 82.3) were all found to be independent predictors of failure to wean from ECMO. Independent predictors of failure of hospital discharge in spite of successful decannulation were ECMO time of 10 or more days (OR, 11.5), a red blood cell transfusion volume greater than 1000 mL/kg during the entire period of ECMO course (OR, 11.5), and sepsis. Patients who underwent single ventricle repair were at higher risk of hospital mortality (OR, 4.9). This study also developed a probability of weaning from ECMO table based on the four previously mentioned predictors. For example, a patient with an ECMO duration of more than 10 days who had renal failure and poor urine output and pH at 24 hours of ECMO would have a predicted mortality rate of 100%. Similar evaluations in larger series of patients to validate such assessments should be performed to refine ECMO care and improve family counseling regarding prognosis.[85]

To obtain more detailed information on cardiac surgical patients who receive ECLS, an addendum to the general ELSO registry data form was developed and should provide more details on these patients. Although ECMO remains the most common method for support of patients with cardiac failure, new and miniaturized mechanical support devices such as the

Berlin Heart and other ventricular assist devices offer alternatives with potential advantages to infants and children.

Extracorporeal Membrane Oxygenation for Resuscitation

Another growing area of the use of ECLS is in support of patients with refractory cardiac arrest.[86-90] This type of support is termed *extracorporeal cardiopulmonary resuscitation (ECPR)*, or ECMO during cardiac arrest. Designed as a resuscitative tool for patients in cardiac arrest, ECPR has been reported in more than 5000 neonates, children, and adults, with an overall survival-to-discharge rate of 35% to 40%. To facilitate expedient access to ECMO support for ECPR, in situations of acute deterioration or whenever there is insufficient time or personnel for routine ECMO, many centers maintain an ECMO circuit setup that is preprimed with a crystalloid solution and stored (usually up to 30 days). Other centers use a portable, centrifugal bypass perfusion system that also is easily set up within 10 to 20 minutes. Both methods often use a hollow-fiber membrane lung.[85-90]

In one meta-analysis of ECPR, 288 patients were identified, with 40% surviving to hospital discharge. Venoarterial ECMO was used in 99% of patients, and 63% underwent cannulation through an open chest. The median length of stay on ECMO was 4.3 days. The overall occurrence of complications was high (59%). The most commonly occurring complications were neurologic (27%), renal (25%), sepsis (17%), bleeding (7%), and multisystem organ failure (9%).

In an analysis of children with cardiac arrest, use of ECMO was noted as one factor associated with improved survival. Another review from the National Registry of CPR found 199 pediatric patients who were treated with ECMO during arrest with an overall survival rate of 44%. In 59 survivors whose neurologic outcome was recorded, 95% had favorable outcomes based on Pediatric Cerebral Performance Scores. By multivariate analysis, renal insufficiency, metabolic or electrolyte abnormality at the time of arrest, and use of sodium bicarbonate or tromethamine were associated with decreased rates of survival. Underlying cardiac illness was associated with an increased rate of survival to discharge.[87]

One cautionary note is that cardiac patients are often reported to have improved outcomes when compared with noncardiac patients. Whether this finding represents disparity in access to ECPR between cardiac and noncardiac patients, underlying pathophysiology or other factors require ongoing study. An addendum to the ELSO registry that has been specifically designed for patients experiencing cardiac arrest may provide more detailed information to answer ongoing questions.

Of interest, several adult reports have found that percutaneous femoral artery and vein cannulation during arrest are efficient and associated with good outcomes.[91,92] The SAVE JAPAN study noted increased survival with such an approach applied in the emergency department to adults patients with out-of-hospital arrest.[93] A review from Australia (the CHEER trial) also found that cannulation of the femoral vessels by critical care physicians, combined with induced hypothermia via a 30 cc/kg bolus of iced saline, in selected patients with in-hospital or out-of-hospital arrest had an overall survival of 54% with good neurologic outcome. Time to establish ECMO once the ECPR team arrived was 20 minutes, and overall CPR duration prior to ECMO initiation averaged 56 minutes.[94] It is likely that similar efforts may expand to

children now that cannulation strategies and equipment have become available.

Although ECPR initiation has become routine in many centers, decision making as to when to *not* offer or to discontinue ECMO efforts if recovery seems futile has opened a new area of ethical discussion. The reluctance of family members to agree with discontinuation of support highlights a dilemma that some clinicians have been faced with. Setting firm goals and decision-making processes, which are explained to the family during the consent process or immediately after initiation in terms of emergent ECLS, may alleviate some of these situations.[95]

Trauma Patients

Trauma patients, particularly those with multiple injuries, are at risk of respiratory failure. Trauma remains the leading cause of death in young adults. Common pathophysiologic mechanisms include direct chest injury causing pulmonary contusion, long bone or pelvic fractures causing fat embolization, or an inflammatory-mediated event following systemic injury known as acute respiratory distress syndrome. Extracorporeal membrane oxygenation provides *lung rest* by permitting reduced ventilator settings and limiting further barotrauma while maintaining tissue perfusion and oxygenation. In a study comprising 28 adult patients treated with ECMO because of trauma-related respiratory failure, 20 patients were successfully weaned off ECMO and discharged. Eight patients died as a result of overwhelming sepsis and irreversible cardiogenic shock. Good outcomes in pediatric patients undergoing ECMO following trauma also have been reported.[62,96]

Other applications of ECMO include management of patients with extreme hypothermia who require gradual extracorporeal rewarming. Trauma patients with massive hemorrhage and ongoing coagulopathy from transfusion-related hypothermia also have received short-term extracorporeal support with bypass to facilitate rewarming to temperatures that help normalize the coagulation process. Once rewarming is achieved, cannulas are withdrawn.

Other Extracorporeal Support

Other advances in membrane lung development have allowed adequate oxygenation without an extracorporeal pump.[97] One device, the Novalung, takes arterial blood from the femoral artery and directs it through a hollow-fiber device for oxygenation and carbon dioxide removal, and then reinfused blood is directed into the femoral vein. Experience with this device is growing, and multiple reports of bridging to lung transplantation or to resolution of lung injury can be found in the literature. Other devices that are effective in removing carbon dioxide with low blood flows are also becoming available.[92-94]

Patient Selection Criteria

Various mortality prediction criteria have been put forth as indicators of when ECMO rescue is best applied. Many of these criteria have been derived from small series of historical data for patients with respiratory failure or were extrapolated from neonatal respiratory failure data. Attempts to provide universally accepted criteria for institution of ECMO have proved difficult.[98-102]

The current state is that almost every patient who receives ECLS is selected on a case-by-case basis. The clinical team discusses the risks and benefits of ECLS in light of the current ICU status and makes a decision about whether or not to offer ECMO to the family as an option. Given the complexity of patients receiving ECLS and the comorbidities often present, clinicians from other services outside the ICU staff (pulmonary, oncology, neurology, etc.) are beneficial in this discussion. Many centers also have smaller teams with special expertise or interest in ECLS within the overall ICU faculty who provide advice on candidacy, ECLS strategy, and patient management.

For the majority of patients who undergo ECMO, less invasive methods of respiratory support have failed. Such methods of support often include conventional mechanical ventilation in pressure control or pressure-regulated volume control modes, high positive end-expiratory pressure (PEEP), high-frequency ventilation (HFV), surfactant, or iNO.[103] One report examined the current utility of respiratory severity indices used in the past for potential ECMO eligibility in 118 children with acute hypoxemic respiratory failure. Indices examined included the $AaDO_2$, OI, PaO_2/FiO_2, ventilation index, and mean airway pressure (Paw), as well as individual ventilator settings and arterial blood gas values. When risk of mortality based on respiratory severity indices predictions were compared with actual mortality observed in these 118 children, survival was much better than would have been predicted based on historical data.[100] As an example, an OI greater than 40 has been associated with more than 80% risk of death in the past. Although only 15 patients reached an OI greater than 40 in this study, the positive predictive risk of mortality in these patients was 40%, significantly lower than predicted by past reports. An $AaDO_2$ greater than 450 for 24 hours, a Paw higher than 23, or an $AaDO_2$ higher than 420 had positive predictive value for mortality rate of 32% to 40%. Using logistic regression, no respiratory parameter ($AaDO_2$, OI, Paw, ventilator settings, or blood gas values) was independently correlated with death. All deaths were associated with multiorgan system failure, coincident pathology, or perceived treatment futility, leading to limitation or withdrawal of care. The overall mortality rate of these 118 children was 22%, with no previously healthy child dying from respiratory failure. Nonconventional therapies applied included HFV in 25 (21%) of 119 (64% survival), surfactant administration in 15 (13%) of 119 (73% survival), iNO in 38 (32%) of 119 (69% survival), and ECMO in 4 (3%) of 119 (75% survival) of patients.[100]

Although severity scores such as PaO_2/FiO_2, shunt fraction, compliance, and others have been used to identify potential ECMO candidates, in children the oxygenation index has remained in favor, as it combines the level of ventilatory support being given and the oxygen level obtained in arterial blood. This measure is calculated as follows:

$$OI = \frac{Mean\ Airway\ Pressure\ (cm\ H_2O) \times FiO_2}{PaO_2\ (torr)}$$

Scores >40 or from 30 to 40 without improvement have been associated with high mortality in the past and were used as ECMO candidacy alerts. Data, however, have noted doubling of mortality from <20% to >40% when OI exceeds 16. When combined with another variable of lung injury, pulmonary dead space, OIs of >16 with dead space of >23% resulted in an observed mortality risk of 60%. In an evaluation of 65 children with serial OI measurements obtained from the electronic medical record from a single center, mortality tripled when the OI exceeded 17. In another review of factors associated with death in children with severe respiratory failure, the peak oxygenation index and pediatric risk of mortality (PRISM) score were found to be independent predictors of outcome, although no definitive OI cutoff that predicted death could be identified. These findings, along with the increased ease of applying ECMO, have led to discussion as to whether ECMO should be applied at OI severity scores much lower than in times past. Indeed, in the adult population, there is now discussion as to whether implementation of ECMO to avert intubation or shortly after the need for mechanical ventilation should be performed.

In an attempt to provide standard definitions for respiratory failure in children and develop consensus regarding pediatric respiratory care guidelines, an expert panel of 19 international clinicians met and examined thousands of published reports by the Rand/University of California at Los Angeles (UCLA) method and achieved consensus results using the modified Delphi method. ECLS was one of the nine areas selected for recommendations. As there were few high-quality report scores for ECMO as scored by the Rand/UCLA method, recommendations were developed primarily by consensus expert opinion. These included the following: (1) serial measurements of severity of illness as criteria for ECMO should be used rather than a single cutoff value; (2) cases should be discussed among treating clinicians as a team; (3) ECMO should not be offered to patients in whom life-sustaining measures were restricted; (4) quality of life and long-term outcome from comorbidities should also be evaluated; (5) all centers should report patients and outcome to a registry, such as ELSO; (6) benchmarking of centers against overall data from such registries is useful to improve quality care.

This consensus report represents baseline agreement on respiratory definitions and care, and it is likely that further refinement of recommendations will occur over time.

Physiology of Extracorporeal Life Support: Gas Exchange and Oxygen Delivery

Oxygenation

The difference between the PO_2 in the gas supplied to the oxygenator and that in the patient's systemic venous blood provides the driving pressure across the membrane lung. As an example, 30% of oxygen blended into the gas entering the oxygenator will result in an estimated PAO_2 of about 228 torr at sea level. The PO_2 of venous blood entering the oxygenator depends on the difference between oxygen delivery and consumption in the patient, but it is usually about 40 torr. The driving pressure for oxygen diffusion into the blood thus would be approximately 188 torr (228 torr − 40 torr = 188 torr), which is adequate to achieve 100% saturation of hemoglobin. Higher oxygen concentrations in the gas phase may be necessary to compensate for loss of membrane surface area over time to maintain hemoglobin saturation. Faster flows through the oxygenator may also decrease the time for gas exchange to occur. At postoxygenator oxygen saturations greater than 95%, increasing the oxygen concentration of the sweep gas has little incremental effect on blood oxygen content. For this reason, oxygen concentration in sweep gas usually is adjusted to maintain an oxygen saturation of approximately 95% in postoxygenator blood.

Carbon Dioxide Exchange

Even though the pressure gradient for carbon dioxide between venous blood and membrane gas is less than that for oxygen, carbon dioxide removal is excellent across the membrane lung. Despite the small pressure difference, the membrane's high diffusion coefficient for carbon dioxide allows excellent carbon dioxide removal, even at low flow rates. To eliminate more carbon dioxide, the gas flow in the membrane must be increased, much as alveolar ventilation must increase to eliminate carbon dioxide from the body under physiologic conditions. Carbon dioxide removal is also limited by the surface area across which gas exchange can occur. Thus increased carbon dioxide clearance may be obtained by using larger oxygenators or using more than one oxygenator in parallel in the circuit. Conversely, to prevent excessive CO_2 removal and hypocapnia in small infants and neonates, the sweep of gas through the membrane lung can be reduced or low levels of carbon dioxide may be blended into the gas mixture to further reduce the partial pressure difference between blood and gas and maintain normocarbia.

Oxygen Delivery

During venoarterial ECMO, both increasing oxygen delivery and increasing the patient's PaO_2 and arterial saturation can be accomplished by increasing the ECMO flow rate. This strategy diverts more of the systemic venous return into the ECMO circuit for oxygenation while at the same time proportionally decreasing the amount of venous blood that enters the diseased pulmonary circuit. Studies have suggested that complete bypass of the pulmonary circuit may lead to pulmonary alkalosis or ischemia and cause direct damage of the pulmonary capillary bed. Microsphere studies have shown that most coronary artery perfusion during venoarterial ECMO comes from native left heart ejection, which is another reason why ECMO is performed in a *partial* bypass state.[104,105] The result of increasing ECMO flow will be an increase in oxygen delivery provided by the circuit and an elevation in measured systemic arterial saturation and PaO_2. Another means to change the proportion of native blood flow to that from the ECMO circuit is to decrease the overall blood volume in the patient. During cardiopulmonary bypass, filling pressures and overall blood volume can be adjusted by removal of blood volume into the bypass circuit. Circulating volume is also frequently decreased by modified ultrafiltration. During ECMO, these same principles can be followed: Excessively high filling pressures can be lowered by simply removing blood volume from the circuit, and diuretics and renal replacement strategies can be used to control fluid balance. Care must be taken, however, to avoid decreasing circulating volume excessively, because this may in turn cause tissue hypoperfusion or an increase in oxygen extraction.

Cardiac output can be altered during ECMO by increasing or decreasing the amount of blood diverted from the patient to the ECMO circuit. As blood returning from the ECMO circuit is already highly saturated with oxygen, oxygen content can be augmented primarily by increasing hemoglobin levels in the patient. Oxygen delivery supplied by the ECMO circuit can be calculated by pump flow as the surrogate for cardiac output and oxygen content by hemoglobin and

postmembrane lung oxygen saturation. Determining the amount of oxygen delivery supplied by the native heart is less clearly calculated. Monitoring of adequate oxygen delivery is aided by following venous saturation. Low venous saturation and other markers such as elevated lactate, poor perfusion, decreased urine output, and mental status changes may indicate the need for improved oxygen delivery. If ECMO flow cannot be increased to provide adequate support, an additional drainage cannula to augment ECMO flow and allow increased support may be needed.

In patients who undergo cannulation via the venovenous route, reduced systemic oxygenation will be observed compared with patients with venoarterial ECMO. This reduced systemic oxygenation is a result of the lower amount of native cardiac output that can be delivered to the circuit, as less native blood can be drained with venovenous cannulation. Several features unique to venovenous cannulation are important to understand. First, because blood is both withdrawn and reinfused into the venous circulation, adequate native cardiac function must exist to provide the "pumping" of oxygenated ECMO return to the patient's systemic circulation. One factor that may influence cardiac function during venovenous ECMO is that well-oxygenated blood returning from the ECMO circuit will enter the right heart. This highly oxygenated blood may reduce pulmonary artery pressure by reducing pulmonary vascular resistance, which may in turn improve right heart function. Likewise, highly saturated blood returning to the left ventricle and pumped to the coronary arteries may improve myocardial blood flow and improve cardiac performance. For these reasons, some clinicians will initiate venovenous ECMO even in patients with cardiac dysfunction and transition to venoarterial ECMO if support is inadequate. Other clinicians prefer to use venoarterial ECMO preferentially if cardiac dysfunction exists. Of note, 30% of children with vasoactive requirements prior to ECMO tolerated venovenous ECMO well in one report.[20]

Another feature of venovenous ECMO is that because blood is withdrawn and reinfused into the venous side of the circulation, some portion of oxygenated blood is likely to be lost into the venous drainage cannula prior to entering the systemic arterial circulation.[33] This phenomenon is known as *recirculation*, and it can be a major limiting factor in providing adequate patient support with venovenous ECMO. With double-lumen cannulas placed via the right IJ vein to the right atrium, careful orientation of the inflow lumen toward the tricuspid valve may limit recirculation. The larger separation of drainage and inflow lumens with the Avalon device seems to be associated with fewer recirculation difficulties than occurs with prior double-lumen cannulas (Fig. 59.6).

With two-site venous cannulation, recirculation can be limited to some degree by ensuring that some distance separates the end tips of the drainage and infusion cannulas in the body. Recirculation also can be reduced by draining from the femoral vein cannula and reinfusing into the right IJ vein cannula. The extent of recirculation can be estimated by following the venous saturation in the ECLS circuit; high levels of recirculation will elevate the displayed venous saturation on the drainage line because some of the highly saturated return from the ECLS circuit is immediately drawn out by the drainage cannula. Following adequacy of oxygen delivery in the patient by means of hemodynamic stability, measures of acid-base balance (lactate) and clinical measures of adequate

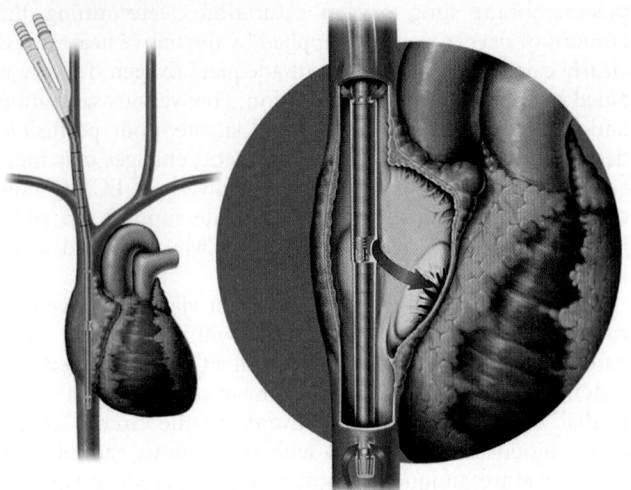

Fig. 59.6. Avalon cannula. (Reproduced from Maquet, Inc., with permission.)

perfusion and oxygenation are required. Whether venovenous cannulation will provide adequate capture of the patient's cardiac output for ECMO support depends on how large the cannulas are, where they lie in the vessel, and how much overall ECMO support the patient requires.

New venovenous cannulas and placement strategies may limit recirculation, but it is unlikely that it can be prevented totally. Persistent signs of inadequate oxygen delivery or continued hemodynamic instability with venovenous ECMO may require conversion to venoarterial ECMO. One indication of recirculation is high measured venous saturations in the ECMO circuit because of mixing of well-oxygenated blood with systemic venous return. Unlike venoarterial ECMO, decreasing the flow rate of blood in this circumstance may decrease the amount of recirculation that is being observed and improve oxygen delivery to the patient. Monitoring venous saturations from another site in the body may be helpful to monitor adequacy of support in this circumstance.

One novel means of improving oxygenation to the head and upper body in patients who have undergone venovenous cannulation through the bilateral femoral veins is to add an additional venous cannula via the right IJ vein to the right atrium. Connecting this cannula to the inflow return side of the ECMO circuit will increase the amount of oxygenated bypass directly returning to the right heart. This procedure may improve overall oxygen delivery to the patient while still avoiding the need for arterial vessel cannulation.

Loose occlusion of the roller heads against the raceway tubing also can lead to less blood being propelled forward through the ECMO circuit and reduce systemic oxygen delivery. In centrifugal pumps, low head revolutions also can result in inadequate forward flow of blood to the patient, and if the patient's arterial blood pressure is higher than that generated within the centrifugal circuit, arterial blood can flow from the patient into the centrifugal circuit. Some circuits contain a one-way valve in the circuit, which prevents backflow. Increasing the revolutions per minute in the pump head will reverse this problem. Persistent vasodilation, which occurs in patients with sepsis, may require the administration of low levels of vasoconstricting agents to maintain adequate central venous

pressures and adequate pump return without massive fluid administration.

Patient Management

Infants who are candidates for ECMO should undergo cranial ultrasonography, if time allows, to identify existing intracranial hemorrhage (ICH) prior to ECMO initiation. Although ICH greater than that confined to the germinal matrix (grade I) has been a contraindication to ECMO in the past, concerns with expansion of existing lesions due to anticoagulation have lessened and successful ECMO with good neurologic outcome has occurred even with infants with larger ICH. Standard care is the performance of repetitive ultrasounds or computed tomography examinations if concerns of intracranial pathology exist and to monitor the extension of known lesions. In many patients, emergent initiation of ECMO precludes any imaging procedures, and clinical neurologic evaluation may be hampered by ongoing sedation or neuromuscular blockade. Older patients may receive computed tomography prior to ECMO if time and patient status allow.

The decision to treat a patient with ECMO is made on the best assessment of neurologic function. Once hemodynamic and gas exchange have been stabilized with ECMO, more informative neurologic testing or examination can be performed. If the patient has evidence of neurologic devastation, then support can be withdrawn.

Echocardiography is usually performed prior to institution of ECMO in infants to determine if hypoxia is a result of structural defects in the heart, which may be better served by surgical repair than by ECMO support. Echocardiography also can identify ventricular dysfunction, pulmonary hypertension, and pericardial effusions; these data are useful to properly manage the patient and to select the optimal form of ECMO or elect less invasive procedures if warranted. ECHO also is used to detect the presence and direction of central shunts within the cardiac system.

Other useful pre-ECMO considerations are to determine where cannulation is optimal to ensure that those vessels are patent by ultrasound and to ensure that planned vascular access is not already in use with an indwelling venous or arterial line. Movement of indwelling catheters to an alternative site in this circumstance should be carried out prior to ECMO if time allows. In patients with a history of repetitive surgical procedures or central line insertions, evaluation of vessel patency at the bedside or from a review of the patient record can be helpful. Information on patients who are critically ill and in whom ECMO *should* or *should not* be considered is useful for the clinical team to include in handoffs. This can avoid confusion in an emergent situation. Consider informing the family if it is deemed that their child is *not* an ECMO candidate and discuss the rationale.[95]

Laboratory measures of blood and platelet counts, electrolyte levels, and coagulation are included in data collection as ECMO is being planned. Correction of existing coagulopathy by infusions of plasma, cryoprecipitate, or platelets may be helpful to prevent early bleeding and to correct baseline dysfunction.

Cannulation and Initiation of Extracorporeal Life Support

Cannulation is usually performed at the bedside, with the patient receiving a combination of local anesthetics and intravenous analgesics, sedatives, and neuromuscular blocking drugs. An initial bolus of heparin (usually 50 to 100 units per kg) and continued heparin infusion ensure systemic anticoagulation for the duration of ECMO. Activated clotting time, measured at the bedside, provides a gauge for adjusting the heparin dose to avoid either catastrophic clotting in the circuit or bleeding complications. The ECMO flow is initiated at 50 mL/kg/min and is increased in 50- to 100-mL increments. In infants, a rate of 100 to 200 mL/kg/min usually provides adequate perfusion and oxygenation, although patients in a state of high cardiac output, such as sepsis, may require a higher rate. Use of high-flow ECMO also is recommended in patients with single ventricle physiology and a systemic-to-pulmonary artery shunt to provide adequate circulation for both systemic and pulmonary organs. Pediatric patients usually require about 90 mL/kg/min of ECMO flow to maintain adequate oxygen delivery, and adult patients require rates of 50 to 70 mL/kg/min. Estimates of flow needs also can be predicted by using cardiac index data based on body surface area (BSA). One caution in estimating ECMO flow in this manner is that patients with sepsis or multiple organ dysfunctions may require flows that are much higher than predicted. These factors must be taken into account when selecting cannula size, as larger cannulas than that predicted by BSA may be required. In venoarterial ECMO, the arterial waveform provides a rough estimation of the degree of bypass provided by the ECMO circuit. ECMO is provided in *partial* bypass form, as total bypass of the pulmonary circuit has been associated with pulmonary ischemia.[106,107] Because ECMO flow is nonpulsatile, increasing flow and decreasing left ventricular output will result in a flattening of the arterial wave contour and a narrowing of the pulse pressure. Severe myocardial dysfunction also may cause a flattened wave contour because left ventricular output may be minimal. This effect must be kept in mind when waveform contour is used to monitor the extent of bypass.

Priming

Priming of the ECMO circuit prior to initiation is accomplished with a crystalloid solution that is then replaced with blood. Because required blood usually has been citrated and stored, it may be acidotic, depleted of calcium, and have a high potassium level. Calcium (usually as calcium chloride), bicarbonate or tromethamine, and heparin are added during the priming procedure. Electrolytes should be measured in the priming blood before bypass is initiated, because disturbances of cardiac rhythm or frank cardiac arrest can occur upon initiation of ECMO. Hyperkalemia exists almost universally in the ECMO primed circuit despite buffering by calcium and bicarbonate. The potassium level rarely causes systemic effects once the ECMO prime is diluted with the patient's intrinsic blood volume. As an example, if a neonatal patient with a blood volume similar to that of the ECMO circuit has a potassium level of three and the ECMO prime has a potassium level of seven, the circulating potassium level may be around five upon ECMO initiation. This scenario is unlikely to cause systemic or cardiac effects. Larger patients having blood volumes much greater than that of the ECMO circuit will have less risk of hyperkalemia or hypocalcemia. Use of the freshest blood available also may lessen the degree of hyperkalemia in the primed circuit. Rarely, hyperkalemia may be of such concern that blood must be washed prior to ECMO use or filtered via a hemofiltration device in the ECMO circuit to reduce the potassium level. Newer centrifugal/hollow fiber systems have a priming volume much lower (<400 cc) than with older roller-pump/silicone lung configurations.

Patient Management During Extracorporeal Life Support

Hypovolemia causes low central venous pressures and results in decreased venous return to the circuit. This situation can be corrected easily with fluid administration. Oxygen delivery also can be raised by increasing the pump flow rate, which increases blood diverted into the ECMO circuit for oxygenation. Anemia can be corrected with transfusion of blood products.[108,109] Hemoglobin must be maintained to sustain adequate oxygen content. Clinicians disagree about the level of hemoglobin needed during ECMO, but the current trend to accept lower levels of hemoglobin in critically ill patients is also followed in ECMO patients, with most centers delaying routine transfusion until the hemoglobin is 10 g/dL or even lower if the patient seems to be doing well. The needs of the patient and the risks of transfusion are a balance that the clinical team assesses on an ongoing basis.

Whatever level of hemoglobin is chosen for "routine" patient management, an intermittent administration of packed red blood cells to maintain adequate blood volume and hematocrit will be required. Fresh frozen plasma also may be given intermittently to provide adequate clotting factors and help prevent excessive bleeding. Platelet sequestration in the ECMO circuit is a constant problem. Historically, platelet counts of 80,000 to 100,000/mm^3 have been maintained routinely for patients undergoing ECMO to deter bleeding, but multiple examples now exist of patients undergoing ECMO with thrombocytopenia of 30,000/mm^3 or lower and in whom massive bleeding was not a problem. Although patients often require frequent platelet transfusions, the capacity of transfusions to increase platelet counts to high levels may be limited in some patients, such as those with cancer. In these patients, lower platelet counts may be allowed and careful monitoring for bleeding is maintained.

Another problem with ECMO, especially for prolonged runs, is heparin-induced thrombocytopenia (HIT). HIT should be suspected in any patient receiving heparin when a drop in platelet count occurs that is unresponsive to platelet transfusion or when the platelet count continues to fall without an identified reason. Although HIT usually develops 5 to 15 days after the initial exposure to heparin, it can occur immediately in patients with previous exposure to heparin, such as patients who have undergone cardiac surgery. HIT associated with immune response to heparin can result in severe thrombocytopenia. The only "cure" is to stop the patient from being exposed to heparin. During ECMO, stopping exposure to heparin necessitates the use of other anticoagulation methods. Currently, lepirudin, biliverdin, and argatroban are alternatives that have been commented on with regard to ECMO, although these treatments are not widely used in the pediatric population in general.

Despite advances in technology, anticoagulation is needed to prevent clotting of the extracorporeal circuit. Heparin remains the mainstay for anticoagulation, but the optimal management scheme to prevent thrombosis without causing bleeding remains elusive. Although the activated clotting time (ACT) remains the most common method for monitoring heparin and anticoagulation, as an improved understanding of the coagulation cascade and the means to measure factors within it have occurred, other regimens now include the anti-Xa level, antithrombin, specific factor analyses, and thromboelastography. No algorithm has proved superior to another in terms of limiting complications or improving outcomes. It is important to understand the pros and cons of each test in terms of the blood volume required for testing, accuracy, and cost. As one example, the use of antithrombin, a protease inhibitor that inactivates factor Xa and thrombin and has markedly enhanced action in the presence of heparin, has increased 9.5-fold to use in over 52% of ECMO patients, despite no evidence it decreases complications or even identifies the correct dose in children. In a similar fashion, anti-Xa measurement, which gives a more direct assessment of heparin level than the whole-blood ACT test, is also used frequently. Although it is not shown to be superior to ACT, it can be monitored intermittently at intervals less than the usual every hour for ACT. Thromboelastography, a technique which produces a visual picture that gives information on the degree of anticoagulation induced by heparin and other information regarding coagulation and platelet defects, is also being used more as new technology makes it easier to perform. Hopefully continued research in this area will yield an optimal anticoagulation regimen that will reduce bleeding and thrombotic complications.[106-110]

Adequate nutrition is essential for healing and is provided as total parenteral nutrition, enteral feeding, or a combination of both. Enteral feeding has been shown to be safe and effective during ECMO in all groups of patients and may limit the need for total parenteral nutrition with its associated complications.[111,112]

Maintaining strict fluid balance in critically ill patients is popular, and patients undergoing ECMO are no exception. The use of diuretics, concentrated drug infusions, and hemofiltration in patients with renal insufficiency is another important aspect of patient care. Renal failure, hypervolemia, and fluid overload are frequently seen in patients undergoing ECMO. The use of continuous renal replacement therapies (CRRTs) has become commonplace during ECMO, to maintain fluid balance, support failing kidneys, and potentially clear "bad humors" from the blood. One of the proposed mechanisms for the development of acute renal failure (ARF) in patients undergoing ECMO is a reduction in the pulsatile character of renal perfusion. Circuit-associated hemolysis in patients receiving CRRT also can perpetuate ARF. Techniques for providing CRRT are to connect a hemofiltration filter into the ECMO circuit and to control the ultrafiltrate volume using an intravenous infusion pump or approved continuous renal replacement systems. Patients receiving CRRT during ECMO have decreased survival, but this is also true in CRRT recipients who do not undergo ECMO. Few survivors have long-term renal failure. One single-center review of 154 ECMO patients who received CRRT found that (1) neonates and pediatric patients had longer ECMO runs than those who did not (248 h versus 97 h neonates, p <0.0001; 211 h versus 173 h, p = 0.026); (2) continuous venovenous hemofiltration (CVVH) use increased from 17% (1997-1999) to 59% (2005-2007); and (3) patients receiving CRRT during ECMO had reduced survival compared to those who did not receive CRRT (88% versus 44%, p <0.0001)[110-117]

Another study that examined acute renal failure in patients who were undergoing ECMO and required CRRT noted that

ARF was present in 70% of patients and CRRT was initiated in 58% of patients. The study concluded that the odds of developing ARF increased with duration of ECMO support. Patients undergoing ECMO in whom ARF developed had a 4.7-fold increase in the odds of in-hospital mortality.

One abstract noted that CRRT with CVVH was used in 27 (32%) of 84 pediatric patients undergoing ECMO, usually to maintain fluid balance. Overall survival was 75% for patients with respiratory failure. Of these 84 patients, 27 were matched for age, diagnosis, and PRISM III score with patients undergoing ECMO who did not receive CVVH. Improved fluid balance over time, less use of diuretics, and the tendency to reach caloric-intake goals more quickly were noted in patients undergoing renal replacement. No difference was found in survival (67% CVVH, 82% non-CVVH, p = .352), duration of ventilation after ECMO, or the need for potassium supplementation between groups. Data from the ELSO registry show that about 30% of pediatric and adult patients undergoing ECMO undergo renal replacement either by hemofiltration or dialysis, although elevations of creatinine greater than 1.5 were reported in only 15% of pediatric patients. Other adjunct extracorporeal therapies such as plasmapheresis or liver support systems also have been used successfully during ECMO.

The optimal ventilatory management for patients undergoing ECMO is not known, and each center may have its own preference for how to treat the lungs during ECMO.[118-120] Minimizing further barotrauma or oxygen toxicity and providing an environment that promotes lung healing are basic goals. For neonatal patients undergoing venoarterial ECMO, most centers use ventilator settings with low peak inspiratory pressure (PIP) (25 to 30 cm H_2O), PEEP (5 cm H_2O), intermittent mandatory ventilation rate (6 to 12 breaths/min), and fraction of inspired oxygen (FiO_2, 0.21–0.30). Lung volume decreases dramatically with such settings in most patients undergoing ECMO, resulting in generalized opacification on the chest radiograph. Maintaining lung expansion and functional residual capacity with higher levels of PEEP (10 to 15 cm H_2O) was associated with shorter ECMO durations in one neonatal study, and this approach is used frequently at many centers. In older patients, use of PEEP with reduced peak airway pressures, low ventilator rates, and low concentrations of inspired oxygen is also the predominant method of support. Commonly, PEEP levels in the range of 5 to 15 cm H_2O, plateau pressures of no more than 25 to 30 cm H_2O, and breath rates of 10 to 12 with inspired oxygen concentrations between 30% and 40% are reported in the pediatric and adult ECMO literature. Spontaneous breathing and even removal of the endotracheal tube or early bedside tracheostomy are gaining popularity as clinicians become more comfortable with allowing their patients on ECMO to be awake and alert. Proponents of spontaneous breathing point out that the natural course of healing in acute respiratory distress syndrome (ARDS) is about 6 weeks, and during the fibroproliferative phase, unmeasurable tidal volumes during ECMO may be unmeasurable for weeks. Thus trying to open these consolidated lungs may create more harm than merely letting these patients recover lung expansion on their own. Bronchoscopy can safely provide intermittent evaluation to remove inspissated secretions or identify airway issues. Computed tomography can also be useful to identify lung pathology. In patients who show no signs of improvement over many weeks or who are being considered for removal from ECMO for futility, lung biopsy may prove useful. Although inherent risks from bleeding exist with biopsy, results can prove useful.[121,122]

Patients with barotrauma and persistent air leaks even at low distending airway pressures on ECMO are among those who may benefit the most from removal from ventilator support or a spontaneous breathing mode. Often, healing of ruptured parenchyma can occur within 48 to 72 hours.

At high flow rates in patients undergoing venoarterial ECMO, a minimal amount of blood is entering the pulmonary circuit. Manipulating ventilator settings, especially in patients with diseased lungs with impaired gas exchange, has little effect on blood gas tensions. Oxygenation and carbon dioxide elimination depend on the function of the ECMO circuit. With venovenous cannulation, less overall bypass is obtained, and the systemic oxygenation provided by ECLS is less than with venoarterial access. Arterial oxygen saturations are thus lower with venovenous support. Although the majority of patients do well with saturations in the 75% to 85% range, monitoring of adequate oxygen delivery by following lactate, venous saturation, urine output, metabolic acid-base balance, and mental status is recommended with these patients.

As the lungs heal, compliance and tidal volume increase. Radiograph of the lung fields gradually improves from atelectatic opacification to increasing lung aeration. Increasing the oxygenation and concentration of expired carbon dioxide also heralds improved alveolar/capillary gas exchange. Evidence of decreasing pulmonary artery pressure (indicated by resolution of right-to-left intracardiac shunting or other echocardiographic information) may also signal that the patient is ready to be weaned from ECMO.

Maintaining patient comfort during ECMO can be a challenge, especially during prolonged ECMO runs. Routine medications such as morphine, fentanyl, midazolam, lorazepam, and other agents provide sedation and analgesia. Medications are known to be absorbed by the membrane lung, although the extent of changes with the newer systems in use today is unclear.[122-125] Patients can also become tolerant to sedatives over time. Drug dependence and withdrawal symptoms become major adverse events and prolong hospital stays in many ECMO survivors. Although anesthesia gas in the membrane oxygenator was used in the silicone lung, hollow fiber membranes are not appropriate for this use, as the gas may pass easily through the device into the room atmosphere. Alpha-2 agonists such as dexmedetomidine have also proved useful to decrease narcotic or benzodiazepine requirements. Multiple reports from European centers on the success of maintaining ECMO patients in an awake state have started a new era of ECMO care. Patient management now promotes maintaining ECMO patients in an awake, alert, and even mobile state to sustain muscle strength and tone. Rehabilitation while on ECMO is especially needed for patients who are bridging to lung or heart transplant. Nursing and family support play a major role in the success of providing ECMO with little sedation.[126]

Weaning From Extracorporeal Membrane Oxygenation

A patient can be weaned from ECMO in several ways.[127,128] The most common venoarterial mode of weaning involves reducing the ECMO flow rate in set increments every 1 to 2 hours,

provided that arterial and mixed venous oxygen saturations remain adequate. Once ECMO flow is reduced to provide only about two-thirds of cardiac output, ventilator support is increased (PIP 20 to 30 cm H_2O, intermittent mechanical ventilation 20–30, PEEP 5 cm H_2O, and FiO_2 30% to 40%). Weaning continues to an ECMO flow of 50 to 100 mL/min in infants or an estimated 10% of cardiac output. If the patient remains physiologically stable with acceptable blood gas tensions at this low flow, the ECMO cannulas are clamped and the infant is observed while off ECMO support for a short time. If respiration and circulation remain stable during the trial, the cannulas are removed and conventional therapy is resumed. Quicker weaning methods involve decreasing ECMO flow in larger increments over shorter periods, similar to the way it is performed during cardiopulmonary bypass in the operating room. For venovenous patients with respiratory failure, FiO_2 to the membrane lung and sweep gas should be decreased to the point where the oxygenator is capped off to allow no gas exchange and to ensure that the native lung can provide adequate oxygenation and ventilation. Although some clinicians also reduce ECMO pump flow during venovenous weaning, it is not necessary to wean flow excessively or clamp a patient off ECMO, as blood flow is already following the native circulation and the heart is providing the pumping to the body.

Decannulation

Decannulation involves removal of surgically placed cannulas and repair of the operative site, with or without vessel repair. Vessels used in traditional, open venotomy or arteriotomy ECMO often can be repaired at decannulation, although this approach is not used universally. Whether avoiding ligation or repairing cannulated vessels results in long-term improvement in blood flow or reduced risk of stroke from thrombosis or infarct is unknown. The longest follow-up study of repaired carotid vessels found restenosis or occlusion in 24%. Patients with reconstructed vessels had fewer neuroradiologic abnormalities and a smaller incidence of cerebral palsy than did unrepaired historical control subjects, although these data represent a small, single-center report and are not the result of a randomized study. Femoral vessels are sometimes accessed via a Gore-Tex or similar graft sewn into the side of the vessel. This graft is tied off at decannulation.

Percutaneously placed cannulas are merely withdrawn at decannulation while gentle pressure is applied to the site until hemostasis is obtained. Vessels accessed percutaneously are not usually ligated either at initiation or decannulation from ECMO. Femoral artery repair often is performed to ensure continued integrity of the vessel and limb perfusion.

Heparin is discontinued at decannulation, and normalization of coagulation usually occurs within a few hours. Protamine is rarely used for the reversal of heparin-induced coagulation effects at decannulation. Venous thrombosis may develop after ECLS has been discontinued, especially if femoral cannulation is used, which may be an additional reason why heparinization should not be reversed. Many clinicians favor some form of anticoagulation or antiplatelet medication following decannulation, especially in adult patients.

Complications

Complications that occur during ECMO can be mechanical or related to the particular patient.

Bleeding

Bleeding as a result of the systemic heparinization required with ECMO is the major complication associated with ECMO.[129-136] Whereas bleeding occurs predominantly from cannulation or surgical sites, intracranial hemorrhage is the most dreaded site for bleeding to occur. Intracranial bleeding occurs in approximately 11% of patients overall, with the rate highest in the neonatal patient and lowest in the adult population. Bleeding that occurs outside of the head that cannot be controlled with medical means requires surgical investigation. Although obvious risks accompany surgical intervention in a bleeding patient who has undergone systemic anticoagulation, many operative repairs have been accomplished during ECMO support. Initial attempts to control bleeding focus on decreasing the rate of heparin infusion and lowering activated clotting time levels. Limitation of heparin may put the circuit at risk for increased clotting, especially at lower flow levels. This risk must be balanced against the bleeding risk.

Medications to help prevent clot breakdown in the patient also are used. Historically, aminocaproic acid, also known by the trade name Amicar, has been the predominant medication used during ECMO. An antifibrinolytic amino acid, Amicar, displaces plasminogen from fibrin and inhibits clot breakdown. Although one survey found that a wide range of doses are used, one common algorithm follows a dosage scheme of 100 mg/kg as a load followed by an infusion of 25 to 50 mg/kg/h. Although it has been used in ECMO centers for many years, a randomized controlled trial of Amicar versus placebo in neonates found no difference between groups in the need for transfusion or the need for circuit changes due to thrombosis.[131] Aprotinin has also been used to prevent or limit bleeding. A serine protease inhibitor, aprotinin is an antifibrinolytic agent that inhibits protein C and factors Va and VIIIa in the extrinsic coagulation pathway and inhibits the intrinsic pathway as well. It also preserves platelet function, reduces vascular permeability, and has been suggested to decrease the inflammatory response to cardiopulmonary bypass. Aprotinin has not been compared in a randomized fashion to Amicar or placebo during ECMO. Aprotinin is administered as a loading dose of 10,000 units/kg and is continued at an infusion rate of 10,000 units/kg/h. Reports in adult patients of an increase in renal failure and poor outcome in cardiac patients receiving aprotinin during bypass surgery have caused it to be removed from the market. Ongoing studies showing its potential anti-inflammatory properties are causing some discussion as to its return to the market. Circuit thromboses may be noted with use of Amicar or aprotinin.[132]

Several reports of intractable bleeding on ECMO have commented on the benefits of factor VIIa, although the data regarding this medication are still too sparse to recommend it without further investigation. In one study, use of factor VIIa was noted to be effective in decreasing chest tube bleeding from 47 to 10 mL/kg/h in four patients with refractory hemorrhage.[133-135] Each patient received two doses of R factor VIIa (dose, 90 to 120 µg/kg) 4 hours apart. In another report, 92% of patients undergoing ECMO with bleeding responded to R factor VIIa therapy. A significant reduction in chest tube bleeding was noted, along with a significant reduction in the administration of blood products. Major thrombosis was noted in two of the patients who received R factor VIIa therapy.

Other centers have reported decreased bleeding with lower doses of R factor VIIa administration; they have administered 40 µg/kg and then increased the dose to 90 µg if bleeding continued. Anecdotal reports of thrombosis with factor VIIa are more frequent than those found in the literature, and thus careful assessment of the risks and benefits should be undertaken prior to factor VIIa use.

Use of antithrombin (AT) during ECMO has also become popular. An increase in off-label use of AT in children of 200%, almost exclusively in patients receiving ECMO, was noted in one report. Although physiologically, replenishment of abnormally low AT levels may make sense, there are few data to show this is effective in limiting bleeding, thrombosis, limiting heparin exposure, or changing outcome, except in small single-center reports. The expense of this medication is also an important factor to consider.

Discontinuation of heparin to help control intractable bleeding also can be beneficial and has been used for variable periods, up to 36 hours or more, without significant clotting in the ECMO circuit. Larger patients with faster ECMO flow rates are more likely to tolerate discontinuation of heparin without significant clotting.[136] However, it is wise to have a backup circuit readily available if clotting does occur and the ECMO system requires an emergent replacement.

Infection

Infection is another potential complication of ECMO.[137-140] Colonization of indwelling catheters, selective adherence of bacteria to polyurethane surfaces, sequestration of bacteria from the body's normal antibody and phagocytic defense mechanisms, and the patient's prior debilitated state are all factors that may increase the risk of infection. Successful therapy may be difficult without eliminating invasive equipment, most significantly the ECMO catheters. Viral infection from blood transfusions may occur rarely. Although sepsis (which was either preexisting or developed as the patient underwent ECMO) was once seen as a reason to exclude patients from ECMO, support for severe septic shock is now common. The most recent guidelines for hemodynamic support of pediatric patients with septic shock note that ECMO should be considered in patients with refractory catecholamine-resistant shock.[140]

Long-Term Outcome

As increasing numbers of critically ill neonates and children survive, attention should be directed to resultant morbidity. Although some studies have been published, most have involved venoarterial neonatal ECMO survivors and few have focused on long-term multidisciplinary evaluations.[142-154]

Medical Outcomes

Despite the fact that severe respiratory failure is the most common indication for ECMO in the neonatal period, airflow obstruction in school-age and adolescent survivors is usually mild.[154] Patients with congenital diaphragmatic hernia (CDH) are a subgroup in which lung function seems to deteriorate as children get older.[161] Risk factors for persistent airflow obstruction after neonatal ECMO are a diagnosis of respiratory distress syndrome, CDH, prolonged duration of ECMO treatment, and chronic lung disease.[154,161,163,164] Sensorineural hearing loss (SNHL) is another physical problem that has been reported in neonatal ECMO survivors. Its prevalence varies among different studies,[150] and risk factors seem to be related to neonatal intensive care treatment such as use of aminoglycosides, neuromuscular blocking agents, and loop diuretics rather than the ECMO treatment itself. In a group of 169 neonatal ECMO survivors (both with and without acute kidney injury), proteinuria as at least one sign of chronic kidney disease or hypertension was observed in 54 children (32%) at a mean age of 8 years.[166]

Neurodevelopmental Outcomes

The greatest burden affecting quality of life and participation in society seems to arise from neurodevelopmental morbidity. This remains an understudied area.

When evaluating the results of different studies on neurodevelopmental outcome, it should be noted that standardized assessments cannot be performed in children with severe disabilities. In general, 5% to 10% of ECMO survivors are unable to fulfill validated assessments that compare developmental outcome with that of healthy peers.

Data on motor function performance after neonatal ECMO are scarce, but problems in this domain occur in approximately 40% of children of preschool age. Most problems are seen with gross motor function. Deterioration of motor function performance has been shown in a longitudinal evaluation: The proportion of children with normal motor function performance declined from 73.7% at 5 years to 40.5% at 12 years.[163] Children with low parental socioeconomic status, those with intracranial abnormalities, and those who need prolonged initial hospitalization are at risk for motor function problems at a later age.

Despite an overall average cognition, however, many children (up to 50%) have special educational needs. Observed problems in neonatal ECMO survivors revealed that at school age children have problems with working speed, memory, impaired visual-spatial abilities, and sustained attention and concentration. Having intracranial abnormalities prior to or during ECMO treatment and severity of critical illness seem to be determinants of neuropsychologic outcome, although standardized and validated scores to express illness severity are currently lacking.[154]

Neonatal ECMO survivors may be at risk for neuropsychologic problems later in life due to impaired development of executive functioning skills, which are developed in early childhood and continue development into young adulthood. These skills are needed to develop academic, behavioral, and social functioning and to prepare for successful daily functioning (eg, starting a career).

Of 4000 pediatric respiratory ECMO patients listed in the registry through July 2009, 9% had intracranial infarct or hemorrhage found on computed tomography examination. Brain death occurred in 6% of the patients, and 6% of patients had reported seizures. Long-term neurologic outcome data are sorely missing in the pediatric population. Few centers maintain regular follow-up clinics, and patients often are referred for ECMO from distant sites, which makes follow-up difficult as well. In one report of 15 pediatric and four adult patients, 58% survived to discharge. Patients were evaluated with use of the Pediatric Cerebral Performance Category (which measures cognitive impairment) and the Pediatric Overall Performance Category (which measures functional morbidity). Overall, 64% of survivors had normal Pediatric Cerebral Performance Category scores, 27% had

mild disabilities, and 9% had moderate cognitive disability. Functional morbidity was normal in 27%, whereas 45% had mild disability, 18% had moderate disability, and 9% were severely disabled. In another small series of 26 patients monitored 1 to 3 years after ECMO, 38% of preschool-age children were described as normal and 31% had observed abnormalities. Four patients (31%) who had prior neurologic dysfunction remained at baseline following ECMO. Among school-age children, 77% were described as normal by parental report. More specific neurologic follow-up in the pediatric age groups is needed.

In a review of patients undergoing cardiac ECMO at <5 years of age who were evaluated 2 years later, a mental score of 73 +/−16 (normal 100 +/−15) was noted, with eight patients (50%) having mental delay. Lactate on admission to the PICU and single ventricle anatomy were associated with death. Time for lactate to normalize on ECMO, inotrope score at 120 hours of support, and chromosomal abnormality accounted for 77% of the variance in mental score when evaluated by stepwise multiple regression. In another report of neonates who received venoarterial ECMO and were tested at 5 years of age, normal development in all domains was noted in only 49%, although severe disability was only found in 13%. Patients with underlying congenital diaphragmatic hernia had the worst outcomes.[171]

Neurologic complications in cardiac patients who undergo ECMO parallel those of patients who have respiratory failure.[172,173] Brain death occurred in 4% of patients, 3% had intracranial infarct, and 6% had intracranial hemorrhage. Because many cardiac patients are in a state of prolonged low cardiac output or sudden cardiac arrest prior to ECMO, the ability to assess neurologic function once ECMO is instituted is vital. Paralysis and sedation should be minimized until a neurologic examination can occur. This information is especially important in patients who are being listed for transplantation to avoid transplanting a viable organ into an inappropriate recipient.

Implications

Because motor function problems deteriorate over time and problems with executive functioning and academic achievement are usually seen at school age and later on, a question arises concerning whether ECMO survivors grow into their deficits. This question cannot be answered from the currently available literature, but prolonged follow-up addressing these issues is of utmost importance to optimize participation in society as ECMO survivors age into adulthood. A proposal for domains that should be addressed during follow-up of ECMO survivors is shown in Table 59.4. Whereas most outcome research has been performed on ECMO survivors who have received venoarterial ECMO cannulation, the impact of venovenous support (which is becoming more frequent in all age groups) on outcome requires further investigation. Additional development of this area is vital for evaluating the quality of life and cost/benefit of ECMO in pediatric patients, and similar issues with long-term outcome in adult ECMO survivors also exist.

The Future

Interhospital transport of patients, either those for ECMO consideration or those for whom ECMO was initiated at a non-ECMO facility, has become more available with the advent of smaller systems that are easier to transport. Currently only a few facilities routinely provide this service; however, ECMO transport companies are emerging that will allow movement from center to center as patient needs dictate. One single-center report found no statistical difference in survival rates in patients for whom ECMO was initiated in their center compared with patients who underwent cannulation at an outside facility and were brought to their center while receiving ECMO support. The typical transport team consisted of an ECMO coordinator, pediatric cardiac surgeon, surgical assistant, and intensivist. The predominant mode of transport was by helicopter (75%). No patient died during transport.[175] Whether the use of ECLS will grow and the need for ECMO transport capabilities throughout the United States will increase is unknown at this time. The logistics involved with maintaining a transport service requires meticulous planning and heavy resource use, and it is expensive to maintain unless the transport volume is high. This is one area where regionalization or contracting with an experienced team of ECMO providers for this service might prove practical.

The use of ECMO in the neonatal patients with respiratory failure has been accepted medical practice for many years, although improved care and management of these patients have reduced the need for ECMO in this population. The current extension of ECLS systems to older pediatric and adult patients in a variety of clinical settings highlights the changes that have occurred in the ECLS environment. Progress in renal replacement, liver support, and plasmapheresis and the development of new cardiac support devices applicable to pediatrics also may expand the use of ECMO or related techniques overall. Additionally, the development of small, portable systems for cardiopulmonary resuscitation may herald a new age of extracorporeal support. Technical advances in ECLS equipment continue to make such support safer and more efficient.[176] Venovenous ECMO techniques have been refined and used successfully in patients from neonatal to adult age groups. Single-cannula, double-lumen catheters for venovenous ECMO may obviate the risks of arterial cannulation and offer the benefit of requiring only one surgical site for venous access. Research and technologic improvements may decrease the need for systemic anticoagulation and the risk of hemorrhagic complications. Until the day when medical science may make the need for extracorporeal life support obsolete, research into ways to make it safer and more efficient should continue.

Key References

2. Hill JD, Gibbon JH Jr. Development of the first successful heart lung machine. *Ann Thorac Surg.* 1982;34:337.
8. Bartlett RH, Gazzaniga AB, Jeffries MR, et al. Extracorporeal membrane oxygenation (ECMO) cardiopulmonary support in infancy. *Trans Am Soc Artif Intern Organs.* 1976;22:80.
9. Short BL, Pearson GD. Neonatal extracorporeal membrane oxygenation: a review. *J Intensive Care Med.* 1986;1:48.
12. Extracorporeal Life Support Organization. *International ECMO registry report of the Extracorporeal Life Support Organization.* Ann Arbor, MI: Extracorporeal Life Support Organization; 2015.
14. Hämmäinen P, Scherstén H, Lemström K, et al. Usefulness of extracorporeal membrane oxygenation as a bridge to lung transplantation: a descriptive study. *J Heart Lung Transplant.* 2011;30:103-107.
19. Gow KW, et al. Extracorporeal life support for support of children with malignancy and respiratory or cardiac failure: the extracorporeal life support experience. *Crit Care Med.* 2009;37:1308-1316.
20. Pettignano R, Fortenberry JD, Heard ML, et al. Primary use of the venovenous approach for extracorporeal membrane oxygenation in pediatric acute respiratory failure. *Pediatr Crit Care Med.* 2003;4:291-298.
22. Pettignano R, Labuz M, Gauthier TW, et al. The use of cephalad cannulae to monitor jugular venous oxygen content during extracorporeal membrane oxygenation. *Crit Care.* 1997;1:95-99.
26. Desai SA, Stanley C, Gringlas M, et al. Five-year follow-up of neonates with reconstructed right common carotid arteries after extracorporeal membrane oxygenation. *J Pediatr.* 1999;134:428-433.
31. Seib PM, Faulkner SC, Erickson CC, et al. Blade and balloon atrial septostomy for left heart decompression in patients with severe ventricular dysfunction on extracorporeal membrane oxygenation. *Catheter Cardiovasc Interv.* 1999;46:179-186.
32. Thomas TH, Price R, Ramaciotti C, et al. Echocardiography, not chest radiography, for evaluation of cannula placement during pediatric extracorporeal membrane oxygenation. *Pediatr Crit Care Med.* 2009;10:56-59.
33. Dalton HJ, Butt WW. Extracorporeal life support: an update of Rogers' Textbook of Pediatric Intensive Care. *Pediatr Crit Care Med.* 2012;13: 461-471.
36. Schreur A, Niles S, Ploessl J. Use of the CDI blood parameter monitoring system 500 for continuous blood gas measurement during extracorporeal membrane oxygenation simulation. *J Extra Corpor Technol.* 2005;37:377-380.
40. Cremers B, Link A, Werner C, et al. Pulsatile venoarterial perfusion using a novel synchronized cardiac assist device augments coronary artery blood flow during ventricular fibrillation. *Artif Organs.* 2015;39:77-82.
45. Pfaender LM. Hemodynamics in the extracorporeal aortic cannula: review of factors affecting choice of appropriate size. *J Extra Corpor Technol.* 1981;13:224-232.
46. Lequier L, et al. Extracorporeal membrane oxygenation circuitry. *Pediatr Crit Care Med.* 2013;14(5 suppl 1):S7-S12.
48. Barrett CS, Jaggers JJ, Cook EF, et al. Pediatric ECMO outcomes: comparison of centrifugal versus roller blood pumps using propensity score matching. *ASAIO J.* 2013;59:145-151.
49. Almond CS, et al. Berlin Heart EXCOR Pediatric ventricular assist device Investigational Device Exemption study: study design and rationale. *Am Heart J.* 2011;162:425-435-e426.
51. Brogan TV, Thiagarajan RR, Rycus PT, et al. Extracorporeal membrane oxygenation in adults with severe respiratory failure: a multi-center database. *Intensive Care Med.* 2009;35:2105-2114.
57. Hebbar KB, Petrillo-Albarano T, Coto-Puckett W, et al. Experience with use of extracorporeal life support for severe refractory status asthmaticus in children. *Crit Care.* 2009;13:R29.
59. Zabrocki LA, Brogan TV, Statler KD, et al. Extracorporeal membrane oxygenation for pediatric respiratory failure: survival and predictors of mortality. *Crit Care Med.* 2011;39:364-370.
63. Preston TJ, Dalton HJ, Nicol KK, et al. Plasma exchange on venovenous extracorporeal membrane oxygenation with bivalirudin anticoagulation. *World J Pediatr Congenit Heart Surg.* 2015;6:119-122.
66. Blum JM, Lynch W, Coopersmith C. Clinical and billing review of ECMO. *Chest.* 2015;147:1697-1703.
67. Deleted in review.
71. Deleted in review.
75. Rajagopal SK, Almond CS, Laussen PC, et al. Extracorporeal membrane oxygenation for the support of infants, children, and young adults with acute myocarditis: a review of the Extracorporeal Life Support Organization registry. *Crit Care Med.* 2010;38:382-387.
77. Kumar TKS, Zurakowski D, Dalton H, et al. Extracorporeal membrane oxygenation in post-cardiotomy patients: predictors of outcome. *J Thorac Cardiovasc Surg.* 2010;140:330-336.
82. Dalton HJ, Tucker D. Resuscitation and extracorporeal life support during cardiopulmonary resuscitation following the Norwood (Stage 1) operation. *Cardiol Young.* 2011;21(suppl 2):101-108.
86. Stub D, Bernard S, Pellegrino V, et al. Refractory cardiac arrest treated with mechanical CPR, hypothermia, ECMO and early reperfusion (the CHEER trial). *Resuscitation.* 2015;86:88-94.
87. Shankar V, Costello JP, Peer SM, et al. Ethical dilemma: offering short-term extracorporeal membrane oxygenation support for terminally ill children who are not candidates for long-term mechanical circulatory support or heart transplantation. *World J Pediatr Congenit Heart Surg.* 2014;5:311-314.

92. Peters MJ, Tasker RC, Kiff KM, et al. Acute hypoxemic respiratory failure in children: case mix and the utility of respiratory severity indices. *Intensive Care Med*. 1998;24:699-705.

99. Secker-Walker JS, Edmonds JF, Spratt EH, et al. The source of coronary perfusion during partial bypass for extracorporeal membrane oxygenation (ECMO). *Ann Thorac Surg*. 1976;21:138-143.

101. Angerstrand CL, Burkart KM, Abrams DC, et al. Blood conservation in extracorporeal membrane oxygenation for acute respiratory distress syndrome. *Ann Thorac Surg*. 2015;99:590-595.

102. Saini A, Spinella PC. Management of anticoagulation and hemostasis for pediatric extracorporeal membrane oxygenation. *Clin Lab Med*. 2014;34:655-673.

104. Piena M, Albers MJ, Van Haard PM, et al. Introduction of enteral feeding in neonates on extracorporeal membrane oxygenation after evaluation of intestinal permeability changes. *J Pediatr Surg*. 1998;33: 30-34.

107. Santiago MJ, Sánchez A, López-Herce J, et al. The use of continuous renal replacement therapy in series with extracorporeal membrane oxygenation. *Kidney Int*. 2009;76:1289-1292.

114. Inwald D, et al. Open lung biopsy in neonatal and paediatric patients referred for extracorporeal membrane oxygenation (ECMO). *Thorax*. 2004;59:328-333.

117. Lemaitre F, Hasni N, Leprince P, et al. Propofol, midazolam, vancomycin and cyclosporine therapeutic drug monitoring in extracorporeal membrane oxygenation circuits primed with whole human blood. *Crit Care*. 2015;19:40.

120. Dalton HJ, Butt WW. Extracorporeal life support: an update of Rogers' Textbook of Pediatric Intensive Care. *Pediatr Crit Care Med*. 2012;13:461-471. Review.

122. Dalton HJ, Garcia-Filion P, Holubkov R, et al. Association of bleeding and thrombosis with outcome in extracorporeal life support. *Pediatr Crit Care Med*. 2015;16:167-174.

127. Agarwal HS, Bennett JE, Churchwell KB, et al. Recombinant factor seven therapy for postoperative bleeding in neonatal and pediatric cardiac surgery. *Ann Thorac Surg*. 2007;84:161-169.

129. Schutze GE, Heulitt MJ. Infections during extracorporeal life support. *J Pediatr Surg*. 1995;30:809-812.

133. The Australia and New Zealand Extracorporeal Membrane Oxygenation (ANZ ECMO) Influenza Investigators: extracorporeal membrane oxygenation for 2009 influenza A(H1N1) acute respiratory distress syndrome. *JAMA*. 2009;302:1888-1895.

140. Bennett CC, et al. UK collaborative randomised trial of neonatal extracorporeal membrane oxygenation: follow-up to age 4 years. *Lancet*. 2001;357:1094-1096.

141. Deleted in review.

142. Cheung PY, Robertson CM. Sensorineural hearing loss in survivors of neonatal extracorporeal membrane oxygenation. *Pediatr Rehabil*. 1997;1:127-130.

143. Cooper JM, et al. Neonatal hypoxia, hippocampal atrophy, and memory impairment: evidence of a causal sequence. *Cereb Cortex*. 2015;25:1469-1476.

144. Ijsselstijn H, van Heijst AF. Long-term outcome of children treated with neonatal extracorporeal membrane oxygenation: increasing problems with increasing age. *Semin Perinatol*. 2014;38:114-121.

145. Joffe AR, et al. Pediatric outcomes after extracorporeal membrane oxygenation for cardiac disease and for cardiac arrest: a review. *ASAIO J*. 2012;58:297-310.

152. Zwiers AJ, et al. CKD and hypertension during long-term follow-up in children and adolescents previously treated with extracorporeal membrane oxygenation. *Clin J Am Soc Nephrol*. 2014;9:2070-2078.

Central Nervous System

Central Nervous System

Structure, Function, and Development of the Nervous System

Michael Shoykhet and Robert S.B. Clark

PEARLS

- In humans, general central nervous anatomy is established by birth. However, the brain undergoes substantial postnatal development including changes in synaptic density and dendritic arborization, maturation of neurotransmitter systems, and experience-dependent modification of neuronal circuits. Thus critical illness– and critical care–related therapeutic and environmental factors can shape ultimate central nervous system development.
- Normal cerebral blood flow (CBF) changes significantly with age. For term human newborns, normal CBF is approximately 40 mL/100 g brain/min. CBF peaks around 4 to 8 years of age at approximately 100 mL/100 g brain/min, declining to adult values of 50 mL/100 g brain/min in late adolescents.
- Normal CBF regulation to changes in blood pressure, CO_2, and O_2 is operative from birth in term human newborns. While cerebrovascular reactivity to CO_2 and O_2 remains relatively unchanged with age, blood pressure–dependent autoregulation operates over a narrower blood pressure range in younger children than older children and adults.

The nervous system, unlike any other organ system in the human body, stands at the intersection of biology and philosophy. While composed of cells and governed by chemical messages like all biological systems, it comprises the essence of each individual as a human being. The former can be quantified and studied; the latter enters the realm of religion, philosophy, and spirituality. Indeed, in a "brain-centric" approach to pediatric critical care, it can be argued that all interventions are ultimately targeted at preserving and protecting the child's nervous system function. Thus knowledge of the structure and function of the nervous system, together with understanding of the developmental processes that are active in children who become patients in the ICU, is essential to the practice of the pediatric intensivist. Furthermore, the impact of disease and injury in the context of the developing nervous system is only now beginning to be understood, with many new advances in diagnosis and treatment undoubtedly yet to come.

Major Cell Types

The nervous system contains two major cell types: neurons and glia. Neurons are responsible for the major operations traditionally ascribed to the nervous system: sensation, movement, thought, memory, and emotion, as well as homeostasis of bodily functions. Interconnected networks of neuronal cells carry out all brain and spinal cord–based behaviors. Glia, although significantly more numerous than the neurons, function to support neuronally based information processing and long-distance information transfer. Both neurons and glia are broad classes of cells, each containing a multitude of specialized cells dedicated to carrying out specific functions in the nervous system.

All neurons, regardless of type and location within the nervous system, contain several standard cellular components that allow them to receive, process, and relay information. The neuronal soma (cell body) contains the nucleus where genes are transcribed into mRNA, the endoplasmic reticulum where mRNA is translated into proteins, and a multitude of mitochondria for cellular respiration and adenosine triphosphate synthesis. Originating from the soma are two types of processes: a number of dendrites and a single axon. Dendrites are short, local processes specialized for receiving information transmitted from other neurons via chemical or electrical synapses (see later). The axon is the output of the neuron, carrying information in the form of action potentials to be received by other neurons, muscles, and many additional body organs, at distances up to meters away.

Glial cells are typically divided into microglia and macroglia. Microglia are phagocytic cells derived from peripheral macrophages and normally exist in a resting or quiescent state in the central nervous system (CNS). Microglia are activated by several physiologically relevant factors, including bacterial lipopolysaccharide in the setting of infection and thrombin in the setting of injury.[1] Whether microglial activation is neurotoxic or neuroprotective in these settings has yet to be fully characterized. In addition, activated microglia play an important role in the neuropathology of Alzheimer disease, HIV-associated dementia, and prion diseases. Therapeutic strategies targeting microglial activation are just now beginning to emerge in animal disease models[2-3] and human clinical trials.[4]

Macroglia comprise several distinct cell subtypes within the nervous system: astrocytes and oligodendrocytes in the CNS and Schwann cells in the peripheral nervous system (PNS). Astrocytes are by far the most numerous cell type in the brain, performing several vital functions. At the synapse, astrocytes regulate ion and neurotransmitter concentrations, contributing to the modern notion that the synapse is a tripartite structure consisting of the presynaptic and postsynaptic neurons and the astrocyte. At the blood-brain barrier (BBB), astrocytes direct their processes toward the endothelial cells and contribute to the proper development of tight junctions (see later). In contrast to the relatively diverse functions of astrocytes, oligodendrocytes' and Schwann cells' primary purpose is to provide myelination for axons in the CNS and the PNS, respectively. Myelination ensures faithful signal propagation along the entire axonal length. Each oligodendrocyte contributes myelin to between 10 and 15 axons in the CNS; each Schwann cell envelops a single axon in the PNS. From a clinical perspective, disorders of myelination contribute significantly to a range of diseases observed in pediatric critical illness, including perinatal asphyxia-induced periventricular leukomalacia, Canavan disease due to mutation in the oligodendrocyte-specific aspartoacylase gene, and Guillain-Barré syndrome, caused commonly by autoimmune-mediated injury to peripheral nerve myelin sheaths.

Intercellular Communication in the Nervous System

Early descriptions of neuronal cell structure by Camillo Golgi and Ramon Cajal in the late 19th century gave rise to two diverging theories of neuronal communication. Golgi proposed that neurons form an interconnected reticulum, much like cardiac muscle cells, and communicate directly with each other via openings in their membranes. Cajal, on the other hand, argued that neurons are individual cells with contiguous cell membranes and that communication takes place chemically at the sites of contact between individual neurons. Despite the radically opposed views, both theories are now known to be correct and both mechanisms contribute to aspects of neuronal communication in the mammalian brain. Direct communication between neurons, known as the electrical synapse, is accomplished via gap junctions. Communication across cell membranes at sites where two neurons contact each other is accomplished using neurotransmitters, with the contact site known as the *chemical synapse*.

Electrical Synapses

At the electrical synapse, cell membranes of the adjoining neurons are tightly bound together into a gap-junction plaque.[5] Each plaque contains numerous channels made of connexin proteins. There are 24 known connexin genes in humans. Each channel consists of two hemichannels, with one on each cell membrane. Two hemichannels join together to form a functional gap junction between two neurons, allowing intercellular diffusion of ions and small molecules such as glucose, cyclic AMP, and ATP. Gap junctions thus allow neurons to share information about their metabolic and excitable states, providing a mechanism for large-scale regulation of energy demands and neuronal network dynamics. Additionally, gap junction channels close in response to lowered intracellular pH or elevated Ca^{2+} levels; because both events occur in damaged cells, paired hemichannels at the gap junction may function to isolate healthy neurons from those damaged during ischemia or trauma. Recent evidence suggests that unpaired hemichannels outside of the gap junction plaques may also contribute to ischemic neuronal cell death.[6]

Glia, like neurons, are also connected by gap junctions. For example, brain astrocytes form an interconnected cellular network, which allows long-distance propagation of calcium signals across many cells. Additionally, layers of myelin generated by oligodendrocytes in the CNS and by Schwann cells in the PNS are linked by gap junctions. Myelin gap junctions provide structural stability to the myelin sheath and allow for rapid diffusion of nutrients and other substances across the sheath toward the underlying axon. In humans, mutations in gap junction protein connexin 32 result in X-linked Charcot-Marie-Tooth disease, a demyelinating neuropathy.[7]

Chemical Synapses

Neuromuscular Junction

The neuromuscular junction (NMJ) is one of the most widely studied examples of chemical synaptic transmission in the nervous system. The overall concept is deceivingly simple: An action potential at the presynaptic neuron releases a neurotransmitter that in turn activates ion channels on the muscle cell membrane, resulting in postsynaptic action potential. Yet every step in this process is exquisitely controlled and modulated in health and may be disrupted in disease. Our evolving understanding of the NMJ provides a critical window into synapse function and pathophysiology.

The NMJ consists of three distinct anatomic components: the presynaptic nerve terminal, the synaptic cleft containing the basement membrane, and the postsynaptic muscle fiber. The presynaptic nerve terminal originates from the myelinated axon of a motoneuron in the spinal cord. Lower motoneurons in the ventral gray matter of the spinal cord send their myelinated axons through the ventral root toward peripheral muscle targets. As the axon approaches the muscle fibers, it loses its myelin sheath and branches into a fine network of terminals, each approximately 2 μm in diameter. Each branch has several swellings along its course, termed *presynaptic boutons*, where the nerve makes synaptic contact with the muscle fiber. Presynaptic boutons are covered by terminal Schwann cells, which provide growth factors, recycle neurotransmitters, and may participate in recovery after nerve and muscle injury. Presynaptic boutons are positioned over specialized regions of the muscle cell membrane called the *end plate regions*. Furthermore, underlying each bouton is a specialized invagination of the cell membrane that contains a high concentration of nicotinic acetylcholine (ACh) receptors and voltage-gated Na^+ channels. The presynaptic bouton and end plate are separated by a 100 nm-wide synaptic cleft containing the basement membrane and extracellular matrix. The basement membrane anchors a number of proteins, including acetylcholinesterase, the enzyme responsible for rapid hydrolysis of ACh in the synaptic cleft.

Several distinct functional steps occur during synaptic transmission at the NMJ. First, the action potential arriving from the motor axon depolarizes the membrane in the presynaptic boutons, causing Ca^{2+} entry via voltage-gated Ca^{2+} channels on the presynaptic membrane. Ca^{2+} entry results in fusion of synaptic vesicles containing ACh with the presynaptic cell membrane and release of ACh into the synaptic cleft. ACh rapidly diffuses toward the postsynaptic membrane and binds to the nicotinic ACh receptor (nACh); two ACh molecules are required to activate the nACh receptor. On activation, the nACh receptor opens and allows both Na^+ and K^+ to flow through the ion pore. The inward Na^+ current, however, dominates over the outward K^+ current, resulting in net depolarization of the muscle membrane at the end plate. This so-called end plate potential propagates a short distance before encountering voltage-gated Na^+ channels. These Na^+ channels open when membrane potential rises to a critical threshold value, allowing only Na^+ ions to flow into the cell and generating the all-or-none muscle action potential. Acetylcholinesterases in the synaptic cleft terminate the depolarizing action of ACh at the postsynaptic membrane by rapidly hydrolyzing ACh into acetate and choline.

A detailed understanding of diseases that affect synaptic transmission at the NMJ, as well as familiarity with clinical pharmacology as it applies to the NMJ, is essential in critical care. Specific diseases affecting the NMJ include toxin-mediated botulism and autoimmune disorders such as myasthenia gravis, Lambert-Eaton syndrome, and neuromyotonia. These are discussed in detail in Chapter 71 (see also Tseng-Ong and Mitchell[8] and Lang and Vincent[9]). Among the pharmacotherapies targeted at the NMJ are some of the most commonly used drugs in the pediatric ICU: neuromuscular blockers. Furthermore, a number of toxins either decrease (anticholinergic agents) or increase (acetylcholinesterase inhibitors) the amount of ACh available at cholinergic synapses, resulting in corresponding toxidromes (see Chapter 128).

Chemical Synapses in the Central Nervous System

Chemical synapses in the CNS operate on basic principles similar to those governing synaptic transmission at the NMJ, although the cadre of neurotransmitters and postsynaptic receptors is significantly more diverse in the CNS. Importantly, a given neuron in the CNS may synthesize and store more than a single neurotransmitter, but it releases the same set of neurotransmitters at all of its synapses (Dale's principle). CNS synapses are generally divided into asymmetric (Gray type I) synapses and symmetric (Gray type II) synapses on the basis of their appearance under electron microscopy. Physiologically, these correspond to excitatory and inhibitory synapses, respectively. Each neuron synthesizes its own complement of neurotransmitters, which are delivered to all synaptic contact sites in the axon and packaged into synaptic vesicles. When an action potential reaches the axon, Ca^{2+} currents cause the synaptic vesicles to fuse with the cell membrane, releasing neurotransmitters into the synaptic cleft. Neurotransmitters then act on their corresponding ionotropic and metabotropic receptors on the postsynaptic membrane. Ionotropic receptor activation leads to either a depolarizing, excitatory current or a hyperpolarizing, inhibitory current. These subthreshold currents are called excitatory and inhibitory postsynaptic potentials (EPSPs and IPSPs), respectively. Temporal and spatial summation of EPSPs in the dendritic tree of the postsynaptic neuron occasionally depolarizes the somatic membrane sufficiently to cross threshold and generate an action potential. One of the distinguishing features of chemical synaptic transmission in the CNS, compared with the NMJ, is its lack of reliability on a single cell level; an action potential in the presynaptic neuron does not necessarily cause a postsynaptic neuron to fire its own action potential. Such lack of determinism likely allows for individual differences in responses to the same stimuli. After interaction with the receptor, the neurotransmitter is cleared from the synapse by diffusion, active reuptake into the terminal, or enzymatic destruction, similar to ACh hydrolysis at the NMJ.

Neurotransmitter Systems

Several substances are employed for communicating information chemically between neurons in the nervous system or

TABLE 60.1   Neurotransmitter Classes

Amines	Amino Acids	Peptides
Acetylcholine	γ-Aminobutyric acid	Substance P
Dopamine	Glutamate	*Vasoactive intestinal peptide*
Norepinephrine	Glycine	Dynorphin
Epinephrine		Enkephalins
Serotonin		*Neuropeptide Y*
Histamine		*Cholecystokinin*

Neurotransmitters that operative exclusively in the central nervous system are in normal font, those used in both the central and peripheral nervous systems are in *italics*, and those used exclusively in the peripheral nervous system are in **bold**.

between a neuron and a muscle at the neuromuscular junction. These substances, called *neurotransmitters,* generally fall into three categories: amines, amino acids, and peptides (Table 60.1). Each neurotransmitter requires its own synthetic machinery and exerts specific actions on the postsynaptic target. Furthermore, neurons tend to be characterized anatomically, immunohistochemically, and functionally by the main neurotransmitter they use, allowing insight into the role of each neurotransmitter system in CNS function.

Neurotransmitters

Acetylcholine

Acetylcholine is an amine that functions as a neurotransmitter at the NMJ, as well as in the CNS. At the NMJ, its actions are quick and precise, whereas in the CNS it functions as a slow, more global modulator of synaptic activity. Cholinergic CNS neurons include all the motoneurons in the spinal cord, as well as a number of cell nuclei in the brainstem reticular formation and the basal forebrain. Cholinergic neurons synthesize ACh using choline acetyltransferase (ChAT), which transfers an acetyl group from acetyl coenzyme A (CoA) to choline (Fig. 60.1A). Choline concentration in the extracellular fluid is the rate-limiting step in the reaction. Cholinergic neurons also synthesize acetylcholinesterase (AChE), the enzyme that breaks down ACh. AChE is released with ACh into the synaptic cleft, where it rapidly hydrolyzes ACh into acetic acid and choline.

Low concentrations of choline in the CNS have been associated with neurologic impairment during fetal[10] and postnatal life.[11] Thus choline supplementation represents an attractive therapeutic strategy in neurologic disorders characterized by decreased CNS choline. Interestingly, patients receiving long-term parenteral nutrition (TPN) occasionally develop choline deficiency, which has been associated with TPN-related liver failure[12] and, possibly, cognitive dysfunction. Hence choline supplementation in TPN-dependent patients may ameliorate some neurologic deficits.[13]

Catecholamines

Catecholamine neurotransmitters include dopamine, norepinephrine, and epinephrine. For all three, the initial starting point in biochemical synthesis is the amino acid tyrosine (Fig. 60.1B). Tyrosine is converted into an intermediate compound, called dopa, by tyrosine hydroxylase (TH). In dopaminergic

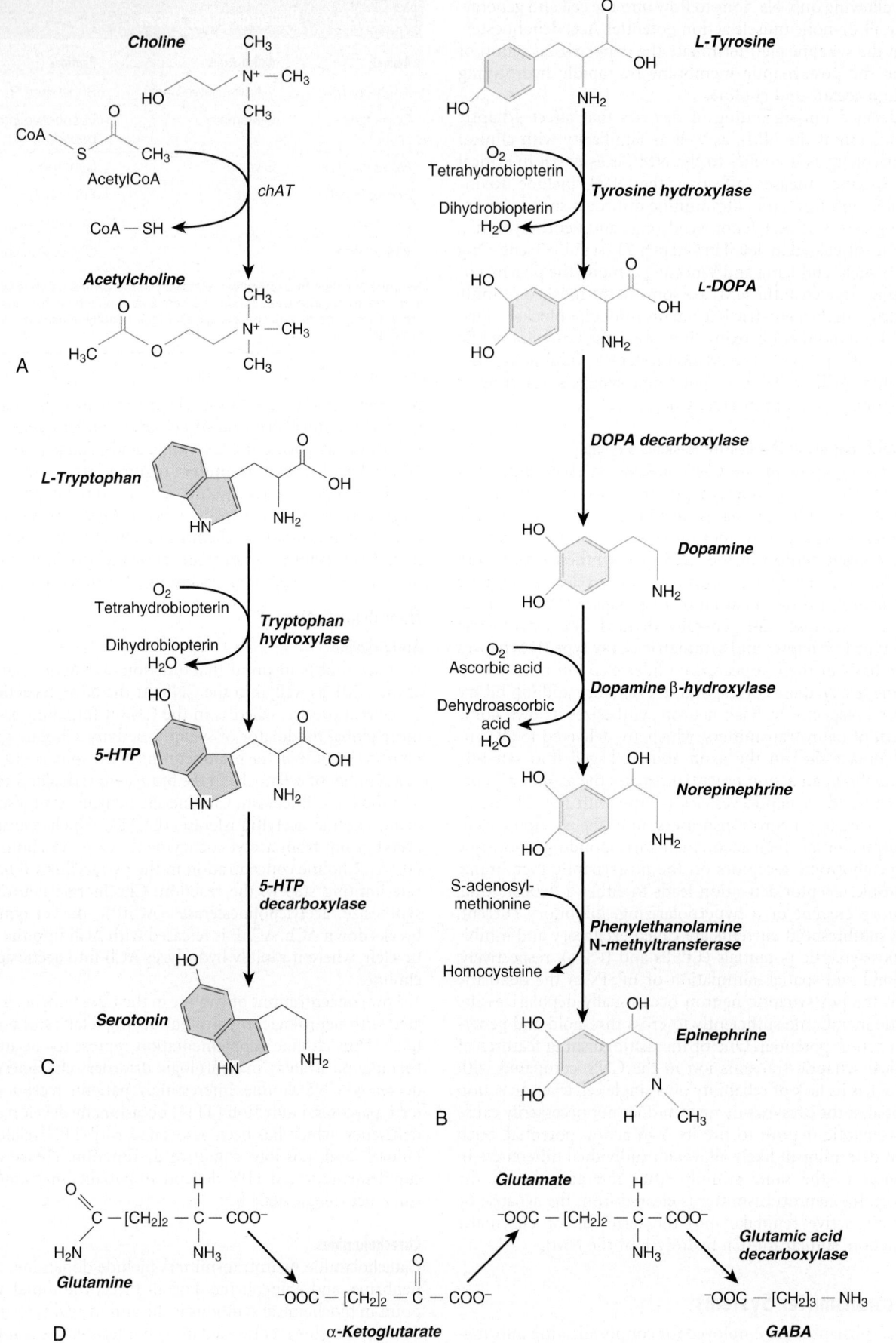

Fig. 60.1. Neurotransmitter structure and synthesis. (A) Acetylcholine. (B) Catecholamines. It should be noted that synthesis of norepinephrine and epinephrine requires dopamine as a precursor. (C) Serotonin, an amine synthesized from tryptophan. (D) Glutamate and gamma-aminobutyric acid, amino acid derivatives.

neurons, dopa is converted into dopamine by dopa decarboxylase. Noradrenergic neurons, which use norepinephrine as a neurotransmitter, further convert dopamine into norepinephrine using dopamine β-hydroxylase. Finally, norepinephrine is converted into epinephrine by an enzyme phentolamine N-methyltransferase, which is found only in adrenergic neurons. Thus all neurons that synthesize catecholamines contain TH and dopa decarboxylase, but only noradrenergic and adrenergic neurons contain the synthetic enzymes required to produce norepinephrine and epinephrine, respectively.

Catecholamine-using neurons reside primarily in the brainstem. Dopaminergic neurons in humans are located in two mesencephalic nuclei: the substantia nigra and its medial neighbor, the ventral tegmental area. Dopaminergic neurons in the substantia nigra project primarily to the basal ganglia, where they are involved with initiation of voluntary movement. Ventral tegmental neurons send dopaminergic fibers to the amygdala and the cerebral cortex and participate in regulation of emotion, reward, and addiction. Brainstem noradrenergic neurons are located in the locus ceruleus and in the reticular formation. They project widely to the thalamus and cortex, as well as to the spinal cord, and play a significant role in arousal and vigilance. Adrenergic CNS neurons are located in the ventrolateral medulla and participate in temperature regulation via their projections to the hypothalamus.

Unlike ACh, which is cleared from the synapse by hydrolysis, catecholamines are cleared from the synaptic cleft by reuptake into the axonal terminal. Once inside the cell, catecholamines are either repackaged into vesicles or destroyed by monoamine oxidase (MAO). Pharmacologic manipulation of synaptic catecholamine concentrations plays a therapeutic role in the management of several disorders, such as depression and attention deficit-hyperactivity disorder (ADHD). Furthermore, recreational drugs affecting catecholamine concentrations at the synapse continue to gain popularity and to grow in number. Therapeutic uses include treatment of severe depression with MAO inhibitors, which inhibit catecholamine breakdown, and treatment of ADHD with amphetamines, which interfere with dopamine transport and increase dopamine concentrations. Recreational drugs include amphetamine and its analogs, along with cocaine, a selective norepinephrine transporter blocker. Excess catecholamine levels at the synapse result in sensations of euphoria, increased energy levels, improved focus, anxiety, paranoia, and jitteriness. Notably, hypertensive crises leading to myocardial infarction and stroke may occur with use of cocaine, amphetamines, and MAO inhibitors.

Serotonin

Serotonin is an amine neurotransmitter synthesized from the amino acid tryptophan in a two-step process (Fig. 60.1C). First, tryptophan is hydroxylated by tryptophan hydroxylase to form 5-hydroxytryptophan (5-HTP). 5-HTP is then decarboxylated by 5-HTP decarboxylase to form serotonin, also known as *5-hydroxytryptamine* (5-HT). After 5-HT is released at the synapse, it is cleared by a specific serotonin reuptake transporter. Serotonergic neurons are located in the rostral and caudal raphe nuclei in the brainstem. Rostral raphe neurons innervate the cerebral cortex, including the limbic system, where serotonin levels help regulate mood and attention. Caudal raphe neurons project to the brainstem and

spinal cord, where they are involved in regulation of general arousal and pain perception, respectively. Importantly, dysfunction of the serotonergic pathways originating in the raphe nuclei has been linked with sudden unexplained infant death (SUID).[14] Additionally, serotonin levels play a key role in depression, giving rise to an entire class of drugs in clinical use called selective serotonin reuptake inhibitors (SSRIs). SSRI abuse or overdose is rare but may result in patients presenting with the potentially life-threatening "serotonin syndrome," characterized by hypertension, tachycardia, mental status changes, myoclonus, and severe hyperthermia. The latter may lead to shock, rhabdomyolysis, renal failure, and death. The serotonin syndrome is particularly likely to occur when SSRIs and MAO inhibitors, inadvertently or intentionally, are taken together. Treatment includes serotonin antagonists, blood pressure control with either adrenergic antagonists or agonists as clinically indicated, and temperature control with benzodiazepines and neuromuscular blockade.

Amino Acids

Neurotransmitters derived from common amino acids include glutamate, gamma-aminobutyric acid (GABA), and glycine. These are among the most widely distributed neurotransmitters in the CNS. Glutamate and glycine exist as amino acids in all cells, where they are used as protein building blocks. Glutamatergic and glycinergic neurons have the additional capacity to package glutamate and glycine, respectively, into synaptic vesicles and release them at the synapse. GABA must be synthesized from glutamate via an additional reaction catalyzed by an enzyme glutamic acid decarboxylase (GAD) (Fig. 60.1D). Only GABA-ergic neurons contain GAD.

Glutamate is generally an excitatory neurotransmitter, whereas GABA and glycine are inhibitory. Excitatory glutamatergic neurons exert their influence both locally and over a long distance, depending on the shape of their axons. Inhibitory neurons, on the other hand, tend to exert local inhibitory control over neuronal circuitry either in the brain (GABA) or spinal cord (glycine). A major exception is cerebellar Purkinje cells, which are GABA-ergic but project over long distances to the brainstem, thalamus, and cerebral cortex (see later).

Adenosine, Peptides, and Nitric Oxide

In addition to the "classic" neurotransmitters described earlier, a number of substances have been documented to mediate or modulate information transfer between neurons. These include adenosine triphosphate (ATP) and adenosine, which at the synapse is a metabolite of ATP released in the synaptic vesicle. ATP modulates neuronal excitability such that energy may be conserved during times of ATP depletion. Adenosine functions as a neurotransmitter in the autonomic nervous system (ANS), in the basal ganglia, and at some cortical synapses. It also modulates the respiratory rate, and adenosine antagonists, such as caffeine, are used to treat apnea and bradycardia of prematurity. In addition to ATP and adenosine, a number of peptides can be released in synaptic vesicles, including substance P, vasoactive intestinal peptide (VIP), endogenous opioids, and endogenous cannabinoids. These peptides are involved in pain sensation and perception (substance P and opioids), modulation of vascular tone (VIP), and as yet uncharacterized processes (cannabinoids).

Finally, several gaseous molecules function as neurotransmitters. These include nitric oxide (NO), carbon monoxide

(CO), and possibly hydrogen sulfide. NO, the most thoroughly studied of the gaseous neurotransmitters, is produced by brainstem neurons in the nucleus tractus solitarius, where it interacts with α-amino-3-hydroxyl-5-methyl-4-isoxazole-propionate (AMPA)-type and N-methyl-D-aspartate (NMDA)-type glutamate receptors and regulates cardiovascular function.[15] Hydrogen sulfide is produced from the amino acid cysteine and may influence cellular redox state and glutamatergic transmission.[16] Intriguingly, hydrogen sulfide induces a suspended animation-like state in animals[17] and may be protective after resuscitation from cardiac arrest.[18]

Neurotransmitter Receptors

Nicotinic Acetylcholine Receptors

Nicotinic ACh receptors are ligand-gated ion channels, related structurally and functionally to GABA$_A$ channels and a subset of serotonin receptors. Five transmembrane subunits comprise the nAChR and form a central pore that allows ionic currents to pass. There are two subunit classes, α and β, with multiple members in each class. nAChR is generally a heteromer, but homomer channels have been described. Each nAChR binds two acetycholine molecules, with affinity for ACh and nicotine dependent on subunit composition. The receptor exists in three distinct states: closed, open, and desensitized. In the closed position, no ionic current passes through the central core. When an agonist, such as ACh or nicotine, binds the nAChR, the receptor opens, becoming permeable to monovalent and divalent cations. After a short period of time, the receptor spontaneously closes. On continued exposure to an agonist, however, the nAChR assumes a permanently closed, or desensitized, conformation.[19] As discussed earlier, nAChRs mediate neuromuscular coupling at the NMJ. In addition, nAChRs are widely distributed in the CNS, where they perform a variety of functions depending on subunit composition and location.

In the CNS, unlike at the NMJ, nAChRs are permeable to both Na$^+$ and Ca^{2+}. In neurons, however, nAChR-evoked Ca^{2+} current exceeds the Na$^+$ current twofold to tenfold. The greater Ca^{2+} permeability indicates that nAChRs mostly modulate synaptic transmission and release of other neurotransmitters. Indeed, although direct nAChR-dependent responses have been observed in the hippocampus and the developing visual cortex, overwhelming evidence points to nicotinic receptors playing the role of modulator in the CNS. Their wide distribution in the CNS with locations presynaptically, postsynaptically, and extrasynaptically further supports that role. Activation of presynaptic nAChRs enhances release of ACh, dopamine, glutamate, and GABA. Coupling of enhanced glutamate release with nAChR-dependent increase in intracellular Ca^{2+} suggests that nAChRs participate in synaptic plasticity during learning. Postsynaptic and extrasynaptic nAChRs regulate excitability and signal propagation in neuronal circuits. In the hippocampus, for example, nAChR activation leads to increased release of GABA from inhibitory interneurons, which decreases the excitability of hippocampal pyramidal neurons. Nicotinic receptors also interact with the dopaminergic system in regulating neuronal circuitry in the basal ganglia and the limbic system. Thus nicotinic receptors have been implicated in not only learning and memory but also regulation of addiction and reward. Furthermore, loss of cholinergic neurons represents one of the distinguishing neuropathologic features of Alzheimer disease, and cholinesterase inhibitors are widely used to improve cognition and memory in Alzheimer patients.[19] In pediatrics, a mutation in nAChR is responsible for a specific clinical epilepsy phenotype, called autosomal dominant nocturnal frontal lobe epilepsy.[20] Seizure onset usually occurs around 12 years of age in otherwise healthy children. Seizures originate in the frontal lobe and occur predominantly during non-REM sleep.[21] The mutant nAChR is more sensitive to ACh than the wild-type receptor, suggesting that cholinergic medications should be avoided in these patients.

Muscarinic Acetylcholine Receptors

Muscarinic ACh receptors (mAChRs) comprise a group of metabotropic receptors that link ACh exposure at the surface with G protein activation inside the cell. There are five distinct subtypes of mAChRs, designated M$_1$ through M$_5$, and these subtypes are divided into two broad classes on the basis of the identity of the G protein with which they interact. M$_2$ and M$_4$ mAChRs couple with G$_i$ proteins, inhibit adenylyl cyclase activity, and reduce intracellular cAMP levels. M$_1$, M$_3$, and M$_5$ receptor subtypes couple with G$_q$ proteins and increase intracellular Ca^{2+} levels via activation of phospholipase C.[22] In the CNS, the M$_1$ mAChR is the most abundant subtype, located on neurons in the cortex, thalamus, and striatum.[23] mAChRs are also present in the PNS in the sweat glands and organs of lacrimation and salivation, as well as in the heart, where they mediate the parasympathetic control of heart rate and contractility. Muscarinic AChRs thus mediate many of the systemic effects of organophosphate exposure and nerve gas poisoning.[24]

Glutamate Receptors

Glutamate is the major excitatory neurotransmitter in the central nervous system. In mammals, it depolarizes postsynaptic neurons by binding to three types of ionotropic glutamate receptors (iGluR), each of which is characterized by different affinities for synthetic analogs, different selectivity to ions, and different time course of the current that is permitted to pass through the cell membrane. The three types of iGluR are the AMPA receptor, NMDA receptor, and kainate receptor. All three channel types are widely present throughout the CNS, with AMPA and NMDA channels mediating the bulk of the excitatory transmission. At present, the function of the kainate channel remains to be clearly defined.

AMPA and NMDA receptors differ from each other with respect to ion permeability and time course of ion flow through the channel. On binding of glutamate, AMPA receptors open their pores, which are permeable to Na$^+$ and K$^+$ ions. At the negative resting potential of the neuronal cell membrane, Na$^+$, driven by the electrochemical gradient, flows into the cell and causes a large, fast depolarization. AMPA receptors are generally impermeable to Ca^{2+}, although more recent findings indicate that Ca^{2+}-permeable AMPA receptors do exist and may significantly contribute to pathology observed in ALS and stroke.[25] In contrast, NMDA receptors are universally permeable to Ca^{2+}, as well as to Na$^+$ and K$^+$, generating a slow inward depolarizing current. NMDA receptors possess a unique property, however, that allows them to pass current only when the neuronal membrane is already depolarized. This property, termed *voltage-dependence,* stems from Mg^{2+} ions blocking the entry pore of the NMDA channel at negative membrane potentials even in the presence of glutamate. As the neuron depolarizes further, mostly due to current flow via the AMPA receptor, the Mg^{2+} block is relieved and Ca^{2+}, as well as Na^+, flows into the cell. Once inside the cell, Ca^{2+} ions mediate a multitude of effects, from modifying protein phosphorylation and gene expression to overt *excitotoxicity* and cell death. NMDA receptors are thus thought to function as coincidence detectors, linking events at the cell membrane (eg, AMPA receptor-mediated depolarization, with long-term changes in synaptic strength and gene expression in the neuron).

In addition to directly modulating current flow via the ionotropic channels, glutamate modulates effector molecules within the neuron by binding to a diversity of G protein–linked metabotropic glutamate receptors (mGluRs). Eight mammalian subtypes of mGluR are divided into three categories on the basis of sequence homology and coupling to secondary effector systems.[26] Group I mGluRs (mGlurR1 and mGluR5) are localized at the edge of the postsynaptic neuronal membrane and are positively coupled with phospholipase C (PLC) via the G_q protein. Group II and III mGluRs are located on the edge of the presynaptic neuronal membrane and are negatively coupled with adenylyl cyclase (AC) via the G_i protein. All three groups are activated only when excess glutamate spills out of the synaptic cleft and diffuses toward mGluRs located at the periphery of the synaptic membrane.

Differential secondary messenger coupling and synaptic localization of the three mGluR groups point to their divergent roles in regulating neuronal function. Binding of glutamate to group I mGluRs leads to activation of PLC, which releases two secondary messengers—diacylglycerol (DAG) and inositol triphosphate (IP_3)—from the membrane phospholipid phosphoinositol 1,4,5-bisphosphate (PIP_2). DAG activates protein kinase C in the neuronal membrane, whereas PIP_2 diffuses toward its receptor on the internal cell membrane and triggers a massive Ca^{2+} release into the cytoplasm. Downstream events lead to (1) modulation of K^+ currents, resulting in increased neuronal excitability, and (2) potentiation of glutamate-dependent current at NMDA receptors specific to the synapses at which excess glutamate release has occurred. Group I mGluRs thus participate in activity-dependent strengthening of synaptic connections and play a significant role in learning and memory.

In contrast, group III, and probably group II, mGluRs on presynaptic neurons provide a negative feedback loop by inhibiting glutamate release. When glutamate binds to group III mGluRs, an inhibitory G protein (G_i) is activated. It then functions to decrease AC-mediated production of cAMP. A decrease in cAMP leads to lower Ca^{2+} concentrations at the presynaptic neuronal membrane and decreased synaptic vesicle fusion. The net effect is a decrease in the amount of glutamate released at the synapse and a reduction in synaptic transmission. Recently, mGluRs have emerged as a major therapeutic target due to the multitude of effects they exert on synaptic transmission. Their extrasynaptic location presumably will allow newly developed pharmaceutic agents to maximize therapeutic value and minimize unwanted side effects.[27]

GABA$_A$ and GABA$_B$ Receptors

GABA is the major inhibitory neurotransmitter in the brain. Like glutamate and ACh, it binds two distinct classes of GABA receptors; GABA$_A$ receptors are ionotropic, and GABA$_B$ receptors are metabotropic. Both receptor classes are involved in regulation of physiologic and pathologic states, and pharmacologic manipulation of GABA receptors plays a major role in the management of pediatric critical illness.

GABA$_A$ receptors are chloride channels. At the normal resting membrane potential, opening of the GABA$_A$ receptor allows chloride ions to flow into the cell down their electrochemical gradient. Influx of negatively charged Cl^- ions results in hyperpolarization of the cell membrane. In neurons, membrane hyperpolarization decreases the probability that the neuron will reach threshold and fire an action potential. Thus on an individual cell level, GABA decreases neuronal activity via the GABA$_A$ receptor.

GABA$_A$ receptors are heteropentamers, similar in structure to the nAChRs. At least eight subunit classes exist in mammals, including humans, and each class consists of several members, allowing for a staggering 150,000 possible subunit combinations to create one functional GABA$_A$ receptor. Only 500 combinations are known to exist, and most receptors contain a various complement of the α, β, and γ subunits.[28] Most GABA$_A$ receptors cluster at postsynaptic densities, and such clustering appears to depend on presence of the γ subunit. However, a subset of the GABA$_A$ receptors, in particular those containing the δ subunit, localize to extrasynaptic sites, mediate tonic levels of inhibition in the brain, and may underlie the pathophysiology of absence seizures.[29]

The pharmacology of the GABA$_A$ receptor is of particular relevance in critical care because the two classes of first-line anticonvulsants and anxiolytics in clinical practice—the benzodiazepines and the barbiturates—allosterically modulate the GABA$_A$ receptor. GABA itself binds the receptor at the junction of the α and β subunits. Benzodiazepines bind the GABA$_A$ receptor at a different site, classically between the α and γ_2 subunits, and, in the presence of GABA, increase the frequency with which the chloride channel opens. Barbiturates, in contrast, bind at yet a different site and increase the duration of the open state in the presence of GABA. Thus both benzodiazepines and barbiturates increase the efficacy of endogenous GABA in hyperpolarizing the cell membrane. A major difference between the two drug classes is that at increasing concentrations, barbiturates, but not benzodiazepines, become direct GABA agonists and can open GABA$_A$ channels independent of endogenous GABA release. Hence barbiturates have a significantly narrower safety window compared with benzodiazepines.

Additional GABA$_A$ receptor ligands of clinical importance include (1) general inhalational anesthetics, which are thought to modulate tonic inhibition via the δ subunit–containing receptors; (2) alcohol, although its mechanistic action is poorly understood; and (3) flumazenil, a competitive benzodiazepine antagonist used clinically to reverse benzodiazepine overdose.

GABA$_A$ receptor mutations contribute to several known disease states in humans. Two different point mutations on chromosome 5, both affecting the γ_2 subunit, are associated with development of febrile seizures and generalized epilepsy, as well as with a link between the two conditions.[30-31] In patients with temporal lobe epilepsy, GABA$_A$ receptor expression is altered in hippocampal neurons[32] and GABA-evoked responses actually depolarize, rather than hyperpolarize, neurons in excised tissue (see also Developmental Processes section later in the chapter).[33] GABA$_A$ receptor dysfunction is also thought to contribute to anxiety, panic disorder, schizophrenia, and sleep disturbances.[34] Thus pharmacologic modulation of GABA$_A$ receptor function represents an active area of research and novel drug development.

GABA$_B$ receptors are heterodimeric proteins that activate G protein–coupled second messenger systems upon interaction with GABA at the membrane.[35] The GABA$_{B1}$ subunit binds GABA at the cell membrane, while the GABA$_{B2}$ subunit interacts with the G protein on the cytosolic surface. GABA$_B$ receptors are widely distributed throughout the CNS but are particularly abundant in the thalamus, cerebellum, and hippocampus. They can be located both presynaptically and postsynaptically. Presynaptic GABA$_B$ receptors allow G protein–coupled Ca^{2+} influx into the cell and lead to feedback inhibition of transmitter release. Postsynaptic GABA$_B$ receptors function as K$^+$ channels by allowing a slow, G protein–dependent K$^+$ current to leak out of the cell and lead to cell hyperpolarization (because positive ions have left the inside of the cell membrane).[36]

Baclofen is the only pharmacologic GABA$_B$ receptor ligand in current clinical use. It directly activates the GABA$_B$ receptor and, through its action in the spinal cord, leads to reduction in muscle tone. Thus it is used primarily to relieve spasticity after CNS injury. When administered systemically, it has a significant side-effect profile, including hypotension and bradycardia.[35] Systemic side effects have been minimized with intrathecal administration via an indwelling catheter and pump.[37,38] Indeed, intrathecal baclofen infusion has emerged as an alternative to the more invasive dorsal rhizotomy in the treatment of spasticity refractory to medical therapy in pediatric patients.[39] Although intrathecal baclofen delivery systems are effective, they have a 10% to 20% failure rate over time. When an intrathecal baclofen pump fails, patients can develop baclofen withdrawal symptoms characterized by agitation, increasing spasticity and dystonia, hypertension, tachycardia, hyperthermia, and potentially death.[39] Thus baclofen withdrawal should be considered in the differential diagnosis of an agitated child with an indwelling baclofen pump.

Major Anatomic Organization of the Nervous System

The nervous system in mammals is organized along an evolutionarily conserved axis. It can be divided anatomically and functionally into the central and peripheral nervous systems. Broadly speaking, the CNS consists of the spinal cord and brain inside the skull. All other components, such as nerves after they leave the spinal canal or exit the brain, as well as autonomic ganglia in the body, comprise the PNS. The general subdivisions are shown in Fig. 60.2. The following sections focus on well-defined functions of these subdivisions as well as on their clinical relevance in pediatric critical care medicine.

Central Nervous System
Spinal Cord
The spinal cord is organized into segments delineated by the exiting spinal nerves. In humans, there are 31 segments: 8 cervical, 12 thoracic, 5 lumbar, 5 sacral, and 1 coccygeal.[40] The first seven cervical nerves exit the spinal canal above the corresponding vertebra, that is, the C1 nerve exits between the occiput and the C1 vertebra (the atlas). Because in humans there are only seven cervical vertebra and eight cervical nerves, the last cervical nerve, C8, exits the spinal canal between C7 and T1. From T1 on, each corresponding spinal nerve exits the spinal cord below its corresponding vertebra, that is, the T12 nerve exits between T12 and L1. Early in fetal life, the spinal cord extends throughout the entire length of the spinal canal. Beginning in gestation week 12, the growth rate of the vertebrae exceeds that of the spinal cord, such that by birth in humans, the spinal cord ends at L3. During postnatal

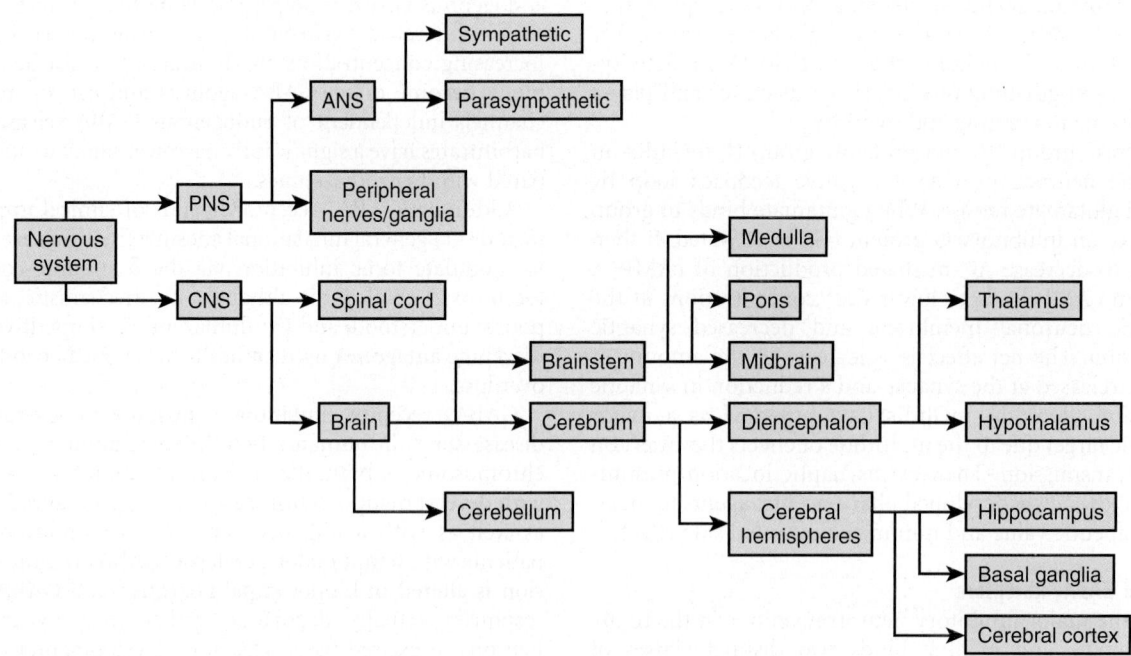

Fig. 60.2. General subdivisions of the nervous system. (Modified from Nolte J. The Human Brain. An Introduction to Its Functional Anatomy. 3rd ed. St. Louis: Mosby–Year Book; 1993.)

development, further differential growth occurs, and in adults, the spinal cord ends more rostrally, between L1 and L2. The nerve roots continue to exit the spinal canal through their corresponding foraminae, such that the caudal spinal roots extend past the end of the spinal cord toward their exit points and form the cauda equina. The end of the spinal cord forms an important landmark during development because the lumbar puncture must be performed below the spinal cord in order to avoid severe injury. Hence in infants, the preferred location of the lumbar puncture is between L4 and L5 vertebrae, with an alternate site between L3 and L4. In adults, it is safe to perform the lumbar puncture between L3 and L4, with both the L2/L3 and the L4/L5 intervertebral spaces as alternative sites.

Spinal cord lesions result in two general subsets of neurologic deficits: those caused by interruption of ascending information flow toward the brain and those caused by interruption of descending brain control of the spinal cord circuitry and the PNS. Thus complete spinal cord transection leads to loss of sensation and muscular paralysis below the level of the lesion due to injury to the ascending sensory pathways and descending motor pathways, respectively. Immediately after the transection, paralysis is flaccid with loss of deep tendon reflexes, characteristic of spinal shock (not to be confused with neurogenic shock, see later). After a period of time, paralysis becomes spastic, with increased muscle tone and hyperactive deep tendon reflexes, due to disrupted inhibitory control of spinal cord circuitry by the brain's motor centers.

Medulla

The medulla extends rostrally from the spinal cord in the rough shape of an ice cream scoop.[40] The closed "handle" portion contains an enclosed central canal contiguous with that in the spinal cord. The open "scoop" portion is located rostrally where the central canal opens into the fourth ventricle. The medulla gives origin to four cranial nerves (CN): the glossopharyngeal (CN IX), vagus (CN X), accessory (CN XI), and hypoglossal (CN XII). It also contains decussations (crossings) of two major fiber tracts. The postsynaptic fibers from the nuclei gracilis and cuneatus, which carry tactile information from the lower and upper parts of the body, respectively, cross the midline in the caudal medulla, giving rise to the sensory decussation. The pyramidal tracts, which contain fibers descending from the motor cortex into the spinal cord, decussate slightly more rostrally, giving rise to the pyramidal, or motor decussation. These decussations are responsible for the fact that the left half of the brain controls and senses the right half of the body, and vice versa. Thus in general, damage to brain structures above the decussation gives rise to contralateral symptoms, whereas damage below the decussation results in ipsilateral symptoms (except for the cerebellum as discussed later). Finally, the medulla contains the brain's respiratory control center, which is of paramount importance in determining brain death (see later). In the absence of neuromuscular blockade, complete apnea in response to rising $PaCO_2$ results only when the medulla has been extensively injured.

Although extensive damage to the medullary structures is often quickly fatal due to ensuing apnea, more localized injury produces a number of recognizable syndromes. Wallenberg, or lateral medullary, syndrome occurs when the territory supplied by posterior inferior cerebellar artery has been compromised and consists of loss of temperature and pain sensation on the contralateral side of the body and ipsilateral side of the face. Additionally, Horner syndrome and varying degrees of vertigo, dysphagia, and dysarthria can be present. The medial medullary syndrome (Dejerine or inferior alternating syndrome) results from injury to the territory supplied by the anterior spinal artery or, occasionally, the vertebral artery. It is characterized by weakness or complete hemiplegia and loss of tactile and vibratory perception on the contralateral side of the body, together with preservation of temperature and pain sensation in the body and full sensation in the face. Medullary injury also occurs as a life-threatening, albeit rare, complication of tonsillectomy and adenoidectomy.[41]

Pons

The pons extends from the medulla to the midbrain and is readily recognized by the massive, bulbous structure with horizontally oriented fibers on its ventral surface that gives rise to its name (from the Latin, *bridge*). The pons begins at the pontine-medullary junction, characterized by a groove from which the abducens (CN VI), facial (CN VII), and vestibulocochlear (CN VIII) nerves emerge. It extends rostrally to the point of emergence of the trochlear nerve (CN IV), where it transitions into the midbrain. The trigeminal nerve (CN V) exits from the lateral aspect of the pons approximately midway between the medulla and midbrain.

In addition to the cranial nerves, the pons contains several other important structures. Its eponymous bulb, called the *basis pontis*, is formed by bundles of corticopontine fibers that connect the cerebral cortex with ipsilateral pontine nuclei. Postsynaptic fibers originating in the pontine nuclei then cross the midline and form the middle cerebellar peduncle, which comprises one of the major input pathways into the cerebellum. Cerebellar output to the thalamus and other structures takes place via the superior cerebellar peduncle contained in the rostral pons. Additionally, the rostral pons contains the locus ceruleus (from the Latin, *blue spot*). Locus ceruleus neurons use norepinephrine as a neurotransmitter, innervate wide-ranging areas of the brain, and likely regulate sleep and arousal.

Injury to pontine structures is of significant relevance in the pediatric ICU (PICU). First, increased intracranial pressure (ICP) from any cause may result in compression of the medially located small abducens nerve (CN VI), leading to paralysis of the lateral rectus eye muscle and associated turning in of the affected eye. Abducens nerve palsy due to increased ICP may precede the notorious fixed and dilated pupil phenomenon observed when CN III is compressed during impending uncal herniation (see later). Second, damage to the rostral pons (or lower midbrain) results in decerebrate posturing, characterized by extension of both upper and lower extremities on painful stimulation. Importantly, decerebrate posturing corresponds to the motor score of 2 on the Glasgow Coma Scale (GCS) score. Finally, infarction of the basis pontis with sparing of the more dorsal pontine structures results in the "locked-in" syndrome. The locked-in state is characterized by complete paralysis of all voluntary muscles except the muscles of ocular movement and by complete cognitive awareness. Because the locked-in patient can communicate only via eye gaze, recognition of the locked-in state by the physician requires extreme diligence in patients with brainstem lesions, lest the patient be misdiagnosed as comatose, with potentially dire consequences.

Midbrain

The midbrain is the most rostral and smallest of the brainstem structures. It is characterized by the presence of the bilateral inferior and superior colliculi on its dorsal surface. Additionally, the oculomotor nerve (CN III) emerges from its ventral surface, immediately below the temporal lobe of the cerebral hemisphere. The midbrain contains structures important for hearing, sound localization, and generation of saccadic eye movements. Furthermore, the substantia nigra in the midbrain contains neurons that use dopamine as their neurotransmitter. These dopaminergic neurons project to the basal ganglia, where dopamine release participates in initiation of voluntary movements, to the limbic system in the cerebral cortex, where dopamine plays a role in reward and emotion, and to the frontal and temporal cortices, indicating that dopamine affects thought and memory. Destruction of dopaminergic substantia nigra neurons underlies the pathology of idiopathic Parkinson disease in older individuals and of Parkinsonian symptoms in drug abusers exposed to 1-methyl-4-phenyl-1,2,3,6-tetrahydropyridine, sometimes a contaminant in heroin preparations.

Two clinical phenomena of significant importance in pediatric critical care medicine arise from damage to midbrain structures. First, global injury to the midbrain results in decorticate posturing, characterized by flexion of upper extremities and extension of lower extremities in response to painful stimulation. Decorticate posturing corresponds to a motor score of 3 on the GCS. Second, the "blown" pupil universally recognized as a sign of increased ICP and impending transtentorial brain herniation results from compression of the oculomotor nerve (CN III) as it exits the midbrain. Pupillary dilatation results from compression and inactivation of the parasympathetic fibers that run on the outer surface of CN III and which are actually responsible for pupillary constriction. When these fibers are damaged, unopposed sympathetic stimulation arising from the cervical sympathetic ganglia results in a constitutively dilated pupil that cannot constrict in response to light stimulation, or in other words, is "fixed." Unilateral fixed and dilated pupil is an emergency that requires immediate medical and/or surgical intervention.

Reticular Formation

The brainstem reticular formation is not a separate anatomic structure but is instead distributed throughout the core of the brainstem from the medulla into the midbrain. It plays a fundamental role in arousal and consciousness, control of movement and sensation, and in regulation of visceral functions. A subset of the reticular formation neurons sends fibers to the intralaminar thalamic nuclei, which in turn project widely throughout the cerebral cortex. Damage to these ascending brainstem fibers, collectively called the *ascending reticular activating system,* results in loss of consciousness and coma, even in the absence of any damage to the cerebral hemispheres. Thus the cerebral cortex requires input from the brainstem to maintain awareness and arousal. In addition, the reticular formation contains neuronal circuits responsible for regulation of respiration, cardiovascular responses to blood pressure and oxygen level modulations, and coordination of swallowing and other oromotor functions. Finally, complex reflexes such as walking and maintenance of body orientation with respect to gravity are coordinated by the brainstem reticular formation and may occur in the absence of input from higher brain regions. Immaturity of the brainstem reticular formation, in particular of its serotonergic component, has been implicated in the etiology of SUID.[14]

Cerebellum

The cerebellum overlies the majority of the brainstem and is separated from the cerebral cortex by a sheetlike reflection of the dura mater, called the *tentorium cerebelli.* Hence the brainstem and cerebellum are referred to as *infratentorial structures* while the cerebral cortex and the diencephalon are referred to as *supratentorial structures.* The cerebellum consists of a midline vermis and two large cerebellar hemispheres.[40] The outer surface of the cerebellum consists of a three-layered cortex, which includes the outer molecular layer, Purkinje cell layer, and granular layer. The molecular layer contains mostly axons and dendrites. The Purkinje cell layer contains the eponymous large GABA-ergic neurons that constitute the sole cerebellar output. Finally, the granular layer contains small granule cells that interact with other granule cells and with Purkinje neurons. In addition to the cerebellar cortex, each cerebellar hemisphere also contains a set of deep nuclei. From lateral to medial, these are the dentate, interposed, and fastigial nuclei.

Cerebellar function has traditionally been confined to regulation and coordination of movement of the eyes, head, and body in space. However, evidence from neuroanatomic and functional neuroimaging studies has suggested that the cerebellum, and in particular the dentate nucleus, plays a significant role in cognition, memory, and language.[42,43] Consequently, lesions in the cerebellum are characterized by ataxia, ipsilateral dysmetria, and intention tremor, as well as by scanning speech, in which each syllable is produced slowly and separately, and by disorders of memory and executive function.[43] In the PICU, cerebellar lesions are seen most frequently in the setting of infratentorial tumors but also occasionally in cerebellar strokes.

Diencephalon

The diencephalon consists of four major structures: thalamus, hypothalamus, subthalamus, and epithalamus. Of these, only the thalamus and the hypothalamus are discussed in detail as they serve crucial functions relevant to pediatric critical care medicine. The thalamus is the major relay station for all sensory information except olfaction as it travels from peripheral sensory organs to the cerebral cortex. For example, optic nerve neurons carrying visual information synapse onto neurons in the lateral geniculate nucleus in the thalamus, which process and transmit the signal to the primary visual cortex in the occipital lobe. Furthermore, the thalamus participates in coordination of motor activity via multiple neuronal loops that connect the cerebellum with the basal ganglia and the cerebral cortex.[43] Lastly, inhibitory thalamic nuclei such as the reticular nucleus (distinct from the brainstem reticular formation) are thought to participate in gating of attention and consciousness.[44]

Injury to the thalamus occurs frequently in both term and preterm neonates exposed to hypoxia-ischemia at birth.[45] Additionally, thalamic necrosis is observed in infectious encephalitis, particularly that associated with the influenza virus[46,47] and *Mycoplasma pneumoniae.*[48] Vascular diseases, such as occlusion of the basilar artery or systemic lupus erythematosus, can result in thalamic injury that can occasionally be reversible.[49] Apparent life-threatening events have been rarely associated with thalamic lesions.[50] Thalamic damage is associated with a wide range of symptoms, including pure sensory loss due to destruction of sensory relay nuclei, acute abnormalities in mental status, labile emotions, and motor dysfunction.

The hypothalamus is located inferior to the thalamus and plays a major role in regulation of emotion, homeostasis, circadian rhythms, and ANS function. Most importantly, it controls hormone release in the pituitary gland via two separate pathways. Large hypothalamic neurons in the supraoptic and paraventricular nuclei project their axons via the pituitary stalk into the posterior pituitary lobe (neurohypophysis), where they release antidiuretic hormone (ADH) and oxytocin directly into the bloodstream. ADH promotes water reabsorption in the kidney, whereas oxytocin participates in parturition and milk secretion. Damage to the posterior pituitary produces diabetes insipidus. Hypothalamic projections into the anterior pituitary (adenohypophysis) also travel down the pituitary stalk and release a multitude of release-promoting or release-inhibiting factors into the pituitary portal vein.[40] These factors then control the release of all anterior pituitary hormones, including adrenocorticotropic hormone, thyroid stimulating hormone, growth hormone, prolactin, and luteinizing/follicle-stimulating hormone. Of these, only prolactin release is constitutively inhibited by the hypothalamus, while the release of all remaining pituitary hormones is under positive control. Thus transection of the pituitary stalk, as can occur during skull base and pituitary surgery,[51] results in panhypopituitary syndrome characterized by diabetes insipidus, hypothyroidism, cortisol deficiency, and hyperprolactinemia.

Damage to hypothalamic nuclei, in addition to disrupting control of the pituitary gland, also results in emotional lability, aggression, and extreme overeating or anorexia leading to rapid weight gain or loss, respectively. Thus overwhelming aggression combined with acute weight changes should raise suspicion for a hypothalamic tumor in a child.

Basal Ganglia

The basal ganglia are a set of deep nuclei that reside below the surface of the cerebral cortex and surround the thalamus. They are composed of the caudate, putamen, globus pallidus, substantia nigra, and subthalamic nucleus. The caudate receives most of its input from the prefrontal cortex and projects via the globus pallidus and thalamus back to the prefrontal cortex. It is thus involved with cognitive function and tends to be one of the nuclei that degenerate slowly over time after a hypoxic-ischemic insult to the cortex. The putamen receives most of its input from the somatosensory and motor cortices and, like the caudate, projects back to these cortices via the globus pallidus and thalamus. The putamen plays a major role in coordination of motor function. The globus pallidus serves as an inhibitory modulator in the cortex–basal ganglia–thalamus–cortex loop. Hence deep brain stimulation in the globus pallidus in patients with Parkinson disease results in resolution of motor symptoms attributable to hyperactivity in the loop, such as tremor and rigidity. The substantia nigra contains dopaminergic neurons that project to the other nuclei in the basal ganglia and participate in initiation and coordination of voluntary movement.

The basal ganglia are the site of injury in multiple processes in pediatrics. They are often injured by hypoxia and hypoglycemia due to interruption of energy supply. Similarly, carbon monoxide poisoning effectively prevents oxygen delivery to the basal ganglia, resulting in characteristic neuroradiologic findings.[52] A number of metabolic diseases, including methylmalonic acidemia, Leigh disease, maple syrup urine disease, and glutaric acidemia type II, also result in degeneration in the basal ganglia. The basal ganglia accumulate iron and copper and consequently can be injured by iron overload or in Wilson disease. Finally, a juvenile form of Huntington disease presents with characteristic degeneration in the caudate nucleus.[52] Clinical signs of injury to the basal ganglia are often nonspecific: lethargy, irritability, and decreased mental status. Movement disorders such as dystonia or chorea can be seen early in the course of injury but are relatively uncommon, being more likely to emerge with chronic deterioration in basal ganglia function.

Cerebral Hemispheres

The cerebral hemispheres are the most rostral part of the CNS, and in humans and some other mammals, they are characterized by extensive folding of the cerebral cortex. The folding greatly expands the area of the cerebral cortex that can fit into the cranial vault. In humans, the cortical sheet has an area of 2.5 square feet when all the folds are flattened, yet the surface area of the adult skull is closer to 0.5 square feet. The folds consist of ridges termed *gyri* (singular, *gyrus*) and spaces separating the ridges termed *sulci* (singular, *sulcus*). Although the detailed organization of each gyrus and sulcus is quite individualized, the larger organizational features are common to all mammals.

Each cerebral hemisphere is divided into four lobes: frontal, parietal, temporal, and occipital (Fig. 60.3). The frontal lobe extends caudally from the rostral pole of the brain to the central sulcus and inferolaterally to the lateral sulcus. The parietal lobe begins at the central sulcus and extends caudally to the parietooccipital sulcus. Inferolaterally, the parietal lobe is bounded by the lateral sulcus and imaginary line connecting the extension of the lateral sulcus with the parietooccipital sulcus. The temporal lobe is delineated primarily by the lateral sulcus. Finally, the occipital lobe resides posteriorly to the parietooccipital sulcus. Each of the four lobes performs dedicated functions, some of which are symmetric, occurring in both hemispheres, whereas others are lateralized, specific to either the right or left cerebral hemisphere.

The frontal lobe is divided into four cortices, reflecting its functional organization. The primary motor cortex, located on the precentral gyrus, directly controls volitional movement on the contralateral side via upper motoneurons projecting to the lower motoneurons in the spinal cord. Moving rostrally, the premotor cortex is involved in planning, coordination, and initiation of movement. The most rostral part of the frontal lobe, the prefrontal cortex, is generally associated with personality and foresight/planning. Additionally, one side of the frontal lobe, usually the left, contains the Broca area on its inferolateral surface. The Broca area participates in the production of spoken and written language.

The parietal lobe contains the primary somatosensory cortex, which is located on the postcentral gyrus and which receives all tactile and proprioceptive sensory information from the contralateral side of the body. The parietal cortex

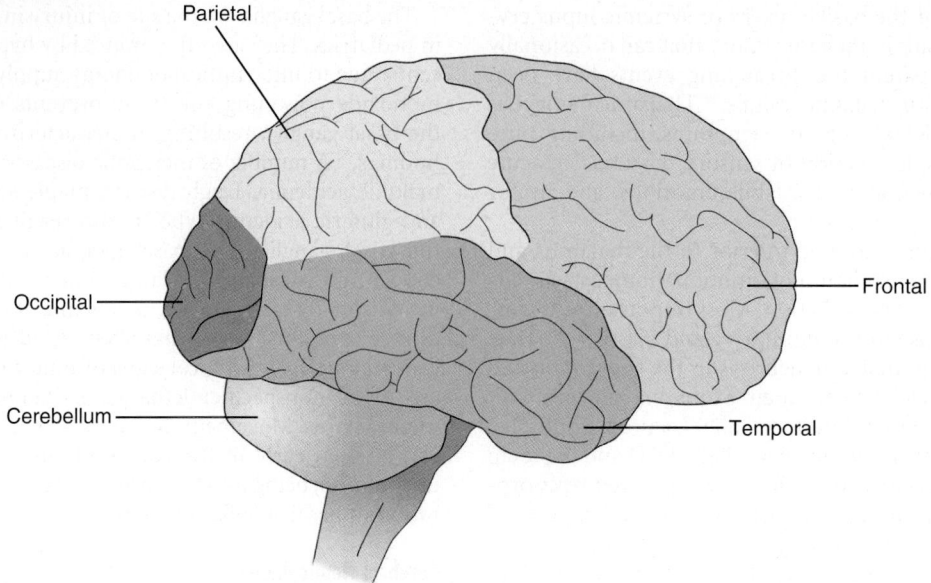

Fig. 60.3. General subdivisions of the human cerebral cortex. Note that the cerebellum is not part of the cortex but is labeled for clarity.

posterior to the primary somatosensory cortex possesses quite lateralized functional areas, with cortex on the left usually involved with language processing and comprehension, and that on the right responsible for perception of space and special orientation. The occipital lobe is generally devoted to vision in humans, containing the primary visual cortex and several secondary visual areas. The temporal lobe, on the other hand, serves more diverse functions. It contains the primary auditory cortex, which receives all auditory stimuli from the periphery. The temporal lobe also encompasses the hippocampus and the limbic system, thus participating in learning, memory, and emotion.

Peripheral Nervous System

The peripheral nervous system is generally divided into two components: the somatic PNS, which includes the peripheral nerves carrying information to and from muscle and skin, and the visceral (or autonomic) PNS, which regulates homeostatic bodily functions and mainly innervates visceral organs such as the heart, lungs, and intestines. Dysfunction of both the somatic and the autonomic systems contributes to the breadth of pathology encountered in pediatric critical care medicine, thus requiring the pediatric intensivist to be familiar with the basic organizational and functional principles of the PNS.

Somatic Peripheral Nervous System

The somatic PNS consists of efferent nerve fibers carrying information to muscle and skin, peripheral sensory receptors, and afferent nerve fibers carrying information from the periphery to the CNS. The efferent fibers emerge from neurons located in the spinal gray matter and exit the spinal cord via the ventral root. The afferent sensory fibers belong to neurons located in dorsal root ganglia, which send an axonal branch into the spinal cord via the dorsal root. The efferent and the afferent fibers travel together between the dorsal root ganglia and the target organ in the peripheral nerve. Diseases of the somatic PNS relevant to pediatric intensive care are generally disorders of myelination, such as Guillain-Barré syndrome, and are discussed in detail in Chapter 71).

Visceral or Autonomic Peripheral Nervous System

The autonomic nervous system regulates bodily functions that do not necessarily require conscious control or awareness, such as heart rate, blood pressure, sphincter function, and digestion. The ANS is divided into three distinct components: the enteric, parasympathetic, and sympathetic nervous systems. The enteric nervous system consists of the myenteric plexus of Auerbach and the submucosal plexus of Meissner, both located in the wall of the alimentary canal. The enteric nervous system interacts with the CNS and parasympathetic and sympathetic components of the ANS but can function entirely independently. It is responsible for sensation and coordination of peristalsis in the gut. Neurons in the enteric nervous system arise from the same progenitors as neurons in the CNS. Hence many neurologic disorders concomitantly affect both the central and enteric nervous systems, including irritable bowel syndrome, anxiety, and depression.[53]

Sympathetic Nervous System

The sympathetic nervous system consists of preganglionic and postganglionic components. Preganglionic fibers originate from neurons in the thoracolumbar region of the spinal cord, giving the sympathetic ANS its anatomic name: the thoracolumbar outflow. Preganglionic fibers exit the spinal cord via the ventral roots with the thoracic and lumbar nerves. After traveling together for a short distance, the preganglionic fibers diverge from the spinal nerves and enter the sympathetic ganglia via the white communicating rami (preganglionic fibers are thinly myelinated; hence, white). The preganglionic fibers carrying output to the head, thorax, and limbs synapse onto neurons in sympathetic ganglia located close to the spinal cord. These ganglia form the paravertebral sympathetic chain that extends from the cervix to the coccyx. The preganglionic fibers carrying output to the abdominal and pelvic viscera synapse onto cells located in sympathetic ganglia farther away from the spinal cord, called the *prevertebral ganglia*. These include the celiac, superior mesenteric, and inferior mesenteric ganglia. Postganglionic neurons from either the paravertebral or prevertebral ganglia send their fibers to the target organs via the gray communicating rami (postganglionic fibers are unmyelinated and hence gray). In the sympathetic ANS, preganglionic neurons use acetylcholine as a neurotransmitter, whereas postganglionic neurons use norepinephrine at the target organs. The exception is the sweat glands, which receive postganglionic sympathetic fibers using acetylcholine.[40]

The sympathetic ANS generally functions to prepare the body for states of increased energy expenditure. Activation of the sympathetic ANS leads to increased heart rate, decreased peristalsis, redistribution of blood from the gut to the peripheral muscles, and pupillary dilatation (mydriasis). Furthermore, the sympathetic ANS directly innervates the adrenal medulla and, when activated, stimulates the medulla to release norepinephrine and epinephrine into the systemic circulation. Systemic catecholamine release produces relatively global and long-lasting effects. In critical care, a significant component of vasopressor support relies on mimicking the effect of sympathetic ANS activation with exogenously administered epinephrine and norepinephrine.

Although autonomous, the sympathetic nervous system is under significant central control. Interruption of the descending control pathways, such as occurs with spinal cord trauma above the level of T1, results in sudden loss of sympathetic tone, causing profound bradycardia and hypotension. This syndrome, termed *neurogenic* or *spinal shock,* emerges early after injury and requires aggressive pharmacologic intervention in order to minimize secondary insults resulting from hypoperfusion of the injured spinal cord.[54,55]

Parasympathetic Autonomic Nervous System

The preganglionic fibers of the parasympathetic ANS originate in the brainstem and sacral spinal cord. Hence the parasympathetic ANS comprises the craniosacral outflow. The brainstem preganglionic fibers travel along cranial nerves III, VII, IX, and X, while the sacral preganglionic fibers travel with the pelvic splanchnic nerves. Parasympathetic ganglia are located close to their targets, unlike the ganglia in the sympathetic ANS. The parasympathetic ANS, also unlike its sympathetic counterpart, uses acetylcholine as a neurotransmitter both in presynaptic and postganglionic neurons. Target organs for the cranial portion of the parasympathetic ANS include the ciliary muscle and pupillary sphincter, innervated by CNIII via the ciliary ganglion; lacrimal and salivary glands; as well as the majority of thoracic and abdominal organs innervated by the vagus nerve (CNX). The sacral portion innervates the bladder and genitalia.

The parasympathetic system, in general, exerts effects opposite to those of the sympathetic ANS. Thus ACh release from parasympathetic fibers causes bradycardia, hypotension, increased gastrointestinal motility, and pupillary constriction. In critical care, atropine, a competitive antagonist of the muscarinic ACh receptor, is used to prevent or treat bradycardia associated with poor perfusion.[56]

Meninges

The CNS is protected by three membranous layers, which anchor the brain within the skull, contain cerebrospinal fluid (CSF), and form the anatomic basis of the cerebral venous sinuses. From the outside in, these are the dura mater, arachnoid, and pia mater. Dura mater, often simply called dura, is physically the most substantial of the three membranes and is called the *pachymeninx.* The arachnoid and pia together are referred to as *leptomeninges.* The dura attaches firmly to the inner surface of the skull and arachnoid. Under normal circumstances, no open space exists either between the dura and skull (the epidural space) or between the dura and arachnoid (the subdural space). Under pathologic conditions, however, blood can dissect the epidural and/or the subdural potential spaces to form potentially life-threatening hematomas. The dura's blood supply is provided by the middle meningeal artery, which traverses between the skull and outer dural surface. Trauma to the skull and the middle meningeal artery can lead to an epidural hematoma. The dura also forms the cerebral venous sinuses into which cerebral veins drain. Rupture of the veins as they leave the brain and enter the venous sinuses can lead to a subdural hematoma.

The arachnoid membrane is significantly thinner than the dura, consisting of several cell layers and a spider web–like collagen network. Whereas it adheres to the dura on the outer surface, on the inner surface it is connected to the pia via thin strands of connective tissue called *arachnoid trabeculae.* The space between the arachnoid and pia (subarachnoid space) forms the only true fluid-filled space around the brain, containing CSF, and forming the basis for CSF cisterns throughout the CNS. CSF from the subarachnoid space returns to the venous circulation via special adaptations in the arachnoid membrane called the *arachnoid villi.* Arachnoid villi protrude from the arachnoid into the dural venous sinuses and contain special channels that allow the CSF to flow out of the subarachnoid space into the venous blood. Additionally, cerebral arteries and veins run in the subarachnoid space before diving below the brain surface. Hence injury to these vessels results in subarachnoid hemorrhage.

The pia mater is the most delicate of the three membranes. Unlike the dura and the arachnoid, it follows the surface of the brain, diving into every sulcus and following blood vessels for some distance as they enter the brain. Around these blood vessels, it gives rise to potential perivascular spaces called the *Virchow-Robin spaces* that serve as a significant reservoir of malignant cells in pediatric leukemia and lymphoma, necessitating CNS irradiation and chemoprophylaxis.

Blood-Brain Barrier

Anatomy

Two experiments more than 100 years ago demonstrated conclusively the presence of a physical barrier between circulating blood and the brain. In 1885, Ehrlich injected a dye intravenously to show that the dye failed to stain the brain while staining almost all other internal organs.[57] In 1909, Goldman conducted the reverse experiment, injecting dye into the CSF to show that the dye stained the brain but did not penetrate into the general circulation,[58] although more contemporary studies have demonstrated an organized pathway for extracellular fluid and macromolecular flux from brain to blood via CNS lymphatics (see later). Modern anatomic studies revealed that, actually, three physical barriers separate the blood and the brain: the BBB, established by the endothelial capillary cells in the brain; the blood-CSF barrier (BCSFB), established by cells in the choroid plexus; and finally, the CSF-brain barrier, composed of ependymal cells lining the surface of the ventricles. All three systems shield the brain from changes in

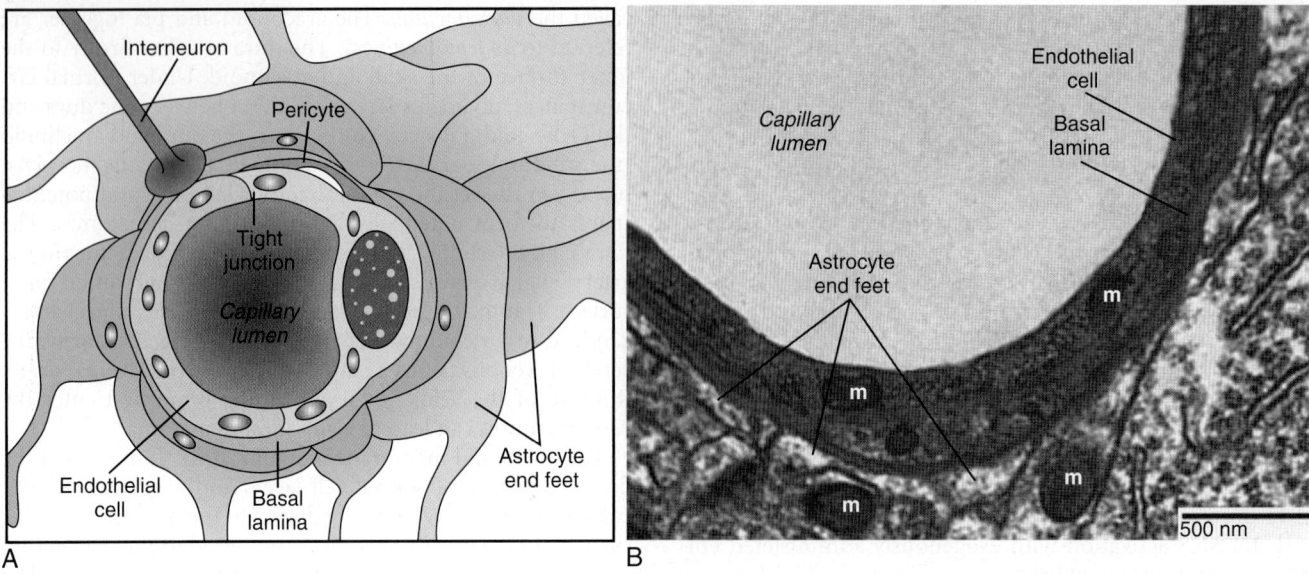

Fig. 60.4. (A) Schematic representation of the major anatomic features contributing to the blood-brain barrier (BBB). It should be noted that endothelial cells surrounding the capillary are linked by tight junctions. (B) An electron micrograph from a mouse brain showing a brain capillary in cross section. The BBB is an active structure, with high energy demands. Hence BBB endothelial cells and astrocytes possess a large number of mitochondria (m).

ionic and biochemical milieu that may jeopardize neuronal function, and all three are important for accomplishing drug transport into and out of the brain parenchyma.[59] However, from the standpoint of clinical relevance to pediatric critical care medicine, the subsequent discussion focuses primarily on the BBB and BCSFB.

The cellular component of the BBB in mammals comprises specialized endothelial cells in brain capillaries, pericytes, and foot processes of brain astrocytes, as well as neurons (Fig. 60.4). Endothelial cells in the brain are linked together by tight junctions, which prevent paracellular diffusion of substances from blood into the brain. The endothelial tight junctions in the brain possess extremely high electrical resistance, resulting in the exclusion of even small ions such as K^+ and Na^+.[60] In addition, the absence of fenestrations, high metabolic rate, and low vesicular transport in endothelial cells severely limit transcellular diffusion of water-soluble substances through the cell membrane. Pericytes surround the endothelial cells and display both contractile and phagocytic properties. Their presence likely contributes to the impermeability of the endothelial tight junctions, as well as to blood vessel reactivity[61] and vessel wall elastic properties in the brain.[62] Pericytes in turn are ensheathed by perivascular astrocytes, which extend cellular processes, known as "end-feet," toward the brain vasculature.[60] The astrocytes are critical for the proper development of the brain-specific phenotype of endothelial cells comprising the BBB.[63] Finally, neurons have been shown to innervate the brain capillary endothelial cells directly, although their exact role in BBB function remains unknown.[64]

In addition to the cellular components, the BBB also contains two distinct and important acellular components: the basement membrane and the extracellular matrix. At present, the role of the extracellular matrix in maintaining or establishing the BBB is unknown. The role of the basement membrane, on the other hand, is better characterized. The basement membrane surrounding small draining venules consists of the endothelial layer, immediately adjacent to the brain capillary endothelium, and the parenchymal layer, which is adjacent to astrocyte end-feet. Interposed between the two basement membranes is a layer of meningeal epithelium. Around the capillaries, however, the meningeal epithelium disappears, and the two layers of the basement membrane fuse to form a composite structure.[60] The basement membrane generally consists of four major types of glycoproteins: collagen type IV, laminin, nidogen, and heparan sulfate proteoglycan. The clinical relevance of these proteins, although not fully understood at this time, is underscored by mutations in collagen type IV that result in intracerebral hemorrhage and porencephaly in rodents and in humans.[65,66]

Selectivity

If the BBB limits the penetration of substances into the CSF, then how is transport of energy sources, signaling molecules, and drugs from blood into the CSF accomplished? Three general transport mechanisms allow chemicals to penetrate from the circulation into the CSF: (1) diffusion of lipid-soluble molecules; (2) receptor-facilitated transport, either energy-dependent or independent; and (3) ion channel-mediated transport. Additionally, several groups of transporters are dedicated to actively pumping substances out of CSF into the circulation.

As a general rule, lipid-soluble substances penetrate into CSF by diffusing across the endothelial plasma membrane, whereas water-soluble substances require active transport to cross the BBB. This property is illustrated by Fig. 60.5, which demonstrates uptake of substances into the brain as a function of their oil-water partition coefficient. Compounds such as benzodiazepines, nicotine, and heroin are highly lipid soluble and penetrate readily into the CSF. The synthetic opiate fentanyl induces the narcotic effect more rapidly than morphine because fentanyl is more lipophilic. The concentration of a lipophilic substance in the CSF is generally directly

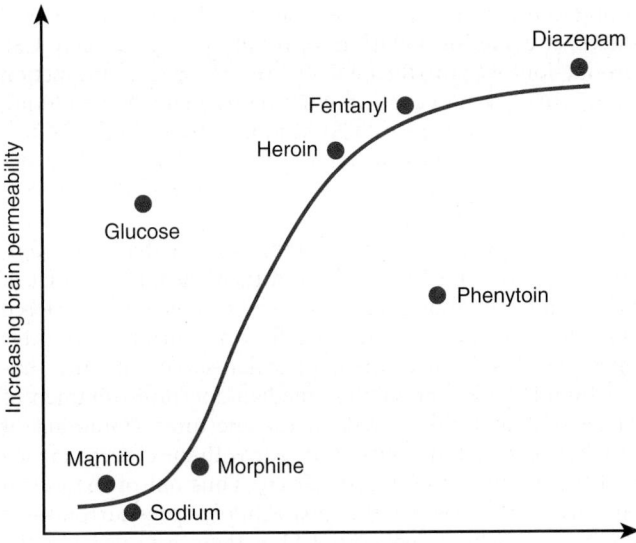

Fig. 60.5. Lipid solubility predicts penetration across the blood-brain barrier *(BBB)*. Substances to the left of the curve, such as glucose, cross the BBB at a higher rate than would be predicted on the basis of their oil solubility. These substances are transported by carriers across the BBB via either an energy-dependent or energy-independent process. In contrast, substances to the right of the curve, such as phenytoin, are highly lipid soluble but are transported across the BBB out of the brain milieu. (Adapted from Laterra J, Goldstein GW. Ventricular organization of cerebrospinal fluid: blood-brain barrier, brain edema, and hydrocephalus. In Kandel ER, Schwartz JH, Jessel TM, editors. Principles of Neural Science. New York: McGraw-Hill; 2000.)

proportional to its concentration in the plasma. In contrast, mannitol and sodium ions are extremely water soluble, do not penetrate into the CSF across the intact BBB, and are thus used clinically to increase serum osmolality relative to that of CSF and to draw water out of the brain in order to decrease ICP. Lipophilic substances with a significant protein-bound fraction (eg, phenytoin) constitute an exception to the generalization that lipid-solubility and plasma concentration determine CSF concentration. Consequently, in the case of phenytoin and its commonly used prodrug fosphenytoin, therapeutic levels are determined by plasma, or free, concentration, rather than the total concentration, which includes the protein-bound fraction.

Receptor-facilitated transport across the BBB can be grouped into processes that require energy and those that do not. The best studied and perhaps most clinically relevant example of receptor-facilitated energy-independent transport is delivery of glucose from plasma into the CSF by the GLUT1 transporter. GLUT1 is a 492 amino-acid membrane protein that resides both on the luminal (facing the plasma) and the abluminal (facing the CSF) surfaces of the endothelial plasma membrane.[67] GLUT1 transports glucose down the concentration gradient and can function in a bidirectional manner. The flow of glucose from plasma into the CSF, rather than in the opposite direction, is ensured by (1) higher plasma glucose concentration ($\approx3:2$ of CSF); (2) high glucose utilization rate by neurons and glia in the CNS such that glucose delivered into the CSF is exhausted rather quickly; and (3) higher density of GLUT1 transporters on the abluminal surface compared with the luminal surface.[68] In addition, metabolic factors

such as hypoxia and ischemia exert transcriptional control over expression and distribution of the GLUT1 transporter, suggesting the existence of tightly controlled mechanisms regulating glucose delivery into the CSF under stressful conditions. Recently, a disorder characterized by GLUT1 deficiency was recognized in a subset of infants with developmental delay, intractable epilepsy, and delayed myelination.[69] Identification of the molecular underpinning of this disorder was driven by the clinical finding of low CSF glucose concentration (hypoglycorrhachia) on repeated lumbar punctures despite normal plasma glucose concentrations in two original patients from the study, highlighting the importance of biochemical BBB function.

While the energy-independent GLUT1 plays an important role in delivering its substrate down the concentration gradient into the CSF, energy-dependent transporters of the ATP-binding cassette (ABC) family function primarily to pump substances against the concentration gradient out of the CSF into plasma.[70] The ABC family of transporters is divided into seven known groups (A through G), of which groups B, C, and G are highly expressed on BBB endothelial cells. The best-described members of this family include the multidrug resistance (MDR) proteins, such as the P-glycoprotein (PgP), and the multidrug resistance-associated proteins (MRP). Human PgP transports a wide range of chemically and structurally diverse substances out of the CSF, including dexamethasone, phenytoin, ondansetron, and chemotherapeutic agents such as etoposide and vincristine.[70] MRPs also contribute to the ATP-dependent efflux of drugs such as 6-mercaptopurine, methotrexate, and, interestingly, pravastatin. The latter belongs to a class of drugs, hydroxymethylglutaryl-CoA (HMG-CoA) reductase inhibitors, that confers protective effects in experimental models of ischemic and traumatic brain injury[71,72] and reduce stroke risk in humans by approximately 30%, to some extent independent of the reduction in cholesterol levels.[73] Thus increasing the intracerebral levels of HMG-CoA reductase inhibitors via reduction in MRP-dependent efflux may represent a therapeutic strategy aimed at ameliorating the effect of trauma and hypoxia on the brain parenchyma. Indeed, the general strategy of inhibiting MDR and MRP transporters to enhance drug delivery into the CNS is currently being explored in clinical trials.

Blood-Brain Barrier–Deficient Areas

Several areas of the brain have special adaptations in the structure of the BBB that allow the CNS control centers to monitor and interact with the rest of the body. These include the posterior pituitary, the subfornical organ, and the area postrema; in all of these areas, capillaries contain fenestrations, and the BBB is quite leaky. The posterior pituitary contains projections of the hypothalamic vasopressin-containing secretory neurons. When salt concentration increases during volume depletion, these neurons are stimulated to release vasopressin (ADH) directly into the bloodstream, leading to increased water retention in the renal tubules and restoration of intravascular volume. The subfornical organ, located at the foramen of Monro on the ventral surface of the fornix, is also involved in maintaining salt-water homeostasis. Angiotensin II production during states of decreased renal perfusion is detected by neurons in the subfornical organ, which then stimulate vasopressin-containing neurons to release vasopressin and also stimulate neurons in the lateral hypothalamus to create an overwhelming sensation of thirst. Finally, neurons in the area postrema are exposed to toxins circulating in the plasma and stimulate the vomiting reflex. Drugs such as ondansetron are thought to prevent nausea and vomiting by blocking serotonin receptors in the area postrema. All brain regions with a leaky BBB are surrounded by specialized cells called *tanycytes*. Tanycytes are connected by tight junctions that prevent uncontrolled diffusion of substances out of these homeostatic brain regions into the rest of the CSF.

Ventricles and Cerebrospinal Fluid
Ventricular System

The ventricular system arises from the hollow space within the developing neural tube and gives rise to cisterns within the CNS, from the brain to the spinal cord. In the brain, the ventricular system consists of paired lateral ventricles that connect to the midline third ventricle via bilateral foramina of Monro. The third ventricle in turn connects to the fourth ventricle located in the pons and the medulla via the aqueduct of Sylvius. The fourth ventricle terminates caudally in the central spinal canal and continues as a miniscule midline structure through the spinal cord. The ventricles contain the choroid plexus, which produces CSF, and serve as conduits for CSF flow in the CNS. Ventricular walls are lined with ependymal cells, which are connected by tight junctions and constitute a CSF-brain barrier.

Cerebrospinal Fluid Production and Flow

CSF is produced by both the choroid epithelial cells and the brain parenchyma, with each system contributing approximately 50% to new CSF production. CSF produced by the choroid plexus flows directly into the ventricles, whereas CSF produced by the brain parenchyma must cross the ependymal

lining to reach the ventricular system. CSF in humans is produced at a rate of 350 μL/min, resulting in total daily CSF production of approximately 500 mL. Daily CSF production rates, when taken in context of the ventricular volume (30 mL in adults) and of the total CSF volume present in the CNS at any given time (130 mL in adults), indicate that CSF circulates out of the ventricular system where it is produced and CSF is continuously reabsorbed.

CSF flows via foramina of Monro out of the lateral ventricles into the third ventricle, and then via the aqueduct of Sylvius into the fourth ventricle. The former two are closed systems, whereas the latter, the fourth ventricle, has three openings that connect the ventricular space with the subarachnoid space. The midline median aperture (foramen of Magendie) and the paired lateral apertures (foramina of Luschka) connect the fourth ventricle with the cisterna magna and the pontine cistern, respectively. Thus out of the fourth ventricle, CSF flows into the subarachnoid space surrounding the brain and the spinal cord. CSF is then reabsorbed by the arachnoid villi into the superior sagittal venous sinus (Fig. 60.6). Knowledge of CSF flow and reabsorption patterns allows for prediction of pathologic findings when either process is interrupted. Obstruction to CSF outflow at any point in the pathway, such as often occurs with tumors, or abnormal CSF reabsorption, such as seen in meningitis or hemorrhage due to cellular debris blocking the arachnoid villi, results in intraventricular CSF accumulation and hydrocephalus. Hydrocephalus may then lead to increased ICP and cerebral herniation, either spontaneous or iatrogenic, for example when a lumbar puncture is performed on a patient with obstruction above the level of the foramen magnum.

Cerebrospinal Fluid Composition and Function

Cells in the choroid plexus actively secrete CSF from the plasma that filters through leaky choroid plexus capillaries.

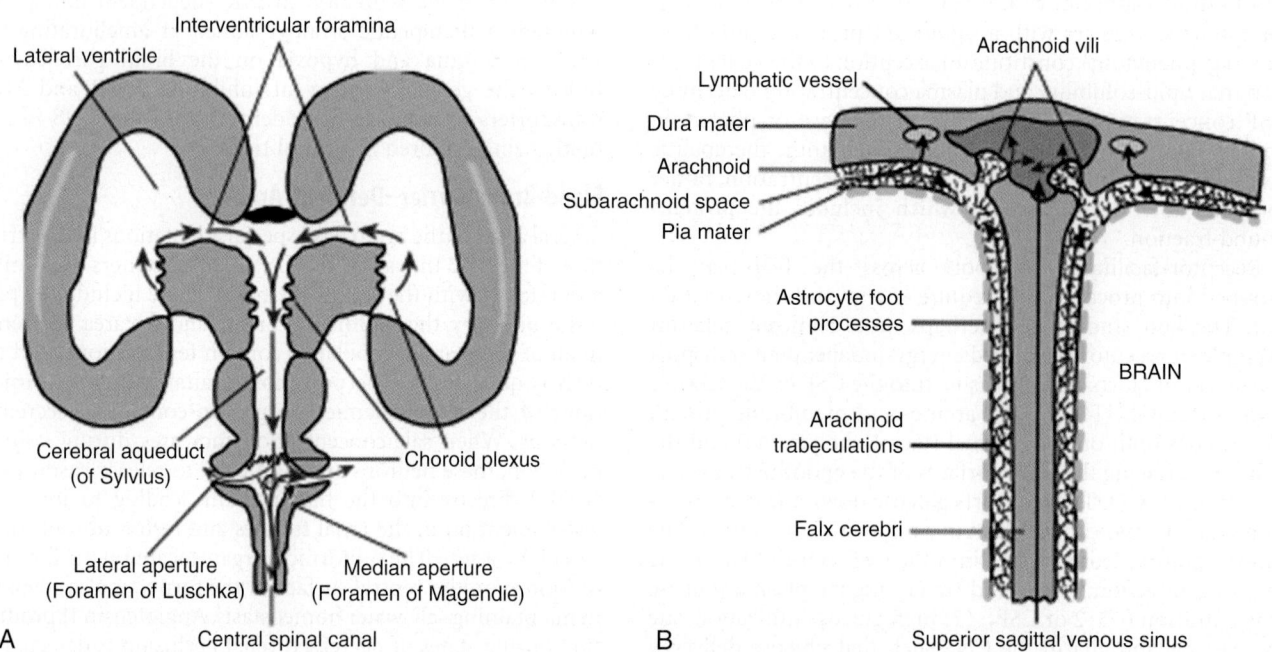

Fig. 60.6. The ventricles and cerebrospinal fluid (CSF) flow. (A) Flow of CSF from choroid plexus through the ventricular system into the subarachnoid space. Note that a portion of the CSF circulating into the distal spinal cord returns to the fourth ventricle. (B) Schematic representation of CSF absorption from the subarachnoid space into the cerebral venous sinus system and perivenous lymphatic vessels.

The process is controlled by multiple mechanisms, resulting in CSF ionic, chemical, and cellular composition that is distinct from blood and plasma. In general, CSF contains higher magnesium and chloride concentrations and lower potassium and calcium concentrations compared with plasma. Glucose concentrations in CSF are approximately two-thirds of plasma levels. CSF has very few cells and a constant protein level. As is well known, these constituents are disrupted in disease. In bacterial meningitis, glucose concentrations are lower than expected and protein concentration is increased. In contrast, in viral meningitis, CSF glucose is usually normal while protein concentration is increased. More recently, levels of various cytokines and proteins leaked from neurons and myelin sheaths have been explored as potential biomarkers of the severity and type of brain injury.[74]

The primary purpose of the CSF is to provide a supportive buoyant environment for the brain. The human brain has the consistency of an incompletely hardened bowl of gelatin. Without the CSF, the human brain flattens significantly under the force of gravity, whereas, suspended in CSF, it retains its native shape. Furthermore, CSF provides a fluid cushion against acceleration-deceleration insults that may be delivered to the brain by the surrounding skull. CSF also functions both as a source of nutrients and a relatively large-volume sink for waste and toxic substances produced in the course of normal neuronal activity. For instance, excess glutamate released at the synapse rapidly diffuses into the CSF, minimizing potential excitotoxicity to both presynaptic and postsynaptic neurons. Excess magnesium ions in the CSF may also participate in the Mg^{2+} block at the NMDA receptors (see section on glutamate receptors), allowing for coincidence detection and learning.

Vasculature in the Central Nervous System
Brain Vasculature

The arterial blood supply to the brain is traditionally divided into an anterior portion supplied by the paired internal carotid arteries and the posterior portion supplied by the paired vertebral arteries. The anterior and posterior arterial circulations are interconnected at the base of the brain via circle of Willis.

The internal carotid artery originates from the common carotid artery at approximately the level of angle of the jaw in humans. It enters the skull through the carotid canal anterior to the jugular foramen, takes a relatively standard but tortuous course through the temporal bone and the cavernous sinus, and then enters the dura mater above the sinus, running horizontally inferolateral to the optic nerve. At this point, it gives off the ophthalmic artery and, a short distance later, the anterior choroidal artery and posterior communicating artery. The former supplies several clinically relevant structures, including parts of the thalamus, hippocampus, optic tract, and internal capsule. The latter, the posterior communicating artery, forms part of the circle of Willis and connects the anterior internal carotid circulation with the posterior vertebral circulation. After generating the posterior communicating artery, the internal carotid bifurcates into major vessels supplying the brain: the anterior and middle cerebral arteries (ACA and MCA, respectively).

The bilateral ACAs connect via the anterior communicating artery at the circle of Willis. Both ACAs then run along the medial surface of the brain and supply the corpus callosum and the medial portions of the cerebral cortex on their respective sides, extending up to and including the postcentral gyrus. Thus ACA occlusion results in damage (among other areas) to the medial portions of the primary sensory and motor cortices, which correspond to the more caudal parts of the human body, such as legs, trunk, and shoulders.

While the ACA supplies blood to the medial cerebral cortex, the MCA provides blood flow to almost the entire lateral portion of the cortex. After diverging from the internal carotid artery, the MCA dives deep into the Sylvian fissure, where it supplies the insula. In addition, within the Sylvian fissure, the MCA gives off small lenticulostriate arteries that supply the thalamus and basal ganglia. The MCA then emerges from the Sylvian fissure and divides into multiple branches responsible for nourishing the lateral components of the frontal, temporal, and parietal lobes. MCA occlusion secondary to ischemic stroke generally results in devastating neurologic deficits. Additionally, in cases of globally decreased perfusion such as seen during cardiac arrest or prolonged hypotension, the border (watershed) zone between the cortical areas supplied by the ACA and the MCA tends to be vulnerable to early injury.

The posterior circulation arises from the paired vertebral arteries, each of which gives rise to a posterior inferior cerebellar artery (PICA) before coalescing into a single basilar artery at the level of the junction between the medulla and the pons. The PICAs supply the inferior portion of the cerebellum, as well as the choroid plexus in the fourth ventricle and the lateral medulla. The basilar artery proceeds rostrally and gives rise to the paired anterior inferior cerebellar and superior cerebellar arteries (AICA and SCA, respectively). At the level of the midbrain, the basilar artery bifurcates into the posterior cerebral arteries (PCA), which supply the occipital lobes and portions of the temporal lobes. In addition, the PCAs nourish a number of thalamic sensory nuclei. Each PCA is connected to the ipsilateral internal carotid artery by the posterior communicating artery. Since the PCA supplies the areas of the thalamus concerned with sensation and cortical areas dedicated to vision, PCA occlusion often results in sensory and/or visual loss on the side contralateral to injury.

Spinal Cord Vasculature

The spinal cord is supplied by two interconnected arterial systems: the longitudinal vasculature that arises from the vertebral arteries and the segmental vasculature that arises from multiple levels along the vertebral arteries and the aorta. The longitudinal arteries consist of a single anterior spinal artery and paired posterior spinal arteries. The anterior spinal artery runs along the anterior median fissure and supplies the ventral two thirds of the spinal cord. Occlusion of the anterior spinal artery, which can occur with traumatic dissection or autoimmune arteritis, results in the anterior spinal syndrome, or Beck syndrome. Beck syndrome is characterized by symmetric weakness and loss of temperature and pain sensation with relative sparing of vibration and position sensation below the level of injury. The paired posterior spinal arteries run along the dorsal columns and supply blood to the posterior one-third of the spinal cord, which includes the dorsal columns and most of the dorsal horns. Posterior spinal arteries are extensively interconnected and receive blood supply from multiple segmental arteries along their course. Thus isolated lesions due to posterior spinal artery occlusion are rare.

The segmental arterial blood supply to the cervical spinal cord arises from the vertebral arteries via the radicular arteries, whereas that to the thoracic and lumbar spinal cord arises from the aorta via the thoracic intercostal arteries and lumbar arteries. Both thoracic and lumbar segmental arteries give rise to smaller radicular arteries that penetrate the intervertebral foramina and supply the spinal cord. In addition, the lower thoracic aorta often gives rise to a single great radicular artery (artery of Adamkiewicz) that supplies the entire lower two-thirds of the spinal column. The artery of Adamkiewicz is often the sole source of blood flow to the lower thoracic spinal cord during surgical repair of coarctation of the aorta. Thus care is taken to ensure adequate distal perfusion pressure during cross-clamp to minimize the risk of paraplegia. In general, spinal cord watershed areas exist at the upper thoracic (T1-T4) and upper lumbar (L1) levels, where interconnections among the segmental arteries are less developed. At any given level, the interior portion of the spinal cord is most susceptible to hypoxic-ischemic injury. For example, in cases of severe cervical hyperextension, hypoxic and/or vascular injury to the central portion of the cervical spinal cord results in central cord syndrome, characterized by muscle weakness in upper extremities to a greater extent than in lower extremities, by urinary retention, and by variable degree of sensory loss.

Regulation of Cerebral Blood Flow

In healthy mammals, the perfusion of cerebral tissues is exquisitely controlled. Blood flow to the brain, as to many other vital organs, is autoregulated by homeostatic mechanisms designed to maintain adequate perfusion. Cerebral autoregulation occurs on the basis of three primary mechanisms: perfusion pressure–based autoregulation, pH-based (PCO_2-based) autoregulation, and metabolic coupling. All three play a major role in determining cerebral blood flow (CBF) in health and in disease, such as trauma and hypoxia-ischemia.

Perfusion Pressure–Related Autoregulation

Experiments in the mid-20th century demonstrated that normal CBF in young adults is 50 to 55 mL/100 g brain/minute, resulting in approximately 750 mL/min total CBF.[75] Thus under resting conditions, the brain receives approximately 15% of total cardiac output. In children, CBF is generally higher than in adults, on the order of 100 mL/100 g brain/min for an 8-year-old child.[76] CBF is kept relatively constant over a range of mean arterial blood pressures (MAPs) by continuous adjustment of vascular tone in brain arterioles (Fig. 60.7A). In adults, CBF remains essentially invariant while MAP is between 50 and 150 mm Hg. Also in adults, CBF decreases and increases passively as a function of MAP when MAP is below 50 or above 150 mm Hg, respectively. The pressure-dependent autoregulatory range is different in newborns, with important clinical implications. The lower limit of autoregulation in neonates appears similar to that in adults at approximately 40 mm Hg; the upper limit, however, is much lower for infants than adults, with CBF increasing linearly as a function of MAP greater than 90 mm Hg.[77] Because infants have an MAP that is much closer to the lower limit of CBF autoregulation, even moderate hypotension in young children may severely impede oxygen delivery to the brain. Similarly, at the upper limit, moderate hypertension may result in unacceptable increases in CBF and damage to the

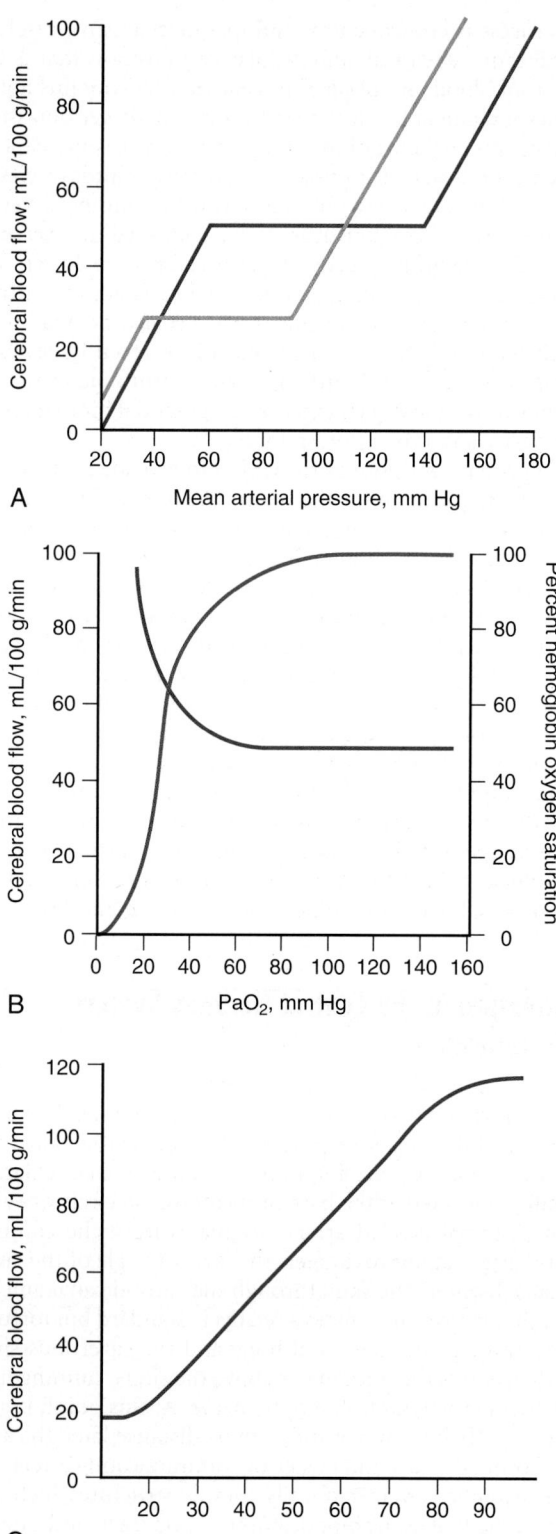

Fig. 60.7. Regulation of cerebral blood flow (CBF). (A) Blood pressure–dependent autoregulation, adult *(red curve)* and infant *(orange curve)*. (B) Oxygen-dependent regulation. *Red curve,* CBF (left ordinate); *blue curve,* hemoglobin-oxygen saturation curve (right ordinate). Note that CBF begins to increase at the PaO_2, at which hemoglobin oxygen saturation begins to decrease. Since oxygen delivery is determined by hemoglobin oxygen saturation to a much larger extent than by PaO_2 and dissolved oxygen in the blood, CBF in humans increases in response to decreasing oxygen delivery, which in turn is correlated with decreasing PaO_2. (C) $PaCO_2$-dependent regulation CBF should increase linearly with $PaCO_2$ except at the extremes of the physiologic range.

BBB. One of the many clinical applications of this principle is the need for meticulous control of MAP in infants on cardiopulmonary bypass in order to minimize the risk of intracranial hemorrhage.

Oxygen-Related Autoregulation

CBF generally remains constant while PaO_2 remains over 60 mm Hg. When PaO_2 decreases below this threshold value, CBF increases almost exponentially as a function of PaO_2 (Fig. 60.7B). Several distinct pathways contribute mechanistically to oxygen-related regulation of CBF, including hydrogen and potassium ions, nitric oxide, arachidonic acid, adenosine, and ATP-sensitive potassium channels.[78,79] The shape of the PaO_2-CBF curve is explained by the hemoglobin-oxygen dissociation curve and the fact that, in humans, CBF depends on blood oxygen content and not on PaO_2.[80] When PaO_2 is less than 60 mm Hg, the percentage of oxyhemoglobin decreases sharply, significantly decreasing the blood oxygen content. CBF rises as a consequence of decreased oxygen delivery. Conversely, increasing PaO_2 above 60 mm Hg does not significantly increase blood oxygen content since hemoglobin is more than 90% saturated with oxygen at these partial pressures. Hence in healthy people, CBF remains constant once PaO_2 crosses the threshold of 60 mm Hg.[81] Furthermore, when inspired oxygen fraction is increased further from 21% to 100%, CBF actually decreases by approximately 15% to 20%.[80] Both hypoxia-related vasodilatation and hyperoxia-related vasoconstriction may be impaired under pathologic conditions such as traumatic brain injury and may portend a poorer outcome. Nevertheless, a PaO_2 less than 60 mm Hg should be rigorously avoided in patients with increased ICP lest hypoxia-related vasodilatation further contribute to decreased compliance within the cranial vault.

Hydrogen Ion-Related Autoregulation

CBF is directly proportional to perivascular pH and, therefore, inversely proportional to the perivascular hydrogen ion concentration. In clinical practice, this relation translates into dependence of CBF on $PaCO_2$ because $PaCO_2$ is related to pH via the bicarbonate buffer system. Within a $PaCO_2$ range from 20 to 100 mm Hg, CBF increases by 2.5% to 4% for every 1 mm Hg increase in $PaCO_2$.[82] No further changes in CBF are observed when $PaCO_2$ is either below 20 mm Hg or above 100 mm Hg (Fig. 60.7C). The observed change in CBF in response to change in $PaCO_2$ is relatively transient, lasting hours. Restoration of intracerebral bicarbonate concentration is thought to be responsible for the temporary nature of the CBF response. Therefore once the brain and CBF have been "reset" to a new $PaCO_2$, acutely restoring $PaCO_2$ into a physiologically normal range actually results in disruption of the acid-base balance in the brain and may exacerbate injury. As such, chronic hyperventilation is not recommended as a therapy for increased ICP. Nevertheless, hyperventilation with concomitant rapid reduction in $PaCO_2$ remains one of the acute treatments for life-threatening increases in ICP and impending brain herniation.

Metabolic Coupling

Local CBF is coupled to the metabolic tissue demands in a relatively small, circumscribed area, reflecting both neuron- and astrocyte-specific energy needs. At rest, areas with greater energy needs, such as the gray matter, receive a greater proportion of CBF than areas with lesser energy needs, such as the white matter. The metabolic rate can be expressed as either cerebral metabolic rate of glucose (CMRGlu) or cerebral metabolic rate of oxygen ($CMRO_2$). Both CMRGlu and $CMRO_2$ have been correlated with CBF. Under conditions of sensory stimulation, however, the increase in CBF to the cortical sensory areas exceeds the increase in $CMRO_2$, suggesting that neuronal activity itself can influence CBF independent of the metabolic demand.[83] Neuronal activity–dependent increases in CBF form the presumed basis of functional magnetic resonance imaging, allowing for detailed studies of brain processes in humans.[84] In children, $CMRO_2$ increases until about 14 years of age and then decreases to adult values.[85] Similarly, CMRGlu increases from infancy until around 9 years of age and then decreases until adulthood.[86] The relationship between disturbances in metabolic coupling of CBF and injury is unclear at this time, although emerging evidence indicates occurrence of metabolic crises in the brain after traumatic injury and cardiac arrest.[76] Whether these crises reflect abnormal CBF regulation and predict outcome remains under investigation.

Emerging Characterization of the "Lymphatic" Circulation in the CNS

Until recently, the CNS has been unique among mammalian organ systems in its supposed absence of a dedicated lymphatic system for regulation of interstitial fluid composition and waste removal. Reexamination of old data and increasing abundance of new data indicate, however, that the mammalian CNS is endowed with a robust two-part lymphatic system—traditional lymphatic system along the dural venous sinuses and a unique "glymphatic" system in the brain parenchyma.

Early studies in multiple mammalian species demonstrated that up to 50% of brain interstitial fluid drains through deep cervical lymph nodes. Injection of radioactive and other tracers into the brain parenchyma resulted in preferential labeling of retropharyngeal lymph nodes.[87] Estimates of draining kinetics suggested that CSF flow through the ventricles into the cisterna magna accounted for less than 20% of total tracer clearance from the brain.[88] In 1981, Cserr and colleagues[88] presciently suggested that proteins in the brain parenchyma are cleared via bulk flow through the perivascular spaces into the deep cervical lymph nodes. These early findings were essentially forgotten for 30 years until discovery of lymphatic vessels in the CNS and rediscovery of bulk interstitial fluid flow along perivascular spaces in the 21st century.

Discovery of lymphatic vessels in the dural venous sinuses occurred during a search for a gateway that allows peripheral T cells to enter and exit the CNS during routine immunologic surveillance and during states of acute inflammation.[89] A novel preparation of mouse meninges revealed an unexpected linear arrangement of T cells in vessel-like structures. These vessel-like structures run along the dural venous sinuses and consist of cells with many immunologic markers of lymphatic endothelial cells. Unlike the systemic lymphatics, however, CNS lymphatic vessels do not contain smooth muscle cells or intraluminal valves. Fluorescent tracers injected into the cerebral ventricles, but not those injected into the systemic circulation, fill these vessels, demonstrating that CNS lymphatic vessels drain CSF. CSF flow in these vessels has a rate and direction similar to those of blood flowing in the venous sinuses.[89] Major drainage occurs via several routes—along the middle meningeal and pterygopalatine arteries, internal jugular veins, and cranial nerves and into nasal mucosa through the cribriform plate.[90] Ultimately, CNS lymphatic vessels appear to drain into deep cervical nodes.

Flow of CSF into the CNS lymphatic vessels occurs at least in part through a "glymphatic" system in the brain parenchyma (Fig. 60.6B). The glymphatic system, so called because of the crucial role of glia in its function, was rediscovered during a search for an answer to a specific question: How does the brain get rid of waste extracellular proteins? To answer this question, Nedergaard and colleagues[91] injected a fluorescent tracer into the cisterna magna of anesthetized mice and imaged its flow through the subarachnoid space using in vivo microscopy techniques. The tracer rapidly diffused throughout the subarachnoid space and then entered the brain parenchyma along the paravascular space, which accompanies the deep penetrating arterioles in the brain. This potential paravascular space has been known to exist for more than 100 years from anatomic and pathologic studies and is called a Virchow-Robin space. Bulk CSF flow along Virchow-Robin spaces occurred with arterial pulsations. Tracers of small molecular size diffused into the brain parenchyma and with time began to accumulate along small venules, ultimately reaching the larger cerebral veins. These experiments demonstrated that CSF circulates from subarachnoid space into Virchow-Robin spaces, crosses the brain parenchyma where it mixes with the interstitial fluid, and exits the brain via paravenous spaces to drain into the cerebral veins.

Remarkably, tracers of large molecular size remained in the Virchow-Robin space. They were trapped between the walls of the arterioles and the perivascular end-feet of astrocytes (hence "glymphatic"). Indeed, astrocyte end-feet cover most of the cerebral microvasculature, with ~20-nm clefts between the end-feet.[92] Astrocytes thus filter macromolecules from the CSF flowing into the brain parenchyma. Decreased oncotic pressure of incoming CSF allows inflow of waste molecules, including proteins, from the interstitial fluid and facilitates waste removal from the brain. In addition, the astrocyte end-feet are enriched for the water channel aquaporin-4 (AQP4).[91] AQP4 preferentially allows free water from the CSF in the Virchow-Robin spaces to enter the interstitial space, further facilitating CSF flow and waste excretion.[91] This "rediscovery" of an anatomic-physiologic means for removal of waste and potentially toxic macromolecules from brain has implications in multiple CNS diseases, including traumatic brain injury, stroke, and inflammatory conditions. Furthermore, it provides a portal for brain-derived biomarkers to be accessible in serum.[93]

Developmental Processes Relevant to Pediatric Critical Care Medicine

Cell Origin and Differentiation

Neurogenesis and gliogenesis in the human begin well before birth, in the eighth gestational week.[94] Neurons are born in the specialized proliferative zones located next to the lateral ventricles and migrate outwards toward the cortical surface during development. The neurons migrate along a subset of glial cells called the radial glia, which span the distance between the ventricular zone and the brain surface early in development. The cortex is generated in an inside-out fashion, such that the deeper cortical layers are formed first. Glutamatergic neurons appear to originate in the dorsal aspect of the ventricular zone, whereas GABA-ergic inhibitory interneurons likely come primarily from the ventral aspect. Thus GABA-ergic neurons have a longer migration path into the cortex than their glutamatergic counterparts and occasionally must migrate tangentially rather than perpendicular to reach their final destination.[94] The process of establishing cortical layers appears complete in humans by the 30th gestational week.[95] Disruption of the radial migration process, due to either genetic or environmental factors, results in lissencephaly and seizures of varying severity.[96]

Synaptogenesis and Synaptic Pruning

By the time of birth in humans, both neurogenesis and neuronal migration have essentially been completed. Thus infants generally have the same neuronal density (number of soma per mm^3) as adults. Yet the human brain undergoes substantial postnatal development, reflected clinically as the maturation of behavioral milestones. The underlying process is evolution of axonal and dendritic processes by neurons in the CNS, together with an explosive increase in the number of synaptic contacts in the brain (Fig. 60.8). Neuronal dendritic arbors increase in complexity, developing more branches and sampling a wider physical space during the first 2 years of life.[40] The number of synapses increases from birth until approximately 2 years of age, when it actually surpasses the number of synapses found in the adult brain. From 2 years until early adolescence, neurons in the CNS undergo synaptic pruning, or elimination. Both synaptic development and pruning are under exquisite control by genetic and experience-dependent factors. For example, a major CNS abnormality found in individuals with fragile X syndrome, the most common cause of mental retardation, is overproduction and impaired pruning of synapses in cortical neurons.[97] Furthermore, a number of drugs used extensively in the PICU, including benzodiazepines, barbiturates, steroids, and opiates, exert a profound effect on synaptogenesis and synaptic function. Steroid use in premature neonates has been associated with worse neurologic outcome,[98] and benzodiazepine use during experience-dependent critical periods in the visual system is associated with premature decline in synaptic plasticity.[99] Thus the true extent of the interaction between the PICU environment and synaptic organization in the developing brain remains to be fully characterized.

Neurotransmitter System Maturation

Maturation of the neurotransmitter systems in the human CNS is a complicated and protracted process. It is complicated because each neurotransmitter system matures along its own developmental time course and because the time course itself may be specific to each brain region. For some neurotransmitters, the process lasts into early adulthood. The complexity of the process is compounded further by the relative lack of human data, requiring extrapolation from animal studies. Nevertheless, some general principles that apply to critically ill children can be derived from current knowledge.

The earliest neurotransmitter system to become apparent in the cortex is ACh. Thalamic afferent fibers contain AChE, and ACh staining in the cortex coincides with arrival

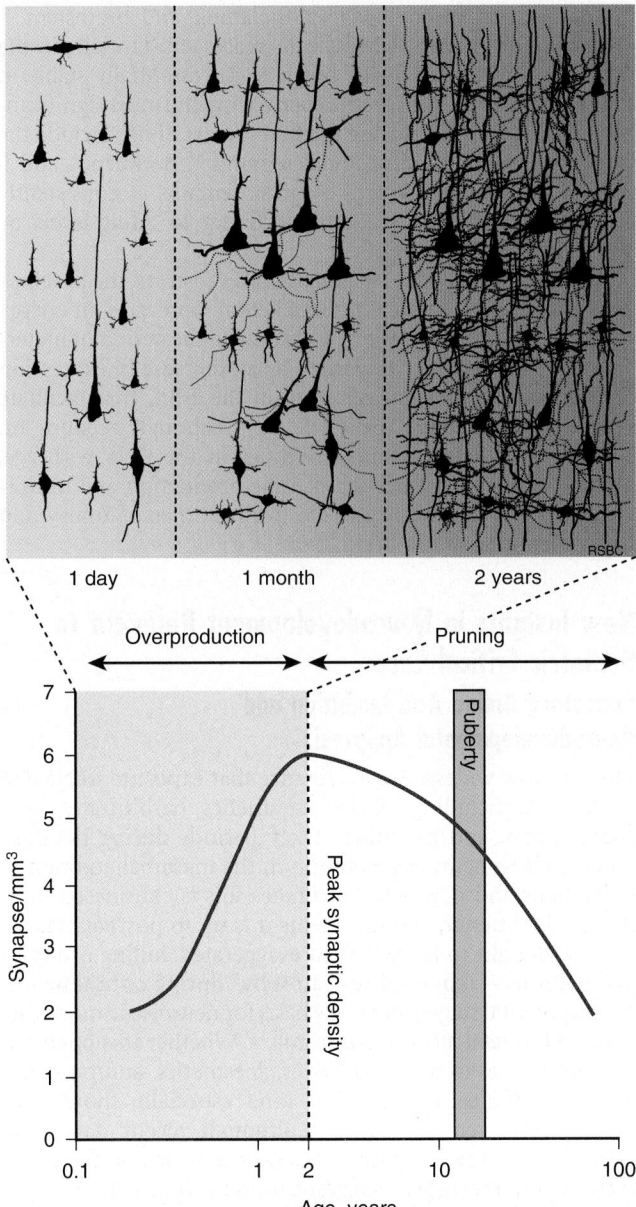

Fig. 60.8. Cortical synaptic density and development of axons and dendrites with age. The synapse density is derived from the visual cortex. Note the logarithmic age scale as abscissa. *Top panel* is a schematic representation of synaptogenesis and dendritic arborization and maturation from birth to 2 years of age. (Modified from Levitt P. Structural and functional maturation of the developing primate brain. J Pediatr. 2003;143:S35-S45 and Nolte J. The Human Brain. An Introduction to Its Functional Anatomy. 3rd ed. St. Louis: Mosby–Year Book; 1993.)

of thalamic input during midgestation.[94,95] Cholinergic innervation in the cortex continues to mature through the third year of life. Development of the GABA-ergic system also begins in midgestation and continues until several months postnatally. GABA receptor α subunits expressed in cortex before birth differ from those expressed after birth.[100] Indeed, in young animals and probably in humans before late gestation, GABA is an excitatory neurotransmitter, evoking large depolarizing currents in postsynaptic neurons.[101] The precise significance of GABA as an excitatory neurotransmitter in

guiding organization of neuronal circuits remains to be determined. Development of the glutamatergic system occurs slightly later, with AMPA-type receptors becoming apparent in the basal ganglia in the 32nd postnatal week. In the cortex, NMDA-type receptors precede the AMPA-type receptors in the course of their appearance at the synapse. Because NMDA receptors do not evoke fast depolarizations leading to an action potential, NMDA-only synapses are functionally silent. Yet these silent synapses contribute to experience-dependent plasticity and possibly injury.[102]

Myelination

Myelination in the human CNS begins 1 to 2 months before birth in the visual system and extends to the other sensory systems over the first year of life.[103] Further myelination of subcortical and cortical tracts continues in the posterior to anterior direction well into the third decade of life, consistent with the time course of maturation of cognitive functions in children and adolescents.[94] Myelination is initiated by the preoligodendrocytes, which are exquisitely sensitive to injury by hypoxia and inflammation. Oligodendrocyte injury, with resulting disruption in axonal myelination, contributes significantly to the development of periventricular leukomalacia in preterm infants.[104]

Development of Cerebrovasculature and Blood-Brain Barrier

Vascularization of the brain begins early during development, with the first vascular plexus surrounding the primitive neural tube before the first heartbeat. Blood vessels then invade the developing brain, growing radially from the pia toward the deeper structures. The process is driven, at least in part, by oxygen sensing. Deeper cortical layers/structures are thought to be relatively oxygen deficient.[105] Relative hypoxia leads to transcription of the hypoxia-inducible factor 1 (HIF1), which in turn leads to release of the vascular endothelial growth factor (VEGF). VEGF drives angiogenesis in the brain both prenatally and postnatally. Interestingly, chronic hypoxia such as is seen in patients with cyanotic heart disease increases the capillary density in the brain via an HIF1-dependent mechanism.[106] The increase is reversed over several weeks by restoring normal oxygenation in animal models, suggesting that brain vasculature has the potential to undergo continuous remodeling.

Development of the BBB coincides with early vascularization of the brain. Immunologic markers of tight junctions redistribute from the cytoplasm to their appropriate locations in the cell membrane by approximately 14 weeks of gestation.[107] Although anatomically intact, the BBB remains more permeable to amino acids, some drugs, and possibly toxins until approximately 6 months of age in humans.[107] However, the exact nature of BBB dynamics during development remains incompletely characterized.

Developmental Aspects of Cerebral Blood Flow, Autoregulation, and Cerebral Metabolism

In humans, gray matter CBF increases several-fold early in development and then decreases gradually after puberty (Fig. 60.9). In normotensive preterm infants, CBF has been measured at 13 to 14 mL/100 g/min.[108] Estimated CBF increases with gestational age from 14 mL/100 g/min at 30 to 32 weeks to 20 mL/100 g/min at 38 to 40 weeks postconception.[109]

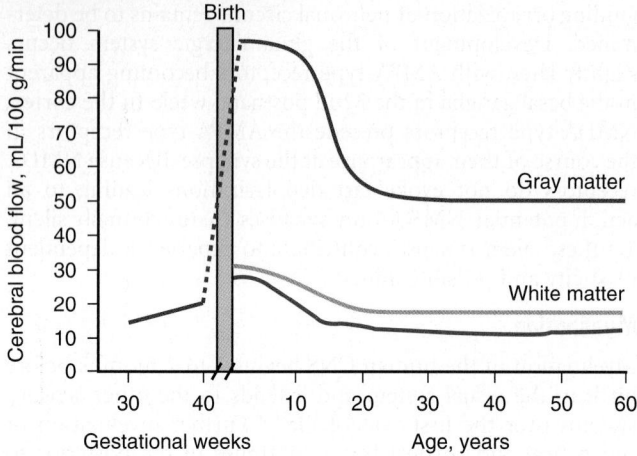

Fig. 60.9. Cerebral blood flow (CBF) as a function of age. Gray matter CBF increases significantly after birth to reach a peak at approximately 4 years of age (note the change from age in gestational weeks to age in years). The *broken line* between the neonatal period and childhood indicates that data are extrapolated from existing experimental data. Gray matter CBF then decreases gradually to adult values. White matter CBF also decreases between 4 years of age and adulthood but not as significantly as that in gray matter. At present, no data exist on the white matter CBF in premature or term newborns.

Furthermore, CBF increases significantly in the first 2 days of life, regardless of gestational age.[110] In children aged 4 to 12 years, gray matter CBF reaches values of 90 to 100 mL/100 g/min and then declines throughout adolescence to reach adult values of 50 to 60 mL/100 g/min by approximately 20 years of age.[111] Interestingly, white matter CBF is only 20% higher in children compared with adults, reflecting perhaps the greater degree of developmental changes in gray versus white matter.[111]

Perfusion pressure–related, $PaCO_2$-related, and PaO_2-related autoregulation of CBF also undergo postnatal maturation. Studies in preterm infants suggest that perfusion pressure–related autoregulation of CBF is present shortly after birth, such that CBF changes by less than 1.5% per 1 mm Hg change in MAP.[112] As mentioned earlier, the upper and lower MAP limits in pressure-related autoregulation in neonates are shifted to the right, compared with adults,[77] leading to different thresholds for intervention in infants. Pressure-related autoregulation may be lost in critically ill infants, resulting in pressure-passive CBF[1] and poor outcome.[113] Similarly, $PaCO_2$-related autoregulation appears present in humans shortly after birth, with CBF changing approximately 1% for every 1 mm Hg change in $PaCO_2$.[108,110,114] In preterm infants, CBF also depends on the interaction between $PaCO_2$-related and MAP-related autoregulation, such that the percent change in CBF as a function of change in $PaCO_2$ increases as MAP increases.[114] Finally, oxygen tension–related CBF autoregulation also appears functional early in life, although much of the current data are derived from animals studies.[115,116] Thus in healthy humans, CBF autoregulation mechanisms are functional at birth and should be taken into account during management of systemic and intracerebral pathologic states, such as sepsis, hypotension, hypoxemia, and hypercarbia.

Cerebral metabolism undergoes substantial maturation during postnatal development in humans with respect to metabolic rate, distribution of metabolic activity, and energy source utilization. Shortly after birth, the CMRGlu is highest

in sensory and motor cortices, thalamus, and brainstem.[117] Over the next 4 years, CMRGlu increases substantially in the thalamus and in the cortex but remains essentially stable in the brainstem. Cortical areas experiencing the most significant increase in CMRGlu during the first 4 years of life include the frontal, temporal, and occipital regions.[117] Between 4 and 9 years of age, CMRGlu in the cortex remains at consistently high values relative to adults, declining to adult levels by approximately 20 years of age.[86]

In addition to relying on glucose as a substrate, the developing brain also extensively utilizes ketone bodies as an energy substrate. Ketone utilization peaks during the period of maternal milk ingestion, accompanied by an increase in expression of monocarboxylate transporters in the BBB, that facilitate ketone entrance into the CNS.[118,119] Although reliance on ketones as an energy source declines in the CNS with age, recent evidence indicates that ketone production and utilization may play a significant role during times of injury and stress even in an adult brain.[118]

New Insights in Neurodevelopment Relevant to Pediatric Critical Care

Excitatory Amino Acid Inhibition and Neurodevelopmental Apoptosis

There is now widespread acceptance that exposure to NMDA antagonists including inhaled anesthetics, barbiturates, benzodiazepines, and ketamine at key periods during development leads to neurodegeneration in the mammalian brain.[120] In humans and nonhuman primates this is considered to be the third trimester, and in rodents it is up to postnatal day 7. This is thought to be related to exaggerated culling of inhibited neurons—akin to "disuse atrophy," during critical neurodevelopmental stages, and is the basis for neurologic morbidity observed in fetal alcohol syndrome.[121] Whether this phenomenon translates to use of sedatives, anesthetics, and/or anxiolytics in infants in the PICU (and especially those born prematurely) remains unclear, although recent data from studies evaluating cognitive consequences of anesthesia for early childhood surgery suggest caution is in order.[122,123]

The Microbiome and Neurodevelopment and Function

Host microbiota and the impact of medical and/or dietary manipulation thereof is emerging as an important aspect of critical illness. Of relevance to this chapter, recent data show that host microbiota regulate maturation and function of CNS microglia.[124] Microglia play key roles in neuronal migration and survival in the developing[125] and adult brain.[126] Microglia can also limit neuronal hyperexcitability by intercalating processes between synaptic clefts[127] and thus may affect neurotransmission in neuroinflammatory conditions such as encephalitis, autoimmune encephalopathies, septic encephalopathy, and traumatic brain injury. In addition to effects on inflammatory cells, gut microbiota can directly influence brain levels of neurotransmitters including GABA and glutamate.[128] Food for thought.

Conclusion

The nervous system is undergoing active development and is often the primarily affected organ when children are hospitalized with a life-threatening illness. Appreciation of normal anatomy and development, as well as knowledge of neurotransmitter systems and homeostatic mechanisms, is required for prompt diagnosis and effective clinical care. Most importantly, ongoing research into the interaction between developmental processes and injury is likely to yield a wealth of new information, implying the need for continuous reevaluation of current knowledge and clinical practice in light of new discoveries.

References are available online at http://www.ExpertConsult.com.

Key References

1. Thameem Dheen S, Kaur C, Ling E-2A. Microglial activation and its implications in the brain diseases. *Curr Med Chem.* 2007;14:1189-1197.
3. Yong VW, Rivest S. Taking advantage of the systemic immune system to cure brain diseases. *Neuron.* 2009;64:55-60.
5. Sohl G, Maxeiner S, Willecke K. Expression and functions of neuronal gap junctions. *Nat Rev Neurosci.* 2005;6:191-200.
9. Lang B, Vincent A. Autoimmune disorders of the neuromuscular junction. *Curr Opin Pharmacol.* 2009;9:336-340.
14. Duncan JR, Paterson DS, Hoffman JM, et al. Brainstem serotonergic deficiency in sudden infant death syndrome. *JAMA.* 2010;303:430-437.
17. Blackstone E, Morrison M, Roth MB. H_2S induces a suspended animation-like state in mice. *Science.* 2005;308:518.
19. Dani JA, Bertrand D. Nicotinic acetylcholine receptors and nicotinic cholinergic mechanisms of the central nervous system. *Annu Rev Pharmacol Toxicol.* 2007;47:699-729.
23. Langmead CJ, Watson J, Reavill C. Muscarinic acetylcholine receptors as CNS drug targets. *Pharmacol Ther.* 2008;117:232-243.
25. Bowie D. Ionotropic glutamate receptors & CNS disorders. *CNS Neurol Disord Drug Targets.* 2008;7:129-143.
26. Conn PJ, Pin J-P. Pharmacology and functions of metabotropic glutamate receptors. *Annu Rev Pharmacol Toxicol.* 1997;37:205-237.
29. Belelli D, Harrison NL, Maguire J, et al. Extrasynaptic GABAA receptors: form, pharmacology, and function. *J Neurosci.* 2009;29:12757-12763.
36. Misgeld U, Bijak M, Jarolimek W. A physiological role for GABAB receptors and the effects of baclofen in the mammalian central nervous system. *Prog Neurobiol.* 1995;46:423-462.
42. Petersen SE, Fox PT, Posner MI, et al. Positron emission tomographic studies of the cortical anatomy of single-word processing. *Nature.* 1988; 331:585-589.
43. Strick PL, Dum RP, Fiez JA. Cerebellum and nonmotor function. *Annu Rev Neurosci.* 2009;32:413-434.
44. Jones EG. Thalamic circuitry and thalamocortical synchrony. *Philos Trans R Soc Lond B Biol Sci.* 2002;357:1659-1673.
45. Lawrence RK, Inder TE. Anatomic changes and imaging in assessing brain injury in the term infant. *Clin Perinatol.* 2008;35:679-693.
52. Ho VB, Fitz CR, Chuang SH, et al. Bilateral basal ganglia lesions: pediatric differential considerations. *Radiographics.* 1993;13:269-292.
54. Dumont RJ, Okonkwo DO, Verma S, et al. Acute spinal cord injury, part I: pathophysiologic mechanisms. *Clin Neuropharmacol.* 2001;24:254-264.
60. Engelhardt B, Sorokin L. The blood–brain and the blood–cerebrospinal fluid barriers: function and dysfunction. *Semin Immunopathol.* 2009;31:497-511.
61. Yemisci M, Gursoy-Ozdemir Y, Vural A, et al. Pericyte contraction induced by oxidative-nitrative stress impairs capillary reflow despite successful opening of an occluded cerebral artery. *Nat Med.* 2009;15:1031-1037.

64. Rubin LL, Staddon JM. The cell biology of the blood-brain barrier. *Annu Rev Neurosci.* 1999;22:11-28.
68. Qutub AA, Hunt CA. Glucose transport to the brain: a systems model. *Brain Res Brain Res Rev.* 2005;49:595-617.
70. Begley DJ. ABC transporters and the blood-brain barrier. *Curr Pharm Des.* 2004;10:1295-1312.
74. Kochanek PM, Berger RP, Bayir H, et al. Biomarkers of primary and evolving damage in traumatic and ischemic brain injury: diagnosis, prognosis, probing mechanisms, and therapeutic decision making. *Curr Opin Crit Care.* 2008;14:135-141.
75. Lassen NA. Cerebral blood flow and oxygen consumption in man. *Physiol Rev.* 1959;39:183-238.
76. Philip S, Udomphorn Y, Kirkham FJ, et al. Cerebrovascular pathophysiology in pediatric traumatic brain injury. *J Trauma.* 2009;67:S128-S134.
80. Johnston AJ, Steiner LA, Gupta AK, et al. Cerebral oxygen vasoreactivity and cerebral tissue oxygen reactivity. *Br J Anaesth.* 2003;90:774-786.
83. Fox PT, Raichle ME. Focal physiological uncoupling of cerebral blood flow and oxidative metabolism during somatosensory stimulation in human subjects. *Proc Natl Acad Sci USA.* 1986;83:1140-1144.
85. Kennedy C, Sokoloff L. An adaptation of the nitrous oxide method to the study of the cerebral circulation in children; normal values for cerebral blood flow and cerebral metabolic rate in childhood. *J Clin Invest.* 1957;36:1130-1137.
86. Chugani HT, Phelps ME, Mazziotta JC. Positron emission tomography study of human brain functional development. *Ann Neurol.* 1987; 22:487-497.
94. Levitt P. Structural and functional maturation of the developing primate brain. *J Pediatr.* 2003;143:S35-S45.
95. Kostovic I, Judas M, Rados M, et al. Laminar organization of the human fetal cerebrum revealed by histochemical markers and magnetic resonance imaging. *Cereb Cortex.* 2002;12:536-544.
100. Brooks-Kayal AR, Pritchett DB. Developmental changes in human gamma-aminobutyric acid A receptor subunit composition. *Ann Neurol.* 1993;34:687-693.
102. Herlenius E, Lagercrantz H. Development of neurotransmitter systems during critical periods. *Exp Neurol.* 2004;190(suppl 1):S8-S21.
103. Paus T, Collins DL, Evans AC, et al. Maturation of white matter in the human brain: a review of magnetic resonance studies. *Brain Res Bull.* 2001;54:255-266.
104. Takashima S, Itoh M, Oka A. A history of our understanding of cerebral vascular development and pathogenesis of perinatal brain damage over the past 30 years. *Semin Pediatr Neurol.* 2009;16:226-236.
111. Biagi L, Abbruzzese A, Bianchi MC, et al. Age dependence of cerebral perfusion assessed by magnetic resonance continuous arterial spin labeling. *J Magn Reson Imaging.* 2007;25:696-702.
116. Szymonowicz W, Walker AM, Cussen L, et al. Developmental changes in regional cerebral blood flow in fetal and newborn lambs. *Am J Physiol.* 1988;254:H52-H58.
117. Kinnala A, Suhonen-Polvi H, Aarimaa T, et al. Cerebral metabolic rate for glucose during the first six months of life: an FDG positron emission tomography study. *Arch Dis Child Fetal Neonatal Ed.* 1996;74:F153-F157.
118. Prins ML. Cerebral metabolic adaptation and ketone metabolism after brain injury. *J Cereb Blood Flow Metab.* 2008;28:1-16.
119. Vannucci RC, Vannucci SJ. Glucose metabolism in the developing brain. *Semin Perinatol.* 2000;24:107-115.
126. Eyo UB, Dailey ME. Microglia: key elements in neuronal development, plasticity, and pathology. *J Neuroimmune Pharmacol.* 2013;8:494-509.
127. Chen Z, Jalabi W, Hu W, et al. Microglia displacement of inhibitory synapses provides neuroprotection in the adult brain. *Nat Commun.* 2014;5:4486.
128. Janik R, Thomason LAM, Stanisz AM, et al. Magnetic resonance spectroscopy reveals oral *Lactobacillus* promotion of increases in brain GABA, N-acetyl aspartate and glutamate. *Neuroimage.* 2016;125:988-995.

Brain Malformations

Robert H. Bonow, Isaac Josh Abecassis, and Samuel R. Browd

PEARLS

- Hydrocephalus is a common brain disease characterized by a buildup of cerebrospinal fluid that requires surgical treatment. Untreated hydrocephalus can be a medical emergency, requiring prompt neurosurgical intervention.
- Arachnoid cysts are generally benign congenital malformations that are frequently identified incidentally; however, they may occasionally hemorrhage or cause mass effect on the brain. They are more likely to require treatment in the very young.
- Chiari I malformations may cause debilitating posttussive headaches that can be relieved with surgery. Chiari II malformations occur in patients with myelomeningocele and may be associated with brain stem compromise.
- Dandy-Walker syndrome is characterized by a posterior fossa cyst and cerebellar hypoplasia. It is associated with hydrocephalus and a number of systemic abnormalities.
- Meningoceles and encephaloceles are characterized by herniation of meninges or brain and meninges through a defect in the skull.
- Myelomeningocele is the most severe form of spinal dysraphism in which failure of primary neurulation leads to herniation of the spinal cord through defects in the vertebrae, soft tissue, and skin. Many children with myelomeningocele also suffer from hydrocephalus.

Hydrocephalus

Background

Hydrocephalus is a complex disease generally defined as a pathologic accumulation of cerebrospinal fluid (CSF) that leads to engorgement of the cerebral ventricles, mechanical deformation of brain structures, and increased intracranial pressure (ICP). Of relevance to the pediatric intensivist, these changes can render the patient critically ill. Thus a fundamental understanding of the condition is important for the clinician caring for these children in the intensive care setting.

Among children, hydrocephalus has an incidence of approximately 1 : 1000.[1-3] In the United States, it accounts for approximately 40,000 hospital admissions and $2 billion in health care expenditures annually.[4] Children with hydrocephalus can be medically complex, and the number of hydrocephalus comorbidities has risen as our ability to care for affected children has improved.[4] These patients frequently require admission to an intensive care unit (ICU) for interventions related to their hydrocephalus and comorbid conditions.

Pathophysiology

CSF physiology and the pathophysiology of hydrocephalus are incompletely understood and remain an area of ongoing research. The prevailing hypothesis describes a *bulk flow* model, in which the CSF produced by the choroid plexus epithelium and the ependymal lining of the ventricles passes through the ventricular system, down the aqueduct of Sylvius, out the foramina of Luschka and Magendie, and into the spinal subarachnoid space. From there, the fluid continues through the subarachnoid spaces of the basal cisterns and the cerebral convexities until it reaches the arachnoid granulations, where it is reabsorbed into the venous system (Fig. 61.1). According to this theory, obstruction at any point in this pathway leads to an accumulation of CSF proximal to the blockage and, consequently, hydrocephalus. The term *noncommunicating* is used when there is an obstruction within the ventricular system; *communicating* hydrocephalus refers to obstruction at the level of the subarachnoid spaces, the arachnoid granulations, or the venous system.[1,5]

With accumulation of CSF, ICP begins to rise. As with any rigid container, pressure within the cranial vault is determined by its contents. In healthy patients, these include the brain, intravascular blood, and CSF. When mass lesions such as tumors or hematomas are present, they constitute an additional compartment and place stress on the system. Under normal circumstances, the body is able to accommodate pressure through the capacitance provided by veins, CSF, and, to a minor extent, the brain itself. The venous structures contain the majority of intracranial blood and have the lowest pressure and greatest compliance of the three; they are readily compressed as other compartments enlarge. Similarly, CSF drains from the ventricles into subarachnoid space and, ultimately, into the venous system in response to mass lesions. The brain itself can also become compressed and provides further accommodation, although this is typically the least compliant compartment. This system is able to minimize pressure changes in response to small challenges, but eventually the ability to compensate is exhausted and ICP elevates. Patients with untreated hydrocephalus are particularly vulnerable, as the CSF compartment offers little to no additional compliance.

Although enlargement of the ventricles because of the accumulation of CSF does cause mechanical deformation of the adjacent brain, the principal concern is control of ICP. Numerous studies have shown a strong association between persistently elevated ICP and poor outcome in the setting of trauma,[6] and intuitively the same association holds true in the case of hydrocephalus. Prompt identification and treatment of intracranial hypertension is therefore imperative.

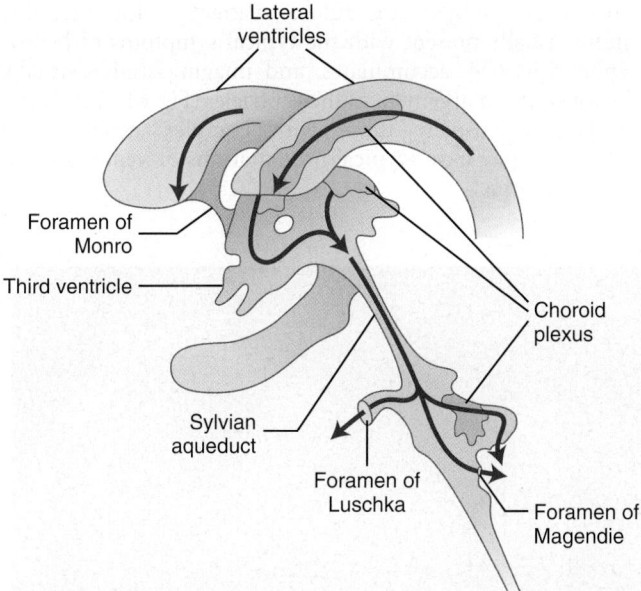

Fig. 61.1. The cerebral ventricular system. Cerebrospinal fluid flows from the lateral ventricles through the foramina of Monro, into the third ventricle, and down the cerebral ("Sylvian") aqueduct. It then passes through the fourth ventricle before finally exiting the ventricular system through the foramina of Magendie and Luschka. (Reproduced with permission from Hdeib A, Cohen AR. Hydrocephalus in children and adults. In: Ellenbogen RG, Abdulrauf SI, Sekhar LN, eds. Principles of Neurological Surgery. 3rd ed. Philadelphia: Saunders; 2012:105-127.)

Clinical Presentation

The clinical manifestations of untreated hydrocephalus depend on the age of the patient. In older children and adults, headache is the most frequent symptom. Nausea, vomiting, and somnolence are also common. Some patients develop an ataxic gait, and visual symptoms such as blurry vision, Parinaud syndrome, or diplopia due to cranial nerve VI palsies may also be seen. Younger children and nonverbal adults may become unusually irritable or intolerant of feeding. Infants with open cranial sutures will demonstrate fullness of the fontanelle and splaying of the suture lines.

Left untreated, these symptoms typically progress to frank lethargy, obtundation, and coma. Late in the course of the disease, bradycardia, hypertension, and abnormal respirations may be seen. This triad, frequently referred to as the Cushing reflex, is a sign of dangerously elevated ICP and frequently heralds impending herniation. These signs are not seen universally, however, so their absence should not necessarily be reassuring in comatose patients. Conversely, patients with bradycardia who are awake and talking are likely not on the verge of herniation, even if they have a history of hydrocephalus.

Causes

In North America, the most commonly identified causes of hydrocephalus are intraventricular hemorrhage (IVH) of prematurity (25%), brain tumors (18%), and myelomeningocele (15%); idiopathic cases account for approximately one-quarter of the total.[7] Postinfectious hydrocephalus is relatively rare in North America (under 4%) but accounts for as many as 60% of cases in sub-Saharan Africa.[7,8]

Diagnosis

Clinical history and physical examination are helpful, but imaging studies with enlarged ventricles are essential to establish the diagnosis. Newborns with IVH of prematurity, myelomeningocele, and other risk factors for hydrocephalus are frequently screened with cranial ultrasounds for ventricular enlargement. In borderline cases not requiring immediate intervention, serial imaging studies and head circumference measurements can be helpful in confirming the need for treatment. The presence of papilledema, a bulging fontanelle, or widely splayed sutures can help to corroborate imaging findings or symptoms concerning for intracranial hypertension and guide treatment decisions.

Management

The principal treatment for hydrocephalus is diversion of cerebrospinal fluid. This goal can be achieved temporarily with an external ventricular drain (EVD) tunneled out through the scalp or permanently with an internalized CSF shunt. In selected patients, endoscopic third ventriculostomy (ETV) with or without choroid plexus cauterization may also be an alternative.

Children with acute hydrocephalus can be critically ill and may require emergent EVD placement, a rapid procedure that is performed at the ICU bedside in some institutions. If the child is deteriorating and an EVD cannot be placed immediately, standard methods for controlling ICP should be employed: elevation of the head of the bed and neutral neck positioning to facilitate venous drainage, administration of analgesics and sedatives, mild hyperventilation with a target $PaCO_2$ of 30 to 35 mm Hg, and hyperosmolar therapy with mannitol or hypertonic saline.[6] Hypotension should be avoided to maintain cerebral perfusion. Because patients with acute hydrocephalus frequently have altered mental status, intubation may be required for airway protection.

An EVD may also be used nonemergently in the setting of a neurosurgical operation to facilitate drainage of debris and blood products from the ventricular system. In this case, the goal is prevention of hydrocephalus.

To place an EVD, a craniostomy is created through a small skin incision behind the hairline, and a catheter is then passed through the brain parenchyma into the lateral ventricle. The other end of the catheter is then tunneled out through the scalp and connected to a bedside collection system, which can be raised and lowered to control the amount of CSF drained. The typical reference point is the patient's external acoustic meatus (EAM). These drains require close monitoring and frequent adjustments to maintain the proper height with changes in patient position; if they are not leveled appropriately, over- or underdrainage of CSF may result, with potentially serious consequences. At some centers, the level of monitoring required is available only in the ICU, and it is not uncommon for patients who are otherwise well to be kept in the ICU for days at a time until their EVDs are removed. When it is thought that the drain is no longer needed, many neurosurgeons "wean" the drain by raising it progressively and ultimately clamping it. If this process is well tolerated without symptoms or imaging evidence of hydrocephalus, the drain is removed; if it is not, a shunt is usually required.

CSF shunting systems are the standard treatment for patients requiring permanent CSF diversion. A variety of shunt constructs are used, but the general form is a ventricular catheter connected in series to a valve and a distal catheter (Fig. 61.2). The distal catheter is tunneled subcutaneously to the peritoneum most commonly, but in some children it is placed in the right cardiac atrium or pleural space. The shunted CSF is then reabsorbed within the distal compartment. Although shunt placement is lifesaving the

devices are subject to failure. Patients with occluded shunts usually present with the typical symptoms of hydrocephalus as CSF accumulates, and imaging studies usually demonstrate enlargement of the ventricles (Fig. 61.3). A subset of patients—usually those with complex neurosurgical histories—may have atypical presentations or ventricles that do not enlarge.

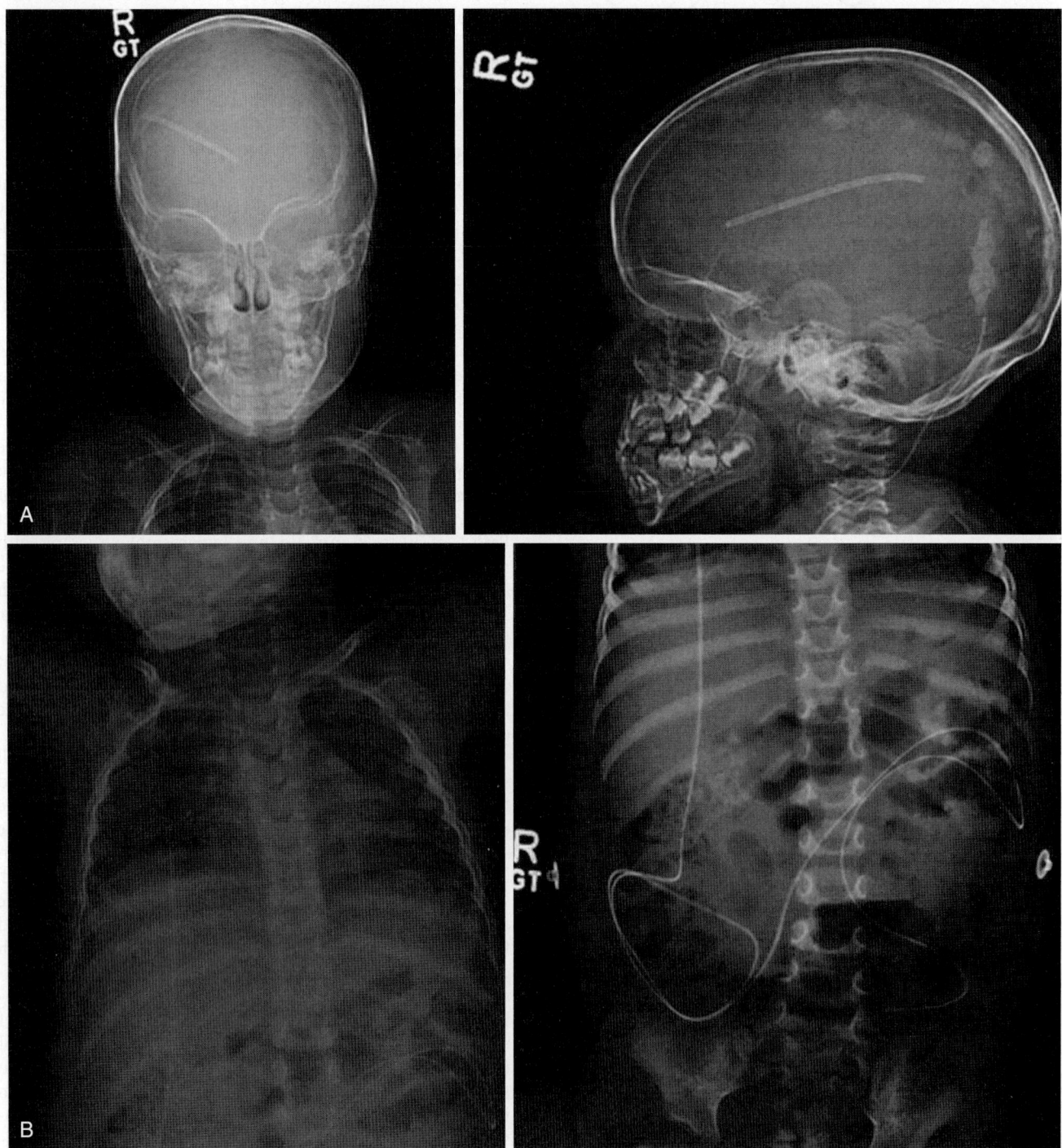

Fig. 61.2. Plain x-rays of a ventriculoperitoneal shunt. (A) Anteroposterior and lateral cranial x-rays show the ventricular catheter connected to a valve with radiolucent tubing. The proximal portion of the peritoneal catheter is seen attached to the distal end of the valve. (B) Anteroposterior chest and abdominal films show the course of the peritoneal catheter down the neck, over the clavicle and ribs, and into the peritoneal cavity. (Reproduced with permission from Hdeib A and Cohen AR. Hydrocephalus in children and adults. In: Ellenbogen RG, Abdulrauf SI, Sekhar LN, eds. Principles of Neurological Surgery. 3rd ed. Philadelphia: Saunders; 2012:105-127.)

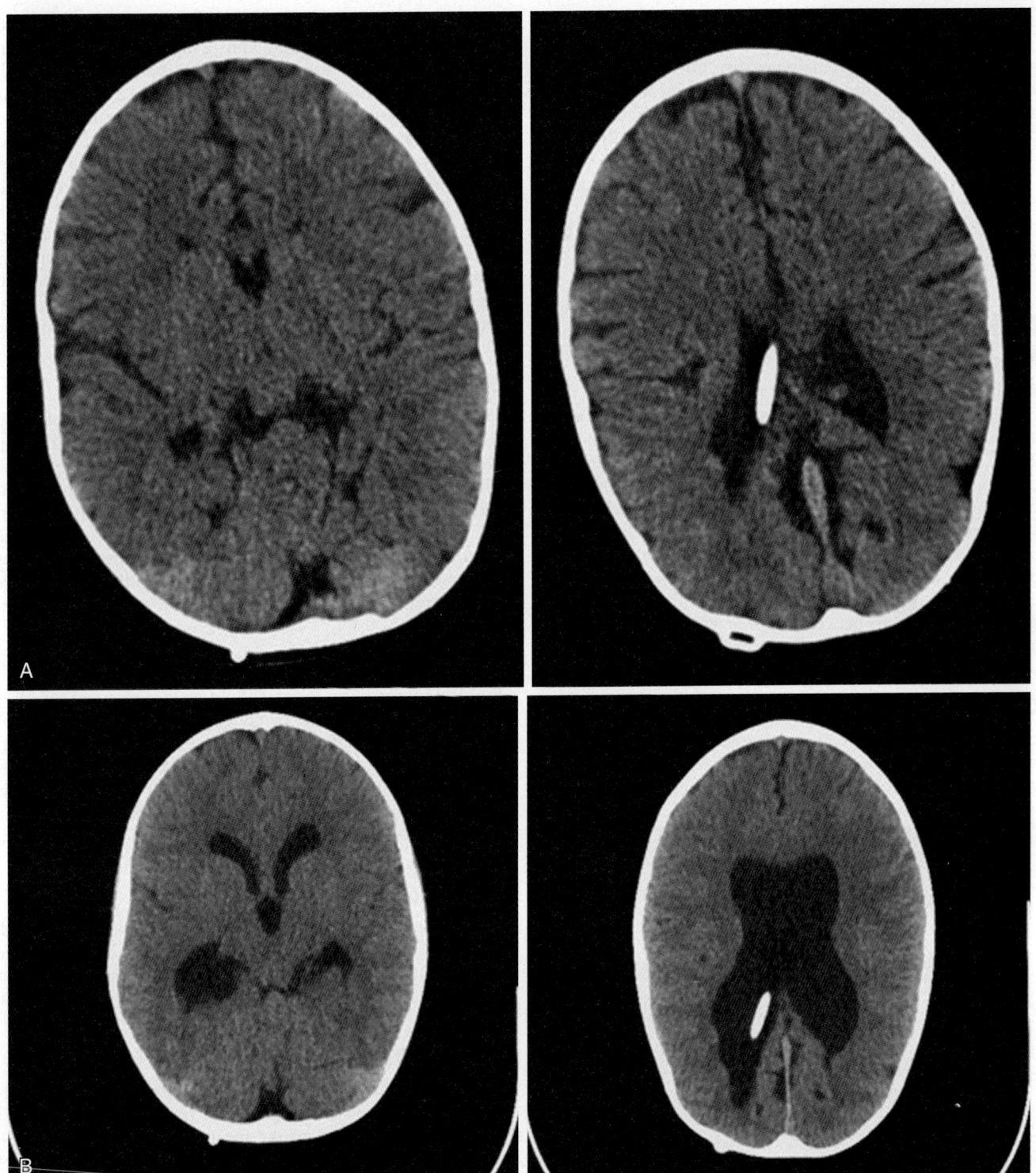

Fig. 61.3. Ventriculoperitoneal shunt malfunction causing ventriculomegaly. (A) Axial computed tomography shows small ventricles with a properly functioning ventriculoperitoneal shunt. (B) With shunt failure, the ventricles are enlarged. (Reproduced with permission from Hdeib A, Cohen AR. Hydrocephalus in children and adults. In: Ellenbogen RG, Abdulrauf SI, Sekhar LN, eds. Principles of Neurological Surgery. 3rd ed. Philadelphia: Saunders; 2012:105-127.)

A failed shunt is a medical emergency requiring immediate neurosurgical intervention for shunt revision. Infection of the shunt hardware can also occur, most commonly due to seeding at the time of surgery. Patients generally present with fever and meningeal symptoms; shunt failure may also be present, and drainage of infectious material into the abdomen may lead to the formation of a pseudocyst or frank peritonitis. If untreated, the infection may progress to ventriculitis, which carries a poor prognosis. Treatment requires surgical removal of the shunt hardware and placement of a temporary EVD until the infection is cleared. After a prolonged course of antibiotics (upward of 2 weeks for some organisms), the shunt may be replaced if CSF cultures remain negative. On average, children with a history of shunt infection have a significantly lower IQ than controls without infection.[9] Fortunately, application of a standardized protocol has been shown to substantially reduce the rate of shunt infection to approximately 5%.[10]

In a selected subset of patients, ETV can provide permanent treatment of hydrocephalus without the need for a shunt.[11,12] In this procedure, a fenestration is made at the floor of the third ventricle, providing an alternative route for CSF drainage.

Arachnoid Cysts

Background

Arachnoid cysts are congenital anomalies filled with fluid similar or identical to CSF and lined by thin membranes of arachnoid (Fig. 61.4). They have an incidence of 0.5% to 2.5%[13] and are more common in males. Although arachnoid cysts can occur anywhere along the neuraxis, they are most commonly found in association with an arachnoid cistern, and approximately half are located in the Sylvian fissure.[14,15]

It was previously thought that arachnoid cysts were related to agenesis of the adjacent brain region; however, modern radiographic techniques have clarified that there is no difference in brain volume between the side with an arachnoid cyst and the side without. Instead, the brain is displaced and, in some cases, the overlying skull is expanded.[16,17]

Clinical Presentation

Generally asymptomatic, most of arachnoid cysts are found incidentally and do not change in size; however, a small subset can progressively enlarge and cause mass effect on adjacent

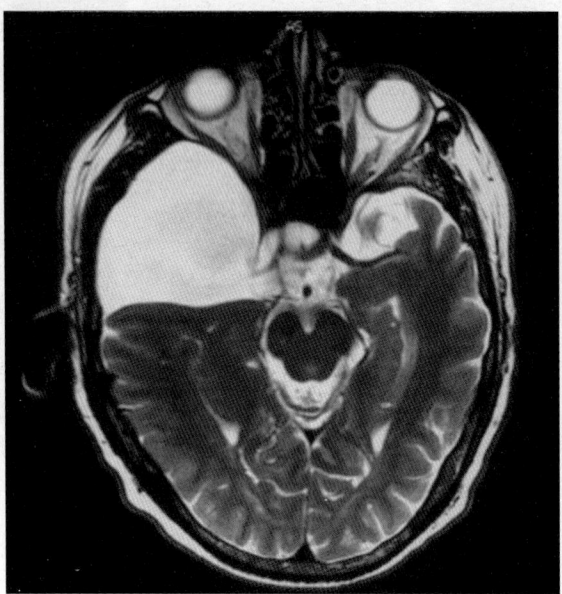

Fig. 61.4. Arachnoid cyst. T2-weighted magnetic resonance image shows a large right middle fossa arachnoid cyst. Note that the signal intensity of the cyst contents is identical to that of cerebrospinal fluid. (Reproduced with permission from Jimenez DF, Gentry Savage J, Samuelson M. Developmental anomalies. In: Ellenbogen RG, Abdulrauf SI, Sekhar LN, eds. Principles of Neurological Surgery. 3rd ed. Philadelphia: Saunders; 2012:129-135.)

structures. In these cases, the effects are generally referable to the location of the lesion, and symptoms of intracranial hypertension may be seen. If the CSF pathway is involved, hydrocephalus can result. In the special case of suprasellar arachnoid cysts, endocrinopathy, visual impairment, and hydrocephalus may result.[18] Fortunately, growth of arachnoid cysts is typically seen only in the very young; in one series of more than 300 cases, no patient over the age of 4 experienced cyst enlargement or required surgical intervention.[16,19]

Rarely, children may present with hemorrhage, either into the cyst itself or into the overlying subdural space. As with any intracranial hemorrhage, these cases represent a medical emergency and require prompt neurosurgical attention. Operative interventions may be required to evacuate the hematoma.

Diagnosis

When a suspected arachnoid cyst is identified, definitive imaging with contrast-enhanced magnetic resonance imaging (MRI) should be performed to rule out other pathology. If the diagnosis of arachnoid cyst is confirmed, close clinical and radiographic follow-up is warranted for young children because of the increased risk of enlargement among this age group.[13] As the patient ages, the need for serial imaging studies decreases. When arachnoid cysts are identified in teenagers and young adults, a single stable follow-up image is often sufficient.

Management

Surgical intervention for arachnoid cysts is reserved for cases with progressive growth or concerning mass effect; asymptomatic, small lesions that do not enlarge are generally left untreated, regardless of their location and size. When an operation is indicated, placement of a cyst-to-peritoneal shunt is usually the procedure of choice, although open or endoscopic operations to fenestrate the cyst wall may also be performed.

Chiari Malformations

Four types of Chiari malformations have been described. Although they share a common name and some morphologic features, they are actually distinct pathologies; they do not represent separate points along the spectrum of a single disease.

Chiari I Malformation

A Chiari I malformation is defined by the presence of cerebellar tonsillar ectopia with the inferior tip of the tonsils at least 5 mm below the level of the foramen magnum (Fig. 61.5). The low-lying tonsils can interfere with the normal flow of CSF across the foramen magnum and cause suboccipital headaches that are brought on by coughing or a Valsalva maneuver. These maneuvers result in transient venous hypertension, which is propagated to the brain parenchyma. In patients without Chiari malformations, CSF egress through the obex of the fourth ventricle accommodates the pressure increase by allowing CSF to exit the ventricles. The Chiari malformation is thought to impede flow through this pop-off valve, resulting in a temporary spike in pressure and, consequently, headaches. Headaches that are not posterior and not elicited by provocative maneuvers are unlikely to be due to the Chiari malformation.[20]

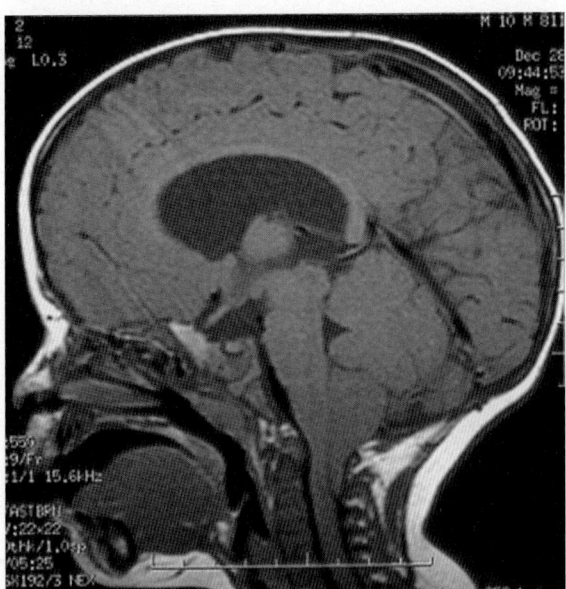

Fig. 61.5. Chiari I malformation. Sagittal T1-weighted magnetic resonance image shows ectopia of the cerebellar tonsils far below the foramen magnum, consistent with a Chiari I malformation. Note the peglike morphology of the tonsils, which are present more commonly in symptomatic lesions. (Reproduced with permission from Tubbs RS, Hankinson TC, Wellons JC. The Chiari malformations and syringohydromyelia. In: Ellenbogen RG, Abdulrauf SI, Sekhar LN, eds. Principles of Neurological Surgery. 3rd ed. Philadelphia: Saunders; 2012:157-168.)

Some patients with Chiari I malformations may also develop syringomyelia.[21] The mechanism by which the syrinx develops is not completely understood, but some have hypothesized that the blockage at the obex redirects CSF flow down the central canal of the spinal cord, resulting in cavitation and cyst formation.[22,23] As a consequence, these patients can have symptoms of myelopathy, including extremity weakness, sensory changes, gait imbalance, and bowel/bladder incontinence. In particularly severe cases, compression of the brain stem by the Chiari I malformation can cause lower cranial nerve dysfunction. These patients may experience dysphagia, dysarthria, or tinnitus.[24] Hydrocephalus is present only rarely.[21]

Chiari I malformation is best diagnosed with an MRI of the brain, which will show in detail the anatomy of the cerebellar tonsils and the brain stem. Patients with round-appearing tonsils close to 5 mm below the foramen magnum are less likely to be symptomatic, whereas those who have more profound tonsillar descent with peg-shaped morphology are more likely to be symptomatic and to benefit from surgery. Cine MRI can also demonstrate obstruction to the normal pulsatile flow of CSF at the foramen magnum.[25,26] Our practice is to routinely obtain an MRI of the spine on all patients with a Chiari I malformation to rule out syringomyelia.

The decision to surgically treat a Chiari I malformation is influenced principally by symptomatology. Patients with lifestyle-limiting headaches and convincing radiographic findings are usually offered an operation, whereas those who are asymptomatic can be observed safely and treated if they develop symptoms.[24,27] Patients with syringomyelia are an exception to this rule; we generally recommend surgical decompression for these patients even in the absence of symptoms to prevent syrinx progression and spinal cord damage.

The goal of surgery is decompression of the cerebellar tonsils and brain stem. To accomplish this objective, a midline suboccipital incision is made, and the posterior arch of C1 and the posterior rim of the foramen magnum are identified and removed. In most patients, the dura is then opened and a dural patch is sewn in place to expand the dural sleeve.[28] If the tonsils are particularly low lying, bipolar cautery can be used to shrink the tonsils. This latter maneuver does not result in lasting neurologic deficits, although patients may experience a subtle, temporary ataxia. Although the postoperative course is generally uneventful, patients are commonly admitted to the ICU overnight to be monitored for neurologic decline or respiratory depression, the latter of which can occur in up to 14% of cases.[24]

Chiari II Malformation

By definition associated with myelomeningocele, the Chiari II malformation is characterized by low-lying cerebellar tonsils with caudal displacement of the brain stem and fourth ventricle. Hydrocephalus is present in most cases because of the associated myelomeningocele. Many developmental abnormalities may be associated with a Chiari II malformation, including a small posterior fossa, polymicrogyria, gray matter heterotopias, and hypoplastic brain stem nuclei.[20]

When symptomatic, neonates and young infants tend to present with signs and symptoms referable to brain stem and lower cranial nerve dysfunction. Neonates may have apneic episodes, which can be due to untreated hydrocephalus or to maldevelopment of the medullary respiratory center. Inspiratory stridor and neurogenic dysphagia may also result from brain stem abnormalities.[29-31] In general, younger patients with more rapid presentations tend to have worse outcomes. In older children, syringomyelia can cause myelopathy and extremity weakness.

Surgical management of Chiari II malformation is similar to that of Chiari I malformation; however, the posterior fossa venous anatomy tends to be atypical in these patients, and our experience is that the expansion duraplasty carries much higher risk in this group. As such, we do not routinely open the dura in these patients.

Chiari III Malformation

Chiari III malformations account for fewer than 1% of all Chiari malformations.[20] They are characterized by occipital or cervical encephaloceles containing tissue from the cerebellum and, in some cases, the brain stem. Hydrocephalus is very common, and severe developmental problems are nearly universal. Surgical treatment for these patients involves repair of the encephalocele.[20]

Chiari IV Malformation

Unlike types I, II, and III, the Chiari IV malformation is not characterized by herniation of brain tissue but is instead an extreme form of cerebellar hypoplasia. Maldevelopment of the brain stem is occasionally seen in this condition. Surgical decompression is not required.

Dandy-Walker Malformation

The Dandy-Walker malformation is defined by an enlarged posterior fossa, cystic dilatation of the fourth ventricle, and vermian hypoplasia or aplasia (Fig. 61.6). It occurs with a

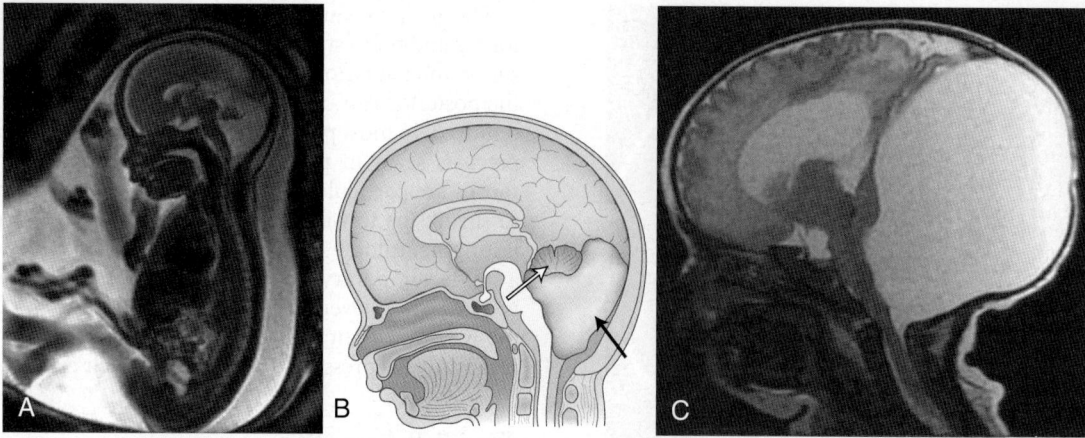

Fig. 61.6. Dandy-Walker syndrome. (A) Prenatal sagittal T2-weighted magnetic resonance image shows a large posterior fossa cyst and abnormal cerebellum, consistent with Dandy-Walker syndrome. (B) The black arrow indicates a large posterior fossa cyst, and the white arrow indicates an abnormal cerebellar vermis. (C) Sagittal T2-weighted magnetic resonance image shows a large posterior fossa cyst with upward displacement of the tentorium. (Reproduced with permission from Choutka O, Mangano FT. Dandy-Walker syndrome. In: Winn HR, ed. Youmans Neurological Surgery. Philadelphia: Elsevier Saunders; 2011:1906-1910.)

frequency of approximately 4 per 100,000, and between 70% and 90% of patients have hydrocephalus, which is the presenting feature in most.[15,32,33] About two-thirds of patients have associated central nervous system (CNS) malformations, with agenesis of the corpus callosum being most common. Meningoceles, encephaloceles, agyria, polymicrogyria, intrinsic brain stem malformations, and others are also seen.[32,34] Some[35-37] but not all [38,39] authors have found a correlation between the presence of these structural abnormalities and intelligence, which is normal in approximately 40% of patients.[36] Epilepsy and sensory disturbances are not infrequent, and these have been consistently shown to correlate with worse cognitive outcome.[35]

Outside of the CNS, Dandy-Walker malformations are associated with a number of systemic anomalies that can be particularly relevant to the pediatric intensivist. For example, tetralogy of Fallot, congenital valve disease, coarctation of the aorta, ventriculoseptal defects, and a patent ductus arteriosus can compromise cardiovascular function in these children. Feeding and the digestive process can be complicated by duodenal atresia, intestinal malrotation, and anorectal malformations. Dysplasia of the kidneys and lungs may also occur. Finally, Dandy-Walker malformation is seen in many children with syndromic disorders.[34]

Management of the condition is neurosurgical. If present, hydrocephalus should be treated by placement of a CSF shunt or ETV.[33,40-45] Fenestration of the fourth ventricular cyst has fallen out of favor as a primary treatment because it is associated with unacceptable morbidity and mortality. It is generally not performed for patients whose hydrocephalus is adequately treated by a shunt; however, several authors have had satisfactory results in patients with recurrent shunt malfunctions.[46-48]

Encephalocele and Meningocele

Encephalocele and meningocele are two related malformations that are characterized by herniation of CNS contents through a skull defect. In an encephalocele, the herniated tissue comprises brain, CSF, and meninges (Fig. 61.7); in a meningocele, only CSF and meningeal tissue are involved.

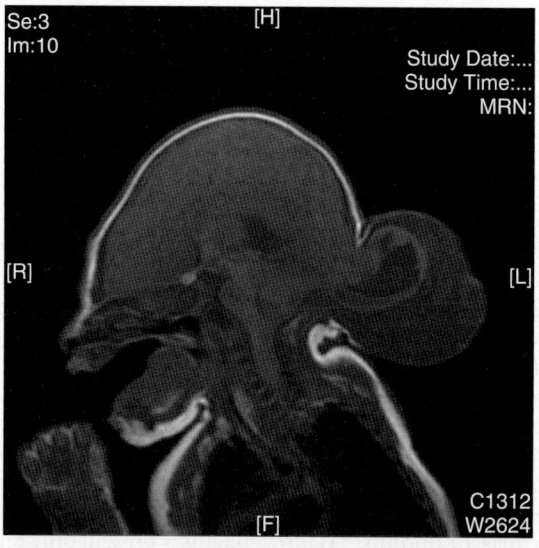

Fig. 61.7. Encephalocele. Sagittal T1-weighted magnetic resonance image shows an occipital encephalocele, with herniation of brain contents through a skull defect and into the sac. (Reproduced with permission from Ghatan S. Encephalocele. In: Winn HR, ed. Youmans Neurological Surgery. Philadelphia: Elsevier Saunders; 2011:1898-1905.)

Encephaloceles occur in approximately 1 to 3 per 10,000 live births and account for 10% to 15% of all neural tube defects.[49-51] Primary encephaloceles are developmental in origin, whereas secondary encephaloceles are acquired, most commonly because of trauma, infection, malignancy, or surgery.[52]

Primary lesions are generally classified based on their location: at the skull base, in the anterior cranial fossa, or along the calvaria. The relative frequency of these lesions varies with the population studied; occipital encephaloceles (along the calvaria at the occiput) account for 80% of all cases in North America and Western Europe, whereas anterior encephaloceles are more common in Southeast Asia and Africa.[52-57] They may occur in isolation or in conjunction with other anomalies as part of a syndrome, such as in Meckel syndrome or amniotic band syndrome.[58-60]

Most of these lesions are now diagnosed prenatally with routine ultrasound examinations, prompting delivery of the fetus by cesarean section. If not seen on prenatal ultrasound, they are frequently obvious at birth.[52] Because clinically significant associated abnormalities are commonly seen throughout the neuraxis, patients with suspected or confirmed encephaloceles should be imaged with an MRI of the brain and spine.[52] As many as one-fifth will have an additional neural tube defect, and hydrocephalus is present in 16% to 65% of cases.[55,61-64] Neurologic function varies with the location of the lesion and the amount of brain matter in the encephalocele; children with small lesions may have no obvious neurologic findings, whereas more significant cases can present with severe deficits, including brain stem dysfunction not compatible with life.[52,65] Among patients with occipital encephaloceles, approximately 17% will have normal neurologic outcomes.[65]

Spinal Dysraphism

Spinal dysraphism refers to a spectrum of related malformations that range in severity from clinically insignificant to life altering. The mildest form, spina bifida occulta, is defined by a congenital absence of all or part of the posterior elements of a lumbar vertebral body. Many of these are found incidentally and cause the patient no harm, although some are associated with other abnormalities that predispose the patient to tethered cord syndrome. Spina bifida aperta is more severe and is divided into two subtypes: meningocele and myelomeningocele. The former is characterized by a more severe defect in the posterior elements than is seen with spina bifida occulta; there is cystic dilatation of the meninges, but the underlying neural structures are normal.[66]

Myelomeningocele is the most severe form, with exposure of the spinal cord and loss of function distal to the affected level (Fig. 61.8). The malformation is caused by failure of the posterior neuropore to close properly, which in turn prevents proper migration of the adjacent ectodermal tissues. As a consequence, the involved segment of the spinal cord is exposed as a *placode* surrounded by fragile arachnoid membranes that tether to the neural tissue to the adjacent skin. These membranes frequently rupture, leading to loss of CSF and increased risk of infection. Chiari II malformations are present in most of these children.[67]

Timely closure of the myelomeningocele is imperative to reduce the risk of infection, which increases after 24 to 36 hours of life because of bacterial colonization.[68] To prevent further loss of function, the newborn should be positioned prone to keep pressure off of the lesion. In addition, the site should be kept moist with saline and covered with saline-soaked Telfa pads.[67] At our center, we commonly place a "donut" of soaked, sterile sponges around the placode, which ensures that the overlying dressing does not apply pressure to the lesion.

Precise surgical techniques for repair vary from center to center. At our institution, the procedure is carried out by a combined team of neurosurgeons and plastic surgeons. The neurosurgeon releases the placode and closes the dura in a watertight fashion to prevent leakage of CSF; the plastic

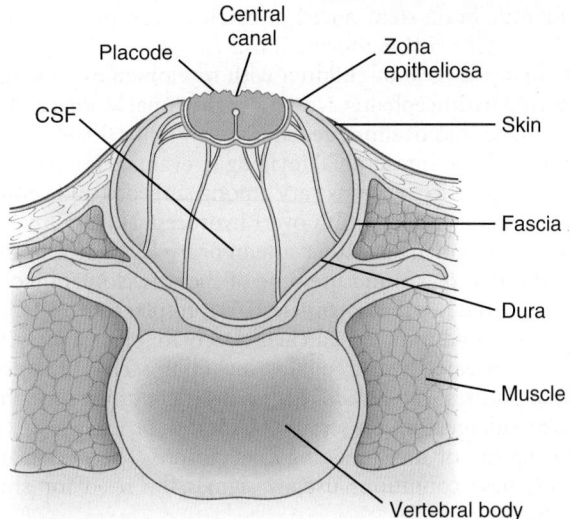

Fig. 61.8. Axial cross-sectional anatomy of a myelomeningocele. Due to failure of primary neurulation, the spinal cord herniates through defects in the vertebrae and soft tissue and is exposed as the placode. The placode is surrounded by the zona epitheliosa, a thin layer of epithelial tissue. (Reproduced with permission from Sutton LN, Bauman JA, Macyszyn LJ. Spinal dysraphism and tethered spinal cord. In: Ellenbogen RG, Abdulrauf SI, Sekhar LN, eds. Principles of Neurological Surgery. 3rd ed. Philadelphia: Saunders; 2012:89-103.)

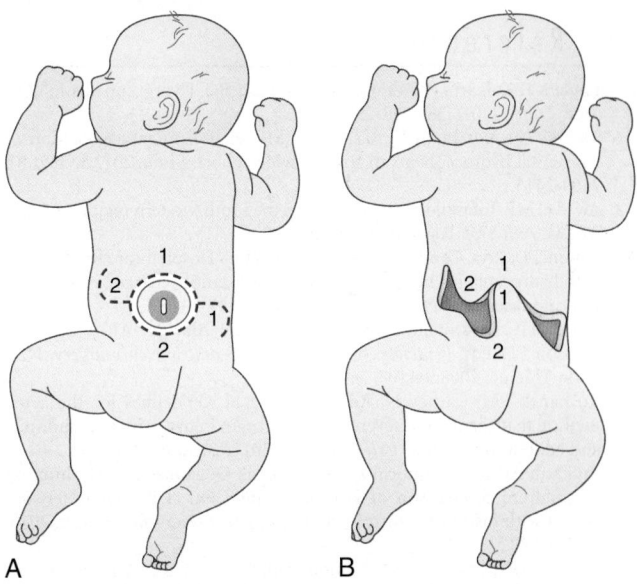

Fig. 61.9. Closure of the myelomeningocele. (A) Once the placode is released and the dura is closed, creation of tissue flaps may be required to close larger defects. Here, an S-shaped incision surrounds the lesion. (B) The tissue flaps are rotated, facilitating a multilayered closure. (Reproduced with permission from Sutton LN, Bauman JA, Macyszyn LJ. Spinal dysraphism and tethered spinal cord. In: Ellenbogen RG, Abdulrauf SI, Sekhar LN, eds. Principles of Neurological Surgery. 3rd ed. Philadelphia: Saunders; 2012:89-103.)

surgery team then mobilizes adjacent soft tissue flaps to perform a layered closure (Fig. 61.9).[69] As in the preoperative period, the patient is kept prone postoperatively to prevent pressure on the wound. Use of narcotics should be limited; many patients are unusually susceptible to the respiratory suppression that these agents cause because of either intrinsically hypoplastic brain stem nuclei or extrinsic compression from associated Chiari II malformations.

As many as 85% of children with myelomeningocele have comorbid hydrocephalus, with more proximal lesions conferring a higher risk of shunt dependence.[67,70] Thus these children should undergo intracranial imaging to evaluate for ventriculomegaly. Practice patterns vary among surgeons and centers, but in general children with overt hydrocephalus on imaging undergo placement of either a temporary EVD or a permanent shunt at or around the time of their myelomeningocele closure. If the neurosurgeon elects not to place an EVD or a shunt, the child must be watched closely for signs and symptoms of untreated hydrocephalus, including a tense fontanelle, splayed sutures, rapidly increasing head circumference, ventricular enlargement on serial ultrasounds, or leakage of CSF from the site of myelomeningocele closure. The presence of any of these conditions usually signals the need for shunt placement.

Ultimately, outcome depends on the level of the lesion and the presence of hydrocephalus. Proximal lesions at T12 or L1 cause complete or nearly complete paralysis of the lower limbs, whereas distal lesions at S1 or S2 may cause only mild distal motor symptoms and sphincter dysfunction. About half of patients have the ability to ambulate with a brace. Seventy percent of patients achieve normal IQ, although that rate is far lower among children who suffer a shunt infection.[68]

Key References

1. Kahle KT, Kulkarni AV, Limbrick DDJ, Warf BC. Hydrocephalus in children. *Lancet.* 2016;387:788-799.
2. Munch TN, Rostgaard K, Rasmussen ML, et al. Familial aggregation of congenital hydrocephalus in a nationwide cohort. *Brain.* 2012;135(Pt 8): 2409-2415.
3. Awad el ME. Infantile hydrocephalus in the south-western region of Saudi Arabia. *Ann Trop Paediatr.* 1992;12:335-338.
4. Simon TD, Riva-Cambrin J, Srivastava R, et al. Hospital care for children with hydrocephalus in the United States: utilization, charges, comorbidities, and deaths. *J Neurosurg Pediatr.* 2008;1:131-137.
5. Rekate HL. Treatment of hydrocephalus. In: Albright AL, Pollack IF, Adelson PD, eds. *Principles and Practice of Pediatric Neurosurgery.* New York: Thieme; 2008:94-108.
6. Kochanek PM, Carney N, Adelson PD, et al. Guidelines for the acute medical management of severe traumatic brain injury in infants, children, and adolescents. *Pediatr Crit Care Med.* 2012;13(suppl 1):S1-S82.
7. Kulkarni AV, Riva-Cambrin J, Butler J, et al. Outcomes of CSF shunting in children: comparison of Hydrocephalus Clinical Research Network cohort with historical controls: clinical article. *J Neurosurg Pediatr.* 2013; 12:334-338.
9. McLone DG, Czyzewski D, Raimondi AJ, Sommers RC. Central nervous system infections as a limiting factor in the intelligence of children with myelomeningocele. *Pediatrics.* 1982;70:338-342.
10. Kestle JRW, Riva-Cambrin J, Wellons JC, et al. A standardized protocol to reduce cerebrospinal fluid shunt infection: the Hydrocephalus Clinical Research Network Quality Improvement Initiative. *J Neurosurg Pediatr.* 2011;8:22-29.
11. Kulkarni AV, Drake JM, Mallucci CL, et al. Endoscopic third ventriculostomy in the treatment of childhood hydrocephalus. *J Pediatr.* 2009; 155:254-259e1.
12. Kulkarni AV, Drake JM, Kestle JR, et al. Predicting who will benefit from endoscopic third ventriculostomy compared with shunt insertion in childhood hydrocephalus using the ETV Success Score. *J Neurosurg Pediatr.* 2010;6:310-315.
13. Al-Holou WN, Yew AY, Boomsaad ZE, et al. Prevalence and natural history of arachnoid cysts in children. *J Neurosurg Pediatr.* 2010;5: 578-585.
14. Rengachary SS, Watanabe I. Ultrastructure and pathogenesis of intracranial arachnoid cysts. *J Neuropathol Exp Neurol.* 1981;40:61-83.
15. Wilkinson CC, Winston KR. Congenital arachnoid cysts and the Dandy-Walker complex. In: Albright AL, Pollack IF, Adelson PD, eds. *Principles and Practice of Pediatric Neurosurgery.* 2nd ed. New York: Thieme; 2008.
17. Shaw CM. "Arachnoid cysts" of the sylvian fissure versus "temporal lobe agenesis" syndrome. *Ann Neurol.* 1979;5:483-485.
18. Pierre-Kahn A, Capelle L, Brauner R, et al. Presentation and management of suprasellar arachnoid cysts. Review of 20 cases. *J Neurosurg.* 1990;73: 355-359.
20. Soleau S, Tubbs RS, Oakes WJ. Chiari malformations. In: Albright AL, Pollack IF, Adelson PD, eds. *Principles and Practice of Pediatric Neurosurgery.* 2nd ed. New York: Thieme; 2008.
21. Guinto G, Zamorano C, Dominguez F, et al. Malformation: part II. *Contemp Neurosurg.* 2004;26:1-7.
22. Pillay PK, Awad IA, Hahn JF. Gardner's hydrodynamic theory of syringomyelia revisited. *Cleve Clin J Med.* 1992;59:373-380.
23. Williams B. Cerebrospinal fluid pressure-gradients in spina bifida cystica, with special reference to the Arnold-Chiari malformation and aqueductal stenosis. *Dev Med Child Neurol Suppl.* 1975;138-150.
24. Paul KS, Lye RH, Strang FA, Dutton J. Arnold-Chiari malformation. Review of 71 cases. *J Neurosurg.* 1983;58:183-187.
26. Ellenbogen RG, Armonda RA, Shaw DW, Winn HR. Toward a rational treatment of Chiari I malformation and syringomyelia. *Neurosurg Focus.* 2000;8:E6.
27. Dyste GN, Menezes AH, VanGilder JC. Symptomatic Chiari malformations. An analysis of presentation, management, and long-term outcome. *J Neurosurg.* 1989;71:159-168.
28. Ellenbogen RG. Duraplasty: a procedure not to fear! *World Neurosurg.* 2011;75:224-225.
29. Pollack IF, Pang D, Kocoshis S, Putnam P. Neurogenic dysphagia resulting from Chiari malformations. *Neurosurgery.* 1992;30:709-719.
30. Pollack IF, Pang D, Albright AL, Krieger D. Outcome following hindbrain decompression of symptomatic Chiari malformations in children previously treated with myelomeningocele closure and shunts. *J Neurosurg.* 1992;77:881-888.
32. Sasaki-Adams D, Elbabaa SK, Jewells V, et al. The Dandy-Walker variant: a case series of 24 pediatric patients and evaluation of associated anomalies, incidence of hydrocephalus, and developmental outcomes. *J Neurosurg Pediatr.* 2008;2:194-199.
35. Bindal AK, Storrs BB, McLone DG. Management of the Dandy-Walker syndrome. *Pediatr Neurosurg.* 1990;16:163-169.
36. Ulm B, Ulm MR, Deutinger J, Bernaschek G. Dandy-Walker malformation diagnosed before 21 weeks of gestation: associated malformations and chromosomal abnormalities. *Ultrasound Obstet Gynecol.* 1997;10: 167-170.
37. Pascual-Castroviejo I, Velez A, Pascual-Pascual SI, et al. Dandy-Walker malformation: analysis of 38 cases. *Childs Nerv Syst.* 1991;7:88-97.
38. Sawaya R, McLaurin RL. Dandy-Walker syndrome. Clinical analysis of 23 cases. *J Neurosurg.* 1981;55:89-98.
39. Naidich TP, Radkowski MA, McLone DG, Leestma J. Chronic cerebral herniation in shunted Dandy-Walker malformation. *Radiology.* 1986; 158:431-434.
40. Fischer EG. Dandy-Walker syndrome: an evaluation of surgical treatment. *J Neurosurg.* 1973;39:615-621.
41. Carmel PW, Antunes JL, Hilal SK, Gold AP. Dandy-Walker syndrome: clinico-pathological features and re-evaluation of modes of treatment. *Surg Neurol.* 1977;8:132-138.
47. Liu JC, Ciacci JD, George TM. Brainstem tethering in Dandy-Walker syndrome: a complication of cystoperitoneal shunting. Case report. *J Neurosurg.* 1995;83:1072-1074.
48. Villavicencio AT, Wellons JC, George TM. Avoiding complicated shunt systems by open fenestration of symptomatic fourth ventricular cysts associated with hydrocephalus. *Pediatr Neurosurg.* 1998;29:314-319.
50. Simpson DA, David DJ, White J. Cephaloceles: treatment, outcome, and antenatal diagnosis. *Neurosurgery.* 1984;15:14-21.
52. Jimenez DF, Barone CM. Encephaloceles, meningoceles, and dermal sinuses. In: Albright AL, Pollack IF, Adelson PD, eds. *Principles and Practice of Pediatric Neurosurgery.* New York: Thieme; 2008:233-253.
53. Suwanwela C. Geographical distribution of fronto-ethmoidal encephalomeningocele. *Br J Prev Soc Med.* 1972;26:193-198.
54. Caviness VS Jr, Evrard P. Occipital encephalocele. *Acta Neuropathol.* 1975;32:245-255.
55. Mealey J, Dzenitis AJ, Hockey AA. The prognosis of encephaloceles. *J Neurosurg.* 1970;32:209-218.
57. Whatmore WJ. Sincipital encephalomeningoceles. *Br J Surg.* 1973;60: 261-270.

59. Cohen MM, Lemire RJ. Syndromes with cephaloceles. *Teratology.* 1982;25:161-172.
60. Mecke S, Passarge E. Encephalocele, polycystic kidneys, and polydactyly as an autosomal recessive trait simulating certain other disorders: the Meckel syndrome. *Ann Genet.* 1971;14:97-103.
61. Fenger C. Basal hernias of the brain. *Am J Med Sci.* 1895;109:1-16.
65. French BN. Midline fusion defects and defects of formation. In: Youmans JR, ed. *Youman's Neurological Surgery.* Philadelphia: Saunders; 1990.
66. McComb JG. Spinal Meningoceles. In: Albright AL, Pollack IF, Adelson PD, eds. *Principles and Practice of Pediatric Neurosurgery.* New York: Thieme; 2008:323-337.
67. Dias MS, McLone DG. Myelomeningocele. In: Albright AL, Pollack IF, Adelson PD, eds. *Principles and Practice of Pediatric Neurosurgery.* New York: Thieme; 2008:338-366.
69. Lien SC, Maher CO, Garton HJL, et al. Local and regional flap closure in myelomeningocele repair: a 15-year review. *Childs Nerv Syst.* 2010;26: 1091-1095.
70. Stein SC, Schut L. Hydrocephalus in myelomeningocele. *Childs Brain.* 1979;5:413-419.

Neurologic Assessment and Monitoring

Mark S. Wainwright

PEARLS

- Much of the practice of brain-directed critical care in children is empirical, but studies in traumatic brain injury support the use of protocol-directed care with multidisciplinary teams in the intensive care unit to reduce mortality.
- The examiner should focus on both localizing a neurologic deficit and identifying mechanisms of injury (or potential injury) as the first steps in developing a treatment approach to reduce brain injury.
- Communication between team members, serial examinations, anticipation, and early recognition of changes in the neurologic exam or other monitoring parameters are essential.
- Metabolic monitoring methods, including partial pressure of oxygen and microdialysis, have great potential to advance the detection of, and therapy for, secondary neurologic injury in pediatric acute brain injury. The application of these tools to neurocritical care and the demonstration of their efficacy in improving outcomes will require advances in data collection, bioinformatics, and methods of data analysis.

Overview and Basic Principles of Pediatric Critical Care Neurology

The approach to the neurologic assessment of the patient in the pediatric or cardiac intensive care unit (ICU) requires an interdisciplinary team involving intensivists, neurologists, neurosurgeons, and specialists from allied disciplines including physiatry and psychiatry. Examples of these programs at different pediatric academic centers have been published.[1-4] Although this method recapitulates elements of the approach to differential diagnosis used in the outpatient setting and inpatient care outside the ICU, there are fundamental differences that are specific to the practice of pediatric critical care neurology.[5,6] In general, these differences involve the need to obtain testing (imaging, neurophysiology, laboratory) on patients who may appear neurologically intact, the need to intervene before a specific neurologic diagnosis has been obtained or mechanism of injury confirmed, and the challenge of determining whether such interventions affect long-term outcome. Indeed, the lack of data from randomized

controlled clinical trials to guide much of the management of children with acute brain injuries is a defining feature of the practice of neurologic critical care in children.

In sum, the practice of pediatric critical care neurology involves the need for serial neurologic examinations, clear communication between nurses and physicians and among practitioners of multiple medical services, the need for an early recognition of changes in the neurologic exam, and the anticipatory management of patients with the potential for progressive neurologic deterioration. The confounding effects of sedation or postoperative anesthesia on neurologic functioning pose an additional set of challenges to the assessment of these patients. Nevertheless, a logical approach to the neurologic examination is possible, using the standard structure of a neurologic examination, combining this exam with attention to the mechanisms of injury (present or potential) and thereby developing a plan for ongoing monitoring and management. Last, it is prudent to regard every patient in the pediatric ICU (PICU) as having the potential for neurologic complications of his or her illness. These patients with primary diagnoses ranging from neurologic complications of solid organ transplant to liver failure to congenital heart disease may suffer neurologic injury from any combination of hypoxic, ischemic, inflammatory, or metabolic cerebral insults.

Recognition of Neurologic Complications of Critical Illness

This is likely an underrecognized population in many PICUs, in part because of the prevalence of nonconvulsive seizures (NCSs)[7,8] or ICU-acquired weakness.[9] In these cases, the recognition of new neurologic deficits relies on the ability of the medical team to recognize changes in the neurologic exam. In general, interventions to treat or attenuate neurologic insults, whether seizures, ischemia, or increasing intracranial pressure (ICP), are more likely to be successful if initiated early in the process of injury. This means that effective neurologic monitoring in the PICU does not rely solely on the availability of a neurologist, electroencephalogram (EEG), or neuroimaging. Rather, the prerequisite to using these monitoring tools is a high index of suspicion for new neurologic injury on the part of the medical team for patients who do not have primary neurologic injuries.

In addition to the physical exam, a number of modalities are used for to monitor neurologic function in critically ill children and adults (some suggestions for review can be found in the references[10,11]). These include continuous EEG monitoring (which is well established as a modality essential for the detection of NCS in the adult and PICU[12-15] ICP), transcranial Doppler (TCD),[16,17] and metabolic tissue oxygen monitoring.[18-20] Thresholds for detecting cerebral ischemic injury have been proposed for brain oxygen tension[21] and near-infrared spectroscopy (NIRS).[22] With respect to pediatric neuromonitoring, as yet there is no consensus on normal values or the age-dependence of these end points.[23]

Anticipatory Planning for New Neurologic Deficits

The ability to recognize changes in the neurologic exam is an essential component of brain-directed critical care for children. Reliance on technology alone is insufficient. Management should include the anticipation of specific changes in the patient's exam, an understanding of the pathophysiology causing that change, and a predetermined plan to intervene and address that mechanism. Common examples include compromise of short-term memory in the patient with acute liver failure (ALF), right leg weakness in the patient with right anterior cerebral artery stroke, and hypophonia in the patient with acute inflammatory demyelinating polyneuropathy. Each example (progression of hepatic encephalopathy, compression of the left anterior cerebral artery caused by increased edema in the right frontal lobe, progression to involve bulbar weakness) requires an escalation in care and cannot be identified by bedside monitors other than an examiner with an understanding of the disease process and the implications of these findings.

An improving exam despite deterioration in other modalities such as EEG, TCDs, ICP, or neuroimaging may change the treatment plan. Similarly, deterioration in the neurologic exam may occur without changes in these other measures. The ability to detect and react to such change requires a consensus on the admission neurologic exam, consensus on the criteria for decline or improvement for each specific patient, and anticipatory planning for the management of changes in the exam. The examiner should first discuss the neurologic findings with the bedside nurse and other members of the medical team. If possible, abnormal findings should be demonstrated to the members of the team. There should be a consensus on the key findings and the approach to be taken for evaluation and management if the neurologic exam changes. The improvements in outcome for children with severe traumatic brain injury (TBI) associated with the introduction of a multidisciplinary care team[24] and adherence to management guidelines[25] suggest that an emphasis on consistent care following established protocols can improve outcome without the need for additional technology (see also Chapter 119).

History and Assessment of Risk Factors

For children in the PICU, the medical history may provide essential information about the mechanisms and timing of neurologic insult. This information is needed for the interpretation of the neurologic exam and assessment of potential mechanisms of neurologic injury. These data are then used to assess the risk for progression of neurologic injury, to prioritize therapeutic interventions, and to determine the need for and timing of additional evaluations including imaging, EEG, and laboratory studies. In many cases, decisions to treat (or not treat) a neurologic injury in the PICU have to be empiric and based on a careful assessment of risk factors, potential mechanisms of injury, and weighing of the risks and benefits of such intervention. For example, the approach to the evaluation of altered mental status presenting to the PICU will be different with children with an established complex partial seizure disorder, those with sickle cell disease, or stem cell transplant recipients on immune suppressant drugs. Before examining the patient, knowledge of salient details of the medical history allows the examiner to begin to formulate a diagnostic approach and to prepare the early steps in management. The patient with a history of epilepsy in the preceding example would likely require an emergent EEG to rule out nonconvulsive seizures, whereas the patient with sickle cell disease and risk factors of vascular injury with the same symptoms may require an imaging study and the immune suppressed patient a lumbar puncture. The presenting neurologic symptoms may be similar, but the history dictates the assessment based on the likely mechanisms producing the deficits found on neurologic examination.

Iatrogenic Complications of Pharmacotherapy

A review of medications should be part of the neurologic assessment of any patient with new neurologic symptoms. The initial assessment of the patient should include attention to medications that cross the blood-brain barrier or that may interfere with the renal or hepatic metabolism of centrally active drugs. In patients in renal or liver failure or in those requiring dialysis, the side effects of a centrally acting drug must be considered in the differential diagnosis for any neurologic symptom. This may occur even in the presence of "normal" doses of drugs or levels of anticonvulsants, as off-target drug toxicities may be due to metabolites, not the drug itself. An example is shown (Fig. 62.1) of a child with a mild static encephalopathy and spasticity, on dialysis as the sequelae of perinatal renal injury, who developed progressive encephalopathy. Treatment with flumazenil and an immediate improvement in mental status confirmed that the accumulation of baclofen in this dialysis-dependent patient was the source of a waxing and waning encephalopathy. Common examples in the PICU include immunophilin-associated seizures, encephalopathy and hypertension, oculogyric crisis, delirium during reduction of sedation, and prolonged sedation and paralysis from overzealous neuromuscular blockade. In many cases, the attribution of the symptoms to a drug side effect (excess level, too rapid withdrawal, idiosyncratic reaction, impairment of clearance) will be a diagnosis of exclusion. Nevertheless, a review of medications and recent changes should be a routine component of the neurologic assessment.

Vital Signs

Therapies that target specific mechanisms of cell injury for acute CNS disease are lacking in adult and pediatric neurocritical care. Nevertheless, the prevention of hyperthermia may significantly reduce secondary neurologic injury. The results of randomized controlled trials of therapeutic hypothermia in children with severe TBI[26,27] and out-of-hospital cardiac arrest[28,29] suggest that early hypothermia, irrespective of ICP, does not improve outcome and in the case of TBI may increase the risk of death.[27,30,31] Despite this observation, the prevention of hyperthermia can be regarded as a safe and effective intervention.[32] Therefore as a general principle for ICU patients with known or suspected CNS injury, fever should be aggressively avoided.

In contrast to the research on adults, there are limited data on the optimum ranges for blood pressure, ICP, and cerebral

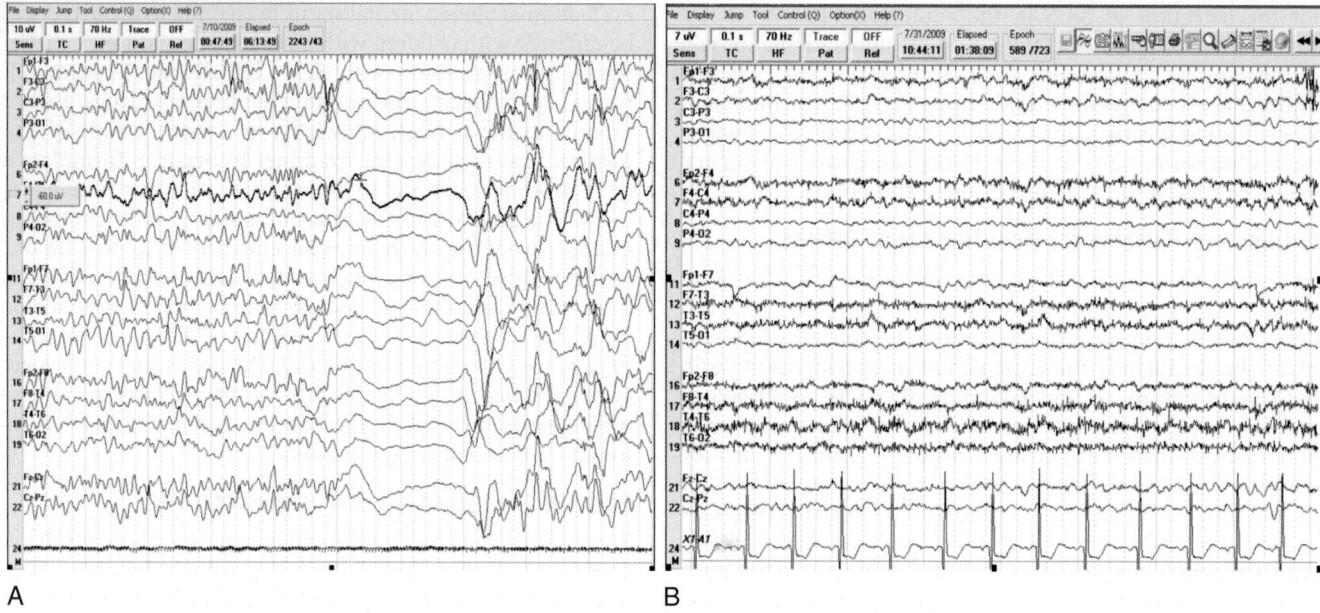

Fig. 62.1. Bipolar EEG montage of a child with a mild static encephalopathy and spasticity, on dialysis as the sequelae of perinatal renal injury, who developed progressive encephalopathy with high amplitude epileptiform discharges (A). Treatment with flumazenil resulted in immediate improvement in mental status and sustained improvement in the EEG (B), confirming that the accumulation of baclofen in this dialysis-dependent patient was the source of a waxing and waning encephalopathy.

perfusion pressure (CPP) for children. For adults, there are goal-directed protocols aimed at improving outcome following TBI. The targets of ICP less than 20 mm Hg and CPP above 60 mm Hg are based on a number of studies.[33-37] In contrast, limited data exist for children with TBI.[38,39] Guidelines suggest an ICP threshold of 20 mm Hg for all ages and a CPP threshold of 40 to 65 mm Hg as an age-related continuum.[40] Although children with TBI who are younger than 2 years of age have a high mortality rate compared with older children, no thresholds for ICP or CPP have been established for this age group.[41] Accordingly, blood pressure, temperatures, and oxygenation must be interpreted in the context of the underlying neurologic insult or risk for further injury. As a general principle, hyperthermia with the attendant increased cerebral metabolic demand should be treated aggressively whatever the primary injury.[42,43]

General Physical Exam

An accurate head circumference measurement is essential in infants and young children and should be documented on admission. This may serve as a baseline for following the development of hydrocephalus in the at-risk infant. In older children, an abnormal (large or small) head circumference may be a previously overlooked sign of pathology. In the infant, the open fontanelle should be palpated and the findings on the exam agreed upon in a quiet, resting state. A bulging fontanelle is an important finding of meningeal irritation or increased ICP. Examination of skin for the cardinal features of the phakomatoses may identify café au lait spots characteristic of neurofibromatosis or shagreen patches, hypopigmented macules, and angiomyofibromas characteristic of tuberous sclerosis. The physical findings associated with inflicted trauma deserve particular mention as these may be subtle,[44] including unusual patterns of bruising, blood in the oropharynx, and burn or belt marks.

Importance of Observation in the Neurologic Exam

The elements of the neurologic examination in the PICU constitute the same features of the neurologic exam for noncritically ill patients. The assessment of mental status, cranial nerves, motor function, reflexes, sensation, and cerebellar function must be adapted to each patient, but the structure of the neurologic exam in the PICU is no different from the outpatient examination. If possible, sedating drugs and paralytic agents should be reduced prior to the exam. If this is not feasible, the exam must be interpreted in the context of these confounds.

The assessment of mental status begins with observation. The examiner should first confirm the drugs used for sedation, if any, and recent changes in dosing. It is not possible to give precise dose ranges for typical sedating agents associated with a mental status exam. For commonly used agents in the PICU (midazolam, morphine, fentanyl, dexmedetomidine), the effects of the drug on arousal and responsiveness will vary with the age of the patient, duration of exposure, nature of the neurologic insult, effect of other drugs on metabolism, and genetically determined ability to clear these drugs. This complex set of interactions underscores the importance of experience in the examination of these patients to determine what is an acceptable level of arousal and the need for serial neurologic examinations.

The observations of the nurses and parents should first be solicited. The examiner should enquire about evidence for changes in arousal or awareness, such as spontaneous eye opening, evidence of a sleep-wake cycle, change in activity, or response to interventions such as suctioning. If family members are present, their observations of the patient's response to their presence or voice are important and may represent the first signs of awareness on the part of the patient. It is appropriate to have a family member carry out part of the exam by asking the patient to follow commands, because these young patients are more likely to respond to their family members than to a stranger.

The pattern of breathing rate and rhythm should be observed. Specific patterns may help localize the site of neurologic dysfunction but not the mechanism involved (Table 62.1). The crescendo-decrescendo pattern alternating with periods of apnea, characteristic of Cheyne-Stokes respiration, may be due to dysfunction of the cerebral hemispheres, thalamus, or hypothalamus with preserved brain stem function, but it can also be found in patients with congestive heart failure or primary respiratory disease. Similarly, the sustained, deep breathing pattern of central neurogenic hyperventilation may be due to structural injury to the midbrain, sepsis, pulmonary disease, or compensated metabolic acidosis.

The conventional neurologic examination proceeds from mental status, cranial nerves, motor (bulk, tone, and strength), reflexes, and sensation to cerebellar exam and gait. In children and in the PICU in particular, the exam must be based on good observation and is often best performed out of sequence. It is easier to assess tone and reflexes in the asleep, relaxed patient before waking the patient up to assess mental status. Although the exam is discussed in the standard order presented next, it may be more informative to begin the hands-on part of the exam with an assessment of tone and reflexes. Once the patient is awake and agitated, subtle asymmetries of tone and reflexes, which may be key findings of the exam, may be obscured.

First, the child is observed. The state of arousal (awake, asleep), responsiveness, (interactive, verbal, nonresponsive), position (tone, asymmetry of limb position), and movement (purposeful, spontaneous, dystonic, choreic, asymmetry of movement) can all be reliably assessed by observation. In a nonintubated, nonsedated patient, the examiner may proceed directly with a standard mental status exam adjusted for age. In the young child who is able to cooperate, the specific cognitive and language skills expected for age can be assessed (Table 62.2).

Assessment of Level of Consciousness and Mental Status

For children with depressed consciousness, the precise stimulus required to elicit a response and the nature of this response should be specified. It is not helpful to describe the patient as lethargic or obtunded. First, the child is called by name to determine if there is a response. If this is not effective, the examiner may ask a family member to speak to the child. Next, the stimulus is increased. It is most helpful to describe the patient's response to specific stimuli and to use the same stimuli for serial examinations. The Glasgow Coma Scale score, though of limited use in preverbal children (Table 62.3), is a rapid, quantitative measure. If the patient's eyes open in response to someone's voice, the response to commands is tested next. This step is discussed in more detail later, but the commands should be increased in complexity from one to two or three steps. If there is no response to voice, a painful stimulus is next applied. Note that in patients with sensory deficits due to neuropathy, spinal cord, or CNS lesions or with focal limb weakness, the extremity or dermatome selected for testing should have intact sensory or motor function. In the sedated or severely impaired patient, the response may constitute only an increase in heart rate. It is important that the stimulus and the specific response, rather than vague descriptors (lethargic, drowsy, sleepy), are documented, as this information will be more helpful in assessing serial examinations. The rate of sedating drugs or recent administration of sedating drugs should be documented with this exam.

The assessment of higher cognitive function and the early recognition of compromise of cognitive function are always challenges when evaluating young children. In the ICU where the additional confounds of sedation, other organ dysfunction, sleep disturbance, and anxiety must be accounted for, this evaluation is somewhat more challenging. Of course, this is usually the most important component of the exam, and the technologies used for neurologic monitoring in the ICU (imaging, EEG, NIRS, microdialysis, optic nerve sheath diameter, tissue oxygenation) all serve the goal of the bedside exam—to detect compromise of cerebral function so as to enable directed therapeutic intervention.

In the older, awake child, a complete mental status exam can be performed. This must be adjusted for age (Table 62.2) but should include an assessment of language (fluency and comprehension) including the ability to name, repeat, write, read, and respond to written commands. Simple mathematical problems should be adjusted to the child's age-dependent ability. Praxis can be assessed quickly, even in the PICU, by asking the child to demonstrate learned behaviors (brush your teeth, brush your hair). Other components of the mental status exam, including memory, fund of knowledge, and reasoning, can be assessed by holding a conversation with the patient.

Most important, the examiner needs to have an appropriate index of suspicion for subtle neurologic deficits of attention, memory, praxis, language comprehension, and reading comprehension, which may be the early sign of new neurologic injury. This is particularly true for patients with metabolic (often liver or renal failure), infectious, or iatrogenic (sedation, immunophilins) risk factors for CNS dysfunction and may easily be missed if not specifically investigated. Again, serial examinations by clinicians familiar with the patient's assessment while sedated are the key to the reliable detection of new deficits of higher cortical function in the ICU.

Funduscopic Examination

Examination of the fundi may reveal hemorrhages or papilledema. Hemorrhages indicate either acute subarachnoid or subdural hemorrhage, cranial trauma from a direct blow or shaking injury, or malignant hypertension. Papilledema indicates raised ICP from any cause. Usually papilledema develops hours after the onset of the elevated ICP. Acute severe increases, however, as with subarachnoid hemorrhage (SAH) from a ruptured saccular aneurysm, can result in almost instantaneous papilledema. Sometimes papilledema never develops, despite prolonged severe elevations of ICP.

Cranial Nerve Examination

The pupillary reaction to light is abolished only by structural damage to the midbrain or third cranial nerve. Loss of the pupillary reflexes is always an ominous finding. Preservation of pupillary reflexes in the presence of deep coma suggests a metabolic-toxic cause. The interpretation of the patterns of pupil reactivity is summarized in Table 62.1.

Pupil size and light response are quantifiable measures of brain stem and autonomic nervous system function, and the absence of pupil reactivity is a poor prognostic sign after TBI or cardiac arrest. To provide a precise measure of pupil size

TABLE 62.1   Approach to the Intensive Care Unit Neurologic Examination: Localization and Mechanism

Exam Finding	Structural-Vascular Insult	Toxic-Metabolic
Consciousness	Stays at same level or deteriorates	Waxes and wanes, milder impairment; toxins may cause progressive decline
Respiration	Cheyne-Stokes (crescendo-decrescendo alternating with apnea): loss of cerebral, thalamic, or hypothalamic control of breathing Neurogenic hyperventilation (sustained, rapid, deep breathing): midbrain disease Gasping respiration (irregularly irregular): dysfunction of lower brain stem or medulla	Cheyne-Stokes: congestive heart failure; primary respiratory disease Neurogenic hyperventilation: metabolic acidosis; sepsis; liver failure Gasping respiration: intoxication (opiates, barbiturates); hypothyroidism
Funduscopy	Papilledema due to increased intracranial pressure	Papilledema does not occur except in hypertensive encephalopathy, lead intoxication, hypoparathyroidism
Eye position	Versive deviation Stroke ipsilateral to direction of deviation Retraction or convergence nystagmus Midbrain Ocular bobbing Pons Intranuclear ophthalmoplegia Pons or midbrain Oculomotor nerve palsy Midbrain or herniation Skew gaze Brain stem	Versive deviation Seizure contralateral to direction of deviation No extraocular movement with preserved pupil reactivity Toxin
Pupil reactivity	Small reactive Thalamus, hypothalamus Midposition, fixed Midbrain Pinpoint, reactive Pons Small, combined with ptosis Horner, lateral medulla, sympathetic chain Large, fixed Oculomotor nerve, tectum	Small reactive Large, fixed Botulism, opthalmic drops
Eye movements	If asymmetric, likely structural Oculomotor nerve palsy Midbrain or herniation syndrome Abducens nerve palsy Unreliable localization Internuclear ophthalmoplegia Midbrain or pons Disconjugate or skew gaze Brain stem Absent vertical and retained horizontal movement Midbrain Absent horizontal and retained vertical movements Pons	Roving more common with metabolic derangements Absence of all movement with intact pupil light reflex
Adventitious movements	Posturing; sign of herniation Myoclonus following severe cerebral ischemia	Restlessness, tremor, spasm, myoclonus, chorea, akathisia
Muscle tone	Asymmetric; increased, normal, or decreased	Symmetric; normal or decreased

and speed of contraction and relaxation, a portable handheld device (pupillometer) illuminates the eye with an infrared light (850 nm) while acquiring images for analysis. The data (pupil size, rate of contraction, and relaxation) are stored on the device and can be downloaded to a computer. In a study of healthy volunteers and adult patients with TBI and ICP monitors in place, a discrepancy in pupil size of more than 0.5 mm appeared to be associated with ICP above 20 mm Hg.[45] In a study of 134 adults with TBI, aneurysmal SAH or intracerebral hemorrhage pupil reactivity decreased an average of 16 hours before the peak ICP was reached.[46] There are as yet

no comparable data for pediatric neurotrauma. In children, no association of age and pupil size has been reported, but the maximum diameter and velocity of constriction are affected by sedation.[47]

Eye movements are assessed first by observation and then elicited in the patient with depressed mental status by application of the doll's head maneuver (oculocephalic response) or cold caloric stimulation (oculovestibular response). The interpretation of eye movements and position is summarized in Table 62.1. In general, coma produced by metabolic dysfunction is initially associated with roving, disconjugate movement

TABLE 62.2   Age-Dependent Motor and Language Patterns

Age (months)	Motor	Language
15	Walks alone; crawls up stairs	Jargon; follows simple commands
18	Runs; sits on chair; walks up stairs with hand held	10 words; names pictures; identifies body parts
24	Runs well; walks up and down stairs	Three-word sentences
30	Jumps	Refers to self as "I"
36	Stands on one foot; goes up stairs with alternating feet	Knows age and gender; counts three objects
48	Hops on one foot; throws ball	Tells a story
60	Skips	Names four colors; repeats 10-syllable sentences

Adapted from Behrman RE, et al. Nelson Textbook of Pediatrics. 14th ed. Philadelphia: WB Saunders; 1994.

TABLE 62.3   Glasgow Coma Scale

Activity	Best Response	Score
Eye opening	Spontaneous	4
	To command	3
	To pain	2
	None	1
Verbal	Oriented	5
	Confused	4
	Inappropriate words	3
	Incomprehensible sounds	2
	None	1
Motor response	Obeys commands	6
	Localizes pain	5
	Withdraws to pain	4
	Abnormal flexion to pain	3
	Abnormal extension	2
	None	1
Total		3-15

and may progress to the cessation of movement. Cold caloric stimulation produces nystagmus with the rapid phase contralateral to the ear that has been stimulated. This rapid phase is the equivalent of saccadic eye movements and indicates intact functioning of the cerebral cortex. The ears are irrigated separately several minutes apart. In comatose patients, the fast, "corrective" phase of nystagmus is lost and the eyes are tonically deflected to the side irrigated with cold water or away from the side irrigated with warm water. These vestibuloocular responses are lost or disrupted in brain stem lesions. Versive eye deviation is a common finding suspicious for seizures. In this case, the eye deviation is contralateral to the hemisphere with the ictal focus. Alternatively, stroke in the ipsilateral hemisphere may also produce versive eye deviation toward the side of the stroke.

An abnormal corneal reflex may indicate either fifth nerve afferent disease (ipsilateral stimulation results in neither a direct nor consensual eye blink) or seventh nerve efferent disease (ipsilateral stimulation results in a brisk consensual but no direct response).

Unilateral weakness of eye closure, forehead movement, and mouth movement indicates peripheral seventh cranial nerve palsy, whereas failure to move only the mouth with preservation of upper face movements indicates a central corticospinal tract lesion rostral to the pons. Facial weakness may be noted during grimacing while responses to painful stimuli are evaluated. Voluntary pharyngeal and laryngeal control is tested by asking the patient to speak and say "ah." In the absence of voluntary movement, a hypoactive gag indicates medullary or vagal dysfunction and a hyperactive gag indicates interruption of corticospinal inhibition to the medulla. In a comatose patient or one whose consciousness is rapidly sinking, one must quickly determine whether the patient is experiencing raised ICP. Papilledema or third cranial nerve palsy are strong evidence of elevated ICP.

Approach to the Motor Exam

In the comatose or obtunded patient, asymmetry of resting tone or spontaneous movement is a simple sign of paresis, which can be detected by first observing the patient. In children this is particularly important, as a subtle weakness may not be apparent once the child is more awake and resisting cooperation with the exam. An externally rotated, partly flexed abducted leg may indicate an ipsilateral hemiparesis due to an upper motor neuron lesion. Facial weakness should also be first evaluated by observation before attempting formal testing (often impossible or unreliable in young, anxious, or sedated children). Signs of facial weakness at rest may include a widened palpebral fissure, diminished nasolabial fold, or flattened corner of the mouth. The examiner should next attend to the initial movement of the face, either spontaneously or in response to a noxious stimulus. Subtle weakness may be apparent only in a delayed response to these stimuli.

Weakness may be due to lesions at any level of the neuraxis. The goal of the examination of the weak patient is to identify the pattern of weakness as that of the upper or lower motor neuron and thereby identify the most likely mechanisms. The upper motor neuron (UMN) comprises the corticospinal tract and its neurons. The corticospinal tract begins in the motor and premotor cortex anterior to the central sulcus, descends through the central white matter of the cerebral hemispheres, decussates in the lower medulla, and terminates on the anterior horn cells or interneurons closely associated with the anterior horn cells. The innervation of muscles that control movement of the jaw, pharynx, larynx, upper half of the face, neck, thorax, and abdomen is derived from both cerebral hemispheres. Consequently, unilateral cerebral lesions lead only to weakness of the contralateral limbs and lower face. The lower motor neuron (LMN) comprises the anterior horn cells, motor roots, peripheral nerves, pre- and postsynaptic components of the neuromuscular junction, and the muscles receiving this innervation. Stereotyped reflex movements may be present despite spinal cord injury because local spinal reflexes below the level of the lesion coordinate these responses. In contrast, movement is absent following injury to the LMN because it is the final common pathway producing muscle activity. If the patient is not able to cooperate with a complete exam testing all muscle groups, in addition to observing for asymmetric posture, the observation of facial movement; testing for neck flexion, grip strength, and pronator drift; and counting the duration (up to 10 seconds) that the patient can maintain a straight leg raise are efficient means of assessment.

A number of key findings on the pattern of weakness can distinguish between UMN and LMN injury, chronic and acute injury, and neuropathy and neuromuscular disorders including ICU-acquired paresis, myasthenia gravis, and Guillain-Barré syndrome (GBS). Acute UMN lesions result in a hypotonic or flaccid pattern of weakness, and in the legs they may be associated with the Babinski sign. In contrast, chronic UMN injury results in a hypertonic limb with associated hyperreflexia. An LMN pattern of weakness is more likely to be associated with a decrease in muscle tone and bulk and decreased or absent reflexes. In general, proximal weakness suggests a myopathic process, whereas a distal pattern of weakness suggests a neuropathy. The precise incidence of ICU-acquired weakness (ICU-AW) is uncertain in children.[9] In a study of the incidence of weakness in 830 critically ill children, only 1.7% had generalized weakness.[48] This is lower than the incidence of ICU-AW in adults.[49] Extensive data from adult studies have identified ICU-AW—manifest as a variable combination of weakness, muscle atrophy, hyporeflexia, and sensory deficits—as a common cause of failure of extubation with a high incidence of long-term morbidity. The contribution of the risk factors in adults (sepsis, hyperosmolarity, neuromuscular blockage, prolonged ventilation, and corticosteroids) to pediatric ICU-AW is not known. ICU-AW is primarily a clinical diagnosis, although nerve conduction and electromyography studies may be confirmatory. Management, particularly in children, is empirical, but this disorder should be suspected in any critically ill child with diminished reflexes and new weakness or difficulty with extubation.

The two most common neuromuscular disorders that require ICU level of care in children are GBS and myasthenia gravis (MG) (discussed in Chapter 71). For patients with known myasthenia admitted to the ICU in crisis, it is essential to note the timing of anticholinesterase treatment and the timing of the neurologic exam in relation to each evaluation of strength. In general, testing should be performed at the nadir of weakness prior to each treatment. This is the only reliable way to detect a decline in strength in these patients. In contrast to GBS, the progression to respiratory failure in MG may be arrested by noninvasive ventilator support with bilevel positive airway pressure (BiPAP). Muscle fatigue in MG is reversible with a combination of anticholinesterase treatment and BiPAP, which may prevent the need for intubation. In the case of GBS, patients who cannot walk unaided should be treated with intravenous immunoglobulin (IVIG).[50] Neither GBS nor myasthenia should alter pupil reactivity. In this case, if the pupils are slow to react or do not react in a weak infant, the diagnosis of botulism should be considered.[51]

Posturing, due to increased ICP, should be distinguished from abnormal movements including chorea and dystonia. Decorticate posturing consists of adduction and stiff extension of the legs, flexion and supination of the arms, and fisting of the hands. This occurs when the midbrain and red nucleus control body posture without inhibition by diencephalon, basal ganglia, and cerebral cortex. Decerebrate posturing

consists of stiff extension of legs, arms, trunk, and head with hyperpronation of lower arms and plantar flexion of the feet. This indicates pontine and vestibular nucleus control of posture without inhibition from more rostral structures. Lesions below the level of vestibular nuclei lead to flaccidity and abolition of all postures and movements. These movements should be distinguished from dystonia or chorea, which may be seen as side effects of medications, the sequelae of basal ganglia injury, or metabolic or neurotransmitter disorders.

Reflexes

Reflexes may be absent in critically ill children, wax and wane during the course of the day, or be elicited by some examiners but not others. This variability can be diminished by performing the exam when the child is in a quiet, resting state and by focusing on key reflexes. In general, the purpose of the exam is to determine whether there are changes in intensity (a reduction or an increase), symmetry, or the development of pathologic reflexes.

At a minimum, reflexes to be tested include the tendon jerks in the upper (if available) and lower extremities and the Babinski sign (dorsiflexion of the great toe, sometimes accompanied by fanning of the toes in response to stimulation of the lateral plantar aspect of the foot) as the cardinal screening test for intact functioning of the pyramidal system. If an extensor plantar reflex is present, this reflects injury along the corticospinal tract. The rest of the neurologic exam is then used to identify the level at which this injury is present. A number of other techniques (Chaddock, Oppenheim, Gordon, Strumpell, Moniz, Gonda-Allen) may be used[52] to elicit the extensor response, but the Babinski is the most reliable.

In patients with decreased or altered mental status, frontal lobe release signs may be tested. These signs reflect diffuse cerebral dysfunction or injury. The grasp reflex involves the patient reflexively gripping the examiner's finger or hand as the palm is brushed. The palmomental reflex is elicited by scratching the thenar eminence and observing for twitching of ipsilateral lower jaw muscles. The snout reflex is elicited by tapping on the mouth and producing puckering of the lips. To elicit the rooting reflex, the mouth is lightly scratched, which causes the patient to turn so as to align the mouth with the finger. The glabellar reflex is elicited by tapping the forehead in the midline (this is done from above the head so as not to confuse the response with the reflex response to visual threat) and observing for repeated blinking each time the forehead above the bridge of the nose is tapped.

Cerebellar Function and Gait Evaluation

Normal coordination requires that both muscle strength and proprioception are intact. The interpretation of the cerebellar exam testing should be done with these systems already evaluated. Abnormal eye movements including dysmetria (overshoots of the target or a series of ratchet-like undershooting movements to reach the target when the eyes are rapidly brought from fixation on one object to another), gaze-evoked or downbeat nystagmus, or speech (slow, impaired prosody, distorted consonants or vowels, mutism) may be the only observable manifestations of cerebellar dysfunction in a patient who is sedated or too weak to cooperate with the remainder of the exam. Truncal ataxia can be detected by sitting the patient up in the bed. If possible, gait should be evaluated and observed for a widened base and the ability to perform rapid turns while maintaining normal balance.

Sensory Examination

Even in the alert patient, this component of the neurologic examination is the least reliable and the first to be discarded if necessary. Of the components of this exam, vibration and joint position sense are the most sensitive. In the sedated patient or patient with a depressed level of consciousness, sensation testing may need to be limited to noting withdrawal or flexion of the stimulated limb or an increase in heart rate. In the cooperative patient, temperature sensation can be evaluated using a tuning fork, which should feel cool. The examiner should be particularly alert to detecting a level at which sensation (pain, temperature, light touch) is lost or diminished in patients with spinal cord injury, TBI (with unrecognized cord injury), or inflammatory (transverse myelitis) or demyelinating disorders of childhood (acute demyelinating encephalomyelitis, multiple sclerosis), which may involve the spinal cord. In patients with cerebral injury, a lack of response to sensory testing should be distinguished from neglect.

Abnormal Movements or Altered Sensorium in the Child With Static Encephalopathy

This is a common issue in the PICU, often because of concern that the patient may be seizing, and may prompt obtaining additional imaging or EEGs because these children have primary neurologic disorders. A stepwise approach is helpful. A limited behavioral repertoire in these patients may mask subtle medical or surgical problems. For a neurologist, this evaluation should also present an opportunity to revisit the diagnosis of cerebral palsy or static encephalopathy, which may be obscuring a diagnosable (and perhaps treatable) disorder such as dopa-responsive dystonia. In such cases, in addition to (often instead of) monitoring for neurologic injury, evaluations should consider other etiologies including pain from unrecognized trauma, hip subluxation, long bone fractures, constipation, urinary infection or retention, volvulus, inguinal hernia, corneal abrasion, otitis media, dental pathology, gastric distention, or bowel adhesions. A systematic approach to evaluation of spells in these patients is essential to avoid missing treatable medical conditions seen in patients with chronic neurologic disorders.

Distinguishing Functional Deficits From Nonorganic Pathology in the Pediatric Intensive Care Unit

Not all neurologic deficits in the PICU are organic. Conversion disorders also occur in critically ill patients or result in patients being admitted to the PICU. In the latter case, this is most often due to a suspicion for nonepileptiform seizures. A number of features of the examination and history may help make this distinction (Table 62.4). In general, and particularly in infants, the eyes are open during a seizure. In one series,[53] over 90% of cases with electrographically confirmed seizures occurred with eye opening. The eyes may look straight ahead, deviate to one side contralateral to the hemisphere from which the seizures originate, or exhibit only nystagmus. Seizures are typically a positive phenomenon and will have movement associated with them unless there has been injury to the corticospinal tracts resulting in a paretic limb. Other features of the exam, or description of the spells including stereotypy, crescendo-decrescendo behavior, or the presence

TABLE 62.4 Clinical Features of Seizures and Nonepileptic Spells

	Seizures	Nonepileptic Spells
Eyes	Open	Closed
Automatisms	Common	Rare
Stereotypical behavior	Common	Rare
Onset is gradual	Rare	Common
Waxing and waning course	Rare	Common
Thrashing movements	Rare	Common

of automatisms, may help to distinguish ictal and nonictal behavior. In most cases, video EEG monitoring is the most definitive means of distinguishing ictal from nonictal events.

Even in the PICU, the examiner should remember that functional deficits may be detectible, and a number of motor signs may help identify the origin of functional symptoms. Given the complex pathophysiology of many critically patients and the multiple potential mechanisms of neurologic injury, the diagnosis of a functional neurologic deficit should be made only after a thorough evaluation for organic causes. Although this is uncommon in the PICU, a functional etiology should not be overlooked, and early identification may minimize diagnostic testing and unnecessary or high-risk treatment. A number of elements of the physical exam may help one to distinguish between organic and functional neurologic deficits.[54] An inconsistent examination may be the first clue, such as that observed in the patient with apparent weakness during bedside strength testing who can change position during sleep or who can walk despite apparent paresis on bedside testing. These observations can help in the assessment of children with weakness thought to be due to a neuromuscular disease. After first observing for inconsistency, the most useful test for functional weakness is the Hoover sign. This test relies on the principle that when flexing one's hip the natural accompanying movement is to extend the contralateral hip.[54] With the patient supine, the examiner places one hand on the weak leg and the other hand under the ankle of the strong leg. The patient is then asked to perform a straight leg raise of the healthy limb. In a functional pattern of weakness, the examiner will feel no downward pressure from the good leg because no effort is being applied to raise the ostensibly weak leg. Other tests include the *arm drop,* in which a paretic or plegic arm is dropped over the patient's face, and a sensory exam that shows exact splitting of sensory or vibration deficits in the midline. A number of functional gait disturbances are also characteristic, including a monoplegic dragging gait (the whole limb is dragged without the circumduction present in pyramidal hemiparesis), a *walking on ice* pattern, excessive slowness, or sudden buckling at the knees with recovery. Of these, none are definitively diagnostic of a functional pathology, and in children in particular they must be interpreted with caution. Importantly, functional and organic deficits may coexist.

Anti–N-methyl-D-aspartate (NMDA) receptor encephalitis is a recently discovered class of disorder that may mimic psychiatric disorders such as depression, catatonia, or viral encephalitis and has important complications including nonconvulsive seizures and autonomic dysfunction requiring ICU care.[55,56] This disorder is one of a family of antibody-associated inflammatory brain diseases in children.[57] Patients may at first appear to have a functional exam before other characteristic features including a movement disorder, sleep disturbance, seizures, and autonomic dysfunction emerge.[58] Early recognition and the initiation of immunosuppression with steroids, IVIG, or plasmapheresis are the keys to improving long-term outcome and reducing complications including cardiac arrhythmia.[59]

Goals of the Neurologic Examination in the Pediatric Intensive Care Unit

At the conclusion of the neurologic examination in the ICU, the examiner should be able to identify the locations of neurologic dysfunction at the very least in terms of injury to gray (encephalopathy, seizures, neglect, aphasia) or white (weakness, spasticity) matter, posterior circulation (brain stem dysfunction, cranial nerve palsy with contralateral weakness), the presence of signs of increased ICP, spinal cord (sensory or motor level), peripheral nerve (decreased or absent reflexes), neuromuscular junction, or muscle injury. This should be established either as the baseline exam or compared to previous examinations and therefore assessed as progressing, improving, or stable. Next, the mechanism producing this injury should be assessed and ranked in order of likelihood. In general, this will involve primary neurologic insult such as TBI, stroke, CNS infection, neurodegenerative disease, autoimmune or parainfectious processes, or the complications of other common pediatric disorders requiring ICU care including sepsis, congenital heart disease, liver failure, organ transplant, diabetic ketoacidosis (DKA), renal disease and dialysis, status epilepticus or iatrogenic complications of commonly used drugs such as immunophilins, or intrathecal chemotherapy.

The goal of the examiner is to combine data from the history, presenting signs, and physical examination (which may need to involve only observing the patient) in order to develop a differential diagnosis for both the site of injury and the mechanism. These mechanisms will involve one or more common etiologies including vascular origins (ischemia, hemorrhage, large or small vessel, arterial or venous, artery-to-artery or cardioembolic); metabolic origins (iatrogenic [often abnormalities of sodium, glucose, or ammonia] or the first presentation of a metabolic disorder); autoimmune origins (CNS lupus, autoimmune encephalopathies and epilepsies); parainfectious origins (ADEM); iatrogenic origins (sedation, neuromuscular blockade, immunophilins); toxic origins (drugs of abuse, drug metabolite accumulation in liver or renal failure); and infectious origins (systemic infection with CNS involvement, meningitis or encephalitis, or reactivation of a latent CNS infection in the immune-suppressed patient).

Based on the postulated location of the insult, stability of the neurologic examination, mechanism of injury, and risk for progression of neurologic injury, the monitoring modalities can then be selected based on the need to establish a diagnosis, monitor for secondary neurologic injury, or both.

Neuroimaging

Computerized tomography (CT) and magnetic resonance imaging (MRI) each have specific advantages (Table 62.5) and should be selected for specific purposes (discussed in Chapter 63). CT can be performed quickly and is a sensitive means of detecting cerebral edema or blood. CT is relatively insensitive to acute ischemic injury and does not provide sufficient resolution in the posterior fossa, where lesions may be missed. Diagnostic CT scans should be performed first without contrast and then with contrast (if not contraindicated). White (dense) lesions on the noncontrast study are either hemorrhage or calcification. In most patients in the PICU, these white areas represent hemorrhage. Contrast enhancement indicates either local breakdown of the blood-brain barrier or excess vascularity and is associated with neoplasms, infections, inflammatory lesions, and subacute stroke.

MRI stimulates tissue with a specific radiofrequency pulse, after which the tissue returns to its preexcited state by processes known as T_1 or T_2 relaxation. In the T_1 sequences, which measure T_1 relaxation, cerebrospinal fluid (CSF) appears dark, and it appears white in the T_2 sequences. Gradient echo (GRE) sequences are most sensitive for detecting hemorrhage on MRI. In these sequences blood appears dark early (4 to 6 hours) after hemorrhage and remains dark in all later stages of hemorrhage. Small infarcts, infections, inflammatory areas, and demyelinating plaques are more readily detected on MRI than on CT. Fluid-attenuated inversion recovery (FLAIR) imaging uses T_2-weighted sequences in which CSF appears dark. For the detection of ischemic conditions, diffusion-weighted images (DWI) are more sensitive than CT scan in the detection of acute cytotoxic edema. This sequence can

TABLE 62.5   Neuroimaging Advantages and Limitations

	Plain CT	MRI	CT Angiogram	MR Angiogram	Conventional Angiogram
Purpose	Detection of edema or blood	Higher anatomic resolution; DWI can detect early ischemic changes	Evaluate large cerebral arteries	Evaluate large cerebral arteries	Gold standard. Obtain if CTA or MRA negative and dissection or vasculitis suspected
Advantage	Fast, widely available	DWI can detect acute ischemia	Better detection of intracranial stenosis and occlusion than MRA	Detects large vessel arteriopathy	Most sensitive to small vessel disease, dissection, vasculitis
Limitations	May not detect acute ischemia; insensitive to posterior fossa lesions	Less available on emergent basis; patient may need sedation	Large radiation dose	Not a measure of flow; not sensitive to small vessel disease	1% risk of complication

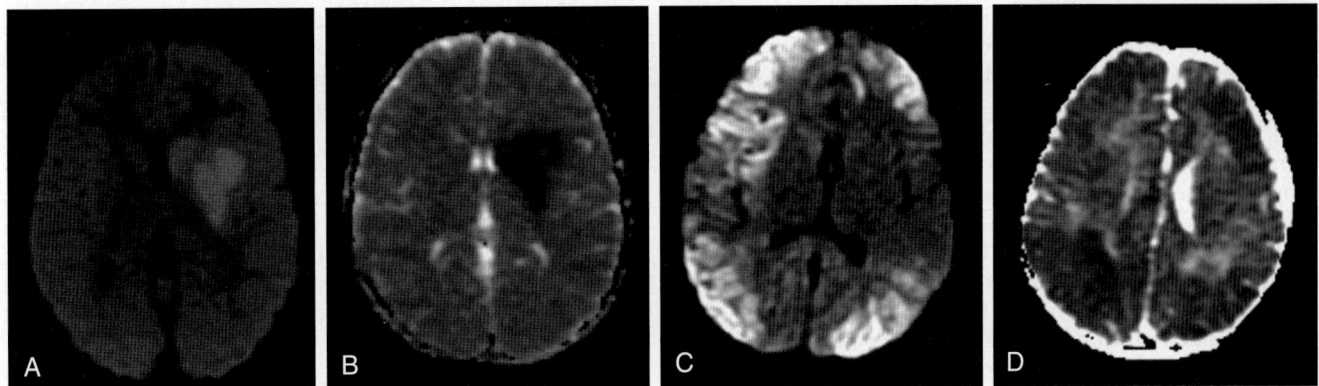

Fig. 62.2. (A) Restricted diffusion manifests as a hyperintense signal in the left caudate, putamen, and globus pallidus in a 5-year-old girl with an acute onset of right-sided weakness due to carotid dissection after a fall. (B) Dark signal on the ADC map supports the mechanism as ischemic in this clinical context. (C) Restricted diffusion in a watershed pattern in a previously healthy 1-year-old child with partial ornithine transcarbamylase deficiency and (D) associated reduced signal in the corresponding ADC map. In this case the mechanism is due to metabolic compromise, not ischemia.

identify acute ischemic strokes as bright lesions within minutes of their occurrence (Fig. 62.2A). Bright lesions on DWI indicate a restriction in the movement of water and thus an increased water content of that region. The degree of water proton mobility is quantified by the apparent diffusion coefficient (ADC). On ADC maps, areas of restricted diffusion appear as hypointense (dark) (Fig. 62.2B). The reason for early decline in ADC is thought to be cytotoxic edema as a result of cellular energy failure causing a loss of ion homeostasis and a subsequent shift of water to the intracellular compartment. Not all restricted diffusion is ischemic in origin (Figs. 62.2C and D) and may instead be associated with inflammation (infection, demyelination) or metabolic derangement as in the case shown, an example of a metabolic stroke due to partial ornithine transcarbamylase deficiency mimicking a watershed stroke. Magnetic resonance angiography (MRA) and magnetic resonance venography (MRV) are used to detect vascular occlusions in large- and medium-size vessels in the head and neck, cerebral aneurysms larger than 5 mm, and arterial dissection (detects the presence of methemoglobin in the false lumen within the vessel wall). If MRA or CT angiography (CTA) is negative and a dissection is suspected, a conventional angiogram should be obtained. Similarly, if small vessel arteriopathy or vasculitis is suspected and MRA or CTA is negative, conventional angiography should also be obtained.

For traumatic diffuse axonal injury (DAI) in particular following TBI, diffusion tensor imaging (DTI) has emerged as a promising means for detecting injury. DAI is thought to be a major contributor to cognitive dysfunction ranging from cognitive difficulty to coma following TBI,[60-63] but it is difficult to diagnose or characterize noninvasively. The cellular mechanisms involved in the long-term sequelae of TBI in children lead to a compromise of neuronal metabolism, perfusion, and axonal function, all components of the neurovascular bundle.[64] Advances in imaging technology using DTI MRI have allowed early detection of axonal injury in patients following TBI and have linked cognitive disability in these patients to white matter signal changes.[62,65-67]

The effect of therapeutic hypothermia on the radiographic evolution of restricted diffusion on DWI in children following cerebral ischemia is not known. In practice, this means that as the use of hypothermia is extended from the asphyxiated

newborn to children with cardiac arrest[68] and TBI, the results of DWI studies may potentially underestimate the degree of ischemia if obtained during or close to treatment with hypothermia. In a retrospective Korean study of adults (lowest age 18 years) with cardiac arrested treated with hypothermia, positive DWI imaging in the first week after arrest was significantly associated with poor outcome (OR, 58.2; 95% CI, 13–255).[69]

As transport of the critically ill child, the increased duration of the scan (compared to CT) and the availability of the scanner are important in the decision to obtain MRI. One approach is to streamline the use of MRI by only obtaining sequences specific to the insult being evaluated. Thus for suspected ischemia, only DWI and ADC sequences are obtained; for hemorrhage, GRE; hydrocephalus, MR of the ventricles; sinus thrombosis, MR venogram; dissection or large vessel vasculitis, MR angiogram; metabolic disease, MR spectroscopy; and for cortical dysplasia in epilepsy patients, standard MRI. This means that a patient admitted with suspected stroke can complete a study (MR ventricles and DWI) in a much shorter time window than is otherwise required and the most important initial question (presence or absence of ischemia) can be addressed so that therapy can be adjusted.

In children in particular, neuroimaging cannot be used as the definitive measure of the presence or absence of intracranial hypertension. Rather, the examiner must rely on a combination of assessment of risk factors and clinical examination (including changes in the examination) combined with imaging findings (which may be unremarkable).

Intracranial Pressure Monitoring

The most common indication for ICP monitoring in critically ill children is TBI (discussed in Chapters 66 and 119), in which the measurement of ICP serves to direct therapy with the goal of preventing the secondary complications of TBI resulting from cerebral hypoperfusion or metabolic stress. For children with severe TBI, a CPP between 40 and 65 mm Hg is recommended,[40] and a CPP of 60 to 70 mm Hg is recommended for adolescents.[70,71] Optimal CPP levels for children under 2 years of age have not been established. The lack of age-specific CPP thresholds for severe TBI was addressed in a study using an online Internet database, TBI-trac containing data from trauma centers in New York State.[72] The investigators measured the survival rates and relative risks of mortality for 317 children with severe TBI based on predefined, age-specific higher and low CPP thresholds (60 and 50 mm Hg for children 12 years old or older, 50 and 35 mm Hg for those 6–11 years, and 40 and 30 mm Hg for those 0–5 years). The results supported age-specific CPP targets above 50 or 60 mm Hg in adults, above 50 mm Hg in 6- to 17-year-olds, and above 40 mm Hg in 0- to 5-year-olds. The authors assumed that the zero points for the ICP and blood pressure transducers were uniform across institutions and that both were set at the level of the foramen of Monro. However, some patients may have had the head of the bed elevated, and this may have led to variability in the calculation of CPP. Because the threshold for increased mortality in this analysis was based on the lowest CPP a patient experienced, comparing these results with the dose of abnormal ICP or CPP as proposed by other investigators is not possible.[30,73]

A multicenter study of 324 patients ages 13 years or older with severe TBI carried out in Bolivia and Ecuador called into question the benefit of monitoring ICP.[74] In this study, patients were randomly assigned to either guidelines-based management using a protocol in which treatment was based on imaging and clinical examination or a protocol for monitoring ICP. There was no significant difference in the primary outcome (a composite measure of functional and cognitive status) or in 6-month mortality between groups; however, non-ICP monitored patients received more ICP-directed therapies than the monitored group. The extent to which these results apply to North American and European practice is uncertain.

The benefits and complications of ICP monitoring are unproven for other conditions in which ICP may be increased (eg, DKA, meningitis, metabolic disorders, ALF, stroke, brain tumors, cardiac arrest, hypoxic-ischemic encephalopathy, drowning). Similarly, data on treatment goals of ICP or CPP specific to each insult are lacking.

In pediatric ALF, neurologic morbidity is a major determinant of outcome[75,76] with compromise of astrocyte metabolism postulated as a pivotal mechanism in the development of cerebral edema associated with hepatic encephalopathy.[77] A single-center retrospective review reported on 14 children with ALF who underwent ICP monitoring of which only one developed a small intracranial hemorrhage,[78] suggesting that invasive ICP monitoring can be performed safely in children with ALF. ICP monitoring is used in approximately 7% of patients with meningitis,[79] and mortality is higher in patients with meningitis and a mean CPP of less than 50 mm Hg.[80] Results of a randomized controlled trial of 110 comatose children with acute CNS infection and raised ICP suggest that a CPP goal is superior to the ICP goal.[81] This study compared a goal CPP of ≥60 mm Hg to a goal ICP of <20 mm Hg,[81,81] and 90-day mortality was significantly lower (18.2%) in the CPP group compared to the ICP group (38.2%; RR = 2.1). This treatment resulted in systolic blood pressures in the 95th percentile for age.

In two children with DKA and cerebral edema, invasive multimodal neuromonitoring, combining ICP and brain tissue oxygen ($PbtO_2$) monitoring, was used to guide therapy.[82] The authors selected a target ICP of ≤20 mm Hg and CPP ≥60 mm Hg, with $PbtO_2$ ≥20 mm Hg. Despite achieving these values for ICP and CPP, there were periods when $PbtO_2$ was below the target value. The study provides a precedent for combining ICP-directed therapy linked to optimizing cerebral metabolism. Whether this approach reduces the neurologic complications of DKA-associated cerebral edema is not known.

In sum, although there is potential for the use of ICP monitoring to direct management of other pediatric CNS injuries beyond severe TBI, there are insufficient data at present to justify its use as a standard of care. Nevertheless, precedent from these and other reports suggests that its use in selected patients may be safe and provide meaningful data to direct care of the injured brain.[83,84]

Electroencephalography Monitoring

The importance of the EEG as a monitoring tool in the PICU derives both from its role in the detection of electrographic seizures and from its potential to identify treatable secondary insults in the critically ill patient. In a full montage, 20 scalp electrodes are placed over the skull to record the electrical activity of the surface of the brain. In general, the EEG is used to detect seizures, electrographic activity alone (nonconvulsive seizures), epileptiform activity, focal slowing, or discharges. Until recently, the use of continuous EEG (cEEG) in pediatric critical care was hampered by a lack of availability, delays in timely interpretation of the EEG tracing, and the absence of data to show that treating seizures in some critically ill populations improves outcome. There is now greater availability of this technology in many PICUs,[13,85] in recognition of both the incidence of seizures[86,87] and data showing the impact[88-90] seizures can have on the long-term outcome from critical illness in children.[88-91]

Consensus criteria for the use of EEG in the ICU have been established.[92,93] cEEG is indicated for the detection of NCS (eg, in the patient not awakening after status epilepticus or the paralyzed sedated patient), for the detection of ischemia in patients at high risk for cerebral ischemia, for the assessment of level of consciousness in sedated or comatose patients, and for prognostication in patients after cardiac arrest.[92,93]

Data in support of these recommendations are robust. NCSs occur in up to 23% of children supported with extracorporeal membrane oxygenation (ECMO)[94] and 8% of neonates after cardiac surgery with cardiopulmonary bypass.[86] NCSs occur in approximately one-third of children with structural brain injuries, prior in-hospital convulsive seizures, or interictal EEG abnormalities.[95] In children with acute encephalopathy, NCSs occurred in 36% to 46%.[90,96] The increasing use of cEEG in pediatric neurotrauma has identified the burden of NCS after TBI. In a prospective study of 87 children with mild to severe TBI, 43% had early post-traumatic seizures (PTS),[97] among which 16% were electrographic only.[97]

For ICU neurology, the EEG cannot be used to determine the etiology of abnormal patterns, discharges, or seizures. Seizures may be the presenting symptom of new ischemic (venous or arterial) or hemorrhagic injury in the critically ill patient. In the PICU, the detection of electrographic or clinical seizures should prompt investigation of common causes such as metabolic derangement, drug reaction, vascular injury, or infection. Often, a change in EEG pattern (loss of complexity, slowing, new epileptiform discharges) in the absence of seizures may also reflect new neurologic insult. The import of these changes can only be interpreted in the context of each patient's risk factors for neurologic injury. Importantly,

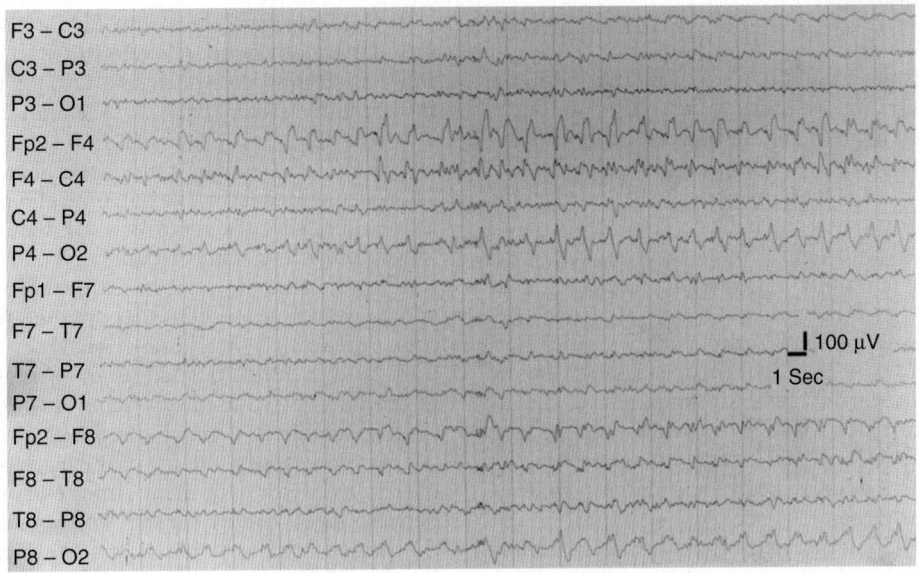

F3 – C3
C3 – P3
P3 – O1
Fp2 – F4
F4 – C4
C4 – P4
P4 – O2
Fp1 – F7
F7 – T7
T7 – P7
P7 – O1
Fp2 – F8
F8 – T8
T8 – P8
P8 – O2

100 μV
1 Sec

Fig. 62.3. Bipolar EEG montage of an 11-year-old girl 4 weeks following umbilical cord transplant for acute myelocytic leukemia. Note the electrographic seizures at F4 and F8. This patient had limbic encephalitis due to reactivation of latent HHV6 infection. The only clinical manifestations of nonconvulsive seizures in this patient were loss of short-term memory and decreased sleep.

routine EEG recording fails to detect NCS in approximately 50% of critically ill patients whose NCSs were detected with cEEG monitoring.[98,99] In patients in which NCSs are suspected, cEEG monitoring for at least 12 hours is required to detect an NCS.[8,99,100] An example of NCS epilepticus is shown in Fig. 62.3 in a patient with limbic encephalitis following cord blood transplant, whose only neurologic deficits were decreased sleep and loss of short-term memory.

Before cEEG monitoring becomes a standard of care in selected critically ill children, studies are needed to show that treatment of NCS improves outcome. Here, too, evidence in support of treatment is accumulating. In a study of 259 patients with a variety of neurologic insults admitted to the PICU and cardiac ICU, these patients underwent cEEG monitoring.[90] Seizure burden was defined as the maximum percentage of any given hour occupied by electrographic seizures. The maximum total seizure burden was much greater in patients with neurologic decline (15.7% per hour) than in patients without such alterations (1.8%). The odds of neurologic decline increased by 1.13 (95% CI = 1.05–1.21; p <0.0016) for every 1% increase in maximum hourly seizure burden. In a study of 300 children with an acute neurologic disorder (137 of whom were neurodevelopmentally normal) who underwent clinically indicated cEEG in the PICU, electrographic seizures and status epilepticus were associated with worse adaptive behavior after discharge than that observed in the previously healthy children.[88] Collectively, these studies suggest that seizures in critically ill children are associated with neurologic decline and may be a therapeutic target.

Transcranial Doppler Measurement of Cerebral Blood Flow

TCD is a noninvasive test that uses ultrasonography to measure the cerebral blood flow velocity (CBFV) in the anterior and posterior circulation. Normal values are described for healthy neonatal, pediatric, and adult populations,[101,102] measured by TCD; CBFV is lower in sedated critically ill children compared to age-matched healthy children.[23]

TCD has been used in adult and pediatric TBI[103-105] neonatal hypoxic-ischemic encephalopathy (HIE),[105] sickle cell disease,[106] and stroke[107] to assess autoregulation, predict mortality, and provide a target for goal-directed therapy. Elevated TCD velocities during pediatric ECMO may occur prior to neurologic injury including intracranial hemorrhage, increased ICP, or ischemia.[108] Vasospasm as measured by TCDs is common in children with moderate and severe TBI.[16] In this study of 69 children, vasospasm (velocities were compared to age- and gender-matched reference values in healthy children) occurred in 21% of those with severe and 8.5% of those with moderate TBI. In children with DKA studied with serial TCDs, autoregulation was compromised in 17% of 32 cases up to 72 hours after the initiation of treatment with insulin.[109] The effect of vasospasm on outcome and the optimal treatment for this complication is not known.

Near Infrared Spectroscopy

Near infrared spectroscopy (NIRS) measures tissue oxygen saturation by determining the difference in intensity between transmitted and received light delivered at specific wavelengths.[110] Commercial cerebral NIRS products measure oxygenation by using light with wavelengths of between 700 and 1000 nm to measure the transparency of tissue to light. Because hemoglobin absorbs NIRS light depending on its oxygenation state, changes in hemoglobin oxygenation can be quantified using the modified Lambert-Beer law. In theory therefore, NIRS may serve as a noninvasive method for detecting cerebral or somatic hypoxia. In practice, the reliability of cerebral NIRS was questioned[111] in a study showing that in infants up to 190 days old, cerebral NIRS values were not reproducible. In adult human cadavers, the cerebral tissue oxygenation measured by NIRS in a third of these subjects was higher than the lowest value of normal controls.[112]

As is the case for many of the technologies reviewed here, the adoption of NIRS as a standard of care has been limited by the retrospective design of many of these single-center studies and the lack of evidence to show that targeting specific NIRS values improves organ function or outcome.[113] Despite this observation, results from studies in children with corrected congenital heart disease suggest that NIRS can detect perioperative cerebral hypoxia and that this reduction is associated with an increased risk for compromise of neurodevelopmental outcome.[114] In a study of postoperative congenital heart disease patients, cerebral and flank regional oxygen saturation were correlated with central venous oxygen saturation in both cyanotic or acyanotic patients and single- or two-ventricle physiology.[115] Change in $PaCO_2$ was associated with a change in cerebral but not flank regional oxygen saturation, suggesting that cerebral NIRS is detecting changes in cerebral oxygenation. A reduction in cerebral oxygen uptake during deep hypothermic cardiac arrest may not be associated with white matter injury, however.[116] NIRS may emerge an effective tool for mitigating perioperative neurologic injury in children with congenital heart disease.[117]

The validity of NIRS in other neurologic insults in children is also not established. A higher regional oxygen saturation may be associated with a greater chance of achieving a return of spontaneous circulation in adults with in-hospital or out-of-hospital cardiac arrest,[118] but such data in children are lacking. In a single-center observational study of infants with cerebral circulatory arrest, cerebral NIRS was significantly reduced in the patients with arrest compared to those with preserved cerebral perfusion.[119] However, the specificity of this difference was low.[118] In a pilot study of 28 children, NIRS was used in combination with head CT to detect the presence of intracerebral hemorrhage (ICH). NIRS (using a difference in optical density of >0.2 between hemispheres or scalp locations) correctly identified all 12 ICH cases.[120] An exciting development in the use of NIRS involves the autocorrelation of cerebral NIRS and mean arterial pressure as a noninvasive measurement of cerebral blood flow autoregulation.[121] A feasibility study of 36 children used autocorrelation of cerebral NIRS and mean arterial pressure (MAP) to identify the optimal MAP for preservation of cerebrovascular reactivity after cardiac arrest.[122] The cumulative evidence suggests that when monitoring for neurologic complications in both postcardiac surgery patients[123,124] and other acute neurologic insults in children, NIRS may contribute to ICU management.

Brain Tissue Oxygen Monitoring

The Neurotrend system, using a colorimetric method with optical fluorescence, measures three variables: O_2, pH, and CO_2; however, it is rarely used in clinical practice in the United States. The Licox system (Integra Neurosciences; Plainsboro, New Jersey) uses a Clark-type electrode and measures both $PbtO_2$ and temperature. The indications for placing the $PbtO_2$ monitor are the same as those for patients requiring ICP monitoring following TBI. Typically, the probe is placed in the white matter of the brain, because it is more metabolically stable than the gray matter. If the region of injury is to be monitored, the catheter is placed adjacent to, but not in, the region of contusion or clot, the insult, or in the ischemic penumbra. A retrospective analysis of 150 evaluable patients with severe TBI found that brain hypoxia ($PbtO_2 <10$ mm Hg) was associated with worse outcome and mortality.[125] There is debate as to whether the $PbtO_2$ monitor is estimating oxygen extraction or CBF.[126-128]

In children, experience with $PbtO_2$ monitoring is increasing, particularly with severe TBI.[20,129,130] In a single-center study of 46 children with severe TBI, the probe was placed in the uninjured frontal cortex.[82] The authors found some cases in which $PbtO_2$ was preserved in the goal range but outcome was poor. CPP was the only factor that was independently associated with a favorable outcome at 6 months. Other pediatric studies have also reported a complex interaction between $PbtO_2$ and other clinical parameters.[131,132] In each of these studies, the analyses were based on hourly values for $PbtO_2$ and daily averages for $PbtO_2$ as opposed to episodes of $PbtO_2$ below predefined thresholds,[129] making comparisons among these studies difficult. Small series at single centers have suggested that $PbtO_2$ monitoring may augment the detection of CNS metabolic crises in children with stroke[133] and DKA.[82]

Differences in the site for probe placement and the thresholds selected for treatment limit meaningful comparisons between these studies. Further, $PbtO_2$ values may reflect both the presence of ischemia and other factors such as PaO_2. Further, $PbtO_2$ measures local tissue conditions and would fail to detect hypoxic-ischemic insults in remote brain regions. The promise of this technology for pediatric neuromonitoring is considerable but a number of caveats remain. For example, the threshold (10–15 mm Hg) for poor outcome is based on mostly adult data, and the dose-dependence of an exposure to cerebral hypoxia and the disease specificity for insults other than TBI remain to be determined.

Optic Nerve Sheath Diameter Measurement

Most of the experience with this technology is also in adults.[134,135] When ICP increases due to expansion of the subarachnoid space, this causes distention of the membrane of the optic nerve sheath, which is contiguous with the dura, and the maximal point of distention can be measured by ultrasound. Transorbital sonographic measurement of the optic nerve sheath diameter (ONSD) has been proposed as a noninvasive means to detect increased ICP in children.[136] A study of 103 healthy volunteers of whom 13% were younger than 16 years found a median ONSD of 4.41 (range 4.24–4.83) mm.[137] Results of studies using ONSD to detect increased ICP in children are equivocal. There was no significant difference of ONSD between children who had ventriculoperitoneal shunt failure (4.5±0.9 mm) and those who did not (5±0.6).[138] Overall, the pediatric data suggest that an ONSD above 4.75 mm may be abnormal, but data are lacking on the correlation with ICP measured by invasive methods and the timing of the increase and recovery of abnormal values related to the initial insult.

Tympanometry

Like ONSD measurement, tympanometry has been proposed as a noninvasive measure of ICP, and it has been subject to the same critiques of lack of accuracy and lack of availability for continuous monitoring.[139] The largest studies have been carried out in Africa in children with acute, nontraumatic coma and excluded children with epilepsy, neurodevelopmental delay, and sickle cell disease.[140,141] Children were more likely to die if tympanometry was abnormal (adjusted odds ratio: 17; 95% confidence interval: 1.9–152.4; p = .01). The majority of the cases (53%) were caused by cerebral malaria and the remainder caused by bacterial meningitis, sepsis, or had no identifiable cause (30%). This technology needs further evaluation in studies that incorporate physiologic monitoring and brain imaging to validate this measurement. Nevertheless, the ease of use and potential in resource-poor countries justify further evaluation.

Cerebral Microdialysis

Cerebral microdialysis uses the capillary technique to measure the concentration of key metabolites (glucose, pyruvate, lactate), excitotoxic amino acids (glutamate and aspartate), and membrane breakdown products (glycerol) in the brain parenchyma in order to detect the evolution of primary and the development of secondary injury.[142] The microdialysis catheter is a fine tube, placed via a burr hole, within a semi-permeable dialysis membrane that permits diffusion of molecules from the extracellular space along the catheter and into a vial. This vial is then placed in the microdialysis analyzer. In general, the catheter is placed via the same burr hole as the PbtO$_2$ and ICP monitors into the normal brain or penumbra of the injured brain. The most common system is the CMA600 microdialysis analyzer (CMA Microdialysis, Stockholm, Sweden). As with PbtO$_2$ monitoring, results will vary depending on the placement of the probe in healthy tissue, tissue adjacent to the primary site of injury (penumbra), or in the injured tissue.[143] A number of adult studies have shown, in TBI and SAH cases, an association between metabolic stress (lactate:pyruvate ratio >40) and poor outcome.[18] In a retrospective analysis of 20 adult patients with severe brain injury, tight systemic glucose control was associated with reduced cerebral glucose and with corresponding evidence (increased lactate/pyruvate ratio) of compromised brain metabolism.[144]

Data from adult studies have supported the use of cerebral microdialysis, primarily for the management of TBI and SAH, and have converged on specific values for each component of brain chemistry. Glucose, lactate, and the lactate/pyruvate ratio appear more useful than glycerol and glutamate. The 2004 consensus statement[143] on its use in neurocritical care was updated in 2015.[145] This expert opinion contains no recommendations about its use in children, and there are no recently published data to assess its risks and utility in the practice of pediatric neurocritical care.

Integrating Neurologic Monitoring Data

The growth in tools for invasive and noninvasive neuromonitoring in the ICU forces the issue of how to collect, integrate, and interpret these data.[146,147] It is clear that the use of physiologic thresholds to define good or bad values is oversimplified for pediatric neurocritical care in particular, based on limited data with no well-established age-dependent parameters.[148] This approach tends to interpret one variable in isolation from others and relies on the skill and experience of the clinician interpreting the data. Further, the volume of data generated on a minute-to-minute basis in the PICU places demands on the network used for storage of these data. The goal of plug-and-play mode for all devices (monitors, infusion pumps, ventilators) that generate potentially clinically important data has not yet been achieved in the PICU. Indeed, these devices typically do not have a common source for recording time, rendering the interpretation of the timing of treatment, changes in ventilator parameters, laboratory results, or physiology open to question even if the obstacles to acquiring these data have been overcome. One approach may be to limit the

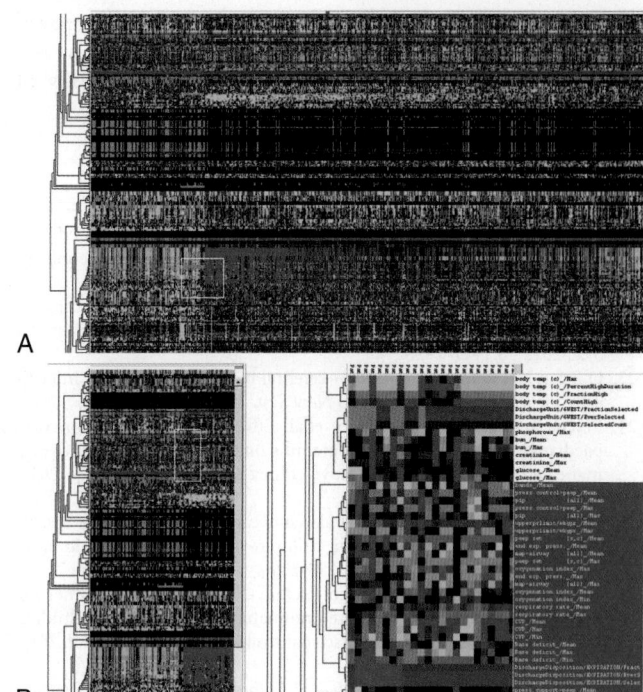

Fig. 62.4. (A) Master view of heat map analysis of all PICU patients over a 5-year period, older than 1 year, who required mechanical ventilation. The differences between survivors *(left)* and nonsurvivors *(right)* can easily be seen. This analysis incorporated thousands of variables ranging from census tract data to laboratory results and ventilator settings. (B) View of a selected cluster of variables highlighting those associated with differences in outcome after ventilation. This approach is proof of the principle of the potential of data mining in the ICU to discover novel relationships and generate hypotheses.

acquisition of data only to those variables best validated for outcomes in TBI. This approach will likely miss unanticipated relationships, which may emerge only using an unbiased non–hypothesis-driven analysis of multiple variables. An example of this approach from a retrospective analysis of PICU data is shown in Fig. 62.4. Using a cluster analysis of all patients older than 1 year who required mechanical ventilation, the differences between survivors and nonsurvivors can easily be seen. This analysis incorporated thousands of variables ranging from census tract data to laboratory results and ventilator settings, and it demonstrates the potential of the application of these tools to the array of data generated in the PICU. Therefore to make use of the data generated by neuromonitoring, to interpret these data in relation to other physiologic and laboratory variables, and to develop new methods of analyses beyond thresholds and values at single time points rather than trends over time, it will be necessary to establish real-time data collection from all devices attached to the PICU patient, link these data (including waveforms) to laboratory and socioeconomic data, direct the flow of this information to new analysis tools, validate the data returning to the bedside, and iteratively develop and test predictive tools for the recognition of new or evolving cerebral injury. Substantial progress has been made in this area in adult neurocritical care[149,150] and in the development of automated algorithms for the detection of septic shock.[151] Thus progress in the application of neuromonitoring for the management of children with brain injury is fundamentally linked to the development of improved (better integrated, higher granularity) data collection and tools for bedside analysis using the emerging methods of bioinformatics.

Key References

7. Abend N, Arndt D, Carpenter J, et al. Electrographic seizures in pediatric ICU patients: cohort study of risk factors and mortality. *Neurology.* 2013;81:383-391.

20. Padayachy LC, Rohlwink U, Zwane E, et al. The frequency of cerebral ischemia/hypoxia in pediatric severe traumatic brain injury. *Childs Nerv Syst.* 2012;28:1911-1918.

23. O'Brien NF. Reference values for cerebral blood flow velocities in critically ill, sedated children. *Childs Nerv Syst.* 2015;31:2269-2276.

24. Pineda J, Leonard J, Mazotas I, et al. Effect of implementation of a paediatric neurocritical care programme on outcomes after severe traumatic brain injury: a retrospective cohort study. *Lancet Neurol.* 2013; 12:45-52.

25. Vavilala M, Kernic M, Wang J, et al. Acute care clinical indicators associated with discharge outcomes in children with severe traumatic brain injury. *Crit Care Med.* 2014;42:2258-2266.

26. Adelson PD, Wisniewski SR, Beca J, et al. Comparison of hypothermia and normothermia after severe traumatic brain injury in children (Cool Kids): a phase 3, randomised controlled trial. *Lancet Neurol.* 2013; 12:546-553.

27. Hutchinson J, Ward R, Lacroix J, et al. Hypothermia therapy after traumatic brain injury in children (for the Hypothermia Pediatric Head Injury Trial Investigators and then Canadian Critical Care Trials Group). *N Engl J Med.* 2008;358:2447-2456.

28. Moler FW, Silverstein FS, Holubkov R, et al. Therapeutic hypothermia after out-of-hospital cardiac arrest in children. *N Engl J Med.* 2015;372: 1898-1908.

33. Bratton S, Chesnut R, Ghajar J, et al. Cerebral perfusion thresholds. *J Neurotrauma.* 2007;24:S59-S64.

39. Chambers I, Stobbart L, Jones P, et al. Age-related differences in intracranial pressure and cerebral perfusion pressure in the first 6 hours of monitoring after children's head injury: association with outcome. *Childs Nerv Syst.* 2005;21:195-199.

43. Elbers J, Wainwright MS, Amlie-Lefond C. The pediatric stroke code: early management of the child with stroke. *J Pediatr.* 2015;167:19-24.

48. Banwell BL, Mildner RJ, Hassall AC, et al. Muscle weakness in critically ill children. *Neurology.* 2003;61:1779-1782.

50. Korinthenberg R, Schessl J, Kirschner J, Schulte J. Intravenously administered immunoglobulin in the treatment of childhood Guillain-Barre syndrome: a randomized trial. *Pediatrics.* 2005;116:8-14.

55. Titulaer MJ, McCracken L, Gabilondo I, et al. Treatment and prognostic factors for long-term outcome in patients with anti-NMDA receptor encephalitis: an observational cohort study. *Lancet Neurol.* 2013;12: 157-165.

61. Veeramuthu V, Narayanan V, Kuo TL, et al. Diffusion tensor imaging parameters in mild traumatic brain injury and its correlation with early neuropsychological impairment: a longitudinal study. *J Neurotrauma.* 2015;32:1497-1509.

64. Bartnik-Olson BL, Holshouser B, Wang H, et al. Impaired neurovascular unit function contributes to persistent symptoms after concussion: a pilot study. *J Neurotrauma.* 2014;31:1497-1506.

70. Kochanek P, Carney N, Adelson P, et al. Guidelines for the acute medical management of severe traumatic brain injury in infants, children, and adolescents-second addition. *Pediatr Crit Care Med.* 2012;13(suppl 1): S1-S82.

72. Allen B, Chiu Y, Gerber L, et al. Age-specific cerebral perfusion pressure thresholds and survival in children and adolescents with severe traumatic brain injury. *Pediatr Crit Care Med.* 2014;15:62-70.

74. Chesnut R, Temkin N, Carney N, et al. A trial of intracranial-pressure monitoring in traumatic brain injury. *N Engl J Med.* 2012;367: 2471-2481.

77. Butterworth RF. Pathogenesis of hepatic encephalopathy and brain edema in acute liver failure. *J Clin Exp Hepatol.* 2015;5:S96-S103.

78. Kamat P, Kunde S, Vos M, et al. Invasive intracranial pressure monitoring is a useful adjunct in the management of severe hepatic encephalopathy associated with pediatric acute liver failure. *Pediatr Crit Care Med.* 2012;13:e33-e38.

81. Kumar R, Singhi S, Singhi P, et al. Randomized controlled trial comparing cerebral perfusion pressure-targeted therapy versus intracranial pressure-targeted therapy for raised intracranial pressure due to acute CNS infections in children. *Crit Care Med.* 2014;42:1775-1787.

82. O'Brien NF, Mella C. Brain tissue oxygenation-guided management of diabetic ketoacidosis induced cerebral edema. *Pediatr Crit Care Med.* 2012;13:e383-e388.

86. Naim MY, Gaynor JW, Chen J, et al. Subclinical seizures identified by postoperative electroencephalographic monitoring are common after neonatal cardiac surgery. *J Thorac Cardiovasc Surg.* 2015;150:169-178, discussion 178-180.

90. Payne ET, Zhao XY, Frndova H, et al. Seizure burden is independently associated with short term outcome in critically ill children. *Brain.* 2014;137:1429-1438.

94. Piantino J, Wainwright M, Grimason M, et al. Nonconvulsive seizures are common in children treated with extracorporeal cardiac life support. *Pediatr Crit Care Med.* 2013;14:601-609.

96. Abend N, Gutierrez-Colina A, Topjian A, et al. Nonconvulsive seizures are common in critically ill children. *Neurology.* 2011;76:1071-1077.

97. Arndt D, Lerner J, Matsumoto J, et al. Subclinical early posttraumatic seizures detected by continuous EEG monitoring in a consecutive pediatric cohort. *Epilepsia.* 2013;54:1780-1788.

101. Vavilala M, Kincaid M, Muangman S, et al. Gender differences in cerebral blood flow velocity and autoregulation between the anterior and posterior circulations in healthy children. *Pediatr Res.* 2005;58: 574-578.

102. Verlhac S. Transcranial Doppler in children. *Pediatr Radiol.* 2011;41(suppl 10):S153-S165.

106. Adams R, McKie V, Hsu L, et al. Prevention of a first stroke by transfusion in children with sickle cell anemia and abnormal results on transcranial Doppler ultrasonography. *N Engl J Med.* 1998;338:5-11.

107. Aries MJ, Elting JW, De Keyser J, et al. Cerebral autoregulation in stroke: a review of transcranial Doppler studies. *Stroke.* 2010;41:2697-2704.

108. O'Brien N, Hall M. Extracorporeal membrane oxygenation and cerebral blood flow velocity in children. *Pediatr Crit Care Med.* 2013;14: e126-e134.

109. Ma L, Roberts J, Pihoker C, et al. Transcranial Doppler-based assessment of cerebral autoregulation in critically ill children during diabetic ketoacidosis treatment. *Pediatr Crit Care Med.* 2014;15:742-749.

115. McQuillen P, Nishimoto M, Bottrell C, et al. Regional and central venous oxygen saturation monitoring following pediatric cardiac surgery: concordance and association with clinical variables. *Pediatr Crit Care Med.* 2007;8:154-160.

119. Blohm ME, Obrecht D, Hartwich J, Singer D. Effect of cerebral circulatory arrest on cerebral near-infrared spectroscopy in pediatric patients. *Paediatr Anaesth.* 2014;24:393-399.

122. Lee JK, Brady KM, Chung SE, et al. A pilot study of cerebrovascular reactivity autoregulation after pediatric cardiac arrest. *Resuscitation.* 2014;85:1387-1393.

130. Stippler M, Ortiz V, Adelson PD, et al. Brain tissue oxygen monitoring after severe traumatic brain injury in children: relationship to outcome and association with other clinical parameters. *J Neurosurg Pediatr.* 2012;10:383-391.

132. Figaji AA, Zwane E, Fieggen AG, et al. Pressure autoregulation, intracranial pressure, and brain tissue oxygenation in children with severe traumatic brain injury. *J Neurosurg Pediatr.* 2009;4:420-428.

135. Dubourg J, Javouhey E, Geeraerts T, et al. Ultrasonography of optic nerve sheath diameter for detection of raised intracranial pressure: a systematic review and meta-analysis. *Intensive Care Med.* 2011;37: 1059-1068.

140. Gwer S, Chengo E, Newton C, Kirkham F. Unexpected relationship between tympanometry and mortality in children with nontraumatic coma. *Pediatrics.* 2013;132:713-717.

144. Oddo M, Schmidt J, Carrera E, et al. Impact of tight glycemic control on cerebral glucose metabolism after severe brain injury: a microdialysis study. *Crit Care Med.* 2008;36:3233-3238.

145. Hutchinson PJ, Jalloh I, Helmy A, et al. Consensus statement from the 2014 International Microdialysis Forum. *Intensive Care Med.* 2015;41: 1517-1528.

149. Cohen M, Grossman A, Morabito D, et al. Identification of complex metabolic states in critically injured patients using bioinformatic cluster analysis. *Crit Care.* 2010;14:R10.

150. Hemphill JC, Andrews P, De Georgia M. Multimodal monitoring and neurocritical care bioinformatics. *Nat Rev Neurol.* 2011;7:451-460.

Neuroimaging

Gisele E. Ishak and Dennis W.W. Shaw

PEARLS

- Multiple imaging modalities are available for evaluation of the brain, head, neck, and spine of the critically ill child. The most appropriate modality depends on consideration of patient pretest probability for the clinically suspected diagnosis, the modality sensitivity, and the patient's age and condition.
- When ordering radiographic studies, particularly computed tomography scans, the physician should keep the radiation burden in mind, especially for infants. When ordering magnetic resonance imaging for young children, one must keep in mind the risk related to sedation and general anesthesia.
- The ever-increasing complexity of imaging modalities and medical problems in the intensive care unit warrants liberal consultation with radiology colleagues to yield an appropriately tailored imaging protocol and a more relevant interpretation.
- In the pediatric population and especially in critically ill patients, noninvasive imaging modalities that are likely to answer the clinical question should carefully be considered as an alternative to a catheter angiogram, which though minimally invasive has a small but nonzero risk of procedure-related complications.

Imaging Modality Overview

Multiple imaging modalities are available to investigate the neurologic status of children in the intensive care unit (ICU). Selection of the most appropriate examination requires weighing factors of modality sensitivity against the suspected pathology, having a degree of suspicion for a particular pathology, and considering the practicalities afforded by the complexity of the examination and the child's condition. This chapter reviews available imaging modalities and the disease processes most likely to be subject to neuroimaging evaluation.

Ultrasound (see also Chapter 20)

Standard cranial ultrasound has been a mainstay in the neonatal ICU. Ultrasound generates grayscale digital images from components of an ultrasound beam reflected off tissue interfaces with no ionizing radiation and with the added advantage that bedside imaging can be performed. However, cranial ultrasound has a restricted window through which to visualize the brain, primarily through an open anterior fontanelle, and therefore it is limited for the most part to the first few months of life. Ultrasound is sensitive to some intracranial pathology, including the detection of germinal matrix hemorrhage, evaluation of ventricular size, and evaluation of severe white matter lesions in premature infants, including cystic periventricular leukomalacia (PVL). It is less sensitive for pathologies such as mild to moderate parenchymal ischemic changes, subarachnoid and punctate parenchymal hemorrhage, dural venous sinus thrombosis, and subtle cerebral malformations. Extraaxial collections, especially those along the lateral cerebral convexities, also can be difficult to appreciate on ultrasound performed through a midline fontanelle.

Color Doppler with the standard ultrasound machine uses the shift in frequency associated with reflection of the sound beam off a moving interface (the "Doppler shift" phenomenon) to detect motion in the image field, most commonly from blood in vessels. Those pixels with movement are assigned a color to distinguish them from pixels without movement. The color assigned (most often red and blue) is different depending on whether movement is away from or toward the transducer, and the color assigned is arbitrary so that arteries and veins are not necessarily red and blue, respectively. Color Doppler allows for some investigation of the cerebral circulation, primarily through the open fontanelle. Transcranial Doppler (TCD) uses the same Doppler shift to produce waveforms that give information about flow velocity and direction. An advantage of TCD is that it can be performed through the thinner portions of the skull, primarily the temporal squamosa, in older children and adults (Fig. 63.1). TCD has been used in the evaluation of cerebral perfusion in patients with sickle cell disease[1] and vasospasm secondary to subarachnoid hemorrhage (SAH).[2] TCD is generally sensitive to vessel stenosis greater than 50% in the central cerebral circulation, with the highest sensitivity and specificity being in the middle cerebral artery (MCA).[3,4]

Computerized Tomography

Computerized tomographic (CT) scanning has higher sensitivity compared with ultrasound for many intracranial pathologies, including most neurosurgical emergencies, and is not limited by closing and closed fontanelles. Imaging on modern scanners with multiarray detectors can be performed rapidly. CT, however, requires transporting the patient from the ICU (although some portable units are available) and uses ionizing radiation (x-rays) to produce digital computer-reconstructed images based on differences in tissue density (which affects x-ray attenuation). The choice of radiation parameters, slice thickness, postprocessing, and image viewing (window width

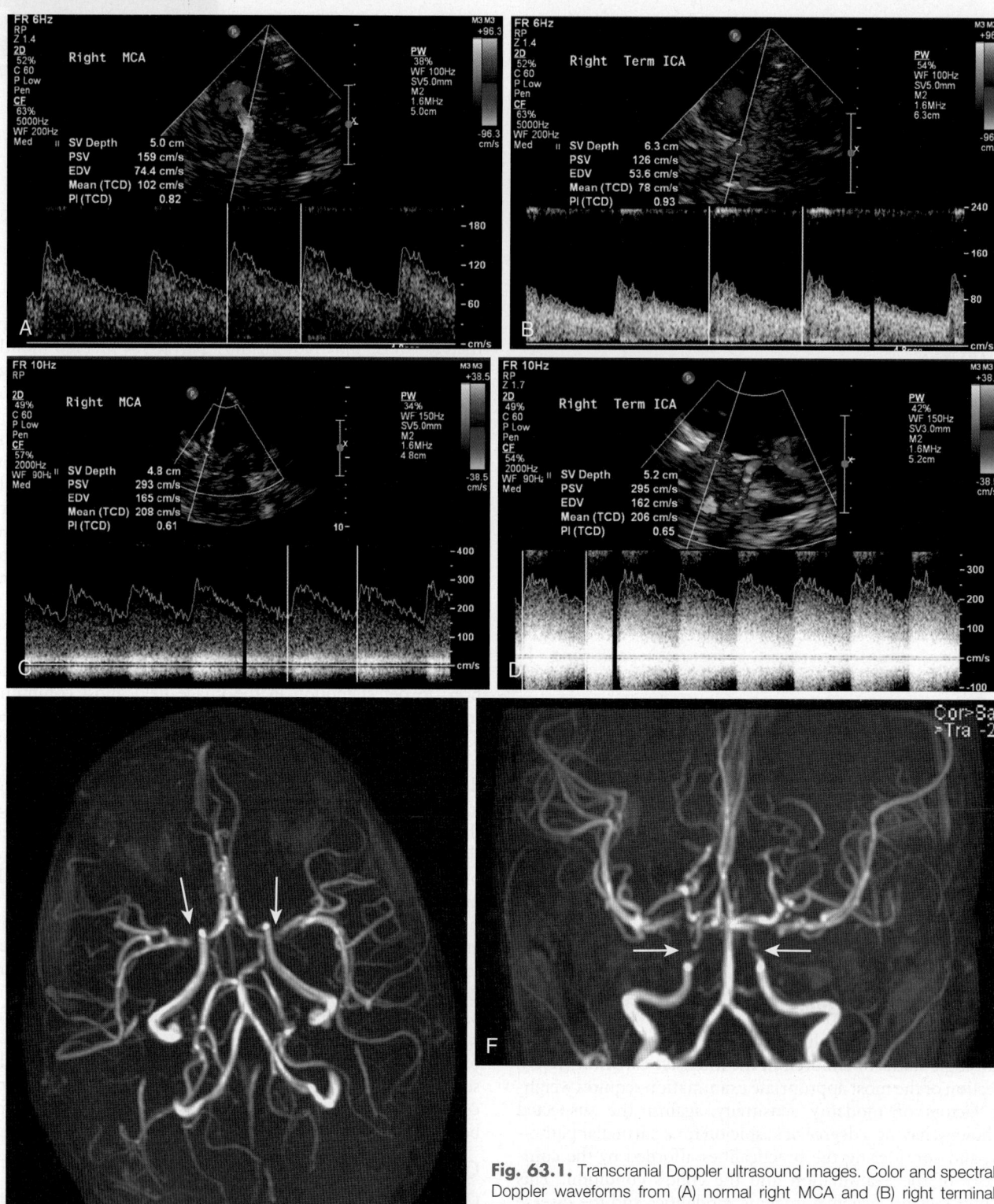

Fig. 63.1. Transcranial Doppler ultrasound images. Color and spectral Doppler waveforms from (A) normal right MCA and (B) right terminal internal carotid artery (ICA). Abnormal right middle cerebral (C) and terminal internal carotid (D) waveforms in another patient with sickle cell disease and prior history of stroke. MR angiographic images (E and F) of this patient with abnormal Transcranial Doppler demonstrate narrowed proximal MCAs and terminal ICA.

and level) must be tailored to the particular clinical question to optimize the images. Newer scanners employing postprocessing algorithms utilizing iterative reconstruction harnessing greater computational power have allowed for decrease in the radiation dose required for any particular degree of image quality. Bone and other calcifications have the highest density, and in decreasing density are (nonadipose) soft tissue (such as the brain), water (eg, cerebrospinal fluid [CSF]), fat, and then air. The difference in density between bone and brain is great, whereas the difference between brain and fat is less. The density difference between gray and white matter is much smaller but is sufficient to be appreciated with the appropriate window and level. Generally, as edema develops in nonfatty tissue, there is a decrease in density. Acute blood (approximately between 12 and 72 hours old) is of higher density than brain, and CT is sensitive in the detection of acute (generally less than 1 week to 10 days old) parenchymal and SAH. CT is also useful in the evaluation of ventricular size, extraaxial collections, and to rule out cerebral herniation in the acute setting, as seen with space-occupying mass and diffuse cerebral edema.

Iodinated intravenous (IV) contrast can be used with CT to evaluate the integrity of the blood-brain barrier (BBB) and differences in tissue perfusion. With injection of IV contrast, vessels demonstrate a transient increase in density, with a variable rate of contrast leak into the tissues, depending on the local pathophysiology. The rate of equilibration of contrast concentration between vessels and parenchyma is much slower in the brain because of the intact BBB. Contrast then is especially useful in the brain, where disruption of the normal BBB can reveal underlying pathology. This increased density from contrast material is also used to image arteries and venous structures with CT angiography (CTA) and CT venography (CTV), respectively. With the appropriate software, postprocessing of the data can produce three-dimensional (3D) images of the vessels.

Magnetic Resonance Imaging

Magnetic resonance imaging (MRI) utilizes a high-field-strength magnet in combination with radiofrequency pulses to produce images based on the nuclear resonance of hydrogen protons in tissue, primarily in water and fat. MRI provides the most sensitive measure of most (but not all) central nervous system (CNS) pathologies, and unlike CT, imaging can be acquired in any plane (although state-of-the-art multidetector CT scanners can acquire volumetric data that can be reformatted in any plane). Imaging, however, requires patient transport to the scanner; increased examination complexity and potential safety concerns are primarily related to the high-field-strength magnet (typically 1.5 or 3.0 Tesla) and generally longer imaging sequences (1 to 10 minutes). MRI provides the greatest tissue characterization, facilitated by several sequences obtained in a complete study. MRI is particularly useful in the evaluation of the posterior fossa (brain stem and cerebellum) and spinal cord, where "beam-hardening" due to bone results in considerable artifact on CT, although this problem has become less of an issue with modern multidetector CT scanners.

Safety associated with MR scanning is an important issue. MRI-compatible monitoring and life support systems must be used. Patients need to be screened for any internal hardware or implants that would preclude scanning, such as MRI-incompatible aneurysm clips. Electronic devices such

as pacemakers are rendered dysfunctional by the changing magnetic field occurring during MRI, and hence patients with such devices generally should not undergo MRI, though some exceptions are being developed. Other devices including extracorporeal membrane oxygenation (ECMO) lines, cochlear implants, and vagus nerve stimulators are also problematic. Many programmable shunts can be scanned but require reprogramming immediately afterward (further details are available at http://www.mrisafety.com). Injuries and deaths have been reported because of the failure to recognize these dangers. Most MRI sequences require imaging times in the range of minutes and are susceptible to motion degradation. Though newer sequences have increased tolerance for (minor) motion, for patients who are unable to cooperate, deep sedation or anesthesia is often required. "Fast and feed" approaches taking advantage of postprandial somnolence are often used successfully in young infants, thereby avoiding sedation. It also is important to screen the renal function of patients who might get an MRI because gadolinium-based contrast may need to be used. Gadolinium has been implicated in the development of nephrogenic systemic fibrosis in some patients with compromised renal function, which is not uncommon in the ICU setting.[5]

MRI exploits nuclear characteristics of hydrogen protons principally in tissue water, referred to as the T1 (longitudinal relaxation) and T2 (spin-spin relaxation) of the tissue. An imaging sequence includes both T1 and T2 components to create an image; however, an individual sequence can be formulated to be predominately one or the other—that is, T1 weighted or T2 weighted (often referred to as simply T1 or T2 sequences). Because most pathobiology results in some disturbance of water, these imaging parameters turn out to be sensitive to many pathologies. On T1-weighted images, water—such as CSF in the ventricles or vitreous in the globes—is dark. This water is bright on T2-weighted images. One point to be aware of is that for the most part the signal intensity of any tissue being imaged on MRI is relative (unlike the absolute density measure in CT). Hence the detection of pathology is dependent on visualizing differences in intensity of one tissue relative to another.

Fluid-attenuated inversion recovery (FLAIR) is a variation of T2-weighted imaging where the CSF is specifically rendered dark or suppressed so as to enhance visibility of hyperintense pathology in parenchyma, especially adjacent to normal CSF spaces. Fat is hyperintense on T1-weighted sequences and is also fairly bright on fast T2-weighted sequences, which is possible with most modern-day scanners. In some situations it is advantageous to suppress the brightness of fat, which can be specifically done at the cost of increased scan time. Gradient-recalled echo (GRE) and susceptibility-weighted (SWI) MRI sequences are often utilized for detection of hemorrhage, although these sequences generally also result in more artifacts. The appearance of acute blood on CT is fairly straight-forward, appearing hyperdense initially (because of the extraction of serum), becoming isodense by about a week, and appearing hypodense thereafter. The appearance of blood on MRI is much more complex, and although generally it is detectable for a much longer period of time, it can be difficult to appreciate hyperacutely (approximately less than 12 hours old) with MRI, especially with SAH. Overall, the detection of calcium and hyperacute blood can be difficult by standard MRI, and CT is often better in this regard, though newer gradient sequences, SWI in particular, are sensitive. IV contrast is also used in MRI, with similar application with CT. In this case the contrast is a gadolinium chelate that shortens the T1 relaxation time of nearby water. The result is that the water near gadolinium is hyperintense on T1-weighted images. This effect can be used to detect BBB disruption, which is seen in various pathologies including ischemia, inflammation/infection, and status epilepticus. Malignant and some benign brain tumors also demonstrate enhanced capillary permeability with enhancement following contrast. MRI with gadolinium is about an order of magnitude more sensitive than CT using iodinated contrast in detecting BBB disruption. Some areas of the brain lack the BBB, including the choroid plexus, pituitary stalk, the median eminence, and the pineal gland, and thus they enhance normally.

Diffusion-weighted imaging (DWI) has assumed an invaluable role, particularly in the intensive care setting. This sequence is now integrated into most brain MRI examinations and is particularly sensitive to areas where brain parenchyma has sustained acute cytotoxic injury, most commonly but not limited to ischemia. DWI is sensitive to the motion of water at the molecular level.[6] Detecting this molecular level motion requires strong fast gradients that have become standard on modern-day MRI scanners to allow sufficiently rapid scanning to effectively "freeze" the gross tissue motion that normally swamps this molecular level motion. Different cerebral pathologies produce different types of edema (eg, cytotoxic, vasogenic, and interstitial) (see also Chapter 66). Evaluation of the molecular (Brownian) motion of water turns out to be a sensitive measure of some pathologic states, the most significant application currently being cytotoxic edema associated with the detection of ischemia.[7] Cytotoxic edema causes "restriction" of water diffusion with a decrease in the apparent diffusion coefficient (ADC). This is seen as hypointensity on the calculated ADC map image but is more easily appreciated as hyperintensity on the DWI "trace" image. In contrast to cytotoxic edema, vasogenic and interstitial edema result in "increased" water diffusion and therefore an increase in the ADC. Care must be taken in interpreting the DWI trace images because they have some T2 weighting, and "T2 shine-through" can result in a focus of increased signal on DWI trace images that does not represent true restricted diffusion. Review of the calculated ADC map images should show a corresponding darkening in a focus of cytotoxic edema to confirm restricted diffusion. Also, the hyperintensity on DWI trace images may "pseudo-normalize" for a period of time several days following the ictus because of the development of associated vasogenic edema. Restricted diffusion due to infarct will generally resolve over the course of 1 to 3 weeks and allows a new infarct to be distinguished from older lesions. It also should be noted that restricted diffusion is not limited to ischemia and can be seen in other acute cerebral pathologies, primarily myelin vacuolization as can be seen in acute demyelination, infection, and highly cellular brain tumors.

Advanced Magnetic Resonance Imaging Techniques
Newer techniques in MRI such as MR perfusion, MR spectroscopy (MRS), and diffusion tensor imaging are providing new information that is being increasingly utilized in the management of critically ill patients.

Perfusion MR is used in the evaluation of cerebral perfusion. The most widely available techniques use rapid scanning associated with a bolus of IV gadolinium contrast to measure first-pass changes in signal intensity. These techniques give a relative measure of perfusion but not quantitative flow. This relative measure can be used to detect diminished cerebral blood flow in one area compared with another. Newer noncontrast MRI techniques such as arterial spin labeling generally have lower signal-to-noise ratio (sensitivity) but are improving and potentially quantifiable. There is some early experience with arterial spin labeling in pediatric stroke cases resulting from sickle cell disease.[8,9]

Conventional MRI is based on the signal intensities derived from the hydrogen bound to oxygen in water and, to a lesser extent, the hydrogen bound to carbon in fat. With the appropriate software, MR can be used as a "probe" for hydrogen bonded to other molecules (termed *MR spectroscopy*). The sensitivity is sufficient to detect metabolite molecules in the millimolar range, although at a much lower resolution than that used to detect water for imaging. The nonwater molecules are most commonly reported as ratios of signal peaks that correspond to one of several molecules. In the brain the most common metabolite peaks detected are N-acetyl aspartate, creatine, choline, and in some physiologic states, lactate. The MRS signal is either obtained from a single voxel (usually several mL in volume; voxel is the "volume element" of the image = pixel × depth) or multiple voxels (as small as 1 to 2 mL in volume). Multivoxel MRS can be used to make low-resolution images using a technique termed *chemical shift imaging* for some of the more prevalent metabolite peaks. The utility of MRS is still in evolution, and newer variants of MRS are constantly being evaluated. Detection of lactate to evaluate newborn ischemia, some metabolic diseases, and brain tumors is one of the ongoing applications and areas of research. MRS also has a role in imaging children with mitochondrial disorders[10] and has been applied in creatine deficiency syndromes as two examples of clinical applications.

Magnetic Resonance Angiography
Fluid motion within tissues can be used by MRI to image flow in vessels and CSF. This imaging can be accomplished with and without contrast, although contrast techniques are generally more sensitive for vascular flow, with some newer contrast angiography sequences also providing temporal/flow information. The MR angiogram can be tailored for artery (MRA) or vein (MRV) visualization, primarily based on flow direction, and is usually most effective if the area of interest can be narrowed—for example, the circle of Willis—although newer techniques have greatly increased the area that can be covered in one scan. The maximum resolution of MRA of slightly under 1 mm is generally less than CTA, where the maximum resolution can be under 0.25 mm.[11] In addition to the source images (the thin angiographic sections obtained during the scan), various reconstructed images can be obtained, including 3D rotational reformations derived from maximum intensity projection reconstructions (Figs. 63.2 and 63.3) and surface renderings, which also can be viewed from multiple projections. Time-resolved MRA techniques (such as TWIST), which utilized the first pass of gadolinium-administered IV, have begun to make inroads in providing temporal information on vascular lesions, previously only available with catheter angiograms, though the latter remain the gold standard. Many clinical cerebral arterial questions, however, are now answered with MRA, and MRV of the superficial and deep

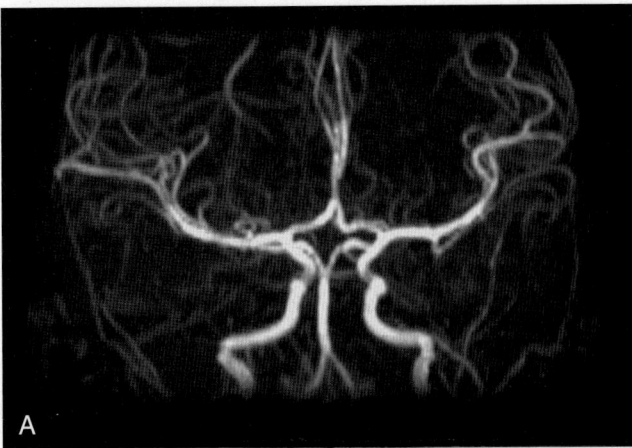

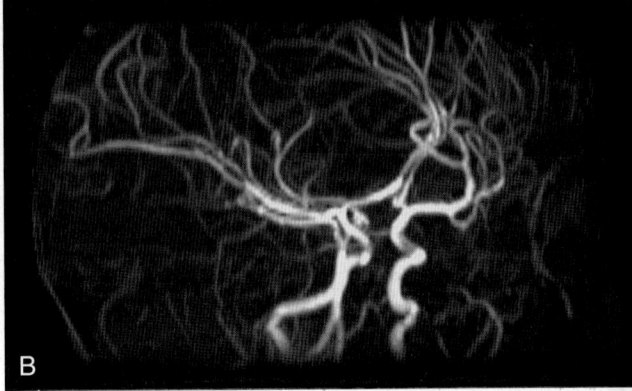

Fig. 63.2. Normal MRA scans. Frontal (A) and oblique (B) maximum intensity projection images from an MRA demonstrate normal anterior and posterior circulations.

venous systems has largely replaced diagnostic catheter venograms.

Catheter Angiograms

Although significant inroads have been made in cerebral vascular evaluation with both CTA and MRA, when indicated, catheter angiography remains the gold standard for most CNS arterial imaging. Catheter angiography also provides temporal/flow data, such as appreciation of early venous drainage with arteriovenous malformations. Angiography is basically a rapid series of radiographs obtained during injection of iodinated contrast directly into the arteries or veins being imaged. Most angiography units produce digital images using digital subtraction (hence the term *digital subtraction angiography*)—that is, images where the background "mask" has been subtracted, leaving an image primarily of the contrast-filled vessels. High-end modern-day units utilize biplane technology that permits acquisition of digital angiographic images from multiple projections using a single contrast injection. This technology also can be used to derive 3D rotational angiograms, images that can be further postprocessed to obtain volume-rendered and surface-shaded images. Catheter angiography requires transport to and patient support in the angiography suite. Vascular access for arterial studies is usually through the femoral artery and generally has a small but "nonzero" risk of vessel injury, including dissection and embolization. In very young patients, injury to the femoral artery is of greater concern, and although any acute risk to the

limb is extremely uncommon, relative diminished leg growth in some cases has been reported. Risks of neurologic complication following cerebral angiography are small but do exist; the incidence of permanent defects in diagnostic angiograms using modern techniques is typically reported in the range of 0.5% to 0.07%.[12,13] Therapeutic endovascular procedures carry higher risks but generally are in lieu of riskier neurosurgical procedures or at times are the only or preferred avenue of treatment.

Myelography

Myelography involves radiographs or CT of the spine following opacification of the subarachnoid space by intrathecal injection of iodinated contrast, most commonly injected at the lumbar level. The myelogram has almost completely been replaced by MRI, especially in the pediatric population, because MRI can depict both extrathecal encroachment and intrathecal masses, as well as evaluate signal characteristics of the spinal cord itself and any intramedullary mass. High-resolution myelographic type contrast can be achieved using MRI with 3D constructive interference in steady state and volume T2 sequences to investigate pathologies where detailed anatomic information is needed, such as with spinal nerve root avulsion and cranial nerve pathologies.

Exceptions where imaging may revert to CT include the inability to obtain an MRI either because of local field disruption, most commonly from ferromagnetic spinal rods, or because of MRI incompatibility due to safety issues (eg, a pacemaker). CT provides better results than MRI in the evaluation of the bony spinal column, particularly in patients with trauma, whereas MRI is used in patients with trauma to evaluate soft tissues in the spinal column, primarily the spinal cord.

Nuclear Medicine

Most nuclear medicine studies involve injection of a very small amount of radioactively labeled substance (radiopharmaceutical tracer compound or radiotracer) and follow either the physiologic uptake and metabolism of the radiotracer or the movement of the radiotracer with a gamma camera.

Technetium pertechnetate and technetium-diethylenetriamine pentaacetic acid (Tc^{99} DTPA) are radiotracers used for radionuclide cerebral angiography to evaluate cerebral perfusion, and they can be used to support a clinical diagnosis of brain death. Single photon emission computed tomography imaging using technetium-hexamethylpropyleneamine oxime (Tc^{99} HMPAO) as the radiotracer is used to monitor for cerebral perfusion defects in patients with SAH who are at risk for vasospasm. With use of acetazolamide (Diamox), a carbonic anhydrase inhibitor, Tc^{99} HMPAO single photon emission CT (SPECT) can be used to evaluate cerebral reserve in patients with stroke.

Ventriculoperitoneal (and ventriculoatrial and ventriculopleural) shunt function evaluation often includes a nuclear medicine shunt study. Flow in the shunt is assessed by injecting a small amount of radiotracer in the shunt reservoir and following the movement of the activity with a gamma camera.

Preterm and Term Neonate Imaging

In the premature infant, ultrasound remains the primary modality for detection and follow-up of germinal matrix hemorrhage and to detect intraventricular extension as well as

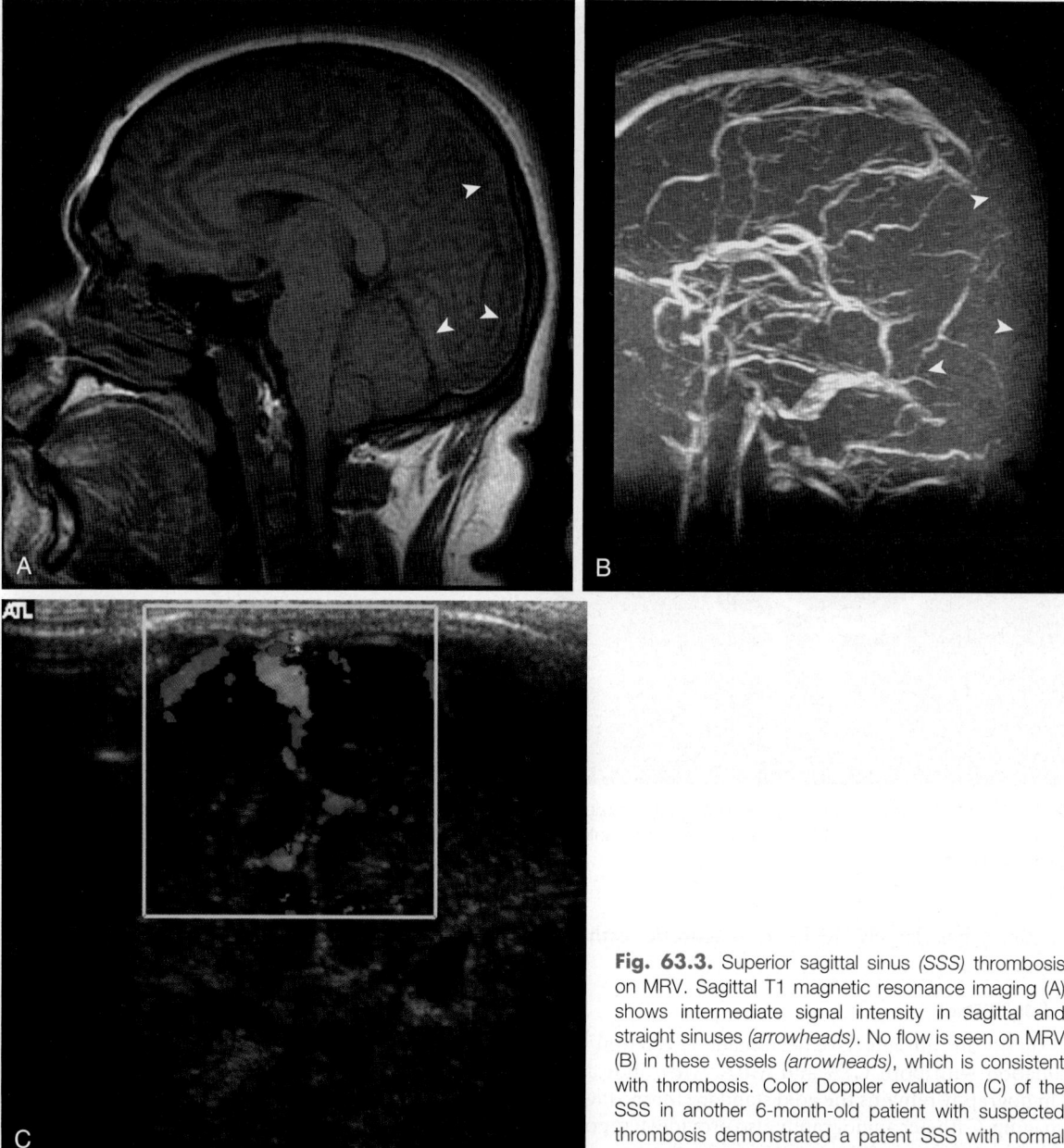

Fig. 63.3. Superior sagittal sinus *(SSS)* thrombosis on MRV. Sagittal T1 magnetic resonance imaging (A) shows intermediate signal intensity in sagittal and straight sinuses *(arrowheads)*. No flow is seen on MRV (B) in these vessels *(arrowheads)*, which is consistent with thrombosis. Color Doppler evaluation (C) of the SSS in another 6-month-old patient with suspected thrombosis demonstrated a patent SSS with normal draining cortical veins (see color inset).

hemorrhagic parenchymal venous infarction; in the neonate, it remains the primary modality to evaluate for hydrocephalus (Fig. 63.4). Furthermore, assessment can be made for white matter injury including periventricular leukomalacia, especially the cystic form, although MRI will be more sensitive for noncystic periventricular leukomalacia, and MRI in preemies performed at about the third week of life has been reported as predictive of outcome at term.[14] Routine screening cranial ultrasound has been recommended for all infants younger than 30 weeks' gestation between day 7 and day 14, optimally repeated at 36 to 40 weeks' gestation.[15] Moderate to large parenchymal and extra axial areas of bleeding also can be detected with ultrasound. As previously mentioned, smaller extra axial collections, especially laterally along the cerebral convexities, can be missed with ultrasound, as can small parenchymal hemorrhages.

As noted in Chapters 60 and 68, understanding of hypoxic-ischemic encephalopathy (HIE) in children is complicated by the developmental status of the child. The pattern of injury seen is determined by the characteristics of the insult and the maturational state of the brain. Metabolic demands and regions of selective vulnerability evolve during development. Grayscale ultrasound, which is widely used for intracranial imaging in the neonate, is relatively insensitive to acute changes associated with HIE.[16] As edema develops, usually after several hours, increased echogenicity of brain parenchyma can be seen, but this measure is nonspecific, relative, and often is difficult to appreciate. Blood associated with a hemorrhagic infarct also will appear as increased echogenicity. As mass effect develops secondary to edema, ventricular and sulcal effacement can be seen. Later, vascular and perivascular mineralization can result in linear thalamic and basal ganglia

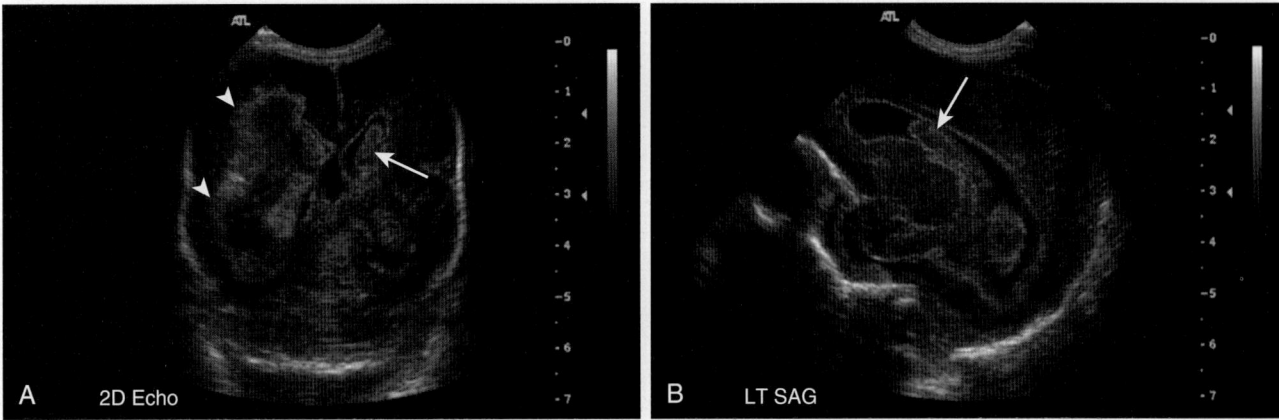

Fig. 63.4. Germinal matrix hemorrhage in a premature infant. Coronal (A) and left parasagittal (B) ultrasound images through the anterior fontanelle demonstrate dilated lateral ventricles with intraventricular extension of clot on the left *(arrows)* and periventricular hemorrhagic venous infarction on the right *(arrowheads)* consistent with a grade 3 hemorrhage on the left and grade 4 hemorrhage on the right (some radiologists would assign this hemorrhage an overall grade of 4).

echogenicities (lenticulostriate vasculopathy or mineralizing angiopathy).[17] Ultrasound Doppler evaluation of newborn ischemia has shown some utility. Brain perfusion can be investigated by determining the resistive index (RI). RI in the normal neonate (0.75 ± 0.1) is higher than that seen in the older infant before (0.65 ± 0.5) and after (0.55 ± 0.5) fontanelle closure.[16] An increase in the RI with a decrease in the peak systolic velocity and end-diastolic velocity in infants with HIE within the first 12 hours of life as measured in the anterior and middle cerebral arteries correlated with a poor prognosis at 1 year of life. A decrease in RI to less than 0.60 at 12 hours (anterior and middle cerebral arteries) and 24 hours (all insonated arteries, including basilar artery) after neonatal asphyxia, which is thought to be a result of the decreased vascular tone associated with loss of autoregulation, has been associated with a poorer outcome at 12 to 18 months of life.[18,19] Approximately half of patients with low RI scores have normal grayscale images. There is a host of other reasons for low RI scores, however, including cardiac disease, extracorporeal membrane oxygenation, ongoing hypoxemia, hypercapnia, and technical issues. It also should be noted that increased fontanelle pressure can increase the RI measure by 20%, hence there is considerable user dependence to this application. If hyperemia persists, and as HIE evolves, cytotoxic edema increases and leads to increased intracranial pressure and increased RI measurements. A high RI score on the first day of life with evidence of neonatal insult suggests an in utero injury. Although some centers have continued to pursue the use of ultrasound, MRI has supplanted much of this evaluation.

CT detection of acute ischemic injury also depends on edema resulting from the injury. Edema is seen as decreased attenuation and loss of gray-white differentiation, usually detected several hours postinsult.[20] Small or early infarcts can be missed with CT, and detection of ischemia in the newborn is made more difficult by the generally lower attenuation of the relatively "watery" unmyelinated newborn brain. For this reason, in some instances of neonatal ischemic injury, there may actually be an increase in the attenuation of this watery unmyelinated white matter because of an outpouring of serum proteins from damaged blood vessels. As brain swelling develops in the first few days, there can be a loss of CSF spaces seen as ventricular compression, sulcal effacement, and loss of perimesencephalic cisterns. Acute thrombotic stroke associated with arterial thrombosis can at times be appreciated acutely as a hyperdense artery, most commonly the middle cerebral artery on noncontrast CT. Acute hemorrhage, such as with hemorrhagic arterial (from reperfusion) or venous infarcts, will be hyperdense initially on CT, evolving to isodense over the first week.

Standard MR sequences exploiting T1 and T2 relaxation times also depend on the development of edema to appreciate acute ischemic injury, which results in hyperintensity on T2-weighted and FLAIR images and hypointensity on T1-weighted images. This change typically takes at least several hours to develop, and although generally more sensitive than CT in adults, evaluation of the newborn is again somewhat difficult by the lack of myelination. As a result, ischemia sometimes can be more conspicuous on CT than on T1- or T2-weighted MRI (Fig. 63.5). The FLAIR sequence has proved to be more sensitive than T1 and T2 to ischemic changes in older myelinated children and adults. DWI is more sensitive than T2 and FLAIR sequences and correlates well with at least short-term neurologic outcome in neonates and infants.[21] These sequences, as previously discussed, have been shown to be acutely sensitive to the cytotoxic edema associated with ischemia.[7] This cytotoxic edema results in diminished diffusion of water in the affected area. DWI in experimental models can detect ischemia in minutes after onset as a region of restricted diffusion.[22,23] These sequences have now become widely implemented in adult and pediatric neuroimaging, where differentiation of acute ischemic stroke from other neurologic disorders permits appropriate and timely implementation of stroke therapies. The restricted diffusion associated with ischemia evolves over a 1- to 3-week period, at which time the diffusion image usually normalizes. If sufficient tissue destruction has occurred, the diffusion ultimately will increase because of the greater amount of free water following necrosis. This change in diffusion is also useful in distinguishing a new stroke (which will show decreased diffusion) from an older lesion (which will have increased diffusion), whereas both lesions may be of similar signal intensity on standard T1 and T2 imaging (Fig. 63.6).

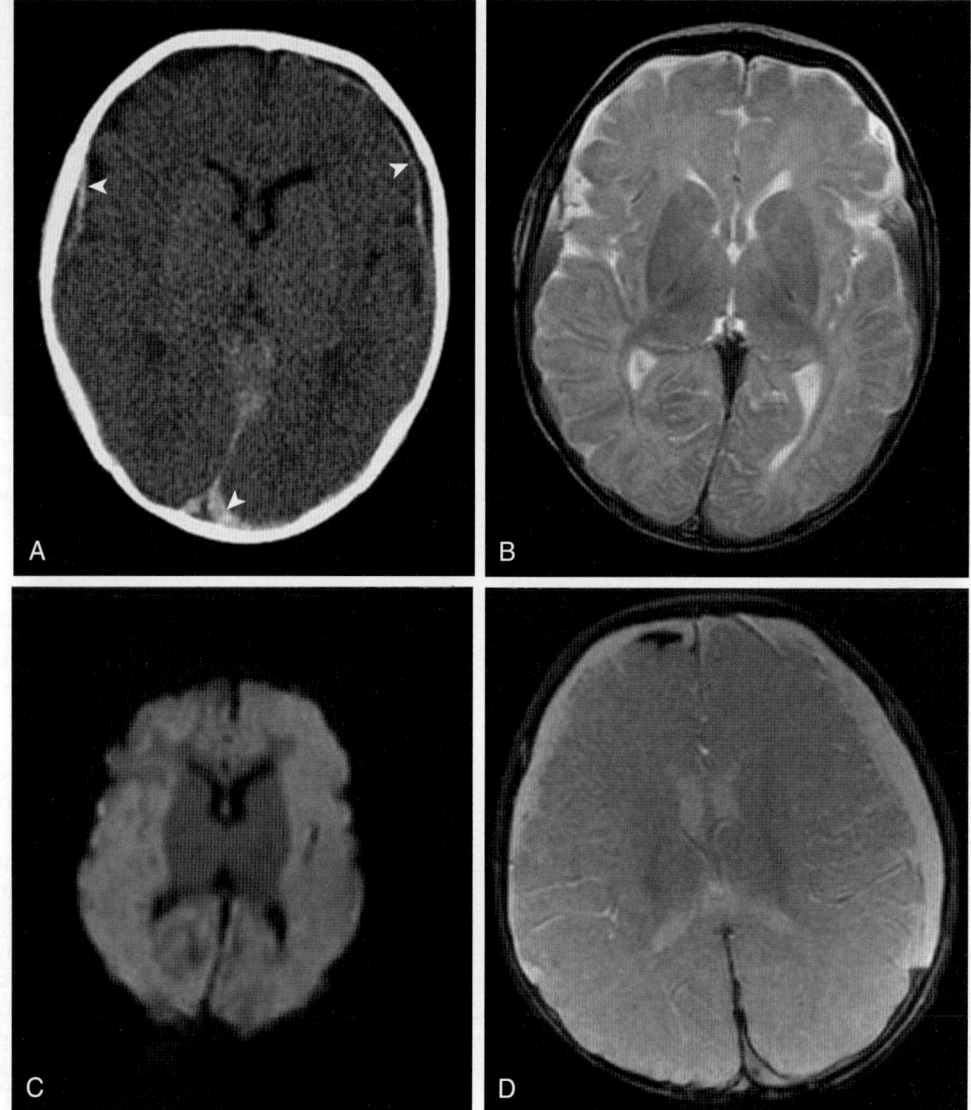

Fig. 63.5. Nonaccidental trauma with diffuse cerebral ischemia. Axial noncontrast CT (A), axial T2-weighted (B), and diffusion-weighted MRI (C). (A) CT shows a thin layer of acute subdural blood *(arrowheads)* and diffuse loss of gray-white demarcation in the cerebral hemispheres. (B) Although the T2 image appears remarkably normal with appropriate lack of myelination in this 3-month-old child, the relative brightness of the cerebral hemi-spheres compared with the central gray on diffusion-weighted images (C) is consistent with a diffuse ischemic insult. (D) Gradient-recalled echo MRI in another 4-month-old with nonaccidental trauma demonstrates dark, low signal areas in the right frontal subdural space and left posterior parafalcine regions, consistent with subdural hematomas.

Timelines for relative T2 and diffusion changes have been shown to differ in neonates and infants versus older children and adults. Animal models have suggested that diffusion changes in neonates and infants with HIE do not necessarily precede T2 changes. This finding is presumably a result of age-dependent differences in brain water content and changes therein as a result of differences in vascular permeability in response to hypoxic-ischemic insult.[24,25] The initial diffusion abnormality may increase over the first day, and the extent of the diffusion abnormality can encompass both the core infarct as well as penumbra and hence potentially overestimate the ultimate infarct. This potential overestimation could be an indication for MR perfusion, which can separate the areas of core infarction and penumbra.[26] The identification of lactate on MRS is also evolving as a useful tool that may serve as a predictor for the severity of perinatal asphyxia, although

considerable complexity is involved, which has limited appli-cation of this technology.[22,27]

As previously mentioned, the pattern of hypoxic-ischemic injury varies with the etiology of the insult, as well as the developmental state of the brain. Early in utero insults result in tissue resorption, without the ability to mount a gliotic response that is not seen until the third trimester. During early brain development, insults can result in congenital malforma-tions. HIE or injury in the early to middle second trimester may result in polymicrogyria with or without associated schizencephaly. In the 24th to 25th week of gestation range, HIE can preferentially injure the deep gray matter nuclei in the setting of total asphyxia. PVL is the pattern of injury seen with prolonged partial hypoxia at 24 to 34 weeks. Typically with PVL on neonatal grayscale ultrasound, there may be increased echogenicity in the periventricular white matter, an

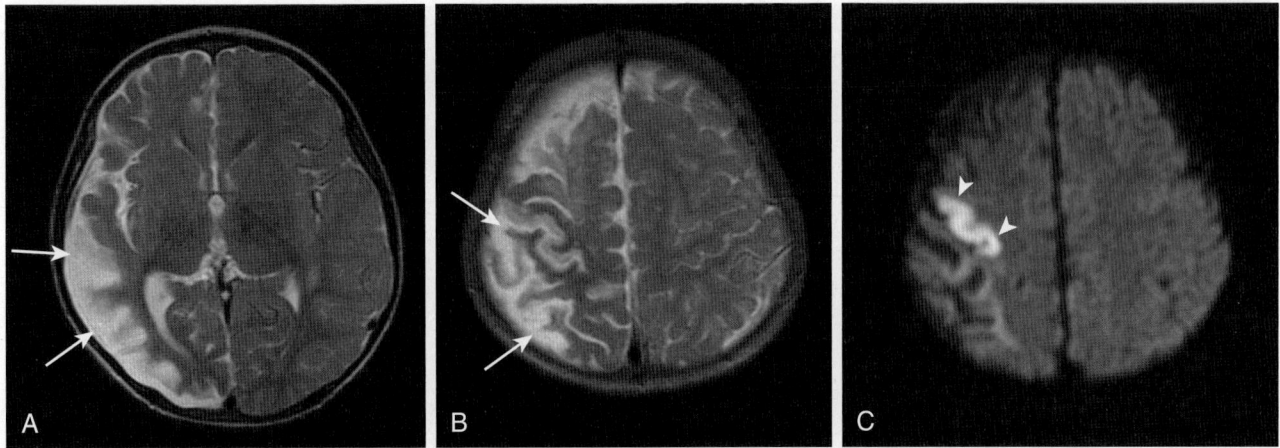

Fig. 63.6. Remote and acute infarcts. Axial T2-weighted MRI (A and B) shows cerebral volume loss with encephalomalacia and gliosis *(arrows)* associated with an old stroke in this child with new onset of progressive left-sided weakness. Diffusion-weighted MRI (C) reveals a new area of infarct *(arrowheads)* at the edge of the remote abnormality.

appearance that is indistinguishable at this stage from edema or from parenchymal hemorrhage, which also may be seen. As PVL progresses, cystic change occurs that progresses to coalescent cavitation of the involved white matter, and collapse of these spaces results ultimately in the thinning and volume loss of the white matter, particularly in the posterior periventricular white matter. Although cranial ultrasound affords better resolution for the visualization of cystic change of early PVL in the premature neonate, MRI has overall greater sensitivity to white matter injury, especially in the more advanced stages of PVL, and demonstrates an undulating ventricular margin with associated periventricular T2/FLAIR signal abnormality with or without a paucity of white matter. However, it is not yet clear if this increased sensitivity is of significant prognostic value. Ischemic insults to the term child demonstrate different patterns of injury, determined by the specifics of the insult and the vulnerability of various areas. Profound hypoxia in the term infant results in injury largely to areas that are most actively myelinating, in particular the perirolandic white matter and the associated corticospinal tracts and the white matter tracts associated with the occipital cortex, as well as other areas with high energy demands such as the putamina, thalami, hippocampi, and brain stem. In contrast, a watershed pattern of injury discussed in the next section develops with prolonged partial ischemia that is not sufficient to cause an infarct of the cerebrum, with shunting to the high-energy demand areas. Current recommendations for the encephalopathic term infant have included early CT to assess for intracranial hemorrhage, with consideration for MRI with DWI and GRE sequences later in the first postnatal week to assess the extent of injury.[15]

Stroke in the Older Infant/Child

Although the imaging picture may not be specific, a diagnosis of acute stroke usually can be made in combination with the clinical history (as discussed in Chapter 69).[28] The imaging pattern can be of help in determining an etiology. A watershed distribution is consistent with a low flow/hypotensive cause (Fig. 63.7). Specifically, changes of ischemic injury are seen at the boundary regions between the major cerebral distributions—that is, between anterior and middle cerebral

territories and between middle and posterior cerebral arterial territories. Lesions involving multiple arterial distributions suggest a central thrombotic source, although other causes such as a vasculitis or demyelinating diseases also can have this multivessel or multifocal picture (Fig. 63.8). Classically, embolic lesions will tend to be seen at the gray-white junction and most commonly in the MCA distribution. Individual variability of boundary regions[29] and pathology-induced alteration in flow limit the definitiveness of arterial distribution categorization following vascular insult.

As previously discussed, diffusion-weighted imaging also proves to be very useful in earlier imaging detection of cerebral infarcts (Fig. 63.9) and separating recent infarcts from a background of abnormality, such as prior infarcts (see Fig. 63.6). The area of restricted diffusion on DWI is generally thought to represent irreversible injury, especially when associated with T2/FLAIR signal abnormality, although there may be some cases in which the lesions are at least potentially reversible. In the setting of acute stroke, perfusion MRI may have a contributory role in demonstrating the total region of brain at risk (penumbra) and predicting the ultimate extent of infarct.[26] The area of perfusion abnormality beyond that of diffusion abnormality is thought to represent the penumbra and to be at risk but potentially salvageable. The presence of hemorrhage with a stroke can represent hemorrhagic conversion of a "bland" stroke or an underlying vascular lesion. A large study found an incidence of hemorrhagic stroke of 1.4 per 100,000 person years in those younger than 20 years of age. An underlying aneurysm was found in 13%, including 57% of those with pure SAH, 2% of those with a pure parenchymal hemorrhage, and 5% of those with a mixed hemorrhage.[30]

Posterior Reversible Encephalopathy Syndrome

Posterior reversible encephalopathy syndrome results from a loss of autoregulation in the older infant and child as seen in hypertensive encephalopathy, cytotoxic and immunosuppressive drug neurotoxicity, and thrombotic thrombocytopenia purpura. Typically posterior reversible encephalopathy syndrome preferentially involves a posterior and parasagittal distribution of the brain with T2 and FLAIR hyperintensities and also less frequently can involve the frontal lobes and brain

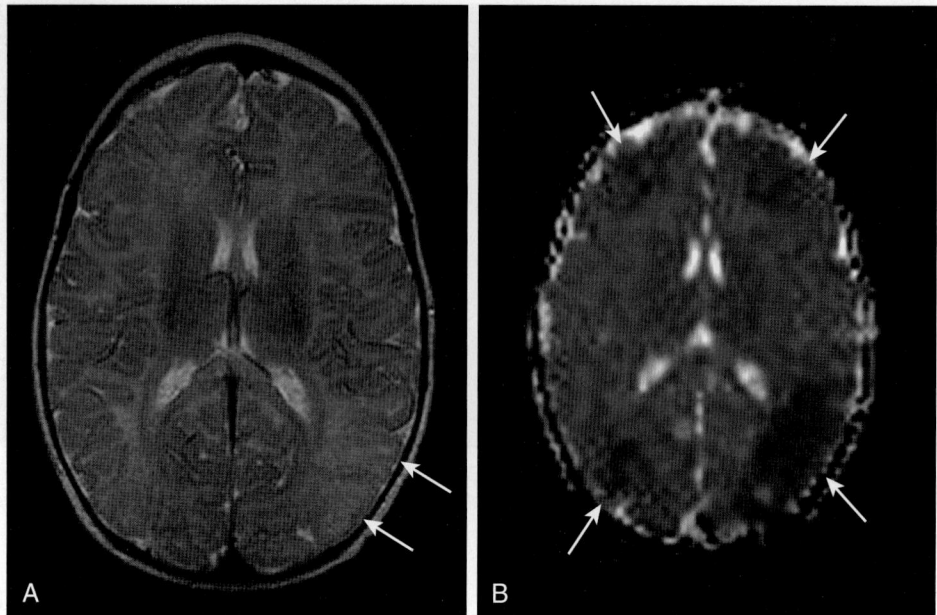

Fig. 63.7. Watershed infarct. (A) Axial T2-weighted MR image shows some loss of the gray-white interface on the left posteriorly *(arrows)*. (B) Diffusion-weighted image shows bilateral restricted diffusion consistent with ischemic injury in a watershed distribution *(arrows)*.

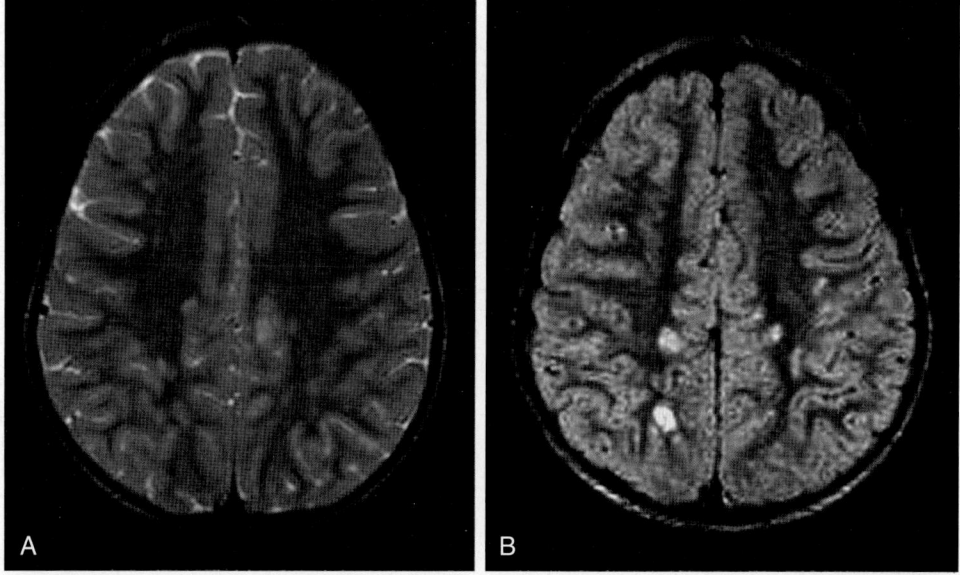

Fig. 63.8. ADEM. T2-weighted (A) and FLAIR (B) images show multiple foci of hyperintensity. In addition to ADEM, vasculitis and multiple emboli could have this imaging appearance.

stem.[31-33] Lesions often are relatively symmetric with confluent lesions centered in the subcortical white matter that rarely demonstrate patchy enhancement (Fig. 63.10). Frequently, because the underlying pathology causes only vasogenic edema, these lesions will not be restricted on DWI. However, ischemia can be triggered by a severe increase in blood pressure, resulting in superimposed cytotoxic edema and therefore diffusion-restricted lesions that usually result in infarctions, the severity of which often correlates with prognosis.

Venous Infarct

The presence of blood in an area of cerebral infarct raises consideration for a venous stroke, although an arterial-induced stroke occasionally can have associated hemorrhage (reperfusion injury). A nonarterial distribution infarct also raises suspicion of a venous stroke. In the setting of suspected venous stroke, evaluation of the cerebral venous system should be undertaken. Ultrasound has limited utility in this setting, although evaluation of superior sagittal sinus flow can be undertaken in the young infant with an open fontanelle (see Fig. 63.3C). CT evidence of a venous clot can be detected as hyperdense venous sinuses acutely on noncontrast scans and as the "empty delta sign" (lower density in area of clot surrounded by enhancing blood) in the superior sagittal sinus on contrast-enhanced scans. This assessment can be problematic in the newborn in whom the normal low-density

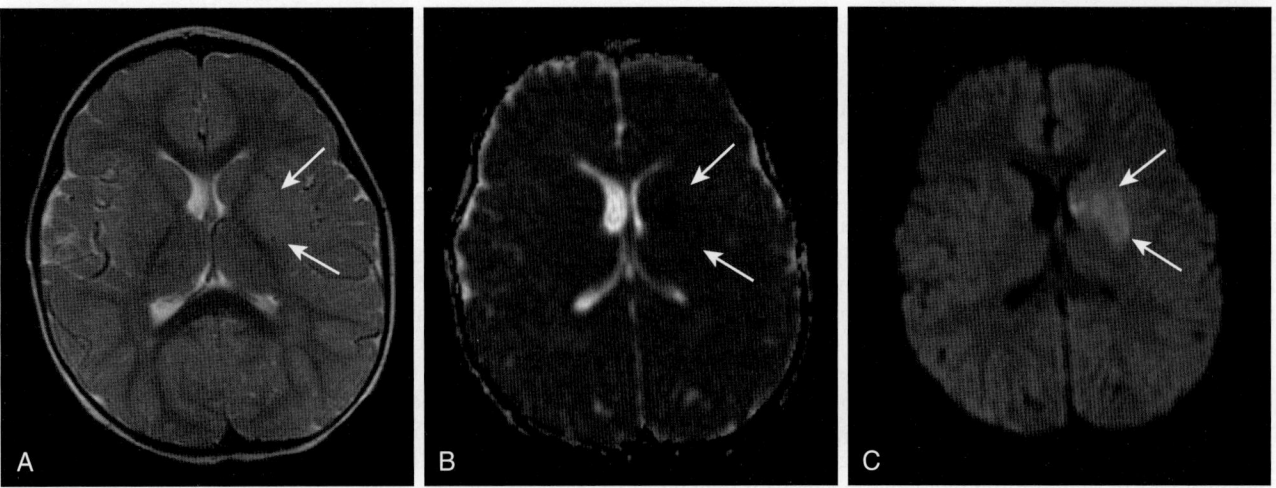

Fig. 63.9. Basal ganglia acute infarct. Axial T2-weighted MR image (A) shows subtle increased T2 signal in left basal ganglia *(arrows)*. More conspicuously shown on the apparent diffusion coefficient map (B) and diffusion-weighted images (C) is restricted diffusion *(arrows)* associated with an early infarct involving the left caudate and lentiform nuclei.

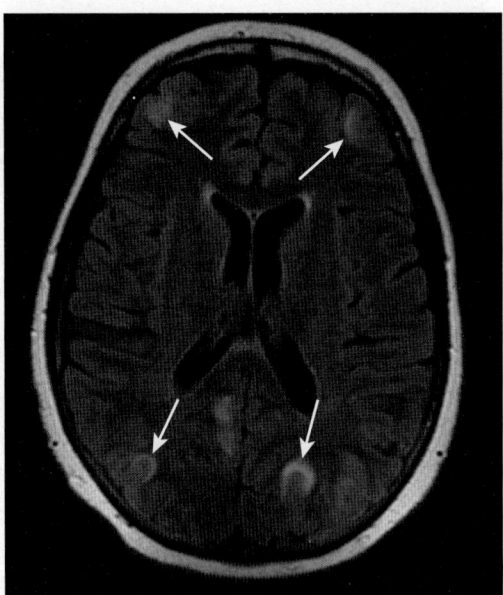

Fig. 63.10. Posterior reversible encephalopathy syndrome. Axial FLAIR MRI showing subcortical foci of hyperintensity *(arrows)* associated with cyclosporin toxicity. Note that abnormalities may have a variable distribution and are frequently, but not always, posterior in location.

unmyelinated brain and typically higher hematocrit make the venous sinuses appear dense normally on CT. Classically, the venous phase of a catheter angiogram has been used to look for venous sinus thrombosis. Catheter evaluation of the venous sinuses, however, has been effectively replaced with MRV techniques. MRV uses flow-sensitive sequences that can delineate the major venous sinuses quite effectively (see Fig. 63.3A and B). A subacute clot in a venous sinus also can be evident on standard T1- and T2-weighted MRI as bright areas in the venous sinuses, although an acute clot can be more difficult to appreciate. On MRI, GRE sequences may demonstrate low signal, and T1 contrast-enhanced sequences may demonstrate areas of nonenhancement of thrombosed venous sinuses.

Etiologic workup of stroke in children includes a broad differential (see also Chapter 69). Although catheter angiogram remains the gold standard and is necessary occasionally, ruling out a vascular lesion has evolved, with greater use of MRA and CTA.

Arterial dissections can be diagnosed with MRI and MRA or with CTA. Visualization of methemoglobin in the false lumen with fat-saturated T1-weighted or proton density–weighted MRI sequences detects most dissections, although subtle lesions may still require catheter angiogram for diagnosis. On CTA, the false lumen is detected by the absent or diminished enhancement compared with the true lumen. Suspicion for dissection is raised in the setting of multiple apparent embolic strokes in a single carotid distribution or within the posterior circulation when there is a history of trauma, although spontaneous dissections are seen occasionally. As previously mentioned, the presence of emboli in multiple circulations raises the question of a more central etiology such as a heart valve vegetation.

Vasculopathy/Vasculitis

Acquired vasculopathies can be a result of known infectious or noninfectious causes or of unknown pathophysiology such as in primary cerebral vasculitis, which tends to involve medium and small vessels, or moyamoya syndrome, which demonstrates greatest involvement of the central cerebral vessels. Vasculopathy involving large and medium-sized vessels can be seen on MRA, although more subtle irregularities and small vessel involvement still requires a catheter angiogram, which remains the gold standard imaging modality.

In transient cerebral angiopathy of childhood, classically a basal ganglia infarct resulting from M1 MCA segment narrowing and occlusion of lenticulostriate vessels is seen, with cortical injury being less common. Narrowing typically of the terminal carotid and proximal M1 MCA segment of the affected side often can be delineated on MRA. A lack of well-developed collaterals also will be noted, in contrast to the typical presentation of moyamoya syndrome, where the vessel occlusion has been more slowly progressive over a longer period. Moyamoya "syndrome" denotes the pattern of vessel involvement that can be associated with type 1 neurofibromatosis, radiation injury, sickle cell disease, Trisomy 21 syndrome, or other pathology. When this pattern is idiopathic, the term moyamoya *disease* is used. More commonly, moyamoya syndrome/disease will be bilateral and MRI will demonstrate evidence of chronic ischemic insult. The enlarged lenticulostriate collaterals generally will be appreciable on both MRA (correlating with the "puff of smoke appearance" initially described with catheter arteriography) and as flow voids through the basal ganglia and basal cisterns on MRI (Fig. 63.11). These apparent flow voids need to be distinguished from enlarged perivascular spaces that also are seen in this region.

Vasculitic changes can accompany infections including meningitis, either through direct invasion of vessels or by an immune response to the particular pathogen. Parenchymal injury, if present, is mediated by ischemic changes. The pattern of involvement in the immune-mediated mechanism may be fairly symmetric, as can be seen in acute disseminated encephalomyelitis (ADEM) or some metabolic diseases. Noninfectious vasculitides, including those associated with systemic disease—for example, systemic lupus erythematosus and, in particular, primary CNS vasculitis—can be more problematic in diagnosis. Classically, a catheter angiogram and occasionally a brain biopsy have been used to evaluate the possibility of primary CNS vasculitis. Most cases of symptomatic vasculitis will demonstrate abnormality on standard MRI (T2, FLAIR, and DWI) sequences, and thus a completely normal MRI makes the likelihood of CNS vasculitis low. Occasionally, however, there can be a vasculitic process in the presence of a normal MRI.[34] Furthermore, cases have been reported of biopsy-proved CNS vasculitis in which the MRI was abnormal and results of a catheter angiogram were normal.[35] Because medium and small vessels often are involved in the setting of CNS vasculitis, to which MRA has less sensitivity, a catheter angiogram may be indicated in the setting of very strong concern for vasculitis with a normal MRA and occasionally even a normal MRI.

Vascular Malformations

Most arteriovenous malformations and aneurysms can be detected with a combination of MRI and MRA or CTA,

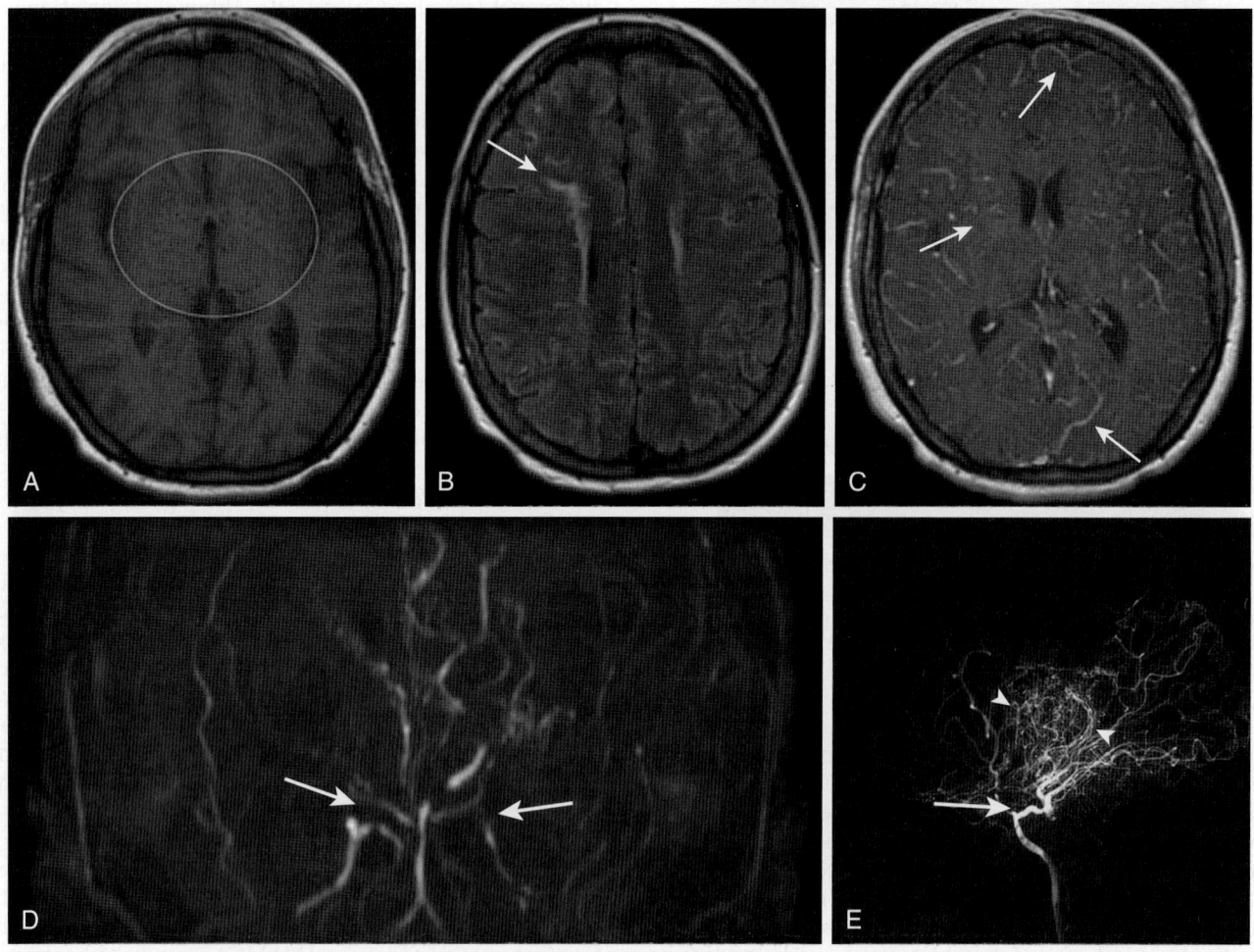

Fig. 63.11. Moyamoya syndrome in a 15-year-old girl. (A) Axial T1-weighted MR image shows flow voids *(circled)* associated with enlarged lenticulostriate collaterals. (B) Axial FLAIR image shows gliosis in the right anterior periventricular white matter *(arrow)* with leptomeningeal linear hyperintensities corresponding to collaterals. (C) Axial T1 postcontrast image demonstrates enhancing right lenticulostriate and leptomeningeal collaterals *(white arrows)*. (D) Coronal maximum intensity projection image from an MRA shows no flow distal to the terminal internal carotid artery and nonvisualization of right and left proximal posterior cerebral arteries (compare with normal frontal MRA image in Fig. 63.2). (E) Lateral view from a right ICA catheter angiogram showing occlusion of the ICA below the siphon *(arrow)* and extensive thalamostriate collateral vessels *(arrowheads)*.

although small lesions can be missed (Fig. 63.12). Catheter angiogram remains the gold standard for arteriovenous malformation diagnosis, confirming flow dynamics and the presence of intranidal aneurysms, and generally will be required before surgical intervention. In the appropriate clinical setting such as a spontaneous SAH without etiology, a negative MRI, MRA, or CTA, however, should not exclude a catheter angiogram. Arterial aneurysms are much less common in children than in adults, with many of those seen likely being congenital or due to infection in contrast to the typical acquired berry aneurysms seen in adults. As in adults, all but the smallest aneurysms can be seen on MRA or CTA, with CTA sensitivity for berry aneurysms in adult series reported in the range of 80% to 97%.[11] These studies, though, need to be of optimum resolution, are generally targeted to the high-risk locations for aneurysms in adults, and may not include less common aneurysm locations, which are seen with greater frequency in children. Angiographically occult lesions including capillary telangiectasia, cavernous malformation, and developmental venous anomalies are seen on MRI but usually are not of consequence except in cases of the occasional large cavernous malformation.

A vein of Galen aneurysmal malformation (VGAM) is a misnomer because it is not the vein of Galen but a persistent embryonic vein that is dilated in association with a large fistula.[36] VGAMs presenting in the newborn period will manifest with cardiac symptoms resulting from the large shunt and high-flow congestive cardiac failure. Although the malformation can be seen with ultrasound, a CT scan is useful as a quick evaluation to visualize the malformation and determine the status of the cerebral cortex, which may be severely affected even at term. A noncontrast CT scan is sufficient because the density of blood (usually with an increased hematocrit) provides good contrast against the relatively less dense newborn brain (Fig. 63.13). In the presence of a VGAM, MRI with MR angiography will give an overall vascular road map for planning endovascular intervention, because the limited amount of contrast that can be used in a neonate necessitates directed intervention.

Central Nervous System Infection

Imaging findings and the role of imaging in cerebral infection will depend on the organism and location of the infection (see

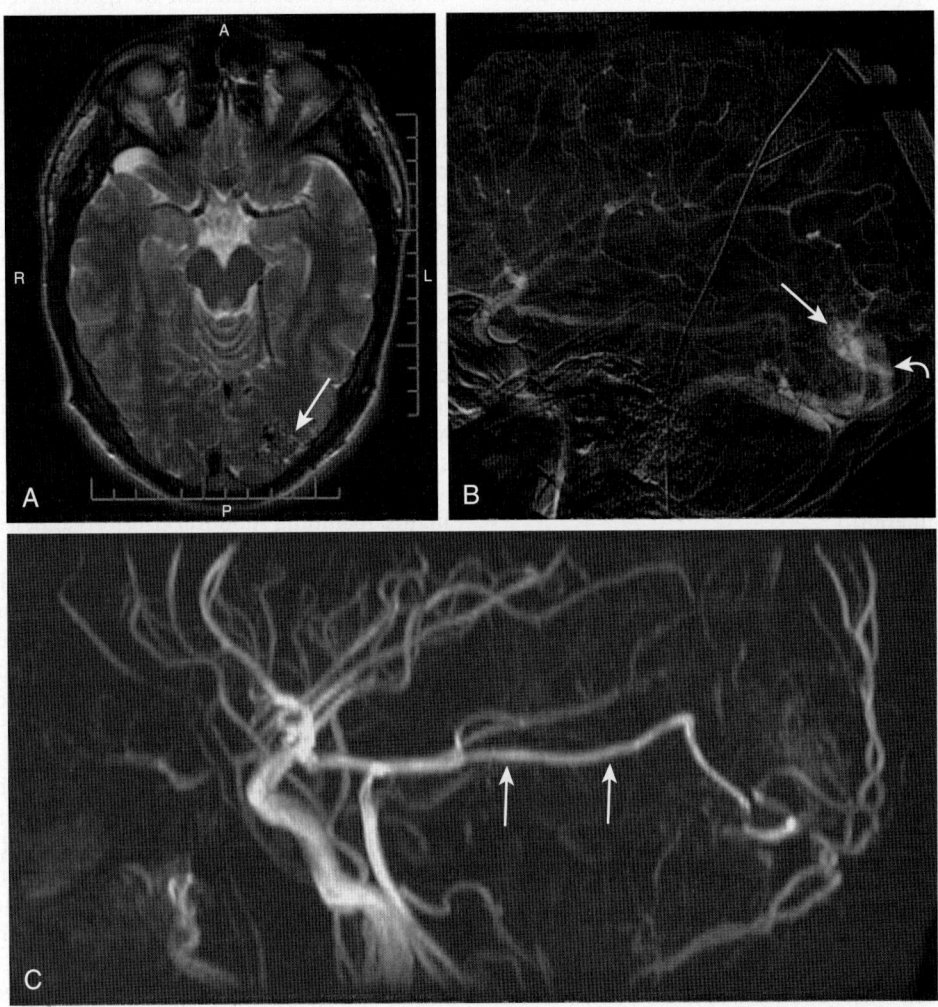

Fig. 63.12. A 14-year-old child with a left occipital arteriovenous malformation (AVM). (A) Axial T2-weighted MRI image shows multiple flow voids in the left occipital lobe *(arrow)*. (B) Lateral view from catheter angiogram confirms the presence of an AVM *(arrow)* and early draining veins *(curved arrow)*. (C) Lateral maximum intensity projection image from an MR angiogram shows an enlarged posterior cerebral artery branch *(arrows)*, which feeds the tangle of abnormal vessels.

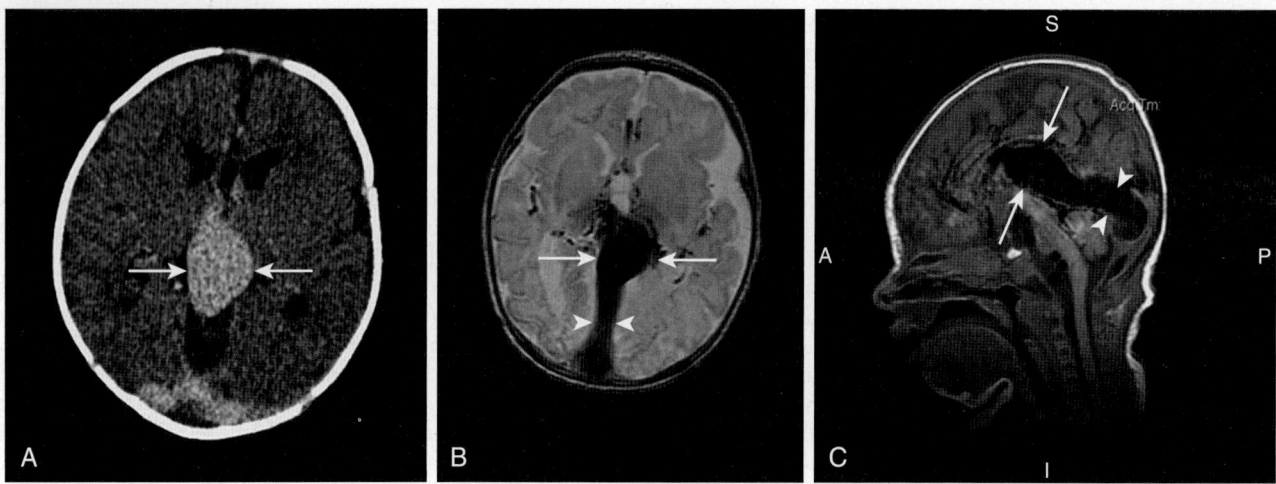

Fig. 63.13. Vein of Galen aneurysmal malformation (VGAM). (A) Axial noncontrast CT shows the dilated embryonic vein *(arrows)*. Axial T2 (B) and sagittal T1 (C) MRI demonstrates the dilated embryonic vein *(arrows)* and the draining vein *(arrowheads)*.

also Chapter 70). The appearance will depend on the cell type infected and the host immune response. Infection can involve the subarachnoid spaces and meninges, the parameningeal spaces, or the brain parenchyma itself either primarily or secondarily. With bacterial meningitis the appearance on CT and MRI may range from normal to diffuse swelling with loss of gray-white differentiation and obliteration of ventricular and cisternal CSF spaces. Coxsackie virus, echovirus, and mumps infect the meninges more than the neurons, whereas poliovirus infects the neurons, particularly the motor neurons. Herpes simplex virus type I has a predilection for the limbic system, most commonly affects the temporal lobes, and is the most common sporadic viral encephalitis.[37] Herpes simplex virus type II encephalitis is most commonly acquired at birth and does not display a predilection for the temporal lobes. Although MRI is more sensitive than CT, a normal MRI still does not entirely exclude viral encephalitis. In the clinical setting of suspected meningeal infection, CT may be indicated prior to lumbar puncture to exclude hydrocephalus or swelling that potentially would preclude lumbar puncture without neurosurgical consultation.

Imaging alone should not be used, however, to exclude meningeal infection. Particularly early in the setting of meningitis, contrast-enhanced CT is often normal. Although MRI with gadolinium is more sensitive, only 55% to 70% of persons with proved meningitis have abnormal CT or MRI scans.[38] Some investigators believe that CSF hyperintensity on the FLAIR sequence is more sensitive than gadolinium-enhanced T1-weighted sequence for meningitis; however, CSF hyperintensity on FLAIR associated with supplemental oxygen and anesthesia as well as noninfectious meningeal irritation and leptomeningeal tumor render this finding less specific.[39,40]

Complications associated with meningeal infection include compromise of the BBB leading to vasogenic edema, arterial spasm that can cause ischemia with cytotoxic edema and eventual infarction, and hydrocephalus potentially with the development of transependymal CSF flow/interstitial edema. Hydrocephalus can be obstructive, typically at the level of the aqueduct (Fig. 63.14) or outlet of the fourth ventricle, or more commonly communicating because of impaired CSF resorption from arachnoid granulation obstruction with exudates.

This impairment of CSF resorption can become permanent because of leptomeningeal-ependymal fibrosis and require shunting. Ultrasound can be used in very young patients; otherwise, CT and more recently half Fourier acquisition single shot turbo spin echo (HASTE) or other rapid, heavily T2-weighted MRI sequences usually are used to follow ventricular dilation. A primary role for imaging in meningitis is to evaluate for these complications. Two patterns of abnormal meningeal enhancement are seen on MRI with meningitis. A pachymeningeal pattern appears as diffuse linear thickening of the normal dural lining. This appearance, however, is not specific because the same pattern can be seen in other settings, including after surgery and occasionally following shunt revision, in some cases because of intracranial hypotension. The other pattern is a leptomeningeal enhancement, where enhancement is seen along the pia-arachnoid membranes, following the sulcal grooves. This pattern also is not specific, with a similar appearance being seen at times with leptomeningeal spread of tumor.

Extraaxial collections can develop in association with meningitis, including subdural effusions and, less commonly, subdural abscesses or empyema. Effusions are crescentic collections that typically are isodense to CSF on CT and isointense to CSF on most MRI sequences, although because the protein level may be increased, the collections may be hyperintense on T1 and FLAIR (Fig. 63.15). Subdural abscesses can be crescentic or lentiform when larger and typically slightly denser than CSF on CT. A rim of enhancement of variable thickness is generally better detected on MRI (Fig. 63.16). DWI can demonstrate restricted diffusion in subdural empyemas. Subdural (and brain) abscess also can occur as a direct extension of paranasal sinus or mastoid infection.

Infection of the brain parenchyma can take the form of a focal abscess(es) or a more diffuse encephalitis. Encephalitis in isolation or associated with meningitis generally will produce nonspecific cerebral parenchymal changes or cerebritis that appear bright on T2 and FLAIR sequences. Differentiation of cerebritis from ischemic changes associated with meningoencephalitis by imaging is problematic, especially because cerebritis also can demonstrate restricted diffusion. Areas of cerebritis evolve into focal abscesses that will

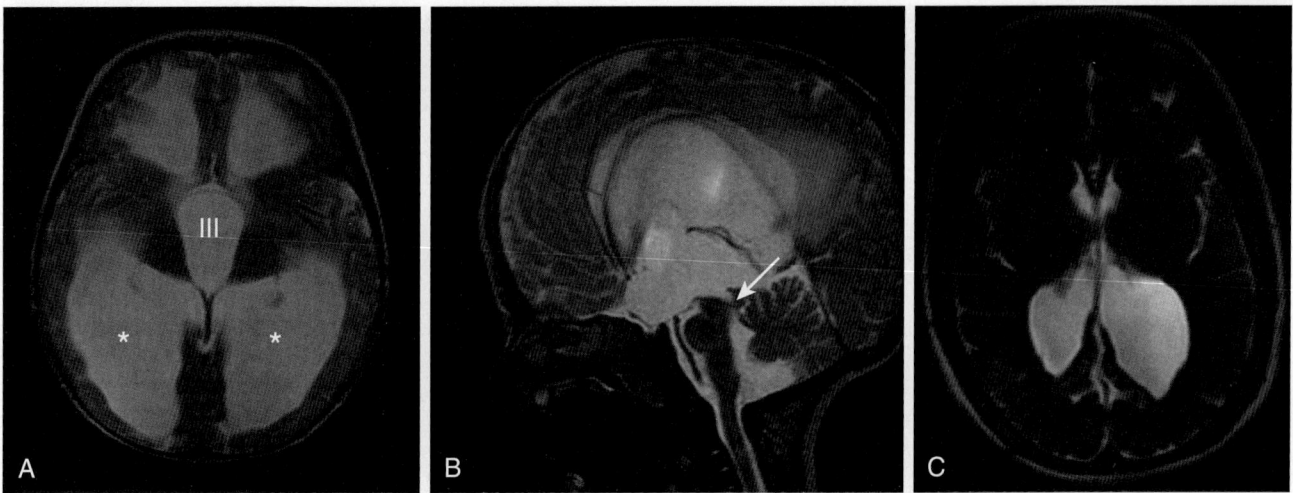

Fig. 63.14. Obstructive hydrocephalus. Axial (A) and midline sagittal (B) T2 MRI shows dilated lateral *(asterisks)* and third *(III)* ventricles that result from aqueductal obstruction *(arrow)*. (C) Chiari II malformation with hydrocephalus. Image demonstrates utility of heavily T2-weighted, half-Fourier acquisition, single-shot, turbo spin-echo MRI in evaluation of ventricles. Sequence can be obtained rapidly without the need for sedation; this avoids the radiation associated with repeated CT scans.

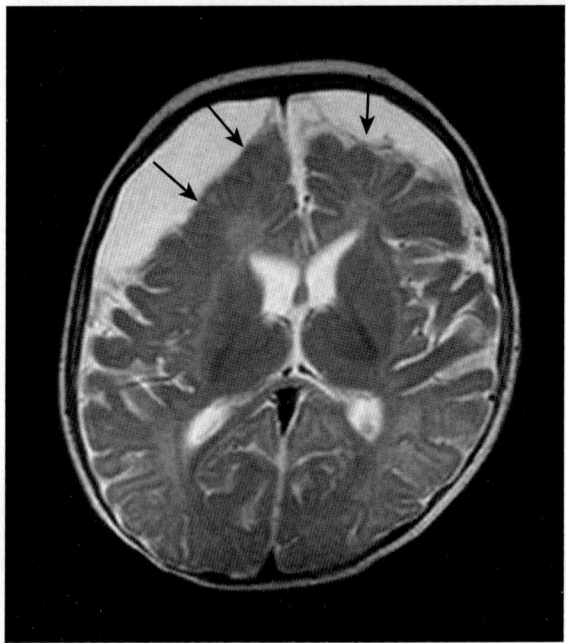

Fig. 63.15. Chronic subdural effusions following meningitis. Axial T2-weighted MRI shows mass effect with sulcal compression associated with bifrontal subdural collections *(arrows))*. Note that these subdural collections can be differentiated from enlarged subarachnoid spaces because the latter would have bridging vessels crossing the CSF in the subarachnoid spaces.

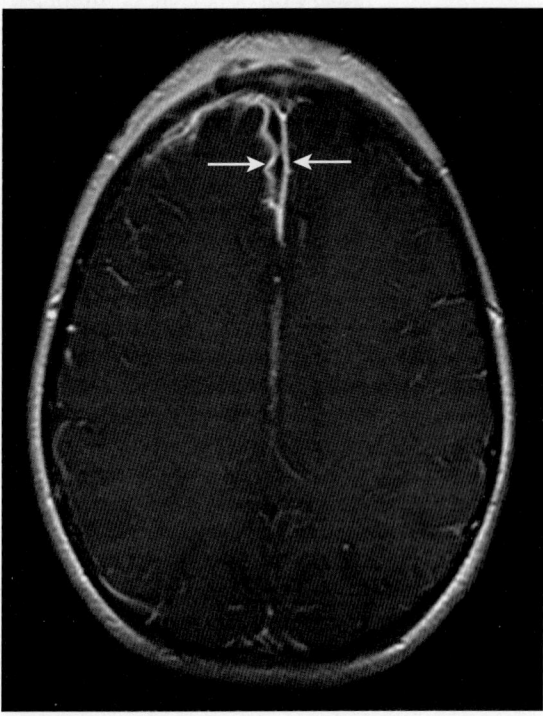

Fig. 63.16. Subdural abscess or subdural empyema. Axial T1-weighted MRI with gadolinium demonstrates a small rim-enhancing right frontal paramedian subdural abscess *(arrows)*. This area was restricted on DWI (not shown).

generally demonstrate a central focus of low density on CT and low T1, high T2, and FLAIR signal on MRI, with a ring of enhancement and variable surrounding edema (Fig. 63.17). More commonly in adults with a ring-enhancing lesion, there can be uncertainty between a brain abscess and necrotic tumor. The brain abscess generally will have a thinner rim of enhancement, and on DWI a pyogenic abscess will demonstrate restricted diffusion. The necrotic tumor often shows a thick, irregular rim with increased diffusion or T2

shine-through. In differentiating pyogenic, tubercular, and fungal abscesses, some studies have described a greater likelihood of homogeneous diffusion restriction with pyogenic and tubercular abscesses but a variable pattern with fungal abscesses.[41,42] Exclusion of a meningeal or parameningeal abscess in the head can be accomplished largely with contrast-enhanced CT, looking for a fluid collection with a surrounding enhancing rim, although occasionally a small collection may be missed on CT but detected by MRI. Evaluation for

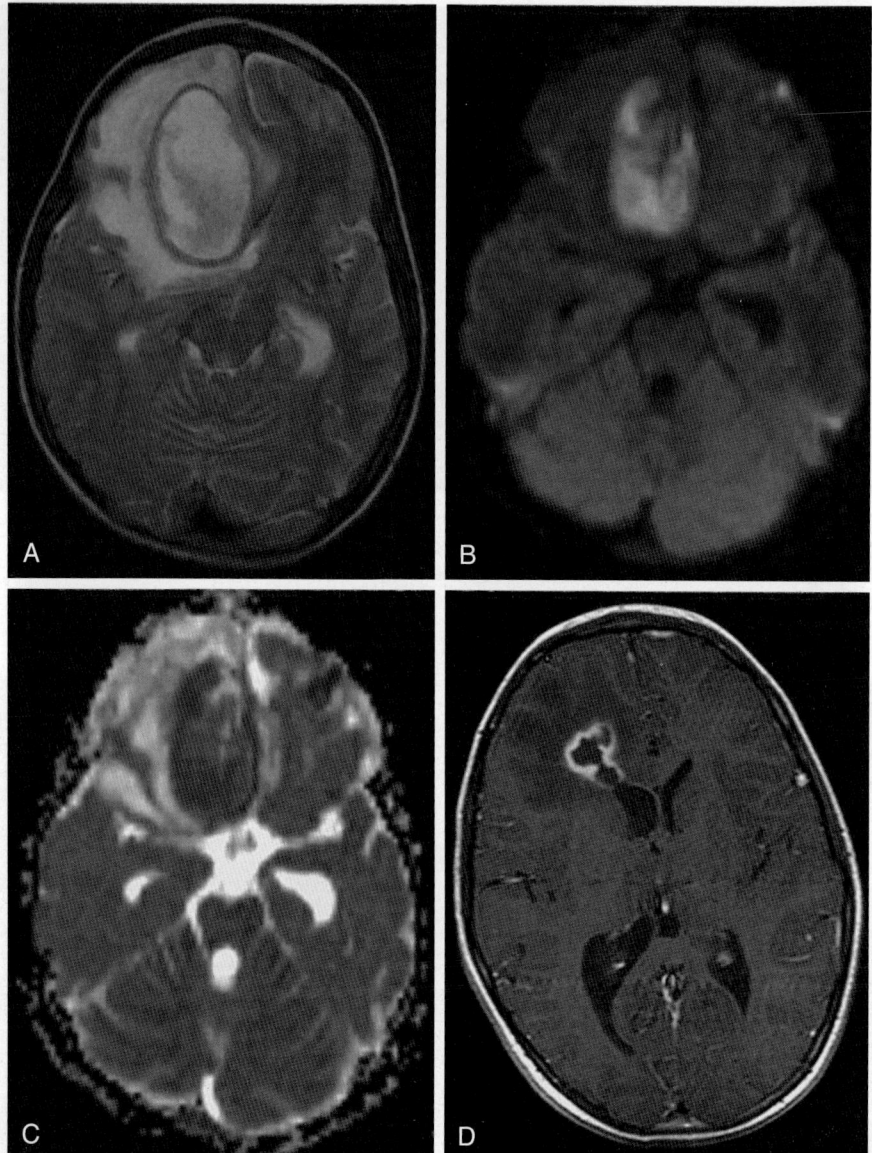

Fig. 63.17. Frontal brain abscesses. Axial T2-weighted MRI (A) demonstrates a right frontal ring-enhancing lesion with a T2 hypointense capsule that has considerable surrounding vasogenic edema and leftward midline shift. The lesion is bright on diffusion (B) and dark on the apparent diffusion coefficient map (C), suggesting that it is diffusion restricted. (D) In another patient, axial postcontrast T1-weighted MR image demonstrates a right frontal periventricular ring-enhancing lesion with T1 hypointense vasogenic edema surrounding it.

meningeal or parameningeal abscess in the spine should be approached with MRI.

Demyelinating Disease

Multiple sclerosis (MS) is much less common in children than in adults, whereas ADEM primarily occurs in children. ADEM can at times manifest with symmetric involvement of central gray matter (Fig. 63.18), with an imaging picture that overlaps with some metabolic diseases. In other cases of ADEM, lesions, typically in the cerebral white matter, can be scattered with a picture similar to vasculitis or embolic infarction. The appearance of MS and ADEM can be similar, though some features such as the perivenule orientation (Dawson fingers) of lesions are more characteristic of MS. The presence of lesions of multiple ages would be consistent with MS (Fig. 63.19) rather than ADEM. Demyelinating lesions are seen most commonly in

white matter but appear in gray matter as well. Acute demyelinating lesions demonstrate enhancement. Acute lesions also can demonstrate restricted diffusion, with an appearance on DWI that mimics an acute ischemic lesion. Often, however, the pattern of involvement is useful in distinguishing demyelinating disease from ischemic disease. The spinal cord can be involved with MS or ADEM (Fig. 63.20), although relatively rarely in isolation, hence imaging the brain to look for additional involvement can be useful in some cases to distinguish between a cord demyelinating process and infarct, which can have a similar imaging appearance.

Trauma

CT remains the primary imaging modality in persons with acute cerebral trauma and has the advantage of relative ease of scanning compared with MRI, including speed of scanning and allowing non-MRI compatible monitoring and life support equipment to be used during imaging (discussed in Chapter 119). CT is usually sufficient for evaluation of most cerebral trauma requiring intervention, including assessment of swelling and acute hemorrhage within the intraaxial and extraaxial compartments. CT is generally more sensitive than MRI in detecting acute SAH and in the evaluation of bony injury (Fig. 63.21). CT is generally sufficient to detect cerebral swelling associated with herniation syndromes and therefore identify the potential need for neurosurgical intervention (Fig. 63.22). MRI is more sensitive for the detection of parenchymal

injury and for more subtle extraaxial collections including more chronic subdural hematomas, a hallmark of inflicted traumatic brain injury associated with child abuse. MRI is indicated when there is doubt as to the presence of a subdural blood collection in the setting of suspected trauma. Also, in the setting of inflicted traumatic brain injury, MRI can detect evidence of old parenchymal or extraaxial hemorrhage not seen with CT using the GRE sequence (see Fig. 63.5D). In particular, gradient sequences and susceptibility-weighted imaging can reveal evidence of old parenchymal hemorrhages. Bony injury of the spine also is better evaluated with CT, although cord compression and injury are better assessed with MRI.

Hydrocephalus

Hydrocephalus can be congenital or caused by hemorrhage, tumor, and meningitis. In the neonatal period, ultrasound is used as a screening tool in evaluating for ventricular enlargement, in particular associated with germinal matrix hemorrhage. Beyond this period, most monitoring of ventricular size and shunts is accomplished with CT. Rapidly acquired heavily T2-weighted half Fourier acquisition single shot turbo spin echo MRI sequences have been used in the evaluation of hydrocephalus. These sequences can be obtained as individual slices in as little as 12 seconds on a 3.0 Tesla scanner and 19 seconds on a 1.5 Tesla scanner for the entire head and hence do not typically require patient sedation. Use of this technique offsets the radiation burden of repeated CT scans. In the initial evaluation of hydrocephalus, MRI can be helpful in determining the level and possible cause of CSF obstruction (see Fig. 63.14). Acute hydrocephalus can be associated with evidence of transependymal CSF flow across the walls of the ventricular system, better appreciated on MRI. The absence of this appearance, however, does not reliably predict the absence of increased pressure. Physiologic/functional evaluation of shunt patency is achieved with nuclear medicine shunt studies, as described previously.

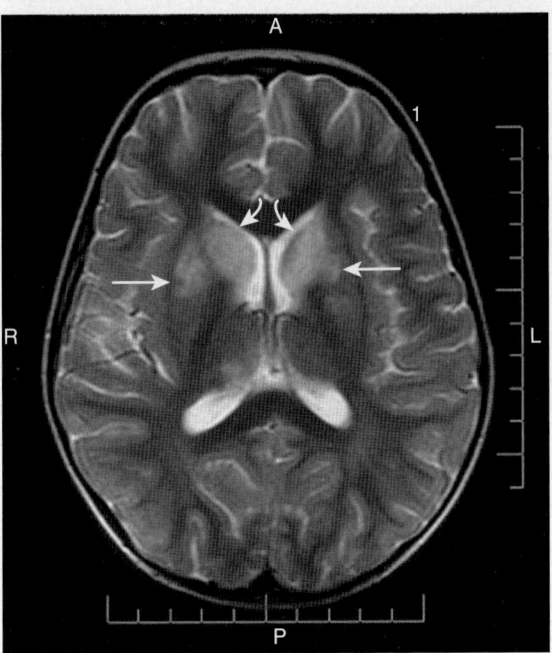

Fig. 63.18. ADEM. Axial T2-weighted MR image shows symmetric increased signal in the head of the caudate nucleus *(curved arrows)* and anterior lentiform nuclei *(straight arrows)* associated with ADEM.

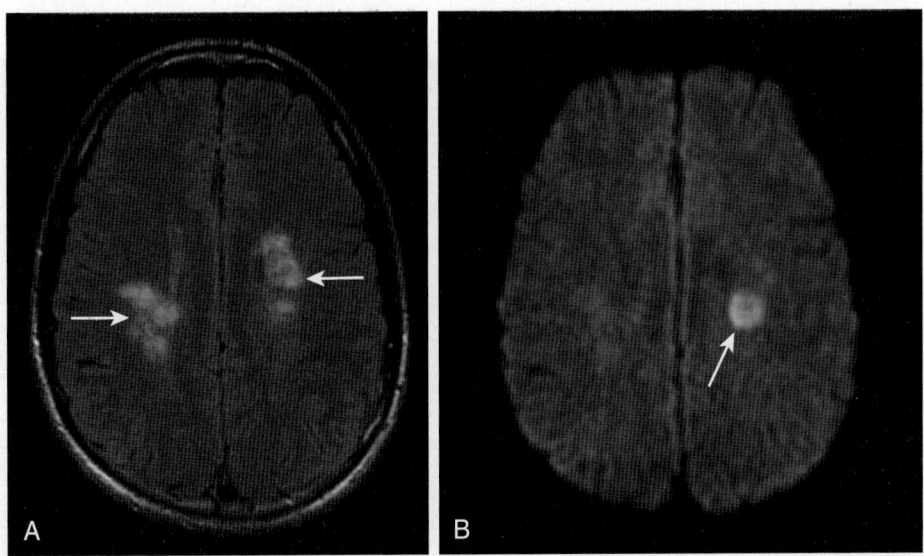

Fig. 63.19. Multiple sclerosis in a 16-year-old child. (A) FLAIR MRI shows bilateral white matter lesions *(arrows)*. (B) DWI demonstrates restriction of the left centrum semiovale lesion that was enhanced on postcontrast T1 MRI (not shown), suggesting an acute or active lesion *(arrow)*.

Tumor

Cerebral tumors are best imaged with MRI (Fig. 63.23). Expedited evaluation of a cerebral mass can be accomplished in the acute setting with CT, which will demonstrate the degree of mass effect and any impending herniation or midline shift. Posterior fossa tumors, which are more common in children and occur more often than supratentorial tumors in the 4- to 11-year age group,[43] and suspected acute spinal cord abnormalities, possibly associated with tumor, are best evaluated with MRI. CT is hampered by beam hardening artifact in the posterior fossa, at the skull base, and within the spinal canal.

Seizures

The CT imaging yield for a single self-limited seizure with no focal neurologic deficit is low, although most children

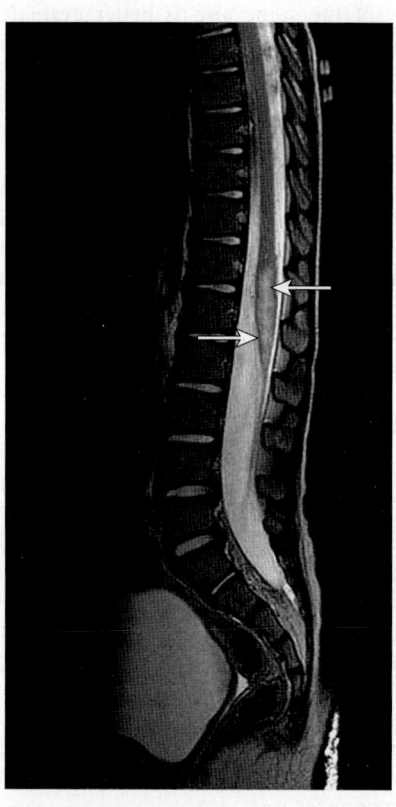

Fig. 63.20. Patient with clinical picture of transverse myelitis. Sagittal T2-weighted MRI of the distal cord shows central T2 hyperintensity within the conus medullaris *(arrows)* in this case of ADEM. An acute spinal cord infarct also could have this imaging appearance.

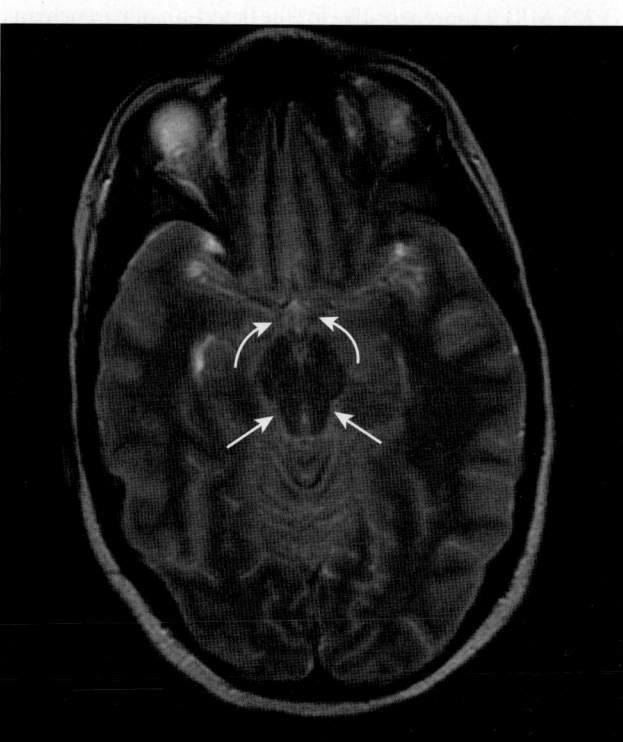

Fig. 63.22. Diffuse brain edema with herniation. T2-weighted MRI shows diffuse cerebral swelling with effacement of cerebrospinal fluid spaces associated with the ambient *(straight arrows)* and suprasellar cisterns *(curved arrows)*.

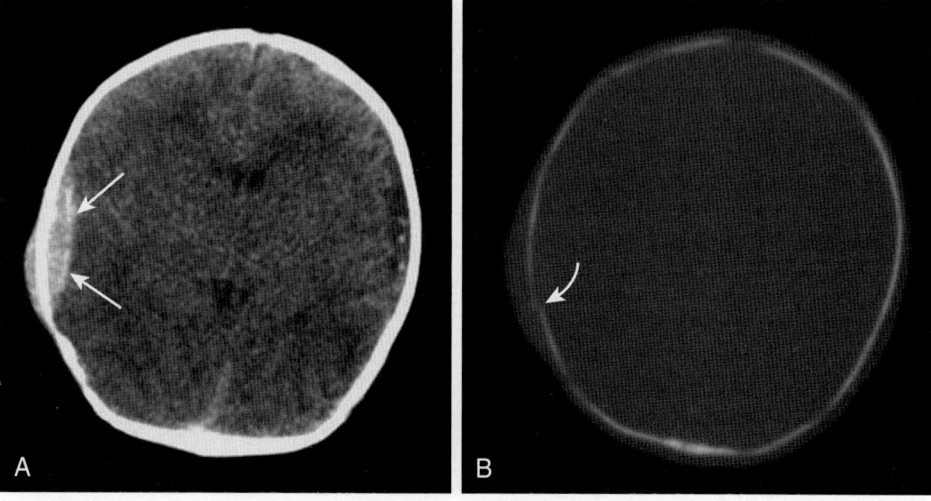

Fig. 63.21. Epidural hematoma with skull fracture. A CT scan in brain (A) and bone (B) windows shows the typical lentiform configuration of right-sided epidural hematoma *(arrows)*. The bone window reveals an associated fracture *(curved arrow)*.

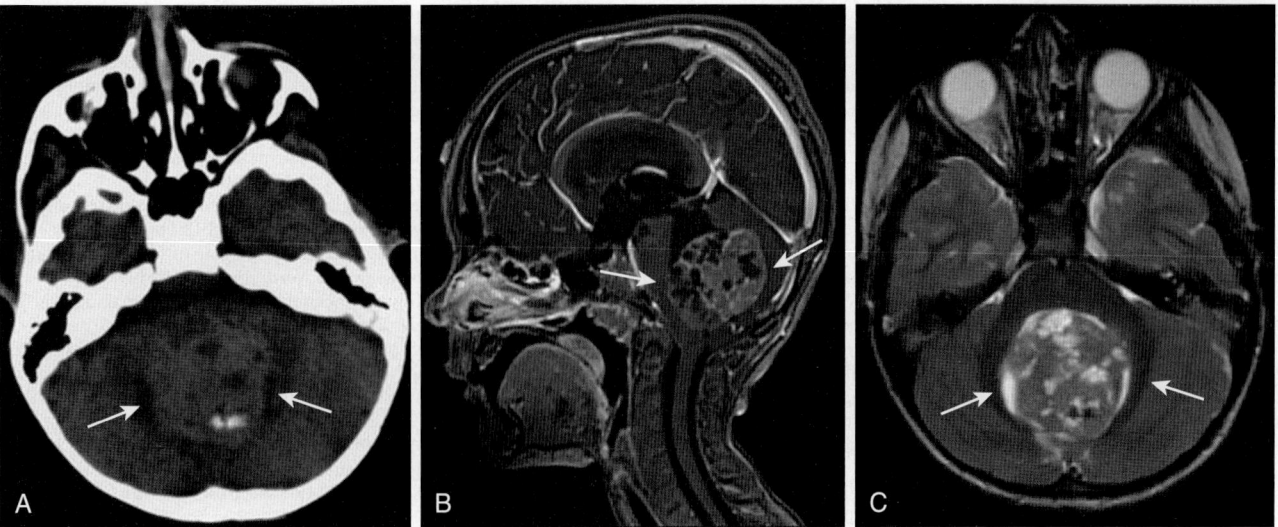

Fig. 63.23. Posterior fossa medulloblastoma. Axial noncontrast CT (A) and sagittal T1-weighted MRI with gadolinium (B) show a midline posterior fossa mass that has heterogeneous enhancement on postcontrast T1 and heterogeneous signal on axial T2-weighted MRI (C).

currently will ultimately be scanned with CT or MRI. With focal neurologic deficit or prolonged seizure activity, the imaging yield increases. As discussed in Chapter 67, after seizures are controlled, MRI is indicated in the absence of a clinically apparent etiology for the seizures. Acute abnormalities on MRI, however, may be secondary to rather than reflecting the underlying cause of seizures. Prolonged seizures can be associated with transient enhancement due to BBB disruption and cytotoxic edema with hyperintensity on DWI that may be confused with stroke. Positron emission tomography can also be used to identify epileptogenic foci by identifying areas of hypermetabolism.

Conclusion

The ultimate selection of imaging modality will depend on clinical question(s), age and condition of the patient, and the locally available imaging technology. Consultation with radiology colleagues is encouraged, and discussion of the clinical scenario and suspicions yields an appropriately tailored imaging protocol and a more relevant interpretation, which is becoming increasingly important with the ever-increasing complexity of imaging modalities.

References

1. Lowe LH, Bulas DI. Transcranial Doppler imaging in children: sickle cell screening and beyond. *Pediatr Radiol.* 2005;35:54-65.
2. Soetaert AM, Lowe LH, Formen C. Pediatric cranial Doppler sonography in children: non-sickle cell applications. *Curr Probl Diagn Radiol.* 2009; 38:218-227.
3. Rasulo FA, De Peri E, Lavinio A. Transcranial Doppler ultrasonography in intensive care. *Eur J Anaesthesiol Suppl.* 2008;42:167-173.
4. Adams RJ. Big strokes in small persons. *Arch Neurol.* 2007;64:1567-1574.
5. Mendichovszky IA, Marks SD, Simcock CM, et al. Gadolinium and nephrogenic systemic fibrosis: time to tighten practice. *Pediatr Radiol.* 2008; 38:489-496.
6. Romero JM, Schaefer PW, Grant PE, et al. Diffusion MR imaging of acute ischemic stroke. *Neuroimaging Clin North Am.* 2002;12:35-53.
7. Mascalchi M, Filippi M, Floris R, et al. Diffusion-weighted MR of the brain: methodology and clinical application. *Radiol Med.* 2005; 109:155-197.
8. Chen J, Licht DJ, Smith SE, et al. Arterial spin labeling perfusion MRI in pediatric arterial ischemic stroke: initial experiences. *J Magn Reson Imaging.* 2009;29:282-290.
9. van den Tweel XW, Nederveen AJ, Majoie CB, et al. Cerebral blood flow measurement in children with sickle cell disease using continuous arterial spin labeling at 3.0-Tesla MRI. *Stroke.* 2009;40:795-800.
10. Saneto RP, Friedman SD, Shaw DW. Neuroimaging of mitochondrial disease. *Mitochondrion.* 2008;8:396-413.
11. Tomandl BF, Kostner NC, Schempershofe M, et al. CT angiography of intracranial aneurysms: a focus on postprocedures. *Radiographics.* 2004; 24:637-655.
12. Cloft HJ, Joseph GJ, Dion JE. Risk of cerebral angiography in patients with subarachnoid hemorrhage, cerebral aneurysm, and arteriovenous malformation: a meta-analysis. *Stroke.* 1999;30:317-320.
13. Willinsky RA, Taylor SM, TerBrugge K, et al. Neurologic complications of cerebral angiography: prospective analysis of 2,899 procedures and review of the literature. *Radiology.* 2003;227:522-528.
14. DeBillon T, Nguyen S, Muet A, et al. Limitations of ultrasonography for diagnosing white matter damage in preterm infants. *Arch Dis Child Fetal Neonatal Ed.* 2003;88:F275-F279.
15. Ment MR, Bada HS, Barnes P, et al. Practice parameter: neuroimaging of the neonate. *Neurology.* 2002;58:1726-1738.
16. Allison JW, Seibert JJ. Transcranial Doppler in the newborn with asphyxia. *Neuroimaging Clin N Am.* 1999;9:11-16.
17. Kashman N, Kramer U, Stavorovsky Z, et al. Prognostic significance of hyperechogenic lesions in the basal ganglia and thalamus in neonates. *J Child Neurol.* 2001;16:591-594.
18. Ilves P, Lintrop M, Metsvaht T, et al. Cerebral blood-flow velocities in predicting outcome of asphyxiated newborn infants. *Acta Paediatr.* 2004;93:523-528.
19. Nishimaki S, Iwasaki S, Minamisawa S, et al. Blood flow velocities in the anterior cerebral artery and basilar artery in asphyxiated infants. *J Ultrasound Med.* 2008;27:955-960.
20. Kucinski T. Unenhanced CT and acute stroke physiology. *Neuroimaging Clin North Am.* 2005;15:397-407, xi-xii.
21. Krishnamoorthy KS, Soman TB, Takeoka M, et al. Diffusion-weighted imaging in neonatal cerebral infarction: clinical utility and follow-up. *J Child Neurol.* 2000;15:592-602.
22. Boichot C, Walker PM, Durand C, et al. Term neonate prognoses after perinatal asphyxia: contributions of MR imaging, MR spectroscopy, relaxation times, and apparent diffusion coefficients. *Radiology.* 2006; 239:839-848.
23. Schaefer PW, Grant PE, Gonzalez RG. Diffusion-weighted MR imaging of the brain. *Radiology.* 2000;217:331-345.

24. Qiao M, Malisza KL, Del Bigio MR, et al. Correlation of cerebral hypoxic-ischemic T2 changes with tissue alterations in water content and protein extravasation. *Stroke*. 2000;32:958-963.

25. Qiao M, Latta P, Meng S, et al. Development of acute edema following cerebral hypoxia-ischemia in neonatal compared with juvenile rats using magnetic resonance imaging. *Pediatr Res*. 2004;55:101-106.

26. Grandin CB, Duprez TP, Smith AM, et al. Which MR-derived perfusion parameters are the best predictors of infarct growth in hyperacute stroke? Comparative study between relative and quantitative measurements. *Radiology*. 2002;223:361-370.

27. Barkovich AJ, Baranski K, Vigneron D, et al. Proton MR spectroscopy for the evaluation of brain injury in asphyxiated, term neonates. *AJNR Am J Neuroradiol*. 1999;20:1399-1405.

28. Provenzale JM, Jahan R, Naidich TP, et al. Assessment of the patient with hyperacute stroke: imaging and therapy. *Radiology*. 2003;229:347-359.

29. van Laar PJ, Hendrikse J, Golay X, et al. In vivo flow territory mapping of major brain feeding arteries. *Neuroimage*. 2006;29:136-144.

30. Jordan LC, Johnston SC, Wu YW, et al. The importance of cerebral aneurysms in childhood hemorrhagic stroke: a population-based study. *Stroke*. 2009;40:400-405.

31. Lamy C, Oppenheim C, Meder JF, et al. Neuroimaging in posterior reversible encephalopathy syndrome. *J Neuroimaging*. 2004;14:89-96.

32. Stott VL, Hurrell MA, Anderson TJ. Reversible posterior leukoencephalopathy syndrome: a misnomer reviewed. *Intern Med J*. 2005;35:83-90.

33. Cooney MJ, Bradley WG, Symko SC, et al. Hypertensive encephalopathy: complication in children treated for myeloproliferative disorders—report of three cases. *Radiology*. 2000;214:711-716.

34. Wasserman BA, Stone JH, Hellmann DB, et al. Reliability of normal findings on MR imaging for excluding the diagnosis of vasculitis of the central nervous system. *AJR Am J Roentgenol*. 2001;177:455-459.

35. Cloft HJ, Phillips CD, Dix JE, et al. Correlation of angiography and MR imaging in cerebral vasculitis. *Acta Radiol*. 1999;40:83-87.

36. Mitchell PJ, Rosenfeld JV, Dargaville P, et al. Endovascular management of vein of Galen aneurysmal malformations presenting in the neonatal period. *Am J Neuroradiol*. 2001;22:1403-1409.

37. Lo CP, Chen CY. Neuroimaging of viral infections in infants and young children. *Neuroimaging Clin North Am*. 2008;18:119-132.

38. Kanamalla US, Ibarra RA, Jinkins JR. Imaging of cranial meningitis and ventriculitis. *Neuroimaging Clin North Am*. 2000;10:309-331.

39. Girard N, Confort-Gouny S, Schneider J, et al. Neuroimaging of neonatal encephalopathies. *J Neuroradiol*. 2007;34:167-182.

40. Frigon C, Jardine DS, Weinberger E, et al. Fraction of inspired oxygen in relation to cerebrospinal fluid hyperintensity on FLAIR MR imaging of the brain in children and young adults undergoing anesthesia. *AJR Am J Roentgenol*. 2002;179:791.

41. Luthra G, Parihar A, Nath K, et al. Comparative evaluation of fungal, tubercular, and pyogenic brain abscesses with conventional and diffusion MR imaging and proton MR spectroscopy. *Am J Neuroradiol*. 2007;28:1332-1338.

42. Mueller-Mang C, Castillo M, Mang TG, et al. Fungal versus bacterial brain abscesses: is diffusion-weighted MR imaging a useful tool in the differential diagnosis? *Neuroradiology*. 2007;49:651-657.

43. Luh GY, Bird CR. Imaging of brain tumor in the pediatric population. *Neuroimaging Clin North Am*. 1999;9:691-716.

Pediatric Neurocritical Care

Michael J. Bell and Mark S. Wainwright

PEARLS

- Neurologic morbidity represents a major determinant of outcome among critically ill children. However, therapies that target specific cellular mechanisms of brain injury in children are lacking.
- Evidence that adult neurocritical care is a viable program in many centers largely rests with its widespread implementation. Such programs have demonstrated an association between their services and improved outcomes.
- Pediatric neurocritical care is no longer a new concept, and there are now published examples of approaches to its implementation and evolving evidence indicating that a neurocritical care service improves outcome.

Neurologic morbidity is a major determinant of outcome in critically ill children,[1] but therapies that target specific cellular mechanisms of brain injury in children with (for example) stroke, refractory seizures, or traumatic brain injury (TBI) are lacking. In the absence of data from randomized controlled trials, much of the clinical practice in the care of children with acute brain injuries or neurologic complications of critical illness is empiric. Moreover, the heterogeneity of disorders and subtleties of the clinical neurologic exam in the critically ill child are often beyond the scope of training for pediatric critical care, neurology, and neurosurgery programs. In response to these challenges, efforts have been made to develop programs to care for children with critical neurologic conditions with teams of dedicated specialists, generally pediatric intensivists and neurologists. These programs, called pediatric neurocritical care programs at present, depend on the ability of dedicated staff members to focus much (if not all) of their clinical and research endeavors toward common or uncommon neurologic conditions in order to improve outcomes for this vulnerable population of children.

This chapter (1) describes the evolution of pediatric neurocritical care as a clinical paradigm from a historical perspective, (2) outlines several rationales for embarking on this new organization of clinical care, and (3) describes challenges for the future development of the discipline. Throughout this chapter and for simplicity, the phrase *adult neurocritical care program* will be used to describe neurocritical care programs developed to treat adults with neurologic disorders. This chapter will *not* review neurocritical care disorders or pathophysiologic principles, such as status epilepticus or the management of intracranial pressure, as these are comprehensively reviewed in other chapters of this text. However, studies of neurocritical care disorders that serve to argue for the further development of a neurocritical care focus in pediatric critical care will be discussed.

Historical Context

Advances in medical care have emerged either as a result of tectonic shifts of the mantel of the health care system or by incremental shifts of the landscape. As an example, military conflicts have contributed to cataclysmic changes in health care, from the development of lifesaving trauma surgical techniques (from the US Civil War to the current conflicts) to the development of effective triage systems for evacuating and treating wounded soldiers (culminating in improved systems developed during World War II through the Korean and Vietnam conflicts).[2] As a specialty, critical care medicine was a product of yet another seismic blast to the health care system—the polio epidemics that raged throughout Europe and the United States in the late 1940s and early 1950s. Advances in ventilation allowed survival from this debilitating affliction, culminating in the organization of the first intensive care unit at the Baltimore City Hospital in 1961 that was staffed by in-house physicians[3] (see also Chapter 1). The director of this first multidisciplinary intensive care unit was Dr. Peter Safar, a founding father of cerebral protection from cardiac arrest who advanced the field of neuroprotection for the duration of his career.

The subspecialty of neurologic critical care has evolved in a more gradual fashion compared to the specialty overall. Dr. D.W. Dandy is credited with developing the first neurosurgical intensive care unit for three patients at the Johns Hopkins Hospital in Baltimore in 1929, whereas the first fully staffed, large-scale neurocritical care unit was formed in 1969 at the University of Colorado by Dr. Michael Earnest.[4] Gradually, similar neurologic critical care units were established in many universities and tertiary care centers, paralleling the development of other subspecialty intensive care units (ICUs) for coronary, cardiovascular, surgical, pulmonary, and other conditions. Currently, neurologic critical care units can be further subdivided in many centers into neurotrauma, neurovascular, neurosurgical, and other specialties. In 2002, several dozen practicing neurointensivists formed the Neurocritical Care Society (with membership now numbering greater than 800) and held its first annual meeting in February 2003. In 2007 the United Council on Neurological Subspecialties offered the first examination in neurocritical care and accredited fellowship programs across the United States.

For pediatrics, caring for neurologically injured children was always at the forefront in establishing critical care programs. In their landmark paper from 1975, Downes and Raphaely[5] begin by writing, "The major objective of intensive care is to provide maximum surveillance and support of vital systems in patients with acute, but reversible life-threatening disease. In pediatric patients, the reversal of life-threatening conditions and preservation of essential functions, especially those of the brain, may result in many years of useful life." During this time, Reye syndrome epidemics were commonly afflicting previously healthy children, and intensive neuroprotective measures were employed with increasing success to restore full neurologic function.[6]

These early years of pediatric critical care led to many advances including (1) management of respiratory failure (eg, the advent of surfactant for respiratory distress syndrome),[7,8] high-frequency oscillatory ventilation,[9] permissive hypercapnia, inhaled nitric oxide,[10] and extracorporeal membrane oxygenation (ECMO)[11]; (2) management of congenital heart diseases including palliative surgery (eg, Blalock-Taussig shunts[12] and the Norwood procedure),[13] definitive repair (eg, the arterial switch procedure for transposition of the great vessels[14] and the Fontan procedure),[15] and supportive care (eg, cardiopulmonary bypass[16,17] and ventricular-assist devices)[18,19]; (3) therapies for sepsis (eg, goal-directed resuscitation therapy[20] and the development of new antibiotics); and (4) supportive therapies for failing organs (eg, extracorporal life support, hemofiltration, hemodialysis, continuous renal replacement therapy, plasmapheresis/plasma exchange, and organ transplantation). The culmination of these and many other clinical advances have led to decreases in mortality in most pediatric critical care units to between 3% and 5%.

With this impressive reduction in mortality, the necessary next step in improving clinical care for critically ill children is to minimize morbidity. It is in this context that pediatric neurocritical care has emerged, as neurologic morbidity was seen as one of the greatest challenges to advancement of the field. In 2000 Dr. Robert Tasker[21] was among the first to write about a conceptual framework of multiple neurologic conditions that might benefit from particular expertise within pediatric neurocritical care when he provided an evidenced-based summary of three important neurologic conditions of critically ill children: the management of severe head injury, the use of benzodiazepines to treat status epilepticus, and the emergence of new forms of encephalopathies in children. In the intervening years, various groups have argued for the introduction of pediatric neurocritical care within the specialty of pediatric critical care medicine. The remainder of this chapter examines the various rationales for advancing pediatric neurocritical care programs and possible future directions for this effort.

Rationales for Development of Pediatric Neurocritical Care

Rationale 1: Sufficient Numbers of Children With Critical Neurologic Conditions Exist to Justify the Establishment of a New Service Specifically for This Population of Children

An important question for the development of pediatric neurocritical care programs involves an assessment of whether there are enough patients to justify the formation of this type of clinical service. As stated earlier, adult neurocritical care units and programs have been in existence for years and have therefore answered this question in the affirmative. During their early period, Bleck and colleagues[22] surveyed admissions to their 14-bed, general medical intensive care unit and found that only 92 of 1850 admissions were related directly to neurologic conditions, mostly stroke and intracerebral hemorrhages. However, they found 217 patients experienced neurologic complications during the admission, including hypoxic/ischemic encephalopathy, seizures, metabolic encephalopathy, and stroke. A more recent analysis demonstrated that brain tumors, strokes, and subarachnoid hemorrhages accounted for more than 50% of admissions to neurocritical care units,[23] but the absolute number of admissions was not reported. In the intervening years, thrombolytic therapy for ischemic stroke, neurovascular procedures for aneurysmal subarachnoid hemorrhage, and the advent of comprehensive TBI and stroke teams have increased the need for intensively cared for adults. The evidence that adult neurocritical care is a viable program in many centers largely rests with its widespread implementation. Although the absolute number of neurocritical care units has not been collated, the United Council of Neurological Subspecialties (UCNS) has certified 60 programs in the United States and more than 1200 diplomates in neurocritical care (see http://www.ucns.org/globals/axon/assets/10301.pdf).

The predominant pediatric experience in subspecialty critical care program development comes from pediatric cardiac intensive care. Large pediatric institutions—Children's Hospital of Boston, Children's Hospital of Philadelphia, and the Hospital for Sick Children in Toronto as some of many examples—have long histories of cardiac intensive care programs.[24] These programs are based on the philosophy that the multidisciplinary team of cardiac intensivists, cardiologists, cardiac surgeons, anesthesiologists, neonatologists, and specially trained nursing and ancillary staff can more effectively treat the unique pathophysiology encountered in the correction of congenital heart disease. The viability of these programs is generally related to the volume of congenital heart surgery cases referred into the institution, and patients admitted to the hospital on this service are generally located in a unique space outside of the general pediatric intensive care unit. As of 2004, there were 132 pediatric cardiac intensive care programs and 250 members of the Pediatric Cardiac Intensive Care Society (PCICS) (http://www.pcics.org), indicating that these types of programs have certainly been viable for many institutions.

Four pediatric academic centers with neurocritical care services have reported their experience and patient volumes. LaRovere and Riviello described developing a pediatric neurocritical care service at Children's Hospital of Boston.[25] In 2006 they reported that 557 neurocritical care consults were obtained over a multiyear period. Little information is provided about the disorders treated and the role of the pediatric neurocritical care team in patient management. Therefore, it is difficult to discern the precise difference between this effort and an active neurologic consult service. At Children's National Medical Center, a neurocritical care consulting service consisting of an intensivist, two neurologists, and the neurosurgical staff was formed within the framework of the pediatric intensive care unit (PICU).[26] This service was designed to improve collaboration between the services and implement evidence-based guidelines for the care of children with TBI, stroke, status epilepticus, and other neurologic disorders. In a 14-month period, 373 neurocritical care consults were obtained among 1423 patient admissions. Approximately two-thirds of the consults were obtained in children with primary neurologic diagnoses at PICU admission, but a substantial portion (34.1%) of the consults were obtained on children admitted with other medical/surgical conditions. The wide variety of diagnoses observed argued strongly that at least the three main specialties (intensivist, neurologist, and neurosurgeon) were required to make a comprehensive clinical team. Weaknesses of this study were the inability to determine if the consulting service led to improved outcomes for patients and lack of analysis on the financial viability of this model of care. A fully independent primary pediatric neurocritical care service staffed by intensivists with extensive neurologic experience began at the University of Pittsburgh in 2009. This service is staffed by attending physicians with experience in clinical or basic research in the field of neurologic injury. Within this service, children with neurosurgical and neurologic emergencies receive care, and protocol-driven research studies are conducted. At Ann & Robert H. Lurie Children's Hospital of Chicago, the neurocritical care service (comprising neurologists, an intensivist, and an advanced practice nurse) reported 1942 consultations over a 7-year period, constituting 19% of all PICU admissions.[27] Precise comparisons of patient volume across centers are not possible because reasons for neurologic consultations varied by institution. Overall the published pediatric experience suggests that 15% to 25% of children in the PICU may require evaluation by a neurocritical care service; however, these data are confounded by variations in institutional definitions of the criteria for mandatory or elective neurocritical care involvement.

Rationale 2: Development of Pediatric Neurocritical Care Programs Will Improve the Overall Outcome of Children Under Their Care

Any successful new program in critical care must lead to improved patient outcomes to justify changing existing approaches. At its basic level, improvements in mortality would provide the ultimate justification for such efforts, with concomitant decreases in neuropsychologic and neurologic morbidity also being important. Seminal work has indicated that adult or pediatric intensivist–led clinical teams are associated with improved outcome[28-31] and serve as models for future innovations in changes in care teams.

Adult neurocritical care programs have demonstrated an association between their services and outcomes in a variety of ways and for several medical disorders. In 2001 Mirski and colleagues[32] reported that admission to a "neuroscience intensive care unit" in a single institution was associated with improved outcome (decreased mortality and decreased length of stay) when compared to the similar institution prior to formation of this new ICU. On a larger scale, Diringer and colleagues[33] analyzed more than 1000 patients admitted with intracerebral hemorrhage from hospitals with and without neurocritical care programs. They found that patients admitted to hospitals without neurointensivists had a 3.4-fold increased risk of in-hospital mortality (OR 3.4; 1.65–7.6) after controlling for patient demographics, severity of intracranial

hemorrhage, and hospital size. Varelas and colleagues[34] demonstrated that patients with stroke also benefited from neurocritical care programs. Specifically, in prospectively studying 433 stroke patients (174 admitted prior to neurocritical care unit development, 259 after unit development), they found no difference in mortality between the groups but decreased length of stay across all stroke subgroups. Lastly, Josephson and colleagues[35] demonstrated that patients with subarachnoid hemorrhage treated in a neurocritical care setting had decreased length of ICU stay (12.4 days versus 10.9 days) and a decreased need for cerebrospinal fluid diversion (23% versus 11.5%) but no change in hospital mortality.

Data from the pediatric neurocritical care services at the University of Pittsburgh,[36] Northwestern University,[27] and from a national survey[37] suggest that critically ill children with primary CNS insults or neurologic complications of critical illness have a significantly increased risk for mortality compared to other children requiring ICU level of care. Neither of these groups reported the impact of their services on mortality. However, a landmark study from the Washington University St. Louis Pediatric Neurocritical Care Program showed that institution of its multidisciplinary neurocritical care service led to a significant reduction in mortality following severe TBI in children.[38] Other indirect evidence supporting the benefits of a protocol-driven, consistent approach to management of pediatric neurotrauma comes from a study examining the impact of adherence to Brain Trauma Foundation guidelines[39] for the management of severe pediatric TBI. In this study from five US centers, each 1% increase in adherence was associated with a 1% decrease in the change of poor functional outcome among survivors. Collectively, these findings suggest that, at least for severe TBI, a multidisciplinary, protocol-driven approach to management can significantly reduce mortality. Whether these findings apply to other pathologies is not known.

Importantly, there are no data that address the impact of any of the published pediatric experience with neurocritical care programs on long-term outcome and neurologic morbidity. It is clear from the authors' clinical experience at Pittsburgh and the precedent from studies of survivors of congenital heart disease[40] that identifying the true burden of neurologic morbidity after ICU discharge requires lengthy follow-up. Of the published pediatric neurocritical care programs only one currently includes long-term follow-up as part of the standard of care.[27]

Despite its significantly longer history, studies demonstrating improved mortality or morbidity after the institution of pediatric cardiac intensive care programs are limited. Data from an ICU survey linked to the Society of Thoracic Surgeons Congenital Heart Disease database did not find overall differences in mortality, ICU length of stay, or complications between 20,922 cardiac patients admitted to either a cardiac intensive care unit (CICU) or a traditional PICU.[40a] In moving forward, it will be important to demonstrate improvements in neurologic outcomes, which will be particularly challenging due to the variety of developmental stages of childhood. In assessing mortality, it will be important to avoid the limitations in the adult neurocritical care studies (comparison to historical controls) and to utilize expected mortality measured by standardized severity of illness measures (such as the Pediatric Risk of Mortality or other scoring systems).

Rationale 3: Advances in Care, Either Technologic or Experimental, Will Be Integrated More Effectively With a Pediatric Neurocritical Care Program Compared to the Standard Approach

Advances in the delivery of neurology-specific care, based on new technologies or standardized guidelines based on new evidence, continue at an increasing rate, and some have argued that this justifies a dedicated team of clinicians to provide such care. As outlined in other chapters within this text, the number of monitoring devices and technical advances for children with neurologic injuries continues to grow (see also Chapters 2, 66, and 67). Digitally acquired electroencephalograms (EEGs) and electronic interpretations that can be gleaned at the bedside in real-time, brain tissue oxygen catheters that provide second-to-second assessments of local cerebral oxygen tension, and noninvasive measures of regional brain saturations by near-infrared spectroscopy devices are now in routine use for children. Other techniques, including cerebral microdialysis and cerebral blood flow (CBF) devices (either catheters to assess local CBF or imaging studies to determine global CBF) are poised to be used in the coming years. Determining the correct combination of monitoring systems and implementing protocols to maximize their potential benefit and minimize possible harm are daunting challenges that all practitioners will face in the coming years. Suarez[41] proposed this argument as a justification for the widespread adoption of adult neurocritical services, and Chang[42] used it to support the development of pediatric cardiac intensive care programs.

Evidence-based guidelines for several neurologic disorders of children continue to emerge, and effective integration of these guidelines, along with technologic advances, into clinical practice in critically ill children will be an important challenge for clinicians. As examples, (1) the Brain Trauma Foundation published guidelines for the management of children after TBI in 2003 and these were revised in 2012,[43] (2) the American Heart Association published guidelines for caring for children after stroke (including the use of antithrombotic therapies),[44] (3) the American Academy of Neurology published a practice parameter to recommend treatment guidelines for children with status epilepticus,[45] and (4) the American Heart Association published guidelines on cardiopulmonary resuscitation and emergency cardiovascular care for children and neonates that includes opinions regarding the neuroprotective strategy of hypothermia.[46-48] All of these general guidelines have important consequences for caring for the critically ill child, and successful incorporation of these recommendations into clinical protocols within the ICU will be an important step in optimizing care.

Several clinical studies also outline the importance of rigorously controlled neuroprotective strategies and argue for specialists that might improve the chances of successful implementation. First, in one of the most significant studies in pediatric critical care, Hutchison and colleagues from the Canadian Critical Care Trials Group tested if early hypothermia—basically the only neuroprotective strategy currently available for testing—would improve outcome after severe TBI in children.[49] In a trial involving 225 children, there was a strong trend toward worse outcome in the treated group, including both death and poor neurologic outcome. However, the authors discerned significant methodological problems with the trial, including the increased number of children with hypotension, an increased incidence of vasoactive agents necessary during the rewarming phase, and an incomplete dose of hypothermia administered (approximately 16 hours based on data within the manuscript compared to 24 hours by the proposed protocol). Second, in a smaller study of a single center, Fink and colleagues[50] found that children receiving hypothermia for cardiac arrest had the same mortality rate compared to those remaining normothermic in an uncontrolled audit of a single center. More important, they found that overshooting of target temperature was common (10% with rectal temperature of <30°C) in this non–protocol-driven care plan. Both of these studies argued that careful control of neuroprotective strategies is essential for both the safety of clinical trials and ultimately clinical care. The Therapeutic Hypothermia After Cardiac Arrest (THAPCA) out-of-hospital cardiac arrest trial reported no benefit of therapeutic hypothermia compared to therapeutic normothermia, in terms of the primary neurocognitive outcome measure, despite good temperature control in both treatment groups.[50a] In the future, in neuroprotective strategies for any of a number of neurologic conditions, it may be the role of the pediatric neurointensivist to effectively implement or provide oversight of the intervention.

Challenges, Controversies, and the Scope of Pediatric Neurocritical Care

The practice of brain-directed critical care in children faces specific challenges compared to that for adults. First, there are limited data to guide practice. For example, there are no randomized controlled trials to guide management of stroke, cardiac arrest, TBI, or refractory status epilepticus. Second, our understanding of the cellular mechanisms of injury in the developing brain is limited and the process for drug development slow. At present, there are no pharmacologic therapies available to the neurointensivist that target the primary cellular mechanisms of injury in, for example, TBI or stroke. Third, the mechanisms of CNS injury in children differ significantly from those in adults, and results of adult studies such as stroke cannot be extrapolated to children. The heterogeneity of disorders in critically ill children that lead to neurologic injury require that management be based on an understanding of fundamental cell biology and cerebral physiology with little evidence-based medicine to support management decisions. Last, the meaningful impact (other than survival) of any therapeutic interventions in children may take months or years to quantify.

Future of Pediatric Neurocritical Care

Pediatric neurocritical care is no longer a new concept, and there are now published examples of approaches to its implementation,[51-56,27] including evidence from the management of TBI that a neurocritical care service improves outcome.[57] There remains debate over staffing and leadership of this effort. Both intensivist-led[58] and neurologist-led approaches[27] have been proposed. Models including pediatric intensivist-led programs (Children's National Medical Center, the University of Pittsburgh Children's Hospital of Boston, and Washington University of St. Louis) and pediatric neurologist-led programs (Northwestern University and Baylor College of Medicine) exist currently. It seems likely at this juncture that an integrative approach with both of these services and neurosurgery will be required for the foreseeable future, as it is as unlikely that an intensivist-trained neurocritical care specialist will feel complete comfort in reading EEGs as it is for a neurologist-trained specialist to manage a critical airway. Although there are variations in structure and leadership by institution, the common theme is the collaborative approach to patient care among the core disciplines of critical care, neurosurgery, and neurology. There is a supportable consensus that there is a need for a specific training program in pediatric neurocritical care,[52,53,59,60] as has been described in adult neurocritical care programs. This has been described as "cross-disciplinary training" between neurology and critical care.[60] The Northwestern Davee Program has adopted this approach with a neurocritical care fellowship program open to intensivists and neurologists, recognizing that conventional

training in critical care or neurology is insufficient preparation for the complexity of the practice of pediatric neurocritical care,[27] and other programs are beginning to offer such opportunities.

The overall organization of pediatric neurocritical care in the future and the scope of its mission remain to be determined, and the authors would suggest that the essential components and disorders that may benefit from this approach are summarized in Tables 64.1 and 64.2. The experience of the pediatric stroke community also suggests that the collaborative multidisciplinary approaches taken by most centers can be successful.[61] Since the previous edition of this text, there is now evidence that a pediatric neurocritical care program can improve survival in an important subset of patients (TBI).[62] Whether the time and expense invested in these programs will help reduce the neurologic morbidity in pediatric critical

TABLE 64.1   Essential and Ideal Components of a Pediatric Neurocritical Care Program

Organization	ICU Care	Follow-Up Care	Education	Administration and Support
Multidisciplinary team of neurologists and intensivists Specialty-trained APN with expertise in NCC Protected time for the NCC service Joint rounds with critical care Stable NCC team for consistency of care Responsible for neonatal, cardiac, and pediatric ICUs	Protocol-driven care Involvement of bedside nurses Iterative modification of care practices based on outcome data Internal guidelines based on best available preclinical and clinical research Use of all available monitoring tools (eg, NIRS, pupillometry, optic nerve ultrasound, brain tissue oxygen monitoring) 24/7 EEG monitoring with interpretation by the NCC service	NCC team follows patients in hospital after leaving the ICU Dedicated NCC follow-up clinic Staffed with neurologist, intensivist, physiatrist, and APN Outcome measures collected for all patients	Create a culture of brain-directed critical care Training rotations in NCC for fellows in critical care, psychiatry, and anesthesia Training rotation in NCC for APNs Weekly NCC teaching conference and joint conference with adult stroke and NCC teams Monthly NCC teaching conference Emphasis on the integration of ICU neurologic exam with fundamental cellular mechanism of cerebral injury	Department or hospital support, recognizing the need to protect team members' time Data collection for all patients used to link long-term outcome to ICU care and to modify practice Participation in multicenter studies Emphasis on publication and sharing of experience and protocols

APN, advanced practice nurse; *EEG,* electroencephalogram; *NCC,* neurocritical care; *NIRS,* near-infrared spectroscopy.

TABLE 64.2   Spectrum of Disease Pathophysiology for Pediatric Neurocritical Care

Acute CNS Injury	Seizures	Neurologic Complications of Common Critical Illness	CNS Infection	Autoimmune Disorders	Neuromuscular Disorders	Neurodegenerative and Metabolic Disorders
TBI Coma and altered mental status CNS tumors Stroke and ICH Cardiac arrest SAH Spinal cord injury Intracranial hypertension	Refractory status epilepticus Nonconvulsive seizures Conversion disorders	Acute liver failure Stem cell and solid organ transplant Diabetic ketoacidosis Septic encephalopathy Medical complications of chronic neurologic disorders	Bacterial meningitis Encephalitis	ADEM and postinfectious neurologic disorders CNS complications of systemic autoimmune disorders (SLE, sarcoid, HLH) Autoimmune encephalopathies	Guillain-Barré syndrome Transverse myelitis Myasthenic crisis ICU-acquired paresis	Gray and white matter disorders Mitochondrial disorders Inborn errors of metabolism

ADEM, acute disseminating encephalomyelitis; *BBB,* blood-brain barrier; *CBF,* cerebral blood flow; *CNS,* central nervous system; *HLH,* hemophagocytic lymphohistiocytosis; *ICH,* intracerebral hemorrhage; *SAH,* subarachnoid hemorrhage; *SLE,* systemic lupus erythematosus; *TBI,* traumatic brain injury.

illness is yet unknown and will require a commitment to the long-term care of these patients and the infrastructure to measure these outcomes. This is a substantial challenge.

In summary, enthusiasm for the practice of pediatric neurocritical care continues to grow across the United States and abroad. At this time, university-affiliated pediatric critical care and neurology divisions have established or are starting clinical services in pediatric neurocritical care. In going forward, it is important to determine if these clinical programs affect important outcomes for children and which team structure allows for the best results. In their landmark paper, Safar and Grenvik[3] argued that a sequence of nine steps must be accomplished when building a successful critical care program: (1) planning and organization, (2) training in basic nursing/ physician skills, (3) building and equipping the unit, (4) opening the unit, (5) developing special standards and protocols, (6) training nonphysician personnel, (7) continuing education of nurses/physicians, (8) developing full-time coverage, and (9) developing research programs. At present, step 3 may not be needed, as there is little effort to build self-standing neurocritical care units for children at this time. Nevertheless, it seems that many programs have accomplished a number of the eight remaining steps with some success. It remains to be seen how implementation of these programs will fare in the coming years and what advances in care may be obtained.

Coma and Depressed Sensorium

Tony Pearson-Shaver and Renuka Mehta

PEARLS

- A Glasgow Coma Scale score less than 15 in children should be taken seriously.
- The ABCs (airway, breathing, and circulation) should be the priority during management of a child with coma.
- A spinal tap should be deferred until the possibility of raised intracranial pressure has been ruled out.
- The patient's blood glucose level should be checked with urgency during the initial presentation of coma.
- When in doubt, it is better to protect the airway and prevent hypoxemia and hypercarbia electively.
- Unequal size of the pupils can be a sign of uncal herniation.
- The goal of therapy should be the prevention of secondary brain injury.

Coma, a state of unresponsiveness and unconsciousness, presents in many disorders ranging from structural central nervous system (CNS) injuries to diffuse systemic abnormalities. As a medical emergency, coma presents a challenge to providers because optimal care requires timely intervention; however, information is frequently limited during the initial evaluation. Knowledge of CNS anatomy and structures responsible for consciousness provides helpful clues as one attempts to interpret physical findings and optimize patient care. A careful general physical examination with a focused neurologic examination can suggest the diagnosis, aid in the location of lesions, guide therapeutic intervention, and determine prognosis. Further adjunctive radiologic and laboratory evaluation will then confirm physical findings. This chapter therefore considers CNS anatomy, the pathophysiology of coma, historical and physical findings that aid in the localization of lesions, the emergent management and evaluation of patients presenting with an altered level of consciousness, and the prognosis of patients who present with coma.

Pathophysiology

The brain tolerates only limited physical or metabolic injury. Coma implies advanced brain failure, and the longer the brain failure lasts, the greater the possibility that the injury will result in permanent neurologic impairment. Coma may be described simplistically as a lack of consciousness. Posner and colleagues[1] described coma as a "state of unresponsiveness in which the patient lies with eyes closed and cannot be aroused to respond appropriately to stimuli even with vigorous stimulation." Comatose patients may grimace in response to pain and the extremities may move in stereotypical withdrawal patterns, but the patient cannot localize responses or make defensive movements. As a coma deepens, responsiveness even to painful stimuli may be lost. Because motor reflexes are preserved, the depth of a coma cannot be assessed based only on motor responses. In many comatose patients, reflex movements will develop in response to stimuli. The depth of coma is best assessed by the patient's level of consciousness.

Consciousness is a set of neural processes that allows an individual to perceive, comprehend, and act on and in the internal and external environment.[1] Two neurophysiologic functions, *arousal* and *awareness,* which rely on discrete neuroanatomic locations, are integrated in the conscious person.[2] *Arousal* or *wakefulness* describes the degree to which an individual appears to be able to interact within the environment. *Awareness* reflects the depth and content of the arousal state. When one is aware, one is alert (or aroused) and cognizant of self and surroundings. The relationship between wakefulness and awareness is hierarchical: Awareness cannot occur without wakefulness, but wakefulness may be observed in the absence of awareness (eg, sleep/wake cycles in a vegetative patient).

Sleeping and waking are common examples of different states of arousal. Although coma and sleep both abolish conscious interaction with the environment, they differ physiologically because sleep is an active physiologic process with several distinct stages, and mechanisms for arousal remain intact. Sleep is dominated by a cortically generated slow wave (electroencephalogram [EEG]) activity within networks of neurons and glia, modulated by extracellular ion currents. Wakefulness is produced through the activation of brain stem and basal forebrain structures that disrupt sleep oscillations and elicit a global change in extracellular ion flow that modifies glial and cerebral blood flow. Coma, however, occurs as a result of an impairment of physiologic components responsible for arousal and an inability to consciously interact.[3-5]

Anatomy of Arousal and Ascending Reticular Activating System

Arousal occurs by physiologic mechanisms that can be selectively impaired by toxins, anesthetics, or physical destruction of the brain stem. Neuroanatomically, the ascending reticular activating system (ARAS) and related structures responsible for arousal are primarily located in the brain stem in the paramedian tegmental gray matter immediately ventral to the

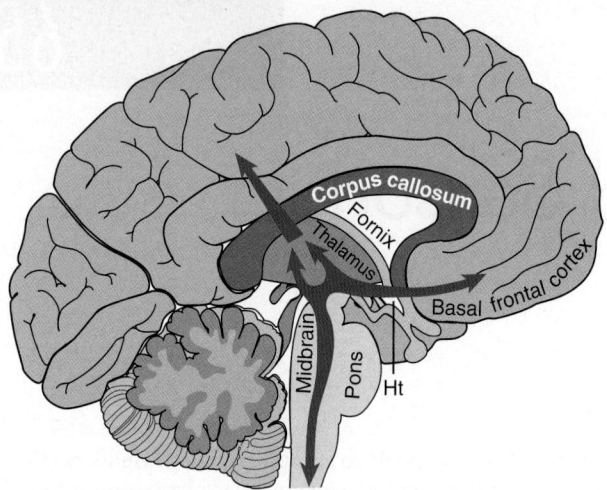

Fig. 65.1. Reticular activating system. (Modified from Hudson AJ. Consciousness: physiological dependence on rapid memory access. Frontiers Biosci 2009;14:2779-2800, 2009.)

BOX 65.1   Traditional Definitions of Levels of Consciousness

1. Clouding of consciousness—impaired capacity to think clearly and to remember current stimuli
2. Delirium—disturbed consciousness with motor restlessness, disorientation, and hallucination
3. Obtundation—reduced alertness; appears to sleep but responds to verbal or tactile stimuli
4. Stupor—markedly reduced alertness; only responds to noxious stimuli
5. Coma—no response to even noxious stimuli and will not utter understandable words

pons. Three ARAS principal pathways have been identified (Fig. 65.1). Communications have been identified between the ARAS and the cortex and the limbic system via the thalamic reticular nucleus, the cortex hypothalamus, the basal forebrain, and the brain stem median raphe (locus caeruleus).[3] Because the ARAS receives collaterals from and is stimulated by every major somatic and sensory pathway directly or indirectly, it is best regarded as a physiologic rather than an anatomic entity. This partly explains why patients with very large discrete lesions (brain tumors) may be entirely alert, whereas patients with anatomically undetectable but biochemically widespread lesions (eg, hepatic encephalopathy) may be deeply comatose.

Primarily, two types of lesions depress the level of arousal: direct brain stem–diencephalic injury involving the reticular formation and nuclei, or bilateral cerebral hemisphere dysfunction. Consequently, conscious behavior depends on the interplay between the cerebral cortex and the ARAS because these neural components are required for arousal and to maintain awareness.[1,3] Because the brain maintains a rich network of connections among the cortex, the ARAS, and the brain stem, patients with large discrete lesions might be alert on presentation, although localized neurologic deficits are noted on physical examination. On the other hand, patients with only minimal exposure to CNS depressants present with a depressed sensorium. Changes in a patient's level of consciousness imply significant dysfunction and can occur with variable degrees of wakefulness.

States of Impaired Sensorium

Precise definitions and descriptions of the various levels of consciousness are helpful in establishing a baseline, communicating with other health care providers, and interpreting changes in a patient's condition. Box 65.1 describes definitions for varying levels of consciousness; however, many terms used to describe alterations in sensorium lack precision and are better avoided. Colloquial use of the terms *lethargy, obtundation, somnolence,* and *stupor* have rendered them imprecise, and health care workers are best served to avoid them when describing patients with altered consciousness. Numerous

scoring systems have been developed to assess acute neurologic conditions. By far the most common is the Glasgow Coma Scale score (GCS). Developed to classify the depth of coma in adults who have sustained a head injury, the use of the GCS has been expanded to evaluate patients who have sustained a variety of neurologic injuries. A GCS score of 8 or less has been used as an alternative definition of coma. Although other scales are used to assess the severity of illness in coma (eg, Liege coma scale, Apache II scale, and Reye syndrome), the GCS has gained wider acceptance because of its ease and familiarity. A modified GCS has been devised that is more applicable to infants.

Several states of depressed consciousness are described and deserve mention. Consciousness disorders should be distinguished from *brain death*, an irreversible loss of all brain and brain stem function.[6,7] *Coma* is a state characterized by the absence of arousal and awareness. To differentiate coma from more transient causes of depressed sensorium (eg, syncope and concussion), coma must last more than 1 hour. Comatose patients do not speak, open their eyes spontaneously, follow commands, move spontaneously, or respond meaningfully to painful stimuli. Spinally mediated stereotypical movements may be made in response to pain, but patients do not actively withdraw. Sleep-wake cycles are not preserved in patients who are in a coma. Patients in a coma are in a transitional state and can either deteriorate to a more permanent state of depressed sensorium, deteriorate to fulfill brain death criteria, or recover.

Identification of Cause

Coma may present as part of the progression of a known neurologic illness or the unpredictable consequence or complication of a known systemic disease, or it may result from a totally unexpected event or illness.[7] An accurate history of the events and circumstances before the onset of the symptoms and information concerning the patient's medical history and use of medications may be invaluable in determining the cause of coma and quickly lead to the most appropriate diagnostic testing and treatment. As with most pediatric disease, the differential diagnosis of coma is age related as described in Table 65.1. Common etiologies of coma seen in the pediatric population are described in Box E65.1.

Initial Assessment and Immediate Resuscitation

The initial assessment of the comatose patient should start with an evaluation of airway patency, the adequacy of ventilation, and the patient's hemodynamic status. Appropriate life support intervention should occur whenever a life-threatening

TABLE 65.1	Common Considerations of Altered Mental Status at Various Ages		
Infant		**Child**	**Adolescent**
Infection		Ingestion	
Inborn error of metabolism		Infection	Ingestion
Metabolic		Intussusception	Intentional
Abusive head trauma		Seizure	Trauma
Trauma		Abusive head trauma Trauma	Drug/alcohol overdose

TABLE 65.2	Respiratory Patterns in Patients With Altered Mental Consciousness	
Pattern	**Description**	**Localization**
Posthyperventilation apnea	Apnea for >10 seconds after 5 deep breaths	Bilateral hemispheric dysfunction
Cheyne-Stokes respiration	Rhythmic waxing and waning of respiratory amplitude	Bilateral hemispheric dysfunction
Central reflex hyperpnea	Continuous deep breathing	Bilateral hemispheric (eg, trauma), lower midbrain, upper pons
Apneustic respiration	Prolonged aspiratory time ("inspiratory cramp")	Pons
Ataxic respiration	Infrequent irregular breaths	Lower pons or upper medulla
Ondine's curse	Failure of involuntary respiration with retained voluntary respiration	Medulla
Apnea	No respiration	Medulla down to C4: peripheral nerves, neuromuscular junction

illness evolves throughout the assessment. Measurement of core temperature is an important adjunct. Many practitioners assign an initial GCS score at this time.

It is important to observe the respiratory pattern. The rate and regularity of respiration depends on a complex interplay of chemical and neural control systems that operate automatically to reset the rate and depth of breathing as changes occur in gas tensions and pH. In the comatose patient, abnormality may occur in rate and in the pattern. A low respiratory rate is associated with CNS depressants—for example, alcohol, barbiturates, benzodiazepines, and narcotics—and leads to hypoventilation. It also can be associated with elevated intracranial pressure (ICP). Tachypnea is far more commonly due to a physiologic response to hypoxia, metabolic acidosis, or fever, but central hyperventilation can be a sign of brain stem herniation.

The hemodynamic disturbance and hypotension leading to shock that occur coincident with coma are mainly seen in systemic diseases (eg, sepsis, drug ingestions, myocardial injury, and adrenal insufficiency), but it is not uncommon to see neurogenic shock related to severe traumatic brain injury (TBI) and spinal cord injury as well. Hypertension in a comatose patient suggests an intracranial structural lesion and raised ICP, but it may be causative related to primary hypertensive encephalopathy.

Once the patient's airway, breathing, and hemodynamics are stabilized, a complete general examination and specific neurologic examination should be performed and any signs of trauma noted. Cervical immobilization should be maintained until trauma has been excluded and the cervical spine has been cleared by radiographic and physical examinations. The patient should be completely exposed to allow a visual appraisal of swelling, lacerations, bruises, and other obvious signs of trauma. Blood or clear fluid noted in the nose or ears suggests a basilar skull fracture. Injuries with characteristic patterns (eg, cigarette burns and glove and stocking burns), characteristic shapes, and characteristic locations (eg, finger marks on the buttocks and bruises over ear lobes) suggest child abuse (see also Chapter 122).

Focused Neurologic Examination

A focused neurologic examination is key to documenting a baseline neurologic status and helps to locate lesions and determine prognosis in patients with a diminished level of conscious (LOC). Because a diminished LOC requires either

ARAS or bilateral hemispheric dysfunction, testing the structures immediately adjacent to the ARAS provides clues to the etiology of coma and directs subsequent investigations. A thorough physical examination must be systematic and is as valuable as radiographic and laboratory studies. The neurologic examination of a comatose patient differs from that of an awake, communicative subject and involves pupillary response, respiratory pattern, stimuli required to illicit a motor response, and the general character of the responses. History and presenting symptoms should be evaluated in the context of neurologic findings. Taken together, the history and presenting symptoms help determine the cause of diminished LOC. The level of neurologic dysfunction can often be defined clinically by the respiratory pattern (Table 65.2), associated eye findings, and motor examination (Table 65.3).

Respiratory Pattern

Breathing abnormalities in rate, depth, or regularity are associated with altered LOC. These abnormalities could be signs of drug overdose, increased ICP, or herniation. Observance of the respiratory pattern also can assist in localizing a lesion. Anatomic correlations between areas of injury and the resultant respiratory patterns are found in Table 65.2 and Fig. 65.2.

Eye Examination

Specific eye findings can help localize the level of lesions and establish prognosis. Pupillary changes are informative during the examination of coma because the brain stem areas that control consciousness are adjacent to those that control

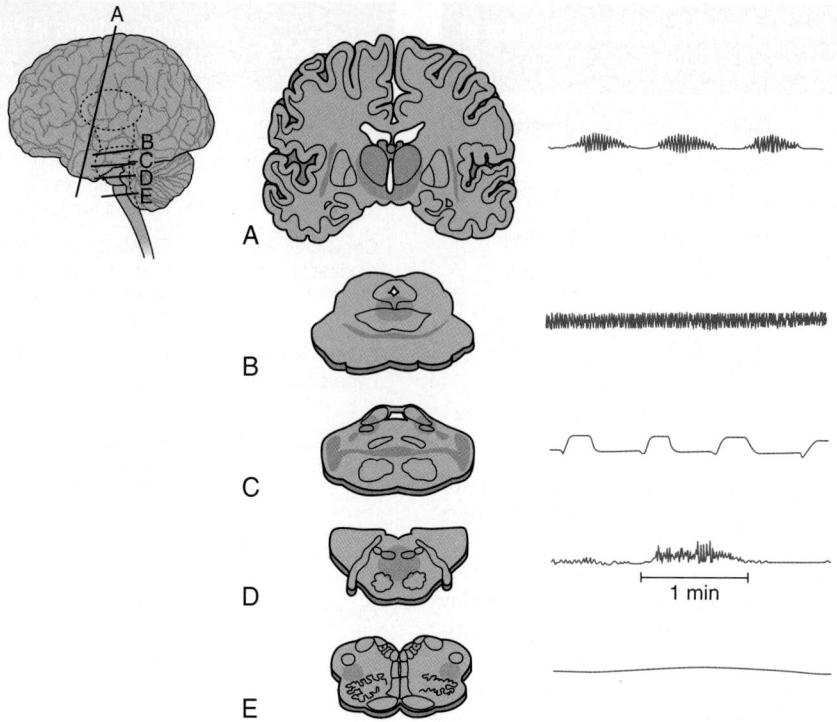

Fig. 65.2. Respiratory patterns and associated levels of injury. (A) Cheyne-Stokes respiration is seen with metabolic injury and lesions in the forebrain and diencephalon. (B) Central neurogenic hyperventilation is most commonly seen with metabolic encephalopathies. (C) Apneustic breathing (inspiratory pauses) is seen in patients with bilateral pontine lesions. (D) Cluster breathing and ataxic breathing are seen in lesions at the pontine medullary junction. (E) Apnea occurs when the medullary ventral respiratory nuclei are injured. (Modified from Posner JB, Saper CB, Schiff ND, et al., eds. The Diagnosis of Stupor and Coma. 4th ed. New York: Oxford University Press; 2007.)

TABLE 65.3	Differentiating Characteristics of Structural and Metabolic Coma		
Supratentorial Lesions	**Infratentorial Lesions**	**Toxic, Metabolic, or Infectious Processes**	
Initial focal signs Retrocaudal progression Asymmetric examination often present early	Brain stem abnormalities often initial signs Sudden onset of coma Cranial nerve abnormality often seen Respiratory pattern often altered, such as central reflex hyperpnea	Confusion/stupor often precede signs Symmetric examination Pupillary reactions preserved Respiratory rate often altered, such as Cheyne-Stokes breathing	

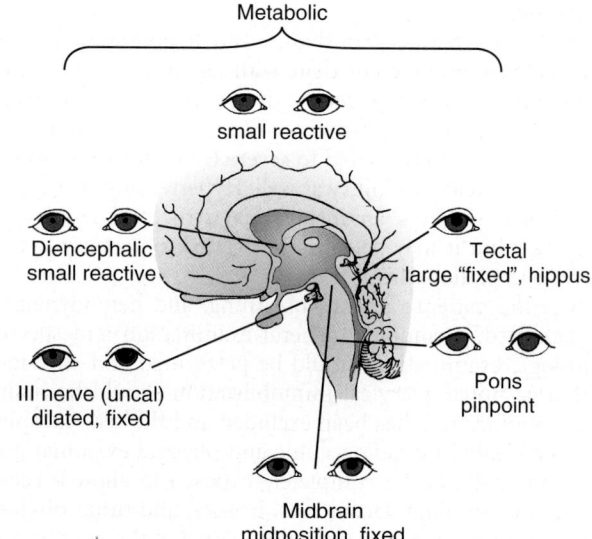

Fig. 65.3. Pupils in comatose patients.

pupillary response. It is important to distinguish between pupillary dilatation caused by disease or injury and that caused by medication. Pupillary changes due to structural lesions depend on the site of the primary lesion and secondarily on the effects of increased ICP as described in Table 65.3 and presented in Fig. 65.3. Because pupillary pathways are relatively resistant to metabolic insults, the presence or absence of a light reflex is the single most important physical finding that distinguishes structural from metabolic disease. Any reactivity is indicative of intact pathways and would rule out brain death.

Pupillary size is the result of a balance in tone between two opposing muscle groups of the iris: the dilator pupillae and the sphincter pupillae muscles. The dilator pupillae is responsible for dilation of the pupils under the control of sympathetic nerve fibers. The sphincter pupillae muscle is responsible for constriction of the pupils under control of parasympathetic nerve fibers. Pupillary size is regulated by reflex mechanisms that occur as a result of ambient light. Size is further affected by age, emotional state, state of arousal, and intraocular pressure.

Anatomically, the pupillary light reflex requires a four-neuron pathway. Light information from retinal ganglion cells travels through the optic nerves, the optic chiasm (where the nasal fibers decussate), the optic tracts, and synapse in the pretectal nuclei of the dorsal midbrain. Pretectal nuclei receive input from both eyes and send axons to both Edinger-Westphal nuclei. The contralateral innervation of the Edinger-Westphal nuclei is the anatomic basis for the consensual light response.

Pupillary constriction occurs as a result of parasympathetic activity (Fig. 65.4). Parasympathetic nerve fibers travel along the third cranial nerve to the ipsilateral ciliary ganglion within the orbit. The pupillary sphincter muscle (and ciliary muscle for lens accommodation) is innervated by the postganglionic parasympathetic fibers. Pupillary constriction to near stimuli occurs as a result of parasympathetic fibers that descend from higher cortical centers directly to the Edinger-Westphal nuclei, bypassing the pretectal nuclei in the dorsal midbrain. This redundancy explains the preservation of the near response when the dorsal midbrain and pretectal nuclei are injured.

Pupillary dilation is mediated through the three-neuron sympathetic (adrenergic) pathways (Fig. 65.5). Sympathetic fibers originate in the hypothalamus and descend caudally to synapse in the cervical spinal cord between levels C8 and T2 at the area of the ciliospinal center of Budge. Neurons then travel from the cervical spinal synapse through the brachial plexus, over the lung apex, and ascend to the superior cervical ganglion near the angle of the mandible at the bifurcation of the common carotid artery. Postganglionic fibers then ascend within the adventitia of the internal carotid artery through the cavernous sinus in close relation to the sixth cranial nerve. Finally, the oculosympathetic pathway joins the ophthalmic division of the fifth cranial nerve (trigeminal nerve) and innervates the dilator pupillae and Müller muscle (a small smooth muscle in the eyelids responsible for a minor portion of the upper lid elevation and lower lid retraction).

Anisocoria is indicative of a lesion in the efferent fibers supplying the pupillary sphincter muscles (dilator pupillae and the sphincter pupillae). Pupillary size is determined by the average amount of illumination detected by each eye. Because the efferent limb of the pupillary reflex is bilateral, both pupils receive the same command and are always the same size. Lesions in the afferent limb of the pupillary reflex do not produce anisocoria if the consensual pupillary response to light is intact. Afferent pupillary defects are noted when the direct and consensual responses to light are different. The examiner will note that the pupil's reaction to direct light is more sluggish, initially slower, or absent. If the afferent defect is severe, the pupil in the affected eye will dilate with direct light. An afferent papillary defect is a sensitive marker for abnormalities of the afferent limb of the visual pathways.

When anisocoria develops, it is important to determine the abnormal pupil (Fig. 65.6). If the small pupil is abnormal, anisocoria is greater in darkness than in light and one will note poor pupillary dilation on the abnormal side. This problem is seen with abnormalities of the sympathetic system. If the larger pupil is abnormal, anisocoria is greater in light than in darkness and one notes poor pupillary constriction on the abnormal side. Poor pupillary constriction is consistent with an abnormality of the parasympathetic system.

Third nerve palsy is the result of lesions anywhere between the oculomotor nucleus and the extraocular muscles. The third cranial nerve originates in the region of the superior colliculus in the midbrain. Fibers travel ventrally in the midbrain and pass the red nucleus and the corticospinal tracts. The nerve exits the midbrain and passes along the brain stem and courses along the lateral wall of the cavernous sinus. The

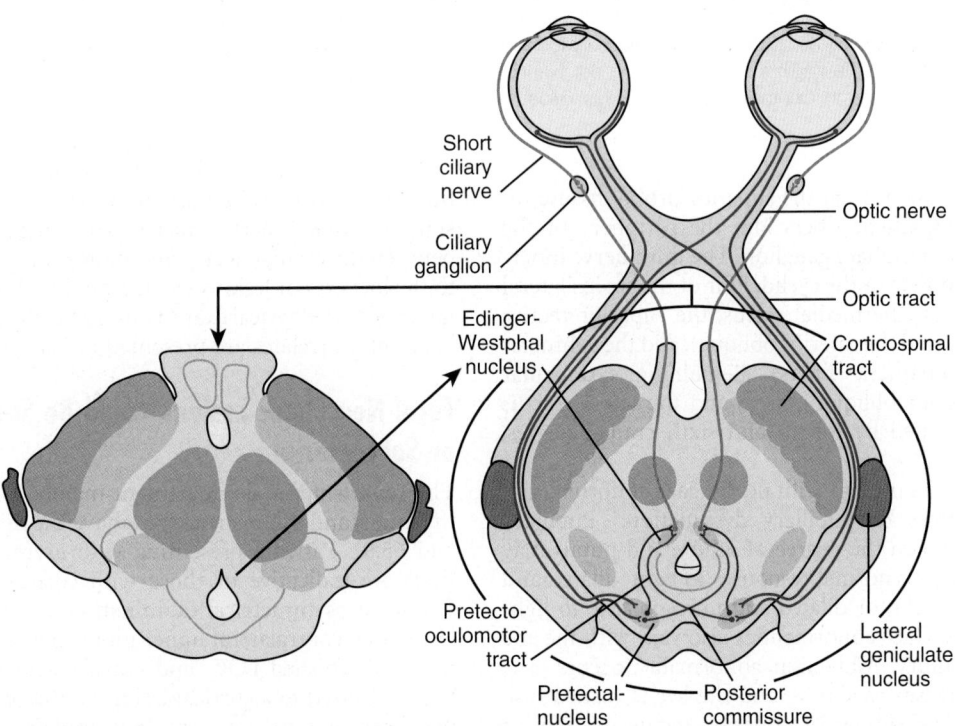

Fig. 65.4. Parasympathetic pathway for pupillary innervations. (Modified from Martin TJ, Corbett JJ. The pupil. In: Krachmer JH, ed. Neuro-ophthalmology: The Requisites in Ophthalmology. St. Louis: Mosby; 2000. Copyright 2000 Elsevier.)

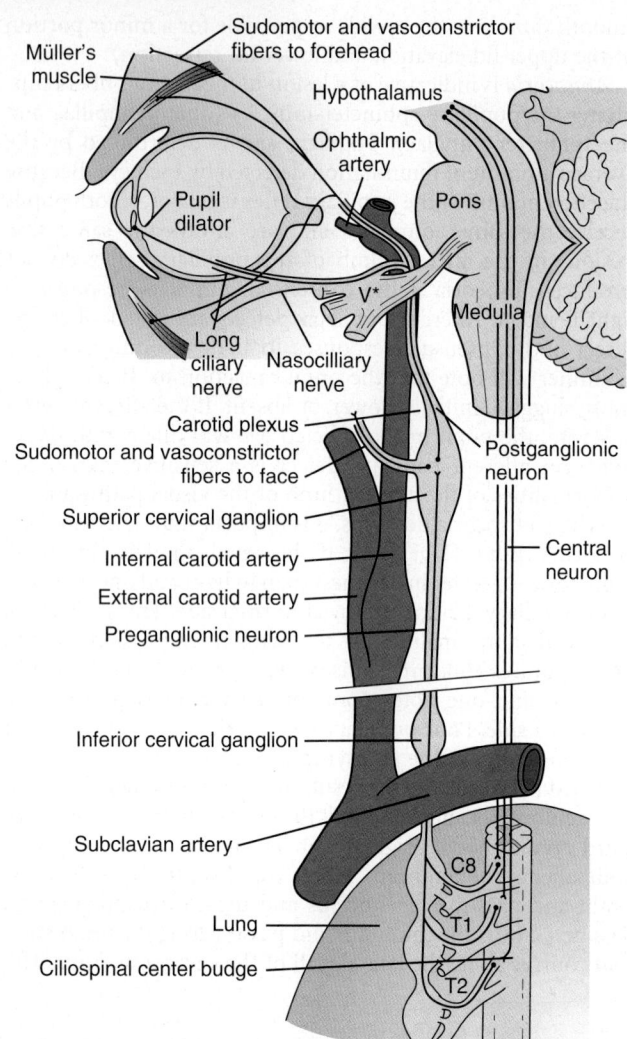

Fig. 65.5. Sympathetic pathway for pupillary innervations. (Modified from Martin TJ, Corbett JJ. The pupil. In: Krachmer JH, ed. Neuro-ophthalmology: The Requisites in Ophthalmology. St. Louis: Mosby; 2000. Copyright 2000 Elsevier.)

third nerve enters the orbit at the superior orbital fissure. In the orbit, parasympathetic fibers join the periphery of the nerve and travel to the ciliary ganglion. The third nerve innervates the levator muscle of the eyelid, four of the six ipsilateral extraocular muscles (the medial rectus, the superior rectus, the inferior rectus, and the inferior oblique), and the sphincter pupillae (parasympathetic fibers). Remaining extraocular muscles, the superior oblique muscle and the lateral rectus muscle, are innervated by fourth and sixth cranial nerves, respectively.

Third nerve palsies present with ptosis, gaze abnormalities, and varying degrees of pupillary dysfunction.[8] Pupillary response will vary with the degree of injury, and pupils may be of normal size with normal responses to light, dilated and poorly reactive to light, or dilated and unresponsive to light and near stimulus. Gaze abnormalities also vary with the site and severity of injury. Adduction abnormality occurs as a result of medial rectus weakness, and the eye is turned out. Injury to the nerve supply of superior rectus or inferior oblique results in elevator muscle weakness, and the eye is turned down. Weak downward gaze results from injury to the nerve supply of the inferior rectus muscle, and the eye is turned up. Classically, third nerve palsy is complete and all muscles are affected, resulting in an eye that is turned down and out.

Fundi should be examined to assess the presence of papilledema and retinal hemorrhages. Papilledema is a late sign of increased ICP, and its absence does not rule out raised ICP. Signs of papilledema include blurring of the margins of the optic disc and a decrease in venous pulsations. Retinal hemorrhages are most commonly associated with abusive head trauma associated with child abuse, although they may be seen following cardiopulmonary resuscitation or acute intracranial hemorrhage. Hemorrhages in the retina appear as perivascular collections of blood that may coalesce to include large areas of the retina. Retinal hemorrhages appear to be associated primarily with significant head injury that disrupts retinal blood vessels between the internal limiting membrane and the ganglion cell layer and vessels in the nerve fiber layer of the retina.

The oculocephalic or so-called doll's eye reflex and the oculovestibular or caloric reflex are the two specific eye maneuvers used in evaluating the comatose child. A positive or normal response to these reflexes indicates that much of the brain stem is intact. Conjugate deviation is noted toward the side of cerebral lesions and away from the side of brain stem lesions. The corneal reflex is a good test for mid- and low-pontine function.

Motor Examination

Motor examination may reveal focal or generalized neurologic deficits. The presence or absence of focal lateralizing neurologic signs sharply shortens the differential diagnosis. If a single anatomic lesion can explain all the signs, then the differential diagnosis shortens to structural CNS causes of coma. If there is neuroanatomic inconsistency, toxic and metabolic causes of coma are most common (Table 65.4). It is important to remember that focal dysfunction may be misinterpreted as altered LOC (eg, a patient with receptive aphasia who is misdiagnosed as confused or psychotic).

Fig. 65.7 describes the path of the corticospinal tracts through the midbrain, pons, and medulla and their relationship to cranial nerve nuclei. The anatomic relationships between the cranial nerves and motor tracts can provide clues to the location of lesions when a careful physical examination is performed. Physical examination findings and their expected anatomic correlates are presented in Table 65.3.

Focal Neurologic Lesions Could Be Supratentorial or Subtentorial

The *supratentorial* compartment mainly contains the cortex, thalamus, and other structures above the midbrain (Figs. 65.8 and 65.9). Patients presenting with asymmetrical examinations are indicative of those with cortical lesions. Given a "focal" or asymmetrical examination, hemiparesis suggests a lesion in a contralateral upper motor neuron pathway. Hypotonia, diminished LOC, and equal reactive pupils are likely to be localized to a cortical lesion on the contralateral side. It has been noted, however, that unilateral cortical lesions often dampen alertness but do not lead to stupor or coma, because ARAS is widely spread in the cerebral cortex region.

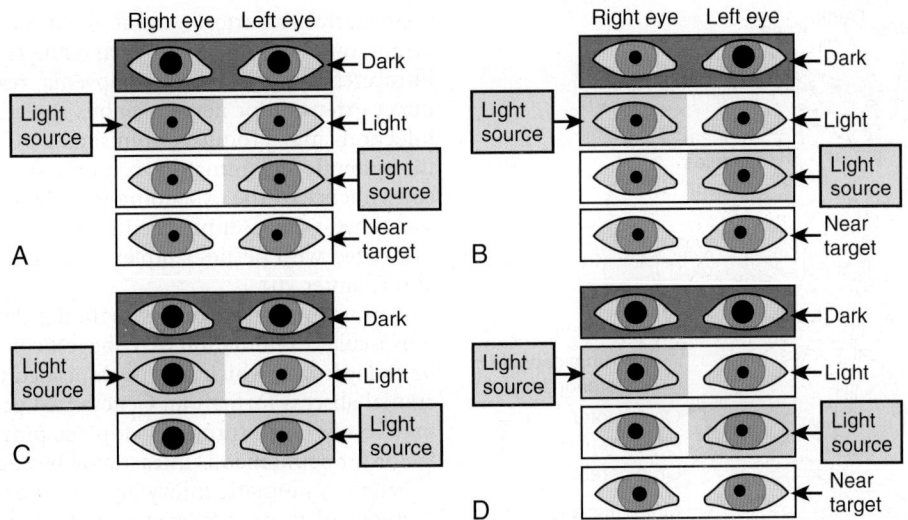

Fig. 65.6. The pupillary examination. Identification of the abnormal pupil when anisocoria is present. (A) Normal pupillary reactions. Both pupils are symmetric in the light and dark. (B) The small pupil is abnormal. The right pupil does not dilate well in the dark. (C) The large pupil is abnormal. The right pupil does not react well to light. (D) Physiologic anisocoria. The amount of anisocoria is the same in light and dark. (Modified from Kedar S, Biousse V, Newman NJ. Approach to the patient with anisocoria. In: Brazis PW, Wilterdink JL, eds. Up to date. Available at www.uptodate.com.)

TABLE 65.4	Clinical Findings With Different Levels of Central Nervous System Dysfunction				
Dysfunction	**Response to Noxious Stimuli**	**Pupils**	**Eye Position and Movements**	**Breathing**	**Motor Findings for Structural Lesions**
Both cortices	Withdrawal	Small, reactive	Extraocular movements can be elicited; ipsilateral deviation in frontal lobe lesion	Posthyperventilation apnea or Cheyne-Stokes respiration	Contralateral hemiparesis
Thalamus	Decorticate posturing	Equal and small, unless the optic tract is also damaged	Eyes deviated down and in toward the side of lesion	Same as above	Contralateral hemiparesis
Midbrain	Decorticate or decerebrate posturing	Midposition, fixed to light, spontaneous fluctuation	Nystagmus may be present; absent vertical but retained horizontal movements; loss of ability to adduct both eyes may be deviated laterally and down in third cranial nerve damage	Usually same as above; potential for central reflex hyperpnea	Hemiplegia with contralateral third cranial nerve palsy
Pons	Decerebrate posturing	Bilateral pinpoint pupils, reactive to light (especially with midline pontine hemorrhage); Horner syndrome with lateral lesions	Ocular bobbing; absent conjugate horizontal movements with retained vertical movements and accommodation; often eyes are deviated medially; seventh cranial nerve damage	May exhibit central reflex hyperpnea, cluster (Biot) breathing, or apneustic breathing	Hemiplegia with contralateral sixth or seventh cranial nerve palsy
Medulla	Weak leg flexion (or none)	Nonreactive, normal size; small, Horner syndrome with lateral lesions	Usually no effect on spontaneous eye movements; may interfere with reflex responses, nystagmus	Rarely ataxic respiration, apnea if respiratory centers involved	Flaccid weakness with difficulty swallowing, phonating, and incoordination
Spinal cord	None	Normal reaction, abnormal response if brain stem affected	Normal response	Normal	Flaccid weakness, loss of bowel and bladder control

Expansion of cortical lesions resulting in raised ICP may reduce cortical blood flow in the other areas of the brain, causing diminished LOC.

Contralateral thalamic lesions and cortical lesions with a retrocaudal progression present with contralateral hemiparesis, decorticate (flexor) posturing, eyes deviated inferiorly and medially, and pupils remaining equal, small, and reactive.

Flexor (decorticate) posturing (ie, tonic flexion of upper extremities and tonic extension, adduction, and internal rotation of lower extremities) reflects a lesion above the midbrain as described in Fig. 65.10.

The history and physical findings are relevant and may help determine the cause of the injury. A sudden change in LOC in an otherwise normal child may be due to a cerebrovascular

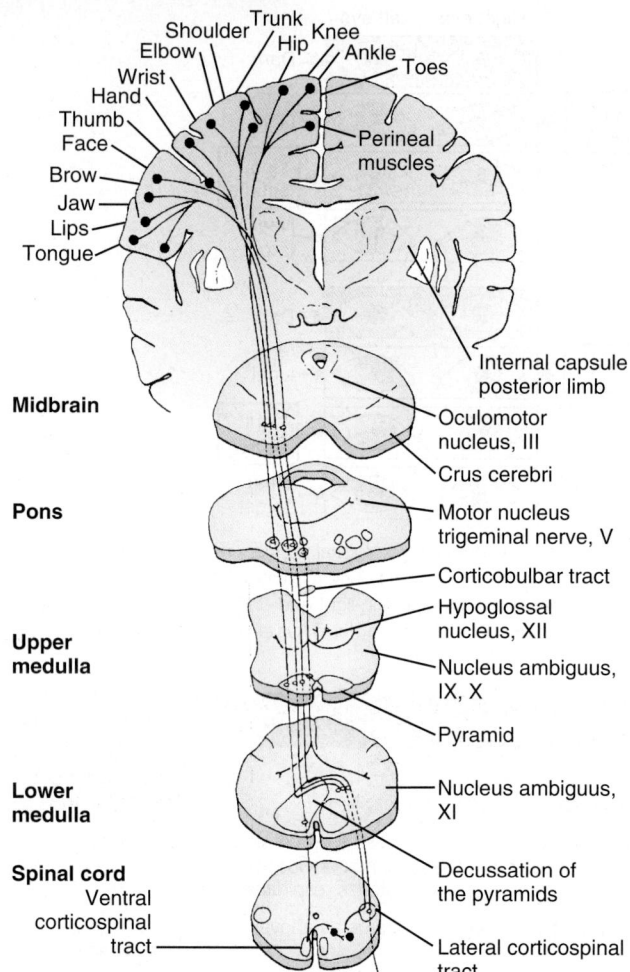

Fig. 65.7. The corticospinal tracts in relation to the cranial nerve nuclei. (Modified from Gilman S, Newman SW. Manter and Gatz's Essentials of Clinical Neuroanatomy and Neurophysiology. 9th ed. Philadelphia: FA Davis; 2003.)

accident from an arteriovenous malformation, a bleeding CNS tumor, or a ruptured aneurysm. Acute sinusitis may result in intracerebral or subdural empyema resulting from either direct extension or hematogenous spread of infection. These infections may produce diminished LOC either as a result of the systemic inflammatory response to the infection or as a consequence of the expanding mass lesion. A history of fever associated with a diminished LOC may suggest encephalitis associated with herpes simplex or arboviruses infections (see also Chapter 70).

A murmur, gallop, or dysrhythmias detected during a cardiovascular examination may suggest congenital heart disease or endocarditis, which may be associated with stroke or intracranial abscess formation. Generalized petechia and purpura may be seen with thrombocytopenic purpura, which is a risk factor for spontaneous intracranial bleeding.

When a traumatic injury occurs, coma may exist from the moment of impact or may be preceded by a lucid interval, suggesting an expanding epidural hematoma. A complete description of TBI is provided in Chapter 119.

Patients presenting with an altered level of consciousness and underlying illnesses such as systemic lupus erythematosus, sickle cell anemia, nephrotic syndrome, homocystinuria, leukemia, or coagulation disorders such as protein C and S deficiency are at risk for cerebral infarction resulting from a vascular obstruction. Patients with diabetic ketoacidosis may have a sudden onset of coma that could be a result of cerebral edema or central venous thrombus (see also Chapter 86). Hypoxic insults and penetrating injuries to vertebral or carotid arteries (as a consequence of vascular disruption) can result in cerebral infarction. Patients with strokes may have a period of lucidity following the acute vascular incident. Stupor and coma develop as swelling increases ICP and the blood supply to the midbrain and brain stem are compromised.

Vomiting and diarrhea leading to severe dehydration and hypercoagulable states may lead to sinus venous thrombosis, particularly in infants. Orbital cellulitis can result in cavernous

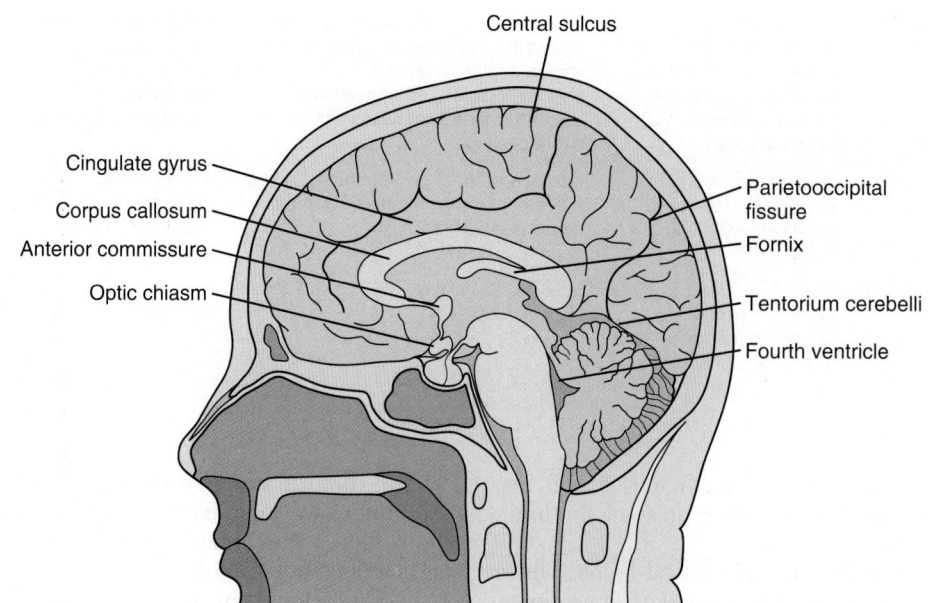

Fig. 65.8. Supratentorial and subtentorial compartments. (Modified from Gilman S, Newman SW. Manter and Gatz's essentials of clinical neuroanatomy and neurophysiology. 9th ed. Philadelphia: FA Davis, 2003.)

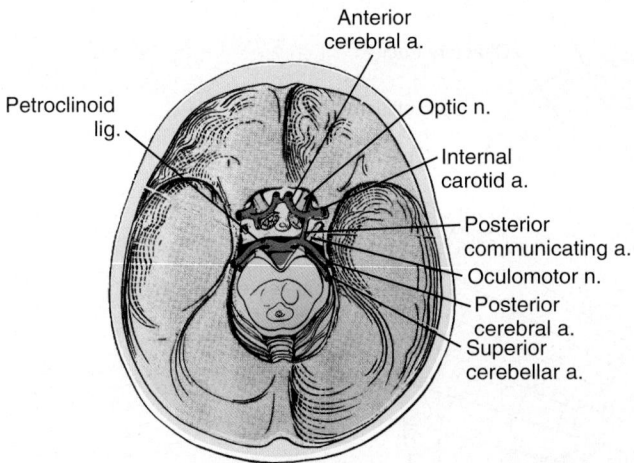

Fig. 65.9. The floor of the anterior and middle fossa, illustrating the tentorial notch and relationship of the third nerve with other intracranial structures. (Modified from Plum F, Posner JB. The Diagnosis of Stupor and Coma. 3rd ed. Philadelphia: FA Davis; 1982.)

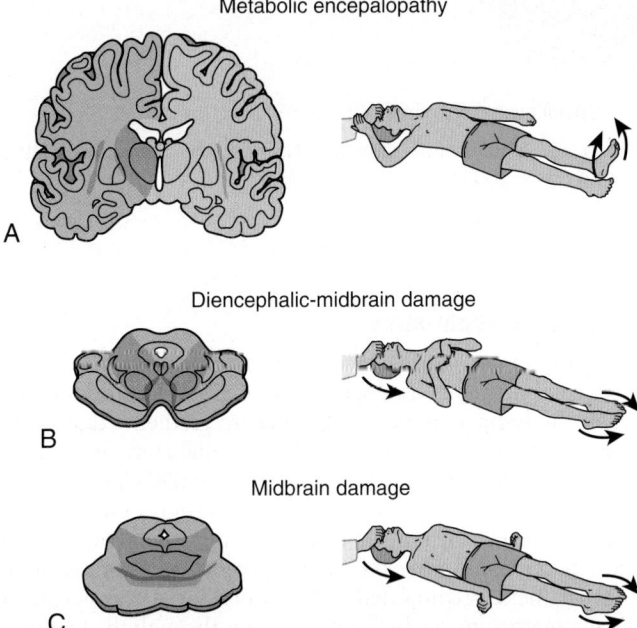

Fig. 65.10. Motor responses to noxious stimulation in patients with cerebral dysfunction. (Modified from Posner JB, Saper CB, Schiff ND, et al., eds. The Diagnosis of Stupor and Coma. 4th ed. New York: Oxford University Press; 2007.)

venous thrombosis. Children with congenital heart disease, especially with right-to-left shunts, are susceptible to cerebral embolism resulting from blood or air thrombus or particles when patients are treated with intravenous therapy.

Diminished LOC also may occur because of bleeding, convulsions, or rapidly rising ICP as a result of a brain tumor. A history of headache may suggest elevated ICP resulting from hydrocephalus or neoplasm but also may be seen in migraine syndrome with impaired consciousness. The presence of neurocutaneous lesions, such as depigmented areas of tuberous sclerosis, can suggest that seizures or intracranial masses are the cause of diminished LOC.

The *subtentorial* compartment is the area beneath the tentorium and contains most of the brain stem, the cerebellum,

the exit sites for most of the cranial nerves, and passages for cerebrospinal fluid (CSF) flow (see Figs. 65.8 and 65.9). Injury and insult can alter function of these components by either destruction or compression. Brain stem lesions are capable of creating immediate LOC because of the close proximity of ARAS. The relationship of cranial nerves to the brain stem is described in Fig. 65.11.

Lesions in the brain stem may be due to demyelinating diseases, cerebrovascular diseases, neoplasm, or head trauma. Uncal herniation can occur following head trauma, which may be due to rapidly expanding subdural or epidural hematoma or diffuse axonal injury. A history of fever, vomiting, and LOC is noted in brain stem and cerebellar infarction. Cerebrovascular lesions disrupt blood supply and result in brain stem dysfunction. A history of headache, vomiting, and gait unsteadiness may suggest a neoplasm.

Midbrain lesions frequently present with ipsilateral weakness and a midposition, nonreactive contralateral pupil due to third cranial nerve palsy. Third cranial nerve palsy generally causes both eyes to deviate laterally or inferiorly and laterally. When gaze is deviated down and out, the patient is said to have the "sun setting sign." Extensor (decerebrate) posturing is elicited in response to noxious stimuli in patients with midbrain lesions. Extensor posturing is the tonic extension of upper extremities as well tonic extension, adduction, and internal rotation of lower extremities (see Fig. 65.10).

Hemiparesis and medial deviation of the contralateral eye are hallmarks of pontine lesions (see Fig. 65.3). Pupils remain small and reactive to light. However, bilateral pinpoint pupils are also seen when midline pontine hemorrhages occur. Horner syndrome with a mildly constricted pupil ipsilateral to the lesion can be seen in lesions affecting pathways between the hypothalamus and brain stem.

Although hypertonia is a feature of preexisting corticospinal tract injury, it can be seen in acute injury to the midbrain or pons, when the more rostral corticospinal tract is disrupted, but the vestibulospinal motor system continues to exert a tonic influence on the spinal cord. These patients exhibit extensor (decerebrate) posturing to noxious stimuli. It should be noted that acute lesions often cause extensor posturing regardless of anatomic location, and both flexion and extensor posturing may occur in combination. These facts render posturing less reliable for localization of CNS lesions. Although not always reliable for localization, posturing suggests that cortical control centers are not functioning.

Patients presenting with flaccid quadriplegia, swallowing difficulties, problems with phonation, nonreactive normal-sized pupils, and normal extraocular eye movements are likely to have an injury in the medulla. The eighth to twelfth cranial nerves exit the brain stem in the area of the medulla. Medullary lesions are associated with problems in bulbar muscles such as speech and swallowing. If respiratory centers are affected, patients may present with apnea. Cerebellar lesions usually produce coma by brain stem compression. Cerebellar signs in confused patients should raise the possibility of intoxication or nutritional deficiency (eg, vitamin B_{12}).

Presentation of Nonfocal Neurologic Lesions

Once causes of focal neurologic lesions have been excluded, further evaluation should proceed to seek causes of coma as described in Box E65.1. Patients with nonfocal lesions and

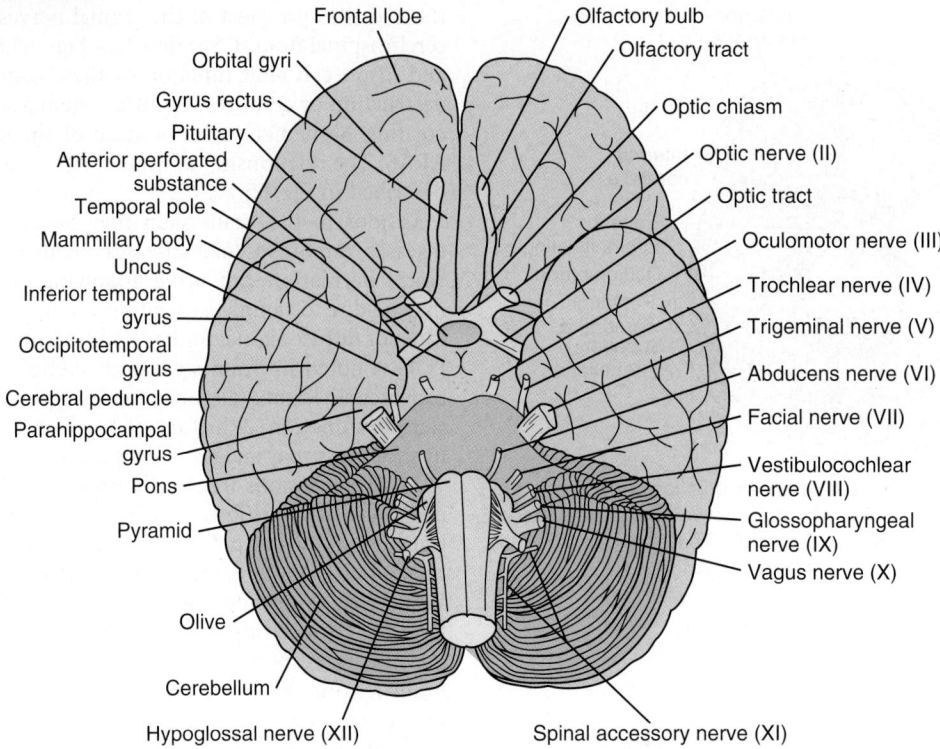

Fig. 65.11. Ventral surface of the brain demonstrating the position of cranial nerves. (Modified from Gilman S, Newman SW. Manter and Gatz's Essentials of Clinical Neuroanatomy and Neurophysiology, 9th ed. Philadelphia: FA Davis; 2003.)

coma commonly lie motionless in an unnatural posture. In most metabolic conditions, pupils are small and reactive to light and extraocular movements are absent. Patients may hyperventilate or present with apnea or Cheyne-Stokes respiration.

Hypoxia and ischemia/reperfusion injury are important causes of coma in pediatric patients. These entities are thoroughly discussed in Chapter 68. Most of the causes of nonfocal neurologic lesions may be obvious. In cases of unusual presentation, a detailed history and physical examination may give a clue to the diagnosis.

Coma preceded by sleepiness or unsteadiness suggests ingestion of a drug or toxin in a previously healthy child. Seizures may lead to a prolonged and deep loss of consciousness if there is an underlying reason for the seizure (eg, cerebral palsy, hypoglycemia, and electrolyte abnormalities) or if metabolic demand during the seizure is not met by a concomitant increase in substrate delivery. A recent history of fever or upper respiratory tract illness may suggest complications of infectious diseases such as acute disseminated encephalomyelitis, Reye syndrome, or mitochondrial disorders.

Intermittent episodes of coma may be due to recurrent drug overdose, inborn error of metabolism, or Munchausen syndrome by proxy. A toddler presenting with intermittent irritability followed by a decreased level of consciousness could be experiencing intussusception.

Inspection of the patient's skin can provide clues to an underlying illness (eg, jaundice in patients with liver failure or a cherry-red color in persons with carbon monoxide poisoning). Generalized increased pigmentation may be seen in cases of Addison disease or adrenoleukodystrophy.

Herniation Syndromes

Expanding mass lesions develop at the expense of one of the CNS compartments (brain, blood, or CSF). Herniation occurs when the brain is subjected to pressure gradients that cause portions of it to flow from one intracranial compartment to another. Although the brain has substantial elasticity, the arteries and veins responsible for its blood supply are relatively fixed in space, creating a risk that brain shifts will cause moving portions to lose their blood supply. The supratentorial compartment is connected to the subtentorial compartment via the tentorium cerebelli, which passes through the tentorial notch (see Fig. 65.9). Located in the tentorial notch are the midbrain, the third cranial nerve, and several arteries including choroidal arteries, the posterior cerebral arteries, and the superior cerebellar arteries. The cerebellum occupies the posterior part of notch. Close proximity of these important structures explains the constellation of symptoms that occurs when supratentorial lesions lead to transtentorial shifts.

Two herniation syndromes are principally important: central herniation and uncal herniation (Fig. 65.12). *Central herniation* occurs when diffuse brain swelling or a centrally located mass causes the diencephalon to move caudally through the tentorial notch. Dysfunction of the ARAS and cerebral hypoperfusion cause the alteration of consciousness. Patients initially become less alert and later progress to stupor and coma. Diencephalic dysfunction initially produces small reactive pupils because sympathetic output from the hypothalamus is lost. At this stage, flexor (decorticate) posturing may be spontaneous or elicited by noxious stimuli, and Cheyne-Stokes respiration is noted (see Fig. 65.2). It is

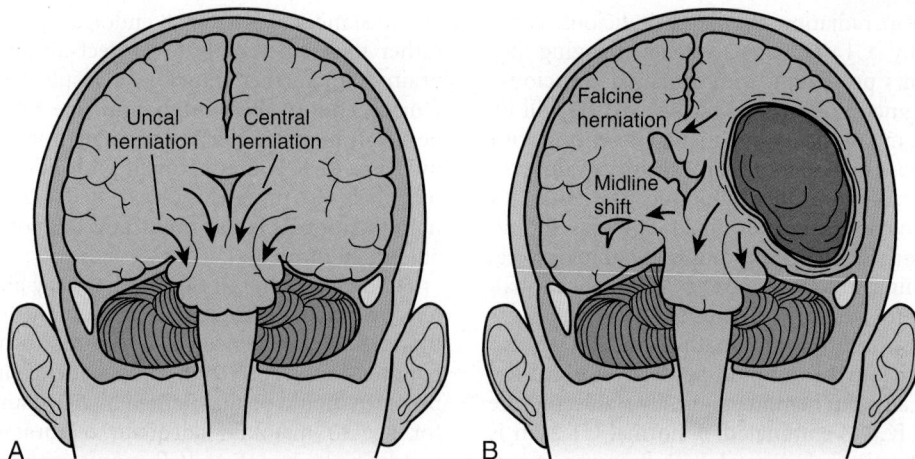

Fig. 65.12. Central (A) and uncal (B) herniation. (Adapted from Posner JB, Saper CB, Schiff ND, et al., eds. The Diagnosis of Stupor and Coma. 4th ed. New York: Oxford University Press; 2007.)

important to recognize this constellation of symptoms because herniation at this stage is reversible. As rostral-caudal progression of central herniation continues into the midbrain and pons, the likelihood of reversibility markedly decreases. As the midbrain begins to fail, pupils enlarge to midposition, and decerebrate (extensor) posturing is noted. Attempts to elicit horizontal eye movements with either cerebroocular reflex or cerebrovestibular reflex fail, and the respiratory rhythm becomes irregular. The patient becomes overtly comatose. Further progression affects the medullary respiratory centers. Virtually all brain stem reflexes are absent and death becomes imminent. The initial cardiovascular response to diminished brain stem perfusion is hypertension, which leads to reflex bradycardia. Classic Cushingoid reflex responses are seen mostly after the development of herniation syndromes. Radiographically, downward herniation is characterized by obliteration of the suprasellar cistern from temporal lobe herniation into the tentorial hiatus with associated compression on the cerebral peduncles.

Uncal herniation occurs when a lateral expanding cerebral mass pushes the uncus and hippocampal gyrus over the lateral edges of the tentorium, putting pressure on the brain stem, especially the midbrain. As the diencephalons begin to shift away from the mass, consciousness begins to diminish, and ipsilateral third cranial nerve palsy develops. When the third cranial nerve is compressed against the tentorial notch, the pupillary fibers controlling the parasympathetic control are primarily damaged, resulting in a large pupil of the affected side, which fails to constrict to the light. A unilateral dilated pupil that is first to appear, often without severe impairment of consciousness, and contralateral hemiparesis are the hallmark findings of uncal herniation. Other findings, such as impaired ocular motility pushing an eye "down and out," may take some time to develop. Cranial arteries may be compressed during herniation. Once present, changes in brain stem function, ipsilateral hemiplegia, and altered oculocephalic reflexes may proceed rapidly. In some patients bilateral pupillary dilatation develops, presumably because of distortion of third cranial nerve anatomy and midbrain ischemia. At this point, uncal herniation begins to affect the midbrain and upper pons, producing fixed pupils and extensor posturing, lethargy, bradycardia, and respiratory abnormalities. Further progression is indistinguishable from central herniation.

Cerebellar tonsillar herniation is seen in patients with posterior fossa masses that cause compression of the brain stem, cranial nerve dysfunction, and obstructive hydrocephalus. As the pressure gradient across the foramen magnum increases, cerebellar tonsils may be pushed through the foramen and also can compress the upper cervical spinal cord. Increased pressure on the brain stem can result in dysfunction of brain centers responsible for controlling respiratory (and cardiac) function, which may result in apnea. Patients with cerebellar tonsillar herniation may complain of neck pain before losing consciousness. *Upward transtentorial herniation* occurs when contents of the posterior fossa herniate into the diencephalic region. This syndrome can be seen in patients who have ventricular drains placed for relief of hydrocephalus or with posterior fossa mass lesions. If a low to high pressure differential is created between the supratentorial and subtentorial regions, respectively, upward transtentorial herniation may occur.

Diagnostic Evaluation

Initial investigation falls into two broad categories: investigation facilitating supportive therapy during the child's illness and investigation to confirm a specific diagnosis (Box E65.2). These investigations, however, should be tailored to the individual child's history and physical examination. Blood chemistry profile should include glucose, sodium, potassium, blood urea nitrogen, calcium, magnesium, carbon dioxide (CO_2), and ammonia. Hypoglycemia may be a presenting feature of some endocrine disorders or inborn errors of metabolism (see also Chapter 82). Therefore all patients with significant impairment of consciousness should have a blood glucose determination performed immediately after presentation. Abnormalities of calcium and magnesium may precipitate unexpected seizures, especially in infants and young children. Hyperammonemia and metabolic acidemia may occur as a result of an inborn error of metabolism. If metabolic acidosis is noted, then lactate and pyruvate levels also should be determined. A complete blood cell count will assist in determining the presence of infection, anemia, and exposure to toxins such as lead. Blood and urine cultures should be obtained if infection is suspected. A urine sample also should be sent for toxicology screening.

Though exposure to radiation should be judicious, computerized tomography (CT) remains a valuable imaging tool for evaluating patients presenting with impaired consciousness. Frequently, magnetic resonance imaging (MRI) will be used as the first imaging modality in patients presenting with impaired consciousness as it offers a more sensitive evaluation without exposure to radiation. Once stable, most patients with impaired consciousness of undetermined etiology should undergo neuroimaging for structural causes of pathology (eg, trauma, tumor, bleeding, infarction, abscess, or calcifications). MRI also is valuable for identifying sinus thrombosis, herpes simplex encephalitis, or acute demyelinating process (see also Chapter 63). Lumbar puncture should be deferred until the patient is neurologically and hemodynamically stable and the possibility of raised ICP is eliminated. A normal CT scan is not a definitive indication of normal ICP; however, it can provide evidence in support of the physical examination. CSF should be collected to rule out bacterial infection as soon as it is deemed safe. Freezing a portion of the sample may assist in identifying viral or metabolic causes later. Additional blood or urine samples also may be obtained for further studies at later stages depending on the patient's clinical course and the initial laboratory evaluation. The electroencephalogram (EEG) is essential to confirm clinically apparent or diagnose subclinical seizures; it also is helpful in determining the prognosis in patients with hypoxic-ischemic encephalopathy (HIE) and in the diagnosis of brain death (see also Chapters 67 and 68).[9]

Therapeutic Intervention

Pathophysiology following brain injury occurs in two phases: primary and secondary. Primary brain injury refers to the initial insult, whether it is ischemic, anoxic/hypoxic, excitotoxic, or shear injury, each potentially resulting in irreversible neuronal cell injury or death. The only available treatment is prevention. Secondary brain injury occurs in otherwise salvageable brain tissue as a result of cerebral hypoxia, hypoperfusion, intracranial hypertension, prolonged excitotoxicity, oxidative stress, or inflammation and may result in further neuronal damage. The goal of therapy is to prevent secondary brain injury.

In neurologic emergencies, evaluation of the patient's airway patency, ventilation, and circulatory status is paramount. Compared with other organs, metabolic activity in the brain is relatively high. The brain has little capacity to store glucose and accordingly depends on constant delivery of substrate and oxygen to maintain normal metabolic functions. Comatose patients often are hypercapnic and have hypoxemia. Thus supplemental oxygen should be provided to the patient with hypoxemia during the initial evaluation.

Upper airway obstruction as a result of decreased muscle tone of the pharyngeal soft tissue is a common problem in unresponsive patients. Once the cervical spine is protected, the clinician should always be prepared to support the airway with maneuvers that improve patency or with endotracheal intubation in unstable patients and in patients likely to become unstable. Once the patient's airway is maintained, adequacy of ventilation must be evaluated by examining the respiratory rate and respiratory effort. It also is common practice to endotracheally intubate patients with a GCS score less than 8, hemodynamic instability, or neurologic instability. In most

circumstances, it is safer to endotracheally intubate electively rather than emergently to protect an already compromised brain from further injury as a result of respiratory failure. During endotracheal intubation, special precautions should be taken to protect cerebral circulation and prevent further increases in ICP. Pretreatment with lidocaine and thiopental may help to diminish raised ICP associated with airway manipulation. It is also important to maintain $PaCO_2$ between 35 and 40 mm Hg.

Following stabilization of the airway and breathing, hypotension must be corrected to reestablish adequate cerebral blood flow and hence oxygen and substrate delivery. Once hypotension is corrected, some evidence indicates that blood pressure should be maintained higher than the 50th percentile for age to maintain adequate cerebral perfusion pressure pending placement of ICP monitoring equipment. Current guidelines suggest that isotonic solutions without dextrose are the preferred fluid for traumatic or ischemic CNS resuscitation in the absence of hypoglycemia.[10] However, any level of hypoglycemia must be avoided (see the next section).

Immediately Treatable Forms of Coma

After initial stabilization, clinicians should rapidly consider the causes of unresponsiveness that could easily and quickly be reversed. Experience gained from unresponsive adults suggests that all unresponsive infants and children should be immediately checked for hypoglycemia. Infants are susceptible to hypoglycemia because of immature glycogen storage and a higher metabolic rate. The blood glucose level can be checked quickly with use of a glucose reagent strip, and abnormalities can be treated immediately with a bolus of dextrose.

An overdose of narcotics should be considered in older children and adolescents. Particularly if the history and physical findings suggest narcotic ingestion, a trial of naloxone is warranted.

Seizures should always be considered, especially when the cause of coma is undetermined. Seizures should be treated immediately because a prolonged status epilepticus has a high mortality rate and has been shown to cause neuronal necrosis. An extensive discussion of seizures and their treatment is provided in Chapter 67.

Rapidly Progressive Reversible Lesions

Space-occupying lesions frequently result in increased ICP, and this situation must be addressed immediately to avoid further damage and death. Therapy must be directed toward limiting the extent of secondary damage and preventing herniation by reducing ICP or surgically addressing the lesion or hydrocephalus if present. When signs of central or uncal herniation are noted, the physician must respond rapidly and attempt to decrease ICP by altering the volume of one of the three intracranial constituents: brain, blood, or CSF. Interventions include elevating the head of bed 30 degrees, keeping the head in midline position, hyperventilation, and administration of mannitol or hypertonic saline solution to rapidly decrease intracranial volume and ICP.[10] A complete discussion of treatment of ICP is presented in Chapter 66.

States Amenable to Prolonged Therapy

Certain brain insults are not readily reversible and require prolonged treatment to obtain the best possible outcome. Although the primary insult may not be reversible or may require extended care, secondary injury such as hypoxia and raised ICP can occur and cause further deterioration, despite the fact that the initial injury may not progress. Examples of primary insults that can have major secondary changes include encephalitis, meningitis, hypoxic-ischemic insults, and certain metabolic abnormalities such as hepatic failure and renal failure. Thus broad-spectrum antibiotics and antiviral therapy should be empirically started when meningitis or encephalitis is suspected, even if the lumbar puncture is deferred. Electrolyte imbalance, especially related to serum sodium either as an underlying cause or as a result of CNS insult due to inappropriate antidiuretic hormone secretion or diabetes insipidus, also should be appropriately corrected. It may be preferable to target high-normal serum sodium levels (~145 mEq/L) if possible for the first 72 hours if intracranial hypertension is confirmed or suspected. Hypoglycemia or hyperglycemia and variation in glucose level are associated with increased morbidity and mortality[11] and should be monitored and prevented, and hypoglycemia should be immediately treated. Adequate blood pressure to maintain cerebral perfusion pressure is immensely important and should be achieved with appropriate fluid resuscitation or inotropic support if necessary. Untreated hypotension in patients with TBI is associated with increased morbidity and mortality. Although therapeutic hypothermia for the initial 24 to 48 hours following anoxia-ischemia has been shown to be beneficial in newborns and adults following ventricular tachycardia/fibrillation cardiac arrest,[12] its utility in children is not established (see Chapter 68). Moreover, data suggest that prevention of fever via targeted temperature management (therapeutic normothermia) may be as efficacious after cardiac arrest in adults. Agitated patients may require sedation to prevent elevations in ICP. Patients should be adequately sedated for comfort and prevention of complications related to ventilation. Analgesia/anxiolysis titration using a standard scoring system can be helpful. Patients at risk of or demonstrating overt or subclinical seizures should be treated appropriately.

Outcome

The major causes of pediatric coma involve HIE and trauma. These conditions are serious and are common reasons for admission to the pediatric intensive care unit. Coma is associated with high morbidity and mortality. It also is hard to predict outcome early in the course. In children, improvement can continue over a very protracted time, even several years, long beyond the time when most adult patients will have reached their plateau of recovery.[13] Thus it is important to provide accurate and timely prognostic information if possible so that appropriate levels of care can be provided. The combination of physical signs, EEG, evoked potentials, and MRI provides useful prognostic information after 24 hours of HIE and can help in predicting outcome. These tests may need to be delayed to rule out compounding factors, or multiple tests may be required to provide the best prognostic information to families.[9]

TBI is a leading cause of death and disability in the pediatric age group. Neuropsychologic and behavioral outcomes depend not only on the severity and type of injury and age at injury but also on premorbid conditions and the families' socioeconomic status.[14-16] Hypotension alone and hypoxemia associated with hypotension are significant predictors of disability and death in patients admitted with moderate to severe TBI. Early fluid resuscitation for hypotension, oxygen supplementation for hypoxemia, and ventilation for apnea in patients with TBI can have a significant impact on outcome. Also, the presence of vascular injury, refractory ICP, elevated ICP, and cisternal effacement at presentation had the highest correlation with subsequent mortality and morbidity. Controlling elevated ICP is an important factor associated with survival following severe pediatric TBI.[17]

The outcome of coma following cardiopulmonary arrest is associated with greater than 80% mortality. Patients with out-of-hospital arrests have a worse outcome than those with in-hospital arrests. Factors associated with mortality were duration of asystole more than 15 minutes and administration of more than one dose of epinephrine.[12] Patients who were alert before resuscitation had better survival beyond 24 hours than did those who were comatose (see Chapter 68).

The precise prognosis of children with severe submersion injuries is difficult to determine within the first few hours of injury. In general, prolonged cardiopulmonary resuscitation, fixed and dilated pupils, and a GCS score of 3 portend a poor outcome (see also Chapter 116).[18,19] Orlowski[19] developed a scoring system for evaluating prognosis in submersion injury based on five unfavorable prognostic factors: age less than 3 years, estimated submersion longer than 5 minutes, no attempts at resuscitation for 10 minutes, coma on admission to the emergency department, and severe acidosis with arterial blood pH 7.1 or less. A total score of 2 or less was associated with 90% chance of recovery, but a score of 3 or greater was associated with only a 5% chance of recovery.[19] Coma following cerebral edema in patients with diabetic ketoacidosis is unpredictable, and outcomes vary and may not be related to any specific management strategy.[20]

Ethical Considerations

The main purpose of coma prognostication is not merely to satisfy a parent's anxiety to know what the future holds but primarily to assist with difficult management decisions. If there is a high probability of death without regaining consciousness, decisions to withdraw life-sustaining technologies often are made. By contrast, a decision to withdraw support based on a high probability of survival with severe motor or mental disability is ultimately a judgment about quality of life, with the implication that "life with severe disability is worse than no life at all." Currently it is not possible to precisely predict outcome in patients in persistent vegetative or minimally conscious states,[21] as distinct from death on the one hand or severe disability on the other. Life and death judgments based on quality of life appear more complex in pediatric versus adult patients.

Terms such as *mild, moderate,* or *severe* disability can subjectively describe levels of neurologic dysfunction. Categories such as *favorable* or *unfavorable* convey value judgments. Thus it is important to use appropriate terminology for coma prognosis. Parents of disabled children tend to strongly disagree with subjective and judgmental terminology, such as life with a *poor* or *unfavorable* outcome. Thus with respect to ethical implications as well as the neurobiology of coma prognosis, the adage holds true: "Children are not miniature adults."

References

1. Posner JB, Saper CB, Schiff ND, et al. *The Diagnosis of Stupor and Coma.* 4th ed. New York: Oxford University Press; 2007.
2. Howsepian AA. The Multi-Society Task Force consensus on the persistent vegetative state: a critical analysis. *Issues Law Med.* 1996;12:3-29.
3. Nieddermeyer E. Consciousness: function and definition. *Clin Electroencephalogr.* 1994;25:86-93.
4. Schwartz RL, Roth T. Neurophysiology of sleep and wakefulness: basic science and clinical implications. *Curr Neuropharmacol.* 2008;6:367-378.
5. Amzica F. Physiology of sleep and wakefulness as it relates to the physiology of epilepsy. *J Clin Neurophysiol.* 2002;19:488-503.
6. Stevens RD, Bhardwaj A. Approach to the comatose patient. *Crit Care Med.* 2006;34:31-41.
7. Hakimi R, McDonagh DL. Unconsciousness in the intensive care unit: a practical approach. *Int Anesthesiol Clin.* 2008;46:171-193.
8. Lee AG, Brazis PW. Third cranial nerve (oculomotor nerve) palsy in children. In: Paysse ES, Fishman MA, Torchia MM, eds. *Up to Date.* Update May 1, 2015. Available at: <www.uptodate.com>.
9. Abend NS, Licht DJ. Predicting outcome in children with hypoxic ischemic encephalopathy. *Pediatr Crit Care Med.* 2008;9:32-39.
10. Zebrack M, Danday C, Hansen K, et al. Early resuscitation of children with moderate-to-severe traumatic brain injury. *Pediatrics.* 2009;124:56-64.
11. Hirshberg E, Larsen G, Van Duker H. Alterations in glucose homeostasis in the pediatric intensive care unit: hyperglycemia and glucose variability are associated with increased mortality and morbidity. *Pediatr Crit Care Med.* 2008;9:361-366.
12. Bernard S. Hypothermia after cardiac arrest: expanding the therapeutic scope. *Crit Care Med.* 2009;37(7 suppl):S227-S233.
13. Topjian AA, Nadkarni VM, Berg RA. Cardiopulmonary resuscitation in children. *Curr Opin Crit Care.* 2009;15:203-208.
14. Keenan HT, Bratton SL. Epidemiology and outcomes of pediatric traumatic brain injury. *Dev Neurosci.* 2006;28:256-263.
15. Keenan HT, Hooper SR, Wetherington CE, et al. Neurodevelopmental consequences of early traumatic brain injury in 3-year-old children. *Pediatrics.* 2007;119:e616-e623.
16. Chaiwat O, Sharma D, Lidomphron Y, et al. Cerebral hemodynamic predictors of poor 6 month Glasgow Outcome score in severe pediatric traumatic brain injury. *J Neurotrauma.* 2009;26:657-663.
17. Jagannathan J, Okonkwo DO, Yeoh HK, et al. Long-term outcomes and prognostic factors in pediatric patients with severe traumatic brain injury and elevated intracranial pressure. *J Neurosurg Pediatr.* 2008;2:240-249.
18. Lee LK, Mao C, Thompson KM. Demographic factors and their association with outcomes in pediatric submersion injury. *Acad Emerg Med.* 2006;13:308-313.
19. Orlowski JP. Prognostic factors in pediatric cases of drowning and near drowning. *JACEP.* 1979;8:176-179.
20. Brown TB. Cerebral oedema in childhood diabetic ketoacidosis: is treatment a factor? *Emerg Med J.* 2004;21:141-144.
21. De Salvo S, Bramanti P, Marino S. Clinical differentiation and outcome evaluation in vegetative and minimally conscious state patients: the neurophysiological approach. *Funct Neurol.* 2012;27:155-162.

Intracranial Hypertension and Brain Monitoring

Robert C. Tasker and Marek Czosnyka

PEARLS

- As intracranial hypertension progresses, changes may occur in the vital signs, with an elevation of blood pressure, a decrease or an increase in pulse, and irregularity in the respiratory rhythm. These signs, sometimes associated with episodes of decerebrate rigidity, indicate the occurrence of transtentorial herniation or "coning" and imply the possibility of impending death if the process cannot be reversed.
- The continuous measurement of intracranial pressure is an essential modality in most brain monitoring systems. After years of enthusiastic attempts to introduce newer modalities for brain monitoring (eg, tissue oxygenation, microdialysis, cortical blood flow, transcranial Doppler ultrasonography, jugular bulb oxygen saturation, and near infrared spectroscopy), the measurement of intracranial pressure remains a robust and only moderately invasive modality, and it can be realistically conducted in most pediatric critical care units.

In most organs in the human body, the environmental pressure for blood perfusion is either low or coupled to atmospheric pressure. The environmental pressure for the brain differs in this respect because the brain is surrounded and protected by a stiff skull. Thus a rise in environmental pressure—intracranial pressure (ICP)—may impede cerebral blood flow (CBF) and cause ischemia. In pediatric critical care, ICP may be of acute significance in a number of instances (eg, traumatic brain injury [TBI], bacterial meningitis, hydrocephalus, and the Fontan circulation). This chapter discusses how information from ICP monitoring and its integration with other forms of monitoring inform the understanding and treatment of brain disorders.

Clinical Background

In critical illness, the early recognition and treatment of intracranial hypertension are important because it is a major cause of mortality and morbidity. Therefore an attempt should be made to collate the clinical evidence for and against its presence. The early symptoms and signs of this complication, however, which are invariably subtle and nonspecific (Table 66.1), make this form of assessment somewhat limited. As will

be discussed later, as intracranial hypertension progresses, changes may occur in the vital signs, with an elevation of systemic arterial blood pressure (ABP), a decrease or an increase in pulse, and irregularity in the respiratory rhythm. These signs, sometimes associated with episodes of decerebrate rigidity, indicate the occurrence of transtentorial herniation or "coning" and imply the possibility of impending death if the process cannot be reversed. Unfortunately, recognition at this stage is often too late to prevent death.

Brain tissue shifts may produce various "syndromes." First, transtentorial or cerebellar herniation may result in midbrain or medullary compression. Many of the clinical signs observed in association with herniation result from direct compression of structures by the impacted tissue or are due to angulation of nerves or arteries against normal structures in the area. These herniations can cause increasingly dense coma, with distortion of the brain stem leading to midbrain and pontine hemorrhages. Cerebellar herniation is likely to occur when the increase in ICP is maximal in the posterior fossa. Such herniation occurs more commonly downward, squeezing one or more of the cerebellar tonsils through the foramen magnum; compressing the medulla; and leading to neck stiffness, head tilt, lower cranial nerve palsies, respiratory irregularities, or sudden cardiorespiratory arrest. Cerebellar herniation may occur upward through the tentorial notch, causing midbrain compression and leading to paralysis of upward gaze, dilated and fixed pupils, and respiratory abnormalities, although this type of cerebellar herniation is uncommon.

When intracranial hypertension is more marked in the supratentorial compartment, for instance, with acute intracerebral hematoma, the temporal lobe on the affected side may be displaced into the tentorial notch and result in unilateral transtentorial herniation. The herniation may be more marked anteriorly (uncal) or posteriorly (hippocampal) and is usually accompanied by displacement of the ipsilateral cingulate gyrus under the falx (cingulate herniation). Clinical manifestations of this condition may include ipsilateral third nerve palsy, contralateral hemiparesis, respiratory irregularities, deepening coma with decerebrate posturing, and ultimately cardiorespiratory arrest.

Finally, when bilateral or a general increase in ICP in the supratentorial compartment occurs, as in diffuse cerebral edema, central transtentorial herniation may occur. This condition leads to impairment of upward gaze, pupillary constriction, hypertonus, and decerebrate posturing. Temperature irregularities and diabetes insipidus may develop, and cardiorespiratory arrest may occur eventually. The clinical features of "central syndrome" are summarized in Tables 66.2 and 66.3.

Physiology of the Intracranial Vault

A physiologic process underlies the clinical picture of intracranial hypertension, and this section of the chapter will familiarize the pediatric intensivist with new approaches to understanding the hydrodynamic function of the intracranial vault. In other words, what happens before brain tissue shifts occur? Most of the developments in this field have occurred in the setting of adult neurosurgery and critical care. In common with any aspect of physiology, the tasks have been straightforward: Can it be measured? Can it be modeled? How do the models help in the understanding of the underlying homeostasis and the mechanism of derangement and perturbation? These topics are highlighted to demonstrate the obvious application to pediatric critical care—that is, use of this form of cerebral monitoring and potential approaches to

ICP assessment. In many specific conditions, however, knowledge is still lacking with regard to which parts of the adult-generated theory may be fully applicable to children.

Cerebrospinal Fluid

Eighty percent of cerebrospinal fluid (CSF) is produced in the choroid plexus of the lateral and fourth (IV) ventricles. The remainder is produced in the interstitial space and ependymal lining. In the adult, the normal CSF volume is 150 mL (50% intracranial and the rest intraspinal). In the neonate, CSF volume is 50 mL. The rate of CSF production across all ages is 0.15 to 0.30 mL/min.

There are two pathways for CSF circulation: a major, "adult," pathway, with CSF absorption through arachnoid villi (arachnoid granulation) into the venous sinuses, and a minor, "infantile," pathway, with CSF drainage through the ventricular ependyma, the interstitial and perivascular space, and recently identified perivenous lymphatics. The need for CSF circulation begins early during intrauterine development because the choroid plexus is formed during the first trimester. Because arachnoid granulations do not appear until just before birth, it is unlikely that CSF reabsorption via the adult route of circulation is the major pathway during infancy. In fact, there is some evidence that arachnoid granulations continue to develop well into the second decade, so the infantile route of circulation may be significant in childhood.

Intracranial Pressure and Cerebrospinal Fluid Circulation

The brain is an expansile structure that expands and contracts with each beat of the heart. Because there are no valves within the venous drainage from the brain, any changes in intrathoracic pressure are transmitted to ICP. Such phenomena can be seen and palpated simply through the examination of a baby's fontanelle and quantified with CSF pressure recording. Once the cranial sutures have fused, any change in cerebral blood volume (CBV) on the arterial-to-arteriolar side of the cerebral circulation must be compensated by either reduction in cerebral venous volume or phasic movement of CSF out of the

TABLE 66.1	Early, Subtle Symptoms and Signs of Raised Intracranial Pressure	
	Infant	**Child**
General state	Poor feeding Vomiting Irritability to coma Seizures	Anorexia and nausea Vomiting Lethargy to coma Seizures
Head/eyes	Full fontanelle Scalp vein distention False localizing signs	False localizing signs
Other	Altered vital signs Hypertension Pulmonary edema	Altered vital signs Hypertension Pulmonary edema

TABLE 66.2	Clinical Features of Central Syndrome or Rostrocaudal Deterioration				
Stage	**Level of Consciousness**	**Respiration**	**Pupil Size and Reactivity**	**Oculocephalic and Oculovestibular Responses**	**Posture and Tone**
Diencephalic (early to late) ↓	Agitation Drowsiness Stupor	Deep sighs or yawns Occasional pauses Cheyne-stokes or periodic breathing	Small (1-3 mm) with brisk reaction to light	Conjugate at rest and respond quickly	Normal or slightly increased Generalized muscular hypertonus
Midbrain to upper pontine ↓	Coma	Central hyperventilation	Midpositon (3-5 mm) with sluggish reaction to light	Dysconjugate	Decorticate posturing and increased tone
Lower pontine to upper medullary ↓	Deep coma		Midposition and fixed	Absent	Flaccid: (1) retained bilateral extensor plantars, (2) occasional flexor responses in the lower limbs
Medullary (terminal)	Deep coma	Irregular breathing interrupted by deep sighs, gasps, and then terminal apnea	May be unequal	Absent	Flaccid

Modified from Plum F, Posner JB. Diagnosis of Stupor and Coma. Philadelphia: 1966; FA Davis.

TABLE 66.3   Brain Tissue Herniation Syndromes

Syndrome	Clinical Features
Foramen Magnum *Herniating tissue:* downward mesial displacement of cerebellar hemispheres *Compression:* unilateral or bilateral medulla by ventral parafollicular or tonsillae through foramen magnum	Episodic tonic extension with opisthotonic posturing, leading to quadriparesis Changes in ABP and heart rate Ataxic breathing Small pupils and disturbance of conjugate gaze
Central Tentorial *Herniating tissue:* downward displacement of one or both cerebral hemispheres *Compression:* diencephalon and midbrain through tentorial notch	ICP is raised Bilateral decorticate or decerebrate posturing Nerve palsy of cranial nerves III and VI Upward herniation occurs if supratentorial ventricles are decompressed in presence of cerebellar mass
Uncal (Lateral Transtentorial) *Herniating tissue:* medial temporal lobe (uncus and parahippocampal gyrus) forced into the incisura *Compression:* midbrain and posterior cerebral artery	ICP is raised Contralateral hemiparesis Ipsilateral pupillary dilatation and ptosis Unilateral or bilateral occipital lobe infarction Obstructive hydrocephalus from compression of aqueduct or perimesencephalic cistern Regions of necrosis and hemorrhage in tegmentum, subthalamus, midbrain, and upper pons
Cingulate *Herniating tissue:* cingulate gyrus herniates under the anterior falx *Compression:* anterior cerebral artery	Infarction of regional tissue Contralateral lower extremity paresis

ABP, arterial blood pressure; ICP, intracranial pressure.
Modified from Plum F, Posner JB. Diagnosis of Stupor and Coma. Philadelphia: 1966; FA Davis.

intracranial vault through the foramen magnum. Such expansion of the cerebral mantle with compression of the lateral ventricles during systole and movement of CSF through the aqueduct of Sylvius and to-and-fro through the foramen magnum was first visualized with pneumoencephalography. These changes now can be seen more easily with dynamic magnetic resonance imaging (MRI). Inevitably a lag phase exists between the systolic increase in CBV and the effect of the compensatory mechanisms so that CSF pressure increases to reflect, in part, the systolic waveform. The CSF pressure waveform is not an exact replica of the arterial waveform because it has been "filtered" by the combined effects of arterial wall compliance of the cerebral arteries, cerebrovascular resistance, and intracranial compliance (Fig. 66.1).[1]

Hydrodynamic Model of Intracranial Pressure

ICP is a function of the circulation of CBF and CSF in which ICP is related to a vascular component ($ICP_{vascular}$) and a CSF component (ICP_{CSF}). There is considerable interest in modeling these relationships as an aid to understanding some of the complex phenomena seen in critically ill patients. The vascular component is difficult to express quantitatively.[2] It is probably derived from the pulsation of CBV that is detected and averaged by nonlinear mechanisms of regulation of CBV. More generally, multiple variables such as the ABP, autoregulation, and cerebral venous outflow contribute to the vascular component and circulation of CSF and movement of interstitial fluid into the ventricles and subarachnoid space contributes the remainder. Drainage is largely passive via arachnoid villi and granulations into the superior sagittal sinus and spinal root sleeve venous drainage. Some drainage, which is

currently unquantifiable, occurs through the olfactory bulb and mucosa into the deep cervical lymphatics.

The equation by Davson and colleagues[3] describes the immediate relationships controlling CSF pressure, in which ICP_{CSF} = (resistance to CSF outflow) × (CSF formation) + (pressure in sagittal sinus). Normal values for sagittal sinus pressure, CSF formation rate, and resistance to CSF outflow are 5 to 8 mm Hg, 0.3 to 0.4 mL/min, and 6 to 10 mm Hg/mL/min, respectively. In most clinical situations, sagittal sinus pressure stays constant or is coupled to central venous pressure. In practice, measured ICP is often greater than the value calculated using the equation. The difference is due to a vascular component, which is probably a result of pulsation in the arterial bed and is determined by the interaction between pulsatile arterial inflow and venous outflow curves, cardiac function, and cerebral vasomotor tone. With these two components—vascular and CSF—taken together, Fig. 66.2 shows the hydrodynamic model of CBF and CSF circulation and the equivalent electrical circuit analog.[4] Such models can be used to interrogate ICP and CSF dynamics clinically. For example, Kashif and associates described a model-based noninvasive estimation of ICP from middle cerebral artery (MCA) blood flow velocity using transcranial Doppler (TCD) and ABP waveforms.[5] Using 35 hours of data from 37 patients with severe TBI, the authors generated ICP estimates and achieved a mean error (bias) of 1.6 mm Hg.

Cerebral Vasodilation and Cerebrospinal Fluid Pressure

Three major factors regulate CBF: cerebral perfusion pressure (CPP), partial pressure of arterial carbon dioxide ($PaCO_2$), and partial pressure of arterial oxygen (PaO_2). Hypercapnia

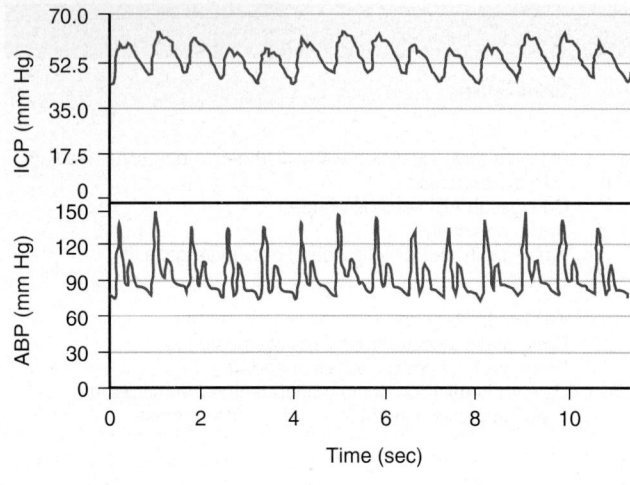

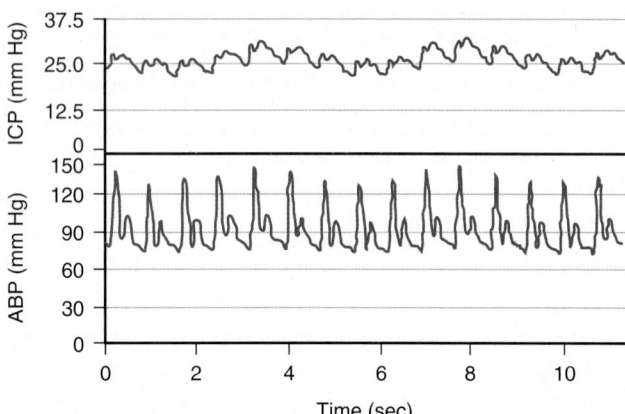

Fig. 66.1. Examples of waveforms of intracranial pressure (ICP) and arterial blood pressure (ABP) recorded at a high level of ICP *(upper plots)* and a lower level of ICP *(lower plots)*. Note that the pattern of ABP waveform is relatively invariant, but ICP changes its shape considerably. (From Pickard JD, Czosnyka M, Steiner LA. Raised intracranial pressure. In: Hughes RAC, ed. Neurological emergencies. London: BMJ Publishing Group; 2003:I.)

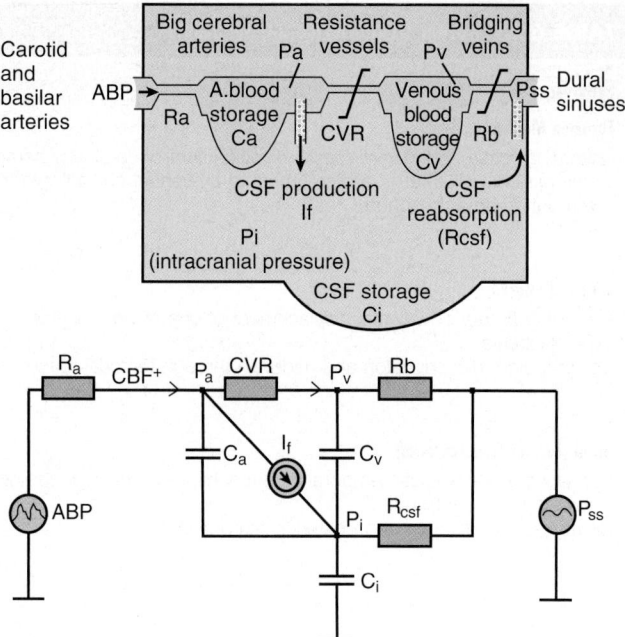

Fig. 66.2. Hydrodynamic model of cerebral blood and cerebrospinal fluid (CSF) circulation *(upper plot)* and its electrical equivalent *(lower plot)*. *ABP,* arterial blood pressure; *CBF,* cerebral blood flow. (From Czosnyka M, Piechnik S, Richards HK, et al. Contribution of mathematical modelling to the bedside tests of cerebrovascular autoregulation. J Neurol Neurosurg Psychiatry. 1997;63:721–731.)

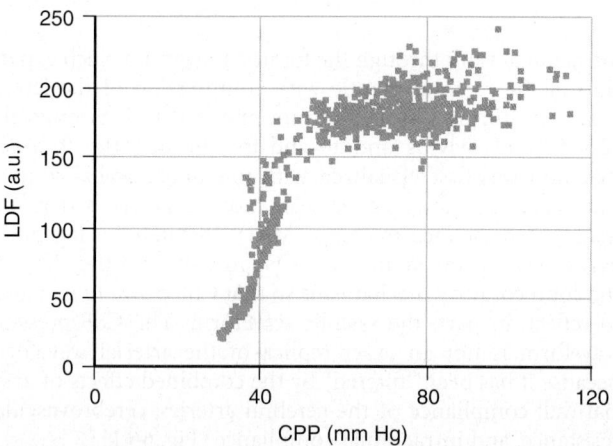

Fig. 66.3. Pressure autoregulation where cerebral blood flow (CBF) stays constant. CBF is measured with laser Doppler flowmetry (LDF) (*y*-axis). During changes in cerebral perfusion pressure (CPP) (*x*-axis), CBF remains constant until a critical threshold is reached, below which CBF falls passively with decreasing CPP.

causes cerebral vasodilatation, increases CBF, and increases ICP. Hypoxia also causes cerebral vasodilatation and a rise in ICP. CPP is taken as the difference between mean ABP and ICP and represents the pressure gradient acting across the cerebrovascular bed; therefore it is an important factor in regulation of CBF.[6] Under normal circumstances, over a wide range of CPP, CBF is autoregulated (ie, it remains constant when CPP or ABP varies). Thus in regard to the effect of this phenomenon on ICP, active cerebral arteriolar constriction occurs and ICP consequently falls to maintain CBF when ABP is increased (ie, hypertension). At the other extreme, systemic hypotension (within the autoregulatory range) provokes cerebral vasodilatation and an increase in ICP. When autoregulation is defective, ICP increases and decreases with ABP (Figs. 66.3 and 66.4).[4,6]

In practice, measurement of ICP can be used to estimate the CPP when it is the most significant "downstream" pressure acting on vascular perfusion. However, in some instances, venous pressure may be of more significance, such as critical Fontan circulation.

Cerebral Perfusion Pressure and Autoregulation

In adults, the lower limit for CPP is taken as a threshold of 60 to 70 mm Hg. In children, however, it is evident from measurement of normal ABP that the lower limit for CPP must be lower than this adult level for much of childhood (Fig. 66.5).[7] A new concept that has arisen in the adult critical care literature is worth considering in this context. The idea is that an autoregulatory reserve exists that is considered to be the difference between current mean CPP and the lower limit of autoregulation.[8] This reserve may become exhausted.

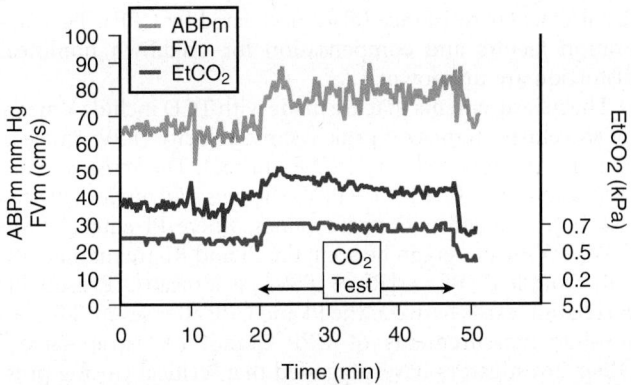

Fig. 66.4. Cerebral vessels dilate when arterial content of carbon dioxide (here measured with end-tidal carbon dioxide [E_tCO_2]) increases. A rise in cerebral blood flow (here assessed with transcranial Doppler velocity [FVm]) also increases.[6] *ABPm,* mean blood pressure.

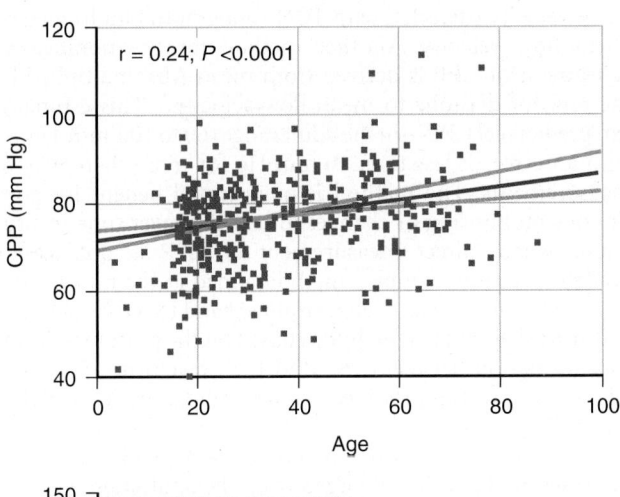

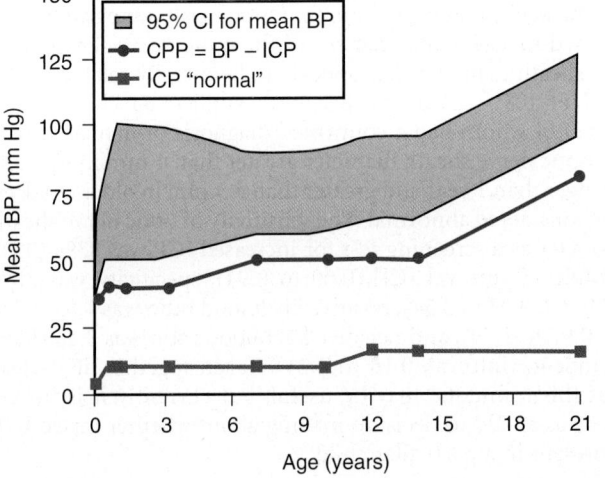

Fig. 66.5. The empiric relation between cerebral perfusion pressure (CPP) and age in nearly 400 adults after head injury *(top panel).* Estimated lower limit of CPP by age in the pediatric range on the basis of normal blood pressure (BP) and intracranial pressure (ICP) data *(bottom panel).*[7]

Alternatively, it may change over time, and it has been argued that the border between adequate and nonadequate CPP should be assessed individually and frequently.

How is this assessment performed? Autoregulation of CBF may be assessed by artificial manipulation of ABP with

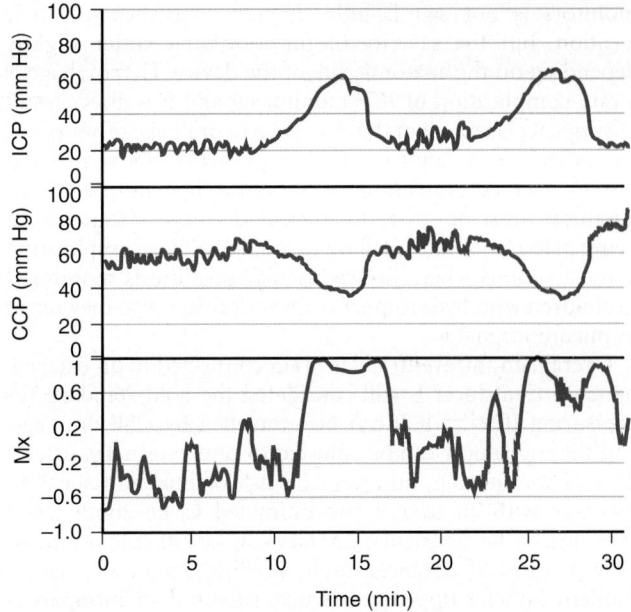

Fig. 66.6. Continuous monitoring of cerebral autoregulation during plateau waves of raised intracranial pressure (ICP). Positive values of the autoregulation index (Mx) indicate faulty autoregulation.[10] Autoregulation fails during the waves, when cerebral vasodilation occurs.[11] *CPP,* cerebral perfusion pressure.

medication, but only at infrequent intervals and with the risk that the drugs used may have a direct cerebrovascular effect. Alternatively, transient hyperemia after transient carotid compression has been used as an all-or-none index of whether autoregulation is intact. A more sophisticated approach is to examine the effect of natural variation in ABP; however, this technique requires precise signal processing. For example, to date, the most robust clinical method is to monitor the slow fluctuations in ABP that last from 30 seconds to a few minutes and are almost always present in patients who undergo ventilation[9,10]; the rate of change observed is usually sufficient to provoke a noticeable vasomotor response. Fig. 66.6 shows that continuous monitoring of cerebrovascular reactivity is possible with this method even during large spontaneous ICP waves (B and plateau waves, discussed later in this chapter).[10,11]

Measurement of Intracranial Pressure

Monitoring Devices

ICP monitoring devices can be categorized according to the anatomic site of placement and the manner in which the pressure record is transduced. For example, in babies, surface tonometry, applied to the anterior fontanelle, was an early method used for noninvasive transduction of the ICP waveform. This method, however, is limited because the force of applanation influences the pressure record. More standard approaches for the measurement of ICP rely on manometry of catheters placed in the ventricular system or in other CSF space. Alternatively, pressure sensors may be placed within the brain.

The complications of ICP monitoring include infection, hemorrhage, CSF over drainage, and monitor malfunction. The overall incidence of infection for the various forms of ICP monitors is not significantly different regardless of their location, but the severity of infection may differ slightly depending on the anatomic site of the device. Hemorrhage is a rare complication of ICP monitoring and is a direct result of surgical placement of the device. Over drainage of ventricular catheters can result in rapid emptying of the ventricular system and accumulation of subdural hematomas. Close attention must be made to prevent drainage systems from being placed too low or falling to the floor. This complication is most serious when intraventricular pressure is monitored in children with hydrocephalus. Over drainage also may result in pneumocephalus.

Overall, an intraventricular drain connected to an external pressure transducer is still considered the gold standard for measuring ICP.[12,13] ICP can be controlled by CSF drainage, and the transducer can be adjusted to zero externally. After 5 days of monitoring, however, the risk of infection starts to increase, with an overall risk estimated to be about 5%.[14] Insertion of the ventricular catheter may be difficult or impossible in cases of advanced brain swelling. As an alternative, modern catheter-tipped ventricular, subdural, or intraparenchymal microtransducers have been used (the most popular types are the Camino ICP Bolt, Camino Laboratories, San Diego, California, and Codman MicroSensor, Johnson and Johnson Professional Inc, Raynham, Massachusetts). These microtransducers are said to reduce the infection rate and risk of hemorrhage and have excellent metrologic properties.[15] One disadvantage of microtransducer systems is that they cannot, in general, be readjusted to zero after insertion, and considerable zero drift sometimes can occur in long-term monitoring.[16]

Regarding other forms of monitoring, contemporary epidural sensors are much more reliable now than they were 10 years ago. Nevertheless, the question as to whether epidural pressure can express ICP with confidence and under all circumstances is still unanswered. Lumbar CSF pressure is seldom measured in patients receiving neurointensive care. This form of assessment of craniospinal dynamics is more often used in the assessment of hydrocephalus and benign intracranial hypertension. It is unreliable if the instantaneous value of the fluid column pressure is recorded; at least 30 minutes averaging in resting conditions (with a period of overnight monitoring as the gold standard) is the desired requirement. Finally, attempts to monitor ICP noninvasively are still in a phase of technical evaluation, with the most promising methods based on TCD of the MCA,[5] ultrasound of the optic nerve sheath,[17,18] and measurement of intraaural pressure waves.[19,20]

Noninvasive Inference of Intracranial Pressure

It would be helpful to measure ICP or CPP without invasive transducers. To this end, TCD examination[5] and tympanic membrane pressure waves[19-21] have been suggested as frontrunners in the field. The description of TCD sonography by Aaslid and colleagues[22] permitted bedside monitoring of one index of CBF noninvasively, repeatedly, and even continuously. The problem has been that it is a "big tube technique" that measures flow velocity in branches of the circle of Willis, most commonly the MCA. Compliant branches of the MCA can be compared with two physiologic pressure transducers. The pattern of blood flow within these vessels is certainly modulated by transmural pressure—that is, CPP and the

distal vascular resistance (also modulated by CPP). The calibration factors and compensation for unknown nonlinear distortion are unknown.

The measurements that are made with TCD include Vmean, mean velocity (cm/sec); peak systolic velocity (PSV; cm/sec); and end-diastolic velocity (EDV; cm/sec). The *resistive index* (RI) is equals [PSV-EDV] ÷ PSV. The *pulsatility index* (PI) can also be calculated with these values, where PI equals [PSV-EDV] ÷ Vmean. As can be seen, the PI and RI are mathematically coupled (PI = [RI × PSV] ÷ Vmean). Reasonable correlation exists between the PI and CPP after severe TBI, but absolute measurements of CPP cannot be extrapolated.[23] Other investigators have suggested that "critical closing pressure" derived from MCA flow velocity and the ABP waveform approximated the value of ICP.[24] The accuracy of this method, however, is far from satisfactory.[25] Aaslid and colleagues[26] suggested that an index of CPP could be derived from the ratio of the amplitudes of the first harmonics of the ABP and the MCA velocity (detected with TCD sonography) multiplied by mean flow velocity. Another method for the noninvasive assessment of CPP is derived from mean ABP multiplied by the ratio of diastolic to mean flow velocity.[27] This estimator can predict real CPP—in the adult range (60 to 100 mm Hg)—with an error of less than 10 mm Hg for more than 80% of measurements. The method is of potential benefit for continuous monitoring of changes in real CPP over time in situations where direct measurement of CPP is not readily available. A more complex method aimed at the noninvasive assessment of ICP has been introduced and tested by Schmidt and coworkers.[28] This method is based on the presumed linear transformation between ABP and ICP waveforms. However, all of these techniques still require validation in pediatric series.

Last, there is one other potential method for predicting increased ICP that has emerged from the adult literature and is now being tested in children. Optic nerve sonography can be used to assess enlargement of the optic nerve sheath, and it is sheath diameter that appears to be directly related to the level of ICP.[29] Le and colleagues[30] studied 64 children, 24 (37%) of whom had a confirmed diagnosis of increased ICP. An optic nerve sheath diameter greater than 4 mm in subjects younger than 1 year and greater than 4.5 mm in older children was considered abnormal. The sensitivity of optic nerve sheath diameter as a screening test for increased ICP was 83% (95% confidence interval [CI], 0.60 to 0.94), specificity was 38% (95% CI, 0.23 to 0.54), positive likelihood ratio was 1.32 (95% CI, 0.97 to 1.79), and negative likelihood ratio was 0.46 (95% confidence interval, 0.18 to 1.23). Taken together, it is clear that this technique may be useful, but currently it is inadequate as an aid to decision making about whether raised ICP is present in a particular child.

Pressure Compartments

In a fluid-filled container, pressure is the same wherever one chooses to measure it within that space. Generally, uniformly distributed ICP can be seen only when CSF is circulating freely among all of its natural pools, equilibrating pressure everywhere. When little or no CSF volume is left (because of brain swelling), the assumption of one uniform value of ICP is questionable. (It is for this reason that brain tissue shift and herniation occur: Tissue shifts in the direction of the pressure gradient.) It is worth remembering that with the commonly used catheter-tipped, intraparenchymal probes, the measurement of pressure is at a particular point in space, an area of cortex within a hemisphere, and the ICP may merely reflect pressure in that compartment rather than be representative of pressure within the ventricular system (ie, real CSF pressure).[31]

Analysis of Intracranial Pressure

Normal Values in Intracranial Pressure Monitoring

Establishing a universal "normal value" for ICP is difficult because it depends on age, body posture, and clinical condition. In the horizontal position, a normal ICP value in healthy adults was reported to be within the range of 7 to 15 mm Hg.[32] In the upright position, ICP is a negative value, with a mean of around ~10 mm Hg but not exceeding ~15 mm Hg.[33] In infants and children, normal values for ICP, usually taken at the time of a "negative" diagnostic lumbar puncture, are lower than the adult values and are probably between 5 and 10 mm Hg.

The definition of a raised ICP value depends on the specific disease. In hydrocephalus, a pressure above 15 mm Hg can be regarded as elevated. After head injury, any pressure above 20 mm Hg is considered abnormal, and aggressive treatment is usually started with values above 25 mm Hg.[34] Also, in most cases, ICP varies with time. Decent averaging for at least 30 minutes is needed to calculate "mean ICP." The patient should be in a horizontal position during the measurement, and movement should be avoided.

Normal Trends in Intracranial Pressure and Waveform Analysis

Overnight monitoring, during natural sleep, provides a "grand average" with a good description of the dynamics of ICP. When monitored continuously in acute states (eg, in the presence of head injury, poor-grade subarachnoid hemorrhage, and intracerebral hematoma), changes in the time-averaged mean ICP may be classified into relatively few patterns (Fig. 66.7).[35] The first pattern, low and stable ICP (below 20 mm Hg), is seen after uncomplicated head injury (Fig. 66.7A). Such a pattern also is seen commonly in the initial period after brain trauma before brain swelling evolves. The second pattern, high and stable ICP (above 20 mm Hg), is the most common pattern to follow head injury (Fig. 66.7B). The third pattern is vasogenic waves—that is, B waves (Fig. 66.7C) and plateau waves (Fig. 66.7D). The fourth pattern is ICP waves related to changes in ABP and hyperemic events (Fig. 66.7E to G). The final pattern, refractory intracranial hypertension (Fig. 66.7H), usually leads to death unless surgical decompression is undertaken.

In addition to these patterns, more information can be gained from analyzing the ICP waveform. The ICP waveform consists of three components, which overlap in the time domain but can be separated in the frequency domain (Fig. 66.8).[35,36] The pulse waveform has several harmonic components; of these, the fundamental component has a frequency equal to the heart rate. The amplitude of this component (AMP) is useful for the evaluation of various indices. The respiratory waveform is related to the frequency of the respiratory cycle (8 to 20 cycles/min). "Slow waves" are usually not as precisely defined as in Lundberg's original work[37]—that is,

all components that have a spectral representation within the frequency limits of 0.05 to 0.0055 Hz (20-second to 3-minute period) are considered slow waves. The magnitude of these waves can be calculated as the square root of the power of the signal, of the passband, or of the equivalent frequency range at the output of the digital filter.

Assessment of Pressure-Volume Compensatory Reserve and Cerebrovascular Pressure Reactivity

Theoretically, the compensatory reserve in intracranial hydrodynamics can be studied through the relation between ICP and changes in volume of the intracerebral space, known as the pressure-volume curve.[38,39] For example, the RAP index, an index of reserve based on the correlation coefficient (R) between AMP amplitude (A) and mean pressure (P), can be derived. This calculation can be done in real time with bedside computing to calculate the linear correlation between consecutive, time-averaged data points of AMP and ICP (usually 40 such samples) acquired over a reasonably long period to average over respiratory and pulse waves (usually 6- to 10-second epochs). The RAP index indicates the degree of correlation between AMP and mean ICP over short periods (~4 minutes). A RAP index close to zero indicates a lack of synchronization between changes in AMP and mean ICP. This index denotes good pressure-volume compensatory reserve at low ICP (ie, a change in volume produces little or no change in pressure) (Fig. 66.9).[40] When the RAP index rises to +1, AMP varies directly with ICP and indicates that the "working point" of the intracranial space shifts to the right toward the steep part of the pressure-volume curve. Here compensatory reserve is low; therefore any further rise in volume may produce a rapid increase in ICP. After head injury and subsequent brain swelling, the RAP index is usually close to +1. With any further increase in ICP, AMP decreases and RAP values fall below zero. This phenomenon occurs when cerebral autoregulatory capacity is exhausted; the pressure-volume curve bends to the right, the capacity of cerebral arterioles to dilate in response to a fall in CPP is exhausted, and the arterioles tend to collapse passively. This phenomenon indicates terminal cerebrovascular derangement with a decrease in pulse pressure transmission from the arterial bed to the intracranial compartment.

Another ICP-derived index is the pressure-reactivity index (PRx), which incorporates the idea of assessing cerebrovascular reaction by observing the response of ICP to slow spontaneous changes in ABP (discussed previously). For example, when the cerebrovascular bed is normally reactive, any change in ABP produces an inverse change in CBV and thus ICP. When cerebrovascular reactivity is disturbed, changes in ABP are transmitted passively to ICP. Again, with the use of computational methods similar to those used for the calculation of the RAP index, PRx is determined with the calculation of the correlation coefficient between 40 consecutive, time-averaged data points of ICP and ABP. A positive PRx signifies a positive gradient of the regression line between the slow components of ABP and ICP, which is suggested as being associated with passive behavior of a nonreactive vascular bed (Fig. 66.10A).[9] A negative value of PRx reflects a normally reactive vascular bed, because ABP waves provoke inversely correlated waves in ICP (Fig. 66.10B). In practice, this index correlates well with TCD ultrasonography indices of autoregulation.[9] Also, abnormal values of both PRx and RAP,

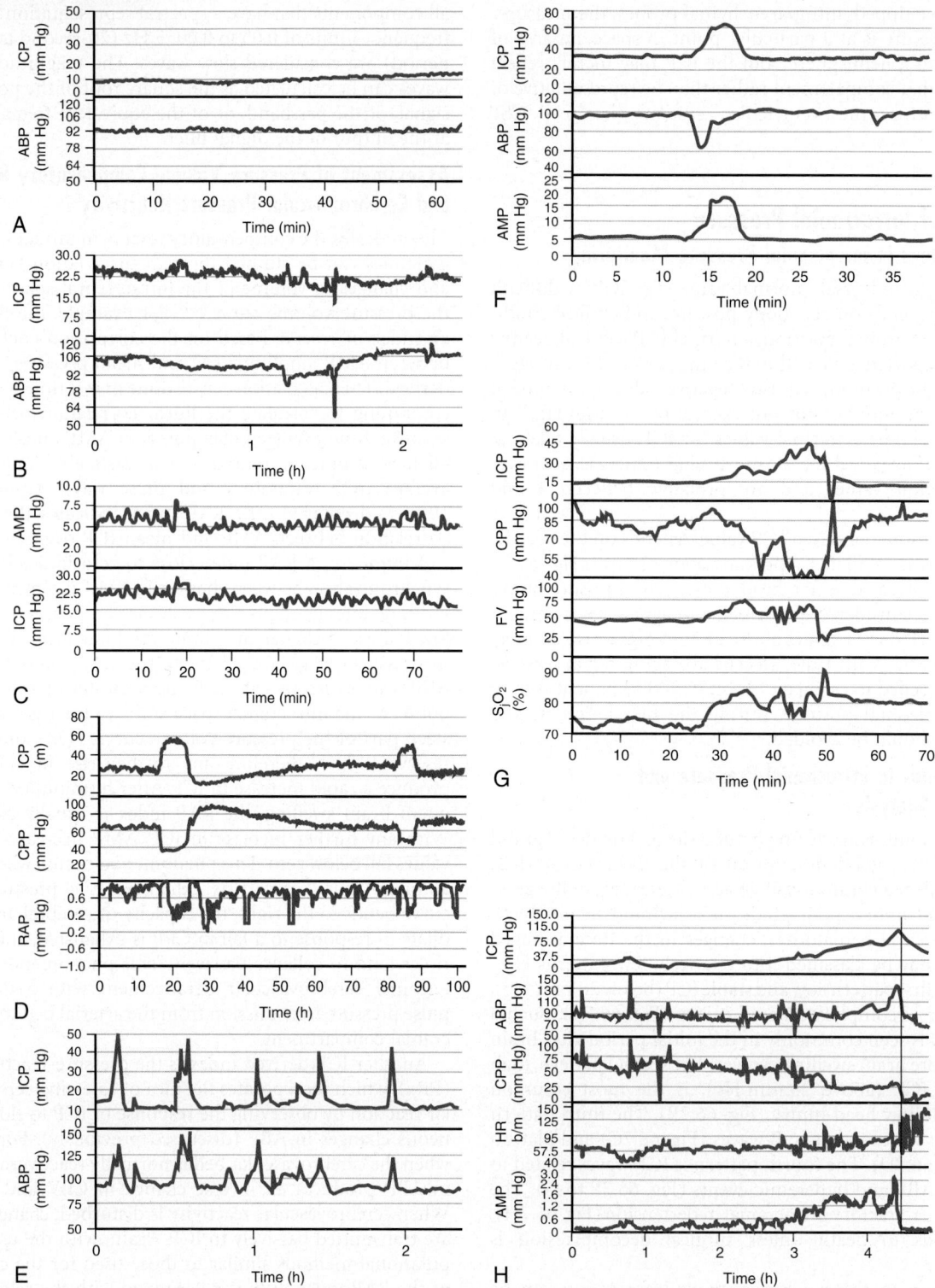

Fig. 66.7. Examples of intracranial pressure (ICP) recording in various clinical scenarios after head trauma[35]; note the different scales. (A) Low and stable ICP: mean arterial blood pressure (ABP) is plotted in the *bottom panel*. (B) Stable and elevated ICP: such a picture can be seen most of the time in patients with head injuries. (C) B waves of ICP: these are seen both in mean ICP and spectrally resolved pulse amplitude of ICP (AMP). They also are usually seen in a plot of time-averaged ABP, but not always. (D) Plateau waves of ICP: cerebrospinal compensatory reserve is usually low when waves are recorded (the correlation coefficient between AMP and mean ABP, RAP, is close to +1). At the top of the waves, during maximal vasodilatation, integration between pulse amplitude and mean ICP fails, as indicated by a fall in RAP. After the plateau wave, ICP usually falls below the baseline level and cerebrospinal compensatory reserve becomes better. *CPP,* cerebral perfusion pressure. (E) High, spiky waves of ICP caused by sudden increases in ABP. (F) Increase in ICP caused by temporary decrease in ABP. (G) Increase in ICP of hyperemic nature: both blood flow velocity (FV) and jugular bulb oxygen saturation (SjO$_2$) increase in parallel with ICP. (H) Refractory intracranial hypertension: ICP increases within a few hours to 100 mm Hg. The *vertical line* denotes the likely moment when the vasomotor centers in the brain stem became ischemic. At this point the heart rate (HR) increased and CPP decreased abruptly. Note that pulse amplitude of ICP (AMP) disappeared around 10 minutes before this terminal event.

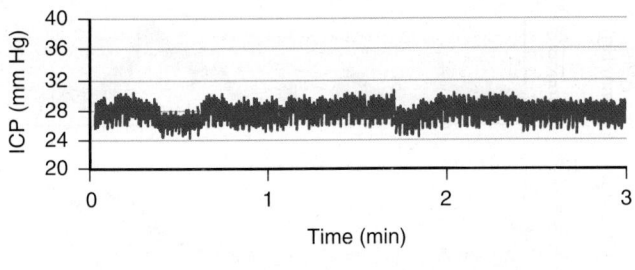

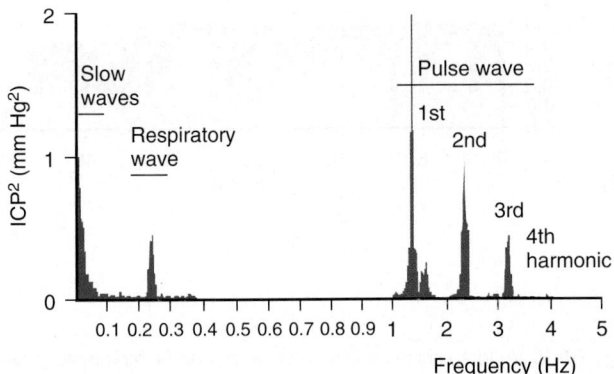

Fig. 66.8. Example of intracranial pressure (cICP) recording showing pulse, respiratory waves, and "slow waves" overlapped in the time domain *(top panel)* and separated in the frequency domain *(bottom panel)*.[36]

which are indicative, respectively, of poor autoregulation or deranged cerebrospinal compensatory reserve, have been shown to be predictive of a poor outcome in adults after head injury.[8]

To date, there are few data on the use of these hydrodynamic indices in children. One report in 32 hydrocephalic children, however, examined maximum ICP, RAP index, magnitude of slow waves, and AMP in individuals presenting with possible ventriculoperitoneal shunt dysfunction.[41] The authors concluded that, because of the association between abnormalities in the parameters studied and improvement in symptoms in patients undergoing shunt revision, such computerized ICP assessments are beneficial. In another study of 21 children with head injuries, Brady and colleagues[42] used continuous monitoring of the PRx and found this parameter to be associated with outcome. In addition, they found that impaired cerebrovascular pressure reactivity was evident at low levels of CPP. The implication is that PRx may be useful for defining age-specific and possibly patient-specific optimal targets for CPP (see the following section).

Monitoring Optimal Cerebral Perfusion Pressure Derived From Intracranial Pressure Parameters

Both the PRx and the RAP index can be used to evaluate secondary variables that combine the value of absolute ICP and CPP with information about the state of autoregulatory and compensatory reserves. In adults with head trauma, PRx plotted against CPP gives a U-shape curve that indicates, for most patients, a value of CPP for which pressure-reactivity is optimal.[8] This optimal pressure can be estimated with the plotting and analyzing of the PRx-CPP curve in sequential 6-hour periods; the greater the distance between the current

and the "optimal" CPP, the more likely outcome will be poor. This potentially useful method attempts to refine the current approach to CPP-oriented therapy: Levels of CPP that are either too low (ischemia) or too high (hyperemia and a resulting increase in ICP) are detrimental. It has been suggested that CPP in adults should be optimized to maintain CPP in the most favorable global state.[8]

Quantifying the Cumulative Intracranial Pressure/Cerebral Perfusion Pressure Insult to the Brain

In adults with severe head injury, the cumulative insult to the brain can be quantified in a number of ways. For example, an average ICP above 25 mm Hg during the entire period of monitoring doubles the risk of death.[8] Averaged values of the RAP index and the PRx also are strong predictors of fatal outcome. Both these indices suggest that good vascular reactivity is an important element of brain homeostasis, which enables the brain to protect itself against an uncontrollable rise in intracerebral volume. Also, a low value of slow waves of ICP also is indicative of a fatal outcome after head injury. Because each of these parameters—ICP, PRx, and the power of ICP slow waves—is an independent predictor of outcome, these three variables, although mutually correlated, should be considered jointly in any analysis. With regard to mean CPP, it is now one of the variables that is actively targeted with treatment; therefore, it may have lost its predictive power for outcome. This fact does not mean that short-term decreases in CPP ("CPP insults") have become any more benign. Reductions in CPP below specific threshold values are associated with poor outcome. In cases of severe pediatric head injury, studies have defined the CPP associated with poor outcome as between 40 and 65 mm Hg. For example, Downard and coworkers[43] studied 118 children (mean age, 7 years) with an overall mortality rate of 28% and found that the CPP associated with survival was greater than 40 mm Hg. No further improvement in outcome was seen with mean CPP in deciles from 40 to 70 mm Hg.

Invasive Intracranial Pressure Monitoring in Clinical Care

Traditionally, ICP monitoring is performed via a ventriculostomy. Newer technologies rely on fiberoptic monitoring, with the catheter sensor-tip placed in the brain parenchyma. On reviewing the literature about ICP monitoring in severe TBI, three key observations emerge.

First, the use of invasive ICP monitoring in management of pediatric severe TBI is by no means universal around the world. In the United States there is variation in practice. For example in a large multicenter database (2001 to 2011) of 4667 children with TBI, there was significant between-hospital variation in ICP monitoring.[44] Overall, 55% of patients ($n = 2586$) received ICP monitoring. Observed hospital ICP monitoring rates were 14% to 83%. After adjustment for patient factors, 13% of the ICP monitoring variation was attributable to between-hospital variation. Hospitals with more observed ICP monitoring, relative-to-expected, and hospitals with higher patient volumes had lower rates of mortality or severe disability. After adjustment for between-hospital variation and patient severity of injury, ICP monitoring was independently associated with age 1 year and older (odds ratio, 3.1; 95% CI, 2.5–3.8) versus age younger than 1 year. Another study, this

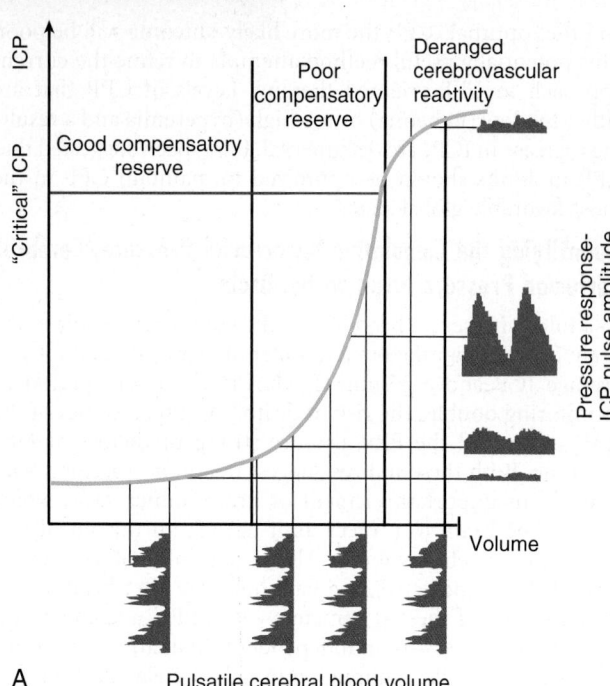

A   Pulsatile cerebral blood volume

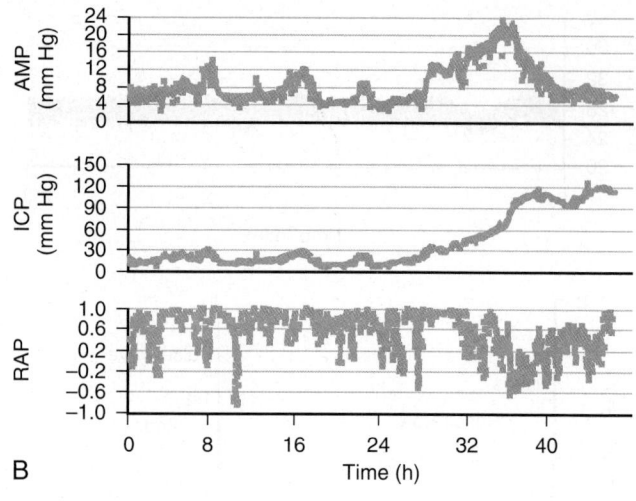

B

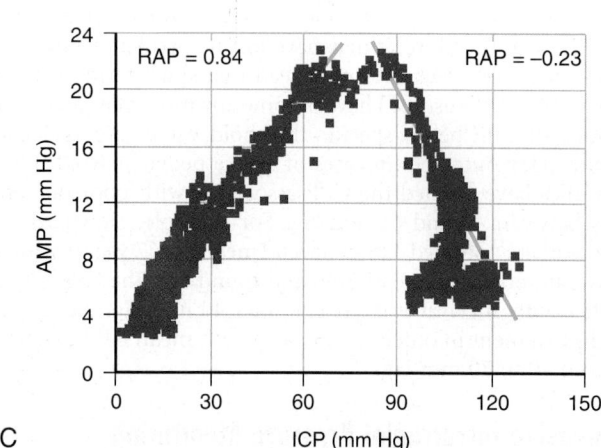

C

Fig. 66.9. (A) In a simple model, pulse amplitude of intracranial pressure (ICP) (AMP, expressed along the *y*-axis on the right side of the panel) results from pulsatile changes in cerebral blood volume (expressed along the *x*-axis) transformed by the pressure-volume curve. This curve has three zones: a flat zone, expressing good compensatory reserve; an exponential zone, depicting poor compensatory reserve; and a flat zone again, seen at very high ICP (above the "critical" ICP), depicting derangement of normal cerebrovascular responses. The pulse amplitude of ICP is low and does not depend on mean ICP in the first zone. The pulse amplitude increases linearly with mean ICP in the zone of poor compensatory reserve. In the third zone, the pulse amplitude starts to decrease with rising ICP. (B) Example of the relation between AMP and mean ICP recorded during a 46-hour period, during which terminal intracranial hypertension developed. Pulse amplitude increased first proportionally to the change in ICP but started to decrease when ICP increased above 80 mm Hg. (C) The regression plot between AMP and ICP indicates a biphasic relation of positive and negative slopes. The correlation coefficient between AMP and ICP (RAP) was positive before 32 hours but negative after that; this indicated terminal cerebrovascular deterioration.[40]

time using the US National Trauma Data Bank of pediatric TBI cases managed in levels I and II centers (2001 to 2006), found that ICP monitoring was undertaken in few pediatric patients with severe TBI.[45] Usage of ICP monitoring was associated with decreased mortality rate in only a small subset of the targeted population. In addition, children who received a monitoring device had longer hospital stay, longer PICU stay, and more ventilator days. These findings suggest that current use of ICP monitoring does not necessarily identify patients who are most likely to benefit from it.

Second, not all patients undergoing invasive ICP monitoring for severe TBI exhibit raised ICP. In a national study in the UK of all pediatric cases of severe TBI managed in the PICU (2001 to 2003), raised ICP was documented in only 49% (98 of 199 cases) of cases undergoing monitoring.[46] The authors found that of the variables significantly associated with raised ICP in univariate analyses (emergency department Glasgow Coma Scale [GCS] score, pupil reactivity, age, and the findings on admission computed tomography scans in relation to presence of subarachnoid hemorrhage, intracerebral hemorrhage,

or traumatic axonal injury (TAI), and lateral ventricle appearance), only the presence of TAI retained an independent association with development of raised ICP in multivariate logistic regression. GCS ≤8 predicted raised ICP with sensitivity 80% and specificity 55% (positive predictive value 59%, negative predictive value 77%). "Any abnormality on CT" predicted raised ICP with sensitivity 91% and specificity 38% (positive predictive value 58%, negative predictive value 82%). And, as also reported by others,[47] the presence of raised ICP despite normal radiology and pupil responses likely reflect the known low sensitivity of CT for clinically significant TAI.

Third, it is now known that aggressive medical treatment of intracranial hypertension complicating severe TBI can be guided by one of two strategies, with no difference in outcome: use of ICP monitoring as a guide to therapy or use of intensive clinical examination and serial CT scans to guide therapy.[48,49] In this 2012 study, in South America, 324 patients (13 years or older, 25% under 22 years of age) were randomly assigned to one of two specific protocols: guidelines-based management in which a protocol for monitoring intraparenchymal

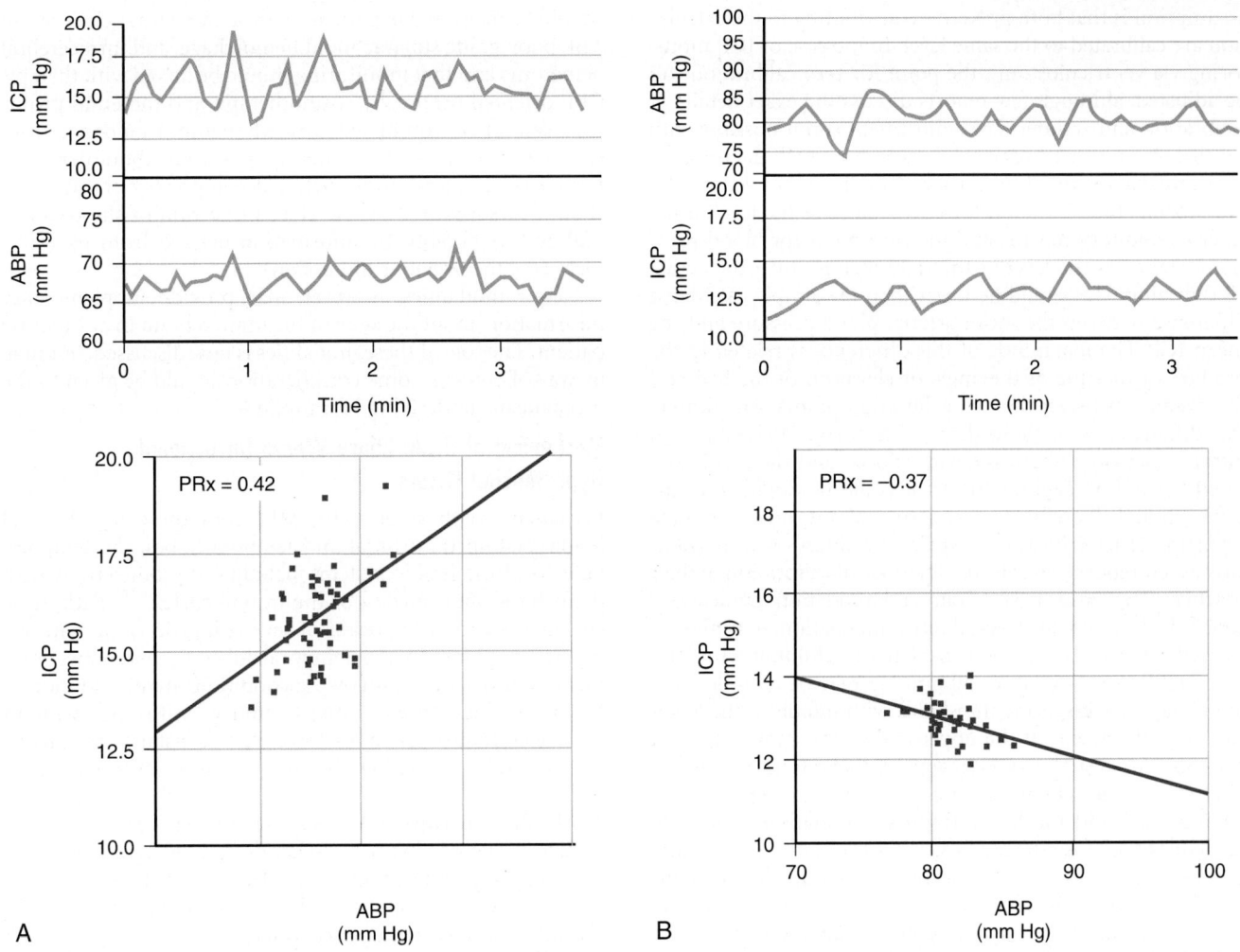

Fig. 66.10. Relation between slow waves of arterial pressure (ABP) and intracranial pressure (ICP). (A) Slow waves in ICP and ABP produce a positive correlation *(lower left panel),* giving a positive value of the pressure-reactivity index (PRx), which indicates loss of cerebrovascular reserve. (B) Coherent waves both in ABP and ICP produced a negative correlation coefficient when plotted on the regression graph *(lower right),* giving values of PRx that were clearly negative.

ICP was used or a protocol in which treatment was based on CT scans and clinical examination. The primary outcome was a composite of survival time, impaired consciousness, and functional status at 3 months and 6 months and neuropsychologic status at 6 months. There was no significant between-group difference in the primary outcome. Six-month mortality was no different between the groups (39% in the pressure-monitoring group and 41% in the imaging-clinical examination group). The median length of stay was similar in the two groups (12 days in the pressure-monitoring group and 9 days in the imaging-clinical examination group), although the number of days of brain-specific treatments (eg, administration of hyperosmolar fluids and the use of hyperventilation) was higher in the imaging-clinical examination group than in the pressure-monitoring group.

Taking everything together, it is clear that there is still much to learn in how we select patients for invasive monitoring and how we use the information from monitoring to guide our therapies. Even so, the authors' practice is to use invasive monitoring to guide treatment, rather than to rely solely on serial clinical examinations and CT imaging.

Intracranial Pressure and Cerebral Perfusion Pressure Target Levels

In adults, the threshold for initiating treatment of intracranial hypertension is taken as 20 to 25 mm Hg. It is likely that the ICP threshold for poorer outcome is similar across all ages and the second edition of the Brain Trauma Foundation's *Guidelines for the Acute Medical Management of Severe TBI in Infants, Children, and Adolescents*[34] concludes that treatment of raised ICP at a threshold of 20 mm Hg may be considered (level III evidence). In this regard, brief increases in ICP that return to normal in <5 min may be insignificant, but sustained increases of ≥20 mm Hg for ≥5 min likely warrant treatment. Despite this practice, it should be noted that the optimal ICP target or targets for pediatric TBI remain to be defined.

Normal values for mean arterial blood pressure and hence CPP are lower in children, particularly in infants and young children. Two assumptions are made when using calculated CPP to guide treatment. The first assumption is that the mean systemic arterial pressure is a good reflection of brain surface arteriolar pressure, and this may not be the case. The second assumption is that both pressures contributing to the calculation are calibrated to the same level. In the case of ICP monitoring via ventriculostomy, the point for zero calibration can be adjusted, although few reports discuss the exact details of calibration and zeroing. This adjustment is not possible with the fiber-tip intraparenchymal devices, for which the pressure is recorded at the tip of the sensor. If, in the case of ventricular monitoring, the zero point for ICP is taken as the level of the external auditory meatus and the zero point for blood pressure is taken as the level of the right atrium, then the actual CPP driving CBF would be lower than the simply calculated difference between the mean arterial blood pressure and the mean ICP. The magnitude of this difference is related to the product of the sine of the angle of elevation of the bed and the distance between the two calibration points. In children, this difference is of the order of 5 mm Hg. However, if an intraparenchymal fiber-tip device is used and the bed is elevated beyond 30 degrees, the error could be doubled. Clinicians should therefore be cautious about how the data reporting exact critical CPP values are interpreted, particularly as few reports describe the methods of calibration in their practice. The 2012 Brain Trauma Foundation guidelines[34] conclude the following level III recommendation: A minimum CPP of 40 mm Hg may be considered in children with TBI, and a CPP threshold 40 to 50 mm Hg may be considered— there may be age-specific thresholds with infants at the lower end and adolescents at the upper end of this range. In adult patients, with respect to CPP, it appears that the critical threshold for cerebral ischemia generally lies in the region of 50 to 60 mm Hg,[50] and the Brain Trauma Foundation adult CPP guidelines therefore suggest "a general threshold in the realm of 60 mm Hg, with further fine-tuning in individual patients based on monitoring of cerebral oxygenation and metabolism and assessment of the status of pressure autoregulation."[51]

In 2014 a report from the Brain Trauma Foundation trac database of 317 pediatric severe TBI cases provided further insight in to age-related CPP thresholds and survival in children and adolescents.[52] The evidence suggests that CPP targets should be age specific: above 50 or 60 mm Hg in adults, above 50 mm Hg in 6- to 17-year-olds, and above 40 mm Hg in 0- to 5-year-olds. Furthermore, because systemic hypotension had an inconsistent relationship with events of low CPP, but elevated ICP did, the authors recommended that ICP should be controlled at all times, while also targeting systolic blood pressure in specific instances. ICP-directed therapies are discussed in the next section.

Clinical Utility of Intracranial Pressure Monitoring With Other Monitoring Modalities

The continuous measurement of ICP is an essential modality in most brain monitoring systems. After enthusiastic attempts to introduce newer modalities for brain monitoring (eg, tissue oxygenation, microdialysis, cortical blood flow, TCD ultrasonography, jugular bulb oxygen saturation, and near infrared spectroscopy), it is becoming increasingly obvious that ICP is robust, only moderately invasive, and can be realistically conducted in most critical care units. As noted earlier, ICP measurement is a complex modality that contains information about compensatory mechanisms intrinsic to the brain and regulation of CBF. Thus continuous monitoring is required to control raised ICP. For example, most authors agree that ICP

should be measured in patients with acute states such as severe TBI, poor-grade subarachnoid hemorrhage, and intracerebral hematoma and that monitoring should be linked with therapy. CPP-oriented protocols,[53] osmotherapy, and the Lund protocol[54] cannot be conducted correctly without guidance from real-time ICP recording. Similarly, a decision about performing a surgical intervention such as decompressive craniectomy should be supported by the close inspection of the trend of ICP and, preferably, by information derived from its waveform (see the previous discussion).

Newer modalities, however, may provide supplementary information about the state of the injured brain in a comatose patient. The role of these modalities is now discussed, but first, by way of context, some consideration should be given to the mechanisms underlying brain injury.

Mechanism of Brain Injury Where Intracranial Hypertension Occurs

In patients with severe TBI, MRI commonly reveals focal lesions within the frontal and temporal lobes, the temporal poles, and the limbic system, including its connections with the orbitofrontal surface of the frontal cortex.[55,56] Pathologic change may occur by means of several injurious mechanisms in these regions. In the temporal lobes or its connections, manifestations of the following conditions may be found:

1. Direct high-speed impact injury with or without acceleration-deceleration forces. In this instance, the medial temporal lobe is vulnerable to mechanical deformation and contusion.[57]
2. Metabolic perturbation resulting from vascular or systemic factors such as hypoxia, ischemia, hypoglycemia, and seizures. In these head injury–related insults, there is a predilection for vulnerability within a structure in the temporal limbic system, the hippocampus.[58]
3. Diffuse axonal injury as a consequence of rotational forces at the time of injury affecting axonal integrity; thereafter, secondary or postacute deafferentation or deafferentation of structures such as the hippocampus occurs.[59,60]
4. Raised ICP with brain swelling resulting in pressure necrosis of the main cortical input to the hippocampus, to the parahippocampal gyrus, and against the free edge of the tentorium cerebelli.[61]
5. Frontal hemodynamic perfusion failure as a consequence of inadequate local CBF, failed local cerebral autoregulation, raised ICP, or anterior compartment syndrome (Fig. 66.11).

When consideration is given to monitoring other modalities besides ICP, two problems are encountered. The first problem is understanding the extent to which these mechanisms contribute to the physiologic derangements that can be followed in the intensive care unit. The second problem is making a difference in patient assessment and outcomes, provided these mechanisms can be influenced.

Monitoring and the Postinsult Natural History

In a patient with severe TBI, the value and utility of monitoring may serve a spectrum of functions. Given the five potential mechanisms outlined in the previous section (ie, direct mechanical effect, metabolic perturbation, axonal injury, brain swelling, and hemodynamic perfusion failure), specific foci, whether for assessment or treatment, can be identified

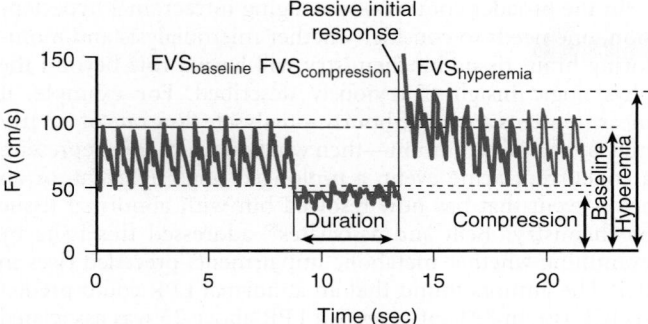

Fig. 66.11. Transient hyperemic response used test to assess autoregulation: middle cerebral artery blood flow velocity (Fv) is measured with transcranial Doppler ultrasonography before, during, and after a 6-second compression of the carotid artery. Hyperemia after release of compression signifies properly functioning vascular reactivity. *FVS,* flow velocities.

for monitoring. The potential for treatment rather than for assessment, however, will be limited by the time course over which the pathophysiologic monitoring is enacted. For example, the following need to be considered: What processes occur at the time of injury, what are the subsequent epiphenomena of these events, and what are the secondary factors that are amenable to treatment and altered outcome?[62-68] Mechanisms 1 and 3 occur at the time of injury, and mechanism 2 starts during the interval between the accident and arrival in the intensive care unit, although this mechanism may, in part, be avoidable with attention to emergency care and life support. Mechanisms 4 and 5 are processes in which treatment that is directed by intensive care monitoring presumably has the potential for altered outcome (ie, focal brain tissue shifts and hemodynamic perfusion failure). One important issue, therefore, is the natural history of brain swelling and local compartment syndrome after severe head injury. In persons with a TBI, intracranial hypertension occurs when there is brain swelling or a hematoma that occupies significant space. In persons with severe TBI and abnormalities shown with CT scans on admission, a greater than 50% chance of raised ICP exists. In adults, this complication may occur in persons whose CT scans appear normal, particularly if two of the following three features are present: age older than 40 years, unilateral or bilateral motor posturing, or systolic ABP below 90 mm Hg.

In children, the occurrence of this complication has been analyzed in a United Kingdom national dataset of all 501 children receiving critical care after sustaining a severe head injury. Forsyth and colleagues[69] found that by modeling demographic, acute physiologic, and cranial imaging variables they could derive an empiric decision rule that predicted the development of raised ICP at any point during intensive care unit admission with a sensitivity of 73% and a specificity of 74% (positive predictive value, 82%; negative predictive value, 63%). Overall raised ICP was present in 25% of those undergoing invasive monitoring. Importantly, the decision rule predicted raised ICP in 20% of children not undergoing ICP monitoring. Natale and associates[70] have shown that the natural history of raised ICP in children not requiring surgery after head injury can be as short as 3 days, but not infrequently it lasts for 7 to 10 days. Thus in regard to brain tissue shifts

and frontal compartment perfusion failure, the potential of a postinsult "therapeutic window" exists, which also implies a goal for therapy directed by monitoring.

Newer Modalities Supplementing Monitoring of Intracranial Pressure

Many of the supplementary, often research-based modalities that are used in monitoring have only been tested in patients with severe TBI, because this is the most common reason for instituting ICP monitoring.

Brain Oxygenation

Jugular bulb oxygen saturation is commonly used to assess cerebral oxygenation. However, this form of monitoring has several shortcomings, not the least of which is that it is a global measure that is insensitive to small, though important, regional changes. The relatively recent development of implantable tissue oxygen and pH microsensors has meant that more direct regional assessments are now being made. The questions, though, are what is normal tissue oxygen tension, and what does it mean? Reports in adults indicate that the threshold for abnormality is around 10 mm Hg,[71,72] although the validity and appropriateness of using such an exact measure has been questioned by Gupta and colleagues.[73,74] These investigators used positron emission tomography scanning in 19 adults with head injuries to validate the reading of brain tissue oxygen pressure (P_tO_2) from a NeuroTrend sensor inserted into the frontal region. End-capillary oxygen tension (P_vO_2) was calculated from oxygen extraction fraction in a 20-mm region of interest around the sensor and compared with P_tO_2. No correlation was found between the absolute values of P_tO_2 and P_vO_2. In contrast, a significant correlation was obtained between the change in P_tO_2 and the change in P_vO_2 produced by a decrease in $PaCO_2$ by approximately 1 kPa (7.5 mm Hg). Therefore these authors could only conclude that such monitoring should be used to assess, in real time, the changes attributable to a particular intervention.

Ushewokunze and Sgouros[75] have reported on five children with head trauma for whom this monitoring has been used. In common with findings in adults, the low P_tO_2 levels that occur during the first 24 hours following severe TBI do not correlate necessarily with poor outcome, and an increase in ICP may be accompanied by a decrease in P_tO_2.

Microdialysis and Brain Tissue Biochemistry

Tissue biochemical metabolic markers—rather than serum or cerebrospinal biomarkers—can be assessed continuously using cerebral microdialysis; essentially, one is potentially sampling cerebral extracellular fluid and using changes to make inferences about cell homeostasis and perturbation. Currently, this approach is used predominantly for research purposes and in adult practice. The technology enables bedside measurement (usually hourly in the case of TBI) of levels of cerebral dialysate glucose, lactate, pyruvate, glutamate, and glycerol. Typically, the glucose level and lactate-pyruvate ratio (LPR) are used as indices of inadequate substrate delivery, altered metabolism, and ischemia. The use of a ratio (ie, LPR), rather than absolute concentrations, means that an alteration in dialysate recovery rate does not result in spurious changes in LPR. A ratio less than 20 suggests uncomplicated cerebral metabolism,[76] and an increase in ratio is a sensitive indicator of a decrease in P_tO_2.[77] Dialysate increases in glutamate and glycerol are used as indices of cumulative tissue responses to secondary ischemic events such as intracranial hypertension, systemic hypotension, seizures, and contusions.

In adults with TBI, an increased ratio results from a 10-fold to 100-fold reduction in pyruvate concentration in association with a 2-fold to 5-fold increase in lactate concentration.[78] Two studies in adults with TBI, however, suggest that the LPR (and levels of the components that make up the ratio) might be revealing more about other forms of cerebral metabolic perturbation besides ischemic crisis. Hlatky and coworkers[79] found that in the first few hours after injury—at a time when P_tO_2 was normal (ie, nonischemic)—the LPR was increased because of low pyruvate concentration and not raised levels of lactate. Later when the P_tO_2 was at its lowest level, signifying "hypoxia/ischemia," increased LPR was due to a combination of increased lactate and decreased pyruvate levels. Vespa and associates[80] found that even though a raised lactate level or LPR was present in 25% of cerebral microdialysis samples, the occurrence of cerebral ischemia—defined as a raised lactate level, LPR, and a low glucose level—was much less frequent (~3%). Furthermore, upon combining these studies with positron emission tomography for assessing the metabolism of oxygen, the incidence of a high oxygen extraction fraction (ie, ischemia) was rare, at approximately 1%. Hillered and colleagues[81] have commented on these clinical reports in adults and suggested that the findings represent two metabolic states:

- *Type 1*, classical cerebral ischemia, is characterized by reduced microdialysis pyruvate and an increased level of lactate, leading to increased LPR (in association with depressed P_tO_2). This state is a result of an overt lack of oxygen and glucose at the mitochondria.
- *Type 2*, cerebral metabolic perturbation, occurs when P_tO_2 is normal (ie, nonischemic) and a reduction in pyruvate is the sole change in dialysis metabolites. The rise in LPR in this state is "perhaps reflecting a limited glucose supply or an impairment of the glycolytic pathway."

However, the mechanism of these early type 1 and type 2 changes are not fully understood, and there is an important difference between the study by Hlatky and coworkers[79] and that reported by Vespa and associates[78,80]: In the first study the microdialysis probes were placed perilesional or pericontusional; in the second study the microdialysis probes were cited as being placed in the nondominant, normal-appearing frontal lobe tissue. This difference is likely to be significant because, as Engstrom and colleagues[82] reported, microdialysis monitoring of normal-appearing tissue is not representative of perilesional tissue. Raised LPR persisted for at least 72 hours in perilesional tissue. In the first 36 hours this rise was associated with raised lactate levels and raised pyruvate concentrations. After that time, raised LPR was a reflection of raised lactate levels with normal pyruvate concentrations. All microdialysis parameters were in the normal range in normal-appearing tissue. These observations suggest that perilesional tissue has features of type 1 cerebral metabolic crisis, but the absence of depressed P_tO_2 suggests that increased lactate occurs as a consequence of increased glycolytic activity, which may be due to perilesional depolarizations.[83] Such hyperglycolysis is marked by increased metabolism relative to utilization and, after trauma, it represents an uncoupling between predominantly glycolytic and oxidative metabolism.[84]

In the broader context of managing intracranial hypertension, one needs to consider whether microdialysis and monitoring brain tissue biochemistry will have a role beyond the physiologic insights previously described. For example, if measurements are made hourly—dialysate flow rate of 0.3 µL/min is the most common—then what does a change represent: a concurrent acute event, a prolonged ongoing event, or an acute event that has now resolved but with abnormal tissue biochemistry? Belli and associates[85] addressed this issue by examining whether metabolic impairments preceded rises in ICP. The authors found that an abnormal LPR could predict an ICP rise in 89% of cases. An LPR above 25 was associated with an odds ratio of 9.8 (95% CI, 5.8 to 16.1) of imminent intracranial hypertension. With regard to the utility of this form of monitoring in children, we know that in the United Kingdom national dataset of critical care for severe TBI, less than 1% of children undergo such monitoring.[86] To date, a case series of only nine children has been reported.[87,88]

Taking all of this metabolic information together, it is unclear whether the real-time cerebral microdialysis data have the potential to direct or influence our practice of ICP/CPP control. What is more intriguing, however, are the reports that indicate how such monitoring can be used to integrate what fuel the distressed brain needs[89,90] and thereby mitigate the severity of ICP/CPP levels.

Transcranial Doppler and Assessment of Autoregulation

TCD ultrasonography provides noninvasive measurement of blood flow velocity in basal cerebral arteries.[22] Most data have been derived from the MCA. This vessel is readily accessible to the ultrasonographer; it is the most convenient for probe fixation and long-term monitoring, and it delivers the largest percentage of supratentorial blood. Although the blood flow velocity cannot express a baseline volume of flow, dynamic changes of CBF are usually reflected in the TCD readings.[22,91] The response of blood flow velocity to a critical decrease in CPP is sensitive and usually immediate (see Fig. 66.11). It is this high-dynamic resolution and close correlation with other hemodynamic modalities that has encouraged the development of the technique in clinical practice.

Increased baseline flow velocity (>100 cm/sec) may indicate cerebral vasospasm or hyperemia.[92,93] Uncoupling between CBF and flow velocity in vasospasm has been documented both experimentally and clinically.[94] For example, if the ratio of flow velocity in the insonated artery to the velocity in the ipsilateral internal carotid artery is greater than 3, vasospasm is likely. A ratio lower than 2 indicates hyperemia as the cause for accelerated blood flow.[95] After a severe TBI is sustained, cerebral autoregulation is frequently disturbed, although the extent of this disturbance may fluctuate with time.[8,9] In a prospective, observational study of 69 children with TBI (GCS score ≤12) and abnormal head imaging, O'Brien and colleagues[96] undertook TCD studies to identify and follow vasospasm. The prevalence of MCA vasospasm with moderate TBI (GCS 9-12) was 8.5%, and it was 33.5% in those with severe TBI (GCS ≤8). Mean time to onset of vasospasm was 4 days and the mean duration of vasospasm was 2 days. Children in whom vasospasm developed were more likely to have been involved in motor vehicle accidents, had higher Injury Severity scores, had fever at admission, and had lower GCS scores.

At present, few pediatric practitioners in critical care medicine are credentialed to undertake TCD for clinical care. This specialization may change in the future as we adopt more adult neurocritical care training requirements. For example, in adult practice it is interesting to note the range of assessments that can be conducted at the bedside:

1. *Static test of autoregulation.* Methods for the static assessment of autoregulation rely on measurement of MCA blood flow velocity during changes in mean ABP induced by a vasopressor infusion. The static rate of autoregulation (SoR) can be calculated as the percentage increase in vascular resistance divided by the percentage rise in ABP. An SoR of 100% indicates fully intact autoregulation, whereas an SoR of 0% indicates fully depleted autoregulation.

2. *TCD reactivity to changes in carbon dioxide concentration.* Testing for CO_2 cerebrovascular reactivity has been shown to have an important application in the assessment of severe head injuries and other cerebrovascular conditions. Many authors have shown that cerebral vessels are reactive to changes in CO_2 when cerebral autoregulation had been impaired.[97] CO_2 reactivity correlates significantly with outcome after a head injury. In patients with an exhausted cerebral compensatory reserve, however, hypercapnia may provoke substantial changes in ICP. Therefore this method cannot be used without consideration of patient safety, particularly if baseline ICP is already elevated.

3. *Dynamic test of autoregulation.* Aaslid and colleagues[98] described a method in which a step decrease in ABP is achieved by the deflation of compressed leg cuffs while TCD flow velocity in the MCA is simultaneously monitored. An index called the dynamic rate of autoregulation describes how quickly cerebral vessels react to the sudden fall in blood pressure. The dynamic rate of autoregulation is thought to express the autoregulatory reserve and, in adult volunteers, has been shown to correlate with blood CO_2 concentration in volunteers.[99]

4. *Transient hyperemic response test.* Short-term compression of the common carotid artery produces a marked decrease in MCA blood flow velocity in the ipsilateral hemisphere. During compression, the distal cerebrovascular bed dilates if autoregulation is intact. On release of the compression, transient hyperemia, which lasts for a few seconds, occurs until the distal cerebrovascular bed constricts to its former diameter. This sequence of events, which underlies the transient hyperemic response test, indicates a positive autoregulatory response (see Fig. 66.11). In persons with a head injury, preliminary results show a positive correlation between the presence of a hyperemic response and outcome.[100]

5. *Continuous analysis of TCD ultrasonography with respiratory waves.* An interesting method of deriving the autoregulatory status from natural fluctuations in MCA blood flow velocity involves the assessment of phase shift between the superimposed respiratory and ABP waves during deep breathing.[101] A 0-degree phase shift indicates absent autoregulation, whereas a phase shift of 90 degrees indicates intact autoregulation. Such an approach may allow for the continuous assessment of autoregulation without performing potentially hazardous test maneuvers on arterial pressure.

6. *Continuous analysis of TCD flow velocity waveform.* In patients with severe head injuries, CPP monitoring can be correlated with mean blood flow velocity continuously. For example, consecutive CPP samples (averaged over 5-second periods) can be assessed with average flow velocity (collected over 5-minute epochs). The correlation coefficient (named mean index) may be positive or negative, and the regression line describing the relationship between the systolic-, mean-, and diastolic-flow velocity and the CPP may be used for assessment. A positive correlation coefficient signifies a positive association of flow velocity with CPP; a negative correlation coefficient signifies a negative association. In persons with a head injury, group analysis has shown that clinical outcome depends on the averaged autoregulation indices.[9] Furthermore, time analysis has shown that failure of autoregulation is a strong independent predictor of fatal outcome after a head injury.[102]

Some data on TCD assessments of cerebral autoregulation in children with TBI are now available. For example, in a series of 36 children, the incidence of impaired cerebral autoregulation was greatest following moderate to severe TBI.[103] Impaired autoregulation was associated with poor outcome, and hyperemia was associated with both impaired autoregulation and poor outcome. In severe cases, cerebral autoregulation often changes over the course of a critical illness, with worsening autoregulation mirroring progression of worsening injury.[104] Importantly, in children, bilateral assessment of cerebral autoregulation is required because hemisphere differences are common in those with an isolated focal injury.[105] Finally, inflicted TBI probably should be considered a special case: In a small case series, Vavilala and coworkers[106] found that none of their critically ill cases had intact autoregulation.

Key References

2. Czosnyka M, Richards HK, Czosnyka Z, et al. Vascular components of cerebrospinal fluid compensation. *J Neurosurg.* 1999;90:752-759.
3. Davson H, Hollingsworth G, Segal MB. The mechanism of drainage of the cerebrospinal fluid. *Brain.* 1970;93:665-678.
4. Czosnyka M, Piechnik S, Richards HK, et al. Contribution of mathematical modelling to the bedside tests of cerebrovascular autoregulation. *J Neurol Neurosurg Psychiatry.* 1997;63:721-731.
5. Kashif FM, Verghase GC, Novak V, et al. Model-based noninvasive estimation of intracranial pressure from cerebral blood flow velocity and arterial pressure. *Sci Transl Med.* 2012;4:129ra44.
6. Miller JD, Stanek A, Langfitt TW. Concepts of cerebral perfusion pressure and vascular compression during intracranial hypertension. *Prog Brain Res.* 1972;35:411-432.
8. Steiner LA, Czosnyka M, Piechnik SK, et al. Continuous monitoring of cerebrovascular pressure reactivity allows determination of optimal cerebral perfusion pressure in patients with traumatic brain injury. *Crit Care Med.* 2002;30:733-738.
11. Czosnyka M, Smielewski P, Piechnik S, et al. Hemodynamic characterization of intracranial pressure plateau waves in head-injured patients. *J Neurosurg.* 1999;91:11-19.
13. Lundberg N. Continuous recording and control of ventricular fluid pressure in neurosurgical practice. *Acta Psychiatr Neurol Scand.* 1960; 36(suppl 149):1-193.
17. Bauerie J, Schuchardt F, Schroeder L, et al. Reproducibility and accuracy of optic nerve sheath diameter assessment using ultrasound compared to magnetic resonance imaging. *BMC Neurol.* 2013;13:187.
18. Launey Y, Nesseier N, Le Malledant Y, et al. Effect of osmotherapy on optic nerve sheath diameter in patients with increased intracranial pressure. *J Neurotrauma.* 2014;31:984-988.
19. Gwer S, Chacha C, Newton CR, Kirkham FJ. Unexpected relationship between tympanometry and mortality in children with nontraumatic coma. *Pediatrics.* 2013;132:e713-e717.
20. Gwer S, Kazungu M, Chengo E, et al. Abnormal intra-aural pressure waves associated with death in African children with acute nontraumatic coma. *Pediatr Res.* 2015;78:38-43.
22. Aaslid R, Markwalder TM, Nornes H. Noninvasive transcranial Doppler ultrasound recording of flow velocity in basal cerebral arteries. *J Neurosurg.* 1982;57:769-774.

29. Soldatos T, Chatzimichail K, Papathanasiou M, et al. Optic nerve sonography: a new window for the non-invasive evaluation of intracranial pressure in brain injury. *Emerg Med J.* 2009;26:630-634.

30. Le A, Hoehn ME, Smith ME, et al. Bedside sonographic measurement of optic nerve sheath diameter as a predictor of increased intracranial pressure in children. *Ann Emerg Med.* 2009;53:785-791.

34. Kochanek PM, Carney NA, Adelson PD, et al. Guidelines for the acute medical management of severe traumatic brain injury in infants, children, and adolescents—second edition. *Pediatr Crit Care Med.* 2012; 13(suppl 1):S1-S82.

37. Lundberg N. Continuous recording and control of ventricular fluid pressure in neurosurgical practice. *Acta Psychiatr Neurol Scand.* 1960;36(suppl 149):1-193.

39. Avezaat CJ, van Eijndhoven JH, Wyper DJ. Cerebrospinal fluid pulse pressure and intracranial volume-pressure relationships. *J Neurol Neurosurg Psychiatry.* 1979;42:687-700.

42. Brady KM, Schaffner DH, Lee JK, et al. Continuous monitoring of cerebrovascular pressure reactivity after traumatic brain injury in children. *Pediatrics.* 2009;124:e1205-e1212.

43. Downard C, Hulka F, Mullins RJ, et al. Relationship of cerebral perfusion pressure and survival in pediatric brain-injured patients. *J Trauma.* 2000;49:654-658.

44. Bennett TD1, Riva-Cambrin J, Keenan HT, et al. Variation in intracranial pressure monitoring and outcomes in pediatric traumatic brain injury. *Arch Pediatr Adolesc Med.* 2012;166:641-647.

46. Forsyth RJ, Parslow RC, Tasker RC, et al. Prediction of raised intracranial pressure complicating severe traumatic brain injury in children: implications for trial design. *Pediatr Crit Care Med.* 2008;9:8-14.

48. Chesnut RM, Temkin N, Carney N, et al. A trial of intracranial-pressure monitoring in traumatic brain injury. *N Engl J Med.* 2012;367: 2471-2481.

49. Chesnut RM. Intracranial pressure monitoring: headstone or a new head start. The BEST TRIP trial in perspective. *Intensive Care Med.* 2013;39: 771-774.

51. Bratton SL, Chestnut RM, Ghajar J, et al. Guidelines for the management of severe traumatic brain injury. IX. Cerebral perfusion thresholds. *J Neurotrauma.* 2007;24(suppl 1):S59-S64.

53. Rosner MJ, Rosner SD, Johnson AH. Cerebral perfusion pressure: management protocol and clinical results. *J Neurosurg.* 1995;83:949-962.

54. Grande PO. The "Lund concept" for treatment of severe brain trauma: a physiological approach. In: Vincent J-L, ed. *Yearbook of Intensive Care and Emergency Medicine.* Springer-Verlag; 2004:806-820.

60. Tasker RC, Salmond CH, Westland AG, et al. Head circumference and brain and hippocampal volume after severe traumatic brain injury in childhood. *Pediatr Res.* 2005;58:302-308.

61. Adams JH, Graham DI. The relationship between ventricular fluid pressure and the neuropathology of raised intracranial pressure. *Neuropathol Appl Neurobiol.* 1976;2:323-332.

62. Slawik H, Salmond CH, Taylor-Tavares J, et al. Frontal cerebral vulnerability and executive deficits from raised intracranial pressure in child traumatic brain injury. *J Neurotrauma.* 2009;26:1891-1903.

66. Shahlaie K, Boggan JE, Latchaw RE, et al. Posttraumatic vasospasm detected by continuous brain tissue oxygen monitoring: treatment with intraarterial verapamil and balloon angioplasty. *Neurocrit Care.* 2009; 10:61-69.

67. Nahed BV, Ferreira M, Naunheim MR, et al. Intracranial vasospasm with subsequent stroke after traumatic subarachnoid hemorrhage in a 22-month-old child. *J Neurosurg Pediatr.* 2009;3:311-315.

69. Forsyth RJ, Parslow RC, Tasker RC, et al. Prediction of raised intracranial pressure complicating severe traumatic brain injury in children: implications for trial design. *Pediatr Crit Care Med.* 2008;9:8-14.

78. Vespa P, McArthur D, Glenn T, et al. Persistently low extracellular glucose correlates with poor outcome at 6 months after traumatic brain injury despite lack of increased lactate: a microdialysis study. *J Cereb Blood Flow Metab.* 2003;23:865-877.

79. Hlatky R, Valadka AB, Goodman JC, et al. Patterns of energy substrate during ischemia measured in the brain by microdialysis. *J Neurotrauma.* 2004;21:894-906.

86. Morris KP, Forsyth RJ, Parslow RC, et al. Intracranial pressure complicating severe traumatic brain injury in children: monitoring and management. *Intensive Care Med.* 2006;32:1606-1612.

96. O'Brien NF, Maa T, Yeates KO. The epidemiology of vasospasm in children with moderate-to-severe traumatic brain injury. *Crit Care Med.* 2015;43:674-685.

97. Steiger HJ, Aaslid R, Stooss R, et al. Transcranial Doppler monitoring in head injury: relationships between type of injury, flow velocities, vasoreactivity and outcome. *Neurosurgery.* 1994;34:79-85.

103. Vavilala MS, Lee LA, Boddu K, et al. Cerebral autoregulation in pediatric traumatic brain injury. *Pediatr Crit Care Med.* 2004;5:257-263.

106. Vavilala MS, Muangman S, Waitayawinyu P, et al. Impaired cerebral autoregulation in infants and young children early after inflicted traumatic brain injury: a preliminary report. *J Neurotrauma.* 2007;24: 87-96.

Status Epilepticus

Edward E. Conway, Jr.

PEARLS

- A seizure is a paroxysmal central nervous system disorder resulting from excessive hypersynchronous discharge of cortical neurons.
- Status epilepticus is a common pediatric neurologic emergency and requires rapid recognition and intervention.
- An operational definition of status epilepticus recommends administration of an antiepileptic agent (AED) after 5 minutes of seizure activity, and a predetermined pathway/guideline can expedite management.
- Management goals include general supportive care, termination of status epilepticus, prevention of recurrence, correction of precipitating causes, and prevention and treatment of potential complications.
- Common errors include underdosing the initial AED and delay in advancing to a second-line AED. A single drug should be maximized to a high therapeutic or supratherapeutic level before adding a second or third drug.
- The longer seizures continue, the more difficult they are to abort with medications. Early diagnosis and aggressive intervention for both convulsive and nonconvulsive seizures are essential for successful treatment.
- Prolonged seizures may cause selective neuronal loss in the hippocampus, cortex, and thalamus, areas rich in glutamate receptors.

A seizure is a paroxysmal disorder of the central nervous system (gray matter) characterized by an abnormal neuronal discharge associated with a change in function of the patient. It results from the excessive hypersynchronous discharge of cortical neurons in the gray matter.

Factors that occur commonly in the pediatric intensive care unit (PICU) and are known to provoke seizures include fever, hyponatremia, hypoglycemia, hypocalcemia, meningitis, head trauma (accidental or nonaccidental), toxin exposure, ethanol, and many other drugs (both legal and illicit). Seizures are a common pediatric entity and occur in almost 5% to 8% of pediatric-aged patients with the highest risk occurring during infancy and early childhood. A seizure must be differentiated from other paroxysmal events, which may include syncope, breath-holding spells, movement disorders, or hyperventilation syndrome.

Status epilepticus (SE) is a common pediatric neurologic emergency estimated to affect between 25,000 to 50,000 children annually, and 40% of all instances of SE will occur in children under age 2. The incidence of convulsive SE in children is approximately 10 to 27/100,000 per year. The definition of SE has undergone revisions, and it was previously defined as a seizure lasting for greater than 30 minutes or recurrent seizures lasting for more than 30 minutes without the patient regaining consciousness between seizures. No clinical data support the 30-minute rule, however, and more recent definitions of SE include a shorter duration of seizure activity. The early definitions were based on animal studies, which suggested that neuronal damage would occur if seizures persisted beyond an established timeline. Much has been learned since these early studies, and it appears that it is the underlying disorder that causes the morbidity and mortality seen in SE. The majority of tonic-clonic generalized seizures will self-terminate in less than 5 minutes.[1] The goal of treating prolonged seizures is to prevent morbidity and mortality, and a new operational definition of SE has been proposed: Generalized convulsive status epilepticus in adults and older children (>5 years old) refers to ≥5 minutes of (1) continuous seizure or (2) two or more discrete seizures between which there is incomplete recovery of consciousness.[2,3]

The authors of this new definition cite a paucity of pediatric data to make recommendations in children younger than 5 years. Although there is general agreement that seizures continuing for longer than 5 minutes should be treated, there exists a concern that overaggressive treatment may lead to avoidable morbidity. A study by DeLorenzo (which included 91 children) compared the outcome of patients with seizures lasting 10 to 29 minutes with that of traditionally defined SE (>30 minutes).[1] Almost 50% of the seizures in the 10- to 29-minute group stopped spontaneously (without therapy), and this group had no mortality. In comparison, the other 50% of patients in the 10- to 29-minute group, who required therapy to stop the seizures, had a mortality of 4.4%. The traditional group (seizures lasting >30 minutes) had a mortality of 19%.[1] Children with SE have an overall mortality of approximately 0% to 3%. Apart from mortality, SE survivors also have an increased risk of subsequent epilepsy, reported to be between 13% and 74%.[4] SE recurs in approximately 20% of cases within 4 years of initial presentation, with most recurrences occurring during the first 2 years.[4] Seizures and SE recurrence are influenced by the underlying etiology, with structural or metabolic lesions associated with the highest risk.[4] Regardless of the definition of SE, there is a consensus

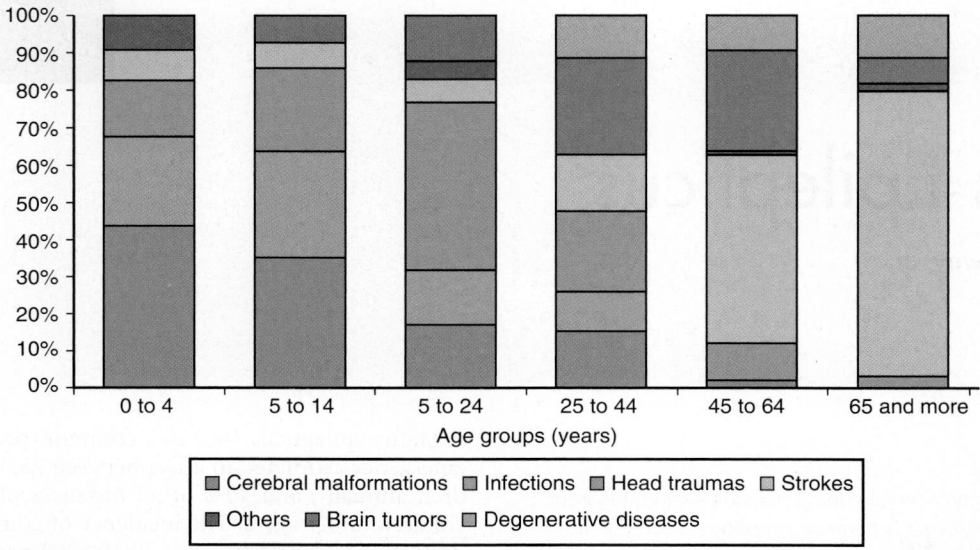

Fig. 67.1. Proportional incidences for symptomatic epilepsies according to age and etiologies. (From Major P, Thiele EA. Seizures in children: determining the variation. Pediatr Rev. 2007;28:363-371.)

in the medical community that continuous or prolonged seizures require urgent intervention. Children with prolonged seizures should receive prompt and aggressive treatment with the aim of stopping seizures as soon as possible.

Two large case series demonstrated similar results showing that SE accounted for 1.6% and 2% of total admissions to the PICU.[5] Although this represented a small total number of patients admitted to the PICU, there was morbidity and mortality associated with SE. SE occurs more frequently in infants and children than adults; the overall mortality is much lower at 3.6%.[5]

SE also may be classified with respect to cause. *Symptomatic* implies a known cause for SE (structural or metabolic) and can be further divided into acute symptomatic and remote symptomatic. Acute symptomatic seizures are those occurring in close temporal association (<7 days) to an acute systemic metabolic or toxic insult or in association with an acute CNS insult. Remote symptomatic refers to seizures owing to a remote CNS injury (>1 week) such as infection, trauma cerebrovascular disease, or cortical dysgenesis, which are presumed to result in a static lesion. Remote symptomatic SE is most often associated with a long-standing history of epilepsy or remote central nervous system (CNS) insult. The term *idiopathic SE* is used when there is no known or suspected cause for the seizures (Fig. 67.1).[6]

Proportional Incidences for Symptomatic Epilepsies According to Age and Etiology

The most common causes of SE reported in pediatric patients include an underlying seizure disorder, fever, meningitis, and encephalitis. One of the largest series of SE in children was published in 1970. This review of 239 cases of SE in children identified 47% of cases to be symptomatic (26% acute symptomatic and 21% remote symptomatic) and the remaining 53% of cases to be idiopathic, including febrile SE.[7] The cause of SE is age dependent; infection plays a larger role in the cause of SE in children than in adults. In a 1996 study in

TABLE 67.1   Physiologic Derangements in Status Epilepticus

	Early <30 min	Late >30 min	Complication
Blood pressure	↑	↓	Hypotension
Pao_2	↓	↓	Hypoxia
$Paco_2$	↑	Variable	↑ Intracranial pressure
Serum pH	↓	↓	Acidosis
Automatic	↑	↔	Arrhythmias
Creatine kinase	Normal	↑	Renal failure
Potassium	Normal	↑	Arrhythmias
Cerebral blood flow	↑ 900%	↑ 200%	Central nervous system bleed
Cerbral metabolic rate of oxygen consumption	↑ 300%	↑ 300%	Ischemia

Modified from Dean JM, Singer HS. Status epilepticus. In: Rogers MC, ed. Textbook of Pediatric Intensive Care Medicine. Baltimore: Williams & Wilkins; 1987:618.

Richmond, Virginia, the three major causes of SE in children were infection with fever, remote symptomatic cause, and low anticonvulsant drug levels (Table 67.1).[8] Three major causes in adults were low antiepileptic drug (AED) levels, remote symptomatic cause, and stroke.[8] The cause also differs among younger and older children. Febrile and acute symptomatic SE are more common in children younger than 2 years, whereas idiopathic and remote symptomatic causes are most common in children older than 4 years.[9,10] In children with a first seizure, 12% present in SE.[11] In a report of 613 children with newly diagnosed epilepsy, 9.1% had provoked or unprovoked SE before the diagnosis of epilepsy and a nearly equal number, 9.5%, had an episode of SE following the diagnosis of epilepsy

(8-year median follow-up).[12,13] Children who had SE before a diagnosis of epilepsy were most likely to have remote symptomatic epilepsy. Younger age of epilepsy onset and symptomatic epilepsy increased the risk of SE.[14]

Epilepsy is a chronic seizure disorder characterized by recurrent (more than two) unprovoked seizures usually in a person who has a predisposition because of an underlying state. It is also a potential long-term complication of SE, refractory status epilepticus (RSE) cEEG, and super-refractory status epilepticus (SRSE).

Refractory SE is defined as continued SE despite the administration of multiple first- and second-line agents with different mechanisms of action including benzodiazepines, fosphenytoin or phenytoin, and phenobarbital. Often these patients have had continuous (clinical or electrographical) seizure activity for hours. The care of these patients should be a collaborative effort between intensive care specialists and neurologists and requires standard invasive intensive care monitoring as well as the 24-hour availability of electroencephalography (EEG). Treatment of refractory status epilepticus requires continuous EEG (cEEG) monitoring because pharmacologic therapy is titrated to EEG seizure suppression or burst suppression. Mortality rates for RSE are as high as 30%.[14]

Super-refractory SE is defined as SE that continues 24 hours or more after the onset of anesthetic therapy for SE, including those cases in which SE recurs during reduction or withdrawal of anesthesia.[14]

Nonconvulsive status epilepticus (NCSE) is defined as clinically subtle or nonconvulsive seizures, which may be common among patients in the intensive care unit, particularly following prolonged convulsive seizures. Postictal stupor or coma due to the sedative effects of medications is often difficult to distinguish from continued nonconvulsive seizures without the aid of cEEG monitoring. Electrographic seizure activity has been reported to occur in up to 15% of patients whose overt clinical seizures are pharmacologically controlled.[12,15,16]

Seizures and SE may occur as common complications in medical and surgical patients in the PICU without an underlying neurologic disorder (Box 67.1).

BOX 67.1	Common Causes of Seizures in the Pediatric Intensive Care Unit
Stroke/arteriovenous malformation/ hemorrhage	Hypoxia and ischemia
Tumor	Fever and febrile seizures
Meningitis/encephalitis/abscess	Drug toxicity and withdrawal
Vasculitis	Renal/hepatic dysfunction
Traumatic brain injury	Metabolic: ↑↓ glucose
Preexisting epilepsy	↑↓ Sodium
Antiepileptic agent withdrawal or change	↑↓ Calcium
Postoperative craniotomy	↑↓ Serum osmol
Genetic CNS disorders	Hypertensive encephalopathy
Cerebral malformation	Neurocutaneous syndromes

Seizure Types and Classification

Seizures are classified based on the clinical presentation and electroencephalographic patterns and are simply divided into partial or generalized seizures. Partial seizures (also referred to as simple, local, or focal) arise in specific areas of the brain, and their presentation depends on the primary function of the affected area (motor, sensory, visual, auditory, gustatory, or affective). Simple partial seizures may remain focal or they can become complex (implying loss of consciousness) and further evolve into a generalized tonic-clonic seizure.

The second group of seizures refers to those labeled as generalized (thus implying that the seizures arise from diffuse cortical areas at one time). Generalized seizures refer to seizures involving both cerebral hemispheres, which are believed to originate within, and rapidly engage, bilaterally distributed neuronal networks. Consciousness is usually impaired. Generalized seizures include seizures with motor movements as well as absence seizures during which no convulsive signs may be present. EEG indicates seizure activity involving both cerebral hemispheres.

Febrile seizures (FSs) are the most common type of pediatric seizure and occur in patients between 6 months and 5 years of age associated with fever but without intracranial infection or defined cause. They are usually transient, age-related responses to noxious stimuli. They occur at a peak incidence of about 18 months and are generalized tonic-clonic and last less than 10 minutes followed by a brief postictal period. Factors associated with the risk of having an FS include a family history of FS, peak temperature, and the nature of the underlying illness. The mean temperature associated with FS is approximately 39°C or greater, and it appears that it is the peak temperature not the rising phase of the fever that is relevant. Studies suggest that cytokines such as interleukin-1, which is a proconvulsant agent, may play a role in febrile seizures. Febrile seizures are classified as simple or complex. FSs are considered simple when they are generalized, do not recur within a defined illness, and last less than 10 to 15 minutes. Complex febrile seizures are defined as those that are focal, last longer than 10 to 15 minutes, or occur multiple times within the same febrile illness.[17-20]

Febrile Status Epilepticus

Approximately 5% of children who present with an FS will have an episode of FSE. Although only a small number of children with an FS will develop SE, this accounts for almost 25% of cases of pediatric SE. Febrile status epilepticus (FSE) rarely stops spontaneously, is fairly resistant to medications, and even with proper treatment may persist for a significant period of time. The FEBSTAT study reported on 199 subjects with FSE with a mean seizure duration of 81 minutes for subjects receiving medications prior to arriving at the emergency department (ED); the median time from the first dose of an AED to the end of the seizure was 38 minutes, and the initial dose of lorazepam or diazepam was suboptimal in 19% of patients (34/166).[17-20]

Seizures Commonly Encountered in the Pediatric Intensive Care Unit

Chemically Induced Seizures

It is difficult at times to determine the immediate precipitant of a seizure/SE in critically ill patients, as multiple factors that can lower the seizure threshold include the underlying medical or surgical process, medications, renal or hepatic dysfunction or failure, fever, hypoxia, metabolic abnormalities, or alkalosis. Medications commonly associated with a decreased seizure threshold include antidepressants, antibiotics, analgesics, antiarrhythmics, baclofen, chemotherapeutic agents, drug withdrawal (barbiturates, alcohol, opiates), immunomodulators (cyclosporine, tacrolimus, interferons), lithium, neuroleptics, radiographic contrast agents, and theophylline. Drugs of abuse associated with seizures/SE include cocaine, amphetamines, phencyclidine, and gamma-hydroxybutyric acid. Less common causes include carbon monoxide, lead, envenomations, camphor, iron, and organophosphates.

Dialysis Disequilibrium Syndrome

Dialysis disequilibrium syndrome is characterized by neurologic symptoms (headache, nausea, disorientation, restlessness, blurred vision, asterixis, confusion, seizures, coma, and even death) seen during or immediately after hemodialysis. The pathophysiology is thought to involve the movement of water into the brain causing cerebral edema following the rapid removal of urea, which lowers the plasma osmolality causing a transient osmotic gradient that favors movement of water into the brain.

Hepatic Mechanisms

Hepatic postulated mechanisms of seizures in liver failure include hyperammonemia, abnormal glutamine metabolism, cerebral ischemia, cerebral edema, accumulation of toxins, or associated electrolyte abnormalities such as hyponatremia, hypomagnesemia, or elevated blood urea nitrogen or creatinine. The management of these seizures and possible SE is the same as in other conditions except one must be cautious with the selection of an antiepileptic medication that is cleared by the liver. The degree of hepatic failure may influence the metabolism of an AED, as early in the process there may be increased blood flow to the liver with normal function where the AED may be normally cleared; however, in the later stages of hepatic failure with necrosis and loss of hepatic cellular function, the AED may not be cleared, leading to a potentially toxic AED level. Hypoalbuminemia may also contribute to AED toxicity, particularly in highly protein-bound drugs such as phenytoin and valproic acid.

Hypertensive Encephalopathy

Patients with hypertensive encephalopathy have disordered cerebral autoregulation and may develop what has been termed *posterior reversible encephalopathy syndrome (PRES)*. Presenting signs and symptoms include headache, visual complaints, vomiting, and seizures. Cerebral autoregulation is the process by which cerebral blood flow (CBF) remains constant across a wide range of cerebral perfusion pressures (CPPs). As the mean arterial pressure (MAP) exceeds 150 to 160 mm Hg, arteriolar vasoconstriction is exhausted and hydrostatic pressure increases continuously resulting in a breakdown of the blood-brain barrier producing cerebral edema (see also Chapters 60 and 66). The increased incidence of vasogenic edema in the parietal and occipital lobes is thought to be due to poor sympathetic innervation of the posterior circulation of the brain.[21,22]

Neonatal Seizures

Neonatal seizures occur secondary to acute brain insults such as vascular, infectious, metabolic, or toxic etiologies during the first 28 days of life. The most common cause is hypoxic-ischemic injury (60%-70%), followed by hemorrhage (~10%), and the remaining causes include sepsis, metabolic disorders, meningitis, hypoglycemia, hypo- and hypernatremia, and hypocalcemia. The incidence is between 1.5 and 5.5/1000 neonates.[23]

Animal data support the concept that newborns are more susceptible to seizures due to excitatory processes developing before inhibitory ones, differences in the microenvironment, and a higher incidence of being exposed to potentially epileptogenic stimuli (hypoxia, fever, infection). Most neonatal seizures occur within the first week of life, and the incidence is highest in low-birth-weight babies. Because the newborn brain is undergoing tremendous growth (it will double in size in 6 months) and there is incomplete development of dendrites, axons, and a lack of myelination, classic generalized tonic-clonic seizures seen in older pediatric patients may not be observed. Neonatal seizures may be subtle and include facial or extremity twitching, posturing, eye deviations, muscle jerking of the extremities, chewing, blinking, bicycling, and apnea. Other autonomic changes that may be seen include hypertension and tachycardia.[23-25]

Posttraumatic Epilepsy

Posttraumatic seizures occur in roughly 25% to 30% of pediatric victims of moderate or severe traumatic brain injury (TBI) and are associated with adverse outcome (see also Chapter 119). The occurrence of posttraumatic seizures or epilepsy increases with injury severity, younger age, and longer follow-up duration. Seizures seen in patients with severe TBI are frequently refractory to medical therapy. Posttraumatic epileptogenesis is a multifactorial process and may involve changes in excitatory and inhibitory networks, altered calcium-mediated second messenger activity, changes in ionotropic receptor function and composition, altered endogenous neuroprotectant activity, or TBI-induced cortical dysplasia.[26-28]

Renal Failure

Acute renal failure is associated with a uremic encephalopathy and seizures that may result from metabolic abnormalities including hyponatremia, calcium disorders, uremia, and hypertensive encephalopathy or disequilibrium syndrome seen with hemodialysis. Treatment of seizures in these patients can be difficult as a result of AED pharmacokinetics in uremia, decreased albumin, and dialysis effects. AEDs that are tightly protein bound (phenytoin, valproic acid) are not significantly dialyzed and usually do not need to be replaced. One should be cautious, however, as the unbound portion of drug may be higher and dosing adjustments may be necessary.

Transplantation

Solid organ transplant is frequently complicated by a spectrum of seizure types, including single partial-onset or generalized tonic-clonic seizures, acute repetitive seizures, or status epilepticus. Seizures may be seen frequently in transplant patients and may result from hyponatremia, hyper/hypoglycemia, immunosuppressive agents, high-dose antibiotics, infections, cerebral edema, infarction, or post-anoxic encephalopathy following hypotension or sepsis. Most seizures occur in the postoperative period on days 4 to 6. The immunosuppressive agents most frequently implicated are the calcineurin inhibitors cyclosporine and tacrolimus. Medication interactions have been described, as phenytoin decreases absorption of cyclosporine, and enzyme inducers (phenytoin, phenobarbital) may increase the clearance of cyclosporine and methylprednisolone.[29]

Pediatric hematopoietic cell transplant (HSCT) is associated with a large spectrum of complications. The most frequent complications are CNS infections, cerebrovascular or metabolic events, and neurotoxicity of immunosuppressive agents manifesting as PRES. Seizures are reported in 7% to 12% of transplanted patients and in 53% to 75% of patients with neurologic complications. There is currently no specific evidence involving the transplant patient population to guide the selection, administration, or duration of AED treatment.[30]

Autoimmune Status Epilepticus

Autoimmune SE is a rare condition but one that has been increasingly recognized by neurologists and PICU physicians. SE may be considered autoimmune if it is refractory to AED treatment and there is no other known cause; this may then lead to empiric immunomodulatory therapy. Major factors that raise the index of suspicion are recent cognitive or behavioral alterations, a history of malignancy or tumor, or the presence of other neurologic features. Treatment may include immunotherapy such as corticosteroids, IV immunoglobulin, plasmapheresis, and other immunosuppressive agents while attempting to maximize AED therapy.[31-33]

Neurophysiology

Seizures result from abnormal synchronous electrical discharge (depolarization) of a group of neurons in the CNS. Depolarization results from the influx of sodium into the neuron, whereas repolarization results from the egress of potassium from the cell resulting in the restoration of the resting negative electrical potential across the cell. This potential is regulated by a sodium-potassium pump that is ATP driven.

Figs. 67.2 and 67.3 provide an excellent overview of the physiology of a normal neuron and the pathophysiology associated with seizures, and the reader is referred to the article by Stafstrom.[34] The ineffective recruitment of inhibitory neurons coupled with excessive neuronal stimulation is a key participant in the initiation and propagation of the electrical disturbance occurring in SE. γ-Aminobutyric acid (GABA) is the major inhibitory neurotransmitter in the CNS. GABA receptors have a chloride ion channel complex and binding sites for barbiturates and benzodiazepines. Activation of these receptors allows for an inward movement of Cl^-, which restores the negative resting potential to the neuron to prevent further firing. The use of GABA agonists and the resultant suppression of seizure activity supports the perception that GABA plays a role in the normal termination of a seizure.

Glutamate is the excitatory neurotransmitter of the CNS and has been implicated in the propagation of seizures by its effects on the N-methyl-D-aspartate (NMDA) and non-NMDA channels and via secondary messenger systems

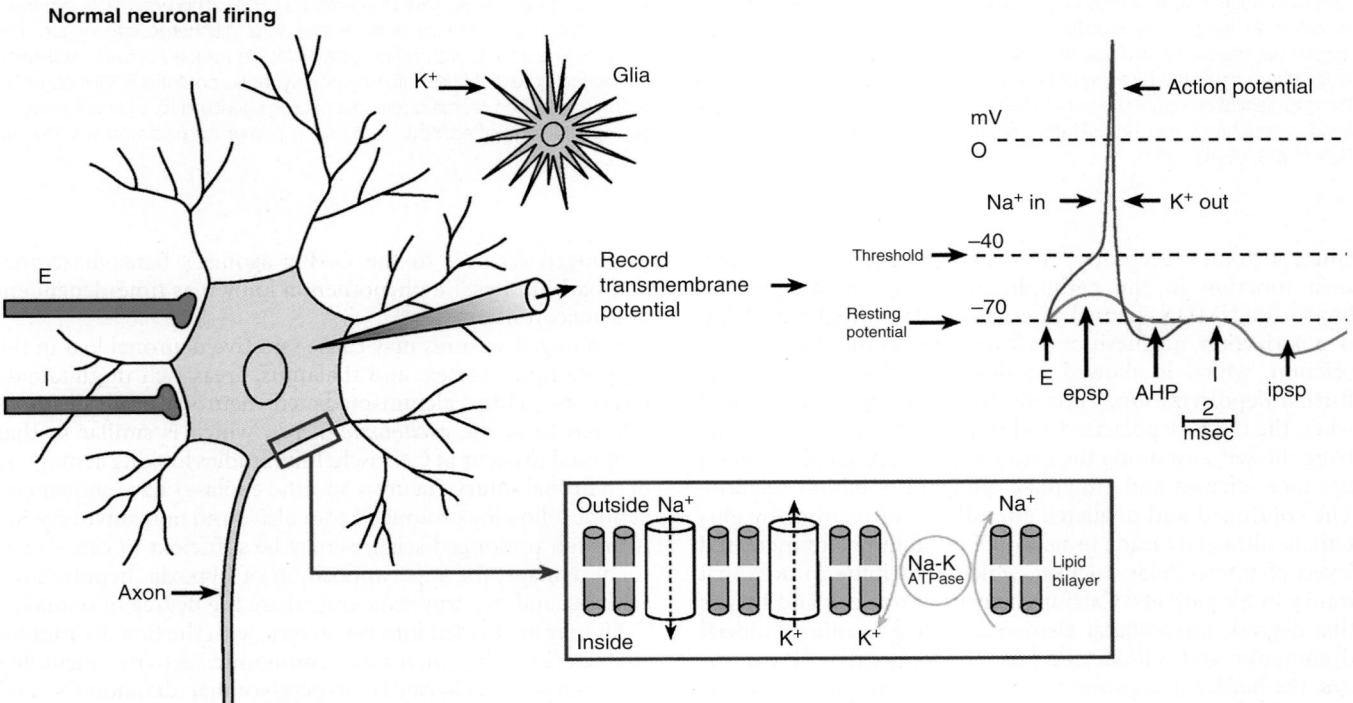

Fig. 67.2. Normal Neuronal Firing. Schematic of a neuron with one excitatory (E) and one inhibitory (I) input. Right side shows membrane potential (in mV), beginning at resting potential (−70 mV). Activation of E leads to graded excitatory postsynaptic potentials, the larger of which reaches threshold (about −40 mV) for an action potential. The action potential is followed by an after hyperpolarization (AHP), the magnitude and duration of which determine when the next action potential can occur. Activation of I causes an inhibitory postsynaptic potential. Inset shows a magnified portion of the neuronal membrane as a lipid bilayer with interposed voltage-gated Na+ and K+ channels; the direction of ion fluxes during excitation is shown. After firing, the membrane-bound Na-K pump and star-shaped astroglial cells restore ionic balance. (Reprinted with permission. Stafstrom CE. The pathophysiology of epileptic seizures: a primer for pediatricians. Pediatr Rev. 1998;19:342-351.)

Abnormal neuronal firing

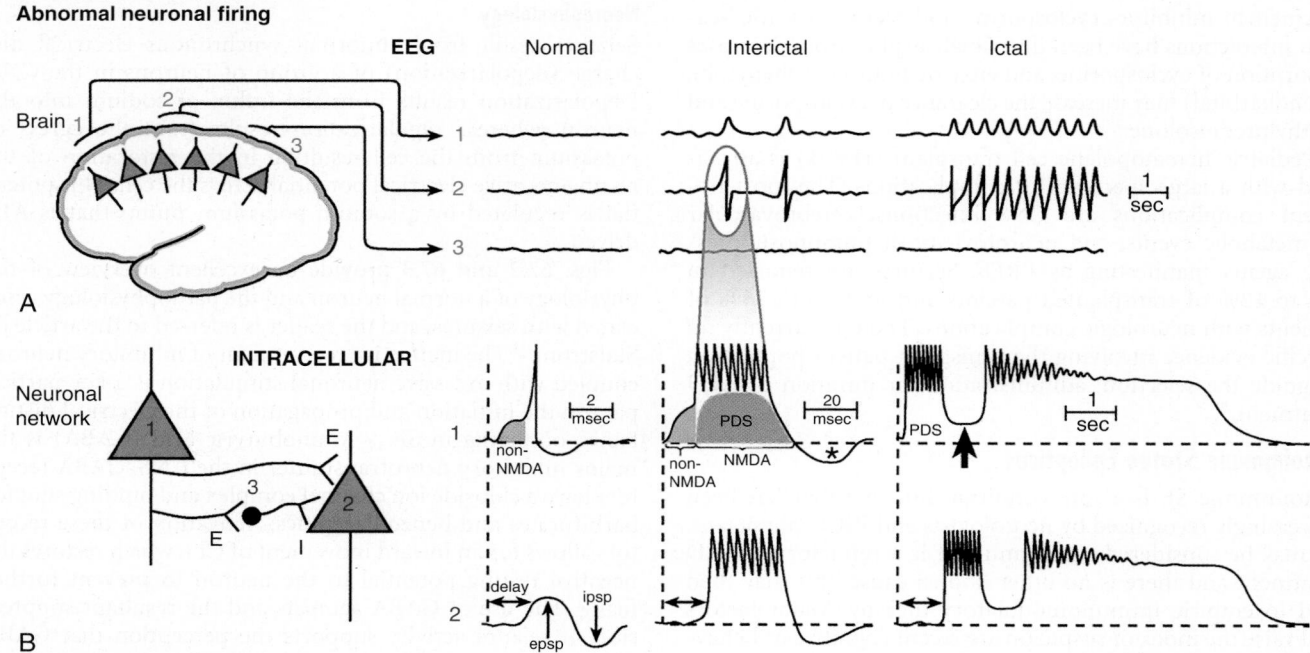

Fig. 67.3. Abnormal Neuronal Firing. Abnormal neuronal firing at the levels of (A) the brain and (B) a simplified neuronal network, consisting of two excitatory neurons (1 and 2) and an inhibitory interneuron (3). EEG *(top set of traces)* and intracellular recordings *(bottom set of traces)* are shown for the normal *(left column)*, interictal *(middle column)*, and ictal conditions *(right column)*. Numbered traces refer to like numbered recording sites. Note time scale differences in different traces. (A) Brain. Three EEG electrodes record activity from superficial neocortical neurons. In the normal case, activity is low voltage and *desynchronized* (neurons are not firing together in synchrony). In the interictal condition, large spikes are seen focally at electrode 2 (and to a lesser extent at electrode 1, where they might be termed *sharp waves*), representing synchronized firing of a large population of hyperexcitable neurons (expanded in time below). The ictal state is characterized by a long run of spikes. (B) Neuronal network. At the neuronal network level, the intracellular correlate of the interictal EEG spike is called the *paroxysmal depolarization shift (PDS)*. The PDS is initiated by a non-NMDA–mediated fast excitatory postsynaptic potential (EPSP) but is maintained by a longer, larger NMDA-mediated EPSP. The post-PDS hyperpolarization (*) temporarily stabilizes the neuron. If this post-PDS hyperpolarization fails *(right column, thick arrow)*, ictal discharge can occur. The lowermost traces, recordings from neuron 2, show activity similar to that recorded in neuron 1, with some delay *(double-headed arrow)*. Activation of inhibitory neuron 3 by firing of neuron 1 prevents neuron 2 from generating an action potential (the inhibitory postsynaptic potential [IPSP] counters the depolarization caused by the EPSP). If it does not reach firing threshold, neuron 2 can then recruit additional neurons, leading to an entire network firing in synchrony (seizure). (Reprinted with permission. Stafstrom CE. The pathophysiology of epileptic seizures: a primer for pediatricians. Pediatr Rev. 1998;19:342-351.)

(metabotropic) receptors.[35] The NMDA receptor may have a dual function in the pathophysiology of SE. Magnesium blocks the NMDA channel when it is in its normal state. With depolarization, magnesium no longer blocks the channel, and calcium, which is allowed to flow into the cell, produces further depolarization. Thus the NMDA receptor is activated when the cell is depolarized and responds by further depolarizing the cell, sustaining the excitation.[35,36] Glutamate agonists produce seizures and glutamate antagonists inhibit seizures. The continued and unabated stimulation of neurons by glutamate ultimately leads to neuronal cell failure and increased levels of intracellular calcium, which contribute to neuronal injury in SE patients. Calcium activates proteases and lipases that degrade intracellular elements, leading to mitochondrial dysfunction and cellular necrosis. The longer that SE continues, the harder it becomes to stop the seizure pharmacologically. This may be due to a shift from inadequate GABAergic inhibitory activity to excessive NMDA excitation.

Prolonged seizures have been associated with deficits in GABA-mediated neuronal inhibition because of the rapid internalization of synaptic GABA$_A$ receptors. Clinically this phenomenon may be demonstrated by the poor response of prolonged seizures to the GABA agonist's benzodiazepines and barbiturates,[37] a phenomenon known as time-dependent pharmacoresistance.[38-40]

Prolonged seizures may cause selective neuronal loss in the hippocampus, cortex, and thalamus, areas rich in glutamate receptors. This calcium-mediated neuronal cell death is referred to as the *excitotoxic theory,* which is similar to that proposed to occur in CNS ischemia. Studies looking at markers of neuronal injury (neuron-specific enolase) have shown elevations following prolonged convulsive and nonconvulsive SE. Although prolonged seizures may be sufficient to cause neuronal damage, the superimposition of hypoxia, hypotension, acidosis, and hyperpyrexia exacerbate the degree of damage.

SE may be divided into two stages, with the first 30 minutes characterized by increased autonomic activity including hypertension, tachycardia, hyperglycemia, diaphoresis, and hyperpyrexia. This is followed by a transition period after approximately 30 minutes when patients enter a second phase, which is characterized by multiorgan involvement and includes respiratory failure (hypoxemia, hypercarbia), decreased CBF, increased intracranial pressure (ICP), and a dropping arterial blood pressure. Severe acidosis ensues and the patients may develop rhabdomyolysis with a leukocytosis, hyperkalemia, and an elevated creatine kinase (secondary to increased muscle activity). These findings are summarized in Table 67.1.

Early in SE, an increase in neuronal metabolic demand occurs with a compensatory increase in CBF and brain oxygenation. Later in SE, these homeostatic mechanisms are unable to keep up with the sustained increase in cerebral metabolic demand. Autoregulation of CBF fails, and consequently a higher mean arterial pressure is required to maintain adequate brain perfusion. As systemic blood pressure falls, a subsequent reduction in brain parenchymal oxygenation occurs. This signals the failure of adaptive mechanisms.

Respiratory failure associated with SE is multifactorial in origin. There is an increase in CO_2 production from the hypermetabolic state, a decrease in respiratory drive, and an increased mechanical load on the respiratory muscles. The decrease in drive (hypoventilation) may be due to muscle fatigue or secondary to medications used to suppress the seizure. There may also be an increase in dead-space ventilation from aspiration or neurogenic pulmonary edema.[41,42]

The cardiovascular changes and initial hyperadrenergic state are due to the release of endogenous catecholamines. Patients will have an initial increase in heart rate and systemic vascular resistance that will decrease over time. Of note, there is an entity called *ictal bradycardia,* which is a rare and probably underestimated manifestation of epileptic seizures whose pathophysiology is still debated. Autonomic modifications may result from either a sympathetic inhibition or a parasympathetic activation probably due to the ictal discharge arising from or spreading to the structures of the central autonomic network.[43]

As the time of the event progresses, it is imperative to prevent hyperpyrexia in these patients as this will contribute to neuronal cell death. Studies in adult patients have shown that there may be a CSF pleocytosis; however, any elevation in the CSF cell count in a pediatric patient should suggest a possible infectious etiology of the seizure. Prolonged muscle activity may produce an elevation in creatine kinase and produce myoglobinuria and acute kidney injury (AKI) so attention to hydration, electrolyte status, and renal function is essential. Acidemia may be worsened by impaired ventilation, hypoxemia, and anaerobic metabolism. At the cellular level, amino acid excitotoxicity leads to cell injury and death through cascades culminating in intracellular calcium influx.[35-37,44-46]

Evaluation and Management

The clinical presentation of SE is variable, depending on seizure type and the baseline developmental and medical status of the child. Diagnosis depends on the identification of continuous or repetitive seizures, which is usually straightforward in the presence of convulsive seizures. However, after prolonged convulsive seizures the motor manifestations often diminish, and the seizures may become subtle or even nonconvulsive. Differentiating between such nonconvulsive seizures and a postictal state can be challenging. Patients with nonconvulsive SE, including absence SE, may be difficult to identify by history and physical examination alone. These patients can have intermittent altered awareness and continuous lethargy or unresponsiveness with or without subtle myoclonic jerks of the face or limbs. In such cases, continuous EEG (cEEG) monitoring is critical for diagnosis. EEG monitoring also can be used to identify nonepileptic (psychogenic) SE.

Although uncommon, prolonged delays in the cEEG-based diagnosis of nonepileptic SE can lead to unnecessary medical intervention.[47]

Common clinical indications for continuous EEG (cEEG) monitoring in the PICU include (1) titration of epileptic drug therapy; (2) screening for subclinical seizures among patients at high risk for conditions such as suspected encephalitis, hypoxic ischemic encephalopathy (postarrest, near drowning), TBI, and stroke; (3) screening for seizures among patients who are paralyzed and at risk for seizures (extracorporeal membrane oxygenation [ECMO]); and (4) characterization of paroxysmal events suspected to represent electrographic seizures. Only half of critically ill children undergoing cEEG monitoring experience their first electrographic seizure during the initial hour of monitoring. Therefore a routine 20- to 30-minute EEG recording will fail to identify the majority of children who go on to develop seizures, justifying the need for cEEG monitoring to accurately diagnose seizures and quantify seizure burden. The majority of electrographic seizures in the PICU are either subclinical or are accompanied by only subtle clinical signs and would likely go undetected without cEEG monitoring.

EEG measures extracellular electrical activity generated by cortical neurons. Data are collected with a standard array of scalp electrodes and presented for visual display onto a paper or digital record.

Because EEG provides real-time information regarding brain activity, it is invaluable in the evaluation of patients with SE, permitting direct correlation between patient behavior and neuronal activity. EEG interpretation should be performed with the assistance of a trained neurologist or neurophysiologist to reduce the potential for both over- and under-identification of seizures.

Abnormal waveforms on EEG can be divided into two categories: epileptiform abnormalities and nonepileptiform abnormalities. Epileptiform abnormalities are abnormal discharges associated with an increased risk of seizures, including sharp waves, spikes, polyspikes, and spike and slow wave discharges. When present between seizures, these waveforms are termed *interictal abnormalities.* Seizures are defined electrographically by the presence of *ictal* EEG abnormalities, whose hallmark is their rhythmicity and their evolution in frequency or distribution over the course of a seizure. Generalized seizures are characterized by widespread bilateral rhythmic epileptiform discharges (Fig. 67.4A). Focal seizures are characterized by rhythmic epileptiform discharges that are confined to one brain region (Fig. 67.4B). Focal seizures may spread to involve both cerebral hemispheres, a process termed *secondary generalization.*

Nonepileptiform abnormalities are not necessarily associated with a risk of seizure but suggest CNS dysfunction. Slow waves are a nonspecific finding, suggesting a structural or functional abnormality, and often are seen after a seizure or SE. The location of slow waves after a seizure may aid in the differentiation between generalized and focal seizures. Generalized slow waves are associated with a diffuse encephalopathy such as a metabolic disturbance, hypoxia-ischemia, or a postictal state.

Two further EEG patterns are of particular relevance to the treatment of prolonged seizures. Burst suppression is characterized by brief bursts containing a mixture of spikes, sharp waves, and slow waves alternating with periods of very low

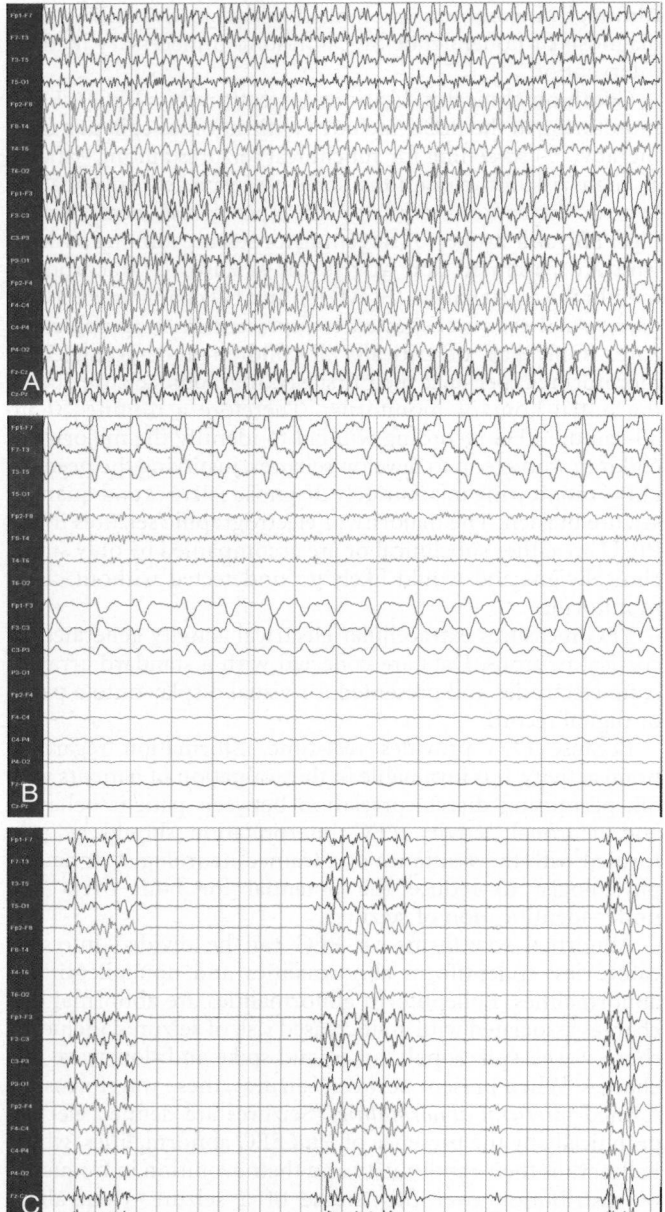

Fig. 67.4. Electroencephalography in status epilepticus (SE). (A) Generalized seizure. (B) Left focal seizure. (C) Burst-suppression pattern in a patient treated with a midazolam infusion for refractory SE.

voltage (Fig. 67.4C). An isoelectric EEG pattern refers to a continuous low-voltage record without any discernable cortical activity. Both burst-suppression and isoelectric EEG patterns can be seen in persons in a coma and may carry a poor prognosis in certain clinical situations. However, in the context of refractory SE, these patterns are often the desired end point for treatment with high-dose barbiturates or benzodiazepines.

Therapeutic goals for SE include (1) general supportive care, (2) termination of SE, (3) prevention of seizure recurrence, (4) correction of precipitating causes, and (5) prevention and treatment of potential complications. Immediate

attention to the airway, breathing, and circulation is essential (ABCs). SE is a situation where simultaneous evaluation and management should be undertaken. A suggested clinical approach is summarized in Fig. 67.5.[48,49]

Although most seizures (~75%)[1] are self-limited and stop in less than 5 minutes, it is reasonable to assume that most children who arrive at the emergency department or PICU have been seizing for a significant length of time. This may include time seizing prior to discovery, time waiting for emergency personnel, time spent en route to the hospital, and time before administration of the first antiepileptic agent. Many patients may have already received potentially sedating medications from family members/EMS personnel that may contribute to respiratory embarrassment on arrival.

The immediate assessment of the airway begins with a check for patency and reflexes. The airway may be secured by simple maneuvers such as suctioning, positioning, and the use of airway adjuncts (nasal trumpets). High-flow oxygen should be administered and pulse oximetry instituted to evaluate oxygenation status. The presence of nasal flaring, poor chest rise, retractions, cyanosis, abdominal paradoxical breathing, diminished breath sounds, or apnea suggests the patient's trachea should be intubated. It is essential to realize that some patients may require the administration of a neuromuscular blocker (NMB) and if so, it should be one with a short half-life. The NMB agent will stop the motor component of the seizure but will not stop the underlying electrographic seizure activity in the brain. Patients who are going to receive continued paralysis should be simultaneously monitored with cEEG. Patients may be hypovolemic, and the continued addition of medications and positive pressure ventilation may actually worsen hypovolemia and perfusion.

Tachycardia, cool extremities, delayed capillary refill, diminished pulses, and poor urine output suggest poor perfusion. One should follow established Pediatric Advanced Life Support (PALS) guidelines to obtain access and once established the patient may receive isotonic fluid blouses (20 mL/kg). Consideration for the administration of antipyretics should be given early in the management of the patient in SE.

Diagnostic testing in children and adolescents with SE varies among centers and likely reflects the limited evidence supporting most diagnostic approaches in SE. Specific studies should be tailored to match the patient history; however, serum glucose should be checked immediately in all pediatric patients, particularly young infants. Other blood work may include serum electrolytes (sodium, calcium, and magnesium), liver function tests, arterial blood gas, urine toxicology, and antiepileptic levels. Approximately 3.8% to 14.8% of seizure patients who arrived to an ED have electrolyte abnormalities.[50,51] In the event of respiratory, cardiovascular, or neurologic concerns or other contraindications such as a coagulopathy or elevated intracranial pressure and if a lumbar puncture is not done immediately, antibiotics and antivirals (if indicated) should be administered. Although blood cultures and a lumbar puncture have a high yield in children with SE and a clinical suspicion of infection, there is insufficient evidence to either support or refute whether these studies should be routinely performed in children in whom there is no clinical suspicion of infection.[52] Currently evidence to support the performance of most diagnostic tests relies on limited data collected in heterogeneous settings with different study objectives.[53]

Immediate management
   Noninvasive airway protection and gas exchange with head positioning
   Intubation if needed
   Monitoring O_2 saturation, blood pressure, heart rate, temperature
   Finger stick blood glucose
   Peripheral IV access
   Medical and neurologic examination
   Labs: BMP, magnesium, phosphate, CBC, LFT, coagulation tests, ABG, anticonvulsant levels

Emergent initial therapy (given immediately)
   IV: Lorazepam 0.1 mg/kg IV (max 4 mg)—may repeat if seizures persist
   No IV:
     Diazepam   2–5 years 0.5 mg/kg, 6–11 years 0.3 mg/kg, 12 years 0.2 g/kg (max 20 mg)
     Midazolam   IM If 13–40 kg then 5 mg. If >40 kg then 10 mg
                 Intranasal 0.2 mg/kg
                 Buccal 0.5 mg/kg
   Consider whether out-of-hospital benzodiazepines have been administered when considering how many doses to administer

Urgent management
   Additional diagnostic testing as indicated: LP, CT, MRI, toxicology labs, inborn errors of metabolism
   Consider EEG monitoring (evaluate for psychogenic status epilepticus or persisting EEG-only seizures)
   Neurologic consultation

Urgent control therapy
   Phenytoin 20 mg/kg IV (may give another 10 mg/kg if needed)—may cause arrhythmia, hypotension, purple glove syndrome
   OR Fosphenytoin 20 PE/kg IV (may be given another 10 PE/kg if needed)
   OR consider phenobarbital, valproate sodium, or levetiracetam

   If <2 years, consider pyridoxine 100 mg IV

Refractory status epilepticus

If seizures continue after benzodiazepines and a second antiseizure medication, the patient is in refractory status epilepticus regardless of elapsed time

Continue management and make plans for ICU admission/transfer. Expect need for continuous EEG monitoring once clinically evident seizures terminate to evaluate for persisting EEG-only seizures

Administer another urgent control anticonvulsant or proceed to pharmacologic coma
   Levetiracetam 20–60 mg/kg IV
   Valproate sodium 20–40 mg/kg IV—contraindicated if liver disease, thrombocytopenia, or possible metabolic disease
   Phenobarbital 20–40 mg/kg IV—may cause respiratory depression and hypotension

Pharmacologic coma medications
   Midazolam 0.2 mg/kg bolus (max 10 mg) and then initiate infusion at 0.1 mg/kg/hr. Titrate up as needed
   Pentobarbital 5 mg/kg bolus and then initiate infusion at 0.5 mg/kg/hour. Titrate up as needed
   Other options: Isoflurane

Pharmacologic coma management
   Titrate to either seizure suppression or burst suppression based on EEG monitoring
   Continue pharmacologic coma for 24–48 hours
   Modify antiseizure medications so additional seizure coverage is in place for infusion wean
   Continue diagnostic testing and implementation of etiology-directed therapy

Add-on options
   Medications: phenytoin, phenobarbital, levetiracetam, valproate sodium, topiramate, lacosamide, ketamine, pyridoxine
   Other: epilepsy surgery, ketogenic diet, vagus nerve stimulator, immunomodulation, hypothermia, electroconvulsive therapy

Fig. 67.5. Guidelines for evaluation and management of SE. (From Abend NS, Loddenkemper T. Pediatric status epilepticus management. Curr Opin Pediatr. 2014;26:668-674.)

One needs to consider nonconvulsive status epilepticus (NCSE) in patients who do not quickly return to their baseline. A study by Allen and colleagues demonstrated that most children regain consciousness within 30 to 40 minutes, although some took many hours to recover without a sinister cause.[54] The two variables determining recovery were seizure etiology and the administration of medications to terminate the seizure. Children recover most quickly from febrile seizures and most slowly from acute symptomatic seizures. The authors stated that "it was surprising that seizure duration did not significantly affect recovery time; clinical dogma is that it does."[54]

Electrographic seizure activity has been reported to occur in up to 15% of patients whose overt clinical seizures are pharmacologically controlled.[55] NCSE presents with altered mentation and absent or subtle motor findings (eg, finger twitch) and is therefore defined by EEG criteria. The ictal episodes must be continuous or recurrent for at least 30 minutes without improvement in the patient's clinical state. The incidence of NCSE in pediatrics is currently unknown; however, adult studies have shown a mortality rate between 30% and 50%.[56] Adult studies have also shown that approximately 8% of patients in coma are in NCSE. Adult etiologies included hypoxia and cerebrovascular accident (CVA) as the most common causes followed by infection, metabolic conditions, traumatic brain injury, tumor, and a low AED level.

Pharmacotherapy

A prospective observational study of 182 children with convulsive SE found that for every minute delay between the SE onset and emergency department arrival there was a 5% cumulative increase in the risk of having SE last more than 60 minutes.[57,58] A retrospective study of 154 children with SE compared children with aborted SE and RSE; it demonstrated that in 71 children who continued to seize despite first- and second-line AEDs, seizures were terminated in 100% of cases in which the third AED was administered within 60 minutes of the first and in only 22% of cases if it was administered more than 1 hour after the original AED.[57,59] The new operational SE definition suggests the administration of medication for seizures lasting longer than 5 minutes. Adult data suggest that only a small portion of seizures will progress to SE; however, the longer the seizure lasts, the more difficult it will be to control. The goal of administering an antiepileptic drug is to terminate the event rapidly and safely and to prevent recurrence. First-line medications commonly administered include the benzodiazepines (valium, lorazepam, and midazolam), and second-line agents include phenytoin, fosphenytoin, and phenobarbital. These agents are summarized in Table 67.2. Common errors in the management of SE include insufficient drug dosages, delay in advancing to a second-line drug, and inadequate supportive care. Third-line medications are indicated to treat RSE and are reviewed later in this chapter. An adult clinical review of the management of status epilepticus stated that there are few randomized controlled trials of status epilepticus and that there are poor data and little evidence to support one treatment regimen over another.[60,61]

In current practice there is substantial variability in the initial management of SE. A survey of physicians in Australia and New Zealand reported that first-line management of SE without intravenous (IV) access included rectal diazepam (49%), intramuscular midazolam (41%), and buccal midazolam (9%), whereas first-line management of SE with IV access included midazolam IV (50%) and diazepam (44%).[57] Benzodiazepines remain the first-line drugs in the treatment of SE.[62] Historically, diazepam had been used as the first-line drug; however, lorazepam now is used more often in both the prehospital and hospital setting due to its minimal side effects. Diazepam and lorazepam were compared in a study funded by the National Institutes of Health (NIH) and coordinated by the Pediatric Emergency Care Applied Research Network (PECARN) to determine which drug is safer and more effective. The results of the randomized clinical trial do not support the hypothesis that lorazepam is superior to diazepam for pediatric SE of at least 5 minutes in duration. Both medications were effective in stopping SE in more than 70% of cases and had rates of severe respiratory depression of less than 20%. Another randomized trial of adults and children, the Rapid Anticonvulsant Medication Prior to Arrival Trial (RAMPART), found, overall, that intramuscular midazolam initiated in the prehospital setting stopped more seizures at arrival to the ED than IV lorazepam; however, a subgroup analysis showed similar results for the two medications. There was also a similar intubation rate of 14% in each group.[63,64]

All three benzodiazepines have an onset of action of less than 5 minutes and enhance inhibitory neurotransmission by binding to a specific benzodiazepine site on the $GABA_A$ receptor. However, diazepam's duration of antiepileptic action appears to be less than 1 hour, making it less attractive than lorazepam. Often patients may have received rectal diazepam prior to arrival to the hospital, and this should be kept in mind as one escalates therapy for SE.[65]

Lorazepam has a slower onset of action than diazepam because it is less lipophilic, but its advantage is its prolonged antiepileptic effect of greater than 6 hours. Currently the Food and Drug Administration (FDA) has approved diazepam for adults and children, whereas lorazepam is approved for adults but is being used off label for children.[66]

Midazolam is a short-acting benzodiazepine used as a first-line agent in prehospital care. It may also be used in the treatment of refractory SE and administered as a continuous infusion. It may be given intravenously, intraosseously, intramuscularly, and per rectum. Small pediatric series have also shown efficacy when given via the buccal or intranasal route as well. The duration of effect is shorter than for lorazepam.[65]

All of the benzodiazepines have the potential to cause respiratory depression and hypotension. Benzodiazepines are less likely to halt seizure activity if multiple dosages are required, and in these situations, additional anticonvulsant medications should be administered. Furthermore, repeated doses of benzodiazepines will have additive sedating effects and may prolong a diminished level of consciousness and prevent adequate neurologic assessment.[65]

Fosphenytoin and phenytoin are preferred second-line, longer-acting AEDs for the treatment of SE. Both drugs exert their effect by stabilizing the neuronal membrane. Each drug takes approximately 20 minutes to achieve a therapeutic effect. Fosphenytoin, a water-soluble disodium phosphate ester of phenytoin, is converted in plasma to phenytoin. Fosphenytoin is compatible with most intravenous solutions, is devoid of propylene glycol, and therefore can be administered at a faster rate and without the cardiovascular risks of phenytoin.

TABLE 67.2   Drugs Used in the Treatment of Status Epilepticus

Drug	Initial Dose	Maximum Single Dose	IV Administration	Onset of Action	Half-Life	Principal Adverse Effects in Short-Term Use
Lorazepam	0.05–0.1 mg/kg IV	4 mg	0.5 mg/min bolus	1–3 min	Neonates: 40 h Children: 10 h	Sedation, hypotension, bradycardia, respiratory depression, paradoxical hyperactivity
Diazepam	0.05–0.3 mg/kg IV	<5 y: 5 mg ≥5 y: 10 mg	0.1 mg/kg/min bolus	1–3 min	Neonates: 50–95 h Infants: 40–50 h Children: 15–20 h	Sedation, hypotension, bradycardia, respiratory depression, paradoxical hyperactivity, thrombophlebitis
Phenobarbital	15–20 mg/kg IV	1 g	1 mg/kg/min bolus to max. 60 mg/min	5 min	Neonates: 45–200 h Infants: 20–133 h Children: 37–73 h	Hypotension, sedation, respiratory depression, paradoxical hyperactivity, immunosuppression
Pentobarbital	5–12 mg/kg	100 mg	1 mg/kg/h infusion, then titrate	1 min	25 h	Sedation, bradycardia, hypotension, cardiac arrhythmia, respiratory depression, laryngospasm, extravasation causes skin necrosis
Phenytoin	15–20 mg/kg IV	1 g	1 mg/kg/min bolus, to max. 50 mg/min		7–42 h (first-order kinetics do not apply)	Dysarthria, ataxia, sedation, hypotension, cardiac arrhythmia, thrombophlebitis, extravasation causes purple glove syndrome
Fosphenytoin	15–20 mg PE/kg IV	1 g PE	3 mg PE/kg/min bolus to max. 150 mg PE/min		12–29 h (first-order kinetics do not apply)	Dysarthria, ataxia, sedation, hypotension, bradycardia, tachycardia
Valproic acid	10–30 mg/kg IV	30 mg/kg	5 mg/kg/min bolus		Children >2 mo: 7–13 h Children 2–14 y: 3.5–20 h	Hypotension, cardiac arrhythmia, hepatitis, pancreatitis
Paraldehyde	200–400 mg/kg PR	10 g	NA		4–10 h	Rectal irritation, lung toxicity
Midazolam	0.15 mg/kg IV	0.15 mg/kg	1 μg/kg/min infusion, titrate to max. 24 μg/kg/min	1–5 min	Neonates: 4–12 h Children: 3–4 h	Sedation, hypotension, bradycardia, respiratory depression, apnea, laryngospasm, paradoxical hyperactivity
Propofol	1–2 mg/kg IV		1–2 mg/kg/h infusion		1.5–12 h	Sedation, hypotension, bradycardia, respiratory depression, bronchospasm, hallucinations, pain when injected, propofol infusion syndrome, metabolic acidosis, rhabdomyolysis, lipemia, cardiac bradyarrhythmias, death
Ketamine	0.5–2 mg/kg IV		2–7 mg/kg/h[a]	30 sec	2.5 h	Hypertension, increased intracranial pressure, hallucinations, vomiting, emergence reactions, laryngospasm
Thiopental	2–4 mg/kg IV		2–4 mg/kg/h infusion	30–60 sec	14–34 h	Sedation, hypotension, respiratory depression, accumulation due to lipid solubility, extravasation causes skin necrosis
Isoflurane	0.5%–1% v/v		NA			Respiratory depression, hypotension, arrhythmias, malignant hyperthermia, laryngospasm, coughing (due to pungent odor)
Lidocaine	2–3 mg/kg IV		2–6 mg/kg/h		1.5–2 h in adults	Sedation, cardiac arrhythmias

[a]Continuous infusion rates for ketamine are not well established in children; refer to institutional guidelines and experience.
IV, intravenous; *NA*, not applicable; *PE*, phenytoin equivalents; *PR*, rectal; *v/v*, volume per volume.

Furthermore, fosphenytoin does not have the deleterious effects on tissue as seen with phenytoin in the event of extravasation, nor does it cause respiratory depression or sedation. In most centers, one must order fosphenytoin in phenytoin equivalent (PE) dosages. Although it remains to be proved that the greater speed of administration of fosphenytoin results in improved seizure control compared with phenytoin, fosphenytoin often is preferred because it is better tolerated at the infusion site, carries a lower risk for cardiac arrhythmia and hypotension, and has not been associated with the purple glove syndrome.[67] The higher cost of fosphenytoin and the lack of definitive evidence for superior efficacy, however, may limit its widespread use, despite the suggestion by pharmacoeconomic analysis that fosphenytoin is cost effective.[68] Although phenytoin is the second-line agent indicated for the treatment of most causes of seizures, it is usually *not* efficacious in the management of drug-induced seizures.

Phenobarbital has a long proven history as an effective antiepileptic drug. It is used commonly to treat neonatal seizures and SE. It may be given intravenously, intraosseously, or intramuscularly. Potential side effects include respiratory depression, hypotension, bradycardia, and prolonged sedation. In particular, prolonged sedation can impair neurologic assessment and is a significant disadvantage of phenobarbital when compared to fosphenytoin and phenytoin. Additionally, the combination of a benzodiazepine and phenobarbital often necessitates tracheal intubation because of respiratory depression.

Propofol is a nonbarbiturate anesthetic agent (GABA agonist) initially approved for rapid induction and maintenance of anesthesia. Its efficacy has been detailed in case reports and small case series and it has been associated with the cessation of seizure activity or burst suppression within seconds of administration.[69] Adverse effects include bradycardia, apnea, and hypotension with rapid infusion. Currently its use has been curtailed in pediatric patients because of the association with the *propofol infusion syndrome,* which includes potentially fatal metabolic acidosis, rhabdomyolysis, and cardiovascular collapse. This agent is not approved for use in status epilepticus in pediatric patients.[70,71]

Valproic acid (VPA) is a common antiepileptic drug with case series describing the use of intravenous VPA for treatment of SE and RSE.[72-76] Possible mechanisms of action include an increase in CNS GABA levels by increased synthesis and decreased catabolism, blockade of T-type Ca^{++} currents, and enhancement of Na^+ channel inactivation. VPA was found to be an effective treatment leading to termination in seizure activity in 78% of 41 children included in the series. Patients were initially loaded with 20- to 40-mg/kg VPA, diluted 1:1 with normal saline or 5% dextrose, and infused over 1 to 5 minutes. An IV infusion of 5 mg/kg/hr followed the loading dose. The infusion was decreased by 1 mg/kg every 2 hours once a 12-hour seizure-free period was attained. Overall, seizures were terminated in 78% with 65.9% responding after the initial bolus. The FDA has not yet approved IV valproic acid for treating SE.[77,78]

Levetiracetam has no effect on voltage-gated Na channels or GABAergic transmission and no affinity for either GABAergic or glutamatergic receptors. Some have proposed that it binds to a presynaptic vesicle glycoprotein (sv2A) to act as a transporter for presynaptic P/Q type voltage-dependent calcium channels. It has been considered a potentially useful agent for SE because, in comparison with other IV AEDs, it has few known side effects, including a low risk of sedation, cardiorespiratory depression, or coagulopathy, and thus it is potentially useful in critically ill children. Clearance is dependent on renal function and completely avoids hepatic metabolism.[79-81]

Lacosamide is a functionalized amino acid that selectively enhances slow inactivation of voltage-gated sodium channels, increasing the proportion of sodium channels unavailable for depolarization. This stabilizes neuronal membranes and inhibits sustained repetitive neuronal firing. In randomized controlled trials in adults, it demonstrated significant benefit in treating refractory seizures, with 30% to 40% of patients achieving a >50% reduction in seizures at doses of 400 to 600 mg/day. Pediatric studies describe similar results in children and young adults with refractory epilepsy.[82] It is generally well tolerated, and the most frequent reactions are dizziness, headache, diplopia, and nausea. These adverse effects are usually dose related and reversible on dose reduction or discontinuance.

There are no controlled, randomized, blinded clinical trials to compare the efficacy and tolerability of currently available treatments for established status epilepticus (ESE), defined as seizures that continue despite the administration of a benzodiazepine. An ongoing study titled the Established Status Epilepticus Treatment Trial (ESETT)[83] is attempting to determine the most effective or the least effective treatment of benzodiazepine-refractory SE among patients older than 2 years. Three active treatment arms are being compared: fosphenytoin, levetiracetam, and valproic acid. Other objectives include comparing the three drugs for secondary outcomes and to describe effectiveness, safety, and rate of adverse reactions to these drugs in children.

Refractory Status Epilepticus

SE that persists beyond 1 hour despite AED therapy is considered refractory (RSE). About 30% of SE cases may prove resistant to standard treatment with one of the benzodiazepines and phenytoin. This subgroup of patients has a higher risk of complications and longer hospital stay and mortality. Most of them have some structural cerebral damage or metabolic disorders or cerebral hypoxia. Other risk factors include delay in receiving treatment, metabolic encephalopathy, hypoxia, and encephalitis.[84]

Conventional AEDs have low efficacy in RSE, and although conventional AEDs (eg, topiramate, levetiracetam, and carbamazepine) should be continued during this treatment phase, higher dose or higher potency agents are required to abort RSE. Therapeutic options include high-dose benzodiazepines, barbiturates, propofol, valproic acid, ketamine, lidocaine, and inhalational anesthetic agents. Currently, insufficient evidence exists to conclude which of these high-dose suppressive medications, either alone or in combination, has superior efficacy in the treatment of RSE.[85]

Goals of Therapy

In the treatment of RSE, as in SE, the goal is termination of all clinical and electrographic seizure activity, and thus cEEG monitoring is required. ICU practitioners should resist the temptation to assess seizure control on the basis of clinical signs alone because the clinical expression of seizures can be subtle and the examination is often confounded by the use of sedative medications. Therefore treatment of RSE should be guided by cEEG monitoring. However, the exact target of cEEG-guided therapy remains controversial. In addition to achieving seizure suppression, it is generally recommended to escalate therapy to achieve a burst-suppression pattern on EEG. The rationale for achieving burst suppression is that profound suppression of brain activity may have a protective effect and break the cycle of seizures, thus reducing the chance of seizure recurrence upon tapering of medications.[86] Debate continues regarding the recommended length of the periods of EEG suppression (the interburst interval) and how long the burst-suppression pattern should be maintained. Furthermore, because of a concern that seizures may persist even when the EEG is interspersed with a burst-suppression pattern, some experts recommend achieving complete EEG suppression—in other words, an isoelectric EEG pattern.[87] As a general approach, once seizure control or a burst-suppression pattern has been achieved, a suggested practice is to maintain the burst-suppression pattern for at least 12 hours before a medication taper is attempted. If seizures recur when medication is tapered, then therapy is reinstated to achieve a burst-suppression pattern for at least another 48 hours.[88,89]

In parallel with high-dose suppressive therapies described in detail in the following sections, conventional AEDs (ie, topiramate, levetiracetam, and carbamazepine) should be titrated to high therapeutic doses, both to assist in aborting RSE and to provide continued anticonvulsant coverage following tapering of high-dose suppressive therapies.

High-Dose Barbiturates

Barbiturates including pentobarbital, thiopental, and phenobarbital are widely used medications for RSE that also may have neuroprotective effects.[90] Pentobarbital is the best-studied drug, and the most data are available on its use. Pentobarbital is administered as an intravenous loading dose of 5 to 10 mg/kg, followed by a continuous infusion of 1 mg/kg/h, increasing as needed to a maximum rate of 10 mg/kg/h. Breakthrough seizures may be treated with additional boluses of 3 to 5 mg/kg.[91] High-dose phenobarbital is an alternative to pentobarbital. Phenobarbital may be given in incremental boluses of 10 mg/kg, without reference to a predetermined maximum level or dose, until seizures are suppressed. There appears to be no maximum dose beyond which further doses are ineffective, and serum levels of up to 344 mg/mL (1490 mmol/L) have been reported.[92] The main drawback of barbiturates in high doses is the risk of cardiovascular depression and hypotension. This situation frequently requires inotropic and vasopressor therapy and, in rare instances, cardiopulmonary resuscitation. In addition, the need for mechanical ventilation and the time to regain consciousness are also greater with barbiturates than with benzodiazepines.[85] Among the barbiturates, phenobarbital probably carries the lowest risk of hypotension and respiratory depression.[92] Finally, evidence indicates that high-dose, prolonged barbiturate therapy is immunosuppressive, thus particular vigilance for nosocomial infections is indicated.[93,94]

High-Dose Benzodiazepines

Midazolam is a short-acting benzodiazepine with an efficacy equal to pentobarbital in controlling RSE.[95] It is administered as a loading dose of 0.15 mg/kg, followed by a continuous infusion beginning at 1 µg/kg/min. The infusion rate may be increased as tolerated to a maximum of 24 µg/kg/min, although even higher infusion rates have been reported. The advantages of midazolam include a rapid onset of action, a short half-life, and a lower incidence of cardiovascular depression and need for vasopressors than with pentobarbital.[85,96] The major disadvantage of midazolam is the need for escalating doses because of tachyphylaxis. High-dose infusions of diazepam and lorazepam represent other alternatives.[97,98]

Propofol

The GABA agonist propofol is an anesthetic agent with potent anticonvulsant properties that has been widely used for the treatment of RSE, particularly in adults. The advantage of propofol is its rapid onset of action and short half-life; however, rapidly tapering propofol can precipitate seizures.[99] The main adverse effects of propofol are respiratory depression and hypotension due to myocardial depression. Early concerns about a possible proconvulsant effect of propofol have been largely allayed.[100,101] The use of propofol, particularly at high doses and with prolonged infusions, has been associated with a so-called propofol infusion syndrome characterized by metabolic acidosis, lipemia, rhabdomyolysis, bradyarrhythmias, and death.[102,103] A retrospective series of 31 adults treated with propofol for RSE found a 6% mortality rate and a 10% rate of cardiorespiratory arrest directly attributable to the propofol infusion syndrome. In addition, 39% of patients developed one or more features of the syndrome.[104] Therefore propofol infusions should be used with caution and should be limited to short duration with careful monitoring for adverse effects. Few data have been published on pediatric dosing of propofol for RSE. One case series reported safety and efficacy using a bolus dose of 1 to 2 mg/kg, followed by a continuous infusion of 1 to 2 mg/kg/h.[105,106]

Valproic Acid

Intravenous valproic acid may have a useful role in RSE, but relatively little evidence exists to support its use.[107] In one case series, the authors reported on the efficacy of intravenous valproic acid for generalized convulsive and nonconvulsive seizures in children. They recommended a loading dose of 20 mg/kg followed by an infusion at 1 to 4 mg/kg/h, depending on the patient's state of hepatic induction (1 mg/kg/h for noninduced, 2 mg/kg/h in the presence of polyanticonvulsant therapy, and 4 mg/kg/h for high-dose pentobarbital).[108] In a subsequent retrospective review of 40 children (18 with SE), the researchers reported on the safety and efficacy of valproic acid when administered at loading doses of 25 mg/kg (in valproate-naive patients) and infused at rates of 2 to 3 mg/kg/min.[109] No significant changes were noted in heart rate or rhythm, blood pressure, or liver enzymes. One patient reported a transient tremor after the infusion.

Inhalational Anesthetics

Several reports describe the efficacy of inhalational anesthetics for SE that is refractory to high-dose benzodiazepines and barbiturates.[110,111] Inhalational anesthetics have the advantage of being easily titratable; however, prolonged use (particularly of halothane) may cause organotoxicity. Hemodynamic compromise is seen with all of these agents, particularly halothane, and all patients in reported studies required vasopressors. In adults, achieving isoelectric EEGs has required isoflurane concentrations of 1.5% to 2%.[112] The use of inhalational anesthetics in the ICU setting is complicated by the need for a proper gas scavenging system and supervision by staff trained in the administration of anesthesia.

Ketamine and Lidocaine

Ketamine is a unique NMDA antagonist reported to have both anticonvulsant and neuroprotective properties. Because of its unique mechanism of action on NMDA receptors, ketamine is an attractive therapeutic option for refractory SE that has failed to respond to high-dose benzodiazepines and barbiturates.[113] Ketamine is commonly used for procedural sedation, but there is no consensus on its dosing for SE, particularly when given as a continuous infusion. Lidocaine, which is given as an intravenous bolus or a continuous infusion, is another treatment option, although it is not widely used in North America.[114]

Pyridoxine

Pyridoxine (vitamin B_6) is a cofactor for both glutamic acid decarboxylase and GABA transaminase, the enzymes required for the synthesis and metabolism of GABA in the brain. Pyridoxine dependency and pyridoxine deficiency are rare disorders (with a prevalence of ~1/300,000 in the United Kingdom) that usually present in the neonatal or infantile period but may present as late as age 2.5 years.[115] Patients with these disorders have intractable seizures that are refractory to conventional anticonvulsant medications but respond promptly to pyridoxine. Therefore a trial of pyridoxine should be considered in any child who is seen before age 3 years with recurrent seizures or SE, particularly if the seizures are refractory to conventional anticonvulsant agents.[115] Isoniazid poisoning is another clinical scenario in which pyridoxine may be the only effective anticonvulsant therapy.

Midazolam as a constant infusion has been reported in children with RSE[116] with surprisingly few adverse effects. Initially the patient is given a 0.15-mg/kg bolus followed by a constant infusion of 1 µg/kg/min. The infusion is increased by 1 µg/kg/min every 15 minutes until seizures are controlled. Continuous EEG monitoring and personnel well skilled in interpretation are essential to the success of therapy. In a case series of children with RSE, seizures were controlled in a mean time of 0.78 hours with infusions ranging from 1 to 18 µg/kg/min. Once seizures are controlled, the infusion rate is decreased after 12 to 24 hours while closely monitoring for seizure recurrence. All prior anticonvulsants should be continued during this phase of treatment. An interesting question is, why would midazolam work after lorazepam and valium have failed?[117,118]

Pentobarbital is often used as the next step in patients with RSE. It is advised that patients be placed on mechanical ventilation and will probably require placement of a central venous catheter and invasive blood pressure monitoring. The goal of pentobarbital therapy is to achieve an EEG pattern of burst suppression. Pentobarbital is a myocardial depressant, and hypotension requiring volume expanders and vasopressors is common. After 12 to 24 hours of burst suppression the infusion is reduced and the patient is monitored for clinical or electrographic seizure activity. If seizures recur, pentobarbital is increased to the rate that achieved burst suppression, more time is allowed to transpire (usually 12–24 hours), and another attempt at dose reduction is made.

Hypothermia

Therapeutic hypothermia has been used to treat RSE and super-refractory SE (SRSE) for many years.[89,118,119] Considering its immediate effect on epileptiform discharges in animal models, its mechanism of action seems to be different from those speculated in other neurologic conditions. Gilliam described its use in 5 children with RSE and reviewed 7 other children reported in the literature. Nine of these 12 had failed to respond midazolam, 4 also failed to respond to pentobarbital, and 1 had not responded to ketamine.[118] In all cases, body cooling to 32° to 35.3°C achieved acute seizure control. Although hypothermia may help control RSE and SRSE, its effect is transient and should be considered a temporizing measure while other AEDs are considered.[119,120]

Ketogenic Diet

The ketogenic diet is a high-fat, low-carbohydrate, and adequate protein diet used to treat pediatric seizures. It has also been used to treat RSE and SRSE. Pediatric series to date demonstrated that 33 of 43 children had responded within 19 days.[121-125]

Surgical Options

Despite exciting developments in the medical management of pediatric epilepsy, a subpopulation of approximately 30% will remain refractory to multiple AEDs. Medically refractory epilepsy threatens the developing brain, thus early identification and treatment will allow for better outcomes in this group of patients. Developments in monitoring (subdural grids) and neuroimaging (CT, MRI, positron emission tomography [PET], and single photon emission computed tomography [SPECT] scans) along with safer surgical techniques have allowed neurosurgeons to consider possible surgical evaluation and management of these patients.

Patients to be considered for epilepsy surgery must have medically refractory and disabling seizures. These patients are then evaluated by an experienced epilepsy team and undergo noninvasive (scalp EEG) and invasive monitoring (subdural grids and strips if needed), structural imaging (MRI), and functional imaging (SPECT, PET).[126,127]

When SE is refractory to multiple medical treatments, including high-dose barbiturates and benzodiazepines, surgical intervention can be considered by centers with experience in pediatric epilepsy surgery. This approach is most easily considered for but not limited to children with a large cortical malformation.[128] Focal cortical resections may be indicated if a focal structural abnormality can be identified on neuroimaging; however, the presence of a lesion on MRI is not sufficient to ensure that seizures are arising from that region. Seizures also may arise from regions remote from a lesion visualized by MRI. Furthermore, in children with prolonged RSE, secondary epileptogenic foci may develop. Typically, multiple investigations will be undertaken to ensure that seizures are arising from the area of potential surgical resection. At a minimum, there should be concordance between the structural lesion and the location of ictal and interictal EEG discharges. If the patient is medically stable, fluorodeoxyglucose positron emission tomography may be used to demonstrate interictal hypometabolism or ictal hypermetabolism of the epileptogenic focus, and magnetoencephalography may be used to support the identification of the epileptogenic focus.[129] Magnetoencephalography is a relatively new functional imaging modality that delineates the epileptogenic zone by detecting magnetic fields produced by interictal epileptiform activity. Implantation of subdural electrodes allows for the most precise localization of the epileptogenic focus; however, this procedure usually is not feasible in the setting of RSE. The evidence for such surgical approaches is limited to case reports and smaller series.[128,130-132]

Specific groups that may possibly benefit from surgical intervention include those with cortical dysplasia, tuberous sclerosis complex, polymicrogyria, hypothalamic hamartoma, hemispheric syndromes, Sturge-Weber syndrome, Rasmussen syndrome, and Landau-Kleffner syndrome. These patients should be referred to a center with expertise in pediatric epilepsy surgery. Surgical procedures may include placement of a vagal nerve stimulator (VNS), resection of a cortical lesion, temporal lobectomy, hemispherectomy, corpus callosotomy (disconnection), or multiple subpial transaction.[133]

VNSs are placed in patients with refractory partial seizures that are not surgical candidates because they lack a resectable seizure focus. The mechanism of action is not known, but it is thought that electrical stimulation may increase the degree of inhibition or decrease the degree of excitation in the CNS. The VNS reduces seizure frequency but does not ablate or destroy a seizure focus, nor does it anatomically disrupt a functional connection from the epileptogenic cortex to surrounding cortex. Outcome data are generally good with a reduction in seizure frequency of more than 50% in 50% to 75% of patients. Postoperative complications include coughing, hoarseness, and throat paresthesias during stimulation.[134-136]

Morbidity and Mortality

The mortality associated with pediatric SE has declined from approximately 11% in 1970 to 3.6% in 1989.[137] The need for admission to a PICU increases the mortality to approximately 6%.[138] Outcome is related to the duration of the seizure, the age of the patient, and the underlying CNS disorder. Patients who remain in SE >1 hour and are less than 1-year-old have the highest risk of mortality. The mortality rate of RSE is approximately 32%, which is much higher than the overall mortality cited earlier for patients with SE. Patients who suffer prolonged seizures also have higher morbidity such as developmental delay and new-onset epilepsy.[139] Overall, children with epilepsy have an increased risk of death; however, most deaths occur in those with severe underlying conditions and are not directly related to the occurrence of seizures.[140-142]

Acknowledgment

I gratefully acknowledge the contribution of Cecil D. Hahn, Sam D. Shemie, and Elizabeth J. Donner who authored this chapter in previous editions.

Key References

1. DeLorenzo RJ, Garnett LK, Towne AR, et al. Comparison of status epilepticus with prolonged seizure activity lasting from 10 to 29 minutes. *Epilepsia.* 1999;40:164-169.
2. Lowenstein DH, Bleck T, Macdonald RL. It's time to revise the definition of status epilepticus. *Epilepsia.* 1999;40:120-122.
4. Raspall-Chaure M, Chin RFM, Neville BG, Scott RC. Outcome of pediatric convulsive status epilepticus: a systematic review. *Lancet Neurol.* 2006;5:769-779.
6. Major P, Thiele EA. Seizures in children: determining the variation. *Pediatr Rev.* 2007;28:363-371.
14. Shorvon S, Ferlisi M. The outcome of therapies in refractory and super refractory convulsive status epilepticus and recommendations for therapy. *Brain.* 2012;135:2314-2328.
15. Sutter R, Kaplan PW. Electroencephalographic criteria for nonconvulsive status epilepticus: synopsis and comprehensive survey. *Epliepsia.* 2012;53(suppl 3):1-51.
16. Freilich ER, Schreiber JM, Zelleke T, Gaillard WD. Pediatric status epilepticus: identification and evaluation. *Curr Opin Pediatr.* 2014; 26:655-661.
18. Ahmad S, Marsh ED. Febrile status epilepticus: current state of clinical and basic research. *Semin Pediatr Neurol.* 2010;17:150-154.
19. Seinfeld S, Shinnar S, Sun S, et al. Emergency management of febrile status epilepticus: results of the FEBSTST study. *Epliepsia.* 2014;55:388-395.
20. Seinfeld DOS, Pellock JM. Recent research on febrile seizure: a review. *J Neurol Neurophysiol.* 2014;165:1-11.
24. Lawrence R, Inder T. Neonatal status epilepticus. *Semin Pediatr Neurol.* 2010;17:163-168.
26. Statler KD. Pediatric posttraumatic seizures: epidemiology, putative mechanisms of epileptogenesis and promising investigational progress. *Dev Neurosci.* 2006;28:354-363.
29. Shepard PW, St. Louis EK. Seizure treatment in transplant patients. *Curr Treat Options Neurol.* 2012;14:332-347.
30. Cordelli DM, Masetti R, Zama D, et al. Etiology, characteristics and outcome of seizures after pediatric hematopoietic cell transplantation. *Seizure.* 2013;23:140-145.
31. LoPinto-Khoury C, Sperling MR. Autoimmune status epilepticus. *Curr Treat Options Neurol.* 2013;15:545-556.
34. Stafstrom CE. Back to basics: the pathophysiology of epileptic seizures: a primer for pediatricians. *Pediatr Rev.* 1998;19:342-351.
38. Treiman DM, Meyers PD, Walon NY, et al. A comparison of four treatments for generalized convulsive status epilepticus. *N Engl J Med.* 1998; 339:792.
44. Lothman E. The biochemical basis and pathophysiology of status epilepticus. *Neurology.* 1990;40(suppl 2):13-23.
48. Abend NS, Loddenkemoer T. Pediatric status epilepticus management. *Curr Opin Pediatr.* 2014;26:668-674.
49. Brophy GM, Bell R, Claassen J, et al. Guidelines for the evaluation and management of status epilepticus. *Neurocrit Care.* 2012;17:3-23.
53. Riviello JJ, Ashwal S, Hirtz D, et al. Practice parameter: diagnostic assessment of the child with status epilepticus (an evidence-based review): report of the Quality Standards subcommittee of the American Academy of Neurology and the Practice Committee of the Child Neurology Society. *Neurology.* 2006;67:1542-1550.
54. Allen JE, Ferrie CD, Livingston JH, Feltbower RG. Recovery of consciousness after epileptic seizures in children. *Arch Dis Child.* 2007;92:39-42.
57. Abend NS, Gutierrez-Colina AM, Dlugos D. Medical treatment of pediatric status epilepticus. *Semin Pediatr Neurol.* 2010;17:169-175.
61. Walker M. Status epilepticus: an evidence based guide. *BMJ.* 2005;33: 673-677.
63. Chamberlain JM, Okada P, Holsti M, et al. Lorazepam vs diazepam for pediatric status epilepticus a randomized clinical trial. *JAMA.* 2014; 311:1652-1660.
65. Trinka E, Hofler J, Leitinger M, Brigo F. Pharmacotherapy for status epilepticus. *Drugs.* 2015;75:1499-1521.
70. Hwang WS, Gwak HM, Seo DW. Propofol syndrome in refractory status epilepticus. *J Epilepsy Res.* 2013;3:21-27.
78. Trinka E, Hofler J, Zerbs A, Brigo F. Efficacy and safety of intravenous valproate for status epilepticus: a systematic review. *CNS Drugs.* 2014;28: 623-639.
79. Abend NS, Monk HM, Licht DJ, Dlugos DJ. Intravenous levetiracetam in critically ill children with status epilepticus or acute repetitive seizures. *Pediatr Crit Care Med.* 2009;10:505-510.
80. Kim JS, Lee JH, Ryu HW, et al. Effectiveness of intravenous levetiracetam as an adjunctive treatment in pediatric refractory status epilepticus. *Pediatr Emerg Care.* 2014;30:525-528.
88. Wilkes R, Tasker RC. Intensive care treatment of uncontrolled status epilepticus in children: systematic literature search of midazolam and anesthetic therapies. *Pediatr Crit Care Med.* 2014;15:632-639.

89. Tasker R, Vitali S. Continuous infusion, general anesthesia and other intensive care treatment for uncontrolled status epilepticus. *Curr Opin Pediatr*. 2014;26:682-689.

104. Iyer VN, Hoel R, Rabinstein AA. Propofol infusion syndrome in patients with refractory status epilepticus: an 11-year clinical experience. *Crit Care Med*. 2009;37:3024-3030.

105. Santillanes G, Luc Q. Emergency department management of seizures in pediatric patients. *Pediatr Emerg Med Pract*. 2015;12:1-27.

118. Motamedi G, Lesser RP, Vicini S. Therapeutic brain hypothermia, its mechanism of action, and its prospects as treatment for epilepsy. *Epilepsia*. 2013;54:959-970.

119. Guilliams K, Rosen M, Butterman S, et al. Hypothermia for pediatric refractory status epilepticus. *Epilepsia*. 2013;54:1586-1594.

120. Alford EL, Wheless JW, Phelps SJ. Treatment of generalized convulsive status epilepticus in pediatric patients. *J Pediatr Pharmacol Ther*. 2015;20:260-289.

121. Kossoff EH, Zupec-Kania BA, Amark PE, et al. Optimal clinical management of children receiving the ketogenic diet: recommendations of the International Ketogenic Diet Study Group. *Epilepsia*. 2002;50:304-317.

123. O'Connor SE, Richardson C, Trescher WH, et al. The ketogenic diet for the treatment of pediatric status epilepticus. *Pediatr Neurol*. 2014;50:101-103.

125. Joshi SM, Singh RK, Shellhaaas RA. Advance treatments for childhood epilepsy: beyond antiseizure medications. *JAMA Pediatr*. 2013;167:76-83.

127. Lee YK, Adelson PD. Neurosurgical management of pediatric epilepsy. *Pediatr Clin North Am*. 2004;51:441-456.

136. De Herdt V, Waterschoot L, Vonck K, et al. Vagus nerve stimulation for refractory status epilepticus. *Eur J Paediatr Neurol*. 2009;13:286-289.

139. Sahin M, Menache CC, Holmes GL, Riviello JJ. Outcome of severe refractory status epilepticus in children. *Epilepsia*. 2001;42:1461-1467.

142. Devinsky O. Sudden unexpected death in epilepsy. *N Engl J Med*. 2011;365:1801-1811.

Hypoxic-Ischemic Encephalopathy: Pathobiology and Therapy of the Postresuscitation Syndrome in Children

Ericka L. Fink, Robert S.B. Clark, Hülya Bayir, Cameron Dezfulian, and Patrick M. Kochanek

PEARLS

- Cardiac arrest in pediatric patients differs from cardiac arrest in adult patients in at least two important aspects: (1) cardiac arrest in pediatric patients is predominantly due to asphyxia, in contrast to adults, where it is more often due to ventricular dysrhythmias, and (2) developmental differences between pediatric and adult patients including ongoing synaptogenesis, lower cerebral blood flow in neonates and higher cerebral blood flow in toddlers and children compared with adults, neurotransmitter receptor maturation, and higher energy expenditure in pediatric patients.

- In 2010, the American Heart Association stated that therapeutic hypothermia (32° to 34°C) may be considered for children who remain comatose after cardiac arrest, although it is reasonable for adolescents resuscitated from sudden, witnessed, out-of-hospital ventricular tachycardia/fibrillation cardiac arrest.[1] A multicenter, randomized clinical trial evaluating 48 hours of hypothermia versus controlled normothermia found no benefit of hypothermia in out-of-hospital pediatric cardiac arrest; results from the in-hospital study are pending.

- At present, there is no clinically proved brain-targeted therapy for hypoxic-ischemic encephalopathy. It is likely that such targeted therapies, spanning field interventions, intensive care, and rehabilitation, will be required to mitigate hypoxic-ischemic encephalopathy in infants and children after cardiac arrest.

Hypoxic-ischemic encephalopathy (HIE) in children surviving cardiac arrest is a significant public health problem and confers a lifelong burden on patients and families. Despite the lack of new targeted therapies for HIE, outcomes for some children after in-hospital pediatric cardiac arrest are improving, which is likely multifactorial.[2] From 2002 to 2005, important clinical trials demonstrated neuroprotective effects of therapeutic hypothermia in adults with cardiac arrest and neonates with moderate to severe HIE.[3-7] Although these studies and an increased understanding of mechanisms of HIE provide hope, challenges remain as the likelihood of intact neurologic survival in children who suffer cardiac arrest remains unacceptably small.[8,9] These trials spurred interest in determining whether therapeutic hypothermia is efficacious in children after cardiac arrest, culminating in a National Institutes of Health–funded multicenter clinical trial of therapeutic hypothermia after pediatric cardiac arrest (THAPCA) in the United States, Canada, and the United Kingdom. Although accrual for this study occurred, questions developed regarding the optimal temperature target for neuroprotection with publication of a randomized clinical trial (RCT) in adults with cardiac cause of cardiac arrest that found similar outcomes when targeting 33°C or 36°C.[10] The out-of-hospital pediatric cardiac arrest THAPCA trial found no difference in survival with favorable outcome; in-hospital results are pending.[11] Thus a proved effective treatment protocol that reliably prevents HIE and improves neurologic recovery after cardiac arrest in infants and children remains elusive. Even the optimal supportive care and monitoring to minimize secondary organ injury and maximize recovery after cardiac arrest are in and of themselves controversial.

A key question is whether or not more advanced monitoring of the brain with titration of supportive care, at least in part, to brain-related pathophysiologic derangements will improve outcomes. This question arises from the pathobiological complexity of cerebral injury and the limitations to monitor key metabolic and physiologic parameters in the brain. This question is beginning to be addressed in both preclinical and clinical investigations via brain tissue oxygen monitoring and intracerebral microdialysis.[12,13] Clinical stumbling blocks in the history of brain resuscitation have also slowed our understanding of HIE after cardiac arrest. Historically, this entity was largely ignored as a specific disease process. Brain resuscitation was dealt with as a single therapeutic paradigm regardless of the etiology.[14] This resulted in the misguided application of results from studies of traumatic brain injury (TBI), stroke, Reye syndrome, and cerebral protection to patients suffering cardiac arrest. Second, within cardiac arrest, etiologies and patient-relevant biological factors are lumped together. Factors influencing neurologic damage and recovery are clearly different depending on the cause (asphyxia, arrhythmia, hemorrhage, trauma, sepsis, etc.), age, comorbidities, genetic factors, interval between arrest and return of spontaneous circulation (ROSC), and effectiveness of cardiopulmonary resuscitation (CPR).

This chapter reviews the pathobiology of HIE with emphasis on cellular mechanisms, pathophysiology, and histopathology. Differences between the most prevalent etiologies of cardiac arrest in children (asphyxia versus cardiac arrhythmia) are examined, and an appraisal of traditional and novel therapies is presented. Finally, any discussion of HIE in children is complicated not only by the specific mode of arrest in children but also by the unique nature of these young patients. The child's brain is still developing, adding another layer of variability in terms of age-specific pathologic and reparative mechanisms, potential for therapies to afford benefit, evaluation of therapeutic effectiveness, and neurologic outcome. Thus the effect of the host's immaturity on the pathobiology of postarrest encephalopathy also is examined.

Epidemiology

In the United States, cardiac arrest occurs in 8 to 20/100,000 children per year in the out-of-hospital setting and in 1.06 of every 1000 pediatric hospital admissions[8,15,16] resulting in roughly two to three many times as many in-hospital as out-of-hospital cases.[9] Males have an increased frequency of cardiac arrest (60% versus 40% for females), but there are no sex differences in mortality.[9] Half of children with cardiac arrest have underlying comorbidities.[9,17]

Asphyxia is the most frequent cause of cardiac arrests and the principal cause of HIE in children.[18,19] In asphyxial arrest, asystole or pulseless electrical activity (PEA) is preceded and precipitated by a period of hypoxemic or anoxic perfusion.[20] Studies are beginning to define the cascade of events that ultimately leads to no flow during asphyxia, and these studies have revealed specific cardiovascular phases and remarkable brain-heart interactions.[21] Hypoxia most commonly results from submersion accidents, airway obstruction, pulmonary aspiration, severe asthma or pneumonia, inhalation injury, or apnea syndromes.[8,9,22] In ventricular fibrillation (VF)-induced cardiac arrest, respiration ceases shortly after loss of perfusion pressure. VF also occurs in children but at an estimated incidence of <10% of pediatric victims of cardiac arrest overall.[9]

Although most in-hospital events are witnessed with bystander CPR performed by health care personnel, less than one-third of out-of-hospital events are witnessed with 30% to 50% of those children receiving bystander CPR, and this distinction influences outcome.[22,23] The largest proportion of unwitnessed out-of-hospital cardiac arrest occurs in infants (86%), the age group with the worst outcomes.[23]

Cellular and Molecular Pathobiology
Mechanisms of Hypoxic-Ischemic Brain Injury

Cerebral neurons in culture can tolerate hours of extreme hypoxia. Although it takes about 160 minutes of exposure to

an anoxic gas mixture for oxygen tension in the culture medium to reach 1 mm Hg, cortical neurons tolerate 1 to 3 additional hours with little histologic change.[24] If 1 mmol/L sodium cyanide is used to simulate immediate anoxia, hippocampal neurons become swollen and vacuolated within 20 to 60 minutes and begin to disintegrate in 4 hours. Similarly, even 1 hour of complete global brain ischemia in monkeys is followed by electrophysiologic recovery of many neurons and significant recovery of some aspects of brain metabolism, such as protein synthesis.[25] Although the time limit for consistently normal outcome after normothermic cardiac arrest is unknown, it is certainly closer to 5 to 10 minutes than 1 to 3 hours. Restoration of integrated brain function—that is, neurologic recovery—differs markedly from physiologic or metabolic brain recovery. In contrast to the relative cellular homogeneity in other organs, the functional specificity and interactions of neurons and glia in the brain make patchy areas of cell death potentially devastating. This is evident in the neuropathology of dogs in persistent coma 1 week after a 10- to 15-minute cardiac arrest. Scattered, regionally dependent neuronal death is evident, but the majority of neurons appear normal.[26] Cardiac arrest is unique from other forms of focal brain ischemia and nonischemic brain injury in that survival requires reperfusion. Reperfusion injury is therefore a mandatory part of the postischemic recovery period and may contribute to the unique phenotype of hypoxic-ischemic brain injury.

Energy Failure

The brain depends on large amounts of substrate (glucose and lactate) because of its tremendous metabolic demands and paltry energy stores. Interruption of cerebral blood flow (CBF) results in loss of consciousness and electroencephalographic silence within seconds. Within 5 to 7 minutes, energy failure occurs, accompanied by disturbances of ion homeostasis in neurons and glial cells. Clinically this rapid depletion of brain high-energy phosphates has been demonstrated after hypoxia-ischemia in neonates using phosphorus magnetic resonance spectroscopy (MRS).[27] Influx of sodium and water and efflux of potassium occur because the cells cannot maintain their energy-dependent electrochemical gradients. When the extracellular potassium concentration reaches 10 to 15 mmol/L, voltage-gated channels open and extracellular calcium influx occurs.[28]

If CBF remains inadequate and energy failure persists, calcium-mediated events such as phospholipase and protease activation can lead to irreversible injury and neuronal cell death. Cerebral acidosis occurs, and intracellular pH decreases from 7 to 6.4.[29] If CBF is restored, however, recovery of basal cellular metabolism (adenosine triphosphate [ATP] levels, protein synthesis, oxygen consumption) and pH occurs. This has been shown in brain tissue samples and intact brain measurements after global ischemic insults that result in a persistent minimally conscious state.[25]

After anoxia or ischemia, the recovery of aerobic metabolism is essential for recovery, but is not in-and-of-itself sufficient. The imbalance between aerobic and anaerobic metabolism and over-dependence of neurons upon lactate as a substrate[30] must be restored. Despite global metabolic recovery, certain neurons progress to cell death. After restitution of CBF and oxidative metabolism after energy failure in the brain cellular and molecular dysfunction can progress and cells may die via immediate necrosis (complete energy failure), programmed cell death (apoptosis, autophagic stress, or regulated necrosis), or a spectrum of these processes (see also Chapter 84).[31-33] Brain MRS demonstrates early (during ischemia) and late (48 hours after reperfusion) depletion of high energy phosphorous compounds and a corresponding lactate peak occurring in the face of normal vital signs, serum glucose, and arterial oxygen saturation after experimental hypoxia-ischemia.[34,35]

Selective Vulnerability

Certain neurons—such as those in the CA_1 region of the hippocampus; basal ganglia; cerebral cortical layers III and V; portions of the amygdaloid nucleus; the cerebellar Purkinje cells; and, in infants, periventricular white matter regions and some brain stem nuclei—are known to be especially vulnerable to global hypoxia-ischemia and reperfusion.[36,37] Five minutes of complete global brain ischemia produces cell death in the regions that begin to appear between 48 and 72 hours, without apparent histologic damage in other brain areas.

Transient calcium accumulation occurs in all cells during ischemia, but secondary irreversible accumulation occurs in the selectively vulnerable zones many hours later.[38] Electrophysiologic studies show that delayed neuronal death is preceded by neuronal hyperactivity. It is hypothesized that ischemic and early postischemic calcium accumulation leads to a complex sequence of derangements in cellular metabolism such as protease activation and oxygen-derived free radical formation.[39] These conditions, in concert with excessive release of excitatory neurotransmitters (glutamate, glycine, aspartate) in these areas, lead to excitotoxicity and cell death. These findings are supported by work in neuronal culture showing that calcium influx accompanies cell death in the presence of anoxia or supraphysiologic levels of excitatory amino acids such as glutamate,[24,40] and that CA_1 cells are the most sensitive to glutamate-mediated injury.[41] Finally, delayed energy depletion, mitochondrial dysfunction, and infarction occur in concert but are regionally distinct, suggesting that metabolic characteristics of brain regions affect recovery from ischemia.[42,43]

Of particular interest is that these intrinsically vulnerable cells do not have a unique vascular distribution.[44] They represent neither vascular watersheds nor hypoperfused zones during reperfusion. Death of these neurons after a threshold ischemic insult occurs in a delayed fashion following reperfusion and thus may be preventable, at least in part, by treatment.

Cell Death Mechanisms

Cell death can occur by multiple distinct pathways, necrosis, apoptosis, or autophagy, but overlap and combination exists, and a number of additional neuronal death pathways including necroptosis, pyroptosis, and ferroptosis have been identified, although their contribution to brain injury after cardiac arrest remains to be defined.[31,45-48] Necrosis, which is characterized by denaturing and coagulation of cellular proteins, is the basic pattern of pathologic cell death that results from a progressive reduction in the cellular content of ATP.[49] Necrosis involves progressive derangements in energy and substrate metabolism that are followed by a series of morphologic alterations including swelling of cells and organelles, subsurface cellular blebbing, amorphous deposits in mitochondria,

condensation of nuclear chromatin, and, finally, breaks in plasma and organellar membranes.[49] Although necrotic cell death was traditionally felt to be entirely irreversible, studies showing that some degree of necrotic cell death responds to treatment after hypoxia-ischemia implicate regulated or programmed necrosis also termed *necroptosis*.[50,51]

Cell death after hypoxic-ischemic insults can also occur by apoptosis.[52] Development of apoptosis usually requires new protein synthesis and the activation of endonucleases. Two distinct types of characteristic cleavage of DNA have been described. The most well described, *caspase-dependent* apoptosis, involves cleavage by caspase-activated deoxyribonuclease at linkage regions between nucleosomes to form fragments of double-stranded DNA.[53] This produces a pattern of DNA cleavage observed on Southern blot analysis termed *DNA laddering*. In contrast, *caspase-independent* apoptosis results in large-scale DNA fragmentation induced by the mitochondrial flavoprotein apoptosis-inducing factor (AIF).[54,55] The stimuli triggering apoptosis are complex and multifactorial, involving extracellular surface receptors, cell signaling pathways, protease cascades, and mitochondrial and other organelle dysfunction. Selective vulnerable cell death in brain regions such as the CA_1 region of the hippocampus after transient global brain ischemia appears to occur by apoptosis,[56] as DNA extracted from the hippocampus of gerbils at 4 days after a threshold global ischemic insult exhibits the characteristic laddering pattern. Thalamic delayed neuronal death was caused by Fas-mediated apoptosis in a model of neonatal hypoxia-ischemia,[57] and durable electrophysiologic disturbances are observed in thalami after asphyxia cardiac arrest in juvenile rats.[58] Li and colleagues[59] reported that apoptosis in the postischemic brain is not limited to scattered neuronal death in what have been traditionally deemed to be selectively vulnerable regions, but it is seen even in penumbral regions around evolving cerebral infarcts (Fig. 68.1). Finally, the proportion of apoptosis in the developing brain after ischemia appears to

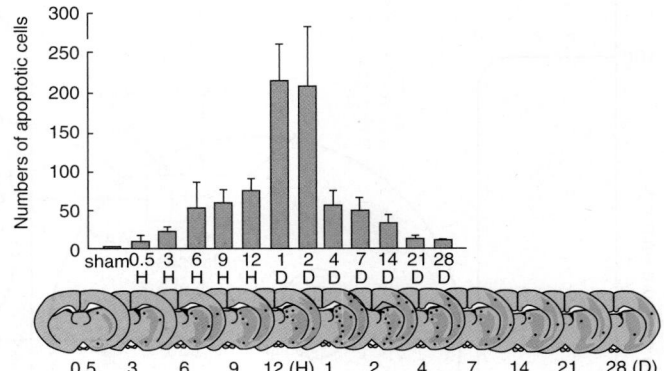

Fig. 68.1. Apoptotic cells in coronal brain sections in rats subjected to 2 hours of middle cerebral artery occlusion and between 0.5 and 28 days of reperfusion. *Top:* Progressive increase in the numbers of apoptotic cells occurs with increasing reperfusion time to peak at 24 hours. However, apoptotic cells are still detectable even after 1 week of reperfusion. *Bottom:* Distribution of apoptosis (*dots*) and necrotic neurons (*hatched areas*). Apoptotic cells are localized predominately to the inner boundary zone of infarction. (From Li Y, Chopp M, Jiang N, Yao F, Zaloga C. Temporal profile of in situ DNA fragmentation after transient middle cerebral artery occlusion in the rat. J Cereb Blood Flow Metab. 1995;15:389-397.)

be sex dependent, as females but not males respond to anti-apoptotic agents after neonatal hypoxia-ischemia.[60]

Autophagy is a homeostatic process that recycles cell resources during periods of nutrient stress.[61] Autophagy is up-regulated after experimental brain ischemia,[62,63] which can be considered profound nutrient stress.[64] Studies show that blocking autophagy after hypoxia-ischemia can be protective or detrimental.[48,65,66] As such, autophagy's role after acute brain injury is controversial, and it may depend on the stage of brain development and sex of the patient, animal, or cell.[64,67] Mouse pups lacking Atg7 (a necessary component for autophagy) or rat pups treated with an inhibitor of autophagy (3-methyladenine) are protected from focal hypoxia-ischemia.[62,63] Knockdown of Atg7 using small interfering RNA (siRNA) was shown to reduce autophagy and Purkinje neuron death in juvenile rats after asphyxia cardiac arrest, with the beneficial effects more prominent in female versus male rat pups.[68]

The proportion of neuronal death that occurs via apoptosis, necrosis, autophagy, or other pathways after cerebral ischemia remains undetermined.[69,70] Although neurons may appear histologically normal in the days after reperfusion, electron microscopy reveals changes present within 6 hours.[70] Moreover, it remains possible that treatments inhibiting apoptosis, for example, may simply convert cell death to necrosis or autophagy, or another pathway.[71,72] Although speculative, it is possible that after cardiac arrest and resuscitation, a continuum exists in neurons from recovery to necrosis[73] that depends on the duration of the insult, the local milieu, and the given brain region.[74-76]

Nevertheless, in any given brain region, irrespective of the neuronal death pathway that is activated, a highly complex series of events occurs during the arrest and after ROSC. A theoretic scheme of the mechanisms involved is given in Fig. 68.2, a scheme that remains remarkably contemporary despite being conceptualized in the 1990s by Bellamy, Safar, and others.[77] Importantly, several molecular and pharmacologic interventions that interrupt apoptosis have been reported to improve outcome after cerebral ischemia, including pediatric models. Although studies showing improved functional recovery with treatments inhibiting apoptosis after cerebral ischemia suggest that some salvaged neurons regain their integrative properties, it is also possible that some of the delayed apoptosis represents appropriate pruning of neurons that have lost their targets. These processes, coupled with the need to restore highly integrated function, explain the clinical scenario of the persistent vegetative (minimally conscious) state despite restoration of normal function in other organ systems. The relationship of these distinct forms of cell death to selective vulnerability of neurons in brain is steadily increasing.

Reperfusion Injury

Reoxygenation and reperfusion are essential to recovery of any organ after ischemia. Experimental evidence suggests, however, that certain aspects of reperfusion result in tissue injury.[78,79] Reperfusion injury is a complex series of interactions between parenchyma and microcirculatory elements, resulting in detrimental effects that negate some fraction of the benefits of reperfusion. The magnitude of reperfusion injury varies with the organ in question, the duration and type of hypoxic-ischemic insult, as well as the timing, duration, and magnitude of reperfusion.[80,81]

In the case of cardiac arrest, ischemia and reperfusion are global events. In the brain, early reperfusion (5–15 min) after asphyxia results in significant hyperemia.[82,83] In many organs and in the brain after focal insults, progressive microcirculatory failure is thought to be an important aspect of reperfusion injury.[84] However, as suggested by the nonspecific vascular distribution of selectively vulnerable neurons, the brain may

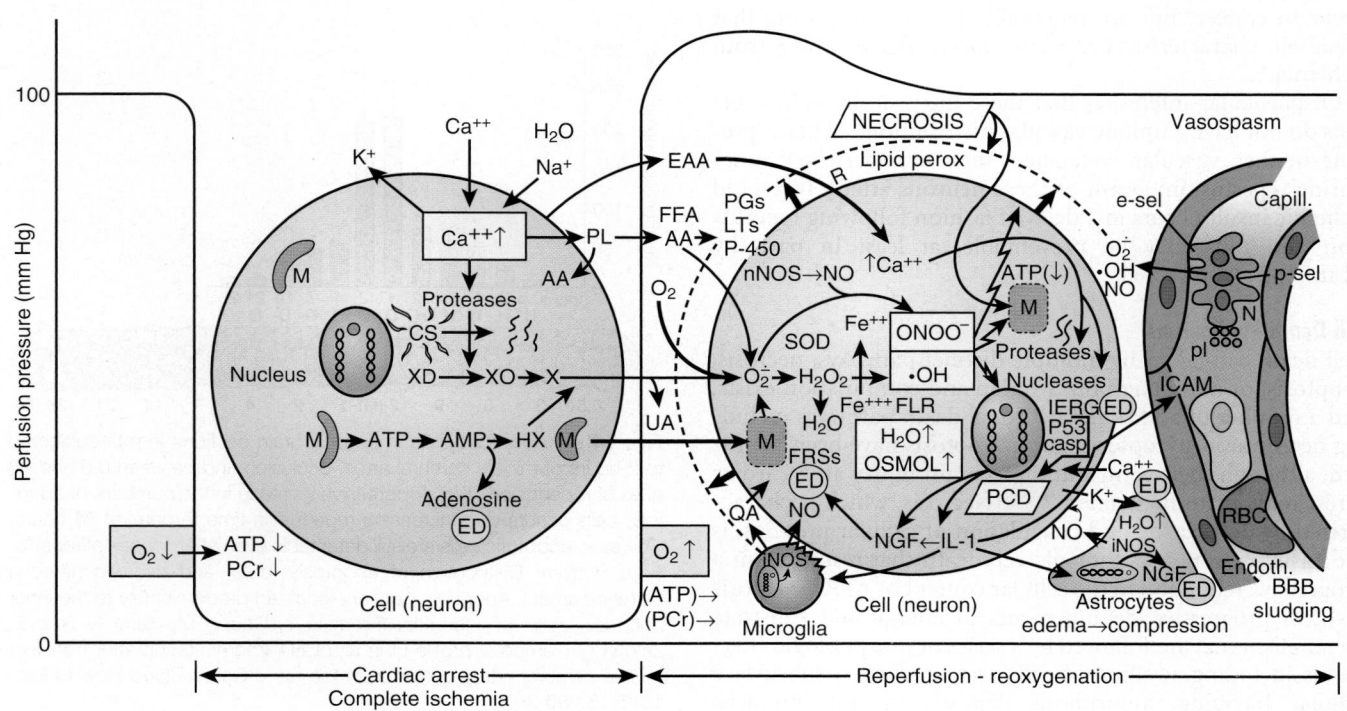

display a second unique setting for the evolution of reperfusion injury, the evolution of selectively vulnerable cell death. Four key mechanisms hypothesized to be important to reperfusion injury in the brain include (1) excitotoxicity and calcium accumulation, (2) protease activation, (3) oxygen radical formation, and (4) membrane phospholipid hydrolysis and mediator formation.

Excitotoxicity and Calcium Accumulation

Glutamate and aspartate are the major excitatory amino acid neurotransmitters in the mammalian central nervous system (CNS), but both also have neurotoxic properties. Pioneering studies by Rothman and associates[85] demonstrated in vitro that hypoxia-induced neuronal death is mediated by synaptic activity. Inhibition of synaptic glutamate release or blockade of glutamate receptors prevented hypoxia-induced neuronal injury. Glutamate is the major neurotransmitter in the selectively vulnerable zones and accumulates extracellularly at supraphysiologic levels in these regions after hypoxic or ischemic insults.[38] In other regions asphyxia induces significant increases in dopamine, serotonin, norepinephrine, and gamma-aminobutyric acid [GABA], which are larger than

Fig. 68.2. Death of cells after temporary ischemia. Diagram of complex, partially hypothesized biochemical cascades in neurons during and after cardiac arrest.[77] Normally the intracellular ($[Ca^{2+}]i$) to extracellular ($[Ca^{2+}]e$) calcium gradient is $1:10,000$. Calcium regulators include calcium/magnesium ATPase, the endoplasmic reticulum (ER), mitochondria, and arachidonic acid (AA). With stimulation, different cell types respond with an increase in $[Ca^{2+}]i$ because of the release of bound Ca^{2+} in the ER and influx of $[Ca^{2+}]e$ or both. During complete ischemic anoxia (cardiac arrest) *(left)*, the level of energy (phosphocreatinine [Pcr] and adenosine triphosphate [ATP]) decreases to near zero in all tissues at different rates, depending on stores of oxygen and substrate; it is fastest in the brain (~5 minutes) and slower in the heart and other vital organs. This energy loss causes membrane pump failure, which causes a shift of sodium (Na^+) ions, water (H_2O), and calcium ions (Ca^{2+}) from the extracellular into the intracellular space (cytosolic edema) and potassium (K^+) leakage from the intracellular into the extracellular space. Increase in $[Ca^{2+}]i$ activates phospholipase A_2, which breaks down membrane phospholipids (PL) into free fatty acids *(FFA)*, particularly arachidonic (AA). Increase in $[Ca^{2+}]i$ also activates proteolytic enzymes, such as calpain, which may disrupt the cytoskeleton (CS) and possibly the nucleus. In mitochondria (M) hydrolysis of ATP to adenosine monophosphate (AMP) leads to an accumulation of hypoxanthine (HX). Increased $[Ca^{2+}]i$ may enhance conversion of xanthine dehydrogenase (XD) to xanthine oxidase (XO), priming the neuron for the production of the oxygen free radical superoxide anion (O_2^-), although this pathway is of questionable importance in neurons (X, Xanthine; UA, uric acid). Excitatory amino acid neurotransmitters (EAA), particularly glutamate and aspartate, increase in extracellular fluid. Increased [EAA]e activates N-methyl-D-aspartate (NMDA) and non-NMDA receptors (R), thereby increasing calcium and sodium influx and mobilizing stores of $[Ca^{2+}]i$. Increased extracellular potassium activates EAA receptors by membrane depolarization. Glycolysis during hypoxia results in anaerobic metabolism and lactic acidosis, until all glucose is used (in the brain, during anoxia after ~20 minutes). This lactic acidosis, plus inability to wash out CO_2, results in mixed tissue acidosis that adversely influences neuronal viability. The net effect of acidosis on the cascades during and after ischemia is not clear. Mild acidosis may actually attenuate NMDA-mediated $[Ca^{2+}]i$ accumulation. Without reoxygenation, cells progress via first reversible, later irreversible structural damage, to necrosis at specific rates for different cell types. During reperfusion and reoxygenation *(right)*, lactate and molecular breakdown products can create osmotic edema and rupture of organelles and mitochondria. Recovery of [ATP] and [Pcr] and of the ionic membrane pump may be hampered by hypoperfusion as a result of vasospasm, cell sludging, adhesion of neutrophils (granulocytes) (N), and capillary compression by swollen astrocytes, which also help to protect neurons by absorbing extracellular potassium. Capillary (blood-brain barrier [BBB]) leakage results in interstitial (vasogenic) edema. Increased concentrations of at least four oxyradical species that break down membranes and proteins, worsen the microcirculation, and possibly also damage the nucleus may be formed: Superoxide anion (O_2^-) leading to hydroxyl radical (·OH) (via the iron-catalyzed $Fe^{+++} \rightarrow Fe^{++}$, Haber-Weiss/Fenton reaction); free lipid radicals (FLR) and peroxynitrite ($OONO^-$). O_2^- may be formed from several sources: (1) directly from eicosanoid metabolism; (2) by the previously described XO system; (3) via quinone-mediated reactions within and outside the electron transport chain (from mitochondria [M]); and (4) by activation of NADPH-oxidase in accumulated neutrophils in the microvasculature or after diapedesis into tissue. Increased O_2^- leads to increased hydrogen peroxide (H_2O_2) production as a result of intracellular action of superoxide dismutase (SOD). [H_2O_2] is controlled by intracellular catalase. Increased O_2^- further leads to increased ·OH, because of conversion of H_2O_2 to ·OH via the Haber-Weiss/Fenton reaction, with iron liberated from mitochondria. This reaction is promoted by acidosis. ·OH and $OONO^-$ damage cellular lipids, proteins, and nucleic acids. Also, AA is metabolized by the cyclooxygenase pathways to prostaglandins (PGs) including thromboxane A_2, or by the lipoxygenase pathway to produce leukotrienes (LTs), and by the cytochrome P-450 pathway. These products can act as neurotransmitters and signal transducers in neuronal and glial cells and can activate thrombotic and inflammatory pathways in the microcirculation. Inflammatory reactions after ischemia have been shown to occur in extracerebral organs, focal brain ischemia, or brain trauma; to date, they have not been demonstrated after temporary complete global brain ischemia. Neuronal injury can signal interleukin-1 and other cytokines to be produced and trigger endogenous activation of microglia, with additional injury (QA, quinolinic acid). In addition, tissue or endothelial injury—particularly associated with necrosis—can signal the endothelium to produce adhesion molecules (intercellular [ICAM], e-selectin [e-sel], p-selectin [p-sel]), cytokines, chemokines, and other mediators, triggering local involvement of systemic inflammatory cells in an interaction between blood and damaged tissue. Reoxygenation restores [ATP] through oxidative phosphorylation, which may result in massive uptake of $[Ca^{2+}]i$ into mitochondria, which are swollen from increased osmolality. Thus mitochondria loaded with bound $[Ca^{2+}]$ may self-destruct by rupturing and releasing additional free radicals. Increased $[Ca^{2+}]i$ by itself and by triggering free radical reactions may result in lipid peroxidation, leaky membranes, and cell death. Neuronal damage can be caused, in part, by increased EAA (excitotoxicity). During reperfusion, $[Ca^{2+}]i$ and increased EAAs normalize. Their contribution to ultimate death of neurons is more likely through the cascades they have triggered during ischemia. During ischemia and subsequent reperfusion, loading of cells and calcium maldistribution in cells are believed to be the key trigger common to the development of cell death. This calcium loading signals a wide variety of pathologic processes. Proteases, lipases, and nucleases are activated, which may contribute to activation of genes or gene products (ie, caspases [Casp] or P53) critical to the development of programmed cell death (PCD, ie, apoptosis, autophagy, or regulated necrosis), or inactivation of genes or gene products normally inhibiting this process. Activation of nNOS by calcium can lead to production of NO, which can combine with superoxide to generate peroxynitrite ($OONO^-$). $OONO^-$ and ·OH both can lead to DNA injury and PCD or protein and membrane peroxidation and necrosis, respectively. Nerve growth factor (NGF) nuclear immediate early response genes (IERG) such as heat shock protein, free radical scavengers (FRSs), adenosine, and other endogenous defenses (ED) may modulate the damage. (Designed in 1995 by P. Safar, MD, and P. Kochanek, MD, with input from N. Bircher, MD, and J. Severinghaus, MD.)

the increases in glutamate in relative though not absolute concentrations.[21]

Glutamate is released at the presynaptic terminal in response to neuronal stimulation and acts by binding to postsynaptic dendritic receptors. Two main classes of excitatory neurotransmitter receptors have been identified. One class consists of the ligand-gated ion channels ("ionotropic" receptors) and includes N-methyl-D-aspartate (NMDA), α-amino-3-hydroxy-5-methyl-4-isoxazole propionic acid (AMPA) or quisqualate, and kainate receptor subtypes. Toxicity caused by NMDA receptor activation is usually rapid, whereas AMPA or kainate receptor-mediated cell death is somewhat slower to develop.[86] Progress in NMDA receptor (NMDAR)–mediated neurotransmission has revealed greater complexity then previously appreciated—and may better inform therapy. NMDARs consist of heterodimeric glutamate receptor (GluR) subunits including NR1, NR2A, and NR2B. NR2A-containing NMDARs are enriched in the synapse (synaptic NMDARs), whereas NR2B-containing NMDARs are enriched at extrasynaptic sites (extrasynaptic NMDARs). Activation of synaptic NMDARs is neuroprotective. They increase nuclear calcium; activate cAMP-response element binding (CREB), brain-derived neurotrophic factor (BDNF), protein kinase B (PKB), and phosphorylated-JACOB (p-JACOB); and up-regulate antioxidants. In contrast, activation of extrasynaptic NMDARs by glutamate spillover in ischemia has the opposite effect. Extrasynaptic NMDARs increase cytoplasmic calcium; inhibit CREB, PKB, p-JACOB, and BDNF; activate calpain; stimulate death-associated protein kinase; and activate autophagy. Thus it appears that it is the extrasynaptic NMDARs that mediate neuronal death. The other class of excitatory neurotransmitter receptors includes the metabotropic receptors, which are coupled with G proteins and modulate intracellular second messengers such as calcium, cyclic nucleotides, and inositol triphosphate.[87] When activated, the ionotropic glutamate receptors open sodium channels and may also initiate membrane depolarization and spreading depression.[88] With ionotropic receptor activation, rapid excitatory amino acid–mediated calcium accumulation occurs. In the face of ischemia this calcium accumulation is exacerbated by cellular energy failure, which disables the Na^+/K^+-ATPase membrane pump and results in further calcium accumulation.[38] Reestablishment of the energy supply can reverse these changes. Delayed glutamate-related neuronal injury is most likely the result of activation of ionotropic receptors and subsequent calcium influx. Calcium influx causes death of neurons in culture under anoxic conditions or in the presence of glutamate.[38] The intracellular accumulation of calcium (1) activates proteases, lipases, and endonucleases resulting in the breakdown of membrane phospholipids; (2) activates neuronal nitric oxide synthase (nNOS), resulting in nitric oxide (NO) production and, in the presence of superoxide, peroxynitrite formation; (3) damages mitochondria; (4) disrupts nucleic acid sequences; and (5) ultimately mediates cell death via necrosis, apoptosis, or autophagy (see Fig. 68.2). The disturbance of the finely regulated intracellular calcium homeostasis is now recognized as a possible final common pathway of neuronal death.[32,38,77,87] Related to this occurrence, studies suggest that novel approaches targeting calcium-calmodulin (CaM)–dependent protein kinase II (CaMKII) may have promise in protecting against neuronal death.[89] NMDA receptor activation has also been shown to stimulate superoxide anion production, which may contribute to cellular injury.[90] The NMDA and AMPA-receptor subtypes have been suggested to play key roles in ischemic brain injury. The potential implications of these mechanisms in regard to therapeutic manipulation of glutamate receptors, as well as calcium and sodium channels, are discussed later.

Protease Activation

One of the candidates for a critical role in neuronal injury as a result of increases in intracellular calcium concentration is protease activation. Protease activation plays a central role in mediating both necrosis and apoptosis. With regard to necrosis, numerous calcium-dependent enzymes can become activated during ischemia and produce important structural injury to neurons. One class of calcium-dependent proteases, calpains, are cytosolic cysteine proteases that have a homeostatic role in cell cycle regulation, differentiation, cell migration, and signal transduction.[91] After injury, calpain-mediated proteolysis of cytoskeletal proteins as well as activation of protein kinase C and phospholipases can occur.[91] Calpains also proteolyze the major plasma membrane sodium/calcium exchanger in neurons during excitotoxicity, allowing enormous secondary influx of calcium into the cell following extrasynaptic NMDA receptor activation and creating a positive feedback environment.[92] In a model of oxygen-glucose deprivation in neuronal cell culture that mimics transient ischemia, calpains induced mitochondrial release of AIF, which translocates to the nucleus to initiate caspase-independent apoptosis.[93]

With regard to apoptosis, the caspase family of cysteine proteases plays an important role after cerebral ischemia and may have a more prominent role in the developing versus mature mammalian brain.[94,95] After unilateral hypoxic-ischemic brain injury, neonatal rats had increased cytochrome c release and caspase-3 activation versus juvenile and adult rats.[67] Regulation of apoptotic machinery also appears to be sex dependent after neonatal hypoxic-ischemic brain injury.[96] Comparatively, female rats had more caspase-mediated apoptosis, whereas male rats had more caspase-independent, AIF-mediated apoptosis.

Oxygen Radical Formation

Toxic oxygen radical species produced during postischemic reperfusion have been implicated as important contributors to reperfusion injury and delayed cell death.[79] The primary species of interest include superoxide anion, hydrogen peroxide, hydroxyl radical, and the reactive nitrogen species peroxynitrite. Very high, pathologic levels of free radical generation occur in brain early in reperfusion with resolution within the first hour.[97-99]

The potential sources of oxygen radicals are many. Two major sources of reactive oxygen species upon reperfusion include electron transport chain components and other proteins such as alpha-ketoglutarate dehydrogenase[100] in mitochondria and NADPH oxidase in the cytosol.[101] Superoxide anion is produced by the electron transport chain during normal mitochondrial respiration. Mitochondrial dysfunction, as may occur under conditions of ischemia, increases the generation of free radicals that may extend beyond the capacity of endogenous antioxidants leading to oxidative stress. Studies have revealed that oxidative stress linked to mitochondria after cardiac arrest and TBI is a highly orchestrated and seminal event in the evolution of oxidative damage, and that the process involves oxidation of the unique mitochondrial lipid cardiolipin by cytochrome c in the inner mitochondrial membrane via a calcium independent pathway.[102,103] Inhibition of this pathway with mitochondrial-targeted nitroxides has been shown to block this pathway and improve outcome specifically in preclinical models of asphyxial cardiac arrest.[103] Studies show that several NADPH oxidase isoforms (Nox1, Nox2, and Nox4) capable of generating significant amounts of superoxide and its dismutation product hydrogen peroxide are expressed in endothelium, neurons, glia, and microglia.[104] Superoxide generation upon stimulation of NMDA receptor can be blocked by the NADPH oxidase inhibitor apocynin and in neurons lacking the p47 (phox) subunit, which is required for NADPH oxidase assembly.[101]

Other sources of reactive oxygen species upon reperfusion may include (1) the cyclooxygenase, lipoxygenase, and cytochrome P-450 pathways, where metabolism of arachidonic may produce superoxide anion as an enzymatic byproduct[79,105]; (2) the xanthine oxidase (XO)[106,107] pathway (however, the importance of XO in contribution to the generation of free radicals in human beings remains unclear)[108,109]; (3) autoxidation of circulating catecholamines or of neurotransmitter catecholamines may represent another potential source of oxygen radicals; and (4) delocalized iron, normally transported in the blood tightly bound to transferrin and stored inside the cell bound to ferritin. In ischemic conditions with accompanying acidosis, however, iron may be displaced from its normal binding sites and can catalyze reactions that promote oxygen radical formation.[110,111] Most commonly implicated is the Haber-Weiss/Fenton reaction, whereby the potent hydroxyl radical is produced from superoxide anion and hydrogen peroxide in the presence of free iron. The iron-chelator, deferoxamine, has been shown to reduce neurologic injury after experimental neonatal hypoxia-ischemia[112,113]; and (5) NO is another free radical that contributes to both nitrosative and oxidative stress. NO increases during ischemia via increased NMDA receptor stimulation, mediated by release of excitatory amino acids and subsequent calcium-mediated activation of nNOS.[114] NO in the presence of superoxide produces peroxynitrite.[115] However, NO can also serve as a potent antioxidant,[116] and beneficial effects of local release of NO and nitrosylation reactions may underlie promising effects of new therapies such as nitrite therapy or remote ischemic postconditioning.[117-119] Free radicals have also been associated directly with an increase release of excitatory amino acids and vice versa.[90,120] Not only do they participate in each other's release and formation but they may act synergistically in causing tissue damage.

The brain may be particularly vulnerable to free radical injury for several reasons. One is the high concentration of polyunsaturated fatty acids, especially arachidonic acid. Release of free fatty acids (FFAs) occurs throughout ischemia. On exposure to oxygen radical species, these FFAs are vulnerable to autocatalytic lipid peroxidation.[121] These free-radical–mediated nonspecific lipid peroxidation reactions are likely a minor contributor and more difficult to target therapeutically compared to enzyme-mediated catalytic lipid peroxidation reactions after reperfusion. Cerebrospinal fluid (CSF) has low concentrations of iron-binding proteins; therefore iron released from injured neurons or glia is likely to contribute to these peroxidation reactions. Byproducts of these reactions,

for example, malondialdehyde and conjugated dienes, although nonspecific, have been used as markers of the extent of lipid peroxidation after brain injury (eg, the thiobarbiturate assay). Lipid peroxides accumulate in the selectively vulnerable zones during reperfusion after transient forebrain ischemia.[110,122] The peroxides do not accumulate during the ischemic period itself or in areas that are not reperfused and thus are implicated in reperfusion injury.[123]

Investigators have also detected oxidative damage to brain proteins after reperfusion.[123] Pyruvate dehydrogenase, a key mitochondrial matrix enzyme that converts pyruvate into acetyl-coenzyme A, undergoes oxidative protein modification after ischemia that impairs enzyme activity, possibly contributing to neuronal cell death,[124] and oxidative damage to DNA could also play a role.[125] Developmental and sex differences exist in terms of the degree of oxidative stress and amount and function of antioxidant enzymes after brain injury. In mice, glutathione and catalase activity in brain are higher in adult female versus male mice, and discrepancies become more exaggerated with age.[126] Furthermore, neurons from male rats have less capacity to replenish glutathione levels after cytotoxic stress in vitro and in vivo after asphyxial cardiac arrest.[127]

Membrane Phospholipid Hydrolysis and Mediator Formation

Membrane phospholipids modulate signaling cascades, affecting the development, differentiation, function, and repair of the CNS, functions that become dysregulated with ischemia and oxidative stress.[128] FFAs are released from neuronal membranes during ischemia, and the amount of FFA released is proportional to the duration of ischemia. FFA release continues to change in proportion to duration of ischemia after the completion of energy failure.[129] FFAs are released by two distinct but related processes. First, phosphatidyl inositol is hydrolyzed by phospholipase C with the production of diacylglycerol (DAG) and inositol phosphates.[130,131] Phospholipase C–mediated hydrolysis begins during the initial moments of the ischemic insult and is related to neurotransmitter receptor stimulation. DAG is then hydrolyzed by lipases to FFAs, predominantly arachidonic and stearic acid. Second, other brain glycerophospholipids are hydrolyzed by phospholipase A_2, which is activated by increases in intracellular calcium concentration. The action of FFA release and metabolism is not a generalized process in the neuronal membrane but is concentrated in the synaptic regions and is thus related to excitotoxicity.[132] As previously discussed, oxidized FFAs can also be released from mitochondrial cardiolipin, and this calcium independent pathway, which is mediated by cytochrome c, has been shown to play an important role in preclinical models of pediatric asphyxial cardiac arrest.[103]

The FFAs released then have potential detrimental effects during the postischemic period by multiple mechanisms: (1) arachidonic acid metabolism via the cyclooxygenase pathway may contribute to oxygen radical production during reperfusion[105]; (2) FFAs and DAG directly increase membrane fluidity, inhibit ATPases, increase neurotransmitter release, and uncouple oxidative phosphorylation; (3) enzymatic oxidation of arachidonic acid during reperfusion by cyclooxygenase, lipoxygenase, or cytochrome P-450 produces a large number of bioactive lipids, including prostaglandins, thromboxanes, leukotrienes, and hydroxy fatty acids, many of which have detrimental effects (see Fig. 68.2); and (4) release of lipid mediators from oxidized cardiolipin by phospholipase $A_2\gamma$. Studies suggest that the cytochrome P-450 metabolite

20-hydroxyeicosatetraenoic acid (HETE) may play a role in producing cortical vasoconstriction after cardiac arrest, and inhibitors of the responsible enzyme are being investigated as a possible therapy for cardiac arrest.[133] This pathway also appears to play a role in the development of brain edema after cardiac arrest.

Endogenous Defenses

In response to the complex sequence of pathobiological events that evolve after brain injury, several endogenous neuroprotectants are produced, induced, or activated after ischemia, and their postulated or proved functions improve cell (specifically neuronal) survival in in vivo and in vitro models. The heat shock proteins are one family of candidate neuroprotectants that are highly conserved among biological species and are induced in cells after a variety of stimuli. Thermal stress is the classic example; however, any insult that damages protein structure, including ischemic[134] and TBI,[135] can produce a heat shock protein (Hsp) response. Simon and colleagues[134] showed that after global ischemia the 72 kDa Hsp72 is temporally expressed in a pattern that mirrors the pattern of selective vulnerability in the model, seen first in the CA_1 region of the hippocampus, followed by CA_3, cortex, and thalamus, and finally in the dentate granule cells. Hsp72 is also induced in both gray and white matter of piglets following mild and severe hypoxia.[136] The Hsps have generated major interest as potential neuroprotectants because their prior induction by a sublethal stress can afford protection from subsequent injury. Transient, subthreshold whole-body hyperthermia reduces subsequent ischemic brain injury in both adult[137] and neonatal rats.[138] Furthermore, exogenous Hsp72 reduces glutamate toxicity in neuronal cell cultures.[139] Importantly, overexpression of Hsp72 reduces ischemic damage and apoptosis after experimental stroke and global ischemia in vivo.[140-142]

Another potential mechanism for endogenous neuroprotection is the up-regulation of genes that inhibit apoptosis and augment neurogenesis. The mammalian gene bcl-2, a proto-oncogene, can block apoptosis[143] and perhaps necrosis as well.[144] The bcl-2 gene is expressed in neurons surviving both focal and global ischemia[145,146] and is reduced in degenerating neurons after cardiac arrest in rats.[147] Viral transfection of bcl-2 reduces infarction after focal ischemia,[148] and up-regulation of bcl-2 via ceramide administered 30 minutes after hypoxia-ischemia reduced the number of cells with DNA damage in immature rat brain.[149] Forced overexpression of the bcl-2 family member bcl-xL also reduces tissue damage after focal cerebral ischemia in adult rats.[150] After TBI in infants and children, CSF levels of bcl-2 are increased in patients that survive compared with those that die.[151] Finally, bcl-2 overexpression promotes neurogenesis in adult mice with and without ischemic injury.[152]

Adenosine is an endogenous biochemical mediator that may serve a protective role after cerebral ischemia, particularly early after injury. It may be produced from ATP breakdown or via the newly discovered 2,3 cAMP adenosine pathway that has been shown to exist in brain.[153] Adenosine is increased in brain tissue after experimental ischemia[154] and in response to hypoxia,[155] hypotension,[156] and hypoglycemia.[157] The release of adenosine after ischemia could afford neuroprotection by a combination of several mechanisms. When bound to A2-receptors, adenosine is a potent cerebrovasodilator and inhibits platelet activation and neutrophil function.[158] Bound to A1-receptors, adenosine reduces neuronal metabolism and excitatory amino acid release and stabilizes postsynaptic membranes.[158] Thus the beneficial effects of adenosine after cerebral ischemia include improved regional CBF, reduced local oxygen demand, attenuation of both excitotoxicity and calcium accumulation, and antiinflammatory and rheologic effects. Finally, adenosine agonists have been shown to improve survival of selectively vulnerable neurons after ischemia in many studies (reviewed in Rudolphi and coworkers[159]).

Clinical Pathophysiology

Cerebral Blood Flow and Metabolism After Resuscitation

The pioneering studies in which global CBF and cerebral metabolic rate for oxygen ($CMRO_2$) were measured in animal models of global ischemia or cardiac arrest focused on the early postresuscitation period. In their classic study, Snyder and colleagues[160] showed that after 15 minutes of global brain ischemia in dogs, CBF transiently increased to levels well above baseline (Fig. 68.3). Then, after 15 to 30 minutes, CBF progressively decreased to a level below normal for the remainder of the monitoring period (90 minutes). This pattern of early transient postischemic hyperemia and subsequent delayed postischemic hypoperfusion has been observed in many global cerebral ischemia models, including both VF and asphyxial arrest, although in adult VF there is some suggestion it is less prominent.[83,161-163] The levels of hyperemia and subsequent hypoperfusion vary in relation to the duration of the insult.[164] Although these phases of increased and decreased CBF characterize the net global effect, regional CBF is often inhomogeneous, particularly during postischemic hypoperfusion, when areas of decreased and increased perfusion may coexist.[165] The ability of antioxidants to blunt reperfusion hyperemia suggests it may be the result of oxidative signaling involving the neurovascular bundle.[99,161]

The heterogeneous- and duration-dependent nature of postarrest CBF was characterized using contemporary imaging techniques allowing for regional assessment and a clinically relevant model of pediatric asphyxial cardiac arrest.[166] Using arterial spin labeling magnetic resonance imaging (MRI), CBF was measured for the first 3 hours after 8.5, 9, or 12 minutes of asphyxial cardiac arrest in postnatal day 17 rats—approximating a 1- to 4-year-old human in terms of brain development (refer to Chapter 60). Although the pattern of early global hyperemia followed by hypoperfusion similar to that observed by Snyder and associates[160] was seen after asphyxial arrests lasting 8.5 and 9 minutes, a pattern of global and persistent hypoperfusion was observed after a 12-minute arrest (Fig. 68.4). Remarkably, CBF disturbances were also found to be region dependent after asphyxial arrests lasting 8.5 and 9 minutes, with subcortical hyperemia but cortical hypoperfusion (see Fig. 68.4). After a 12-minute asphyxial arrest, hypoperfusion was observed in both cortical and subcortical regions, and CBF was pressure-passive with epinephrine infusion, perhaps indicating loss of autoregulation after a prolonged arrest. This is consistent with descriptions of increased loss of neurovascular coupling with longer global ischemic durations.[167] In the same model using a 9-minute asphyxial arrest duration, intravenous (IV) infusion with polynitroxyl albumin, an antioxidant, during resuscitation decreased early (5-minute) hyperemia whereas albumin augmented and prolonged hyperemia. Both interventions led to

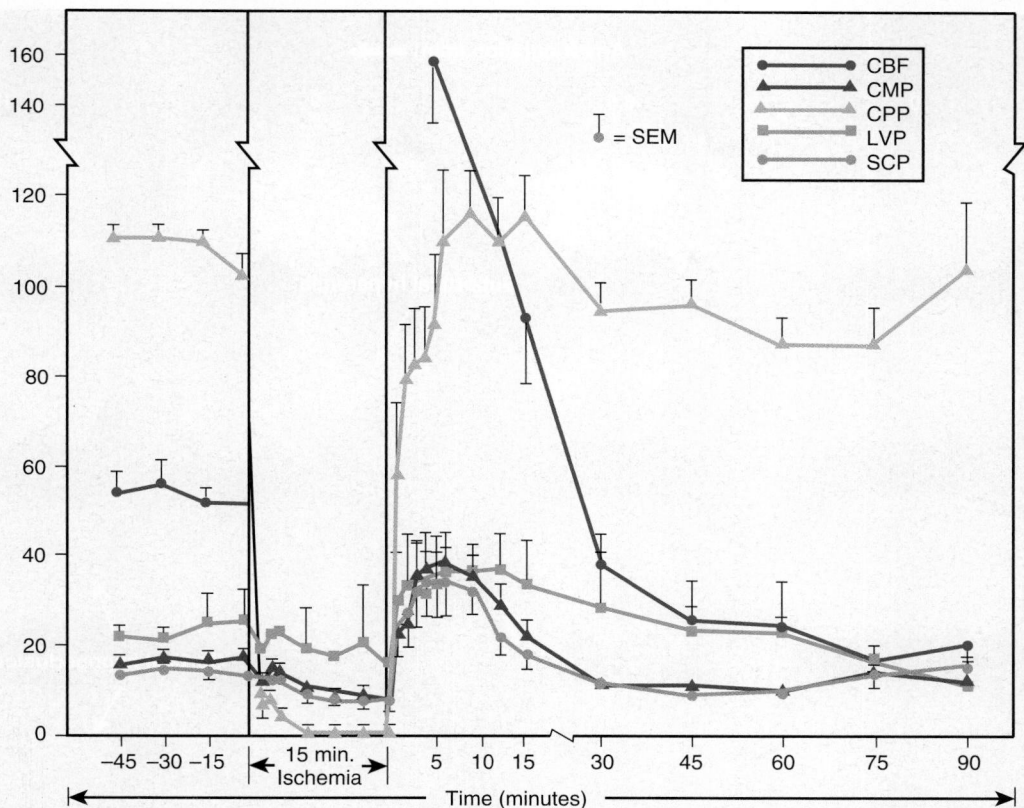

Fig. 68.3. Global cerebral blood flow *(CBF)*, cisterna magna pressure *(CMP)*, cerebral perfusion pressure *(CPP)*, lateral ventricular pressure *(LVP)*, and supracortical pressure *(SCP)* measured before, during, and for 90 minutes after a 15-minute circulatory arrest in dogs. CBF data demonstrate that early postresuscitation hyperemia occurs, followed by hypoperfusion. (Adapted from Snyder JV, Nemoto EM, Carroll RG, Safar P. Global ischemia in dogs: intracranial pressures, brain blood flow and metabolism. Stroke. 1975;6:21-27.)

improved spatial memory performance in male rats only.[82] The optimal CBF target postresuscitation is not known and may be brain region and time dependent.

Invasive measurement of brain tissue oxygenation (PbtO$_2$) is a marker of local oxygen extraction fraction and surrogate marker of CBF. In the rat pediatric asphyxial cardiac arrest model, postresuscitation cortical PbtO$_2$ values decreased below baseline by 30 minutes and remained low at 2 hours. In contrast, significant hyperoxia was observed in the thalamus 5 minutes after ROSC, decreasing to normal values over 2 hours.[12] Notably, PbtO$_2$ was FiO$_2$ dose responsive in both brain regions. In a swine model of VF arrest, marked hyperoxia is observed in the cortex 15 minutes after ROSC using an FiO$_2$ of 1 and 1 hour after ROSC with reduced FiO2 to 0.5 (PbO$_2$ > 3× and 2× baseline, respectively).[168] It is unclear whether differences in postresuscitation PbO$_2$ seen in these two studies are related to differences between asphyxia and VF arrest, species, developmental age, injury severity, or any combination of these factors.

In patients with good outcomes, global CBF recovers over the subsequent 24 to 72 hours and CO$_2$ reactivity remains intact. Patients who do not regain consciousness or progress to brain death develop absolute or relative CBF hyperemia with impaired CO$_2$ reactivity.[169,170] A theoretic scheme of postarrest global CBF and its relation to neurologic outcome is presented in Fig. 68.5. Most studies in experimental animal models of asphyxial arrest suggest a similar pattern of CBF and CMRO$_2$ to that observed after VF cardiac arrest and global ischemia in the early postresuscitation period in humans.[162,169] However, there are some exceptions.[171] Results from clinical studies of pediatric asphyxial arrest are scarce and somewhat conflicting with regard to the prognostic implications of high or low values of postarrest CBF based on a single measurement; however, loss of CO$_2$ reactivity appears to be associated with poor outcome in all studies. In studies of children between 24 and 48 hours after near-drowning, Ashwal and colleagues[172] observed low CBF in the seven nonsurvivors and no relationship between CBF and PaCO$_2$ in these patients—again suggesting loss of CBF reactivity to changes in PaCO$_2$. In this study, hyperemia was not routinely observed in either survivors in a persistent vegetative state or children who died, but only a single CBF measurement was made in these patients. Beyda[173] obtained serial measurements of postarrest [133]Xenon in a series of children who suffered asphyxial arrest from submersion accidents. Children with good neurologic outcomes had slightly decreased CBF values at 12 hours that increased to normal during the subsequent 24 to 60 hours. In these children, CBF reactivity to CO$_2$ was intact. Children with eventual vegetative outcome or brain death exhibited hyperemia with loss or attenuation of CO$_2$ reactivity. This hyperemia progressed to low or normal flow over the following 12 to 72 hours in children with vegetative outcome and

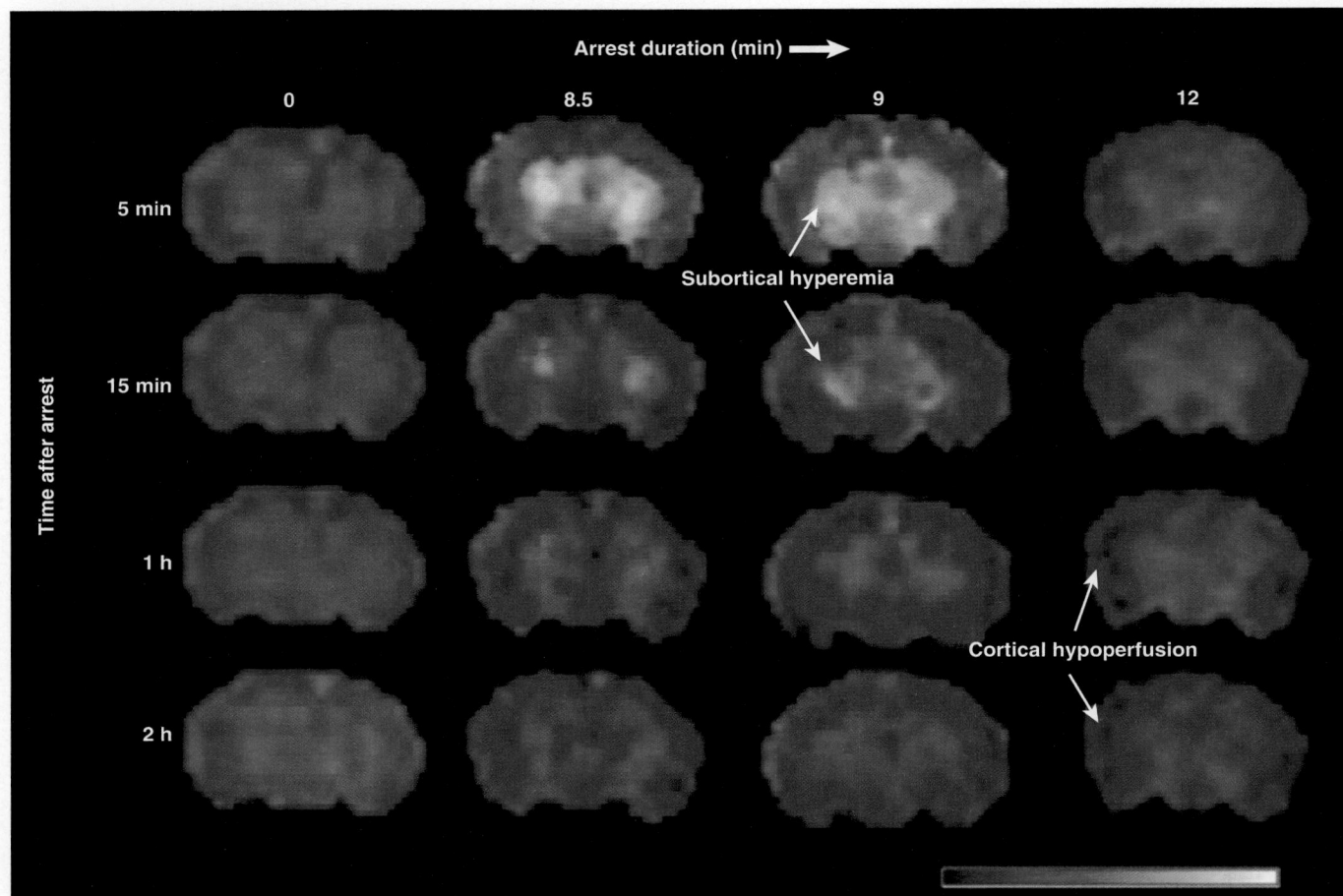

Fig. 68.4. Duration and regional dependency of cerebral blood flow (*CBF*) disturbances acutely after asphyxial cardiac arrest in postnatal day 17 rats. CBF data demonstrate that early postresuscitation hyperemia occurs in subcortical regions after an 8.5- and 9-minute but not a 12-minute asphyxial cardiac arrest and that duration-dependent hypoperfusion occurs in cortical regions. (Adapted from Manole MD, Foley LM, Hitchens TK, et al. Magnetic resonance imaging assessment of regional cerebral blood flow after asphyxial cardiac arrest in immature rats. J Cereb Blood Flow Metab. 2009;29:197-205.)

progressed to low and then no flow with the development of brain death. A pilot pediatric study found that time spent under the optimal mean arterial pressure range where autoregulation was present, based on an infrared cerebral oximetry-arterial pressure–based system, was predictive of poor outcomes.[174] Arterial spin labeling MRI techniques have been developed that do not require contrast material injections. In a small study that included both adults and children, global hyperemia was demonstrated after cardiac arrest at varying time points.[175] In neonates with HIE, hyperperfusion occurred in regions with concurrent water diffusion abnormalities, implying a potential pathophysiologic linkage between the two observations, but patient outcomes were not reported.[176]

Brain metabolism, as assessed by $CMRO_2$, is reduced during the early postischemic period and then progressively recovers to a level that varies, depending on the model used and on the duration of ischemia.[164,177] In some models, including VF arrest in dogs, significant recovery of $CMRO_2$ may occur during the first few hours, despite persistent postischemic hypoperfusion—creating the potential for a secondary ischemic insult during reperfusion. Whether this increase in $CMRO_2$ represents appropriate synaptic activity, seizures, or basal metabolism is not certain. In other models and in descriptions of adult cardiac arrest, global CBF and $CMRO_2$ were matched during the first few hours after ischemia with delayed relative global hyperperfusion.[169]

Cerebral microdialysis has been used in pilot studies to assess for alterations in metabolism after cardiac arrest. Using microdialysis in a porcine model of cardiac arrest, increased lactate/pyruvate ratios were found during arrest and again in a delayed fashion especially if kept normothermic versus hypothermic.[178] This same group found increased lactate/pyruvate ratios and glutamate using microdialysis in adult survivors after cardiac arrest, all of whom were treated with hypothermia.[179] Prolonged increases in brain lactate detected using proton MRS after global hypoxia-ischemia in children have also been reported.[35,180,181] Oxidative stress decreases the function of the pyruvate dehydrogenase complex, a key enzyme in oxidative metabolism, possibly contributing to the shift to anaerobic metabolism.[182] Although routine monitoring of CBF, CMR, or $PbtO_2$ has not been applied extensively to the postarrest setting in children, their routine assessment using contemporary methods may possibly lead to an improved understanding of pathophysiology.

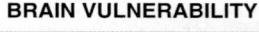

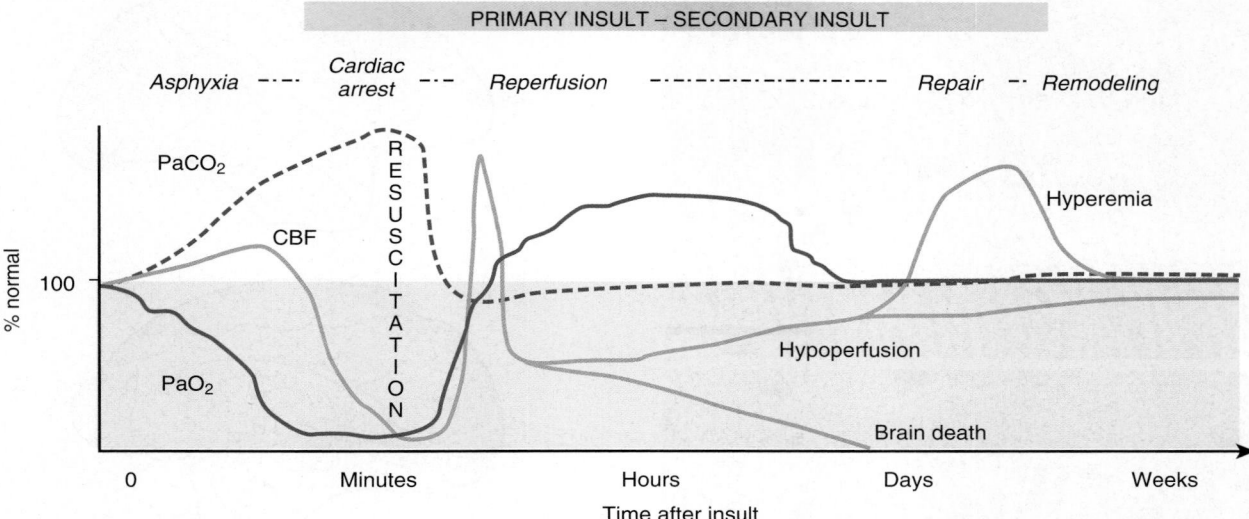

Fig. 68.5. Hypothetical diagram illustrating the patterns of *global* cerebral blood flow *(CBF)* during and after cardiac arrest of moderate duration in humans. Immediately after resuscitation, "early postischemic hyperemia" occurs for about 15 minutes in subcortical brain regions. This is followed by patchy multifocal "delayed postischemic hypoperfusion" in cortical brain regions lasting from a few hours to days. Progressive return of CBF to normal is seen in patients with intact neurologic outcome. In contrast, "delayed postischemic hyperemia" can be observed hours to days postarrest in patients with more severe insults.[170,173] This delayed hyperemia appears to be associated with disabled or vegetative outcome (where CBF gradually decreases to near normal or below normal) or brain death (where CBF decreases to no flow). It is unclear, however, if all patients with vegetative outcome or eventual brain death develop delayed hyperemia.

Drugs such as nimodipine can increase CBF during the early postischemic hypoperfusion phase after global cerebral ischemia, though outcomes were not affected.[183] $CMRO_2$ recovery generally is not affected by treatment.[184] The testing of strategies targeting early postarrest hypoperfusion deserves further study. Safar and coworkers[185] have reported that a multifaceted treatment strategy to increase CBF ("flow promotion") and reduce CMR or $CMRO_2$ early after VF in dogs improved outcome. This was accomplished by use of cardiac bypass (CPB), mild hypothermia, hemodilution, and transient hypertension. However, more selective therapies may be needed, and potential agents targeting CBF currently being explored, as previously stated, include nitrite, remote ischemic postconditioning, and 20-HETE inhibitors, among others.

An important limitation in all existing studies on CBF/ $CMRO_2$ is that the spatial resolution of the techniques used (positron emission tomography [PET], Xe CT, MRI) permits examination of regional CBF heterogeneity but does not resolve to the level of the microcirculation. At this level, studies using two photon microscopy have yielded important findings. First, a microvascular no-reflow phenomenon may be present on the basis of pericyte contraction, with ischemia and cell death that is not amenable to increasing cerebral perfusion pressure.[186] Second, microvascular shunts at the level of small arterioles may redirect blood flow toward or away from capillary beds with either beneficial or detrimental effects on microcirculatory flow, respectively.[187] The implication of these findings is that cerebral perfusion pressure though adequate as a measure of global CBF may not provide adequate perfusion on the microcirculatory level due to these issues. At present the only clinically useful method to detect such disturbance would be microdialysis, which is limited to only a small area of tissue interrogation.

Histopathology of Hypoxic-Ischemic Encephalopathy

Ischemic neuronal change (Fig. 68.6), as first described by Sommer in 1880 and later by Spielmeyer, involves a progression from extensive cellular microvacuolation to a cell that resembles a naked shrunken nucleus.[25] As described by Brierley and colleagues,[44] "this type of neuronal damage is neither ubiquitous nor randomly distributed but is found in regions which exhibit selective vulnerability to hypoxic stress." As discussed previously, death of selectively vulnerable neurons (eg, hippocampal CA_1) cannot be explained by vascular distribution. Remarkably, these clinical descriptions of cell shrinkage were consistent with apoptosis rather than necrosis. However, the connection between selective vulnerability and apoptosis was made 100 years later.[56] Neuronal death after cardiac arrest is seen not only in the selectively vulnerable neurons but also as a subtle histopathologic finding in the arterial boundary zones. These neurons (not otherwise selectively vulnerable) are in the most poorly perfused areas during or after resuscitation.[41] Neuronal death in the arterial boundary zones was elegantly described by Nemoto and associates in a monkey model of 16 minutes of complete global brain ischemia followed by 7 days of intensive care.[188] Maximal damage appeared to be in the classically described selectively vulnerable zones, but neuronal death was also observed in the most distal distribution of the posterior cerebral artery and in the watershed zones of the anterior and middle cerebral arteries (Fig. 68.7). With sufficient injury in the arterial boundary zone, more severe findings such as microinfarction or laminar necrosis can be seen.[26,188] As previously discussed, even in stroke, neuronal death in an ischemic penumbra can occur either by necrosis or apoptosis. Thus it appears that there may be a continuum between apoptosis and necrosis that may depend on a large number of factors, such as duration of the insult

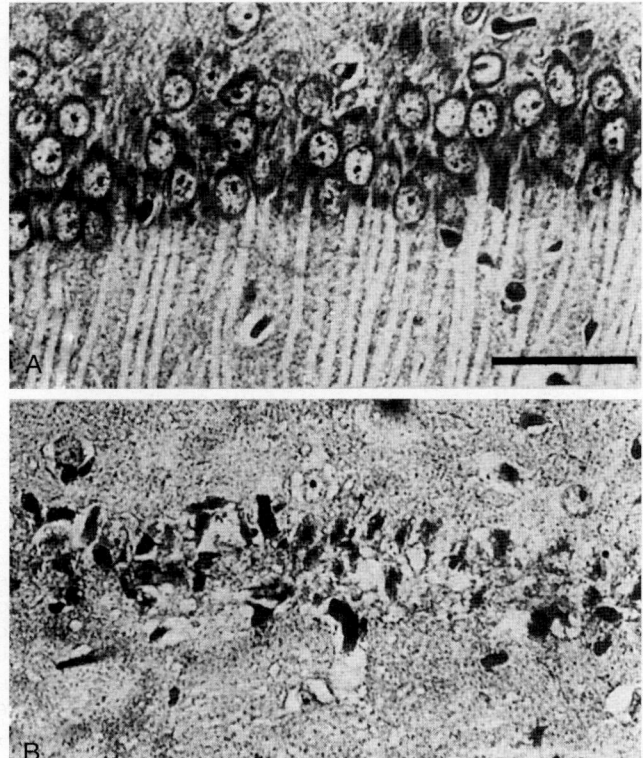

Fig. 68.6. Light micrograph of dorsal hippocampus in gerbils 7 days after 5 minutes of sham ischemia (A) or global ischemia by carotid occlusion (B). Ischemic neuronal change is seen with CA_1 neurons appearing as dark, shrunken nuclei without cytoplasm (B) by contrast with the normal-appearing nonischemic neurons (A). Investigations by Nitatori and colleagues[56] indicate that neuronal death in selective areas, after threshold ischemia insults, occurs via apoptosis. (From Kuroiwa T, Bonnekoh P, Hossmann KA. Therapeutic window of CA1 neuronal damage defined by an ultrashort-acting barbiturate after brain ischemia in gerbils. Stroke. 1990;21:1489-1493.)

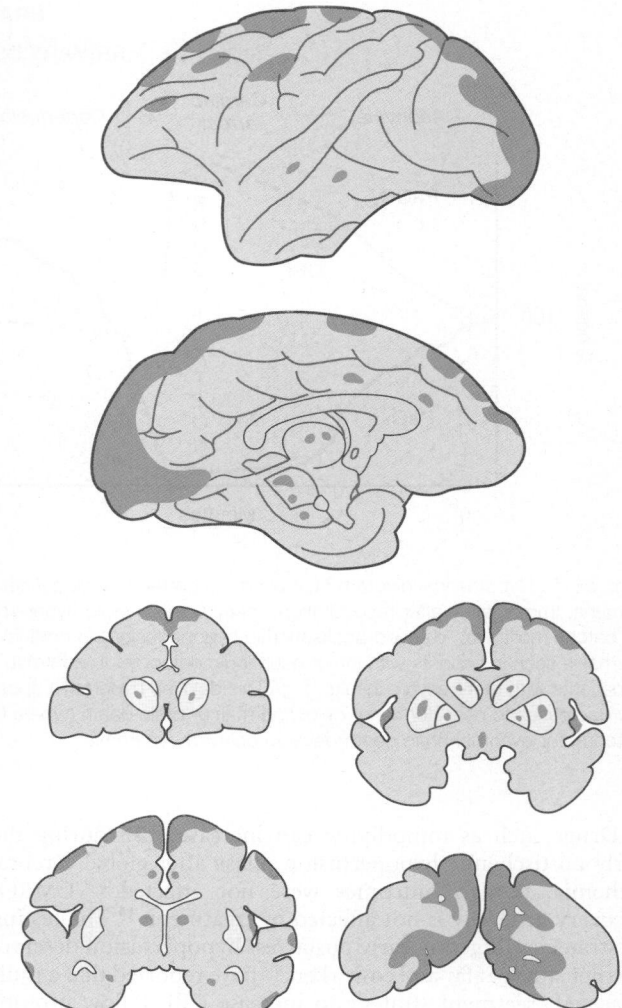

Fig. 68.7. Topographic distribution of cortical lesions 7 days after 16 minutes of global brain ischemia in rhesus monkeys. Neuronal death in areas with intrinsic selective vulnerability was most apparent in the distal distribution of the posterior cerebral artery. Damage in the watershed distributions of the anterior and middle cerebral arteries was less consistent. (Adapted from Nemoto EM, Bleyaert AL, Stezoski SW, Moossy J, Rao GR, Safar P. Global brain ischemia: a reproducible monkey model. Stroke. 1977;8:558-564.)

and brain region in question.[73] Whereas apoptosis in a given area often affects only a select percentage of neurons, infarction affects all neurons and glia. Obviously, if the arrest time is long or if the postischemic conditions are sufficiently poor, infarction of the entire brain can occur.

Vaagenes and colleagues studied neuropathology after primary VF arrest of 10 minutes in dogs.[26] Despite vegetative outcome at 96 hours, only scattered ischemic neuronal changes in the selectively vulnerable neurons and to a much lesser extent in the vascular watersheds were observed. Microinfarct formation was seen in only 5 of 18 dogs, suggesting that patchy ischemic neuronal change is sufficient for vegetative outcome. They then compared this 10-minute VF arrest with an asphyxial episode (airway occlusion) resulting in cardiac arrest with 7 minutes of no flow. Related either to differences in the initial insult or to postischemic events, asphyxial arrest resulted not only in ischemic neuronal change in the selectively vulnerable regions but also in marked microinfarct formation (30 of 32 dogs) and scattered petechial hemorrhages. This more severe histologic injury was seen despite significantly *easier* ROSC in the asphyxial arrest group (Fig. 68.8). In addition, unlike VF arrest, asphyxial arrest caused some ischemic neuronal changes even after no flow of only 2

minutes. These findings may explain the poor outcome generally observed in cardiac arrest in children (usually asphyxial arrest) compared with that in adult series (VF arrest). After asphyxial cardiac arrest that results in long-term survival in both adult and pediatric-aged animals,[189-191] the pattern of neuronal death produced is similar to that reported in human studies[192] including that of the young victim of asphyxial cardiac arrest, Karen Ann Quinlan,[193] where a predilection for basal ganglia injury resulting in a persistent vegetative state is observed. Finally, studies by Hogler and associates[194] demonstrated the expansion of damage comparing 7 versus 10 minutes of VF cardiac arrest in pigs. Substantial expansion of neuronal death across multiple brain structures such as cortex, caudate, and cerebellum was seen between the 7- and 10-minute durations, and edema appeared in the 10-minute group. These studies shed additional light on the impact of

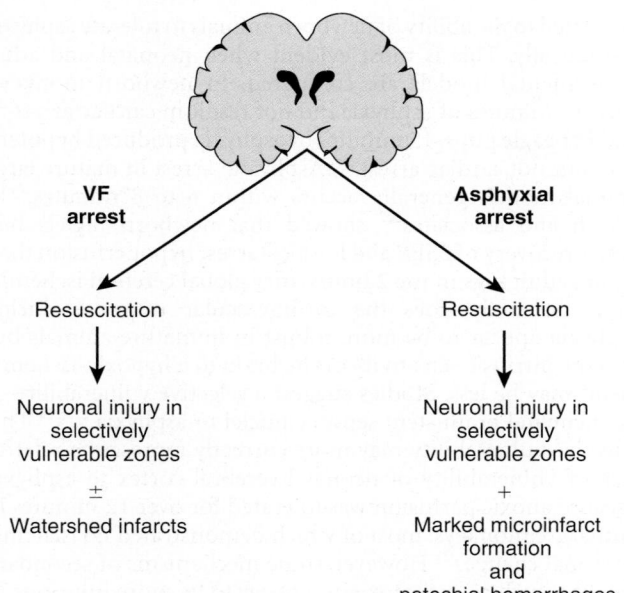

VF arrest

Asphyxial arrest

Resuscitation

Resuscitation

Neuronal injury in selectively vulnerable zones

Neuronal injury in selectively vulnerable zones

±

+

Watershed infarcts

Marked microinfarct formation
and
petechial hemorrhages

Fig. 68.8. Schematic diagram based on the work of Vaagenes and colleagues[26] comparing the histologic outcome of VF cardiac (adult) and asphyxial (pediatric) arrest. (From Kochanek PM. Novel pharmacologic approaches to brain resuscitation after cardiorespiratory arrest in the pediatric patient. In Holbrook P, ed. Critical Care Clinics. Philadelphia: W.B. Saunders; 1988:661-777.)

cardiac arrest duration on the extent of neuronal damage, given the challenges of defining arrest duration in the human condition.

Clinical Outcome After Pediatric Cardiac Arrest

Survival and neurologic outcome after cardiac arrest in infants and children are remarkably poor.[8] One review summarizing the results from 44 studies totaling 3094 pediatric patients after cardiac arrest showed survival at hospital discharge in only 13% of patients, 8% for out-of-hospital and 24% for in-hospital cardiac arrest, respectively.[19] Survival to hospital discharge after out-of-hospital arrest ranges from 8% to 25% and after in-patient arrest is 24% to 51% in several studies, with an overall survival of 13%.[9,15,16,19,22] However, if the child had a pulse by hospital arrival after out-of-hospital cardiac arrest, survival increases to 38%.[9] The most common cause of death is neurologic injury for out-of-hospital arrests and cardiovascular failure for in-hospital arrests.[9] Although survival to hospital discharge is higher in pediatric than adult cardiac arrest, the proportion of patients with good neurologic outcomes is lower, which may reflect in part lesser limitations of life-sustaining therapies in children compared to adults.[22] Good neurologic outcome in pediatric patients surviving cardiac arrest is often overestimated using traditional categorical outcome measures such as the Glasgow Outcome Scale score and Pediatric Cerebral Performance Category Scale.[195-197] Furthermore, contemporary longer-term outcome studies evaluating overall functional status, neuropsychologic function, and quality of life do not exist. One observational study focusing on late improvements in functional outcome noted improved mobility in 22% of children after cardiac arrest versus 66% of children after TBI 2 years after the initial event.[198]

High mortality and poor outcome after cardiac arrest in children generally represent out-of-hospital or unwitnessed cardiac arrests. The outcomes are worst in infants and preschool children where the proportion of witnessed arrests, bystander CPR, and nonasphyxial arrests are the lowest.[23,199] Recovery is much better in children who had witnessed arrests, cold water submersion, or isolated respiratory arrest, after which intact survival rates as high as 44% to 75% have been reported.[9,18,200-202] Nevertheless, these clinical data seem to bear out the severe neuropathology observed in asphyxia-induced arrest in animal models because asphyxial arrest is the most common mode of arrest in all of the clinical pediatric series.[18,19,195,200-202]

Clinical factors such as initial pH, number of epinephrine doses, and arrest duration have been examined in an attempt to prognosticate outcome from cardiac arrest. Although sometimes predictive, this information can be misleading. For example, the time delay before analysis of the first blood sample can vary, as can estimates of arrest duration. With asphyxial arrest, even controlled experimental animal studies show that the time from asphyxia until cardiac arrest varies considerably. Currently, the most powerful individual predictor of neurologic outcome after cardiac arrest is the neurologic examination.[203] As noted in one review, abnormal pupillary reactivity and motor response after 24 hours postcardiac arrest in the absence of sedation and muscle relaxation medications are useful for prognostication.[204]

The electroencephalogram (EEG) can also provide prognostic information for patients after cardiac arrest. Scollo-Lavizzari and Bassetti[205] retrospectively examined the relation between first postarrest EEG and clinical outcome in 408 cases. A five-grade classification was used to categorize EEGs. Although permanent severe neurologic damage was observed in some patients with grade I EEG, none of the 208 patients with grade IV or V EEGs had a good neurologic recovery. A single-center retrospective case series in children showed that having a burst suppression or electrocerebral silence pattern was associated with poor outcome at hospital discharge, with a positive predictive value of 90% and negative predictive value of 91%.[206] In children who underwent hypothermia postarrest, seizures were common, largely nonconvulsive, and occurred most frequently during the rewarming period.[207] Detailed quantitative EEG may also have a role in the prediction of neurologic outcome after cardiac arrest.[208] EEG reactivity may be an important prognostic tool after cardiac arrest in children.[209]

Adjunctive prognostic information also can be derived from brain-derived protein levels in serum or CSF. Serum brain biomarker trajectories, including S100b (from astrocytes), neuron specific enolase (NSE, from neurons), and myelin basic protein (MBP, from myelin), were noted to differ by brain insult.[210] Biomarker levels peaked earlier after accidental TBI, later after hypoxia, and were in-between for children with abusive head trauma. Two single-center prospective studies in children with cardiac arrest found that serum S100b and NSE had excellent prognostication accuracy.[211,212] NSE and other biomarkers may be useful in determining responsiveness to therapeutic interventions—that is, it has been reported that decreasing serum NSE occurs mainly in hypothermic (versus normothermic) adults after cardiac arrest and is predictive of outcome.[213]

Studies have used somatosensory-evoked potentials (SSEPs) in an attempt to provide early prognostic information about outcome after cardiac arrest resuscitation. Madl and colleagues tested median nerve SSEP in 66 adults after successful resuscitation from cardiac arrest. They reported that the presence or absence and the latency of the cortical N70 peak reliably differentiated between bad and favorable outcome with 100% predictive ability.[214] Testing was performed within 48 hours of resuscitation, which is a clinically relevant time frame. Auditory-evoked response testing has been used in children with cardiac arrest after a submersion accident.[215] Normal evoked responses were observed in all children who recovered neurologically intact. Children who recovered with significant handicaps demonstrated a reduction in wave V amplitude over time and prolonged wave I-V interpeak latencies. In adults, bilaterally absent N20 waves at 24 and 48 hours have a reported specificity of 100% in predicting poor outcome after cardiac arrest, but note that in many studies the SSEP results were used to guide medical decision making.[216] Summary recommendations from Abend and coworkers have suggested that the absence of bilateral cortical SSEPs are most reliably predictive of outcome when peripheral SSEP responses are present.[203]

The prospective utility of computed tomography (CT) of the head and other neuroimaging modalities after cardiac arrest is unknown (Fig. 68.9). Head CT takes only a few minutes and is useful for ruling out intracranial lesions contributing to the cause of arrest. In a large retrospective case series of children with near-drowning experiences, children with any abnormal CT finding (eg, loss of gray-white differentiation, infarction) within the first 24 hours of admission died.[217] Ninety-six percent of children with an initially normal CT on the first day who had a subsequent abnormal CT either died or remained in a coma. A new single-center retrospective study in children with cardiac arrest and brain CT within 24 hours found that loss of gray-white differentiation and basilar cistern effacement were associated with unfavorable outcomes.[218]

Brain MRI can provide excellent regional evidence of brain injury after cardiac arrest without radiation, but it requires long transports outside of the ICU. It is typically employed for prognostication subacutely after the patient stabilizes, but findings evolve over time. In one study that utilized a novel scoring system, damage seen in the cortex and basal ganglia correlated well with neurologic outcome.[219] Cortical lobe abnormalities in diffusion-weighted imaging and injury to the basal ganglia on conventional MRI were predictive of unfavorable outcome after pediatric cardiac arrest.[220] Using brain MRS, decreases in the brain metabolite N-acetylaspartate and increases in lactate in the basal ganglia and cortex can assist in outcome determination in children after near drowning and cardiac arrest.[180,221,222]

However, no one test or clinical variable will have sufficient accuracy to prognosticate on its own. Combining clinical variables with testing results improves accuracy of outcome prediction.[223,224] Development and prospective validation of tests and panels of tests obtained early after cardiac arrest, that reliably predict ultimate outcome, would be valuable.

Response of the Immature Brain to Cardiac Arrest

Clinical and laboratory studies suggest that the neurologic outcome of newborn animals after a hypoxic-ischemic insult is favorable compared with that of adults, although this may be related to the ability of newborn animals to tolerate asphyxia systemically. This is most evident when neonatal and adult experimental models are compared. In newborn monkeys, even 12 minutes of asphyxia did not result in cardiac arrest,[225] and in beagle pups, 15 minutes of asphyxia produced hypotension but not cardiac arrest.[226] Asphyxial arrest in mature large animal models generally occurs within 6 to 8 minutes.[26,161] Kirsch and associates[227] showed that newborn piglets had better recovery of SSEP and less postarrest hypoperfusion than young adult pigs in the 2 hours after global cerebral ischemia. Thus not only does the cardiovascular response during asphyxia appear to be more robust in immature animals but also the intrinsic sensitivity of the brain to a hypoxic-ischemic insult may be less. Studies suggest a selective vulnerability of the neonatal brain stem sensory nuclei to asphyxia.[225,228] This selective vulnerability may more correctly represent a relative lack of vulnerability of neonatal cerebral cortex to asphyxia because anoxic perfusion was tolerated for over 12 minutes in immature monkeys, most of which demonstrated no ischemic neuronal change.[225] However, some mechanisms of secondary damage, such as excitotoxicity, appear to be more injurious in the immature.[229,230] Further complexity is added to processes such as excitoxicity when the immature brain is involved, as some degree of excitatory stimulation is essential for neuronal survival and normal development.[231] That fact may underscore the recognized vulnerability of developing neurons to sustained (6–8 hours or longer) exposure to certain anesthetics—a process that occurs in developing primates.[232] Finally, greater plasticity in the immature brain may also allow for improved long-term recovery of function, although this may be more important in focal insults.[233,234]

The poor clinical outcome of infants and children presenting in cardiac arrest is probably more related to specific mechanisms operating in the special setting of the asphyxial arrest. As the asphyxial arrest is developing, cardiac standstill is preceded by a variable period of severe hypoxia with increased CBF. During this period, severely hypoxic perfusion, a form of incomplete ischemia is produced, which can markedly increase cerebral lactate production.[235] The initial phase of asphyxia can also be accompanied by extreme stress during struggling, which could increase $CMRO_2$ and may be accompanied by systemic hyperglycemia.[172] The combination of hypoxic perfusion or incomplete hypoxia-ischemia and hyperglycemia can increase cerebral lactate concentration to 30 to 35 µmol/g and decrease tissue pH to levels as low as 6.05.[236-238] These lactate levels are much higher than those observed during even 30 minutes of complete ischemia (11 to 14 µmol/g) and are above the threshold of 20 to 25 µmol/g, at which lactic acid can produce local coagulation necrosis.[239] In addition, it has been shown that a veritable storm of neurotransmitters is released to extremely high levels during the asphyxiation prior to reperfusion.[21] Thus the no-flow period in asphyxial cardiac arrest—in contrast to VF—is occurring in a brain that is already in a severely biochemically compromised state. As suggested by the histopathologic outcome studies previously discussed,[26] cardiac arrest or reperfusion may be particularly devastating to the brain in this milieu. Also, because of the relative resistance of the immature myocardium to asphyxia, it is easier to restore cardiovascular function in younger patients after longer durations of cardiac arrest than would be possible in adults. Total insult time (hypoxia plus anoxia plus cardiac arrest) is often very long. In adults with asystole or a

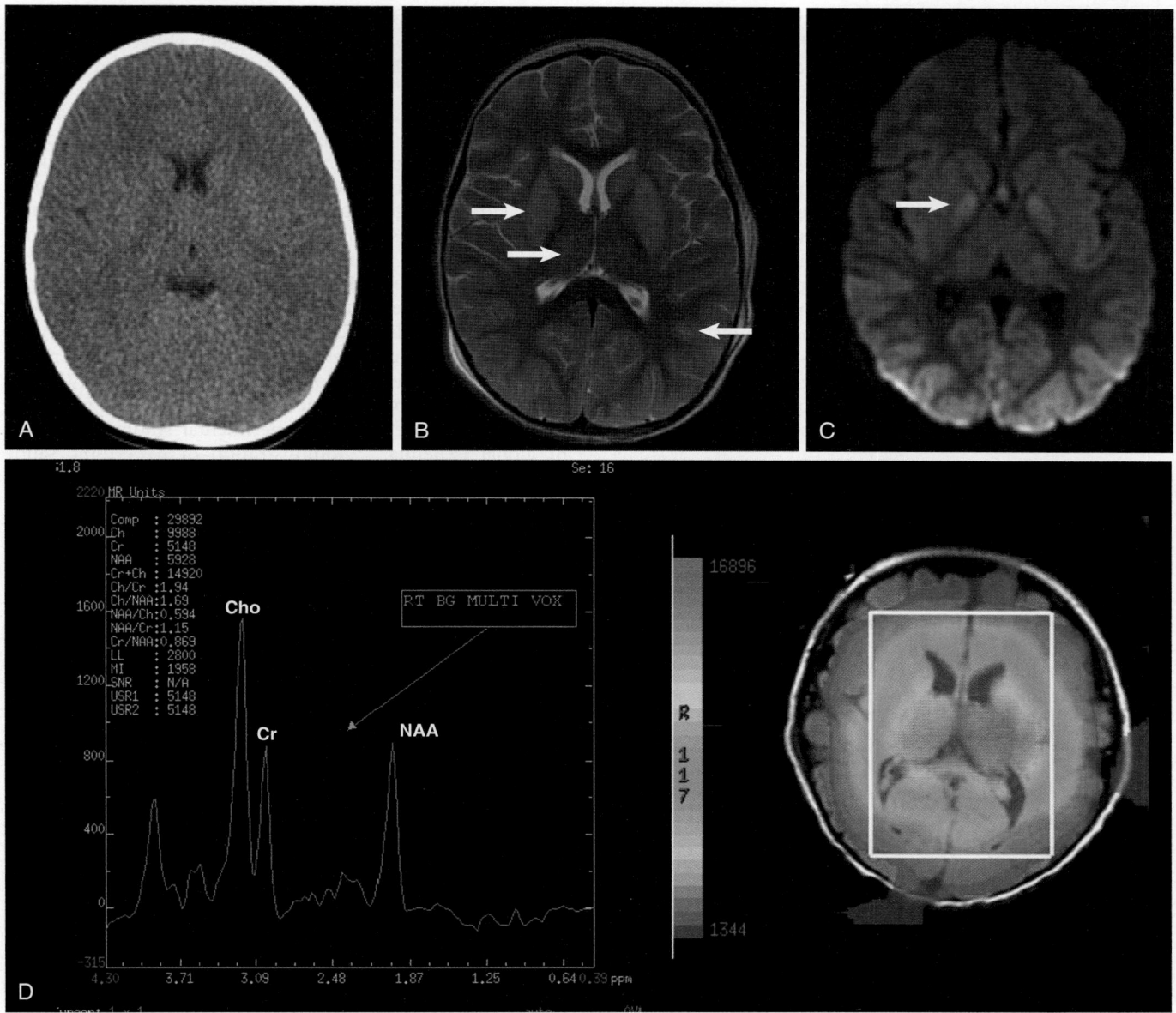

Fig. 68.9. Neuroimaging after asphyxial cardiac arrest in children. (A) Computerized tomography scan of the head on day 1 showing decreased gray-white differentiation, consistent with cerebral edema. (B) T2-weighted magnetic resonance image using a 3-Tesla magnet on day 10 showing enhancement of the basal ganglia, thalamus, and parietal lobes *(arrows)*. (C) Diffusion-weighted imaging shows corresponding edema of the globus pallidus *(arrow)*. (D) Multivoxel magnetic resonance spectroscopy showing the whole brain chemical analysis of *N*-acetylaspartate *(NAA)*, choline *(Cho)*, and Creatine *(Cr)*. A regional color map for NAA is provided.

pulseless bradycardia rather than VF, outcome is also poor.[240] Thus although pediatric intensivists have the apparent luxury of dealing with a somewhat resistant and more resilient brain, with capacity for plasticity, this advantage is often trivial compared to the devastating pathobiology of the asphyxial arrest.[191,241]

Treatment of Cardiac Arrest

Adequate understanding of the pathobiology of HIE after cardiac arrest in children is possible given the development of contemporary models of pediatric asphyxial arrest. These models will hopefully lead to more etiology-specific evalua-

tion of the postresuscitation syndrome in terms of mechanisms and relevant therapies.[190,191] Prospective study of clinical targets for supportive postresuscitation care to optimize outcomes is vital.

Field Interventions

Pediatric cardiac arrests are usually not sudden in onset as in adults, and thus a window of opportunity exists during which interventions could potentially prevent cardiac arrest and subsequent poor outcome. As discussed, children sustaining isolated respiratory arrest have a mortality rate as low as 25%, whereas patients with cardiac arrests as a result of hypoxemia have a high mortality.[8,19] Thus the sooner the recognition and interventions, the better are the chances for a good outcome. Aside from witnesses with knowledge of CPR or the capacity to follow instructions provided by telephone emergency services, prehospital emergency medical services (EMS) are capable of providing the earliest medical interventions and hold the greatest promise for improving outcome from prehospital pediatric cardiac arrest. Emergency medical services have developed sophisticated methods for dispatch and transport, but there are logistical limits to the rapidity with which they can provide basic interventions. Nationwide the average response time is well over 8 minutes, greater than the time required for an infant to progress from apnea to cardiac arrest. As a result, more advanced, traditionally hospital-based, and investigational interventions must also be administered in the prehospital setting in attempts to optimize outcome. Toward this end, use of medical simulation has greatly improved both the understanding of the mechanics of quality CPR as well as teaching and training (see also Chapters 41 and 42).

Intracranial Pressure Interventions

Controlled experimental or prospective clinical studies of intracranial pressure (ICP) monitoring or treatment after asphyxial arrest have not been performed. It could be predicted that ICP elevation would be more common after asphyxial arrest than after isolated global brain ischemia or VF arrest, given the severe histopathology seen after asphyxial arrest and the long insult times from which the myocardium can recover in children. Sustained elevation of ICP (>20 mm Hg) has been shown uniformly to predict poor outcome in four series of pediatric submersion accidents.[242-245] Unfortunately, as in VF arrest, the threshold for poor outcome from asphyxial arrest appears to be below the threshold for the occurrence of intracranial hypertension because some patients experience poor outcome despite normal ICP.[245] Although anecdotal cases of asphyxial arrest in patients with intact neurologic outcome despite elevated ICP are occasionally discussed, in the series cited previously the ability to control ICP elevation did not result in meaningful survival.[243,245] Routine ICP monitoring and ICP-directed treatment are not currently recommended after asphyxial arrest[243,245,246]; however, studies using ICP-directed therapy in the era of contemporary neurointensive care have yet to be performed.

The use of hyperventilation for cerebral resuscitation after cardiac arrest is currently out of favor. Only one laboratory study of cardiac arrest has demonstrated a beneficial effect of hyperventilation. Vanicky and colleagues[247] reported that 8 hours of hyperventilation reduced neuronal damage after cardiac arrest in dogs. However, histology was examined at 3 hours after arrest, and no long-term outcome was studied. The blind application of hyperventilation early after severe TBI in adults worsened outcome.[248] The failure of ICP-directed therapy to improve outcome after cardiac arrest and the commonly observed period of hypoperfusion in the first hours to days after arrest seriously question the application of an intervention with the potential to further reduce CBF.[249,250] Although irreversible ischemic brain damage has never been demonstrated with hyperventilation,[251] these data suggest that it is probably not wise to intentionally or unintentionally hyperventilate patients routinely after arrest, particularly during the period of postischemic hypoperfusion.[160,173,188] Clinical studies suggest that postischemic hyperemia is accompanied by loss or severe attenuation of the CBF response to alterations in $PaCO_2$ resulting from severe ischemic insult.[170,173] However, some postresuscitation patients with delayed hyperemia but intact CBF response to $PaCO_2$ have been observed (Fig. 68.10).

The traditional approach to cerebral resuscitation has also recommended the use of hyperosmotic agents in the postarrest period[252]; although similar to hyperventilation, the use of hyperosmotic agents after cardiac arrest is currently out of favor. However, again studies in the setting of cardiac arrest are lacking. In dogs subjected to 6 minutes of global ischemia, mannitol (2 g/kg) further reduced CBF during the postischemic hypoperfusion phase.[253] This unwanted effect of mannitol likely represents a result of dehydration because with more conventional doses, decreased blood viscosity after mannitol administration lowers cerebral blood volume but maintains CBF.[254] A few anecdotal reports in support of the use of albumin as an osmotic agent after cardiac arrest exist,[255,256] supported by several more experimental studies in models of global ischemia.[257] Administration of hypertonic saline improves myocardial blood flow and survival versus standard resuscitation after VF in pigs.[258] These studies suggest that clinical trials examining the effect of hypertonic solutions on outcome after cardiac arrest are warranted.

In clinical practice, patients are encountered who have been successfully resuscitated from an arrest of unknown etiology, have a clinical history suggestive of trauma, or demonstrate focal pupillary findings. In this setting it is appropriate to hyperventilate or to administer mannitol until CT and clinical examination confirm the absence of trauma or a mass lesion.

Supportive Care in the Intensive Care Unit

A hypothetical algorithm for the management of infants and children after cardiac arrest is provided in Fig. 68.11. In addition to maintenance of normal ventilation, arterial oxygenation, temperature, and blood pressure, several other aspects of supportive care are important to discuss because suboptimal treatment might adversely affect outcome.

There is an association between hyperoxia and outcome in both in vitro and in vivo models of brain injury, thought to be a result of increased oxidative stress.[259,260] In neonates, two systematic reviews showed a mortality benefit to resuscitating infants with room air versus 100% oxygen.[261,262] No long-term developmental outcomes were available; however, these and other data resulted in changes in the approach of neonatal resuscitation.[263]

Although neonates have lower PaO_2 prior to delivery, findings in adults with cardiac arrest may provide more insight for children. Kilgannon and colleagues found that hyperoxia (PaO_2 >300 mm Hg) and hypoxia (PaO_2 <60 mm Hg) on first arterial blood gas post-ROSC were associated with mortality in adults with cardiac arrest.[264] A study in children followed, finding an association of extreme hypoxemia (odds ratio, 1.92; 95% confidence interval, 1.80 to 2.21 at PaO_2 of 23 mm Hg) and hyperoxia (odds ratio, 1.25; 95% confidence interval, 1.17 to 1.37 at PaO_2 of 600 mm Hg) on first arterial blood gas with PICU mortality.[265] A single-center retrospective analysis found no relationship between hyperoxia or hypoxia within the first 24 hours post-ROSC with mortality.[266] Similarly, a multicenter retrospective analysis found that although derangements in oxygenation and ventilation were common, there was no association between blood gas parameters in the first 6 hours post-ROSC and survival with favorable neurologic outcome.[267]

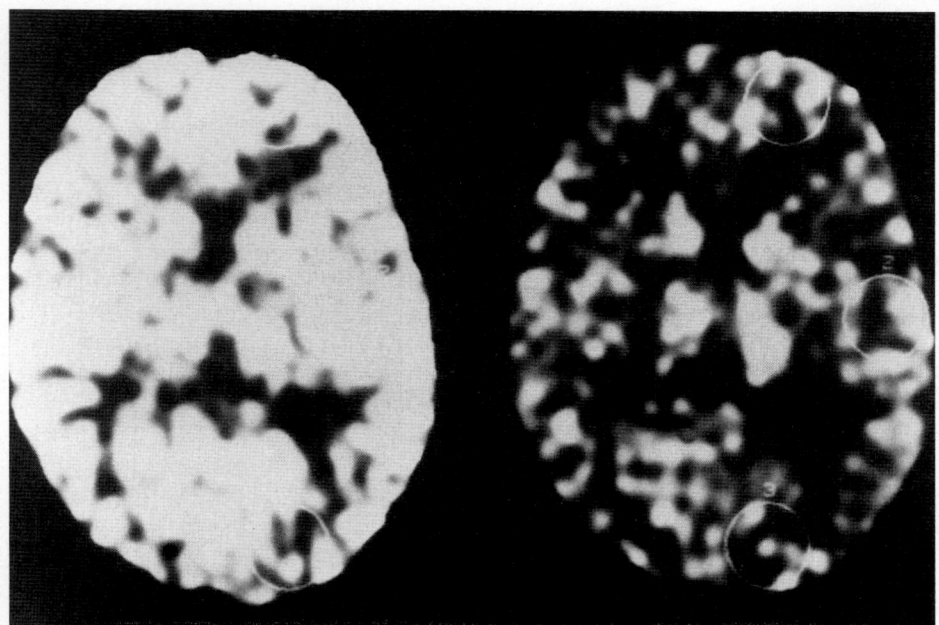

Fig. 68.10. Stable-xenon CT cerebral blood flow study in a comatose 6-year-old 3 days after cold-water submersion accident with asphyxial cardiac arrest. Delayed CBF hyperemia is represented as high-density white areas through the CT brain section shown on the left (PaCO$_2$ ~40 mm Hg). Flows (calculated from this scan) are in excess of 100 ml/100 g/min throughout the brain. Normal values are ~60 to 70 ml/100 g/min. Despite diffuse hyperemia, CBF reactivity to changes in PaCO$_2$ remain intact. CBF values ranged from 50 to 60 ml/100 g/min *(right)* in areas sampled when PaCO$_2$ was reduced to 29 mm Hg with hyperventilation. Six months after the arrest, the child was moderately disabled but not in a vegetative state.

A prospective multicenter study found that oxygenation was not associated with mortality, but hypocapnia (PaCO$_2$ <30 mm Hg) and hypercapnia (PaCO$_2$ >50 mm Hg) were associated with mortality after pediatric cardiac arrest.[268] However, in a large study from Australia and New Zealand, only hypocapnia (PaCO$_2$ <35 mm Hg) was associated with mortality.[269] Pediatric guidelines written prior to availability of these pediatric data recommend resuscitation with 100% oxygen with subsequent titration of oxygen saturations to ≥94% post-ROSC.[1]

Although the optimal cerebral perfusion pattern for neuronal recovery remains to be defined,[252] blood pressure fluctuations, both high and low, adversely affect outcome. In their classic study of the neuropathology of systemic circulatory arrest in immature monkeys, Miller and Myers[225] found that systolic blood pressures at or below 50 mm Hg during the reperfusion period had devastating effects on survival and neuropathology. This occurred even when the ischemic time was less than the 12-minute minimum that caused brain injury in their model. In contrast, Bleyaert and coworkers[270] showed that intermittent episodes of hypertension (MAP 150 to 190 mm Hg) induced with norepinephrine during the first 24 hours after 16 minutes of global brain ischemia in monkeys worsened neurologic outcome. A beneficial effect of transient hypertension during the immediate postresuscitation period has been suggested,[14] hypothesizing that this improves flow in areas with microvascular sludging. Safar and colleagues[185] suggested that transient hypertension was beneficial after cardiac arrest in dogs. However, it was applied as part of a multifaceted treatment protocol, and its specific benefit remains controversial. Newer data show that in a multicenter, observational cohort of children with cardiac arrest, having a blood pressure <5% for age (56% of cohort) within the first 6 hours post-ROSC was associated with increased mortality and worse neurologic outcomes.[271] No data exist on optimal blood pressure adjuvants after pediatric cardiac arrest.

Although seizures may be seen in 30% to 50% of children after cardiac arrest, the use of prophylactic antiepileptics is also controversial. A prospective study showed that 9 of 19 children who received therapeutic hypothermia and continuous EEG monitoring had seizures, many occurring near or during the rewarming period.[207] A small case series in children surviving cardiac arrest observed how a 7-channel EEG test evolved from the first few hours to days after resuscitation.[272] EEGs were grouped into normal, impaired, grossly impaired, and death of the brain, and the authors posited that the first EEG may not be valid for outcome prediction. The independent association between poor outcome and the presence and severity of seizures after birth asphyxia is better established.[273] There is strong rationale for treating clinical seizures postarrest; however, whether or not to aggressively treat subclinical seizures or use antiepileptics prophylactically remains to be determined.

Although transient hyperglycemia commonly occurs after resuscitation from cardiac arrest,[274] the optimal therapy or need for controlling blood glucose after resuscitation has not been established. Current recommendations are for the use of glucose-containing solutions during newborn resuscitations[275] because of evidence that hypoglycemia has synergistic deleterious effects coupled with perinatal asphyxia.[276] Dextrose-containing solutions are generally avoided in the resuscitation of the older child, given the association between hyperglycemia and poorer outcome after near drowning and TBI in pediatric patients.[172,277] Although a cause and effect

POSTRESUSCITATION ALGORITHM

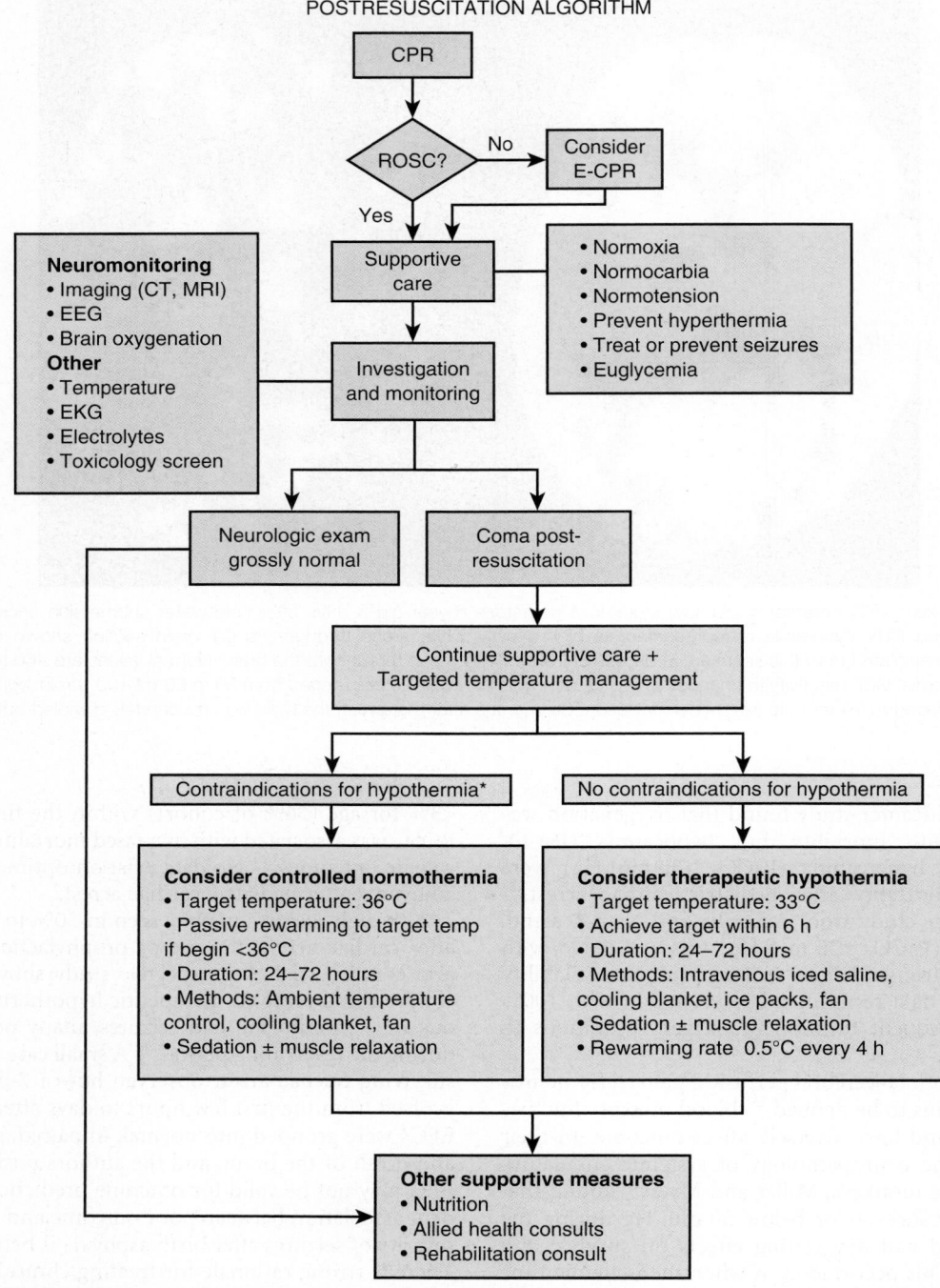

Fig. 68.11. A hypothetical algorithm for the management of infants, children, and adolescents after cardiac arrest. *Contraindications to use of hypothermia include active hemorrhage, uncorrected coagulopathy, sepsis, and certain dysrhythmias.

relationship between hyperglycemia and outcome in humans has not been established, it is curious to note that in one of the clinical trials showing beneficial effects of hypothermia in adults after cardiac arrest, hyperglycemia was associated with hypothermic treatment.[6] However, reports of tight glucose control versus standard care in adults with VF arrest showed no difference in outcome.[278] The optimal resuscitation fluid has not been established, particularly in pediatric patients beyond the neonatal period and prior to adolescence, but is likely to be age and perhaps mechanism dependent.

Current and Novel Therapies
Postresuscitative Hypothermia

Therapeutic hypothermia has been used to treat acute brain injury for over a century.[279] Classically, the beneficial effect of hypothermia was thought to be primarily related to a reduction in oxidative metabolism. Rosomoff and Holaday demonstrated that with each decrement of 1°C, brain oxidative metabolism slows by 6.7%,[280] a finding also seen in immature rats.[281] More recently it was reported that 36°C favorably altered cellular biochemistry in cultured neurons and astrocytes, with potential for clinical translational.[282] Moderate hypothermia (31°C) during neonatal hypoxia-ischemia maintains brain glucose and ATP concentration and reduces lactate production compared with normothermia (37°C) or mild hypothermia (34°C).[281] Taken together with the well-documented effects of hypothermia on neurologic outcome in experimental models, at least a partial contribution of the effect of hypothermia on cellular energetics in affording neuroprotection after cardiac arrest is supported. However, given that mild hypothermia, which does not significantly lower oxygen consumption, provides some degree of neuroprotection, it seems more likely that hypothermia affects multiple mechanisms that influence outcome after cardiac arrest. These mechanisms include, but are not limited to, excitotoxicity, calcium fluxes, oxidative stress, and inflammation.[283]

Although the composition of mechanisms by which hypothermia confers neuroprotection after cardiac arrest is still under debate, numerous experimental studies support further preclinical and clinical studies designed to optimize its application in humans. For instance, both applied mild hypothermia, reducing temperature by as little as 2°C,[284] and delayed spontaneous hypothermia[285] reduce neuronal death seen after cerebral ischemia in rats. Leonov and colleagues[286] reported improved neurologic recovery in dogs subjected to ice-water immersion of the cranium beginning 3 minutes after the onset of 12.5 minutes VF arrest, using CPB to maintain core temperature at 34°C for 1 hour. In this same canine VF arrest model, mild (34°C) or moderate (30°C) hypothermia was found to be protective whereas deep (15°C) hypothermia worsened cerebral and cardiac outcome.[287] Relevant to pediatric cardiac arrest, post treatment with brief (1-hour) and prolonged (24-hour) hypothermia improved neurologic outcome in a juvenile rat model and piglet model of asphyxial cardiac arrest, respectively.[190,288]

The effectiveness of hypothermia as a cerebral protective intervention (ie, prearrest) is unquestioned. The beneficial effects of hypothermia applied immediately before and during cardiac arrest are also clearly demonstrated by the clinical experience with cold-water submersion (near drowning) accident victims.[246] By contrast, complications from the use of moderate hypothermia (30°–34°C) post arrest and the apparent lack of a beneficial effect led to the abandonment of its routine application in the 1980s.[289] Randomized clinical trials in adults published in 2002 who were comatose after resuscitation from ventricular-arrhythmia–induced out-of-hospital cardiac arrest showed a beneficial effect of hypothermia (32°–34°C).[5,6] These studies prompted the International Liaison Committee on Resuscitation and the American Heart Association to recommend 12 to 24 hours of hypothermia (32°–34°C) for adult victims of VF or VT out-of-hospital cardiac arrest.[290,291] There was concern that the lack of temperature control in the normothermia or placebo groups in these two landmark studies resulted in many subjects having fever, which is known to be detrimental following cardiac arrest.[292,293] Thus a new trial was performed in adults remaining comatose after resuscitation from presumed cardiac etiology out-of-hospital cardiac arrest using active targeted temperature management (TTM) for both arms (33°C versus 36°C). They found no difference in mortality between the two groups.[10] It was noteworthy that the outcome of the control arm of this study was similar to that of the hypothermia arm

in the prior hypothermia after cardiac arrest trial that demonstrated benefit of hypothermia a decade earlier. Thus a key question raised by this study is whether the prevention of fever is all that is necessary to improve outcome or whether clamping temperature at a slightly hypothermic level of 36°C confers benefit.[10] It is, as discussed, clear that even a single degree of hyperthermia produces detrimental effects on outcomes after cardiac arrest in newborns.[294] Thus this important question remains to be addressed for optimized TTM in children. Although somewhat different from a pathophysiologic standpoint, studies in neonates at risk for HIE from birth asphyxia have similarly shown that local head or whole body mild hypothermia applied for 72 hours improves survival and neurologic outcome.[3,4,295] One trial demonstrated superior outcomes using 33.5°C for 72 hours versus longer duration (120 hours) or deeper hypothermia (32°C) for either duration.[296]

The efficacy of hypothermia for neuroprotection in neonates with birth asphyxia and in adults with VF arrest prompted some clinicians to treat pediatric victims of asphyxial or arrhythmia-induced cardiac arrest with hypothermia.[297] Two retrospective studies found that clinicians were applying hypothermia to patients with historically poor outcomes: out-of-hospital and unwitnessed arrests that required multiple doses of epinephrine for ROSC.[298,299] A multicenter, randomized prospective trial was published (Therapeutic Hypothermia after Pediatric Cardiac Arrest; THAPCA) and demonstrated no difference in survival with favorable outcome between active normothermia (36.8°C) and hypothermia (33°C) groups for children with out-of-hospital cardiac arrest (relative likelihood 1.54; 95% CI, 0.86 to 2.76; p = 0.14).[11] However, it should be noted that in contrast to the adult TTM out-of-hospital study where the outcomes were nearly equivalent between groups (hazard ratio, 1.06; 95% confidence interval [CI], 0.89 to 1.28; p = 0.51, 33°C vs. 36°C),[10] THAPCA recruited only 25% as many subjects and demonstrated a favorable point estimate for the hypothermic group. Additionally, the prevalence of asphyxia in THAPCA (72%), compared to TTM, which recruited out-of-hospital arrests of presumed cardiac etiology, may provide an explanation for the observed differences. Results for THAPCA's in-hospital pediatric cardiac arrest study, with similar randomized interventions, are pending.

Prehospital hypothermia using cold saline in adults increased the incidence of recurrent arrest and pulmonary edema and did not improve outcomes.[300] Although intraarrest cooling has shown promise in preclinical models of cardiac arrest,[301] the results of clinical trials have been disappointing[302] and the lack of clear benefit of hypothermia in pediatric cardiac arrest should limit enthusiasm for any temperature manipulation in the field unless the patient is febrile.

Therapy Directed by Grouped Characteristics

It is increasingly clear within critical care that appropriate phenotyping of heterogenous processes on the basis of physiologic, biochemical, and genetic attributes may be needed to better target therapies to the individual's situation. Within pediatric out-of-hospital cardiac arrest, infants are unlikely to have their cardiac arrests witnessed resulting in longer no-flow ischemia.[8,23] As previously described, longer no-flow times increase the risk of threshold hypoperfusion and loss of autoregulation. Thus these patients may be in greatest need of closer cerebral monitoring, although it remains uncertain this will improve outcomes. In these infants the most common cause of out-of-hospital cardiac arrest is sudden unexpected infant death (SUID). Although the pathophysiology of SUID is not singular, a substantial number of these children have evidence of autonomic dysfunction as well as neurochemical and structural brain anomalies.[303-305] Present technology precludes therapy directed at these anomalies. Preclinical studies demonstrate important differences in the pathology of brain injury,[26] which in turn may imply different neuronal cell death pathways and alterations in CBF[83] after asphyxial versus VF cardiac arrest. In addition, differences in myocardial dysfunction[306,307] and ventilation[308] between these different forms of cardiac arrest may require different management strategies to prevent secondary brain injury. In the case of asphyxia it is clear the brain senses the insult and has a neurochemical and electrical response long before no flow,[21] which may increase the risk for excitotoxicity after resuscitation, suggesting a role for therapies such as NMDA antagonisms in these forms of arrest. Further studies of targeted therapies in targeted subpopulations of cardiac arrest are needed to better define the differences suggested by these preliminary studies.

Inhibition of Postischemic Excitotoxicity

The observation in animal models that hypermetabolism accompanies postischemic hypoperfusion formed the basis for early clinical cerebroprotective strategies in the postarrest setting. Therapies directed at attenuating active cerebral metabolism (resulting from synaptic transmission) were applied in the hope of reducing this secondary insult of hypoperfusion plus hypermetabolism. The cerebral protective effects of interventions that decrease cerebral metabolic rate *before* the onset of ischemia, such as barbiturates and hypothermia, are well established and clinically important.[309,310] The selective inhibitory effect of barbiturates on active $CMRO_2$ was particularly attractive. However, therapeutic reductions in brain metabolism when applied *after* the insult, as in the *HYPER* therapy of the 1970s and 1980s, did not improve outcome.[289,311] This may have been the result of the relative lack of postarrest hypermetabolism in human beings.[169] In addition, adverse hemodynamic consequences of barbiturates and the ill effects of sustained hypothermia on immune function and blood rheology may have counteracted any beneficial effects. More targeted therapies may need to be developed. As previously outlined, agents inhibiting extrasynaptic neuronal death pathways or CaMKII may have promise in protecting against neuronal death.[89,312]

Futuristic Approaches
Mitochondria Targeting Strategies

Therapies targeting mitochondria can be divided into (1) alternative fuels, (2) inhibitors of mitochondrial permeability transition (MPT), and (3) mitochondria-targeted electron scavengers and antioxidants. Among the first category, acetyl-L-carnitine was shown to potentiate normalization of brain energy metabolites and improve neurologic outcome after complete global cerebral ischemia reperfusion.[313] Experimental studies in cardiac arrest report improved myocardial function and reduction in neuronal damage with an MPT inhibitor cyclosporine when administered at the time of reperfusion or shortly thereafter.[314-316] In contrast to the first two strategies,

the third class of therapies will selectively accumulate in mitochondria and bind targets within the organelle to exert their effects.[102] Several strategies have been used to effectively target mitochondrial localization of small molecules including conjugation to lipophilic cations such as triphenylphosphonium that take advantage of negative membrane potential of mitochondria[102] and bind to a specific mitochondrial target such as cardiolipin, a phospholipid exclusively found in the inner mitochondrial membrane.[70] Only one compound in the first category has been tested in cardiac arrest. Administration of mitochondria-targeted sulfide donor AP39 at the time of CPR or 1 minute after ROSC was shown to improve neurologic function and long-term survival rates after an 8-minute cardiac arrest induced by potassium chloride in adult mice.[317] Compounds in the second category include Szeto-Schiller (SS) peptides.[104] Their uptake into mitochondria is thought to be independent of membrane potential with a high affinity binding to the inner membrane.[104] They contain four alternating aromatic amino acids and some have antioxidant activity. One of these peptides, SS-31, protects mitochondria, accelerates ATP recovery, and reduces infarct size in the heart.[104] Another class of compounds in the second category promising for pediatric cardiac arrest is made up of the hemigramicidin-nitroxides (GS-nitroxide) inspired by the shared ancestry between mitochondria and bacteria, taking advantage of chemical moieties used in antibacterial agents (the antibiotic gramicidin S) with high affinity for the cardiolipin-rich inner mitochondrial membrane.[105] One GS-nitroxide, XJB-5-131, was shown to partition almost exclusively into neuronal mitochondria in vitro, penetrate the blood-brain barrier, prevent cardiolipin oxidation and caspase activation, and improve neurocognitive outcome after asphyxial cardiac arrest in juvenile rats.[103]

Erythropoietin

Erythropoietin (EPO) is better known for its bone marrow stimulation effect,[318] but it is also required for normal brain development, stimulating neural progenitor cells.[319,320] EPO used therapeutically in experimental models of neonatal hypoxia-ischemia has multiple potential mechanisms of neuroprotection, including prevention of apoptosis, protection from oxidative stress, modulation of cellular water permeability, and promotion of neurogenesis and angiogenesis.[319,321,322]

Therapeutic hypothermia has become standard of care for newborns with moderate/severe HIE,[323] leading investigators to find other therapies that complement or synergize with hypothermia. Combination therapy with hypothermia and EPO shows promise in experimental models, improving sensorimotor function, with 7-day-old female rats benefiting more than males.[324] In a nonhuman primate model of perinatal asphyxia, combination therapy produced superior results over placebo and hypothermia alone in terms of the primary outcome, death, or moderate-severe cerebral palsy.[325] Pilot studies have demonstrated pharmacokinetics, feasibility, safety, and, in some instances, improved outcomes.[326-330] Efficacy of combination therapy is now being explored in a multicenter randomized controlled trial (RCT; NCT01913340).

Stem Cell Therapy

Pluripotent stem cells have the capacity to differentiate into cells with antiinflammatory, immune-modulating, and potentially neuroprotectant properties.[331] In experimental brain injury models, stem cells have been shown to localize to injury regions, express neuronal and glial markers, reduce cell death, increase CNS cellularity, and improve outcomes.[332-335] Treatment efficacy was affected by method of delivery (ie, intracerebral, intravenous), timing, frequency, type of stem cell, and model, with some reports having neutral effects on outcome and others having adverse effects such as brain tumor development.[336,337]

A pilot study in which autologous umbilical cord blood was transfused in neonates with birth asphyxia who also received hypothermia therapy did not reveal serious safety issues.[338] At least one RCT is actively recruiting newborns to determine further safety and feasibility of stem cells in this cohort (NCT00593242). Preliminary studies in children with cerebral palsy show promise in safety and feasibility.[339-341] An RCT evaluating umbilical cord blood transfusions in combination with EPO showed improvement in motor and cognitive functioning.[342] One RCT using autologous umbilical cord blood for treatment of cerebral palsy is actively recruiting patients (NCT01147653).

Extracorporeal Support

Extracorporeal support in the form of CPB initiated immediately after VF arrest in dogs (with cannulae already in place) improves outcome when compared to standard advanced cardiac life support–guided resuscitation.[343] CPB produced 64% survival after even 20 minutes of VF arrest, although all dogs were neurologically impaired. This supports the concept that cerebral and coronary perfusion during CPR extends tolerated insult time, although studies with vascular cannulation during resuscitation have not been reported. These studies would be important in light of the difficulty in obtaining this type of vascular access during arrest in children. Nevertheless, extracorporeal support allows control of postarrest blood flow and temperature, and the cardiovascular support provided might allow use of otherwise contraindicated therapies.

Many studies have shown that rescue extracorporeal life support (ECLS) or E-CPR is feasible under varied circumstances. This intervention is detailed in Chapter 59.

Summary

The social and economic impact of children left with persistent neurologic injury after cardiac arrest remains staggering. Preventive approaches to this problem are unlikely to reduce significantly the occurrence of these multifactorial and largely unanticipated events. However, it is worthwhile for the general public to become more knowledgeable of child CPR, safety measures (eg, pool and road safety), and the enormous benefit of quality CPR[344] and to consider implementation of systems that recognize a hospitalized child in distress before an arrest is imminent, such as pediatric medical emergency teams.[345] Improvements in prognostication after cardiac arrest are on the horizon with a more concerted application of existing methods and new techniques. The successful application of novel brain-oriented therapeutic approaches is somewhat more speculative, but it is likely to require intervention beginning in the prehospital setting or emergency department. Improved, pathophysiology-guided stratification of postarrest patients is essential to determine which patients have resuscitable insults and, with optimal supportive care and prevention of secondary neuronal deterioration, potential for a good

rather than devastating outcome. Unfortunately, this group is unlikely to include most patients with prolonged asphyxial arrest and in any single institution represents a small number of cases per year. Biochemically and physiologically guided, multifaceted pharmacologic and mechanical approaches will almost certainly be required, with their application based on the temporal sequence of pathologic events.

Acknowledgment

This chapter remains dedicated to Peter J. Safar, the "father of modern-day CPR," who passed away on August 3, 2003. *Rest in Peace.*

Key References

1. Kleinman ME, Chameides L, Schexnayder SM, et al. Part 14: pediatric advanced life support: 2010 American Heart Association Guidelines for Cardiopulmonary Resuscitation and Emergency Cardiovascular Care. *Circulation.* 2010;122:S876-S908.
2. Girotra S, Spertus JA, Li Y, et al. Survival trends in pediatric in-hospital cardiac arrests: an analysis from Get With the Guidelines-Resuscitation. *Circ Cardiovasc Qual Outcomes.* 2013;6:42-49.
4. Shankaran S, Laptook AR, Ehrenkranz RA, et al. Whole-body hypothermia for neonates with hypoxic-ischemic encephalopathy. *N Engl J Med.* 2005;353:1574-1584.
7. Hypothermia after Cardiac Arrest Study Group. Mild therapeutic hypothermia to improve the neurologic outcome after cardiac arrest. *N Engl J Med.* 2002;346:549-556.
9. Moler FW, Meert K, Donaldson AE, et al. In-hospital versus out-of-hospital pediatric cardiac arrest: a multicenter cohort study. *Crit Care Med.* 2009;37:2259-2267.
10. Nielsen N, Wetterslev J, Cronberg T, et al. Targeted temperature management at 33 degrees C versus 36 degrees C after cardiac arrest. *N Engl J Med.* 2013;369:2197-2206.
11. Moler FW, Silverstein FS, Holubkov R, et al. Therapeutic hypothermia after out-of-hospital cardiac arrest in children. *N Engl J Med.* 2015; 372:1898-1908.
25. Bodsch W, Barbier A, Oehmichen M, et al. Recovery of monkey brain after prolonged ischemia. II. Protein synthesis and morphological alterations. *J Cereb Blood Flow Metab.* 1986;6:22-33.
26. Vaagenes P, Safar P, Moossy J, et al. Asphyxiation versus ventricular fibrillation cardiac arrest in dogs. Differences in cerebral resuscitation effects—a preliminary study. *Resuscitation.* 1997;35:41-52.
34. Lorek A, Takei Y, Cady EB, et al. Delayed ("secondary") cerebral energy failure after acute hypoxia-ischemia in the newborn piglet: continuous 48-hour studies by phosphorus magnetic resonance spectroscopy. *Pediatr Res.* 1994;36:699-706.
39. Katz LM, Callaway CW, Kagan VE, Kochanek PM. Electron spin resonance measure of brain antioxidant activity during ischemia/reperfusion. *Neuroreport.* 1998;9:1587-1593.
43. Sims NR, Pulsinelli WA. Altered mitochondrial respiration in selectively vulnerable brain subregions following transient forebrain ischemia in the rat. *J Neurochem.* 1987;49:1367-1374.
48. Au AK, Bayir H, Kochanek PM, Clark RS. Evaluation of autophagy using mouse models of brain injury. *Biochim Biophys Acta.* 2010;1802: 918-923.
49. Buja LM, Eigenbrodt ML, Eigenbrodt EH. Apoptosis and necrosis. *Arch Pathol Lab Med.* 1993;117:1208-1214.
57. Northington FJ, Ferriero DM, Flock DL, Martin LJ. Delayed neurodegeneration in neonatal rat thalamus after hypoxia-ischemia is apoptosis. *J Neurosci.* 2001;21:1931-1938.
58. Shoykhet M, Simons DJ, Alexander H, et al. Thalamocortical dysfunction and thalamic injury after asphyxial cardiac arrest in developing rats. *J Neurosci.* 2012;32:4972-4981.
60. Renolleau S, Fau S, Goyenvalle C, et al. Specific caspase inhibitor Q-VD-OPh prevents neonatal stroke in P7 rat: a role for gender. *J Neurochem.* 2007;100:1062-1071.
76. Northington FJ, Ferriero DM, Graham EM, et al. Early neurodegeneration after hypoxia-ischemia in neonatal rat is necrosis while delayed neuronal death is apoptosis. *Neurobiol Dis.* 2001;8:207-219.

82. Manole MD, Kochanek PM, Foley LM, et al. Polynitroxyl albumin and albumin therapy after pediatric asphyxial cardiac arrest: effects on cerebral blood flow and neurologic outcome. *J Cereb Blood Flow Metab.* 2012;32:560-569.

83. Drabek T, Foley LM, Janata A, et al. Global and regional differences in cerebral blood flow after asphyxial versus ventricular fibrillation cardiac arrest in rats using ASL-MRI. *Resuscitation.* 2014;85:964-971.

103. Ji J, Baart S, Vikulina AS, et al. Deciphering of mitochondrial cardiolipin oxidative signaling in cerebral ischemia-reperfusion. *J Cereb Blood Flow Metab.* 2015;35:319-328.

117. Dezfulian C, Shiva S, Alekseyenko A, et al. Nitrite therapy after cardiac arrest reduces reactive oxygen species generation, improves cardiac and neurological function, and enhances survival via reversible inhibition of mitochondrial complex I. *Circulation.* 2009;120:897-905.

127. Du L, Bayir H, Lai Y, et al. Innate gender-based proclivity in response to cytotoxicity and programmed cell death pathway. *J Biol Chem.* 2004;279:38563-38570.

151. Clark RS, Kochanek PM, Chen M, et al. Increases in bcl-2 and cleavage of caspase-1 and caspase-3 in human brain after head injury. *FASEB J.* 1999;13:813-821.

166. Manole MD, Foley LM, Hitchens TK, et al. Magnetic resonance imaging assessment of regional cerebral blood flow after asphyxial cardiac arrest in immature rats. *J Cereb Blood Flow Metab.* 2009;29:197-205.

174. Lee JK, Brady KM, Chung SE, et al. A pilot study of cerebrovascular reactivity autoregulation after pediatric cardiac arrest. *Resuscitation.* 2014;85:1387-1393.

176. Pienaar R, Paldino MJ, Madan N, et al. A quantitative method for correlating observations of decreased apparent diffusion coefficient with elevated cerebral blood perfusion in newborns presenting cerebral ischemic insults. *Neuroimage.* 2012;63:1510-1518.

179. Nordmark J, Rubertsson S, Mortberg E, et al. Intracerebral monitoring in comatose patients treated with hypothermia after a cardiac arrest. *Acta Anaesthesiol Scand.* 2009;53:289-298.

180. Ashwal S, Holshouser BA, Tomasi LG, et al. 1H-magnetic resonance spectroscopy-determined cerebral lactate and poor neurological outcomes in children with central nervous system disease. *Ann Neurol.* 1997;41:470-481.

195. Robertson CM, Joffe AR, Moore AJ, Watt JM. Neurodevelopmental outcome of young pediatric intensive care survivors of serious brain injury. *Pediatr Crit Care Med.* 2002;3:345-350.

203. Abend NS, Licht DJ. Predicting outcome in children with hypoxic ischemic encephalopathy. *Pediatr Crit Care Med.* 2008;9:32-39.

206. Nishisaki A, Sullivan J 3rd, Steger B, et al. Retrospective analysis of the prognostic value of electroencephalography patterns obtained in pediatric in-hospital cardiac arrest survivors during three years. *Pediatr Crit Care Med.* 2007;8:10-17.

210. Berger RP, Adelson PD, Richichi R, Kochanek PM. Serum biomarkers after traumatic and hypoxemic brain injuries: insight into the biochemical response of the pediatric brain to inflicted brain injury. *Dev Neurosci.* 2006;28:327-335.

212. Fink EL, Berger RP, Clark RSB, et al. Serum biomarkers of brain injury to classify outcome after pediatric cardiac arrest. *Crit Care Med.* 2014;42:664-674.

217. Rafaat KT, Spear RM, Kuelbs C, et al. Cranial computed tomographic findings in a large group of children with drowning: diagnostic, prognostic, and forensic implications. *Pediatr Crit Care Med.* 2008;9:567-572.

220. Fink EL, Panigrahy A, Clark RS, et al. Regional brain injury on conventional and diffusion weighted MRI is associated with outcome after pediatric cardiac arrest. *Neurocrit Care.* 2013;19:31-40.

246. Biggart MJ, Bohn DJ. Effect of hypothermia and cardiac arrest on outcome of near-drowning accidents in children. *J Pediatr.* 1990;117:179-183.

265. Ferguson LP, Durward A, Tibby SM. Relationship between arterial partial oxygen pressure after resuscitation from cardiac arrest and mortality in children. *Circulation.* 2012;126:335-342.

271. Topjian AA, French B, Sutton RM, et al. Early postresuscitation hypotension is associated with increased mortality following pediatric cardiac arrest. *Crit Care Med.* 2014;42:1518-1523.

274. Neumar RW, Nolan JP, Adrie C, et al. Post-cardiac arrest syndrome: [?] epidemiology, pathophysiology, treatment, and prognostication a consensus statement from the International Liaison Committee on Resuscitation (American Heart Association, Australian and New Zealand Council on Resuscitation, European Resuscitation Council, Heart and Stroke Foundation of Canada, InterAmerican Heart Foundation, Resuscitation Council of Asia, and the Resuscitation Council of Southern Africa); the American Heart Association Emergency Cardiovascular Care Committee; the Council on Cardiovascular Surgery and Anesthesia; the Council on Cardiopulmonary, Perioperative, and Critical Care; the Council on Clinical Cardiology; and the Stroke Council. *Circulation.* 2008;118:2452-2483.

282. Jackson TC, Manole MD, Kotermanski SE, et al. Cold stress protein RBM3 responds to temperature change in an ultra-sensitive manner in young neurons. *Neuroscience.* 2015;305:268-278.

284. Busto R, Dietrich WD, Globus MY, et al. Small differences in intraischemic brain temperature critically determine the extent of ischemic neuronal injury. *J Cereb Blood Flow Metab.* 1987;7:729-738.

293. Bembea M, Nadkarni V, Diener-West M, et al. Temperature patterns in the early post-resuscitation period after pediatric in-hospital cardiac arrest. *Pediatr Crit Care Med.* 2010;11:723-730.

296. Shankaran S, Laptook AR, Pappas A, et al. Effect of depth and duration of cooling on deaths in the NICU among neonates with hypoxic ischemic encephalopathy: a randomized clinical trial. *JAMA.* 2014;312:2629-2639.

323. Papile LA, Baley JE, Benitz W, et al. Hypothermia and neonatal encephalopathy. *Pediatrics.* 2014;133:1146-1150.

331. Fleiss B, Guillot PV, Titomanlio L, et al. Stem cell therapy for neonatal brain injury. *Clin Perinatol.* 2014;41:133-148.

338. Cotten CM, Murtha AP, Goldberg RN, et al. Feasibility of autologous cord blood cells for infants with hypoxic-ischemic encephalopathy. *J Pediatr.* 2014;164:973-979.e1.

344. Kitamura T, Iwami T, Kawamura T, et al. Conventional and chest-compression-only cardiopulmonary resuscitation by bystanders for children who have out-of-hospital cardiac arrests: a prospective, nationwide, population-based cohort study. *Lancet.* 2010;375:1347-1354.

345. Tibballs J, Kinney S. Reduction of hospital mortality and of preventable cardiac arrest and death on introduction of a pediatric medical emergency team. *Pediatr Crit Care Med.* 2009;10:306-312.

Pediatric Stroke and Intracerebral Hemorrhage

Catherine Amlie-Lefond and Jeffrey Ojemann

PEARLS

- Childhood stroke includes arterial ischemic stroke, cerebral sinus venous thrombosis, and intracranial hemorrhage.
- Diagnosis of acute stroke in childhood is often delayed due to failure to detect neurologic deficit in a child, low clinical suspicion of stroke, frequency of stroke mimics, and delays in diagnostic imaging.
- Compared with adults, the causes of pediatric stroke are much more heterogeneous, and often risk factors, rather than definitive causes, are identified.
- Supportive care in an intensive care unit, with careful attention to optimizing cerebral perfusion and oxygenation, decreasing metabolic demands on the brain, and preventing early stroke recurrence, is critical.

Significance

The incidence of childhood stroke ranges from 2.3 to 13 per 100,000 children.[1,2] Following an episode of stroke, 10% of children die, approximately 10% to 20% will have another stroke, and most survivors will have long-term neurologic or neuropsychologic deficits, including emerging deficits over time. Childhood stroke encompasses arterial ischemic stroke, hemorrhagic stroke, and cerebral sinus venous thrombosis. Approximately half of childhood strokes are ischemic and half are hemorrhagic. The diverse etiologies, risk factors, presentations, treatments, and potential complications of acute stroke in childhood must be considered to minimize morbidity and mortality in the intensive care setting.

Arterial Ischemic Stroke

Acute arterial ischemic stroke (AIS) is defined as the acute onset of a neurologic deficit consistent with infarction in a vascular territory, with imaging or pathologic confirmation. Secondary hemorrhage due to tissue and vascular injury within the ischemic core can occur (*hemorrhagic conversion*), but unlike hemorrhagic stroke, the initial event is ischemic.

Etiologies and Risk Factors

Approximately half of all children presenting with initial AIS have an underlying condition that increases the risk of stroke (symptomatic stroke) and the other half have cryptogenic

stroke. After extensive evaluation, most children will have at least one risk factor for stroke identified. It is likely that most instances of AIS in childhood are multifactorial.

Cerebral Arteriopathy

Cerebral arteriopathy is well associated with primary and recurrent stroke.[3,4] In the Vascular Effects of Infection in Pediatric Stroke (VIPS) study, definite or possible arteriopathy was present on vascular imaging in 46% of all patients and in 55% of the subset of patients who were previously healthy—that is, had no previously known risk factors for stroke.[5] In addition, cerebral arteriopathy has been found in children with acute AIS who have other stroke risk factors such as congenital heart disease.[6]

Focal cerebral arteriopathy (FCA) is a discrete intracranial arterial stenosis that accounts for approximately one-quarter of arteriopathies in childhood AIS.[7,8] FCA has been well associated with varicella zoster virus infection.[9] A subset of FCA is transient cerebral arteriopathy (TCA), which is defined as FCA that improves or shows no progression after 6 months.[8]

Moyamoya is a progressive steno-occlusive disease of the distal internal carotid arteries and proximal middle cerebral arteries, and not infrequently the anterior cerebral arteries, associated with collateral formation at the base of the brain, producing the *moyamoya* (Japanese for "puff of smoke") configuration seen on a catheter cerebral angiogram. Moyamoya usually presents with AIS in childhood, whereas adults frequently present with hemorrhagic stroke. Moyamoya may be idiopathic, termed *moyamoya disease,* or occur in association with predisposing syndromes, such as sickle cell disease, trisomy 21, or neurofibromatosis type 1, termed *moyamoya syndrome* (Fig. 69.1). Moyamoya disease is likely a genetic disease, most probably polygenic, based on the high prevalence of moyamoya in Asia, as well as familial aggregation in 5% to 10% of cases.[10,11] The only effective treatment for moyamoya is surgical revascularization to decrease the risk of further transient ischemic attacks (TIAs) and ischemic and hemorrhagic stroke.[12,13]

Cervicocephalic arterial dissection (CCAD) accounts for 7.5% to 20% of childhood AIS.[7,8,14] Because children with CCAD are at risk for recurrent stroke, anticoagulant therapy is recommended,[15] although antiplatelet therapy such as aspirin is also used, which is consistent with the recommendation of antiplatelet or anticoagulant treatment of CCAD in adults.[16] Often a history of trauma to the head or neck is obtained in children presenting with CCAD, such as can occur

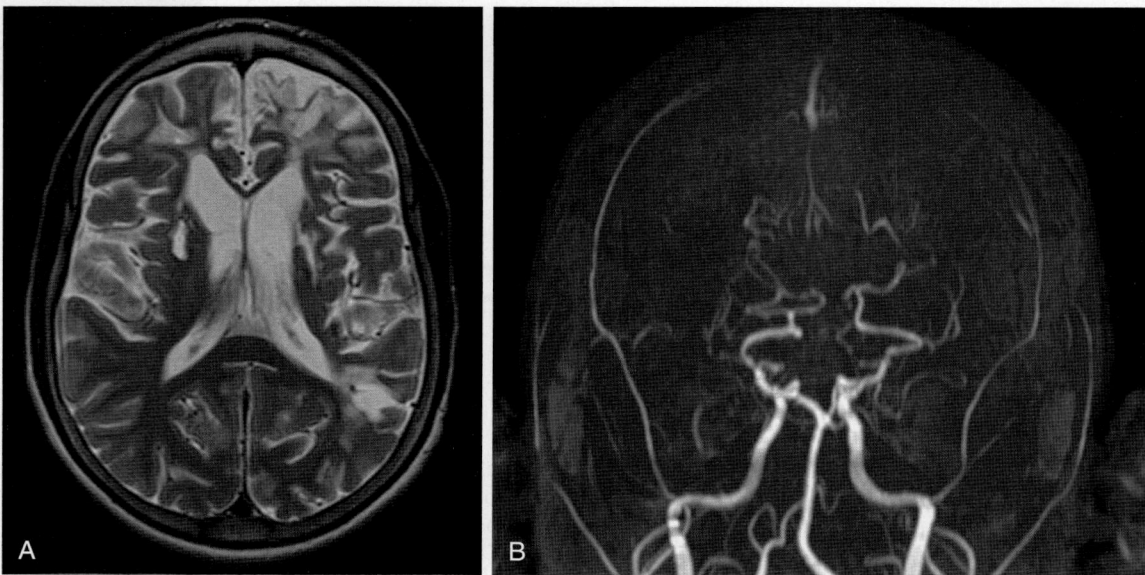

Fig. 69.1. A 13-year-old boy with SCD and bilateral moyamoya. High T2 signal and parenchymal volume loss represents sequelae of multiple infarcts seen in the bilateral anterior circulation (A). There is occlusion of the bilateral distal internal carotid arteries (B) and associated bilateral lenticulostriate and thalamoperforator collaterals consistent with moyamoya.

with sports injuries; however, CCAD can also present spontaneously. Dissection can also be complicated by subarachnoid hemorrhage due to aneurysmal dilation and recurrent dissection. Children with collagenopathies or elastinopathies such as Ehlers-Danlos syndrome, Marfan syndrome, Loeys-Dietz syndrome, and arterial tortuosity syndrome are at increased risk for initial and recurrent CCAD.[17]

Central nervous system (CNS) vasculitis is an inflammatory cerebral arteriopathy that can be primary, or idiopathic, or secondary to a systemic cause, most commonly systemic rheumatologic disease or infection. In childhood primary angiitis of the CNS (cPACNS), inflammation only involves the arteries of the CNS.[18] cPACNS can be divided into large-medium vessel disease, in which arteriopathy can be detected on cerebral catheter angiogram, and small vessel cPACNS, in which it is not visible on a catheter angiogram. Children with large-medium vessel cPACNS typically present with hemiparesis or aphasia, and stuttering onset of symptoms is common. Systemic inflammatory markers are often unremarkable in large-medium vessel cPACNS, and cerebrospinal fluid (CSF) pleocytosis or elevated protein is present in only one-third of children. Treatment of progressive large-medium vessel cPACNS requires immunosuppression. The use of anticoagulation or antiplatelet treatment may decrease the risk of stroke.[19]

In small vessel cPACNS, patients often present with diffuse neurologic deficits and headache. Brain magnetic resonance imaging (MRI) is usually abnormal, but findings are nonspecific. Biomarkers including C-reactive protein (CRP), erythrocyte sedimentation rate (ESR), leukocytosis, anemia, and thrombocytosis are frequently, but not consistently, abnormal. Brain biopsy is necessary to diagnose small vessel CNS vasculitis; however, this may yield a false-negative result in a significant number of patients.[19]

Secondary CNS vasculitis is a common manifestation of underlying systemic inflammatory diseases such as Takayasu arteritis, polyarteritis nodosa, and systemic lupus erythematosus. Arteritis is also commonly seen with acute bacterial meningitis, and heparin and aspirin have been used to prevent recurrent stroke in childhood bacterial meningitis.[20]

Varicella zoster virus (VZV) infection, both primary infection and reactivation, is associated with vasculopathy and stroke in children and adults.[9,21-23] VZV vasculopathy is diagnosed by the detection of VZV DNA or anti-VZV IgG antibody in CSF or both.[22] Treatment of VZV vasculopathy with both acyclovir and corticosteroids is recommended.[24]

Sickle Cell Disease

Stroke is a common complication of sickle cell disease (SCD), and without treatment, 11% of children will have a stroke by 20 years of age[25] (see also Chapter 90). The incidence of initial stroke is markedly decreased by regular red blood cell transfusions in children with elevated transcranial Doppler (TCD) velocity in the middle cerebral artery.[26,27] Following initial stroke, the risk of a recurrent stroke is approximately 20%, even with the use of chronic red blood cell transfusion. Many patients with SCD-associated stroke have an underlying cerebral arteriopathy, a risk factor for primary and recurrent stroke.[28-30] In addition, patients with SCD are at risk for aneurysmal hemorrhage.

The possibility of stroke needs to be considered in any child with SCD with transient or persistent focal weakness or deficit in addition to a history of new seizures or severe headache regardless of presence of pain. Blood should be sent for type and cross-match sickle negative, antigen selected, leuko-reduced (minor antigen-matched red blood cells if available) for exchange transfusion. Risk factors for stroke include increased blood pressure, lower hemoglobin concentrations, high leukocyte count, prior transient ischemic attacks, history of meningitis, presentation with seizure, surgery, priapism, acute anemia, recent acute chest syndrome and transfusion within the past 2 weeks, and a history of overt or silent stroke.[25,31,32]

An emergent head computerized tomography (CT) scan without contrast can be used to assess for possible hemorrhage or other intracranial process. Head MRI and magnetic resonance angiography (MRA) with diffusion-weighted imaging are the best ways to assess for possible acute stroke in a child with SCD and clinical presentation of possible stroke. Current guidelines recommend urgent erythrocyte transfusion in neuroimaging-confirmed stroke[33]; however, some recommend that transfusion not be delayed while awaiting confirmatory neuroimaging. There is a risk of ischemia due to increased viscosity if hemoglobin rises to >13 g/dL following transfusion.

Oxygen supplementation is used to maintain oxygen saturation greater than 93% through the completion of the transfusion and through the first night following to minimize nocturnal hypoxemia. Cooling blankets should be avoided in patients with sickle cell disease. Cardiology consultation should be obtained prior to exchange transfusion if there is clinical suspicion of cardiac dysfunction, to assist with cardiac monitoring during exchange transfusion.

Although SCD is not an established contraindication to intravenous tissue plasminogen activator (tPA) in adults, there are no data with which to guide the use of tPA for stroke in children with SCD. As the pathophysiology of stroke in children with SCD may not be particularly responsive to thrombolysis, it is currently not recommended in this setting.

Congenital and Acquired Heart Disease

Cardioembolic stroke secondary to congenital and acquired cardiac disease accounts for almost one-third of AIS in children, with children with complex congenital heart disease (CHD) and right-to-left shunts at highest risk.[4] Among children with heart disease and stroke, one-quarter of strokes occurred in the setting of cardiac surgery or catheterization.[4] Not infrequently, the child with cardiac disease and stroke is acutely ill and sedated, and the stroke is not discovered until sedation or paralytics are weaned. Prothrombotic factors increase the risk of both initial[34] and recurrent stroke in the setting of CHD.[35] The risk of recurrent stroke in children with CHD is 27% at 10 years, with the highest risk immediately following the initial stroke.[35]

Hypercoagulable States

A prothrombotic state is identified in 13% of children with AIS,[4] and the risk of AIS increases when multiple thrombophilias are present or when combined with other risk factors such as CHD. Protein S deficiency, protein C deficiency, factor V Leiden mutation, antithrombin III deficiency, elevated lipoprotein (a), homocystinuria, and antiphospholipid antibodies have been associated with AIS in childhood[4,36] (Table 69.1).

Pathophysiology

Ischemic stroke occurs when blood supply to an area of the brain is not adequate for metabolic needs. This may occur due to occlusion of flow resulting from thrombus or embolus or due to critical stenosis. Decreased cerebral blood flow (CBF) below a critical threshold results in neuronal injury and potentially neuronal death. The central region with absence of CBF ("no flow") is the ischemic core, which will not survive. The surrounding area of ischemic penumbra is

TABLE 69.1	Risk Factors Reported in Acute Arterial Ischemic Stroke in Childhood
Cerebral Arteriopathy	Focal cerebral arteriopathy Moyamoya Cervicocephalic arterial dissection Primary CNS vasculitis Secondary vasculitis Varicella-associated vasculopathy
Hematologic Disorders	Sickle cell disease Iron deficiency anemia Thrombocytosis Leukemia
Heart Disease	Congenital heart disease Acquired heart disease
Hypercoagulable State	Protein C deficiency Protein S deficiency Factor V Leiden Homocystinemia Anticardiolipin antibodies Elevated lipoprotein (a)
Infection	Bacterial meningitis Varicella Mycotic meningitis Tuberculous meningitis
Drugs	Asparaginase Estrogen Illicit drugs (cocaine, methamphetamine)
Inflammatory/Autoimmune	Systemic lupus erythematosus Rheumatoid arthritis Vasculitis (as above)

not irreversibly injured and potentially viable, but it will not survive without prompt restoration of blood flow (see also Chapter 68). The goal of reperfusion using intravenous tPA or acute endovascular intervention is to "rescue" the penumbra by restoring adequate perfusion to prevent cell death. The size of infarction is determined by the extent and duration of ischemia, cerebral perfusion pressure, and extent of collateral circulation. Fever may increase infarction size due to increased metabolic demands. Therefore strategies to minimize injury include ensuring adequate cerebral perfusion pressure and aggressively treating fever.

As energy failure at the cellular level results in neuronal hyperexcitability, seizures including status epilepticus can occur following acute stroke. Although prophylactic antiepileptic medication is not recommended, close monitoring for seizures, including the use of electroencephalography monitoring for subclinical seizures, is recommended. Seizures can be refractory in the immediate poststroke period.

Presentation

Recognition of stroke in childhood is challenging, as identifying neurologic deficits in children, particularly young children, is difficult and stroke is often not considered in the child presenting with acute neurologic deficit. In addition, mimics of childhood stroke are common, and the differential diagnosis is broad, including other diagnoses requiring urgent diagnosis and treatment such as brain tumors, hypertensive encephalopathy, demyelinating disorders, infection, postictal hemiparesis, and metabolic disorders.[37,38] Signs and symptoms of anterior circulation stroke in childhood include hemiparesis, hemisensory loss, aphasia, visual field cuts with gaze preference, and neglect. Posterior circulation strokes can present with ataxia, vomiting, vertigo, dysarthria, diplopia, and dysmetria. Diagnosis of cerebellar stroke is particularly challenging, as cerebellar stroke often presents with nonspecific symptoms such as headache and vomiting, or with ataxia, which mimics acute cerebellar ataxia. From 10% to 20% of childhood AIS cases are heralded by seizures. New neurologic deficit following a seizure in a child with acute stroke may be mistaken for postictal paresis.

Critical initial data to be collected in a child presenting with possible stroke include history of predisposing factors, time since the child was last seen well, recent trauma or infection, and medications. A baseline neurologic assessment such as the pediatric version of the National Institutes of Health (NIH) Stroke Scale (PedNIHSS)[39] should be performed.

Neuroimaging

The potential for acute treatment and intervention will determine the urgency of neuroimaging studies. Head CT is usually the imaging modality used for a child presenting with acute neurologic symptoms or signs, due to speed and availability, and sensitivity for acute intracranial hemorrhage (ICH) and cerebral edema and impending herniation. Head CT is the first-line imaging study for the child with suspected ICH, trauma, or if MR is contraindicated; however, it is much less sensitive for early ischemic stroke than MRI using diffusion-weighted imaging (DWI).[40]

Although head CT and brain MRI will both evaluate for acute hemorrhage in children, the need to confirm AIS and rule out stroke mimics and the desire to limit radiation

exposure results in MRI as the optimal first-line study in most cases. A rapid stroke MR protocol that can be done in 20 to 30 minutes may be used. Sequences should include DWI/ apparent diffusion coefficient (ADC), which is sensitive for early ischemia, although not specific, and T1- and T2-weighted (or T2 fluid attenuation inverse recovery [FLAIR]) sequences and MRA of the head and neck (Fig. 69.2). FLAIR is less useful in children under 2 years of age due to immature cerebral myelination. Susceptibility weighted (SWI) or gradient echo (GE) will increase the sensitivity for detection of hemorrhage. Young children and those unable to cooperate will require sedation for acquired neuroimaging, which requires maintenance of blood pressure to optimize brain perfusion, particularly in the setting of flow-limiting arteriopathy.

MRA will reveal arteriopathy including stenosis and dissection in half to three-quarters of children with acute stroke,[3,7,41,42] but MRA cannot detect lesions in smaller arteries. Related imaging of the cerebral venous system is indicated if there are concerns about cerebral venous thrombosis. Vessel wall imaging is increasingly used in adults to evaluate the arterial wall itself, including for the presence of inflammation, rather than just the lumen as seen with MRA, CT angiography (CTA), and catheter angiograms, and is being used more often in children as well.

CTA of the head and neck can diagnose arteriopathy but requires sedation in the younger child and entails significant radiation exposure. For the latter reason, if a head MRA can be obtained, CTA may be avoided in some instances. If cerebral arteriopathy is strongly suspected despite a normal MRA, cerebral catheter angiography may be preferable to CTA due to greater sensitivity in diagnosing cerebral arteriopathy, particularly medium and small vessel arteriopathy.[43] It requires radiation and anesthesia; however, periprocedural complications are rare with experienced angiographers.[44] A cerebral catheter angiogram can be used for diagnosis of arteriopathy

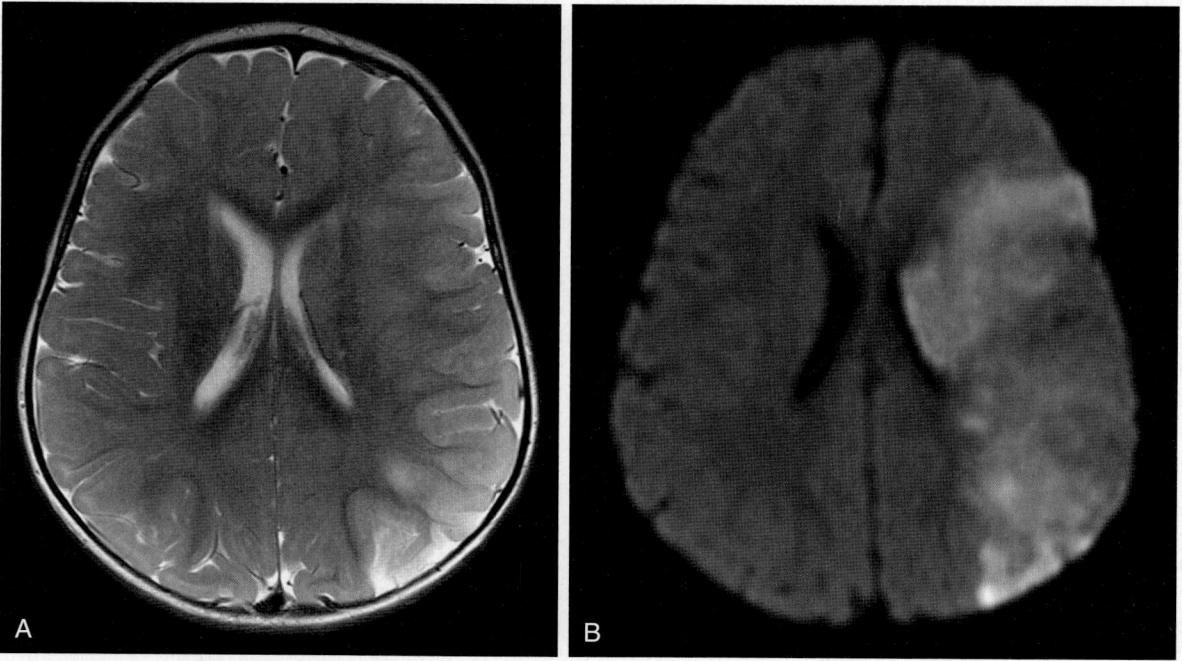

Fig. 69.2. Head MRI of a 1-year-old boy with acute onset of right-sided hemiplegia, with edema on T2 imaging (A) and restricted diffusion on DWI (B) in the left MCA territory.

as well as for mechanical thrombectomy, treatment of aneurysm, and other neurointerventions.

Even when hyperacute treatment is not being considered, diagnosis of underlying etiologies such as CCAD, cardiac embolus, and cerebral sinus venous thrombosis (CSVT) will modify immediate treatment. Cerebral arteriopathy is an important predictor of primary and recurrent arterial ischemic stroke in childhood, and depending on etiology, treatment with antithrombotic medications, immunosuppressive agents, and antiviral medication may be indicated.

Laboratory Evaluation

Initial laboratory studies include complete blood count (CBC), electrolytes, blood urea nitrogen (BUN), creatinine, glucose, prothrombin time (PT), partial thromboplastin time (PTT), international normalized ratio (INR), ESR, blood gas and type, and screen or cross-match if intracranial hemorrhage is suspected, the child has SCD, or thrombolysis or thrombectomy is being considered (Table 69.2). Initial laboratory studies are initiated in a child with possible acute stroke. If the child is on anticoagulation, studies to assess therapeutic range include low-molecular-weight heparin (LMWH) activity and anti-Xa for LMWH, PTT for unfractionated heparin (UFH), and PT/INR for warfarin. Tests to rule out a hypercoagulable state should also be included (Table 69.3).

Laboratory tests considered in childhood AIS do not need to be sent urgently when maintaining an optimal hematocrit is critical, and not all patients require exhaustive testing. Urgent evaluations may include screening for systemic inflammatory disease (ESR, CRP, antinuclear antibodies), and a lupus inhibitor screen, antiphospholipid panel, and pregnancy test. Lumbar puncture may be indicated if there are concerns about infection; however, this may need to be delayed until the risk of intracranial hypertension has passed. If a cardioembolic etiology is suspected, urgent echocardiogram is indicated.

TABLE 69.2 Initial Laboratory Studies in Child With Possible Acute Stroke

Complete blood count
Coagulation studies: PT, PTT, INR
For child on anticoagulation:
— Low-molecula-weight heparin (LMWH) activity and anti-Xa for LMWH — PT/INR for warfarin
Electrolyte panel
Glucose
ESR
Renal and liver function studies
If clinically indicated:
— Pregnancy test — Urine or serum toxicology — Blood gas
Type and screen or cross if intracranial hemorrhage is suspected, the child has sickle cell disease, or thrombolysis or thrombectomy is being considered

TABLE 69.3 Laboratory Tests Considered in Childhood Arterial Ischemic Stroke

Laboratory Tests	Caveat
Hemoglobin S percentage	If child has known or suspected sickle cell disease
Iron and total iron-binding capacity	Severe iron deficiency anemia is a risk factor for stroke
Antinuclear antibodies (ANA)[a]	If clinical concern about underlying rheumatologic disease
Rheumatoid factor[a]	If clinical concern about underlying rheumatologic disease
Antiphospholipid antibody studies	Includes anticardiolipin antibody IgM, IgG, and IgA; anti–beta-2 glycoprotein IgM, IgG, IgA; and lupus anticoagulant
Factor V Leiden (FVL) mutation[a]	Most common cause of activated protein C (APC) resistance; 3%-8% of people with European ancestry carry one copy of the mutation
Prothrombin gene mutation (factor II/G20210A)[a]	More common in Caucasian population
Protein C activity and antigen	Can be lowered by warfarin, vitamin K deficiency, liver disease, disseminated intravascular coagulation (DIC)
Protein S activity and free antigen	Can be lowered by warfarin, vitamin K deficiency, liver disease, DIC, pregnancy; only the free protein S is functional as a c-factor for protein C
Activated protein C resistance (APCR)[a]	Rarely indicated as FVL accounts for most cases of APC resistance
5,10-Methylene tetrahydrofolate reductase (MTHFR)[a]	Only needs to be sent if homocysteine is elevated
Prothrombin time (PT), activated partial thromboplastin time (aPTT), andinternational normalized ratio (INR)	PT and INR measure extrinsic pathway of coagulation; PTT measures intrinsic pathway of coagulation
Antithrombin III (AT III) activity	Heparin and direct thrombin inhibitors can affect results; AT III should be checked if a patient is requiring higher heparin doses than expected, as anti-Xa activity is dependent on patient's AT III level
D-Dimer	May reflect clot burden
C-reactive protein (CRP)	Acute phase reactant to inflammation
Erythrocyte sedimentation rate (ESR)	Nonspecific measure of inflammation
Homocysteine[a]	Fasting sample preferred
β-HCG (pregnancy test)	Strongly consider in any female of childbearing age
Toxicology screen	Cocaine, methamphetamine, other vasoactive drugs, and cannabis associated with stroke
Lipoprotein (a)[a]	Does not need to be a fasting sample

[a]Rarely indicated in the acute period.

Treatment

Initial management includes optimizing cerebral perfusion and preventing hypoxemia, rescuing and minimizing expansion of the penumbra, and preventing complications. Children with acute stroke should be admitted to the pediatric intensive care unit (PICU) for a minimum of 48 hours for neurologic and medical monitoring and aggressive management of complications. Neurologic status should be followed by the bedside nurse (hourly pediatric Glasgow Coma Scale and pupils until stable) as well as by medical staff. Ideally, the pediatric NIHSS[39] should be used to serially assess the patient. Urgent neuroimaging should be obtained for any neurologic deterioration.

Supportive Therapy

For the most part, therapy for childhood stroke is based on extrapolation from adult-based guidelines. Endotracheal intubation and mechanical ventilation are indicated for children with inadequate oxygenation or respiratory drive or an inability to protect their airway and may be needed to facilitate diagnostic or therapeutic procedures. Keeping the head of the bed flat may optimize cerebral perfusion. Blood pressure should be maintained with careful attention to adequate blood volume to avoid hypotension. Many children have transient hypertension following stroke, possibly representing a compensatory mechanism to maintain CBF, and permissive hypertension is usually recommended. If hypertension requires treatment, blood pressure should be lowered cautiously with close attention to worsening of neurologic status. Clinical and electrographic seizures should be treated, but there are no data to support seizure prophylaxis with antiepileptic medications. Fever should be treated aggressively to decrease metabolic demands on the brain. Cooling blankets should not be used in patients with sickle cell anemia.

Thrombolysis

There are minimal data on the use of tPA in acute childhood stroke, and currently the American Heart Association (AHA) recommends against the use of tPA in younger children outside of a clinical trial.[45] Due to the challenge of determining time of stroke onset and limitations of extrapolation from adult data to very young children, tPA for AIS should be used with great caution in children younger than 2 years of age and avoided in neonates. For older children and adolescents, data on safety and efficacy are limited, but tPA could be considered in selected patients. Published consensus-based guidelines and safety monitoring recommendations exist.[37]

Endovascular/Neurosurgical Treatment

If the patient was last seen at baseline within 6 hours and MRA or CTA shows occlusion in the internal carotid or M1 segment of the middle cerebral artery (MCA) or the vertebral and basilar artery, thrombectomy could be considered, particularly in an older adolescent. Although not approved by the Food and Drug Administration for use in children, studies of the safety and efficacy of mechanical thrombectomy in adults have been promising.[46-48] This procedure should be approached with caution, including full disclosure of the lack of data in children, and should only be performed by neuro-interventionalists or interventional radiologists with pediatric experience. Urgent neurosurgical consultation for possible decompressive hemicraniectomy should be obtained promptly in children with malignant middle cerebral artery infarct (Fig. 69.3). Suboccipital craniectomy with dural expansion should be considered in patients with neurologic deterioration due to edema from cerebellar infarction. In malignant infarction, monitoring of intracranial pressure (ICP) has not been shown to be helpful and may delay surgical treatment in these patients.

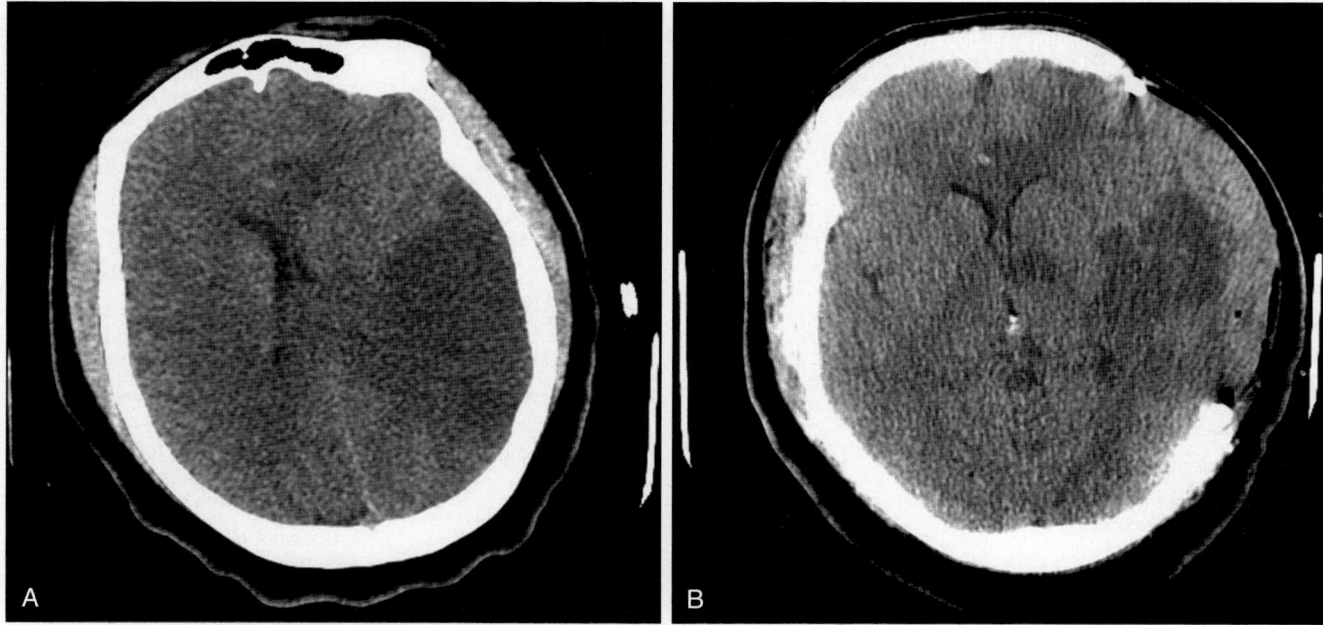

Fig. 69.3. Head CT of a 17-year-old girl with complete left middle cerebral infarct prior to (A) and following (B) decompressive hemicraniectomy.

Antithrombotic Therapy

A full review of the use of antithrombotic therapies in children is available in the *Chest* guidelines.[15] Anticoagulation is typically used in children with acute AIS without hemorrhage pending complete workup of potential etiologies to prevent recurrent stroke, which can occur early, particularly in the setting of dissection or cardioembolic stroke. Anticoagulation is usually initially achieved with continuous intravenous heparin, which can be reversed if necessary by protamine or fresh frozen plasma, with transition to LMWH when the child is stable. LMWH has more predictable pharmacokinetics and reduces the risk of heparin-induced thrombocytopenia, a serious antibody-mediated complication of heparin[49]; however, it cannot be reversed rapidly and has renal clearance, necessitating dosage adjustment in the setting of impaired renal function. For long-term anticoagulation, LMWH or warfarin is used. Warfarin has difficult-to-manage pharmacokinetics, and oftentimes LMWH is the anticoagulant of choice, despite the need for subcutaneous injection. Newer anticoagulants are currently being studied to treat adult stroke but have not been used widely in cases of pediatric stroke. Anticoagulation is usually continued in children with presumed cardioembolic stroke, significant thrombophilic states such as antiphospholipid syndrome, and cervical artery dissection.[15,45]

Aspirin inhibits platelet activity by irreversibly inhibiting cyclooxygenase-1 and is used based on consensus for stroke prevention in children not felt to require anticoagulation. A dose of 3 to 5 mg/kg/day is recommended acutely after contraindications such as ICH have been excluded.[45] Aspirin is often used for long-term stroke prophylaxis in children as well; however, optimal doses and duration are unknown. The doses used for stroke prophylaxis are less than those associated with Reye syndrome[50] (Table 69.4).

Cerebral Sinus Venous Thrombosis

Cerebral sinus venous thrombosis (CSVT) occurs when thrombosis is present in the major venous sinuses draining the brain. Headache is the most common presenting symptom of CSVT. CSVT can result from multiple processes including venous stasis, hypercoagulable state, dehydration, and direct damage to the vessel wall in the venous system, which has slower blood flow. CSVT can involve the dural venous sinuses (superior sagittal, transverse, or sigmoid sinus), deep venous system (internal cerebral veins), or cortical dural veins. Multiple sinuses are involved in most children, with the transverse sinus most commonly affected followed by the sagittal sinus.[51] Potential complications due to CSVT include venous infarction, which occurs secondary to venous outflow obstruction, intracranial hypertension, cranial nerve palsies, and cerebral hemorrhage.

The incidence of CSVT in children age 1 month to 18 years is approximately 0.4/100,000/year,[52] although with advances in neuroimaging, this reported incidence may rise. Children with CSVT often present with nonspecific findings such as headache, seizures, increased ICP, and lethargy, although localizing signs such as cranial nerve palsies and hemiparesis may be present.

Etiologies and Risk Factors

Most children with CSVT have underlying risk factors identified, and multiple risk factors are often present.[51-57]

TABLE 69.4	Published Guidelines for Antithrombotic Treatment of Childhood Acute Arterial Ischemic Stroke	
Indication	American College of Chest Physicians (ACCP) guidelines, 2012[15]	American Heart Association Guidelines for Management of Stroke in Infants and Children, 2008[45]
Initial treatment	UFH or LMWH or aspirin 1–5 mg/day until cardiac etiology or arterial dissection ruled out	UFH or LMWH until etiology determined; aspirin 3–5 mg/kg/day for children without known risk of recurrent embolism or severe hypercoagulable disorder
Cardiac embolism with risk of recurrence (excluding native valve endocarditis)	LMWH	UFH or LMWH
Extracranial cervicocephalic arterial dissection	LMWH	UFH or LMWH
Sickle cell disease	Exchange transfusion with goal HbS <30%	Exchange transfusion and hydration
Intravenous tPA	Not recommended for children outside of research protocol	Generally not recommended outside of a clinical trial

Prothrombotic disorders are found in approximately half of children with CSVT.[52,53,57,58] The AHA guidelines note that children with CSVT may benefit from thrombophilia screening, which may impact care decisions (class IIb, level of evidence C).[45] Laboratory studies should be directed based on the medical history, and a family history of thrombophilia and thrombosis should be obtained. An abbreviated thrombophilia screen may be adequate in children with triggered CSVT, for example, following surgery involving the dural sinuses or following head trauma (Table 69.5).

Neuroimaging

CSVT can be seen in some cases on CT scan and in particular contrast-enhanced CT scan; however, the sensitivity is poor. A clot may be visible on a nonenhanced CT scan as a dense clot sign. The delta sign, a triangular area of high contrast enhancement with a low attenuating center, may be present on enhanced CT scan. This is best seen with sagittal sinus thrombosis. CT venography is sensitive for CSV\T but requires radiation and does not assess parenchyma well for venous congestion or infarct.

Head MRI and magnetic resonance venography (MRV) are the preferred diagnostic modalities. MRI is the best modality to detect associated parenchymal abnormalities. The head MRI and MRV should be ordered with and without contrast, with the caveat that contrast is not needed if the radiologist is satisfied with the noncontrast images. Contrast may be particularly helpful in borderline or unusual cases or with suspected infection as the etiology. Rarely, a high-resolution CT venography or catheter angiogram will be indicated.

| TABLE 69.5 | Risk Factors Reported in Pediatric Cerebral Sinus Venous Thrombosis |

Inherited Thrombophilias
G20210A mutation[54]

Factor V Leiden[54,66]

Protein C deficiency[54,66]

Protein S deficiency[54,119]

Antithrombin III deficiency[53,54,66]

Homocysteine[120,121]

Acquired Thrombophilias
Asparaginase[52,57,122]

Exogenous estrogen[52,123]

Infection[51,53]
Sinusitis[57]

Otitis media[51]

Mastoiditis[51,66]

Lemierre syndrome[124]

Primary varicella[57]

Autoimmune/Inflammatory Disorders
Systemic lupus erythematosus[51,52]

Inflammatory bowel disease[57,125]

Celiac disease[126]

Antiphospholipid antibodies[52,53,119]

Lupus anticoagulant[54]

Behçet disease[127]

Acute Illness[52]
Dehydration[52,53,66]

Chronic Illness[52]
Nephrotic syndrome[51,52,128]

Anemia[53]

Hematologic malignancy[51,129]

Obesity[130]

Other
Sickle cell disease[51,53]

Head trauma[131]

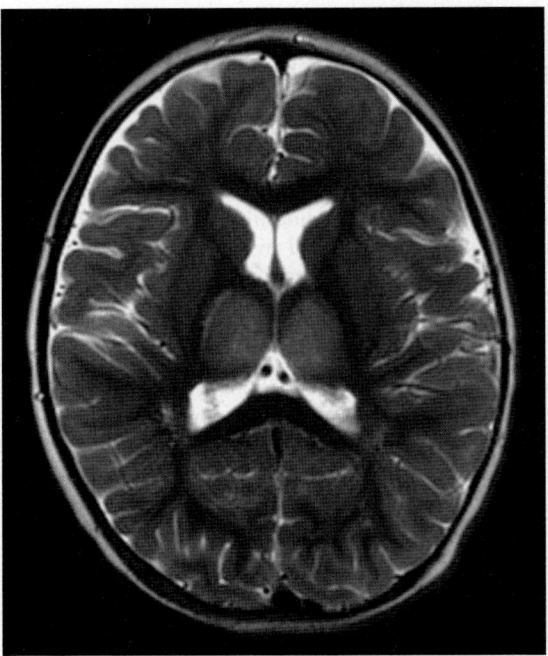

Fig. 69.4. A 15-month-old boy with a week of irritability who presents with a generalized tonic-clonic seizure followed by sleepiness with extensive thrombosis of the inferior sagittal sinus, straight sinus, internal cerebral veins, and vein of Galen. Laboratory studies showed severe iron deficiency (hemoglobin 6.2 g/dL, microcytic anemia, and high total iron-binding capacity). There is symmetric T2 hyperintensity within the bilateral thalami associated with involvement of the deep venous system.

Laboratory Evaluation

Initial laboratory studies include CBC, electrolytes, BUN, creatinine, glucose, PT/PTT, ESR, and antithrombin III activity in preparation for possible heparin administration, as well as a pregnancy test in females of childbearing age. Urgency of evaluation for risk factors for CSVT will be determined by history and presentation.

Treatment

Supportive measures include adequate ventilation, hydration, treatment of infection if indicated, and control of seizures. Children with CSVT may rapidly progress to obtundation, particularly when the deep venous system is involved (Fig. 69.4), and even death. Signs and symptoms of infection of the head and neck should be sought and broad-spectrum antibiotics started when appropriate. Seizures have been reported in over half of children with CSVT.[52] Children with acute symptomatic CSVT should be cared for in the PICU, particularly while anticoagulation is being initiated.

Both UFH and LMWH are recommended in adults with CSVT.[59] With close monitoring, UFH and LMWH can be administered to children, and this likely improves outcome.[60-63] Recommendation from the International Paediatric Stroke Study (IPSS) group is that older children without hemorrhage should receive anticoagulation. In a single-center study, worse clinical outcome and propagation of thrombus were associated with a lack of anticoagulation. Hemorrhagic complications were relatively rare (5%); however, children with "significant intracranial hemorrhage" were excluded from anticoagulation treatment[62] (Table 69.6).

Thrombolysis, thrombectomy, or surgical decompression may be considered in children with severe CSVT in whom there is no improvement with UFH.[15] Studies of thrombolysis and thrombectomy for CSVT have not been performed but case reports and series exist, particularly of children who are comatose or have declining mental status.[55,64]

Many patients with CSVT have increased intracranial pressure and are at risk for vision loss.[53] Lumbar puncture is the most effective way to lower ICP; however, this option requires interruption of anticoagulation to decrease the risk of bleeding.

Prognosis

The mortality following CSVT in childhood is approximately 4% to 7%,[51,65] and CSVT is frequently associated with long-term neurologic sequelae.[66] Recurrence has been reported in

TABLE 69.6	Guideline for Anticoagulation in Cerebral Sinus Venous Thrombosis	
Guideline	**Population**	**Recommendation**
American College of Chest Physicians (ACCP) guidelines, 2012[15]	Children	Initial UFH or LMWH, then LMWH or vitamin K antagonist for minimum 3 months plus another 3 months if occlusion persists or symptoms ongoing. For children with CSVT with significant hemorrhage, anticoagulation as above or follow-up neuroimaging at 5-7 days and anticoagulation if thrombus propagation has occurred.
American Heart Association Guidelines for Management of Stroke in Infants and Children, 2008[45]	Children	Consider initial UFH or LMWH followed by warfarin for 3-6 months, whether or not intracranial hemorrhage is present.
Diagnosis and Management of Cerebral Venous Thrombosis, AHA, 2011[59]	Adults	Initial UFH or LMWH in full anticoagulant doses is reasonable, followed by vitamin K antagonists, regardless of the presence of ICH. With provoked CSVT, vitamin K antagonists may be continued for 3-6 months. With unprovoked CVT, vitamin K antagonists may be continued for 6-12 months.

TABLE 69.7	Spetzler-Martin Grading Scale for Arteriovenous Malformations

Size 0-3 cm: 0 points
Size 3-6 cm: 1point
>6 cm: 2 points
Eloquent (yes = 1, no = 0)
Deep drainage (yes = 1, superficial only = 0)
Grades 1-3 generally considered operative

6% of children following CSVT at an average follow-up of 36 months. Predictors of recurrence included persistent occlusion from CSVT, presence of heterozygosity for G20210A mutation, lack of anticoagulant therapy, and initial thrombosis occurring after 2 years of age.[60]

Vision loss can occur due to elevated ICP after CSVT,[53] and accordingly ophthalmology follow-up is warranted. Children with ongoing thrombophilia are at increased risk of recurrent pathologic thrombosis, particularly with triggers such as immobilization, pregnancy and puerperium, prolonged plane travel, and oral contraceptive use; preventive precautions should be discussed with the patient and family. Recurrent thrombosis can occur in the absence of identified thrombophilia as well.[60]

Spontaneous Intracranial Hemorrhage

Although spontaneous ICH, or hemorrhagic stroke, accounts for less than 20% of strokes in adults, it accounts for almost half of all pediatric stroke.[67-69] Spontaneous ICH includes intraparenchymal hemorrhage accounting for approximately 75% of cases,[68] intraventricular hemorrhage (IVH), and subarachnoid hemorrhage (SAH) of nontraumatic origin. Following ICH, approximately 10% to 25% of children will die,[70,71] and over 70% will have neurologic deficits.[72]

The three most common vascular malformations of the CNS are arteriovenous malformations (AVMs), cerebral cavernous malformations (CMs), and venous malformations.

AVMs account for approximately half of intraparenchymal ICH.[64,67] CMs account for approximately one-quarter of ICH, with higher numbers found in later studies that included MRI assessment. Other vascular malformations, brain tumors, and coagulation defects (thrombocytopenia, hemophilia, hepatic failure, anticoagulation) account for most of the remaining cases of spontaneous ICH in childhood.

Arteriovenous Malformations

AVMs are abnormal tangles of vessels (Fig. 69.5) that connect arteries directly to veins, resulting in abnormally high flow and pressures in vessels with weak walls. This disrupts normal blood flow and leads to hemorrhage and the formation of aneurysms. Eighty percent of AVMs are supratentorial, and three-quarters of those that become symptomatic present with ICH. Children with ruptured AVMs present with altered mental status including coma and seizures. Multiple AVMs are more common in children than adults and suggest hereditary hemorrhagic telangiectasia (Osler-Weber-Rendu),[73] familial AVMs, and Wyburn-Mason syndrome. Vein of Galen malformation is a distinct AVM that appears in newborns and is associated with congestive heart failure due to left-to-right cardiovascular shunting.

The risk of hemorrhage in children with known AVMs is 2% to 4% per year, and 25% of the hemorrhages are fatal.[74-76] Although children have a lower annual risk of hemorrhage than adults, they have a greater lifetime risk. Although AVMs are traditionally considered to be congenital without the potential for growth, recurrence of AVM has been reported in children following complete obliteration, and long-term follow-up is indicated.[77] Larger AVMs may be less likely to hemorrhage than small AVMs, perhaps because of increased pressure in the smaller malformations.[78-80] As AVMs are often diagnosed at the time of hemorrhage, there may be a bias toward diagnosis of lesions with a higher incidence of hemorrhage. The incidentally found AVM may have a different natural history, but there are insufficient data to make this determination.[81]

MRI will demonstrate AVMs, and cerebral catheter angiograms will establish the arteriovenous shunt, as well as feed arteries and drain veins. The Spetzler-Martin grading system accounts for size, involvement of eloquent brain, and pattern of venous drainage.[82] AVMs under 3 cm in maximal diameter, with superficial drainage and away from critical areas (eg, language, motor, and visual areas), have the lowest risk associated with intervention and the best overall prognosis (Table 69.7). When possible, AVMs should be treated with total surgical resection. The annual risk of rebleeding following AVM hemorrhage is 20% in children, approximately fourfold the risk in adults.[83] Deep-seated AVMs and AVMs with a recent (5-year) history of hemorrhage are at higher risk of bleeding.[81]

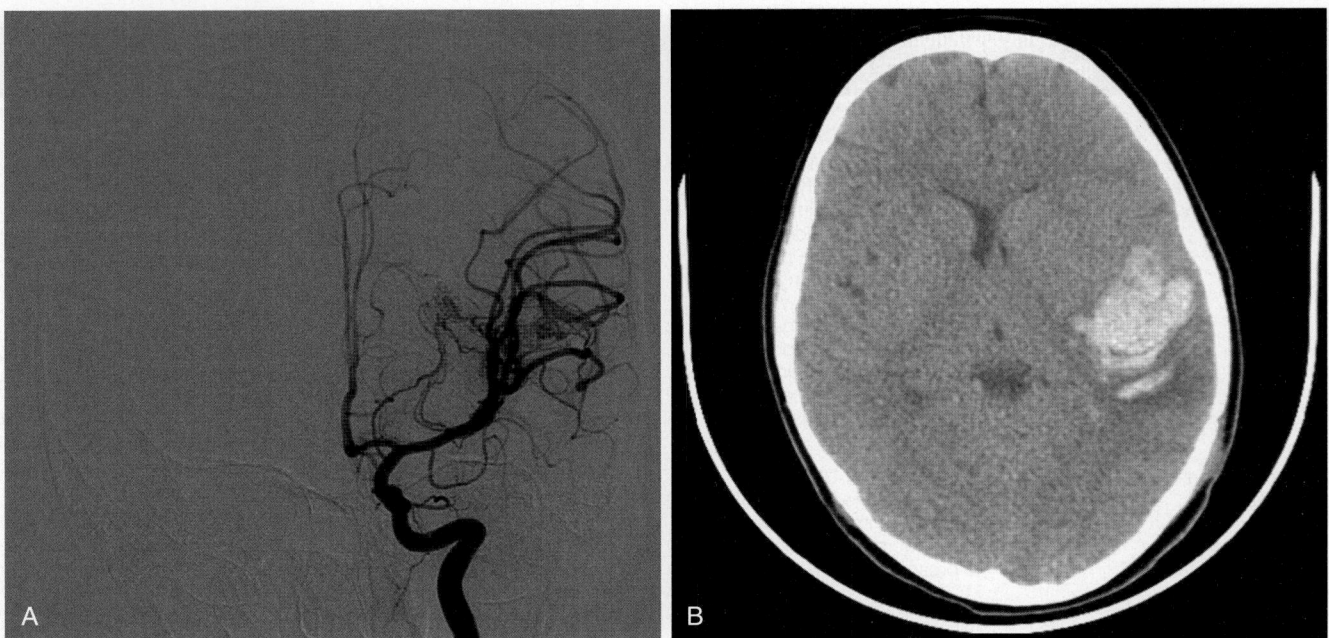

Fig. 69.5. A 7-year-old girl had presented with a small hemorrhage. A sylvian fissure AVM is seen on left carotid injection during conventional cerebral angiogram (A). Head CT shows a large hemorrhage requiring emergent evacuation 1 month following the initial angiogram (B). A small residual was treated with radiosurgery, and the lesion is obliterated at 10-year follow-up.

Surgical treatment is associated with a very high success rate but is not universally curative. A series[84] of pediatric AVMs resected surgically found about a 1% recurrence at 5 years suggesting some degree of postoperative surveillance is warranted.

Partial treatment with embolization does not decrease risk of hemorrhage.[85] Complete obliteration with embolization is not possible, but embolization has been used as an option to reduce the size prior to surgical resection or radiosurgery. Gamma knife has been used to treat pediatric AVM with an obliteration rate of 71.3% after one treatment and 62.5% for patients requiring another treatment. The mean time to obliteration was 32.4 and 79.6 months, respectively.[86] AVMs with a nidus diameter less than 2.5 cm and with a single draining vein were most likely to respond completely to radiosurgery,[87] but these same characteristics also predispose to a favorable outcome with microsurgical resection. Ischemic changes presenting as clinical stroke at the site of radiation can occur following radiation.

Aneurysms

Aneurysms account for 10% of hemorrhagic strokes in childhood[88] and usually have symptomatic onset in children younger than 2 years or older than 10 years of age.[89] Ruptured aneurysms usually present with SAH but can present with IVH or intraparenchymal hemorrhage. The most common location for aneurysm in children is a saccular aneurysm at the internal carotid artery bifurcation followed by the middle cerebral artery bifurcation.[90] Infants and children are more likely than adults to have giant aneurysms and posterior circulation involvement, and they are less likely to have aneurysms of the anterior communicating artery and posterior communicating artery,[91] although most giant aneurysms in infants involve the middle cerebral artery.[92] Approximately 5%

of children with aneurysms have multiple aneurysms, as opposed to 20% in adults.

There are multiple genetic disorders associated with the development of aneurysms, including coarctation of the aorta,[93,94] fibromuscular dysplasia,[95,96] Ehlers-Danlos syndrome,[97] pseudoxanthoma elasticum,[98] autosomal dominant polycystic kidney disease, and a family history of aneurysms. Aneurysms can also be associated with AVMs[99,100] and can form following radiation for pediatric brain tumors and AVMs.

Intracerebral locations, as opposed to SAH, suggest an aneurysm due to infection, or mycotic aneurysms. Infective endocarditis, meningitis, chronic pulmonary infection, and intravenous drug use are commonly predisposing infections. Mycotic aneurysms tend to be more distal and are often multiple.

Cerebral catheter angiography is the study of choice for cerebral aneurysms, although CTA is often the initial imaging study performed with head CT on presentation, and it may be useful in emergency situations when urgent operative decompression of the hemorrhage is needed. Head MRI and MRA can be used for screening of aneurysms but are less sensitive than angiography, which provides more detail of the vascular anatomy.[101] Cerebral catheter angiography can be diagnostic and preparatory for endovascular treatment as well.

The annual risk of aneurysmal rupture is estimated at 0.1% to 8%, with larger aneurysms at higher risk. In patients with unruptured aneurysm, symptoms can be related to expanding size. Common symptoms include third nerve palsy, afferent pupillary defect, and other cranial nerve deficits, depending on the location of the aneurysm.

Frank rupture of an aneurysm results in catastrophic ICH, with sudden severe headache, altered mental status, nausea and vomiting, and loss of consciousness. The mortality rate in children following aneurysmal rupture is 20%.[102] Some patients will have a recent history of *sentinel bleed* with a severe headache. The sudden onset of severe headache requires a neuroimaging evaluation for possible SAH. The most common complication following SAH is cerebral vasospasm resulting in ischemic stroke. Vasospasm usually presents within 5 to 10 days following the hemorrhage but can present for up to 2 weeks. In adults, euvolemia and nimodipine, a calcium channel blocker, are recommended following aneurysmal SAH to prevent delayed cerebral ischemia, with induction of hypertension if delayed cerebral ischemia has occurred.[103] Nimodipine and Pravachol have been used together to prevent or minimize vasospasm. Hypervolemia using intravenous fluids has not been shown to be effective in preventing vasospasm, and currently maintaining patients in a euvolemic state is recommended, with hypovolemia carefully avoided. Hypertension may be useful in treating symptomatic vasospasm. Approximately one-third of patients will exhibit cerebral salt wasting and as such, serum sodium should be monitored. Hydrocephalus is common and CSF diversion often necessary.

As recurrent hemorrhage from a ruptured aneurysm is a frequent and early event, with 15% of adults suffering a recurrent hemorrhage in the first 24 hours,[104] treatment of the aneurysm must be prompt. Options for treatment include endovascular therapy, ligation, and clip placement. Long-term follow-up is indicated, as over 40% of children with aneurysms will develop new aneurysms later in life.[105] For adults, the 10-year risk of SAH in a patient with one first-degree relative with SAH was 0.8%, and with two first-degree relatives the risk was 7.1%.[106] The risk to other family members of children with nonsyndromic aneurysms is unknown.

Cavernous Malformations

Cerebral CMs are vascular malformations with thin-walled sinusoidal spaces lined with endothelial tissue without intervening parenchyma, often containing calcifications. CMs cause approximately one-fifth of ICH in childhood.[67,107] For untreated CMs, the risk of recurrent hemorrhage is 4% to 5% per year. CMs occur in approximately 1 in 200 adults and account for approximately 10% of vascular malformations of the CNS. Most occur in the brain, usually supratentorially, although infratentorial and brain stem involvement can occur. Less frequently, the spinal cord is involved. There is no arteriovenous shunting, so the degree of hemorrhage tends to be smaller than with AVMs, often with hemosiderin staining in the absence of a clinical hemorrhage.

Most CMs are asymptomatic with 20% to 30% of patients having symptoms. CM can present with headache, seizures, focal neurologic deficit, and hemorrhage. Seizures are the most common presenting symptom, especially with involvement of the frontal and temporal lobes (Fig. 69.6). CMs often increase in size over time, with a progressing and regressing course due to resorption of blood and reorganization followed by recurrent hemorrhage. Although CMs are low-flow lesions, severe hemorrhage can occur. One study of patients age 25 years and younger found that the hemorrhage rate was 1.6% per patient-year and 0.9% per cavernoma-year. The hemorrhage rate in the symptomatic group was 8% annually and 0.2% in the asymptomatic group where CM was found incidentally.[108] In a series of 292 patients diagnosed at age 3.5 to 88.9 years (mean 45.8 years), 74 presented with hemorrhage. The annual risk of hemorrhage in patients presenting with

hemorrhage was 6.2%, with risk decreasing over time. The risk of hemorrhage increased in the setting of multiple CMs.[109]

CM can be either familial or sporadic, and the incidence of CM on imaging increases during childhood with age. Multiple CMs occur in 13% of sporadic cases and half of familial cases,[110] with greater number of lesions predicting familial CM. Multiple genetic mutations have been associated with familial CM, including CCM1/KRIT1, CCM2/MGC4607, and CCM3/PDCD10, accounting for three-fourths or more of families.[111] In one series of 92 children with CM, 30% had multiple CMs and 9% had a family history of CMs.[108] In another series of 66 children with CM, 7 (11%) had multiple CMs.[112]

On MRI, CMs are described as having a popcorn appearance due to the mixture of high and low T1 and T2 signal surrounded by hemosiderin from chronic, recurrent hemorrhage. Findings on CT are nonspecific, and CMs are not detectable on catheter angiography. CMs can be associated with the developmental venous anomalies that are seen on angiography, however.

If complete resection of a particular CM lesion is possible, this is curative. Most patients with symptomatic localization epilepsy associated with the CM will be seizure free following resection as well, especially if the associated hemosiderin rim is also removed (see Fig. 69.5). Functional considerations may limit surgery or define the surgical approach. Preoperative assessment may include functional MRI or other mapping tools if the location is suspected to be near the motor or language cortex. Such mapping tools are possible in patients as young as age 5 or 6 years.[113]

Resection is not always an option and can be associated with increased neurologic deficit. Brain stem CMs in childhood are particularly problematic, as they tend to be larger with a higher rate of recurrence following incomplete resection than seen in adults.[114] Radiosurgery has been considered for patients in whom surgery is not an option. Radiosurgery does not appear to be curative and can be associated with significant complications. The adaptation of stereotactic laser ablation has also been applied to the treatment of CMs, though the experience with this approach is extremely limited to date.[115]

The risk of intervention needs to be balanced against the risk with natural history. A posterior fossa CM is associated with a greater risk of hemorrhage, as well as rebleeding, than other locations. Brain stem CMs are high risk if untreated, although surgical resection is also high risk in this location, often requiring skull base approaches to access the lesion where it comes to the surface. Surgical management of patients with multiple lesions, particular familial CM where lesions may be numerous, is possible if the symptomatic lesion is identified and resectable. In these cases, risk of recurrence, or of a new lesion arising in adjacent or distant areas, is possible (see Fig. 69.6C).

Genetic screening for patients with familial CM has been debated and currently identified genes account for 96% of familial cases. Nevertheless, if a causative gene is found in a pedigree, this could be used to screen other family members. Family members of patients with CM should be imaged if there are any symptoms causing a concern for CM such as headache, seizures, or neurologic deficit.

Symptomatic epilepsy will need appropriate antiepileptic treatment. Seizures may be medically refractory or intractable. Follow-up MR imaging should be pursued every 1 to 2 years to assess for growth or hemorrhage of the CM.

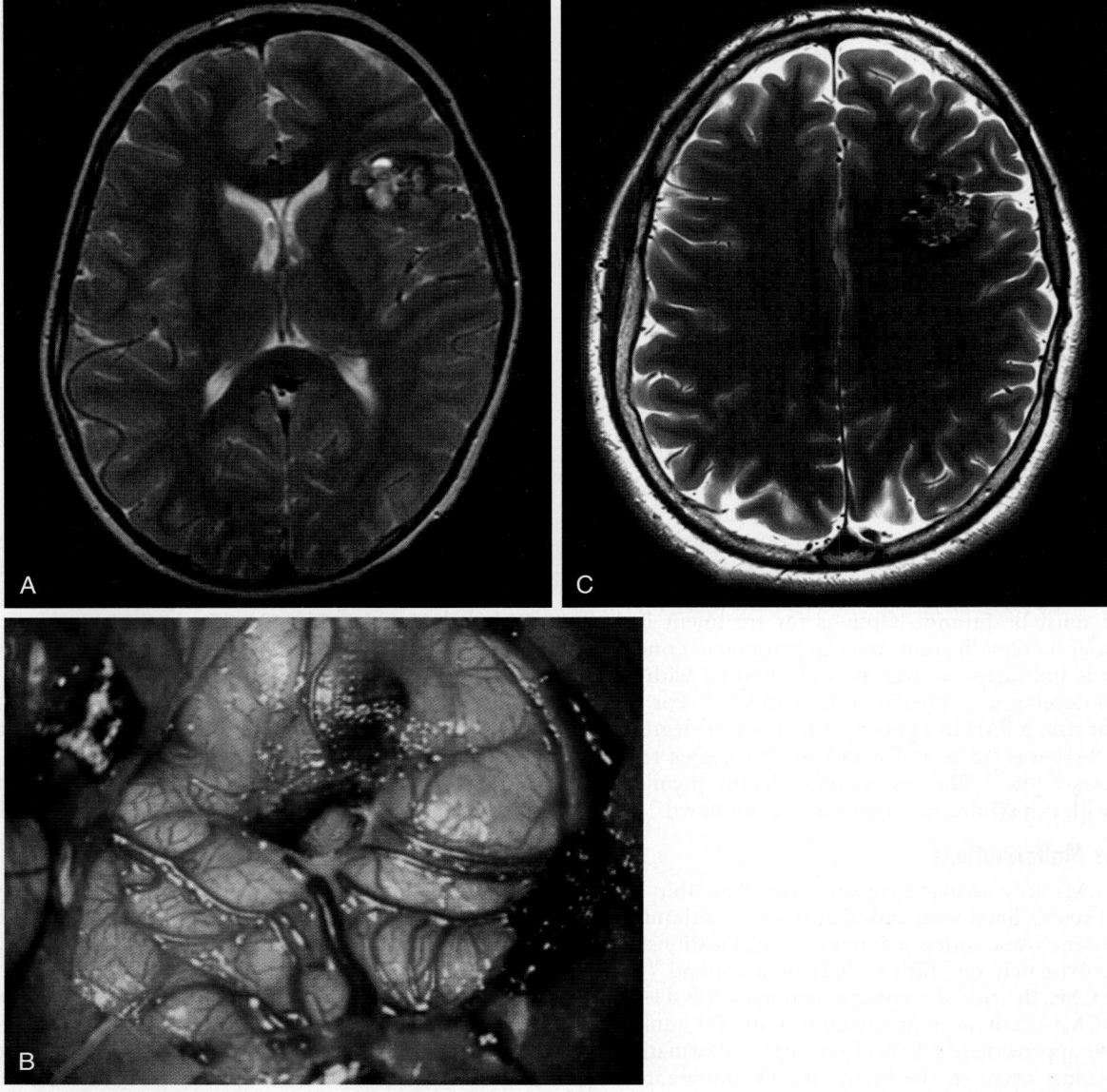

Fig. 69.6. A left frontal cavernous malformation (A) was resected in an 8-year-old with intractable focal motor seizures, resulting in 10 years of seizure freedom. The lesion was entered from within the sulcus (B). Seizures recurred in the setting of a new lesion superior to the first (C) along with a new lesion in the right cerebellum (not shown).

Coagulation Disorders

Hemophilia A and B can result in spontaneous ICH, as can severe thrombocytopenia and coagulopathy due to liver failure. ICH associated with vitamin K deficiency occurs in infants who do not receive vitamin K prophylaxis at birth due to omission or parental choice.[116] Late ICH associated with vitamin K deficiency peaks at 3 to 8 weeks and can be catastrophic.[117]

General Care of the Child With Intracerebral Hemorrhage

A child with ICH can present with emesis, severe headache, seizures, and declining mental status, and children with ICH can deteriorate rapidly to coma and death. Rapid

diagnosis and stabilization of the child with ICH is critical. Head CT can detect ICH as well as mass effect and impending herniation. A CBC, coagulation profile and type and hold or cross should be sent. Initial stabilization will include ensuring control of the airway and ventilation, treatment of seizures with antiepileptic drugs, and prevention of fever. Specific coagulopathy should be identified and corrected.

Urgent evacuation of hemorrhage may be indicated, as well as decompressive hemicraniectomy. Management of elevated ICP may include hyperosmolar therapy such as mannitol or hypertonic saline, hyperventilation for induced hypocapnia and cerebral vasoconstriction, and elevation of the head of the bed up to 30 degrees. A ventriculostomy drain allows drainage of CSF as well as ICP monitoring and is indicated in the setting of obstructive hydrocephalus as a consequence of IVH.

Prognosis

Prognosis following ICH depends on the etiology and severity of the initial hemorrhage, risk of recurrence, and morbidity associated with treatment of the underlying lesion. A study of 56 children followed for a mean of a decade after ICH found that 13 children died acutely, 9 suffered recurrent hemorrhage (which was fatal in 3 children), and only a quarter of the survivors were without neurologic or cognitive deficit.[118]

Conclusion

Childhood stroke, including AIS, CSVT, and ICH, is a significant cause of childhood morbidity and mortality. Children presenting with acute stroke require intensive care to address urgent management, supportive care, neuroprotection, and prevention of early recurrence and complications.

Key References

3. Fullerton HJ, Wu YW, Sidney S, Johnston SC. Risk of recurrent childhood arterial ischemic stroke in a population-based cohort: the importance of cerebrovascular imaging. *Pediatrics*. 2007;119:495-501.
4. Mackay MT, Wiznitzer M, Benedict SL, et al. Arterial ischemic stroke risk factors: the International Pediatric Stroke Study. *Ann Neurol*. 2011;69:130-140.
5. Wintermark M, Hills NK, deVeber GA, et al. Arteriopathy diagnosis in childhood arterial ischemic stroke: results of the vascular effects of infection in pediatric stroke study. *Stroke*. 2014;45:3597-3605.
14. Rafay MF, Armstrong D, Deveber G, et al. Craniocervical arterial dissection in children: clinical and radiographic presentation and outcome. *J Child Neurol*. 2006;21:8-16.
15. Monagle P, Chan AK, Goldenberg NA, et al. Antithrombotic therapy in neonates and children: Antithrombotic Therapy and Prevention of Thrombosis, 9th ed: American College of Chest Physicians Evidence-Based Clinical Practice Guidelines. *Chest*. 2012;141:e737S-801S.
16. Kernan WN, Ovbiagele B, Black HR, et al. Guidelines for the prevention of stroke in patients with stroke and transient ischemic attack: a guideline for healthcare professionals from the American Heart Association/American Stroke Association. *Stroke*. 2014;45:2160-2236.
17. Vanakker OM, Hemelsoet D, De Paepe A. Hereditary connective tissue diseases in young adult stroke: a comprehensive synthesis. *Stroke Res Treat*. 2011;2011:712903.
18. Moharir M, Shroff M, Benseler SM. Childhood central nervous system vasculitis. *Neuroimaging Clin N Am*. 2013;23:293-308.
22. Nagel MA, Cohrs RJ, Mahalingam R, et al. The varicella zoster virus vasculopathies: clinical, CSF, imaging, and virologic features. *Neurology*. 2008;70:853-860.
23. Sebire G, Meyer L, Chabrier S. Varicella as a risk factor for cerebral infarction in childhood: a case-control study. *Ann Neurol*. 1999;45:679-680.
24. Gilden DH, Kleinschmidt-DeMasters BK, LaGuardia JJ, et al. Neurologic complications of the reactivation of varicella-zoster virus. *N Engl J Med*. 2000;342:635-645.
25. Ohene-Frempong K, Weiner SJ, Sleeper LA, et al. Cerebrovascular accidents in sickle cell disease: rates and risk factors. *Blood*. 1998;91:288-294.
26. Adams RJ, McKie VC, Hsu L, et al. Prevention of a first stroke by transfusions in children with sickle cell anemia and abnormal results on transcranial Doppler ultrasonography. *N Engl J Med*. 1998;339:5-11.
30. Hulbert ML, McKinstry RC, Lacey JL, et al. Silent cerebral infarcts occur despite regular blood transfusion therapy after first strokes in children with sickle cell disease. *Blood*. 2011;117:772-779.
32. Miller ST, Macklin EA, Pegelow CH, et al. Silent infarction as a risk factor for overt stroke in children with sickle cell anemia: a report from the Cooperative Study of Sickle Cell Disease. *J Pediatr*. 2001;139:385-390.
34. Strater R, Vielhaber H, Kassenbohmer R, et al. Genetic risk factors of thrombophilia in ischaemic childhood stroke of cardiac origin. A prospective ESPED survey. *Eur J Pediatr*. 1999;158(suppl 3):S122-S125.

37. Rivkin MJ, deVeber G, Ichord RN, et al. Thrombolysis in pediatric stroke study. *Stroke*. 2015;46:880-885.
39. Ichord RN, Bastian R, Abraham L, et al. Interrater reliability of the Pediatric National Institutes of Health Stroke Scale (PedNIHSS) in a multicenter study. *Stroke*. 2011;42:613-617.
42. Buerki S, Roellin K, Remonda L, et al. Neuroimaging in childhood arterial ischaemic stroke: evaluation of imaging modalities and aetiologies. *Dev Med Child Neurol*. 2010;52:1033-1037.
43. Husson B, Lasjaunias P. Radiological approach to disorders of arterial brain vessels associated with childhood arterial stroke-a comparison between MRA and contrast angiography. *Pediatr Radiol*. 2004;34:10-15.
45. Roach ES, Golomb MR, Adams R, et al. Management of stroke in infants and children: a scientific statement from a Special Writing Group of the American Heart Association Stroke Council and the Council on Cardiovascular Disease in the Young. *Stroke*. 2008;39:2644-2691.
51. Wasay M, Dai AI, Ansari M, et al. Cerebral venous sinus thrombosis in children: a multicenter cohort from the United States. *J Child Neurol*. 2008;23:26-31.
53. Sebire G, Tabarki B, Saunders DE, et al. Cerebral venous sinus thrombosis in children: risk factors, presentation, diagnosis and outcome. *Brain*. 2005;128:477-489.
54. Kenet G, Lutkhoff LK, Albisetti M, et al. Impact of thrombophilia on risk of arterial ischemic stroke or cerebral sinovenous thrombosis in neonates and children: a systematic review and meta-analysis of observational studies. *Circulation*. 2010;121:1838-1847.
59. Saposnik G, Barinagarrementeria F, Brown RD Jr, et al. Diagnosis and management of cerebral venous thrombosis: a statement for healthcare professionals from the American Heart Association/American Stroke Association. *Stroke*. 2011;42:1158-1192.
60. Kenet G, Kirkham F, Niederstadt T, et al. Risk factors for recurrent venous thromboembolism in the European collaborative paediatric database on cerebral venous thrombosis: a multicentre cohort study. *Lancet Neurol*. 2007;6:595-603.
62. Moharir MD, Shroff M, Stephens D, et al. Anticoagulants in pediatric cerebral sinovenous thrombosis: a safety and outcome study. *Ann Neurol*. 2010;67:590-599.
65. Ichord RN, Benedict SL, Chan AK, et al. Paediatric cerebral sinovenous thrombosis: findings of the International Paediatric Stroke Study. *Arch Dis Child*. 2015;100:174-179.
67. Broderick J, Talbot GT, Prenger E, et al. Stroke in children within a major metropolitan area: the surprising importance of intracerebral hemorrhage. *J Child Neurol*. 1993;8:250-255.
70. Al-Jarallah A, Al-Rifai MT, Riela AR, Roach ES. Nontraumatic brain hemorrhage in children: etiology and presentation. *J Child Neurol*. 2000;15:284-289.
72. Beslow LA, Licht DJ, Smith SE, et al. Predictors of outcome in childhood intracerebral hemorrhage: a prospective consecutive cohort study. *Stroke*. 2010;41:313-318.
74. Smith ER, Butler WE, Ogilvy CS. Surgical approaches to vascular anomalies of the child's brain. *Curr Opin Neurol*. 2002;15:165-171.
75. Kondziolka D, Humphreys RP, Hoffman HJ, et al. Arteriovenous malformations of the brain in children: a forty year experience. *Can J Neurol Sci*. 1992;19:40-45.
76. Fullerton HJ, Achrol AS, Johnston SC, et al. Long-term hemorrhage risk in children versus adults with brain arteriovenous malformations. *Stroke*. 2005;36:2099-2104.
77. Lang SS, Beslow LA, Bailey RL, et al. Follow-up imaging to detect recurrence of surgically treated pediatric arteriovenous malformations. *J Neurosurg Pediatr*. 2012;9:497-504.
81. Niazi TN, Klimo P Jr, Anderson RC, Raffel C. Diagnosis and management of arteriovenous malformations in children. *Neurosurg Clin N Am*. 2010;21:443-456.
82. Spetzler RF, Martin NA. A proposed grading system for arteriovenous malformations. *J Neurosurg*. 1986;65:476-483.
84. Gross BA, Storey A, Orbach DB, et al. Microsurgical treatment of arteriovenous malformations in pediatric patients: the Boston Children's Hospital experience. *J Neurosurg Pediatr*. 2015;15:71-77.
87. Sheth SA, Potts MB, Sneed PK, et al. Angiographic features help predict outcome after stereotactic radiosurgery for the treatment of pediatric arteriovenous malformations. *Childs Nerv Syst*. 2014;30:241-247.
88. Jordan LC, Johnston SC, Wu YW, et al. The importance of cerebral aneurysms in childhood hemorrhagic stroke: a population-based study. *Stroke*. 2009;40:400-405.

90. Mehrotra A, Nair AP, Das KK, et al. Clinical and radiological profiles and outcomes in pediatric patients with intracranial aneurysms. *J Neurosurg Pediatr.* 2012;10:340-346.

99. Anderson RC, McDowell MM, Kellner CP, et al. Arteriovenous malformation-associated aneurysms in the pediatric population. *J Neurosurg Pediatr.* 2012;9:11-16.

101. Liu AC, Segaren N, Cox TS, et al. Is there a role for magnetic resonance imaging in the evaluation of non-traumatic intraparenchymal haemorrhage in children? *Pediatr Radiol.* 2006;36:940-946.

103. Connolly ES Jr, Rabinstein AA, Carhuapoma JR, et al. Guidelines for the management of aneurysmal subarachnoid hemorrhage: a guideline for healthcare professionals from the American Heart Association/American Stroke Association. *Stroke.* 2012;43:1711-1737.

106. Teasdale GM, Wardlaw JM, White PM, et al. The familial risk of subarachnoid haemorrhage. *Brain.* 2005;128:1677-1685.

108. Al-Holou WN, O'Lynnger TM, Pandey AS, et al. Natural history and imaging prevalence of cavernous malformations in children and young adults. *J Neurosurg Pediatr.* 2012;9:198-205.

114. Abla AA, Lekovic GP, Garrett M, et al. Cavernous malformations of the brainstem presenting in childhood: surgical experience in 40 patients. *Neurosurgery.* 2010;67:1589-1598, discussion 1598-1589.

115. McCracken DJ, Willie JT, Fernald BA, et al. Magnetic resonance thermometry-guided stereotactic laser ablation of cavernous malformations in drug-resistant epilepsy: imaging and clinical results. *Neurosurgery.* 2015;[Epub ahead of print].

116. Schulte R, Jordan LC, Morad A, et al. Rise in late onset vitamin K deficiency bleeding in young infants because of omission or refusal of prophylaxis at birth. *Pediatr Neurol.* 2014;50:564-568.

Central Nervous System Infections and Related Conditions

Erin P. Reade, Dennis W. Simon, and Mark E. Rowin

PEARLS

- Despite the success of vaccination for common bacterial meningitis pathogens, intensivists must continue to look for and treat both vaccine and nonvaccine serotypes of *S. pneumoniae* and Neisseria.
- Viral meningitis is a diverse disease process with a broad range of presentations and outcomes and little specific therapy.
- Inflammatory and autoimmune causes of CNS disease are emerging as important entities in the pediatric ICU and require a high index of suspicion.

Introduction

Infections of the central nervous system (CNS) and other conditions that often mimic CNS infections are life-threatening indications for admission to the pediatric intensive care unit (PICU). The diversity of infectious agents causing CNS disease includes bacteria, viruses, fungi, parasites, and amebas. In addition, posttraumatic and postsurgical infections, though relatively uncommon, can be fatal. Inflammatory diseases such as acute disseminated encephalomyelitis (ADEM) and autoimmune processes such as acute hemorrhagic leukoencephalitis, anti–N-methyl-D-aspartate (NMDA) receptor-mediated encephalitis, and CNS hemophagocytic lymphohistiocytosis (HLH) feature diverse presentations and require a high index of suspicion. The pediatric intensivist must integrate knowledge of epidemiology, signs and symptoms, predisposing factors, and host defenses as well as utilize appropriate cerebrospinal fluid analysis, pathology, and imaging in order to diagnose and treat CNS infections and related diseases.

Bacterial Meningitis

Acute bacterial meningitis is a relatively common and potentially severe infection in children. Bacterial meningitis often results from the hematogenous dissemination of microorganisms from a distant site of infection. More than two-thirds of cases of meningitis occur in the first 2 years of life, owing in part to an immature immune system and developmental differences in the vascularity of the brain. These children are often admitted to a PICU for supportive care.

Many microorganisms have the ability to cause meningitis. Most are acquired through a hematogenous route, others

through direct extension from nasal cavities, paranasal sinuses, mastoids, or the middle ear. CNS infections can also be associated with trauma, surgery, and placement of foreign materials.

Epidemiology

The epidemiology of bacterial meningitis continues to shift with the development of conjugate vaccines for the most common bacterial pathogens. In the 1980s, five etiologic agents, namely *Haemophilus influenzae, Neisseria meningitidis, Streptococcus pneumoniae, Listeria monocytogenes,* and *Streptococcus agalactiae,* accounted for almost 80% of meningitis cases in the United States. A conjugate vaccine against *Haemophilus influenzae* type b (Hib) was introduced in the early1990s. During the first decade of the 21st century, a pivotal change occurred in the management of acute bacterial meningitis with the introduction of the conjugate vaccines for *S. pneumoniae* (Prevnar) in 2000 and *N. meningitidis* (Menactra) in 2005. These bacterial conjugate vaccines have dramatically altered the epidemiology of childhood meningitis, with viral agents now becoming increasingly predominant. In addition, nonvaccine serotypes have emerged as "newly recognized" pathogens.[1,2] The isolation of nonvaccine serotypes of *S. pneumoniae* has increased since the introduction of the conjugate vaccine. Of great therapeutic concern, approximately one-quarter of these invasive isolates were penicillin-resistant, and more than 10% were resistant to cephalosporins.

The introduction of vaccines against *Haemophilus, Pneumococcus,* and *Neisseria* has had an undeniable impact on the incidence and etiology of meningitis. A study using the Kids' Inpatient Database and the National Inpatient Database examined trends in bacterial meningitis over the 19 years since routine vaccinations against these organisms were instituted in the United States.[3] Over this period, the authors noted approximately 15,000 cases per year. However, there has been a 47% reduction in cases of meningitis in children (and elderly patients) since the introduction of the conjugate vaccines. When all ages are considered, the incidence of both pneumococcal and meningococcal meningitis decreased by ~10%. However, during this same period, an increase in the incidence of staphylococcal and streptococcal meningitides was observed.

S. pneumoniae continues to be a leading cause of bacterial meningitis both internationally and in the United States. In a study of children presenting to the emergency department with bacterial meningitis, roughly one-third of cases were caused by *S. pneumoniae*. Of interest, 62% of the pneumococcal isolates were nonvaccine serotypes.[4] An epidemiologic study from the United States showed the incidence of *S. pneumoniae* meningitis fell from 0.8 per 100,000 people in 1997 to 0.3 per 100,000 people in 2010. Among infants younger than 1 year of age, the incidence is even less, estimated at 0.2 per 100,000. The case mortality from pneumococcal meningitis decreased from 0.049 per 100,000 people in 2004 to 0.024 per 100,000 people in 2008.[5]

Neisseria meningitidis is the second most common cause of sepsis and meningitis beyond the neonatal period.[5] Following the introduction of the conjugated meningococcal vaccine, the incidence of *Neisseria meningitidis* meningitis decreased from 0.7 per 100,000 people in 1997 to 0.1 per 100,000 people in 2010. Globally, *Neisseria meningitidis* causes around 500,000 cases of meningitis and septic shock every year, although incidence rates vary from <1 per 100,000 per year in North America to 10 to 1000 per 100,000 per year in sub-Saharan Africa. The peak incidence of invasive meningococcal disease occurs in children between 6 months and 2 years of age, with a second smaller peak in adolescents and young adults. Capsular group B is the major disease-causing group in most countries and causes the highest rates of disease in North America and Europe. In a 9-year Canadian study of invasive meningococcal disease, the authors noted that this organism presented as meningitis in over 50% of cases and, in children, had a case fatality rate of 2%.[6]

During the first months of life, *Escherichia coli* and other gram-negative organisms cause one-fifth of sepsis and meningitis cases. Because of targeted intrapartum antibiotic prophylaxis, *Streptococcus agalactiae* (group B streptococcus) meningitis is increasingly less common in newborns in the United States.[7,8] However, in a study from the United Kingdom evaluating the epidemiology of meningitis in children in the postvaccine age, group B streptococcus was the most frequently identified bacterial pathogen.[9] Additionally, a bacterial pathogen was detected in only 19% of children with meningitis. A virus was identified in 37% of cases, with enterovirus as the most common viral pathogen identified. In greater than 40% of cases, no pathogen was identified.

Mycobacterium tuberculosis is a rare cause of pediatric meningitis, but it is well recognized for its high degree of morbidity and mortality. Tuberculous (TB) meningitis disproportionately affects young children and, after scrofula, is the most common form of childhood extrapulmonary tuberculosis. Before antituberculosis drugs, TB meningitis invariably caused death, usually within weeks. One meta-analysis showed that risk of death from TB meningitis was 19.3%, and risk of neurologic sequelae among survivors was greater than 50%.[10] As with acute bacterial meningitis, later diagnosis in TB meningitis is associated with poorer outcomes. Morbidity and mortality have improved with effective antimicrobials, corticosteroid use, and advances in management of intracranial hypertension. However, early diagnosis remains a substantial challenge because stage 1 (the earliest stage of TB meningitis) presents with nonspecific signs and symptoms.

Pathogenesis

Tissue injury and subsequent morbidity in acute bacterial meningitis is caused by multiple factors including bacterial proliferation in the subarachnoid space, release of bacterial products, local immune response from CNS tissue, and leukocyte migration into infected tissue. Colonization of the nasopharynx is frequently the antecedent event in clinical meningitis. Organisms in the nasopharynx penetrate respiratory epithelial cells as a preamble to disease. Organisms then enter the bloodstream and undergo intravascular multiplication and eventually penetrate the blood-brain barrier (BBB). A lack of immune defenses in the subarachnoid space allows for the rapid multiplication of bacteria within the CNS.

Certain predisposing factors are clearly associated with increased risk for development of acute bacterial meningitis. Children with asplenia, humoral immunodeficiencies, cochlear implants, human immunodeficiency virus, and cerebrospinal fluid (CSF) leakage secondary to trauma are at increased risk for pneumococcal meningitis. Asplenic children and those with complement deficiencies are at increased risk for meningococcal meningitis. On rare occasions, otitis media has been associated with *Streptococcus pyogenes* meningitis.[11] Infections by *Staphylococcus aureus* and coagulase-negative staphylococci are generally associated with neurosurgery or trauma. Many studies have explored the genetic determinants of infectious diseases. In invasive meningococcal disease, several mutations and polymorphisms have been associated with a higher susceptibility and severity of illness. To date, the genetic markers with the strongest supportive evidence are specific polymorphisms in the coding genes of plasminogen activator inhibitor 1 (PAI-1) and receptors of the Fc fraction of immunoglobulins.[12]

Clinical Manifestations

The classic clinical presentation of meningitis is characterized by fever, headache, nuchal rigidity, and altered mental status. Clinical symptoms are often ambiguous in the pediatric patient. In fact, the triad of fever, neck stiffness, and a change in mental status is present in less than 50% of pediatric cases. Nuchal rigidity is frequently absent, and changes in mental status such as irritability can often be dismissed as normal behavior in a newborn. Similarly, Kernig and Brudzinski signs frequently go unrecognized or are absent. The presence of petechiae and purpura may suggest meningococcus as the causative agent. However, similar findings have been observed in children with *S. pneumoniae* and *H. influenzae* type a sepsis.[13] A meta-analysis evaluating clinical prediction rules for meningitis showed that no constellation of clinical signs and symptoms was 100% predictive of meningitis.[14] Thus the clinician must have a high index of suspicion when considering this diagnosis in pediatric patients.

Poorly reactive pupils, a bulging fontanel, diplopia, papilledema, and uncontrollable vomiting are signs of increased intracranial pressure (ICP). Elevated ICP is frequently noted in bacterial meningitis, most likely due to obstruction of the arachnoid tissue by leukocyte migration, as a consequence of CNS inflammation or obstruction of CSF flow by purulent debris of the lateral, third, or fourth ventricles. However, frank hydrocephalus visible on computed tomography (CT) of the brain is rare.

A multiyear retrospective study from South America evaluated risk factors in pediatric patients with confirmed bacterial meningitis for the subsequent development of seizure activity. Risk factors for seizure development included age less than 2 years, pneumococcal etiology, altered mental status at admission, and CSF leukocyte count less than 1000 cells.

Generalized seizures were present in 20% to 30% of patients within the first 3 days of illness. The presence of focal seizures and onset past the third day of illness were associated with long-term neurologic sequelae. Development of seizure activity in these patients was associated with a ninefold increase in mortality.[15]

Diagnosis

Meningitis is a serious medical emergency in which the microbiology laboratory plays a critical role in early identification of the causative bacterium. When clinically feasible, the diagnosis of meningitis requires the examination of CSF. In most cases of bacterial meningitis, the diagnosis relies on the isolation of bacteria from a CSF specimen. Cell count and differential, protein, glucose, Gram stain, and cultures are essential tests to be performed. In bacterial meningitis, about 80% of patients will have concurrent bacteremia, but the use of blood culture alone as an initial screening test is not appropriate. Prior oral antimicrobial therapy will not significantly alter CSF cell counts, differential, and chemistries in children with bacterial meningitis. However, Gram stain and culture sensitivity are greatly reduced.[16]

Lumbar puncture should be postponed in children with an ongoing coagulopathy, concern for elevated ICP (such as altered mental status or hydrocephalus seen on CT or MRI), cardiorespiratory difficulty, and patients with suspected mass-occupying lesions. Although not required in all children with suspected meningitis, CT scan is indicated prior to lumbar puncture in those with focal neurologic findings or signs of elevated ICP. It is important to remember that even when CT scans are normal, herniation may still occur in both children[17] and adults with meningitis.[18]

Antibiotic therapy and other supportive measures must be started early when meningitis is suspected and should not be delayed while awaiting CSF results. Delays in antibiotic administration have been repeatedly shown to increase mortality. A delay of antibiotics initiation for as little as 3 hours can be associated with an unfavorable outcome. The risk for poor outcome increases by up to 30% per hour of antibiotic treatment delay.[19] Routine end-of-treatment lumbar punctures are no longer recommended. However, meningitis caused by multidrug resistant S. pneumoniae or gram-negative bacilli meningitis may require a repeat lumbar puncture at 48 hours after initiating therapy to document sterilization.

CSF with pleocytosis, usually greater than 1000/uL, and a predominance of polymorphonuclear leukocytes (PMN) is highly suggestive of bacterial meningitis. High protein and low glucose (usually $< \frac{1}{2}$ serum value) concentrations also support the diagnosis. A predominance of lymphocytes and monocytes suggests a viral pathogen. These can also be observed in patients with rickettsial and tuberculous meningitis. CSF eosinophils are commonly observed in patients with CSF shunt devices, but also this can be observed in parasitic CNS infections such as baylisascariasis and Angiostrongylus species.

Clinicians must remember that a PMN-predominance may be observed early in enteroviral meningitis as well. Frequently, these patients have normal protein and glucose concentrations. Interestingly, hypoglycorrachia can be observed with certain viral pathogens such as enterovirus and mumps virus. On occasion, a small percentage of patients may have an initial "normal-appearing" CSF analysis, especially with N. meningitidis.

Positive CSF cultures remain the gold standard of meningitis diagnosis. Gram stains have been reported to demonstrate organisms in 50% to 75% of patients with bacterial meningitis. The clinician must be cautioned not to make significant changes in antimicrobial therapy solely based on a Gram stain result, as this may reflect difference in CSF staining during slide preparation. Routine use of rapid bacterial antigen detection assays has been shown to be of limited clinical relevance.[20] In children, the combination of CSF gram staining and latex agglutination studies can detect 85% of cases of acute bacterial meningitis. However, the addition of CSF cultures to Gram stains and latex agglutination studies increases the sensitivity and specificity of meningitis detection to almost 100%.[21]

Antibiotic pretreatment often results in a clinical dilemma, related to identification of the pathogen causing meningitis. However, several new laboratory tools are now available to pediatric intensivists. A multicenter study from Asia and Africa demonstrated high sensitivity and specificity for immunochromatographic analysis of pneumococcal antigen.[22] Similarly, real-time fluorescent quantitative polymerase chain reaction (PCR) amplification of the bacterial 16S rRNA gene is a useful clinical tool for the rapid diagnosis of bacterial meningitis. Compared to bacterial culture controls, sensitivity for S. pneumoniae and N. meningitidis as the etiologic agents was 86% to 100%.[23-25] In a clinical setting, a real-time PCR for N. meningitidis was found to have high sensitivity, specificity, and predictive values.[26] Serum procalcitonin assays have been used to differentiate between bacterial and aseptic meningitis. In a small study, procalcitonin determination had 99% sensitivity and 83% specificity for distinguishing bacterial meningitis from other causes.[27] Additional clinical studies will be needed to assess the ultimate clinical roles for these assays.

Treatment

An effective antimicrobial agent for the treatment of bacterial meningitis must be bactericidal and must achieve high concentrations in the CSF. In addition, initial empiric therapy should take into consideration antimicrobial resistance among the most likely meningeal pathogens. Hospital antibiograms that demonstrate resistance among local community flora are an invaluable resource. Once meningitis is suspected, antimicrobial therapy must be initiated promptly.

All critical care clinicians should be familiar with recommendations for antibiotic management in bacterial meningitis.[28] Tables 70.1 through 70.3 provide a listing of most frequent meningeal pathogens and recommended antimicrobial regimens along with dosage information. The Infectious Disease Society of America and the British National Institute for Clinical Evidence have both published guidelines on duration of therapy for bacterial meningitis in children. These recommendations are similar but not identical (Table 70.4). Guidelines such as these are useful tools in pediatrics. However, the emphasis on fixed durations of IV antibiotics needs to take into account the patient's clinical response. Studies suggest that the currently established length of antibiotic therapies for meningitis may soon be redefined.[29]

The duration of antimicrobial therapy will vary according to causative pathogen. Children with gram-negative bacterial meningitis require a minimum of 3 weeks. Classically, infants with group B streptococcal meningitis require 14 to 21 days; S. pneumoniae, 10 to 14 days; N. meningitidis, 7 days; and

TABLE 70.1	Initial Antimicrobial Therapy for Bacterial Meningitis Based on Presumptive Pathogen(s)	
Age or Predisposing Condition	**Likely Pathogens**	**Antimicrobial Therapy**
<1 month	Escherichia coli, Streptococcus agalactiae, Klebsiella species, Listeria monocytogenes	Ampicillin plus cefotaxime +/− aminoglycoside
1-2 months	Streptococcus pneumoniae, Neisseria meningitidis, Streptococcus agalactiae, Haemophilus influenzae, Escherichia coli	Vancomycin plus third-generation cephalosporin[a]
2 months to 5 years	Streptococcus pneumoniae, Neisseria meningitidis, Haemophilus influenzae	Vancomycin plus third-generation cephalosporin[a]
>5 years	Streptococcus pneumoniae, Neisseria meningitidis	Vancomycin plus third-generation cephalosporin[a]
Humoral immunodeficiency, HIV, asplenia	Streptococcus pneumoniae, Neisseria meningitidis, Haemophilus influenzae, Salmonella species	Vancomycin plus third-generation cephalosporin[a]
Complement deficiencies	Neisseria meningitidis, Streptococcus pneumoniae	Vancomycin plus third-generation cephalosporin[a]
Basilar skull fractures	Streptococcus pneumoniae, Neisseria meningitidis, Streptococcus pyogenes	Vancomycin plus third-generation cephalosporin[b]
Cerebrospinal fluid shunt related	Coagulase-negative staphylococci, Staphylococcus aureus, Pseudomonas aeruginosa, Propionibacterium acnes	Vancomycin plus ceftazidime or vancomycin plus cefepime or vancomycin plus meropenem[b]
Cochlear implants	Streptococcus pneumoniae	Vancomycin plus third-generation cephalosporin[a]

[a]Cefotaxime or ceftriaxone.
[b]The choice of anti–gram-negative bacillary agent should be based on the institution's susceptibility patterns.

TABLE 70.2	Antimicrobial Therapy for Specific Meningeal Pathogens
Streptococcus agalactiae	Penicillin G +/− gentamicin or ampicillin +/− gentamicin
Haemophilus influenzae, β-lactamase-negative	Ampicillin
H. influenzae, β-lactamase-positive	Third-generation cephalosporin[a]
Streptococcus pneumoniae, penicillin-susceptible	Penicillin G or ampicillin
S. pneumoniae, penicillin-resistant, cephalosporin-susceptible	Third-generation cephalosporin[a]
S. pneumoniae, drug-resistant (multiply-resistant)	Vancomycin plus rifampin
Neisseria meningitidis	Third-generation cephalosporin[a]
Neisseria meningitidis, penicillin-susceptible	Penicillin G or ampicillin
Escherichia coli Other aerobic enteric gram-negative bacilli (not including Pseudomonas aeruginosa)	Cefotaxime or ceftriaxone (if >1 month of age) plus aminoglycoside
Pseudomonas aeruginosa	Meropenem plus aminoglycoside or cefepime plus aminoglycoside or ceftazidime plus aminoglycoside
Coagulase-negative staphylococci, methicillin-resistant Staphylococcus aureus	Vancomycin +/− rifampin
Methicillin-susceptible S. aureus	Nafcillin

[a]Cefotaxime or ceftriaxone.

H. influenzae, 7 to 10 days. However, in certain clinical circumstances, a shorter duration may be feasible. A meta-analysis on duration of therapy in pediatric meningitis evaluated the three most common pathogens and compared short-course (4–7 days) versus long-course (7–14 days) therapy. There was no significant difference in clinical success or long-term neurologic complications between groups.[30] Subsequently, a multicountry trial enrolled more than 1000 children with meningitis caused by *H. influenzae* type b, *S. pneumonia*, or *N. meningitidis* who were stable after 5 days of intravenous (IV) ceftriaxone therapy and randomized them to receive placebo or an additional 5 days of ceftriaxone.[31] Again, there were no significant differences in bacteriologic failures, clinical failures, or clinical sequelae in survivors. The authors concluded that ceftriaxone could be discontinued in children with bacterial meningitis who are clinically stable after 5 days of IV therapy. Of note, patients with persistent seizures, bacteremia, brain abscesses, other infections, or who were judged to be severely ill at the 5-day mark were excluded.

The initial antibiotic regimen for community-acquired meningitis depends on the bacterial antibiotic resistance patterns in the area. In regions with less than 1% of *S. pneumoniae* isolates resistant to third-generation cephalosporins, ceftriaxone (plus ampicillin in areas with *L. monocytogenes*) should be

TABLE 70.3   Dosages of Antimicrobial Agents for Treatment of Bacterial Meningitis Expressed as mg/kg/day[a]

Antibiotic	Neonates 0 to 7 days > 2000 grams[b]	Neonates > 7 days > 2000 grams	Infants and Children	Maximum Daily Adult Dose
Ampicillin	150	200	300-400	12 grams
Cefepime	-	-	150	6 grams
Cefotaxime	150	200	200-300	12 grams
Ceftriaxone	-	-	100	4 grams
Gentamicin	5	7.5	7.5	5 mg/kg
Meropenem	-	-	120	6 grams
Penicillin G	150,000	200,000	300,000	24 million units
Rifampin	-	10-20	10-20	600 mg
Vancomycin	30	45	60	45 mg/kg

[a]Exception: Penicillin G is expressed as units/kg/day.
[b]Dosages of agents for neonates < 2000 grams can be obtained from Lexi-Comp, Inc. Online or from Bradley JS, 2016 Nelson's Pediatric Antimicrobial Therapy, 22nd edition. American Academy of Pediatrics., Elk Grove Village, IL.

TABLE 70.4   Comparison of Recommended Durations of Antibiotic Therapy for Meningitis From the Infectious Disease Society of America (IDSA) and the National Institute for Clinical Excellence (NICE)

Organism	IDSA Recommendations	NICE Recommendations
Streptococcus pneumoniae	10-14 days	14 days
Neisseria meningitidis	7 days	7 days
Group B streptococcus	14-21 days	14 days
Haemophilus influenzae	7 days	10 days

initiated. In areas with more than 1% cephalosporin-resistant *S. pneumoniae*, ceftriaxone plus vancomycin is the empiric therapy of choice at present. Among newborns, cefotaxime plus ampicillin remains the treatment of choice. It is the opinion of many clinicians that ampicillin or penicillin G plus gentamicin are the agents of choice for group B streptococcal meningitis in the young infant. Alterations to these regimens may be influenced by Gram stain, culture, and drug susceptibility results. Additional empiric agents could be added according to epidemiologic exposures, underlying conditions, and the presence of resistant organisms in the community or hospital. Once a specific pathogen has been identified and susceptibility (antibiogram) data are available, antimicrobial therapy could be "narrowed" to specifically target the offending pathogen.

There are increasing numbers of newer antibiotics that may have a role in meningitis management. Carbapenems may offer a treatment option in antibiotic-resistant strains causing meningitis. Imipenem is not recommended for CNS infections due to its proconvulsive association, but meropenem is as effective as ceftriaxone or cefotaxime as empiric therapy for bacterial meningitis. It can be considered for use in nosocomial meningitis either as a single agent or in combination with vancomycin. Linezolid, from the antibiotic class oxazolidinones, readily enters the CSF and is active against gram-positive organisms. Although primarily a bacteriostatic agent, it has been used successfully for CNS infections caused by multidrug-resistant organisms. Daptomycin, fluoroquinolones, tigecycline, and newer cephalosporins such as ceftaroline and ceftobiprole cannot be recommended as empiric therapy at this time but may have a role in individual cases of meningitis based on the organism's antibiograms.

Optimum therapy for childhood TB meningitis is unclear. No randomized controlled trials have been conducted. In drug-susceptible mycobacteria, the World Health Organization recommends 2 months of isoniazid, rifampicin, pyrazinamide, and ethambutol, with a subsequent 10-month course of isoniazid and rifampin. However, treatment length is controversial, with various experts advocating for 6 to 9 months of initial therapy.

Supportive Care

In addition to provision of an effective antimicrobial regimen, correction of hyponatremia, hypoxemia, and hypotension should also be included in the treatment plan of CNS infections. Rapid placement of an external ventriculostomy is indicated in patients with radiographic or clinical evidence of obstructive hydrocephalus. The presence of any of these along with a delay in CSF sterilization is associated with poor outcomes and neurologic sequelae.

In patients who present in shock or dehydration, administration of IV fluids is critical for the maintenance of normal blood pressure and proper perfusion. There has been disagreement regarding IV fluid management in patients with meningitis. There are potential risks from giving too much fluid (especially brain swelling) as well as too little fluid (especially shock). In a Cochrane review, the authors evaluated differing volumes of fluid given in the initial management of bacterial meningitis. Sadly, only three trials could be compared. All three trials were on pediatric patient groups. The meta-analysis found no significant difference between the maintenance-fluid and restricted-fluid groups in number of deaths, acute severe neurologic sequelae, or in mild to moderate sequelae.[32] However, when neurologic sequelae were further defined, there was a statistically significant difference in favor of the maintenance-fluid group for decrease in seizure activity at both 72 hours and 14 days, as well as less neurologic sequelae at 3 months. It must be noted that the reviewers mention the quality of evidence regarding fluid therapy in children with acute bacterial meningitis is marginal and there is a need for further research.

In patients with altered mental status, airway protection and assisted ventilation may be required. Patients who present in septic shock may require inotropes or vasopressors. Anticonvulsant therapy is indicated in patients with seizures. Consultation with infectious disease and pharmacy colleagues is often invaluable.

Adjunctive Therapy

The search for therapeutic adjuncts designed to improve therapy in meningitis is ongoing but often hampered by the difficulty in conducting randomized clinical trials due to the acuity of the disease, the narrow time frame in which adjuncts can influence outcome, and the increasingly small number of cases in this postvaccine era. Immunomodulation, hypothermia, free radical scavengers, C5 monoclonal antibodies, neutrophil proapoptosis agents, and toll-like receptor antagonists have all shown benefit in experimental models of meningitis.

Two agents, glycerol and dexamethasone, have been evaluated in pediatrics as possible adjuvant therapy in meningitis. The addition of adjunctive corticosteroids prior to antibiotic treatment in bacterial meningitis was endorsed by the Infectious Diseases Society of America (IDSA) guidelines in 2004. However, use of corticosteroids, such as dexamethasone, in meningitis has not been universally adopted among clinicians.

Oral glycerol has been shown to reduce neurologic sequelae in children with bacterial meningitis.[33] Its mechanism of action is unknown but possibly occurs through a reduction in serum viscosity, allowing for vasoconstriction with maintenance of cerebral blood flow and a subsequent reduction in cerebral blood volume.[34] Some clinicians believe glycerol may be more beneficial than corticosteroids as an adjuvant in decreasing neurologic sequelae.[35] Although promising, further investigations are required before empiric therapy with this agent can be recommended.

Corticosteroids are well studied in meningitis, although their exact beneficial mechanism of action remains obscure. In early studies in children with Hib meningitis, dexamethasone-treated children had a lower incidence of moderate-to-severe hearing deficits when compared to placebo.[36] However, one of the study's antimicrobial agents, cefuroxime, was later shown to be associated with increased neurologic sequelae. In adults with pneumococcal meningitis, the early administration of dexamethasone, 15 to 20 minutes before or with the first dose of antibiotic, was associated with a reduction in mortality and unfavorable outcomes.[37,38] In pediatric studies, dexamethasone did not demonstrate the same improvement in mortality noted in adults, but it was associated with an improvement in moderate-or-severe hearing loss.[39,40] There is no evidence that corticosteroid use is beneficial in viral or neonatal bacterial meningitis.[41]

A Cochrane database review examined the effect of adjuvant corticosteroid therapy on meningitis in both adults and children.[42] This meta-analysis included studies from 1966 through 2013. It reviewed 25 studies and demonstrated no reduction in mortality in either adult or pediatric-aged patients who received corticosteroids at some point in their meningitis management. However, subgroup analyses for causative organisms showed corticosteroids reduced mortality in S. pneumoniae meningitis but not in meningitis caused by H. influenzae or N. meningitidis. Additionally, corticosteroid recipients showed a significant reduction in hearing loss and neurologic sequelae. Interestingly, the benefit of corticosteroids was noted only in countries with higher socioeconomic classes. The Cochrane study ultimately recommended a 4-day regimen of dexamethasone, but it also remarked that the strength of evidence is not optimal.

Adjunctive steroid therapy reduces vasculitis associated with TB meningitis. In addition, patients with TB meningitis treated with steroids have improved survival compared to nonrecipients. However, the severity of neurologic disability observed with TB meningitis is not altered.[43]

In summary, studies of adjuvant corticosteroid therapy in children have not unequivocally demonstrated beneficial effects. Study design flaws and the fact that most studies were done in the era of Hib disease limits the applicability of these results to today's practice. Meta-analysis and retrospective studies have demonstrated beneficial effects in Hib and pneumococcal meningitis. However, these were conducted at a time when drug-resistant S. pneumoniae (DRSP) was not a serious problem. The data could support a beneficial effect in Hib meningitis, but because this organism is an uncommon pathogen at this time, empiric therapy would not be warranted in most cases. In the era of DRSP, where an isolate may be resistant to the third-generation cephalosporin, it has been suggested that dexamethasone may impair the diffusion of vancomycin through the BBB, thus delaying CSF sterilization. Thus, caution is merited. Some clinicians recommend the addition of rifampin under these circumstances. Lastly, because maximal beneficial effect would be gained by administering dexamethasone prior to antibiotic therapy, children previously treated with antibiotics should not receive dexamethasone.

Prevention

Individuals with significant, prolonged, or close exposures (ie, household members and caregivers, daycare center playmates) to children with N. meningitidis meningitis should receive antimicrobial prophylaxis with ceftriaxone, ciprofloxacin, or rifampin.[44] However, ciprofloxacin resistance has been reported in the United States.[45] Thus antibiogram data are important in making antibiotic prophylaxis decisions.

Routine childhood vaccinations against Hib, S. pneumoniae, and N. meningitidis type A, C, W-135, and Y have significantly decreased the incidence of bacterial meningitis. Clinicians should recommend their use without hesitation. However, N. meningitidis type B continues to account for a majority of invasive meningococcal disease. In 2013, a vaccine against N. meningitidis type B was approved for use in Europe. Its effect on meningitis epidemiology is yet to be determined.

Outcomes

With aggressive support and appropriate antimicrobial therapy, the mortality rate of bacterial meningitis remains low. Unfortunately, neurologic sequelae still occur. When compared to other pathogens, pneumococcal, TB, and gram-negative bacillary meningitis are most commonly associated with neurologic sequelae. Seizures, hearing loss, hydrocephalus, and learning disabilities are the most common sequelae reported.

It is difficult to predict individual outcomes for a patient with meningitis admitted to the PICU. No single factor is entirely predictive. Among bacteria, *S. pneumoniae* is associated with the highest mortality. Interestingly, antimicrobial resistance in pneumococcal meningitis was not associated with death, ICU admission, need for mechanical ventilation, focal neurologic deficits, seizures, secondary fevers, or increased duration of hospital stay.[46] In a retrospective study of 15 PICUs in the United States, patients with both bacterial and nonbacterial meningitis had an unadjusted mortality rate of 7%. Nonsurvivors had a significantly higher Pediatric Risk of Mortality III score. Mortality was threefold higher in patients with bacterial-confirmed meningitis. The presence of coma upon initial presentation to the PICU increased mortality 10-fold.[47] In another study evaluating only pneumococcal meningitis, the presence of shock, hyponatremia, or coma upon admission to the ICU was associated with a higher use of invasive medical devices and higher mortality.[48] A third pediatric study of all causes of meningitis showed factors associated with increased mortality included low Glasgow Coma Score, respiratory distress at presentation, seizures at any point during admission, and, in third world countries, malnutrition.[49] Among laboratory findings, the presence of low leukocyte blood cell and platelet counts was associated with increased mortality.[50,51]

The hippocampal formation is a region of the brain frequently affected in bacterial meningitis, a region of the brain known to be important in learning and memory.[52] A significant portion of meningitis survivors demonstrate neuropsychologic deficits and cognitive issues later in life. An educational outcomes evaluation showed that children recovering from CNS infections significantly underperformed on neuropsychologic evaluations in comparison to healthy controls.[53] Teachers noted children who recovered from CNS infections performed worse on educational assessments and had more problems with schoolwork. This group of children performed below average in both areas of executive function and attention. Analysis revealed that aspects of neuropsychologic function, such as memory function, and teacher-rated academic performance were most reduced in children with a history of meningoencephalitis.

Subdural Empyema

Subdural empyemas (SDEs) are serious central nervous system infections defined as purulent fluid collections outside the brain parenchyma but contained under the dura. They are usually encapsulated and often loculated. Historically, otorhinolaryngeal infections were an important predisposing factor to SDEs in older children. In a retrospective study over 24 years, the medical records of children with extraaxial CNS infection at a single children's hospital were analyzed. Over this time course, 70 children developed SDEs. Sinusitis was the most common etiology, followed by bacterial meningitis.[54] In this study, all patients were older than 7 years of age at diagnosis. However, another study that included infants demonstrated only 10% of SDE were related to otorhinolaryngeal infection.[55] This relatively low percentage is presumed to be from increased antibiotic use in this group of patients. In this study, meningitis, head trauma, or neurosurgery was identified as more common predisposing conditions for SDE. A third study, from 2001 through 2011, showed neurosurgical procedures were the most commonly identified source of infection.[56]

The pathophysiology of extraaxial CNS infections is well understood. Multiple predisposing etiologies are responsible, including extension of infection from regional sinuses, otitis, mastoiditis, and hematologic spread of pathogens from distant sites. In young infants, SDE is usually a complication of purulent meningitis wherein the infection extends through the arachnoid and into the subdural space.[57] Reactive subdural effusions can also occur following meningitis in infants. Though often a source of fever, these fluid collections are typically sterile.

Certain presenting characteristics were specific to the various etiologic subgroups. Potts puffy tumors are found frequently among patients with prior sinusitis. In the pediatric population, extraaxial CNS infections are most common in two distinct age groups, corresponding to known etiologies. SDEs following meningitis are more common in infants, whereas sinus-related infections are most common in those older than 6 years of age.[58]

Fever, headaches, eye pain, and altered level of consciousness are common presenting features in SDE. Not unexpectedly, many of these symptoms are common to those suffering from sinusitis. An altered level of consciousness and focal neurologic deficits are frequently observed. Seizures and cerebral edema from cortical vein thrombosis are common complications among patients presenting with subdural empyemas.[59] Prolonged fever (90%), seizures (70%), and focal neurologic signs (60%) are the most common clinical signs noted in the pediatric population.[55] The sequelae of SDE may be more severe in young infants than in any other age group.[60]

Historically, in children, SDE was often secondary to *H. influenzae* type b or *S. pneumoniae* meningitis. SDE also occurs with *Salmonella, N. meningitides, E. coli,* and TB. Streptococcus species and *S. aureus* were the most common pathogens identified.[54,56] The most common pathogen in infants younger than 4 months of age is group B streptococcus.[55]

The diagnosis is often made with radiologic assistance and evaluation of the subdural fluid collection. It is often difficult to distinguish an SDE from a sterile reactive subdural effusion (RSE).[61] The differentiation of SDE from sterile RSE may not be possible if contrast enhancement of the inner membrane is not seen on CT. MR imaging is superior to CT in the demonstration of both the extraaxial fluid and the enhancement of the inner membrane with a paramagnetic contrast medium. Still, no MR imaging characteristics are specific for SDE compared to a sterile RSE. Analysis of the subdural fluid is often required to establish the diagnosis of SDE. Serial cranial ultrasounds may be the modality of choice for the evaluation of response to medical management.[62]

The goal of treatment is evacuation of pus and eradication of the source of infection. Management choice should be related to the clinical condition. Medical treatment may be adequate if the empyema is small. A surgical approach is suggested in those patients who are not responding well to medical treatment or in those who have massive subdural pus accumulation. Craniotomy is the preferred procedure in most cases (Fig. 70.1). In young infants, a subdural tap through the anterior fontanel or bur hole is the preferred mode of intracranial pus evacuation because of ease of access. Many patients require repeated surgical procedures due to empyema recurrence.

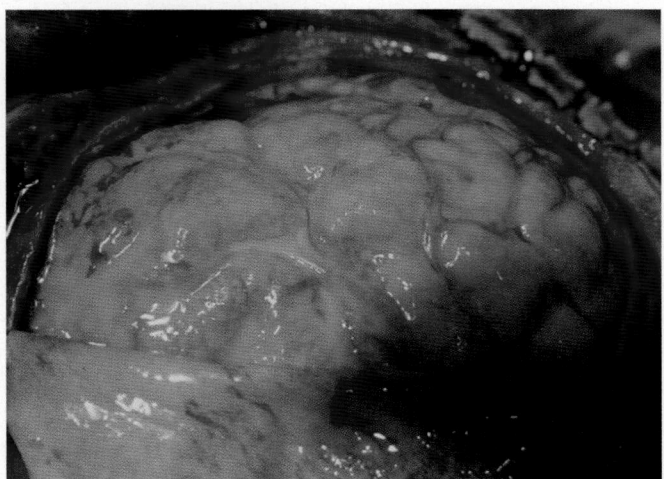

Fig. 70.1. Operative photograph of a patient with cranial subdural empyema. (Courtesy Alan R. Turtz, MD, Cooper University Hospital, Camden, NJ.)

The keys to an optimal outcome are early, accurate diagnosis, timely intervention, and appropriate antibiotic therapy. The reported mortality rates of SDE are approximately 10% following meningitis and up to 20% following untreated sinus infections.[63]

Germiller and colleagues reported a 4% mortality rate in a pediatric series of intracranial suppurative infections.[64] Survivors often had significant long-term morbidity with persistent seizures, hemiparesis, or residual neurologic deficits. Age, initial level of consciousness, timing and aggressiveness of treatment, and the rapidity of disease progression all influence outcome.

SDEs are rare and difficult to diagnose because initial symptoms may be vague. Patients with sinus infections and progressive headaches or any neurologic deficits should be evaluated with CT or MRI imaging to rule out intracranial spread. Because SDEs have serious morbidity and mortality if not recognized and treated promptly, the ICU physician must have a low threshold for requesting emergency neurosurgical intervention.

Brain Abscesses

The brain parenchyma is remarkably resistant to microbial infections. Despite the relative frequency of occult bacteremia in the pediatric-age patient, cerebral abscess formation is a rare occurrence. A brain abscess is an intraparenchymal infection that begins as a localized area of cerebritis and evolves through various stages until finally organizing into a collection of encapsulated purulent material. Among intracranial masses, the incidence of brain abscess is ~8% in developing countries and ~1% to 2% in Europe and North America.[65] Incidence of brain abscesses in children is 4 cases per million, with a peak age of presentation between 4 and 7 years of age.[66] Certain medical conditions, especially those that impair the immune response, predispose patients for an increased incidence of brain abscess formation. These include prolonged steroid use, diabetes mellitus, alcoholism, and primary immunodeficiencies.[67] At a single children's hospital over a 19-year period, congenital heart disease and sinus/otic infections were

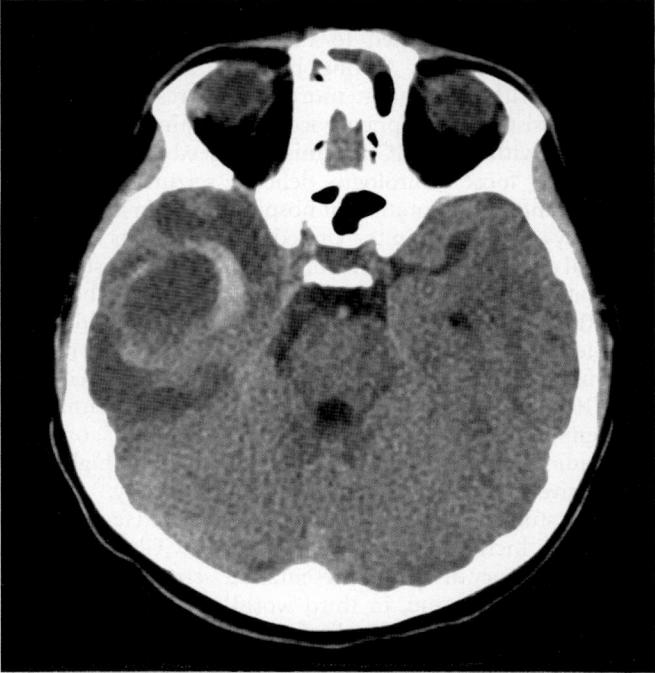

Fig. 70.2. Head CT demonstrating a large brain abscess in the parietal lobe associated with sinusitis. Cultures grew *Streptococcus* spp.

the most common predisposing factors to development of cerebral abscesses.[68]

Brain abscesses are often classified according to their likely point of entry. The most common origin of CNS abscesses in children is direct or indirect extension from the middle ear, paranasal sinus, or dental abscesses.[69] Brain abscesses are sequelae in 65% to 8% of untreated sinusitis cases and up to 10% of mastoiditis cases.[66] Abscesses in the temporal lobe or cerebellum are typically linked to ear or mastoid air cell points of entry and tend to be solitary. Frontal and parietal lobe abscesses are often due to sinus or dental infections (Fig. 70.2).

Abscesses of hematogenous origin are often noted in specific CNS parenchymal areas, especially in the middle cerebral artery distributions including the parietal and occipital regions (Fig. 70.3). The etiology of these multiple foci is often from distant sources in children with cardiac or pulmonary right-to-left shunts. Not surprisingly, cyanotic heart disease increases the risk of brain abscess formation.[66,70] In patients diagnosed with a brain abscess, a third will have an underlying heart defect.[71] Of these, tetralogy of Fallot, transposition of the great vessels, atrial septal defects, ventricular septal defects, and the Eisenmenger complex are reported to predispose children to brain abscesses. This increased predisposition may be due to the presence of areas of brain ischemia caused by decreased arterial oxygen saturation and increased hemoglobin, which may act as a focus for infection to develop. Right-to-left shunting may also predispose to brain abscess, as the removal of organisms from the systemic circulation by the lungs is bypassed. Hematogenous spread can also occur by way of the veins that drain into the cavernous sinus, resulting in frontal lobe abscesses that correlate with infections of the facial tissues or ethmoid sinuses.

Extensions from cranial osteomyelitis, scalp infections, endocarditis, and meningitis are other known causes of CNS

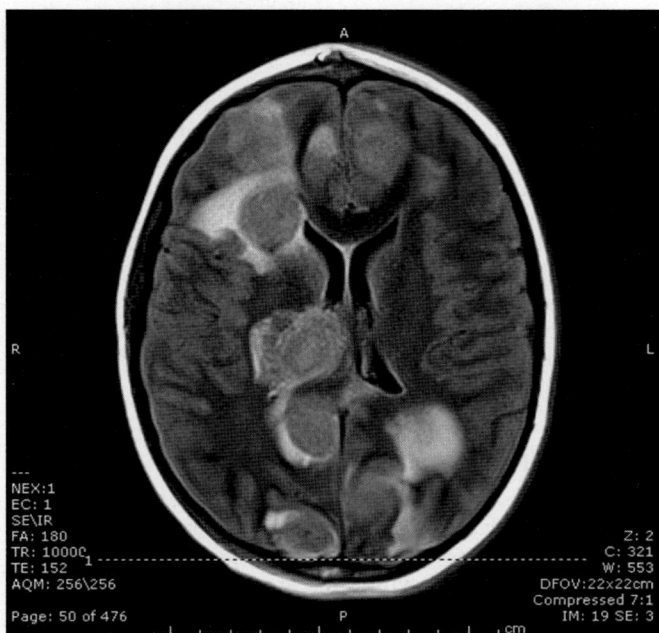

Fig. 70.3. MRI demonstrating multiple brain abscesses in a patient with cyanotic heart disease and single ventricle physiology. (Image courtesy of John Christenson, Indiana University.)

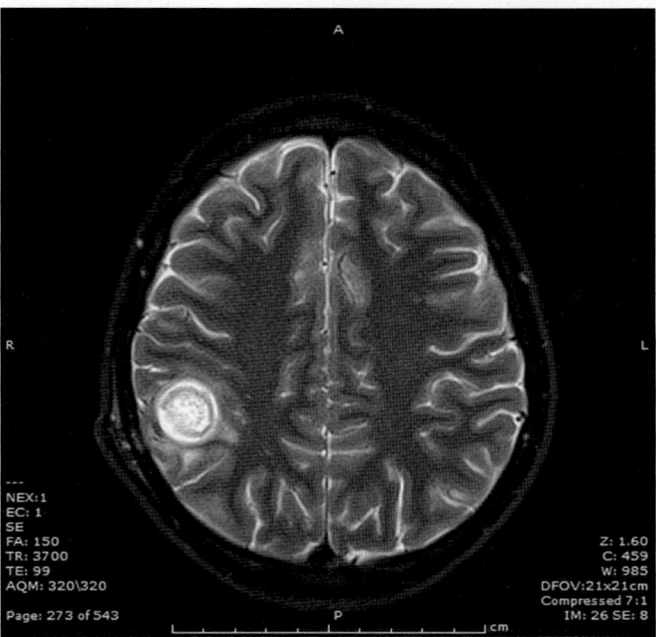

Fig. 70.4. Solitary brain abscess on MRI demonstrating evidence of liquefaction necrosis and a well-vascularized collagenous capsule. (Image courtesy of John Christenson, Indiana University.)

abscess formation. Several studies examined the etiology of brain abscesses in noncardiac patients. Incidence is reported as endocarditis in 10% of patients, bacteremia in 8%, immune deficiency in 12%, pulmonary anomalies in 5%, and skin folliculitis in 3%.[72,73] Infants and toddlers are more susceptible than other age groups to brain abscesses arising as complications of bacterial meningitis or bacteremia.[74] Historically, penetrating head trauma and neurosurgery represent a small proportion of the predisposing causes of CNS abscess, but the proportion is increasing, possibly as other predisposing factors such as middle ear infection become less important. In roughly one quarter of brain abscess cases, no identifiable route or predisposing factors are identified.[69]

Abscess formation results from the seeding of the parenchyma as the result of hematogenous spread from remote sources, direct invasion from contiguous infection of nonneural tissues, or from implantation of pathogens following penetrating wounds or surgery. Histologically, brain abscesses typically begin as areas of cerebritis with foci of acute inflammation. Vascular dilation, microthrombus formation, and rupture of small vessels are all noted. After 4 to 9 days, the center of the lesion undergoes liquefaction necrosis. By 10 to 14 days, a well-vascularized collagenous capsule with peripheral gliosis or fibrosis is typically present (Fig. 70.4).

The clinical presentation varies, depending on the size, multiplicity, and location of the lesion. Most patients are symptomatic within a week of the onset of abscess formation. Symptoms in adults are nonspecific and include headache (70%), fever (60%), vomiting (50%), focal neurologic deficits (45%), and seizures (40%).[69,75] Clinical symptoms occur even less commonly in pediatric cases. The triad of fever, headache, and focal deficits occurs in less than 30%, whereas meningeal signs occur in less than 25%.[76] Among clinical signs, over half of the cases will have papilledema. The sudden worsening of

a preexisting headache can indicate rupture of the brain abscess into the ventricular space or impending herniation from the lesion's mass effect. Significant alteration in mental status is an ominous clinical finding. Children with abscesses located within their brain stem typically present with fever, headaches, hemiparesis, and often have cranial nerve palsies of III, VI, and VII.

The most important microbiologic investigation in the management of patients with brain abscess is culture of the abscess fluid. The widespread acceptance of CT-guided stereotactic aspiration of brain abscesses, a minimally invasive procedure with low morbidity and mortality, is often indicated. This procedure allows both rapid and effective surgical drainage of the brain abscess and obtains material for culture. Lumbar puncture to obtain CSF may be contraindicated in a patient with a brain abscess, as raised ICP may lead to brain stem herniation in these patients. Additionally, CSF culture does not contribute significantly to the identification of the organism. Blood cultures can be helpful in a small percentage of patients, especially in those in whom the abscess is thought to be the result of hematogenous spread.

The microorganisms cultured from the brain abscess are variable and often depend on the original source. *S. aureus*, *Streptococcus* spp., and gram-negative anaerobic bacilli tend to predominate. *Citrobacter* and *E. sakazakii* are frequently associated with brain abscesses in neonates. In children with impaired host defenses, fungi and uncommon pathogens such as *Toxoplasma*, *Nocardia*, and *Mycobacterium* can be identified. Mixed aerobic and anaerobic flora are isolated in up to a third of patients, especially children with chronic otitis and sinusitis.[77] A quarter of abscess samples may demonstrate no bacterial growth.

Because the clinical presentation of brain abscess is often nonspecific, the diagnosis is often made by CT. Without imaging, it may be difficult to differentiate between brain abscess and other intracerebral pathologic processes. The advent of CT has altered the prognosis of brain abscess by improving diagnosis. MRI is also a useful tool in diagnosis but has not yet been shown to be superior to CT in establishing diagnosis. MRI may have a diagnostic advantage over CT by better differentiation of edema from liquefaction necrosis and greater sensitivity for early detection of satellite lesions.[78] Both CT and MRI are able to locate the position of the abscess accurately, thus enabling a focused surgical intervention. Serial CT scanning may provide additional information about response to treatment.

There have been no randomized, controlled trials comparing the various treatments for brain abscesses. The neurologic status of the patient, the location of the abscess, the number/size of the abscesses, and the stage of abscess formation should influence medical management. Stereotactic CT-guided drainage of the abscess, followed by antibiotic therapy, is the treatment of choice in most patients. Typically, abscesses >2.5 cm require surgical drainage.[79] Even in the critically ill PICU patient, a stereotactic procedure is minimally invasive and the risk-benefit profile will often support its use. Aspiration of the abscess allows both removal of infected nidus and likely identification of the causative organism. Endoscopic drainage may be useful in lesions located in a periventricular distribution.

Craniotomy and excision are usually reserved for abscesses that enlarge after 2 weeks of antibiotic therapy or that fail to shrink after 3 to 4 weeks of antibiotics.[80] Craniotomy is also recommended for multiloculated abscesses and larger lesions with significant mass effect. Craniotomy and direct surgical drainage are required in some cases of fungal or helminthic infections or after failed stereotactic drainage. Also, brain abscesses secondary to traumatic brain injury should be considered strongly for surgical excision because of the possibility of retained foreign bodies or bone fragments. Lesions located in the cerebellum may have a lower mortality, incidence of developing obstructive hydrocephalus, and shorter hospital stays if primary excision is chosen over stereotactic aspiration.[81]

There are few indications for the nonoperative management of brain abscesses. These include patients with surgically inaccessible lesions, early cerebritis, multiple small abscesses, or medical comorbidities that would classify the patient as high risk. In specific cases where there is a small lesion and the infecting organism is known, medical treatment alone may be considered appropriate.

A combination of a third generation cephalosporin and metronidazole is a reasonable combination for initial antibiotic therapy in brain abscesses. Vancomycin can be added if *S. aureus* is identified or suspected as the causative organism. Vancomycin is also a reasonable choice if the abscess is believed to have occurred as a consequence of a neurosurgical procedure. There are no prospective studies in children to guide antibiotic therapy. Duration of treatment is typically based on clinical response. Duration can be as short as 1 to 2 weeks of IV antibiotic therapy followed by 2 to 4 weeks of an oral antibiotic after surgical drainage. Some clinicians recommend duration of IV therapy as long as 4 to 6 weeks.[78] If antibiotics alone are utilized, duration of IV therapy is typically longer, with some clinicians recommending up to 6 to 8 weeks.[79]

Mortality attributed to brain abscess was 60% prior to 1970. Since the advent of newer radiologic procedures such has high-resolution head CT or MRI, detection of brain abscesses is more efficient. With earlier detection, mortality has dropped and currently is about 10% to 15%.[75,76] Long-term neurologic morbidity attributed to the abscess and therapy ranges from 10% to 30% depending on both size and location of the lesion as well as response to therapy. The patient's neurologic status at presentation is a significant predictor of outcome with an increased mortality rate in those who present to the PICU with an altered mental status or rapid neurologic deterioration.[82] Brain abscesses resulting from a contiguous focus of infection and those developing after a traumatic injury tend to have a good prognosis. Those resulting from patients with immunologic or cardiac predisposing factor are more likely to have a poorer outcome.

Viral Meningoencephalitis

The incidence of bacterial meningitis has decreased significantly in the vaccine era. However, viral meningoencephalitis continues to be a common neurologic problem in the PICU. The initial signs and symptoms are often indistinguishable from bacterial meningitis, and a diagnosis of a viral, rather than bacterial, CNS infection does not correlate with decreased morbidity or mortality.

Whereas meningitis implies that the meninges are primarily involved, encephalitis indicates brain parenchymal involvement. The presence or absence of normal brain function is important in distinguishing between meningitis and encephalitis. Patients with meningitis typically have fever, meningeal signs, CSF pleocytosis, and no associated neurologic dysfunction unless related to seizure activity or elevated ICP. Abnormal neurologic findings such as focal neurologic signs, cranial nerve involvement, motor deficits, sensory deficits, or speech difficulties suggest brain parenchymal involvement and encephalitis. Patients presenting with seizures may have meningitis or encephalitis. Making the distinction between meningitis and encephalitis is often difficult, and patients may present with both a parenchymal and meningeal process. Therefore, some authors prefer the term *meningoencephalitis* to recognize the inherent overlap between the two clinical entities.

Epidemiology

A survey of hospital discharge records from 1988 to 1997 showed approximately 19,000 hospitalizations per year (7.3 hospitalizations per 100,000 population), 230,000 hospital days, and 1400 deaths annually due to viral encephalitis in the United States.[83] Children under the age of 1 year had the highest risk for hospitalization due to encephalitis. Between 1989 and 1998, there were approximately 1100 deaths due to encephalitis in children under the age of 19 in the United States. The highest rate of death was in children less than 1 year of age (9.3 per 100,000 population).[83] Although the causative agent in encephalitis can be difficult to isolate, most cases are attributed to enteroviruses, herpesviruses, and arboviruses. The enteroviruses and arboviruses in particular display seasonality in infection, being seen most frequently in the summer and autumn months. Herpesviruses, cytomegalovirus (CMV), varicella-zoster virus (VZV), and Epstein-Barr virus (EBV) often show a predilection for the winter and spring. Herpes simplex, however, does not demonstrate any seasonality. With this epidemiology in mind, the evaluation of children with suspected viral meningoencephalitis is guided by many factors including age, geographic location, season of the year, vaccination status, chronic conditions or immunosuppression, history of tick or mosquito exposure, and travel history.

Pathophysiology/Pathogenesis of Viral Meningoencephalitis

Infection of the CNS by most neurotropic viruses begins with multiplication of the virus at the port of entry (mucosal surfaces of the skin, gastrointestinal tract, or respiratory tract). The viruses then travel to extraneural sites in the body. They then migrate to vascular tissue, further multiply, and, finally, infect the CNS. Viruses may reach the CNS by several mechanisms. Although most directly invade across cerebral capillary endothelial cells that comprise the BBB, they may also (1) directly infect cerebral microvascular endothelial cells before infection of adjacent glia and neurons, (2) be carried between cerebral endothelial cells in infected leukocytes after BBB disruption, (3) initially infect glia without evidence of endothelial cell infection, (4) enter the choroid plexus epithelium, or (5) spread along olfactory nerve or peripheral nerve pathways.[84] Once a virus has invaded the CNS, it attaches within susceptible cells and induces the cellular changes and inflammatory responses that manifest as meningitis or encephalitis.

Clinical Evaluation

Bacterial and other causes of meningoencephalitis as well as other causes of encephalopathy such as trauma, hepatic failure, electrolyte abnormalities, and toxic ingestions must be ruled out before viral encephalitis is diagnosed. A careful history will yield important information such as immunization status, recent viral or other infections, history of immune diseases, travel history, tick or mosquito exposure, and the history of maternal herpes infection in the case of neonates. Physical exam should focus on evaluation of the mucous membranes and skin as well as a complete neurologic examination including the funduscopic examination. A high level of suspicion and vigilance, with serial neurologic examinations, is essential because viral injury may result in the development of cerebral edema and even brain stem herniation. As in meningitis, antibiotics or antiviral medications should not be withheld while the laboratory and imaging workup of encephalitis is pursued.

Laboratory Manifestations

Lumbar puncture with an opening pressure is essential in the evaluation of the patient with suspected meningoencephalitis. Initial evaluation of CSF includes cell count, protein, glucose, culture, herpes simplex virus (HSV) PCR, enteroviral PCR, and oligoclonal bands.[85] CSF findings in viral encephalitis include pleocytosis with white blood cell counts in the 100 to 1000 cells/uL range. Polymorphonuclear cells are often predominant in early infection and even up to 48 hours of infection; lymphocytes typically become more predominant later in the time course.[86] There is usually at least mild elevation in CSF protein, and there may be mildly decreased glucose; however, glucose is often normal. Elevated red blood cells are often seen with herpesvirus. In addition to CSF, blood should be obtained for complete blood count and culture, erythrocyte sedimentation rate or C-reactive protein, and electrolytes. If suggested by the history, additional studies for viral studies should be obtained. These often include CSF and serum

arboviral titers (virus-specific IgM) and serum, urine, or nasal specimens for viruses such as HSV, varicella, EBV, CMV, adenovirus, influenza, and parainfluenza.

As a more rapid alternative to tissue culture, PCR techniques allow for relatively sensitive and specific diagnosis of enteroviruses and herpesviruses in the clinical setting. For enteroviruses, PCR is directed at genomic RNA in the highly conserved regions of the 5′ noncoding region. PCR allows for accurate diagnosis of enteroviruses in a few hours, and sensitivity has been shown to be approximately 98%.[87] Specific virologic diagnosis of enteroviruses requires recovery of virus from CSF or tissue culture, with a sensitivity of 65% to 75%.[88] For HSV, CSF PCR is the test of choice, with approximately 98% sensitivity and 94% specificity.[89,90] PCR for VZV DNA has been found to be 95% specific but only 30% sensitive. Therefore, it is recommended that in cases of suspected VZV encephalitis the CSF be tested for intrathecal synthesis of VZV-specific antibody (IgM and CSF-to-serum IgG ratio).[91,92] PCR testing is also available for EBV and CMV from the CSF. For HHV-6 infection, which may present as severe encephalitis in immunocompromised patients, PCR has been shown to be somewhat sensitive; however, it may unreliably detect the virus, and viral isolation may be required.[93,94]

Arboviruses in the CSF and serum are detected by IgG and IgM antibody testing. According to criteria of the Centers for Disease Control and Prevention (CDC), confirmed cases of arboviral disease must demonstrate (1) a fourfold or greater change in virus-specific antibody titer; (2) isolation of virus from or demonstration of specific viral antigen or genomic sequences in tissue, blood, or CSF; (3) virus-specific IgM in CSF by antibody-capture enzyme immunoassay (EIA); or (4) virus-specific antibodies demonstrated in serum by antibody-capture EIA and confirmed by IgG antibodies in either the same or a later specimen.[95] Many states have epidemiologic programs to provide surveillance of arboviral infections, and consultation with local and state health departments will help guide serologic testing.

In some rare cases, brain biopsy is required for definitive diagnosis and remains the gold standard to diagnose viral infections of the CNS.

Neuroimaging

The initial noncontrast head CT may be normal in patients with meningoencephalitis. Although most patients will undergo a CT scan in the early period of illness, MRI is most sensitive for detecting inflammation, edema, and hemorrhage in viral encephalitis. If there is concern for spinal cord involvement (transverse myelitis, enterovirus), then the MRI should also include the spine.[95] Depending on disease severity, patients with viral encephalitis may show focal or diffuse cerebral edema and even uncal or transtentorial herniation on either CT or MRI.

Specific infections often show characteristic MRI findings that may be helpful in formulating a diagnosis. The MRI appearance of viral encephalitis is generally that of diffuse scattered or confluent areas of T2-weighted hyperintensity. There is a variable degree of mass effect and edema. Inflammation often involves meninges, and gadolinium enhancement is diffuse. The classic finding in HSV and HHV-6 encephalitis is hemorrhagic inflammation, often bilateral, of the temporal lobe, which manifests as T2-weighted hyperintensity on MRI and usually spares the deep nuclear structures

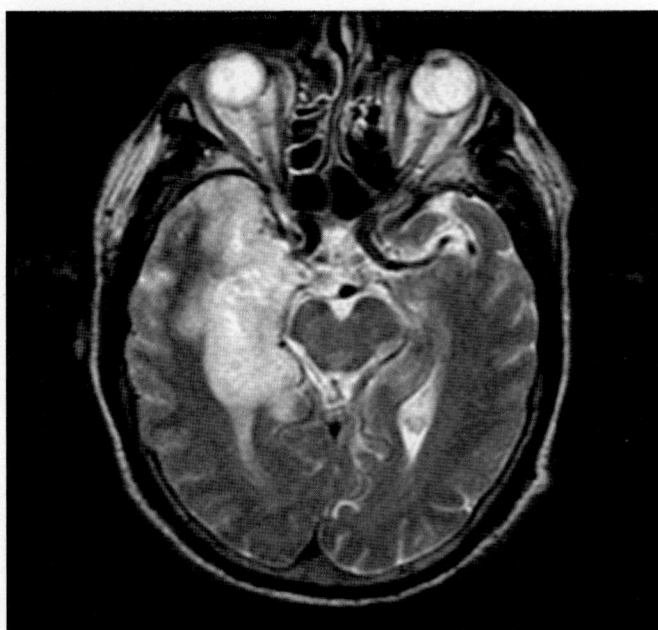

Fig. 70.5. Classic temporal lobe enhancement noted on a head T2-weighted MRI in a patient with herpes simplex virus encephalitis. (Image courtesy of Karen Bloch, Vanderbilt Medical Center.)

(Fig. 70.5).[96,97] Neonates with HSV encephalitis may demonstrate less defined areas of inflammation on MRI and may have a loss of gray-white matter distinction only.[95] Among other herpesviruses, VZV encephalitis may demonstrate multifocal ischemia and infarction as well as demyelinating lesions in the white matter and at gray-white junctions. CMV often shows characteristic enhancement in the ependyma around the lateral ventricles.[97] Togaviruses, including West Nile virus, St. Louis encephalitis virus, Japanese encephalitis virus, and Eastern and Western equine encephalitis viruses, show involvement in the subcortical white matter, thalami, and substantia nigra.[97] In particular, Eastern equine encephalitis has been shown to produce focal lesions in the basal ganglia, thalami, and brain stem.[98] MRI findings in enterovirus encephalitis are less clearly defined and may be highly variable. However, patients with enterovirus 71 infection have demonstrated increased T2 and fluid-attenuated inversion recovery (FLAIR) signal intensity in the midbrain, pons, medulla, and even the spinal cord.[99]

Clinical Presentation and Course

The clinical course of viral meningoencephalitis is highly variable, ranging from mild disease to death. Children with viral meningoencephalitis or encephalitis usually present with a prodrome of fever, headache, irritability, malaise, decreased oral intake, nausea, and possibly neck pain or nuchal rigidity. These signs and symptoms are essentially identical to the presentation of viral meningitis. However, a child with encephalitis also shows a decline in the level of consciousness and may demonstrate confusion, ataxia, seizures, aphasia, visual changes, and focal motor deficits or sensory deficits corresponding to the affected areas of the brain. In general, the most common focal neurologic deficits seen in encephalitis

are hemiparesis, aphasia, ataxia, cranial nerve palsies, seizures, and myoclonus. Patients may also demonstrate autonomic dysregulation or hypothalamic dysfunction resulting in diabetes insipidus or syndrome of inappropriate antidiuretic hormone (SIADH). Seizures are possible, especially in infants and children with herpes encephalitis. At the most extreme end of the encephalitis spectrum, focal or diffuse cerebral edema and even brain stem herniation may occur.

HSV, from either a new infection or a latent reinfection, remains the most common cause of fatal sporadic encephalitis in humans, despite specific antiviral therapy.[100] HSV encephalitis is particularly severe in children with immunocompromise due to chemotherapeutic regimens, genetic immune defects, or human immunodeficiency virus infection. Children and adolescents with HSV encephalitis present with nonspecific neurologic signs and often have seizures. Support for the diagnosis of HSV encephalitis may be bolstered by findings of temporal lobe involvement on MRI as well as spike and slow-wave activity on EEG.[101] Adults and children typically present with HSV-1 infection. In neonates, the majority of encephalitis cases are caused by HSV-2 due to perinatal transmission and shedding of virus in the maternal genital tract. Neonates presenting with encephalitis due to HSV often do not demonstrate fever. Skin lesion findings are variable. The most common presenting signs for neonates with HSV CNS disease are seizures and lethargy.[102] Infants with HSV infection may also have disseminated disease, which increases the risk of morbidity and mortality significantly. However, as the majority of infants with HSV encephalitis are <21 days of age, testing for HSV without specific symptoms or radiologic findings and broad use of empiric acyclovir in older infants and children may be unnecessary.[103,104]

Enteroviral encephalitis may be highly variable in its presentation. The majority of cases are self-limited, but a large proportion of patients experience at least short-term morbidity. Although HSV has predilection for the temporal lobes in many cases, the enteroviral infections are more global in nature in general. Patients with enteroviral encephalitis often present with fever, headache, nausea, vomiting, and nuchal rigidity. They may also demonstrate confusion or delirium as well as have seizures or focal neurologic signs.[105]

Enterovirus 71, the cause of hand-foot-mouth disease/ herpangina, usually causes flulike symptoms and a characteristic rash on hands, feet, and buttocks and oral ulcers. It can also cause flaccid paralysis, inflammation and necrosis of the tissues of the brain stem, and death in about 16% of cases.[106] In addition, myocarditis and heart failure have also been reported with enterovirus 71 infections. Severe enterovirus 71 outbreaks were originally described in Asia. High fever and lethargy predict severe disease, and myoclonus often indicates early brain stem involvement. PCR of throat swabs and vesicle fluid, if available, is among the diagnostic tests of choice. Features of inflammation, particularly in the anterior horns of the spinal cord, the dorsal pons, and the medulla can be seen on MRI. Although there is no established antiviral treatment, intravenous immunoglobulin (IVIG) seems to be beneficial in severe disease, perhaps through nonspecific antiinflammatory mechanisms.[107] This virus may represent an important worldwide emerging pathogen.[108] Unfortunately, the neurodevelopmental follow-up of children with severe enterovirus 71 brain stem encephalitis reveals significant long-term cognitive and motor deficits.[109,110]

Neuroinvasive arboviral infections include the California serogroup viruses, Eastern and Western equine encephalitis viruses, Powassan virus, St. Louis encephalitis virus, and West Nile virus. Their incidence increases when mosquito vectors are most active, usually in the summer months, and incidence varies significantly based on geographic region. This group causes encephalitis as well as myelitis. In fact, West Nile virus infection has been misdiagnosed as Guillain-Barré syndrome due to flaccid paralysis. Arboviral encephalitis is characterized by fever, headache, and altered mental status ranging from confusion to coma, with or without additional signs of brain dysfunction. Arboviral myelitis causes acute bulbar or limb paresis or a flaccid paralysis.[111] A review of data from ArboNET, the national arboviral surveillance system in the United States, published in 2014 found 1217 cases and 22 deaths due to pediatric neuroinvasive arboviral infections from 2003 through 2012. La Crosse virus (665 cases, 55%) and West Nile virus (505 cases, 41%) were the most common viruses identified. However, Eastern equine encephalitis was the most deadly, causing 10 deaths out of 30 cases identified.[112] West Nile virus occurred throughout the United States, whereas La Crosse virus was most common in the Appalachian and Midwestern regions (Tennessee, West Virginia, North Carolina, and Ohio). Eastern equine encephalitis virus is most common along the Atlantic and Gulf coasts of the United States. Many arboviruses show increased incidence in boys, and it is unclear whether this is related to increased outdoor activity in boys or a true sex-based predilection.

Other zoonoses can cause encephalitis. Exposure to tick populations may suggest infection with Colorado tick fever in the western United States or nonviral etiologies such as Lyme disease or Rocky Mountain spotted fever. Nipah virus encephalitis has been seen in Malaysia, Singapore, and Bangladesh and may be associated with bat or pig exposures.[113-115] Lymphocytic choriomeningitis virus is caused by a rodent-borne arenavirus and is transmitted via mice, rat, and hamster secretions. Rabies, while rare in the United States, should be suspected in patients with prodromal symptoms of encephalitis followed by hydrophobia and pharyngeal spasms as well as exposure to bats or other reservoirs. The incubation period is typically 20 to 60 days but can be in the 5-day to 6-month range.[116] In the developing world, canine rabies transmission to humans remains a significant public health problem, with an estimated (but probably severely underestimated) 55,000 deaths annually in Africa and Asia.[117]

Influenza virus infection has been associated with a number of neurologic complications such as seizures and mild encephalopathy.[118] The neuroimaging of many of these patients demonstrates a distinct pattern of bilateral, multifocal lesions of the thalami that have been described as acute necrotizing encephalopathy.[119,120] In addition, many patients with influenza-associated encephalitis and necrotizing encephalitis progress to multisystem organ failure. In a survey of more than 140 cases in Japan during the 1998–1999 influenza A (H3N2) outbreak, 31.8% of patients with influenza-associated encephalitis or encephalopathy died and another 27.7% experienced either short- or long-term disability.[121] Brain CT revealed abnormalities in 66% of patients, with the most frequent findings being cerebral edema and hypodensities in the thalamus, brain stem, and brain parenchyma. Approximately 10% of the patients in the 1998–1999 case series showed the characteristic findings of acute necrotizing encephalopathy.

Only a small number of these patients have had influenza RNA isolated from CSF, and autopsies demonstrate a lack of direct viral invasion in the central nervous system. Many of the cases have been described in Japan and other parts of Asia, leading to some speculation that there may be a genetic susceptibility to developing influenza-associated encephalitis/encephalopathy, but cases are also described in Europe and North America.[122-124]

Treatment

With the exception of herpesviruses, therapy for patients with HSV encephalitis is largely supportive. Those with severe neurologic dysfunction or status epilepticus may require airway, respiratory, and circulatory support. Clinicians should maintain careful attention to fluid and electrolyte status due to the risk of diabetes insipidus, SIADH, and cerebral salt wasting. ICP monitoring has been used at some centers, and therapies to decrease intracranial pressure may be required.[125] Several small case series and case reports have discussed the use of decompressive craniotomy or craniectomy in the setting of severe encephalitis-induced intracranial hypertension in both adults and children.[126] However, to date there have been no large studies on the outcomes of children with severe viral encephalitis and intracranial hypertension managed with ICP monitoring or decompressive craniectomy. Seizures, both clinical and subclinical, should be treated and subsequently prevented as much as possible. Continuous EEG monitoring and barbiturate coma have been used in selected cases; however, the literature suggests that patients with refractory status epilepticus and viral encephalitis have extremely poor outcomes.[127]

Medical treatment of viral encephalitis is most effective in treatment of herpesvirus. In neonates with HSV encephalitis, antiviral therapy has significantly improved survival and decreased disease progression. The current recommended treatment for patients from infancy to age 12 years with HSV encephalitis is "high-dose" acyclovir (20 mg/kg IV every 8 hours) given for 21 days for both encephalitis and disseminated disease. Those over 12 years of age should receive acyclovir at 30 mg/kg per day in three divided doses for 21 days.[128] Acyclovir-resistant HSV infections, though rare, have been reported and treated with foscarnet.[129]

Infants born to mothers who contract primary varicella infection from 5 days prior to delivery until 2 days after delivery are at increased risk for severe varicella encephalitis. Exposed newborns may be candidates for VZV specific immunoglobulin prophylaxis (VariZIG) if the mother has severe skin involvement. There is a paucity of data, but the use of IV acyclovir at doses identical to treatment for HSV infection is recommended for neonates with clinical signs of varicella due to the risk of severe disease. Intravenous acyclovir therapy is also recommended for other pediatric patients with encephalitis as well as immunocompromised patients with any form of varicella disease. Children with varicella should not receive salicylates due to the increased risk for Reye syndrome, and those on chronic salicylate therapy for other conditions should have their salicylate suspended. Like HSV, acyclovir-resistant varicella has been treated with foscarnet.

Case reports of immunocompromised patients with human herpesvirus 6 (HHV-6) encephalitis suggest that this may be an emerging pathogen, particularly among transplant recipients.[130] Encephalitis may be caused by either a new infection or a reactivation of latent HHV-6. Isolation of HHV-6 from the blood or detection of viral DNA in serum or plasma via PCR indicates active viral infection. Serology is considered unreliable, particularly in immunocompromised patients. Foscarnet, ganciclovir, and cidofovir have been shown to have efficacy against HHV-6, and the International Herpes Management Forum recommends foscarnet and ganciclovir, either alone or in combination, for treatment of HHV-6-related central nervous system illness.[131]

CMV has caused encephalitis in immunocompromised patients and is particularly fatal in HIV disease. Foscarnet-ganciclovir combination therapy has been used with limited success.

Influenza encephalitis remains a challenge because often the virus is not detected in the CSF or even in brain tissue specimens. The neuraminidase inhibitor oseltamivir as well as the ion channel blocker amantadine were both used in the largest prospective study of acute encephalitis/encephalopathy and influenza. It is unknown whether these agents change the outcome of this particularly clinically diverse and evolving entity.[132] Despite antiviral therapy, influenza encephalitis is frequently fatal.

Prognosis

The prognosis for patients with meningoencephalitis is extremely variable and depends on the causative agent and the degree of CNS injury. Some patients with relatively mild disease may experience only short-term sequelae of their infection. Although antiviral therapy has significantly improved mortality for HSV encephalitis in neonates, studies suggest that the long-term cognitive and neurodevelopmental consequences for survivors of HSV encephalitis and disseminated HSV disease include static encephalopathy, mental retardation, autism, cortical blindness, and epilepsy. Focal signs on neurologic exam, multiple seizures or status epilepticus on admission, leukopenia, and focal slow waves or continuous generalized delta waves on EEG are all associated with poor neurologic outcomes.[133] Serial neuroimaging studies and close neurologic follow-up may aid in counseling families regarding the prognosis for individual patients, but predicting neurologic functional outcomes in this group of patients remains a challenge for clinicians.

Central Nervous System Amebic Infections

Free-living amebas found in freshwater environments cause rare, often fatal forms of meningoencephalitis affecting both the brain and spinal cord. The three most common organisms are *Naegleria fowleri*, *Acanthamoeba* species, and *Balamuthia mandrillaris*. *Naegleria* causes primary amebic meningoencephalitis (PAM). *Acanthamoeba* and *Balamuthia* cause granulomatous amebic encephalitis (GAE).

PAM is a rare, often fatal disease most commonly caused by infection with *Naegleria fowleri*, a thermophilic, free-living ameba found in freshwater environments. *N. fowleri* is the causal agent of most PAM infections, but other species of *Naegleria* having pathogenic potential have been described (*N. australiensis, N. italica*). Currently, more than a dozen species of *Naegleria* are recognized based on small subunit ribosomal DNA.[134] The habitat for *N. fowleri* is natural or man-made freshwater lakes or an inadequately chlorinated swimming pool where the amebas can feed on bacteria and proliferate. In the United States, *N. fowleri* is commonly found in warm

freshwater environments in 15 southern tier states (Arizona, Arkansas, California, Florida, Georgia, Louisiana, Mississippi, Missouri, Nevada, New Mexico, North Carolina, Oklahoma, South Carolina, Texas, and Virginia).

In the United States, 111 PAM patients were diagnosed, reported, and verified by state health officials between 1962 and 2008. These infections occurred primarily in previously healthy young males exposed to warm recreational waters, especially lakes and ponds, during summer months. The annual number of PAM case reports varied but did not appear to be increasing over time. The fatality rate was approximately 95%.[135] However, in 2013, there were two pediatric survivors of PAM in the United States. One was a 12-year-old girl, one an 8-year-old boy. Both received similar treatment regimens, with the exception being that the 12-year-old girl was also managed with hypothermia. The 12-year-old girl who received the combination therapy and therapeutic hypothermia made a full neurologic recovery, whereas the 8-year-old boy, who was diagnosed and treatment begun several days after presentation, suffered permanent neurologic complications.[136]

Naegleria species typically cause PAM in children and healthy adults who have been swimming in infected water. *N. fowleri* enter through the olfactory neuroepithelium at the level of the cribriform plate and invade the submucosal nervous plexus. Symptoms begin after a 3- to 7-day incubation period. PAM presents in a manner similar to acute bacterial meningitis, but physicians often miss the diagnosis initially. History is vital for making the diagnosis. Recent exposure to diving, swimming, or splashing in warm freshwater should suggest the possibility of amebic meningoencephalitis. Prompt examination of the CSF for *N. fowleri* is fundamental to establishing this diagnosis. The onset of PAM is abrupt but nonspecific. Patients may complain of sore throat, headache, nausea, vomiting, malaise, and fever. Early findings may also include irritability, hallucinations, meningismus, cerebellar ataxia, and cranial nerve palsies, although focal neurologic defects are usually absent. Alterations in taste and smell may occur, likely due to involvement of the olfactory nerve.[137] Brain imaging should be obtained, but findings of CT and MR imaging may be normal early in the disease, with evidence of brain edema, basilar meningeal enhancement, and sometimes infarcts seen later in the disease process.[138]

Differential diagnosis for PAM includes acute bacterial meningitis, HSV-1 or other viral encephalitis, and fungal meningitis. With immunosuppressed patients, PAM might be confused with toxoplasmosis, CMV infection, and other opportunistic pathogens. The diagnosis is made by examination of centrifuged CSF wet mounts for motile trophozoites. However, failure to visualize these amebae does not exclude PAM. The diagnosis is often missed when *Naegleria* organisms are mistaken for atypical leukocytes, specifically monocytes or lymphocytes.[139]

PAM infections tend to be fulminant, with seizures progressing to coma and death within 4 to 6 days. Autopsy findings typically demonstrate acute hemorrhagic necrotizing meningoencephalitis with purulent exudates in the brain, brain stem, and cerebellum.

The extremely low incidence of PAM makes epidemiologic study difficult. Questions concerning why certain individuals become infected with the amebae while many others are exposed to the same freshwater sources remain. Attempts are under way to determine what concentration of *N. fowleri* in the environment poses an unacceptable risk to swimmers, how a standard might be set to protect human health, and how regulators might measure and enforce such a standard.

The free-living amebas *Acanthamoeba* spp. and *Balamuthia mandrillaris* cause a subacute CNS infection, GAE. More so than the *Naegleria* organism, *Acanthamoeba* is ubiquitous in the environment, with amebas widely disseminated in soil and water. Unlike the healthy individuals acquiring *Naegleria* infections, *Acanthamoeba* infections of the CNS are typically in compromised hosts, such as those with AIDS, those with IgA deficiency, or those undergoing suppressive therapy for organ transplant or autoimmune diseases. However, cases in immunocompetent individuals have also been reported. Making this diagnosis requires a high index of suspicion, as it is easily confounded by potential manifestations of the underlying disease. The portal of entry of this species of ameba can vary. It may be intranasal, allowing amebas to migrate directly to the CNS, via a break in the skin or through the respiratory tract, with subsequent spread of amebas to the CNS by a hematogenous route. The disease assumes a chronic status, leading to slow deterioration. Gadolinium-enhanced TI-weighted MR images of the brain show multiple punctate focal areas of enhancement bilaterally throughout the cerebellar hemispheres, with some scattered foci supratentorially.[140] These lesions may represent focal cerebritis or microabscesses. Diagnosis is most often made by postmortem examination of brain tissue showing patchy, chronic granulomas encephalitis with trophozoites and cysts in the lesions. Brain biopsy, often required to make a definitive diagnosis, reveals numerous trophozoites with round nucleus, prominent nucleolus, and thin nuclear membrane. Methenamine silver stain shows encysted ameba. Specific serum antibodies may not be a reliable measure in immunocompromised patients, and trophozoites in CSF can be confused with monocytes.[141]

Based on the treatment regimens used in the most recent survivors of PAM, the CDC currently recommends the following drug therapy in CNS infections caused by *N. fowleri* as well as *B. mandrillaris* and *Acanthamoeba* species: (1) IV amphotericin B, (2) intrathecal amphotericin B, (3) azithromycin, (4) fluconazole, (5) rifampin, (6) miltefosine, and (7) dexamethasone. Miltefosine is an investigational drug previously used to treat breast cancer and leishmaniasis shown to have amebicidal activity against *Balamuthia, N. fowleri,* and *Acanthamoeba.*[142] The CDC has an investigational drug protocol (IND) in effect with the FDA to make miltefosine available directly from the CDC for the treatment of free-living amebas.[143,144] For diagnostic assistance, specimen collection guidance, shipping instructions, and treatment recommendations, clinicians are to contact the CDC Emergency Operations Center at (770) 488–7100.

Acute Disseminated Encephalomyelitis

Acute disseminated encephalomyelitis (ADEM) is an acute inflammatory demyelinating disorder of the central nervous system. Though it is not typically associated with primary CNS infection, patients with ADEM often have a preceding febrile illness (93%) or vaccination (5%) that is thought to trigger an autoimmune response.[145] The inflammatory response of ADEM may result in a clinical picture that is similar to infectious meningitis or encephalitis, and therefore advanced neuroimaging and an infectious workup are often performed. Population-based epidemiologic studies have

estimated that between 0.1 and 0.8/100,000 cases of ADEM occur in children annually, at a median age of 5 to 8 years.[145-147] Although ADEM may be diagnosed with mild symptoms such as headache and lethargy, children often present with more severe and progressive symptoms with up to 25% of cases requiring admission to a PICU.[148]

ADEM is an immune-mediated process likely triggered by antigenic stimulation. According to this hypothesis, called "molecular mimicry," certain amino acid sequence homologies and antigenic epitopes are shared between an invading pathogen or inoculated vaccine and host CNS proteins such as myelin basic protein. Initially, the pathogenic material is processed at the site of infection or inoculation. The adaptive immune response causes T-cell activation and ultimately the production of antigen-specific B cells. If these cells encounter the homologous myelin protein, local reactivation and immune reaction against the presumed foreign antigen are elicited. Thus, a physiologic immune response causes autoimmunity distant from the original site of infection or inoculation. Histologically, the lesions of ADEM appear similar to those of patients with multiple sclerosis (MS), though ADEM can often be distinguished by the finding of perivenous demyelination of similar age as opposed to the more confluent demyelination and heterogeneous appearance characteristic of MS.[149] In patients with ADEM, demyelination may not be present in the acute lesion(s) but tends to develop later in the disease process, often in a sleevelike pattern confined to the area of inflammation. Damage to the axon itself is rare.

The combination of altered consciousness or behavior and multifocal neurologic deficits, especially in close relation to an infection or vaccination, should raise the clinician's suspicion of ADEM. Patients may present with nonspecific symptoms such as headache, vomiting, lethargy, and low-grade fever. Apart from neurologic findings, the remainder of the physical examination is most often normal. Distinct functional cognitive deficits are present in the majority of patients at the time of admission. Motor deficits and cranial neuropathies (particularly of extraocular movements) are the most common focal finding. Clinical deterioration and development of new neurologic deficits are prominent features in the hospital course of many patients with ADEM. When ICU management is needed, patients often require mechanical ventilation, typically due to brain stem involvement or severely impaired consciousness, with the median duration of mechanical ventilation of 3 days (Table 70.5).[148]

Specific laboratory criteria do not exist for the diagnosis of ADEM. Similar to other demyelinating conditions, patients with ADEM typically have increased levels of CSF protein and a mild lymphocytic CSF pleocytosis. In contrast to MS, oligoclonal bands are rarely detected.[150] EEG will often be abnormal and typically shows diffuse slowing consistent with encephalopathy. Focal lesions may be present on neuroimaging, but the finding of focal epileptiform activity is rare. A CT scan is often the initial neuroimaging study obtained to rule out conditions such as a space-occupying lesion or acute hydrocephalus. However, the radiologic study of choice to diagnose ADEM is an MRI of the brain and spinal cord. The T2-weighted and fluid-attenuated inversion recovery (FLAIR) sequences are most useful for identifying ADEM-associated lesions (Fig. 70.6). Although there is no lesion pattern pathognomonic for ADEM, they are most typically large (≥1–2 cm), asymmetric, poorly demarcated, and involve the subcortical and central

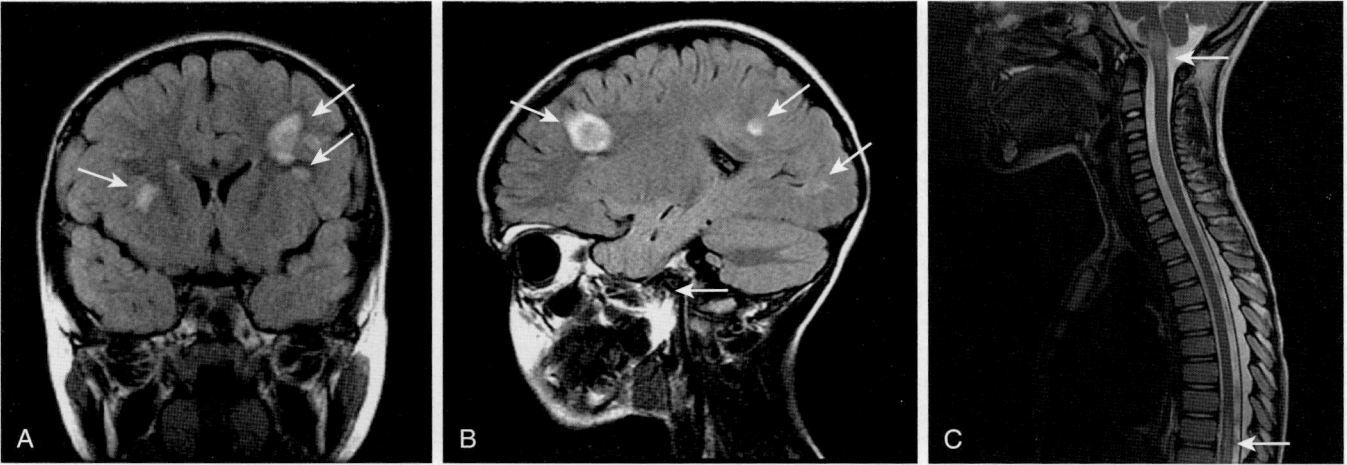

Fig. 70.6. A 6-year-old patient affected by ADEM. Coronal *(left)* and sagittal *(middle)* FLAIR images of the brain show confluent T2-FLAIR hyperintense lesions in the subcortical white matter of the cerebral hemispheres bilaterally *(arrows)*. Sagittal T2 image of the cervical and thoracic spine *(right)* shows medullary involvement extending from brain stem to cervical cord. Beginning at T8-9 disc space, there is another lesion with abnormal T2 signal *(arrows)*.

TABLE 70.5	Clinical Features of Children With Acute Disseminated Encephalomyelitis Requiring Intensive Care	
Feature/Symptom		**Prevalence (%)**
Encephalopathy/encephalitis/encephalomyelitis		100
Multifocal neurologic deficit		22
Seizure		19
Mechanical ventilation (typically due to brain stem involvement or severely impaired consciousness)		78
Inotrope/vasopressors		15
Invasive intracranial pressure monitoring		4

Data from Absoud M, Parslow RC, Wassmer E, et al. Severe acute disseminated encephalomyelitis: a paediatric intensive care population-based study. Mult Scler. 2010;17: 1258-1261.

white matter and the gray-white matter junction of the cerebral hemispheres, cerebellum, brain stem, and spinal cord. Gray matter involvement may be seen, particularly in the thalamus and basal ganglia. Using diffusion-weighted imaging (DWI) and apparent diffusion coefficient (ADC) maps, most patients will demonstrate vasogenic edema (increased signal intensity in both sequences), as opposed to cytotoxic edema.[151]

Given the presumed autoimmune pathogenesis of ADEM, high-dose corticosteroid therapy is the recommended first-line therapy. Typically, methylprednisolone 10 to 30 mg/kg/day is administered for 3 to 5 days, followed by an oral taper over 4 to 6 weeks.[146] A taper less than 4 weeks is associated with a greater risk of relapse. Of note, there are no randomized clinical trials of steroids for the treatment of ADEM. A retrospective study of 84 children comparing treatment with methylprednisolone to dexamethasone found improved disability scores in the children who received methylprednisolone. IVIG may be used, either alone or more commonly in combination with corticosteroids, at a dose of 2 g/kg divided over 2 to 5 days. In cases refractory to high-dose steroids, plasmapheresis has been shown to have a 42% response rate. In fulminant cases with severe cerebral edema and elevated ICP, successful decompressive craniectomy has been reported in children.[152] Although relapses may occur, most children make a complete neurologic recovery within 6 months of the initial presentation. Patients with large or bithalamic lesions on MRI are more likely to have residual disability.[153]

Acute Hemorrhagic Leukoencephalitis

Acute hemorrhagic leukoencephalitis (AHLE) is a rare, and often fatal, demyelinating disorder of the CNS seen in adults and children. It is often considered to be a severe presentation on a spectrum of autoimmune demyelinating disorders with ADEM (Table 70.6). In each case, patients may have a history of recent illness or vaccination, they typically present with or develop alterations in mental status and multifocal neurologic deficits, and neuroimaging demonstrates large poorly demarcated areas of demyelination and edema. However, compared to ADEM, patients with AHLE typically have (1) higher CSF and peripheral leukocytosis with neutrophilic predominance, (2) elevated ICP, and (3) a rapidly progressive and often fatal course. Additionally, AHLE may be more common in young adults and patients of Asian or Pacific Island ancestry with several reported cases in patients of Filipino descent.[154,155]

Despite extensive clinical workup in most cases, the pathogenesis of AHLE remains unknown. Brain biopsy or autopsy from children with AHLE classically shows hemorrhagic perivascular demyelination, edema, and neutrophilic inflammatory infiltrates. Biopsies taken within the first 48 hours of symptom onset may not yet show demyelination. Instead, early biopsy may demonstrate widespread dystrophic astrocytes with swollen perivascular end feet. This suggests that demyelination in AHLE might be secondary to astrocyte injury similar to that observed in patients with neuromyelitis optica and central pontine myelinolysis.[156] Complement activation may have a role in the pathophysiology of AHLE. Two patients with recurrent AHLE and a fulminant course were

TABLE 70.6 Clinical and Laboratory Features of Acute Disseminated Encephalomyelitis (ADEM) and Acute Hemorrhagic Leukoencephalitis (AHLE)

Feature	ADEM	AHLE
Rapidly progressive and fatal	3%	60%
Typical age	Children	Young adults
Prodromal illness or vaccination	Often	Often
CSF WBC, median (range), cell/uL	15 (0-340)	145 (2-11,900)
CSF protein, median (range), mg/dL	32 (14-672)	115 (12-1290)
Elevated CSF opening pressure or ICP	8%	71%
Peripheral WBC, median (range), cells/uL	13,000 (3300-28,100)	17,000 (15,000-40,000)
Pathologic features	Focal demyelination, perivascular neutrophilic infiltrates, hemorrhage absent	Focal demyelination, perivascular neutrophilic infiltrates, focal perivascular hemorrhage

Data from Leake JA, Billman GF, Nespeca MP, et al. Pediatric acute hemorrhagic leukoencephalitis: report of a surviving patient and review. Clin Infect Dis. 2002;34: 699-703.

each found to have a significant decrease in complement inhibition. The patients had a genetic mutation in complement factor I gene that led to increased C3b, membrane attack complex deposition on neuronal cell surfaces, and interleukin-1β (IL-1β) mediated inflammation. A similar deficiency of complement inhibition is known to cause atypical hemolytic uremic syndrome. In addition to ICP-directed therapies, each patient received immunomodulatory treatment with high-dose corticosteroids, IVIG, and anakinra (IL-1 receptor antagonist). Anakinra was continued long term to prevent relapse, and each patient had a good functional outcome.[155]

Approximately 20 cases of pediatric AHLE have been reported, and overall mortality is ~50%.[157] The patients who have survived received ICP-directed therapy including hyperosmolar therapies and craniectomy, high-dose corticosteroids, and in some cases additional immunomodulatory therapies such as IVIG and anakinra. If possible, most clinicians will perform lumbar puncture to exclude active CNS infection prior to giving high-dose steroids. A lumbar puncture with elevated opening pressure, leukocytosis with neutrophilic predominance, and elevated CSF protein that may mimic a bacterial or fulminant herpetic infection may be seen in cases of AHLE. In this case, neuroimaging may be beneficial to limit delays in therapy if the characteristic large, multifocal, white matter AHLE lesions are observed.

Anti–N-Methyl-D-Aspartate Receptor–Mediated Encephalitis

In 2007, a case series was published of 12 women with prominent psychiatric symptoms, amnesia, dyskinesias, seizures, and autonomic dysfunction caused by antibodies to the N-terminal extracellular domain of the NR1 subunit of the NMDA receptor (NMDAR). These women all had ovarian or mediastinal teratoma, and resection of the tumor and immunotherapy proved curative.[158] More recent population-based studies have established anti-NMDAR encephalitis as the cause for many cases of idiopathic encephalitis and even diagnosed patients thought to have primary psychiatric disorders admitted to the ICU. For example, in epidemiologic studies from California, Australia, and the United Kingdom, 4% to 6% of patients with encephalitis have anti-NMDAR antibodies.[159-161] This finding makes anti-NMDAR encephalitis the second most common cause of immune-mediated encephalitis (behind ADEM), and four times more common than HSV-1, WNV, and VZV. Additional antigenic targets on the neuronal surface have been identified such as the voltage-gated potassium channel complex (VGKC), α-amino-3-hydroxy-5-methyl-4-isoxazoleproprionic acid receptor, and glycine receptor, but apart from anti-VGKC encephalitis, these rarely cause illness in pediatric patients.

Anti-NMDAR antibodies act by decreasing the surface density and synaptic localization of NMDAR clusters, by mechanisms including antibody-mediated capping and internalization, without affecting other synaptic proteins or receptors.[162] The effect is dose-dependent—higher antibody titers that cause a greater decrease in NMDAR density, and a reduction of antibody titers reverses this effect. The loss of synaptic NMDARs impairs glutamatergic synaptic transmission and may cause the cognitive and behavioral changes characteristic of autoimmune encephalitis. In 55% of adults, anti-NMDAR antibodies are associated with a tumor, typically an ovarian teratoma that contains nervous tissue and expresses NMDARs. In children, the presence of tumor is less common. Current theories suggest antigenic stimulation by infection or tumor that activates lymphocytes, disrupts the BBB, and allows clonal expansion of B cells within the CNS. The NMDAR antibodies can be detected in serum but are often higher in CSF, suggesting intrathecal antibody synthesis.[163]

The diagnosis of anti-NMDAR encephalitis is suggested by a characteristic clinical progression: prodrome of fever, headache, and gastrointestinal or respiratory symptoms followed by psychiatric and behavioral changes, language deficits, and seizures, progressing to dysautonomia, movement disorders, altered consciousness, and central hypoventilation. This pattern suggests an initial cortical disease process progressing to involve subcortical structures.[163] In children older than 12 years old, psychiatric or behavioral symptoms often present first; whereas children younger than 12 often present with new-onset seizures or movement disorder. Orofacial dyskinesias are characteristic and described as fish- or rabbit-like movements, although many other movements are described and can be self-injurious. The seizures of anti-NMDAR encephalitis can be difficult to diagnose and treat with traditional anti-epileptic drugs. One case report describes a woman who was in a nonconvulsive status epilepticus and pentobarbital coma for months before a prophylactic oophorectomy found a microscopic ovarian teratoma. The patient improved within a week following the procedure.[164] Many children with anti-NMDAR encephalitis will require critical care as symptoms progress to include autonomic instability, hypoventilation, and altered consciousness. Up to one-quarter of patients will require mechanical ventilation.

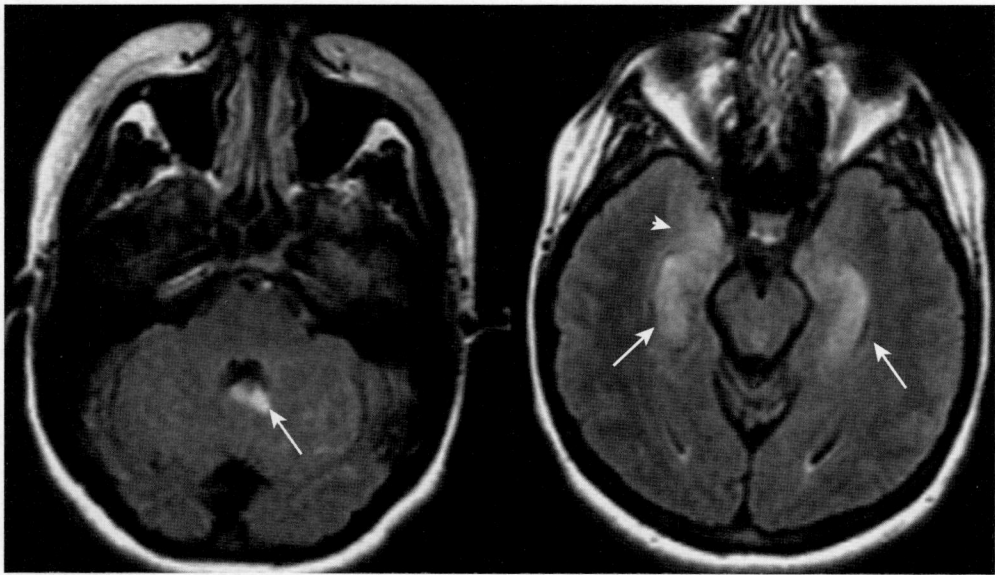

Fig. 70.7. A 26-year-old patient with anti-NMDAR encephalitis and ovarian teratoma. Axial T2-FLAIR images show increased signal in the cerebellar vermis *(left, arrow)*, bilateral hippocampus *(right, arrows)*, and right temporal uncus *(right, arrowhead)*. (From Simon DW, Da Silva YS, Zuccoli G, et al. Acute encephalitis. Crit Care Clin. 2013;29:259-277.)

MRI is normal in 50% of patients with anti-NMDAR encephalitis, but it may show T2 signal intensity in the frontotemporal region, hippocampus, basal ganglia, brain stem, or spinal cord (Fig. 70.7). Initial lumbar puncture typically shows variable CSF lymphocytic pleocytosis, elevated protein, and oligoclonal bands. Clinical tests for NMDAR antibodies are available and should be sent from serum and CSF. Low serum titers should be interpreted cautiously and are not 100% specific. All patients should be tested for an underlying ovarian teratoma or testicular germ cell tumor, although other malignancies such as Hodgkin lymphoma and neuroblastoma, as well as infectious etiologies, have been associated with anti-NMDAR antibodies.[163]

A large-multicenter cohort study of 577 patients with anti-NMDAR encephalitis (including 212 children) found that only 53% of patients responded to first-line therapy, including tumor removal or immunotherapy (steroids, IVIG, or plasma exchange). There were no differences according to age of the patient. Of patients who failed first-line therapy, treatment with second-line therapy (rituximab, cyclophosphamide) improved outcomes versus no additional therapy.[165] The strongest predictors of good outcome were early treatment (Fig. 70.8) and lack of ICU admission. Persistent deficits are more likely if a tumor is not detected, and they are primarily in executive function and memory, where NMDAR function is most influential.

Central Nervous System Hemophagocytic Lymphohistiocytosis

Hemophagocytic lymphohistiocytosis (HLH) is severe sepsis-like disease that primarily affects infants and young children. Caused by autosomal recessive mutation in the genes that control perforin and granzyme signaling required for natural killer and cytotoxic T-lymphocyte cytotoxicity (also called familial HLH, or fHLH), patients are unable to turn off the

immune response leading to cytokine storm and multiorgan failure (see Chapter 112 for additional details). Postmortem studies have shown that CNS HLH has a large severity spectrum, with mild cases having a lymphocytic and macrophage infiltration of the meninges, to severe cases in which there is tissue infiltration and multifocal necrosis.[166] Hemophagocytosis was observed in most of the brains at all injury severity levels.

Neurologic symptoms are common and may even precede systemic symptoms of HLH. In these cases, distinguishing CNS HLH from primary CNS disorders such as meningitis and ADEM can be a challenge. Patients with fHLH commonly present with neurologic deficits or abnormal CSF values: 63% of children presenting with fHLH have neurologic symptoms and an additional 24% have abnormal findings on CSF analysis.[167] The presenting symptoms of CNS HLH include seizure (35%), impaired consciousness (31%), meningismus (31%), hypotonia (21%), motor deficit (17%), and cranial nerve palsy (7%). CSF analysis typically shows only mild elevation in protein or leukocytosis. Similarly, half of the children with CNS HLH will have normal MRI findings early in the course. When changes are detected on MRI, in comparison to ADEM, they are more likely to be symmetric, periventricular, and involving a large area of the brain.[167] Patients presenting with neurologic findings or abnormal CSF have a greater risk of long-term neurologic sequelae and higher mortality rate than patients without neurologic features and normal CSF.

Treatment of fHLH is guided by the HLH-2004 protocol.[168] In children with persistent symptoms of CNS involvement despite systemic chemotherapy, intrathecal chemotherapy (often methotrexate) is often added. Dexamethasone, which has better BBB penetration than other systemic corticosteroids, is often used in place of methylprednisolone or prednisone. Perhaps the best way to reduce long-term neurologic deficits is hematopoietic stem cell transplant (HSCT) once

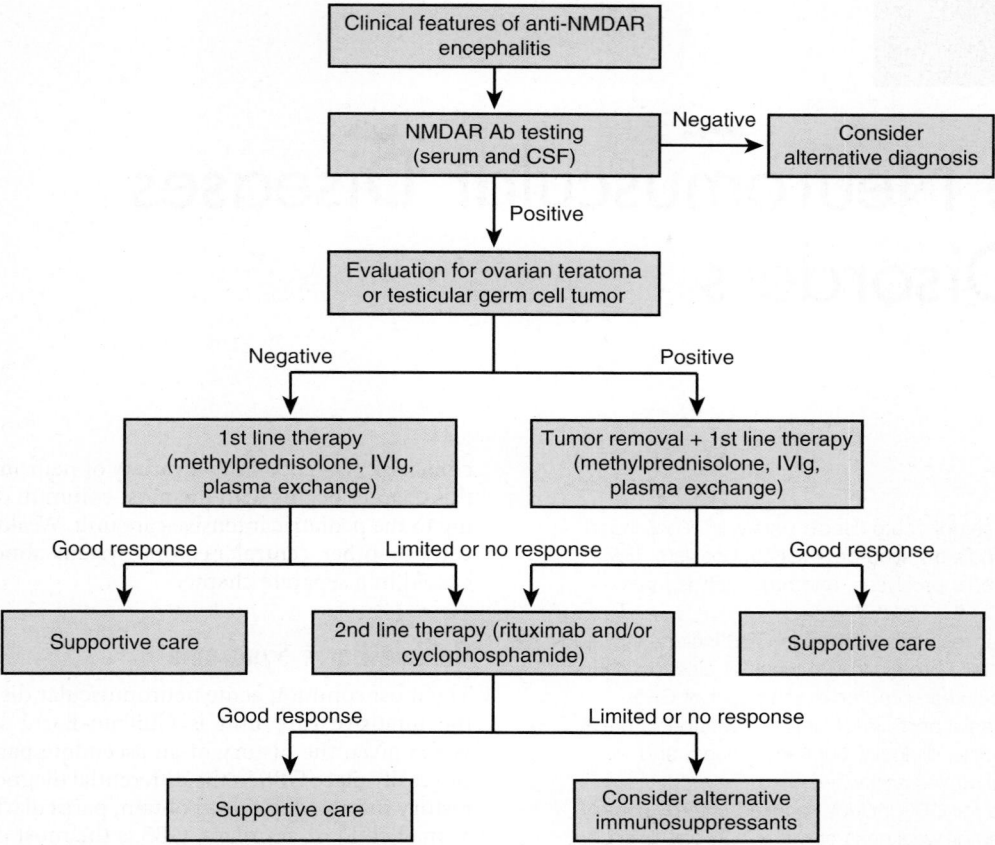

Fig. 70.8. Proposed treatment approach for anti-NMDAR encephalitis. (Adapted from Florence-Ryan N, Dalmau J. Update on anti-*N*-methyl-D-aspartate receptor encephalitis in children and adolescents. Curr Opin Pediatr. 2010;22:739-744.)

remission is obtained.[169] Unfortunately, despite significant improvements since the 1990s in the treatment of patients with fHLH using multimodal chemotherapy and HSCT, outcomes for patients with CNS HLH remain poor with greater than 25% mortality and 60% long-term neurologic sequelae (27% with severe deficits).

Conclusion

CNS infectious and parainfectious diseases represent an important cause of mortality among PICU patients. Prompt recognition of CNS disease is essential in order for the intensivist to initiate specific medical and surgical treatment. Although the lack of specific therapy for many viral causes of meningoencephalitis remains frustrating, appropriate supportive care can improve mortality and functional outcomes for all patients with CNS infections and related conditions.

Key References

1. Hsu HE, Shutt KA, Moore MR, et al. Effect of pneumococcal conjugate vaccine on pneumococcal meningitis. *N Engl J Med.* 2009;360:244-256.
18. Hasbun R, Abrahams J, Jekel J, Quagliarello VJ. Computed tomography of the head before lumbar puncture in adults with suspected meningitis. *N Engl J Med.* 2001;345:1727-1733.
23. Chen LH, Duan QJ, Cai MT, et al. Rapid diagnosis of sepsis and bacterial meningitis in children with real-time fluorescent quantitative polymerase chain reaction amplification in the bacterial 16S rRNA gene. *Clin Pediatr (Phila).* 2009;48:641-647.

30. Karageorgopoulos DE, Valkimadi PE, Kapaskelis A, et al. Short versus long duration of antibiotic therapy for bacterial meningitis: a meta-analysis of randomised controlled trials in children. *Arch Dis Child.* 2009;94:607-614.
36. Lebel MH, Freij BJ, Syrogiannopoulos GA, et al. Dexamethasone therapy for bacterial meningitis. Results of a two-double-blind placebo-controlled trials. *N Engl J Med.* 1988;319:964-971.
68. Goodkin HP, Harper MB, Pomeroy SL. Intracerebral abscess in children: historical trends at Children's Hospital Boston. *Pediatrics.* 2004;113:1765-1770.
86. Silvia MT, Licht DJ. Pediatric Central Nervous System Infections and Inflammatory White Matter Disease. *Pediatr Clin North Am.* 2005;52:1107-1126.
117. Whitley RJ, Gnann JW. Viral encephalitis: familiar infections and emerging pathogens. *Lancet.* 2002;359:507-514.
120. Mizuguchi M. Acute necrotizing encephalopathy of childhood: a novel form of acute encephalopathy prevalent in Japan and Taiwan. *Brain Dev.* 1997;19:81-92.
136. Yoder JS, Eddy BA, Visvesvara GS, et al. The epidemiology of primary amoebic meningoencephalitis in the USA, 1962-2008. *Epidemiol Infect.* 2010;138:968-975.
145. Leake JA, Albani S, Kao AS, et al. Acute disseminated encephalomyelitis in childhood: epidemiologic, clinical and laboratory features. *Pediatr Infect Dis J.* 2004;23:756-764.
158. Dalmau J, Tuzun E, Wu HY, et al. Paraneoplastic anti-N-methyl-D-aspartate receptor encephalitis associated with ovarian teratoma. *Ann Neurol.* 2007;61:25-36.
165. Titulaer MJ, McCracken L, Gabilondo I, et al. Treatment and prognostic factors for long-term outcome in patients with anti-NMDA receptor encephalitis: an observational cohort study. *Lancet Neurol.* 2013;12:157-165.
168. Henter JI, Horne A, Arico M, et al. HLH-2004: diagnostic and therapeutic guidelines for hemophagocytic lymphohistiocytosis. *Pediatr Blood Cancer.* 2007;48:124-131.

Acute Neuromuscular Diseases and Disorders

Ann H. Tilton

PEARLS

- Common causes of acute flaccid paralysis in childhood include Guillain-Barré syndrome (GBS), botulism, tick paralysis, periodic paralyses, and organophosphate poisoning.
- Risk factors for respiratory failure in GBS include elevated cerebrospinal fluid protein in first week of disease, short time interval between prodrome and onset of GBS symptoms, cranial nerve involvement, myasthenia gravis symptoms, ptosis, diplopia, pupillary sparing, and weakness that waxes and wanes.
- Asbury criteria for GBS include required criteria, namely progressive motor weakness of more than one limb and areflexia, and supportive criteria, namely symmetry of symptoms, mild sensory changes, cranial nerve involvement, and autonomic symptoms. Recovery begins 2 to 4 weeks after symptom progression discontinues.
- Classic botulism symptoms include weak cry, poor suck and swallow, decreased tone, decreased reflexes, weakness in descending pattern, constipation, and autonomic symptoms especially tachycardia and fluctuating blood pressure, urinary retention, decreased tears and saliva, and flushed skin or pallor.

Neuromuscular diseases that encompass the entire motor unit may have similar presentations initially and must be deciphered in a methodical manner. The motor unit consists of the anterior horn cell, which is located in the spinal cord and terminates in a motor nerve; the myelin associated with the nerve; the neuromuscular junction; and the muscle that the nerve innervates. Any disruption of function in this pathway may produce weakness of some variety. Neuropathies and myopathies have similar clinical findings, including weakness and decreased or absent reflexes. These disease processes may be distinguished, however, by sensory abnormalities and the distribution of the weakness. Neuromuscular junction defects may have reflexes present, as in myasthenia gravis, or absent, as seen in tick paralysis. The clinician can narrow the etiologic possibilities by considering the clinical presentation, family history, recent illness, travel, inciting factors, and the clinical course.

This chapter is devoted to acute neuromuscular diseases that present to a pediatric intensive care unit. Although

clinicians may encounter a variety of neuromuscular illnesses, this chapter begins with the most common disorders presenting to the pediatric intensive care unit. Weakness due to spinal cord or other central nervous system abnormalities is discussed in a separate chapter.

Guillain-Barré Syndrome

The most common acute neuromuscular disease to present to the intensive care unit is Guillain-Barré syndrome (GBS). When given the history of an ascending paralysis, a clinician can easily place GBS in the differential diagnosis; however, this history may be difficult to obtain, particularly if the patient is a small child or an infant. GBS is the most common cause of acute flaccid paralysis in children with an incidence estimated to be 0.38 to 1.1 per 100,000 in a population younger than 15 years.[1,2] A prodromal respiratory or gastrointestinal illness is commonly reported. These illnesses may include *Campylobacter jejuni* and cytomegalovirus (CMV). In one study, 70% of patients reported an illness before the onset of symptoms with 26% having documented CMV.[3]

The neurologic symptoms typically present with progressive paralysis that is relatively symmetric and may evolve to all extremities. Other symptoms include varying degrees of hyporeflexia or areflexia or even respiratory embarrassment. Presentations may include acute ataxia, pain, or cranial neuropathies.[4,5] Of note, pain is often a major complaint in the young child and makes the examination difficult. In one study, risk factors for patients requiring ventilation included cranial nerve involvement, elevated cerebrospinal fluid (CSF) protein during the first week of illness, and a short period between antecedent illness and onset of symptoms.[6] Autonomic symptoms may be overlooked. Autonomic instability, particularly cardiac arrhythmias, increases the morbidity of this disease. Cardiac monitoring of the R-R interval with reduction of beat-to-beat variability may possibly identify patients at risk for fatal arrhythmia.[7] Cardiac arrhythmias induced by tracheal tube manipulation have been reported.[8]

Symptoms that are strongly supportive of GBS include the relative symmetry of symptoms, mild sensory symptoms, cranial nerve involvement, autonomic symptoms, and recovery that usually begins 2 to 4 weeks after symptom progression discontinues. Sphincter disturbances rarely occur early in the course of GBS and are usually transient.[9,10]

Diagnostic studies include examination of the CSF and nerve conduction studies. The CSF reveals elevated protein

(>45 mg/dL) amid a relative paucity of white blood cells (WBCs), usually less than 10 cells/mL with the protein increasing after the first week of symptoms.[9] Electrodiagnostic testing reveals motor conduction velocities in the demyelinating range, conduction block, temporal dispersion, and prolonged F waves. Bradshaw and Jones[4] reported that conduction block and temporal dispersion occurred in 74% of the patients.

It is important to recognize that the patients may need an intensive care setting. Criteria for ICU care include rapidly advancing weakness, flaccid quadriparesis, bulbar symptoms, vital capacity less than 20 mL/kg, and autonomic instability (cardiac).[10] If the symptoms are severe, treatment options for GBS primarily include plasmapheresis and intravenous immunoglobulin (IVIG). Based predominantly on adult literature, the American Academy of Neurology has published practice guidelines providing treatment recommendations.[11,12] First, plasmapheresis and IVIG both hasten recovery, and neither is more efficacious. Using these two treatments sequentially is not superior to either treatment alone. Finally, steroids do not seem to help.[13] The decision of which therapy to apply to children is controversial because no large randomized study has yet been performed. Plasmapheresis may be technically difficult in young or very small children; therefore immunoglobulin is often used as the first choice. Favorable improvement in pediatric patients treated with immunoglobulin has been reported in several small series and on Cochrane review.[14-17] A randomized trial in children showed that fewer relapses occurred if 2 g/kg of IVIG were divided over 5 days instead of 2 days.[17] If additional courses of IVIG are necessary, a 2-day protocol is often well tolerated.

Several GBS variants exist. The best known are the Miller-Fisher variant and acute inflammatory axonal polyneuropathy, the axonal form of GBS. The neurologic triad found in the Miller-Fisher syndrome includes ataxia, areflexia, and ophthalmoparesis. Miller-Fisher syndrome has been linked to immunoglobulin G (IgG) antibodies against ganglioside GQ1b.[18] In some *C. jejuni* strains, molecular mimicry exists between the surface epitopes and ganglioside GQ1b.[19] The GQ1b ganglioside is thought to cross-react in the brain stem area of the ophthalmic cranial nerves.[20] The axonal form of GBS has been associated with a more prolonged recovery than the classic form of GBS due to axonal involvement. Early research suggests that CSF levels of neurofilament correspond to levels of axonal damage on electromyography (EMG) testing and may complement EMG studies to help predict patients with more prolonged recoveries.[21,22]

Myasthenia Gravis

Myasthenia gravis (MG) has many forms that may present in the pediatric population. The juvenile form of MG is the most common and is clinically identical to the autoimmune adult form of MG. Overall, however, juvenile MG is rare and constitutes 10% of all cases of MG in Western populations. Antibodies directed toward the acetylcholine receptor (AchR) at the postsynaptic neuromuscular junction cause this form of the disease. These antibodies result in blockade of the AchR, increase the degradation of the AchR, and also result in complement damage to the AchR.[23] AchR antibodies are found less frequently in juvenile MG compared with adult autoimmune MG and are more easily demonstrated in the postpubertal patient population.[24] Anticholinesterase antibody levels

should be drawn, however, in all patients with suspected MG. Newer assays are identifying antibodies previously missed in older anticholinesterase antibody assays, including binding, blocking, and modulating antibodies, but these may need to be ordered separately.[25-27]

The most common heralding symptoms of weakness in MG include ptosis (with pupillary sparing) and diplopia from restricted eye movements. These symptoms wax and wane, and the weakness may generalize to the extremities. The two clinical forms of juvenile MG are ocular and generalized. In ocular MG, symptoms include ptosis and diplopia, but the weakness does not progress to other areas of the body. Generalized MG may begin with ocular symptoms and progress to generalized weakness, usually within 1 year of onset; however, generalized weakness may be the initial presentation. As in adults with MG, pediatric patients have fewer symptoms in the morning or after rest. Increasing fatigability with exercise is an important hallmark of this disorder. The most troublesome symptoms in generalized MG are those involving bulbar muscles (difficulty chewing and swallowing), respiratory muscles, and exercise intolerance.

When a patient is suspected to have MG, the classic diagnostic bedside test is the edrophonium (Tensilon) challenge. Edrophonium is an intravenous short-acting anticholinesterase preparation that has limited availability in many hospitals. The dosing in infants is 0.15 mg/kg and 0.20 mg/kg in older children. Only 10% of the entire dose is given initially so that the clinician can observe for muscarinic side effects. Atropine (0.015 to 0.040 mg/kg) should be available for these possible side effects, which include bradycardia and respiratory distress secondary to bronchial secretions and bronchospasm. After the trial dose is tolerated, the entire dose is then given. In lieu of edrophonium, neostigmine is given at a dose of 0.025 to 0.050 mg/kg intramuscularly (IM). The patient should be observed during the trial for changes in ptosis or fatigability. The onset of action with edrophonium is approximately 30 to 90 seconds after intravenous delivery and remains for approximately 5 minutes. Neostigmine has an onset of action within 15 minutes, and effects may last for 1 hour. Many clinicians also perform a blinded placebo trial of normal saline.

The neurodiagnostic study used in patients with suspected MG is repetitive nerve stimulation. This study is best performed on proximal muscles, although distal muscles are often studied. The confirmatory finding on repetitive nerve stimulation is a 10% decrement in amplitude of the compound muscle action potential.

Antibodies have been found that can block, bind, or modulate AChR. Approximately 80% of patients will have antibodies to AChR found in standard assays. Antibodies directed against muscle specific kinase (MuSK) appear to account for some of the remaining 20%.[25] Newer, more sensitive assays can also identify antibodies with low affinity for AChR.[27] Clinically, MuSK-positive patients tend to have more frequent bulbar involvement and respiratory crises than AChR-positive patients and require larger doses of maintenance corticosteroids, though there is no clear difference in clinical outcomes.[28] Seronegative (AChR-negative and MuSK-negative) patients have a disease severity between the other two groups but appear to have better clinical outcomes.[28]

Treatment of MG begins with anticholinesterase medications. The symptoms of MG usually respond to pyridostigmine bromide (Mestinon), the most common oral form of anticholinesterase medication. The dosage of pyridostigmine bromide is 7 mg/kg per day divided four to six times daily as needed for symptoms. Immunosuppressant agents, including prednisone, azathioprine, cyclophosphamide, tacrolimus, and rituximab, may be added to the regimen for pyridostigmine nonresponders.[29] Mycophenolate mofetil may also be prescribed, though it has not proved more efficacious than placebo in two randomized trials of patients already on prednisone.[30-32] However, a subsequent study with an extended outcome duration, >25 months compared to 9 months in the previously mentioned studies, demonstrated that mycophenolate mofetil might be effective as either adjunctive therapy with prednisone or monotherapy, but maximum results may not be seen for greater than a year.[30] Prednisone is usually initiated at 1 to 2 mg/kg per day. Clinicians must be careful with the use of prednisone because it may exacerbate weakness on initiation.

Many studies have suggested that beneficial effects of thymectomy are best when performed early in the course of MG.[24,33,34] Because of the spontaneous remission rate reported by Rodriquez and colleagues as 22.4 per 1000 person-years, however, many clinicians are reluctant to proceed with early thymectomy, particularly with young children.[35]

Myasthenic crisis is an exacerbation of myasthenic symptoms requiring ventilatory assistance. In adult MG, myasthenic crisis has been reported to occur in 15% to 20% of patients, with 74% having their first crisis within 2 years of disease presentation.[36,37] Anlar and coworkers reported that one-third of patients with juvenile MG had at least one episode of crisis.[38] Initial therapy during crisis includes mechanical ventilation, which provides rest for the weakened patient.

Anticholinesterase medications should be discontinued during a crisis because they increase secretions that could lead to mucous plugging. Myasthenic crisis is most commonly heralded by infection in 38% of patients; however, 30% of patients have no obvious trigger for their crisis other than respiratory or bulbar weakness.[37] A thorough investigation for the cause of crisis should be undertaken.

Plasmapheresis and IVIG (2 g/kg over 2 to 5 days) also play a role in the treatment of myasthenic crisis and acute exacerbation of myasthenic symptoms. In adult crisis, plasmapheresis has been shown to be more efficacious than IVIG; however, plasmapheresis has more deleterious side effects, including cardiovascular and infectious complications.[39] IVIG has been shown superior to placebo in a randomized controlled trial with significant improvements seen as early as 14 days after infusion and lasting through 28 days.[40] Evidence supports the use of IVIG for treatment in myasthenic crisis or exacerbation in patients for whom plasmapheresis is not feasible.

Cholinergic crisis must also be a consideration in a patient with an MG exacerbation. Cholinergic crisis occurs with an overdose of anticholinesterase drugs in patients with MG. The overdose causes depolarization of skeletal muscles and muscarinic side effects, including increased secretions, diarrhea, lacrimation, sweating, and bradycardia. These symptoms will improve on withdrawal of the anticholinesterase medications. Some authors argue that cholinergic crisis is rarely the cause for worsening myasthenic symptoms.[36,41]

The clinician must always be cautious when initiating new medications in the patient with MG. Many drugs interfere with the neuromuscular junction; the best known are the aminoglycoside medications. Although not well recognized,

steroids can also exacerbate weakness in a patient with MG. For this reason, one must be cautious when beginning prednisone in the patient with refractory MG, observing closely for any initial increased weakness. Other antibiotics that have been implicated in the worsening of myasthenic symptoms include ampicillin, ciprofloxacin, clindamycin, erythromycin, sulfonamide, tetracycline, and the peptide antibiotics (polymyxin A and B and colistin). Cardiovascular medications including the antiarrhythmics (quinidine, procainamide, and lidocaine) and beta-blockers have also been reported to worsen symptoms. Thyroid replacement medications and phenytoin may also cause problems. The neuromuscular junction blockers, including vecuronium, rocuronium, and pancuronium, as well as succinylcholine, should be used with caution because the effects of these medications are prolonged in patients with MG.[41,42] On its website at www.myasthenia.org, the Myasthenia Gravis Foundation of America maintains a list of medications to avoid and to use with caution.

Additional immune diseases have been associated in approximately 16% of patients with juvenile MG.[35] The autoimmune diseases may include asthma, rheumatoid arthritis, juvenile diabetes mellitus, hyperthyroidism, chronic inflammatory demyelinating polyneuropathy, and CNS demyelination.[35,43,44] Seizures have also occurred in 4% to 12% of patients with juvenile MG, although the exact cause is not known.[35]

Congenital and Transient Neonatal Myasthenia Gravis

The other forms of MG are congenital MG and neonatal transient MG. Neonatal transient MG is unique in neonates who are born to mothers with autoimmune MG. Neonates can manifest symptoms of neonatal transient MG even if the mothers were symptom free during pregnancy and delivery. Neonatal transient MG occurs in approximately 12% of infants born to mothers with MG.[45] If a mother with MG gives birth to an infant with neonatal MG, her subsequent neonates are also at increased risk of having this transient disorder. Neonatal MG usually resolves in the first few weeks after birth, when the maternally derived antibody level diminishes in the neonate. Results from several studies have shown that even symptom-free infants born to mothers with MG have elevated titers of AchR antibodies.[46] Additionally, the same phenomenon has been reported in infants born to mothers with anti-MuSK.[38] The antibody concentration of the symptom-free neonate rapidly decreases when compared with the antibody concentration of a neonate with symptoms.[47] The symptoms of neonatal transient MG usually include hypotonia, feeding problems (particularly fatigue), weak cry, and respiratory difficulty. The treatment of these symptoms is supportive, with anticholinesterase medications used for severe symptoms.

Congenital MG usually presents in childhood, with symptoms similar to those of juvenile MG. Many defects are responsible for causing symptoms in congenital MG, including congenital abnormalities resulting in presynaptic, synaptic, or postsynaptic defects of the neuromuscular junction.[48] Congenital MG is always negative for Ach antibody, and a family history of congenital MG may or may not be present. The inheritance of congenital MG may be autosomal recessive or dominant or sporadic.[48] Treatment of congenital MG is different from the treatment of juvenile MG because immunosuppression obviously does not play a role. Symptoms of congenital MG may or may not respond to anticholinesterase medications.

Tick Paralysis

The clinician must always entertain tick paralysis in the differential diagnosis of acute flaccid paralysis in children. On presentation, patients with tick paralysis may be mistakenly diagnosed with GBS. The treatment of the two diseases is distinct; therefore, a high index of suspicion for tick paralysis should be maintained.

Affected patients are usually between the ages of 1 and 5 years. A review of 33 patients with tick paralysis reported 82% were younger than age 10 years, and 76% were female.[49] Longer hairstyles have been speculated to be the cause of this female preponderance. A thorough search of the patient should ensue because more than one tick may be attached. The ticks most commonly implicated in North America are *Dermacentor andersoni* (wood tick) and *Dermacentor variabilis* (dog tick); however, other types of ticks have also been documented.[50] In Australia, the most common tick variety to cause paralysis is *Ixodes holocyclus*.[50] The cause of the weakness is a neurotoxin that is secreted in the saliva of the gravid female tick. The neurotoxin is produced during the engorgement phase of feeding after mating. The neurotoxin inhibits the release of acetylcholine at the presynaptic terminal.[50]

The symptoms in North American hosts begin with vague complaints of fatigue, irritability, and pain. Vague symptoms may not begin until approximately 5 days after tick attachment, but they progress rapidly.[51] Symptoms may also include cerebellar signs, such as ataxia.[51] If the tick remains attached, a symmetric ascending flaccid paralysis with areflexia develops. Subsequently, bulbar and facial weakness as well as respiratory involvement occur. No systemic features are seen in tick paralysis. Patients are afebrile with normal vital signs, erythrocyte sedimentation rate (ESR), CSF, and mental status. The removal of the tick rapidly reverses symptoms, usually within 24 hours.

On discovery, the tick needs to be promptly removed. The tick is removed with blunt curved forceps or tweezers. The tick should be grasped at the point of attachment, as close to the skin as possible. The tick should be pulled upward with steady pressure. Twisting or jerking motions may cause parts of the tick to break off, particularly the mouthparts. The tick should not be handled with bare hands. Needham[52] evaluated various methods of tick removal including fingernail polish, petroleum jelly, 70% isopropyl alcohol, and a hot kitchen match. None of these passive techniques induced tick detachment.

Tick paralysis is more severe in Australia than in North America. The presenting symptoms are similar to those in the North American cases; however, ocular involvement with nonreactive pupils has been described.[53] Flaccid paralysis may take days to evolve, unlike in North American hosts. The major difference in Australian tick paralysis occurs after the tick is removed. Australian patients must be carefully observed because maximal weakness may not occur until 48 hours after tick removal.[53]

Periodic Paralyses

Clinicians may encounter various forms of periodic paralysis (PP), including hypokalemic and hyperkalemic. Most forms of the periodic paralyses have a family history of the disease. The weakness, that eventually results in paralysis, is associated with potassium response as demonstrated in hyperkalemic PP or potassium serum levels in hypokalemic PP. Periodic paralysis may also be accompanied by abnormal cardiac rhythms including prolonged QT, as in Andersen-Tawil syndrome; checking an electrocardiogram may be prudent, regardless of the serum potassium level.[54] Andersen-Tawil consists of a triad of ventricular dysrhythmia, periodic paralysis, and dysmorphic features.[55]

Hypokalemic Periodic Paralysis

Hypokalemic periodic paralysis (HypoPP) is the most common form of the periodic paralyses. The presentation of HypoPP usually occurs within the second decade of life. The number of attacks, which may be frequent, usually decreases as patients get older. Occurrence of HypoPP is 1 in 100,000 people. The inheritance pattern of HypoPP is autosomal dominant with males more frequently affected, but one-third of cases are sporadic.[56] The most common mutation in familial HypoPP is the dihydropyridine receptor in the voltage sensitive Ca^{++} channel, located on chromosome 1q.[57] Another common mutation is a voltage-sensitive sodium channel, SCN4A.[56,58,59] In a minority of cases no mutation is found.[59,60]

The onset of symptoms in HypoPP usually occurs after the consumption of a high-carbohydrate meal or after vigorous exercise followed by rest. Other provoking factors include cold temperature, emotional stress, menses, and pregnancy. Weakness usually begins during sleep with the patient noticing weakness on awakening; initially the weakness is proximal in the legs then progresses distally before involvement in the upper extremities. It may progress to flaccid paralysis of all limbs with areflexia and normal sensation. Cranial nerve function remains normal with swallowing and respiratory function rarely affected. The patient remains alert with a normal mental status during the attack, and sensation remains intact. Weakness typically lasts a few hours but may last several days. On noticing the initial symptoms of mild muscle cramping or heaviness, some patients are able to abort an attack with light exercise.[60,61] Sudden death from cardiac arrhythmias or respiratory failure has been reported.[61-63] During paralytic attacks, patients have minimal urine output with decreased potassium excretion and absent defecation.[60,64] In HypoPP, myotonia confined to the eyelids has been described.[65] Before this report, myotonia was described as occurring only with hyperkalemic periodic paralysis.

Diagnosis of HypoPP can be confirmed with the identification of hypokalemia during an attack. Laboratory testing during HypoPP reveals a markedly diminished potassium level. Although serum potassium levels are decreased, the total body amount of potassium remains normal. The decreased potassium level is due to a shift of the potassium into the muscle cells, resulting in inexcitable muscle cells.[66] During an attack, potassium levels usually fall below 3, but levels below 2 have been reported.[67] Secondary causes of hypokalemia such as Bartter syndrome, corticosteroids, diuretics, hyperaldosteronism, laxatives, licorice, renal tubular acidosis, amphotericin B, p-aminosalicylic acid, alcoholism, and villous adenoma must be ruled out.[68]

The paralytic attack may be reversed with normalization of the potassium level. The clinician must be careful when correcting the potassium level, remembering that the total body amount of potassium remains normal. Correction with oral potassium (0.2 to 0.4 mmol/kg every 15 to 30 minutes) should be considered. Patients with cardiac symptoms or an inability to swallow, however, require parental potassium.[55] While the potassium level is corrected, vigilant cardiac monitoring, serial potassium levels, and muscle strength examinations should be used. Intravenous fluids with dextrose or physiologic saline should be avoided because they may prolong an attack or even induce cardiac arrhythmias.[68,69] Griggs, Resnick, and Engel [68] reported that 5% mannitol solution should be considered as a diluent for intravenous potassium replacement.

Links and colleagues[60] studied a large kindred with HypoPP and showed that all family members older than 50 years had permanent muscle weakness. The authors concluded that although all patients eventually exhibit permanent muscle weakness, only 60% may have paralytic attacks.

Once a patient is known to have HypoPP, prophylactic medications should be initiated. Acetazolamide has been shown to prevent future attacks in patients with and without a family history of the disease when they take daily doses of 250 to 750 mg.[70] Some patients, however, have been reported to have an exacerbation of attacks when taking acetazolamide.[71] Another report revealed acetazolamide prophylaxis improved strength between attacks in 80% of patients who displayed persistent weakness between paralytic attacks.[70] Daily oral potassium chloride does shorten the duration of the attacks but does not appear to prevent attacks.[70] Other medications used for prophylaxis of attacks include triamterene and spironolactone in patients not responsive to acetazolamide.[70,71] Considerations for the prevention of attacks include avoidance of high-sodium, high-carbohydrate meals, prolonged rest, and arduous exercise.

Thyrotoxic periodic paralysis is another entity of weakness with concomitant hypokalemia. As the name implies, a thyrotoxic state is the impetus of this disease. It is mostly found in adult Asian males, although it has been reported in the Asian-American pediatric population.[72] The purpose of treatment of this disease is to alleviate the hyperthyroid state (see also Chapter 85).

Hyperkalemic Periodic Paralysis

The term *hyperkalemic periodic paralysis (HyperPP)* may be misleading because high, normal, and low levels of potassium have been reported in these attacks.[73] The name *HyperPP* actually correlates to the response these patients have to potassium. HyperPP is also referred to as potassium-sensitive PP, which may be more appropriate and less confusing. HyperPP is autosomal dominant with a common gene located on chromosome 17q affecting the alpha subunit of the sodium channel, but other sodium channels may also be affected.[56,74,75] Sporadic cases have also been reported.[56,76] HyperPP usually presents in the first decade of life.

Rest after exercise is the most common provoking feature. Other provoking factors include cold temperatures and meal skipping. The pattern of weakness is similar to that for HypoPP: The legs are usually affected before the arms, with symmetric weakness. Weakness during the attacks varies from mild to flaccid quadriplegia with areflexia, but respiratory weakness rarely occurs. The sensory examination is normal.

The length of attacks is typically shorter than that of HypoPP attacks, usually resolving in a few hours, but may persist for days. Myotonia and Chvostek sign are often found in these patients.

Attacks may be provoked by potassium intake and relieved by glucose intake. Light exercise can prevent an attack. Most attacks do not require treatment. In the rare severe attack, intravenous glucose, thiazides, acetazolamide, and beta-adrenergics can be used.[77] Cardiac monitoring is important if medical intervention is needed because cardiac arrhythmias may occur.[78] Prophylactic therapy should be considered in these patients because permanent muscle weakness does develop over time.[79] Acetazolamide and thiazides have also been used for prophylaxis of this disease.[80]

Botulism

Infantile botulism is a syndrome predominately found in infants 6 days to 12 months of age.[81] In infantile botulism, *Clostridium botulinum* enters the body as a spore through ingestion, germination occurs, and the organism begins to produce the neurotoxin that is the cause of the symptoms.[82] It differs from food-borne botulism, in which the preformed toxin is actually ingested. In mouse models, the relationship of the gut and the spores is important, with the pH of the gut and the transient lack of competitive intestinal flora being essential in allowing the spores to germinate.[81] Infants appear to be susceptible, as are adults who have abnormal intestinal flora from abdominal surgery, gut abnormalities, or antibiotic use.[83-86]

Most cases of infantile botulism occur in California, Pennsylvania, and Utah. In one report, more than 75% of the patients with botulism had *C. botulinum* in their home environment.[87] Other sources include soil disruption from cultivation or construction and parental occupations that involve soil exposure.[88] The consumption of honey and corn syrup is a risk factor. Children younger than 12 months should not be fed these products. The disease modifying role of breast-feeding remains controversial.[89,90]

The botulinum toxin irreversibly binds at the presynaptic segment of the neuromuscular junction, inhibiting acetylcholine release and causing neuromuscular weakness. The autonomic system is also affected because the toxin binds the acetylcholine-mediated preganglionic parasympathetic and sympathetic synapses, as well as the postganglionic parasympathetic synapse.[91]

The most common symptoms include weak cry, poor suck and feeding, decreased tone with decreased reflexes, weakness in a descending pattern, and constipation.[91] Autonomic symptoms, often the first to appear, include constipation, tachycardia, fluctuating blood pressure, urinary retention, decreased tears and saliva, and flushed skin or pallor.[81,92] L'Hommedieu and Polin[92] proposed an algorithm of symptoms beginning with tachycardia and constipation progressing to loss of head control, difficulty feeding, and weak cry. A depressed gag reflex is followed by peripheral muscle weakness and, finally, diaphragmatic weakness. Because of the combination of autonomic and neuromuscular symptoms, the infant with botulism may be mistaken to be septic or dehydrated. Enlarged, sluggishly reactive pupils may also be present but are less common than the other autonomic symptoms.[93]

The most concerning consequence of botulism is respiratory embarrassment. Schreiner, Field, and Ruddy[91] reported only 24% of the patients reviewed did not require ventilation or an artificial airway. Patients with botulism have also become apneic during certain procedures, including lumbar puncture and intravenous catheter placement.[91] Hypoxic ischemic encephalopathy resulting from respiratory arrest has been described, as well as syndromes of inappropriate secretion of antidiuretic hormone (SIADH), urinary tract infections, pneumonia, and autonomic instability.[91,93] Aminoglycosides exacerbate the neuromuscular blockade and should be avoided in botulism.[94]

The diagnosis of botulism is clinical but confirmed by isolation of the organism or toxin in stool. EMG in patients with botulism reveals decreased compound motor action potential (CMAP) amplitude and facilitation of the CMAP amplitude with high-frequency repetitive motor nerve stimulation.[95]

The management of patients with botulism has advanced. Previously, clinicians could offer only supportive care until axonal sprouting could reestablish the neuromuscular junction. The median length of hospital stay was 27 to 37 days, and patients typically required mechanical ventilation for a median of 13 to 16 days.[87,93,96] In respiratory compromise, mechanical ventilation should be instituted until the patient regains protective reflexes and respiratory strength. If patients are unable to tolerate oral feeds, nasogastric or nasojejunal feeding should be initiated. Human botulism immune globulin (BIG) has provided the first direct pharmacologic treatment. A randomized, controlled trial has shown that BIG decreased mean hospital stay (5.7 weeks to 2.6 weeks), mean duration of mechanical ventilation, mean duration of feeding through tube or IV, and mean hospital charges with no adverse effects related to BIG.[97] A retrospective article spanning 30 years complemented the randomized trial.[98] Resolution of symptoms occurs in the reverse pattern of presentation, with return of head control appearing to be a reliable measure of improving muscle function.[92]

Diphtheria

Although diphtheria was the leading killer of children in the early 20th century, the United States currently reports fewer than 10 cases of diphtheria annually. Epidemics still occur in developed and developing countries.[99-100]

The most common form of diphtheria in children is the upper respiratory tract infection. Initial mild infection of the pharynx is followed by tonsillar pseudomembrane formation. The pseudomembrane consists of necrotic epithelium, fibrin, and numerous bacterial colonies, covering the airways and pharynx to the main bronchi down into the smaller bronchi. It can lead to aspiration and complete obstruction of the airway. Extensive soft tissue edema and lymph node enlargement occur.[99-101]

Toxic cardiomyopathy is estimated to occur in 10% to 25% of patients and is responsible for 50% to 60% of deaths.[102] It often arises in the second to third week of illness when the affected individual appears to be clinically improving. Abnormalities of the myocardium, the conductive system, and the pericardium occur. The conductive disturbances are in response to the toxin.[103] Cardiac ectopy is 100% sensitive and specific to predict fatal outcome in children with severe diphtheria.[102]

When there is severe disease, neuropathy is seen in approximately three-fourths of the patients.[99,101] In a classic case of diphtheria, local paralysis of the soft palate occurs 2 to 3 weeks after the beginning of the oropharyngeal infection. Weaknesses of the pharyngeal, facial, and ocular nerves follow. The symmetric polyneuropathy occurs in a stocking-glove distribution and begins between 10 days to 3 months following the oropharyngeal infection.[99,101,102]

The distal ascending weakness and spinal fluid findings may be indistinguishable from GBS.[102] Additionally, rare cases can have dysfunction of the autonomic function with associated hypertension and cardiac failure. Typically, there is complete recovery.

Diagnostically, cultures should be obtained from the nose, throat, and the infected mucocutaneous area. Giving the antitoxin is critical even if the diagnosis is only presumptive. If the antitoxin is administered on the first day, the mortality is 1% compared with a mortality of 20% if administration is delayed until the fourth day.[102] Immunoglobulin preparations have also been hypothesized as helpful. The only antimicrobials that have had prospective studies proving efficacy are penicillin and erythromycin.[102]

One should anticipate airway complications, congestive heart failure, and malnutrition. Studies have revealed no difference in the occurrence of carditis, neuritis, or death in those receiving steroids. Digitalis is associated with an increased occurrence of arrhythmias. Overall prognosis depends on multiple variables, including the delay in the administration of the antitoxin, immunization status, and age. The mortality rate of 10% for respiratory tract diphtheria has not changed since the 1960s.[102]

Acute Intermittent Porphyria

The most common of the four types of porphyria is acute intermittent porphyria (AIP). Clinical symptoms in acute attacks span multiple medical subspecialties and may be precipitated by numerous medications, hormonal variations, calorie restrictions, and alcohol. AIP most commonly occurs in females with the age of onset between 15 and 40 years and rarely occurs before puberty.[103,104]

An acute neuropathy is found in approximately 40% of acute AIP attacks.[104-106] The neuropathy typically follows the onset of the attack by 1 to 4 weeks but may do so as late as 11 weeks. Although paresthesias and distal sensory changes may be a prodromal finding, the motor signs are much more prominent. Classically, the patient has symmetric upper extremity proximal weakness, but it may advance to involve the lower extremities. Generalized weakness is documented in approximately 42% of patients.[104] In AIP's most dramatic setting, the patient can have a rapid progression of weakness that leads to a flaccid involvement of all four extremities and respiratory compromise. When cranial nerves are involved, VII and X are the most frequently affected. Vascular compromise has been documented in individuals with vision loss, which may be monocular or total. Although this vision loss is usually transient, it can be permanent.[104]

AIP is often difficult to diagnose. The chief complaints are typically nonspecific abdominal and back pain. This colicky abdominal pain often leads to the consideration of surgical intervention. Notably, AIP is not associated with temperature elevation, leukocytosis, or rebound tenderness.[104,105]

Neurologic and psychiatric symptoms often accompany the onset of attack. Of note, many antiepileptic medications can worsen or induce an attack. Worsening has been reported with phenytoin, carbamazepine, phenobarbital, valproate, lamotrigine, and potentially tiagabine and topiramate. Gabapentin and levetiracetam have been successfully used to alleviate symptoms. Oxcarbazepine is a consideration, but there are concerns regarding hyponatremia.[104,105]

Another important management issue in AIP is the significant hyponatremia and associated seizures that may be further precipitated by the use of intravenous fluids containing dextrose and water. Cardiovascular complications include hypertension and tachycardia. In its most extreme case, there may be significant hypertension with associated hypertensive encephalopathy and ischemic changes. An intravenous infusion of magnesium sulfate may be helpful.[104] Nutritional support is important in order to avoid a catabolic state, which will further complicate the clinical picture. In the event that nutrition is required intravenously, high-glucose solutions with dextrose are recommended. Enteral feeding is preferred, with carbohydrates providing 50% to 60% of the energy needs.[104]

Diagnostically in AIP, urine and stool can be tested for alpha aminolevulinic acid (ALA). Also, there is a marked elevation of urinary porphobilinogen (PBG). In the blood, PBG deaminase is helpful in that its level is abnormal even between the acute attacks.[104] AIP should be a consideration in the differential diagnosis of progressive weakness. It is most often confused with GBS. The ascending weakness that is classic in GBS is rare in acute porphyria. Additionally, acute porphyria does not have elevation of the CSF protein or abnormalities of the cellular contents. The associated abdominal discomfort and tachycardia that are seen in porphyria would not be anticipated in GBS. Differential considerations should also include lead intoxication and hereditary tyrosinemia. Elder and Hift[104] provided a review of AIP therapy. The two recommended approaches are carbohydrate loading and administration of heme to replenish the depleted heme, which is the principal product of porphyrin metabolism. If the patient has severe symptoms such as seizures, hyponatremia, and initial signs of neuropathy, aggressive therapy should begin as early in the crisis as possible.[106] In mild attacks it may be possible to wait 24 hours to determine if the attack will resolve spontaneously. Carbohydrate loading is delivered as a 20% glucose solution provided via a central venous catheter. Studies that support the use of heme are primarily noncontrolled and have difficulty reaching statistical significance, but the overall consensus is that it does provide benefit. Daily measurements of urinary ALA or PBG may be a helpful clinical monitor.

Spinal Muscular Atrophy

Spinal muscular atrophy (SMA), a disease of the anterior horn cell, is most commonly inherited in an autosomal recessive manner. The responsible gene is the survivor motor neuron gene on chromosome 5q13.[107,108] SMA has three subtypes that present in childhood, and both autosomal dominant and X-linked inheritance have been reported. The combined incidence of all forms of SMA has been estimated as 1 case in 6000 to 25,700 live births.[109,110] After cystic fibrosis, SMA is the next most common fatal disease with an autosomal recessive pattern of inheritance.[109] The most severe form was

previously known as Werdnig-Hoffmann disease but is now more commonly referred to as SMA type I. It classically presents shortly after birth. The findings should be apparent before age 6 months, and type I SMA is often clinically defined by the patient's inability to achieve independent sitting. SMA type II usually presents between ages 6 and 18 months and is characterized by the patient sitting but never standing or walking. In SMA type III, patients do stand independently and walk.

In patients with SMA type I, the examination reveals a floppy baby with proximal weakness greater than distal. The lower extremities are more affected than the upper extremities, and the only spontaneous movement in these infants may be in the hands and feet. When supine, the infant will assume a frog-legged position. Polyminimyoclonus, a fine tremor most easily visualized in the hands, may also be present in these patients. Areflexia, tongue fasciculations, facial weakness, and normal sensation are also found.[111,112] Retrospectively, some mothers will report decreased fetal movement during the pregnancy with the affected infant. Death often occurs before 2 years of age as a result of respiratory problems.[109] Patients with clinical symptoms within the first day of life have a life expectancy between 2 and 6 months with a mean age at death slightly before 4 months.[113]

Patients with SMA type II usually have delayed motor milestones after having normal motor development in infancy. Polyminimyoclonus is also present in these patients. Life expectancy is variable, with many patients not surviving past adolescence.[109] Life expectancy can be enhanced, however, with fastidious respiratory care.[114] Not surprising was the correlation that patients with an earlier onset of the disease had an earlier death.[115]

In SMA type III, weakness is again more proximal than distal with the lower extremities being more severely affected. The gait exhibited in these patients has a waddling quality, and lumbar lordosis is also prominent.[116] If symptoms begin after age 2 years, ambulation may continue to a median age of 44 years.[116] If symptoms begin before age 2 years, ambulation continues to a median age of 12 years.[116] Life expectancy for patients with SMA type III may be the same as in the normal population because muscle weakness appears to stabilize in these patients.

Electrodiagnostic studies on these patients reveal normal motor conduction velocities. Over time, the amplitude of the compound muscle action potential may be decreased. Results from sensory nerve conduction studies are normal. EMG reveals evidence of acute denervation with spontaneous activity and chronic denervative changes with polyphasic motor units. Muscle biopsy specimens reveal angulated fibers suggestive of denervation. The creatine phosphokinase (CPK) level may or may not be increased. Genetic testing is utilized to confirm the diagnosis.

Respiratory complications are the most concerning aspect of this disease and include aspiration, pneumonia, and respiratory failure. Respiratory failure may even be the presenting symptom in SMA type I.[117] Respiratory muscle weakness results in restrictive lung disease with a weak cough and hypoventilation.[112] Hypercapnia is also a consequence of restrictive lung disease, and as a result supplemental oxygen may have devastating consequences including apnea and death.[112] If supplemental oxygen is needed, conventional ventilation or noninvasive ventilation should be instituted.

Other complications may also occur over time including scoliosis and contractures. Scoliosis also complicates pulmonary function over time because of chest wall alterations. In addition, feeding difficulties play a prominent role, particularly in the developing infant with SMA type I. If concerns arise, feeding evaluation should be performed to rule out aspiration. Supplemental feeding through nasogastric tube or gastrostomy may be necessary.[115]

Aggressive symptomatic treatment, including more frequent use of ventilation and gastrostomy, has been associated with longer life spans. Specific pharmacologic treatments have not been successful.[118]

Poliomyelitis

The paralytic form of polio represents only 1% to 2% of the actual infections. Aseptic meningitis represents less than 10% and is often thought to be a nonspecific illness; the remainder of those affected have no apparent infection. Patients with the paralytic disorder present with very high fevers, significant muscle pain, and lack of reflexes. Paralysis rapidly progresses over a few hours to a complete asymmetric loss of motor use in one or more extremities. Classically, the weakness peaks at 5 days. The distribution of weakness is predominantly proximal and in the lower extremities, with cranial nerve abnormalities reported in 5% to 35% of the patients. Bowel and bladder problems may occur over the initial 3 days. Sensory abnormalities are rare. Classically, the "head drop" may occur on exam: As the examiner lifts the patient's shoulders and raises the trunk from supine, the head falls backward in a limp fashion. It is thought that this is not due to paralysis of the neck muscles because it can occur in the nonparalytic form. The clinical course may include significant respiratory muscle weakness. Involvement of the bulbar muscles, brain stem, and the respiratory center results in respiratory compromise. Cranial nerve involvement leads to paralysis of the pharynx and vocal cords and further poses difficulties in breathing. Respiratory compromise leads to most deaths in the paralytic form.[119] Typically, 50% of patients with any paralysis exhibit some degree of residual deficits, although most do improve. A 10% mortality is now reported in the patients with the paralytic form. Before mechanical ventilation, 60% of the individuals died.[119]

Early in the course of the pharyngeal infection throat cultures may reveal the poliovirus. Later in the course, the stool culture becomes increasingly helpful. Spinal fluid culture has lower sensitivity. Usually, the results of routine laboratory tests are unremarkable. Cerebral spinal fluid findings are characteristic of aseptic meningitis. In the first few hours after the onset of symptoms, polymorphonuclear leukocytes may predominate, but within 12 hours the predominance of lymphocytes is seen.[119]

Numerous other clinical manifestations may occur. In the viral myocarditis, the heart is extremely sensitive to development of arrhythmias. Hypertension is well recognized and can be severe enough to cause encephalopathy. Analgesics, including opiates, may be required for pain relief. Hot packs have been noted to be effective when applied every 2 to 4 hours. Constipation and bladder paralysis are major issues early in the course and should be monitored closely. The risk of aspiration and airway compromise necessitates a high level of vigilance. If the patient demonstrates respiratory compromise, a tracheostomy is indicated with accompanying mechanical ventilation.[119] Use of antiviral agents is debated. Additionally, some authors argue that steroids are not indicated in enteroviral infections.[119]

Children with mild weakness generally have full recovery. If paralysis is present, the recovery is ongoing for 2 years with 80% realized by 6 months.[119] Adults may have new symptoms long after the infection resolves, including weakness and muscle atrophy that are related to continued normal attrition of anterior horn cells.[120]

Polio-Like Syndromes

Polio-like syndromes have been reported, with West Nile virus and multiple subtypes of enterovirus (most notably D68) being prominent agents.[121-123] These cases are often associated with a prior illness (either gastrointestinal or respiratory) and may present with respiratory failure and an acute flaccid paralysis of one or more limbs consistent with anterior horn cell disease. Clusters of cases with acute flaccid myelitis have been described in California and Colorado (http://www.cdc.gov/ncird/downloads/acute-flaccid-myelitis.pdf). Encephalopathy and cranial nerve abnormalities are common, as is CSF pleocytosis. Some authors have suggested the use of interferon-α based on small case studies, but no blinded and randomized studies have been published.[122-125] Prognosis may be more optimistic with some viruses. However, several series report poor motor recovery with enterovirus D68, likely due to significant motor neuron damage.[122,123]

Organophosphate and Carbamate Poisoning

The clinician must always maintain a high index of suspicion and consider poisoning in the differential diagnosis in patients with altered mental status, respiratory symptoms, or weakness (see also Chapters 127 and 128). Zweiner and Ginsburg[126] reported in their study of 37 children with organophosphate or carbamate poisonings that 43% of these patients were evaluated by their primary care doctor, and pesticide toxicity was not suspected. Patients commonly do not have a known history of exposure. Exposure to these substances may occur as inhalation, ingestion, or dermal contact. In one study of 37 infants and children with organophosphate and carbamate poisonings, 76% of these patients ingested these substances (which were improperly stored), 16% had transcutaneous exposure (through contact with treated carpets, linens, and lawns), and 8% were poisoned by an unknown etiology.[126] Cholinesterase, which is present in the neuromuscular junction, is irreversibly inhibited by organophosphates and reversibly inhibited by carbamate compounds. Therefore, a constellation of muscarinic, nicotinic, and central nervous system symptoms may occur.

Symptoms may originate from various systems. Muscarinic symptoms include miosis, excessive salivation, sweating, lacrimation, diarrhea, urination, and bradycardia. In severe poisonings, flaccid paralysis with areflexia is common. In moderate poisonings, muscle fasciculations may be present. Central nervous system symptoms include coma and seizures; however, seizures are less common in carbamate toxicity.[127] Pulmonary symptoms including bronchoconstriction, increased pulmonary secretions, and wheezing have been reported.[128] In one study of 52 children with organophosphate or carbamate poisoning, 100% of these patients exhibited hypotonia, stupor, or coma.[129] With further analysis of the 16 patients with organophosphate poisoning, the other common symptoms included miosis (56%), salivation (37%), pulmonary edema (37%), diarrhea (30%), and bradycardia (25%).[129] Various cardiac rhythms may occur with pathologic signs of cardiotoxicity.[130] Overall, carbamate poisonings are usually less severe and shorter in duration, although the symptoms are essentially the same as those found in organophosphate poisonings.[131]

If organophosphate and carbamate compounds are ingested, gastric lavage and activated charcoal should be initiated. If contaminated, the patient's skin and hair should be rinsed and cleansed thoroughly with soap, and clothes should be changed to reduce further exposure.[127]

In both forms of poisonings, atropine is used as an antidote for the muscarinic symptoms. Treatment with atropine, however, does not reverse the nicotinic symptoms, which include muscle weakness and respiratory failure. Atropine should be administered as quickly as possible and in adequate doses. In children older than 12 years, the dosing is 1 to 2 mg intravenously every 10 to 30 minutes. In children younger than 12 years, the initial dose is 0.05 mg/kg with maintenance doses of 0.02 to 0.05 mg/kg over 10 to 30 minutes.[128] In organophosphate and carbamate poisonings, the atropine dose is five to ten times greater than conventional atropine dosing.[128] Atropine should be continued until the muscarinic symptoms begin to abate. The signs of atropinization include mydriasis, tachycardia, and xerostomia, and they help provide parameters for adequate dosing.[132] Atropine should be continued for at least 24 hours after severe exposures and then tapered if symptoms are improving.[128]

Pralidoxime chloride, the only cholinesterase reactivator in the United States, is an antidote for only the nicotinic symptoms of organophosphate poisonings; therefore atropine must be used concomitantly. Pralidoxime chloride does not help in carbamate exposures. Various doses have been reported for pralidoxime in patients older than 12 years. A conservative dose is 0.5 to 1 g IV over 15 to 30 minutes, repeated every 10 to 12 hours, beginning 1 to 2 hours after the initial dose. Another study suggests a 2-g loading dose with a continuous infusion of 1g/h for 48 hours. These doses have not been directly compared to each other. In patients younger than 12 years, the dose is 25 to 50 mg/kg IV over 15 to 30 minutes, repeated every 10 to 12 hours, beginning 1 to 2 hours after the initial dose.[128,133,134]

After the antidotes are given, the mainstay of treatment is supportive. If necessary, ventilation should be provided until the patient regains respiratory strength. Suctioning of secretions in both the oropharynx and in the respiratory tree is essential. Seizures should be treated with diazepam or lorazepam. Cardiac monitoring should be implemented because complex ventricular arrhythmias may occur.[130,135] Early feeding may prolong hospital stay.[136] Death usually occurs as a result of respiratory arrest and pulmonary complications, including excessive secretions, edema, and bronchoconstriction.[128]

Diagnosis is based on clinical findings and response to antidote medications. Serum and red blood cell cholinesterase levels should be obtained to assist in the diagnosis of organophosphate poisoning. Treatment should be initiated immediately and not delayed while waiting for cholinesterase level results. Cholinesterase levels do not assist in the diagnosis of

carbamate exposure because the reversal of the enzyme occurs too rapidly to be quantified.

Key References

3. Ammache Z, Afifi A, Brown C, et al. Childhood Guillain-Barre syndrome: clinical and electrophysiologic features predictive of outcome. *J Child Neurol.* 2001;6:477-483.
4. Bradshaw D, Jones H. Guillain-Barre syndrome in children: clinical course, electrodiagnosis, and prognosis. *Muscle Nerve.* 1992;15:500-506.
7. Dimario FJ Jr, Edwards C. Autonomic dysfunction in childhood Guillain-Barre syndrome. *J Child Neurol.* 2012;27:581-586.
9. Asbury A, Cornblath D. Assessment of current diagnostic criteria for Guillain-Barre syndrome. *Ann Neurol.* 1990;27(suppl):S21-S24.
12. Patwa HS, Chaudhry V, Katzberg H, et al. Evidence-based guideline: intravenous immunoglobulin in the treatment of neuromuscular disorders: report of the Therapeutics and Technology Assessment Subcommittee of the American Academy of Neurology. *Neurology.* 2012;78:1009-1015.
13. Hughes RA, van Doorn PA. Corticosteroids for Guillain-Barre syndrome. *Cochrane Database Syst Rev.* 2012;(8):CD001466.
14. Hughes RA, Swan AV, van Doorn PA. Intravenous immunoglobulin for Guillain-Barre syndrome. *Cochrane Database Syst Rev.* 2014;(9):CD002063.
20. Chiba A, Kusunoki S, Obata H, et al. Serum anti-GQ1b IgG antibody is associated with ophthalmoplegia in Miller Fisher syndrome and Guillain-Barre syndrome: clinical and immunohistochemical studies. *Neurology.* 1993;43:1911-1917.
21. Petzold A, Brettschneider J, Jin K, et al. CSF protein biomarkers for proximal axonal damage improve prognostic accuracy in the acute phase of Guillain-Barré Syndrome. *Muscle Nerve.* 2009;40:42-49.
23. Drachman D. Myasthenia gravis. *N Engl J Med.* 1994;330:1797-1810.
25. Bartoccioni E, Scuderi F, Minicuci GM, et al. Anti-MuSK antibodies: correlation with myasthenia gravis severity. *Neurology.* 2006;67:504-507.
28. Deymeer F, Gungor-Tuncer O, Yilmaz V, et al. Clinical comparison of anti-MuSK- vs anti-AChR-positive and seronegative myasthenia gravis. *Neurology.* 2007;68:609-611.
29. Chiang LM, Darras BT, Kang PB. Juvenile myasthenia gravis. *Muscle Nerve.* 2009;39:423-431.
30. The Muscle Study Group. A trial of mycophenolate mofetil with prednisone as initial immunotherapy in myasthenia gravis. *Neurology.* 2008;71:394-399.
31. Hehir MK, Burns TM, Alpers J, et al. Mycophenolate mofetil in Ach-R-antibody-positive myasthenia gravis: outcomes in 102 patients. *Muscle Nerve.* 2010;41:593-598.
37. Thomas C, Mayer S, Gungor Y, et al. Myasthenic crisis: clinical features, mortality, complications, and risk factors for prolonged intubation. *Neurology.* 1997;48:1253-1260.
39. Qureshi A, Choudhry M, Akbar M, et al. Plasma exchange versus intravenous immunoglobulin treatment in myasthenic crisis. *Neurology.* 1999;52:629-632.
41. Mayer S. Intensive care of the myasthenic patient. *Neurology.* 1997;48(suppl 5):S70-S75.
42. Adams S, Mathews J, Grammer L. Drugs that may exacerbate myasthenia gravis. *Ann Emerg Med.* 1984;13:532-538.
44. Gotkine M, Fellig Y, Abramsky O. Occurrence of CNS demyelinating disease in patients with myasthenia gravis. *Neurology.* 2006;67:881-883.
48. Engel A, Ohno K, Milone M. Congenital myasthenic syndromes caused by mutations in acetylcholine receptor genes. *Neurology.* 1997;48(suppl 5):S28-S35.
50. Greenstein P. Tick paralysis. *Med Clin North Am.* 2002;86:441-446.
53. Grattan-Smith P, Morris J, Johnston H, et al. Clinical and neurophysiological features of tick paralysis. *Brain.* 1997;120:1975-1987.
54. Donaldson MR, Yoon G, Fu YH, Ptacek LJ. Andersen-Tawil syndrome: a model of clinical variability, pleiotropy, and genetic heterogeneity. *Ann Med.* 2004;36(suppl 1):92-97.
55. Tawil R, Ptacek LJ, Pavlakis SG, et al. Andersen's syndrome: potassium sensitive periodic paralysis, ventricular ectopy and dysmorphic features. *Ann Neurol.* 1994;35:326-330.
56. Miller TM, Dias da Silva MR, Miller HA, et al. Correlating phenotype and genotype in the periodic paralyses. *Neurology.* 2004;63:1647-1655.

59. Matthews E, Labrum R, Sweeney MG, et al. Voltage sensor charge loss accounts for most cases of hypokalemic periodic paralysis. *Neurology.* 2009;72:1544-1547.

60. Links T, Smit A, Molenaar W, et al. Familial hypokalemic periodic paralysis clinical, diagnostic and therapeutic aspects. *J Neurol Sci.* 1994;122:33-43.

70. Griggs R, Engel W, Resnick J. Acetazolamide treatment of hypokalemic periodic paralysis: prevention of attacks and improvement of persistent weakness. *Ann Intern Med.* 1970;73:39-48.

80. Layzer R, Lovelace R, Rowland L. Hyperkalemic periodic paralysis. *Arch Neurol.* 1967;16:455-472.

81. Long S. Infant botulism. *Pediatr Infect Dis J.* 2001;20:707-709.

93. Thompson J, Glasgow L, Warpinski J, et al. Infant botulism: clinical spectrum and epidemiology. *Pediatrics.* 1980;66:936-942.

95. Cornblath D, Sladky J, Sumner A. Clinical electrophysiology of infantile botulism. *Muscle Nerve.* 1983;6:448-452.

97. Arnon SS, Schechter R, Maslanka SE, et al. Human botulism immune globulin for the treatment of infant botulism. *NEJM.* 2006;354:462-471.

99. Both L, Collins S, de Zoysa A, et al. Molecular and epidemiologic review of toxigenic diphtheria infections in England between 2007 and 2013. *J Clin Microbiol.* 2015;53:567-572.

100. Camello TCF, Pereira GA, Hirata R Jr, et al. Diphtheria outbreak in Maranhao, Brazil: microbiological, clinical and epidemiological aspects. *Epidemiol Infect.* 2015;143:791-798.

104. Elder GH, Hift RJ. Treatment of acute porphyria. *Hos Med.* 2001;62:422-425.

105. Kuo HC, Huang CC, Chu CC, et al. Neurological complications of acute intermittent porphyria. *Eur Neurol.* 2011;66:247-252.

106. Albers JW, Fink JK. Porphyric neuropathy. *Muscle Nerve.* 2004;30:410-422.

108. Oskoui M, Levy G, Garland CJ, et al. The changing natural history of spinal muscular atrophy type 1. *Neurology.* 2007;69:1931-1936.

114. Gozal D. Pulmonary manifestations of neuromuscular disease with special reference to Duchenne muscular dystrophy and spinal muscular atrophy. *Pediatr Pulmonol.* 2000;29:141-150.

118. Bosboom WM, Vrancken AF, van den Berg LH, et al. Drug treatment for spinal muscular atrophy type I. *Cochrane Database Syst Rev.* 2009;(1):CD006281.

122. Messacar K, Schreiner TL, Maloney JA, et al. A cluster of acute flaccid paralysis and cranial nerve dysfunction temporarily associated with an outbreak of enterovirus D68 in children in Colorado, USA. *Lancet.* 2015;385:1662-1671.

123. Ayscue P, Van Haren K, Sheriff H, et al. Acute flaccid paralysis with anterior myelitis—California, June 2012–June 2014. *MMWR Morb Mortal Wkly Rep.* 2014;63:903-906.

130. Anand S, Singh S, Saikia UN, et al. Cardiac abnormalities in acute organophosphate poisoning. *Clin Toxicol.* 2009;47:230-235.

133. Pawar KS, Bhoite RR, Pillay CP, et al. Continuous pralidoxime infusion versus repeated bolus injection to treat organophosphorus pesticide poisoning: a randomised controlled trial. *Lancet.* 2006;368:2136-2141.

134. Peter JV, Moran JL, Graham P. Oxime therapy and outcomes in human organophosphate poisoning: an evaluation using meta-analytic techniques. *Crit Care Med.* 2006;34:502-510.

Renal, Fluids, Electrolytes

Renal Structure and Function

Maury N. Pinsk and Victoria F. Norwood

PEARLS

- The efferent blood supply from a single glomerulus will contribute to the capillary vascular supply of tubules from different nephrons. This arrangement of the vascular supply explains the patchy distribution of tubular damage after ischemic injury.
- Combinations of angiotensin-converting enzyme inhibitors and nonsteroidal antiinflammatory drugs inhibit afferent arteriolar vasodilation and efferent arteriolar vasoconstriction. In low flow states, these agents can cause a precipitous loss of glomerular filtration pressure and kidney function.
- Tubular dysfunction in the setting of acute kidney injury results in the inability to transport sodium into the medulla to establish concentration gradients, impairing the concentration of urine and resulting in diuresis. Furosemide and other loop diuretics, which also impair sodium transport into the medulla, are often ineffective at increasing urine output in this setting.

Renal Development

The human kidneys begin development in the third week of gestation, at which time they are primitive organs called pronephroi. These early kidneys are functional but regress as development unfolds. As gestation continues in the fourth week, the secondary kidney elements, the mesonephroi, form from parallel strips of mesoderm along the paravertebral axis. The mesonephroi begin functioning between the sixth and tenth week of gestation before involution in a cranial-caudal direction beginning at 10 weeks gestation. The definitive kidneys, or metanephroi, begin development at the fifth week of gestation and begin functioning between the tenth and fourteenth week. This kidney develops in the pelvis as the branching ureteric bud and undifferentiated metanephric mesenchyme interact in a complex series of reciprocal inductions.[1-3] These interactions lead to the formation of glomeruli, whereas vessels and tubules form from mesenchymal precursors, and distal tubules and collecting ducts derive from ureteric bud epithelium. This process occurs in a centrifugal fashion so that deeper corticomedullary nephrons form earliest in organogenesis, whereas the more peripheral cortical nephrons form later. As the metanephros develops, the maturing kidney ascends into the retroperitoneal space to its final location with the upper poles at the T12 vertebra. During the ascent, the systemic blood supply is derived from more cranial aspects of the aorta and from the lumbar renal arteries at the final position of the kidney. The ureters elongate and canalize during the ascent to maintain drainage to the bladder. By the time human nephrogenesis is complete at 34 to 36 weeks of gestation, repeated cycles of mesenchymal induction, ureteric branching, and morphogenesis result in approximately 1 million nephrons per kidney.

Renal Anatomy

Normal human kidneys reside in the retroperitoneal space at the level of the T12 vertebra. The liver is superior to the right kidney and thus displaces it lower than the kidney on the left side. The spleen and stomach overlie the superior aspect of the left kidney. Kidneys, however, can be found in a variety of other locations and have altered morphologies as a result of alterations of the normal developmental program (reviewed by Schedl[4]). For example, failure of the kidney to ascend normally results in a pelvic kidney that has abnormal vascular supplies from the aorta and iliac vessels. Mesenchymal regions of the two kidneys coming in contact during early development likely cause fused kidneys, most commonly the horseshoe kidney. Partial or complete renal duplications comprise a variety of abnormalities that may arise from aberrant branching of the ureteric bud into the developing mesenchyme. Unilateral agenesis likely results from failure of ureteric bud development or abnormal mesenchymal induction, leading to regression of the metanephric mesenchyme and failed renal development.

Renal Vasculature
Vascular Development

Markers of early vascular development are expressed in undifferentiated metanephric mesenchyme, which suggests that the blood supply to the nephron develops at least partially from precursors inherent to the maturing kidney.[5] Migration of committed endothelial cells into the developing glomerulus occurs in response to secreted factors such as vascular endothelial growth factor, which is secreted under the transcriptional regulation of the oxygen-sensitive hypoxic inducible factor.[6] Control of the corresponding branching of extraglomerular vessels is an area of active study and may involve branching from existing vessels, de novo vessel formation, or both processes. These actions appear to be regulated in part by the renin-angiotensin system.[7]

Vascular Anatomy

The arterial supply of the kidney branches from the main renal artery and enters the kidney in a series of rays called interlobar arteries. The interlobar vessels branch at the corticomedullary junction to run parallel to the surface of the kidney as arcuate arteries. Arcuate arteries penetrate the cortex as interlobular arteries, which ascend into the cortex in a radial pattern. It is from the interlobular arteries that afferent arterioles of the glomeruli arise. After filtration across the glomerular tuft, blood exits the glomerulus by efferent arterioles, which travel to the surface of the cortex and eventually feed the peritubular capillary vascular beds, the vasa rectae. The efferent arteriole of a single nephron can supply blood to multiple vasa rectae. The postglomerular vasculature of the cortex is supplied by efferent arterioles from midcortical and superficial cortical nephrons, whereas the blood supply to the medulla is entirely derived from juxtamedullary efferent arterioles. The vasa rectae of the medulla branch as they descend toward the papilla of the kidney and form the complex meshwork of the medullary capillary vascular beds. Only a few vessels of the vasa rectae eventually reach the papillary tip.

Venous drainage of the vasa rectae is divided into two types: the vessels of the deep medulla ascend to join the arcuate veins at the corticomedullary junction, and those of the superficial medulla ascend into the cortex to join the cortical capillary network and ultimately the interlobular and arcuate veins (Fig. 72.1). The arcuate veins join with the interlobar veins via the interlobular veins and finally drain into the main renal vein to join the main circulation.

Vascular Function

The kidneys are extraordinarily vascular organs; they receive 15% to 18% of cardiac output in the neonate and up to 20% of cardiac output in the adult.[8] Blood flow to the kidney is tightly regulated to ensure continued renal function over a range of blood pressures. Sympathetic α_1-receptors, myogenic contraction, and vasoactive mediators control vascular resistance and provide autoregulation of renal blood flow. Maintenance of glomerular filtration rate at the level of the glomerulus occurs by vasoconstriction of efferent arterioles in response to vasopressors such as angiotensin II, whereas afferent arterioles relax in response to vasodilators such as prostacyclin. Circulating angiotensin II is elevated in the neonate,[9] as are corresponding vasodilators.[10,11] Therefore infants have a decreased capacity to regulate renal blood flow, which explains their increased susceptibility to renal ischemia in hypotensive states.

Nephron Unit

The nephron unit consists of a glomerular tuft, proximal tubule, loop of Henle, distal tubule, and collecting duct (Fig. 72.2). The proximal tubule is an extension of the urinary space of the glomerulus and courses into the loop of Henle. Two types of nephrons are characterized on the basis of the location of the glomerulus and the path of the loop of Henle: the juxtamedullary nephrons and the cortical nephrons. Most nephrons are cortical in location, have short loops of Henle that extend into the superficial medulla, and have a relatively low capacity to reabsorb solute and water. Juxtamedullary nephrons are fewer in number but have longer loops of Henle

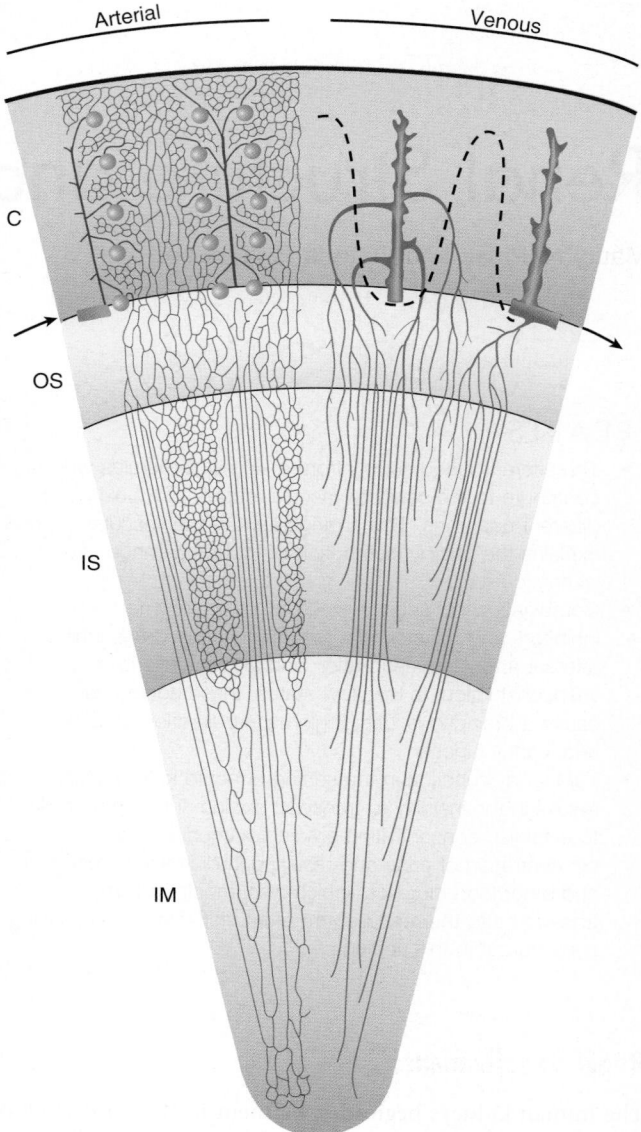

Fig. 72.1. The microvasculature of the mammalian kidney. Arterial supply *(left):* The arcuate artery *(arrow)* travels parallel to the surface of the kidney, branching into interlobular arteries that travel toward the kidney surface and further branching into afferent arterioles supplying each glomerulus. The efferent arterioles travel to the medulla forming the vasa rectae. Venous drainage *(right):* Interlobular veins receive blood from the vasa rectae of the medulla and superficial cortex. Interlobular veins drain into arcuate veins and ultimately rejoin the systemic circulation via the renal vein. *C,* cortex; *IM,* inner medulla; *IS,* inner stripe; *OS,* outer stripe. (Modified from Kriz W, Lever AF. Renal countercurrent mechanisms: structure and function, Am Heart J. 1969;78:101-118; Rollhäuser H, Kriz W, Heinke W. Das Gefässsystem der Rattenniere [The vascular system of the rat kidney]. Z Zellforsch Mikrosk Anat. 1964;64:381-403; and Naylor RW, Davidson AJ. Hnf1beta and nephron segmentation. Pediatr Nephrol. 2014;29:659-664.)

that extend deep into the medulla. Consequently, these nephrons absorb larger amounts of salt and water, generate steep osmotic gradients, and produce highly concentrated urine. Regardless of the location of the nephron, the loop of Henle returns to the cortex to become a distal tubule. The distal tubule then continues on to form the collecting duct, the final

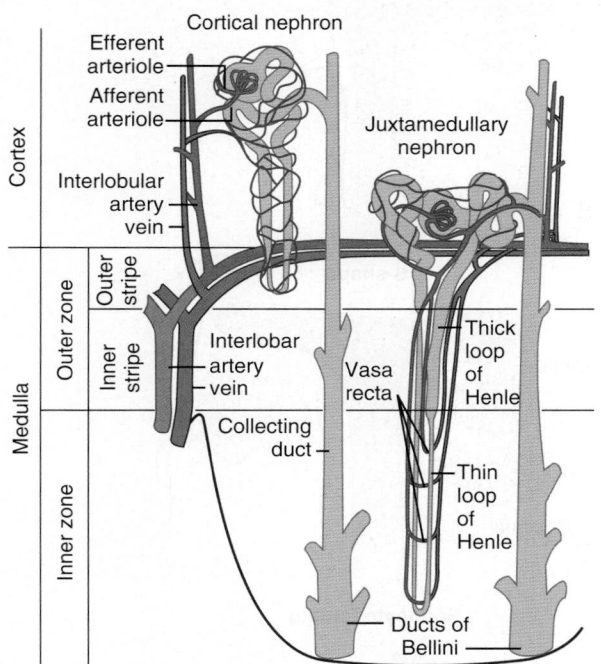

Fig. 72.2. The nephron structure. (From Guyton A. Formation of urine by the kidney: I. Renal blood flow, glomerular filtration, and their control. In: Wonsiewicz M, ed. Textbook of Medical Physiology. ed 8. Philadelphia: WB Saunders; 1991.)

common pathway for several nephrons draining into the renal papilla.

Nephron Development

Nephron development occurs through a complex, interactive series of processes.[1-3] Nephron development begins with the out-pouching of ureteric epithelium, the ureteric bud. This precursor to the collecting duct encroaches on undifferentiated mesenchyme in the caudal retroperitoneal space and induces the development of an epithelial cell condensate, the precursor to the glomerulus and tubule (Fig. 72.3). Simultaneously, factors within the metanephric mesenchyme induce the ureteric bud to continue branching. The epithelial condensate forms a vesicle that convolutes progressively into a comma-shaped body and then an S-shaped body, signifying the development of the urinary space and early tubule segments. The terminal portion of the tubule is contributed by the ureteric bud derivatives and forms the collecting duct. The mechanisms by which the ureteric bud epithelial derivatives link to the corresponding mesenchymal derivatives in the distal nephron remain unknown but may involve mesenchymal to epithelial cell transitioning (reviewed in Naylor). The glomerular capillary loops form through the angiogenic processes of committed endothelial cells,[5] and supporting mesangial cells develop from committed metanephric mesenchyme with myoblastic characteristics.[12] Nephrogenesis in the human is essentially complete by the thirty-fourth week of gestation, but functional maturation continues into the second year of life.[1-3]

Glomerular Anatomy

The glomerular tuft consists of endothelial cells, specialized epithelial cells (podocytes), and supporting mesangial cells.

Epithelial cells also form the urinary compartment into which ultrafiltrate passes (Bowman space). Endothelial cells and podocytes sit on opposite sides of the glomerular basement membrane, the entirety of which forms the filtration apparatus. The epithelial side is characterized by fingerlike extensions of the podocyte cell membrane that interdigitate to form a mesh on the glomerular basement membrane. Glomerular endothelial cells on the blood side of the filtration barrier are highly fenestrated, thereby enhancing solute and fluid transfer. Mesangial cells form the supporting network of the glomerular structure, provide some phagocytic function, and participate in control of glomerular filtration.

Glomerular Function

Filtration is the primary function of the glomerulus. For filtration to occur, there must be a gradient across the glomerular basement membrane favoring the movement of filtrate to a low-pressure area. There are generally four factors that determine the quantity of filtrate obtained across the glomerular basement membrane (Fig. 72.4). First, hydrostatic pressure in the glomerular capillary drives filtration of fluid across the glomerular basement membrane. If the blood flow to the glomerulus decreases, the hydrostatic pressure also drops, which necessitates an increase in efferent vascular resistance to maintain glomerular perfusion pressure. Angiotensin II, prostaglandins, and renal sympathetic activity control afferent and efferent vascular tone to carefully regulate glomerular vascular resistance.

The second factor controlling filtration is the oncotic pressure of the blood entering the glomerulus. As blood is filtered and water leaves the vascular compartment, the oncotic pressure in the blood compartment rises, retarding the further passage of fluid across the glomerular basement membrane. In situations of low oncotic pressure, such as nephrotic syndrome, the initial rate of ultrafiltrate formation is increased because of low oncotic pressure. Low oncotic pressure can also cause a redistribution of intravascular volume into peripheral tissue spaces, resulting in decreased vascular hydrostatic pressure and forcing ultrafiltrate production to drop.

The third factor determining the efficiency of ultrafiltrate formation is tubular hydrostatic pressure, or the resistance within the urinary space. In urinary tract obstruction, tubular hydrostatic pressure limits ultrafiltrate generation as it rises above the hydrostatic pressure of the blood compartment and arrests ultrafiltrate generation.

The last important factor in the determination of ultrafiltrate formation is the available glomerular basement membrane available surface area and the filtration efficiency. Physiologically, the functional size of the glomerular basement membrane can be determined at the whole kidney level or at the glomerular level. At the whole kidney level, the number of nephrons receiving adequate blood supply determines glomerular basement membrane area available for filtration. For example, shunting of blood from the cortex into the medulla, as seen in hepatorenal syndrome, effectively decreases the available glomerular basement membrane area by reducing the number of actively filtering nephrons. At the glomerular level, glomerular basement membrane area can be altered by mesangial cell function. In hypovolemic states, mesangial cell contraction is thought to decrease glomerular basement membrane area in response to hormonal mediators, resulting in decreased filtration and preservation of intravascular

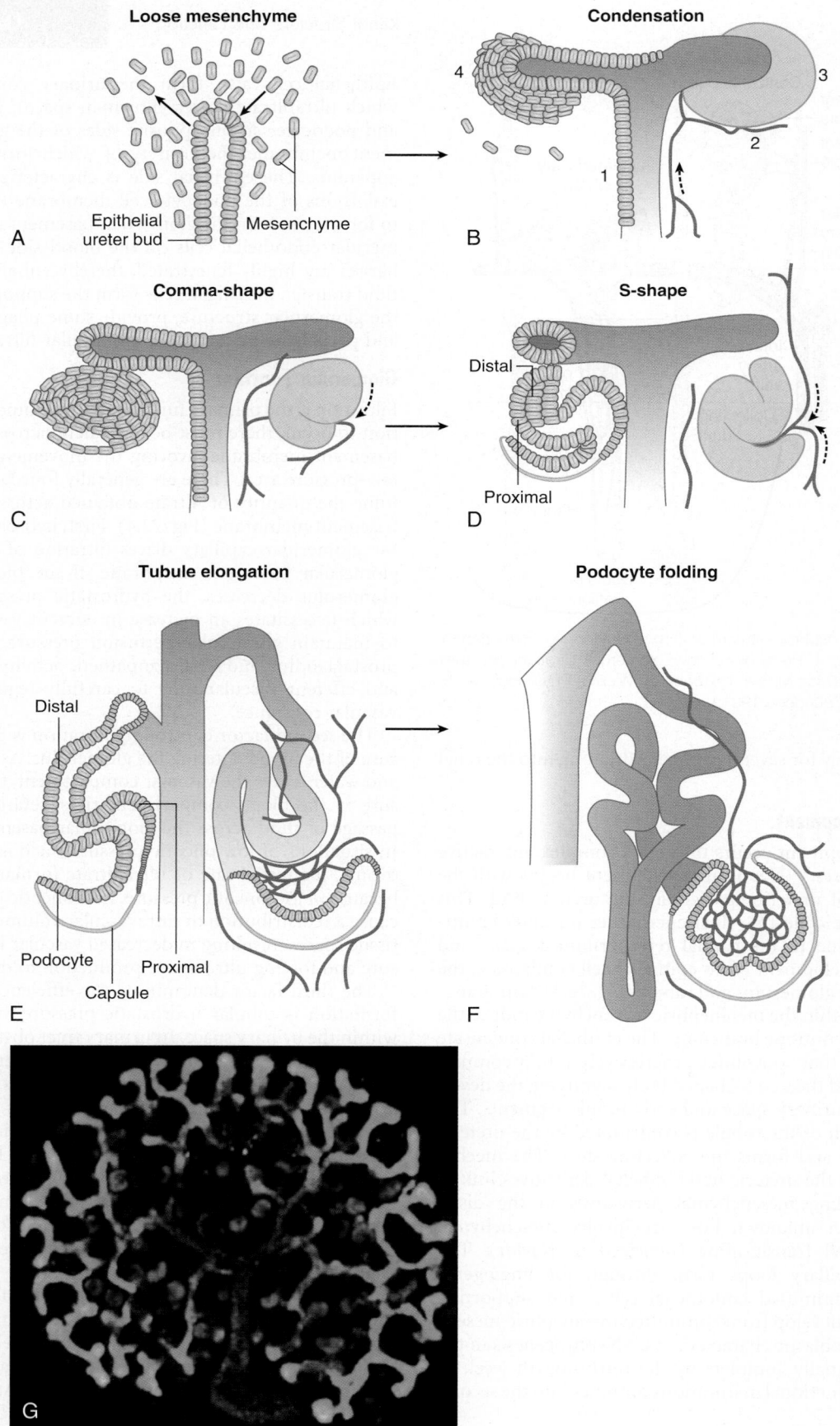

Fig. 72.3. Branching morphogenesis of the developing kidney. (A and B) The ureteric epithelium interacts with the metanephric mesenchyme, inducing condensation of the mesenchyme (1 = ureteric epithelium, 2 = vasculature, 3 = undifferentiated mesenchyme, 4 = condensed mesenchyme [precursor to epithelium]). (C and D) Infolding of the glomerular epithelium forms a comma-shaped body, followed by development of an S-shaped body. (E and F) Infolding of the glomerular epithelium and vascular structures and elongation of the tubular elements form the completed nephron. The mature glomerular capillary network is likely initiated during C and D. (G) Fluorescent microscopy of branching morphogenesis in organ culture. (A to F, From Gomez RA, Norwood VF. Recent advances in renal development. Curr Opin Pediatr. 1999;11:136. G, Courtesy John Bertram, Kidney Development and Research Group.)

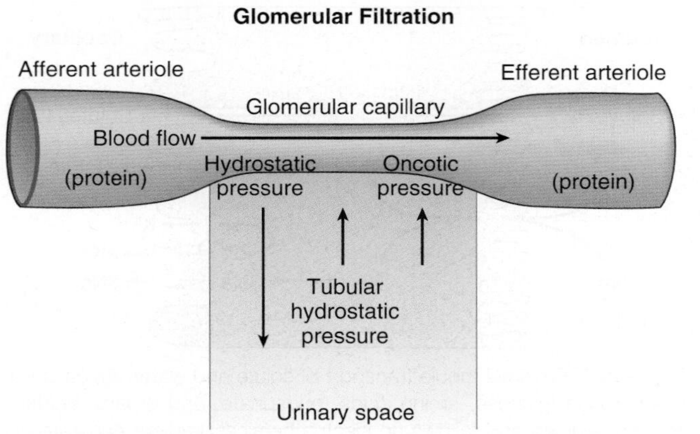

Glomerular Filtration

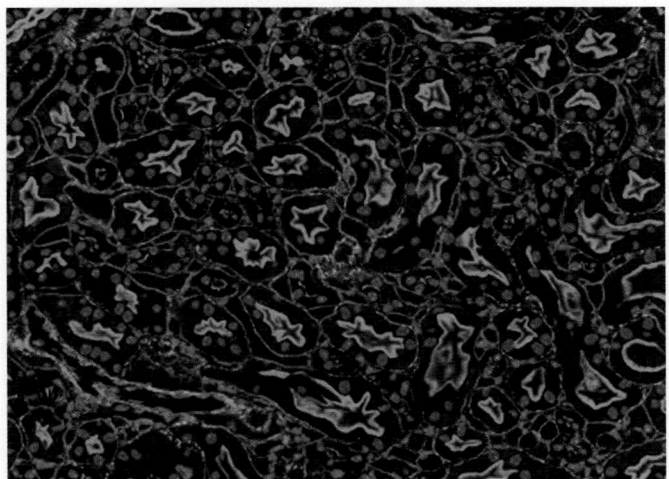

Fig. 72.4. Forces affecting ultrafiltrate formation in the isolated nephron.

Fig. 72.5. Proximal and distal tubules. (Courtesy Thomas J. Deerinck, National Center for Microscopy & Imaging Research.)

volume.[13] The efficiency of basement membrane filtration is also affected by disease states including immune complex deposition, fibrosis, or complement activation, which disrupt the integrity and efficiency of the membrane. Finally, selectivity of the filtration barrier is determined by the ability of the basement membrane to permit some materials to pass into the urinary space while restricting others to stay in the blood compartment. Selectivity appears to be the result of both size discrimination of the glomerular basement membrane and the orientation of podocyte foot processes on the glomerular basement membrane. Disruption of the normal podocyte physiology results in nephrotic range proteinuria.[14,15]

Tubular Anatomy
Proximal Tubule

The proximal tubule consists of polarized epithelia with a distinctive apical brush border not seen in other parts of the tubule (Fig. 72.5). The brush border increases the surface area of the luminal side of the cell so that maximal contact with the ultrafiltrate is made. Increased surface area facilitates reabsorption of solute and water, which occurs through an abundant variety of sodium-coupled transport proteins. Also on the brush border membrane are ion channels and ion exchange proteins that maintain electrochemical gradients across the apical membrane. On the basolateral aspect of the proximal tubular cells are located sodium-potassium adenosine triphosphatase (Na/K-ATPase) proteins and a high density of mitochondria. It is through the Na/K-ATPase that favorable sodium and electrochemical gradients are generated to facilitate transcellular and paracellular transport of solutes and water. The lateral membranes of the proximal tubule cells are characterized by the presence of cell-cell adhesion complexes called tight junctions. Tight junctions maintain the polarity of the proximal tubule cells by separating transport proteins on the apical side from the gradient-generating basolateral membrane proteins.

Loop of Henle

The cortical and juxtamedullary nephrons are defined by their position within the cortex but also by the length of the loop of Henle. The juxtamedullary nephrons have loops of Henle that extend deep into the hyperosmolar medulla, whereas most nephrons are cortical and have loops that reach only the mildly hyperosmolar outer medulla. The properties of the epithelial cells change throughout the length of the loop of Henle. The proximal portions have cells with prominent microvilli and permeable cell junctions that permit passage of fluid via aquaporin-1 channels.[16] The distal sections of the loop of Henle consist of flat epithelia lacking microvilli and are devoid of aquaporin-1 channels; the thin ascending limb of the loop of Henle is impermeable to water and urea but transports other solutes, particularly chloride, and is important in assisting with the establishment of medullary gradients.[17]

An abrupt transition occurs at the beginning of the thick ascending limb of the loop of Henle (TALH). The TALH is impermeable to water but transports solute in an active, ATP-dependent manner. These cells do not have prominent microvilli but do have dense tight junctions. These tight junctions allow solute, but not water, to move among cells into the basolateral space. TALH cells have dense localization of mitochondria and Na/K-ATPase at the basolateral membrane that generate gradients for solute transport across the luminal surface. Compared with the proximal tubule, the TALH basolateral surface is larger than the luminal surface and accommodates a larger number of Na/K-ATPase pumps.[18] At the distal end of the TALH, the tubule courses back toward its originating glomerulus. Here a small plaque of tall, narrow cells, the macula densa, contacts the vascular pole and extraglomerular mesangial cells (Fig. 72.6). The primary function of the macula densa cells appears to be the detection of tubular chloride content and the regulation of glomerular filtration.

Distal Nephron

The distal nephron segment from the TALH to the beginning of the collecting duct has three distinct morphologic regions. The first region is the distal convoluted tubule, the cells of which contain the luminal sodium chloride transporter (NCC2, or thiazide-sensitive transporter) and the highest density of mitochondria in the nephron. The basolateral membrane of this segment is composed of interdigitating membranes from adjacent cells, giving the appearance of membranous convolutions. This composition maximizes the

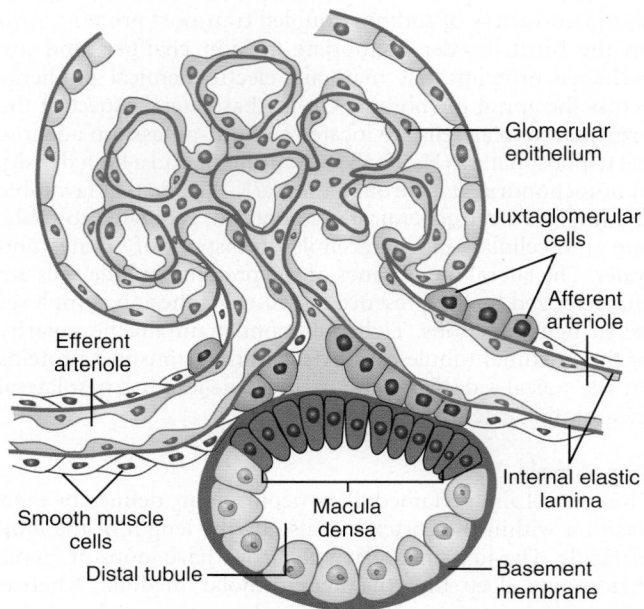

Fig. 72.6. Structure of the juxtaglomerular apparatus. (From Guyton A. Formation of urine by the kidney: I. Renal blood flow, glomerular filtration, and their control. In: Wonsiewicz M, ed. Textbook of Medical Physiology. ed 8. Philadelphia: WB Saunders; 1991.)

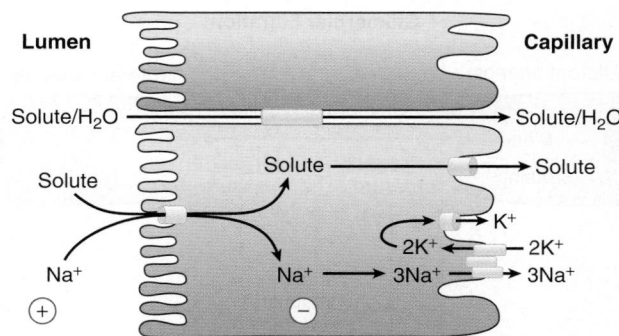

Fig. 72.7. Proximal tubule transport of solute and water. Apical solute reabsorption (glucose, amino acids, phosphate, and organic acids) is sodium coupled and follows an electrochemical gradient generated by basolateral sodium-potassium adenosine triphosphatase (Na/K-ATPase) activity.

basolateral surface area to accommodate the high density of mitochondria and allow for high levels of Na/K-ATPase function. Moving distally, the tubule contains transitional cells that have a smaller basolateral surface area and fewer mitochondria at the basolateral membrane. Transitional cells express both the NCC2 channel and the luminal epithelial sodium channel (ENaC), with the quantities of ENaC increasing and NCC2 decreasing with distal progression along the segment.

The next segment is the connecting tubule, where cells show even fewer mitochondria and smaller basolateral membranes. These cells are distinguished by a more flattened appearance, an expression of ENaC, and a luminal potassium channel (ROMK), but not NCC2. The basolateral membrane is expanded to some degree by infoldings of the basal membrane, but there is no interdigitation from neighboring cells. Because of the presence of magnesium transporters (TRPM6) and calcium transporters (TRPV6), there is also a role for divalent cation regulation.[19,20]

The last segment in the distal nephron is the collecting duct. The primary cells of this segment, the principal cells, have apical vacuoles, some of which store aquaporin-2 channels. They also contain mineralocorticoid receptors and apical sodium channels that function in sodium and potassium balance. The basolateral membrane is infolded but to a lesser degree than other cells in the region. These folds diminish in cells of the medullary collecting duct compared with those in the cortical collecting duct. In the medullary portions of the collecting duct, urea transporters again appear.

Two forms of intercalated cells, "type A" and "non–type A," exist as single cells interspersed throughout the distal nephron. These cells have prominent microfolds in the apical membrane, have high densities of mitochondria, and express several important membrane proteins such as the luminal H+-ATPase and H+/K+-ATPase, as well as cytoplasmic carbonic anhydrase, serving an integral role in acid-base balance. The essential difference between type A and non–type A intercalated cells is that cell polarity is opposite in the two cell types. In "type A" intercalated cells, the apical membrane contains an H+/K+-ATPase, whereas the basolateral membrane contains AE1, a bicarbonate/chloride exchanger that provides a mechanism for proton secretion. The non–type A intercalated cell has vacuolar H+-ATPase on the basolateral and apical surfaces and a chloride bicarbonate exchanger, pendrin, on the apical surface, allowing for both bicarbonate secretion and proton reabsorption.[21] Generally, the number of type A and non–type A intercalated cells can vary to accommodate the acid-base status in the blood.[22]

Tubular Function

Although the function of the glomerulus is filtration, the function of the tubule is to modify the ultrafiltrate to maintain metabolic balance.

Proximal Tubule

Solute and water are transported in the proximal tubule via both paracellular and transcellular routes (Fig. 72.7). Paracellular transport is a high-flux means of moving water and solute between cells along chemical or electrical gradients generated by the basolateral Na/K-ATPase. The mechanism for high flux movement of sodium out of the lumen is explained by a net luminal positive charge generated by the basolateral Na/K-ATPase and net anion reabsorption. The bulk of the sodium therefore follows an electrochemical gradient through paracellular pathways into the blood space. The same principle applies to other cations, such as calcium, which are reabsorbed down electrochemical gradients in the proximal tubule. Neutrally charged solutes move between cells following concentration gradients, the transport becoming less effective more distally as the gradient dissipates. Water movement generally follows sodium movement and is facilitated by the high oncotic pressure of the peritubular capillary network. This favorable osmotic gradient allows for reabsorption of approximately 70% of the filtered water in the adult proximal tubule.

Transcellular movement of solute is a high-resistance method of sodium-coupled transport that results from electrochemical and concentration gradients established by the basolateral Na/K-ATPase (see Fig. 72.7). The Na/K-ATPase pumps three sodium molecules into the basolateral extracellular milieu against a concentration gradient and imports two potassium molecules into the cell against a concentration gradient. The process, which is ATP dependent, establishes a low intracellular sodium concentration and permits luminal sodium entry along a concentration gradient coupled with solutes such as phosphate, glucose, amino acids, and organic acids. In a similar fashion, protons are exported from the luminal membrane by a Na/H+ exchanger that exploits the intracellular movement of sodium to facilitate the export of protons. Bicarbonate is indirectly absorbed through the activity of luminal carbonic anhydrase and the Na/H+ exchanger. The high oncotic pressure of the blood in the arterioles and early vasa recta drives transcellular water reabsorption in the proximal tubular cells via constitutively expressed aquaporin-1 channels that permit water to flow from lumen to vasculature.[23] Some proximal solute reabsorption is modifiable by hormone activity. Parathyroid hormone binding to the proximal tubule receptors activates several second messenger systems that ultimately result in decreased sodium-phosphate transporter activity and phosphate excretion.[24] The proximal tubule is also a site of hormone production, with 1α-hydroxylase activity converting 25-hydroxyvitamin D to the active 1,25-dihydroxy form. This conversion permits vitamin D to act in calcium and phosphate metabolism.[24]

Maturational development of the proximal tubule imparts functional differences in neonatal proximal tubules compared with those in adult kidneys. The relatively low outer cortical nephron blood flow in infancy results in a generalized decrease in proximal tubule resorptive capacity because fewer nephrons participate in active solute and water reabsorption. In the neonate, the proximal tubule also expresses specific neonatal isoforms of the Na/H+ exchanger, has decreased chloride permeability, and expresses different permeability proteins (claudins) in the transcellular space. As a result, neonatal reabsorptive capacity is reduced compared with adults.[25] In addition, hormone receptors are expressed in fewer numbers or may have higher thresholds for activation in the neonate. For example, isoforms of sodium-phosphate transporters of the premature neonate exhibit a relatively low sensitivity to parathyroid hormone but a high transport capacity for phosphate, resulting in lower urinary excretion of phosphate and higher serum phosphate levels than those seen in adults.[26]

Loop of Henle

The loop of Henle plays an important role in establishing the osmotic gradients facilitating water reabsorption in the kidney. In the descending limb of the loop of Henle, the tubular epithelium is impermeable to solute but not water. Therefore as ultrafiltrate passes down the descending loop of Henle, ultrafiltrate becomes increasingly hyperosmolar as water leaves the luminal space. Water permeability decreases, however, in the ascending loop, and solute transporters become more prevalent, allowing the filtrate to become hypoosmolar by the time it reaches the outer cortex.

The thick ascending loop of Henle is responsible for roughly 25% of the total sodium reclamation in the kidney, primarily by the NKCC2 channel, that allows one sodium, one potassium, and two chloride ions to move from the tubular lumen into the cell.[27] Potassium subsequently leaks back into the lumen via the ROMK potassium channel, causing the lumen to become positively charged. This electrochemical gradient permits paracellular reabsorption of cations such as calcium and magnesium as they are propelled out of the tubular lumen.

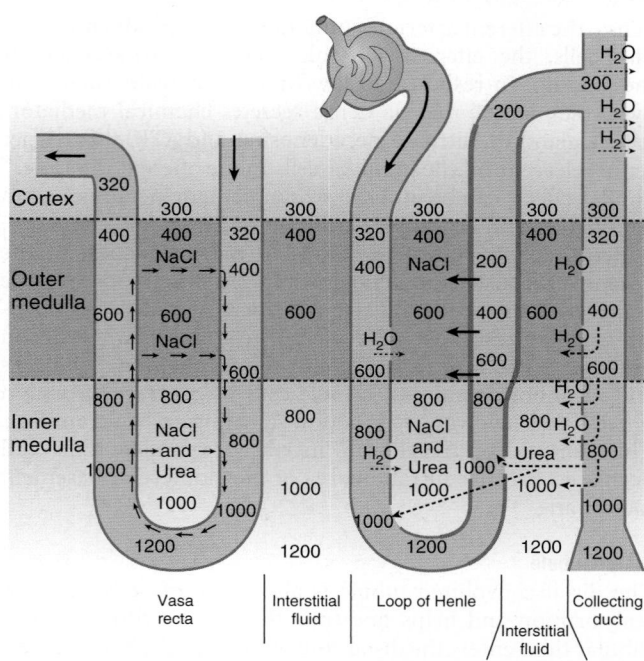

Fig. 72.8. The countercurrent amplification mechanism permitting urinary concentration. (From Guyton A. Renal and associated mechanisms for controlling extracellular fluid osmolality and sodium. In: Wonsiewicz M, ed. Textbook of Medical Physiology. ed 8. Philadelphia: WB Saunders; 1991.)

The reabsorption of sodium in the TALH also helps establish osmotic gradients in the renal interstitium by the countercurrent amplification mechanism (Fig. 72.8). Although sodium, potassium, and chloride are absorbed into the interstitium, back leak of ions occurs into the descending limb of the loop of Henle, thereby increasing the concentration of solute in the descending limb tubular fluid. As this fluid passes into the ascending loop of Henle, the higher sodium content is also reabsorbed into the interstitium, augmenting the osmotic gradient in the medulla. Under normal conditions, ultrafiltrate leaving the ascending loop of Henle is more dilute than that entering the descending loop because of the proficient solute reabsorption in the late ascending limb. Loop diuretics such as bumetanide or furosemide block the NKCC2 channel function and impair the ability both to establish osmotic gradients and to reabsorb solute. The result is the production of large volumes of urine that is isotonic to plasma. In the immature kidney, the loop of Henle is relatively short and impedes the ability to set up steep osmotic gradients. In the setting of stable vasopressin levels, neonatal urinary concentrating ability is relatively weak compared with that of the mature adult kidney.[28]

The thick ascending loop of Henle returns to its glomerulus of origin where the tubular epithelium is attached to the triangle between the efferent and afferent arteriole. The tubular epithelium in contact with the glomerulus contains about 15 to 20 cells in the form of a plaque, called the macula densa (see Fig. 72.6). The macula densa actively reabsorbs sodium, potassium, and chloride through the NKCC2 channel and, in doing so, acts as a sensor of tubular chloride concentration.[29] This sensing mechanism is integral to the functioning of the juxtaglomerular apparatus, which consists of the macula densa, the afferent arteriole containing renin-producing granular cells, the efferent arteriole, and the extraglomerular mesangium. In response to low tubular chloride, such as in hypovolemia, the macula densa secretes chemical mediators (prostaglandins, nitric oxide, adenosine, and ATP) that trigger renin release from the granular cells in the afferent arteriole.[30] Similar effects can be induced by sympathetic nervous system stimulation and arteriolar baroreceptor activation.[31]

Renin activity ultimately leads to the production of the potent vasoconstrictor angiotensin II, vascular smooth muscle contraction in the efferent arteriole, increased efferent arteriolar vascular resistance, and a rise in glomerular perfusion pressure.[31] The macula densa also signals the mesangial cells and neighboring smooth muscle cells to contract through a process that involves gap junction signaling and calcium flux. This contraction results in increased vascular tone and decreased effective filtration area of the glomerular basement membrane.[32,33]

Distal Tubule

The distal convoluted tubule is also a site of active sodium reabsorption and helps fine-tune the urinary filtrate. When tubular fluid enters the distal convoluted tubule, it is relatively dilute because of active solute reabsorption in the TALH. Thus reabsorption of sodium and chloride in this segment occurs against a concentration gradient. Sodium and chloride are actively reabsorbed through the luminal thiazide-sensitive cotransporter (NCCT) following electrochemical gradients generated by the basolateral Na/K-ATPase. However, regulation of the NCCT, and hence sodium flux, is modifiable through a series of modulator kinases (WNK-1 and WNK-4).[34] Approximately 10% of filtered calcium is also reabsorbed from the luminal space in the distal convoluted tubule through parathyroid hormone activation of ATP-dependent TRPV5 calcium channels.[35] Once inside the cell, calcium is sequestered by calbindin-D28k, a protein that facilitates the transport of calcium to the basolateral membrane. Calcium exits the cell through either a basolateral Na-Ca exchanger, NCX1, or the plasma membrane Ca efflux ATPase.[35]

Collecting Duct

The collecting duct also fine-tunes the final composition of the renal ultrafiltrate adjusting sodium, potassium, water content, and acid-base balance. Approximately 5% of the filtered sodium is reabsorbed at this location and occurs through active transport. Sodium enters the cell through apical epithelial sodium channels (ENaCs) and generates a luminal electronegative gradient.[36] Consequently, the excretion of cations such as potassium (principal cell) or protons (a-type intercalated cell) is favored (Fig. 72.9). Because relatively little potassium is in the tubular fluid when it reaches this segment, potassium excretion down a concentration gradient is facilitated. As potassium is excreted, urine flow keeps the concentration in the tubular fluid low, and the favorable gradient is

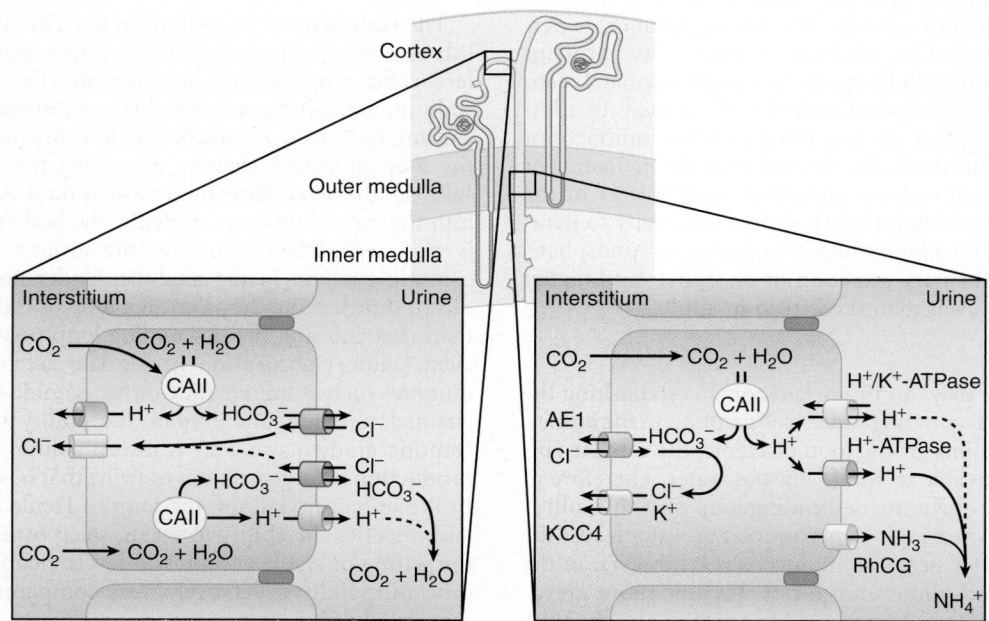

Fig. 72.9. Two types of intercalated cells. Intercalated cells are expressed from the late distal convoluted tubule to the initial third of the inner medullary collecting duct *(shaded red)*. *Left,* Cell model of non–type A intercalated cell. These cells express on the luminal membrane the chloride/bicarbonate exchanger pendrin mediating bicarbonate excretion and chloride absorption. Bicarbonate is produced from CO_2 and H_2O catalyzed by carbonic anhydrase II (CAII). Non–type A intercalated cells express also V-type H^+-adenosine triphosphatases (ATPases), which can be found on the basolateral or luminal membrane and may drive pendrin transport activity. Chloride is released across the basolateral membrane through chloride channels that consist of ClC-kb and Barttin subunits. *Right,* Cell model of type a intercalated cell. Bicarbonate and proton generation is catalyzed by CAII, providing protons for luminal V-type H^+-ATPases and bicarbonate for basolateral chloride/bicarbonate exchangers, including AE1. Type A intercalated cells also express basolateral KCC4 KCl-cotransporters, which may function in maintaining in low intracellular chloride. Type A intercalated cells also express on their luminal membrane H^+/K^+-ATPases that are not further discussed in this review and serve mostly for preservation of potassium during potassium deficiency. Moreover, both type A and non–type A intercalated cells participate in ammonium excretion. (Adapted from Wagner CA, Devuyst O, Bourgeois S, et al. Regulated acid-base transport in the collecting duct. Pflugers Arch. 2009;458:137-156.)

maintained. In states of low urine flow the tubular potassium concentration rises, the gradient is reduced, and potassium excretion decreases.

Potassium excretion and sodium reabsorption are also enhanced by the presence of aldosterone. Binding of aldosterone to its receptor and subsequent translocation to the cell nucleus induces transcription of the luminal sodium channel and basolateral Na/K-ATPase.[37] Increased efficiency and numbers of ENaCs on the luminal membrane tend to increase cell permeability to sodium, and this increase allows the tubular fluid to become more negatively charged after the influx of sodium. This process is facilitated by the increased activity and number of Na/K-ATPase pumps at the basolateral membrane, which creates larger electrical gradients. The net result is an increased capacity to excrete potassium or, in the hypokalemic state, an increased capacity to excrete protons.

The electrical gradient in the collecting duct also favors proton secretion into the tubular lumen, but the chemical gradient does not; the pH in the lumen can be as low as 5, whereas that of the intracellular space is 7.3. Excretion of protons occurs through an apical H-ATPase in the a-type intercalated cells and is also increased by aldosterone action in principal cells, as previously described. Protons secreted into the lumen are bound by ammonia (NH_3) to form NH_4^+ or are bound by other titratable acids such as phosphate or sulfate. This sequestration lowers the concentration of free protons in the ultrafiltrate, prevents diffusion of protons back into the intracellular space, and ultimately promotes acid secretion.

The collecting duct is also responsible for establishing the final concentration of the urine by controlling water reabsorption. At the beginning of the medullary collecting duct, the ultrafiltrate remains relatively dilute and the cells are relatively impermeable to water and solute (see Fig. 72.8). In the setting of hypovolemia or hyperosmolarity, arginine vasopressin binds to V2 vasopressin receptors on the basolateral membrane of the medullary collecting duct cell. V2 receptor signaling results in aquaporin-2 channel migration from intracellular vesicles to the apical surface, and this migration increases tubular permeability to water. Because of the high interstitial osmolality, water is reabsorbed through the aquaporin channels along an osmotic gradient into the blood space causing increased urinary concentration.[38]

Although largely established by active sodium reabsorption in the TALH, the medullary osmotic gradient is also maintained by the presence of urea gradients generated in the collecting tubule (see Fig. 72.8). As tubular fluid moves down the collecting duct, the water entering the interstitium allows the urine to become more concentrated and the urea concentration to rise. The interstitium, however, becomes less hyperosmolar with the influx of water. As the distal tubular permeability to urea increases distally, urea moves from an area of high concentration (the lumen) into an area of lower urea concentration (the interstitium) via the UT-1 urea transporters.[39] The interstitium becomes more hypertonic with the influx of urea, and the concentrating mechanism of the interstitium is partially restored.

Interstitium

Development

The tubular interstitium remains a poorly understood region of the kidney, both from developmental and functional standpoints. From a developmental perspective, the interstitium arises from cells that surround the ureteric bud and condensing mesenchyme and are possibly of mesenchymal origin. As the metanephros develops, the primordial interstitium differentiates to form the larger inner and outer medullary interstitium and the smaller cortical interstitium. In the inner medulla, the interstitium is involved in growth and branching of the collecting duct. In the outer medulla, the interstitium is involved in the elongation of the loops of Henle of the corticomedullary nephrons. Although the mechanisms for both processes remain unclear, the role of the interstitium appears to be in the promotion of growth/branching and attachment, respectively occurring through the secretion of growth factors and matrix proteins.[40]

Structure and Function

The interstitium is a composite of cells, fluid, matrix proteins, and fibrils that form a network supporting the function of tubules. In the cortex, the interstitium contains two dominant components: fibroblasts and dendritic cells. Cortical interstitial fibroblasts provide both structural support of the kidney and a synthetic role in the synthesis of erythropoietin.[41] The dendritic cells appear to originate from bone marrow and function largely in an immune capacity, presenting antigen in major histocompatibility complex (MHC) class II molecules to surveying cells of the immune system.[40,41] In the medulla, the interstitium is the site where the steep osmotic gradients are maintained. Additionally, some evidence supports a role for medullary interstitium in the secretion of vasodepressors. The role of these depressors, on either a local or systemic effect, requires further study.[40]

The interstitium is also a target of disease, with the result often being interstitial fibrosis. The development of interstitial fibrosis in response to injury is modulated by dendritic cell activity and subsequent cytokine release, as well as the synthesis of matrix by fibroblasts, most notably transforming growth factor β. A number of chronic inflammatory processes may induce chronic renal insufficiency through the development of interstitial fibrosis, a phenomenon that remains an area of active study.[41]

Summary

Structural development of the human kidney supports the observation that renal physiologic processes change with maturation. Perfusion, tubular function, and hormonal responses are unique in young patients and affect the renal response in health and disease. Understanding the functions of the pediatric kidney at various stages of development is important for predicting therapeutic responsiveness in the critically ill child and for monitoring recovery from illness.

Key References

1. Costantini F. Renal branching morphogenesis: concepts, questions, and recent advances. *Differentiation*. 2006;74:402-421.
2. Dressler GR. The cellular basis of kidney development. *Annu Rev Cell Dev Biol*. 2006;22:509-529.
3. Michos O. Kidney development: from ureteric bud formation to branching morphogenesis. *Curr Opin Genet Dev*. 2009;19:484-490.
4. Schedl A. Renal abnormalities and their developmental origin. *Nat Rev Genet*. 2007;8:791-802.

5. Robert B, Abrahamson DR. Control of glomerular capillary development by growth factor/receptor kinases. *Pediatr Nephrol.* 2001;16:294-301.

8. Musso CG, Ghezzi L, Ferraris J. Renal physiology in newborns and old people: similar characteristics but different mechanisms. *Int Urol Nephrol.* 2004;36:273-276.

13. Brenner BM, Humes HD. Mechanics of glomerular ultrafiltration. *N Engl J Med.* 1977;297:148-154.

14. Braun N, Grone HJ, Schena FP. Immunological and non-immunological mechanisms of proteinuria. *Minerva Urol Nefrol.* 2009;61:385-396.

18. Sands JM, Layton HE. The physiology of urinary concentration: an update. *Semin Nephrol.* 2009;29:178-195.

21. Wagner CA, Devuyst O, Bourgeois S, et al. Regulated acid-base transport in the collecting duct. *Pflugers Arch.* 2009;458:137-156.

23. Nielsen S, Frokiaer J, Marples D, et al. Aquaporins in the kidney: from molecules to medicine. *Physiol Rev.* 2002;82:205-244.

25. Baum M. Developmental changes in proximal tubule NaCl transport. *Pediatr Nephrol.* 2008;23:185-194.

26. Spitzer A, Barac-Nieto M. Ontogeny of renal phosphate transport and the process of growth. *Pediatr Nephrol.* 2001;16:763-771.

28. Nyul Z, Vajda Z, Vida G, et al. Urinary aquaporin-2 excretion in preterm and full-term neonates. *Biol Neonate.* 2002;82:17-21.

29. Singh P, Thomson SC. Renal homeostasis and tubuloglomerular feedback. *Curr Opin Nephrol Hypertens.* 2009;19:59-64.

30. Rosivall L. Intrarenal renin-angiotensin system. *Mol Cell Endocrinol.* 2009;302:185-192.

31. Welch WJ. The pathophysiology of renin release in renovascular hypertension. *Semin Nephrol.* 2000;20:394-401.

33. Yao J, Zhu Y, Morioka T, et al. Pathophysiological roles of gap junction in glomerular mesangial cells. *J Membr Biol.* 2007;217:123-130.

34. Golbang AP, Cope G, Hamad A, et al. Regulation of the expression of the Na/Cl cotransporter by WNK4 and WNK1: evidence that accelerated dynamin-dependent endocytosis is not involved. *Am J Physiol Renal Physiol.* 2006;291:F1369-F1376.

35. Boros S, Bindels RJ, Hoenderop JG. Active Ca(2+) reabsorption in the connecting tubule. *Pflugers Arch.* 2009;458:99-109.

36. Loffing J, Korbmacher C. Regulated sodium transport in the renal connecting tubule (CNT) via the epithelial sodium channel (ENaC). *Pflugers Arch.* 2009;458:111-135.

37. Butterworth MB, Edinger RS, Frizzell RA, et al. Regulation of the epithelial sodium channel by membrane trafficking. *Am J Physiol Renal Physiol.* 2009;296:F10-F24.

38. Hasler U. Controlled aquaporin-2 expression in the hypertonic environment. *Am J Physiol Cell Physiol.* 2009;296:C641-C653.

39. Wang Y, Klein JD, Blount MA, et al. Epac regulates UT-A1 to increase urea transport in inner medullary collecting ducts. *J Am Soc Nephrol.* 2009;20:2018-2024.

40. Alcorn D, Maric C, McCausland J. Development of the renal interstitium. *Pediatr Nephrol.* 1999;13:347-354.

41. Kaissling B, Le Hir M. The renal cortical interstitium: morphological and functional aspects. *Histochem Cell Biol.* 2008;130:247-262.

Fluid and Electrolyte Issues in Pediatric Critical Illness

Robert Lynch, Ellen Glenn Wood, and Tara M. Neumayr

PEARLS

- Hypotonic maintenance IV fluids are associated with mild to moderate hyponatremia in postoperative patients. Anesthesia, stress, and inflammatory mediators probably contribute. Electrolyte monitoring in patients at risk is essential for detection and management of the occasional patient who develops severe hyponatremia. This critical effect of the syndrome of inappropriate antidiuretic hormone may occur even in patients on isotonic IV fluids.

- Medical patients with high levels of inflammatory mediators appear to be at increased risk of significant hyponatremia. Interleukin effects on antidiuretic hormone release may contribute.

- Albumin infusions have been generally safe but may introduce increased mortality risk in patients with traumatic brain injury. Those given albumin had increased intracranial pressure, which may contribute to the apparent risk.

- After septic patients achieve hemodynamic stabilization, avoiding or correcting excessive fluid volume overload will assist in liberating patients from ventilators and the intensive care unit.

- Proton pump inhibitors may cause hypomagnesemia, particularly in patients on concurrent diuretics. Although usually mild, this may be of significance in critically vulnerable patients.

Overview

Traditional fluid and electrolyte management in critical illness is being refined by science, observations of clinical experience, and expert opinion. Particular attention is drawn to intravenous fluid (IVF) composition, appropriate uses and choices of colloids, extracellular fluid (ECF) volume targets from resuscitation to maintenance, and approaches to removal of excessive ECF volume using diuresis, continuous renal replacement therapy (CRRT), and intermittent hemodialysis (IHD).

Fluid and electrolyte management often begins at resuscitation, but important choices are also made at anesthesia induction and at initial postoperative maintenance. Resuscitative normal saline imposes an acid load, largely related to the chloride content.[1] Although physiologically effective and cost effective in almost all circumstances,[2] concerns regarding chloride toxicity warrant further clarification.[3] Similarly,

intraoperative fluids influence acid-base and electrolyte status, particularly of vulnerable patients.[4] The choice of Na+ content and balancing ions of IVF for postoperative or critical care maintenance may be important for some patients thus justifying additional expense. Clearly 0.18 and 0.225 mM saline is associated with a higher incidence of mild hyponatremia,[5,6] although controlled trials do not show this effect for 0.46 mM saline.[7,8] Severe hyponatremia has been associated with pulmonary or CNS illness in pediatrics and is infrequent even within those categories, with the exception of children with traumatic brain injury (TBI). Among patients with those and other illnesses, the evolving study of the influence of inflammatory mediators directly on the hypothalamus and indirectly on vasopressin secretion may further clarify which patients are at most risk of clinically significant hyponatremia.[9,10]

Evidence for and against the use of colloids in specific groups of critical patients is accumulating. Intriguing but less than definitive studies suggest benefit in severe sepsis[11-14] and possible harm in patients with TBI, perhaps associated with increased intracranial pressure.[15] Consideration of albumin use in selected patients remains appropriate.[16,17] Albumin does appear useful in stabilizing patients with severe hepatic failure and in prevention of hepatorenal syndrome.[18-20]

Evidence for albumin use with or without diuresis among those with acute respiratory distress syndrome (ARDS) suggests improved oxygenation but minimal effect on outcomes.[21] In general, in patients with relatively intact vascular endothelium, 10 to 15 mL/kg of 4% or 5% albumin may be used for intravascular volume expansion with slower leakage into the ECF space compared to crystalloids. Albumin concentrate at 25% may be useful in temporarily redistributing ECF volume from the extravascular to the intravascular space to facilitate organ perfusion and spontaneous or drug-assisted diuresis with minimal additional infused fluid volume. There are currently no formulations of hydroxyethyl starch that can be recommended for use in critically ill patients.[22,23]

Adult and pediatric studies have raised concern regarding damaging effects of fluid volume overload particularly in patients with sepsis or ARDS.[24,25] Patients with less fluid gain early in their illness have more ventilator-free days and shorter ICU stays than those with greater than 10% to 15% early positive fluid balance. It remains unclear if mortality rates are affected.[26-29]

This effect of fluid volume on morbidity and perhaps mortality has led to proposals of a phased approach to fluid management including aggressive resuscitation using appropriate fluids guided by careful clinical measurement and evaluation, prompt reduction of resuscitation fluid rates when hemodynamically tolerated, gradual correction of volume excesses using fluid restriction, colloid dosing to adjust fluid space distribution, continuous infusion diuresis, and CRRT or IHD when needed.[30-33]

As ICU patients progress from stabilization to maintenance, ECF volume overload may spontaneously resolve, or it may warrant active intervention due to the association of persisting major overload with increased morbidity. Loop diuretics do not prevent or ameliorate acute kidney injury[34] but may be useful in mobilizing excess ECF volume.[35] Studies of this measure are variable as to dosages, patient diagnoses, and renal conditions. Carefully titrated continuous infusion of loop diuretics may be superior to bolus dosing.[36-39] In ARDS, continuous infusion plus albumin have enhanced fluid mobilization.[40-42] Careful studies of approaches to fluid removal are needed. Accompanying loss of K+, Ca++, and Mg++ should be anticipated and replaced appropriately. For patients unresponsive to diuresis, either CRRT or IHD can provide electrolyte management and gradual ECF fluid correction[43-45] (see also Chapter 78).

Sodium

Sodium distribution is 90% extracellular and, with its associated anions, largely determines the osmotic condition of the extracellular fluid (ECF). Disturbance of ECF osmolality affects cell volume with critical clinical significance in the central nervous system (CNS). Neurologic symptoms, therefore, dominate the clinical picture in both hyponatremia and hypernatremia. In pediatric patients in the intensive care unit (ICU), young age, underlying neurologic conditions, developmental delay, cerebral hypoperfusion, and medication effects may obscure subtle neurologic findings, and judicious laboratory monitoring along with careful clinical assessment is essential.

Emerging evidence in both adult and pediatric patients suggests an association between disturbances in sodium balance and adverse outcomes, including mortality, ICU length of stay (LOS), use of both noninvasive and invasive mechanical ventilation, and long-term neurologic sequelae.[46-52] It is unclear at this time whether these adverse effects are a direct consequence of the sodium imbalance, are a reflection of a greater severity of illness, or are related to other underlying pathologic processes. Mild disturbances of sodium may serve as a warning of an ongoing process of greater significance. More severe hyponatremia or hypernatremia may be life threatening.[53] These disturbances may result from the disproportionate gain or loss of either sodium or water. Pathologic sodium retention may occur in disorders such as congestive heart failure (CHF), cirrhosis, and nephrotic syndrome without causing a significant change in ECF concentration, but the concomitant expansion of the ECF volume may be damaging.

Hyponatremia

Sudden, severe hyponatremia is life threatening, and its management demands prompt, measured action with ongoing monitoring and therapeutic adjustment. The syndrome of inappropriate antidiuretic hormone secretion (SIADH) and cerebral salt wasting (CSW) are the most common causes of severe hyponatremia, although gross feeding or iatrogenic misadventures also should be considered. Severe hyponatremia, which is variably defined as a serum sodium concentration of either <125 mEq/L or <120 mEq/L, is uncommon and is usually associated with known risk factors such as pulmonary or CNS disease or injury or the use of certain drugs. Mild hyponatremia is common among hospitalized pediatric patients and occurs predictably in postoperative patients. Patients with renal, hepatic, or cardiac disease and those exposed to prolonged general anesthesia are particularly at risk. Accurate identification of patients at risk will inform decisions on frequency of laboratory monitoring and will allow an early evaluation of and response to evolving hyponatremia, whether related to water retention or sodium excretion.

Pathophysiology and Etiology

Hyponatremia may occur in the presence of decreased, increased, or normal amounts of total body sodium.

Decreased Total Body Sodium

Loss of total body sodium results in hyponatremia if total body water is retained in relative excess of the sodium loss. Hypovolemic stimulation of antidiuretic hormone (ADH) release may overwhelm osmotic ADH control, maintaining water retention despite hyponatremia and hypoosmolality. A decrease of as little as 5% in circulating volume may be sufficient to trigger this response.[54] Sodium deficit and volume loss may occur through extrarenal or renal losses. In children, extrarenal losses most often occur from vomiting and diarrhea. In critically ill patients, large extrarenal losses may result from fluid sequestration that occurs with septicemia, peritonitis, pancreatitis, ileus, rhabdomyolysis, ventriculostomy drains, and burns. Renal losses include diuretic use, osmotic diuresis, various salt-losing renal diseases, CSW, and adrenal insufficiency.[55]

Renal Sodium Losses

Renal salt-wasting states are generally identified by a urinary sodium excretion in excess of 20 mEq/L and a fractional excretion (FE_{Na}) of more than 1%. The use of thiazide diuretics can exacerbate hyponatremia and hypovolemia and lead to a characteristic hypokalemic metabolic alkalosis (ie, "contraction alkalosis"). In normally functioning kidneys, concentrated urine is produced by the equilibration of fluid in the collecting tubules with the hyperosmotic medullary interstitium, which in turn is generated by sodium chloride (NaCl) reabsorption without water in the ascending limb of the loop of Henle. Thiazides act in the cortical distal tubule and do not impair the ability of ADH to increase water reabsorption in the collecting tubules and collecting duct,[56] resulting in thiazide-associated hyponatremia. Osmotic sodium and water losses occur in a child with uncontrolled hyperglycemia with glucosuria, with mannitol use, and during urea diuresis following relief of urinary tract obstruction. Hyperglycemia and mannitol, in addition to inducing urinary sodium and water losses, produce osmotic water movement from the intracellular fluid (ICF) to the extracellular fluid (ECF), further lowering serum sodium. Sodium levels drop about 1.5 mEq/L for every 100 mg/dL rise in blood glucose level. Significant salt wasting may occur with several intrinsic renal diseases (Box 73.1). Adrenal insufficiency is distinguished by hyponatremia

BOX 73.1 Causes of Hyponatremia

Decreased Total Body Sodium

Extrarenal

Vomiting/diarrhea
Sequestration: sepsis, peritonitis, pancreatitis, rhabdomyolysis, ileus
Cutaneous: burns, cystic fibrosis
Ventriculostomy drainage

Renal

Cerebral-renal salt wasting (CRSW)
Diuretics
Thiazides, loop diuretics (listed in order of severity of salt wasting)
Osmotic diuretic agents: mannitol, glucose, urea
Tubulointerstitial diseases
Medullary cystic disease, obstructive uropathy, tubulointerstitial nephritis, chronic pyelonephritis, renal tubular acidosis, Kearns-Sayre syndrome
Adrenal insufficiency
Congenital adrenal hyperplasia, Addison disease
Adrenal insufficiency
Congenital adrenal hyperplasia, Addison disease

Increased Total Body Sodium

Congestive heart failure
Cirrhosis
Nephrotic syndrome
Advanced renal failure

Normal Total Body Sodium

Syndrome of inappropriate antidiuretic hormone secretion (SIADH)
Glucocorticoid deficiency
Hypothyroidism
Infantile water intoxication
Abusive water intoxication

TABLE 73.1 Cerebral-Renal Salt-Wasting Syndrome

Cerebral Salt	Wasting Syndrome
Trigger	Acute intracranial injury or illness (subarachnoid hemorrhage, trauma, etc.)
Onset	Typically a few days after the injury occurs
Signs	Falling serum Na$^+$, high urine output, high urine Na$^+$
Course	Without treatment, proceeds to intravascular volume depletion, hypotension, and hypoperfusion
Treatment	Replace salt and water losses; may require 3% NaCl +/− loop diuretics; fludrocortisone in refractory cases
Resolution	Days to weeks
Differential diagnosis	Syndrome of inappropriate antidiuretic hormone (SIADH), adrenal insufficiency, osmotic diuresis

TABLE 73.2 Cerebral Salt Wasting (CSW) Versus Syndrome of Inappropriate Antidiuretic Hormone (SIADH)

	CSW	SIADH
Urine Na$^+$	Very high, often >100 mEq/L	Variable, but usually >30 mEq/L
Urine output	Inappropriately high, leading to volume depletion	Variable; may be normal or decreased
Response to saline challenge	Improvement in volume deficit and serum Na$^+$	No improvement
Response to fluid and salt restriction	No improvement; volume deficit and hyponatremia may worsen	Improvement in serum Na$^+$

in association with hyperkalemia and decreased urinary potassium excretion.

Cerebral Salt Wasting

Cerebral salt wasting (CSW) is a clinical entity that continues to generate controversy. First described by Peters and coworkers in 1950, it was superseded by the description of SIADH by Schwartz and coworkers in 1957 and then rediscovered in 1981 when Nelson and associates studied hyponatremia in a series of neurosurgical patients with isotopically measured low blood volumes.[57] Despite lingering skepticism, its distinct clinical identity continues to be supported (Table 73.1).[58-61] Patients typically have an acute neurologic injury with hemorrhage, trauma, infection, or a mass and may have undergone neurosurgical procedures. CSW differs from SIADH in that large urine volumes contain very high sodium concentrations, leading to rapid depletion of both sodium and ECF volume (Table 73.2). An otherwise unexplained intravascular volume contraction is central to the diagnosis and may cause a secondary boost in ADH release. Left untreated, CSW results in intravascular volume depletion, hypotension, and hypoperfusion or hypovolemic shock as well as hyponatremia. Untreated SIADH, in contrast, leads to progressive hyponatremia and the clinical consequences thereof with maintenance or mild expansion of fluid balance. The pathophysiologic link between intracranial injury and renal salt wasting has yet to be elucidated, contributing in no small part to the controversy. Both brain natriuretic peptide (BNP) and atrial natriuretic peptide (ANP) are attractive as potential mediators, but neither has a proved etiologic role.[62,63] Decreased sympathetic input to the

kidneys is another postulated mechanism.[61] Distinguishing CSW from SIADH may be difficult in many complex clinical scenarios. In cases of severe or symptomatic hyponatremia, however, this may be temporarily unnecessary because the initial therapy is the same.[57] Administration of enough concentrated sodium to result in a small increase in osmolality is appropriate, and support of intravascular volume is required. A reasonable approach might begin with the administration of 5 mL/kg of hypertonic (3%) NaCl followed by isotonic repletion of the remaining volume deficit. Once this is achieved, sufficient sodium and fluid administration to account for daily maintenance requirements as well as ongoing losses is necessary. Administration of fludrocortisone, a mineralocorticoid, has been reported to aid in CSW management in severe or prolonged cases that are refractory to initial therapy.[61] In less severe cases, infusion of isotonic saline represents a reasonable first step in management, and the observed response may help to differentiate between CSW and SIADH. In CSW, saline administration addresses volume depletion and hyponatremia. It is of limited or no benefit in patients with SIADH, who are more effectively managed with fluid restriction.[59] Throughout, the absolutely essential part of therapy is the frequent reassessment of sodium levels and volume status with treatment adjustments as indicated.

Increased Total Body Sodium

Hyponatremia with increased total body sodium occurs when the increase in total body water exceeds the sodium retention. Four clinical situations are commonly seen: congestive heart failure, cirrhosis, nephrotic syndrome, and advanced renal failure. In all four conditions, hyponatremia tends to be mild or moderate, asymptomatic, and nonprogressive or slowly progressive. These patients typically present to the ICU primarily for care related to these underlying conditions rather than for symptoms related to hyponatremia.

Congestive Heart Failure

Hyponatremia in heart failure is associated with a worse prognosis.[64,65] Low cardiac output states are characterized by a decrease in effective circulating volume that is detected by vasoreceptors in the carotid sinus, the aortic arch, and the renal juxtaglomerular apparatus. Activation of various neurohormonal modulators promotes vasoconstriction along with sodium and water retention. Increased sympathetic activity and stimulation of the renin-angiotensin-aldosterone system (RAAS) produce increased afferent and efferent arteriolar vascular resistance and decreased glomerular filtration rate (GFR) with a resultant decrease in urinary sodium excretion. Nonosmotic ADH release is stimulated, further impairing water excretion. In addition, decreased aldosterone degradation, along with altered levels of other vasoactive and nonvasoactive substances, leads to a primary increase in tubular sodium reabsorption. A deleterious positive feedback loop is created, in which the vasoconstrictive and fluid retentive effects of these neurohormonal systems promote further vasoconstriction and worsening renal perfusion.[66] The complex interactions between renal and cardiovascular pathophysiology have been described as the "cardiorenal syndromes" with five subtypes based on the primary organ affected and the acuity of the physiologic derangement.[67]

Cirrhosis

Early in cirrhosis, increased intrahepatic pressure may initiate renal sodium retention before ascites formation. The development of portal hypertension leads to nitric oxide–mediated peripheral vasodilation and to the formation of arteriovenous fistulae. The result is a decrease in effective circulating volume. These decompensated patients have higher levels of renin, aldosterone, ADH, and norepinephrine than do compensated patients with cirrhosis. Hyponatremia arises in the setting of persistent renal sodium and water retention.[68]

Nephrotic Syndrome

Hyponatremia is an occasional finding in patients with nephrotic syndrome. It may be present, however, in patients with apparently normal or decreased central volume. The humoral factors involved in patients with decreased central volume appear to be similar to those with decompensated cirrhosis.

Renal Failure

As a diseased kidney loses nephrons, the remaining nephrons exhibit a dramatically elevated fractional sodium excretion in efforts to maintain sodium balance. Edema develops when larger quantities of sodium are ingested than can be excreted. The ability to excrete water is also impaired, primarily because of the progressive decrease in GFR. Hyponatremia occurs when water intake exceeds insensible losses plus the maximum volume that can be excreted.

Normal Total Body Sodium

Hyponatremia without evidence of hypovolemia or edema in the pediatric population is usually associated with SIADH. Renal concentrating and diluting ability ultimately depends on the presence or absence of ADH to modulate water permeability in the collecting duct. Osmoreceptors for ADH reside in the anterior hypothalamus, responding to changes of as little as 1% in plasma osmolality. The nonosmotic stimuli that induce release of ADH are associated with changes in autonomic neural tone due to physical pain or trauma, emotional stress, hypoxia, cardiac failure, nausea and vomiting, adrenal insufficiency, volume depletion, and exposure to general anesthesia (Box 73.2). Nonosmotic stimuli, as the name implies, are active even in the face of normal plasma osmolality, and a decrease in plasma volume of as little as 5% is sufficient to trigger a strong ADH response.[54] Vasopressin (ADH) synthesized in the hypothalamus is transported in neurosecretory granules to the axonal bulbs in the median eminence and posterior pituitary gland and is released by exocytosis in the presence of appropriate stimuli. Increasing evidence indicates that inflammatory mediators facilitate release and contribute to the high incidence of hyponatremia in Rocky Mountain spotted fever, Kawasaki, and other inflammatory illnesses.[10] After release, ADH binds to V2 receptors in the basolateral membrane of the renal collecting duct, increasing cyclic adenosine 3′,5′-monophosphate formation and facilitating phosphorylation of aquaporin-2. Incorporation of aquaporin-2-containing vesicles in the apical (luminal) membrane increases cell permeability to water and provides a pathway for water reabsorption.[69]

Clinically, SIADH is characterized by (1) hyponatremia, (2) euvolemia or mild hypervolemia, (3) hypoosmolality, (4) inappropriately elevated urine osmolality, and (5) elevated urine sodium concentration. It has been associated with several categories of clinical disease, including CNS and pulmonary disorders, malignancies, and as an adverse effect of numerous drugs (Box 73.2).[70] Underlying renal function is normal. Under normal physiologic conditions, a decrease in serum sodium of 4 to 5 mEq/L below normal (with a serum osmolality of less than 270 mOsm) should maximally inhibit ADH secretion with a resultant urine osmolality of less than 100 mOsm. It is frequently difficult to determine, however, whether urine osmolality and urine sodium are inappropriately elevated, particularly in critically ill patients receiving IV fluids. Variable sodium and water administration rates, isotonic or hypertonic fluid boluses, fluctuations in hemodynamic status and urine output, and a history of diuretic use can all confound laboratory interpretation. The key consideration is the relative relationship between the degree of hyponatremia and hypoosmolality and the robustness of the dilutional response in the urine. Failure to maximally dilute urine in the face of hypoosmolality represents inappropriate ADH response so that a urine osmolality of 200 to 250 mOsm may reflect SIADH in hyponatremic patients. The urinary sodium level is generally more than 30 mEq/L but may be

BOX 73.2 **Nonosmotic Stimuli Associated With Syndrome of Inappropriate Antidiuretic Hormone**

CNS Disorders
Infection
Meningitis
Encephalitis, including HIV/AIDS encephalitis
Brain abscess
Rocky Mountain spotted fever
Mass lesions
Subarachnoid or subdural hemorrhage
Cerebral thrombosis or hemorrhage
Brain tumors
Head trauma with cerebral edema
Hydrocephalus
Cavernous sinus thrombosis
Other
Guillain-Barré syndrome
Multiple sclerosis
Hypoxic encephalopathy, including neonatal hypoxic-ischemic
     encephalopathy (HIE)
Pituitary disease
Acute psychosis

Pulmonary Disease
Infection
Bacterial and viral pneumonias
Pulmonary abscess
Tuberculosis
Aspergillosis
Asthma
Respiratory failure with positive pressure ventilation

Tumors
Carcinomas of the lung, oropharynx, gastrointestinal tract
     (including the pancreas), and genitourinary tract
Lymphoma, thymoma
Ewing sarcoma, mesothelioma

Drugs
Antidiuretic hormone analogs (vasopressin, desmopressin/1-
     deamino-8-D-arginine vasopressin [DDAVP], oxytocin)
Vincristine
Salicylates
Chlorpropamide
Cyclophosphamide
Carbamazepine
Barbiturates
Colchicine
Haloperidol
Fluphenazine
Tricyclic antidepressants and selective serotonin reuptake inhibitors
     (SSRIs)
Clofibrate
Indomethacin and nonsteroidal antiinflammatory drugs (NSAIDs)
Interferon
Ecstasy (3,4-methylenedioxy-methamphetamine [MDMA])

Miscellaneous
High levels of inflammatory mediators general anesthesia
Nausea/vomiting
Pain or emotional stress
General anesthesia
Marathon running or endurance exercise
Hereditary (gain-of-function mutations in the vasopressin V2
     receptor)

much less in patients who are provided a low sodium intake.[71] When the urinary sodium concentration is very high, it is the net balance between intake and output that differentiates between SIADH and a renal salt-wasting syndrome. Renal salt wasting is favored when the urinary sodium excretion grossly exceeds sodium intake.

Signs and Symptoms

The severity of signs and symptoms depends on the rapidity of the development of hyponatremia. Neurologic symptoms predominate as plasma hypoosmolality causes a shift in fluid from the ECF to the ICF compartment, leading to generalized cellular swelling. The rigidity of the intracranial space leaves little room for cellular expansion, resulting in increasing intracranial pressure. Brain cells prevent massive swelling in the early phases of hyponatremia by extrusion of electrolytes and other cellular osmolytes. Acute decreases in sodium concentration are associated with lethargy, apathy, and disorientation, often accompanied by nausea, vomiting, and muscle cramps. No predictable correlation exists between the degree of hyponatremia and its resultant symptoms, as severe hyponatremia that develops gradually may present with minimal symptoms. Acute decreases in sodium to less than 120 mEq/L, however, generally produce severe symptoms such as seizures or coma. Other findings may include decreased deep tendon reflexes, pathologic reflexes, pseudobulbar palsy, and a Cheyne-Stokes respiratory pattern. Cerebral edema and intracranial hypertension may be severe enough to result in herniation, permanent neurologic injury, and death.[72]

Treatment

Prevention

Stimuli for ADH release are frequently present in both surgical and nonsurgical ICU patients, putting them at risk for hyponatremia. Use of hypotonic intravenous (IV) maintenance fluids increases the risk for development of hyponatremia. The appropriate administration of isotonic IV fluids in these patients will decrease the incidence of hyponatremia.[73-78] For patients with severe SIADH or CSW, however, the use of isotonic fluids alone may not be adequate to prevent life-threatening disturbances in sodium and water balance. Thoughtful monitoring of sodium levels along with avoidance of large volumes of hypotonic fluids is mandatory.

Therapy

The time course over which hyponatremia develops is a key determinant of the therapeutic approach. Severe hyponatremia is associated with significant morbidity and mortality and requires urgent attention. As described previously, acute hyponatremia produces significant cerebral edema when initial compensation mechanisms are overwhelmed and more chronic adaptive mechanisms are not yet fully developed. Hyponatremia that has been present less than 4 hours can safely be corrected promptly. When the evolution of hyponatremia is gradual, however, brain cells respond adaptively to prevent cerebral edema.

Thus there are two essential questions in constructing a therapeutic plan: (1) Did hyponatremia evolve rapidly or slowly, and (2) does the patient have CNS symptoms or imaging suggestive of cerebral edema? CNS cellular swelling and its symptoms are more likely with acute hyponatremia or with severe chronic hyponatremia.[79,80] Symptomatic hyponatremia that develops suddenly—that is, in fewer than 4 hours—can be rapidly reversed without incurring risk. If asymptomatic hyponatremia has developed over many hours, days, or weeks (ie, chronic hyponatremia), a gradual, conservative approach is likely to be uncomplicated. Symptomatic chronic hyponatremia, on the other hand, requires a small but rapid increase in serum sodium to stabilize or begin to reverse cerebral swelling and to avoid impending herniation, followed by a more gradual correction to normalize sodium balance. An increase of 5 mEq/L is usually sufficient to halt the progress of symptomatic cerebral edema and can be achieved with an initial bolus of 5 to 6 mL/kg of 3% saline. The subsequent correction rate for patients with either acute symptomatic hyponatremia or any chronic hyponatremia should not exceed 0.5 mEq/L/h. In acute hyponatremia without CNS symptoms, rates of 0.7 to 1 mEq/L/h have been reported without patient morbidity or mortality. A regimen of hypertonic 3% saline infused at 1 to 2 mL/kg/h with intermittent administration of a loop diuretic results in an appropriate correction for those patients for whom "rapid" correction is safe. Further correction may require isotonic fluids or a mixture of isotonic and hypertonic fluids, particularly in patients with CSW. In resistant, severe CSW, mineralocorticoid (fludrocortisone) treatment has been helpful in several reports.[61,81,82] Other protocol approaches are available.[83]

Prolonged hyponatremia in animal studies is notable for a striking decrease in total brain amino acid content as well as lower brain water content.[84] When this brain cell adaptation has occurred, a rapid rise in serum sodium concentration may induce a shift of water from the ICF to the ECF compartment, resulting in brain dehydration, brain injury, and the osmotic demyelination syndrome (ODS).[85] Both central pontine and extrapontine myelinolysis have been reported in children.[86-89] Extrapontine sites include the cerebellum, thalamus, basal nuclei, hippocampus, midbrain, and subcortical white matter.[41] Traditional risk factors for ODS include chronic alcoholism, malnutrition, and rapid correction of hyponatremia.[90] Osmotic demyelination can occur, however, without hyponatremia as a starting point.[88,89,91] Large bolus doses of hypertonic saline may place the patient at risk regardless of starting sodium concentration. Electrolyte fluctuations around the time of liver transplantation may account for the risk of myelinolysis noted in these patients.[92] Rarely, ODS has been reported in patients with diabetic ketoacidosis but without hyponatremia on admission, including one case in an 18-month-old child.[87,89] Even rapid correction of hypernatremia is a possible cause of myelinolysis and suggests that pressure effects may be capable of causing damage to myelinated structures. Symptoms of osmotic demyelination may include obtundation, quadriplegia, pseudobulbar palsy, tremor, amnesia, seizures, and coma.[93,94] Classically, the clinical presentation is that of a brief period of recovery from encephalopathy followed by emergence of a "locked in" state or various movement disorders.[90] When CNS symptoms concerning for ODS emerge during therapy, long-term neurologic sequelae may be avoided by decreasing serum sodium to its nadir followed by a slower rate of correction.[95-97]

In cases of SIADH where fluid restriction is a feasible option, a decrease in fluid intake, occasionally with the use of oral sodium supplements, may be all that is required to normalize serum sodium gradually and safely. In a patient with hypovolemia, volume status clearly must be corrected in addition to the hyponatremia. Patients with SIADH or fluid-retaining states may respond to treatment with an ADH receptor antagonist. This receptor blocker group increases urine volume and reduces urine osmolality, creating a water diuresis that leads to an increase in serum sodium concentration.[98,99] Evidence for improvement in other clinical outcomes such as

mortality or ICU length of stay, however, is currently lacking. Conivaptan is an intravenous ADH V1 and V2 receptor antagonist that is approved for the treatment of euvolemic and hypervolemic hyponatremia in adults.[100] Tolvaptan, an oral ADH V2 receptor antagonist, was approved in 2009 as therapy for euvolemic or hypervolemic hyponatremia in adult patients with heart failure, cirrhosis, or SIADH.[99] Pediatric usage of the ADH receptor blockers has been reported in the settings of SIADH and cardiac disease,[99-103] but further study of kinetics, safety, and efficacy will be needed to clarify the clinical role in pediatrics.

Hypernatremia

As with hyponatremia, hypernatremia can develop with low, normal, or high levels of total body sodium. History and weights are particularly important in evaluating the hydration state of patients with hypernatremia because a shift in the ICF to the ECF tends to obscure the physical findings of dehydration. Accurate assessment of total body sodium and water aids considerably in planning management, although the most important management principle is the frequent monitoring of the patient's progress with treatment adjustments as needed.

Pathophysiology and Etiology

Low Total Body Sodium

Patients with a low total body sodium level have a loss of water in relative excess of sodium losses. Because the ECF space is hyperosmolar, water movement from the ICF occurs with resulting cellular dehydration. The ECF space, therefore, is somewhat preserved until an extreme degree of hypovolemia is present. Losses of sodium and water may be extrarenal or renal (see Box 73.3).

In the pediatric patient, extrarenal losses are commonly seen from vomiting and diarrhea, although hospital-acquired hypernatremia from insufficient free water administration is

---

BOX 73.3   Causes of Hypernatremia

Decreased Total Body Sodium
Extrarenal
Vomiting/diarrhea, excessive sweating
Administration of 70% sorbitol

Renal
Osmotic diuresis: mannitol, glucose, urea

Inadequate Intake
Insufficient lactation

Normal Total Body Sodium
Extrarenal
Respiratory insensible water losses
Cutaneous insensible water losses
Fever, burns, phototherapy
Radiant warmers, especially with premature infants

Renal
Diabetes insipidus (DI)
Central DI
Nephrogenic DI
Hypodipsia (reset osmostat)

Increased Total Body Sodium
Administration or ingestion of large sodium loads
Improperly diluted formula

a major concern.[104,105] Renal causes include osmotic diuresis from mannitol, hyperglycemia, or increased urea excretion. Infants are particularly susceptible to hypernatremic dehydration due to their high surface area/weight ratio and their relative renal immaturity, which necessitates greater water losses for excretion of a solute load compared with older children and adults.[106] Insufficient maternal lactation places young infants at risk of hypernatremic dehydration.

Normal Total Body Sodium

Loss of water occurs without excessive sodium losses in some conditions. Extrarenal losses include (1) increased respiratory losses as may occur with tachypnea, hyperventilation, or mechanical ventilation with inadequate humidification and (2) transcutaneous losses associated with fever, burns, extreme prematurity, or use of phototherapy or radiant warmers in the neonate without adequate water replacement. Renal losses result from congenital or acquired diabetes insipidus (DI), either central or nephrogenic. Acquired forms of DI are more commonly seen in the ICU. Major insults resulting in central DI include head trauma, tumors, infections, hypoxic brain injury, neurosurgical procedures, and nontraumatic brain death. Classically, in experimental animals and in humans, three stages occur: (1) an initial polyuric phase (hours to several days), (2) a period of antidiuresis probably due to ADH release from injured axons (hours to days), and (3) a second period of polyuria that may or may not resolve.[107,108] Sudden onset of polyuria is characteristic, and the conscious patient will often experience a concomitant polydipsia. In the critically ill patient, the inability to access increased water intake—whether from altered mental status, impaired thirst regulation, or other causes—may result in life-threatening hypernatremia.[109] Patients with the rare congenital forms of nephrogenic DI, resulting from X-linked alteration of the ADH V2 receptor or from autosomal recessive changes in the aquaporin II water channel itself, may have repeated bouts of hypernatremic dehydration.[110] Causes of DI are shown in Box 73.4.

Increased Total Body Sodium

Hypernatremia with an increased total body sodium level is most often an iatrogenic problem. In the ICU, hypertonic solutions of sodium bicarbonate are administered during resuscitation efforts or as therapy for intractable metabolic acidosis, excessive hypertonic saline administration, ingestion by infants of improperly diluted formula, and dialysis against a high sodium concentration. Normonatremic patients with massive edema who undergo a forced diuresis frequently become mildly hypernatremic because the induced urine may be hypotonic, with water loss exceeding sodium loss.

Hypernatremia is intentionally induced in patients with traumatic brain injury as a form of osmotherapy for control of intracranial hypertension associated with cerebral edema.[111,112] Such patients have tolerated serum sodium as high as 175 mEq/L when carefully managed. When the ECF osmolality of these patients is manipulated, the risks involved with rapid changes in either direction must be kept in mind (see also Chapter 119).

Signs and Symptoms

Clinical manifestations of hypernatremia, as is the case with hyponatremia, relate predominantly to the CNS. Marked irritability, a high-pitched cry, altered sensorium varying from

---

BOX 73.4   Causes of Diabetes Insipidus

Central
Congenital
Arginine vasopressin (AVP) antidiuretic hormone (ADH) gene mutations, autosomal dominant or (rarely) autosomal recessive inheritance
Idiopathic (30% to 50% of cases)

Acquired
Head trauma, orbital trauma
Tumors, suprasellar and intrasellar
Encephalitis
Meningitis
Guillain-Barré syndrome
Hypoxic injury, including neonatal hypoxic-ischemic encephalopathy (HIE)
Postneurosurgical procedures
Cerebral aneurysms, thrombosis, hemorrhage
Histiocytosis
Granulomas
Nontraumatic brain death

Nephrogenic
Congenital
VR_2 mutation, X-linked
AQP-2 mutation

Acquired
Chronic renal failure
Renal tubulointerstitial diseases
Hypercalcemia
K^+ depletion
Drugs
Alcohol, lithium, diuretics, amphotericin B, methoxyflurane, demeclocycline
Sickle cell disease
Dietary abnormalities
Primary polydipsia
Decreased sodium chloride intake
Severe protein restriction or depletion

---

lethargy to coma, increased muscle tone, and overt seizure activity may occur in children with the development of severe hypernatremia over 48 hours or more. Hyperglycemia and hypocalcemia also may occur. In infants with acute hypernatremia, vomiting, fever, respiratory distress, spasticity, tonic-clonic seizures, and coma are common. Death from respiratory failure occurred in experimental animals when serum osmolality approached 430 mOsm/kg.[113] Mortality in children with severe hypernatremia has ranged from 10% to 45% with chronic and acute hypernatremia, respectively.

Anatomic changes seen with the hyperosmolar state include loss of volume of brain cells with resultant tearing of cerebral vessels, capillary and venous congestion, subcortical or subarachnoid bleeding, and venous sinus thrombosis. During the first 4 hours of experimental acute hypernatremia, brain water significantly decreases, while the concentration of solutes (electrolytes and glucose) increases.[114] This leads to a partial restitution of brain volume within a few hours' time. Over several days, brain volume normalizes as a result of intracellular accumulation of organic osmolytes consisting of polyols, amino acids, and methylamines.[108,115]

Treatment

Whenever possible, therapy of hypernatremia should address correction of the underlying disease process as a primary goal.

Correction of dehydration with slow hypernatremia correction is the target. When sodium exceeds 165 mEq/L, isotonic fluid or colloid may be used for correction of shock or circulatory collapse and initial reversal of hypernatremia. When hypernatremia has been present for more than a few hours, the presence of intracellular organic osmolytes dictates a slow rate of correction. Numerous fatal cases of cerebral edema and herniation have occurred with correction over a 24-hour period, leading to recommendations for correction over no less than 48 hours.[116,117] There is general agreement that plasma osmolality should not be decreased more rapidly than 2 mOsm/h, correlating with a rate of sodium decline that does not exceed 1 mEq/h. In cases of very severe or long-standing hypernatremia, a more conservative correction rate of 1 mOsm/h (0.5 mEq/hr of sodium) may be appropriate. Thus, normalization from extreme hypernatremia may take several days. This slower rate of correction appears to allow time for dissipation of the organic osmolytes without development of cerebral edema. Estimated deficits, ongoing maintenance requirements, and additional excessive losses must be accounted for in calculations of the amount of fluid replacement required.

Central DI is a likely cause of hypernatremia in an ICU patient with high urine volume and low urine osmolality, particularly in patients who have head trauma or who have undergone a recent intracranial operation. In these patients, a trial of vasopressin is in order. Either aqueous vasopressin given subcutaneously or intravenously (0.5 to 10 milliunits/kg/h) or 1-deamino-8-D-arginine vasopressin (DDAVP) given orally or intranasally may be used. Oral dosing is limited to tablet form at this time with a recommended dosing range of 0.05 to 0.4 mg administered twice daily. Intranasal DDAVP is generally begun in a dosage ranging from 0.05 to 0.1 mL once or twice daily. An increase in urine osmolality to values exceeding that in serum after vasopressin administration supports the diagnosis of central DI. Hyponatremia has been reported after vasopressin administration in patients with central DI as well as in patients receiving vasopressin for hemodynamic support and for bleeding disorders in the perioperative period.[118,119] In the outpatient setting, symptomatic hyponatremia, including seizures and altered mental status, has been reported in patients receiving DDAVP for enuresis, particularly in periods of intercurrent illness or with excess fluid intake.[120] Careful attention to the IV fluid prescription, serial monitoring of sodium levels, and timely adjustment in therapy are necessary to avoid severe complications in patients receiving any type of vasopressin therapy.

In patients with an increased total body sodium level and, often, hypervolemia, the goal is sodium removal. In patients with intact renal function, sodium removal may be accomplished with diuretics and a decrease in sodium administration. If renal failure is present, dialysis may be required.

Potassium

The total body K+ of about 50 mEq/kg is divided with about 98% being intracellular. The transmembrane concentration gradient is large with the intracellular concentration of 150 mEq/L being maintained by sodium-potassium adenosine triphosphatase (Na+/K+-ATPase) pumps. The resultant transmembrane potential is normally tightly regulated but physiologically dynamic in contractile or conductive cells.

Changes in extracellular or intracellular K+ concentration may alter the critical transmembrane potential of cardiac, skeletal, or smooth muscle cells with serious results.

Hypokalemia is relatively common in pediatric intensive care unit (PICU) patients but generally is detectable and manageable.[121] Severe hyperkalemia is much less frequent but much more likely to be life threatening with minimal warning.

Factors involved in total body distribution include acid-base status, insulin, catecholamines, magnesium, and aldosterone.[122-125] Acidemia tends to increase the serum potassium, and alkalemia lowers it. The type of acid-base disturbance (metabolic or respiratory), the duration of the disturbance, and the nature of the anion accompanying the hydrogen ion in metabolic acidosis are important in determining what effect a particular acid-base disorder may have on potassium concentration.

Diabetic ketoacidosis (DKA) may occasionally present with severe hypokalemia[126] due to losses. Hyperosmolality and decreased circulating insulin will preserve or even elevate serum K+ in most cases.[127,128] Epinephrine, albuterol,[129] and other beta-agonists decrease serum potassium, moving it into cells. β-adrenergic blocking drugs abolish this effect. Change in intracellular magnesium (Mg++) may affect the sodium-potassium adenosine triphosphatase (ATPase) pump and alter the transcellular distribution. All of these mechanisms, however, are generally representative of fine-tuning in potassium homeostasis. Ultimately, potassium balance is regulated through excretion by the kidney and to a lesser extent the gastrointestinal (GI) tract. Massive cell lysis may overwhelm these and require aggressive management of the sudden shift of intracellular K into the ECF, particularly in the presence of compromised renal function.

Most of the filtered potassium is absorbed before the distal nephron in normal kidneys. The potassium excreted in the urine then is mainly due to secretion in the distal convoluted tubule and cortical collecting duct. As with sodium, the kidney's capacity to vary potassium excretion is profound, ranging from a low of approximately 5 mEq/L to amounts exceeding 100 mEq/L of urine. Factors influencing renal potassium excretion include mineralocorticoid and glucocorticoid hormones, acid-base balance, anion effects, tubular fluid flow rate, sodium intake, potassium intake, ICF and plasma potassium concentrations, and diuretics.[130] Aldosterone is a major kaliuretic hormone. Metabolic acidosis decreases and metabolic alkalosis increases intracellular potassium activity in cells of the distal tubule, causing enhanced potassium secretion during alkalosis and reabsorption during acidosis. Fluid delivery to the distal tubule probably enhances potassium secretion by two mechanisms: (1) the faster fluid moves past the secretory site, and a greater amount of potassium can be secreted, and (2) because tubular fluid potassium concentration decreases as flow rate increases, a favorable gradient for potassium movement is maintained at high flow rates.

Hypokalemia

Causes of Hypokalemia
Hypokalemia Without Potassium Deficit
The detection of a low serum potassium level may reflect a true deficit in total body stores or an apparent deficit from the shift of this ion from the ECF to the ICF pool. A shift to the

ICF pool may occur in alkalemia,[131] administered or endogenous release of beta-agonist,[129,132] familial or thyrotoxic periodic paralysis,[133,134] barium poisoning,[135] and excess insulin. In the case of alkalemia, potassium moves into the cell in exchange for H+ in an attempt to maintain extracellular pH. The pediatric patient with alkalemia may have a true potassium deficit in addition due to decreased potassium intake or increased losses.

Periodic paralysis is a rare autosomal dominant disorder presenting with intermittent episodes of profound muscle weakness associated with a sudden fall in serum potassium concentration precipitated high-carbohydrate/low-potassium diet, exercise, infection, stress, or alcohol ingestion. Barium poisoning can produce hypokalemic weakness and paralysis, probably by competitive blockade of inward rectifying K+ channels. Insulin shifts potassium into muscle and liver cells in association with glycogen formation.

Hypokalemia With Potassium Deficit

A deficit in total body potassium may occur from decreased intake, from renal losses, or from GI losses. GI loss occurs with pyloric stenosis or other persistent vomiting, diarrhea, or binding of enteric K+ by ingested clay in patients with pica.[136]

Renal Losses

Major categories seen in the ICU include loop, thiazide, and osmotic diuretics, renal tubular acidosis, hyperaldosteronism, magnesium deficiency, and recovery from acute renal failure (ARF). Osmotic diuresis from glucosuria can cause severe renal potassium wasting in prolonged DKA predisposing to ventricular arrhythmia. The severity of K+ loss may be masked by the shift of potassium from the ICF to the ECF space related to insulin deficiency, metabolic acidosis, and hypertonicity.

Primary aldosteronism, congenital adrenal hyperplasia, adrenal adenoma, and familial idiopathic hyperaldosteronism[137,138] are rare in children and even rarer in the pediatric ICU setting. Secondary hyperaldosteronism is common, however, either from volume depletion or from CHF, cirrhosis, or nephrotic syndrome. Patients with the latter conditions, however, rarely have severe hypokalemia unless they are additionally treated with diuretics. Infants with Bartter or Gitelman syndrome[139] may initially come to the ICU because of multiple metabolic derangements including hypokalemia, metabolic alkalosis, hypomagnesemia, and hyperuricemia. Other findings include weakness, polyuria, and failure to thrive, with elevated renin and aldosterone levels in the absence of hypertension. Additional conditions associated with elevated renin secretion, secondary hyperaldosteronism, and hypokalemia include renal artery stenosis, malignant hypertension, renin-producing tumor, or Wilms tumor. Additional mechanisms include secondary hyperaldosteronism and increased distal tubular fluid delivery.

Other agents that induce excessive renal losses include amphotericin B (kaliuresis with reduced renal function and tubular injury); aminoglycosides, particularly gentamicin; and high-dose penicillin and carbenicillin, which produce an osmotic load in addition to acting as non-reabsorbable anions. Renal tubular acidosis, hypomagnesemia, and caffeine toxicity may cause renal potassium wasting.[140-142]

Gastrointestinal Losses

Upper GI losses from vomiting or from nasogastric (NG) suction are frequently associated with hypokalemia. The gastric concentration of potassium ranges from 5 to 10 mEq/L.

Concomitant volume depletion and metabolic alkalosis associated with NaCl and hydrogen ion losses often result in secondary aldosteronism, however, and an increased filtered load of bicarbonate with resultant renal potassium losses. Diarrhea, regardless of cause, may result in large potassium losses, the amount lost being related to the volume of fluid lost. Other GI causes are listed in Box 73.5.

Signs and Symptoms

For the intensivist, cardiovascular and neuromuscular effects of potassium deficiency are of particular concern, although metabolic, hormonal, and renal effects may also occur.

Electrocardiographic (ECG) changes include T-wave flattening or inversion, ST depression, and the appearance of a U wave. Resting membrane potential is increased, as are both the duration of the action potential and the refractory period. The decreased conductivity predisposes to arrhythmias, as do increased threshold potential and automaticity.[143]

Hypokalemia diminishes skeletal muscular excitability. This can present as a dynamic ileus or a skeletal muscle weakness resembling Guillain-Barré syndrome. It can eventually affect the trunk and upper extremities, becoming severe enough to result in quadriplegia and respiratory failure.[144] Hypokalemia can lead to severe rhabdomyolysis in a variety of underlying conditions,[145-148] and may progress to ARF and hyperkalemia.[149] Autonomic insufficiency may also occur, generally manifested as orthostatic hypotension. In patients with severe liver disease, hypokalemia may precipitate or exacerbate encephalopathy. Glucose intolerance in the presence of primary hyperaldosteronism and in certain patients receiving

---

BOX 73.5   Causes of Hypokalemia

Hypokalemia without potassium deficit
    Alkalosis
    β-agonist, exogenous or endogenous
    Familial periodic paralysis
    Thyrotoxic periodic paralysis
    Barium poisoning
    Excessive insulin
Hypokalemia with potassium deficit
    Decrease intake
    Renal losses
    Hyperaldosteronism
    Primary or secondary
    Barter, Liddle, Gitelman syndrome
    Laxative or diuretic abuse
    Licorice ingestion
    Osmotic agents
Drugs
    Caffeine
    Diuretics
    Amphotericin B
    Aminoglycosides
    High-dose penicillin, carbenicillin
Miscellaneous
    Hypomagnesemia
    Renal tubular acidosis
    Toluene toxicity
Extrarenal losses
Gastrointestinal
    Vomiting, nasogastric suction
    Diarrhea
    Laxative abuse
    Ureteral sigmoidostomy
    Obstructed or long ileal loop

thiazide diuretics has been corrected with potassium repletion. Renal effects of hypokalemia include polyuria and polydipsia, renal structural changes and functional deterioration with cellular vacuolization in the proximal tubule, and occasional interstitial fibrosis.

Treatment

Because of the wide spectrum of abnormalities resulting from marked potassium depletion, judicious correction is generally in order. In most pediatric ICUs, patients with cardiovascular disease are given NG or IV supplements at serum levels of 3 to 3.5 mEq/L. In the patient without life-threatening complications, the oral route is generally preferred for treatment, if possible, because this route is rarely associated with "overshoot" hyperkalemia if normal renal function exists. Oral dosage is frequently 1 mEq/kg up to a maximum of 20 mEq per dose, repeated if necessary. If, however, depletion is associated with digoxin use or with life-threatening complications, including cardiac arrhythmias, rhabdomyolysis, extreme weakness with quadriplegia, or respiratory distress, then urgent IV therapy is generally needed. Recommendations for IV dosage in the pediatric patient have ranged from infusions of 0.25 mEq/kg/hr to those as high as 1 to 2 mEq/kg/hr in the face of severe hypokalemia associated with DKA, arrhythmias, or quadriparesis and respiratory insufficiency. Ventricular tachycardia clearly associated with hypokalemia may initially require more rapid administration. Continuous ECG monitoring is essential, as well as frequent physical examination and determination of serum potassium levels to avoid hyperkalemic complications. Highly concentrated K solutions given IV should only be administered centrally. Patients who receive albuterol continuously are frequently mildly hypokalemic, but they rarely warrant potassium chloride replacement.

The potential for catastrophic drug error in replacing potassium is real. In most pediatric ICUs, patients with cardiovascular disease frequently require NG or IV supplements. Steps to decrease the chance of error include satellite pharmacy dosing, use of a mandatory drug request form, NG replacement when possible, use of a single solution concentration for all doses, and small aliquot solution containers. Continuing education regarding this risk for the pediatric ICU staff is essential.

Hyperkalemia

Causes

Hyperkalemia may result from artifactual elevation; from redistribution of potassium from ICF to ECF space; or from increased intake, decreased losses, or both (Box 73.6).

Artifactual

Tight, prolonged tourniquet use produces spurious potassium elevation due to potassium release from ischemic muscle. Even more common is hemolysis of red cells with potassium release associated with capillary sampling or aspiration or delivery under pressure through a small needle. The lab may note hemolysis, but artifactual normality or actual elevation should always be considered.[150] Less commonly, in vitro release of potassium occurs from white blood cells (WBCs) (>100,000/uL) or platelets (>1,000,000/uL) and may result in increased levels.

BOX 73.6	Causes of Hyperkalemia

Artifactual
Ischemic potassium loss from muscle due to tourniquet use
In vitro hemolysis, profound leukocytosis, thrombocytosis

Drugs
Digoxin toxicity, β-blockers (b_2-inhibitory activity), succinylcholine, arginine, or lysine hydrochloride, chemotherapeutic agents, sodium fluoride, epsilon-amino caproic acid

True Potassium Excess
Increased Load
IV infusion, PO supplements, potassium-containing salt substitutes, potassium penicillin, blood transfusion

Redistribution and Tissue Necrosis
In vivo red cell injury
Change in pH
Hypertonicity
Burns, trauma, rhabdomyolysis, intravascular coagulation
Gastrointestinal bleeding
Tumor cell lysis
Reabsorption of hematoma
Diabetes mellitus, diabetic ketoacidosis (DKA)

Decreased Excretion
Acute renal failure
Chronic renal failure
Mineralocorticoid deficiency
    Addison disease
    21-Hydroxylase deficiency
    Desmolase deficiency
    3-b-OH-dehydrogenase deficiency
Renal tubulointerstitial disease

Renal Tubular Secretory Deficit
Pseudohypoaldosteronism
Sickle cell disease
Systemic lupus erythematosus
Renal allograft rejection
Urinary tract obstruction
Very-low-birth-weight infants

Inhibition of Tubular Secretion
Drugs
    Spironolactone, triamterene, amiloride
    Indomethacin, converting enzyme inhibitors, heparin, cyclosporine, tacrolimus trimethoprim, pentamidine, amphotericin B

Redistribution

In general, when extracellular pH falls, potassium exits from cells; the result is an increase in serum potassium. As mentioned earlier, metabolic acidosis from mineral acids has a more pronounced effect than that of organic acids. Respiratory acidosis does not usually cause a marked change in potassium concentration.

Hypertonicity per se produces a shift of potassium from ICF to ECF. Studies of anephric animals show potassium increasing by 0.1 to 0.6 mEq/L for each increment of 10 mOsm/kg H_2O in tonicity. Hypertonicity causes cellular dehydration and therefore an increase in ICF potassium that favors increased passive diffusion out of cells. A very small percentage shift of IC potassium delivers a significant potassium load to the ECF. In the hyperkalemic patient in the ICU who has acute oliguria, mannitol should not be used for diuresis as further K+ elevation may result. In the patient with hyperglycemia, hypertonicity is likely only one of several mechanisms resulting in elevated serum levels.

Several commonly used drugs result in net movement of potassium from ICF to ECF. Digoxin inhibits the net uptake of K by cells by inhibiting Na/K-ATPase, with hyperkalemia commonly occurring in severe digitalis poisoning.[151] Other drugs include beta-blockers with β_2 activity and the muscle relaxant succinylcholine. This drug induces a prolonged dose-related increase in the ionic permeability of muscle, with subsequent efflux of potassium from muscle cells. Normal serum potassium concentration rises about 0.5 mEq/L. Succinylcholine should be avoided in patients with burns, muscle trauma, spinal injuries, certain neuromuscular diseases, near drowning, and closed head trauma, as up-regulated and new forms of acetylcholine receptors may respond with life-threatening hyperkalemia.[152] New examples of patients at risk will continue to be reported.[153,154] Hyperkalemia may result in nonsuspect patients via rhabdomyolysis or malignant hyperthermia following succinylcholine. Rhabdomyolysis has many causes including influenza, severe exercise, drugs, ischemia, and many more.[155-157] Familial hyperkalemic periodic paralysis appears to be related to potassium redistribution related to changes in ion channel function. Rebound hyperkalemia may be life threatening after coma-inducing barbiturate is stopped or surgical insulinoma removal.

Increased Load

Hyperkalemia due to an increased potassium load is unusual as long as renal function is normal. Serious elevations may be seen with inappropriate IV infusion, large volume blood transfusions,[158] bypass circuit initiation,[159] oral potassium supplements, salt substitutes containing potassium, or large doses of potassium penicillin. Strict measures to guard against accidental K overdoses are mandatory.[160] Large endogenous loads of potassium are more likely in the patient who is in the ICU. The release of cellular potassium associated with tissue necrosis from burns, trauma, rhabdomyolysis including that from spider bites[161] or the propofol syndrome,[162,163] massive intravascular coagulopathy, rapid hemolysis, or GI bleeding may lead to hyperkalemia.

Tumor lysis syndrome (TLS) is classically associated with drug or radiation treatment of sensitive lymphoid malignancies and results in hyperkalemia often accompanied by hypocalcemia, hyperphosphatemia, acidosis, and compromised renal function.[164] Many fatalities have been reported. The list of TLS-producing events or therapies includes transcatheter chemical and embolic tumor necrosis, monoclonal antibody treatment with rituximab, and enzyme-inhibiting agents bortezomib, imatinib, and sorafinib. Cases have occurred in tumor patients with surgical stress or dexamethasone given for potential airway edema (see also Chapter 94).

Manifestations of Hyperkalemia

Life-threatening complications are most likely to result from the cardiac changes caused by hyperkalemia. ECG signs include tall, peaked T waves in the precordial leads, followed by a decrease in amplitude of the R wave, bradycardia, widened QRS complexes, prolonged PR intervals, and decreased amplitude and disappearance of the P wave.[165] Finally, the classic sine wave of hyperkalemia from the blending of the QRS complex with the P wave may appear. ECG changes do not necessarily correlate with specific levels of serum K+.[166] Realizing that ventricular arrhythmias or cardiac arrest may occur at any point in this progression and that

progression may occur over a matter of minutes is extremely important.

Treatment

Treatment of hyperkalemia depends on the level of plasma potassium and the state of cardiac irritability.[47] If the potassium concentration is more than 6.5 mEq/L with associated ECG changes, additional measures are indicated. In the absence of digitalis toxicity, hyperkalemia with ECG changes should be treated with a secure and rapid IV infusion of calcium chloride or calcium gluconate. Hand injection with ECG monitoring is reasonable beginning with the administration of 10 mg/kg of calcium chloride (or gluconate equivalent) over 1 to 5 minutes. Infusion may be stopped if the electrocardiogram has normalized or if deterioration of the electrocardiogram seems to be precipitated by the potassium, suggesting a clinical scenario more complex than simple hyperkalemia. If the electrocardiogram improves but is not normalized by this calcium dose, additional calcium chloride may be given at a lower rate. It should be anticipated that ECG changes will recur in 15 to 30 minutes unless additional measures are taken immediately to treat the hyperkalemia. The effective calcium dose may be repeated as necessary to preserve cardiac function while additional treatments are in progress. Additional, rapidly effective treatments include nebulized albuterol (rapid neb or continuous neb of 0.3 to 0.5 mg/kg) or salbutamol (IV dose of 4 to 5 µg/kg over 20 minutes and repeated after 2 hours).[168,169]

Insulin and glucose are also rapidly helpful in redistributing potassium to the ICF. Glucose (1 g/kg) and insulin (0.2 U/g of glucose) may be given over 15 to 30 minutes and then infused continuously with a similar amount per hour. A premixed combination glucose and insulin solution has been successfully demonstrated in a 21 patient series.[170] Blood glucose monitoring is essential because the relative glucose and insulin amounts may need adjustment.

Sodium bicarbonate (1–2 mEq/kg given intravenously) has been a part of the classic treatment of hyperkalemia. Its benefit, however, is more difficult to predict and slower in onset than that of the measures mentioned earlier.

Sodium polystyrene sulfonate removes potassium and may be administered while dialysis arrangements are made. Sodium polystyrene sulfonate administered rectally must be retained for 15 to 30 minutes to be effective. If the oral route is available, it is generally more efficient.

Hemodialysis is the treatment of choice for removal of K+ in emergent conditions. In the patient with severely compromised renal function, the measures above generally allow stabilization of potassium long enough to institute dialysis. Although hemodialysis is much more efficient for potassium removal than peritoneal dialysis, the latter may be more quickly instituted in many centers, particularly in the small infant in whom vascular access to support reasonable blood flow may be difficult to accomplish. In the absence of renal failure, loop diuretics or thiazide diuretics or both are useful for the increase of renal excretion. If mineralocorticoid activity is deficient, the administration of fludrocortisone may be indicated. In patients with severe hyperglycemia and moderate hyperkalemia, early steps to improve glucose control should decrease ECF potassium shifts from hyperosmolality and decrease ECF potassium shifts from hyperosmolality and decreased insulin.

If the potassium is less than 6.5 mEq/L without ECG changes, discontinuation of exogenous potassium and drugs that decrease its excretion with close follow-up of potassium levels may be all that is necessary. In the patient with renal compromise, extra potassium may be eliminated with use of the potassium-binding agent sodium polystyrene sulfonate (Kayexalate, resonium) (oral, NG, or rectal doses of 1 to 2 g/kg in a sorbitol or dextrose solution). When administered rectally, sorbitol may not be necessary, and it should certainly not be given rectally in concentration greater than 20%. Highly concentrated sorbitol may cause severe proctitis and colonic injury. Increasing reports of colonic injury particularly in hemodynamically compromised or premature patients suggest caution be exercised in using this preparation. However, when needed, having the pharmacy stock a pre-mixed 10% to 20% suspension of sodium polystyrene sulfonate and sorbitol allows either oral or rectal administration on short notice.

Magnesium

Magnesium plays a key role in numerous metabolic processes, including cellular energy production, storage, and utilization involving adenosine triphosphate (ATP); the metabolism of protein, fat, and nucleic acids; and the maintenance of normal cell membrane function. It is also involved in neuromuscular transmission, cardiac excitability, and cardiovascular tone.[171]

Magnesium balance is maintained through intestinal absorption and renal excretion; 25% to 65% of ingested Mg is absorbed in the ileum. Absorption varies inversely with intake and is also affected by paracellular water reabsorption. Increased bowel water from any cause results in decreased magnesium absorption. Regulation of renal excretion occurs by glomerular filtration and reabsorption. The majority of filtered magnesium is reabsorbed in the ascending limb of the loop of Henle, resulting from active NaCl reabsorption and susceptible to loop diuretic inhibition. The threshold value for magnesium excretion varies between 1.5 and 2 mg/dL in different species. Thus if serum magnesium levels fall even slightly, renal excretion dramatically decreases under normal circumstances. Primary factors that increase renal magnesium excretion include ECF volume expansion; hypermagnesemia; hypercalcemia; metabolic acidosis; phosphate depletion; and various drugs including loop and osmotic diuretics, cisplatin, aminoglycosides, cyclosporin, and digoxin. Decreased excretion occurs with ECF volume depletion, hypomagnesemia, hypocalcemia, hypothyroidism, and metabolic alkalosis to a lesser extent. Parathyroid hormone (PTH) may decrease magnesium excretion but that effect may be offset by the opposite effect of causing hypercalcemia.

Hypomagnesemia

Free, ionized magnesium and intracellular magnesium may be the critical concentrations, but determination of total magnesium is still clinically effective. Critically ill children have been reported to frequently have low ionized magnesium despite normal total magnesium levels.[172] Evidence supporting obligatory ionized magnesium measurement remains elusive.[173]

Magnesium depletion may result in hypocalcemia, via suppression of PTH secretion. Hypokalemia also occurs in patients with hypomagnesemia. Magnesium deficiency impairs the Na/K pump, allowing potassium loss from the ICF to the ECF and urinary excretion. Magnesium repletion is important to resolution of these secondary disturbances.

Causes

Intensivists deal with hypomagnesemia most often in patients receiving loop diuretics or transplant immunosuppressives.[174] Other causes must be considered.

Magnesium deficiency may be caused by decreased intake or increased losses. Although slight falls in serum magnesium levels may occur after 1 week of a deficient diet, a more sustained period of deprivation is generally necessary for significant hypomagnesemia to occur. In children, magnesium deficiency has been particularly common in protein-energy malnutrition and in anorexia nervosa, where refeeding syndrome is a particular risk.[175,176] Intestinal malabsorption is a major cause of magnesium deficiency. Isolated familial primary hypomagnesemia occurs from selective malabsorption of magnesium with patients generally having symptoms in infancy. These include tetany and convulsions as a result of severe hypomagnesemia with consequent hypocalcemia and respond well to supplemental magnesium. Other causes associated with magnesium malabsorption include regional enteritis, ulcerative colitis, massive small bowel resection, generalized malabsorption syndromes, pancreatic insufficiency, and cystic fibrosis. In some, the formation of insoluble soaps due to the complexing of magnesium with unabsorbed fat is the postulated mechanism for hypomagnesemia.

Increasing use of induced hypothermia may increase hypomagnesemia occurrence.[177] Epidermal growth factor blocking antibodies are associated with a small incidence of induced hypomagnesemia.[178,179] Hypomagnesemia may be more common than appreciated in patients presenting with hematologic malignancies.[180]

Intrinsic renal tubular disorders associated with hypomagnesemia are rare in the ICU setting (Box 73.7).

Drugs that induce renal magnesium wasting are more common causes and include aminoglycosides,[181] cisplatin,[182] amphotericin B,[183] diuretics,[184] cyclosporin A,[185] tacrolimus,[185] and proton pump inhibitors.[186,187] Magnesium supplementation is often needed in transplant recipients who receive cyclosporine or tacrolimus. Fractional excretion of magnesium and total excretion are elevated. Patients with DKA may also have marked renal magnesium wasting during the acidotic period, as well as in early treatment. An increased urine calcium level, from whatever cause, is often associated with magnesium wasting from competitive inhibition of renal tubular reabsorption of magnesium in the ascending limb.

Signs and Symptoms

In addition to biochemical derangements associated with hypomagnesemia, a wide spectrum of other clinical disorders has been attributed to its depletion, including cardiac arrhythmias, increased sensitivity to digoxin, coronary spasm, hypertension, seizures, and neuromuscular derangements. Hypomagnesemic arrhythmias include ventricular premature beats, ventricular tachycardia, torsades de pointes, and ventricular fibrillation.[188] Supraventricular arrhythmias are less common. Following magnesium infusion, improvement in resistant ventricular arrhythmias including torsades has been reported,[189] although other metabolic derangements often coexist in such patients. Magnesium deficiency enhances

BOX 73.7	Causes of Hypomagnesemia

Decreased intake
  Low Mg++ TPN, IVF, eating disorders
Increased losses
  Gastrointestinal
  Malabsorption
  Familial primary hypomagnesemia
  Small bowel disease
  Regional enteritis, ulcerative colitis, massive bowel resection
  Pancreatic insufficiency, pancreatitis
  Cystic fibrosis
Renal
  Congenital renal magnesium wasting
  Diffuse tubular disorders
  Hypophosphatemia
  Drugs: aminoglycosides, cisplatin, amphotericin B, diuretics, cyclosporine, tacrolimus, pentamidine, foscarnet, GM-CSF
  Hypercalciuria
  Diabetic ketoacidosis
  Barter syndrome
  Hyperaldosteronism
  Inappropriate ADH secretion
Miscellaneous
  Epinephrine, β-agonists
  Thyrotoxicosis
  Citrated blood transfusion (massive)
  Burns
  Alcoholism

ADH, antidiuretic hormone; *GM-CSF,* granulocyte-macrophage colony-stimulating factor; *IVF,* intravascular fluid; *TPN,* total parenteral nutrition.

myocardial cell uptake of digoxin and toxicity. Both inhibit Na/K-ATPase with resultant ICF potassium depletion.

Depletion is thought to contribute to the development or worsening of hypertension by increasing vascular smooth muscle tone and reactivity. Increased cellular influx of calcium and decreased reuptake by sarcoplasmic reticula occur; the result is increased cytosolic calcium for activation of actin-myosin contractile proteins. Similar effects in coronary and cerebral vessels have also been observed.

Seizures may be the first symptom noted in an ICU setting. Other neuromuscular changes may include tremors, fasciculations, spontaneous carpopedal spasm, muscle cramps, paresthesias, seizures, and coma.[190,191,192] Personality changes, including apathetic behavior and depression, have also been associated.

Treatment

Patients undergoing or at immediate risk of hypomagnesemic malignant ventricular arrhythmias (such as torsades) or seizures can be given magnesium sulfate intravenously with careful monitoring. An IV infusion of 25 to 50 mg/kg per dose diluted to 10 mg/mL can be administered over 15 to 60 minutes. The rate of infusion should not exceed 150 mg/min. Doses may be repeated as needed depending on patient response. Complications of parenteral magnesium therapy include neuromuscular and respiratory depression, rare arrhythmias, flushing, hypotension, and prolonged bleeding times.[193] Other routes of therapy include intramuscular magnesium sulfate, injections of which are painful, and oral therapy with magnesium oxide or citrate. In situations known to be associated with the development of hypomagnesemia, it seems particularly important to attempt to avoid deficiency

by adequate magnesium intake before development of life-threatening symptoms. The use of supplemental magnesium infusions in perinatal asphyxia[177] remains to be fully tested or extended to other hypoxic-ischemic encephalopathies.

Hypermagnesemia

Hypermagnesemia is less common than hypomagnesemia, but they can be life threatening when extreme.[194] Magnesium infusions in pediatric status asthmaticus have become common, despite remaining controversial in adult pulmonology.[195] Large doses clearly produce elevated blood levels,[196] but side effects are not common.

Cause

Hypermagnesemia occurs in patients with renal failure and is generally associated with iatrogenic administration of magnesium as antacids, cathartics, or enemas or through total parenteral nutrition (TPN) containing magnesium. In the absence of renal failure, the administration of large quantities of magnesium cathartics in the management of constipation[197] or overdoses[198] and antacid use with increased peritoneal absorption of magnesium in the presence of a perforated viscus[199] are causes. Magnesium levels as high as 10 to 12 mEq/L have been reported. Megadose vitamin-mineral supplementation, including magnesium oxide, has been fatal.[200]

Signs and Symptoms

Acute elevations of magnesium depress the CNS and the peripheral neuromuscular junction. Pseudocoma with fixed, dilated pupils has been reported. Deep tendon reflexes are depressed at levels greater than 4 mEq/L with total disappearance along with flaccid quadriplegia at levels greater than 8 to 10 mEq/L. Hypotension, hypoventilation, and cardiac arrhythmias may also occur.[201-204] Moderate hyperkalemia has resulted from prolonged magnesium infusions in occasional patients.

Treatment

Calcium acts as a direct antagonist to magnesium. In life-threatening situations associated with severe magnesium intoxication, intravenous calcium should be used as the initial therapy. An initial dose of calcium chloride at 10 mg/kg or an equivalent amount of calcium gluconate has been suggested for infants and children. Magnesium-containing medications obviously should be discontinued. If renal function is normal, IV furosemide may be administered to increase magnesium excretion while urine output is replaced with half-normal saline. In patients with renal failure or severe toxicity, dialysis may be necessary for removal.

Calcium

Hypocalcemia is a common issue in pediatric critical care.[205,206] Hypercalcemia is an uncommon challenge in the PICU. Extracellular fluid (ECF) calcium concentration is best estimated with measurement of ionized calcium (Ca++) concentration. Total serum calcium includes physiologically accessible Ca++ plus that bound to protein or complexed with anions such as citrate of phosphate. The Ca++ concentration is under dual hormone control with PTH mobilizing Ca++ and calcitonin acting in bone and cartilage to retain fixed calcium. The concentration of Ca++ is particularly critical for cardiac, vasomotor, and neurologic function but is susceptible to disturbance by many factors including drugs, sepsis, major surgery, enteric disease, malignancy, pancreatitis, endocrinopathy, genetic misfortune, and many others.

Entry of Ca++ into cardiac and skeletal muscle cell mediates conversion of electrochemical into mechanical energy with resultant muscle contraction. Adenylate cyclase, phosphodiesterase and protein kinases are regulated by the interaction of Ca++ with calmodulin. A similar interaction stimulates myosin kinase in vascular smooth muscle so that Ca++ influx (enhanced by α-adrenergic and inhibited by β-adrenergic stimuli) causes vasoconstriction. Ca++ also plays a critical role in the clotting system and various membrane transport systems.

Extracellular Ca++ is monitored by Ca++-sensing receptors[207,208] on the surface of the chief cells of the parathyroid glands, the juxtaglomerular apparatus, the proximal tubule, the cortical thick ascending limb of the loop of Henle, the inner medullary collecting duct, the intestine, parts of the brain, thyroid C cells, breast cells, and the adrenal glands. Binding of Ca++ to this calcium sensor activates phospholipase C and the accumulation of inositol triphosphate, which leads to inhibition of the secretion and synthesis of PTH and inactivation of its proteolysis.

Regulation of Calcium

In the ICU, many changes in calcium activity result from changes in protein binding and chelation, excessive or deficient hormonal action, or excessive losses or intake of calcium. A majority of total serum calcium is bound to proteins, and this binding is pH dependent. Acidic pH decreases calcium binding and increases Ca++, whereas alkalemia increases binding and reduces Ca++. Blood products, renal failure, or massive cell lysis may result in increased chelation. Fortunately, direct measurement of Ca++ is now readily available in PICUs.

Hormonal Regulation of Calcium

Hormonal control of calcium homeostasis involves PTH, vitamin D, and calcitonin. Secretion of PTH by the parathyroid chief cell varies inversely with the serum Ca++ and is inhibited by hypomagnesemia and 1,25(OH)2-vitamin D. Rapid proteolytic degradation of PTH yields a physiologically inactive C-terminal fragment and an active NH_2-terminal fragment. PTH binds to cell surface receptors in bone osteoblasts and kidney and exerts its effects through binding of a subunit of a membrane-associated heterotrimeric protein, which mediates increased formation of cyclic adenosine 3′,5′-monophosphate.

In the kidney, PTH inhibits proximal tubular phosphate reabsorption and promotes phosphaturia. This loss of phosphate inhibits bone mineralization and tends to shift the flow of calcium from bone to the ECF. PTH also increases distal tubular reabsorption of filtered calcium. PTH stimulates 1α-hydroxylation of 25(OH)-vitamin D, resulting in production of metabolically active 1,25(diOH)-vitamin D that stimulates intestinal absorption of calcium and phosphate. The overall effect of PTH is to raise serum calcium levels and lower serum phosphate levels. This characteristic reciprocal relationship is helpful in distinguishing PTH disorders from those involving vitamin D alone.[209]

Hyperphosphatemia lowers Ca++ by chelation, by shifting the equilibrium in calcium flux from ECF toward bone and by inhibiting 1α–hydroxylation activity. Calcitonin is a 32-amino acid, calcium-lowering hormone elaborated by C cells of the thyroid in response to rising Ca++ levels.[210] Although it rapidly reduces the bone resorptive function of osteoclasts and promotes calciuria and phosphaturia, its excess or absence causes no known disorder.

Hypocalcemia

Clinical and Laboratory Concerns

Hypocalcemia in pediatric critical illness may be associated with PTH deficiency, hypercalcitoninemia, or hypomagnesemia. Multiple mechanisms may act simultaneously. In children with severe burns, hypocalcemia, magnesium depletion, hypoparathyroidism, and renal resistance to PTH may all develop.

Cardiovascular manifestations are of particular ICU concern and may include hypotension, myocardial depression, CHF, and dysrhythmias. Cardiac contractility may be compromised acutely as in postoperative hypocalcemia. However, subacute cardiac myopathy from vitamin D deficiency and hypocalcemia may also be life threatening and reversible.[211-213]

Hypocalcemia inhibits acetylcholine release in both sensory and motor nerves. Accordingly, a variety of peripheral and CNS effects may result, including seizures, tetany, carpopedal spasms, muscle cramps and twitching, paresthesias, laryngeal stridor, and apnea in the newborn.

Somatic changes accompanying prolonged hypocalcemia include dry coarse skin, eczematous dermatitis, brittle hair with areas of alopecia, brittle nails with smooth transverse grooves, and dental enamel hypoplasia.

Determination of the free ionized Ca++ level is diagnostic, although the rate of decline also contributes to the development of symptoms. Estimations of Ca++ correcting for protein binding are not appropriate for managing critical illness.

The causes of hypocalcemia are summarized in Box 73.8.

Reduced PTH effect can result from parathyroid gland failure (autoimmune or surgical or radiotherapy thyroidectomy),[214-216] insensitivity to PTH (pseudohypoparathyroidism), or suppression of PTH release (hypomagnesemia, maternal hypocalcemia, burns). Hyperphosphatemia is frequently present. Clinical features may be distinguishing, but measurement of immunoreactive PTH is diagnostic.

Reduced vitamin D effect results from vitamin D deficiency seen in malabsorption in enteric diseases[217-219] or impaired conversion of 25(OH) to 1,25 (diOH) vitamin D seen in renal insufficiency. Certain drugs such as phenytoin can increase vitamin D metabolic degradation and cause deficiency.

Infusion of large amounts of citrate-preserved blood and acute phosphorus overload or retention can rapidly deplete ECF Ca++. Various drugs, particularly loop diuretics, also contribute to the development of hypocalcemia (see Box 73.8).[220-221]

Treatment

Correction of hypocalcemia should be preceded by consideration of readily treated or confounding factors such as respiratory alkalemia. Rapid development of hyperphosphatemia suggests acute renal failure, cell lysis, or excessive supply. As

BOX 73-8 Causes of Hypocalcemia

Reduced PTH Effect

Parathyroid Gland Failure

Hypoparathyroidism—idiopathic or autoimmune
Trauma
Postsurgery
Post–^{131}I therapy
Infarction
Infiltration (eg, sarcoid hemosiderosis)

Insensitivity to PTH

Pseudohypoparathyroidism
Hypomagnesemia

Suppression of PTH Release

Hypomagnesemia
Neonatal, resulting from maternal hypercalcemia
Burns
Sepsis
Drugs
- Aminoglycosides
- Cimetidine
- Cisplatin
- β-Adrenergic blockers

Reduced Vitamin D Effect

Vitamin D Deficiency

Dietary insufficiency
Increased losses related to:
    Malabsorption
    Nephrotic syndrome
    Phenytoin, phenobarbital

Impaired Activation of Vitamin D

Renal disease
Hypoparathyroidism
Liver failure
Rhabdomyolysis

Changes in Ca^{++} Binding or Chelation

Alkalosis

Respiratory alkalosis
Bicarbonate infusion

Hyperphosphatemia

Renal failure
Phosphate administration (eg, high-phosphate formulas, enemas)
Chemotherapy
Rhabdomyolysis
Malignancy
Pancreatitis
Fat embolism
Transfusion with citrate-preserved blood

Drug/Toxins

Glucagon
Mithramycin
Calcitonin
EDTA
Protamine
Sodium fluoride
Colchicine
Theophylline
Ethylene glycol

EDTA, ethylenediamine tetraacetic acid.

appropriate, efforts should be made to reduce serum phosphate levels, because intravenous calcium therapy may cause metastatic deposition of calcium phosphate salts. Hypomagnesemia impairs PTH release, response to PTH, and, consequently, correction of hypocalcemia. Hypomagnesemia may develop in critically ill patients by several mechanisms previously discussed.

Urgency of therapy is determined by the child's clinical status. Asymptomatic hypocalcemia is appropriately treated with oral calcium salts and vitamin D if needed. For the seriously ill patient with overt or evolving hypocalcemia, replacement therapy is accomplished with IV calcium chloride, 5 to 20 mg/kg, or an equivalent calcium gluconate infusion. Potential bradycardia and asystole with infusion of calcium should be anticipated with cardiac monitoring and atropine readily available. Care is required to prevent tissue damage by extravasation or precipitation with concomitantly administered bicarbonate. In patients receiving digitalis, IV calcium is particularly dangerous as the arrhythmia potential is great. Hyperkalemia in digitalis toxicity should be treated with antidigitalis FAB therapy and not IV calcium infusion.

Oral administration of calcium salts is efficient for control of most persistent hypocalcemia and is preferable to prolonged infusion (although some patients with DiGeorge hypocalcemia require aggressive multi-modal treatment). Liberal amounts can be administered orally (eg, calcium 50 mg/kg/day in 4–5 divided doses), with attention paid to the differing calcium content of various oral preparations. For patients with fat malabsorption, supplementation of calcium therapy with magnesium or vitamin D may be needed. In the setting of hypoparathyroidism secondary to magnesium depletion, magnesium replenishment must occur.

Hypercalcemia

In contrast to dramatic manifestations of hypocalcemia, the effects of hypercalcemia may be subtle. However, a serum total calcium greater than 15 mg/dL represents a medical emergency. Renal, cardiovascular, and CNS disturbances predominate and reflect both the degree and duration of calcium elevation. Increased filtered load of calcium creates hypercalciuria and accompanying polyuria, reduced concentrating ability, dehydration, and eventual renal lithiasis. Hypertension is common, mediated through increased renin production and peripheral vasoconstriction. Alterations in the cardiac conduction system include a shortened QT interval and a tendency to dysrhythmias. Impaired nerve conduction creates hypotonia, hyporeflexia, and paresis in severe cases. Changes in CNS function include lethargy, confusion, and even coma. Constipation, anorexia, and abdominal pain resulting from reduced intestinal motility are frequent. Promotion of gastrin release by calcium may account for an increased incidence of peptic ulcer disease. Soft tissue deposition of calcium phosphate can impair function of lungs, kidneys, cardiac conduction tissue, blood vessels, and joints.

In the absence of hyperproteinemia, determination of elevated serum total calcium levels reliably indicates increased Ca++ concentrations. Because hyperparathyroidism and malignancies are less common in children, the pediatric intensivist encounters hypercalcemia less frequently. Diagnostic possibilities may be approached by considering the underlying mechanisms of hypercalcemia as outlined in Table 73.3.

TABLE 73.3   Tumor Lysis Syndrome

High risk	Lymphoid malignancies, large tumor mass, B-cell lymphoma concurrent renal compromise
Initiating event	Cytolytic chemotherapy
	Radiation therapy
	Embolic tumor infarction
Prophylaxis	Hydration, urinary alkalinization, allopurinol
	Gradual chemotherapy initiation, rasburicase
Serious disturbances	Hyperkalemia, hypocalcemia, acidosis, renal failure, hyperuricemia, hyperphosphatemia
Management	Obsessive electrolyte monitoring, Hemodialysis available stat, CVVHD helpful, may not be adequate

CVVHD, continuous venovenous hemodialysis; *stat,* immediately.

Increased bone resorption reflects excess PTH effect, immobilization, or bone lysis by metastatic malignancy. PTH-mediated hypercalcemia is distinguished by a depressed serum phosphate concentration, decreased renal tubular reabsorption of phosphate ($TmPO_4$/GFR), and an iPTH level inappropriately elevated for the simultaneous serum Ca++. In the child with hyperparathyroidism, evaluation for multiple endocrine neoplasias is warranted. Heightened vitamin D effect is manifested by increased intestinal calcium absorption and can be related to vitamin D intoxication,[222,223] increased sensitivity to vitamin D, or ectopically produced 1,25(diOH)-vitamin D, as seen in sarcoidosis. Serum phosphate levels and $TmPO_4$/GFR ratios are normal or increased, and iPTH levels are suppressed in these disorders. Detection of an elevated 25(OH)-vitamin D level may be helpful. High levels of vitamin A can also cause hypercalcemia and are particularly likely in patients with excessive intake or those with renal insufficiency.[224,225]

Decreased excretion of calcium occurs with dehydration or treatment with thiazide diuretics, aggravating the severity of hypercalcemia in hyperparathyroidism. Familial hypocalciuric hypercalcemia, an autosomal dominant disorder resulting from partially deactivating mutations in the Ca++-sensing receptor, is characterized by normal to slightly elevated iPTH levels and decreased urinary calcium excretion.[226] Thus determination of serum Ca++, phosphate, iPTH, vitamin D levels, and urinary calcium and phosphate excretion allows differentiation of most hypercalcemic disorders.

Treatment

A serum calcium level greater than 15 mg/dLc may be life threatening and requires direct Ca-lowering therapy in addition to attention to the underlying disorder. Hydration with isotonic saline (200 to 250 mL/kg/day) and furosemide diuresis results in calciuresis and amelioration of hypercalcemia in the majority of cases. Excessive losses of sodium, potassium, magnesium, and phosphate may require replacement.

Adjunct therapy is directed at the specific cause of hypercalcemia. Drugs that inhibit bone resorption include calcitonin (10 U/kg IV every 4–6 hours), mithramycin (25 mg/kg IV over 4 hours), and indomethacin (1 mg/kg/day). Recombinant calcitonin blocks PTH-induced bone resorption, facilitates calciuria, is relatively nontoxic, and has peak effect by 1 hour. Mithramycin is a toxic antibiotic that inhibits osteoclastic activity but has potential adverse effects including thrombocytopenia, hepatotoxicity, and renal injury. Indomethacin is useful when excessive prostaglandin E_2 production is suspected as in some cases of malignancy hypercalcemia.

Bisphosphonates have been used successfully in pediatrics for treatment of various disorders including hypercalcemia.[227-229] Corticosteroids are useful for treatment of vitamin D–related hypercalcemia, although the onset of action is not rapid.

Phosphorus

Virtually all of plasma phosphorus is in the inorganic form, with a small organic component composed entirely of phospholipids bound to protein. Serum levels vary with age; approximate normal values (specific to the analytical instrument) are 4.8 to 8.2 mg/dL for neonates, 3.8 to 6.5 mg/dL for children aged 1 week to 3 years, 3.7 to 5.5 mg/dL for children aged 3 years to 12 years, and 2.9 to 5 mg/dL for adolescents aged 12 to 19 years.[230] Differences are thought to be related to more rapid rates of skeletal growth in the pediatric population. Most total body phosphorus resides in bone. As much as 60% to 80% of ingested phosphorus is absorbed, primarily in the jejunum. Absorption occurs by two pathways, one passive and one active. Passive paracellular transport is nonsaturable, so the greater the dietary intake, the higher is the net absorption. Active transport accounts for only 20% of total absorption via a vitamin D–dependent transporter, the Na-dependent phosphorus transporter 2b (NPT2b). Increased excretion of phosphorus from the kidneys after increased dietary intake is dependent on inhibition of the Na-phosphorus cotransporters 2a and 2c (NPT2a and NPT2c) in the luminal membrane of the proximal tubule. These transporters are inhibited from increased secretion of fibroblast growth factor 23 (FGF23). FGF23 is secreted by osteocytes and osteoblasts in response to oral phosphorus loading or an increase in serum 1,25 dihydroxy vitamin D levels. FGF23 induces an increase in the fractional excretion of phosphorus in the proximal tubule and decreases the efficiency of phosphorus absorption in the gut by lowering 1,25 vitamin D levels. PTH is also stimulated by increased intake of phosphorus by the fall in ionized calcium induced by transient hyperphosphatemia. Increased PTH causes a decrease in the expression of NPT2a and NPT2c in proximal tubules.[231] Absorption may also be decreased by a high calcium intake or by ingestion of antacids such as calcium carbonate or acetate, which bind phosphorus in the bowel. Glucose competitively inhibits phosphorus reabsorption. Glucocorticoids produce phosphaturia by a decrease in sodium-dependent transport in the proximal tubule.

Phosphorus plays an important role in cellular structure and function, bone mineralization, and urinary acid excretion. The development of severe phosphorus depletion affects the availability of intracellular ATP, depletes the erythrocyte of 2,3-diphosphoglycerate (2,3-DPG), with resultant tissue hypoxia, and impairs urinary acid excretion. The major acute effect of hyperphosphatemia is hypocalcemia; the long-term consequence is soft tissue calcification.[232]

Hypophosphatemia

Hypophosphatemia as measured by serum or plasma levels may or may not indicate true phosphorus deficiency. Severely depressed levels of serum-measurable phosphorus may occur in the absence of true deficiency after transcellular shifts from the ECF to the ICF, whereas a moderate phosphorus deficiency may be indicated only by slightly decreased serum levels.[233] Other processes that lead to true hypophosphatemia include increased excretion from the kidneys and decreased intestinal absorption. Hypophosphatemia may also result from a combination of these three mechanisms. Moderate hypophosphatemia has been defined as levels between 1.5 and 2.5 mg/dL and severe hypophosphatemia as levels less than 1.5 mg/dL on serum determination. In general, only with severe deficiency of phosphorus do multiple symptoms occur, as well as overt cell dysfunction or necrosis. Risk is greatest when superimposed additional cellular injury exists.

Cause of Severe Hypophosphatemia

Although numerous abnormalities may result in moderate decreases in phosphorus levels, severe hypophosphatemia has been associated with only a handful of clinical syndromes. These syndromes include significant respiratory alkalosis, prolonged use of phosphate-deficient TPN, the nutritional refeeding syndrome, thermal burns, DKA, pharmacologic binding of phosphorus in the gut, alcohol withdrawal, and several medications.[233-235] An association with continuous renal replacement therapy and bone recovery after renal transplant also has been reported.[236,237] The increase in the ICF pH associated with acute respiratory alkalosis stimulates the enzymes of glycolysis, with subsequent depletion of ICF phosphorus, which is replaced by an influx from the ECF space. Although carbon dioxide diffuses across membranes much more readily than bicarbonate does, metabolic alkalosis rarely produces a decrease in phosphorus levels, whereas very low levels may be seen with respiratory alkalosis.[238] An absolute deficiency from malnutrition and transcellular shifts from the ECF to the ICF with an anabolic response to increasing caloric intake are the causes associated with TPN use.[239] In the pediatric population, the preterm infant is particularly susceptible. Nearly 80% of calcium-phosphorus assimilation in the fetus occurs in the last trimester of pregnancy. The preterm infant is therefore born deficient in total body phosphorus. When reasonable nutrition has been absent for even short periods or when phosphorus has not been provided in TPN, severe hypophosphatemia has occurred, associated in several cases with the development of hypercalcemia.[240] A similar situation may occur with the refeeding of patients who have significant protein calorie malnutrition including anorexia patients.[241] As previously noted, an absolute phosphorus deficiency and transcellular shifts from the ECF to the ICF in the face of an anabolic response are responsible.

Significant hypophosphatemia in burn patients during their recovery phase has been associated with the presence of respiratory alkalosis, diuresis of initially retained sodium and water, and acceleration of glycolysis.[231,233] As previously described, ECF phosphorus shifts to the ICF compartment when intracellular-free phosphorus has been used in phosphorylation of organic compounds such as occurs during glycolysis, oxidative phosphorylation, glycogenolysis, and synthesis of glycogen, protein, and phosphocreatine. Acidosis decomposes organic compounds within the cell with subsequent movement of inorganic phosphorus from ICF to ECF and excretion in the urine. Osmotic diuresis augments these losses. Decreased intake also commonly occurs. During treatment of DKA, renal phosphorus clearance generally increases with fluid administration. In addition, insulin therapy results in stimulation of glycolysis and anabolism with a shift of phosphorus back to the ICF. If the acidosis has been present for only a few days, then rarely is there a severe phosphorus deficiency. Although levels may decrease, they generally return to normal without extra phosphorus therapy. In the patient whose symptoms have been present for a number of days to weeks, however, severe deficiency may exist at the time of admission. These patients may have life-threatening complications of hypophosphatemia if they are not treated. In general, this subset of patients has low phosphorus levels on admission, whereas phosphorus levels are normal or increased at admission in less severely affected patients. Patients undergoing continuous renal replacement therapy (CRRT) who become hypophosphatemic may be at higher risk for mortality.[242] In burn patients with >19% total body surface area burns, patients receiving preemptive infusions of intravenous (IV) phosphorus beginning at 24 hours after injury had less hypophosphatemia and fewer complications versus those treated once hypophosphatemia developed.[243]

Signs and Symptoms

Multiple organ systems may be affected by severe hypophosphatemia, including CNS, cardiac, respiratory, musculoskeletal, hematologic, renal, and hepatic abnormalities.[244-251] Decreased diaphragmatic contractility in patients with hypophosphatemia with acute respiratory failure significantly improved as measured by transdiaphragmatic pressures during phrenic stimulation with treatment of hypophosphatemia.[252] Respiratory muscle weakness in patients with hypophosphatemia but with or without respiratory failure also has been documented and shown to normalize with phosphorus repletion.[248,250,251,253]

Neurologic symptoms may initially include irritability and apprehension followed by weakness, peripheral neuropathy with numbness, and paresthesias. Dysarthria, confusion, obtundation, seizures, and coma may occur in more profound cases.[246,249,254] Reports in the literature include Guillain-Barré–like syndrome,[255] diffuse slowing on electroencephalogram, and congestive cardiomyopathy[256] that significantly improved with correction of phosphorus depletion. In dogs, decreased cardiac output, decreased ventricular ejection velocity, and increased left ventricular end-diastolic pressure reversed with phosphorus repletion. In humans, rhabdomyolysis has been predominantly seen in alcoholic patients, in whom subtle myopathy was likely present, and rarely in patients with DKA or after TPN therapy. Decreased levels of 2,3-DPG in red blood cells (RBCs) may depress P-50 (oxygen half-saturation pressure) values so that the release of molecular oxygen to peripheral tissues is decreased, with resultant tissue hypoxia.[244] Structural defects of RBCs associated with hypophosphatemia have included rigidity and rarely hemolysis and have generally occurred when additional metabolic stresses such as metabolic acidosis or infection were placed on the RBC. Decreased levels of ATP in neutrophils may result in decreased chemotaxis, phagocytosis, and bacterial killing.[257] The mechanisms underlying the development of metabolic acidosis include decreased phosphorus excretion that thereby limits titratable acid excretion and decreased ammonia levels.

Treatment

As with other minerals and electrolytes, when oral therapy is potentially possible it is the preferable route for administration. In patients with severe hypophosphatemia, IV therapy is often indicated, though there remain no evidence-based recommendations for IV replacement.[258-260] Few data exist in the pediatric literature regarding dosage. Therefore most data are extrapolated from adult literature.[260-263] Reasonable recommendations in children with severe phosphorus depletion are to use 0.15 to 0.33 mmol/kg per dose, given as a continuous infusion over 4 to 6 hours. Subsequent doses are generally calculated on the basis of response to this initial dosage. Either potassium or sodium phosphate may be administered with the attendant potential complications of hypernatremia or hyperkalemia. A common recommendation is to use potassium phosphate if potassium (K) is <4 meq/L and sodium phosphate if the K is >4 meq/L. Other potential complications of therapy include hyperphosphatemia, metastatic deposition of calcium phosphate, hypocalcemia, potential nephrocalcinosis with renal failure, and hypotension. Both sodium and potassium phosphate contain 3 mmol of phosphate per mL and 4 or 4.5 mEq of sodium or potassium, respectively. For oral administration, a combination product of sodium with potassium phosphate (Neutra-Phos) has been used commonly in children. One capsule supplies 8 mmol of phosphorus along with 7.1 mEq of sodium and potassium. Capsules can be reconstituted in water as well. In infants the IV preparations may be used enterally with smaller volumes needed. Hypophosphatemia associated with continuous renal replacement therapy provides a special case. IV replacement is required in many such patients.[236]

Hyperphosphatemia

Causes of Hyperphosphatemia

Acute and chronic renal failure with decreased phosphorus excretion are the most common causes of hyperphosphatemia, with elevation in serum phosphorus occurring when the GFR is less than 30 mL/min/1.73 m^2. Extreme hyperphosphatemia associated with several deaths has been reported from the use of either oral sodium phosphate or enemas containing sodium phosphate in infants and children.[264,265] Abnormalities of intestinal anatomy or motility predisposing to retention of enemas or renal insufficiency represent risk factors, but no risk factors are identified in 30% of reported patients. Previous treatment does not guarantee safety with these agents, as 30% of reported patients had previously received enemas or oral therapy without complications. Average time to recognition has ranged from 12 minutes to 24 hours, with mean of 6.53 hours. Mean phosphorus levels were 27.9 mg/dL with plasma total calcium mean of 4.95 mg/dL. Unless there was kidney disease when older children and adolescents have also been affected, all reported patients have been <5 years of age.[264] The administration of IV boluses of sodium or potassium phosphate rather than slow infusion may result in symptomatic hyperphosphatemia. An error in parenteral nutrition resulted in hyperphosphatemia in multiple infants,[266] and severe hyperphosphatemia has been reported related to use of liposomal amphotericin B.[267]

Tumor lysis syndrome represents an additional cause of hyperphosphatemia along with hyperkalemia, acidosis, hypocalcemia, and renal failure. It results from induced lysis of tumor cells and is always a concern in a child with a lymphoid malignancy and substantial cellular mass, but it can occur in a variety of settings (see also Chapter 94). Initial chemotherapy or radiation of B-cell lymphoma is particularly likely to produce cell lysis and hyperphosphatemia along with hyperuricemia, acute renal failure (ARF), hyperkalemia, metabolic acidosis, and hypocalcemia. Aggressive hydration and careful initiation of chemotherapy usually will result in a manageable degree of electrolyte abnormality. Urinary alkalinization to increase urate solubility is usually recommended but is being reexamined. Rasburicase is replacing allopurinol in the control of urate levels. Hemodialysis or CRRT is an essential resource to have available if managing such a patient (see Table 73.2).

Signs and Symptoms

The major clinical consequence of severe hyperphosphatemia is its associated hypocalcemia, as well as soft tissue deposition of calcium phosphate salts. Seizures, coma, and cardiac arrest have been reported, generally in the presence of both hypocalcemia and hyperphosphatemia. In one case report, however, seizures, malignant ventricular arrhythmias, and cardiac arrest with acute hyperphosphatemia alone were described.[268] Hyperphosphatemia may be a proximate cause of ARF via precipitation in renal tissue.[269,270]

Treatment

In patients with life-threatening complications or multiple additional electrolyte disturbances or in the presence of renal failure, dialysis may be required. Intravenous fluid loading to increase renal phosphorus losses and intravenous calcium may increase excretion. Mannitol diuresis will inhibit proximal phosphorus reabsorption and theoretically should expedite phosphaturia. If oral administration is possible, Sevelamer has been used in patients with TLS to bind phosphorus and perhaps decrease the need for more invasive therapy.[271]

Key References

1. Kaplan L, Kellum J, et al. Fluids, pH, ions and electrolytes. *Curr Opin Crit Care.* 2010;16:323-331.
5. Kannan L, Lodha R, Vivekanandhan S, et al. Intravenous fluid regimen and hyponatraemia among children: a randomized controlled trial. *Peidatr Nephrol.* 2010;25:2303-2309.
8. Friedman JN, Beck CE, DeGroot J, et al. Comparison of isotonic and hypotonic intravenous maintenance fluids: a randomized clinical trial. *JAMA Pediatr.* 2015;10:1001.
9. Mastorakos G, Weber JS, Magiakou MA, et al. Hypothalamic-pituitary-adrenal axis activation and stimulation of systemic vasopressin secretion by recombinant interleukin-6 in humans: potential implications for the syndrome of inappropriate vasopressin secretion. *J Clin Endocrinol Metab.* 1994;79:934-939.
10. Park SJ, Shin JI, et al. Inflammation and hyponatremia: an underrecognized condition? *Korean J Pediatr.* 2013;56:519-522.
13. Caironi P, Tognoni G, Masson S, et al. Albumin replacement in patients with severe sepsis or septic shock. *N Engl J Med.* 2014;370:1412-1421.
25. Arikan AA, Zappitelli M, Goldstein SL, et al. Fluid overload is associated with impaired oxygenation and morbidity in critically ill children. *Pediatr Crit Care Med.* 2012;13:253-258.

26. Sinitsky L, Walls D, Nadel S, et al. Fluid overload at 48 hours is associated with respiratory morbidity but not mortality in a general PICU: retrospective cohort study. *Pediatr Crit Care Med*. 2015;16:205-209.

27. Wiedemann HP, Wheeler AP, Bernard GR, et al. Comparison of two fluid-management strategies in acute lung injury. *N Engl J Med*. 2006;354:2564-2575.

57. Stern RH, Silver SM. Cerebral salt wasting versus SIADH: what difference? *J Am Soc Nephrol*. 2008;19:194.

61. Celik T, Orkun T, Ilknur T, et al. Cerebral salt wasting in status epilepticus: two cases and review of the literature. *Pediatr Neurol*. 2014;50:397.

69. Schrier RW. Vasopressin and Aquaporin 2 (AQP2) in clinical disorders of water homeostasis. *Semin Nephrol*. 2008;28:289.

85. Kallakatta RN, Radhakrishnan A, Fayaz RK, et al. Clinical and functional outcome and factors predicting prognosis in osmotic demyelination syndrome (central pontine and/or extrapontine myelinolysis) in 25 patients. *J Neurol Neurosurg Psychiatry*. 2011;82:326.

103. Jones RC, Rajasekaran S, Rayburn M, et al. Initial experience with conivaptan use in critically ill infants with cardiac disease. *J Pediatr Pharmacol Ther*. 2012;17:78.

121. Cummings BM, Macklin EA, Yager PH, et al. Potassium abnormalities in a pediatric intensive care unit: frequency and severity. *J Intensive Care Med*. 2014;29:269-274.

151. Woof AD, Wenger T, Smith TW, et al. The use of digoxin-specific fab fragments for severe digitalis intoxication in children. *N Engl J Med*. 1992;326:1739-1744.

152. Racca F, Mongini T, Wolfler A, et al. Recommendations for anesthesia and perioperative management of patients with neuromuscular disorders. *Minerva Anestesiol*. 2013;79:419-433.

164. Rajendran A, Bansal D, Marwaha RK, et al. Tumor lysis syndrome. *Indian J Pediatr*. 2013;80:50-54.

170. Janjua HS, Mahan JD, Patel HP, et al. Continuous infusion of a standard combination solution in the management of hyperkalemia. *Nephrol Dial Transplant*. 2011;26:2503-2508.

171. De Baaij JH, Hoenderop JG, Bendels RJ, et al. Magnesium in man: implications for health and disease. *Physiol Rev*. 2015;95:1-46.

177. Horn A, Thompson C, Woods D, et al. Induced hypothermia for infants with hypoxic-ischemic encephalopathy using a servo-controlled fan: an exploratory pilot study. *Pediatrics*. 2009;123:e1090-e1098.

196. Egelund TA, Wassil SK, Edwards EM, et al. High-dose magnesium sulfate infusion protocol for status asthmaticus: a safety and pharmacokinetics cohort study. *Intensive Care Med*. 2013;39:117-122.

205. Cias CR, Leite HP, Nogueira PC, et al. Ionized hypocalcemia is an early event and is associated with organ dysfunction in children admitted to the intensive care unit. *J Crit Care*. 2013;28:810-815.

207. Ward BK, Magno AL, Walsh JP, et al. The role of the calcium-sensing receptor in human disease. *Clin Biochem*. 2012;45:943-953.

213. Yilmaz O, Olgun H, Ciftel M, et al. Dilated cardiomyopathy secondary to rickets-related hypocalcaemia: eight case reports and a review of the literature. *Cardiol Young*. 2015;25:261-266.

225. Manickavasagar B, McArdle AJ, Yadav P, et al. Hypervitaminosis A is prevalent in children with CKD and contributes to hypercalcemia. *Pediatr Nephrol*. 2015;30:317-325.

234. Amanzadeh J, Reilly RF Jr. Hypophosphatemia: an evidence-based approach to its clinical consequences and management. *Nat Clin Pract Nephrol*. 2006;2:136.

236. Santiago MJ, Lopez-Herce J, Urbano J, et al. Hypophosphatemia and phosphate supplementation during continuous renal replacement therapy in children. *Kidney Int*. 2009;75:312.

241. de Meneses JF, Leite HP, de Carvalho WB, et al. Hypophosphatemia in critically ill children: prevalence and associated risk factors. *Pediatr Crit Care Med*. 2009;10:234.

251. Sprung J, Weingarten TN. Severe hypophosphatemia: a rare cause of postoperative muscle weakness. *J Clin Anesth*. 2014;26:584.

265. Mendoza J, Legido J, Rubio S, et al. Systematic review: the adverse effects of sodium phosphate enema. *Aliment Pharmacol Ther*. 2007;26:9.

271. Abdullah S, Diezi M, Sung L, et al. Sevelamer hydrochloride: a novel treatment of hyperphosphatemia associated with tumor lysis syndrome in children. *Pediatr Blood Cancer*. 2008;51:59.

Tests of Kidney Function in Children

Ayesa N. Mian and George J. Schwartz

PEARLS

- As a marker of glomerular function, serum creatinine provides a crude assessment because it is influenced by several factors other than glomerular filtration, of which the amount of muscle mass is clinically most significant.
- Serum cystatin C, another endogenous filtration marker not significantly affected by muscle mass, may provide a more accurate assessment of renal function, particularly in individuals with reduced muscle mass.
- Prediction formulas in children provide a better estimate of glomerular filtration rate (GFR) than serum creatinine alone because they incorporate surrogate variables for muscle mass.
- Current pediatric GFR estimating equations are not universally applicable. Appropriate use and interpretation of GFR prediction formulas require knowledge about the physiology of the marker, assays/auto-analyzers used to measure the marker, and characteristics of the population in whom the equation was developed.
- Neither serum creatinine nor the prediction formula is valid when renal function changes rapidly, yet both are used clinically, as better alternatives are not available. Changes in serum creatinine lag behind changes in GFR. It is essential to recognize that use of serum creatinine or creatinine-based equations in the setting of developing acute kidney injury (AKI) and before the establishment of a new steady state will result in an overestimation of GFR. Conversely, during the recovery phase of AKI, their use will result in an underestimation of GFR.
- Formal clearance studies are still clinically essential to assess renal function in select patients with atypical body habitus or diet.
- Novel biomarkers for AKI are still in the research phase but hold promise to facilitate earlier diagnosis of AKI, as well as to help distinguish among AKI phenotypes.

Renal dysfunction and injury are not unusual in the critically ill child and may develop as a consequence of the underlying disease process (eg, hypoperfusion secondary to sepsis, progressive glomerulonephritis) or its therapy (eg, aminoglycoside toxicity). The ability to accurately, precisely, and rapidly assess renal function is essential for the early detection of acute kidney injury (AKI), for dose adjustments of medications excreted by or toxic to the kidney, in risk assessment for imaging studies involving intravenous contrast agents or gadolinium, and for monitoring for medication-related nephrotoxicity. AKI is now recognized to encompass a spectrum of disease ranging from mild, reversible, renal dysfunction to severe, potentially irreversible organ failure with need for dialysis support. In the past 10 to 15 years, standardized classification schemes for AKI based on an acute increase in serum creatinine or decrease in urine output [RIFLE (Risk, Injury, Failure, Loss, End-Stage Renal Disease); AKIN (Acute Kidney Injury Network); and KDIGO (Kidney Disease: Improving Global Outcomes)] have been proposed and validated in adults[1-3] with modified versions proposed for children[4,5] (Table 74.1). An increase in serum creatinine as small as 0.3 mg/dL is now well recognized to be associated with increased morbidity and mortality underscoring the need for precise, sensitive, and timely measures of renal function.[5,6] Notably, however, none of these definitions addresses AKI in the neonate. Jetton et al.[7] recently proposed a modification of the KDIGO classification for use in neonates (Table 74.2). The authors and others have found that preterm infants frequently experience a serum creatinine elevation of 0.3 mg/dL and that such increases can be associated with increased morbidity and mortality.[8] The true incidence of AKI in the pediatric intensive care unit (PICU) is not well established, but recent studies suggest it is increasing as advances in critical care medicine have led to improved patient survival and salvage of more critically ill individuals.[4,9] However, morbidity and mortality rates associated with AKI remain high.[4] Therapeutic intervention trials for AKI have had disappointing results in part related to delays in diagnosis, as well as the heterogeneity of patients enrolled.[10,11] The focus is therefore on earlier recognition and intervention for AKI, which should provide greater potential for recovery and/or stabilization of renal function. However, the early detection of incipient AKI is severely limited by the lack of sensitive and specific tools currently available to assess renal function.

Assessment of Glomerular Function and Injury

Glomerular filtration rate (GFR) is considered the best overall indicator of kidney function but remains challenging to accurately and efficiently measure in clinical practice. Functionally, the total kidney GFR is determined by the cumulative number of nephrons and the GFR within each nephron (single nephron glomerular filtration rate, or SNGFR). Conceptually, it represents the volume of plasma that could be completely cleared of a substance per unit of time. Kidney function may therefore decline due to hypoperfusion, resulting in a decrease in SNGFR, or due to nephron injury, resulting in fewer functioning nephrons; often both factors are present. The kidney has

TABLE 74.1   KDIGO Acute Kidney Injury Criteria

Stage	Change in Serum Creatinine	Urine Output
1	↑ ≥0.3 mg/dL over 48 h or ↑ 150%-200% over 7 days	<0.5 mL/kg/h for 8 h
2	↑ ≥200-300%	<0.5 mL/kg/h for 16 h
3	↑ ≥300%, S cr ≥4 mg/dL, or dialysis or eGFR ≤35 mL/min/1.73 m^2 for pts <18 yo	<0.5 mL/kg/h for 24 h or anuria for 12 h

From Kidney Disease: Improving Global Outcomes (KDIGO). Acute Kidney Injury Work Group. KDIGO clinical practice guidelines for acute kidney injury. Kidney Int Suppl. 2012;2:19.

TABLE 74.2   Proposed Neonatal Acute Kidney Injury Classification

Stage	Serum Creatinine	Urine Output
0	No change in S_{cr} or ↑ ≤0.3 mg/dL	≥0.5 mL/kg/h
1	S_{cr} ↑ ≥0.3 mg/dL within 48 h or ↑ ≥1.5-1.9 × reference S_{cr}[a] within 7 days	<0.5 mL/kg/h for 6-12 h
2	S_{cr}↑ ≥2-2.9 × reference S_{cr}[a]	<0.5 mL/kg/h for ≥12 h
3	S_{cr} ↑ ≥3 × reference S_{cr}[a] or S_{cr} ≥2.5 mg/dL[b] or receipt of dialysis	<0.3 mL/kg/h for ≥24 h or anuria for ≥12 h

[a]Baseline S_{cr} is defined as the lowest previous S_{cr} value.
[b]S_{cr} value of 2.5 mg/dL represents <10 mL/min/1.73 m^2.
From Jetton JG and Askenazi DJ. Acute kidney injury in the neonate. Clin Perinatol. 2012;41:487-502.

TABLE 74.3   Normal Glomerular Filtration Rate Values for Children

Age	GFR (mL/min/1.73 m^2)	Range (mL/min/1.73 m^2)
Preterm (<34 wk)		
2-8 days	11	11-15
4-28 days	20	15-28
30-90 days	50	40-65
Term (>34 wk)		
2-8 days	39	17-60
4-28 days	47	26-68
30-90 days	58	30-86
1-6 mo	77	39-114
6-12 mo	103	49-157
12-19 mo	127	62-191
2-12 yr	127	89-165

Modified from Heilbron DC, Holliday MA, al-Dahwi A, et al. Expressing glomerular filtration rate in children. Pediatr Nephrol. 1991;5:5-11.

a certain degree of reserve and attempts to adapt to nephron loss by increasing the SNGFR of the remaining nephrons, thus maintaining total kidney GFR initially and masking early renal injury. Indeed, by the time the GFR actually falls, significant injury has already occurred. Loss of this renal reserve is one of the earliest manifestations of renal injury but is even more challenging to measure than GFR.[12-14]

Glomerular filtration is a dynamic variable that can fluctuate in a given individual by as much as 7% to 8% from day to day on the basis of differences in hydration status, activity, and protein consumption.[15,16] GFR is also influenced by age, gender, and body size and therefore varies between individuals as well. Therefore to facilitate comparison of GFR among children and adults of considerably different size, absolute GFR is normalized to body surface area (BSA), which correlates well with kidney weight, the most direct standard of reference.[17] Appreciation of the maturational increase in GFR that occurs during infancy is also necessary for proper assessment of kidney function in children. At birth, the mean GFR is quite low (20 mL/min/1.73 m^2 in term infants) due to renal immaturity yet sufficient to meet the metabolic demands of a healthy infant. The GFR doubles within the first 2 weeks of life and then continues to gradually increase to reach a mean of 77 mL/min/1.73 m^2 between 1 and 6 months of age and

adult levels of 120 to 130 mL/min/1.73 m^2 by approximately 2 years of age (Table 74.3).[18]

GFR itself cannot be directly measured but can be assessed by measuring the clearance of an ideal filtration marker or estimated using predictive formulas. Urinary or plasma clearance studies provide the greatest accuracy but are expensive, time consuming, and labor intensive. Consequently, they are used mainly for research and in select clinical situations where an accurate assessment of kidney function is necessary (eg, chemotherapy dosing). For the daily clinical management of patients, serum creatinine and GFR estimating equations are used most commonly. They offer the advantage of being convenient, noninvasive, and inexpensive with timely accessibility of results. However, accuracy and sensitivity to small changes in renal function are sacrificed, making the detection of acute, early renal dysfunction difficult. The search for novel biomarkers of renal function (such as cystatin C) and early renal injury (eg, neutrophil gelatinase-associated lipocalin [NGAL]) has therefore been a major focus in the field of AKI.

Renal Clearance Techniques
Inulin

The renal clearance of inulin remains the gold standard for measuring GFR. Inulin is an inert, uncharged 5.2-kDa polymer of fructose that possesses many characteristics of an ideal filtration marker. It is not protein bound and is freely filtered at the glomerulus without being reabsorbed, secreted, or metabolized by the kidney. Further, it is eliminated exclusively by the kidney.[19] In the steady state the filtered load of inulin (GFR × P_{in}) is therefore equal to its urinary excretion (U_{in} × V) where P_{in} and U_{in} are the plasma and urine concentrations of inulin (mg/dL), respectively, and V is the urine flow rate (mL/min). The renal clearance of inulin (C_{in}) can be calculated:

$$C_{in} = GFR = (U_{in} \times V)/P_{in} \qquad \text{Eq. 74.1}$$

C_{in} is usually scaled for BSA:

$$C_{in} = GFR = [(U_{in} \times V)/P_{in}] \times [1.73\,m^2/BSA] \qquad \text{Eq. 74.2}$$

The classic protocol for inulin clearance is cumbersome, involving an intravenous infusion of inulin over several hours and serial timed blood and urine specimens. Properly done, inulin clearances provide the most accurate measure of GFR; however, the complexity of the protocol introduces a potential for significant error. Incomplete urine collections diminish the accuracy of the test and can be particularly problematic in children who are not yet toilet-trained or who have urologic disease (eg, vesicoureteral reflux, bladder dyssynergia) affecting their ability to spontaneously void to completion. Placement of a bladder catheter or use of a bladder scanner may improve accuracy, although the former may pose a small risk of infection and the latter may be of limited benefit in children with vesicoureteral reflux. Limited availability of inulin, technical issues pertaining to its assay, and the laborious nature of the protocol make it impractical for routine clinical use.

Iothalamate

Iothalamate (614 Da) is also freely filtered by the glomerulus and has been studied extensively as an alternative exogenous marker for GFR measurements. Unlike inulin, however, iothalamate has some protein binding (<8%) and proximal tubular secretion (10%), raising concern for overestimation of GFR. Reported correlations between iothalamate and inulin renal clearances in the literature have been variable, with some studies demonstrating good correlation, whereas most suggest that iothalamate overestimates inulin clearance.[20-22]

Creatinine Clearance

Clearance studies that make use of endogenous markers such as serum creatinine obviate the need for a constant infusion and make the study more amenable to clinical practice. However, the problems associated with timed urine collections persist and accordingly limit the usefulness of this technique, particularly in children. Further, creatinine is a flawed filtration marker. Although it is predominantly eliminated by glomerular filtration, a small but variable amount (~10%) is eliminated by tubular secretion. As renal function deteriorates, the proportion of secreted to filtered creatinine progressively increases, leading to an overestimation of GFR and a less reliable measure of GFR.[16] Administration of oral cimetidine beginning 2 days before the study can at least partially circumvent this issue by inhibiting the tubular secretion of creatinine.[23] Although timed urine collections are still necessary, they are typically obtained over a 2-hour period facilitating performance in a monitored clinic setting.

Guidelines from the National Kidney Foundation no longer recommend routine performance of creatinine clearance studies to estimate GFR, as prediction formulas are considered more accurate.[24] Nonetheless, creatinine clearance-based studies can still be helpful when assessing renal function in individuals with atypical body composition (eg, anorexia, malnutrition) or dietary intake (eg, vegetarian diet).[24,25]

Plasma Disappearance Techniques

Plasma disappearance techniques further simplify the measurement of GFR and avoid the need for urine collections. They are most commonly performed using a single intravenous injection technique, although constant infusion and subcutaneous protocols are also available.[20,26,27] Serial blood samples collected at specified times over a several-hour period following injection of the filtration marker are used to generate a plasma disappearance curve. This curve can be well approximated by a double exponential curve that is characterized by an initial "fast" curve and a later "slow" curve as illustrated in Fig. 74.1. The initial "fast" curve represents the distribution phase and reflects renal elimination, as well as diffusion of the marker into the extravascular space, whereas the late "slow" curve reflects only the renal elimination phase. Renal clearance can be calculated by dividing the delivered dose by the entire area under the plasma disappearance curve.[28] Modification from a two-compartment model to a one-compartment model focusing on the renal elimination phase simplifies the procedure, reducing the number of required blood specimens to two. GFR can then be derived from the slope of the slow curve but requires incorporation

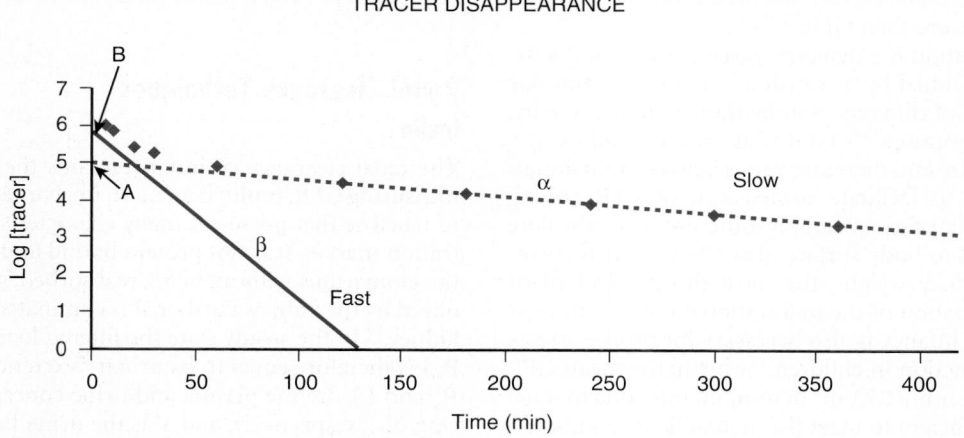

TRACER DISAPPEARANCE

Fig. 74.1. Plasma disappearance of filtration marker as a function of time after injection into blood. The curve is composed of two components: the slow curve with slope α and intercept A and the fast curve with slope β and intercept B. (Modified from Schwartz GJ, Furth SL. Glomerular filtration rate measurement and estimation in chronic kidney disease. Pediatr Nephrol. 2007;22:1839-1848.)

of a correction factor to compensate for overestimation of the GFR, which results from exclusion of the area under the fast curve.[28-31] Appropriate timing of the specimens is critical to ensure an accurate estimation of GFR. The first sample must be obtained after the marker has equilibrated, typically 2 hours after injection. The second specimen is obtained approximately 5 hours after injection, but in subjects with more advanced chronic kidney disease (CKD), this may need to be delayed further to minimize overestimation of the GFR, which can result from an inaccurate depiction of the lower slope of the plasma disappearance curve.[30] The validity of the single-compartment model may also be compromised in edematous states where the volume of distribution is increased, or with extravasation of the tracer at the injection site, as this decreases the actual dose delivered.[29] Although plasma disappearance studies are time consuming and too complex for routine clinical care, they are useful in cases for which GFR estimates do not appear to be accurate.

Radioisotopes

Plasma clearance studies are most commonly performed with radioisotopes that are more readily available and easier to assay than inulin. Their major disadvantage is, of course, radiation exposure, which limits their use, particularly in children.[32] ^{51}Cr-ethylenediaminetetraacetic acid (EDTA), ^{99m}Tc-DTPA, and ^{125}I-Iothalamate have been extensively studied and compared with inulin renal clearance.[20,33] All are low-molecular-weight compounds that are freely filtered by the glomerulus but differ slightly in protein binding and renal disposition. ^{51}Cr-EDTA (292 Da) appears to have little protein binding, and its plasma clearance correlates well with inulin clearances. It is commonly used in Europe but unavailable in the United States.[30] ^{99m}Tc-DTPA (393 Da) is most frequently used in the United States but demonstrates variable accuracy in GFR measurements on the basis of product source, differences in protein binding, and potential dissociation of the chelate ($t_{1/2}$ = 6 hours) during the study.[34] ^{125}I-Iothalamate (614 Da) is a high-osmolar anionic contrast agent with some protein binding that also undergoes active secretion by the proximal tubule, contributing to overestimation of plasma clearance compared with inulin or EDTA.[22] Nuclear GFR studies can also be performed using a gamma camera, which measures the renal uptake of the tracer 2 to 3 minutes after injection and can provide information regarding differential kidney function; however, the estimated GFR obtained this way is not as accurate as with the plasma-sampling technique.[30] To reduce radiation exposure, plasma clearance studies can also be performed using nonradiolabeled iothalamate, which can be measured by high-performance liquid chromatography (HPLC).[35,36]

Iohexol

Iohexol is now widely accepted as an excellent alternative to inulin and radioisotopes for clearance studies. Iohexol (Omnipaque) is a low-molecular-weight (821 Da), nonionic, relatively low-osmolar intravenous contrast agent used routinely in the United States for radiologic studies at doses appreciably higher than that required for GFR studies.[37,38] It is almost entirely eliminated through glomerular filtration and is not reabsorbed, secreted, or metabolized by the kidney, thus fulfilling many of the desired traits of an ideal filtration marker. Further, it has minimal protein binding and negligible

extrarenal elimination even in advanced chronic kidney failure.[37,39] It can easily be measured by high-performance liquid chromatography or mass spectroscopy.[38,40-42] Iohexol has been safely used for clearance studies for many years in Scandinavia[37,43,44] and the United States.[31,45] Iohexol plasma clearance results appear to be comparable with renal inulin clearance and plasma EDTA disappearance studies across a broad range of GFR.[38,46,47] Schwartz et al.[48,49] recently demonstrated the feasibility of conducting iohexol clearance studies using the finger prick technique with filter paper technology in adults, a procedure which would alleviate the need for repeated venipunctures or placement of a second IV from which to collect serum samples making it attractive for use in children.[48] However, additional studies are necessary before it is ready for widespread clinical use.

Renal Inulin Clearance Compared With Other GFR Measurement Techniques

Soveri et al.[50] recently performed a comprehensive, systematic literature review examining the accuracy of GFR measurement techniques using renal inulin clearance as the gold standard. The renal clearance of EDTA and iothalamate, as well as the plasma disappearance of EDTA and iohexol, were considered suitable alternatives with an associated bias less than 10% (mean difference between renal inulin clearance and that obtained using other techniques), P_{30} >80% and P_{10} >50% (percentage of GFR measurements within 30% and 10%, respectively, of inulin GFR). Creatinine clearance was not accurate and there was insufficient data to accurately assess the use of the plasma clearance of DTPA.[50]

Plasma Markers
Creatinine

Serum creatinine is the most commonly used laboratory study to assess renal function in clinical practice. It is simple, convenient, and practical—requiring a single blood sample—and therefore well suited for serial examination. However, the relationship between serum creatinine and GFR is quite complex, being influenced by several factors other than GFR. Therefore, at best, creatinine provides a crude estimate of the GFR. As illustrated in Fig. 74.2, serum creatinine bears an inverse, nonlinear relationship with GFR and lacks sensitivity to acute and small changes in GFR. Notably, at low levels of serum creatinine corresponding to normal renal function, a substantial decrease in GFR may occur before being reflected by even a small increase in serum creatinine. In contrast, at higher levels of serum creatinine associated with renal failure, the same absolute rise in creatinine reflects a much smaller loss of remaining renal function. To a first approximation, every doubling of the serum creatinine represents a 50% decline in remaining GFR.

Ideally, an endogenous marker such as creatinine can serve as a useful surrogate for GFR if it is produced at a constant rate and eliminated only via the kidney at a rate equivalent to its production rate such that a steady state exists. Fig. 74.3 illustrates the relationship between the plasma level of an endogenous filtration marker, its generation (from cells and diet), and its elimination (renal and extrarenal). The serum level of the marker would then be expected to rise with renal impairment. Serum creatinine, however, does not strictly fulfill these criteria. Although creatinine production is relatively constant, it varies among and within individuals.[51] It is derived from the nonenzymatic dehydration of muscle creatine and hence is highly dependent on muscle mass. Consequently, in children, creatinine generation is affected by growth in addition to diet and illness, as seen with adults.[51] The reference range for serum creatinine levels representing normal GFR will thus vary with age, size, and gender after puberty. The relationship between GFR and serum creatinine is therefore particularly complex in children. Maturational changes in serum creatinine and GFR do not parallel one another. GFR is physiologically low at birth, whereas serum creatinine is elevated; however, because of fetal-maternal-placental equilibration of creatinine, the elevated creatinine is not indicative of the infant's renal function but rather the mother's. Following birth, GFR steadily increases, reaching adult levels over the next 2 years. Serum creatinine, on the other hand, declines over the first few weeks, becoming reflective of the infant's renal function. The creatinine level then remains stable until approximately 2 years of age as muscle mass accrues proportionally to the increase in GFR. Beyond 2 years of age, when GFR per BSA has fully matured, the ongoing accretion of muscle results in a progressive rise in serum creatinine until adolescence, when adult levels are achieved (0.7 mg/dL for adolescent females and 0.9 mg/dL for adolescent males). Superimposition of a severe or chronic illness associated with malnutrition and muscle wasting makes the interpretation of GFR from serum creatinine alone even more difficult in the pediatric patient. For example, at first glance, maintenance of a stable creatinine in a patient with a prolonged ICU course may be reassuring for preservation of renal function; however, if significant muscle atrophy has occurred, this actually suggests deterioration of renal function. In the steady state when height is used as a surrogate for growth, there is a strong correlation of the parameter Ht/S_{Cr} and GFR.[52-54]

The second requirement, that excretion of the marker occurs only by glomerular filtration, is also flawed in the case of creatinine. Although the majority of serum creatinine is eliminated by glomerular filtration, a small but unpredictable amount is eliminated by tubular secretion and gastrointestinal degradation. Proximal tubular secretion of creatinine typically accounts for approximately 10% of its elimination, although considerable interindividual and intraindividual variability exist.[55] At normal levels of GFR, the impact of tubular secretion on GFR is minimal. However, with deteriorating renal

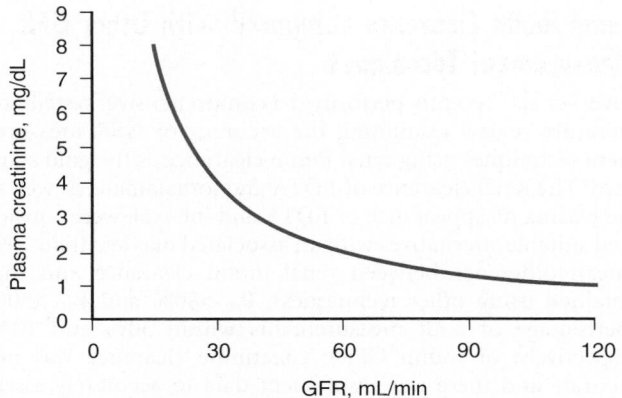

Fig. 74.2. Idealized relation between the steady-state levels of serum creatinine and glomerular filtration rate (GFR) in adults. When renal function is normal, a marked decrease in GFR can be associated with only a mild increase in serum creatinine.

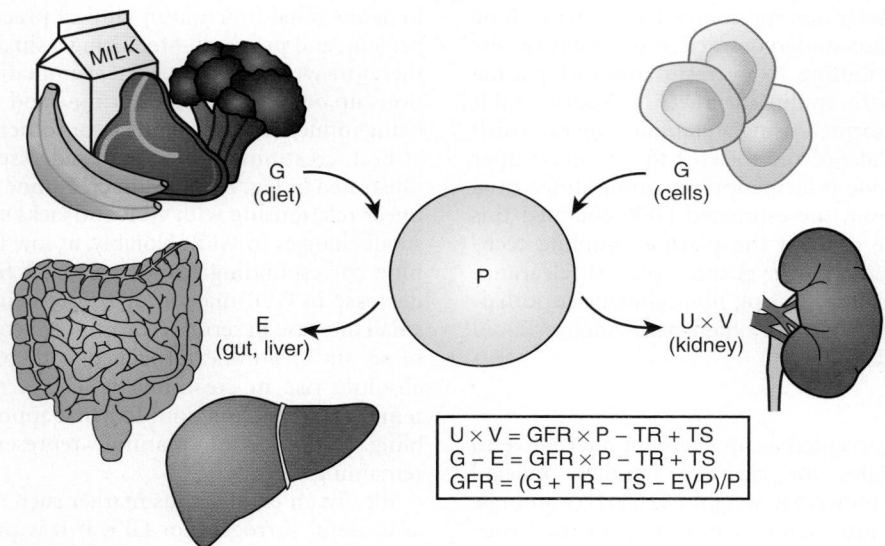

$$U \times V = GFR \times P - TR + TS$$
$$G - E = GFR \times P - TR + TS$$
$$GFR = (G + TR - TS - EVP)/P$$

Fig. 74.3. Determinants of the serum level of endogenous filtration markers. The plasma level *(P)* of an endogenous filtration marker is determined by its generation *(G)* from cells and diet, extrarenal elimination *(E)* by gut and liver, and urinary excretion *(U + V)* by the kidney. Urinary excretion is the sum of filtered load *(GFR × P)*, tubular secretion *(TS)*, and reabsorption *(TR)*. In the steady state, urinary excretion equals generation minus extrarenal elimination. By substitution and rearrangement, GFR can be expressed as the ratio of the non-GFR determinants (G, TS, TR, and E) to the plasma level. (Modified from Stevens LA and Levey AS. Measured GFR as a confirmatory test for estimated GFR. J Am Soc Nephrol. 2009;20:2305-2313.)

function, the proportion of secreted versus filtered creatinine increases, resulting in a lower serum creatinine than predicted for the true level of GFR, thus decreasing the sensitivity for serum creatinine to detect mild decreases in renal function.[55] A similar phenomenon occurs in the setting of moderate-to-severe renal failure, when the bacterial degradation of creatinine within the gastrointestinal tract can become clinically significant, leading to a decrease in serum creatinine concentration.[56,57] Failure to recognize the influence of tubular secretion and gastrointestinal elimination on serum creatinine values can result in overestimation of renal function and may lead to higher, inappropriate dosing of medications. Conversely, in patients with advanced kidney failure, administration of medications (eg, cimetidine, trimethoprim) that inhibit the tubular secretion of creatinine or administration of antibiotics that mitigate the gastrointestinal degradation of creatinine may result in an elevation of serum creatinine and subsequent underestimation of GFR without any true change in renal function. If not appreciated, this may be misconstrued as worsening renal function and lead to potential underdosing of medications.

Third, the requirement for a steady state cannot be overemphasized. When GFR abruptly declines with AKI, the production rate of creatinine exceeds its clearance rate leading to a gradual rise in serum creatinine that lags behind the true GFR (Fig. 74.4). During this period, serum creatinine does not accurately reflect the true GFR. Nonetheless, serum creatinine is still typically used to estimate renal function as better alternatives do not currently exist. However, use of the serum creatinine or creatinine-based estimating equations (see later) to estimate GFR before the establishment of a new steady state will result in overestimation of the renal function. Similarly, during the recovery phase of AKI, serum creatinine will underestimate GFR as it will again lag behind the true GFR until the kidney clears the accumulated creatinine and reaches a new steady state.

Finally, analytic factors related to the creatinine assay itself provide another potential source of error when assessing GFR.

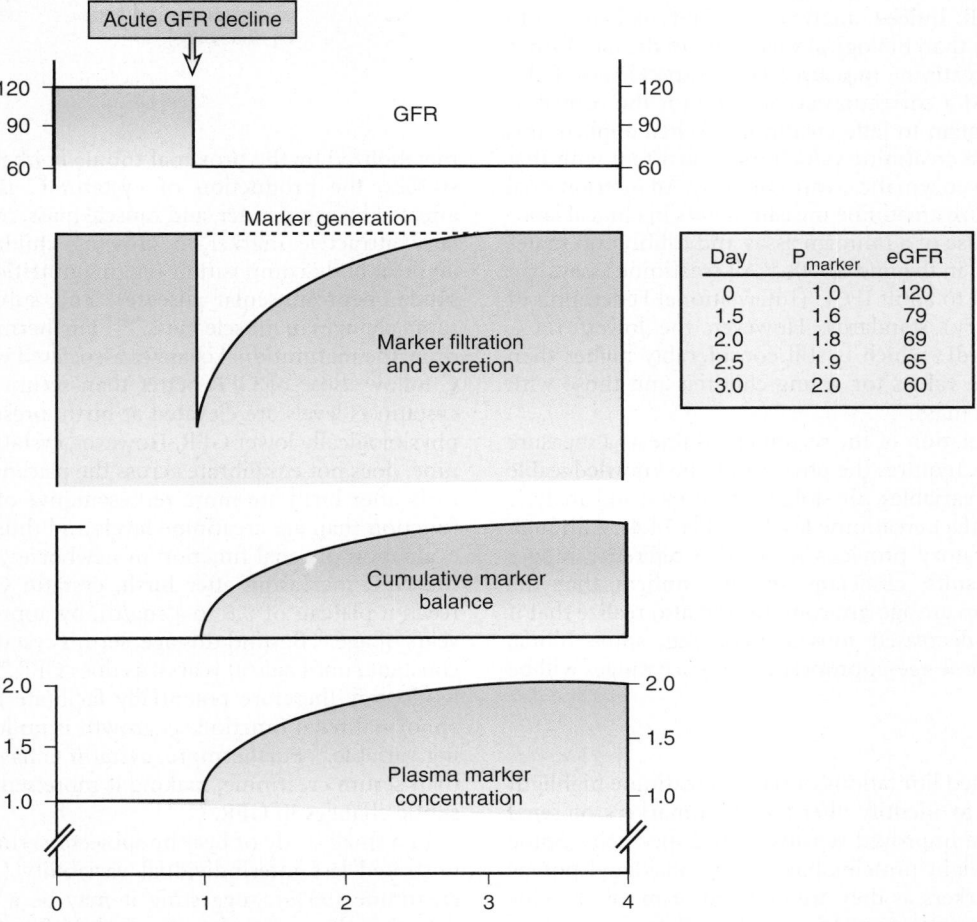

Day	P_marker	eGFR
0	1.0	120
1.5	1.6	79
2.0	1.8	69
2.5	1.9	65
3.0	2.0	60

Fig. 74.4. Following an acute decline in glomerular filtration rate (GFR), filtration and excretion of an endogenous marker (eg, creatinine) decrease while production of the marker remains constant, leading to a gradual rise in serum marker concentration over several days. During this period, use of the serum level of the marker to assess GFR will result in an overestimate, as illustrated earlier (where eGFR is expressed in mL/min/1.73 m²). The increase in serum marker level results in a higher filtered load until a new steady state is achieved, such that the production and filtration rates of the marker are again equivalent, assuming tubular secretion and extrarenal elimination are negligible. Once a new steady state is achieved, eGFR approaches GFR. (Modified from Stevens LA, Levey AS: Measured GFR as a confirmatory test for estimated GFR. J Am Soc Nephrol. 2009;20:2305-2313; and Kassirer JP. Current concepts: clinical evaluation of kidney function: glomerular function. N Engl J Med. 1971;285:385-389.)

True creatinine levels can be measured by isotope dilution mass spectroscopy (IDMS) or HPLC, but these are expensive and not readily available for routine clinical use.[58] Enzymatic creatinine assays, now available in many laboratories, exhibit greater specificity for creatinine than the conventional Jaffe (alkaline picrate) assay resulting in 10% to 30% lower creatinine levels. Enzymatic creatinine levels approximate high-performance liquid chromatography (HPLC) values but can differ in their performance, some being more influenced by interfering substances than others. Although problems with accuracy and precision still persist, the coefficient of variation using new autoanalyzers is now approximately 3% and significantly lower than for the Jaffe assay.[51,59] Nonetheless, according to the 2007 College of American Pathologists, many laboratories continue to use a modified version of the Jaffe assay because it is less expensive than enzymatic assays.[60] The Jaffe method, based on an alkaline picrate colorimetric reaction, tends to falsely elevate the true creatinine by up to 20% (for creatinine ~1 mg/dL) due to the presence of interfering, noncreatinine chromagens, the most significant of which is serum total protein.[61] This effect is greatest at the lower levels of creatinine typically observed in infants and children.[62] By falsely elevating the true creatinine, the Jaffe creatinine underestimates the GFR. Indeed, analytic variability is believed to play a greater role than biological variability in the day-to-day fluctuations of creatinine measurements.[51] Speeckaert et al.[61] recently published a correction accounting for the contribution of serum protein to Jaffe creatinines. When applied, this correction yields a creatinine value more consistent with that obtained using an enzymatic creatinine assay. An international effort to standardize creatinine measurements in clinical laboratories through use of a uniform assay and calibration materials was launched in the mid-2000s.[63] All creatinine assays can now be calibrated to adult IFCC (International Federation of Clinical Chemistry) standards. However, the lowest IFCC standard is 1 mg/dL, which is still considerably higher than normal creatinine values for young children and those with decreased muscle mass.[58]

Proper interpretation of the serum creatinine as a measure of GFR, therefore, requires the physician to be knowledgeable about the clinical variables, physiologic processes, and analytic factors that can affect creatinine levels (Table 74.4). Although the clinical laboratory provides normative reference ranges alongside the results, clinicians should confirm that the reported references are age-appropriate and also realize that if the patient has decreased muscle mass (eg, spina bifida, anorexia), even these age-appropriate reference ranges will be incorrect.

Cystatin C

The well-established limitations of serum creatinine highlight the critical need to identify alternative biomarkers of renal function that have improved sensitivity and specificity. Some low-molecular-weight proteins have been considered potential candidate markers as they are excreted primarily by glomerular filtration and are produced at a relatively constant rate. Several low-molecular-weight proteins have been considered but cystatin C, a 13-kDa cationic cysteine protease inhibitor produced at a constant rate by all nucleated cells, has shown the greatest promise. Like creatinine, it is freely filtered at the glomerulus[64] but, unlike serum creatinine, it is not secreted by the tubules; rather, it is completely reabsorbed and

	SERUM CREATININE LEVEL	
Factor	**Increase**	**Decrease**
Affecting creatinine generation	Age (infancy through adolescence)	Chronic illness; anorexia, malnutrition; neuromuscular disease (spina bifida, muscular dystrophy); liver disease
	Male gender (after puberty)	Body habitus (amputation)
	Body habitus (muscular)	Diet (vegetarian)
	Diet; consumption of cooked meat; creatine supplements	
Affecting creatinine elimination	Impaired tubular secretion (trimethoprim, cimetidine)	Tubular secretion
	Impaired extrarenal elimination (sterilization of gastrointestinal flora by antibiotics)	Extrarenal elimination (gastrointestinal degradation)

TABLE 74.4 Non–Glomerular Filtration Rate Factors Affecting Creatinine Levels in Children

metabolized by the proximal tubule epithelial cells.[65] In most studies, the production of cystatin C is not significantly affected by age, gender, and muscle mass, making it a particularly attractive marker in growing children, subjects with atypical body composition (eg, malnutrition, anorexia, spina bifida, neuromuscular disease), and subjects experiencing rapid changes in muscle mass.[66-68] Furthermore, in young children, the maturational changes associated with serum cystatin C follow those of GFR better than serum creatinine. Serum cystatin C levels are elevated at birth, presumably due to the physiologically lower GFR. However, cystatin C, unlike creatinine, does not equilibrate across the placenta; hence the levels early after birth are more representative of the infant's renal function than are creatinine levels and thus may facilitate the evaluation of renal function in newborns.[69] Concurrent with the GFR increasing after birth, cystatin C levels decline to reach a plateau of 0.8 to 1 mg/dL by approximately 1.5 to 2 years of age.[70] Beyond this age, serum cystatin C levels remain constant (until age 50 years), as does GFR.[66] Serum cystatin C levels may therefore potentially facilitate the recognition of abnormal renal function, as growth is no longer a confounding variable.[68] Furthermore, cystatin C has a shorter half-life than serum creatinine, making it more sensitive to acute and subtle changes in GFR.[71,72]

In a small study of healthy subjects, serum cystatin C demonstrated less interindividual variability (25%) than serum creatinine (93%), suggesting it may be a better marker for detecting the onset of acute renal dysfunction. However, the intraindividual variability greatly exceeded that of serum creatinine, limiting its usefulness to monitor the progression of CKD.[73]

Studies comparing the use of cystatin C to serum creatinine as a diagnostic marker of kidney function have yielded conflicting results. Nonetheless, two meta-analyses including adult and pediatric studies suggest cystatin C is superior or equivalent to serum creatinine as a marker of renal function.[74,75] Specifically, cystatin C may be advantageous in populations with low or atypical muscle mass (eg, spina bifida)[76,77] and mild renal impairment.[78] Changes in serum cystatin C levels may also potentially allow earlier detection of AKI. Herget-Rosenthal[79] found that cystatin C levels rose 1 to 2 days earlier than serum creatinine in critically ill adults with AKI. A meta-analysis in 2011 involving mainly adults concluded that serum cystatin C seems to be a good predictor of AKI.[80] However, more recent studies in children have yielded conflicting results.[81,82] Further investigation regarding the use of cystatin C to predict and define AKI is clearly necessary.

Although promising, cystatin C also has limitations for estimating GFR. Cystatin C levels can be affected by several potentially confounding variables including age, gender, race,[83] obesity,[84] nonrenal elimination,[85] glucocorticoids,[70] and thyroid dysfunction,[70] as well as differences in cystatin C assays.[86] At least two automated immunoassays are available (particle-enhanced turbidimetric immunoassay [PETIA] and particle-enhanced nephelometric immunoassay [PENIA]) but differ by as much as 20% to 30% in reported values.[86] Nephelometry is more sensitive than turbidimetry, particularly when dilute solutions are assayed.[53,87] Standardized reference materials for cystatin C became available in 2010, following which an international effort to standardize cystatin C measurements has been launched.[88-90] Because cystatin C is completely reabsorbed by the proximal tubular cells, urinary clearance studies are not possible. However, cystatin C has been noted in the urine of patients with glomerular and tubular disease, raising questions about its accuracy in estimating GFR.[91]

Estimating Equations

Empiric formulas (Cockcroft-Gault for adults; Schwartz and Counahan-Barratt for children) were first developed in the 1970s to enhance the physician's ability to estimate GFR (eGFR) and, in particular, to facilitate the recognition of chronic renal impairment.[92-94] This is especially helpful in children for whom the serum creatinine corresponding to normal renal function progressively increases during childhood until adult levels are achieved during adolescence. The equations were developed in CKD populations and based on serum creatinine but incorporate clinical variables such as height, weight, age, and gender as surrogates for muscle mass. However, because they are creatinine based, they are subject to some of the same constraints as use of serum creatinine alone; for example, tubular creatinine secretion and technical issues related to the creatinine assay itself will influence eGFR results. Nonetheless, these equations perform better than serum creatinine alone. Current national guidelines now recommend that estimated GFR (eGFR) be routinely reported alongside the creatinine value using the 2009 CKD-EPI (Chronic Kidney Disease Epidemiology Collaboration) formula for adults and the updated "bedside" Schwartz formula for children. Both formulas were developed using creatinine measurements calibrated to be traceable to an IDMS reference standard.[95] Within the past decade, routine reporting of eGFR has been implemented for adults but has been more challenging to implement for children because the equation is based on height, a parameter not routinely

available in the laboratory electronic medical record.[71] According to the College of American Pathologists, as of 2013, 90% of laboratories surveyed were reporting eGFR along with creatinine for adults but less than 10% of laboratories surveyed were reporting eGFR for children.[96]

The ideal GFR estimating equation would be based on a standardized creatinine measurement, applicable across the full spectrum of renal function, and generalizable to a diverse population. In 2009, the CKD-EPI creatinine equation was developed using standardized creatinine measurements in a diverse population of adults with and without renal dysfunction. This was a substantial improvement over the 2006 MDRD (Modification of Diet in Renal Disease) equation, which was developed in adults with moderate CKD (GFR <60 mL/min/1.73 m^2) and therefore systematically underestimated eGFR in patients with normal renal function or mild CKD.[97] Limited studies assessing the application of these adult formulas in children have shown them to be inaccurate.[98-101]

In pediatrics, the Schwartz formula has been most commonly used to predict GFR. The original Schwartz formula was developed in the 1970s and based on a modified Jaffe creatinine, using inulin clearance as the reference standard. GFR is related to serum creatinine, using length as a surrogate for muscle mass and an empiric constant to account for age- and gender-related differences in body composition:

$$eGFR = k \times L/S_{Cr} \qquad \text{Eq. 74.3}$$

where *eGFR* is estimated GFR in mL/min/1.73 m^2, *L* is length in cm, S_{Cr} is serum creatinine in mg/dL, and *k* is an empiric constant (ie, 0.45 for term infants through the first year of life, 0.55 for children and adolescent females, and 0.7 for adolescent males).[62,94] The simplicity of the formula makes it convenient and practical for use at the bedside, although knowledge of the patient's height is required. Counahan-Barratt developed a similar formula using ^{51}Cr-EDTA plasma disappearance as the reference standard.[93] This formula, however, uses a single constant with a lower value, attributed to a difference in creatinine assays:

$$eGFR \,(mL/min/1.73\,m^2) = 0.43 \times L/S_{Cr} \qquad \text{Eq. 74.4}$$

It is now well recognized that Schwartz's original formula systematically overestimates GFR, most likely due to a change in creatinine methodology over the years from the Jaffe assay to an IDMS referenced enzymatic assay.[45] As noted earlier, enzymatic creatinine levels in infants and children tend to run lower than Jaffe creatinine levels.

In 2009 using data from the CKiD Study (Chronic Kidney Disease in Children Study), Schwartz et al. developed an updated "bedside" formula on the basis of an IDMS traceable enzymatic creatinine assay using the plasma disappearance of iohexol as the reference standard:

$$eGFR = 0.413 \times L/S_{Cr} \qquad \text{Eq. 74.5}$$

where length is in centimeters and serum creatinine is in mg/dL.[52] Notably, this is the first multicenter study to generate an estimating formula in children with moderate CKD (GFR range 15–75 mL/min/1.73 m^2). Using the updated Schwartz formula, approximately 80% of eGFR values fell within 30% of the GFR measured by iohexol plasma disappearance and 37% fell within 10%.[71] However, similar to the situation with the MDRD equation developed in adults with CKD, the accuracy of the updated bedside Schwartz equation in predicting eGFR for children with mild CKD or normal renal function is unclear.[52] In a cohort of children who had measured GFRs by inulin ranging from 17 to 150 mL/min/1.73 m^2, Gao et al.[102] found the Schwartz formula performed well within the GFR range (15–103 mL/min/1.73 m^2) but overestimated GFR at higher levels of measured GFR. Staples et al.[103] compared the updated Schwartz formula with GFRs measured by iothalamate in a broad pediatric range and found good agreement, even at higher levels of GFR. Other investigators have found the updated Schwartz formula does not perform as well when renal function is normal, but the direction of bias varied by study.[101,103,104]

Other pediatric estimating formulas have been proposed in the past decade.[105,106] Some are considerably more complex, not more accurate, and not easily used at the bedside.[105,106] Pottel's group[107] recently developed an estimating equation for children on the basis of a population normalized serum creatinine value Q (average creatinine for healthy children of a specific age) generated from a large Belgian hospital database:

$$eGFR = 107.3/(S_{Cr}/Q) \qquad \text{Eq. 74.6}$$

Using the concept of a population normalized serum creatinine, they developed and validated two new eGFR equations for use in children, adolescents, and young adults.[108] In one, Q is based on height (Q_{height}), whereas in the other, Q is height independent and based on age and gender (Q_{age}). Though both equations have been validated in a Belgian cohort, the Q_{height}-based equation was more accurate across all ages and levels of renal function; it also performed better in underweight subjects, further supporting the premise that height can be used as a good surrogate for muscle mass. The height-independent Q_{age}-based equation, however, may potentially allow development of a screening tool for renal dysfunction in children.[54] Further studies are necessary to assess the applicability of this formula and validity of the technique in other pediatric populations.

Given the limitations of creatinine, cystatin C–based GFR-estimating equations have also been developed in an effort to improve accuracy. Several have been published for use in both adults and children.[90,97,105,109] They vary in accuracy and precision but appear at least as good as the creatinine-based equation[97] for the general population. In high-risk populations with reduced muscle mass such as oncology patients, hematopoietic stem cell transplant recipients, spina bifida/muscular dystrophy, and spinal cord injury patients, cystatin C–based formulas seem to more accurately estimate the measured GFR than creatinine-based equations.[76,110-113] However, cystatin C is not readily available in many hospital laboratories, it is more expensive, and assays have not been standardized in the United States.[70] Incorporation of both creatinine and cystatin C into the estimating formula appears to provide a better estimate than either one alone.[54,97] Using data from the CKiD study, Schwartz et al.[53] developed a new multivariate eGFR equation incorporating both cystatin C and serum creatinine in addition to height, BUN, and gender:

$$eGFR = 39.8 \times [\text{height (m)}/S_{Cr} \text{ (mg/dL)}]^{0.456}$$
$$\times [1.8/\text{cystatin C (mg/dL)}]^{0.418} \times [30/\text{BUN (mg/dL)}]^{0.079}$$
$$\times [1.076]^{gender} \times [\text{height (m)}/1.4]^{0.179}$$

$$\text{Eq. 74.7}$$

where *gender* = 1 for male and 0 for female. Using this formula, over 90% of the eGFRs were within 30% of the GFR measured by iohexol, the reference standard for this study, and 48% were within 10%.[52,53] The equation is valid in the range of 15 to 75 mL/min/1.73 m^2 and uses a standardized creatinine measurement and nephelometric assay for cystatin C.[53] The cystatin C values have not yet been referenced to an IFCC calibration. A bedside cystatin C formula has also been generated, eGFR = 70.69 × [cystatin C]$^{-0.931}$, to facilitate use in the clinical setting.[53]

Summary of Recommendations Regarding Use of GFR Estimating Equations

Serum creatinine alone does not reliably indicate renal function and should be replaced by a GFR prediction formula, as this accounts for the non-GFR determinants of serum creatinine. For adults, KDIGO recommends the 2009 CKD-EPI creatinine-based equation be used to routinely assess renal function. For individuals in whom the creatinine-based equation may be inaccurate (eg, malnourished patient), cystatin C and combined cystatin C–creatinine-based estimates are recommended as confirmatory tests. For children, KDIGO recommends use of the updated bedside Schwartz formula (creatinine based). For those in whom a more precise estimate is needed or in whom the use of a creatinine-based formula may be inaccurate, Grubb and CKiD et al.[54] suggest confirmation with a cystatin C–based formula. If the two estimates are similar (within 10%-15% agreement), use of the more complex multivariate cystatin C–creatinine formula provides an estimated GFR, which approximates the measured GFR. If, however, the univariate creatinine-based and cystatin C–based eGFRs are discrepant, a measured GFR is recommended.

Proper use of a GFR estimating formula requires the clinician to be cognizant of the population from which it was derived and its range of measured GFR, as well as the analytes and assay methods used. Finally, it should be reemphasized that none of the GFR estimating equations is truly appropriate for assessing renal function in the non–steady state such as AKI. However, a more suitable alternative does not exist leading to their ongoing use in nonsteady state situations where the imprecision will be even greater.

Neonatal Renal Function

Accurate assessment of renal function is even more challenging in the neonate. Renal clearance and plasma disappearance studies are not practical. The limitations to the interpretation of serum creatinine discussed earlier are further confounded by the unique physiology of newborns. As noted previously, due to maternal-fetal equilibration of creatinine across the placenta, serum creatinine at birth reflects the mother's renal function. For full-term infants, serum creatinine begins falling after birth as GFR increases, resulting in excretion of the maternal load of creatinine. Serum creatinine becomes reflective of the full-term infant's renal function by approximately 1 week of age. On the other hand, premature infants born before the completion of nephrogenesis at 36 weeks gestation have significantly lower GFR at birth than full-term infants and experience a slower maturational increase in GFR, which can result in an initial rise in serum creatinine during the first few days of life.[114] Serum creatinine thus takes longer to become reflective of the preterm infant's renal function. Use of a creatinine-based definition for AKI therefore becomes especially challenging in neonates as renal dysfunction may manifest not only as the traditional rise in serum creatinine but also as a failure for the creatinine to decline at an appropriate rate. Additionally, there are methodologic issues as Jaffe creatinines are less accurate at lower concentrations typical for a neonate.

In this regard, cystatin C may hold more promise as a marker of neonatal renal function. Cystatin C is not thought to equilibrate across the placenta and is therefore considered more reflective of the neonate's renal function from birth.[115] Similar to creatinine, serum cystatin C levels are high at birth but presumably due to a physiologically lower GFR. Levels gradually decline over the next 18 to 24 months to reach a plateau ~0.8 to 1 mg/dL. Reference values for neonatal cystatin C levels are now available for full-term and preterm infants, but studies are limited and small and do not fully document the normal postnatal course.[116,117]

Given the challenges associated with developing estimating equations in neonates, Abitbol et al.[118] sought to validate existing pediatric GFR estimating formulas in the neonatal population making use of historical controls with GFR measured by inulin clearance. Creatinine-based pediatric equations underestimated GFR when applied to neonates, whereas cystatin C–based and the Zappitelli combined cystatin C–creatinine-based equations correlated best with the measured GFR. Treiber et al.[119] recently developed a neonatal cystatin C–based eGFR equation, which incorporates body surface area and kidney volume as measured by renal ultrasound. They also used historic reference values to validate their equation. Additional research in the field of neonatal renal function and AKI is clearly needed.

Other Novel Biomarkers of Acute Kidney Injury Under Investigation

The currently available tools for assessing AKI are inadequate for detecting the onset of renal cellular damage, as well as the onset of renal functional impairment. Advances in molecular biology have significantly enhanced our understanding of the pathogenesis of AKI, leading to the identification of several potential candidate biomarkers for AKI. NGAL is the most extensively studied and one of the most promising.[120] NGAL is a ubiquitous 25-kDa protein bound to gelatinase from human neutrophils and constitutively expressed at low levels in the kidneys, as well as lung, liver, and gastrointestinal tract.[121] Following ischemia and epithelial cell injury such as after cardiac bypass, NGAL expression is upregulated, leading to marked increases in serum and urine NGAL levels that precede a rise in serum creatinine.[122,123] In a heterogeneous group of critically ill children and adults for whom the onset of renal injury is unknown, Zappitelli et al.[124] found that urine NGAL concentrations increased 48 hours before a serum creatinine increase of 50% or more. They also found that sepsis-related AKI was associated with higher urinary NGAL levels than AKI unrelated to sepsis, a finding also confirmed in adults.[125] Urinary NGAL may thus have variable specificity for predicting AKI on the basis of subtype of AKI. Despite this variability, a meta-analysis including adult and pediatric studies concluded that NGAL levels appear to have diagnostic value.[126]

The expression of kidney injury molecule-1 (KIM-1), a transmembrane receptor with unclear function, also appears to be significantly upregulated in proximal tubular cells following ischemic or nephrotoxic injury. After undergoing cleavage, the extracellular domain is shed into the urine, where it can be detected approximately 12 to 24 hours following the injury. Urinary interleukin-18 (IL-18), a proinflammatory cytokine induced in proximal tubular cells following AKI, appears to be more specific to ischemic AKI and other types of acute tubular necrosis than to other forms of acute renal disease (eg, urinary tract infection or prerenal azotemia).[127] Liver-type fatty acid binding protein (L-FABP), another promising new biomarker expressed in several organs including the liver and kidney, is involved with fatty acid metabolism and intracellular signal transduction; it may also play a role in both kidney injury and repair. Expression within the kidney occurs in both normal and disease states. Urine levels of L-FABP have been reported to increase significantly within 6 hours after cardiac surgery in children and adults who subsequently developed AKI by serum creatinine criteria.[128] Significant increases have also been noted in patients developing contrast-induced nephropathy.[128]

The role of biomarkers for diagnosing AKI remains in the preclinical/research stages. It is a promising field as use of novel biomarkers offers the potential to localize the site of injury within the kidney (glomerular vs. tubular), as well as the potential to differentiate subtypes of AKI. Indeed, the use of biomarkers in addition to serum creatinine, the traditional marker for AKI, may lead to a new paradigm for AKI: (1) hemodynamic AKI associated with a decrease in GFR but no structural changes within the kidney, (2) subclinical AKI associated with structural injury to the kidney without any apparent loss of function, and (3) AKI in which structural injury to the kidney is associated with a loss of function[129] (Fig. 74.5).

Tubular Function

Disorders of electrolyte balance, acid-base homeostasis, and volume regulation are also encountered in the ICU and require assessment of renal tubular function. Although the techniques required to assess tubular function may be easier to perform than techniques needed to assess GFR, the interpretation of test results is not always straightforward. Whereas a result may fall within the usual limits reported by the laboratory, this may not represent an appropriate response given the clinical context.

Urine Electrolytes (Sodium and Chloride)

Urine sodium (U_{Na}) and chloride (U_{Cl}) are commonly used to assess intravascular volume status and to help differentiate prerenal azotemia from acute tubular necrosis (ATN). With prerenal azotemia, U_{Na} is typically less than 20 mEq/L and U_{Cl} less than 15 mEq/L as the kidney avidly tries to reclaim sodium, chloride, and water in an effort to restore the extracellular fluid volume, whereas with ATN, the U_{Na} is typically greater than 40 mEq/L due to structural tubular damage. However, overlap can occur as the final concentration of sodium in the urine will depend on not only the amount of sodium reclaimed by the tubules but also the amount of water reabsorbed in the distal tubule under the influence of antidiuretic hormone. Thus the U_{Na} could exceed 20 mEq/L even in a prerenal state, particularly if oliguria is present.

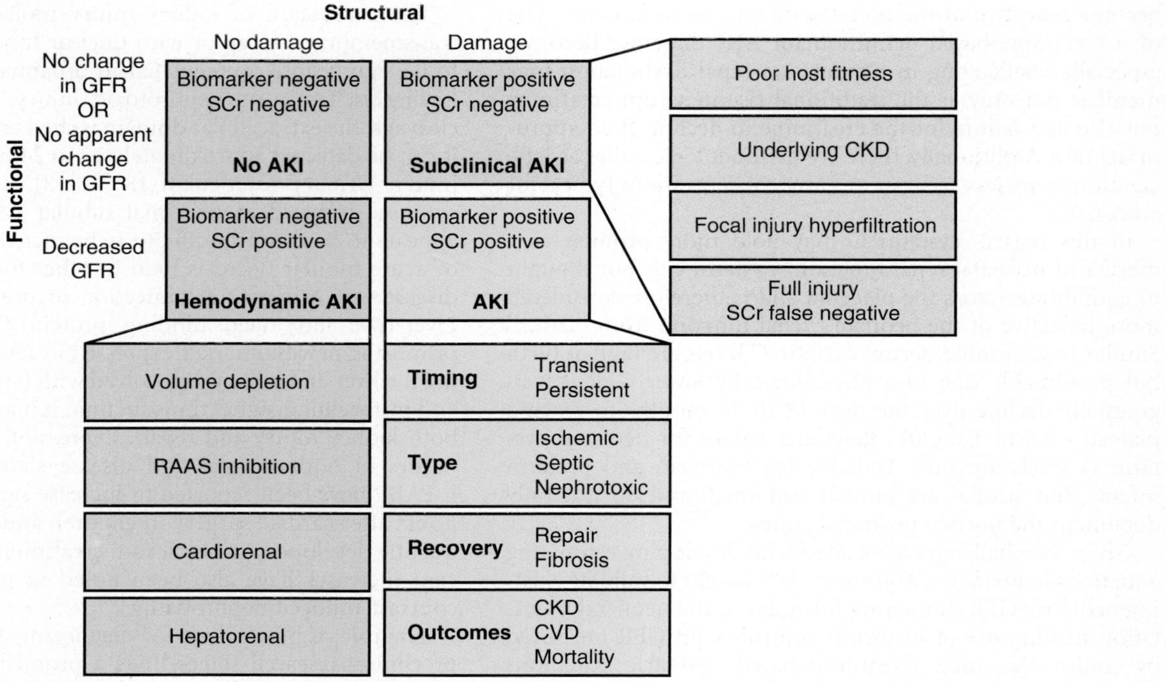

Structural

Fig. 74.5. Phenotyping acute kidney injury (AKI) by biomarkers. Identification of clinically relevant structural kidney damage using biomarkers. Concurrent use of intrinsic kidney injury biomarkers and serum creatinine-based estimation of glomerular filtration rate (GFR) identifies at least four clinically relevant categories differentiating prerenal declines in GFR without structural injury and structural injury by biomarker positivity with and without changes in serum creatinine. Establishing AKI biomarker signatures that can further refine and subtype AKI on multiple dimensions has the potential to better identify treatment targets and therapeutic windows. *CKD,* chronic kidney disease; *CVD,* cardiovascular disease; *RAAS,* renin angiotensin-aldosterone system; S_{Cr}, serum creatinine. (Reprinted with permission from Huen SC and Parikh CR. Molecular phenotyping of clinical AKI with novel urinary biomarkers. Am J Physiol Renal Physiol. 2015;309:F408.)

The fractional excretion of sodium (FE_{Na}) accounts for this differential degree of water reabsorption and therefore provides a more accurate reflection of the kidney's ability to conserve sodium. FE_{Na} represents the fraction of filtered sodium that is excreted into the urine:

$$FE_{Na} = (U_{Na}/S_{Na})/(U_{Cr}/S_{Cr}) \times 100 \qquad \text{Eq. 74.8}$$

where U_{Na} and S_{Na} correspond to the urine and serum sodium (mmol/L), respectively, and U_{Cr} and S_{Cr} (mg/dL) correspond to the urine and serum creatinine, respectively. With prerenal azotemia, the FE_{Na} is generally less than 1%, whereas with ATN it is greater than 1%. In premature infants, due to tubular immaturity, this threshold for FE_{Na} is approximately 3%, not 1%. It should be noted that FE_{Na} is really only meaningful in the setting of oliguric AKI. In euvolemic patients, the urinary excretion of sodium will be more dependent on dietary sodium intake. The accuracy of U_{Na} and FE_{Na} is further compromised when urinary salt-wasting conditions are present (eg, diuretic use, renal dysplasia, chronic renal failure, cerebral salt wasting, as well as mineralocorticoid deficiency such as congenital adrenal hyperplasia secondary to 21-hydroxylase deficiency). These conditions are associated with elevated urinary chloride levels as well.[130]

Urine Concentration Capacity

The urine specific gravity (U_{SG}) and urine osmolality (U_{Osm}) assess the kidney's ability to concentrate the urine. U_{SG} and U_{Osm} bear a linear relationship, with U_{SG} rising approximately 0.001 for every 30 to 40 mOsm/kg. When urine is iso-osmotic

to serum, the U_{SG} is approximately 1.010. In a healthy kidney, the limits of U_{SG} range from 1.003 to 1.035 and U_{Osm} from 50 to 1400 mOsm/kg. However, due to renal immaturity, infants have a reduced urinary concentration capacity of about 600 mOsm/kg for preterm and 800 mOsm/kg for full-term infants. U_{SG} can be easily measured by refractometer and is therefore clinically used more often than U_{Osm}, which requires an osmometer. In general, U_{SG} provides a good estimate of the kidney's concentration ability. However, because U_{SG} compares the density of urine to that of water, the presence of heavier solutes such as glucose, contrast dye, or protein can increase the urine specific gravity without affecting the urine osmolality. Urine osmolality therefore provides a more accurate assessment of the kidney's response to antidiuretic hormone (ADH). With prerenal azotemia, the appropriate renal response is to retain sodium and water. Classically, the U_{SG} exceeds 1.020, U_{Osm} exceeds 500, and the urine output decreases, with the patient often becoming oliguric (urine output <1 mL/kg/h). With ATN, on the other hand, the conservation of water is impaired secondary to tubular injury resulting in isosthenuria (U_{SG} ~1.010, U_{Osm} ~300–350 mOsm/kg). It is crucial to remember, however, that children with underlying urinary concentration defects and tubular resistance to ADH (eg, renal dysplasia, nephrogenic diabetes insipidus, chronic kidney failure) may have a low U_{SG}, low U_{Osm}, and high urine output despite life-threatening intravascular volume depletion.

Urine osmolality is also helpful in evaluation of the child with polyuria. A low osmolality (<150 mOsm/kg) suggests a urinary concentration defect such as central or nephrogenic diabetes insipidus, whereas a urine osmolality of 300 to 350, associated with a high specific gravity, suggests an osmotic diuresis. The urinary concentrating capacity can be assessed by (1) checking the osmolality of a first morning urine after overnight fluid restriction with close monitoring or (2) a water deprivation test.

Serum Blood Urea Nitrogen/Creatinine Ratio

The ratio of serum blood urea nitrogen (BUN) to creatinine is also frequently used to help differentiate prerenal AKI from ATN. Urea, like creatinine, is freely filtered at the glomerulus but, unlike creatinine, has significant tubular reabsorption that further increases with hypovolemia. In prerenal states, therefore, the BUN/creatinine ratio generally exceeds 20:1, while it is lower than this with ATN. However, this ratio becomes inaccurate in clinical conditions where the BUN is elevated for nonrenal reasons such as a gastrointestinal bleed, catabolic state, or corticosteroid use; nor is it accurate in clinical conditions associated with a low BUN, such as protein calorie malnutrition or liver disease. The ratio may also be misleading in conditions associated with a particularly low muscle mass and serum creatinine such as muscular dystrophy.

Urine Microscopy

Urine microscopy can aid in determining the etiology for AKI. The presence of muddy brown or renal cellular casts and renal tubular epithelial cells is consistent with ATN. However, the absence of such findings does not rule out less severe ATN. In the setting of prerenal azotemia, urine microscopy is bland; hyaline and granular casts may be seen. Hematuria with dysmorphic red blood cells (RBCs) and red cell casts is consistent with glomerulonephritis, whereas hematuria with eumorphic RBCs suggests lower tract bleeding and hematuria in the absence of RBCs on a freshly examined urine suggests hemoglobinuria or myoglobinuria. Leukocyturia with white cell casts suggests pyelonephritis or interstitial nephritis. Eosinophils in the urine can be detected using special stains and are classically associated with interstitial nephritis but can also be seen with pyelonephritis and urinary tract obstruction.[131] Examination of a fresh, concentrated (or first morning) urine specimen optimizes the opportunity for detecting these cellular elements.

Proteinuria

Protein excretion in healthy individuals is minimal (<4 mg/m^2/hour in children) but can increase with renal injury. Glomerulopathies are associated with albuminuria and nonspecific proteinuria, while tubulointerstitial disease results in low-molecular-weight proteinuria (eg, β_2-microglobulin, retinol binding protein). Urinary protein excretion can be detected qualitatively by reagent strips. However, these strips only detect albumin and are therefore helpful for assessing glomerular proteinuria but not tubular or low-molecular-weight proteinuria. Low-level proteinuria by dipstick (30–99 mg/dL) can be a false positive in alkaline urine or can signify more significant disease if the patient is polyuric. Quantitative assessments of proteinuria can be obtained using a random urine total protein/creatinine ratio (normal <0.2 for children older than 3 years) measured by the biuret method[132] and are preferred for following glomerular and tubular proteinuria. First morning urine specimens are often recommended as this can distinguish orthostatic proteinuria, which is benign, from fixed proteinuria, which is pathologic. Twenty-four-hour urine collections for protein and creatinine can also be performed but are not believed to be advantageous over the random urine protein/creatinine ratio, particularly in children.

In diabetics, the development of overt proteinuria detectable by reagent strips is preceded by the presence of microalbuminuria, defined as persistent albumin excretion between 30 and 300 mg/g creatinine.[133] Use of the microalbumin/creatinine ratio allows for early detection of glomerular damage in diabetic kidney disease.[25]

Renal Acidification

Metabolic acidosis is also commonly encountered in the PICU. When associated with a normal serum anion gap, the major diagnostic consideration is renal tubular acidosis versus gastrointestinal loss of bicarbonate. The appropriate renal response to a metabolic acidosis is to increase proton secretion and ammonium production, which will allow increased net acid excretion (also see Chapter 76). The urine pH in this case should fall below 5.3, ideally measured with a pH meter after collecting a fresh specimen in an airtight syringe. Whereas a urine pH greater than 5.3 in the setting of systemic acidemia is consistent with renal tubular acidosis, a urine pH less than 5.3 does not exclude the diagnosis. Proximal RTA is characterized by bicarbonaturia secondary to a reduced threshold for bicarbonate reabsorption. At low levels of serum bicarbonate (<14 mEq/L), the filtered bicarbonate is able to be reabsorbed, resulting in a low urine pH. However, under conditions of bicarbonate loading, the reabsorptive capacity of the proximal tubule is exceeded leading to fractional excretion of bicarbonate greater than 15% to 20%:

$$FE_{bicarb} = (U_{HCO3}/S_{HCO3})/(U_{Cr}/S_{Cr}) \times 100 \qquad \text{Eq. 74.9}$$

where U_{HCO3} and S_{HCO3} are the urine and serum bicarbonate concentrations in mmol/ L and U_{Cr} and S_{Cr} are the urine and serum creatinine concentrations in mg/dL. Assessment of distal acidification includes calculation of the urine net charge and osmolal gap, both of which provide an indirect assessment of ammonium production, which cannot be routinely measured. The former is simpler to calculate:

$$\text{Urine Net Charge} = (U_{Na} + U_K - U_{Cl}) \qquad \text{Eq. 74.10}$$

where U_{Na} is the urine sodium concentration (mEq/L), U_K is the urine potassium concentration (mEq/L), and U_{Cl} is the urine chloride concentration (mEq/L). Assuming chloride is the major anion excreted, an appropriate urine net charge in the setting of acidosis should be negative (−30 to −50), indicating the presence of ammonium, an unmeasured cation. A positive net charge would therefore suggest impaired ammonium production or proton secretion. The urine net charge, however, has limited utility when the urine sodium concentration is low (<25 mEq/L), as occurs with hypovolemia. In this setting, the kidney avidly conserves sodium and chloride (urine chloride <15 mEq/L), leaving less anion available for excretion with ammonium and resulting in a reversible impairment of urinary acidification. The urine net charge is also misleading in the presence of unmeasured anions (eg, beta hydroxybutyrate and acetoacetate in diabetic ketoacidosis, hippurate from toluene ingestion/glue sniffing, or penicillins). In this setting, the urine net charge is positive and underestimates ammonium excretion because the cations—ammonium, sodium, and potassium—are excreted with the unmeasured anion instead of chloride. In infants, the validity of the urine net charge is also compromised due to considerable variability in the unmeasured ionic composition of the urine.[134] The urinary osmolal gap is more informative because it accounts for the excretion of the unmeasured anions. It represents the difference between the measured and calculated urine osmolalities where the calculated osmolality is:

$$U_{Osm} = \{2 \times [U_{Na} \text{ (mmol/L)} + U_K \text{ (mmol/L)}]\}$$
$$+ [U_{urea} \text{ (mg/dL)}/2.8] + [U_{glucose} \text{ (mg/dL)}/18]^{135}$$

$$\text{Eq. 74.11}$$

Assuming urinary ammonium is the predominant unmeasured cation, the concentration of excreted ammonium is approximately half of the urine osmolal gap. During periods of systemic acidosis, urinary ammonium excretion increases to concentrations greater than 75 mEq/L; a level less than 25 mEq/L in this setting suggests impaired ammoniagenesis.[136]

More sophisticated tests are available to assess distal tubular acidification (proton secretion). Traditional tests include (1) measuring the difference in PCO_2 between the urine and blood during bicarbonate loading and (2) an NH_4Cl loading test. However, these can be difficult to perform and may not be well tolerated. More recently, simultaneous administration of furosemide to enhance distal sodium delivery and fludrocortisone to enhance distal sodium reabsorption, as well as stimulate proton secretion, has been used as an alternative test for distal acidification. In the presence of intact distal acidification, the urine pH should decrease to less than 5.3. This test has the advantages of being easy to perform and well tolerated.[137]

Potassium Regulation

Unlike urine sodium, which can be extremely efficiently reclaimed by the tubules, there is an obligate K excretion of at least 5 to 10 mmol/day due to K secretion that occurs in the distal tubule. Potassium excretion is primarily dependent on the aldosterone activity and serum K concentration but also requires an adequate urine flow rate and delivery of sodium to the distal nephron. The TTKG (transtubular potassium gradient) provides an assessment of potassium excretion secondary to mineralocorticoid activity and is calculated:

$$\text{TTKG} = [U_K \times S_{Osm}] / [S_K \times U_{Osm}] \qquad \text{Eq. 74.12}$$

where U_K and S_K represent urine and serum concentrations of potassium (mEq/L), respectively, and S_{Osm} and U_{Osm} represent serum and urine osmolalities (mOsm/kg). In the setting of hyperkalemia, the TTKG should be elevated; therefore a low TTKG (<4.1 in children; <7 in adults) suggests hypoaldosteronism. In the setting of hypokalemia, on the other hand, the TTKG would be expected to be quite low; levels greater than 2 suggest aldosterone activity is not appropriately suppressed.[130,138]

Generalized Proximal Tubulopathy

Generalized proximal tubulopathies (Fanconi syndrome) can be congenital (ie, cystinosis, tyrosinemia) or acquired (eg, aminoglycoside toxicity, ifosfamide, severe ATN) and may be partial or complete. Biochemical abnormalities associated with a complete Fanconi syndrome include hypokalemia, metabolic acidosis, hypophosphatemia, hypouricemia, and low serum carnitine associated with urinary wasting of sodium, potassium, bicarbonate, phosphorus, uric acid, carnitine, glucose, amino acids, and low-molecular-weight proteins. A generalized proximal tubulopathy should be suspected when electrolyte wasting is profound and/or involves several electrolytes.

Key References

3. Kellum JA, Lameire N, KDIGO AKI Guideline Work Group. Diagnosis, evaluation, and management of acute kidney injury: a KDIGO summary (Part 1). *Crit Care.* 2013;17:204.
12. Bosch JP. Renal reserve: a functional view of glomerular filtration rate. *Semin Nephrol.* 1995;15:381-385.
17. Smith H. Renal function in infancy and childhood. In: *The Kidney: Structure and Function in Health and Disease.* New York, NY: Oxford University Press; 1951:492-519.
18. Heilbron DC, Holliday MA, al-Dahwi A, Kogan BA. Expressing glomerular filtration rate in children. *Pediatr Nephrol.* 1991;5:5-11.
24. Levey AS, Coresh J, Balk E, et al. National Kidney Foundation practice guidelines for chronic kidney disease: evaluation, classification, and stratification. *Ann Intern Med.* 2003;139:137-147.
25. Hogg RJ, Furth S, Lemley KV, et al. National Kidney Foundation's Kidney Disease Outcomes Quality Initiative clinical practice guidelines for chronic kidney disease in children and adolescents: evaluation, classification, and stratification. *Pediatrics.* 2003;111(6 Pt 1):1416-1421.
28. Brochner-Mortensen J. Current status on assessment and measurement of glomerular filtration rate. *Clin Physiol.* 1985;5:1-17.
29. Piepsz A, Colarinha P, Gordon I, et al. Guidelines for glomerular filtration rate determination in children. *Eur J Nucl Med.* 2001;28:BP31-BP36.
31. Schwartz GJ, Abraham AG, Furth SL, et al. Optimizing iohexol plasma disappearance curves to measure the glomerular filtration rate in children with chronic kidney disease. *Kidney Int.* 2010;77:65-71.
38. Gaspari F, Perico N, Ruggenenti P, et al. Plasma clearance of nonradioactive iohexol as a measure of glomerular filtration rate. *J Am Soc Nephrol.* 1995;6:257-263.
40. Stake G, Monn E, Rootwelt K, et al. Glomerular filtration rate estimated by X-ray fluorescence technique in children: comparison between the plasma disappearance of 99Tcm-DTPA and iohexol after urography. *Scand J Clin Lab Invest.* 1990;50:161-167.
41. Dixon J, Lane K, Dalton R, et al. Validation of a continuous infusion of low dose Iohexol to measure glomerular filtration rate: randomised clinical trial. *J Translat Med.* 2015;13:58.
43. Stake G, Monn E, Rootwelt K, Monclair T. The clearance of iohexol as a measure of the glomerular filtration rate in children with chronic renal failure. *Scand J Clin Lab Invest.* 1991;51:729-734.
45. Schwartz GJ, Furth S, Cole SR, et al. Glomerular filtration rate via plasma iohexol disappearance: pilot study for chronic kidney disease in children. *Kidney Int.* 2006;69:2070-2077.
47. Brown SC, O'Reilly PH. Iohexol clearance for the determination of glomerular filtration rate in clinical practice: evidence for a new gold standard. *J Urol.* 1991;146:675-679.
50. Soveri I, Berg UB, Bjork J, et al. Measuring GFR: a systematic review. *Am J Kidney Dis.* 2014;64:411-424.
52. Schwartz GJ, Munoz A, Schneider MF, et al. New equations to estimate GFR in children with CKD. *J Am Soc Nephrol.* 2009;20:629-637.
53. Schwartz GJ, Schneider MF, Maier PS, et al. Improved equations estimating GFR in children with chronic kidney disease using an immunonephelometric determination of cystatin C. *Kidney Int.* 2012;82:445-453.
54. Schwartz GJ. Height: the missing link in estimating glomerular filtration rate in children and adolescents. *Nephrol Dial Transplant.* 2014;29:944-947.
58. Schwartz GJ, Kwong T, Erway B, et al. Validation of creatinine assays utilizing HPLC and IDMS traceable standards in sera of children. *Pediatr Nephrol.* 2009;24:113-119.
59. Cobbaert CM, Baadenhuijsen H, Weykamp CW. Prime time for enzymatic creatinine methods in pediatrics. *Clin Chem.* 2009;55:549-558.

60. Srivastava T, Alon US, Althahabi R, Garg U. Impact of standardization of creatinine methodology on the assessment of glomerular filtration rate in children. *Pediatr Res.* 2009;65:113-116.

61. Speeckaert MM, Wuyts B, Stove V, et al. Compensating for the influence of total serum protein in the Schwartz formula. *Clin Chem Lab Med.* 2012;50:1597-1600.

62. Schwartz GJ, Brion LP, Spitzer A. The use of plasma creatinine concentration for estimating glomerular filtration rate in infants, children, and adolescents. *Pediatr Clin North Am.* 1987;34:571-590.

63. Myers GL, Miller WG, Coresh J, et al. Recommendations for improving serum creatinine measurement: a report from the Laboratory Working Group of the National Kidney Disease Education Program. *Clin Chem.* 2006;52:5-18.

66. Finney H, Newman DJ, Thakkar H, et al. Reference ranges for plasma cystatin C and creatinine measurements in premature infants, neonates, and older children. *Arch Dis Child.* 2000;82:71-75.

70. Andersen TB, Eskild-Jensen A, Frokiaer J, et al. Measuring glomerular filtration rate in children; can cystatin C replace established methods? A review. *Pediatr Nephrol.* 2009;24:929-941.

71. Schwartz GJ, Work DF. Measurement and estimation of GFR in children and adolescents. *Clin J Am Soc Nephrol.* 2009;4:1832-1843.

72. Dworkin LD. Serum cystatin C as a marker of glomerular filtration rate. *Curr Opin Nephrol Hypertens.* 2001;10:551-553.

74. Dharnidharka VR, Kwon C, Stevens G. Serum cystatin C is superior to serum creatinine as a marker of kidney function: a meta-analysis. *Am J Kidney Dis.* 2002;40:221-226.

75. Roos JF, Doust J, Tett SE, Kirkpatrick CM. Diagnostic accuracy of cystatin C compared to serum creatinine for the estimation of renal dysfunction in adults and children—a meta-analysis. *Clin Biochem.* 2007;40:383-391.

80. Zhang Z, Lu B, Sheng X, Jin N. Cystatin C in prediction of acute kidney injury: a systemic review and meta-analysis. *Am J Kidney Dis.* 2011;58:356-365.

82. Lagos-Arevalo P, Palijan A, Vertullo L, et al. Cystatin C in acute kidney injury diagnosis: early biomarker or alternative to serum creatinine? *Pediatr Nephrol.* 2015;30:665-676.

86. Madero M, Sarnak MJ, Stevens LA. Serum cystatin C as a marker of glomerular filtration rate. *Curr Opin Nephrol Hypertens.* 2006;15:610-616.

89. Blirup-Jensen S, Grubb A, Lindstrom V, et al. Standardization of cystatin C: development of primary and secondary reference preparations. *Scand J Clin Lab Invest Suppl.* 2008;241:67-70.

90. Levey AS, Fan L, Eckfeldt JH, Inker LA. Cystatin C for glomerular filtration rate estimation: coming of age. *Clin Chem.* 2014;60:916-919.

93. Counahan R, Chantler C, Ghazali S, et al. Estimation of glomerular filtration rate from plasma creatinine concentration in children. *Arch Dis Child.* 1976;51:875-878.

94. Schwartz GJ, Haycock GB, Edelmann CM Jr, Spitzer A. A simple estimate of glomerular filtration rate in children derived from body length and plasma creatinine. *Pediatrics.* 1976;58:259-263.

95. Kidney Disease: Improving Global Outcomes (KDIGO) CKD Work Group. KDIGO 2012 Clinical Practice Guideline for the Evaluation and Management of Chronic Kidney Disease. *Kidney Int Suppl.* 2013;3:1-150.

97. Levey AS, Inker LA, Coresh J. GFR estimation: from physiology to public health. *Am J Kidney Dis.* 2014;63:820-834.

98. Azzi A, Cachat F, Faouzi M, et al. Is there an age cutoff to apply adult formulas for GFR estimation in children? *J Nephrol.* 2015;28:59-66.

100. Chehade H, Girardin E, Iglesias K, et al. Assessment of adult formulas for glomerular filtration rate estimation in children. *Pediatr Nephrol.* 2013;28:105-114.

101. Selistre L, De Souza V, Cochat P, et al. GFR estimation in adolescents and young adults. *J Am Soc Nephrol.* 2012;23:989-996.

103. Staples A, LeBlond R, Watkins S, et al. Validation of the revised Schwartz estimating equation in a predominantly non-CKD population. *Pediatr Nephrol.* 2010;25:2321-2326.

104. Bacchetta J, Cochat P, Rognant N, et al. Which creatinine and cystatin C equations can be reliably used in children? *Clin J Am Soc Nephrol.* 2011;6:552-560.

105. Deng F, Finer G, Haymond S, et al. Applicability of estimating glomerular filtration rate equations in pediatric patients: comparison with a measured glomerular filtration rate by iohexol clearance. *Transl Res.* 2015;165:437-445.

106. Rink N, Zappitelli M. Estimation of glomerular filtration rate with and without height: effect of age and renal function level. *Pediatr Nephrol.* 2015;30:1327-1336.

107. Pottel H, Hoste L, Martens F. A simple height-independent equation for estimating glomerular filtration rate in children. *Pediatr Nephrol.* 2012;27:973-979.

108. Hoste L, Dubourg L, Selistre L, et al. A new equation to estimate the glomerular filtration rate in children, adolescents and young adults. *Nephrol Dial Transplant.* 2014;29:1082-1091.

129. Huen SC, Parikh CR. Molecular phenotyping of clinical AKI with novel urinary biomarkers. *Am J Physiol Renal Physiol.* 2015;309:F406-F413.

Glomerulotubular Dysfunction and Acute Kidney Injury

Cristin D.W. Kaspar and Timothy E. Bunchman

PEARLS

- Acute kidney injury (AKI) has replaced the term *acute kidney failure*. There are more than 30 definitions of AKI in children. Use of the pediatric Risk, Injury, Failure, Loss, End stage renal disease (pRIFLE), Acute Kidney Injury Network (AKIN), or Kidney Disease Improving Global Outcomes (KDIGO) scores for AKI may help in streamlining the definition. In the future, biomarkers may add clarity to this definition at an earlier time frame than when they are presently used.
- In the critically ill child, AKI is often associated with cardiovascular instability, which, if prolonged, exhausts the normal kidney compensatory responses to maintain kidney blood flow and glomerular filtration.
- Because tubular blood flow, and thus oxygen delivery to this vital epithelium, depends on postglomerular blood flow, prolonged vasoconstriction of glomerular arterioles results in tubular necrosis.
- Nephrotoxic drugs, sepsis, and overzealous use of diuretics are common comorbid conditions that further contribute to AKI.
- Attention to cardiovascular status and the avoidance of unnecessary nephrotoxic agents such as aminoglycosides, nonsteroidal antiinflammatory drugs, and contrast agents may avoid further AKI.

Acute kidney injury (AKI) is a frequent problem in the pediatric intensive care unit (PICU), but an accurate incidence is difficult to establish due to the ongoing evolution of a clear definition of renal failure. The classic definition was a 50% reduction of glomerular filtration rate (GFR) accompanied by a 50% increase in creatinine. A RIFLE classification of renal injury to allow earlier appreciation of renal dysfunction is now utilized in adults and a modification of this system (pRIFLE) can also be applied to children.[1-3] However, use of serum creatinine level in the diagnostic criteria is problematic for several reasons including variability of creatinine based on muscle mass and a delay in the rise of creatinine after kidney injury.

Early detection of renal dysfunction by biomarkers is needed to allow a more timely awareness of injury and thereby allow modifications to alleviate the renal stress. Investigations in this area, although early in their development, postulate that a panel approach (plasma panel of neutrophil gelatinase-associated lipocalin [NGAL] and cystatin C or a urine panel

of NGAL, interleukin 18, and kidney injury molecule-1 [KIM-1]) may be of help in the future to provide more sensitive and specific detection of early AKI.[4-6]

Acute Kidney Injury Pathophysiology
Physiology of Glomerular Filtration

GFR is the product of the filtration rate of the individual nephron and the number of functioning nephrons.[7] A single nephron glomerular filtration rate (SNGFR) is defined by the Starling forces of the glomerular capillaries and the properties of the glomerular capillary wall,

$$SNGFR = Kf\,(\Delta P - \Delta \pi) = KfP_{uf} \qquad \text{Eq. 75.1}$$

where Kf is a capillary wall property known as the ultrafiltration coefficient and is the product of the surface area available for filtration and the hydraulic conductivity of the membrane. The Starling forces (or pressures) that affect filtration are the hydraulic pressure in the glomerular capillary (P_{gc}), the hydraulic pressure in the Bowman space (P_{bs}), the oncotic pressure of the glomerular capillary (π_{gc}), and the oncotic pressure in the Bowman space (π_{bs}), which is usually zero because the ultrafiltrate is essentially protein free.[8] P_{gc} favors filtration; P_{bs} and π_{gc} are opposing forces to filtration. The mean ultrafiltration pressure (P_{uf}) is the difference between the net change in hydraulic pressure and the net change in the oncotic pressure. Thus SNGFR may be modified by alterations in the glomerular capillary pressures, glomerular membrane characteristics, or the surface area available for filtration.

The kidneys are responsible for plasma water and electrolyte balance through filtration at the glomerular membrane and then reabsorption of this filtrate from the renal tubular epithelium. The loss of filtration and tubular reabsorption in AKI is the result of renal adaptive changes that initially function to preserve renal perfusion and glomerular filtration; however, when these are exhausted, the kidney's compensatory mechanisms fail and renal dysfunction ensues.

Glomerular filtration depends on adequate renal perfusion; the kidneys receive approximately 25% of total cardiac output. The fraction of cardiac output perfusing the kidneys is related to the ratio of renal vascular resistance (RVR) and systemic vascular resistance.[9] Renal blood flow (RBF) is determined by systemic blood pressure (SBP) and RVR, expressed by the formula RBF = SBP/RVR.[9] Kidney autoregulation, which maintains a constant renal perfusion pressure, occurs through alterations in RVR in response to changes in systemic vascular resistance or intravascular volume. When SBP is within the normal physiologic or autoregulatory range, the kidney can maintain constant blood flow and GFR by dilation of the preglomerular or afferent arteriole, which reduces RVR and increases RBF. This afferent arteriole dilation is accomplished by two known mechanisms, smooth muscle relaxation of the afferent arteriole in response to sensing a transmural pressure drop (the myogenic reflex[3]) and the tubuloglomerular feedback system. The tubuloglomerular feedback system is operational following a reduction of plasma flow. When solute and water deliveries to the macula densa are reduced, the juxtaglomerular apparatus responds by relaxing the smooth muscle of the adjacent afferent arteriole. Thus a reduction in cardiac output or effective renal plasma flow is accompanied by vasodilation at the preglomerular arteriole, which in turn reduces RVR, thereby restoring RBF.

During states of reduced cardiac output or intravascular volume depletion, the systemic vasoconstrictors, angiotensin II and vasopressin, are released to help preserve vascular tone. The kidney counteracts the renal vasoconstrictor activity of angiotensin II and increased sympathetic tone through the intrarenal production of vasodilatory prostaglandins such as prostaglandin I_2.[10] These locally produced substances may attenuate renal vasoconstrictive forces and help preserve renal perfusion. Animal model data of congestive heart failure have provided evidence that enhanced prostaglandin synthesis is required for preservation of renal perfusion and GFR. Patients receiving prostaglandin synthetase inhibitors such as nonsteroidal antiinflammatory drugs (NSAIDs) have potentiation of renal ischemia because of an increase in renal vasoconstriction not antagonized by intrarenal prostaglandin synthesis.[11] Endothelium-derived relaxation factors (EDRFs), which are vasodilatory, and the potent vasoconstrictor endothelin, produced by the endothelium, may also affect the regional vascular tone.[12]

Constriction of the postglomerular capillary sphincter, the efferent arteriole, in the face of reduced RBF increases the filtration fraction and preserves GFR, although this occurs at the expense of renal plasma flow, which may be further reduced. Vasoconstriction at the efferent arteriole is mediated by angiotensin II and, to a lesser extent, by the action of the adrenergic system by epinephrine.[13] Elevation in postglomerular arteriolar resistance may be blocked by the angiotensin-converting enzyme inhibitors. When converting enzyme inhibitors are administered to the patient who requires efferent arteriolar constriction to maintain GFR, renal decompensation often results.[14]

As previously noted, reductions in effective intravascular volume and cardiac output are accompanied by increased activity of the sympathetic nervous system and the renin-angiotensin-aldosterone system and increased circulating levels of vasopressin (see also Chapter 81).[15] Hormonal and neural systems signal the kidneys to increase the reabsorption of sodium and water to help restore the deficient intravascular volume, increase cardiac output, and consequently improve RBF. These and the kidney's homeostatic mechanism, by afferent arteriolar vasodilation and efferent arteriolar constriction, maintain the kidney's glomerular filtration. The kidney's homeostatic mechanisms, however, are not without limitation. The autoregulatory ability of the afferent arteriole is

maximal once the mean SBP falls below 80 mm Hg. The renal autoregulatory range appears to be age dependent, because younger animals can autoregulate over lower pressure ranges. The range of perfusion pressure over which the kidney can autoregulate may be limited in certain conditions so that vasodilation is maximal with a minor reduction in mean arterial blood pressure. Examples include extracellular fluid depletion, renal ischemia, or renal vascular disease (eg, hypertension, diabetes, atherosclerosis).

As the stimulus for release of vasoconstrictors continues, afferent arteriolar constriction rather than vasodilation may predominate, and the result is a decrease in renal plasma flow and filtration rate.

Constriction of the afferent arteriole may be stimulated by increased sympathetic nervous system activity and increased levels of endogenous or exogenous circulating catecholamines such as dopamine or norepinephrine. Thus the administration of these vasoactive-inotropic agents may actually compromise the kidney's adaptive mechanisms. Excessive vasoconstriction eventually results in diminished filtration rate and oxygen delivery to the kidney.

Pharmacologic agents may alter renal perfusion by changing SBP through an action on systemic vasculature or by direct effects on renal vasculature (Box 75.1). Vasodilators, such as hydralazine, lower SBP without changing renal perfusion pressure because the decrease in SBP is accompanied by decreased RVR. Conversely, epinephrine increases SBP but decreases RBF by its vasoconstrictor effect on intrarenal blood vessels.

Morphologic Changes in Renal Injury

Morphologic changes seen in acute renal injury, especially those in the tubules, depend on the duration of injury as well as the eliciting mechanism.

The kidney's complex structure, with heterogeneous segments within the kidney receiving differential regional perfusion and thereby oxygenation, sets up a common form of renal failure, that of the tubulointerstitium. This region is at greatest risk for ischemia because of its gradient of regional perfusion and oxygenation. In addition, vascular disease, including glomerular disease, often occurs in children and results in AKI, but there are studies that suggest the extent of damage to the tubulointerstitium has the greatest prognostic implication to the degree of final renal recovery.[16]

Initial structural changes in tubular cells are seen as apical and basal surface changes of simplification, with microvilli of

| **BOX 75.1** | **Vasoactive Substances in the Kidney Vasculature** |

1. ↑ Kidney Vascular Resistance/↓ Kidney Blood Flow
   - Epinephrine
   - Norepinephrine
   - Angiotensin II
   - Arachidonic acid
   - Thromboxane A_2
2. ↓ Kidney Vascular Resistance/↑ Kidney Blood Flow
   - Prostaglandin E_1
   - Prostaglandin E_2
   - Dopamine
   - Furosemide
   - Angiotensin-converting enzyme inhibitors
   - Bradykinin
   - Isoproterenol
   - Acetylcholine

the brush border shortening and disappearing by either detachment from the apical surface or being internalized within the tubular cells.[17]

In this scenario, enzymes of the brush border (alkaline phosphatase and gamma glutamyl transpeptidase) may be found in the urine and may be used as markers of early tubular injury.[18] The loss of microvilli surface area leads to loss of enzymes and transport sites for transcellular absorption and apical uptake. Additionally, loss at the basolateral interdigitating infoldings of the tubular cells then results in further reduction of surface area for transport and loss of the Na^+/K^+-adenosine triphosphatase (ATPase) that is localized to this membrane and involved in many transport processes.[19]

Morphologic changes in distal tubules and outer medulla also occur and may be found even when proximal tubular injury is not readily identified on biopsy. Experimentally, the outer medulla has been identified as sensitive to hypoxia, including that induced by toxins such as radiocontrast agents and cyclosporine.[20]

Injury at this outer medulla region may be missed on biopsy since this site often is not sampled. Tubular cell detachment with exposed, denuded regions of the basement membrane can be found on biopsies, as a result of altered cell-matrix attachments.[21]

Renal tubular sensitivity to ischemic injury is primarily influenced by the individual renal cell's energy requirements, its glycolytic capacity, and the extent of hypoxic stress upon the cell. Glycolysis and oxidative phosphorylation both supply the adenosine triphosphate (ATP) required by the cell to drive its metabolism, and it follows that cells with a greater capacity for glycolysis (distal tubular cells) are less sensitive to oxygen deprivation than the cells that rely mainly on mitochondrial-derived energy (proximal tubular cells).[22]

In vivo and in vitro studies may be discordant in identifying susceptibility to hypoxia. Medullary straight portions of the proximal tubule have a higher glycolytic capacity than the cortical segments of the proximal tubule but, due to the regional distribution of perfusion within the kidney, the medullary portions operate in a lower oxygen-tension environment and therefore are more susceptible to hypoxia/ischemic injury.[23] The individual cell's energy requirements to conduct its transport activities further influences its risk to hypoxic injury. The outer medullary proximal tubular cell (pars recta), due to the high energy requirements for its transport functions, has a greater injury risk than the deep inner medullary tubular cell with its low-oxygen and low-energy requirement to maintain its transport function.[24]

When energy stores are rapidly depleted, the normal Na^+/K^+ ATPase pump begins to fail and the most basic of cell function, membrane integrity, is jeopardized, with resultant accumulation of Na^+, Cl^-, and water within the cell; this cell swelling (oncosis) is a hallmark feature of necrosis.[25] Not all cells that fail to maintain their energy requirements die through necrosis. Apoptosis, which appears morphologically as cell shrinkage, is also a result of inadequate energy support. Apoptosis is an asynchronous cell death triggered over hours to days, with the earliest cellular element involving mitochondrial changes including loss of transmembrane potential and release of mitochondrial cytochrome c into the cytosol.[30] It is mitochondrial function/dysfunction that primarily determines the fate of the cell for recovery and survival or death and by what form: apoptosis or necrosis[11] (see also Chapter 84).

Pathogenesis of Reduced Glomerular Filtration Rate in Acute Kidney Injury

The mechanisms responsible for GFR reduction in acute renal injury have been studied extensively with experimental models of AKI. Multiple mechanisms are often operational in mediating hypofiltration. Whereas one factor may have greater importance in the initiation of injury and decreased filtration, others are involved in the sustained reduction in GFR during the maintenance phase of AKI. Four major mechanisms result in reduced GFR during AKI: reduced blood flow, decreased Kf, tubular obstruction, and back leakage of tubular fluid.[31] Each factor is discussed regarding its role in both the initiation and maintenance phases of AKI.

A reduction in RBF can be demonstrated during the initiation phase of many forms of AKI and seems to play a predominant role in ischemic injury and rhabdomyolysis.[31] Proposed theories for the reduction of RBF include (1) a proportional increase in the afferent and efferent arteriolar resistances in response to activation of the renin-angiotensin system, (2) vascular endothelial cell swelling and damage with release of vasoactive peptides such as endothelin, and (3) hyperemic congestion of the medullary peritubular capillaries.

Kf may be reduced in both nephrotoxic and ischemic forms of renal failure. Endothelial or mesangial cell swelling reduces the surface area available for filtration; altered permeability induced by humoral factors such as angiotensin II and vasopressin may also decrease Kf. Circulating levels of both hormones are increased during AKI.

Renal tubular cells are the primary site of injury in both ischemia and nephrotoxin-induced renal injury. Tubular cell injury may be sublethal or lethal and result in cell necrosis or apoptosis. Once this injury occurs, cells detach from the supporting basement membrane and obstruct the tubule lumen. In addition, even with sublethal injury, tight junctions may be disrupted, and the intact layer may be lost. The loss of epithelial integrity allows back leakage of ultrafiltrate, which contains creatinine and urea, through paracellular pathways into the renal interstitium, creating further diminution of excretory function and reduced urine formation. Necrosis of a selected region of the renal tubule is accompanied by tubular obstruction and eventual filtration failure by that entire unit or nephron.

Intratubular obstruction occurs in most forms of acute renal injury, either as a contributing factor in the initiation phase or during the maintenance phase.[31] Tubular obstruction with cellular debris and precipitated protein is a prominent finding in both the initiation and maintenance phases of ischemic injury. In the case of nephrotoxic injury, the degree of injury may determine the extent of tubular obstruction. In an experimental model of gentamicin nephrotoxicity, the drug dose was positively correlated with the contribution of tubular obstruction to reduced GFR.[31] Tubular obstruction and loss of epithelial integrity caused by tubular cell injury result in the back leakage of tubular fluid and solutes. Excretion of solute and fluid is decreased, and this decrease possibly signals a further reduction in the GFR by stimulation of the tubuloglomerular feedback mechanism.[31] Back leakage of fluid involves tubular factors and is not a result of hypofiltration, although it does impair the excretory function of the kidney. Consequently, a falsely low estimation of actual GFR may occur because tubular fluid containing urea and creatinine leaks back into the vascular space and interstitium. Prevention of the tubular obstruction may alter the course of renal failure, even in those states in which the primary mechanism of injury is not obstruction.

AKI may be viewed as an evolving process into three phases[32]: (1) an initiation phase in which the primary mechanism of injury is operational, (2) a maintenance phase during which renal function remains poor and other factors may contribute to sustained injury, and (3) a recovery phase during which there is regeneration of cells and restoration of function. Although the primary initiating event may be hypoperfusion with ischemia, often it involves multiple contributing factors that mediate additional cellular damage, usually through alterations in energy supply. From a clinical perspective, it may be most helpful to consider acute renal dysfunction syndromes according to the cause of the inciting event; however, it is equally vital to understand the other contributing mechanisms that ultimately affect outcome.

Endothelial injury and vascular dysfunction have been postulated to occur during the initiation and particularly during the maintenance phases of AKI. Although most studies have focused on the tubular cell as the primary site of injury leading to dysfunction, studies have provided insight into the potential role for endothelial injury in continued reduced RBF and altered vascular function.[33] Sutton and colleagues proposed that an additional phase be added to the current model for AKI: After the initiation phase, an extension phase occurs that is due to microvascular injury related to ischemic damage to endothelial cells, infiltration of leukocytes, and activation of the coagulation system. This process is thought to predominate in the corticomedullary and outer medullary microvessels and may occur in the face of early tubular cell regeneration so that limiting the extension process provides a potential mechanism for aiding recovery.

Mechanisms of Renal Cell Injury

The renal tubular cell expends energy in the form of ATP to maintain a high intracellular concentration of potassium and a low intracellular concentration of sodium. This concentration gradient depends on the continuous activity of the Na^+/K^+-ATPase and is the driving force for the reabsorption of sodium. Active reabsorption of sodium is the primary driving force for water reabsorption and the coupled transport of amino acids, carbohydrates, organic acids, and other compounds. Thus all transport functions, as well as many other vital cell functions, depend on normal activity of the Na^+/K^+ pump, which, in turn, depends on an adequate supply of energy. In addition, membrane fluidity or integrity is important to transport functions in tubular cells. Processes that result in alterations in the membrane or in the supply of energy are common final pathways for renal tubular cell death.

A decrease in the cellular ATP content occurs in many forms of renal injury, possibly as the result of primary alterations in the cell's ability to perform oxidative phosphorylation or as the end result of other perturbations. Heterogeneity exists in the susceptibility of nephron segments to oxygen deprivation with more distal segments being relatively resistant. This is related to the greater glycolytic capacity of the distal tubule compared with the proximal tubule, which relies on oxygen-consuming pathways for ATP generation. Therefore the net result of renal injury is usually a depletion of energy in the form of ATP, with the inability of the cell to perform vital functions, including transport and maintenance of cell integrity.

Cellular injury may be modified by the requirements made on its energy stores. If more transport is required of the cell, more energy is consumed, and less energy is left for cell maintenance. Evidence exists to support this theory. If transport requirements are reduced by the administration of diuretics or by the stimulation of the glomerulotubular feedback mechanism, then further injury may be attenuated. The feedback mechanism, whereby there is reduction of GFR in the face of reduced reabsorption by the proximal tubule, is a protective signal that conserves cell energy by reducing metabolic demands made on the cell.

Heat shock proteins (HSPs) are a family of proteins that appear to protect cells from injury as a result of hyperthermia, ischemia, or toxins. The HSP induction by sublethal thermal stress has been found to attenuate subsequent injury in the kidney.[34] Renal transplants from animals that underwent short-term hyperthermia had better initial function and subsequent survival. Furthermore, in cultured inner medullary collecting-duct cells, induction of HSP-1 by preconditioning hyperthermia attenuated the alterations in mitochondrial function and glycolysis that were observed after cells were exposed to high temperatures. Investigations into potential mechanisms to use this natural cell defense mechanism are under way.

The ability of renal tubular epithelial cells to undergo regeneration determines in large part the degree of renal recovery. Therefore much work has been done to study ways that cells regenerate and mechanisms that might enhance recovery. Early in ischemic injury there is induction of early response genes such as c-fos and Egr-1.[35] By 2 days after ischemia, the proliferating cell nuclear antigen is detected, followed by expression of other dedifferentiated cell markers, which seem to be a sign of early recovery. Other cells appear to undergo apoptosis or cell death. Postischemic regeneration seems to be a recapitulation of early renal tubular cell development. Growth factors such as insulin-like growth factor-1 (IGF-1) and epidermal growth factor 1 (EGF-1) have been associated with enhanced recovery as well. Renal levels of hepatocyte growth factor (HGF) increase after two models of renal failure, postnephrectomy, and following CCL4 (chemokine [C-C motif] ligand 4) injection, and this increase supports a role for HGF in renal repair.[36] Exogenous EGF has been shown to enhance renal tubular cell regeneration and to lessen the severity and duration of hypoxia and toxin-induced renal failure. EGF receptor levels increase within hours of ischemic injury in the rat. Elevation of soluble EGF occurs along with morphologic evidence of tubular injury within 12 hours of ischemia, which is followed by cell proliferation and a decrease in soluble EGF by 24 to 48 hours after ischemia.

Alterations in Cell Membranes

Membrane phospholipids have a structural function and affect membrane permeability, as well as the activity of membrane transport systems.[37] These compounds are regulated in part by the activity of phospholipases, which release free fatty acids from phospholipids. Several mechanisms related to acute cell injury may alter phospholipase activity and thereby change membrane phospholipids and membrane integrity: altered intracellular calcium homeostasis, depletion of ATP, and lipid peroxidation.[33] Increased phospholipase activity has been associated with an abnormal increase in permeability of the inner mitochondrial membrane, which ultimately results in disruption of mitochondria and loss of the ability to produce adequate energy.

Cellular Calcium Homeostasis

Increased intracellular calcium is commonly found in cell injury. It is not, however, a consistent finding in all models of renal injury.[38] Techniques to study changes in the subcellular distribution of calcium have allowed time-related changes to be assessed. In the rat proximal tubule, steady-state hypoxia is accompanied by a prompt increase in cytosolic free calcium that precedes the appearance of membrane damage.[29] The increase in calcium is reversed with reoxygenation. Increased cellular calcium may activate phospholipases, as previously mentioned; alter the cytoskeleton and cause injury by allowing cell swelling; or affect membrane permeability at the plasma membrane, the mitochondrial membrane, or the endoplasmic reticulum. Alterations in mitochondrial function that occur as a result of calcium loading of this organelle have been extensively studied. Excess mitochondrial calcium is associated with changes in the permeability of the inner mitochondrial membrane with loss of the electrochemical gradient and the capacity for oxidative phosphorylation. In addition, changes in enzyme activity and mitochondrial levels of nucleotides may exist.

Production of Free Radicals

Renal cell damage induced by inflammation or oxygen deprivation may be mediated, in part, by oxygen free radicals that are generated by several cell processes, including accumulation of long chain acyl-CoA as a result of mitochondrial dysfunction. The net result is increased intracellular calcium and, ultimately, changes in membrane-related functions.[32]

Tubular Cell Energy Metabolism

After exposure to a variety of nephrotoxins or ischemia, renal cortical ATP levels are reduced even before changes in membrane integrity and cell death occur.[39] In ischemic injury, alterations in renal perfusion may result in decreased oxygen delivery to tubular epithelium. Direct mitochondrial damage has been postulated to be the primary event in many forms of nephrotoxic injury.[32] Other nephrotoxins interfere with energy production by the inhibition of enzymes along the citric acid cycle. In this way, toxins impair energy production. ATP levels decrease immediately after ischemia, with concomitant increases in ATP hydrolysis products. Reperfusion is associated with a gradual increase in cell ATP levels.

Classification of Acute Glomerulotubular Dysfunction

Hemodynamically Mediated Acute Kidney Injury

Renal hypoperfusion with ischemia is a common form of acute renal damage, especially in the setting of the ICU. This form of renal injury is often accompanied by oliguria and results from alterations in renal perfusion after a period of hypoxia, hypotension, cardiac dysfunction, or any condition that promotes hemodynamic instability, decreased effective

plasma volume, or both states. This condition is commonly referred to as *acute tubular necrosis* because it is characterized by necrosis of tubule cells; however, this is a nonspecific term that may also define nephrotoxic injury. A preferred term is *vasomotor nephropathy* or *hemodynamically mediated renal failure*.[40] The same physiologic alterations that initiate renal injury in this form of nephropathy may potentiate renal failure in conditions whose primary inciting event may not have been vascular.

Vasomotor nephropathy commonly follows a period of renal compensatory changes that may be termed *prerenal failure*,[9] which are discussed in the preceding section on physiology. When the kidney has fully used normal compensatory mechanisms, renal oxygen delivery is critically impaired, and this impairment results in cell damage or tubular cell necrosis. Thus it is apparent that acute tubular necrosis is the end result of a continuum of renal adaptive mechanisms. Acute cortical necrosis is an exaggerated and more advanced form of renal ischemia.

When vascular or hemodynamic abnormalities persist or are profound, renal compensatory mechanisms are unable to preserve RBF and maintain sufficient oxygen delivery and GFR. At a mean renal perfusion pressure of 80 mm Hg, afferent arteriolar dilation is maximal, and below these systemic pressures, RBF dramatically declines.[9,40] In addition, loss of the ability to autoregulate as a result of ischemia may cause further damage. Renal cell injury develops as the result of deficient oxygen delivery, depletion of cellular energy, loss of membrane integrity, and release of reactive oxygen species. Without sufficient oxygen, the kidney cannot support cell functions that maintain architectural integrity and complex transport functions.

Although total RBF is decreased in vasomotor nephropathy, outer cortical blood flow is preferentially reduced. The medulla is not spared, however, because of its increased susceptibility to alterations in renal perfusion.[41] Oxygen delivery to this segment of the kidney is precarious. Medullary partial pressure of oxygen (PO_2) is approximately 10 mm Hg in the rat and dog. This oxygen level approaches the critical minimum level required to support oxidative phosphorylation and ATP synthesis for cell function. In general, the proximal tubule sustains the greatest injury. The renal arteriogram of human subjects with vasomotor nephropathy reveals marked narrowing of the arcuate arteries and absence of peripheral vasculature, providing further evidence for the marked vascular resistance enhancement.[40]

The primary event in vasomotor nephropathy is injury of the renal tubule. The initiation of this injury, however, is microvascular in origin. Maximal renal compensation with marked efferent and afferent arteriolar vasoconstriction reduces glomerular plasma flow with resulting hypofiltration and compromises postglomerular blood supply to the renal tubule. Tubular cell necrosis with sloughing of tubular cells into the lumen results in obstruction of flow and back leakage of filtrate through the injured epithelium. Alterations in tubular cell function in cells receiving sublethal or lethal injury increase fluid and salt delivery distally, and this increase signals the glomerulotubular feedback system to cause vasoconstriction of the afferent arteriole and limit the fraction of plasma filtered at the glomerulus.[40] Although the initial reduction in GFR is the result of decreased RBF and tubular factors such as obstruction and back leakage, continued hypofiltration during the maintenance phase is related primarily to continued vasoconstriction and renal hypoperfusion.[40] Recovery from postischemic AKI is biphasic. Initially, an increase in GFR occurs with relief of tubular obstruction and, subsequently, improved filtration in association with renal vasodilation.

Oliguria in the presence of renal hypoperfusion has been referred to as acute renal success by investigators who propose that the response of an intelligent organ to a perceived reduction in blood flow is to reduce fluid and electrolyte losses by vasoconstriction to reduce the fraction of plasma filtered and by maximal reabsorption of fluid and salt to restore the circulation. In addition, increased distal delivery of water and solutes because of tubular cell necrosis reflects failure of the renal tubule to absorb what is filtered. The appropriate response of an intact nephron is to reduce filtration by release of angiotensin II into the interstitium. Angiotensin II mediates arteriolar vasoconstriction, which decreases glomerular plasma flow, and retraction of the glomerular tuft, which reduces Kf, the net effect being decreased glomerular filtration.[41]

The classic form of hemodynamically mediated AKI was oliguric by definition; however, nonoliguric acute vasomotor nephropathy is increasingly recognized.[41,42] This form of less severe disease has been referred to as attenuated acute tubular dysfunction and has allowed the recognition of three stages of AKI that actually represent a continuum of worsening disease: First, abbreviated renal insufficiency occurs after a single event of renal hypoperfusion, such as aortic cross-clamping, in the face of adequate volume repletion and systolic blood pressure (SBP). This syndrome is characterized by an acute drop in the GFR with gradual return to normal within a few days. The inability to concentrate the urine or to conserve sodium provides evidence of tubular injury. The second phase or form is referred to as overt renal failure. An example of this situation is aortic cross-clamping followed by continued renal hypoperfusion because of poor cardiac function. A more prolonged period of hypofiltration lasts for several days to weeks with a gradual return of the GFR. If recovery of renal perfusion is impaired by repeated episodes of ischemia/hypotension, sepsis, or hypoxia, the third pattern may be observed in which a protracted course may be observed and chances for recovery may be doubtful.[42] One situation in which the last example could exist is aggressive hemodialysis (ultrafiltration) with hypovolemia and, consequently, renal hypoperfusion in the recovering phase of renal failure. Clinical experience has supported this theory. Patients with multiple renal insults have a more protracted course and increased morbidity.[43]

Using the updated Schwartz formula for estimate of creatinine clearance (eGFR) in infants and children, a modified RIFLE classification (pRIFLE) has been developed. The updated Schwartz formula is as follows[44,45]:

$$eGFR = 0.413 \cdot [height\,(cm)]/[sCr\,(mg/dL)]   Eq. 75.2$$

The pRIFLE classification is defined by the percentage reduction in eCrCl or the amount of diminishing urine output[2] (Table 75.1).

Treatment of Acute Kidney Injury
Prevention/Attenuation of Acute Renal Failure

Prevention or attenuation of ARF has been the subject of numerous studies, as most agree that protection of the kidney

TABLE 75.1   pRIFLE Classification

pRIFLE	Estimated CrCL	Urine Output
Risk	25% decrease	<0.5 mL/kg/h for 8 hours
Injury	50% decrease	<0.5 mL/kg/h for 16 hours
Failure	75% decrease	<0.3 mL/kg/h for 24 hours or anuric for 12 hours
Loss	Persistent failure >4 weeks	
End-stage renal disease	Persistent failure >3 months	

from damage or enhancing recovery after damage would be preferable to the currently available supportive therapies. Primary prevention of AKI in the ICU is limited to those conditions in which the timing of injury is predictable, such as exposure to radiocontrast dye, cardiopulmonary bypass, nephrotoxic medications, or chemotherapy. In contrast to most cases of community-acquired AKI, nearly all cases of ICU-associated AKI result from more than a single insult.[46] Protective agents have been studied extensively with animal models of acute renal injury. Some of these agents have ultimately been used in clinical situations with variable success. In general, methods to reduce renal injury have been aimed at manipulation of RVR or alteration of the metabolic processes of the renal tubular cell.

Dopamine

Dopamine, when infused in low intravenous doses, increases RBF, GFR, and sodium excretion. In the past, clinicians frequently used "renal dose" dopamine in the hopes that such a maneuver might attenuate renal injury and improve survival. In addition, clinicians often interpret an increase in urinary output as proof that these two assumptions are valid. Dopamine stimulates both dopaminergic and adrenergic receptors. As such, dopamine may affect renal blood flow by direct vasodilation (dopamine receptors), by increasing cardiac output (β-receptors), or by increasing perfusion pressure. Of particular interest is its action on dopamine 1 (D1) receptors, which are abundantly distributed throughout the renal vasculature.[47] Stimulation of D1 receptors results in vasodilation by means of receptor coupling with cyclic adenosine monophosphate (cAMP) and calcium flux generated by protein kinase A. In addition, D1 receptors are also found within the brush border and basolateral membranes of the proximal tubule; medullary ascending limb of the loop of Henle; distal tubule; and cortical collecting ducts where agonist induces a decrease in sodium, phosphate, and bicarbonate absorption. D1 receptors have also been localized to the macula densa where they may modify renin production.[47] Dopamine inhibits the Na/K-ATPase along the nephron. Interestingly, this action would be expected to decrease the oxygen consumption of the renal tubule; thus it would be less susceptible to ischemic or hypoxic injury. Dopamine 2 (D2) receptors are present along the renal tubule. In the inner medulla, a subclass, D2k is coupled to prostaglandin E2 and attenuates the action of antidiuretic hormone (ADH) in this segment.

Dopamine in the dosage range of 0.5 to 2 μg/kg/min increases RBF by 20% to 40%. The GFR increases by 5% to

20%, an effect related to enhanced glomerular ultrafiltration by a preferential vasodilation at the afferent arteriole. This is thought to be related to a dopamine-induced increase in local angiotensin production, which attenuates the dopamine-induced vasodilation at the efferent but not the afferent arteriole. The increase in medullary blood flow observed with dopamine results in a decrease in the urea concentration within the medullary interstitium and contributes to the limited concentrating ability of the dopamine-stimulated renal tubule.

The observed increase in urinary flow is thought to be related primarily to the tubular actions rather than the vascular actions of dopamine. At higher doses, dopamine stimulation of receptors results in decreased sodium and fluid excretion, as well as renal vasoconstriction. Dopamine clearance is decreased in the presence of renal or liver dysfunction.

Despite these descriptive studies suggesting the possible benefit of low-dose dopamine infusion in the setting of evolving AKI, the 2012 iteration of the Surviving Sepsis Campaign guidelines state with a GRADE methodology grading of 1A (strong recommendation, strong evidence) that low-dose dopamine should not be used for renal protection.[48] A large randomized trial and meta-analysis comparing low-dose dopamine to placebo found no difference in either primary outcomes (peak serum creatinine, need for renal replacement, urine output, time to recovery of normal renal function) or secondary outcomes (survival to either ICU or hospital discharge, ICU stay, hospital stay, arrhythmias).

Dopamine may inhibit thyrotropin hormone release from the hypothalamus and have immunosuppressive effects through its inhibition of release of the lymphotropic factor prolactin. Dopamine should be used cautiously in neonates because the renal vascular response to dopamine is age dependent,[49] although administration of dopamine (0.5 to 2 μg/kg/min) to premature neonates with respiratory distress syndrome and renal insufficiency was reported to result in improved creatinine clearance without major side effects.

Diuretics

Intravenous diuretics have been frequently used in the intensive care unit to ameliorate fluid overload by increasing urine output.[50] This widespread use of loop diuretics in the face of impending renal failure has been ascribed to a combination of animal and human data. Loop diuretics decrease renal vascular resistance and increase renal blood flow.[51] In addition, loop diuretics inhibit the sodium/potassium chloride cotransporter system (NKCC2), thereby reducing active oxygen transport and potentially reducing oxygen consumption and thus limiting ischemic injury to the outer medullary tubules. Indeed, furosemide has been shown to decrease renal oxygen consumption in critically ill patients.

Mannitol may attenuate renal failure if it is given before the insult or immediately afterward.[52] Loop diuretics, such as furosemide, if given along with a potentially nephrotoxic agent, may increase the renal excretion of the agent and reduce associated nephrotoxicity. Mannitol has been shown to ameliorate nephrotoxicity related to gentamicin, amphotericin B, cisplatin, and myoglobin. A specific beneficial effect is doubtful, however, because acute saline loading alone provides similar protection. When tubular obstruction plays a major role, mannitol may increase tubular flow enough to wash obstructing debris downstream. It seems reasonable to use mannitol and potentially furosemide in the initial phases of oliguria when AKI may not be established; however, these agents provide little benefit and may increase toxicity in sustained oliguria as a result of tubular necrosis.

Calcium Entry Blockers

These agents may prevent renal insufficiency through their vasodilatory action on renal vasculature, as well as inhibition of calcium entry. The calcium channel blockers verapamil, nitrendipine, diltiazem, and nisoldipine have been administered to various animal models of ischemic injury with some success in the prevention or attenuation of renal failure. Minimal protection is observed, however, if they are administered after ischemia.[52] Calcium entry blockers had a beneficial effect in endotoxin-mediated AKI. This effect was postulated to be a result of an antagonism of platelet-activating factor.[53] The perfusion of cadaveric renal grafts before transplantation with diltiazem was associated with improved graft survival compared with control subjects.[54] Preoperative administration of calcium channel blockers to adults undergoing cardiac surgical procedures did not provide any obvious protection from the development of AKI.[55]

Prostaglandins

Vasoconstrictive forces in the renal vasculature may result from the action of vasoconstrictor prostaglandins and are counteracted by the vasodilatory substances.[56] Infusion or stimulation of the vasodilatory prostaglandins or inhibition of the vasoconstrictor prostaglandins seems to be a reasonable approach. Prostacyclin provided protection during ischemia in a rat model.[56] Administration of the thromboxane synthetase inhibitor OKY-046 partially ameliorated hypofiltration in a rat model of ischemic renal failure.[57] In addition, the administration of the free radical scavenger's dimethylthiourea and superoxide dismutase attenuated renal insufficiency and reduced thromboxane levels.

Renin-Angiotensin Antagonists

Administration of saralasin, an angiotensin II receptor antagonist, either before or after ischemia was not beneficial in the rat model. Blockade of angiotensin production by the conversion of enzyme inhibition with enalapril or captopril was not successful in preventing AKI.[58] Whereas captopril did prevent a fall in RBF, it also results in a drop in GFR.

Adenosine and Adenosine Triphosphate

Renal ischemia results in the depletion of cellular adenine nucleotides and increased levels of adenosine, an agent implicated as a mediator of local renal vasoconstriction.[59] Adenosine may also have protective tubular effects during ischemia because it inhibits solute reabsorption in the medullary thick ascending limb of the loop of Henle. Theophylline, a competitive inhibitor of adenosine receptors, partially prevents the hypofiltration following ischemia in the rat.

Infusion of ATP-magnesium chloride ($ATP-MgCl_2$) after renal ischemia promotes more rapid cellular recovery and attenuates renal injury.[59] In animal models, exogenous ATP, adenosine diphosphate (ADP), adenosine monophosphate (AMP), and adenosine preserve renal tubular cell metabolism during anoxia by protecting the membrane from disruption and providing precursors for rapid synthesis of ATP during reperfusion.

Atrial Natriuretic Factor

Atrial natriuretic factor (ANF) has direct effects on glomerular hemodynamics and GFR.[60] ANF dilates arcuate, interlobular, and proximal afferent arterioles, and it relaxes mesangial cells.[61] In a rat model of rhabdomyolysis, administration of ANF improved GFR and enhanced sodium and water excretion. In addition, ANF improved GFR and maintained cell energy levels during ischemic injury.[62] ANF preserves glomerular filtration and cellular ATP levels in experimental models of AKI by its effect on glomerular hemodynamics.

Free Radical Scavengers

Reactive oxygen species have been proposed as a cause of cellular injury in many forms of AKI. The conversion of xanthine to hypoxanthine during reoxygenation produces reactive oxygen species. Antioxidants and xanthine oxidase inhibition (allopurinol) have proved to attenuate renal injury in many models of AKI.

Thyroxine

Thyroxine reduces renal injury in a number of experimental models when given before the injury, immediately after, or 24 hours after ischemia. The mechanism by which thyroxine preserves both glomerular and tubular function is not completely understood; however, the rate of recovery of cellular ATP levels was much more rapid in animals given thyroxine after ischemic AKI. Isolated mitochondria from rats subjected to 45 minutes of ischemia exhibited decreased mitochondrial ADP transport. Administration of thyroxine was associated with significantly enhanced ADP transport.[63] The investigators speculated that part of the ATP depletion associated with ischemic injury might be the result of decreased mitochondrial uptake of the ATP precursor, ADP. The administration of thyroxine at 5 to 6 ng/kg/day for 5 to 10 days in eight children with AKI resulted in the recovery of renal function in all but one child, who died of the original disease.[64]

Glycine and Alanine

The amino acids glycine and alanine have been shown to have cytoprotective effects against injury in anoxia-hypoxia and chemotherapy-induced renal failure. The mechanism of cytoprotection is not understood but does not appear to involve preservation of intracellular ATP levels. Studies performed in cultured proximal tubular cells indicate that glycine and alanine may stimulate the expression of HSP genes and increase HSP proteins, which protect cells from injury. The cytoprotective effect was not observed with other amino acids and was independent of cellular ATP levels in this model of renal injury.[65] Incubation of isolated renal tubules with glycine during hypoxia was associated with increased levels of glutathione, as well as increased cell ATP, although these did not appear to account fully for the protective effect of glycine. In addition, administration of glycine prevented renal injury in rats treated with nephrotoxic doses of cisplatin.[66]

Acute Kidney Injury: Clinical Impact

Severe deterioration of kidney function can have a profound effect on body fluid homeostasis and on blood pressure. The nature of these alterations often requires intensive care management regardless of the precise underlying diagnosis. A wide variety of kidney diseases may result in AKI. The most urgent aspects of AKI are (1) hyperkalemia, (2) severe hypertension, (3) severe plasma and extracellular volume expansion leading to heart failure and pulmonary edema, (4) unremitting metabolic acidosis, (5) hypocalcemia/hyperphosphatemia. Each of these can be viewed as an indication for intensive care and consideration of dialysis.[67] Additionally, the presence and degree of fluid overload (FO) has been shown to be a predictor of survival at the initiation of renal replacement therapy (RRT) and is now considered an important indication for intervention.[68-71]

Hyperkalemia

The major reason for the development of hyperkalemia (serum potassium concentration more than 6 mEq/L) is the release (or infusion, or both) of potassium into the extracellular space at a rate greater than the kidney's ability to excrete potassium. Further, the intracellular potassium is in the concentration range of 140 to 150 mEq/L, adding to the total source of potassium. The fact that AKI and oliguria have developed does not mean that hyperkalemia will develop. By the same token, hyperkalemia may develop rapidly in situations of extensive tissue destruction even without oliguria and "full-blown" AKI. Thus in the clinical situation of a crush injury or the tumor lysis syndrome, hyperkalemia should be anticipated and careful anticipatory monitoring begun.

Severe Hypertension

Hypertension is frequently associated with kidney disease. The two main mechanisms by which kidney disease leads to hypertension, especially accelerated hypertension, are (1) plasma volume expansion caused by the failure to excrete sodium chloride and water and (2) hyperreninemia associated with decreased kidney perfusion.

Plasma and Extracellular Volume Expansion

Plasma and extracellular volume expansion are associated with kidney failure. With an abrupt decline in GFR, even "normal" amounts of sodium and water intake expand the extracellular and plasma volumes. Depending on the cardiac status of the patient, the serum albumin level, and the degree of capillary permeability, this extracellular and plasma volume expansion may be manifest as peripheral edema, hypertension, or congestive heart failure and pulmonary edema. In situations of hypertension or congestive heart failure, the treatment involves two principles. The first is to reduce to as low a level as possible the amount of sodium and fluid the patient receives. This requires attention to diet, intravenous or hyperalimentation solutions, and drugs. The second principle is to remove extracellular fluid. If the patient's kidney function permits (glomerular filtration of approximately 15 mL/min or higher), then diuretics, especially loop diuretics such as furosemide, bumetanide, or ethacrynic acid, will help to stimulate a diuresis that should improve the blood pressure or the congestive heart failure. The addition of thiazide diuretics prior to the use of loop diuretics may potentiate the effectiveness of loop diuretics allowing for a greater diuresis.[72] In children with more severe kidney disease, diuretic therapy does not result in diuresis, and dialysis will be necessary.

Severe Metabolic Acidosis

The kidney is responsible for the excretion of hydrogen ion and the regeneration of bicarbonate. When kidney function rapidly deteriorates, then the extracellular concentration of hydrogen ion increases, and this increase leads to acidosis and low serum bicarbonate concentrations. This problem is exacerbated by conditions that increase the production of hydrogen ion and its release into the extracellular fluid. Conditions such as sepsis, severe trauma, burns, extensive abdominal disease or surgery, high chloride-containing intravenous fluids, and hemolysis are all examples in which hypoxia, high hydrogen ion production or release into the extracellular space, and a decline in RBF and the GFR are combined. The result is severe metabolic acidosis (see also Chapter 76).

Hypocalcemia/Hyperphosphatemia

Hypocalcemia arises from hyperphosphatemia as a result of dietary load, cellular breakdown, and reduced kidney phosphate excretion; reduced synthesis of calcitriol; downregulation of skeletal cell receptors for parathyroid hormone; and acidosis.[73]

Hyperphosphatemia may not be recognized, for the plasma phosphorus level is not contained on any of the classic "lab panels" as directed by Medicare; it therefore needs to be thought of and sought out for identification.

Uremia

The symptoms of uremia are frequently vague and difficult to quantitate. They include central nervous system (CNS) manifestations such as lethargy, confusion, seizures, and obtundation and also gastrointestinal manifestations such as anorexia, nausea, and vomiting. These symptoms plus metabolic derangements often lead to the initiation of dialysis.

Renal Disposition of Endogenous and Exogenous Compounds

An important consideration in AKI is the role of the kidney in the metabolism, elimination, and detoxification of endogenous and exogenous materials. Any drugs given must be reviewed because the dosing interval or the dose of drug may need to be altered in AKI. Endogenous substances generally are more slowly metabolized or excreted. For example, the hormone gastrin is metabolized by the proximal tubule after being filtered by the glomerulus. The resultant persistent high circulating levels of gastrin may explain the higher incidence of gastritis and ulcer disease seen in patients with kidney failure.

Specific Kidney Diseases That May Lead to Acute Kidney Injury
Hemolytic Uremic Syndrome

Hemolytic uremic syndrome (HUS) is considered to be the most common cause of AKI in children in the world.[74] Whereas this may be correct, it should be recognized that within "westernized" medical systems, AKI is more commonly a consequence of sepsis, cardiac disease, and other comorbid and chronic underlying conditions.[75]

HUS is characterized by thrombotic microangiopathy with platelet aggregation and fibrin deposition in small vessels in the kidney, intestine, CNS, and elsewhere. The hemolytic anemia is related predominantly to shearing of red blood cells as they pass through involved vessels. The syndrome is defined by the triad of microangiopathic hemolytic anemia, thrombocytopenia, and impaired kidney function. In the typical form of the disease, a triggering infectious agent has frequently been reported and is usually accompanied by diarrhea, hence "typical" HUS is usually synonymous with the term *diarrhea-positive* HUS. *Escherichia coli* (0157:H7) has been implicated in a large number of cases of typical (epidemic) forms of HUS.[76] It should be understood that there exist a myriad of causes of HUS (*Streptococcus pneumoniae* infection, usually severe; *Shigella dysenteriae; Citrobacter;* etc.) and that in the absence of verotoxin-secreting *E. coli*, HUS can still occur. Atypical HUS is usually used to describe diarrhea-negative or atypically presenting cases (positive family history, early presentation less than 6 months), although it is increasingly applied to cases of suspected or confirmed complement pathway mutation. A third entity, thrombotic thrombocytopenic purpura (TTP), presents as a pentad of symptoms that overlap with HUS: microangiopathic hemolytic anemia, thrombocytopenia, mild renal impairment, fever, and neurologic disease. HUS may also present with fever and neurologic involvement, making the clinical diagnosis difficult to distinguish. TTP has now been linked to a deficiency or inactivation of the protease that cleaves von Willebrand factor, ADAMTS13, which can be used to differentiate the two diagnoses.

Clinical Signs

Typical HUS usually presents in "epidemics" and is characterized by a prodrome of bloody diarrhea. Children with HUS are older than 1 year and younger than 10 years (typically, 18 months to 3 years). The important presenting features of bloody diarrhea, fever, lethargy, decreased urine output, and pallor should lead to a suspicion of HUS. Laboratory evaluation will verify the diagnosis. Atypical HUS is caused by complement pathway mutations (most commonly factor H or factor I but also membrane cofactor protein, C3-convertase, and factor B), which are responsible for promoting the decay of the spontaneously activating alternative complement pathway. The alternative complement pathway normally assists the body in discriminating between host and foreign cells, and mutations lead to an uncontrolled activation. The development of HUS has also been associated with oral contraceptives and calcineurin inhibitors.[76,77] The final common pathway, regardless of the initiating agent, is endothelial cell injury, platelet activation, and activation of the alternative complement pathway.[78]

Once the endothelium is injured and the subendothelial region is exposed, a sequence of events is set into motion that amplifies the initial endothelial damage. Platelets adhere to the subendothelial space, and a release reaction follows that activates additional platelets and initiates fibrin deposition. Both endothelial cell and platelet factors are involved in the propagation of intraglomerular fibrin deposition and coagulation. Direct injury of the endothelial cell may initiate coagulation by release of tissue factor or exposure of the basement membrane. Evidence suggests that the endothelial cells in patients with HUS have reduced ability to produce prostacyclin (PGI_2), a potent vasodilator and inhibitor of platelet aggregation. Some patients with HUS lack a plasma factor that stimulates PGI_2 production. In addition, there is decreased glomerular fibrinolytic activity because of a circulating inhibitor of plasminogen activator. Interestingly, this fibrinolysis inhibitor is removed from the circulation by dialysis.[79] Platelet count and survival time is decreased in patients with HUS, and occasionally there is evidence of platelet activation.

Hemolysis may be brisk and may require transfusions on a daily basis. The aim of transfusions during the period of hemolysis should be to prevent heart failure and not to return the hematocrit value to normal. Thrombocytopenia may be severe but only rarely results in significant bleeding, and therefore platelets should not be given unless clearly needed to stop bleeding or in anticipation of invasive (especially vascular) procedures. Some have suggested that platelets play an important role in the pathophysiology of this disorder. It is further suggested that infusing platelets may actually prolong or worsen the intravascular deposition characteristic of HUS.

Complications
Other organ system involvement may lead to serious complications. CNS involvement may reflect the metabolic effects of uremia and can be manifested by lethargy, somnolence, stupor, or coma. Seizures, paresis, and even CNS hemorrhages can result from vascular damage and CNS vessel occlusion. Gastrointestinal involvement has also been well documented. Liver enzyme elevations, abdominal pain, intestinal obstruction, and bowel perforation have all been reported. These possibilities must be considered and evaluated when appropriate. In some instances, the diagnosis of HUS has been made after abdominal exploration.

Therapy
Therapy has been supportive, aimed at preventing deterioration and carefully managing complications such as AKI, anemia, CNS, and abdominal symptoms. Heparin, fibrinolytics, and antiplatelet drugs (aspirin, dipyridamole) have all been attempted. In general, reports demonstrate lack of benefit and, in the cases of heparin and fibrinolytics, increased harm from increased bleeding. Platelet transfusions can enhance thrombosis in microvasculature, so they are not indicated unless there is active bleeding. The HUS outbreak in Germany that resulted in a large number of deaths has shed light on the understanding of treatment interventions regardless of classic or atypical types of HUS.[80]

In severe cases of HUS, plasma exchange (PE) may be indicated, with various studies citing an increase in survival between 10% and 78%[81-83] versus supportive care alone. However, complete hematologic (normalization of lactate dehydrogenase [LDH], platelet count) and renal response rates are lower in patients with identified complement mutations, as the underlying complement dysregulation and thrombotic microangiopathic processes likely persist despite PE.[84] Eculizumab, a C5 complement inhibitor that prevents downstream formation of the membranolytic membrane attack complex (MAC), has been used in atypical HUS with good and promising efficacy. The medication is costly, and randomized controlled trials have not been completed to determine optimal pediatric dosing intervals or duration, although several studies are ongoing. The majority of published data use an eculizumab induction dose of 900 mg once a week for 4 weeks, followed by maintenance 1200 mg every 2 weeks for 1 year in patients >40 kg.[84] Cataland and Wu[83] proposed a treatment schema in adults of suspected atypical HUS or TTP cases beginning with PE and continuing if the patient is deemed a good responder by hematologic and renal recovery criteria. If the patient is a nonresponder after a period of 3 to 5 days on PE, they recommend then basing treatment on ADAMTS13 activity; if normal, the patient is treated as atypical HUS with eculizumab, and if ADAMTS13 is deficient, the patient is treated with immunosuppressive therapies. Case series in the pediatric literature report good neurologic and renal outcomes after use of eculizumab; however, dosage and duration are not uniform. Further prospective studies are needed to determine the most cost-effective pediatric dosing regimen and whether outcomes in pediatric patients are improved.

Prognosis
The prognosis for the "typical" form of HUS is good. Most series report 3% to 5% mortality rates and an additional 3% to 5% with chronic changes such as chronic kidney disease, persistent hematuria/proteinuria, and chronic hypertension. Thus more than 90% of children with the typical form of HUS recover completely.

In the face of AKI, many of the therapies (red blood cell [RBC], platelet infusion, fresh frozen plasma) result in volume to the children, potentially increasing the risk of fluid overload. Further, the plasma components of packed red blood cells (PRBCs) are hyperkalemic, acidotic, and hypocalcemic. Therefore, transfusing PRBCs to a patient with AKI may induce not only fluid overload but also significant and even lethal electrolyte disturbances. The use of RRT may be needed to offset these potential risks.

Acute Glomerulonephritis
Nearly every form of glomerulonephritis has been reported to present as AKI (Box 75.2). In some instances the kidney insufficiency may be the result of an immunologic process leading to acute inflammation (eg, acute postinfectious glomerulonephritis). In others, intravascular volume depletion may play a prominent role in AKI (eg, minimal change nephrotic syndrome).

In general, glomerulonephritis is initiated by immunologic events within the glomerulus followed by mechanisms that result in damage to the glomerulus.[85] Glomerular disease results from the deposition of immune complexes composed of (1) antibodies to nonkidney antigens that localize within the glomeruli and form in situ immune complexes; (2) circulating soluble immune complexes that are trapped within the mesangium or subendothelial space; or (3) antibody to antigens within the glomerulus, either as normal glomerular antigens or as neoantigens induced by inflammation or infection.

BOX 75.2	Glomerular Disease Associated With Acute Kidney Injury

Hypocomplementemic (low C3)
- Acute postinfectious glomerulonephritis
- Membranoproliferative glomerulonephritis
- Systemic lupus erythematosus

Normocomplementemic (normal C3)
- Henoch-Schönlein purpura
- Immunoglobulin A nephropathy
- Wegener granulomatosis
- Goodpasture syndrome
- Membranous nephropathy

Hemolytic-uremic syndrome
Minimal-change nephrotic syndrome

Antibody deposits promote injury by activation of inflammatory cells or by their direct interaction with glomerular cells. The result is mesangial cell proliferation, capillary wall and basement membrane injury, and extracapillary proliferation of epithelial cells, a process known as crescent formation.

Immune complexes mediate glomerular injury in two ways: through direct membrane damage by the MAC complex or by stimulation of glomerular localized inflammatory cells.

Salt and water retention commonly observed with acute glomerulonephritis is the result of a decreased GFR, not increased tubular reabsorption, as once proposed. The renin-angiotensin system is thought not to play a role in the positive salt and water balance. In general, the presentation of glomerulonephritis as AKI implies a virulent form of disease known as rapidly progressive or crescentic glomerulonephritis. Although rapidly progressive refers to a clinical characteristic and crescentic to a pathologic feature, the two are commonly coincidental in the presentation of AKI. A classification of rapidly progressive glomerulonephritis is presented in Box 75.3. Four prototypical conditions serve as examples of acute kidney disease that may result in the need for intensive care.

Acute Postinfectious (Streptococcal) Glomerulonephritis

This condition is well known to pediatricians. An association between glomerulonephritis and scarlet fever was known in the 18th century. In the early 20th century, however, a clear connection between streptococcal infections and glomerulonephritis was established. The disease most frequently occurs between the ages of 2 and 12 years. It is seen as a sporadic event or in epidemics. It appears that only certain strains of streptococci lead to glomerulonephritis, thus the term *nephritogenic streptococcus*.[86] The more recent term is *postinfectious glomerulonephritis (PIGN)* due to the fact that no longer does *Streptococcus* cause the majority of the cases of PIGN cases.

The mechanisms by which nephritogenic streptococci cause glomerular injury are similar to that seen with "shunt nephritis." It is generally accepted that immune complexes, with the participation of complement and other inflammatory mediators, cause glomerular inflammation. The precise nature of the bacterial antigen and its site of formation (circulation compared with in situ in the glomerulus) remain areas of study.

Clinical Signs

The usual sites of infection are the upper respiratory tract, skin, or both. A long-standing observation is that the latent period is 7 to 14 days if the infection is in the upper respiratory tract and 21 to 40 days if the infection is on the skin.

BOX 75.3	**Classification of Rapidly Progressive Crescentic Glomerulonephritis**

Pulmonary renal syndromes
- Antiglomerular basement membrane antibody-mediated (Goodpasture syndrome)
- Systemic lupus erythematosus
- Polyarteritis nodosa
- Granulomatosis polyangiitis (Wegener granulomatosis)
- Churg-Strauss syndrome

Postinfectious
Henoch-Schönlein purpura
Immunoglobulin A nephropathy
Membranoproliferative glomerulonephritis

Subclinical cases may be common; they are estimated to be 2 to 19 times as frequent as clinical cases. Symptomatic cases usually present with an acute nephritic syndrome: edema, hypertension, hematuria, and oliguria. Other important clinical features include proteinuria, red cell casts, and abnormal urinary red cell morphologic findings, all markers of glomerular injury. Pulmonary edema may also be present, especially if significant salt and water retention are present and if hypertension is severe. Nonspecific findings include malaise, anorexia, abdominal pain, nausea, and vomiting. (This presentation is seen with other forms of acute glomerulonephritis.) Patients may have AKI.

Laboratory Findings

Laboratory findings at the time of presentation or early in the course include high serum IgG levels and low serum complement levels, especially C3 and CH50. In general, the alternate pathway of complement is the mechanism of complement activation, although on occasion C2 and C4 may be depressed as well. Complement levels return to normal in 4 to 6 weeks. Therefore if complement levels remain depressed for 6 to 8 weeks after the onset of acute glomerulonephritis, another diagnosis should be strongly entertained (systemic lupus erythematosus or membranoproliferative glomerulonephritis). The definitive diagnosis is based on renal biopsy that can be performed easily adding clarity to the diagnosis.

Treatment

Treatment is based on the patient's symptoms and is directed at preventing or reducing salt and water retention and hypertension. All patients should have salt and water restriction unless dehydration is obvious (an unusual situation). Approximately 50% to 60% of patients require treatment for hypertension. Diuretics, angiotensin-converting enzyme inhibitors, and potent vasodilators should be considered. Five percent of patients may require dialysis for congestive heart failure, hypervolemia, or encephalopathy.

Prognosis

The long-term prognosis in acute postinfectious glomerulonephritis is a matter of debate. The mortality rate is approximately 0.5%, and death usually results from severe hypertension and encephalopathy or heart failure. A study by Potter and colleagues[87] suggested that the long-term prognosis generally thought to be excellent was in fact not necessarily so. Studies with follow-up of 10 to 15 years suggest that chronic kidney injury develops in approximately 1% of patients. A second consensus conclusion is that the prognosis is better in children than in adults. Longer-term follow-up is needed.

Systemic Lupus Erythematosus

Systemic lupus erythematosus (SLE) is a protean illness affecting many organ systems. In some instances, intensive care is needed for aspects of SLE such as nephritis, cerebritis, carditis, serositis, or sepsis.

Even within a relatively narrow aspect of SLE such as nephritis, great heterogeneity exists. Glomerulonephritis develops in approximately 75% of patients with SLE.[88] This may range from mild hematuria and proteinuria to nephrotic syndrome and rarely to rapidly progressive kidney failure. The patterns of lesions in lupus nephritis are varied. The World Health Organization (WHO) has classified lupus nephritis based on light microscopy into five categories: (1) minimal disease, (2) mesangial disease, (3) focal proliferative glomerulonephritis, (4) diffuse proliferative glomerulonephritis, and

(5) membranous nephropathy. These five categories have been further subdivided to reflect activity (eg, cellular proliferation, crescents, thrombi, presence of tubulointerstitial disease) and chronicity (eg, sclerosis, fibrosis, tubular atrophy). Combining these pathologic categories with a small number of clinical predictors of poor outcome such as age younger than 24 years, male gender, and decreased kidney function on presentation has permitted a more careful assessment of therapeutic interventions.

Clinical Signs

The broad variation in clinical manifestations may reflect individual expression of similar immunopathologic mechanisms or different immunopathologic mechanisms presenting as a similar constellation of clinical manifestations.[89] It is clear that SLE represents the overproduction of antibodies against multiple "self"-antigens. Patients with lupus have high titers of antinuclear antibodies and in particular anti-double-stranded DNA antibodies, which are often seen in SLE nephritis. Work by Hobbs and associates demonstrated a high presence of antiphospholipid antibodies placing the child at risk for clotting. This clotting risk may be accentuated in the face of nephrotic syndrome or the use of birth control pills.[90] The factors that lead to the abundant production and activation of relevant B cells are unclear. Certainly hormonal influence must be important because most patients with SLE are women. Environmental factors may be important in cases of SLE induced by drugs or viruses and the known association of SLE with ultraviolet light exposure. Other important factors are suggested by the higher than normal T helper/T suppressor cell ratio. Many of these act in concert to result in abundant antibody production and the deposition of complexes in target organs such as the kidney.

Clinically, patients with SLE nephritis who require intensive care probably have rapidly progressive glomerulonephritis or AKI. Their presentation includes many of the following features: hypertension; active urinary sediment with proteinuria, hematuria, and casts; oliguria or rarely anuria; intravascular volume expansion; and declining kidney function with rising serum creatinine, hyperkalemia, and metabolic acidosis. Unlike the glomerulonephritis described previously, treatment should include management of kidney dysfunction as previously outlined and management aimed at the SLE itself. Kidney biopsy is useful not only to assess the degree of glomerular involvement as classified by the WHO grading system but also to evaluate for acute tubular necrosis or drug toxicity with tubular damage.[91]

Treatment

In the intensive care setting, treatment directed at rapidly progressive or diffuse proliferative SLE nephritis consists of high-dose bolus corticosteroid (usually methylprednisolone) at a dosage of 10 to 20 mg/kg intravenously (IV) given 3 to 5 times in a daily or every-other-day regimen. This therapy is associated with hypertension. Other treatments have included plasmapheresis, immunosuppressives including azathioprine, cyclophosphamide, mycophenolate mofetil or other alkylating agents, and methotrexate. Over the past decade the use of rituximab and other immune-modulators such as belimumab have been studied in children of varying results, with detailed review elsewhere.[92] Data from the National Institutes of Health and others have suggested significant benefit from cyclophosphamide or mycophenolate mofetil in maintaining kidney function.[93]

Prognosis

The long-term prognosis for children with SLE nephritis is unclear.[89] Regardless, patients and families must expect persistent evidence of kidney injury such as hematuria, proteinuria, hypertension, and even reduced kidney function such as a diminished GFR. Further, patients may have relapsing episodes of nephrotic syndrome or acute glomerulonephritis.

Other Glomerulonephritides

Two other forms of glomerulonephritis may result in the need for intensive care therapy. These are antiglomerular basement membrane (anti-GBM) antibody disease (Goodpasture syndrome) and granulomatosis with polyangiitis (GPA, formerly known as Wegener granulomatosis). Although rare in children, both conditions can result in AKI. Therapy should be directed at the general condition of AKI as discussed previously in addition to specific therapy.

In the case of anti-GBM antibody disease, patients may have both kidney disease and pulmonary disease, often pulmonary hemorrhage. Treatment includes corticosteroids, plasmapheresis, and immunosuppressives, mainly alkylating agents. Despite therapy, end-stage kidney disease develops in some patients. Recurrences of anti-GBM antibody disease in kidney allografts have also been reported but are rare.[94] Vasculitic syndromes associated with kidney disease include GPA and microscopic polyangiitis (MPA), associated with antineutrophil cytoplasm antibody (ANCA).[95] ANCA is an autoantibody that is found in one of two patterns in many forms of vasculitis and serves as a potentially useful diagnostic tool. GPA, or Wegener granulomatosis, is characterized by granulomatous vasculitis that attacks the respiratory tract including sinuses, trachea and lungs, and the kidneys. This condition may be difficult to diagnose, and biopsy may be the only means of determining the diagnosis if the plasma ANCA is negative. Children often present with nonspecific constitutional symptoms, with glomerulonephritis and pulmonary disease also common at presentation. Cyclophosphamide induction with azathioprine maintenance has been shown to be beneficial in the treatment of the kidney disease of Wegener granulomatosis, and plasmapheresis is also of potential benefit in crescentic forms, although it is not widely used because of frequent complications. Rituximab, a monoclonal antibody to CD20 on B cells, has been approved for the treatment of severe ANCA-associated vasculitis on the basis of the adult rituximab in ANCA-associated vasculitis (RAVE) trial,[96] which showed that a single course of rituximab plus steroid for induction was noninferior to cyclophosphamide followed by azathioprine.

Nephrotic Syndrome and Acute Kidney Failure

AKI is an uncommon complication of primary nephrotic syndrome in children but may occur as a result of intravascular volume depletion, bilateral kidney venous thrombosis, or drug-induced kidney toxicity.[97]

The clinical scenario is one in which the child has a low serum albumin level and edema (increased extracellular volume). These patients have stable and often normal plasma volumes despite low oncotic pressure. Should an acute illness (eg, gastroenteritis) occur, however, intravascular volume depletion and AKI may develop rapidly. Patients with nephrotic syndrome who have fluid losses or are unable to take in fluids should be admitted to the hospital, and intravenous administration of albumin plus maintenance and replacement fluids should be considered. The use of intravenous albumin helps to maintain the intravascular volume and reduces the edema that might develop during fluid therapy. Removal of fluid with diuretics or dialysis/hemofiltration can assist with recovery of function. Placing a vascular access for dialysis in a child with nephrotic syndrome is not without risk. In general, children with nephrotic syndrome have a high risk of clotting, independent of vascular access. The large bore vascular access commonly used for dialysis may potentiate this risk. Use of heparin for thrombosis prevention should be considered in certain high-risk situations.

Tubulointerstitial Disease

Acute Tubulointerstitial Nephritis

Acute tubulointerstitial nephritis (ATIN) is a clinical syndrome characterized by inflammation of the kidney interstitium accompanied by interstitial edema and kidney tubular injury. ATIN may be caused by numerous drugs, infectious agents, and systemic illnesses.[98] A partial list of causes can be found in Box 75.4.

In most cases, ATIN is immunologic in origin. Most understanding of the pathogenesis has been obtained from animal models. Three phases have been described for ATIN. The initial phase involves recognition of a nephritogenic antigen located in the interstitium. The antigen may be a normal component of the interstitium, a modified constituent, drug induced, or infection induced. Loss of host tolerance is thought to be required for the initial phase to occur. The immune regulatory phase is characterized by the activation of T-helper lymphocytes, which induce differentiation of T and B cells that directly injure the interstitium. The inability of the host to counteract this response with T-suppressor cells permits T- and B-cell activation to go unabated. In the effector phase, both humoral and cell-mediated components contribute to tissue injury. Antibodies to tissue antigens promote injury by activation of the complement cascade, chemotaxis, and cell-mediated cytotoxicity. IgE is also produced, which may recruit eosinophils or mast cells. Mononuclear cell infiltration produces tissue injury by release of proteases and lymphokines. Eosinophils also damage surrounding tissue by release of proteases, leukotrienes, and toxic oxygen species.

Several theories have been proposed to explain the reduced GFR: (1) the "clogged drain," (2) the capillary bed, and (3) vascular tone hypotheses. The clogged drain theory proposes that tubular obstruction caused by luminal debris and interstitial edema results in increased pressure in the Bowman space and decreased pressure favoring filtration. Interstitial inflammation results in injury to the blood supply of the tubules (capillary bed hypothesis). Because these vessels are postglomerular, the increased resistance and reduced surface area associated with vessel injury result in an increase in efferent arteriolar pressure and a reduction in the pressure gradient across the glomerulus with a resultant drop in the GFR. Decreased sodium reabsorption by injured proximal tubular epithelial cells reduces the medullary interstitial osmolality and impairs the ability to concentrate the urine. Thus an increased volume of filtrate is delivered distally, stimulating the juxtaglomerular apparatus to increase angiotensin II production (vascular tone hypothesis). The net result is vasoconstriction and a diminished GFR.

Pathologically, diffuse or patchy infiltration of the kidney interstitium by lymphocytes, plasma cells, and eosinophils and edema of the interstitial space is observed. Eosinophils are usually indicative of an acute phase, whereas epithelioid granulomas with giant cells and fibroblasts or fibrosis indicate chronic disease. Tubules may have mild structural alterations or marked necrosis with loss of brush border. Drug-induced interstitial nephritis is the most common form of ATIN in adults and children. Eight of 13 pediatric patients described in one series[98] and 38 of 57 in another series of children[99] with interstitial nephritis had drug-related causes of ATIN. Numerous drugs have been associated with ATIN. The β-lactam antibiotics are the most frequently associated with ATIN with methicillin being the prototype, although ampicillin is the most common offending drug in pediatric series. NSAIDs are increasingly recognized as a cause of acute kidney dysfunction.

Clinically apparent disease usually develops days to weeks after exposure to the inciting drug or agent but may be immediate.[100] Drug-induced tubulointerstitial disease is localized predominantly to the cortex, whereas infectious or infiltrative disorders more commonly localize to the medulla. The functional abnormality often indicates the primary site of tubular injury. Damage involving mainly the proximal tubule results in the wasting of bicarbonate, phosphate, glucose, amino acids, and uric acid. Distal tubular involvement may be manifest as hyperkalemic kidney tubular acidosis as a result of impaired secretion of both K^+ and H^+. Nephrogenic diabetes insipidus can result with medullary involvement.

Although ATIN is primarily a disease of the kidney interstitium and tubule with lack of glomerular structural alterations, the GFR may also be reduced. Of 13 children described by Ellis and colleagues[98] and Andreoli,[101] 12 had a creatinine clearance of less than 50 mL/min/1.73 m². AKI resulting from ATIN may be oliguric. Other clinical signs of ATIN are fever and rash. ATIN usually resolves with removal of the offending agent, although occasionally chronic kidney insufficiency may result.

Cardiorenal Syndrome

Renal insufficiency occurs commonly in adult and pediatric patients with heart failure. Although the mechanisms are not fully understood, diminished cardiac function coupled with renal dysfunction, or the cardiorenal syndrome, has been observed in both the acute and chronic care settings. The phenomenon remains better characterized in adult medicine.

BOX 75.4   Primary Causes of Acute Tubulointerstitial Nephritis

Drugs
Infections
Septicemia
Leptospirosis
Candidiasis
Malignant infiltration
Lymphoma
Leukemia
Systemic diseases
Systemic lupus erythematosus
Sarcoidosis

Decreased urine output and resultant fluid retention can aggravate heart failure symptoms and contribute to clinical deterioration. Even a modest increase in serum creatinine (ie, >0.2 mg/dL) can predict mortality in adult patients hospitalized for heart failure.[102] The relationship of renal function and heart failure in children has not been well examined. Retrospective data analysis has shown a high incidence of cardiac disease among children who exhibit renal insufficiency while hospitalized, and clinical experience suggests that as in adults, worsening renal function is associated with worse outcomes among children with heart failure.[103]

Basis for Deteriorating Renal Function

The physiologic interaction of the heart and kidney is complex and not well understood, although it is recognized that disease of one organ system frequently complicates the other. Some have termed this combined cardiac and renal dysfunction the *cardiorenal syndrome*. Renal insufficiency occurring in heart failure patients is usually attributed to a "prerenal state" resulting from diminished cardiac output and renal perfusion. It is hypothesized that deteriorating cardiac output and decreasing renal blood flow trigger neurohormonal activities that lead to fluid retention and increased systemic vascular resistance, causing further progression of ventricular dysfunction. Data from animal studies show that isolated renal ischemia leads to increased pulmonary vascular permeability, suggesting a bidirectional pathophysiologic interaction between the renal and cardiopulmonary systems.[104] Other mechanisms may also contribute to a decline in renal function, including medications being used to support cardiovascular function, such as vasoactive drugs. A study by Price and coworkers[105] reported worsening renal function with the use of dopamine and nesiritide.

There is evidence that right ventricular (RV) dysfunction may be associated with renal venous congestion. Using echocardiographically derived measurements, Testani and colleagues showed that in 151 patients, RV dysfunction remained a significant predictor of change in glomerular filtration rate after controlling for heart rate, hemoglobin, admission serum urea nitrogen, B-type natriuretic peptide level, diuretic dose, length of stay, ejection fraction, cardiac output, tricuspid regurgitation severity, and inferior vena cava inspiratory collapse.[106]

Cardiac Surgery—Related Acute Kidney Injury

AKI is not uncommon following cardiac surgery, and its presence portends a worse prognosis. In a survey of 542 patients who underwent cardiopulmonary bypass to fix their congenital cardiac disease, the rate of acute kidney injury after congenital cardiac surgery was shown to be about 11%.[107] Other studies have found mortality rates to be four times higher in patients with renal failure compared to those without. Studies have shown that a small rise (less than 50%) in creatinine in the first 48 hours could predict a greater than 50% increase in serum creatinine in the next 48 hours. Significant independent risk factors for AKI were bypass time and longer vasopressor use; there was a tendency toward younger age as a risk factor.[108] Cardiac surgery—related AKI has been characterized and described in adult medicine; however, at this time it remains difficult to characterize the exact nature of the injury in the pediatric population. Cardiac surgery—associated acute kidney injury (CSA-AKI) is a significant clinical problem. It results from the interactions between the complicated interventions required in the process of congenital cardiac surgery such as cardiac bypass, use of blood products, the anatomic variability of the congenital cardiac abnormality such as single ventricles, and the surgical correction/palliation of the lesion. It likely involves at least six major mechanisms: exogenous toxins and cytokines, metabolic factors, ischemia and reperfusion, neurohormonal activation, inflammation, and oxidative stress.[109] These mechanisms of injury are likely to be active at different times with different intensity and probably act synergistically. There are also some data that suggest that at least some of the injury may be pigment related, but this is yet to be substantiated.[110] There have also been attempts at ameliorating the injury with interventions such as *N*-acetyl cysteine, but this has resulted in an increase in bleeding with any benefit yet to be established.[111]

There are, however, newer markers of renal injury such as plasma neutrophil gelatinase-associated lipocalin (NGAL) that are more sensitive than serum creatinine in predicting acute kidney injury. In fact, plasma NGAL at 2 hours after cardiopulmonary bypass (CPB) was the most powerful independent predictor of AKI in patients post-CPB.[112,113] Serum creatinine is an inadequate marker because nearly 50% of renal function has to be lost before its levels are elevated, and serum creatinine does not accurately depict kidney function until a steady state has been reached, which may require several days. Biomarkers such as plasma NGAL may provide for earlier clinical intervention, thereby preventing significant mortality or morbidity. The renal histologic changes in cardiac surgery—related AKI are yet to be well characterized.

Porcine data utilizing experimental cardiopulmonary bypass revealed higher tubular injury scores in kidneys post-CPB relative to controls (median score 1.0 [IQR 1.0-1.0], p = .019). AKI was associated with endothelial injury and activation, as demonstrated by reduced *Dolichos biflorus* agglutinin (DBA) lectin and increased endothelin-1 and vascular cell adhesion molecule (VCAM) staining.[114]

Tumor Lysis Syndrome

Tumor lysis syndrome (TLS) is an oncologic emergency that is usually seen when tumor cells undergo rapid decomposition spontaneously or, more often, in response to cytoreductive therapy with the release of large amounts of potassium, phosphate, and nucleic acids into the systemic circulation (see also Chapter 94). Catabolism of the nucleic acids to uric acid leads to hyperuricemia, and a marked increase in uric acid excretion can result in the precipitation of uric acid in the renal tubules and mediate acute renal failure. Despite advances in treatment and diagnosis of cancer patients, large population-based studies have cited a 1-year risk of AKI of 17.5% and a 5-year risk of 27%.[115] Even mild AKI that does not require renal replacement therapy has been associated with increased long-term risk for renal failure and mortality. The levels of phosphorus in malignant cells can be up to four times the levels found in normal cells, and rapid release of these stores can result in hyperphosphatemia, with an increase in serum levels by as much as 2.1 mmol/L in children. Initially, the kidneys respond by increasing urinary excretion and decreasing tubular resorption. However, tubular transport mechanisms eventually become saturated, leading to increasing serum phosphorus levels. Acute renal insufficiency caused by uric acid or other complications may further exacerbate the development of hyperphosphatemia. In 2008, a group of researchers published evidence-based guidelines for the prevention and treatment of tumor lysis syndrome.[116]

Management

Vigorous IV hydration with diuresis has long been the cornerstone to prevention and treatment of tumor lysis syndrome (to achieve urine output of 80 to 100 mL/m²/h). Increasing intravascular volume and urine output increases the renal excretion of uric acid and phosphate. Alkalinization of the urine is no longer recommended, due to the lack of supporting evidence and the potential for enhancing the precipitation of xanthine in the urine.[117] Allopurinol works to lower serum uric acid levels by reducing the production of uric acid from purine precursors by inhibiting xanthine oxidase. Because it does not alter the uric acid already formed, it works best when initiated at least 48 hours prior to chemotherapy.[117] It is generally well tolerated and can be given orally or intravenously; the dose needs adjustment for preexisting renal impairment.

Rasburicase

Recombinant urate oxidase exerts its pharmacologic activity by enzymatic oxidation of uric acid into allantoin. It works rapidly, often dropping the uric acid level to less than normal within hours. Although contraindicated in patients with glucose-6-phosphate dehydrogenase deficiency, it is overall well tolerated. The traditional recommended dosage is 0.15 to 0.20 mg/kg per dose IV daily for up to 7 days. Investigators recommend the use of rasburicase as the first line intervention for high-risk patients (see Box 75.1) and as backup therapy for moderate-risk therapy for those patients who go on to develop hyperuricemia despite allopurinol and hydration (Table 75.2).[116]

Work by Hobbs and associates showed partial reversal of AKI associated with elevated uric acid when treated with rasburicase in infants.[119] Rasburicase is remarkably well tolerated. The rare, but serious, adverse events that require prompt and permanent discontinuation of rasburicase are methemoglobinemia and hemolysis. Glucose-6-phosphate dehydrogenase (G6PD) deficiency is regarded as the main predisposing factor for hemolysis and remains a contraindication to its use (the mechanism is related to oxidative stress from the hydrogen peroxide [H_2O_2] produced as uric acid is converted to allantoin), justifying, when possible, the screening for patients at high risk for G6PD deficiency (eg, African or Mediterranean ancestry).

Role of Renal Replacement Therapy

The understanding of the optimal start time, method, and dosage of renal replacement therapies (RRTs) has evolved (see also Chapter 78). Early intervention is favored, because most AKI survivors leave the hospital with independent kidney function.[120] Once the process of cell turnover is uncoupled, the rapid release of intracellular contents into the bloodstream, including anions, cations, proteins, and nucleic acids, occurs. In this clinical paradigm, the early institution of renal replacement interrupts the cascade before the occurrence of tumor lysis–related AKI with life-threatening complications. Therefore, the group recommended that for pediatric patients at high risk of TLS, cytotoxic chemotherapy should only be administered in a facility with ready access to dialysis. Although dialysis usage has been reduced since the introduction of rasburicase, as many as 3% of patients (1.5% of pediatric patients and 5% of adult patients) still require RRT.[121] In line with this observation, the panel recommended that renal consultation be obtained immediately if urine output is low, if there are persistently elevated phosphate levels, or in the case of hypocalcemia.[116]

Pigment Nephropathy

Rhabdomyolysis is a dissolution of skeletal muscles that produces a nonspecific clinical syndrome that causes extrusion of toxic intracellular contents from myocytes into the circulatory system. The possible causes of rhabdomyolysis are myriad; with direct muscle injury remaining the most common cause, additional causes include hereditary enzyme disorders, drugs, toxins, endocrinopathies, malignant hyperthermia, neuroleptic malignant syndrome, heatstroke, hypothermia, electrolyte alterations, diabetic ketoacidosis and nonketotic hyperosmolar coma, severe hypothyroidism or hyperthyroidism, and bacterial or viral infections. Most of the data remain adult based. In a study of 210 pediatric patients, the most common causes of rhabdomyolysis were viral myositis (38%), trauma (26%), and connective tissue disease (5%). Higher initial creatine kinase levels (>6000 IU/dL) and higher fluid administration rates were associated with higher maximal creatinine levels.[122]

TABLE 75.2 Patient Stratification by Risk

Type of Cancer	RISK		
	High	Intermediate	Low
NHL	Burkitt lymphoblastic, B-ALL	DLBCL	Indolent NHL
ALL	WBC ≥100,000	WBC 50,000-100,000	WBC ≤50,000
AML	WBC ≥50,000, monoblastic	WBC 10,000-50,000	WBC ≤10,000
CLL		WBC 10,000-100,000 Tx w/fludarabine	WBC ≤10,000
Other hematologic malignancies (including CML and multiple myeloma) and solid tumors		Rapid proliferation with expected rapid response to therapy	Remainder of patients

ALL, acute lymphoblastic leukemia; *AML,* acute myeloid leukemia; *B-ALL,* Burkitt acute lymphoblastic leukemia; *CLL,* chronic lymphocytic leukemia; *CML,* chronic myeloid leukemia; *DLBCL,* diffuse large B-cell lymphoma; *NHL,* non-Hodgkin lymphoma; *Tx,* treatment; *WBC,* white blood cell count.
Data from Coiffier BJ. Guidelines for the management of pediatric and adult tumor lysis syndrome: an evidence-based review. Clin Oncol. 2008;26:2767-2778.

Pathophysiology

Rhabdomyolysis, which literally means "dissolution of striped [skeletal] muscle," is the final pathway of many different processes. Regardless of the underlying mechanism, myocyte dissolution triggers a cascade of events that leads to the rapid release of calcium ions into muscle cells resulting in a pathologic interaction between actin and myosin and activation of cell protease, with subsequent myocyte necrosis of muscle fibers, release of potassium, phosphates, myoglobin, creatine kinase (CK), and urates into the extracellular space and into the bloodstream. As such, myoglobin can precipitate in the glomerular filtrate, particularly in an acidic environment, causing tubular occlusion and severe kidney damage. Pigmented myoglobin casts, which characterize the rhabdomyolysis syndrome, are the result of the interaction between myoglobin and Tamm-Horsfall protein in an acid environment.[123] Additional mechanisms causing renal damage include (1) a direct cytotoxic effect of myoglobin on renal cells; (2) urate precipitation, leading to intraluminal casts, increased intratubular pressure, and subsequent decreased glomerular filtration rate; (3) renal vasoconstriction and ischemia due to the heme group of myoglobin causing activation of the cytokine cascade; and (4) oxidant injury through heme-induced reactive oxygen species such as superoxide anion, hydrogen peroxide, or hydroxyl radicals causing direct oxidative damage.[124]

The classic triad of symptoms of rhabdomyolysis includes myalgia, weakness, and dark urine, although these findings may be inconsistent.[122]

The definitive diagnosis of rhabdomyolysis requires an elevation of CK levels to greater than five times normal in the absence of significant elevations of brain or cardiac CK fractions. The most dangerous sequela of rhabdomyolysis is AKI, the exact mechanisms of which are unclear but may be attributable to vasoconstriction/hypoperfusion, renal tubular dysfunction/cast formation, or myoglobin-induced tubular cytotoxicity.

The mainstay of treatment for rhabdomyolysis, directed at preventing AKI, is fluid therapy.[122] Many clinicians advocate alkalinization of urine with sodium bicarbonate (sometimes with concomitant forced diuresis with mannitol). Once the patient has reached the hospital, fluid infusion should be continued, with the goal of maintaining a brisk urinary flow and a urine pH above 6.5 and plasma pH below 7.50.[125] The rate of infusion should be at 150% of maintenance rate, with hemodynamic parameters and urine output monitored closely. Some authors also suggest administering mannitol. This is done to induce osmotic diuresis and to remove liquids from the damaged muscular interstitium, thus relaxing the compartments involved.[126] To force diuresis, some clinicians also recommend the addition of furosemide.

There is little clinical evidence to support the use of bicarbonate, mannitol, and furosemide. It is important to understand that the treatment benchmark is aggressive forced hydration with saline and glucose solutions. Studies in humans show that alkalinization and osmotic and diuretic treatment add little to the beneficial effect of hydration.[123] Forced hydration should be continued until the disappearance of myoglobinuria, which typically occurs after the third day. Hyperkalemia must be managed using the usual techniques, considering that treatment with glucose and insulin may prove to be ineffective in this context due to the damaged muscle's inability to capture potassium from the extracellular space. It is often necessary to treat severe hyperkalemia with renal replacement therapy.

Hypocalcemia

Secondary sequestration of calcium into damaged muscle cells must be viewed critically. Administration of intravenous calcium (either chloride or gluconate) should be used only to treat life-threatening electrocardiographic alterations, secondary to hyperkalemia or extreme hypocalcemia.

Drug-Induced Nephrotoxicity

Many different drugs and agents may cause AKI in children. In the ICU, factors such as age, pharmacogenetics, underlying disease, the dosage of the toxin, and concomitant medication all interact and influence the severity of nephrotoxic insults. Pediatric retrospective studies have reported incidences of AKI in PICUs of between 8% and 30%.[127] It is widely recognized that neonates have higher rates of AKI, especially following cardiac surgery, severe asphyxia, or premature birth. Although in most cases the etiology of AKI in the ICU is multifactorial (eg, sepsis, ischemia/hypoperfusion), several large epidemiologic studies have shown that nephrotoxic drugs were contributing factors in 19% to 25% of cases of severe acute renal failure in critically ill adult patients.[128]

NSAIDs, antibiotics, amphotericin B, antiviral agents, angiotensin-converting enzyme (ACE) inhibitors, calcineurin inhibitors, radiocontrast media, and cytostatics are the most important drugs implicated in the etiology of AKI in children. The mechanisms of nephrotoxicity include constriction of intrarenal vessels, acute tubular necrosis, acute interstitial nephritis, and, more infrequently, tubular obstruction.[127]

Aminoglycoside Nephrotoxicity

Aminoglycosides (AGs) are non–protein-bound drugs that are primarily excreted unmetabolized by glomerular filtration. Their cationic nature facilitates binding to the tubuloepithelial membrane in the proximal tubule, resulting in rapid intracellular transport.[129] The molecular number of cationic groups determines the facility with which these drugs are transported across cell membranes and is an important determinant of toxicity.[130,131] Neomycin is associated with the most nephrotoxicity; gentamicin, tobramycin, and amikacin are intermediate, and streptomycin is the least nephrotoxic.[132] Several hypotheses have been proposed to explain the nephrotoxic effects of aminoglycosides. Intracellular accumulation of AG within lysosomes is thought to interfere with normal cellular function such as protein synthesis and mitochondrial function, eventually leading to cell death.[133] Aminoglycosides also are known to stimulate the calcium-sensing receptor on the apical membrane thereby inducing cell signaling and eventual cell death.[134]

Risk factors for aminoglycoside nephrotoxicity include the type of AG, high peak serum levels, cumulative dose, the duration and frequency of administration, and patient-related factors such as age, preexisting renal dysfunction, hypoalbuminemia, liver dysfunction, decreased renal perfusion, and the concomitant use of nephrotoxic drugs.[132]

Several approaches have been evaluated in both animals and humans as potential treatments to attenuate the nephrotoxicity of aminoglycosides. Investigators have demonstrated that calcium supplementation reduces the nephrotoxic effect, likely through competitive inhibition of calcium channels in the proximal tubule.[135] Similarly, calcium channel blockers also have been shown to attenuate AG nephrotoxicity.[136] Also the protective effect of concomitant use of β-lactam antibiotics has been recognized for several years, although the mechanism by which this may occur is somewhat unclear.[137,138] More recent investigations have evaluated a possible role for antioxidants in renoprotection.[139] Once-daily dosing of aminoglycosides is the only clinical approach that is commonly used to reduce nephrotoxicity.[140] The rationale for the efficacy of consolidated AG dosing against gram-negative bacteria is based on two pharmacodynamic properties of aminoglycosides: (1) the bacteriocidal mechanism of action is concentration-dependent and (2) there is a prolonged post-antibiotic effect.[132]

Clinical evidence of AG-induced acute tubular necrosis is seen within a week of initiation of aminoglycoside treatment. AG-induced acute renal failure is generally nonoliguric and may be associated with decreased urine concentrating ability and urinary magnesium wasting. It is generally reversible after discontinuation of the drug; however, supportive renal replacement therapy may be required. Alternative antimicrobials may be considered when possible in patients at high risk for AG nephrotoxicity. If required and consolidated AG dosing is used, renal function should be assessed daily to monitor for changes in renal function, and trough levels should be followed to guide dosage.

Amphotericin B

The use of antifungals has become more commonplace in intensive care units, as the prevalence of fungemia (specifically candidemia) has increased in critically ill patients. For decades, amphotericin B was the drug of choice because of its broad spectrum of activity and its wide availability; however, its use has been sharply curtailed because of its considerable side effects (specifically, nephrotoxicity) and the availability of newer, less-toxic agents.

Approximately 80% of patients who receive treatment with amphotericin B will experience some renal dysfunction.[141] There are several mechanisms by which amphotericin B is thought to induce renal dysfunction: (1) by directly binding to tubular epithelial cells in the cortical collecting duct, resulting in altered cell permeability; (2) by causing sodium, potassium, and magnesium wasting; and (3) by directly causing afferent arteriolar (preglomerular) vasoconstriction.[142] Risk factors for amphotericin B nephrotoxicity include preexisting renal insufficiency, hypokalemia, volume depletion, the use of concomitant nephrotoxins, and large individual and cumulative dosages.[143]

A number of strategies have been studied to minimize the associated nephrotoxicity, including sodium loading and longer infusion rates.[144] Although some have shown a reduction in nephrotoxicity, these studies are very small and typically enroll low-risk patients. Lipid-based formulations of amphotericin B also are available, which may produce less nephrotoxicity. However, these agents are considerably more expensive. The introduction of alternative antifungal agents such as itraconazole, voriconazole, and caspofungin has largely supplanted the use of amphotericin B in high-risk patients with renal impairment; however, it continues to be used widely in patients with normal renal function because of its relatively low cost and broad spectrum of activity.

Given the presence of many underlying risk factors for nephrotoxicity in critically ill patients, it is recommended that amphotericin B should be avoided in this patient population if alternative therapies are available. When it is used, sodium loading with intravenous hydration is recommended to attenuate vasoconstrictive effects, and longer infusion times should also be considered. Renal function and serum electrolytes (specifically potassium) should be monitored during treatment.

Vancomycin

The use of vancomycin hydrochloride has increased considerably as it has become the standard therapy for treatment of methicillin-resistant *Staphylococcus aureus* infections. Data from the 2004 Centers for Disease Control and Prevention, National Nosocomial Infections Surveillance System indicate that the prevalence of methicillin-resistant *S. aureus* exceeds 50% in US hospitals. The synergistic nephrotoxicity of combination therapy involving vancomycin and aminoglycosides is well established, with a reported frequency of acute renal failure in the range of 20% to 30%. However, the nephrotoxicity of vancomycin alone increasingly is being recognized as high-dose therapy has become more common for the treatment of methicillin-resistant *S. aureus*.[146] In addition, adult studies showed administration of vancomycin plus piperacillin-tazobactam may lead to higher rates of AKI.[147] An analysis by our group had similar findings in children: The incidence of AKI when vancomycin and piperacillin-tazobactam were administered together was fourfold greater compared to either medication alone (unpublished data).

Vancomycin is excreted by glomerular filtration, 80% to 90% in an unaltered form.[148] It is hard to determine the exact rates of vancomycin-related toxicity because most reported cases have had additional risk factors for acute renal failure, which makes it difficult to determine the true risk of treatment. The mechanism by which it exerts its nephrotoxicity is unknown. Independent risk factors for nephrotoxicity include the use of concomitant nephrotoxic agents, age, duration of therapy, and drug levels achieved.[147] Trough levels higher than 15 μg/mL are associated with increased risk of nephrotoxicity, and peak levels also have been associated with increased nephrotoxicity. The dosing of vancomycin requires careful consideration of renal function and estimated glomerular filtration rate. Trough levels should be monitored frequently in patients with fluctuating renal function.

Calcineurin Inhibitors

The introduction of calcineurin inhibitors (CNIs) for transplant recipients has led to dramatic improvement in both allograft and patient survival. The clinical use of CNIs often is limited by their nephrotoxic effect, which can present as two distinct and well-characterized forms: acute and chronic nephrotoxicity. Calcineurin inhibitor-induced AKI may occur as early as a few weeks or months after initiation of therapy. The clinical manifestations of CNI-induced renal dysfunction include reduction of GFR, hyperkalemia, hypertension, renal tubular acidosis, increased resorption of sodium, and oliguria. The acute adverse effects of calcineurin inhibitors on renal hemodynamics are thought to be directly related to the cyclosporine (CsA) or tacrolimus dosage and blood concentration and can be managed by dose reduction. This is in contrast to calcineurin inhibitor-induced chronic nephropathy, which is largely irreversible and can occur independently of acute renal dysfunction, CNI dosage, or blood concentration.

Although the exact mechanism of nephrotoxicity is not fully understood, several factors have been implicated in the pathogenesis of CNI nephrotoxicity.[149] Experimental models of acute CsA toxicity revealed that CsA administration is associated with afferent and efferent arteriolar vasoconstriction, which results in a significant reduction of renal plasma flow and GFR.[150,151] The precise mechanism by which CsA induces renal vasoconstriction has not been established clearly. Results from several studies indicate that vascular dysfunction induced by CsA results from an increase in vasoconstrictor factors that include endothelin, thromboxane, and angiotensin II, as well as a reduction of vasodilator factors such as prostacyclin and nitric oxide.[151,152]

Cyclosporine and tacrolimus differ with respect to side effects; however, the available data comparing nephrotoxicity are conflicting. Whereas some studies have suggested that tacrolimus may be associated with a decreased severity of renal dysfunction in comparison to CsA,[132] other investigators have demonstrated no difference between the two CNIs.[153]

Studies have been conflicting on the protective effect of calcium channel blockers on the preservation of renal function for patients receiving CNIs. In a multicenter, prospective, randomized, placebo-controlled study in 118 cadaveric renal transplant recipients receiving CsA, the use of a calcium channel blocker resulted in a significantly better allograft function at 2 years and demonstrated an improvement in graft function, as assessed by serum creatinine and GFR, that was independent of lowered blood pressure.[154] More research is being done with goals of improving the safety profile of CNIs and identifying safer alternatives.

Sirolimus

Sirolimus is a mammalian target of rapamycin (mTOR) inhibitor that is becoming increasingly used in allograft preservation. Its target protein, mTOR, is a serine/threonine protein kinase that regulates cell growth, cell proliferation, cell motility, cell survival, protein synthesis, and transcription in transplantation.[155] As its use in transplant medicine is increasing, it was hoped that its lack of nephrotoxicity in animal models would be translated in humans to improve immunosuppression with minimal effect on renal function. Unfortunately, several studies suggest that sirolimus has inherent nephrotoxicity, such as the development of proteinuria and a delay in recovery from ischemia-reperfusion injury. In addition, several studies have shown that the nephrotoxicity associated with CNIs is exacerbated when used in combination with sirolimus.[156]

Nonsteroidal Antiinflammatory Drugs

In most circumstances, nonsteroidal antiinflammatory drugs (NSAIDs) do not pose a significant risk to patients with normal renal function. However, in situations in which renal perfusion is compromised (which is relatively common with critically ill patients), the inhibition of prostaglandin-induced vasodilation with the use of NSAIDs may further compromise renal blood flow and exacerbate ischemia. The renal effects of NSAIDs do seem to be dependent on the type, dose, and duration of treatment. Indomethacin is thought to be the most likely drug to impair renal function, and aspirin the least likely.[157] Patients at high risk of NSAID-induced nephrotoxicity include patients with preexisting renal dysfunction, those

with severe cardiovascular or hepatic failure, or the concomitant use of other potentially nephrotoxic medications, such as aminoglycosides, angiotensin-converting enzyme inhibitors, and angiotensin receptor blockers.[157]

Contrast-Induced Nephropathy

Contrast-induced nephropathy (CIN) acute kidney injury is an important complication in the use of iodinated contrast media that accounts for a significant number of cases of hospital-acquired AKI. The occurrence of AKI as a result of contrast will continue to increase, as there is growing use of imaging and interventional procedures in pediatric intensive care patients.[158] At the same time, many patients in intensive and critical care units have compromised renal function, representing the most important risk factor for contrast-induced AKI.

Three core elements are intertwined in the pathophysiology of CIN: (1) direct toxicity of iodinated contrast to nephrons, (2) microshowers of atheroemboli to the kidneys, and (3) contrast- and atheroemboli-induced intrarenal vasoconstriction.[159] Direct toxicity to nephrons with iodinated contrast has been demonstrated and seems to be related to the osmolality of the contrast.[160] Hence, low-ionic or nonionic, and low-osmolar or iso-osmolar contrast agents were shown to be less nephrotoxic in vitro. Microshowers of cholesterol emboli are believed to occur in up to 50% of percutaneous interventions where a guiding catheter is passed through the aorta. Most of these showers are clinically silent; however, in approximately 1% of high-risk cases, acute cholesterol emboli syndrome (CES) can develop, which is manifested by AKI, mesenteric ischemia, decreased microcirculation to the extremities, and, in some cases, embolic stroke.[161] Finally, intrarenal vasoconstriction as a pathologic vascular response to contrast media, and perhaps an organ response to cholesterol emboli, is a final hypoxic/ischemic injury to the kidney.[162] Hypoxia triggers activation of the renal sympathetic nervous system and results in a reduction in renal blood flow, especially in the outer medulla.[161] There is disagreement about the direct vasoconstrictor or vasodilator effects in the kidney of contrast agents when given to animals.[163] It is likely that in completely normal human renal blood vessels, contrast agents provoke a vasodilation and an osmotic diuresis. When there is vascular disease, endothelial dysfunction, and glomerular injury, however, contrast and the multifactorial insult of renal hypoxia provoke a vasoconstrictive response and hence mediate, in part, an ischemic injury.[163] The most important predictor of CIN is underlying renal dysfunction. The "remnant nephron" theory postulates that after sufficient chronic kidney damage has occurred, the remaining nephrons assume the remaining filtration load, require increased oxygen demands, and are more susceptible to ischemic and oxidative injury. Understanding the pathophysiology of CIN is key to devising a preventive strategy.

Role of Renal Replacement Therapy

Contrast media are removed by dialysis, but there is no clinical evidence that prophylactic dialysis reduces the risk of AKI, even when carried out within 1 hour or simultaneously with administration. Hemofiltration performed before and after contrast administration deserves further investigation given reports of reduced mortality and need for hemodialysis, but the high cost and need for prolonged ICU care will also limit the utility of this prophylactic approach.[164]

There are no currently approved pharmacologic agents that will prevent CIN AKI. With iodinated contrast, the pharmacologic agents tested in small trials that deserve further evaluation include theophylline, statins, ascorbic acid, and prostaglandin E_1.[165] Although popular, N-acetylcysteine has not been consistently shown to be effective. Nine published meta-analyses document significant heterogeneity between studies and pooled odds ratios for N-acetylcysteine approaching unity.[166] Importantly, only in those trials in which N-acetylcysteine reduced serum creatinine below baseline values because of decreased skeletal muscle production did renal injury rates seem to be reduced. Thus N-acetylcysteine seems to falsely lower creatinine and not fundamentally protect the kidney against injury. However, a study suggested that the use of volume supplementation with sodium bicarbonate together with N-acetylcysteine was more effective than N-acetylcysteine alone in reducing the risk of CIN. Fenoldopam, dopamine, calcium channel blockers, atrial natriuretic peptide, and L-arginine have not been shown to be effective in the prevention of contrast-induced AKI. Furosemide, mannitol, and an endothelin-receptor antagonist are potentially detrimental.[166]

Acute Renal Failure After Stem Cell Transplantation

One of the most frequent complications of bone marrow transplant (BMT) is renal failure, with 5% to 15% of all BMT patients developing AKI and 5% to 20% of the survivors developing chronic renal failure (CRF).[167] Hematopoietic stem cell transplantation is a common procedure for the treatment of malignancies and some nonmalignant hematologic disorders. The process of stem cell transfusion predisposes these patients to renal failure because of prior chemotherapy, irradiation, sepsis, and exposure to nephrotoxic agents. Complicating outcomes are newer conditioning regimens that allow for reduced intensity and nonmyeloablative regimens, thereby allowing patients with significant comorbidities to undergo transplantation with reduced morbidity and mortality. These have led to challenges in the ICU management of these patients, because they already have residual organ injury. A study of 29 pediatric patients who required continuous renal replacement therapy (CRRT) in the ICU showed an almost 100% mortality at 6 months post-ICU admission due to transplant-related illness. This study demonstrated the management and ethical difficulties being posed by hematopoietic stem cell transplant patients becoming critically ill and requiring organ support at tertiary care centers. In contrast with the improving survival rates following stem cell transplantation, there are greater numbers of children surviving and progressing to end-stage renal disease (ESRD). Some of these patients are being treated with renal transplantation.[168]

A better understanding of the underlying histopathologic changes in renal morphology would perhaps lead to a better control of the renal insults that occur during the process of stem cell transfusion. Some histopathology-based studies have shown a variety of findings in patients post–stem cell transplantation, including features of tubulitis and peritubular vasculitis. These studies also show that kidneys from adult patients who had grade III-IV graft-versus-host disease (GVHD) were more likely to have tubulitis and peritubular capillaritis.[169] Other studies have shown membranous glomerulonephritis and thrombotic microangiopathy to be common histologic features post–stem cell transplantation.[170] However, there remains a paucity of pediatric studies examining renal histopathology in patients posttransplantation (see also Chapter 95).

Urinary Tract Obstruction

Obstruction of urine flow may result in AKI, although unilateral obstruction rarely causes AKI unless there is a single kidney or disease in the other kidney. Both unilateral and bilateral ureteral obstructions are accompanied by an initial increase in RBF caused by afferent arteriolar vasodilation.[171] Relaxation of the preglomerular capillary sphincter is mediated by the local release of vasodilatory prostaglandins.[172] Administration of indomethacin, a cyclooxygenase inhibitor, results in a marked reduction in the GFR after a decrease in glomerular plasma flow and an increase in both afferent and efferent arteriolar resistances.[173] This indicates an important role of vasodilatory prostaglandins in the maintenance of the GFR.

If the obstruction persists, RBF progressively decreases as afferent arteriolar resistance increases because of the overriding action of angiotensin II and thromboxane. This vasoconstriction may actually protect the kidney from damage during the period of obstruction. Intratubular pressure rises after ureteral obstruction; this pressure is translated to the glomerulus as increased pressure in the Bowman space. The contribution of this increased force opposing filtration to the decrease in the GFR is probably inconsequential because the intratubular pressure rise is transient.[171] In addition, the elevation in Bowman space pressure is negated by an increase in the glomerular capillary pressure that increases the GFR. RBF is redistributed from the outer to the inner cortex and results in relative ischemia of the kidney medulla.[171]

Various clinical causes of urinary tract obstruction are listed in Table 75.3. The most important factors determining recovery of kidney and tubular function are the degree and severity of the obstruction. Treatment consists of decompression of the urinary collecting system by removal of the obstruction or by urinary diversion. Relief of obstruction is accompanied by a marked diuresis resulting from increased RBF and abnormal tubular function. The increase in urine volume is related to a concentrating defect caused by loss of the medullary gradient and unresponsiveness of the kidney tubule to vasopressin.[174] Hydrogen ion and potassium secretion may also be impaired, and the result is a distal type of kidney tubular acidosis with hyperkalemia.[175]

Conclusions

This chapter has reviewed the major factors that contribute to the development of AKI, both in its oliguric and nonoliguric forms. Also indicated are the clinical settings in which AKI may occur. In addition, treatment modalities have been discussed. Clearly, the challenge in AKI is the development of novel therapeutic strategies that will more directly intervene in the disease process and that can have an impact on the cellular and metabolic mechanisms that contribute to kidney cell injury. Certain current investigations were discussed because they may lead to clinical trials in the coming years. Included among these agents are calcium channel blockers, adenine nucleotides, thyroid hormone, and oxyradical scavengers because they may modulate the full expression of kidney cell injury. Only with an understanding of the pathophysiologic mechanisms in AKI can these potential therapeutics be applied in a clinical setting to the care of pediatric patients.

TABLE 75.3   Management of Electrolyte Abnormalities

Abnormality	Management Recommendation
Hyperphosphatemia	
Moderate (≥2.1 mmol/L)	Avoid IV phosphate administration Administration of phosphate binder
Severe	Dialysis, CAVH, CVVH, CAVHD, or CVVHD
Hypocalcemia (≤1.75 mmol/L)	
Asymptomatic	No therapy
Symptomatic	Calcium gluconate 50-100 mg/kg IV administered slowly with ECG monitoring
Hyperkalemia	
Moderate and asymptomatic (≥6 mmol/L)	Avoid IV and oral potassium ECG and cardiac rhythm monitoring Sodium polystyrene sulfonate
Severe (>7 mmol/L) or symptomatic	Same as above, plus: Calcium gluconate 100-200 mg/kg by slow IV infusion for life-threatening arrhythmias Regular insulin (0.1 U/kg IV) + D25 (2 mL/kg) IV Sodium bicarbonate (1-2 mEq/kg IV push) can be given to induce influx of potassium into cells; however, sodium bicarbonate and calcium should not be administered through the same line Dialysis
Renal dysfunction (uremia)	Fluid and electrolyte management Uric acid and phosphate management Adjust renally excreted drug doses Dialysis (hemodialysis or peritoneal) Hemofiltration (CAVH, CVVH, CAVHD, or CVVHD)

CAVH, continuous arteriovenous hemofiltration; *CAVHD,* continuous arteriovenous hemodialysis; *CVVH,* continuous venovenous hemofiltration; *CVVHD,* continuous venovenous hemodialysis.
Data from Zaffanello M, Antonucci R, Cuzzolin L, et al. Early diagnosis of acute kidney injury with urinary biomarkers in the newborn. J Matern Fetal Neonatal Med. 2009;3(suppl 22):62-66; and Coiffier BJ. Guidelines for the management of pediatric and adult tumor lysis syndrome: an evidence-based review. Clin Oncol. 2008;26:2767-2778, 2008.

Key References

2. Akcan-Arikan Zappitelli M, Loftis LL, et al. Modified RIFLE criteria in critically ill children with acute kidney injury. *Kidney Int.* 2007;71:1028-1035.
3. Plotz FB, Bouma AB, van Wijk JA, et al. Pediatric acute kidney injury in the ICU: an independent evaluation of pRIFLE criteria. *Intensive Care Med.* 2008;34:1713-1717.
4. Wasung MT, Chawla LS, Madero M. Biomarkers of renal function, which and when? *Clin Chim Acta.* 2015;438:350-357.
5. Zaffanello M, Antonucci R, Cuzzolin L, et al. Early diagnosis of acute kidney injury with urinary biomarkers in the newborn. *J Matern Fetal Neonatal Med.* 2009;22(suppl 3):62-66.
9. Badr KF, Ichikawa I. Prekidney failure: a deleterious shift from kidney compensation to decompensation. *N Engl J Med.* 1988;319:623.
18. Wedeen PR, Udasin I, Fiedler N, et al. Urinary biomarkers as indicator of renal disease. *Ren Fail.* 1999;21:241-249.
20. Brezis M, Rosen S. Hypoxia of the renal medulla-its implications for disease. *N Engl J Med.* 1995;32:647-655.
23. Epstein F, Agmon Y, Brezis M. Physiology of renal hypoxia. *Ann N Y Acad Sci.* 1994;718:72-81.
31. Neill MA, Tarr PI, Clausen CR, et al. Escherichia coli 0157:H7 as the predominant pathogen associated with the hemolytic uremic syndrome: a prospective study in the Pacific Northwest. *Pediatrics.* 1987;80:37.

40. Oken DE. Hemodynamic basis for human acute AKI (vasomotor nephropathy). *Am J Med.* 1984;76:702.
44. Schwartz GJ, Munoz A, Schneider MF, et al. New equations to estimate GFR in children with CKD. *JASN.* 2009;20:629-637.
48. Kellum JA, et al. Use of dopamine in acute renal failure: a meta-analysis. *Crit Care Med.* 2001;29:1526-1531.
50. Karajala V, Mansour W, Kellum JA. Diuretics in acute kidney injury. *Minerva Anestesiol.* 2009;75:251-257.
54. Wagner K, Albrecht S, Neumayer HH. Prevention of delayed graft function in cadaveric kidney transplantation by a calcium antagonist: preliminary results of two prospective randomized trials. *Transplant Proc.* 1986;18:510.
67. Barletta GM, Bunchman TE. Acute renal failure in children and infants. *Curr Opin Crit Care.* 2004;10:499-504.
68. Goldstein SL, Somers MJ, Baum MA, et al. Pediatric patients with multiorgan dysfunction syndrome receiving continuous renal replacement therapy. *Kidney Int.* 2005;67:653-658.
69. Goldstein SL, Currier H, Graf CD, et al. Outcome in children receiving continuous venovenous hemofiltration. *Pediatrics.* 2001;107:1309-1312.
70. Gillespie RS, Seidel K, Symons JM. Effect of fluid overload and dose of replacement fluid on survival in hemofiltration. *Pediatr Nephrol.* 2004;19:1394-1399.
71. Foland JA, Fortenberry JD, Warshaw BL, et al. Fluid overload before continuous hemofiltration and survival in critically ill children: a retrospective analysis. *Crit Care Med.* 2004;32:1771-1776.
75. Bunchman TE, McBryde KD, Mottes TE, et al. Pediatric acute renal failure: outcome by modality and disease. *Pediatr Nephrol.* 2001;16:1067-1071.
78. Noris M, Mescia F, Remuzzi G. STEC-HUS, atypical HUS and TTP are all diseases of complement activation. *Nat Rev Nephrol.* 2012;8:622-633.
80. Kielsten JT, et al. Best supportive care and therapeutic plasma exchange with or without eculizumab in Shiga-toxin producing E. coli O104:H4 induced haemolytic-uraemic syndrome: an analysis of the German STEC-HUS registry. *Nephrol Dial Transplant.* 2012;27:3807-3815.
83. Cataland SR, Wu HM. How I treat: the clinical differentiation and initial treatment of adult patients with atypical hemolytic uremic syndrome. *Blood.* 2014;123:2478-2484.
84. Legendre CM, et al. Terminal complement inhibitor eculizumab in atypical hemolytic-uremic syndrome. *N Engl J Med.* 2013;368:2169-2181.
85. Jennette JC, Falk RJ. Diagnosis and management of glomerulonephritis and vasculitis presenting as acute kidney failure. *Med Clin North Am.* 1990;74:893.
90. Hobbs DJ, Barletta GM, Rajpal JS, et al. Severe paediatric systemic lupus erythematosus nephritis-a single-centre experience. *Nephrol Dial Transplant.* 2010;25:457-463.
92. Sinha R, Raut S. Pediatric lupus nephritis: management update. *World J Nephrol.* 2014;3:16-23.
93. Ginzler EM, Dooley MA, Aranow C, et al. Mycophenolate mofetil or intravenous cyclophosphamide for lupus nephritis. *N Engl J Med.* 2005;353:2219-2228.
96. Stone JH, et al. Rituximab versus Cyclophosphamide for ANCA-associated vasculitis. *N Engl J Med.* 2010;363:221-232.
97. Sakarcan A, Timmons C, Seikaly MG. Reversible idiopathic acute renal failure in children with primary nephrotic syndrome. *J Pediatr.* 1994;125:723.
99. Hawkins EP, Beray P, Silva F. Tubulointerstitial nephritis in children: clinical, morphologic, immunohistochemical and lectin studies. Southwest Pediatric Nephrology Study Group. *Am J Kidney Dis.* 1987;14:466.
102. Praught ML. Are small changes in serum creatinine an important risk factor? *Curr Opin Nephrol Hypertens.* 2005;14:265-270.
103. Hui-Stickle S, Brewer ED, Goldstein SL. Pediatric ARF epidemiology at a tertiary care center from 1999 to 2001. *Am J Kidney Dis.* 2005;45:96-101.
105. Price JF, et al. Worsening renal function in children hospitalized with decompensated heart failure: evidence for a pediatric cardiorenal syndrome? *Pediatr Crit Care Med.* 2008;9:279-284.
106. Testani AJ, et al. Effect of right ventricular function and venous congestion on cardiorenal interactions during the treatment of decompensated heart failure. *Am J Cardiol.* 2010;105:511-516.
107. Pedersen KR, et al. Clinical outcome in children with acute renal failure treated with peritoneal dialysis after surgery for congenital heart disease. *Kidney Int Suppl.* 2008;S81-S86.
108. Zappitelli M, et al. A small post-operative rise in serum creatinine predicts acute kidney injury in children undergoing cardiac surgery. *Kidney Int.* 2009;76:885-892.

110. Haase M, Haase-Fielitz A, Bagshaw SM, et al. Cardiopulmonary bypass-associated acute kidney injury: a pigment nephropathy? *Contrib Nephrol.* 2007;156:340-353.

112. Mishra J, et al. Neutrophil gelatinase-associated lipocalin (NGAL) as a biomarker for acute renal injury after cardiac surgery. *Lancet.* 2005; 365:1231-1238.

113. Dent CL, et al. Plasma neutrophil gelatinase-associated lipocalin predicts acute kidney injury, morbidity and mortality after pediatric cardiac surgery: a prospective uncontrolled cohort study. *Crit Care.* 2007;11:R127.

115. Lam AQ, Humphrey BD. Onco-nephrology: AKI in the cancer patient. *Clin J Am Soc Nephrol.* 2012;7:1692-1700.

116. Coiffier B, Altman A, Pui CH, et al. Guidelines for the management of pediatric and adult tumor lysis syndrome: an evidence-based review. *J Clin Oncol.* 2008;26:2767-2778.

117. Goldman SC, et al. A randomized comparison between rasburicase and allopurinol in children with lymphoma or leukemia at high risk for tumor lysis. *Blood.* 2001;97:2998-3003.

123. Cervellin G, Comelli L. Lippi G: Review: rhabdomyolysis: historical background, clinical, diagnostic and therapeutic features. *Clin Chem Lab Med.* 2010;Epub.

126. Sever MS, Vanholder R, Lameire N. Management of crush-related injuries after disasters. *N Engl J Med.* 2006;354:1052-1063.

128. Oliveira JF, et al. Prevalence and risk factors for aminoglycoside nephrotoxicity in intensive care units. *Antimicrob Agents Chemother.* 2009;53: 2887-2891.

147. Burgess LD, Drew RH. Comparison of the incidence of vancomycin-induced nephrotoxicity in hospitalized patients with and without concomitant piperacillin-tazobactam. *Pharmacotherapy.* 2014;34:670-676.

149. Campistol JM, Sacks SH. Mechanisms of nephrotoxicity. *Transplantation.* 2000;69(suppl 12):SS5-SS10.

166. Stacul F, et al. Strategies to reduce the risk of contrast-induced nephropathy. *Am J Cardiol.* 2006;98:59K-77K.

167. Detaille T, Anslot C, de Clety SC. Acute kidney injury in paediatric bone marrow patients. *Acta Clin Belg Suppl.* 2007;2:401-404.

Acid-Base Disorders

Hector Carrillo-Lopez, Adrian Chavez, and Alberto Jarillo

PEARLS

- Plasma and intracellular fluid can be viewed as a complex aqueous solution with multiple cations and anions that interact with each other and with the solvent, water. Until recently, water was viewed as a passive element in the acid-base balance, but it is now envisioned as a physicochemical active participant, because it represents a virtually inexhaustible source of hydrogen ions.

- The principles of electroneutrality, constancy of the ionic product for water, and the law of mass action all influence acid-base equilibrium.

- PCO_2, pH, standard base excess, and HCO_3^-, with the addition of anion gap, are the tools used in a classical acid-base assessment.

- According to the physicochemical approach to acid-base balance, PCO_2 and the balance between cations and anions are the main determinants of pH, through water dissociation and regulatory responses of lung ventilation and the kidneys.

- Because PCO_2 is regulated by ventilation, changes in PCO_2 result in respiratory acid-base disorders, in both the classical and physicochemical acid-base models, but in the latter HCO_3^- is considered as primarily determined by PCO_2 and not vice versa.

- *Strong ion* (fully dissociated) *difference (SID)* and plasma nonbicarbonate (nonvolatile) weak acids (A_{TOT}) are the determinants of metabolic acid-base balance.

- The apparent gap between the sum of all strong cations and all the strong anions is called *apparent strong ion difference (SID_{APP})*, which is calculated as $([Na^+] + [K^+] + [Ca^{2+}] + [Mg^{2+}]) - ([Cl^-] + [lactate^-])$. The difference between $[Na^+]$ and $[Cl^-]$ is an effective surrogate of the more cumbersome calculation of SID_{APP}.

- According to the principle of electroneutrality, there must be remaining negative charges balancing the *excess* of plasma strong cations in relation to the strong anions. These balancing negative charges come from weak anions or acids that include total CO_2 ($\sim[HCO_3^-]$), albumin, and dihydrogen phosphate. Once weak acids are quantitatively taken into account, the SID_{APP} to SID_{EFF} difference should equal zero (electrical charge neutrality) unless there are unmeasured charges to explain this *ion gap*.

- Clinical assessment of an acid-base disorder should utilize all the tools of the classical approach, in addition to some merging concepts from the physicochemical approach. Anion gap must always be *corrected* for albumin and lactate levels in order to surrogate SIG, and the sodium-chloride difference can be used to surrogate SID_{APP}. These two indexes are particularly important in the setting of high-volume resuscitation, if the presence of unmeasured anions is expected, or if a complex or mixed pattern of acid-base metabolic derangement is suspected.

- Among all metabolic acidoses, lactic acidosis signals trouble.

- Acid-base disorders must be considered more important for what they tell the clinician about the patient than for any harm that is directly provoked by the acid-base imbalance. Mortality is more closely related to the nature of an acid-base disorder than to the magnitude of the derangement of the pH, whether acidotic or alkalotic.

Acid-base disorders are common in the critically ill of every age.[1] Acid-base homeostasis remains one of the best examples of the close correlation between basic and clinical sciences. To master acid balance physiology and pathophysiology is not an easy task, because it is patently integrative.[2-5] This implies that understanding the data in a blood gas panel requires an appreciation of not only acids and bases but also ventilation, gas exchange, dynamics of electrolyte and water movement, plasma composition, hemodynamics, respiratory control, and renal mechanisms of hydrogen ions, electrolytes, and water excretion. In addition, it is essential to have an understanding of a number of other organic, metabolic, and structural dysfunctions that can potentially contribute to deficits or loads of acid or base in the extracellular or intracellular spaces, including sepsis, acute kidney injury, different types of shock and tissue damage, severe metabolic dysregulation (eg, inborn errors, diabetic ketoacidosis), and the toxic effects of certain compounds and medications. Thus it is not uncommon that many physicians seem to display only a superficial knowledge of this field.[5-8] Although most of the acid-base unbalances do not cause harm and are self-limiting after appropriate resuscitation and management of the associated clinical condition, many physicians and critical care practitioners tend to think about an acid-base disturbance as a disease, and they unfortunately spend long hours treating numbers rather than the patient. This response probably relates to the fact that traditional teaching emphasizes data interpretation rather than pathophysiology. Thus a sizable number of critical care physicians experience difficulty in interpreting the significance or understanding of various acid-base disturbances.[6-9] Hence it is not a surprise to find easily available software for computers, handheld devices and smartphone applications, along with Internet-available blood-gas calculators, videos, tutorials, and primers for the interpretation of blood gases and acid-base status, with a variable level of quality and accuracy.[9-17] This is because some clinicians lack a logical stepwise learning approach or they are not organized to maximize ease of learning.[18] Numerous so-called practical solutions for understanding the acid-base physiology and its clinical implications seem to imply that many health workers, physicians included, seem to need some assistance to truly master the acid-base balance and its derangements. As a paradox, it is likely that such quick solutions contribute to the situation, as they provide practitioners with a fast-track interpretation of the arterial and venous blood gases and acid-base status, even when all the complexities are not fully understand.[2-8]

Because intensivists spend much of their time managing problems related to fluids, electrolytes, and acid-base balance, a thorough but practical understanding of the physiology and pathophysiology of acid-base disorders is a central aspect of the expertise of critical care practitioners in both pediatric and adult fields.

Overview of Acid-Base Physiology
Defining Acids and Bases

Most of the concepts of acid-base physiology are founded on the accepted definitions of acids and bases. These definitions and understanding of acid-base physiology were profoundly transformed at the end of the 19th and in the early 20th centuries. Between 1887 and 1903 Svante Arrhenius outlined the theories of ionization and dissociation, and Ostwald described the ability of water to dissociate, generating hydrogen (H^+) and hydroxide or hydroxyl (OH^-) ions. Arrhenius defined an acid as any substance that, when dissolved in water, produces an increased concentration of hydrogen ions, H.[19-21] In this definition it is not mandatory for a given substance to have hydrogen atoms, as the water itself can be the source of the hydrogen ions, in agreement with the works from Ostwald.[20-21] Accordingly, an Arrhenius base is a substance that, when dissolved in water, decreases the concentration of H^+ ions.[19,22] Consequently, by 1900 Naunyn and others proposed that the acid-base status in biological systems was, at least partially, determined by the concentration of electrolytes, mainly sodium and chloride, which had been formerly described by Faraday as "base-forming cation" and "acid-forming anion," respectively.[21] In 1923, Brønsted in Denmark and Lowry in England, working independently, stated that an acid is a substance that contains hydrogen atoms and that is able to release them—that is, an acid is a proton-donor substance.[21,22] Thus an acid (HA) may dissociate and donate a proton (ie, an hydrogen ion, H^+) to the solution, forming the conjugate base (or anion) A^- in a reversible manner, according to the law of mass action:

$$[HA] \xleftrightarrow{K_a} [H^+] + [A^-] \qquad \text{(Eq. 1)}$$

where K_a (or K_{eq}) is the equilibrium or dissociation constant, particular to every different substance and influenced by the characteristics of the particular solution in which the reaction is taking place. Therefore a base is a substance with the ability for binding or *trapping* free hydrogen ions ("proton acceptor substance").[22-25] Examples include bicarbonate, hemoglobin, proteins, and phosphates. The Brønsted-Lowry definition led to the concept of conjugate acid-base pairs. Whatever

definition of acid is used, its validity depends on the given situation in which one is trying to understand or explain some event. The broader definitions of acids and bases from Brønsted and Lowry and others were designed for chemistry, as they extend the concepts of acidity and alkalinity beyond the aqueous systems, to which the Arrhenius definitions are restricted.[22-26] In the context of the body fluids, the two definitions are not only valid but are both necessary to understand the complete picture in complex biological solutions. The Arrhenius definitions acknowledge the paramount participation of chloride, sodium, and other strong (fully dissociated) ions, whereas Brønsted-Lowry's definition recognizes the importance of the conjugate acid-base pairs, such as the bicarbonate/carbonic acid system. In spite of the fact that some of the most important developments in the evolution of acid-base physiology occurred before the publication of the Brønsted-Lowry theory in 1923, this definition gradually became the most popular among acid-base physiologists, and the Arrhenius definitions became outdated, as many thought that this approach to acid-base balance did not include the central and direct role of hydrogen ions. However, with this approach, the concept of chloride as an acid-forming anion and sodium as a base-forming cation became obsolete.[21-24] It was argued that there was an insufficient link between electrolytes such as sodium and chloride and subsequent changes in hydrogen ions. However, the role of water as a hydrogen ion source was neglected.

Role of Water and Electrolytes in Acid-Base Balance

All body fluids are water-based solutions. It seems rather surprising to find that water was rendered as a passive component of the body fluids until somewhat recent times.[26-28] From the work of Arrhenius and Ostwald, it is now well known that water molecules exhibit self-ionization or auto-dissociation. The hydrogen ion, H^+, immediately protonates another water molecule to form the so-called hydronium ion, H_3O^+ (also known as hydroxonium ion or oxonium ion):

$$H_2O + H_2O \leftrightarrow H_3O^+ + OH^- \qquad \text{(Eq. 2A)}$$

This equilibrium applies both to pure water and to any aqueous solution.

The symbol H^+ is interpreted as a shorthand for H_3O^+ because it is now known that a bare proton does not exist as a free species in aqueous solution. Accordingly, in medical biochemistry water dissociation is usually written as follows:

$$H_2O \leftrightarrow H^+ + OH^- \qquad \text{(Eq. 2B)}$$

Because water can supply a virtually inexhaustible natural reservoir of hydrogen (and hydroxyl) ions, acid-base balance must include the chemical properties of water. Acid-base unbalance can be viewed as an alteration of water dissociation. Although pure water dissociates only slightly, in plasma the presence of electrolytes, CO_2, and other weak acids produces powerful electrochemical forces, influencing water dissociation.[29,30] Human plasma is an aqueous solution that has to comply with certain physicochemical laws and principles, such as the *principle of electrical neutrality*, the *law of mass action* (which explains the dissociation equilibrium of partially dissociated substances such as electrolytes and others), and the *constancy of the ionic product for water*. The state of ionization of plasma water varies according to the plasma ionic composition to maintain these chemical rules.[29-33]

Principle of Electroneutrality

In physiologic conditions, there is little dissociation of water molecules into its components (Eqs. 2A and 2B). Electrical charge and temperature represent the main determinants for its eventual dissociation. Electrolytes and other substances, mainly organic acids, dissociate in water, forming cations (positively charged ions) and anions (negatively charged ions). In humans, plasma cations include hydrogen ion (H^+), sodium, potassium, calcium, magnesium, and ammonium. Sodium ion contributes quantitatively the greatest positive charge to plasma, with a concentration of approximately 140 mEq/L or millimoles per liter (mmol/L, mM). Plasma anions include hydroxide ion (OH^-, also termed *hydroxyl ion*), chloride, bicarbonate (HCO_3^-), albumin, phosphate, lactate, β-hydroxybutyrate, acetoacetate, sulphate, urate, and other organic anions such as pyruvate and propionate. The most abundant anion in human plasma is chloride with a concentration of approximately 100 mEq/L or mmol/L, mM. The plasma bicarbonate level is approximately 25 mEq/L (or mmol/L, mM) and therefore also contributes significantly to the plasma negative charge in quantitative terms.

In aqueous solutions, electrical neutrality is always constant—that is, the sum of all positively charged ions (cations) must be equal to the sum of all negatively charged ions (anions). Both extra- and intracellular fluids are an ionic mix of electrolytes, proteins, and other substances, whose charges tend to modify the electrical balance and then can have an influence on the dissociation of water. To preserve normal plasma ionic composition and to keep electroneutrality, the kidneys produce urine with different concentration of ions depending on body requirements. Urine cations include sodium, potassium, calcium, magnesium, ammonium, and hydrogen ions. Urine anions include chloride, bicarbonate, phosphate, sulphate, citrate, oxalate, and hydroxide ions. Plasma and urine are electrically neutral and the sum of anions (negative electrical charge) equals the sum of cations (positive electrical charge).[29,30,33] So that electroneutrality can be maintained, water molecules dissociate. In other words, the determinants of $[H^+]$ are the determinants of water dissociation, and the quantification of the water dissociation is made through the measurement of the hydrogen ion concentration $[H^+]$.[29]

Normal concentration of hydrogen ions in the extracellular fluid is extremely low, in the nanoequivalent (nEq) or nanomole (nmol) range. The usual arterial blood $[H^+]$ is about 40 nEq/L (or nmol/L).[34] In other words, serum $[H^+]$ is about 3 million times less than the serum sodium concentration.[35] For convenience, the $[H^+]$ value is usually expressed as pH units, which are obtained from the negative $\log_{10}$ of the hydrogen ion concentration in nanoequivalents per liter. This concept was developed by Sörensen and adapted by Karl Hasselbalch into clinical medicine in 1909.[36,37] A normal pH of 7.4 corresponds to a blood hydrogen ion concentration of 40 nEq/L, at 37°C. The relationship between pH and serum $[H^+]$ is nonlinear, but it is almost linear over the narrow normal pH range of 7.35 to 7.45 (corresponding to 45 to 35 nEq/L of $[H^+]$).[35,37] When the hydrogen ion concentration increases, pH will decrease, and vice versa. Nevertheless, the logarithmic scale of pH can be somewhat confusing, because it has the negative effect of obscuring the magnitude of deviations from normal. For example, a change in pH from a normal value of 7.4 to 7.2, a decrease of *only* 0.2, results in a 60% increase in $[H^+]$

from 40 to 63 nEq/L or nmol/L.[29,37] Although the use of pH instead of nanomoles of H^+ has been repeatedly challenged, pH has survived, as pH provides a measurement of the *activity* of the H^+, rather than simple H^+ concentration.[36-38]

The term *acidosis* is used to describe the process that tends to produce an increase in $[H^+]$, whether or not there is a change in blood pH. *Alkalosis* is the opposite—that is, the process that tends to produce a decrease in $[H^+]$, with or without changes in blood pH. *Acidemia* and *alkalemia* are the corresponding terms for those situations in which blood pH actually changes.[34,35]

Constancy of the Ionic Product for Water

Any reversible chemical reaction at a specific temperature has a specific equilibrium constant. The law of mass action, which defines the final equilibrium concentrations of reactants and products, can be applied to the water dissociation reaction (Eqs. 2A and 2B), and therefore an equilibrium constant (K_{eq} or K_a) for the reversible ionization of water can be defined[33,39,40]:

$$K_{eq} = \frac{[H^+][OH^-]}{[H_2O]} \qquad \text{(Eq. 3)}$$

At any given time, the number of hydronium (hydrogen) ions and hydroxide ions present in water is extremely small and consequently the concentration of undissociated water molecules ($[H_2O]$) is virtually unchanged by this minute ionization and may be considered a constant:

$$K_{eq} \times [H_2O] = [H^+][OH^-] \qquad \text{(Eq. 4)}$$

The product $K_{eq} \times [H_2O]$ is a constant termed the *ionic product for water* (K_w), which therefore is expressed as follows:

$$K_w = [H^+][OH^-] \qquad \text{(Eq. 5)}$$

The concentration of molecules in pure water is 55.5 M and the value for the equilibrium constant, determined by electrical conductivity measurements, is 1.8×10^{-16} M at 25°C of temperature. Substituting these values in the equilibrium constant equation (Eq. 5):

$$K_w = (1.8 \times 10^{-16}) \times 55.5 = 99.9 \times 10^{-16} \approx 1 \times 10^{-14} \qquad \text{(Eq. 6)}$$

Therefore,

$$K_w = [H^+][OH^-] = 10^{-14[33,39,40]} \qquad \text{(Eq. 7)}$$

In pure water, the concentration of hydrogen ions is equal to the concentration of hydroxide ions: ($[H^+] = [OH^-]$). Hence at 25°C, both concentrations are equal to 10^{-7} M. The ionic product for water ($[H^+][OH^-]$) is always constant in any aqueous solution, regardless of the presence of dissolved solutes.[33,40] If the presence of other electrically charged molecules provokes a change in the concentration of either hydrogen ions or hydroxide ions, a concomitant change of the same magnitude must occur in the other ion to maintain constant the ionic product for water.[30-33,39]

Variations in the concentration of plasma ions, either anions or cations, organic acids or electrolytes, may modify the relative proportion of anions and cations and predictably lead to a change in the plasma concentration of hydrogen ions by driving changes and adjustments in water ionization, thus allowing plasma electroneutrality while maintaining constant the ionic product for water.[30-33,39]

Acids, Bases, and Buffers

Clinical acid-base base balance includes a combination of the Arrhenius approach (acid = H^+ increased in aqueous solution) and the Brönsted-Lowry approach (acid = proton donor).[21,41] In a similar way, bases are compounds that decrease the concentration of hydrogen ions, either by accepting the protons directly in their own molecules or by decreasing [H^+] as a result of the electrochemical effect of certain solutes on water dissociation. For instance, hydrochloric acid (HCl) dissociates into H^+ and chloride (Cl^-) when dissolved in water, whereas ammonia (NH_3) becomes protonated when dissolved in water producing ammonium ion (NH_4^+). Each acid or base, as proton donor or acceptor, has a characteristic tendency to release or to catch hydrogen ions in an aqueous solution, according to the reversible reaction depicted in Eq. 8.[1]

$$K_a = \frac{[H^+][A^-]}{[HA]} \qquad \text{(Eq. 8)}$$

The tendency of an acid to dissociate releasing hydrogen ions and anions may be assessed from equilibrium or dissociation constant (K_a). The larger the value of the equilibrium constant, the greater the tendency of the acid to dissociate and the stronger the acid. An acid is considered strong when it dissociates its hydrogen ion easily because the corresponding base has a low affinity for it (high K_a value). The relative strength of a base can be assessed in a similar way: The lower the value of its dissociation constant, the higher the tendency of the base to capture hydrogen ions (protons) and the higher the concentration of the protonated molecule.[22,23,33,42]

The dissociation constant K_a, as in the case of pH, can be expressed as $-\log_{10}K_a$ and is termed pK_a, which is the most used measure of the tendency of the acid-base pair to ionize. The well-known Henderson-Hasselbalch equation is the logarithmic transformation of the equilibrium constant equation, in which pH is the $-\log$ of [$H+$] and pK_a is the $-\log$ of Ka:

$$pH = pK_a + \log\frac{[A^-]}{[HA]} \quad \text{in the case of an acid} \qquad \text{(Eq. 9)}$$

or

$$pH = pK_a + \log\frac{[B]}{[HB^+]} \quad \text{in the case of a base} \qquad \text{(Eq. 10)}$$

The pK_a estimates the relative strength of an acid or base. Strong acids have a low pK_a (high K_a) and weak acids have high pK_a (low K_a). The tendency of a base to join hydrogen ions also is reflected in the pK_a value. The stronger the base, the greater its tendency to bind protons and the higher its pK_a (and lower the K_a).[33,42] When the concentration of the undissociated moiety of both acids and bases is equal to the concentration of the dissociated moiety, then pH equals pK_a as log 1 = 0. Therefore the pK_a of an acid or a base is the pH at which the concentration of dissociated and undissociated forms is the same, as can be understood with a quick view to Eqs. 9 and 10.

When the pK_a of an acid is lower than the pH of the aqueous solution in which it is dissolved, the acid tends to dissociate itself, at least in a certain proportion, and releases hydrogen ions, being transformed into an anion. Strong acids have low pK_a values, usually below 3, and completely dissociate in

aqueous solutions, yielding strong anions. Such is the case of the pair constituted by phosphoric acid (H_3PO_4)/dihydrogen phosphate ($H_2PO_4^-$), with a pK_a of 1.97, which means that phosphoric acid is virtually not present in the human body but as its anion form $H_2PO_4^-$. Acids with pK_a values of around 4 or less also generate rather strong anions at physiologic pH values. Many organic acids existing in the human body have pK_a values around 4 and therefore appear predominantly in their anionic form, such as the pair carbonic acid/ bicarbonate (H_2CO_3/HCO_3^-) with pK_a = 3.7; lactic acid/ lactate, pK_a= 3.86; pyruvic acid/pyruvate, pK_a = 2.49; citric acid/citrate, pK_a = 3.09; acetoacetic acid/acetoacetate, pK_a = 3.58; and β-hydroxybutyric acid/β-hydroxybutyrate, pK_a = 4.39.[33] When the pH of the aqueous solution is lower than the pK_a value of a dissolved base, the base captures hydrogen ions and becomes protonated. Strong bases have high pK_a values and therefore they remain protonated at physiologic plasma pH. For instance, the pK_a value for the pair NH_3/NH_4^+ is 9.3, indicating that virtually only the protonated moiety (NH_4^+) is present in the human body. Something similar occurs with the pair monohydrogen phosphate (HPO_4^{2-})/phosphate (PO_4^{3-}), which has a pK_a of 12.35.

Weak acids only partially dissociate because their corresponding base has high affinity for hydrogen ions (high pK_a, low K_a values). When this is the case, both the acid and base forms of the parental molecule are present in the resulting solution in near-equimolar proportions. Thus weak acids and bases are those with pK_a values closer to approximately 7. These solutions have the ability to resist changes in pH after the addition of a strong acid or base. This solution, constituted by an acid-base pair, was designed with the word *puffer* (in German), which was first introduced in the scientific lexicon in the first decade of the 20th century, and popularized as *buffer,* to refer to the property of weak acid-base pairs that tends to minimize changes in pH by reversibly *producing* or *consuming* hydrogen ions.[43]

An ideal buffer is a weak acid in equilibrium with its corresponding weak base. This weak acid-base pair is more effective as a buffer in living systems when its pK_a is close to physiologic pH.[22,33,42,43] At physiologic pH values, their degree of dissociation or protonation, respectively, is variable. Weak anions in the human body include the pair dihydrogen phosphate/monohydrogen phosphate ($H_2PO_4^-$/HPO_4^{2-}), with a pK_a of 6.86, and uric acid/urate (pK_a 5.75).

Physiologic buffering systems may be classified into two general categories: the bicarbonate/carbonic acid (HCO_3^-/H_2CO_3) buffering system, which acts in both the extracellular space and inside the erythrocytes, and the nonbicarbonate buffers, which include hemoglobin and oxyhemoglobin, organic phosphates, inorganic phosphates (in intracellular space), and plasma proteins. Extracellular buffers (HCO_3^-, plasma proteins) represent the body's first, more abundant and immediate line of defense against any alteration of pH of the body fluids. In the bicarbonate/carbonic acid (HCO_3^-/H_2CO_3) buffering system, the acid part is actually constituted by the sum of both the volatile [CO_2] and nonvolatile [H_2CO_3] forms of the carbonic acid, which is a moderately strong acid with a pK_a of 3.7. However, most of the acid moiety of the bicarbonate/carbonic acid buffering system is CO_2, with only about one-thousandth as the full H_2CO_3 molecule. Thus when [CO_2] is included in the dissociation equation (Eqs. 8-10), the pK_a shifts to 6.1, which is equivalent to a dissociation constant

(K_a) about a thousand times smaller and much closer to the physiologic pH, which makes the $[HCO_3^-]/[CO_2]$ system a powerful buffer.

After extracellular buffering occurs, a second intracellular phase takes place, as long as intracellular buffers (intracellular proteins, dibasic phosphates, hemoglobin-oxyhemoglobin, and carbonate in bones) reach buffering capacity over the next several hours.[43,44] The buffering systems (with the exception of HCO_3^-/CO_2) cannot truly eliminate hydrogen ions from the body, but they tamper sudden changes in $[H^+]$ (or pH) and buy time until a new balance can be achieved. Altogether, extracellular and intracellular buffers provide a volume of distribution close to that of the total body water to any exogenous acid load (or deficit). This represents a formidable capacity for resisting changes in pH.

The major acid-base buffering system in the blood, the bicarbonate/carbonic acid system, has the tremendous advantage of its interconversion with CO_2, the volatile form of H_2CO_3, which means this is an *open system* buffer:

$$CO_2 + H_2O \leftrightarrow H_2CO_3 \leftrightarrow H^+ + HCO_3^- \qquad \text{(Eq. 11)}$$

Any increase in $[H^+]$ (or drop in pH) will shift the preceding reaction to the left, including an increase in alveolar ventilation to eliminate the resultant increase in CO_2. This respiratory response begins within minutes, but it may not reach a steady state for 12 to 24 hours. This method of achieving a fast and actual decrease of the acid component is a unique characteristic of the bicarbonate/carbonic acid buffering system. For the other buffers, the addition or removal of hydrogen ions has the corresponding opposite effects on the buffer components, limiting the maximum buffering capacity. However, the capacity of the bicarbonate-CO_2 system is greatly increased because the lungs can eliminate a vast amount of CO_2 per day. Similarly, the kidneys can eliminate or regenerate bicarbonate, as needed, although its response is slower than that of the lungs. This respiratory response is particularly useful to the tissues, because of its rapid effect on intracellular pH as well as extracellular pH. Carbon dioxide crosses cell membranes easily, so changes in PCO_2 affect intracellular pH rapidly and in a predictable direction.

Tight regulation of the H^+ is mandatory for the body, because nearly every metabolic pathway includes moieties such as phosphate, ammonium, or carboxylic acid, which undergo variable ionization with changes in pH.[38,41,45] The body has a relatively large capacity to tolerate severe shifts in the levels of pH. For example, from a pH of 7.4 (40 nEq/L or nmol/L) to a severe acidosis of pH 6.7 (equivalent to 175 nEq/L or nmol/L), the $[H^+]$ increases by a factor of 4, and this could not be tolerated with other ions such as potassium, calcium, or chloride.[41] Nevertheless, the range of pH compatible with life, of about 6.9 (0.126 mEq/L or mmol/l H^+) to 7.6 (0.025 mEq/L or mmol/L H+), implies a difference in $[H^+]$ of barely 0.1 mEq/L or mmol/L. It is amazing that an ion with such a low concentration plays such a major role in body homeostasis. Hydrogen ion concentration and, more important, hydrogen ion activity have a strong influence on the function of almost all enzymatic systems of the body.[41,43,45]

In the body, normal metabolism continuously produces both anions and cations, (ie, acids and bases) in two major ways. The first one involves CO_2 production during oxidative metabolism of carbohydrates, fat, and amino acids, which is then hydrated by the cytoplasmic and erythrocytic carbonic anhydrase to produce carbonic acid (H_2CO_3), which dissociates in hydrogen ion and bicarbonate (Eq. 11).

The second pathway involves cations such as ammonium and anions such as nonvolatile metabolic acids that are produced by the normal daily catabolic load (oxidation of sulfur [SO_4^{2-}] containing amino acids, hydrolysis of pyrophosphate, and orthophosphate esters) or during situations with incomplete catabolism of carbohydrates and fat, such as lactic acidosis or diabetic ketoacidosis (DKA), with increased aceto-acetate and β-hydroxybutyrate, or in cases with defective processing or excretion of certain metabolites, as occurs in some inborn errors of metabolism and in uremic acidosis. The free hydrogen ions are neutralized by extracellular and intracellular buffers, but because these acids are not in equilibrium in the normal plasma, they must be metabolized, mainly in the liver, and then excreted by the kidneys.[43,44] In addition, other charged molecules circulate in human plasma, including anions such as albumin and cations such as immunoglobulins. Anomalous plasma ions may be derived from exogenous substances, including cations such as lithium and anions such as salicylates, and formate generated from methanol, for example. All of these may potentially change the plasma pH when modifications in their concentration alter the normal relative proportion of plasma anions and cations. According to the electroneutrality principle and the constancy of the ionic product for water, the plasma concentration and activity of hydrogen ions depend on the plasma level of other ions, and variations in the plasma ionic composition predictably lead to a change in plasma pH.[26,29,33,40]

CO$_2$ and Bicarbonate-Physiologic Relationship and Effect on Acid-Base Balance

Plasma bicarbonate is a circulating anion that contributes substantially to the plasma negative charge in quantitative terms and therefore plays a role in defining plasma pH. Unlike other plasma ions, bicarbonate concentration is determined by the lung ventilatory activity besides the kidney handling of bicarbonate. Several isoenzymes of carbonic anhydrase are ubiquitously expressed in the human body and catalyze the reversible conversion of carbon dioxide into bicarbonate.[46] Carbon dioxide formed during cell metabolism continuously diffuses across the plasma membrane into the tissue capillary network, being transported by blood in a number of ways. Approximately 5% of the carbon dioxide remains as a gas in the aqueous phase of blood, measured as the partial pressure of carbon dioxide (PCO_2). An even smaller proportion of carbon dioxide binds to plasma proteins. Most of the carbon dioxide (90%-95%) arriving in capillary blood diffuses into the red blood cells, where it is hydrated to bicarbonate (HCO_3^-) by the cytosolic enzyme carbonic anhydrase II, generating hydrogen ions that bind to oxyhemoglobin.[33] As a result, oxygen is released from oxyhemoglobin and leaves the erythrocyte, reaching the tissues (see also Chapter 89). Bicarbonate formed inside the red blood cells by carbonic anhydrase II moves into the plasma in exchange for chloride through the plasma membrane transporter anion exchanger–1 (AE1). Erythrocytes with protonated deoxyhemoglobin formed in the tissue capillaries travel to the lungs, where the uptake of oxygen transforms deoxyhemoglobin into oxyhemoglobin, releasing hydrogen ions that are combined with bicarbonate diffusing back from plasma by carbonic anhydrase II, generating water and carbon dioxide, which is exhaled as a gas.[47]

Henderson clearly noticed the quantitative importance of the bicarbonate/carbonic acid buffering system when he developed his famous equation, a simple formula linking hydrogen ion concentration and the composition of an acid-base pair.[48] Henderson's equation was modified by Hasselbalch shortly after (Eqs. 9 and 10). The Henderson-Hasselbalch equation expresses the relationship of the bicarbonate/carbonic acid buffering system to pH:[21,33,36,48,49]

$$pH = pK_a + \log([HCO_3^-]/[H_2CO_3]) \quad \text{(Eq. 12)}$$

The pH is equal to the $^-\log_{10}$ of the dissociation constant (pK_a) for H_2CO_3, plus the log of the ratio of HCO_3^- (proton acceptor) to H_2CO_3 (proton donor). The modified Henderson-Hasselbalch equation takes into consideration that most H_2CO_3 exists as dissolved CO_2 and is rewritten as follows[33,35,49]:

$$pH = pK_a + \log([HCO_3^-]/0.03 \times PCO_2) \quad \text{(Eq. 13)}$$

where 0.03 is the solubility coefficient for carbon dioxide in blood at 37°C, and PCO_2 the partial pressure of CO_2 in blood.

The Henderson-Hasselbalch equation expresses how pH is affected by the change in the ratio of the concentration of undissociated acid HA (in this case carbonic acid or PCO_2) to the concentration of the conjugated base or anion A^- (in this case HCO_3^-). At the physiologic values of pH, the ratio between HCO_3^- and the acidic component (CO_2—ie, carbonic acid) is 20:1. Knowing that HCO_3^-/H_2CO_3 (CO_2) is the only buffer system with a volatile component that can be regulated through the respiration, it is possible to have a clear appreciation of the pH alterations related to changes in PCO_2. When pH is altered as the result of changes in the volatile component (increases or decreases of PCO_2), the change is referred to as *respiratory*, because the primary alteration in the volatile component is always associated with either hypoventilation or hyperventilation.[34,35] When pH is modified by any other cause (ie, changes in nonvolatile acids [eg, lactic acid, keto-acids] or by changes in serum cations or anions [eg, hyper/hypochloremia]), the alteration is referred to as *metabolic* in origin.[21,29,34,35,49] Therefore this equation allows disorders to be classified according to the primary type of acid being increased or decreased. For example, if a patient's pH is low (acidemia), then the patient may have either an increased PCO_2 or a PCO_2 within normal or decreased values. If the PCO_2 is increased or at least higher than expected (alveolar hypoventilation), the condition is classified as *respiratory acidosis;* if this is not the case, the condition cannot be a respiratory acidosis. Therefore either some nonvolatile acid or a mineral-derived anion *must be* the cause of the acidemia, which is then referred to as *metabolic acidosis.* If these examples are reversed, then alkalemia conditions can also be classified as resulting from either respiratory or metabolic alkalosis.[34,35,44]

Thus the main usefulness of the Henderson-Hasselbalch equation is that it allows quantification of the severity of the respiratory component of the acid-base balance. For example, in a respiratory acidosis, the increase in the PCO_2 quantifies the derangement even when there are mixed disorders. The relationship between PCO_2 and HCO_3^- may provide a useful clinical guide for uncovering the metabolic origin of a given derangement in many rather simple acidosis cases, mainly the ones associated to the presence of organic acids; however, this is complicated by the fact that PCO_2, H_2CO_3, and HCO_3^- are

all interlinked (Eqs. 11 to 13), so when bicarbonate increases, PCO_2 increases, and vice versa.[21,26,29,33,36,49] When taken as a mathematical expression of the relationship among its three variables, the equation is a valid statement of the dissociation equilibrium for carbonic acid. But the equation does not indicate, as is sometimes suggested, that pH is physically as well as mathematically determined by the values of $[HCO_3^-]$ and PCO_2. For this to be true, $[HCO_3^-]$ and PCO_2 would have to be able to vary independently of each other. In reality, both pH and $[HCO_3^-]$ are determined by PCO_2 in conjunction with other variables that are not included in the Henderson-Hasselbalch equation. Thus the Henderson-Hasselbalch equation does not provide information about acids other than CO_2/H_2CO_3, which means that only the HCO_3^-/CO_2 buffering system is being assessed, and the influence of other buffering systems and mineral anions and cations is overlooked.[21,26,41,48,49] In addition, the Henderson-Hasselbalch equation, as Henderson himself knew, was derived assuming that the concentrations of both the acid and the base were not modified by dissociation or hydrolysis, which is not necessarily true in physiologic conditions.[26,48,49] In systems with significant concentrations of nonvolatile weak acids, a change in PCO_2 causes a change in $[HCO_3^-]$—that is, it varies not only with metabolic but also with respiratory acid-base state. Hence the metabolic component can only be approximated through the change in HCO_3^-.

The understanding that a rise in plasma CO_2 causes increased plasma HCO_3^- set the pace for the development of various refinements to quantify the metabolic component of acid-base disturbances, from the direct determination of pH and partial pressure of CO_2 (PCO_2), to the development of several tools for quantifying the metabolic component.[8,36,50,51] Because plasma bicarbonate is the principal means of transportation of carbon dioxide in blood, plasma bicarbonate level increases as carbon dioxide rises, whereas plasma bicarbonate concentration falls as carbon dioxide declines. Hence both carbon dioxide and plasma bicarbonate reflect mainly ventilatory status. Hypoventilation results in hypercapnia and a rise in plasma bicarbonate concentration, whereas hyperventilation leads to hypocapnia and a subsequent reduction in the plasma bicarbonate level. A quantitative relationship between carbon dioxide and plasma bicarbonate has been demonstrated in a number of situations, further highlighting this physiologic relationship.[33,36,50-57] Close attention must be paid to PCO_2, to pH, and to the clinical data and expected physiology and pathophysiology before an increased or decreased bicarbonate can be labeled as having a *metabolic* origin.[36,53-57])

Bicarbonate levels in blood are the result of the respiratory control of CO_2 elimination (quantitatively the largest influence), but they are also influenced by renal function, the presence of abnormal anions and acids in blood, liver function, and the potential abnormal loss of bicarbonate-rich fluids, as in diarrhea or renal tubular acidosis.[43,51,52,54-60] Therefore to rely only on the bicarbonate levels for the estimation of the metabolic component of an acid-base unbalance is an oversimplification that could be misleading in certain complex cases. For a single solution containing several weak acids (such as human plasma), all the weak acids are equilibrated with a single pool of hydrogen ions. In other words, all buffering systems, which participate in keeping the acid-base balance, are in equilibrium with each other. This is called the *isohydric principle.*[21] It may be illustrated with two buffer systems: bicarbonate/carbonic acid and phosphate/phosphoric acid:

$$H_2CO_3 \leftrightarrow HCO_3^- + H^+ + HPO_4^{2-} \leftrightarrow H_2PO_4^- \quad \text{(Eq. 14)}$$

In this equilibrium H⁺ will eventually form both carbonic acid and phosphoric acid from the single H^+ plasmatic pool. Expressing the same concept in the Henderson-Hasselbalch way:

$$pK_{a1} + \log([HCO_3^-]/[H_2CO_3]) = pH$$
$$= pK_{a2} + \log([HPO_4^{2-}/[H_2PO_4^-]) \quad \text{(Eq. 15)}$$

Thus according to the isohydric principle, the ratio of *any pair* of conjugate base or anion and its undissociated acid will be able to describe the [H⁺] or pH.[21,26] This means that although the ratio of PCO_2 to bicarbonate can describe the pH and the respiratory component of the acid-base status, this buffering system is not necessarily the primary or underlying mechanism for explaining by itself all the changes in pH, nor may the changes in bicarbonate explain by themselves all the possible derangements of the metabolic component.[21,29] This is particularly true in the so-called mixed or complex cases.

Many physiologists focused on the plasma bicarbonate concentration and the Henderson-Hasselbalch equation, neglecting almost entirely all other influences on acid-base status.[21,41,49] This was the beginning of the still dominant concept that plasma bicarbonate is not only the best indicator of acid-base status but also the main determinant of it. Immersed in the bicarbonate-centered approach, investigators yielded basically two solutions for analyzing the metabolic side of the equation: the base excess method and the six bicarbonate rules of thumb. The role of the mineral anions was also taken into account, albeit not in an integrated way, by the use of anion gap (AG). Stewart's physicochemical approach appeared later.[21,35,36,61-63]

Tools for Interpreting Acid-Base Disorders

The understanding that a rise in plasma CO_2 causes increased plasma HCO_3^- set the pace for the development of various refinements to quantify the metabolic component of acid-base disturbances. In an attempt to identify acid-base changes independent of carbon dioxide, Singer and Hastings advanced the concept of a *buffer base (BB),* which is the sum of weak acids (buffer anions) in plasma—that is HCO_3^- and all nonvolatile weak acid buffers, albumin included; they also defined fixed acids as nonbuffer anions, chloride being one.[8,21,26,64,65] Other research groups later proposed several PCO_2-independent indicators of nonrespiratory acid-base disturbances. One is the *standard bicarbonate,* which is measured plasma HCO_3^- at a $PaCO_2$ of 40 mm Hg (5.33 kPa).[66] *Base excess or deficit (BE),* developed by Siggard-Andersen in 1963, is another indicator, which is a measure of the deviation of BB from its normal value.[67] Two trends developed, one relying on plasma [HCO_3^-] and the other on BE for detection of metabolic acidosis or alkalosis. Both base excess and bicarbonate rules of thumb use a bicarbonate-centered approach. Indeed, both approaches can detect metabolic disturbances, mostly the simple ones, but if PCO_2 varies, the picture may be blurred.[8,21,26] A singular change in either [HCO_3^-] or BE does not differentiate among the various possible sources of nonrespiratory acid-base disturbances. Such a determination is often important in clinical medicine.

Base Excess and Standard Base Excess

The change in pH of a given buffered solution is dependent on both the amount of strong acid (or strong base) that is added and the buffering capacity of the system. As acid is added, for every H⁺ that is buffered, one molecule of conjugate base of the buffer is consumed. Therefore quantifying the changes in the concentration of the conjugate base of the buffer is more useful than the degree of change in the pH in estimating the number of nonvolatile acids present. Siggaard-Andersen, from Copenhagen, developed the *base excess method* in the late 1950s and early 1960s.[26,36,66-68]

Base excess (BE) is defined as the amount of strong acid (or strong base) in mol/L that must be added in vitro to a whole blood sample to return the pH of the sample to 7.4 while the PCO_2 is kept constant at 40 mm Hg.[8,21,26,66-69] Therefore if the blood sample is normal (ie, pH is 7.4 and PCO_2 is about 40 mm Hg), the BE will be 0 mmol/L. Positive values mean literally an excess of metabolic bases; negative values mean an excess of metabolic acids.[35,68-70] To apply the BE to the clinical setting, a nomogram was developed, which was later mathematically transcribed to allow BE calculation by blood gas analyzers.[68,70-73] BE, even though calculated, comes closest to being the parameter that is least influenced by changes in $PaCO_2$. However, several limitations appeared.[70,73-75] For clinical accuracy, other assumptions had to be incorporated (correction factors, adjusted formulas, nomogram modifications),[21,68,70,72,76] and remarkably an empiric estimate of hemoglobin concentration throughout the entire extracellular fluid space (whole blood plus interstitial fluid) had to be established. The original BE was calculated only for plasma buffers. As Hb is the main buffer in blood, changes in Hb can significantly affect BE. To take into account the net effect of all the buffers of the body, the three compartments relevant to acid-base balance—plasma, erythrocytes, and interstitial fluid—had to be considered, including the influence of hemoglobin.[26,33,76] The chosen hemoglobin concentration was 50 g/L (5 g/dL) as an estimation of the concentration of hemoglobin as it is diluted throughout the body. This estimation is, of course, somewhat arbitrary. For example, in a patient with a hemoglobin concentration of 5 mg/dL from the outset, the impact of the interstitium is not actually taken into account.[70,76] BE calculated this way is called *standard base excess (SBE),* a parameter reported nowadays by modern gas analyzers and used in the classical approach to acid-base balance (Table 76.1). Although SBE has good correlation with bicarbonate levels and quantifies the change in metabolic acid-base status in vivo, its accuracy depends on the 5 g/dL of hemoglobin assumption. It does not provide information about the origin or mechanisms of the metabolic acid-base derangement because SBE is not a substance that can be regulated, absorbed, or excreted by the body.[29] Perhaps the main drawback is that SBE value represents the net effect of all metabolic acid-base abnormalities. Therefore the effect of coexisting metabolic acidosis and alkaloses may cancel each other, and the "normal figure" of the SBE will mistakenly suggest that no acid-base derangement exists. Actually, 15% to 18% of critically ill adults with acid-base disorders have normal SBE.[61,77] In practice, SBE is calculated by well-established formulas or derived from nomograms.[68,69] Nomograms are widely incorporated in blood-gas analyzer software and SBE calculated from variables like pH, HCO_3^-, and Hb.

TABLE 76.1   Classical Acid-Base Parameters

pH	Log_{10} H^+. Measured directly by electrode. Normal = 7.35-7.45.
PCO_2	Partial pressure of gaseous CO_2. Measured directly by electrode. Usually expressed in mm Hg. Normal value: 35-45 mm Hg (sea level, arterial blood).
HCO_3^-	Bicarbonate concentration. A calculated parameter, derived from pH and PCO_2 values using a nomogram or the Henderson-Hasselbalch equation, or equal to the difference between serum total CO_2 (CO_{2TOT}) and the dissolved CO_2. ($PCO_2 \times 0.03$). Normal value: 22-28 mEq/L.
Base excess (BE or BE/D)	Also known as base excess/deficit. Defined as the amount of strong base (negative base excess, or "base deficit") or strong acid (positive base excess) in mmol/L that would be needed to restore a pH of 7.4 to a liter of whole blood equilibrated at PCO_2 = 40 mm Hg. It is calculated by a nomogram or equation that was derived from an experimental series of in vitro titrations of strong acid and base in whole blood samples at various PCO_2 levels. It excludes the effect of acute changes in PCO_2, so it loses accuracy if PCO_2 is abnormal. It should not be used in critically ill patients.
Standard base excess (SBE)	An improvement of base excess to allow equilibration across the entire extracellular fluid space (whole blood interstitial fluid) and thus preserve accuracy at variable PCO_2 values. The new equation assumes an average concentration of hemoglobin through that space of 5 g/dL. Despite being a somewhat arbitrary figure, it indeed works in vivo.
CO_{2TOT} or CO_2	Total CO_2 or CO_2 concentration. A serum chemistry measured value. Its components include HCO_3^-, dissolved gaseous CO_2, carbonic acid (H_2CO_3), carbamino CO_2, and carbonate (CO_3^{2-}). About 95% exists as HCO_3^-, and 4% to 5% as dissolved gaseous CO_2. Remaining species are negligible. Because the difference between CO_{2TOT} and HCO_3^- is about 1 mEq/L at physiologic pH, for clinical purposes they are taken almost as equivalents.
Anion gap (AG)	A calculated value that, taking advantage of the electroneutrality principle that rules plasmatic ions (total number of cations should be the same as the total number of anions), indicates the presence of unmeasured anions (mostly organic acids). AG = $(Na^+ + K^+) - (Cl^- + HCO_3^-)$. Normal values are 16 mEq/L (if K^+ is included) or 12 mEq/L (without K^+, with variations of ± 2 to 4 mEq/L). These values may be influenced by the way the values of some of the parameters are measured, so it is always better to consult each institution's own expected normal AG.
Corrected anion gap (AG_{CORR})	An improvement in the calculation of AG that acknowledges that an increase in AG from organic acids may be masked by a decrease in AG from low protein (albumin) levels. AG is corrected for the patient's own albumin concentration as follows: $AG_{CORRECTED} = AG_{OBSERVED} \times 2.5$[normal albumin (g/dL)] – [observed albumin (g/dL)], considering normal albumin from 3.2 to 4.5 g/dL. To avoid [$lactate^-$] influence on AG_{CORR} that could mask the detection of other unmeasured anions, it has been suggested that AG should be corrected not only for albumin but also for lactate. This is simply made by subtracting the serum lactate concentration (in mmol/L) from the already albumin-corrected AG: $AG_{CORRLACT}$ = Albumin-corrected AG – [$lactate^-$ (mmol/L)].
Urinary anion gap (uGap)	The same principle of the anion gap applied to urinary ions—that is, uGap estimates unmeasured urinary ions. It has also been designated by some as the urine strong ion difference (uSID), a functionally correct name, as all the involved ions are strong ions: uGap = uSID = [$uNa^+ + uK^+$] – [uCl^-]. The most important unmeasured urinary strong anion (Ur^-) is SO_4^{2-} (derived from the metabolism of sulfur amino acids), whereas the most important unmeasured cation (Ur^+) is ammonium (NH_4^+). In physiologically normal conditions, uSID must equal the plasmatic SID_{APP}, or 38-42 mEq/L.

Simple mathematical rules can be applied for using SBE in common acid-base disturbances.[8,9,69] Thus SBE does not change in acute respiratory acidosis or alkalosis. In metabolic acidosis, SBE decreases and becomes negative (−BE or base deficit), whereas it becomes positive in metabolic alkalosis (simply called BE or +BE). However, calculating SBE is not without its inconveniences. SBE can still vary with changes in $PaCO_2$, albeit only slightly, and may be unreliable in the presence of low albumin or phosphate levels. Other drawbacks include inaccuracy due to in vitro measurement and that it does not take into account the respiratory status or the volume of distribution of bicarbonate.[9]

Bicarbonate Rules of Thumb

Strong criticism of the SBE in the great transatlantic debate[21,41,49,72-75] yielded the six bicarbonate rules of thumb[72,73] (Table 76.2). Because the body always seeks to tightly control [H^+], when an acid-base derangement tends to appear, several physiologic responses become active over time, and then the

relationship between PCO_2 and HCO_3^- expressed in the Henderson-Hasselbalch equation is modified so pH changes can be minimized. On the observation of many patients with clearly defined alterations of the acid-base balance, Schwartz and Relman[73] concluded that several global patterns could be detected. With this Boston school *six rules of thumb* approach, it is possible to predict to what extent changes in pH and PCO_2 modify the concentration of bicarbonate in an acute alteration or a chronic respiratory disorder. Similarly, even primary metabolic disorders can be predicted, based on changes in the PCO_2 in the context of a normal respiratory compensation (assuming normal respiratory function).[70] These rules are useful for uncovering mixed disorders, to differentiate acute from chronic respiratory unbalances, and to describe the physiologic compensation to acid-base changes to optimize acid-base homeostasis (Tables 76.2 and 76.3). [H^+] is related to CO_2 in respiratory and to CO_2/HCO_3^- in metabolic acid-base disturbances. This approach is easy to use in stable patients exhibiting simple acid-base disturbances, where the

TABLE 76.2   Classical Acid-Base Approach: Observational Acid-Base Patterns

Primary Disorder	Expected Changes [HCO$_3^-$] (mEq/L or mmol/L)	Expected Changes PCO$_2$ (mm Hg)*	Expected Changes SBE (mmol/L)
Metabolic acidosis[a]	Primary decrease <22	**Bicarbonate Approach** PCO$_2$ = (1.5 × HCO$_3^-$) + (8 ± 2) or PCO$_2$ ↓ 1.2 – 1.5 mm Hg for each mEq/L [HCO$_3^-$] ↓ **SBE Approach** PCO$_2$ = 40 ± SBE, or PCO$_2$ ↓ 1 mm Hg for each mEq/L SBE ↓	Base deficit <−3
Metabolic alkalosis[b]	Primary increase >26	**Bicarbonate Approach** PCO$_2$ = (0.7 × HCO$_3^-$) + (21 ± 2) or PCO$_2$ ↑ 0.7 mm Hg for each mEq/L HCO$_3^-$] ↑ **SBE Approach** PCO$_2$ = 40 ± (0.6 × SBE), or PaCO$_2$ ↑ 0.6 mm Hg for each mEq/l [HCO$_3^-$] ↑	Base excess >+3
Acute respiratory acidosis	= [(PCO$_2$ − 40)/10] + 24 or [HCO$_3^-$] ↑ 0.1 mEq/L for each mm Hg PCO$_2$ ↑	Primary PCO$_2$ increase >45 ΔpH = 0.008 × (PCO$_2$ − 40)	0
Chronic respiratory acidosis	= [(PCO$_2$ − 40)/3] + 24 or [HCO$_3^-$] ↑ 0.3 mEq/L for each mm Hg PCO$_2$ ↑	Primary PCO$_2$ increase >45 ΔpH = 0.003 × (PCO$_2$ − 40)	0.4 × (PCO$_2$ − 40) or SBE ↑ 0.4 mEq/L for each mm Hg PCO$_2$ ↑
Acute respiratory alkalosis	= [(40 − PCO$_2$)/5] + 24 or [HCO$_3^-$] ↓ 0.2 mEq/L for each mm Hg PCO$_2$ ↓	Primary PCO$_2$ decrease <35 ΔpH = 0.008 × (40 − PCO$_2$)	0
Chronic respiratory alkalosis	= [(40 − PCO$_2$)/10] + 24 [HCO$_3^-$] ↓ 0.4 mEq/L for each mm Hg ↓ PCO$_2$	Primary PCO$_2$ decrease <35 ΔpH = 0.017 × (40 − PCO$_2$)	0.4 × (PCO$_2$ − 40) or ↓ 0.4 mEq/L for each mm Hg ↓

*Always adjust PCO$_2$ values to the height above sea level. Empirical rules for expected values and compensation are minimally affected.
[a]In metabolic acidosis, hyperventilation PCO$_2$ decreases in a highly predictable fashion, if respiratory and CNS function are normal.
[b]In metabolic alkalosis, compensatory respiratory hypoventilation is highly variable even if respiratory and CNS function are normal.
Acute = minutes to hours; chronic = several days or longer.
See Table 76.3.
SBE, standard base excess.

magnitude of increase in unmeasured anions parallels the drop in [HCO$_3^-$]. However, as [HCO$_3^-$] varies with changes in PaCO$_2$, the severity of the nonrespiratory (metabolic) component of acid-base disorders and the nature of acids other than carbonic are difficult to assess. The CO$_2$/HCO$_3^-$ approach is mostly applied to determine resting PaCO$_2$ in patients with chronic respiratory failure.[8,9]

Anion Gap and Corrected Anion Gap

The anion gap (AG) was first suggested by Emmet and Narins as a complementary diagnostic tool for either SBE or bicarbonate rules of thumb approaches of metabolic disturbances, particularly the metabolic acidoses.[77] It is based on the principle of electroneutrality, which states that in an aqueous solution like plasma and intracellular fluid there is no net electrical charge.[33] Accordingly, serum positive-charged cations must equal serum negative-charged anions[26,35] (see Table 76.1):

$$[Na^+]+[K^+]+[Ca^{2+}]+[Mg^{2+}]+[H^+]$$
$$=[Cl^-]+[HCO_3^-]+[proteins^-]+[PO_4^{2-}]$$
$$+[SO_4^{2-}]+[OH^-]+[CO_3^{2-}]+[lactate^-]+[XA^-]) \quad (Eq. 16)$$

where [XA$^-$] equals the unmeasured acid anions (UMAs). The plasma concentrations of SO$_4^{2-}$, OH$^-$, CO$_3^{2-}$, and H$^+$ (H$_3$O$_2^+$) are quite small and can be neglected, whereas Ca^{2+} and Mg^{2+} are omitted by convention.

Concentrations of Na$^+$, K$^+$, Cl$^-$, and HCO$_3^-$ (in the form of total CO$_2$) are reported in a standard chemistry panel, and hence they are used for AG calculation. Thus AG is commonly defined as follows:[8,35]

$$AG = ([Na^+]+[K^+])-([Cl^-]+[HCO_3^-]) \quad (Eq. 17A)$$

If [K$^+$] is omitted and its effect neglected,[78]

$$AG = [Na^+]-([Cl^-]+[HCO_3^-]) \quad (Eq. 17B)$$

TABLE 76.3   Classical Acid-Base Approach: Additional Clues

1. A metabolic acid-base derangement exists if any of the following occurs:
   a. pH is abnormal.
   b. pH and PCO$_2$ have changed in the same direction (both increased or both decreased).
   c. Respiratory compensation is intact if PaCO$_2$ resembles last two digits of pH (eg, pH 7.23 and PaCO$_2$ ≤23 mm Hg).
2. A respiratory acid-base derangement is overlapped if any of the following occurs:
   a. pH is abnormal but PCO$_2$ is reported within normal limits.
   b. PCO$_2$ reported is higher than expected PCO$_2$ (respiratory acidosis overlapped).
   c. PCO$_2$ reported is lower than expected PCO$_2$ (respiratory alkalosis overlapped).
3. A respiratory acid-base derangement exists if any of the following occurs:
   a. PaCO$_2$ is abnormal.
   b. PCO$_2$ and pH have changed in opposite directions (ie, raised PCO$_2$ and decreased pH or vice versa).
4. If the change of pH is ... (see formulas in Table 76.2)
   a. 0.008 × change in PCO$_2$, there is no compensation; then the derangement is acute.
   b. >0.003 but <0.008 × change in PCO$_2$, there is a partial compensation.
   c. 0.003 × change in PCO$_2$, there is full compensation; then the derangement is chronic.
   d. >0.008 × change in PCO$_2$, there is an overlapping metabolic derangement.
5. There is a mixed derangement (acidosis and alkalosis) if any of the following occurs:
   a. PaCO$_2$ is abnormal and pH has not changed as expected or is within normal values.
   b. pH is abnormal and PaCO$_2$ has not changed as expected or is within normal values.

Modified from Marino PL. Acid-base interpretations. In: The Little ICU Book of Facts and Figures. Philadelphia: Lippincott Williams & Wilkins; 2009:349-362.

The sum of the difference in charge carried by these four commonly measured extracellular cations and anions reveals a gap of about 12 to 16 mmol/L or mEq/L. The gap value accounts for unmeasured anions (lactate, ketones, sulfate, etc.). Typically, normal values are 16 mEq/L or mmol/L if [K$^+$] is included or 12 mEq/L without it, with variations of ±2 to 4 mEq/L. However, this classical reference value is now lower and narrower because of the use of the ion-selective electrode, which provides higher chloride values than previous techniques. Several studies have reported "normal" AG values (K$^+$ not included) as 6.6 ± 2 mEq/L (range, 2.6 to 10.6 mEq/L).[79-81] Because AG value may be highly influenced by the way the concentrations of the parameters are measured, it is always better to consult each institution's own expected normal AG.[8,79]

It must be realized that calculated AG is affected by any change in the concentrations of either the UMAs or the cations not included in Eqs. 17A and 17B.[82] If AG increases, this is due to the accumulation of anions, like lactate or ketones, that are not measured, which cause a compensatory drop in chloride or bicarbonate levels, for the sake of electroneutrality. This condition is termed *widened anion-gap acidosis* or just *gap acidosis*. The AG approach is actually the principal method for detecting unmeasured anions as the cause of metabolic acidosis (lactic acidosis, acidosis caused by specific substances, ketoacids, etc.).[82] However, some considerations must be kept in mind.[83]

Plasma proteins and phosphate levels can be significantly decreased in the critical care setting. Reduced protein and phosphate levels result in a decreased UMA and hence in a decreased AG. Therefore an increase in AG from organic acids may be masked by a decrease in AG from low protein and phosphate levels, and therefore it is wise to make the proper corrections.[78,83] This is particularly true in the pediatric critical care setting, where hypoalbuminemia is nearly ubiquitous.[84,85] Phosphate and globulin influence is rather small because their pK_a is much greater than plasma pH (they do not easily dissociate) and hence they do not have a significant charge contribution. Figge and colleagues showed that in most patients, the AG could be corrected (AG$_{CORR}$) as follows[78]:

$$AG_{CORR} = AG_{OBSERVED} + 2.5[\text{normal albumin g/dL}] \\ - [\text{observed albumin g/dL}] \quad \text{(Eq. 18A)}$$

or

$$AG_{CORR} = AG_{OBSERVED} + 0.25[\text{normal albumin g/L}] \\ - [\text{observed albumin g/L}] \quad \text{(Eq. 18B)}$$

considering normal albumin 3.2 to 4.5 g/dL.

The albumin-corrected AG (AG$_{CORR}$) can unmask an organic acidosis previously undetected in the setting of hypoalbuminemia, and it adds sensitivity for detecting unmeasured anions, including lactate, although the specificity for hyperlactatemia is poor.[8,86-88] Thus lactate must be directly determined.

Despite the fact that it is not useful for quantifying the metabolic derangement, AG is a powerful tool for the clinician in the categorization of metabolic acidoses, as not all metabolic acidoses result in an elevated AG.[83] As a hypothetical example, consider that acid in the form of HCl is added to the circulation. Upon dissociation, Cl$^-$ remains as the conjugate base while the plasmatic bicarbonate buffer is "consumed" by the hydrogen ion. The result is that an increase in [Cl$^-$] is balanced by a decrease in [HCO$_3^-$] (ie, there is metabolic acidosis without a change in the AG). Employing the AG$_{CORR}$ it is possible to differentiate hyperchloremic acidosis (normal AG) from gap acidoses (increased AG).[78,83] The last category includes all conditions of metabolic simple acidosis caused by increased concentrations of nonvolatile anions other than chloride, usually unmeasured (or unmeasurable), such as lactate, ketoacids, phosphate, sulfates (and other anions in renal failure setting), salicylate, some β-lactam antibiotics, organic acids from congenital errors of metabolism, and acetate from parenteral nutrition[83,86] (Table 76.4). Non-AG, hyperchloremic acidoses include an excessive infusion of chloride salts (saline or parenteral nutrition) and increased renal or gastrointestinal bicarbonate losses. Alternatively, metabolic alkalosis may stem from hypochloremia resulting from chloride loss or bicarbonate gain and from hypoalbuminemia.[86] AG performance is not so good in mixed acid-base physiology despite several attempts to improve it. This represents an important limitation for its use in critical care patients, in whom single metabolic acid-base disorders are more the exception than the rule. Bicarbonate itself represents another

TABLE 76.4 Causes of Metabolic Acidosis in Critically Ill Patients

I. Accumulation of Unmeasured Anions: The Anion Gap Acidoses

A. Endogenous Source of Acids

1. Type A hyperlactatemia (decreased tissue O_2 delivery)
2. Type B hyperlactatemia (not associated with tissue hypoxia)
   a. Adrenalin infusion
   b. Reactive hyperglycemia
   c. Liver failure
   d. Drug-induced mitochondrial inhibition (eg, linezolid)
   e. Miscellaneous
3. Ketoacidosis (diabetic, alcoholic, starvation, inborn errors of metabolism)
4. Renal failure: accumulation of phosphates, sulfates, and organic ions
5. Unidentified anions in sepsis other than lactate
6. Organic acids from inborn errors of metabolism
7. Late metabolic acidosis of prematurity

B. Exogenous Source of Acids

1. Ingested toxins and drugs that directly provoke acidosis
   a. Methanol, formic acid, keto acids, lactate
   b. Ethylene glycol, glycolic acid, oxalic acid, paraldehyde
   c. Ethanol
   d. Salicylate, salicylic acid, acetic acid
   e. Nonlegal drugs
2. Total parenteral nutrition[a]

II. Hyperchloremic Acidoses: The Nonanion Gap Acidoses

A. Exogenous Chloride Load

1. Normal saline or hypertonic saline resuscitation
2. HCl, NH_4Cl, arginine-HCl administration
3. Total parenteral nutrition[a]

B. Loss of Cations From the Lower Gastrointestinal Tract (Postpyloric Gastrointestinal Fluid Losses)[b]

1. Infectious secretory diarrhea and dehydration
2. Short bowel syndrome
3. Drainage from ostomies, tubes, fistulas (small bowel, pancreatic, or biliary drainage)
4. Sulfamylon, cholestyramine

C. Renal Causes[c]

1. Chronic renal insufficiency (impaired ammonium [NH_4^+] generation)
2. Renal tubular acidoses
3. Hypoaldosteronism
4. Recovery phase of diabetic ketoacidosis
5. Urinary tract obstruction
6. Drug-mediated loss of cations and tubulopathies
   a. Acetazolamide
   b. Amphotericin B
   c. K^+-sparing diuretics

D. Urinary Reconstruction Using Bowel Segments

[a]Total parenteral nutrition may cause both anion gap and nonanion gap acidosis. In the first case, an excessive amount of exogenous acid is the cause, mainly if liver or renal functions are impaired; in the latter, an unbalanced, excessive chloride content in the formulation provokes the derangement, which is easily produced in the setting of renal failure.
[b]This class corresponds to the gastrointestinal loss of the bicarbonate type of acidosis, according to the classical approach to A-B.
[c]This class corresponds to the renal loss of the bicarbonate type of acidosis, according to the classical approach.

potential unstable variable in the AG equation, as it can potentially be influenced by certain therapeutic interventions, such as furosemide infusion, deliberate hyperventilation in head trauma, or permissive hypercapnia in acute respiratory distress syndrome.[8]

Physicochemical Approach: Interacting Chemical Mechanisms Regulate pH

In the late 1970s and early 1980s, Peter Stewart developed a mathematical model of acid-base balance through the application of several basic principles of physical chemistry, particularly electroneutrality, conservation of mass, and dissociation equilibrium of partially dissociated substances (law of mass action).[8,21,26,29,61,89] Electroneutrality states that in aqueous solutions the sum of all positively charged ions must equal the sum of all negatively charged ions. In pure water for the system, $H_2CO_3 \leftrightarrow HCO_3^- + H^+$, the concentration of H^+ ions should be equal to the concentration of HCO_3^- ions. But biological fluids are complex and dynamic systems, in which multiple mechanisms are involved in influencing the particular concentration of any single chemical species. Hydrogen ion is an example of one of these species whose concentration depends on several interacting chemical mechanisms that must equilibrate so the [H+] (or pH) in the solution at that point in time can be determined. To calculate the equilibrium concentration of any species, one must take into account all the mechanisms involved. In plasma, for example, the other charged ions present also have an effect on the relative proportions of H^+ and HCO_3^-. Plasma is an aqueous solution that contains strong ions that are completely dissociated at physiologic pH, weak acids that are partially dissociated at physiologic pH, and carbon dioxide that is in equilibrium with an external partial pressure of carbon dioxide. These other charged molecules, which affect the dissociation of water to generate H^+, can be classed into three independent controlling variables of H^+ concentration[8,21,26,27]:

1. *Partial pressure of carbon dioxide (PCO$_2$).* In arterial blood plasma, PCO_2 is primarily regulated by PCO_2 in alveolar gas, with the consequence that all fluid compartments of the body can be considered as open systems with regard to CO_2.

2. *The strong ion difference (SID).* Blood plasma contains numerous ions, which may be classified not only in regard to their electrical charge (cations are positive, anions are negative) but also according to their tendency to dissociate. Some ions are fully dissociated in aqueous solutions and are called *strong ions,* such as Na^+, K^+, Ca^{2+}, Mg^{2+}, and Cl^-. Others, such as albumin, phosphate, and HCO_3^-, can exist both as charged (ie, dissociated) and uncharged forms and are called *weak ions.* Certain organic acids, such as lactate and others, are nearly completely dissociated under physiologic conditions, and so they are considered strong ions. In blood plasma, strong cations outnumber strong anions. The difference between the sum of all of the strong cations and that of all of the strong anions is called *strong ion difference (SID),* which represents the net electric charge on the strong ions (ie, electrolytes, lactate, and certain highly dissociated acids). Sodium and chloride are the two most important plasmatic strong ions. In plasma, strong ions are primarily regulated by the kidneys so that body fluids are an open system for water and electrolytes.[8,21,26]

3. *The total concentration of nonvolatile weak acids (A_{TOT}).* That is, for each of them this variable represents the sum of its dissociated and undissociated forms ($A_{TOT} = A^- + HA$).[26,27,32] Weak acids are not fully dissociated at physiologic pH; the most important of them is albumin, with a minor effect from phosphate. The system H_2CO_3/HCO_3^- is

also a weak acid, but it has already been considered as a part of the PCO_2.

According to Stewart's calculations, *independent variables* mean that PCO_2, SID, and A_{TOT} are *causally* related to the hydrogen ion, rather than being merely correlated.[26,27] The traditional acid-base analysis makes the implicit assumption that $[H^+]$ is an independent variable, but this is not a physicochemically solid statement.[12,13,26,35,36,38] Normal acid-base status occurs when the independent variables have normal values. Abnormality of one or more of the independent variables underlies all acid-base disturbances. Adjustment of the independent variables is the essence of all therapeutic interventions because none of the dependent variables (eg, pH, BE, or $[HCO_3^-]$) can be changed primarily or individually; the dependent variables change all of them simultaneously if, and only if, one or more of the independent variables change.[26,29,61] Because PCO_2 is regulated by respiration, its changes result in respiratory acid-base disorders. Metabolic acid-base disorders stem from changes in either SID or A_{TOT}, regulated by kidney and physical-chemical interactions in body fluids.

CO_2 and Bicarbonate in Stewart's Approach

In Stewart's approach, CO_2 is an independent determinant of pH. However, the role of bicarbonate is reduced from being causative to a mere indicator, as hydrogen ion and bicarbonate concentrations are totally dependent on the three independent controlling variables noted earlier. Hence, according to Stewart, the major use for the bicarbonate rules of thumb and SBE is to determine the extent of the clinical acid-base disorder, rather than the mechanism.[8,21,26,29]

The rise of the PCO_2, according to the Henderson-Hasselbalch equation (Eq. 13), will increase both H^+ and HCO_3^- concentrations. Therefore the change in HCO_3^- concentration is mediated by chemical equilibrium (Eq. 11) and not by any systemic adaptive response.[29] The total CO_2 concentration (and hence the $[HCO_3^-]$) is determined by the PCO_2, which is in turn determined by the balance between alveolar ventilation and CO_2 production at the tissue level. Therefore HCO_3^- cannot be regulated independently of PCO_2. Plasma bicarbonate concentration will always increase if PCO_2 increases, but this is not an alkalosis. Therefore the increased bicarbonate concentration is not *buffering* the rise of $[H^+]$, and there will be no change in the SBE. As CO_2 easily diffuses through membranes, when PCO_2 increases there is always tissue acidosis. If PCO_2 remains high, the body will attempt to compensate by increasing renal bicarbonate production.[26,29] The same response, but in the opposite direction, occurs when PCO_2 drops.[89]

Strong Ion Difference: Apparent and Effective

SID is defined as the charge difference between the sum of all strong cations and the sum of all strong anions. When SID is calculated from direct measurement of serum-strong ions, it is termed *apparent* SID (SID_{APP}),[29,86,90] with the understanding that more unmeasured (or unmeasurable) ions might also be present (Table 76.5):

$$SID_{APP} = ([Na^+]+[K^+]+[Ca^{2+}]+[Mg^{2+}])-([Cl^-]) \quad \text{(Eq. 19A)}$$

Unless elevated, lactate is ignored, as its contribution to total SID is negligible. In the critical care setting, the sicker the patient, the higher the chance that lactate or other strong anions are increased; thus lactate should be include in those cases:

$$SID_{APP} = ([Na^+]+[K^+]+[Ca^{2+}]+[Mg^{2+}])-([Cl^-]+[lactate^-])$$
$$\text{(Eq. 19B)}$$

From actual measurements in healthy volunteers, the "normal" range of SID_{APP} has been estimated to be from 38 to 42 mEq/L.[21,29,61,91] In critical illnesses, SID_{APP} may be substantially reduced, even when there is no evidence (by the traditional approach) of a metabolic acid-base derangement.[79,92,93] In "stable" critical care patients, SID_{APP} values have been reported to be between 33 ± 5.6 mEq/L[92] and 41.5 ± 5.1 mEq/L.[79] Thus in spite of the lack of consensus about what value of SID_{APP} one should expect in an ICU population, it is clear that SID_{APP} values are lower than they are for healthy volunteers.[91-93] The lower the baseline of the SID_{APP}, the greater the susceptibility to a subsequent acid load.[91-93]

SID has a powerful electrochemical effect on water dissociation, and hence on $[H^+]$. Both H^+ and OH^- behave as a weak cation and anion, respectively. Because practically all the cations in plasma are strong ions, except for H^+, only H^+ concentration can vary in response to changes in anions. On the other hand, there are several anions that are weak ions, and thus there are several options of anion molecules that can change their charges if cations change.[29,94] As the SID_{APP} increases (strong cations in excess over strong anions), plasma tends to become positively charged. Hence H^+, a weak cation, decreases and pH increases to maintain electrical neutrality, and alkalosis is produced. On the other hand, if the SID_{APP} decreases (strong anions in relative excess over strong cations), plasma tends to become negatively charged, more water is dissociated to have more H^+ for keeping electroneutrality, and acidosis is produced.[26,29,95] Changes in SID result from either a relative or an absolute change in strong ion concentrations. A change in the free water content alters the relative concentration of the strong ions, and hence a change in SID. If, as a result, $[Na^+]$, $[K^+]$, and $[Cl^-]$ decrease, the absolute figure for SID will decrease proportionately. Thus an excess of free water lowers SID and results in a tendency toward metabolic acidosis. In a similar manner, a free water deficit causes metabolic alkalosis by increasing the SID through a relative increase in concentration of all strong ions. Relative and absolute changes in sodium concentration primarily result from osmoregulation, and thus they are reflective of changes in free water. The remaining strong cations, potassium, magnesium, and calcium, as they are tightly regulated by the body for other functions (coagulation, membrane excitability, neuromuscular plates, muscle contraction, etc.), do not vary significantly enough to directly cause alterations in acid-base balance.[61] On the other hand, changes in strong anion concentrations are significant to acid-base status. Hypochloremia (from gastrointestinal or renal losses) is associated with metabolic alkalosis. Hyperchloremia (eg, from resuscitation with normal saline infusion) is associated with metabolic acidosis.

As the SID requires an actual change in the relative concentrations of strong cations or anions to be modified, the kidneys are the primary organs in charge of SID regulation by the body. As the kidneys can excrete only small amounts of strong ion into the urine each minute, several minutes to hours are required for achieving a significant change of the SID. Control of the kidney is important and precise because every chloride ion filtered and not reabsorbed increases the SID.

TABLE 76.5   Tools for the Assessment of the Acid-Base Balance

Tool	BICARBONATE-CENTERED APPROACHES		PHYSICOCHEMICAL APPROACH
	Bicarbonate "Rules of Thumb"	Base Excess/Deficit (BE)	PCO_2/SID-SIG/A_{TOT}
Foundation	Henderson-Hasselbalch equation; "rules" and figures empirically derived Brønsted-Lowry acids	Henderson-Hasselbalch equation and chemical principles of acid-base titration Brønsted-Lowry acids	Principles of electrical neutrality and product ionic for water, law of mass action, behavior of cations and anions in mixed aqueous solutions Arrhenius (Van Slyke) and Brønsted-Lowry acids
Determinations	pH and PCO_2 only parameters actually measured	Calculated from measured pH, PCO_2 (BE), and hemoglobin (SBE) Needs several assumptions	pH, PCO_2 measured SID_{APP} SID_{EFF}, SIG, A_{TOT} calculated from measured cations and anions $SID_{APP} = ([Na^+] + [K^+] + [Ca^{++}] + [Mg^{++}] + [lactate^-] + [\text{other strong anions}])$ $SID_{EFF} = \{HCO_3^-\} + [Alb^-] + [Pi^-]$ $[Alb^-] = [Alb^-] \times [(0.123 \times pH) - 0.631]$ $[Pi] = [Pi, mmol/L] \times [(0.309 \times pH) - 0.469]$ $SIG = SID_{APP} - SID_{EFF}$ $A_{TOT} = 2.43 \times [\text{total protein, g/dl}]$
Application	Simple acid-base derangements Bedside and point-of-care gas analyzers	Simple acid-base derangements Bedside and point-of-care gas analyzers	Simple and complex acid-base derangements Lab info available bedside with most blood analyzers; full lab required for albumin and phosphate
Caveats	"Rules" of PCO_2 and HCO_3^- are valid only in not so extreme pH values "Rules" must be adjusted for chronic situations Mixed and complex derangements are empirically interpreted	Does not give direct information about mixed or complex derangements Not reliable in patients with extreme values of Hb or severely edematous "Normal" values reported between +/-2 up to +/-5	Original equations complex and no suitable for bedside; needs consultation online or specific app Abridged equations (presented here) still complex and cumbersome Needs total proteins, albumin, and every electrolyte available Need more lab determinations, higher chance for analytic error More expensive
Need complement?	Yes. Anion gap: $([Na^+] + [K^+] - [Cl^-] + HCO_3^-])$ PCO_2 and HCO_3^- do not change independently from one another (neither physiologically nor mathematically)	Yes. Anion gap: $([Na^+] + [K^+] - [Cl^-] + HCO_3^-])$ Both BE and SBE are artificial chemical indexes (body does not secrete or excrete them); in order to be calculated, blood sample must be kept at 37°C and PCO_2 is assumed to be in 40 mm Hg; for SBE it is assumed an average Hb of 5 g/dl throughout the body fluids	No, but surrogates are convenient for bedside: —$[Na^+] - [Cl^-]$ for SID_{APP} —$AG_{CORRLACT}$ for SIG Applies only for plasma
Expected "normal" values	Well defined, need adjustment according to height above sea level	+/-3 dimensionless	—$SID_{APP} = 38\text{-}42$; 33 ± 5.6 in most "stable" critical care patients —SID_{EFF} = Sum of HCO_3^- plus expected electric charges of nonbicarbonate buffers (albumin + Pi) —SIG = <8 mEq/L or mmol/L

All variables expressed in mEq/L unless expressed otherwise.
Alb^-, in g/L; A_{TOT}, total concentration of weak acids in plasma; *BE*, base excess; *Hb*, hemoglobin (g/dl); Pi^-, inorganic phosphate, in mmol/L; *SBE*, standard base excess; SID_{APP}, strong ion difference (apparent); SID_{EFF}, strong ion difference (effective); *SIG*, strong ion gap.
Ca^{++} and Mg^{++} in ionized concentrations.
Surrogates can be used: $[Na^+] - [Cl^-]$ for SIDAPP; Anion gap corrected for albumin and lactate for SIG. (See Fig. 76.1.)

Acid handling of the kidney has traditionally focused on H^+ excretion and the role of ammonia (NH_3) and ammonium (NH_4^+) as hydrogen ion carriers.[35,44,96,97] Because water provides an essentially infinite source of H^+, its excretion per se is possibly not as relevant as formerly taught. In fact, the H^+ net excretion by the kidney as water molecules is larger than the excretion as NH_4^+. Therefore the purpose of renal NH_4^+ production is to allow the excretion of Cl^- without the excretion of Na^+ or K^+. Thus NH_4^+ is important to systemic acid-base balance, not only for its role as an H^+ carrier or for its direct action in the plasma (normal $[NH_4^+]$ is <0.01 mmol/L) but because it allows a safe excretion of Cl^-.[29,97]

Additional strong anions may become significant (hyperlactatemia, sulfate, ketoacids, anions from Krebs cycle, etc.), appear de novo in disease states (several organic acids from inborn errors of metabolism), or enter the body as medications or toxic substances (salicylates, certain β-lactam antibiotics, etc.). They may eventually influence the value of SID_{APP}.[91-93,98,99] Because it is usually not possible to have a direct measure of $[XA^-]$ at bedside (with the exception of lactate), it is not always convenient to use SID_{APP} for assessing the strong ions status, particularly among the most critically ill patients. According to the principle of electroneutrality (Eq. 16), blood plasma cannot be charged, so there should be remaining negative charges balancing the excess of plasma strong cations in relation to the strong anions, which is the origin of SID_{APP}. These balancing negative charges do not come from other strong anions but from weak anions. SID_{APP} (Eqs. 19A and 19B) does not take into account the role of weak acids (HCO_3^-, albumin, and dihydrogen phosphate), which have concentrations in plasma large enough that their changes can produce significant acid disturbance. This is expressed through the calculation of the effective strong ion difference (SIDe):

$$SID_{EFF} = 1000 \times 2.46 \times 10^{-11} \times PCO_2/10^{-pH} + [\text{albumin in g/dL}]$$
$$\times (0.123 \times pH - 0.631) + [PO_4 \text{ in mmol/L}]$$
$$\times (0.309 \times pH - 0.469)$$

$$(\text{Eq. 20})$$

The original calculation proposed by Figge and colleagues[94,100] is complex and cumbersome for use in the clinical arena.[86,101-103] Several simplifications have been proposed.[8,45,86,104,105] Although there is no consensus and no data about what equation should be used, the following is one of the most frequently cited[106]:

$$\{[HCO_3^-] + (\text{albumin} \times 0.123 \times [pH - 0.631])$$
$$+ \text{phosphate} \times 0.309 \times [pH - 0.469]\} \quad (\text{Eq. 21})$$

where HCO_3^- is in mEq/L, albumin in g/L, and phosphate in mmol/L.

The SID_{EFF} formula quantitatively accounts for the contribution of weak acids to the electrical charge equilibrium in plasma. Once weak acids are quantitatively taken into account, the SID_{APP} to SID_{EFF} difference should equal zero (electrical charge neutrality) unless there are unmeasured charges to explain this ion gap.

Strong Ion Gap

In the healthy individual, SID_{APP} and SID_{EFF} are nearly identical and therefore are adequate estimates of the true SID and of the acid-base status.[29,78] However, in disease states, this might not be true, as several unmeasured ions (mainly anions) may be present in plasma.[99,100,107-109] To address this situation, Jones[110] and Figge[98] independently proposed a similar scanning tool. Kellum and coworkers coined the term *strong ion gap (SIG)* to name this new tool,[111,112] a far from ideal term, because the unmeasured anions creating the gap can be either strong or weak[99,100,113] (see Table 76.5). Nowadays, a modern clinical lab can easily measure all the components of the SID_{APP} and SID_{EFF} equations, including lactate. As a result, $[XA^-]$ is easily approximated through SIG, which is calculated as follows:

$$SIG = SID_{APP} - SID_{EFF} \quad (\text{Eq. 22})$$

By convention, SIG is positive when unmeasured anions exceed unmeasured cations (acidosis) and negative when unmeasured cations exceed unmeasured anions (alkalosis). In ideal theoretic conditions, it would be possible for the sum of strong cations and weak anions to cancel each other out, with a SIG equal to zero. In the real world, most SIGs are positive (anions > cations). The use of SIG is advocated in situations in which SID_{APP} and SID_{EFF} are not equal.[111,112] SIG different to zero may also be explained, at least in part, by the difference between *ionic molar concentration* (the basis for SID_{APP}) and *ionic activity* itself (the basis for SID_{EFF}). Ionic molar concentration is a measure of the actual number of ions in solution. On the contrary, ionic activity is a measure of the effective concentration of electrolytes that results from the charge interaction on dissociated species. The difference between ionic concentration and ionic activity is important because the molar concentration of any electrolyte will not affect the molar concentration of any other electrolyte. But ionic activities are mutually interactive. The principle of electrical neutrality only refers to the latter.[33] Both SID_{EFF} and SIG have been evaluated as prognostic markers in both children and adults. Both indexes have shown good predictive capability in most publications, but there is not universal agreement regarding its clinical usefulness.[8,61,85,101,114-123] If one would like to increase the precision of SIG, one should include as many factors as possible in the calculation of SID_{EFF}. However, a theoretic downside is that each additional analyte may increase imprecision,[113] and the calculations remain cumbersome in the clinical arena, but appropriate online calculators are available. Perhaps the main advantage of SIG is that it remains stable with severe pH stress (<6.85, >7.55), a clear advantage when compared to AG. The well-known AG increase parallel with pH has been related to altered albumin and phosphate dissociation in extremes of pH.[111]

Nonvolatile Weak Acids (Albumin and Phosphate)

Unlike H_2CO_3 through its conversion to CO_2, nonvolatile weak acids cannot be eliminated by respiration; most have a pK_a near the physiologic pH of 7.4. Therefore weak acids (A_{TOT}), as opposed to strong ions, can exist at physiologic pH as dissociated (A^-) or associated with a proton (AH). Weak acids are often referred to as buffers. The concentration of each one of these weak acids is the sum of its dissociated and undissociated forms:

$$A_{TOT} = AH + A^- \quad (\text{Eq. 23})$$

The two nonvolatile weak acids with great enough concentrations in plasma to have an influence on acid-base status are albumin and inorganic phosphate, the latter having a minor effect. Although the loss of weak acid (A_{TOT}) from the plasma space is an alkalinizing process, there is no evidence that the body regulates A_{TOT} directly to maintain acid-base balance. For example, there is no evidence that clinicians should treat hypoalbuminemia as an acid-base derangement.[29] What is observed in hypoalbuminemic patients is that SID tends to be decreased in relation to healthy individuals. This means that the kidney has already compensated for the alkalinizing effect of hypoalbuminemia by increasing the reabsorption of Cl^-, increasing plasma strong anions and reducing the SID.[29] There remains controversy about whether or not albumin fluctuations provoke a change in the pH.[41,120] Although albumin is a prominent acid in serum, there is no documented respiratory compensation with changes in albumin concentration.[124]

Strong Ions and Urinary Anion Gap

A urinary anion gap (uGap) was described some time ago to compare the loss of measured strong cations (sodium and potassium) with the loss of chloride.[125] This urinary gap has also been designated by some authors as the *urine strong ion difference (uSID)*[29,35] or the *urinary net charge gap*[122]:

$$uGap = uSID = [uNa^+ + uK^+] - [uCl^-] \qquad (Eq.\ 24)$$

Certainly, sodium, potassium, and chloride are all strong ions, so the name is, at least, functionally correct. As its serum analog, the uSID estimates the unmeasured urinary ions. The excretion patterns of urinary electrolytes reflect the ability of the kidney to counteract nonrenal acid-base disorders. The capacity of the kidney to excrete ammonium chloride in acidosis allows for the elimination of anions with conservation of sodium for volume and potassium for potassium balance. This potassium-sparing effect of urinary ammonium is evident in the hypokalemic stimulation of ammoniagenesis. The traditional physiologic approach interprets the urine electrolytes to deduce the presence of ammonium and bicarbonate with less emphasis on the strong ion pathogenesis of acid-base disorders. The physicochemical model emphasizes the relative losses of the actual measured quantities to determine the cause of the disturbance. Both perspectives are complementary and enlightening for the critical care field.[96,97,122]

In terms of quantity, the most important unmeasured urinary strong anion (Ur^-) is SO_4^{2-} (derived from the metabolism of sulfur amino acids), whereas the most important unmeasured cation (Ur^+) is ammonium (NH_4^+). In physiologically normal conditions, uSID must equal the plasmatic SID_{APP} (ie, 38-42 mEq/L). When a strong ion enters the plasma (eg, lactate, or a chloride load), plasmatic SID obviously will decrease. Normal kidneys will react by increasing its excretion of chloride, thereby decreasing the plasma chloride concentration, whereas $[Na^+]$ and $[K^+]$ must be maintained within normal ranges. This is accomplished by increasing the excretion rate of NH_4^+, which is the more efficient way for increasing chloride elimination without losing sodium or potassium.[96,97] The increased excretion of chloride will decrease the uSID.[103] Thus a negative value for the uSID indicates the presence of the unmeasured cation, ammonium (excretion of ammonium chloride). The loss of ammonium chloride in the urine of a patient with metabolic acidosis is a normal renal response to nonrenal causes of metabolic acidosis, because the losses of urinary chloride result in an increased plasma strong ion difference, which in turn permits the formation of more bicarbonate. However, in the situation of a metabolic alkalosis, a relative excess of chloride in the urine strongly suggests

that the losses of urinary chloride are causally related to the metabolic alkalosis process by increasing the plasma strong ion difference. This is a typical situation in patients receiving furosemide, which inhibits the sodium-potassium-chloride cotransporter in the thin ascending limb of the loop of Henle. This causes proportionately more chloride than sodium loss in the urine. Thus there is a direct explanation for the hypochloremic metabolic alkalosis in such cases. Inhibition of the sodium-chloride cotransporter of the distal tubule by thiazides is another cause of metabolic alkalosis because of the proportionally greater loss of chloride than sodium from the extracellular fluid. In addition to chloride wasting by diuretics, many hereditary disorders of sodium and chloride transport by the renal tubules (the so-called channelopathies) may cause acid-base disorders.

A positive value for the uSID indicates excretion of an unmeasured anion. The lost, unmeasured anion may be bicarbonate or nonbicarbonate anions such as ketones, lactate, and hippurate among persons who sniff glue.[122,126] This loss of anions will decrease the plasma strong ion difference and acidify the extracellular fluid as the process returns chloride to the circulation. If the urinary clearance of these nonchloride anions is high enough that they do not accumulate as a plasma anion gap, then the hyperchloremia may be mistaken for renal tubular acidosis.[125] Without those nonbicarbonate anions, metabolic acidosis with the loss of urinary sodium and potassium and retention of chloride (the positive-charge gap) will result in a decreased plasma strong ion difference, constituting a renal cause of acidosis (eg, carbonic anhydrase inhibition by acetazolamide, or renal tubular acidosis). If metabolic alkalosis is present, a positive urinary gap suggests that the renal loss of strong cations (sodium and potassium) and conservation of chloride will try to acidify the extracellular fluid because of a decrease in the plasma strong ion difference and in the bicarbonate concentration.[122] In the presence of volume and potassium depletion, metabolic alkalosis is maintained, not corrected, by the kidneys.[127] Low extracellular fluid volume and low blood pressure increase angiotensin II and aldosterone levels. Increased sodium reabsorption through proximal tubular sodium-hydrogen exchange and the collecting-duct sodium channel, accompanied by hydrogen secretion by the hydrogen ATPase and the potassium-hydrogen ATPase, in turn increases bicarbonate reabsorption until the urinary pH decreases as it becomes free of bicarbonate. This paradoxical aciduria in the middle of alkalemia is evidence that blood pH depends on strong ion balance. The alkalemia will be corrected only with sufficient replacement of sodium, chloride, and potassium.[122]

In respiratory conditions, the $PaCO_2$ is the initial abnormality leading to sudden changes in pH, with little change in strong ion concentrations. Over time, however, the change in the level of chloride and reciprocal changes in the level of bicarbonate are the major factors that allow pH to return toward normal values. The hyperchloremic renal compensation for respiratory alkalosis is the excretion of filtered sodium and potassium with bicarbonate, because low $PaCO_2$ decreases proximal and distal hydrogen secretion. As the plasma strong ion difference decreases, the plasma bicarbonate concentration will decrease. In respiratory acidosis, high $PaCO_2$ increases production of ammonia by the kidney, and the excretion of ammonium chloride with a negative uSID results in hypochloremia, an increased plasma strong ion difference, and an elevated plasma bicarbonate concentration. The elevated $PaCO_2$ increases the renal reabsorption of sodium and bicarbonate, so the compensation is maintained. If the $PaCO_2$ is abruptly lowered through mechanical ventilation, the compensatory response shifts to posthypercapnic hypochloremic metabolic alkalosis, which will not resolve until the chloride that is lost as ammonium chloride is replenished.[96,122]

In addition to the kidney, both the liver and the gastrointestinal tract may have an influence on SID. In the stomach, Cl^- is pumped out of the plasma and into the lumen, reducing the SID (and pH) of the gastric fluids, but increasing the SID (and pH) in the plasma side ("alkaline tide"), because of the exit of Cl^- to the stomach. However, only a slight change in plasma pH becomes evident, because Cl^- is reabsorbed in the duodenum just as fast as it was pumped out. However, if gastric secretions are removed, either by vomiting or suction catheter, the SID will progressively increase, as will the pH, as a result of Cl^- loss. Although H^+ is excreted as HCl, it is also lost with every water molecule that exits the body. When the body loses Cl^-, a strong ion, without also losing a strong cation, SID is increased and therefore $[H^+]$ is decreased and alkalosis ensues. When H^+ is excreted as H_2O rather than as HCl, there is no change in SID, and consequently there is no change in $[H^+]$. It remains unknown whether the gastrointestinal tract, the liver, and the pancreas are capable of compensatory actions for regulating strong ion uptake.[128]

Conceptual and Practical Integration of the Tools for Assessing Acid-Base Balance

Three methods are currently applied to measure acid-base disorders: the bicarbonate/CO_2 physiologic approach, the base excess approach, and the physicochemical approach. The first two approaches, which are based on the analysis of plasma concentration of bicarbonate and standard base excess (SBE), and further by the use of plasma anion gap (AG), are the most widely used methods to evaluate the metabolic component of acid-base disturbances. One advantage of these methods is that they are easy to understand and apply in common clinical situations. However, the SBE is a calculated figure derived from $PaCO_2$ and arterial pH, but reliance on its use alone to quantify metabolic disturbances has a number of pitfalls. First, it cannot identify whether an acidosis is due to increased tissue acids, hyperchloremia, or a combination of both. Second, its calculation assumes normal plasma protein, which may limit its accuracy in critically ill patients.[61,98] AG is grossly underestimated in the presence of hypoalbuminemia, which is a frequent occurrence in critically ill patients.[78] An alternative evaluation is the mathematical model based on physicochemical principles described by Stewart[32] and modified by Figge.[78,94,100] This method allows the clinician to quantify individual components of acid-base abnormalities and provides insight into their pathogenesis.[61] Many studies have shown that this approach, compared to the traditional approaches, works best to identify acid-base disorders in the population of critically ill patients.[129,130] Nevertheless, Stewart's approach is a time-consuming method and unsuitable at the bedside.

Table 76.5 presents an overview of the available tools for the assessment of the metabolic component of acid-base balance. Table 76.6 summarizes the classification of acid-base derangements according with the tools and assumptions of the different approaches.

Despite apparent differences between the traditional bicarbonate-centered and the physicochemical approaches to the acid-base physiology, they are complementary. At the present time, most clinicians accept a bimodal categorization of acid-base disorders as either *respiratory* or *metabolic,* but after more than a century, there is still no universally agreed upon method of defining and quantifying the metabolic component. This is perhaps not surprising, if one considers not only the conceptual controversies but the human passion rather than rationale involved in this controversy.[8,36,41,49,72-75] For example, Stewart's classification of HCO_3^- and H^+ as *dependent* variables is felt to be a sacrilege by many physiologists as well as clinicians.[8,41,49] All available methods (bicarbonate, SBE, AG, and Stewart's) have been heavily criticized,[41,131-133] and all of them have been advocated as the gold standard, whereas others claim that they all yield virtually identical results.[41,65,134] Perhaps the major merit of the physicochemical approach is that it became attractive to the intensivist because it offered a comprehensive explanation for some metabolic derangements associated with ionic alterations, such as the so-called hyperchloremic acidosis. The evidence connecting acid-base balance with electrolyte balance is apparent at the cellular level (ion transporters, their stoichiometric balance, and the hormones that regulate them) and in clinical practice. The fact that transporters often couple a strong ion such as sodium or potassium with hydrogen, or chloride with bicarbonate, suggests an ultimate coherence between the two systems.[59,122,135,136] Since the 1920s and 1930s, Peters and Van Slyke defined acid-base balance in the blood as the chemical state resulting from the balance between cations and anions.[24] This means that metabolic acid-base disorders can be visualized as the predicted consequences of a primary fluid and electrolyte imbalance. In keeping with the laws of electroneutrality, all charged species must balance. This requires that any change in the concentration of one of the charged variables (the strong ion difference) must be matched by a change in the concentration of another charged species. Thus all metabolic acid-base disorders are associated with either a change in the concentration of sodium, potassium, calcium, chloride, hydrogen, phosphate, or albumin or a change in the anion gap.[122] Therefore the first step in understanding how an acid-base disorder develops is to know or assume the specific electrolyte content of any gained fluids (eg, intravenous fluids) or lost fluids (eg, gastrointestinal fluids, sweat, or urinary fluids). Because the normal concentration ratio of sodium to chloride in extracellular fluid is approximately 140:100, an increase in the sodium level, a decrease in the chloride level, or both will increase the strong ion difference and the bicarbonate concentration will increase (metabolic alkalosis), according to electroneutrality requirements.[137] When the strong ion difference decreases, pH and the bicarbonate level will decrease (metabolic acidosis). Any developed difference in the ionic charge, or strong ion difference, determines the bicarbonate concentration. The traditional acid-base approach tacitly overlaps with aspects of the strong ion theory (Table 76.7). Both experimental and clinical observations can be explained with the use of either model. Yet the physicochemical model is useful in revealing individual processes in the development of an acid-base disturbance because it associates the abnormality with specific electrolyte disturbances.[26,122]

The major inconvenience of the physicochemical approach is the complexity and potential inaccuracies in correctly

TABLE 76.6   Classification of Acid-Base Derangements According to Several Approaches

Derangement	BICARBONATE-CENTERED APPROACHES		PHYSICOCHEMICAL APPROACH
	Bicarbonate Rules of Thumb	Base Excess/Deficit (BE)	PCO_2/SID-SIG/A_{TOT}
Metabolic Acidosis			
—Primary problem	↓ [HCO_3^-] and ↓ pH	Base deficit (-BE, -SBE), ↓ pH	↓ SID_{EFF}, and ↓pH
—Secondary response	↓ PCO_2[a]	↓ PCO_2[a]	↓ PCO_2[a]
Unmeasured anions	Needed[b] Normal AG = hyperchloremic acidosis High AG = normochloremic acidosis	Needed[b] Normal AG = hyperchloremic acidosis High AG = normochloremic acidosis	Included by default SID acidosis (↓ SID_{APP} = ↓ SID_{EFF}), so SIG = 0 (*equivalent to* hyperchloremic acidosis) SIG acidosis (SID_{APP}, no change ↓ SID_{EFF}) so SIG = ↑ (*equivalent to* normochloremic acidosis)
Effect of non HCO_3^- plasma weak acids mainly albumin	Not assessed	Not assessed	↑ primary in A_{TOT} ("hyperalbuminemic acidosis")
Metabolic Alkalosis			
—Primary problem	↑ [HCO_3^-] and pH	Primary base excess (+BE, +SBE), ↑ pH	↑ primary SID_{APP} and SID_{EFF} ↑ pH (SID alkalosis)
—Secondary response	↑ PCO_2	↑ in PCO_2	Not contemplated
Effect of non-HCO_3^- plasma weak acids mainly albumin	Not assessed	Not assessed	↓ Primary in A_{TOT} ("hypoalbuminemic alkalosis")
Respiratory Acidosis			
—Primary problem	↑ in PCO_2 and ↓ pH	↑ PCO_2 and ↓ pH	↑ PCO_2 and ↓ pH
—Secondary response	↑ [HCO_3^-] Acute or chronic	Acute: ΔSBE = 0 Chronic: +SBE	Not considered
Respiratory Alkalosis			
—Primary problem	↓ PCO_2 and ↑ pH	↓ PCO_2 and ↑ pH	↓ PCO_2 and ↑ pH
—Secondary response	↓ [HCO_3^-] Acute or chronic	Acute: ΔSBE = 0 Chronic: ΔSBE = −SBE	Not considered

[a]Always adjust PCO_2 values to the height above sea level of your city. Empirical rules for compensation are minimally affected.
[b]Anion gap correction for albumin and lactate not usually performed. It is now recommended to do so (see text for details).
Acute, minutes to hours; *AG,* anion gap; A_{TOT}, total anions in plasma (non HCO_3^- weak acids); *BE,* base excess; *chronic,* several days or longer; ↓, decrease; HCO_3^-, bicarbonate; ↑, increase; PCO_2, carbon dioxide partial pressure (always arterial for calculating deltas); *SBE,* standard base excess; SID_{APP}, strong ion difference (apparent); SID_{EFF}, strong ion difference (effective); *SIG,* strong ion gap.
Adapted from Seifter JL. Integration of acid-base and electrolyte disorders. N Engl J Med 2014;371:1821-1831; Adrogué HJ, Gennari FJ, Galla JH, Madias NE. Assessing acid-base disorders. Kidney Int 2009;76:1239-1247.

calculating SID_{APP}, SID_{EFF}, and SIG.[8,41,49,79] Nevertheless, because the Stewart method evaluates all major serum ions, and many of these variables are measured daily in the intensive care setting, many critical care practitioners, particularly in the adult field, have adopted this concept to describe complex acid-base derangements.[104] To help simplify things, there are now surrogates of some of the complex physicochemical equations. With PCO_2 analysis and the Henderson-Hasselbalch equation, it is possible to describe and quantify the respiratory side of the acid-base balance. To describe the metabolic side requires more complex analysis. The traditional tools for approaching the metabolic side, AG and SBE, now have been augmented by Stewart's physical-chemical concepts, with improved performance.[84-86,138,139] In spite of the apparent differences among these three methods, they all share a common theoretic foundation based on the principle of electroneutrality and the role of plasma weak acids (Fig. 76.1). Prompt identification of unmeasured anions is essential in any acid-base analysis in the critical care setting, because mortality associated with strong ion acidosis, both lactic and nonlactic, is significantly higher than that associated

with hyperchloremic acidosis (56%, 39%, and 29%, respectively).[1,86,119] Accordingly elevated unmeasured anion is a predictor of mortality. The best diagnostic tools for the early detection of the unmeasured anions (XA^-) are AG_{CORR} (not AG), SIG, and physicochemical adjusted SBE (also known as partitioned SBE or the BE gap).[86,139]

Surrogates of Strong Ion Difference and Strong Ion Gap: Corrected Anion Gap and Na^+–Cl^- Difference

In addition to correcting the anion gap for hypoalbuminemia (AG_{CORR}) additional corrections may be warranted.[83] Hyperchloremic acidosis may go undetected with the AG_{CORR} method, in the setting of a dilutional alkalosis.[86] Hence a "corrected" value of chloride would theoretically be needed. However, the very concept of "corrected chloride" is criticized by some authors, as no other element of AG equation (nor of SID or SIG's) is "corrected" for water excess or deficit,[113,139] and because the "sodium correction" of the chloride assumes a fixed sodium-chloride relationship that does not occur in vivo.[140-143] Hence there is no uniform acceptance of "corrected"

TABLE 76.7   Integrated Clinical Approach to Acid-Base Derangements in Critical Care

Step	1. Inquiry	2. Assessment	3. Action
1	Clinical suspicion of metabolic derangement?	No CVC: Check peripheral venous blood sample for tCO_2 and pH Already in PICU or ER? Direct to action!	Obtain ABG if peripheral tCO_2 or pH are abnormal or if clinical picture justifies it
2	pH?	pH <7.35 → acidosis with acidemia pH >7.45 → alkalosis with alkalemia If pH = 735-7.45, unbalance is not yet ruled out	Check PCO_2 and SBE
3	Respiratory side?	PCO_2 and pH have moved in opposite directions	There is a respiratory problem Use traditional approaches (bicarbonate rules of the thumb or SBE) (see Table 76.6)
4	Metabolic side?	PCO_2 and pH have moved in the same direction OR SBE <-3? OR Clinical suspicion of ACIDOSIS in spite of inconclusive pH, PCO_2, SBE (and HCO_3^-)?	There is a metabolic problem with respiratory compensation There is a metabolic acidosis Check lactate and albumin Calculate $AG_{CORRLACT}$ Will need Na^+ and Cl^-
5	Anions?	Use surrogates of SID and SIG: a. For SID_{APP} use $[Na^+] - [Cl^-]$ b. For SIG use $AG_{CORRLACT}$ c. Lactate >2 mmol/l or >50% of SBE? d. Lactate <2 mmol/l; normal Cl^-? e. SIG >50% of SBE?	a. $[Na^+] - [Cl^-] - $<42.7 mEq/L = SID acidosis (hyperchloremic acidosis) – >47.5 mEq/L = SID alkalosis (hypochloremic alkalosis) b. $AG_{CORRLACT}$ >8 mEq/L = SIG acidosis (normochloremic or gap acidosis) c. Predominant lactic metabolic acidosis d. Check A_{TOT} and full calculation of SID_{APP}, SID_{EFF}, and SIG e. Yes: Predominant SIG metabolic acidosis (normochloremic acidosis, Gap acidosis) No: Predominant SID metabolic acidosis (hyperchloremic acidosis, nonGap acidosis) IF no single anion group accounts >50% of SBE, there is probably a mixed disorder
6	Compensations?	Use bicarbonate or SBE observational patterns	Warnings! 1. Under ventilatory support or with neural or respiratory problems, respiratory compensation can be modified or not completed 2. Hypoalbuminemia is common in PICU. Extreme low levels (<2 g/dl) may modify AG and, potentially, pH 3. Diuretics may modify metabolic response to acidosis through Na^+ and Cl^- losses in urine; uGap can be useful to assess renal response
7	Final analysis?	Define the A-B derangement: Simple versus mixed? Compensated versus noncompensated?	Construct differential diagnosis of the possible underlying causes
8	Treatment?	Focus on the underlying disorder Compensate every electrolyte unbalance Consider bicarbonate and mechanical ventilation in severe cases (pH <7.1)	Follow PALS guidelines Reassessment according to progress

Note: Please read each line from left to right (Inquiry → Assessment → Action) before proceeding to the next step, starting again from the left side, in the same order.

ABG, arterial blood gas; $AG_{CORRLACT}$, anion gap corrected for albumin and lactate; A_{TOT}, total nonbicarbonate plasma anions (weak acids); *CVC*, central venous catheter; HCO_3^-, bicarbonate; Na^+ *and* Cl^-, Na^+ and Cl^- blood levels; *PALS*, pediatric advanced life support; PCO_2, carbon dioxide partial pressure; *SBE*, standard base excess; SID_{APP}, strong ion difference (apparent); SID_{EFF}, strong ion difference (effective); *SIG*, strong ion gap; tCO_2, total CO_2; *uGap*, urinary anion gap.
(See text for calculation of $AG_{CORRLACT}$, SID_{APP}, SID_{EFF}, SIG, uGap; for bicarbonate and SBE rules of thumb, see Tables 76.2, 76.3, and 76.6.)

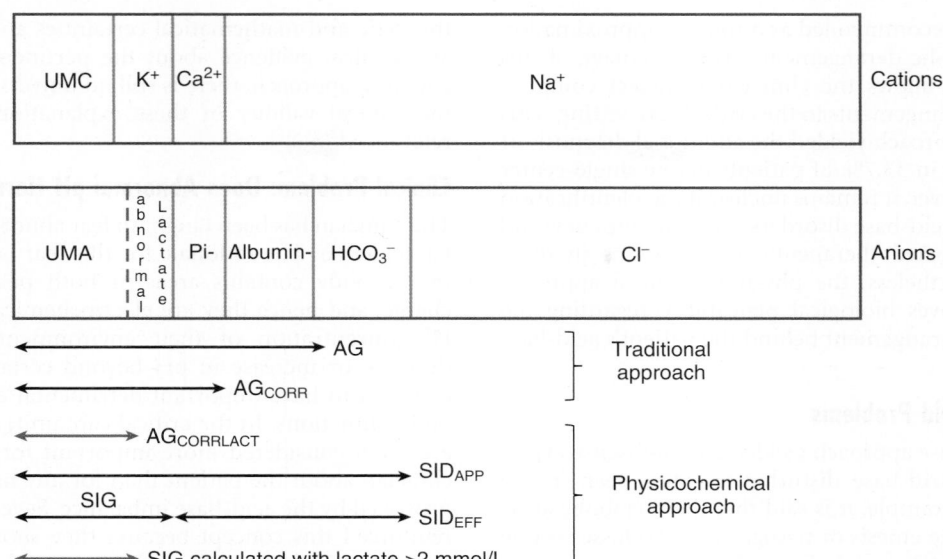

Fig. 76.1. Indexes used for detection of unmeasued anions in both approaches: traditional and physicochemical. If lactate levels are higher than normal, then its value should be added to SID$_{EFF}$ and included in the calculation of SIG. When this is the case, note that SIG and AG$_{CORRLACT}$ are very similar, as ocurrs with SID$_{APP}$ and the [Na$^+$] − [Cl$^-$] difference. *AG*, Anion Gap; *AG$_{CORR}$*, Anion Gap corrected for albumin; *Ca^{2+}*, Calcium (ionic); *Cl$^-$*, Chloride; *K$^+$*, Potassium; *Na$^+$*, Sodium; *Pi$^-$*, Inorganic phosphate; *SID$_{APP}$*, Strong Ion Difference (apparent); *SID$_{EFF}$*, Stron Ion Difference (effective); *SIG*, Strong Ion Gap; *UMA*, Unmeasured or unidentified anions; *UMC*, Unmeasured or unidentified cations.

Cl$^-$ values for calculating AG. On the other hand, in order to avoid [lactate$^-$] influence on AG$_{CORR}$ that could mask the detection of other unmeasured anions, it has been suggested that AG should be corrected not only for albumin but also for lactate. This is simply made by substracting the serum lactate concentration (in mmol/L) from the already albumin-corrected AG (Eq. 18A and 18B)

$$AG_{CORRLACT} = \text{Albumin-corrected AG} - [\text{lactate (mmol/L)}]$$

$$(\text{Eq. 25})$$

This albumin- and lactate-corrected AG (AG$_{CORRLACT}$) seems to correlate well with the SIG.[108,140,144] AG$_{CORRLACT}$ is an easy bedside measurement that may approximate the SIG in critically ill patients. Using uncorrected value AG in critically ill patients, is often unwise given the high prevalence of hypoalbuminemia. If AG needs to be determined, it should be corrected for hypoalbuminemia and lactate as appropriate (AG$_{CORR}$ or AG$_{CORRLACT}$).[83-88,138,139]

As sodium and chloride are the ions with the highest plasma concentration, the difference between them ([Na$^+$]−[Cl$^-$]) can be used as surrogate for the apparent SID.[85,145,146] In a cohort of 341 critically ill patients, researchers demonstrated that the difference between sodium and chloride ([Na$^+$] − [Cl$^-$]) and anion gap corrected for albumin and lactate (AG$_{CORRLACT}$) can be used as apparent strong ion difference (SID$_{APP}$) and strong ion gap (SIG) surrogates, respectively.[106] Substitution of [Na$^+$] − [Cl$^-$] and AG$_{CORRLACT}$ for SAD$_{APP}$ and SIG, respectively, simplifies the diagnosis and management of acid-base disorders in critically ill patients. Similarly, there have been suggestions for improving the SBE. Partitioned SBE, or *base excess gap*, is an attempt to combine the approaches of Siggaard-Andersen and Stewart in

a kind of physicochemical adjusted SBE, which seeks to quantify the metabolic component of acid-base disorders.

Based on an analysis of Stewart's model, Gilfix[147] proposed that only four conditions may create nonrespiratory acid-base disturbances, which are as follows: (1) free water deficit or excess (BE$_{fw}$), as determined by changes in sodium concentration; (2) changes in chloride concentration (first corrected for the free water effect) (BE$_{Cl}$); (3) changes in protein charges, mainly albumin (BE$_{alb}$); and (4) the presence of organic unmeasured anions (BE$_{XA}$). Accordingly SBE may be "partitioned" (using abridged Stewart equations)[144,148-150] into four "physical-chemical" segments. Gilfix showed that the lab-reported SBE, or total SBE (SBE$_{TOTAL}$) should equal the sum of the BE for each one of the four conditions. This approach has received some criticism for small but potentially important inaccuracies.[113] In spite of these physiologic and conceptual caveats, this approach was first tested in children in a pediatric intensive care unit in 1999, with apparent success.[144] Reported successful applications in mortality prediction, and classification of acidosis in several settings, including sepsis and septic shock, cardiac surgery, diabetic ketoacidosis, and others, soon followed.[8] Unfortunately, lack of standardization in regard to the formulas employed for BE partitioning has been associated with large and clinically important discrepancies between several studies.[139,147-150]

Tools of the traditional approach are the first line for choice assessing respiratory acid-base disturbances and for the initial appraisal of the metabolic problems (bicarbonate and SBE) (see Table 76.7). For in-depth metabolic analysis, the proved surrogates of SID$_{APP}$ and SIG, AG$_{CORRLACT}$ and the difference [Na$^+$] − [Cl$^-$], are recommended. At present time, SBE partitioning is not recommended as a routine approximation to acid-base metabolic derangements. The advantage of this approach is that it allows the clinician to detect complex, mixed acid-base derangements in the critical care setting. This physicochemical approach yielded the additional diagnosis of metabolic disorders in 33.7% of patients in one single-center adult study.[151] However, it remains unclear if the identification of these additional acid-base disorders translates into new and otherwise unanticipated therapeutic interventions in these patients.[120,134] Nevertheless, the physical-chemical approach undoubtedly improves biological plausibility regarding the physiopathologic derangement behind the patient's acid-base status.[31]

New Insights for Old Problems

The classical acid-base approach yielded commonsense explanations for some acid-base disturbances often seen in the clinical arena. For example, it is said that the metabolic alkalosis seen with severe emesis or nasogastric tube losses is due to a *loss of H+*, that the metabolic acidosis seen in persistent postpyloric fluid losses is due to a *loss of bicarbonate*, that an acidosis caused by large volume fluid administration is caused by *dilution of bicarbonate*, and that sodium bicarbonate (NaHCO$_3$) therapy corrects metabolic acidosis by contributing bicarbonate ion (HCO$_3^-$) to the body. These time-honored explanations have been challenged by the new view of the acid-base balance, in which water dissociation and the ionic composition of body fluids represent a core principle.[28,29,33,122] According to these new concepts, pH has no direct relationship with any total body direct loss or gain of H+ or HCO$_3^-$ but rather reflects the change of the proportion in cations and anions (strong ions and weak acids), their effect on water dissociation, and possibly other mechanisms controlling ion flux through cell membranes.[122] Kidney function, and possibly other organs such as liver, also participates in the control of the pH and HCO$_3^-$, but the fundamental physicochemical principles are the same.

For example, it is well recognized that the acute expansion of extracellular volume with normal saline solution (sodium chloride [NaCl] 0.9%) or with any unbalanced synthetic colloid solution (6% hydroxyethyl starch solution or 4% gelatin) may result in hyperchloremic acidosis.[148,152-160] The understanding of this condition has improved through the physicochemical comprehension of the acid-base equilibrium: Saline causes acidosis not through dilution of bicarbonate but rather by its Cl$^-$ content, which increases the anion chloride out of proportion of the cation sodium, which decreases the SID$_{APP}$ and increases water dissociation and [H+].[152-157] This occurs despite equal amounts of Na+ and Cl$^-$ in saline solution, because in plasma sodium and chloride concentrations are different. Therefore when large amounts of NaCl in solution are infused, they have a proportionally greater effect on total body chloride than on total body sodium.

Elevated gastric fluid losses seen with severe emesis or nasogastric drainage are the opposite example: The loss of high amounts of chloride leads to an increase in SID$_{APP}$ and to alkalosis.[161] In addition to these examples, Stewart's water dissociation-centered model may provide new insight into the molecular biology and transport physiology of the renal tubule. For example, renal tubule acidosis (RTA) and Bartter syndrome may be redefined as *chloride channelopathies*, rather than disorders of net acid excretion.[104,122,162] In spite of the

theoretic and mathematical certainties and the experimental and clinical evidence about the pertinence of the physicochemical approach, there is still no universal agreement about the clinical validity of these explanations or their clinical relevance.[121,163,164]

Clinical Problem: Does Abnormal pH Harm?

The clinician has been taught to fear abnormal pH, in particular acidemia. The rationale for this fear is that every protein in the body contains areas of both positive and negative charge, and hence they are electrochemically sensitive to the H+ concentration of their environment.[8,33,41] Therefore a decrease or increase in pH beyond certain limits might be expected to have important detrimental effects on a host of bodily functions. In the critical care unit, acid-base disorders are often considered more important for what they tell the clinician about the patient than for any harm that is directly provoked by the acid-base imbalance. Several studies[29,165] have reinforced this concept because they showed that mortality was more closely related to the nature of acid-base disorders than to the magnitude of metabolic acidosis (estimated by partitioned SBE). Hyperlactatemia, more than the elevation of unmeasured anions (AG$_{CORR LACT}$, SID$_{APP}$, SIG) or SBE, is predictive of a poor outcome. Despite these reliable data from children with shock, it is generally accepted that acid-base derangement itself may cause harm in certain circumstances.[44,62,166] The obvious examples are the extreme conditions of pH (<7 or >7.7). It is also important, however, to consider how fast the acid-base derangement is evolving, along with the specific expected consequences of the alteration in specific patients. For example, in a patient who depends on vasopressors, vasodilation due to alkalosis—either respiratory and iatrogenic in origin for overzealous hand bagging of the patient or metabolic as a consequence of gastric fluid losses caused by a mechanically obstructed jejunum—can be catastrophic. Another typical example is the spontaneously breathing patient with metabolic acidosis who tries to compensate by increasing minute ventilation; if the patient gets tired, there is the possibility that hypoxemia will develop along with respiratory acidosis. In such cases, the underlying disorder must be treated, but one must also provide immediate treatment for the acid-base derangement itself.

The main expected physiologic effects of acidemia and alkalemia are as follows. Acidemia initially causes sympathetic and adrenal stimulation, an effect that is counterbalanced as the drop in pH becomes more and more severe, by a depressed responsiveness of adrenergic receptors to circulating catecholamines.[62,167-169] In isolated animal heart preparations and in isolated human ventricle muscle, there is no doubt that acidosis reduces contractile function.[169-171] The net influence of acidosis in the whole animal and in real patients, however, is more complicated to discern, and depending on the experimental or clinical model, it has been found that acidosis caused myocardial contractility to remain constant, decrease marginally, or transiently rise and then fall.[172] Hence the whole-body response to acidosis is less clearly detrimental in real individuals. In many preclinical and clinical studies of patients undergoing permissive hypercapnia, a pH less than 7.2 was well tolerated,[173,174] as it is in youngsters with diabetic ketoacidosis,[175] children and adults with supercarbia,[176] and those with grand mal seizures.[177] Thus it is now clear that the effect of acidosis may differ according to type, magnitude, and time of onset.[119,176] Three types of extracellular acidosis—inorganic, respiratory, and lactic—may have disparate effects on left ventricular function in a model of isolated rabbit hearts.[178] Lactic acidosis caused a significant increase in the time to peak left ventricular pressure while retarding ventricular relaxation. This reinforced the concept that lactate ions have an independent and deleterious effect on myocardial function.[171,178] These findings make sense when they are extrapolated (with some reserve) to the clinical setting. Despite the frequent coincidence of clinical shock and metabolic acidosis, the striking discordance between the clinical course and outcome of patients with lactic acidosis compared with those who have ketoacidosis or ventilatory failure suggests that the low pH itself is important but not crucial for the presentation of the hemodynamic collapse of these patients.[168,172] Therefore the net effect on ventricular performance, heart rhythm, and vascular tone depends on the relative effects of many, sometimes competing, influences. In general terms, severe acidemia (pH <7.1-7.2)[1,35,44,62,171] is associated with decreased cardiac performance that provokes a drop in cardiac output, along with decreased vascular reactivity that manifests itself as arterial vasodilatation and venous constriction.[167] An important effect in the critical care setting is the marked increase in cerebral blood flow due to acute respiratory acidemia and its abrupt decrease with respiratory alkalosis (see also Chapters 60, 62 and 66).[179,180]

When PCO_2 acutely rises in excess of 70 mm Hg, loss of consciousness and seizures can be seen, probably due to the abrupt lowering of intracellular pH. Cultured lung epithelial cells exposed to cyclic stretch similar to that seen with mechanical ventilation produced a lactic acidosis that markedly enhanced the growth of *E. coli*.[181] In contrast, alkalinizing the pH abolished this effect. The demonstration that clinically relevant levels of metabolic acidosis enhance bacterial growth is of concern. However, in patients with acute respiratory distress syndrome (ARDS) treated with permissive hypercapnia mechanical ventilation, the gradual rise of the PCO_2 and the consequent drop of the pH are well tolerated in general terms, with no significant negative effects on systemic cardiac output, oxygen delivery, or vascular resistances, both pulmonary and systemic.[173,174] Actually, the hypercapnic acidosis has been shown to provide beneficial effects on pulmonary function by interacting with reactive oxygen species, the immune system, and the alveolar-capillary barrier.[180,181] However, evidence gathered through a multivariate analysis showed that changes in arterial pH, but not in positive end-expiratory pressure (PEEP) levels, were significantly correlated with impaired right ventricular function, whereas the left ventricle was spared.[182] Thus the net effect of respiratory acidemia to the patient, beneficial or detrimental, may be complex to elucidate. Other potential effects of acidemia include endogenous catecholamine, aldosterone, and parathyroid hormone stimulation; insulin resistance; increased free radical formation; increased protein degradation; gut barrier dysfunction; further respiratory depression; decreased sensorium; hyperkalemia; hypercalcemia; and hyperuricemia.[29,62] In regard to the effect of extracellular acidemia on inflammatory response and immune function, research has indicated that different acids produce different effects, despite similar extracellular pH.[166]

When associated with severe alkalemia (pH >7.6), both metabolic and respiratory alkalosis lower blood pressure and cardiac output. The potential deleterious effects of this drop

in systemic and regional blood flow may be aggravated by the increased hemoglobin oxygen affinity (shift to the left of the oxyhemoglobin dissociation curve), particularly in acute alkalosis. In chronic alkalemia this effect is counterbalanced by an increase in the 2,3-diphosphoglyceric acid concentration in red cells.[44] Cerebral circulation responds dramatically to alkalemia with marked vasoconstriction. Acute hyperventilation to PCO_2 of 20 mm Hg may drop cerebral blood flow to 50% of the basal flow. This effect has been used as an emergency management response to a rise in intracranial pressure, but it carries the risk of producing an excessive drop of blood flow in the most affected areas of the brain, with the increased possibility of ischemia and subsequent cerebral infarct (see also Chapter 66).[180] Because both metabolic and respiratory alkalemia may provoke abrupt transcellular membrane shifts of several electrolytes, mainly potassium and calcium, the net effect is an increase in neuromuscular irritability and excitability. Occurrence of seizures and cardiac arrhythmias has been reported, if pH exceeds 7.7.[161]

Therefore in terms of whether abnormal pH causes harm, the answer is complex: Potential harm always exists, but the occurrence of real damage depends on many factors, including the clinical setting of the patient; type of derangement (metabolic versus respiratory); timing of presentation (gradual versus sudden); renal, lung, and liver functional status; and type of metabolic acidosis and magnitude (mild, moderate, or severe). The answer regarding the possible benefit of acidosis is also complex, with similar caveats.

Blood Gases: Arterial, Central Venous, or Capillary Samples?

Considering the diversity of microcirculations and tissue metabolism throughout the body, the clinician must be aware that the value of a single arterial blood pH is limited, particularly as most functional proteins are intracellular.[168,172] There is a significant correlation in pH, PCO_2, partial pressure of oxygen (PO_2), SBE, and HCO_3^- among arterial, central venous, and capillary blood gases in healthy volunteers and in stable patients. However, in the presence of hypotension or shock, there is very poor or no correlation at all in PO_2 but some correlation of acid-base parameters.[183] Thus capillary and central venous blood gas measurements may be useful alternatives to arterial samples when an arterial line is not in place, in particular for acid-base evaluation.[184] However, in the severe circulatory failure setting, such as in decompensated, catecholamine-resistant septic shock and cardiac arrest, significant widening of the arteriovenous differences in pH, PCO_2, and lactate may occur. In the presence of severe hypoperfusion, hypercapnia and acidemia of peripheral tissues are best detected in central venous blood rather than in arterial blood samples.[185] In the setting of ARDS, the lungs may become important lactate producers, leading to significantly larger levels of lactate in the arterial blood gases than in the venous blood gases. Therefore both arterial and central venous blood samples are needed to assess acid-base status in patients with severe hemodynamic compromise.

Metabolic Acidosis

The classical approach to metabolic acidosis is to classify the disorders as those with either *elevated AG* or *normal AG*, which continues to be a practical although not a pathophysiologically based classification (see Table 76.4). Using the physicochemical approach, metabolic acidosis can be classified as due to an *imbalance of strong ions* (decreased SID) or due to the presence of *abnormal nonvolatile weak acids* (increased A_{TOT}). In turn, decreased SID acidosis can be classified in two categories: that due to an excess of unmeasured anions (excess [XA^-]) (which grossly corresponds to the elevated AG acidosis) and that due to an excess of chloride or relative or absolute deficit of sodium-water excess (which corresponds to the non-AG acidosis) (see Tables 76.6 and 76.7). There appears to be a complex regulation of cations and anions (hence, for SID) for acid-base purposes, but no such mechanisms are known to control [A_{TOT}]. For this reason, there is no agreement as to whether or not changes in [A_{TOT}] should be accepted as acid-base disorders, despite their influence on pH.[41] The classical approach will be used as the main frame for addressing metabolic acidoses, with additional information, mainly about pathophysiology, from the physicochemical approach.

Elevated Anion Gap Acidoses

These are a group of disorders in which there is the accumulation of an acidic anion. There are three clinically relevant examples: lactic acidosis, ketoacidosis, and acidosis secondary to the ingestion or administration of a toxin or drug.

Lactic Acidosis

The popular classification of hyperlactatemia as type A (*associated with or caused by* inadequate tissue oxygen delivery) or type B (adequate tissue oxygen delivery) is sustained because of its simplicity, even though it is not necessarily a reflection of the pathophysiologic mechanism underlying this alteration, as considerable overlap exists between types A and B[186] (Table 76.8). Type B was originally further subdivided into types B1, B2, and B3 acidoses: B1 associated with an underlying disease (eg diabetes mellitus, asthma, malignancies); B2 due to drugs or toxins (cyanide, metformin, epinephrine, etc.); and B3 due to inborn errors of metabolism. Type A seems to be the most frequent cause of lactic acidosis encountered in critically ill patients.[186,187]

Among all metabolic acidoses, lactic acidosis in the pediatric intensive care unit (PICU) signals trouble, regardless of patient age.[187-193] Depending on the source, hyperlactatemia is defined as a lactate level between 2 and 5 mmol/L, whereas lactic acidosis is said to be present when the lactate level exceeds 5 mmol/L and the arterial pH is less than 7.35.[194] The lower limit of the normal range for the blood lactate level, 0.5 mmol/L, is consistent among clinical laboratories, but the upper limit can vary substantially, from 1 to 2.2 mmol/L. Levels at the upper tier of normal values have been associated with increased poor outcomes among seriously ill patients.[194-196] Previously, the definition of lactic acidosis included a blood pH of ≤ 7.35 or a serum [$HCO3^-$] ≤ 20 mmol/L.[197] However, the absence of one or both of these features because of coexisting acid-base disorders does not rule out lactic acidosis. For example, coexisting respiratory alkalosis can increase the blood pH into the alkalemic range, whereas the exogenous administration of furosemide or bicarbonate itself can result in both hyperbicarbonatemia and alkalemia. In contrast, coexisting respiratory acidosis can cause severe acidemia. Lactic acidosis during grand mal seizures is associated with normokalemia, because the concurrent entry of lactate and protons

TABLE 76.8	Causes of Metabolic Alkalosis in Critically Ill Patients

I. Chloride-Responsive (Decreased Urine [Cl⁻])ᵃ

A. Gastrointestinal Losses of Cl⁻
1. Gastric drainage or persisting vomiting
2. Chloride-wasting acute diarrheas

B. Renal Losses of Cl⁻ and K⁺
1. Diuretics (mainly acute use)
2. High dose of certain penicillin-derivative antibiotics
3. Posthypercapnia

II. Chloride-Resistant (Increased Urine [Cl⁻])ᵇ

A. Excess Mineralocorticoid Activity: Ongoing Losses of K⁺ and Cl⁻
1. Primary and secondary hyperaldosteronism
2. Congenital adrenal hyperplasia (17α-hydroxylase or 11β-hydroxylase deficiency)
3. Cushing syndrome
4. Primary renin-secreting tumors
5. Steroid treatment

B. Genetic Renal Tubular Defects of Electrolyte Transport
1. Problem in chloride reabsorption
   a. Bartter and Gitelman syndromes
2. Defective epithelial sodium channel (decreased sodium elimination)
   b. Liddle syndrome

C. Drug-Induced Hypokalemic Alkalosis
1. Diuretics administered for prolonged time
2. High-dose glucocorticoids
3. Fludrocortisone
4. Aminoglycosides
5. Toxic effects of licorice (*Glycyrrhiza glabra*)
6. Ion exchange resin

D. Excess Cation (Alkali) Gain
1. Massive blood transfusion
2. Massive infusion of lactated Ringer solution
3. Parenteral hyperalimentation with excessive sodium acetate
4. Alkali ingestion/treatment and milk-alkali syndrome
5. Magnesium depletion

III. Miscellaneous Group (Variable Urine [Cl⁻])ᵇ

A. Hypoproteinemia
B. Cystic Fibrosis
C. Congenital Chloride Diarrhea
D. Salt-Losing Nephropathy

ᵃ<20 mEq/L, usually <15 mE/L.
ᵇ>20 mEq/L, usually >40 mEq/L.

into neural cells precludes potassium exit from cells to maintain electroneutrality.[194] An increase in the anion gap can mirror the blood lactate level, but a close relationship might not always be present, because anions other than lactate often contribute to the AG. Thus a normal anion gap does not rule out lactic acidosis. As many as 50% of patients with a serum lactate level of 5 to 10 mmol/L did not have an elevated anion gap.[198] Correction of the anion gap for the effect of serum albumin can improve its sensitivity, but many cases will still escape detection. Therefore the serum anion gap lacks sufficient sensitivity or specificity to serve as a screening tool for lactic acidosis. Physicochemical indexes, such as SID_{EFF} and SIG, have a better performance[199] but always below the direct determination of lactate levels.

Blood lactate concentration, in terms of both the magnitude and the persistence of lactate elevation, has been shown to correlate with mortality in pediatric and adult patients in many situations, including septic and hemorrhagic shock, neonates receiving ventilation, and necrotizing enterocolitis,[119,165,187-192] and it has been used for the titration of inotropes and blood cell transfusions during early goal-directed therapy for severe sepsis and septic shock with a performance not inferior to the mixed venous saturation.[193] Others, however, found no correlation between simultaneously measured $ScvO_2$ and lactate levels in patients with severe systemic inflammatory response syndrome and severe sepsis, but normalization of lactate levels within 48 hours was a predictive factor for survival.[200] Hyperlactatemia may also be present in children following cardiac surgery.[201] Therefore lactate measurement has become a common attribute in point-of-care blood gas analyzers used at bedside in modern ICUs.[202] A new lactate-based categorization of septic shock in adult patients has been proposed: Hyperlactatemia is associated with risk of death independent of vasopressor need resulting in different phenotypes within the classic categories of severe sepsis and septic shock.[203,204]

Lactate represents the end product of anaerobic metabolism (ie, it is a product of pyruvate reduction via the enzyme lactate dehydrogenase and the reduced nicotinamide hypoxanthine dinucleotide/nicotinamide hypoxanthine dinucleotide [NADH/NAD] cofactor system[187,205,206] [see also Chapters 80 and 81]). It derives primarily from skeletal muscle, gut, brain, and circulating erythrocytes, with a production of about 1 mmol/kg/h. The healthy liver uptakes most lactate and recycles it via three primary options: conversion back to glucose (Cori cycle); oxidation back to pyruvate, which subsequently can be oxidized to CO_2 via the Krebs cycle; or transamination into alanine.[205,206] A decrease in oxygen availability at tissue and cellular levels impairs oxidative phosphorylation, which increases the intracellular levels of NADH, the cofactor that facilitates the conversion of pyruvate to lactate. Because of its close relationship with anaerobic metabolism, increased lactate concentration has been largely considered a dead-end waste product of glycolysis due to hypoxia. However, using blood lactate concentration as evidence of tissue hypoperfusion, hypoxia, and hyperactive anaerobic glycolysis is, at best, an oversimplification.[185,196,206]

Evidence now supports the view that sepsis-associated hyperlactatemia is not due only to tissue hypoxia or anaerobic glycolysis and that this response may actually facilitate bioenergetic efficiency through an increase in lactate oxidation. In this sense, the characteristics of lactate production best fit the notion of an adaptive survival response that increases in intensity as disease severity increases.[207-211] Skeletal muscle appears to be a leading source of lactate formation as a result of exaggerated aerobic glycolysis through Na^+/K^+-ATPase stimulation by circulating epinephrine, both endogenous and exogenous.[207-210] Increased lactate as a result of hypoxia or dysoxia may be more the exception than the rule, at least in the hyperdynamic, hypermetabolic phase of sepsis.[199,206-208] Lactate is an important intermediary in numerous metabolic processes, a highly mobile fuel for aerobic metabolism through cell-to-cell shuttles, allowing the coordination of intermediary metabolism in different tissues and between cells within those tissues.[206] Accordingly, high lactate concentration in septic shock patients can still be interpreted as a marker of the disease's severity, but it should not be taken as an irrefutable proof of oxygen debt or hypoperfusion, needing increases in

systemic or regional perfusion or oxygenation to supranormal values.[207,208,211]

During systemic hypoperfusion several tissues are a clear source of lactic acid. For example, underperfused intestine can release lactate but not if mesenteric perfusion is maintained.[107,212] Causes of hyperlactatemia and lactic acidosis are numerous in the critical care setting[186,187,191] (see Table 76.8). Lactate levels may fluctuate in response to exogenous catecholamines, particularly epinephrine, which thereby clearly increases lactate levels through stimulation of glycogenolysis and glycolytic flux with a resultant increase in pyruvate production. This effect does not occur with norepinephrine or dobutamine infusions and is not related to decreased tissue perfusion.[205,213-215] Several studies have shown that the lung is a major source of lactate in severe sepsis/septic shock[214,216] and that decreased lactate clearance by the liver is also an important component of sepsis-associated hyperlactatemia and lactic acidosis.[214,217]

On the other side, the brain is a lactate-consuming organ. Lactate is thought to be an alternative and supplemental fuel for the injured brain and is important for regulating glucose metabolism and cerebral blood flow. Exogenous lactate supplementation may be neuroprotective after experimental acute brain injury. Hypertonic lactate solutions may be a valid therapeutic option for secondary energy dysfunction and elevated intracranial pressure among patients with specific conditions, such as glucose transporter type-1 deficiency syndrome and glycogen-storage disease.[218,219] Therefore instead of just being a biomarker of cellular oxygen debt, persistent lactate elevation often seen in patients with sepsis (and in patients after trauma resuscitation) may be the consequence of more complex physiologic, inflammatory, and metabolic processes.

Although the source and pathophysiologic interpretation of lactic acidosis are matters of discussion, no question exists about the ability of lactate accumulation to produce acidemia. Given its pK_a of 3.9, lactic acid behaves as a strong ion within clinically encountered pH. Therefore the accumulation of lactate (a strong anion) without the addition of an important strong cation such as sodium will be expected to lower the SID, increase $[H^+]$, and decrease the pH. Lactic acidosis would also be expected to be associated with increased adenosine triphosphate (ATP) hydrolysis, another source of hydrogen ions. Because the body can produce and clear lactate rapidly, it functions as one of the most dynamic components of the SID.[205]

Type B lactic acidoses are probably operative in many clinical circumstances where the so-called type A lactic acidoses have traditionally been invoked.[205,207-217] A potentially useful method for distinguishing anaerobically produced lactate from other sources is to measure the whole blood pyruvate concentration. The normal lactate-to-pyruvate ratio is 10 : 1. Because pyruvate is reduced to lactate during anaerobic metabolism, the ratio of lactate to pyruvate increases. If this ratio is higher than 25 : 1, it is considered evidence of anaerobic metabolism.[213] Unfortunately, pyruvate is unstable in solution, and an accurate measurement in the clinical setting is therefore challenging.

In many settings, including septic shock and liver failure, the magnitude of the accumulation of lactate does not always account for the whole of the acid-balance derangement observed.[85,119,165] In fact, the increase in the AG, SID, and SIG seen in severe sepsis is often substantially greater than the actual lactate concentration. This finding has led to the active search of the so-called unexplained or unmeasured anions (abbreviated [XA⁻] or [UMAs]).[29,107,119] Donnan equilibrium alterations due to sepsis-mediated endothelial damage and a switch from a hepatic anion-uptake state to an anion-release state during endotoxemia have been the main proposals for explaining the fact that as much as 15% to 50% of the increased AG, SID, and SIG are not related to the increased lactate.[29,107,214,216,217] The accumulation of molecules such as succinate, citrate, and formate has also been implicated.[98,99,108,113]

In addition to epinephrine, numerous drugs and toxins encountered in critical care medicine may cause or contribute to increased lactate, with or without acidemia. Likewise, drugs associated with the release of endogenous catecholamines, such as cocaine, can stimulate lactate production.[220] A similar mechanism is advocated in patients with pheochromocytoma.[221] Sodium nitroprusside remains a key vasodilator drug. Because it is metabolized to cyanide and thiocyanate, these toxins may accumulate if excessive drug is administered or cyanide clearance is impaired as occurs in hepatic and renal failure (see also Chapters 126, 127 and 128). In such cases, mitochondrial respiratory chain activity may be inhibited and lactate production increased.[222] Thus nitroprusside toxicity is usually heralded by the rise in lactate levels, with or without a drop in the pH.[205] Similarly, propofol toxicity resulting in lactic acidosis, rhabdomyolysis (including the cardiac muscle), or myocardial, renal, and hepatic failure seems to involve mitochondrial toxicity, which occurs more often with continuous and prolonged infusion, hence the designation *propofol infusion syndrome*.[223,224] As noted previously, in ARDS, lactate levels may be high even in the absence of shock or sepsis.[216] In acute lung injury (ALI)/ARDS, the lung is an important source of lactate.[216,225] This was first evidenced by higher lactate levels in arterial blood than in the mixed blood obtained from patients with ALI/ARDS. A similar phenomenon has been observed in patients receiving mechanical ventilation after cardiopulmonary bypass.[226,227] Potential mechanisms of lactate production by the injured lung may include not only the onset of anaerobic metabolism in hypoxic zones but also direct cytokine effects on pulmonary cells and a stress-induced enhancement of glycolysis and lactate synthesis by both the parenchymal and nonparenchymal cells (eg, endothelial cells and inflammatory cells infiltrating lung tissue such as macrophages and neutrophils).[216,225-227] A similar mechanism is operative in wound tissue, the intestine, and the liver in patients with trauma.[217] Hyperlactatemia occurs in about 80% of cases of acute liver failure.[228,229] Both decreased hepatic clearance of systemically produced lactic acid and increased hepatic production of lactate are involved.[217,228,229] Hypermetabolism associated with lactate accumulation has been found in organs rich in mononuclear phagocytes, especially the liver and spleen. In patients with severe hepatic failure, both the liver and intestine behave as net producers of lactate.[228,229] After transplantation, the grafted liver becomes a net consumer of lactate as evidenced by a negative lactate gradient between hepatic and portal venous blood.

A key concept acknowledges that lactate can be considered a waste product when released from one cell, but it becomes a useful substrate when taken up by another cell. Lactate turnover in vivo in humans is similar to that of glucose, alanine,

or glutamine, which means that lactate has one of the highest recycling rates in intermediary metabolism. Accordingly, increased lactate levels can be viewed as an adaptive response, by which some lactate-producing cells are providing other group of cells with an energy substrate via the so-called lactate shuttle.[206,230]

Lactic acidosis in status asthmaticus seems to be multifactorial and includes contributions from lactate production by overwhelmed respiratory muscles, tissue hypoxia, a hyperadrenergic state, and the metabolic effect of pharmacologic β_2 agonists.[231-236] Non-lactic, non-AG acidosis has been described in adults presenting with status asthmaticus and seems to be related to hyperchloremia associated with exacerbated chronic hypocapnia.[237] In multiple trauma, lactic acidosis can occur as an effect of polytrauma and hemorrhagic shock and as a manifestation of severe traumatic brain injury, and it is a risk factor for adverse outcomes.[238] Salicylate intoxication is a special situation in which lactic acidosis may play an important role (see also Chapters 127 and 128). Although salicylate toxicity occurs less frequently now than in the past because of the increased use of alternative antipyretics in young children, it must still be considered in certain therapeutic situations (eg, rheumatic diseases), as well as in cases of intentional or iatrogenic overdose. It remains as a potential pediatric health hazard, rising concern as children are more fragile to salicylate poisoning because of their reduced ability of buffer the acid stress.[239] Salicylates directly or indirectly affect most organ systems in the body by uncoupling oxidative phosphorylation, inhibiting Krebs cycle enzymes, and inhibiting amino acid synthesis. These derangements can result in variable acid-base patterns: respiratory alkalosis, mixed respiratory alkalosis plus metabolic acidosis, or (less commonly) simple metabolic acidosis.[240] A *paradoxical aciduria* may occur despite respiratory alkalosis and aggravate the clinical manifestations because a higher percentage of salicylate in acidic urine remains in the unionized form, which is reabsorbed from the glomerular filtrate. Metabolic acidosis is mainly due to lactic acid, but ketoacids and other metabolic acids also participate. Chronic salicylate poisoning has been described, in which the patients usually have metabolic acidosis and a pseudosepsis syndrome, similar to some inborn errors of metabolism, with high rate of permanent organ dysfunctions and mortality.[241]

Elevation of blood lactate up to the 5 mmol/L level may be seen in about 25% of human immunodeficiency virus (HIV)-positive patients who receive nucleoside reverse transcriptase inhibitors (mainly stavudine). Most patients remain asymptomatic, but a small proportion may present with dyspnea and abdominal pain, as manifestations of lactic acidosis, 3 to 4 months after starting the treatment. If the drug is discontinued and fluids are replaced, the process is reversible. The mechanism appears to involve uncoupled oxidative phosphorylation due to an inhibition of DNA polymerase-gamma.[242]

As a result of the worldwide problem of obesity, increasing numbers of school-age children receive some treatment for the peripheral resistance to insulin. Thus metformin, formerly limited to adult patients, is now being used with increasing frequency in children. The incidence of metformin-associated lactic acidosis is low, but it has a high mortality rate. Obese children and adolescents who receive metformin in the setting of intercurrent illnesses that may predispose to accumulation of the drug (eg, renal function impairment) are at risk of developing metformin-associated lactic acidosis.[243] It also may occur as a consequence of accidental ingestion or a suicidal attempt. Survival depends on the nadir pH and the maximum concentration of lactate and metformin. The mechanism involves uncoupling of the oxidative-phosphorylation with acceleration of the glycolytic flux, which increases lactate production. From 1960 to 2000 the overall mortality rate for metformin-associated lactic acidosis was around 50%, but it has since fallen to around 25%.[244]

A curious form of lactic acidosis is the so-called D-lactic acidosis. Lactic acid produced by mammals is a levo-isomer. Dextroisomer (D)-lactate derived from bacterial fermentation in the bowel lumen may reach systemic circulation and lead to metabolic acidemia, especially if liver function (and thus lactate clearance) is suboptimal.[245] D-lactic acidosis must be considered in patients with a history of intestinal disease who have neurologic findings such as confusion and ataxia, and high AG metabolic acidosis, with normal L-lactate levels. Symptoms worsen after high-carbohydrate meals or tube hyperalimentation. In patients with short bowel syndrome, there may be not only an overgrowth of bacteria but also an accumulation of carbohydrates in the colon. Treatment focuses on decreasing gut bacteria overgrowth with antibiotics and the avoidance of high-carbohydrate or lactose feeding. Some studies have advocated the use of probiotics for treating and preventing this problem,[246] but the reports are conflicting.[247,248]

The use of linezolid has increased with the emergence of multidrug-resistant bacteria, including *Staphylococcus aureus* and *Mycobacterium tuberculosis*. Serum lactic acidosis has been reported as a serious side effect of linezolid. Prolonged administration of linezolid (>6 weeks) is one of the risk factors for metabolic acidosis. Studies confirm that this adverse drug event may be predicted with genetic testing.[249,250]

Ketoacidosis

Ketones are formed by beta-oxidation of fatty acids, a process that increases substantially in insulin-deficient states. In the pediatric intensive care setting, this is most often seen in patients with DKA with overproduction and underutilization of acetone, β-hydroxybutyric (βOH-B), and acetoacetic acids (ketone bodies), which accumulate in plasma (see also Chapter 86). Ketoacidosis is also seen in various inborn errors of amino acid and organic acid metabolism, and a mixed ketoacidosis and lactic acidosis are seen with glycogen storage disease type I (glucose-6-phosphate deficiency) (see also Chapter 82). The urinary dipstick for ketones uses a nitroprusside reagent, hence it detects acetoacetate but not βOH-B. If a patient with DKA develops shock, βOH-B may be produced in ratios up to 3:1. Hence the urinary dipstick will mistakenly appear to have few ketones, and their concentration may paradoxically rise as perfusion improves and the patient gets better.[251,252] Capillary blood determination of βOH-B is a better alternative for DKA treatment guidance.[252,253] As the renal threshold for the ketone bodies is low, they are readily filtered, with no reabsorption mechanism, and the kidneys can eliminate a significant number of ketones. This loss can shift the AG, which may appear less than expected, because of the anions eliminated though the urine, with renal retention of chloride and bicarbonate. The picture can be even more complicated if hypocapnia from hyperventilation is present. Therefore AG (even corrected AG) may not be instructive; SIG may be more useful in such complicated

scenarios.[111] Alcoholic ketoacidosis (AKA) is most frequent in patients with chronic ethanol intake and liver disease, and it usually occurs after a period of heavy drinking in association with reduced food intake. AKA is quickly responsive to fluid administration, with faster resolution when dextrose and saline are infused together.[254]

Toxic Compounds That Directly Provoke Acidosis

Alcohol intoxications, including methanol, ethylene glycol, diethylene glycol, and propylene glycol, may present with a high anion gap metabolic acidosis, a decrease in serum bicarbonate, and an increased serum osmolality and osmolal gap (see also Chapter 127). The acidosis and cellular dysfunction are direct effects of the metabolites of these substances, whereas the parent compounds are associated with an increase in serum osmolality. These are rather infrequent problems in pediatric cases, but adolescents who ingest alcohol or illicit drugs (including inhalants) or have suicidal risks are potential victims.[254] The clinical presentation may range from mild subclinical poisoning to an unexpected and rather sudden onset of high anion gap acidosis, renal failure, and encephalopathy, with an increased risk for mortality and neurologic sequelae.[255] The intoxication is best treated with supportive critical care including alkalinization and early continuous hemofiltration or hemodiafiltration. A competitive inhibitor of alcohol dehydrogenase (4-methylpyrazole [or fomepizole]) is available for use in ethylene glycol and methanol poisoning (possibly also useful in diethylene glycol and propylene glycol intoxications), but extracorporeal removal should always be employed for serious poisoning. For methanol and ethylene glycol, ethanol infusion is an alternative competitive inhibitor of the alcohol-dehydrogenase ezyme.[254,256]

Other Forms of Metabolic Acidosis Associated With an Increased Anion Gap

Late metabolic acidosis of prematurity[257] occurs more frequently in the premature infant when compared with the term infant (20% versus 5%). Limited capacity of less well developed renal tubules to excrete H^+ and Cl^- and to concentrate is a fairly common situation during the first month of life. Although this level of renal tubular development is adequate for the breast-fed infant, if the protein intake or solute load is excessive, the renal capacity may be exceeded and a metabolic acidosis may develop, particularly during periods of stress. In the setting of renal disease generally, the clinician must anticipate the occurrence of metabolic derangements. When chronic renal insufficiency develops, hyperchloremic metabolic acidosis, a nonanion gap acidosis, may initially occur because of impaired ammonium (NH_4^+) generation and excretion. When the glomerular filtration rate (GFR) falls below 20 mL/min, the kidneys are incapable of excreting fixed acids. The resulting accumulation of sulfates among other acids may increase the AG. These acidoses are usually mild, producing an excess AG of approximately 10 mEq/L. A mixed metabolic acidosis (high and normal AG mechanisms) is not uncommon in this setting.[63,251] If the patient has sepsis or another condition associated with hypermetabolism, however, the rate of acid generation increases and the acidosis may become severe. The SID decreases, and because of the lack of renal compensation, some intervention is required. Patients who do not yet require dialysis and those who are between their dialytic sessions are often given sodium bicarbonate (provided there is no hypernatremia) or sodium potassium citrate.[258] When bicarbonate is contraindicated, dialytic therapy is indicated.

Hyperchloremic Acidoses: The Nonanion Gap Metabolic Acidoses

In the classical view, hyperchloremia was considered an epiphenomenon of a drop of the concentration of bicarbonate, due to its *abnormal loss* through urine or stools (see Table 76.4). The rise in chloride concentration is responsible for maintaining a "normal" anion gap, in spite of the drop in bicarbonate levels (ie, a *nonanion gap* acidosis is produced). When bicarbonate is *consumed* to buffer an acid load, hyperchloremia is not produced, because there are other anions, deriving from the acid load, that will preserve electroneutrality as bicarbonate falls. In this case, the anion gap increases because of the presence of these new (and unmeasured) anions.[63,124] However, physiologic thought is moving from kidneys that directly sense and regulate [H^+] to kidneys that react to Cl^- balance and therefore control directly the independent variable SID in the acid-base regulation. This change is supported by identification of several ion transporters in the renal tubules.[95-97,144,162,259-262] Thus hyperchloremic acidoses occur either as a result of an increase in chloride concentration relative to strong cations (especially sodium) or because of the loss of cations with a retention of chloride (see Table 76.6). When the pH drops, the normal response by the kidney is to increase chloride excretion as ammonium chloride (NH_4Cl) in order to increase the SID and raise back the pH. Thus the role of the formation of ammonium (NH_4^+) and its eventual tubular excretion is not so much the elimination of H^+ but rather Cl^- excretion without the loss of sodium or potassium. Failure of this mechanism identifies the kidney as the problem, as in renal tubular acidosis (RTA).[63,199,251] There are four main causes of nonanion gap acidoses: (1) exogenous chloride loads (saline boluses, parenteral nutrition, etc.); (2) loss of cations from the lower gastrointestinal tract without proportional losses of chloride, as in secretory diarrhea, but also in conditions in which alkaline loss of small bowel, biliary, or pancreatic secretions are present (such as drainage from ostomies, tubes, or fistulas); (3) renal tubular acidoses and drug-mediated tubulopathies; and (4) urinary reconstruction using bowel segments.

Exogenous Chloride Load

In the critical care unit there are often mandatory therapeutic interventions associated with hyperchloremic metabolic acidosis. The more common interventions are the rapid infusion of isotonic saline (0.9% NaCl) and the infusion of parenteral nutrition. As stated before, the classical explanation for acidosis following saline administration was the so-called bicarbonate dilution. This mechanism probably can play a role in certain conditions.[143,163] Healthy, metabolically stable individuals have a plasma SID of around 40 mEq/L, and it is around 30 mEq/L in critically ill patients. But the SID of normal saline is *zero* mEq/L, because sodium and chloride are both strong ions. Therefore IV administration of 0.9% NaCl necessarily will decrease plasma SID, creating a strong ion acidosis, as long as the infusion does not cause a change in PCO_2 or albumin or phosphate concentrations. Hyperchloremic acidosis should be expected whenever large volumes of normal saline are rapidly administered, such as in fluid boluses

for treating shock or during surgical procedures.[148,152,156,159] Even the acid-base status of disorders in which one or more unmeasured anions will be participating (septic shock [lactate], DKA [ketones]) is influenced by the chloride infused with resuscitation fluids.[150,152,155,157,263] In one study of 81 children with meningococcal sepsis, metabolic acidosis was common and prolonged (persisted for 48 hours), but the pathophysiology changed from one of unmeasured anions at admission to predominant hyperchloremia by 8 to 12 hours.[152] There is no doubt about the relationship between normal saline resuscitation and the development of hyperchloremia and acidosis (not necessarily acidemia).[152,163,262,264] However, it is not clear if this hyperchloremic acidosis is really detrimental.[115,118,157-160,264] Actually, in a group of 97 children evaluated in their postoperative period following open cardiac surgery, the occurrence of hyperchloremia was associated with a reduced requirement for epinephrine therapy, so the authors suggested that hyperchloremic metabolic acidosis is a benign finding.[148] A review concluded that there is an accumulating trend in scientific evidence showing that both hyperchloremia and hyperchloremic acidoses have subtle but potentially significant adverse physiologic and clinical effects.[158] It is unclear whether the acidosis or the high chloride levels should be of concern. The effects of hyperchloremia and hyperchloremic acidosis may not influence outcome for most patients. Given that hyperchloremic acidosis is often iatrogenic and it is associated with proved morbidity (increased ICU length of stay, delayed DKA recovery, increased incidence of postoperative nausea/emesis),[263] it has been suggested that normal saline should be avoided whenever possible.[158,265]

Several groups have assessed the use of the so-called balanced fluids—that is, fluids with SID nearer to the SID of human plasma.[156,259,265,266] However, this suggested change of practice is still inconclusive. At least one prospective study in adults suggested that the amount of fluids given, rather than the types of fluid, had the stronger effect on the changes in base excess.[267] It is probably wise to view normal saline as a potential hazard, especially in patients with previously known renal or liver dysfunction, those with shock, and surgical patients needing high amounts of intraoperative saline for resuscitation.[268] It has been suggested that intraoperative serial chloride determinations may unmask or exclude hyperchloremia as a cause of acidosis, undetectable through SBE alone.[159]

Parenteral nutrition formulas contain weak anions, such as acetate, in addition to chloride, and thus they are buffered. However, with an insufficient number of weak anions, plasma [Cl^-] will increase, SID will decrease, and acidosis may result.[97]

Postpyloric Gastrointestinal Fluid Losses

The gastrointestinal (GI) tract, liver, and pancreas can be conceptualized as a giant ion exchanger organ. Throughout all the sequential segments of the GI tract, a distinct group of ion transporters and channels interact with one another to determine the electrolyte content, pH, and volume of the fluid in the gut lumen. The main transport system is driven primarily by Na^+/K^+-ATPase across the basolateral membrane of the epithelial cells, with the participation of several key apical membrane electrolyte transporters, including Cl^-/HCO_3^- and Na^+/H^+ ion exchangers and the so-called *cystic fibrosis transmembrane conductance regulator, or CFTR Cl^- channel.* Large numbers of cations and anions traverse the specialized epithelia of the gut every day. This transport is adjusted for achieving an efficient absorption of dietary components, rather than for acid-base homeostasis. Under normal conditions, only a small net amount of alkali (30-40 mmol per day) is lost in stool, so the kidney and lungs have no problem compensating for pH. However, the disruption of normal gut function can provoke disorders that vary from severe acidosis (most of postpyloric losses) to severe alkalosis (prepyloric losses, congenital chloridorrhea), depending on the segment of the GI tract affected and the nature of the losses that ensue.[269] For acid-base and electrolytes abnormalities to occur in diarrheal diseases, the volume of fluid lost must be large enough to exceed the kidney's ability to adjust excretion to maintain acid-base balance. With large losses, any form of diarrhea may lead to a significant fall in extracellular fluid volume, reducing the GFR and limiting the ability of the kidneys to compensate for the problem. Secretory diarrheas (cholera, enteropathic *E. coli,* rotavirus, and other infectious diarrheas) most commonly produce this clinical scenario, with the typical presentation of hypovolemia, hypotension, acute renal failure, hyperchloremic metabolic acidosis (lost stools are usually rich in sodium, potassium, and bicarbonate, so SID decreases), and hypokalemia. If the hypovolemia and hypotension are not corrected, lactic acidosis superimposes, as a result of tissue hypoperfusion. AG_{CORR}, initially normal, may increase gradually, but more frequently it will remain normal in spite of lactacidemia, hence the value of measuring lactate levels. The mechanism of the acidosis is well defined for cholera diarrhea but is less defined for other pathogens. *Vibrio cholera* produces a toxin that increases cAMP levels in intestinal crypt cells, producing a sustained activation of the apical membrane CFTR Cl^- channel and thereby leading to excessive Cl^- secretion into the ileum and colon. This increased chloride secretion in turn stimulates the apical Cl^-/HCO_3^- exchanger, increasing the bicarbonate concentration in stools, which results in increased paracellular Na^+ and water entry, resulting in high-volume losses that contain a large amount of HCO_3^-, as well as Na^+, Cl^-, and K^+. The lost fluid and electrolytes can be replaced with oral solutions (100 mL/kg body weight of a solution with 60 to 90 mEq/L of sodium).[270] In cases of excessive losses or emesis, vigorous intravenous volume repletion must be implemented. Diarrhea due to laxative abuse can be seen in bulimic or anorexia nervosa adolescents, but it is usually not associated with acid-base derangements; however, if excessive diarrheal losses are induced, metabolic acidosis can occur, as with any severe diarrhea.[269]

Both biliary and pancreatic secretions have alkaline pH. When pancreatic or biliary drainages are required after surgery, usually the volume is low, so despite the loss of a $NaHCO_3$-rich fluid, significant metabolic acidosis does not occur. In the rare occasions in which such drainage is excessive (>30 mL/kg/ day), metabolic acidosis will develop and be maintained by concomitant volume depletion. Replenishment with sodium solutions will restore SID. Bicarbonate administration is equally effective.[269] Patients with well-functioning ileostomies usually adapt to the extra fluid obligatory loss through subtle changes in salt and water intake, as well as changes in urine volume and electrolyte and acid excretion. If the ileostomy drainage abruptly increases, resultant salt and water losses can easily lead to clinically significant volume depletion. In this setting, the development of metabolic acidosis is common, because $[HCO_3^-]$ in ileostomy fluid is usually higher than in plasma, causing disproportionate sodium and alkali loss.

Hyperkalemia usually presents with this metabolic acidosis, indicating that K^+ is not secreted into the ileum. In addition, renal K^+ excretion is decreased with volume depletion.

Renal Tubular Acidoses and Drug-Mediated Tubulopathies

RTA comprises a group of disorders characterized by a low capacity for net acid excretion (NAE) and persistent hyperchloremic, as well as metabolic, acidosis with normal anion gap and normal or minimally affected filtration rate (GFR). On the basis of functional studies, RTA has traditionally been separated into three main categories: (1) proximal RTA, or type 2; (2) distal RTA, or type 1; and (3) hyperkalemic RTA, or type 4. Sometimes a fourth kind is added: combined proximal and distal RTA (mixed RTA), or type 3.[271] Type 4 RTA is of special interest in the critical care setting, as the hyperkalemia may be triggered by some drugs used in intensive care units, such as converting enzyme inhibitors, heparin, trimethoprim, α-adrenergic agonists, β-adrenergic antagonists, digoxin, and others. Classical RTA teaching states that metabolic acidosis arises from a lack of urine excretion of protons (hydrogen ions) or an excessive loss of bicarbonate due to a variety of tubular disorders.[271] Molecular studies have identified genetic or acquired defects in transporters of protons and bicarbonate in most varieties of RTA.[271,272] This classical physiologic view has been challenged by the physicochemical acid-base interpretation; it is supported by the fact that these transporters are also involved in Cl^- and Na^+ transport and that at least certain cases of RTA are clearly associated with primary defects in electrolyte transporters alone. In an illustrative study, 12 children with alkali-treated distal RTA were compared with healthy controls. Both groups received a load of hypotonic saline (0.45%), but only the RTA patients exhibited subsequent hyperchloremia and metabolic acidosis, associated with the high total and distal fractional absorption of chloride. However, urinary excretion of bicarbonate did not correlate with changes in either blood pH or plasma bicarbonate concentration. Thus renal tubular avidity for chloride absorption was primarily increased in RTA.[162,261,273] These tubular transport mechanisms determine the excretion of strong ions, Na^+, K^+, and Cl^- and hence the balance of the concentration of SID, both in the extracellular compartment dominated by Na^+ and Cl^- and in the intracellular compartment dominated by K^+. SID determines pH, and by way of sensor and effector mechanisms it must provide feedback to tubular activity. Thus acid-base homeostasis is directly regulated by electrolyte transport in renal tubules, and hydrogen ions and bicarbonate movement represent the balancing requirement imposed by physical chemistry.[104,162,261,273] This reasoning supports the notion that the role of NH_4^+ is more related to the elimination of Cl^- without losing Na^+ or K^+ rather than to the titration of urinary H^+.[104,261,273] According to the physicochemical approach, the underlying defect in all RTA types is an inability to excrete chloride in proportion to sodium, although the transporter involved dictates the specific type of RTA.[162,261,273] In the critical care setting, the presence of RTA may complicate management of the resuscitation fluids including acid-base balance. Previously unknown RTA must be suspected whenever a patient's clinical condition does not improve as expected with the proper therapeutic interventions. Treatment largely depends on whether there are losses of sodium that can be replaced with $NaHCO_3$ or whether the kidney will require mineralocorticoid replacement. It is worth mentioning that urinary AG (uGAP = [uNa$^+$ + uK$^+$] − [uCl$^−$]),[195] more recently termed the *urine strong ion difference*,[97,199] is useful in the diagnostic workup of the patient with hyperchloremic acidosis. If it is negative (uCl$^−$ > uNa$^+$ + uK$^+$), it suggests GI bicarbonate loss, acute infusion of a high volume of saline isotonic fluid (NaCl 0.9%), or a proximal RTA. On the other hand, if the uGAP is positive (uCl$^−$ < uNa$^+$ + uK$^+$), it suggests the presence of a distal renal defect.

Also of importance to the intensivist is iatrogenic renal tubular acidosis caused by the nephrotoxicity of amphotericin B, aminoglycosides, and other drugs. Kidney alterations due to amphotericin B include decreased GFR, distal tubulopathy with urinary loss of potassium and magnesium, RTA, loss of urine concentration ability, and sometimes the Fanconi syndrome. Nephrotoxicity is related to treatment duration, dosing schedule, cumulative dosage, concurrent diuretics treatment, and the administration of other nephrotoxic drugs (aminoglycosides, cyclosporin A, tacrolimus, cisplatin, ifosfamide). Each dose increment of 0.1 mg/kg/day has been found to be associated with a 1.8-fold increase in the risk of nephrotoxicity.[274] Mechanisms of amphotericin nephrotoxicity include the deoxycholate vehicle for amphotericin B, reduction in renal blood flow and GFR, increased salt concentration at the macula densa, interaction of amphotericin B with ergosterol in the cell membrane, and apoptosis in proximal tubular and medullary interstitial cells. Salt loading, with a daily sodium intake >4 mEq/kg/day, is the only measure proved by a controlled prospective study to ameliorate amphotericin B nephrotoxicity in humans, including extremely low-birth-weight infants.[275] Proper hydration must be assured prior to administration of the drug. Lipid formulations of amphotericin B (liposomal, lipid complex, colloidal dispersion) are indicated in children receiving other nephrotoxic drugs, those with already reduced GFR, or those with previously documented amphotericin adverse events. Total dose ≥35 mg, chronic renal disease, concomitant use of cyclosporine or amikacin, and male gender have been identified in adults as risk factors. Patients with more than two risk factors showed an incidence of moderate-to-severe nephrotoxicity of 29%.[276]

Trimethoprim-sulfamethoxazole is another antimicrobial that has been related to RTA and hyperchloremic metabolic acidosis.[277] Topiramate, one of the new anticonvulsant drugs, has been reported to cause hyperchloremic metabolic acidosis in children and adults. Topiramate inhibits the enzyme carbonic anhydrase, and thus a type 3 or mixed RTA is produced.[278] Another rare cause of normal AG metabolic acidosis that may be seen in the ICU is acetazolamide, a carbonic anhydrase inhibitor used occasionally to decrease cerebral spinal fluid production in conditions of hydrocephalus and to stimulate renal bicarbonate wasting.[279] This drug decreases hydrolysis of H_2CO_3 to CO_2 and H_2O, resulting in a decrease of renal $HCO_3^−$ reabsorption. Rarely acetazolamide can produce a severe lactic acidosis with elevated anion gap, increased lactate-to-pyruvate ratio, ketosis with a low β-hydroxybutyrate-to-acetoacetate ratio, and a urinary organic acid profile typical of pyruvate carboxylase deficiency.[280] This acquired enzymatic injury stems from the inhibition of mitochondrial carbonic anhydrase type V.

Urinary Reconstruction Using Bowel Segments

Children with irreversible lower urinary tract dysfunction due to developmental abnormalities involving the genitourinary (GU) system, neurogenic and myogenic bladder, may require urologic surgical procedures for their management, including urinary diversion and enterocystoplasty. Various techniques and bowel segments can be used depending on the clinical situation. The GI tract is a relatively poor substitute for urothelium, and its semipermeability allows nonphysiologic fluid and electrolyte absorption leading to metabolic abnormalities.[281] The significance of these problems is related to the portion of the GI tract used and the length of time the urine is exposed to the bowel surface. In addition, if the loss of some portions of the GI tract results in chronic diarrhea, there may be further metabolic consequences. Jejunal substitution is typically associated with hyponatremic/hypochloremic/hyperkalemic acidosis, clinically manifested by nausea, vomiting, anorexia, and muscular weakness. Hyperchloremic/hypokalemic metabolic acidosis can also occur when the ileum or colon is used for the GU reconstruction. In less severe cases, a chronic metabolic acidosis may go undetected, resulting in growth retardation. In one series, 41% of children with bowel segment urinary reconstruction required chronic prophylactic alkaline substitution.[282,281] Thus although acute decompensations may require intravenous correction of the acidosis with bicarbonate or fluid administration, most cases will maintain electrolyte balance with lifelong alkalinization with enteral bicarbonate, sodium citrate, or citric acid solutions.

Treating Metabolic Acidosis

Treatment of metabolic acidosis should focus on the underlying cause. Certain acidoses have specific therapies, such as insulin and fluids for the patient with DKA, NaHCO$_3$ and citrate for patients with the classic distal RTA, and fomepizole for methanol or ethylene glycol intoxication. The following discussion focuses on lactic acidosis, unless otherwise mentioned.

Sodium Bicarbonate

NaHCO$_3$ administration has long been the standard therapy for metabolic acidosis including lactic acidosis.[63,168,251] There is consensus regarding the advantages of alkali and sodium bicarbonate therapy of normal anion gap acidosis. However, in the presence of high anion gap acidosis, especially lactic acidosis (in shock and cardiopulmonary resuscitation) and diabetic acidosis, there is negative safety and efficacy evidence for use of sodium bicarbonate. Justification for the persistent use of bicarbonate comes from a variety of sources, many based more in philosophy than in science.[63,168,172,251,283,284] In agreement with Eqs. 20 and 21, administration of NaHCO$_3$ increases the SID (which tends to raise the pH) because sodium is a strong cation and bicarbonate is a weak anion, but in agreement with Eq. 11, bicarbonate is an anion that rapidly converts to carbonic acid and then to CO_2, which tends to lower the pH.[172,285,286] Therefore NaHCO$_3$ may increase arterial pH if, and only if, alveolar ventilation is adequate.[168,172,283-290] *Paradoxical intracellular acidosis* following bicarbonate administration does not always occur, nor is it always detrimental to the cell.[128,172,286,287] The ultimate effect of NaHCO$_3$ on intracellular pH depends on changes in PCO$_2$ in the medium bathing the cells, which is influenced by the extracellular nonbicarbonate buffering capacity.[286] In addition, bicarbonate administration may promote metabolic reactions that may themselves alter not only PCO$_2$ but also the total concentration of weak acids and the SID. It has been documented that bicarbonate can increase the production of lactic acid in both animals and humans.[172] Mechanisms to explain this reaction remain speculative but include a shift in the oxyhemoglobin-saturation relationship, enhanced anaerobic glycolysis probably mediated by the pH-sensitive enzyme phosphofructokinase, and changes in hepatic blood flow or lactate uptake.[172,214] Clinical experience has confirmed that arterial pH can be raised and even normalized with $NaHCO_3$.[63,168,172,251] However, even when $NaHCO_3$ added to central venous blood reliably elevates the arterial pH, its effect can be erratic at tissue and cellular levels. For example, in the cerebrospinal fluid and intracellular spaces, pH may drop further, without concordance with an already alkalemic arterial blood sample. In fact, in most animal models and in most organs studied to date, including the brain in healthy human volunteers, intracellular pH decreases with bicarbonate administration.[172,185,286,287] Results of human studies examining the impact of bicarbonate administration during cardiopulmonary resuscitation have uniformly shown no benefit in terms of survival and hemodynamic recovery.[168,172,185,285] Accordingly the American Heart Association no longer recommends routine administration of sodium bicarbonate during cardiopulmonary resuscitation. Its use may be considered only after effective ventilation, chest compressions, and epinephrine administration have occurred and for cases in which bicarbonate is a specific therapeutic intervention (eg, hyperkalemia, hypermagnesemia, tricyclic antidepressant poisoning, cocaine cardiac effects, and sodium channel blocker poisoning).[291] Similarly there is also no evidence of benefit with sodium bicarbonate infusion during resuscitation of neonates.[292,293] Reported hemodynamic responses to bicarbonate administration in patients treated with inotropic/vasoactive drug infusions may simply be due to preload augmentation rather than enhanced catecholamine responsiveness.[168,172]

Data suggesting increased mortality with bicarbonate administration continue to appear.[294-296] Even with severe acidosis (pH <7) the role of bicarbonate is unclear, as no reliable argument exists to prove that this acidosis is harmful under these conditions in humans.[211,289,290] However, the 2007 update of the Clinical Practice Parameters for hemodynamic support of pediatric and neonatal septic shock from the American College of Critical Care Medicine[297] stated that sepsis-induced acidosis and hypoxia can increase pulmonary vascular resistance. Although inhaled nitric oxide is the treatment of choice, the committee concluded that metabolic alkalinization remains an important initial resuscitative strategy during shock, as pulmonary hypertension in the setting of septic shock can reverse when acidosis is corrected. A small, adult observational study applied a quantitative acid-base analysis approach to clarify the components of sepsis-associated metabolic acidosis.[298] The study subjects presented with a complex pattern of metabolic acidosis, caused predominantly by hyperchloremic acidosis. Acidosis resolution among survivors was attributable to a decrease in strong ion gap and lactate levels. This study suggested that a subset of sepsis/septic shock patients (those with hyperchloremic acidosis identified by SIG and $AG_{CORRLACT}$) may indeed benefit from sodium bicarbonate administration.

Adverse side effects of $NaHCO_3$ relate to fluid and sodium loads that can cause hypervolemia, hyperosmolarity, and hypernatremia.[283] Given as a rapid intravenous (IV) bolus, $NaHCO_3$ can cause a transient decrease in arterial blood pressure and a transient rise in intracranial pressure, probably related to its hypertonicity.[172] Intravenous bicarbonate administration can cause sudden shifts of several cations through cell membrane–mediated mechanisms. Although advantageous in treating hyperkalemia,[291] this strategy can be dangerous because bicarbonate lowers ionized calcium. Overshoot alkalosis can result from overly aggressive bicarbonate correction.[288-290] If used, the amount of bicarbonate administered should raise the pH up to 7.2.[290]

Salicylate intoxication represents a special setting. Because the risk of death and the severity of neurologic manifestations depend on the concentration of salicylates in the central nervous system, therapy is directed at limiting further drug absorption by administering activated charcoal in the emergency department and promoting the exit of the drug from the cerebral tissue by increasing the alkalinity of the blood, which will also raise urine pH and therefore inhibit salicylate reabsorption by ion trapping (see also Chapters 127 and 128). The target pH of the urine is 7 to 7.5. Hemodialysis is utilized for severe salicylate intoxication, especially that involving renal dysfunction.

If a decision is made to administer $NaHCO_3$, some time-honored clinical clues are valuable. $NaHCO_3$ dose is best estimated using either the SBE or the bicarbonate level derived from PCO_2 measured by the blood gas analyzer:

$$\text{Total body base deficit} = SBE \times \text{body weight (kg)} \times 0.3 \quad (Eq.\ 26)$$

$$HCO_3^- \text{ deficit (mEq)} = 0.3 \times \text{body weight (kg)} \\ \times [HCO_3^- \text{ expected} - HCO_3^- \text{ observed}]$$
$$(Eq.\ 27)$$

Distribution volume of bicarbonate is 30% of the lean body weight. The theoretic distribution volume of $NaHCO_3$ equals the extracellular fluid volume, which grossly represents 60% of the body weight (70% in young infants), and therefore it can be argued that the correct arithmetic factor should be 0.6 rather than 0.3. Experience has shown, however, that as a starting point, bicarbonate or SBE correction with 0.3 ("half correction") will suffice in most cases and will avoid unnecessary risks from an excessive load of solutes and fluid as well as the overshoot alkalemia.

Alternative Alkalinizing Agents

Concern about the CO_2-producing effect of bicarbonate led to the development of carbicarb, which consists of equimolar concentrations of sodium bicarbonate ($NaHCO_3$) and sodium carbonate (Na_2CO_3).[168,222,299,300] Carbicarb raises the SID and thus increases the pH far more than bicarbonate, with much less rise in PCO_2. Risks of hypervolemia and hypertonicity are similar to those of bicarbonate. Although carbicarb more consistently increases intracellular pH, studies of its effects on hemodynamics have yielded conflicting results.[222] Carbicarb is not currently available for clinical use, pending further clinical research.

THAM (tris[hydroxymethyl]aminomethane), also known as tromethamine and tris-buffer, is an amino alcohol that behaves as a weak base (pK_a 7.8). It exists in neutral form at physiologic pH. Protonated THAM is excreted by the kidneys.[301] It crosses lipid membranes and penetrates cells easily. Therefore it has the potential to raise both intracellular and central nervous system pH. In addition, THAM's buffering action occurs without producing CO_2 and thus is not dependent on pulmonary function.[302] Even though THAM has been commercially available for several decades, there are few studies establishing its clinical efficacy. In animal models, THAM incompletely buffered metabolic acidosis but significantly improved contractility and relaxation in an isolated rabbit heart model.[168] A small adult ICU study showed that THAM had an equivalent but shorter-lasting alkalinizing effect in comparison to that of bicarbonate, but it produced no decrease in potassium and did not increase sodium.[303] A paucity of clinical information and the report of several serious side effects, including hyperkalemia, hypoglycemia, local extravasation injury, and hepatic necrosis in neonates, have limited its widespread clinical use.

Of particular relevance for lactic acidosis is dichloroacetate (DCA), a simple compound that reduces plasma lactic acid concentration. DCA is not a buffer but a stimulator of pyruvate dehydrogenase, the enzyme that catalyzes the oxidation of pyruvate to acetylcoenzyme A (CoA), facilitating its entry to the Krebs cycle and thus decreasing lactate production and promoting the clearance of accumulated lactate.[168,304] In addition, DCA promotes myocardial glucose utilization and contractility. Initial data from both children and adults were promising,[286] but a large controlled clinical trial in adults with severe lactic acidosis showed that DCA treatment resulted in statistically significant but clinically unimportant changes in arterial blood lactate concentrations and pH. It also failed to alter hemodynamics or survival. Renewed interest in DCA has arisen from its potential applications for attenuating lactic acidosis in certain congenital errors of metabolism[305] and lactic acidosis due to severe malaria in children.[306]

Dialysis Management of Metabolic Acidosis

Dialytic procedures may be indicated in some cases of metabolic acidosis that are refractory to bicarbonate or in cases in which there are serious limitations in the amount of fluid or sodium load that can be administered to the patient, a common situation in the pediatric critical care unit (see also Chapter 78). Uncompensated metabolic acidosis (pH <7.1) remains one of the acknowledged criteria for the initiation of renal replacement therapy in the pediatric ICU.[284] Peritoneal dialysis is often not the best choice, particularly in lactic acidosis associated with hypoperfusion. In this setting the hypoperfused peritoneal membranes may not be efficient for supporting enough peritoneal flux, and the increase in intraabdominal pressure may contribute to a further drop of cardiac output. If peritoneal dialysis is chosen, bicarbonate-buffered peritoneal dialysis solution provides some advantages over the conventional lactate-buffered peritoneal dialysis solution in terms of both pH control and mesothelial cell preservation. Most critically ill patients lack the hemodynamic stability to tolerate intermittent hemodialysis. Hemofiltration and hemodiafiltration are better options. Acute renal replacement therapy may be needed for critically ill patients with metabolic acidosis that is multifactorial in origin. Once continuous hemofiltration is started, it becomes the dominant force in controlling metabolic acid-base status and profound changes are rapidly achieved. The result is the progressive resolution of acidemia and acidosis, with lowering concentrations of phosphate and unmeasured anions. Hemofiltration techniques replace plasma water, which is low in bicarbonate concentration and has decreased SID, with a solution that contains an above-normal sodium bicarbonate (or lactate or

acetate) concentration. Such weak anions free their sodium (which increases SID), buffer hydrogen ions, and then are transformed into CO_2 (lactate and acetate must convert first to bicarbonate in the liver), which is removed by ventilation. This exchange contributes to the correction of acidosis, along with the increase in SID through the sodium contribution. If these oxidizable anions are not fully extracted and metabolized by the liver, they accumulate in plasma and their ability to correct acidosis is lost, as they fail to increase the SID.

Metabolic Alkalosis

Metabolic alkalosis is defined as an elevation of plasma HCO_3^- with an arterial pH above 7.45. There is no accurate estimate of the incidence or prevalence of metabolic alkalosis. However, in the critical care setting, it is estimated that metabolic alkalosis is the more common form of acid-base disorder, as it may be present in about 50% of all acid-base disorders. A study in pediatric patients undergoing open-heart surgery found that 72% of children younger than 12 months of age developed metabolic alkalosis, in contrast with 30% of those older than 12 months of age. It is difficult to attribute a figure of mortality or morbidity directly to metabolic alkalosis. However, at least one study in adults found that mortality progressively rose with the pH: 47% with pH 7.57 to 7.59, 65% with pH 7.60 to 7.64, and 80% with pH 7.65 to 7.70.[307,308] An increased incidence of metabolic alkalosis in patients with severe sepsis and trauma is due to factors related to a vigorous correction of shock, hypotension, and acidosis, where large quantities of citrated blood or lactated Ringer solution are given, as well as the administration of bicarbonate itself[307] (Table 76.9). Other subsets of patients may arrive to the PICU with preexisting metabolic alkalosis associated with the chronic use of diuretics, excessive exogenous or endogenous steroids, high-dose antacids, elevated gastrointestinal fluid losses (emesis, suction, or chloride-rich diarrhea), and a posthypercapnic state, the typical pattern of a chronic lung disease after the resolution of an acute episode of decompensation.[308,309] Alkalemia has been classified as mild (pH 7.45-7.50), moderate (pH 7.50-7.55), or severe (pH >7.55).[307]

According to the physicochemical approach, metabolic alkalosis results from an increase in SID, or a decrease in A_{TOT}, due to a lost of anions (Cl$^-$ from the digestive tract or through the kidneys, albumin from the plasma) or rarely to an excess of cations.[199] In the classic approach to acid-base derangements, metabolic alkalosis is generated by net gain of base (primarily bicarbonate) or loss of nonvolatile acid from the extracellular fluid.[63,310] The excess of base may be gained through oral or parenteral bicarbonate administration or by the administration of other weak anions such as lactate, acetate, or citrate. Actually, however, it is the gain of strong cations (mainly sodium) that causes pH to increase. The acid deficit may be due to the hydrochloric acid loss by vomiting or enhanced renal acid excretion promoted by diuretics or aldosterone excess and is often accompanied by hypochloremia and hypokalemia.[307-309] In a similar way, it is the loss of strong anions (mainly chloride) rather than the direct loss of hydrogen ions that actually increases pH. There may also be a concurrent contraction of the extracellular fluid volume secondary to the chloride loss. Concomitant changes in the intracellular fluid do occur, including a loss of intracellular potassium along with a net gain of sodium and hydrogen.

TABLE 76.9 Causes of Respiratory Acid-Base Derangements

Acidosis (↑ PaCO₂)	Alkalosis (↓ PaCO₂)
Central nervous system depression: Severe head trauma, brain edema, metabolic diseases, infectious diseases, intentional sedation, pharmacologic effect of drugs	**Hypoxemia:** High altitudes, pulmonary disease
Neural (peripheral), muscular, and skeletal structures:	**Pulmonary disorders:** Pneumonia, interstitial pneumonitis, fibrosis, edema, pulmonary embolism, vascular disease, bronchial asthma, pneumothorax
Electrolyte disturbances: hypophosphatemia, hypokalemia	**Cardiovascular disorders** Congestive heart failure, hypotension
Specific diseases: myasthenia gravis, Guillain-Barré syndrome, spinal cord injury, Werdnig-Hoffmann disease, Duchenne muscular dystrophy, etc.	**Metabolic disorders:** Acidosis (diabetic, renal, or lactic), hepatic failure
Ventilatory restriction: rib fractures and flail chest, patients with intraabdominal hypertension from ascites, from closure of congenital abdominal wall defects, etc.	**Central nervous system disorders:** Psychogenic or anxiety-induced hyperventilation, central nervous system infection, central nervous system tumors
Lungs (airway and alveoli):	**Drugs:** Salicylates, methylxanthines, β-adrenergic agonists, progesterone
Respiratory obstructive disease, either acute or chronic: croup, asthma, bronchiolitis, bronchopulmonary dysplasia	**Miscellaneous:** Fever, sepsis, pain, pregnancy
Alveolar injury: pneumonia, acute lung injury, acute respiratory distress syndrome, cardiogenic pulmonary edema	

Hence metabolic alkalosis in the extracellular fluid is usually accompanied by acidosis and potassium depletion in the intracellular compartment. Bicarbonate or base loading is rarely the single cause of metabolic alkalosis, although this may transiently occur after an IV infusion of NaHCO₃ or an equivalent base (eg, citrate anticoagulant in transfused packed red blood cells). This situation may also occur after the successful treatment of ketoacidosis or lactic acidosis, because these organic anions are metabolized to bicarbonate, and after the resolution of hypercapnia, either permissive or as a part of unintentional respiratory acidosis, before the kidney can excrete the bicarbonate previously retained for compensation. It is generally accepted that metabolic alkalosis involves a *generative* stage, during which the relative concentration of alkali within the body increases, and a *maintenance* stage,[308,309] during which the kidneys fail to compensate by excreting strong cations and HCO₃⁻. Three major factors underlie the maintenance phase in most clinical situations: (1) depletion of circulating volume, changes in generalized hemodynamics (eg, heart failure) and in intrarenal hemodynamics, which combine to reduce the filtered load of bicarbonate traversing the proximal tubule despite the increase in bicarbonate concentration; (2) increased aldosterone secretion (and probably endothelin-1), due to volume contraction and increased angiotensin-II, that stimulates acid secretion; and (3) total

potassium depletion and hypokalemia, which alter glomerular hemodynamics, stimulate the renal H⁺-K⁺-ATPase, and secondarily increase renal acid secretion in the presence of aldosterone.[310] In other words, the regulation of pH through strong cation (mainly sodium) and bicarbonate elimination is sacrificed to preserve volume and potassium stores. If volume and potassium are normalized, metabolic alkalosis self-corrects.

Metabolic alkalosis has been classified by the primary organ system involved, the response to therapy, or the underlying disease.[309,311] In the critical care setting it may be more convenient to classify it according to the response to therapy and to use the serum chloride concentration as the key variable for this classification.[29,44,89,63,199] Sometimes the loss of Cl⁻ is temporary and can be treated effectively by replacing it; this type of metabolic alkalosis is known as *chloride responsive.* It represents the most frequently encountered metabolic alkalosis in the pediatric critical care unit that is also the most severe.[307-311] These disorders are usually the result of Cl⁻ losses from gastric drainage or persisting vomiting, as in pyloric hypertrophy and other causes of upper gastrointestinal obstruction.[29,161,307-309] This type of metabolic acidosis also may occur as a consequence of the administration of diuretics.[44] Both persisting vomiting and excessive diuretics generate some degree of dehydration, with volume contraction and secondary stimulation of aldosterone release, which in turn leads to increased tubular Na⁺ reabsorption, an alkalinizing process, because it increases the SID, and to increased urinary loss of K⁺, which may result in hypokalemia.[309]

In other cases, hormonal mechanisms leading to an excess of mineralocorticoid activity directly produce ongoing losses of K⁺ and Cl⁻, or such a loss is associated with genetic renal tubular defects of electrolyte transport, mainly in chloride reabsorption. Decreased plasma levels of Cl⁻ and K⁺ lead to an increased SID, which in turn yields metabolic alkalosis. In this setting, the Cl⁻ deficit can be offset only temporarily, at best, by Cl⁻ administration. Therefore this form of metabolic alkalosis is said to be *chloride resistant*[29,44,63,199,307-311] (see Table 76.9). The hallmark of this group of disorders is an increased urine Cl⁻ concentration, more than 20 mEq/L (usually >40 mEq/L).[307-311] Treatment requires a search for the underlying disorder and, if possible, a specific therapeutic intervention. Among the most important causes of chloride-resistant disorders are (1) the group of diseases with mineralocorticoid excess, which includes primary and secondary aldosteronism, congenital adrenal hyperplasia renin-secreting tumors, and Cushing syndrome; (2) the group of tubulopathies, including chloride wasting tubulopathies (Bartter and Gitelman syndromes) and a defective epithelial sodium channel (ENaC) leading to a decreased sodium elimination (Liddle syndrome); (3) the group of drug-induced hypokalemic alkaloses including diuretics, high-dose glucocorticoids, fludrocortisone, aminoglycosides, and the toxic effects of licorice *(Glycyrrhiza glabra);* and (4) the miscellaneous group, which includes 11β-hydroxylase deficiency, salt-losing nephropathy, cystic fibrosis, and congenital chloride diarrhea, among others.[161,308-315]

Random urine chloride determination may useful: uCl⁻ <20 mEq/L is consistent with chloride-responsive metabolic alkalosis; uCl⁻ >20 mEq/L is consistent with chloride-unresponsive metabolic alkalosis.[308-313] However, this general rule may not apply to other special causes of metabolic alkalosis, which include the extrarenal chloride-resistant forms, such as cystic fibrosis,[314] and congenital chloride diarrhea, a recessively inherited disorder of chloride transport in the distal ileum and colon.[315] In both disorders a huge extrarenal chloride loss occurs (through sweat or diarrhea), and urine chloride may be low, normal, or high, depending on the patient's renal function and the clinical situation. Finally, metabolic alkalosis may occur as the SID increases as a consequence of the gain of cations rather than strong anion depletion. The most common clinical situation in the critical care setting is the IV administration of strong cations without strong anions, such as occurs with a massive blood transfusion. In this case, sodium is administered predominantly with citrate (a weak anion) instead of chloride. A similar mechanism of metabolic alkalosis occurs when the parenteral nutrition contains excess sodium acetate (another weak anion) and insufficient chloride to balance the sodium load. The excessive infusion of some gelatins used as plasma volume expanders and sodium lactate (as in Ringer solution) can also cause metabolic alkalosis. The milk-alkali syndrome is now a rare cause of this disorder.

Treating Metabolic Alkalosis

Alkalosis and alkalemia are important because they may increase morbidity and mortality. An increase in blood pH increases neuromuscular excitability, probably related to a decrease in ionized calcium concentration and potassium shifts, leading to an alteration of consciousness, increased seizure activity, increased cardiac arrhythmias, decreased oxygen release to tissue from hemoglobin, tetany secondary to hypocalcemia, increased ammonia generation by the kidney, and, in some instances, depression of ventilatory drive. Because mortality is especially high when a pH in excess of 7.6 develops, intervention at a pH of 7.55 and greater is recommended.[307,310] Regardless of the type of metabolic alkalosis, the first step for its proper management is to moderate or stop the process that generated the problem, even if only temporarily.[307] For example, if continuation of gastric drainage is required, the loss of gastric fluid can be reduced though the administration of H_2 receptor blockers or inhibitors of the gastric H^+/K^+-ATPase. If it is not possible to withdraw diuretics, it may be possible to use potassium-sparing compounds (eg, spironolactone or amiloride), which decrease distal tubule acidification and curtail potassium excretion. The administration of bicarbonate or its precursors such as lactate, citrate, and acetate should be discontinued. If drugs with mineralocorticoid activity are being administered, their indication and dose should be reassessed.

Up to 10% of the total bicarbonate filtered is reabsorbed or lost to urine in the distal renal tubule. In most patients with metabolic alkalosis, extracellular fluid, together with chloride, potassium, and magnesium concentrations, is decreased. Hence the blood flow to the kidneys is also decreased, and secretion of both aldosterone and endothelin-1 is stimulated, bicarbonate urine loss is reduced, chloride wasting increases, and urinary hydrogen ions and potassium are reduced even more. Because potassium, chloride, and magnesium concentrations limit bicarbonate excretion, their low concentrations will make metabolic alkalosis refractory to correction. Thus the restoration of circulating volume and electrolyte composition will allow renal excretion of bicarbonate and the correction of metabolic alkalosis.[307] Or in accordance with the physicochemical approach, it really does not matter if

bicarbonate excretion is enhanced, but it is the replacement of Cl^- that corrects the increased SID.[199] Saline plus KCl infusion is usually the best choice because of the typical coexisting volume depletion and hypokalemia. The administration of normal saline is effective despite the release of equal amounts of Na^+ and Cl^- because this results in larger relative increases in Cl^- concentration compared with Na^+ concentration. Patients who have developed metabolic alkalosis as a result of the effects of diuretics will be best treated by the provision of potassium chloride, because their previous treatments have rendered them potassium depleted. For renal failure patients, decreasing or adjusting the diuretic regimen, adding acetazolamide (a carbonic anhydrase enzyme inhibitor that enhances renal sodium bicarbonate loss, increasing urinary SID and decreasing blood SID),[279] and cautiously administering NaCl and potassium chloride may suffice.[307] If the pace of correction of the alkalemia needs to be accelerated, hydrochloric acid (HCl) can be infused intravenously as a 0.1 to 0.2 N solution (ie, 100-200 mmol/L of H^+). This intervention, which is rarely needed, is safe and effective for the symptomatic rapid relief of severe metabolic alkalosis. Because of its sclerosing properties and its hyperosmotic concentration, HCl must be infused through a central venous line at an infusion rate of no more than 0.2 mmol/kg/h up to 20 to 50 mmol/h,[307] with arterial pH monitoring every hour. Calculation of the amount of HCl solution to be infused is based on a distribution volume equivalent to 30% of the body weight. Thus the HCl dosage can be calculated with either the SBE or the bicarbonate difference in a manner similar to the bicarbonate administration formula (Eq. 26 and 27):

$$Total\ body\ BE = SBE \times body\ weight\ (kg) \times 0.3 \quad (Eq.\ 28A)$$

$$HCO_3^-\ ``excess"\ (mEq) = 0.3 \times body\ weight\ (kg)$$
$$\times [HCO_3^-\ observed - HCO_3^-\ desired]$$
$$(Eq.\ 28B)$$

In both formulas, the result is expressed in millimoles of HCl to be administered. If this intervention is contraindicated, not effective, or not available, and the alkalemia is severe with no hope of quick control, hemodialysis or hemodiafiltration can rapidly correct severe alkalemia and volume overload, but a dialysis solution low in lactate or bicarbonate must be used to prevent worsening of the alkalemia. The only specific treatment available to date for Liddle syndrome is a decreased dietary sodium intake or a sodium channel blocker, such as amiloride or triamterene.[310]

Respiratory Acid-Base Derangements

Although the underlying pathologic process may vary, the respiratory acid-base derangements always have the same mechanism: Alveolar ventilation is increased or decreased out of proportion to CO_2 production. CO_2 arises either from the cellular metabolism or by the titration of HCO_3^- by metabolic acids. Normal CO_2 production by the body (and its excretion by the lungs) is impressive: about 220 mL/min or about 317 L/day in a 70-kg adult, which is equivalent to 15,000 mmol of carbonic acid per day, compared with the 500 mmol/day of all nonrespiratory acids that are handled by the kidneys and gut.[44] Pulmonary ventilation is adjusted by the respiratory center in the brain stem in response to changes in $PaCO_2$, pH, and PaO_2, although respiratory drive can be influenced by other neural (anxiety, wakefulness) and non-neural factors (eg, exercise, muscle strength) and also can be altered in some pathologic situations (cystic fibrosis, asthma, and congenital central hypoventilation syndrome).[316] A precise and real-time match of alveolar minute ventilation to CO_2 production allows stable $PaCO_2$ levels of 35 to 45 mm Hg at sea level. Accuracy of the central control allows the body to adjust PaO_2 in compensation for alterations in arterial pH produced by metabolic acidosis or alkalosis in predictable ways (see Tables 76.2 and 76.3). When this normal respiratory system is disrupted or overwhelmed, $PaCO_2$ deviates from normal and respiratory acid-base disturbances are initiated. Respiratory acidosis is produced by CO_2 retention leading to hypercapnia (elevation of $PaCO_2$). Respiratory alkalosis is produced by hyperventilation, leading to a drop in $PaCO_2$ (ie, hypocapnia). As soon as $PaCO_2$ increases or decreases, plasma and intracellular buffers change their dissociation to maintain a stable pH, the effect of which is fully manifested within 15 to 30 minutes. If the alteration in $PaCO_2$ is sustained for more than 6 hours, renal mechanisms induce far larger changes in bicarbonate concentration, reaching maximal impact within 3 to 5 days. These renal effects lead to a new steady state for the pH. The two responses to the primary alterations in $PaCO_2$, plasma plus tissue buffers and the renal response, permit description of the respiratory acid-base derangements into acute and chronic phases.[44,63,19]

Respiratory Acidosis

Respiratory acidosis occurs whenever the CO_2 elimination by the lungs is lower than the CO_2 production by the tissues, resulting in a positive balance of CO_2, which in turn increases $PaCO_2$ to a new equilibrium. Because the increase in CO_2 production alone is not sufficient to overcome the normal ability of the lungs to increase alveolar ventilation,[44,63,199] what is central to all forms of respiratory acidosis is a failure of alveolar ventilation and CO_2 excretion to increase in response to a rising $PaCO_2$. However, an increase in CO_2 production in the face of fixed ventilation can result in respiratory acidosis and may occur in the critical care setting in patients receiving mechanical hypoventilation and a high carbohydrates load in their parenteral nutrition or in a hypoventilated patient with fever-induced acute hypermetabolism. The increase in $PaCO_2$ immediately increases both the hydrogen ion and bicarbonate concentrations in blood (Eqs. 11 to 13). The increase in [HCO_3^-] occurs as a consequence of physical chemical principles and not as a consequence of an adaptive response in order to *buffer* the increase in [H^+].[21,29,61] The only immediate buffering activity in hypercapnia comes from the nonbicarbonate plasma and intracellular buffers.[286] Because of the increase in bicarbonate (a weak anion), no change in the SID is produced, and thus no change occurs in the SBE. Because CO_2 is produced within the cells and can freely diffuse across the lipophilic cellular membranes, intracellular acidosis always occurs with respiratory acidosis.[286,287] If the $PaCO_2$ remains increased, active compensatory mechanisms are activated, and the SID increases to restore [H^+] toward normal. Primarily, respiratory acidemia compensation is accomplished by removal of Cl^- from the plasma space. Because movement of Cl^- into the tissues or red blood cells results in a drop of intracellular pH, Cl^- must be removed from the body to achieve a lasting effect on the SID. The kidneys are the most important organs for this task. Because every chloride ion that

is filtered and not reabsorbed increases the SID (and the pH), Cl^- removal by the kidney must be accurate. Again the role of ammonium in this process is preeminent, not as a hydrogen ion carrier or as a potential buffer but as a cation for the excretion of Cl^- without losing Na^+ or K.[29,96] Thus when renal function is intact, Cl^- is eliminated in the urine, and after a few days, the SID increases to the level necessary to return blood pH near 7.35. This amount of time is required by the physiologic constraints of the system, but this is not entirely a disadvantage because this rate of response is useful to avoid being oversensitive to transient changes in alveolar ventilation. In any case, the compensation results in an increased pH for any degree of hypercarbia. According to the Henderson-Hasselbalch equation (Eqs. 12 and 13), the increased pH will result in an increased HCO_3^- concentration for a given PCO_2. Therefore the so-called adaptive increase in [HCO_3^-] to hypercapnia actually results *from* the increase in pH, and it *is not the cause of* the increase in the pH, which actually occurred from the increase in the SID as a consequence of the removal of chloride. Although the change in HCO_3^- concentration is a convenient and reliable marker for the metabolic compensation (Tables 61.2 and 61.3), it is not the mechanism.

Acute respiratory acidosis develops as a consequence of the impaired function of one or more of the three participants in the ventilatory function: central nervous system; neural (peripheral), muscular, and skeletal structures; and lungs (airway and alveoli) (see also Chapters 45 and 47). Airway and parenchymal lung disease are the most common causes of acute CO_2 retention. This last group of conditions also produces primary hypoxemia, not only hypercapnia. It is hypoxemia, not hypercapnia or acidemia, that poses the principal threat to life. Conditions that cause the failure of the lungs to eliminate CO_2 can also be grouped into two types of ventilatory disorders.[44,63,199] The first or "pure" hypoventilation occurs as a result of brain stem or neuromuscular dysfunction or because of extrapulmonary restrictive lung compromise. In this setting, the lung simply fails to move enough air in and out to exchange CO_2 and oxygen. As a result, PaO_2 falls in proportion to the rise in $PaCO_2$. In the second and more common situation in the critical care setting, alveolar hypoventilation is the result of the imbalance between perfused and hypoventilated segments of a damaged lung (ie, ventilation-perfusion [V/Q] inequality) (see also Chapter 48). In this case, a fall in PaO_2 often precedes hypercapnia, and when hypercapnia finally develops, the reduction in PaO_2 is proportionally greater than the rise in $PaCO_2$. With both types of ventilatory defects, however, hypoxemia is a concurrent finding when hypercapnia is present.[44]

Chronic respiratory acidosis is most often associated with chronic lung disease (eg, bronchopulmonary dysplasia) or chest diseases with abnormal chest wall mechanics (chest congenital deformities, kyphoscoliosis), but it can also be caused by chronic upper airway obstruction (eg, obstructive sleep apnea syndrome and craniofacial disorders),[316] chronic neuromuscular diseases, or chronic central nervous system problems (congenital central hypoventilation syndrome).[317] Respiratory decompensation in patients with these conditions usually results from recently acquired infection, use of narcotics, or uncontrolled oxygen therapy.[318] These additional factors superimpose an acute element of CO_2 retention and acidemia on the already elevated baseline CO_2. Progressive narcosis and coma (ie, hypercapnic encephalopathy) may ensue. On the basis of the preeminent renal participation in the ultimate compensation of hypercapnia, one should expect that patients with renal disease (with difficulties excreting chloride) will have a defective adaptation to chronic hypercapnia.

Treating Respiratory Acidosis

As the main threat to life in respiratory acidosis comes from associated hypoxemia, and not from the level of hypercapnia or acidemia, oxygen administration represents a critical element in the management of respiratory acidosis. Caution must be taken when uncontrolled concentrations of oxygen are administered to some patients with hypercarbia, particularly those with chronic lung disease, in whom exaggerated oxygen supplementation could depress respiratory drive and provoke a further increase in $PaCO_2$.[318] This occurs because chronic hypercapnia is thought to down regulate CO_2 chemoreceptor sensitivity, which means that these patients are more dependent on hypoxic drive to maintain adequate spontaneous ventilation. It should be emphasized, however, that the correction of hypoxia overrides strategies to avert oxygen-related hypercapnia, which normally tends to be of small clinical significance in children. Whenever feasible, treatment of hypoventilation must be directed to the underlying cause. Sometimes it is possible to solve the primary cause of hypoventilation rather quickly (eg, relief of obstruction from croup with racemic epinephrine, reversal of narcotics with naloxone, or resolution of bronchial spasm with a β_2 agonist). Generally speaking, mechanical ventilation is indicated when the patient is at risk of instability, the patient is already unstable, or central nervous system function is deteriorating.[319] It is not the absolute value of $PaCO_2$ (or PaO_2) that is important but rather the clinical condition and perceived trajectory of the patient. If the patient is obtunded or unable to cough and if hypercapnia and acidemia are worsening, mechanical ventilation should be instituted. Application of noninvasive mechanical ventilation in children is growing both in acute situations within the ICU and in cases of chronic hypercapnic and hypoxemic respiratory failure of various causes.[320] When $PaCO_2$ is increased and minute ventilation is low, level of consciousness is generally impaired. These patients usually require intubation for airway protection in addition to ventilatory assistance, unless the hypercapnia can be quickly reversed.[321] Hypoxemia is treated with FiO_2 augmentation and recruitment of airspaces, whereas the usual ventilatory strategy for hypercapnia is to increase minute ventilation. When the ventilator is used to correct respiratory acidosis, the end-inspiratory plateau and auto-PEEP pressures should be monitored routinely to detect any adverse effects of hyperventilation. Overly rapid reduction in the $PaCO_2$ risks development of *posthypercapnic alkalosis,* with potentially serious consequences. One possible option not yet routinely available for intractable hypercapnia is intratracheal pulmonary ventilation, in which an intratracheal catheter with a reversed continuous flow of gas at its tip (away from the lungs) facilitates flushing CO_2 from the proximal dead space.[322] Another possible approach is the extracorporeal removal of CO_2 (see also Chapter 59).[323]

Permissive hypercapnia may be indicated in patients with severe ARDS to minimize ventilator-associated lung injury (see also Chapters 51 and 57).[173,324] Use of permissive hypercapnia as part of a lung-protective strategy in children should be utilized, provided it does not result in significant hemodynamic instability or there is a coexisting contraindication,

such as intracranial hypertension.[324,325] It has been suggested that hypercapnia be targeted to maintain pH >7.2,[324] and this strategy appears to be safe for any age.[324-330]

In adult patients undergoing permissive hypercapnia, a pH well below 7.2 has been tolerated.[329] In terms of the limits of hypercarbia in otherwise healthy children, even transient $PaCO_2$ in the range of 200 to 300 has been tolerated without long-term sequellae.[176,331] This might not be the case for a critically ill child with multiple system involvement, particularly brain injury.[332]

Animal studies have demonstrated hypercarbic acidosis may protect against lung and systemic injury, even when instituted after the initiation of the lung or systemic injury process.[325,329] The mechanism involving inhibition of cytokine and chemokine production seems to be mediated, at least partially, through the inhibition of nuclear factor-κB (NFκB).[325,329,333] Hypercapnic acidosis also appears to inhibit repair of pulmonary epithelial injury.[333-336]

There is evidence that the protective effects of hypercarbic acidosis in acute lung injury are more a function of the acidosis rather than of elevated carbon dioxide *per se.*[337-339] In a recent and elegantly designed animal experiment,[340] it was found that moderate hypercapnia ($PaCO_2$ 80-100 mm Hg, pH 7.13 ± 0.09) was neuroprotective after transient global cerebral ischemia/reperfusion injury. The protective effect was attributed to the modulation of apoptosis-regulating proteins. In contrast, severe hypercapnia ($PaCO_2$ 100-120 mm Hg, pH 7.05 ± 0.1) was associated with increased brain injury. These results suggest a potential role for "therapeutic hypercapnic acidosis" after global cerebral ischemia, a potential paradigmatic therapeutic change.

Respiratory Alkalosis

If alveolar ventilation rises out of proportion to CO_2 production, then $PaCO_2$ falls. For any given rate of CO_2 production, an increase in alveolar ventilation always reduces $PaCO_2$. In the ICU environment, hyperventilation occurs in a number of pathologic conditions, including salicylate intoxication, early sepsis, hypoxic respiratory disorders including early phase of ARDS, Kussmaul respiration, hepatic failure, fever, certain central nervous system alterations, and pain or anxiety. The presence of respiratory alkalosis is a bad prognostic sign because mortality increases in direct proportion to the severity of the hypocapnia.[341] The detrimental effects of hypocapnia have been described in many settings: in premature infants in whom it has been associated with poor neurologic outcome; in children after severe traumatic brain injury, in whom a relationship between hypocapnia and cerebral ischemia and infarcts have been described[341]; and in children after a cardiopulmonary bypass procedure.[342]

As in acute respiratory acidosis, acute respiratory alkalosis elicits a secondary change in plasma bicarbonate that has two components. The first is the occurrence of a small to moderate acute decrease in the bicarbonate concentration; this fall is dictated by the Henderson-Hasselbalch equation (Eqs. 12 and 13) and is also due to some tissue buffering.[29,341,343] With the persistence of the hypocapnia, the second component appears: SID will begin to decrease as a result of renal chloride reabsorption, which is associated with a larger decrease of bicarbonate and a rise in urine pH.[5,9,10,21,35,44] By 48 to 72 hours, SID assumes a new, lower, steady state. This occurs because renal adaptation to hypocapnia *backtitrates* the nonbicarbonate buffers, an action that decreases SID and tends to return pH toward normal values, usually with an increased chloride serum concentration.[21] Usually, blood pH does not exceed 7.55 in most cases of respiratory alkalosis, and severe manifestations of alkalemia are unusual. Marked alkalemia can occur in certain circumstances: inappropriate mechanical ventilation parameters, central nervous system disorders, and some psychiatric diseases, not often seen in children.

Pseudorespiratory Alkalosis

Arterial hypocapnia does not necessarily imply respiratory alkalosis or the secondary and compensatory response to metabolic acidosis. The presence of arterial hypocapnia in patients with profound circulatory shock has been termed *pseudorespiratory alkalosis,* or simply *venoarterial carbon dioxide gradient.*[185] This condition can be seen when alveolar ventilation is relatively preserved but profound cardiovascular depression exists. In such conditions, the severely reduced pulmonary blood flow limits the CO_2 delivered to the lungs for its excretion. On the other hand, the increased ratio of ventilation to perfusion and the increased pulmonary transit time result in the removal of a larger-than-normal amount of CO_2 per unit of blood traversing the pulmonary circulation.[344] Thus despite decreased CO_2 delivery to the lungs, a situation that provokes a significant elevation of the mixed venous blood CO_2, arterial normocapnia or frank hypocapnia may be noted. Overall, CO_2 excretion is markedly decreased, however, and the CO_2 balance of the body is positive, a phenomenon that is the hallmark of respiratory acidosis. Marked tissue acidosis is reflected in mixed venous blood acidemia, usually involving both metabolic and respiratory components. The metabolic component derives from tissue hypoperfusion and hyperlactatemia. This is accompanied by an arterial pH that ranges from mildly acidic to frankly alkaline. This venous-arterial PCO_2 gradient increases as cardiac index decreases.[185,344,345] In animal models, both venous-arterial PCO_2 gradient and venous-arterial pH difference increase as oxygen delivery declines. In septic shock, an elevated venous-arterial PCO_2 gradient is seen in patients with low cardiac output and in those with pulmonary disease who cannot eliminate CO_2.[346] In patients with cardiogenic and septic shock, the venous-arterial PCO_2 gradient decreases as hemodynamic variables improve.

Mixed Acid-Base Derangements

Coexisting metabolic acidosis and respiratory acidosis can be seen in cardiopulmonary arrest, bronchopulmonary dysplasia complicated with pneumonia and septic shock, renal and pulmonary insufficiency, and as a consequence of certain toxic agents that may provoke both neural depression (and hypoventilation) and cardiocirculatory collapse (and metabolic acidosis).[44,63,90,95,199] As usual, treatment must be targeted to the underlying causes. In addition, both components of the acid-based derangement must be addressed.

Alkalemia of both metabolic and respiratory origin may occur in several complex settings, such as in patients with chronic liver disease in whom hyperventilation ensues as the initial manifestation of pneumonia.[347] This hypocapnia appears in a patient in whom metabolic alkalosis is common because of vomiting or gastric drainage, hypokalemia, diuretics, or alkali administration.[90,347] Mixed alkalosis may also

occur in patients with chronic renal insufficiency in whom primary hypocapnia develops. In this setting, inappropriately high plasma bicarbonate levels occur as a consequence of the nonexistent renal adaptive response. This situation is seen despite the patient's dialysis program because the dialytic procedures are an alkalinizing influence and are much less effective in compensating alkalemia than acidemia.[348,349] This effect can be minimized by switching the patient from peritoneal dialysis to hemodiafiltration or hemodialysis.

Both the physicochemical (SIG and SID_{EFF}) and the modified SBE approaches are well suited for unmasking coexisting, mixed acid-base disorders.

Acid-Base Balance in Special Situations: Hypothermia

Systemic hypothermia is one of the strategies employed for brain preservation and end-organ protection in global ischemia scenarios. Hypothermia is routinely applied in cardiopulmonary bypass for cardiac surgery, and thus anesthesiologists deal with most acid-base derangements during profound hypothermia in the operating room (see also Chapter 37).[350] Hypothermia can occur accidentally after near-drowning in ice water or other environmental exposures. As temperature decreases, $[H^+]$ decreases and pH increases in aqueous systems. Hence the measured pH in an electrochemically neutral cell at 37°C is 7.4, whereas in an electrochemically neutral cell at 20°C, the measured pH will be 7.8. Changes in cellular pH during hypothermia are mediated through PCO_2 homeostasis. As temperature decreases, the solubility of CO_2 in blood increases, which in turn reduces PCO_2. For example, if the total CO_2 content is held constant, and the measured PCO_2 at 37°C is 40 mm Hg, then the measured PCO_2 at 20°C will be 16 mm Hg. When a blood sample is introduced into a blood-gas analyzer, the sample is warmed to 37°C before measurement. The values obtained at 37°C are called the *temperature-uncorrected* values. These values are converted by the blood-gas analyzer to *temperature-corrected* values (actual patient's temperature) using a nomogram, which accounts for temperature-induced changes in pH, and in O_2 and CO_2 solubility. If pH and PCO_2 are measured at 37°C and then corrected to a lower temperature, the corrected pH will be higher and the corrected PCO_2 will be lower than the values at 37°C.

Alpha-stat and *pH-stat* are acid-base management methods that directly influence blood flow to the brain and other organs, and they both can be applied using either corrected or uncorrected blood gases. At a patient temperature of 37°C, there is no difference between alpha-stat and pH-stat management. The difference between these two strategies becomes apparent as patient temperature progressively decreases below 37°C and is not clinically relevant until patient temperature is around 30°C and below. Alpha-stat strategy has solid theoretic foundations. It is well known that functions of proteins are critically dependent on their tertiary and quaternary structures, which in turn depend on the ionic charges of individual amino acid constituents. Thus intracellular proteins must have a buffer of their own in order to keep a constant ionizing state in spite of pH change. The imidazole moiety of the amino acid histidine has a pK_a that is similar to the pK_a of the water, and hence it undergoes ionization with temperature changes in a similar proportion as water. The portion of the histidine imidazole group that loses a proton, acting as a buffer to maintain electrical neutrality, is designated alpha-imidazole. Thus whereas changes in temperature will affect the degree of dissociation (ie, pH) of water, the ionization state of the proteins will remain the same because it will adapt to the new temperature-influenced pH. Hence proteins will maintain their structure and function regardless of the temperature. So according to this alpha-stat hypothesis, the alpha-stat management is simple: Electrochemical neutrality is maintained by keeping pH in the alkalotic range in temperature-corrected blood gases and normal in temperature-uncorrected gases. For practical purposes, it is easier to use uncorrected gases and make any necessary adjustment in order to keep pH at 7.4 and $PaCO_2$ at 40 mm Hg at 37°C, regardless of the patient's body temperature.

On the contrary, in the pH-stat approach, interventions are directed toward maintaining pH 7.4 and $PaCO_2$ 40 mm Hg, irrespective of patient's core body temperature. This means that the goal is to keep pH and PCO_2 at normal values for 37°C when the patient's body temperature-corrected gases are used and at acidotic values when temperature-uncorrected gases are used. For practical purposes, pH-stat is maintained by adding CO_2 to the ventilating gas during hypothermic cardiopulmonary bypass to increase PCO_2 and decrease the pH. In contrast to the alpha-stat approach, in which CO_2 content is held constant, pH-stat regulation results in an increase in total CO_2 content.

There is still debate as to whether pH-stat or alpha-stat management should be used during deep hypothermia and circulatory arrest in neonates, infants, and children. Based on the theoretic advantages of maintaining electrochemical neutrality during hypothermia, in the early 1980s the strategy at Boston Children's Hospital switched from pH-stat management to alpha-stat management. Within a short period of time, the incidence of severe neurologic injury in the form of choreoathetosis increased markedly following procedures under deep hypothermia cardiac arrest.[350,351] After this negative experience and the clinical trial that resulted from it, and on the basis of other preclinical and clinical data, the current best evidence suggests that the best technique to follow in the management of acid-base in patients undergoing deep hypothermic circulatory arrest during cardiac surgery is dependent on the age of the patient, with better results using pH-stat in the pediatric patient and alpha-stat in the adult patient.[351,352] This is not surprising, as the mechanisms of cerebral injury between adults and young children are quite different.

Summary

When one approaches a critically ill child with an acid-base imbalance, the first step is to define the nature of the disorder—that is, acidosis versus alkalosis, acidemia versus alkalemia, simple versus mixed, acute versus chronic, or severe and harmful versus neither severe nor harmful. The easiest way for screening the acid-base status is to examine the venous bicarbonate (or CO_{2TOT}) concentration. However, a normal concentration does not rule out the possibility of an acid-base derangement. So if the clinical setting suggests an illness known to be associated with acid-base imbalances, at least serum electrolytes and albumin concentrations should be obtained in order to calculate the AG_{CORR}. If the bicarbonate (or tCO_2) or AG_{CORR} is abnormal, or if a complex, potentially harmful, mixed acid-base disorder is suspected, an arterial blood analysis must be performed, which will provide information on pH, $PaCO_2$, and SBE. If possible, lactate concentration should also be obtained. This is mandatory if metabolic acidosis exists (with or without acidemia). If the presence of unmeasured anions or a mixed acid-base problem is suspected, it is advisable to calculate SID_{APP}, SID_{EFF}, and SIG, directly or through surrogates. If the patient's history documents resuscitation with large volumes of normal saline, special attention must be given to chloride concentrations. There is compelling evidence that abnormal pH by itself may not be as dangerous as once thought. However, an individualized approach must be taken to decide if a given patient may benefit or not from modifying his or her pH and acid-base status. Finally, none of the approaches for interpreting acid-base homeostasis are without flaws. However, the physicochemical approach offers better identification and cause-related diagnosis for complex acid-base problems. Perhaps the paramount merit of this approach relates to increased awareness of the close interactions between acid-base balance and the electrolytes, anions, and cations in the body fluids.

"We are still confused—but on a much higher level" (W. Churchill).[41]

Key References

5. Friis UG, Plovsing R, Hansen K, et al. Teaching acid/base physiology in the laboratory. *Adv Physiol Educ.* 2010;34:233-238.
6. Broughton JO Jr, Kennedy TC. Interpretation of arterial blood gases by computer. *Chest.* 1984;85:148-149.
8. Kishen R, Honoré PM, Jacobs R, et al. Facing acid-base disorders in the third millennium: the Stewart approach revisited. *Int J Nephrol Renovasc Dis.* 2014;7:209-217.
20. Malkin HM. Historical review: concept of acid-base balance in medicine. *Ann Clin Lab Sci.* 2003;33:337-344.
21. Story DA. Bench-to-bedside review: a brief history of clinical acid-base. *Crit Care.* 2004;8:253-258.
26. Fencl V, Leith DE. Stewart's quantitative acid-base chemistry: applications in biology and medicine. *Respir Physiol.* 1993;91:1-16.
27. Stewart PA. Independent and dependent variables of acid-base control. *Respir Physiol.* 1978;33:9-26.
29. Kellum JA. Determinants of plasma acid-base balance. *Crit Care Clin.* 2005;21:329-346.
33. Adeva-Andany MM, Carneiro-Freire N, Donapetry-García C, et al. The importance of the ionic product for water to understand the physiology of the acid-base balance in humans. *BioMed Res Inter.* 2014, Article ID 695281.
36. Severinghaus JW, Astrup P, Murray JF. Blood gas analysis and critical care medicine. *Am J Respir Crit Care Med.* 1998;157(4 Pt 2):S114-S122.
40. Geissler PL, Dellago C, Chandler D, et al. Autoionization in liquid water. *Science.* 2001;291:2121-2124.
41. Berend K. Acid-base pathophysiology after 130 years: confusing, irrational and controversial. *J Nephrol.* 2013;26:254-265.
46. Geers C, Gros G. Carbon dioxide transport and carbonic anhydrase in blood and muscle. *Physiol Rev.* 2000;80:681-715.
49. Aiken CGA. History of medical understanding and misunderstanding of acid base balance. *J Clin Exp Res.* 2013;7:2038-2041.
53. Kartal M, Eray O, Rinnert S, et al. ETCO2: a predictive tool for excluding metabolic disturbances in nonintubated patients. *Am J Emerg Med.* 2011;29:260-267.
55. Feldman M, Alvarez NM, Trevino M, Weinstein GL. Respiratory compensation to a primary metabolic alkalosis in humans. *Clin Nephrol.* 2012;78:365-369.
58. Cohen RD. Roles of the liver and kidney in acid-base regulation and its disorders. *Br J Anaesth.* 1991;67:154-164.
60. Weiner ID, Verlander JW. Renal ammonia metabolism and transport. *Compr Physiol.* 2013;3:201-220.
61. Fencl V, Jabor A, Kazda A, Figge J. Diagnosis of metabolic acid-base disturbances in critically ill patients. *Am J Respir Crit Care Med.* 2000; 162:2246-2251.

63. Al-Jaghbeer M, Kellum JA. Acid-base disturbances in intensive care patients: etiology, pathophysiology and treatment. *Nephrol Dial Transplant.* 2015;30:1104-1111.

78. Figge J, Jabor A, Kazda A, et al. Anion gap and hypoalbuminemia. *Crit Care Med.* 1998;26:1807-1810.

83. Kraut JA, Madias NE. Serum anion gap: its uses and limitations in clinical medicine. *Clin J Am Soc Nephrol.* 2007;2:162-174.

85. Hatherill M, Waggie Z, Purves L, et al. Correction of the anion gap for albumin in order to detect occult tissue anions in shock. *Arch Dis Child.* 2002;87:526-529.

97. Karim Z, Szutkowska M, Vernimmen C, et al. Recent concepts concerning the renal handling of NH_3/NH_4^+. *J Nephrol.* 2006;19(suppl 9): S27-S32.

106. Mallat J, Barrailler S, Lemyze M, et al. Use of sodium-chloride difference and corrected anion gap as surrogates of Stewart variables in critically ill patients. *PLoSONE.* 2013;8:e56635.

108. Moviat M, Terpstra AM, Ruitenbeek W, et al. Contribution of various metabolites to the "unmeasured" anions in critically ill patients with metabolic acidosis. *Crit Care Med.* 2008;36:752-758.

114. Durward A, Tibby S, Skellett S, et al. The strong ion gap predicts mortality in children following cardiopulmonary bypass surgery. *Pediatr Crit Care Med.* 2005;6:281-285.

117. Murray DM, Olhsson V, Fraser JI. Defining acidosis in postoperative cardiac patients using Stewart's method of strong ion difference. *Pediatr Crit Care Med.* 2004;5:240-245.

119. Hatherill M, Waggie Z, Purves L, et al. Mortality and the nature of metabolic acidosis in children with shock. *Intensive Care Med.* 2003; 29:286-291.

122. Seifter JL. Integration of acid-base and electrolyte disorders. *N Engl J Med.* 2014;371:1821-1831.

123. Antonogiannaki EM, Mitrouska I, Amargianitakis V, Georgopoulos D. Evaluation of acid-base status in patients admitted to ED-physicochemical vs traditional approaches. *Am J Emerg Med.* 2015;33:378-382.

127. Luke RG, Galla JH. It is chloride depletion alkalosis, not contraction alkalosis. *J Am Soc Nephrol.* 2012;23:204-207.

139. Kellum JA. Clinical review: reunification of acid-base physiology. *Crit Care.* 2005;9:500-507.

145. Nagaoka D, Nassar APJ, Maciel AT, et al. The use of sodium-chloride difference and chloride-sodium ratio as strong ion difference surrogates in the evaluation of metabolic acidosis in critically ill patients. *J Crit Care.* 2010;25:525-531.

154. Kellum JA. Saline-induced hyperchloremic metabolic acidosis. *Crit Care Med.* 2002;30:259-261.

172. Forsythe SM, Schmidt GA. Sodium bicarbonate for the treatment of lactic acidosis. *Chest.* 2000;117:260-267.

174. Laffey J, Honan D, Hopkins N, et al. Hypercapnic acidosis attenuates endotoxin-induced acute lung injury. *Am J Respir Crit Care Med.* 2004;169:46-56.

183. Yildizdaş D, Yapicioğlu H, Yilmaz HL, et al. Correlation of simultaneously obtained capillary, venous, and arterial blood gases of patients in a paediatric intensive care unit. *Arch Dis Child.* 2004;89:176-180.

186. Mizock BA, Falk JL. Lactic acidosis in critical illness. *Crit Care Med.* 1992;20:80-93.

194. Kraut JA, Madias NE. Lactic acidosis. *N Engl J Med.* 2014;371:2309-2319.

201. Jackman L, Shetty N, Davies P, et al. Late-onset hyperlactataemia following paediatric cardiac surgery. *Intensive Care Med.* 2009;35:537-545.

211. Garcia-Alvarez M, Marik P, Bellomo R. Sepsis-associated hyperlactatemia. *Crit Care.* 2014;18:503.

215. Suetrong B, Walley KR. Lactic acidosis in sepsis: it's not all anaerobic: implications for diagnosis and management. *Chest.* 2016;149:252-261.

251. Kamel KS, Halperin ML. Acid-base problems in diabetic ketoacidosis. *N Engl J Med.* 2015;372:546-554.

259. Constable PD. Hyperchloremic acidosis: the classic example of strong ion acidosis. *Anesth Analg.* 2003;96:919-922.

272. Pereira PC, Miranda DM, Oliveira EA, et al. Molecular pathophysiology of renal tubular acidosis. *Curr Genomics.* 2009;10:51-59.

289. Boyd JH, Walley KR. Is there a role for sodium bicarbonate in treating lactic acidosis from shock? *Curr Opin Crit Care.* 2008;14:379-383.

294. Kim HJ, Son YK, An WS. Effect of sodium bicarbonate administration on mortality in patients with lactic acidosis: a retrospective e analysis. *PLoS ONE.* 2013;8:e65283.

310. Laski ME, Sabatini S. Metabolic alkalosis, bedside and bench. *Semin Nephrol.* 2006;26:404-421.

329. O'Croinin D, Ni Chonghaile M, Higgins B, et al. Bench-to-bedside review: permissive hypercapnia. *Crit Care.* 2005;9:51-59.

348. Naka T, Bellomo R. Bench-to bedside review: treating acid-base abnormalities in the intensive care unit: the role of renal replacement therapy. *Crit Care.* 2004;8:108-114.

Renal Pharmacology

Douglas L. Blowey

PEARLS

- For a goal of maintaining of a serum concentration close to the steady state throughout the dosing interval, decreasing the size of the dose while maintaining the normal dosing interval will decrease the variation between the serum drug concentration peak and trough.
- With the exception of spironolactone and arginine vasopressin antagonists, diuretics must reach the renal tubular fluid to produce a pharmacologic effect.
- Loop diuretics decrease sodium reabsorption by inhibiting the electroneutral $Na^+/K^+/2Cl^-$ cotransporter located in the ascending limb of Henle.
- Spironolactone prevents the binding of aldosterone to a cytosolic receptor resulting in a decrease in the number of apical sodium channels.
- Continuous infusion of a loop diuretic is more efficient than intermittent high doses and avoids the high and low serum concentrations associated with toxicity and resistance.

The kidney plays a central role in many physiologic processes that have a direct impact on drug action and disposition, and it is also an important target for drug therapy in the critically ill child. Key functions of the kidney are elimination of endogenous and exogenous substances from the body, including drug and drug metabolites, and maintenance of body fluid composition and volume. Glomerular and tubular mechanisms that affect these functions are directly and indirectly influenced by the function of other organs. For example, congestive heart failure decreases the adequacy of arterial blood flow and is detected by sensors located throughout the circulatory system. Sensed reduction in effective arterial blood volume triggers a complex neurohormonal response that decreases kidney blood flow, increases sodium and water retention by the kidney, and further aggravates the edema associated with congestive heart failure. Conversely, the accumulation of drugs, drug metabolites, metabolic waste products, and alterations in body fluid composition and volume associated with kidney failure may have deleterious effects on the function of other vital organs and physiologic systems.

Kidney Function and Drug Disposition

Many drugs are eliminated by the kidney, and abnormal kidney function can affect the amount of drug present at the site of action and the magnitude of the drug response.

Understanding of the effects of abnormal kidney function on drug disposition and action is important because abnormal kidney function is common in the critically ill child and alterations in drug disposition or action may result in suboptimal therapeutic efficacy or serious adverse events.

The pharmacologic effect of a therapeutic agent is determined by the amount, and time, that the active drug component (eg, parent drug or drug metabolite) is present at the site of action and the responsiveness of the target organ to the drug. Only the free, unbound form of a drug can exert a pharmacologic effect through interaction with receptors. Disposition of a drug after administration is determined by the drug formulation and route of administration, rate and extent of absorption from the site of administration, extent of distribution in the body fluids and tissues, rate and extent of metabolism, and rate and route of elimination. Drug disposition and response are further influenced by the genetic, physiologic, and pathologic constitution of the ill child.[1,2] Pharmacokinetics is the mathematic expression of drug disposition, and pharmacodynamics describes the magnitude of response to a drug. Determination of pharmacokinetic parameters is an invaluable tool for designing individualized drug-dosing regimens in children with kidney failure or critical illnesses that may alter drug disposition.

Although decreased kidney elimination of drugs and drug metabolites is the most obvious consequence of altered kidney function, kidney failure or the associated coexisting conditions may affect drug absorption, distribution, and metabolism (Table 77.1).[3-5] The mechanisms that govern drug removal by the kidneys are glomerular filtration, tubular secretion, and tubular reabsorption. These processes are altered in children with kidney disease, as well as other organ dysfunction. Each of the kidney's 1 million nephrons consists of a tuft of capillaries (glomerulus) enveloped by an epithelial-lined capsule (Bowman space) that drains into a contiguous tubular system (see also Chapter 72). As blood flows through the glomerular capillaries, fluid and small solutes, including drugs and drug metabolites not bound to plasma proteins, pass through the glomeruli into the Bowman space. The volume of water and accompanying solute that is filtered through the glomeruli per unit time is the glomerular filtration rate (GFR) and is the most important measure of kidney function (see Chapter 74). The GFR is estimated with the measurement of the rate that the kidney removes a substance from the blood (eg, renal clearance). The measured substance may be an endogenous compound (eg, creatinine [Cr] or cystatin C), an exogenous compound that is specifically administered to measure the GFR (eg, inulin, isotope, or iohexol), or a compound primarily eliminated by glomerular filtration that is administered as part

TABLE 77.1	Potential Alterations of Drug Distribution in Kidney Failure		
PK Parameter	**Effect**	**Proposed Mechanism**	
Absorption	↓	Edema of GI tract, uremic N/V, delayed gastric emptying Drug interaction—phosphate binders, H_2 blockers Altered GI pH	
Distribution	↑	Increased unbound drug fraction Hypoalbuminemia (nephrosis, malnutrition) Uremic changes in albumin structure	
Metabolism	↓ ↑	Inhibition of CYP-450 metabolism (liver, intestine, kidney) Drug interaction Direct inhibition by "uremic" milieu Induced CYP-450 metabolism	
Excretion	↓	Decreased GFR Decreased tubular secretion Increased tubular reabsorption	

CYP-450, cytochrome P-450; *GFR*, glomerular filtration rate; *GI*, gastrointestinal; *N/V*, nausea and vomiting; *PK*, pharmacokinetic.

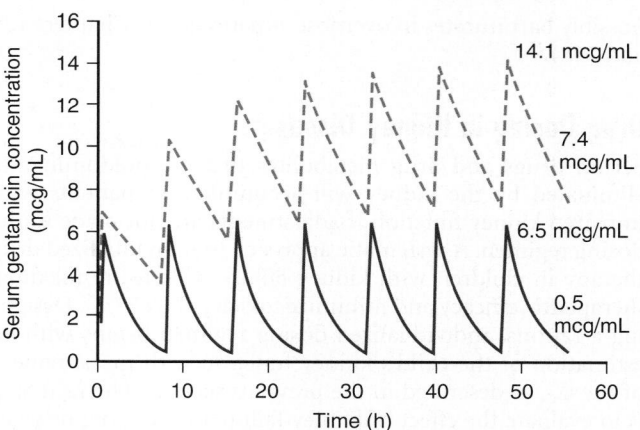

Fig. 77.1. Gentamicin time-concentration profile in a 5-year-old child receiving 2.5 mg/kg intravenously every 8 hours. The *solid line* represents the plasma concentration-time profile in a child with normal kidney function (eg, 120 mL/min/1.73 m²) and the *dashed line* represents the plasma concentration-time profile in a child with a creatinine clearance of 30 mL/min/1.73 m².

of clinical care (eg, gentamicin).[6] The clearance of Cr corrected for body surface area is the most common method used to estimate the GFR. Creatinine clearance (C_{Cr}), expressed in mL/min/1.73 m², is calculated with the measurement of the amount of Cr in an accurately timed urine collection and a midcollection plasma Cr.

$$C_{cr} = \frac{[\text{Urine CR (mg/dL)} \times (\text{Urine volume [mL]/Time [min]})]}{\text{Plasma Cr (mg/dL)}}$$
$$\times \frac{1.73\,\text{m}^2}{\text{BSA (m}^2)}$$

C_{Cr} is low at birth and rapidly increases during the first 2 weeks of life, followed by a steady rise until adult values are reached by 8 to 12 months.[7,8]

Although not as accurate as a timed urine collection, for children aged 1 to 18 years, C_{Cr} can be quickly estimated with the measurement of the child's serum Cr and length with the following equation[9]:

$$C_{cr} = \frac{\text{Length (cm)} \times 0.41}{\text{Plasma Cr (mg/dL)}}$$

The total amount of drug eliminated from the body by the kidneys is a composition of the amount of drug filtered across the glomeruli, the amount actively secreted into the filtrate by the renal tubules, and the amount reabsorbed by the renal tubules. Because albumin and other large molecules do not pass through the glomeruli, large drugs and drugs bound to plasma proteins normally do not pass through the glomeruli and are not effectively removed by glomerular filtration but may be efficiently eliminated by the kidney through renal tubular secretion (eg, furosemide). For drugs and drug metabolites that are primarily eliminated by glomerular filtration, the rate of elimination mirrors kidney function (C_{Cr}). As such, when kidney function declines, the reduced drug elimination

results in drug accumulation in the body. For example, gentamicin is an aminoglycoside that is eliminated primarily by glomerular filtration with an elimination half-life of around 2 hours in children and adults with normal kidney function and 4 to 12 hours in infants because of the well-characterized developmental immaturity of kidney function.[7,8] A 75% reduction of the GFR (eg, C_{Cr} = 30 mL/min/1.73 m²) in a 5-year-old child receiving intravenous (IV) gentamicin will prolong the elimination half-life to 8 hours. Unless adjustments are made in the dosing regimen to account for the decreased kidney elimination, gentamicin will accumulate to toxic serum concentrations (Fig. 77.1).

Active renal tubular secretion of drugs and drug metabolites by relatively nonspecific anionic and cationic transport systems in the proximal tubule can contribute substantially to the amount of drug eliminated by the kidney. Renal tubular secretion of a drug may be inhibited by other drugs or endogenous substrates that use the same nonspecific transport systems. For example, probenecid blocks the tubular secretion of many drugs by the organic anion transporter and is useful as an adjuvant to antibiotic therapy and the prevention of drug-induced nephrotoxicity.[10-12] Coadministration of probenecid and penicillin-type antibiotics results in higher and more prolonged serum penicillin levels because of the inhibition of penicillin secretion by the renal tubule. The resultant increased penicillin exposure may enhance its therapeutic efficacy.[13,14] Nephrotoxicity is the major dose-limiting adverse effect of the antiviral agent cidofovir that is in part mediated by the proximal tubular transport of cidofovir by the organic anion system. Coadministration of probenecid restricts the proximal renal tubular uptake of cidofovir and decreases nephrotoxicity.[11] Reabsorption is the passive diffusion of nonionized (noncharged) drug from the filtrate into the renal tubular cell. Basic urine (eg, urine pH >7.5) favors the ionized form of acidic drugs and limits reabsorption, whereas reabsorption of basic drugs is enhanced in basic urine because the nonionized form of the drug is favored. Urinary alkalinization is used to enhance the renal elimination of salicylates and possibly barbiturates in overdose situations (see Chapters 127 and 128).[15]

Drug Dosing in Kidney Disease

Serum drugs and drug metabolites that are predominantly eliminated by the kidney will accumulate in patients with impaired kidney function if adjustments are not made to the dosing regimen. A systematic approach to individualized drug therapy in children with kidney failure will ensure maximal therapeutic efficacy and minimize toxicity (Box 77.1). Designing a rational individualized dosing regimen begins with an estimation of the child's kidney function with measurement of the C_{Cr} as described in the previous section. The next step is to evaluate the effect of kidney failure on the drug disposition characteristics for all of the drugs prescribed to the child. Reference books such as the *Pediatric Dosage Handbook,*[16] *Physicians Desk Reference,* and *Micro Medex* are excellent beginning sources for information about drug disposition in kidney failure. Unfortunately, because there is little pharmacokinetic information about drug disposition in children with kidney failure, estimates from adult patients with kidney failure are cautiously used, keeping in mind the potential changes in drug disposition that occur with development.[17] The most important information for designing an optimal dosing regimen is the amount of drug that is eliminated by the kidneys in persons with normal kidney function. If one assumes that drug protein binding, distribution, and metabolism are not greatly altered in kidney failure, an assumption that is likely true for most drugs,[5] then a dosage adjustment factor (Q) can be estimated:

$$Q = 1 - \left[\% \text{ excreted unchanged} \times 1 - \frac{(\text{Child's creatine clearance [mL/min/1.73 m}^2])}{\text{Normal creatine clearance (120 mL/min/1.73 m}^2)} \right]$$

Once the need for a dosage adjustment has been established and the adjustment factor (Q) calculated, the best method of adjustment, whether it be a change in the size of the dose or the length of the dosing interval, is selected on the basis of the known relationships between the peak and trough drug concentrations and clinical response or toxicity. Fig. 77.2 illustrates the concentration-time profiles for two different IV gentamicin dosing regimens in a child with a measured C_{Cr} of 30 mL/min/1.73 m[2]. About 95% of gentamicin is excreted unchanged in the urine, and the dosage adjustment factor is calculated as follows:

$$Q = 1 - \left[0.95 \times 1 - \frac{(30 \text{ mL/min/1.73 m}^2)}{120 \text{ mL/min/1.73 m}^2} \right] = 0.30$$

BOX 77.1	Guidelines for Drug Dosing in Kidney Failure

1. Estimate the glomerular filtration rate.
2. Determine the percentage of drug eliminated by the kidney.
3. Calculate the dosage adjustment factor (Q).
4. Adjust the dose size or dosing interval.
5. Monitor response.
6. Monitor the therapeutic drug (when available).

When the dosing interval is increased and the size of the drug dose remains unchanged (see Fig. 77.2, *solid line*), the steady-state peak and trough drug concentration are similar to those seen in children with normal renal function; however, there is a prolonged period when the serum gentamicin concentration is above and below the average steady state concentration. This dosing regimen may be inappropriate for drugs that should be maintained at a relatively stable serum concentration, such as cephalosporins or antihypertensive medications. When the goal is maintenance of a serum concentration close to the steady-state level throughout the dosing interval, decreasing the size of the dose while maintaining the normal dosing interval will decrease the variation between the serum drug concentration peak and trough (see Fig. 77.2, *solid line*). Dosing adjustments are estimates based on many assumptions, and the final step in individual therapy is close monitoring of clinical efficacy and toxicity. When available, the measurement of serum drug concentrations and determination of pharmacokinetic parameters are invaluable for individual drug therapy, especially in agents with a narrow therapeutic index.

Dialysis

Some form of dialysis is utilized in about 3% of children admitted to the intensive care unit. Drug elimination in children receiving dialysis is a composite of nonrenal drug elimination, residual kidney elimination, and the added elimination provided by dialysis. Efficiency of a given dialysis modality to eliminate a drug depends on the physiochemical characteristics of the drug and the form and characteristics of the dialysis procedure. Hemodialysis, peritoneal dialysis, and the varied forms of continuous renal replacement therapies that include continuous venovenous hemodialysis and continuous venovenous hemodiafiltration are all used in the intensive care setting (see also Chapter 78). It is beyond the scope of this chapter to

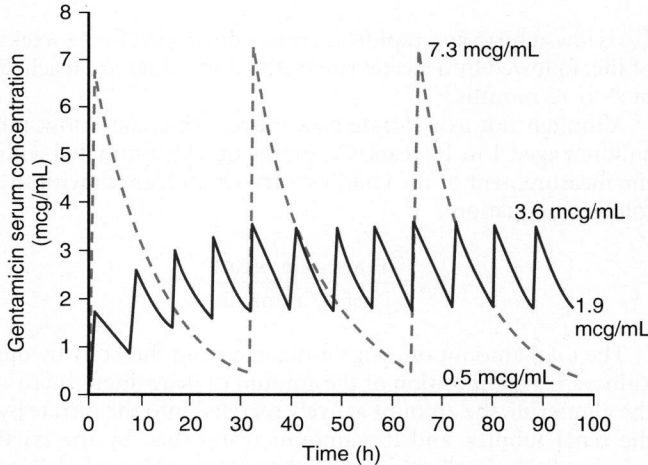

Fig. 77.2. Gentamicin concentration-time profile in a child with a creatinine clearance of 30 mL/min/1.73 m[2] receiving intravenous gentamicin. The *solid line* represents the plasma concentration-time profile when the dose remains unchanged (2.5 mg/kg) and the dosing interval is adjusted to 32 hours [normal dosing interval (8 hour) ÷ dosing adjustment factor (0.3)]. The *dashed line* represents the plasma concentration-time profile if the dosing interval remains unchanged (8 hours) and the dose is adjusted to 0.625 mg/kg [normal dose (2.5 mg/kg) × dosing adjustment factor (0.3)].

detail drug disposition in the various forms of dialysis, and the reader is referred to other excellent sources for further information.[4,18] In general, highly protein-bound drugs and drugs with a large volume of distribution are not well removed by dialysis.

Kidney as a Therapeutic Target: Diuretics

Diuretics are a diverse group of drugs that act on the kidney to increase salt or water excretion. In the intensive care setting, diuretics are commonly prescribed for mobilization of excess body fluid and treatment of cerebral and pulmonary edema, ascites, and hypertension. Less common indications include congestive heart failure, disorders of calcium metabolism, glaucoma, and drug overdoses. Diuretics are grouped into six classes according to the primary site of action: Osmotic diuretics and carbonic anhydrase inhibitors act in the proximal tubule; loop diuretics act in the thick ascending limb of Henle; thiazide and thiazide-like diuretics act in the distal tubule; potassium-sparing diuretics act in the cortical collecting ducts; and vasopressin receptor antagonists act in the medullary collecting duct.

Renal tubular cells transport solute and water from the apical cell membrane (tubular fluid) to the basolateral cell membrane (blood side). Reabsorption of sodium is central to the kidney's ability to reabsorb water and other solutes (eg, glucose, amino acids, and bicarbonate). Apical cell sodium entry is mediated by channels that permit sodium to enter by diffusion or transport by specific proteins located on the apical cell membrane. In all renal tubular cells, the sodium-potassium adenosine triphosphatase (ATPase) located on the basolateral membrane maintains the low intracellular sodium concentration that favors sodium movement from the tubular fluid into the renal tubular cell. Diuretics inhibit sodium reabsorption by blocking sodium channels or sodium transport proteins located on the apical cell membrane at discrete sites along the nephron. Because sodium reabsorption occurs in a sequential manner along the nephron, the combination of diuretics with different sites of action (eg, loop diuretic plus a thiazide diuretic) has a synergistic effect on sodium reabsorption. The additional osmotic force associated with the increased urinary sodium causes a rise in urine volume. Diuresis is associated with a decrease in vascular volume that stimulates movement of sodium and water from the interstitial space into the vascular space, as well as stimulation of counterregulatory pathways (eg, the renin-angiotensin-aldosterone system) that serve to maintain an adequate extracellular fluid volume.

With the exception of spironolactone and the vasopressin receptor antagonists, diuretics must reach the renal tubular fluid to produce a pharmacologic effect. Because diuretics are extensively bound to plasma proteins, their entry into the tubular fluid depends primarily on proximal tubular secretion. Organic anion transporters actively secrete carbonic anhydrase inhibitors, loop diuretics, and thiazide diuretics, whereas the organic cation transporters actively secrete amiloride and triamterene. Mannitol is freely filtered at the glomerulus, and spironolactone has a complex mechanism of action that does not require entry into the tubular fluid for pharmacologic effect. Finally, the nephron delivers a hypotonic fluid to the medullary collecting duct where water is either excreted or reabsorbed based on the presence or absence

of apical water channels (eg, aquaporins). In response to increased plasma osmolality or reduced plasma volume, the posterior pituitary releases vasopressin into the blood that interacts with vasopressin receptors on the basolateral membrane of the collecting duct. Vasopressin mediates the insertion of water channels and the reabsorption of water (see also Chapters 81, 85).

The response to diuretics is determined by the amount and time course of drug reaching the site of action and the sensitivity of the active site to the diuretic. The concentration-response curve (Fig. 77.3) depicts the relationship between the urinary excretion rate of loop and thiazide diuretics and diuretic response. As indicated by the S-shaped curve for each diuretic, there exists a therapeutic threshold (minimal concentration) that must be reached at the site of action before any response is noted and a maximal response (ceiling) above which no further response will occur even if more drug reaches the site of action. The amount and time course of drug reaching the site of action, tubular response to the diuretic, are influenced by the route and frequency of administration, as well as drug and disease states that modify the amount of diuretic reaching the tubular fluid. An example is the twofold to threefold increase in loop diuretic dosage required for response in patients with decreased kidney function. In kidney failure, the entry of loop diuretics into the tubular fluid is limited by decreased drug delivery to the organic anion transporters due to decreased renal blood flow and competitive inhibition of diuretic transport by "uremic toxins." Adequate tubular fluid diuretic concentration and response can be achieved with the administration of high doses of diuretic,[19] but at the risk of increasing ototoxicity, particularly with concurrent aminoglycoside administration.[20,21]

Loop diuretics, such as furosemide, bumetanide, and torsemide, are the most potent diuretics because a large percentage of the filtered sodium is reabsorbed (25%) in the ascending limb of Henle. Loop diuretics decrease sodium reabsorption by inhibiting the electroneutral $Na^+/K^+/2Cl^-$ cotransporter located on the apical cell membrane in the ascending limb of Henle. Loop diuretics increase sodium delivery to the distal tubular segments and diminish water reabsorption by increasing the tubular fluid osmotic force and disrupting the generation of a hypertonic medullary interstitium. The potential for profound fluid and electrolyte loss with loop diuretics man-

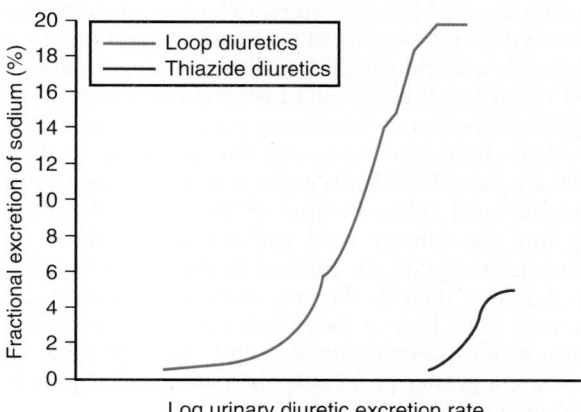

Fig. 77.3. Concentration-response curve depicting the relationship between the urinary diuretic excretion rate and the excretion of sodium in the urine.

dates close monitoring of body fluid volume and serum electrolytes during therapy.

Increased delivery of sodium to the distal nephron segments has three significant physiologic consequences. First, because sodium reabsorption in the thick ascending limb results in a lumen-positive transepithelial voltage that drives passive magnesium and calcium reabsorption, inhibition of sodium reabsorption by loop diuretics diminishes the transepithelial voltage and causes an increase in the urinary excretion of calcium and magnesium. Accordingly long-term use of loop diuretics is associated with hypomagnesemia, hypercalciuria, and calcium-based kidney stones.[22-24] On the other hand, the enhanced urinary excretion of magnesium and calcium observed with loop diuretics is clinically beneficial in the treatment of hypercalcemia and hypermagnesemia.[25,26]

The second physiologic consequence of increased sodium delivery to the distal nephron segments is enhanced potassium secretion. Sodium reabsorption by the principal cell in the collecting duct favors potassium secretion into the tubular fluid and promotes hypokalemia.[27,28] Finally, the increased sodium delivery to the distal nephron is associated with acute and chronic adaptive processes that enhance distal sodium reabsorption and diminish diuretic efficacy.[29]

Loop diuretics display similar efficacy but differ slightly in pharmacokinetic characteristics. Bumetanide and torsemide are almost completely absorbed after oral administration, whereas the absorption of furosemide is extremely variable, with an average bioavailability of 50%.[30,31] Therefore when furosemide is switched from IV to oral dosing, the dose is increased to account for the decreased absorption. The onset of diuretic effect is within minutes of IV administration of a loop diuretic and 30 to 60 minutes after oral administration. The duration of diuretic effect is short (2-6 hours),[27,32,33] and this short duration often results in the need for multiple doses or a continuous infusion to achieve the desired effect.

Thiazide and thiazide-like diuretics, such as chlorothiazide, hydrochlorothiazide, metolazone, and chlorthalidone, decrease sodium reabsorption by inhibiting the Na^+/Cl^- cotransporter located on the apical membrane in the distal tubule. The thiazide diuretics are less effective than the loop diuretics (see Fig. 77.3) because less sodium reabsorption occurs in the distal tubule (5% to 10%) compared with the ascending limb of Henle. Thiazide diuretics have a synergistic effect on fluid and electrolyte excretion when combined with loop diuretics.[34-36] Thiazide diuretics have similar efficacy, and the main difference resides in potency and duration of action. Metolazone and chlorthalidone display a longer duration of effect than chlorothiazide and hydrochlorothiazide; however, the biological effect of thiazide agents is prolonged compared with their elimination rates, and thus dosing is usually once or twice a day. Thiazide drugs are relatively ineffective in the setting of renal failure because of the decreased delivery of drug into the tubular fluid and the limited distal tubule sodium reabsorption. In contrast to the calcinuric effect of loop diuretics, thiazide diuretics enhance calcium reabsorption and may have a beneficial effect in children with nephrocalcinosis/nephrolithiasis and hypercalciuria. Thiazides have a greater propensity than other diuretics to cause hypokalemia.

The potassium-sparing diuretics triamterene and amiloride decrease sodium reabsorption by blocking the apical membrane sodium channel in the principal cells of the cortical-collecting duct. Sodium reabsorption in the cortical-collecting duct results in a transepithelial voltage that favors the secretion of potassium and hydrogen ions. Although potassium-sparing diuretics can enhance diuresis, particularly in patients receiving loop or thiazide diuretics, the main clinical benefit of these agents is a reduction in the potassium excretion induced by loop and thiazide diuretics. Spironolactone prevents the binding of aldosterone to a cytosolic receptor, resulting in decreased activity of Na^+/K^+ adenosine triphosphatase and a decrease in the number of apical sodium channels. Spironolactone is effective in primary and secondary hyperaldosteronism (eg, liver disease). Potassium-sparing diuretics are not recommended in patients with renal failure because of the propensity for the development of hyperkalemia.

Osmotic diuretics are nonelectrolytes that are freely filtered at the glomerulus and poorly reabsorbed or, in the case of glucose, present in amounts that exceed the tubular reabsorptive capacity. Mannitol is the prototypical osmotic diuretic, and its therapeutic effectiveness is directly related to the mannitol dose being large enough to raise the plasma and tubular fluid osmolality. Extraction of water from the intracellular compartments to the extracellular fluid volume that is associated with mannitol administration is clinically useful in cerebral edema, glaucoma, and the prevention of dialysis dysequilibrium syndrome. Mannitol-induced expansion of the extracellular fluid volume may be sufficient to perpetuate congestive heart failure, pulmonary edema, and significant hyponatremia in patients with renal failure in whom the half-life of mannitol is prolonged and the ability to excrete free water is limited.[37]

Carbonic anhydrase catalyzes the dehydration of carbonic acid to water and carbon dioxide, as well as the reverse hydration reaction. Acetazolamide is the prototypical carbonic anhydrase inhibitor and is more clinically useful for its extrarenal effects than its diuretic effects. Acetazolamide is used to treat glaucoma, acute mountain sickness, and occasionally epilepsy. The effectiveness of the carbonic anhydrase inhibitor is limited by the metabolic acidosis that develops because of the bicarbonate loss in the urine.

Vaptans (eg, conivaptan) are nonpeptide arginine vasopressin antagonists that inhibit the arginine vasopressin–stimulated absorption of free water in the medullary collecting duct. In contrast to other diuretics, the vasopressin antagonists increase urine flow without increasing the renal elimination of sodium. Conivaptan has been used in patients with euvolemic, or hypervolemic, hyponatremia associated with the inappropriate secretion of antidiuretic hormone or congestive heart failure.[38]

Diuretic Resistance

An inadequate diuretic response results from disease- or drug-related alterations in diuretic pharmacokinetics or pharmacodynamics, high dietary salt intake,[39] or adaptive processes[29] (Box 77.2). During diuretic-induced extracellular volume depletion, short-term and long-term adaptive processes protect the intravascular volume; however, when these adaptive processes interfere with the diuretic responsiveness before the desired reduction in the extracellular fluid volume is achieved, they contribute to diuretic resistance.

Short-term adaptation results from enhanced postdiuretic sodium retention. The brisk diuresis associated with diuretics

BOX 77.2   Causes of Diuretic Resistance

Noncompliance
- Medication, salt restriction

Poor absorption of medication
- Poorly absorbed formulation (eg, furosemide oral)
- Disease-induced changes in absorption

Impaired excretion of diuretic
- Renal failure, renal transplant
- Drug interactions: NSAIDs, probenecid

Protein binding in renal tubule
- Nephrotic syndrome

Hemodynamic
- Shock, hypoxemia
- Drugs: NSAIDs, antihypertensive drugs

Change in dose response
- CHF, nephrotic syndrome, cirrhosis

Adaptive responses

CHF, congestive heart failure; NS, nephrotic syndrome; NSAID, nonsteroidal anti-inflammatory drug.

BOX 77.3   Intensive Diuretic Therapy

1. High-dose diuretic therapy
2. Combination of diuretic therapy
3. Continuous infusion diuretic therapy

BOX 77.4   Common Adverse Effects Associated With Diuretics

1. Volume depletion
2. Electrolyte abnormalities
   - Hyponatremia
   - Hypokalemia (loop and thiazide diuretics)
   - Hypomagnesemia (loop diuretics)
   - Hypercalciuria (loop diuretics)
   - Ototoxicity (loop diuretics, especially furosemide)

activates counterregulatory pathways that enhance sodium reabsorption and maintain extracellular fluid volume. Counterregulatory mechanisms involved in the short-term adaptation to diuretics include a decrease in atrial natriuretic peptide, increased renal sympathetic activity, increased antidiuretic hormone, stimulated renin-angiotensin-aldosterone system, and a reduced GFR. The balance favors sodium and water excretion when the diuretic concentration in the renal tubular fluid is sufficient to inhibit sodium reabsorption. When the concentration of diuretic in the tubular fluid is below the threshold needed to elicit sodium excretion, the balance favors sodium and water reabsorption. In patients receiving a generous salt intake, which may be either dietary or associated with obligate fluids or medications, the postdiuretic sodium reabsorption may compensate entirely for the diuretic-induced sodium losses, resulting in no change in the extracellular fluid volume. Long-term adaptation occurs after several days of diuretic use and is characterized by a diminished response to each successive dose of diuretic.[39] Adaptation occurs because of the persistence of short-term counterregulatory mechanisms, as well as functional and structural changes that enhance the sodium reabsorptive capability of the distal tubule.[40,41]

If the response to moderate doses of a diuretic fails to be adequate in patients, several dosing strategies may help overcome the apparent diuretic resistance including high-dose diuretic therapy, combination diuretic therapy, or a continuous diuretic infusion (Box 77.3).

In patients with edema, the dose-response curve may be shifted to the right, indicating that a greater amount of drug is needed in the renal tubule to produce the desired diuretic response. In patients who have renal failure or patients who receive drugs that inhibit the secretion of diuretic from the blood into the renal tubule, the dose-response curve is normal, but the problem lies in the inability to get a sufficient concentration of diuretic into the renal tubule. In both situations, an intermittent high-dose diuretic regimen may overcome the impaired rate of tubular secretion and increase the urinary diuretic concentration sufficient to elicit a response. High-dose therapy is associated with an increased risk of fluid and electrolyte abnormalities and a risk of toxicity related to high blood concentrations. Loop diuretic ototoxicity is more common with rapid infusion of high doses, especially when furosemide is combined with other ototoxic drugs.[36]

Because sodium reabsorption in the kidney is sequential and many of the adaptive processes increase sodium reabsorption distal to the site of diuretic action, combination therapy with diuretics that inhibit the distal tubule with loop inhibitors may be effective. Part of the effectiveness of combination diuretic therapy resides in the longer duration of effect for thiazides that prevents the postdiuretic sodium reabsorption noted with the shorter-acting loop diuretics. Fluid and electrolyte abnormalities are more common with combination drug therapy (Box 77.4).

The final strategy to overcome diuretic resistance, continuous infusion of a loop diuretic, is more efficient than intermittent high doses and avoids the high and low serum concentrations associated with toxicity and resistance.[42-45] Continuous infusions result in steady diuretic effect and may avoid the rapid hemodynamic changes and stimulation of counterregulatory processes associated with rapid changes in extracellular fluid volume. A loading dose of diuretic is recommended at initiation and with each upward dosing adjustment to ensure a prompt response. Diuretic response may be further augmented by the addition of a distally acting diuretic.

Prevention/Reversal of Acute Renal Failure

Acute renal failure in the pediatric intensive care unit is generally associated with diminished renal perfusion caused by hypovolemia, hypotension, or decreased cardiac output. In addition, acute renal failure is also associated with nephrotoxins such as radiocontrast agents, antibiotics (eg, vancomycin), and chemotherapeutic agents (eg, cisplatin). With the exception of simple saline hydration, little evidence suggests that in humans, mannitol, furosemide, or dopamine prevents the development of acute renal failure in high-risk patients or changes the outcome in patients with established acute renal failure.[46-49] Nevertheless, the use of high-dose furosemide alone or in combination with low-dose dopamine might increase urine output and ease patient care by improving fluid management and permitting increased nutrition.

References

1. Leeder JS, Kearns GL. Pharmacogenetics in pediatrics. *Pediatr Clin North Am.* 1997;44:55-77.

2. MacLoed S. Drug disposition and action in disease. In: Radde I, MacLoed S, eds. *Pediatric Pharmacology and Therapeutics*. Chicago: Mosby; 1993.

3. Blowey D, Kearns G, Lalkin A. Special considerations in the prescribing of medications for the pediatric CAPD/CCPD patient. In: Fine R, Alexander S, Warady B, eds. *CAPD/CCPD in Children*. Boston: Kluwer Academic Publishers; 1998.

4. Olyaei A, de Mattos A, Bennett W. Prescribing drugs in renal disease. In: Brenner B, ed. *The Kidney*. Philadelphia: WB Saunders; 2000.

5. Dreisbach AW. The influence of chronic renal failure on drug metabolism and transport. *Clin Pharmacol Ther*. 2009;86:553-556.

6. Koren G, James A, Perlman M. A simple method for the estimation of glomerular filtration rate by gentamicin pharmacokinetics during routine drug monitoring in the newborn. *Clin Pharmacol Ther*. 1985;38:680-685.

7. Arant BS Jr. Developmental patterns of renal functional maturation in the human neonate. *J Pediatr*. 1978;92:705-712.

8. van den Anker JN, Schoemaker R, Hop W, et al. Ceftazidime pharmacokinetics in preterm infants: effects of renal function and gestational age. *Clin Pharmacol Ther*. 1995;58:650-659.

9. Schwartz GJ, Munoz A, Schneider MF, et al. New equations to estimate GFR in children with CKD. *J Am Soc Nephrol*. 2009;20:629-637.

10. Jacobs C, Kaubisch S, Halsey J, et al. The use of probenecid as a chemoprotector against cisplatin nephrotoxicity. *Cancer*. 1991;67:1518-1524.

11. Lacy S, Hitchcock M, Lee W, et al. Effect of oral probenecid coadministration on the chronic toxicity and pharmacokinetics of intravenous cidofovir in cynomolgus monkeys. *Toxicol Sci*. 1988;44:97-106.

12. Lalezari J, Holland G, Kramer F, et al. Randomized, controlled study of the safety and efficacy of intravenous cidofovir for the treatment of relapsing cytomegalovirus retinitis in patients with AIDS. *J Acquir Immune Defic Syndr Hum Retrovirol*. 1998;17:339-344.

13. Holmes K, Karney W, Harnisch J, et al. Single-dose aqueous procaine penicillin G therapy for gonorrhea: use of probenecid and cause of treatment failure. *J Infect Dis*. 1973;127:455-460.

14. Odugbemi T. An open evaluation study of sulbactam/ampicillin with or without probenecid in the treatment of gonococcal infections in Lagos. *Drugs*. 1988;35(suppl 7):89-91.

15. Prescott L, Balali-Mood M, Critchley J, et al. Diuresis or urinary alkalinisation for salicylate poisoning. *Br Med J (Clin Red Ed)*. 1982;285:1383-1386.

16. Taketomo CK, Hodding JH, Kraus DM. *Pediatric Dosage Handbook*. 15th ed. Hudson, OH: Lexi-Comp; 2008.

17. Kearns G. Pediatric pharmacokinetics. In: Ritschel W, Kearns G, eds. *Handbook of Basic Pharmacokinetics, Including Clinical Applications*. 7th ed. Washington, DC: American Pharmaceutical Association; 2009.

18. Reetze-Bonorden P, Bohler J, Keller E. Drug dosage in patients during continuous renal replacement therapy. *Clin Pharmacokinet*. 1993;24:362-379.

19. Voelker J, Cartwright-Brown D, Anderson S, et al. Comparison of loop diuretics in patients with chronic renal insufficiency. *Kidney Int*. 1987;32:572-578.

20. Brummett R, Bendrick T, Himes D. Comparative ototoxicity of bumetanide and furosemide when used in combination with kanamycin. *J Clin Pharmacol*. 1981;21(11-12 Pt 2):628-636.

21. Gallagher K, Jones J. Furosemide-induced ototoxicity. *Ann Intern Med*. 1979;91:744-745.

22. Downing G, Egelhoff J, Daily D, et al. Furosemide-related renal calcifications in the premature infant. A longitudinal ultrasonographic study. *Pediatr Radiol*. 1991;21:563-565.

23. Ryan M, Devane J, Ryan M, et al. Effects of diuretics on the renal handling of magnesium. *Drugs*. 1984;28(suppl 1):167-181.

24. Sutton R. Diuretics and calcium metabolism. *Am J Kidney Dis*. 1985;5:4-9.

25. Bilezikian J. Clinical review 51: management of hypercalcemia. *J Clin Endocrinol Metab*. 1993;77:1445-1449.

26. Suki W, Yium J, Von Minden M, et al. Acute treatment of hypercalcemia with furosemide. *N Engl J Med*. 1970;283:836-840.

27. Engle M, Lewy J, Lewy P, et al. The use of furosemide in the treatment of edema in infants and children. *Pediatrics*. 1978;62:811-818.

28. Flamenbaum W, Friedman R. Pharmacology, therapeutic efficacy, and adverse effects of bumetanide, a new "loop" diuretic. *Pharmacotherapy*. 1982;2:213-222.

29. Ellison D. Adaptation to diuretic drugs. In: Seldin D, Giebisch G, eds. *Diuretic Agents: Clinical Physiology and Pharmacology*. Boston: Academic Press; 1997.

30. Grahnen A, Hammarlund M, Lundqvist T. Implications of intraindividual variability in bioavailability studies of furosemide. *Eur J Clin Pharmacol*. 1984;27:595-602.

31. Peterson R, Simmons M, Rumack B, et al. Pharmacology of furosemide in the premature newborn infant. *J Pediatr*. 1980;97:139-143.

32. Marshall J, Wells T, Letzig L, et al. Pharmacokinetics and pharmacodynamics of bumetanide in critically ill pediatric patients. *J Clin Pharmacol*. 1998;38:994-1002.

33. Repetto H, Lewy J, Braudo J, et al. The renal functional response to furosemide in children with acute glomerulonephritis. *J Pediatr*. 1972; 80:660-666.

34. Arnold W. Efficacy of metolazone and furosemide in children with furosemide-resistant edema. *Pediatrics*. 1984;74:872-875.

35. Segar J, Robillard J, Johnson K, et al. Addition of metolazone to overcome tolerance to furosemide in infants with bronchopulmonary dysplasia. *J Pediatr*. 1992;120:966-973.

36. Sica D, Gehr T. Diuretic combinations in refractory oedema states: pharmacokinetic-pharmacodynamic relationships. *Clin Pharmacokinet*. 1996;30:229-249.

37. Borges H, Hocks J, Kjellstrand C. Mannitol intoxication in patients with renal failure. *Arch Intern Med*. 1982;142:63-66.

38. Decaux G, Soupart A, Vassart G. Non-peptide arginine-vasopressin antagonists: the vaptans. *Lancet*. 2008;371:1624-1632.

39. Wilcox C, Mitch W, Kelly R, et al. Response of the kidney to furosemide. I. Effects of salt intake and renal compensation. *J Lab Clin Med*. 1983;102:450-458.

40. Kobayashi S, Clemmons D, Nogami H, et al. Tubular hypertrophy due to work load induced by furosemide is associated with increases of IGF-1 and IGFBP-1. *Kidney Int*. 1995;47:818-828.

41. Loon N, Wilcox C, Unwin R. Mechanisms of impaired natriuretic response to furosemide during prolonged therapy. *Kidney Int*. 1989;36:682-689.

42. Klinge J, Scharf J, Hofbeck M, et al. Intermittent administration of furosemide versus continuous infusion in the postoperative management of children following open heart surgery. *Intensive Care Med*. 1997;23:693-697.

43. Rudy DW, Voelker JR, Greene PK, et al. Loop diuretics for chronic renal insufficiency: a continuous infusion is more efficacious than bolus therapy. *Ann Intern Med*. 1991;115:360-366.

44. Singh N, Kissoon N, Al Mofada S, et al. Comparison of continuous versus intermittent furosemide administration in postoperative cardiac patients. *Crit Care Med*. 1992;20:17-21.

45. van der Vorst M, Ruys-Dudok van Heel I, Kist-van Holthe J, et al. Continuous intravenous furosemide in haemodynamically unstable children after cardiac surgery. *Intensive Care Med*. 2001;27:711-715.

46. Brown C, Ogg C, Cameron J. High dose furosemide in acute renal failure: a controlled trial. *Clin Nephrol*. 1981;15:90-96.

47. Gubern J, Sancho J, Simo J, et al. A randomized trial on the effect of mannitol on postoperative renal function in patients with obstructive jaundice. *Surgery*. 1988;103:39-44.

48. Minuth A, Terrell J Jr, Suki W. Acute renal failure: a study of the course and prognosis of 104 patients and of the role of furosemide. *Am J Med Sci*. 1976;271:317-324.

49. Solomon R, Werner C, Mann D, et al. Effects of saline, mannitol, and furosemide to prevent acute decreases in renal function induced by radiocontrast agents. *N Engl J Med*. 1994;331:1416-1420.

Pediatric Renal Replacement Therapy in the Intensive Care Unit

Raj Munshi and Jordan M. Symons

PEARLS

- Patients receiving renal replacement therapy require careful monitoring of fluid and electrolyte balance and nutritional needs.
- Coordination between the critical care and nephrology staff is essential for the successful care of patients requiring renal replacement therapy.
- Earlier initiation of renal replacement therapy may improve outcome.
- Peritoneal dialysis remains an excellent form of acute pediatric renal replacement therapy.
- Hemodialysis is the modality of choice for rapid correction of fluid or metabolic imbalance.
- Continuous renal replacement therapy can establish and maintain fluid and metabolic control in unstable patients.

Renal replacement therapy (RRT) has an established role in the pediatric intensive care unit (ICU).[1] Indications for RRT include volume overload, azotemia, electrolyte and metabolic imbalance, intoxication, or inability to provide adequate nutrition due to renal compromise. Acute kidney injury (AKI), however severe, is highly correlated with poor outcome in hospitalized adults and children (see also Chapter 75).[2-5] In pediatric patients, studies demonstrate increased mortality in critically ill children with excessive fluid overload with concomitant AKI.[6-10] These observations, coupled with advanced capabilities for renal replacement therapy and growing evidence that early supportive therapy may improve outcomes, lead many clinicians to consider early initiation of renal support.[11-13] Earlier intervention, either with renal replacement therapy or perhaps through careful conservative management, may prevent complications associated with serious metabolic disarray and volume overload and permit vigorous nutritional and medical support.

Although all modalities of renal replacement therapy can correct these abnormalities, certain modalities may be better suited for specific pediatric clinical situations. To date, there is no evidence that the choice of RRT modality has an effect on mortality.[14-17] However, growing evidence favors continuous renal replacement therapy (CRRT) as compared to intermittent renal replacement therapy for renal recovery.[18,19]

Basic Physiology of Dialysis and Ultrafiltration

The physical principles of molecular movement across a semipermeable membrane underlie peritoneal dialysis, hemodialysis, and CRRT modalities. The following brief review summarizes the basic mechanisms of particle and water removal for all forms of renal replacement therapy.

Diffusion describes the movement of dissolved particles across a semipermeable membrane from an area of high concentration to an area of low concentration (Fig. 78.1). This physical principle operates in all renal replacement modalities in which dialysate is used. Diffusion favors the movement of smaller particles and is most rapid when the concentration gradient across the semipermeable membrane is greatest; diffusion stops when the concentrations achieve equilibrium.

Convection occurs when dissolved particles pass across a semipermeable membrane because of the effects of a pressure gradient (Fig. 78.2). Particles that are smaller than the pores of the membrane can pass freely, whereas larger particles are restricted. Because particles and water are moving together, the removed solution is isotonic to the original.

Ultrafiltration describes the movement of water across the semipermeable membrane due to pressure. Convection occurs with ultrafiltration.

Peritoneal Dialysis

Peritoneal dialysis (PD) has been successfully used as a therapy for AKI since 1946.[20] It is a frequent choice for chronic dialysis support, especially in children. There has been a shift in developed countries of using hemodialysis and hemofiltration for renal replacement therapy in AKI,[21] though observational studies in children and systematic review in adults show no difference in mortality between PD and hemodialysis and hemofiltration.[22-24] Today acute PD is a modality most often used in the developing world where its simplicity, effectiveness, and low cost make it attractive.[25] PD is also the ideal modality in patients with difficult vascular access and in those where the risk of complication from anticoagulation therapy is significant. Early initiation of PD in children, especially infants, who suffer AKI following cardiac surgery has been associated with improved outcomes.[26-28]

Physiology

It has been known for many years that the peritoneum can be used as a dialyzing membrane.[29] Instillation of dialysate into

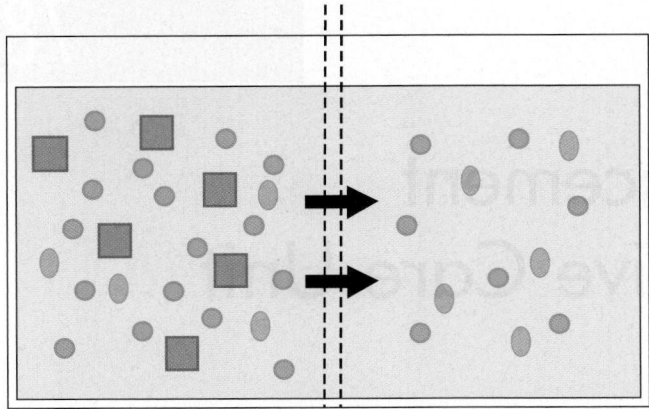

Fig. 78.1. Diffusion. Particles move across the semipermeable membrane from an area of higher concentration to an area of lower concentration. Smaller particles diffuse more freely, whereas larger particles are relatively restricted.

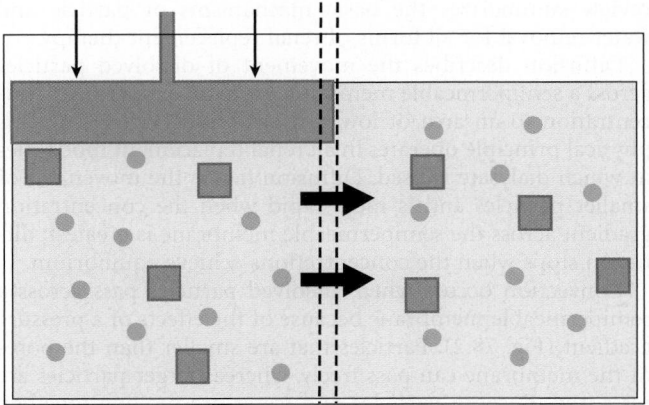

Fig. 78.2. Convection. Particles move across the semipermeable membrane, carried by ultrafiltered water, because of the effect of pressure. All particles up to the cutoff size of the membrane move relatively equally. The concentration of the effluent is equal to that of the original solution.

the peritoneal space permits diffusion of particles out of the blood and into the fluid across the peritoneum, which acts as a semipermeable membrane. Hypertonic solution, causing an osmotic gradient, generates an ultrafiltrate. Water movement will also tend to drag particles across the peritoneum by convection. After the dwell is complete, the spent dialysate is drained from the abdomen and fresh dialysis fluid is introduced.

Indications

PD can remove excess fluid and provide volume control in patients with oligoanuria. Compared with fluid removal by intermittent hemodialysis, fluid removal with PD is much slower. Manipulation of dialysis fluid osmolality and dwell time can adjust the quantity of volume removed. The slow, steady ultrafiltration achieved with PD may be preferable to the rapid fluid removal that occurs in intermittent hemodialysis, particularly in hemodynamically unstable, critically ill patients.

Similar to volume control, PD provides slow and relatively continuous metabolic control. It is an effective method for correction of uremia. Manipulation of the PD prescription can improve molecular clearance.

Technique

The basic technique for PD involves instilling a sterile dialysate into the peritoneal cavity and allowing it to dwell for a specified period, during which particles diffuse across the peritoneal membrane and water moves across by ultrafiltration. At the end of the dwell time, the fluid is removed from the peritoneal space and the process is repeated.

Flexible catheters are most often used for chronic PD in pediatric patients. For acute PD, either this form of a surgically placed catheter or percutaneously inserted temporary PD catheters may be used. Data suggest that fewer complications occur with surgically placed catheters.[30] Catheters come in a variety of sizes, depending on the size of the patient. Local practice often determines who will insert the catheters when they are needed; the procedure requires expertise to ensure proper functioning of the catheter. The International Society for Peritoneal Dialysis recommends a surgically placed Tenckhoff catheter, currently the most utilized flexible PD catheter.[31]

PD fluid comes in standardized, sterile bags with premixed formulations; pharmacy preparation is usually unnecessary. The solutions consist of electrolytes (such as sodium, calcium, magnesium), dextrose as the primary osmotic agent, and base (either lactate or bicarbonate). Lactate absorption can lead to confusion regarding acid/base interpretation, especially in critically ill infants. In such settings bicarbonate-based dialysis fluid may be preferable,[32] although this fluid may require extemporaneous preparation by the local pharmacy, as premade solutions that use bicarbonate as a base are not available in all countries.

Ultrafiltration in PD is accomplished by osmotic pressure, usually through the presence of dextrose in the dialysis fluid. Peritoneal dialysate contains standardized concentrations of dextrose; the choices vary somewhat between the United States and other countries. Dialysate with higher concentrations of dextrose yields greater ultrafiltration for each exchange of fluid.

Peritoneal dialysate should be warmed to body temperature before instillation. This step is particularly important in small patients, in whom cold dialysate infusion can cause hypotension.

Initial exchanges with a new PD catheter should use relatively lower volumes of dialysate (10 to 20 mL/kg; <500 mL/m^2) to limit the chance of leakage from the catheter entrance operative site. Volumes may increase gradually during the next few days or weeks to 30 to 40 mL/kg; 800-1100 mL/m^2.[33]

Longer dwell periods between exchanges provide more time for equilibration of dialyzable particles and for ultrafiltration. Although shorter dwell times may not maximize mass transport for given dwell periods, they may permit more dialysis and ultrafiltration in a 24-hour period by allowing more exchanges per day. Initial dwell periods of 30 to 60 minutes can be adjusted later on the basis of clinical status.

PD fluid can be instilled by hand (manual PD) or with the use of a cycler (automated PD), a device that will automatically fill and empty the patient's abdomen with dialysate on a preprogrammed schedule. The cycler also contains a warmer for the fluid and monitoring systems to record effluent volumes. Several brands of cyclers are currently available. Programming limitations may prevent the use of a cycler for some patients who require very small fill volumes or very short dwell times.

When solute clearance or ultrafiltration is suboptimal with conventional PD or the patient cannot tolerate high fill volumes, one may consider the technique of continuous flow peritoneal dialysis (CFPD). CFPD requires two dialysis catheters placed in the peritoneum, one for inflow and the other for outflow of peritoneal fluid.[34] There is no dwell time per se as the peritoneal fluid is in constant transit through the peritoneum. CFPD can result in a fivefold increase in clearance and a ninefold increase in ultrafiltration.[35] Experience with CFPD is limited and it cannot at this time be considered a standard technique in pediatrics, although it may hold promise in the future.

Disadvantages and Complications

The PD technique requires placement of a peritoneal catheter and a sufficiently maintained intraabdominal status to permit infusion of dialysate with successful diffusion and ultrafiltration. Patients who have undergone an abdominal operation or have had abdominal complications may be poor candidates for PD.

Invasion of the peritoneal space puts the patient at risk for peritonitis, a potentially serious complication. The importance of sterile technique when performing PD cannot be overemphasized. Appropriate technique limits the risk of infectious complications, which could be fatal in a critically ill patient, but does not eliminate the risk.

Peritonitis must always be considered in a patient undergoing PD who has a fever or cloudy effluent. Dialysate should be analyzed for cell count, Gram stain, and bacterial culture if infection is suspected. Empirical or specific antibiotics can be placed in the dialysate to treat peritonitis via the intraperitoneal route.[36]

Dialysate can fail to fill or drain through the PD catheter because of a number of potential problems, including kinking of the catheter, fibrin plugs, omental obstruction, and catheter malposition. Percutaneously inserted temporary dialysis catheters are more prone to malfunction than are surgically placed catheters.[37] Abdominal x-ray images can confirm appropriate positioning and permit checks for kinks in the catheter. Some success has been reported with thrombolytic agents to treat fibrin plugging.[38-40] Revision or replacement of the catheter may need to be considered if simple maneuvers do not correct the malfunction.

Perforation of abdominal or pelvic structures can occur, either at the time of initial catheter placement or later.[37] Although this event is relatively uncommon, significant morbidity can result.

PD is a suboptimal choice for patients who require rapid correction of metabolic abnormalities, immediate removal of circulating toxins, or rapid ultrafiltration for acute complications of fluid overload. For the latter indications, hemodialysis would be the preferred modality. Effectiveness of PD may be suboptimal in settings of low cardiac output where splanchnic circulation is compromised. However, this does not preclude the use of PD in selected cases, such as for infants following surgery for congenital heart disease.[26-28]

Fluid leakage is seen most often with dwell volumes that are too large, especially in the period immediately after catheter placement.[41] Lower fill volumes should be used. Fluid leakage into the thorax can compromise respiration. External fluid leakage around the catheter increases the risk of infection.

Intensive Care Unit Issues

Patients undergoing PD can lose protein into the dialysate. Nutritional support must provide sufficient protein to compensate for this loss. High dextrose concentrations in the dialysate can cause hyperglycemia; administration of insulin may be necessary. Indwelling dialysis fluid causes increased intraabdominal pressure that can complicate care of the critically ill patient. Diaphragmatic excursion may be limited and venous return can be reduced. Stomach compression can lead to gastroesophageal reflux. Although patients undergoing long-term PD who receive fewer daily exchanges usually require maximal fill volumes to achieve adequate dialysis, patients undergoing short-term PD may do better using submaximal fill volumes with more frequent exchanges provided around the clock.

Intermittent Hemodialysis

Intermittent hemodialysis (IHD) is a well-established technique for pediatric patients.[42] IHD offers the advantage of high efficiency for rapid metabolic correction and fluid removal. Efficient fluid and toxin removal requires rapid blood and dialysate flow. Factors that prevent achievement of high blood flow include systemic hypotension and a narrow vascular access. IHD for infants and small children can be technically demanding due to access difficulties and relatively large extracorporeal blood volume. IHD may be the preferred modality for some critically ill pediatric patients that require rapid removal of a specific toxin; successful treatment in this setting requires experienced personnel.

Physiology

The dialyzer used in IHD is an artificial semipermeable membrane. The most common design used today is the hollow-fiber dialyzer. It consists of a plastic cartridge traversed by several thousand thin hollow fibers, each with microscopic fenestrations that permit the passage of water and other small molecules. Dialyzers vary in surface area, permeability, priming volume, and membrane composition; numerous dialyzers are available commercially. Choosing different dialyzer characteristics permits adjustment of the dialysis prescription to the clinical situation.

While blood flows through the hollow fibers of the dialyzer, dialysate flows through the cartridge in the space surrounding the hollow fibers. Particles move by diffusion from the blood across the semipermeable membrane into the dialysate. Use of high-flow dialysate with maximal blood flow through the dialyzer permits intermittent hemodialysis to remove particles more efficiently than any other renal replacement therapy.

Increasing blood flow, dialysate flow, or dialyzer size will increase the rate of diffusion. Because diffusion favors the movement of small particles over large particles, large molecules or small molecules bound to larger molecules (such as albumin) will not dialyze well. In addition, intracellular particles will move into the vascular compartment on the basis of individual cell membrane transport characteristics, which may limit the rate at which dialysis can remove particles that do not reside within the vascular compartment.

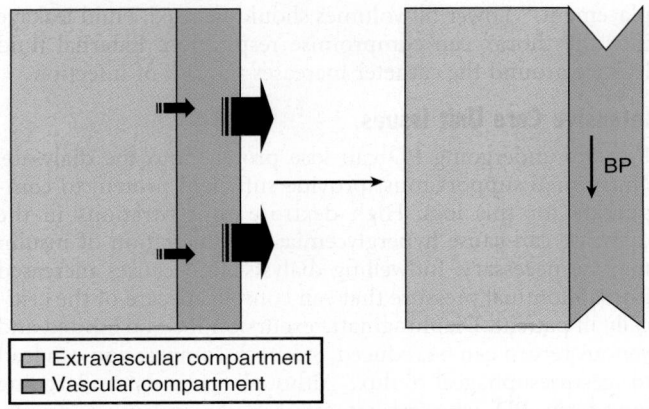

Fig. 78.3. Two-compartment model of ultrafiltration. The rate of water removal from the vascular compartment by ultrafiltration *(large arrows)* exceeds the rate of refilling from the extravascular compartment *(smaller arrows),* and this process leads to relative vascular volume depletion and hypotension.

Ultrafiltration on hemodialysis occurs because of hydrostatic pressure across the membrane that forces water out of the blood. Dissolved particles will travel with the water, leaving by convection. With use of IHD, dialysis staff can control the rate of ultrafiltration with precision and can achieve high rates of ultrafiltration.

Analogous to the process of diffusion, ultrafiltration during IHD removes fluid only from the vascular compartment. Extravascular or "third space" fluid must move into the vascular compartment for removal by ultrafiltration. When the rate of movement from the extravascular space is slower than the rate of ultrafiltration, intravascular depletion can occur even though total body water remains elevated (Fig. 78.3). This "two-compartment" model represents a potential limitation of rapid ultrafiltration during IHD, especially in the critically ill patient.

Indications

Due to its high efficiency, hemodialysis is the best modality for rapid particle removal. IHD is indicated for the treatment of toxic ingestions, many serious drug overdoses, and metabolic derangements that lead to the overproduction of endogenous toxins such as ammonia (see Chapters 82 and 128).[43-46]

The IHD system can perform ultrafiltration more rapidly than any other renal replacement modality. Consequently it is often the best choice for the treatment of critical volume overload but may be limited by the patient's ability to tolerate rapid fluid removal. Technology to guide ultrafiltration by the noninvasive monitoring of hematocrit changes during IHD may prevent or mitigate hypotension associated with ultrafiltration.[47]

Profound metabolic imbalance, such as that seen with critical hyperkalemia, can be corrected most quickly with IHD. Patients with oncologic problems such as tumor lysis syndrome may require IHD to rapidly correct the multiple metabolic abnormalities and to aid clearance of uric acid, which can cause AKI (see Chapter 94).[48,49]

Technique

Vascular access is the first step for successful hemodialysis. Double-lumen catheters for hemodialysis come in a variety of sizes; occasionally, two single-lumen catheters at separate sites are needed for small infants, although data suggest that these catheters do not perform as well.[50,51] Catheters can be placed in jugular, femoral, or subclavian positions (see Chapter 19). The most desirable site for a double-lumen hemodialysis catheter is the right internal jugular vein; it provides access to a high flow area in the superior vena cava/right atrium, permits a straight venous path for the operator from insertion site to the target location, can be readily accessed for insertion of either tunneled or nontunneled catheters depending on the indication, allows ambulation and reduces discomfort for the patient as compared to the femoral site, and is less susceptible to complicating venous stenosis that will limit future permanent vascular access creation such as arteriovenous (AV) fistula. By contrast, subclavian access is associated with increased risk of stenosis that would result in loss of potential sites for AV fistula formation in the ipsilateral arm and therefore is not recommended. In neonates, umbilical catheters have been utilized if other access has failed but are often not successful due to poor flow dynamics and are not recommended.

Most patients receiving IHD will require anticoagulation therapy to prevent clotting within the dialysis circuit. Any anticoagulant can be used, with goal-activated clotting time to be 1.5 to 2 times normal if clinically appropriate. Unfractionated heparin is the most common anticoagulant used for IHD. Some may be able to undergo successful dialysis with little or no heparin because of coagulopathy related to their systemic disease. If regional anticoagulation (anticoagulation of the dialysis circuit without systemic effects) is preferred, dialysate containing citrate is available.[52] The citrate in the dialysate will bind calcium locally at the dialyzer membrane, limiting clotting within the dialyzer. Monitoring of ionized calcium is not required as the concentration of citrate is low, and thus the patient is not at risk for hypocalcemia. Clinical experience thus far shows citrate containing dialysate to be effective as an anticoagulant, but some centers have found that additional reduced doses of systemic heparinization were required.[53]

The blood pump rate is chosen based on the patient's clinical status and the quality of the vascular access. In smaller patients with smaller catheters, blood pump speeds often must run at less than 100 mL/min; in infants, speeds may run as low as 25 to 50 mL/min. Larger patients can tolerate faster blood pump speeds. Higher blood flow rates permit greater mass transfer of particles out of the patient in a given period.

The chosen dialyzer should provide sufficient clearance to achieve the goals of the dialysis session. Smaller patients receive dialysis with smaller dialyzers to limit extracorporeal blood volume and reduce the risk of dialyzer clotting with slower blood flow rates.

Small patients or those with unstable blood pressure may require priming of the IHD circuit with saline solution, albumin, or reconstituted whole blood. Dialysis machines with precise volumetric ultrafiltration control permit accurate and safe IHD in neonates and infants, for whom small inaccuracies in ultrafiltration volumes could potentially lead to severe fluid imbalances. Dialysis fluid concentrations of electrolytes can be adjusted to some extent on the basis of the clinical situation. The length of the IHD session will vary depending on the clinical situation and goals of the therapy. Mathematical models permit estimation of dialytic clearance and can be used to structure session length. The rate at which the patient can tolerate ultrafiltration is often the limiting factor in IHD for critically ill patients. Sessions may need to be extended to achieve ultrafiltration goals without significant hypotension.

Disadvantages and Complications

The principal disadvantage of IHD is the requirement for vascular access. Acceptable access can be difficult to achieve in critically ill children. Complications related to the access can include infection, bleeding, and thrombosis.

IHD's benefit of high efficiency with rapid fluid and particle removal can lead to difficulties in the ICU setting. Critically ill patients may not tolerate the rapid ultrafiltration and metabolic shifts of IHD.

Smaller patients or those with unstable blood pressure may require priming of the extracorporeal circuit to limit hemodynamic stress at dialysis initiation. For infants in whom the extracorporeal volume is relatively much larger, priming may need to be done with a blood/albumin mix, which exposes the patient to blood products.

Most IHD sessions require systemic anticoagulation with heparin, which can be difficult to manage in a critically ill child. Heparin exposure can complicate bleeding and cause heparin-induced thrombocytopenia. With careful monitoring of clotting times and circuit performance during the session, it is possible to perform IHD without any anticoagulation. Regional anticoagulation is also available with dialysate containing citrate.

Intensive Care Unit Issues

Patients receiving IHD as ongoing renal replacement therapy in the ICU require special attention to fluid and electrolyte balance. One should limit potassium and phosphorus delivery and may need to limit total daily fluids because ultrafiltration only occurs intermittently. Packed red blood cells should ideally be administered while on dialysis to dialyze off the excess potassium. Medication doses and schedule may require adjustment because of poor excretion with renal failure and subsequent rapid removal with dialysis (see Chapters 77 and 124).

Continuous Renal Replacement Therapy

CRRT is a generic term applied to several techniques of extracorporeal renal support. Similar to IHD in the use of a blood pump and hemofilter, the various subcategories of CRRT differ in their reliance on diffusion, convection, or a combination of the two for molecular clearance.

CRRT has become more popular as a method of renal support for pediatric patients.[1,51] Technologic improvements in catheters, blood pumps, and ultrafiltration control mechanisms permit the application of CRRT to even the smallest infants.[54,55] Compared to IHD, data suggest continuous modalities of renal replacement therapy may increase the likelihood of recovery of renal function in critically ill survivors of AKI.[18,19]

Physiology

The CRRT hemofilter is similar to that used for IHD. CRRT membranes traditionally have been more porous to permit greater removal of water. Numerous hemofilters are available commercially.

Both convection and diffusion can be used to remove particles during CRRT. Dialysate allows diffusion, which favors the movement of smaller molecules. High rates of ultrafiltration will remove both small and larger particles by convection, up to the limits of the membrane. With high ultrafiltration rates to achieve better convective clearance, the patient may need to receive replacement of volume and electrolytes to compensate for that lost in ultrafiltrate.

Because of slower flow rates, the clearance achieved with CRRT may be lower than that of IHD. Continuous therapies, however, make up for this lower efficiency through the extended time of the treatment. Compared with a 3- or 4-hour IHD session, CRRT running 24 hours a day can achieve equivalent daily clearance with less metabolic variation. Newer CRRT devices can run at flow rates approaching those seen in IHD, greatly increasing the potential for rapid molecular clearance.

Nomenclature for the various subcategories of CRRT is based on the vascular access and the primary method of particle clearance (convection, diffusion, or both). Because most CRRT in pediatric patients uses a pump-assisted venovenous method, the most commonly used terms are *continuous venovenous hemofiltration* (CVVH), which uses high convective clearance requiring replacement fluids; *continuous venovenous hemodialysis* (CVVHD), which uses dialysis fluid for diffusion but minimal additional convection; and *continuous venovenous hemodiafiltration* (CVVHDF), which uses both dialysis fluid and replacement fluids for combined diffusion and high-grade convection.

Indications

As a result of the slow, continuous removal of fluid, CRRT is particularly well suited to the treatment of volume overload in critically ill patients. Whereas IHD will attempt to reach an ultrafiltration goal within a relatively short therapeutic session, CRRT allows continuous ultrafiltration that can help maintain cardiovascular stability.

CRRT is useful to maintain metabolic balance through ongoing removal of unwanted particles. Although it is less efficient than IHD, CRRT's continuous nature can avoid daily fluctuations inherent in the use of an intermittent modality. In addition, CRRT can be used as a secondary method to maintain metabolic balance after rapid correction with IHD.[56]

For patients with diminished renal function and decreased urinary output, CRRT can allow administration of the daily load of fluids and clearance required to deliver medication, nutrition, and blood products. With this modality the patient can be maintained in a more stable balance compared with IHD, in which the patient has progressive volume overload between IHD sessions and then must achieve the ultrafiltration goal in a brief treatment period.

Technique

As in IHD, successful CRRT requires adequate vascular access (see Chapter 19). Given the relatively large extracorporeal volume, smaller patients may require priming of the CRRT circuit with blood/albumin mix. In larger, more stable patients, CRRT can be initiated successfully with saline prime.

Earlier methods that entailed arteriovenous access have largely been abandoned in favor of venovenous CRRT. Older systems with adapted blood and fluid pumps linked together extemporaneously have been replaced by dedicated CRRT machinery. Several CRRT systems are available at this time; this latest generation of CRRT machines permits much greater accuracy for blood pump speed, fluid delivery, and ultrafiltration control.

Anticoagulation

Adequate anticoagulation is essential for successful CRRT. Similar to IHD, any anticoagulant can be used, with goal activated clotting time to be 1.5 to 2 times normal if clinically appropriate. Currently, most patients treated with CRRT receive systemic heparin, regional citrate, or no added anticoagulation.

Systemic heparinization has been the traditional form of anticoagulation used in CRRT. This method is proven and functions well. Disadvantages include systemic anticoagulation with risk of bleeding, risk of heparin-induced thrombocytopenia, and the need for frequent monitoring and adjustment of the heparin dose.

Regional citrate anticoagulation has become popular for CRRT in both adult and pediatric patients. Citrate, introduced into the CRRT circuit, chelates calcium, which is a required cofactor in both the intrinsic and extrinsic arms of the clotting cascade. Calcium is infused back into the patient through a central access to prevent systemic hypocalcemia. Citrate is metabolized to bicarbonate, acting as a source of base. Several protocols have been developed for regional citrate anticoagulation in CRRT.[57-60] The systems are stable and require less monitoring than heparin-based anticoagulation. Disadvantages include the potential for acid/base imbalance, the risk of hypercalcemia or hypocalcemia, citrate excess due to poor metabolism or diminished clearance, and the need for additional central access for high rates of calcium delivery.

Many critically ill patients have disorders of coagulation as a part of their multiple organ system injury and can undergo CRRT without exogenous anticoagulation. Increased clotting of the CRRT circuit in such patients may be a sign of improving clinical status. A study of pediatric CRRT suggested that circuits that are run without anticoagulation have a significantly shorter life span; thus it may be appropriate to consider the use of anticoagulation even in the coagulopathic patient to ensure continued delivery of the therapy.[61]

Patient and vascular access size can limit blood pump rate. The current generation of CRRT machines can run at lower blood pump speeds with greater accuracy than did earlier systems.

Many brands of hemofilter are available for CRRT. Larger surface areas will permit more rapid ultrafiltration and clearance by convection. Of particular interest in the pediatric patient are reports of profound hypotensive events related to the use of a type of polyacrylonitrile hemofilter known as the acrylonitrile AN-69 membrane.[62] This reaction, occurring rapidly when the patient's blood comes in contact with the hemofilter, is thought to be related to the release of bradykinin in response to the low pH of blood used to prime the CRRT circuit. Smaller patients and those with metabolic acidosis seem to be at greatest risk. Maneuvers to adjust pH within the circuit and limit this reaction have been described.[62-64] Some practitioners prefer to avoid use of the AN-69 membrane to limit the risk of complication, while others choose to tolerate this potential complication in patients with sepsis in light of the relatively high interleukin-6 clearance provided by AN-69 membranes.[65]

Dialysate and Infused Fluids

Nearly all of the current CRRT machines use premade, fully compounded dialysate or hemofiltration fluid rather than generating dialysis fluid online from concentrates (during IHD the dialysate is generated online). Commercially available dialysis and hemofiltration fluid, compounded under quality-controlled conditions and delivered in premixed sterile bags, have largely replaced the use of extemporaneously prepared fluid from local pharmacy services. Several manufacturers offer solutions for CRRT; the products come in a variety of electrolyte concentrations to suit differing clinical needs. It has been suggested that the use of commercial CRRT solutions, rather than those made by a local pharmacy, can reduce the likelihood of errors related to solution preparation.[66]

Replacement fluids are infused to the CRRT system either before the hemofilter ("prefilter" or "predilution") or after ("postfilter" or "postdilution"). Prefilter delivery reduces convective clearance at a given ultrafiltration rate because the blood entering the hemofilter will be diluted by the replacement fluid. This reduction, however, can be easily overcome with an increase of the ultrafiltration rate. Furthermore, prefilter replacement may permit higher ultrafiltration rates because it limits hemoconcentration within the hemofilter and thus lessens the chances of filter clotting; this may be less of a concern with citrate anticoagulation, which is very effective at preserving filter life. Some CRRT machines will permit either prefilter or postfilter delivery of replacement fluids, whereas others have a fixed location for replacement fluids.

Clearance

CRRT blood pump, dialysate, and replacement fluid rates traditionally have been lower overall than those used in IHD. Consequently, clearance rates are lower but total daily clearance increases because the therapy is continuous. In most prescriptions, the limiting factor in CRRT clearance is the solution flow rate; greater rates of clearance often can be achieved with an increase in the rate of dialysate or replacement fluid. Newer CRRT machines are capable of higher solution rates than in the past. Slower blood pump speeds can also potentially limit clearances; some newer devices are capable of higher blood pump speeds. Controversy exists in adult patients regarding appropriate goals for clearance. An influential single-center study suggested better outcomes with higher rates of clearance,[67] but this finding has not been reproduced in subsequent multicenter trials.[68,69] This question has not been fully studied in children.

Slow, steady ultrafiltration to gradually achieve fluid balance and then maintain it is the hallmark of CRRT. Slow ultrafiltration can permit movement of extravascular fluid into the vascular space at a rate roughly equal to the ultrafiltration rate, which allows greater mobilization of fluid while the risk of acute intravascular volume depletion and hypotension is limited. Ultrafiltration rates must be chosen on the basis of clinical status of the patient and fluid balance goals; frequent reevaluation is often necessary.

Disadvantages and Complications

Like IHD, CRRT requires vascular access, which can be difficult to obtain in infants and small children. Data suggest that 5-Fr single-lumen catheters should not be used for CRRT because they are associated with significantly shorter functional CRRT circuit survival.[50] Continuous extracorporeal perfusion and anticoagulation carry risks of bleeding and infection. Some patients experience blood pressure instability despite the slow method of ultrafiltration. Continuous exposure to heparin can lead to heparin-induced thrombocytopenia. Patients receiving citrate anticoagulation are at risk for acid/base disturbance or hypocalcemia. Citrate excess can cause low patient ionized calcium with normal or high total calcium levels, the so-called *calcium gap* or *citrate lock*,[58,70] which occurs when excess citrate binds free calcium in the patient. Under these circumstances, citrate delivery should be reduced or clearance through the CRRT system should be increased.

Intensive Care Unit Issues

Continuous clearance on CRRT, particularly with convective modalities, can cause profound electrolyte deficiencies. Careful attention must be paid to appropriate replacement of electrolytes lost through CRRT. Similarly, nitrogen losses on CRRT can be high.[71] Patients require increased nutritional support during CRRT therapy, and careful consideration of the nutritional prescription is required.[72] Medication dosages often require adjustment because of losses through the CRRT system. Coordination between the ICU staff and nephrology staff is essential to establish appropriate goals for fluid removal and metabolic control.

Extended Daily Dialysis

IHD sessions can be extended in length to provide therapy that approaches CRRT. Variously referred to as slow low-efficiency dialysis or slow extended daily dialysis, such techniques can provide improved molecular clearance with better tolerance of ultrafiltration when compared with conventional schedules for IHD. Sessions may run 6 to 8 hours or more on a daily basis.[73]

Some institutions may prefer extended daily dialysis methods because they obviate the need to purchase and maintain separate, dedicated CRRT equipment, using instead standard IHD machines that have been adapted for longer session length. In addition, disposable materials for IHD are usually less expensive than are those for CRRT, potentially leading to cost savings. Because the patient is not connected to the device 24 hours a day, patient mobility for tests or surgical procedures may be facilitated and risk of treatment-related complications may be reduced. Online generation of dialysate, as for standard IHD, greatly simplifies the question of solutions compared with premixed bags that must be frequently exchanged for CRRT. However, most online dialysate is not sterile, raising a theoretic risk for the critically ill patient. Newer devices capable of extended therapies can be adapted to provide ultrapure dialysis fluid, which may mitigate this potential concern. Individual institutions may need to consider staffing requirements related to tending an IHD device for extended sessions.

Although use of extended intermittent hemodialysis (EIHD) techniques for both adult and pediatric patients is growing, the literature has a dearth of information regarding efficacy in the pediatric population. This modality is often chosen for pragmatic reasons rather than because of proven superiority. Meta-analysis of adult studies comparing EIHD and CRRT limited to randomized control trials found no differences in recovery in renal function, fluid removal, days in the intensive care unit, or mortality.[74] It remains a reasonable option under the appropriate circumstances.

Outcomes of Renal Replacement in Critically Ill Children

Outcome data comparing modalities for pediatric renal replacement are sparse. Most studies are from single centers and are limited by small numbers of subjects.

Studies in pediatric renal replacement therapy have centered on CRRT. Findings from five studies, comprising an aggregate of more than 400 patients, demonstrate an association of higher mortality for patients with more severe levels of volume overload.[6-9,75] A multicenter observational registry has provided insight on outcomes in pediatric CRRT.[55] Overall survival on CRRT in this cohort of more than 300 critically ill children was 58%; this percentage is superior to previously reported outcomes and likely represents improvement in CRRT techniques as well as overall critical care for the pediatric patient. Outcomes in the subpopulations of children with multisystem organ dysfunction and stem cell transplant who required CRRT also were noted to be improved compared with historical reports.[6,76] Because these studies did not compare CRRT to other interventions, no specific evidence-based comments can be made regarding choice of modality in the modern era, and this decision is largely based on experience and opinion.

Overall mortality of patients with AKI was determined to be 15.3% in a cross-sectional analysis of the 2009 Kids Inpatient Database comprising 2,644,263 children of whom 10,322 had developed AKI.[77] The study also demonstrated that children younger than 1 month of age, children requiring critical care, and those requiring dialysis had the highest rate of inpatient mortality.

Advances in Pediatric Renal Replacement Therapies

Pediatric renal replacement therapy traditionally has come from adaptation of adult technologies to the smaller pediatric patient. Advancement in technology has resulted in smaller filter size, permitting lower blood flow rate and smaller extracorporeal blood volume. Despite these advancements, renal replacement therapy for smaller patients remains a challenge; some consider manual PD as the only option in patients who are less than 3 kg. Two therapies have been developed specifically for neonates and small children. The first is a CRRT machine developed in Italy by Dr. Claudio Ronco. Named CARPEDIEM (Cardio-Renal Pediatric Dialysis Emergency Machine), it has low extracorporeal blood volume of <30 mL and accurate ultrafiltration control with a precision of 1 gram. Four- and seven-French double-lumen catheters can be utilized for access. The therapy has been used successfully in patients <3 kg.[78] The second device is a hemodialysis machine developed by Dr. Malcom G. Coulthard's group in Newcastle, United Kingdom, named NIDUS (Newcastle Infant Dialysis and Ultrafiltration System). Using a syringe-based system, the machine withdraws 5- to 12.5-mL aliquots of blood from a single-lumen central venous catheter and passes it through a dialyzer filter before returning it to the patient. Extracorporeal blood volume is limited to 9.3 mL, and ultrafiltration precision is controlled to 3.2 μL.[79] Both of these devices offer the hope of providing renal replacement therapies safely to neonates and small children.

Summary

Pediatric patients who require renal replacement therapy represent a special challenge. Multiple modalities are available, and the best choice may be dictated by the clinical situation and local expertise. Careful attention to fluid and electrolyte balance and appropriate nutritional support and close interaction between critical care and nephrology personnel will yield the best outcomes.

Key References

1. Walters S, Porter C, Brophy PD. Dialysis and pediatric acute kidney injury: choice of renal support modality. *Pediatr Nephrol.* 2009;24: 37-48.
3. Akcan-Arikan A, Zappitelli M, Loftis LL, et al. Modified RIFLE criteria in critically ill children with acute kidney injury. *Kidney Int.* 2007;71: 1028-1035.
4. Plotz FB, Bouma AB, van Wijk JA, et al. Pediatric acute kidney injury in the ICU: an independent evaluation of pRIFLE criteria. *Intensive Care Med.* 2008;34:1713-1717.
6. Goldstein SL, Somers MJ, Baum MA, et al. Pediatric patients with multiorgan dysfunction syndrome receiving continuous renal replacement therapy. *Kidney Int.* 2005;67:653-658.
10. Sutherland SM, Zappitelli M, Alexander SR, et al. Fluid overload and mortality in children receiving continuous renal replacement therapy: the prospective pediatric continuous renal replacement therapy registry. *Am J Kidney Dis.* 2010;55:316-325.
11. Karvellas CJ, Farhat MR, Sajjad I, et al. A comparison of early versus late initiation of renal replacement therapy in critically ill patients with acute kidney injury: a systematic review and meta-analysis. *Crit Care.* 2011;15:R72.
12. Wang X, Jie Yuan W. Timing of initiation of renal replacement therapy in acute kidney injury: a systematic review and meta-analysis. *Ren Fail.* 2012; 34:396-402.
13. Modem V, Thompson M, Gollhofer D, et al. Timing of continuous renal replacement therapy and mortality in critically ill children. *Crit Care Med.* 2014;42:943-953.
15. Rabindranath K, Adams J, Macleod AM, et al. Intermittent versus continuous renal replacement therapy for acute renal failure in adults. *Cochrane Database Syst Rev.* 2007;CD003773.
16. Pannu N, Klarenbach S, Wiebe N, et al. Renal replacement therapy in patients with acute renal failure: a systematic review. *JAMA.* 2008;299: 793-805.
18. Schneider AG, Bellomo R, Bagshaw SM, et al. Choice of renal replacement therapy modality and dialysis dependence after acute kidney injury: a systematic review and meta-analysis. *Intensive Care Med.* 2013;39: 987-997.
24. Chionh CY, Soni SS, Finkelstein FO, et al. Use of peritoneal dialysis in AKI: a systematic review. *Clin J Am Soc Nephrol.* 2013;8:1649-1660.
25. Mishra OP, Gupta AK, Pooniya V, et al. Peritoneal dialysis in children with acute kidney injury: a developing country experience. *Perit Dial Int.* 2012;32:431-436.
26. Kwiatkowski DM, Menon S, Krawczeski CD, et al. Improved outcomes with peritoneal dialysis catheter placement after cardiopulmonary bypass in infants. *J Thoracic Cardiovasc Surg.* 2015;149:230-236.
27. Bojan M, Gioanni S, Vouhe PR, et al. Early initiation of peritoneal dialysis in neonates and infants with acute kidney injury following cardiac surgery is associated with a significant decrease in mortality. *Kidney Int.* 2012;82:474-481.
31. Cullis B, Abdelraheem M, Abrahams G, et al. Peritoneal dialysis for acute kidney injury. *Perit Dial Int.* 2014;34:494-517.
34. Raaijmakers R, Schroder CH, Gajjar P, et al. Continuous flow peritoneal dialysis: first experience in children with acute renal failure. *Clin J Am Soc Nephrol.* 2011;6:311-318.
35. Amerling R, DeSimone L, Inciong-Reyes R, et al. Clinical experience with continuous flow and flow-through peritoneal dialysis. *Semin Dial.* 2001;14:388-390.

36. Warady BA, Bakkaloglu S, Newland J, et al. Consensus guidelines for the prevention and treatment of catheter-related infections and peritonitis in pediatric patients receiving peritoneal dialysis: 2012 update. *Perit Dial Int.* 2012;32(suppl 2):S32-S86.
40. Krishnan RG, Moghal NE. Tissue plasminogen activator for blocked peritoneal dialysis catheters. *Pediatr Nephrol.* 2006;21:300.
42. Fischbach M, Terzic J, Menouer S, et al. Hemodialysis in children: principles and practice. *Semin Nephrol.* 2001;21:470-479.
47. Michael M, Brewer ED, Goldstein SL. Blood volume monitoring to achieve target weight in pediatric hemodialysis patients. *Pediatr Nephrol.* 2004;19:432-437.
50. Hackbarth R, Bunchman TE, Chua AN, et al. The effect of vascular access location and size on circuit survival in pediatric continuous renal replacement therapy: a report from the PPCRRT registry. *Int J Artif Organs.* 2007;30:1116-1121.
52. Davenport A. Alternatives to standard unfractionated heparin for pediatric hemodialysis treatments. *Pediatr Nephrol.* 2012;27:1869-1879.
53. Hanevold C, Lu S, Yonekawa K. Utility of citrate dialysate in management of acute kidney injury in children. *Hemodial Int.* 2010;14(suppl 1): S2-S6.
54. Symons JM, Brophy PD, Gregory MJ, et al. Continuous renal replacement therapy in children up to 10 kg. *Am J Kidney Dis.* 2003;41:984-989.
55. Symons JM, Chua AN, Somers MJ, et al. Demographic characteristics of pediatric continuous renal replacement therapy: a report of the prospective pediatric continuous renal replacement therapy registry. *Clin J Am Soc Nephrol: CJASN.* 2007;2:732-738.
56. McBryde KD, Kershaw DB, Bunchman TE, et al. Renal replacement therapy in the treatment of confirmed or suspected inborn errors of metabolism. *J Pediatr.* 2006;148:770-778.
57. Mehta RL, McDonald BR, Aguilar MM, et al. Regional citrate anticoagulation for continuous arteriovenous hemodialysis in critically ill patients. *Kidney Int.* 1990;38:976-981.
59. Tolwani AJ, Campbell RC, Schenk MB, et al. Simplified citrate anticoagulation for continuous renal replacement therapy. *Kidney Int.* 2001;60: 370-374.
60. Tolwani AJ, Prendergast MB, Speer RR, et al. A practical citrate anticoagulation continuous venovenous hemodiafiltration protocol for metabolic control and high solute clearance. *Clin J Am Soc Nephrol: CJASN.* 2006;1:79-87.
61. Brophy PD, Somers MJ, Baum MA, et al. Multi-centre evaluation of anticoagulation in patients receiving continuous renal replacement therapy (CRRT). *Nephrol Dial Transplant.* 2005;20:1416-1421.
62. Brophy PD, Mottes TA, Kudelka TL, et al. AN-69 membrane reactions are pH-dependent and preventable. *Am J Kidney Dis.* 2001;38:173-178.
63. Pasko DA, Mottes TA, Mueller BA. Pre dialysis of blood prime in continuous hemodialysis normalizes pH and electrolytes. *Pediatr Nephrol.* 2003; 18:1177-1183.
64. Hackbarth RM, Eding D, Gianoli Smith C, et al. Zero balance ultrafiltration (Z-BUF) in blood-primed CRRT circuits achieves electrolyte and acid-base homeostasis prior to patient connection. *Pediatr Nephrol.* 2005;20:1328-1333.
65. Honore PM, Matson JR. Hemofiltration, adsorption, sieving and the challenge of sepsis therapy design. *Crit Care.* 2002;6:394-396.
66. Barletta JF, Barletta GM, Brophy PD, et al. Medication errors and patient complications with continuous renal replacement therapy. *Pediatr Nephrol.* 2006;21:842-845.
67. Ronco C, Bellomo R, Homel P, et al. Effects of different doses in continuous veno-venous haemofiltration on outcomes of acute renal failure: a prospective randomised trial. *Lancet.* 2000;356:26-30.
68. Palevsky PM, Zhang JH, O'Connor TZ, et al. Intensity of renal support in critically ill patients with acute kidney injury. *N Engl J Med.* 2008; 359:7-20.
69. Bellomo R, Cass A, Cole L, et al. Intensity of continuous renal-replacement therapy in critically ill patients. *N Engl J Med.* 2009;361:1627-1638.
70. Meier-Kriesche HU, Gitomer J, Finkel K, et al. Increased total to ionized calcium ratio during continuous venovenous hemodialysis with regional citrate anticoagulation. *Crit Care Med.* 2001;29:748-752.
71. Maxvold NJ, Smoyer WE, Custer JR, et al. Amino acid loss and nitrogen balance in critically ill children with acute renal failure: a prospective comparison between classic hemofiltration and hemofiltration with dialysis. *Crit Care Med.* 2000;28:1161-1165.
72. Zappitelli M, Goldstein SL, Symons JM, et al. Protein and calorie prescription for children and young adults receiving continuous renal replacement therapy: a report from the Prospective Pediatric Continuous

Renal Replacement Therapy Registry Group. *Crit Care Med.* 2008;36: 3239-3245.

73. Tolwani AJ, Wheeler TS, Wille KM. Sustained low-efficiency dialysis. *Contrib Nephrol.* 2007;156:320-324.

74. Zhang L, Yang J, Eastwood GM, et al. Extended daily dialysis versus continuous renal replacement therapy for acute kidney injury: a meta-analysis. *Am J Kidney Dis.* 2015;66:322-330.

75. Goldstein SL, Currier H, Graf C, et al. Outcome in children receiving continuous venovenous hemofiltration. *Pediatrics.* 2001;107:1309-1312.

76. Flores FX, Brophy PD, Symons JM, et al. Continuous renal replacement therapy (CRRT) after stem cell transplantation. A report from the prospective pediatric CRRT Registry Group. *Pediatr Nephrol.* 2008;23: 625-630.

77. Sutherland SM, Ji J, Sheikhi FH, et al. AKI in hospitalized children: epidemiology and clinical associations in a national cohort. *Clin J Am Soc Nephrol.* 2013;8:1661-1669.

78. Ronco C, Garzotto F, Brendolan A, et al. Continuous renal replacement therapy in neonates and small infants: development and first-in-human use of a miniaturised machine (CARPEDIEM). *Lancet.* 2014;383: 1807-1813.

79. Coulthard MG, Crosier J, Griffiths C, et al. Haemodialysing babies weighing <8 kg with the Newcastle infant dialysis and ultrafiltration system (Nidus): comparison with peritoneal and conventional haemodialysis. *Pediatr Nephrol.* 2014;29:1873-1881.

Acute Severe Hypertension

Joseph T. Flynn

PEARLS

- Acute severe hypertension, defined as symptomatic blood pressure elevation with evidence of acute hypertensive target organ damage, requires prompt therapy to prevent or ameliorate further target organ damage.
- The most common causes of acute severe hypertension in children are renal and cardiac conditions, and the central nervous system is the most commonly affected target organ.
- Although hypervolemia is common in many patients with acute severe hypertension, the high perfusion pressure may lead to pressure diuresis, rendering some patients relatively hypovolemic, with hemoconcentration and activation of the renin-angiotensin-aldosterone system. Consequently, persistent hypovolemia may trigger a vicious cycle of further stimulation of the renin-angiotensin-aldosterone system, thus increasing systemic vascular resistance.
- Treatment of acute severe hypertension requires continuous monitoring of blood pressure and administration of intravenous antihypertensive medication(s), most commonly labetalol or nicardipine.
- In clinical practice, mean arterial pressure during a hypertensive crisis should be lowered no more than 25% within the first 8 hours to prevent harm from dropping blood pressure and thus organ perfusion too rapidly (eg, cerebral, coronary, or renal ischemia).

Introduction

Systemic hypertension (HTN) is a major lifelong condition that begins in childhood and is one of the leading causes of premature death in both developed countries and developing nations. The current pediatric obesity epidemic along with other lifestyle choices has likely led to the increasing numbers of children now being diagnosed with HTN.[1] Current estimates suggest that up to 5% of children have HTN compared with estimates of approximately 1% in the early 2000s, and another 10% to 25% have prehypertension.[1-3] Although most hypertensive patients in the pediatric intensive care unit (PICU) will have underlying causes for their blood pressure (BP) elevation, the increasing prevalence of pediatric primary HTN may ultimately increase the frequency with which such patients present to the PICU.

Several questions are commonly posed to the intensivist when managing a patient with acute severe HTN: What constitutes acute severe HTN in the PICU? Is this level of HTN dangerous? Does the HTN represent a transient acute response, or is there an underlying chronic process to be uncovered? Is it important to manage the high BP at this moment? How aggressively should it be managed? The objective of this chapter is to establish the foundation for understanding the deleterious effects of systemic HTN, recognizing when invasive versus noninvasive monitoring is warranted, and developing a prompt but measured approach to management.

Terminology

The most recent clinical practice guidelines for diagnosing and managing HTN in children and adolescents were published in 2004 by the National High Blood Pressure Education Program[4] and were designed to mirror adult guidelines published in the Seventh Report of the Joint National Committee on Prevention, Detection, Evaluation, and Treatment of High Blood Pressure.[5] Using a statistical definition based on the distribution of BP values in the pediatric population, HTN in children and adolescents is defined as sustained systolic or diastolic BP elevation greater than or equal to the 95th percentile for age, gender, and height.[4] Its severity can be further classified according to the scheme in Table 79.1, which also provides the adult HTN staging criteria,[5] which should be applied to adolescents aged 18 years and older.

Severe HTN, however, has not been as rigorously defined, which has led to some confusion with respect to terminology. The clinical state of a "malignant sclerosis" or "bösartig hypertension" was first reported by Volhard and Fahr in 1914 in patients with HTN and "hypernephrosclerosis."[6] In 1928, Keith and colleagues described 81 cases of what was termed "the malignant hypertension syndrome," which was a diagnosis made before end-stage damage of retinal, cerebral, cardiac, or renal function occurred.[7,8] It was also the first description of pediatric patients with significantly uncontrolled HTN. Subsequently, the terms *hypertensive crisis* and *hypertensive emergency* have appeared interchangeably in the literature, usually to denote a rapidly elevated level of either systolic or diastolic BP that is associated with end-organ damage. Organs commonly affected include the central nervous system (CNS; hypertensive encephalopathy, retinal vasculopathy-induced visual changes, cerebral infarction, and hemorrhage), the cardiovascular system (congestive heart failure, myocardial ischemia, aortic dissection), and the kidneys (proteinuria, hematuria, and acute renal insufficiency).

Traditionally, severe HTN has been divided into hypertensive emergencies and hypertensive urgencies, the former associated with life-threatening symptoms or target-organ injury and the latter associated with less significant symptoms and

TABLE 79.1	Classification of Blood Pressure Levels in Children and Adolescents	
Blood Pressure Classification	**Children and Adolescents <18 Years of Age**	**Adolescents ≥18 Years of Age**
Normal	SBP and DBP <90th percentile	SBP <120 mm Hg and DBP <80 mm Hg
Prehypertension	SBP or DBP 90th-95th percentile; or if BP is >120/80 even if <90th percentile	SBP 120-139 mm Hg or DBP 80-89 mm Hg
Stage 1 hypertension	SBP or DBP ≥95th to 99th percentile plus 5 mm Hg	SBP 140-159 mm Hg or DBP 90-99 mm Hg
Stage 2 hypertension	SBP or DBP >99th percentile plus 5 mm Hg	SBP ≥160 mm Hg or DBP ≥100 mm Hg

DBP, diastolic blood pressure; *SBP,* systolic blood pressure.
Adapted from National High Blood Pressure Education Program Working Group on High Blood Pressure in Children and Adolescents. The fourth report on the diagnosis, evaluation, and treatment of high blood pressure in children and adolescents. Pediatrics. 2004;114(2 suppl):555-576; and Chobanian AV, Bakris GL, Black HR, et al. The Seventh Report of the Joint National Committee on Prevention, Detection, Evaluation, and Treatment of High Blood Pressure: the JNC 7 report. JAMA. 2003;289:2560-2572.

TABLE 79.2	Drug-Induced Hypertension

Drug withdrawal (narcotic, benzodiazepine)[a]
Cyclosporine and tacrolimus[a]
Erythropoietin
Glucocorticoids and mineralocorticoids
Heavy metals
Maternal drug use (cocaine, heroin)
MDMA ("Ecstasy")[a]
Nonsteroidal antiinflammatory agents
Oral contraceptive agents
Rebound after withdrawal of antihypertensives (especially clonidine, methyldopa, and β-blockers)[a]
Sympathomimetic drugs (amphetamines, cocaine, ephedrine, lysergic acid diethylamide, phenylephrine)[a]
Theophylline/caffeine

[a]More likely to present acutely.

TABLE 79.3	Causes of Severe Hypertension in Children and Adolescents	
Renal Disease		**Malignancy**
Glomerulonephritis, especially membranoproliferative glomerulonephritis		Pheochromocytoma
Reflux nephropathy		Wilms tumor
Obstructive uropathy		Neuroblastoma
Acute kidney injury		
Polycystic kidney disease		
Hemolytic-uremic syndrome		
End-stage renal disease at presentation		
Vascular		**Other**
Aortic coarctation (thoracic, abdominal)		Medication noncompliance in a patient with known hypertension
Renal artery stenosis		Drug-induced (see Table 79.2)
Vasculitis		Primary hypertension (rare)

no target-organ injury.[9] For example, an adolescent with seizures and hypertensive encephalopathy would be considered to be experiencing a hypertensive emergency, whereas a hypertensive child with nausea and vomiting would be classified as a hypertensive urgency. This distinction is not absolute and depends somewhat on clinical judgment. Given the lack of clear distinction in terminology, the term *acute severe hypertension* will be utilized in this chapter. This can be defined as an acute BP elevation that fulfills (and usually exceeds) the definition of stage 2 HTN and that is accompanied by severe symptoms; physical exam or laboratory findings of accelerated HTN are frequently also present.[10]

Etiology

HTN may be either primary (also known as "essential") or secondary to another underlying medical condition. Children with primary HTN are frequently overweight and have positive family histories for HTN and cardiovascular disease.[11] The prevalence of HTN increases progressively with a rise in body mass index, with approximately 30% of overweight children (body mass index >95th percentile) exhibiting HTN.[12] That said, although the frequency of primary HTN has been increasing,[1] it is unusual in the PICU, with almost all cases of acute severe HTN being secondary to another condition.[10]

Secondary causes of HTN can be both transient and sustained. The most common reasons for transiently elevated BP in a critical care unit are inadequately treated pain and agitation. Without a high degree of suspicion, this can be difficult to detect, particularly if neuromuscular blockade is administered. Tachycardia as well as eye tearing with noxious interventions is a useful clue to this condition. Drug-induced HTN is also common in the critical care setting, especially when high-dose corticosteroids are used in patients with organ transplantation and other immunologic conditions. A number of other

drugs associated with elevated BP are listed in Table 79.2. A review of all medications taken by the patient, as well as considering illicit drug use, is therefore indicated for all patients with an elevated BP. A patient's fluid balance should also be reviewed when HTN develops while in the ICU. Apparently innocuous discrepancies between input and output for a single day can cumulatively produce significant fluid overload after several days, although this alone is not typically enough to cause HTN in the absence of other renal, cardiovascular, or CNS problems that raise systemic vascular resistance (SVR), cardiac output (CO), or both. Finally, postoperative HTN is common in the ICU setting, occurring in up to 75% of patients. Initially, factors such as hypoxia, hypercarbia (through its sympathomimetic effects), and pain should be promptly and adequately addressed.[13] Afterward, pharmacologic therapy is indicated if HTN is refractory or sustained despite adequate ventilation, sedation, and analgesia.

Renal disease predominates in most pediatric case series of acute severe HTN (Table 79.3). Deal and coworkers from Great Ormond Street Hospital retrospectively reviewed their experience with severe HTN in children in 1992.[14] The most common causes of severe HTN in their series included reflux nephropathy, glomerular disease, renovascular disease, obstructive uropathy, and hemolytic-uremic syndrome, which together accounted for 76% of the cases. In a relatively large series of children with severe HTN treated with intravenous nicardipine,[15] causes included complications of organ transplantation, multiorgan failure, renovascular disease, and acute kidney injury. Renal disease accounted for 48% of patients included in a more recent case series focusing on the use of intravenous labetalol in severely hypertensive infants.[16]

Severe fluid overload in dialysis patients, or noncompliance with antihypertensive therapy in patients with established HTN of any cause, may also result in severe, symptomatic HTN requiring immediate treatment. This was clearly demonstrated in a case series of adults presenting to the emergency department of a teaching hospital in the United States.[17] In that study, 90% of patients requiring intervention for a hypertensive urgency had a known diagnosis of HTN; the most common contributing factors to the severe BP elevation included running out of prescribed medications and medication noncompliance. Although no similar pediatric data exist, this is likely a not infrequent situation in the young as well, particularly for hypertensive children and adolescents followed at referral centers. Finally, abrupt withdrawal of clonidine, dexmedetomidine, or a beta-adrenergic blocker may result in severe "rebound" HTN that may require prompt intervention.

Pathophysiology

The mechanisms responsible for generating and maintaining acute severe HTN crisis continue to be elucidated. What seems plausible in many cases is that there is a triggering event that precipitates a dramatic increase in BP over a short time period in a patient who is hypertensive at baseline. This event then leads to further arteriolar damage that prolongs the hypertensive state.

Mean arterial pressure (MAP) is approximately equal to the product of CO and SVR, as expressed mathematically by the following equation: $MAP \cong CO \times SVR$ (central venous pressure should be subtracted from the MAP in this equation but is usually so small it can be ignored). Thus factors that increase either CO or SVR lead to elevated BP if the other does not decrease proportionally. In addition, chronically, these factors have an interdependent interaction that is still poorly understood. For example, while the initiating event leading to HTN may cause a rise in CO, a compensatory rise in peripheral vascular resistance often develops that may persist even after CO returns to baseline.[18]

Endothelial Homeostasis

The endothelium seems to play a crucial role in the development of severe symptomatic HTN (see also Chapter 27). The endothelium is on the receiving end of the excessive pressures and shear stress generated from high blood flows along with concomitant increased resistance imparted by the vascular architectural scaffolding and surrounding smooth muscle cells. Aside from structural trauma, endothelial cell function is also affected. For instance, the stressed endothelial cell increases intracellular levels of nuclear factor-κB (NF-κB).[19] In turn, NF-κB results in expression of vascular cell adhesion molecule-1, which binds to monocytes and T lymphocytes (facilitating invasion through the vascular wall that normally

does not occur) and contributes to the inflammatory state.[19,20] The proinflammatory mediators interleukin-1β and tumor necrosis factor-α also induce vascular cell adhesion molecule-1 expression in endothelial cells through the NF-κB pathway.[19] In addition to vasoconstrictor mediators, the coagulation system also has been implicated in the pathogenesis of HTN; injured endothelial cells locally activate the coagulation cascade and promote platelet aggregation that leads to a prothrombotic surface.[19,21,22]

Adults with primary HTN who experienced acute severe HTN demonstrated a significant decline in BP when given L-arginine (a precursor of nitric oxide [NO]) compared with patients who also had primary HTN but had not experienced a similar event. This observation underscores the importance of the endothelium in the pathogenesis of acute severe HTN because an intact functional endothelial cell surface is necessary to respond to L-arginine.[23] Von Willebrand factor (an endothelial cell surface marker), P-selectin (platelet activation), and fibrinogen serum levels were all increased in hypertensive adult patients with acute severe HTN compared with control hypertensive subjects, suggesting that alterations in the homeostasis of the endothelial or the coagulation system occur during an episode of acute severe HTN.[24]

Sympathetic Nervous System Activation

A common cause of increased CO in hypertensive individuals is sympathetic nervous system (SNS) activation, often in concert with an increase in intravascular volume. At the same time, SNS activation further increases SVR, exacerbating the rise in BP. The therapeutic approach to HTN depends on reducing SVR and often suppressing or reducing SNS activation. Without the latter being suppressed, the drop in SVR mediated by a vasodilator may be compensated by an increase in sympathetic activation with a resultant increase in CO and no net reduction in BP.

The SNS can also be the cause of severe HTN. This is particularly seen in children with pheochromocytomas and other tumors that produce vasoactive substances, including neuroblastoma.[25] Hemodialysis can contribute to a substantial increase in catecholamines and also of renin, which thus can contribute to HTN.[26] Increased sympathetic activity can worsen severe HTN in several conditions, including renovascular HTN and polycystic kidney disease, and seems to be unrelated to the level of kidney function. Renal ischemia triggered by these diseases seems to cause the systemic overactivation.[27] Activation of the SNS leading to systemic vasoconstriction is generally accepted as the mechanism of severe postoperative HTN.[28]

Renin-Angiotensin-Aldosterone System

The renin-angiotensin-aldosterone system (RAAS) is thought to play a prominent role in many patients during an episode of acute severe HTN.[22,29] Renin is a proteolytic enzyme synthesized in the juxtaglomerular cells of the afferent renal arterioles that cleaves angiotensinogen (an α_2-globulin synthesized in the liver) to create angiotensin I (a decapeptide). In turn, angiotensin-converting enzyme (ACE) coverts angiotensin I to angiotensin II (an octapeptide), which acts at the angiotensin type 1 receptor (a G-coupled receptor found in renal afferent and efferent arterioles) to cause vasoconstriction, increased aldosterone release, and enhanced sodium and water reabsorption (see also Chapter 81).[18]

Increased serum renin levels can reflect a primary condition, such as renovascular disease, or be secondary to renal parenchymal ischemia, hypotension, hypovolemia, increased sympathetic effects, β-adrenergic agonists, or a combination of these factors.[18,30] Ultimately, increased renin levels raise BP through a number of mechanisms primarily mediated through angiotensin II. Aside from its vasoconstrictive properties, angiotensin II increases the expression of aldosterone that leads to increased renal sodium and water retention, thus augmenting CO by increasing intravascular volume. Angiotensin II also induces the expression of interleukin-6 and NF-κB that in turn leads to elevated levels of tumor necrosis factor-α and increases nicotinamide adenine dinucleotide phosphate oxidase activity; the latter generates reactive oxygen species, promoting oxidative stress, and inhibits the cytokine-mediated activation of inducible-nitric oxide synthase (iNOS) that attenuates vasodilation.[18] Over time the collective result of these processes is enhanced and sustained endothelial cell trauma, vascular dysfunction, and ultimately end-organ damage.

Focal impairment of renal blood flow with release of renin and a subsequent increase in circulating angiotensin II underlie many types of childhood HTN.[31] For example, thromboemboli from umbilical or central vascular catheters may impair renal perfusion, and coarctation of the aorta is associated with high peripheral renin activity.[31,32]

Nitric Oxide

NO, now recognized as a ubiquitous biological effector, is a labile, short-lived chemical produced from arginine via NO synthases.[33] These synthases are distinguished by cellular distribution and by the requirement for calcium as a cofactor. The constitutive isoform of NOS is believed most responsible for basal vasomotor tone, although iNOS may have a role. NO is released continuously from arteries and arterioles but not from veins. In addition, other mediators function through the NO system. For instance, bradykinin stimulates the release of NO to produce vasodilation. NO diffuses from the endothelium to the vascular smooth muscle cell, where it produces its vasodilatory effect in part by increasing the intracellular concentration of cyclic guanosine monophosphate (cGMP) through stimulation of soluble guanylate cyclase. NO that diffuses from the local endothelial environment reacts with hemoglobin, forming nitrosohemoglobin and methemoglobin. Thus HTN need not be attributed only to a direct vasoconstrictor effect but also may be related to loss of basal NO vasodilation. Therapeutic agents such as sodium nitroprusside and nitroglycerin produce their systemic vasodilator action by stimulating NO production (see HTN management section that follows).

Volume Overload

An acute increase in intravascular volume is a frequent cause of acute decompensation of BP control in a patient with chronic HTN, particularly in the setting of stimuli that increase sympathetic nervous system and/or renin-angiotensin-aldosterone system activation. Volume overload is the most common mechanism leading to HTN in children with renal diseases. It is often caused by acute kidney injury with oliguria or anuria in those without preexisting renal disease.

Although volume overload is a common cause of acute severe HTN, pressure diuresis may render some patients relatively hypovolemic, producing hemoconcentration and further marked activation of the RAAS.[29] Further volume depletion may actually worsen HTN by stimulating a further increase in SVR with the potential for organ ischemia. Thus diuretics and fluid restriction are not standard therapy for patients who present with acute severe HTN; they are reserved for patients with clinically apparent fluid overload.[21,29,34]

In children on dialysis, fluid overload is probably the most important contributing factor to episodes of severe HTN. Fluid overload in dialysis patients often results from poor adherence to dietary sodium and fluid restrictions. Chronic underdialysis and failure to consistently reach "dry weight" may lead to gradual fluid accumulation that can be clinically imperceptible until the child presents with severe HTN. This may happen even in the best dialysis center due to the difficulty in assessment of fluid status in children and also because differences in body weight may be attributed to growth instead of to fluid accumulation.[35]

Clinical Presentation

The presentation of a patient with acute severe HTN depends on underlying medical conditions, baseline systemic BP, rate of rise and degree of BP elevation, as well as effects on end organs. Headache, dizziness, and nausea/vomiting are common presenting complaints in patients with acute severe HTN, as was demonstrated in a case series of Chinese children presenting to an emergency department with acute severe HTN.[36] Visual impairment is another common presenting complaint in patients with acute severe HTN and may signal the presence of cerebral involvement.[37] A small number of severely hypertensive children may manifest isolated abdominal pain with or without vomiting.[38] Although exceedingly rare in the pediatric age group, aortic dissection may present with severe HTN along with the abrupt onset of chest or back pain.[39]

Neurologic manifestations of acute severe HTN are probably most common in children; symptoms may include seizures, lethargy, confusion, headache, and visual disturbances. Hypertensive encephalopathy (increased blood flow with pressures exceeding the autoregulatory range) typically presents as a severe headache with dizziness and changes in mental status ultimately culminating as seizures; other reported symptoms include facial palsies and visual changes that may lead to blindness and coma.[14,40,41] Hypertensive encephalopathy may occur with a mean arterial pressure below 200 mm Hg in the normotensive individual, but it may require a much higher mean arterial pressure in patients who have sustained hypertension (Fig. 79.1).

Cardiac manifestations of severe acute HTN are relatively common in adults and may include asymptomatic left ventricular hypertrophy, acute congestive heart failure with pulmonary edema, and myocardial ischemia.[42,43] Unfortunately, extensive pediatric data are lacking. In two case series of children with severe HTN from the Great Ormond Street Hospital, the incidence of left ventricular hypertrophy ranged from 13% to 66%, and the incidence of congestive heart failure was 9%.[14,44] Clearly, a high index of suspicion for an underlying cause of HTN should be maintained in a patient who presents acutely with cardiac symptoms and severe HTN, and appropriate investigation should be initiated.

Severely hypertensive children can also exhibit evidence of acute renal damage such as hematuria, albuminuria, and uremia (Fig. 79.2). However, in many cases, attempts to determine the acute renal effects of severe HTN may be complicated by the frequent association of renal parenchymal or renovascular disease with systemic HTN. Moreover, hypertensive pathology is not usually limited to a single organ like the kidney; other end-organ abnormalities usually can be seen, such as left ventricular hypertrophy and neurologic sequelae

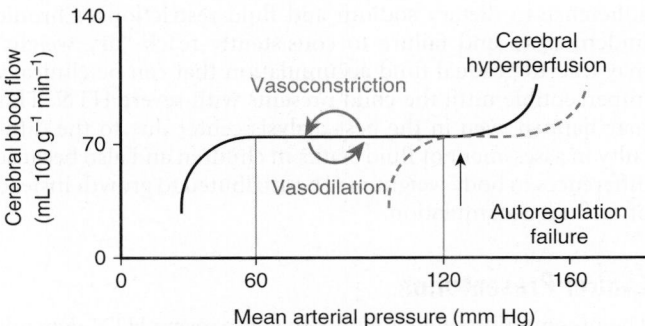

Fig. 79.1. Altered cerebral blood flow autoregulation in chronic hypertension.

(such as mental status changes, seizures, and cerebrovascular accidents).[45] Nevertheless, children with severe HTN resulting from vasculitis have been found to have nephrotic range proteinuria, microscopic hematuria, elevated serum creatinine levels, and diminished glomerular filtration rates.[45-47]

Patient Evaluation and Monitoring

Evaluation should be targeted at identifying both the etiology as well as any potential signs of injury to the cardiovascular, neurologic, renal, and ocular systems. A detailed history and review of systems should be obtained for all patients, with special care paid to symptoms suggestive of an underlying hypertensive disorder or target-organ damage (Table 79.4). Signs and symptoms are often reflective of the severity and rapidity of onset of HTN. Chronic HTN is more commonly asymptomatic or characterized by low-grade generalized symptoms such as fatigue and recurrent headaches. As already discussed, acutely hypertensive patients may present with a wide range of symptoms, with headache, nausea, seizures, and other neurologic complaints among the most common.

Physical examination should include BP measurements in all four extremities (or at least both arms and one leg) as a screening for coarctation of the aorta, which should be suspected if upper extremity pressures are higher than lower extremity pressures and lower extremity pulses are weak or absent. Special attention also should be paid to pulse rate because HTN with associated bradycardia is suggestive of increased intracranial pressure (ICP). Rapidly lowering BP in

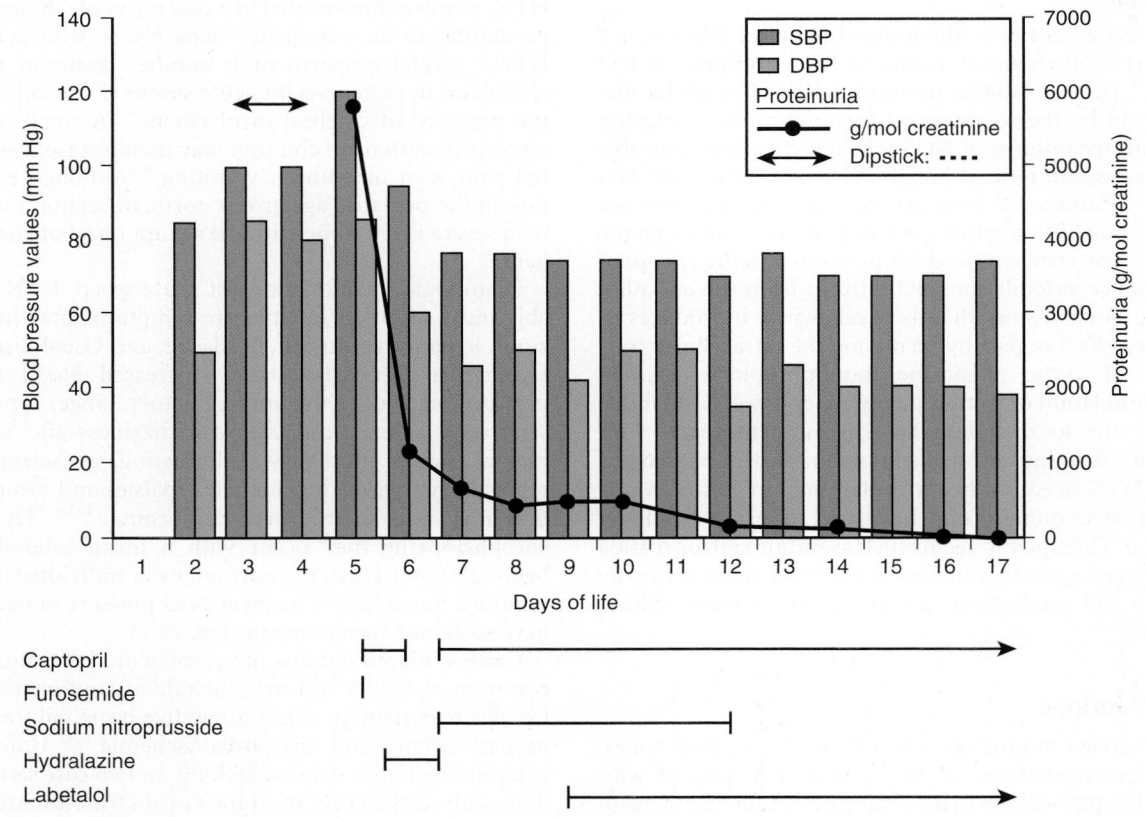

Fig. 79.2. Effects of BP control on proteinuria in an infant with renal artery stenosis. The infant also had left ventricular failure that resolved according to echocardiography performed 3 months after discharge. (Reprinted with permission from Cachat F, Bogaru A, Micheli JL, et al. Severe hypertension and massive proteinuria in a newborn with renal artery stenosis. Pediatr Nephrol. 2004;19:544-546.[126])

TABLE 79.4 History and Physical Examination Findings in Hypertension

Finding	Possible Significance	Finding	Possible Significance
Historical Findings		**Head and Neck**	
Complaint/Review of Systems		Moon facies	Cushing disease
Headaches, dizziness, epistaxis, visual changes	Nonspecific with respect to etiology of HTN	Elfin facies	Williams syndrome
		Proptosis/goiter	Hyperthyroidism
Abdominal/flank pain with hematuria	Renal artery or vein thrombosis	Web neck	Turner syndrome
Hematuria, swelling, decreased urine output	Acute glomerulonephritis	Adenotonsillar hypertrophy	Sleep disorders
		Fundal changes	Chronic or severe HTN
Dysuria, frequency, urgency, nocturia, enuresis	Underlying renal disease	**Cardiovascular**	
		Friction rub	Systemic lupus erythematosus, collagen vascular disease, uremia
Joint pains/swelling, edema, rashes	Autoimmune mediated disease/ glomerulonephritis		
Weight loss, sweating, flushing, palpitations	Pheochromocytoma or hyperthyroidism	Apical heave	Left ventricular hypertrophy
		Disparity in pulses	Coarctation
Muscle cramps, weakness, constipation	Hypokalemia associated with hyperaldosteronism	**Lungs**	
		Crackles/rales	Heart failure
Delayed puberty	Congenital adrenal hyperplasia	**Abdomen**	
Snoring	Sleep apnea	Masses	Obstructive nephropathy, Wilms tumor, neuroblastoma, pheochromocytoma, polycystic kidney disease
Prescription, over-the-counter, or illicit drug use	Drug-induced HTN		
Medical History			
Umbilical artery catheterization	Renal artery thrombosis/renal embolus	Hepatomegaly	Heart failure
		Bruit	Renal artery stenosis, abdominal coarctation
Previous urinary tract infections	Renal scarring		
Thyroid cancer, neurofibromatosis, von-Hippel Lindau disease	Pheochromocytoma	**Genitalia**	
		Ambiguous, viralized	Congenital adrenal hyperplasia
		Extremities	
Family History		Edema	Underlying kidney disease
HTN	Inherited forms of hypertension (AME, Gordon syndrome, Liddle syndrome, GRA), essential HTN	Joint swelling	Autoimmune disease
		Rickettsial changes	Chronic kidney disease
		Dermatologic	
Renal disease	Polycystic kidney disease, Alport syndrome	Neurofibromas	Neurofibromatosis
Tumors	Familial pheochromocytoma, multiple endocrine neoplasia type II	Tubers, ash leaf spots, adenoma sebaceum	Tuberous sclerosis
		Bronzed skin	Excessive adrenocorticotropic hormone
Physical Examination Findings			
Vital Signs		Acanthosis nigricans	Insulin resistance/metabolic syndrome
Tachycardia	Hyperthyroidism, pheochromocytoma, neuroblastoma, primary HTN		
		Striae, acne	Cushing disease
		Rashes	Vasculitis/nephritis
Bradycardia	Increased intracranial pressure (tumor, hydrocephalus)	Needle tracks	Drug-induced HTN
		Neurologic	
Drop in blood pressure from upper to lower extremities	Coarctation of aorta	Mental status changes	Severe HTN
		Cranial nerve palsy	Severe HTN
General			
Growth retardation	Chronic kidney disease		
Truncal obesity	Cushing disease, insulin resistance		

AME, apparent mineralocorticoid excess; *GRA,* glucocorticoid-remediable aldosteronism; *HTN,* hypertension.

this scenario could lead to decreased cerebral perfusion and its associated sequelae. A thorough cardiac examination to identify signs of heart failure, a search for carotid or abdominal bruits, a funduscopic examination, evaluation of cutaneous lesions, and a neurologic examination also are essential in the initial evaluation of patients with severe HTN.

With respect to the funduscopic exam, evidence indicates that the pattern of retinal lesions can offer some information related to the onset of HTN. For instance, generalized arteriolar narrowing and arteriovenous nicking were associated with long-standing systemic HTN, whereas focal arteriolar narrowing, retinal hemorrhages, microaneurysms, and cotton-wool spots were indicative of recent significant increases in BP.[48] Papilledema may also be present in some patients.

As with any hypertensive child or adolescent, the remainder of the physical exam should be focused on identifying clues to underlying secondary causes of HTN such as renal disease or a genetic syndrome.[4] Specific examples can be found in Table 79.4.

Initial laboratory studies for all patients with acute severe HTN should include electrolytes, blood urea nitrogen, creatinine, complete blood cell count with peripheral smear, and urinalysis. Renal disease is the most common cause of secondary HTN in children, and both chronic and acute renal conditions may present with severe HTN. Anemia associated with chronic disease or a microangiopathic anemia resulting from disseminated activation of the coagulation system or hemolytic uremic syndrome may be seen as well. Finally, a hypokalemic metabolic alkalosis may develop with volume depletion and secondary hyperaldosteronism. Similar laboratory findings may be seen in children with inherited monogenic forms of HTN.[49] Further laboratory evaluation for the cause of HTN should be targeted, based on the history and physical exam findings. In selected patients, thyroid studies, a drug screen, cortisol levels, and plasma or urinary catecholamines/metanephrines may help elicit the cause of elevated BP.

Renal ultrasonography is indicated for most patients to evaluate for renal parenchymal lesions such as small scarred kidneys, polycystic kidney disease, obstruction, or other structural anomalies. Doppler evaluation of blood flow to the kidneys also should be performed, although this evaluation is less sensitive than in adults at identifying subtle renal artery stenosis in smaller children and is therefore not always helpful if negative.[50] Although both computed tomography (CT) and magnetic resonance (MR) angiography have shown some promise as screening tools for renal artery stenosis, renal arteriography, sometimes in conjunction with renal vein renin sampling, remains the gold standard for identifying this lesion.[32,50,51] Further renal imaging such as a dimethylsuccinic acid (DMSA) scan may be indicated in children who are suspected of having renal scarring; plasma renin and aldosterone levels also may help discern the etiology of HTN, although typically they are not rapidly available.

A chest radiograph and electrocardiogram should be obtained at presentation to look for signs of heart failure and electrocardiographic evidence of ventricular hypertrophy, strain, or both. An echocardiogram is now recommended for all children with acute severe HTN to assess for congenital anomalies such as a coarctation of the aorta as well as for left ventricular hypertrophy and should be performed emergently if the child has signs of congestive heart failure.

A head CT scan should be done in patients with concern for increased ICP. In children with cerebral edema or increased ICP, increased BP may develop as a strategy to preserve cerebral perfusion due to the increased resistance to cerebral blood flow. Initially, a child with traumatic brain injury will often maintain sufficient cerebral blood flow over a range of BPs because of the brain's capacity for autoregulation, as depicted in Fig. 79.2.[10,21] However, if the resistance to cerebral blood flow increases, such as when ICP rises from cerebral edema, then the patient may compensate through cerebral vasodilation or increased CO to meet the metabolic needs of the brain. Cerebral vasodilation, however, will only increase ICP further. To attempt to maintain adequate cerebral blood flow, the perfusion pressure must increase as noted in the following mathematical relationship: Cerebral perfusion pressure = mean arterial pressure (MAP) − ICP. In such situations, it is prudent to undertake measures to control brain edema through hyperosmolar therapy, judicious sedation/analgesia, and avoiding maneuvers that might inadvertently increase ICP while cautiously securing the airway to control oxygenation and ventilation. Efforts to directly lower systemic BP can undermine the patient's ability to support injured but viable cerebral tissue (see also Chapter 66).

MR imaging of the brain should be considered for patients with other neurologic symptoms. The most common brain-associated finding in children with acute severe HTN has been termed "posterior reversible encephalopathy syndrome (PRES)." PRES is characterized by the sudden onset of severe HTN, headaches, altered mental status, seizures, visual loss, and even cortical blindness.[52,53] Neuroimaging studies during PRES typically demonstrate cerebral edema affecting the white matter in a parietooccipital distribution.[54] PRES is associated with immunosuppressive therapy (especially cyclosporine and tacrolimus), acute glomerulonephritis, eclampsia of pregnancy, and hypertensive encephalopathy (Fig. 79.3).[53,55] Hypertensive emergencies and tonic-clonic seizures were presenting features in 59% of renal transplant patients who were found to have PRES on further workup.[56] In addition, nearly half of the patients with PRES had no history of uncontrolled chronic HTN. This constellation of symptoms and pathology, which has also been called reversible posterior leukoencephalopathy by other authors, typically resolves once the HTN is treated, but it may take weeks to months for the imaging abnormalities to normalize.[37,56]

Blood Pressure Measurement and Other Monitoring

The most critical component of identifying and monitoring patients with acute severe HTN is accurately measuring BP. Both noninvasive and invasive techniques may be used in the ICU setting and are commonly used together. The main techniques available to determine BP in the ICU are the auscultatory method, oscillometric method, Doppler method, and invasive hemodynamic monitoring.

Auscultatory, oscillometric, and Doppler BP (DBP) methods are noninvasive techniques that are based on the return of blood flow through a major artery after compression by an inflatable cuff. *Auscultatory methods* require the observer to listen to the Korotkoff sounds generated as the sphygmomanometer cuff deflates. Korotkoff sounds 1 and 5 should be used to represent systolic blood pressure (SBP) and DBP, respectively. It should be noted that the current pediatric

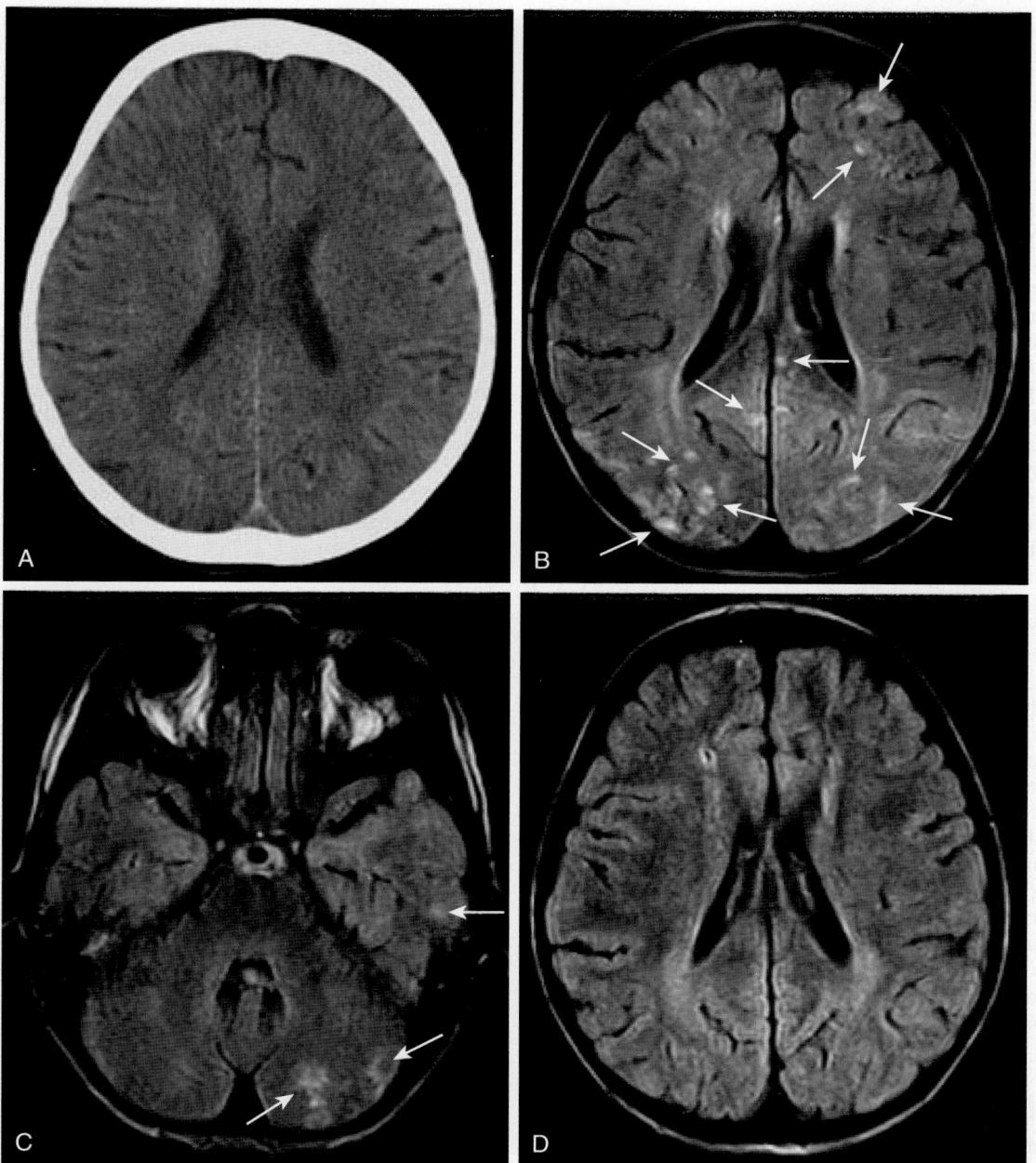

Fig. 79.3. A 6-year-old female patient with sickle cell disease, acute chest syndrome complicated with acute kidney injury, and severe hypertension. (A) Axial CT image of the brain during the episode is normal. (B, C) Axial FLAIR MR images at the same level performed the same day as the CT scan show multiple supratentorial and left cerebellar lesions *(arrows)*. (D) Follow-up FLAIR image after the episode shows resolution of the lesions. *CT*, computed tomography; *FLAIR*, Fluid-attenuated inversion recovery; *MR*, magnetic resonance. (Reprinted with permission from Onder AM, Lopez R, Teomete U, et al. Posterior reversible encephalopathy syndrome in the pediatric renal population. Pediatr Nephrol. 2007;22:1921-1929.[56])

normative BP values were generated using this technique over the brachial artery, and it is therefore the preferred site of BP measurement in children. To obtain accurate measurements, it is important that an appropriately sized cuff size be used, which should cover 80% to 100% of the upper arm circumference.[4] *Oscillometric techniques* utilize a similar technique except that the MAP is first determined from oscillometric wave forms generated as blood flow returns through the artery. SBP and DBP are then calculated using a proprietary formula specific to the brand of monitor. *Doppler devices* use changes in ultrasound frequency to infer velocity of blood

flow. The Doppler shift corresponds to the turbulent flow, as signified by the Korotkoff sounds, that diminishes as laminar flow predominates.[57] As with the auscultatory method, selection of an appropriate cuff size is paramount for both the oscillometric and Doppler BP methods.

Invasive arterial lines are fluid-filled tubes attached to a pressure transducer, a device consisting of a thin flexible diaphragm connected to a strain gauge and capable of converting the pressure transmitted to an electrical signal (see Chapter 19). The most common source of inaccuracy is the influence of electrical damping on reported BP. An overdamped signal underestimates both SBP and DBP, although MAP may be accurate. On the other hand, an underdamped system overestimates SBP, especially with a hyperdynamic circulation, but does not affect MAP. This phenomenon is recognized as a narrow peaked pressure wave and wide pulse pressure. Moreover, invasive BP measured in the lower extremity is higher than in the upper extremities because of the nature of BP wave transmission, which results in an increase in SBP reading the further away from the heart it is measured.

Generally, children with acute severe HTN need to be closely monitored in a controlled setting such as the ICU, and the ideal way to continuously follow BPs is with the aid of an indwelling arterial catheter. Arterial lines can be placed in a variety of locations, but usually they are placed in peripheral arteries that supply areas with robust collateral blood flow; common sites include the radial, dorsalis pedis, and posterior tibial arteries. Continuous intraarterial BP monitoring is generally preferred for patients with acute severe HTN because of the lability of BP when continuous infusions of intravenous (IV) medications are utilized. However, using noninvasive techniques to confirm that transduced values are accurate is a common practice because electrical damping of the transduced signal can cause inaccuracies in SBP and DBP, although MAP is likely to be less affected. Additionally, modern oscillometric devices can be programmed to take repeated measurements of BP at short intervals and may therefore sometimes be acceptable for short time periods or for patients without life-threatening symptoms.

Other important aspects of monitoring the patient with acute severe HTN include pulse oximetry and frequent neurologic assessment. Appropriate IV access should be established; ideally there should be an IV line placed that is used only for administration of antihypertensive medications. Monitoring of central venous pressure may also be helpful in selected patients, especially when volume status is otherwise difficult to assess. Finally, an indwelling Foley catheter may be needed for urine output monitoring, especially in severely hypertensive patients with known or suspected acute or chronic renal disease.

Pharmacologic Therapy
General Considerations

The therapeutic strategy for patients with acute severe HTN depends on the clinical context of the BP elevation. Hypertensive children returning from surgery need to be adequately sedated and given sufficient analgesia postoperatively for comfort and to control sympathetic activation. It is not uncommon for children to return to recovery areas, general care floors, and ICUs with variable levels of anesthetics still circulating that can permit pain, anxiety, and emergence phenomena that could be accompanied by elevated BPs. This situation by no means minimizes the potential detrimental effects of severely elevated systolic or diastolic pressures if they are inadequately treated or ignored.

It is prudent to ascertain the patient's volume status while determining the best management approach. Some clinical situations, such as the presence of pulmonary edema and renal failure, clearly identify the child with probable fluid overload. On the other hand, other children with significant HTN may exhibit a pressure-induced diuresis associated with secondary

activation of the RAAS, and these patients may actually need judicious volume replenishment while managing their HTN.

The child with altered mental status, unequal (anisocoria) pupils, and systemic HTN needs agents directed at managing increased ICP such as mannitol or hypertonic saline solution, along with careful rapid sequence intubation and controlled ventilation. The goal here is to prevent cerebral herniation and not to directly lower BP too rapidly, which may be deleterious.

Finally, the strategic pharmacologic goal for a patient experiencing a hypertensive crisis is to aim for a controlled decrease in BP as opposed to a sudden rapid fall. Lowering BP to the "normal range" of MAP too rapidly may produce a clinically significant decrease in cerebral blood flow, especially in patients with preexisting chronic HTN (see Fig. 79.1). This can lead to cerebral ischemia. One group reported the occurrence of permanent neurologic deficits in adults treated with bolus antihypertensive therapy resulting in rapid BP reduction,[58] and similar catastrophes have occurred in children as well.[59,60] Thus it is normally recommended that the BP should be reduced by 25% of the planned BP reduction over first 8 to 12 hours, a further 25% over the next 8 to 12 hours, and the final 50% over the 24 hours after that.[10]

The indications, pharmacology, and adverse effects of medications available for treatment of acute severe HTN are reviewed in the following section. Dosing for recommended agents is summarized in Table 79.5. Some agents are included in the following section but not in the table; reasons for their exclusion from the table will be evident from the discussion. Finally, a suggested algorithm for the pharmacologic management of pediatric patients with acute severe HTN can be found in Fig. 79.4.

Clonidine

Clonidine is a centrally acting oral α2-adrenergic agonist that reduces BP by reducing cerebral sympathetic output. Clonidine is a mixed agonist that stimulates both central α2-adrenergic and imidazoline (I1) receptors.[61] The stimulation

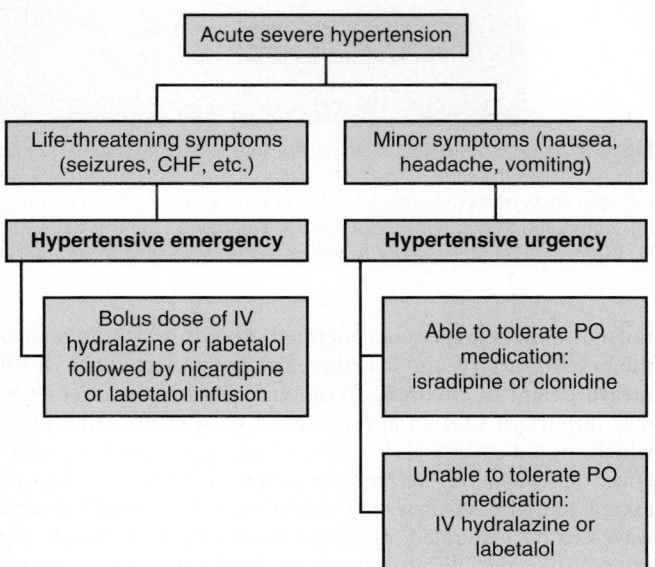

Fig. 79.4. Algorithm for initial management of children with acute severe HTN. *CHF,* congestive heart failure; *IV,* intravenous; *PO,* oral.

TABLE 79.5   Recommended Antihypertensive Agents for Acute Severe Hypertension

		USEFUL FOR SEVERELY HYPERTENSIVE PATIENTS WITH LIFE-THREATENING SYMPTOMS		
Drug	**Class**	**Dose**	**Route**	**Comments**
Esmolol	β-adrenergic blocker	100-500 mcg/kg/min	IV infusion	Very short-acting—constant infusion preferred. May cause profound bradycardia.
Hydralazine	Direct vasodilator	0-1-0.2 mg/kg/dose up to 0.6 mg/kg/dose	IV, IM	Should be given q4hr when given IV bolus.
Labetalol	α- and β-adrenergic blocker	Bolus: 0.20-1 mg/kg/dose, up to 40 mg/dose Infusion: 0.25-3 mg/kg/hr	IV bolus or infusion	Asthma and overt heart failure are relative contraindications.
Nicardipine	Calcium channel blocker	Bolus: 30 mcg/kg up to 2 mg/dose Infusion: 0.5-4 mcg/kg/min	IV bolus or infusion	May cause reflex tachycardia. Increases cyclosporine and tacrolimus levels. Increases cerebral blood flow.
Sodium nitroprusside	Direct vasodilator	Starting: 0-3-0.5-10 mcg/kg/min Maximum: 10 mcg/kg/min	IV infusion	Monitor cyanide levels with prolonged (>72 hr) use or in renal failure or co-administer with sodium thiosulfate. Increases cerebral blood flow.
		USEFUL FOR SEVERELY HYPERTENSIVE PATIENTS WITH LESS SIGNIFICANT SYMPTOMS		
Drug	**Class**	**Dose**	**Route**	**Comments**
Clonidine	Central α2-agonist	2-5 mcg/kg/dose, up to 10 mcg/kg/dose given q6-8hr	PO	Side effects include dry mouth and drowsiness.
Fenoldopam	Dopamine receptor agonist	0.2-0.5 mcg/kg/min up to 0.8 mcg/kg/min	IV infusion	Higher doses worsen tachycardia without further reducing BP.
Hydralazine	Direct vasodilator	0.25 mg/kg/dose up to 25 mg/dose given Q6-8 hours	PO	Half-life varies with genetically determined acetylation rates.
Isradipine	Calcium channel blocker	0.05-0.1 mg/kg/dose up to 5 mg/dose given Q6-8 hours	PO	Exaggerated fall in BP can be seen in patients receiving azole antifungals.
Minoxidil	Direct vasodilator	0.1-0.2 mg/kg/dose up to 10 mg/dose given Q8-12 hours	PO	Most potent oral vasodilator; long acting.

ACE, angiotensin-converting enzyme; *BP*, blood pressure; *IM*, intramuscular; *IV*, intravenous; *kg*, kilogram; *mcg*, microgram; *mg*, milligram; *PO*, oral.

of α_2-adrenergic receptors in the CNS inhibits peripheral sympathetic activity that results in vasodilatation. Its effects are targeted primarily toward arterioles at lower doses.[62] Clonidine is well known as an antihypertensive agent with a favorable hemodynamic profile, especially because of the infrequency of postural hypotension. Compared to other centrally acting agents, clonidine has a relatively rapid onset of effect, approximately 15 to 30 minutes following oral administration,[63] making it attractive for use in management of acute HTN. It is metabolized hepatically into inactive forms and excreted unchanged in the urine with some gastrointestinal excretion because of enterohepatic recirculation.

Adverse effects of clonidine include bradycardia, dry mouth, and sedation.[61] In addition, severe rebound HTN may occur in patients treated chronically with clonidine (including those treated with the transdermal preparation) if the drug is abruptly stopped.

Esmolol

Esmolol is an IV pure β_1-adrenergic blocker that decreases BP by reducing CO. In a study of 17 children (6 months to 14 years), esmolol was shown to lower BP along with cardiac index, shortening fraction, and heart rate, whereas SVR remained unaffected.[64] It has a rapid onset of action and short

half-life (2 to 4 minutes), which makes it ideal for critically ill patients with labile HTN who require frequent titration for BP management.[64,65] Because esmolol is rapidly hydrolyzed by esterases in the cytosol of red blood cells, its clearance is not dependent on organ blood flow or function.[66]

Like labetalol, esmolol has the advantage of not increasing ICP. It should not be used in patients with obstructive lung disease, such as asthma, and should be used with caution if the patient has congestive heart failure. It can cause profound bradycardia. In addition, the use of β-blockers alone should be avoided in children with suspected neuroendocrine catecholamine secreting tumors because the stimulation of α-receptors from these catecholamines without opposing β-stimulation can severely worsen BP.

A large multicenter, double-blind, randomized, dose-ranging study of 116 pediatric patients (younger than 6 years) with postoperative HTN after coarctation of the aorta repair studied one of three doses of esmolol (125, 250, or 500 μg/kg/min, after respective loading doses of 125, 250, and 500 μg/kg). The results showed a decrease in systolic BP in all three dose groups, but there was no statistically significant difference between groups in either the change from baseline or percentage change from baseline.[67] Despite the lack of dose response in the clinical trial setting, it is likely that esmolol can be effectively titrated to achieve control of BP in children with severe HTN. Esmolol has been used successfully for the intraoperative management of HTN during pheochromocytoma resection in children.[68] Other published experience with esmolol therapy in children without cardiovascular lesions is limited.

Hydralazine

Hydralazine, available in both IV and oral preparations, is a direct vasodilator of arteriolar smooth muscle with an unclear mechanism of action, most likely an alteration of intracellular calcium metabolism, leading to interference with the calcium movements within the vascular smooth muscle that are responsible for initiating or maintaining the contractile state. It does not affect coronary arteries or venous smooth muscle, but its effects on arteriolar smooth muscle stimulate the sympathetic nervous system, leading to tachycardia, increased renin activity, and sodium retention.[69] The positive inotropic effects of hydralazine exhibit both cyclic adenylate monophosphate–dependent and independent mechanisms, yet the importance of each remains elusive.[70] Nevertheless, it is known that intracellular calcium homeostasis is altered when hydralazine mediates its effects.[71]

Hydralazine, when given orally, has low systemic bioavailability (16% in fast acetylators and 35% in slow acetylators). Consequently, the dose needed to achieve therapeutic levels is higher in fast acetylators because the acetylated form is inactive. *N*-acetylation of hydralazine occurs in the bowel or the liver. The half-life is a function of genetically determined acetylation rates, but on average it is approximately 60 minutes; it is cleared hepatically, and elimination is a function of hepatic blood flow. The onset of action after IV administration is 5 to 20 minutes, with a duration of 1 to 4 hours. Although hydralazine's half-life is variable, its effect on BP generally persists for 2 to 4 hours.[72,73] When administered orally, hydralazine has an onset of action of 30 minutes to 2 hours and an unpredictable duration of action of 6 to 12 hours. Hydralazine also may be given intramuscularly; dosing is similar to IV administration.

Despite its long history of use in children,[74] no prospective pediatric clinical trial of hydralazine has been conducted. However, two retrospective case series of hydralazine use in hospitalized children with acute HTN suggest that this agent can produce effective BP reduction after IV administration and that adverse effects are relatively infrequent.[75,76] However, the BP response to IV hydralazine was erratic in both reports, likely reflecting the retrospective study designs. There are no published pediatric data on the efficacy of oral hydralazine.

Adverse effects are related to the reflexive increase in sympathetic activity and include tachycardia, palpitations, flushing, headache, and dizziness. Additionally, there appears to be an increased risk of excessive BP reduction following IV hydralazine administration in children[76]; thus caution is advised when using this agent.

Isradipine

Isradipine is an oral second-generation dihydropyridine calcium channel blocker (CCB) that is specific for the L-type calcium channel found in smooth muscle. It lowers BP by relaxing arteriolar smooth muscle, leading to decreases in peripheral vascular resistance. As a result, the CCBs elicit a sympathetic discharge that causes stimulation of the sinoatrial node and

consequent tachycardia.[77] It has a relatively rapid onset of action, with a peak effect that can last as long as 3 hours.

Several retrospective case series of pediatric isradipine use have established its utility for both acute and chronic HTN.[78-81] In a study of 282 hospitalized children with acute HTN treated with oral isradipine, BP reductions of 16.3 ± 11.6% (mean ±SD) for systolic BP and 24.2 ± 17.2% for diastolic BP were observed.[81] Another study examined isradipine use in 80 children with secondary HTN over a 5-year period and found that isradipine monotherapy decreased SBP by a mean of 13 mm Hg and DBP by 10 mm Hg over a broad range of ages from 1 week to 16.8 years.[79] Similar responses to isradipine (a decrease in systolic pressure of 11.8% and diastolic pressure of 17.4%) were seen retrospectively in 53 children (ages 1 day to 16 years) treated with an average dose of 0.4 mg/kg/day.[80]

Isradipine undergoes extensive first-pass metabolism in the liver by the cytochrome 4-50 isoenzyme CYP3A4.[77] It is highly protein bound and is excreted essentially as inactive metabolites in the urine (two-thirds) and feces (one-third). Adverse events attributed to isradipine occurred in 9.5% of patients in one case series and included headache, dizziness, flushing, and tachycardia.[79] Of note, an exaggerated BP response to isradipine has been observed in patients receiving concomitant treatment with azole antifungal agents,[81] so caution is advised when using isradipine in such patients.

Labetalol

Labetalol is a combined α- and β-adrenergic blocker that can be administered as a continuous IV infusion or as an IV bolus. It lowers systemic vascular resistance with minimal effect on CO.[82] It provides nonselective β-adrenergic blockade, which reduces reflex tachycardia and increased cardiac contractility that may be seen with vasodilators. β_2-adrenergic blockade would increase SVR, but this effect is counterbalanced by its α-adrenergic blockade, which is selective for the α_1-receptor, resulting in vasodilation. The α-to-β blocking ratio of the oral preparation is 1:3, whereas it is 1:7 for the IV form. Labetalol is therefore most useful in situations where HTN is produced by excessive SNS activity. Labetalol has an onset of action of 2 to 5 minutes with a peak at 5 to 15 minutes, and it can last up to 4 hours, a longer duration of action than nitroprusside or nicardipine, and does not increase heart rate or CO as does nitroprusside.[83] It is metabolized in the liver through glucuronide conjugation and excreted in the urine, bile, and stool.

Published experience with IV labetalol in severely hypertensive children is limited to several small case series.[14,16,84] In all of these reports, labetalol was felt to be an effective antihypertensive agent; in the most recent report, labetalol was felt to have a similar antihypertensive effect as nicardipine and sodium nitroprusside. Adverse effects include bradycardia and bronchospasm, although in one report a pediatric patient with a history of asthma experienced no respiratory difficulty when given labetalol for HTN.[83] Unfortunately, no prospective pediatric trial of labetalol has been conducted.

Nicardipine

Nicardipine is an intravenous dihydropyridine CCB that is specific for L-type calcium channels and is primarily an arteriolar vasodilator. It is selective for L-type calcium channels in vascular smooth muscle as opposed to cardiac myocytes. Moreover, nicardipine has profound coronary and cerebral vasodilatory activity.[77] Its potent BP actions are without negative inotropic effects or suppression of cardiac conduction; it has minimal effects on automaticity and causes no appreciable venodilation.[77]

Many pediatric case series of IV nicardipine use in infants and children with severe HTN have been published[15,85-88]; and in all of these studies, it has been reported to be effective and well tolerated. The vasodilatory effects appear to be greater in patients with HTN than in patients with normal BP.[89] In addition, it has gained a role in various cardiovascular, neurosurgical, and general surgery procedures as well as in the postoperative period.[90]

In head-to-head trials for treatment of severe HTN in adults, nicardipine was as effective as nitroprusside.[13] Unlike nitroprusside, nicardipine does not pose the risk for cyanide or thiocyanate toxicity and can be used for a longer duration than nitroprusside. It does have a slightly longer onset of action and a much longer elimination half-life compared with nitroprusside.[89] Plasma levels of nicardipine increase rapidly in the first few hours of a continuous infusion but then reach a steady state thereafter. The elimination half-life is a few hours with normal renal function and prolonged with decreased clearance during renal failure. Given its metabolism by the hepatic P-450 enzyme system, there is the potential for clinically significant drug interactions[77]; the most important of these include decreased clearance of cyclosporine, tacrolimus, and vecuronium.

Because nicardipine may cause thrombophlebitis when given through a peripheral intravenous line, central venous administration is recommended. Like other arterial vasodilators, nicardipine has the potential to increase ICP, although another dihydropyridine CCB (nimodipine) is neuroprotective and is often used in patients with subarachnoid hemorrhage. Conversion of nicardipine infusions to oral dosing has been reported in adults,[91] but no similar reports have been published for children.

Sodium Nitroprusside

Sodium nitroprusside (SNP) lowers systemic BP both as an arteriolar (peripheral resistance vessel) and venous (peripheral capacitance vessel) dilator. Consequently, this effect often results in a reflex tachycardia because of the fall in arteriolar BP. SNP lowers right atrial pressures through relaxation of venous capacitance vessels, thus increasing venous compliance. In addition, SNP reduces right ventricular afterload through its pulmonary arterial vasodilator activity.[92] Its potent pulmonary vasodilation inhibits hypoxic-mediated pulmonary vasoconstriction.[93] Generally, when used in acutely hypertensive patients with normal left ventricular function, SNP reduces CO through its venous pooling (eg, increased venous capacitance) effects. On the other hand, SNP improves CO in patients with poor left ventricular function and diastolic ventricular distention mainly by decreasing afterload by means of relaxing arteriolar resistance vessels.[94]

SNP has a prompt onset of action and a very short half-life, making it ideal for frequent titration. It is an unstable compound that breaks down under alkaline conditions and when exposed to ambient light. Immediately during infusion, SNP interacts with oxyhemoglobin to yield methemoglobin, cyanide, and NO. In contrast to the organic nitrates (eg, nitroglycerin) that require thiol-containing compounds to generate NO, SNP spontaneously generates NO, thus functioning as a

prodrug.[95] Once generated, NO activates the enzyme guanylate cyclase found within vascular smooth muscle, resulting in increased levels of cGMP, which inhibits calcium entry into vascular smooth muscle cells, producing vasodilation. Its onset of action is 30 seconds, it peaks at 2 minutes, and it is eliminated 3 minutes after cessation.

The cyanide that is produced is rapidly cleared by nonenzymatic means by reacting with sulfhydryl groups on proteins in surrounding tissue and in erythrocytes.[93] In addition, the liver enzymatically metabolizes cyanide to thiocyanate by means of rhodanese. Because the liver is the major source of rhodanese, in patients with liver failure, signs and symptoms of cyanide intoxication may develop upon nitroprusside administration. Adverse effects from methemoglobinemia generated by SNP metabolism are rare, even in patients with a congenital inability to convert methemoglobin to hemoglobin (ie, methemoglobin reductase deficiency). In any event, any patient receiving SNP in whom CNS dysfunction, cardiovascular instability, or increasing metabolic acidosis develops should be evaluated for cyanide toxicity.[93] If cyanide toxicity is suspected, SNP infusion should be stopped and therapies directed toward cyanide toxicity should be considered. Because the rate-limiting step of cyanide detoxification to thiocyanate usually entails the need for a sulfur donor, co-administration of sodium thiosulfate as a sulfur donor increases the rate of reaction of rhodanese, removing cyanide from the circulation.[89] A solution of 0.1% sodium nitroprusside and 1% sodium thiosulfate or a 1:10 ratio by weight in light-protected tubing is administered according to the usual dosing guidelines for sodium nitroprusside.[96-97] Alternatively, hydroxocobalamin (vitamin B_{12a}) can be used to trap the cyanide ion by exchanging the hydroxyl group for cyanide and forming cyanocobalamin, which is excreted unchanged in the urine.[98] Cyanocobalamin is the synthetic form of vitamin B_{12} (cobalamin) that is used for food additives and is nontoxic. Of note, IV methylene blue is contraindicated in treating methemoglobinemia attributable to cyanide toxicity because the conversion of methemoglobin to hemoglobin may liberate large amounts of cyanide.[98]

Thiocyanate is eliminated in the urine with an elimination half-life of 3 days in patients with normal renal function. Because thiocyanate accumulates in patients with renal failure and can result in renal toxicity, nitroprusside should usually be avoided in children with renal failure. In fact, a significant proportion of children with normal renal function treated with SNP may develop elevated cyanide levels,[99] so widespread use of SNP in pediatric patients is probably not advisable. Clinically, patients with thiocyanate toxicity exhibit anorexia, nausea, fatigue, disorientation, and psychosis. Thiocyanate also inhibits iodine uptake by the thyroid and may produce hypothyroidism. Thus thiocyanate levels should be monitored with prolonged infusion (>24 hours).

In one study evaluating the effectiveness of nitroprusside in children presenting with acute severe HTN of renal origin, target levels of BP were achieved within 1 to 20 minutes in all patients. In addition, symptoms of cardiac failure resolved in all patients, and neurologic symptoms abated in 80% of children within 24 to 48 hours.[100] In a clinical trial in children requiring prolonged hypotension, SNP was significantly more effective than placebo in maintaining BP control.[99] The disadvantages of SNP include not only the potential for cyanide and thiocyanate toxicity but also acute hypotension, rebound

HTN, increasing cerebral blood flow/ICP, oxygen desaturations (via inhibition of hypoxic vasoconstriction), and, in time, tachyphylaxis.[22]

Other Available Agents

Clevidipine is an ultra–short-acting IV dihydropyridine CCB with high specificity for vascular smooth muscle. Unlike oral dihydropyridine CCBs such as amlodipine that have long durations of action, clevidipine administration lowers BP within 2 minutes after initiation of a continuous infusion and has a rapid offset once the infusion is discontinued, with a half-life of just a few minutes.[101] This makes its pharmacokinetics similar to those of SNP; indeed, comparative studies of clevidipine and SNP in adults following coronary artery bypass have confirmed similar clinical efficacy of these two agents.[102] Clevidipine may be superior to both SNP and IV nicardipine due to its decreased tendency to produce tachycardia compared to nitroprusside and its more rapid offset of action compared to nicardipine.

Although originally developed for control of BP during surgical procedures, clevidipine has also found a role in the management of postoperative severe HTN in adults following cardiac surgery.[103] Pediatric use of clevidipine has been reported in several clinical situations, primarily in patients requiring intraoperative BP reduction.[104] In an open-label trial, clevidipine was administered to 30 children undergoing spinal fusion in whom controlled hypotension was needed. All patients achieved the desired reduction in MAP without significant adverse effects such as tachycardia.[105]

Enalaprilat is an IV form of the angiotensin-converting enzyme (ACE) inhibitor enalapril. ACE inhibition blocks the conversion of angiotensin I to angiotensin II, a potent vasoconstrictor. Thus ACE inhibition leads to vasodilation because of decreased levels of angiotensin II.[18] Interestingly, ACE also metabolizes bradykinin; hence bradykinins increase during ACE inhibition, and this effect may contribute to vasodilation as well.[106] In any event, ACE inhibitors decrease SVR and thus afterload and systolic wall stress. Consequently, CO and stroke volume improve.

All ACE inhibitors are cleared predominantly by the kidneys. Therefore doses of these agents need to be reduced in patients with renal insufficiency. ACE inhibitors are most potent in patients with high renin levels; significant decreases in BP can occur in this population. Enalaprilat should not be used in patients with myocardial infarction, bilateral renal artery stenosis, pregnancy, or preeclampsia/eclampsia.

There is no established pediatric dose for enalaprilat. A dose range of 5 to 10 μg/kg/dose IV every 8 to 24 hours was reported as effective in one small case series of hypertensive neonates[107]; however, no further pediatric reports of this agent have been published and it is therefore probably best avoided in severely hypertensive children, many of whom will have renovascular forms of HTN, where use of an ACE inhibitor is not recommended in the acute setting.[10]

Fenoldopam is the first available peripheral dopamine$_1$ receptor (DA1) agonist, the newest class of antihypertensive agents available to treat acute severe HTN. Stimulation of the DA1 receptor causes vasodilation of peripheral arteries as well as the mesenteric and renal vasculature, with less effect in the cerebral and coronary circulations. Thus it lowers BP and peripheral vascular resistance while maintaining renal blood flow.[108] DA1 receptor stimulation leads to vasodilatation by increasing cyclic AMP (cAMP), which promotes smooth muscle relaxation. cAMP also inhibits the sodium-hydrogen exchanger and the sodium/potassium-adenosine triphosphatase pump in the renal tubule.[18] This feature gives fenoldopam the advantage of maintaining or increasing renal perfusion; its use is associated with short-term increases in urine output, sodium excretion, and creatinine clearance.

Fenoldopam has an onset and duration of action similar to that of IV nicardipine[109] and has a half-life ranging from 5 to 10 minutes.[108] It has been shown to be generally equivalent to SNP in the management of acute severe HTN in adults.[110] Pediatric experience with this agent for severe HTN is limited to a few case reports.[111,112] However, it has found use in children requiring perioperative BP control. In a blinded, randomized, prospective study of children ranging from 3 weeks to 12 years of age who were scheduled for surgery with a planned induction of hypotension, fenoldopam rapidly lowered MAP compared with placebo.[109] A retrospective analysis of 13 patients aged 4 months to 18 years with primarily cardiac lesions demonstrated increased urine output with fenoldopam without the need to increase fluid intake; no increase in serum creatinine levels or adverse hemodynamic effects were observed.[113]

Like other drugs that act through adrenergic receptor stimulation, tolerance develops in patients who take fenoldopam for longer than 48 hours. Fenoldopam has the potential to increase intraocular pressure and is known to cause a dose-dependent tachycardia.[108,109]

Minoxidil is a direct vasodilator that opens potassium channels in smooth muscle cells, causing potassium efflux, which in turn leads to hyperpolarization and relaxation.[114] It acts primarily on arterioles and does not produce venous dilation. Minoxidil generally acts within 1 hour and its effects may last as long as 8 to 12 hours. It is renally excreted and easily removed by dialysis; therefore dose adjustment may be needed in patients with severe renal insufficiency, and it should be dosed after dialysis.[114]

Minoxidil has been shown to be effective in children with severe chronic HTN refractory to other oral agents[115] and also in children with chronic HTN experiencing acute BP elevations.[116] It has well-known side effects of hirsutism and fluid retention that are primarily seen with chronic use, so these should not be a significant consideration in the acutely hypertensive patient.

Nitroglycerin is principally a venodilator, although arteriolar dilation occurs at higher doses. Once nitroglycerin is converted to NO, it activates guanylate cyclase within smooth muscle (similar to SNP) and stimulates the production of cGMP. The result is increased venous capacitance with a predictable decrease in myocardial preload.[117] In volume-depleted patients, reduction of myocardial preload reduces CO and is undesirable, especially in patients with compromised myocardial, cerebral, or renal perfusion.[118]

Onset of action of IV nitroglycerin is 1 to 2 minutes, with a duration of action of 3 to 5 minutes.[119] Common adverse effects include headache, orthostatic hypotension, nausea, palpitations, and flushing. The hemodynamic effects of nitroglycerin may be deleterious in patients with anatomically restrictive cardiac lesions such as aortic stenosis or other left-sided obstructive cardiac lesions. Furthermore, nitroglycerin should be avoided in patients with increased ICP because of its cerebral vasodilatory properties.

Special Situations

Preeclampsia

Pregnancy associated with preeclampsia also must be considered in female adolescents experiencing acute severe HTN. Preeclampsia is a state of hypertensive proteinuria in a pregnant woman who is at greater than 20 weeks gestation.[120] Clinically, the classic triad of preeclampsia consists of HTN, proteinuria, and edema, although now it is accepted that edema should no longer be considered a prerequisite for making the diagnosis of preeclampsia. Under these circumstances, an elevated BP separated by a minimum of 4 hours (maximum 7 days) is considered adequate for making a diagnosis for HTN (>140/90 mm Hg) or severe HTN (>160/100 mm Hg). Proteinuria is considered significant when two random urine samples collected at least 4 hours (but <7 days) apart have a level of 30 mg/dL or higher (1+) or 300 mg or more of protein are present in a 24-hour urine collection.[120] In the absence of proteinuria, pregnancy-induced HTN, gestational HTN, or chronic HTN must be considered.

The goal of managing preeclampsia is to meticulously control the BP in order to protect the fetus from insufficient placental-uterine blood flow via overly aggressive antihypertensive therapy and to avoid development of eclampsia (the condition characterized by tonic-clonic seizure activity culminating in coma). IV antihypertensives that are commonly used for acute severe HTN in pregnancy include labetalol and hydralazine, but other drugs, including esmolol and nicardipine, have been safely used.[121]

Pheochromocytoma

Although rare as a cause of HTN in childhood,[122] pheochromocytomas present a unique set of management challenges to the intensivist. Many children with pheochromocytomas initially present with severe, symptomatic HTN of unknown etiology.[123] Such children require careful immediate stabilization and gradual BP reduction as described in the preceding sections until such time as the necessary studies can be obtained to establish the diagnosis. Although theoretically the α- and β-adrenergic blocker labetalol may seem uniquely well suited for treatment of HTN caused by a pheochromocytoma, in practice a continuous infusion of any of the intravenous antihypertensives listed in Table 79.5 could be utilized for initial BP management. Phentolamine has also been advocated in such patients,[124] although pediatric experience with this agent is extremely limited.

Once the diagnosis of pheochromocytoma has been made, the child's blood pressure should be stabilized with oral antihypertensives until the tumor can be surgically removed. Phenoxybenzamine, a potent α-adrenergic blocker, is usually recommended as the primary agent for this phase of management, although there has been a recent trend toward use of doxazosin for α blockade.[125] β-adrenergic blockade is frequently advocated as adjunctive therapy to counter tachycardia in patients treated with phenoxybenzamine. In the ICU setting, it is likely that these oral agents will need to be overlapped with IV therapy, followed by gradual discontinuation of IV therapy. Goal BP does not need to be reached prior to patient transfer out of the ICU, but the BP should be sufficiently controlled so that the patient is no longer experiencing symptoms of severe HTN.

The patient with pheochromocytoma may present back to the ICU following surgical removal of the tumor, usually for a brief period to ensure that the BP has stabilized. Intraoperatively, BP surges and arrhythmias may occur due to manipulation of the tumor. These complications are typically treated with use of rapidly acting intravenous antihypertensive agents and beta-adrenergic blockade. Volume resuscitation may be required immediately following removal of the tumor, but postoperative volume overload is not a significant concern.

Summary

Severe HTN is a potential medical emergency that needs to be addressed immediately. After a brief evaluation of the possible etiology, antihypertensive treatment should be initiated. This is mostly done with intravenous agents, of which a number of options, albeit many not well studied in children, exist. The intensivist needs a heightened awareness for factors that predispose children to severe hypertensive events as well as an understanding of the clinical symptoms that may reflect end-organ damage from critically high BPs.

Acknowledgment

The contributions of Karen McNiece Redwine, Ronald Sanders, and Arnold Zartitsky, authors of the prior version of this chapter, are gratefully acknowledged.

Key References

1. Flynn JT. The changing face of pediatric hypertension in the era of the childhood obesity epidemic. *Pediatr Nephrol*. 2013;28:1059-1066.
4. National High Blood Pressure Education Program Working Group on High Blood Pressure in Children and Adolescents. The fourth report on the diagnosis, evaluation, and treatment of high blood pressure in children and adolescents. *Pediatrics*. 2004;114(2 suppl):555-576.
9. Marik PE, Varon J. Hypertensive crises: challenges and management. *Chest*. 2007;131:1949-1962.
10. Flynn JT, Tullus K. Severe hypertension in children and adolescents: pathophysiology and treatment. *Pediatr Nephrol*. 2009;24:1101-1112.
15. Flynn JT, Mottes TA, Brophy PB, et al. Intravenous nicardipine for treatment of severe hypertension in children. *J Pediatr*. 2001;139:38-43.
16. Thomas CA, Moffett BS, Wagner JL, et al. Safety and efficacy of intravenous labetalol for hypertensive crisis in infants and small children. *Pediatr Crit Care Med*. 2011;12:28-32.
18. Yamaguchi I, Flynn JT. Pathophysiology of hypertension. In: Avner E, Harmon W, Niaudet P, Yoshikawa N, eds. *Pediatric Nephrology*. 7th ed. Philadelphia, PA: Lippincott Williams and Wilkins; 2005 in press.
36. Yang WC, Zhao LL, Chen CY, et al. First-attack pediatric hypertensive crisis presenting to the pediatric emergency department. *BMC Pediatr*. 2012;12:200.
37. Lee VH, Wijdicks EF, Manno EM, Rabinstein AA. Clinical spectrum of reversible posterior leukoencephalopathy syndrome. *Arch Neurol*. 2008; 65:205-210.
49. Vehaskari VM. Heritable forms of hypertension. *Pediatr Nephrol*. 2009; 24:1929-1937.
50. Marks SD, Tullus K. Update on imaging for suspected renovascular hypertension in children and adolescents. *Curr Hypertens Rep*. 2012; 14:591-595.
53. Ishikura K, Hamasaki Y, Sakai T, et al. Posterior reversible encephalopathy syndrome in children with kidney diseases. *Pediatr Nephrol*. 2012;27: 375-384.
67. Tabbutt S, Nicolson SC, Adamson PC, et al. The safety, efficacy, and pharmacokinetics of esmolol for blood pressure control immediately after repair of coarctation of the aorta in infants and children: a multicenter, double-blind, randomized trial. *J Thorac Cardiovasc Surg*. 2008;136:321-328.

75. Ostrye J, Hailpern SM, Jones J, et al. The efficacy and safety of intravenous hydralazine for the treatment of hypertension in the hospitalized child. *Pediatr Nephrol*. 2014;29:1403-1409.

77. Flynn JT, Pasko DA. Calcium channel blockers: pharmacology and place in therapy of pediatric hypertension. *Pediatr Nephrol*. 2000;15:302-316.

81. Miyashita Y, Peterson D, Rees JM, Flynn JT. Isradipine for treatment of acute hypertension in hospitalized children and adolescents. *J Clin Hypertens (Greenwich)*. 2010;12:850-855.

99. Hammer GB, Lewandowski A, Drover DR, et al. Safety and efficacy of sodium nitroprusside during prolonged infusion in pediatric patients. *Pediatr Crit Care Med*. 2015;doi:10.1097/PCC.0000000000000383.

105. Kako H, Gable A, Martin D, et al. A prospective, open-label trial of clevidipine for controlled hypotension during posterior spinal fusion. *J Pediatr Pharmacol Ther*. 2015;20:54-60.

113. Moffett BS, Mott AR, Nelson DP, et al. Renal effects of fenoldopam in critically ill pediatric patients: a retrospective review. *Pediatr Crit Care Med*. 2008;9:403-406.

121. Too GT, Hill JB. Hypertensive crisis during pregnancy and postpartum period. *Semin Perinatol*. 2013;37:280-287.

122. Waguespack SG, Rich T, Grubbs E, et al. A current review of the etiology, diagnosis, and treatment of pediatric pheochromocytoma and paraganglioma. *J Clin Endocrinol Metab*. 2010;95:2023-2037.

Metabolism, Endocrinology, and Nutrition

Cellular Respiration

Scott L. Weiss, Clifford S. Deutschman, and Lance B. Becker

"In every one of us there is a living process of combustion going on very similar to that of a candle, and I must try to make that plain to you. For it is not merely true in a poetical sense."
Michael Faraday, A Course of Six Lectures on the Chemical History of a Candle (1861)

PEARLS

- Cellular respiration is largely coordinated in the mitochondria and normally aligns energy demand with energy production. In critical illness, disruption of cellular bioenergetic homeostasis may be a final common pathway for organ dysfunction and death.
- Cellular respiration consists of three related series of biochemical reactions:
  - Glycolysis of carbohydrates, β-oxidation of fatty acids, and catabolism of amino acids to produce acetyl-coenzyme A (acetyl-CoA)
  - Metabolism of acetyl-CoA in the Krebs cycle to produce electron-rich nicotinamide dinucleotide (NADH) and flavin adenine dinucleotide ($FADH_2$)
  - Shuttling of electrons from NADH and $FADH_2$ to oxygen in order to synthesize adenosine triphosphate (ATP) in the mitochondria
- Shock is an imbalance balance between oxygen (and substrate) delivery and oxygen (and substrate) utilization such that cellular metabolic demands are not met. If oxygen delivery is not rapidly restored, ATP turnover will decrease and an altered state of bioenergetic homeostasis will lead to cell injury and organ dysfunction. Persistent mitochondrial dysfunction may contribute to a clinical state of *cytopathic hypoxia* in which cellular respiration remains abnormal even despite restoration of oxygen delivery.
- Bedside measures of cellular respiration remain challenging. The two most commonly used measures, lactate and venous oxygen saturation, provide important information about global oxygen utilization and have proved useful to guide acute resuscitation, but they have important limitations. More direct measures of cellular respiration may be available in the near future.
- A therapeutic approach that better aligns oxygen (and substrate) utilization with oxygen (and substrate) delivery may help to restore bioenergetic homeostasis and improve cellular—and thus organ—function. Several existing and novel therapies may help to improve mitochondrial function in particular.

In 1920 Haldane was credited with the observation that hypoxemia not only stops the (respiration) machine but wrecks the (respiration) machinery as well.[1] Indeed, the priorities of pediatric advanced life support and cardiopulmonary resuscitation are to restore oxygen and substrate delivery to tissues and cells. Critical care extends these basic principles of restoration of oxygen and substrate delivery to also support oxygen utilization and cellular respiration with the goal to reestablish and maintain bioenergetic homeostasis.

Although early resuscitation targeted toward prespecified hemodynamic end points improves outcomes in children with critical illness, this strategy does not benefit all patients at all time points in disease. Alterations in cellular respiration can contribute to a bioenergetic imbalance that results in cell—and ultimately—organ dysfunction.[2] Oxygen availability and utilization are vital for cells to efficiently convert the chemical energy of nutrient molecules into useful energy in the form of adenosine triphosphate (ATP).[3] This process involves a highly regulated network of multienzyme reactions, largely coordinated in the mitochondria, which normally closely align energy demand with energy production. In critical illness, this delicate homeostatic balance may be disrupted and has been identified as a possible final common pathway for organ failure and death.[4,5] Consequently, a working knowledge of cellular respiration is a key tenet of critical care medicine.

This chapter reviews (1) major pathways of cellular respiration with a focus on the mitochondria, (2) the role of impaired cellular respiration in critical illness, particularly in shock and multiple organ dysfunction syndrome (MODS), (3) clinical assessment of oxygen utilization, and (4) potential therapeutic strategies to improve mitochondrial respiration and restore bioenergetic homeostasis.

Pathways of Cellular Respiration

Plants harness the sun's energy to split water into hydrogen and oxygen (Fig. 80.1). The hydrogen is then attached to carbon to create glucose and starch, while the oxygen is released into the atmosphere. Animals, including humans, eat plants to acquire carbohydrates (as well as other animals to obtain protein and fat), ultimately removing the hydrogen and combining it with oxygen to regenerate water. Through this cyclical process, humans convert energy in the form of photons from the sun to usable cellular energy in the form of ATP (Fig. 80.2) through a process called *oxidative phosphorylation*.[6] As will be discussed, an interconnected and alternative pathway of *anaerobic respiration* also exists within the cytoplasm, but in the absence of oxygen it is not sufficient to sustain human life.[7]

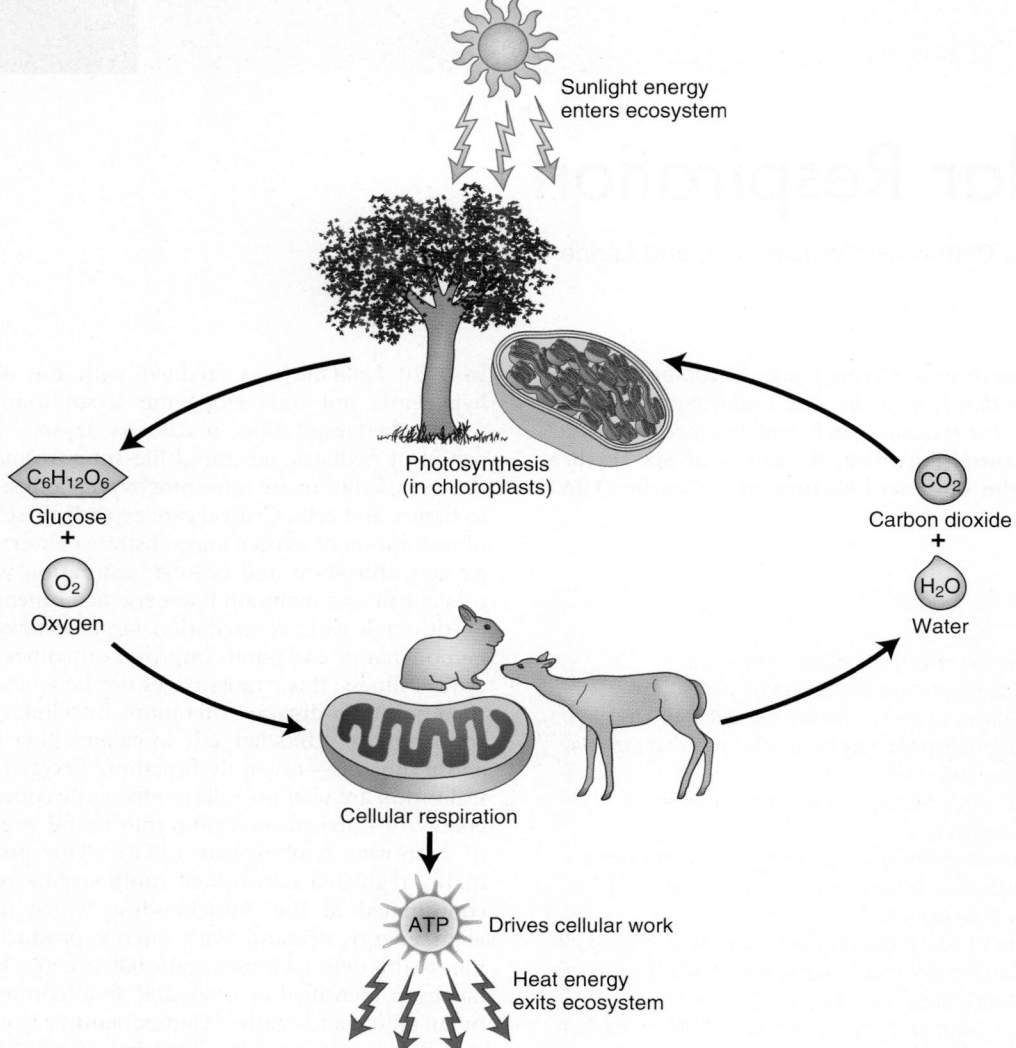

Fig. 80.1. Cyclical process through which plants help animals to convert the sun's energy into usable cellular energy in the form of ATP.

Apart from erythrocytes, all human cells possess mitochondria. These organelles account for nearly all of total body oxygen consumption and are responsible for >90% of ATP production.[8] Although mitochondria participate in many cellular processes other than ATP production, this chapter focuses on their role as the bioenergetic powerhouse of the cell. An alternative end production of oxygen consumption is the formation of reactive oxygen species (ROS); this too will be discussed. Mitochondrial involvement in cell signaling, heat production, calcium regulation, hormone synthesis, cell death pathways, and genomic/epigenomic expression are reviewed elsewhere.[8,9]

A typical human adult male consumes approximately 380 liters of oxygen per day, with well-conditioned athletes achieving rates up to 10 times higher.[10] Oxygen serves as the final electron receptor at the terminal complex of the mitochondrial electron transport system (ETS). Through a series of oxidation-reduction (redox) reactions, electrons are transferred through the ETS to oxygen, pumping protons from the mitochondrial matrix to the intermembrane space producing a proton motive force that is coupled to ATP production by ATP synthase (ETS complex V). Mitchell first described this *chemiosmotic principle*—the coupling of biological electron transfer to ATP synthesis—in the 1960s.[11] It is now recognized that 3×10^{21} protons per second are transferred across all of the inner mitochondrial membranes in an adult male producing ATP at a rate of 9×10^{20} molecules per second. This is equivalent to a turnover rate of 65 kg of ATP per day, with even higher rates during periods of activity.[10]

The phosphorylation of adenosine diphosphate (ADP) to form ATP through aerobic and, to a lesser extent, anaerobic processes provides the currency for cells to perform a wide range of energy-consuming activities, such as the active pumping of solutes against a concentration gradient across a membrane barrier. The first law of thermodynamics states that the total amount of energy in a system remains constant during a chemical reaction. The second law of thermodynamics states that even though total energy does not change, the net amount of usable or *free energy* (termed *Gibbs free energy* and designated by the letter G) is always decreased—that is, a negative ΔG.[5] Chemical reactions are characterized either as those that produce energy (*exergonic* or $\Delta G < 0$) or those that

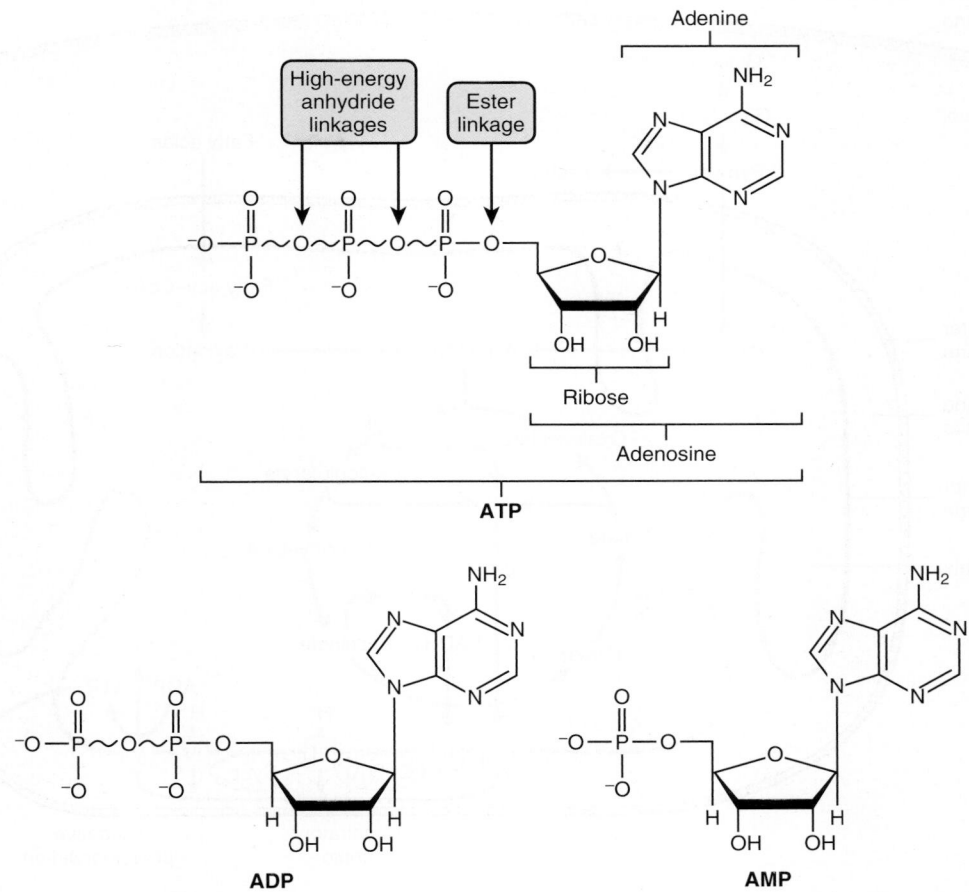

Fig. 80.2. Structure of ATP. (Modified from Baynes JW, Dominiczak MH. Medical Biochemistry. New York: Mosby Elsevier; 2009.)

consume energy (*endergonic* or ΔG >0). In living organisms, the highly complex, ordered state of homeostasis would naturally degrade to a less complex disordered state (ie, toward a negative overall ΔG) without continual cellular maintenance. By coupling energy-consuming endergonic processes to the hydrolysis of ATP to yield ADP and inorganic phosphate—an energetically favorable exergonic reaction—cells are able to drive forward critical chemical reactions that would otherwise not be possible.

Complete oxidation of nutrient fuels is accompanied by a large release of free energy that is used to produce ATP. In general, cellular respiration consists of three related series of biochemical reactions (Fig. 80.3):

1. Chemical reactions resulting in the formation of two-carbon acetyl-coenzyme A (acetyl-CoA) through glycolysis of carbohydrates, β-oxidation of fatty acids, and catabolism of amino acids
2. Metabolism of acetate to carbon dioxide in the Krebs cycle with generation of the electron-rich reducing equivalents nicotinamide dinucleotide (NADH) and flavin adenine dinucleotide (FADH₂)
3. Shuttling of electrons from the reducing equivalents in NADH and FADH₂ along the mitochondrial ETS leading to ATP synthesis and ultimately reducing oxygen to water

Although the initial catabolic steps vary among the different fuels (eg, carbohydrates, fats, and amino acids), all nutrient molecules eventually converge to a common mitochondrial pathway (Fig. 80.4).

Glycolysis (Anaerobic Respiration)

Glucose is the principal metabolic substrate for glycolysis and the primary fuel for many organ systems, including the central nervous system. Glucose is transported into cells via glucose transporter (GLUT) receptors and down osmotic gradients. Once in the cell, glucose enters the glycolytic pathway and is rapidly phosphorylated by the enzyme hexokinase to glucose-6-phosphate. Consequently, cellular glucose concentrations are low, allowing for a substantial favorable osmotic gradient for glucose to enter cells.[12]

Ten enzymatic reactions within the cell cytoplasm define the metabolic pathway of anaerobic respiration, termed *glycolysis*. Overall, the full sequence of glycolysis is irreversible and exergonic such that the free energy extracted from glucose is used to synthesize two net molecules of ATP, two molecules of NADH, and two molecules of pyruvate. Under aerobic conditions (ie, when oxygen is available), pyruvate is shuttled into the mitochondrial matrix through a specific low K_m transporter where it is metabolized by *pyruvate dehydrogenase (PDH)* to acetyl-CoA and carbon dioxide (CO_2) and NAD^+ is converted to NADH. PDH is thus a key enzyme that links cytoplasmic glycolysis to mitochondrial respiration, and its activity is controlled by the overall energy state of the cell

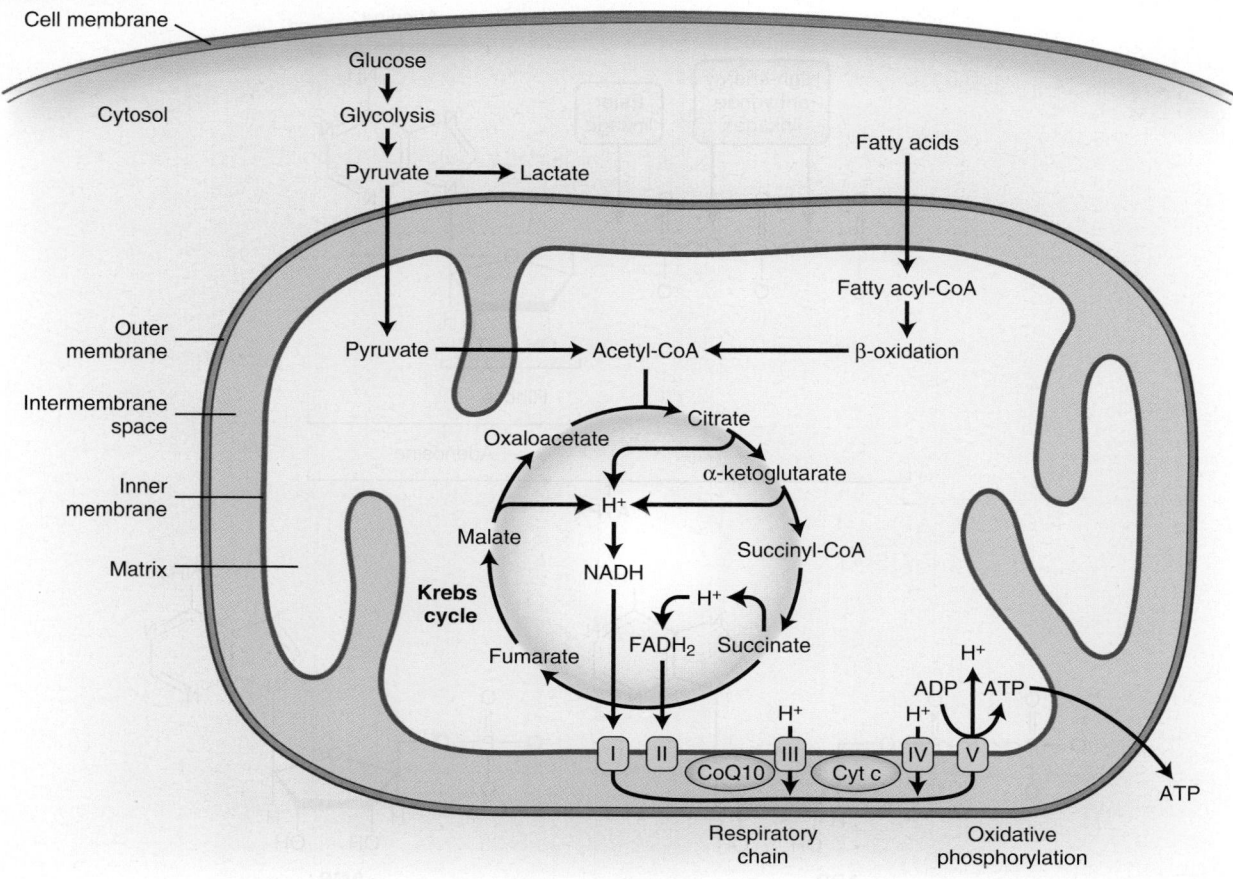

Fig. 80.3. Overview of the pathways of cellular respiration. (Modified from Genge A, Massie R. Mitochondrial structure, function, and genetics. Up-To-Date; 2013.)

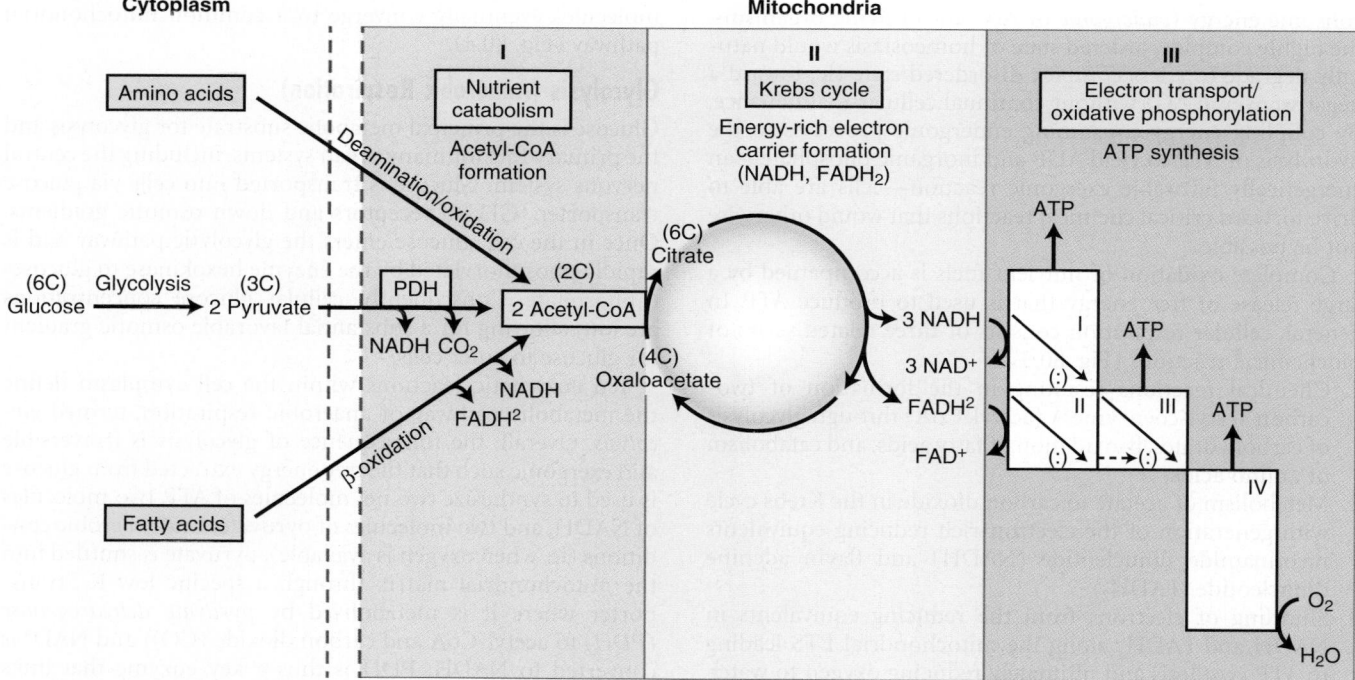

Fig. 80.4. Metabolic fates of pyruvate, the end product of glycolysis. (Modified from Baynes JW, Dominiczak MH. Medical Biochemistry. New York: Mosby Elsevier; 2009.)

through feedback regulation by both PDH kinase and PDH phosphatase. Inhibition of PDH activity occurs with elevated ratios of NADH/NAD$^+$, ATP/ADP, and acetyl-CoA/CoA ratios indicating an energy-replete state, thus helping to maintain bioenergetic homeostasis. Alternatively, under anaerobic conditions, pyruvate is reduced by NADH to lactate by *lactate dehydrogenase (LDH)* in order to regenerate the NAD$^+$ needed to continue glycolysis. During periods of hypoxemia, anaerobic respiration through glycolysis can be increased for a limited time to generate ATP in the absence of oxygen. However, glycolysis alone results in a net generation of only two ATP molecules compared to the much more efficient process of oxidative phosphorylation described later.[13]

Fatty Acid β-Oxidation

Fatty acids are primarily oxidized through β-oxidation in the mitochondrial matrix. Entry of long-chain free fatty acids into the mitochondria is dependent on the carnitine transport system, while medium-chain fatty acids and ketone bodies enter the mitochondria without carnitine. Catabolism of fatty acids by β-oxidation sequentially removes two-carbon units from the carboxyl terminal to generate one molecule of acetyl-CoA, one FADH$_2$, and one NADH for each two-carbon fatty acid fragment cycle. Like carbohydrate metabolism through glycolysis, lipid metabolism is a tightly regulated process. Lipid stored in adipose tissue cycles continuously between triglycerides and free fatty acids. When glucose and insulin concentrations are high (eg, after a meal), fatty acid uptake into adipocytes is increased, resulting in the synthesis and storage of triglycerides. In contrast, when glucose levels are low (eg, during starvation), up-regulation of catecholamines and glucagon stimulate lipases that release free fatty acids into the circulation to be used directly by peripheral tissues as fuel for the Krebs cycle or are transported to the liver to be converted into ketone bodies in the liver. The ketone bodies, acetoacetate and β-hydroxybutyrate, are important substrates for oxidative phosphorylation in most tissues, including the heart, brain, kidney, and skeletal muscle. Because generation of acetyl-CoA by fatty acid β-oxidation (either directly or through catabolism of ketone bodies) occurs independent of pyruvate dehydrogenase, lipids provide an alternative fuel for oxidative phosphorylation when glucose metabolism is rate limited.[14]

Protein Catabolism

Although typically protected as a fuel source, amino acids can be mobilized for energy production in times of energy need (such as starvation or critical illness).[15] As part of the metabolic stress response mediated by a decrease in insulin and up-regulation of cortisol, catecholamines, tumor necrosis factor-α, and interleukins (IL)-1 and IL-6, protein degradation can occur with release of amino acids from skeletal muscle (see also Chapter 81). Ten of the 20 amino acids enter the Krebs cycle by way of acetyl-CoA, whereas others enter through various Krebs cycle intermediates, usually α-ketoglutarate and succinyl-CoA.[13] Alternatively, amino acids (alanine and glutamine in particular) can feed gluconeogenesis, a costly process that requires four ATP molecules plus two guanosine triphosphate (GTP) molecules and two NADH molecules to regenerate one molecule of glucose from two molecules of pyruvate. The ATP and GTP for these series of reactions are provided through β-oxidation of fatty acids.

Krebs Cycle

The Krebs cycle summarizes a circular series of nine reactions that occur in the mitochondrial matrix in which acetyl-CoA derived from glycolysis, β-oxidation, or protein catabolism is metabolized to two molecules of CO_2, one molecule of GTP, three molecules of NADH, and one molecule of FADH$_2$ (see Fig. 80.3). GTP is equivalent to ATP in terms of energy charge and is ultimately converted to ATP by the enzyme nucleoside diphosphokinase. Although oxygen itself is not part of the Krebs cycle, its presence at the end of the mitochondrial electron transport system ensures recycling of NAD$^+$ and FAD required in the Krebs cycle.

The first step in the Krebs cycle catalyzes the formation of the six-carbon citrate molecule (hence the alternative name of the Krebs cycle is the *citric acid cycle*) from the two-carbon acetyl-CoA and four-carbon oxaloacetate. This reaction is catalyzed by the enzyme citrate synthase and is the rate-limiting step of the Krebs cycle. With each revolution of the cycle, the fuel substrate that entered the cycle as acetyl-CoA is completely oxidized to CO_2 and water and oxaloacetate is regenerated to again react with a new acetyl-CoA molecule.

Mitochondrial Oxidative Phosphorylation

Some 2 billion to 4 billion years ago, aerobic bacteria invaded and subsequently colonized a form of primordial eukaryotic cells that lacked the ability to use oxygen. Over the ensuing millions of years, a critical symbiotic relationship developed between the cell and the aerobic bacteria that have remained steadfast through evolution.[16,17] The cell nucleus has evolved to regulate structure and overall cell function, while the oxygen-consuming bacteria formed mitochondria specialized in the energy production necessary for the development of increasingly complex species, including humans. Despite extensive intercommunication between mitochondria and its nuclear-cytosol host, mitochondria have retained many features characteristic of their bacterial origins: (1) mitochondria only arise from other mitochondria; (2) mitochondria maintain their own genome that, in contrast to eukaryotic nuclear DNA, is circular in structure, lacking in associated histones, and is replicated up to dozens of times; (3) mitochondria synthesize their own proteins that, like bacterial proteins, exhibit *N*-formyl methionine; and (4) many antibiotics that inhibit protein synthesis in bacteria are also toxic to mitochondria.[10] The independent mitochondrial genome, located within the mitochondrial matrix, contains genes that encode 37 proteins involved in the ETS, enzymes comprising the Krebs cycle, fatty acid β-oxidation, and pyruvate oxidation and the machinery needed for mitochondrial gene translation.[17] Notably, nuclear DNA encodes approximately 1500 additional mitochondrial proteins, including 79 of the 92 subunits of the ETS complexes.[18]

Mitochondrial oxidative phosphorylation is fueled by pairs of elections originating from NADH and FADH$_2$ that are produced through the series of metabolic pathways described previously (Fig. 80.5). These electrons are shuttled along the mitochondrial ETS, ultimately reducing oxygen to water.[8] To capture as much of the energy released in a usable form when strong reducing agents such as NADH and FADH$_2$ react with a powerful oxidizing agent such as oxygen, mitochondria "step down" the reducing potential of these molecules through a controlled series of intermediate compounds in the ETS with progressively lower reducing potentials.[5] Five complexes of

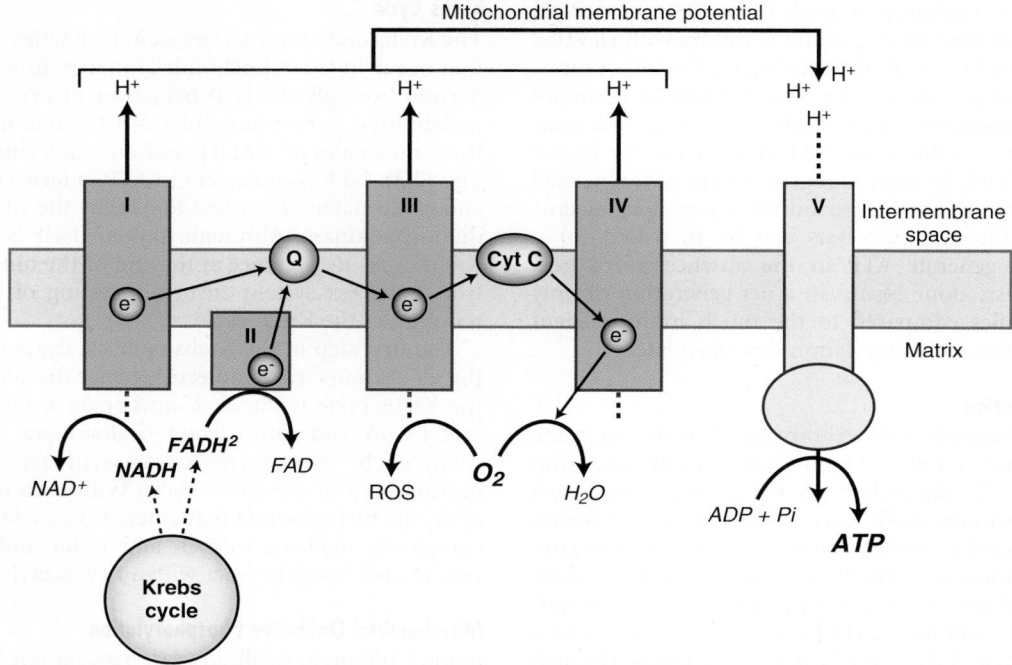

Fig. 80.5. Oxidative phosphorylation and ROS production through the mitochondrial electron transport chain. (Modified from Protti A, Singer S. Bench-to-bedside review: potential strategies to protect or reverse mitochondrial dysfunction in sepsis-induced organ failure. Crit Care. 2006;10:228.)

proteins and cytochromes embedded within the inner mitochondrial membrane comprise the ETS, including NADH dehydrogenase–ubiquinone oxidoreductase (complex I), succinate dehydrogenase–ubiquinone oxidoreductase (complex II), ubiquinone–cytochrome c oxidoreductase (complex III), cytochrome c oxidase (complex IV), and ATP synthase (complex V). The cofactors ubiquinone (coenzyme Q10) and cytochrome c facilitate the transfer of electrons from complexes I and II to complex III and from complex III to complex IV, respectively. Electrons in the form of hydride ions from NADH and $FADH_2$ cascade along these protein/cytochrome complexes toward complex IV where they are finally passed to molecular oxygen, generating water. Protons generated during these reactions are pumped across the inner mitochondrial membrane by complexes I, III, and IV, generating a proton motive force. The resulting electrochemical gradient across the inner mitochondrial membrane drives ATP synthesis by the *chemiosmotic principle.* Energy for ATP synthesis arises from an influx of these protons back into the matrix through the rotary motor of ATP synthase (complex V).[19] For each pair of electrons involved in one hydride equivalent, three molecules of ATP are produced. This process is termed *oxidative phosphorylation* because the reduction of molecular oxygen to water is linked to the addition of inorganic phosphate to ADP producing the high-energy terminal pyrophosphate in ATP. Aerobic respiration through oxidative phosphorylation is up to 15 times more efficient than anaerobic metabolism, producing 30 to 34 ATP molecules compared to only 2 ATP molecules per 1 molecule of glucose through glycolysis alone. ATP molecules are transferred out of the mitochondria through a specific adenine nucleotide translocase (ANT) antiporter on the inner mitochondrial membrane and through a voltage-dependent anion channel (VDAC) on the outer mitochondrial membrane for use as energy currency for all cellular functions.

The overall metabolism of glucose through cellular respiration can be summarized as follows (the negative ΔG indicates that the overall reaction can occur spontaneously):

$$Glucose + 6\,O_2 \rightarrow 6\,CO_2 + 6\,H_2O + heat$$

$$\Delta G = -2880 \text{ kJ per molecule of glucose}$$

Although multiple regulatory steps exist along the pathways of cellular respiration, the following three are preeminent:
1. Oxygen availability to serve as the ultimate electron acceptor
2. Availability of nutrient metabolism to generate reducing equivalents in the form of NADH and $FADH_2$
3. The overall cellular energy state defined by the ratios of $NADH/NAD^+$, ATP/ADP, and acetyl-CoA/CoA

Oxygen Toxicity

In health, approximately 1% to 2% of oxygen consumption is directed toward the production of reactive oxygen species (ROS) and an even greater amount is "uncoupled" from energy production and lost as heat.[2] Heat production varies substantially from tissue to tissue, being low in the heart and much higher in skeletal muscle and brown fat.[20] Despite the terminology, uncoupling is itself a controlled process regulated by a series of uncoupling proteins (UCPs) that insert within the inner mitochondrial membrane and provide an alternative pathway for protons to move back into the matrix bypassing ATP synthase. For example, UCP-1 present in brown fat provides a vital source of heat generation for neonates and hibernating mammals.[21]

Successive one-electron additions to molecular oxygen result in the production of superoxide anion, hydrogen peroxide (H_2O_2), hydroxyl radical, and water, respectively.[22] The partially reduced oxygen compounds are referred to as *reactive oxygen species* and are responsible for the so-called *antagonistic pleiotropy* characteristic of oxygen.[23] Under normal conditions, small amounts of constitutively produced ROS, primarily in the form of H_2O_2, are necessary for a variety of intracellular signaling pathways. Production of ROS occurs by multiple mechanisms, but the following four are prominent:

1. Mitochondrial electron transport bleed (approximately 1% to 2% of all electrons shuttled across mitochondrial complexes I, II, and III produce partially reduced oxygen species)[24]
2. Nicotinamide adenine dinucleotide phosphate (NADPH) oxidoreductases and the related cytochrome P450 oxidation reactions[25]
3. Xanthine oxidase (primarily during reperfusion following ischemic events)[26]
4. Cyclooxygenase and lipoxygenase pathways in the metabolism of arachidonic acid[27]

It has been estimated that approximately 2 billion molecules of superoxide anion and hydrogen peroxide are produced per cell per day. An antioxidant repertoire that includes superoxide dismutase, catalase, glutathione peroxidase, uric acid, vitamin C, and vitamin E counteracts this oxidant stress. Under conditions of metabolic, infectious, or inflammatory stress, ROS production can increase substantially. Although the majority of cellular ROS is sequestered within the mitochondria—thereby protecting the redox state of other intracellular molecules—such an increase can quickly outstrip availability of antioxidant defense mechanisms and cause oxidant injury to cellular proteins, lipids, and DNA.[22]

Nitrogen is also involved in the generation of another group of toxic metabolic moieties known as *reactive nitrogen species (RNS)*. Nitric oxide (NO) is known to be generated from at least four NO synthase (NOS) isoenzymes, including constitutive, inducible, neuronal, and mitochondrial forms.[28] NO is believed to play a role in mitochondrial respiration through the formation of nitrosyl complexes with various iron-sulfur center enzymes in the ETS as well as through direct competition with oxygen for binding at the heme *a,a3* active site of cytochrome oxidase. In addition to direct toxicity, NO can react with the superoxide anion to form the powerful oxidant peroxynitrite. Peroxynitrite has been demonstrated to be involved in lipid peroxidation of cell and organelle membranes, damage to various elements of the mitochondrial electron transport chain and ATP synthase, inhibition of glyceraldehyde 3-phosphate dehydrogenase, injury of the sodium-potassium ATPase pump, disruption of sodium channels, production of DNA strand breaks, and activation of the poly-adenosine ribosyl phosphate system. Peroxynitrite can also irreversibly inhibit the Krebs cycle enzyme aconitase and increase mitochondrial proton leak.[28]

Increased ROS- and RNS-mediated stress can promote the formation of the mitochondrial permeability transition pore (MPTP) leading to release of pro-apoptotic proteins, including cytochrome c, into the cytoplasm.[22,29,30] This can help to trigger activation of the apoptotic pathway orchestrating cell death. Integrity of the mitochondrial ETS complexes defines a fine line between maintaining mitochondrial homeostasis and efficient respiration versus excessive ROS/RNS production, mitochondrial dysfunction, and cell death. This balance is maintained through multiple feedback signals related to mitochondrial proton and calcium concentrations, reactive oxygen species, overall mitochondrial redox state, mitochondrial membrane potential, and mitochondrial matrix pH, all of which affect the cascade of electron transfer along the mitochondrial ETS.[10]

Impaired Cellular Respiration in Critical Illness

Mitochondrial ATP production relies on a complex series of chemical reactions that, overall, are controlled by metabolic demand. During periods of rest, metabolic needs are generally reduced and less energy is required. Conversely, during periods of activity and stress, metabolic requirements increase with a concurrent rise in cellular oxygen utilization and ATP production. An increase in ATP production ensures sufficient energy is available to respond to the activity or stress and prevents the cell from depleting ATP levels below a critical threshold that can trigger apoptotic and necrotic cell death pathways. With an acute decrease in oxygen delivery to tissues, such as with cardiac arrest, shock, or hemorrhage, mitochondrial energy output will necessarily fall. A concurrent increase in anaerobic respiration through glycolysis will attempt to partially offset the decline in ATP production through oxidative phosphorylation, but if oxygen delivery is not rapidly restored, bioenergetic homeostasis will be perturbed, leading to eventual cell injury and organ dysfunction.[2]

In critical illness, shock represents the imbalance balance between oxygen (and substrate) delivery and oxygen (and substrate) utilization such that cellular metabolic demands are not met. Early in the course of shock and other inflammatory conditions, the total body metabolic rate rises with the surge in catecholamine and catabolic hormones. In healthy volunteers, injection of endotoxin leads to a systemic inflammatory response characterized by fever and a rapid rise (within hours) in total-body oxygen consumption.[31] Over time, total body oxygen consumption and energy expenditure decrease with increasing illness severity in both animal models and critically ill patients.[32] Following trauma, failure to attain a low-normal level of oxygen consumption has been associated with increased risk of multiorgan dysfunction.[33] Survivors of critical illness subsequently demonstrate a return of oxygen consumption toward baseline levels.[32]

Changes in total body oxygen consumption and energy expenditure suggest that mitochondrial respiration is altered in critical illness. The inability of cells to effectively utilize oxygen to generate ATP is termed *cytopathic hypoxia*.[3,5] To date, most studies have focused on sepsis, though increasing evidence supports the development of cytopathic hypoxia after trauma, brain injury, and cardiac arrest. Ultrastructural mitochondrial abnormalities in a variety of organ systems have been recognized in in vivo, ex vivo, and in vitro models of sepsis for over 30 years.[34] For example, Crouser and associates demonstrated marked swelling and disruption of mitochondrial architecture in the liver following cecal ligation and puncture (CLP) in a mouse model (Fig. 80.6).[4] Morphologic abnormalities have also been noted in mitochondria taken from heart, kidney, liver, endothelial cells, intestinal epithelial cells, and skeletal muscle in animal models of sepsis.[35] In human sepsis, heart and liver biopsies obtained immediately postmortem from adult nonsurvivors similarly show swollen and damaged mitochondria.[36]

Functional alterations in mitochondrial respiration have been more variably reported as increased, decreased, or unchanged in short-term sepsis models. However,

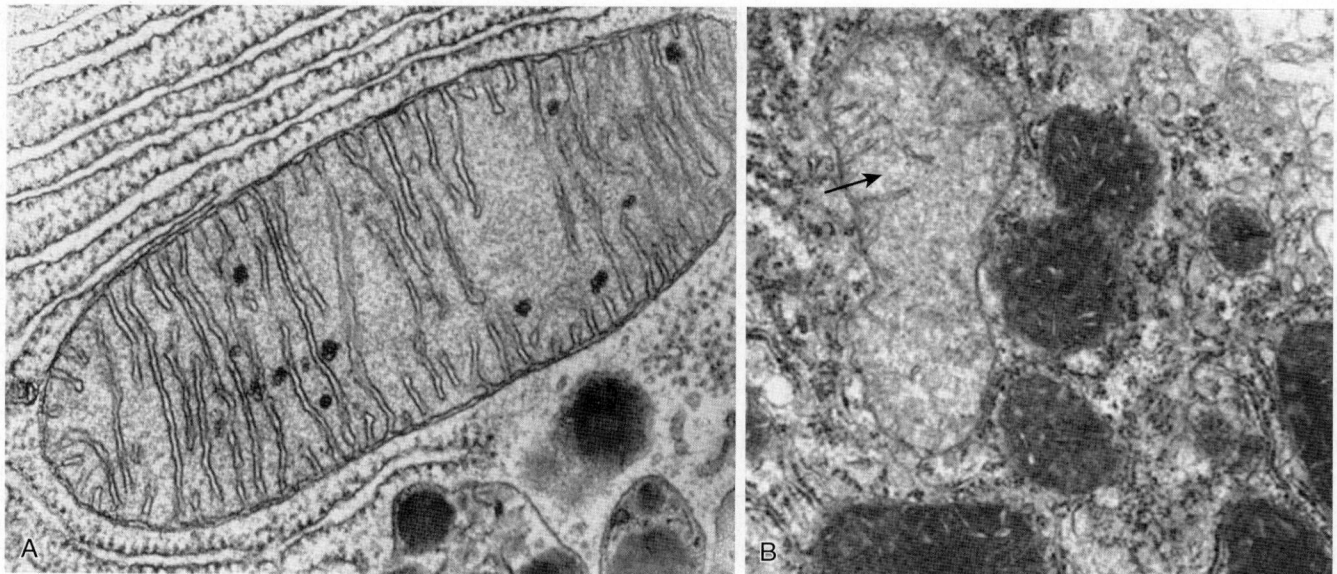

Fig. 80.6. Electron micrograph of a mitochondrion at the site of cellular respiration. (A) A normal invaginated cristae membrane provides the scaffolding for components of the electron transport chain. (B) Disrupted and edematous mitochondrial architecture observed in the liver 24 hours after cecal ligation and puncture in a mouse. (Modified from Crouser ED. Mitochondrial dysfunction in septic shock and multiple organ dysfunction syndrome. Mitochondrion. 2004;4:729-741.)

longer-term models that may better align with human critical illness more consistently demonstrate depressed mitochondrial function. In human sepsis, most—but not all—studies demonstrate decreased mitochondrial oxygen consumption in both immune and nonimmune cells.[2,37,38] For example, in a study of pediatric patients with septic shock and multiorgan dysfunction, direct measurements of mitochondrial respiration in peripheral blood mononuclear immune cells (PBMCs) showed that spare respiratory capacity—which reflects the ability of the ETS to keep pace with a rise in energy demand—was decreased and mitochondrial uncoupling was increased compared to noninfected controls.[38] Similar findings have been reported in PBMCs in adults with sepsis,[39] though one study demonstrated a progressive increase in mitochondrial respiration from day 1 to day 2 through day 6 to day 7 of sepsis compared to healthy controls.[37]

When considering bioenergetic impairment in sepsis, investigators have most commonly focused on NADH dehydrogenase–ubiquinone oxidoreductase (complex I) and cytochrome oxidase (complex IV). As the largest complex of the ETS, complex I is subject to impairment from changes in a variety of protein subunits. Multiple studies have demonstrated decreased activity of ETS complex I in sepsis models and in humans.[40,41] Complex IV contains two heme subgroups (cytochrome a and $a3$) that assist in the final transfer of electrons to reduce oxygen to water. A reduced cytochrome $a,a3$ redox state in the absence of tissue hypoxia indicates a defect in mitochondrial oxygen use and suggests impaired oxidative phosphorylation. A number of investigators have demonstrated reduced cytochrome $a,a3$ redox status during endotoxemia and gram-negative bacteremia in the heart, brain, skeletal muscle, and intestine in a variety of animals.[42,43] In addition, decoupled cytochrome $a,a3$ was more likely in adults who did versus did not develop multiorgan system dysfunction following trauma, despite normalization of

oxygen delivery.[44] In baboons following *Escherichia coli* infusion, myocardial cytochrome oxidase activity decreased to 51% of baseline.[45] Steady-state levels of cytochrome oxidase subunit I messenger RNA (mRNA) and protein are also decreased in the murine heart following CLP.[43] Interestingly, Verma and colleagues demonstrated that when complex IV activity is stimulated by administration of caffeine, myocardial function and survival improved after cecal ligation and puncture in a rodent model.[46]

Despite structural, biochemical, and functional evidence for mitochondrial dysfunction in sepsis, trauma, and other critical illness, the literature is less clear regarding these effects on tissue ATP availability. Several studies have reported preservation of ATP levels in septic myocardium, but others have shown decreased high-energy phosphates with endotoxemia.[2,5] In a study of 28 human adults with severe sepsis, 12 (43%) of whom died of sepsis-related MODS, nonsurvivors had lower levels of ATP in skeletal muscle compared to survivors.[40] However, even preservation of ATP does not imply an absence of mitochondrial dysfunction in sepsis.[47] When oxygen delivery and cellular hypoxia are limited (as in shock), cells may adapt to maintain viability by down-regulating oxygen consumption, energy requirements, and ATP demand.[2,5,9] Thus, a fall in ATP utilization may help to preserve ATP even if energy production is diminished. In the heart, this response is referred to as *myocardial hibernation* and classically occurs following an acute coronary syndrome. If cellular metabolic activity continued unchanged despite mitochondrial dysfunction, then ATP levels would inevitably diminish and cell death pathways would be activated. Because cell death does not appear to be a primary feature of sepsis-induced organ dysfunction, it follows that cells may instead adapt to cope with the falling energy supply.[34,48] Thus, finding preserved ATP during sepsis reveals little about the integrity of oxidative phosphorylation.

Though experimental data demonstrate an association of pro-inflammatory cytokines and ROS/RNS production with mitochondrial dysfunction, the precise etiology by which mitochondrial function is altered in critical illness remains unclear. A number of mutually compatible mechanisms may contribute to a clinical state of cytopathic hypoxia under pathologic conditions, including the following:

1. Decreased tissue oxygen (and substrate) delivery impairing oxidative phosphorylation
2. Inhibition of PDH with decreased flux of acetyl-CoA through the Krebs cycle
3. NO-mediated inhibition of ETS complexes
4. Peroxynitrite-mediated inhibition of the Krebs cycle and ETS complexes I, II, and V
5. Depletion of cellular NADH due to activation of the enzyme poly(ADP-ribose) polymerase (PARP)-1 in response to ROS-mediated nuclear DNA damage
6. Insufficient mitochondrial turnover due to impaired mitochondrial biogenesis, fission/fusion, or mitophagy
7. Hormonal alterations, including relative hypothyroidism
8. Pharmacologic inhibition of mitochondrial function as a side effect of many drugs commonly used in the intensive care unit setting, including some antibiotics, catecholamines, and sedatives (propofol in particular)

Injection of lipopolysaccharide (LPS) endotoxin into healthy human volunteers also results in widespread suppression of genes regulating mitochondrial energy production and protein synthesis.[49] Differential expression of mitochondrial genes in blood cells has been reported for several diseases in which bioenergetic failure is a postulated mechanism.[50,51] In a study of adult sepsis, decreased ETS gene expression correlated with impaired activity of ETS complexes I and IV in skeletal muscle.[52] In pediatric sepsis, suppression of nuclear-encoded mitochondrial genes was greatest in the subgroup of patients with the highest rates of MODS and death.[53]

Accumulating evidence also supports a propagative role for mitochondrial damage to feed-forward the systemic inflammatory response and contribute to distant organ injury in trauma and sepsis.[9] Oxidative injury due to an increase in mitochondrial ROS and RNS can fragment mitochondrial DNA (mtDNA). Oxidatively damaged mtDNA fragments can be exported from the mitochondrial through the MPTP to the cytosol or the extracellular space. In the cytosol, mtDNA promotes the formation of the Nod-like receptor-P3 (NLRP3) inflammasome, a supramolecular platform that activates caspase-1 and increases the release of the proinflammatory cytokines IL-1β and IL-18.[54] In the circulation, mitochondria are recognized by the innate immune systems as a danger-associated molecular pattern (DAMP) via the pattern recognition receptor, TLR [toll like receptor]-9, due to their evolutionary similarities with bacterial pathogens.[55] Several studies in human sepsis and trauma have demonstrated that an increase in circulating levels of mtDNA is associated with adverse outcomes.[55,56] Consequently, mtDNA has been proposed as a potential novel biomarker linked to mitochondrial dysfunction in critical illness.

Despite demonstration of altered mitochondrial structure and function, there is actually little evidence that impaired mitochondrial respiration *causes* organ dysfunction in critical illness. In fact, the decrease in oxygen utilization and overall metabolic rate seen in sepsis parallels similar physiologic changes observed in hibernating mammals that reduce their metabolism to promote survival amid decreased substrate availability.[48] Indeed despite physiologic and biochemical mitochondrial dysfunction in many tissues recovered from animal models and human patients with sepsis, there tends to be minimal evidence of cell death in dysfunctional organ systems. Moreover, survivors of critical illness rapidly recover organ function. Therefore, although a profound and prolonged metabolic down-regulation can trigger cell death, the observation that mitochondrial hibernation is a conserved physiologic response across models and species suggests that some degree of transient energetic swoon early in sepsis (and other critical illnesses) could be an adaptive response to ischemia, hypoxemia, and shock.[2,48,57] The use of induced hypothermia to decrease metabolic demand and protect vital organs during cardiopulmonary bypass and following cardiac arrest supports the notion that a decrease in metabolic demand may help to restore bioenergetic homeostasis when oxygen (and substrate) delivery—and thus ATP production—is limited. Although this may manifest clinically as organ dysfunction, protected bioenergetic homeostasis may help to prevent cell death and offer the prospect of organ recovery once oxygen (and substrate) supply is restored.[2]

Clinical Assessment of Oxygen Utilization

Biochemical pathways and cellular energetics may seem far removed from the daily care of patients in the pediatric intensive care unit, where discussions about the respiratory and circulatory systems seem to dominate. However, at its core, the goal of critical care medicine is to maintain and support the basic physiologic functions of the patient until his or her own homeostasis returns. This means that the underlying goal of cardiopulmonary and other organ support is to optimize cellular function, and that function requires energy derived from the metabolism of oxygen.

Inherent in this goal is the need to assess the adequacy of oxygen delivery and utilization at the bedside. Traditional markers, such as blood pressure, capillary refill, and urine output, are used to evaluate hypoperfusion but are not sensitive or specific indicators of tissue metabolic stress or impaired oxygen utilization. Several monitoring techniques are available, but all have important physiologic or practice limitations.

Lactate

Lactate is a commonly used surrogate for tissue hypoxia, as it is produced as a byproduct of anaerobic metabolism. In general, lactic acidosis occurs when there is an imbalance between production and clearance of lactate. Measurement of lactate in human blood was first described in 1843 in a lethal case of fulminant septic shock due to puerperal fever in a young woman.[58] Blood lactate monitoring is frequently performed in critically ill patients, usually with the aim of detecting tissue hypoxia leading to anaerobic respiration, traditionally termed *type A lactic acidosis*. In this case, increased lactate production is presumed to reflect impaired oxidative phosphorylation in the absence of sufficient oxygen available to the mitochondria such that glycolysis-derived pyruvate is shuttled through LDH to lactate to regenerate the NAD^+ needed to continue anaerobic ATP production.[59] However, other processes not related to tissue hypoxia can also result in increased blood lactate levels, such as with excess adrenergic stimulation that increases aerobic glycolysis and pyruvate production beyond the rate of mitochondrial metabolism (termed *type B lactic acidosis* and common in severe asthma or therapy with epinephrine), impaired PDH activity, or delayed lactate clearance seen in patients with hepatic dysfunction.[60-62] Although lactic acidosis is often associated with a high anion gap and is generally defined as a lactate level greater than 5 mmol/L and a serum pH less than 7.35, the presence of hypoalbuminemia may mask the anion gap and concomitant alkalosis may raise the pH. As originally reported by Huckabee, normal arterial blood lactate is approximately 0.620 mmol/L and venous lactate is slightly higher at 0.997 mmol/L.[63]

During anaerobic conditions, pyruvate derived from the conversion of glucose cannot enter the Krebs cycle via acetyl-CoA to produce energy. Instead, pyruvate is converted into lactate, known as the *Pasteur effect*. The normal lactate/pyruvate ratio is approximately 20:1, and it rises under hypoxic conditions as lactate production increases. The causal relationship between anaerobic hyperlactatemia and tissue hypoxemia has been confirmed by experimental and clinical studies demonstrating that limiting oxygen consumption (VO_2) by decreasing oxygen delivery (DO_2) below a threshold coincides with a sharp increase in lactate levels.[59,64] Accordingly, in the early phase of septic shock, hyperlactatemia is accompanied by oxygen supply dependency,[65] and several studies have found that initial lactate correlates with increased mortality.[66,67] Moreover, lactate clearance of 10% or more during the early hours of sepsis resuscitation predicts survival,[67,68] and an elevated blood lactate concentration may be sufficient evidence that tissue perfusion is inadequate, even if hypotension is not present (so called *cryptic shock*).[69] On the other hand, in a study of 123 adult patients with vasopressor-dependent septic shock, 45% were found to be "nonlactate expressers" (defined as a lactate <2.4 mmol/L), but mortality remained high at 20% in these patients.[70] In pediatrics, hyperlactatemia appears to be less common overall than in adults with septic shock.[71] Thus, though hyperlactatemia has been associated with increased risk of organ dysfunction, need for resuscitative therapies, and has been independently associated with in-hospital mortality,[72,73] the absence of an elevated lactate should not slow ongoing aggressive resuscitative efforts in children with other indices of altered perfusion.

Despite wide availability and an association with both global tissue hypoxia and poor outcome, no data are currently available to support monitoring lactate levels beyond the immediate resuscitative period, especially once DO_2 has been restored. The numerous etiologies of increased lactate and the lack of sensitivity and specificity for regional tissue perfusion and respiration remain important limitations in using lactate to monitor cellular bioenergetics. A common clinical scenario occurs during volume resuscitation of patients (iatrogenic hyperchloremia) or epinephrine infusions, in which a chloride load and type B lactic acidosis are interpreted as ongoing shock, thus prompting additional fluid and more vasoactive-inotropic support. This scenario may initiate a vicious cycle with the potential for overresuscitation.[74] The treatment of the patient with lactic acidosis should therefore be aimed at the underlying disease, with resuscitation guided by the overall clinical improvement of the patient and not just the lactate concentration itself. Accordingly, the routine daily measurement of serum lactate levels in critically ill patients remains controversial.

Venous Oxygen Saturation

DO_2 is defined as the product of the arterial oxygen content of the blood and the cardiac output (1):

$$DO_2 = CO \times CaO_2$$
$$\text{where } CaO_2 = (1.34 \times Hb \times SaO_2) + (0.003 \times PaO_2)$$

and CO is cardiac output, CaO_2 is arterial oxygen content, Hb is the hemoglobin concentration, SaO_2 is the arterial oxyhemoglobin saturation, and PaO_2 is the arterial oxygen tension. Given that the amount of dissolved O_2 is so small, it is often dropped from the calculation for simplicity. Derivation of cardiac output is described elsewhere in this text (see Chapter 85). VO_2 is defined as the amount of oxygen extracted by the body from the blood and, according to the Fick principle, is calculated by the difference between the CaO_2 and the CvO_2 (the oxygen contents of arterial and mixed venous blood) multiplied by the cardiac output (2):

$$VO_2 = CO \times (CaO_2 - CvO_2)$$
$$\text{where } CvO_2 = (1.34 \times Hb \times SvO_2) + (0.003 \times PvO_2)$$

In the normal, healthy state DO_2 is in significant excess of VO_2. That is, the blood is carrying an excess of oxygen compared with the amount of oxygen the body needs. The ratio of consumption to delivery is called the oxygen extraction ratio (ERO_2) and is calculated as follows (3):

$$ERO_2 = (CaO_2 - CvO_2)/CaO_2$$

Given that typical SvO_2 is approximately 65% to 75%, the ERO_2 is typically 0.25 to 0.35. This means that delivery normally exceeds consumption by a factor of 2 to 3. Thus, a buffer exists where decreases in cardiac output are well tolerated across a certain range such that an increase in ERO_2 ensures that VO_2 remains unaffected by changes in DO_2. There is a point, however, at which the oxygen extraction capabilities of the tissues are exceeded. At that point, VO_2 becomes dependent on DO_2. This biphasic relationship of DO_2 and VO_2 is shown in Fig. 80.7.

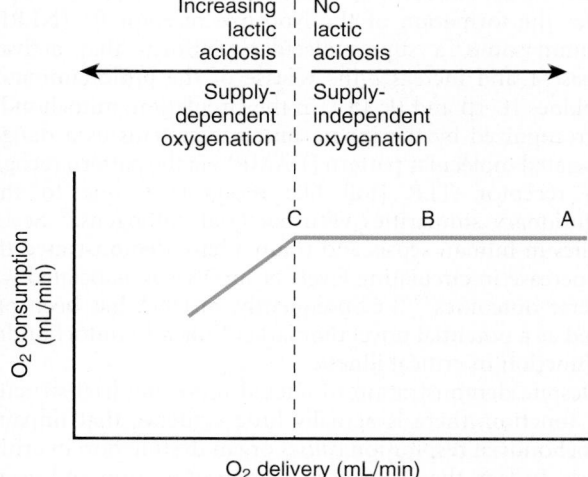

Fig. 80.7. Biphasic relationship between oxygen delivery and oxygen consumption.

Bedside evaluation of DO_2 and VO_2 would be of great value to the clinician. Unfortunately, most of the methods of calculating VO_2 rely on cardiac output (via the Fick principle), which results in a situation where a single measured variable is included in two parts of a regression analysis, so-called mathematical coupling. This dependency leads to amplification of any error in that measurement and may result in an apparent relationship between variables that does not truly exist. Other methods to measure VO_2 in intubated critically ill patients require use of a metabolic cart,[75] but routine use is currently lacking. As in many areas of critical care medicine, when something cannot be measured directly, a surrogate measure must be used.

In practice, the central venous or mixed venous oxygen saturation ($ScvO_2$ or $SmvO_2$) can be used as a continuous or intermittent measure to assess the global balance of oxygen delivery and consumption in a patient with septic shock.[76] As central venous catheters have largely replaced the use of pulmonary arterial catheters, particularly in pediatrics, $ScvO_2$ is now more commonly measured than $SmvO_2$.[77] $ScvO_2$ is ideally measured from a catheter with its tip at the superior vena cava–right atrial junction. Measurements taken from a femoral catheter with its tip in the inferior vena cava are thought to be less reliable due to greater variability in splanchnic oxygen utilization.[78] An $ScvO_2$ <70% indicates that tissue oxygen extraction is increased from normal, suggesting inadequate oxygen delivery due to either low cardiac output, decreased arterial oxygen content, or both.[76] Such a finding should prompt one to consider therapies to improve oxygen delivery either through additional fluid administration, vasoactive therapy, or an increase in arterial blood oxygen content.[79] However, $ScvO_2$ may also be low if oxygen utilization is increased, as in states of high metabolic demand (eg, fever in sepsis, seizure, or hyperthyroidism). Alternatively, elevated $ScvO_2$ >80% suggests that oxygen utilization may be impaired due to mitochondrial dysfunction, reflecting a global state of cytopathic hypoxia.[5]

In a trial of early goal-directed therapy in adult septic shock by Rivers and colleagues,[79] an $ScvO_2$ >70% was targeted as a primary hemodynamic end point. Although three more recent trials failed to demonstrate benefit from routine $ScvO_2$ monitoring,[80-82] an $ScvO_2$ >70% remains the recommended target in current pediatric shock guidelines.[41] A pediatric trial in children with fluid refractory shock found that targeting an $ScvO_2$ >70% for 72 hours compared to standard therapy reduced mortality from 39.2% to 11.8% ($p = 0.002$).[71] Furthermore, in a pediatric prospective cohort trial evaluating the effect of intermittent $ScvO_2$ monitoring on 120 children with fluid refractory septic shock, children who had intermittent $ScvO_2$ monitoring performed at 1, 3, and 6 hours had significantly lower in-hospital mortality (33% versus 55%, $p = 0.02$) and a reduction in the number dysfunctional organs (two versus three, $p <0.001$).[83]

An important limitation of $ScvO_2$ is the need for central venous access, making this laboratory value difficult to obtain in many children who may not otherwise require such an invasive procedure. In addition, continuous $ScvO_2$ measurements require a specialized catheter that may not be available in all centers. A prospective cohort study of adult patients diagnosed with severe sepsis at three different hospitals found that mean arterial pressure and central venous pressure were still the most important hemodynamic variables in initial hemodynamic resuscitation and that low postresuscitation SvO_2 was not associated with a worse outcome.[84] Other studies have failed to show an advantage of using $ScvO_2$ over other markers, including lactate, in predicting in-hospital mortality.[67,85] Three large randomized trials also recently failed to show that routine $ScvO_2$ monitoring improved outcomes during resuscitation of adults with septic shock.[80-82] Consequently, although both low (<70%) and high (>80%) $ScvO_2$ may provide general insight into the global state of DO_2-VO_2 mismatch, this measure, much like lactate, cannot detect tissue-specific changes in bioenergetic homeostasis.

Microdialysis

Microdialysis allows for the measurement of energy-related metabolites within the interstitial space of a regional tissue bed. This is most commonly performed using a thin, flexible catheter with a semipermeable membrane inserted into skeletal muscle. A solution of a known solute concentration is slowly pumped into the catheter, and soluble small molecules, such as glucose, lactate, pyruvate, and glycerol, equilibrate across the membrane. The fluid is then collected and analyzed as a regional measurement of cellular metabolic activity. Although it provides a more tissue-specific measure, the degree to which respiration in skeletal muscle reflects other vital organs is not clear.[86] Because blood and oxygen delivery are diverted away from skeletal muscle to critical organs (brain, heart, and kidneys) in shock, changes in muscle cellular respiration have be a sensitive indicator of inadequate systemic perfusion. Indeed, animal and human studies in sepsis and hemorrhage have demonstrated an association between microdialysis lactate/pyruvate ratios and outcome.[87,88] Further studies are needed to validate the utility of microdialysis as a clinically useful measure of cellular respiration.

Near-Infrared Spectroscopy

Near-infrared spectroscopy (NIRS) enables continuous, noninvasive bedside monitoring of regional tissue oxygenation and mitochondrial complex IV redox state. As with pulse oximetry, NIRS is based on the principle that the oxygen-carrying pigments hemoglobin and myoglobin and cytochrome $a,a3$ have well-defined absorption spectra that are influenced by oxygen binding. NIRS technology thus uses a modification of the Beer-Lambert law, which describes the relationship between absorption of light and the concentration of deoxygenated hemoglobin [Hb], oxygenated hemoglobin [HbO$_2$], and intracellular chromophores (cytochrome a,a_3).

Clinical utilization of NIRS to date has generally focused on monitoring tissue-specific oxy- and deoxyhemoglobin concentrations, most commonly in brain, kidney, and skeletal muscle.[89-91] Available NIRS monitors are mathematically weighted toward venous blood, thus largely reflecting deoxygenated Hb levels, and display a number (referred to as *regional SO$_2$* or *rSO$_2$*) that varies with local oxygen delivery and extraction. A decrease in NIRS rSO$_2$ has been correlated with a fall in local tissue perfusion in animal models of shock, decreased cardiac output in infants following cardiac surgery, and predicted fluid responsiveness in dehydrated children.[89-91] However, large variations in "normal" rSO$_2$ levels, the lack of defined "critical threshold" for rSO$_2$, and the inability of rSO$_2$ to differentiate between changes in DO_2 or VO_2 have limited the universal acceptance of NIRS monitoring.

In addition to hemoglobin, NIRS can assess the cytochrome a,a_3 redox state of complex IV in the mitochondrial ETS.[92] Cytochrome a,a_3 is the terminal component along the ETS that reduces oxygen to water, and it remains in a reduced state during hypoxemia. The absorption spectrum of cytochrome a,a_3 in its reduced state shows a weak peak at 700 nm, whereas the oxygenated form does not. Therefore monitoring changes in the cytochrome a,a_3 redox state can provide a measure of the adequacy of oxidative metabolism.[93] To date, however, NIRS assessment of mitochondrial redox state, while promising, remains technologically challenging and has therefore been limited to research settings.

Optical Spectroscopy

Similar to NIRS, optical spectroscopy uses absorption of light by tissues to assess concentration of various analytes of interest. By using an entire spectral region in the visible or near-infrared spectral region that includes many (up to hundreds) of wavelengths of light, it is possible to improve distinction between similar molecules. In particular, advances in optical spectroscopy have made it possible to measure the oxygenation state of myoglobin independently from that of hemoglobin despite similar absorbance spectra.[94] Myoglobin is an intracellular protein found in skeletal and cardiac muscle cells and is involved in the transport of oxygen from the cytoplasm to the mitochondria. Quantification of myoglobin saturation (percentage of total myoglobin bound with oxygen) provides a direct measure of *intracellular* oxygen availability.

Measurements of myoglobin saturation in the presence of hemoglobin, hemoglobin saturation in the presence of myoglobin, and cytochrome oxidation states have been recorded from optical reflectance spectra acquired from muscle.[95] These measurements remove the ambiguity present in conventional near-infrared spectroscopic methods in which hemoglobin and myoglobin absorbances are combined. In a guinea pig endotoxin model, ex vivo perfused hearts were noted to have higher levels of intracellular oxygenation and lower rates of oxygen consumption compared to controls supporting the concept of impaired oxygen utilization.[96] Optical spectroscopy thus has the potential to separately identify the oxygenation state in anatomically and physiologically distinct tissue regions, including the vascular (hemoglobin), cellular (myoglobin), and mitochondrial (cytochromes) levels.

Tissue Oxygen Tension

Tissue oxygen tension (tPO_2) measures the partial pressure of oxygen within the interstitial space. Traditional probes use Clark electrodes, but newer techniques are now available that can more accurately measure tPO_2 without themselves consuming oxygen. A decrease in DO_2 would be expected to lower tPO_2 whereas a decrease in VO_2 would raise tPO_2 (so long as DO_2 levels were not concurrently diminished).[86] In sepsis models, several studies have demonstrated that skeletal muscle and mucosal tPO_2 are unchanged or increased, suggesting a fall in VO_2 either concurrent with or greater than the decrease in DO_2.[97,98] In human studies, brain tPO_2 monitoring has been demonstrated to improve outcomes following traumatic brain injury.[99] More studies are needed to determine the benefits of tPO_2 monitoring in pediatric critical illness.

NADH Fluorometry

Reduced NADH has the useful property of fluorescing in response to 340-nm excitation light, whereas the oxidized form, NAD+, does not. Changes in the emitted light are therefore proportional to the turnover NADH, which is predominately related to mitochondrial function. When oxygen utilization slows, NADH will accumulate and fluorescence will rise, though this may also occur under hypoxemic conditions. As with NIRS, however, only changes relative to an arbitrary baseline measurement can be obtained, as absolute values are not possible.[86]

Magnetic Resonance Spectroscopy

Magnetic resonance spectroscopy (MRS) uses radiolabeled molecules to noninvasively measure in vivo tissue metabolite concentrations. MRS has been used clinically for more than two decades in neurologic disorders to measure blood vessel distribution and architecture, blood flow velocity, regional perfusion and blood volume, blood and tissue oxygenation, lactate production and intracellular pH, Krebs cycle activity, and mitochondrial oxidative phosphorylation in the brain. For bioenergetic studies, phosphorus-31 MRS is primarily used to detect changes in phosphocreatine, ATP and inorganic phosphate, and certain compounds related to membrane synthesis and degradation.[100] Because phosphocreatine is the primary ATP buffer in muscle, depletion in this molecule leads to a drop in ATP levels.[100] Proton MRS can also be used to measure four markers related to oxygen metabolism: the peak of N-acetyl-aspartate (NAA), an amino acid present in neurons that reflects the status of neuronal tissue; creatine, found in glia and neurons, which serves as a point of reference because its level is believed to be stable; choline, a constitutive component of cell membranes that reflects glial proliferation or membrane breakdown; and lactate, a marker of anaerobic metabolism and therefore of ischemia. Elevated lactate and decreased NAA are associated with worse neurologic outcome in neonates with asphyxial injury.[101,102] Although MRS is useful for diagnosis and prognosis, it is not currently practical as a method to guide minute-to-minute patient management.

Blood Mitochondrial DNA

Under conditions of hypoxemia, ischemia, inflammation, and oxidative stress, mitochondrial damage can lead to fragmentation of mtDNA and release into the circulation. It has therefore been proposed that blood levels (both cellular and free plasma concentrations) of mtDNA may be a biomarker of mitochondrial dysfunction and overall severity of illness.[55,103] Increased levels of blood mtDNA have been reported in adult patients with sepsis and trauma,[56,104] though methodological variability may underlie important differences between studies.[103] Circulating mtDNA may also serve as DAMP, propagating inflammation and contributing to distant organ injury as noted previously.[57]

Mitochondrial- and Bioenergetic-Targeted Therapy in Critical Illness

With increasing recognition of the central role of altered cellular respiration—and mitochondrial dysfunction in particular—in the pathogenesis of organ failure in critical illness, there has been concurrent emerging interest in the potential for metabolic- and mitochondrial-targeted therapeutic strategies to improve patient outcomes. A therapeutic strategy that partners an up-regulation or down-regulation of oxygen utilization to better match oxygen delivery may restore bioenergetic homeostasis and improve cellular—and thus organ—function. Several existing and novel agents have demonstrated potential to optimize cellular respiration and improve mitochondrial function, though questions of clinical utility remain largely unanswered at this time.

Antioxidants

As discussed earlier, ROS and RNS play essential roles in cell signaling and, as such, their activity is normally tightly regulated by a network of intracellular antioxidants. In sepsis, cardiac arrest, and other severe illnesses, the production of ROS and RNS increases sharply (largely due to alterations of the mitochondrial ETS), leading to a wide array of local cellular damage and systemic inflammation. The natural cellular antioxidant defense system includes manganese dismutase (MnSOD), glutathione (GSH), thioredoxin (TSH), catalase, peroxidase, peroxiredoxins, sulfiredoxins, cytochrome c, and peroxidase. With a large increase in ROS and RNS, these molecules may be rapidly depleted, leading to an overall imbalance of oxidative and nitrosative stress.

A wide variety of exogenous antioxidant supplements have been studied in animal models and humans with critical illness, including vitamin A, vitamin E, vitamin C, coenzyme A, selenium, melatonin, and N-acetylcysteine, among others. Although antioxidant supplementation can successfully reduce oxidative stress, thus far clinical trials have failed to convincingly demonstrate an outcome benefit.[105] A strategy that better targets antioxidants to the mitochondria, however, has shown some promise in preclinical studies and may be better suited for use in critically ill patients.[106,107] One example involves antioxidant molecules that are covalently joined with a lipophilic cation concentrate within the mitochondria. Such molecules, including MitoQ and MitoVitE, have been shown in vitro to protect mitochondria and whole cells from oxidative stress and have demonstrated utility to reduce organ dysfunction in animal models.[106] Similarly, a series of small synthetic positively charged peptides less than 10 amino acids in length, termed *Szeto-Schiller (SS) peptides,* can freely penetrate cell and mitochondrial membranes and have been shown to be effective in some ischemia-reperfusion oxidative stress models.[108] Several early-phase human trials of mitochondrial-targeted antioxidants and SS peptides are ongoing.

Nitric Oxide Synthase Inhibitors

Sepsis and other inflammatory illnesses have long been associated with a marked increase in inducible NOS-production (iNOS) of nitric oxide. In addition to its role in decreasing vascular resistance in distributive shock, NO directly inhibits ETS complex IV activity and indirectly disrupts several cellular respiration pathways through up-regulation of ROS/RNS, chiefly peroxynitrite. Despite the failure of a nonselective NOS inhibitor to improve outcomes in a randomized trial in adult sepsis,[109] selective iNOS inhibitors such as NG-nitro-L-arginine methyl ester (L-NAME), have demonstrated beneficial effects on mitochondrial respiration, hemodynamic function, and organ function in animal models.[110,111]

Glycemic Control

Hyperglycemia and insulin resistance are common findings in critically ill patients. The inability of cells to utilize glucose to generate pyruvate can lead to downstream limitations of oxidative phosphorylation and results in mobilization of fat and protein stores. Since the 1990s, there has been substantial interest in the use of exogenous insulin to restore normoglycemia in adult and pediatric critical illness. Despite widespread enthusiasm following an adult trial of insulin to achieve tight glycemic control (80–110 mg/dL) that reduced ICU mortality from 8% to 4.6%,[112] subsequent studies have failed to replicate the overall benefit, including two randomized pediatric trials.[113,114] Interestingly, insulin has been shown to stimulate mitochondrial ATP production in human skeletal muscle ex vivo,[115] and maintenance of normoglycemia with insulin preserves hepatic mitochondrial structure and function in adult critical illness.[116] Thus the potential for targeted insulin therapy and glycemic control to improve cellular bioenergetic homeostasis remains unclear.

Substrate Provision

Several studies suggest that despite decreased activity complex I of the mitochondrial ETS, complex II is relatively preserved in sepsis. Complex II transfers electrons from $FADH_2$ produced from the oxidation of succinate to coenzyme Q. Consequently, supplementation of succinate may help to restore overall ETS activity and ATP production, as has been suggested in animal models of sepsis.[117] However, different insults may be prone to distinct pathophysiology and thus variable therapies. For example, in a porcine model of pediatric traumatic brain injury, mitochondrial ETS complex II exhibited the most profound decrease in activity.[118] Alternative fuels for cellular respiration, including carnitine supplementation, have shown promising results in animal models,[119] but direct evidence for benefit in humans has not yet been demonstrated. Similarly, supplementation with coenzyme Q, cytochrome c, and caffeine improves mitochondrial function in vitro and in animal models.[43,46,120,121]

Mitochondrial Biogenesis and Mitophagy

All cells that undergo oxidative phosphorylation have robust quality control mechanisms to ensure a full complement of healthy mitochondria. Cells optimize the overall mitochondrial number, distribution, and function through a network of interrelated processes of biogenesis, fission, fusion, and mitophagy.[57] Mitochondrial biogenesis is the process of synthesizing new functional mitochondria and can be induced by oxidative stress and inflammation.[9] Depending on the stimulus, mitochondrial biogenesis is executed through several signaling pathways that converge on a common set of coactivators and transcription factors, including peroxisome proliferator-activated receptor gamma-1 coactivator alpha (PGC-1α), nuclear respiratory factors (NRF-1 and NRF-2), nuclear factor erythroid 2-related factor 2 (Nrf2), and mitochondrial transcription factor A (TFAM).[9] These proteins either increase transcription of nuclear-encoded mitochondrial proteins or are imported into the mitochondria to directly up-regulate expression of mtDNA to promote ETS complex assembly.

Data from both animal studies and septic patients have shown that mitochondrial biogenesis is associated with recovery of organ function and survival. Haden and colleagues showed that mitochondrial biogenesis is evident over 1 to 3 days following a nonlethal exposure to *Staphylococcus aureus* in a rodent model, with a subsequent recovery of oxidative phosphorylation.[122] The same group further showed that sepsis survival could be improved in rodents treated with daily exposure to a low dose of carbon monoxide.[123] Similarly, removal of dysfunctional mitochondria—termed *mitophagy*—has also been shown to be protective in sepsis. For example, in both liver and kidney of hyperglycemic critically ill rabbits, biochemical markers indicating insufficient mitophagy were more pronounced in nonsurviving animals.[124] Interestingly, after 3 and 7 days of illness, mitophagy was better preserved in animals treated with insulin to preserve normoglycemia, which correlated with improved mitochondrial function and less organ damage.[124] Pharmacologic agents that induce mitochondrial biogenesis, such as pioglitazone,[125] resveratrol,[126] and recombinant human TFAM (rhTFAM),[127] and that simulate mitophagy, such as rapamycin,[124] are currently being explored as potential therapeutic strategies to recover mitochondrial function and restore bioenergetic homeostasis in critical illness.

Membrane Stabilizers

Ultrastructural evidence of mitochondrial injury in critical illness includes damage to the inner mitochondrial membrane and organelle swelling. These features are associated with loss of the electrochemical gradient that drives ATP production through oxidative phosphorylation. Although the mechanisms underlying these physiologic changes remain incompletely understood, opening of the MPTP is believed to be involved. A number of compounds that inhibit pore opening, including cyclosporine A and melatonin, are being investigated as another approach to restore mitochondrial function through membrane stabilization.[120] For example, in a piglet model of nonimpact rotational brain injury, administration of cyclosporine A at a clinically relevant time point ameliorated mitochondrial dysfunction and promoted a 42% decrease in injured brain volume.[118]

Hibernation

Another potential strategy to restore bioenergetic homeostasis that could be pursued in the presence of impaired cellular respiration is to suppress metabolic energy expenditure. In many hibernating mammals, a purposive metabolic down-regulation is a crucial response that facilitates tolerance to a lack of energetic substrates during harsh environmental conditions and promotes survival.[128,129] The hibernating state prevents a cellular bioenergetic crisis by reducing demand for

ATP when substrate or oxygen supply is low and decreases mitochondrial oxidative stress. Although humans do not hibernate and have only a limited tolerance to diminished oxygen or substrate delivery to vital organs, the impairment in cytochrome oxidase activity observed during sepsis mimics that of true hibernation, suggesting that, at least early on, such impairment may be an adaptive response to an inflammatory insult.[48] Following myocardial ischemia, as in adult coronary artery disease, a transient decrease in myocardial contractility—termed *myocardial hibernation*—has been well described, with subsequent functional recovery if adequate perfusion is promptly restored.

Attempts to reduce metabolic demand through induced moderate hypothermia after neonatal hypoxic-ischemic injury, cardiac arrest, traumatic brain injury, and hyperammonemic metabolic crises have demonstrated variable success. Challenges to induced hypothermia include unclear optimal timing, depth, and duration of this therapy. Other strategies to reduce metabolic demand include use of low-dose carbon monoxide and hydrogen disulfide, though the extreme toxicity of these agents limits the therapeutic window for such agents.

Conclusions

Although the restoration of tissue perfusion and oxygen/substrate delivery remains a primary goal in critical illness, alterations in cellular respiration contribute to a bioenergetic imbalance that results in cell—and ultimately—organ dysfunction. As discussed, impaired oxygen delivery can decrease the ability of cells to produce ATP. However, metabolic alterations that affect overall bioenergetic homeostasis may develop, and even persist, irrespective of the state of oxygen delivery. Indeed, it may well be the case that *utilization* of oxygen—or some other metabolic substrate—is of even greater importance to cell survival, organ function, and patient outcomes than normalization of oxygen delivery. Although shock is classically defined as an imbalance between oxygen (and substrate) delivery and demand, ultimately it is the state of cellular respiration rather than circulatory dysfunction that determines outcome from critical illness.

Key References

5. Fink MP. Bench-to-bedside review: cytopathic hypoxia. *Crit Care*. 2002;6:491-499.
34. Singer M. The role of mitochondrial dysfunction in sepsis-induced multi-organ failure. *Virulence*. 2014;5:66-72.
40. Brealey D, Brand M, Hargreaves I, et al. Association between mitochondrial dysfunction and severity and outcome of septic shock. *Lancet*. 2002;360:219-223.
48. Levy RJ. Mitochondrial dysfunction, bioenergetic impairment, and metabolic down-regulation in sepsis. *Shock*. 2007;28:24-28.
85. Jones AE, Shapiro NI, Trzeciak S, et al. Lactate clearance vs central venous oxygen saturation as goals of early sepsis therapy: a randomized clinical trial. *JAMA*. 2010;303:739-746.
106. Galley HF. Bench-to-bedside review: targeting antioxidants to mitochondria in sepsis. *Crit Care*. 2010;14:230.

Biology of the Stress Response

Stephen Standage and Jerry J. Zimmerman

PEARLS

- The stress response is a universal, stereotypical, and integrated neurogenic, endocrine, inflammatory, and metabolic systems response with multiple feed forward and feed backward modulation signaling designed to maximize host survival.
- The brain is the paramount organ of the stress response, as it determines what constitutes a stress and what is the appropriate reaction and extent of reaction. Multiple afferent stress signals are integrated at the level of the hypothalamus where the stress response is initiated.
- Excessive or prolonged stress stimuli can precipitate a dysregulated stress response.
- A complicated critical illness course may reflect elements of an ongoing stress response manifested as protein catabolism with poor wound healing, diffuse weakness, and immunosuppression associated with hospital-acquired infections.
- Therapeutic intervention must respect the physiologic alterations necessary to accommodate the stress response. Pursuing "normal" values as physiologic target parameters may ultimately be counterproductive.

Introduction

Human beings demonstrate tremendous adaptability, which has allowed them to inhabit and flourish in all sorts of climates and environments. The resilience of human physiology has permitted the achievement of tremendous feats of endurance and survival under the most inhospitable circumstances. The biological systems that facilitate our detection and response to stresses in our internal and external environments have been crucial to our success as a species. These same systems are at play in the intensive care unit when children confront life-threatening conditions and affect how they respond to both injury and treatment. This chapter discusses the nature and function of the various physiologic systems that constitute the stress response as it applies to critical illness.

Definitions and Historical Perspectives

Stress may be defined as any force or influence on an organism that perturbs its usual state of equilibrium. Strain is the magnitude of deviation from baseline norms that the organism

experiences in response to the inciting stressor. Resiliency is the organism's ability to adapt to or cope with the stresses and strains imposed on it. The process of host adaptation to an environmental, biological, or psychosocial insult is referred to as the stress response.

All life requires a relatively high degree of stability to maintain vital functions. Enzymes perform optimally at specific temperatures and hydrogen ion concentrations. Action potentials are promulgated along cell membranes based on a narrow range of ion concentrations. There are two competing principles relating to stability: homeostasis and allostasis. Homeostasis is the process of achieving stability through maintaining systemic variables within a fairly narrow dynamic range. Allostasis is the process of achieving stability through physiologic or behavioral changes.[1] Whereas normal physiology imposes homeostatic forces on vital functions to maintain constancy within an optimal range, the stress response facilitates a change in physiology to adapt to 85 stressors that would otherwise be fatal. This allostatic response, however, is designed to be temporary so that once the stressor has resolved, the organism can return to its baseline physiologic function. Prolonged exposure to stress or an abnormal stress response induces chronic allostasis, which is pathologic.

To illustrate this concept, the reader may consider a skyscraper built in an earthquake-prone area. Rising high above the earth and bearing thousands of tons of steel, concrete, and glass, the structure normally moves very little. However, in the event of an earthquake the building is engineered to tolerate a significant amount of swaying and rocking to avoid breaking and tumbling to the ground. The attributes of its structural elements that allow it to bend without breaking constitute the resilience of the building, which allow it to accommodate the strain imposed by the stress of the earthquake. Likewise, the stress response in humans provides resilience to adapt to various internal and external stressors without catastrophic physiologic decompensation. Strain is evident in the physiologic changes undertaken in response to stress, which fosters survival.[2]

As a concept, stress was first considered a perturbation of normal intracellular physiology by Claude Bernard in 1892 as part of his classic discussion of constancy of the "environment within" (milieu inte'rieur). At that time he noted that stressors to the cell result in an immediate compensation and equilibrium response and that this property of responding to change was essential for free and independent life. Later in 1932 Walter Cannon actually defined the concept of homeostasis; the stress response was noted to typically occur when homeostasis was disrupted.[3] Clinically the stress response was described as actions facilitating freeze, fright, flight, and fight.

With the benefit of ongoing research in physiology and biochemistry, the stress response was ultimately recognized to be a rather universal, stereotypical, and integrated set of biological activities that respond to both internal and external stimuli.[2] Stressors that were recognized to activate this response included physiologic, biochemical, emotional, and physical stimuli. In 1936, Selye described chronologic development of the stress response in terms of alarm, resistance, and exhaustion, the latter associated with morbidity and death as opposed to enhanced survival.[4] This dynamic view of the stress response was termed the *general adaption syndrome* and was continued to be viewed as an attempt to reestablish homeostasis and protect the organism during acute stress. Recognized essential clinical aspects of the stress response included adaptive functions such as arousal, vigilance and focused attention, general inhibition of vegetative functions, and increased delivery of both oxygen and nutrients to the brain, heart, and skeletal muscles to facilitate increased metabolic activity. Later, stress response activity was described schematically in terms of a U-shaped graphic, where both insufficient as well as excessive or maladaptive responses might be pathologic.[5]

Subsequently, a perhaps more sophisticated view of the stress response was formulated by McEwen and colleagues employing the concept of allostasis described earlier.[6] In allostasis, the body responds to a particular challenge or stress by adjusting to a new steady state (strain), but it terminates this activity once the stress has stopped. Again, such change may be appropriate and adaptive or, alternatively, maladaptive, particularly if the stress and its associated strain are extreme or prolonged.[1]

A mathematical model of the stress response is depicted as follows[2]:

$$F_n = \int_{t_i}^{t_f} (\rho t_n) \times L(t_n) \times dt$$

Here stress is depicted as a force (F) generated by a stressor that is equal to the host's resilience (ρ) over time multiplied by the response (L) of the body, which can alternatively be described as strain. Fn, a force generated by a stressor; ρ, resiliency during evolution of the stress response; L, response of the body; t_n, particular point in time; t_i, time initial; t_f, time final. In real life, strain might be represented by a multiple organ dysfunction score such as PELOD.[7] An individual's resilience is affected by genetic predispositions, comorbid conditions, and environmental influences. A simplified depiction of this integral is the equation that equates the stress force F to the body's resiliency (ρ) times the change in strain, or $F = \rho \times \Delta L$.[2]

Stress System Primary Elements

The stress response is mediated by the stress system that reestablishes homeostasis or alternatively maintains stability through change, allostasis. The stress system has an afferent, sensory limb allowing it to detect stress signals as well as an efferent, effector limb, which brings about physiologic responses to address the stressors. Initiation and regulation of the stress response occur in the brain. In this regard the brain is the paramount organ of the stress response, as it determines what constitutes a stress and what is the appropriate reaction and extent of reaction.[8] The brain integrates multiple afferent signals and appraises the degree of threat presented by

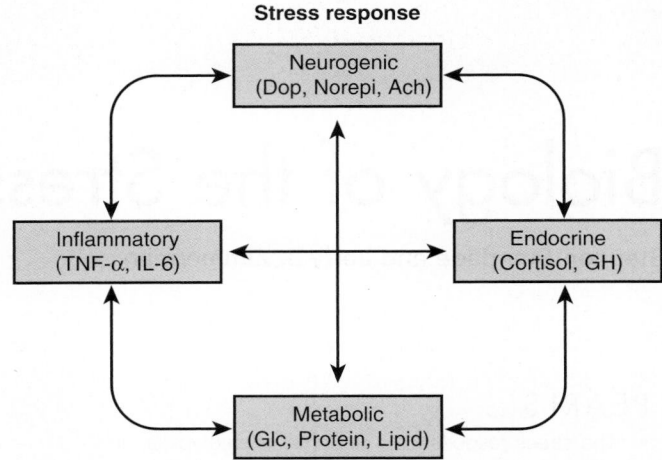

Stress response

Fig. 81.1. Schematic depiction of the major elements of the stress response. *Ach,* acetyl choline; *Dop,* dopamine; *GH,* growth hormone; *Norepi,* norepinephrine; *TNFα,* tumor necrosis factor alpha; *IL-6,* interleukin-6; *Glc,* glucose.

potential stressors. When the brain perceives stimuli as stress, it triggers allostatic mechanisms through its efferent pathways to maintain physiologic stability in the face of the threat.

Fig. 81.1 depicts the stress system as an integrated network of neurogenic, endocrine, inflammatory, and metabolic subsystems that interact through multiple feed forward and feed backward signaling channels. Ultimately, this system is responsible in eliciting four major responses to stress signals including (1) activation of both the sympathetic and parasympathetic nervous systems; (2) enhanced release of the various counter regulatory hormones, particularly cortisol, and vasopressin with activation of the renin-angiotensin-aldosterone axis; (3) synthesis of both pro- and antiinflammatory mediators; and (4) mobilization of metabolic substrate from physiologic depots to provide energy and molecular building blocks for the highly energetic functions of the stress response. All of these activities are essential for an integrated stress response that maximizes host survival. However, if these activities become dysregulated or prolonged (chronic critical illness), the result may involve evolution from the stress response to the distress response.

Stress Response

The effector stress response can be compartmentalized into central, peripheral, and cellular components.[9] The interaction of all these subsystems is coordinated to achieve three primary objectives: (1) maintain perfusion of the heart, brain, and other vital organs; (2) deploy energy resources from body fuel storage depots; (3) optimize adenosine triphosphate (ATP) availability to vital cells and tissues at the expense of nonessential tissues.

Central Activation and Integration

A multitude of signals may activate a stress response.[10,11] Examples of afferent stressors include pain, visual, auditory and olfactory stimuli, and psychologic distress. In critical illness, common stressors include hypoperfusion, hypoxia, tissue injury, and infection. Hypotension is sensed as a decreased stretch of baroreceptors located in the carotid sinus and aortic arch. Peripheral chemoreceptors in the carotid and aortic bodies sense oxygen levels. Tissue injury and infection are detected by the innate immune system that recognizes both pathogen-associated molecular patterns (PAMPs) as well as host damage-associated molecular patterns (DAMPs) that may occur as a result of direct tissue injury from trauma, critical illness in general, or as collateral damage from inflammatory responses.[12,13] Innate immune cells elaborate cytokines that signal stress to the rest of the body. These cytokines, and various other soluble mediators that provide afferent signaling for the stress response, are transported to the brain and across the blood-brain barrier through fenestrated capillaries as well as by active transport mechanisms. In addition, the vagus nerve facilitates bidirectional communication between the brain and the immune system as well as the various organs that it innervates.[14]

The diencephalon, including the arcuate nucleus, paraventricular nucleus, dorsal vagus complex, catecholamine cell group, and the brain stem, all receive afferent signals activated from both internal as well as external stressors. Multiple afferent stress signals are integrated at the level of the hypothalamus where the stress response is initiated.[10,15,16] Intercommunications between brain stem nuclei, hypothalamus, hippocampus, and limbic systems represent important circuits through which the stress response is coordinated.[8,17]

Peripheral Responses

Efferent signaling from the brain involves descending neuroendocrine and autonomic pathways that ultimately control hemodynamic, immune, and metabolic aspects of the stress response. Activation of the stress system triggers release of the corticotropin-releasing hormone (CRH) from the hypothalamus, which in turn induces release of adrenocorticotropic hormone (ACTH) from the anterior pituitary. Other stimulants of ACTH secretion include vasopressin, catecholamines, angiotensin II, serotonin, vasoactive intestinal peptide, and inflammatory cytokines (IL-1[interleukin-1], IL-2, IL-6, TNFα). ACTH in turn stimulates the adrenal cortex to produce cortisol, which is essential to the stress response to critical illness and injury.[18] Cortisol affects the transcription of approximately 25% of the entire genome,[19] and hence it mediates a wide range of hemodynamic, immunologic, and metabolic actions. A detailed discussion of cortisol metabolism in critical illness is provided in Chapter 85. CRH also induces the secretion of proopiomelanocortin and other opioid peptides—the latter (including β-endorphin) mediate analgesia and provide negative feedback to the stress response.[20]

The parvicellular neurons of the hypothalamus secrete thyrotropin-releasing hormone, which acts on the anterior pituitary gland to release thyroid-stimulating hormone (TSH). Early in critical illness, TSH and T_4 levels increase transiently, but this is associated peripherally with a rapid decline in T_3 levels and an increase in rT_3 levels due to alterations to peripheral conversion of T_4.[21–23] The elevated TSH levels quickly return to the normal range, but T_3 levels remain low, resulting in the nonthyroidal illness or sick-euthyroid syndrome, which is also discussed in more detail in Chapter 85.

Two other hormones from the anterior pituitary are released by the stress response: growth hormone and prolactin. Like most other components of the stress response, both of these hormones are under control of the hypothalamus. Growth hormone is released from the anterior pituitary in response to

hypothalamic growth hormone–releasing hormone (GHRH) secretion. Prolactin release, which facilitates the immune response by augmenting lymphocyte activation, is under tonic inhibition from dopaminergic neurons in the hypothalamus. Its secretion is enhanced with decreased dopaminergic signaling from the hypothalamus. Secretion of both of these hormones is stimulated by activation of the stress response.

Vasopressin release is another early response to stress that is crucial to survival in critical illness.[24,25] The magnocellular neurons of the hypothalamic supraoptic and paraventricular nuclei project their axons through the pituitary stalk and onto the capillary bed of the posterior pituitary gland where they release vasopressin directly into the circulation. Additionally, corticotropin-releasing hormone and vasopressin signaling pathways mutually innervate and stimulate each other.[26] Vasopressin release is stimulated dramatically by decreased arterial blood pressure, but it can also be activated by increased serum osmolality. Vasopressin induces peripheral vasoconstriction by signaling through the V_1 receptor and thus helps to maintain blood pressure. Activation of V_2 receptors by vasopressin in the renal collecting ducts results in the insertion of aquaporin channels into the luminal membrane of the renal tubular epithelial cells. This mechanism facilitates the reabsorption of free water into the vasculature to maintain or restore circulating blood volume, which is particularly important in shock states.

Receiving inputs from the hypothalamus and the limbic system, the autonomic nervous system is also activated in the stress response. The locus ceruleus, located in the posterior area of the rostral pons, is an important center of sympathetic outflow. Within the central nervous system, sympathetic activation results in increased arousal, concentration, and alertness. Additionally, noradrenergic signals originating in the locus ceruleus descend through autonomic efferent pathways to stimulate a peripheral sympathetic response.[10] Simultaneously, a parasympathetic response is initiated to balance the magnitude of the initial proinflammatory stress response. This balancing aspect of the stress response has been termed the *inflammatory reflex*.[27] Increased vagal efferent signaling suppresses peripheral cytokine release through macrophage nicotinic receptors and the cholinergic antiinflammatory pathway.[28]

The peripheral effects of the stress response are seen most quickly with activation of the sympathetic arm of the autonomic nervous system. The heart, blood vessels, bronchioles, and most endocrine cells are richly innervated with adrenergic nerve fibers. Norepinephrine release from sympathetic axon terminals in the adrenal medulla stimulates secretion of epinephrine into the blood. The combination of circulating epinephrine and release of norepinephrine from adrenergic neurons increases heart rate and blood pressure augmenting cardiac output and maintaining perfusion to vital organs.

An important peripheral system that works in concert with the adrenergic and vasopressin responses is the renin-angiotensin-aldosterone system. The primary purpose of this system is to help regulate sodium and water balance in the body. Renin is produced and stored in the juxtaglomerular granular cells of the afferent renal arterioles. Renin release is mediated by three primary control mechanisms: (1) decreased afferent renal arteriole blood pressure, (2) sympathetic stimulation from noradrenergic autonomic input, and (3) signaling from macula densa cells that sense decreased flow rate and sodium composition of the fluid flowing through the nephron. Renin is an enzyme that cleaves angiotensinogen, a protein produced in the liver, to generate the 10 amino acid polypeptide angiotensin I. Angiotensin I is further cleaved to an 8 amino acid polypeptide, angiotensin II, by the angiotensin-converting enzyme localized predominantly in the pulmonary vascular endothelium. Angiotensin II has several important effects. It is a potent vasoconstrictor and thereby increases blood pressure. Its vasoconstrictor effects also reduce renal blood flow and the glomerular filtration rate, which serves to prevent urinary fluid losses. Angiotensin II directly stimulates proximal tubular sodium reabsorption in the nephron. One of its most important effects, however, is to stimulate secretion of aldosterone from the adrenal cortex. Aldosterone increases sodium reabsorption in the kidneys, predominantly in the distal convoluted tubule, and also facilitates potassium and hydrogen ion secretion. The increased reabsorption of sodium from the nephron pulls water with it into the vascular space, ultimately increasing the intravascular volume without significantly increasing plasma sodium levels.

Counterregulatory hormones mediate important aspects of the stress response. Adrenergic stimulation also triggers the release of glucagon from alpha cells in the pancreatic islets while inhibiting the release of insulin from the beta cells. This effect of the sympathetic response has important metabolic ramifications. Glucagon—in concert with cortisol, growth hormone, and circulating epinephrine—initiates widespread catabolic mechanisms that affect essentially every tissue in the body. The overarching objective of imposing this catabolic state is to provide energetic substrate and molecular building blocks for the highly resource-intensive functions of the stress response.

These counterregulatory hormones stimulate hepatic gluconeogenesis and glycogenolysis and thereby increase blood glucose levels. Peripheral tissues become resistant to the effects of insulin under the influence of glucagon and growth hormone, which leads to critical illness–associated hyperglycemia. This phenomenon, associated with a decrease in the thyroid hormone T_3, may have as its purpose to reduce the metabolism and energy consumption of nonessential tissues, allowing circulating glucose to be used primarily by those cells and tissues directly involved in the immune response and tissue repair.[22]

In adipose tissue, epinephrine and glucagon activate hormone sensitive lipase, which catalyzes the first step in triglyceride hydrolysis and liberates free fatty acids and glycerol into the circulation. Glycerol is utilized as a gluconeogenic substrate in the liver, and the fatty acids are taken up by metabolically active cells to support their function or to provide structural components necessary for cellular growth and division. Leukocytes, for example, undergo rapid clonal expansion in inflammatory states and require significant amounts of lipid substrate both for activation as well as structural components of cell membranes.[29,30]

Skeletal muscle is also significantly affected. Epinephrine, cortisol, and glucagon initiate glycogenolysis in the muscle, but because myocytes lack glucose-6-phosphatase they cannot release glucose into the bloodstream like the liver. Whatever glucose liberated from glycogen that is not utilized for the energetic demands of the muscle itself is converted into lactate and released into the bloodstream. Indeed, significant β-adrenergic stimulation (eg, exogenous epinephrine) can induce the production of lactate even in the presence of adequate oxygen by inhibiting pyruvate decarboxylase, the final step of glycolysis that converts pyruvate into acetyl-CoA for

incorporation in the mitochondrial citric acid cycle.[31] Some tissues, like the myocardium, can use lactate as a primary energy source, but most of the lactate is taken up by the liver and used as gluconeogenic substrate to further increase circulating glucose levels. Protein catabolism in the muscle also releases amino acids into the circulation, which too are used by the liver for gluconeogenesis and for the elaboration of acute phase proteins necessary for the stress response. This protein catabolism is significantly enhanced by cytokine stimulation from the inflammatory response.[32]

Cellular Responses

Mitochondria represent the final common cellular pathway for the stress response,[33] as these organelles are primarily responsible for generating the enormous energy demands necessary to fuel the fight or flight response. However, in addition to respiration, mitochondria are also involved in thermogenesis, lipid metabolism, calcium regulation, intracellular signaling, and initiation of cell silencing pathways. The latter may involve apoptosis or mitochondrial hibernation (metabolic shutdown), either of which may provide an overarching mechanism for multiple organ dysfunction syndrome (see Chapter 112). It is of interest that short-term exposure to stress concentrations of corticosteroids is associated with induction of mitochondrial biogenesis and enzymatic activity, whereas prolonged exposure is associated with respiratory chain dysfunction, increased reactive oxygen species generation, mitochondrial structural abnormalities, apoptosis, and cell death.[33] A detailed discussion of mitochondrial biology related to critical illness may be found in Chapter 80.

Stress Response in Critical Illness

Critical illness reflects the ultimate manifestation of severe stress. Three phases of the stress response may be observed in the intensive care unit:

1. *Acute phase.* During this early time period after exposure to the critical stressor, analogous to the "Golden Hour" of resuscitation, the stress response comprises primarily those rapidly acting mechanisms designed to preserve tissue perfusion and oxygenation. Blood pressure, cardiac output, and intravascular volume are all maintained through adrenergic signaling, vasopressin secretion, and activation of the renin-angiotensin-aldosterone system. The response time in these systems is so rapid because they rely on preformed mediators to bring about their physiologic effects.

2. *Established phase.* As time elapses, the full breadth of the stress response is brought to bear as endocrine and metabolic mechanisms come into play. These are slower to activate because they rely predominantly on neuroendocrine regulation of gene transcription and protein translation. The focus of this phase of the response is to adapt host physiology to preserve vital functions while directing resources toward resolving the inciting stressor. Nonessential systems are deactivated. To achieve their desired ends, these allostatic changes may permit, or even seek, physiologic parameters that are not congruent with baseline homeostasis. For example, cytokines stimulate the hypothalamic thermostat to increase body temperature. Though abnormal relative to baseline conditions, fever is an important physiologic adaptation that facilitates leukocyte eradication of infectious agents. This ability to adapt

to the needs of the circumstances is the physiologic resilience we referred to at the outset of this chapter.

3. *Recovery or repair phase.* When the inciting stressor is removed, the stress response is attenuated, the strain on host systems is relieved, and the body returns incrementally to normal homeostatic parameters.

From a teleologic point of view, the acute stress response is intended to be self-terminating within hours to a few days at most, rather than a prolonged condition persisting weeks or more. Clearly, failure to mount an adequate stress response is associated with worse outcomes. However, excessive or chronic stress compromises the body's allostatic responses and may itself promote pathology.[1] Due to the magnitude and nature of life-threatening conditions, the stress response in critical illness can become dysregulated and prolonged. When this occurs the stress response devolves into the distress response as pathologic results emerge from misdirected or excessive allostatic adaptations. This is observed frequently in the intensive care unit (ICU).

Decreased neurologic function secondary to the inciting disease process itself or iatrogenic sedation precludes appropriate threat appraisal and stress system regulation by the central nervous system. Excessive adrenergic output can directly impair cardiac function.[34,35] The antiinflammatory neurogenic reflex may play a role in the immunoparalysis seen so often after trauma and sepsis.[27,36]

Both very high and low cortisol levels are observed in critically ill children and are associated with increased mortality.[21,22] Elevated levels of cortisol likely contribute to immune dysfunction as well as metabolic dysregulation, whereas insufficient cortisol secretion is associated with cardiovascular collapse. The debate over steroid administration in critical illness has raged for decades and will likely continue for several more.[37] These topics are reviewed in much greater depth in Chapter 85.

The overall tone of the stress system in severe or prolonged critical illness is one of generalized depression. As noted earlier, thyroid hormone levels are suppressed, which may be an adaptive response, to a degree, by allowing energetic resources to be consumed by more vital processes. When taken to an extreme, however, very depressed thyroid levels are associated with mortality.[38,39] Growth hormone and prolactin release surges early in the stress response but drops to very low levels with persistent critical illness resulting in dysregulated metabolism and immunity.[21,22]

Vasopressin is elevated early in the acute phase of shock states, but it rapidly declines and remains quite low through prolonged critical illness.[24,40] Vasopressin deficiency has been observed among children treated with cardiopulmonary bypass.[41] In septic shock, regulation of vasopressin is characterized by decreased plasma concentrations, unaltered clearance, depleted neurohypophyseal vesicles, and altered osmolar signaling.[42] Likewise the renin-angiotensin-aldosterone system can be dysregulated in critical illness. Elevated renin and angiotensin are observed in sepsis and correlate with measures of microvascular dysfunction and organ system failure.[43] In a subset of critically ill patients, however, aldosterone levels are inappropriately low despite elevated plasma renin activity.[44-46] Mineralocorticoid deficiency may therefore contribute to the hyponatremia sometimes observed in pediatric intensive care unit (PICU) patients.

Significant metabolic dysregulation can be seen with severe and persistent stress responses. The combined effect of increased glucose production and peripheral insulin resistance can result in extremely elevated blood sugar levels, which correlate with organ system dysfunction and survival.[47-49] Intense hypercytokinemia and adrenergic stimulation both mobilize lipid and amino acid substrate from adipose tissue and skeletal muscle, which can result in hypertriglyceridemia and severe muscle wasting.[50,51,32] The clinical significance of elevated serum triglyceride levels is uncertain, but muscle wasting leads to critical illness–related weakness and prolonged mechanical ventilation with all of their comorbidities.[52]

Analogous to inflammation, stress is beneficial acutely but when prolonged may generate collateral damage. Complicated or prolonged critical illness may represent a stress-related decompensation syndrome.[2] A complicated ICU course may reflect elements of an ongoing stress response manifested as protein catabolism with poor wound healing and diffuse weakness and immunosuppression associated with hospital-acquired infections, all of this reflecting a persistent inflammation immunosuppression catabolism syndrome (PICS).[53] When stress evolves into distress, allostatic overload occurs resulting in mitochondrial hibernation as an antecedent of metabolic shutdown and widespread energy failure associated with multiple organ dysfunction syndrome (MODS).[54] Maladaptive response to stress can outlast the actual stress phase by months or even years, and chronic stress can lead to the development of the metabolic syndrome long after discharge from the PICU.[55]

Recommendations and Conclusions

An understanding of the stress response should influence how we care for children in the PICU. Because pathophysiology can change rapidly in critical illness and varies along the continuum from injury to resolution, we need to adapt our clinical posture to fluctuating physiologic parameters in the different phases of the stress response:

1. *Acute phase.* In this "Golden Hour" period, emphasis is directed at avoiding hypoxemia and ischemia. Attention must also be paid to removing the inciting stressor that has precipitated the stress response as quickly as possible. For example, in infectious causes of critical illness, achieving early source control is paramount. Likewise, aggressive interventions to stop seizures in status epilepticus or to relieve bronchoconstriction in severe asthma are crucial. The longer the stimulus persists, the more intense and prolonged the stress response it elicits.

2. *Established phase.* During this interval, clinicians should focus on permissive treatment that respects the stress response and avoids iatrogenic injury, recognizing that many ICU interventions can exacerbate stress system dysregulation (vasoactive infusions, systemic steroids, etc.). Healthy physiologic values routinely targeted in the critically ill may not be appropriate in light of the adaptations necessary for the stress response. The therapeutic implication here is that most of the acute endocrine and metabolic responses are likely to be adaptive and thus should probably not be aggressively treated.[21] In many situations providing less intervention may provide greater long-term benefit.[56]

3. *Recovery or repair phase.* In this phase, clinicians refocus on targeting normal physiologic values. Here the environment of the ICU plays a key role in terms of avoiding prolongation or reinitiation of an acute stress response.

In addition to providing critical care interventions targeted at removing the primary pathophysiologic stressors, the multidisciplinary care team can optimize long-term outcomes by implementing interventions to de-stress their critically ill patients: avoiding supraphysiologic resuscitation; facilitating sleep; reestablishing circadian rhythms; decreasing noise levels; avoiding pain, anxiety, and delirium; promoting early mobilization; providing natural light; and restoring entitlement.

References

1. Brame AL, Singer M. Stressing the obvious? An allostatic look at critical illness. *Crit Care Med.* 2010;38:S600-S607.
2. Cuesta JM, Singer M. The stress response and critical illness: a review. *Crit Care Med.* 2012;40:3283-3289.
3. Cannon WB. *The Wisdom of the Body.* New York: W.W. Norton; 1932.
4. Selye H. Stress and the general adaptation syndrome. *Br Med J.* 1950;1:1383-1392.
5. Chrousos GP. Stress and disorders of the stress system. *Nat Rev Endocrinol.* 2009;5:374-381.
6. McEwen BS, Wingfield JC. What is in a name? Integrating homeostasis, allostasis and stress. *Horm Behav.* 2010;57:105-111.
7. Leteurtre S, Duhamel A, Salleron J, et al. PELOD-2: an update of the PEdiatric logistic organ dysfunction score. *Crit Care Med.* 2013;41:1761-1773.
8. McEwen BS. Physiology and neurobiology of stress and adaptation: central role of the brain. *Physiol Rev.* 2007;87:873-904.
9. Charmandari E, Tsigos C, Chrousos G. Endocrinology of the stress response. *Annu Rev Physiol.* 2005;67:259-284.
10. Molina PE. Neurobiology of the stress response: contribution of the sympathetic nervous system to the neuroimmune axis in traumatic injury. *Shock.* 2005;24:3-10.
11. Baumann H, Gauldie J. The acute phase response. *Immunol Today.* 1994;15:74-80.
12. Abreu MT, Arditi M. Innate immunity and toll-like receptors: clinical implications of basic science research. *J Pediatr.* 2004;144:421-429.
13. Zhang Q, Raoof M, Chen Y, et al. Circulating mitochondrial DAMPs cause inflammatory responses to injury. *Nature.* 2010;464:104-107.
14. Ulloa L. The vagus nerve and the nicotinic anti-inflammatory pathway. *Nat Rev Drug Discov.* 2005;4:673-684.
15. Besedovsky HO, del Rey A. Immune-neuro-endocrine interactions: facts and hypotheses. *Endocr Rev.* 1996;17:64-102.
16. Turnbull AV, Rivier CL. Regulation of the hypothalamic-pituitary-adrenal axis by cytokines: actions and mechanisms of action. *Physiol Rev.* 1999;79:1-71.
17. Annane D. Hippocampus: a future target for sepsis treatment! *Intensive Care Med.* 2009;35:585-586.
18. Chrousos GP. The hypothalamic-pituitary-adrenal axis and immune-mediated inflammation. *N Engl J Med.* 1995;332:1351-1362.
19. Galon J, Franchimont D, Hiroi N, et al. Gene profiling reveals unknown enhancing and suppressive actions of glucocorticoids on immune cells. *FASEB J Off Publ Fed Am Soc Exp Biol.* 2002;16:61-71.
20. Rhen T, Cidlowski JA. Antiinflammatory action of glucocorticoids: new mechanisms for old drugs. *N Engl J Med.* 2005;353:1711-1723.
21. Boonen E, Van den Berghe G. Endocrine responses to critical illness: novel insights and therapeutic implications. *J Clin Endocrinol Metab.* 2014;99:1569-1582.
22. Vanhorebeek I, Langouche L, Van den Berghe G. Endocrine aspects of acute and prolonged critical illness. *Nat Clin Pract Endocrinol Metab.* 2006;2:20-31.
23. Shih JL, Agus MSD. Thyroid function in the critically ill newborn and child. *Curr Opin Pediatr.* 2009;21:536-540.
24. Choong K, Kissoon N. Vasopressin in pediatric shock and cardiac arrest. *Pediatr Crit Care Med J Soc Crit Care Med World Fed Pediatr Intensive Crit Care Soc.* 2008;9:372-379.
25. Russell JA. Bench-to-bedside review: vasopressin in the management of septic shock. *Crit Care Lond Engl.* 2011;15:226.
26. Chrousos GP, Gold PW. The concepts of stress and stress system disorders. Overview of physical and behavioral homeostasis. *JAMA.* 1992;267:1244-1252.
27. Tracey KJ. Physiology and immunology of the cholinergic antiinflammatory pathway. *J Clin Invest.* 2007;117:289-296.
28. Levy G, Fishman JE, Xu D, et al. Parasympathetic stimulation via the vagus nerve prevents systemic organ dysfunction by abrogating gut injury and lymph toxicity in trauma and hemorrhagic shock. *Shock.* 2013;39:39-44.
29. Pearce EJ, Everts B. Dendritic cell metabolism. *Nat Rev Immunol.* 2014;15:18-29.
30. Buck MD, O'Sullivan D, Pearce EL. T cell metabolism drives immunity. *J Exp Med.* 2015;212:1345-1360.
31. Meert KL, Clark J, Sarnaik AP. Metabolic acidosis as an underlying mechanism of respiratory distress in children with severe acute asthma. *Pediatr Crit Care Med J Soc Crit Care Med World Fed Pediatr Intensive Crit Care Soc.* 2007;8:519-523.
32. Puthucheary ZA, Rawal J, McPhail M, et al. Acute skeletal muscle wasting in critical illness. *JAMA.* 2013;310:1591-1600.
33. Manoli I, Alesci S, Blackman MR, et al. Mitochondria as key components of the stress response. *Trends Endocrinol Metab TEM.* 2007;18:190-198.
34. Wittekind SG, Yanay O, Johnson EM, et al. Two pediatric cases of variant neurogenic stress cardiomyopathy after intracranial hemorrhage. *Pediatrics.* 2014;134:e1211-e1217.
35. Boland TA, Lee VH, Bleck TP. Stress-induced cardiomyopathy. *Crit Care Med.* 2015;43:686-693.
36. Hotchkiss RS, Coopersmith CM, McDunn JE, et al. The sepsis seesaw: tilting toward immunosuppression. *Nat Med.* 2009;15:496-497.
37. Patel GP, Balk RA. Systemic steroids in severe sepsis and septic shock. *Am J Respir Crit Care Med.* 2012;185:133-139.
38. Peeters RP, Wouters PJ, van Toor H, et al. Serum 3,3',5'-triiodothyronine (rT3) and 3,5,3'-triiodothyronine/rT3 are prognostic markers in critically ill patients and are associated with postmortem tissue deiodinase activities. *J Clin Endocrinol Metab.* 2005;90:4559-4565.
39. Wang F, Pan W, Wang H, et al. Relationship between thyroid function and ICU mortality: a prospective observation study. *Crit Care Lond Engl.* 2012;16:R11.
40. Landry DW, Levin HR, Gallant EM, et al. Vasopressin deficiency contributes to the vasodilation of septic shock. *Circulation.* 1997;95:1122-1125.
41. Mastropietro CW, Rossi NF, Clark JA, et al. Relative deficiency of arginine vasopressin in children after cardiopulmonary bypass. *Crit Care Med.* 2010;38:2052-2058.
42. Siami S, Bailly-Salin J, Polito A, et al. Osmoregulation of vasopressin secretion is altered in the postacute phase of septic shock. *Crit Care Med.* 2010;38:1962-1969.
43. Doerschug KC, Delsing AS, Schmidt GA, et al. Renin-angiotensin system activation correlates with microvascular dysfunction in a prospective cohort study of clinical sepsis. *Crit Care Lond Engl.* 2010;14:R24.
44. Findling JW, Waters VO, Raff H. The dissociation of renin and aldosterone during critical illness. *J Clin Endocrinol Metab.* 1987;64:592-595.
45. Lichtarowicz-Krynska EJ, Cole TJ, Camacho-Hubner C, et al. Circulating aldosterone levels are unexpectedly low in children with acute meningococcal disease. *J Clin Endocrinol Metab.* 2004;89:1410-1414.
46. Tolstoy NS, Aized M, McMonagle MP, et al. Mineralocorticoid deficiency in hemorrhagic shock. *J Surg Res.* 2013;180:232-237.
47. Faustino EV, Apkon M. Persistent hyperglycemia in critically ill children. *J Pediatr.* 2005;146:30-34.
48. Yung M, Wilkins B, Norton L, et al. Glucose control, organ failure, and mortality in pediatric intensive care. *Pediatr Crit Care Med J Soc Crit Care Med World Fed Pediatr Intensive Crit Care Soc.* 2008;9:147-152.
49. Weiss SL, Alexander J, Agus MSD. Extreme stress hyperglycemia during acute illness in a pediatric emergency department. *Pediatr Emerg Care.* 2010;26:626-632.
50. Klein S, Peters EJ, Shangraw RE, et al. Lipolytic response to metabolic stress in critically ill patients. *Crit Care Med.* 1991;19:776-779.
51. Tappy L, Chioléro R. Substrate utilization in sepsis and multiple organ failure. *Crit Care Med.* 2007;35:S531-S534.
52. Hermans G, Van den Berghe G. Clinical review: intensive care unit acquired weakness. *Crit Care Lond Engl.* 2015;19:274.
53. Vanzant EL, Lopez CM, Ozrazgat-Baslanti T, et al. Persistent inflammation, immunosuppression, and catabolism syndrome after severe blunt trauma. *J Trauma Acute Care Surg.* 2014;76:21-29, discussion 29-30.
54. Singer M, De Santis V, Vitale D, et al. Multiorgan failure is an adaptive, endocrine-mediated, metabolic response to overwhelming systemic inflammation. *Lancet Lond Engl.* 2004;364:545-548.
55. Schmidt MV, Sterlemann V, Müller MB. Chronic stress and individual vulnerability. *Ann N Y Acad Sci.* 2008;1148:174-183.
56. Singer M. The key advance in the treatment of sepsis in the last 10 years ... doing less. *Crit Care Lond Engl.* 2006;10:122.

Inborn Errors of Metabolism

Cary O. Harding

PEARLS

- Unexpected and unexplained clinical deterioration in a previously healthy infant or child is an important clue to the presence of an inborn error of metabolism (IEM).
- Loss of previously attained developmental milestones during childhood is an important clue to the presence of a neurodegenerative disorder such as lysosomal storage disease.
- Blood glucose less than 40 mg/dL is distinctly unusual after the first 24 hours of life, particularly in infants who have started feeding, and should be thoroughly investigated.
- Laboratory evaluation for inborn error of metabolism should be undertaken in any child with a suggestive clinical history regardless of the results of newborn screening. A normal newborn screen, although perhaps reassuring, does not rule out the possibility of an IEM.
- With catastrophic illness in a previously well child without signs of any particular IEM, the "shotgun" diagnostic evaluation should minimally include plasma amino acid analysis, plasma acylcarnitine profile, urine organic acid analysis by gas chromatography-mass spectrometry, and urine-reducing substances.

Metabolism can be defined as the sum of all biochemical processes that convert food to smaller molecules and energy for the purposes of structure and function. An inborn error of metabolism (IEM) is an inherited deficiency of any critical step in metabolism. Although genetic deficiency of catalytic enzymes in intermediary metabolic pathways is the classic paradigm for IEM, the pathophysiology of metabolic disorders may involve abnormalities of any number of cellular processes, including transmembrane transport, cell signaling, cell differentiation and development, energy production, and others. Many IEMs are individually rare, although a few, including phenylketonuria (PKU)[1] and medium-chain acyl-coenzyme A (acyl-CoA) dehydrogenase deficiency (MCADD),[2] a defect in fatty acid oxidation, exhibit a population incidence approaching 1:10,000 live births. Specific IEMs may be more common in certain ethnic groups with a history of relative reproductive isolation. Collectively, the population incidence of all IEMs may approach 1:1500 live births, depending on how broadly IEM is defined. Many IEMs are associated with catastrophic illness necessitating advanced life support. Although IEM may present rarely within the professional lifetime of the average medical practitioner, critically ill children

with IEM will not be uncommon visitors to the pediatric intensive care unit, especially in a tertiary care center.

Other published textbooks on the diagnosis and treatment of IEM provide an exhaustive list of known disorders.[3,4] Rather than recapitulate an encyclopedia of possible diseases, this chapter presents a diagnostic rationale based on specific clinical symptom complexes that are likely to occur in the critically ill child. Algorithms for the differential diagnosis of specific clinical scenarios are given in support of this rationale. Symptoms often begin during early infancy in the biochemically most severe IEM; naturally, these IEMs with neonatal onset are the focus of the discussion in this chapter. However, "milder" or late-onset variants of virtually every IEM have been described with onset of symptoms occurring at all ages, even during adulthood. Some IEMs uniformly present after the neonatal period; age of symptom onset (late infancy, childhood, or adulthood) often is an important clue to the specific diagnosis. The clinical presentation, diagnostic workup, and treatment of neonatal onset disorders provide a paradigm for the evaluation and management of possible IEM in a child of any age.

Pathophysiology of Inborn Errors of Metabolism

Under the classic paradigm, an IEM is associated with deficiency of a specific protein, often a catalytic enzyme, involved in a critical metabolic pathway (Fig. 82.1). This deficiency leads to a block in the pathway and the accumulation of the enzyme substrate. In this model, three distinct pathogenic mechanisms are possible proximate causes of the symptoms associated with an IEM. The specific pathogenic mechanism involved in any given IEM dictates the appropriate treatment strategy. First, accumulation of the substrate may lead to toxic effects at very high levels; successful therapy requires effective elimination of the substrate or a method to block its toxic effects. An example for this mechanism is PKU, in which elevated phenylalanine levels adversely affect neuronal development, and the reduction of tissue phenylalanine content through dietary phenylalanine restriction largely prevents the major clinical features of PKU.[5] Second, deficiency of the reaction product, should it be a critically important metabolite, may lead to disease. Supplementation with the essential metabolite, if possible, may cure the disease. Biotin is a required cofactor for four distinct carboxylase enzymes. Deficiency of free biotin develops in the face of genetic biotinidase deficiency and leads to symptoms of multiple carboxylase deficiency. Supplementation with oral biotin completely prevents the clinical manifestations of biotinidase deficiency.[6] The final pathogenic mechanism involves the conversion of the enzyme substrate, through normally

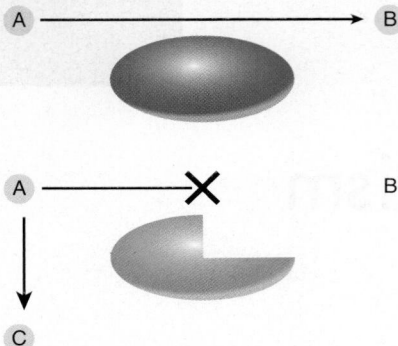

Fig. 82.1. Inborn error of metabolism paradigm. Normally, in a given step of intermediate metabolism with intact enzymatic activity, the substrate A is efficiently converted to the product B. In an inborn error of metabolism, a deficiency of enzyme activity may lead to excessive accumulation of the substrate; critical deficiency of the product; or production of an alternative, potentially toxic metabolite C through normally quiescent pathways.

TABLE 82.1	Signs and Symptoms of Inborn Errors of Metabolism

Acute illness after period of normal behavior and feeding (hours to weeks)
Recurrent decompensation with fasting, intercurrent illness, or specific food ingestion
Unusual body odor
Persistent or recurrent vomiting
Failure to thrive
Apnea or tachypnea
Jaundice
Hepatomegaly or liver dysfunction
Lethargy or coma
Sepsis
Unexplained hemorrhage or strokes
Developmental delay with unknown etiology
Developmental regression
Seizures, especially if seizures are intractable
Hypotonia
Chronic movement disorder (ataxia, dystonia, choreoathetosis)
Family history of unexplained death or current illness in siblings
Parental consanguinity

BOX 82.1	Screening Metabolic Laboratory Studies for Children With Suspected Inborn Errors of Metabolism

- Plasma amino acid analysis
  Minimum 2 mL blood in a heparin tube
- Plasma acylcarnitine profile
  Minimum 2 mL blood in a heparin tube
- Urine organic acid analysis
- Urine screening—reducing substances, qualitative mucopolysaccharide screening
  Minimum 10 mL urine

quiescent alternative pathways, to toxic secondary metabolites. Elimination or decreased production of these secondary metabolites may improve disease symptoms. For example, tyrosinemia type I (fumarylacetoacetate hydrolase [FAH] deficiency) is associated with recurrent attacks of abdominal pain and paresthesias reminiscent of acute intermittent porphyria. The accumulating substrate, fumarylacetoacetic acid, is converted through secondary pathways to succinylacetone, and succinylacetone in turn inhibits the heme synthetic pathway and causes porphyria-like symptoms. Pharmacologic inhibition of the tyrosine catabolic pathway proximal to the block at FAH decreases the production of fumarylacetoacetic acid and succinylacetone and alleviates the pathology associated with these toxic compounds.[7]

Inheritance of Inborn Errors of Metabolism

IEMs are heritable disorders. The majority of diseases are inherited in an autosomal recessive pattern, yielding a 25% recurrence risk in future offspring. The gene defects associated with several IEMs are located on the X chromosome. These IEMs, such as ornithine transcarbamoylase deficiency and glycerol kinase deficiency, are inherited in an X-linked pattern. These IEMs are most severe in males, but carrier females may be symptomatic, although usually with less severe or late-onset disease as a result of skewed X chromosome inactivation. Mutations for several mitochondrial disorders are found on mitochondrial deoxyribonucleic acid (mtDNA). Because mtDNA is exclusively passed from mothers to their offspring, these IEMs exhibit a maternal inheritance pattern but often with variable penetrance and expressivity. Prenatal diagnosis is possible for many IEMs. In addition to allowing for appropriate medical therapy, the timely diagnosis of an IEM in a sick infant or child is important for genetic counseling purposes.

Signs and Symptoms of Inborn Errors of Metabolism

Clinical signs and symptoms frequently associated with IEM are listed in Table 82.1. The symptom repertoire of the

critically ill infant is limited, and the clinical presentation of metabolic disorders often is nonspecific. It is for this reason that the diagnosis of an IEM may be easily missed. To maintain maximum diagnostic sensitivity for IEM, the clinician must maintain a high level of suspicion and be willing to initiate screening metabolic laboratory studies with little provocation (Box 82.1). As was true for appendectomies in the era prior to the advent of ultrasound-based diagnosis of appendicitis, a certain number of nondiagnostic metabolic laboratory workups in sick children must be performed to ensure ascertainment of individuals with inherited metabolic disorders. In particular, IEM should be a strong diagnostic consideration in any neonate who has become catastrophically ill following a period of normalcy. This presentation may be clinically indistinguishable from bacterial or viral sepsis, and the nonspecific supportive therapy provided to potentially septic infants (fluid and glucose administration) may alleviate the symptoms and mask the presence of an IEM. Diagnostic metabolic laboratory studies are most likely to provide definitive information if performed on clinical samples obtained at initial presentation and before any therapy is initiated. Failure to obtain the necessary specimens at this time may miss an important diagnostic window of opportunity. Many children with IEM have been saved initially by intensive but nonspecific treatment but then suffered clinical relapse or even death in the absence of the correct diagnosis. Certainly, the possibility of an IEM should be considered in any child for whom the clinical picture suggests sepsis, but the laboratory evaluation for sepsis is negative. Unfortunately, bacterial sepsis is often a complicating factor in critically ill children with IEM. For example, *Escherichia coli* infection (including pyelonephritis, bacteremia, or meningitis) is frequently detected at presentation in infants with galactosemia. The astute clinician remains ever vigilant for the signs and symptoms that may suggest an inherited metabolic disorder.

Recurrent episodes of vomiting and dehydration in response to fasting or intercurrent illness are an important clue to IEM in older infants and children. Feeding difficulties and failure to thrive are common chronic complications. Children with unexplained hypotonia, developmental delay, or movement disorder should be evaluated for possible IEM. Inherited neurodegenerative disorders, such as the lysosomal storage diseases, stereotypically cause developmental regression, specifically loss of previously attained developmental milestones. Several IEMs are associated with major physical anomalies (Table 82.2). When present, these anomalies are exceedingly valuable in suggesting a specific diagnosis and directing the diagnostic evaluation. More commonly, the child with IEM is morphologically normal, and the presenting symptoms are nonspecific. The clinician must then rely on screening laboratory tests to evaluate the potential for IEM.

Laboratory Evaluation of Suspected Inborn Errors of Metabolism

Abnormal results of routine laboratory studies may provide clues to the presence and type of IEM (Table 82.3). Highly informative but sometimes subtle laboratory abnormalities are often overlooked, especially in a busy intensive care unit or hospital ward. For instance, a clinically relevant newborn screening result may have been sent to the primary care provider or birth hospital but not efficiently communicated to the intensive care unit in a different hospital, to which the now critically ill infant has been admitted. It is imperative to verify the infant's screening results with the primary care provider or newborn screening laboratory. Calculation of the anion gap, another example of a routine and highly informative result, is key to the differential diagnosis of metabolic acidosis (see also Chapter 76). The absence of urine ketones in hypoglycemic children older than 2 weeks strongly suggests impaired ketogenesis as a consequence of either hyperinsulinism or fatty acid oxidation disorder. On the other hand, fatty acid oxidation and ketogenesis are incompletely developed in neonates. The presence of ketones in urine of infants younger than 2 weeks is unusual, even during fasting or hypoglycemia, and suggests the presence of an unusual ketoacid, such as those excreted in maple syrup disease or the organic acidemias. Ketoacids, organic acids, and sugars such as galactose or fructose increase urine specific gravity. Urine specific gravity >1.020 in any neonate or in well-hydrated older children suggests the unexpected presence of an osmotically active substance. Routine urinalysis at many hospitals may not include use of the Clinitest to detect reducing substances. Urine Chemstrips utilize a colorimetric glucose oxidase-based method to specifically detect glucose. This test does not react with any other sugar (galactose or fructose). However, some bedside glucose monitoring systems do react with galactose or fructose; inappropriately elevated capillary blood "glucose" accompanied by a normal venous glucose as measured by chemistry analyzer suggests the presence of a sugar other than glucose in the blood. A comatose infant with a blood urea nitrogen (BUN) level below the limits of detection may have an inherited defect in the urea cycle. Blood ammonia measurement is crucial to confirming that suspicion. Failure to check the blood ammonia level has caused missed diagnoses, failure to appropriately treat hyperammonemia, and morbidity and mortality in comatose infants with urea cycle disorders or organic acidemias. Finally, bacterial sepsis and meningitis are more common causes of severe lethargy and coma in infants than is IEM, but bacterial infection may also be a complicating feature in severely ill infants with IEM. Infants with galactosemia, for example, are particularly prone to pyelonephritis, bacteremia, sepsis, or meningitis, often with *E. coli*, as noted previously. Antibiotic therapy without diagnosis and specific treatment of the underlying disorder may be useful in the short term but does not mitigate long-term IEM-specific effects.

Suspicion of an IEM based on clinical and routine laboratory findings should initiate specialized biochemical testing (Table 82.4). In the case of severely ill infants or when the clinical suspicion of IEM is very high, consultation with a biochemical geneticist, even if only by phone, is strongly advised

TABLE 82.2	Physical Anomalies Associated with Inborn Errors of Metabolism
Dysmorphic facial features	Peroxisomal disorders Glutaric aciduria type II Smith-Lemli-Opitz syndrome Menkes syndrome Lysosomal storage disorders
Structural brain anomalies	Glutaric aciduria type II (cortical cysts) Pyruvate dehydrogenase deficiency (cortical cysts, agenesis of the corpus callosum) Glycosylation disorders (cerebellar agenesis)
Macrocephaly	Glutaric aciduria type I (with subdural effusions) Canavan disease Alexander disease
Cataracts	Galactosemia Peroxisomal disorders Mitochondrial disorders Lowe syndrome
Lens dislocation	Homocystinuria Sulfite oxidase deficiency Molybdenum cofactor deficiency
Pigmentary retinopathy	Peroxisomal disorders Lysosomal storage disorders (cherry red spots) Long chain 3-hydroxyacyl-CoA dehydrogenase deficiency
Renal cysts	Glutaric aciduria type II Peroxisomal disorders Mitochondrial disorders
Ambiguous genitalia	Congenital adrenal hyperplasia Smith-Lemli-Opitz syndrome
Skeletal abnormalities	Menkes disease Homocystinuria Peroxisomal disorders Lysosomal storage diseases
Hair or skin abnormalities	Menkes disease Holocarboxylase synthetase deficiency Biotinidase deficiency Argininosuccinic aciduria Phenylketonuria

TABLE 82.3   Initial Laboratory Evaluation of Suspected Inborn Errors of Metabolism

Laboratory Test	Abnormality	Disorder
Complete blood count	Neutropenia	Organic acidemias Glycogenosis type 1b
	Macrocytic anemia	Cobalamin processing defects
	Pancytopenia	Congenital lactic acidoses
Serum electrolytes	Metabolic acidosis	Glycogenoses Organic acidemias FAO disorders MSUD Congenital lactic acidoses
Blood gas	Metabolic acidosis	Same as above
	Metabolic alkalosis	Urea cycle disorders
Blood urea nitrogen (BUN)	Low or undetectable BUN (with hyperammonemia)	Urea cycle disorders
Transaminases (ALT, AST)	Liver dysfunction	Galactosemia Fructosemia Tyrosinemia Alpha-1-antitrypsin deficiency FAO disorders Organic acidemias Congenital lactic acidoses Congenital disorders of glycosylation
Total and direct bilirubin	Hyperbilirubinemia	Galactosemia Fructosemia Tyrosinemia Alpha-1-antitrypsin deficiency Congenital lactic acidoses
Serum uric acid	Hyperuricemia	Glycogenoses Purine disorders
Blood ammonia	Hyperammonemia	Urea cycle disorders FAO disorders Organic acidemias
Blood lactate	Lactic acidemia	Congenital lactic acidoses Glycogenoses Fructosemia Gluconeogenesis disorders
Urinalysis Odor Color pH Specific gravity Ketones Reducing substances	Unusual odor Inappropriately high specific gravity due to metabolites Ketosis Positive reducing substances	PKU, MSUD, organic acidemias Organic acidemias, galactosemia, fructosemia MSUD, organic acidemias Galactosemia, fructosemia

FAO, fatty acid oxidation; *MSUD,* maple syrup urine disease; *PKU,* phenylketonuria.

to help direct the laboratory investigation and initial therapy. When the clinical presentation is nonspecific—that is, catastrophic illness in a previously well child without signs of any particular IEM—the "shotgun" diagnostic evaluation should minimally include plasma amino acid analysis, urine organic acid analysis by gas chromatography-mass spectrometry, and a so-called urine metabolic screen. The battery of qualitative assays included in a urine metabolic screen differs among laboratories, and the ordering clinician should be aware of which tests and disorders are included in the repertoire of the diagnostic laboratory chosen. Furthermore, although diagnostic laboratories in the United States must meet Clinical Laboratory Improvement Amendment (CLIA) requirements and often are accredited by the College of American Pathologists (CAP), the testing methodologies used, the quality of diagnostic testing for IEM, and more problematically the availability

of laboratory-associated consultants with experience in the diagnosis and treatment of IEM vary widely among laboratories. Although the ability of clinicians to direct clinical specimens toward specific diagnostic laboratories may be inhibited by contractual arrangements between the hospital and large referral laboratories, the critically ill patient is best served by diagnostic evaluation carried out in a timely manner by an experienced biochemical genetics laboratory, with laboratory staff available by phone for expert consultation on interpretation of test results.

The specific clinical presentation or specific screening laboratory findings may direct the intensivist or biochemical geneticist to order other more specialized metabolic tests (see Table 82.4). These analyses may provide diagnostic confirmation for specific disorders and supportive evidence alone for others. For several IEMs, confirmation of diagnosis may

TABLE 82.4   Biochemical Genetic Laboratory Studies

Specimen	Test	Disorder
Blood	Plasma amino acid analysis	Aminoacidopathies
	Plasma carnitine	Organic acidemias FAO disorders
	Plasma acylcarnitine profile	Organic acidemias FAO disorders
	Serum transferrin electrophoresis	Congenital disorders of glycosylation
Urine	Metabolic screen	
	Ketones	Organic acidemias
	Reducing substances	Galactosemia, fructosemia
	Mucopolysaccharide screen	Mucopolysaccharidoses
	Organic acid analysis	Organic acidemias FAO disorders
	Acylglycine profile	Organic acidemias FAO disorders
	Quantitative mucopolysaccharide measurement and electrophoresis	Mucopolysaccharidoses
	Qualitative sulfites (Sulfitest) or quantitative sulfocysteine	Sulfite oxidase deficiency Molybdenum cofactor deficiency
	Quantitative succinylacetone	Tyrosinemia type 1
	Quantitative purines	Purine synthesis disorders

FAO, fatty acid oxidation.

require enzyme activity analysis in tissue (red blood cells, lymphocytes, cultured skin fibroblasts, liver, or skeletal muscle depending on the specific disorder in question) or molecular DNA testing for a specific gene defect. In general, these tertiary tests, which are often difficult, labor intensive, and expensive, should be ordered following consultation with a biochemical geneticist. In some instances, confirmatory diagnostic biochemical or molecular tests are available only through specialized research laboratories. Molecular DNA analysis has become a prevalent and powerful weapon in the arsenal of available diagnostic tools. Whole exome sequencing—that is, DNA sequencing of all regions of the genome known to code functional proteins, using novel high throughput DNA sequencing platforms—has proved utility in the diagnosis of complex phenotypes.[8] Biochemical testing, which is more rapidly accomplished than DNA sequencing in most clinical laboratories and which is necessary to confirm the pathogenicity of sequence variants detected by molecular DNA analysis, remains vital to the process of disease diagnosis and treatment management.

Postmortem Evaluation of a Child With Suspected Inborn Errors of Metabolism

Some IEMs, particularly those exacerbated by fasting, may present as sudden infant death. For many IEMs, acute metabolic compensation may be rapid and lethal despite intensive medical intervention. The time after clinical presentation but prior to death may be insufficient to execute an adequate metabolic evaluation. Disease diagnosis is still possible postmortem and is important for fully understanding the cause of death and determining recurrence risk in the family. A protocol for postmortem evaluation of an infant or child with suspected IEM is provided in Table 82.5. Many of the biochemical genetic analyses recommended for acutely ill children are still valid on postmortem specimens. Valuable information may be learned from amino acid, carnitine, and acylcarnitine analyses in blood and from metabolic screening and organic acid analysis in urine (Box 82.2). However, collection of blood and urine may not be possible postmortem, especially if the autopsy is performed many hours after death. In these instances, metabolic testing may be obtained on alternative specimens such as vitreous humor or bile. In the event that screening biochemical studies suggest a specific diagnosis, disease confirmation by enzyme analysis in tissue is highly desirable. Many enzymes can be assayed in cultured fibroblasts; viable fibroblasts may be cultured from skin or Achilles tendon samples obtained as late as 24 hours after death. Biopsies of other organs may be necessary for analysis of certain other enzymes. Muscle, liver, and kidney specimens may be obtained postmortem for enzymatic analysis, but most enzymatic activities in solid organs deteriorate rapidly following death. Collection of specimens as soon as possible after death is critical for valid enzyme analyses.

Emergency Treatment of Children With Suspected Inborn Errors of Metabolism

Laboratory investigation of suspected IEM may require several days to complete, given that the biochemical genetics laboratory may be physically remote from the treating hospital and many of the tests involve complex specimen preparation and analysis. A general approach to emergency treatment of children with suspected IEM while awaiting diagnostic studies is outlined in Table 82.6. For many IEMs associated with acute catastrophic illness, elimination of the offending metabolite is the key to therapy. Immediate cessation of oral feedings, to stop protein or fat intake, will begin to limit toxin production in disorders of amino acid or fatty acid metabolism. Adequate energy intake as carbohydrate must be supplied, usually parenterally, until a specific diagnosis and definitive treatment plan are available. Dextrose infusion at a high rate suppresses catabolism and reduces the consumption of endogenous protein or fatty acid stores. In extremely recalcitrant cases, insulin infusion drives anabolism and further decreases toxin production. Acute metabolic decompensation in some IEMs (eg, maple syrup disease) is associated with mild peripheral insulin resistance. Insulin administration (often as little as 0.01–0.05 units/kg/hour given by continuous intravenous [IV] infusion or subcutaneous bolus injection) overcomes this resistance and has an immediate impact on metabolic control. Some clinicians also use anabolic agents such as growth hormone or testosterone to acutely suppress protein and fat catabolism. In certain types of congenital lactic acidosis, particularly defects of pyruvate metabolism, carbohydrate infusion worsens lactic acidosis. Replacement of some carbohydrate with fat as an intralipid infusion may partly reduce blood lactate levels, but infants with this degree of sensitivity to glucose infusion often are difficult to treat and suffer high mortality. Severe hyperammonemia that does not respond to dietary protein restriction and dextrose infusion must be treated by hemodialysis. Ammonia clearance with exchange

TABLE 82.5	Postmortem Biochemical Genetic Evaluation

To be performed on any deceased infant <1 year for which the cause of death is not apparent or any child with suspected IEM. Analyses are most reliable if obtained within 6 hours after death.

1. Contact newborn screening laboratory for results of neonatal screening.
2. Obtain a 3-mm punch biopsy of skin or Achilles tendon for fibroblast culture.
   A. Prepare skin with chlorhexidine (Hibiclens) or alcohol. Do not use Betadine because it may inhibit fibroblast growth.
   B. Use sterile technique.
   C. Store biopsy specimen in sterile RPMI culture media (if available) at room temperature. May be stored in sterile nonbacteriostatic saline for up to 24 hours prior to culture if culture media are not readily available.
   D. Send to cytogenetics or biochemical genetics laboratory for culture, possible enzyme analyses, and frozen storage.
3. Collect blood via cardiac puncture (~5 ml per tube).
   A. One red top tube at room temperature. Collect and store serum at −70°C.
      —I. Comprehensive metabolic panel (potassium, lipids, uric acid may not be accurate postmortem)
      —II. If hypoglycemic, insulin, growth hormone, and cortisol levels
   B. One green top (sodium heparin) at room temperature. Collect and store plasma at −70°C.
      —I. Plasma amino acid analysis
      —II. Plasma carnitine levels
      —III. Plasma acylcarnitine profile
   C. One green top (sodium heparin) at room temperature for cytogenetic (karyotype) analysis.
   D. If storage disorder suspected, one green top (sodium heparin) at 4°C (wet ice) for leukocyte isolation and diagnostic enzyme analyses.
   E. One lavender top (EDTA) tube at room temperature for complete blood count.
   F. One yellow top (ACD) tube for DNA isolation and possible mutation analysis.
   G. If infant <1 year, spot whole blood onto newborn screening filter paper card for repeat screen.
   H. Blood lactate and ammonia may not be accurate postmortem.
4. Collect urine (10–20 mL) by suprapubic tap or by swabbing the bladder interior with cotton swab.
   A. Urinalysis
   B. Urine-reducing substances
   C. Urine organic acid analysis
   D. If storage disorder suspected, quantitative urine mucopolysaccharide and oligosaccharide analysis
5. If urine is unobtainable, organic acid analysis may be performed on vitreous humor collected by needle aspiration from an eye. Freeze vitreous humor at −70°C
6. If blood is unobtainable, collect bile (2–3 mL) via puncture of the gallbladder for acylcarnitine profile. Store at −20°C.
7. Collect several biopsies (2 g each) from skeletal muscle, cardiac muscle, kidney, and liver.
   A. For routine histology, biopsies should be submitted fresh to the pathology laboratory.
   B. For enzyme analyses, biopsies should be wrapped in aluminum foil, placed in a labeled small specimen container, and immediately frozen in liquid nitrogen. Store at −70°C.

Modified from Steiner RD, Cederbaum SD. Laboratory evaluation of urea cycle disorders. *J Pediatr.* 2001;138(suppl 1):S21-29.

BOX 82.2	Postmortem Metabolic Evaluation

- **Blood**
  Electrolytes, glucose
  Amino acid analysis
  Organic acid analysis
  Acylcarnitine profile
- **Bile**
  Acylcarnitine profile
- **Vitreous humor**
  Organic acid analysis
  Acylcarnitine profile
- **Urine**
  Urinalysis
  Organic acid analysis
  Reducing substances
- **Liver and skeletal muscle:**
  Samples frozen at −80°C for possible enzyme analysis
- **Skin biopsy or Achilles tendon**
  Fibroblast culture for enzyme or DNA studies

transfusion or peritoneal dialysis is insufficient to adequately decrease blood ammonia levels. If the results of specialized biochemical genetic diagnostic tests are expected within 2 to 3 days, then parenteral dextrose infusion alone should be adequate to maintain nutrition until a more definitive treatment plan is available. Beyond 3 days, developing essential amino acid and fatty acid deficiencies may induce catabolism of endogenous protein and fat. To prevent this occurrence, enteral or parenteral nutrition with minimal amounts of protein (0.5 g/kg body weight/day) and lipid (20% of total energy intake) should be considered. Empiric administration of cofactors such as the B vitamins is not harmful and may improve metabolite clearance, particularly in disorders caused by deficiency of enzymes that require specific cofactors. Carnitine is required for transport of long-chain fatty acids across the mitochondrial membrane and serves a secondary role in the disposal of excess and potentially toxic acyl-CoA species. Secondary carnitine deficiency is commonly associated with acute metabolic decompensation in organic acidemias and fatty acid oxidation defects. L-Carnitine administration prevents secondary carnitine deficiency and may improve clearance of toxic metabolites; it is lifesaving in specific inherited dilated cardiomyopathies.

Classification of Inborn Errors of Metabolism by Clinical Presentation

As mentioned previously, the clinical presentation of IEM in neonates provides a paradigm for the suspicion and evaluation of potential IEM at all ages. The classification outlined here is adapted and expanded to include late-onset disorders from a neonatal IEM classification system first described by Jean-Marie Saudubray and colleagues.[4,9]

IEM can be classified into one of three groups by pathogenic mechanism. In group 1 IEMs, the production or catabolism of complex molecules is disturbed. The lysosomal storage and peroxisomal disorders are included in this group. The symptoms of these disorders include permanent and progressive somatic and neurologic abnormalities that develop in utero, are often clinically apparent at birth, and are unaffected by food intake. This group is often distinguished by the presence of somatic abnormalities such as dysmorphic features or hepatosplenomegaly. Typical clinical features,

TABLE 82.6   Emergency Treatment of Suspected Inborn Error of Metabolism

Goal	Action
Suppress toxic metabolite production	Discontinue oral feedings
Correct fluid imbalance and electrolyte abnormalities	Appropriate intravenous fluid management
Correct hypoglycemia	Intravenous dextrose-containing fluid infusion
Correct metabolic acidosis	Intravenous hydration if pH >7.2 Add IV bicarbonate if pH <7.2 Sodium bicarbonate (1 mEq/ml solution), 1 mEq/kg IV push at <1 mEq/min. May repeat ×3 until pH >7.2; maximum dose 7 mEq/kg/24 hours
Correct hyperammonemia	Suppress protein catabolism Hemodialysis
Treat infection	Appropriate infectious disease laboratory evaluation and antibiotic therapy
Suppress protein and lipid catabolism	Infuse D_{10}1/2NS at 1.5–2× maintenance rate Add insulin infusion if hyperglycemic If severe, unrelenting acidosis, consider growth hormone or testosterone therapy to promote anabolism.
Empiric cofactor administration	L-carnitine, 25–50 mg/kg/every 6 hours IV if organic acidemia suspected or cardiomyopathy present. B vitamin complex, 100 mg each vitamin every day Vitamin B_{12}, 1 mg IM ×1 if macrocytic anemia
Maintain nutritional status (if without enteral feeds ×2 days and without diagnosis of a specific IEM)	Enteral feeds or parenteral hyperalimentation to include the following: Protein, 0.5 g/kg/day only Lipid, 20% of total energy intake Carbohydrate to provide at least the minimum necessary energy intake

TABLE 82.7   Features of Group 1 Inborn Errors of Metabolism

Clinical Features	Laboratory Findings	Possible Diagnoses	Specialized Diagnostic Tests

Hepatosplenomegaly
Coarse facies
Macroglossia
Fetal hydrops
Macular cherry red spots
Bone changes
Hypotonia or hypertonia
Chronic rhinorrhea
Failure to thrive
	Liver dysfunction
	No acidosis
	Normal ammonia
	Normal glucose
		Neonatal onset
		  GM1 gangliosidosis
		  I cell disease
		  Sialidosis
		  Galactosialidosis
		  Niemann-Pick type A
		  MPS VII
		  CDG
		Later onset
		  Tay-Sachs disease
		  Krabbe disease
		  Other MPS syndromes
		  Niemann-Pick B or C
			Urine mucopolysaccharides
			Urine oligosaccharides
			Serum transferrin electrophoresis
			Enzyme analysis in molecular DNA analysis serum, lymphocytes, or fibroblasts

Hepatomegaly
Dysmorphic facies
Severe hypotonia
Large anterior fontanelle
Seizures
Epiphyseal calcific stippling on x-ray
	Liver dysfunction
	No acidosis
	Normal ammonia
	Normal glucose
	Adrenal insufficiency
		Peroxisomal disorders
		  Zellweger syndrome
		  Neonatal adrenoleukodystrophy
		  Others
			Plasma very-long-chain fatty acid analysis
			Functional and genetic analysis of fibroblasts
			Molecular DNA analysis

CDG, congenital disorders of glycosylation; *MPS*, mucopolysaccharidosis; *MPS VII*, Sly syndrome.

potential neonatal and late-onset diagnoses, and confirmatory diagnostic tests are listed in Table 82.7.

In group 2 IEMs, the symptoms are caused by defects in the production or utilization of energy. This group includes the congenital lactic acidoses, glycogenoses, gluconeogenic defects, and fatty acid oxidation disorders. In group 3 IEMs, clinical symptoms are caused by progressive intoxication in a previously well infant because of accumulation of toxic metabolites proximal to a metabolic block. Often, neonatal onset IEM in groups 2 and 3 can be distinguished by the time of clinical onset relative to birth. The symptoms of a block in energy production or utilization (group 2) may present within hours after birth, whereas symptoms of intoxication (group 3) develop over the first week of life with increasing food intake and accumulation of toxic metabolites. However, variants of many of these disorders may not become clinically apparent for several months or even years after birth.

Group 2 Inborn Errors of Metabolism

Systemic or tissue-specific impaired energy production from food substrates is the unifying feature of disorders classified in group 2. Generalized profound neurologic dysfunction, including severe central hypotonia, coma, and seizures, sometimes with peripheral spasticity or abnormal movements, typifies the clinical presentation. Children with these disorders present with similar clinical phenotypes but are easily separated into four subgroups (A-D) based on associated results of routine laboratory studies (Table 82.8). Severe refractory generalized motor seizures, often beginning within the first hours after birth, sometimes even prenatally, are the hallmark of subgroup A. Routine laboratory studies (glucose, blood pH, electrolytes, ammonia) are generally normal unless the infant is near extremis and secondary metabolic abnormalities are present. Several inherited disorders are associated with this phenotype; diagnostic differentiation depends on clinical evaluation by an experienced pediatric neurologist or geneticist and the judicious use of specialized diagnostic laboratory tests.

The amino acid glycine is an abundant neurotransmitter within the central nervous system (CNS). Inherited deficiency of the glycine cleavage system, which removes glycine from its receptor in the neuronal synapse, causes severe unrelenting generalized seizures and profound developmental arrest. The only ubiquitous laboratory finding is an elevated cerebrospinal fluid (CSF/plasma glycine ratio).[10] Sulfite oxidase deficiency, either as a primary genetic defect or secondary to generalized deficiency of its molybdenum-containing cofactor, is another rare but important cause of neonatal-onset seizures. Infantile-onset pyridoxine- or folinic acid-dependent seizure disorders have both been found to be caused by recessively inherited deficiency of α-aminoadipic semialdehyde (α-AASA) dehydrogenase, an intermediate enzyme in the metabolism of the amino acid lysine.[11] Consequently, all neonates with refractory seizures should be screened for these treatable disorders either through measurement of α-AASA in urine or sequencing of the *ALDH7A1* (antiquitin) gene. Profound neurologic dysfunction with seizures is one of

TABLE 82.8   Features of Group 2 Inborn Errors of Metabolism

Clinical Features	Associated Laboratory Findings	Possible Diagnoses	Specialized Diagnostic Testing
Subgroup A			
Profound neurologic dysfunction Severe hypotonia Seizures	No acidosis Normal ammonia Normal glucose	Nonketotic hyperglycinemia Sulfite oxidase or molybdenum cofactor deficiency Pyridoxine- or folinic acid-responsive seizures Peroxisomal disorders Respiratory chain disorders CDG Cholesterol synthesis defects Neurotransmitter synthesis defects	Plasma and CSF amino acid analysis Urine sulfocysteine Urine oxypurines Urine α–aminoadipic semialdehyde Plasma very-long-chain fatty acid analysis Blood and CSF lactate Plasma acylcarnitine Urine organic acids Serum transferrin electrophoresis Plasma sterols CSF neurotransmitters Neonatal onset epilepsy gene sequencing panel
Subgroup B			

Neurologic dysfunction
Hypotonia
Seizures
With severe acidosis
  ± liver dysfunction
  ± dilated cardiomyopathy
	Severe acidosis
	Lactic acidosis
	± ketosis
	± hypoglycemia
	± anemia
		Congenital lactic acidoses
		Pyruvate dehydrogenase
		Pyruvate carboxylase
		Respiratory chain disorders
			Blood and CSF lactate
			Plasma and CSF amino acid analysis
			Urine organic acids
			Diagnostic muscle biopsy to include histology, enzyme analysis

Subgroup C			

Neurologic dysfunction
Vomiting
Dehydration
Hypotonia
Coma
  ± hepatomegaly, liver dysfunction
  ± dilated cardiomyopathy
Triggered by fasting or intercurrent illness
	Hypoglycemia
	No ketones in urine
	Acidosis
	± hyperammonemia
	± lactic acidosis
		Fatty acid oxidation defects
		  MCAD
		  LCHAD
		  VLCAD
		  CPT II
		  CAT
		  MACD
		Ketogenesis defects
		  HMG-CoA lyase
		  MCKAT
		  SCOT
			Urine organic acids
			Plasma carnitine
			Plasma acylcarnitine profile
			Diagnostic fasting study
			Fatty acid oxidation studies in cultured skin fibroblasts
			Gene-specific mutation analysis

Subgroup D			

Neurologic dysfunction triggered by short fast
Hepatomegaly
	Severe fasting hypoglycemia
	Lactic acidosis
	Normal ammonia
	± ketosis
	± hyperuricemia
	± hypophosphatemia
		Glycogen storage
		  Glycogenosis 1
		  Glycogenosis 3
		Fructose 1,6-bisphosphatase deficiency
			Diagnostic fasting study
			Enzyme studies in liver
			Gene-specific mutation analysis

CAT, carnitine acylcarnitine translocase; *CDG,* congenital disorders of glycosylation; *CPT II,* carnitine palmitoyltransferase II; *HMG-CoA lyase,* 3-hydroxy-3-methylglutaryl-CoA lyase; *LCHAD,* long chain 3-hydroxyacyl-CoA dehydrogenase; *MACD,* multiple acyl-CoA dehydrogenase deficiency (also known as glutaric aciduria type 2); *MCAD,* medium chain acyl-CoA dehydrogenase; *MCKAT,* medium chain ketoacyl-CoA thiolase; *SCOT,* succinyl-CoA:oxaloacetate transferase; *VLCAD,* very-long-chain acyl-CoA dehydrogenase.

many possible clinical presentations of infants with peroxisomal or respiratory chain disorders. Some subtypes of a still expanding list of congenital disorders of glycosylation present with seizures,[12] as do disorders of sterol production such as Smith-Lemli-Opitz syndrome,[13] but these diagnoses are often associated with stereotypic dysmorphic features and anomalies. Finally, disorders of neurotransmitter synthesis should be considered in any infant with idiopathic seizures and neurologic dysfunction, especially if a movement disorder, most commonly dystonia, is also present. Abnormal CSF neurotransmitter levels (5-methyltetrahydrofolate, 5-hydroxyindoleacetic acid, homovanillic acid, 3-methyl-DOPA) are the only associated laboratory diagnostic clue in this latter category of disease.

Severe persistent lactic acidosis is the hallmark of the disorders in subgroup B of early-onset energy deficiency diseases. The presence of metabolic acidosis with an elevated anion gap suggests the possibility of lactic acidosis (subgroup B) or an organic acidemia (see group 3, intoxication types); these are differentiated by measurement of blood lactate and urine organic acid analysis. Blood lactate is most reliably measured on arterial blood or a free-flowing sample drawn from an indwelling central venous catheter. Artifactual elevation of lactate in peripheral venous blood samples is nearly ubiquitous and should be confirmed by lactate measurement in a more appropriate sample. Secondary lactic acidosis resulting from asphyxia, poor tissue perfusion, or tissue necrosis is much more common and may be difficult to differentiate from the congenital lactic acidoses (see also Chapters 76 and 80). Occult cardiac disease, intracranial hemorrhage, or bowel necrosis must considered and ruled out in infants with severe lactic acidosis. Congenital lactic acidosis generally persists despite adequate life support measures, including fluid resuscitation and ventilatory assistance. In certain enzyme deficiencies, the blood lactate level may further increase with IV dextrose infusion. Simultaneous measurements of blood and CSF lactate and amino acids are useful for differentiating primary from secondary lactic acidoses. In congenital lactic acidosis, the CSF lactate level often is higher than the blood lactate level, whereas the CNS is relatively protected from systemic acidosis in secondary lactic acidemias. The blood pyruvate level is elevated in some congenital lactic acidoses such as pyruvate dehydrogenase deficiency. However, accurate measurement of blood pyruvate is difficult and fraught with false-positive elevations. Elevated plasma alanine (which is measured as part of a plasma amino acid analysis) is a more stable and reliable indicator of pyruvic acidosis, as alanine and pyruvate are in equilibrium. Enzymatic analysis in cultured skin fibroblasts or mitochondria isolated from a fresh muscle biopsy often is necessary to confirm a specific enzyme deficiency.

Children with subgroup C defects present with hypoketotic hypoglycemia, triggered by fasting, metabolic stress, or intercurrent illness. In these disorders, utilization of fatty acids as fuel is impaired. The most common of the fatty acid oxidation defects is MCADD, which occurs in up to 1:10,000 Caucasian births. Although fatty acid oxidation and ketogenesis defects may present in the newborn period, particularly in the setting of delayed maternal milk production for exclusively breast-fed infants, the first clinically significant episode may not occur for weeks to months or even years after birth. With extended fasting or intercurrent illness where metabolic demand exceeds

available energy supply, severe lethargy acutely develops and then progresses to coma. Recurrent vomiting and consequent dehydration may be associated. Sudden infant death after an overnight fast is an all too frequent initial presentation in up to one-third of infants with fatty acid oxidation defects. Infants who survive may suffer recurrent episodes of fasting or illness-induced coma, leading to progressive CNS damage and permanent disability. Metabolic acidosis (resulting from accumulation of partially oxidized fatty acids or secondary lactic acidosis), hyperammonemia, hepatomegaly and liver dysfunction, and hypertrophic cardiomyopathy may occur during acute metabolic decompensation episodes. Liver histology is typified by severe steatosis. Chronically affected children may exhibit recurrent vomiting, failure to thrive, developmental delay, and muscular hypotonia. Certain disorders that affect oxidation of long-chain fatty acids are frequently associated with recurrent rhabdomyolysis and myoglobinuria (long-chain 3-hydroxyacyl-CoA dehydrogenase [LCHAD] deficiency, trifunctional protein deficiency, very-long-chain acyl-CoA dehydrogenase [VLCAD] deficiency, or carnitine-palmitoyl transferase [CPT]-II deficiency) or pigmentary retinopathy and slowly progressive vision loss (LCHAD or trifunctional protein deficiency). Mothers of infants with fatty acid oxidation disorders (particularly LCHAD or trifunctional protein deficiency) may present with acute liver dysfunction during pregnancy with an affected fetus. This may manifest as acute fatty liver of pregnancy or maternal hemolysis, elevated liver enzymes, or low platelets (HELLP) syndrome. In the affected infant, hypoglycemia (serum glucose <40 mg/dL) with inappropriately low or absent ketone production during a symptomatic episode is the key laboratory finding that leads to suspicion of a disorder in this subgroup. Differentiation of the specific defects requires analysis of urine organic acids and plasma acylcarnitine species. Between episodes, when the child is clinically well, the urine organic acid profile may be completely normal. Acylcarnitine profiles are more consistently abnormal, but both tests, if normal initially, should be repeated on samples obtained during a symptomatic period to absolutely rule out the possibility of a fatty acid oxidation defect. Carnitine is required for normal fatty acid oxidation; long-chain fatty acids are activated to fatty acyl-CoA, then esterified to carnitine by CPT-I on the outer mitochondrial membrane. These acylcarnitine esters are then transported into mitochondria to complete the oxidation process. In fatty acid oxidation defects, the metabolic block leads to accumulation of the fatty acyl-CoA substrate specific to the deficient enzyme; these species appear in blood as acylcarnitine esters. Analysis of plasma acylcarnitine profiles by tandem mass spectrometry often suggests a specific enzyme deficiency in children with suspected fatty acid oxidation disorders.[14] In the past, diagnostic confirmation may require enzyme analysis in liver tissue or radiometric evaluation of fatty acid oxidation in cultured skin fibroblasts. For the most part, however, these assays have been replaced by sequencing of genes encoding enzymes in the fatty acid oxidation pathway. Two disorders, namely, MCADD[15] and LCHAD deficiency,[16] are associated with relatively common disease-causing mutations. Treatment of all disorders in this subgroup is based on the provision of adequate nonfat calories and prevention of fasting. Generous IV glucose infusion is lifesaving and essential during acute episodes of metabolic decompensation. Chronic dietary therapy is tailored to the specific enzyme deficiency involved. Many practitioners prescribe carnitine supplementation, initially intravenously during an acute episode and later orally, but the efficacy of this intervention has not been formally investigated in any controlled clinical trial, and its use in disorders of long-chain fatty acid oxidation remains controversial.

Hypoglycemia following a short fast of only 4 to 6 hours is highly suggestive of a glycogen storage disease or disorder of gluconeogenesis such as fructose 1,6-bisphosphatase deficiency. These disorders of energy deficiency are classified in subgroup D. These infants appear healthy while fed but quickly become obtunded and hypotonic with fasting hypoglycemia. Hepatomegaly is a prominent physical feature. During acute hypoglycemia, other biochemical derangements, including lactic acidosis, hypophosphatemia, hyperuricemia, and hypertriglyceridemia, are frequently present. Confirmation of the diagnosis may require a provocative fast under controlled conditions with continuous monitoring and, sometimes, measurement of glycogen content or enzymatic analysis on a liver biopsy specimen. Molecular DNA analyses are commonly available for a less invasive approach to diagnostic confirmation in this class of diseases.

Group 3 Inborn Errors of Metabolism

Infants with group 3 IEM display symptoms and a progressive clinical course suggestive of intoxication. In these infants, who appear completely healthy at birth and for the first few days of life, neurologic dysfunction appears as toxic metabolites accumulate with increasing food intake. Initial symptoms may include vomiting and lethargy that progress, perhaps over only a few hours, to complete coma or shock. This specific clinical presentation in particular suggests the possibility of bacterial or viral sepsis; evaluation for infectious disease is entirely appropriate. However, the clinician must remain alert to the possibility of an underlying IEM in a previously healthy infant suffering catastrophic illness within the first days of life. Group 3 IEMs can be subdivided into four subgroups (A-D) based on specific clinical and laboratory findings (Table 82.9).

Maple syrup urine disease ([MSUD] branched-chain ketoacid dehydrogenase [BCKD] deficiency) affects the catabolism of the branched-chain amino acids leucine, isoleucine, and valine and is the only disorder in subgroup A. Affected infants present with coma; abnormal body movements including seizures; and, in contrast to many IEMs, hypertonia and opisthotonus. A severe burst-suppression pattern is the typical EEG abnormality. A sweet body odor, concentrated particularly in urine and cerumen, is often present. Mothers with previously affected children can often diagnose MSUD in a new infant by the presence of this odor. Routine laboratory studies may document mild metabolic acidosis and mild ketosis but normal lactate and ammonia. The branched-chain ketoacids that accumulate in MSUD react only slightly with the urine dipstick test for ketones but readily form a flocculent white precipitate with 2,4-dinitrophenylhydrazine (DNPH) in

---

TABLE 82.9 Features of Group 3 Inborn Errors of Metabolism

Clinical Features	Associated Laboratory Findings	Possible Diagnoses	Specialized Diagnostic Studies
Subgroup A			
Neurologic deterioration Coma Abnormal movements Hypertonia Sweet odor	Mild acidosis Normal lactate ± ketonuria Normal ammonia + urine DNPH test	Maple syrup disease (branched chain ketoacid dehydrogenase deficiency)	Plasma amino acid analysis Urine organic acid analysis
Subgroup B			

Neurologic deterioration
Coma
Dehydration
	Severe acidosis
	Severe ketonuria
	± hyperammonemia
	± lactic acidosis
	± hypoglycemia
	± neutropenia
	– urine DNPH test
		Organic acidemias
		  Propionic acidemia
		  Methylmalonic acidemia
		  Isovaleric acidemia
		  MCD deficiency
		  Others
			Urine organic acid analysis
			Plasma carnitine levels
			Plasma acylcarnitine profile
			Urine acylglycine profile
			Molecular DNA analysis

Subgroup C			
Neurologic deterioration Coma Seizures Hypotonia ± liver dysfunction	Severe hyperammonemia No acidosis + alkalosis Low BUN Normal glucose Normal lactate	Urea cycle disorders (CPS, OTC, ASS, ASL deficiencies) Triple H syndrome (hyperornithinemia-hyperammonemia-homocitrullinuria)	Plasma amino acid analysis Urine organic acid analysis Urine orotic acid Enzyme studies in liver or fibroblasts Molecular DNA analysis
Subgroup D			
Neurologic deterioration Hepatomegaly Liver dysfunction Cholestatic jaundice	Direct hyperbilirubinemia ± hypoglycemia ± acidosis ± lactic acidosis ± ketosis	Galactosemia Fructosemia Tyrosinemia type 1 Neonatal hemochromatosis Respiratory chain disorders	Urine-reducing substances Plasma amino acid analysis Urine organic acid analysis Urine succinylacetone Enzyme studies Molecular DNA analysis

ASL, Argininosuccinate lyase; *ASS,* argininosuccinate synthetase; *BUN,* blood urea nitrogen; *CPS,* carbamyl phosphate synthetase; *DNPH,* dinitrophenylhydrazine; *MCD,* multiple carboxylase deficiency; *OTC,* ornithine transcarbamoylase.

a urine metabolic screen. The presence and specific identities of branched-chain ketoacids in urine are confirmed by urine organic acid analysis. Plasma amino acid analysis reveals tremendous elevation of leucine with lesser accumulations of valine and isoleucine. The neurologic symptoms associated with MSUD result entirely from leucine intoxication. Valine and isoleucine, which do not cross the blood-brain barrier as readily as leucine, seem to contribute little to the neurologic phenotype. Reduction of leucine levels in the body is the goal of MSUD treatment.[17] Emergency therapy during the initial clinical episode includes dietary protein restriction and IV infusion of dextrose-containing fluids. Hyponatremia is a common associated feature; IV hydration with hypotonic fluids easily exacerbates this problem. Additionally, leucine accumulates in CSF and brain and is strongly osmotically active. Rapid IV infusion of hypotonic solutions in several instances has led to acute cerebral edema and death. Dextrose solutions containing a minimum of 0.45% saline (one-half normal saline) are essential, but 10% dextrose with normal saline is preferred if the serum sodium is <135 mEq/L. With administration of IV dextrose, mild hyperglycemia secondary to insulin resistance may occur; inclusion of regular insulin (often only 0.05 units/kg body weight/hour) by either IV infusion or subcutaneous injection promotes anabolism, suppresses endogenous protein catabolism, and accelerates leucine clearance. The vitamin thiamine is a cofactor for BCKD; some individuals with BCKD deficiency (usually with a late rather than neonatal presentation) may respond clinically to thiamine supplementation. Oral thiamine (100 mg/day) is often given empirically to determine whether there is any effect on leucine levels. Once the diagnosis of MSUD is confirmed by plasma amino acid analysis, enteral feedings with a medical food that is free of branched-chain amino acids should be initiated even if the infant is comatose and nasogastric feedings are necessary. Parenteral hydration should continue until results of urine ketone and DNPH tests are negative and full enteral feeds are reestablished. On this regimen, plasma valine and isoleucine levels plummet rapidly, but several days may be required before plasma leucine normalizes. Valine and isoleucine deficiencies that frequently develop on this regimen stimulate endogenous protein catabolism, which impairs reduction of blood leucine, prolongs neurologic impairment, and chronically may be associated with symptoms of protein insufficiency (hair loss, skin breakdown, growth failure). Therefore valine and isoleucine supplementation (50–100 mg/kg/day) is required. Chronic lifelong therapy involves dietary protein restriction and provision of sufficient energy and amino acids in a leucine-free synthetic medical food. Despite this effort, infants who suffered prolonged severe leucinosis as neonates often exhibit significant developmental disability. Early diagnosis and appropriate therapy critically enhance neurodevelopmental outcome.

Severe ketoacidosis is the hallmark of IEMs in subgroup B, the organic acidemias. Methylmalonic, propionic, and isovaleric acidemias are the most common disorders in this subgroup. Infants with organic acidemia present with catastrophic episodes of vomiting, dehydration, and coma. Hypoglycemia, lactic acidosis, hyperammonemia, neutropenia, or pancytopenia may be associated findings depending on the specific IEM. The urine dipstick test for ketones is strongly positive, but in contrast to MSUD, little precipitate forms following the addition of DNPH reagent to the urine. Identification of the specific offending organic acid is accomplished by urine organic acid analysis using gas chromatography–mass spectrometry. Diagnostic confirmation may require enzymatic analysis in tissues such as leukocytes, liver, or cultured skin fibroblasts. Molecular DNA analysis is increasingly available as a diagnostic modality as well. Cessation of protein intake, vigorous rehydration with dextrose-containing fluid, and management of acidosis with sodium bicarbonate infusion are the mainstays of emergency management. In severely acidotic patients, especially with associated hyperammonemia, hemodialysis may be useful for quickly removing both ammonia and the offending organic acid with the goal of minimizing CNS damage. IV infusion of l-carnitine (100–300 mg/kg/day) assists with the removal of the offending organic acid and prevents secondary carnitine deficiency. Oral l-glycine supplementation has a similar role in certain IEMs, most notably isovaleric acidemia. Chronic therapy is tailored to the specific enzyme deficiency but often involves dietary protein restriction and provision of a synthetic medical food supplying sufficient energy and amino acids. Recurrent episodes of life-threatening ketoacidosis and coma, generally triggered by fasting or intercurrent illness, are often the greatest long-term clinical difficulties.

Advancing dietary protein intake and normal protein catabolism during the first few days of life lead to severe hyperammonemia in infants with urea cycle and allied disorders (subgroup C). The clinical presentation is nonspecific, with progressive vomiting and neurologic dysfunction. Routine laboratory studies are generally deceptively normal, although the BUN often is below the limits of detection in infants who are unable to synthesize urea. No acidosis is present unless the infant is apneic or hypoperfused and secondary lactic acidosis has developed. Most severely hyperammonemic infants demonstrate respiratory alkalosis secondary to Kussmaul-like hyperventilation triggered by cerebral edema. Detection of hyperammonemia is the critical diagnostic key. The blood ammonia level must be measured in any child with acute-onset obtundation without a clear etiology such as trauma. Determination of the specific IEM involved requires analysis of blood amino acids and urine organic acids. Diagnostic confirmation is now often accomplished through molecular DNA analysis of specific genes involved in the urea cycle, but in rare instances, enzyme analysis in liver or for a few defects in cultured skin fibroblasts may yet be necessary if molecular testing is inconclusive. Provision of nonprotein energy and suppression of protein catabolism through IV dextrose infusion are essential, as in the organic acidemias, but emergency hemodialysis to rapidly decrease blood ammonia is absolutely required if any possibility of favorable neurodevelopmental outcome is to be preserved. Ammonia clearance by exchange transfusion or peritoneal dialysis is insufficient to accomplish this goal. Even with prompt hemodialysis, the metabolic derangement in some infants is so severe that little sustained decrease in blood ammonia is observed. Despite aggressive therapy, neonatal-onset urea cycle disorders are frequently lethal. The few infants exposed to hyperammonemia for a prolonged period who, because of extraordinary life support efforts, survive are often profoundly neurologically impaired. On the other hand, clinical outcome is favorable in cases where blood ammonia levels rapidly correct on hemodialysis. This dichotomy in outcome presents a considerable dilemma to the intensivist faced with these critical treatment decisions.

In practice, hemodialysis should be attempted as soon as possible after the discovery of hyperammonemia unless clinical signs of severe permanent CNS damage are already present. Disorder-specific therapy should continue for infants whose blood ammonia levels immediately normalize with hemodialysis. Aggressive life support measures should be limited for infants with recalcitrant hyperammonemia. Following dialysis, generous IV hydration and provision of nonprotein calories should continue. The amino acid arginine, normally synthesized through the urea cycle, becomes an essential amino acid that must be provided exogenously in urea cycle disorders. l-Arginine hydrochloride is available for IV administration as 10% solution and should be added to the IV fluid bag to give 0.66 g arginine HCl/m^2/day (6 mL/kg/day in infants). The ammonia scavenging agents sodium phenylacetate and sodium benzoate are available as a combined IV solution. Administration of this solution dramatically improves ammonia clearance and is indicated for the acute management of the proximal urea cycle disorders, but it is associated with severe adverse effects including metabolic acidosis and erosive gastritis if administered inappropriately. This solution should be used only in consultation with a provider experienced with its administration and with careful monitoring. Long-term therapy is based on dietary protein restriction and oral l-arginine or l-citrulline supplementation. Oral administration of sodium benzoate, sodium phenylbutyrate, or glycerol triphenylbutyrate as ammonia scavengers is often prescribed. Episodes of fasting or illness-induced hyperammonemic coma frequently recur. Management of recurrent hyperammonemia in a patient known to have a urea cycle disorder is similar to that outlined earlier but can be tailored to the specific defect. Liver transplantation is a viable treatment option for individuals suffering recurrent hyperammonemia and chronic clinical and developmental difficulties despite adequate nutritional and medical therapy.

Hepatomegaly, liver dysfunction, and cholestatic jaundice in association with neurologic deterioration are the central presenting features of IEM in subgroup D. For all of these disorders, the accumulating toxin is particularly damaging to hepatocellular function. Hypoglycemia, acidosis, and mild ketosis may be present. Bacterial infection, particularly urinary tract infection, bacteremia, or meningitis, often caused by *E. coli* or other gram-negative enteral flora, is a frequent occurrence in infants with galactosemia. The specific diagnosis is suggested by the clinical scenario and by the results of screening laboratory studies. Infants with this clinical presentation who are breast-fed or receiving cow's milk–based infant formula are at risk for symptoms of galactosemia, given that lactose (milk sugar) is a disaccharide of galactose and glucose. Infants receiving exclusively soy milk–based formula ingest little galactose. The predominant dietary carbohydrates in soy formula are fructose and glucose, so infants fed soy formula who have this clinical presentation are likely to have fructosemia rather than galactosemia. More typically, infants with fructosemia present clinically after the introduction of fruit to their diet. In either galactosemia or fructosemia, reducing sugars are detected in urine following ingestion of the offending sugar by the urine-reducing substance test (Clinitest). Plasma tyrosine level is elevated, urine organic acid analysis displays metabolites from the tyrosine pathway, and succinylacetone is detected in the urine of children with tyrosinemia type I (fumarylacetoacetate hydrolase deficiency).

Neonatal hemochromatosis can be diagnosed only on liver biopsy by staining for iron. Diagnostic confirmation differs for each disorder but may include further metabolite analyses, enzymatic analysis in tissue, or molecular DNA testing. Initial therapy is nonspecific: cessation of enteral feeding and IV infusion of dextrose-containing fluid. Once the exact diagnosis is known, a specific therapy plan can be developed. For the carbohydrate disorders, the offending sugar must be reduced or eliminated from the diet. Galactosemic infants are fed soy milk–based formulas only. After weaning, ingestion of dairy products, including baked goods prepared with dairy products, is strictly avoided. Similarly, fructosemic individuals must strenuously avoid any fructose-containing foods. In prior eras, cirrhosis and liver failure were the inevitable outcome in children with tyrosinemia type I unless they received a liver transplant. Effective therapy that prevents liver degeneration in tyrosinemia has now been developed. The oral drug 2-(2-nitro-4-trifluoro-methylbenzoyl)-1,3-cyclohexanedione (NTBC) blocks tyrosine metabolism upstream from FAH and prevents accumulation of the intermediate metabolites that are toxic to hepatocytes.[18] This medication was highly successful in preventing cirrhosis in two separate clinical trials and has been approved by the US Food and Drug Administration for general use. The long-term efficacy of NTBC therapy, particularly with regard to the incidence of hepatic adenoma, a common complication of tyrosinemia I, has yet to be proved.[19]

Summary

Most IEMs with symptom onset in the neonatal period emerge as one of the clinical presentations described. As mentioned previously, many of these IEMs have milder or late-onset forms that present with identical symptoms as described, but months or years after birth and often following the stress of fasting or intercurrent illness. These clinical scenarios provide a framework for the recognition, initial evaluation, and emergency treatment of infants with IEM. The remainder of this chapter focuses on the differential diagnosis of select clinical situations encountered in the pediatric intensive care unit.

Metabolic Acidosis

The key to the differential diagnosis of metabolic acidosis is calculating the serum anion gap (Na – [Cl^- + HCO_3]). This calculation, normally 10 to 15 mM, represents the unmeasured negative ions, predominantly albumin, in blood. Normal anion gap acidosis (low serum HCO_3 but normal anion gap) is caused by excess bicarbonate loss from either the gut (diarrhea) or kidney (renal tubular acidosis). An elevated or so-called positive anion gap suggests the presence of another unmeasured anion. Incidentally, a low serum anion gap may be seen in extreme hypoalbuminemia, as occurs in nephrotic syndrome (see Chapters 75 and 76).

The differential diagnosis of positive anion gap metabolic acidosis in children is similar to that of adults (eg, a favorite mnemonic may be applied, such as MUDPILES or KETONES), but with the addition of another class of acidoses, the IEMs. Poisoning with methanol, ethanol, paraldehyde, isoniazid, or salicylates can be readily ruled out by history or drug screen. Uremia is also easily discovered by laboratory evaluation. The most common etiologies of a positive anion gap acidosis in children are ketosis, lactic acidosis, or a combination of the two. Extreme dehydration can cause both ketosis and lactic acidosis; these abnormalities are readily corrected with vigorous parenteral rehydration with dextrose-containing fluids. Persistent lactic acidosis suggests ongoing tissue damage from hypoxemia, hypoperfusion, or, more rarely, an inborn error of mitochondrial metabolism. It should be remembered that several organic acids, such as propionic and methylmalonic acids, react with the urinary ketones dipstick. These pathologic organic acids can be differentiated only from the more typical ketones, 3-hydroxybutyric and acetoacetic acids, by urine organic acid analysis. Severe positive anion gap metabolic acidosis that cannot be easily explained by the clinical context, especially if it occurs recurrently or is recalcitrant to parenteral fluid therapy, suggests an inborn error of organic acid metabolism and should be evaluated with a battery of screening metabolic studies including plasma amino acid analysis, urine organic acid analysis, and urine qualitative metabolic screen.

Hypoglycemia

Hypoglycemia can be defined as a blood glucose concentration less than 40 mg/dL.[20] Low blood glucose may be present within the first few hours after birth, especially in preterm or low-birth-weight infants, but the capacity for effective gluconeogenesis and fatty acid oxidation is induced within the first day after birth. Therefore blood glucose less than 40 mg/dL is distinctly unusual after the first 24 hours of life, particularly in infants who have started feeding, and should be thoroughly

investigated (Fig. 82.2). A review of hypoglycemia in infants and children along with a useful diagnostic algorithm has been published.[21] A detailed medical history and careful physical examination are essential to discovering the cause of hypoglycemia. The timing of hypoglycemia relative to feeding is a critical item of historical information. Persistent or postprandial hypoglycemia suggests hyperinsulinism. Hypoglycemia after a short fast (3–6 hours) along with permanent hepatomegaly suggests a glycogen storage disorder. Hypoglycemia following a longer fast (8–12 hours) suggests a defect in gluconeogenesis or a problem with utilization of fatty acids. The presence of ketones in urine (as measured qualitatively by urine dipstick) or in serum (quantitative measurement of 3-hydroxybutyrate or acetoacetate) is an important clue to the etiology of hypoglycemia. Ketosis during hypoglycemia demonstrates that insulin secretion is appropriately suppressed and that fatty acid mobilization and oxidation are intact. Glycogen storage disorders, gluconeogenic defects, and defects of ketone utilization all are associated with ketosis. The absence of ketogenesis during hypoglycemia suggests that either insulin levels are inappropriately elevated or fatty acid oxidation is blocked. An important caveat to this rule is that infants younger than approximately 1 week cannot normally produce enough ketones during fasting to trigger a positive urine dipstick test for ketones. The absence of urine ketones in an infant younger than 1 week does not contribute to the differential diagnosis of hypoglycemia. On the other hand, serum ketones increase with fasting even in neonates, and this test provides

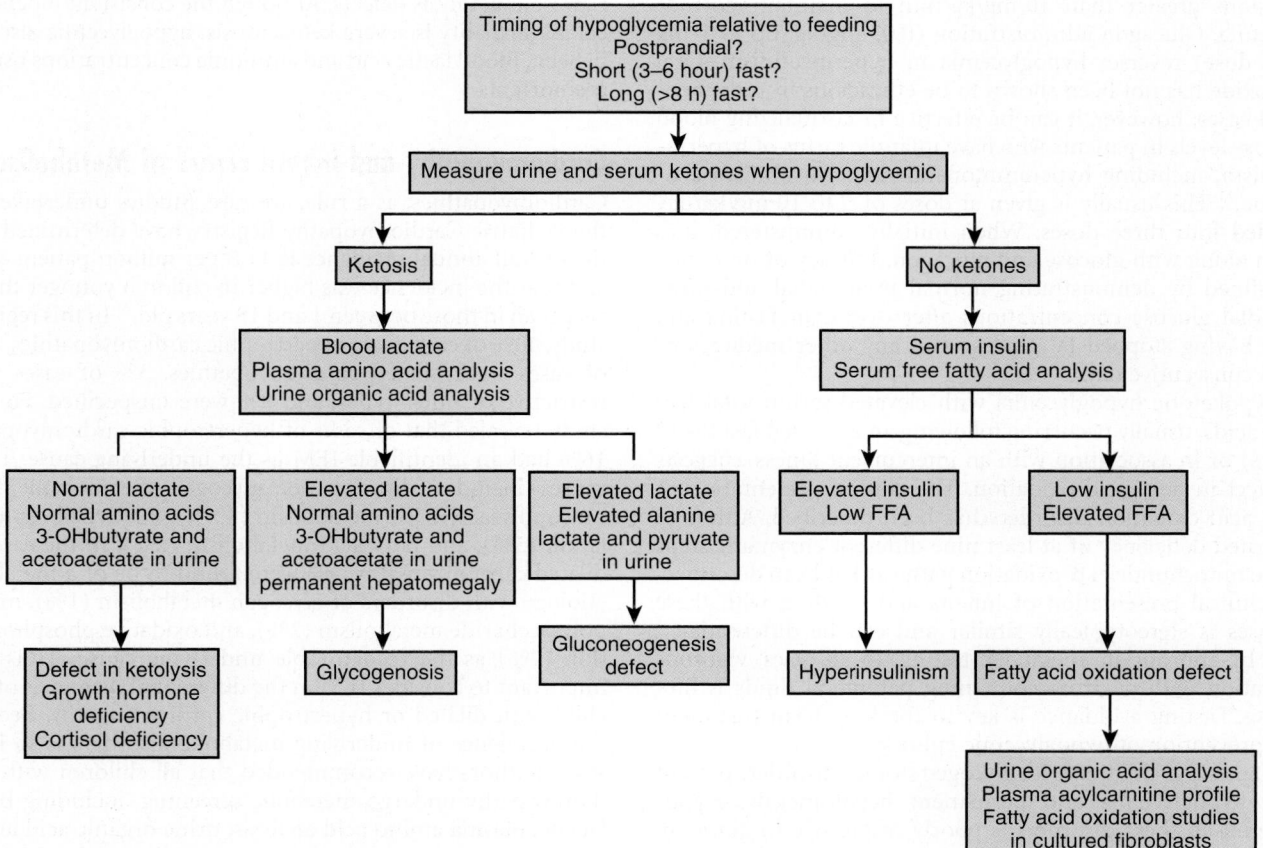

Fig. 82.2. Algorithm for evaluation of hypoglycemia in children. *FFA*, free fatty acid; *SCOT*, succinyl-CoA oxoacid transferase.

a valuable result in the investigation of hypoglycemia. In hypoketotic hypoglycemia, measurement of total serum free fatty acids provides further useful diagnostic information. During fasting, insulin secretion normally is suppressed, free fatty acids are mobilized into circulation from peripheral adipose tissues, and ketones are produced by oxidation of fatty acids in liver. A low serum total free fatty acid level during hypoketotic hypoglycemia strongly suggests inappropriate insulin secretion, even if insulin levels do not appear to be dramatically elevated. Hypoketotic hypoglycemia in association with elevated serum total free fatty acids suggests a defect in fatty acid oxidation.

The importance of treating hypoglycemia cannot be overemphasized as affected individuals are at high risk for seizures and permanent brain damage.[22] After appropriate diagnostic studies are obtained, hypoglycemia should be treated with IV glucose administration at the rate of normal hepatic glucose production, approximately 10 mg glucose/kg body weight per minute or 150 mL/kg per day of a 10% solution until the underlying disorder is identified and more appropriate therapies can be initiated.

Hypoketotic hypoglycemia with low serum total free fatty acids suggests hyperinsulinism. Hyperinsulinism presenting in the newborn period may be caused by intrauterine exposure to elevated glucose levels (maternal diabetes mellitus), familial hyperinsulinemic hypoglycemia (defect in the sulfonylurea receptor), or hyperammonemia/hyperinsulinism syndrome (abnormality in regulation of insulin secretion secondary to mutation in glutamate dehydrogenase). Infants with hyperinsulinism often are obese and require glucose infusions greater than 10 mg/kg/min to maintain normoglycemia. Glucagon administration (0.03 mg/kg, up to 1-mg total dose) reverses hypoglycemia in hyperinsulinism. Oral diazoxide has not been shown to be efficacious in most neonatal cases; however, it can be effective in normalizing blood glucose levels in patients who have infantile forms of hyperinsulinism, including hyperammonemia/hyperinsulinism syndrome.[23] This usually is given at doses of 5 to 10 mg/kg/day divided into three doses. When initially administered, it is given along with glucose and glucagon. Efficacy of diazoxide is defined by demonstrating normal preprandial and postprandial glucose concentrations after overnight fasting and after having stopped IV glucose and any other medications for 5 consecutive days.

Hypoketotic hypoglycemia with elevated serum total free fatty acids, usually occurring following an extended fast (8–12 hours) or in association with an intercurrent illness, suggests a defect in fatty acid oxidation. The clinical presentation of fatty acid oxidation disorders has been described. Although inherited deficiency of at least nine different enzymatic steps in the mitochondrial β-oxidation pathway has been described, the clinical presentation of infants and children with these diseases is stereotypically similar and can be differentiated only by appropriate metabolic testing. In all cases, vigorous hydration with dextrose-containing parenteral fluids is lifesaving. Fasting avoidance is key to the long-term treatment and prevention of hypoglycemic episodes.

Infants and children with glycogen storage disorders present with hypoglycemia and permanent hepatomegaly. Hypoglycemia in these disorders is poorly responsive to glucagon administration. Enzymatic defects affecting glycogen synthesis, including glycogen synthase deficiency (GSD-0), as well as

defects in glycogen breakdown, such as debranching enzyme deficiency (GSD-III), result in hypoglycemia. Glycogen synthase deficiency usually presents as severe morning hypoglycemia with hyperketonemia and low lactic acid and alanine. Debranching enzyme deficiency results in hypoglycemia secondary to limitation of glucose release from the outer branches of the glycogen molecule. Ketosis is present in GSD-III as the body attempts to generate fuel by increased fatty acid oxidation. Furthermore, the gluconeogenesis pathway is intact; thus hypoglycemia is much milder. In glucose 6-phosphatase deficiency (GSD-1a) and glucose 6-phosphate translocase deficiency (GSD-1b), hypoglycemia usually is apparent 2.5 to 3 hours postprandial as these disorders not only affect glucose release from glycogen but also disrupt gluconeogenesis. Individuals with these disorders have lactic acidosis, ketosis, and hyperuricemia in addition to hepatomegaly.

Hypoglycemia following a longer fast (8–12 hours) suggests a defect in gluconeogenesis, ketogenesis, ketolysis, or fatty acid oxidation. Fructose 1,6-bisphosphatase, a disorder of gluconeogenesis, presents as fasting hypoglycemia but also with metabolic decompensation following fructose ingestion. Ketonemia and lactic acidemia are major features, in addition to the hypoglycemia. The ketone synthesis defects that present with fasting hypoketotic hypoglycemia include 3-hydroxy-3-methylglutaryl-CoA synthase deficiency and 3-hydroxy-3-methylglutaryl-CoA lyase deficiency. These patients have hypoglycemia in combination with normal blood lactate but no ketonuria. Infants with 3-hydroxy-3-methylglutaryl-CoA lyase deficiency also are hyperammonemic. Defects in succinyl-CoA oxoacid transferase and methylacetoacetyl-CoA thiolase represent ketolysis defects. Although the consistent biochemical abnormality is severe ketoacidosis, hypoglycemia also can be seen. Blood lactic acid and ammonia concentrations usually are normal.

Cardiomyopathy and Inborn Errors of Metabolism

Cardiomyopathies, as a rule, are rare. Studies undertaken by the Pediatric Cardiomyopathy Registry have determined that the overall annual incidence is 11.8 per million patient-years and that the incidence was higher in children younger than 1 year than in those between 1 and 18 years old.[24] In this regional study, 40% of cases were hypertrophic cardiomyopathies, 49% of cases were dilated cardiomyopathies, 3% of cases were restrictive or other types, and 8% were unspecified. Further study revealed that of cases of hypertrophic cardiomyopathy, 16% had an identifiable IEM as the underlying cause. These causes included disorders of glycogen metabolism (5%), mucopolysaccharide metabolism (4%), oxidative phosphorylation (5%), and fatty acid metabolism (2%). In the cases of dilated cardiomyopathy, 5% were found to be of a metabolic etiology with disorders of glycogen metabolism (1%), mucopolysaccharide metabolism (2%), and oxidative phosphorylation (2%) as the recognizable underlying cause. Thus it is important to consider IEM in the differential diagnosis of any child with dilated or hypertrophic cardiomyopathy. Because the prevalence of underlying metabolic disorders is so high, some authors have recommended that all children with cardiomyopathy undergo metabolic screening, including blood lactate, plasma amino acid analysis, urine organic acid analysis, urine metabolic screening (particularly for the detection of excessive urinary mucopolysaccharides), plasma carnitine levels, and plasma acylcarnitine profile (Box 82.3).[25] Additionally, serum creatine kinase (CK) should be measured to exclude muscular dystrophy.

Autosomal dominant hypertrophic cardiomyopathy has an incidence of 1:500 but demonstrates extremely variable penetrance. Mutation in genes encoding structural sarcomeric proteins is a frequent cause of dominant hypertrophic cardiomyopathy. More than 140 mutations in 15 different genes have been identified.[26]

Cardiomyopathy may be a complicating feature of several IEMs (Table 82.10), but with a few exceptions, other associated symptoms or physical examination findings at the time of presentation point toward the appropriate diagnosis. Broadly, the pathogenesis of cardiomyopathy in IEMs is either myocardial energy deficiency, as occurs in the dilated cardiomyopathy associated with several organic acidemias, or excessive storage of complex molecules in the heart, as occurs in the hypertrophic cardiomyopathy of mucopolysaccharidoses such as Hurler syndrome. Cardiomyopathy occurs as the sole initial clinical manifestation in a relatively restricted list of metabolic diseases, including autosomal recessively inherited deficiency of the cellular carnitine transporter, fatty acid oxidation disorders, glycogenosis types II and IX, and disorders of oxidative phosphorylation. The carnitine transporter defect is caused by deficiency of the sodium-dependent transporter

---

BOX 82.3   Screening Laboratory Studies for Evaluation of Cardiomyopathy

- Blood lactate
- Serum creatine kinase
- Plasma amino acid analysis
- Urine organic acid analysis
- Urine mucopolysaccharide screen
- Plasma carnitine levels
- Plasma acylcarnitine profile

TABLE 82.10   Cardiomyopathy and Inborn Errors of Metabolism

Cardiomyopathy as the sole or key presenting feature	Carnitine transport defect
	Fatty acid oxidation defects including:
	  VLCAD deficiency
	  Mitochondrial trifunctional protein deficiency
	  Carnitine palmitoyltransferase deficiency
	Glycogen storage disease type II (Pompe)
	Glycogen storage disease type IX (phosphorylase B kinase deficiency)
	Disorders of oxidative phosphorylation (Mitochondrial myopathy)

Cardiomyopathy as a secondary feature	Organic acidemias including:
	  Propionic acidemia
	  Methylmalonic acidemia
	  3-methylglutaconic aciduria
	  D-2-hydroxyglutaric aciduria
	  Biotinidase deficiency
	Glycogen storage disease type III
	Glycogen storage disease type IV
	Mucopolysaccharidoses
	Congenital disorders of glycosylation
	Congenital myotonic dystrophy
	Congenital muscular dystrophies

VLCAD, very-long-chain acyl-CoA dehydrogenase.

OCTN2, which is responsible for transporting carnitine from the circulation into tissues including cardiac and skeletal muscle.[27] Dilated cardiomyopathy with symptoms of heart failure generally presents within the first years of life and is associated with severely low plasma total carnitine levels. Cardiac function improves dramatically after carnitine supplementation, and cardiomyopathy rarely recurs if carnitine is continued.

Hypertrophic cardiomyopathy resulting from myocardial steatosis may be an isolated presenting feature in several disorders of fatty acid oxidation, particularly those affecting long-chain fatty acid metabolism such as VLCAD or mitochondrial trifunctional protein deficiencies. Saudubray and colleagues[28] examined a series of 109 patients with fatty acid oxidation defects and found that cardiac involvement, including hypertrophic cardiomyopathy or arrhythmia, was apparent at presentation in 51% of cases. Fatty acid oxidation disorders are most reliably detected by analysis of plasma acylcarnitine profiles by tandem mass spectrometry. Long-chain fatty acids are activated to CoA derivatives and then esterified to carnitine prior to transport into mitochondria for β-oxidation. In fatty acid oxidation disorders, especially during acute metabolic decompensation, acylcarnitine species accumulate in plasma and provide a diagnostic profile that is specific to a given enzyme deficiency. Confirmation of the diagnosis may require enzymatic analysis in cultured fibroblasts or mutation analysis. Once the diagnosis of a long-chain fatty acid oxidation disorder has been established, restriction of dietary long-chain fat intake and provision of medium-chain triglyceride oil as an alternative fuel source for the myocardium often reverses cardiomyopathy. Cardiac support measures, including extracorporeal membrane oxygenation, may be necessary for as long as 1 to 2 weeks after presentation before heart function improves.

Glycogen storage disease type II (acid α-glucosidase deficiency; Pompe disease) is a disorder of lysosomal glycogen accumulation that frequently presents as hypertrophic cardiomyopathy, yielding the classic boot-shaped radiographic appearance of the cardiac silhouette. Skeletal myopathy manifesting as severe hypotonia may complicate the presentation. Confirmation of the diagnosis requires measurement of enzyme activity in skeletal or cardiac muscle or cultured fibroblasts. In the past, treatment has only been supportive, but enzyme replacement therapy is now available. Intravenous infusion of recombinant acid α-glucosidase every other week has led to improved cardiac function, neuromuscular development, and survival in infants with Pompe disease.[29] However, antibody formation against the drug in some infants with subsequently decreased treatment effectiveness remains a clinical problem.

Myocardial function is highly dependent on mitochondrial oxidative phosphorylation; up to 30% of the total myocardial volume is composed of mitochondria.[30] Dilated or hypertrophic cardiomyopathy is a frequent presenting feature in infants with severe defects of mitochondrial oxidative phosphorylation. Skeletal muscle myopathy, liver dysfunction, renal tubulopathy, bone marrow failure, or CNS abnormalities may occur. Chronic lactic acidosis, if present, is an important indicator of mitochondrial dysfunction. Screening metabolic laboratory studies demonstrate nonspecific abnormalities associated with chronic lactic acidosis. Definitive diagnosis requires histologic evaluation of skeletal muscle and measurement of respiratory chain enzyme activities. Isolated deficiency of cytochrome c oxidase (COX or complex IV) and reduced nicotinamide adenine dinucleotide (NADH)-ubiquinone oxidoreductase (complex I) of the mitochondrial respiratory chain are the most common oxidative phosphorylation defects presenting with cardiomyopathy. Although some protein subunits of complexes I and IV are encoded by mtDNA, most infant-onset isolated complex deficiencies probably are the result of autosomal-recessively inherited deficiency of nuclear-encoded respiratory chain subunits or of chaperone proteins that ensure proper assembly of functional complexes. For instance, hypertrophic cardiomyopathy caused by functional COX deficiency has been associated with mutations in nuclear COX subunit genes[31,32] or nuclear genes for COX-associated proteins SCO1 and SCO2.[33]

Cardiomyopathy may be seen in several other IEMs, but in these disorders, other physical or biochemical features are generally apparent at initial clinical presentation. For instance, dilated cardiomyopathy may complicate propionic acidemia during acute metabolic decompensation, but features of severe metabolic acidosis, vomiting, dehydration, coma, and possibly hyperammonemia are part of the initial clinical presentation.

Metabolic Myopathies and Rhabdomyolysis

Rhabdomyolysis is a clinical syndrome resulting from skeletal muscle injury and release of potentially toxic substances into the circulatory system. Acute onset of severe muscle pain associated with increased serum CK levels is the hallmark of the disorder. In extreme cases, massive myoglobinuria may cause acute renal insufficiency. Although trauma and direct muscle injury are by far the most common causes of rhabdomyolysis, inborn errors of muscle metabolism should be considered in the differential diagnosis of rhabdomyolysis occurring at any age. In the absence of a history of trauma, the differential diagnosis of acute rhabdomyolysis should include drug or toxin exposure, muscle hypoxia (often associated with seizures), temperature alterations, inflammatory diseases, and IEMs. Because muscle contraction depends on adenosine triphosphate (ATP) generated by the mitochondrial electron transport chain, it follows that any process that impairs muscle ATP synthesis or that results in energy expenditure that surpasses ATP production could lead to rhabdomyolysis. The clinical history should lead toward the appropriate diagnosis. A family history that includes rhabdomyolysis or a history in which more than one episode of exercise-induced rhabdomyolysis has been observed should induce suspicion of a metabolic disorder. Along with muscular dystrophy and endocrine etiologies (hypothyroidism, hyperthyroidism, diabetic ketoacidosis, pheochromocytoma), glycolytic defects, fatty acid oxidation disorders, purine biosynthetic disorders, and disorders of mitochondrial oxidative phosphorylation should be considered if historical elements do not direct toward the more common etiologies. As described previously, the fatty acid oxidation disorders can be detected by urine organic acid analysis and plasma acylcarnitine profile. Chronic lactic acidosis may be a clue to a disorder of oxidative phosphorylation. Measurement of blood lactate level before and after an exercise treadmill protocol may help detect a respiratory chain defect if the postexercise lactate level is severely elevated. Definitive diagnosis of a mitochondrial disorder requires histologic and enzymatic analysis of a fresh muscle biopsy. The glycolytic defects of phosphofructokinase and phosphoglycerate mutase deficiencies along with myophosphorylase deficiency (glycogen storage disease type V or McArdle disease) cause severe recurrent rhabdomyolysis; their detection requires enzymatic analysis of muscle tissue. Likewise, myoadenylate deaminase deficiency, a defect in purine catabolism, and CPT-II deficiency are also diagnosed by measurement of the enzyme activities in muscle.

Neonatal Screening

Newborn screening for IEMs was first introduced in the 1960s, with screening for phenylketonuria. Technologic advances, most significantly the introduction of tandem mass spectrometry for mass screening, have greatly increased the number of disorders that can be identified by analysis of a dried blood spot on a filter paper card.[34] An expert review conducted by the American College of Medical Genetics led to the recommendation that 29 core conditions, including several aminoacidopathies, fatty acid oxidation defects, and organic acidurias detectable by tandem mass spectrometry, should be included in the panel of disorders screened.[29] As of 2009, all states in the United States and most of Europe have now adopted this recommendation. The cost versus benefits of expanded screening, whether to include specific rare or poorly treatable disorders in the screening panel, and the availability of adequate follow-up resources continue to be debated, but a general consensus has emerged that expanded newborn screening is an effective tool for identifying IEM early in life, allowing for the initiation of therapy, often before the infant becomes symptomatic, and for preventing morbidity and mortality associated with IEM.[35] It must be remembered, however, that newborn screening is just that—a screen—and both false-positive and false-negative results are possible. Thus the astute clinician must remain cognizant of the fact that in an ill infant, a normal newborn screen is reassuring but should not be taken as absolute proof-positive that an IEM identifiable on newborn screening is not present. Appropriate screening laboratory evaluation and emergency treatment should be instituted if clinical signs and symptoms of an IEM are present in a sick child.

Conclusion

Inborn errors of metabolism are individually rare but collectively will make not-infrequent appearances in a busy pediatric intensive care unit. The signs and symptoms of IEM may be nonspecific and often overlap extensively with more common disorders. When clinical suspicion of an IEM arises, screening biochemical genetic laboratory studies must be ordered. Further confirmatory testing often is necessary if screening laboratory tests point toward a specific disease. Confirmatory testing and disease-specific therapy should be instituted following consultation with a biochemical genetics specialist. If detected and treated early, the clinical outcome for many IEMs can be favorable.

References

1. Eisensmith RC, Woo SL. Population genetics of phenylketonuria. *Acta Paediatr Suppl.* 1994;407:19-26.

2. Hoffmann GF, von Kries R, Klose D, et al. Frequencies of inherited organic acidurias and disorders of mitochondrial fatty acid transport and oxidation in Germany. *Eur J Pediatr.* 2004;163:76-80.

3. Nyhan WL, Ozand PT. *Atlas of Metabolic Diseases.* London, UK: Chapman & Hall; 1998.

4. Fernandes J, Saudubray J-M, van den Berghe G, Walter J. *Inborn Metabolic Diseases.* 4th ed. Heidelberg: Springer; 2004.

5. Phenylketonuria: screening and management. *NIH Consens Statement.* 2000;17:1-27.

6. Baumgartner ER, Suormala T. Multiple carboxylase deficiency: inherited and acquired disorders of biotin metabolism. *Int J Vitam Nutr Res.* 1997;67:377-384.

7. Russo PA, Mitchell GA, Tanguay RM. Tyrosinemia: a review. *Pediatr Dev Pathol.* 2001;4:212-221.

8. Stark Z, Tan TY, Chong B, et al. A prospective evaluation of whole-exome sequencing as a first-tier molecular test in infants with suspected monogenic disorders. *Genet Med.* 2016; [Epub ahead of print].

9. Saudubray JM, Narcy C, Lyonnet L, et al. Clinical approach to inherited metabolic disorders in neonates. *Biol Neonate.* 1990;58(suppl 1):44-53.

10. Hayasaka K, Tada K, Fueki N, et al. Nonketotic hyperglycinemia: analyses of glycine cleavage system in typical and atypical cases. *J Pediatr.* 1987;110:873-877.

11. Gallagher RC, Van Hove JL, Scharer G, et al. Folinic acid-responsive seizures are identical to pyridoxine-dependent epilepsy. *Ann Neurol.* 2009; 65:550-556.

12. Marquardt T, Denecke J. Congenital disorders of glycosylation: review of their molecular bases, clinical presentations and specific therapies. *Eur J Pediatr.* 2003;162:359-379.

13. Opitz JM, Gilbert-Barness E, Ackerman J, Lowichik A. Cholesterol and development: the RSH ("Smith-Lemli-Opitz") syndrome and related conditions. *Pediatr Pathol Mol Med.* 2002;21:153-181.

14. Millington DS, Kodo N, Norwood DL, Roe CR. Tandem mass spectrometry: a new method for acylcarnitine profiling with potential for neonatal screening for inborn errors of metabolism. *J Inherit Metab Dis.* 1990;13:321-324.

15. Yokota I, Indo Y, Coates PM, Tanaka K. Molecular basis of medium chain acyl-coenzyme A dehydrogenase deficiency. An A to G transition at position 985 that causes a lysine-304 to glutamate substitution in the mature protein is the single prevalent mutation. *J Clin Invest.* 1990;86:1000-1003.

16. Sims HF, Brackett JC, Powell CK, et al. The molecular basis of pediatric long chain 3-hydroxyacyl-CoA dehydrogenase deficiency associated with maternal acute fatty liver of pregnancy. *Proc Natl Acad Sci USA.* 1995;92:841-845.

17. Morton DH, Strauss KA, Robinson DL, et al. Diagnosis and treatment of maple syrup disease: a study of 36 patients. *Pediatrics.* 2002;109:999-1008.

18. Grompe M. The pathophysiology and treatment of hereditary tyrosinemia type 1. *Semin Liver Dis.* 2001;21:563-571.

19. Luijerink MC, Jacobs SM, van Beurden EA, et al. Extensive changes in liver gene expression induced by hereditary tyrosinemia type I are not normalized by treatment with 2-(2-nitro-4-trifluoromethylbenzoyl)-1,3-cyclohexanedione (NTBC). *J Hepatol.* 2003;39:901-909.

20. LaFranchi S. Hypoglycemia of infancy and childhood. *Pediatr Clin North Am.* 1987;34:961-982.

21. Lteif AN, Schwenk WF. Hypoglycemia in infants and children. *Endocrinol Metab Clin North Am.* 1999;28:619-646, vii.

22. de Lonlay P, Giurgea I, Touati G, Saudubray JM. Neonatal hypoglycaemia: aetiologies. *Semin Neonatol.* 2004;9:49-58.

23. Stanley CA. Hyperinsulinism in infants and children. *Pediatr Clin North Am.* 1997;44:363-374.

24. Lipshultz SE, Sleeper LA, Towbin JA, et al. The incidence of pediatric cardiomyopathy in two regions of the United States. *N Engl J Med.* 2003;348:1647-1655.

25. Bonnet D, de Lonlay P, Gautier I, et al. Efficiency of metabolic screening in childhood cardiomyopathies. *Eur Heart J.* 1998;19:790-793.

26. Ackerman MJ, VanDriest SL, Ommen SR, et al. Prevalence and age-dependence of malignant mutations in the beta-myosin heavy chain and troponin T genes in hypertrophic cardiomyopathy: a comprehensive outpatient perspective. *J Am Coll Cardiol.* 2002;39:2042-2048.

27. Nezu J, Tamai I, Oku A, et al. Primary systemic carnitine deficiency is caused by mutations in a gene encoding sodium ion-dependent carnitine transporter. *Nat Genet.* 1999;21:91-94.

28. Saudubray JM, Martin D, de Lonlay P, et al. Recognition and management of fatty acid oxidation defects: a series of 107 patients. *J Inherit Metab Dis.* 1999;22:488-502.

29. Newborn screening: toward a uniform screening panel and system. *Genet Med.* 2006;8(suppl 1):1S-252S.

30. Page E, Polimeni PI, Zak R, et al. Myofibrillar mass in rat and rabbit heart muscle. Correlation of microchemical and stereological measurements in normal and hypertrophic hearts. *Circ Res.* 1972;30:430-439.

31. Antonicka H, Leary SC, Guercin GH, et al. Mutations in COX10 result in a defect in mitochondrial heme A biosynthesis and account for multiple, early-onset clinical phenotypes associated with isolated COX deficiency. *Hum Mol Genet.* 2003;12:2693-2702.

32. Antonicka H, Mattman A, Carlson CG, et al. Mutations in COX15 produce a defect in the mitochondrial heme biosynthetic pathway, causing early-onset fatal hypertrophic cardiomyopathy. *Am J Hum Genet.* 2003;72:101-114.

33. Leary SC, Kaufman BA, Pellecchia G, et al. Human SCO1 and SCO2 have independent, cooperative functions in copper delivery to cytochrome c oxidase. *Hum Mol Genet.* 2004;13:1839-1848.

34. Schulze A, Lindner M, Kohlmuller D, et al. Expanded newborn screening for inborn errors of metabolism by electrospray ionization-tandem mass spectrometry: results, outcome, and implications. *Pediatrics.* 2003;111(6 Pt 1):1399-1406.

35. Fearing MK, Marsden D. Expanded newborn screening. *Pediatr Ann.* 2003;32:509-515.

Genetic Variation in Health and Disease

David Jardine

PEARLS

- The DNA from two unrelated humans differs by approximately 0.1%.
- Genetic variation occurs on many different scales, with the smallest being single nucleotide polymorphisms (SNPs) and the largest being chromosomal nondisjunction.
- Mutations originating in somatic cells are not inherited; only those mutations occurring in germline cells are inherited.
- Mutations occurring in somatic cell lines are responsible for a number of disorders, including many nonhereditary cancers.
- Monogenic traits tend to follow Mendelian patterns of inheritance. A relatively small proportion of the inherited burden of disease is attributed monogenic traits. A much larger portion of the inherited burden of disease is caused by complex traits in which many genes contribute to a disease phenotype.
- Genome-wide association studies (GWASs) have great potential to reveal genetic variants that are associated with disease phenotypes; however, GWAS may be difficult and expensive to conduct because a large number of patients may be required to achieve adequate study power.
- Population stratification refers to systematic differences in allele frequencies among subpopulations with different ancestries. This must be carefully considered before determining the applicability of the results of a genetic study to a new population.

Introduction

After the discovery of the structure of DNA in 1953,[1] progress in understanding the genetic basis of human disease was painfully slow. Almost 40 years later, in 1989, the sequence for the cystic fibrosis gene was published, making it one of the first disease-associated genes to be fully sequenced. Automated sequencing of DNA made this process faster and cheaper, but managing the flood of data provided new challenges. The incorporation of computer technology addressed these problems by performing the tedious work of sequence alignment and managing the ever-increasing volume of sequence data. In the last decade of the 20th century, the continued improvement of these two innovations made feasible the Human Genome Project. By 2003, five years after this broad international collaboration was fully under way, sequencing of the first complete version of the human genome was publicly available.[2,3] Subsequent work has been directed at refining the information contained in the reference human genome and in understanding genetic variation in the population. Continued improvements in sequencing technologies have made this endeavor faster, cheaper, and more accurate. The public cost of sequencing the first human genome was estimated to have been approximately $3 billion (the Human Genome Project). The current cost of sequencing a human genome is now $1,000 and is declining rapidly. As information about human genetic variability becomes more readily available, it will have major implications for science and medicine. In an example that is particularly relevant to pediatric critical care, the understanding of the genetic basis of sepsis is rapidly expanding.[4] Translating these findings to relevant clinical interventions will require time; however, it is certain that knowledge of a patient's genetic makeup will be an important therapeutic consideration within the next few years. Although the era of genetic medicine may seem far off, the feasibility of using rapid whole genome sequencing for the diagnosis of monogenic diseases in an ICU has already been demonstrated.[5] Understanding the potential and limitations of high-throughput genetic screening will have increasing relevance to the practice of medicine, especially in the critical care setting where the illnesses are life threatening and risks of complications and toxicity are great.

Sequence Variation in Health and Disease

The human genome consists of approximately 3 billion DNA base pairs partitioned into 23 chromosome pairs. In spite of the seemingly great differences between individual human beings (phenotype), the genetic differences between individuals is approximately 0.1%.[6] Nevertheless, human genetic variability accounts for a large portion of the differences in susceptibility to disease, rates of aging, and longevity. To understand human genetic variability, genomes from people of varying ethnic origins have been sequenced. These genomes serve as references to understand genetic variations between and within different human subpopulations.

Scale of Mutational Event

Variation can occur on several different scales (Table 83.1). With a few exceptions, before the widespread availability of

TABLE 83.1

Variation	Size	Change Compared With Reference Genome
SNP (single nucleotide polymorphism)	1 base pair	A single base pair is altered
Indel (insertion or deletion)	1-1000 base pairs	A small region of DNA is inserted or deleted
CNV (copy number variation)	1000-3 million base pairs	The number of copies of a section of DNA is increased or decreased

sequencing technology, the only chromosomal changes that could be documented were those that were observable through a light microscope. These variants can include chromosomal aneuploidies, rearrangements, heteromorphisms, and fragile sites[7] and are referred to as a cell's karyotype. In general, these structural variants must encompass sections of DNA greater than 3 million base pairs in size in order to be visible microscopically. Compared with DNA variants detectable by sequence analysis, the microscopically detectable structural variants are relatively uncommon.

After the first two reference versions of the human genome were published in 2001, an intensive effort was launched to detect variation at the single nucleotide polymorphism (SNP) level. Soon afterward, improved analytic techniques enabled efficient detection of submicroscopic structural variants (1–3 million base pairs). It now appears that submicroscopic structural variants contribute at least as much variability to the human genome as SNPs.[7,8]

SNP: A single nucleotide polymorphism (SNP) is the smallest change that can occur within a DNA sequence. This change occurs when one nucleotide is substituted for another in the DNA sequence. By convention, a change in a single nucleotide is referred to as an SNP if the change is found in ≥1% of the subpopulation to which the individual belongs. If the altered nucleotide is found in <1% of the reference subpopulation, it is referred to as a *mutation*. The frequency of occurrence of variation at the single nucleotide level (SNP vs. mutation) does not correlate with the risk of an altered phenotype. Both common and rare variants can have profound effects on the phenotype or can be silent.

Nucleotide level variation is heterogenous in different human subpopulations. In other words, the SNPs in people of African, Asian, and European origin differ markedly from one group to another. For this reason, it is important to consider the population structure when interpreting studies on genetic variation.

Indel: When one or more nucleotides are *in*serted or *del*eted from a specific point in the DNA, this change is referred to as an *indel*. The length of an indel is between 1 and 10,000 base pairs and can include either insertions, deletions, or both.[9] Deletions occur with approximately three times the frequency of insertions.[10] Small indels (1–50 base pairs) are much more frequent than larger indels. The number of indels in the human genome is thought to be in excess of 2

million. Of these, more than 800,000 map to known human genes, affecting approximately 5.8% of all known human genes.[11] Consequently, indels are a significant source of genetic variation. Indels within coding and regulatory regions (promoters) are more likely to produce identifiable human phenotypes than indels in other parts of the genome.

Copy number variation (CNV): This refers to a segment of the genome 50 to 1 million base pairs that shows greater or fewer copies than the reference genome. Compared with SNPs and CNVs, this sort of variation has been more challenging to detect. As a result, the phenotypes associated with CNVs are still being defined. It appears that CNV is a relatively common form of genetic variation, especially those CNVs of relatively small size. Although CNV may be associated with disease, not all CNVs are pathogenic. It appears that normal individuals have multiple small CNVs.[12] Larger CNVs are less common and are more likely to be pathogenic. Nevertheless, even relatively large CNVs are still common. Approximately 65% to 80% of individuals harbor CNVs of at least 100,000 base pairs and up to 10% harbor CNVs of at least 500,000 base pairs. Although CNVs are not always pathogenic, multiple illness phenotypes have been associated with CNVs, including Prader-Willi syndrome, Charcot-Marie-Tooth disease, Williams syndrome, and DiGeorge syndrome.[13,14]

Chromosome alterations: Chromosomal aneuploidy and translocation are detectable with microscopy and have been well characterized. Although balanced translocations in which the total amount of genetic material within the cell is unchanged may not be pathogenic, chromosomal abnormalities are frequent causes of genetic illness.

Because genetic variation within an individual occurs on multiple scales, all of these must be considered in order to understand the contribution of genetic variation to illness.

Genetic Variation and Protein Synthesis

If the genotype is a blueprint for the building of an organism, proteins are the important building blocks. Genetic variation produces changes in the blueprint and may produce important changes in the protein building blocks. Proteins structure may be altered by changes in the amino acid sequence, altered splicing, and early termination. Genetic variation may also affect rates of protein synthesis or change protein stability. Although neither of these mechanisms alter protein structure, they may produce important changes in the quantity of proteins present within a cell or secreted by a cell. Because protein function is dependent on both structure and concentration, any of these changes may have profound effects on the phenotype.

Although the purpose of our DNA is to encode proteins, only about 1% of the genome is dedicated to this purpose. Some of the noncoding portions of the genome serve regulatory functions, but little is still understood about a large portion of the noncoding DNA. Genes themselves contain both coding regions (exons) and noncoding regions (introns). On average, each gene contains 8.8 exons and 7.8 introns.[15] During RNA processing, the introns are removed and the remaining pieces of RNA are spliced together so that an intact protein may be transcribed from the messenger RNA. The location of a genetic variant (eg, SNP, CNV) is the primary determinant of the effect that will be produced by the variant.

Depending on where it occurs, an SNP can have different effects on protein levels and protein function. SNPs that occur in promoter regions of a gene may alter the rate of protein synthesis. The availability of mRNA from a given gene may be changed if an SNP alters the rate of RNA degradation. Increased RNA degradation would diminish protein synthesis while decreased RNA degradation could be expected to result in increased protein synthesis. SNPs occurring in introns can alter post-translational processing of the nascent protein, resulting in different protein splice variants. Many proteins have several splice variants that show differing levels of function. Indeed, it appears that splice site variation may be responsible for a significant portion of the burden of human disease.[10]

SNPs that occur within exons may be silent if they do not produce a change in the amino acid encoded by a codon (synonymous SNPs) or they may alter protein function if they result in substitution of a different amino acid within the protein sequence (nonsynonymous SNPs). If a nonsynonymous SNP changes an amino acid codon to a stop codon, protein synthesis undergoes early termination. Because the gene is only partially transcribed, the resulting protein is likely to function poorly, if at all.

Indels can alter protein function by many of the mechanisms indicated earlier. Indels may also produce frameshift mutations. Amino acids in a protein are encoded by a series of nucleotide triplets (codons) in the DNA. If an indel disrupts one of these triplets by inserting or deleting an amino acid, the reading frame of all subsequent nucleotides is altered. In addition to changing many of the amino acids encoded after the mutation, frameshift mutations frequently result in an early stop codon causing early termination of protein synthesis.

Copy number variations and chromosomal alterations (eg, aneuploidy) are associated with a variety of disease states. Although the phenotypes produced by chromosomal alterations have long been recognized, the mechanism by which these large-scale changes in genome structure produce disease is not yet fully understood. An explanation to account for a portion of the observed phenotypic changes is that these events alter "gene dosing," with the result that certain gene products (proteins) are increased or decreased compared with the normal phenotype. Experimental evidence from several model organisms indicates that there is a correlation between gene copy number and mRNA levels.[16,17] A number of human genes that produce dosage-sensitive phenotypes have been identified.[18] Although this is an attractive mechanism for explaining the effects of copy number variations and chromosomal alterations, other effects may be important.

Finally, although epigenetic changes in DNA (methylation, histone modification, etc.) are beyond the scope of this discussion, these phenomena can produce important changes in phenotypes. Although many epigenetic traits are not heritable, some are transgenerational and will alter the phenotype of offspring. Such epigenetic changes may help to explain a portion of complex traits that are not easily understood in terms of classical genetics.

Developmental Timing of Mutations and Consequences

All mutations result from replication errors or DNA damage that is unrepaired or incorrectly repaired. In the latter case, environmental factors that injure DNA increase the risk of mutations. Changes in the sequence and structure of DNA can occur in germ cells or somatic cells. Depending on the cell type in which a mutation occurs, the ramifications for that mutation are quite different. Mutations inherited through the germline are transmitted to all the somatic cells of the offspring. In contrast, de novo mutations in somatic cells are transmitted only to the progeny of the original cell in which the mutation first occurred. Because somatic mutations do not involve germline cells, they are not inherited.

Mutations Occurring in Germline Cells (Prezygotic Mutations)

On average, every human being inherits approximately 60 new SNPs from their parents, although this figure may vary widely among individuals.[19] These inherited mutations occur in the germ cells of the parents and are transmitted to their offspring. Although somatic cell mutations may have serious consequences for an organism, only germline mutations have a long-term effect on population fitness. The frequency and type of mutation are influenced by gender and age of the parents. Germline SNPs increase sharply with paternal age, with approximately two new mutations per year.[20] Consequently, a 40-year-old father will carry approximately twice the number of germline SNPs as a 20-year-old father. The effect of age exerts a much smaller influence on increasing maternal germline SNPs. Approximately 95% of the variation in de novo SNPs among offspring is attributable to paternal age effect. Similarly, de novo copy number variations also correlate strongly with paternal age.[21] Increases in paternal age have been associated with an increased risk of autism, schizophrenia,[22] neurofibromatosis,[23] achondroplasia, and Apert syndrome among others.[24] Because humans have a long life relative to other species, the effects of paternal age may play a larger role in humans than in shorter-lived animals.

In contrast, maternal age correlates strongly with the risk of chromosomal structural mutations such as aneuploidy and chromosomal nondisjunction errors. In the past, because these large-scale events were detectable with light microscopy, the effect of maternal age on germline mutations was more readily appreciated compared with the effect of paternal age. Several disorders caused by chromosomal nondisjunction are frequently encountered in the critical care setting, including Down syndrome (trisomy 21), Klinefelter syndrome, Turner syndrome (monosomy X), Edward syndrome (trisomy 18), and Pautau syndrome (trisomy 13).

Mutations Occurring in Somatic Cells (Postzygotic Mutations)

Somatic cell mutations (those mutations that do not arise in germline cells) are not inherited from parents. These mutations can arise at any time during the life span of an individual. Human cells undergo trillions of cell divisions during the normal life span, with each division constituting a risk for somatic mutation. Somatic cell mutations that occur early in embryogenesis may become widespread through the organism leading to mosaicism. Recent evidence suggests that early fetal somatic cell mutations lead to substantial genetic variation within different tissues from the same individual.[25] Unlike germline mutations, which must result in a viable organism in order to be manifest, somatic cell mutations must only be compatible with producing a viable cell. Consequently, the spectrum of somatic cell mutations is broader than germline mutations.

Most somatic mutations are harmless; however, when one of these mutations causes a cell to escape from normal mechanisms regulating its growth and survival, the phenotype of this mutation may be cancer, which is the clonal expansion of a single abnormal cell. Usually, more than one mutation is required before a clone of cells fully escapes from normal biological regulation. The initial mutation may result in a precancerous condition, which becomes cancer when one or more subsequent mutations permit the cell clone to escape fully from normal regulation. An example of this stepwise progression is adenomatous polyps of the colon that pose a risk for progression to colon carcinoma.[26] Because the accumulation of somatic mutations increases over the lifetime of an individual, the risk of developing cancer also increases as one ages.

Mutations in over 350 genes (approximately 1.6% of all genes) have been associated with an increased risk of cancer.[27] In more than 90% of these genes, the mutation is dominantly acting, which means that mutation of only one allele can contribute to cancer development. Many of these mutations operate quite differently from each other, which is consonant with the recognition that cancer may be caused by multiple molecular derangements. Scientists have discovered the genetic basis for many pediatric cancers including neuroblastoma, many leukemias, and brain stem medulloblastoma, among others.[28-30] Understanding of these derangements has suggested novel therapeutic targets, many of which are highly specific. Consequently, identification of the genetic mechanism of a particular cancer may be of paramount importance in selecting the optimal therapy.

Genetic Variation in Mendelian and Complex Traits

Human genetic traits may be classified as monogenic or complex, although there is often overlap between these two categories. Monogenic traits are those in which the phenotype is strongly influenced by a single gene. These traits follow Mendelian inheritance patterns and are the basis of "classical" genetics. Complex traits refer to phenotypes that are influenced by multiple genes. As the sequence and structure of the genome have been explored, it has become increasingly apparent that monogenic traits are relatively uncommon and that complex traits in which more than one gene influences a phenotype are more frequently encountered. Many commonly encountered illnesses that are phenotypes of complex traits include obesity, heart disease, hypertension, schizophrenia, Alzheimer disease, sepsis, and epilepsy, to name only a few. When several genetic loci contribute to the phenotype, the relative strength of each contribution must be determined in order to understand the disease phenotype.[31] Often, only a limited amount of the heritable component of a complex trait may be identified, which further complicates the understanding of the genetic basis for complex disease phenotypes. The power of genetic studies to detect disease-genotype associations is further impaired by the need to correct for multiple hypothesis testing, discussed in the following section.

High-Throughput Technologies—the Good and the Bad

Modern analysis of DNA and RNA relies heavily on high-throughput technologies in which thousands of chemical analyses are conducted in parallel. Such technologies are intensively reliant on computational data analysis and data management. High-throughput technologies have been used with great success in DNA sequencing and in quantitating gene expression. The appeal of being able to conduct thousands of experiments at the same time is obvious: It is highly efficient. With some approaches, it is possible to assess the entire human genome in a single experiment consisting of thousands of individual analyses. When multiple analyses are conducted on the same sample, the analysis must adjust for multiple comparisons. Careful statistical analysis with attention to robust correction for multiple testing is essential to reduce the probability of false-positive results (type I error). Such adjustments come at a price. These statistical corrections decrease the power of the study and elevate the possibility of false negatives (type II error). This problem may be overcome by increasing the number of subjects in an investigation, but enrollment of additional subjects may be difficult and additional high-throughput analyses may be expensive. Because of these issues, high-throughput studies are at risk of being underpowered. Studies that lack sufficient statistical power are more likely to miss real associations between genetic variation and disease. When interpreting the results from high-throughput studies, it is important to keep in mind these caveats. Although high-throughput studies offer great potential because of their ability to survey the entire genome, this promise is accompanied by noteworthy challenges.

Genome-Wide Association Studies

Genome-wide association studies (GWASs) examine the association between SNPs and disease phenotypes. Such studies are possible because the HapMap project, which was completed in 2003, identified the frequency and location of SNPs in the human genome.[32] With the advent of high-throughput SNP genotyping technologies, GWASs have flourished. Since 2005, more than 2300 GWASs have been published,[33] providing insights into the heritable aspects of many human diseases. SNPs underlie a number of common monogenic and complex diseases.

SNPs occur once in approximately every 300 nucleotides, so there are approximately 10 million SNPs within the human genome. Fortunately, because a given SNP is usually in linkage disequilibrium with other SNPs, it is not necessary to test every SNP in the human genome to determine its association with a disease phenotype. Instead, in GWASs, a marker SNP is usually used as a surrogate for a genomic region that may contain hundreds of other SNPs. Because GWASs rely heavily on marker SNPs (called "tag" SNPs), an SNP that is found to be associated with a disease phenotype is often not the causative SNP. Instead, all that can be known with certainty is that the tag SNP is in linkage disequilibrium with the causative variant. This variant could be another SNP or could be a structural variant. Although this approach eliminates the need to test all 10 million SNPs within the genome, the greater the number of SNPs that are tested, the higher the resolution of the results. It is common for current SNP analyses to test more than 100,000 SNPs in each study subject.

Individuals of European ancestry are overrepresented in GWASs.[34] Because of the differences in SNP distributions in different ancestral populations, it is important to consider the populations examined in a GWAS before generalizing the results to other populations. Other issues must also be considered in interpreting GWASs. Because of the large number of genetic loci that are screened for their association with disease, GWASs have an increased risk of type II error (false-negative errors). Unless a study is adequately powered, failure to find an association between a genetic locus and a disease may represent a false-negative finding. The high cost of GWAS analyses and the challenges of enrolling a large number of subjects constitute formidable hurdles to achieving sufficient power in GWASs.

Positive findings in a GWAS should be replicated in a separate investigation with a different group of patients (with appropriate attention to population structure of the new cohort). Positive findings may be replicated in another GWAS, or they may be replicated in a targeted analysis that tests only a small number of SNPs that are in linkage disequilibrium with the SNP identified in the original study. A targeted approach tests fewer SNPs, so the loss of power from multiple hypothesis testing is much less of a problem. Accordingly, it may be possible to enroll fewer patients and conduct a more cost-efficient study. Once the findings have been replicated, other challenges must be addressed such as determining the causative variant and determining the mechanism by which this variant causes disease susceptibility.

Although GWASs have great potential to expand the understanding of sepsis and other diseases commonly encountered in critical care, this promise is offset somewhat by the limited power of GWASs.[35] To overcome this obstacle requires the enrollment of large numbers of patients, which is a difficult and expensive undertaking in the critical care setting. Furthermore, many of the disease processes in critical care are likely to be caused by complex genetic traits, which are known to pose special challenges for GWASs. The promise of GWASs is great; however, a substantial investment in time and money may be necessary to begin to realize this promise.

Looking Toward the Future

Using information about a patient's unique genetic makeup to create an optimal care plan is the long-sought goal of personalized medicine. While progress has been made toward this goal, the full complexity of variation within the human genome is still being defined. Many human phenotypes are complex and involve contributions from multiple genetic loci, making this goal difficult to achieve. As clinicians gain a better understanding of the relationship between human genetic variation and states of health and disease, they will be presented with a host of opportunities to improve health care.

References

1. Watson JD, Crick FH. Molecular structure of nucleic acids; a structure for deoxyribose nucleic acid. *Nature.* 1953;171:737-738.
2. Pennisi E. Human genome. Reaching their goal early, sequencing labs celebrate. *Science.* 2003;300:409.
3. Thomas G, Cann H. Irruption of genomics in the search for disease related genes. *Gut.* 2003;52(suppl 2):ii1-ii5.
4. Wong HR. Genetics and genomics in pediatric septic shock. *Crit Care Med.* 2012;40:1618-1626.
5. Saunders CJ, Miller NA, Soden SE, et al. Rapid whole-genome sequencing for genetic disease diagnosis in neonatal intensive care units. *Sci Transl Med.* 2012;4:154ra35.
6. 1000 Genomes Project Consortium, Auton A, Brooks LD, et al. A global reference for human genetic variation. *Nature.* 2015;526:68-74.
7. Feuk L, Carson AR, Scherer SW. Structural variation in the human genome. *Nat Rev Genet.* 2006;7:85-97.
8. Stankiewicz P, Lupski JR. Structural variation in the human genome and its role in disease. *Annu Rev Med.* 2010;61:437-455.
9. Mullaney JM, Mills RE, Pittard WS, et al. Small insertions and deletions (INDELs) in human genomes. *Hum Mol Genet.* 2010;19:R131-R136.
10. Lynch M. Rate, molecular spectrum, and consequences of human mutation. *Proc Natl Acad Sci USA.* 2010;107:961-968.
11. Mills RE, Pittard WS, Mullaney JM, et al. Natural genetic variation caused by small insertions and deletions in the human genome. *Genome Res.* 2011;21:830-839.
12. Lupski JR. Genomic rearrangements and sporadic disease. *Nat Genet.* 2007;39(suppl 7):S43-S47.
13. Girirajan S, Campbell CD, Eichler EE. Human copy number variation and complex genetic disease. *Annu Rev Genet.* 2011;45:203-226.
14. Riggs ER, Ledbetter DH, Martin CL. Genomic variation: lessons learned from whole-genome CNV analysis. *Curr Genet Med Rep.* 2014;2: 146-150.
15. Sakharkar MK, Chow VT, Kangueane P. Distributions of exons and introns in the human genome. *In Silico Biol.* 2004;4:387-393.
16. Birchler JA, Veitia RA. Gene balance hypothesis: connecting issues of dosage sensitivity across biological disciplines. *Proc Natl Acad Sci USA.* 2012;109:14746-14753.
17. Weischenfeldt J, Symmons O, Spitz F, et al. Phenotypic impact of genomic structural variation: insights from and for human disease. *Nat Rev Genet.* 2013;14:125-138.
18. Dang VT, Kassahn KS, Marcos AE, et al. Identification of human haploinsufficient genes and their genomic proximity to segmental duplications. *Eur J Hum Genet.* 2008;16:1350-1357.
19. Shendure J, Akey JM. The origins, determinants, and consequences of human mutations. *Science.* 2015;349:1478-1483.
20. Kong A, Frigge ML, Masson G, et al. Rate of de novo mutations and the importance of father's age to disease risk. *Nature.* 2012;488:471-475.
21. Hehir-Kwa JY, Rodriguez-Santiago B, Vissers LE, et al. De novo copy number variants associated with intellectual disability have a paternal origin and age bias. *J Med Genet.* 2011;48:776-778.
22. Malaspina D, Gilman C, Kranz TM. Paternal age and mental health of offspring. *Fertil Steril.* 2015;103:1392-1396.
23. Snajderova M, Riccardi VM, Petrak B, et al. The importance of advanced parental age in the origin of neurofibromatosis type 1. *Am J Med Genet A.* 2012;158A:519-523.
24. Ramasamy R, Chiba K, Butler P, et al. Male biological clock: a critical analysis of advanced paternal age. *Fertil Steril.* 2015;103:1402-1406.
25. O'Huallachain M, Karczewski KJ, Weissman SM, et al. Extensive genetic variation in somatic human tissues. *Proc Natl Acad Sci USA.* 2012;109: 18018-18023.
26. Martincorena I, Campbell PJ. Somatic mutation in cancer and normal cells. *Science.* 2015;349:1483-1489.
27. Stratton MR, Campbell PJ, Futreal PA. The cancer genome. *Nature.* 2009;458:719-724.
28. Downing JR, Wilson RK, Zhang J, et al. The Pediatric Cancer Genome Project. *Nat Genet.* 2012;44:619-622.
29. Cheung NK, Dyer MA. Neuroblastoma: developmental biology, cancer genomics and immunotherapy. *Nat Rev Cancer.* 2013;13:397-411.
30. Stieglitz E, Loh ML. Genetic predispositions to childhood leukemia. *Ther Adv Hematol.* 2013;4:270-290.
31. Abiola O, Angel JM, Avner P, et al. The nature and identification of quantitative trait loci: a community's view. *Nat Rev Genet.* 2003;4:911-916.
32. Thorisson GA, Smith AV, Krishnan L, et al. The international HapMap project website. *Genome Res.* 2005;15:1592-1593.
33. Burdett T, Hall P, Hasting E, et al. The NHGRI-EBI Catalog of published genome-wide association studies. Available at: <www.ebi.ac.uk/gwas>; Accessed 20.11.15.
34. Leslie R, O'Donnell CJ, Johnson AD. GRASP: analysis of genotype-phenotype results from 1390 genome-wide association studies and corresponding open access database. *Bioinformatics.* 2014;30:i185-i194.
35. Skibsted S, Bhasin MK, Aird WC, et al. Bench-to-bedside review: future novel diagnostics for sepsis—a systems biology approach. *Crit Care.* 2013;17:231.

Molecular Foundations of Cellular Injury: Apoptosis and Necrosis

Rohit Mittal, John D. Lyons, and Craig M. Coopersmith

PEARLS

- Cell death is an important physiologic homeostatic mechanism critical for host survival.
- Apoptosis and autophagy are evolutionarily conserved processes.
- Alterations in the machinery driving apoptosis and autophagy play an important role in the pathogenesis of critical illness.
- Necroptosis appears relevant to a number of clinical disease processes, although its role in critical illness is still being defined.
- Targeting the mechanisms of cell death may play an important role in the future treatment of human disease and critical illness.

Cell Death

Each day, the human body produces and eradicates billions of cells, a rate of cell death of nearly 1 million per second.[1] Cell death is therefore an integral homeostatic process to the survival of a living organism, but when perturbed it can also lead to sickness or mortality. Cell death, both physiologic and pathologic, occurs through distinct mechanisms, including apoptosis, necrosis, necroptosis, and autophagy.[2] These mechanisms are regulated by molecular signals that culminate in morphologically different modes of cell death.

Apoptosis is a programmed form of cell suicide that morphologically results in nuclear condensation (pyknosis) and fragmentation (karyorrhexis), organelle shrinkage and removal, and cytoplasmic blebbing without alterations in the integrity of the cellular plasma membrane.[1,3,4] As cells undergo apoptosis, they shrink and form apoptotic bodies, which are subsequently engulfed by nearby phagocytic cells and cleared by lysosomes.[5] Orderly DNA fragmentation is identifiable on electrophoretic gels as a characteristic "ladder" pattern. Apoptosis is an evolutionarily conserved process that is vital during fetal development in shaping limbs, the intestinal tract, and other vital organs and persists throughout life in tisses undergoing high cell turnover. Notably, because cytosolic contents are not released into the interstitial space, apoptosis is not accompanied by an inflammatory response.

Unlike the orderly process of apoptosis, necrosis is a form of cell death due to extrinsic stress or damage, resulting in nuclear and organelle swelling and eventual cell lysis.[2] Morphologically, a necrotic cell swells and has a random pattern of DNA and cellular fragmentation, which is a stark contrast to the controlled shrinkage of an apoptotic cell.[1,2,6] As cell membranes break down, intracellular contents are released into the interstitial space and may be detected by neighboring immune cells, triggering an inflammatory host response. These molecules or fragments are referred to as damage-associated molecular patterns (DAMPs).[6-8]

Though the process of necrosis has traditionally been considered accidental or uncontrolled, forms of regulated necrosis or "necroptosis" have recently been described.[9-11] Necroptosis is similar to apoptosis in that it is a receptor-mediated process driven by highly regulated intracellular signaling pathways. However, an important distinction from apoptosis is that necroptosis results in cell permeabilization, swelling and release of intracellular contents that more closely resemble traditional necrosis.[9,10] As with more "classical" forms of necrosis, the release of intracellular contents associated with regulated cell death in necroptosis is highly inflammatory.[7]

Similar to apoptosis, autophagy is a conserved cell death pathway; however, autophagy is a mechanism of cytoprotection that takes place during states of cellular stress.[4] This process involves sequestration of cellular contents within vesicles called autophagosomes, which then proceed to lysosomal degradation.[3] In physiologic situations, this highly regulated process serves to maintain homeostasis within a cell by eliminating excessive, dysfunctional, or wasteful organelles and allowing their catabolic end products to be recycled to meet the energy needs of a cell.[12] Although this is an adaptive cytoprotective response, if it persists uncontrolled, the end point is loss of vital cell components and eventual cell death.

Mechanisms of Cell Death

Apoptosis is regulated by a complex and conserved set of pathways (Fig. 84.1). The process is initiated either by an extrinsic (receptor-mediated) pathway or an intrinsic (mitochondrial) pathway. The extrinsic pathway is regulated through Fas ligand, tumor necrosis factor TNFα, or TNF-related apoptosis-inducing ligand (TRAIL) signaling via their respective receptors (Fas, TNFR1, TNFR2, TRAIL-R1, TRAIL-R2) on the cell surface. This leads to activation of cysteine aspartyl protease (caspase)-8 intracellularly.

In contrast, the intrinsic pathway is regulated through intracellular mitochondrial signaling. In this pathway, DNA

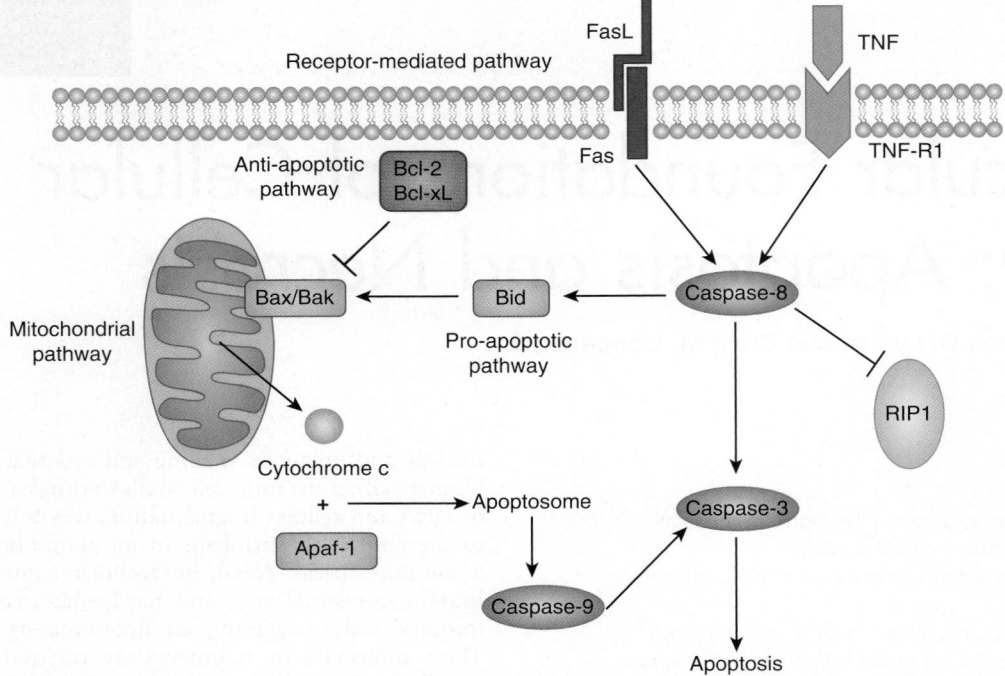

Fig. 84.1. Diagram of complex and conserved set of pathways that regulates apoptosis.

damage from reactive oxygen species, radiation, chemotherapy, or other pathologic insults results in the release of cytochrome c from the mitochondria into the cytoplasm, which allows apoptotic protease activating factor (APAF)-1 to interact with adenosine triphosphate (ATP) to form an apoptosome, which triggers caspase-9 activation[13] (see also Chapter 80). Within the mitochondrial pathway, the Bcl-2 family of molecules plays a critical role. This group of proteins includes more than 20 proapoptotic and antiapoptotic molecules, many of which physically interact with each other. Their primary function appears to be regulation of cytochrome c release from the mitochondria with proapoptotic family members promoting and antiapoptotic members suppressing its release. Prototypical proapoptotic proteins in this family include Bax and Bak, whereas prototypical antiapoptotic proteins include Bcl-2 and Bcl-xL[3,13-16]

Caspase-8 and caspase-9 ultimately both converge on the final common pathway of apoptosis, via induction of the death effector caspase-3, ultimately leading to the death of the cell. Additionally, activation of caspase-8 facilitates crosstalk between both pathways via activation of Bid.[16,17]

Necroptosis is also initiated via a receptor-mediated pathway (Fig. 84.2) via intracellular signaling primarily through the serine-threonine protein kinases receptor-interaction proteins 1 and 3 (RIP1 and RIP3). When caspase-8 activity is compromised, binding of TNFα (or other extrinsic death ligands) to its cell surface receptors allows RIP1-RIP3 interaction and phosphorylation, leading to RIP3-mediated phosphorylation of mixed lineage kinase domain-like protein (MLKL).[18-22] Activated MLKL is then trafficked to the cellular membrane, which it then permeabilizes, facilitating cell swelling, calcium influx, and necrotic cell death.[23,24] Several initiating factors have been shown to be capable of inducing necroptosis under varying cellular conditions, including TNFα, Fas, IFNγ, and signaling via TLR3 and TLR4.[18,19,25,26]

Research has begun to unravel the mechanisms that lead to autophagosome formation in autophagy. Although autophagy serves an important adaptive role during stress, excessive cellular degradation can lead to or propagate states of disease. During states of stress, autophagy can be induced via interruptions in the interaction between the antiapoptotic protein Bcl-2 or Bcl-xL and beclin-1, a protein important for autophagosome formation and signaling.[3] The crosstalk between the machinery driving autophagy is complex and byproducts of the autodegradation process, such as autophagy protein (Atg)-5, can stimulate cytochrome c release and apoptosome activation via the intrinsic pathway or though Atg-5 and caspase-8 interactions resulting in a proapoptotic complex.[3,4,27]

How Do Cellular Death Mechanisms Propagate Critical Illness?

Human Studies

The role of cell death, especially apoptosis, in critical illness has become increasingly understood. In 1999, Hotchkiss and colleagues showed that septic patients who died in a surgical intensive care unit and underwent immediate autopsy had markedly increased lymphocytic and gut epithelial apoptosis.[28] In addition, necrosis was detectable in the liver a third of the time but was minimal or absent in all other tissues examined. Similar findings have been shown in both neonates and pediatric patients with sepsis.[29,30] Subsequently, Takasu and coworkers examined what role cell death might play in sepsis-induced cardiac and renal dysfunction and noted little evidence of cardiac myocyte death.[31] Although there was some evidence of necrosis in renal tissue, the extent of overall cellular death noted did not explain the degree of organ dysfunction. Liver autophagy is also increased in autopsy studies of septic patients with sepsis.[32] Increased lymphocyte apoptosis

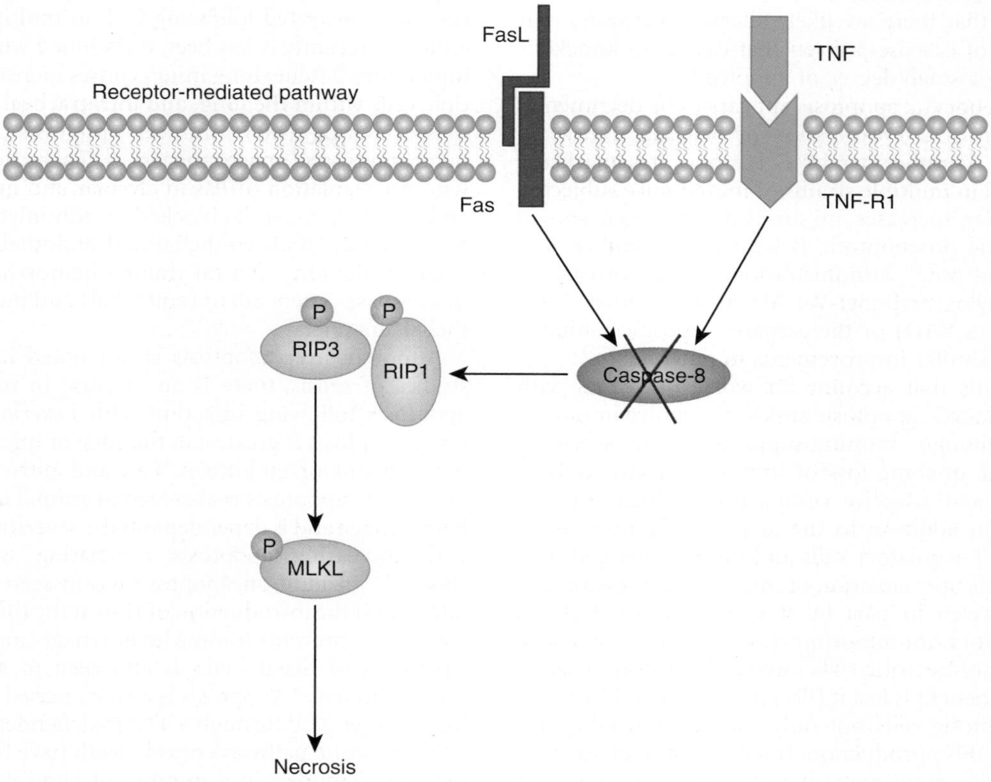

Fig. 84.2. Diagram of a receptor-mediated pathway that initiated necroptosis.

in septic patients has also been demonstrated to be associated with an increase in active caspase-3 activity. Further, B and CD4+ T lymphocytes are disproportionately lost in septic patients,[33] and B and CD4+ T-lymphocyte apoptosis is caspase-9 dependent, with the degree of cell death greater the longer the patient is septic. Antigen-presenting dendritic cells are also decreased in spleens of septic patients.[34] Notably, spleen biopsies from patients who died in a surgical intensive care unit demonstrated significant immune cell loss, including decreased populations of CD4+ and CD8+ T cells as well as biochemical findings of immune suppression including impaired T-cell effector function and cytokine production.[35] In contrast, apoptosis is significantly decreased in bronchoalveolar lavage (BAL) macrophages in septic patients compared with nonseptic controls,[36] associated with lower levels of Bcl-2 than in control patients. Minimal macrophage necrosis has been detected in BAL fluid. In addition, apoptosis is decreased in neutrophils in septic patients through up-regulation of tyrosine phosphorylation by circulating mediators.[37]

Increased apoptosis is also seen in circulating T lymphocytes of patients following blunt trauma or burn injury,[38,39] and increased apoptosis in circulating T cells of trauma patients correlates with T-cell anergy. In contrast, neutrophil apoptosis is low in BAL fluid from patients with acute respiratory distress syndrome (ARDS) as well as those at risk for ARDS.[40,41] Notably, in vitro human polymorphonuclear leukocytes from healthy volunteers have less apoptosis when incubated with BAL fluid from ARDS patients as compared to BAL fluid from healthy controls. Further evaluation of this antiapoptotic effect on normal neutrophils showed it to be highest during the early stages of ARDS with subsequent decreases over time. The change in apoptotic response to BAL fluid from ARDS patients correlates with levels of granulocyte colony-stimulating factor and granulocyte-macrophage colony-stimulating factor.[42] Soluble Fas ligand is also higher at the onset of ARDS in patients who eventually die, and BAL fluid from patients with ARDS induces a Fas-dependent apoptosis in distal lung epithelial cells, whereas BAL fluid from patients at risk for ARDS but without the disease does not have an effect on distal lung epithelial cell death. BAL fluid also has elevated concentrations of the apoptosis-related molecules perforin, granzyme A, and granzyme B in critically ill patients with early ARDS compared with those not having lung injury or late ARDS.[43]

Animal Studies

Similar to human autopsy studies, apoptosis is primarily localized to lymphocytes, dendritic cells, and the gut epithelium in animal models of sepsis. In both cecal ligation and puncture (CLP), a murine model of fecal peritonitis and *Pseudomonas aeruginosa* pneumonia, maximal lymphocytic and intestinal apoptosis occur 24 hours after the onset of septic insult.[44-47] Both intrinsic and extrinsic pathways play a role in sepsis-induced apoptosis, and pathways differ depending on which model of sepsis is examined.[48] Animals with gene specific knockouts of multiple members of the proapoptotic Bcl-2 family members (mitochondrial pathway) or Fas-associated death domain transgenic mice (receptor mediated) demonstrate significant decreases in sepsis-induced splenocyte apoptosis.[49,50] Although apoptosis, whether initiated by the mitochondrial or the receptor-mediated pathway, converges into a single common pathway mediated by caspase-3, it should be noted that there are likely alternate pathways that are independent of caspase-3 given that caspase-3 knockout mice exhibit only a small degree of apoptosis.[51]

Increased lymphocytic apoptosis appears to be detrimental to survival in sepsis. Overexpression of Bcl-2 in transgenic mice in either T lymphocytes or B lymphocytes markedly improves survival in multiple strains of inbred mice subjected to CLP.[51,52] Similar increases in survival have been shown in mice where the proapoptotic Bcl-2 family member Bim has been knocked out.[50] Administration of the polycaspase inhibitor N-benzyloxycarbonyl-Val-Ala-Asp(O-methyl) fluoromethyl ketone (z-VAD) or the caspase-3 specific inhibitor M-971 results in similar improvements in outcome.[52,53]

The mechanisms that account for worse outcomes with increasing lymphocytic apoptosis appear to involve immunosuppression. Although immunosuppression in sepsis is multifactorial, the ongoing loss of immune effector cells in both the innate and adaptive compartments likely plays a significant role. In addition to the loss of cells, there is an up-regulation of T regulatory cells and myeloid-derived suppressor cells.[53] This up-regulation of immunosuppressive cells appears to be driven in part by the production of IL-10, an antiinflammatory, immunosuppressive cytokine. Notably, adoptive transfer of necrotic cells improves survival in septic animals, and this benefit is lost if IFNγ production is blocked.[54] In contrast, apoptotic cells not only increase mortality but they also prevent IFNγ production. Interestingly, a preexisting immunosuppressive state may alter the immune apoptotic response. Septic mice with preexisting pancreatic adenocarcinoma tumors have a higher mortality when compared to non-cancer septic mice,[55] and the presence of malignancy not only impairs tumor-specific immune responses but also pathogen-specific responses as well resulting in a state of generalized immune suppression.[56] Notably, either lymphocyte overexpression of Bcl-2 or germline deletion of Bim in cancer mice results in elevated mortality, contrary to what is seen in septic hosts that were previously healthy.[57]

Prevention of gut epithelial apoptosis also improves survival in preclinical models of sepsis as overexpression of Bcl-2 in gut epithelium decreases mortality in mice subjected to CLP or *P. aeruginosa* pneumonia.[47,58] In addition, giving systemic epidermal growth factor (EGF) normalizes intestinal Bid expression and apoptosis and mortality following CLP,[59,60] and these protective effects appear to be modulated through the intestinal epithelium as similar results are seen if EGF is selectively overexpressed in intestinal enterocytes.[61-63] Notably, the immune system directly impacts apoptosis in the intestinal epithelium in critical illness. Rag$^{-/-}$ mice, which lack lymphocytes, have a fivefold higher level of gut epithelial apoptosis after CLP compared to WT mice, and adoptive transfer of CD4+ T cells in Rag$^{-/-}$ mice restores apoptosis back down to WT levels.[64]

Respiratory epithelial cells are resistant to apoptosis when exposed to *P. aeruginosa,* undergoing cell death in vitro.[65] However, *P. aeruginosa* pneumonia induces respiratory epithelial apoptosis in mice through activation of the Fas/Fas ligand system,[66] and respiratory apoptosis appears to be essential for survival in this study, with rapid sepsis-induced mortality in Fas or Fas ligand–deficient mice that lack bronchial apoptosis. Alveolar and bronchiolar apoptosis are also present in rats with *Streptococcus sanguis* or *Streptococcus pneumoniae* type 25 pneumonia.[67,68] Lung apoptosis has also

been demonstrated following CLP in multiple mouse strains although recently it has been questioned whether CLP causes lung injury.[69] Acute lung injury causes increased death in multiple cells within the lung, and intratracheal injection of lipopolysaccharide (LPS) induces apoptosis in alveolar cells, neutrophils, and macrophages.[68,70] This process is associated with up-regulation of Fas in alveolar and inflammatory cells, and lung injury can be blocked by administration of an anti-Fas antibody. Both epithelial and endothelial apoptosis also occur in the lung in a rat trauma-hemorrhagic shock model in a caspase-3 dependent (epithelial) and independent (endothelial) manner.[71]

Although liver apoptosis is not noted in human autopsy studies of sepsis, there is an increase in murine hepatocyte apoptosis following infection with *Listeria monocytogenes*.[72] Liver apoptosis is greatest at the edge of microabscesses and is independent of endotoxin, Fas, and nitric oxide. Extensive hepatocyte apoptosis is also seen in animal models of trauma/hemorrhage and is dependent on the severity of shock induced with increasing apoptosis correlating with duration of shock.[73,74] In addition, apoptosis is only seen following resuscitation, and the introduction of IL-6 at the time of resuscitation completely prevents trauma hemorrhage–induced apoptosis.[74] Apoptosis of hepatocytes is also seen in animal models of thermal injury.[75] Apoptosis is also increased in murine granulocytes after CLP through a TNFα-dependent pathway.[76]

Necroptotic pathways of cell death have been implicated in preclinical models in a number of clinical disease processes including sepsis, viral infections, stroke, myocardial infarction, pancreatitis, acute kidney injury, and inflammatory bowel disease.[26,77-81] Notably, deletion of RIP3 results in a substantial survival advantage in mice undergoing CLP.[82] When mice deficient in apoptosis-inhibitors are subjected to influenza infection, they suffer significant lung epithelial cell destruction via RIP3 and display mortality compared to WT controls.[83] Further, mice deficient in the apoptotic adaptor Fas-associated death domain (FADD) develop a severe and erosive colitis, similar to that seen in Crohn colitis, and like human colitis, the inflammation in FADD-deficient mice is largely TNFα driven. Interestingly, inflammatory colon lesions in these animals are prevented by deletion of the necroptotic protein RIP3.[58] TNFα-dependent skin conditions can also be cured in animals by deleting necroptotic proteins, suggesting that these pathways may be involved in a host of human disease that prominently feature TNFα as a mediator.[84,85] Beyond tissue-specific processes, deletion of RIP1 has been shown to cause perinatal lethality associated with severe systemic inflammation at birth with cell necrosis via RIP3-MLKL.[86]

There is a growing body of literature characterizing the role of autophagy in animal models of critical illness. Hepatocytes have a decline in autophagy in the later stages of sepsis following CLP,[87] and mice treated with carbamazepine have a more complete activation of the autophagic response and attenuated liver injury following CLP.[88] Similarly, septic animals have an attenuated autophagic response in renal tubules following sepsis.[89] In the heart, rapamycin treatment induces autophagy and restores CLP-induced cardiac dysfunction.[90] Autophagy may also play a role in immune dysfunction as T cells in septic mice have decreased autophagy (in addition to increased apoptosis).[91]

Globally, the balance of cell production and loss is critical to homeostasis, and normal physiologic cell death plays a vital role in maintaining this balance. However, cell death is also centrally implicated in multiple human diseases and can result in significant pathology when left unchecked. Therapeutic agents that target and manipulate cell death pathways may be attractive targets to treat critically ill patients. However, it is important to note, though, that blocking one pathway of cell death may simply trigger another. Necroptosis was first identified in cell cultures with inhibited apoptotic machinery, and animal models have confirmed that blocking apoptosis can unleash necrotic cell death.[18,20,92] In vivo myocardial infarction modeling has also indicated that outcomes are most improved not by limiting just apoptosis or necrosis but by limiting both simultaneously.[93] If novel drug therapies are to one day treat human disease and critical illness, a thorough and complete

understanding of the intricate, interconnected pathways of cell death must first be established.

Key References

9. Linkermann A, Green DR. Necroptosis. *N Engl J Med*. 2014;370:455-465.
10. Vanden Berghe T, Linkermann A, Jouan-Lanhouet S, et al. Regulated necrosis: the expanding network of non-apoptotic cell death pathways. *Nat Rev Mol Cell Biol*. 2014;15:135-147.
14. Mittal R, Coopersmith CM. Redefining the gut as the motor of critical illness. *Trends Mol Med*. 2014;20:214-223.
35. Boomer JS, To K, Chang KC, et al. Immunosuppression in patients who die of sepsis and multiple organ failure. *JAMA*. 2011;306:2594-2605.
52. Hotchkiss RS, Coopersmith CM, McDunn JE, Ferguson TA. The sepsis seesaw: tilting toward immunosuppression. *Nat Med*. 2009;15:496-497.

Common Endocrinopathies in the Pediatric Intensive Care Unit

Ofer Yanay and Jerry J. Zimmerman

PEARLS

- Cortisol, produced in the adrenal *zona fasciculate,* is a key mediator of the stress response and influences much more than hemodynamics and inflammation by modulating the transcription of perhaps 20% of the entire genome.
- Relative adrenal insufficiency and critical illness–related corticosteroid insufficiency are poorly understood concepts in terms of both pathophysiology and therapeutic intervention.
- Critical illness hyperglycemia is the result of inflammation-mediated increased endogenous glucose production and decreased utilization secondary to insulin resistance.
- Although the evidence on glycemic control and its benefits is controversial, it is difficult to ignore the convincing association that exists between hyperglycemia and morbidity and mortality, as well as the results of initial trials reporting a significant decrease in mortality when critically ill adult and pediatric patients were maintained euglycemic.
- Sick euthyroid syndrome, common among critically ill patients, is characterized by a rapid decrease in T3 and variable increase in rT3 that appears to be proportional to the intensity of illness severity and concentration of TNF-α.

As discussed in Chapter 81 the endocrine system is closely aligned with the neurogenic and inflammatory systems, particularly as an aspect of the stress response. Multiple servo feed-forward and feed-back signaling normally provide precise control over this integrated system, but critical illness and its treatment may generate unique endocrinopathies. In addition, the intensivist may encounter patients with primary deficiency or excess endocrinopathies as the underlying cause of critical illness.

Hypothalamic-Pituitary-Adrenal Axis

A schematic overview of the classic regulation of cortisol synthesis and secretion is provided in Fig. 85.1.

A variety of stimuli converge on the paraventricular nucleus of the hypothalamus, resulting in release of corticotropin-releasing hormone (CRH).[2-4] Similar stimuli also increase release of antidiuretic hormone (ADH, arginine vasopressin).[5] ADH and aldosterone, generated via activation of the renin-angiotensin-aldosterone axis,[6] control salt and water balance as discussed in Chapter 73. As summarized in Table 85.1, angiotensin II also mediates a number of other neurogenic-endocrine-inflammation–related actions relevant to critical illness.

CRH is transported via hypophyseal portal capillaries to the anterior pituitary, facilitating the production of pro-opiomelanocortin, a 239 amino acid peptide that includes primary protein sequences for adrenocorticotropic hormone (ACTH), beta-lipotropin, beta-endorphin, and melanocyte-stimulating hormone. The hypothalamic-pituitary stalk is susceptible to shear injury, and this may be associated with long-term pituitary dysfunction following head trauma.[7] ACTH is transported by the blood to the *zona fasciculata* of the adrenal gland, where it binds to type 2 melanocortin receptors (MC2R). Bioinactive ACTH (the p.R8C ACTH mutant that lacks bioactivity but conserves immunoreactivity) has recently been demonstrated as a cause of adrenal insufficiency.[8] Familial cortisol deficiency is a lethal condition associated with hypoplastic adrenal glands and is caused by another mutation in the *MC2R* gene.[9] Single nucleotide polymorphisms in *MC2R* may be responsible for some of the variability in cortisol response to pediatric critical illness.[10] *MC2R* is a seven-transmembrane domain protein coupled with G proteins that uses intracellular cyclic adenosine monophosphate signaling to modulate adrenal steroidogenesis.[11]

During critical illness, activation of the HPA axis frequently reflects activation of the systemic inflammatory response syndrome (eg, by interleukin-6).[12] Interleukins 1, 2, and 6 are generally thought to stimulate cortisol production, whereas tumor necrosis factor–alpha (TNF-α), macrophage inhibitory protein (MIP), and corticostatin, a peptide defensin with anti-ACTH activity, are generally considered to be inhibitory for cortisol production.

Cortisol Biochemistry

A schematic overview of the biosynthesis of adrenal cortical hormones is summarized in Fig. 85.2.[13]

Synthesis of pregnenolone from cholesterol represents a rate-limiting step in cortisol production and requires both mobilization of cholesterol from storage depots, as well as a transfer to a specific cytochrome P-450 located on the inner mitochondrial membrane that catalyzes side chain cleavage.[14] The second rate-limiting step in cortisol production involves the conversion of 11-deoxycortisol to cortisol by

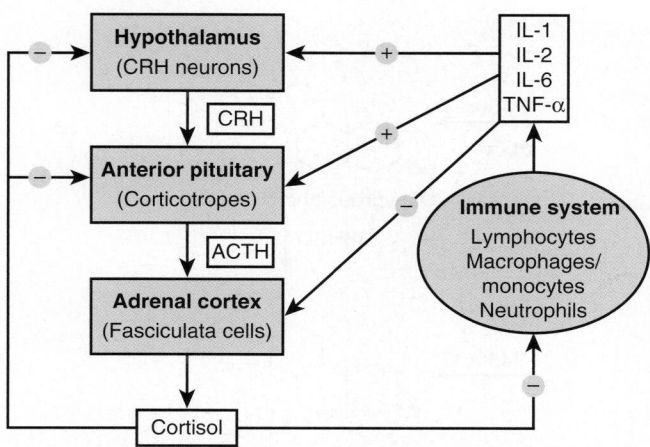

Fig. 85.1. Signaling for hypothalamic-pituitary-adrenal axis.[1]

TABLE 85.1	Activities of Angiotensin II

- Increases systemic vascular resistance and blood pressure
- Stimulates aldosterone release
- Increases plasminogen activator inhibitor–1, promoting prothrombotic state
- Enhances thirst and salt craving
- Increases antidiuretic hormone, adrenocorticotropic hormone, and norepinephrine release
- Facilitates Na reabsorption at proximal convoluted tubule
- Stimulates renal afferent/efferent vasoconstriction
- Increases nuclear transcription factor NF-κB, resulting in increased proinflammatory cytokine production
- Mediates cardiomyocyte hypertrophy

the enzyme 11β-hydroxysteroid dehydrogenase, another specific cytochrome P-450 isoenzyme.[15] Generation of a unique hydroxyl group at carbon 11 is essential for cortisol-mediated antiinflammatory and glucose homeostasis functions. A diurnal rhythm of cortisol production is noted among healthy (but not critically ill) patients with peak cortisol production typically 0800 to 0900 and a nadir of cortisol production typically around midnight. Normal adrenal production of cortisol is approximately 9 mg/m²/day. Stress production of cortisol may reach 200 to 300 mg/day, resulting in a plasma total cortisol concentration occasionally exceeding 60 µg/dL. Among critically ill patients, plasma cortisol–cortisone ratios increase due to an increase in 11β-hydroxysteroid dehydrogenase activity.[16] In addition, reduced cortisol breakdown, related to suppressed expression and activity of cortisol catabolic enzymes, contributes to hypercortisolemia and associated ACTH suppression.[17] If the latter is maintained during prolonged critical illness, adrenal lipid depletion and reduced ACTH-regulated gene expression may occur in conjunction with adrenal atrophy and insufficiency.[18] Hypercortisolemia in critical illness is correlated with severity of illness.[19] Mean and range of plasma cortisol concentrations as a function of age have been reported for normal children and may be found in Table 85e.1.[20]

Although the plasma half-life for cortisol ranges 80 to 115 minutes, biological duration of action of cortisol is approximately 8 hours. Cortisol is catabolized by reduction of the

steroid nucleus C4-C5 double bond, reduction of the C3 ketone to a hydroxyl, oxidation of the C11 hydroxyl group, or conjugation of the C11 hydroxyl group with either sulfate or glucuronic acid. Cortisol exhibits mineralocorticoid activity approximately 1% that of aldosterone.

Actions of Cortisol

Cortisol is transported from the adrenal gland to various tissues via cortisol binding proteins, namely transcortin with high affinity but low capacity and albumin with low affinity but high capacity.[21] Transcortin with a molecular weight of 58,000 Da is a member of the serpin serine protease super family, with a plasma concentration of approximately 1 µM. Cortisol concentration is locally increased at sites of inflammation through degradation of transcortin by neutrophil elastase, as well as local upregulation of 11β-hydroxysteroid dehydrogenase.[22]

Cortisol diffuses through the plasma membrane binding to the glucocorticoid receptor (GCR), which is flanked by heat shock proteins for transport to the cell nucleus, where cortisol subsequently binds to glucocorticoid responsive elements.[23,24] Commonly occurring GCR polymorphisms may explain individualized patient responses to corticosteroids.[25] Children with septic shock demonstrate a transient depression of GCR mRNA in their neutrophils[26] that may reflect an adaptive cortisol resistance response. On the other hand, septic patients may demonstrate a transient increased[27] or decreased[28] expression of GCR on mononuclear cells. Corticosteroid treatment induces expression of microRNA-124 that downregulates GCR-alpha with resultant modulation of antiinflammatory effects.[29] A common polymorphism of the GCR has been associated with posttraumatic stress disorder following critical illness.[30] Glucocorticoid receptors represent a potential drug target for treatment of severe inflammation and the consequences of excess endogenous or exogenous corticosteroid.[31]

Cortisol also affects nuclear migration of transcription factors NF-κB, as well as activator protein-1 (AP-1).[32,33] Ultimately, cortisol modulates the transcription of thousands of genes, perhaps 20% of the entire genome.[34,35] Although the majority of corticosteroid action is related to changes in gene transcription mediated through chromatin remodeling, corticosteroids also affect protein synthesis by decreasing the stability of messenger RNA. A number of inflammatory proteins appear to be regulated by this posttranscriptional mechanism.[34] Even with appropriate cortisol production by the adrenal gland, cortisol resistance syndrome can occur by multiple mechanisms including depletion of corticosteroid-binding globulins, activation of 11β-hydroxysteroid dehydrogenase, decreased glucocorticoid receptor density and activity, and elevated antiglucocorticoid compounds and receptors.[32,36,37]

Cortisol affects three general areas of physiology: immunity, metabolism, and hemodynamics.

Immunity[32,38-40]

Much of critical illness may involve disturbance of the balance between systemic inflammatory responses (SIRs) versus compensatory antiinflammatory responses (CARs).[41-43] As depicted in Fig. 85.3, cortisol biochemistry represents a key regulatory mechanism for virtually all aspects of antiinflammation.

In this respect, cortisol increases the synthesis of IκB, trapping NF-κB in the cytoplasm and effectively thwarting

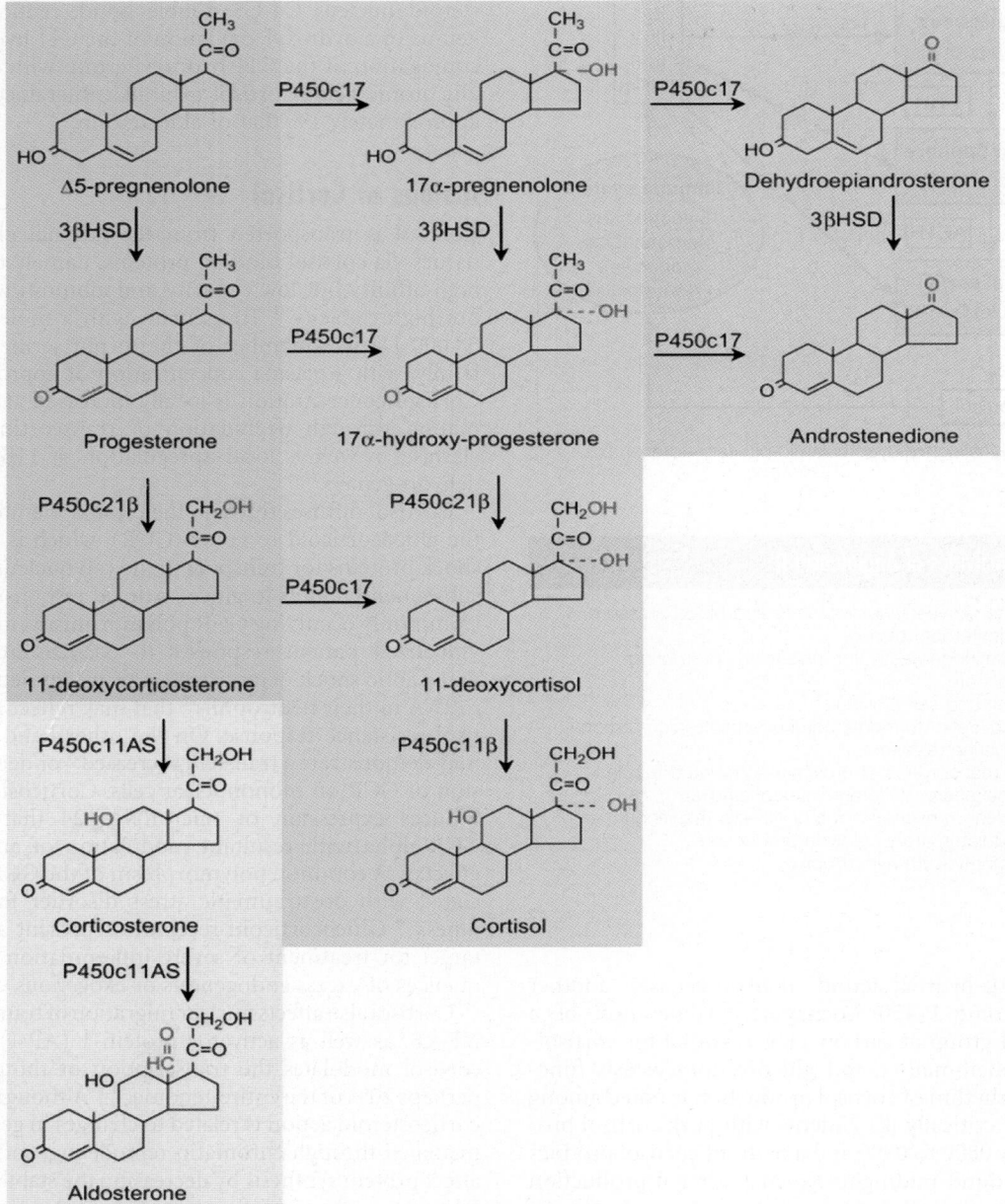

Fig. 85.2. Biosynthetic pathways for adrenal cortical hormones. Reactions highlighted in yellow are unique to the zona glomerulosa. Reactions highlighted in blue occur in the zona fasciculata. Reactions highlighted in green are seen in both the zona glomerulosa and reticularis. Reactions highlighted in pink are largely confined to the zona reticularis. Structural changes produced in each reaction are shown in red. (From Goodman HM. Basic Medical Endocrinology. Boston: Elsevier; 2009, p 65.)

synthesis of a variety of proinflammatory mediators. Similarly, cortisol blocks NF-κB and AP-1 binding to appropriate DNA promoter regions. In addition, cortisol increases the production of annexin that inhibits phospholipase A$_2$, resulting in modulation of both cyclooxygenase and lipoxygenase inflammatory lipid pathways. Sepsis induces widespread immunosuppression.[44] Among septic children administered corticosteroids, further repression of gene networks related to adaptive immunity has been reported.[39]

Metabolism[45-48]

A schematic summary of the effects of cortisol on metabolism is displayed in Fig. 85.4.[13]

As a key mediator of the stress response, cortisol facilitates lean muscle catabolism to provide substrate for hepatic gluconeogenesis, synthesis of acute phase reactants, and expansion of the immune system. Hypercortisolemia represents a key mediator in hyperglycemia of critical illness discussed later.[49] Both protein catabolism and hyperglycemia, if prolonged in the ICU, can become maladaptive and associated with increased risk for adverse outcomes including death (see also Chapter 81).

Hemodynamics[50-52]

Cortisol's permissive effects on maintaining a normal hemodynamic status includes augmenting cardiac contractility,

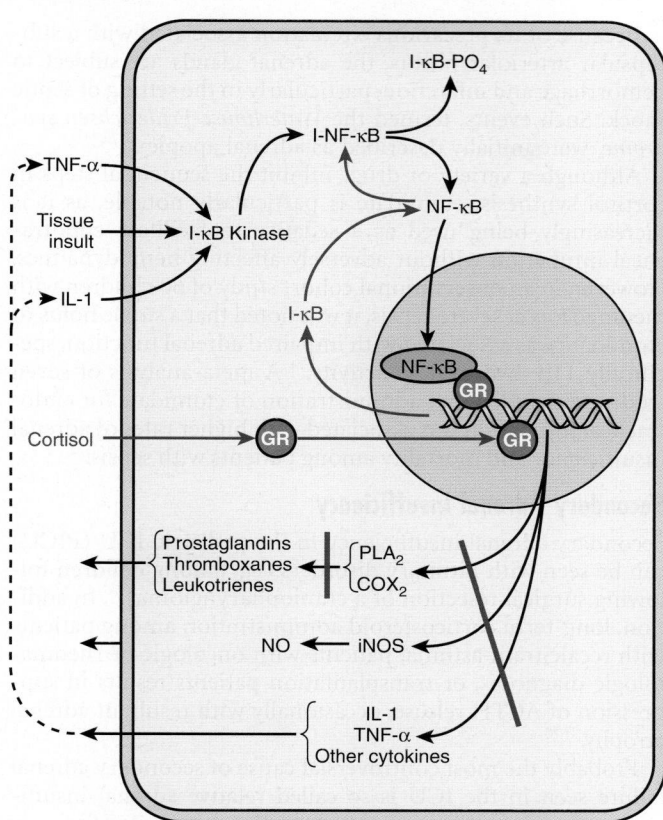

Fig. 85.3. Signaling for the antiinflammatory actions of cortisol.[13] (From Goodman HM. Basic Medical Endocrinology. Boston: Elsevier; 2009, p 80.)

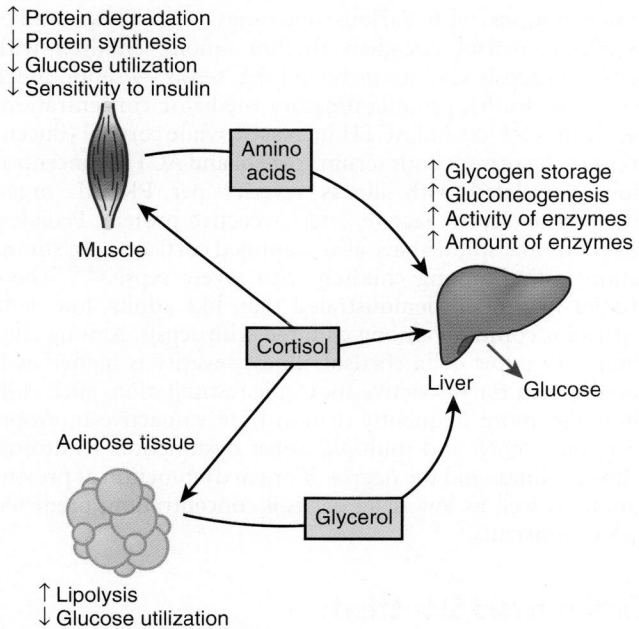

Fig. 85.4. Schematic overview of metabolic actions of cortisol. (From Goodman HM. Basic Medical Endocrinology. Boston: Elsevier; 2009, p 76.)

maintaining vascular tone, promoting endothelial integrity, upregulating vasoactive receptors, and increasing catecholamine synthesis.

Assessing the Cortisol Stress Response

Historically, adrenal function during critical illness has been quantified by random total plasma cortisol concentrations or by calculating the difference between a corticotropin-stimulated plasma cortisol concentration minus a baseline cortisol concentration. In the latter case a so-called delta value less than 9 μg/dL was previously considered evidence of adrenal insufficiency (AI) or inadequate adrenal reserve.[53] Depending on the cutoff value chosen (10, 15, 18, 20, 25 μg/dL), critically ill patients may demonstrate a wide range of adrenal insufficiency occurrence when random baseline total plasma cortisol concentrations are evaluated.[54]

Examples of cortisol testing approaches are illustrated in Table 85e.1.

A detailed evaluation of critically ill adults with sepsis indicated that those patients with a high baseline plasma cortisol concentration but delta cortisol concentration less than 9 μg/dL exhibited the highest risk for hemodynamic instability and mortality.[55] In fact, a subsequent interventional trial of adjunctive hydrocortisone for adult septic shock was designed on the basis of these findings.[56] However, a confirmatory trial failed to replicate this finding and concluded that corticotropin stimulation testing provided no information regarding which patients with septic shock would benefit from hydrocortisone replacement therapy.[57] Although the overnight metyrapone test is not generally applicable to critically ill patients, it has been employed as a gold standard in an attempt to identify an adult population with an apparent inadequate adrenal response to the stress of critical illness. Metyrapone administration will result in increased ACTH and the cortisol precursor 11β-deoxycortisol. Among adult patients with severe sepsis, approximately 60% exhibited an abnormal cortisol stress response per the overnight metyrapone test. The best predictors of this scenario included a baseline total cortisol of less than or equal to 10 μg/dL, a delta total cortisol of less than or equal to 9 μg/dL, or a free cortisol less than 2 μg/dL.[53]

Serial low-dose corticotropin stimulation testing in addition to comprehensive ACTH, dehydroepiandrosterone, and cytokine measurements in a cohort of critically ill Turkish children revealed that 28% exhibited AI that was largely resolved by 2 weeks.[58] Baseline cortisol levels of the patients were significantly higher than those of healthy children. Patients with multiple organ dysfunction syndrome (MODS) had significantly higher concentrations of baseline and stimulated cortisol, as well as higher procalcitonin, TNF-α, and IL-6 concentrations compared with those without MODS. Cortisol, ACTH, and dehydroepiandrosterone concentrations were higher among the children with AI compared with those without AI. Interestingly, sepsis as an antecedent of critical illness was not associated with an increased risk of AI. Similarly, among 381 critically ill Canadian children also evaluated by low-dose corticotropin stimulation testing, AI was noted in 30.2%.[59] Children with AI exhibited higher baseline cortisol concentrations, were significantly older, and demonstrated an increased need for volume resuscitation and vasoactive-inotropic support.

Free Cortisol

Although most cortisol is bound to transcortin or serum albumin, the free fraction comprising 10% to 15% of the total is actually responsible for the protean effects of cortisol. Accordingly, it has been suggested that perhaps free cortisol rather than total cortisol concentrations might be more reliable in terms of identifying a population that would most benefit from cortisol replacement therapy.[60] For most critically ill patients, cortisol-binding globulin is typically decreased and the percent of cortisol as the free fraction increased. Moreover, with corticotropin adrenal stimulation, free cortisol increases substantially more than total cortisol.[61-63] Assessing total cortisol concentrations may be especially problematic in critically ill patients with low albumin.[60] Multiple limitations of corticotropin stimulation testing to assess total cortisol during critical illness have been summarized.[64] Free cortisol may be assessed in urine and saliva,[65] but blood contamination of either specimen may limit this approach. Free cortisol concentrations may be determined among critically ill children using microdialysis or centrifugal ultrafiltration plasma fractionation.[63] In an investigation that measured both total and free cortisol concentrations in a general population of critically ill children, the majority exhibited both total and free cortisol concentrations that would be considered inadequate by the metyrapone testing criteria mentioned earlier. However, none of these children demonstrated evidence of corticosteroid insufficiency (hypotension, hyponatremia, hypoglycemia).[19] These results question the use of current thresholds for assigning diagnoses of AI or critical illness–related corticosteroid insufficiency in critically ill children and further suggest that clinicians currently are unable to reliably define adequacy of the adrenal response to the stress of critical illness.

Adrenal Insufficiency in the Intensive Care Unit

Adrenal insufficiency may be classified under two major categories: primary, in which direct malformation or destruction of the adrenal glands occurs, and secondary, in which there is typically loss of HPA axis integrity. The latter situation is most often encountered among critically ill patients.

Primary Adrenal Insufficiency

Primary adrenal insufficiency or Addison disease is typically encountered in adult patients and is included in a group of disorders termed *autoimmune adrenalitis*.[66,67] Signs and symptoms of Addisonian crisis include intercurrent illness with a history of chronic weight loss and anorexia, dizziness, lethargy, and chronic pigmentation. Symptoms more likely to be associated with admission to the ICU include sudden hypovolemic shock, hyperkalemia, vomiting, diarrhea, abdominal pain, and coma. Other causes of primary adrenal failure include congenital adrenal hyperplasia, an autosomal recessive disorder, with approximately 90% of cases secondary to 21 hydroxylase deficiency (CYP21A2 mutation).[68,69] The next most common congenital inborn error of metabolism is 11-hydroxylase deficiency.[70] Primary congenital adrenal failure can also occur among infants with adrenoleukodystrophy associated with a metabolic defect in metabolism of very-long-chain fatty acids. Other causes of congenital adrenal failure include Wollman disease and familial unresponsiveness to ACTH involving altered *MC2R* as previously discussed.[71]

Because of its precarious circulation associated with a subcapsular arteriolar plexus, the adrenal glands are subject to hemorrhage and infarction, particularly in the setting of septic shock. Such events, termed the *Waterhouse-Friderichsen syndrome*, were initially described as adrenal apoplexy.[72,73] Although a variety of drugs inhibit the sequential steps in cortisol synthesis, etomidate is particularly notable, as it is increasingly being used as a sedative to facilitate endotracheal intubation without adversely affecting hemodynamics. However, in an observational cohort study of 60 children with meningococcal severe sepsis, it was noted that a single bolus of etomidate was associated with impaired adrenal function, specifically 11β–hydroxylase activity.[74] A meta-analysis of seven studies concluded that administration of etomidate for endotracheal intubation was associated with higher rates of adrenal insufficiency and mortality among patients with sepsis.[75]

Secondary Adrenal Insufficiency

Secondary adrenal insufficiency in the pediatric ICU (PICU) can be seen with pituitary disorders (eg, among children following surgical resection of a craniopharyngioma).[76] In addition, long-term corticosteroid administration among patients with recalcitrant asthma, patients with oncologic or rheumatologic diagnoses, or transplantation patients results in suppression of ACTH release, occasionally with resultant adrenal atrophy.[77,78]

Probably the most controversial cause of secondary adrenal failure seen in the ICU is so-called relative adrenal insufficiency or critical illness–related corticosteroid insufficiency (CIRCI).[79] A seemingly inadequate adrenal response relative to the magnitude of stress characterizes CIRCI. This situation is a dynamic, typically reversible state that is thought to be secondary to both decreased cortisol production and tissue resistance to cortisol, as discussed previously. Multiple pediatric observational studies, most associated with sepsis, have examined associations with random, baseline serum cortisol concentrations with various outcomes.[74,80-83] These studies ascertain cortisol circadian rhythm among children with sepsis. As sepsis severity increased (eg, sepsis → septic shock → sepsis death), proinflammatory mediator concentrations (eg, IL-6, TNF-α) and ACTH increased, while cortisol concentrations decreased. Both serum cortisol and ACTH concentrations correlated with illness severity per PRISM, organ dysfunction scores, lactate, and C-reactive protein. Pediatric observational studies have also examined corticotropin stimulation testing among children with severe sepsis.[84-88] These studies in general demonstrated that, like adults, low delta cortisol is common among children with sepsis. Among children with a low delta cortisol, illness severity is higher, as is requirement for vasoactive-inotropic resuscitation. Such children also more frequently demonstrate vasoactive-inotropic resistance shock and multiple organ dysfunction syndrome. Chronic illness and the degree of organ dysfunction at presentation, as well as low delta cortisol concentration, predicted risk of mortality.

Corticosteroid Side Effects

Corticosteroid therapy has been associated with increased risk for hospital-acquired infection among a general population of critically ill children[89] and in children following surgery for congenital heart disease.[90] In the latter investigation, children who received hydrocortisone were nearly 30 times more likely to develop a central catheter–associated infection as compared with children who did not receive hydrocortisone. With increasing recognition of the key role of immunosuppression in the pathogenesis of sepsis, it is noteworthy that children with sepsis demonstrate widespread repression of gene programs associated with adaptive immunity and that this gene repression is further enhanced with concurrent corticosteroid administration.[39] Loss of HLA-DR (the antigen presentation protein motif) on monocytes appears to be an early event in sepsis, and persistence of HLA-DR downregulation is associated with sepsis severity and sepsis prognosis. Endogenous cortisol mediates transcriptional regulation of this process; the role of exogenous corticosteroids in this setting has not been detailed.[91]

Dissolution of lean body mass mediated by both endogenous and exogenous[45] corticosteroids represents a key element of the stress response.[47] Although this may be beneficial in the short term, prolonged corticosteroid mediated muscle catabolism can be associated with ICU weakness (including the diaphragm) and hyperglycemia. Muscle weakness has been associated with prolonged mechanical ventilation weaning.[48,92-94] Hyperglycemia has been associated with a variety of adverse events in the PICU as detailed later.[49] Additional important clinical consequences of protein catabolism that may be exaggerated by exogenous corticosteroid administration include impaired wound healing, hypoalbuminemia, disordered coagulation, and impaired gut function with bacterial translocation.[95]

In the CORTICUS sepsis interventional trial,[57] transient hypernatremia was also noted among patients receiving hydrocortisone. Although gastrointestinal hemorrhage represented an important side effect in previous clinical trials examining the potential utility of high-dose methylprednisolone as adjunctive therapy in sepsis, this side effect has not been problematic in later investigations using low-dose hydrocortisone. Among adult critically ill patients with acute lung injury, corticosteroid administration is associated with transition to delirium.[96]

Long-term exposure to corticosteroids results in characteristic side effects (eg, as manifested in children with bronchopulmonary dysplasia).[97] In the absence of obvious exogenous steroid administration, true Cushing's syndrome is diagnosed as a high 24-hour urine-free cortisol concentration that is not suppressed by administration of dexamethasone.[98] Clinical characteristics of Cushing syndrome include hypertension, hypokalemic alkalosis, proximal myopathy, hyperglycemia, osteoporosis, opportunistic infections, psychiatric problems, and central obesity with characteristic striae.

Alterations of Glucose Homeostasis
Glucose Homeostasis in Health

Under normal conditions, glucose concentration is tightly regulated by the neuroendocrine system. Control of blood glucose is complex, involving interaction among liver, pancreas, muscle, adipose tissue, pituitary, adrenals, and bone. The brain and periphery conduct a constant biochemical conversation by which the periphery informs the brain about its metabolic needs and the brain addresses these needs through its control of somatomotor, autonomic, and neurohumoral pathways involved in energy intake, expenditure, and storage.[99,100]

Glucose is obtained from three sources: intestinal absorption of food, glycogenolysis, and gluconeogenesis. Once transported into cells, glucose can be stored as glycogen or it can undergo glycolysis to pyruvate. Pyruvate can be reduced to lactate, transaminated to form alanine, or converted to acetyl coenzyme A (CoA) (see also Chapter 80). Acetyl CoA can be oxidized in the mitochondrial tricarboxylic acid cycle to carbon dioxide and water, converted to fatty acids for storage as triglyceride, or serve as substrate for ketone body or cholesterol synthesis. Although glycogenolysis can occur in most tissues in the body, only liver and kidneys express the enzyme glucose-6-phosphatase, which is required for release of cellular glucose into the bloodstream. The liver and kidneys also contain the enzymes required for gluconeogenesis. Of the two organs, the liver is responsible for the bulk of glucose output; the kidney supplies only 10% to 20% of glucose production during fasting.

Current understanding of glucose homeostasis is centered on glucose-induced secretion of insulin from pancreatic beta cells and insulin effect on glucose metabolism in peripheral tissues. The switch from glycogen synthesis during and immediately after meals to glycogen breakdown and gluconeogenesis is orchestrated by hormones of which insulin is centrally important. Plasma insulin concentrations increase to peak levels of 50 to 100 μU/mL after meals. This surge in insulin activates glycogen synthesis, enhances peripheral glucose uptake, and inhibits glucose production. In addition, lipogenesis is stimulated while lipolysis and ketogenesis are suppressed. During fasting, plasma insulin level falls to less than or equal to 5 to 10 μU/mL. Hormones including glucagon, catecholamines, cortisol, and growth hormone (GH) counteract the effects of insulin and promote glycogenolysis, gluconeogenesis, lipolysis, and ketogenesis.

Insulin binds to its receptor, a tyrosine kinase expressed in many cell types. It then triggers a complex series of events that lead to insulin receptor substrate binding, recognition of the activated insulin receptor substrate by intracellular signal transducing proteins, and activation of postreceptor signaling pathways. This action activates phosphatidylinositol-3 kinase and nuclear gene expression modulating proteins. These in turn stimulate glycogen synthesis and inhibit glycogenolysis in liver and muscle, increase glucose uptake by increasing glucose transporter (GLUT)-4 on the cellular membrane, downregulate the expression of phosphoenolpyruvate carboxykinase (PEPCK), and inhibit fructose 1,6-bisphosphatase, the key rate-limiting steps of hepatic gluconeogenesis. Response to insulin is tissue specific (see Fig. 85.5).

Recent findings support the concept of even more complex mechanisms for glucose homeostasis. These include the "gut-brain-liver" axis, hepatic independent glucose sensing, and a bone-pancreas loop. Brain neurons are equipped with mechanisms allowing them to detect and respond to changes in circulating levels of several hormones and metabolites. Following ingestion of food, presence of nutrients in the gastrointestinal tract initiates complex neuronal and hormonal responses, informing the brain of ongoing change in nutritional status. The gut is richly supplied with both sympathetic and parasympathetic afferent fibers of the autonomic nervous system. Metabolic sensing neurons (previously called "glucosensing") respond to glucose, fatty acids, and metabolites from the periphery. These neurons use glucose and other

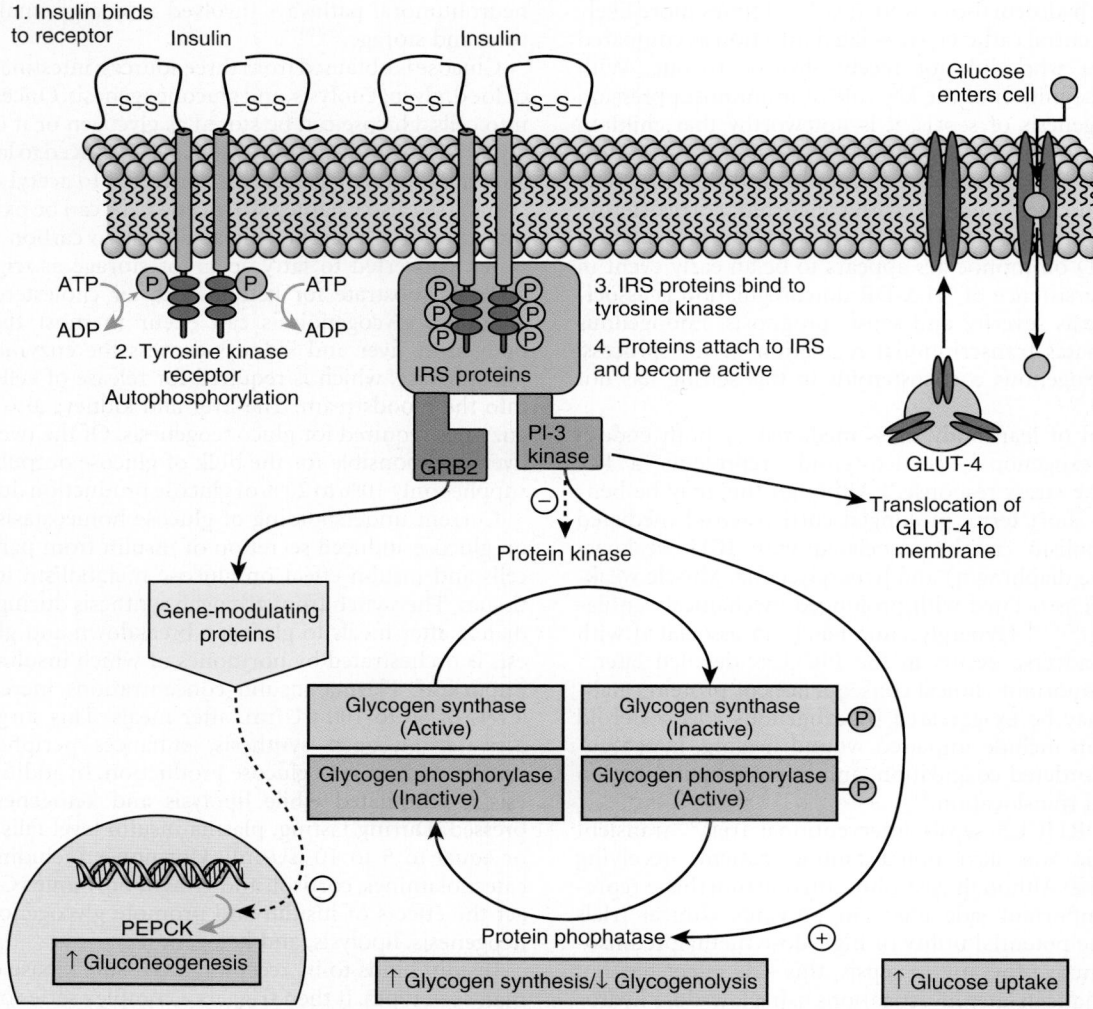

Fig. 85.5. Insulin receptor signaling pathways. After insulin attaches to the receptor, it activates tyrosine kinase activity, causing the enzyme to autophosphorylate. Insulin receptor substrate (IRS) proteins bind to the now active tyrosine kinase receptor. IRS then serves as a loading dock for several different proteins. Growth factor receptor–bound protein 2 (GRB2) is one of the proteins involved in signal transduction and will activate gene-modulating proteins that inhibit phosphoenolpyruvate carboxykinase (PEPCK) expression in the nucleus, thereby decreasing gluconeogenesis. PI-3 kinase also becomes active after attaching to IRS, and this leads to inhibition of protein kinases and stimulation of protein phosphatases. This results in increased glycogen synthesis and decreased glycogenolysis. Activated PI-3 kinase also results in translocation of glucose transporter 4 (GLUT-4) to the membrane, facilitating glucose uptake.

metabolites as signaling molecules to regulate their membrane potential and neuron signaling. In glucose-excited neurons, the increase in extracellular glucose leads to augmentation of the ATP-to-ADP ratio and closure of the K_{ATP} channels, which leads to plasma membrane depolarization and Ca^{2+} entry through voltage-gated channels, thereby increasing neuronal activity and neurotransmitter secretion.

The gut also informs the brain of these changes by secreting a host of gut peptides including ghrelin, cholecystokinin (CCK), and glucagon-like peptide-1 (GLP-1).[101] Signals from the gut are integrated by the hindbrain and projected to the hypothalamus.[102] The brain can then signal peripheral tissues to alter their glucose uptake and/or secretion appropriately, by both insulin-dependent and independent mechanisms. A functional network of enzymes and transcription factors enables independent glucose sensing in the liver, which

is also an essential component of systemic glucose and energy homeostasis.[103]

Recently, bone has emerged as another endocrine "gland." Osteocalcin, a bone-specific protein, was identified as a hormone that stimulates insulin sensitivity in peripheral tissues (liver, muscle, and adipose tissue) and insulin secretion by the pancreas. The latter is accomplished by direct effect on beta cells and indirectly by promoting gut secretion of GLP-1.[104]

In the current era, obesity is an increasingly prevalent disease in the pediatric population. Glucose metabolism in patients with obesity is altered in health with chronic inflammation and dysregulated immune pathways, leading toward impaired glucose metabolism.[105]

Current understanding of the impact of obesity on children during critical illness is limited. This subset of patients may require special attention when dealing with stress hyperglycemia.

Glucose Metabolism

Sugars are essential for cellular function. They serve five main purposes: source of energy (utilization and storage), source of carbon skeletons, osmolality activity, signaling, and transport function. Glucose is a polar molecule, and its transport into cells occurs largely by active transport or facilitated diffusion.

The human genome codes for more than 20 sugar transporters (7 sodium-glucose symporters [SGLTs], 14 glucose transporters [GLUTs], 1 NaGLT1, and 1 SWEET).[106] Of the 14 members of the GLUT family, 13 are facilitative transporters. One or more GLUT proteins are expressed in virtually every cell type of the human body. Within the GLUT family members, 11 of 14 are capable of transporting glucose, although it is highly likely that the principal physiologic substrates for some of these proteins have not been identified. GLUT-1 to GLUT-4 facilitate the glucose uptake in myriad of cell types and are well summarized in Table 85.2. The redundancy of proteins transporting glucose can be easily explained by the critical nature of this sugar as circulating fuel in humans and the consequent need for multiple glucose transporters with different kinetics and regulatory properties that are expressed in a cell-type specific fashion.[107] Transporter activity can be efficiently controlled through transporter delivery or endocytosis, as best exemplified in the case of GLUT-4 trafficking by insulin.

Hyperglycemia

Hyperglycemia has been defined by the World Health Organization as blood glucose levels greater than 126 mg/dL when fasting. There are no specific age-adjusted levels for infants and children. No guidelines specifically define stress hyperglycemia, although a common definition describes it as transient hyperglycemia resolving spontaneously after dissipation of acute severe illness. Stress hyperglycemia (SHG) was first described by Thomas Willis in the 17th century. Initially identified as an appropriate adaptive harmless or even beneficial short-term physiologic response to critical illness, it is now considered a risk factor, especially because advanced critical care has improved survival and extended ICU length of stay (LOS).[108] Hyperglycemia is common in nondiabetic, critically ill children and occurs in up to 86% of patients.[109]

Stress Hyperglycemia and Outcomes

Studies in children have challenged the assertion that hyperglycemia is beneficial or inconsequential, by observing that SHG is associated with worse clinical outcomes. A retrospective study from a single PICU examined 1173 admissions. Hyperglycemia was prevalent and associated with increased

---

TABLE 85.2   Characteristics of Glucose Transporters

GLUT-1 and GLUT-3 are responsible for maintaining basal rate of glucose uptake. Their high glucose affinity facilitates constant uptake from the bloodstream. GLUT-2 has low affinity, which allows glucose sensing and glucose entry proportional to blood levels (glucose enters only when blood levels are high). Because the bulk of blood glucose is taken up by skeletal muscle in the presence of elevated insulin and GLUT-4 transport activity is rate limiting for this process, GLUT-4 plays a critical role in the regulation of whole-body glucose homeostasis.

GLUT Receptor	Distribution	Glucose Affinity	Significant Glucose Uptake	Insulin Dependence	Additional Remarks
GLUT-1 (55-kDa, 45-kDa isoforms)	All human tissues, often in conjunction with ≥1 additional GLUT isoforms	High	Basal glucose uptake	Insulin independent	Highly expressed in brain endothelial cells. Different isoform expressed in astrocytes, choroid plexus, and ependymal cells. Common in erythrocytes
GLUT-2	Beta cells, liver, renal tubules, small intestine, some CNS cells	Low	Postprandial glucose uptake	Insulin independent	Major basolateral glucose transporter isoform in intestine. Absolutely required for renal glucose reabsorption in kidney. Associated with glucose-sensing mechanisms in brain (mostly in the hypothalamus)
GLUT-3	All human tissues. Widely expressed in parenchymal neurons, placenta and leukocytes	High	Basal glucose uptake	Insulin independent	Major transporter in CNS neurons
GLUT-4	Skeletal muscles, myocardium, adipocytes		Glucose uptake typically postprandial transporter expression is insulin dependent	Insulin dependent, translocation from cytosol to cell membrane	
GLUT-5	Brush border of intestinal cells, liver, spermatozoa	N/A		Primarily transports fructose	

CNS, central nervous system; GLUT, glucose transporter.

morbidity as characterized by increased LOS and mortality.[110] Association between hyperglycemia and worse outcome in children was also demonstrated in specific disease processes such as traumatic brain injury,[111] general trauma,[112] severe burns,[113] septic shock,[114] meningococcal sepsis,[115] and postoperative congenital heart disease.[116,117] Hyperglycemia is common in infants with necrotizing enterocolitis admitted to the NICU and is associated with increased late mortality and NICU LOS.[118] SHG is also associated with specific complications such as increased risk of venous thromboembolism in nondiabetic children[119] and more frequent nosocomial infections including surgical site infection.[120]

While clearly prevalent in critically ill children, some studies were unable to show clear association between hyperglycemia and worse outcomes. One retrospective study found that hyperglycemia within 24 hours of PICU admission was associated with increased rate of mechanical ventilation, ICU LOS, and mortality, but when controlled for disease severity, it was not independently associated with increased morbidity or mortality.[121] Another retrospective study evaluated the association between blood glucose level and duration of mechanical ventilation and ICU LOS in mechanically ventilated patients with bronchiolitis. Hyperglycemia was a frequent event in this patient population, yet results failed to show independent association with worse outcomes.[122] Such studies support the notion that hyperglycemia may be a marker of severity of illness rather than a cause.

Preexisting nutritional status may also impact outcomes associated with hyperglycemia in the critically ill child. A prospective study from Brazil reported that compared with those well nourished, malnourished patients with hyperglycemia were at greater risk of mortality independent of severity of illness.[123] Obesity is prevalent among critically ill pediatric patients, but the available literature on the relationship between obesity and clinical outcome is limited.[124] There exist no available studies examining the relationships between obesity and SHG.

With current knowledge, it is clear that hyperglycemia is prevalent in critically ill children and is associated with worse outcome in some disease processes but not in others. Many studies are not controlled for severity of illness, making it difficult to interpret results. Different definitions for SHG used by different authors (range of 126–250 mg/dL, in 9 key pediatric studies of association of SHG and mortality)[125] make it even harder to compare results and create thresholds for treatment. Moreover, thus far, all studies have failed to establish cause-and-effect relationships, yet many suggest that aggressive maneuvers should be used to normalize plasma glucose levels. Younger patients (<1 year) are at higher risk for spontaneous hypoglycemia and require special consideration when treating hyperglycemia with insulin.[126]

Pathophysiology of Stress Hyperglycemia

During stress the normal mechanisms that counteract hyperglycemia are overwhelmed, causing a persistent unchecked state of high glucose blood levels. These changes help the body provide glucose to meet increased metabolic demands. SHG results from increased levels of counter regulatory hormones (epinephrine and norepinephrine, glucagon, cortisol, and growth hormone) and proinflammatory cytokines (TNF-α, IL-1, and IL-6) (see also Chapter 81). The overall effect is increased hepatic and renal glucose production. Peripheral

and hepatic insulin resistance is a well-recognized phenomenon in critically ill patients. It is characterized by organ-specific alteration in glucose utilization/production and impaired insulin mediated uptake.[108] Insulin concentrations may be elevated or decreased. Use of carbohydrate-based feeds, glucose-containing fluids, and drugs like epinephrine and corticosteroids may exacerbate the picture.

High hepatic output of glucose, especially through gluconeogenesis, is the most important contributor to SHG. Glycogen stores are limited and rapidly depleted during stress. Lactate, pyruvate, and alanine are the main precursors used by the liver for gluconeogenesis. Often overlooked, renal-derived gluconeogenesis is a significant contributor (up to 40%) of glucose production during stress, mostly in response to epinephrine.[127] The principal precursors for renal gluconeogenesis are lactate and glycerol (see Fig. 85.6).

Mechanisms underlying insulin resistance occur at several levels. Insulin receptor levels are unchanged in most short-term animal models of sepsis. However, reduction in insulin receptors is seen in longer-term models.[128] Although the level of insulin receptor may be unchanged, TNF-α activates protein kinase B, inducing serine phosphorylation of insulin receptor substrate 1, and inhibits insulin receptor tyrosine kinase, thereby reducing cellular utilization of glucose through GLUT-4. TNF-α, hypoxia, and insulin-like growth factor binding protein 3 (IGFBP-3) inhibit peroxisome proliferator activator (PPARγ), which impacts gene expression including adiponectin, a hormone capable of sensitizing cells to insulin effect. Inhibition of PPARγ has significant impact on cell metabolism in sepsis and other stress conditions, including insulin resistance during SHG.

A different mechanism for hepatic insulin resistance is associated with increase in growth hormone (GH) and reduction in insulin growth factor–1 (IGF-1). Effects of IGF-1 are similar to insulin in terms of cell growth promotion. During critical illness, GH levels increase significantly, but there is a fall in hepatic GH receptor with disruption of downstream signaling. IGF-1 levels drop in response to proinflammatory cytokines, especially TNF-α with decreased IGF-1 synthesis. In addition, low IGF-1 may result from upregulation and increased affinity of its binding protein IGFBP-3, reducing the free active protein.[129]

Elevated insulin levels are common in adults. The critically ill child may present with insulin deficiency due to beta cell dysfunction and impaired insulin production (direct effect of proinflammatory cytokines), which contributes to stress hyperglycemia.[130,131]

Despite insulin resistance, critical illness is associated with increased glucose utilization, mostly through the insulin-independent transporter, GLUT-1. Additionally, impaired nonoxidative glucose disposal results from reduced skeletal muscle glycogen synthesis.

Insulin resistance ultimately promotes a catabolic state in which lipolysis is activated. Lipotoxicity, glucotoxicity, and inflammation are key components of global SHG.

Hyperglycemia itself further exacerbates the inflammatory and oxidative stress response and proinflammatory cytokine storming, promoting a vicious cycle whereby SHG leads to further SHG.

During critical illness, specific interventions can mediate development of SHG. Use of vasoactive-inotropic drugs such as epinephrine, norepinephrine, and dopamine is frequently

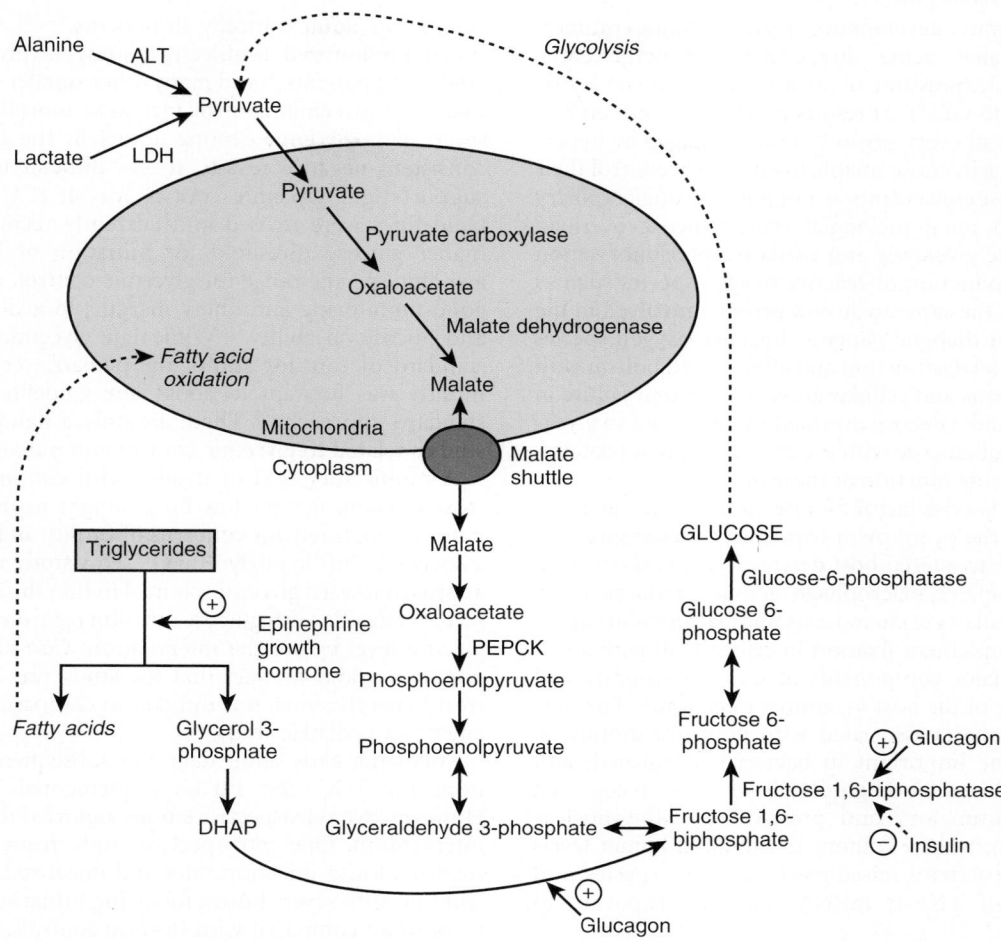

Fig. 85.6. Schematic overview of gluconeogenesis. Pyruvate is generated from glycolysis, lactate, or alanine through pyruvate kinase, lactate dehydrogenase (LDH), and alanine-amino transferase (ALT), respectively. Pyruvate enters the mitochondria freely and is converted into oxaloacetate, which is then converted into malate in order to enter the malate shuttle and cross the mitochondrial membrane into the cytoplasm, where it is again converted into oxaloacetate and through phosphoenolpyruvate carboxykinase (PEPCK) is converted into phosphoenolpyruvate that serves as substrate for a series of enzymatic-driven reactions and is finally converted into glucose. It should be noted that the rate-limiting step of gluconeogenesis is the conversion of fructose biphosphate into fructose 6-phosphate and is regulated by the actions of glucagon (stimulates) and insulin (inhibits) on fructose 1,6-biphosphatase. Triglycerides also contribute to gluconeogenesis by their breakdown into fatty acids and glycerol 3-phosphate. The latter is then transformed into dihydroacetone phosphate and then into fructose 1,6-biphosphate to follow the rest of the gluconeogenic pathway and result in the generation of glucose.

associated with SHG. Epinephrine stimulates β_2 receptors, promoting glycogenolysis and gluconeogenesis, and increases insulin resistance by release of glucagon and cortisol. It also reduces insulin secretion via stimulation of α_2 receptors. Effects of dopamine and norepinephrine are less prominent due to lesser activity at the β_2 receptors. Several medications commonly used in the ICU setting may result in development of SHG (eg, patients frequently receive antifungal and antibiotic medications in large volumes of dextrose-containing fluids). Corticosteroids can increase the risk of SHG, especially when given in bolus doses. Thiazide diuretics are also associated with the occurrence of SHG. Calcineurin inhibitors such as tacrolimus and cyclosporine can result in SHG and posttransplant diabetes due to decreased insulin biosynthesis and release.

Nutritional support practices strongly influence SHG (see also Chapter 87). Critically ill children are frequently prescribed parenteral nutrition (PN). Provision of excess carbohydrate calories in PN can result in SHG. Overfeeding is common in critically ill children, regardless of whether PN or enteral nutrition is employed. Studies have shown that commonly used predictive equations to calculate caloric needs are inferior to targeted indirect calorimetry and frequently result in overprescription of calories.[132]

Mechanisms of Stress Hyperglycemia Adverse Outcomes

Postulated mechanisms by which SHG cause harm include direct cellular damage and alterations of essential organ function. In diabetic patients, four main molecular mechanisms have been identified in glucose-mediated complications: (1) increased polyol pathway flux; (2) increased advanced glycation end product formation; (3) activation of protein kinase C isoforms; and (4) increased hexosamine pathway flux. Each of the four pathogenic mechanisms reflects a hyperglycemia-induced process, namely overproduction of superoxide anion by the mitochondrial electron-transport chain.[133]

Diabetes-related injury develops over years, but some common mechanisms parallel acute stress-related hyperglycemia. During SHG, overexpression of insulin independent transporters (GLUT-1 to GLUT-3) results in glucose overload and toxicity essentially in every organ.[134] Cells damaged by hyperglycemia are primarily those unable to effectively control their intracellular glucose concentration, notably neuronal, capillary endothelium, and renal mesangial cells. Glucose overload results in excessive glycolysis and oxidative phosphorylation with increased production of reactive oxygen species such as superoxide anion, the same toxic end product involved in the injury pathway for diabetic patients. Reactive oxygen species cause mitochondrial dysfunction and altered metabolism with subsequent apoptosis and cellular and organ system failure in the critically ill child. Glucose overload can also lead to glycation, the reaction of glucose with the amine group of proteins, which may impair the function of these proteins.

Hyperglycemia is a risk factor for infection in acute illness.[108] The relative bacterial overgrowth witnessed in hyperglycemia may be partly due to altered host defenses. Acute, short-term hyperglycemia impairs macrophage activity, reduces polymorphonuclear leukocyte chemotaxis and bactericidal capacity, and alters complement fixation in critically ill patients.[135] SHG affects all major components of innate immunity and impairs the ability of the host to combat infection.[135] Furthermore, hyperglycemia is associated with poor gut motility, a factor that may be important in bacterial overgrowth and translocation. A raised blood glucose level is also recognized as being proinflammatory and pro-oxidant. Mononuclear cells isolated from healthy volunteers exhibited higher levels of NF-κB binding activity, raised reactive oxygen species, and increased levels of TNF-α mRNA following exposure to hyperglycemia.[136]

Hyperglycemia also results in a hypercoagulable state partly through the increased expression of tissue factor, which is both procoagulant and proinflammatory.[137] SHG is implicated in other abnormalities such as endothelial dysfunction and alteration in vascular smooth muscle tone, commonly observed during critical illness.[138] Likewise, hyperglycemia has been associated with deleterious effects on the nervous system. Underlying mechanisms in critical illness remain largely speculative and are often extrapolated from knowledge in diabetic patients. Hyperglycemia-induced blood-brain barrier permeability, oxidative stress, and microglia activation may play a role and compromise neurons and glial cell integrity.[139]

Clinical Trials Examining Management of Critical Illness Hyperglycemia

In 2001, a single-center adult study reported reduction of hospital mortality by more than 30% using a tight glycemic control (TGC) protocol.[140] The effect was attributed to the actual glycemic control rather than the infused insulin dose. These impressive results brought the issue of SHG into clinical attention and fostered considerable discussion. Previously seen as an aspect of a normal stress response, physicians now started viewing SHG differently, considering it as a major cause or contributor to pathophysiology that must be aggressively addressed and treated. The appeal of such straightforward intervention was too great to resist.[141] Subsequent studies failed to reproduce these results, yet guidelines generated by professional societies warmly recommended tight glycemic

control for adult critically ill patients.[142,143] A large international randomized multicenter study involving more than 6000 adult patients[144] and many other smaller studies reported that tight glycemic control increased mortality and risk for severe hypoglycemia among adults in the ICU. With such consistent negative results, it was difficult to continue and support tight glycemic control for all ICU adult patients. Guidelines were revised and currently recommend using a higher glucose threshold for initiation of insulin therapy, avoiding specific range for glycemic control, and focusing on good monitoring and safety margins to avoid hypoglycemia and glucose variability.[145] While tight glycemic control became standard of care for adults, the pediatric critical care community was hesitant to adopt any guidelines or consistent standard approach.[146] There are only a handful of pediatric studies related to glycemic control and outcome.

A multicenter trial of insulin with continuous 20% dextrose infusion in very-low-birth-weight neonates was terminated prematurely for concerns of futility and potential harm associated with hypoglycemia.[147] This study took a proactive approach toward glycemic control in that the treatment group received insulin with glucose infusion regardless of their blood glucose level before the intervention. Considering the study population and the fact that the study was not designed to treat hyperglycemia, it is difficult to compare the results with any other pediatric study.

Following early adult data and subsequent recommendations for TGC, few PICUs implemented TGC protocols. However, two retrospective studies reported the impact of this intervention. One retrospective study from a single center reported lower infection rates and improved survival among children with severe burns, following initiation of a TGC protocol when compared with historic controls.[148] A second retrospective study from two centers compared all nondiabetic PICU patients who presented with hyperglycemia of greater than 150 mg/dL and treated with insulin with historic controls who were not treated with insulin. The authors concluded that blood glucose control with insulin appeared to be associated with worse outcome.[149]

Four randomized prospective studies have examined the association between TGC and clinical outcomes. The first study published in 2009, derived from a single center in Belgium, enrolled a mixed medical/surgical patient population, although 75% of the subjects had undergone cardiac surgery.[150] The study targeted age-adjusted glycemic range for infants and children. Results showed improved short-term outcome including mortality in the TGC group, despite the fact that the TGC group had an unacceptable rate (25%) of severe hypoglycemia (<40 mg/dL). The concern for impact of hypoglycemia on neurodevelopment cognitive long-term outcome was addressed by the same group with 4-year neurocognitive follow-up that ascertained that brief hypoglycemia evoked by TGC was not associated with worse neurocognitive outcome.[151] Three subsequent subgroup analyses were conducted using the parent investigation[150] database. The first examined the effects of the TGC protocol on the somatotropic axis and reported that intensive insulin therapy did not reverse the catabolic state of critical illness.[152] The second, focused on the thyroid axis, concluded that TGC further accentuated the peripheral inactivation of thyroid hormone.[153] In addition, a predefined small subgroup analysis (14 neonates) found that TGC in neonates undergoing cardiac surgery appeared to protect the myocardium and reduce inflammation.[154]

In 2010, a single-center study focusing on pediatric patients with severe burns concluded that intensive insulin therapy significantly decreased infections and sepsis and improved organ function by decreasing inflammation.[155] A two-center prospective randomized trial published in 2012 enrolled 980 children who underwent surgery with cardiopulmonary bypass. The authors reported that TGC can be achieved with a low hypoglycemia rate; however, the study found no clinical benefit for TGC in terms of infection rate, mortality, LOS, or measures of organ failure when compared with standard care.[156] A post hoc analysis of this study demonstrated that TGC may, in fact, lower the rate of infection in children older than 60 days of age at the time of cardiac surgery when compared with standard care.[157] In a secondary analysis of this trial, insulin appeared to have no discernible impact on skeletal muscle degradation.[158] In 2014, a large multicenter randomized trial involving 13 centers in England reported that TGC in critically ill children had no significant effect on major clinical outcomes (number of days alive and free from mechanical ventilation at 30 days after enrollment), but patients in the TGC arm had lower need for renal replacement therapy and reduced total hospital stay and cost. These effects were mostly notable in the noncardiac patient population.[159]

A summary of prospective randomized pediatric studies of tight glycemic control with intense insulin therapy for stress hyperglycemia may be found in Table 85e.2.

TGC with the use of intensive IV insulin therapy significantly reduced morbidity, mortality, or both in two randomized control trials involving children[150,155] but not in two others.[156,159] The patient population differed among the four studies with one involving children with severe burns, one involving children who were in the ICU following cardiac surgery, and two involving children who were in the ICU for a variety of reasons, although these studies included a significant portion of patients postcardiac surgery. The intervention increased the rate of severe hypoglycemia, although to a lesser extent in one study where continuous glucose monitoring was performed[156] and in another when nursing-directed glucose monitoring protocol was used.[159] These interventional trials are justified given that an association between pediatric hyperglycemia and mortality has been repeatedly reported.[109,116,161-164] Interestingly, hypoglycemia encountered in application of TGC was not associated with increased risk of neurocognitive disability in a 4-year follow-up study.[151]

Various reasons have been put forth to explain the observed differences in results in these studies. These include disparities in patient population and targeted age groups, difference in glucose control targets, variability in attaining these targets, differences in ICU-specific protocol, glucose control and glucose monitoring protocols, and different nutrition support practices. With current data, the pediatric critical care provider remains conflicted when treating a patient with hyperglycemia. At this time the evidence for (or against) using TGC protocols with intensive insulin therapy to improve outcome (especially mortality) is inconclusive. Moreover, there is little knowledge about long-term outcomes. Large-scale multicenter studies, with strategies that combine continuous glucose monitoring with TGC, may yet afford the best chance to evaluate whether TGC using intensive insulin therapy in critically ill children is associated with improved

outcome while limiting the risks associated with hypoglycemia.[165] There is also a need to identify patients who are at high risk for hyperglycemia-mediated harm. These patients are most likely to benefit from intervention.

Whether hyperglycemia should be addressed or left untreated has never been evaluated by any prospective clinical trial.

Glucose Measurement

Until recently, intermittent blood glucose levels (using point of care, blood gas analyzer, or central laboratory measurement) were the only means of blood glucose monitoring. Accuracy is probably the most important metric in selecting the best glycemic management device for critically ill children, but rapidity/turnaround time, cost, and sample volume are also important factors.[166] Intermittent measurements are limited by the workload associated with the sampling process and with the potential that "between measurements" events will be missed. A simulation study modeling adult patients on TGC protocol demonstrated that increasing the frequency of glucose measurements reduced the adverse impact of glucose measurement imprecision on glycemic control.[167] A mathematical simulation in a cohort of critically ill patients suggested that glycemic control is more optimal with a blood glucose measurement interval no longer than 1 hour, with further benefit obtained with use of a measurement interval of 15 minutes. These findings have important implications for the development of glycemic control standards and future studies.[168] With growing interest in glycemic control and the possible beneficial effect of frequent glucose measurements, continuous glucose monitoring systems have been developed. Although termed *continuous,* current systems still sample glucose intermittently with a measurement interval of a few milliseconds up to 15 minutes. The Clinical and Laboratory Standard Institute uses 15 minutes as the cutoff for definition of continuous measurement.[169] This frequency may not be sufficient to detect trends and prevent harm in critically ill patients.

One of the key advantages of continuous glucose monitoring is the ability to identify and display trends in blood glucose measurements. High-quality continuous glucose monitoring devices enable us to assess the complexity of the glycemic signal—how one point in time changes relative to neighboring measurements.[170] The clinical significance of these datasets in the pediatric population is unknown at this time. Continuous glucose monitoring has the potential to improve blood glucose control and patient outcome. Continuous glucose monitoring mandates new approaches to the analysis of parameters of glucose regulation. Different goals can be achieved including maintenance of specified target range, avoidance of hypoglycemia, assessment of glucose variability, and determining the degree of glucose complexity.[171]

Future Directions

TGC with intensive insulin therapy in the pediatric population remains controversial. Large multicenter studies with intensive insulin therapy and continuous glucose monitoring are necessary in order to determine whether this strategy can improve outcome. Hypoglycemia rate has been reported and discussed, but other domains of the glycemic control (glucose variability and complexity) have not. In a retrospective analysis of prospectively collected data from more than 3000 adult patients with ICU LOS of longer than 1 day, it was shown that time in blood glucose range of 70 to 140 mg/dL was strongly associated with survival independently of ICU LOS and severity of illness.[172] Current clinical practice and future studies may need to consider methods to define the ideal age-appropriate glucose range and improve the time each patient spends within that range. Most studies reported in the literature have focused on insulin therapy for hyperglycemia. A different potential direction would be to use other medications that may improve glycemic control with lower risk for hypoglycemia and glucose variability.[173,174]

Hypoglycemia

Although the determination of which glucose levels represent hypoglycemia is controversial, a glucose level less than 40 mg/dL is generally accepted to be in the hypoglycemic range. However, this concentration is well below the level at which counterregulatory responses occur. As plasma glucose levels reach 80 to 85 mg/dL, insulin secretion decreases, and as levels approximate 65 mg/dL, glucagon, epinephrine, cortisol, and growth hormone are released.[175] In addition, a decrease in mental efficiency may be seen when levels fall below 50 to 60 mg/dL. Because a delay in the recognition and management of hypoglycemia may lead to long-term neurologic sequelae,[176] it is important to make a distinction between the laboratory diagnosis of hypoglycemia (<40 to 50 mg/dL) and an interventional threshold at which therapies to raise serum glucose should be applied. Setting the interventional threshold at a level similar to that which elicits counterregulatory responses seems appropriate, and as such, treatment should be offered for hypoglycemia when levels fall below 60 mg/dL to prevent complications, especially in young children. An even higher interventional threshold (<70 mg/dL) is warranted for children who are at increased risk of hypoglycemia.

Clinical Manifestations

Diaphoresis, tremor, tachycardia, anxiety, weakness, hunger, nausea, and vomiting are all autonomic manifestations caused by the adrenergic stress response that occurs with a rapid decline in blood glucose levels. Other symptoms associated with hypoglycemia are a result of a deficiency of the brain's primary energy substrate and as such are known as neuroglycopenic symptoms. These symptoms include headache, visual disturbances, lethargy, restlessness, irritability, dysarthria, confusion, somnolence, stupor, coma, hypothermia, seizures, and motor and sensory disturbances. The glycemic ranges at which these symptoms manifest vary, as critically ill patients cannot recognize or communicate symptoms. The picture is further masked by sedation and analgesia.

Pathogenesis

Imaging studies of infants who sustained neonatal hypoglycemic brain injury display diffuse cortical and subcortical white matter damage that is most prominent in the parietal and occipital lobes. This pattern differs from the neuroimaging features of other neonatal insults, including hypoxic-ischemic encephalopathy.[177] Interestingly, this pattern does not resemble the glucose uptake pattern of neonatal brains by positron emission tomography, which may indicate that neuronal damage is not simply due to cerebral deprivation of its primary substrate for energy production. Evidence indicates that hypoglycemia activates receptors for excitatory amino acids within the brain and causes cell depolarization, with subsequent cellular edema and apoptosis.[178]

Fasting Adaptation

Consumption of glucose is largely dependent on the brain-to-body ratio. This phenomenon explains the reduced fasting tolerance of infants whose glucose utilization rate (approximately 6 mg/kg/min) is significantly higher than that of older children and adults (1 to 2 mg/kg/min). This reality places younger patients at increased risk of hypoglycemia. In addition, their ability to maintain euglycemia through glycogenolysis and gluconeogenesis is reduced because glycogen stores and muscle bulk are small, thus reducing the pool of available gluconeogenic substrates. Within the brain, astrocytes but not neurons are capable of storing glycogen. The brain contains <1 mmol/kg of free glucose reserve. Fasting tolerance increases rapidly in the first days of life. Neonates may fast up to 18 hours after 1 week of age. By 1 year a 24-hour fast is tolerated, and by 5 years a child may fast for up to 36 hours without experiencing hypoglycemia.

Understanding fasting physiology is crucial to the logic and methodologic approach required for diagnosing the etiology of hypoglycemia. Normally in the postabsorptive state, metabolism is governed primarily by counterregulatory hormones. In the first 4 hours of a fast in infants or in the first 8 hours in older children, glucagon is released and euglycemia is maintained primarily by glycogenolysis. Following glycogen store depletion, gluconeogenesis gains importance in the maintenance of normal glucose levels (Fig. 85.6).

Muscle provides amino acids, particularly alanine and glutamine, as gluconeogenic substrates. Glycerol 3-phosphate derived from triglyceride hydrolysis is also a gluconeogenic precursor. Fatty acids resulting from triglyceride hydrolysis are transported to the liver, where they are oxidized to generate acetyl coenzyme A and ketones. The latter may then be used as alternative fuel by skeletal and cardiac muscle to help ensure availability of glucose to the brain and to erythrocytes that are strictly dependent on glucose for energy production. The brain may also use ketones as an alternative fuel source, but it does so only during a prolonged fast (see also Chapter 87).

Hypoglycemia that occurs early during fasting may indicate hormonal imbalance or a primary disorder of glycogenolysis. Disorders of gluconeogenesis will not manifest during early fast. They become apparent only after glycogen stores have been depleted; hence typically they present later in infancy once feeding intervals become increasingly prolonged. The same is true for fatty oxidation disorders. These disorders generally require a more prolonged fast to manifest, nearing 12 to 18 hours in infants and 18 to 24 hours in older children. A comprehensive approach to diagnosing pediatric hypoglycemia is provided in Chapter 82. However, the most common cause of childhood hypoglycemia is ketotic hypoglycemia.[179] This illness most frequently occurs in toddlers and preschoolers and is uncommon after 8 to 9 years. It is typically triggered by intercurrent infection and caloric restriction, both common events in the PICU. A defect in protein catabolism, transamination, or amino acid efflux from skeletal muscle, as well as impaired autonomic regulation of epinephrine secretion, has been postulated.

Hypoglycemia has been observed in association with a variety of critical illness diagnoses, including sepsis, congestive heart failure, renal failure, liver failure, and pancreatitis, and it has been associated with increased mortality among critically ill children.[180,181] Critically ill patients are at risk of hypoglycemia, not only because of their underlying illness but because of factors unique to their hospitalization, such as muscular atrophy from prolonged immobilization and gluconeogenic substrate depletion, undernutrition often resulting from the limitation of caloric intake because of fluid restriction, increased glucose consumption, adrenal insufficiency, loss of IV access or inadvertent disconnection of infusion lines, or iatrogenic factors related to drugs and therapies, including the practice of strict glycemic control.

Hypoglycemia Treatment

After obtaining the "critical" blood/urine samples (see also Chapter 82), administration of 2 mL/kg of 10% dextrose water solution is indicated for patients with hypoglycemia. Subsequently, an IV maintenance fluid regimen should be initiated to provide a glucose infusion rate of 8 mg/kg/min. Serum glucose should be rechecked 15 minutes after the initial bolus, and if hypoglycemia persists, a bolus of 5 mL/kg of 10% dextrose water should be administered and the glucose infusion rate increased by 50%. If the volume of fluid required to maintain glucose concentrations greater than 70 mg/dL is excessive, a higher dextrose concentration should be used. Glucagon (0.03 mg/kg for patients <20 kg, or 1 mg for patients >20 kg) can reverse hypoglycemia in patients with adequate glycogen stores and normal glycogenolytic pathways. Definitive treatment will depend on the underlying etiology.

In summary, hypoglycemia is a manifestation of iatrogenic, intentional, or accidental drug ingestion or administration or the manifestation of an underlying disorder. All critically ill patients with hypoglycemia should raise a high index of suspicion because many defects that cause hypoglycemia remain silent until an intercurrent illness or stress overwhelms the compensatory capacity of the individual. Unless certitude of the etiology of the hypoglycemia exists before therapy, a "critical" blood/urine sample should be obtained to guide diagnosis and further management. Prompt recognition and treatment are necessary to prevent neurologic injury. A multidisciplinary approach is often necessary.

Alterations of Thyroid Hormone in Critical Illness
Thyroid Biochemistry

Thyroid-stimulating hormone (TSH) derived from the anterior pituitary is a pleotropic hormone that modulates all aspects of thyroid hormone synthesis.[182] TSH action within the thyroid follicular cells facilitates the sodium iodide symporter, resulting in (1) enhanced iodine concentration in the thyroid gland; (2) increased synthesis of thyroglobulin, the site of tyrosine residues destined for iodination; and (3) activated thyroid peroxidase that catalyzes iodination of tyrosine residues, as well as tyrosine coupling. It is important to note that autoantibodies may bind to TSH receptors and stimulate a response similar to TSH, resulting in a hyperthyroid state. Leptin is likely to mediate an important role in

the regulation of the thyroid axis, as suggested by the close correlation between the circadian rhythm of leptin secretion and TSH.[183]

An overview of thyroid hormone biosynthesis and secretion is provided in Fig. 85.7.[13] In this schematic diagram, iodide is transported into the thyroid follicular cell by the action of the sodium-iodide symporter (NIS). Subsequently, this iodide diffuses passively through the iodide channel termed *pendrin* (P). Thyroglobulin (TG) is synthesized within the rough endoplasmic reticulum (ER) and subsequently packaged by the Golgi apparatus into thyroglobulin secretory vesicles that are released into the follicular cell lumen. Thyroid oxidase (TO) produces hydrogen peroxide that is subsequently used by thyroid peroxidase (TPO) to oxidize iodide to iodine, which subsequently reacts with the tyrosine residues within thyroglobulin to produce monoiodotyrosine (MIT) and diiodotyrosine (DIT) residues within the thyroglobulin peptide.

Thyroid peroxidase also catalyzes coupling of adjacent iodotyrosines to form thyroxin (T4), as well as lesser amounts of triiodothyronine (T3). Secretion of thyroxin from the thyroid follicular cell begins with thyroglobulin phagocytosis with a subsequent fusion of thyroglobulin endosomes containing proteolytic enzymes capable of digesting thyroglobulin to peptide fragments (PF), as well as monoiodotyrosine, diiodotyrosine, and thyroxin. While thyroxin is released from the cell at the basal membrane, both monoiodotyrosine and diiodotyrosine are deiodinated by iodotyrosine deiodinase (ITDI) and subsequently recycled (see Fig. 85.8).

Thyroxine is transported to peripheral tissues via transport hormones thyroxine-binding globulin, transthyretin, and albumin. Because all of the thyroxine transport proteins are moderate sized, thyroxine is not filtered by the kidney.

In peripheral tissues, thyroxine (T4) is metabolized to triiodotyrosine (T3) and reverse T3 (rT3) by the action of various isoforms of iodothyrosine deiodinases.[184] Transcription and translation of this enzyme are highly dependent on cytokine stimulation. Selenocysteine residues characterize the active site of this iodine cleavage enzyme. As indicated in Fig. 85.8, if monodeiodination occurs on the outer tyrosine ring, the product is T3, and if the monodeiodination occurs on the inner tyrosine ring, the resultant product is rT3.[13]

In peripheral tissues, T3 binds to thyroid hormone receptors that subsequently undergo homodimerization with other thyroid hormone receptors or heterodimerization with retinoid receptors. Thyroid hormone receptors can bind to specific nucleotide sequences termed *thyroid responsive elements* within promoter regions of genes that they regulate whether or not the thyroid hormone is present. Presence or absence of T3 on the thyroid receptor dictates a corepressor or coactivator activity.[185]

Thyroid Hormone Actions

Box 85.1 summarizes the effects of thyroid hormone on metabolism.[186]

Thyroid hormone significantly affects skeletal and central nervous system growth and maturation. Unrecognized hypothyroidism in infancy results in marked physical, motor, and mental delay termed *cretinism*.[187] Hemodynamically thyroid hormone is known to increase beta-adrenergic receptor density and activity, as well as upregulate genes encoding calcium channels (ryanodine receptor) and sodium potassium ATPase. In a general way, thyroid hormone provides gain control for

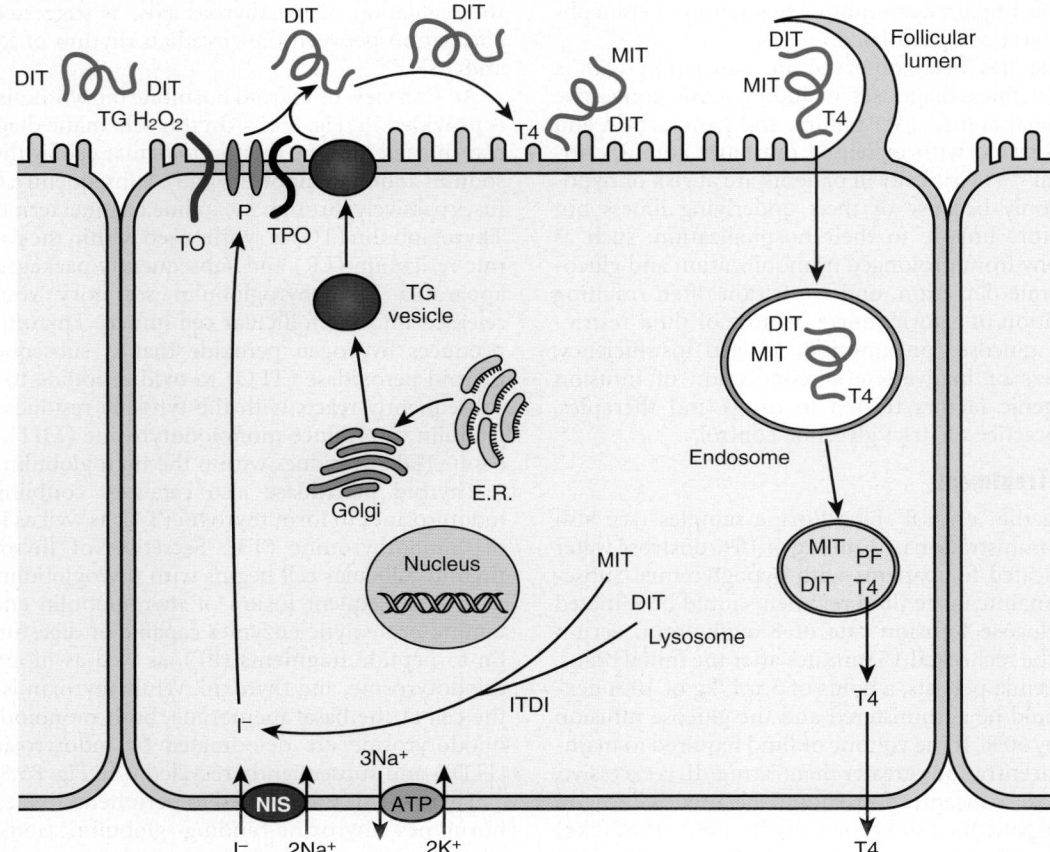

Fig. 85.7. Thyroid hormone biosynthesis and secretion (abbreviations explained in text). (From Goodman HM. Basic Medical Endocrinology. Boston: Elsevier; 2009, p 45.)

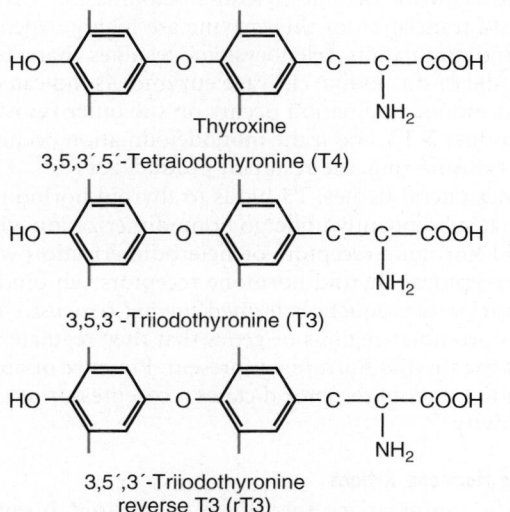

Fig. 85.8. Thyroid hormone chemical structures. (From Goodman HM. Basic Medical Endocrinology. Boston: Elsevier; 2009, p 44.)

BOX 85.1	Thyroid Effects on Metabolism

1. Increased oxygen consumption
2. Enhanced thermogenesis
3. Accelerated amino acid and lipid metabolism
4. Facilitated water and ion transport
5. Enhanced tissue growth and development
6. Altered cortisol and insulin catabolism
7. Modulated growth hormone and parathormone activity
8. Enhanced respiratory response to hypoxia and hypercarbia
9. Increased β-adrenergic receptor affinity and responsiveness to catecholamines

Hyperthyroidism

Manifestations of thyrotoxicosis reflect increased thyroid hormone concentration, and thyroid storm represents the most severe manifestation of hyperthyroidism. Grave disease is probably the best known example of hyperthyroidism and classically is associated with a diffusely enlarged thyroid gland (goiter), exophthalmos, and cardiac palpitations. Pathophysiology of Grave disease involves thyroid-stimulating autoantibodies that bind to TSH receptors.[190] Hypertrophy and hyperplasia of the thyroid accompanying Grave disease are associated with lymphocytic infiltration.[191] Grave disease typically occurs in adults and chronically is associated with nervousness, fatigue, tremor, heat intolerance, and weight loss.[192]

carbohydrate and lipid metabolism and significantly accelerates both protein synthesis and degradation. Through its effects on uncoupling of ATP production, thyroid hormone can significantly affect energy metabolism and homeostasis, as well as heat production.[188,189]

BOX 85.2	Signs and Symptoms of Thyrotoxicosis

1. Hyperactivity, tremor, agitation, hyperreflexia
2. Sinus tachycardia, palpitations, arrhythmias, systolic hypertension, heart failure
3. Perspiration
4. Abdominal pain, diarrhea
5. Bulging eyes (exophthalmos)
6. Thirst
7. Proximal myopathy
8. Apathy, stupor, coma

TABLE 85.3   Euthyroid Sick Syndrome Laboratory Data

Variable	Value
Free T4	Normal
T4 → T3 Conversion	Decreased
T3	Markedly decreased
rT3	Variable
TSH	Normal

Clinical Grave disease can also occur via increased production of TSH secondary to a pituitary adenoma. Painful thyroiditis (DeQuervain) can occur following a viral illness and be associated with hyperthyroidism.[193] A more likely presentation of hyperthyroidism in a teenager is likely to be caused by Hashimoto thyroiditis.[194] Amiodarone with a structure similar to thyroxine can be associated with either hyperthyroidism or hypothyroidism.[195]

Patients admitted to the ICU with exaggerated hyperthyroidism (thyrotoxicosis) will typically exhibit either sinus tachycardia or supraventricular tachycardia, nausea, vomiting and diarrhea, weakness, as well as confusion, delirium, or even coma.[196] Classic findings of a diffusely enlarged thyroid with a overlying bruit or murmur may not be present. Neonatal thyrotoxicosis is similar to Grave disease and involves transplacental passage of TSH-like autoantibodies from the mother to the fetus. Thyrotoxicosis pathophysiology is more common among patients with Down syndrome, diabetes mellitus, and McCuen Albright syndrome. Signs and symptoms of thyrotoxicosis are summarized in Box 85.2.

Treatment of thyroid storm involves a four-pronged approach: (1) controlling thyroid gland production of T4 using thionamides such as propylthiouracil and methimazole, which interfere with thyroid peroxidase iodination; (2) blocking T3 activity in peripheral tissues using thionamides, iopanoic acid, beta-adrenergic blockage, and corticosteroids; (3) providing supportive measures such as antipyretics, anxiolytics, and volume resuscitation as needed; and (4) identifying and treating identifiable precipitating antecedents. In severe cases of recalcitrant thyroid storm, plasmapheresis with charcoal hemoperfusion has been used to reduce circulating thyroxine.[197] Occasionally, subtotal thyroidectomy may be required for chronic thyrotoxicosis. Postsurgical complications in such patients that intensivists should anticipate include recurrent laryngeal nerve damage, hypocalcaemia with tetany secondary to inadvertent parathyroid gland resection, and hypothyroidism.[198]

Hypothyroidism

The most common cause of hypothyroidism is iodine deficiency, affecting approximately 800 million people worldwide.[199] As noted previously, unrecognized neonatal hypothyroidism is of particular concern given the consequences if appropriate intervention is not initiated. In the PICU, Down syndrome children with unstable hemodynamics following cardiovascular surgery should be particularly suspect for hypothyroidism. Signs and symptoms of neonatal hyperthyroidism include prolonged neonatal jaundice, coarse features, protruding tongue, apathy, poor feeding, and umbilical hernia. True hypothyroidism secondary to thyroid gland failure or maldevelopment will manifest with an elevated TSH concentration, although this response may be blunted in the ICU by malnutrition and administration of dopamine and corticosteroids.

Euthyroid Sick Syndrome in Critical Illness

As previously noted, monodiodination of the inner tyrosine residue of thyroxine leads to production of reverse T3. Euthyroid sick syndrome is characterized by a rapid decrease in T3 and variable increase in rT3 that appears to be proportional to the intensity of illness severity and concentration of TNF-α.[200] In addition, a decline in various thyroid hormone-binding proteins is evident. Conversion of T4 to T3 is suppressed secondary to decreased 5'-deiodinase activity. Because of decreased thyroid-releasing hormone (TRH) gene expression in the hypothalamus, TRH is decreased with a resultant reduced TSH messenger RNA. Euthyroid sick syndrome (nonthyroidal illness syndrome) has been detailed among pediatric cardiac surgery patients.[201,202] Laboratory finding characteristics of euthyroid sick syndrome are summarized in Table 85.3.[203]

Significance of euthyroid sick syndrome in critical illness remains controversial. Evidence indicating overt pathology in this setting is sparse. Some argue that this scenario reflects an effort of the body to conserve energy expenditure during one aspect of the stress response (see Chapter 81). Thyroid hormone alterations characteristic of euthyroid sick syndrome would also be expected to modulate protein catabolism.[204] Euthyroid sick syndrome should be differentiated from true hypothyroidism. The latter can occasionally occur among patients administered dopamine and high-dose corticosteroids, both secondary to inhibition of TSH. Various drug effects on thyroid hormone metabolism are summarized in Table 85.4.

Thyroid Hormone Supplementation in PICU

Patients with true hypothyroidism should obviously receive replacement thyroxine. Treatment of euthyroid sick syndrome is more controversial. Although the basis for the observation is not clear, adult investigators have previously demonstrated that low serum T3 levels represent the single most significant predictor of cardiovascular and all-cause mortality among adults with heart disease.[205] Triiodothyronine replacement in adults with impaired left ventricular function resulted in improved left ventricular function, as well as restored cardiomyocyte gene expression to euthyroid levels.[206] Among adult patients with heart failure, infusion of T3 for 72 hours resulted in normalization of serum T3 levels with concomitant

TABLE 85.4	Effects of Various Drugs on Thyroid Hormone Metabolism
Drug	**Effect**
Dopamine	Blunts TSH response to TRH
Corticosteroids	Suppresses basal and TRH-stimulated TSH release
Iodinated contrast agents	Decreases hepatic conversion of T4 to T3
Amiodarone	Decreases hepatic conversion of T4 to T3 and decreases servo feedback T3 binding at the pituitary
Phenytoin	Enhances T4 to T3 conversion (low free T4 and low total T4)

TRH, thyroid-releasing hormone; *TSH,* thyroid-stimulating hormone.

improvement in stroke volume, as well as left ventricular end-diastolic volume.[207] Such findings have stimulated interest in thyroid hormone pathophysiology among children with cardiovascular disease. Thyroid function and clinical outcomes were assessed serially among children undergoing cardiac bypass surgery. All subjects demonstrated euthyroid sick syndrome characterized by reduced TSH, total T3, free T3 index, and T3 uptake. These changes were correlated with prolonged need for mechanical ventilation, degree of organ dysfunction, and vasoactive-inotropic scores.[208]

One interventional trial reported the effect of T3 supplementation among children undergoing cardiovascular surgery. In this investigation, replacement dosing of T3 following cardiopulmonary bypass resulted in increases in plasma T3 concomitant with measures of improved myocardial performance, particularly among those children exhibiting low postoperative cardiac output.[209] A subsequent multicenter, double-blind, randomized, placebo-controlled trial enrolling children younger than 2 years old undergoing cardiac surgery requiring cardiopulmonary bypass examined the effect of IV T3 ($n = 98$) or placebo ($n = 95$). Overall the primary outcome, time to tracheal extubation, was similar between groups. However, for patients younger than 5 months, the hazard ratio (chance of extubation) for extubation was 1.72 ($P = 0.0216$), with median time to extubation in the T3 group 55 hours compared with 98 hours in the placebo group. Shorter duration of mechanical ventilation corresponded to a reduction in inotropic agent use and improvement in cardiac function. There were no differences in adverse event rates, including arrhythmia between groups.

Acknowledgment

The authors acknowledge the considerable contributions of Dr. Kalia Ulate for this chapter in the fourth edition of *Pediatric Critical Care.*

Key References

2. Chrousos GP. The hypothalamic-pituitary-adrenal axis and immune-mediated inflammation. *N Engl J Med.* 1995;332:1351-1362.

5. Chrousos GP, Gold PW. The concepts of stress and stress system disorders. Overview of physical and behavioral homeostasis. *JAMA.* 1992; 267:1244-1252.

6. Ferrario CM. Importance of the renin-angiotensin-aldosterone system (RAS) in the physiology and pathology of hypertension. An overview. *Drugs.* 1990;39(suppl 2):1-8.

9. Chida D, Nakagawa S, Nagai S, et al. Melanocortin 2 receptor is required for adrenal gland development, steroidogenesis, and neonatal gluconeogenesis. *Proc Natl Acad Sci USA.* 2007;104:18205-18210.

10. Jardine D, Emond M, Meert KL, et al. A single nucleotide polymorphism in the corticotropin receptor gene is associated with a blunted cortisol response during pediatric critical illness. *Pediatr Crit Care Med.* 2014;15: 698-705.

17. Boonen E, Vervenne H, Meersseman P, et al. Reduced cortisol metabolism during critical illness. *N Engl J Med.* 2013;368:1477-1488.

18. Boonen E, Langouche L, Janssens T, et al. Impact of duration of critical illness on the adrenal glands of human intensive care patients. *J Clin Endocrinol Metab.* 2014;99:4214-4222.

24. Vandevyver S, Dejager L, Libert C. Comprehensive overview of the structure and regulation of the glucocorticoid receptor. *Endocr Rev.* 2014;35:671-693.

26. van den Akker EL, Koper JW, Joosten K, et al. Glucocorticoid receptor mRNA levels are selectively decreased in neutrophils of children with sepsis. *Intensive Care Med.* 2009;35:1247-1254.

28. Shibata AR, Troster EJ, Wong HR. Glucocorticoid receptor expression in peripheral WBCs of critically ill children. *Pediatr Crit Care Med.* 2015;16:e132-e140.

31. Patel R, Williams-Dautovich J, Cummins CL. Minireview: new molecular mediators of glucocorticoid receptor activity in metabolic tissues. *Mol Endocrinol.* 2014;28:999-1011.

37. Adcock IM, Barnes PJ. Molecular mechanisms of corticosteroid resistance. *Chest.* 2008;134:394-401.

40. Rhen T, Cidlowski JA. Antiinflammatory action of glucocorticoids—new mechanisms for old drugs. *N Engl J Med.* 2005;353:1711-1723.

44. Hotchkiss RS, Monneret G, Payen D. Sepsis-induced immunosuppression: from cellular dysfunctions to immunotherapy. *Nat Rev Immunol.* 2013;13:862-874.

50. Annane D, Bellissant E, Sebille V, et al. Impaired pressor sensitivity to noradrenaline in septic shock patients with and without impaired adrenal function reserve. *Br J Clin Pharmacol.* 1998;46:589-597.

51. Boonen E, Van den Berghe G. Endocrine responses to critical illness: novel insights and therapeutic implications. *J Clin Endocrinol Metab.* 2014;99:1569-1582.

53. Annane D, Maxime V, Ibrahim F, et al. Diagnosis of adrenal insufficiency in severe sepsis and septic shock. *Am J Respir Crit Care Med.* 2006;174: 1319-1326.

68. Delle Piane L, Rinaudo PF, Miller WL. 150 years of congenital adrenal hyperplasia: translation and commentary of De Crecchio's classic paper from 1865. *Endocrinology.* 2015;156:1210-1217.

74. den Brinker M, Joosten KF, Liem O, et al. Adrenal insufficiency in meningococcal sepsis: bioavailable cortisol levels and impact of interleukin-6 levels and intubation with etomidate on adrenal function and mortality. *J Clin Endocrinol Metab.* 2005;90:5110-5117.

76. Muller HL. Craniopharyngioma. *Endocr Rev.* 2014;35:513-543.

77. Broersen LH, Pereira AM, Jorgensen JO, Dekkers OM. Adrenal insufficiency in corticosteroid use: systematic review and meta-analysis. *J Clin Endocrinol Metab.* 2015;100:2171-2180.

78. Sacre K, Dehoux M, Chauveheid MP, et al. Pituitary-adrenal function after prolonged glucocorticoid therapy for systemic inflammatory disorders: an observational study. *J Clin Endocrinol Metab.* 2013;98: 3199-3205.

98. Findling JW, Raff H. Cushing's syndrome: important issues in diagnosis and management. *J Clin Endocrinol Metab.* 2006;91:3746-3753.

104. Faienza MF, Luce V, Ventura A, et al. Skeleton and glucose metabolism: a bone-pancreas loop. *Int J Endocrinol.* 2015;2015:758148.

105. Brestoff JR, Artis D. Immune regulation of metabolic homeostasis in health and disease. *Cell.* 2015;161:146-160.

106. Chen LQ, Cheung LS, Feng L, et al. Transport of sugars. *Annu Rev Biochem.* 2015;84:865-894.

107. Mueckler M, Thorens B. The SLC2 (GLUT) family of membrane transporters. *Mol Aspects Med.* 2013;34:121-138.

108. Brealey D, Singer M. Hyperglycemia in critical illness: a review. *J Diabetes Sci Technol.* 2009;3:1250-1260.

131. Hacihamdioglu B, Kendirli T, Ocal G, et al. Pathophysiology of critical illness hyperglycemia in children. *J Pediatr Endocrinol Metab.* 2013;26: 715-720.

134. Van den Berghe G. How does blood glucose control with insulin save lives in intensive care? *J Clin Invest.* 2004;114:1187-1195.

139. Sonneville R, Vanhorebeek I, den Hertog HM, et al. Critical illness-induced dysglycemia and the brain. *Intensive Care Med.* 2015;41:192-202.

140. van den Berghe G, Wouters P, Weekers F, et al. Intensive insulin therapy in the critically ill patients. *N Engl J Med.* 2001;345:1359-1367.

141. Kavanagh BP. Glucose in the ICU—evidence, guidelines, and outcomes. *N Engl J Med.* 2012;367:1259-1260.

150. Vlasselaers D, Milants I, Desmet L, et al. Intensive insulin therapy for patients in paediatric intensive care: a prospective, randomised controlled study. *Lancet.* 2009;373:547-556.

155. Jeschke MG, Kulp GA, Kraft R, et al. Intensive insulin therapy in severely burned pediatric patients: a prospective randomized trial. *Am J Respir Crit Care Med.* 2010;182:351-359.

156. Agus MS, Steil GM, Wypij D, et al. Tight glycemic control versus standard care after pediatric cardiac surgery. *N Engl J Med.* 2012;367:1208-1219.

159. Macrae D, Grieve R, Allen E, et al. A randomized trial of hyperglycemic control in pediatric intensive care. *N Engl J Med.* 2014;370:107-118.

163. Kyle UG, Coss Bu JA, Kennedy CE, Jefferson LS. Organ dysfunction is associated with hyperglycemia in critically ill children. *Intensive Care Med.* 2010;36:312-320.

165. Srinivasan V, Agus MS. Tight glucose control in critically ill children—a systematic review and meta-analysis. *Pediatr Diabetes.* 2014;15:75-83.

168. Krinsley JS, Bruns DE, Boyd JC. The impact of measurement frequency on the domains of glycemic control in the critically ill—a Monte Carlo simulation. *J Diabetes Sci Technol.* 2015;9:237-245.

173. Galiatsatos P, Gibson BR, Rabiee A, et al. The glucoregulatory benefits of glucagon-like peptide-1 (7-36) amide infusion during intensive insulin therapy in critically ill surgical patients: a pilot study. *Crit Care Med.* 2014;42:638-645.

179. Lteif AN, Schwenk WF. Hypoglycemia in infants and children. *Endocrinol Metab Clin North Am.* 1999;28:619-646, vii.

181. Wintergerst KA, Buckingham B, Gandrud L, et al. Association of hypoglycemia, hyperglycemia, and glucose variability with morbidity and death in the pediatric intensive care unit. *Pediatrics.* 2006;118:173-179.

182. Fekete C, Lechan RM. Central regulation of hypothalamic-pituitary-thyroid axis under physiological and pathophysiological conditions. *Endocr Rev.* 2014;35:159-194.

183. Mantzoros CS, Magkos F, Brinkoetter M, et al. Leptin in human physiology and pathophysiology. *Am J Physiol Endocrinol Metab.* 2011;301:E567-E584.

184. Maia AL, Goemann IM, Meyer EL, Wajner SM. Deiodinases: the balance of thyroid hormone: type 1 iodothyronine deiodinase in human physiology and disease. *J Endocrinol.* 2011;209:283-297.

185. Yen PM. Physiological and molecular basis of thyroid hormone action. *Physiol Rev.* 2001;81:1097-1142.

188. Joseph-Bravo P, Jaimes-Hoy L, Charli JL. Regulation of TRH neurons and energy homeostasis-related signals under stress. *J Endocrinol.* 2015;224:R139-R159.

189. McAninch EA, Bianco AC. Thyroid hormone signaling in energy homeostasis and energy metabolism. *Ann N Y Acad Sci.* 2014;1311:77-87.

Diabetic Ketoacidosis

Ildiko H. Koves and Nicole Glaser

PEARLS

- Diabetic ketoacidosis (DKA) results either from absolute insulin deficiency or from relative insulin deficiency in the setting of high levels of counterregulatory hormones stimulated by infection or other illness.
- DKA is characterized by hyperglycemia, ketosis, and acidosis.
- Treatment of pediatric DKA involves intravenous insulin administration, intravenous fluid administration to correct dehydration, and replacement of electrolyte deficits.
- Cerebral edema is the most frequent serious complication of DKA in children and is the most frequent cause of morbidity and mortality resulting from DKA.

Etiology, Definition, and Presentation

Diabetic ketoacidosis (DKA) occurs when serum insulin concentrations are very low in relation to concentrations of glucagon and other counterregulatory hormones (epinephrine, norepinephrine, cortisol, and growth hormone). This situation occurs most commonly in new onsets of type 1 diabetes mellitus (T1DM) and in patients with known diabetes during infections or other intercurrent illnesses or with insulin omission (discussed later). In the setting of low insulin concentrations in relation to counterregulatory hormone concentrations, the normal physiologic mechanisms responsible for maintaining adequate fuel supply during fasting and physiologic stress are exaggerated, resulting in hyperglycemia, ketosis, and acidosis. A diagnosis of DKA can be made when the serum glucose concentration is greater than 200 mg/dL (>11 mmol/L) and venous pH is less than 7.30 (or the serum bicarbonate concentration is less than 15 mmol/L) in the presence of elevated urine or serum ketone concentrations.

In a child with new onset of T1DM, declining insulin production results from autoimmune destruction of pancreatic beta cells. The concentration of insulin is decreased relative to glucagon causing excess hepatic glucose production and decreased peripheral glucose uptake in muscle and adipose tissue.[1,2] When the serum glucose concentration rises above approximately 180 to 200 mg/dL, the renal threshold for glucose reabsorption is exceeded causing glycosuria, which leads to osmotic diuresis and compensatory polydipsia. Low insulin concentrations also stimulate the release of free fatty acids (FFAs) from adipose tissue to fuel ketogenesis.[3] This, in combination with activation of the hepatic β-oxidative enzyme sequence resulting from relative excess of glucagon in relation to insulin, results in markedly increased hepatic ketone production.[2-4]

Progressive dehydration and increasing acidosis eventually stimulate release of the counterregulatory ("stress") hormones, cortisol, catecholamines, and growth hormone, which accelerate hepatic glucose output and ketone production.[5,6] Infection or other illness or injury can likewise contribute to this process by stimulating release of counterregulatory hormones. Elevated cortisol concentrations augment FFA release from adipose tissue and decrease peripheral glucose uptake. Increased epinephrine concentrations directly increase glycogenolysis and stimulate the release of gluconeogenic precursors from muscle.[7,8] Both epinephrine and norepinephrine also stimulate lipolysis and β-oxidation of FFAs.[9,10] Catecholamines may also directly inhibit insulin secretion, thereby accelerating DKA in those with endogenous insulin capacity, such as those with a new diagnosis of T1DM or those with type 2 diabetes.[11,12] Growth hormone also decreases peripheral glucose uptake and enhances ketone production by increasing FFA release.[13] Elevated concentrations of counterregulatory hormones thus result in increased acidosis, hyperglycemia, and dehydration. This in turn stimulates further counterregulatory hormone release, thereby creating a vicious cycle resulting in rapid worsening of DKA (Fig. 86.1).

During DKA, intestinal ileus results from potassium depletion, acidosis, and diminished splanchnic perfusion, causing abdominal pain and vomiting and thereby limiting fluid intake. Progressive dehydration eventually leads to diminished tissue perfusion sufficient to cause an accumulation of lactic acid, enhancing acidosis.[14] In addition, poor perfusion may result in diminished renal function, limiting the capacity for clearance of glucose and ketones. Ongoing osmotic diuresis and ketonuria in the setting of acidosis also results in urinary losses of electrolytes (potassium, sodium, chloride, calcium, phosphate, and magnesium).

Classical symptoms of DKA include polyuria, polydipsia, polyphagia, weight loss, abdominal pain, nausea, and vomiting. Abdominal tenderness, absence of bowel sounds, and guarding are frequent and may even mimic the acute abdomen.[15] Tachycardia and signs of hypoperfusion, such as delayed capillary refill time and cool extremities, are also common as well as dry mucous membranes, absence of tears, and poor skin turgor. Despite substantial volume depletion, however, hypotension is unusual in children with DKA and occasional children may present with hypertension. Kussmaul breathing and tachypnea are the result of metabolic acidosis and respiratory compensatory mechanisms. Fruity breath

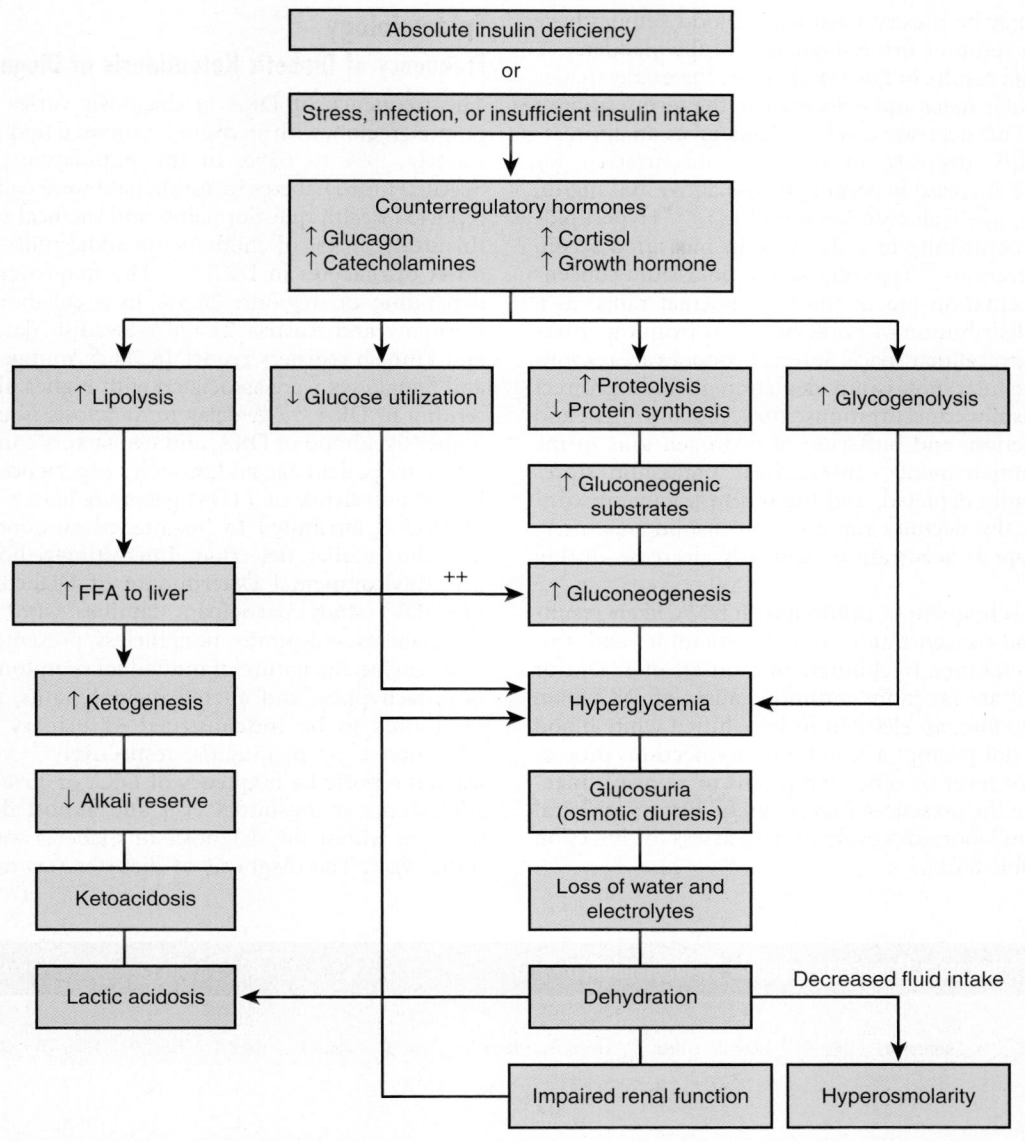

Fig. 86.1. Pathophysiology of DKA. (Reprinted with permission from Wolfsdorf J, Glaser N, Sperling MA. Diabetic ketoacidosis in infants, children, and adolescents: a consensus statement from the American Diabetes Association. Diabetes Care. 2006;29:1150-1159.)

odor (acetone) may be present. Hypothermia has also been described.[16]

Although hyperglycemia is part of the definition of DKA, in rare cases, the serum glucose concentration may be nearly normal, so-called euglycemic DKA. This situation has been reported most frequently in pregnant women.[17-19] Normal glucose concentrations or even hypoglycemia despite ketosis may also occur in children with known diabetes who administer insulin to treat DKA prior to arrival in the emergency department. In general, however, the persistence and severity of hyperglycemia reflect the severity of dehydration. In the absence of preexisting renal disease or unusually high carbohydrate intake just prior to presentation, blood glucose concentrations in excess of 500 to 600 mg/dL imply that dehydration is of sufficient severity to diminish the glomerular filtration rate and thereby diminish the capacity for renal clearance of excess glucose.[20]

Concentrations of ketone bodies (beta-hydroxybutyrate [βOHB] and acetoacetate [AcAc]) are elevated in DKA resulting in acidosis. Hyperchloremic acidosis frequently coexists with increased anion-gap acidosis, and the anion gap reflects the combination of these processes.[21] The ratio of βOHB:AcAc (typically 1:1 in the normal state) is increased during DKA and may be as high as 10:1.[22] During treatment, this ratio returns to normal. The nitroprusside reaction used to test urine ketone concentrations detects only AcAc and not βOHB. As a result, urine testing cannot be relied on to determine DKA severity or treatment response. Bedside blood ketone meters provide a rapid means for measuring βOHB and may be useful in place of or in addition to urine testing particularly in patients with anuria or oliguria who produce insufficient amounts of urine for ketone testing.[23] Blood ketone measurements are also useful for determining the timing of transition from intravenous to subcutaneous insulin administration.

Urine ketones may be present even when blood ketones have normalized as a result of urine stagnating in the bladder.

Hyperglycemia results in fluid shifts from the extravascular to the intravascular space and a decrease in the serum sodium concentration. This decrease can be calculated as an approximately 1.6 mEq/L decrease in sodium concentration for every 100 mg/dL increase in serum glucose above 100 mg/dL ($Na_{corrected} = Na_{actual} + [glucose-5.5\ mmol/L]$).[24,25] Hyperlipidemia may also contribute to a decrease in measured serum sodium concentrations.[26] Typically, serum potassium concentrations at presentation are in the high-normal range as a result of the redistribution of potassium ions from the intracellular to the extracellular space. Several processes are responsible for intracellular potassium depletion including direct effects of low insulin concentrations, intracellular protein and phosphate depletion, and buffering of hydrogen ions in the intracellular compartment.[27] Intracellular potassium stores may be profoundly depleted, and the serum potassium concentration typically declines rapidly with insulin treatment. Serum phosphate concentrations similarly decrease during treatment.

Leukocytosis is frequent in children with DKA, likely resulting from elevated concentrations of catecholamines and pro-inflammatory cytokines. In children, new onsets of T1DM or insulin omission are far more common causes of DKA than infection.[28] Therefore, an elevated or left-shifted white blood cell count need not prompt a search for an infectious process in the absence of fever or other symptoms or signs of infection. However, in the presence of fever, careful history, physical examination, and laboratory evaluation to assess for infection are prudent (Table 86.1).

Epidemiology
Frequency of Diabetic Ketoacidosis at Diagnosis

The frequency of DKA at diagnosis varies widely by geographic region, with an overall estimated frequency of approximately 20% to 67%. In the population-based US study SEARCH for Diabetes in Youth, data were collected from self-reported health questionnaires and medical record review. In this study, 36.4% of children and adolescents presented at the onset of diabetes in DKA.[29,30] The frequency of DKA varies depending on regions: 26.3% in a collaborative cohort in Germany and Austria 21.1%[31]; Swedish data report 16.9%; and Finnish registers report 18.7%.[32] Younger age (<5 years) and female sex were associated with higher likelihood of presenting in DKA.[33,34] A delay in diagnosis is associated with a higher likelihood of DKA, and two factors contributing to this result are patient age and provider experience. Regions with a higher prevalence of T1DM generally have a lower frequency of DKA,[35] attributed to heightened awareness in providers and thus earlier detection. Interestingly, however, three of The Environmental Determinant of Diabetes in the Young (TEDDY) study participant families who were counseled on diabetes symptoms nonetheless presented with DKA.[36] The nonspecific nature of individual symptoms, such as polyuria, tachypnea, and altered mental status, may cause such symptoms to be misconstrued as urinary tract infection, pneumonia, or meningitis, respectively.[37] Mallare and colleagues reported a frequency of DKA of 33% in children and adolescents at the initial visit and almost double (59%) in those in whom the diagnosis of diabetes was missed at the initial visit. The diagnosis of diabetes was more likely to be

TABLE 86.1	Laboratory Monitoring Schedule Recommendation												
Laboratory Analysis	DKA Confirmed	Hour 1	Hour 2	Hour 3	Hour 4	Hour 5	Hour 6	Hour 7	Hour 8	Hour 9	Hour 10	Hour 11	Hour 12
Glucose[a]	X	X	X	X	X	X	X	X	X	X	X	X	X
Sodium[b]	X	X	X		X		X		X		X		X
Potassium	X		X		X				X				
Chloride	X		X		X				X				
Bicarbonate	X		X		X				X				
BUN	X												
Creatinine	X												
Magnesium[c]	X				X				X				
Calcium[c]	X				X				X				
Phosphorus[c]	X				X				X				
Blood gas (capillary blood gas, venous blood gas, arterial blood gas)	X				X								
β-hydroxybutyrate[b]	X		X		X		X		X		X		X
Blood culture[d]	X												
Urinalysis[d]	X												

[a]Repeat glucose every hour while on insulin drip; send first glucose to the lab as well for serum glucose.
[b]Repeat sodium and β-hydroxybutyrate (BOHB) every 2 hours while on insulin drip.
[c]May repeat these labs every 4 hours until normalized, especially while on insulin drip.
[d]Only if febrile or concern for infection, and do not repeat if done at referral hospital.

missed in very young children (34% of children ≤5 years of age compared to 8.5% in those older than 10 years of age),[38] particularly when these very young children are evaluated by family practitioners rather than pediatricians.[39] Usher-Smith and coworkers found protective factors of a first-degree relative with T1DM, higher parental education, and higher background incidence of T1DM in a systemic review of 46 studies involving 24,000 children from 31 countries.[40]

Frequency of Diabetic Ketoacidosis in Children and Adolescents After Diagnosis

Although there are several population-based studies reporting the frequency of DKA at presentation, fewer data are available describing the incidence of DKA in children and adolescents with established diabetes. Reported frequencies range from 1 to 10 per 100 patient-years.[41] In the Diabetes Control and Complications Trial, the incidence of DKA in adolescents treated with intensive management regimens was 2.8 per 100 patient-years, significantly lower than the incidence in those treated conventionally (4.7 per 100 patient-years). Although this is an older study, it was a time- and resource-intensive study and represents a more idealized situation than often encountered in the overall pediatric diabetes population.[42] In a more recent study from the Barbara Davis Center for Childhood Diabetes in Denver, Colorado, the overall incidence of DKA was 8 per 100 person-years. In that study, factors associated with higher incidence included older age, higher HbA1C (relative risk [RR] of 1.68 per 1% increase in HbA1C in younger children, RR of 1.43 in older children), higher reported insulin dose, DSM4 psychiatric diagnoses, and "underinsurance" reflected lower socioeconomic status.[43] DKA is also observed more often in children and adolescents on continuous subcutaneous insulin infusion therapy (CSII) than on subcutaneous injections, particularly in the first year of initiation of CSII.[44] However, lower rates of DKA are achievable for those on CSII with adequate training and resources.

T2DM has been occurring with increasing frequency in older children and adolescents. Certain racial/ethnic groups in the United States are disproportionately affected, including Native Americans, Hispanics, and African Americans. DKA can be the clinical presentation of T2DM in youth estimated at 5% to 10%.[45] Youth with T2DM may also present with hyperglycemic hyperosmolar state (HHS), also referred to hyperosmotic hyperglycemic nonketotic coma (HHNK, described more fully later).

Morbidity and Mortality Associated with Diabetic Ketoacidosis

Mortality in children presenting with DKA is approximately 0.25% to 0.30%.[41] Most of the mortality in DKA occurs in children with cerebral edema, accounting for 57% to 87% of deaths. Neurologic sequelae of DKA are described later. Other causes of morbidity and mortality include sepsis and secondary infection, electrolyte abnormalities (eg, hypokalemia), arrhythmias, rhabdomyolysis, cerebral infarction, thrombosis, pneumomediastinum, subcutaneous emphysema, and pulmonary edema.

Management Guidelines (Fig. 86.2)
Fluids
Restoration of adequate peripheral perfusion and hemodynamic stability with bolus administration of intravenous

fluids (0.9% saline or other isotonic fluids) should begin as soon as possible. Typical patients require an initial fluid bolus of 10 mL/kg and repeated boluses if ongoing hemodynamic instability is present. Studies have shown that clinical assessments of dehydration severity in children with DKA tend to be inaccurate (Fig. 86.3).[46-48] The average degree of dehydration for most patients is approximately 7% to 9% of body weight, and this figure should be used as a basis for determining the total volume of fluids to be replaced. The estimated fluid deficit, along with maintenance fluid requirements, should be replaced over 36 to 48 hours using 0.45% to 0.90% saline, generally initially with 0.90% saline then transitioning to 0.45% saline after several hours. Replacement of ongoing urinary fluid losses is usually unnecessary because osmotic diuresis typically resolves rapidly after beginning DKA treatment. However, in circumstances of persistently high urine output, or profuse vomiting or diarrhea, replacement of ongoing losses may be considered. Large multicenter studies are under way comparing rapid and slower rehydration regimens.[49] Some guidelines (national and international publication by the International Society of Pediatric and Adolescent Diabetes [ISPAD] British and Australasian Endocrine Group) have favored more gradual rehydration, with attention to effective osmolality,[30,50] but prospective data are lacking at present.

Insulin
Low-dose insulin should be administered intravenously at a rate of 0.05 to 0.10 units/kg/hour. Insulin administration results in resolution of acidosis and hyperglycemia via suppression of ketogenesis and hepatic glucose output and promotion of peripheral glucose uptake. An initial bolus or loading dose of insulin is not recommended. Maximal suppression of ketogenesis is achieved rapidly with an insulin infusion (0.05–0.10 unit/kg/hour).[51-53] Even in the absence of insulin administration, the serum glucose concentration often decreases substantially with initial rehydration, reflecting improvements in renal perfusion and decreased counterregulatory hormone concentrations.[14] This decline in glucose concentration during the initial period of rehydration should not be interpreted as indicating excessive insulin administration.

Serum glucose concentrations typically normalize before ketosis and acidosis resolve. To continue insulin administration at dosages sufficient to allow resolution of ketosis, dextrose should be added to the intravenous fluids. Transition to dextrose-containing fluids should occur when the serum glucose concentrations decline below approximately 250 mg/dL. The "two bag system" for dextrose administration allows a rapid response to changes in serum glucose concentration and is cost effective.[54] Two bags of intravenous fluids with identical electrolyte content, but different dextrose content (0% and 10%), are administered simultaneously with the relative rates of administration frequently adjusted to increase or decrease the dextrose concentration while maintaining a constant overall rate of administration of fluid and electrolytes.

Electrolytes
Serum potassium concentrations often decline rapidly during treatment and potassium replacement is mandatory. Typical patients require potassium administration at concentrations of 30 to 40 mEq (occasionally up to 80 mEq) per liter of intravenous fluids. Potassium chloride may be used alone or

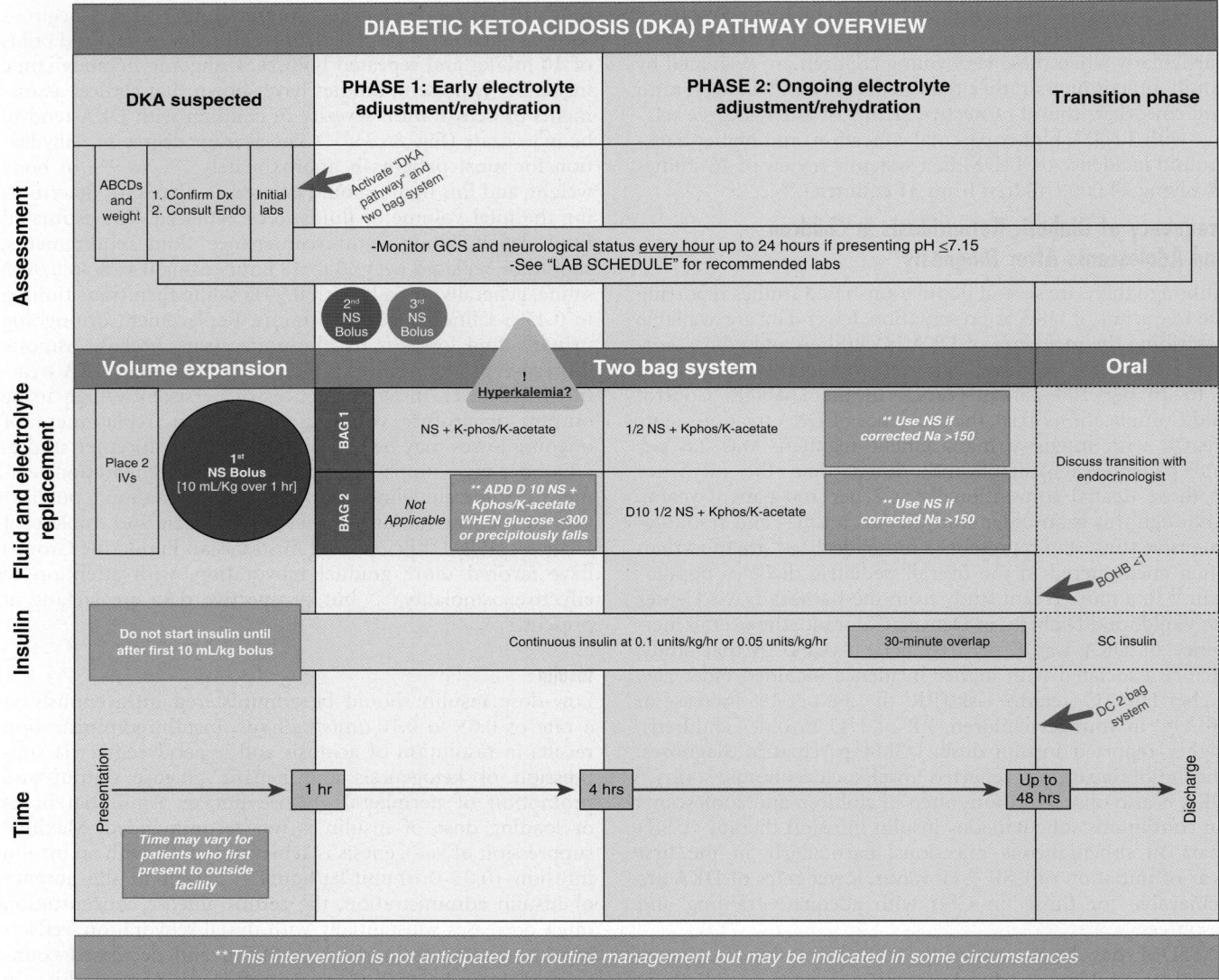

Fig. 86.2. DKA treatment algorithm in children and adolescents.

in combination with other potassium salts (potassium phosphate or potassium acetate), allowing for lower chloride administration. Adequacy of renal function should be considered before administration of potassium.

Phosphate replacement in children with DKA is controversial. Theoretically, low 2,3-diphosphoglycerate (DPG) levels in red blood cells may occur in association with hypophosphatemia leading to decreased tissue oxygen delivery.[55,56] Occurrence of this effect to a clinically relevant degree, however, has not been shown. Although the risk of hypocalcemia during DKA treatment is increased with phosphate replacement, symptomatic hypocalcemia is uncommon when phosphate is administered slowly and in the more modest concentrations recommended in most DKA treatment protocols.[57,58] Severe hypophosphatemia during DKA has been shown to be associated with rhabdomyolysis and hemolytic anemia, suggesting that monitoring of serum phosphate concentrations is necessary and treatment of severe hypophosphatemia is essential.[59,60]

Hypomagnesemia and hypocalcemia may also occur during DKA treatment but are generally mild, rarely requiring treatment. Monitoring of serum calcium and magnesium concentrations, however, is recommended.

Correction of Acidosis

Routine bicarbonate administration is contraindicated in children with DKA, as acidosis generally corrects rapidly with insulin and fluid administration, and hemodynamic instability resulting from acidosis is rare. Bicarbonate administration is associated with several possible adverse effects including an increase in the risk of hypokalemia and a theoretic increase in tissue hypoxia resulting from a leftward shift in the hemoglobin-oxygen dissociation curve.[55,61] Paradoxical acidosis of the cerebrospinal fluid has also been documented with bicarbonate administration, likely resulting from diminished respiratory drive and a rise in the partial pressure of CO_2, which readily crosses the blood-brain barrier generating CSF acidosis.[62,63] Bicarbonate administration has also been associated with an increased risk of DKA-related cerebral edema.[64] In very rare circumstances (severe hemodynamic instability not responding to standard measures or potentially life-threatening hyperkalemia), bicarbonate administration may be considered.

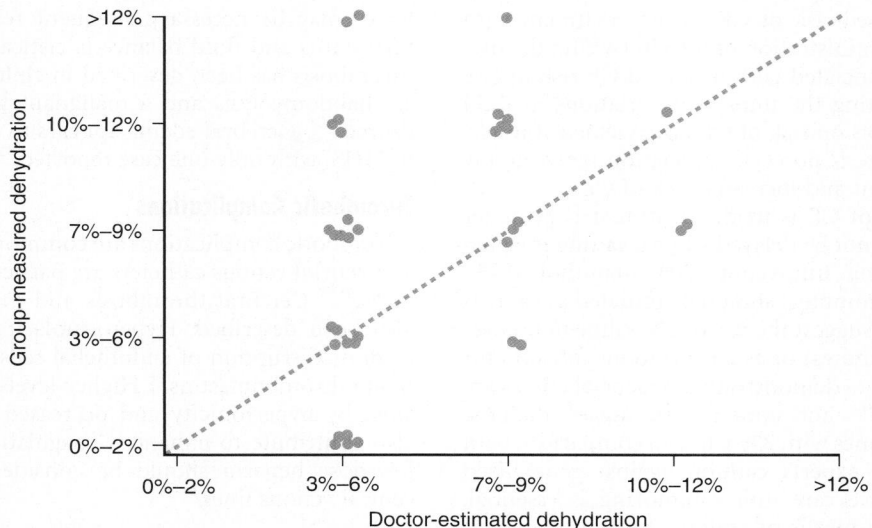

Fig. 86.3. Estimated versus measured dehydration in children with DKA. (Reprinted with permission from Koves IH, Neutze J, Donath S, et al. The accuracy of clinical assessment of dehydration during diabetic ketoacidosis in childhood. Diabetes Care. 2004;27:2485-2487.)

Monitoring

Intensive monitoring is essential for children with DKA, and most should be treated in a pediatric intensive care unit or other unit with similar capacities.[65,66] Blood glucose concentrations are typically measured hourly and electrolyte concentrations every 2 to 4 hours. Determinations of serum pH (every 2 to 4 hours) are helpful, particularly because serum bicarbonate concentrations may not increase during the first several hours. Free-flowing venous blood gas samples generally are sufficient and arterial samples are rarely needed. Failure of acidosis to improve during treatment should prompt evaluation of the adequacy of insulin infusion, fluid balance, and a search for other causes such as hyperchloremia, renal failure, sepsis, or even appendicitis. Monitoring of the βOHB level during DKA is prudent as its clearance (to <1 mmol/L) provides an end point for ongoing intensive DKA care.[50,67]

All fluid intake and output should be accurately recorded. Consideration of fluids and other management that may have occurred prior to admission to a pediatric intensive care unit is important. Vital signs and mental status should be monitored hourly. One study showed a high frequency of prolonged QT interval corrected for heart rate (QTc) in children with DKA, and arrhythmias have been described in rare cases.[68] Therefore, cardiac monitoring is recommended.

Diabetic Ketoacidosis–Associated Complications

Cerebral edema (CE) has been recognized as a complication of T1DM in children since 1936. It is essentially a clinical diagnosis, based on the deterioration of mental state during resuscitation for DKA. Signs and symptoms that should prompt consideration of CE include the Cushing triad (inappropriate slowing of heart rate, hypertension, and widening pulse pressure), severe headache, recurrence of vomiting, irritability, lethargy, or other mental status changes.[69] Some patients progress to coma, respiratory arrest, and cerebral herniation. Most episodes of CE occur several hours after the initiation of DKA treatment; however, 5% to 20% of cases occur at the time of presentation, prior to the initiation of therapy. Cerebral edema remains the leading cause of death

and morbidity in children with T1DM. The frequency of CE associated with DKA remains unchanged despite clinical efforts to the contrary.[34]

The reported mortality from CE varies widely and is in part dependent on the criteria used to define CE. Rates as high as 50% to 90% have been reported, but more recent studies[64,70] report lower rates of 21% to 24%. Overall, the incidence of CE is approximately 0.7% to 0.9% within DKA presentations. In other words, approximately 1 in 400 children with DKA die as a result of CE. Morbidity is significant; in particular debilitating neurologic sequelae occur in 21% to 26% of children with DKA-related CE.[64,70] Although frank CE is uncommon, there is substantial data to suggest that subclinical or asymptomatic CE occurs in many children with DKA, perhaps even in the majority. Limited data suggest that subtle brain injury may also be associated with DKA, even in the absence of clinically apparent CE.[71]

The pathophysiology of CE remains enigmatic. Several causative theories have been proposed for the occurrence of CE during DKA. Idiogenic, osmotically active substances that regulate cell volume have been thought to play a role in causing DKA-related CE. Taurine, 2-aminoethane sulfonic acid, is thought to have a critical role in neuro-osmoregulation during DKA.[72] Alternatively, cerebral hypoperfusion (caused by hypocapnia and volume depletion) prior to DKA treatment and the effects of reperfusion during DKA therapy have been hypothesized to result in CE and cerebral injury.[73,74] Direct effects of ketone bodies and inflammatory cytokines on blood-brain barrier function, increased activity of brain ion transporters, and activation of brain microglia have also been hypothesized to be involved.[75-78] To date, however, the precise pathophysiology of CE remains unresolved, and multiple factors may be involved with individual susceptibility.

Epidemiologic studies of risk factors for CE show that children with higher initial blood urea nitrogen (BUN) concentrations, lower initial PCO_2 concentrations, and greater acidosis at the time of presentation of DKA seem to be at greatest risk for CE.[64,74,79,80] A lesser rise in measured serum sodium concentration during DKA treatment has also been associated with increased risk of CE, as has treatment with bicarbonate.[64] Early administration of insulin (within the first hour) has also been associated with increased CE risk in one study.[79] Studies evaluating the impact of variations in fluid administration protocols on risk of CE have yielded conflicting results. As yet, there is no clear association between any aspect of fluid treatment and increased risk of CE.

Once the diagnosis of CE is made, treatment is a matter of urgency and should not be delayed while awaiting imaging studies or further testing. Intravenous 20% mannitol (0.25–1 g/kg infused over 15 minutes) should be initiated as soon as possible. Some reports suggest the use of 3% saline in boluses (5 mL/kg over 5–10 minutes) or as a continuous infusion for treatment of CE, but data demonstrating beneficial effects are limited to case reports[81,82] and some reports suggest the possibility of poorer outcomes with 3% saline in comparison with mannitol.[83] Therefore, experts caution against generalized use.[84] Ongoing intensive care unit monitoring is essential. Respiratory support by means of endotracheal intubation is likely to be required due to severe alterations in mental status and impaired airway reflexes. Therapeutic hyperventilation in intubated patients, however, has been associated with poorer outcomes.[85] Therefore, decreasing PCO_2 below the patient's own compensation for metabolic acidosis should be avoided in children with DKA except where absolutely necessary to treat impending cerebral herniation. A reasonable approach would be to initially maintain the patient's current PCO_2 level and then gradually allow the PCO_2 to increase as acidosis corrects. CNS imaging in patients with suspected CE should be used to exclude other etiologies of altered mental status such as CNS thrombosis or infarction. Imaging may not be necessary if there are improvements after CE therapy.[30,30]

Hyperglycemic Hyperosmolar Syndrome

Hyperglycemic hyperosmolar syndrome (HHS) is characterized by extreme elevations in serum glucose (>600 mg/dL) and hyperosmolarity (serum osm >330 mOsm/kg) in the absence of significant ketosis or acidosis (urine ketone concentration <1.5 mmol/L and serum bicarbonate >15 meq/L). Although HHS is defined as a condition separate from DKA, 30% of cases occur in combination with substantial ketosis and acidosis meeting criteria for both HHS and DKA. Until recently HHS was thought to occur infrequently in pediatrics. An increase in case reports of HHS in children suggests that the frequency may be increasing.[86,87] As in adults, HHS in children has a relatively high mortality of 10% to 35%.[88,89] The majority of HHS reports in children are in patients who have acanthosis nigricans, are obese, are African American, and have a family history of type 2 diabetes. Most cases of HHS are the initial presentation of diabetes, and most of these youths will subsequently have a clinical diagnosis of type 2 diabetes.

The occurrence of HHS during DKA poses challenges in terms of recognition and treatment. Generally dehydration is more profound than the clinical assessment would suggest, reflecting difficulties in clinical evaluation due to obesity and relative preservation of intravascular volume due to hyperosmolarity. Electrolyte losses similarly exceed those of DKA as a result of more prolonged osmotic diuresis. Patients who meet criteria for both DKA and HHS require more prolonged and aggressive fluid and electrolyte replacement therapy than typical children with DKA. Replacement of ongoing urinary

losses may be necessary. Frequent reassessment of circulatory status and fluid balance is critical. A high frequency of thrombosis has been described in children with HHS as well as rhabdomyolysis and a malignant hyperthermia-like syndrome.[90,91] Cerebral edema appears to be a rare complication of HHS, with only one case reported.[92]

Thrombotic Complications

Thrombotic complications are common in children with DKA and central venous catheters are particularly prone to thrombosis.[93,94] Cerebral thrombosis and pulmonary emboli have also been described. Hyperosmolarity may result in direct osmotic disruption of endothelial cells leading to a release of tissue thromboplastins.[95] Higher levels of vasopressin stimulated by hypertonicity and decreased vascular volume may also contribute to enhanced coagulation.[96] Prophylaxis with low-dose heparin should be considered for children with central venous lines.[97-99]

Other Complications

Rhabdomyolysis[100,101] is potentially life threatening. It is characterized by elevated serum creatine kinase, lactate dehydrogenase, and amino alanine transferase concentrations due to muscle injury. Rhabdomyolysis may result in renal failure, compartment syndrome, severe hyperkalemia, and other electrolyte disorders leading to arrhythmias. Hyperosmolarity has been thought to be one causative factor, and the risk is higher in children who have DKA complicated by features of HHS.[100]

Acute pancreatitis has been described in case reports of both children and adults with DKA, but it occurs rarely. Far more frequent are benign elevations in serum amylase or lipase occurring in 24% to 40% of children with DKA. These elevated pancreatic enzyme concentrations typically normalize rapidly with DKA treatment and are not associated with clinical features of pancreatitis.[102]

Although neurologic deterioration in children with DKA is most frequently caused by cerebral edema, cerebral infarctions with and without hemorrhage and cerebral thrombosis have also been described.[103] Other rare complication of DKA in children include pulmonary edema,[104] cardiac arrhythmias,[105] renal failure,[106] intestinal necrosis,[107-109] and rhinocerebral mucormycosis.[110,111]

Neuropsychologic Sequelae

Adverse neurodevelopmental outcomes in children with diabetes have in large part been attributed to recurrent hypoglycemia, and this area has been extensively investigated. Hyperglycemia and hyperglycemic extremes such as occur with DKA have been attracting increasing attention and interest for their potential neuropsychologic sequelae. Short-term effects on neurocognitive performance involving complex skills, such as inhibiting an over-learned response and learning of complex novel information, have been described.[112] Long-term deficits in memory,[71] mental state scores on standardized, validated testing, poorer sustained attention, and poorer delayed memory recall[113] have been found to be associated with DKA.

Health Care Costs Associated With Diabetic Ketoacidosis

Health care costs for DKA vary by geographic regions in the United States, and comparing costs is often complicated by variations in health care systems, methods of reporting costs (eg, hospital costs versus payer costs), and contractual arrangements. Several studies document that admissions for DKA are an important driver of diabetes-related health care costs in the United States.[114-116] In addition, among patients with known diabetes admitted for DKA, readmissions within 1 year of discharge are common.[114] One strategy to decrease the frequency of DKA is to promote awareness in the general population, in communities, and among providers. A successful campaign to heighten awareness of signs and symptoms of DKA took place in Parma, Italy. In the Parma campaign, simple messages regarding signs and symptoms of diabetes were provided to practitioners and schools, and free access to care was arranged. Compared to neighboring regions where the frequency of DKA was quite high at 78%, the Parma region observed a very low frequency of 12.5% during the 8 years of the campaign. Of note, the campaign was relatively inexpensive, costing $23,000 for the 8 years of the campaign.[35]

Another more targeted strategy is linked to recognition of diabetes risk. In children enrolled in prevention studies (mainly siblings of probands with type 1 diabetes), the frequency of DKA is far less than that of the general population; less than 4% of those participating in the Diabetes and Prevention Trial 1 presented in DKA, and 63.3% were asymptomatic.[117] For children and adolescents with diagnosed diabetes, multidisciplinary and intensive team management approaches have been shown to decrease the frequency of DKA. Unfortunately, obtaining sufficient reimbursement for intensive case management in the United States has been challenging, despite demonstrated savings to the health care system. In a relatively small study, the costs for emergency and hospital visits for those not involved in intervention more than exceeded (125%) the costs of intensive case management.[118] This included only hospital charges and did not include additional costs, such as missed days of work and school, patient and family anxiety, and cognitive and long-term health impact of recurrent DKA and poor glycemic control. In a larger study of home-based psychotherapy for adolescents with poorly controlled diabetes, admissions for DKA were reduced by almost half over a 2-year period, resulting in a cost savings of $23,886 to $72,226 (the range reflecting hospital costs and third-payer costs, respectively).[119] These examples emphasize the need for preventive rather than crisis-based approaches to the pediatric diabetes population.

Very young children with diabetes are the most likely to present in DKA and constitute the age group with the most rapid rise in incidence of diabetes. These data suggest that there are important opportunities for prevention strategies in this age group. Major efforts are needed to address health care disparities overall in children with diabetes, and prevention of DKA is no exception.

Key References

12. Porte D. Sympathetic regulation of insulin secretion. *Arch Intern Med.* 1969;123:252-620.
15. Valerio D. Acute diabetic abdomen in children. *Lancet.* 1976;1:66-68.
19. Jenkins D, Close C, Krentz A, et al. Euglycemic diabetic ketoacidosis: does it exist? *Acta Diabetol.* 1993;30:251-253.
22. Laffel L. Ketone bodies: a review of physiology, pathophysiology and application of monitoring to diabetes. *Diabetes Metab Res Rev.* 1999;15: 412-426.
23. Ham M, Okada P, White P. Bedside ketone determination in diabetic children with hyperglycemia and ketosis in the acute care setting. *Pediatr Diab.* 2004;5:39-43.
24. Katz MA. Hyperglycemia-induced hyponatremia–calculation of expected serum sodium depression. *N Engl J Med.* 1973;289:843-844.
25. Oh G, Anderson S, Tancredi D, et al. Hyponatremia in pediatric diabetic ketoacidosis: reevaluating the correction factor for hyperglycemia. *Arch Pediatr Adolesc Med.* 2009;163:771-772.
29. Rewers A, Klingensmith G, Davis C, et al. Presence of diabetic ketoacidosis at diagnosis of diabetes mellitus in youth: the Search for Diabetes in Youth Study. *Pediatrics.* 2008;121:e1258-e1266.
30. Wolfsdorf J, Craig ME, Daneman D, et al. Diabetic ketoacidosis in children and adolescents with diabetes. *Pediatr Diabetes.* 2009;10(suppl 12): 118-133.
31. Neu A, Hofer S, Karges B, et al. Ketoacidosis at diabetes onset is still frequent in children and adolescents: a multicenter analysis of 14,664 patients from 106 institutions. *Diab Care.* 2009;32:1647-1648.
32. Watts W, Edge JA. How can cerebral edema during treatment of diabetic ketoacidosis be avoided? *Pediatr Diabetes.* 2014;15:271-276.
33. Neu A, Willasch A, Ehehalt S, et al. Ketoacidosis at onset of type 1 diabetes mellitus in children–frequency and clinical presentation. *Pediatr Diab.* 2003;4:77-81.
34. Bui T, Werther G, Cameron F. Trends in diabetic ketoacidosis in childhood and adolescence: a 15-yr experience. *Pediatr Diab.* 2002;3:82-88.
35. Vanelli M, Chiari G, Ghizzoni L, et al. Effectiveness of a prevention program for diabetic ketoacidosis in children. *Diab Care.* 1999;22:7-9.
38. Mallare J, Cordice C, Ryan B, et al. Identifying risk factors for the development of diabetic ketoacidosis in new onset type 1 diabetes mellitus. *Clin Pediatr.* 2003;42:591-597.
41. Dunger D, Sperling M, Acerini C, et al. ESPE/LWPES Consensus statement on diabetic ketoacidosis in children and adolescents. *Arch Dis Child.* 2003;89:188-194.
43. Rewers A, Chase H, Mackenzie T, et al. Predictors of acute complications in children with type 1 diabetes. *JAMA.* 2002;287:2511-2518.
44. Hanas RLF, Lindblad B. A 2-yr national population study of pediatric ketoacidosis in Sweden: predisposing conditions and insulin pump use. *Pediatr Diabetes.* 2009;10:33-37.
45. Wolfsdorf J, et al. Diabetic ketoacidosis in children and adolescents with diabetes. *Pediatr Diabetes.* 2009;10:118-133.
46. Koves I, Neutze J, Donath S, et al. The accuracy of clinical assessment of dehydration druing diabetic ketoacidosis in childhood. *Diab Care.* 2004;27:2485-2487.
47. Fagan MJ, Avner J, Khine H. Initial fluid resuscitation for patients with diabetic ketoacidosis: how dry are they? *Clin Pediatr (Phila).* 2008; 47:851-855.
48. Sottosanti M, Morrison GC, Singh RN, et al. Dehydration in children with diabetic ketoacidosis: a prospective study. *Arch Dis Child.* 2012;97: 96-100.
49. Glaser NS, Ghetti S, Casper TC, et al. Pediatric diabetic ketoacidosis, fluid therapy, and cerebral injury: the design of a factorial randomized controlled trial. *Pediatr Diabetes.* 2013;14:435-446.
50. Koves IH, Leu MG, Spencer S, et al. Improving care for pediatric diabetic ketoacidosis. *Pediatrics.* 2014;134:e848-e856.
53. Nallasamy K, Jayashree M, Singhi S, Bansal A. Low-dose vs standard-dose insulin in pediatric diabetic ketoacidosis: a randomized clinical trial. *JAMA pediatrics.* 2014;168:999-1005.
54. Grimberg A, Cerri R, Satin-Smith M, Cohen P. The "two bag system" for variable intravenous dextrose and fluid administration: benefits in diabetic ketoacidosis management. *J Pediatr.* 1999;134:376-378.
56. Fisher J, Kitabchi A. A randomized study of phosphate therapy in the treatment of diabetic ketoacidosis. *J Clin Endocrinol Metab.* 1983; 57:177-180.
63. Bureau M, Begin R, Berthiaume Y, et al. Cerebral hypoxia from bicarbonate infusion in diabetic acidosis. *J Pediatr.* 1980;96:968-973.
64. Glaser N, Barnett P, McCaslin I, et al. Risk factors for cerebral edema in children with diabetic ketoacidosis. *N Engl J Med.* 2001;344:264-269.
65. Sperling M, Dunger D, Acerini C, et al. ESPE/LWPES consensus statement on diabetic ketoacidosis in children and adolescents. *Pediatrics.* 2003;113:e133-e140.
66. Wolfsdorf J, Glaser N, Sperling M. Diabetic ketoacidosis in infants, children and adolescents: a consensus statement from the American Diabetes Association. *Diab Care.* 2006;29:1150-1159.
67. Noyes KJ, Crofton P, Bath LE, et al. Hydroxybutyrate near-patient testing to evaluate a new end-point for intravenous insulin therapy in the treatment of diabetic ketoacidosis in children. *Pediatr Diabetes.* 2007;8: 150-156.
70. Edge J, Hawkins M, Winter D, Dunger D. The risk and outcome of cerebral oedema developing during diabetic ketoacidosis. *Arch Dis Child.* 2001;85:16-22.

72. Cameron F, Kean M, Wellard R, et al. Insights into the acute cerebral metabolic changes associated with childhood diabetes. *Diabet Med.* 2005;22:648-653.

73. Glaser N. Cerebral injury and cerebral edema in children with diabetic ketoacidosis: could cerebral ischemia and reperfusion injury be involved? *Pediatr Diab.* 2009;10:534-541.

78. Isales C, Min L, Hoffman W. Acetoacetate and B-hydroxybutyrate differentially regulate endothelin-1 and vascular endothelial growth factor in mouse brain microvascular endothelial cells. *J Diab Comp.* 1999;13:91-97.

79. Edge J, Jakes R, Roy Y, et al. The UK case-control study of cerebral oedema complicating diabetic ketoacidosis in children. *Diabetologia.* 2006;49:2002-2009.

80. Lawrence S, Cummings E, Gaboury I, Daneman D. Population-based study of incidence and risk factors for cerebral edema in pediatric diabetic ketoacidosis. *J Pediatr.* 2005;146:688-692.

81. Curtis J, Bohn D, Daneman D. Use of hypertonic saline in the treatment of cerebral edema in diabetic ketoacidosis (DKA). *Pediatr Diabetes.* 2001;2:191-194.

83. Decourcey DD, Steil GM, Wypij D, Agus MS. Increasing use of hypertonic saline over mannitol in the treatment of symptomatic cerebral edema in pediatric diabetic ketoacidosis: an 11-year retrospective analysis of mortality*. *Pediatr Crit Care Med.* 2013;14:694-700.

84. Tasker RC, Burns J. Hypertonic saline therapy for cerebral edema in diabetic ketoacidosis: no change yet, please. *Pediatr Crit Care Med.* 2014; 15:284-285.

85. Marcin J, Glaser N, Barnett P, et al. Clinical and therapeutic factors associated with adverse outcomes in children with DKA-related cerebral edema. *J Pediatr.* 2003;141:793-797.

88. Rosenbloom A. Hyperglycemic crises and their complications in children. *J Pediatr Endocrinol Metab.* 2007;20:5-18.

93. Davis J, Surendran T, Thompson S, Corkey C. DKA, CVL and DVT. Increased risk of deep venous thrombosis in children with diabetic ketoacidosis and femoral central venous lines. *Ir Med J.* 2007;100:344.

94. Gutierrez J, Bagatell R, Sampson M, et al. Femoral central venous catheter-associated deep venous thrombosis in children with diabetic ketoacidosis. *Crit Care Med.* 2003;31:80-83.

112. Spencer-Smith M, Northam E, Koves I. Neurocognitive changes over a 6 month period in children newly diagnosed type 1 diabetes mellitus and diabetic ketoacidosis ISPAD conference. Abstract 2007.

113. Cameron FJ, Scratch SE, Nadebaum C, et al. Neurological consequences of diabetic ketoacidosis at initial presentation of type 1 diabetes in a prospective cohort study of children. *Diabetes Care.* 2014;37:1554-1562.

114. Tieder JS, McLeod L, Keren R, et al. Variation in resource use and readmission for diabetic ketoacidosis in children's hospitals. *Pediatrics.* 2013;132:229-236.

116. Shrestha SS, Zhang P, Barker L, Imperatore G. Medical expenditures associated with diabetes acute complications in privately insured U.S. youth. *Diabetes Care.* 2010;33:2617-2622.

119. Ellis D, Naar-King S, Templin T, et al. Multisystemic therapy for adolescents with poorly controlled type 1 diabetes: reduced diabetic ketoacidosis admissions and related costs over 24 months. *Diabetes Care.* 2008;31:1746-1747.

Nutrition in the Critically Ill Child

Nilesh M. Mehta

PEARLS

- Provision of individually tailored optimal nutrition to the critically ill child is an important goal of pediatric critical care.
- Malnutrition is prevalent in the pediatric intensive care unit (PICU) and is associated with increased physiologic instability and resource utilization.
- Failure to accurately estimate or measure energy expenditure during critical illness may result in unintended underfeeding or overfeeding. Indirect calorimetry may help prevent energy imbalances.
- The metabolic response to critical illness results in glucose and lipid intolerance and increased protein breakdown. Protein catabolism and nitrogen loss is a characteristic feature of the metabolic stress response to critical illness, resulting in net negative protein balance and loss of lean body mass.
- Failure to deliver optimal energy and protein has been associated with poor outcomes in critically ill adults and children.
- Enteral nutrition (EN) is the preferred mode of nutrient delivery in patients in the PICU with a functioning gastrointestinal tract. Early EN has been associated with positive outcomes in critically ill patients.
- The gastric route is preferred for enteral nutrition. Postpyloric (small bowel) feeding may improve nutrient delivery and may be considered for patients at risk of aspiration or when gastric feeding is not feasible or has not been tolerated.
- Use of EN algorithms and the presence of a dedicated dietitian in the PICU may decrease the barriers to EN and facilitate optimal nutrient delivery.
- Parenteral nutrition is associated with mechanical, infectious, and metabolic complications and should be used in carefully selected patients where EN is contraindicated, not tolerated, or has failed to provide adequate nutrition.

Introduction

Malnutrition is prevalent in critically ill children at the time of admission to the pediatric intensive care unit (PICU).[1,2] Further nutritional deficiencies during their illness course are often incurred due to the burden of illness or suboptimal nutrient intake and may result in poor outcomes. Safe provision of optimal nutrients during hospitalization is an important goal of pediatric critical care. The prediction, estimation, and measurement of true energy expenditure in the PICU patients can be challenging, resulting in unintended underfeeding or overfeeding. Although underfeeding has long been recognized as a problem, a significant proportion of critically ill children are at the risk of being overfed.[3] The enteral route is preferred, and the role and timing of parenteral nutrition continue to be evaluated. However, there exist a myriad of barriers that impede the delivery of prescribed nutrients to the critically ill child and result in a delay or a failure to achieve the prescribed energy and protein goal. Although the complexities of critical care or the nature of illness frequently conflicts with nutrient provision, many perceived barriers to bedside nutrient delivery may be avoidable. Studies have shown significant associations between energy and protein intake during critical illness and outcomes. Future studies will clarify the nature and the role of optimal nutritional therapies in improving patient outcomes in the PICU. Until then, careful screening for malnutrition, awareness of the metabolic state during illness course, accurate assessment of energy demands with attention to energy balance, optimal protein delivery, multidisciplinary efforts to overcome common barriers to nutrient intake at the bedside, and commitment to prioritizing nutritional support during critical illness are desirable.

Malnutrition in the Pediatric Critically Ill Patient

Critical illness increases metabolic demand on the host in the early stages of the stress response when nutrient intake may be limited (see also Chapter 81). As a result, children admitted to the PICU are at risk of deteriorating nutritional status and anthropometric changes with increased morbidity.[1] This effect is more pronounced in a subgroup of patients who are already malnourished or at risk of malnutrition on admission. The prevalence of malnutrition in children admitted to the ICU has remained largely unchanged since the 1990s. One in every four children admitted to the PICU shows signs of acute or chronic malnutrition on admission.[1,2] Malnutrition is associated with increased physiologic instability and the need for increased quantity of care in the ICU.[4] Despite its high prevalence and consequences, medical awareness of malnutrition is lacking. The nutritional status of hospitalized patients is not routinely assessed, and only a minority of patients are referred for expert nutritional consultation or support.[5] Careful nutritional evaluation at admission to the PICU will allow identification of children at risk for further nutritional deterioration and hence candidates for interventions to optimize nutrient intake. Efforts by organizations such as the American Society of Parenteral and Enteral Nutrition (A.S.P.E.N.) have renewed the focus on malnutrition and facilitated a uniform approach toward detecting and managing malnutrition in hospitalized adults and children.[6,7]

Assessment of Nutritional Status

In a proposed concept by A.S.P.E.N., the definition of malnutrition was expanded beyond anthropometric thresholds to include etiology and pathogenesis of malnutrition and its impact on patient outcomes.[7] Uniform use of reference charts and statistics was proposed to compare individual patient measurements to the reference population and thereby classify malnutrition. The association of malnutrition with disease states, in particular inflammation, was highlighted. Assessment of the nutritional status in the critically ill child is vital but often challenging. Clinicians use a combination of anthropometric and laboratory data to diagnose undernourishment. Carefully elicited past history with details of weight gain, dietary history, recent illness, and medications allows identification of risk factors for preoperative malnutrition. Weight on admission to the hospital is important and may be the only measure of the actual dry weight before capillary leak syndrome results in edema and weight gain. Unless regular and accurate weights are obtained, acute changes in nutritional status may be missed or detected late.[8] Children in the PICU are often not weighed as the procedure is deemed to be unsafe or not important. The lack of availability of reliable weight trends in PICU patients reflects the overall low priority among health care workers for nutritional assessment, and as a result the true incidence of malnutrition in this cohort may indeed be underestimated. Physical examination should be directed toward specific signs of nutritional and metabolic deficiencies. Hair, skin, eyes, mouth, and extremities may reveal stigmata of protein-energy malnutrition or vitamin and mineral deficiencies.

A variety of other measurements including arm anthropometry (mid-upper arm circumference and triceps skin fold), body length, and body mass index have been used to monitor growth in children. Recommendations for anthropometric variables and thresholds to classify malnutrition in children are shown in Table 87.1.[9] Although bedside anthropometric methods are inexpensive, they are sporadically applied in hospitalized children, may be insensitive in the setting of critical illness, and are limited by significant interobserver variability. Weight changes and other anthropometric measurements in critically ill children should be interpreted in the context of edema, fluid therapy, volume overload, and diuresis. In the presence of ascites or edema, ongoing loss of lean body mass may not be evident using weight monitoring alone.

Body Composition

Body composition is emerging as a primary determinant of health and a predictor of morbidity and mortality in children. Preservation and accrual of lean body mass during illness are important predictors of clinical outcomes in patients with sepsis, cystic fibrosis, and malnutrition.[10,11] Body composition is measured by a variety of techniques including body densitometry by underwater weighing, neutron activation analysis, total body potassium determination, bioelectrical impedance assessment (BIA), and dual-energy x-ray absorptiometry (DXA). DXA is a radiographic technique that can determine the composition and density of different body compartments (fat, lean tissue, fat-free mass, and bone mineral content) and their distribution in the body. DXA has been used extensively in pediatric practice for determining fat-free mass, fat mass, and lean mass, and it is recognized as a reference method for body composition research.[12] However, DXA is not practical for application in the PICU. BIA, in contrast, is a bedside technique that can be applied to pediatric patients without exposure to radiation and with ease.[13-15] Electrical current is conducted by body water and is impeded by other body components. BIA estimates the volumes of body compartments, including extracellular water and total body water (TBW). TBW measures can be used to estimate lean body mass by applying age-appropriate hydration factors. BIA has not been validated in critically ill populations; hence, its use outside clinical studies is not recommended in the PICU. The ideal bedside body composition measurement technique in critically ill patients remains elusive.

Biochemical Assessment

The nutritional status can also be assessed by measuring the visceral (or constitutive) protein pool, the acute-phase protein pool, nitrogen balance, and resting energy expenditure. Visceral proteins are rapid turnover proteins produced in the liver. Low circulating levels of visceral protein are seen in the setting of malnutrition, inflammatory states, and impaired hepatic synthetic function. The reliability of serum albumin as a marker of visceral protein status is questionable. Albumin has a large pool and a half-life of 14 to 20 days, and it is not an indicator of the immediate nutritional status. Serum albumin may be affected by changes in fluid status, albumin infusion, sepsis, trauma, and liver disease, and these changes are independent of nutritional status. Prealbumin (also known as transthyretin or thyroxine-binding prealbumin) is a stable circulating glycoprotein synthesized in the liver. It binds with retinol-binding protein and is involved in the transport of thyroxine and retinol. Prealbumin, so named because of its

TABLE 87.1	Indicators of Pediatric Malnutrition Based on Single Anthropometric Measurements		
Primary Indicators	**Mild Malnutrition**	**Moderate Malnutrition**	**Severe Malnutrition**
Weight for height Z score	−1 to −1.9 Z score	−2 to −2.9 Z score	−3 or lower Z score
Body mass index (BMI) for age Z score	−1 to −1.9 Z score	−2 to −2.9 Z score	−3 or lower Z score
Length/height Z score	No data	No data	−3 Z score
Mid-upper arm circumference	−1 to −1.9 Z score	−2 to −2.9 Z score	−3 Z score or lower

proximity to albumin on an electrophoretic strip, is readily measured in most hospitals and is a good marker for the visceral protein pool.[16,17] It has a half-life of 24 to 48 hours and reflects more acute nutritional changes. Prealbumin concentration is diminished in liver disease. Acute-phase reactant proteins are elevated proportional to the severity of injury in response to cytokines released during stress response and have been be used to longitudinally monitor the inflammatory response. Serum levels of acute-phase protein are elevated in children within 12 to 24 hours after burn injury due to hepatic reprioritization of protein synthesis.[18] When measured serially, serum prealbumin and C-reactive protein (CRP) are inversely related (ie, serum prealbumin levels decrease and CRP levels increase with the magnitude proportional to injury severity and then return to normal as the acute injury response resolves). In infants after surgery, decreases in serum CRP values to less than 2 mg/dL have been associated with the return of anabolic metabolism and are followed by increases in serum prealbumin levels.[19] Proinflammatory cytokines such as interleukin 6 (IL-6) are recognized as early markers of the systemic inflammatory response syndrome (SIRS) in several disease models. Serum concentrations of IL-6 may be useful in identifying patients at risk for nutritional deterioration and to determine whether the inflammatory response is intact. Chemistry profiles should be monitored on admission and repeated periodically. Serum electrolytes, blood urea nitrogen, glucose, coagulation profile, iron, magnesium, calcium, and phosphate levels are routinely monitored. Adequacy of cellular immunity can be estimated through the measurement of total lymphocyte count and by delayed-type hypersensitivity testing with a series of common antigens (eg, candida, Trichophyton, tuberculin).

Metabolic Consequences of Critical Illness

The energy burden imposed by the metabolic response to injury, surgery, or inflammation may be proportional to the severity and duration of the stress but cannot always be accurately estimated and varies in intensity and duration between individuals. Importantly, nutritional support itself cannot reverse or prevent the metabolic stress response but rather offsets the catabolic losses during this state. Failure to provide optimal calories and protein during the acute stage of illness can exaggerate existing nutritional deficiencies or further exacerbate underlying nutritional status. Respiratory compromise involving loss of respiratory muscle mass, cardiac dysfunction and arrhythmias involving loss of myocardial muscle tissue, and intestinal dysfunction involving loss of the gut barrier contribute to the morbidity and mortality of critical illness. In some cases, overestimation of this energy cost of metabolic stress may result in provision of energy in excess of requirement. Hence, large energy imbalances attributable to underfeeding and overfeeding in critically ill children must be avoided.[3] This can be prevented by individualized nutritional regimens that are tailored for each child and reviewed regularly during the course of illness. In a trial of a 12-week individualized nutritional intervention in home-ventilated children, significant improvements were observed in respiratory and body composition variables.[20] A basic understanding of the metabolic events that accompany critical illness and surgery is essential for planning appropriate nutritional support in critically ill children.

The unique hormonal and cytokine profile manifested during critical illness is characterized by an elevation in serum levels of insulin, glucagon, cortisol, catecholamines, and proinflammatory cytokines.[21] Increased serum counterregulatory hormone concentrations induce insulin and growth hormone resistance, resulting in the catabolism of endogenous stores of protein, carbohydrate, and fat to provide essential substrate intermediates and energy necessary to support maintenance energy and micronutrient needs in addition to the ongoing metabolic stress response. Fig. 87.1 illustrates the basic pathways involved in the metabolic stress response. In general, the net increase in muscle protein degradation, characteristic of the metabolic stress response, results in a large number of free amino acids in the circulation. Free amino acids are used as the building blocks for the rapid synthesis of proteins that act

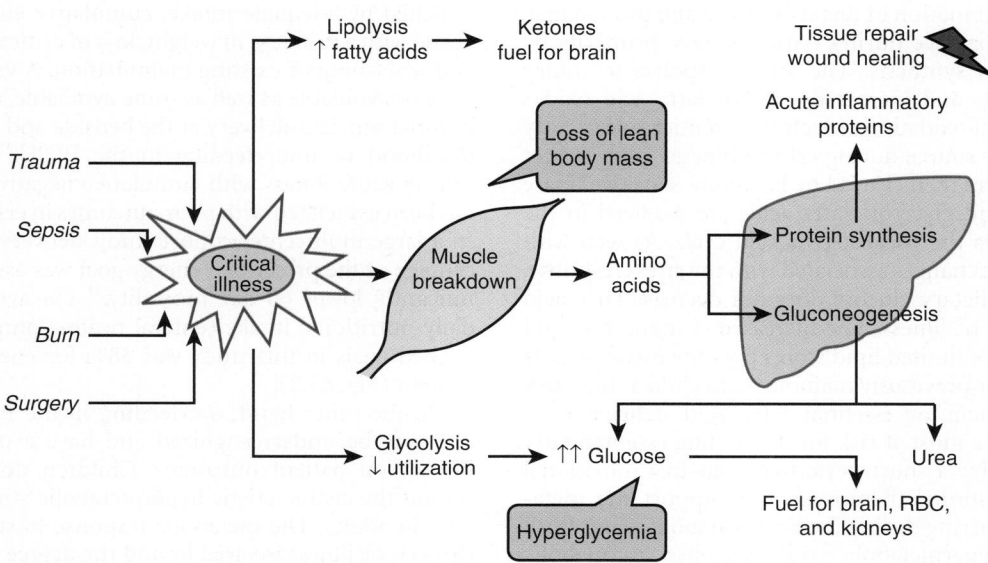

Fig. 87.1. The metabolic response to stress. (Reproduced with permission from Mehta N, Jaksic T. The critically ill child. In: Duggan C, Watkins JB, Walker WA, eds. Nutrition in Pediatrics. 4th ed. Hamilton, Ontario, Canada: BC Decker; 2008:663–673.)

as inflammatory response mediators and are used for tissue repair. Protein breakdown may continue for an extended period of time, in an attempt to channel the amino acids through the liver, wherein their carbon skeletons are used to create glucose through gluconeogenesis and for production of glucose as the preferred energy substrate for the brain, erythrocytes, and renal medulla. Reprioritization of protein during the metabolic stress increases the synthesis of acute-phase reactant proteins such as C-reactive protein, alpha$_1$-acid glycoprotein, haptoglobin, alpha$_1$-antitrypsin, alpha$_2$-macroglobulin, ceruloplasmin, and fibrinogen. Plasma concentrations of other proteins, including transferrin and albumin, decrease with injury or sepsis. Overall, the intense protein catabolism during critical illness outstrips anabolism with net negative protein balance. This condition results in weight reduction and rapid loss of lean body mass. The intense catabolism seen in metabolic stress cannot be suppressed by supplying calories, and negative protein balance continues relentlessly. This is one of the principal differences between stress response and starvation.

Starvation, or protein-calorie malnutrition, may be caused by socioeconomic, psychosocial, disease-related, or iatrogenic factors. The metabolic response to starvation involves decreased secretion of insulin and thyroid hormones, normal secretion of glucocorticoids and catecholamines, and decreased oxygen consumption. In starvation states, the body tries to preserve itself by using less energy for basic metabolic functions; thus, overall metabolic rate decreases. Metabolism shifts to use fat as a primary energy source, and the corresponding ketones help provide fuel for the brain and spare glucose and protein utilization. However, body tissues still must be broken down to supply amino acids for other critical functions, eventually leading to a loss of lean body mass, vital organ wasting, and possibly death. Table 87.2 summarizes the basic differences between starvation and metabolic stress.

Carbohydrate turnover is simultaneously increased during the metabolic stress response, with a significant increase in glucose oxidation and gluconeogenesis. The administration of exogenous glucose does not blunt the elevated rates of gluconeogenesis, however, and net protein catabolism continues unabated.[22] A combination of dietary glucose and protein may improve protein balance during critical illness, primarily by enhancing protein synthesis. The stress response to injury stimulates lipolysis and increased rates of fatty acid oxidation.[23] Increased fat oxidation reflects the premier role of fatty acids as an energy source during critical illness. Triglycerides in adipose tissue are then cleaved by hormone-sensitive lipase into fatty acids and glycerol. Fatty acids are oxidized in the liver for energy via the tricarboxylic acid cycle. As seen with the other catabolic changes associated with the stress response, the provision of dietary glucose does not decrease fatty acid turnover in times of illness. The increased demand for lipid use in the setting of limited lipid stores puts the metabolically stressed neonate or previously malnourished child at high risk for the development of essential fatty acid deficiency.[24,25] Preterm infants are most at risk for developing essential fatty acid deficiency after a short period of a fat-free nutritional regimen.[25,26] Nutritional therapy should support the metabolic changes occurring during the acute catabolic stage. With resolution of a hypermetabolic stress response, an anabolic phase typically follows, with increased release of growth hormone (GH) and insulin-like growth factor-1 (IGF-1).

TABLE 87.2	Metabolic Stress Versus Starvation	
	Metabolic Stress	**Starvation**
BMR	⇑⇑⇑	⇔⇓
Oxygen consumption (VO$_2$)	⇑⇑⇑	⇓
Protein catabolism	⇑⇑⇑⇑	⇔
UUN	⇑⇑⇑	⇔
Weight loss	Rapid	Slow
LBM loss	Early	Late
Response to caloric intake	Protein catabolism continues	Protein catabolism halted
Insulin, cortisol, and catecholamines	⇑⇑⇑	⇓
Ketones	⇑⇑⇑	⇔
Gluconeogenesis	⇑	⇓

BMR, basal metabolic rate; *LBM*, lean body mass; *UUN*, urinary urea nitrogen.

Supply of adequate nutrition is essential for this recovery phase. In summary, the metabolic response to critical illness results in glucose and lipid intolerance and increased protein breakdown.

Underfeeding and Overfeeding in the Pediatric Intensive Care Unit

Individual assessment of energy requirements and provision of optimal energy should be the standard of care in the PICU. Both underfeeding and overfeeding are prevalent in the PICU, with resultant nutritional deficiencies that are associated with complications.[4,27] True energy expenditure during acute illness may not be easily predicted, and several studies have documented discrepancies in measured versus equation-estimated energy expenditure.[28-30] Unless increased energy requirements during the acute stage of illnesses are accurately measured and matched by adequate intake, cumulative energy deficits will ensue with a decrease in weight, loss of critical lean body mass, and worsening of existing malnutrition. A variety of barriers, both unavoidable as well as some avoidable, exist that impede optimal nutrient delivery at the bedside and contribute to the likelihood of underfeeding in the PICU.[31,32] Underfeeding during acute illness with cumulative negative energy balance has been associated with poor outcomes in critically ill adults.[33] In a large multicenter cohort study, delivery of a higher percentage of the prescribed energy goal was associated with significantly lower 60-day mortality.[34] On average, percentage daily nutritional intake (enteral route) compared to the prescribed goals in this study was 38% for energy and 43% for protein (Fig. 87.2).

On the other hand, overfeeding in the PICU is prevalent but may be underrecognized and have a potential negative impact on patient outcomes. Children do not predictably mount the characteristic hypermetabolic stress response as is seen in adults. The metabolic response to stress from injury, surgery, or illness is variable, and the degree of hypermetabolism is unpredictable and unlikely to be sustained during a prolonged course in the PICU.[35] Critically ill children cannot

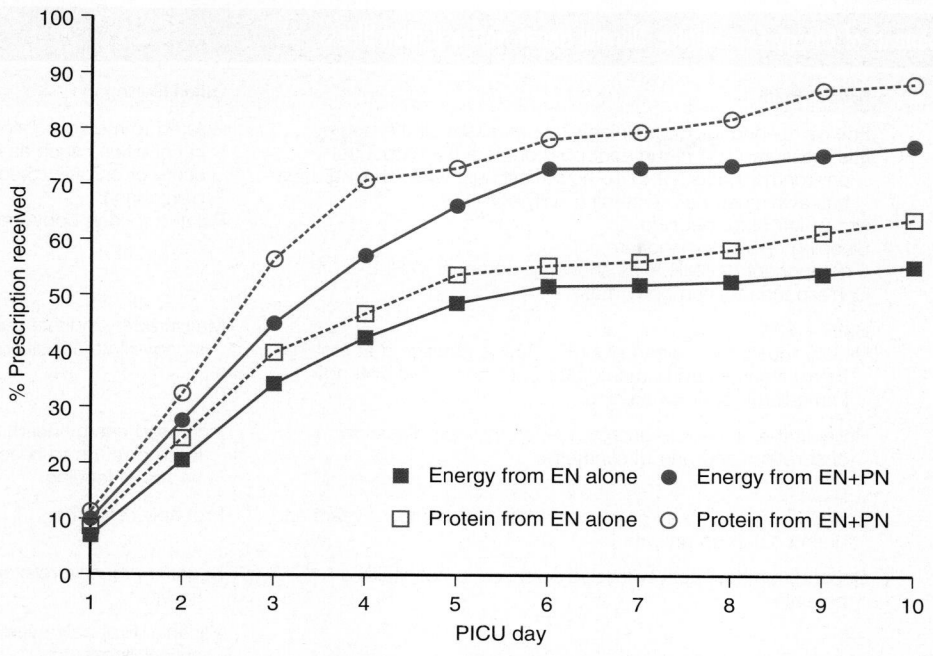

Fig. 87.2. Daily mean cumulative energy intake (as percentage of prescribed goal) for the cohort. *EN,* enteral nutrition; *PN,* parenteral nutrition; *PICU,* pediatric intensive care unit.

be presumed to be hypermetabolic following acute illness or injury, and energy expenditure may actually be decreased in some groups of patients.[36-39] Children on extracorporeal life support or after surgery have failed to show any significant hypermetabolism, and measured energy expenditure is close to resting energy expenditure in these populations.[40] Critically ill children who are sedated and mechanically ventilated may have a significant reduction in actual total energy expenditure, due to multiple factors. Stress or activity correction factors factored into basal energy requirement estimates, in an attempt to account for the perceived hypermetabolic effects of the illness, may result in overfeeding in hypometabolic patients.[41,42] Overfeeding may have deleterious consequences for the critically ill child.[27,43] Overfeeding critically ill children is associated with net lipogenesis, hepatic steatosis, liver dysfunction, and increased CO_2 production and difficulty in ventilator weaning.[44] Investigators have proposed hypocaloric diets in critically ill adults.[45,46] Hypocaloric diets may have a protein-sparing effect and have demonstrable benefits in critically ill obese patients. However, it is uncertain if administration of energy intake lower than the measured expenditure is appropriate for the critically ill pediatric patient. There is not enough evidence to recommend its general use in critically ill children. In general, the energy goals in critically ill children should be individualized and based on accurate and serial assessment of energy requirement during the illness course.

Current recommendations for nutritional requirements of the critically ill child are derived from limited data, based on studies in healthy children and based on limited methodological approaches. Table 87.3 summarizes the recommended energy and protein intake for critically ill children. The components of total energy expenditure in children include (1) basal metabolic rate (BMR) 70%, (2) diet-induced thermogenesis (DIT) 10%, (3) energy expended during physical activity (PA) 20%, and (4) energy expended for growth. The

TABLE 87.3	Recommended Energy and Protein Allowances During Critical Illness		
	Age (years)	Energy (kcal/kg/day)	Protein (g/kg/day)
Infants	0-0.5	115	2.2
	0.5-1	105	2.0
Children	1-3	100	1.8
	4-6	85	1.5
	7-10	86	1.2
Males	11-14	60	1.0
	15-18	42	0.8
Females	11-14	48	1.0
	15-18	38	0.8

From the Food and Nutrition Board, National Academy of Science, National Research Council. 9th ed. Washington, DC: National Academy of Science; 1980.

sum of these components determines the energy requirement for an individual. These traditional components of energy expenditure in healthy children may not apply during critical illness (Table 87.4). Thus prescribing optimal energy for the critically ill child requires careful review of each component of total energy expenditure. Recommendations for energy requirements were based on estimates of basal metabolic rate or resting energy expenditure (REE) derived by either indirect calorimetry or standard equations.[37,47] REE estimates have a large individual variability, and predictive equations are unreliable, particularly in underweight, overweight, or critically ill children.[30,48,49] Newer equations have attempted to improve the prediction of REE in children by accounting for weight-based groups or including pubertal staging, with variable success.[49,50] These equations have not satisfactorily been

TABLE 87.4 Components of Energy Expenditure: Normal Health versus Critical Illness

Component	Normal Health	Critical Illness
BMR (60%-70%)	Energy needed for maintaining vital processes of the body. It is measured in a recumbent position, in a thermoneutral environment after 12 to 18 hours fast, just when the individual has awakened before starting daily activities. Not practical for bedside Sleeping energy expenditure, a component of BMR, was shown to be equal to REE 3 0.9 Corresponds to lean body mass.	Related to metabolic state. May be increased in conditions such as inflammation, fever, acute or chronic disease (ie, cardiac, pulmonary). Related to lean body mass.
REE (50%-60%)	BMR + 10% Usually measured instead of BMR. REE is measured at rest in a thermoneutral environment, after 8-12 hours fast and not immediately after awakening.	Measured by indirect calorimetry with steady-state conditions.
DIT or TEF (10%)	Reflects the amount of energy needed for food digestion, absorption, and part of synthesis.	Increased energy needs following enteral feeding return to baseline approximately >4 hrs of feeding.
Growth (variable)	Energy for growth may be higher in healthy infants <2 years and during catch-up growth.	Probably halted?
Physical activity (PA) (variable)	Depends on age, activity level. Decreased in hospitalized patients.	Sedation, muscle relaxants, decreased activity.
Stress	—	Variable. Probably overestimated during critical illness.
Total energy expenditure	REE + DIT + PA + Growth	Probably close to REE in most critically ill children. Addition of stress factors may be necessary where relevant.

BMR, basal metabolic rate; *DIT,* diet-induced thermogenesis; *REE,* resting energy expenditure; *TEF,* thermic effect of food.

validated in critically ill children.[51] The variability of the metabolic state may be responsible for the failure of estimation equations in accurately predicting the measured REE in critically ill children. The A.S.P.E.N. guidelines recommend indirect calorimetry when available for the most accurate assessment of energy expenditure in critically ill children.[52]

Indirect Calorimetry

Historically, indirect calorimetry (IC) has been regarded as the gold standard for accurate measurement of REE. Energy expenditure is obtained by measuring the volume of oxygen consumed (VO_2) and the volume of CO_2 produced (VCO_2) over a period of time.[53] VO_2 and VCO_2 values are used to calculate REE using the modified Weir equation: REE = [VO_2 (3.941) + VCO_2 (1.11)] × 1440. This technique has been validated in healthy children by using a whole-body chamber to allow 24-hour measurement. For obvious reasons, the whole-body chamber cannot be used in critically ill children. The application of IC in different PICU populations has shown the variability in energy expended during illness. In the past, studies have demonstrated a relatively higher resting metabolic rate in critically ill children (37% higher than the resting metabolic rate of age-matched healthy controls).[54] However, contrary to beliefs held for years, studies have shown that the total energy expenditure is not increased in head-injured children, postoperative general surgical patients, or children after major cardiac surgery.[55-57] The muted metabolic responses to major surgeries and injuries in studies may reflect advances in surgical and intensive care over the years. In critically ill mechanically ventilated children, use of sedation and muscle paralysis decreases the component of energy requirement related to physical activity,[44] and caloric needs in the critically

TABLE 87.5 Factors Associated With Inaccurate or Unreliable Indirect Calorimetry Measurements

Error in VCO_2 Measurement	Limitations or Mechanical Issues With the Device	Failure to Reach Steady State
Air leak >10% around endotracheal tube	High inspired Fio2 (>60%)	Recent interventions (suctioning, painful procedure)
Air leak in the circuit	Calibration issues	Fever, seizures, dysautonomia
Chest tube for pneumothorax	Moisture or obstruction due to water in the circuit	Recent change in ventilator settings
		Study period too short

ill child may be lower than previously considered. IC remains sporadically applied in critically ill children despite mounting evidence of the inaccuracy of estimated basal metabolic rate using standard equations. This could potentially subject a subgroup of children in the PICU to the risk of underfeeding or overfeeding. However, IC application is not feasible in all patients due to (1) specific subject requirements, (2) device limitations, and (3) the need for expertise and resources. Table 87.5 describes some of the common problems associated with IC testing in critically ill children. In the era of resource constraints, IC may be applied or targeted for certain high-risk groups in the PICU.[3] Selective application of IC may allow many units to balance the need for accurate REE measurement and limited resources (see Table 87.6 for suggested criteria for targeted IC).[52] Although IC application has illuminated our understanding of energy expended during critical illness, this is yet to be translated into improving patient outcomes. Studies examining the role of simplified IC technique, its role in optimizing nutrient intake, its ability to prevent overfeeding or underfeeding in selected subjects, and the cost-benefit analyses of its application in the PICU are desirable. The effect of energy intake on outcomes needs to be examined in pediatric populations, especially in those on the extremes of body mass index (BMI).

Another method of energy expenditure determination is based on the use of doubly labeled water. However, at this time the technique remains confined to research settings. Stable isotope technique has been available for many years and was first applied for energy expenditure measurement in humans by Schoeller and van Santen[58] in 1982. Isotope studies using doubly labeled water have since been validated and following intense and skeptical scrutiny have now been established as a gold standard for total energy expenditure estimation with widespread application.[43,59-62] In this method, stable isotopes of water (^2H_2O and $H_2^{18}O$) are administered enterally. They mix with the body water and the ^{18}O is lost from the body as both water and CO_2, whereas the ^2H is lost from the body only as water. The difference in the rates of loss of the isotopes ^{18}O and ^2H from the body reflects the rate of CO_2 production, which can be used to calculate the total energy expenditure. This method has advantages in children because of its noninvasive nature. However, isotope decay is measured over two half-lives of the isotope, and hence the technique only gives an average estimate of total energy expenditure over a period of a few days. Analytic errors in the mass spectrometric estimation of isotope enrichment, isotope fractionation during CO_2 formation or vaporization of water, and the calculation of total body water or respiratory quotient are factors that might introduce errors in the estimation of total energy expenditure with this technique. If the necessary conditions are met, the doubly labeled water technique is currently the best method for estimating energy expenditure because expired gas analysis is not required, and serial measurements of stable isotopes in urine samples provide an objective assessment of energy expenditure over a period of 4 to 21 days. However, the doubly labeled water technique for determining energy expenditure is difficult to use in critically ill children because it requires fluid balance in the steady state. This is a major problem in the critically ill child with active capillary "leak" syndrome. Hence, decreased urinary output, capillary leak syndrome, use of diuretics, and fluid overload exclude the use of this technique. The isotope costs and availability may be concerns, and the doubly labeled water technique cannot measure brief periods of peak energy expenditure.

In summary, energy expenditure must be carefully evaluated throughout the course of critical illness, using actual measurements when available. In patients meeting the requirements for this test, IC provides an accurate measurement of REE. IC may need to be targeted to specific patient groups due to the risk of metabolic instability, but it may help prevent unintended underfeeding and overfeeding in these patients. In the absence of measured REE, equation estimated REE may be used. However, the uniform application of stress factors is not advisable and must only be used in individual cases after careful evaluation. Once energy needs are determined, the optimal substrate required for maintenance of energy needs is mixed fuel (glucose and fat). The proportion of each varies according to the clinical situation.

Protein Requirements

Protein turnover and catabolism are increased several-fold in critically ill children. This is one of the most characteristic features of the metabolic stress response and probably represents an adaptive response that was critical to survival of human prehistoric ancestors as a race. An advantage of high-protein turnover is that a continuous flow of amino acids is available for synthesis of new proteins. Specifically, this process involves a redistribution of amino acids from skeletal muscle to the liver, wound, and other tissues involved in the inflammatory response. This allows for maximal physiologic adaptability at times of injury or illness. The catabolism of muscle protein to generate glucose and inflammatory response proteins is an excellent short-term adaptation, but it is ultimately limited in children and neonates because of the limited protein reserves available. Children, especially preterm infants, have reduced macronutrient reserves with less than half the protein content of adults.[63] Although children with critical illness have increases in both whole-body protein degradation and whole-body protein synthesis, it is the former that predominates during the stress response and results in a net negative protein balance. Infants and malnourished children with already decreased or depleted lean body mass reserves may not tolerate the ill effects of cumulative negative protein balance. In a large international cohort study of more than 1200 mechanically ventilated children, 60-day mortality was lower in children who received a higher proportion of their daily prescribed protein goal.[64] Fig. 87.3 depicts the linear relation between enteral protein intake adequacy (percentage of the protein goal delivered) and 60-day mortality in mechanically ventilated patients in this cohort. A similar association between

---

TABLE 87.6   Suggested Criteria for Targeted Indirect Calorimetry[3,52]

Children at High Risk for Metabolic Alterations Who Are Suggested Candidates for Targeted Measurement of Resting Energy Expenditure (REE) in the PICU Include the Following:

- Underweight (body mass index [BMI] <5th percentile for age), at risk of overweight (BMI >85th percentile for age) or overweight (BMI >95th percentile for age)
- Children with >10% weight gain or loss during ICU stay
- Failure to consistently meet prescribed caloric goals
- Failure to wean, or need to escalate respiratory support
- Need for muscle relaxants for >7 days
- Neurologic trauma (traumatic, hypoxic, or ischemic) with evidence of dysautonomia
- Oncologic diagnoses (including children with stem cell or bone marrow transplant)
- Children with thermal injury
- Children requiring mechanical ventilator support for >7 days
- Children suspected to be severely hypermetabolic (status epilepticus, hyperthermia, systemic inflammatory response syndrome, dysautonomic storms, etc.) or hypometabolic (hypothermia, hypothyroidism, pentobarbital or midazolam coma, etc.)
- Any patient with ICU LOS >4 weeks may benefit from indirect calorimetry to assess adequacy of nutrient intake.

LOS, length of stay; *PICU,* pediatric intensive care unit.

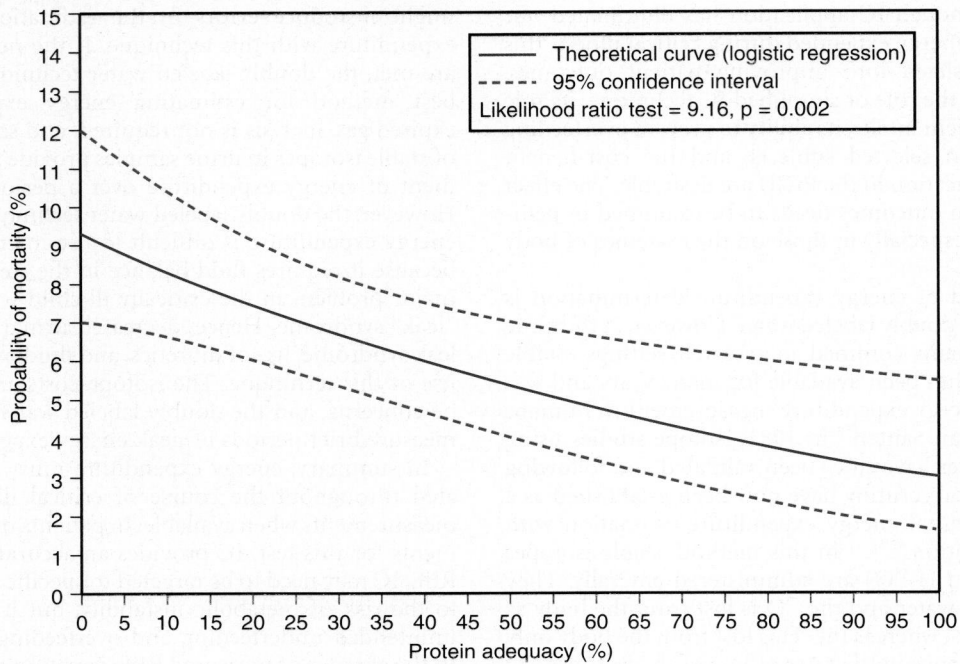

Fig. 87.3. Linear relation between enteral protein intake adequacy (percentage of the protein goal delivered) as a continuous variable and 60-d mortality. (With permission from Mehta NM, et al. Adequate enteral protein intake is inversely associated with 60-d mortality in critically ill children: a multicenter, prospective, cohort study. Am J Clin Nutr. 2015;102:199-206.)

lower protein intake and mortality was also shown in a large international study of adult critically ill patients.[45] These reports suggest a strong association between protein intake and outcomes, which is both biologically plausible and independent of energy intake.

Unlike starvation, the provision of dietary carbohydrate alone is ineffective in reducing the protein catabolism or endogenous glucose production via gluconeogenesis in the metabolically stressed state.[22] Therefore, without elimination of the inciting stress for catabolism (ie, the critical illness or injury), the progressive breakdown of muscle mass from critical organs may result in loss of diaphragmatic and intercostal muscle (leading to respiratory compromise) and the loss of cardiac muscle.[65,66] The amount of protein required to optimally enhance protein accretion is higher in critically ill than in healthy children. Infants demonstrate 25% higher protein degradation after surgery and a 100% increase in urinary nitrogen excretion with bacterial sepsis.[65,66] Following burn injury, protein catabolism and whole body protein turnover are increased and may persist for up to several months after the inciting event.[67] The provision of dietary protein sufficient to optimize protein synthesis, facilitate wound healing and the inflammatory response, and preserve skeletal muscle protein mass is the most important nutrition intervention in critically ill children. Supply of adequate proteins and energy intake improves protein balance by increasing protein synthesis, although protein breakdown is not affected. The amount of protein required to maintain a positive nitrogen balance may vary according to the severity of illness. Nitrogen balance is used as a surrogate for protein balance. In a systematic review of protein supplementation trials, a minimum of 1.5 g/kg/day protein intake was required to achieve a positive nitrogen balance.[68] This threshold of 1.5 g/kg/day protein intake was again shown to be the minimum required to achieve a positive

protein balance in studies of critically ill children.[69,70] Despite these studies, the current prescription for protein in the PICU remains low. It is clear that the requirements of protein in a critically ill child exceed those for a healthy child. The dietary reference intake (DRI) recommendations for protein intake for healthy children are inadequate to meet the demands in critically ill children and should not be used to guide protein prescription in the PICU population.[64] Failure to deliver the prescribed protein due a variety of barriers at the bedside further increases the gap between requirement and actual delivery. Further studies to determine the individual requirement of specific amino acids under catabolic conditions are necessary, particularly in view of the important functions of amino acids, not only in protein synthesis but as signaling molecules[71] and precursors for important substrates such as glutathione[46] and methyl group donors.[72] Alternatively, excessive protein administration could be deleterious, particularly in children with marginal hepatic or renal function. Neonates with higher protein intakes have been shown to develop azotemia, pyrexia, and possible long-term detrimental effects on cognitive development.[73,74] Hence, future studies on specific nutritional and functional requirements of amino acids and their impact on functional outcomes are needed.

Lipid Requirements

Nonprotein calories are commonly provided as carbohydrates (55% to 65%) and fat (35% to 45%). In the absence of adequate lipid supplementation in the diet, critically ill children, who have depleted lipid stores at baseline, are likely to suffer essential fatty acid deficiency.[72] Lipid administration is generally restricted to 30% to 40% of the total calories, and after an initial prescription of 1 g/kg/day it may be gradually increased to 2 to 4 g/kg/day, depending on the tolerance level.

Triglyceride levels should be regularly monitored for lipid tolerance. Concentrated lipid formulas (Intralipid 20%) should be used, given the limitation on fluid volume for administration of nutritional support. The potential role for omega-2 fatty acids during critical illness is discussed further in the parenteral nutrition section.

Micronutrient Requirements

Micronutrients play significant physiologic roles. Beneficial effects of micronutrients such as fat-soluble vitamins (A, D, E, and K), water-soluble vitamin (C), zinc, selenium, and folic acid have been described in selected groups of patients in well-defined settings. Presumed safety of micronutrients and probably exaggerated efficacy and generalized applicability to heterogeneous populations are factors that may be responsible for the widespread prescription of these compounds.[75] Commercially available antioxidant nutrients need to be scrutinized for optimal dosage and side effects in the clinical setting where they are most likely to be beneficial. Hospitalized patients, especially those with critical illness, currently receive these additives in accordance with Food and Nutrition Board recommendations for daily allowances. The antioxidant properties of certain micronutrients have renewed interest in their role during critical illness.[76] Vitamins C and E have important antioxidant properties. Selenium has also been shown to be a critical micronutrient with antioxidant functions in patients with thermal injury and trauma.[77] A complex system of special enzymes, their cofactors (selenium, zinc, iron, and manganese), sulfhydryl group donors (glutathione), and vitamins (E and C) form a defense system to counter the oxidant stress seen in the acute phase of injury or illness. Critically ill patients may have variable deficiencies of micronutrients in the early phase of illness. Vitamins and trace elements are redistributed from central circulation to tissues and organs during systemic inflammatory response syndrome (SIRS).[76] Levels of trace elements, such as iron, selenium, and zinc, and water-soluble vitamins are decreased, whereas copper and manganese levels may be increased.[78] In addition, trauma and thermal injuries are characterized by extensive losses of biological fluids through wound exudates, drains, and hemorrhage, which cause negative micronutrient balances. The reduced stores of these enzyme cofactors, vitamins, and trace elements decrease rapidly after injury and remain at subnormal levels for weeks. Low endogenous stores of antioxidants are associated with an increase in free radical generation, augmented systemic inflammatory response, cell injury, and increased morbidity and mortality in the critically ill.[59,60]

Preliminary studies have shown low plasma zinc levels in critically ill children, associated with inflammatory markers and degree of organ failure.[61,62] These observations have driven dosing studies to examine the efficacy of zinc supplementation in critically ill children.[58] There has been increased interest in the role of vitamin D as an antioxidant. Serum levels of vitamin D are decreased in children with severe burns.[79] Vitamin D status may be compromised for months after burn injury. Indeed studies show a much larger incidence of vitamin D deficiency in the general population.[80-84] Significantly low levels of vitamin D have been reported in critically ill children.[85,86] In a study of more than 500 critically ill children, the median 25(OH)D level was 22.5 ng/mL and over 40% of the cohort was deficient (level <20 ng/mL).[86] In another prospective multicenter observational study of critically ill children from Canada, low levels of vitamin D were independently associated with severity of illness, catecholamine utilization, need for fluid boluses, and PICU length of stay.[87] The concept of early micronutrient supplementation to prevent the development of acute deficiency, to rectify the oxidant-antioxidant balance, and to reduce oxidative-mediated injuries to organs has driven trials in critically ill patients.[88] Antioxidant research in the critically ill has focused on copper, selenium, zinc, vitamins C and E, and the vitamin B group. Most of these studies were performed in relatively small patient populations presenting with heterogeneous diseases, such as trauma, burns, sepsis, or acute respiratory distress syndrome, however, and thus are underpowered to detect a treatment effect on clinically important outcomes. Based on a systematic review of trials, supplementing critically ill patients with antioxidants, trace elements, and vitamins was deemed safe and associated with a reduction in mortality in critically ill patients.[76] However, a trial of glutamine and antioxidant supplementation in critically ill adults did not show any benefit from antioxidant supplementation for the primary outcome, 28-day mortality, or any of the secondary outcomes.[89]

Electrolyte management in critically ill children can be complicated because of existing deficiencies, fluid shifts, increased insensible losses, drainage of bodily secretions, and renal failure (see also Chapter 73). Intravenous fluids or parenteral nutrition (PN) prescriptions need to be reviewed daily in light of the basic electrolytes and blood sugar levels. In children with significant gastrointestinal fluid loss (gastric, pancreatic, small intestinal, or bile), the actual measurement of electrolytes from the drained fluid may assist in prescribing replacement fluids. Acute changes in serum electrolytes that require urgent electrolyte replacement must not be managed by changes in the PN infusion rate or composition, because this method may be imprecise and potentially dangerous. Phosphate and magnesium levels are often abnormal in critically ill children, especially in those with existing nutritional deficiencies, sepsis, or ongoing nutritional deprivation.

Refeeding Syndrome

Aggressive nutritional rehabilitation in malnourished patients or those with prolonged fasting results in a constellation of biochemical and clinical features with cardiopulmonary complications. This well-described entity is called refeeding syndrome and is often unrecognized. Hypophosphatemia is the hallmark of refeeding syndrome, which is also associated with hypomagnesemia, hypokalemia, and fluid retention. Patients admitted to the PICU with nutritional deficiencies, those with chronic conditions causing malnutrition, or those fasted for 10 to 14 days are at risk of refeeding syndrome following aggressive oral, enteral, or parenteral nourishment. The introduction of nutrition in these patients stimulates anabolism, with a switch from protein and fat catabolism to predominantly carbohydrate metabolism. Glucose becomes the primary energy source leading to insulin release. Insulin-mediated cellular uptake of glucose causes an intracellular shift of phosphate, potassium, and magnesium, thus rapidly lowering their serum levels. Insulin also causes sodium and fluid retention with rapid expansion of extracellular fluid volume. The clinical manifestations of refeeding syndrome are a result of the dyselectrolytemia and fluid overload involving the cardiorespiratory, neuromuscular, and hematologic complications. Hypotension, respiratory failure, muscular weakness, confusion, seizures, coma, and even death may result from refeeding syndrome.

Awareness of this syndrome, identification of at-risk patients, and gradual introduction of nutrition in these individuals help prevent the refeeding syndrome. Calories may be introduced at 25% to 50% of requirement and increased 10% to 25% daily until the caloric goal is met. Careful monitoring of electrolytes and vigilance for clinical manifestations of the syndrome allow early detection of complications, and feeds are advanced in the setting of biochemical stability. Prompt correction of electrolyte abnormalities, close attention to fluid balance, and supplementation with multivitamins will help avoid the cardiorespiratory sequelae from refeeding in the critically ill child.

Enteral Nutrition in Critically Ill Children

Enteral nutrition (EN) is the preferred mode of nutrient intake in critically ill patients with a functional gastrointestinal system due to its lower cost and complication rate when compared to PN.[52] Early institution of EN is associated with beneficial outcomes in animal models and human studies[76] and has been increasingly implemented during critical illness, often using nutrition guidelines or protocols.[90] Early enteral nutrition has been shown to decrease infectious episodes and decrease length of hospital stay in critically ill patients.[91] In a multicenter retrospective study including 12 PICUs, early EN was associated with lower odds of mortality.[92] Early EN, defined as delivery of at least 25% of energy goal in the first 48 hours after admission, was achieved in 27% of the 5105 patients in this study. Centers have achieved successful implementation of early enteral nutrition using institutional protocols.[90,93]

Although early EN has been adopted in a majority of the units, subsequent maintenance of enteral nutrient delivery remains elusive, as EN is frequently interrupted in the intensive care setting for a variety of reasons, some of which are avoidable.[32,94] Frequent interruptions in enteral nutrient delivery may affect clinical outcomes secondary to suboptimal provision of calories and reliance on PN. This author has reported EN interruptions in a third of patients in the PICU who were started on EN.[31] EN was frequently interrupted for avoidable reasons. Patients experiencing avoidable EN interruptions had more than a threefold increase in the use of PN and significant delay in reaching caloric goals. This collaborative study, examining bedside nutrition practice, illustrates some of the challenges to the provision of nutrition support and highlights opportunities for practice modification. Fasting for procedures and intolerance to EN were the most common reasons for prolonged EN interruptions. Interventions aimed at optimizing EN delivery must be designed after examining existing barriers to EN and directed at high-risk individuals who are most likely to benefit from these interventions. Knowledge of existing barriers to EN, such as those identified in this study, will allow appropriate interventions to be planned. Intolerance to enteral feeds may be a limiting factor, and supplementation with PN in this group of patients allows earlier optimal nutritional intake. Taylor and colleagues reviewed nutritional delivery in a group of 95 children in a PICU over a 12-month period and made similar observations.[95] Children received a

median of 58.8% (range 0% to 277%) of their estimated energy requirements in this review. Enteral feeding was interrupted on 264 occasions to allow clinical procedures. Rogers and colleagues reviewed nutritional intake in 42 patients admitted to an Australian tertiary-level PICU over 458 ICU days.[32] When actual energy intake was compared with estimated energy requirement, only 50% of patients had received full estimated energy requirements after a median of 7 days in the ICU. Fluid restriction is a major factor hindering the achievement of estimated energy requirements despite maximizing the energy content of feeds. Table 87.7 summarizes some of the barriers to successful enteral feeding in the PICU.

Protocols or algorithms have been employed in the PICU to ensure prompt institution of EN in eligible patients, followed by advancement of feeds to the goal and management of feeding intolerance. Fig. 87.4 describes an EN initiation and advancement protocol at a tertiary center. The implementation of this algorithm resulted in a significant increase in the number of patients reaching energy delivery goal in this PICU.[96] A significant decrease in the number of avoidable EN interruptions and use of PN was recorded after the implementation of this algorithm. Stepwise algorithms have been used by other investigators to facilitate optimal EN delivery in the PICU.[97,98] However, they are used in a minority of centers, and the actual components of the algorithms vary significantly.[99] The use of postpyloric feeding has been compared to gastric feeding in the PICU population. In a randomized control trial of mechanically ventilated children, the use of a postpyloric tube for feeding allowed a higher amount of nutrient delivery (percentage of caloric goal) compared to gastric tube feeding.[100] The incidence of aspiration of gastric contents as well as symptoms of EN intolerance was similar in the two groups. Postpyloric tubes provide the opportunity to feed a subset of children for whom intragastric feeding has not succeeded or is deemed unsafe. The use of the postpyloric route for feeding critically ill children is limited to centers with the appropriate resources and expertise for placement and management of

TABLE 87.7	Barriers to Enteral Nutrient Delivery in the Pediatric Intensive Care Unit

Fasting before procedures
   Endotracheal tube–related procedures (intubation, extubation)
   Major operative procedures
   Other procedures requiring general anesthesia
   Bedside procedures requiring sedation
   Radiology suite or interventional radiology procedures
Fluid restriction
Delay in establishing enteric tube for feeding
   Delay or difficulty in enteric tube placement
   Malpositioned, obstructed, or displaced enteric tube
Gastrointestinal dysfunction
   Malabsorption, diarrhea, or severe constipation
   Ileus associated with opioid use or postoperative
Patients at risk of aspiration of gastric contents
Holding EN for perceived intolerance
   High gastric residual volume
   Abdominal distension or discomfort
   Vomiting or diarrhea
Failure to implement evidence-based uniform algorithmic approach to EN
   Delay in initiating EN

EN, enteral nutrition.

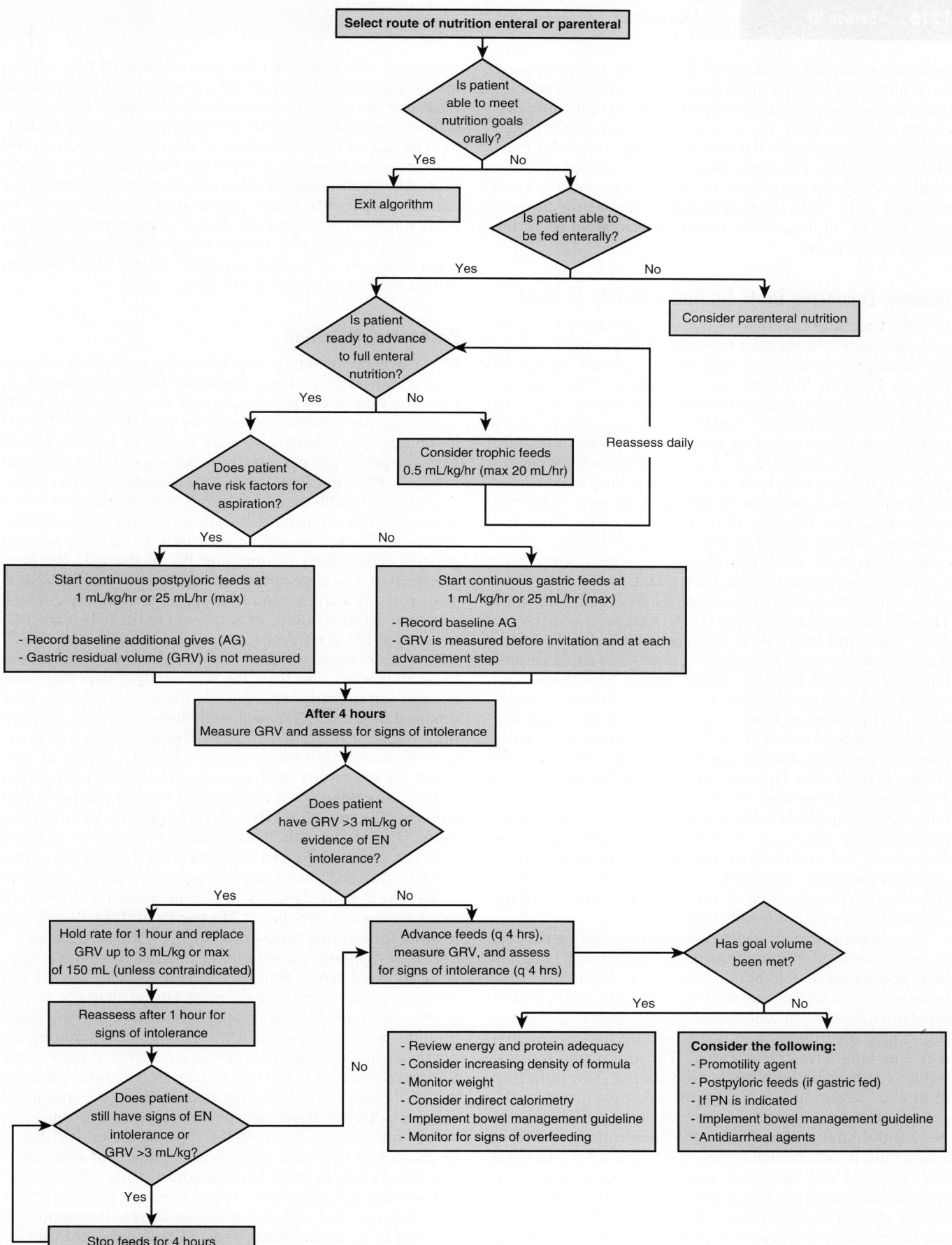

Fig. 87.4. Enteral nutrition support algorithm. (With permission from Hamilton S, et al. A stepwise enteral nutrition algorithm for critically ill children helps achieve nutrient delivery goals. Pediatr Crit Care Med. 2014;15:583-589.)

these tubes. Surgical placement of gastrostomy or jejunostomy tubes allows long-term enteral feeding and administration of drugs in selected patients during intensive care and after discharge from the ICU. The advent of percutaneously placed gastric and jejunal tubes has minimized cost, time, and morbidity. Stoma site infection, obstruction, and tube dislodgment are common complications and must be identified and managed early. Tube tip malposition is frequently encountered with any of these devices either at placement or during the course of its use.

Immune-Enhancing Diets for the Critically Ill Child

In 1996, Bone and colleagues[101] outlined the role of the compensatory antiinflammatory response (CARS), which follows the initial proinflammatory response by the body challenged with an insult or infection (see Chapters 81, 101, 102, and 105). The antiinflammatory response was believed to be the second phase of a biphasic, highly coordinated inflammatory response and was aimed at keeping the proinflammatory response under control. It is clear that immunomodulation plays a significant role in the nature of response to infectious insult and impacts outcome in children with sepsis admitted to the ICU (see Chapter 105). The role of nutrition has expanded beyond that of growth and rehabilitation. Newer components have been introduced in enteral feeds such L-arginine, glutamine, taurine, nucleotides, w-3 and w-6 fatty acids, carnitine, growth factors, probiotics, and prebiotics. These immune-enhancing diets (IEDs) have been available for many years, and their role in the care of critically ill patients remains controversial. An increasing number of studies examining the effect of IEDs in various clinical populations and related meta-analyses continue to provide conflicting conclusions. Methodological flaws in conducting initial studies and the heterogeneous nature of the IED formulations used do not allow for dispelling current doubts regarding the safety and efficacy of these diets. The commercially available diets contain a mixture of compounds in varying doses, and the role of individual compounds is impossible to interpret. The immunomodulating effects of individual compounds are dose dependent, and mixtures of different immunomodulating nutrients may have synergistic but also antagonistic effects. However, the compositions of the products compared in the meta-analysis are considerably different.

There are insufficient pediatric studies evaluating the role of nutrition-based immunonutrition in critically ill children. In a randomized double-blind comparative effectiveness trial, investigators sought to examine the impact of nutraceutical supplementation with zinc, selenium, glutamine, and metoclopramide on preventing nosocomial infection in children requiring long-term critical care.[102] The group who received immune-enhancing supplementation did not show difference in time to acquiring infection/sepsis when compared to the group with whey supplementation. In a subset of the cohort (9%) with immunocompromise, the intervention resulted in a reduction of nosocomial infection rates. In a 2 × 2 factorial trial, Heyland and colleagues randomized more than 1200 adults with multiorgan failure and mechanical ventilation to receive glutamine, antioxidants, both, or placebo.[89] The trial was stopped early as there was a trend toward increased 28-day mortality, significantly increased in-hospital mortality, and 60-month mortality in the patients who received glutamine as compared with those who did not receive glutamine. Glutamine supplementation was not associated with decrease in rates of organ failure or infectious complications. Antioxidant supplementation in this trial had no effect on 28-day mortality. The lack of beneficial effect of glutamine and association with increased mortality in this study has resulted in a significant lack of enthusiasm for the immunonutrition strategy for critically ill patients. Future studies may examine the role of other micronutrients and the impact of immunonutrition in improving outcomes in immunocompromised patients. The generalized use of immunonutrition in the PICU children cannot be recommended at this time.

Parenteral Nutrition

PN or hyperalimentation bypasses the gut, allowing intravenous administration of macronutrients and micronutrients to meet the nutritional requirements of the body, either partly (as a supplement to enteral feeds) or entirely (total PN). PN is indicated for children who are unable to tolerate enteral feeds for prolonged periods. In the setting of intact intestinal function, PN is not indicated if enteral feeds alone can maintain nutrition. Although widespread in its application, PN is associated with mechanical, infectious, and metabolic complications and hence should be used only in carefully selected patients. The timing of imitating PN in the ICU has been investigated. In a large randomized controlled trial (EPaNIC), 4640 patients were randomly assigned to receive parenteral nutrition within 48 hours of admission to the ICU (early PN) or received PN at 8 days or later after admission (late PN).[103] Patients from the group that received late PN were more likely to be discharged alive from the ICU within 8 days than were patients given early PN. No significant differences were reported in the ICU, hospital, and 90-day mortality between the groups. Furthermore, the late PN group had shorter duration of mechanical ventilation and hospital length of stay. Based on the results of this study, PN is used when EN is contraindicated or when EN is unable to meet macronutrient demands for approximately 7 days. In preterm infants, newborns, and those with malnutrition, PN may be initiated earlier. A randomized trial examining the role of early versus late PN (initiated after 7 days) in patients who are unable to reach caloric goals via the enteral route in the PICU environment is currently ongoing.[104] The results of this trial will help instruct the optimal timing of PN in critically ill children.

PN prescription, compounding, and delivery require vigilance to avoid errors that are inherent to each stage of this complex process. Institutions must ensure that PN is prescribed by individuals with appropriate competency, and a multidisciplinary approach with communication among the physician, dietitian, and pharmacist is essential to achieve safe PN delivery in the PICU. Fluid and electrolyte status guide the initial PN prescription. Fluid restrictions limit the amount of calories delivered despite use of a concentrated formula. PN should not be used for replacing ongoing losses. PN should be prescribed daily and after reviewing levels of electrolytes and blood sugar in order to allow adjustments in the macronutrient and micronutrient composition. The patient's hydration, size, age, and underlying disease dictate the amount of the fluid to be administered. Table 87.8 describes the calculations used to determine calories provided from macronutrients in PN.

TABLE 87.8 Calculating Parenteral Nutrition calories

Total carbohydrate (CHO) in g/day x 3.4 kcals/g = CHO calories
1 g dextrose provides 3.4 kcals (most other CHOs provide 4 kcals/g)
10% dextrose = 10 g dextrose/100 mL
Total protein in g pro/day x 4 kcals/g = protein calories
1 g protein provides 4 kcals
Total fat (20% lipids) in mL x 2.0 kcals/mL = lipid calories
(10% lipids = 1.1 kcal/mL)
Total calories = CHO + protein + lipid calories
Total nonprotein calories = CHO + lipid calories

Carbohydrates

Carbohydrates are the major nonprotein source of energy. D-Glucose is provided in the monohydrate form for intravenous administration and yields 3.4 kcal/g. The concentration of the dextrose solution should not exceed 10% for peripheral administration. In the setting of central venous access, a range of concentrations (5% to 40%) can be prepared. Higher glucose concentration makes the solutions hyperosmolar and may cause phlebitis or thrombosis and decrease the life span of the vessel when PN is administered peripherally through a vein. Blood glucose estimations must be followed carefully given the increased incidence of hyperglycemia, especially in young infants. Carbohydrate is started at 5 to 8 mg/kg/min. Gradually increasing the carbohydrate load allows appropriate endogenous insulin response and prevents fluctuations in blood sugar. Abrupt cessation of PN may result in hypoglycemia and should be anticipated and avoided.[105] Fat is supplied as Intralipid, which provides the other source of calories in PN and reduces the carbon dioxide production and water retention that is seen when carbohydrate is the sole source of calories.

Amino Acids

One gram of protein yields 4 kcal. Initial recommended dosages range from 0.5 to 3 g/kg/day based on age, disease state, and individual requirements. Usual concentrations available are between 1% and 4%, although patients with hepatic disease, renal insufficiency, and children with metabolic diseases (eg, maple syrup urine disease) should receive appropriately modified concentrations. Trophamine contains a higher percentage of branched-chain amino acids and a small amount of glycyl-cysteine. This solution is mainly used in the neonatal population. It is recommended and used in patients with hepatic encephalopathy and in children on long-term PN (eg, short bowel), although data supporting this application are scarce. There is an increasing interest in the use of glutamine in PN. Glutamine and cysteine as glycyl-cysteine are precursors for glutathione, which is a major antioxidant. Glutamine is also a precursor for nucleotide synthesis, and although it is a nonessential amino acid, it can become conditionally essential, especially in catabolic states such as sepsis and trauma. Glutamine has a short shelf life. However, its applicability has been widespread. It has been introduced in PN solutions for its presumed benefits, such as restoration of protein and nitrogen balance, attenuation of gastrointestinal mucosal atrophy, reduction of bacterial translocation, and bacteremia after chemotherapy. The National Institute of Child Health and Development (NICHD) neonatal research network did not find significant differences in outcomes when a multicenter study randomized 1430 extremely low-birth-weight neonates to PN containing 20% glutamine or an isonitrogenous control. However, pediatric burn patients have been shown to have deficient peripheral glutamine production. In a double-blinded randomized control trial, glutamine-enhanced PN reduced gram-negative bacteremia in severely burned patients.[106]

Lipids

Lipids are an integral part of PN and provide energy through fatty acid oxidation. Lipids are usually started at 0.5 to 1 g/kg and advanced to a maximum intake of 3 g/kg or a maximum 60% of total kilocalories. Lipid calories allow for lower concentration of carbohydrate (lower osmolarity of PN). Lipid emulsions are available as 10% (1.1 kcal/mL) or 20% (2 kcal/mL). Intralipid prevents or treats essential fatty acid deficiency. The total lipid usually is delivered over an 18- to 24-hour period through separate tubing using a Y connector near the infusion site. Delivery of amino acid, glucose, and lipid (three-in-one) is no longer recommended for neonatal patients because of the risk of calcium phosphate precipitation being obscured by lipid in the preparation.

Lipids are a crucial source of nutrition in parenteral formulas. Traditionally considered a calorie-dense nutrient and a source of essential fatty acids, lipids in intravenous feeding regimens have added advantages, such as providing a more balanced energy expenditure and facilitating better respiratory function parameters. Fatty acid derivatives are major biological modulators.[107] Fig. 87.5 illustrates the basic pathways and inflammatory effects of fatty acid metabolites. The linoleic acid load, as a consequence of predominantly soy-based lipid in current formulations, results in increased arachidonic acid production and decreased production of eicosapentaenoic acid (EPA) and docosahexaenoic acid (DHA).[108] Increased arachidonic acid levels may increase the proinflammatory cytokine production and activity. EPA levels may influence the production of antiinflammatory cytokines,[107] and DHA has been shown to lower blood pressure, improve endothelial function, and elevate levels of high-density and low-density lipoproteins.[109] Thus DHA and EPA, found in fish and fish oils, are essential fatty acids for humans. In an attempt to decrease the linoleic acid intake, soy-based oil has been partly replaced by medium-chain triglycerides, olive oil, or fish oil in intravenous emulsions. Based on the putative advantages of fish oils as immune modulatory agents, they have been applied in clinical trials across a wide spectrum of critically ill patients.[34,86] The OMEGA trial was a double-blinded multicenter placebo-controlled trial where subjects received twice-daily enteral supplementation with omega-3 fatty acids, γ-linolenic acid, and antioxidants compared with an isocaloric control.[110] The trial was stopped early due to futility. The supplemented group did not show any improvement in the primary outcome of ventilator-free days and rather appeared to have a higher incidence of harm compared to the control group. There are currently no pediatric data to support the use of omega-3 fatty acid supplementation in the PICU.

Electrolytes/Minerals and Trace Elements

All solutions typically are prepared with minimum acetate (ie, all salts are added as chloride) unless prescribed otherwise. It is possible to prescribe an all-acetate solution with no

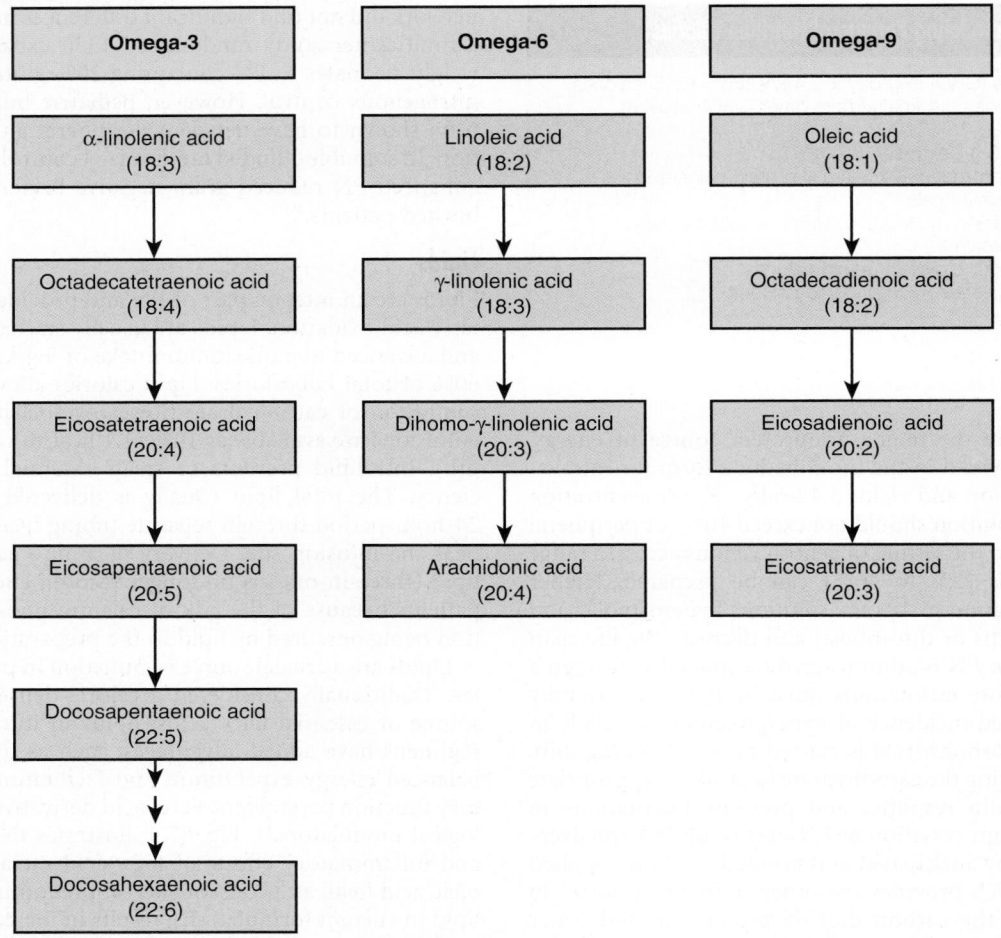

Fig. 87.5. Omega-3 and omega-6 fatty acid metabolites.[120] (Adapted from Lee S, et al. Current clinical applications of omega-6 and omega-3 fatty acids. Nutr Clin Pract. 2006;21:323-341.)

chloride. Calcium and phosphorus precipitate when their concentrations exceed an allowable limit, related to the solubility index of $(Ca)_3(PO_4)_2$ and the pH of the solution. Selenium may not be routinely added to PN. A serum selenium level is obtained if a patient requires PN for more than 30 days without enteral intake. Multivitamins and trace elements are routinely added to the PN, and recommended intakes are elucidated elsewhere.[111] Heparin usage in PN is practiced in many centers and has been shown to decrease catheter-related sepsis.[112] Heparin in concentrations of 0.5 to 1 U/mL are thought to prevent thrombosis and possibly phlebitis in peripheral lines, although there are no controlled trials showing significant benefit of heparin usage in PN.

Biochemical Monitoring

A PN profile is recommended at initiation of therapy and weekly thereafter. The profile includes serum levels of sodium, potassium, chloride, glucose, carbon dioxide, blood urine nitrogen, creatinine, albumin, magnesium, phosphate, total and direct bilirubin, and transaminases. For children requiring PN for more than 30 days, selenium, iron, zinc, copper, and carnitine levels should be checked. Daily vital statistics and routine anthropometry must be monitored to ensure adequate growth and development. Critical care units benefit from the expertise of a dedicated nutritionist, who

should be consulted on a regular basis to guide optimal nutritional intake of patients.

Central venous access is required for delivery of hyperosmolar PN solutions into a large-bore vein with high-volume blood flow to prevent thrombosis and phlebitis (see Chapter 19). The incidences of infective and life-threatening complications related to indwelling central lines have necessitated extreme caution with central PN use.[113,114] Central lines should be placed by experienced operators and line tip position confirmed by radiography before the lines are used for PN delivery. It is recommended that central line tips be positioned outside the cardiac chambers at all times. Central lines are recommended for delivery of infusates with osmolarity greater than 900 mOsm/L (10% dextrose, 2% amino acids with standard additives).

Nutritional Support of Obese Critically Ill Children

Overweight/obesity continues to increase in children and adolescents, and annual obesity-related hospital costs in 6- to 17-year-olds have reached $127 million per year. Obesity may be a risk factor for higher mortality in children with critical illness, particularly those with oncologic diseases or undergoing organ transplantation.[115] The severity of obesity is classified based on BMI into the following three categories: (1)

overweight = BMI 25 to 30 kg/m^2, (2) obesity = BMI 30 to 40 kg/m^2, and (3) morbid obesity = BMI >40 kg/m^2. Overweight children and adolescents are increasingly being diagnosed with impaired glucose tolerance and type II diabetes, and they show early signs of the insulin resistance syndrome and cardiovascular risk. Centralized distribution of body fat is associated with the risk of metabolic syndrome. Metabolic syndrome is observed in obese children and is characterized by visceral obesity, insulin resistance, and dyslipidemia. There is a high risk for type II diabetes and cardiovascular complications in patients with metabolic syndrome. Grossly overweight patients are prone to sleep apnea syndrome, restrictive lung disease, venous thrombosis, musculoskeletal degenerative disorders, hepatic steatosis, and metabolic disorders associated with bariatric surgery. The metabolic response to stress in obese critically ill patients is complex, given that it occurs in a population with preexisting major metabolic and endocrine alterations. In critically ill obese patients, the pattern of substrate oxidation is mainly protein and glucose, with decreased fat oxidation.[116] The extent of protein breakdown is greater than in nonobese critically ill adults. No data on metabolic abnormalities of obese children are available. In the adult critically ill population, hypocaloric nutrition estimated for ideal weight has been recommended.[117] The limited adult literature suggests that protein requirements are higher in critically ill adult obese patients. It is recommended that fat be administrated sparingly, mainly to prevent essential fatty acid deficiency.[118] Evidence for the best nutritional support strategy for critically ill obese children is not currently available.

Routine equations for tend to overestimate energy expenditure in obese patients.[119] Energy requirements in this group should be guided by IC measurement of REE, where available. When REE is estimated, there is no consensus on the use of ideal body weight versus adjusted body weight. As the incidence of obesity in children admitted to the PICU is rising, future research aimed at addressing some of these knowledge gaps is desirable.

Guidelines for Pediatric Critical Care Nutrition

Due to the complexities of critical care, nutrient intake during critical illness is challenging. The lack of robust evidence for many of the bedside decision making around nutrition support in the PICU has resulted in heterogeneity in practice. Optimal nutrition support in the PICU cannot be achieved unless there is some uniformity in practice based on evidence or consensus and an attempt to systematically evaluate practice parameters for feasibility, efficacy, and impact on patient outcomes. However, the direct effect of nutritional strategies in a heterogeneous cohort of patients with varying degrees of illness severity is difficult to assess. Multiple factors influence outcome during critical illness. Due to these challenges, current literature is scarce and guidelines for pediatric critical care nutrition have been based on few good studies but mainly smaller studies of expert opinion. In 2009, the American Society of Parenteral and Enteral Nutrition published the revised guidelines for pediatric critical care nutrition practice (Table 87.9).[52] These guidelines were based on best available

TABLE 87.9   Guidelines for Pediatric Critical Care Nutritional Support[52]

	NUTRITION SUPPORT GUIDELINE RECOMMENDATIONS IN THE CRITICALLY ILL CHILD	
#	**Guideline Recommendations**	**Grade**
1	1A. Children admitted with critical illnesses should undergo nutrition screening to identify those with existing malnutrition and those who are nutritionally at risk.	D
	1B. A formal nutrition assessment with the development of a nutrition care plan should be required, especially in those children with premorbid malnutrition.	E
2	2A. Energy expenditure should be assessed throughout the course of illness to determine the energy needs of critically ill children. Estimates of energy expenditure using available standard equations are often unreliable.	D
	2B. In a subgroup of patients with suspected metabolic alterations or malnutrition, accurate measurement of energy expenditure using indirect calorimetry (IC) is desirable. If IC is not feasible or available, initial energy provision may be based on published formulas or nomograms. Attention to imbalance between energy intake and expenditure will help to prevent overfeeding and underfeeding in this population.	E
3	There are insufficient data to make evidence-based recommendations for macronutrient intake in critically ill children. After determination of energy needs for the critically ill child, the rational partitioning of the major substrates should be based on understanding of protein metabolism and carbohydrate and lipid handling during critical illness.	E
4	4A. In critically ill children with a functioning gastrointestinal tract, enteral nutrition (EN) should be the preferred mode of nutrient provision, if tolerated.	C
	4B. A variety of barriers to EN exist in the pediatric intensive care unit (PICU). Clinicians must identify and prevent avoidable interruptions to EN in critically ill children.	D
	4C. There are insufficient data to recommend the appropriate site (gastric vs. postpyloric/transpyloric) for enteral feeding in critically ill children. Postpyloric or transpyloric feeding may improve caloric intake when compared to gastric feeds. Postpyloric feeding may be considered in children at high risk of aspiration or those who have failed a trial of gastric feeding.	C
5	Based on the available pediatric data, the routine use of immunonutrition or immune-enhancing diets/nutrients in critically ill children is not recommended.	D
6	A specialized nutrition support team in the PICU and aggressive feeding protocols may enhance the overall delivery of nutrition, with shorter time to goal nutrition, increased delivery of EN, and decreased use of parenteral nutrition. The effect of these strategies on patient outcomes has not been demonstrated.	

From Mehta NM, Compher C. A.s.p.e.N. Clinical guidelines: nutrition support of the critically ill child. JPEN J Parenter Enteral Nutr. 2009;33:260-276.

evidence and help clarify the principles guiding nutrition therapy in the PICU population. Early enteral nutrition is recommended in critically ill children with a functional gastrointestinal tract. Careful assessment or measurement of energy expenditure with attention to unintended energy imbalance (due to underfeeding or overfeeding) seems prudent. Health care workers must work in a collaborative fashion to identify and prevent common barriers to nutrition support in the PICU. The application of indirect calorimetry and postpyloric feeding is currently limited to centers with available expertise and resources.

Conclusions

Accurate assessment of nutritional needs and the provision of individually tailored optimal nutrition support to the critically ill child are important goals of pediatric critical care. Malnutrition and obesity are prevalent in the PICU and have significant influence on the outcome of critical illness. Furthermore, the hypermetabolic stress response places demands on the critically ill child that must be met with evidence-based nutrient supplementation. Intensivists must remain alert to the possibility of both underfeeding and overfeeding in order to prevent unintended cumulative energy imbalances in critically ill children. Evidence suggests a significant relationship between inadequate protein intake and poor outcomes from critical illness. A multidisciplinary effort to overcome common barriers to nutrient delivery and the use of evidence-based algorithms will help achieve nutrition goals in the PICU.

Interest in the immune-modulating effects of nutrients, micronutrient supplementation, and the role of newer sources of lipid formulations has introduced the concept of pharmaconutrients, but the benefits on outcome in the PICU have not been realized yet. The feasibility of strict glycemic control in the PICU is currently being examined in the setting of a randomized control study. In the future, patients will benefit from individually tailored nutritional regimens suited to the type and stage of their illness. There are a number of knowledge gaps in the field of critical care nutrition that need to be addressed by collaborative research. Until then a multidisciplinary effort must be made to increase awareness of nutritional issues and prioritization of nutrition support in the PICU.

Key References

1. Hulst J, Joosten K, Zimmermann L, et al. Malnutrition in critically ill children: from admission to 6 months after discharge. *Clin Nutr.* 2004;23:223-232.
3. Mehta NM, Bechard LJ, Leavitt K, Duggan C. Cumulative energy imbalance in the pediatric intensive care unit: role of targeted indirect calorimetry. *JPEN J Parenter Enteral Nutr.* 2009;33:336-344.
7. Mehta NM, Corkins MR, Lyman B, et al. Defining pediatric malnutrition: a paradigm shift toward etiology-related definitions. *JPEN J Parenter Enteral Nutr.* 2013;37:460-481.
9. Becker PJ, Nieman Carney L, Corkins MR, et al. Consensus statement of the Academy of Nutrition and Dietetics/American Society for Parenteral and Enteral Nutrition: indicators recommended for the identification and documentation of pediatric malnutrition (undernutrition). *J Acad Nutr Diet.* 2014;114:1988-2000.
11. Brambilla P, Rolland-Cachera MF, Testolin C, et al. Lean mass of children in various nutritional states. Comparison between dual-energy X-ray absorptiometry and anthropometry. *Ann N Y Acad Sci.* 2000;904:433-436.
12. Elberg J, McDuffie JR, Sebring NG, et al. Comparison of methods to assess change in children's body composition. *Am J Clin Nutr.* 2004;80:64-69.
14. Eisenmann JC, Heelan KA, Welk GJ. Assessing body composition among 3- to 8-year-old children: anthropometry, BIA, and DXA. *Obes Res.* 2004;12:1633-1640.
15. Mehta NM, Raphael B, Guteirrez IM, et al. Comparison of body composition assessment methods in pediatric intestinal failure. *J Pediatr Gastroenterol Nutr.* 2014;59:99-105.
19. Letton RW, Chwals WJ, Jamie A, Charles B. Early postoperative alterations in infant energy use increase the risk of overfeeding. *J Pediatr Surg.* 1995;30:988-992, discussion 992-983.
20. Martinez EE, Smallwood CD, Bechard LJ, et al. Metabolic assessment and individualized nutrition in children dependent on mechanical ventilation at home. *J Pediatr.* 2015;166:350-357.
23. Coss-Bu JA, Klish WJ, Walding D, et al. Energy metabolism, nitrogen balance, and substrate utilization in critically ill children. *Am J Clin Nutr.* 2001;74:664-669.
27. Askanazi J, Rosenbaum SH, Hyman AI, et al. Respiratory changes induced by the large glucose loads of total parenteral nutrition. *JAMA.* 1980;243:1444-1447.
28. Framson CM, LeLeiko NS, Dallal GE, et al. Energy expenditure in critically ill children. *Pediatr Crit Care Med.* 2007;8:264-267.
29. Hardy CM, Dwyer J, Snelling LK, et al. Pitfalls in predicting resting energy requirements in critically ill children: a comparison of predictive methods to indirect calorimetry. *Nutr Clin Pract.* 2002;17:182-189.
31. Mehta NM, McAleer D, Hamilton S, et al. Challenges to optimal enteral nutrition in a multidisciplinary pediatric intensive care unit. *JPEN J Parenter Enteral Nutr.* 2010;34:38-45.
34. Mehta NM, Bechard LJ, Cahill N, et al. Nutritional practices and their relationship to clinical outcomes in critically ill children–an international multicenter cohort study. *Crit Care Med.* 2012;40:2204-2211.
37. White MS, Shepherd RW, McEniery JA. Energy expenditure in 100 ventilated, critically ill children: improving the accuracy of predictive equations. *Crit Care Med.* 2000;28:2307-2312.
38. Jaksic T, Shew SB, Keshen TH, et al. Do critically ill surgical neonates have increased energy expenditure? *J Pediatr Surg.* 2001;36:63-67.
40. Shew SB, Keshen TH, Jahoor F, Jaksic T. The determinants of protein catabolism in neonates on extracorporeal membrane oxygenation. *J Pediatr Surg.* 1999;34:1086-1090.
43. Chwals WJ. Overfeeding the critically ill child: fact or fantasy? *New Horiz.* 1994;2:147-155.
44. Goran MI, Kaskoun M, Johnson R. Determinants of resting energy expenditure in young children. *J Pediatr.* 1994;125:362-367.
47. Schofield WN. Predicting basal metabolic rate, new standards and review of previous work. *Hum Nutr Clin Nutr.* 1985;39(suppl 1):5-41.
52. Mehta NM, Compher C. A.s.p.e.N. Clinical guidelines: nutrition support of the critically ill child. *JPEN J Parenter Enteral Nutr.* 2009;33:260-276.
56. Mehta NM, Costello JM, Bechard LJ, et al. Resting energy expenditure after Fontan surgery in children with single-ventricle heart defects. *JPEN J Parenter Enteral Nutr.* 2012;36:685-692.
57. Mtaweh H, Smith R, Kochanek PM, et al. Energy expenditure in children after severe traumatic brain injury. *Pediatr Crit Care Med.* 2014;15:242-249.
58. Cvijanovich NZ, King JC, Flori HR, et al. A Safety and dose escalation study of intravenous zinc supplementation in pediatric critical illness. *JPEN J Parenter Enteral Nutr.* 2015;[Epub ahead of print].
64. Mehta NM, Bechard LJ, Zurakowski D, et al. Adequate enteral protein intake is inversely associated with 60-d mortality in critically ill children: a multicenter, prospective, cohort study. *Am J Clin Nutr.* 2015;102:199-206.
66. Keshen TH, Miller RG, Jahoor F, Jaksic T. Stable isotopic quantitation of protein metabolism and energy expenditure in neonates on- and post-extracorporeal life support. *J Pediatr Surg.* 1997;32:958-962, discussion 962-953.
67. Borsheim E, Chinkes DL, McEntire SJ, et al. Whole body protein kinetics measured with a non-invasive method in severely burned children. *Burns.* 2010;36:1006-1012.
68. Bechard LJ, Parrott JS, Mehta NM. Systematic review of the influence of energy and protein intake on protein balance in critically ill children. *J Pediatr.* 2012;161:333-339, e331.
69. Bairdain S, Khan FA, Fisher J, et al. Nutritional outcomes in survivors of congenital diaphragmatic hernia (CDH)-factors associated with growth at one year. *J Pediatr Surg.* 2015;50:74-77.

70. Jotterand Chaparro C, Laure Depeyre J, Longchamp D, et al. How much protein and energy are needed to equilibrate nitrogen and energy balances in ventilated critically ill children? *Clin Nutr*. 2016;35: 460-467.

85. Abrams SA, Coss-Bu JA. Vitamin D deficiency in critically ill children: a roadmap to interventional research. *Pediatrics*. 2012;130: 557-558.

86. Madden K, Feldman HA, Smith EM, et al. Vitamin D deficiency in critically ill children. *Pediatrics*. 2012;130:421-428.

87. McNally JD, Menon K, Chakraborty P, et al. The association of vitamin D status with pediatric critical illness. *Pediatrics*. 2012;130:429-436.

90. Chellis MJ, Sanders SV, Webster H, et al. Early enteral feeding in the pediatric intensive care unit. *JPEN J Parenter Enteral Nutr*. 1996;20: 71-73.

92. Mikhailov TA, Kuhn EM, Manzi J, et al. Early enteral nutrition is associated with lower mortality in critically ill children. *JPEN J Parenter Enteral Nutr*. 2014;38:459-466.

93. Briassoulis GC, Zavras NJ, Hatzis MT. Effectiveness and safety of a protocol for promotion of early intragastric feeding in critically ill children. *Pediatr Crit Care Med*. 2001;2:113-121.

96. Hamilton S, McAleer DM, Ariagno K, et al. A stepwise enteral nutrition algorithm for critically ill children helps achieve nutrient delivery goals. *Pediatr Crit Care Med*. 2014;15:583-589.

98. Petrillo-Albarano T, Pettignano R, Asfaw M, Easley K. Use of a feeding protocol to improve nutritional support through early, aggressive, enteral nutrition in the pediatric intensive care unit. *Pediatr Crit Care Med*. 2006;7:340-344.

99. Martinez EE, Bechard LJ, Mehta NM. Nutrition algorithms and bedside nutrient delivery practices in pediatric intensive care units: an international multicenter cohort study. *Nutr Clin Pract*. 2014;29:360-367.

100. Meert KL, Daphtary KM, Metheny NA. Gastric vs small-bowel feeding in critically ill children receiving mechanical ventilation: a randomized controlled trial. *Chest*. 2004;126:872-878.

102. Carcillo JA, Dean JM, Holubkov R, et al. The randomized comparative pediatric critical illness stress-induced immune suppression (CRISIS) prevention trial. *Pediatr Crit Care Med*. 2012;13:165-173.

104. Fivez T, Kerklaan D, Verbruggen S, et al. Impact of withholding early parenteral nutrition completing enteral nutrition in pediatric critically ill patients (PEPaNIC trial): study protocol for a randomized controlled trial. *Trials*. 2015;16:202.

110. Rice TW, Wheeler AP, Thompson BT, et al. Enteral omega-3 fatty acid, gamma-linolenic acid, and antioxidant supplementation in acute lung injury. *JAMA*. 2011;306:1574-1581.

115. Bechard LJ, Rothpletz-Puglia P, Touger-Decker R, et al. Influence of obesity on clinical outcomes in hospitalized children: a systematic review. *JAMA Pediatr*. 2013;167:476-482.

119. Martinez EE, Ariagno K, Arriola A, et al. Challenges to nutrition therapy in the pediatric critically ill obese patient. *Nutr Clin Pract*. 2015.

120. Lee S, Gura KM, Kim S, et al. Current clinical applications of omega-6 and omega-3 fatty acids. *Nutr Clin Pract*. 2006;21:323-341.

Hematology-Oncology

Structure and Function of Hematopoietic Organs

Seth J. Corey and Julie Blatt

PEARLS

- Normal ranges for blood cell numbers or function depend on the age of the patient.
- Hematopoiesis in a given bone varies with age and must be considered for successful bone marrow aspiration or biopsy.
- Because the marrow circulation connects with the general circulation, fluids and medications injected into bone marrow are absorbed as rapidly as when they are administered intravenously.
- For major invasive procedures such as surgery or placement of arterial lines or endotracheal tubes, platelet count should be maintained at ≥50,000/μL.
- Clinical application of small molecule regulators of hematopoiesis is increasing.

Poised to maintain homeostasis, the hematopoietic system must respond quickly to changes in oxygen tension, bleeding, or infection by increasing the production of erythrocytes, platelets, or neutrophils. When stressed, especially in a very ill neonate or child, hematopoiesis and blood cell function may be insufficient. Alternatively, excessive or poorly controlled leukocytes lead to autoimmunity, macrophage activation syndromes, or chronic inflammation. The extensive use of red blood cell (RBC) or platelet transfusions and antimicrobials supports the importance of the blood system as a vital organ affected in the pediatric intensive care unit setting. This chapter reviews the anatomy and physiology of the hematopoietic system to provide a basis for understanding the repercussions of primary hematologic abnormalities, as well as hematopoietic manifestations of nonhematologic diseases. Aspects that are of practical importance to the intensivist are emphasized.

Structure and Function of the Bone Marrow

During embryogenesis and fetal development, hematopoiesis shifts from the yolk sac (primitive hematopoiesis) to the liver and, after 20th week of gestation, to the bone marrow (definitive hematopoiesis).[1] Although extramedullary erythropoiesis may persist for several weeks after birth, in the term infant hematopoiesis takes place almost entirely in the bone marrow. A defining feature of hematopoietic stem cells is their ability

to home to the bone marrow. This homing occurs via chemoattractants such as stromal cell-derived factor-1 and its cognate receptor CXCR4 on the stem cell, as well as interaction between a variety of stem cell adhesion molecules and their ligands on stroma and endothelial cells. Compartments of hematopoietic stem, progenitor, and precursor cells may be identified by the presence of cell surface markers. In particular, the hematopoietic stem cells are identified by the cell surface expression of CD34 and the ability to exclude Hoechst dye 33342 via a multidrug transporter.[2]

Grossly, two types of bone marrow can be recognized in normal individuals: yellow marrow, so called because of the predominance of adipocytes, and red marrow, in which blood cells predominate. White marrow, consisting predominantly of stromal cells and intercellular matrix, may result from atrophy or starvation. Red marrow proportionately is a much greater component of body weight and volume in the infant than in the adult (Fig. 88.1).[3] Early in life, it is contained in the medullary cavities of the long bones, which gradually fill with fat such that by late puberty, the adult distribution of hematopoiesis (sternum, pelvis, vertebrae, cranium, ribs, epiphyses of long bones) is achieved. That the degree of hematopoiesis in a given bone varies with age is an important consideration in selecting a site for bone marrow aspiration or biopsy; for example, although the anterior and posterior iliac crests can be used at any age, the tibia can be used only until the age of 2 years. In disease states characterized by excessive destruction of blood cells, such as severe hemolytic anemias, hematopoiesis may increase twofold to eightfold. Active sites of hematopoiesis may expand and can result in frontal bossing of the skull, which is characteristic in children with untreated thalassemia major. Extramedullary hematopoiesis may be found, particularly in the liver and spleen.

Microscopically, the marrow is a network of vascular channels (sinuses) separating islands of fat, hematopoietic cells, and rare osteoblasts and osteoclasts (which are important for bone remodeling).[4,5] The vasculature and cells are joined by a reticulin (fiber) network or scaffolding. By light microscopy, bone marrow aspirate specimens demonstrate hematopoietic elements; however, a bone marrow biopsy provides a more accurate measure of cellularity. Reticulin can be seen by light microscopy with histochemical staining, and it suggests myelofibrosis, either a primary or secondary.

The blood vessels that feed the marrow are branches of those that feed the surrounding bone.[4,6] Large central arteries run longitudinally within the marrow and send radial branches

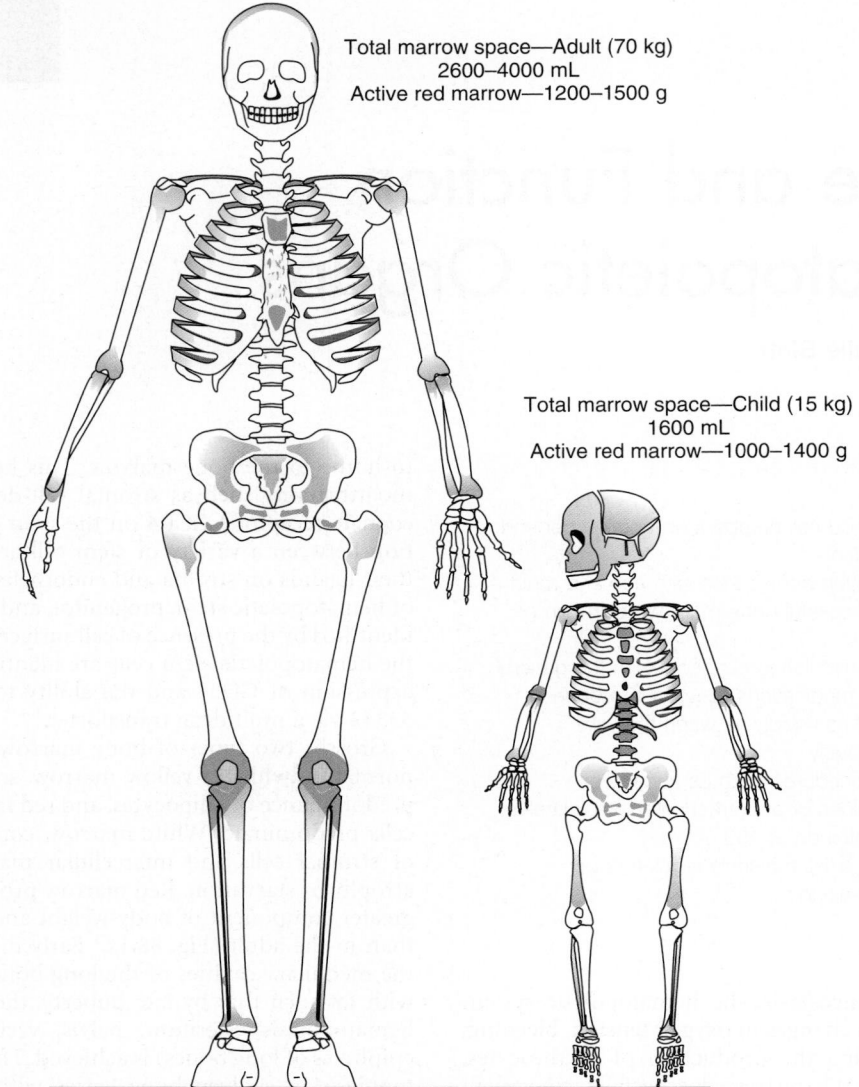

Total marrow space—Adult (70 kg)
2600–4000 mL
Active red marrow—1200–1500 g

Total marrow space—Child (15 kg)
1600 mL
Active red marrow—1000–1400 g

Fig. 88.1. Comparison of active red marrow–bearing areas in the child and the adult. Note the almost identical amount of active red marrow in the child and adult despite a fivefold discrepancy in body weight. (Modified from MacFarlane RC, Robb-Smith AHT. Functions of the Blood. Oxford: Blackwell; 1961.)

that penetrate the endosteum and form capillaries in the Haversian and Volkmann canals of the bony cortex.[4] These capillary systems drain into the bone marrow sinuses, which in turn drain into a central sinus or vein. Because the marrow circulation connects with the general circulation in this fashion, fluids and medication injected in bone marrow are absorbed as rapidly as through intravenous routes. Unlike peripheral veins, intramedullary vessels supported by their bony shell do not collapse in shock; therefore intraosseous (either tibial or iliac crest) infusion is appropriate when peripheral intravenous access is not available (see also Chapter 19).[7] It is also noteworthy that the connection between the marrow and general circulation provides the mechanism by which bone marrow may embolize to the lung after osseous trauma or fracture. This has not been demonstrated to be of clinical significance in the case of intraosseous infusion.[8]

The concept of the stem cell has expanded recently,[9,10] and its ex vivo manipulation has raised much interest by a wide group of physicians and scientists studying nonhematologic systems. One essential feature of the stem cell is its plasticity.[11] Provocative studies have shown that stem cells isolated from the bone marrow can be driven to differentiate to muscle, liver, cardiac, or neuronal tissue. In addition, differentiated cells may be isolated from patients and be reprogrammed to become an induced pluripotent stem cell (iPSC) through transient expression of stem cell transcription factors. These approaches raise the possibility that the marrow may be a convenient and ethically less challenging source of stem cells for stem cell engineering and tissue replacement. Although the clinical applications to nonhematologic tissues remain distant, the use of hematopoietic stem cells to replace a diseased marrow is a common practice (ie, stem cell transplantation) (see also Chapter 95). Alternative sources of hematopoietic stem cells have been found in peripheral blood following growth factor–induced mobilization or from placental cord blood.

Hematopoiesis

Bone marrow cells include the RBCs, granulocytes (neutrophils, eosinophils, basophils), monocytes and macrophages, platelets, lymphocytes, and their precursors. Hematopoietic stem and progenitor cells look like small lymphocytes and are not usually distinguishable from them by microscopy. Their existence, which constitutes less than 1% of the marrow population, was best confirmed by in vitro culture assays in which nucleated cells from bone marrow aspirate specimens plated onto tissue culture dishes layered with methylcellulose generate colonies (aggregates of cells) of one or more lineages. Now, immunophenotyping provides rapid identification of cell lineage and stage of development.[12] The first morphologically identifiable precursor cells are the proerythroblast, myeloblast, monoblast, megakaryoblast, and lymphoblast. These committed precursors and their terminally differentiated counterparts sit within the hematopoietic islands. Megakaryocytes (which make up <1% of hematopoietic cells) generally are located next to marrow sinusoids and shed platelets (fragments of megakaryocyte cytoplasm) directly into the lumen. Erythroblasts also are produced near the walls of the vascular sinuses in clusters with macrophages called erythroblast islets. As the erythroblasts develop, they extrude their nuclei, which are phagocytosed by the macrophages. During severe stress-induced erythropoiesis (eg, hypoxia and severe hemolytic anemia) or when the marrow space is disrupted by tumor cell infiltration, circulating nucleated RBCs may be observed. In contrast, granulocytes (the most numerous cell found in the bone marrow), monocytes, and lymphocytes are produced throughout the marrow away from vascular sinuses. The mature white blood cells (WBCs) are motile and migrate to the sinuses.

Within the peripheral circulation, the number of cells of each type is maintained in a narrow range in the normal individual. Adults and postpubertal adolescents have approximately 5000 granulocytes, 2000 lymphocytes, 500 monocytes, 5×10^6 RBCs, and 150,000 to 300,000 platelets per microliter of whole blood. Age-dependent values for younger children are shown in Table 88.1.[13] To a lesser extent, values are also a function of race and sex, so that African Americans (especially males) normally may have granulocyte counts less than 1500/µL. Normative values for Latinos are less clear but have been reported to be closer to those of Caucasians.[14] Under normal conditions the rate of production of each cell type equals the rate of destruction. Because the life span of mature RBCs in adults is 100 to 120 days, 5×10^4 RBCs/µL are produced daily. The average platelet life span is 7 to 10 days so that approximately 2×10^4 platelets/µL are produced daily. Granulocytes production occurs at a rate of 10^4 cells/µL/day, but their life span remains unsettled with estimates from hours to up to 5.4 days. The very slow rate of production of lymphocytes reflects their long life span, measured in years.

The mechanisms that regulate this steady state are incompletely understood. However, evidence strongly suggests the existence of a pluripotent stem cell that is capable of self-renewal, from which progenitor cells committed to hematopoiesis (RBCs, granulocytes, megakaryocytes, and monocytes) and to lymphopoiesis develop (Fig. 88.2).[13] The "trilineage myeloid" stem cell has been designated *colony forming unit-stem* (CFU-S) on the basis of bone marrow culture assays and experiments in which the spleens of lethally irradiated mice infused with donor marrow cells are found to contain colonies each consisting of precursors of RBCs, granulocytes, monocytes, and megakaryocytes.[15] The existence of CFU-S in humans is supported by chromosomal studies in

TABLE 88.1	Normal Values for Hematology								
Age	Hemoglobin (g %)	Hematocrit (%)	Mean Corpuscular Volume (fl)	MCHC (g/%RBC)	Reticulocytes (%)	WBC/µL × 100 Range (avg)	% Neutrophils	Platelet (10³/µL)
28-week gestation	14.5	45	120	31	5-10	—	—	275 ± 60
32-week gestation	15.0	47	118	32	3-10	—	—	290 ± 70
1 day*	16.8-21.2	57-68	110-128	29.7-33.5	1.8-4.6	7-35 (18)	45-85	310 ± 68
1 week*	15.0-19.6	46-62	107-129	30.4-33.6	0.1-0.9	4-20 (10)	30-50	
1 month*	11.1-14.3	31-41	93-109	33.3-36.5	0.1-1.7	6-18 (10)	30-50	
3-5 months	10.4-12.2	33	80-96	31.8-36.2	0.4-1.0	6-17 (10)	30-50	300 ± 50
6-11 months	11.8	35	77	33	0.7-2.3	6-16 (10)	30-50	
1 year	11.2	35	78	32	0.6-1.7	6-15 (10)	30-50	
2-10 years	12.8	37	80	34	0.5-1.0	7-13 (9)	35-60	
11-15 years	13.4	39	82	34	0.5-1.0	5-12 (8.5)	40-60	
Adult								300 ± 50
Male	16.0 ± 2.0	47 ± 7	91	34	0.8-2.5	4.3-10 (7)	25-62	
Female	14.0 ± 2.0	42 ± 5	(82-101)	(31.5-36)	0.8-4.1			

Absolute eosinophil count: average 250/µL (100-600/µL).
*Under 1 month of age, capillary hemoglobin exceeds venous hemoglobin: 1 hour, 3.6 g difference; 5 days, 2.2 g difference; 3 weeks, 1.1 g difference.
MCHC, mean corpuscular hemoglobin count.
Data from Guest GM, Brown EW. Erythrocytes and hemoglobin of the blood in infancy and childhood. III. Factors in variability, statistical studies. Am J Dis Child. 1957;93:486; Matoth Y, et al. Postnatal changes in some red cell parameters. Acta Paediatr Scand. 1971;60:317; Wintrobe MN. Clinical Hematology. ed 7. Philadelphia: Lea & Febiger; 1974; Mauer AM. Pediatric Hematology. New York: McGraw-Hill; 1961; Oski FA, Naiman JL. Hematologic Problems in the Newborn Infant. Philadelphia: WB Saunders; 1972; and Nathan D, Oski F. Hematology of Infancy and Childhood. Philadelphia: WB Saunders; 1981.

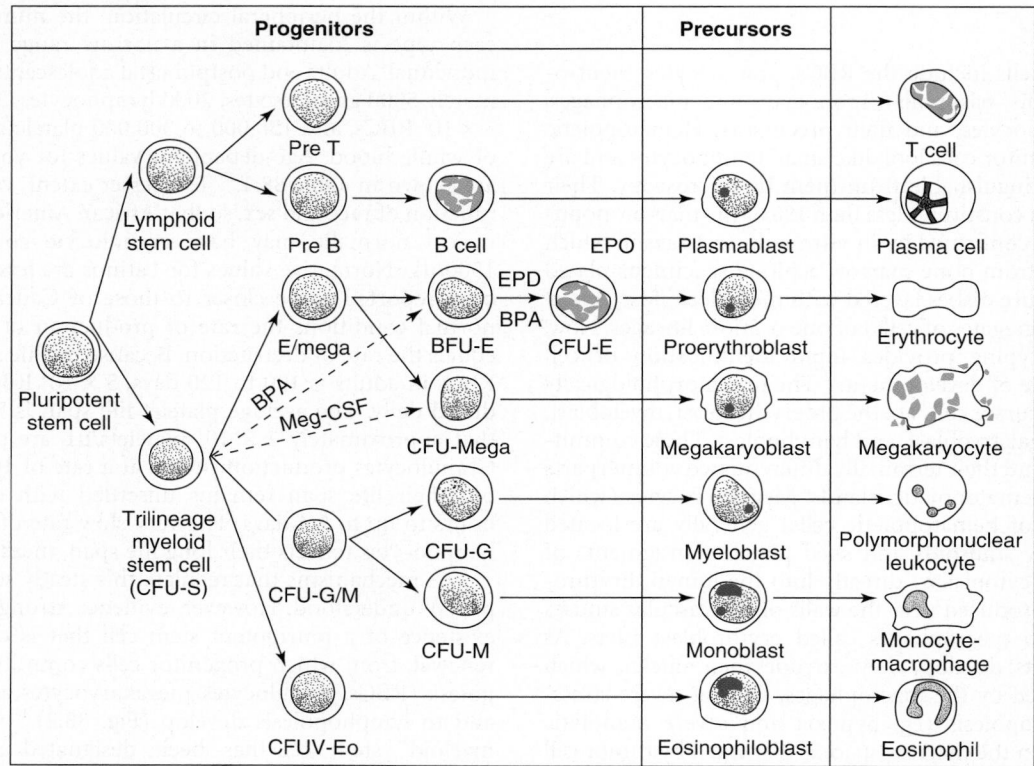

Fig. 88.2. Schematic outline of the progenitor basis of hematopoiesis. Not shown in this outline is the process of self-renewal of fractions of the progenitor cell populations, particularly the immature progenitors. Also not shown is the progressive amplification of progenitors and precursors as they mature and differentiate. The bipotential erythroid-megakaryocyte progenitor shown in this drawing has been demonstrated in the mouse but not definitively in humans. *Dotted arrows* indicate an alternative scheme. (Modified from Nathan DG. Introduction: hematologic diseases. In: Wyngaarden JB, Smith JH, eds. Cecil's Textbook of Medicine. Philadelphia: WB Saunders; 1988.)

myeloproliferative disorders. Lymphoid development appears to arise from a separate progenitor. Although the CFU-S is found predominantly in the bone marrow, there probably are small numbers of circulating pluripotent stem cells because it has long been known that marrow of lethally irradiated animals can be reconstituted with unmanipulated peripheral blood.[16]

The number of committed progenitor cells that differentiate in any time period is dependent on feedback from humoral regulators that are produced within the marrow microenvironment and by extramedullary sources, including T cells, macrophages, endothelial cells, and fibroblasts. These hematopoietic growth factors are cytokines. Many of the cytokines have overlapping functions. However, gene targeting in the mouse ("knockout mouse") of cytokines or their cognate receptors has identified the essential nonredundant functions for several hematopoietic growth factors. Mice deficient in erythropoietin (Epo), thrombopoietin (Tpo), and granulocyte colony-stimulating factor (G-CSF) suffer from severe anemia, thrombocytopenia, or neutropenia, respectively.

The list of cytokines and small molecules that regulate hematopoiesis and their clinical application continue to grow. Chemical modification of Epo and G-CSF has resulted in two longer-acting forms, darbepoetin alpha and pegfilgrastim, respectively. Their primary advantage is longer half-lives. In lieu of thrombopoietin, two platelet-stimulating agents, romiplostim and eltrombopag, have been approved by the Food and Drug Administration (FDA) for use in adults with

TABLE 88.2   Recombinant Hematopoietic Growth Factors

CSF	Target	Clinically Available
SCF	HSC, mast cells	No
IL-3	HSC	No
Epo	Erythroid progenitors	Yes
G-CSF	Granulocytes and their precursors	Yes
GM-CSF	Phagocytes and their precursors, dendritic cells	Yes
M-CSF	Monocytes and their precursors	No
Tpo*	Megakaryocytes	Yes*
IL-11	Megakaryocytes	Yes

*Thrombopoietin receptor agonists, romiplostim and eltrombopag, are approved.
Epo, erythropoietin; G-CSF, granulocyte colony-stimulating factor; GM-CSF, granulocyte-macrophage colony-stimulating factor; HSC, hematopoietic stem cells; IL, interleukin; M-CSF, macrophage colony-stimulating factor; SCF, stem cell factor; Tpo, thrombopoietin.

chronic immune thrombocytopenic purpura (ITP). Eltrombopag has also been approved for treatment of severe aplastic anemia in adults. Both drugs have been used in phase II clinical trials in pediatrics.[17] Characteristics of specific hematopoietic growth factors, discussed in the following sections, are summarized in Table 88.2.

Erythropoiesis

On its way toward RBC maturation (see Fig. 88.2), the CFU-S sequentially differentiates into burst-forming units-erythroid (BFU-E) and colony forming units-erythroid (CFU-E), which are identifiable experimentally on the basis of growth characteristics in culture. These phases of development, which involve amplification of cell number, are extensively reviewed elsewhere.[18] As noted earlier, the proerythroblast is the earliest morphologically identifiable precursor and presumably is the successor to the CFU-E. The subsequent sequence of RBC production normally takes 3 to 4 days in the marrow and involves multiple cell divisions with increasing differentiation, characterized chiefly by globin messenger RNA, cytoplasmic synthesis of hemoglobin, and ultimately extrusion of the RBC nucleus. The enucleated cell is large and, because it contains residual RNA, stains deeply by the Wright-Giemsa technique (ie, polychromatophilic macrocyte). Normally at this stage the erythrocyte is released into the circulation where it can be demonstrated as a reticulocyte. In newborns younger than 1 week of age, reticulocytes in the blood can comprise more than 5% of the total RBCs. At any older age, the normal reticulocyte count is less than 2%. From this uncorrected reticulocyte count, the absolute reticulocyte count can be calculated by multiplying by the RBC count. The normal absolute reticulocyte count would be 0.02 to 5×10^6 RBC/μL. Alternatively, a corrected reticulocyte count is used, as determined by multiplying the reticulocyte percentage by the observed hematocrit divided by the normal hematocrit. If the corrected reticulocyte count is less than 1%, one must suspect bone marrow failure or insufficiency. Because the reticulocytes lose their RNA within 24 to 30 hours, their quantitation provides a rough estimate of the rate of erythropoiesis during the past 24 hours. This can be more accurately measured by ferrokinetic studies, but these are not readily available. The proportion of erythroid precursors in a bone marrow aspirate also provides a more convenient estimate of total erythropoiesis that is valid if a cellular specimen is obtained and if granulopoiesis is normal. In the older child or adult, erythroid precursors normally are one-third as plentiful as myeloid precursors (ie, the myeloid/erythroid ratio is about 3 : 1). Approximately 10% of erythroid precursors do not produce circulating RBCs (ineffective erythropoiesis).

Maturation of RBC precursors is regulated by a number of humoral and nutritional factors. Epo appears to act predominantly by increasing proliferation of CFU-E (see Table 88.2 and Fig. 88.2). Its production is stimulated by hypoxemia or acute hemorrhage. During fetal development, it is mainly produced in the liver, but this site shifts later to the juxtamedullary region in the kidneys. Humoral factors less well characterized than Epo that are derived from multiple sources (spleen cells, peripheral blood monocytes, and mononuclear bone marrow cells) appear to act at an earlier stage of differentiation to amplify the number of progenitors committed to Epo responsiveness. Among these are burst-promoting activity, which enhances production and proliferation of BFU-E. Within the marrow, normal RBC maturation requires both folate and vitamin B_{12}; a deficiency of either results in abnormal nucleic acid synthesis and the production of an abnormal precursor, the megaloblast. Iron is required for hemoglobin synthesis, and deficiency results in poorly hemoglobinized small (hypochromic, microcytic) RBCs.

Once in the peripheral blood, the life span of the normal RBC in the adult or older child is 100 to 120 days. In the term newborn, the RBC life span is about 60 days, which progressively diminishes with increasing prematurity.[15] Presumably these differences in age-dependent RBC longevity reflect differences in membrane stability and oxidative stress. Removal of RBCs from the circulation is not a random process. Senescent RBCs are removed selectively from the circulation by the macrophages of the reticuloendothelial system. Although this is primarily a function of the spleen (see the following section), asplenic patients with normal RBCs accomplish this process in the liver and other sites and do not exhibit an increased RBC life span. In subjects with hemolytic anemias who undergo therapeutic splenectomy, the red cell life span increases, but not to normal levels.

The primary function of the circulating RBC is to carry O_2 from the lungs to the tissues. Hemoglobin (Hb) must be packaged within the RBC membrane to prolong its plasma half-life. Interference with the reversible binding of O_2 by Hb can occur by several mechanisms, including (1) methemoglobinemia, the inability to maintain ionic iron within the Hb molecule in the reduced (ferrous, Fe^{++}) state; (2) the presence of abnormal hemoglobins, among which are the methemoglobins, which have an abnormal affinity for O_2; (3) age- or disease-related differences in the percentage of structurally normal HbF, which has a high affinity for oxygen; and (4) changes in the microenvironment that alter the intracellular concentration of 2,3-diphosphoglycerate (2,3-DPG).[18] The oxyhemoglobin interaction also is complicated by the Bohr effect (at a lower pH, Hb binds O_2 with less affinity) independent of 2,3-DPG concentration. Patients with severe acidosis have low concentrations of 2,3-DPG, which results in an oxygen dissociation curve that shifts to the left. However, the in vivo curve may be normally placed because the Bohr effect counterbalances the reduction in red cell 2,3-DPG. If metabolic acidosis is rapidly corrected, the prompt rise in blood pH is reflected in a proportional increase in oxygen affinity (the Bohr effect). However, there is a lag of several hours before the red cell 2,3-DPG increases to normal. During this time, there is a shift to the left in both the in vivo and the in vitro O_2 dissociation curves. This phenomenon may compromise tissue oxygenation in patients who have diminished cardiovascular reserves.

Premature infants with respiratory failure may have a left-shifted O_2 affinity curve both because of the high levels of HbF and because of an acidosis-induced decrease in 2,3-DPG levels. Exchange transfusions with fresh adult blood have been found to reduce mortality, perhaps by providing blood with "normal" O_2 affinity.[19] Other reasons for impaired O_2 delivery are decreased RBC mass (anemia, which leads to a compensatory increase in 2,3-DPG) and decreased blood flow, either because of vascular anatomic abnormalities or because of increased blood viscosity (eg, in sickle cell disease). In addition to Hb-bound O_2, the oxygen dissolved in plasma (which normally amounts to less than 2% of the total oxygen carried in the blood) increases linearly with increases in PO_2. For this reason, very anemic patients, who have insufficient Hb with which to carry O_2, benefit from administration of O_2. Extensive research into the design of artificial blood has focused both on "red blood" (repackaged Hb from senescent RBCs or of Hb produced with genetic engineering) and "white blood" or perfluorocarbons (emulsions that dissolve large amounts of O_2), but their use is still limited and investigational. For now, RBC transfusions ameliorate anemia acutely, otherwise Epo may be used to elevate Hb over several weeks (see also Chapter 93). Although antibody-mediated Epo-associated pure red cell aplasia is infrequent,[20] familiarity with possible Epo toxicity should accompany its use.

Granulopoiesis

As shown in Fig. 88.2, in addition to BFU-E, CFU-S also gives rise to several other distinct cell populations. The best characterized of these are the CFU-GM (also known as *granulocyte macrophage progenitor cell*, which in turn generates both CFU-G [granulocyte colony-forming units] and CFU-M [monocyte-macrophage colony-forming units]) and the CFU-Eos (eosinophil colony-forming units). As with the CFU-E, these are not morphologically recognizable and probably masquerade in the bone marrow as small lymphocytes. They are identified on the basis of growth characteristics in in vitro bone marrow culture assays.

Subsequent stages of granulocytic (neutrophilic, eosinophilic, and basophilic) and monocytic differentiation can be visualized by routine histochemical stains of bone marrow aspirates.[21] In the neutrophilic polymorphonuclear (PMN) series, the transition from myeloblast to mature PMN involves an overall decrease in cell size; coarsening, indentation, and ultimately separation of nuclear chromatin, with loss of nuclear chromatin, with loss of nucleoli; and replacement of azurophilic granules (whose contents include myeloperoxidase [MPO]), prominent in promyelocytes, by the specific granules (containing a number of secretory factors important for neutrophil function but not MPO) in mature PMNs. Other structural changes during the course of PMN maturation include the disappearance of certain surface antigens, which can be identified by specific monoclonal antibodies, and the appearance of receptor sites for complement (C3) and for the Fc portion of the immunoglobulin molecule. These

stages in development are accompanied by functional changes, including increases in cell motility, responsiveness to chemoattractants, deformability, and phagocytic capabilities.

Parallel morphologic and functional changes occur with eosinophilic granulocyte differentiation. It is noteworthy that the peroxidase in eosinophil granules is different from that in neutrophils or monocytes so that congenital deficiencies of myeloperoxidase in the latter cells leave eosinophil function intact. The blood basophil (which histologically is similar to the tissue mast cell) also is presumed to arise in the bone marrow from the CFU-GM. In contrast to the CFU-Eos, there is no evidence as yet for a separate basophil CFU. DNA labeling studies have demonstrated the kinetics of neutrophil development within the bone marrow. As shown in Fig. 88.3, there is a mitotic pool (myeloblast and myelocyte) that allows for amplification of cell number and a storage or reserve pool (metamyelocyte and PMN) that in older children and adults contains roughly 100 times the number of granulocytes normally found in the peripheral blood.[22] This reserve is mobilized and leads to mature neutrophilia at times of stress (eg, sepsis, exercise, tachycardia, and pregnancy) or on administration of pharmacologic doses of corticosteroids or exposure to endotoxin. In neonates, the storage pool is only two to three times the circulating pool of PMNs and can be depleted, for example, by overwhelming sepsis.[23] Sepsis-related neutropenia may be due to apoptosis of neutrophils and their progenitors as well as a block in their maturation.[24] Thus, sepsis results in both neutropenia and neutrophilia.

Eosinophilic granulocytes also have mitotic and storage pools in the marrow that are about 300 times that seen in the periphery. After less than a week, they are released from the marrow in response to hypoxia and eosinophilic factors (eg, heparin, histamine). In contrast to their effects on neutrophils, corticosteroids and epinephrine block mobilization of eosinophils from the marrow. The effect of epinephrine can be blocked by propranolol, suggesting mediation by β-adrenergic

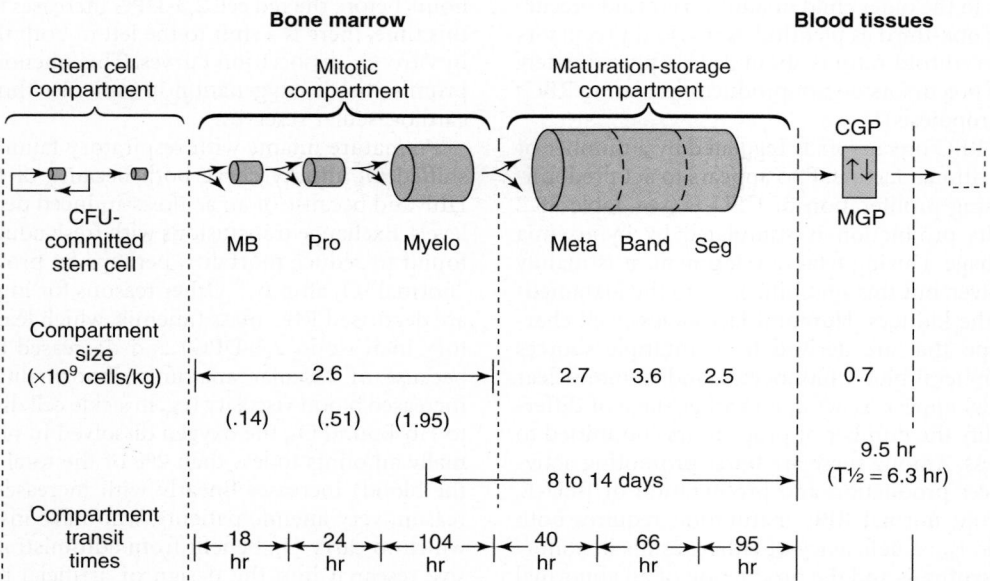

Fig. 88.3. Model of the production and kinetics of neutrophils in humans. The marrow and blood compartments have been drawn to show their relative sizes. The compartment transit times, as derived from DF^{32}P studies, are shown on the next to last line. Values derived from tritiated thymidine studies are shown on the last line. (Modified from Wintrobe MN, et al. Clinical Hematology. ed 8. Philadelphia: Lea & Febiger; 1981.)

receptors. Little is known about basophil development in the bone marrow. Monocyte development, which, as previously suggested, is closely related to myelopoiesis, is also poorly understood. However, there does not appear to be a storage pool.

The mature neutrophil escapes from the marrow into the circulation by migration through reversible gaps between the endothelial cells lining the sinuses and capillaries. Factors known to influence this process include chemoattractants, such as products of the serum complement system. Those factors noted previously that mobilize the storage pool may cause an egress of less mature granulocytes with a resultant "shift to the left" in the peripheral blood. Once in the periphery, approximately half of the polymorphs adhere to the endothelium of blood vessels as the marginating pool while the other half actually circulate. Stress and epinephrine release the marginating cells and therefore double the absolute granulocyte count. Eosinophils have a similar arrangement of circulating and marginating cells, whereas the marginating pool of monocytes is three times that of the circulating pool.

The life span of the neutrophil once in the periphery may be as long as 5.4 days but can be hours in the presence of inflammation, fever, or infection. Neutrophils are irreversibly removed from the circulation into the liver, lungs, bowel, or bladder, back to the bone marrow, or to sites of infection where they contribute to the acute inflammatory response. Their extravascular half-life also is on the order of hours. Although the circulating half-life of eosinophils is comparable with that of neutrophils, eosinophils can persist in the tissues for many days. Under pathologic conditions, eosinophils may cycle back and forth between the tissues and circulation.

Monocytes also have a circulating half-life measured in hours. Once in the tissues, however, they mature into macrophages. Their precise functions depend on the organ of residence; for example, in the liver they are identified as Kupffer cells and in the lung as alveolar macrophages. Macrophages may be "polarized" by cytokines or ligands for the toll-like receptors into two categories: either an antiinflammatory (M1) or a proinflammatory (M2) macrophage.

The CSFs that regulate myelopoiesis are diverse, and their biological specificities may overlap.[25] Cytokines such as interleukin (IL)-1, tumor necrosis factor, granulocyte-macrophage colony-stimulating factor (GM-CSF), and G-CSF expand the PMN precursor compartment and mobilize them by promoting their diapedesis from the marrow and from vascular endothelium. Endotoxin promotes the host inflammatory response by stimulating endothelial cells, macrophages, and fibroblasts to produce cytokines.

Both GM-CSF and G-CSF prime PMNs for enhanced phagocytosis and superoxide production in vitro, modulate cell surface expression of adhesion receptors, inhibit apoptosis, and promote antibody-dependent cellular cytotoxicity. However, GM-CSF inhibits chemotaxis, whereas G-CSF promotes it. G-CSF acts only on the granulocytic lineage. GM-CSF affects macrophages and eosinophils, which accounts for its side effects of eosinophilia and, at high doses, capillary leak syndrome. Because of stickiness and margination along vascular endothelium, a transient drop in O_2 saturation may occur within minutes after administration. GM-CSF can result in transient fever. Bone pain may occur with administration of either drug, if marrow production is high. WBCs must be monitored, and the drug typically is discontinued

TABLE 88.3 Comparison of Granulocyte-Macrophage Colony-Stimulating Factor and Granulocyte Colony-Stimulating Factor

Factor	Additional Uses	Starting Dose
G-CSF	Chemotherapy-induced suppression, severe congenital neutropenia, peripheral stem cell harvest, drug-induced neutropenia	5 µg/kg/d SQ or IV
GM-CSF	Autologous SCT, enhanced antigen presentation, drug-induced neutropenia	250 µg/m²/d SQ or IV

SCT, stem cell transplantation.

when the absolute neutrophil count exceeds 1500 /µL. When it is discontinued, the number of circulating PMNs decreases. Multiple trials have demonstrated the efficacy of growth factors in decreasing the time interval of profound neutropenia or length of antibiotic coverage and hospitalization; however, their use has not changed overall survival. Clinical uses of G-CSF and GM-CSF are summarized in Table 88.3. Although nonhematopoietic tumor cell lines can display receptors for GM-CSF or G-CSF, administration of these drugs has not led to an appreciated increase in relapse or progressive disease. There has been concern that erythroid stimulating agents might stimulate cancer growth.[26] These agents can be given to patients with myeloid leukemias or myelodysplastic syndromes without adverse effects. Based on *adult* studies, the FDA now warns that erythropoiesis stimulating agents may lead to serious cardiovascular and stroke events when Hgb is greater than 11 g/dL and may lead to tumor progression and decreased survival.

As in the case of RBC and platelet development, normal myelopoiesis also requires the presence of vitamin and mineral growth factors. One hallmark of megaloblastic anemia (vitamin B_{12} and folate deficiencies) is the hypersegmented PMN. The hypochromic microcytic anemia of copper deficiency is characteristically associated with neutropenia. Among the nonlymphoid WBCs, clinical sequelae of quantitative or qualitative deficiencies of neutrophils have been particularly well studied. Systemic or mucocutaneous bacterial infections (gram-positive and gram-negative organisms) are frequent. They occur with an incidence that increases with the degree and duration of neutropenia and in the presence of indwelling catheters, intravascular lines, and endotracheal tubes.

Recommendations for prevention of infections in neutropenia include strict handwashing, changing sites of percutaneous lines as often as every 48 hours, and use of recombinant CSFs in limited situations (as noted previously). The use of prophylactic antibiotics and reverse isolation is controversial and will vary among centers and divisions within centers. In addition to clearing bacteria and fungi, monocytes secrete a variety of inflammatory cytokines.

Megakaryocyte and Platelet Production

The CFU-S gives rise to a committed megakaryocyte progenitor, the CFU-Mega (see Fig. 88.2) identifiable in in vitro clonogenic assays and by the presence of platelet glycoprotein surface antigens. Unlike RBC and granulocyte differentiation in which cell division keeps up with mitosis, the next phase of development of megakaryocytes is characterized by endo-reduplication, a process of mitosis without cell division that leads to increased DNA content up to a ploidy of 32N (where 2N is a diploid cell). With increasing ploidy comes increased cell volume, degree of nuclear lobulation, and granules containing factors that influence platelet function. A system of "demarcation membranes" identified by electron microscopy separates the megakaryocyte cytoplasm into several thousand anucleate platelets, which are shed into the lumens of the marrow sinusoids. The entire process takes about 5 days. Although megakaryocytes can be visualized on bone marrow aspirates and biopsy specimens, their quantitation by these techniques is approximate and correlates only loosely with platelet production. Factors controlling platelet shedding have not been studied extensively. With exceptions, however, large platelets or megathrombocytes (increased mean platelet volume) are seen in thrombocytopenia caused by increased platelet destruction. Normal platelet volume occurs more frequently in thrombocytopenia resulting from decreased platelet production.

Some platelets move directly from the marrow to the blood, where they remain; others go temporarily to the spleen, which possibly contributes to their further maturation. Normally one-third of the total body platelet mass is sequestered there, although the number can go as high as 90% in pathologic states. Once in the peripheral blood, platelets have a life span of about 10 days. Chromium studies, useful to assess platelet life span, have severe limitations in estimating the extent of organ-specific uptake of platelets and response to splenectomy.

Thrombopoietin (TPO) is the critical growth factor for the production of platelets.[27] Whereas IL-3, GM-CSF, Epo, IL-11, and IL-6 stimulate CFU-Mega growth in vitro, none of these factors has proved to be highly effective in increasing platelet counts in clinical trials. Instead, there are two FDA-approved thrombopoietin receptor activators, romiplostim and eltrombopag. TPO potently stimulates the expression of CFU-Mega and megakaryocytes, resulting in an increased platelet mass. Because knockout mice have been created that lack the gene for the thrombopoietin receptor but still produce some platelets, other cytokines must contribute to platelet production. These factors, such as IL-3 and IL-11, most likely synergize with thrombopoietin. Although iron deficiency anemia is often associated with thrombocytosis, increases in Epo may not be the immediate mechanism, and not all disease states associated with elevated Epo levels are characterized by increased platelet number. As with the other cell lines, megakaryopoiesis is also dependent on vitamins; severe megaloblastic anemia may be associated with thrombocytopenia and bizarre platelet and megakaryocyte morphology.

Spontaneous bleeding is unlikely unless there are fewer than 20,000/µL normally functioning platelets. However, for major invasive procedures such as surgery or placement of arterial lines or endotracheal tubes, the platelet count should be maintained at a level more than 50,000/µL or even 100,000/µL. The minimum platelet count for performing a spinal tap is less clear, but most clinicians would ask that the platelet count be at least 30,000/µL. Other indications for platelet transfusions are discussed in Chapter 93. In the rare patient with idiopathic thrombocytopenic purpura and intracranial hemorrhage,

optimum control of bleeding requires cooperation among neurosurgery, general surgery, hematology, and intensive care clinicians and some combination of splenectomy, high-dose gamma globulin, steroid therapy, and platelet transfusions.

Lymphopoiesis

The bone marrow and thymus are the primary lymphoid organs, the site of lymphocyte production. The secondary lymphoid organs, to which the B and T cells migrate, include the spleen, lymph nodes, and gut-associated lymphoid tissue (tonsils, appendix, and Peyer patches of the small intestine).

Spleen

The spleen is enclosed in a thick, fibromuscular capsule. Numerous trabeculae spring from the capsule to divide the interior pulp into lobules, within which is a scaffolding of reticular cells and fibers. Unlike the thymus, the spleen has a hilum through which the splenic artery and its branches enter and then branch further to course along the trabeculae. Collaterals from the gastric artery enter through the splenic capsule so that splenic artery ligation does not result in infarction. The branches of the splenic artery pass into the parenchyma to form central arteries that are surrounded for much of their length by a dense sheath of T lymphocytes and macrophages. Lymphoid follicles, some with germinal centers containing B cells from the bone narrow (as noted previously), are also present in the periarterial lymphatic sheath. Together the B-cell– and T-cell–dependent areas compose the white pulp of the spleen. The rest of the splenic parenchyma is the red pulp. It contains radial branches of the central arteries that carry hemoconcentrated blood (plasma is skimmed off and runs in other arterial branches), well-defined endothelial lined venous sinuses that ultimately drain into the splenic vein, and an anatomically separate reticulin network, the splenic vein, which functions as endothelial-lined blood vessels. Most of the circulation runs from the arterial system into the cords and then into the venous system, probably by squeezing through gaps in the endothelium. After the neonatal period, a marginal zone of the red pulp that abuts the white pulp becomes more prominent. It contains antigen-processing macrophages that are needed for B-cell function. It is believed to be the initial site of interactions between antigen and lymphocytes. Small numbers of efferent lymphatic vessels lie at the proximal end of the central arteries and leave the spleen through the trabeculae.

Normally the spleen is found in the left-upper quadrant of the abdomen. Its weight increases linearly with body weight until puberty, after which it shrinks somewhat. A spleen tip is palpable in 10% of normal children. On the basis of data from splenectomy cases, small accessory spleens occur in almost 20% of individuals. Generally they are located near the hilum of the main spleen, with which they share their vascular supply.

The spleen has many functions. The red pulp filters damaged and old RBCs from the systemic circulation by several mechanisms: (1) The cells are distorted and disrupt as they pass through the small lumens of the arterial capillaries or between the endothelial cells of the sinuses: In particular, cells with HbS undergo increased sickling, and cells with abnormalities of glycolytic metabolism or senescent cells become increasingly fragile in the face of decreased O_2 tension with lactic acidosis and decreased adenosine triphosphate production.

(2) Cells are entrapped in the viscous blood within the fine mesh reticulin. (3) Cells undergo antibody-mediated (especially immunoglobulin G) hemolysis or phagocytosis, as seen in some autoimmune hemolytic anemias. Damaged cells or their debris produced by any of these mechanisms are removed by macrophages of the red pulp or may escape back into the circulation. Rigid inclusions such as Howell-Jolly bodies may be pitted without destroying the parent RBC on passage through the sinus endothelium. Therefore the presence of even small numbers of Howell-Jolly bodies is a subtle indicator of impaired splenic function except in the term and especially in the premature neonate, where they also are seen and thought to be a normal developmental stage.

As mentioned earlier, the spleen also is a temporary reservoir for platelets and to a small extent for WBCs. Thus after splenectomy there is a usually transient thrombocytosis that resolves within 3 to 6 months. In children it does not appear to carry a predisposition to thrombosis even with platelet counts as high as $10^9/\mu L$. In the presence of antiplatelet or anti-WBC antibody (some synthesized by the spleen) and in hypersplenism without antibody, the spleen may also function as a filter and result in thrombopenia and neutropenia, which may be reversible by surgical or pharmacologic (steroids, high-dose gamma globulin) splenectomy (see the "Megakaryocyte and Platelet Production" section).

The spleen, predominantly the white pulp and marginal zone, also plays a number of roles in host defense, elegantly and elaborately discussed elsewhere.[15] In short, splenectomy has been associated with an increased incidence of serious infections with encapsulated bacteria, intraerythrocytic parasites, and possibly leukemia in patients who have splenectomy as part of the management of Hodgkin disease. Most clinicians recommend use of *Haemophilus influenzae* type b, meningococcal, and pneumococcal vaccines 1 to 3 weeks before splenectomy (in previously unimmunized individuals), with boosters against pneumococcal disease every 5 to 10 years, and prophylactic antibiotics for variable times but at least through adolescence. Although it is not a site of hematopoiesis beyond fetal life under normal conditions, in certain disease states the spleen can reactivate its hematopoietic potential. These states include some congenital hemolytic anemias and acquired diseases, such as myeloid metaplasia. All are associated with splenomegaly and usually with hepatomegaly, signifying a more general expansion of hematopoiesis. The liver can fulfill some of these functions so that in functionally or literally asplenic patients RBC life span, for example, is not increased. However, the liver is less effective at other functions, including pitting and host defense.

Lymph Nodes

Like most of the rest of the lymphoreticular system, lymph nodes are surrounded by capsules and have architecturally distinct cortices and medullary zones, functionally distinct B-cell– and T-cell–dependent areas, and macrophages—all compartmentalized by a reticular meshwork. Many of the small lymphocytes, especially the T cells, continually are recycled through the systemic circulation by the thoracic duct. They function primarily as a site of interaction between the immune system and invading antigens. Mediastinal lymph node enlargement as a result of invasion by lymphoid or nonlymphoid tumors or from endogenous antigenic stimulation may compromise the airway and present anesthetic risks.

References

1. Orkin SH, Zon LI. Hematopoiesis: an evolving paradigm for stem cell biology. *Cell.* 2008;132:631-644.
2. Weissman IL, Shizuru JA. The origins of the identification and isolation of hematopoietic stem cells, and their capability to induce donor-specific transplantation tolerance and treat autoimmune diseases. *Blood.* 2008;112:3543-3553.
3. Gurevitch O, Slavin S, Feldman AG. Conversion of red bone marrow into yellow: cause and mechanisms. *Med Hypotheses.* 2007;69:531-536.
4. Weiss L. The hematopoietic microenvironment of the bone marrow: an ultrastructural study of the stroma in rats. *Anat Rec.* 1976;186:161-184.
5. Adams GB, Scadden DT. The hematopoietic stem cell in its place. *Nat Immunol.* 2006;7:333-337.
6. Lo Celso C, Fleming HE, Wu JW, et al. Live-animal tracking of individual haematopoietic stem/progenitor cells in their niche. *Nature.* 2009;457:92-96.
7. Fiorito BA, Mirza F, Doran TM, et al. Intraosseous access in the setting of pediatric critical care transport. *Pediatr Crit Care Med.* 2005;6:50-53.
8. Orlowski JP, Julius CJ, Petras RE, et al. The safety of intraosseous infusions: risks of fat and bone marrow emboli to the lungs. *Ann Emerg Med.* 1989;18:1062-1067.
9. Dick JE. Stem cell concepts renew cancer research. *Blood.* 2008;112:4793-4807.
10. Lane SW, Scadden DT, Gilliland DG. The leukemic stem cell niche: current concepts and therapeutic opportunities. *Blood.* 2009;114:1150-1157.
11. Goodell MA. Stem-cell "plasticity": befuddled by the muddle. *Curr Opin Hematol.* 2003;10:208-213.
12. Gratama JW, Sutherland DR, Keeney M. Flow cytometric enumeration and immunophenotyping of hematopoietic stem and progenitor cells. *Semin Hematol.* 2001;38:139-147.
13. Robertson J, Shilkofski MN, eds. *Harriet Lane Handbook.* Philadelphia: Elsevier; 2005.
14. Iosub S, Naik M, Bhalani K, Gromisch DS. Leukocyte and neutrophil counts in healthy Puerto Rican children and children with acute appendicitis. *Clin Pediatr (Phila).* 1986;25:366-368.
15. Sieff CA, Zon LI. Anatomy and physiology of hematopoiesis. In: Orkin S, Fisher D, Look AT, et al., eds. *Nathan and Oski's Hematology of Infancy and Childhood.* 7th ed. Philadelphia: Saunders Elsevier; 2009.
16. Barnes DW, Loutit JF. Haemopoietic stem cells in the peripheral blood. *Lancet.* 1967;25:1138-1141.
17. Ramaswamy K, Hsieh L, Leven E, et al. Thrombopoietic agents for the treatment of persistent and chronic immune thrombocytopenia in children. *J Pediatr.* 2014;165:600-605.
18. Steinberg MH, Benz EJ, Adewoye HA, et al. Pathobiology of the human erythrocyte and its hemoglobins. In: Hoffman R, Benz EJ, Shattil SJ, eds. *Hematology, Basic Principles and Practice.* 4th ed. Philadelphia: Elsevier; 2005.
19. Delivoria-Papadopoulos M, Miller LD, Forster RE 2nd, Oski FA. The role of exchange transfusion in the management of low-birth-weight infants with and without severe respiratory distress syndrome. I. Initial observations. *J Pediatr.* 1976;89:273-278.
20. McKoy JM, Stonecash RE, Cournoyer D, et al. Epoetin-associated pure red cell aplasia: past, present, and future considerations. *Transfusion.* 2008;48:1754-1762.
21. Dinauer MC, Newburger PE. The phagocyte system and disorders of granulopoiesis and granulocyte function. In: Orkin S, Fisher D, Look AT, et al., eds. *Nathan and Oski's Hematology of Infancy and Childhood.* 7th ed. Philadelphia: Saunders Elsevier; 2009.
22. Wintrobe MN, Lee RG, Boggs DR, et al. *Clinical Hematology.* 8th ed. Philadelphia: Lea & Febiger; 1981.
23. Christensen RD, Rothstein G. Exhaustion of mature marrow neutrophils in neonates with sepsis. *J Pediatr.* 1980;96:316-318.
24. Rodriguez S, Chora A, Goumnerov B, et al. Dysfunctional expansion of hematopoietic stem cells and block of myeloid differentiation in lethal sepsis. *Blood.* 2009;114:4064-4076.
25. Vose JM, Armitage JO. Clinical applications of hematopoietic growth factors. *J Clin Oncol.* 1995;13:1023-1035.
26. Rizzo JD, Somerfield MR, Hagerty KL, et al. Use of epoetin and darbepoetin in patients with cancer: 2007 American Society of Clinical Oncology/American Society of Hematology clinical practice guideline update. *J Clin Oncol.* 2008;26:132-149.
27. Kaushansky K. Thrombopoietin. *N Engl J Med.* 1998;339:746-754.

Erythron in Critical Illness

Ahmed Said, Stephen Rogers, and Allan Doctor

PEARLS

- Together, all red blood cells (RBCs) at each stage of development may be considered an organ (termed the *erythron*) now appreciated to participate in active regulation of regional blood flow distribution as well as O_2 and CO_2 transport.
- RBCs are subject to intense biochemical, biomechanical, and physiologic stress during repeated circulatory transit; as such, they possess unique properties and robust energetic and antioxidant systems to maintain functionality for a 3- to 4-month lifetime.
- RBCs actively regulate blood flow and distribution to maintain coupling between O_2 delivery and demand. The trapping, processing, and delivery of nitric oxide by RBCs have emerged as a conserved mechanism through which regional blood flow is linked to biochemical cues of perfusion sufficiency.
- A new paradigm for O_2 delivery homeostasis has emerged, based on coordinated gas transport and vascular signaling by RBCs. By coordinating vascular signaling in a fashion that links O_2 and nitric oxide flux, RBCs couple vessel caliber (and thus blood flow) to O_2 need in tissue. Malfunction of this signaling system is implicated in a wide array of pathophysiologies and may be, in part, explanatory for the dysoxia frequently encountered in the critical care setting.

Introduction

The erythron includes red blood cells (RBCs) at all stages of development, from progenitors to senescent forms, and is the organ (composed of anucleated cells in suspension) responsible for oxygen (O_2) transport from lungs to tissue.[1] This role is newly appreciated to include active vasoregulation (by RBCs) that links regional blood flow to O_2 availability in the lung and to consumption in the periphery.[2] Considerable energy is devoted to maintaining a robust RBC population (20 trillion to 30 trillion cells circulate in the average adult, and approximately 25% of the cells in the body are RBCs); 1.4 million RBCs are released into the circulation per second, replacing ~1% of the circulating mass per day. Mature RBCs have a life span of ~4 months, the majority of which is spent traversing the microcirculation. It is estimated that an RBC travels approximately 400 km during this interval, having made 170,000 circuits through the vascular tree. Circulating RBCs demonstrate unique physiology and are adapted to withstand significant biomechanical and biochemical stress.

As RBCs age, energy and antioxidant systems fail; key proteins (including hemoglobin [Hb] and lipids) suffer oxidative injury, negatively impacting performance (rheology, adhesion, gas transport, vascular signaling). Such cells acquire marks of senescence and are cleared by the spleen or by undergoing eryptosis (a process unique to RBCs, similar to apoptosis). Of importance, this process may be accelerated in the course of critical illness and thereby, by limiting O_2 delivery, influence organ failure progression and outcome.

Moreover, it is essential to note that in the setting of insufficient O_2 delivery, blood flow (rather than content) is the focus of O_2 delivery regulation: O_2 content is relatively fixed, whereas flow can be increased by several orders of magnitude. Thus, blood flow volume and distribution are actively regulated to maintain coupling between O_2 delivery and demand. The trapping, processing, and delivery of nitric oxide (NO) by RBCs have emerged as a conserved mechanism through which regional blood flow is linked to biochemical cues of perfusion sufficiency. This chapter reviews conventional RBC physiology influencing O_2 delivery (O_2 affinity and rheology) and introduces a new paradigm for O_2 delivery homeostasis based on coordinated gas transport and vascular signaling by RBCs. By coordinating vascular signaling in a fashion that links O_2 and NO flux, RBCs couple vessel caliber (and thus blood flow) to O_2 need in tissue. Malfunction of this signaling system is implicated in a wide array of pathophysiologies and may in part explain the dysoxia frequently encountered in the critical care setting.

Oxygen Transport

Hemoglobin (Hb) is formed by 2 α and 2 β globin chains, each carrying a heme prosthetic group composed of a porphyrin ring bearing a ferrous atom that can reversibly bind an oxygen (O_2) molecule. In the deoxygenated state, the Hb tetramer is electrostatically held in a tense (T) conformation. Binding of the first O_2 molecule leads to mechanical disruption of these bonds, an increase in free energy, and transition to the relaxed (R) conformation. Each successive O_2 captured by T-state Hb shifts the Hb tetramer closer to the R state, which has an estimated 500-fold increase in O_2 affinity. This concept of thermodynamically coupled "cooperativity" in O_2 binding was first described by Perutz and explains the sigmoidal appearance of the O_2-Hb binding curve, also known as the oxy-hemoglobin dissociation curve (ODC) (Fig. 89.1). Moreover, understanding of allosteric influence of protein function by "heterotropic effectors" was first achieved following description of the variation in Hb~O_2 affinity. For example, for Hb~O_2, which binds to the heme "active" site, is the

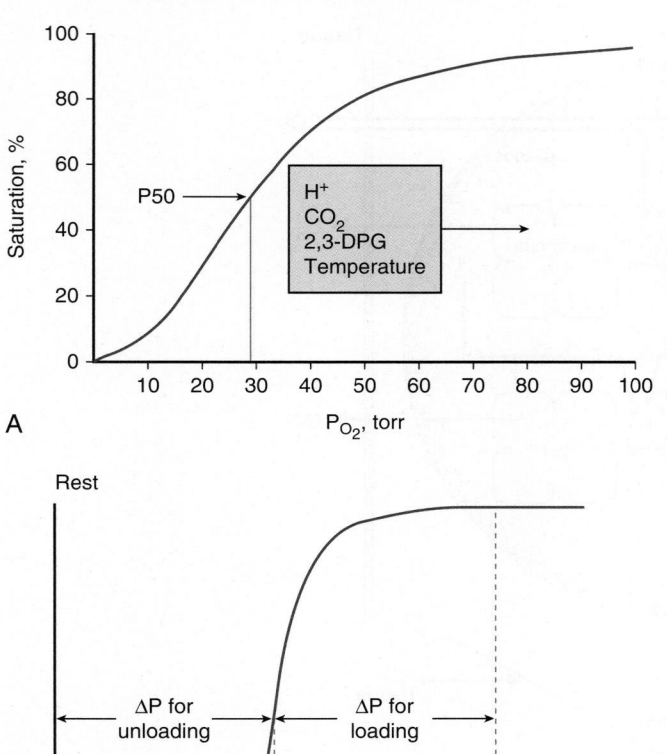

Fig. 89.1. Oxyhemoglobin Dissociation Curve. (A) The normal whole blood oxygen dissociation curve (ODC). P_{50} is the PO_2 at which hemoglobin is half-saturated with O_2. The principal effectors that alter the position and shape of the curve under physiologic conditions are indicated. (B) Changes in P_{50} optimize O_2 loading in the lungs and unloading in tissue. The difference in O_2 tension (ΔP) between the alveolar air and the pulmonary-capillary blood provides the gradient for loading in the lungs. The difference in O_2 tension between the blood leaving the lungs and perfusing tissue provides the gradient for O_2 unloading in the periphery. Optimal O_2 transport is achieved through P_{50} shifts that match the gradients for loading and unloading to the respective diffusing capacities of the lungs and tissues. (A, Adapted from Winslow RM. The role of hemoglobin oxygen affinity in oxygen transport at high altitude. Respir Physiol Neurobiol. 2007;158:121-127; B, Adapted from Hsia CCW. Respiratory function of hemoglobin. N Engl J Med. 1998;338:239-247.)

homotropic ligand, and all other molecules influencing the Hb~O_2 binding relationship are termed *heterotropic effectors*. In addition to the homotropic effects of ligand binding on quaternary conformational changes (eg, cooperativity), primary ligand binding affinity (O_2) is also affected by multiple heterotropic effectors of significant physiologic relevance (also known as allosteric effectors). The major heterotropic effectors that influence Hb O_2 affinity are hydrogen ion (H^+), chloride ion (Cl^-), carbon dioxide (CO_2), and 2,3-diphosphoglycerate (DPG).

P_{50}, the oxygen tension at which 50% of Hb binding sites are saturated, is the standard metric employed to quantify change in Hb~O_2 affinity and is inversely related to the binding affinity of Hb for O_2.[3,4] Elevated levels of H^+, Cl^-, and CO_2 reduce O_2 binding affinity (eg, raise P_{50}). This allosteric shift in O_2 affinity, called the Bohr effect, arises from the interactions among the above heterotropic effectors bound to different sites on hemoglobin, all of which serve to stabilize the low-energy, low-affinity, T-state Hb conformation. This effect is achieved by complex interactions between carbonic anhydrase (CA) and the anion exchange protein 1 (AE1) (also known as the Band 3 [B3] membrane protein) (Fig. 89.2). Specifically, CA generates H^+ and HCO_3^- from CO_2 encountered in the microcirculation; HCO_3^- then exchanges for Cl^- across the RBC membrane through AE1. As a consequence, extra erythrocytic CO_2 is converted into intraerythrocytic HCl by the CA-AE1 complex, thus acidifying RBC cytoplasm and raising P_{50} (lowering affinity, also termed *right shifting* the ODC). Additionally, through the Haldane effect, CO_2 more directly lowers O_2 affinity (by binding to the *N*-terminus of the globin chains to form a carbamino, further stabilizing T-state Hb); carbamino formation also releases another hydrogen ion (further reinforcing the *right shift* in ODC) (see Fig. 89.2). This set of reactions is reversed in the alkaline (and low CO_2) milieu in the pulmonary circulation, leading to increased Hb~O_2 binding affinity (lower P_{50}). In sum, this physiology vastly improves O_2 transport efficiency by enhancing gas capture in the lung and release to tissue, and it does so in proportion to perfusion sufficiency (in the setting of impaired perfusion, acidosis and hypercapnea improve O_2 release). In the setting of impaired O_2 delivery that results in anaerobic glycolysis, lactate diffusion into capillary blood (by lowering pH) further increases O_2 dissociation and facilitates O_2 delivery. Of note, this tightly regulated modulation of O_2 affinity requires coordinated interaction of a complex intraerythrocytic protein network and may fail consequent to acquired RBC injury in the setting of critical illness,[5-8] thereby partially explaining the dysoxia commonly observed in this setting.

Less acute modulation of P_{50} is achieved by DPG, a glycolytic intermediate that binds in an electrically charged pocket between the β chains of hemoglobin, which stabilizes the T conformation, decreasing O_2 affinity and elevating P_{50}. DPG binding also releases protons, lowering intracellular pH and further reinforcing the Bohr effect. DPG in RBCs increases whenever O_2 availability is diminished (as in hypoxia or anemia) or when glycolytic flux is stimulated. Lastly, temperature significantly influences Hb~O_2 affinity. As body temperature increases, affinity lessens (P_{50} increases, ODC shifts right); the reverse happens in hypothermia. This feature is of physiologic importance during heavy exercise, fever, or induced hypothermia. It should be noted that clinical co-oximetry results and blood gas values are reported at 37°C and not at true in vivo temperature and can lead to either under- or overestimation of true HbSO2% values and blood O_2 tension.

Carbon Dioxide Transport

As a lipophilic molecule, carbon dioxide (CO_2) produced from tissue respiration readily diffuses into capillary blood and through the RBC membrane.[9] A minority (5%-10%) of diffused CO_2 binds to the α-amino terminus of Hb globin chains as carbaminohemoglobin, lowering O_2 affinity (raising P_{50}); this P_{50} shift is termed *the Haldane effect*.[9,10] The majority of the CO_2 is hydrated by the two intraerythrocytic carbonic

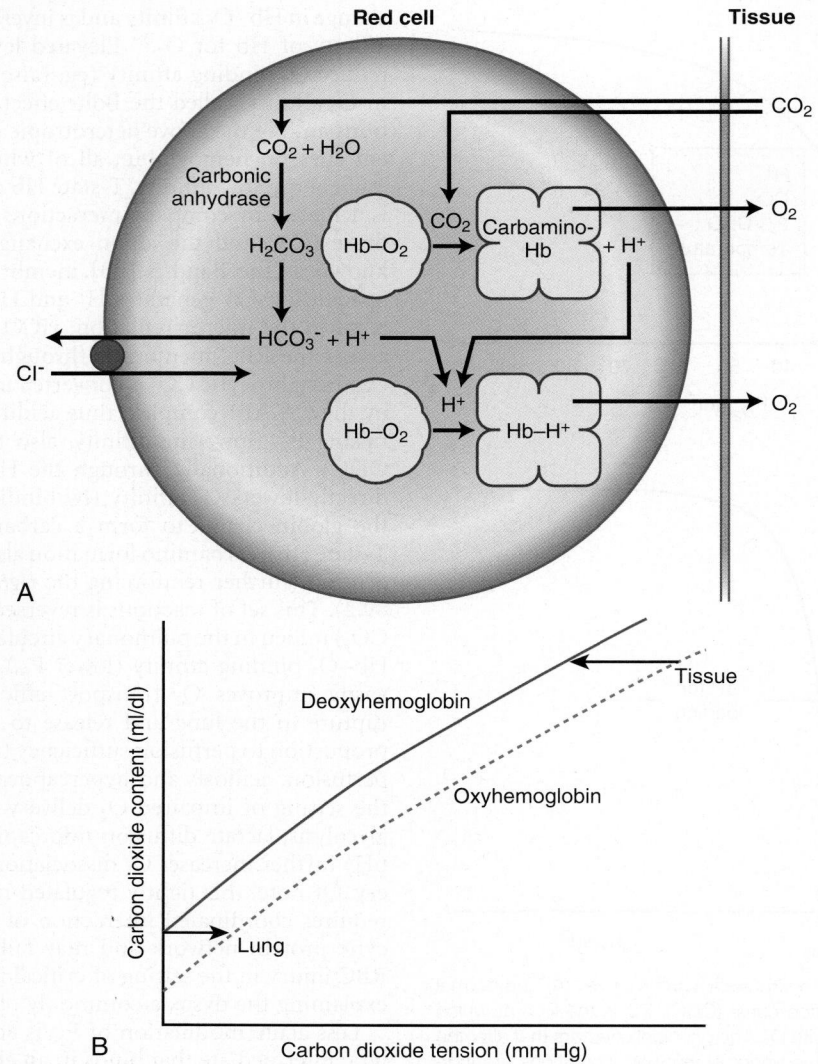

Fig. 89.2. Coupled O$_2$ and CO$_2$ Transport Within RBCs. (A) In the periphery, CO$_2$ uptake by RBCs, processing by the carbonic anhydrase system (Bohr effect), and carbamino-Hb formation (Haldane effect) stabilize T conformation and facilitate O$_2$ release. (B) Binding of O$_2$ to Hb reduces binding affinity for CO$_2$, leading to a rightward shift of the CO$_2$ dissociation curve and facilitating CO$_2$ release in the lung. This interaction reverses upon deoxygenation in the periphery tissues, facilitating CO$_2$ uptake and minimizing the arteriovenous CO$_2$ difference. (Adapted from Hsia CCW. Respiratory function of hemoglobin. N Engl J Med. 1998;338:239-247.)

anhydrase (CA) isoforms, CA I (low turnover rate) and CA II (high turnover rate); this conversion into bicarbonate (and a proton, as discussed earlier) is essential for efficient CO$_2$ transport and for maintaining the venous-arterial difference in total CO$_2$ (see Fig. 89.2). The released protons stabilize the T conformation of hemoglobin and thereby facilitate O$_2$ offloading in proportion to CO$_2$ genesis (and thus, regional tissue respiration). Carbaminohemoglobin also acts to directly stabilize T-state conformation. The process reverses during pulmonary transit (because the lungs act as a CO$_2$ sink), raising intraerythrocytic pH and enhancing O$_2$ affinity in proportion to regional alveolar ventilation (CO$_2$ removal).

Biophysical Factors Influencing Gas Transport

Blood Rheology

Disease-based variation in blood fluidity has been recognized since the early 20th century,[11] and there is substantive evidence that this property strongly influences tissue perfusion.[12] Plasma is a newtonian fluid (viscosity is independent of shear rate); its viscosity is closely related to protein content and in critical illness, physiologically significant changes in viscosity may vary with concentration of acute phase reactants.[13-15] Whole blood, however, is considered a non-newtonian suspension (fluidity cannot be described by a single viscosity value); whole blood fluidity is determined by combined rheologic properties of plasma and the cellular components.

The cellular components of blood, particularly RBCs, influence blood viscosity as a function of both number and deformability. RBC concentration in plasma (hematocrit) has an exponential relationship with viscosity and meaningfully diminishes tissue perfusion when Hct exceeds ~60 to 65. RBC deformability, or behavior under shear stress, also strongly influences blood fluidity. Normal RBCs behave like fluid drops under most conditions, are highly deformable under shear, and orient with flow streamlines. However, during inflammatory stress, RBCs tend to aggregate into linear arrays like a stack of coins (rouleaux); fibrinogen and other acute phase reactants in plasma stabilize such aggregates, significantly increasing blood viscosity. Such a change in viscosity most impacts O_2 delivery during low-flow (eg, low-shear) states (such as in critical illness) in the microcirculation.[16] RBC biomechanics and aggregation impact blood viscosity, strongly influencing the volume and distribution of O_2 delivery (again, more so in the low-shear microcirculation or when vessel tone is abnormal).[17] This hemorheologic physiology is perturbed by oxidative stress (common in critical illness)[18,19] and in sepsis.[20-25] This has been attributed to increased intracellular 2,3-DPG concentration,[26] intracellular free Ca^{2+},[27] and decreased intraerythrocytic ATP with subsequent decreased sialic acid content in RBC membranes.[28] Both increased direct contact between RBCs and WBCs and reactive oxygen species released during sepsis have also been shown to alter RBC membrane properties.[29,30]

Red Blood Cell Aggregation and Adhesion

As noted previously, in the absence of shear, RBCs suspended in autologous plasma stack in large aggregates, known as rouleaux. Acute phase reactants, especially fibrinogen, C-reactive protein, serum amyloid A, haptoglobin, and ceruloplasmin, have been shown to increase RBC aggregation.[31] Pathophysiologic conditions such as sepsis and ischemia-reperfusion injury have been shown to alter RBC surface proteins and increase RBC "aggregability."[19] Activated white blood cells (WBCs) are also thought to cause structural changes in the RBC glycocalyx and increase RBC aggregability.[32]

Under normal conditions, RBC adherence to endothelial cells (ECs) is insignificant, and RBC deformability permits efficient passage through the microcirculation. Again, under normal conditions, enhanced EC adherence plays a role in the removal of senescent RBCs in the spleen. However, during critical illness, RBC~endothelial interactions are altered by RBC injuries associated with sepsis[22,23,33,34] or oxidative stress.[19] This is more prominent with "activated" endothelium, as

frequently occurs in critical illness.[34-36] Such RBC~endothelial aggregates create a physiologically significant increase in apparent blood viscosity.[17] Moreover, RBC adhesion directly damages endothelium[37-40] and augments leukocyte adhesion,[41-44] further impairing apparent viscosity and microcirculatory flow. This phenomenon is commonly appreciated in the pathophysiology of vasoocclusive crises in sickle cell disease patients, malaria, diabetic vasculopathy, polycythemia vera, and central retinal vein thrombosis, but it may be more widespread than originally appreciated.

Red Blood Cell Deformability

Tissue deformation can be defined as the relative displacement of specific points within a cell or structure. Mature RBCs are biconcave disks ranging from 2 to 8 μm in thickness, which act like droplets that deform reversibly under the shear encountered during circulatory transit.[17,45] Unique RBC geometry and deformability arises from (1) cytoplasmic viscosity and (2) specific interactions between the plasma membrane and underlying protein skeleton[28] (Fig. 89.3). Cytoplasmic viscosity is mainly determined by hemoglobin concentration, which varies with intraerythrocytic hydration, which is actively regulated by ATP-dependent cation pumps.[46] The integral transmembrane membrane proteins AE-1 (also known as B3) and glycophorins are reversibly anchored to a submembrane filamentous protein mesh composed of spectrin, actin, and protein 4.1. The linear extensibility of this mesh defines the limits of RBC deformability.[47] Maintenance of membrane-mesh interactions and robust RBC mechanical behavior is dependent on ATP-dependent ion pumps as well as support from NADPH-dependent antioxidant systems.[46] The sole energy source (for both) in RBCs is anaerobic glycolysis, which is discussed in detail later. RBC geometric and mechanical alterations secondary to impaired metabolism (leading to RBC dehydration, elevated intraerythrocytic calcium, and ATP/NADPH depletion) are well-described consequences in blood stored for prolonged periods[48] and in RBCs subjected to significant metabolic stress during critical illness.[49,50]

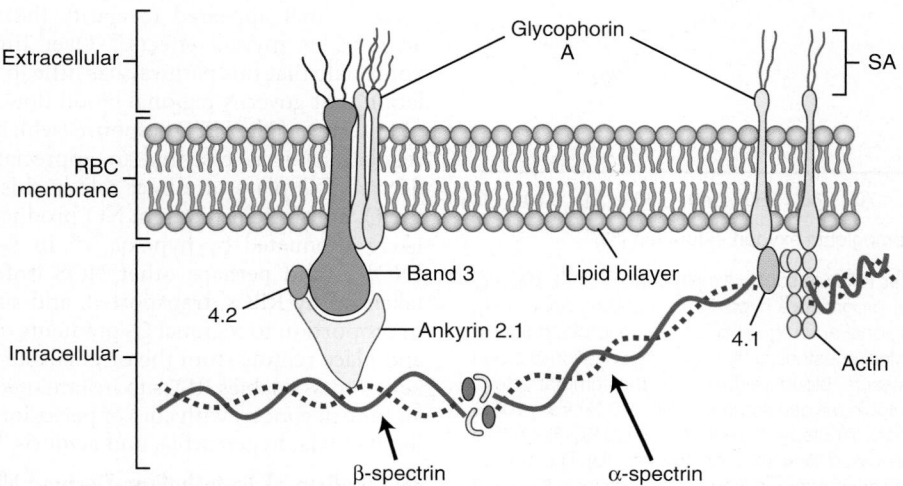

Fig. 89.3. Schematic Representation of RBC Membrane. The membrane is composed of a phospholipid membrane bilayer and transmembrane proteins including glycophorin A and Band 3 proteins. Glycophorin A is the major sialoglycoprotein of the RBC. Sialic acid (SA) bound to glycophorin A is responsible for the negative charge of the RBC membrane. The intracellular compartment (IC) is constituted by spectrin (α and β subunits), actin, protein 4.1, and ankyrin. (Adapted from Piagnerelli M, et al. Red blood cell rheology in sepsis. Intensive Care Med. 2003; 29(7):1052-1061.)

Regulation of Blood Flow Distribution by Red Blood Cells

Microcirculatory blood flow is physiologically regulated to instantaneously match O_2 delivery to metabolic demand. This extraordinarily sensitive programmed response to tissue hypoperfusion is termed *hypoxic vasodilation (HVD)*.[51] This process involves the detection of point-to-point variations in arteriolar O_2 content[52] with the subsequent initiation of signaling mechanism(s) capable of immediate, regionally specific, modulation of vascular tone (Fig. 89.4).

In the 1980s, intracellular RBC Hb was identified as a potential circulating O_2 sensor, following demonstration that in severe hypoxia, O_2 content was more important than partial pressure of O_2 (PO_2) in the maintenance of regional

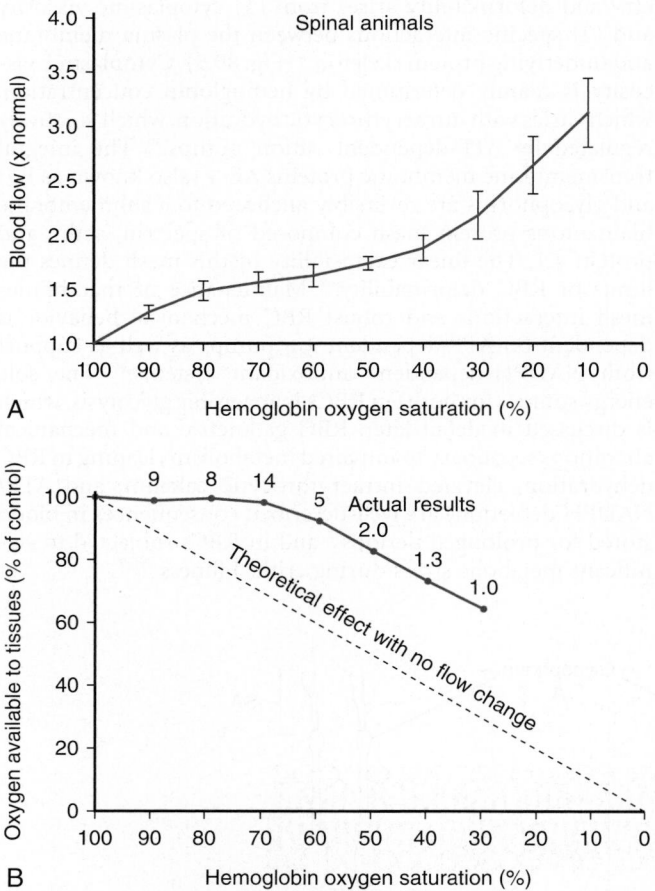

Fig. 89.4. Local vascular reflexes support maintenance of O_2 delivery to tissue in the setting of progressive hypoxia. In a classic paper (51), Guyton demonstrated regional autoregulation of systemic blood flow in normal dogs (following spinal anesthesia) by observing variation in blood flow during constant pressure blood perfusion of the femoral artery, while reducing the hemoglobin oxygen saturation (Hb SO_2%) from 100% to 0% in the perfusing blood. (A) Stepwise reduction in Hb SO_2% caused a progressive increase in blood flow through the leg. (B) These data demonstrate that autoregulation of blood flow occurs at a local level and this regulation serves to improve oxygen supply when blood oxygen content falls. In addition, effects on blood flow were replicated by injecting partially deoxygenated versus oxygenated red blood cells into the artery, demonstrating that effects could be elicited during arteriovenous transit (<1 s).

O_2 supply.[53] It was later demonstrated in vivo that Hb O_2 saturation (HbSO$_2$) directly correlated with blood flow in a fashion independent of plasma or tissue PO_2.[54] These findings implicated a role for RBCs in the regulation of O_2 supply, given the following evidence: (1) the Hb molecule within the RBC is the only component in the O_2 transport pathway directly influenced by O_2 content, and (2) the level of O_2 content of the RBC at a particular point in the circulation is linked to the level of O_2 utilization.[55]

With the vascular O_2 sensor identified, the mechanism involved in mediating the vasoactive response has remained in debate. To date, three HbSO$_2$-dependent RBC-derived signaling mechanisms have been proposed, the first two linked to the vasoactive effector NO and the third to RBC adenosine triphosphate (ATP): (1) formation and export of S-nitrosothiols, "catalyzed" by Hb (SNOHb hypothesis)[56-58]; (2) reduction of nitrite (NO_2^-) to NO by deoxygenated Hb (nitrite hypothesis)[59]; and (3) hypoxia responsive release of ATP (ATP hypothesis).[55,60] Each of these hypotheses will be addressed further.

Role of Red Blood Cell–Nitric Oxide Interactions in Vasoregulation

Interest in the free radical NO began with its identification as endothelium-derived relaxing factor (EDRF), first reported in 1980,[61] which resolved the apparent paradox as to why acetylcholine, an agent known to be a vasodilator in vivo, often caused vasoconstriction in vitro. Experiments performed with dissected segments of rabbit thoracic aorta mounted on a force transducer demonstrated that handling of the tissue in a fashion that preserved endothelium always resulted in acetylcholine having relaxant properties. However, removal of the endothelium eradicated this action.[61,62] Identification of EDRF consequently led to a race to discover its chemical identity. It was not until 7 years later that two groups simultaneously published definitive studies characterizing and identifying EDRF as NO.[63,64] However, the means by which NO exerted its physiologic effects remained unknown, and effort focused upon identifying the "NO receptor(s)." This effort characterized the "classical" signaling pathway for NO via soluble guanylate cyclase (sGC) and cyclic guanosine 3′,5′-monophosphate (cGMP) that appeared to clarify the means by which NO achieves its myriad effects.[65] Over time, however, we now appreciate that this pathway has little to do with the vasoregulation that governs regional blood flow distribution.

In terms of the HVD response (which underlies blood flow regulation) it is essential to appreciate that endothelium-derived NO plays no direct role in this reflex.[54,66] Because of the O_2 substrate limitation, NO production by eNOS is most likely attenuated by hypoxia.[67,68] In fact, NO derived from eNOS[56] (and perhaps other NOS isoforms[69] or nitrite[70]) is taken up by RBCs, transported, and subsequently dispensed in proportion to regional O_2 gradients to effect HVD at a time and place remote from the original site of NO synthesis. This key process enables RBCs to instantaneously modulate vascular tone in concert with cues of perfusion insufficiency, including hypoxia, hypercarbia, and acidosis.[56,57]

Metabolism of Endothelium-Derived Nitric Oxide by Red Blood Cells: Historical View

In the original NO paradigm, NO derived from endothelial nitric oxide synthase (eNOS) was felt to play a purely paracrine role in the circulation, acting within the vicinity of its release.[71] Its metabolic fate was explained by the diffusion of the "gas" in solution and its terminal reactions (1) in vascular smooth muscle cells with the ferrous heme iron (Fe^{2+}) of soluble guanylate cyclase (sGC)[72] and (2) in the vessel lumen, with the heme group (Fe^{2+}) of oxyHb (the resultant oxidation reaction forming MetHb and nitrate), or deoxyHb (the resultant addition reaction forming iron nitrosyl Hb; HbNO), or in plasma with dissolved O_2 (the resultant autoxidation reaction),[73] or O_2-derived free radicals including superoxide (O_2^-), hydrogen peroxide (H_2O_2), or hydroxyl radicals (OH^-). Several "barriers" were presumed to retard NO diffusing into the blood vessel lumen to react avidly with the abundance of Hb, including the RBC membrane, the submembrane protein matrix, and an unstirred layer around the RBC,[74,75] in addition to laminar blood flow.[76] These barriers were thought to limit these luminal reactions, thus allowing the local concentration of NO adjacent to endothelial cells to increase sufficiently to provide a diffusional gradient for NO to activate the underlying vascular smooth muscle sGC. Reactions of NO in the bloodstream were assumed only to scavenge/inactivate NO via the formation of metabolites unable to activate sGC.[72]

Metabolism of Endothelium-Derived Nitric Oxide by Red Blood Cells: Modern View

A much broader biological chemistry of endothelial NO (than in the above paradigm) has been elucidated.[77-79] Most notable is the covalent binding of NO^+ to cysteine thiols, forming S-nitrosothiols (SNOs). This paradigm developed following the discovery that endogenously produced NO circulated in human plasma primarily complexed to the protein albumin (S-nitrosoalbumin[80]), which transformed the understanding of bloodborne NO signaling. SNO proteins thus offered a means to conserve NO bioactivity, allowing the storage, transport, and potential release of NO remote from its location of synthesis.[81] The SNO hypothesis was extended to include a reactive thiol of Hb (Cysß93) that was demonstrated to undergo S-nitrosylation and sustain bioactivity under oxygenated conditions and NO release under low O_2 conditions (see HbSNO hypothesis).[56,57]

In this SNO paradigm, the NO radical must be oxidized to an NO^+ (nitrosonium) equivalent, which can then be passed between thiols in peptides and proteins, thereby preserving NO bioactivity.[77,78] S-nitrosylation then is akin to protein phosphorylation in terms of regulating protein function. SNO biochemistry offers NO a far broader signaling repertoire and has enabled awareness that the heme in sGC is not the sole, or even the principal, target of NO generated by endothelium. A wide array of alternative sGC (cyclic guanosine monophosphate)-independent reactions following endothelial NOS (eNOS) activation have been identified.[79,82]

Processing and Export of S-Nitrosothiols by Red Blood Cells

Hb S-nitrosylation (HbSNO), which has been characterized by both mass spectrometry[83] and x-ray crystallography,[84] provides an explanation as to how NO circumvents terminal reactions with Hb, enabling RBCs to conserve NO bioactivity and transport it throughout the circulation[56,57] (Fig. 89.5). The formation and export of NO groups by Hb is governed by the transition in Hb conformation that occurs in the course of O_2 loading/unloading during arteriovenous (A-V) transit. This is due to conformational dependent change in reactivity of the Cysß93 residue toward NO, which is higher in the R (oxygenated) Hb state and lower in the T (deoxygenated) Hb state.[56,57]

In a tightly regulated fashion, Hb captures and binds NO at its β-hemes and then passes the NO group from the heme to a thiol (Cys-β93-SNO).[70,85] Transfer of NO between heme and thiol requires heme-redox coupled activation of the NO group, which is controlled by O_2 capture-induced conformational transition across the lung.[86] Once in R state, the Cys-β93-SNO is protected through confinement to a hydrophobic pocket.[84] NO group export from Cys-β93-SNO occurs when steep O_2 gradients are encountered in the periphery (HVD). The R- to T-state conformational transition that occurs upon Cys-β93-SNO deoxygenation (or oxidation) results in a shift in the location of the β chain from its hydrophobic niche toward the aqueous cytoplasmic solvent.[84] This allows the Cys-β93-SNO to be "chemically available" for transfer to target thiol-containing proteins, including those associated with the RBC membrane protein AE-1 (Band 3)[87] and extraerythrocytic thiols.[88,89] Resultant plasma or other cellular SNOs then become vasoactive at low nM concentrations.[56,57] Importantly, all NO transfers in this process involve NO^+,[56,58] which protects bioactivity from Fe^{2+} heme recapture or inactivation. S-nitrosothiols are the only known endogenous NO compounds that retain bioactivity in the presence of Hb.[56,89,90]

Extensive evidence supports SNO-Hb biology, whereby RBCs exert graded vasodilator and vasoconstrictor responses across the physiologic microcirculatory O_2 gradient. RBCs dilate preconstricted aortic rings at low PO_2 (1% O_2), while constricting at high PO_2 (95% O_2).[57,90-92] The vasodilatory response at low O_2 is enhanced following the addition of NO (or SNO) to RBCs, commensurate with SNO-Hb formation.[56,87,90,93] Additionally, the vasodilatory response is enhanced in the presence of extracellular free thiol,[90] occurs in the absence of endothelium[58,90] (which is consistent with in vivo observation that HVD is endothelium independent[94]), and transpires in the time frame of circulatory transit, as confirmed by measurements of A-V gradients in SNO-Hb.[56,88,91,92] In addition to these ex vivo experiments, numerous groups have also demonstrated bioactivity of inhaled NO, commensurate with SNO-Hb formation.[95-99]

Metabolism of Nitrite by Red Blood Cells

Nitrite (NO_2^-), formed mainly via hydration reactions involving N-oxides, was long viewed as an inactive oxidation product of NO metabolism. More recently it has been proposed as circulating pool of bioactive NO.[100] Some have suggested that the reduction of nitrite by deoxyHb may serve as the RBC-derived signaling mechanism regulating HVD.[101] However, this hypothesis has two major shortcomings in terms of known NO chemistry/biochemistry and HVD physiology. First, to influence vascular tone, the NO radical produced from NO_2^- must escape RBCs at low O_2 tension in order to elicit a vasodilatory response. Experimental evidence, however, unambiguously refutes the possibility of NO escaping RBCs as an authentic radical, especially given the proximity, high concentration, and rapid reaction kinetics ($10^7 M^{-1} s^{-1}$) of authentic NO with deoxyHb. The only plausible reconciliation would be that bioactivity from this reaction may derive from heme captured NO (HbFe^{2+}NO) being further converted into SNO-Hb,[70,85] as HbFe^{2+}NO itself acts as a vasoconstrictor rather than vasodilator.[102] The second shortcoming relates to the fact that the NO_2^- reductase activity of deoxyHb

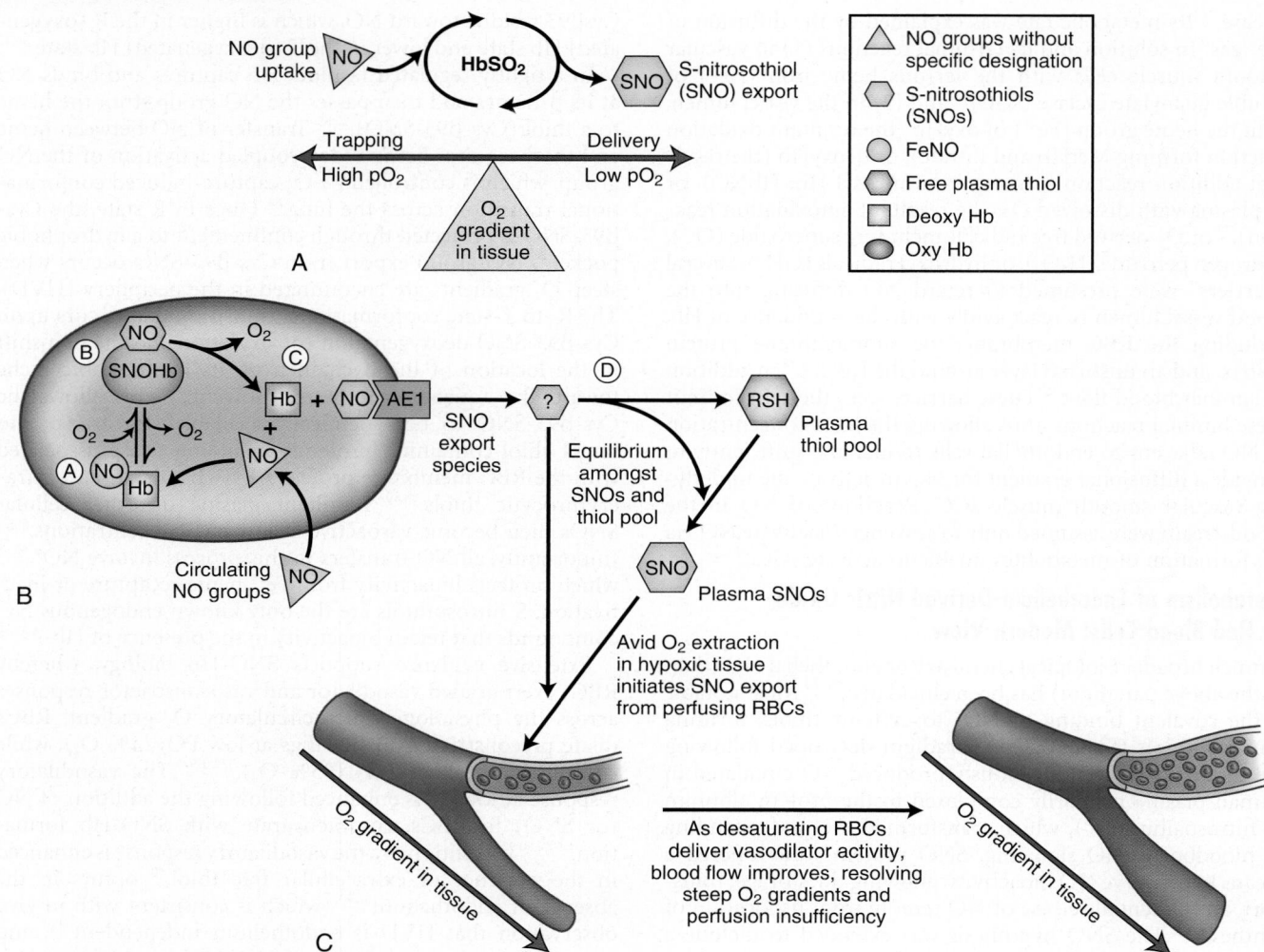

Fig. 89.5. RBCs transduce regional O_2 gradients in tissue to control nitric oxide (NO) bioactivity in plasma by trapping or delivering NO groups as a function of hemoglobin (Hb) O_2 saturation. (A) In this fashion, circulating NO groups are processed by Hb into the highly vasoactive (thiol-based) NO congener, S-nitrosothiol (SNO). By exporting SNOs as a function of Hb deoxygenation, RBCs precisely dispense vasodilator bioactivity in direct proportion to regional blood flow lack. (B) O_2 delivery homeostasis requires biochemical coupling of vessel tone to environmental cues that will match perfusion sufficiency to metabolic demand. Because oxy- and deoxy-Hb process NO differently (see the text), allosteric transitions in Hb conformation afford context-responsive (O_2-coupled) control of NO bioavailability, thereby linking the sensor and effector arms of this system. Specifically, Hb conformation governs the equilibria among deoxy-HbFeNO (A; NO sink), SNO-oxy-Hb (B; NO store), and acceptor thiols including the membrane protein SNO-AE-1 (C; bioactive NO source). Direct SNO export from RBCs or S-transnitrosylation from RBCs to plasma thiols (D) or to endothelial cells directly (not shown) yields vasoactive SNOs, which influence resistance vessel caliber and close this signaling loop. Thus, RBCs either trap (A) or export (D) NO groups to optimize blood flow. (C) NO processing in RBCs (A and B) couples vessel tone to tissue PO_2; this system subserves hypoxic vasodilation in the arterial periphery and thereby calibrates blood flow to regional tissue hypoxia.

is purportedly symmetrical across the physiologic O_2 gradient,[103,104] with maximal activity occurring at the P_{50} of Hb (~27 mm Hg).[103,105] This reaction profile does not match the HVD response, which increases in a steadily graded fashion as PO_2 falls in the physiologic range from 100 mm Hg down to approximately 5 mm Hg (HbSO$_2$ ~1%-2%).[51,54] If RBC-based vasoactivity were maximal at Hb's P_{50}, then blood flow would be diverted away from regions with PO_2 below 27 mm Hg, where it would be needed most. Additionally, based on the symmetry of Hb nitrite reductase activity at the P_{50}, RBCs traversing vascular beds with PO_2 at 25 or 75 would generate equal NO-based activity,[101] whereas it should be obvious that at such gas tensions different blood flow demands are required.

Vasoregulation by Red Blood Cell–Derived Adenosine Triphosphate

Adenosine triphosphate (ATP) has long been known to act as an endothelium-dependent vasodilator in humans,[55] binding to P_2Y purinergic receptors to induce local and conducted vasodilation via stimulation of vasoactive signals including endothelial NO, prostaglandins, and endothelial-derived hyperpolarization factors (EDHFs). More recently, RBCs have been identified as sources of vascular ATP,[55,106] with release stimulated by conditions associated with diminished O_2 supply relative to demand, hypoxia, hypercapnia, and low pH.[55,107] O_2 offloading from membrane-associated Hb is thought to initiate RBC ATP release,[106] stimulating heterotrimeric G protein,[108] as a result of membrane deformation. This leads to activation of adenylyl cyclase and an increase in cAMP,[109] which activates protein kinase A (PKA).[109] PKA stimulates cystic fibrosis transmembrane conductance regulator (CFTR),[110] which activates release of ATP from the RBC via pannexin 1.[111] Release of ATP via this pathway requires an increase in intracellular cAMP, which is controlled by the relative activities of adenylyl cyclase and phosphodiesterase 3 (PDE3B).[60]

Despite potential as a HVD mediator, RBC-derived ATP falls short on two fronts. First, HVD is unaltered by both endothelial denudation and eNOS deletion[58]; however, ATP vasoactivity is endothelium dependent. Second, blood levels of ATP rise and fall over a period of minutes, which is not commensurate with the HVD response that occurs in the course of A-V transit over a couple of seconds. Despite its shortcomings in terms of acting as a primary mediator of HVD, it is likely that Hb and ATP serve complementary vasoactive roles, in acute local and prolonged systemic hypoxia, respectively.[58]

Energy Metabolism in Red Blood Cells

The mature RBC, devoid of the organelles and enzymes required for oxidative energy production, relies on the relatively inefficient anaerobic glycolytic pathway for ATP generation (Fig. 89.6). This pathway, also known as the Embden-Meyerhof pathway (EMP), shares the same initial substrate (glucose-6-phosphate; G6P) as its sister pathway the pentose shunt, otherwise known as the hexose monophosphate pathway (HMP). These two metabolic pathways fulfill different cellular requirements. The EMP furnishes RBCs with ATP, 2,3-DPG (aiding in O_2 unloading), and NADH (necessary to reverse formation of metHb). The HMP ensures efficient NADPH recycling, necessary to maintain the antioxidant capacity required to protect RBCs from oxidative stress.

Glucose is the principal RBC energy source; however, other substrates including inosine, fructose, mannose, and galactose can also be metabolized. Glucose enters RBCs by energy-independent facilitated diffusion via the insulin-independent glucose transporter GLUT-1. Upon entry, it is immediately phosphorylated to glucose-6-phosphate (G6P), thus preventing escape from RBCs.

Regulation of Red Blood Cell Energetics by Hemoglobin

Historically, the regulation of RBC energetics was thought to be under the control of covalent modifications or feedback inhibition/activation of key enzymes. However, more recently it has been demonstrated that RBC metabolism is under the control of an O_2-sensitive reciprocal binding relationship between key EMP enzymes and Hb for the cytoplasmic domain of the Band 3 (cdB3) membrane protein.[112-116] EMP enzyme binding to cdB3 is inhibitory, decelerating this pathway in oxygenated RBCs.[117,118] Specifically, it has been demonstrated that (1) deoxygenated Hb displays a higher affinity for cdB3 than oxygenated Hb,[119] (2) phosphorylation of specific tyrosine residues (positions 8 and 21) on cdB3 displaces EMP enzymes from the membrane,[112,120] and (3) tyrosine phosphorylation up-regulates the EMP and down-regulates the HMP.[121]

O_2-sensitive regulation of glucose flux perfectly suits RBC requirements. Under fully oxygenated conditions, inhibition of glycolytic enzymes (due to their binding to cdB3) releases substrate constraint on G6P, allowing greater HMP flux and ensuring efficient NADPH recycling, necessary to protect RBCs from oxidative stress derived from the high O_2 load/environment. Conversely, the displacement and activation of EMP enzymes from cdB3 under low O_2 conditions up-regulates EMP activity, furnishing RBCs with ATP, 2,3-DPG (aiding in O_2 unloading), and NADH (necessary to reverse formation of metHb), which occurs subsequent to O_2 unloading.[114]

In unstressed conditions, 90% to 95 % of total erythrocytic glucose is metabolized via the EMP. Under such conditions, the G6PD reaction operates at less than 1% of its capacity,[122] largely due to inhibition of the enzyme by NADPH. Exposure of RBCs to oxidant stress results in the oxidation of NADPH (to NADP$^+$), releasing the inhibition on G6PD. In such situations, the HMP can account for 80% to 100% of total glucose consumed.[123,124] This ability to up-regulate the HMP serves to maintain levels of the reducing equivalent NADPH, which protects the cell by preserving functionality of several antioxidant systems. Loss of ability to accelerate EMP flux plays a significant role in RBC dysfunction in a variety of conditions, including critical illness.[125-127]

Role of Embden-Meyerhof Pathway

The 2 mol of ATP per mole of glucose generated via the RBC EMP is used almost exclusively in and on the plasma membrane to maintain electrochemical and ion gradients, phosphorylation reactions, and turnover of phospholipid phosphates. Cytosolic processes account for less than 10% of total ATP utilization.[128] These minor components include the maintenance of glycolysis and reduction reactions involving Hb, enzyme, and membrane protein sulfhydryls.

In addition to ATP generation, the EMP also generates the allosteric effector 2,3-diphosphoglycerate (2,3-DPG), via the subsidiary Luebering–Rapoport shunt (L-RS). 2,3-DPG stabilizes the deoxygenated Hb "T-state" conformation, thereby decreasing Hb affinity for O_2 and facilitating O_2 release to tissue, effectively raising P_{50}, or shifting the oxyhemoglobin dissociation curve to the right. Flux through the L-RS is O_2 and pH dependent: At an RBC intracellular physiologic pH of 7.2, this pathway accounts for approximately 20% of glycolytic flux. However, greater flux is observed in response to hypoxia and increases in pH. The glyceraldehyde phosphate dehydrogenase (GAPDH) reaction of the EMP also furnishes the cells with NADH, which is utilized by the enzyme methemoglobin reductase to reduce the heme group of Hb from its oxidized ferric state (Fe^{3+}) to its reduced ferrous state (Fe^{2+}),[129] thus maintaining the ability of Hb to reversibly bind O_2. This system maintains metHb concentrations in healthy individuals at less than 1% of total Hb.[128]

Role of Hexose Monophosphate Pathway

The HMP, which shares G6P (with the EMP) as initial substrate, does not generate any high-energy phosphate bonds. Instead, its primary function is reduction of NADP$^+$ to NADPH. This is achieved via the glucose-6-phosphate dehydrogenase (G6PD) reaction. The reducing equivalent NADPH is highly relevant in terms of cellular antioxidant capacity, as it serves as the electron source for several enzymes including

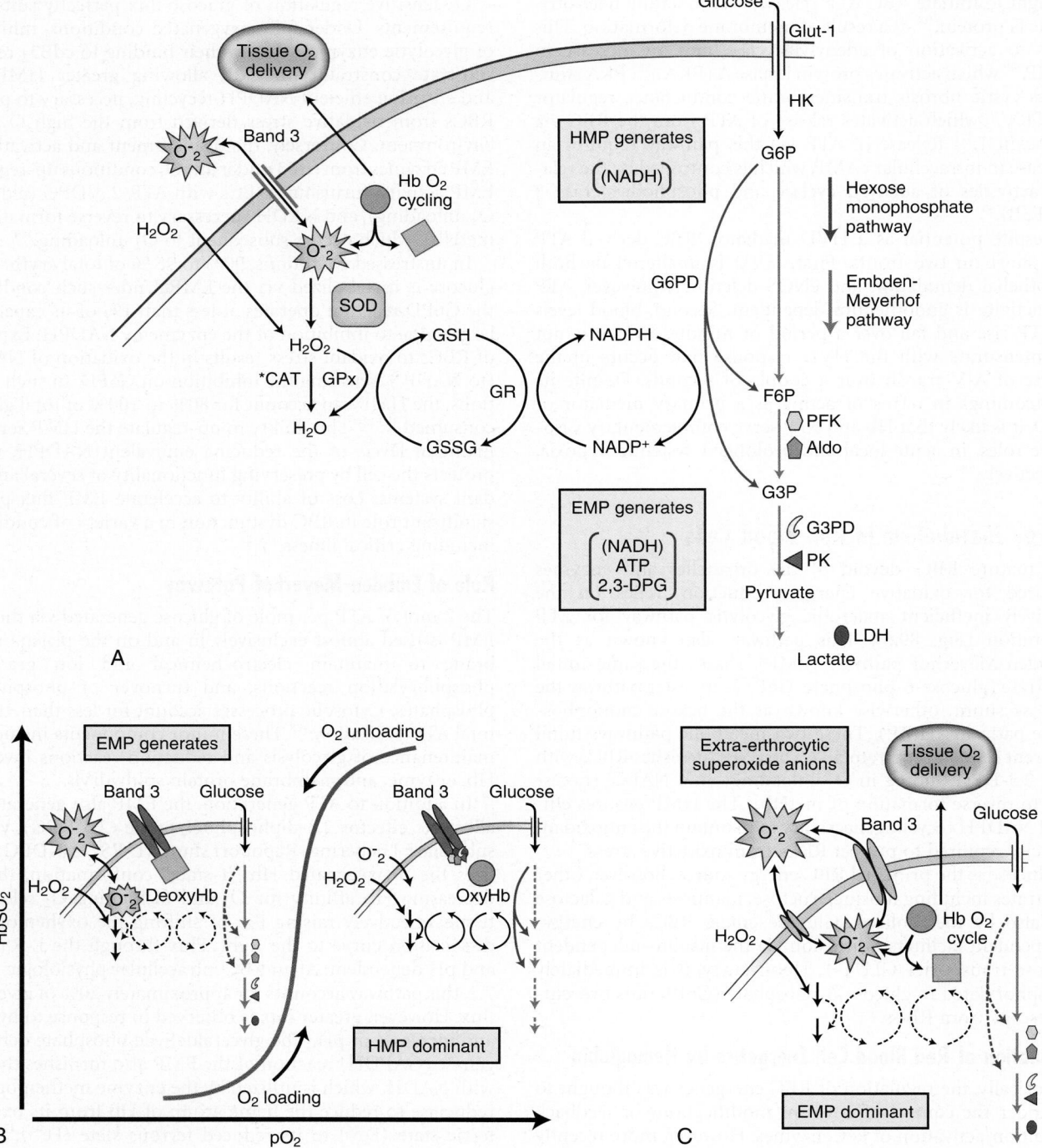

Fig. 89.6. Simplified scheme of cdB3-based control of RBC metabolism and proposed causal path for SiRD. (A) Energy metabolism in RBCs proceeds through either the Embden-Meyerhof pathway (EMP, *orange arrows*) or the hexose monophosphate pathway (HMP, *blue arrows,* also known as the "pentose shunt"). Both share glucose-6-phosphate (G6P) as initial substrate. The HMP is the sole source of NADPH in RBCs and generates fructose-6-phosphate (F6P) or glyceraldehyde-3-phosphate (G3P), which will rejoin the EMP prior to glyceraldehyde-3-phosphate dehydrogenase (G3PD/GAPDH), a key regulatory point. The EMP generates NADH (utilized by metHb reductase), as well as ATP (to drive ion pumps) and 2,3-DPG (to modulate hemoglobin P_{50}). Hydrogen peroxide (H_2O_2) and superoxide anion (O_2^-) are the principal endogenous reactive O_2 species (ROS) that are generated/encountered by RBCs. Both ROS are generated internally in the course of HbO_2 cycling.[176-178] Notably, only H_2O_2 can cross the membrane directly. O_2^- enters/departs RBCs via the Band 3 channel (anion exchange protein 1, or AE-1). O_2^- and H_2O_2 are ultimately reduced to water by catalase (CAT) or glutathione peroxidase (GPx). (B) O_2 content modulates EMP/HMP balance via reciprocal binding for cdB3 between deoxyHb and key EMP enzymes (PFK, Aldo, G3PD, PK, and LDH). In oxygenated RBCs (right half of stylized O_2 dissociation plot), EMP enzyme sequestration to cdB3 inactivates this pathway, resulting in HMP dominance and maximal NADPH (and thus GSH) recycling capacity. In deoxygenated RBCs (left half of O_2 dissociation plot), deoxyHb binding to cdB3 disperses bound EMP enzymes, activating the EMP, creating G6P substrate competition, constraining HMP flux, limiting NADPH and GSH recycling capacity, and weakening resilience to ROS, such as O_2^-. (C) In sepsis, data suggest cdB3-complex assembly may be prevented (particularly, with coincident hypoxia, see text). As in settings similarly impacting the cdB3 complex, it appears that this disturbs normal EMP/HMP balance (disfavoring HMP), depowering antioxidant systems and rendering RBCs vulnerable to oxidant attack. *Aldo,* aldolase; *GSH,* glutathione; *GR,* glutathione reductase; *NADPH,* nicotinamide adenine dinucleotide phosphate; *PFK,* phosphofructokinase; *PK,* pyruvate kinase; *LDH,* lactate dehydrogenase.

glutathione reductase, catalase, and thioredoxin reductase, which are central to RBC antioxidant systems.

Red Blood Cells, Free Radicals, and Reactive Oxygen Species

During circulation, RBCs encounter a variety of naturally produced free radicals. These chemical species, which contain one or more unpaired electrons, play a number of important signaling roles and include superoxide, O_2^-; hydroxyl radical, $HO\bullet$; and nitric oxide, $NO\bullet$.[58,130] RBCs also encounter various reactive oxygen species (ROS), including nonradical derivatives of O_2 such as hydrogen peroxide (H_2O_2). Although low concentrations of these species are essential for normal function, uncontrolled accumulation is damaging. The specific fate of ROS in RBCs is subject to their specific reaction rates, reactant concentration, and competing reaction rates. Consequently, ROS compartmentalization plays a significant role in protection strategies. For example, uncharged molecules such as H_2O_2 freely cross the RBC membrane, whereas charged molecules such as O_2^- enter only via transmembrane anion channels. For this reason, O_2^- is often concentrated in the intracellular compartment. Additionally, H_2O_2 and O_2^- are more selective in terms of their reactivity with biological molecules. For example, the main reactions of O_2^- are with itself (dismutation), with other radical species, or with transition metals. On the other hand, $HO\bullet$ is a much more aggressive oxidizing species and reacts with numerous biological targets, making it potentially much more damaging.

By virtue of the environment to which they are exposed, which is rich in O_2 and heme-iron, RBCs are continuously exposed to oxidant stress. During reversible O_2 binding, occasional spontaneous conformational fluctuations in the heme pocket of oxygenated Hb allow water or a small anion to enter, resulting in transfer of an electron from the iron to O_2 to produce metHb and the O_2^- radical. In fact, approximately 2% to 3% of total Hb undergoes auto-oxidation daily.[104] In addition to scavenging endogenously produced oxidants, due to their ubiquitous distribution, RBCs are also ideally positioned to act as circulating detoxification agents, neutralizing other oxidants produced throughout the circulation.[131]

Red Blood Cell Antioxidant Systems

RBCs require robust antioxidant systems, with the ability to rapidly counter the detrimental effects of oxidative insult. Oxidant damage occurring to RBCs may result from either an increase in ROS production or a reduction in antioxidant capacity. Generally, such situations are mainly observed under pathologic conditions, leading to disruption of membrane transport systems, enzymes, proteins, and lipids and the premature removal of the RBC from the circulation. Classically, the RBC antioxidant system comprises components to scavenge and detoxify ROS and prevents generation of radical chain reactions.[132] However, additional secondary mechanisms are also important and selectively rid the RBC of damaged proteins,[133,134] thereby prolonging circulation time.

Several enzymatic antioxidants are found in RBCs, including superoxide dismutase (SOD), catalase (Cat), glutathione peroxidase (GSHPx), glutathione reductase (GR), periredoxin (Prx), TrxR, plasma membrane oxidoreductases (PMOR), and metHb reductase (metHbR). Ongoing functionality of these enzymatic antioxidant systems requires recycling of the reducing equivalents NADPH and NADH, which are recycled in RBCs via glucose metabolism through the HMP and EMP, respectively.

In healthy RBCs, most metHb reduction is achieved through an NADH-linked system.[135] NADH, furnished via the EMP (glycolytic) pathway in the G3PD reaction, is utilized by the enzyme metHbR. NADH reduces cytochrome b_5, which in turn reduces the iron of metHb from its ferric trivalent (+3) state to its ferrous divalent (+2) state. GSH and ascorbic acid also play a role in metHb reduction, although their contribution is minimal. Ongoing functionality of metHbR requires metabolic flux via the EMP, which is the main route via which RBCs recycle NAD+ to its reduced form (NADH).

In addition to the enzymatic antioxidant systems, RBCs also contain numerous nonenzymatic antioxidants, including glutathione (GSH); vitamins A, C (ascorbate), and E (alpha tocopherol); and other less familiar species such as uric acid and melatonin.

GSH (L-y-glutamyl-L-cysteinylglycine) is the most abundant low-molecular-weight thiol found in RBCs (concentration ~2 mM). GSH can act as a direct scavenger of free radicals or as a substrate for GSHPx during the detoxification of H_2O_2 and lipid hydroperoxides. GSH also directly reduces protein sulfhydryls, generating glutathione disulfide (GSSG), which is recycled by GR. Steady-state GSH levels reflect a balance between synthesis (including both de novo synthesis and GR-mediated regeneration of GSH from GSSG) and loss due to GSSG efflux from the cell. The RBC membrane is permeable to GSSG, but not GSH. GSSG removal from the cell occurs as a result of active transport, in a process that is temperature sensitive and dependent on metabolic energy.[136,137] When the cell is no longer able to maintain GSH content, irreversible damage occurs.

Three vitamins (A, C, and E) provide important defense against oxidant stress in RBCs. Carotenoids, the precursors to vitamin A, also exert antioxidant effects in RBCs. In total, six carotenoid species have been detected in RBCs including lutein, zeaxanthin, β-cryptoxanthin, α-carotene, β-carotene, and lycopene. Vitamin C (ascorbic acid or ascorbate) readily donates one or two electrons to a variety of oxidants, including O_2 free radicals, peroxides, and superoxide. Additionally vitamin C functions to recycle vitamin E (alpha tocopherol) in a nonenzymatic pathway involving dihydrolipoic acid. Each stage of vitamin C oxidation is reversible, thus permitting recycling. RBCs lack an active transporter for vitamin C. Uptake occurs by simple diffusion and is consequently very slow, with a half-time of hours. Dehydroascorbic acid (DHA), however, is taken up by RBCs by facilitated diffusion through the glucose transporter (GLUT-1), after which it is rapidly converted to ascorbate and trapped within the cells.[138] RBCs also have enzymes that can facilitate GSH-dependent reduction of DHA, including the thioltransferase glutaredoxin. Vitamins A and E are both lipophilic and reside in the RBC membrane. Vitamin E acts as the major radical chain-breaking antioxidant. In the process of scavenging lipid and nonlipid radical species, vitamin E is oxidized to a tocopheroxyl radical. This radical can be recycled back to vitamin E in an NADH cytochrome b_5-dependent reaction or via a nonenzymatic pathway involving vitamin C. Melatonin (N-acetyl-5-methoxytryptamine), the chief secretory product of the pineal gland, is also synthesized in RBCs. This synthetic product functions as a direct ROS scavenger for O_2^-, H_2O_2, and $HO\bullet$, in addition to lipid peroxides. Furthermore, melatonin has also been demonstrated to stimulate other antioxidant enzymes, including Cu-Zn-SOD, catalase, GSHPx, glutathione reductase, and G6PD.

Acquired Red Blood Cell Injury, Eryptosis, and Clearance

After maturation to an anucleated cell furnished with the metabolic systems described earlier, the estimated normal life span of a mature RBC is 110 to 120 days.[139] To date, clearance of normal senescent RBC is not clearly understood. Two mechanisms have been proposed, clustering of the Band 3 (B3) membrane protein[140-143] and externalization of membrane phosphatidyl serine (PS),[144-147] both of these processes may be accelerated in the setting of critical illness, impairing oxygen transport capacity. Oxidatively modified hemoglobin (Hb) forms hemichrome aggregates, which associate with the cytoplasmic domain of the abundant membrane protein B3. Subsequent clustering of B3 exofascial domains increases affinity of naturally occurring anti-B3 autoantibodies, which activate the complement system, leading to RBC uptake and destruction by macrophages.[148] Normally, PS is asymmetrically distributed in the plasma membrane (a process regulated by flippases). Disruption of this pattern is a well-documented mark of RBC senescence,[144-147] signaling RBC removal by the reticuloendothelial system.[147] Alternatively, RBCs may proceed through a form of "stimulated suicide" similar to apoptosis (termed *eryptosis*), which is characterized by cell shrinkage and cell membrane scrambling that is stimulated by Ca^{2+} entry through Ca^{2+}-permeable, PGE_2-activated cation channels, by ceramide, caspases, calpain, complement, hyperosmotic shock, energy depletion, oxidative stress, and deranged activity of several kinases (eg, AMPK, GK, PAK_2, $CK1\alpha$, JAK_3, PKC, p38-MAPK). Eryptosis has been described in the setting of ethanol intoxication, malignancy, hepatic failure, diabetes, chronic renal insufficiency, hemolytic uremic syndrome, dehydration, phosphate depletion, fever, sepsis, mycoplasma infection, malaria, iron deficiency, sickle cell anemia, thalassemia, G6PD deficiency, and Wilson disease.[147,149,150]

Blood Flow Disruption During Critical Illness by Maladaptive Red Blood Cell–Based Signaling

Evidence is mounting in support of a causal relationship between acquired RBC dysfunction and a host of perfusion-related morbidities that complicates critical illness.[20,92,151-165] It has been observed that levels of SNO-Hb are altered in several disease states characterized by disordered tissue oxygenation.[92,93,166-173] In addition, where examined, RBCs from such patients exhibit impaired vasodilatory capacity.[88,92,93,170,172-174] These data suggest that altered RBC-derived NO bioactivity may contribute to human pathophysiology. Specifically, alterations in thiol-based RBC NO metabolism have been reported in congestive heart failure,[92] diabetes,[93,169] pulmonary hypertension,[91,168] and sickle cell disease,[170,175] all of which are conditions characterized by inflammation, oxidative stress, and dysfunctional vascular control. Moreover, known cross-talk between SNO signaling and cellular communication via carbon monoxide, serotonin, prostanoids, catecholamines, and endothelin may permit broad dispersal of signals initiated by dysfunctional RBCs. Precise understanding of the roles of dysregulated RBC-based NO transport in the spread of vasomotor dysfunction in stressed vascular beds may open novel therapeutic approaches to a range of pathologies.

Key References

2. Doctor A, Stamler JS. Nitric oxide transport in blood: a third gas in the respiratory cycle. *Compr Physiol.* 2011;1:541-568.
3. Hsia CCW. Respiratory function of hemoglobin. *N Engl J Med.* 1998; 338:239-247.
4. Hsia CCW. Coordinated adaptation of oxygen transport in cardiopulmonary disease. *Circulation.* 2001;104:963-969.
9. Geers C, Gros G. Carbon dioxide transport and carbonic anhydrase in blood and muscle. *Physiol Rev.* 2000;80:681-715.
17. Baskurt OK, Meiselman HJ. Blood rheology and hemodynamics. *Semin Thromb Hemost.* 2003;29:435-450.
20. Reggiori G, Occhipinti G, De Gasperi A, et al. Early alterations of red blood cell rheology in critically ill patients. *Crit Care Med.* 2009;37:3041-3046.
22. Aird WC. The hematologic system as a marker of organ dysfunction in sepsis. *Mayo Clin Proc.* 2003;78:869-881.
23. Goyette RE, Key NS, Ely EW. Hematologic changes in sepsis and their therapeutic implications. *Semin Respir Crit Care Med.* 2004;25:645-659.
34. Tissot Van Patot MC, MacKenzie S, Tucker A, Voelkel NF. Endotoxin-induced adhesion of red blood cells to pulmonary artery endothelial cells. *Am J Physiol.* 1996;270(1 Pt 1):L28-L36.
41. Munn LL, Melder RJ, Jain RK. Role of erythrocytes in leukocyte-endothelial interactions: mathematical model and experimental validation. *Biophys J.* 1996;71:466-478.
45. Evans EA, La Celle PL. Intrinsic material properties of the erythrocyte membrane indicated by mechanical analysis of deformation. *Blood.* 1975;45:29-43.
49. Kayar E, Mat F, Meiselman HJ, Baskurt OK. Red blood cell rheological alterations in a rat model of ischemia-reperfusion injury. *Biorheology.* 2001;38:405-414.
50. Baskurt O. Activated granulocyte induced alterations in red blood cells and protection by antioxidant enzymes. *Clin Hemorheol Microcirc.* 1996; 16:49-56.
51. Ross JM, Fairchild HM, Weldy J, Guyton AC. Autoregulation of blood flow by oxygen lack. *Am J Physiol.* 1962;202:21-24.
53. Stein JC, Ellsworth ML. Capillary oxygen transport during severe hypoxia: role of hemoglobin oxygen affinity. *J Appl Physiol.* 1985;75:1601-1607.
54. Gonzalez-Alonso J, Richardson RS, Saltin B. Exercising skeletal muscle blood flow in humans responds to reduction in arterial oxyhaemoglobin, but not to altered free oxygen. *J Physiol.* 2001;530(Pt 2):331-341.
55. Ellsworth ML, Forrester T, Ellis CG, Dietrich HH. The erythrocyte as a regulator of vascular tone. *Am J Physiol.* 1995;269(6 Pt 2):H2155-H2161.
56. Jia L, Bonaventura C, Bonaventura J, Stamler JS. S-nitrosohaemoglobin: a dynamic activity of blood involved in vascular control. *Nature.* 1996;380:221-226.
57. Stamler JS, Jia L, Eu JP, et al. Blood flow regulation by S-nitrosohemoglobin in the physiological oxygen gradient. *Science.* 1997;276:2034-2037.
58. Singel DJ, Stamler JS. Chemical physiology of blood flow regulation by red blood cells: the role of nitric oxide and S-nitrosohemoglobin. *Annu Rev Physiol.* 2005;67:99-145.
60. Ellsworth ML, Ellis CG, Goldman D, et al. Erythrocytes: oxygen sensors and modulators of vascular tone. *Physiology (Bethesda).* 2009;24:107-116.
61. Furchgott RF, Zawadzki JV. The obligatory role of endothelial cells in the relaxation of arterial smooth muscle by acetylcholine. *Nature.* 1980;288:373-376.
62. Furchgott RF. Endothelium-derived relaxing factor: discovery, early studies, and identification as nitric oxide. *Biosci Rep.* 1999;19:235-251.
63. Ignarro LJ, Buga GM, Wood KS, et al. Endothelium-derived relaxing factor produced and released from artery and vein is nitric oxide. *Proc Natl Acad Sci USA.* 1987;84:9265-9269.
64. Palmer RM, Ferrige AG, Moncada S. Nitric oxide release accounts for the biological activity of endothelium-derived relaxing factor. *Nature.* 1987;327:524-526.
65. Arnold WP, Mittal CK, Katsuki S, Murad F. Nitric oxide activates guanylate cyclase and increases guanosine 3′:5′-cyclic monophosphate levels in

various tissue preparations. *Proc Natl Acad Sci USA*. 1977;74:3203-3207.

66. Gonzalez-Alonso J, Mortensen SP, Dawson EA, et al. Erythrocytes and the regulation of human skeletal muscle blood flow and oxygen delivery: role of erythrocyte count and oxygenation state of haemoglobin. *J Physiol*. 2006;572(Pt 1):295-305.

70. Angelo M, Singel DJ, Stamler JS, An S. nitrosothiol (SNO) synthase function of hemoglobin that utilizes nitrite as a substrate. *Proc Natl Acad Sci USA*. 2006;103:8366-8371.

71. Schechter AN, Gladwin MT. Hemoglobin and the paracrine and endocrine functions of nitric oxide. *N Engl J Med*. 2003;348:1483-1485.

75. Huang KT, Han TH, Hyduke DR, et al. Modulation of nitric oxide bioavailability by erythrocytes. *Proc Natl Acad Sci USA*. 2001;98:11771-11776.

76. Liao JC, Hein TW, Vaughn MW, et al. Intravascular flow decreases erythrocyte consumption of nitric oxide. *Proc Natl Acad Sci USA*. 1999;96:8757-8761.

78. Hess DT, Matsumoto A, Kim SO, et al. Protein S-nitrosylation: purview and parameters. *Nat Rev Mol Cell Biol*. 2005;6:150-166.

79. Stamler JS, Singel DJ, Loscalzo J. Biochemistry of nitric oxide and its redox-activated forms. *Science*. 1992;258:1898-1902.

80. Stamler JS, Jaraki O, Osborne J, et al. Nitric oxide circulates in mammalian plasma primarily as an S-nitroso adduct of serum albumin. *Proc Natl Acad Sci USA*. 1992;89:7674-7677.

86. Gow AJ, Stamler JS. Reactions between nitric oxide and haemoglobin under physiological conditions. *Nature*. 1998;391:169-173.

87. Pawloski JR, Hess DT, Stamler JS. Export by red blood cells of nitric oxide bioactivity. *Nature*. 2001;409:622-626.

88. Doctor A, Platt R, Sheram ML, et al. Hemoglobin conformation couples erythrocyte S-nitrosothiol content to O2 gradients. *Proc Natl Acad Sci USA*. 2005;102:5709-5714.

89. Palmer LA, Doctor A, Chhabra P, et al. S-nitrosothiols signal hypoxia-mimetic vascular pathology. *J Clin Invest*. 2007;117:2592-2601.

90. Diesen DL, Hess DT, Stamler JS. Hypoxic vasodilation by red blood cells: evidence for an S-nitrosothiol-based signal. *Circ Res*. 2008;103:545-553.

91. McMahon TJ, Moon RE, Luschinger BP, et al. Nitric oxide in the human respiratory cycle. *Nat Med*. 2002;8:711-717.

106. Jagger JE, Bateman RM, Ellsworth ML, Ellis CG. Role of erythrocyte in regulating local O2 delivery mediated by hemoglobin oxygenation. *Am J Physiol Heart Circ Physiol*. 2001;280:H2833-H2839.

112. Harrison ML, Rathinavelu P, Arese P, et al. Role of band 3 tyrosine phosphorylation in the regulation of erythrocyte glycolysis. *J Biol Chem*. 1991;266:4106-4111.

113. Low PS, Rathinavelu P, Harrison ML. Regulation of glycolysis via reversible enzyme binding to the membrane protein, band 3. *J Biol Chem*. 1993;268:14627-14631.

114. Messana I, Orlando M, Cassiano L, et al. Human erythrocyte metabolism is modulated by the O2-linked transition of hemoglobin. *FEBS Lett*. 1996;390:25-28.

115. Castagnola M, Messana I, Sanna MT, Giardina B. Oxygen-linked modulation of erythrocyte metabolism: state of the art. *Blood Transfus*. 2010; 8(suppl 3):s53-s58.

116. De Rosa MC, Alinovi CC, Galtieri A, et al. Allosteric properties of hemoglobin and the plasma membrane of the erythrocyte: new insights in gas transport and metabolic modulation. *IUBMB Life*. 2008;60:87-93.

120. Campanella ME, Chu H, Low PS. Assembly and regulation of a glycolytic enzyme complex on the human erythrocyte membrane. *Proc Natl Acad Sci USA*. 2005;102:2402-2407.

121. Lewis IA, Campanella ME, Markley JL, Low PS. Role of band 3 in regulating metabolic flux of red blood cells. *Proc Natl Acad Sci USA*. 2009;106:18515-18520.

125. Rogers SC, Ross JG, d'Avignon A, et al. Sickle hemoglobin disturbs normal coupling among erythrocyte O2 content, glycolysis, and antioxidant capacity. *Blood*. 2013;121:1651-1662.

126. Rogers SC, Said A, Corcuera D, et al. Hypoxia limits antioxidant capacity in red blood cells by altering glycolytic pathway dominance. *FASEB J*. 2009;23:3159-3170.

127. van Wijk R, van Solinge WW. The energy-less red blood cell is lost: erythrocyte enzyme abnormalities of glycolysis. *Blood*. 2005;106:4034-4042.

132. Cimen MY. Free radical metabolism in human erythrocytes. *Clin Chim Acta*. 2008;390:1-11.

Hemoglobinopathies

M.A. Bender and Gabrielle Douthitt Seibel

PEARLS

- The pathophysiology of sickle cell disease is multifactorial, involving hemoglobin polymerization, oxidative damage to cell membrane proteins, white blood cell activation and inflammation, activation of the clotting cascade, and chronic hemolysis resulting in disturbances in nitric oxide metabolism.
- Acute chest syndrome is responsible for up to 25% of deaths in sickle cell disease, and its management should include antibiotic therapy with both a cephalosporin and a macrolide, oxygen to maintain saturations greater than 94%, prevention of atelectasis with incentive spirometry and potential biphasic positive airway pressure, diligent fluid management, adequate pain control, and bronchodilators.
- The default should always be to trust a patient's self-assessment of sickle cell pain.
- Up to 30% of patients with sickle cell disease have pulmonary hypertension, and the threshold to treat must be lower than for other etiologies as even mild elevations in pulmonary arterial pressure (>25 mm Hg) correlate with a significantly increased risk of death.
- A major cause of death in thalassemia major is cardiac failure secondary to iron overload; therefore a thalassemic patient presenting with cardiac failure must be assessed for cardiac iron content and, if present, undergo continuous chelation therapy.

Perspective

The evolution of animals is dependent on high concentrations of hemoglobin in red cells, which relies on the extraordinarily robust and coordinated synthesis of the α- and β-like globin polypeptide chains and iron-containing heme rings. Each has a highly evolved structure essential for optimal pairing of α- and β-like chains, as unpaired peptides are unstable and initiate cellular damage. The resultant $\alpha2\beta2$ hemoglobin plays a critical role in the transport and regulation of carbon dioxide, pH, and nitric oxide (NO) in addition to O_2. Thus hemoglobin synthesis is a high-stakes process in which any mutation may affect hemoglobin production, stability, function, or result in unpaired globin chains leading to devastating downstream effects. The approach to any hemoglobin alterations must consider the qualitative effects (how the plethora of hemoglobin's functions are altered) and quantitative effects (the amount of hemoglobin and unpaired globin chains).

Globin Gene Loci

The α- and β-like genes reside within multigene loci and are transcribed at unparalleled levels in both tightly tissue-specific and developmentally specific patterns.[1] This, and their involvement in human disease, has made these loci paradigms for gene regulation and pathophysiology. The five genes of the β-globin locus reside in a cluster on chromosome 11. The genes are expressed in an erythroid and developmentally stage-specific manor, the ε, Aγ and Gγ, and δ and β genes being expressed primarily during the embryonic, fetal, and postnatal periods, respectively. At birth, the majority of β-like chains are γ and the rest are β. This ratio inverts during the first year of life, explaining why phenotypes limited to the β-globin gene such as sickle cell and most β-thalassemias often do not manifest until several months of age. Expression of the chromosome 16–based α-like genes differs; the embryonic ζ-gene parallels the expression of ε, but the twin α-genes are expressed from the fetal period onward. Thus α abnormalities manifest in utero, potentially with devastating consequences (eg, hydrops fetalis). The resultant hemoglobin α-, β-heterotetramers (Hb) are developmentally expressed (eFig. 90.1).

Sickle Cell Disease
Molecular Description and Epidemiology

Sickle cell disease (SCD) refers to a group of single gene, autosomal recessive disorders most common in people originating from specific regions of Africa or India and in those of Hispanic descent. SCD encompasses a group of disorders characterized by the presence of the sickle mutation (substitution of an adenine [A] for a thymidine [T] in codon 6) and a second abnormal allele allowing the sickle hemoglobin to polymerize. This mutation results in replacement of a hydrophilic glutamic acid residue with a hydrophobic valine residue. With deoxygenation, allosteric changes in hemoglobin expose a destabilizing valine-containing pocket that aligns with others, leading to polymerization (crystallization), transition to the classic sickle cell morphology (Fig. 90.1), and the initiation of downstream events leading to pain and chronic end-organ damage (Fig. 90.2). In the United States, approximately 1 in 12 and 1 in 500 African Americans have sickle trait and SCD, respectively, with approximately 100,000 cases and approximately 2000 new birth cases per year (in contrast to approximately 200,000 birth cases per year in Africa). With increased ethnic mixing, compound heterozygous forms of SCD are increasingly being observed (eg, S/β-thalassemia or HbS/E).

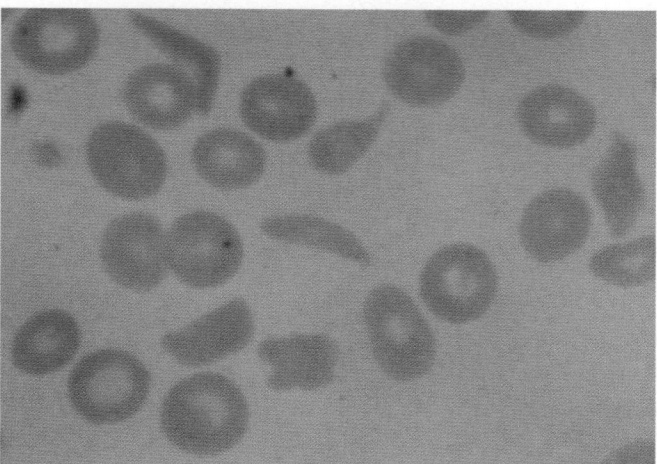

Fig. 90.1. Morphology of sickled cells. Note that although a subset of cells has a high degree of polymerized HbS and has taken on the classic sickle shape, the majority of cells maintain normal morphology. (Courtesy Dr. Min Xu, Seattle Children's Hospital.)

Sickle Cell Trait

Sickle cell trait (SCT) is distinguished from SCD by the presence of a normal β-globin allele and more HbA than HbS (typically 40% HbS) (Table 90.1). SCT does not result in the classic spectrum of sickle-related complications or alter red cell indices, but it can lead to clinical abnormalities.[2,3] Most notable is the concern that extremes of aerobic physical exertion, dehydration, and humidity may induce sudden death in rare student athletes with sickle cell trait.[3,4]

Spectrum of Sickle Cell Disease Genotypes and Natural History

The clinical manifestations of SCD result from intermittent episodes of vascular occlusion leading to tissue ischemia/reperfusion injury and variable degrees of hemolysis, both of which contribute to multiorgan dysfunction. Although homozygous sickle cell (Hb S/S, often called sickle cell anemia) is most common, it is essential to be aware of additional genotypes that result in a spectrum of disease severity

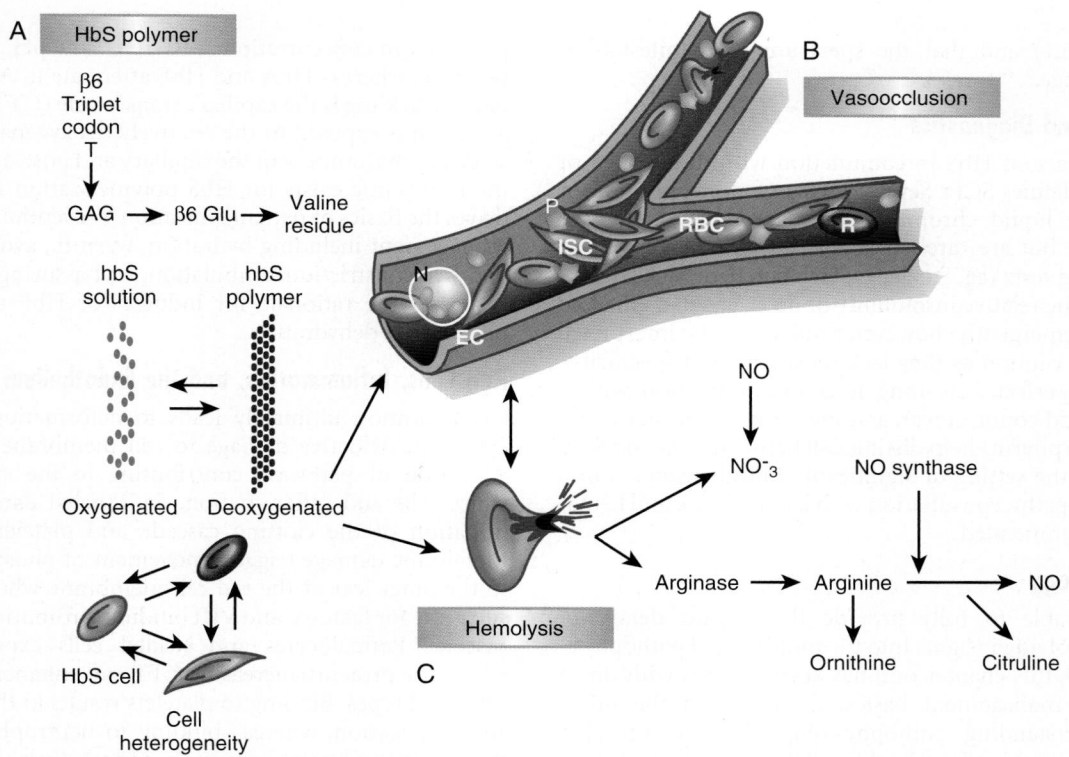

Fig. 90.2. Summary of multiple interacting steps contributing to the pathophysiology of sickle cell disease. Although this is an oversimplification and additional pathways are involved, the three predominant pathophysiologic steps are summarized. (A) Polymerization of HbS. A single nucleotide change results in HbS, which polymerizes upon prolonged deoxygenation, leading to sickled cells. (B) Red cells, inflammation, and the endothelium. Activation of adherence receptors, coagulation, platelet aggregation, and inflammatory pathways lead to slowed flow, increased capillary transit time, sickling of red blood cells, and eventual occlusion of blood flow. (*EC,* endothelial cell; *ISC,* irreversibly sickled cell; *N,* neutrophil; *P,* platelet; *RBC,* red blood cell; *R,* reticulocyte.) (C) Hemolysis and NO homeostasis. Hemolysis releases free hemoglobin, which breaks down NO, whereas release of arginase converts the substrate for NO, arginine, to ornithine. Thus less NO is generated and more is destroyed. (Modified courtesy Dr. Martin Steinberg, Boston University School of Medicine.)

TABLE 90.1   Hematologic Characteristics of Sickle Hemoglobinopathies

Diagnosis[a]	Predominant Hemoglobins After Age 1 Year[b]	Phenotype[c]	HEMATOLOGIC STUDIES AFTER AGE 1 YEAR[D]		
			Hgb	MCV[e]	HbA$_2$ (%)[f]
HbA	A	nl	nl	nl	nl
HbA/S (trait)	A > S[g]	nl[h]	nl	nl	nl
HbS/S	S	Hemolysis and anemia by age 6–12 mo	↓↓	nl	nl
HbS/β^0-thalassemia	S	Hemolysis and anemia by age 6–12 mo	↓↓	↓↓	nl or ↑
HbS/β$^+$-thalassemia	S > A	Milder hemolysis and anemia	↓	↓	nl or ↑
HbS/C	S ≅ C	Milder hemolysis and anemia	↓	nl or ↓	nl
HbS/E	S > E	Milder hemolysis and anemia[i]	↓	↓	nl[j]

Table shows typical results; exceptions occur.
[a]The β-thalassemias are divided into β$^+$-thalassemia, in which reduced levels of normal β-globin chains are produced, and β^0-thalassemia, in which there is no β-globin chain synthesis.
[b]Hemoglobins are reported in order of quantity. Only the most prominent hemoglobins are listed.
[c]Overview of phenotype.
[d]Values vary during the first year of life. Some patient's values continue to change after age 1 year.
[e]Must use age-specific values. MCV can be lowered by α-thalassemia trait and increased by hydroxyurea.
[f]HbA$_2$ results vary depending on laboratory method.
[g]In sickle trait, HbS is ~40% of total hemoglobins.
[h]Although patients do not have severe sequela, patients may have subtle abnormalities.
[i]Although patients have hemolysis and anemia, the severity of sickle cell–related complications tends to be less than HbS/C.
[j]Although HbA$_2$ is typically normal, this is often difficult to discern as HbE and HbA2 comigrate in some assays.
Hb, hemoglobin type; *Hgb*, hemoglobin concentration; *nl*, normal; ↑, increased; ↓, decreased; ↓↓, significantly decreased.
From Bender MA, Seibel GD. Sickle cell disease GeneReviews at GeneTests: Medical Genetics Information Resource. Seattle: University of Washington; 2014.

(see Table 90.1) and that the spectrum of manifestations change with age.[5]

Laboratory and Diagnostics

The prominence of HbS in conjunction with diminished or absent HbA defines SCD. Several forms of electrophoresis or high-pressure liquid chromatography are most often used diagnostically but are rarely available on an emergent basis. HbS screening tests (eg, Sickledex, Sickleprep, or Sicklequick) make use of the relative insolubility of deoxygenated HbS and are available emergently; however, results must be interpreted with extreme caution as they lack sensitivity and specificity.[6] Although imperfect, screening tests in conjunction with a complete blood count, smear, and measure of iron status (eg, zinc-protoporphyrin) help distinguish between SCD and SCT. Therefore in the setting of significant clinical suspicion of a hemoglobinopathy, consultation with lab medicine and hematology is recommended.

Pathophysiology

Although unable to fully provide the elegant details of the rapidly evolving insights into the multifaceted pathophysiology of SCD, this chapter outlines key pathways with direct relevance to management basics. Even though the initial era of understanding pathophysiology focused on HbS polymerization and red cell "sickling," this was followed by an awareness of the critical role of endothelial interactions, inflammation, and, later, of hemolysis and perturbations of NO metabolism (see Fig. 90.2).[7-12]

Hemoglobin Polymerization

The aforementioned crystallization of hemoglobin is enhanced by a high hemoglobin concentration (mean corpuscular hemoglobin concentration [MCHC]), low pH, and low temperature, whereas HbA and HbF attenuate it. A key determinant of sickling is the capillary transit time (CTT). The longer a red cell is exposed to the relatively deoxygenated, cold, and acidotic environment of the capillary and postcapillary venule, the more time exists for HbS polymerization to occur. This drives the basics of patient education, prevention, and medical management including hydration, warmth, avoiding acidosis and vasoconstriction, ambulation, and assuring oxygenation. It also is the rationale for inducers of HbF and agents to prevent cell dehydration.

Red Cells, Inflammation, and the Endothelium

Crystallization ultimately leads to deformation of erythrocytes and oxidative damage to cell membrane proteins, the activation of pathways contributing to the stimulation of white cells and inflammation, endothelial damage, and the initiation of the clotting cascade and platelet aggregation. Membrane damage triggers movement of phosphatidylserine to the outer leaf of the red cell membrane where it acts as a substrate for factor V and VIII binding, promoting the clotting cascade. Reticulocytes and sickled cells expose increased adherence proteins, increasing CTT and enhancing binding to other cell types. Binding to platelets results in their activation and aggregation, whereas binding to neutrophils stimulates the oxidative burst, damaging endothelium and exposing tissue factor, further promoting coagulation, platelet aggregation, and clot formation. Bound white cells release cytokines, increasing inflammatory cell recruitment and division and thereby perpetuating the process. Thus sickle cell represents an activated, inflammatory state in which the CTT is prolonged, propagating the cycle. This activation and integration of multiple pathways explains the tremendous clinical

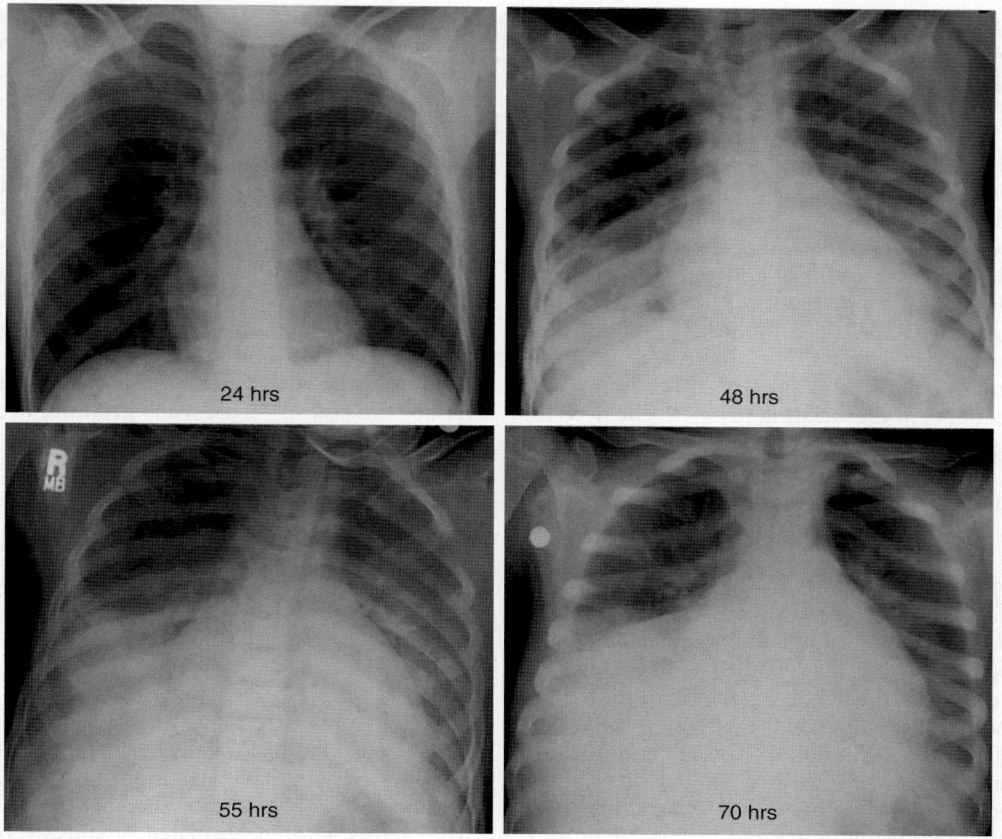

Fig. 90.3. Rapid progression of acute chest syndrome. Serial chest radiographs of a 13-year-old male with homozygous sickle cell disease admitted for pain. Hours from admission are noted. Notably acute chest syndrome typically presents 2 to 3 days into an admission for a vasoocclusive event.

heterogeneity observed in people with the same hemoglobin genotype, as well as why patients can show rapid clinical decline (Fig. 90.3). Consistent with the clinical importance of these pathways, an elevated white blood cell (WBC) count is a risk factor for pain episodes, acute chest syndrome, and early death.[13,14] Therapeutically, this points to the benefits of nonsteroidal antiinflammatory drugs (NSAIDs) in affecting the underlying pathophysiology as well as providing analgesia and why clinical response to hydroxyurea is correlated with a decrease in WBC count.[15,16]

Hemolysis and Nitric Oxide Homeostasis

In contrast to the vasoocclusive complications that correlate with a high WBC count and diminished HbF, a subset of complications—including pulmonary hypertension, skin ulcers, and priapism—was found to correlate with increased lactate dehydrogenase and bilirubin and reticulocyte count and is associated with a hemolytic phenotype arising and disturbances in NO hemostasis.[8-10,12] Hemolysis releases red blood cell (RBC) sequestered hemoglobin (Fe^{++}), allowing it to diffuse to the site of NO production (the endothelium) where it catalyzes the destruction of NO several thousand-fold, decreasing NO to nitrate metabolism with resultant formation of methemoglobin (Fe^{+++}). In addition, hemolysis releases arginase, depleting arginine, the precursor for NO synthesis. Thus chronic hemolysis leads to decreased NO synthesis and increased destruction, resulting in altered NO

hemostasis and increased tone of small vessels, slowing flow, and increasing sickling. Optimal management of hemolysis-related pathophysiology remains uncertain. Hemolysis prevention with hydroxyurea is appropriate and well accepted. NO metabolism is directly modified with class 5 phosphodiesterase inhibitors (eg, sildenafil) or by administering NO, its precursors, or related metabolites, approaches being actively investigated for both acute and chronic use.[12]

Clinical Manifestations

Although a summary of clinical problems and management is listed in the following section, the reader is referred to the National Heart Lung and Blood Institute standard of care guidelines[17] for more details (http://www.nhlbi.nih.gov/health-pro/guidelines/sickle-cell-disease-guidelines).

Pain

See eFig. 90.2 for a detailed care plan and eFigs. 90.3 and 90.4 for overviews of pain management.[18] Pain management in SCD is particularly difficult, as there are numerous etiologies (eg, vasoocclusive events [VOEs], dactylitis, avascular necrosis, acute chest syndrome, priapism, splenic sequestration and infarcts, hepatic crisis, and leg ulcers) and pathways involved (eg vasoocclusion, inflammation, and alterations in pain processing).[19-26] VOEs, defined as the acute onset of severe pain due to ischemia and reperfusion injury, are a hallmark of SCD. The complexities of SCD pain are best summarized by Shapiro and Ballas: "Vaso-occlusion is a physiologic process, but the resultant pain is a biopsychosocial phenomenon. Psychosocial issues such as coping skills, social context, personality, mood, and interactions with the health care system mingle with the biologic factors and contribute to the expression of the illness."[27] In the ICU, there must be an awareness of potential alterations in pain processing as well as awareness of the acute, neuropathic, inflammatory, psychologic, and social-cultural components of pain. Too often there is a primary focus opiate receptor blockade to the exclusion of addressing the inflammatory and neuropathic components. Pain can be acute, recurrent, or persistent, and it is complicated by coexisting chronic disease and racial overlays.[19-21,28] Too often racial attitudes and concerns of drug seeking prevent sufficient medication delivery to patients in excruciating pain.[28,29] The need for aggressive and rapid treatment is critical and well documented in guidelines of the American Pain Society and British Society of Hematology and is essential for humane care and physiologic improvements (eg, improving respiratory mechanics when having rib infarct pain).[30-32]

Pathophysiology, Diagnosis, and Presentation

Individual risk factors for VOE pain include a higher WBC count, lower HbF, coexisting alpha thalassemia, and older age.[26] Physiologic factors that may lend to VOE include Hb polymerization, rheology of RBCs, cellular dehydration, RBC deformability and fragility, whole blood viscosity, WBC activation, endothelial factors, adhesion of RBCs to endothelium intimal hyperplasia, hemostatic factors, altered nitric oxide metabolism, and vascular factors.[8,11,22-26] Vessel occlusion results in ischemic/reperfusion injury and the release of multiple inflammatory mediators that activate nociceptors, evoking a pain response. Recurrent episodes lead to altered pain processing making assessment and management more complex. Diagnosis is based on a detailed qualitative description (typically two components: a deep fatiguing, unrelenting ache with a component of biting, gnawing or throbbing) and location (eFig. 90.5). The description is essential to help rule out other etiologies of pain, as there is no definitive test to differentiate sickle pain from other sources of pain. Physical findings can include swelling, warmth, erythema, and tenderness, but exams may be normal and it must be reenforced that patients can appear in no apparent distress. The role of laboratory and radiologic studies is to rule out other etiologies of pain. It is essential to perform quantitative pain assessments every several hours using a developmentally appropriate pain scale, followed by a reassessment of the pain plan. Pain assessment is difficult but pain is subjective and self-reports should be trusted. As pain becomes more chronic, the focus should move toward functional assessments.

Management

See eFig. 90.2 for a detailed care plan and eFigs. 90.3 and 90.4 in the appendix for overviews of pain management.[18] An effective management strategy considers not only the underlying tissue damage and nociception but also the history of pain episodes, doses of medications required to achieve acceptable analgesia, baseline pain medications, history of tolerance, mental state, how the patient processes pain, coexisting depression, as well as the presence of anxiety or fear. A multimodal approach is outlined in eFigs. 90.3 and 90.4 but essential components include (1) environmental manipulation; (2) complementary methods; (3) addressing pathophysiology and triggers (fluids to maintain euvolemia, warmth, and NSAIDs to

decrease CTT); and (4) adjunctive interventions such as physical therapy, ambulation, and incentive spirometry to maintain blood flow and prevent atelectasis and acute chest syndrome (ACS). After these issues have been addressed, providers may focus on opiates and additional medications.

Initial pharmacologic management of severe pain episodes includes the initiation of around-the-clock NSAIDs (many children will have resolution of pain with intravenous ketorolac[33]) followed by rapid and repeated doses of opiates (dosed every 20 minutes), transitioning to continuous infusion or patient-controlled analgesia (if developmentally appropriate).[30-32,34] Although the absence of pain is not a goal, the aim is to relieve pain and suffering and allow rest and health-promoting activities (incentive spirometry and ambulation to reduce the risk of ACS), while avoiding oversedation, which can contribute to the development of pulmonary complications. As cannabinoids have multiple effects on inflammation and neuropathic components of pain and can attenuate hyperalgesia, there is strong rationale for its use in SCD, although this remains controversial socially.[35] Use of L-arginine (a precursor of NO) has resulted in a 50% reduction in overall opiate use in SCD,[36] and there is increasing evidence for the use of glutamine.

Sepsis

Detailed sepsis care plans are presented in eFigs. 90.6 and 90.7.[18] Sepsis has historically been a major cause of morbidity and mortality in SCD. Strikingly, in the 1970s, 20% of SCD patients in the United States died before age 6 years, primarily from sepsis with encapsulated organisms, particularly *Streptococcus pneumoniae*.[5] With the initiation of universal newborn screening in the United States leading to early identification, early prophylactic penicillin, and education on the importance of fever response and immunizations, deaths from sepsis have plummeted.[37] Currently, the presence of a central line is the biggest risk factor for bacteremia.[38]

Pathophysiology and Etiology

The developmental timing of sepsis risk correlates with decreased splenic function due to infarcts leading to functional asplenia, which can be observed as early as 3 months. The resultant defects in cellular immunity, the alternate complement pathway and decrease in memory cells, and opsonizing antibodies will reduce clearance of encapsulated organisms. Children with SCD have a 100 to 400 times increased risk of bacteremia from encapsulated pathogens.

Management

The pathophysiology, diagnosis, and management of sepsis are presented in Chapter 111. Several aspects of sepsis that are unique to SCD are noted in eFig. 90.7.

Acute Chest Syndrome

Table 90.2 and eFig. 90.8 show detailed care plans.[18] ACS is clinically heterogeneous, and its definitions vary in the literature and among institutions, making comparisons of studies difficult. The most general definition is a new nonatelectatic infiltrate on chest radiograph in a patient with SCD, although others add requirements for fever, full lung segment involvement, or respiratory symptoms. ACS, the second leading cause of hospitalization in SCD and the leading cause of intensive care unit, admits among those 12 years and older.[39]

ACS can progress in mere hours, resulting in a mortality rate of 1% in children (4% in adults), with most deaths

TABLE 90.2	**Management of Acute Chest Syndrome**
(1) Antibiotics	A cephalosporin to cover encapsulated organisms, particularly *S. pneumoniae*, and a macrolide such as *Mycoplasma* and *Chlamydia* are the most common infectious pathogens.
(2) Oxygen	Maintain saturations greater than 94%.
(3) Judicious fluid resuscitation	Maintain euvolemia while avoiding overly aggressive fluid resuscitation that may worsen cardiac and respiratory status due to a combination of severe anemia and decreased cardiac function.
(4) Prevention of atelectasis	Incentive spirometry (IS) has been shown to prevent development of ACS, thus IS and its alternatives.[142] Chest physiotherapy and ambulation may be of benefit once atelectasis and consolidation are present.[142,143] Bilevel positive airway pressure (BiPAP) or continuous positive airway pressure (CPAP) as a preventive measure is untested but appropriate as early intervention may prevent atelectasis and minute areas of collapse, preventing progression and the need for intubation.
(5) Pain management	Opiates should be carefully titrated to minimize splinting and allow IS, while minimizing respiratory depression (small opiate boluses before IS may be helpful). Unfortunately opiates are often withheld due to concerns of respiratory depression. In fact, pain relief can improve respiratory mechanics, significantly improving clinical status.
(6) Bronchodilators	Are indicated as asthma is common in sickle cell disease (SCD) and its presence increases the risk of acute chest syndrome (ACS), and a subset of patients respond independent of documented wheezing.[144]
(7) Corticosteroids	Use remains controversial as they tend to improve ACS but lead to rebound pain. Tapering of even pulsed steroids may reduce the rebound.[45-47]
(8) Transfusion	For multilobar disease, worsening pulmonary status despite conservative methods of treatment, or those who are critically ill.
(9) BiPAP or CPAP	For worsening pulmonary status, clinical decline, or those who are critically ill.

occurring in children younger than age 3 years[40] (see Fig. 90.3). ACS accounts for 25% of all deaths in SCD.[40] Risk factors include a history of asthma, high baseline Hgb, and low HbF. Factors associated with mortality include a prior episode of ACS, development of respiratory failure within 48 hours of presentation, sepsis, and simultaneous presentation with pain.[40] Etiologies vary by age with multiple etiologic factors often present and include bacterial infections with typical and atypical organisms, viral infections, and fat emboli, as well as pulmonary infarction and hemorrhage (see also eFig. 90.9).[41] In addition, a functionally based etiology is chest or other extreme pain resulting in poor lung expansions and increased areas of atelectasis that then can lead to vasoocclusion and inflammation.

Presentation

ACS frequently occurs 2 to 3 days into a VOE. ACS should be suspected when there is fever, chest pain, cough, or other pulmonary symptoms; however, notably, there is no single pattern of signs and symptoms that predicts ACS, and up to 35% of patients will have a normal pulmonary exam.[40,42] As a result, there should always be a low threshold to obtain a chest radiograph to rule out ACS. Leukocytosis and significant drops in hemoglobin and platelets are common.[40] Significant morbidity is associated with ACS, including pneumothorax and empyema, and 14% of patients developed respiratory failure in one study.[41] Risk factors for respiratory failure include (1) extensive lobar involvement, (2) platelet count less than 199,000/µL, and (3) a history of cardiac disease.[41]

Management

Detailed care plans are presented in Table 90.2 and eFig. 90.8.[18] Management of ACS can be addressed in stages. Although there are not many randomized controlled trials to guide care of ACS,[43,44] suggestions for an approach to care are presented in Table 90.2. All patients should receive conservative care (highlighted in green in the table). The use of steroids (highlighted in yellow) deserves special attention. Although their use in ACS is controversial (see Table 90.2), due to the risk of rebound pain with steroid withdrawal a taper is indicated, even if only pulsed therapies are used (as in asthma or prior to extubation).[45-47] Transfusion (highlighted in red in the table) has been shown to significantly improve oxygenation and clinical status in ACS.[41] Although transfusion is usually effective at reversing ACS, because of the risks, including alloimmunization, transfusion is not part of initial management unless the patient is severely ill. Although 20% to 70% of patients with ACS are transfused, views differ on performing a simple transfusion targeting an Hgb of 10 g/dL or an exchange transfusion targeting the same Hgb while lowering the HbS to under 30%.[40,41] Both approaches improve oxygenation and are safe and effective; however, exchange transfusion requires exposure to more donors, increases alloimmunization, is more time consuming, and may require central access in this population with increased thrombotic risk. Thus a simple direct transfusion is recommended for most situations.[48,49] The benefit of direct transfusion in ACS patients with a high Hgb (>9 g/dL) is less clear, as a minimal number of red cells can be transfused, and exchange may be more advantageous in this circumstance.

Although lacking formal studies, the use of bilevel positive airway pressure (BiPAP) or CPAP in an attempt to stave off intubation makes sense pathophysiologically. One small study determined that BiPAP use was successful in staving off respiratory failure,[50] whereas another found improvement in gas exchange and respiratory rate but not in hypoxemia or patient comfort.[51] There is no consensus as to when to intubate or the optimal ventilation strategy in ACS, thus patients are often treated as children with acute lung injury or acute respiratory distress syndrome (ARDS). For patients with refractory hypoxemia, both high-frequency oscillatory ventilation and venovenous extracorporeal membrane oxygenation have been successful.[52-54] A promising approach to ACS is to improve NO metabolism with inhaled NO or oral arginine, a precursor of NO.

Stroke

Clinical guidelines for stroke (eFig. 90.10) provide elements of a detailed care plan.[18] This section focuses on acute, clinically apparent cerebrovascular accident (CVA)–related to SCD; a detailed discussion of stroke can be found in Chapter 69. Before screening and prevention programs, 11% of children with HbS/S or HbS/β-thalassemia developed overt strokes (peak, 2 to 9 years), with another 20% to 35% having silent infarcts.[55-57] Risk factors include anemia, moyamoya, history of previous CVA, and abnormal transcranial Doppler (TCD) (discussed later).[58] Patients with HbS/C disease and other compound heterozygotic states do not have this significantly increased risk, although it may be higher than that in the general population. Strokes may be due to ischemia, hemorrhage, or thromboembolic events involving large, medium, and small vessels.

Natural History
Prior to screening and preventive transfusion therapy, approximately 11% of patients with SCD had an overt stroke. Untreated, 50% have a recurrent stroke in the first 2 years, and 66% have recurrence within 9 years.[59] Maintaining the HbS under 30% reduces the recurrence rate to 10%, with many if these "resistant" patients having moyamoya.[60-62] Screening TCDs using a standardized approach identify patients with high cerebral vessel flow, associated with an excessively high stroke risk within 3 years.[63] Screening TCDs coupled with chronic prophylactic transfusion therapy have decreased the prevalence of stroke from 11% to 1%.[59]

Diagnosis
Although diagnosis is suggested by a history of acute neurologic changes and abnormalities on neurologic physical exam, magnetic resonance imaging (MRI) and magnetic resonance angiogram (MRA) confirm it. *Although an MRI/MRA is needed, it should never delay definitive therapy (transfusion or surgery) if stroke has been diagnosed clinically.*[64] Notably, headache and signs of increased cranial pressure are more common in hemorrhagic stroke (see Chapter 69). Neurosurgical intervention for a hemorrhagic lesion should never be delayed; thus an emergent noncontrast CT is obtained to immediately rule out any surgically amenable lesions, and MRI/MRA may be deferred. Other etiologies of childhood stroke must be considered and ruled out including infection, thrombosis (thrombosis panel and anticardiolipin antibodies), cardiac embolic disease, masses, and trauma with vascular damage.

Management
A detailed stroke management plan is provided in eFig. 90.10.[18] Acute care and monitoring are similar to that for other children with CVAs (see Chapter 69) except that emergent exchange transfusion is accepted as the standard of care in SCD.[17] The goal is an HbS under 30% and a final Hgb of 10 g/dL, which is most efficiently accomplished with exchange transfusion. Care must be taken to avoid hypotension with blood withdrawal during the exchange. Due to the importance of transfusing emergently, an initial direct transfusion followed by exchange transfusion to avoid delays in treatment may be appropriate, especially if the Hgb is under 8.[59] Seizures should be treated, but there is no role for seizure prophylaxis. Although tissue plasminogen activator (t-PA) has a role in non-SCD stroke, t-PA or anticoagulant therapy is not recommended in children, in part due to the different pathophysiology. Addition of low-dose aspirin is controversial but is started for some with concerns of an active cerebral vasculopathy.[65] Once stabilized, extensive evaluation by physical, occupational, and speech therapy as well as a neurocognitive

evaluation is essential to define new postevent baselines and guide future needs.

Aplastic Crisis
An approach to evaluation and care is provided in eFig. 90.11.[18] An acute worsening of baseline anemia (by 1 to 2 g/dL of Hgb) associated with decreased reticulocyte count (typically <1%) suggests aplastic crises and is caused by acute infection such as parvovirus B19. Sickle RBCs survive 10 to 14 days (versus 60 to 100 days for normal cells); thus patients are dependent on a significantly increased reticulocyte production and any decrease can lead to a transient red cell aplasia with rapid development of a profound anemia. Monitoring of Hgb (both absolute and compared with the individual's baseline), reticulocyte count, and cardiovascular status is essential. Most parvovirus B19 infections will spontaneously resolve. However, intravenous gamma globulin should be considered to hasten viral clearance if reticulocytopenia persists. Transfusion may be required if the patient demonstrates hemodynamic instability and may be considered if the hemoglobin acutely falls more than 2 g/dL. Profound anemia or cardiac compromise may require a slow transfusion (2 mL/kg/hr), possibly with diuretics, or even exchange transfusion to avoid congestive heart failure.

Splenic Sequestration
An approach to evaluation and care is presented in eFig. 90.12.[18] Sequestration is characterized by an acutely enlarging spleen with an Hgb more than 2 g/dL below an individual's baseline value. Mild to moderate thrombocytopenia may also be present. Splenic sequestration occurs in 10% to 30% of children with SCD, most commonly between the age 6 months and 3 years, often following a febrile illness. Abdominal pain, nausea, and vomiting are common, and severe episodes of sequestration may progress rapidly to cardiovascular collapse and death.[66] Transfusion is indicated when signs of cardiovascular instability are present and, as with aplastic crises, caution should be taken to avoid contributing to congestive heart failure. If the patient is transfused, it is important to be aware that with transfusion some patients release RBCs from their spleen, resulting in an unexpectedly high Hgb. Care must be taken not to overshoot the desired target, avoiding an Hgb of over 11g/dL. Though rare, emergent splenectomy may be required. Elective splenectomy is indicated for recurrent episodes of sequestration with cardiovascular compromise.

Pulmonary Hypertension
Pulmonary artery hypertension (PAH) confirmed by right heart catheterization affects approximately 6% to 11% of adults and children with sickle cell disease. Elevated tricuspid regurgitation velocity indicating PAH occurs in approximately 30% of adults with sickle cell disease and is associated with increased mortality.[67] With approximately 100,000 people with SCD in the United States, this translates into about 30,000 cases of PAH, making sickle cell the leading cause of PAH nationally. Although there has been concern for overdiagnosing PAH in SCD by an elevated tricuspid regurgitant jet velocity (TRV) on transthoracic echocardiography (TTE), it is increasingly understood that adults with estimated PAPs greater than 25 mm Hg or a tricuspid regurgitation velocity jet velocity (TR jet) of greater than 2.5 m/sec have a strikingly higher mortality rate.[12,68,69] Thus it is essential to have a

significantly lower threshold for aggressive intervention for PAH in the hemoglobinopathy patient than in others.

Pathophysiology and Etiology

Multiple pathways contribute to PAH in the sickle cell patient. Hemolysis leads to nitric oxide dysregulation, vascular dysfunction, injury, and inflammation, which can ultimately lead to PAH.[8,12,70] Progressive increases in pulmonary vascular resistance related to decreases in nitric oxide (NO) availability and dysregulation ultimately lead to right ventricular failure and decreased cardiac output. The 2014 American Thoracic Society Guidelines for PAH in SCD define PAH as a resting mean pulmonary arterial pressure equal to or exceeding 25 mm Hg.[67] Frequently confounding factors in the PH of SCD include (1) hypoxic PAH due to the high incidence of enlarged tonsils, obstructive sleep apnea, asthma, and chronic lung disease; (2) arterial obstructive PAH secondary to increased coagulation and embolic disease; and (3) pulmonary venous hypertension due to cardiomyopathy. Contributing to the high morbidity in SCD are the protean manifestations of mild pulmonary hypertension (>25 mm Hg). The majority of patients with SCD and PAH will be asymptomatic or have mild decreases in exercise tolerance (eg, 6-minute walk) yet have a 10-fold increased risk of death.[69] Increased mortality has been associated with a TRV of 2.5 m/second or higher in adults (10 times greater mortality risk), NT-pro-BNP levels of >160 in adults (at least 5 times greater mortality risk), and pulmonary artery pressure >25 mm Hg on right ventricular heart catheterization in adults. Sufficient data in children are lacking, thus some suggest using the American Thoracic Society (ATS) adult criteria, though this is controversial as it has be suggested that there is no increased risk of death within 3 years of diagnosis.[71]

Diagnosis

Though cardiac catheterization is the gold standard for determination of PAH, it is invasive and expensive. Catheterization is reserved for a subset of the patients initiating PAH-specific therapies.[67] Current diagnostic recommendations include TRV as measured by echocardiogram, using a TRV of 2.5 m/sec as a criterion for diagnosis.

Management

Although there is minimal evidence for specific therapies in the treatment of PAH in SCD, a multitiered approach is accepted by many: (1) identifying and reversing factors potentially contributing to PH (eg, tonsil- and adenoidectomy, bilevel positive airway pressure [BiPAP] or continuous positive airway pressure [CPAP], and nighttime O_2 if contributing to obstructive sleep apnea [OSA]), (2) optimizing of sickle cell specific care (eg, hydroxyurea or chronic transfusions), and (3) applying PH-specific therapies. Hydroxyurea (HU) is the first-line treatment for SCD-specific care, as it decreases hemolysis and sickle cell formation, it decreases ACS and VOE (both of which are associated with acute increases in pulmonary pressures), and it is recommended for most adults and most pediatric patients. Chronic transfusion therapy is the second-line therapy for PAH in SCD, reserved for those who do not respond to HU. Although controversial and lacking data, the mortality risk of PAH is felt to outweigh the potential side effects of transfusion therapy. For those with right heart catheterization defined PAH additional therapies are recommended. For those with venous thromboembolism and no additional risk factors for bleeding, indefinite anticoagulant therapy is recommended. Targeted PAH therapies such as

prostacyclin agonists (eg, iloprost), endothelin receptor antagonists (eg, bosentan), soluble guanylate cyclase stimulators (eg, riociguat), or phosphodiesterase-5 inhibitors (eg, tadalafil), and other PH therapies should be tried, but limited data exist for their use (see also Chapter 56). Despite considerable enthusiasm for the use of sildenafil, a randomized controlled trial (RCT) was halted early do to an increase in VOE in the treatment group, emphasizing caution in applying accepted PH therapies to SCD.[72]

A mainstay of treatment of PAH in the ICU is inhaled NO (iNO), which provides both direct vasodilation of the pulmonary vasculature and simultaneous reversal of the underlying disruption in NO metabolism. The major challenge with iNO is the development of rebound PAH on discontinuation of therapy and difficulty in administration, thus driving a focus on alternative therapies. Oral arginine, a precursor of NO, was shown to reduce PAP within 5 days of therapy in a small number of patients with SCD and PHTN[73] and is being further investigated.

Multiorgan Failure

Multiorgan failure syndrome is defined as severe pain associated with failure of at least two of the following organs: liver, lung, and kidney. It is often associated with severe pain in patients with previously mild disease and a relatively high Hgb.[74] Widespread vasoocclusion is thought to be responsible, though data are lacking. Patients present with an atypically severe VOE, fever, and sudden deterioration including a drop in Hgb and platelets, diffuse encephalopathy, and rhabdomyolysis. Death has been reported in up to 25% of patients.[75] Exchange transfusion should be considered early and can result in rapid recovery of organ function as well as survival. Antibiotics are often used, though many patients are culture negative. There are isolated reports of success with NO or plasma exchange in those with transfusion-resistant disease, consistent with the idea that this may represent a thrombotic thrombocytopenia (TTP)–like state.[76]

Renal Conditions

Renal injury is caused by sickling in the renal microvasculature.[77,78] The normal renal medullary environment is hypoxic, acidotic, and hypertonic. In the face of sickle cell disease and sometimes even the sickle trait, these conditions lead to sickling, increased viscosity, and ischemia, causing damage to the renal medulla such as segmental scarring and interstitial fibrosis, which can progress to infarction and necrosis including papillary necrosis:

1. Hyposthenuria is an inability to concentrate urine. It is critical to remain aware of this condition in the ICU, as the production of dilute urine cannot be used as a marker for being euvolemic, and patients are prone to dehydration, leading to vasoocclusive episodes.

2. Hematuria can range from micro- to gross hematuria associated with papillary necrosis due to medullary infarction. Conservative management with bed rest, IV fluids, and maintenance of high-urine output to avoid the development of clots usually suffices. Transfusions may be needed if blood loss is significant. Vasopressin has been used with some success, as has ε-amino caproic acid, though the latter should be used with caution as it can lead to clot. If recurrent transfusions are required or bleeding becomes life threatening, resection of the involved region may be indicated.

3. Tubule dysfunction may occur, including an incomplete renal tubular acidosis worsened by the hyposthenuria, and hyperkalemia secondary to impaired urinary potassium excretion, the use of potassium-sparing diuretics, angiotensin-converting enzyme inhibitors, or β-blockers.

4. Chronic renal failure is associated with glomerular injury and proteinuria and can include nephrotic syndrome. End-stage renal disease develops in 40% of patients with nephrotic syndrome, thus persistent proteinuria is an indication for an in-depth evaluation. Risk factors include hypertension, hematuria, proteinuria, and worsening anemia. Although there is no clear cure, angiotensin-converting enzyme inhibitors can reduce the proteinuria, and NSAIDs should be avoided. Worsening anemia can be treated with erythropoietin, though sickle cell patients often need higher doses than others.

Iron Overload

Unlike thalassemia, the iron overload of sickle cell is primarily related to transfusion.[79] Sickle cell and thalassemic patients show different patterns of iron deposition, and the heart accumulates iron far less readily in SCD. The acute management in the ICU is similar and is discussed in the "Thalassemia" section.

Sleep Conditions

Children with SCD have a higher prevalence of obstructive sleep apnea (OSA) than the general pediatric population (20%-41%), likely due to greater airway crowding related to increased tonsillar, adenoid, and cervical node size.[80-82] Sleep disturbances and OSA contribute to decreased oxygen saturation levels, further increased endothelial dysfunction and inflammatory process leading to increased VOE, decreased pulmonary function, increased risk of pulmonary hypertension, and depression.[82,83] Although tonsillectomy and adenoidectomy may be helpful in OSA, noninvasive ventilation with CPAP or BiPAP may be necessary and may be initiated in the pediatric intensive care unit (PICU). CPAP has been well tolerated in SCD and shown to improve sleep and cognitive function.[84]

Depression and Suicide

With recurrent pain and complications that can occur without warning, it is not surprising that anxiety and depression are increased in patients with SCD.[85,86] Interestingly, rates are higher than in cystic fibrosis, spina bifida, or diabetes, with 49% having anxiety symptoms in one study, and the risk of suicide in adults is increased.[86-89] Anxiety and depression as well as suicidal ideation if present should be addressed in the acute care setting.

Surgery and Anesthesia

A detailed care plan for the sickle cell patient scheduled for surgery and anesthesia is provided in eFig. 90.13.[18] Major surgery in sickle cell patients is associated with increased perioperative risks including VOE pain, acute chest syndrome, and death, but these can be minimized with specific perioperative care. Preoperative direct transfusion targeting an Hgb of 10 minimizes these risks and is preferred over an exchange transfusion in most cases because of the exposure to fewer units of blood and less alloimmunization.[90,91] Communication and coordination between the anesthesiologist, surgeon, and hematologist are essential, and institutions are encouraged to have a standard perioperative care plan for SCD. Most patients are admitted overnight following surgery for oxygen, pain management to assure the ability to deep breathe and perform incentive spirometry, and monitoring for pain and pulmonary complications, even if cleared to return home from a surgical standpoint. Because of poor compliance with incentive spirometry, the use of BiPAP in the immediate postoperative period may be beneficial.[92] Specific recommendations should be followed (see eFig. 90.13).

Disease-Modifying Therapies and Interventions

The impact of public health policy and family education focused on prevention, early detection, and early intervention cannot be overstated. The preventive measures have led to dramatic improvement in morbidity, mortality, and quality of life. Additional therapies for prevention or the long-term treatment of complications targeting specific mechanisms involved in the pathophysiology of SCD follow (see eFig. 90.14 for an overview).

Hydroxyurea

Although hydroxyurea is not an acute intervention, the intensivist should be aware that most SCD patients should be on hydroxyurea.[17,93-95] Hydroxyurea ameliorates sickle cell disease by decreasing pain, ACS episodes, and transfusion needs while increasing hemoglobin, quality of life, and life span.[17,93-95] Originally used in SCD to stimulate HbF production, the primary clinical benefits may stem from the relative leukopenia induced by this oral chemotherapeutic as well as decreasing hemolysis (see "Pathophysiology" and "Etilogy," presented earlier). When assessing complete blood counts (CBCs), clinicians should remain aware that hydroxyurea can decrease all cell lineages and lead to a red cell macrocytosis with mean corpuscular volumes (MCVs) into the 115 range. There is no recommendation to routinely discontinue hydroxyurea during acute illness or hospitalizations. The intensivist should be aware that hydroxyurea can cause a transaminitis and is renally cleared so it should be adjusted or held with hepatic or renal compromise, or with clinically significant cytopenias.

Transfusion

Though a mainstay of therapy, guidelines for transfusions in SCD are complex and vary by indication. The reflective tendency to transfuse SCD patients should be avoided. Because of alloimmunization and other risks, attempts should be made to avoid transfusion unless there is a clear clinical indication, and consultation with hematology is advised. Table 90.3 summarizes guidelines, and additional information is provided in specific sections presented earlier.[17,96-100] General guidelines for transfusion are provided in Chapter 93 for general information regarding blood transfusion. SCD-specific issues follow.

Choice of Product

Packed RBCs should be leuko-depleted to minimize febrile reactions and alloimmunization. Although transfusion from sickle trait donors is safe and effective, HbS-negative blood should be requested as it complicates assessment of posttransfusion HbS levels. An extended cross-match for antigens of clinical significance that vary between racial groups should always be requested, as it reduces alloimmunization and should include Rh (Cc, D, Ee) and Kell in addition to ABO.[17,101,102] The intensivist must be aware that matching or

TABLE 90.3 Indications for Transfusion in Sickle Cell Disease

	Duration	Consensus	Method	Goal[a]
Stroke, acute	Single	+	Ex	HbS <30%
Stroke, ongoing care	Chronic	+	Either	HbS <30%
High-velocity TCD	Chronic	+	Either	HbS <30%
ACS, initial episode	Single	+ (for severe or progressive ACS)	Dir > Ex	Hgb 10
ACS, recurrent	6-12 months	+	Either	
PHTN	Chronic	+	Either	
Multiorgan failure	Single	+	Ex	
Major surgery	Single	+	Dir	Hgb 10
Acute anemia	Single	+	Dir	
Recurrent spleen sequestration	Chronic	+		
Sepsis/meningitis	Single	+	Dir	
Severe chronic pain	6-12 months	+		
Congestive heart failure	Chronic	+		
Silent infarct	Chronic	–		
Pregnancy		–		
Anemia/renal failure	Chronic	–		
Leg ulcers	6-12 months	–		
Severe growth delay		–		
Severe eye disease		–		
Priapism		–		

[a]Goal of transfusion if a consensus has been reached.
Dir, direct; *Ex,* exchange; *Hb,* hemoglobin type; *Hgb,* hemoglobin concentration; +, consensus reached; –, consensus not reached.

finding compatible units for highly immunized patients may take considerable time, thus a type and cross should be sent well before blood is needed, and in some emergencies extended matching may need to be forgone. Unlike the protocol used for patients with hematologic malignancies, there is no need for blood product irradiation or CMV negative selection unless the patient is waiting for or undergoing transplant.

Type and Goals of Transfusion
Goals of transfusion in SCD include increasing O_2 carrying capacity or decreasing HbS. Different modes of transfusion can be utilized to reach the intended goal. The target hemoglobin concentration or HbS percentage varies with indication (see Table 90.3), but in most cases the final Hgb should never be higher than 11 because whereas oxygen carrying capacity increases, O_2 delivery may fall.[103] Formulas for calculating blood volumes for routine and exchange transfusions are available (eFig. 90.15). In many cases, a direct transfusion is as effective as an exchange transfusion and is therefore preferred to minimize alloimmunization. One significant exception is acute stroke, where an automated exchange (erythrocytapheresis) to bring the HbS level down quickly while raising the Hgb is standard of care.[17] This requires either two large-bore peripheral IVs (which can be difficult in some patients) or a pheresis-compatible central line that can accommodate flow rates and pressures required during red cell erythrocytapheresis (RCE). Good coordination and

communication about the specific line to be placed should occur with the blood center or program operating the pheresis machine. Children under 10 kg may not be able to tolerate automated RCE and may require a manual exchange transfusion, which requires significant nursing time to complete but can be effective and requires only one large-bore peripheral IV. A brief summary table of recommendations for mode of transfusion is provided for reference (see Table 90.3).

Hematopoietic Stem Cell Transplantation
Hematopoietic stem cell transplantation (HSCT) remains the one cure for SCD, and the role of the ICU is supportive care posttransplant (see Chapter 95). Because of striking results with a matched sibling transplant after a myeloablative-conditioning regime (85% event-free survival and a 94% overall survival with approximately 10% graft failure and 12% to 20% significant graft-versus-host disease [GVHD]) increasingly children with less severe disease are being transplanted.[104-108] Multiple SCD research transplant studies are available and address optimizing the conditioning regime, extending transplants to older patients, and using alternate donors (unrelated, cord blood, haploidentical).[106-109]

Gene Therapy
Modification of autologous HSCs to correct the sickle mutation or add a normal gene avoids many of the problems of routine HSCT but remains experimental with a limited

number of clinical trials (see "Thalassemia" presented later). Go to clinicaltrials.gov for currently open trials.

Induction of β-Like Chains

See the "Thalassemia" section for more detailed information on this topic.

Novel Therapies

The numerous pathophysiologic paths contributing to SCD are providing targets for novel therapeutics, too numerous to be reviewed here but discussed elsewhere.[110,111] Similarly, multiple mechanisms involved in the classic approach, such as induction of HbF, are actively being pursued.[112-114]

Thalassemia
Molecular Description and Epidemiology

In contrast to a single mutation being responsible for sickle cell and the mutant peptide directly leading to the pathophysiology, a textbook compendium of mutations can lead to thalassemia and it is the residual unpaired phenotypically normal globin chains that incite damage. The hallmark of thalassemia is an imbalance in the ratio of α- and β-chains, not necessarily a deficiency in chains. The distinction becomes important when one considers α-/β-thalassemia compound heterozygotes or duplicated (excess) globin genes. Gene deletions account for the majority of α-thalassemias, leading to quantum incremental changes in phenotype depending on whether one, two, three, or all four adult α-globin genes are missing. In contrast, the broad range of mutations that leads to β-thalassemia result in a continuum of clinical phenotypes. As with the sickle cell trait, the thalassemia trait is thought to provide increased fitness in malaria zones. The coexistence of α- and β-thalassemia in the same geographic regions leads to compound heterozygotes being common, resulting in a huge spectrum of disease and complicating diagnostics.

Laboratory and Diagnostics

Although the sine qua non of diagnostics is a microcytic anemia with the demonstration of an α- to β-globin chain imbalance, this is not practical for routine testing, thus most clinical laboratories rely on a variation of a thalassemia screen. The screen helps distinguish thalassemia from iron deficiency, and α- from β-thalassemia. Due to the wide range of defects

and frequent mixed α- and β-thalassemia patients, it is impossible to state absolutes for diagnostic interpretation, and there should be a low threshold to consult with a hematologist. Components of the screen include (1) a complete blood count where emphasis is placed on the MCV, which is decreased in proportion to hemoglobin production, the RBC to assess the degree of compensation for the decreased cell size, the hemoglobin, and the smear; (2) a hemoglobin electrophoresis or high pressure liquid chromatography (HPLC) to quantitate normal and variant hemoglobins; (3) an inclusion body or Brilliant Cresyl Blue preparation to semiquantitatively assess excess β-like chains and distinguish α- and β-thalassemia; and a (4) zinc-protoporphyrin or similar screen to exclude iron deficiency. α-Thalassemia results in excess β-like chains that form tetramers (β4: Hb H, γ4: Hb Barts) that precipitate in proportion to the number of missing α-genes, resulting in a positive inclusion body prep (Table 90.4). The diagnosis of β-thalassemia is less direct. Excess α-chains are less stable and degrade so no α-tetramers are detectable on electrophoresis or HPLC. Thus a microcytic anemia with negative inclusion body prep in the face of adequate iron is suggestive of β-thalassemia. Frequently β-thalassemia results in up regulation of HbA2 or HbF; thus the presence of either is suggestive of the diagnosis.

DNA testing is increasingly available and cost effective, though it remains problematic as no single assay or panel detects all abnormalities. With the increasing application of high throughput genome sequencing to clinical medicine, it will not be long before comprehensive sequence-based assays will be available.

Pathophysiology

The pathophysiology of thalassemia is complex but in brief, unpaired globin chains lead to ineffective erythropoiesis and hemolysis, the degree of which depends on the specific form of thalassemia and the patient's genetic background (eFig. 90.16).[115] Free globin chains increase reactive oxygen species, whereas decreased glutathione and antioxidant stores result in oxidative damage to the fragile red cell membrane, as well as to apoptosis in a Fas-mediated process. The result is a cadre of processes contributing to the heterogeneity of disease presentation. Phosphatidyl serine moves to the outer leaf of the red cell membrane, enhancing macrophage-mediated destruction in the spleen and marrow and acting as a substrate for factors V and VIII binding, enhancing the generation of

TABLE 90.4 Distinguishing Laboratory Features of α- and β-Thalassemias

Diagnosis[a]	BCB Prep[b]	HbA2[c]	HbF	HbH	Hb Barts in Newborn[d]
Normal	−	nl	nl	nl	−
α-Thalassemia	+	nl	nl	nl or ↑	+
β-Thalassemia	−	nl or ↑	nl or ↑	nl	−

Table shows typical results; exceptions occur.
[a]All forms of α- or β-thalassemia are pooled; specific results will vary.
[b]Brilliant cresyl blue (BCB) or inclusion body prep. Results vary by lab, but this can be done semiquantitatively and increases with the degree of α-thalassemia. This can be negative when a one α-globin deletion is present (silent carrier). This assay is unreliable in the presence of other hemoglobins (eg, HbS or HbE). This can be negative when α- and β-thalassemia are simultaneously present.
[c]HbA2 results vary depending on laboratory method.
[d]Hb Barts increases with the degree of α-thalassemia.
Hb, hemoglobin type; *nl*, normal; ↑, increased; −, negative; +, positive.

thrombin, which together with decreased protein C and S levels and increased platelet activation and adhesion leads to increased thrombosis. In an attempt to compensate for the hemolysis and ineffective erythropoiesis, medullary and extramedullary erythropoiesis lead to skeletal abnormalities such as the thalassemic facies (eFig. 90.17) and thinning of the cortex of long bones, which, along with endocrine abnormalities (see the following section), lead to increased fractures. High levels of nontransferrin-bound iron from red cell destruction, increased intestinal absorption from inappropriately low levels of hepcidin, and transfusions lead to iron deposition, resulting in liver, cardiac, and endocrine dysfunction.

Forms and Variations

α-Thalassemia

Typical laboratory findings are summarized in eFig. 90.18. Although alpha thalassemia leads to a tremendous burden on health worldwide and is well reviewed elsewhere, it is not a major cause of ICU admits in the United States, thus the focus will be on β-thalassemia major.[116]

β-Thalassemia

In contrast to α-thalassemia, the plethora of β-gene mutations leads to a continuous spectrum of disease. β0-thalassemia denotes nonexpressing alleles, whereas β+-thalassemia is used for genes that express a reduced amount of normal protein. Most mutations do not eliminate ε- or γ-gene expression, thus it is unusual for clinical complications to occur until several months of life, when infants become dependent on adult β-globin chains. Nomenclature is based on this continuum of phenotypic severity rather than genotype. β-thalassemia trait, also referred to as thalassemia minor, is due to a single silent allele and is benign and only of note for primary care and genetic counseling. The term *thalassemia major* (also known as Cooley anemia) is reserved for transfusion-dependent phenotypes, whereas those with clinical sequelae, but who are not dependent on transfusions for survival, are referred to as having thalassemia intermedia. The latter require the most clinical decision making as there is increasing awareness of the high morbidity in many of these patients, as many benefit from transfusion.[117]

HbE/β0-Thalassemia

Of the numerous hemoglobin variants, this compound heterozygous state is worth special mention. The HbE mutation is common throughout Southeast Asia and results in an RNA splicing abnormality and a destabilizing amino acid substitution, leading to a thalassemic allele. When combined with another β-thalassemic allele the phenotype is extraordinarily variable, with some thriving, and a subset being transfusion dependent.[118,119] Management is similar to that for other thalassemias and guided by clinical presentation, not genotype.

Natural History

Natural history is highly variable depending on the genotype, modifying genetic factors, and, critically, if and at what interventions such as transfusion and chelation are available. If not diagnosed by newborn screening or from a known familial risk, children can present with anemia, growth delays, bony abnormalities, iron overload (even if untransfused), and, most common for the intensivist, congestive heart failure.

Assessment of Iron Overload

Direct tissue measurement of iron is essential. Though inexpensive, serum ferritin is a poor indicator of iron stores; it is elevated with inflammation and does not correlate well with tissue iron content, especially in chelated patients.[120,121] MRI-based assessment of iron overload is based on relaxation times correlating with iron content and is now widely accepted.[121,122] Techniques evolve rapidly, and standards and practices vary greatly, making it essential to discuss options with local radiologists. Ferriscan is a commercially available test where data are sent out for analysis, and it is limited to the assessment of hepatic iron.[123] In contrast, T2* imaging is increasingly available and allows simultaneous assessment of hepatic and cardiac iron and, potentially, other target organs.[121,124] A lower T2* correlates with higher degrees of iron overload (see "Cardiac Complications," presented later).

Spectrum of Disease

Although a summary of clinical problems and management is listed here and in eFig. 90.19, the reader is referred to the Northern California Comprehensive Thalassemia Center standard of care guidelines[125] for more details (http://thalassemia.com/documents/SOCGuidelines2012.pdf).

Anemia

Although there is much debate as to the optimal Hgb that should be targeted, in the ICU one must factor in the acuteness of the anemia, the degree of cardiovascular compromise, and the patient's baseline Hgb. A baseline level of under 6 g/dL is often the threshold for initiating chronic transfusions, though a higher threshold is used if growth, skeletal malformations, or extramedullary erythropoiesis becomes problematic. The goal should be to maintain an Hgb of 9 to 10 g/dL pretransfusion (10 to 12 g/dL if cardiac disease is present) but no higher than 14 g/dL posttransfusion. As with SCD, profound anemia or cardiac compromise may require a slow transfusion, diuretics, or even an exchange transfusion to avoid congestive heart failure. Blood products should be leuko-reduced to minimize alloimmunization, febrile nonhemolytic transfusion reactions, and CMV transmission. As with SCD, blood should be matched for ABO, Rh (Cc, D, Ee), and Kell. Family and related donor transfusion should be avoided if a hematopoietic stem cell transplant is to be considered, as alloimmunization to donor antigens increases graft rejection.

Transfusion-Related Complications

Chronic or frequent transfusions increase iron overload, the risk of alloimmunization, and infectious risk[126] (also described in Chapter 94). Because of inappropriately low hepcidin levels, the ability of the body to absorb iron is unopposed, leaving blood loss and sloughing of endothelial and skin cells as the only mechanism to decrease iron in the face of iron overload. This is estimated to lead to a loss of 1 mg/day in an adult, which pales in comparison to the approximately 200 mg of iron in each unit of blood. Although previous focus was on hepatic iron overload and cirrhosis, there is increasing awareness of iron overload in the heart, pituitary, and endocrine organs leading to dysfunction (see the following section) and excessive melanin production leading to bronze pigmentation. Iron overload requires chelation; a summary of chelation drugs and potential toxicities can be found in eFig. 90.20.

Cardiac Complications

Cardiac failure due to iron overload, defined as a low ejection fraction with a component of cardiomyopathy, is the major cause of ICU admission and death in thalassemic patients.[127,128] A thalassemic patient in failure should be assumed to have cardiac iron overload until proved otherwise.[125] Risk factors include transfusion history and underchelation. Untreated overload can also lead to dysrhythmias including atrial fibrillation and ventricular tachycardia, as well as conduction disturbances and heart block.[127,128] Excess unbound iron from transfusion and inappropriate gastrointestinal absorption freely penetrates cardiac myocytes leading to progressive tissue damage. Iron accumulates predominantly in the epicardial portion of the ventricular septum and ventricular free walls, stimulating the production of free radicals and resulting in peroxidative tissue damage, decreased cardiac contractility, and dysrhythmias. This, in combination with the high output state from chronic anemia, results in the early development of cardiac failure. Cardiac iron overload occurs well after the liver becomes overloaded. Initial cardiac iron deposition increases the influx of additional iron resulting in a rapid accumulation and the potential for rapid decline, a wide range of dysrhythmias, and failure after years of normal function. The clinical presentation is that of congestive heart failure; however, some present solely with abdominal pain due to liver distenion. Clinicians should maintain a low threshold to evaluate for cardiac dysfunction. With advances in both transfusion and chelation therapy, survival is increasing but is highly dependent on the underlying thalassemia as well as access to transfusion and chelation.

Assessments

Cardiac iron accumulation and function must both be assessed. Ferritin and assessments of liver iron concentration (LIC) cannot be used to assess cardiac risk because kinetics of iron deposition and unloading differ between the organs. Iron assessment by T2* is invaluable as one can assess cardiac iron, as well as LIC.[124] A T2* of over 20 ms is not associated with increased cardiac risk. In contrast, a value of 10 to 20 ms denotes overload and increased cardiac risk, and a T2* of under 10 ms portends a high risk of cardiac dysfunction and an emergent situation requiring aggressive chelation (eFig. 90.21).[120,125,127-129] Echocardiography is essential, and left ventricular dysfunction is highly suggestive of iron overload.[130] Given the high output state, some suggest the cutoff for a normal ejection fraction in thalassemics should be 60%.[131] Electrocardiogram often revels biventricular dysfunction with left ventricular hypertrophy, a prolonged PR interval, bradycardia, ST-T wave change, and T-wave inversions. Iron-related parathyroid and thyroid and adrenal dysfunction, as well as vitamin D and thiamine status, should be investigated, as they may impact cardiac function.

Management

The key to management of iron-related cardiac dysfunction is chelation. For details see the Standards for Care Guidelines for Thalassemia and eFig. 90.21 in the appendix.[125] High-risk cardiac patients (failure, arrhythmias, a cardiac T2* <10 ms, or an LIC >30 μg/g dry weight) demand emergent intervention with deferoxamine at higher dosing than for routine chelation. Optimal chelation strategies in emergent situations are evolving rapidly, thus an expert on chelation should be consulted. Conservative therapy consists of 24-hour continuous deferoxamine infusion at 50 to 100 mg/kg/day, 7 days a week,

given intravenously or subcutaneously depending on access and comfort.[125] Deferoxamine can lead to histamine-mediated hypotension when given intravenously, so blood pressure should be monitored closely. After the initiation of continuous deferoxamine, deferiprone or deferasirox should be considered as addition of either can be beneficial.[132] Arrhythmias often resolve promptly with chelation and are commonly treated with amiodarone. Due to the diffuse injury and reversibility with chelation, ablation is not recommended. Although ascorbic acid releases iron, facilitating chelation, it should not be used initially as the increased release of iron may lead to cardiac damage. Total iron must be assessed to avoid toxicity from overchelation. Afterload reduction, diuresis, and inotropic support should be considered, and serial echoes to follow shortening and ejection fractions are indicated. Additional measures to optimize cardiac function include maintaining a pretransfusion Hgb of 12 g/dL, protecting oxidative damage with carnitine, correcting thyroid and parathyroid deficiencies, and administering intravenous calcium with oral vitamin D to maintain cardiac contractility. Unless emergent, interventions such as pacemakers and cardiac transplant should not be considered until after cardiac iron has been reduced because dysfunction is often reversible with chelation.

Hepatic Dysfunction

The intensivist should remain aware that liver damage and dysfunction from iron overload, transfusion-related viral hepatitis, medications, autoimmune disease, and genetic factors such as α1-antitrypsin deficiency and Wilson disease are common in thalassemia. Assessment of liver damage is often multimodal, requiring a T2* for LIC, and CT or routine MRI to assess tissue damage and cirrhosis. Liver biopsy may be necessary to more fully assess the underlying damage.

Thrombosis and Pulmonary Emboli

Thrombotic complications of pulmonary emboli, arterial occlusion, portal thrombosis, deep vein thrombosis, and stroke are increased in thalassemia, especially after splenectomy. Enhanced thrombin generation due to factor V and VIII alterations as well as decreased protein C and S levels and increased platelet aggregation lead to a thrombotic state resulting in increased venous thrombosis and emboli (see eFig. 90.16).

Pulmonary Hypertension

Although pulmonary hypertension is common in thalassemia, the true prevalence is not known. As with SCD (discussed previously), NO destruction secondary to free hemoglobin from hemolysis contributes to pulmonary hypertension, as do the direct effects of iron overload on the vascular endothelium and myocardium stiffness and function. In addition, cell fragments or debris can cause vasoconstriction in the pulmonary vasculature, which is worsened with splenectomy. As in SCD, screening by transthoracic echo is common, with concerns raised for a TR jet of over 2.5 m/sec and a diagnostic catheterization if over 3 m/sec.[125,133,134] Treatment should address the various pathways contributing to pulmonary hypertension.[125,133] Maintaining the Hgb over 9.5 g/dL helps suppress ineffective erythropoiesis and the resultant hemolysis and NO destruction and decrease cell debris. If evidence of cardiac dysfunction from iron overload chelation is critical, oxygenation should be maintained, keeping saturations over 95%, and anticoagulation should be considered. For persistent disease, sildenafil should be considered, though there are some data for the use of bosentan and epoprostenol.[125,133]

Therapies and Interventions

Interventions for specific complications are described previously, in the Northern California Comprehensive Thalassemia Center standard of care guidelines,[125] and in eFig. 90.19. Although transfusions are the mainstay of therapy for severe thalassemia, guidelines for when to initiate transfusions and what Hgb to target vary with each individual's presentation and among centers. In the acute setting it is essential to remain aware of the patient's recent baseline Hgb, maintain a higher Hgb (10 to 12 g/dL) for cardiac failure, and consult with the hematologist. Although HSCT and gene therapy are potentially curative and inducers of nonadult globin genes are actively being optimized, none are currently useful in the acute ICU setting.

Hematopoietic Stem Cell Transplantation

Currently hematopoietic stem cell transplantation (HSCT) is the most available cure for thalassemic patients, though a handful have been cured by gene therapy. For HSCT, long transfusion histories increase the chance of graft failure, necessitating an aggressive myeloablative conditioning regimen, which in turn can lead to a high treatment-related toxicity, especially if significant end-organ damage is present. Thus success depends on having an adequate donor and the degree of end-organ damage. The latter is assessed using the Lucarelli staging system that factors in the degree of hepatomegaly, the degree of portal fibrosis, and the quality of the chelation treatment given before the transplant.[135,136] With improved pretransplant care and increased myeloablation and immunosuppression, even the highest risk groups have done well with matched-sibling donors with 90% event-free survival, 96% overall survival, and 7% rejection rates.[136-139]

Gene Therapy

Gene therapy addresses three major barriers to HSCT: graft failure from rejection, the difficulty of finding a suitable donor, and graft-versus-host disease. Though many novel strategies are being evaluated, the open clinical trials use viral vectors containing β-like globin genes to infect a patient's CD34+ hematopoietic progenitors, followed by autologous transplantation. Several patients have become transfusion independent.[140,141] Although numerous approaches are being investigated, most excitingly the technology to perform genome editing to correct thalassemic and SCD mutations is rapidly improving.

Inducers of Other β-Like Genes

Induction of HbF remains the holy grail of β-thalassemia and SCD therapy. After decades of limited success, understanding the multiple pathways involved in globin gene regulation is facilitating the development of multiple classes of novel regulators of HbF.[112-114] Additional approaches are reviewed elsewhere.[110]

Key References

1. Stamatoyannopoulos G. Molecular and cellular basis of hemoglobin switching. In: Steinberg MH, Forget BG, Higgs HR, Weatherall DJ, eds. *Disorders of Hemoglobin*. 2nd ed. Cambridge: Cambridge University Press; 2009:86-100.
3. Key NS, Connes P. Derebail VK. Negative health implications of sickle cell trait in high income countries: from the football field to the laboratory. *Br J Haematol*. 2015;170:5-14.
5. Gill FM, Sleeper LA, Weiner SJ, et al. Clinical events in the first decade in a cohort of infants with sickle cell disease. Cooperative Study of Sickle Cell Disease. *Blood*. 1995;86:776-783.
6. Bender MA, Douthitt Seibel G. Sickle cell disease. In: Pagon RA, Adam MP, Ardinger HH, et al., eds. *GeneReviews® [Internet]*. Seattle, WA: University of Washington, Seattle; 2014.
8. Kato GJ, Gladwin MT, Steinberg MH. Deconstructing sickle cell disease: reappraisal of the role of hemolysis in the development of clinical subphenotypes. *Blood Rev*. 2007;21:37-47.
9. Morris CR. Mechanisms of vasculopathy in sickle cell disease and thalassemia. *Hematology Am Soc Hematol Educ Program*. 2008;177-185.
10. Steinberg MH. Sickle cell anemia, the first molecular disease: overview of molecular etiology, pathophysiology, and therapeutic approaches. *ScientificWorldJournal*. 2008;8:1295-1324.
12. Potoka KP, Gladwin MT. Vasculopathy and pulmonary hypertension in sickle cell disease. *Am J Physiol Lung Cell Mol Physiol*. 2015;308: L314-L324.
17. Yawn BP, Buchanan GR, Afenyi-Annan AN, et al. Management of sickle cell disease: summary of the 2014 evidence-based report by expert panel members. *JAMA*. 2014;312:1033-1048.
18. Bender MA, Douthitt Seibel G. *Sickle Cell Disease: Critical Elements of Care*. 5th ed. Seattle: Seattle Children's Hospital; 2012 January 2012.
20. Ballas SK, Gupta K, Adams-Graves P. Sickle cell pain: a critical reappraisal. *Blood*. 2012;120:3647-3656.
21. Darbari DS, Ballas SK, Clauw DJ. Thinking beyond sickling to better understand pain in sickle cell disease. *Eur J Haematol*. 2014;93:89-95.
25. Ballas SK. Current issues in sickle cell pain and its management. *Hematology Am Soc Hematol Educ Program*. 2007;97-105.
29. Todd KH, Green C, Bonham VL Jr, et al. Sickle cell disease related pain: crisis and conflict. *J Pain*. 2006;7:453-458.
30. Solomon LR. Treatment and prevention of pain due to vaso-occlusive crises in adults with sickle cell disease: an educational void. *Blood*. 2008;111:997-1003.
31. Benjamin LJ, Dampier CD, Jacox AK, et al. *Guideline for the Management of Acute and Chronic Pain in Sickle-Cell Disease*. Glenville, IL: American Pain Association; 1999.
32. Rees DC, Olujohungbe AD, Parker NE, et al. Guidelines for the management of the acute painful crisis in sickle cell disease. *Br J Haematol*. 2003;120:744-752.
40. Vichinsky EP, Styles LA, Colangelo LH, et al. Acute chest syndrome in sickle cell disease: clinical presentation and course. Cooperative Study of Sickle Cell Disease. *Blood*. 1997;89:1787-1792.
41. Vichinsky EP, Neumayr LD, Earles AN, et al. Causes and outcomes of the acute chest syndrome in sickle cell disease. National Acute Chest Syndrome Study Group. *N Engl J Med*. 2000;342:1855-1865.
51. Fartoukh M, Lefort Y, Habibi A, et al. Early intermittent noninvasive ventilation for acute chest syndrome in adults with sickle cell disease: a pilot study. *Intensive Care Med*. 2010;36:1355-1362.
59. Kassim AA, Galadanci NA, Pruthi S, DeBaun MR. How I treat acute strokes and long-term management in sickle cell disease. *Blood*. 2015;125:3401-3410.
65. Venkataraman A, Adams RJ. Neurologic complications of sickle cell disease. *Handb Clin Neurol*. 2014;120:1015-1025.
67. Klings ES, Machado RF, Barst RJ, et al. An official American Thoracic Society clinical practice guideline: diagnosis, risk stratification, and management of pulmonary hypertension of sickle cell disease. *Am J Respir Crit Care Med*. 2014;189:727-740.
69. Gladwin MT, Sachdev V, Jison ML, et al. Pulmonary hypertension as a risk factor for death in patients with sickle cell disease. *N Eng J Med* 2004;350:886-895.
70. Morris CR, Gladwin MT, Kato GJ. Nitric oxide and arginine dysregulation: a novel pathway to pulmonary hypertension in hemolytic disorders. *Curr Mol Med*. 2008;8:620-632.
73. Morris CR, Sidney M, Morris J, et al. Arginine therapy: a new treatment for pulmonary hypertension in sickle cell disease? *Am J Respir Crit Care Med*. 2003;168:63-69.
74. Hassell KL, Eckman JR, Lane PA. Acute multiorgan failure syndrome: a potentially catastrophic complication of severe sickle cell pain episodes. *Am J Med*. 1994;96:155-162.
78. Nath KA, Hebbel RP. Sickle cell disease: renal manifestations and mechanisms. *Nat Rev Nephrol*. 2015;11:161-171.

79. Porter J, Garbowski M. Consequences and management of iron overload in sickle cell disease. *Hematology Am Soc Hematol Educ Program.* 2013;2013:447-456.

80. Rosen CL, Debaun MR, Strunk RC, et al. Obstructive sleep apnea and sickle cell anemia. *Pediatrics.* 2014;134:273-281.

90. Vichinsky EP, Haberkern CM, Neumayr L, et al. A comparison of conservative and aggressive transfusion regimens in the perioperative management of sickle cell disease. The Preoperative Transfusion in Sickle Cell Disease Study Group. *N Engl J Med.* 1995;333:206-213.

91. Howard J, Malfroy M, Llewelyn C, et al. The Transfusion Alternatives Preoperatively in Sickle Cell Disease (TAPS) study: a randomised, controlled, multicentre clinical trial. *Lancet.* 2013;381:930-938.

95. Wong TE, Brandow AM, Lim W, Lottenberg R. Update on the use of hydroxyurea therapy in sickle cell disease. *Blood.* 2014;124:3850-3857. quiz 4004.

99. Smith-Whitley K, Thompson AA. Indications and complications of transfusions in sickle cell disease. *Pediatr Blood Cancer.* 2012;59:358-364.

100. Chou ST. Transfusion therapy for sickle cell disease: a balancing act. *Hematology Am Soc Hematol Educ Program.* 2013;2013:439-446.

107. King A, Shenoy S. Evidence-based focused review of the status of hematopoietic stem cell transplantation as treatment of sickle cell disease and thalassemia. *Blood.* 2014;123:3089-3094, quiz 3210.

111. Vichinsky E. Emerging "A" therapies in hemoglobinopathies: agonists, antagonists, antioxidants, and arginine. *Hematology Am Soc Hematol Educ Program.* 2012;2012:271-275.

115. Rund D, Rachmilewitz E. Beta-thalassemia. *N Engl J Med.* 2005;353: 1135-1146.

120. Kwiatkowski JL. Oral iron chelators. *Pediatr Clin North Am.* 2008;55:461-482, x.

121. Wood JC. Impact of iron assessment by MRI. *Hematology Am Soc Hematol Educ Program.* 2011;2011:443-450.

125. Vichinsky E, Levine L, et al. *Standards of Care Guidelines for Thalassemia.* Oakland: Children's Hospital & Research Center Oakland; 2012.

128. Walker JM. Thalassaemia major and the heart: a toxic cardiomyopathy tamed? *Heart.* 2013;99:827-834.

132. Porter JB, Wood J, Olivieri N, et al. Treatment of heart failure in adults with thalassemia major: response in patients randomised to deferoxamine with or without deferiprone. *J Cardiovasc Magn Reson.* 2013;15:38.

136. Lucarelli G, Isgro A, Sodani P, Gaziev J. Hematopoietic stem cell transplantation in thalassemia and sickle cell anemia. *Cold Spring Harb Perspect Med* 2012;2:a011825.

142. Bellet PS, Kalinyak KA, Shukla R, et al. Incentive spirometry to prevent acute pulmonary complications in sickle cell diseases. *N Engl J Med.* 1995;333:699-703.

Coagulation and Coagulopathy in Critical Illness

Robert I. Parker

PEARLS

- Hemostasis is a dynamic process; once bleeding occurs, clot formation and degradation (fibrinolysis) are also initiated.
- Coagulation is an integral part of inflammation and will often lead to microvascular thrombosis.
- A consumptive coagulopathy should always be considered in a patient with diffuse or generalized bleeding; however, liver disease and vitamin K deficiency are much more common.
- The international normalized ratio is not an appropriate surrogate for the prothrombin time in patients not on vitamin K antagonist anticoagulation, and a prolonged prothrombin time in the presence of liver disease is not an accurate predictor of bleeding risk.
- Localized bleeding in a trauma or postoperative patient is generally the result of an anatomic lesion rather than a systemic coagulopathy.
- Thrombotic events are being recognized with increased frequency in the pediatric intensive care unit; no more than 60% of children with documented thromboses will be found to have an identifiable underlying hematologic abnormality.
- The presence of a central venous catheter is the most common identified thrombotic risk factor in critically ill children.
- rhF.VIIa is effective in controlling bleeding unresponsive to other measures, but its use has not yet been shown to improve outcome.
- The absence of a prolonged prothrombin time or activated partial thromboplastin time does not rule out the possibility of an abnormality in hemostasis.
- Clot formation in vivo is critically dependent on factor VII and tissue factor.

Introduction

Abnormalities in hemostasis often accompany critical illnesses whether as an intrinsic component of the illness (eg, sepsis, trauma) or merely a byproduct or a comorbidity not directly related to the critical illness that resulted in pediatric intensive care unit (PICU) admission. Although many of the abnormalities noted in critical illness may lead to excessive bleeding, not all hemostatic alterations produce the same result. In some, the bleeding may be severe and systemic or relatively mild; in others the imbalance in hemostasis may favor excessive clot formation. In some conditions the abnormality may in fact represent a laboratory artifact that is without clinical manifestations (Table 91.1). For the practicing intensivist to adequately and accurately assess the patient with a potential or clinically apparent hemostatic defect, it is necessary to briefly review the initiation and regulation of hemostasis and how it is measured in the clinical lab.

Overview of Hemostasis

Hemostasis and coagulation are not synonymous. Although coagulation is the process by which blood transforms from a liquid to a solid state (ie, the process of clot formation), hemostasis includes all of the processes in the arrest of bleeding. Additionally, the working definition of hemostasis often includes the restoration of blood to its liquid state through the process of fibrinolysis. Traditionally, coagulation has been presented as a set of discrete units, the "intrinsic," "extrinsic," and "common" pathways, that progress in an orderly nonoverlapping sequence (Fig. 91.1). This depiction is useful when explaining the various tests employed to assess clot formation (eg, prothrombin time [PT], activated partial thromboplastin time [aPTT], thrombin time [TT]). However, this representation of coagulation does not include any involvement of inflammatory mediators, platelets, endothelial cells, adhesive glycoproteins, or thrombolytic factors in the process of hemostasis.

Historically, the "intrinsic" pathway, beginning with the activation of factor XII (F.XII) to activated factor XII (F.XIIa) in contact with some biological or foreign surface, was believed to be physiologically the most important in the initiation of clot formation because deficiencies of either factor VIII (F.VIII) (hemophilia A) or F.IX (hemophilia B) produced a severe bleeding diathesis. However, we now understand that the activation of F.X to F.Xa through the action of the F.VIIa/tissue factor (TF) complex plays a more central role in this process.[1,2] The elements of the clotting cascade act in concert, hence the use of the term *tenase* to describe the action of F.VIIa/TF complex, along with the F.IXa/F.VIIIa complex on the activation of F.X to F.Xa, and the use of the term *prothrombinase* to describe the F.Xa/F.Va complex, which cleaves prothrombin (F.II) to form thrombin (F.IIa). In addition, several points of "crosstalk" exist between the two arms of the clotting cascade, with F.VIIa being able to enhance the activation of F.IX (to F.IXa) and F.XI (to F.XIa), further highlighting the

TABLE 91.1   Overview of Coagulation Disorders Seen in the Intensive Care Unit

Conditions Associated With Serious Bleeding or a High Probability of Bleeding

Disseminated intravascular coagulation
Liver disease/hepatic insufficiency
Vitamin K deficiency/depletion
Massive transfusion syndrome
Anticoagulant overdose (heparin, warfarin)
Thrombocytopenia (drug induced, immunologic)
Acquired platelet defects (drug induced, uremia)

Thrombotic Clinical Syndromes (see Chapter 92)

Thrombotic thrombocytopenia purpura/hemolytic uremic syndrome
Deep venous thrombosis
Pulmonary embolism
Coronary thrombosis/acute myocardial infarction

Laboratory Abnormalities Not Associated With Clinical Bleeding

Lupus anticoagulant
Reactive hyperfibrinogenemia

Other Selected Clinical Syndromes

Hemophilia (A and B)
Specific factor deficiencies associated with specific diseases
    Amyloidosis–factor X, Gaucher disease–factor IX, nephritic syndrome–factor IX, antithrombin III
    Cyanotic congenital heart disease (polycythemia, qualitative platelet defect)
Depressed clotting factor levels (newborns)

central role of F.VIIa and TF in vivo (Fig. 91.2). Furthermore, various "positive feedback" loops involving thrombin enhance the "upstream" activation of the clotting process. The activation of coagulation is initiated from TF, which is found in the subendothelial matrix, on cellular elements (eg, monocytes) and circulating freely in plasma as soluble TF. However, clotting does not occur in free-flowing blood but rather on surfaces. Platelets, endothelial cells, the subendothelial matrix, and biological polymers (catheters, grafts, stents, etc.) provide these surfaces for clot formation, and each plays a critical role in clot formation.

Platelets not only initiate the clot formation through the formation of a platelet plug, but more important, they provide specific proteins that regulate the clotting response (F.VIII, inhibitors of fibrinolysis, etc.) to the area of bleeding and provide a surface on which co-localization of clotting factors occurs for efficient clot formation (Fig. 91.3). Under "normal" (ie, resting, unstimulated) conditions, platelets do not adhere to the vascular endothelium, but upon stimulation or when the endothelium is mechanically disrupted (eg, cut) or activated by inflammation, platelets will adhere to the endothelial cell or subendothelial matrix via a von Willebrand factor-dependent mechanism. Once adherent, activated platelets secrete various molecules that further enhance platelet adherence and aggregation, vascular contraction, clot formation, and wound healing.[3]

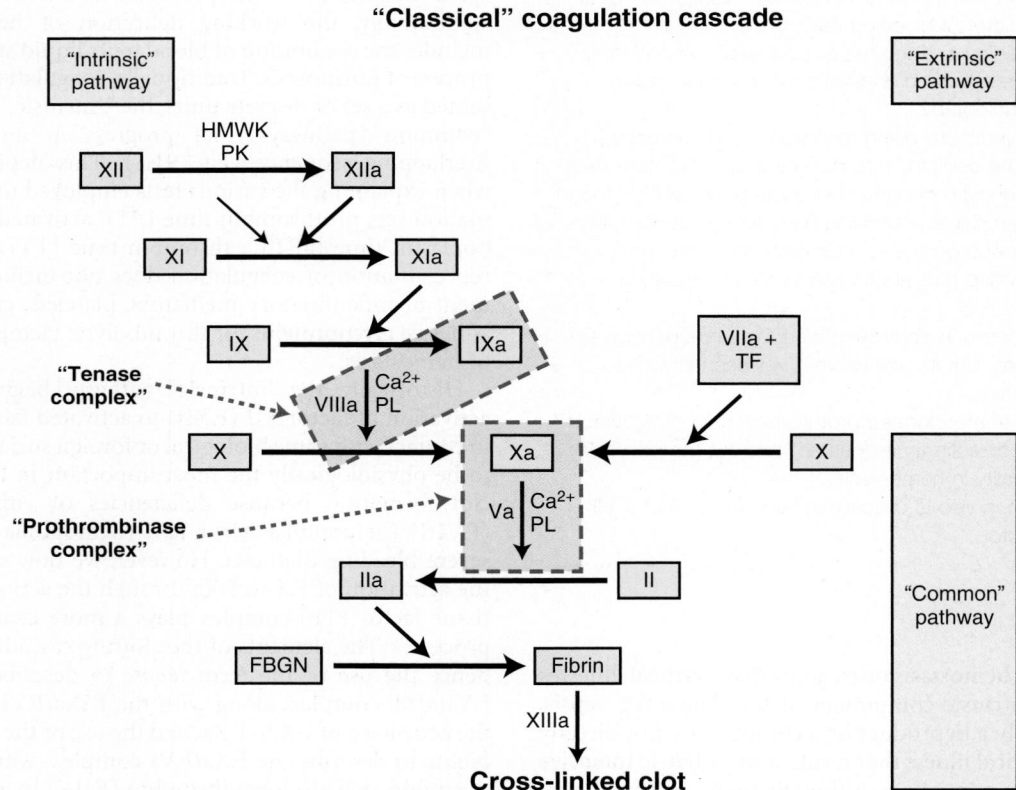

Fig. 91.1. Coagulation is initiated either through the "intrinsic" pathway by activation of factor XII in the presence of high-molecular-weight kininogen (HMWK) and prekallikrein (PK) or through activation of the "extrinsic" pathway by tissue factor. Roman numerals indicate zymogen clotting factors; "a" indicates activated forms of the clotting factors. (Factor II is prothrombin and F.IIa is thrombin); *FBGN,* fibrinogen

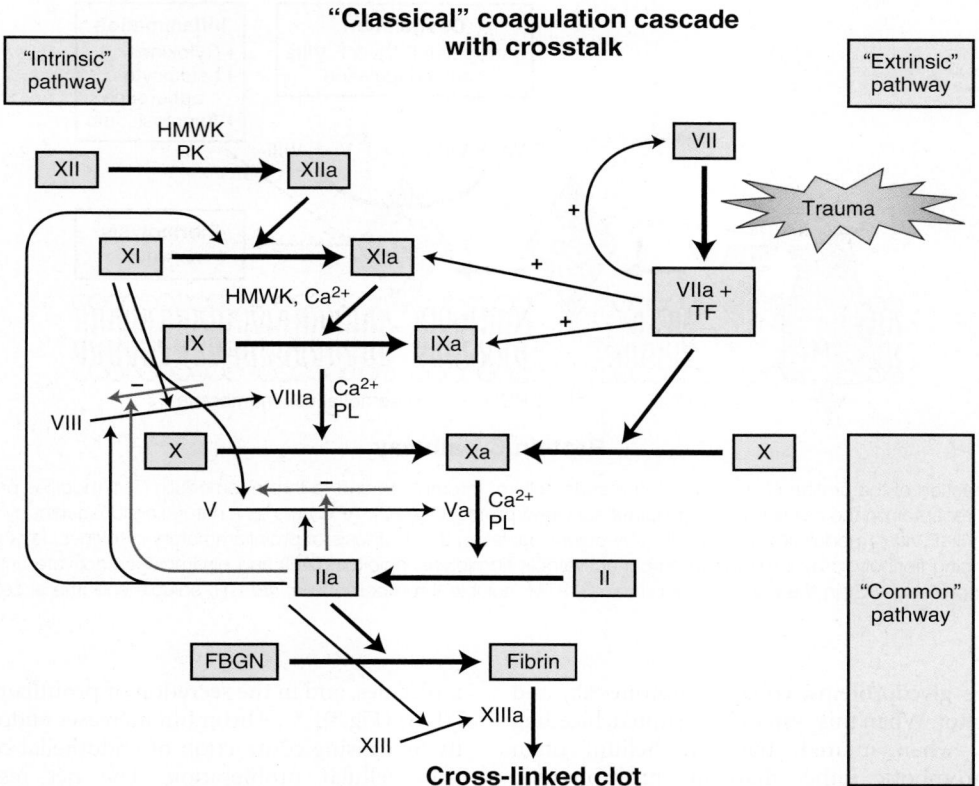

Fig. 91.2. Modified clotting cascade indicating crosstalk between the intrinsic and extrinsic pathways by the action of factor VIIa/tissue factor (TF) enhancing the conversion of factor XI to activated factor XI (XIa) and factor IX to IXa. *HK,* high-molecular-weight kininogen; *PK,* prekallikrein; *PL,* phospholipid.

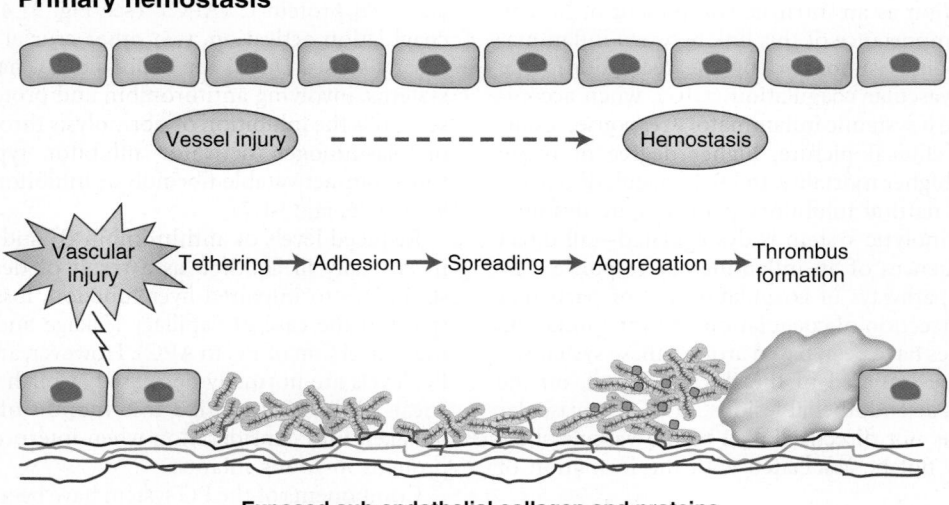

Fig. 91.3. The role of platelets in mediating primary hemostasis at sites of vascular injury. Platelets are initially activated and express specific adhesion receptors on their surface, followed by adhesion to activated endothelial cells and exposed subendothelial components (eg, collagen, von Willebrand factor). Subsequent platelet aggregation occurs with the development of a primary platelet plug. Coagulation occurs on the developing platelet plug with the creation of a fibrin clot.

The endothelium is a specialized organ that is integral to the regulation of hemostasis; it presents a nonthrombogenic surface to flowing blood and enhances clot formation when the endothelium is disrupted by trauma or injured by infection or inflammation[4,5] (see also Chapter 27). This process involves multiple components of the protein C pathway (Fig. 91.4). The normal endothelium produces inhibitors of blood coagulation and platelet activation and modulates vascular tone and permeability. Endothelial cells also synthesize and secrete components of the subendothelial extracellular matrix,

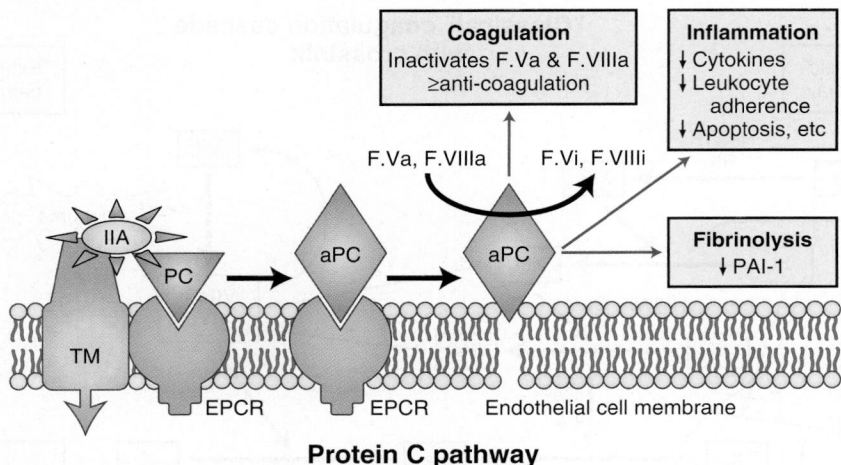

Protein C pathway

Fig. 91.4. The interaction of the protein C system with the endothelium: thrombin bound to thrombomodulin (TM) modifies protein C bound to the endothelial protein C receptor on the cell surface to generate activated protein C (APC). APC acts as a natural anticoagulant by inactivating activated factors V (F.Va) and VIII (F.VIIIa), modulating inflammation by down-regulating the synthesis of proinflammatory cytokines, leukocyte adherence, and apoptosis and enhancing fibrinolysis by inhibiting thrombin-activatable fibrinolysis inhibitor (TAFI) and plasminogen activator inhibitor type 1 (PAI-1). *C4Bbp,* C4b binding protein; *+PS,* in the presence of protein S; *sTM,* soluble thrombomodulin; *sEPCR,* soluble endothelial cell protein C receptor.

including adhesive glycoproteins, collagen, fibronectin, and von Willebrand factor. When this system is disrupted, bleeding occurs. However, when injured, the endothelium often becomes a prothrombotic rather than an antithrombotic organ, and unwanted clot formation may occur.

Interaction of Coagulation and Inflammation

Coagulation has been identified as an integral part of the immune response, and evidence exists that this system developed during evolution as an intrinsic component of human host defense. The importance of this link between inflammation and coagulation is supported by the recognition that disseminated intravascular coagulation (DIC), when accompanied by sepsis and a systemic inflammatory response, results in a more severe clinical picture, higher degree of organ dysfunction, and a higher mortality. In DIC, coagulation pathways are activated, natural inhibitory pathways are dysfunctional, and the fibrinolytic system is dysregulated—all direct or indirect consequences of an inflammatory response. The natural inhibitory pathways of coagulation are of particular interest in this intersection of coagulation and inflammation, as potential therapies have been based around these systems.[6,7] Coagulation may be initiated in the flowing blood, on the endothelial surface, at endothelial lesions, in the perivascular tissues, and in areas not directly linked to the vascular bed, and it may or may not be associated with the formation of fibrin clots.[6]

During sepsis, TF expression is up-regulated in activated monocytes and endothelial cells as a response to endotoxin and other pathogen-associated/pathogen-initiated events, with the consequence being the secretion of proinflammatory cytokines and activation of coagulation leading to increased thrombin generation. Prior to its neutralization by antithrombin, thrombin plays a central role in coagulation and inflammation through the induction of procoagulant, anticoagulant, inflammatory, and mitogenic responses.[8] Thrombin results in the activation, aggregation, and lysis of leukocytes and platelets, in increased expression of endothelial adhesion

molecules, and in the secretion of proinflammatory cytokines (IL-6) (Fig. 91.5). Thrombin increases endothelial permeability by causing contraction of endothelial cells; it also stimulates cellular proliferation. The net result of thrombin generation is production of a procoagulant state; it leads to the formation of fibrin; activates coagulation factors V, VIII, IX, XI; and leads to the expression of TF and von Willebrand factor and the aggregation of platelets. However, thrombin also has antiinflammatory effects through the production of activated protein C (APC)[8] (see Fig. 91.4). Concurrent with coagulation activation, two other crucial mechanisms occur during sepsis. One is the depression of natural anticoagulant systems, involving antithrombin and protein C (PC), and the second is the inhibition of fibrinolysis through the production of plasminogen activator inhibitor type 1 (PAI-1) and thrombin-activatable fibrinolysis inhibitor (TAFI) (Figs. 91.4, 91.5, 91.6, and 91.7).

Reduced levels of antithrombin III and PC may also occur in critically ill children as a result of decreased production secondary to impaired liver function, loss from the vascular space in the case of capillary leakage and consumption (eg, the conversion of PC to APC). However, antithrombin-III and PC levels are normally decreased at birth and do not achieve "near-adult" levels until 3 to 6 months of age; this fact must be taken into consideration when interpreting levels of these proteins in young infants.

Components of the PC system have been shown to be major regulators of coagulation (ie, natural anticoagulants) with decreased activity of this pathway resulting in pathologic thrombosis, and they have been shown to possess intrinsic immunomodulating properties (see Fig. 91.4). In vitro, APC inhibits tumor necrosis factor-α elaboration from monocytes, blocks leukocyte adhesion to selectins, and influences apoptosis.[8] The PC pathway is engaged when thrombin binds to thrombomodulin on the surface of the endothelial cells. In vivo, binding of PC to the endothelial cell PC receptor (EPCR) augments PC activation by the thrombin-thrombomodulin complex more than 10-fold. This receptor is shed from

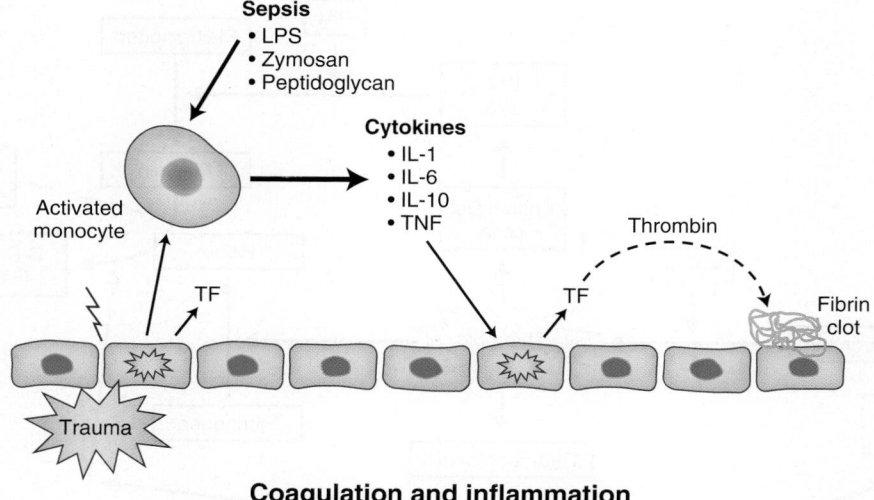

Coagulation and inflammation

Fig. 91.5. Inflammation enhances coagulation through the induction of proinflammatory cytokines that induce tissue factor formation, which in turn decreases activated protein C (APC) formation, leading to enhanced thrombin and fibrin generation. In addition, the decrease in APC allows for greater inhibition of fibrinolysis through the action of plasminogen activator inhibitor type 1 (PAI-1).

PAI-1 in coagulation and fibrinolysis

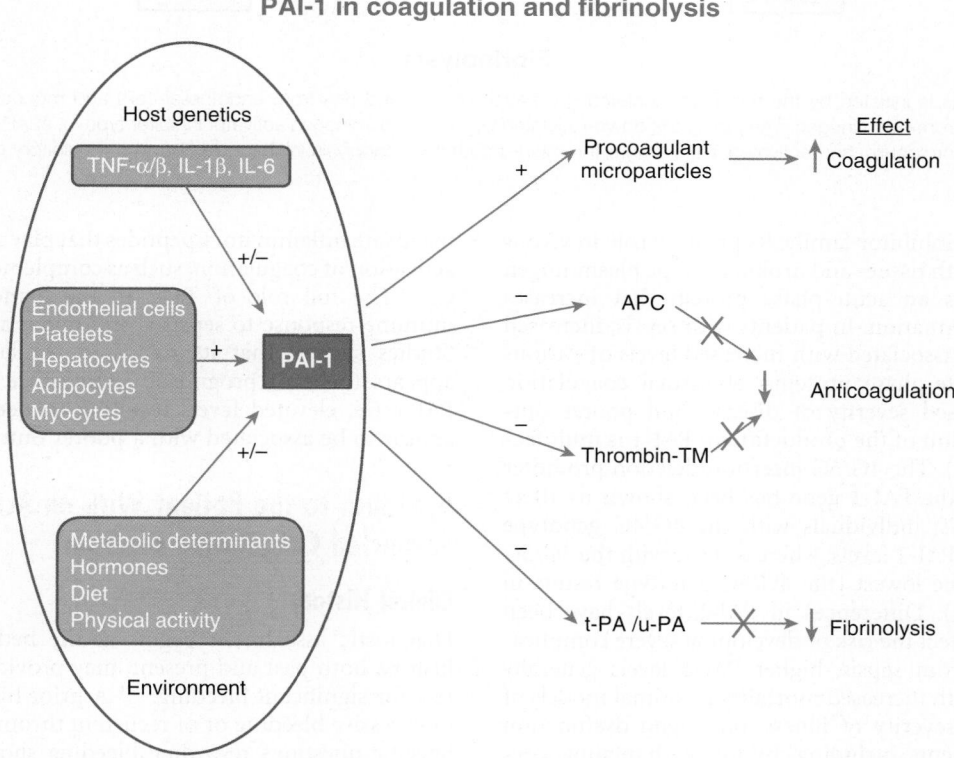

Fig. 91.6. Genetic and environmental influences on the expression of plasminogen activator inhibitor type 1 (PAI-1) and the importance of PAI-1 in the coagulation and fibrinolysis pathways. *TNF-α,* tumor necrosis factor-α; *APC,* activated protein C; *TM,* thrombomodulin; *t-PA,* tissue-type plasminogen activator; *u-PA,* urokinase-type plasminogen activator. (Modified from Hermans PW, Hazelzet JA. Plasminogen activator inhibitor type 1 gene polymorphism and sepsis. Clin Infect Dis. 2005; 41[suppl 7]:S453-458, with permission.)

endothelial cells upon exposure to inflammatory mediators and thrombin, thereby down-regulating PC activation in sepsis and inflammation. Additionally, it may also translocate from the plasma membrane to the nucleus, where it redirects gene expression. During translocation it can carry APC to the

nucleus, possibly accounting for the ability of APC to modulate inflammatory mediator responses in the endothelium.[8]

The third important property of APC is its influence on fibrinolysis. APC is capable of neutralizing the fibrinolysis inhibitors PAI-1 and TAFI. PAI-1 is a 50-kDa glycoprotein of

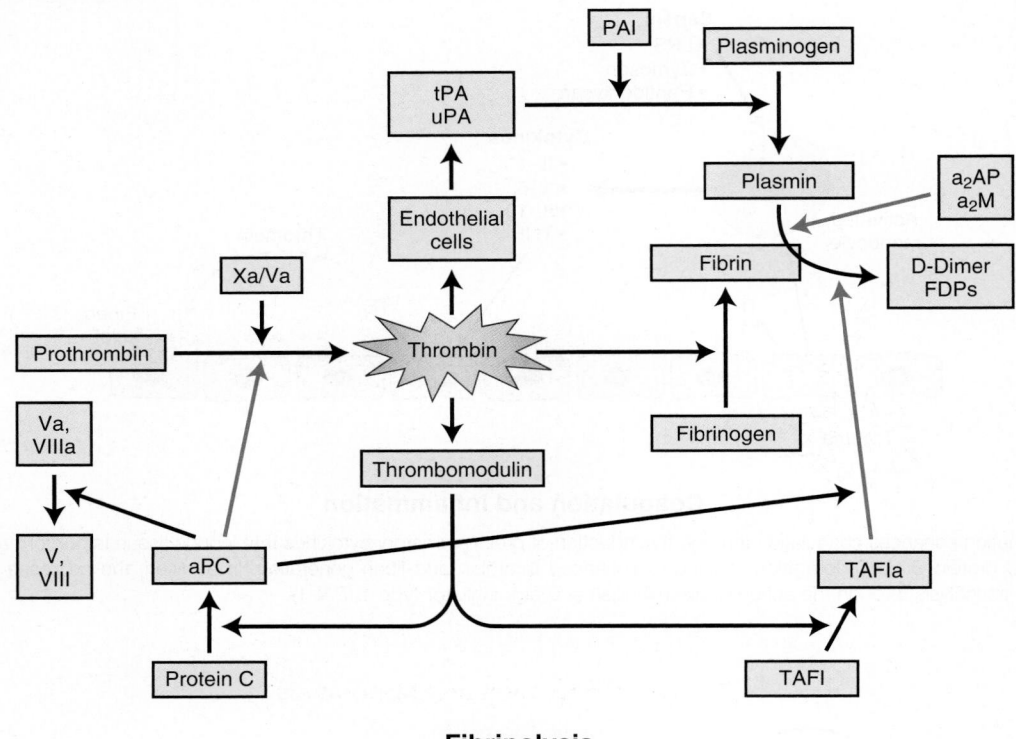

Fibrinolysis

Fig. 91.7. Fibrinolysis is initiated by the thrombin-mediated generation of uPA and tPA from endothelial cells and monocytes with subsequent generation of plasmin from plasminogen. The process is down-regulated by PAI-1 (plasminogen activator inhibitor type 1), a2AP (alpha-2-antiplasmin), and a2M (alpha-2-micorglobulin) and activated TAFI. *TAFIa,* thrombin-activatable fibrinolysis inhibitor; red arrows = inhibitory pathways.

the serine protease inhibitor family. Its primary role in vivo is the inhibition of both tissue- and urokinase-type plasminogen activators. PAI-1 is an acute-phase protein that increases during acute inflammation. In patients with sepsis, increased levels of PAI-1 are associated with increased levels of various cytokines and acute-phase proteins, abnormal coagulation parameters, increased severity of disease, and poorer outcomes. The regulation of the production of PAI-1 is multifactorial (see Fig. 91.6). The 4G/5G insertion/deletion promoter polymorphism of the PAI-1 gene has been shown to affect PAI-1 plasma levels; individuals with the 4G/4G genotype display the highest PAI-1 levels, whereas those with the 5G/5G genotype display the lowest (the 4G/5G genotype results in intermediate levels). Differences in PAI-1 levels have been demonstrated to affect the risk of developing severe complications and death from sepsis, higher PAI-1 levels generally being associated with increased mortality in animal models of sepsis and higher severity of illness and organ dysfunction scores in septic patients, including children with meningococcal sepsis.[9-11] However, the regulation of PAI-1 levels is complex involving not only promoters of synthesis. Activated protein C can stimulate fibrinolysis by forming a tight 1:1 complex with PAI-1, leading to inactivation of this fibrinolysis inhibitor. High levels of thrombin lead to increased levels of activated protein C, which can complex to PAI-1. This complex is subsequently cleared from the circulation, resulting in PC depletion.[10]

Thrombin generation also increases the levels of TAFI, also known as carboxypeptidase R. TAFI is an important negative regulator of the fibrinolytic system and has been shown to

inactivate inflammatory peptides that play a role in the contact activation of coagulation, such as complement factors C3a and C5a. The full role of TAFI in the hemostatic and innate immune response to sepsis is still under active investigation. Studies suggest that its role as a regulator of fibrinolysis appears to be of prognostic significance similar to that of PAI-1 (ie, elevated levels resulting in decreased fibrinolysis appear to be associated with a poorer outcome in sepsis).[12-14]

Approach to the Patient With an Actual or Suspected Coagulation Disorder

Clinical History

Diagnostic assessment begins at the bedside. The medical history, both past and present, may provide insights into the risk for significant bleeding.[15,16] A prior history of prolonged or excessive bleeding or of recurrent thrombosis is important. Specific questions regarding bleeding should investigate the occurrence of any of the following: spontaneous, easy, or disproportionately severe bruising; intramuscular hematoma formation (either spontaneous or related to trauma); spontaneous or trauma-induced hemarthrosis; spontaneous mucous membrane bleeding; prior problems with bleeding related to surgery (including dental extractions, tonsillectomy, and circumcision); the need for unanticipated transfusions in the past; menstrual history; and, finally, current medications.

In spite of the decreased general use of aspirin in children, there remain numerous over-the-counter aspirin-containing medications that can potentially interfere with platelet-mediated primary hemostasis. Patients (and parents) may not be aware of the aspirin contained in these products. High doses of over-the-counter and prescription nonsteroidal antiinflammatory medications (eg, ibuprofen, naproxen-sodium) may also impair platelet function. However, unlike aspirin, which produces a noncompetitive inhibition of platelets, the inhibition caused by these other NSAIDs is competitive and resolves once the drug is no longer present. Many of the drugs used in the ICU are also associated with bleeding abnormalities and are discussed later. In trauma situations (either surgical or accidental), it is important to determine the severity of injury relative to the magnitude of bleeding that follows. A prior personal history (or strong family history) of significant thrombosis (eg, deep venous thrombosis, pulmonary embolus, stroke) also suggests the possibility of the presence of a hypercoagulable condition. As thrombotic events are generally uncommon in children, the occurrence of thrombotic events, particularly early cardiovascular events such as myocardial infarction in young adult relatives should cause the clinician to consider the presence of a congenital thrombophilic abnormality in the patient. These abnormalities include antithrombin-III deficiency, PC or S deficiency, the presence of the factor V Leiden R506Q mutation, the prothrombin G20210A polymorphism/mutation, and (possibly) the C677T mutation/polymorphism of the methylenetetrahydrofolate reductase (MTHFR) gene (discussed later). In addition, vasculitis associated with an autoimmune disorder such as systemic lupus erythematosus must always be considered in the evaluation of a child with an unexplained pathologic clot. In all cases, the family history is important in attempting to separate congenital from acquired disorders.

In a general sense, defects in primary or secondary hemostasis can be separated according to the nature of the bleeding. Patients with primary hemostatic defects tend to manifest "capillary-type bleeding"—oozing from cuts or incisions, mucous membrane bleeding, or excessive bruising. This type of bleeding is seen in patients with quantitative or qualitative platelet defects or von Willebrand disease. In contrast, patients with dysfunction of secondary hemostasis (ie, fibrin clot formation) tend to display "large-vessel bleeding," characterized by hemarthrosis, intramuscular hematomas, and the like. This type of bleeding is most often associated with specific coagulation factor deficiencies or inhibitors. However, patients with severe platelet-type defects may also manifest this type of bleeding. Consequently, the presence of only mucosal bleeding is more helpful as this would point to a platelet-type defect affecting mainly primary hemostasis rather than an abnormality of fibrin clot formation (ie, a coagulopathy).

Physical Examination

Development of generalized bleeding in critically ill patients in the ICU presents a special problem. Such bleeding is often a marker of severe underlying multiorgan system dysfunction. Thus correction of the coagulopathy usually requires improvement in the patient's overall clinical status. Supportive evidence or physical findings of other concurrent organ system dysfunction (eg, renal failure, respiratory failure, hypotension) often are readily apparent. With the exception of massive transfusion syndrome (discussed later), generalized bleeding in critically ill children and infants is often caused by sepsis-related DIC.[17,18] However, the clinician must also consider the coagulopathy of severe liver dysfunction,

undiagnosed congenital bleeding disorders (eg, hemophilia, von Willebrand disease), nonaccidental injury, or vitamin K deficiency in newborns or older children with malabsorption in the differential diagnosis.[17-19] In young infants (<3 months of age), the coagulation system is often not yet mature, and prolongation of the prothrombin time (PT) or activated partial thromboplastin time (aPTT) may not reflect an abnormality in hemostasis.[20] Consequently, the intensivist must also take this into consideration when interpreting "abnormal" results. In these cases, consultation with a pediatric hematologist may be indicated.

The physical examination of the patient with a bleeding disorder should address several basic questions. Is the process localized or diffuse? Is it related to an anatomic or surgical lesion? Is the bleeding primarily mucocutaneous? Finally, when appropriate, are there signs of thrombosis (either arterial or venous)? The answers to these questions may provide clues to the cause of the problem (primary versus secondary hemostatic dysfunction).

During the general examination, particular attention should be paid to the presence of several specific physical findings that may be helpful in determining the etiology of a suspected hemostatic abnormality. For example, the presence of an enlarged spleen coupled with thrombocytopenia suggests that splenic sequestration may be a contributor to the observed thrombocytopenia. Splenomegaly accompanied by prolongation of the PT or aPTT may be a consequence of underlying liver disease, whereas splenomegaly in the presence of normal PT and aPTT may indicate that a marrow infiltrative process may be present. Further, evidence of liver disease (eg, portal hypertension, ascites) points to decreased clotting factor synthesis as a possible etiology of a prolonged PT or aPTT. When lymphadenopathy, splenomegaly, or other findings suggestive of disseminated malignancy are detected, acute or chronic DIC should be suspected as the cause of prolonged coagulation times, hypofibrinogenemia, or thrombocytopenia. Purpura that are palpable suggest capillary leak from vasculitis. In contrast, purpura associated with thrombocytopenia or qualitative platelet defects are generally not elevated and cannot be distinguished by touch. Finally, venous and arterial telangiectasia may be seen in von Willebrand disease and liver disease, respectively. When selective pressure is centrally applied to an arterial telangiectasia, the entire lesion fades, whereas a venous telangiectasia requires confluent pressure across the entire lesion (as with a glass slide) for blanching to occur.

Diagnostic Laboratory Evaluation

Before discussion of the appropriate tests that enable the clinician to interpret information from the history, physical examination, or previously obtained (and often confusing) laboratory data, the importance of correct specimen collection for hemostatic evaluation must be emphasized. In the PICU, it is common for laboratory samples to be drawn through an indwelling arterial or central venous cannula, often because other access is no longer available. Therefore, heparin may be present, either in solutions used to flush the cannula or transduce a waveform or as a component of the IV infusion. Depending on the concentration of heparin in the infusing fluid and the volume of blood withdrawn, several tests can be influenced. Fibrin degradation products (FDPs) can be falsely elevated and fibrinogen falsely low. Likewise, the PT, aPTT, and thrombin time (TT) can be spuriously prolonged. Therefore, a minimum of 20 mL of blood in adolescents and adults (10 mL of blood in younger children) should be withdrawn through the cannula and either discarded or used for other purposes before obtaining a specimen for laboratory hemostasis analysis.[21] This practice should minimize any influence of heparin on the results. In young children and infants, it may not be reasonable to withdraw this volume of blood (even with the use of blood conservation techniques), and a peripheral venipuncture may be necessary. Because the aPTT is sensitive to the presence of small amounts of heparin, the presence of an unexpected prolonged aPTT obtained through a heparinized catheter should raise the suspicion of sample contamination. In this setting, the TT will also be prolonged but will normalize if the contaminating heparin is neutralized (eg, with toluidine blue or Hemasorb).

The presence of most suspected bleeding disorders can be confirmed using routinely available tests, including evaluation of the peripheral blood smear (including an estimate of the platelet count and platelet and red blood cell morphologic features); measurement of the PT, aPTT, and the TT; and assays for fibrinogen, the presence of FDPs, or the D-dimer fragment of polymerized fibrin. This latter test is more specific for the fibrinolytic fragment produced when polymerized fibrin monomer, produced through the action of thrombin on fibrinogen, is cleaved by the proteolytic enzyme plasmin. In contrast, the older assays for FDPs or fibrin split products will be positive even if fibrin is not produced and the fragments are the result of proteolytic degradation of native fibrinogen. Discretion should be used in determining which of these tests

are most appropriate for assessment; they need not be ordered as a blanket panel on all patients with known or suspected bleeding disorders. Several major categories of hemorrhagic disorders and the tests that are characteristically abnormal in each are summarized in Table 91.2. In most instances, measurement of the platelet count, fibrinogen level, PT, aPTT, and TT should provide sufficient information for determining the correct diagnosis—or at least for making an educated guess. By using these five screening tests and assessing other, more specific tests only when an absolute diagnosis is necessary, inappropriate use of laboratory resources may be avoided.

Patients who present with a thrombotic event will generally not display abnormalities of usual "clotting" studies—that is, their PT, aPTT, TT, and fibrinogen will usually be within normal ranges. The finding of a shortened PT or aPTT is not necessarily indicative of a prothrombotic or thrombophilic process being present. Although hyperfibrinogenemia and persistent elevations of F.VIII have been associated with an increased risk of thrombosis, both may be elevated by acute inflammation. Consequently, the finding of elevations of these clotting factors in a patient who has experienced an unexpected thrombotic event may not necessarily indicate that the cause of the event was an elevation in either factor; without prior samples, it is impossible to determine if the elevation is the consequence of the thrombosis or was present prior to its development and potentially causative.

Several inherited or acquired abnormalities that place an individual at increased risk for thrombosis have been identified, and determination of these factors should be undertaken when a thrombotic event is suspected or documented. Prior to initiation of anticoagulation, plasma levels of PC (antigen

TABLE 91.2	**Hemorrhagic Syndromes and Associated Laboratory Findings**	
Clinical Syndrome	**Screening Tests**	**Supportive Tests**
Disseminated intravascular coagulation	Prolonged PT, aPTT, TT; decreased fibrinogen, platelets; microangiopathy	(+) FDPs, D-dimer; decreased factors V, VIII, and II (late)
Massive transfusion	Prolonged PT, aPTT; decreased fibrinogen, platelets ± prolonged TT	All factors decreased; (−) FDPs, D-dimer (unless DIC develops); (+) transfusion history
Anticoagulant Overdose		
Heparin	Prolonged aPTT, TT; ± prolonged PT	Toluidine blue/protamine corrects TT; reptilase time normal
Warfarin (same as vitamin K deficiency)	Prolonged PT; ± prolonged aPTT (severe); normal TT, fibrinogen, platelets	Vitamin K–dependent factors decreased; factors V, VIII normal
Liver Disease		
Early	Prolonged PT	Decreased factor VII
Late	Prolonged PT, aPTT; decreased fibrinogen (terminal liver failure); normal platelet count (if splenomegaly absent)	Decreased factors II, V, VII, IX, and X; decreased plasminogen; ± FDPs unless DIC develops
Primary fibrinolysis	Prolonged PT, aPTT, TT; decreased fibrinogen ± platelets decreased	(+) FDPs, (−) D-dimer; short euglobulin clot lysis time
Thrombotic thrombocytopenic purpura	Thrombocytopenia, microangiopathy with mild anemia; PT, aPTT, fibrinogen generally within normal limits/mildly abnormal	ADAMTS13 deficiency/inhibitor, unusually large von Willebrand factor multimers between episodes; mild increase in FDPs or D-dimer
Hemolytic uremic syndrome	Microangiopathic hemolytic anemia, ± thrombocytopenia; PT, aPTT generally within normal limits	Renal insufficiency; FDPs and D-dimer generally (−)

aPTT, activated partial thromboplastin time; *FDPs,* fibrin degradation products; *PT,* prothrombin time; *TT,* thrombin time.

and activity), protein S (antigen and activity; total and free), and antithrombin-III (antigen and activity) should be obtained. In addition, polymerase chain reaction (PCR) analysis for mutations in the F.V (F.V Leiden; R506Q, and prothrombin [G20210A]) genes should be performed. In addition, a baseline serum homocysteine may be obtained, as the thrombosis risk of the MTHFR mutation may be related to elevations of homocysteine caused by alterations in the metabolism of folic acid rather than the mutation per se. Analysis of population-based data has called into question the prior interpretation that the MTHFR C677T polymorphism/ mutation is an independent risk factor for thrombosis in the absence of an elevated serum homocysteine.[22-24] However, as there are numerous well described cases of idiopathic thrombosis occurring in patients for whom the only identified risk factor is the presence of the C677T mutation, it cannot be conclusively stated that the presence of the MTHFR C677T mutation without elevations of serum homocysteine results in no increased risk for pathologic thrombosis. In adult populations, ~40% of patients with thrombosis will not display one of the known thrombophilic risk factors, and it is likely that the percentage in children who are negative for these abnormalities is at least as high or higher. The intensivist must look for confounding clinical conditions, such as dehydration (particularly in the case of central venous sinus thrombosis in infants and young children), indwelling catheters, vascular compression (eg, cervical ribs), type-II heparin-induced thrombocytopenia (see below), and the like in evaluating a patient with thrombosis.

Potentially Serious Acquired Bleeding Disorders

Disseminated Intravascular Coagulation and Other Microangiopathic Consumptive Disorders

Pathogenesis

Because it often occurs in conjunction with other life-threatening disorders, DIC is one of the most serious hemostatic abnormalities seen in the PICU. The clinical syndrome itself results from the activation of blood coagulation, which then leads to excessive thrombin generation. The result of this process is the widespread formation of fibrin thrombi in the microcirculation, with resultant consumption of certain clotting factors and platelets. Ultimately, this consumption is largely responsible for the development of significant bleeding, as the rate of consumption outpaces the rate at which the clotting factors and platelets are produced.[25] Several specific conditions associated with the development of DIC are presented in Table 91.3. In general, the conditions associated with DIC are the same in adults and children and include a wide variety of disorders, the common feature of which is their ability to initiate coagulation to varying degrees. The mechanisms involved generally can be considered in two categories: (1) those intrinsic processes that enzymatically activate procoagulant proteins and (2) those that cause the release of TF, which then triggers coagulation. These are complex events that can lead to significant bleeding and often complicate the management of an already critically ill child.

Fibrinolysis invariably accompanies thrombin formation in DIC,[25] and thrombin generation or release of the tissue plasminogen activator usually initiates this process. Plasmin is generated and then digests fibrinogen and fibrin clots as they

TABLE 91.3	Underlying Diseases Associated With Disseminated Intravascular Coagulation
Sepsis	Retained placenta
Liver disease	Hypertonic saline abortion
Shock	Amniotic fluid embolus
Penetrating brain injury	Retention of a dead fetus
Necrotizing pneumonitis	Eclampsia
Tissue necrosis/crush injury	Localized endothelial injury
Intravascular hemolysis	(aortic aneurysm, giant
Acute promyelocytic leukemia	hemangiomata, angiography)
Thermal injury	
Freshwater drowning	Disseminated malignancy
Fat embolism syndrome	(prostate, pancreatic)

form. Plasmin also inactivates several activated coagulation factors and impairs platelet aggregation. As such, DIC represents an imbalance between the activity of thrombin, which leads to microvascular thrombi with coagulation factor and platelet consumption, and plasmin, which degrades these fibrin-based clots as they form. Therefore, thrombin-induced coagulation factor consumption, thrombocytopenia, and plasmin generation contribute to the presence of bleeding. Globally, DIC represents an imbalance between clot formation (coagulation) and clot breakdown (fibrinolysis). Initially, DIC is a thrombotic disorder characterized by microvascular thrombosis with bleeding occurring only when the consumption of platelets and clotting factors outpaces the ability to replace these critical elements.

In addition to bleeding complications, the presence of fibrin thrombi in the microcirculation can lead to ischemic tissue injury. Pathologic data indicate that renal failure, acrocyanosis, multifocal pulmonary emboli, and transient cerebral ischemia may be related clinically to the presence of such thrombi. The presence of fibrinopeptides A and B (resulting from enzymatic cleavage of fibrinogen) leads to pulmonary and systemic vasoconstriction, which can potentiate an existing ischemic injury. In a given patient with DIC, either bleeding or thrombotic tendencies may predominate; in most patients, bleeding is usually the predominant problem. However, in up to 10% of patients with DIC, the presentation is exclusively thrombotic (eg, pulmonary emboli with pulmonary hypertension, renal insufficiency, altered mental status, acrocyanosis) without hemorrhage. Whether the presentation of DIC is thrombotic, hemorrhagic, or "compensated" (that is, laboratory results are consistent with DIC without overt bleeding), microthrombosis likely contributes to the development and progression of multiorgan failure.

Clinical Presentation and Diagnosis

DIC is often suspected when there is unexplained, generalized oozing or bleeding; unexplained, abnormal laboratory parameters of hemostasis; or both. This usually occurs in the context of a suggestive clinical scenario or associated disease (see Table 91.3). Although infection and multiple trauma are the most common underlying conditions associated with the

TABLE 91.4	Laboratory Tests for the Diagnosis of Disseminated Intravascular Coagulation

Test	Discriminator Value
Platelet count	<80-100,000 or a decrease of >50% from baseline
Fibrinogen	<100 mg/dL or a decrease of >50% from baseline
Prothrombin time	>3-sec prolongation above upper limit of normal
Fibrin degradation products	>80 mg/dL
D-dimer	"Moderate" increase

development of DIC, certain other organ system dysfunctions predispose to DIC, including hepatic insufficiency and splenectomy.[17,18] Both of these conditions are associated with impaired reticuloendothelial system function and consequent impaired clearance of activated coagulation proteins and fibrin/fibrinogen degradation fragments, which may inhibit fibrin polymerization and clot formation.

The clinical severity of DIC has traditionally been assessed by the severity of bleeding and coagulation abnormalities. Scoring tools that employ a panel of laboratory tests along with severity of illness scores to assess the likelihood and severity of DIC have been proposed in an attempt to determine prognosis at the time of diagnosis to better direct initial therapy. The tests most commonly employed in many of these scoring systems for the diagnosis of DIC are listed in Table 91.4. Although no data exist for pediatric patients, this approach does have prognostic value, particularly in patients with sepsis.[26-28] The more commonly employed scoring systems identify those patients at higher or lesser risk for having DIC based on either a qualitative or quantitative score.[29,30] Although each has been shown to be useful in identifying patients with suspected or confirmed DIC, they have not been fully validated for critically ill children. Limited studies have shown that early identification of DIC, before the onset of a gross hemorrhagic diathesis, improves survival in critically ill children.[29,30]

The combination of a prolonged PT, hypofibrinogenemia, thrombocytopenia, and evidence of microangiopathic hemolysis on peripheral blood smear (ie, RBC schistocytes) in the appropriate clinical setting is sufficient to suspect the diagnosis of DIC in most instances. Severe hepatic insufficiency (with splenomegaly and splenic sequestration of platelets) can yield a similar laboratory profile and must be ruled out. In addition to liver disease, several other conditions have presentations similar to DIC and must be considered in the differential diagnosis; they include the coagulopathy of massive transfusion, primary fibrinolysis, thrombotic thrombocytopenic purpura (TTP), atypical hemolytic uremic syndrome (aHUS), heparin therapy, and dysfibrinogenemia.

Although TTP and HUS demonstrate findings consistent with a microangiopathy, the coagulation profile noted with these disorders generally does not strongly suggest DIC. Conversely, the conditions that may present a coagulation profile suggestive of DIC generally do not manifest peripheral blood findings of microangiopathic hemolysis. A comparison of the laboratory findings in these disorders is noted in Table 91.2.

To confirm a diagnosis of suspected DIC, tests that indicate increased fibrinogen turnover (ie, elevated FDPs or D-dimer assay) may be necessary. The D-dimer assay, which measures the D-D fragment of polymerized fibrin, has been shown to be both highly sensitive and specific for proteolytic degradation of polymerized fibrin (fibrin clot that has been produced in the presence of thrombin). Consequently, this test is employed with increasing frequency in patients with suspected DIC and is often stated to be the preferred test of fibrin/fibrinogen consumption. However, remembering that thrombin is produced whenever coagulation is activated in the presence of bleeding, the clinician must interpret a modest elevation of D-dimer in a postoperative or trauma patient with some degree of caution. The presence of a marked elevation of D-dimer in a nonbleeding patient essentially excludes primary fibrinogenolysis as the sole cause of measurable FDPs in the serum. The TT is a less sensitive test for DIC, but it may be useful in cases of suspected heparin overdose, because it corrects in the test tube with the addition of protamine sulfate or toluidine blue. Similarly, the euglobulin clot lysis time may not be sensitive to fibrinolysis associated with DIC but is significantly shortened in most cases of primary fibrino(geno) lysis. Other tests of purported value, such as soluble fibrin monomer or thrombin-antithrombin complex formation, either have problems with sensitivity or are impractical for widespread use outside of a research setting.

Meningococcal Purpura Fulminans

Purpura fulminans is a systemic coagulopathy similar, if not identical, to DIC that classically accompanies meningococcal sepsis and is sporadically noted with other similarly severe infections. The hallmark of this syndrome is tissue ischemia and necrosis due to marked microvascular thrombosis. Patients are generally noted to have severely depressed levels of PC; the degree of suppression has been shown to correlate with mortality. The presence of the PAI-1 4G/4G genotype associated with the highest plasma levels of PAI-1 has been described in patients with meningococcal sepsis and has been shown to be associated with increased sepsis and mortality but not with an increased incidence of meningococcal meningitis.[13] As mentioned before, APC can stimulate fibrinolysis by forming a tight 1:1 complex with PAI-1 thereby leading to inactivation of this fibrinolysis inhibitor. Thus because APC complexes to PAI-1, the reported findings of increased PAI-1 and decreased PC are probably interrelated. High levels of thrombin lead to high levels of APC, APC complexes to PAI-1, and, finally, PC is depleted.[9] This mechanism is possibly the explanation for the extremely low levels of PC found in meningococcal disease. The purpura seen in this disease is similar to that seen in congenital PC deficiency. From a therapeutic point of view, meningococcal sepsis has been considered as a model for sepsis-associated PC deficiency, and many open-label studies of PC replacement therapy have been published in this patient population. The suggestion of one study—that a disturbed activation process of PC on the basis of semiquantitative analysis of expression of thrombomodulin and the endothelial PC receptor in the dermal microvasculature of children with severe meningococcemia and purpuric or petechial lesions[31]—calls into question the benefit of PC concentrates. A randomized, placebo-controlled, dose-finding study of PC concentrate in the same patient population demonstrated adequate activation of PC to APC, even in the most severely ill patients, with a dose-dependent improvement in coagulation parameters following PC replenishment.[32]

Thrombocytopenic Purpura and Hemolytic Uremic Syndrome

Although neither TTP nor HUS generally produces a coagulopathic state, both are characterized by marked microangiopathy and microvascular thrombosis. In spite of this similarity, these two entities are not merely different end points of the same pathophysiologic process manifesting different end-organ effects.[33] HUS is more commonly seen in children and is characterized by a prodrome of fever and diffuse diarrhea (often bloody). Endemic cases of HUS are generally caused by verotoxin expressing enteropathic strains of *Escherichia coli* (O157:H7) or Shigatoxin-expressing strains of *Shigella*. Sporadic cases are generally not associated with diarrhea and are felt to represent atypical HUS resulting from familial defects in complement factor H. Therapy is supportive, including renal replacement measures when indications exist. Although some benefit from plasma exchange has been reported, the role of plasma exchange is unclear. However, aggressive treatment with an anti-complement monoclonal antibody (eculizumab) has been reported to be beneficial in these patients.[33,34]

TTP is characterized by the pentad of microangiopathic hemolytic anemia, thrombocytopenia, neurologic symptoms, fever, and renal dysfunction. Although only 40% of patients will display the full pentad, up to 75% will manifest a triad of microangiopathic hemolytic anemia, neurologic symptoms, and thrombocytopenia. This disorder has been shown to result from the absence of a von Willebrand factor–cleaving protease (ADAMTS-13), resulting in the circulation of unusually large von Willebrand factor multimers that can induce or enhance the pathologic adhesion of platelets to the endothelium. The therapy of choice for TTP is plasma exchange by apheresis. Platelet transfusions are generally not recommended, except in the case of major bleeding due to the risk of inducing vascular (arterial) occlusion.

Septic patients with thrombocytopenia-associated multiple organ failure (TAMOF) have been described, and in many a decrease in ADAMST-13 has been documented. Intensive plasma exchange by apheresis has been shown to reverse the course of disease and multiorgan failure in many of these children.[35] In some patients, prolongation of PT suggested activation of coagulation and fibrin consumption, and on autopsy patients were noted to have fibrin- and vWf-rich thrombi similar to those seen in classical DIC.

Management

The primary treatment for DIC is correction of the underlying problem that led to its development. Specific therapy for DIC should not be undertaken unless the patient has significant bleeding or organ dysfunction secondary to DIC, significant thrombosis has occurred, or treatment of the underlying disorder (eg, acute promyelocytic leukemia) is likely to increase the severity of DIC.

Supportive therapy for DIC includes the use of several component blood products.[36,37] Packed red blood cells are given according to accepted guidelines in the face of active bleeding. Fresh whole blood (ie, <24–48 hours old) may be given to replete both volume and oxygen-carrying capacity, with the potential additional benefit of providing coagulation proteins, including fibrinogen and platelets. FFP is of limited value for the treatment of significant hypofibrinogenemia because of the inordinate volumes required to make any meaningful contribution to plasma fibrinogen concentration. Cryoprecipitate contains a much higher concentration of fibrinogen than does whole blood or fresh frozen plasma (FFP) and therefore is more likely to provide the quantity of fibrinogen necessary to replenish fibrinogen that is consumed by DIC. Commercial fibrinogen concentrate contains even greater amounts of fibrinogen (by volume) than does cryoprecipitate and has the advantage of being processed to reduce the risk of viral transmission and also enables the clinician to infuse a known amount of fibrinogen. FFP infusions may effectively replete other coagulation factors consumed with DIC, such as PC, although the increase in these proteins may be quite small unless large volumes of FFP are infused. The use of cryoprecipitate or FFP in the treatment of DIC has been open to debate in the past because of concern that these products merely provide further substrate for ongoing DIC and thus increase the amount of fibrin thrombi formed. However, clinical (autopsy) studies have failed to confirm this concern.

The goal of blood component therapy is not to produce normal "numbers" but rather to produce clinical stability. If the serum fibrinogen level is <75 to 50 mg/dL, repletion with cryoprecipitate (or fibrinogen concentrate) to raise plasma levels to ≥100 mg/dL is the goal. A reasonable starting dose is 1 bag of cryoprecipitate for every 10 kg of body weight every 8 to 12 hours. As cryoprecipitate is not a standardized component (ie, its content varies from bag to bag), the fibrinogen level should be rechecked after an infusion to assess the increase. The amount and timing of the next infusion is then adjusted according to the results. Infusions of commercial fibrinogen concentrate are dosed based on the formula included in the manufacturer's package insert. Platelet transfusions also may be used when thrombocytopenia is thought to contribute to ongoing bleeding. Many of the fibrin/fibrinogen fragments produced in DIC have the potential to impair platelet function by inhibiting fibrinogen binding to platelets, which may be clinically significant at the concentration of FDPs achieved with fulminant DIC. Platelet transfusions in patients with DIC should be considered to maintain platelet counts up to 40,000 to 80,000/uL depending on the clinical specifics of the patient. In the case of children with sepsis-associated TAMOF and low ADAMST-13, plasma exchange may represent an intervention that is simultaneously supportive and therapeutic.

Pharmacologic therapy for DIC has two primary aims: to "turn off" ongoing coagulation so that repletion of coagulation factors may begin and to impede thrombus formation and ensuing ischemic injury. Recombinant activated factor VII (rhF.VIIa), a recombinant hemostatic factor, has been used to treat bleeding in DIC refractory to other therapies as well as in trauma and in other medical and surgical causes of severe, life-threatening bleeding. Most of these studies have demonstrated efficacy in the control of hemorrhage, but most have not demonstrated a decrease in mortality.[38-41] With the exception of those patients with acquired inhibitors to F.VIII, no controlled trials have been conducted in children. Recombinant activated factor VII has also been shown to correct the hemostatic defect caused by the antiplatelet agents aspirin and clopidogrel.[42] Reports have noted that use of rhF.VIIa may result in an increase in thrombosis and thromboembolic events, although the incidence appears to be small and the severity of most events mild.[43]

Various synthetic and natural modulators of hemostasis have shown some efficacy in moderating multiorgan dysfunction in animal models of sepsis. These include anticoagulant molecules (eg, heparin, antithrombin III, tissue factor pathway inhibitor [TFPI], activated protein C [APC]) and thrombolytic modulators (eg, tissue plasminogen activator [tPA], thrombin-activatable fibrinolysis inhibitor [TAFI]). Although initial reports of the use of recombinant human APC in sepsis demonstrated a benefit on survival in septic adults, there was increased bleeding in the elderly, and the pediatric trial was stopped because of futility and increased bleeding in infants. Subsequent reanalysis of data demonstrated no benefit of this agent in the treatment of sepsis and it was withdrawn from the US market. Clinical trials addressing the use of other natural modulators of thrombosis and fibrinolysis have not consistently demonstrated benefit in septic patients,[44-48] although results from ongoing clinical studies (particularly in Japan) continue to show some benefit worth exploring.[49]

Liver Disease and Hepatic Insufficiency

Abnormal Hemostasis in Liver Disease

Liver disease is a common cause of abnormal hemostasis in patients in the ICU, with abnormal coagulation studies or overt bleeding occurring in ~15% of patients who have either clinical or laboratory evidence of hepatic dysfunction. It is a common cause of a prolonged PT or aPTT, often without any clinical sequelae. The hemostatic defect associated with liver disease is multifactorial, with multiple aspects of hemostasis being affected.[50,51] In liver disease, synthesis of several plasma coagulation proteins, including factors II, V, VII, IX, and X, is impaired. Fibrinogen synthesis by the liver is usually maintained at levels that prevent bleeding until terminal liver failure is present. Factor VIII and von Willebrand factor levels are generally normal to increased in acute and chronic liver disease.

In addition to these deficiencies in plasma coagulation protein synthesis, many patients with liver disease, particularly cirrhosis, have increased fibrinolytic activity. Increase in fibrinolysis potential is a frequent occurrence in patients who have undergone portacaval shunt procedures. The mechanism for this heightened fibrinolytic state is not clear, although increased amounts of plasminogen activator can often be demonstrated. It may be difficult to discern whether fibrinolysis occurs solely because of underlying severe liver disease or as a result of concurrent DIC, as patients with cirrhosis are at increased risk for the development of DIC. The clinical distinction can be virtually impossible if active bleeding is present. In liver disease, increased levels of FDPs may result from increased fibrinolysis and by decreased hepatic clearance.

Thrombocytopenia may be present to a variable degree in patients with hepatic dysfunction—usually ascribed to splenic sequestration. It is rarely profound and as a solitary defect generally does not produce clinically significant bleeding. In vitro platelet aggregation is often affected, however. Increased plasma concentrations of FDPs are a possible cause of these abnormalities. The thrombocytopenia of liver disease in conjunction with other coagulation/hemostatic defects secondary to liver disease may result in bleeding that is difficult to manage, particularly if all aspects of the problem are not addressed.

Patients with synthetic liver disease may also exhibit decreased synthesis of the vitamin K–dependent anticoagulant proteins protein C and protein S, as well as antithrombin III.[51] Decreased levels of these natural anticoagulants may increase the risk of thrombosis. The PT, aPTT, and TT will not be affected by the levels of any of these naturally occurring anticoagulants.

Many clinicians utilize the international normalized ratio (INR) as a surrogate measure of the PT. The INR was developed to compare the intensity of vitamin K antagonist (VKA) anticoagulant therapy between clinical labs employing reagents of differing sensitivities, and, although it is calculated from the PT, it is not a surrogate for the PT. It has only been standardized and validated for the purpose of quantifying the intensity of VKA anticoagulation. As INR is calculated from the PT, any condition that produces a prolonged PT will give an increased INR. Many clinicians have assumed that the presence of an elevated INR indicates an increased risk for bleeding, as in a patient on vitamin K antagonist therapy. However, no data exist to confirm this assumption. Multiple studies on patients with liver disease and prolonged PT have demonstrated maintenance of thrombin generation and increased risk for thrombosis rather than an increased risk of bleeding.[52-55] Some of these studies have documented a decrease in fibrinolytic potential in liver disease by thromboelastography presumably accounting for the increased risk of thrombosis. However, other investigators have shown an increase in global fibrinolytic potential in patients with liver disease, but this finding has not been linked to an increase in bleeding.[56] The lack of correlation of PT (and consequently INR) with bleeding risk in patients with liver disease may be explained by the fact that, in contrast to vitamin K antagonist therapy in which only one pathway involved in hemostasis is affected, liver disease has effects on essentially all phases of hemostasis: primary (platelet-dependant) hemostasis, fibrin clot initiation, coagulation inhibition, and fibrinolysis. Of these, the PT and (coincidentally) the INR measure only fibrin clot production. The net result of these multiple effects is a "rebalancing" of hemostasis in patients with liver disease. As a consequence, neither the PT (nor INR) accurately reflects the risk of bleeding in these patients.[57-60] However, patients with liver disease may still experience clinically significant bleeding as a consequence of severe thrombocytopenia, a rebalanced hemostatic system that does not adequately compensate for a decrease in procoagulant clotting factors or increased fibrinolysis. Anatomic lesions such as esophageal varices due to portal hypertension also represent a significant risk for upper gastrointestinal hemorrhage in these patients. Consequently, the intensive care clinician must carefully and thoroughly assess his or her patient for these risks. However, the role traditional measures of coagulation (ie, PT, aPTT) play in this assessment is limited at best.

Presentation

The hemostatic defect in liver disease is multifactorial, and each patient should be approached accordingly. The most common scenario is a patient with liver disease and a prolonged PT without overt bleeding in whom the potential for bleeding is a concern. In patients with liver disease and impaired synthetic capabilities, particularly those who are critically ill, F.VII activity levels are usually the first to decrease due to its short half-life of 4 to 6 hours and increased turnover, which results in a prolonged PT and can be noted even when usual markers of hepatocellular injury/hepatic insufficiency remain relatively normal.[50,51] A prolonged TT in the setting of liver disease may indicate the presence of dysfibrinogenemia as a result of altered hepatic fibrinogen synthesis. As the severity of liver disease increases, the aPTT may also be affected, reflecting more severely impaired synthetic function. In this setting, plasma concentrations of the vitamin K–dependent coagulation proteins decrease, as do those of F.V (which is synthesized in the liver but not vitamin K dependent). Although fibrinogen synthesis occurs in the liver, its plasma level is maintained until the disease approaches end stage. When fibrinogen levels are severely depressed as a consequence of decreased synthesis and not increased degradation (fibrinolysis) or consumption (conversion to fibrin), liver failure has typically reached the terminal phase.

In more severe forms of liver disease, fibrinolysis may complicate clinical management. The differentiation between concomitant DIC and fibrinolysis attributable to liver disease alone may be difficult. The D-dimer assay result should be negative in the patient who has liver disease, elevated FDPs, and fibrinolysis but no active bleeding because thrombin is not being generated. Further clinical distinction usually is not possible, and in practice it is difficult to distinguish between a patient with fibrinolysis alone and not activation of coagulation and one who has a DIC-like process.

Management

If the patient is not actively bleeding, no specific therapy is required, with certain provisos. In patients with a prolonged PT who are in a postoperative state or are scheduled for an invasive procedure, correction of the PT may be considered; FFP is the component of choice for this purpose. However, studies have shown inconsistent and incomplete correction of the PT in liver disease and also call into question the need to correct this parameter at all. Multiple studies have shown that invasive procedures can be performed safely without correction of a prolonged PT.[57,61,62] When a correction of the PT is desired, a decrease of the PT to a value ≤3 seconds above the upper limit of normal for the testing lab is considered adequate.[62-64]

Supplementation of fibrinogen, in the form of cryoprecipitate or fibrinogen concentrate, is required only if fibrinogen levels are <50 to 100 mg/dL or if significant dysfibrinogenemia is documented. Vitamin K deficiency is also relatively common in this patient population, and replacement may be necessary. In contrast to children with dietary vitamin K deficiency and normal liver function, correction of the PT in vitamin K–responsive critically ill patients typically requires longer than 12 to 24 hours. Patients with significant hepatic impairment may manifest a partial response or may not respond at all. The immediate use of FFP prothrombin complex concentrates (PCC) is therefore appropriate when rapid correction is necessary. rhF.VIIa infusions have been shown to control bleeding in severe liver disease, although reduced mortality does not necessarily result.[65,66] To date, no studies have conclusively shown rhF.VIIa concentrate to be superior to prothrombin complex concentrates (PCCs) for the management of bleeding.[67]

When the synthetic capability of the liver becomes more profoundly impaired and the aPTT is prolonged, greater volumes of FFP or more specific therapy may be necessary. The use of F.IX concentrates (prothrombin complex concentrates; PCC) or rhF.VIIa has been advocated, particularly if

bleeding is present. The products produced from plasma pooled from multiple donors carry a relatively low but still measurable risk of hepatitis (both types B and C) and HIV. In addition, they may initiate thromboembolic events, provoke DIC, and worsen hemostasis.[68] A comprehensive therapeutic approach is required in the patient with active bleeding as a result of liver disease. Initially, FFP, 10 to 15 mL/kg body weight, may be given every 6 to 8 hours until bleeding slows significantly; it should then be continued at maintenance levels as dictated by clinical status and coagulation studies. Continuous infusions of FFP (starting dose 2–4 mL/kg/hr) have also been used with success to control bleeding following a bolus infusion.[69] rhF.VIIa or prothrombin complex concentrates may be used in those patients who are unresponsive to FFP infusions.[66,70] PCCs containing three factors (F.II, IX, X) and four factors (F.II, VII, IX, X) are the preferred products for those patients who do not manifest a good response to FFP infusions as greater amounts of clotting factors can be infused in smaller volumes when compared to FFP. However, if therapy is designed to replace a known deficiency of a factor not contained in a pooled concentrate, then FFP infusion is indicated. Cryoprecipitate, or commercial fibrinogen concentrate, should be infused for fibrinogen levels <50 to 100 mg/dL. Platelet transfusions also may be required if the platelet count is <40 to 80,000/μL, depending on the clinical situation. Vitamin K should be empirically administered on the presumption that part of the synthetic defect may result from a lack of this cofactor. However, a poor response to vitamin K in the presence of severe liver disease should be anticipated. Transfusions of packed cells are administered as deemed appropriate by the clinician.

Vitamin K Deficiency

The most common cause of a prolonged PT in the ICU is vitamin K deficiency. Vitamin K is necessary for the γ-carboxylation of factors II, VII, IX, and X, without which these factors cannot bind calcium and are not efficiently converted into their activated forms. F.VII has the shortest half-life of these coagulation proteins; accordingly, the PT is the most sensitive early indicator of vitamin K deficiency.

Vitamin K deficiency is relatively common in critically ill patients for several reasons, including the use of broad-spectrum antibiotics, poor nutrition preceding or subsequent to ICU admission, and the use of parenteral nutrition without vitamin K supplementation. Many of the second- and third-generation cephalosporins directly interfere with vitamin K absorption from the gut lumen. The metabolites of these antibiotics may even act as competitive inhibitors of vitamin K. In addition, these and other antibiotics may kill or inhibit the growth of gut bacteria and limit the amounts of vitamin K that they normally produce and excrete into the gut lumen. Although malnutrition also may contribute to the development of vitamin K deficiency, it usually requires 1 to 2 weeks to develop in the complete absence of vitamin K intake. However, the use of parenteral alimentation without vitamin K supplementation coupled with antibiotic use may result in rapid vitamin K depletion, and prolongation of the PT can occur within only 2 to 3 days. Finally, fat malabsorption states, including cystic fibrosis, may be associated with vitamin K deficiency. Vitamin K is fat soluble and is not absorbed well in some conditions of biliary tract and intrinsic small bowel disease. In the ICU, vitamin K deficiency usually results from the interaction of several of these factors and is rarely limited to only one of the conditions mentioned. It is the responsibility of the clinician to maintain an awareness of the potential for vitamin K deficiency and to treat accordingly.

The differential diagnosis of an isolated prolongation of the PT, with or without bleeding, includes both vitamin K deficiency and liver disease. The clinical presentation of these patients is often quite similar. In fact, the distinction sometimes can be made only on the basis of the response (or lack thereof) to empirical vitamin K therapy. Warfarin administration (either overt or covert) also should be excluded as a cause of a prolonged PT. Newer, long-acting vitamin K antagonist rodenticides (so-called "superwarfarin"), which when ingested, produce a profound, prolonged, vitamin K–resistant reduction in vitamin K–dependent clotting factors, may produce an isolated prolongation of the PT initially. Treatment of poisoning with these agents requires aggressive, prolonged use of vitamin K and, in the bleeding patient, support with 4-factor PCC, FFP infusions, or rhF.VIIa. Confirmation of warfarin exposure as the cause of a prolonged PT is possible by toxicologic methods to detect the drug or its metabolites or the presence of non-carboxylated forms of vitamin K–dependent clotting factors (**p**roteins **i**nduced by **v**itamin **K a**ntagonist; PIVKAs) in plasma. In addition, the presence of a specific inhibitor or congenital deficiency of F.VII will also result in an isolated prolongation of the PT. Acquired inhibitors of F.VII are rare, and homozygous deficiency of F.VII has not been described. Individuals who are heterozygous for F.VII deficiency tend to have F.VII levels in the 25% to 35% range and do not appear to be at significant increased risk for bleeding. Lupus-like anticoagulants that result from inflammation may also lead to an isolated prolongation of the PT; these are generally of no clinical significance and are not associated with an increased risk of bleeding.

Infants who fail to receive vitamin K in the immediate postnatal period may develop a systemic coagulopathy manifested by bruising and gastrointestinal bleeding, generally occurring between 1 and 2 weeks of age. The first manifestation is often prolonged bleeding following circumcision. Infants with malabsorption or breast-fed infants who ingest medications that interfere with vitamin K in breast milk may develop similar manifestations beyond 2 weeks of age.

The laboratory findings of an isolated vitamin K deficiency, in addition to a prolonged PT, include a normal fibrinogen level, platelet count, and F.V level. F.V is not a vitamin K–dependent protein and should therefore be normal, except in cases of DIC (consumption) or severe liver disease (decreased production). Prolongation of the aPTT from vitamin K deficiency, warfarin therapy, or liver disease is a relatively late event and occurs initially as a result of F.IX depletion.

Management
The management of vitamin K deficiency consists primarily of its repletion, usually by IV or subcutaneous routes in critically ill patients. Therapy should not await the development of bleeding or oozing but should be administered when the PT abnormality is detected and vitamin K deficiency is thought to be responsible. As with other drugs administered subcutaneously (eg, insulin), adequate blood pressure and subcutaneous perfusion are necessary to ensure reliable absorption from the soft tissues. Concern exists regarding the possibility of anaphylactoid reactions with the IV use of vitamin K. This risk

is minimized when the drug is given as a piggyback infusion over 30 to 45 minutes in a small volume of fluid rather than as a bolus or "slow-push" dose; IV-piggyback infusion is the preferred method of drug administration in hemodynamically unstable patients. The usual dose of vitamin K in children is 1 to 5 mg IV or subcutaneously (up to 10 mg in larger children). In an otherwise healthy person, the PT should correct within 12 to 24 hours after this dose. However, serial dosing of critically ill patients is often utilized, and the PT may require up to 72 hours to normalize. If the PT does not correct within 72 hours after three daily doses of vitamin K, intrinsic liver disease should be suspected. Further administration of vitamin K is of no additional benefit in this setting.

When the patient is actively bleeding, it is not sufficient to give vitamin K alone. A more immediate restoration of coagulation is required. FFP has traditionally been employed in this setting. To restore hemostasis to an acceptable level (30%-50%) of normal enzyme activity, 10- to 15-mL/kg body weight of FFP is typically required. A similar approach is used in patients who were previously given warfarin. rhF.VIIa (15–20 mcg/kg) has been used with success to reverse the bleeding noted in vitamin K deficiency and in warfarin overdose.[39,66,70,71] Four-factor PCCs that contain significant amounts of F.VII are effective in correcting both PT and aPTT values in these patients and have become the treatment of choice to correct a patient with warfarin overdose–associated bleeding.[68]

Iatrogenic Coagulopathy

Massive Transfusion Syndrome
Transfusion of large quantities of blood can result in a multifactorial hemostatic defect. The genesis of this problem is related to the "washout" of plasma coagulation proteins and platelets, and it may be exacerbated by the development of DIC with consequent factor consumption, hypothermia, acidosis, or rarely, by citrate toxicity or hypocalcemia. These variables often act in combination to cause a coagulopathic state.[72]

A washout syndrome can result from the transfusion of large amounts of stored blood products that are devoid of clotting factors and platelets and develops exclusively in patients who receive large volumes of packed red blood cells (eg, trauma victims, patients with massive gastrointestinal hemorrhage or hepatectomy, or those undergoing cardiopulmonary bypass) without also receiving FFP and platelets. Factors V and VII have short shelf half-lives and are often deficient in blood that has been banked longer than 48 hours. In addition, a qualitative platelet defect can be demonstrated in whole blood within hours of its storage, especially if an acid-citrate-dextrose solution is used. Consequently, transfusion of large quantities of stored whole blood may produce limited improvement in the bleeding that results from decreased clotting factors and platelets. The development of a washout coagulopathy is directly dependent on the volume of blood transfused relative to the blood volume of the patient. As a general rule, residual plasma clotting activity after single-blood-volume exchange falls to 18% to 37% of normal; after a double-blood-volume exchange, residual activity is only 3% to 14% of normal; and after a triple-blood-volume exchange, <5% of normal clotting function remains.

The patient who is bleeding as a consequence of massive transfusion or washout presents with diffuse oozing and bleeding from all surgical wounds and puncture sites. Laboratory abnormalities include prolonged PT, aPTT, and TT. Fibrinogen levels and platelet counts are typically decreased; FDPs are not usually increased unless concurrent DIC is present (see Table 91.2). The likelihood that the clinicolaboratory picture is a direct result of the massive transfusion can be estimated from the amount of bleeding that has occurred and the blood volume that has been administered relative to the patient's blood volume (ie, the number of blood volume exchanges that have been given). The more stored blood (eg, packed red blood cells) transfused relative to the patient's blood volume, the greater the chance of the development of coagulopathy due to massive transfusion.

Management

Children with severe trauma frequently present with massive bleeding and acidosis secondary to hypoperfusion (see also Chapter 118). Aggressive transfusion support through the implementation of a formal transfusion protocol that would provide multiproduct support with red blood cells (RBCs), plasma, and platelets in a set ratio closer to 1:1:1 has been hypothesized to improve the outcome in these children.[74-77] However, to date prospective studies have not clearly demonstrated an improvement in outcome, and concern for an increase in transfusion-related organ dysfunction exists. However, blood product use and blood bank–related costs have been shown to be less with such transfusion regimens. Some centers have investigated the use of rotational elastometry to guide blood product transfusion in trauma patients.[3,71-73] Although this methodology offers the potential advantage of evaluating several different aspects of hemostasis and not merely fibrin clot formation (as is measured by the PT and aPTT), these methods have not yet been widely accepted in clinical practice.

Prospective identification of those at risk to develop a coagulopathy from massive transfusion is important. When the magnitude of the insult and the anticipated need for blood are large, both platelets and FFP should be given before a coagulopathy develops; the exact ratio of packed red blood cells to other blood components (ie, platelets, plasma, or cryoprecipitate) to prevent the development of massive transfusion coagulopathy has not been established.[78-80] However, studies in adults suggest that 1 unit of FFP for every unit of packed RBCs transfused effectively replaces plasma clotting factors.[81] In larger children (eg, weight ≥30 to 40 kg or body surface area ≥1 m^2), half of a unit of apheresis-collected platelets (generally equivalent to 4 to 5 units of platelets derived from whole blood donation) and 1 unit of FFP should be given for each 5 units of whole blood or packed cells transfused. In smaller children, 10 mL/kg of platelets and 10- to 15-mL/kg FFP should be given for each 40 to 50 mL/kg of blood transfused. These amounts should prevent washout and its attendant bleeding. The therapeutic approach to patients who develop a coagulopathy from massive transfusion is supportive.

Anticoagulant Overdose

Anticoagulant therapy is not unusual in the PICU, and the possibility of errors in administration exists. Methods of prophylactic anticoagulant use, systemic anticoagulation, and thrombolytic therapy are sometimes poorly standardized and can lead to overdose.

Heparin

Heparin is a repeating polymer of two disaccharide glycosaminoglycans and is commercially prepared from either porcine intestinal mucosa or bovine lung. Heparin is currently available in two types of preparations: unfractionated heparin (UH) and low-molecular-weight heparin (LMWH). It is important to understand the differences between these two forms of the drug, as they have different mechanisms of action and associated precautions. UH has an immediate effect on coagulation that is mediated primarily through its association with antithrombin III. The resulting heparin-antithrombin III complex possesses a much greater affinity for thrombin than antithrombin III alone, and it inactivates thrombin, thereby damping down clot formation. In addition, heparin has an anti-F.Xa effect that is also dependent on an association with AT-III, although this represents a smaller anticoagulant component. Achieving a therapeutic aPTT with UH is very difficult in the face of low levels of antithrombin III. The degree of anticoagulation produced by heparin is monitored by the prolongation of the aPTT. In contrast, LMWH, produced by controlled enzymatic cleavage of heparin polymers, affects anticoagulation almost exclusively through inhibition of F.Xa. This also requires association with AT-III, but the anticoagulant effect is less dependent on variation in AT-III plasma levels. Consequently, a more stable degree of anticoagulation is produced. Due to its longer half-life (~3–5 hours) and biological activity (~24 hours), LMWH allows for intermittent bolus therapy (ie, every 12 or 24 hours) while maintaining a steady-state effect. However, LMWH does not produce consistent prolongation of the aPTT and requires assay of anti-Xa activity for monitoring.

Heparin is metabolized in the liver by the heparinase enzyme in a dose-dependent fashion, with excess heparin then being excreted through the kidneys. As the rate of heparin administration is increased, the half-life of the drug is prolonged due the increase in the percentage of the drug being excreted by the kidney. For example, when a 100-U/kg bolus of heparin is infused IV, the average half-life of the drug is 1 hour. If the bolus is increased to 400 or 800 U/kg, the half-life is prolonged to 2.5 and 5 hours, respectively. The nonlinear response results in greater drug effects on coagulation with smaller dosage increments. When one "re-boluses" or increases a heparin infusion rate in response to insufficient anticoagulation (ie, inadequate prolongation of the aPTT), a point will be reached when further small increments in the heparin infusion rate may result in a substantially greater prolongation of the aPTT. The risk of pathologic bleeding associated with heparin increases when the prolongation of the aPTT is beyond the therapeutic window (generally considered to be 1.5–2.5 times the patient's baseline aPTT, corresponding to a plasma heparin concentration of 0.2–0.4 units/mL or anti-Xa level of 0.3–0.7 units/mL). As a corollary, administration of heparin as a continuous infusion rather than in an intermittent bolus dose regimen is less likely to be associated with pathologic bleeding.

Management

Serious bleeding associated with heparin overdose can be rapidly reversed by protamine sulfate. Protamine binds ionically with heparin to form a complex that lacks any anticoagulant activity. As a general rule, 1 mg of protamine neutralizes ~100 U of heparin (specifically, 90 US Pharmacopeia (USP) units of bovine heparin or 115 USP units of porcine heparin). The dose of protamine required is calculated from the number of units of active heparin remaining in the patient's system. This, in turn, is estimated from the original heparin dose and the typical half-life for that infusion rate. The aPTT is used to gauge the residual effects of heparin. During and after cardiopulmonary bypass surgery, the activated clotting time (ACT) is frequently used to measure the heparin effect and to judge the effectiveness of and need for protamine neutralization. This methodology is sometimes employed in the ICU. However, the equipment used for this measurement is poorly standardized and different systems give different results.[82] Consequently, care must be taken when employing one of these methods in the ICU.

Protamine itself potentially has anticoagulant effects, and precautions are necessary during its administration. The drug should be given by slow IV push over 8 to 10 minutes. A single dose should not exceed 1 mg/kg (50-mg maximum dose). This dose may be repeated, but no more than 2 mg/kg (100-mg maximum dose) should be given as a cumulative dose without rechecking coagulation parameters. The dose of protamine should always be monitored by coagulation studies. Significant side effects are most commonly seen in situations of overly rapid drug administration and include hypotension and anaphylactoid-like reactions. The allergic reactions to protamine represent type I anaphylactic reactions between an antigen (protamine) and antibody (IgE or IgG) and result in histamine release. Consequently, H2 blockers have been shown to be effective in treating and minimizing these reactions. In addition, complement activation, thromboxane, and nitric oxide production have all been shown to play some role in the pathogenesis of these reactions.[83,84] Risk factors for protamine hypersensitivity reactions include prior exposure to protamine, insulin-dependent diabetes (with NPH exposure), fish allergy, and vasectomy. In that LMWH is not predictably neutralized by protamine, invasive procedures should not be performed within 24 hours of administration. Bleeding following LMWH therapy has been treated effectively with rhF.VIIa.

Warfarin

Warfarin and vitamin K are structurally similar in their respective 4-hydroxycoumarin nucleus and naphthoquinone ring. The mechanism of action of warfarin is through competitive inhibition of vitamin K epoxide reductase, which is necessary to regenerate the reduced form of vitamin K. This form of vitamin K is a necessary cofactor in the postribosomal modification of the vitamin K–dependent coagulation proteins (factors II, VII, IX, and X) γ-carboxylation. This postsynthetic modification produces a calcium-binding site on the molecule, which, when occupied, allows for the efficient activation of the zymogen clotting factor into its enzymatically active form. When warfarin is present in sufficient plasma concentrations, the active (γ-carboxylated) forms of vitamin K–dependent factors are depleted.

The PT (INR) is an accurate indicator of the effects of warfarin when its use has continued beyond 2 or 3 days. F.VIIa (the active form) has a half-life of only 4 to 6 hours and is rapidly depleted after one or two doses of warfarin. The remainder of the vitamin K–dependent factors may take up

TABLE 91.5	Drugs That Potentiate the Anticoagulant Effects of Warfarin

Antibiotics
Broad-spectrum antibiotics (especially cephalosporins)
Griseofulvin (oral)
Metronidazole
Sulfonamides
Trimethoprim-sulfamethoxazole

Antiinflammatory Drugs
Steroids (anabolic, in particular)
Acetylated salicylates
Phenylbutazone (oxyphenbutazone)
Sulfinpyrazone

Other Drugs
Clofibrate
Disulfiram
Phenytoin
Thyroxine (both D- and L-isomers)
Tolbutamide

to a week to become depleted. The PT becomes prolonged with F.VII depletion alone but does not reflect an overall state of anticoagulation until an equilibrium period of several days has passed, generally once the INR is at or near target value for 2 to 3 days. Over this interval, the other vitamin K–dependent factors become depleted, and PT prolongation, as measured by the INR, can then be used to assess the anticoagulant effects of warfarin. In severe cases of warfarin overdose, the aPTT also becomes prolonged as a result of a marked reduction of the active forms of factors II, IX, and X.

Several drugs and pathophysiologic conditions are associated with potentiation of warfarin's effects on coagulation. Many of the drugs known to prolong the effects of warfarin are listed in Table 91.5. These drugs have a variety of mechanisms that generally include either inhibition of function or competitive binding of the enzymes that are responsible for active warfarin metabolism. Aspirin does not seem to have any direct influence on warfarin metabolism but so profoundly influences qualitative platelet function that it increases the bleeding risk resulting from warfarin's anticoagulant effects. The same is true for clofibrate. Ingestion of large doses of aspirin may also impair prothrombin (F.II) synthesis, further increasing the effects of warfarin administration. Warfarin is metabolized by the liver. Conditions of acute and chronic hepatic dysfunction can alter warfarin metabolism and vitamin K–mediated γ-carboxylation of the vitamin K–dependent coagulation proteins. Broad-spectrum antibiotics also may limit vitamin K availability through their alteration of the gut flora (in addition to any direct effect on vitamin K metabolism). All of these factors may ultimately influence a patient's response to warfarin.

A clinical syndrome referred to as "warfarin (Coumadin) necrosis" has been noted during the initial stages of anticoagulation with a vitamin–K antagonist. It is characterized clinically by the development of skin and subcutaneous necrosis, particularly in areas of subcutaneous fat, and pathologically by the thrombosis of small blood vessels in the fat and subcutaneous tissues. This syndrome is caused by the rapid depletion of the vitamin K–dependent, anticoagulant PC prior to achieving depletion of procoagulant proteins and occurs predominantly in individuals who are heterozygous for PC deficiency. Although anticoagulation generally requires a decrease in procoagulant protein levels to ~20% to 25%, a prothrombotic milieu is created with PC levels of ≤40%. Consequently, individuals who are heterozygous for PC deficiency and have baseline PC levels of 50% to 60% may develop a prothrombotic environment during the first few days of warfarin therapy. The risk of developing warfarin necrosis appears to be greater when an initial dose of warfarin >10 to 15 mg is administered. The development of this syndrome generally can be avoided if heparin and warfarin therapy are overlapped until "coumadinization" is complete and if large loading doses of warfarin (>15 mg) are avoided.

Management

When over-anticoagulation with warfarin presents with bleeding, immediate reversal is usually mandated.[71] The treatment of choice is FFP, which provides prompt restoration of the deficient vitamin K–dependent coagulation proteins, along with restoration of hemostatic function. Ten to 15 mL/kg of FFP is usually sufficient to produce significant correction of the PT, although repeat infusions of FFP may be necessary for continued correction of the PT due to the short half-life of F.VII.[78] Vitamin K also may be administered, particularly in situations that are less acute although this will make it more difficult to "recoumadinize" the patient afterward. For severe bleeding or bleeding not controlled by FFP infusions, rhF.VIIa and 4-factor PCC have been used successfully (see the "Vitamin K Deficiency" section, presented earlier). The "3-factor" PCCs currently available in the United States are not approved for the treatment of factor VII deficiency (either congenital or secondary to VKA treatment) owing to the limited amount of F.VII contained in them.[68]

Platelet Disorders

Platelets are necessary for efficient clot formation. They not only produce a physical barrier at the site of vascular injury (the so-called "platelet plug"); they also serve to focus the clotting process at the point of bleeding by delivering vasoconstrictors, clotting factors to the bleeding site, and provide a surface on which clot development occurs (see Fig. 91.3). Quantitative and qualitative platelet disorders are a common cause of clinical bleeding in the PICU. An overview of platelet disorders based on this classification scheme is presented in Table 91.6.

Quantitative Platelet Disorders

A decrease in the number of circulating platelets reflects the presence of increased peripheral destruction or sequestration, decreased marrow production, or a combination of these factors. Examples of increased peripheral destruction include immune-mediated processes (both autoimmune and drug induced), abnormal consumption (as in DIC), and mechanical destruction (eg, cardiopulmonary bypass, hyperthermia). Autoimmune processes such as idiopathic thrombocytopenic purpura (ITP; now referred to as immune thrombocytopenia), systemic lupus erythematosus, or acquired immunodeficiency syndrome can result in increased peripheral destruction and increased splenic sequestration of platelets. Autoimmune destruction also may occur in conjunction with lymphocytic leukemia or lymphoma.

TABLE 91.6 Platelet Disorders Seen in the Intensive Care Unit

Quantitative	Qualitative
Increased Destruction	**Drugs**
Immune	Antiinflammatory agents
Idiopathic thrombocytopenic purpura	Aspirin (irreversible)
Systemic lupus erythematosus	Nonsteroidal antiinflammatory agents
Acquired immunodeficiency syndrome	Corticosteroids
Drugs (gold salts, heparin, sulfonamides, quinidine, quinine)	Antibiotics
Sepsis	Penicillins (eg, ampicillin, carbenicillin, ti.carcillin, penicillin-G)
Nonimmune	Cephalosporins (eg, cephalothin)
Thrombotic thrombocytopenic purpura/hemolytic uremic syndrome	Nitrofurantoin
Mechanical destruction (eg, cardiopulmonary bypass, hyperthermia)	Chloroquine, hydroxychloroquine
	Phosphodiesterase inhibitors
	Dipyridamole
Consumption (ie, disseminated intravascular coagulation)	Methylxanthines (eg, theophylline)
Decreased Production	Other drugs
Marrow suppression	Antihistamines
Chemotherapy	α-blockers (eg, phentolamine)
Viral illness (eg, cytomegalovirus Epstein-Barr virus, herpes simplex, parvovirus)	β-blockers (eg, propranolol)
	Dextran
Drugs (thiazides, ethanol, cimetidine)	Ethanol
	Furosemide
Marrow replacement	Heparin
Tumor	Local anesthetics (eg, lidocaine)
Myelofibrosis	
Other conditions	Phenothiazines
Splenic sequestration	Tricyclic antidepressants
Dilution (see massive transfusion syndrome)	Nitrates (eg, sodium nitroprusside, nitroglycerin)
	Metabolic Causes
	Uremia
	Stored whole blood
	Disseminated intravascular coagulation (ie, fibrin degradation product-mediated inhibition)
	Hypothyroidism

The prototypic example of immune thrombocytopenia is ITP, in which immunoglobin (generally IgG) directed against specific platelet antigens results in platelet destruction by a cell-mediated mechanism. Acute ITP is usually self-limited; in contrast, chronic ITP generally requires immunosuppressive therapy to maintain an acceptable platelet count. Although life-threatening bleeding may occur in either acute or chronic

ITP, it is a rarity; the incidence of intracranial hemorrhage in ITP is estimated to be less than 1%, and in most series it is between 0.1 and 0.2%.[85,86] Most episodes of severe bleeding occur when the platelet count is less than 10 to 20,000/uL, but a decision to institute therapy should be based on the overall clinical setting and not just the platelet count. Steroids may be given (2–4 mg/kg/day of prednisone or its equivalent). High doses of IV γ-globulin (1–2 g/kg given over 2–5 days) and infusions of anti-RhD antigen antibody (WinRho; 25–60 mcg/kg) are equally efficacious in producing at least transient elevations in platelet counts. Note, however, that WinRho should only be used in patients who are Rh (+) and have a functioning spleen. Agents such as vincristine/vinblastine, cyclophosphamide, and, with increasing frequency, rituximab (anti-CD20 monoclonal antibody) also have been used as immunosuppressants, with variable success, although responses are generally not immediate. Splenectomy may be required to avert serious bleeding complications in patients who do not respond to medical management, although this approach is chosen much less often in children than in adults. In ITP, the degree of bleeding attributed to thrombocytopenia is generally less than that noted when thrombocytopenia results from decreased platelet production. In general, severe bleeding is not noted until the platelet count is <10,000/μL, although levels below 40,000 to 50,000/uL may increase the risk of bleeding associated with invasive procedures. The use of thrombopoietin-like drugs to stimulate platelet production in chronic ITP generally does not play a role in the management of immune thrombocytopenia in the ICU, as platelet counts only demonstrate a significant increase after several weeks of therapy.

The development of drug-induced, immune-mediated platelet destruction should always be considered in the thrombocytopenic PICU patient. When present, it is usually reversible; withdrawal of the offending drug prevents further immune-mediated platelet destruction. The exact mechanism of platelet destruction may be related to the binding of drug to the platelet membrane, with subsequent binding to the platelet, platelet-drug complex, or both, of a specific antibody. The resulting platelet-drug-antibody complexes are then cleared by the reticuloendothelial system (eg, the spleen), and thrombocytopenia develops. Drugs used in the ICU that are most commonly associated with this clinical picture include quinidine, quinine, heparin, gold salts, various penicillin and cephalosporin antibiotics, and the sulfonamides. The anticonvulsant valproic acid frequently produces a dose-dependent thrombocytopenia that is, at least in part, immunologic in nature.

A variety of drugs are associated with the nonimmune development of thrombocytopenia by bone marrow suppression. Most cancer chemotherapeutic agents produce thrombocytopenia as a consequence of marrow suppression. The thiazide diuretics, cimetidine, ethanol, and several of the cephalosporin and penicillin antibiotics may suppress platelet production. Generalized infection (such as bacterial sepsis) and many viral illnesses are also associated with bone marrow suppression and thrombocytopenia, even if an element of immune platelet destruction is present. Disorders such as Gaucher disease may produce a mild-to-moderate thrombocytopenia as a result of marrow replacement by nonhematopoietic cells.

Consumption of platelets can also cause thrombocytopenia. Mechanical destruction invariably occurs during cardiopulmonary bypass or the use of ventricular assist devices. It is not uncommon to note a 50% drop in platelet count postbypass when compared to preoperative platelet levels. Platelet counts generally recover toward preoperative levels by 48 to 72 hours after bypass. The high body temperatures seen in severe hyperthermic syndromes may also destroy platelets, and they are consumed during microvascular coagulation in DIC. In many of these circumstances, the thrombocytopenia may be the sole or a contributing cause of significant bleeding.

Heparin-Induced Thrombocytopenia

Heparin is widely used in ICUs to maintain vascular access or as a therapy for acute thrombosis. Exposure to heparin may result in thrombocytopenia and in a small number of cases this may result in arterial thrombosis. Thrombocytopenia may develop upon exposure to heparin in one of two ways. Acute nonidiosyncratic thrombocytopenia is seen in 10% to 15% of patients who receive heparin. The degree of thrombocytopenia is usually mild and usually remits despite continued use of the drug. This has previously been referred to as type I heparin-induced thrombocytopenia (HIT). The thrombocytopenia results from the direct binding of the heparin molecule to the platelet surface, does not involve an immune mechanism, and has no clinical significance. Heparin need not be stopped in these patients. Idiosyncratic HIT is of much greater clinical consequence. Although it is a less frequent occurrence (typically seen in <5% of patients who receive heparin), it has a much greater potential for clinical morbidity. Arterial thrombosis is the most significant risk of this form of HIT (previously referred to as type II HIT) and may be life threatening, causing myocardial infarction, cerebrovascular accident, pulmonary embolism, or renal infarction. The thrombosis is the consequence of the deposition of platelet aggregates in the microcirculation.[87,88] Thrombocytopenia in this disorder involves the formation of platelet aggregates mediated by the binding of a specific antibody, directed against a heparin-platelet factor-4 complex, to platelets in the presence of heparin. This results in the activation of platelets and appears to require minuscule amounts of heparin. Clinical bleeding is an infrequent problem in these patients. Severe thrombocytopenia (ie, <15–20,000/μl) is unusual in this disorder.

From a practical perspective, the diagnosis of HIT is usually one of exclusion. Clinical scoring systems to assess the probability of HIT have been developed, but they are more useful for identifying those individuals who are less likely to have HIT and are less sensitive in their ability to accurately identify patients with HIT.[89,90] None of these scoring systems have been validated in pediatric patients. Diagnostic markers do exist (eg, heparin-dependent platelet antibodies, platelet aggregation, or serotonin release), but these tests are best considered confirmatory and not exclusionary. An ELISA assay for heparin-dependent platelet antibodies is the most common test obtained to investigate a possible diagnosis of HIT, but because of a relatively high "false-positive" rate, it is generally recommended that a more specific heparin-induced platelet injury assay, such as a serotonin release assay, be performed for confirmation. The diagnosis may be difficult to recognize because coexisting clinical illnesses with the potential to cause thrombocytopenia also may be present. Although HIT may be more likely to be associated with the use of bovine lung heparin, it can occur after exposure to porcine heparin or, much less commonly, LMWH. When type II HIT is suspected or confirmed, all exposure to heparin, including heparin flushes, heparin in total parenteral nutrition, and heparin-coated catheters, must be removed, and anticoagulation with an alternate agent must be initiated because of the risk of delayed thrombosis, which can occur up to 30 days after removal of heparin exposure.[88,91] Patients with type II HIT should receive continued anticoagulation with direct thrombin inhibitors (argatroban, bivalirudin) or with the heparinoid danaparoid (currently not available in the United States). Production of the direct thrombin inhibitor lepirudin was discontinued in 2012 and is no longer available. Although anti-Xa agents, such as fondaparinux, may also be used, the direct thrombin inhibitors are preferred, as they carry no risk of cross-reacting with the heparin-dependent antibodies already present.[91,92] Of the members of this class of anticoagulants, bivalirudin is gaining increasing preference for anticoagulation in children at high risk for or with suspected or documented HIT.[93-97] Bivalirudin is largely cleared by proteolysis in the plasma; argatroban is cleared by the liver and lepirudin by the kidney. Consequently, the choice and dose of drug may be affected by the presence of hepatic or renal insufficiency. Although there are pharmacokinetic and safety data for use in children for bivalirudin and argatroban, there are no similar data pertaining to the use of lepirudin in children.[98,99] Warfarin alone is not adequate therapy for suspected type II HIT because of the risk of thrombosis from depression of PC levels. However, warfarin can be utilized in conjunction with a direct thrombin inhibitor and subsequently continued as a single agent once therapeutic suppression of vitamin K–dependent clotting factors has been achieved.

Qualitative Platelet Disorders

Many of the drugs frequently used in the ICU have the potential to impair platelet function. Frequently, the sicker patients are more likely to be exposed to one of these drugs. These patients often have other underlying pathophysiologic conditions that in and of themselves can predispose to bleeding. An abbreviated list of the drugs that can affect at least in vitro platelet function is presented in Table 91.6.

All unnecessary drugs should be viewed as suspect and discontinued in patients with evidence of qualitative platelet dysfunction or in those in whom it is strongly suspected. In most cases, terminating the offending drugs usually restores normal platelet activity. Aspirin is a notable exception as it irreversibly inhibits platelet cyclooxygenase, resulting in a defect that lasts for the duration of the platelet life span (8–9 days). The effect is profound: A single 325-mg aspirin tablet results in a qualitative platelet defect that remains in 50% of the circulating platelets 5 days after its ingestion. Ideally, all aspirin ingestion should be avoided for at least 7 days prior to an elective invasive procedure. New drugs that target the adenosine diphosphate $P2Y_{12}$ receptor on the surface of platelets (eg, clopidogrel, prasugrel, ticagrelor) also produce a prolonged inhibition of platelet reactivity that may last up to 2 weeks following discontinuance of the drug depending on the duration of therapy.[100]

Nonsteroidal antiinflammatory agents similarly affect the platelet cyclooxygenase enzyme. However, their effects are reversible, and normal platelet function is usually restored within 24 hours of the last dose. Under most circumstances, the degree of platelet inhibition produced by these agents is not clinically significant, and patients can receive these drugs for analgesia and fever control. However, it is reasonable to

minimize their use in the bleeding severely thrombocytopenic patient. The β-lactam antibiotics can sterically hinder the binding of a platelet aggregation agonist (eg, adenosine diphosphate [ADP]) to its specific platelet receptor, resulting in impaired platelet aggregation under circumstances of normal physiologic stimulation. This, too, is reversed on removal of the drug. Fortunately, only a minority of patients exposed to these antibiotics will exhibit clinically significant platelet inhibition.

In the PICU, the possibility must always be considered that a patient with bleeding suggestive of a platelet defect might have an inherited disorder of platelet function. Though rare, these disorders are encountered from time to time and include Glanzmann thrombasthenia (abnormal platelet GPIIb/IIIa), Bernard-Soulier syndrome (abnormal GP Ib/IX), Wiskott-Aldrich syndrome, platelet storage pool deficiency (abnormal platelet-dense bodies), and the gray platelet disorder (abnormal platelet α-granules). Individuals with vitamin C deficiency (scurvy) or those with collagen disorders (eg, Ehlers-Danlos syndrome) will present with mucocutaneous bleeding but have normal platelet number and in vitro function. The defect in these conditions is the production of abnormal collagen that is unable to support platelet adhesion, resulting in poor clot initiation and tensile strength. Vitamin C deficiency is an acquired defect in collagen structure, whereas Ehlers-Danlos syndrome is congenital. Individuals with scurvy typically have hypertrophied purpuric gums, whereas those with Ehlers-Danlos syndrome (and related disorders) have a lifelong history of joint dislocations and poor wound healing. Individuals with von Willebrand disease will also present with mucocutaneous bleeding, but many will also have a variably prolonged aPTT as a result of the secondary decrease in F.VIII in this disease.

Management

Because many of the adverse drug-related platelet effects are reversible, all unnecessary medications should be discontinued promptly when platelet function seems impaired. The more controversial issue is deciding whether platelet transfusions are warranted in a particular patient. The relationship of thrombocytopenia to clinical bleeding is relative—that is, it is difficult to identify a specific, arbitrary platelet count (threshold) below which bleeding is likely to occur. Several conditions, such as massive transfusion syndrome and DIC, may respond to empirical platelet transfusion at counts as high as 80,000 or even 100,000 platelets/uL, although significant bleeding in the presence of a platelet count of 40,000 to 50,000/uL (or greater) is unlikely to be a result of the thrombocytopenia. With other causes such as thrombocytopenia seen with cancer chemotherapy and bone marrow aplasia, prophylactic therapy may not be required until counts fall below 10,000 to 20,000/uL. As previously stated, rhF.VIIa has been used to reverse the hemostatic defect caused by aspirin or clopidogrel.[42]

The morbidity and mortality related to bleeding increase measurably in patients who undergo induction chemotherapy for acute leukemia when the platelet count falls below 10,000 to 20,000/uL. Empirical administration of platelets to these patients significantly limits both morbidity and mortality. This finding has resulted in the practice of most patients receiving cancer chemotherapy receiving prophylactic platelet transfusions once their platelet count falls below this threshold. However, the application of this practice for all other patients with platelet counts in this range is unclear. A major concern that should temper the empirical use of platelet transfusion is the development of alloimmunization to transfused platelets, potentially negating any future benefit from platelet transfusion in a time of need. Patients with aplastic anemia appear to have a particularly high incidence of platelet alloimmunization following transfusion. Patients with autoimmune disorders associated with increased peripheral platelet destruction, drug-related thrombocytopenia, and disorders causing splenic sequestration are unlikely to benefit from platelet transfusion and routine platelet transfusions should be avoided. An exception is related to planned, invasive procedures with an increased risk of bleeding. In this situation, empirical platelet transfusion immediately before the procedure may be reasonable.

Uremia

Uremia is commonly seen in the ICU and is associated with an increased risk of bleeding.[101,102] Uremia has been shown to cause a reversible impairment of platelet function, although the "toxin" responsible for this defect is not well defined.[103] Some studies have demonstrated an impairment of platelet-vessel wall interactions and suggest defects in von Willebrand factor. The degree of platelet impairment appears to be related to the severity of uremia for a given patient. In addition, thrombotic events are also increased in patients with uremia. These, too, appear to be multifactorial in etiology but in part reflect the increased renal loss of antithrombin III and protein S in nephritic-range proteinuria.[102]

Several therapeutic approaches may modulate the qualitative platelet defect associated with uremia. The primary therapy in this setting is dialysis. Cryoprecipitate, 1-deamino-8-D-arginine vasopressin (DDAVP; 0.3 mcg/kg, maximum dose 21 mcg), and conjugated estrogens (10 mg/day in adult patients) have been given with good results to patients with severe uremia and an acquired defect in primary hemostasis. The benefit derived by treatment with cryoprecipitate or DDAVP appears to be related to the consequent increase in the plasma concentration of the large multimeric forms of von Willebrand factor, thus greatly improving platelet adhesion. However, the duration of action of these agents is limited, reaching their zenith at between 2 and 6 hours. Additional doses of DDAVP during the same 24-hour period may result in a diminished response to the drug (tachyphylaxis) with little or no further benefit. Patients who exhibit tachyphylaxis to DDAVP may require 48 to 72 hours before again responding to this agent. Repeated administration of DDAVP may result in significant hyponatremia, particularly in infants and young children. The mechanism of action of the conjugated estrogens is not known. In contrast to infusion of cryoprecipitate or DDAVP, the effect of estrogen is more protracted and does not diminish with repeat dosing, although a benefit is frequently not apparent until 3 to 5 days after therapy begins.

Selected Disorders

Systemic Diseases Associated With Factor Deficiencies

Patients with amyloidosis, Gaucher disease, or nephrotic syndrome are occasionally admitted to the pediatric ICU for the care of a severe acute illness. Each may have one or more associated factor deficiencies that may complicate patient management and result in bleeding. Patients with either amyloidosis or Gaucher disease may develop F.IX deficiency. F.X deficiency has also been associated with amyloidosis. These deficiencies generally result from the adsorption of the specific clotting factor by the abnormal proteins present in each disorder. In the nephrotic syndrome, F.IX deficiency may develop. Although it was originally thought that proteinuria was responsible for the development of F.IX deficiency, this does not appear to be the case. The deficiency typically remits with corticosteroid therapy.

Key References

1. Eilertsen KE, Osterud B. Tissue factor: (patho)physiology and cellular biology. *Blood Coagul Fibrinolysis*. 2004;15:521-538.
4. Aird WC. The role of the endothelium in severe sepsis and the multiple organ dysfunction syndrome. *Blood*. 2003;101:3765-3777.
8. Esmon CT. Crosstalk between inflammation and thrombosis. *Maturitas*. 2004;47:305-314.
17. Chuansumrit A, Hotrakitya S, Sirinavin S, et al. Disseminated intravascular coagulation findings in 100 patients. *J Med Assoc Thai*. 1999; 82(suppl 1):S63-S68.
18. Oren H, Cingoz I, Duman M, et al. Disseminated intravascular coagulation in pediatric patients: clinical and laboratory features and prognostic factors influencing survival. *Pediatr Hematol Oncol*. 2005;22:679-688.
21. Barton JC, Poon MC. Coagulation testing of the Hickmann catheter blood in patients with acute leukemia. *Arch Intern Med*. 1986;146:2165-2169.
25. Bick RL, Arun B, Frenkel EP. Disseminated intravascular coagulation. Clinical and pathophysiological mechanisms and manifestations. *Haemostasis*. 1999;29:111-134.
26. Cauchie P, Cauchie Ch, Boudjeltia KZ, et al. Diagnosis and prognosis of overt disseminated intravascular coagulation in a general hospital—meaning of the ISTH score system, fibrin monomers, and lipoprotein-C-reactive protein complex formation. *Am J Hematol*. 2006;81: 414-419.
28. Voves C, Wuillemin WA, Zeerleder S. International Society on Thrombosis and Haemostasis score for overt disseminated intravascular coagulation predicts organ dysfunction and fatality in sepsis patients. *Blood Coagul Fibrinolysis*. 2006;17:445-451.
29. Gando S. The utility of a diagnostic scoring system for disseminated intravascular coagulation. *Crit Care Clin*. 2012;28:373-388.
30. El-Nawawy A, Abbassy AA, El-Bordiny M, et al. Evaluation of early detection and management of disseminated intravascular coagulation among Alexandria University pediatric intensive care patients. *J Trop Pediatr*. 2004;50:339-347.
33. Fakhouri F, Fremeaux-Bacchi V, Loirat C. Atypical hemolytic uremic syndrome: from the rediscovery of complement to targeted therapy. *Eur J Intern Med*. 2013;24:492-495.
34. Kaplan BS, Ruebner RL, Spinale JM, Copelovitch L. Current treatment of atypical hemolytic uremic syndrome. *Intractable Rare Dis Res*. 2014;3: 34-45.
35. Nguyen TC, Han YY, Kiss JE, et al. Intensive plasma exchange increases a disintegrin and metalloprotease with thrombospondin motifs-13 activity and reverses organ dysfunction in children with thrombocytopenia–associated multiple organ failure. *Crit Care Med*. 2008;36:2878-2887.
37. Goldenberg NA, Manco-Johnson MJ. Pediatric hemostasis and use of plasma components. *Best Prac Res Clin Haematol*. 2005;19:143-155.
38. Boffard KD, Riou B, Warren B, et al. Recombinant factor VIIa as adjunctive therapy for bleeding control in severely injured trauma patients: two parallel randomized, placebo-controlled, double blind clinical trials. *J Trauma*. 2005;59:8-15, discussion 15–18.
39. Mathew P, Young G. Recombinant factor VIIa in paediatric bleeding disorders—a 2006 review. *Haemophilia*. 2006;12:457-472.
42. Altman R, Scazziota A, De Lourdes Herrera M, et al. Recombinant factor VIIa reverses the inhibitory effect of aspirin or aspirin plus clopidogrel on in vivo thrombin generation. *J Thromb Haemost*. 2006;4: 2022-2027.
44. Afshari A. Evidence based evaluation of immune-coagulatory interventions in critical care. *Dan Med Bull*. 2011;58:B4316.

49. Iba T, Gando S, Thachil J. Anticoagulant therapy for sepsis-associated disseminated intravascular coagulation: the view from Japan. *J Thromb Haemost.* 2014;12:1010-1019.

51. Lisman T, Caldwell SH, Leebeck FWG, et al. Hemostasis in chronic liver disease. *J Thromb Haemost.* 2006;4:2059.

53. Roberts LN, Patel RK, Arya R. Haemostasis and thrombosis in liver disease. *Br J Haematol.* 2009;148:507-512.

54. Lisman T, Potre RJ. Rebalanced hemostasis in patients with liver disease: evidence and clinical consequences. *Blood.* 2010;116:878-885.

55. Lisman T, Bakhtiari K, Adelmeijer J, et al. Intact thrombin generation and decreased fibrinolytic capacity in patients with acute liver injury or acute liver failure. *J Thromb Haemost.* 2012;10:1312-1319.

57. Townsend JC, Heard R, Powers ER, Reuben A. Usefulness of international normalized ratio to predict bleeding complications in patients with end-stage liver disease who undergo cardiac catheterization. *Am J Cardiol.* 2012;110:1062-1065.

59. Tripodi A, Baglin T, Robert A, et al. Reporting prothrombin time results as international normalized ratios for patients with chronic liver disease. *J Thromb Haemost.* 2010;8:1410-1412.

62. Segal JB, Dzik WH. Paucity of studies to support that abnormal coagulation test results predict bleeding in the setting of invasive procedures: an evidence-based review. *Transfusion.* 2005;45:1413-1425.

63. Dasher K, Trotter JF. Intensive care unit management of liver-related coagulation disorders. *Crit Care Clin.* 2012;28:389-398.

64. Youssef WI, Salazar F, Dasarathy S, et al. Role of fresh frozen plasma infusion in correction of coagulopathy of chronic liver disease: a dual phase study. *Am J Gastroenterology.* 2003;98:1391-1394.

65. Ganguly S, Spengel K, Tilzer LL, et al. Recombinant factor VIIa: unregulated continuous use in patients with bleeding and coagulopathy does not alter mortality and outcome. *Clin Lab Haematol.* 2006;28:309-312.

66. Ramsey G. Treating coagulopathy in liver disease with plasma transfusions or recombinant factor VIIa: an evidence based review. *Best Prac Res Clin Haematol.* 2005;19:113-126.

68. Goodnough LT. A reappraisal of plasma, prothrombin complex concentrates, and recombinant factor VIIa in patient blood management. *Crit Care Clin.* 2012;28:413-426.

70. Brady KM, Easley RB, Tobias JD. Recombinant activated factor VII (rFVIIa) treatment in infants with hemorrhage. *Paediatr Anaesth.* 2006;16:1042-1046.

71. Dentali F, Ageno W, Crowther M. Treatment of coumarin-associated coagulopathy: a systemic review and proposed treatment algorithms. *J Thromb Haemost.* 2006;4:1853-1863.

72. Hardy JF, de Moerloose P, Samama CM, et al. Massive transfusion and coagulopathy: pathophysiology and implications for clinical management. *Can J Anaesth.* 2006;53(6 suppl):S40-S58.

73. Nosanov L, Inaba K, Okoye O, et al. The impact of blood product ratios in massively transfused pediatric trauma patients. *Am J Surg.* 2013;20:655-660.

80. Theusinger OM, Madjdpour C, Spahn DR. Resuscitation and transfusion management in trauma patients: emerging concepts. *Curr Opin Crit Care.* 2012;18:661-670.

83. Carr JA, Silverman N. The heparin-protamine interaction: a review. *J Cardiovasc Surg (Torino).* 1999;40:659-666.

85. Neunert C, Noroozi N, Norman G, et al. Severe bleeding events in adults and children with primary immune thrombocytopenia: a systematic review. *J Thromb Haemost.* 2015;13:457-464.

87. Frost J, Murbee L, Russo P, et al. Heparin-induced thrombocytopenia in the pediatric intensive care unit population. *Pediatr Crit Care Med.* 2005;6:216-219.

88. Warkentin TE, Kelton JG. A 14-year study of heparin-induced thrombocytopenia. *Am J Med.* 1996;101:502-507.

89. Cuker A, Arepally G, Crowther MA, et al. The HIT Expert Probability (HEP) Score: a novel pre-test probability model for heparin-induced thrombocytopenia based on broad expert opinion. *J Thromb Haemost.* 2010;8:2642-2650.

90. Cuker A, Gimotty PA, Crowther MA, Warkentin TE. Predictive value of the 4Ts scoring system for heparin-induced thrombocytopenia: a systematic review and meta-analysis. *Blood.* 2012;120:4160-4167.

91. Risch L, Huber AR, Schmugge M. Diagnosis and treatment of heparin-induced thrombocytopenia in neonates and children. *Thromb Res.* 2006;118:123-135.

93. Takemoto CM, Streiff MB. Heparin-induced thrombocytopenia screening and management in pediatric patients. *Am Soc Hematol.* 2011;2011:162-169.

98. Young G, Tarantino MD, Wohrley J, et al. Pilot dose-finding and safety of bivalirudin in infants <6 months of age with thrombosis. *J Thromb Haemost.* 2007;5:1654-1659.

99. Young G, Boshkov LK, Sullivan LJ, et al. Argatroban therapy in pediatric patients requiring nonheparin anticoagulation: an open-label, safety, efficacy, and pharmacokinetic study. *Pediatr Blood Cancer.* 2011;56:1103-1109.

100. Hall R, Mazer CD. Antiplatelet drugs: a review of their pharmacology and management in the perioperative period. *Anesth Analg.* 2011;112:292-311.

Thrombosis in Pediatric Intensive Care

Sally Campbell and Paul Monagle

PEARLS

- Vascular access devices are the most common cause of thromboembolic disease in children, and every attempt should be made to limit their use based on real clinical need.
- Thrombophilia is rarely the major cause of thrombosis in critically ill children, and multiple tests to identify thrombophilic states are rarely useful to patient management.
- For reasons that remain uncertain, heparin-induced thrombocytopenia is rarely seen in children.
- Care must be taken in the diagnosis of thrombosis in children, as assumptions made in adult diagnostic strategies may not be true in children.
- Unfractionated heparin is the most useful anticoagulant in critically ill children; however, dosing errors are common, and pediatric intensive care units should spend considerable resources on training and systems to ensure safe management of heparin.

Dramatic improvements in pediatric intensive care have led to the improved survival of critically ill children and to the emergence of previously rare complications. To achieve this improved survival, there has been a dramatic increase in the invasiveness of supportive care. The use of central venous access, invasive arterial monitoring, and circulatory support including ventricular assist devices (VADs) and extracorporeal membrane oxygenation (ECMO), as well as processes such as hemofiltration and hemodialysis that are performed through large-bore vascular access devices, will increase the likelihood of vascular endothelial damage or direct vascular obstruction. These insults to the vascular system are often combined with prolonged hypotension, systemic inflammatory states, and infection, all of which may alter endothelial and vascular responsiveness. Finally, a multitude of drugs and fluids are administered during the periods of critical illness, which can impact directly on plasma proteins and endothelial function or which may lead to dilution of critical plasma proteins involved in the coagulation system. Not surprisingly, therefore, thromboembolism is an increasingly common problem

faced in the pediatric intensive care unit (PICU) setting, and it contributes significantly to morbidity and mortality.

This chapter describes key issues related to thrombosis in the PICU. Developmental hemostasis is a crucial concept both to the understanding of the etiology of thrombosis in children and to the application of diagnostic and therapeutic strategies. The etiology, epidemiology, clinical features, diagnosis, and management of the major types of thrombosis encountered in children in the PICU will be discussed. However, thromboses of the central nervous system (CNS), including arterial ischemic stroke and cerebral sinovenous thrombosis, are beyond the scope of this chapter (see Chapter 69). As in many areas of pediatrics, high-level evidence is often lacking; however, best-available evidence will be drawn upon where possible. Extrapolation from adult studies resulting in suboptimal treatment outcomes in children highlights the need for pediatric-specific trials and guidelines.

Developmental Hemostasis

The hemostatic system is a dynamic, evolving entity that not only affects the frequency and natural history of thromboembolic disease in children but also the response to therapeutic agents.[1-5] The global functioning of the coagulation system in neonates and children is different from that in adults, as are the plasma levels of many coagulation proteins. Overall the levels of most coagulation proteins increase with age, and neonates compared with adults have significantly lower levels of these proteins.[6] The exceptions are FV, FVIII, FXIII, and vWF, which are elevated at birth compared with adults. In addition to quantitative differences, there is evidence (mostly from animal models) of qualitative differences in many coagulation proteins, especially in neonates.[7,8] Although ongoing research in this area is desperately needed, current knowledge regarding the differences between adults and children in plasma proteins most likely to impact on anticoagulation therapy is as follows.

Plasma concentrations of antithrombin (AT) are physiologically low at birth (~0.50 U/mL) and do not increase to adult values until 3 months of age. Sick premature neonates frequently have plasma levels of AT of less than 0.30 U/mL. This likely has a profound effect on the action of heparin, whose antithrombotic activity is dependent on the catalysis of AT to inactivate specific coagulation enzymes, in particular thrombin. Some studies suggest children in pediatric intensive care

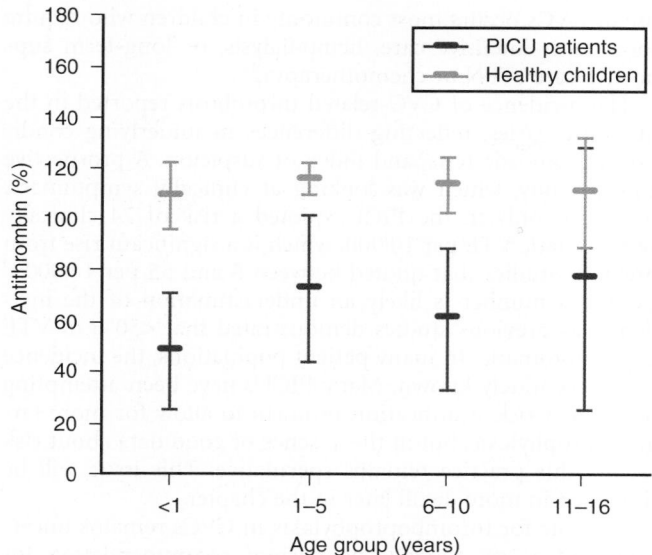

Fig. 92.1. Antithrombin levels by age group in samples obtained from children in a pediatric intensive care unit (PICU) compared to age-matched controls. Note the reduction in antithrombin levels in sick children. (Courtesy P. Monagle.)

units have markedly reduced AT levels compared to age-matched controls, potentially further enhancing this effect (Fig. 92.1). The capacity of plasmas from neonates to generate thrombin is both delayed and decreased compared to adults, and it is similar to plasma from adults receiving therapeutic amounts of heparin.[9] Both an increased sensitivity and an increased resistance to unfractionated heparin's anticoagulant activities have been reported in vitro in plasma from neonates. Increased sensitivity to unfractionated heparin is observed in systems based on assays dependent on thrombin generation (eg, activated partial thromboplastin time [APTT]). The in vitro effects of unfractionated heparin (0.25 U/mL) on neonates, children, and adults were compared, and thrombin generation was delayed and reduced in children compared to adults and virtually absent in neonates.[10] Resistance to unfractionated heparin is observed in systems based on assays that measure the inhibition of exogenously added factor Xa or thrombin and that are dependent on plasma concentrations of AT.

In vitro, thrombin generation is similar in adults and children at the same concentration of low-molecular-weight heparin (LMWH). However, at 0.25 U/mL LMWH, thrombin generation was delayed and reduced by approximately half in newborns compared to adults. These differences were matched by reductions in rates of prothrombin consumption.[10]

The vitamin K–dependent clotting factors are the most extensively studied group of factors in infants. Factors II, VIII, IX, and X have been demonstrated to be one-half to one-third of that of adults, despite receiving vitamin K prophylaxis at birth. The levels of the vitamin K–dependent factors and the contact factors (factors XI and XII, prekallikrein, and high-molecular-weight kininogen) gradually increase to values approaching adult levels by 6 months of life. For children receiving vitamin K antagonists, the capacity of their plasmas to generate thrombin is delayed and decreased by 25% com-

pared to plasmas from adults with similar international normalized ratios (INRs).[11]

Whether the overall activity of the protein C/protein S system varies with age is unknown. However, at birth, plasma concentrations of protein C are very low, and they remain decreased during the first 6 months of life. Although total amounts of protein S are decreased at birth, functional activity is similar to that in the adult because protein S is completely present in the free, active form because of the absence of C4-binding protein.[12,13] Furthermore, the interaction of protein S with activated protein C in newborn plasma may be regulated by the increased levels of α_2-macroglobulin. Plasma concentrations of thrombomodulin are increased in early childhood and decrease to adult values by the late teenage years. However, the influence of age on endothelial cell expression of thrombomodulin has not been determined.[14]

Despite the changes in individual protein levels and in global tests of coagulation, the hemostatic system in neonates and children does not seem disadvantageous compared to the "normal" coagulation system as measured in adults. There are no data to support either an increased bleeding or thrombotic risk during infancy and childhood for any given stimulus; on the contrary, one could argue that the hemostatic system in neonates and children is protective against bleeding and thrombotic complications compared to adults. This is despite the fact that when considering individual proteins, many proteins exist at levels during stages of infancy that would be associated with disease in adults. There clearly remains much to be learned about the evolution of the coagulation system with age, and this is an area in which there is much ongoing active research. As a better understanding of the neonatal and child coagulation system is achieved over coming years, thinking may change regarding many aspects of thrombosis development and management in this patient population.

Etiology and Epidemiology

Unlike adults, 95% of venous thromboembolism (VTE) cases in children are secondary to an identifiable risk factor,[15] and although there are a variety of risk factors to consider, perhaps the most useful concept for the clinician to understand remains the Virchow triad.[16] The Virchow triad recognizes that three factors are involved in the development of thrombosis: the blood vessel wall, the blood constituents, and blood flow[17] (Fig. 92.2). Patients in the PICU often demonstrate abnormalities in one, two, or all of these factors, and the recognition of this information can be a useful guide to therapy. For example, in a patient with a cardiac lesion, either primary or postsurgical, where there is extremely poor blood flow in one part of the cardiovascular system, the optimal management is to improve the blood flow. Although anticoagulation may have an important role, progressively increasing the intensity of anticoagulation will significantly increase the risk of bleeding and yet may not substantially further reduce the risk of thrombosis, which is being driven primarily by flow. Alternatively, patients with disseminated intravascular coagulation (DIC) have a marked perturbation of function of the vascular endothelium; therefore anticoagulation alone is unlikely to prevent thrombotic complications, which will only be avoided by treatment of the primary illness and subsequent resolution of the DIC.

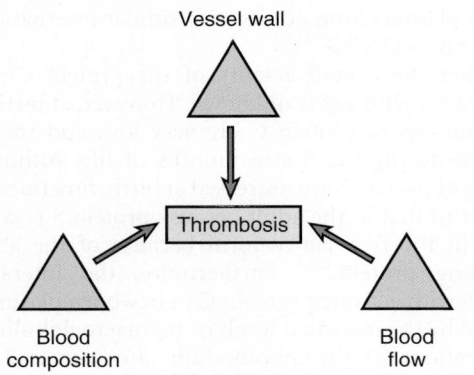

Fig. 92.2. Virchow's triad, highlighting the importance of each factor in contributing to thrombosis formation.

Combinations of these factors are important in many instances. For example, central venous access is a common precipitant of thrombosis, most typically through interruption to flow (especially in small infants where the catheter-to-vein diameter ratio is close to 1:1) and through disruption of the vessel wall at the insertion site. However, thrombosis is seen more commonly when there is an additional abnormality in the blood constituents as well, for example, in protein-losing states like nephrotic syndrome or enteropathy, through inflammatory or septic conditions, or via drugs such as oral contraceptives. Consideration of the etiologic factors in this way often enables clinicians to make some attempt at risk stratification and to modify care to reduce some of the multifactorial drivers of thrombosis on an individual basis, even though there may not be clear numeric data from large studies on the actual level of risk.

Table 92.1 summarizes the epidemiology and known risk factors for most etiologies of common non-CNS thrombosis seen in critically ill children. The most important risk factors for thrombosis in the pediatric intensive care unit remain the presence of vascular access devices and recent cardiac surgery. Two additional risk factors worth discussing, although they are not often particularly relevant in children, are thrombophilias and heparin-induced thrombocytopenia.

Central Venous Access Devices

The most common risk factor for venous thrombosis in children appears to be the presence of a central venous catheter (CVC), although most children have several concomitant risk factors.[18] Over 50% of venous thromboembolisms in children occur in the upper venous system secondary to the use of CVCs. Three types of CVC-related thrombosis are described in the literature: clots at the tips of CVCs that impair infusion or withdrawal of blood; fibrin sleeves that are not adherent to vessel walls but may occlude CVCs; and CVC-related thrombi that adhere to vessel walls, with partial or complete obstruction of vessels where the CVC is located. This discussion refers to this third type of thrombosis only—that is, obstructive CVC-related thrombosis. A number of mechanisms may contribute to the development of CVC-related thrombosis, including damage to the vessel wall by the CVC or by substances infused through the CVC (total parenteral nutrition [TPN], chemotherapy), disrupted blood flow due to the presence of the CVC, and thrombogenic catheter materials. The

use of CVCs occurs most commonly in children who require short-term intensive care, hemodialysis, or long-term supportive care (TPN or chemotherapy).[16]

The incidence of CVC-related thrombosis reported in the literature varies, reflecting differences in underlying conditions, diagnostic tests, and index of suspicion. A prospective cohort study, which was looking at clinically symptomatic thrombus only in the PICU, quoted a risk of 74 clinically symptomatic VTE per 10,000, which is a significant rise from previous studies that quoted between 5 and 55 per 10,000.[19] Even this number is likely an underestimation of the incidence, as previous studies demonstrated that <50% of VTE are symptomatic. In many patient populations, the incidence is not accurately known. Many PICUs have been attempting to create a risk stratification protocol to allow for more targeted prophylaxis, but in the absence of good data about risk factors this practice remains speculative. This issue will be discussed in more detail later in the chapter.

The role for thromboprophylaxis in CVCs remains uncertain, and as yet there is no current recommendation for routine systemic prophylaxis for short- to medium-term CVC. One of the many issues with studying this area is the difference in nomenclature about "prophylaxis." VTE prophylaxis with unfractionated heparin (UFH) or LMWH is often confused with "line prophylaxis" or "line patency prophylaxis" (usually UFH but at very different doses).

Arterial Access

The most common type of arterial thrombosis in children occurs as a result of placement of arterial catheters. Non–catheter-related arterial thrombosis may be congenital (familial hyperlipidemia and hyperhomocysteinemia) or acquired (Takayasu arteritis, Kawasaki disease, congenital heart disease, and arterial thrombosis in transplanted organs). There are, in general, three types of arterial catheterizations that are used in children that may result in arterial thrombosis: umbilical arterial catheterization in neonates (which will not be discussed in this chapter), cardiac catheterization, and peripheral catheterization. Arterial occlusion causes tissue ischemia resulting in tissue necrosis if the vascular occlusion persists. Organ and tissue damage at remote sites may result from embolic events occurring due to fragmentation of the original thrombus.

Often, in the PICU, short-term femoral artery access will be required, emergency femoral artery puncture will be performed, or, alternatively, the femoral artery will be inadvertently accessed during attempts at femoral venous access. In terms of understanding the implications of this approach, one can only really extrapolate from the cardiac catheterization literature, recognizing that diagnostic and therapeutic cardiac catheterization via the femoral artery have significant differences in terms of thrombosis risk.

Adverse events occurring as a result of femoral artery puncture include arterial spasm and arterial thrombosis. Clinically, vascular spasm and thrombosis are indistinguishable in the initial phases of presentation with the following symptoms: decreased or absent pulses, pale or mottled limb, and decreased capillary refill. Arterial spasm usually resolves within a few hours in the absence of therapy, whereas arterial thrombosis usually requires therapy. The incidence of femoral artery thrombosis following cardiac catheterization without thromboprophylaxis is approximately 40%. The incidence is inversely proportional to patient age and weight, with infants at highest risk.[20] The frequency of femoral artery thrombosis in PICUs is unclear. Similarly with peripheral arterial catheterization, the mechanism of injury is endothelial damage and blood vessel occlusion. The exact frequency of peripheral arterial occlusion in the PICU remains unknown.

Cardiac Surgery

Children with congenital heart disease constitute a major proportion of children seen in tertiary hospitals with thrombosis. Data show that almost 50% of infants less than 6 months old and 30% of older children who suffer venous thromboembolic disease have underlying cardiac disorders. Similarly, almost 70% of infants (less than 6 months) and 30% of children who suffer arterial thrombosis have underlying cardiac defects. In addition, the majority of children receiving primary anticoagulant prophylaxis are being treated for complex congenital heart disease or severe acquired cardiac illness.[20] Presumably, the mechanisms underlying this increased risk of thrombosis are alterations to blood flow (for example, following Fontan surgery, where venous return is driving the pulmonary blood flow) and disturbances of the vascular endothelium related to intravascular sutures or vascular manipulation. Whether a postsurgical inflammatory state induces changes in the blood constituents that predispose to thrombosis is also unknown. Two classic examples of cardiac surgery–related thrombosis are the Blalock Taussig (BT) shunt and the Fontan procedure.

The natural history of BT shunts has been assessed using angiography. Godart and colleagues[21] assessed BT shunt growth and development of stenosis and distortion in 78 patients at a mean follow-up time of 51 months. They found that growth of the pulmonary arteries occurred but did not exceed the normal growth of the pulmonary arterial tree. However, a shunt procedure could cause distortion and stenosis of the pulmonary artery that might have important implications for future corrective surgical intervention. Risk factors for patency and stenosis include the age of the patient and graft size.[22,23]

The incidence of thrombotic occlusion of BT shunts in the literature ranges from 1% to 17%.[24-27] This risk might be increased in children having first-stage Norwood surgery, as these children are small and unstable and often have labile blood pressures as well.

There have been a number of reviews regarding anticoagulation after Fontan surgery.[28,29] The Fontan procedure, or a modified version, is the definitive palliative surgical treatment for most congenital univentricular heart lesions. Thrombosis remains a major cause of early and late morbidity and mortality. Reported incidences of venous thrombosis and stroke ranged from 3% to 16% and 3% to 19%, respectively, in retrospective cohort studies where thrombosis was the primary outcome, and from 1% to 7% in retrospective studies assessing multiple outcomes. Thrombosis may occur anytime following Fontan procedures, but it often presents months to years later. No predisposing factors have been identified with certainty, although this may be due to inadequate power and the retrospective nature of the studies.

Thrombophilia

Congenital thrombophilia is usually defined as having the following features: (1) positive family history, (2) early age of onset of thromboembolism, (3) recurrent disease, and (4) multiple or unusual thrombosis locations. Clinically, the most significant inherited prothrombotic conditions are deficiencies of antithrombin (AT), protein C (PC), and protein S (PS), because of the large increase in relative risk these deficiencies confer. Activated protein C resistance/factor V Leiden (FV-R506Q) and prothrombin G20210A (IIG20210A) polymorphism, while having less impact on individual risk, are significant because of their frequencies in certain populations. A large number of other candidate genes have been proposed as risk factors for congenital thrombophilia.[30] However, most of these candidates have not undergone careful segregation or population studies to define their pathogenic role. In fact, some of the seemingly obvious candidates such as abnormalities in fibrinolysis do not appear to confer thrombotic risk.[31] These latter studies are, however, hampered by the low prevalence of most of these inherited abnormalities in the general population.

Reports demonstrate an increased risk for thrombosis in families with a second genetic abnormality.[32] Most reports have described a combination of FV-R506Q with abnormalities of PC, PS, or AT. These findings begin to shed light on the marked variability in clinical expression of these syndromes. The effect of more severe deficiencies has long been evident from the severely affected neonates with homozygous PC and PS deficiency. Apart from the well-defined homozygous cases, the risk and severity of thrombosis appear to vary with the type and number of underlying genetic abnormalities.[32-34]

The role of these congenital prothrombotic states in childhood thrombosis remains controversial. Despite meta-analyses suggesting that thrombophilia is a significant risk factor in childhood thrombosis, there are serious limitations to the published literature on which these meta-analyses are based.[35]

The reported incidence of congenital prothrombotic disorders in children with venous thrombosis varies from less than 1% to over 60%.[33,34,36-64] If one considers the deficiencies of AT, PC, and PS in addition to the factor V Leiden and prothrombin gene mutations, large family studies found negligible rates of thrombosis in children younger than 15 years.[65] A number of cohort studies have failed to identify AT deficiency in children with both arterial and venous thrombosis.[53,54,56,57] Those studies that reported higher frequencies of AT deficiency did not distinguish between acquired and inherited deficiency. In children with cancer and venous thrombosis, the reported incidences of thrombophilias are 3%.[52,57] The variability in incidence reported in all these studies reflects small sample sizes, variability in study design, differing definitions of prothrombotic disorders, and different patient selection criteria.[66] A prospective study of an unselected cohort of children with venous thrombosis found that with the exception of teenagers with spontaneous thrombosis, inherited thrombophilic markers did not contribute significantly to the pathogenesis of venous thrombosis in children.[67]

Screening for congenital prothrombotic disorders in children with venous thrombosis is of unproved benefit, regardless of the presence or absence of acquired risk factors. At this time, uniform screening of children with major illnesses, or those who require CVCs, for congenital prothrombotic disorders in order to provide prophylactic therapy cannot be recommended. The contribution of congenital prothrombotic disorders to venous thrombosis in pediatric patients remains to be clarified. Few children develop thrombosis due to a heterozygote congenital prothrombotic condition without also having an acquired risk factor.[51,68-76]

TABLE 92.1   Summary of the Epidemiology, Clinical Features, Diagnosis, and Complications of the Most Common Types of Non-CNS Thromboembolism in Children

	Type/Location	Age/Sex	Incidence	Underlying Illness or Risk Factors	Clinical Features	Diagnosis	Complications
Spontaneous VTE	Lower limb	M = F Teenagers	1.2 per 10,000 hospital admissions		Leg, inguinal, or abdominal pain Leg swelling or discoloration	Doppler US	Immediate: PE Cardiac extension Chylothorax SVC syndrome Long-term: Recurrent VTE PPS
	Axillary	M = F Teenagers	Very rare	Mass lesion Thoracic inlet obstruction New sport involving arms	Arm swelling, pain, and discoloration	Doppler US	
CVAD-related VTE	Line tip thrombosis	Higher in neonates		Cancer, sepsis, trauma, surgery, immobility, long-term lines, congenital heart disease, burns, cardiac catheterization	Inability to flush or draw from line	Linogram Echocardiogram if tip in RA	Variceal hemorrhage
	Fibrin sleeve				Asymptomatic	Linogram, venography	
	CVAD-related DVT Iliofemoral, IVC, jugular, subclavian		1%–75%		Asymptomatic Limb or facial swelling, pain, discoloration SVC syndrome, chylothorax	Doppler US for neck, limb, and abdominal TE Venography (radiograph, CT, or MR) for intrathoracic TE	
PE			Up to 30% children with CVC-related DVT	CVAD-related DVT RA thrombus, cancer, CHD, cardiomyopathy, burns, sepsis, trauma, nephrotic syndrome, APLA, transplantation	Asymptomatic (up to 50%) Tachycardia Chest pain Respiratory distress Increased oxygen requirements Acute right heart failure Collapse Sudden death	V/Q scan Pulmonary angiography Plain radiography, CT, MR ECG Autopsy most common diagnostic test in children	Death Pulmonary hypertension and heart failure Recurrence
Arterial TE	Peripheral arterial catheter Radial artery, occasionally foot arteries			Peripheral arterial catheter	Acute limb ischemia: blanching, pallor, diminished pulses/CR Loss of patency	Doppler US	Ischemia (hand)
	UAC Celiac, mesenteric, renal, and lower limb arteries			Umbilical arterial catheter	Loss of patency Lower limb ischemia NEC/organ ischemia	Doppler US Contrast angiography	Organ ischemia NEC Lower limb TE CNS TE (via PFO)

Site	Incidence	Risk factors	Clinical features	Diagnosis	Complications
Cardiac catheter / Femoral artery	Up to 10%; Increased in younger children	Repeated manipulations, balloon dilatations, raised hematocrit	Limb ischemia	Doppler US	Reduced limb growth; Claudication; Loss of future access
Congenital and acquired arterial disease / Coronary, cerebral, peripheral arterial disease	Rare	Hyperlipidemia, homocystinuria, acquired arteritis (Takayasu, Kawasaki)	Xanthomata; Features of vasculitis or underlying disease	Echocardiography; Doppler US; Angiography	Myocardial infarction; Stroke
Cardiac valve		Mechanical heart valves	Murmur, valvular dysfunction	Echocardiography; Angiography, CT, MR	Stroke; Limb TE; PE
Cardiac shunt including Fontan	19% post-Fontan patients	Shunts including Fontan	Acute loss of pulmonary blood flow		
Renal vein thrombosis (Neonates: Unilateral 70%, Bilateral 30%; Older children)	M = 64%	Asphyxia, polycythemia, and dehydration, sepsis, cyanotic CHD, infant of diabetic mother; Nephrotic syndrome, burns, SLE, transplant	Flank mass; Hematuria, proteinuria; Thrombocytopenia; Renal failure; Diarrhea and vomiting; Dehydration, hypovolemia	Doppler US (CT, MRI)	Adrenal hemorrhage; Renal failure; Hypertension
Portal vein thrombosis		Neonates: UVC; Children: Liver transplant, abdominal sepsis, splenectomy, sickle cell disease, APLA; Up to 50% idiopathic	Acute abdomen; Portal hypertension, GI bleeding, splenomegaly	Doppler US; MRI/MRA; CT	Death; Portal hypertension and variceal hemorrhage
Hepatic artery thrombosis			Asymptomatic	Pulsed Doppler + real time US; Angiography; CT/MRI	
Renal artery thrombosis			Anuria, renal failure; Other signs of acute rejection	Doppler US	

APLA, antiphospholipid antibody; *CHD*, congenital heart disease; *CNS*, central nervous system; *CR*, capillary return; *CT*, computed tomography; *CVAD*, central venous access device; *CVC*, central venous catheter; *DVT*, deep vein thrombosis; *ECG*, electrocardiogram; *F*, female; *IVC*, inferior vena cava; *M*, male; *MRA*, magnetic resonance angiography; *MRI*, magnetic resonance imaging; *NEC*, necrotizing enterocolitis; *PE*, pulmonary embolus; *PFO*, patent foramen ovale; *PPS*, postphlebotic syndrome; *RA*, right atrium; *SLE*, systemic lupus erythematosus; *SVC*, superior vena cava; *TE*, thromboembolism; *UAC*, umbilical arterial catheter; *UVC*, umbilical venous catheter; *US*, ultrasound; *V/Q*, ventilation/perfusion; *VTE*, venous thromboembolism.

In summary, the data supporting inherited thrombophilia as a major factor in thrombosis in childhood are conflicting. In the PICU, it is likely that the dominant factors are clinical risk factors for thrombosis and that, if it contributes at all, thrombophilia may act as an additional hit in a multihit pathogenesis. However, there remains no evidence to support routine screening for thrombophilia, and there are certainly no data to support primary prophylaxis of children with inherited heterozygous thrombophilia. Further, there is no evidence that the presence or absence of thrombophilia changes acute treatment once a thrombosis is diagnosed. Given the inherent difficulties in interpreting at least the functional assays of protein levels in acutely sick children, there seems little role for thrombophilia testing in the PICU.

Heparin-Induced Thrombocytopenia

Heparin-induced thrombocytopenia (HIT) occurs in approximately 3% to 5% of adults exposed to UFH and is typically associated with a reduced platelet count, occurrence 5 to 10 days after heparin exposure, and an increased risk of thrombosis despite the thrombocytopenia. HIT is the result of a complex antigen-antibody interaction, and the most important therapeutic intervention once HIT is diagnosed is the immediate withdrawal of all heparinoid anticoagulants and substitution with nonheparinoid drugs until the risk of thrombosis is ameliorated.[77]

A number of case reports of pediatric HIT have described patients ranging in age from 3 months to 15 years.[15,78-82] UFH exposure in these cases ranged from low-dose exposure during heparin flushes used in maintaining patency of venous access devices, to supratherapeutic doses given during cardiopulmonary bypass and hemodialysis. Studies specifically examining the frequency of HIT in children have varied in their reported results, likely related to differences in patient inclusion and laboratory techniques.[83-87] Reported rates vary from almost nonexistent in unselected heparinized children[86] to up to 2.3% in children in the PICU.[87] However, HIT appears to occur far less frequently in children than in adults, and the rationale for this is unclear.[86] Many patients in the neonatal intensive care unit/PICU who are exposed to UFH have multiple potential reasons for thrombocytopenia or thrombosis, and papers confirm that many positive HIT tests are in fact false positives.[88] Danaparoid, hirudin, and argatroban are alternatives to UFH in children with HIT[80-82,89-91]; however, these drugs have significant risks in children.[92] Until such time as the true clinical incidence of HIT in children is understood, the diagnostic tests have higher sensitivity and specificity, and there are safe and reliable alternatives to heparin therapy in acutely sick children, the diagnosis of HIT in children should be made with caution. Careful attention to the diagnostic criteria, exclusion of other causes, and rational use of test results are all required.

Clinical Features

The clinical symptoms and complications of venous thrombosis in children can be classified as acute or long term. The acute clinical symptoms include loss of CVC patency; swelling, pain, and discoloration of the related limb; swelling of the face and head with superior vena cava syndrome; and respiratory compromise with pulmonary embolus (PE). The long-term complications include prominent collateral circulation in the skin (face, back, chest, and neck as sequelae of upper venous thrombosis, and abdomen, pelvis, groin, and legs as sequelae of lower venous thrombosis), repeated loss of CVC patency, repeated requirement for CVC replacement, eventual loss of venous access, CVC-related sepsis, chylothorax, chylopericardium, recurrent thrombosis necessitating long-term anticoagulation and its risk of bleeding, and postthrombotic syndrome.

In adults, asymptomatic thromboses are not necessarily treated, and thrombosis experts argue that these thrombi are probably inconsequential. Symptomatic thrombi are treated to prevent embolism and extension. Asymptomatic thromboses in pediatric patients may carry significance for many reasons, namely the risk of sepsis, a potential source for a pulmonary embolus, and loss of access that may be life threatening for children requiring organ transplant. The relationship between VTE and infection remains complex, as each one appears to be risk factor for the other, and although it is appreciable that VTE can be a nidus for infection, having a bloodstream infection particularly with staphylococcus aureus is a potent stimulator for the development of VTE.[93] PE in children is frequently not diagnosed during life due to the subtle symptoms and the presence of other illnesses, but it can cause sudden respiratory compromise. However, PE most commonly results from CVC-related thrombosis and can cause death.[62] Additionally, in a child with a patent foramen ovale (or any cardiac right-to-left shunt) and venous thrombosis, stroke may occur as a result of the right-to-left intracardiac connection. Sudden death has been described in a few case reports from rupture of an intrathoracic collateral vessel thought to have resulted from CVC placement years earlier. Loss of venous access is a devastating complication of CVC-related thrombosis in children requiring vascular access for organ transplant, lifelong TPN, or dialysis. The exact rate of complications from asymptomatic CVC-related deep vein thrombosis (DVT) in critically ill children is unknown. Despite the aforementioned theoretic reasons for why asymptomatic thromboses in children have raised concerns about the need for treatment, a study examining the acute complications of asymptomatic CVC-related DVT in critically ill children found no increase in complications.[83] This raises the question as to whether asymptomatic thromboses that are CVC related should be treated, and further research to answer this question is needed.

The clinical presentation of pulmonary embolus in children is often masked. In critically ill children, sudden cardiorespiratory deterioration can be due to a multitude of causes, and the difficulty in performing appropriate imaging to confirm the diagnosis of PE often means the diagnosis is either not considered or unable to be substantiated. Further, previously healthy children tend to tolerate large pulmonary embolus remarkably well, so often shortness of breath or dyspnea is transient, and the resolution of symptoms betrays the significance of the underlying pathology. Many children with substantial PE have no symptoms at all, until they demonstrate those of chronic venous hypertension or a subsequent further PE has fatal consequences. Clinical suspicion for PE must be high in all critically unwell children, especially those with central venous access devices in situ.

The clinical presentation of arterial thrombosis in children is often more straightforward, with cold, pale, pulseless limbs acutely related in time to the placement of an arterial catheter. However, other systemic arterial thrombosis, for example, emboli to abdominal organs, may present with vague and nondiscriminatory symptoms. Arterial thrombosis related to transplanted vessels may present as sudden graft loss.

Diagnosis
Venous Thrombosis

Little is known about the precision and accuracy of the noninvasive imaging techniques that are commonly used to make the diagnosis of venous thrombosis in neonates. There are few studies comparing currently used diagnostic tests. The low pulse pressure and small vessels in premature newborns can make ultrasound more difficult to interpret. Similarly, the presence of CVCs makes compressibility difficult to assess and, accordingly, greatly reduces the sensitivity of ultrasound. In neonates with umbilical vein catheters, Doppler ultrasound was shown to be poor compared to contrast venography in detecting asymptomatic thrombi.

The exception is renal vein thrombosis (RVT), where ultrasound is the radiographic test of choice because of its sensitivity in detecting an enlarged kidney, as distinct from the ability to detect intravascular thrombosis. Color Doppler ultrasound may demonstrate absent intrarenal and renal venous flow in the early stages of RVT. Magnetic resonance imaging (MRI) and computerized tomography (CT) have also been used for RVT, but they have no apparent advantages over ultrasound.

In summary, in neonates with suspected venous thrombosis, venography remains the gold standard where possible. Clinicians will often be forced to use a combination of clinical assessment and suboptimal imaging to make clinical decisions, because the gold standard is practically unachievable. This issue must be factored into progressive decision making.

In older children, there are a few more data about diagnostic strategies. A well-designed substudy of the PAARKA investigation compared venography versus ultrasound for the diagnosis of asymptomatic upper venous system CVC-related venous thromboembolism. Ultrasound was demonstrated to have a sensitivity of 20% for intrathoracic thrombosis, yet it diagnosed jugular thrombi that were missed on venography.[94] The Linogram, Ultrasound, and Venogram (LUV) study compared linogram, ultrasound, and venography for the diagnosis of symptomatic upper venous system CVC-related thrombosis.[95] Most of the thrombi in this study were located in the jugular veins and diagnosed by ultrasound (80% sensitivity) but not venography.[96] Another study compared magnetic resonance venography (MRV) to ultrasound and linogram in 25 children with multiple CVC insertions who were suspected of having major central venous thrombosis.[96] Linogram consistently underestimated the extent of thrombosis. Ultrasound detected only 7 of 18 thromboses seen on MRV and underestimated the extent of 4 of the 7. In all cases, ultrasound identified jugular thrombosis but failed to identify more central thrombosis. Further, MRV identified a patent vein for reinsertion of CVC in 22 of 25 children. At operation, venous patency was confirmed in 20 patients (91%). There are no studies determining the sensitivity and specificity of diagnostic testing for lower venous system CVC-related thrombosis in children.

In summary, for children with suspected upper system thrombosis, a combination of ultrasound (jugular veins) and bilateral upper limb venography (subclavian and central veins) is recommended. The temptation to extend ultrasound imaging below the clavicles should be resisted. MRV may be a viable alternative to formal venography depending on local expertise. For children with suspected lower system thrombosis, ultrasound is a reasonable alternative for veins distal to the groin, based on adult experience. As in adults, serial ultrasound may be required to exclude thrombosis in specific circumstances. For more proximal veins, venography or MRV should be considered. Of importance, although there is considerable literature about the value of sensitive D-dimer assays in excluding DVT in adults, there are no such data in children. Furthermore, given the preceding medical and surgical therapies that most children with DVT have received, D-dimer is unlikely to be of use. At this time, D-dimer is not part of the recommended diagnostic strategy for venous thrombosis in children.

Pulmonary Embolus

There are no studies determining the sensitivity and specificity of diagnostic testing for PE in children. However, literature would support the conclusion that PE is significantly underdiagnosed in children, especially those in intensive care settings. A number of potential difficulties with interpreting ventilation/perfusion (V/Q) scans in children at risk from PE have been identified. This is particularly the case in children following specific cardiac surgeries such as Fontan surgery, where total pulmonary blood flow may not be assessed by isotope injected into an upper limb. The true impact of these difficulties on diagnostic accuracy remains to be determined. In addition, there are concerns about the safety of perfusion scanning in children with significant right-to-left cardiac shunts, as it is likely that significant amounts of macroaggregated albumin will lodge in the cerebral circulation, and the impact of this factor is unknown.[97] Ventilation-perfusion scanning remains the recommended first-line investigation for PE in neonates and children. Pulmonary angiography remains the gold standard. Clinicians will frequently need to make a presumptive diagnosis based on clinical findings and the presence or absence of source thrombosis. CT pulmonary angiography may be an alternative, especially in the specific populations in whom V/Q scanning is more worrisome (eg, large right-to-left shunts), but CT may miss small peripheral pulmonary emboli. Further, repeated CT angiogram may cause significant radiation exposure to breast tissue in young female patients.[62]

Arterial Thrombosis

There is little specific information related to diagnostic strategies in neonates. Contrast angiography remains the gold standard. Peripheral arterial thrombosis is usually diagnosed clinically. Ultrasound remains unproved, although serial measurements may provide useful information. Aortic thrombosis, usually secondary to umbilical artery catheterization, requires radiologic diagnosis. Contrast angiography is rarely feasible in critically ill newborns. Noninvasive imaging techniques have not been validated. In fact, in one of the only comparative studies, ultrasound failed to visualize aortic thrombosis in four patients, three of whom had complete aortic obstruction by contrast angiography. Thus clinicians must often use clinical findings and suboptimal imaging to make clinical decisions.

In older children, many arterial thromboses are diagnosed on clinical grounds alone, for example, after femoral artery puncture. False negatives are reported using ultrasound to diagnose spontaneous femoral artery thrombosis in children. False-positive magnetic resonance angiography has been reported for chronic femoral artery obstruction when compared with formal angiography. In suspected peripheral artery thrombosis, clinicians should consider the possibility of intramural or external hematoma causing arterial compression as a differential diagnosis, and for peripheral arteries, ultrasound may be sufficiently sensitive to exclude this phenomenon.

Other important arterial thromboses are those that occur in the arterial supply to transplanted organs. For hepatic artery thrombosis after liver transplant, serial testing with pulsed Doppler combined with real-time ultrasound of the liver parenchyma has a sensitivity of approximately 70%. Both false-positive and false-negative results occur, such that angiography is usually required to confirm the diagnosis. Computerized tomography of the liver may be of aid in equivocal cases. Spiral CT has been shown to be sensitive and specific in adults. The value of MRI is yet to be fully determined.

Intracardiac Thrombosis

Three studies have specifically compared transthoracic echocardiography (TTE) to transesophageal echocardiography (TEE) in the diagnosis of intracardiac thrombosis following Fontan surgery.[98-100] Stumper and colleagues, in a cross-sectional survey of 18 patients, found three intracardiac thromboses using TEE, only one of which was detected by TTE. Fyfe and associates, in a similar study, found six thrombi in four pediatric patients using TEE, only one of which was detected by TTE. Balling and coworkers performed a cross-sectional study of 52 patients after Fontan surgery. Seventeen patients (33%) had thromboses seen on TEE, only one of which was identified on TTE. Several other publications reported intracardiac thromboses diagnosed by TEE or angiography that were not detected using TTE. Thus transthoracic echocardiography is likely insufficient to exclude intracardiac thrombosis in children after Fontan surgery, although the studies published had a number of design flaws.

The validity of transthoracic echocardiography in other clinical situations is unknown, and clinicians should consider the local expertise, availability of TEE, and the clinical situation before determining the diagnostic approach in any individual child. Right atrial and intracardiac thromboses are most common in children with CVCs extending into the right atrium. Risk stratification based on clot size and mobility is suggested. For low-risk patients with clot size <2 cm, nonmobile and attached to atrial wall, removal of the CVC without anticoagulation may be appropriate.[101]

Management

Overall, the management of thrombosis in children is based around anticoagulation. There are a multitude of reasons why anticoagulation therapy in children is more difficult to manage than anticoagulation therapy in adults, and some of these reasons are listed in Table 92.2. The indications for surgical intervention or thrombolysis are few and far between. A limited drug arsenal exists in terms of drugs for which there is experience in children. No anticoagulants are formally approved for use in children, so all anticoagulants are used off label. In critically unwell children, there are often multiple relative or even absolute contraindications to anticoagulation,

TABLE 92.2	Factors That Increase the Complexity of Anticoagulant Therapy in Children Compared With Adults
Factor	**Impact**
Epidemiology of thrombosis	Increased proportion of sick children with multiple comorbidities
Developmental hemostasis	Affects response to therapeutic agents
Pharmacokinetic differences	Volume of distribution, binding, and clearance of drugs varies with age
Concurrent illnesses	Increased frequency of intercurrent infections (and hence medications) in children
Less diagnostic certainty	Requirement for general anesthetic to perform diagnostic studies impairs ability to investigate and monitor thrombosis in children
Limited vascular access	Delivery of intravenous therapy and monitoring of anticoagulant therapy more difficult
Drug formulations	All anticoagulants are "off label" in children and there are no specific pediatric preparations, making accurate dosing difficult
Dietary differences	Formula-fed versus breast-fed infants have vastly different responses to certain drugs (eg, vitamin K antagonists)
Compliance	Age significantly affects ability to understand and cooperate with therapy
Parental supervision	Children in dysfunctional families present special management issues not seen in adults

and the balance of risk versus benefit is difficult to ascertain due to the lack of well-designed studies. In general, anticoagulation is best managed by a pediatric hematologist experienced in thrombosis and anticoagulation, in consultation with the critical care team. At all times, the overall management of the child's underlying condition must be kept in perspective versus the management of an individual thrombosis.

In terms of specific guidelines for managing thrombosis in children, the American College of Chest Physicians regularly publishes evidence-based guidelines, and the reader is referred to the most up-to-date version of these guidelines as the best overall guide to antithrombotic therapy in children.[15]

The most common drug used in critically unwell children is unfractionated heparin. Of all currently available anticoagulants, it is the only intravenous preparation with a short half-life and rapid onset and offset for which there is a known antidote. Low-molecular-weight heparins such as enoxaparin, tinzaparin, and dalteparin are all indicated for subcutaneous use in children. Although there are many situations in which low-molecular-weight heparins are advantageous, their long half-life and lack of reversibility with protamine usually make them poor anticoagulants for critically unwell children. Oral anticoagulation with coumarin derivatives such as warfarin is suitable for long-term anticoagulation, but the need for oral administration, slow onset of action, and long half-life make them unsuitable for acute anticoagulation of critically unwell children. A multitude of newer anticoagulants are available for use in adults, and their use in children has been reviewed.[92] To date, the outcome of these newer drugs when used in children has been poor. The lack of antidote for most of them is an important limitation when considering their use in critically ill children. Thus until further research identifies an alternative anticoagulant that has the advantageous properties of UFH, it will remain the anticoagulant of choice in PICUs.

Unfractionated Heparin in Children

UFH can be used as a first-line intervention to treat arterial and venous thromboses in infants and children. In addition, UFH also has numerous indications for primary thromboprophylaxis in infants and children, including cardiac angiography, artificial circuits (eg, cardiopulmonary bypass, hemodialysis, extracorporeal membrane oxygenation), arterial cannulation, and venoocclusive disease prevention during bone marrow transplantation. The short half-life of UFH makes it the ideal antithrombotic agent for use in critically ill children who are at greater risk of bleeding complications but who nonetheless require antithrombotic therapy.[102]

Unfractionated heparin is a complex glycosaminoglycan capable of binding to many circulating proteins as well as to the vascular endothelium.[103-105] The anticoagulant effect of therapeutic doses of UFH is largely limited to its interaction with antithrombin and tissue factor pathway inhibitor. Unfractionated heparin binding to AT occurs via a unique pentasaccharide sequence present in approximately one-third of UFH molecules.[105] The UFH:AT complex produces a thousandfold increase in AT inhibition of coagulation protein activity compared to AT alone.[106] Following intravenous administration of UFH, tissue factor pathway inhibitor (TFPI) release from the vascular endothelium increases in a dose- and concentration-dependent manner.[107] Unfractionated heparin is believed to increase the antithrombotic effect of TFPI by increasing its affinity for factor Xa by simultaneously binding to both proteins (Table 92.3).

The monitoring of UFH therapy in the PICU is a major problem. For many indications, there is no clear therapeutic range and certainly no clinical outcome data in pediatrics to support any particular therapeutic range. In addition, each of the monitoring tests available has significant limitations, particularly in children. Clearly, global measures of hemostasis such as the APTT will always be limited by confounding variables that affect results. Direct measurement of UFH's ability to inhibit specific coagulation proteins (eg, factor Xa), while producing definitive values, only represents one component

of UFH's inhibitory effect on in vivo coagulation. Protamine titration has been viewed as the gold standard with respect to the measurement of UFH; however, the lack of automation renders protamine titration less clinically practical. A summary of the available tests for monitoring UFH and their shortcomings in pediatrics is presented in Table 92.4.

The most important adverse effect from heparin therapy in children is bleeding. One cohort study reported bleeding in 1.5% (95% CI, 0.0% to 8.3%) of children treated with UFH for DVT/PE. However, many children were treated with subtherapeutic doses of UFH (compared to the target APTT) in this study.[108] A single-center cohort study reported a major bleeding rate of 24% in children in PICUs receiving UFH therapy.[109] Further studies are required to determine the true frequency of UFH-induced bleeding in optimally treated children. There are only three case reports of pediatric UFH-induced osteoporosis. In two of these, the patient received concurrent steroid therapy. However, given the convincing relationship between UFH and osteoporosis in adults, clinicians should avoid long-term use of UFH in children when alternative anticoagulants are available. HIT was discussed previously in this chapter.

When considering bleeding as an adverse effect of UFH, clinicians frequently view this complication as a consequence of trying to manage the balance between bleeding and clotting in critically ill children. However, in reality, one of the most common reasons for heparin-associated bleeding is an accidental overdose of UFH. This often occurs in children who are receiving low-dose UFH flushing of vascular access devices, intended, for example, to be 50 units UFH/5 mL. Errors in vial selection and failure of bedside checking procedures result in 5000 units UFH/5 mL being injected, and in small infants this results in a massive overdose of UFH. Although reports of such events rarely occur in the medical literature, and in fact there are no specific reports of this outcome in the literature for more than 20 years, the popular press is littered with reports of medicolegal activity and deaths of children due to such errors. A Google search of heparin overdose in children will highlight many incidents, several with fatal outcomes. Fig. 92.3 summarizes the range of heparin preparations found in a typical PICU. It is not hard to see how such errors occur in busy units that operate 24 hours per day. Units should actively manage the choices of UFH preparations available to their staff to minimize the risk of confusion. Staff should be educated in the dangers of UFH and encouraged to be vigilant at all times when administering a drug that consistently ranks in hospital lists of the drugs most commonly involved in medication errors.

Another adverse event from UFH is anaphylaxis, which in 2007–2008 accounted for more than 80 deaths due to an unintended contaminant introduced in the manufacturing process. Again, although there is almost nothing in the medical literature describing these events, the US Food and Drug Administration (FDA) released a number of warning statements, and one impact has been the move to make changes to the labeling of UFH. The potential for contamination of drug products made from biological sources will always be real. An important mechanism to minimize this risk is to ensure that children only receive UFH when the risks are clearly outweighed by the benefits. UFH has been described as being ubiquitous in PICUs, and clinicians should actively minimize unnecessary exposure.

TABLE 92.3	Factors in Children That Affect the Action of Unfractionated Heparin	
UFH Factor	**Age-Related Difference**
UFH acts via AT-mediated catabolism of thrombin and factor Xa	Reduced levels of AT [3,4] Reduced capacity to generate thrombin[10,11] Age-related difference in anti-Xa/anti-IIa activity
UFH is bound to plasma proteins, which limits free active UFH	Alterations in plasma binding
Endothelial release of TFPI	Age-related differences in amount of TFPI release for same amount of UFH

UFH, unfractionated heparin.

TABLE 92.4   Assays Used in the Monitoring of Unfractionated Heparin Therapy

Assay	Common Uses	Advantages	Disadvantages in Children
APTT F-Clot	Coagulation screening assay Therapeutic UFH monitoring	Low cost Easy to perform Widely available	Baseline APTT often prolonged in children Wide variability in reagent sensitivity to age-related differences Nonphysiologic measure of UFH effect No validation of therapeutic ranges in children
TCT F-Clot	Coagulation screening assay Therapeutic UFH monitoring (rarely)	Easy to perform	Patients previously exposed to topical thrombin may have antibodies causing prolongation of the clotting time Optimal concentration of thrombin used for the assay is unknown No validated reference range for UFH in children
ACT F-clot	CPB, extracorporeal circuits	Easy bedside whole blood test Extensive experience in most PICUs	Does not correlate with any specific measures of heparin activity Analyzer dependent
Anti-Xa F-Ch	Calibration of APTT reference ranges Therapeutic UFH monitoring	Direct measure of UFH inhibition of Xa Easy to perform	Not as widely available as APTT and costs significantly more Does not measure other mechanisms of UFH effect (eg, anti-IIa) and assumes constant ration of effect, which is not true in children Some kits have exogenous AT, others have dextran sulphate, both of which will introduce in vitro error in small children for different reasons
Protamine titration Q	Not used clinically Used by reference laboratories	Only assay that directly measures UFH concentration Low cost	Not widely available Automated methods have not been validated for management of therapeutic UFH and manual methods labor intensive

ACT, activated clotting time; *APTT,* activated partial thromboplastin time; *AT,* antithrombin; *F-Ch,* functional, chromogenic assay; *F-Clot,* Functional, clot-based assay; *Q,* quantitative assay; *TCT,* thrombin clotting time; *UFH,* unfractionated heparin.

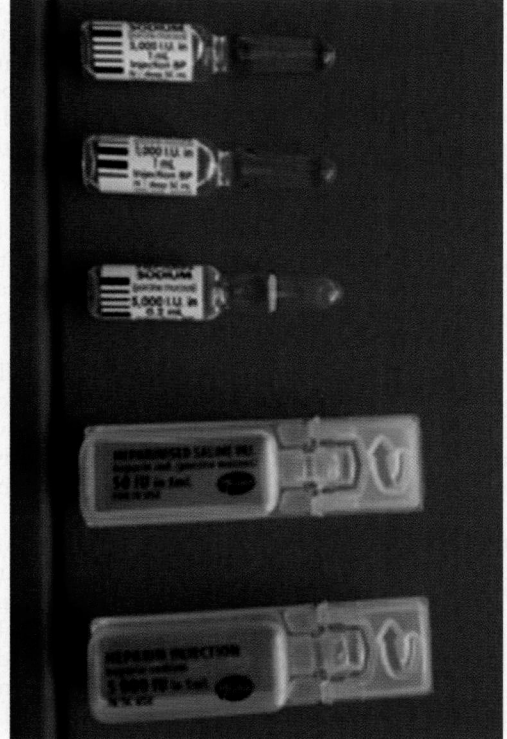

Fig. 92.3. Preparations of UFH commonly found on an Australian pediatric ward. Note the minimal differences in packaging, and the significant differences in UFH concentration, such that there is potential for a 100-fold overdose should a selection error be made.

In summary, anticoagulation in children in PICU is common, and UFH is the most common agent currently utilized. Although there remain many concerns about the potential adverse effects of UFH, there are currently no real alternative anticoagulant agents available for intravenous use in sick children. Many adverse events are related to dosing errors, and it is likely that PICUs can significantly improve the safety of UFH by developing systems to prevent medication errors. In addition, there is emerging evidence that our understanding of the pharmacokinetics of UFH in children and of the assays used to monitor UFH in children is far from ideal. Urgent research is required to improve the safety and utility of UFH in critically ill children.

Thromboprophylaxis in the Pediatric Intensive Care Unit

In critically ill adults, pharmacologic thromboprophylaxis is highly recommended due to its proved efficacy and safety in the prevention of DVT. It remains unclear if the same can be applied to the pediatric population. The increasing incidence of thromboembolism in the PICU patient has led several institutions to develop risk stratification protocols to target patients at the highest risk.[110,111] The most common risk factors continue to be the presence of CVC, cardiac disease, and infants <1 year.[19] There are various practices depending on the center, and currently between 0% and 50% of children receive thromboprophylaxis. A prospective study looking at pediatric trauma patients developed a risk stratification protocol and found a decrease by 65% in VTE with implementation of this protocol.[111] Of note, in this study of 76 patients determined to be at high risk for VTE, only 2 received pharmacologic thromboprophylaxis as per their protocol.

Routine thromboprophylaxis is unlikely to be of benefit in the PICU, as this area remains poorly studied and carries significant risk. The development of risk assessment tools and their effectiveness remains an area of research that is desperately needed. Nonpharmacologic thromboprophylaxis should be encouraged, which revolves around removing risk factors where possible, such as early mobilization and removal of CVC as soon as feasible.

Conclusions

Thromboembolic disease is now a major cause of mortality and morbidity in critically ill children, in the context of children having marked differences in the hemostatic system compared to adults, which appear to be age related. There remains much to be learned about the etiology and clinical presentations of thrombosis. Diagnostic strategies are mostly extrapolated from adult studies but are likely suboptimal. Similarly, management strategies and the use of anticoagulants in children for either treatment or primary prophylaxis are guided by minimal evidence, and there is a desperate need for further research. In the meantime, clinical decisions must be made, and for the time being these decisions require considerable consideration of the individual risk-benefit ratios for each patient.

Acknowledgment

We gratefully acknowledge the contribution of John Roy, who authored this chapter in previous editions.

Key References

1. Andrew M, et al. Development of human coagulation system in the full term infant. *Blood.* 1987;70:165-172.
3. Andrew M, Paes B, Milner R, et al. Development of the human coagulation system in the healthy premature infant. *Blood.* 1988;72:1651-1657.
4. Andrew M, Vegh P, Johnston M, et al. Maturation of the hemostatic system during childhood. *Blood.* 1992;80:1998-2005.
5. Reverdiau-Moalic P, Delahousse B, Body G, et al. Evolution of blood coagulation activators and inhibitors in the healthy human fetus. *Blood.* 1996;88:900-906.
6. Attard C, van der Straaten T, Karlaftis V, et al. Developmental hemostasis: age-specific differences in the levels of hemostatic proteins. *J Thromb Haemost.* 2013;11:1850-1854.
10. Chan AKC, Berry LR, Monagle PT, Andrew M. Decreased concentrations of heparinoids are required to inhibit thrombin generation in plasma from newborns and children compared to plasma from adults due to reduced thrombin potential. *Thromb Haemost.* 2002;87:606-613.
15. Monagle P, Chan AK, Goldenberg NA, et al. Antithrombotic therapy in neonates and children: Antithrombotic Therapy and Prevention of Thrombosis, 9th ed: American College of Chest Physicians Evidence-Based Clinical Practice Guidelines. *Chest.* 2012;141(2 suppl):e737S-e801S.
18. Chalmers EA. Epidemiology of venous thromboembolism in neonates and children. *Thromb Res.* 2006;118:3-12.
19. Higgerson R, Lawson K, Christie L, Brown A. Incidence and risk factors associated with venous thrombotic events in pediatric intensive care unit patients. *Pediatr Crit Care Med.* 2011;12:628-634.
20. Monagle P. Thrombosis in pediatric cardiac patients. *Semin Thromb Hemost.* 2003;29:547-555.
21. Godart F, Qureshi SA, Simha A, et al. Effects of modified and classic Blalock-Taussig shunts on the pulmonary arterial tree. *Ann Thorac Surg.* 1998;66:512-517, discussion 518.
22. Gladman G, McCrindle BW, Williams WG, et al. The modified Blalock-Taussig shunt: clinical impact and morbidity in Fallot's tetralogy in the current era. *J Thorac Cardiovasc Surg.* 1997;114:25-30.
23. Tsai KT, Chang CH, Lin PJ. Modified Blalock-Taussig shunt: statistical analysis of potential factors influencing shunt outcome. *J Cardiovasc Surg (Torino).* 1996;37:149-152.

32. Seligsohn U, Zivelin A. Thrombophilia as a multigenic disorder. *Thromb Haemost.* 1997;78:297-301.
33. Koeleman BP, Reitsma PH, Allaart CF, Bertina RM. Activated protein C resistance as an additional risk factor for thrombosis in protein C-deficient families. *Blood.* 1994;84:1031-1035.
34. Zoller B, et al. Resistance to activated protein C as an additional genetic risk factor in hereditary deficiency of protein S. *Blood.* 1995;85:3518-3523.
35. Young G, Albisetti M, Bonduel M, et al. Impact of inherited thrombophilia on venous thromboembolism in children: a systematic review and meta-analysis of observational studies. *Circulation.* 2008;118:1373-1382.
38. Bonduel M, Sciuccati G, Hepner M, et al. Prethrombotic disorders in children with arterial ischemic stroke and sinovenous thrombosis. *Arch Neurol.* 1999;56:967-971.
39. Charuvanij A, Laothamatas J, Torcharus K, Sirivimonmas S. Moyamoya disease and protein S deficiency: a case report. *Pediatr Neurol.* 1997;17:171-173.
40. Debus O, et al. Factor and genetic defects of thrombophilia in childhood porencephaly. *Arch Dis Child Fetal Neonatal Ed.* 1998;78:F121-F124.
41. Fabri D, Belangero VM, Annichino-Bizzacchi JM, Arruda VR. Inherited risk factors for thrombophilia in children with nephrotic syndrome. *Eur J Pediatr.* 1998;157:939-942.
42. Ganesan V, McShane MA, Liesner R, et al. Inherited prothrombotic states and ischaemic stroke in childhood. *J Neurol Neurosurg Psychiatry.* 1998;65:508-511.
51. Nowak-Gottl U, et al. Inherited defects of the protein C anticoagulant system in childhood thrombo-embolism. *Eur J Pediatr.* 1996;155:921-927.
52. Nowak-Gottl U, et al. Resistance to activated protein C (APCR) in children with acute lymphoblastic leukaemia-the need for a prospective multicentre study. *Blood Coagul Fibrinolysis.* 1995;6:761-764.
53. Nowak-Gottl U, et al. Ischaemic stroke in infancy and childhood: role of the Arg506 to Gln mutation in the factor V gene. *Blood Coagul Fibrinolysis.* 1996;7:684-688.
54. Nuss R, Hays T, Chudgar U, Manco-Johnson M. Antiphospholipid antibodies and coagulation regulatory protein abnormalities in children with pulmonary emboli. *J Pediatr Hematol Oncol.* 1997;19:202-207.
55. Nuss R, Hays T, Manco-Johnson M. Childhood thrombosis. *Pediatrics.* 1995;96(2 Pt 1):291-294.
62. Van Ommen CH, Peters M. Acute pulmonary embolism in childhood. *Thromb Res.* 2006;118:13-25.
63. Vielhaber H, Ehrenforth S, Koch HG, et al. Cerebral venous sinus thrombosis in infancy and childhood: role of genetic and acquired risk factors of thrombophilia. *Eur J Pediatr.* 1998;157:555-560.
66. Sutor AH. Screening children with thrombosis for thrombophilic proteins. Cui bono? *J Thromb Haemost.* 2003;1:886-888.
67. Revel-Vilk S, Chan A, Bauman M, Massicotte P. Prothrombotic conditions in an unselected cohort of children with venous thromboembolic disease. *J Thromb Haemost.* 2003;1:915-921.
87. Schmugge M, Risch L, Huber AR, et al. Heparin-induced thrombocytopenia-associated thrombosis in pediatric intensive care patients. *Pediatrics.* 2002;109:E10.
88. Lo GK, Sigouin CS, Warkentin TE. What is the potential for overdiagnosis of heparin-induced thrombocytopenia? *Am J Hematol.* 2007;82:1037-1043.
89. Klenner AF, Lubenow N, Raschke R, Greinacher A. Heparin-induced thrombocytopenia in children: 12 new cases and review of the literature. *Thromb Haemost.* 2004;91:719-724.
90. Risch L, Fischer JE, Herklotz R, Huber AR. Heparin-induced thrombocytopenia in paediatrics: clinical characteristics, therapy and outcomes. *Intensive Care Med.* 2004;30:1615-1624.
91. Saxon BR, Black MD, Edgell D, et al. Pediatric heparin-induced thrombocytopenia: management with Danaparoid (Orgaran). *Ann Thorac Surg.* 1999;68:1076-1078.
92. Chan VHT, Monagle P, Massicotte P, Chan AKC. Novel paediatric anticoagulants: a review of the current literature. *Blood Coagul Fibrinolysis.* 2010;21:144-151.
93. Polikoff L, Faustino EV. Venous thromboembolism in critically ill children. *Curr Opin Pediatr.* 2014;26:286-291.
94. Male C, Chait P, Ginsberg JS, et al. Comparison of venography and ultrasound for the diagnosis of asymptomatic deep vein thrombosis in the upper body in children: results of the PARKAA study. Prophylactic antithrombin replacement in kids with ALL treated with asparaginase. *Thromb Haemost.* 2002;87:593-598.
95. Chait P, Dinyari M, Massicotte MP. The sensitivity and specificity of lineograms and ultrasound compared to venography for the diagnosis

of central venous line related thrombosis in symptomatic children: the LUV study. *Thromb Haemost.* 2001;(suppl):697.

96. Shankar KR, Abernethy LJ, Das KS, et al. Magnetic resonance venography in assessing venous patency after multiple venous catheters. *J Pediatr Surg.* 2002;37:175-179.

97. Andrew M, Monagle P, Brooker L. Pulmonary embolism in childhood. In: *Thromboembolic complications during infancy and childhood.* Hamilton/London: BC Decker Inc; 2000:147-164.

98. Balling G, Vogt M, Kaemmerer H, et al. Intracardiac thrombus formation after the Fontan operation. *J Thorac Cardiovasc Surg.* 2000;119(4 Pt 1):745-752.

99. Fyfe DA, Kline CH, Sade RM, Gillette PC. Transesophageal echocardiography detects thrombus formation not identified by transthoracic echocardiography after the Fontan operation. *J Am Coll Cardiol.* 1991;18:1733-1737.

100. Stumper O, et al. Transesophageal echocardiography in evaluation and management after a Fontan procedure. *J Am Coll Cardiol.* 1991;17:1152-1160.

101. Yang J, Williams S, Chan LRB, Neonatal A. and childhood right atrial thrombosis: recognition and risk stratified treatment approach. *Blood Coagul Fibrinolysis.* 2010;21:301-307.

102. Newall F, Johnston L, Ignjatovic V, Monagle P. Unfractionated heparin therapy in infants and children. *Pediatrics.* 2009;123:e510-e518.

103. Lane D, Lindahl U. Heparin: Chemical and Biological Properties. In: *Clinical Applications.* Boca Raton: CRC Press; 1989:1-23.

108. Andrew M, et al. Heparin therapy in pediatric patients: a prospective cohort study. *Pediatr Res.* 1994;31:78-83.

109. Kuhle S. A clinically significant incidence of bleeding in critically ill children receiving therapeutic doses of unfractionated heparin: a prospective cohort study. *Haematologica.* 2007;92:244-247.

110. Atchison CM, Arlikar S, Amankwah E, et al. Development of a new risk score for hospital-associated venous thromboembolism in noncritically ill children: findings from a large single-institutional case-control study. *J Pediatr.* 2014;165:793-798.

111. Hanson S, Punzalan R, Arca M. Effectiveness of clinical guidelines for deep vein thrombosis prophylaxis in reducing the incidence of venous thromboembolism in critically ill children after trauma. *J Trauma.* 2014;72:1292-1297.

Transfusion Medicine in the Pediatric Intensive Care Unit

Jacques Lacroix, Marisa Tucci, Oliver Karam, and Philip C. Spinella

PEARLS

- The decision to prescribe the transfusion of any blood product must be based on individualized indications and must take into account specific health problems.
- Acute severe anemia (hemoglobin concentration <5 g/dL) may increase the risk of death in critically ill patients.
- There is no evidence that a red cell transfusion improves outcomes in stable critically ill children if their hemoglobin concentration is >7 g/dL. A hemoglobin concentration higher than 7 g/dL may be required in unstable critically ill children and in pediatric intensive care patients with heart disease, particularly those with cyanotic heart disease, but the best threshold is unknown.
- Plasma can be useful to treat severe coagulopathy.
- Plasma should not be used as a volume expander.
- Platelets can be useful to treat bleeding caused by low platelet counts or platelet dysfunction.
- In pediatric intensive care units, most transfusion-related adverse events are linked to immunomediated effects of blood products rather than to transfusion-transmitted infectious diseases.

Red Blood Cells

Native red blood cells (RBCs) contain hemoglobin (Hb), which carries oxygen (O_2) to cells, thus allowing efficient adenosine triphosphate (ATP) production and ensuring cell survival. Because energy expenditure is high in critically ill patients, it would seem rational to maintain their Hb level in the normal range. Anemia is observed in 74% of critically ill children.[1] The transfusion of RBC units is the only effective way to rapidly increase the Hb level. However, the efficacy and safety of transfused RBCs have been questioned. Infections transmitted by blood products were the most important concern in the 1980s. In the 1990s, noninfectious serious hazards of transfusion (NISHOT), like transfusion-related immune modulation (TRIM),[2] transfusion-related acute lung injury (TRALI), transfusion-associated circulatory overload (TACO),[3-5] and multiple organ dysfunction syndrome (MODS)[6-8] have become significant concerns.

This chapter discusses anemia and O_2 delivery (DO_2), reviews evidence on the effectiveness of RBC transfusion in the intensive care setting, discusses the recommendations found in guidelines on RBC transfusion in critically ill children, and reviews the most frequent transfusion reactions.

Red Blood Cell Transfusion: Why and Why Not

Anemia and O_2 Delivery

O_2 Delivery in the Critically Ill

Anemia decreases the capacity of blood to deliver O_2 because of lower Hb content. Systemic (global) DO_2 is dependent on cardiac output and the arterial concentration of O_2 (CaO_2): DO_2 = cardiac output (stroke volume × heart rate) × CaO_2. CaO_2 is defined by the formula:

$$CaO_2 (mL\ O_2/dL) = \{(Hb \times SaO_2 \times 1.34) + (0.003 \times PaO_2)\} \quad \text{Eq. 93.1}$$

Because systemic DO_2 is directly linked to Hb concentration, the most rapid and effective way of increasing DO_2 (within minutes) is by giving an RBC transfusion. This presumes that the Hb in a transfused unit of RBCs is functional and able to deliver O_2 to the tissues (see also Chapter 89). More modest augmentation in systemic DO_2 can be attained by increasing cardiac output or SaO_2.

An adequate O_2 delivery to cells does not imply necessarily that O_2 consumption (VO_2) is adequate and that cells produce enough energy. VO_2 depends on substrate availability and on metabolic demands; it can be amplified by increasing cellular O_2 extraction rate (O_2ER) or by increasing DO_2 if there is VO_2/ DO_2 dependence.

The relationship between O_2 delivery and consumption is characterized by two phases: a directly linear relationship between VO_2 and DO_2 up to a "critical threshold" (often referred to as the critical DO_2) and a flat section above this threshold (Fig. 93.1). Below the threshold, VO_2 diminishes if DO_2 decreases. Above this threshold, a fall in DO_2 does not cause a drop in VO_2 because it is compensated by mechanisms like an increase in O_2ER; these mechanisms are limited though, which explains why there is a critical threshold of DO_2 under which O_2ER cannot increase any further, and below which VO_2 begins to fall.

The stress of critical illness increases metabolic rate and VO_2, which shifts the critical level of DO_2 to the right and upward. However, compensatory mechanisms are limited in anemic critically ill patients.

Adaptive Mechanisms With Anemia

Anemia significantly decreases blood O_2 carrying capacity. However, in the normal host, the amount of O_2 delivered to

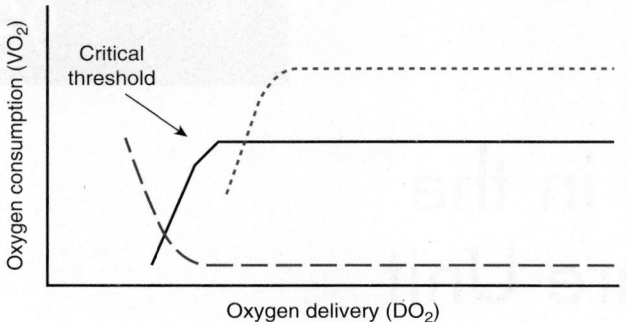

Fig. 93.1. This figure illustrates the relationship between oxygen delivery (DO_2) and O_2 consumption (VO_2) in normal patients *(black line)*, of DO_2 and blood lactate level in normal patients *(hatched blue line)*, and of DO_2 and VO_2 in septic critically ill patients *(red dotted line)*. Under the "critical threshold" marked by an arrow, VO_2 diminishes and blood lactate level increases if DO_2 decreases. Over this threshold, a fall in DO_2 does not cause a drop in VO_2 because it is compensated by an increase in O_2 extraction or an increased cardiac index. In critically ill patients, the VO_2 is frequently higher than normal. Then the level of the DO_2/VO_2 curve *(red dotted line)* is shifted upward; the critical threshold may also be shifted to the right, which may explain why pathologic O_2 supply dependence is reported in some critically ill patients.

tissues exceeds resting O_2 requirements by a two-to-fourfold factor. While the Hb concentration is dropping, several adaptive processes maintain VO_2. These processes include (1) increased O_2ER; (2) increased heart rate and stroke volume, which increase cardiac output; (3) redistribution of blood flow from nonvital organs toward the heart and brain, at the expense of O_2 delivery to less important vascular beds, like the splanchnic vasculature; and (4) right shift of the oxy-Hb-dissociation curve, which decreases affinity between Hb and O_2, thereby increasing the amount of O_2 released to cells.

Increasing O_2ER is an important way to adapt to anemia. The upper range of normal O_2ER is 30%; O_2ER increases if O_2 requirements are not met. Higher O_2ER is frequently observed in severely ill patients, which translates into low $SmvO_2$ (mixed venous O_2 saturation and $ScvO_2$ (central venous O_2 saturation). When maximal O_2ER is attained and other adaptive mechanisms are overwhelmed, VO_2/DO_2 dependence appears and may result in O_2 debt, which is associated with mortality. O_2 requirements are increased in patients with sepsis and MODS. Impaired left ventricular function and abnormal regulation of their vascular tone can restrict DO_2 and disturb redistribution of regional blood flow. Moreover, the mitochondria of patients with severe sepsis and MODS are dysfunctional and cannot adequately produce ATP.[9] A severe energy crisis may result (see also Chapter 80).

A number of host characteristics specific to children and infants may also impair their adaptive mechanisms. Although an increase in cardiac output generally compensates for anemia, this may not occur in the first few weeks of life due to lower myocardial compliance during this period and a significant impairment in diastolic filling, which limits stroke volume increase. In addition, an elevated resting heart rate in newborns also limits their ability to increase cardiac output. Greater energy requirements in young infants and children mostly attributable to growth imply a greater need for substrates including O_2. Issues affecting O_2 transport and release in children also include a higher proportion of fetal Hb during

the first months of life, which caused a left shift of the oxy-Hb saturation curve, and a physiologic anemia.

O_2 Kinetics in the Critically Ill

Tissue hypoxia from low DO_2 may be due to low Hb concentration (anemic hypoxia), low cardiac output (stagnant hypoxia), or low Hb saturation (hypoxic hypoxia). A significant number of intensivists use RBC transfusion to increase DO_2 in critically ill children.[10] RBC transfusion indeed increases DO_2, but it does not always increase tissue VO_2 in ICU patients.[11] Several mechanisms may explain this outcome.[12] Mitochondrial dysfunction can impede O_2 utilization in critically ill patients.[9] Moreover, peripheral O_2 delivery is impaired in ICU patients, and there is some evidence that RBC transfusion may worsen that problem.[13]

Regulation by Red Blood Cells of DO_2 to Tissue

Although RBC transfusion certainly increases systemic DO_2 in the central circulation, this does not imply that regional O_2 delivery improves. There is indeed evidence that RBC transfusion may disturb local DO_2.[14] However, data on regional DO_2 are inconsistent, their clinical significance remains to be determined, and the underlying mechanisms, which may involve blood viscosity, microcirculatory flow, local DO_2, and cellular respiration, are not well characterized.

RBC transfusion increases blood viscosity, which can lead to microcirculatory stasis and impaired DO_2 to tissues.[15] No hard data indicate that blood viscosity is a clinically important problem unless the Hb level is above 20 g/dL.

Activation of white blood cells (WBCs) in packed RBC units and cytokine generation in the supernatant of transfused RBC units may also have a microcirculatory effect: Some cytokines can mediate vasoconstriction or thrombosis of small vessels and cause local ischemia. Most packed RBC units are now prestorage leukocyte reduced, which significantly decreases cytokine levels in the supernatant. The clinical impact of cytokines on regional DO_2 remains to be determined.

There is evidence that RBC transfusion can cause vasoconstriction of microvasculature via an interaction between intracellular Hb and uptake by RBCs of nitric oxide released by blood vessels. With local tissue hypoxia, Hb in the microvasculature releases nitric oxide and triggers local vasodilatation; conversely, if there is sufficient O_2 in the microvasculature, Hb traps nitric oxide and causes vasoconstriction. This regulatory mechanism is almost immediately lost once RBCs are stored: It has been shown that in vitro exposure of blood vessels to RBC units stored 3 hours or more causes vasoconstriction.[16,17] The clinical significance of these observations is not clear; nonetheless they suggest that regional DO_2 can be disturbed by RBC transfusion.

Packed RBC units undergo several changes during storage, which are generally referred to as "storage lesion."[12,18] For example, the level of 2,3-DPG in stored RBCs decreases over time and can induce a left shift in the oxy-Hb dissociation curve, which impedes O_2 release to tissues even if systemic DO_2 is increased.[17] In addition, RBC deformability decreases after 2 or 3 weeks of storage, which may alter their capacity to pass through the capillary bed. Furthermore, hemolysis in older packed RBC units releases substantial amounts of free Hb ranging from 0.5 mg/dL in a 1-day-old RBC unit to 250 mg/dL in a 25-day-old unit.[19] Moreover, microparticles are released by RBC stored more than 2 or 3 weeks. Free intravascular Hb and microparticles have the ability to tightly bind nitric oxide and therefore cause vasoconstriction.[20]

Thus, although RBC transfusions certainly increase systemic DO_2, some available evidence suggests that impaired microcirculatory flow and O_2 availability can occur, which may have adverse effects on tissue oxygenation and cellular respiration.

Transfusion of Red Blood Cells: Indications (When)

A prospective cohort study involving 30 North American pediatric intensive care units (PICUs) reported that the proportion of patients who received at least one RBC transfusion while in the PICU ranged from 15% to 75%.[1]

RBC transfusions are clearly indicated for the treatment of hemorrhagic shock.[11] In such instances, the decision to prescribe RBC transfusions should be based on the physiologic state, the estimated amount of blood loss, and the risk of ongoing hemorrhage and not on the Hb concentration.

RBC transfusion is more questionable if there is no clinically significant hemorrhage or bleeding. Pediatric intensivists have stated in two surveys that their decision to prescribe an RBC transfusion would be based on reasons such as a low DO_2 or VO_2, cardiovascular insufficiency, respiratory failure, or use of certain specific technologies such as extracorporeal membrane oxygenation (ECMO), hemodialysis, hemofiltration, plasmapheresis, or exchange transfusion; nonetheless the most frequent reason to transfuse RBCs was reported to be a low Hb concentration.[1,10] The Hb level that should prompt a pediatric intensivist to prescribe an RBC transfusion remains a matter of debate, but there is some evidence in the medical literature that can guide practitioners.

Anemia

Severe anemia is associated with a higher risk of mortality. Carson and associates combined the data of two studies involving bloodless surgery in adults; the unadjusted mortality rate was 0.9% when the nadir Hb level was ≥ 7 g/dL, 9% if it was between 5 and 7 g/dL, 29.8% if it was between 4 and 5 g/dL, and 41% if it was <4 g/dL[21-23] Clearly, the risk of mortality augments when the Hb level falls below 5 g/dl. It is less obvious when to transfuse if the nadir Hb level is between 5 and 7 g/dL. It is important to recognize that the relationship between anemia and outcomes does not mean that transfusion to treat anemia will necessarily improve outcomes.

There are fewer data on the relationship between anemia and adverse outcome in children. Lackritz and colleagues[24] followed 2433 anemic African children among whom 20% received RBCs in the form of a whole blood transfusion; whole blood transfusion seemed beneficial if the Hb level was below 4.7 g/dL and if the patient presented some respiratory distress. Given these data, local guidelines were implemented recommending that RBCs should be transfused to hospitalized children if their Hb level was <5 g/dL. Lackritz and colleagues[25] subsequently enrolled 303 children with a Hb level <5 g/dL; 116 (38%) did not receive a transfusion, mostly because blood products units were not available. Each child with severe anemia was matched with the next child hospitalized with a Hb >5 g/dL. Death rates were 19.5% in 303 patients with a Hb >5 g/dL who were not transfused, 21.4% in 187 patients with a Hb <5 g/dL who were transfused, and 41.4% in 116 patients with a Hb <5 g/dL who were not transfused. English

and coworkers[26] completed a prospective cohort study of 1269 children with malaria hospitalized in Kenya; blood transfusion seemed to decrease mortality if anemia was severe (Hb level <4 g/dL) or if a Hb level <5 g/dL was associated with dyspnea. These studies suggest that the risk of mortality increases significantly in children ill enough to require hospitalization if their Hb concentration is lower than 5 g/dL, particularly if respiratory symptoms are present.

Evidence on Red Blood Cell Transfusion

Four case series assessed hemodynamic parameters before and after a 10- to 20-mL/kg RBC transfusion; those studied were children with septic shock, postoperative pediatric cardiac surgery patients, and children with cyanotic heart disease undergoing elective cardiac catheterization.[27-30] These articles reported a greater systemic DO_2 after transfusion, but only one study reported an increase in calculated VO_2.[27] RBC transfusion increases systemic DO_2, but it does not increase VO_2 in many instances.

Two randomized controlled trials evaluated RBC transfusion strategies in children. The first trial was performed in 106 African children with malaria crisis (hematocrit: 12% to 17%). Whole blood transfusion did not improve the mortality rate (1/53 versus 2/53) in patients without respiratory or cardiovascular compromise.[31] In the transfusion requirement in PICU (TRIPICU) study, a randomized controlled trial involving 637 stable critically ill children with Hb level <9.5 g/dL, 320 patients were allocated to an RBC transfusion threshold of 7 g/dL of Hb (restrictive group) and 317 to a threshold of 9.5 g/dL (liberal group). A statistically significant noninferiority was found: 38 and 39 patients, respectively, developed new or progressive MODS, and there were 14 deaths in both strategy groups within 28 days postrandomization. The conclusion was that a restrictive strategy is as safe as a liberal strategy in stable critically ill children. Moreover, given that 174 patients (54%) in the restrictive group received no RBC transfusion compared to 7 (2%) in the liberal group (p <0.0001) and that patients in the restrictive group received 54% fewer RBC transfusions, the findings supported adopting a restrictive transfusion strategy for stabilized critically ill children.[32] Three subgroup analyses, respectively, on patients with sepsis,[33] on postoperative cardiac patients,[34] and on noncardiac surgery cases[35] showed trends identical to those reported in the original TRIPICU study.

Red Blood Cell Transfusion: Current Recommendations
Noncardiac Patients

RBC transfusion in PICU is associated not only with a low Hb level (multivariate odds ratio if Hb <7 g/dL: 61.3; 95% confidence interval [CI]: 27.75, 134.7) but also with congenital heart disease (3.61; 1.99, 6.55), age <12 months (2.43; 1.19, 4.96), higher severity of illness (daily PELOD score >20: 6.33; 1.72, 23.25), and presence of some organ dysfunctions (cardiovascular, hematologic, neurologic, or hepatic).[36] In a cohort study,[1] pediatric intensivists declared that they might consider prescribing an RBC transfusion based on the following markers: Hb concentration, low SaO_2, low PaO_2, low cardiac output (poor DO_2), high blood lactate level, low central venous ($ScvO_2$) or mixed venous saturation of O_2 ($SmvO_2$), poor VO_2, high severity of illness, active bleeding, and emergency surgery. However, how these determinants of RBC transfusion interacted with each other was unclear.

In the TRIPICU study, 234 and 246 patients with respiratory dysfunction were enrolled in the restrictive and liberal group (threshold Hb for RBC transfusion: 7 and 9.5 g/dL, respectively).[6] The number of cases of new/progressive MODS was similar (33 and 35), respectively. Duration of mechanical ventilation was also comparable in these 480 patients (6.4 ± 6 versus 6.3 ± 5.3 days; absolute risk difference: −0.16; 95% CI: −1.2, 0.9, p = 0.75), including 73 with an acute lung injury (ALI) (7.2 ± 6.5 versus 7.1 ± 6.2 days; absolute risk difference: −0.12; 95% CI: −3.1, 2.9, p = 0.94) and 48 with an acute respiratory distress syndrome (ARDS) (10.5 ± 9.2 versus 8.5 ± 7.2 days; absolute risk difference: −2; 95% CI: −6.8, 2.8, p = 0.40). Thus targeting higher Hb thresholds does not improve outcome in stable critically ill children with respiratory problems if their Hb level is >7 g/dL.

Although many physicians believe that a higher Hb level is required in severely ill septic patients, there is little evidence to support this belief. The outcome of 137 septic children (34 in septic shock, 31 with severe sepsis) allocated in the TRIPICU study to a restrictive or a liberal transfusion strategy was similar with 13/69 versus 13/68, respectively, developing new/progressive MODS (absolute risk difference: 0.3%; 95% CI: −12%, +14%).[37] Holst and colleagues[38] randomized 1005 adults with septic shock to receive an RBC transfusion only if their Hb level fell below 7 or 9 g/dL. Some of these patients were not hemodynamically stable. The 90-day mortality was similar (43% versus 45%; relative risk: 0.94; 95% CI: 0.78, 1.09; p = 0.44). Thus a threshold Hb of 7 g/dL can probably be safely applied in critically ill children with sepsis.

Guidelines from many organizations emphasize that the decision to administer RBC should not be based solely on Hb levels but should involve sound clinical judgment.[39,40] Goal-directed transfusion therapy is also frequently advocated.[41,42] Although it is theoretically rational to base the decision to transfuse RBCs on physiologic need, it is still a matter of debate what parameters best determine that need. It has been suggested that an RBC transfusion is indicated for patients with symptomatic anemia, but most critically ill children are unable to report these symptoms. Some have suggested that systemic markers of oxygenation deficit (eg, systemic VO_2, VO_2/DO_2 dependence, blood lactate level, $ScvO_2$ or $SmvO_2$) or O_2ER, might be more useful.[43] Others have proposed that parameters reflecting regional oxygenation deficit, such as brain tissue O_2 pressure ($PbtO_2$),[44] gastric tonometry,[45] tissue O_2 saturation (StO_2) measured by near-infrared spectroscopy (NIRS),[14] or digital O_2 extraction rate measured by noninvasive devices, may be more reliable. Actually, it is presently not known which markers are best suited for this purpose and what cutoff values should be used to determine the need for RBC transfusion. The concept of goal-directed transfusion therapy is laudable, but it is presently vaguely defined and not supported by hard data. Specific recommendations for goal-directed transfusion therapy remain undetermined at the present time.[46]

In practice, a low Hb concentration remains the most frequent and the primary justification for pediatric intensivists to prescribe an RBC transfusion.[1] Therefore, it makes sense that the Hb concentration be the first parameter assessed when an RBC transfusion is considered. Given the available evidence, critically ill children should receive an RBC transfusion if their Hb level is below 5 g/dL. In stable patients, including septic patients,[37] patients having undergone noncardiac surgery,[35] severely burned children[47] and trauma patients,[48] it is suggested to consider RBC transfusion if the Hb concentration is <7 g/dL, but a transfusion is not recommended if the Hb concentration is above this level. However, determinants other than the Hb concentration must be considered including age, severity of illness, or evidence of organ dysfunction or O_2 dependency, such as elevated blood lactate level or low $ScvO_2$. For example, it would seem appropriate to consider a higher threshold and a more aggressive RBC transfusion strategy in unstable patients for whom the optimal and safe lower limit of the transfusion threshold has not been established. Moreover, any recommendations made must also factor in specific considerations for disorders like sickle cell disease[49] and cardiac conditions.

Cardiac Patients

Critically ill children with cardiac disease receive more RBC transfusions than other PICU patients.[36] There is no strong evidence that indicates this strategy improves outcomes.

Few clinical studies have addressed RBC transfusion in cyanotic heart disease. Experience with bloodless cardiac surgery for congenital heart disease in children whose families refuse transfusion seems to suggest that a lower Hb level may be well tolerated. This theory is supported by a randomized controlled trial involving 59 children undergoing bidirectional Glenn or Fontan procedures in which patients were allocated to either a restrictive or a liberal transfusion strategy (respective threshold: Hb concentration of 9 and 12 g/dL). The mean postoperative Hb was 11.1 ± 13 versus 13.9 ± 0.5 g/dL, and the mean number of RBC transfusions was 0.47 ± 0.6 versus 2.03 ± 1.2 per patient in the restrictive and liberal groups, respectively. No difference was noted with regard to surrogate outcomes such as peak blood lactate level (3 ± 1.5 versus 3.1 ± 1.3 mmol/L), ventilator support, duration of vasoactive agent administration, ICU or hospital length of stay, or survival.[50] More data are required before a restrictive transfusion strategy can be safely implemented in patients with cyanotic heart disease.

On the other hand, there is some evidence that using a 7-g/dL threshold is safe in the postoperative care of noncyanotic congenital heart disease in stabilized patients older than 28 days. Willems and associates[34] analyzed a subgroup of 125 postoperative cardiac patients enrolled in the TRIPICU study after a cardiac surgery. No significant difference in the incidence of new or progressive MODS (12.7% versus 6.5%; p = 0.36), PICU length of stay (7 ± 5 versus 7.4 ± 6.4 days), or 28-day mortality (2 versus 2 deaths) was found between the restrictive and liberal groups. Another randomized controlled trial compared outcome in pediatric cardiac surgery patients aged more than 6 weeks allocated to receive an RBC transfusion if their Hb level dropped below 8 g/dL (restrictive) or 10.8 g/dL (liberal group).[51] Patients with cyanotic cardiac disease were excluded. Randomization occurred before surgery; the research protocol with respect to RBC transfusion was initiated in the operating room and maintained up to PICU discharge. In the 107 patients enrolled and retained for analysis, duration of mechanical ventilation, PICU length of stay, and the incidence of adverse events were similar in both groups, whereas hospital length of stay was shorter in the restrictive group (median: 8; [interquartile range: 7–11] versus 9 [7–14] days, p = 0.063). The British Society of Haematology[39] supports the acceptance of a postoperative Hb level of 7 g/dL in children when there is good postoperative cardiac function in the absence of persisting cyanotic heart disease. The Society of Thoracic Surgeons makes a similar recommendation for all cardiac surgery patients.[52] The data reported by Willems and associates[34] and de Gast-Bakker[51] support these recommendations.

Data in adults suggest that RBC transfusions may be detrimental in patients with cardiac conditions.[53] RBC transfusions must be used cautiously in children with cardiac disease. Given the currently available evidence, an Hb level of 7 g/dL can be considered safe for hemodynamically stable children older than 28 days who have noncyanotic heart disease and a level of 9 g/dL for children with cyanotic heart disease.[6,50] Further studies are needed to better characterize appropriate determinants for RBC transfusion in critically ill children with heart disease.

Prevention of Anemia and of Red Blood Cell Transfusion

Bloodless medicine is a popular concept; it refers to all the strategies that can be used to provide medical care without allogeneic RBC transfusion, including blood conservation. Many strategies can prevent or significantly decrease the number of RBC transfusions and exposure to transfusion. Adopting a restrictive RBC transfusion strategy in stable critically ill children is one of them; other strategies could include raising the Hb concentration before elective surgery, using blood products only when necessary, limiting blood loss, and administering the patient's own blood.

Bloodless medicine begins before surgery, when applicable. In the preoperative period, the use of erythropoietin and iron supplementation can be considered to optimize the preoperative Hb level, collection of autologous donations can take place to minimize or prevent allogeneic transfusion, medications that increase the risk of bleeding should be avoided, including herbal medicine (garlic, ginseng, ginger, etc[42]), and optimal control of any existing coagulation disorders should be attained just prior to surgery.

During surgery, maximal attention should be given limiting blood loss[54] and ensuring good hemostasis and rapid control of any bleeding. In some instances, desmopressin, fibrin sealants, or antifibrinolytic agents such as aprotinin or tranexamic acid may be used to stop a hemorrhage. Recombinant activated factor VII (rFVIIa) is advocated by some practitioners, but it is associated with a significant risk of thrombosis; the cost-benefit ratio of rFVIIa in children is not well evaluated, and its use should be limited to situations involving uncontrolled life-threatening bleeding. Prothrombin complex and fibrinogen concentrates are also potential agents that can improve hemostasis in children with significant bleeding, but the appropriate indications for these agents and their safety profile in children are not well established. The safety and cost-effectiveness of intraoperative blood conservation strategies like normovolemic hemodilution, autologous blood cell salvage modalities, intraoperative autotransfusion, and deliberate hypotension remain to be determined.

Postoperative and ICU management of anemia and bleeding are also important. A restrictive transfusion strategy is in line with the concept of "permissive anemia" supported by the British Committee for Standards in Haematology Transfusion Task Force.[39] A prospective study reported that 73% of blood loss in the PICU is attributable to blood draws.[1] The number and frequency of blood tests must be limited, and the amount of blood collected reduced. Many devices can help to minimize blood loss, including the use of loop sampling, pediatric blood collection tubes, microanalysis techniques requiring small volumes of blood, and in-line measurement of parameters like blood gases and Hb concentration.

Erythropoietin response to anemia is blunted and poorer than expected in critically ill patients.[55] In spite of this response, erythropoietin can prevent anemia in critically ill adults,[56] in low-birth-weight preterm infants,[57] and in the postoperative care of neonates.[58] In critically ill children, there are no data to support the use of erythropoietin as a preventive measure because most RBC transfusions are administered within 2 or 3 days after PICU admission,[1,36,59] a period of time too short to allow for a response to erythropoietin, which generally occurs after several days. The standard use of erythropoietin is presently not recommended in the PICU.

Iron supplementation is also not indicated. In critically ill patients, it had no discernible effect on iron-deficient erythropoiesis, Hb concentration, and RBC transfusion requirement,[60] and it can even be harmful.[61]

Conclusion

RBC transfusion should be administered only if the anticipated benefits outweigh the potential risks. A threshold Hb concentration of 7 g/dL is adequate in most stable critically ill children.[6,46] The optimal Hb concentration or transfusion threshold above which the benefits outweigh the risks and costs remains to be determined in unstable patients and in patients with congenital heart disease.

Types of Packed Red Blood Cell Products
Standard Red Blood Cell Products
Packed Red Blood Cell Units
Storage of RBC units is made possible by refrigeration at about 4°C and by storage in preservative anticoagulant solutions that contain dextrose, sodium citrate, citric acid, and sodium diphosphate. RBCs use dextrose and phosphate to generate ATP, which is essential for their survival. Citrate blocks coagulation by chelating calcium; it is also metabolized to bicarbonate, which stabilizes the stored RBC unit pH above 6.4. RBCs in CPDA–1 (citrate-phosphate-dextrose-adenine) solution can be stored up to 35 days because the level of ATP is normal after 21 days of storage and is about 50% after 35 days. Packed RBC units are prepared by removing 200 to 250 mL of plasma from one unit of whole blood after centrifugation. To support the nutrient needs of RBCs after plasma is removed, additive solutions were developed, such as AS–1 (Adsol), AS–3 (Nutricel), and AS–5 (Optisol), and saline-adenine-glucose (SAG) or SAG-mannitol (SAGM)[62]; these additive solutions further decrease RBC lysis and allow for storage up to 42 days.

The volume of a CPDA–1 unit is about 250 mL, including 63 mL of preservative solution; it must be diluted with 75 mL of NaCl 0.9% before transfusion (final volume: 325 mL). The volume of an AS–3 unit is about 350 mL, and the volume of a SAGM unit is about 300 mL; both include approximately 100 mL of preservative solution and do not require any dilution.

Whole Blood
The use of whole blood has been advocated mostly for first-line therapy in hemorrhagic shock, as it contains RBCs,

coagulation factors, and platelets.[63] However, it is generally not available. Approximately 15% of children's hospitals in the United States provide whole blood to children, predominantly for cardiac surgery, liver transplantation, and massive transfusion protocols. Some also uses whole blood units for neonatal exchange transfusions.[64] Whole blood is stored at 2° to 6°C for up to at least 21 days based on the storage solution. Barriers to whole blood availability have been based on the concepts that the platelets in whole blood will not be functional when stored at 2° to 6°C, whole blood cannot be leukocyte-reduced without removing platelets, and it must be ABO specific when transfused. These concepts have been challenged.[65,66] Platelets actually have increased hemostatic function when stored at 2° to 6°C compared to 20° to 24°C.[67,68] Function has been classically defined as circulation time, which may not be an appropriate measure of function in a patient with severe bleeding. Interestingly, two randomized controlled trials in humans have indicated that there is less blood loss or improved functional hemostatic measures for platelet-containing blood products stored at 2° to 6°C compared to 20° to 24°C.[69] Platelet-sparing leukoreduction filters are now available for whole blood units and in clinical use at children's hospitals. Lastly, when data from the UK Serious Hazards of Transfusion (SHOT) database were analyzed, it was inferred there is less risk of severe hemolytic reactions when group O whole blood is transfused compared to the use of ABO type specific whole blood.[62]

The use of whole blood is very controversial and it should only be considered for patients with hemorrhagic shock. Whole blood is not recommended in normovolemic patients because it can cause cardiac overload. The volume of a typical whole blood unit is about 450 mL.

Other Types of Red Blood Cell Units

Many other types of RBC units are available: leukocyte-reduced, washed, irradiated, cytomegalovirus (CMV) negative, autologous, and directed.

Leukocyte-Reduced Red Blood Cell Units

Packed RBC units contain some nonviable platelets, small amounts of coagulation factors, and WBCs, which can release pro- and antiinflammatory mediators during storage. Prestorage leukocyte reduction is a standard procedure for all blood components in many countries, like Australia, Canada, and the United Kingdom; it can decrease the number of WBCs in packed RBC units from 1×10^9 to less 1×10^6 per product, the concentration of cytokines in the supernatant, as well as some T-cell–regulated immunomodulation.[70] In 2005 88% of packed RBC units given in US PICUs were leukocyte-reduced at collection.[1] Transmission of intracellular viruses like CMV and herpes is less frequent if there are fewer WBCs.

Washed Red Blood Cell Units

RBCs can be washed with sterile saline; the process removes not only 98% of plasma but also up to 20% of RBCs. RBC washing increases the hematocrit to 0.8, but the procedure takes up to 2 hours; thus it is impossible to use washed packed RBC units on an emergency basis unless they are prepared in advance. Washed units must be used within 24 hours after processing. Multiple wash cycles are required. The procedure may not completely remove all proteins and therefore does not prevent hypersensitivity reactions (eg, hypersensitivity to

IgA). The overall volume of a washed RBC unit is significantly decreased (about 200 mL rather than 350 mL for an AS–3 RBC unit), making them sometimes useful to limit the volume administered in some patients. Washed RBC units should not be considered leukocyte-reduced.

A randomized controlled trial that included 161 children reported that washing RBC transfused in cardiac PICU patients reduces postoperative inflammation and number of transfusions.[71] A randomized trial of washed RBC and platelet transfusions in 43 adults with acute leukemia reported similar trends.[72] However, the washing process is not without consequences; for example, it increases hemolysis and decreases 2,3-DPG content.[73] Further studies are required before washing of all RBC units can be recommended for PICU patients.

Washed RBC units can be considered for patients with severe, recurrent allergic reactions to blood, patients with an anti-IgA deficiency, and some patients with a high risk or circulatory overload.

Irradiated Red Blood Cell Units

Some WBCs remain in RBC and platelets units, even in prestorage leukocyte-reduced units. The objective of irradiation is to induce enough DNA damage to prevent leukocyte proliferation.[74] Irradiation destroys the ability of transfused lymphocytes to divide and therefore to respond to host foreign antigens, thereby decreasing the risk of developing transfusion-associated graft-versus-host (TAGVH) disease in susceptible recipients. However, irradiation is not without drawbacks. For example, it can damage the RBC membrane causing the release of significant amounts of free Hb and potassium. Moreover, the shelf life of irradiated RBC units is reduced from 42 to 28 days.[75]

Irradiated RBCs are indicated for all children with congenital or acquired cellular immune deficiency (eg, allogeneic stem cell transplant recipients, certain hematologic malignancies, myeloablative chemotherapy recipients) to prevent TAGVH disease. Because di George syndrome is not rare among infants with congenital heart disease undergoing cardiac surgery, these patients should receive irradiated units. Irradiation is also indicated in patients receiving directed donation from family members. Irradiation is not mandatory for patients with most solid tumors, routine immunosuppressive therapy (corticosteroids) solid organ transplantation, nonmyeloablative chemotherapy recipients, or humoral immunodeficiency.

Cytomegalovirus-Negative Red Blood Cell Units

RBC transfusion can transmit CMV infection. A large proportion (30% to 70%) of blood donors are CMV positive. Although it would be ideal to administer only CMV-negative RBC units to CMV-negative patients, the high prevalence of CMV infection among donors does not permit this. Nevertheless, prestorage leukocyte reduction of blood products decreases transmission of CMV to 1% to 2% (similar to the rate of infection following the transfusion of CMV-negative units) compared to standard products for which transmission is 13% to 37%.

Administration of a CMV-positive RBC unit is generally not an issue for immunocompetent patients. Established indications for CMV-negative units include CMV-negative recipients of organ or bone marrow transplants from CMV-negative donors, CMV-negative bone marrow transplant recipients, and intrauterine transfusions. Less well-established indications include CMV-negative patients who are potential candidates for autologous or allogeneic bone marrow transplant, CMV-negative patients undergoing splenectomy, potential seronegative donors for bone marrow transplant, and CMV-negative patients with HIV.

Directed Red Blood Cell Units

Directed blood is donated by family members or friends. Parents frequently believe that giving their own blood decreases the risks of transfusion, which, in practice, is not the case. A small increase of transfusion-transmitted infectious diseases has been reported.[76] Moreover, the risk of contracting a TAGVH is increased even in immunocompetent patients. Regardless, directed blood donation remains popular. Good clinical studies to better estimate the risk-benefit ratio of this practice are warranted. All directed RBC units must be irradiated pretransfusion.

Autologous Red Blood Cell Units

Older healthy children can give their own blood a few weeks before elective surgery. It is frequently believed that autologous RBC units are free of risk, which is untrue. These units are usually quite old by the time transfusion is required, which raises concerns with respect to RBC unit length of storage. Moreover, autologous RBC units are not leukocyte-reduced, at least in Canada. The risk-benefit ratio of autologous RBC units remains to be determined.

Red Blood Cell Substitutes and Other Alternatives to Red Blood Cell Transfusion

Hb-based O_2 carrier solutions (semisynthetic or synthetic preparations of Hb) and perfluorocarbon derivatives can carry O_2.[77] Both were developed as alternatives to RBCs, but there are serious concerns about their safety and usefulness. None can be recommended presently.

Transfusion of Red Blood Cells: How

RBC transfusion is the best way to rapidly increase the Hb concentration. Once a practitioner decides an RBC transfusion is warranted, several issues need to be decided including the type of RBC unit (discussed previously), the blood type, the volume necessary, how the unit must be perfused, and what monitoring is required.

Blood Types

Table 93.1 describes the compatibility of different blood products. A complete cross-match is mandatory before any transfusion is given, with few exceptions. Transfusion of group O Rh-negative RBC or group AB Rh-positive plasma can be life saving, but this must be reserved for severe and acute situations. It takes 15 to 20 minutes to type a patient for ABO and Rh. If there are no RBC antibodies, fully compatible blood or immediate spin cross-match may be issued quickly. In the case of RBC antibodies or other anomalies, a full serologic cross-match is required, which is lengthier. The risk of severe reaction to typed, but not cross-matched blood RBC units, is about 1/1000 if the patient has never received a transfusion; the risk is decreased 10-fold if a cross-match is done. It is recommended that similar units be used until patient recovery if a

TABLE 93.1	Compatibility of Blood Products		
Blood Product		**Receiver**	**Donor**
Packed RBC unit and whole blood		A	A, O
		B	B, O
		O	O
		AB	AB, A, B, O
		Rh⁺	Rh⁺ or Rh⁻
		Rh⁻	Rh⁻
Plasma or platelets		A	A, AB
		B	B, AB
		O	O, A, B, AB
		AB	AB
Platelets		Rh⁺	Rh⁺ or Rh⁻
		Rh⁻	Rh⁻ or Rh⁺ᵃ

ᵃGive an anti-D vaccine (WinRho SDF) if the receiver is Rh⁻ and the platelet concentrate is Rh⁺.
RBC, red blood cells.

patient receives more than 20% of his or her blood volume with non–cross-matched packed RBC units. However, this practice is a little outdated, as there is little plasma in AS–3 and SAGM RBC units. If anti-A/B antibodies are detected on blood typing, then antigen-negative blood should be provided; otherwise ABO-identical units should be used when available. Repeat verification that the correct blood unit has been delivered to a given patient is essential because blood mismatch is the most important cause of severe transfusion reaction.

For high-risk elective procedures, type and cross-matching done prior to any bleeding allows for compatible RBC units to be reserved. If an unforeseen emergency transfusion is required for an actively bleeding patient, it is impossible to deliver RBC units that are typed and cross-matched within a reasonable time frame and group O Rh-negative RBC units must be administered (some hospitals outside the United States also deliver O Rh-positive RBC units for men and for women after menopause, but this is not a common practice). Ordering a transfusion stat means transfusion is required within a few minutes; this is not indicated unless the patient is actively bleeding.

Volume and Number of Red Blood Cell Units

Prescribing the right volume of packed RBC units is important, as this prevents cardiac overload and limits exposure to several donors. An easy albeit simplistic rule of thumb exists that suggests administration of 10 mL/kg of packed RBC units increases the Hb level by 2 to 3 g/dL. If the Hb concentration is stable in a patient who is not actively bleeding, it is better to calculate the difference between the Hb concentration observed before transfusion and the targeted Hb level using the following formula:

$$\text{Volume (mL)} = [(\text{Hb}_{\text{targeted}} - \text{Hb}_{\text{observed}}) \times \text{blood volume}]/[\text{Hb}_{\text{RBC unit}}]$$
Eq. 93.2

where $\text{Hb}_{\text{targeted}}$ is the Hb concentration targeted post transfusion (for example, 10 g/dL), where $\text{Hb}_{\text{observed}}$ is the most recently measured Hb concentration (g/dL), and where $\text{Hb}_{\text{RBC unit}}$ is the average Hb concentration in the packed RBC units (g/dL) delivered by the blood bank. Hb concentration in RBC units may vary depending on the center and the preservative solution. For example, the hematocrit of RBC units with AS–3 (Nutricel) is approximately 0.55, and $Hb_{RBC\ unit}$ concentration is about 19.5 g/dL (range: 18 to 21 g/dL); the hematocrit of CPDA–1 is 0.75 to 0.65, and the $Hb_{RBC\ unit}$ is about 25 g/dL. The blood volume can be calculated according to the following formula:

$$\text{Total body blood volume} = \text{weight} \times \text{blood volume}\qquad \text{Eq. 93.3}$$

where weight is expressed in kg and blood volume in liter/kg (0.08 L/kg for a less than 2-year-old child, 0.07 L/kg for 2 to 14 years of age). For example, if the $Hb_{observed}$ in a 2-week-old 3-kg baby is 6.5 g/dL, the baby's blood volume is 0.24 L (0.08 L/kg × 3 kg), and the $Hb_{RBC\ unit}$ is 19.5 g/dL (AS–3), and if the physician targets a Hb concentration ($Hb_{targeted}$) of 10 g/dL, the volume of RBC unit to be transfused would be as follows:

$$\text{Volume} = \{(10\ g/dL - 6.5\ g/dL) \times 0.24\ L\}/\{19.5\ g/dL\}$$
$$= 0.043\ L = 43\ mL. \qquad \text{Eq. 93.4}$$

If the volume needed to reach the $Hb_{targeted}$ is greater than the volume of one unit of packed RBCs, blood should be transfused one unit at a time to minimize exposure to multiple donors. Prior to the administration of additional packed RBCs, the Hb concentration should be measured after allowing at least 30 minutes post transfusion for Hb and hematocrit values to equilibrate. The transfusion can be completed with another unit or partial unit if a reasonable Hb level is not attained.

If the volume of packed RBCs required is less than one unit, a partial unit can be given. Whole packed RBC units can be divided in half (standard division) or in small pediatric 75-mL transfer packs (Pedi-Pak). Partial units prepared nonsterilely expire 24 hours after preparation. On the other hand, partial units prepared sterilely can be kept as long as the original unit (up to 42 days for AS–3). A small volume of packed RBC unit placed in a syringe must always be administered within 24 hours.

Length of Storage

Regulatory agencies and scientific societies, such as the Food and Drug Administration and the American Association of Blood Banks, mandate that packed RBC units can be stored up to 42 days based on the premise that at least 75% of transfused RBC will be alive 24 hours post transfusion and that hemolysis will be <1%.[78] However, a *storage lesion* occurs over time, which raises many concerns.[18,79] These storage lesions involve a number of biochemical and biomechanical RBC changes including a depletion of adenosine triphosphate (ATP) and 2,3-DPG, membrane phospholipid vesiculation and loss, protein oxidation, lipid peroxidation of red cell membranes, and loss of RBC deformability.

Prolonged storage changes the supernatant as well as RBC. Studies have noted the generation of cytokines and other bioreactive substances in the storage medium, including histamine, complement, lipids, and cytokines. These bioactive substances may stimulate proinflammatory pathways and perhaps change flow patterns in the microcirculation.[14,16] Other well-documented time-dependent changes to the storage medium are described, including a progressive fall in pH, an increase in plasma potassium, and release of free Hb from hemolyzed RBCs.[17]

It is uncertain that fresher blood products are perfectly safe. The risk of transmission of some infectious diseases, such as malaria, Chagas disease, and intracellular viruses including CMV, herpes type 8, and Epstein-Barr virus, may be greater with fresher blood. Microchimerism is another concern.[80] The risk of contracting a TAGVH is greater with blood stored less than a week.[81,82]

Data from descriptive studies in human beings on the relationship between RBC storage time and outcomes are inconsistent: Some studies suggest that the outcome of transfused critically ill patients is better if transfused with fresher RBC units, whereas other studies do not support this option.[83,84] The Age of Blood Evaluation (ABLE) study, a double-blind randomized controlled trial, enrolled 2510 critically ill adults who were allocated to receive either RBC stored less ≤7 days or standard issue RBCs (the oldest compatible RBC units available in the blood bank were delivered according to a first-in, first-out policy).[85] RBCs in the fresh group were stored 6.1 ± 4.9 days, whereas RBCs in the standard group were stored for 22 ± 8.4 days (p <0.0001). Mortality at 90 days after randomization was 35.3% in the standard group (430 patients) versus 37% in the fresh group (448 patients) (absolute risk difference: 1.7%; 95% CI: −2.1%, 5.5%). The same trends were observed for all secondary outcomes (major morbidities; length of respiratory, hemodynamic, and renal support; ICU length of stay; and red cell transfusion reactions) or in any subgroups. The trial concluded that fresher RBCs do not decrease adverse outcome in critically ill adults. The RECESS study randomized 1600 participants ≥12 years of age who were undergoing elective complex cardiac surgery and among whom 1098 received RBCs.[86] The shorter-term storage group received RBCs stored ≤10 days, and the longer-term storage group received RBCs stored ≥21 days; the mean durations of RBC storage were 7.8 ± 4.8 days in the shorter-term storage group and 28.3 ± 6.7 in the longer-term storage group. Change in multiple organ dysfunction score was the same in both groups. In addition, 7-day and 28-day mortality and adverse events (except for hyperbilirubinemia, which was more common in the longer-term storage group) did not differ significantly. This large trial also concluded that fresher RBCs were not superior. Three other large randomized controlled trials addressing the same question are ongoing: the Red Cell Storage Duration and Outcomes in Cardiac Surgery (NCT00458783), which will enroll 2600 adults after an elective cardiac surgery; the TRANSFUSE study, which will include 6000 transfused critically ill adults,[87] and the INFORM trial, which will recruit 24,400 hospitalized adults.[88]

Although all of the adult studies may demonstrate that using fresher RBC units does not improve the outcomes of transfused critically ill adults, one can question whether this will hold true in children. Two prospective descriptive studies undertaken in critically ill children suggest that outcome is less favorable with transfusion of packed RBC units stored for more than 2 or 3 weeks.[33,89] A large randomized controlled trial, the Age of Blood in Children in PICU (ABC-PICU) study (NCT01977547) that will enroll 1538 transfused PICU patients should provide definitive evidence. Presently, there is no justification to require fresh RBC units in critically ill children.

Perfusion, Warming, and Filtration

An RBC transfusion must be completed within 4 to 6 hours (4 hours in the United States) after the unit is delivered by the hospital blood bank. A packed RBC unit is usually transfused over 1 to 3 hours, but it can be given more slowly (up to 4 hours) or divided in two transfusions if there is some risk of cardiac overload.[76]

The viscosity of packed RBC units is high, which implies it is preferable to use larger bore needles to administer them. No drugs should be given in the line used for packed RBC unit perfusion. There is in theory a risk of hemolysis if RBCs are given with 0.2% saline or dextrose 10%, but the coinfusion of RBC and hypo- or hypertonic solution seems safe if it is short lasting (a few minutes).[90] It is inappropriate to mix RBC units with Ringer's lactate (risk of coagulation) or calcium.

Packed RBC units must be warmed before administration to diminish the viscosity of the blood product and to avoid hypothermia. Blood viscosity decreases by about 7% for each 1°C increase, thus reducing resistance and making it easier to administer blood products through catheters. RBC units are stored at 1° to 6°C and could cause significant hypothermia if given to a patient without warming. All blood products are warmed to room temperature (about 20°C) before delivery to the bedside. Warming to body temperature (37°C) may be required for patients weighing less than 10 kg or if large amounts need to be given corresponding to more than 20% to 30% of the circulating blood volume. Standard blood-warming devices must be used to raise the temperature of whole blood or packed RBC units, not microwave ovens that can cause severe hemolysis.

Because all packed RBC units (even prestorage leukocyte-reduced RBC units) contain fibrin, platelets, and WBC aggregates, a filter (with 80-, 179-, or 260-micron pores) must always be used to bind these aggregates before they are administered. Although their cost usefulness has not been determined, filter with 20- to 40-micron micropores are more effective, and some evidence suggests that they can prevent some cases of TRALI. Filters with smaller micropores are not considered standard treatment.

Plasma

Types of Plasma

Plasma is separated from RBCs after collection of whole blood or it is collected using an apheresis machine; it is then frozen for storage to preserve the levels of coagulation factors. The name *fresh frozen plasma* is used if the unit is refrigerated within 8 hours of collection, and the term *frozen plasma* is used if refrigerated within 24 hours of collection. There is a slight reduction in factor VIII levels in frozen plasma, but in clinical practice these two types of plasma are essentially interchangeable.[91] We will use the acronym FP (frozen plasma) in this section to designate both types of plasma units.

FP units are collected from a single donor, whereas units of solvent detergent (SD) plasma (Octaplas, Octapharma) are constituted from a pool of FP collected from approximately 700 donors and processed using the SD process for inactivation of lipid-enveloped viruses. In some countries, only FP may be available, but in many countries fresh FP was still available in the year 2015.

FP units are systematically leukocyte reduced by filtration before storage in many countries, but not in the United States. FP volume is about 200 to 250 mL/unit,[76] whereas the volume of SD plasma is about 200 mL/unit. On average, FP contains

one unit/mL of all coagulation factors, but there is significant variability among individual units, which is attributable to biological variation in factor levels among individual donors and differences in processing, storage, and preparation for transfusion.[92] The levels of coagulation factors in SD plasma are more standard with little variation among units, as it is a pooled plasma product. FP is stored at −18°C for up to 1 year after collection. SD plasma can be stored for up to 48 months.

Epidemiologic studies reported that adults transfused with FP are more prone to contract ventilator-associated pneumonia, bloodstream infection, and septic shock (relative risk for all infections: 2.99; 95% CI: 2.28–3.93, p = 0.02).[93] A prospective cohort study involving 831 critically ill children reported an increased incidence rate of morbidity and nosocomial infections: The adjusted odds ratio was 3.2 (95% CI: 1.6, 6.6) and 2.3 (95% CI: 1, 5.3), respectively; there was also a significant difference in the adjusted length of PICU stay.[94] FP transfusions are associated with adverse clinical outcomes; this might be attributable to their immunomodulative properties.

Transfusion of Plasma: Indication (When)

Generally, plasma is transfused to correct multiple coagulation factor deficiencies (or single factor deficiencies when no recombinant or plasma-derived coagulation factor concentrates are available) in patients with active bleeding or prior to invasive procedures when no alternative therapies are available or appropriate. Common coagulopathies for which FP may be given include liver disease and symptomatic disseminated intravascular coagulation (DIC). However, the use of plasma to treat DIC is controversial because thrombosis is frequently a component of this disorder.[76] FP can also be given for the emergency reversal of warfarin or vitamin K deficiency when prothrombin complex concentrates are not available.[95] FP is also given to prevent bleeding in patients with abnormal coagulation tests. Guidelines suggest transfusing FP only when the international normalized ratio (INR), the prothrombin time (DIC), or the activated partial thromboplastin time (aPTT) is more than 1.5 × normal, as coagulation factors are generally adequate for hemostasis below this level. However, some data suggest that FP is not effective at normalizing mild abnormalities of coagulation tests, and the potential clinical benefit of FP transfusion seems minimal when the INR is <2.5 or an aPTT is <60.[96]

FP may also be administered during massive transfusion of packed RBC units. Some experts advocate early replacement of FP in a 1:1 ratio with RBC units in trauma patients with massive bleeding whereas others suggest that FP transfusions should be guided by the presence of abnormal coagulation test results as previously listed. However, according to a systematic review, application of a thromboelastography (TEG or ROTEM)-guided transfusion strategy did reduce the amount of bleeding in patients with massive transfusion but failed to improve morbidity and mortality.[97] FP or whole blood should be administered in patients who have received more than 150% of their circulating blood volume, even if there is no bleeding, or in patients who have received more than one circulating blood volume and who have clinical evidence of oozing or microvascular bleeding.[95,98]

Plasma exchange is used for thrombotic thrombocytopenic purpura (TTP).[95] There is no evidence that FP should be given in prophylaxis to nonbleeding patients. Plasma should not be used as a volume expander; crystalloids, synthetic colloids, or purified human albumin solutions are preferred.

Transfusion of Plasma: How

One mL of FP contains about one unit of each of the coagulation factors. For most deficiencies, 30% of normal factor activity is enough to ensure hemostasis. Surgical hemostasis may be achieved with factor II levels 5% to 50% of normal, factor V approximately 30% of normal, factor VII 25% of normal, and factor VIII 30% to 60% of normal.[42] It should be appreciated that these data were generated from single factor deficiencies and have never been analyzed in the setting of multiple factor deficiencies that are seen in the vast majority of bleeding patients in the PICU. Practitioners usually administer 10 to 20 mL/kg of plasma initially; this should increase the level of the individual coagulation factors above 30%. As the levels of coagulation factors vary among units, the response to FP is not consistent. Therefore, the effectiveness of FP transfusion should be estimated by clinical judgment of ongoing bleeding and, if necessary, repeat coagulation testing. Additional doses of FP may be required for ongoing bleeding with persistently elevated coagulation tests. Karam and associates reported that a dose-response relationship was only found in patients with an INR >2.5; patients with lower INR had no significant change in coagulation tests.[96] Normalization of coagulation tests often does not occur and therefore should not be used as the only guide for additional FP transfusions.

FP transfusions should be ABO compatible but are not required to be identical. In contrast to RBC, group AB positive plasma is the universal plasma donor and can be given in emergency situations when a blood group is not available. Cross-matching is not required as FP units are screened for antibodies against non-ABO and Rh antibodies, which may cause hemolytic reactions.

FP must be thawed (20 to 30 minutes) prior to transfusion. Warming FP can be shortened to 7 minutes using microwave ovens specifically constructed for this task (a standard microwave oven can disable coagulation factors). A thawed unit of FP is ideally transfused within 4 hours, but thawed plasma can be relabeled and stored for up to 5 days (American Association of Blood Banks [AABB] Technical Manual). The clinical indications for thawed plasma are similar to FP but there is some decrease in the labile coagulation factors (factor V and VIII). An 80- or 170-micron pore filter must be used.

Platelets

Platelet Transfusion: Why and Why Not

More than 1.5 million platelet products are transfused in the United States each year.[99] Most platelet transfusions are given to increase platelet count. The prevalence of thrombocytopenia, defined by a platelet count <150,000/uL (<150 × 10^9/L), is 17.3% on admission into the PICU; 25.3% of children are thrombocytopenic at some point during their PICU stay.[100] Thrombocytopenia arises from decreased platelet production, increased platelet destruction, and dilutional or distributional causes. In the PICU, most thrombocytopenia is caused by sepsis, disseminated intravascular coagulation, MODS, or hemolytic uremic syndrome. However, heparin-induced thrombocytopenia, massive transfusion, and reactive hemophagocytic syndrome are not so rare. In critically ill children,

thrombocytopenia at PICU entry is associated with increased mortality (17.6% versus 2.5%), bleeding complications, thrombosis, and prolonged PICU and hospital length of stay.[100]

Pediatric subjects are at higher risk of bleeding over a wide range of platelet counts, indicating that their excess bleeding risk may be because of factors other than platelet counts.[101] Platelet dysfunction might be the problem, at least in some instances. In PICU patients, it is caused most of the time by specific treatments (cardiopulmonary bypass, hypothermia, pentastarch, and hetastarch) or antiplatelet drugs (low-dose aspirin, nonsteroidal antiinflammatory drugs), but it can also be caused by hereditary disease (eg, Bernard-Soulier disease, etc.). Platelets are important actors in hemostasis. They also have inflammatory functions and can influence both innate and adaptive immune response.[102]

Types of Platelet Products

Standard Platelet Products

Different methods can be used to obtain platelet products: they may be whole blood–derived platelets—either by the platelet-rich plasma (United States and UK) or the buffy-coat method (Europe and Canada)—or by apheresis (single-donor) platelets (United States, Europe, and Canada). For whole blood–derived platelets, platelet concentrates are often pooled (up to six units) for a single platelet transfusion.

The maximum in vivo platelet life span is 10.5 days.[103] When stored at 20° to 24°C and gently agitated in a continuous manner, stored platelets can be used up to 5 days (up to 7 days in some European countries) after they were collected, but they will become active only 4 hours post transfusion. If they are stored at 4°C, they are active immediately but cannot be stored for more than 48 hours. In practice, most platelets units are stored at 20°C.

Special Platelet Concentrates

Leukocyte-Reduced Platelets

A platelet concentrate must contain <8.3 × 10^5 WBCs to be labeled leukocyte reduced. Prestorage leukocyte reduction is a standard procedure in many countries. A bedside leukocyte reduction filter should not be used when prestorage leukocyte reduction was done because it is useless and can decrease the number of platelets.

Irradiated Platelets

The risk of TAGVH is increased in patients who receive human leukocyte antigen (HLA)–compatible platelets. Therefore, pretransfusion irradiation is mandatory for all HLA-compatible platelet concentrates. Irradiation is also recommended for intrauterine transfusion and infants at risk of TAGVH.[76]

Cytomegalovirus Negative Platelets

Platelet concentrates can transmit CMV. The indications for CMV-negative platelets and RBCs are similar.

Platelets Substitutes

There is no alternative to platelets transfusion. However, cryoprecipitate can be used to treat platelet dysfunction caused by uremia if therapy as dialysis is not successful.[76]

Transfusion of Platelets: Indication (When)

Platelet transfusions are indicated for the prevention or treatment of bleeding in patients with thrombocytopenia or platelet dysfunction. As platelet transfusions will only result in modest elevations for 1 to 3 days in patients with persistent thrombocytopenia, the purpose of platelet therapy is not to eliminate all bleeding but to prevent or stop major hemorrhagic events.

Therapeutic platelet transfusions are given to treat clinically significant bleeding associated with a low platelet count. There is evidence that correction of thrombocytopenia reduces the mortality of critically ill patients,[100,104] but a platelet transfusion should be considered only if the platelet count in an actively bleeding patient is <50,000 to 100,000/uL.

More than 50% of platelet transfusions are given to prevent bleeding, even though the need for prophylactic transfusions has not been conclusively proved. There is insufficient evidence to support a particular threshold for prophylactic platelet transfusion in children. Most recommendations come from guidelines developed for adults, based on expert opinion. For patients with hypoproliferative thrombocytopenia (eg, chemotherapy induced), a platelet transfusion threshold of 10,000/uL is recommended.[76] This is based on two clinical trials in adults: Slichter and colleagues[103] reported no increases in bleeding rates when comparing platelet transfusion thresholds of 10,000 versus 20,000/uL[103]; on the other hand, Stanworth and coworkers[105] reported more bleeding in patients with hematologic cancer and a platelet count <10,000/uL who did not receive prophylactic platelet transfusion versus those who did.

In the ICU, higher platelet transfusion thresholds are usually employed. Intensivists generally prescribe platelets for patients on ECMO if their platelet count is <100,000/uL; the same threshold is frequently used when a central nervous system procedure is undertaken. When the platelet count is <50,000/uL, platelets are usually given just prior to an invasive procedure (surgery, insertion of central venous catheter, etc.); they can also be considered in mechanically ventilated patients because the risk of pulmonary hemorrhage is significant. A threshold of 10,000 or 20,000/uL is recommended for lumbar puncture.

The platelet count must be monitored closely if a large amount—more than one blood volume—of crystalloids or packed RBC units is given because this can significantly dilute the circulating platelet volume.

The platelet count is not the only element to consider when deciding whether to administer platelets: Increasing the threshold that triggers platelet transfusion may be appropriate if a rapid decrease in the platelet count is observed, if the risk of bleeding is high, or if platelets are dysfunctional. Platelets are contraindicated in patients with thrombotic thrombocytopenic purpura and heparin-induced thrombocytopenia because of the increased thrombotic risk.

The capacity of platelets to stop a hemorrhage is related not only to their number but also to their function. Many tests can be used to estimate platelet function like thromboelastography and devices or systems such as the Sonoclot coagulation analyzer, the Plateletworks analyzer, the Hemostatus platelet function test, the Platelet function analyzer, and VerifyNow (Ultegra) System.[42] However, the results of these tests are not available on an emergency basis in most hospitals.[106] Measurement of platelet mass may be a practical alternative. There is evidence that larger platelets exhibit increased hemostatic activity.[107] The results of a randomized controlled trial conducted in a neonatal ICU suggest that using platelet mass (platelet count × mean platelet volume) rather than platelet

count to trigger a platelet transfusion may reduce the number of transfusions.[108] Nevertheless, it must be underlined that the clinical usefulness of all these tests remains undetermined in the PICU.

There is a significant diversity in the stated practice pattern with respect to platelet transfusion.[109] Most guidelines are based on experts' opinion, not on hard data.[39,95,110] Additional research must be conducted to better determine when platelets should be given to critically ill children.

Transfusion of Platelets: How

There are about 55×10^9 platelets per unit. A simple rule of thumb suggests giving one or two platelet units per 10 kg but not more than six units per transfusion. For children weighing less than 10 kg, the platelet dose can be 5 to 10 mL/kg of pooled or apheresis platelet unit. Transfusion of one platelet concentrate per m^2 of body surface generally increases the platelet count by 7000 to 11,000/uL. By body weight, the administration of one unit per 10 kg should increase the platelet count by 30,000 to 50,000/uL. However, a clinical trial, where platelet dose was estimated by body surface area, evaluated low- (1.1×10^{12} platelets/m^2), medium- (2.2×10^{12}/m^2), and high-dose (3.3×10^{12}/m^2) prophylactic platelet transfusions and did not find any differences in bleeding among adult or pediatric patients.[111] Platelets must be used within 4 hours after delivery from the blood bank, but there is some evidence that the platelet count rises more if the unit is given within an hour. A filter with 80- or 170-micron pores must be used to remove aggregates that can form between harvesting and transfusion.

The volume of a platelet-rich unit is about 50 to 70 mL, whereas that of an apheresis platelet unit ranges from 200 to 300 mL; 90% to 95% of this volume is plasma. It is important to note that this plasma is not an adequate source of coagulation factors because their concentration drops rapidly during platelet storage. Platelet units can be volume reduced (removal of plasma) prior to transfusion, but this process can decrease the platelet count by 15% to 20%, shortens the storage time to 4 hours, and delays platelet release from the blood bank by approximately 1 hour. Volume reduction should only be considered if there is a risk of severe cardiac overload, but it is not recommended as a standard procedure because it can activate platelets.[76]

Unlike RBC units, ABO compatibility is not mandatory with platelets. However, it is better to use ABO compatible platelet units in young patients with small blood volume. Moreover it is recommended to deliver ABO compatible platelets when inventory and time permit, unless the plasma component has been substantially reduced. In addition, Rh compatibility is desired because all platelet units contain some RBCs. Transfusion of an Rh-positive unit to an Rh-negative patient can cause Rh alloimmunization; an anti-D immunoglobulin (WinRho) should be administered within 48 hours to prevent this complication when Rh-positive platelets are given to an Rh-negative patient, particularly if female.[99]

The percentage platelet increment (difference between post- and pretransfusion platelet count) should be higher than 20% if the dose is adequate and if a platelet count is performed 10 to 60 minutes post transfusion; it should be higher than 10% if measured 18 to 24 hours post transfusion.[99] Platelet refractoriness can occur due to nonimmune factors such as disseminated intravascular coagulation, in which platelet consumption can be high, acquired hemophagocytic syndrome, with drugs like amphotericin or heparin, or secondary to immune factors involving antiplatelet antibodies.[99] Treatment of the underlying problem is mandatory in such instances (eg, discontinuing all heparin administration in heparin-induced thrombocytopenia). Patients with anti-IgA antibodies should receive washed platelets or platelets collected from IgA-deficient donors.

Cryoprecipitate

Cryoprecipitate is a concentrated source of fibrinogen, factor VIII, factor XIII, and von Willebrand factor. It is stored at a minimum of −18°C for a maximum of 1 year. It is used in patients with congenital or acquired hypofibrinogenemia and patients with coagulopathy and significant bleeding. It can also be used in patients with von Willebrand disease and hemophilia A if specific factor concentrates are not available. The dose is 1 or 2 units/10 kg (maximum: 12 units), which should increase fibrinogen level about 60 to 100 mg/dL.[76] A blood filter (80 or 180 micron) should be used. The recommended rate of delivery is 30 minutes (maximum: 4 hours).

Transfusions Reactions and Complications

Transfusion of labile blood products (RBC, plasma, platelets) can cause immediate or delayed transfusion reactions and various complications. Immediate reactions usually occur during the transfusion or within 6 hours after the end of the transfusion. Delayed reactions can occur after a few days, weeks, or even months or years later.

Transfusion Reactions to Red Blood Cells, Plasma, and Platelets

Immediate Transfusion Reactions

The incidence of typical immediate transfusion reactions after RBC, FP, and platelet transfusion is reported in Table 93.2. The risk of transfusion reactions is higher in children. The SHOT report on transfusion reactions observed in children in the United Kingdom from 1996 to 2005 estimated the incidence of transfusion-related adverse events to be 13 per 100,000 RBC units issued for adults, 18:100,000 for children younger than 18 years, and 37:100,000 for infants younger than 12 months.[112] Among the 321 adverse reports in children, 82% were instances of incorrect blood component transfusion and 50 cases (14%) were acute transfusion reactions.

Transfusion reactions are probably underdiagnosed in critically ill children. In a study conducted in the PICU of Sainte-Justine Hospital, all transfusions between February 2002 and February 2004 were prospectively monitored.[113] A total of 2509 transfusions were administered to 305 patients; 40 acute transfusion reactions (1.6%) occurred: 24 nonhemolytic febrile reactions, 6 minor and 1 major (anaphylactic shock) allergic reactions, 4 isolated hypotensive reactions, 3 bacterial contaminations, 1 hemolytic reaction, and 1 TRALI.

The most important acute transfusion reactions are described next.

Respiratory System

TRALI (transfusion-related acute lung injury) is one of the most dangerous transfusion reactions. Two pathophysiologic mechanisms are currently proposed.[114,115] (1) According to the antibody hypothesis, TRALI is caused by an antigen-antibody reaction.[116] The antibodies (granulocyte antibodies or HLA class I or II antibodies) are present in the donor plasma and react with the recipient's WBC antigens (or rarely vice versa). The administration of such antibodies can directly injure the lung or can activate neutrophils, monocytes, and complement, creating an inflammatory reaction that may result in pulmonary damage. (2) According to the *two-hit* or *neutrophil priming* hypothesis, recipients must first have a predisposing factor, which *primes* their neutrophils, like a septic state or a MODS; then, the recipient's neutrophils are activated again by donor plasma that contains leukocyte antibody or proinflammatory molecules like cytokines and bioactive lipids.[117]

A panel of experts suggested a consensus definition of TRALI in 2004[118]; the list of diagnostic criteria advocated by these experts is detailed in Table 93.3. The diagnosis of TRALI is made on the basis of clinical signs and symptoms, chest x-ray suggestive of pulmonary edema, and time relationship with transfusion (onset per transfusion or within 6 hours post transfusion). Experts defined TRALI as a new ALI for which no other risk factor than the transfusion can be found. They suggested the term *possible TRALI* if another risk factor can be temporally related to the ALI. TRALI is a clinical syndrome, and no laboratory test is pathognomonic, but the presence of HLA or neutrophil antibodies in the donor plasma is highly suggestive[114]; however, the absence of such antibodies does not exclude a typical case of TRALI. Causes of pulmonary edema other than TRALI should also be excluded, like fluid overload or cardiac dysfunction.

The incidence rate of TRALI in the PICU is unknown, but there is evidence that it is underreported.[119,120] Over a 3-year period, Gauvin and colleagues[113] observed one case of TRALI among 305 transfused PICU patients.

All blood products that contain plasma, even in minute quantities, can cause a TRALI. When such a reaction occurs, the transfusion must be stopped immediately and supportive therapy administered. Associated hypotension may be unresponsive to fluid administration and may require the use of inotropes/vasopressors. Diuretics are not useful and are contraindicated in hypotensive patients. All suspected TRALI reactions must be reported to the blood bank, because the donor's other blood products have to be withdrawn.

The prognosis of cases of TRALI is usually good if the patient survives, but a mortality rate of 6% has been reported. In survivors, resolution is usually rapid (within 96 hours) and there are no long-term sequelae.[121]

The diagnostic criteria advocated by the panel of experts in 2004 exclude the possibility that a TRALI appears more than 6 hours post transfusion or in patients who already present an ALI or ARDS, a frequent occurrence in the PICU. Marik and coworkers[122] suggested expanding the definition of TRALI in ICU to ALI/ARDS observed within 72 hours after the transfusion of a blood product: They reported that such "delayed TRALI syndrome" occurred in up to 25% of transfused critically ill adults. Church and associates[123] also reported an association between the transfusion of plasma or packed RBC units and ALI/ARDS. There is also some evidence that TRALI should also be considered in some patients with ALI/ARDS before a transfusion if their respiratory dysfunction deteriorates significantly during or after a transfusion.[124] The bioactive substances contained in packed RBC and plasma units can cause or add to the severity of cases of ALI/ARDS.[123,125] Actually, there is a synergistic effect of anemia and RBC transfusion

TABLE 93.2   Incidence of Transfusion Reactions (Adults and Children)

	RISK PER 1 UNIT OF BLOOD COMPONENT[a]			
	All products	RBC	FP	Platelets[b]
A. Early Transfusion Reactions (Onset Usually <6 Hours Post Transfusion)				
Cardiorespiratory systems:				
—Transfusion-related acute lung injury (TRALI)[a,168]	1:31,960	1:23,350	1:19.783	1:15,595
—Transfusion-associated circulatory overload (TACO)[a,168]	1:34,091	1:32,690	1:32,971	–
—Hypotension[a,c,168]	1:102,273	1:108,968	1:98,914	+
—Cardiac arrhythmias[d,169]	+	+	–	–
Hematologic and immunologic systems:				
—Acute hemolytic reactions[a,168]	1:26,914	1:18,161	–	1:31,189
—ABO incompatibility[a,168]	1:85,227	1:108,968	1:98,914	1:15,595
—Major allergic reaction (anaphylaxis)[a,168]	1:11,117	1:23,350	1:6182	1:3889
—Minor allergic reaction (urticaria)[148]	1:100	+	+	+
Other acute transfusion reactions and complications:[e]				
—Febrile nonhemolytic reaction[170,171]	1:50 to 1:200	1:300	–	1:10
—Bacterial contamination[a,168]	1:51,136	1:65,381	1:49,457	1:31,189
B. Delayed Transfusion Reactions (Onset Usually Days After Transfusion)				
Transfusion-associated graft-versus-host disease[81]	1:1 million	+	+	+
Delayed hemolytic transfusion reactions[a,168]	1:255,682	1:163,452	–	–
Post transfusion purpura[a,168]	1:85,227	1:108,968	–	1:31,189
Transfusion-transmitted nonbacterial infections	See Table 93.4	+	+	+

[a]Reported in 2003.
[b]Risk per pool of five units of platelet.
[c]Hypotension can be caused by allergic or hemolytic reactions, septicemia, citrate toxicity, reaction to leukocyte reduction filters, and bradykinins in the supernatant of blood products.
[d]One retrospective study involving 143 critically ill adults with sepsis or septic shock reported more atrial fibrillation (p = 0.04), cardiac arrest (p = 0.03), and "all cardiac events" (p = 0.001) in recipients of packed RBC units.[169]
[e]Metabolic complications include hypothermia, metabolic alkalosis,[172] hypocalcemia,[173] hypomagnesemia,[172] hyperkalemia,[173] hyponatremia,[17] and hyperglycemia.[174]
FP, frozen plasma; RBC, red blood cell.

TABLE 93.3   Diagnostic Criteria of Transfusion-Related Acute Lung Injury (TRALI) and Possible TRALI[175]

Diagnostic Criteria of TRALI (All Four Criteria Must Be Present):

1. Diagnostic criteria of acute lung injury (ALI):
   —Acute onset
   —Hypoxemia: PaO_2/FiO_2 ≤300 or SpO_2 <90% on room air
   —Bilateral infiltrates on frontal chest radiograph
   —No evidence of left atrial hypertension (ie, no circulatory overload)
2. No preexisting ALI before transfusion
3. Onset during or within 6 hours post transfusion
4. No temporal relationship to an alternative risk factor of ALI (see list of factors[a])

Diagnostic Criteria of Possible TRALI:

Acute lung injury (ALI)
No preexisting ALI before transfusion
Onset during or within 6 hours posttransfusion
A clear temporal relationship to an alternative risk factor for ALI

[a]Risk factors of direct lung injury: aspiration, pneumonia, toxic inhalation, lung contusion, near drowning. Risk factors of indirect lung injury: severe sepsis, shock, multiple trauma, burn injury, acute pancreatitis, cardiopulmonary bypass, drug overdose.

on inflammation and lung injury.[126] Further investigation is required to better characterize the epidemiology, the mechanisms, and the clinical impact of transfusion-related ALI/ARDS in the PICU.

Respiratory Dysfunction Associated With Transfusion. Respiratory complications associated with RBC transfusions may be underestimated in the PICU because current definitions exclude patients with preexisting respiratory dysfunction (RD). Emeriaud and colleagues[124] undertook a prospective cohort study to determine the epidemiology of new or progressive RD observed after RBC transfusion in critically ill children. A respiratory dysfunction associated with transfusion (RDAT) was considered new if it appeared after the first RBC transfusion in the PICU. A progressive RDAT was diagnosed if an RD was present before the transfusion and the PaO_2/FiO_2 or SpO_2/FiO_2 ratio dropped by at least 20% thereafter. Among 136 transfused patients, 58 cases of RDAT (43% of transfused patients) were detected, including 9 (7%) new RDAT and 49 (36%) progressive RDAT. Higher severity of illness, MODS prior to transfusion, and volume (mL/kg) of RBC transfusion were independently associated with RDAT. A dose-response relationship was observed between transfusion volume (mL/kg) and the incidence of RDAT. Patients with

RDAT developed more MODS, had a longer duration of intubation and PICU length of stay, and had higher mortality. The conclusion was that RDAT is frequent in the PICU and occurs mainly in patients with prior RD, who would not be identified using current definitions for transfusion-associated respiratory complications. RDAT is not recognized as a transfusion reaction by the hemovigilance system, but it seems to be a clinically significant transfusion complication. RDAT should be further studied, given the high incidence and the serious adverse outcomes associated with it.

Cardiovascular System

Transfusion-Associated Circulatory Overload. Transfusion-associated circulatory overload (TACO) is presently the leading cause of transfusion-related morbidity and mortality in North America.[127] From 2000 to 2009, 730 cases of TACO were reported to the Quebec Hemovigilance System.[128] In 2013, 96 cases of TACO were collected by the British Haemovigilance Scheme; none were reported in children.[127]

TACO in critically ill adults is underreported to hemovigilance systems.[125,129-133] There are almost no data on TACO in the PICU.[89,94,113,119,120,134-137] The risk of contracting a TACO is likely higher in children in the PICU because cardiac dysfunction, a well-recognized risk factor for TACO, is common in PICU patients.[127,138] Indeed, it may be that TACO is not reported to the hemovigilance system in critically ill children probably because the diagnostic criteria of TACO are not well suited to children.

Two sets of diagnostic criteria of TACO are presently used:

1. TACO definition, according to the US Biovigilance Network (www.aabb.org/programs/biovigilance/Documents/diagnose_full.html)—New onset or exacerbation of three or more of the following within 6 hours of cessation of transfusion: (1) acute respiratory distress (dyspnea, orthopnea, cough), (2) evidence of positive fluid balance, (3) elevated brain natriuretic peptide (BNP), (4) radiographic evidence of pulmonary edema, (5) evidence of left heart failure, (6) elevated central venous pressure.

2. TACO definition, according to the British Haemovigilance Scheme (Serious Hazards of Transfusion [SHOT]) and the International Society of Blood Transfusion (ISBT)[139]— TACO is present if at least four or the five following criteria are met within 6 hours of transfusion: (1) acute respiratory distress, (2) tachycardia, (3) increased blood pressure, (4) acute or worsening pulmonary edema, (5) evidence of positive fluid balance.

In 2009, no TACO was reported in a prospective cohort study of 136 consecutive PICU patients transfused with RBC.[140] A subsequent chart review was undertaken to ascertain whether TACO cases had been missed. Attempts to use the criteria advocated by the British Haemovigilance Scheme[119] were problematic because terms such as *tachycardia* and *increased blood pressure* were vaguely defined and did not provide age-adjusted reference ranges. When using diagnostic criteria that compared heart rate or blood pressure with normal pediatric values or that assessed change between pre- and posttransfusion value, it was noted that the incidence rate of TACO could have ranged from 1.5% to 46% depending on the set of diagnostic criteria used. TACO is probably frequent in the PICU. Its epidemiology can differ significantly if appropriate diagnostic criteria are not used; this implies that better diagnostic criteria must be developed.

TACO is most commonly associated with a rapid or massive transfusion that causes pulmonary edema secondary to heart failure.[141] Reduced cardiac reserve, chronic and severe anemia (Hb <5 g/dL), and age (infants and elderly patients) are risk factors. The main symptoms are respiratory distress, hypoxemia, tachycardia, and hypertension. When TACO is suspected, transfusion must be stopped and supportive treatment provided. Slow transfusion (≤1 mL/kg/h) for at-risk patients can prevent TACO.

Hypotensive reactions are increasingly recognized,[142] but their etiology remains uncertain. They are probably attributable to bradykinin generation, which can happen when a blood product is exposed to negatively charged surfaces (eg, filters). The risk of hypotensive reaction is increased in patients receiving angiotensin conversion enzyme inhibitors (ACEI) or with diminished bradykinin metabolism. Hypotensive reactions are more frequently associated with platelets than with RBC and plasma. However, the authors observed only five platelet-related hypotensive episodes among 3672 consecutive PICU admissions.[143] Transfusion-related hypotension may happen alone or with some flushing; it occurs rapidly after the transfusion begins. The treatment is straightforward: The transfusion must be stopped and supportive treatment (ie, fluid bolus) should be undertaken.

Other Acute Transfusion Reactions. *Nonhemolytic febrile reaction* is the most frequent and benign acute transfusion reaction (1 in 300 RBC and 1 in 20 platelet transfusions).[144] In addition to fever, it can be accompanied by chills, discomfort, headache, nausea, or vomiting. The symptoms usually occur toward the end or soon after a transfusion. These reactions are mediated by pyrogenic substances that accumulate during storage or by the recipient's antibodies that bind with leukocytes from the donated blood, which allow activation of the complement system and production of cytokines. Acetaminophen can be used to minimize fever, but premedication with acetaminophen, diphenhydramine, or steroids is not useful. A decrease in the incidence of these reactions is reported with prestorage leukocyte reduction.[145,146]

Acute hemolytic reactions may be much more serious. They are caused by lysis or accelerated destruction of RBCs due to immunologic incompatibility between donor and recipient blood. The mortality rate associated with transfusion errors is <10%.[147] ABO mismatch is the most frequent and most severe of the blood group incompatibilities, with hemolysis and death as the results. In most instances, mistransfusion is the cause—that is, the patient receives a packed RBC unit that was prepared for another patient. The risk that such errors happen is obviously higher in the context of emergency transfusion; its prevention warrants careful verification by medical staff of all blood products administered. The reaction is characterized by fever, chills, discomfort, diffuse pain, and hemoglobinuria; hypotension, shock, renal failure, and disseminated intravascular coagulation are also observed in some cases. When such a reaction is suspected, the transfusion must be stopped immediately and supportive treatment administered. To avoid these hemolytic reactions, donor and recipient compatibility must be thoroughly checked (ABO and Rh types, unit identification number) and the recipient must be properly identified (name and medical record number) when the sample is taken for pretransfusion analyses as well as before the transfusion begins. Several centers have instituted double verification by two different individuals for every assessment made.

Nonimmune hemolysis can be caused by mechanical trauma to RBCs, rapid administration through a small catheter, excessive warming or freezing, or contact with hypotonic solution.

Allergic transfusion reactions result from the interaction between donor allergens and recipient antibodies (IgE) that provokes a type I hypersensitivity reaction.[148] Other possible mechanisms include preexisting class-specific anti-IgA in patients with IgA deficiency, preexisting antibodies to polymorphic forms of other serum proteins (IgG, albumin, haptoglobin, etc.) that the patient is lacking, transfusion of allergens to which a patient is presensitized (drugs, chemicals, etc.), and passive transfer of IgE antibodies to transfused patients.[148] The reaction can be minor (eg, isolated urticaria) or major (eg, hypotension, anaphylactic shock, respiratory distress, digestive disorders). A severe reaction usually occurs quickly, whereas a benign reaction may occur up to 4 hours after the transfusion has been completed. When an allergic reaction is suspected, the transfusion must be stopped and supportive treatment undertaken with antihistamines, corticosteroids, and epinephrine if required. Prevention must be considered. Premedication of patients with antihistamines is suggested if they have already presented two minor episodes. In patients with major reactions, premedication can be used with corticosteroids and antihistamines. Washed RBC and platelets units can also be used. Patients with anti-IgA antibodies must receive blood products from donors with IgA deficiency or products that have been washed several times. Leukocyte reduction does not offer any benefit.

Bacterial contamination is more frequent with platelets than with RBC units or plasma because platelet concentrates are stored at 20° to 24°C. Contamination may be due to unsuspected bacteremia in the donor, skin flora contamination when taking a blood sample from the donor, or issues related to product handling. The most common microorganisms identified are gram-negative bacteria such as *Klebsiella pneumoniae*, *Serratia marcescens,* and *Pseudomonas species,* and gram-positive bacteria such as *Staphylococcus aureus, Staphylococcus epidermidis,* and *Bacillus cereus.* The reaction is characterized by fever and chills and may lead to septic shock. Symptoms usually appear during or within 4 hours after transfusion. When bacterial contamination is suspected, transfusion must be stopped immediately, wide-spectrum antibiotics must be given (third-generation cephalosporin or beta-lactam in combination with aminoglycoside), and supportive treatment administered. The blood bank must be informed immediately, as other blood products from the same donor may need to be withdrawn.

Many descriptive studies have reported an association between RBC transfusion and necrotizing enterocolitis (NEC) in very low-birth-weight neonates.[149,150] The relevance of *transfusion-related acute gut injury (TRAGI)* in PICU patients is undetermined.

Delayed Transfusion Reactions. Among the 321 adverse events reported in children by SHOT in UK from 1996 to 2005,[112] there were five cases of severe delayed transfusion reactions, including two cases of TAGVH disease. *TAGVH* is rare but very serious.[81,82] It may occur when viable lymphocytes from a donor are infused to a recipient who is unable to reject them because of immune suppression or partial HLA matching (closed-donor genetic profile). Donor leukocytes can then persist in the recipient, because these lymphocytes recognize the recipient's HLA antigens as foreign and an immune reaction is triggered. Signs and symptoms (generalized skin rash, diarrhea, abnormal liver function, or fever) appear 8 to 10 days after transfusion.[151] Associated complications are aplastic anemia with pancytopenia, which may lead to hemorrhage and severe infections. The mortality rate is 90%. The risk of TAGVH is higher in premature babies and if a patient with a congenital or acquired immunodeficiency receives a nonirradiated RBC unit or if the blood was a directed donation collected from a relative. Neoplasia (eg, leukemia, solid tumors), chemotherapy and transplantation (stem cell, bone marrow, solid organ),[144] intrauterine transfusions, and exchange transfusions are other risk factors. No effective treatment is recognized. Prevention can be accomplished by irradiating blood products.

Delayed (extravascular) hemolytic reactions result from the interaction between recipient irregular alloantibodies and donor RBCs. They involve either antibodies that were present prior to transfusion, but were missed because they were undetectable by cross-matching, or antibodies that appear after the transfusion. Involved antibodies are usually E, Jk^a, c, Fy^a, or K.[144] These reactions occur 3 days to 2 weeks after the transfusion. Symptoms include anemia and jaundice. The outcome is usually good except in some patients with sickle cell anemia. There is no specific treatment.

Posttransfusion purpura is characterized by dramatic, sudden, and self-limiting thrombocytopenia. The pathogenesis is unclear but is presumably related to the development of platelet-specific antibody following transfusion. The platelet count drops below <10,000/uL 5 to 10 days after transfusion was given in a patient with a history of sensitization by pregnancy or prior transfusion.[152] Purpura and diffuse hemorrhages (mucosal, gastrointestinal, urinary, cerebral) may be observed. The thrombocytopenia is refractory to platelet transfusion. The mortality rate is 8%. Treatment includes corticosteroids, plasmapheresis, and immunoglobulins.

Complications Related to Massive Transfusion

Massive transfusion is defined as the administration of more than one circulating volume of blood products within 24 hours, or more than 50% of the circulating blood volume in 3 hours or less, or 10 RBC units in adults.[153] A number of complications may occur: (1) coagulopathy and dilutional thrombocytopenia, which may trigger bleeding; (2) hypothermia due to a rapid infusion of cold blood products, which can lead to arrhythmias, platelet dysfunction, and cardiac dysfunction; (3) citrate toxicity that may trigger hypocalcemia, hypomagnesemia, and metabolic alkalosis; and (4) hyperkalemia.[144] These complications can be avoided by various measures including the use of a blood warmer if the transfusion rate exceeds 50 mL/kg/h, close monitoring of the coagulation profile, platelet transfusion to maintain a count >50,000/uL, plasma administration to attain an INR <1.5 to 2, cryoprecipitate administration to attain a fibrinogen level over 0.1 g/dL, monitoring of hypocalcemia, and calcium supplementation, as required.

Transfusion-Transmitted Infections

In the United States, blood donation is tested at least for the following infectious agents: hepatitis A, B, and C; human immunodeficiency virus (HIV); human T-cell lymphotropic virus (HTLV); West Nile virus (seasonal); and syphilis.[76] These

TABLE 93.4	Transfusion-Transmitted Infectious Diseases in Canada
Infection	**Risk per Units Component[a]**
Human immunodeficiency virus (HIV)[176]	1 in 8 to 12 million
Hepatitis B[176]	1 in 1.1 to 1.7 million
Hepatitis C[176]	1 in 5 to 7 million
Parvovirus B19[176]	1 : 5000 to 1 : 20,000
Cytomegalovirus[176]	Rare
Syphilis[176]	<1 in 100 million
Other infections[b]	Low

[a]Most transfusion-transmitted infections are attributable to red blood cell units. However, there is historical evidence that the following infectious agents can be transmitted by plasma-derived products: HIV, hepatitis B and C, and parvovirus B19 but not cytomegalovirus or parasites.[168]
[b]Many other agents can be transmitted by a transfusion, like West Nile virus, insect-borne zoonoses (for example, malaria,[177] babesiosis,[178] Bartonella quintana[179]), and variant Creutzfeldt-Jakob disease[180]).

tests and better donor selection have resulted in a significant decrease in the risk of transfusion-transmitted infectious diseases. However, there will always be some residual risk, attributable to the *window period* (the time from the beginning of an infection to the time when tests can detect the infection) and to false-negative results. Emerging pathogens can also be a problem.[154] Table 93.4 lists the risks of contracting specific infections with transfusion.

Transfusion-Related Immunomodulation

There is strong evidence that transfusions might generate or enhance both anti- and proinflammatory reactions. Clinically important immune suppression is described in recipients of RBC units. This immune suppression might explain the increased rates of nosocomial infections reported in transfused critically ill patients.[93,155-157]

On the other hand, many proinflammatory molecules are found in plasma-rich blood products, which may initiate, maintain, or enhance an inflammatory process. The WBC and these substances may trigger or maintain a systemic inflammatory response syndrome (SIRS) in the transfusion recipients. Administering a transfusion to a critically ill patient with SIRS may stimulate the patient's inflammatory syndrome and constitute a *second hit,* which can cause additional organ dysfunction, contribute to MODS,[158] and perhaps ultimately result in higher mortality rates.[53,83,159-161] Some clinical data suggest that these risks decrease significantly if the blood product is leukocyte reduced prior to storage.[162] However, in vitro data suggest that some inflammatory mediators are active even in leukocyte-reduced packed RBC units.[163] One pediatric prospective study indicated that the immune response to RBC transfusion was altered according to the storage age of the cells transfused, although in this small study there were no differences in clinical outcomes.[163a] The clinical impact of transfusion on the immunologic responses of critically ill children remains to be determined.

Complications Specific to Plasma Transfusion

Overall the noninfectious and infectious complications associated with FP are similar to those of RBC transfusions, excluding hemolysis. The most notable risks associated with FP transfusion are TRALI. There are antibodies and other biologically active substances in plasma, but hemovigilance data suggest that SD plasma and a male-predominant plasma transfusion strategy are associated with a reduced incidence of TRALI.[164] FP is known to have immunomodulatory properties,[165] which may explain why plasma is associated with an increased risk of complications associated with transfusion-related immunomodulation. Epidemiologic studies have shown that adults and children transfused with plasma are more prone to contract nosocomial infections.[94] Additionally, large volumes of FP transfused can result in TACO. Allergic reactions are also relatively common with FP transfusions (1%–3%).

The risk of transfusion-transmitted viral infections is the same for FP and RBC units. SD plasma has a reduced risk of infection related to enveloped viral pathogens, and SD donors are tested for nonenveloped viruses, but the risk could be higher with regard to emerging nonenveloped viruses.

Complications Specific to Platelet Transfusion

Major allergic reactions and bacterial contamination are the most frequent severe complications associated with platelet transfusion.[166] Serious noninfectious complications of platelet transfusion are similar to those reported with plasma and RBC with the exception of hemolytic transfusion reactions. Rarely, hemolytic transfusion reactions can be seen after the transfusion of non-ABO identical platelets, which contain anti-A or anti-B antibodies. Platelet transfusion may also be associated with specific adverse effects including platelet refractoriness due to HLA alloimmunization. Prestorage leukocyte-reduced platelet products are available in most North American blood banks, which significantly decreases the risk of HLA alloimmunization and platelet refractoriness, nonhemolytic febrile reactions, and CMV transmission.

The most important infectious complication associated with platelet transfusion is bacterial infection. As platelet concentrates are stored at room temperature, the incidence of bacterially contaminated platelet products is higher than with RBCs. The risk of bacterial infection can be significantly reduced, but not eliminated, by bacterial testing (eg, routine culture). Pathogens can also be inactivated by different methods using ultraviolet light.[167] The risk of other transfusion-transmitted infections is similar for platelets and other blood components.

Treatment of Transfusion Reactions

Patients should be monitored closely while receiving a transfusion. Vital signs should be taken before transfusion as well as within the first 15 minutes and every hour up to 4 hours after transfusion. The following symptoms and signs suggest that an acute blood reaction has occurred: fever, shivering (rigors), pain, anxiety, agitation, dyspnea, hypotension, hypertension, hemorrhage, shock, and hemoglobinuria (pink or red urine).

If a transfusion reaction is suspected, the transfusion must be stopped immediately, an intravenous access with NaCl 0.9% must be maintained, all measures to ensure patient stability must be undertaken, verification that the patient received the correct unit must be ascertained, a visual inspection of the unit must be conducted and described in the patient hospital chart, clinical data on the event must be detailed in the hospital chart, and the patient should be monitored for at least a few hours. In many centers, the unit that was being transfused, the filter and the tubing being used, and the remaining blood product are returned to the blood bank. A workup must be done to assess for infection as well as to measure antibodies, antigens, free Hb, and sometimes other markers of metabolic disturbance (acidosis, hyperkalemia, hypocalcemia, etc.). All possible transfusion reactions must be reported to the appropriate blood agency or hemovigilance system, which is the blood blank in many hospitals.

Conclusion

A transfusion can save a life but can also cause significant problems. The risk of death attributable to transfusion of a labile blood product is low: Only 1 death over 2,845,459 blood component units was reported in the United Kingdom in 2008.[4] However, serious reactions and severe complications can happen. A transfusion is a serious matter: It should be prescribed only if deemed necessary. Closed monitoring of the recipient is mandatory while a transfusion is given.

Key References

1. Bateman ST, Lacroix J, Boven K, et al. Anemia, blood loss and blood transfusion in North American children in the intensive care unit. *Am J Respir Crit Care Med*. 2008;178:26-33.
5. Bolton-Maggs PHB, Poles D, Watt A, Thomas D, on behalf of the Serious Hazards of Transfusion (SHOT) Steering Group. *The 2013 Annual SHOT Report*. London: Serious Hazards of Transfusion; 2014.
6. Lacroix J, Hébert PC, Hutchison JH, et al. Transfusion strategies for patients in pediatric intensive care units. *N Engl J Med*. 2007;356:1609-1619.
13. Doctor A, Stamler JS. Nitric oxide transport in blood: a third gas in the respiratory cycle. *Compr Physiol*. 2011;1:611-638.
21. Carson JL, Noveck H, Berlin JA, Gould SA. Mortality and morbidity in patients with very low postoperative Hb levels who decline blood transfusion. *Transfusion*. 2002;42:812-818.
26. English M, Ahmed M, Ngando C, et al. Blood transfusion for severe anaemia in children in a Kenyan hospital. *Lancet*. 2002;359:494-495.
38. Holst LB, Haase N, Wetterslev J, et al. Lower versus higher hemoglobin threshold for transfusion in septic shock. *N Engl J Med*. 2014;371:1381-1391.
39. Gibson BE, Todd A, Roberts I, et al. Transfusion guidelines for neonates and older children. *Br J Haematol*. 2004;124:433-453.
46. Lacroix J, Tucci M, Du Pont-Thibodeau G. Red blood cell transfusion decision making in critically ill children. *Curr Opin Pediatr*. 2015;27:286-291.
49. Riddington C, Wang W, eds. *Blood Transfusion for Preventing Stroke in People With Sickle Cell Disease (Cochrane Review)*. The Cochrane Library; Oxford: Update Software; 2002.
53. Du Pont-Thibodeau G, Harrington K, Lacroix J. Anemia and red blood cell transfusion in critically ill cardiac patients. *Ann Intensive Care*. 2014;4:16.
85. Lacroix J, Hébert PC, Fergusson DA, et al. Age of transfused blood in critically ill adults. *N Engl J Med*. 2015;372:1410-1418.
86. Steiner ME, Ness PM, Assmann SF, et al. Effects of red-cell storage duration on patients undergoing cardiac surgery. *N Engl J Med*. 2015;372:1419-1429.
105. Stanworth SJ, Estcourt LJ, Powter G, et al. A no-prophylaxis platelet-transfusion strategy for hematologic cancers. *N Engl J Med*. 2013;368:1771-1780.
112. Stainsby D, Jones H, Wells AW, et al.; on behalf of the SHOT Steering Group. Adverse outcomes of blood donation in children: analysis of UK reports to the serious hazards of transfusion scheme 1996-2005. *Br J Haematol*. 2008;141:73-79.
172. Popovsky MA. *Transfusion Reactions*. 2nd ed. Bethesda: AABB Press; 2001.
176. MacDonald NE, O'Brien SF, Delage G, Canadian Paediatric Society, Infectious Diseases and Immunization Committee. Transfusion and risk of infection in Canada: update 2012. *Paediatr Child Health*. 2012;17:e102-e111.

Hematology and Oncology Problems in the Intensive Care Unit

Jesse Wenger, Rebecca Gardner, and Joan S. Roberts

PEARLS

- Proactive treatment measures for tumor lysis syndrome include hydration with hypotonic or isotonic saline solution, alkalinization, use of allopurinol or urate oxidase, avoidance of exogenous potassium, close monitoring of fluid status, and frequent monitoring of serum potassium, sodium, chloride, bicarbonate, calcium, phosphorus, uric acid, blood urea nitrogen, and creatinine concentrations.
- Clinically significant hyperleukocytosis occurs with a white blood cell count greater than 200,000/μL in acute myeloid leukemia and greater than 300,000/μL in acute lymphocytic leukemia.
- Concurrent thrombocytopenia and hyperleukocytosis increase risk of adverse outcomes including intracranial hemorrhage and death. Aggressive therapy to correct coagulopathy with fresh-frozen plasma and vitamin K and to maintain platelet count greater than 20,000/μL is critical.
- Oxygen consumption may become delivery dependent when the hemoglobin concentration falls below 5 g/dL.
- Signs of significant cardiovascular compromise may not become evident until the child has acutely lost at least 25% of total blood volume.
- In the absence of other hemorrhagic risks, platelet counts 10,000/μL and greater are associated with little risk of serious bleeding.
- Gastrointestinal bleeding is an important cause of morbidity and mortality in patients with end-stage renal disease.
- Intravenous administration of desmopressin acetate at a dosage of 0.3 μg/kg over 30 minutes improves platelet dysfunction caused by uremia within 1 hour, and the effect is maintained for 4 to 8 hours.
- Childhood mediastinal masses produce few symptoms until they have occluded a substantial portion of the cross-sectional area of the trachea or main stem bronchi or the superior vena cava. Diagnosis should be established with the least invasive means available, because these patients are at significant risk for anesthetic complications.
- Spinal cord compression most frequently occurs as metastatic disease and requires emergent treatment with 1 mg/kg of dexamethasone over 30 minutes.
- Hemophagocytic lymphohistiocytosis (HLH) produces severe illnesses that may be confused with other forms of systemic inflammatory response syndrome, such as sepsis. Appropriate diagnosis is tantamount as untreated HLH is almost always fatal.

Hematologic Emergencies

Anemia

Anemia results from a deficiency in the oxygen-carrying capacity of the blood. The deficit may be in the number of red blood cells (RBCs), the RBC hemoglobin concentration, or both. Because hemoglobin serves as the primary transport molecule for oxygen, anemia may affect the delivery of oxygen (O_2) to the tissues with wide-ranging potential complications (see also Chapters 89 and 93).

Under steady-state conditions, oxygen consumption remains constant and is independent of oxygen delivery until it falls below a critical level, which varies for each organ system. When the hemoglobin concentration decreases to approximately 5 g/dL or less, oxygen delivery and consumption may be altered. Below this level, O_2 consumption becomes delivery dependent.

The body responds to acute, normovolemic anemia by increasing cardiac output, through increases in stroke volume, heart rate, or both. As the hematocrit falls, blood viscosity diminishes, thus increasing venous return and augmenting preload. In the patient with chronic anemia, increases in cardiac output are supplemented by increased levels of 2,3-diphosphoglycerate shifting the oxyhemoglobin curve to the right and augmenting O_2 delivery at the tissue level.

Anemias generally are classified either by the mechanism resulting in the hemoglobin deficit—decreased production, accelerated destruction, or loss of erythrocytes—or by the morphologic appearance of the erythrocyte (Box 94.1).[1]

Morphologic classifications of anemia are based on either erythrocyte size, as defined by mean corpuscular volume and mean corpuscular hemoglobin concentration, or abnormalities in the erythrocyte shape (Box 94.2).[1] The normal values for mean corpuscular volume and mean corpuscular hemoglobin concentration vary with the child's age. A wide variety of conditions, some intrinsic to the erythrocyte and others related to extrinsic factors, may result in abnormal RBC morphology. The more common causes of profound anemia encountered in the pediatric intensive care setting are reviewed here.

Hemorrhagic Anemia

Bleeding may be either acute or chronic. Chronic bleeding generally causes anemia through depletion of iron stores. In response, patients adopt mechanisms to increase O_2 delivery and to avoid hypovolemia, permitting them to tolerate hemoglobin levels well below the normal range, with mild clinical

BOX 94.1   Physiologic Classification of Anemia

A. Disorders of Red Cell Production in Which the Rate of Red Cell Production Is Less Than Expected for the Degree of Anemia
1. Marrow failure
   a. Aplastic anemia
      (i) Congenital
      (ii) Acquired
   b. Pure red cell aplasia
      (i) Congenital
      (ii) Diamond-Blackfan syndrome
      (iii) Aase syndrome
      (iv) Acquired
      (v) Transient erythroblastopenia of childhood
      (vi) Other
   c. Marrow replacement
      (i) Malignancies
      (ii) Osteopetrosis
      (iii) Myelofibrosis
      (iv) Chronic renal disease
      (v) Vitamin D deficiency
   d. Pancreatic insufficiency–marrow hypoplasia syndrome
2. Impaired erythropoietin production
   a. Chronic renal disease
   b. Hypothyroidism, hypopituitarism
   c. Chronic inflammation
   d. Protein malnutrition
   e. Hemoglobin mutants with decreased affinity for oxygen

B. Disorders of Erythroid Maturation and Ineffective Erythropoiesis
1. Abnormalities of cytoplasmic maturation
   a. Iron deficiency
   b. Thalassemia syndromes
   c. Sideroblastic anemias
   d. Lead poisoning
2. Abnormalities of nuclear maturation
   a. Vitamin B_{12}; deficiency
   b. Folic acid deficiency
   c. Thiamine-responsive megaloblastic anemia
   d. Hereditary abnormalities in folate metabolism
   e. Orotic aciduria
3. Primary dyserythropoietic anemias (types I, II, II, IV)
4. Erythropoietic protoporphyria
5. Refractory sideroblastic anemia with vacuolization of marrow precursors and pancreatic dysfunction deficiency

C. Hemolytic Anemias
1. Defects of hemoglobin
   a. Structured mutants
   b. Synthetic mutants (thalassemia syndromes)
2. Defects of the red cell membrane
3. Defects of red cell metabolism
4. Antibody mediated
5. Mechanical injury to the erythrocyte
6. Thermal injury to the erythrocyte
7. Oxidant-induced red cell injury
8. Infectious agent-induced red cell injury
9. Paroxysmal nocturnal hemoglobinuria
10. Plasma lipid-induced abnormalities of the red cell membrane

BOX 94.2   Classification of Anemias Based on Red Cell Size

A. Microcytic Anemias
1. Iron deficiency (nutritional, chronic blood loss)
2. Chronic lead poisoning
3. Thalassemia syndromes
4. Sideroblastic anemias
5. Chronic inflammation
6. Some congenital hemolytic anemias with unstable hemoglobin

B. Macrocytic Anemias
1. With megaloblastic bone marrow
   a. Vitamin B_{12} deficiency
   b. Folic acid deficiency
   c. Hereditary orotic aciduria
   d. Thiamine-responsive anemia
2. Without megaloblastic bone marrow
   a. Aplastic anemia
   b. Diamond-Blackfan syndrome
   c. Hypothyroidism
   d. Liver disease
   e. Bone marrow infiltration
   f. Dyserythropoietic anemias

C. Normocytic Anemias
1. Congenital hemolytic anemias
   a. Hemoglobin mutants
   b. Red cell enzyme defects
   c. Disorders of the red cell membrane
2. Acquired hemolytic anemias
   a. Antibody mediated
   b. Microangiopathic hemolytic anemias
   c. Secondary to acute infections
3. Acute blood loss
4. Splenic pooling
5. Chronic renal disease (usually)

maintaining ventilation, and initiating volume replacement via an adequate intravenous catheter.

RBC transfusion should be given if O_2 delivery to the end organ is impaired. Either whole blood or packed RBCs can be used, but the former has many difficulties related to storage and transport (see also Chapter 93). If packed RBCs or plasma-poor red cells are used to correct O_2-carrying capacity during massive blood loss, deficits of coagulation factors develop earlier than during transfusion of whole blood. Hypofibrinogenemia generally develops first, followed by deficits in other clotting factors and later by thrombocytopenia. Fresh-frozen plasma should be used to treat coagulopathy that develops during replacement of massive blood loss with packed RBCs. Other clinical abnormalities associated with replacement of large volumes of RBCs include hyperkalemia, hypocalcemia, and transfusion reactions. Transfusion of platelets should be guided by serial platelet counts. Central venous pressure should be monitored to allow for rapid administration of RBCs and volume replacement while decreasing the risks of hypervolemia. Blood and other fluids may be administered rapidly until central venous pressure rises to 6 to 7 mm Hg.

Anemia Secondary to Bone Marrow Failure

Several hematologic diseases are associated with diminished blood cell production. Acquired aplastic anemia, characterized by pancytopenia and hypocellular or acellular bone marrow, is defined by at least two of the three following: granulocytes less than 500/µL, platelets less than 20,000/µL,

findings. Signs and symptoms of acute hemorrhage result from poor end-organ perfusion, with consequent diminished O_2 delivery. Diagnosis of the presence and degree of blood loss may be difficult in an otherwise healthy child. Signs of impending shock, such as pallor, anxiety, and tachypnea, may be subtle. Signs of significant cardiovascular compromise may not become evident until the child has lost at least 25% of total blood volume when patients usually manifest age-related systolic hypotension.[2] Initial management should include achieving hemostasis, establishing a secure airway, and anemia with a corrected reticulocyte count less than 1%, in conjunction with markedly hypocellular bone marrow.[3] The majority of cases have no definable cause but the pathophysiology appears immune mediated with destruction of blood-forming cells by lymphocytes. Excessive production of interferon-γ, tumor necrosis factor, and interleukin-2 has been noted. Altered immunity results in CD34 cell death and in intracellular pathways leading to cell cycle arrest.[4] Cases may follow chemical or drug exposure, as well as a posthepatitis aplastic anemia typically seen in young males, with pancytopenia presenting several weeks after severe liver inflammation. Acquired aplastic anemia can be distinguished from bone marrow failure resulting from Fanconi anemia by specific assays, called *chromosomal breakage studies*, that quantify chromosomal susceptibility to chemical cross-linking agents that characterize Fanconi anemia.[5] Cytogenetic studies usually are normal in aplastic anemia, whereas aneuploidy or structural abnormalities are relatively common in myelodysplasia. Myelodysplasia may evolve in patients treated for aplastic anemia. Some patients with paroxysmal nocturnal hemoglobinuria develop bone marrow failure; conversely, paroxysmal nocturnal hemoglobinuria may evolve years after aplastic anemia is diagnosed.

Irrespective of the etiology of bone marrow failure, life-threatening complications may arise from blood cytopenias. The most common causes of death are bacterial sepsis and fungal infection secondary to refractory granulocytopenia. Broad-spectrum antibiotics should be used to treat suspected infection in the granulocytopenic patient. Historically, gram-negative organisms were the most frequent cause of fulminant infection in this patient population. With the increased use of central venous catheters, gram-positive organisms now predominate.[6] Antifungal therapy should be instituted in patients who fail to defervesce within 3 to 5 days of treatment with antibiotics. Persistent, unexplained fever requires thorough evaluation to look for evidence of invasive fungal infection.

Platelet transfusions should be used judiciously in an effort to avoid alloimmunization to platelet antigens and are generally reserved for episodes of active bleeding. Similarly, RBC transfusions should be reserved for patients whose oxygen delivery may be compromised as a result of profound anemia. The patient should not receive blood products donated by family members to avoid sensitization to leukocyte and platelet antigens of potential bone marrow donors. All blood products should be irradiated and leukodepleted to decrease the risk of graft-versus-host disease, with preference given to single-donor apheresis units. Treatment of severe acquired aplastic anemia involves either the use of immunosuppressive therapy or replacement of bone marrow through stem cell transplantation. The treatment of choice, bone marrow or peripheral blood stem cell transplantation from a histocompatible sibling, produces long-term survival rates of 75% to 80%.[7] Unfortunately, up to 70% of patients may lack a suitably matched sibling donor. Stem cells harvested from a matched unrelated donor, or umbilical cord blood, produce poorer outcomes because of the higher rate of graft-versus-host disease. For these patients, immunomodulation, which usually includes a combination of antithymocyte globulin and cyclosporin, often with use of hematopoietic growth factors, has resulted in response rates of 70% to 80%.[8] Not all responders achieve a complete remission. Late relapses, as well as evolution to myelodysplasia and leukemia, are reported.

Hemolytic Anemia

Hemolysis, the destruction of RBCs with liberation of hemoglobin, may occur within either the blood vessels (intravascular hemolysis) or the reticuloendothelial system (extravascular hemolysis). Anemia results when the rate of RBC destruction exceeds new RBC production in the bone marrow. Laboratory findings in patients with hemolytic anemia usually include increased reticulocyte count and elevated serum concentrations of unconjugated bilirubin and lactate dehydrogenase. Intravascular hemolysis usually results in decreased serum haptoglobin concentrations.

Premature destruction of RBCs may result from intrinsic RBC abnormalities, such as hemoglobinopathies, from red cell membrane defects, or from a variety of extrinsic factors (Fig. 94.1).[1] Numerous hemoglobin variants resulting in shortened RBC survival have been identified. Individuals with sickling hemoglobinopathies may suffer a variety of complications that require treatment in an ICU (see Chapter 90). Abnormalities in the structure of the RBC membrane, as in hereditary spherocytosis, or decreased quantities of RBC enzymes, as in G6PD deficiency, also decrease red cell survival. Hemolysis in these settings occurs primarily extravascularly. Mechanical disruption of the red cell membrane secondary to factors extrinsic to the RBC may lead to macroangiopathic hemolytic anemia, as with turbulent flow around a prosthetic heart valve, or microangiopathic hemolytic anemia, caused by fibrin deposition in the microvasculature. The latter process is seen in consumptive disorders, including disseminated intravascular coagulation (DIC), hemolytic uremic syndrome, and thrombotic thrombocytopenic purpura.[9] In these entities, hemolysis is primarily intravascular, with characteristic schistocytes seen on the blood smear.

The hemolytic processes that result from abnormal interactions between erythrocytes and the immune system are known collectively as *autoimmune hemolytic anemia* (AIHA).[1] AIHA can be classified as either primary, in which there is no identifiable systemic illness except possibly a history of a recent viral-like illness, or secondary, in which the hemolytic anemia is present in the context of another illness. AIHA has been reported as a manifestation of autoimmune disorders (eg, lupus erythematosus), immunodeficiency disorders, malignancies, specific infections, or as a drug reaction (Box 94.3).[9] AIHA also may be classified by the thermal sensitivity of the autoantibodies. The most common form is the result of warm-reactive immunoglobulin (Ig) G

BOX 94.3 **Classification of Autoimmune Hemolytic Anemia in Children**

A. Primary AIHA
1. Warm-reactive autoantibodies, usually IgG
2. Paroxysmal cold hemoglobinuria, usually IgG
3. Cold-agglutinin disease, usually IgM

B. Secondary AIHA
1. Systemic autoimmune disease (eg, lupus)
2. Malignancy (Hodgkin and non-Hodgkin lymphoma)
3. Immunodeficiency
4. Infection (*Mycoplasma*, viruses)
5. Drug induced

autoantibodies directed against RBC membrane proteins. Extravascular hemolysis occurs, with sensitized erythrocytes cleared primarily in the spleen. Cold-agglutinin disease, the second most common form of AIHA, most frequently occurs with *Mycoplasma pneumoniae* infections, but it also is associated with other infectious agents, including Epstein-Barr virus, cytomegalovirus, and mumps virus. In this disorder, IgM autoantibody binds to the RBC and fixes complement. The erythrocytes may undergo intravascular hemolysis, or they may be cleared by the reticuloendothelial system, primarily in the liver. Paroxysmal cold hemoglobinuria is a rare variant of AIHA that usually occurs following a viral illness and in which an IgG autoantibody binds at cold temperature to the P-antigen of the erythrocyte, fixing complement (the Donath-Landsteiner antibody) and producing intravascular hemolysis. Although drug-induced autoantibodies occur uncommonly in children, they may follow exposure to some antibiotics, including penicillins and cephalosporins. Mechanisms of drug-induced hemolysis may include autoantibody formation and adsorption of the drug onto the red cell membrane, with immune complex formation with IgG or IgM.

Patients with AIHA usually present with pallor, jaundice, and splenomegaly on physical examination. The reticulocyte count is generally elevated, although initially it may be low or normal. The direct antiglobulin test (Coombs test) demonstrates the presence of antibodies or complement on the red cells. The indirect antiglobulin test measures the presence of unbound antierythrocyte antibodies in the patient's serum.

Therapy depends on the type of AIHA and the severity of clinical symptoms. Profound anemia, usually with a hemoglobin level of less than 5 g/dL, may result in cardiovascular compromise and requires erythrocyte transfusion to increase O_2-carrying capacity. The presence of autoantibodies often makes cross-matching blood difficult, and the patient may require transfusion with "least incompatible" blood. Significant hemolytic transfusion reactions are infrequent. However, severe hemolysis occurs on rare occasions, with hemoglobinemia and hemoglobinuria resulting in renal failure. Therefore transfusions should be started at a slow rate, and both plasma and urine samples should be checked regularly for free hemoglobin. Patients with cold-reactive antibodies should be kept warm, and a blood warmer should be used for the transfused blood. Even in the absence of transfusion, significant intravascular hemolysis may occur in patients with cold-reactive antibodies. Maintaining good renal blood flow and careful monitoring of urine output in this setting may help obviate renal injury. Corticosteroids appear to slow the hemolytic process, particularly in patients with IgG autoantibodies, in whom this drug class appears to inhibit Fc receptor-mediated clearance of sensitized erythrocytes. The usual dosage is 1 to 2 mg/kg methylprednisolone administered intravenously every 6 hours until the patient is clinically stable. The patient then can be switched to oral prednisone (2 mg/kg/day for 2 to 4 weeks, followed by a slow taper over 1 to 3 months).

Corticosteroids may also be effective in cold agglutinin disease, although the response is less predictable. High-dose intravenous γ-globulin (IVIG, 1 g/kg/day for 5 days) produces response in approximately one-third of patients with warm-reactive disease. Plasmapheresis and plasma exchange may be beneficial, particularly in patients with IgM autoantibodies. The overall prognosis for children with AIHA is good.

Cold-reactive AIHA generally resolves completely. Some patients with warm-reactive antibodies have a chronic course, marked by remissions and exacerbations.

Thrombocytopenia

Thrombocytopenia may be secondary to either decreased platelet production or increased platelet destruction. Decreased platelet production may result from primary bone marrow failure states or from bone marrow infiltration by malignant cells as in leukemia, lymphoma, and metastatic solid tumors. Bone marrow suppression, a common side effect of antineoplastic therapy including both chemotherapy and radiotherapy, frequently leads to periods of thrombocytopenia. Thrombocytopenia or platelet dysfunction may result in bleeding, usually involving the skin and mucous membranes. Clinical manifestations include petechiae and purpura, epistaxis, gastrointestinal bleeding, hematuria, and menorrhagia. Intracranial hemorrhage is an infrequent manifestation of thrombocytopenia.

Indications for platelet transfusion in these settings vary with the underlying cause of thrombocytopenia and the patient's clinical status. Patients with primary bone marrow failure, who likely will experience prolonged thrombocytopenia, generally receive transfusions only for active bleeding because of the risk of alloimmunization. In addition, exposure to multiple platelet donors may jeopardize the success of bone marrow transplantation by increasing the risk of graft rejection. The threshold for transfusion may need to be higher in patients with sepsis, decreased humoral coagulants, or other risk factors. In the perioperative setting, platelet counts should be maintained at higher than 50,000/dL and greater than 100,000/dL for neurologic or ophthalmologic surgery. Use of ABO-compatible donors and leukoreduction diminishes the risk of platelet alloimmunization. Single-donor apheresis units reduce donor exposure compared with pooled platelet concentrates, but whether such usage reduces the incidence of platelet alloimmunization remains unclear.

Immune Thrombocytopenia

Immune platelet destruction may be caused by autoantibodies, drug-dependent antibodies, or alloantibodies. Alloantibodies result from exposure to polymorphic epitopes expressed on foreign platelets to which the patient has been exposed (see the previous section). Drug-induced thrombocytopenia may be suggested by the patient's medication history. Laboratory tests for specific drug-associated antiplatelet antibodies are available.

In immune thrombocytopenia purpura (ITP), autoantibodies to platelets may be associated with other autoimmune disorders, immune deficiency states, or after viral illness or immunization. The incidence of childhood ITP was found to range from 5 to 7 per 100,000 per year, with 25% of the children subsequently developing chronic ITP.[10] Frequently no predisposing condition is identified (idiopathic thrombocytopenia purpura). Regardless of cause, the reticuloendothelial system removes antibody-coated platelets, with the bulk of the destruction occurring in the spleen. These children typically present with petechiae, purpura, bleeding from mucous membranes, and isolated thrombocytopenia. The bone marrow responds with increased platelet production. The rapid turnover in platelets results in younger, somewhat larger platelets entering the blood. Hence, serious bleeding rarely occurs because of the increased effectiveness of platelets. Low admission mean platelet volume value (<8 μL) and a history of viral prodrome have been found to be independent prognostic variables that predicted durable remission.

The primary goal of therapy in children with ITP is to limit bleeding, especially from the central nervous system. Therapy does not appear to affect the natural history of the illness. There is no consensus regarding the management of acute ITP, and the need for intervention in the absence of significant hemorrhage remains the subject of debate. Intracranial hemorrhage remains rare, and there are no data that treatment actually reduces the incidence of intracranial hemorrhage. Therapy is directed at slowing clearance of sensitized thrombocytes in the spleen and reducing antibody production. Initial medical management usually involves the use of corticosteroids (methylprednisolone 30 mg/kg/dose × 3 doses) or IVIG (1 g/kg/dose × 2) resulting in increased platelet counts within 48 hours.[11] Meta-analysis of randomized controlled trials (RCTs) comparing high-dose to low-dose IVIG showed no difference in outcomes, with significantly reduced risk of side effects with low-dose IVIG (total dose less than 2 g/kg).[12] Bone marrow evaluation to rule out malignancy before corticosteroid therapy should occur. Infusion of anti-Rh(D) immunoglobulin (50 to 75 μg/kg) for individuals who have Rh(D)-positive RBCs prolongs survival of antibody-coated platelets in patients with ITP but should be avoided in patients who present with anemia. As with IVIG, the major mechanism appears to include blockage of Fc receptors on reticuloendothelial cells. Use of these agents usually halts bleeding and raises platelet counts to safe levels within a few days, although evidence indicating their influence on the course of the disease remains lacking.

Intracranial hemorrhage, a devastating but rare complication of ITP, requires immediate intervention. Consequently, patients presenting with headaches, persistent vomiting, or neurologic symptoms require an emergent computed tomography (CT) scan of the head. Therapy for intracranial hemorrhage usually includes IVIG, corticosteroids, and emergency splenectomy.[13] Platelet transfusions in ITP rarely result in an increase in the platelet count because of rapid consumption of transfused platelets. Nevertheless, intermittent (2 to 4 IU/m² every 6 to 8 hours) or continuous (0.5 to 1 IU/m²/hr) platelet transfusions have been administered for life-threatening hemorrhage, with decreases in bleeding reported. Plasmapheresis may be beneficial in patients who do not respond to these interventions. A splenectomy should be performed if a craniotomy is required, to maximize the perioperative platelet count.[14]

Nonimmune Thrombocytopenia

DIC occurs when generalized activation of the plasma coagulation pathways occurs within small blood vessels with formation of fibrin and depletion of circulating levels of clotting factors and platelets. DIC usually follows a systemic insult, most often sepsis or shock. Treatment should be directed to the underlying cause. Hemorrhage frequently occurs at platelet counts greater than 10,000/μL because of concomitant depletion of clotting factors. Control of bleeding may necessitate platelet and plasma transfusions. DIC had been thought to be the etiology of much of the multiorgan system failure in ICU patients, with formation of a large number of microthrombotic foci leading to organ microcirculation failure and subsequent failure of the organ itself (see Chapter 112). More recently, some studies have suggested that vascular endothelial damage induced by humoral mediators is the primary cause of thrombocytopenic multiorgan system failure. In these instances, thrombocytopenia may be a marker of poor prognosis rather than a cause of ICU mortality.

Increased platelet consumption with resultant thrombocytopenia occurs in diseases associated with extensive vascular endothelial damage, including hemolytic uremic syndrome and thrombotic thrombocytopenic purpura. Aggregates of activated platelets become trapped in small blood vessels, causing a microangiopathic hemolytic anemia. Schistocytes usually are present on the peripheral blood smear. Platelet transfusions should be given only for life-threatening bleeding because they may worsen the thrombotic process.[15]

Thrombocytopenia caused by splenic sequestration develops in individuals with massive splenomegaly. The etiology of splenomegaly includes infectious, infiltrative, neoplastic, obstructive, and hemolytic causes. The Kasabach-Merritt syndrome is an association of a giant hemangioma with localized intravascular coagulation causing thrombocytopenia and hypofibrinogenemia. Rare congenital thrombocytopenic syndromes include congenital amegakaryocytic thrombocytopenia, thrombocytopenia-absent radius, and Wiskott-Aldrich syndrome.

Bleeding in Uremia

Hemorrhagic manifestations in patients with renal failure are characterized by purpura and bleeding from mucous membranes and puncture sites. Gastrointestinal bleeding may contribute to morbidity and mortality in patients with end-stage renal disease. Concurrent hypertension increases the risk of subdural hematoma. The hemostatic defect in uremia is multifactorial, resulting in part from altered metabolism of platelets and vascular endothelial cells and from abnormal interactions between platelets and vascular endothelium.[16]

When uremia is present, clinical bleeding may be increased relative to the degree of thrombocytopenia resulting from secondary platelet dysfunction. Intravenous administration of desmopressin acetate (0.3 μg/kg over 30 minutes) improves platelet dysfunction caused by uremia within 1 hour with an effect for 4 to 8 hours.[17] Tachyphylaxis may occur after two to three doses. Intravenous or transdermal conjugated estrogens or oral estrogens cause slower but more sustained improvements in bleeding time.[18] Dialysis improves platelet function through reduction of azotemia.

When severe anemia is present, platelets travel closer to the blood midstream and are less likely to interact with the vascular endothelium. In addition, RBCs exert metabolic effects on platelets by enhancing adenosine diphosphate and thromboxane A2 release. Therefore use of red cell transfusions or erythropoietin to increase the hematocrit to 30% helps to correct the bleeding time.[19] Further increase in hematocrit increases the risk of thrombosis, particularly of arteriovenous shunts and the extracorporeal hemodialysis circuit.

Oncologic Emergencies
Tumor Lysis Syndrome

Tumor lysis syndrome (TLS) results from the death of tumor cells resulting in the rapid extravasation of intracellular contents into the blood.[20] The release of intracellular contents may cause metabolic derangements and produce end-organ damage. Careful monitoring and rigorous attention to organ function may help to obviate the majority of complications from this syndrome. Although the lysis of malignant cells usually begins after the institution of chemotherapy, spontaneous TLS can occur.[21] Important considerations in TLS include the level of tumor burden and the sensitivity of the cells to the antitumor agents.[22] In children, hematologic malignancies such as acute lymphoblastic leukemia (ALL), acute myelogenous leukemia (AML), and Burkitt lymphoma account for the majority of cases of TLS.[23] TLS usually occurs with new-onset disease, preexisting renal dysfunction, in the setting of nephrotoxic drugs, and with dehydration. Conventionally, the diagnosis of TLS requires some combination of hyperkalemia, hyperphosphatemia, hyperuricemia, and hypocalcemia in the face of a tumor; however, no definitive classification or grading system exists. Although some differentiate between laboratory and clinical TLS, the value of published classifications has not been established.

On cell lysis, tumor cells release normal or supranormal quantities of many intracellular contents that pour into the circulation on cell death including potassium, nucleic acids, inorganic phosphates, and proteins.[20] The metabolism of nucleic acids results in the production of uric acid. With high tumor burden and highly effective chemotherapy, a massive release of these chemicals may overwhelm normal homeostatic mechanisms, threatening the patient with hyperkalemia, hyperphosphatemia, hyperuricemia, hypocalcemia, and end-organ damage.

Hyperkalemia can acutely threaten cardiovascular status by altering cardiac rhythm. Levels of potassium greater than 6.5 to 7 mmol/L may lead to widening of the QRS complex and peaked T waves that can progress to disorganized ventricular rhythms and severe cardiac dysfunction. Other symptoms include irritability, fatigue, muscle weakness and cramps, paresthesias, nausea, emesis, and diarrhea. Hyperkalemia must be addressed emergently.

Phosphate released during TLS avidly binds to calcium, depleting serum calcium levels. The resultant calcium phosphate may precipitate in the renal tubules, exacerbating renal dysfunction, and producing fatigue, lethargy, weakness, nausea, and emesis. Hypocalcemia may also result in muscle cramps, tetany, seizures, and dysrhythmias. Counterintuitively, low levels of calcium must be addressed by treating the elevated phosphate rather than by administering intravenous calcium.

Uric acid, the final product of purine nucleotide metabolism, is excreted in the urine but has low solubility, especially in acidic urine. Production of uric acid depends on the enzyme xanthine oxidase. Hyperuricemia may injure renal tubules through various mechanisms including deposition of urate crystals in renal tubules causing microobstruction, altering kidney hemodynamics through vasoconstriction, and possible direct toxic effects on the nephron through various mechanisms, especially in the context of dehydration and administration of nephrotoxic medications.[24,25] Increasing serum uric acid levels have been associated with increasing risk for TLS.

Uremia may also occur in patients at risk for TLS either from TLS itself, from preexisting renal injury, or from a combination of these factors. In TLS, the most common cause of renal injury is precipitation of uric acid crystals in the renal

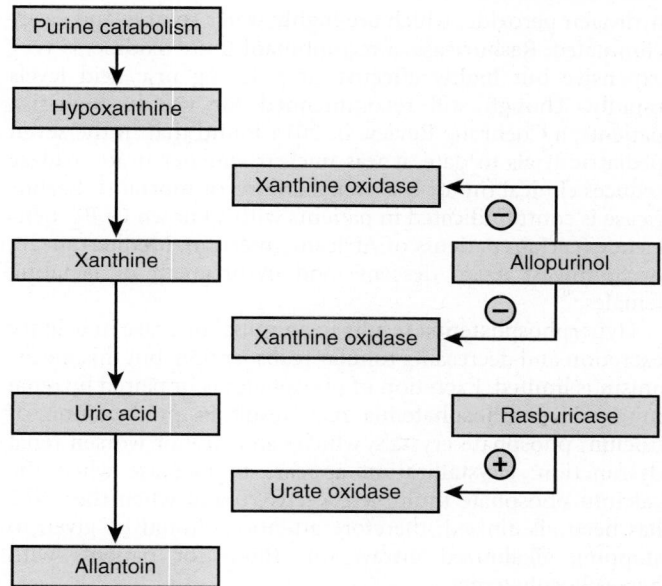

Fig. 94.1. Diagram showing purine degradation and mechanism of action of allopurinol and rasburicase. *CU,* copper; *DIC,* disseminated intravascular coagulation; *G6PD,* glucose 6-phosphate dehydrogenase; *HS,* hereditary spherocytosis; *PK,* pyruvate kinase; *PNH,* paroxysmal nocturnal hemoglobinuria.

tubule, but it can be due to calcium phosphate or xanthine crystals, nephrotoxic drugs, tumor infiltration, or obstruction and infection.[26]

The bedrock of therapy is volume expansion to assure adequate end-organ perfusion and a robust urine flow rate. Sometimes, in order to protect end organs, additional medications are needed to alter uric acid production or to more rapidly bind or eliminate abnormal electrolytes.

Hyperkalemia is a medical emergency, especially when the level exceeds 6.5 to 7 mEq/dL. Therapy includes oral or rectal cation exchange resins, intravenous calcium (gluconate or chloride) to antagonize the action of K^+ on the cardiac myocyte, and sodium bicarbonate to correct acidosis and increase the gradient of K^+ into the cells. Insulin and glucose encourage the movement of K^+ into cells. Diuretic therapy or dialysis may be used to help the excretion of K^+ (see also Chapter 78).

Treatment of hyperuricemia is accomplished by optimizing elimination through alkalization of the urine and decreasing uric acid production through allopurinol or urate oxidase (rasburicase). The solubility of uric acid is highly pH dependent. With an increase in pH from 5 to 7, urine concentrations of uric acid increase from 15 mg/dL to 200 mg/dL.

Allopurinol, a xanthine analogue, inhibits the conversion of xanthine and hypoxanthine to uric acid by competitively blocking the enzyme xanthine oxidase and thus reduces the incidence of obstructive uropathy caused by uric acid.[27,28] Allopurinol cannot, however, lower elevated uric acid levels that may precede therapy, and inhibition of xanthine oxidase may increase the levels of xanthine, which may also produce renal tubular damage.

Hyperuricemia that persists after volume expansion and allopurinol or that is dangerously elevated on presentation requires aggressive therapy. Urate oxidase, a nonhuman lytic enzyme, cleaves uric acid to allantoin, carbon dioxide, and hydrogen peroxide, which are highly water soluble and easily eliminated. Rasburicase, a recombinant urate oxidase, is very expensive but highly effective at reducing uric acid levels rapidly. Though still recommended for use in high-risk patients, a Cochrane Review in 2014 found that in the seven pediatric trials to date, it was unclear whether urate oxidase reduces clinical tumor lysis, renal failure, or mortality. Rasburicase is contraindicated in patients with a known G6PD deficiency (certain patients of African-American, Mediterranean, or Southeast Asian descent) and in pregnant or lactating females.[29]

Hyperphosphatemia results in an initial increase in urinary excretion and decreasing tubular reabsorption, but this mechanism is limited. Excretion of phosphates is impaired by renal injury. Hyperphosphatemia may result in precipitation of calcium phosphate crystals, which can cause or worsen renal dysfunction. Crystallization appears to increase when the calcium phosphate multiple exceeds 70 and when the urine has been alkalinized; therefore attention should be given to stopping alkalinized intravenous fluids for patients with hyperphosphatemia.

Hyperleukocytosis

Hyperleukocytosis, arbitrarily defined as a white blood cell (WBC) count greater than 100,000/μL, is seen in 5% to 20% of children diagnosed with leukemia, most often in patients with ALL.[30] Hyperleukocytosis causing symptomatic leukostasis usually occurs with WBC counts greater than 200,000/μL in AML, greater than 300,000/μL in ALL, and greater than 600,000/μL in chronic myeloid leukemia.[31] Leukostasis seems to happen at lower WBCs in AML because myeloblasts and monoblasts tend to be larger and more rigid than lymphoblasts and granulocytes and are more likely to obstruct vessels.

The viscosity of the blood is dependent on the leukocyte and erythrocyte volumes as well as the deformability of the cells.[32] Substantial increases in WBC counts produce aggregates of leukocytes, which may obstruct small blood vessels. Leukostasis results in local hypoxia, and invasion of the blood vessels by leukemic cells can produce organ and vascular damage or hemorrhage. Leukemic cells' variable expression of adhesion molecules and cytokines, such as interleukin-1 and tumor necrosis factor-alpha, may explain the variability of WBC and clinical presentation of patients with leukostasis.[30]

Children with hyperleukocytosis have higher rates of morbidity and mortality than other children with leukemia. Children with AML and hyperleukocytosis have a higher risk of early morbidity and mortality than patients with nonhyperleukocytosis AML or ALL and hyperleukocytosis, but the true incidence of these complications is not well elucidated.[33] Based mostly on adult data, there is a 20% to 40% mortality associated with symptomatic leukostasis within the first week of presentation. Hyperleukocytosis most frequently causes neurologic leukostasis, pulmonary leukostasis, and tumor lysis syndrome.

Signs and symptoms of neurologic leukostasis may include headache, altered mental status, visual disturbances, or seizures. The most concerning neurologic complication is an intracranial hemorrhage, which typically is limited to the white matter. The risk for intracerebral hemorrhage can persist even after reduction of the WBC count. Clinicians should consider urgent neuroimaging with any changes in a patient's neurologic status with judicious use of intravenous contrast. Central nervous system hemorrhage with high WBC counts occurs in 5% to 33% of patients with AML and hyperleukocytosis, usually correlating with the degree of hyperleukocytosis.[32]

Respiratory symptoms found with pulmonary leukostasis may include dyspnea, hypoxemia, respiratory failure, and acute respiratory distress syndrome. Arterial measurement of oxygenation should be interpreted with caution because pseudohypoxemia from so-called leukocyte larceny can occur even with samples immediately placed on ice. Pulse oximetry may be a more reliable measure of oxygenation. Chest radiograph findings of pulmonary leukostasis may be normal or reveal diffuse interstitial infiltrates. Immediate cytoreduction is indicated when excessive O_2 metabolism of leukocytes causes tissue hypoxemia. Elevated serum lactate levels have been described as an early sign of microcirculatory failure.[30]

Therapy for hyperleukocytosis has not undergone rigorous analysis. Diuretic therapy and packed red cell transfusion both increase viscosity and are best avoided. Concurrent thrombocytopenia and hyperleukocytosis increase risk of death from bleeding complications. Aggressive therapy with fresh frozen plasma and vitamin K to correct coagulopathy and maintenance of platelet count greater than 20,000/μL are critical.[30] Hydration, alkalinization, and allopurinol have been used in patients with WBC counts higher than 100,000/μL.[31] More aggressive therapies must be considered for symptomatic patients, especially those with laboratory evidence of hypoxia or ischemia, or in certain patients depending on malignancy type and WBC count. Exchange transfusion, leukapheresis, or chemotherapy can be used to rapidly lower WBC. No randomized trials of cytoreduction have been performed, and although a reduced incidence of electrolyte abnormalities has been shown, no improvement in pulmonary status, central nervous system outcome, or mortality has been demonstrated.[34] Complications of leukapheresis include difficulty with vascular access, rapid rebound of WBC count, and the need for anticoagulation. Cytoreduction by leukapheresis, exchange transfusion, or other methods may modulate cell-cycle distribution and nucleoside transporters in leukemic cells by increasing the fraction of the S-phase. No beneficial role has been demonstrated for use of corticosteroids or emergency cranial radiation.[32] Leukapheresis should never be undertaken in a patient with suspected acute promyelocytic leukemia due to hemorrhagic complications.

Spinal Cord Compression

Compression of the spinal cord by malignancy occurs uncommonly but still represents an important cause of morbidity in children, affecting between 2.7% to 5% of children with cancer. Most frequently, compression occurs as metastatic disease spreads rather than as primary spinal cord tumors themselves. Ewing sarcoma, neuroblastoma, and primitive neuroectodermal tumors appear to be the most frequent diagnoses, although compression may be found with lymphoma, nephroblastoma, and germ cell tumors.[35]

Most cord compression results from epidural compression due to extension of paravertebral tumor through the intervertebral foramina or, less commonly, extension of the tumor in the vertebral column. Compression of the vertebral venous plexus by epidural tumor causes vasogenic cord ischemia, edema, venous hemorrhage, and myelin loss.[36] Spinal cord compression usually localizes to the dorsal and lumbosacral regions (42% each). Patients frequently develop back pain, motor dysfunction, sphincter abnormalities, and alteration in sensation. Such findings represent harbingers of potential permanent loss of neurologic function, necessitating emergent evaluation including magnetic resonance imaging.

Confirmation of tumor compression of the spinal cord requires emergent medical action. Treatment requires 1 mg/kg dexamethasone intravenously over 30 minutes and next mandates a decision between immediate surgical decompression, radiation therapy, or chemotherapy. This decision is influenced by a number of factors, including the presence of a histologic diagnosis, likelihood of response to chemotherapy or radiotherapy, as well as degree and rate of progression of neurologic deficit. Although controversy exists, decompressive laminectomy is indicated for tumors without a diagnosis, patients with small cell tumors with rapid neurologic deterioration or complete loss of motor function, and sarcoma, with the exception of osteogenic sarcoma.[35] Laminectomy in children often leads to scoliosis, kyphosis, and anterior subluxation. Consequently, the decision must be made with this issue in mind, as laminectomy patients often require subsequent treatment for orthopedic sequelae of the initial surgery. Among children with complete sensory and motor loss below the level of spinal cord compression, 30% to 60% of treated children experience neurologic recovery.[36]

Acute Airway Compromise in Anterior Mediastinal Tumors

Childhood mediastinal masses pose difficult diagnostic and therapeutic challenges. Such masses often produce few symptoms until they have occluded a substantial portion of the trachea or main stem bronchi or the superior vena cava. Complete airway occlusion in these children represents a potentially fatal complication, a risk that increases at the time of sedation for diagnostic procedures. An estimated 9% to 15% of pediatric patients with anterior mediastinal masses and airway obstruction have been reported to develop life-threatening complications with anesthesia.[37-39] Since the 1990s, increased awareness of the potential for airway or cardiovascular collapse in pediatric patients with anterior mediastinal masses has led to improved management. Major airway complications are now more likely to occur in the postanesthetic period.[40] Superior vena cava syndrome, left atrial compression, and pericardial effusion may lead to a state of fixed cardiac output.

Mediastinal masses are classified by their anatomic compartment, and anterior mediastinal masses represent 46% of all such masses in children.[41] The most common tumors found in the anterior mediastinal compartment include hematologic malignancies: T-cell lymphoblastic leukemia, Hodgkin disease, and T-cell lymphoblastic non-Hodgkin lymphoma.[42,43] Children with an anterior mediastinal mass often present with nonspecific findings including orthopnea, dyspnea, cough, pleural effusion, wheezing, superior vena cava (SVC) syndrome, pain, and stridor.[44] Mediastinal masses are far more common in older children and teenagers than in children younger than 5 years. Barking cough and stridor in an older child or teenager rarely occur with croup and therefore require further investigation.

Important risk factors for airway compromise include computed tomography findings of more than 50% decrease in a cross-sectional area of the trachea, peak expiratory flow less than 50% of predicted value, anterior mediastinal mass, tracheal compression, main stem bronchus compression, larger

median mediastinal mass ratio, lymphoma, vena cava syndrome, pericardial effusion, pleural effusion, history of recurrent chest infections, stridor, orthopnea, cough, wheeze, and shortness of breath.[37,38] The predictive value of these risk factors remains controversial, however. Unfortunately, compression at the level of the carina or bronchi may contribute appreciably to respiratory compromise, even in patients with a cross-sectional area above 50% of predicted.[43] A computed tomography scan will provide evidence of airway compression at a tracheal or bronchial level as well as the existence of exacerbating factors such as pleural effusion that may limit a patient's physiologic reserve.

The preoperative evaluation of patients with critical airway from compression by an anterior mediastinal mass should include an experienced multidisciplinary pediatric team made up of an oncologist, anesthesiologist, interventional radiologist, surgeon, and intensivist. Computed tomography provides the most useful, rapid step in the assessment for airway compromise; unfortunately, severe or rapid progressive symptoms may preclude lying supine for the scan (Fig. 94.2). In such cases, the risks and benefits of performing a diagnostic procedure under local anesthesia with ultrasound guidance, beginning preoperative treatment prior to pathologic diagnosis, or proceeding with general anesthesia need to be discussed by the team and with the family. Empiric treatment is controversial because it can distort the histopathologic appearance and hinder a definitive diagnosis. However, in one study an accurate diagnosis was made in 95% of patients receiving corticosteroids prior to biopsy.[42] Bone marrow or lymph node biopsy and pleural fluid analysis may be helpful in patients who are not unstable. Complete blood count and α-fetoprotein, β-human chorionic gonadotropin, and lactate dehydrogenase levels should be obtained. Image-guided needle biopsy performed under local anesthesia for mediastinal mass or lymph node by a skilled interventional radiologist remains the diagnostic test of choice.[43]

Superior Vena Cava Syndrome

SVC syndrome encompasses the signs and symptoms related to compression or obstruction of the SVC, which in childhood most commonly results from anterior mediastinal mass, middle mediastinal lymph nodes, or occlusion of the SVC itself. SVC obstruction may be accompanied by compression of other mediastinal structures, large airways, pulmonary vessels, and aorta. SVC syndrome is most often caused by lymphoid malignancy, including non-Hodgkin lymphoma, acute lymphocytic leukemia, and Hodgkin disease. In addition to malignancies, indwelling catheters, previous cardiac surgery, previous extracorporeal life support, right-sided congenital diaphragmatic hernia, and ventriculoperitoneal shunts are other causes of SVC syndrome in pediatric patients.

In children, respiratory symptoms usually predominate; air hunger, dyspnea, wheezing, and anxiety occur, particularly with position change. The gradual development of SVC syndrome may manifest with periorbital edema, conjunctival suffusion, facial swelling, dizziness, syncope, and cough. SVC syndrome may occur in conjunction with spinal cord compression (Rubin syndrome), where significant venous obstruction usually develops before the spinal cord compression. Patients with SVC syndrome and back pain should be evaluated with magnetic resonance imaging of the vertebral spine when their condition is stable.

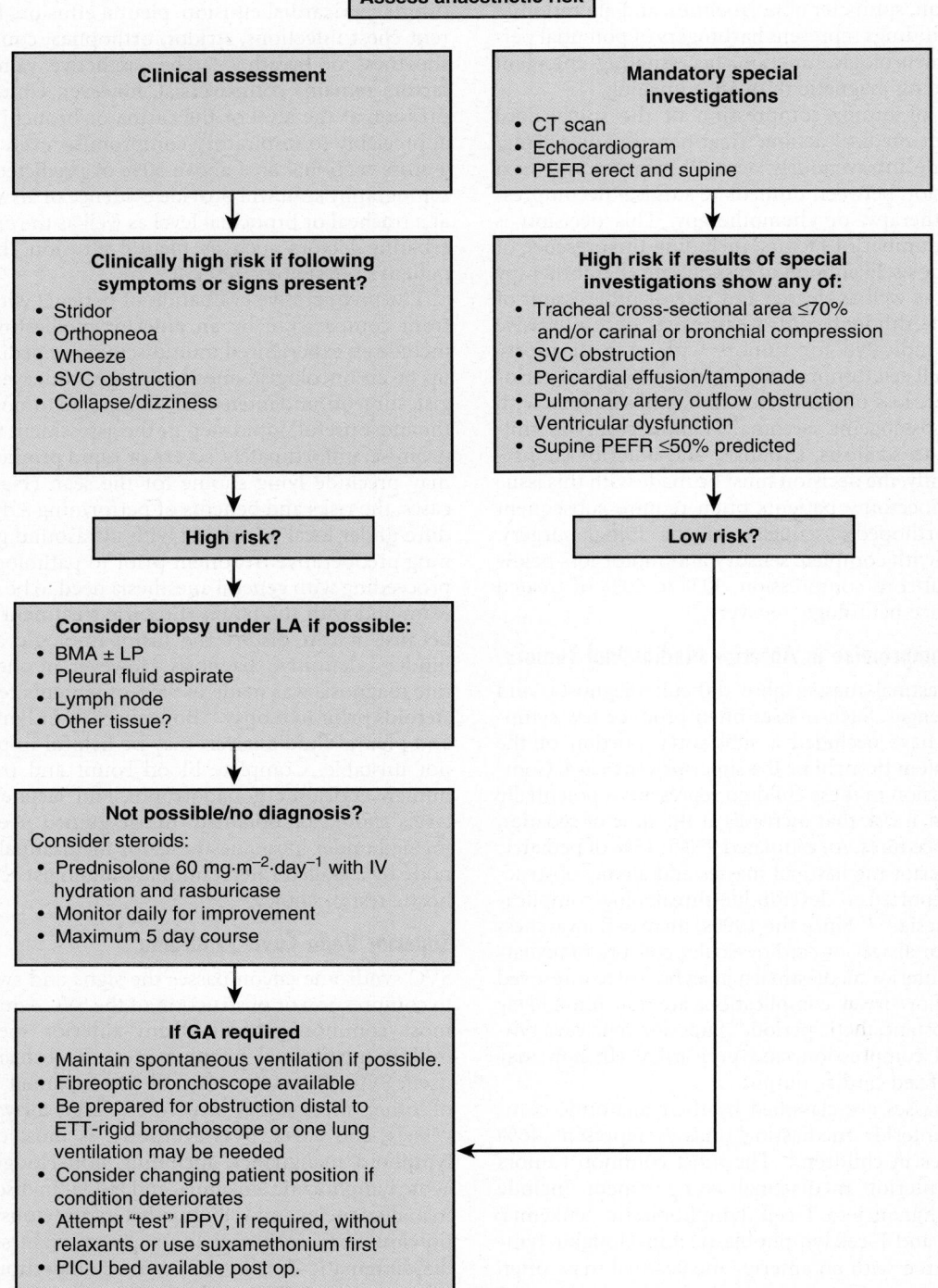

Fig. 94.2. Preoperative anesthetic guidelines for a child with a mediastinal mass. (From Hack HA, Wright NB, Wynn RF. The anaesthetic management of children with anterior mediastinal masses. Anaesthesia 2008;63:837-846; with permission.)

Evaluation of an anterior mediastinal mass was described previously. As in airway compression, SVC syndrome places a patient at significant risk for anesthetic complications during diagnostic procedures. CT should be pursued without sedation and may require prone positioning because compression of the great vessels may occur despite a patent airway, resulting in profound hypoxia and reduced cardiac output. In addition, echocardiography can evaluate cardiac motility and the degree of venous return. Diagnosis should be established with the least invasive means available, but empiric anticancer therapy may be required if no histologic sample can be obtained safely. Tissue for definitive diagnosis should be obtained as soon as the patient's clinical status allows in order to decrease the likelihood that empiric therapy will permanently obscure the diagnosis.

Hemophagocytic Lymphohistiocytosis

Hemophagocytic lymphohistiocytosis (HLH) describes a syndrome of conditions rather than a specific disease entity that is marked by hyperinflammation resulting from riotously elevated circulating cytokines.[45] HLH represents an emergency because it shares many clinical features with the systemic inflammatory response syndrome (SIRS) or sepsis syndrome. These similarities make the diagnosis difficult; however, identifying HLH results in a much different treatment algorithm.[46] Inadequately treated HLH results in very poor outcomes. Classically, HLH is thought to occur as a consequence of acquired or inherited defects in cytotoxic activity, but emerging data suggest that HLH should be viewed as a single syndrome with a continuum of risk factors.[47] Generally, these defects diminish elimination of cellular targets and impair down-regulation of the immune response.[45] HLH arises from abnormalities involving the process by which cytotoxic vesicles migrate to contact, attach, fuse, and release their contents with a target cell. Familial HLH is usually an autosomal recessive condition and is caused by one of several mutations in the natural killer (NK)/T-cell cytotoxic pathway.[48] Perforin is a cytotoxic protein stored in secretory granules of cytotoxic cells, and defects in this protein account for 50% of all familial HLH cases in North America.[49] Familial HLH is associated with and can be the initial presentation of an immunodeficiency syndrome such as Chediak-Higashi syndrome, Griscelli syndrome, and X-linked lymphoproliferative syndrome.

Acquired HLH most frequently occurs in the setting of infections, malignancy, or rheumatologic conditions; however, the mechanism of impairment of natural killer cells and cytotoxic lymphocytes in secondary HLH remains unclear but occurs in all age groups.[45] Less common associations include Kawasaki disease, metabolic diseases such as lysinuria protein intolerance, multiple sulfatase deficiency, and Wolman disease. *Macrophage activation syndrome* is a term commonly used to describe HLH in the setting of an underlying autoimmune disorder, most commonly rheumatoid arthritis.

Patients typically present with signs and symptoms of systemic infection or SIRS including prolonged fever (usually unresponsive to antibiotics), hepatosplenomegaly, and cytopenias. In some patients, neurologic symptoms, seizures, and cranial nerve palsies may occur. Because HLH often mimics other conditions, a high index of suspicion remains paramount. Fortunately, diagnostic guidelines exist (Box 94.4), but each clinical situation must be considered carefully because of the substantial overlap with severe sepsis, SIRS, and multiple organ dysfunction syndromes.

Laboratory studies often aid in diagnosis but may not be routinely obtained in patients who may have provisional diagnoses such as severe sepsis. Diagnostic criteria require a ferritin level higher than 500 ng/mL, but the levels are usually much higher, exceeding 10,000, unlike in sepsis where serum ferritin is elevated but appears to be generally below 2000. Serum triglycerides often are elevated. Soluble interleukin-2 receptor (sCD 25) and soluble Fas (CD178) are elevated. Although helpful in making the diagnosis of HLH, hemophagocytosis may be absent early in the disease, can be missed on bone marrow aspirates, and is a nonspecific finding.

BOX 94.4 Diagnostic Criteria for Hemophagocytic Lymphohistiocytosis

Familial Disease/Known Genetic Defect
Clinical and Laboratory Criteria (Five of Eight Criteria)

1. Fever
2. Splenomegaly
3. Cytopenia ≥2 cell lines
4. Hemoglobin <90 g/L (below 4 weeks <120 µg/L)
5. Platelets <100 × 10^9/L
6. Neutrophils <1 × 10^9/L
7. Hypertriglyceridemia or hypofibrinogenemia
   a. Fasting triglycerides >3 mmol/L
   b. Fibrinogen <1.5 g/L
8. Ferritin >500 lg/L
9. sCD25 = >2400 U/mL
10. Decreased or absent natural killer cell activity
11. Hemophagocytosis in bone marrow, CSF, or lymph nodes

Treatment depends on whether HLH is genetic or acquired. Initial treatment is meant to suppress hyperinflammation using immunosuppressive and cytostatic treatment with corticosteroids, cyclosporine A, or etoposide.[45] Identification of infection or malignancy should prompt immediate treatment of the underlying disease. Evidence of macrophage activation syndrome should prompt rheumatologic consultation.

Patients with primary HLH or underlying immune deficiency may require stem cell transplantation.

Anthracycline-Induced Cardiogenic Shock

The anthracyclines daunorubicin, doxorubicin, epirubicin, mitoxantrone, and idarubicin are used for chemotherapy for a wide variety of solid tumor and hematopoietic malignancies of childhood. Unfortunately, 15% of all pediatric cardiomyopathies occur in patients treated for childhood or adolescent malignancies.[50] In one prospective study, after anthracycline treatment, 5% of the children developed heart failure and 19% presented abnormal left ventricular function.[51] Shortening fractions declined proportionally to cumulative doses. Furthermore, differential susceptibility to cardiotoxicity became apparent early in treatment. Hence, patients at high risk for important anthracycline cardiotoxicity may be identifiable early in treatment by regular echocardiography. Pediatric age and female gender are known risk factors for anthracycline cardiotoxicity.

Anthracycline-induced acute myocardial injury is a rare form of cardiotoxicity that may occur immediately after a single dose or after a course of anthracycline therapy, with clinical symptoms usually occurring within a week of treatment.[52] Acute cardiotoxicity ranges from relatively benign arrhythmias to serious conditions such as fatal ventricular arrhythmias, myocardial ischemia/infarction, congestive heart failure, and cardiomyopathy.

The pathophysiology of anthracycline-induced cardiotoxicity may include free-radical–mediated myocyte damage, adrenergic dysfunction, intracellular calcium overload, and release of cardiotoxic cytokines. The myocardium appears susceptible to free radical damage from low levels of superoxide dismutase, catalase, and glutathione peroxidase activity. Cardiac mitochondria contain a unique enzyme (reduced nicotinamide adenine dinucleotide dehydrogenase) in their inner membrane that reduces anthracyclines to their semiquinones, producing severe oxidative damage to mitochondrial DNA, reductions in cellular energy production, and myocyte apoptosis.

Prevention of cardiotoxicity remains the ultimate goal. There is evidence that dexrazoxane reduces the cardiotoxicity associated with some anthracyclines without affecting the efficacy of anthracycline therapy.[53] The antioxidant CoQ10 is an integral component of the mitochondrial respiratory chain and has successfully been used in the treatment of cardiac failure.

The outcome of anthracycline-induced cardiogenic shock during chemotherapy remains poor. The myocardium has limited regeneration ability. The mortality rate related to anthracycline-associated heart failure is substantial; heart transplantation is often the only option for long-term survival.[5] Supportive treatment including mechanical support (eg, extracorporeal life support or ventricular assist devices) may stabilize patients while decisions about longer term care can be made.[54]

Posterior Reversible Encephalopathy

Posterior reversible encephalopathy syndrome (PRES) is a clinicoradiographic syndrome that classically presents with clinical signs and symptoms of headache, visual acuity disturbances, abrupt changes in mental status, and seizures with neuroimaging showing posterior white matter edema. The reversible posterior leukoencephalopathy syndrome was initially characterized by Hinchey and colleagues in 1996 in a case series that included patients aged 15 to 62 and was closely associated with hypertensive encephalopathy, preeclampsia/eclampsia, cyclosporine A neurotoxicity, and uremic encephalopathy.[55] As more cases were reported and neuroimaging improved, the name PRES was introduced in 1999 by Casey as a better description of the syndrome because the radiographic lesions were not felt to be consistent with a leukoencephalopathy.[56] Since the 1990s, PRES has become more clinically recognized in pediatric populations, especially in those pediatric populations who are exposed to immunomodulatory or cytotoxic therapy.[57] Although the exact incidence of PRES is unknown, in the context of tacrolimus or CSA used after solid organ transplant, PRES developed in 1% to 6% of all recipients. The exact precipitating factor for PRES is unknown but it is felt that the syndrome is associated with a disorder of cerebrovascular autoregulation likely from multiple etiologies. It is believed that the severe hypertension or other causes of PRES disrupt cerebrovascular autoregulation with a resulting leakage of fluid into brain parenchyma. Compared to the carotid system, the vertebrobasilar system has fewer adrenergic innervations, which may make it more prone to disruption of its autoregulation. This may explain the predominance of lesions in the posterior cerebral area seen in PRES. Although lesions can be seen in the cortex, the cortex is thought to be more "resistant" to edema because it is structurally more tightly packed, and thus most PRES lesions are seen in the white matter. There is also a proposed direct cytotoxic effect of various chemotherapeutic and immunomodulatory agents on the vascular endothelium.

PRES is a clinicoradiographic syndrome without specific diagnostic criteria. A high index of suspicion is required to help guide appropriate neuroimaging in a suggestive clinical context. Whereas abnormalities consistent with PRES can be seen on computed tomography (CT) scans, magnetic resonance imaging (MRI), especially FLAIR sequences, are most sensitive for PRES lesions.[56] MRI is also helpful in distinguishing PRES from ischemia and guiding appropriate therapy. The treatment for PRES is mostly supportive with reduction of hypertension, treatment of seizures, and withdrawal or reducing the dose of the offending agent. It is important to distinguish PRES lesions from ischemia because PRES requires aggressive treatment of hypertension, whereas ischemia is permissive of mild to moderate hypertension. The seizures associated with PRES usually respond well to benzodiazepines, but most case series report using multiple doses and sometimes requiring loading doses of another anti-epileptic medication (eg, phenytoin, phenobarbital) in order to break the seizure.[57,58] Most patients require admission to a pediatric intensive care unit for continued monitoring and optimization of support for vital functions. Rarely, seizures associated with PRES require more aggressive antiepileptic medication in the context of status epilepticus.

Chimeric Antigen Receptor T-Cell–Mediated Toxicity

Clinical trials using T-cell–engaging immunotherapies have shown promise to improve the survival of relapsed leukemia and lymphoma.[59] For pediatrics, chimeric antigen receptor modified T cells (CAR T cells) with specificity against CD19 have especially improved survival in relapsed pre–B-cell acute lymphocytic leukemia (ALL).[60] This unique therapy, however, has unique toxicities. Patients treated with CAR T cells experience a sudden increase in multiple cytokines as the T cells engage the immune system and eliminate leukemic cells. This cytokine release syndrome (CRS), or cytokine storm, is defined as a disorder characterized by fever, nausea, headache, tachycardia, hypotension, rash, and shortness of breath caused by the release of cytokines from cells.[61] CRS is part of the efficacy of the CAR T-cell treatment; however, it can become severe, affecting nearly every organ system including fluid refractory hypotension, tachycardia, cardiomyopathy, acute respiratory failure, neurologic toxicity, and disseminated intravascular coagulation (Fig. 94.3).[59]

The timing of symptom onset and CRS severity is likely dependent on tumor burden, baseline cytokine levels, and the underlying genetic predisposition of each patient. The onset of CRS usually happens days to as late as 2 to 3 weeks after the initial infusion and coincides with the maximal in vivo T-cell expansion.[59] The manifestation of CRS in pediatric patients can mimic the clinical presentation of HLH/macrophage activation syndrome (MAS) with highly elevated serum ferritin, D-dimer, aminotransferases, lactate dehydrogenase, triglycerides, hypofibrinogenemia, and hepatosplenomegaly. CRS occurs in about two-thirds of patients treated with CAR T cells.[62] When the syndrome becomes severe or life threatening, inhibition of the inflammatory cascade outweighs further expansion of CAR T cells. Cytokine levels drawn during CAR T-cell therapy indicate IL-6 as a central mediator of toxicity in CRS and have been shown to be a possible target for down regulating the inflammatory cascade.

Tocilizumab is a humanized immunoglobulin antihuman IL-6R mAb approved for treatment of rheumatoid arthritis,[63] juvenile idiopathic arthritis,[64] and polyarticular juvenile rheumatoid arthritis. Clinical experience at several institutions conducting CAR T-cell trials has indicated that tocilizumab is an effective treatment for severe or life-threatening CRS.[65,66] Initial dosing is 8 mg/kg, which is administered over 1 hour. This dose can be repeated in 24 to 48 hours if clinical

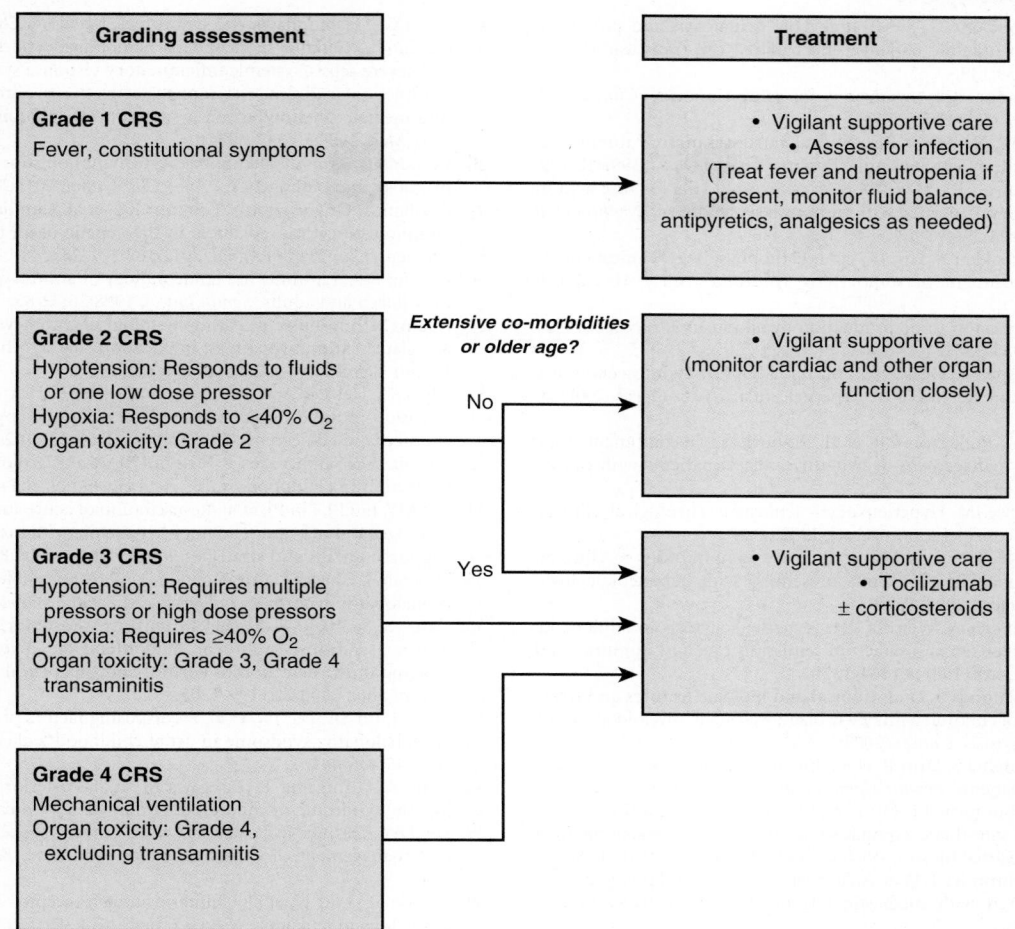

Fig. 94.3. Treatment algorithm for management of cytokine release syndrome. (From Lee DW, Gardner R, Porter DL, et al. Current concepts in the diagnosis and management of cytokine release syndrome. *Blood* 2014;124:188-194; with permission.)

improvement does not occur. Clinical response is usually seen within a few hours, with resolution of hypotension and fever allowing for weaning of supportive measures and pressors. If clinical response is not achieved 24 to 48 hours after the administration of tocilizumab, another immunosuppressive agent, such as corticosteroids, should be considered. Corticosteroids are usually avoided because of their probable adverse effect on the antitumor activity of the CAR T cells, although this remains debatable. Dosing and choice of corticosteroid can vary among patients, but an initial dose of methylprednisolone of 2 mg/kg/day can be considered and then weaned over several days, with a preference of dexamethasone in patients experiencing neurotoxicity. As more children are treated with highly active T-cell–engaging therapies, we will continue to gain clinical experience with managing the toxicities of this novel treatment. The continued challenge will be to control the toxicity without interfering with the efficacy.

Key References

1. Oski FA, Brugnaro C, Nathan DG. A diagnostic approach to the anemic patient. In: Nathan DG, Orkin SH, eds. *Nathan and Oski's Hematology of Infancy and Childhood.* 5th ed. Philadelphia: WB Saunders; 1998:2.
3. Kirkpatrick DV. Aplastic anemia: pathogenesis, complications and treatment. *Cancer Bull.* 1985;37:221.
5. Sieff CA, Nisbet-Brown E, Nathan DG. Congenital bone marrow failure syndromes. *Br J Haematol.* 2000;111:30-42.
6. Zinner SH. Changing epidemiology of infections in patients with neutropenia and cancer: emphasis on gram-positive. *Clin Infect Dis.* 1999;29:490.
7. Deeg HJ, Leisenring W, Storb R, et al. Long-term outcome after marrow transplantation for severe aplastic anemia. *Blood.* 1998;91:3637.
8. Rosenfeld SJ, Kimball J, Vining D, et al. Intensive immunosuppression with anthithymocyte globulin and cyclosporine as treatment for severe acquired aplastic anemia. *Blood.* 1995;85:3058.
9. Payne LG, Haywood CPM, Kelton JG. Destruction of red cells by the vasculature and reticuloendothelial system. In: Nathan DG, Orkin SH, eds. *Nathan and Oski's Hematology of Infancy and Childhood.* 5th ed. Philadelphia: WB Saunders; 1998.
11. Acona KG, Parker RI, Atlas MP, et al. Randomized trial of high-dose methylprednisolone versus intravenous immunoglobulin for the treatment of acute idiopathic thrombocytopenic purpura in children. *J Pediatr Hematol Oncol.* 2002;24:540.
12. Qin YH, Zhou TB, Su LN, et al. The efficacy of different doses intravenous immunoglobulin in treating acute idiopathic thrombocytopenic purpura. *Blood Coag Fib.* 2010;21:713.
13. Woerner SJ, Abildgaard CF, French BN. Intracranial hemorrhage in children with idiopathic thrombocytopenic purpura. *Pediatrics.* 1981;67:453.
14. Psaila B, Petrovic A, Page LK, et al. Intracranial hemorrhage of children with immune thrombocytopenia: study of 40 cases. *Blood.* 2009;114:4777.
15. Gordon Li, Kwaan HC, Ross EC. Deleterious effects of platelet transfusions and recovery thrombocytosis in patients with thrombotic microangiopathy. *Semin Hematol.* 1987;24:194.
16. Weigert AL, Shafer AI. Uremia bleeding: pathogenesis and therapy. *Am J Med Sci.* 1998;316:94.

19. Fernandez F, Goudable C, Sie P, et al. Low hematocrit and prolonged bleeding time in uraemic patients: effect of red cell transfusions. *Br J Haematol.* 1985;59:139.

22. Gemici C. Tumour lysis syndrome in solid tumours. *Clin Oncol.* 2006;18:773-780.

23. Kedar A, Grow W, Neiberger RE. Clinical versus laboratory tumor lysis syndrome in children with leukemia. *Pediatr Hematol Oncol.* 1995;12:129.

24. Shimada M, Johnson RJ, May WS Jr, et al. A novel role for uric acid in acute kidney injury associated with tumour lysis syndrome. *Nephrol Dial Transplant.* 2009;24:2960-2964.

26. Davidson MB, Thakkar S, Hix JK, et al. Pathophysiology, clinical consequences, and treatment of tumor lysis syndrome. *Am J Med.* 2004; 116:546-554.

27. Spector T. Inhibition of urate production by allopurinol. *Biochem Pharmacol.* 1977;26:355-358.

28. Smalley RV, Guaspari A, Haase-Statz S, et al. Allopurinol: intravenous use for prevention and treatment of hyperuricemia. *J Clin Oncol.* 2000;18: 1758-1763.

29. Bosly A, Sonet A, Pinkerton CR, et al. Rasburicase (recombinant urate oxidase) for the management of hyperuricemia in patients with cancer. *Cancer.* 2003;98:1048.

30. Lictman MA, Rowe JM. Hyperleukocytic leukemias: rheological, clinical, and therapeutic considerations. *Blood.* 1982;60:279.

32. Lowe EJ, Pui C-H, Hancock ML, et al. Early complications in children with acute lymphoblastic leukemia presenting with hyperleukocytosis. *Pediatr Blood Cancer.* 2005;45:10-15.

33. Dutcher JP, Schiffer CA, Wiernik PH. Hyperleukocytosis in adult acute nonlymphocytic leukemia: impact on remission rate and duration, and survival. *J Clin Oncol.* 1987;5:1364-1372.

34. Inaba H, Fan Y, Pounds S, et al. Clinical and biologic features and treatment outcomes of children with newly diagnosed acute myeloid leukemia and hyperleukocytosis. *Cancer.* 2008;113:522-529.

36. Pollono D, Tomarchia S, Drut R, et al. Spinal cord compression: a review of 70 pediatric patients. *Pediatr Hematol Oncol.* 2003;20:457.

37. Anghelescu DL, Burgoyne LL, Liu T, et al. Clinical and diagnostic imaging findings predict anesthetic complications in children presenting with malignant mediastinal masses. *Paediatr Anaesth.* 2007;17:1090-1098.

38. Ng A, Bennett J, Bromley P, et al. Anaesthetic outcome and predictive risk factors in children with mediastinal tumours. *Pediatr Blood Cancer.* 2007;48:160-164.

39. King DR, Patrick LE, Ginn-Pease ME, et al. Pulmonary function is compromised in children with mediastinal lymphoma. *J Pediatr Surg.* 1997;32: 294-300.

41. Lee EY. Evaluation of non-vascular mediastinal masses in infants and children: an evidence-based practical approach. *Pediatr Radiol.* 2009;39(suppl 2):S184-S190.

43. Perger L, Lee EY, Shamberger RC. Management of children and adolescents with a critical airway due to compression by an anterior mediastinal mass. *J Pediatr Surg.* 2008;43:1990-1997.

44. Saraswatula A, McShane D, Tideswell D, et al. Mediastinal masses masquerading as common respiratory conditions of childhood: a case series. *Eur J Pediatr.* 2009;168:1395-1399.

45. Janka GE. Hemophagocytic syndromes. *Blood Rev.* 2007;21:245-253.

46. Castillo L, Carcillo J. Secondary hemophagocytic lymphohistiocytosis and severe sepsis/systemic inflammatory response syndrome/multiorgan dysfunction syndrome/macrophage activation syndrome share common intermediate phenotypes on a spectrum of inflammation. *Pediatr Crit Care Med.* 2009;10:387-392.

48. Rosado FG, Kim AS. Hemophagocytic lymphohistiocytosis: an update on diagnosis and pathogenesis. *Am J Clin Pathol.* 2013;139:713-727.

49. Gholam C, Grigoriadou S, Gilmour KC, et al. Familial haemophagocytic lymphohistiocytosis: advances in the genetic basis, diagnosis and management. *Clin Exp Immunol.* 2011;163:271-283.

50. Grenier MA, Lipshultz SE. Epidemiology of anthracycline cardio-toxicity in children and adults. *Semin Oncol.* 1998;25:72-85.

51. Adams MJ, Lipshultz SE. Pathophysiology of anthracycline- and radiation-associated cardiomyopathies: implications for screening and prevention. *Pediatr Blood Cancer.* 2005;44:600-606.

52. Chen C, Heusch A, Donner B, et al. Present risk of anthracycline or radiation-induced cardiac sequelae following therapy of malignancies in children and adolescents. *Klin Padiatr.* 2009;221:162-166.

53. Lipsultz SE, Sambatokos P, Maguire M, et al. Cardiotoxicity and cardioprotection in childhood cancer. *Acta Haematol.* 2014;132:391.

54. Wu MY, Liu PJ, Lin PJ, et al. Resuscitation of acute anthracycline-induced cardiogenic shock and refractory hypoxemia with mechanical circulatory supports: pitfalls and strategies. *Resuscitation.* 2009;80:385-386.

55. Hinchey J, Chaves C, Appignani B, et al. A reversible posterior leukoencephalopathy syndrome. *N Engl J Med.* 1996;334:494-500.

56. Casey S, Sampaio R, Michel E, Truwit C. Posterior reversible encephalopathy syndrome: utility of fluid-attenuated inversion recovery MR imaging in the detection of cortical and subcortical lesions. *AJNR Am J Neuroradiol.* 2000;21:1199-1206.

57. Kim SJ, Im SA, Lee JW, et al. Predisposing factors of posterior reversible encephalopathy syndrome in acute childhood leukemia. *Pediatr Neurol.* 2012;47:436-442.

58. Endo A, Fushigama T, Hasegawa M, et al. Posterior reversible encephalopathy syndrome in childhood. *Pediatr Emerg Care.* 2012;28:2.

59. Lee DW, Gardner R, Porter DL, et al. Current concepts in the diagnosis and management of cytokine release syndrome. *Blood.* 2014;124:188-194.

60. Maude SL, Frey N, et al. Chimeric antigen receptor T cells for sustained remissions in leukemia. *N Engl J Med.* 2014;371:1507-1517.

64. Yokota S, Miyamae T, Imagawa T, et al. Therapeutic efficacy of humanized recombinant anti-interleukin-6 receptor antibody in children with systemic-onset juvenile idiopathic arthritis. *Arthritis Rheum.* 2005;52:818-825.

65. Grupp SA, Kalos M, Barrett D, et al. Chimeric antigen receptor-modified T cells for acute lymphoid leukemia. *N Engl J Med.* 2013;368:1509-1518.

66. Winkler U, Jensen M, Manzke O, et al. Cytokine-release syndrome in patients with B-cell chronic lymphocytic leukemia and high lymphocyte counts after treatment with an anti-CDD20 monoclonal antibody (rituximab, IDEC-C2B8). *Blood.* 1999;94:2217-2224.

Critical Illness Involving Children Undergoing Hematopoietic Cell Transplantation

Jennifer McArthur, Christine Duncan, Prakad Rajapreyar, Julie-An Talano, and Robert T. Tamburro, Jr.

PEARLS

- Patients undergoing allogeneic hematopoietic cell transplant (HCT) experience prolonged immune dysregulation and are at risk for both opportunist infection and graft-versus-host disease (GVHD).
- HCT patients experiencing respiratory symptoms including a new oxygen requirement deserve prompt evaluation by the critical care team as they are at risk for rapid development of respiratory failure.
- Outcomes for HCT patients requiring intensive care unit care have improved since the 1990s.
- Patients who develop GVHD are at high risk for developing other transplant-related toxicities.

Overview

Hematopoietic progenitor cell transplantation has evolved as the treatment for a variety of congenital and acquired malignant and nonmalignant disorders. Over the years the name of this procedure has changed in an attempt to be more accurate. Throughout the literature, it has been referred to as bone marrow transplant (BMT), hematopoietic progenitor cell transplant (HPCT), hematopoietic stem cell transplant (HSCT), and, more recently, hematopoietic cell transplant (HCT).

The first successful pediatric bone marrow transplant occurred in a child with combined immunodeficiency. Reported in 1968, the patient received marrow from a human leukocyte antigen (HLA)-matched sibling.[1] Presently, in adults and children, the majority of allogeneic transplants are performed for the treatment of malignant disorders such as leukemias and lymphomas, although the field continues to expand to include nonmalignant disorders such as autoimmune disorders, metabolic diseases, immune deficiencies, and hemoglobinopathies. Since its inception, the field of pediatric HCT has demonstrated vast improvements in morbidity and mortality related to transplantation; however, there are still

many hurdles to overcome. The major contributors to morbidity and mortality of allogeneic transplantation continue to be relapse of disease, transplant-related toxicity, infection, and graft-versus-host disease (GVHD).

Sources of Hematopoietic Progenitor Cells and Identification of Donors

HCT involves transplanting hematopoietic progenitor cells from a donor source into a recipient. These stem cells are capable of self-renewal and terminal differentiation that ultimately give rise to myeloid cells, lymphocytes, erythrocytes, and platelets (Fig. 95.1). The donor source of these stem cells can be from the patients/recipients themselves (autologous) or from another individual (allogeneic). The source of the donor (autologous versus allogeneic) depends on the indication for which the transplant is being performed. Traditionally, HCT has been performed using stem cells obtained from bone marrow. However, stem cells can be mobilized into the peripheral blood and harvested for transplant. These peripheral blood stem cells (PBSCs) allow for faster hematopoietic recovery and possibly less tumor contamination than bone marrow when used in autologous transplantation. However, there may be more side effects in the allogeneic setting, particularly increased incidence of GVHD.[2]

Umbilical cord blood has also been shown to contain large numbers of stem cells capable of reconstituting hematopoiesis. The first HCT using cord blood was performed in 1988 for a child with Fanconi anemia.[3] Since then, unrelated cord blood stem cells have been used and numerous public cord blood banks have been established worldwide. These cord blood banks are now regulated by the National Marrow Donor Program.

When no matched unrelated donor or cord blood can be found in a timely fashion, haploidentical transplantation can be performed using a parent or a sibling as donor. Histoincompatibility barriers of a mismatched transplantation are overcome by using megadoses of stem cells. However, for this to be successful, a majority of the T cells have to be removed from the graft to prevent severe GVHD. Unfortunately, this increases the risk for severe infection and relapse of the patient's original disease.[4,5] Centers are utilizing a T-cell replete haploidentical transplantation approach, which incorporates high-dose, posttransplantation cyclophosphamide to promote graft-host tolerance after allogeneic hematopoietic stem cell transplantation.[6]

HLAs are expressed on the surface of various cells, in particular white blood cells (WBCs). These antigens are also known as the major histocompatibility complex with relevant genes on the short arm of chromosome 6.[7] This genetic region has been divided into chromosomal regions, called classes. Classes I and II are important in transplantation. Class I is made up of HLA-A, HLA-B, and HLA-C, and class II is made up of HLA-DR, HLA-DP, and HLA-DQ, as well as variations on these genes. Traditionally, the loci critical for matching for a bone marrow donor are HLA-A, HLA-B, and HLA-DR. HLA-C and HLA-DQ have gained importance and are now considered in determining the best available donor.[7,8]

Ideally a matched sibling donor is the best donor for a patient. However, only 25% of patients with siblings are fortunate to have a matched sibling donor. If there is no sibling donor, an alternative donor is identified using the National Marrow Donor Program (NMDP), which has approximately 12.5 million potential donors and nearly 150,209,000 cord blood units available for patients who need an HCT.[9] As the degree of mismatch between patient and donor increases, so do the risks of complications from transplant, especially GVHD and graft failure.

Indications and Outcomes

HCT has been used for a variety of diseases. Autologous transplantation has traditionally been used to treat nonhematologic malignant diseases by escalating the doses of chemotherapy to myeloablative doses in hopes of eradicating the cancer. Successive (two or three) autologous transplants have been performed with nonmyeloablative doses of chemotherapy, particularly in brain tumors. The rationale of giving hematopoietic stem cells after the chemotherapy has been completed is to minimize the period of neutropenia, which will hopefully reduce the number of infections and life-threatening complications.[2]

Allogeneic HCT is performed for hematologic cancers. In children these are most commonly acute lymphoblastic leukemia (ALL) and acute myelogenous leukemia (AML). It is also used to treat hematologic diseases including sickle cell anemia, thalassemias, and severe aplastic anemia. A variety of immune deficiencies and metabolic disorders are cured by allogeneic transplant, including severe combined immune deficiency and hemophagocytic lymphohistiocytosis (Table 95.1).[2]

Survival from HCT has improved. In autologous transplantation the incidence of treatment-related mortality is less than 10%. However, the majority of treatment failures are due to recurrent disease. Specifically the event-free survival rate for autologous HCT for high-risk neuroblastoma ranges from

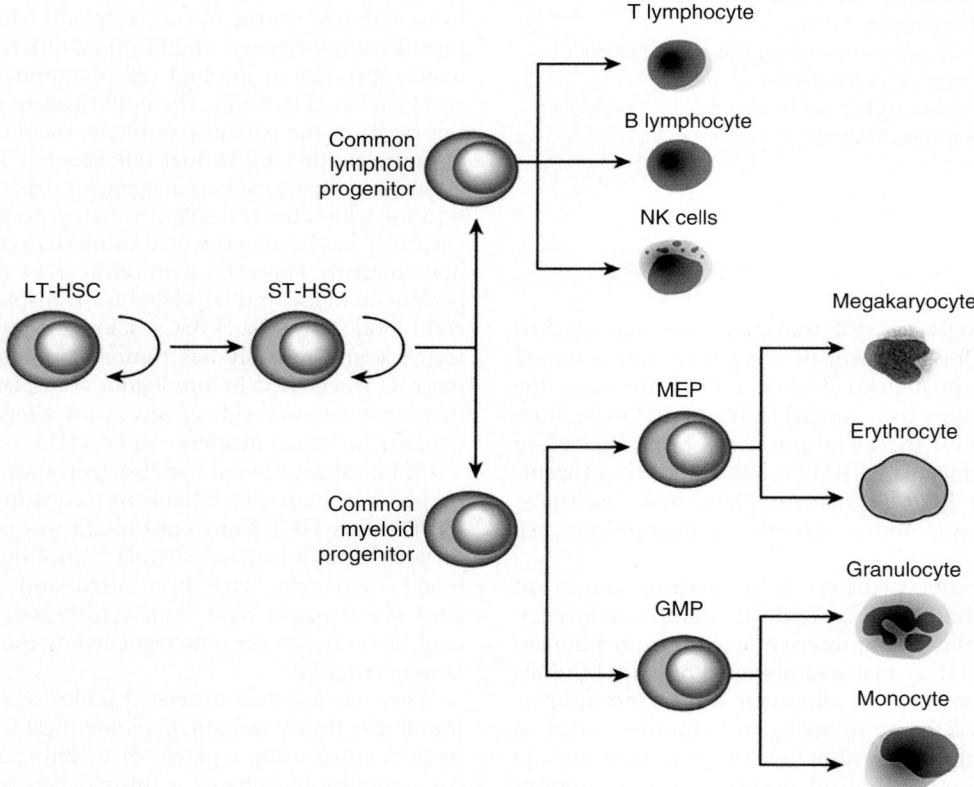

Fig. 95.1. As hematopoietic stem cells divide, they give rise to common lymphoid and common myeloid precursor cells that eventually generate all mature blood lineages of the body. *GMP,* granulocyte-monocyte precursors; *LT-HSC,* long-term hematopoietic stem cells; *MEP,* megakaryocyte-erythrocyte precursors; *NK,* natural killer; *ST-HSC,* short-term hematopoietic stem cells. (Modified from Leung AYH, Verfaillie CM. Stem cell model of hematopoiesis. In: Hematology: Basic Principles and Practice. 4th ed. Philadelphia, 2001, Elsevier.)

TABLE 95.1	Indications for Pediatric Hematopoietic Progenitor Cell Transplantation

Autologous Transplantation

Malignant Disorders

High-risk neuroblastoma
Relapsed non-Hodgkin lymphoma
Relapsed Hodgkin disease
Medulloblastoma
Germ cell tumors
Brain tumors
Relapsed Ewing sarcoma

Nonmalignant Disorders

Autoimmune disorders

Allogeneic Transplantation

Malignant Disorders

Acute myelogenous leukemia
Acute lymphoblastic leukemia
Chronic myeloid leukemia
Myelodysplastic syndromes
Juvenile myelomonocytic leukemia

Nonmalignant Disorders

Aplastic anemia
Fanconi anemia
Severe combined immunodeficiency
Thalassemia major
Diamond-Blackfan anemia
Sickle cell anemia
Wiskott-Aldrich syndrome
Osteopetrosis
Inborn errors of metabolism
Hemophagocytic lymphohistiocytosis
Shwachman-Diamond syndrome
Congenital immune deficiencies

33% to 66%.[10-14] For recurrent or refractory non-Hodgkin lymphoma the event-free survival in autologous HCT ranges from 27% to 59%.[15] In relapsed or refractory Hodgkin disease the event-free survival ranges from 20% to 62%.[15]

Among children with ALL, allogeneic transplantation is generally reserved for patients with high-risk disease, patients who fail to achieve remission, or patients who relapse after chemotherapy. Among the 2096 patients younger than 20 receiving an HLA-matched sibling transplant for ALL between 2002 to 2012, the 3-year survival rates range from 26% to 67% depending on their disease status going into transplant. The corresponding survival rates among the 3291 recipients of an unrelated donor transplant range from 31% to 66%.[16] For pediatric patients with AML transplanted with matched siblings donors between 2002 and 2012, the 3-year survival rates following transplant range from 30% to 66%.[16] For unrelated donor transplants the 5-year overall survival rates range from 20% to 50%.[16]

Allogeneic HCT is the treatment of choice for young patients with severe aplastic anemia and an available HLA-matched sibling donor. These patients have excellent outcomes with survival rates ranging from 73% for unrelated donor transplants to 88% for matched sibling transplants.[16] Transplant outcomes for other nonmalignant diseases are also improved, with Fanconi anemia patients having a 5-year overall survival of 60% to 75%,[17-19] Wiskott-Aldrich disease at 90%, and severe combined immune deficiency at 71%.[20] For inherited metabolic disorders, the overall survival of pediatric

patients with adrenoleukodystrophy/metachromatic leukodystrophy is approximately 60% and for Hurler syndrome it is approximately 70% when using unrelated donor transplants facilitated by the NMDP from 2001 to 2010.[21-23]

Transplant Procedure
Conditioning Regimen

Patients undergoing HCT are subjected to a treatment regimen referred to as a conditioning regimen or preparative regimen prior to infusion of the hematopoietic progenitor cells. The purpose of this preparative regimen is multifold. In cases of malignant disorders, it eradicates disease. In addition, the preparative regimen must be immunosuppressive in allogeneic transplantation to allow the donor cells infused to establish themselves in the marrow cavity and overcome host rejection. The precise conditioning regimens can include chemotherapy alone or in combination with radiation. Numerous regimens have been explored and are dependent on the disease for which the transplant is required and the research interests of the institution performing the transplant.

Stem Cell Harvesting/Collection/Cryopreservation

Stem cells can be collected or harvested from either bone marrow or peripheral blood. For patients or donors undergoing bone marrow harvest, general anesthesia or regional anesthesia is given. Bone marrow is generally aspirated using special bone marrow harvest needles percutaneously from the posterior iliac crests using numerous passes. The amount of marrow taken is based on the size of the recipient. If there is a significant size discrepancy between the donor and the recipient (recipient larger than the donor), the donor may lose a significant amount of blood. Donors can be placed on iron therapy after harvest, or they can electively store autologous blood ahead of time. A newer technique allows for the collected marrow to be processed with removal of red blood cells (RBCs) (particularly necessary in cases of major ABO incompatibility between donor and recipient), and these RBCs can be transfused to the donor postoperatively.

Peripheral blood stem cells can be mobilized in patients recovering from chemotherapy (autologous) or by giving allogeneic donors cytokines such as G-CSF. Their stem cells then can be collected using an apheresis machine in an outpatient setting. Collection of sufficient cells for transplantation may require several apheresis procedures. Stem cells for allogeneic transplantation usually are collected on the day they are anticipated to be reinfused into the patient. Autologous collection of stem cells requires cryopreservation of the cells until the day of reinfusion. Dimethyl sulfoxide (DMSO) is added to the collection product to ensure cell viability, and the cells are frozen in liquid nitrogen until needed.

Stem cells can be collected from umbilical cord blood. After delivery of the infant, sterile umbilical venous access is obtained and the blood is collected into anticoagulated tubes. This can be done either before or after delivery of the placenta. A sample of this cord blood is used for HLA typing and infectious disease testing; the remainder is cryopreserved.

Reinfusion

The day of stem cell reinfusion is referred to as day 0 for the transplant period. Cryopreserved stem cells are thawed in a water bath under sterile conditions and may be washed to remove the DMSO cryopreservant. Stem cells then are infused into the patient though the indwelling central venous catheter. These cells are capable of migrating into the bone marrow on their own. Blood transfusion–like complications can occur with reinfusion of stem cells, and patients are generally placed on cardiac monitors with emergency medications available at the bedside during the infusion. The infusion procedure is generally short, lasting anywhere from approximately 10 minutes to 4 hours, depending on the volume of cells infusing.

Recovery Period

After the reinfusion of stem cells, patients wait for count recovery to occur and receive treatment for any toxicities. Allogeneic transplant patients receive immunosuppressive medicines to prevent GVHD. Most patients are hospitalized for the entire transplant procedure, starting with the conditioning regimen. However, there is a trend toward outpatient HCT, particularly in the autologous setting. A typical hospitalization for HCT is 4 to 6 weeks, but it may be prolonged if umbilical cord blood is used or shortened for autologous transplants.

Complications

Patients undergoing HCT are at high risk for complications that may require a stay in the pediatric intensive care unit (PICU). In one series, 19% of pediatric HCT patients required a PICU admission.[24] In other published series, 6% to 25% of pediatric HCT patients required mechanical ventilation.[25,26] Because of the high use of critical care services by HCT patients, it is beneficial for the pediatric intensivist to be familiar with their complications.

The reasons for these patients being at high risk for critical illness are multifactorial. Many of these patients are undergoing HCT for an underlying disease that places them at risk for critical illness such as malignancies, severe immunodeficiencies, and metabolic disorders. To make room for the new hematopoietic progenitor cells, patients are given conditioning regimens with high doses of toxic chemotherapy or radiation. This makes them severely immunocompromised, placing them at high risk for opportunistic infections. The conditioning agents themselves cause significant oxidative stress and may be the common denominator behind many of these complications.[27]

Although mortality rates for HCT patients requiring ICU care are quite high in comparison to the general ICU population, they appear to be improving. Data from the 1980s showed mortality rates for mechanically ventilated pediatric HCT patients to be near 90%.[26,28] However, more recent data indicate the mortality rates to be closer to 60%.[29-31] In a single institution report, HCT patients requiring vasoactive-inotropic support due to sepsis had PICU mortality rates of 30%. In the subgroup of septic patients requiring both vasoactive-inotropic support and mechanical ventilation, mortality rates were 74%.[32] Some of the improvements seen in outcomes over the years may be due to differing characteristics of the patients, as few studies reported severity of illness scores.[28] In any case, no series reporting on mortality of pediatric HCT patients was able to predict with 100% certainty that a given patient would not survive. Therefore the critical care and transplant teams must work together and use their best judgment when making recommendations to families regarding the appropriateness and duration of critical care services for this complex patient population.

Cardiac Complications

Cardiac complications following HCT can occur during the immediate transplant period or be late sequelae in survivors. The heart may be injured during the transplant process from a variety of pathophysiologic etiologies.[33,34] First, previous cardiotoxic treatments and therapies such as anthracyclines and iron overload from frequent red cell transfusions may predispose the heart to subsequent injury during transplantation. In addition, cardiotoxic therapies such as cyclophosphamide and irradiation used as part of the preparative regimen may further injure the recipient heart.[35-37] Moreover, hyperhydration therapies, blood product transfusions, and impaired renal function may place further stress on the heart. Sepsis, which commonly affects the HCT patient, has also been found to decrease cardiac contractility.[38] More specific to the HCT patient, there are rare reports of acute GVHD affecting the heart and cardiovascular system.[39] Further, transplant-associated thrombotic microangiopathy has been associated with cardiovascular complications such as pericardial effusions and pulmonary arterial hypertension.[40,41] Additionally, in a small series of children treated for a primary immunodeficiency with HCT (n = 10), cardiac chamber hypertrophy was reported to occur in those transplanted at less than a year of age and who received high-dose corticosteroids for acute GVHD.[42] Finally, there is evidence to suggest that genetic susceptibility may also play a role in HCT-related heart failure. For example, using a nested case-control study design, it was noted that polymorphisms in the NAD(P)H oxidase subunit RAC2 as well as carbonyl reductase CBR1 were associated with a significant increase in the risk of acute heart failure among HCT recipients. These findings suggest that acute heart failure occurs as a result of oxidative stress or metabolic derangements induced by cardiotoxic alcohol metabolites of anthracyclines and that variants of RAC2 and CBR1 modulate this risk.[43]

Although the heart and cardiovascular system are at risk from these various processes, cardiac complications are relatively rare in the early posttransplant period after HCT. In an analysis of 2821 adult and pediatric patients, only 26 (0.9%) experienced a major or fatal cardiac complication in the first 100 days after transplant.[44] Seven of the 26 cardiac complications occurred in children. Given the median age of 22 years in that trial, an incidence of approximately 0.5% may be inferred for pediatric HCT recipients. Among the 26 patients with significant cardiac complications, 11 had evidence of heart failure, 5 had pericardial tamponade, and 10 had dysrhythmias.[44] All 11 patients with heart failure died compared with only one each with tamponade or a dysrhythmia. All cases of heart failure occurred between day −6 and day +35. Four of the seven pediatric patients had heart failure. In another report, the Associazione Italiana Ematologia Oncologia Pediatrica-BMT Group described its transplant-related toxicities in 636 pediatric patients transplanted for acute leukemia.[45] In the group's experience, the incidence of moderate or severe cardiac toxicity in the first 90 days posttransplant varied by the type of transplant with autologous recipients experiencing an incidence of 1.9% (4 in 216, two deaths) and allogenic recipients of a compatible related donor experiencing a comparable incidence of 2.4% (7 in 294, four deaths). However, recipients of an allogeneic alternative donor experienced a 6.4% rate of these cardiac complications (8 in 126) with all eight experiencing an early death. In that study, the presence of moderate or severe cardiac toxicity increased the relative risk of an early posttransplant death more than ninefold (relative risk, 9.1; 95% confidence interval, 2.8 to 29.6) and more so than toxicity to any other organ system. The manifestations of the cardiac disease are varied and include myocardial ischemia, dysrhythmias, pericardial effusion, pericarditis, and progressive congestive heart failure. One particular cardiovascular complication that merits special attention in the pediatric HCT patient is the occurrence of pulmonary hypertension.

Pulmonary arterial hypertension in the setting of pediatric HCT is reported with increased frequency. In one report, a routine day +7 echocardiogram detected elevated right ventricular pressures in 13% of the patients.[46] In that report, and others, the pulmonary arterial hypertension is found to be associated with transplant-associated thrombotic microangiopathy.[41,46] Additionally, pulmonary arterial hypertension is reported to occur in the setting of patients undergoing transplant for malignant infantile osteopetrosis.[47] Pulmonary venoocclusive disease may also account for episodes of pulmonary arterial hypertension.[48] The incidence of pulmonary venoocclusive disease in HSCT patients is speculative given the limited available data.[48] Pulmonary hypertension is reported to be the proximate cause of death in pediatric patients undergoing HCT for hemophagocytic lymphohistiocytosis and idiopathic myelofibrosis.[49,50] Independent of the cause, pulmonary arterial hypertension should always be suspected in the pediatric HCT patient with unexplained cardiopulmonary dysfunction as emergent therapy may be lifesaving.

An accepted scoring system based on previously published grading of cardiac toxicities following stem cell transplantation consists of the following[44]:

Grade I: (1) Cardiomegaly on chest radiograph without symptoms, (2) mild electrocardiogram changes not requiring treatment, (3) asymptomatic pericardial effusion
Grade II: (1) Moderate electrocardiogram changes requiring and responding to medical intervention, (2) congestive heart failure requiring and responding to afterload reduction, diuretics, and digitalis, (3) pericarditis
Grade III: (1) Severe electrocardiogram abnormalities with no or only partial response to medical intervention, (2) congestive heart failure requiring inotropic support, (3) cardiogenic shock, (4) a decrease in QRS voltage by more than 50%, (5) pericardial tamponade
Grade IV: Fatal toxicity

Late cardiovascular toxicity occurring a year or more after HCT has also been reported.[51-53] Late cardiovascular complications following HCT included heart failure, dysrhythmias, hypertension, and cerebrovascular accidents. Several pathologic mechanisms of late congestive heart failure have been offered including the same mechanisms causing acute heart failure such as previous cardiotoxic agents (anthracyclines, alkylating agents, thoracic irradiation) in conjunction with cyclophosphamide and total body irradiation during conditioning regimens. A report evaluating long-term health outcomes in three groups revealed that survivors of childhood

HCT had a 13-fold increased risk of severe cardiovascular complications when compared to healthy sibling controls but had an equivalent risk to that observed in conventionally treated childhood cancer survivors.[43,54] In one report of 155 long-term pediatric survivors of HCT with a median length of follow-up of 9 years, 14 were found to have hypertension, 4 were found to have abnormal asymptomatic electrocardiograms, and 4 were found to have abnormal asymptomatic echocardiograms.[53] All patients in that report had a left ventricular shortening fraction greater than 30%. In another report of 112 children who received an allogeneic HCT and survived at least 1 year, 11 had abnormal echocardiographic findings, 8 had hypertension, and 2 had cerebrovascular accidents.[55] The probability of developing a cardiovascular complication at 10 years was 11% ± 3% in that report. Moreover, among patients who developed a cardiac complication, all had received total body irradiation. Other factors such as the presence of chronic GVHD and patient characteristics such as age, size, and gender may play a role in late congestive heart failure. Total body irradiation, both alone and in conjunction with pretransplant anthracycline use, was also associated with a negative impact on cardiac function 5 years after transplant in a cohort of 162 pediatric patients who underwent allogeneic HCT for both malignant and nonmalignant diseases.[56] In that study, 14 (12%) of the 119 patients with pretransplant echocardiograms were found to have abnormal shortening fractions at the time of transplant. The cumulative incidence of shortening fraction abnormalities increased to 26% by the fifth year of follow-up in that report. In another study, assessing cardiac function during cardiopulmonary exercise testing revealed a significantly decreased maximal cardiac index in 33 children who had undergone HCT in longitudinal follow-up.[57] Although no patient experienced a dysrhythmia or had electrocardiographic evidence of ischemia, four patients were found to have a shortening fraction less than 28%. Based on the finding of a decreased maximal cardiac index and a normal peak heart rate, the authors concluded that this provided evidence of long-standing subclinical cardiac dysfunction in this patient population. In a long-term follow-up (median = 12 years) of 204 pediatric allogeneic HCT patients, the most common cardiovascular complications were hypertension (7%) and left ventricular dysfunction (3%).[51]

Despite the relatively low incidence of overt cardiac dysfunction, subclinical cardiac dysfunction appears relatively common in pediatric HCT recipients and may portend a poor outcome. For example, in a case control study of 40 consecutive pediatric HCT patients, HCT patients were found to have similar left ventricular ejection fractions as controls.[58] However, the HCT recipients were found to have significantly decreased rate-corrected velocity of circumferential fiber shortening, mitral inflow E velocity, and mitral septal annular E' velocity. Using speckle tracking echocardiography, HCT patients were also noted to have decreased left ventricular global circumferential systolic strain, strain rate, circumferential diastolic strain rate, and longitudinal diastolic strain rate. Also, pericardial effusion, which has been reported to occur in approximately 17% of pediatric HCT recipients, is asymptomatic in approximately half of the cases and is rarely the proximal cause of death.[40] Despite that observation, HCT patients with a pericardial effusion have a significantly increased risk of mortality. A pretransplant prolonged corrected QT dispersion may help identify patients at risk for a pericardial effusion.[40,59] In another report, 100 pediatric HCT patients underwent a routine, scheduled echocardiogram at day +7.[46] At least one abnormality was noted in 30% of the children, most commonly a pericardial effusion or an elevated estimated right ventricular pressure. Survival was decreased in children with any abnormality detected. In addition to echocardiography and electrocardiography, biomarkers may also identify patients at risk for cardiac dysfunction. Elevations in NT-proBNP concentrations at day 14 after stem cell transplant can identify patients at risk of developing cardiac events during the first 6 months after HCT.[60,61]

In summary, cardiac toxicity appears to be an uncommon, although serious, complication following HCT. It may present as an acute finding in the immediate posttransplant period with evidence of progressive heart failure, dysrhythmias, and pericardial effusions with tamponade. Late cardiovascular complications are also being studied. Although clinically evident late cardiac complications are being reported, there appears to be a number of subclinical findings detected by use of more involved testing. The importance of these subclinical findings is likely to be better understood as these children age further.

Pulmonary Complications

The incidence of HCT-related pulmonary complications in children is reported between 12% and 25%.[62,63] The need for mechanical ventilation support is the most frequent reason for admission of HCT patients to the PICU.[24,31] Pulmonary complications can be divided into early and late complications (Table 95.2). Early complications occur within the first 100 days after transplant. The division into early and late complications is not absolute but may help the clinician in developing a differential diagnosis. Early complications include infection, peri-engraftment respiratory distress syndrome (PERDS), pulmonary cytolytic thrombi (PCT), diffuse alveolar hemorrhage (DAH), and idiopathic pneumonia syndrome.[64] Late-onset complications occur beyond 3 months after HPCT and include bronchiolitis obliterans (BO), bronchiolitis obliterans organizing pneumonia (BOOP), and idiopathic pneumonia syndrome (IPS).[65]

Early Pulmonary Complications
Periengraftment Respiratory Distress Syndrome
Periengraftment respiratory distress syndrome (PERDS) occurs just as patients begin to show signs of neutrophil recovery. This syndrome is likely caused by pulmonary leukoagglutination and inflammatory cytokines. Patients may develop fever, rash, fluid retention, capillary leak, and pulmonary edema. In severe cases patients can develop multiorgan involvement.[66] Engraftment syndrome may be related to a graft-versus-host response or in some cases a host-versus-graft response. In mild cases no treatment is necessary.[66] In more severe cases, particularly if there is lung involvement, corticosteroids can be beneficial.[66-68] Survival from PERDS is quite good in comparison to other pulmonary complications of HCT, in excess of 90%.[69]

Pulmonary Cytolytic Thrombi
Pulmonary cytolytic thrombi (PCT) is a rare pulmonary complication of HCT. It was first described in a small case series of 13 patients published in 2000.[70] Patients in this series presented with fever at a median of 72 days after HCT (range, 8–343 days). Two of the 13 patients also had a cough at presentation. Chest CT performed on these patients revealed pulmonary nodules. Pathologic exam showed necrosis and basophilic thromboemboli in the nodules. Immunohistochemical staining showed the nodules to contain entrapped leukocytes and disrupted endothelium.

Further publications of PCT describe the pulmonary nodules seen on CT as being bilateral and located primarily in the periphery, subpleural, and basilar areas of the lungs.[71] Further investigation of pathologic samples discovered the leukocytes to be monocytes[72] and described the lung parenchyma adjacent to the nodules to often be infarcted, likely secondary to entrapped debris in surrounding vessels.[71] PCT seems to be responsive to treatment with cyclosporine and corticosteroids. Both radiologic and clinical improvement may be seen within 1 to 2 weeks of beginning treatment.[70,73] Development of PCT in leukemia patients undergoing HCT may be associated with the benefit of decreased risk of relapse.[71]

Diffuse Alveolar Hemorrhage
Alveolar hemorrhage may be infectious or noninfectious in etiology. However, the term *DAH* in an HCT patient generally refers to a noninfectious etiology. The reported incidence ranges from 1% to 21% of HCT patients, with the highest incidence seeming to be in patients with mucopolysaccharide storage diseases.[74,75] It usually occurs in the early posttransplant period and is characterized by widespread alveolar injury, absence of infection, and progressively bloodier return of bronchoalveolar lavage fluid during bronchoscopy.[76] Patients commonly present with respiratory distress and fever and less commonly have hemoptysis.[76] It can occur in both

TABLE 95.2	Pulmonary Complications of Hematopoietic Progenitor Cell Transplantation	
Complications	**Characteristics**	**Treatment**
Early-Onset Pulmonary Complications		
Infection	Positive test for infection	Antimicrobials
Diffuse alveolar hemorrhage	Progressive bloody return on BAL	Corticosteroids, FFP, plasmapheresis
Idiopathic pneumonia syndrome	Diffuse noninfectious lung injury	Etanercept
Engraftment syndrome	Periengraftment pulmonary edema	Corticosteroids
Late-Onset Pulmonary Complications		
Bronchiolitis obliterans	Obstructive lung disease	Corticosteroids, macrolides
Bronchiolitis obliterans organizing pneumonitis	Restrictive lung disease	Corticosteroids
Idiopathic pneumonia syndrome	Diffuse noninfectious lung injury	Etanercept
Pulmonary venoocclusive disease	Pulmonary hypertension	Sildenafil, prostacyclin, defibrotide

BAL, bronchoalveolar lavage; *FFP,* fresh frozen plasma.

autologous and allogeneic transplants.[76] The exact etiology of DAH is unknown, but like other noninfectious pulmonary complications it is associated with GVHD and engraftment.[77-79] Endothelial injuries from chemotherapy and radiation, inflammation, undiagnosed infections, and immune-mediated damage related to GVHD have all been postulated as the cause.[76,78]

Successful use of high-dose corticosteroids has been reported in case reports of DAH.[76,80] However, no prospective studies have proved the benefit of this therapy.[76,78] Despite this observation, they remain standard of care for DAH. Fresh frozen plasma transfusions and plasmapheresis have been tried but are of uncertain benefit.[76] Recombinant factor VIIa has been used for refractory bleeding in these patients[81] but has not been shown to have an impact on survival.[82] Aminocaproic acid used in conjunction with corticosteroids has been described in a series of eight patients with DAH refractory to corticosteroids. The overall 100-day mortality for these eight patients was 44%, an improvement over those treated with corticosteroids alone where the 100-day mortality was 83%.[83]

Idiopathic Pneumonia Syndrome

The incidence of IPS in pediatric HCT patients has been reported to be between 2% and 15%.[63,65,84-86] IPS is usually considered an early complication of transplant, but it has also been described as a late complication. The diagnosis is made by meeting the diagnostic criteria set by an expert panel convened by the National Institutes of Health (NIH) in 1993. Patients must show evidence of widespread lung injury as confirmed radiographically by bilateral lung disease, signs and symptoms of pneumonia (cough, dyspnea, or rales), abnormal lung function (increased alveolar to arterial oxygen gradient, pulmonary function testing with restrictive lung disease), and the absence of an infectious etiology.[87]

The term *IPS* is often used interchangeably with idiopathic pneumonitis and interstitial pneumonitis in the literature. However, interstitial pneumonitis is the histopathologic description in some cases of IPS. Other cases of IPS will show histopathologic findings consistent with DAH or BOOP.[87] IPS, interstitial pneumonitis, DAH, BOOP, and BOS are all considered noninfectious pulmonary complications of transplant. As prevention and treatment of infectious pulmonary complications have improved, these noninfectious complications are now the more troublesome.[88]

The literature continues to be confusing regarding the nomenclature of these noninfectious pulmonary complications of transplant. It is important for the critical care physician at the bedside to treat his or her patient appropriately without becoming anguished over the particular name of the disease. Though corticosteroids and etanercept, a tumor necrosis factor-alpha (TNFα) receptor antagonist, may prove to be beneficial in some cases, at the present time there is no definitive treatment for any of the noninfectious pulmonary complications. Therefore providing excellent supportive care in the ICU by paying close attention to fluid balance and utilizing lung protective strategies during mechanical ventilation are likely the most important aspects of care we can provide.

Inflammation plays a significant role in the development of IPS. GVHD is known to be associated with high levels of inflammatory cytokines. GVHD has consistently been shown to be associated with IPS.[65,84,89] Because of this association, there is debate in the literature as to whether IPS actually represents GVHD of the lung.[87] However, the histopathology of IPS often does not resemble that of acute GVHD, which typically involves epithelial cell apoptosis.[85]

In the mouse models of IPS when TNFα knockout mice are used as recipients, the mice develop IPS like wild-type mice. However, when TNFα knockout mice are used as donors for wild-type recipients, the severity of IPS is significantly less. In this model, TNFα is derived from donor T cells.[90] This animal model fits the clinical observation that patients who receive T-cell–depleted grafts have a lower incidence of pulmonary complications.[91,92]

Some cases of IPS may be caused by an unidentified infection. A retrospective study of stored BAL samples from HCT patients with pulmonary complications detected human metapneumovirus in 5 (3%) of 163 patients. Three of the 5 patients were diagnosed with IPS. On review of these patients' medical records, they initially presented in the first 40 days after transplant with typical upper respiratory symptoms: fever, cough, nasal congestion, and sore throat. Four of the five patients died of rapidly progressive acute respiratory failure. Three of the 5 had DAH.[93]

Because of the role of inflammation in IPS, corticosteroids have been used as therapy but have not been shown to be universally efficacious.[65,94] Therefore because TNFα has been shown to be an important mediator in mouse models of IPS, the soluble TNFα-binding protein, etanercept, has been used. Etanercept showed promise in an early phase I/II trial when given with systemic corticosteroids to patients with IPS. Ten of 15 patients treated on the protocol were able to be weaned from supplemental oxygen.[95] A retrospective study comparing etanercept and corticosteroids versus corticosteroids alone showed improved survival in the patients receiving etanercept.[96] These promising results lead to a phase II trial of etanercept in pediatric IPS patients. These results were also encouraging with a response rate of 71%, 28-day survival of 89%, and 1-year survival of 63%.[97] These results were in contrast, however, to the parallel adult study where the 1-year survival was <25%.[98] There were significant transplant-related differences between the adult and pediatric patients that could explain the differences in outcomes. The adult patients were also much less compliant with the etanercept dosing in comparison to the pediatric patients.[85]

Continuous venovenous hemofiltration has also been used in patients with acute lung injury after chemotherapy and HCT (see also Chapter 78). In a series of 10 patients, 7 had a noninfectious lung injury. Four of these 7 were HCT patients. All patients were mechanically ventilated and met criteria for ARDS. Three of the four HCT patients with noninfectious lung injury survived to extubation.[99]

Lung transplantation has been reported in children who have developed chronic respiratory failure as a complication of HCT in multiple case series in the literature.[100-104] Of the patients reported, survival appears to be comparable to lung transplantation in the general populations. Therefore this may be an appropriate option in select patients.

Calfactant (calf lung–derived surfactant) may play a role in the treatment of acute lung injury after HCT. A post-hoc analysis of a multicenter trial of calfactant in mechanically ventilated pediatric patients with acute lung injury showed possible benefit in the subgroup of immunocompromised patients. Twenty-seven of the 52 immunocompromised patients analyzed had undergone HCT. In this subgroup analysis, patients who received calfactant had a 50% mortality rate, whereas those receiving placebo had a 60% mortality rate.[105] A trial of calfactant in pediatric patients with acute lung injury with leukemia, lymphoma, or history of HCT is currently under way.

Extracorporeal membrane oxygenation (ECMO) has infrequently been used as a heroic measure for HCT patients with severe lung injury. In reviews of the Extracorporeal Life Support Organization (ELSO) database published in 2008, there were no ECMO survivors with a history of recent HCT.[106] However, there was one case report in the literature of an 8-month-old girl with severe combined immunodeficiencies who was transplanted while symptomatic with bronchiolitis. ECMO was used successfully as a bridge to engraftment.[107] A review of the ELSO database reported 3 survivors to hospital discharge of the 29 pediatric HCT patients who received ECMO support after HCT.[108] The authors of this report concluded that although outcomes of ECMO in HCT patients are poor, it should be considered in select patients who received HCT for a nonmalignant condition or a malignancy with a low risk of relapse.

Late Pulmonary Complications
Bronchiolitis Obliterans Syndrome/Bronchiolitis Obliterans Organizing Pneumonia

Bronchiolitis obliterans syndrome (BOS) and BOOP are late-onset noninfectious pulmonary complications of HCT. Both of these complications are associated with chronic graft-versus-host disease and are much more commonly seen after allogeneic transplant as opposed to autologous transplant.[92,109,110] The NIH developed consensus criteria for BOS in 2005, with a proposed amendment in 2009, to facilitate communication in the literature. The amended criteria include (1) absence of an infectious etiology, (2) evidence of chronic GVHD at another site, (3) forced expiratory volume <75% predicted or a decline of >10% from previous, and (4) forced expiratory volume in 1 sec/forced expiratory vital capacity <0.7 or residual volume/total lung capacity >120% and computerized tomography findings of air trapping or bronchiectasis.[110]

The pathophysiology of BOS likely involves donor T cells causing an immune-mediated injury to lung epithelial cells. This injury then causes the release of inflammatory mediators leading to fibroblast migration, smooth muscle cell proliferation, and eventual deposition of collagen and fibrin in the airway lumens.[110] Risk factors for the development of BOS include busulfan conditioning,[111] allogeneic transplant,[110] recurrent pulmonary infections,[112] and chronic graft-versus-host disease.[113-115]

Patients with BOS typically present 6 to 12 months after HCT, are afebrile, and have nonspecific symptoms such as a nonproductive cough and exertional dyspnea.[110] They may have a history of recurrent respiratory infections and graft-versus-host disease. Radiographic findings, pulmonary function testing, and pathology findings from lung biopsy are used to make the diagnosis.[110] Patients with BOS have an obstructive pattern on pulmonary function testing. On high-resolution chest computed tomography (CT) both high and low attenuation areas are seen, as are bronchial dilatation, bronchial thickening, vascular attenuation, and expiratory air trapping. Biopsy specimens show submucosal bronchiolar fibrosis and luminal narrowing and obliteration.[109]

BOOP is also known as cryptogenic organizing pneumonia. Patients with BOOP may present 2 to 6 months after HCT,

which is earlier than BOS.[110] They also tend to present more acutely than patients with BOS, presenting with fever, cough, dyspnea, and rales.[110] Patients with BOOP have patchy air space disease on chest radiograph. High-resolution chest CT shows ground-glass opacifications, areas of consolidation, and pulmonary nodules.[109] As opposed to patients with BOS, pulmonary function testing in BOOP shows a restrictive lung disease pattern. Biopsy specimens of BOOP show granulation tissue in the distal airways, alveolar ducts, and peribronchial alveolar space.[88,116] Similar to BOS, the pathophysiology seems to involve T cells and inflammatory cytokines leading to alveolar epithelial cell injury.[110]

For both BOS and BOOP it is recommended that patients undergo bronchial alveolar lavage to rule out infection. BOS may be diagnosed on clinical grounds to avoid open lung biopsy and its associated risks. The diagnosis of BOOP generally requires biopsy. However, a transbronchial specimen is often sufficient.[109]

The number of patients with BOS or BOOP reported in the literature is small. Therefore it is difficult to make firm recommendations regarding treatment or prognosis. BOOP seems to have a better prognosis than BOS and may be reversible, whereas the goal of therapy in BOS is stabilization of disease. It is thought that making the diagnosis early in order to begin therapy when the disease is less severe may be of benefit. Therefore serial pulmonary function tests are currently recommended in HCT patients at risk for pulmonary complications.[113] BOS and BOOP may respond better to corticosteroids than other noninfectious pulmonary complications of HCT.[65,88] First-line therapy for these complications remains a systemic corticosteroids burst with a prolonged taper over several months. There may be some role for combination therapy with inhaled fluticasone, azithromycin, and montelukast to enable a decrease in the dose of systemic corticosteroids.[110] Macrolide therapy may benefit patients with BOS after HCT but requires further study.[117] Other therapies such as inhaled cyclosporine, etanercept, infliximab, and extracorporeal photochemotherapy have been described in case reports for BOS and require further study.[109]

Pulmonary Veno-occlusive Disease

Case reports of pulmonary veno-occlusive disease (PVOD) in HCT patients have been infrequently described. Patients have presented both early and late after HCT with increasing dyspnea and signs of right heart failure. Cardiomegaly and pulmonary edema are seen on chest x-ray. Pulmonary hypertension is seen on echocardiogram. In patients who have undergone cardiac catheterization, high right atrial pressure, right ventricular pressure, and pulmonary artery pressures are seen, whereas the pulmonary artery wedge pressure is frequently normal. Pathologic specimens show fibrosis of the venules and small pulmonary veins, whereas the larger pulmonary veins are typically normal. Because the resistance to flow in the pulmonary veins is typically normal in PVOD, the pulmonary artery wedge pressure appears normal despite having increased resistance through pulmonary venules and small pulmonary veins. Pulmonary arterial intimal fibrosis and hypertrophy may also be seen.[48,118] Pulmonary function testing (PFT) is normal for forced expiratory lung volume, functional vital capacity, and total lung capacity, but carbon monoxide diffusing capacity is typically <50%.[119]

Lung biopsy has historically been the gold standard for diagnosis for PVOD; however, this procedure carries a high risk of complication. Mineo and coworkers reported that the presence of two of three characteristic CT findings (ground glass appearance, septal thickening, and mediastinal lymphadenopathy) was able to diagnose PVOD with 95.5% sensitivity and 89% specificity.[119] Therefore clinical suspicion, PFT, and CT findings may be sufficient to make the diagnosis. There may be a genetic predisposition to PVOD as abnormalities in the bone morphogenetic receptor type II are reported in both PVOD and pulmonary hypertension patients.[110] Corticosteroids, other immunosuppressive agents, and anticoagulation have been used without notable benefit. Sildenafil with prostacyclin has been reported to be of some benefit in treating the pulmonary hypertension. However, these should be used with caution as they may make some patients worse by causing an increase in pulmonary edema.[110] Theoretically, defibrotide may be beneficial given its efficacy in hepatic veno-occlusive disease (VOD), but there are no available reports of its use in patients with pulmonary VOD.[48,118]

Dilemmas in the Diagnosis of Pulmonary Complications

As HCT patients with pulmonary complications are frequently tenuous, placing these patients at risk for complications from diagnostic procedures is a difficult decision. Although it is difficult to treat these critically ill patients without a firm diagnosis, it is also unpalatable to worsen the patient's condition while performing a diagnostic procedure that does not result in a diagnosis. Therefore the debate continues in the literature and at the bedside regarding the risk/benefit ratio of invasive diagnostic procedures such as bronchial alveolar lavage (BAL) and lung biopsy.

St. Jude Children's Hospital published data regarding the diagnostic yield of BAL at the institution.[120] BAL identified the cause of respiratory symptoms in 53 (67.9%) of 78 allogeneic patients and 7 (63%) of 11 autologous patients. The most common finding diagnosed on BAL was bacterial infection (52%). The patients tolerated the procedure well with complications noted in less than 20%. In this series, transbronchial biopsy added information in only 2 of 7 patients. The researchers also noted that 14 of 16 patients who underwent open-lung biopsy already had a positive BAL. The authors concluded that BAL had a beneficial risk/benefit profile and was useful in identifying patients who had an infectious etiology to their lung injury. However, biopsy did not add significantly more information but carried an unacceptable morbidity rate of 47%.

A meta-analysis including 72 studies of BAL and 31 studies of lung biopsy in both pediatric and adult patients found that BAL was superior to lung biopsy for diagnosing an infectious etiology of lung injury, whereas lung biopsy was superior for diagnosing noninfectious lung injury.[121] Either technique led to a diagnosis in over 50% of procedures. Complications were reported at 8% for BAL and 15% for biopsy. Complications of lung biopsy were higher in children than adults (p = .003). It was also noted that the addition of BAL galactomannan significantly improved the ability to detect invasive fungal infections. The authors concluded that a reasonable approach was to begin the diagnostic workup with BAL, particularly if infection was suspected, and proceed to biopsy if a noninfectious etiology became more suspect.

Hepatic Complications

Hepatic complications of hematopoietic cell transplantation have been a common cause of morbidity and mortality

since the inception of the procedure.[122-126] The complications include hepatic infections (viral, fungal, and bacterial), cholestasis, drug toxicity, sinusoidal obstruction syndrome (SOS) (which is more commonly known as veno-occlusive disease [VOD]), and GVHD. HCT patients may also have an underlying liver disease going into HCT such as tumor infiltration, chronic hepatitis, iron overload, or extramedullary hematopoiesis.[122,126-128]

Viral hepatitis can be caused by any viral pathogen, including hepatitis C, cytomegalovirus (CMV), Epstein-Barr virus (EBV), hepatitis B, adenovirus, herpes simplex, and varicella zoster. The diagnosis of these pathogens is based on clinical manifestations, with identification of the virus determined (1) histologically, (2) by culture of blood or tissue, or (3) by the presence of viral antigen or nucleic acid within serum or liver tissue. Treatment is dependent on identification of the viral pathogen. Herpes simplex and varicella zoster are treated with acyclovir, whereas CMV is treated with ganciclovir or foscarnet. Epstein-Barr virus–induced donor lymphocytes have been used to treat Epstein-Barr virus–associated lymphoproliferative disorders after allogeneic bone marrow transplantation.[129]

Fungal involvement of the liver is often seen in conjunction with widespread dissemination. There may be granulomas, abscesses, cysts, fungus in biliary ducts, or infarcts from vascular occlusion. Typically, *Candida* species are seen; however, any fungal pathogen can occur. Fungal infection often presents with right upper quadrant abdominal pain. Workup then discovers positive serum tests for fungal antigens or DNA, radiologic findings of fungal infection, and, if necessary, histology (including special stains).[127,130] If there is a suspicion of active infection in the liver, liposomal amphotericin, voriconazole, or caspofungin should be given until engraftment is established.[127,131] Bacterial infections of the liver occur less commonly but present similarly.

Gallbladder stones from poor oral intake, cytoreductive therapy causing exfoliation of gallbladder mucous-containing cells, and increased biliary excretion of precipitable material (cyclosporine A [CSA], antibiotics) all contribute to a 70% incidence of gallbladder sludge.[132,133] Sepsis can also lead to cholestasis and hyperbilirubinemia. This is mediated by endotoxins, interleukin 6 (IL-6) and TNFα.[127,134] Rarely, persistent biliary obstruction can be caused by lymphoproliferation from EBV or CMV-related biliary disease, duodenal hematoma as a complication of endoscopy, inspissated biliary sludge, or leukemic relapse in the head of pancreas.[127,135] Numerous medications required for HCT can have direct toxicity on the liver, including antibiotics, fluconazole, and CSA. Histologically, drug effect should be suspected when there is significant hepatocellular necrosis and minimal inflammation.

Veno-occlusive disease (VOD) after allogeneic HCT was first reported in 1979[136] and now is recognized as a major cause of morbidity and mortality in the first 100 days of transplant. The disease process begins in the sinusoids due to endothelial injury and affects venules only late in the course of the disease.[127] The pathogenesis is believed to result from hepatic venule and sinusoidal endothelial injury.[137] Histologically, subendothelial edema, endothelial cell damage with microthrombosis, fibrin deposition, and expression of factor VIII and von Willebrand factor within venular walls are seen.[138] Hepatic necrosis occurs, and collagen deposition in the sinusoids, venular wall sclerosis, and collagen deposition in the venular lumen are seen as the disease progresses.[139] Risk factors can include elevated transaminases before the conditioning regimen,[140-142] age <6 to 7 years,[143] use of methotrexate for GVHD prophylaxis,[144] presence of oral mucositis,[145] interstitial pneumonitis,[146] or transfusional iron overload.[147] Certain preparative regimens have also been found to have a higher incidence of VOD, including those with high doses of total body irradiation, cyclophosphamide, or the combination of busulfan and cyclophosphamide, or etoposide and carboplatin.[141,142,148,149] A trial of adults undergoing HCT using everolimus and sirolimus for GVHD prophylaxis was terminated prematurely because of an unacceptably high rate of severe VOD and thrombotic microangiopathy.[150] The authors felt that busulfan use in conditioning may have been a contributing factor.

Clinically, VOD presents with hyperbilirubinemia, painful hepatomegaly, and fluid retention. The incidence varies based on risk factors and the criteria used but reportedly are as high as 55%,[140] with mortality rates ranging from 3% to 67%.[151] Significant variability in mortality results from differing conditioning regimens and definitions of VOD. Two sets of criteria have been used for VOD. Jones and associates[141] first described VOD and modified this criterion as hyperbilirubinemia greater than 2 mg/dL within 21 days of transplant with at least two of three other findings: hepatomegaly, ascites, or 5% or greater weight gain. McDonald and colleagues[140] in Seattle defined VOD in their series as two of the following criteria occurring within 20 days of transplant: hyperbilirubinemia greater than 2 mg/dL, hepatomegaly or right upper quadrant pain, or sudden weight gain greater than 2% of body weight. Clinically, most patients with VOD develop symptoms between days 6 and 7 after transplant, peak around 10 days after onset, and return to baseline 10 days later if they are going to recover.[141] Multiorgan failure is seen more frequently in patients with VOD.[140,142] Pulmonary dysfunction, pleural effusions, hepatorenal syndrome, sodium retention with subsequent edema, and congestive heart failure all can occur and contribute to the high mortality rate. Liver ultrasound with Doppler study showing reversal of portal flow is a late finding in VOD[143] but is not part of the diagnostic criteria. Liver biopsy can be performed to diagnose VOD, but it is recommended that it be reserved for patients in who the diagnosis is uncertain and other diagnoses must be excluded such as hepatic GVHD.[152]

In some patients it is difficult to differentiate between VOD and hepatic GVHD, and more invasive procedures are needed. Transvenous liver biopsy and hepatic venous pressure gradient measurements can be performed safely[153] and have been found in a limited setting to have predictive value, with a hepatic venous pressure gradient greater than 30 mm Hg associated with poor outcome.[154] Hepatic venous pressure gradient levels greater than 10 mm Hg have been shown to be highly specific for diagnosis of VOD.[155,156]

Given that the pathogenesis of VOD is thought to involve endothelial injury and coagulation factor deposition, attempts have been made to reduce the hypercoagulable state with several agents, including heparin, prostaglandin, and bile salts. A systematic review and meta-analysis by Imran and coworkers[157] evaluated 12 studies using low-molecular-weight heparin or unfractionated heparin as prophylaxis for VOD and found that the decrease in risk of VOD was statistically not significant. A prospective study compared antithrombin III in 91 children to 71 historic controls and reported no significant difference in the incidence between the two groups.[158] Ursodiol in historical studies and randomized trials has been shown to cause mild to moderate reduction in VOD occurrence.[159,160] More promising is the use of defibrotide for prophylaxis, and several studies have been published describing its efficacy.[161-163] A phase 3 randomized controlled, multicenter trial published in 2012 showed a lower incidence of VOD (12% versus 20% p value of 0.05) and VOD-associated renal failure with no difference in the risk of hemorrhagic events.[164] The joint working group by the hemato-oncology subgroup of the British Committee Standards in Hematology (BCSH) and the British Society for Blood and Marrow Transplantation (BSBMT) published guidelines in 2013 recommending (strength 1A) the use of defibrotide for the prevention of VOD in children with specific preexisting risk factors.

N-acetylcysteine, a thiol antioxidant, and nitric oxide have been tried in anecdotal reports as treatment for VOD.[165,166] Thrombolytic therapy with recombinant tissue plasminogen activator has been used successfully.[167,168] However, this is accompanied by the risk of bleeding, with one of these studies reporting an 88% incidence of bleeding and 28% incidence of severe bleeding.[167] Defibrotide has been evaluated in phase II trials showing 30% to 60% remission rates, even in patients with severe VOD.[169] A multicenter prospective study of 333 patients published as an online abstract showed a statistically improved outcome in complete response to defibrotide treatment (29% versus 9%, p = 0.0019) and D+100 survival (49% versus 25%, p = 0.0016) compared with historical controls (303 subjects had received HCT, whereas 28 were non-HCT patients who developed VOD). There was an 18% incidence of bleeding with a 2% incidence of life-threatening hemorrhage with defibrotide therapy in these patients. Due to the risk of hemorrhage, defibrotide therapy requires close monitoring.[170] There is currently a multicenter study in the United States of defibrotide for patients diagnosed with VOD. The study is titled "Defibrotide for Patients with Hepatic Venoocclusive Disease: A Treatment IND Study."[171] Defibrotide is no longer available in the United States for compassionate use. Further work is required to investigate the optimal dose and route in the treatment of these patients. The joint working group by BCSH/BSBMT also recommended the use of defibrotide in treatment of VOD in children (strength 1B).[152] Supportive treatment for fluid retention and multiorgan failure is an important part of management of these patients.

Colitis and Other Gastrointestinal Complications

Gastrointestinal (GI) complications that arise after transplantation often result from mucosal damage secondary to radiotherapy and chemotherapy regimens, together with immunosuppression following transplant.[172] Upper GI complications include diffuse mucositis, nausea, vomiting, and nonspecific abdominal pain. Barker and colleagues reported a 90.1% incidence of mucositis and an 85.2% incidence of posttransplant vomiting in a retrospective study of 142 patients who underwent HCT.

Lower GI/intestinal acute complications include *C. difficile* colitis, viral and other gastroenteritis, typhlitis, intestinal GVHD, and intestinal thrombotic microangiopathy.[173] In this case series, *C. difficile* colitis was seen in 8.5% of patients, viral enteritis in 7.0%, typhlitis in 3.5%, and intestinal GVHD in

27.4%.[173] The incidence of typhlitis in this series was much lower than the 32% incidence previously reported in the literature for AML patients.[174]

Viruses such as CMV, adenoviruses, and rotaviruses can cause diarrhea in the immediate posttransplant period. Imaging findings include nonspecific bowel wall thickening, ascites, and adjacent inflammatory change especially in the ileocecal region.[172]

Neutropenic enterocolitis or typhlitis is a necrotizing inflammation of the colon in an immunocompromised patient. There is a predilection for the cecum, thought to be due to the marked distensibility of the cecum along with lower vascularity. The clinical manifestations are a triad of abdominal pain/tenderness, fever, and neutropenia.[172] The incidence of typhlitis can vary depending on the aggressiveness of chemotherapy and prophylactic antibiotics used.[175] The typical time frame to be diagnosed with typhlitis, after HCT, appears to be around 15.5 ± 7 days.[175] Plain x-ray or ultrasounds of the abdomen appear to be good initial imaging modalities. CT scan can be utilized if the diagnosis is questionable with initial imaging. Plain x-ray of the abdomen will likely show dilation of small bowel loops with a paucity of gas in the right side of the abdomen. In advanced cases with perforation, one may see free intraabdominal air. Ultrasound of the abdomen will likely show asymmetric, echogenic wall thickening of the cecum and terminal ileum. If utilized, CT will show luminal narrowing and stranding in the pericecal fat.[172] Management includes bowel rest, antibiotic coverage to include gram-negative organisms, G-CSF to treat neutropenia, and providing optimal parenteral nutrition. Consideration for antifungals should be considered if there is no clinical improvement on initiation of antibiotics. Persistent GI bleeding despite resolution of neutropenia and coagulopathy, evidence of perforation with peritonitis, and uncontrolled sepsis are potential surgical indications.[174]

Pneumatosis intestinalis can be seen in typhlitis, in which case it implies imminent bowel perforation.[172] Corticosteroid therapy appears to be a significant factor, inducing atrophy of the Peyer patches in the intestine with resultant mucosal defects and dissection of intraluminal air into the submucosal or subserosal regions. If detected in an asymptomatic patient it will most often be resolved with conservative management.[172,176]

Intestinal acute GVHD usually develops after 3 to 5 weeks and can be accompanied by skin and hepatic GVHD. Chronic GVHD occurs several months after transplantation.[177,178] Symptoms include secretory diarrhea, fever, nausea, vomiting, abdominal pain, and intestinal hemorrhage.[179] CT in addition to nonspecific findings may show bowel wall enhancement correlating with mucosal destruction and replacement with granulation tissue.[172]

Thrombotic microangiopathy (TMA) of intestines can occur after HCT and is caused by intimal injury to the microvasculature followed by formation of microthrombi. The injury is presumed to be due to chemotherapy, total body irradiation or pretransplant conditioning regimen, and the addition of drugs known to be associated with this disease such as tacrolimus and cyclosporine A. This is a rare complication but can mimic GVHD by presenting with fever and refractory diarrhea. Laboratory findings include elevated LDH and fragmented erythrocytes on a peripheral blood smear. Treatment is challenging and often requires removal of the possible offending immunosuppressant medication. Daclizumab has shown some promising results in experimental studies.[180]

Pancreatitis can also be seen in HCT patients. Barker and colleagues reported a 4.9% incidence of pancreatitis. This was not associated with any specific induction chemotherapy regimen.[173] Werlin and associates reported a similar 3.5% incidence of pancreatitis and recommended testing for pancreatitis prior to attributing GI symptoms to mucositis.[181]

Myelosuppression and Hematologic Complications

Myelosuppression and Immune Dysregulation

Stem cell transplant conditioning results in an extended period of neutropenia, anemia, and thrombocytopenia. Neutrophil engraftment is defined as an absolute neutrophil count (ANC) of greater than or equal to $0.5 \times 10^3/\mu L$ on 3 consecutive days following the postconditioning nadir. Neutrophil engraftment typically occurs 2 to 4 weeks following stem cell infusion. The duration of time from stem cell infusion to engraftment depends on numerous transplant-related factors.[182] When peripheral blood progenitor cells are used, engraftment typically occurs 1 to 6 days sooner than when bone marrow is used as the stem cell source.[183] Engraftment occurs slower when umbilical cord blood is used compared to PBSC and bone marrow.[184] Granulocyte stimulating factors are commonly used following autologous HPT and umbilical cord blood transplant to reduce the time to neutrophil engraftment.[185] Platelet engraftment generally occurs 1 to 2 weeks following neutrophil engraftment but can take weeks to months. A platelet count less than 100,000 on day 100 following transplant is associated with poor outcome.[185]

Neutrophil engraftment does not signify the reconstitution of a fully functional immune system. It is crucial to remember that engrafted post-HCT patients remain significantly immunocompromised and are at risk for life-threatening opportunistic infections. The restoration of normal immune function can take as long as a year in patients without significant post-HCT complications and longer in patients with chronic GVHD.[186] Typically, natural killer cell recovery takes approximately 1 month and T-lymphocyte recovery takes 6 to 12 months.[187] Restoration of normal B-cell function takes approximately 3 to 6 months in the absence of GVHD.[188]

Infectious Complications

Patients undergoing HCT have increased susceptibility to infection because of a combination of (1) neutropenia, (2) breakdown of physical barriers (mucositis, indwelling venous catheters, skin lesions), and (3) defects in cellular and humoral immunity as a result of the conditioning regimen and immunosuppressive therapy given. The susceptibility to any particular organism varies according to the stem cell source (for example, umbilical cord blood recipients are at increased risk for viral infection) and over the course of the transplant period. During the first 2 to 4 weeks of the posttransplant period while the patient is neutropenic, bacterial infections account for approximately 90% of the infections. Enteric gram-negative bacilli (eg, *Escherichia coli, Klebsiella, Enterobacter, Pseudomonas aeruginosa*) can cause rapid hemodynamic instability. The gram-positive infections (*Staphylococcus* and *Streptococcus*) are frequent causes of infections when central venous catheters are present. Therefore empiric antibiotic coverage for fevers during this time must be broad spectrum and provide adequate coverage for these organisms.[189-191]

Fungal infections are increasing in frequency with better treatment and prophylaxis of bacterial and viral infections, particularly after allogeneic transplantation. Fungal pathogens in HCT patients include the yeasts (eg, *Candida* spp., *Cryptococcus neoformans*), molds (eg, *Aspergillus, Fusarium, Mucormycosis*), and dimorphic fungi (eg, *Coccidioides, Histoplasma, Blastomyces*). Of these, *Candida* and *Aspergillus* are most common. *Candida* spp. colonize the gastrointestinal tract in more than half of healthy people,[192] but they become opportunistic infections in HCT patients.

Candidal infections can occur as superficial mucosal infections (eg, thrush) or deeply invasive (hepatosplenic candidiasis). Esophageal candidiasis is associated with dysphagia and retrosternal pain. This may be difficult to distinguish from chemotherapy or radiation-induced mucositis or herpetic mucositis. Endoscopy may be necessary to diagnose and appropriately treat. Candidemia may present with fever and systemic symptoms and is frequently not associated with tissue involvement. Because many HCT patients receive fluconazole prophylaxis, candidemia should be treated with amphotericin B. Traditionally, patients with documented candidemia or persistent/recurrent fevers should have undergone evaluation for multiorgan involvement, including CT or magnetic resonance imaging (MRI) of the brain, chest, and abdomen, and an ophthalmologic examination. However, given that more attention is being focused on the radiation risk of CT for the development of future cancers and the improvement in antifungal prophylaxis, the use of abdominal and pelvic CT scans as screening tools (not in cases of documented fungemia) for invasive fungal disease is now being called into question. A quality improvement project from St. Jude Children's Research Hospital showed very low yield of abdominal CT in detecting undiagnosed fungal infections in patients with prolonged fever and neutropenia.[193] The group recommends that routine abdominal CT as a screening tool for invasive fungal disease no longer be performed. Instead they recommend ultrasound or limited MRI in patients with clinical suspicion for invasive fungal disease in the abdomen.

Aspergillus spores are routinely inhaled and in immunocompromised or HCT patients can cause invasive infections. Neutropenia and GVHD with immunosuppressive treatment are risk factors for this. Outbreaks of aspergillus can occur in areas of construction or with contaminated ventilation. Invasive aspergillosis occurs most commonly in the lungs with fever, cough, dyspnea, and ultimately hemoptysis as the disease progresses. The characteristic radiographic appearance is a cavitary lesion, but nodular infiltrates and bronchopneumonia are also seen.[194] BAL should be performed initially. However, up to 50% of patients have a negative BAL, and open-lung biopsy should be considered if suspicion remains after a negative BAL.[195]

CMV is one of the most problematic viral infections for HCT patients posttransplant. CMV may emerge in the allogeneic patient between 1 to 3 months posttransplantation if either the patient or donor was CMV positive before transplant. CMV lays dormant after the initial clinical infection. However, in immunosuppressed patients, this virus can reactivate and result in interstitial pneumonitis, enteritis, encephalitis, retinitis, or bone marrow suppression. CMV infection is defined as the identification of CMV from any site or the

seroconversion to CMV positivity on PCR or antigenemia testing. CMV disease is defined as the clinical manifestations seen in the presence of CMV infection. The use of CMV-negative blood products and leukofiltration of blood products along with routine screening during the first 100 days posttransplant with PCR or antigen testing has helped reduce the risk of CMV infections in patients undergoing transplant. Monitoring of CMV with antigenemia testing and PCR testing is the standard of care for 100 days posttransplant and allows for preemptive therapy if results of these tests become positive before onset of clinically apparent disease. Ganciclovir, valganciclovir, or foscarnet treatment is then given for 7 to 14 days followed by prophylaxis or screening through 100 days posttransplantation.[196] Interstitial pneumonitis from CMV presents with hypoxia and fever and an interstitial pattern on chest x-ray film. Untreated, there is an 80% mortality rate.[197] Ganciclovir and intravenous (IV) immunoglobin are the recommended treatments for CMV interstitial pneumonitis.[198] Ganciclovir is dosed at 10 mg/kg daily for 21 days followed by 5 mg/kg/day 5 days per week until day 180 posttransplantation. IV immunoglobin is given at 500 mg/kg every other day for 21 days, followed by 500 mg/kg weekly until day +180. With this regimen, survival is 80%. For patients resistant to ganciclovir or unacceptable medication toxicity, foscarnet may be given at 60 mg/kg three times daily for 7 days, then 90 mg/kg/day until day +180.[17,199] Ganciclovir can cause neutropenia, and administration of growth factor (eg, G-CSF, granulocyte macrophage–CSF) should be considered if the absolute neutrophil count falls below 1000/uL. If the absolute neutrophil count falls below 500/µL, holding the drug should be considered. In addition, renal adjustment may be necessary, as both ganciclovir and foscarnet can be renal toxic. CMV prophylaxis with ganciclovir is prohibited by its marrow-suppressive effects.

CMV enteropathy presents with dysphagia, abdominal pain, nausea, vomiting, diarrhea, or gastrointestinal bleeding. These symptoms can be seen with GVHD as well, and endoscopy should be performed to aid in the diagnosis. Treatment is similar to that of CMV pneumonia.

EBV, HHV6, herpes simplex virus, adenovirus, varicellazoster virus, human metapneumovirus, and BK virus infections are all common posttransplantation and cause a range of clinic findings including hemorrhagic cystitis, colitis, retinitis, encephalitis, and pneumonitis. The diagnostic and treatment options for each of these viruses and clinical presentations are beyond the scope of this chapter. The reader is referred to multiple published reviews of this topic.[200-204]

Study has focused on the role of adoptive transfer of virus-specific T cells from seropositive donors. Translational and clinical research have focused on the role of this immunotherapeutic approach to the treatment of CMV, EBV, and adenovirus. Broad application of this biotechnology is evolving.[205-207]

Graft Failure

Graft failure is an uncommon, potentially lethal complication of HCT. Primary graft failure is defined as failure of the stem cell graft to recover hematopoietic function by day 30, though some patients successfully engraft later than day 30. Secondary graft failure is the loss of the donor stem cell graft after initial engraftment. The risk of graft failure is increased with HLA-disparity between donor and host, when reduced-intensity conditioning regimens are used, with the use of umbilical cord blood stem cells, and when transplant is performed for a non-malignant hematologic condition.[208] It is rare in HLA-matched sibling donor transplants. Graft failure is treated with the infusion of hematopoietic cells either alone or in combination with growth factors, chemotherapy, or immunosuppression.[209,210] Graft failure is an emergency as the risk of death increases with the duration of neutropenia and because there are few effective therapies.

Hematologic Complications

HCT recipients commonly require frequent blood product transfusions during the acute transplant phase due to conditioning-associated myeloablation and potentially increased consumption of platelets and RBCs. For most patients, the need for blood product transfusions declines rapidly following engraftment and hospital discharge. However, some patients need transfusion support for months after transplant. All blood products should be gamma-irradiated to rid the product of competent donor T-cells that can cause transfusion-associated GVHD.[211] Additionally, blood products must be CMV negative to prevent transmission of the virus to nonimmune patients. This can be achieved by using blood from CMV seronegative donors or with leukofiltration.[212]

There is no commonly accepted standard transfusion parameter for either packed RBCs or platelets (see also Chapter 93). Studies have investigated the use of a platelet transfusion threshold of 10,000. Most studies have found the use of this lower trigger safe for nonbleeding patients, but it is not supported in all studies.[213-216] A Cochrane review of prophylactic transfusion at thresholds of $10 \times 10^3/\mu L$, $20 \times 10^3/\mu L$, and $30 \times 10^3/\mu L$ was reported.[217] The review found no difference in mortality rate or severe bleeding events among the groups. Similar studies are needed to assess the transfusion parameters of RBCs. Although transfusion parameters can be clinically useful, they do not replace clinical judgment.

Donors and recipients who are HLA matched are not necessarily ABO matched. ABO matching is not required for successful transplant and is a secondary consideration when choosing a donor. However, ABO mismatching puts the recipient at risk for immune-mediated hemolytic anemia. The risk for and severity of the potential hemolytic anemia depends on the degree of compatibility and is divided into four groups: (1) ABO-matched; (2) minor ABO mismatch, in which there is potential for hemolysis of the recipient RBCs by donor isoagglutinins (eg, donor blood type O+ and recipient A+); (3) major ABO mismatch, in which case the recipient isoagglutinins are directed against donor RBCs after engraftment (eg, donor blood type A+ and recipient O+); and (4) bidirectional mismatch, which combines minor and major ABO mismatch (eg, donor blood type A+ and recipient blood type B+).[218] When there is a major or bidirectional mismatch, the stem cell product must be RBC depleted or the patient must have the offending isoagglutinins removed by pheresis prior to infusion to prevent a hemolytic reaction. Minor incompatibility, in which the recipients RBCs are incompatible with components of the donor's plasma, puts the recipient at risk for an immune-mediated transfusion reaction. Plasma depletion of the product prior to infusion reduces the risk. Even when plasma depletion is used, mild hemolysis can exist for weeks to months due to antibody production from newly produced B lymphocytes against residual recipient RBCs.

There are many described late hemolytic complications of transplant, and most are uncommon. Autoimmune hemolytic anemias, thrombocytopenia, and neutropenias from post-HCT immune dysregulation can occur months to years after transplant and are typically managed with immune suppression, immune modulation, or IV immunoglobin.

Post-HCT thrombotic microangiopathy (TMA) processes include hemolytic uremic syndrome (HUS) and thrombotic thrombocytopenic purpura (TTP).[219,220] Both are reported with increased frequency in patients who received calcineurin inhibitors as part of their GVHD prophylaxis regimen.

HUS is a potentially life-threatening, uncommon post-HCT complication. It presents with hemolysis and mild to moderate renal dysfunction at a median time of 5 months post-HCT.[221] Patients may also have seizures and hypertension. Many cases of post-HCT HUS gradually self-resolve, although patients may be left with residual renal dysfunction. Post-HCT TTP classically presents earlier than HUS with thrombocytopenia, schistocytes on the peripheral blood smear, and elevated LDH. Endothelial damage from transplant conditioning, GVHD, and calcineurin inhibitors is thought to contribute to the development of post-HCT TTP.[222] It differs from classic TTP of childhood in that ADAMTS13 deficiency is not present.[220,222] Additionally, standard therapies for idiopathic TTP, such as plasma exchange, do not appear to be effective for the treatment of post-HCT treatment. The role of eculizumab in posttransplant TMA is currently investigational, but it may be helpful.[223]

Iron Overload

Iron overload has been recognized as an important transplant complication as well as a risk factor for the development of other transplant-related complications.[224] HCT patients are at risk for increased iron burden due to repeated blood transfusions pre- and post-HCT and disturbed iron metabolism.[224,225] Adverse effects from iron overload may include increased susceptibility to infection, VOD, chronic liver disease, and cardiac dysfunction.[1,161,226] Studies show that iron overload has an adverse impact on survival in patients undergoing HCT for beta-thalassemia major and hematologic malignancies.[225,227,228] However, it is less clear what impact iron overload has on the risk for transplant-related toxicities in patients transplanted for other reasons.[229]

There are multiple ways to diagnose iron overload. Liver biopsy remains the gold standard, but frequently the diagnosis is made with imaging and laboratory studies. The serum ferritin is elevated in iron overload. However, ferritin is a nonspecific marker of inflammation that makes this a sensitive but not specific indicator of iron overload. Serum iron studies are useful adjuncts for diagnosis and are often used when monitoring the efficacy of therapy. MRI can provide a quantification of organ specific iron burden.[230] Phlebotomy is a standard treatment for iron overload.[231,232] However, it may have limited utility given that many patients may be anemic after HCT. Iron chelation is effective but limited by the practical considerations in the case of deferoxamine infusion and potential toxicities of the treatments.[233]

Graft-Versus-Host Disease

GVHD is the most common complication of allogeneic HCT. GVHD develops when donor T lymphocytes respond to proteins on recipient cells.[234] Activated donor T lymphocytes, monocytes, and macrophages trigger a self-propagating cycle of cytokine production and inflammation.[234,235] GVHD was historically categorized by the time of occurrence following transplant, with acute GVHD diagnosed if symptoms developed before day 100 or chronic if the presentation was after day 100. The traditional definitions of acute and chronic GVHD do not fully address the pathophysiology of the diseases and have evolved. The current National Institutes of Health (NIH) consensus recommends classification based on the clinical presentation rather than posttransplant day.[236] This classification recognizes two main categories of GVHD—acute and chronic—each with subcategories. Acute GVHD includes classic acute GVHD that develops within 100 days after transplant and persistent, recurrent, or late-onset acute GVHD that clinically resembles acute GVHD but occurs greater than 100 days after transplantation. Chronic GVHD includes classic chronic GVHD occurring greater than 100 days after HCT with manifestations specific to chronic GVHD and an overlap syndrome, which has features of chronic GVHD and features typical of acute GVHD.[236] A follow-up NIH consensus conference has been convened and further change in definitions may be recommended.

The skin, gastrointestinal tract, and liver are the most common involved systems in acute GVHD. The cutaneous presentation is typically an erythematous maculopapular rash, although there are various possible skin findings. Diffuse bullous lesions with skin sloughing are the most severe manifestations of cutaneous GVHD. Acute gastrointestinal GVHD is characterized by diarrhea that is often bloody, may contain tissue, and is accompanied by severe abdominal pain and cramping. Hepatic acute GVHD typically presents with a cholestatic pattern of elevated bilirubin and alkaline phosphatase. Isolated transaminase elevation is uncommon. Less common presentations of acute GVHD are oral inflammation with possible ulceration and ocular inflammation. Acute GVHD is graded according to severity of the systems involved (Table 95.3).

The clinical presentation of chronic GVHD is more varied. The skin is the most commonly involved system. Patients may have persistent erythematous rash, severely dry skin, atrophy, changes in skin pigmentation, hair loss, or nail changes. The most severe clinical presentation of chronic cutaneous GVHD is sclerodermatous fasciitis. Chronic hepatic GVHD is clinically similar to acute hepatic GVHD. The differential diagnosis includes viral infection, iron overload, and medication toxicity. A liver biopsy can aid diagnosis, but it must be performed with caution in patients with increased bleeding risk.[29]

In 2005, the NIH published a consensus paper defining chronic pulmonary GVHD as (1) biopsy-proved BOS or (2) BOS diagnosed by pulmonary function and radiologic testing in conjunction with chronic GVHD at an extrapulmonary site.[236] There is discussion in the literature that other late pulmonary complications such as BOOP, idiopathic pneumonitis, and late-onset diffuse alveolar hemorrhage may represent varied presentations of chronic GVHD. However, chronic pulmonary GVHD being manifested as anything other than BOS is not yet widely accepted.[110]

Gastrointestinal tract chronic GVHD may present as anorexia, nausea, vomiting, diarrhea, malabsorption, or weight loss. Other manifestations of chronic GVHD are sicca syndrome, oral scarring with salivary gland scarring, fasciitis, immune dysfunction, protein losing renal disease, and

TABLE 95.3	Consensus Criteria for Clinical Staging and Grading of Acute Graft-Versus-Host Disease		
Skin	**Liver**	**Gut**	
Stage			
1	Rash[1] <25% or persistent nausea[2]	Bilirubin 2-3 mg/dL[3]	Diarrhea >500 mL/day[4]
2	Rash 25%-50%	Bilirubin 3-6 mg/dL	Diarrhea >1000 mL/day
3	Rash >50%	Bilirubin 6-15 mg/dL	Diarrhea >1500 mL/day
4	Generalized erythroderma with bullae	Bilirubin >15 mg/dL	Severe abdominal pain with or without ileus
Grade[5]			
I	Stage 1-2	None	None
II	Stage 3 or	Stage 1 or	Stage 1
III	—	Stage 2-3 or	Stage 2-4
IV	Stage 4 or	Stage 4 or	Stage 4[6]

[1]Use rule of nines or burn chart to determine extent of rash.
[2]Persistent nausea with histologic evidence of graft-versus-host disease in the stomach or duodenum.
[3]Range given as total bilirubin. Downgrade one stage if an additional cause of elevated bilirubin can be documented.
[4]Volume of diarrhea applies to adults. For pediatric patients, the volume of diarrhea should be based on body surface area. Downgrade one stage if an additional cause of diarrhea has been documented.
[5]Criteria for grading given as degree of organ involvement required to confer that grade.
[6]Grade IV may include lesser organ involvement with Karnofsky performance status <50%, so patients with stage 4 gut graft-versus-host disease usually are grade IV.
From Przepiorka D, Weisdorf D, Martin P, et al. 1994 consensus conference on acute GVHD grading. Bone Marrow Transplant. 1995;15:825-828.

genitourinary scarring. Immune dysfunction independent of immunosuppressive medications is characteristic of chronic GVHD. Patients with chronic GVHD have abnormal splenic function and often need prophylaxis against encapsulated bacteria.[237]

GVHD prevention regimens differ between institutions and are chosen based on the donor and recipient pairing, underlying disease, stem cell source, recipient comorbidities, conditioning regimen used, and potential stem cell manipulation. Agents commonly used for prevention include cyclosporine, tacrolimus, methotrexate, rapamycin, mycophenolate mofetil, and corticosteroids. Depletion of the T-cell component of the stem cell graft effectively eliminates the risk of GVHD.

Corticosteroids are the mainstay of treatment for GVHD. Other upfront treatments that specifically target affected systems are oral dexamethasone and tacrolimus rinses and corticosteroid or tacrolimus topical therapies. There are many available second-line agents and treatment strategies for corticosteroid refractory GVHD, but none are considered standard. The choice of second-line therapy depends on the individual clinical situation. Due to prolonged treatment with corticosteroid, some patients with chronic GVHD are adrenally insufficient. When a patient with chronic GVHD needs intensive care, one should consider the use of stress dose hydrocortisone.

Neurologic Complications

Neurologic complications contribute significantly to the morbidity and mortality following HCT and are more common following HCT than in nontransplant oncology patients.[45,181,238,239] Seizures appear to be the most common clinical manifestation following HCT, occurring in approximately half of the reported cases of neurologic complications.[181,238] Other symptoms include encephalopathy, motor function deficits, cranial nerve palsies, visual disturbances, and impaired coordination.[45,181,238,239] In one account, encephalopathy was reported in 26 (6.4%) of 405 pediatric patients following allogeneic HCT.[239] In that report, the encephalopathy developed within the first 100 posttransplant days in all but one patient. Leukoencephalopathy was commonly reported in that study and others.[181,239-241]

Leukoencephalopathy primarily occurs in HCT patients who receive cranial radiation or intrathecal chemotherapy before and after transplantation. Clinically, this condition manifests days to months after transplantation and may present with dysarthria, ataxia, dysphasia, confusion, or decreased sensorium in severe cases. The white matter changes can be detected with either CT or MRI. Peripheral nervous system neurotoxicity also occurs posttransplantation as an immune-mediated complication. Inflammatory degenerating polyneuropathy, myasthenia gravis, and polymyositis have all been described posttransplant.[242-244] These conditions present with muscle flaccidity, hypoactive deep tendon reflexes, and absence of extensor plantar reflexes.

Depending on the complications assessed, the length of follow-up time, and the patient population studied, clinical analyses report a wide range of neurologic complications in pediatric HCT patients with more recent studies reporting a range of 10% to 24%.[45,181,239,240,245,246] However, an autopsy study of both children and adults (age range, 1 to 48 years; average, 23.7 years) demonstrated neuropathologic abnormalities in more than 90% of patients who died after HCT.[247] In one pediatric report, 11 (10%) of 133 children experienced a life-threatening neurologic complication within the first 3 months following HCT.[245] In a more recent analysis, 40 (24%) of 165 pediatric HCT patients were found to experience neurologic complications.[181] In that study, neurologic complications were categorized as either (1) transient and nonrepetitive symptoms lasting less than 24 hours and without abnormalities on MRI or on CSF analysis or (2) persistent (lasting more than 24 hours) or repetitive symptoms associated with radiographic cerebral imaging or CSF analysis abnormalities. Nineteen (12%) of the 165 patients satisfied the criteria of the second group, approximating the incidence of the earlier study.

In that report, neurologic complications occurred most commonly in children who had undergone unrelated allogeneic transplantation (39%), more than related allogeneic transplants (21%) or autologous transplantations (11%). The finding of neurologic complications occurring more commonly in allogeneic rather than autologous HCT recipients has been previously noted.[240,248,249] These data support the finding that neurologic complications following HCT are related to the presence of GVHD and immunosuppression.[181,240,245,250-252] GVHD and the need for prolonged immunosuppression are clearly associated with many of the etiologies of neurologic complications in this patient population. Common etiologies of neurologic complications in these children include CNS infections, intracranial hemorrhage and stroke, metabolic disturbances, medication toxicity, and CNS involvement of the underlying disease.[181,238,239]

CNS infections are a consequence of neutropenia and immunosuppression. Depending on the time period after transplant, patients may develop bacterial meningitis, aspergillus invasion of the brain parenchyma and vessels, cerebral toxoplasmosis, or viral encephalitis. These CNS infections contribute significantly to the morbidity and mortality following HCT.[253] In addition to the association of GVHD with CNS infections, the medications used to treat GVHD are common causes of neurologic complications in this patient population. Neurotoxicity from CSA or tacrolimus can include tremor, seizures, headaches, cortical blindness, neuropathy, or mental status changes. Frequently, these symptoms are observed with levels above the therapeutic range, but this is not always the case. These effects usually are reversible with elimination of the drug. From 5% to 6% of HCT patients taking CSA may experience seizures.[254,255] Phenytoin, phenobarbital, or carbamazepine, often used to treat seizures, can alter cytochrome P-450 activity and interfere with CSA or tacrolimus levels. Valproic acid or levetiracetam may be a better alternative in this situation.[256-258]

Several chemotherapy agents that may be used in the HCT conditioning regimen can have neurotoxicity. High-dose carmustine, frequently used for autologous transplants for Hodgkin disease or lymphomas, has been associated with seizures. Busulfan, frequently used in allogeneic transplants, can also cause seizures. In fact, phenytoin is often given prophylactically during busulfan administration. Levetiracetam may be a better alternative in this situation as well due to its lack of effect on cytochrome P-450 activity. Through phenytoin's induction of cytochrome P-450, it can alter busulfan metabolism (which is also metabolized through cytochrome P-450) lowering the patient's exposure to busulfan and potentially increasing the risk of relapse.[257,258]

CSA and tacrolimus are associated with the posterior reversible encephalopathy syndrome (PRES) seen in HCT patients.[181] PRES is a clinical entity that presents with headache, mental status changes, visual disturbance, and seizures. Neurologic imaging shows subcortical vasogenic edema preferentially involving the posterior regions of the brain. This syndrome is not unique to HCT patients and can be seen in patients with acute hypertension, preeclampsia, and renal disease (see also Chapter 94).[259] Treatment includes control of blood pressure, management of seizures, and replacement of calcineurin inhibitors such as tacrolimus or CSA with a different class of immunosuppressive agent.[259] If appropriately recognized and promptly treated, the neurologic changes in PRES are reversible. However, it is worth mentioning that this entity can present with life-threatening complications such as cerebral hemorrhages, cerebellar herniation, hydrocephalus, and status epilepticus.[260]

CSA, tacrolimus, and chemotherapeutics may also cause renal wasting of magnesium resulting in hypomagnesemia and lowering of the seizure threshold. In addition to hypomagnesemia, other metabolic abnormalities may occur in this setting, contributing to seizures. Moreover, metabolic derangements resulting in encephalopathy are the most common neurologic complications following HCT with an incidence estimated to be as high as 37%.[261] A more recent pediatric analysis suggests that metabolic derangements remain a significant cause of encephalopathy after HCT but with a much lower incidence (14%) than this earlier study.[239] Hypoxia, ischemia, hepatic failure, electrolyte imbalance, and renal failure have all been found to be etiologies of these metabolic derangements resulting in encephalopathy. Idiopathic hyperammonemia can occur in patients after high-dose chemotherapy used in transplant conditioning regimens. Altered mental status and respiratory alkalosis with elevated plasma ammonia occur acutely. Left untreated, irreversible cerebral edema may result.

Neurovascular complications are not uncommonly reported as neurologic toxicities associated with HCT. Thromboembolic episodes, subdural hemorrhages, and intracerebral hemorrhages are common examples. Thrombotic thrombocytopenic purpura has also been reported as a cause of encephalopathy following pediatric HCT.[239] In one report, 2 (10%) of 21 children with a definitive diagnosis of encephalopathy following HCT were found to have TTP and 1 other (5%) had evidence of a stroke.[239] In that report, 1 (5%) of the 22 children with intracranial imaging was found to have a subdural hematoma, and 2 (10%) were noted to have infarctions. In another report, 2 (11%) of the 19 children with persistent neurologic symptoms (>24 hours) after HCT were diagnosed with intracranial hemorrhage.[181] In a study of patients receiving HCT or conventional chemotherapy alone in a pediatric oncology center, 9 (12%) of the 76 patients who experienced a neurologic complication were found to have a vascular event.[238]

Neurologic complications appear to portend a poor prognosis. Nearly 60% of the children with persistent/repetitive symptoms and either radiographic or cerebrospinal fluid abnormalities following HCT died, more than a third of them as a result of their neurologic complication.[181] In another study of 113 pediatric allogeneic HCT patients, children with a neurologic complication following HCT were significantly more likely to die than those who did not experience such a complication.[245] Thirty-three (32%) of 102 patients without a neurologic complication had died at 6 years of follow-up as compared with 10 (91%) of the 11 patients with a neurologic complication (p < .001). In another study, neurologic complications were also associated with a higher mortality among pediatric HCT patients, but only in the early posttransplant period.[240] Similarly, in the Associazione Italiana Ematologia Oncologia Pediatrica's prospective study of 636 pediatric patients transplanted for acute leukemia, CNS toxicity was associated with early treatment-related death.[45] In that report, severe CNS toxicity was related to a threefold increase in the risk of treatment-related death as compared with absent or mild toxicity (p = 0.02). However, in a logistic regression model of all organ toxicities, the relationship between CNS toxicity and early treatment-related death was not statistically significant (relative risk, 2.2; 95% confidence interval, 0.8 to 5.5; p = .11). Finally, in a study of encephalopathy after pediatric HCT, 17 (65%) of 26 patients died; 12 never recovered from their encephalopathy.[239] In that report, only 4 (15%) of the 26 patients experienced a full recovery of their encephalopathy.

Late Effects

A complete discussion of the late effects of HCT is beyond the scope of this chapter. However, some potential late effects are relevant to intensive care providers. Patients who have been treated with total body irradiation, focal lung radiation, and some chemotherapeutic agents are at risk for chronic lung disease, including pulmonary fibrosis, obstructive lung disease, and restrictive changes.[53] Post-HCT cardiac late effects include cardiomyopathy, congestive heart failure, and arrhythmia. Anthracycline chemotherapy is a primary cause of cardiomyopathy. Anthracycline-related cardiomyopathy is dose dependent, and treatment given before transplant contributes largely to the risk of developing cardiac dysfunction though radiation may also play a role. Cardiac late effects related to radiation include fibrosis, arrhythmia (related to fibrosis), and restrictive cardiomyopathy. Children who received radiation are at an increased risk for myocardial infarction and congestive heart failure.[262]

Nutritional Support in the Critically Ill Hematopoietic Progenitor Cell Transplantation Patient

HCT patients may begin their course in malnourished state, which could put them at risk for the development of micronutrient deficiencies during transplant.[263,264] Deficiencies of micronutrients including magnesium, phosphorus, zinc, selenium, vitamin E, vitamin D, and β-carotene have been described during conditioning.[263,265-268] HCT patients are also at significant risk for the development of severe mucositis and vomiting, making oral enteral nutrition difficult. Standardized feeding protocols may improve the chances of enteral nutrition being successful. In a study of 79 pediatric HCT patients who were followed closely on an enteral nutrition protocol, the majority of patients could be successfully fed enterally. In this protocol, the patient's oral caloric intake was measured daily. When it fell below 75% of the recommended intake for 3 consecutive days, an nasogastric tube was inserted and enteral feedings initiated. Seventy-one of the 79 patients required only enteral nutrition to maintain weight, 5 patients required a combination of enteral and parenteral nutrition, and only 3 patients were fed by parenteral nutrition alone.[269] Enteral nutrition may be the preferred method of nutrition when possible, as there is evidence that patients fed enterally are at decreased risk for developing GVHD.[270-272]

A few studies have shown an association between micronutrient deficiencies and transplant complications. Low zinc levels during the transplant course were associated with more febrile episodes, longer duration of febrile episodes, and more positive blood cultures.[273] Persistently low vitamin D levels were associated with more severe GVHD.[268] Low vitamin D levels have also been associated with worse overall survival after HCT as well as increased risk of graft rejection and relapse.[274]

Biochemical markers of oxidative stress during conditioning have been seen in HCT patients. Decreased glutathione and α- and γ-tocopherol levels have been documented during conditioning.[275] Increased serum Fe levels and a decreased total radical trapping antioxidant parameter of plasma (a measure of antioxidant reserve) and linoleic acid concentrations have also been documented in HCT patients.[276]

There is also increasing evidence for oxidative stress in critically ill patients with sepsis, systemic inflammation, and lung injury—all common reasons for ICU admission of HCT patients.[277-283] Therefore it is likely that the critically ill HCT patient who has recently undergone conditioning may be under a significant amount of oxidative stress.

There are a handful of published trials of antioxidant supplementation during HCT. In one trial, 37 pediatric HCT patients were given ursodeoxycholic acid, vitamin E, folinic acid, and total parenteral nutrition with traditional amounts of vitamins, minerals, and trace elements. There was no control group. The main outcome of the study was the feasibility of patients taking oral supplements. Most patients tolerated the oral medications well, and the authors were able to prove feasibility. In these patients they also noted less mucositis, less hepatic toxicity, and a shorter time to engraftment in comparison to a historical control group.[284] Another group performed a double-blind, randomized, placebo-control trial of selenium supplementation to 77 adults undergoing HCT. The researchers were able to show improvement in selenium and glutathione peroxidase levels in the group receiving selenium supplements. Those receiving selenium supplements also had less severe oral mucositis as well as a shorter duration of mucositis.[285]

Although common sense dictates that some type of nutrition is good and prolonged lack of any nutrition would lead to death, little is known about the optimal nutrition for critically ill pediatric HCT patients[286] (see also Chapter 87). Critical illness and HCT cause significant oxidative stress. Therefore it is possible that critically ill HCT patients may benefit from specialized nutritional strategies that optimize antioxidant capacity. This is a field that begs for further study.

Key References

16. Pasquini MC, et al. Current use and outcome of hematopoietic stem cell transplantation: CIBMTR Summary Slides, 2014. <http://www.cibmtr.org2014>.

26. Tamburro RF, Barfield RC, Shaffer ML, et al. Changes in outcomes (1996-2004) for pediatric oncology and hematopoietic stem cell transplant patients requiring invasive mechanical ventilation. *Pediatr Crit Care Med.* 2008;9:270-277.

28. van Gestel JP, Bollen CW, van der Tweel I, et al. Intensive care unit mortality trends in children after hematopoietic stem cell transplantation: a meta-regression analysis. *Crit Care Med.* 2008;36:2898-2904.

29. Duncan CN, Lehmann LE, Cheifetz IM, et al. Clinical outcomes of children receiving intensive cardiopulmonary support during hematopoietic stem cell transplant. *Pediatr Crit Care Med.* 2013;14:261-267.

32. Fiser RT, West NK, Bush AJ, et al. Outcome of severe sepsis in pediatric oncology patients. *Pediatr Crit Care Med.* 2005;6:531-536.

39. Tichelli A, Bhatia S, Socie G. Cardiac and cardiovascular consequences after haematopoietic stem cell transplantation. *Br J Haematol.* 2008;142:11-26.

41. Jodele S, Hirsch R, Laskin B, et al. Pulmonary arterial hypertension in pediatric patients with hematopoietic stem cell transplant-associated thrombotic microangiopathy. *Biol Blood Marrow Transplant.* 2013;19:202-207.

43. Nieder ML, McDonald GB, Kida A, et al. National Cancer Institute-National Heart, Lung and Blood Institute/Pediatric Blood and Marrow Transplant Consortium First International Consensus Conference on late effects after pediatric hematopoietic cell transplantation: long-term organ damage and dysfunction. *Biol Blood Marrow Transplant.* 2011;17:1573-1584.

45. Balduzzi A, Valsecchi MG, Silvestri D, et al. Transplant-related toxicity and mortality: an AIEOP prospective study in 636 pediatric patients transplanted for acute leukemia. *Bone Marrow Transplant.* 2002;29:93-100.

51. Wilhelmsson M, Vatanen A, Borgstrom B, et al. Adverse health events and late mortality after pediatric allogeneic hematopoietic SCT-two decades of longitudinal follow-up. *Bone Marrow Transplant.* 2015;50:850-857.

54. Armenian SH, Sun CL, Kawashima T, et al. Long-term health-related outcomes in survivors of childhood cancer treated with HSCT versus conventional therapy: a report from the Bone Marrow Transplant Survivor Study (BMTSS) and Childhood Cancer Survivor Study (CCSS). *Blood.* 2011;118:1413-1420.

65. Nishio N, Yagasaki H, Takahashi Y, et al. Late-onset non-infectious pulmonary complications following allogeneic hematopoietic stem cell transplantation in children. *Bone Marrow Transplant.* 2009;44:303-308.

70. Woodard JP, Gulbahce E, Shreve M, et al. Pulmonary cytolytic thrombi: a newly recognized complication of stem cell transplantation. *Bone Marrow Transplant.* 2000;25:293-300.

75. Kharbanda S, Panoskaltsis-Mortari A, Haddad IY, et al. Inflammatory cytokines and the development of pulmonary complications after allogeneic hematopoietic cell transplantation in patients with inherited metabolic storage disorders. *Biol Blood Marrow Transplant.* 2006;12:430-437.

76. Afessa B, Tefferi A, Litzow MR, et al. Diffuse alveolar hemorrhage in hematopoietic stem cell transplant recipients. *Am J Respir Crit Care Med.* 2002;166:641-645.

84. Keates-Baleeiro J, Moore P, Koyama T, et al. Incidence and outcome of idiopathic pneumonia syndrome in pediatric stem cell transplant recipients. *Bone Marrow Transplant.* 2006;38:285-289.

87. Cooke KR, Yanik G. Acute lung injury after allogeneic stem cell transplantation: is the lung a target of acute graft-versus-host disease? *Bone Marrow Transplant.* 2004;34:753-765.

88. Afessa B, Peters SG. Noninfectious pneumonitis after blood and marrow transplant. *Curr Opin Oncol.* 2008;20:227-233.

92. Ditschkowski M, Elmaagacli AH, Trenschel R, et al. T-cell depletion prevents from bronchiolitis obliterans and bronchiolitis obliterans with organizing pneumonia after allogeneic hematopoietic stem cell transplantation with related donors. *Haematologica.* 2007;92:558-561.

97. Yanik GA, Grupp SA, Pulsipher MA, et al. TNF-receptor inhibitor therapy for the treatment of children with idiopathic pneumonia syndrome. A Joint Pediatric Blood and Marrow Transplant Consortium and Children's Oncology Group Study (ASCT0521). *Biol Blood Marrow Transplant.* 2015;21:67-73.

105. Tamburro RF, Thomas NJ, Pon S, et al. Post hoc analysis of calfactant use in immunocompromised children with acute lung injury: impact and feasibility of further clinical trials. *Pediatr Crit Care Med.* 2008;9:459-464.

106. Gupta M, Shanley TP, Moler FW. Extracorporeal life support for severe respiratory failure in children with immune compromised conditions. *Pediatr Crit Care Med.* 2008;9:380-385.

107. Leahey AM, Bunin NJ, Schears GJ, et al. Successful use of extracorporeal membrane oxygenation (ECMO) during BMT for SCID. *Bone Marrow Transplant.* 1998;21:839-840.

115. Sakaida E, Nakaseko C, Harima A, et al. Late-onset noninfectious pulmonary complications after allogeneic stem cell transplantation are significantly associated with chronic graft-versus-host disease and with the graft-versus-leukemia effect. *Blood.* 2003;102:4236-4242.

121. Chellapandian D, Lehrnbecher T, Phillips B, et al. Bronchoalveolar lavage and lung biopsy in patients with cancer and hematopoietic stem-cell transplantation recipients: a systematic review and meta-analysis. *J Clin Oncol.* 2015;33:501-509.

126. Sakai M, Strasser SI, Shulman HM, et al. Severe hepatocellular injury after hematopoietic cell transplant: incidence, etiology and outcome. *Bone Marrow Transplant.* 2009;44:441-447.

128. Shulman HM, et al. In: Gershwin ME, Vierling JM, Manns M, eds. *Hepatic Complications of Hematopoietic Cell Transplantation.* Totowa, NJ: Humana Press; 2007.

137. Miano M, Faraci M, Dini G, Bordigoni P. Early complications following haematopoietic SCT in children. *Bone Marrow Transplant.* 2008;41(suppl 2):S39-S42.

143. Cesaro S, Pillon M, Talenti E, et al. A prospective survey on incidence, risk factors and therapy of hepatic veno-occlusive disease in children after hematopoietic stem cell transplantation. *Haematologica.* 2005;90:1396-1404.

147. Jastaniah W, Harmatz P, Pakbaz Z, et al. Transfusional iron burden and liver toxicity after bone marrow transplantation for acute myelogenous leukemia and hemoglobinopathies. *Pediatr Blood Cancer.* 2008;50:319-324.

150. Platzbecker U, von Bonin M, Goekkurt E, et al. Graft-versus-host disease prophylaxis with everolimus and tacrolimus is associated with a high incidence of sinusoidal obstruction syndrome and microangiopathy: results of the EVTAC trial. *Biol Blood Marrow Transplant.* 2009;15:101-108.

152. Dignan FL, Wynn RF, Hadzic N, et al. BCSH/BSBMT guideline: diagnosis and management of veno-occlusive disease (sinusoidal obstruction syndrome) following haematopoietic stem cell transplantation. *Br J Haematol.* 2013;163:444-457.

170. Richardson PG, et al. Defibrotide Study Group (2011) Defibrotide (DF) in the treatment of hepatic veno-occlusive disease (VOD) in stem cell transplant (SCT) and non-SCT patients (pts): early intervention improves outcome: updated results of a treatment IND expanded access protocol. *Blood.* 2011;118:487.

180. Stavrou E, Lazarus HM. Thrombotic microangiopathy in haematopoietic cell transplantation: an update. *Mediterr J Hematol Infect Dis.* 2010;2:e2010033.

181. Weber C, Schaper J, Tibussek D, et al. Diagnostic and therapeutic implications of neurological complications following paediatric haematopoietic stem cell transplantation. *Bone Marrow Transplant.* 2008;41:253-259.

185. Smith TJ, Khatcheressian J, Lyman GH, et al. 2006 update of recommendations for the use of white blood cell growth factors: an evidence-based clinical practice guideline. *J Clin Oncol.* 2006;24:3187-3205.

188. Avigan D, Pirofski LA, Lazarus HM. Vaccination against infectious disease following hematopoietic stem cell transplantation. *Biol Blood Marrow Transplant.* 2001;7:171-183.

192. Slavin MA, Osborne B, Adams R, et al. Efficacy and safety of fluconazole prophylaxis for fungal infections after marrow transplantation–a prospective, randomized, double-blind study. *J Infect Dis.* 1995;171:1545-1552.

194. Jung J, Kim MY, Lee HJ, et al. Comparison of computed tomographic findings in pulmonary mucormycosis and invasive pulmonary aspergillosis. *Clin Microbiol Infect.* 2015;21:684.e11-684.e18.

200. Weigt SS, Gregson AL, Deng JC, et al. Respiratory viral infections in hematopoietic stem cell and solid organ transplant recipients. *Semin Respir Crit Care Med.* 2011;32:471-493.

213. Nevo S, Fuller AK, Hartley E, et al. Acute bleeding complications in patients after hematopoietic stem cell transplantation with prophylactic platelet transfusion triggers of 10 x 10 and 20 x 10 per L. *Transfusion.* 2007;47:801-812.

216. Lightdale JR, Randolph AG, Tran CM, et al. Impact of a conservative red blood cell transfusion strategy in children undergoing hematopoietic stem cell transplantation. *Biol Blood Marrow Transplant.* 2012;18:813-817.

220. Hale GA, Bowman LC, Rochester RJ, et al. Hemolytic uremic syndrome after bone marrow transplantation: clinical characteristics and outcome in children. *Biol Blood Marrow Transplant.* 2005;11:912-920.

223. de Fontbrune FS, Galambrun C, Sirvent A, et al. Use of eculizumab in patients with allogeneic stem cell transplant-associated thrombotic microangiopathy: a study from the SFGM-TC. *Transplantation.* 2015;99:1953-1959.

229. Trottier BJ, Burns LJ, DeFor TE, et al. Association of iron overload with allogeneic hematopoietic cell transplantation outcomes: a prospective cohort study using R2-MRI-measured liver iron content. *Blood.* 2013;122:1678-1684.

238. Schmidt K, Schulz AS, Debatin KM, et al. CNS complications in children receiving chemotherapy or hematopoietic stem cell transplantation: retrospective analysis and clinical study of survivors. *Pediatr Blood Cancer.* 2008;50:331-336.

239. Woodard P, Helton K, McDaniel H, et al. Encephalopathy in pediatric patients after allogeneic hematopoietic stem cell transplantation is associated with a poor prognosis. *Bone Marrow Transplant.* 2004;33:1151-1157.

245. Uckan D, Cetin M, Yigitkanli I, et al. Life-threatening neurological complications after bone marrow transplantation in children. *Bone Marrow Transplant.* 2005;35:71-76.

258. Soni S, Skeens M, Termuhlen AM, et al. Levetiracetam for busulfan-induced seizure prophylaxis in children undergoing hematopoietic stem cell transplantation. *Pediatr Blood Cancer.* 2012;59:762-764.

260. Cordelli DM, Masetti R, Ricci E, et al. Life-threatening complications of posterior reversible encephalopathy syndrome in children. *Eur J Paediatr Neurol.* 2014;18:632-640.

Section **VIII**

Gastrointestinal System

Gastrointestinal System

Gastrointestinal Structure and Function

David M. Steinhorn

"All the diseases begin in the gut" and *"death sits in the bowel."*
Hippocrates[1]

PEARLS

- The alimentary tract is responsible for mechanical and enzymatic degradation of nutrients, absorption of biochemical substrates, hormone regulation of substrate flow, separation of the external from internal environments, and excretion of waste.
- The pancreas exhibits both endocrine and exocrine functions. Four distinct cell types facilitate endocrine function: B cells, which secrete insulin; A cells, which secrete glucagon; D cells, which secrete somatostatin; and PP cells, which secrete pancreatic polypeptide.
- The liver is composed of hepatocytes, endothelial cells, Kupffer cells (reticuloendothelial cells), bile duct cells, hepatic stellate cells, and oval cells. It has a dual vascular supply derived from the hepatic artery branches of the celiac axis providing about 30% of the blood supply with the portal vein providing approximately 70%.
- Cells of the gut-associated lymphoid tissue (GALT) are organized into three compartments: diffusely scattered through the lamina propria, within the epithelium itself, and as an aspect of lymphoid follicles called Peyer patches.
- Bacterial translocation is defined as the migration of bacteria or bacterial products from the intestinal lumen to mesenteric lymph nodes or other extra intestinal organs, and represents a disruption of the normal host flora equilibrium that leads to a self-perpetuating inflammatory response and ultimately to infection.

Introduction

Whether from primary gastrointestinal (GI) disease, sequelae of surgery, or complications of systemic disease, restoration of hepatic and GI function are central to successful discharge from the pediatric intensive care unit (PICU). The GI tract subserves multiple functions beyond digestion that impact systemic immunology, endocrinology, and microbiology.[2] New insights into the role of gut innervation are emerging as well as the compelling importance of the intestinal microbiome in drug metabolism and host protection.[3,4] The interactions among the gut, liver, and lung and between the liver and kidneys have led to the view that the gut may play a role as an *engine* of multiple organ dysfunction[5-7] as well as a regulator of metabolic and immunologic homeostasis. This chapter provides a comprehensive overview of basic gastrointestinal and hepatobiliary function for clinicians dealing with critically ill children.

Intestinal Structure, Digestion, Absorption of Nutrients, Water, and Electrolytes[8]

The alimentary tract is responsible for mechanical and enzymatic degradation of nutrients, absorption of biochemical substrates, hormone regulation of substrate flow, separation of the external from internal environments, and excretion of waste. Its primary role is to alter nutrients to be compatible with the internal environment of the body.

The functional absorptive unit of the intestine consists of villi and crypts. The cells of the small intestine are separated from one another by specialized junctions that serve as gaskets to prevent back diffusion of material into the intestinal lumen. A mucus layer secreted by goblet cells in crypts separates enterocytes from direct contact with the luminal contents.

Stem cells in crypts produce enterocytes and other specialized epithelial cells that differentiate as they migrate up the villi, a process that takes 48 to 72 hours (Table 96.1). Mature villous cells live ~6 days and are covered by microvilli making up the brush border containing digestive enzymes and membrane-bound transport systems for nutrients and electrolytes. Villous tips are predominantly absorptive, whereas crypt cells are primarily secretory. Rotavirus infections cause villous loss resulting in small intestinal mucosa composed largely of crypts and immature villi, leading to malabsorption and osmotic diarrhea. Malabsorption of nutrients is another manifestation of villous injury as is seen in gluten-sensitive enteropathy. In patients with poor tissue perfusion, mucosal ischemia and diminished flow to villi lead to ischemic injury and sloughing of the epithelium with an associated loss of barrier and transport functions.

Water and Solute Transport Across Intestinal Epithelium

Surface area and integrity of intercellular junctions are the major determinants of water and solute flux across epithelium. Microvilli increase the luminal surface area up to 40-fold. Transport of solute and water across epithelium occurs either by active or passive transport or by facilitated diffusion (Table 96.2). The average luminal fluid input of the adult gut is about 9 L per day and is composed of oral intake and endogenous secretions. Approximately 8.8 L is absorbed, about 7 L in the small intestine and 1.8 L in the colon. Less than 0.2 L is excreted as a component of the normal stool output. When rapid changes in dietary intake or endogenous secretions occur, the intestinal mucosa can adapt transport functions to compensate for the changes. The loss of mucosal surface area through disease or surgical resection alters net flux of solute and water in the GI tract. Loss of specialized absorptive function may occur following loss of specific areas of gut. An example of this reaction occurs in the setting of resection of terminal ileum, with loss of ability to absorb bile acids and

intrinsic factor. Malfunction of absorptive mechanisms may lead to a life-threatening loss of fluid and electrolytes.[9]

Nutrients consist of macronutrients, such as carbohydrates, protein, and lipids, and micronutrients including minerals, electrolytes, trace elements, vitamins, and other metabolic cofactors such as biotin and carnitine. Critical illness leads to reduced intake of all nutrients and important alterations in substrate requirements and utilization. The fasting state in a healthy individual is characterized by a conservation of lean body tissue and reduction in energy expenditure with a shift to fatty acids for energy sources. In contrast, critical illness is associated with an increased metabolic rate and gluconeogenesis in excess of that needed to maintain serum glucose. Breakdown of lean tissue and peripheral oxidation of amino acids with increased ureagenesis leads rapidly to malnutrition as a result of so-called autocannibalism. These changes are mediated by the classic stress hormones including cortisol, catecholamines, and relative excess of glucagon versus insulin levels (see also Chapter 81). Additionally, children with burn injury, septic shock and systemic inflammatory response syndrome (SIRS), those on dialysis, patients with extremely short intestine, or those receiving catecholamines or neuromuscular blocking agents are at risk for ICU-associated malnutrition and myopathy.

Enteral nutrition is the preferred method of feeding for critically ill children.[10,11] Early transpyloric enteral nutrition is well tolerated in critically ill children and is not associated with an increased incidence of complications. Many skilled PICU nurses can reliably place transpyloric tubes at the bedside, and placement is confirmed by abdominal x-ray. Small-bowel feeding allows a greater amount of nutrition to be successfully delivered to critically ill children compared to gastric feeds but may not eliminate the risk of occult gastric contents aspiration.[12] The institution of a feeding protocol has been found to achieve goal feedings quickly and also improve the tolerance of enteral feedings in patients admitted to the pediatric intensive care unit (see also Chapter 87).

Digestion of Carbohydrates[13] (Box 96.1)

Dietary carbohydrates include monosaccharides (glucose and fructose present in fruits, sweet corn, corn syrup, and honey), disaccharides, (sucrose, maltose, and lactose), and the principal mammalian milk sugar. Polysaccharides, such as starch, are polymers of glucose and are abundantly present in wheat, grains, potatoes, peas, beans, and vegetables. Fiber consists of nondigestible complex polysaccharides of plant origin. This includes both water-insoluble and water-soluble fiber. The average American diet is 3:1 soluble to insoluble fiber, and this may be markedly altered by the diets fed to ICU patients. Insoluble fibers affect fecal bulk, whereas soluble fibers have viscous effects in the upper GI tract including delayed gastric emptying, decreased postprandial glycemic response, and constipating effect. Furthermore, indigestible fiber is now known to be an important source of nutrition for the microbiome of the gut.[14]

TABLE 96.1	Functional Unit of Intestine
Structure	**Function**
Enterocyte	Formed in crypts, migrate to villus over 2-3 days; life span 6 days
Villi	Absorption
Crypts	Secretion
Microvilli	Amplifies surface area, contains enzymes and transport systems

TABLE 96.2	Intestinal Transport Mechanisms[33-35]
Active	Against electrochemical gradient Saturable kinetics Requires ATP
Passive	Ionic specificity May be associated with transport of a nonelectrolyte Proceeds down electrochemical gradient Steady-state based upon concentration differences Displays first-order kinetics May occur by convection via osmotic or hydrostatic gradient
Facilitated diffusion	Saturable kinetics Substrate specific Depends on carrier molecules (glucose, amino acid)
Na^+-H^+ exchanger	1:1 exchange of Na^+ or K^+ for H^+
K^+-H^+ exchanger (colon)	(regulates intracellular pH, cell volume, growth)
Coupled transport (Na movement down electrochemical gradient)	Na-Cl Na-K-Cl co-transport Na-glucose co-transport
Acidosis	Na^+ and Cl^- absorption
Aldosterone	Ileal and colonic Na^+ and water absorption
Glucocorticoids	Na^+ and water absorption in colon
VIP, PGE_1	Electrolyte and water secretion by intestinal epithelia

PGE1, prostaglandin E1; *VIP,* vasoactive intestinal protein.

BOX 96.1	Conditions Impairing Dietary Carbohydrate Uptake

- Disaccharidase deficiency (acquired or congenital)
- Pancreatic insufficiency
- Membrane-associated transporter defect

Carbohydrates are a major source of calories in healthy children and enter metabolic pathways via glycolysis and the Krebs cycle pathway. They may be stored as glycogen and lipids when ingested beyond momentary energy needs or converted to structural materials. A person's requirement for energy is highly dependent on activity level or, in hospitalized patients, the degree of hypermetabolism accompanying illness. In critically ill patients, the maximal ability to utilize carbohydrates may be limited during periods of high physiologic stress as a result of unbridled gluconeogenesis.

In the critically ill patient and those receiving tube feedings, the mechanical impact of chewing and salivary enzymes is absent. However, the liquid or elemental nature of enteral formulas circumvents that issue. For infants receiving breast milk, mammary amylase facilitates starch digestion because of their low levels of endogenous salivary and pancreatic amylase.[15] Pancreatic amylase is the major enzyme of starch digestion resulting in short oligosaccharides, maltotriose, maltose, and α-limit dextrins. The amylase concentration in the duodenum becomes limiting in cases of pancreatic insufficiency (eg, severe cystic fibrosis or major resection) when amylase levels become less than 10% of normal.[16]

The enterocyte is incapable of absorbing carbohydrates larger than monosaccharides. Therefore, further hydrolysis to monosaccharides is performed by intestinal *brush border disaccharidases*. Lactase and sucrase are the most clinically relevant disaccharidases and are synthesized in the enterocyte with insertion into the apical brush border membrane. With the exception of lactase and occasionally sucrase, the disaccharidases are rarely rate limiting for complete carbohydrate digestion. Deficiencies of any of the disaccharidase enzymes, either acquired or hereditary, may result in carbohydrate malabsorption. This is characterized by osmotic diarrhea with elevated fecal reducing sugars, abdominal distention, and flatulence secondary to fermentation of undigested oligosaccharides by colonic bacteria. An example is congenital sucrase isomaltase deficiency, an autosomal recessive disorder that is associated with absence of sucrase and maltase.[17,18]

Carbohydrates are absorbed by simple diffusion of monosaccharides or via brush border–associated transport mechanisms. Glucose, galactose, and xylitol are transported with sodium by the Na^+/glucose cotransporter leading to movement of luminal sodium across the apical membrane, bringing with it glucose or galactose in a one-to-one molar ratio. Glucose-galactose malabsorption is a deficiency of this transport mechanism leading to neonatal onset of severe diarrhea.[19] The second mechanism is a non–energy-dependent facilitated transport system for fructose. The general intestinal transport mechanisms are summarized in Table 96.2. The capacity to absorb fructose is limited in most humans, and excess ingestion has been found to cause symptoms of carbohydrate malabsorption.[20]

Loss of the epithelium and brush border frequently leads to symptoms of carbohydrate malabsorption. Common clinical conditions include rotaviral gastroenteritis, inflammatory bowel disease, celiac disease, sprue, ischemia/hypoxia, bacterial overgrowth of the proximal gut as a result of either stasis or use of antacids, and malnutrition. Severe mucosal damage requires 7 to 10 days for recovery of brush border function. Several infant and enteral formulas rely on starch as a carbohydrate source to minimize reliance on lactase.

The digestion of carbohydrates is generally very efficient, ranging from 80% to 100% of absorption from starch depending on the source of the starch. Bacterial fermentation of fiber and undigested carbohydrates produces short-chain fatty acids, used as fuel by the enterocytes, as well as gaseous hydrogen and methane, contributing to the flatulence associated with increased dietary fiber and malabsorption syndromes.

Digestion of Proteins[13] (Box 96.2)

The GI tract processes exogenous proteins with great efficiency as well as recycling endogenous proteins such as digestive enzymes, mucus, sloughed cells, and plasma proteins that leak into the alimentary tract.[21] The enteral processing of proteins entails a digestive and transport phase.

In the digestive phase, gastric acid denatures complex proteins making them more susceptible to the actions of proteolytic enzymes. The chief cells of the stomach release pepsinogens that are converted to active pepsins under acidic conditions. The pepsins are endopeptidases that release relatively large peptides and are inactivated when the pH rises above 4 as the food enters the duodenum. The completeness of gastric proteolysis depends in part on the rate of gastric emptying, the pH of intragastric contents, and the types of protein ingested.[21] There is, however, no evidence that patients with achlorhydria or those receiving antacids, H_2 blockers, or both agents have impaired protein digestion. In addition to initiating protein digestion in the mature subject, pepsins act as milk clotting factors, which are important in the neonate for curd formation and provide bulk to the infant's stools.

Luminal digestion proceeds in the small intestine mediated by five pancreatic peptidases, which are secreted by the pancreatic acinar cells as proenzymes and activated by enterokinase and trypsin. Each peptidase possesses proteolytic activity at specific internal or external peptide bonds. Proteins are degraded typically into mixtures of one-third free amino acids and two-thirds peptides containing two to six amino acid residues, which are suitable substrates for the brush border peptidases. The brush border peptidases convert the oligopeptides into monopeptides, dipeptides, and tripeptides suitable for transport into the enterocyte.

In the transport phase, specific membrane-associated transport mechanisms exist for the uptake of amino acids and dipeptides. They involve *simple diffusion, facilitated transport, and carrier-mediated active transport* (see Table 96.2). Na^+ coupled active transport is an energy-dependent process associated with the uptake of luminal Na^+ and an amino acid (or glucose) and exchange of the sodium and associated molecule for K^+ through the basolateral membrane on the serosal side.[22] Peptide transport may also occur using an H^+/peptide transport protein, which moves according to an H^+ gradient in the acidic pH microclimate of the intestinal brush border. Na^+-H^+ exchange in the brush border and Na^+-K^+-ATPase in the basolateral membrane[23] maintain the necessary gradient. It is important to note that many amino acids are absorbed more rapidly as dipeptides than as free amino acids. This fact has

---

BOX 96.2   Conditions Impairing Dietary Protein Uptake

- Ineffective pancreatic protease secretion
- Abnormal epithelial transport
  (Hartnup lysinuric protein intolerance)

been capitalized on in the development of enteral nutritional formulas for critically ill patients because oligopeptide mixtures have a lower osmolarity and are more efficiently absorbed than single amino acid solutions of equal nitrogen content. Because of the efficient gastrointestinal absorption of dipeptides, patients with specific amino acid transport defects such as Hartnup disease (defective tryptophan transport) and lysinuric protein intolerance (defect in dibasic amino acid transport—lysine, arginine) infrequently have gastrointestinal symptoms related to dietary protein malabsorption and instead more commonly manifest with nongastrointestinal symptoms such as aminoaciduria.

Once inside the enterocyte, peptides are quickly degraded into their constituent amino acids by cytoplasmic peptidases. Only minute quantities of intact peptide and protein gain access to the systemic circulation. The cytoplasmic amino acids derived from digested proteins are a major source of free amino acids used directly by the enterocyte. When absorbed beyond cellular needs, the free amino acids are released to the portal venous circulation for hepatic and systemic use. Only 23% of absorbed amino acids will pass to the periphery without modification.[24] Of the remaining nitrogen, 57% is converted to urea with the carbon skeleton salvaged for synthesizing other substances, and 20% of the total ingested amino acids will be used directly for hepatic protein synthesis.

During periods of fasting, the enterocyte derives the majority of its nourishment from the mesenteric arterial vascular supply, whereas during digestion, the enterocyte derives a significant part of its nutrient requirements from the luminal contents. Experience with mucosal recovery and adaptation after injury reveals that an enteral route of nutrition permits optimal recovery.[25] In the premature infant and neonate, the small intestine is capable of absorbing intact milk proteins by pinocytosis. These proteins may include secretory immunoglobulins from breast milk as well as food antigens. Peptidase inhibitors have been demonstrated in colostrum and breast milk, partially explaining the failure of normal digestive mechanisms to degrade some of these complex dietary proteins. Both antibodies and antigens ingested with maternal milk create an important part of the immune repertory developed during early infancy (see later section on gut immunology). Although the exact time of "closure" of the intestinal mucosa to the uptake of macromolecules has not been defined in human infants, other mammals demonstrate marked intestinal impermeability to foreign proteins by the time of weaning from breast-feeding.

Digestion of Lipids[26] (Box 96.3)

Dietary fat accounts for approximately 50% to 70% of the nonprotein calories consumed by infants and ~30% of

---

BOX 96.3 **Conditions Impairing Dietary Lipid Uptake**

- Decreased bile salt pool in gut (biliary obstruction, short bowel syndrome)
- Impaired pancreatic secretions (pancreatic insufficiency, pancreatitis)
- Suboptimal pH in gut (gastric hypersecretion)
- Rapid transit time (short gut syndrome, diarrheal states)
- Mucosal diseases (celiac disease, inflammatory bowel disease, bacterial overgrowth)
- Impaired enterocyte function (abetalipoproteinemia)

---

nonprotein calories consumed after age 2 years.[27] Dietary fat is ingested principally in the form of triglycerides containing the fatty acids palmitate and oleate (C16:0 and C18:1, respectively). Dietary triglycerides of animal origin predominantly contain long-chain (ie, longer than C14 chain length) saturated fatty acids. Polyunsaturated fatty acids are mostly of vegetable origin and include linoleic and linolenic acid, also referred to as essential fatty acids because of absent de novo synthesis in humans. Other dietary lipids include fat-soluble vitamins, cholesterol, prostaglandins, waxes, and phospholipids.

In healthy adults, digestion and absorption of fat are complete with only 5% to 7% of ingested fat escaping absorption. Under normal physiologic conditions, healthy infants up to age 9 to 12 months fail to absorb 15% to 35% of dietary fat. Digestion and absorption of dietary fat are generally completed by the middle third of the jejunum; however, the presence of dietary fiber may reduce the rate and extent of absorption. Loss of dietary fat places children at significant risk for calorie and fat-soluble vitamin malnutrition.

Fat Digestion

Fat digestion begins with the formation of emulsions, which increase the surface area for enzyme interaction. Emulsification begins with the release of fat by mastication and gastric milling of chyme. Bile salts and coating by phospholipid derived from the diet result in a stable emulsion droplet with a hydrophobic center consisting of triglyceride, cholesterol esters, and diglyceride in a hydrophilic envelope. Mammary, lingual, and gastric lipases play an important role in direct lipolysis of long- and medium-chain triglycerides that are present in maternal milk.[28] Lingual and gastric lipases are active at pH <5 and begin digestion of fat in the stomach; however, overall they play only a limited role in the digestion of lipids. Intragastric lipolysis is consistent across all age groups.[29]

Most of the enzymatic degradation of dietary lipids to fatty acids and monoglyceride occurs by the action of pancreatic lipase and colipase, and it requires an alkaline environment (pH 6 to 8). This underscores the importance of secretion of bicarbonate by the pancreas and biliary tract in order to neutralize gastric acid. Colipase is an essential cofactor for lipase action. Colipase's role is to displace the bile salt-triglyceride interaction in emulsion droplets and micelles in order to facilitate lipase hydrolysis of the triglyceride. Triglyceride hydrolysis occurs at the interface between the emulsion droplet and aqueous phase within the lumen. This is a two-step process. The first step is the enzymatic hydrolysis of long-chain triglycerides and liberation of fatty acids from the glycerol backbone. The second step is formation of fatty acid micelles, which is most efficiently done with the aid of bile salts[30] to move the fatty acids across the unstirred water layer to the epithelium for absorption.

The transit through the unstirred water layer adjacent to the epithelial surface is considered the rate-limiting step in lipid absorption. Brush border lipase enzymes are involved as well. The milieu of the unstirred water layer is acidic (pH 5 to 6) owing to the activity of the brush border membrane sodium-hydrogen (Na^+/H^+) exchanger. The acid environment facilitates dissociation of fatty acids from micelles resulting in a high concentration of fatty acids necessary for diffusion across the mucosal membrane.

Once inside the enterocyte, long-chain fatty acids and monoglycerides are resynthesized into triglycerides and packaged as chylomicrons. Lipoproteins (eg, apo-A, apo-B) and cholesterol are attached to the intestinal chylomicrons and confer important properties for the subsequent systemic uptake and metabolism of the chylomicrons. This process appears to be defective in cystic fibrosis and may account for some of the fat malabsorption seen in this disease.[31] The chylomicrons are exported into the intercellular space and transported through the intestinal lacteals to become part of the intestinal lymph. On entering the bloodstream through the thoracic duct, the chylomicrons are associated with other apolipoproteins that allow them to be recognized by specific peripheral tissues.[32]

Dietary lipids containing short- and medium-chain (C6-C12) triglycerides (MCTs) are handled differently from those of long-chain triglycerides. As much as 30% of MCTs may be absorbed intact into enterocytes by passive diffusion and enter the portal venous blood directly. MCTs are hydrolyzed by pancreatic and mammary lipases to fatty acids and monoglycerides and rapidly enter the enterocytes where they emerge into the portal venous system without reesterification as occurs with long-chain fatty acids.

Intestinal Lymphatics

The intestinal lymph *chyle* is composed of chylomicrons and lipoproteins secreted by the intestinal epithelium in the postprandial state together with nonresorbed interstitial fluid. Chyle follows the intestinal lymphatic channels along the mesentery and enters regional lymph nodes from which it flows cephalad through the thoracic duct and ultimately enters the central venous circulation. In the fasting state, intestinal lymph production is relatively low. It increases 20-fold during the active absorption of a typical meal. The intestinal chyle is joined by lymphatic drainage from other tissues including liver and pancreas. The protein content of chyle is 2.2 to 5.9 g/dL with a triglyceride content of 0.4 to 6 g/dL and 400 to 6800 lymphocytes/dL. During digestion of a meal containing long-chain fats, chyle has a typical milky white appearance because of the presence of chylomicrons. The rate of formation of chyle depends on the state of nutrient absorption, portal venous pressure, and the rate of lymphatic uptake. Conditions that create portal hypertension (eg, portal vein thrombosis, cirrhosis, congestive heart failure) or impair the flow of lymph back to the central circulation (eg, increased central venous pressure, superior vena cava syndrome) predispose to the collection of chylous ascites in the abdomen.

Regulation of Electrolyte and Water Movement[33-35]

The movement of water is primarily coupled to the movement of solute in the form of electrolytes and nutrients. It is largely passive, occurring through paracellular routes in the intestine coupled with solute movement. Expression of transporters involved in intestinal water and electrolyte transport is regionally defined in the intestines. Electrolytes are taken up by enterocytes at the apical membrane and extruded through the basolateral membrane into the paracellular space. The relatively hypertonic paracellular fluid pulls water into this space, increasing the hydrostatic pressure locally. Because the tight junction between enterocytes is more impermeable to fluid flux than the capillary membranes, fluid and electrolytes are preferentially driven in the direction of the vascular space.

Tight junctions are selective and dynamic in function and are regulated by a number of signaling pathways and cellular processes that can determine the size, selectivity, and flow of molecules across this barrier.[33,36]

The gut responds to both systemic and local stimuli to regulate motility, transport, and digestive functions. Secretion and motility are mediated through typical agonist membrane receptor mechanisms, by local autocrine and paracrine action, or through remote endocrine and neurocrine actions.[37] Regulation of intestinal motility is crucial for keeping the chyme in contact with the epithelial surface long enough for efficient absorption of nutrients while permitting removal of unusable material and bacteria from the alimentary tract on a regular basis. GI smooth muscle demonstrates phasic and tonic patterns of contraction. Numerous factors affecting the frequency of contractions include changes in autonomic tone, stimulation of the gut by neurohormonal peptides or pharmacologic agents, and noxious stimuli associated with infectious or inflammatory processes. Hypoxia and ischemia decrease motility, frequently leading to paralytic ileus. Neural regulation of the GI tract integrates the processes of intestinal water and electrolyte transport, motility, and blood flow. The augmentation of water and electrolyte absorption after a meal in the jejunum is neurally mediated.[38] The enteric nervous system is capable of functioning independently but also may be modified by the autonomic nervous system.[37,39]

Many other factors alter the functions of the gut. The terminal ileum and colon are particularly important in this respect. The presence of an ileostomy increases the risk of excessive sodium losses, dehydration, and electrolyte abnormalities. Terminal ileal resection or other diseases of the terminal ileum such as Crohn disease or radiation enteritis may result in bile acid malabsorption. In patients with bile acid malabsorption, bile acids reach the colon, which stimulates electrolyte and chloride secretion. Patients with mild to moderate malabsorption present with watery diarrhea and may respond to a bile acid binder such as cholestyramine.[40] Impairment of water and ion absorption in inflammatory bowel disease may occur due to numerous mechanisms including alteration of epithelial integrity, augmented secretion, and reduced absorption. Intestinal inflammation is associated with defects in epithelial barrier function and has a major impact on fluid and electrolyte flux.[41] Hyperosmolality of the ileal and colonic contents and the presence of unresorbed bile acids in the colon lead to a diarrheal state. This state is seen when unabsorbed nutrients enter the distal alimentary tract and are broken down by enteric bacteria, resulting in increased luminal osmotic activity and osmotic diarrhea.

Electrolyte Transport[33-35]

Several basic mechanisms exist for the transport of electrolytes by the epithelia, as summarized in Table 96.2. The presence of glucose in the lumen of the small intestine stimulates increased sodium absorption through coupled transport. Backflow of sodium into the lumen is a passive process, as a major task for the GI tract is sodium conservation. Systemic acidosis increases Na^+ and Cl^- absorption in the ileum and colon, whereas alkalosis has the opposite effect. As seen in other epithelial tissues, aldosterone increases ileal and colonic absorption of Na^+ and can increase absorption of water in colon three- to fourfold.[42] Spironolactone blocks this effect. Glutamine has been shown to stimulate water and electrolyte absorption in the jejunum[43]; however, its overall value in intestinal rehabilitation remains uncertain. Glucocorticoids increase sodium and water absorption in the distal colon. Opiate receptor stimulation increases active sodium and chloride absorption in the ileum, and opiate antagonists decrease basal absorption of water and electrolytes. The primary antidiarrheal effect of opiates, however, is mediated through a slowing of transit time.[44,45]

In the colon, active absorption and secretion of K^+ occur in a manner consistent with K^+-H^+ exchange and are electroneutral and independent of Na^+-Cl^- exchange. The process of sodium extrusion depends on the Na^+-K^+ ATPase pumping function located at the basolateral membranes. Oxidative stress inhibits water and electrolyte absorption in the jejunum through inhibition of Na-K-ATPase on the basolateral membrane.[46]

The extrusion of Cl^- follows an electrochemical potential difference. The intraluminal secretion of water and other electrolytes appears to follow active secretion of Cl^- from the crypt cells of the jejunum, ileum, and colon with the cystic fibrosis transmembrane conductance regulator (CFTR) mechanism playing an important role.[33-35] This is a common physiologic pattern in the liver, pancreas, and kidney. Numerous substances, such as muscarinic receptor agonists, serotonin, and substance P, work through second messengers and signaling cascades to induce active chloride secretion. Vasoactive intestinal peptide (VIP) mediates increased secretion of electrolytes and water by increased cyclic adenosine monophosphate production that stimulates active chloride secretion and inhibits sodium-chloride absorption. Certain arachidonic acid metabolites, such as prostaglandins (eg, prostaglandin E_1), have been shown to increase active chloride secretion leading to increased loss of electrolytes and fluid. Many laxatives and antacids may affect fluid and electrolyte balance by stimulating active electrolyte and fluid secretion in the terminal ileum. In addition, these agents may increase mucosal permeability and stimulate motility.

Disruption of normal Na^+-K^+ ATPase activity results in the net secretion of fluid and electrolytes. This mechanism is the final common pathway in a number of secretory diarrheal states such as ischemia-reperfusion, cholera, enterotoxigenic *E.coli, Salmonella, Campylobacter jejuni,* and *Clostridium perfringens,* which appear to act via second messenger pathways via their toxins.[47] Rotavirus appears to have several mechanisms of causing diarrhea. The first appears to be a mechanism of increasing chloride secretion with a resulting secretory diarrhea mediated by Ca^{++}, a different mechanism than most bacterial mediated diarrheal diseases. The second is an osmotic diarrhea caused by villus destruction and resultant malabsorption.[48] In addition, the effects of various paracrine and endocrine mediators alter intestinal adenyl cyclase activity and lead to changes in electrolyte and water balance.

Zinc[49,50]

Zinc bears special comment because of its pluripotent effects throughout the body. Intact zinc metabolism is required for a wide range of cellular responses including immune competence, adequate antioxidant capacity, glucose homeostasis, and wound healing. Zinc is a required cofactor for many enzymes, transcription factors, and replication factors. In noncritically ill patients, zinc supplementation may be associated with an improvement in markers of immune function. Plasma zinc concentrations are low in critically ill children, correlate with measures of inflammation, and are associated with the degree of organ failure.[51] Large intestinal losses of zinc with and without complexed proteins often occur in association with high intestinal fluid losses through stomas and fistulae. Some patients with sepsis have demonstrated significantly faster recovery with zinc supplementation among other antioxidants.[52] Thus, most PICUs tend to supplement zinc during critical illness based on experiences with adults and the burn population.[53-55]

Gastric Acid

Hydrochloric acid secretion by the gastric parietal cell is necessary for pepsinogen activation (pH <5) and to reduce bacterial colonization. H+ and bicarbonate are produced from water and carbon dioxide by the action of carbonic anhydrase within the parietal cell. The bicarbonate is secreted into the bloodstream in exchange for chloride at the basolateral membrane. Chloride and potassium are both secreted along with H+ across the apical membrane against a large concentration gradient. This is an active process, mainly due to the action of the proton pump, H^+/K^+ ATPase, which is the final step in gastric acid secretion and the site of action of proton pump inhibitor antacids (PPIs).

Histamine, gastrin, and acetylcholine are the main stimulants of gastric acid secretion. Gastric distention, dietary amino acids, and amines stimulate gastrin hormone secretion by G cells located in the gastric antrum. Gastrin is the most potent endogenous stimulant of gastric acid secretion and stimulates the release of histamine by the enterochromaffin-like cells. Histamine then binds to histamine-2 (H_2) receptors on parietal cells leading to acid secretion. Prostaglandins and somatostatin have an inhibitory effect on gastric acid secretion via specific receptors located on the parietal cell.[56]

H_2 receptor antagonists (H2RA) block histamine-mediated gastric acid secretion found in postprandial acid secretion, Zollinger Ellison syndrome, and other disorders associated with hypergastrinemia. PPIs block gastric acid secretion by inhibiting the parietal cell H^+/K^+ ATPase. They bind irreversibly to the enzyme, and subsequent secretion of acid can occur only with the synthesis of new proton pump enzyme, a process that takes 12 to 24 hours. For these reasons, PPIs have revolutionized gastric acid suppression therapy. H2RAs and PPIs are similarly effective in many patients for preventing bleeding in the upper part of the gastrointestinal tract in patients receiving mechanical ventilation.[57] Studies have shown that some oral PPIs suppress acid in ICU patients to a greater extent than intravenous preparations.[58] ICU patients at risk of stress ulcer-related bleeding are most likely to benefit from prophylaxis,[59] although the increased presence of gram-negative organisms in the upper GI tract due to antacid therapies has been implicated in ventilator-associated pneumonias.[60,61]

Pancreas

The pancreas has both endocrine and exocrine functions. The pancreas acts in concert with the liver to regulate blood glucose levels. Endocrine-secreting cells of the pancreas are aggregated in the islets of Langerhans. There are approximately 1 million islets in the human pancreas. Four distinct cell types in the islets, which serve the endocrine function, include B cells, which secrete insulin (50%-80%); A cells, which secrete glucagon (5%-20%); D cells, which secrete somatostatin (5%); and PP cells, which secrete pancreatic polypeptide.[62,63]

Branches of the celiac, superior mesenteric, and splenic arteries supply the pancreas. Venous drainage is via the pancreaticoduodenal veins, the splenic veins, and ultimately the portal vein, providing direct hormonal influence over hepatic metabolism. Both parasympathetic and sympathetic innervation of the pancreas occurs by means of the vagal nerve and abdominal plexuses, respectively. The vagal innervation of acini, islets, and ducts facilitates secretory function, whereas sympathetic innervation occurs primarily to vascular structures. Functional ectopic pancreatic tissue may be found commonly throughout the upper gastrointestinal tract.

Pancreatic Exocrine Secretory Function

The functional unit of the exocrine pancreas is the acinus composed of specialized cells containing secretory granules that drain into ductules leading to the pancreatic duct. In contrast to the pancreatic endocrine cells that demonstrate specialized function, each acinar cell is capable of secreting all the pancreatic digestive enzymes. The basolateral membrane has receptors for hormones and neurotransmitters that stimulate pancreatic secretion of the digestive enzymes stored in zymogen granules near the apical membrane of each acinar cell.[64] Ultimately, the pancreatic duct joins with the common bile duct and drains into the duodenum through the ampulla of Vater. Anatomic variation exists. Although 74% of people have a common channel, 19% have a separate opening and 7% have an interposed septum.[65]

Pancreatic juice is an isotonic fluid, containing primarily Na^+, K^+, Cl^-, and HCO_3^-. The total volume of secretion is 2.5 L daily. CFTR is the main channel for chloride secretion in the pancreas and may be involved in other ion transport.[66] Secretion of bicarbonate and water is mediated through the actions of the gut hormones secretin, cholecystokinin, and vasoactive intestinal peptide. Stimulation of the vagus nerves or the administration of acetylcholine induces digestive enzyme secretion. These effects may be blocked with atropine.

There are four phases of pancreatic secretion. *Basal secretion* represents approximately 2% of the potential maximum HCO_3^-. The *cephalic phase* is mediated by the vagal nerves in response to the sight and smell of food. The *gastric phase* consisting of secretion of a protein-rich pancreatic juice of low volume and HCO_3^- occurs following either distention of the stomach or after the ingestion of food. The *intestinal phase* is characterized by marked output of digestive enzymes, fluid, and HCO_3^-.[67,68]

The presence of bicarbonate is essential to achieve an optimal pH (pH >5) for pancreatic digestive enzyme activity and to ensure solubility of bile salts. In addition to bicarbonate, the primary secretory products of the exocrine pancreas are amylase, lipase, and the proteases. The secondary digestive enzymes consist of nucleases, colipase, and lecithinase. The roles of the pancreatic digestive enzymes are discussed in the sections on carbohydrate digestion (amylase), lipid digestion (lipase), and protein digestion (proteases). Cholecystokinin (CCK) is the major humoral mediator of meal-stimulated enzyme secretion. It is released from the small intestinal mucosa in response to presence of fat, protein, and starch. The response is related to total load rather than concentration. CCK activates afferent neurons in duodenal mucosa, which leads to secretin release via a vasovagal reflex.[69] Inhibitors of exocrine pancreatic secretion include somatostatin, pancreatic polypeptide, and peptide YY.[67,70] Octreotide, a somatostatin analog, has been used for its antisecretory effect in clinical management of pancreatic pseudocysts and fistulae, but its use in acute or chronic pancreatitis remains controversial. It is widely used for chylous effusions and upper GI bleeding. Inflammation of the pancreas (acute pancreatitis), from both infectious and noninfectious causes, can produce a dramatic systemic inflammatory response resulting in generalized permeability changes and acute lung injury.[71]

Hepatobiliary System
Physical Examination

A complete physical examination of all children admitted to a PICU should include inspection, palpation, and auscultation of the abdomen with particular attention to hepatic or splenic enlargement, distended superficial veins, abdominal masses, the characteristics of the bowel sounds, and finally visual inspection of the perianal region for signs of trauma, fistulae, and venous distention (see also Chapters 97 and 100).

Palpation of the liver provides information about the hepatobiliary tract as well as function of the right side of the heart. Normally, the liver is palpable roughly 1 to 3 cm below the right costal margin in the midclavicular line; however, assessment of liver *span*, and not palpation alone, is the only reliable nonradiologic method for determining liver size. Liver span is determined by percussion, palpation, and auscultation along the right midclavicular line with the patient supine and breathing quietly. The dullness of the upper border is determined by percussion. Either palpation or auscultation is used to establish the lower border. The liver span increases with body weight and age in both sexes, ranging from 4.5 to 5 cm at 1 wk of age to 7 to 8 cm in boys and 6 to 6.5 cm in girls by 12 years of age.[72]

Examination of the liver should note consistency, contour, tenderness, the presence of any masses or bruits, and assessment of spleen size. Documentation of the presence of ascites and stigmata of chronic liver disease is important. Tenderness over the liver suggests inflammation or stretching of the fibrous capsule through rapid enlargement. Conditions associated with downward displacement of a normal liver include hyperinflated lungs, pneumothorax, retroperitoneal masses, and subdiaphragmatic abscess. End-stage liver disease and cirrhosis are associated with a reduced liver span corresponding to decreased hepatic cell mass. The spleen tip may be palpable normally in children, especially during inspiration. Enlargement of the spleen generally represents elevated portal venous pressures or invasive processes such as sequestration, malignancy, extramedullary hematopoiesis, or hyperplasia of the reticuloendothelial system.[73]

Anatomy: Microanatomy, Structure, and Function

The liver is the largest organ in the body and is composed of 60% hepatocytes, approximately 17% to 20% endothelial cells and Kupffer cells (reticuloendothelial cells), 3% to 5% bile ducts, and 1% hepatic stellate cells (HSCs) and oval cells. The liver has a dual vascular supply derived from the hepatic artery branches of the celiac axis providing about 30% of the blood supply and the portal vein providing approximately 70%. Innervation of the liver is by the parasympathetic branches derived from both vagal nerves and sympathetic branches, which also carry afferent fibers deriving from thoracic segments. Denervation of the liver, such as seen after liver transplantation, does not affect function.[74]

The *liver lobule,* the functional unit of the liver, is composed of interconnected hepatocytes (hepatic plates) 1 to 2 cells thick and 20 to 25 cells in length separated by a venous sinusoidal space and radiating around the central vein–like spokes in wheel (Fig. 96.1). The narrow tissue space between the endothelial cells and hepatic plates, the space of Disse, connects with lymphatic vessels in the interlobular septa. Hepatic sinusoidal endothelial cells are flat cells that do not form intracellular junctions and overlap one another. They are fenestrated, allowing plasma to enter into the space of Disse and come into direct contact with the surface of hepatocytes.[36] This facilitates bidirectional exchange between the hepatocytes and the sinusoidal space. Macrophage-derived Kupffer cells line the sinusoidal space. These cells have a phagocytic function and contribute to the hepatic inflammatory response.

HSCs, also known as *ito* cells, lie within the space of Disse. HSCs serve as the hepatic storage site of vitamin A, are effectors of fibrogenesis, and play a role in extracellular matrix remodeling after recovery from injury. Chronic activation and proliferation of HSCs may lead to noncirrhotic portal hypertension, fibrosis, and cirrhosis.[75] Bile canaliculi lie between adjacent hepatocytes and drain into small terminal bile ducts, which successively drain into larger bile ductules, intralobular bile ducts, and eventually the extrahepatic bile ducts. Tight junctions between the hepatocytes at the canalicular space permit unidirectional transport of substances from the hepatocytes into the canalicular space. Several different carriers, receptors, and transport proteins facilitate movement of compounds across the sinusoidal, hepatocyte, and canalicular membranes. ATP-binding cassette (ABC) proteins are expressed in the canalicular membrane and play an important role in transportation of organic ions.[76] Alkaline phosphatase, leucine aminopeptidase, and γ-glutamyl transpeptidase are transaminase enzymes selectively localized in the bile canaliculi and are released with injury to cells as markers of biliary disease.

The microcirculatory "path" within the lobules leads along a declining hydrostatic pressure gradient from the terminal hepatic arterioles and portal venules within the portal triad toward the central vein representing the beginning of the hepatic vein, resulting conceptually in three hepatocyte functional zones (see Fig. 96.1). Zone 1 hepatocytes closest to the portal triad are exposed to sinusoidal blood containing the highest concentration of solutes (nutrients, pancreatic hormones) and oxygen. In contrast, zones 2 and 3 represent hepatocytes more distant from the portal blood supply and are exposed to a declining oxygen and solute gradient. In addition, zone 3 hepatocytes actively participate in drug metabolism and disposition. Ischemic injury and drug hepatotoxicity impact zone 3 hepatocytes to the greatest degree.[77] Following irreversible injury in zone 3, fibrosis occurs in a pattern bridging the terminal hepatic venules leading to the stellate pattern of bridging fibrosis seen histologically.

Portal Circulation

The portal venous system drains the intestines, pancreas, and spleen with numerous collateral anastomoses to other venous beds of the abdomen. There is a mixing of portal and systemic blood circulation within the sinusoids, and all the blood eventually drains from the liver via the hepatic veins to the inferior vena cava. The liver has a high blood flow (~27% of the resting cardiac output) and low vascular resistance. The portal pressure gradient (PPG) is the pressure difference between the inferior vena cava and the portal vein. The average PPG is 0 to 5 mm Hg. Portal hypertension is defined as a PPG of between 6 and 10 mm Hg. A PPG >10 mm Hg carries risk for the development of esophageal varices, and a PPG >12 mm Hg predisposes toward ascites formation.[77,78] Obstruction of the portal venous drainage at any level leads to portal hypertension. Portal hypertension may be classified as prehepatic,

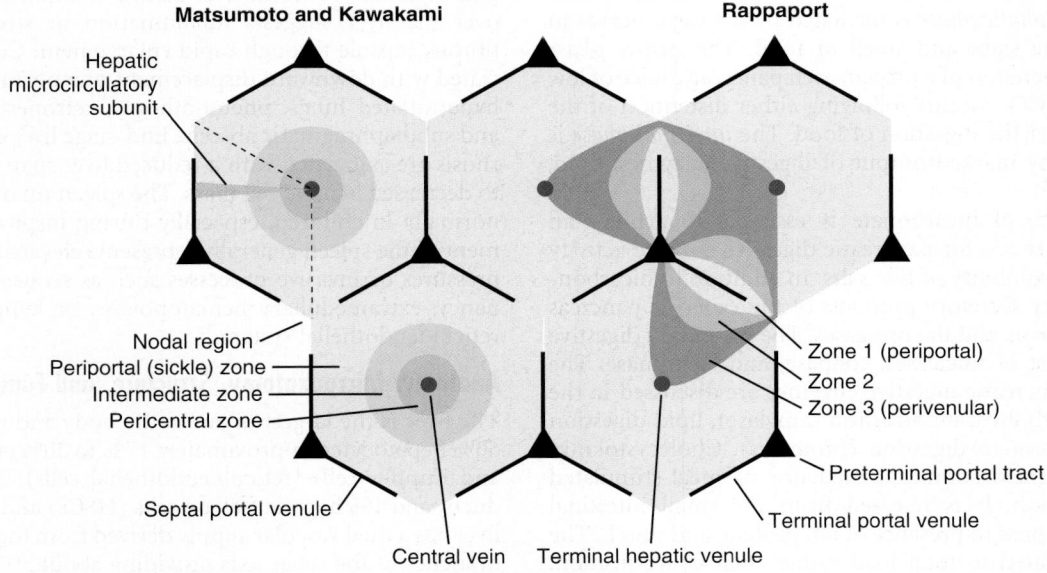

Fig. 96.1. Microanatomy of the liver depicting the hepatic acinus and microcirculatory subunits. (From Young B, et al. *Wheater's Functional Histology: A Text and Colour Atlas.* Philadelphia: Elsevier Livingstone; 2014:281.)

intrahepatic, or posthepatic, according to the level at which the obstruction to flow occurs. The determination of the location of obstruction is critical for instituting appropriate therapy.

Ascites formation is multifactorial. The central event in ascites formation in cirrhosis is splanchnic arterial vasodilatation secondary to portal hypertension. This creates an increase in capillary pressure due to increased blood inflow leading to leakage of fluids based on classic Starling forces. Additionally, impairment of systemic hemodynamics and renal function leads to sodium and water retention with intravascular volume expansion.[79-81] Ascites may form in the absence of portal hypertension as the result of low plasma oncotic pressure associated with malnutrition, with renal or enteral protein losses, or through impaired thoracic duct lymph drainage. Rarely, arterial-portal venous malformations may lead to portal hypertension as a result of excess portal blood flow and must be investigated when other causes of ascites are not found. One additional factor predisposing to ascites is an elevated central venous pressure that increases formation and impairs resorption of interstitial fluid often associated with generalized anasarca or other signs of right heart failure.

Hepatic Function

The function of the liver may be broadly characterized in terms of (1) production of substances uniquely made in the liver; (2) the degradation, elimination, and detoxification of biological materials; (3) the maintenance of biochemical homeostasis; and (4) storage of nutritional materials.

Substances Produced in the Liver With Pediatric Intensive Care Unit Relevance

The liver occupies an ideal place in the scheme of digestion. Hepatocytes are exposed to large quantities of absorbed nutrients after ingestion of a meal, with 20% of the total absorbed nitrogen used for hepatic protein synthesis. Of the large number of plasma proteins synthesized by the liver, several are of major significance in the PICU.

Albumin has a half-life of 18 to 20 days and is a significant contributor to colloid oncotic pressure.[82] It is synthesized solely in the liver, and decreased serum levels may predispose to edema formation and decreased binding of bilirubin, calcium, xenobiotics, and other highly protein-bound molecules. Low serum albumin levels can be secondary to impaired synthesis from protein-calorie malnutrition, chronic liver disease, cachexia, or cytokines. Alternatively, increased losses from proteinuria, protein-losing enteropathy, burns, or other iatrogenic losses including paracentesis or chest tube losses may cause hypoalbuminemia and hypogammaglobulinemia.

Prealbumin, also known as transthyretin, is a visceral protein with a short half-life of ~1.9 days. Because hepatic synthesis is exquisitely sensitive to both the adequacy and levels of protein and energy intakes, it may be used as a nutritional marker and for monitoring short-term response to nutritional intervention.[83]

α_1-Antitrypsin is an important antiprotease with regulatory activity for elastase and other plasma proteases. α_1-Antitrypsin is important in regulating elastase-induced tissue injury in certain lung diseases, and its absence leads to uncontrolled proteolytic activity in the lung.[84] Because α_1-antitrypsin is an endogenous protein that is relatively resistant to hydrolysis

by enteric bacteria, it is a useful marker of protein-losing enteropathy.[85]

Hepatic synthesis of transferrin facilitates iron transport in the plasma by binding two molecules of iron. Ferritin is the primary storage molecule of iron with each molecule storing up to 4500 atoms of iron. Many coagulation factors are synthesized in the liver. They include plasminogen, fibrinogen, and factors II, V, VII, IX, X, XI, XII, and XIII. Factors II, VII, IX, and X are the so-called vitamin K–dependent factors that require vitamin K for synthesis and secretion in active form.[86] In addition, the anticlotting proteins antithrombin III, protein C, and protein S are synthesized largely in the liver and may be vitamin K dependent (see also Chapter 91). Several additional common plasma proteins are synthesized by the liver, including haptoglobin, ceruloplasmin, lipoproteins, α-fetoprotein, and the C3 component of complement.

Alterations in plasma proteins frequently occur during acute and chronic liver disease. Although the levels of many of these proteins may rise (acute-phase reactants) as part of the systemic inflammatory response (SIRS), plasma levels are generally reduced during liver disease, depending on the duration of hepatic insufficiency and the half-lives of the specific proteins. Thus a decrease in albumin generally represents a chronic disease state, whereas a prolonged prothrombin time may be seen within hours of acute hepatic failure because of the short half-life of factor VII (~6 hours).[87]

Degradation and Elimination by the Liver

Detoxification and catabolism of ammonia, bilirubin, and xenobiotics are essential to life. Ammonia arises through bacterial degradation of nitrogenous compounds in the intestine, as well as from other physiologic sources including the kidneys and peripheral tissues such as skeletal muscle and the brain. Ammonia is transported to the liver via the portal vein in high concentrations. Ammonia is quickly metabolized in the liver to urea. High levels of ammonia are incompatible with life, and during hepatic failure, hyperammonemia represents a life-threatening aspect of liver disease.[88]

Bilirubin is derived mainly from hemoglobin degradation, and its elimination is a critical excretory function of the liver. Smaller amounts are made through the breakdown of cytochromes and myoglobin. Heme is broken down into bilirubin in the reticuloendothelial system. Hepatic metabolism of bilirubin involves several steps, including transport to the hepatocyte and cellular uptake, cytosolic transport within the hepatocyte, conjugation, active cellular export, and elimination. Impairment at any step becomes manifest as hyperbilirubinemia and ultimately clinical jaundice. It may be defined as prehepatic if production is increased beyond the ability to clear or cholestatic if the conjugated bilirubin cannot not be excreted.

Enterohepatic Circulation

Bile acids represent a family of steroid molecules derived from cholesterol. They eliminate cholesterol from the body and solubilize dietary fats through a detergent-like action. Enterohepatic circulation conserves bile acids because a minimum concentration of bile acids is required for micelle formation. Bile salts are secreted into the duodenum with 97% reuptake in the terminal ileum, undergoing recycling 4 to 12 times per day. The distal and terminal ileum have specialized transport mechanisms for absorption of bile salts and vitamin B_{12}, which are adversely affected by terminal ileal resection, jejunostomies, inflammatory bowel disease, or other acquired lesions in this anatomic region (eg, necrotizing enterocolitis). Functional loss of the distal and terminal ileum results in malabsorption of vitamin B_{12}, bile salt deficiency, and impaired digestion and absorption of fat-soluble vitamins and long-chain fats. Furthermore, unresorbed bile acids entering the colon play a major role in secretory diarrhea.

Hepatic insufficiency, either from immaturity or as a result of disease, affects the elimination of many drugs. A large number of commonly used drugs of all classes including aminophylline preparations, narcotics, barbiturates, H_2-blockers, vasodilators, antidysrhythmics, and others demonstrate significant hepatic elimination. The hepatic P-450 (CYP) system plays a central role in many of the mixed-function oxidative reactions responsible for converting lipophilic compounds into more water-soluble ones.[89,90] The liver may conjugate drug metabolites to form hydrophilic products that can be eliminated easier in bile or through the kidney. The half-life of many drugs may be prolonged during hepatic insufficiency as a result of a decrease in the total number of functioning hepatocytes. In addition, the half-life of many drugs may be prolonged through competitive inhibition by the presence of other drugs, or it may be shortened by the induction of rate-limiting elimination pathways. For example, phenobarbital decreases the half-life of xanthines and may increase the toxicity of acetaminophen. Adjustment of medication dosage and schedule must be considered for those drugs with significant hepatic elimination when impaired liver function exists.[36]

Hepatic Regulatory Function

The liver provides major counterregulation through (1) interconversion of amino acids to maintain physiologic plasma levels, (2) gluconeogenesis to maintain adequate serum levels for glucose-dependent tissues, and (3) regulation of numerous plasma hormones (Box 96.4). The direct secretion of insulin and glucagon into the portal circulation exposes the liver to concentrations up to 10-fold greater than peripheral tissues. This relationship amplifies the hepatic influence over carbohydrate metabolism. Approximately 50% of secreted insulin

and a large portion of glucagon are degraded on a first-pass basis by the liver. Both of these hormones are known to have hepatotrophic effects and are thought to be important for differentiation and regeneration of hepatocytes. Intensive insulin therapy in the critical care setting has been shown to have a beneficial effect on liver function.[91]

Storage Function

The last category of hepatic function involves storage of glycogen, triglycerides, folic acid, vitamin B_{12}, and vitamins A and D. The liver uses glycogenolysis to mobilize hepatic glycogen stores and provide an almost immediate source of glucose to maintain serum levels. The liver glycogen stores contain up to a 2-day supply of glucose,[92] although these can be depleted rapidly by infants who become ill and have a decrease in oral nutrition. Synthesis of vitamin D_3 (cholecalciferol) occurs in the skin with subsequent accumulation of D_3 in the liver. Hydroxylation in the 25-position that occurs in the liver results in a large pool of circulating 25-$(OH)D_3$, the precursor of the active 1, 25-(dihydroxy) D_3. Defective storage and absorption of dietary vitamin D and 25-hydroxylation may be present in chronic liver failure.[93,94]

Host-Defense Mechanisms of the Gut: Immunology and Microbiology

Both the intestine and the hepatic-based macrophages can serve as major sources of nitric oxide following injury or stimulation[95] and contribute to the gastrointestinal tract's role in systemic responses. The frequent association of hepatic dysfunction with the acute respiratory distress syndrome has led to intensive investigation of the lung-liver axis during critical illness.[96] A major unifying theme in these organ interactions is the regional activation of macrophages and platelets and damage to the endothelium after injury leading to both localized and remote organ function disturbance. The gut has become one of the important focuses in our evolving understanding of multiple organ dysfunction syndrome (MODS) (see also Chapter 112).[7]

The gastrointestinal tract is the largest immunologic organ in the body and is where 80% of the body's entire immune system resides. [97] As such, the gut is in a constant state of controlled inflammation, serving essentially three immunologic functions: (1) to achieve tolerance to commensal microbiota and dietary proteins, (2) to induce destruction or elimination of pathogenic organisms and antigens, (3) to suppress the tendency toward dysplasia in this chronically "controlled" inflammatory environment. Although these processes develop from birth to adulthood, the gut also undergoes developmental changes in the microbiome.[98] Based on multiple studies, it is clear that the components of the microbiome have affects on health and disease of the gut immune system as well as the rest of the body.[99,100]

Immunologic Processes of Gut

When an antigen is presented to the gut, it must survive exposure to several nonimmune protective measures (referred to as innate immunity) including salivary and pancreatic enzymes, low gastric pH, the detergent effect of bile acids, the "house cleaning" function of intestinal motility, and the protective effects of the mucus layer above the epithelium. Once antigen reaches the epithelium, dendritic cells "sample" the antigen, process it, and then a response occurs involving either

---

BOX 96.4 | Hepatic Endocrine Regulation

Catabolism Primarily by Liver
- Insulin
- Glucagon
- Growth hormone
- Glucocorticoids
- Estrogens
- Progesterone
- Parathyroid hormone
- Some gut hormones

Catabolism by Liver and Other Tissues
- Thyroid hormone
- Luteinizing hormone
- Antidiuretic hormone
- Testosterone
- Aldosterone
- Oxytocin
- Adrenocorticotropic hormone
- Thyroid-stimulating hormone
- Thyroid-releasing hormone

TABLE 96.3   Innate and Adaptive Immunity

Innate Immune System	Adaptive Immune System
Naively responds to invading pathogens/antigens	Allows for memory and suppression, T- and B-cells
Phylogenetically older defenses (eg, lectins, surfactants, chetlidicins, defensins)	Provides rapid response to known antigens
Antigen presenting cells: phagocytes, dendritic cells	Adapts and suppresses reaction to future exposure

(See also Chapters 101 and 102.)

destruction/elimination of the antigen or tolerance of the antigen. The cells of the gut-associated lymphoid tissue (GALT) involved in this highly complex and coordinated dance are roughly organized into three compartments: diffusely scattered through the lamina propria, within the epithelium itself, and into lymphoid follicles called Peyer patches. A key theme in this complexity is the understanding that these cells have developed from evolutionary archaic *innate* cell function to more advanced *adaptive* functions. They have evolved to form both innate and adaptive immune responds (Table 96.3). The cellular basis of immunity in the gut depends on the production of mucus by goblet cells, alpha-defensins by Paneth cells, and tight junctions preventing penetration by large peptides once gut "closure" occurs. IgA is produced in response to gut flora binding to bacteria and sweeping them out in the feces.

Lymphocytes play a central role in the balanced inflammatory response within the intestine and recapitulate patterns of control common to specialized lymphocyte population elsewhere in the body (see also Chapter 102).[101,102] In the infant, lymphocytes in fresh breast milk can invade the GALT and confer the mother's immunologic memory to the naive infant's immune system. Similarly, intact protein can permeate the epithelium and lead to sensitization to foreign proteins as is seen in cow's milk protein sensitivity. The intestinal lymphocytes depend on vitamins A and D as well as zinc for generation of T lymphocytes, suggesting the importance of micronutrients in intestinal immune function.

The intestinal flora or microbiota are extremely important for systemic health and are frequently disrupted by the broad-spectrum antibiotics used in critically ill patients.[99,100] For example, early studies of mice raised in a germ-free environment suggested the importance of a healthy balance of intestinal bacteria, whereas small bowel bacterial overgrowth is a well-recognized source of chronic diarrhea and morbidity in children.[103] Dysbiosis is a known factor in several common diseases seen in the PICU including *C. difficile* colitis, Crohn disease, ulcerative colitis, and necrotizing enterocolitis.

The continual crosstalk between the GALT and intestinal contents provides a critical feedback mechanism for counter-regulation of the lymphocyte pools.[104] This area of intestinal immunology is under active investigation, although the importance of the intestinal flora in restoring and maintaining health is beyond question. Evidence for this effect comes from the 90% cure rate for *C. difficile* colitis achieved through fecal material transplantation.[105,106] In addition, the role of the intestinal bacteria in drug and bile salt metabolism has only become appreciated.[107]

The interaction between gut and brain has come under investigation with numerous small series studies demonstrating important effects of the intestinal microbiome with behavioral and psychologic conditions (depression, autism, etc.).[39] This observation has led to the concept of the gut-brain axis.[108,109] Its implications for the intensivist are far less clear than the data on restoring healthy gut flora but may have implications for a range of issues dealt with in the PICU including delirium, muscle wasting, and the like.

Bacterial translocation is defined as the migration of bacteria or bacterial products from the intestinal lumen to mesenteric lymph nodes or other extraintestinal organs, representing a disruption of the normal host flora equilibrium that leads to a self-perpetuating inflammatory response and ultimately to infection.[110] This process is increasingly being recognized as a potential source of pathogens producing bacteremia and sepsis in a variety of premorbid disease conditions such as cirrhosis and prematurity.[111,112] Translocation may occur directly through the M cells that cover the Peyer patches or it may occur by ingestion of viable pathogenic material by the mobile phagocytic system with transport into the host bypassing the previously outlined barrier mechanisms. Alteration in intestinal microbiome, host immune defenses, and damage to the microcirculation predispose to bacterial translocation. *E. coli*, *Proteus mirabilis*, and *Klebsiella pneumoniae* appear to be more commonly associated with translocation from the gastrointestinal tract.

Kupffer cells, which account for the largest pool of mononuclear phagocytes with direct access to the blood, play a major role in clearing portal bacteria. In addition, Kupffer cells are key participants in response to tissue injury or organ invasion through the elaboration of cytokine mediators, such as tumor necrosis factor (TNF) and interleukin (IL)-1, and the release of nitric oxide, leading to many of the systemic responses seen in sepsis.[95] Through their intimate proximity to the hepatocyte, Kupffer cells interact directly with hepatocytes by means of cell-cell and paracrine interactions. In response to TNF and IL-1, well-documented alterations in hepatic function occur, including the inhibition of albumin synthesis, gluconeogenesis, and P-450–mediated detoxification. Acute-phase reactant synthesis is also induced by TNF, IL-6, and IL-1.[113]

Gastrointestinal and Hepatobiliary Testing in the Intensive Care Unit

Diagnostic testing in the ICU permits the identification of organ system injury and dysfunction and assists in monitoring the course of a disease as well as its response to therapies. Laboratory testing is helpful in detecting and monitoring hepatocellular injury and dysfunction. In the ICU setting, impaired synthetic function is the hallmark of liver failure. This is of more immediate concern than hepatocellular injury alone. Decreased synthesis of the liver-dependent clotting factors I (fibrinogen), II (prothrombin), V, VII, IX, and X, results in a prolonged prothrombin time (PT). In the absence of vitamin K deficiency or related inhibitors, this represents liver failure. Because factor VII has the shortest half-life (2 to 6 hours) compared to the other factors, it acts as the rate-limiting step for conversion of prothrombin to thrombin. The use of recombinant activated factor VII in acute liver failure remains under debate.[87,114] Other less specific measures of liver dysfunction include increased bilirubin, decreased serum albumin, and decreased prealbumin.

Liver failure may also be associated with life-threatening hypoglycemia due to decreased hepatic synthesis and release of glucose, hyperinsulinemia from impaired hepatic degradation, and increased glucose utilization secondary to anaerobic metabolism. Plasma ammonia is frequently elevated resulting from urea cycle defects, portal systemic shunting, and events such as gastrointestinal bleeding that lead to increased ammonia production by enteric bacteria

Liver disease can be broadly categorized into hepatocellular, cholestatic, and infiltrative processes. The biochemical tests commonly used to detect cholestasis, which is impaired bile flow and hepatocellular injury, are serum bilirubin and aminotransferase activities (alanine transaminase [ALT], aspartate transaminase [AST]). Cholestasis, reduced bile excretion or transport, and biliary obstruction in the bile canaliculi or large ducts are represented by elevations in serum conjugated bilirubin, bile acids, alkaline phosphatase (ALK), γ-glutamyltransferase (GGT), or 5′-nucleotidase (5-NT).

The van den Bergh reaction assesses conjugated (direct fraction) bilirubin levels. The unconjugated (indirect) fraction represents the difference between the total bilirubin and the direct fraction. Elevated levels of indirect bilirubin result from (1) increased bilirubin load to the liver (eg, hemolysis), (2) diminished uptake and intracellular transport, and (3) reduced conjugation (eg, immaturity, fulminant necrosis).

In children, elevations in ALK may be seen with rickets or during periods of rapid skeletal growth. Isoenzymes of ALK may distinguish between liver or bony sources. Alanine transaminase (ALT or SGPT) and aspartate transaminase (AST or SGOT) are hepatic cytosolic enzymes that catalyze the reversible transfer of the α-amino group of the amino acids alanine and aspartic acids to the α-keto group of α-ketoglutaric acid producing pyruvic and oxaloacetic acids, respectively, plus glutamate. Elevations in serum activities of ALT and AST suggest hepatocellular injury (Table 96.4). AST is also present in myocardial tissue, skeletal muscle, kidney, pancreas, and erythrocytes; therefore increased AST is not specific for hepatocellular injury. ALT is present in only relatively low concentrations in tissues other than liver, providing greater specificity for hepatocellular injury than AST. Falling levels of AST and ALT in the setting of rising levels of conjugated bilirubin and ammonia represent increased destruction of hepatocytes rather than recovery. Elevated serum lactate dehydrogenase activity (LDH) lacks specificity and may be seen in association with hepatocellular injury, hemolysis, and myopathy; however, when in association with elevated serum creatinine phosphokinase (CPK) or aldolase, elevated LDH indicates myopathy or a rhabdomyolysis (Table 96.5).

TABLE 96.5 Diagnosis of Selected Hepatobiliary Disorders

Form of Liver Injury	Supportive History/Laboratory Data
Predominantly Hepatocellular	
Viral hepatitis	Viral serologies: hepatitis A, B, C, E, EBV, CMV, VZV, HSV
Drug-induced hepatitis	History of toxic/excess ingestion, ± elevated Eosinophil count
Ischemia	Shock, postcardiac surgery
Autoimmune hepatitis	Increased globulin ratio, antinuclear antibody, antismooth muscle antibody, antiliver kidney microsomal antibody
Wilson disease	Serum ceruloplasmin, 24-hour urine copper
α-antitrypsin deficiency	Pi typing
Cholestatic	
Bacterial sepsis	*Proteus, E. coli,* UTI
Galactosemia	Urine-reducing substances, *E. coli,* sepsis, red blood cell galactose-1-phosphate uridyltransferase
Tyrosinemia	Urine succinylacetone
Biliary atresia	Intraoperative cholangiogram
Anatomic anomalies: choledochal cysts, biliary stricture, cholelithiasis, congential hepatic fibrosis, Caroli disease	Ultrasonography, cholangiogram
Alagille syndrome	Butterfly vertebrae, posterior embryotoxon on eye exam, echocardiogram
Cystic fibrosis	Sweat test, genetic testing
GVHD, veno-occlusive disease	History of bone marrow transplant, high-dose busulfan
Ischemia	ECLS
Infiltrative	
Hepatocellular carcinoma, hepatoblastoma	α-Fetoprotein
Predominantly Coagulopathy	
Neonatal hematochromatosis	Serum iron and ferritin

CMV, cytomegalovirus; *EBV,* Epstein Barr virus; *ECLS,* extracorporeal life support; *HSV,* herpes simplex virus; *VZV,* varicella zoster virus.

TABLE 96.4 Pattern of Biochemical Tests Based on Category of Liver Disease

Biochemical Test	Hepatocellular Necrosis	Cholestasis	Infiltrative Process
ALT, AST	++ to +++	0 to +	0 to +
ALK, GGT	0 to +	++ to +++	+
Total/conjugated bilirubin	0 to +++	0 to +++	0 to +
PT	Prolonged	Prolonged; responsive to vitamin K	0
Albumin	Decreased in chronic disorders	Decreased in chronic disorders	0
Cholesterol	0	0 to +++	0
Bile acids	+ to +++	+ to +++	0

0, normal; + to +++, degrees of elevation.
ALK, alkaline phosphatase; *ALT,* alanine transaminase; *AST,* aspartate transaminase; *GGT,* g-glutamyltransferase; *PT,* prothrombin time.

Imaging of the hepatobiliary system has become easier, safer, and more reliable. Ultrasonography is particularly useful in the ICU and allows rapid, safe, bedside evaluation of (1) hepatic vascular structures and patterns of blood flow; (2) structural abnormalities such as tumors, abscess, hematoma, or dilated intrahepatic bile ducts; (3) the gallbladder, extrahepatic, pancreatic, and common biliary system; (4) the pancreas; (5) the genitourinary system; and (6) the abdomen and retroperitoneum (see also Chapter 20). In addition, ultrasound can provide guidance for therapeutic interventions such as drainage of abscesses.

Computed tomographic (CT) scan with and without contrast has become the diagnostic procedure of choice for evaluating the abdomen following trauma and in the ICU. Magnetic resonance imaging (MRI) provides an additional method for evaluating the abdominal and retroperitoneal organs for masses, abscesses, and fluid collections as well as vascular structures when contrast is administered.[115] A downside to both modalities is that they usually require a prolonged period away from the ICU, although rapid sequence CT and MRI procedures have reduced acquisition time for unstable patients.

Many of the radioisotope studies can be performed in the ICU when a portable scintillation camera is available. Technetium-99m (^{99m}Tc) IDA compounds are handled by the hepatobiliary system much like bilirubin and provide a qualitative and semiquantitative image of function and structure. These compounds may be used diagnostically to evaluate infants with persistent jaundice and also used in follow-up after the Kasai procedure or liver transplantation.

Of the available biochemical markers of pancreatic disease, serum amylase and lipase determinations are the most widely available. Serum lipase is elevated in about 87% of patients with acute pancreatitis and demonstrates fewer false-positive results than amylase testing. Transient hypocalcemia (<8 mg/dL) occurs in about 30% of patients with pancreatitis. Mild to moderate hyperglycemia as a result of islet cell damage is seen in up to 25% of cases, often necessitating the administration of exogenous insulin.

Evaluation of the alimentary tract consists of examining gastric aspirates and stool samples for gross bleeding or occult blood with the guaiac test (hemocult). A positive result mandates further evaluation and surveillance to determine the source and severity of gastrointestinal tract blood loss. Nasogastric lavage may be used to distinguish a source of bleeding as being proximal or distal to the pylorus. ^{99m}Tc sulfur colloid or red blood cells labeled with ^{99m}Tc may provide information regarding the site of active mucosal bleeding and are less invasive than arteriography.

Esophageal pH monitoring is useful for evaluating the efficacy of antisecretory therapy. It may be useful to correlate symptoms (eg, cough, chest pain) with acid reflux episodes and to select those infants and children with wheezing or respiratory symptoms in whom gastroesophageal reflex (GER) is an aggravating factor. The sensitivity, specificity, and clinical utility of pH monitoring for diagnosis and management of possible extraesophageal complications of GER are not well established.[116]

Imaging studies are of primary importance in acutely ill patients in a number of circumstances. Plain radiographs can be reliably used to locate radiopaque objects and to diagnose intestinal ileus, mechanical obstruction, and perforated viscus. Contrast studies are required to diagnose organ and soft tissue inflammation including appendicitis, pancreatitis and its complications, mesenteric and retroperitoneal masses, abscesses/fluid collections, intussusceptions, and anatomic anomalies.

Gastrointestinal bleeding from sites distal to the ligament of Treitz and proximal to the terminal ileum—sites that are inaccessible to video endoscopy, such as Meckel diverticulum, vascular malformations, and altered anatomy post gastrointestinal surgery—is best assessed using radio nuclide scans and angiography. Because of the need to perform the more sophisticated imaging studies away from the controlled environment of the ICU, the studies must be tailored to the patient's diagnostic needs according to the priorities of the initial stabilization of life-threatening illness and subsequent treatment of the underlying pathologic condition.

Video and or fiberoptic endoscopy in the hands of operators skilled in managing small children has found a place in ICU management to diagnose the source of upper gastrointestinal tract bleeding, to control and sclerose bleeding varices, to place percutaneous gastrostomy tubes for feeding, and for the placement of stents to maintain patency of the distal biliary and pancreatic tract.

Key References

4. Patterson E, et al. Gut microbiota, the pharmabiotics they produce and host health. *Proc Nutr Soc.* 2014;73:477-489.
6. Deitch EA. Gut-origin sepsis: evolution of a concept. *Surgeon.* 2012; 10:350-356.
7. Sertaridou E, et al. Gut failure in critical care: old school versus new school. *Ann Gastroenterol.* 2015;28:309-322.
8. Chang E, Leung P. Regulation of gastrointestinal functions. In: Leung P, ed. *The Gastrointestinal System: Gastrointestinal, Nutritional, and Hepatobiliary Physiology.* New York: Springer; 2014:3-58.
25. Wales P, et al. A.S.P.E.N. clinical guidelines: support of pediatric patients with intestinal failure at risk of parenteral nutrition-associated liver disease. *JPEN J Parenter Enteral Nutr.* 2014;38:538-557.
39. Carabotti M, et al. The gut-brain axis: interactions between enteric microbiota, central and enteric nervous systems. *Ann Gastroenterol.* 2015;28:203-209.
78. Iwakiri Y. Pathophysiology of portal hypertension. *Clin Liver Dis.* 2014; 18:281-291.
96. Hilliard KL, et al. The lung-liver axis: a requirement for maximal innate immunity and hepatoprotection during pneumonia. *Am J Respir Cell Mol Biol.* 2015;53:378-390.
107. Klaassen CD, Cui JY. Review: mechanisms of how the intestinal microbiota alters the effects of drugs and bile acids. *Drug Metab Dispos.* 2015;43:1505-1521.
108. Mayer EA, Tillisch K, Gupta A. Gut/brain axis and the microbiota. *J Clin Invest.* 2015;125:926-938.
116. Vandenplas Y, et al. Pediatric gastroesophageal reflux clinical practice guidelines: joint recommendations of the North American Society of Pediatric Gastroenterology, Hepatology, and Nutrition and the European Society of Pediatric Gastroenterology, Hepatology, and Nutrition. *J Pediatr Gastroenterol Nutr.* 2009;49:498-547.

Disorders and Diseases of the Gastrointestinal Tract and Liver

Claire Stewart and Samuel A. Kocoshis

PEARLS

- So much reliance is placed on electronic monitoring of patients that physicians are often tempted to perform only a cursory examination or go days without laying hands on the patient. Regrettably, adopting such an approach deprives the clinician of an adequate perspective on the patient's day-to-day condition and deprives the patient of optimal care.
- When compared with a scintiscan of the lungs after administration of a radiolabeled meal or with the discovery of lipid-laden macrophages after bronchoalveolar lavage, the use of colorants to monitor for aspiration pneumonitis is notoriously inaccurate.
- Several antireflux barriers exist in the region of the lower esophageal sphincter. Beyond intrinsic myogenic tone, barriers such as the cardioesophageal angle, the abdominal esophagus (which acts as a flutter valve), the mucosal rosette of the sphincter (which acts as a choke valve), and the diaphragmatic crura themselves act to prevent reflux of gastric contents.
- The association between *Helicobacter pylori* infection and both chronic gastritis and duodenal ulcer is well established, but the role of *H. pylori* in the pathogenesis of gastric ulceration remains somewhat speculative.
- Intravenous administration of somatostatin or its synthetic analogue, the active octreotide moiety, has been effective in stemming variceal hemorrhage and may work for other causes of gastrointestinal bleeding. In addition to their hemodynamic effects, these agents inhibit gastric acid production.
- Crohn disease and ulcerative colitis are chronic, relapsing disorders without known causes. The transmural inflammation of Crohn disease may affect any portion of the alimentary tract in a patchy distribution, whereas the inflammation of ulcerative colitis is confined to the mucosa of the colon.
- An abdominal plain film showing pneumatosis intestinalis, hepatic portal air, or both confirms the diagnosis of necrotizing enterocolitis. Because the pathogenesis is unknown, treatment must be symptomatic. In most centers, feedings are discontinued for 48 hours to 2 weeks depending on the severity of symptoms. Fluid resuscitation and broad-spectrum parenteral antibiotics are the bases of medical therapy. Surgical resection is reserved for severe

cases when medical management fails and gangrenous bowel develops.
- Abdominal compartment hypertension and syndrome are two distinct entities becoming increasingly recognized in the intensive care setting. Prompt recognition of clinical symptoms and signs may prevent vital organ compromise.

Gastrointestinal Evaluation of the Critically Ill Child

Dramatic advances in pediatric critical care have improved outcomes for children admitted to pediatric intensive care units (PICUs). Indeed, the technology available today has improved management strategies for a variety of conditions. So much reliance is placed on electronic monitoring of patients that physicians are often tempted to perform only a cursory examination or go days without laying hands on the patient. Regrettably, adopting such an approach deprives the clinician of an adequate perspective on the patient's day-to-day condition and deprives the patient of optimal care. Daily physical examination is of paramount importance in the assessment of children with either life-threatening gastrointestinal disease or gastrointestinal manifestations of multisystem disease. This chapter therefore reviews the current approach to gastroenterologic diagnosis and therapy as well as the principles of gastroenterologic physical examination.

Abdominal Examination

Astute clinicians recognize that the abdomen extends from the neck to the knees. A thorough examination of the head, neck, and chest is essential when patients with abdominal symptoms are evaluated. For example, pneumonia may be discovered by chest auscultation in the child who has abdominal pain.

The abdominal examination, which can be difficult to perform on young children without life-threatening illness, is made more difficult in the ICU setting. Pain and fear limit cooperation. Patients who are obtunded by narcotics, sedatives, or an underlying central nervous system (CNS) disorder display inconsistent responses to abdominal palpation. Neuromuscular blockade abolishes abdominal guarding. Children with multisystem trauma may not localize pain. These impediments notwithstanding, the observant clinician can glean a great deal of information from a carefully performed examination. Simple inspection of the child's abdomen can reveal generalized distention, abnormally prominent abdominal wall veins (which signify portal hypertension), or anterior and lateral abdominal wall ecchymoses, such as Cullen sign or Grey Turner sign (which herald acute pancreatitis). In addition, because of the child's relatively undeveloped abdominal musculature, visceromegaly or abdominal masses may be apparent on inspection.

Auscultation will ascertain the frequency and quality of peristaltic sounds. They normally occur every 10 to 30 seconds and are low pitched. High-pitched, frequent bowel sounds suggest enteritis or obstruction. In obstruction, bowel sounds characteristically reverberate and seem to originate from a deep well. Bowel sounds are absent in paralytic ileus or peritonitis. Ancillary findings include venous hums, which suggest portal obstruction, or bruits that may denote arteriovenous malformations.

In pediatric patients, palpation should generally precede percussion because it is less threatening. The child should be in the supine position, and when possible the hips and knees should be comfortably flexed to enhance abdominal wall relaxation. The abdomen should be palpated through all phases of respiration in all four quadrants. The examiner should lightly palpate to judge guarding and tenderness and should use gentle ballottement. Deeper palpation better localizes organomegaly or masses.

Percussion permits estimation of visceral size and helps to diagnose obstruction, peritonitis, or ascites. Excessive tympany implies that bowel loops are distended with air, whereas dullness suggests that excessive fluid or a solid mass is present. Shifting dullness is relatively easy to detect in cooperative children with percussion of the abdomen with the child in the supine, left lateral, and right lateral positions. When the child with ascites is in the supine position, dullness is found primarily over the flanks. The dullness moves to a new level nearer the midline when the child is moved to each lateral position. It is essential to perform a digital examination of the rectum in children with gastrointestinal dysfunction. Inspection of the perineum may reveal perianal or perirectal abscesses, which may be the first sign of acute leukemia, chronic granulomatous disease of childhood, or Crohn disease. Similarly, deep fissures or sentinel piles suggest ulcerative colitis or Crohn disease, and hemorrhoids can be found in portal hypertension. The digital examination should be performed in the alert, older child only after its purpose is explained. Any material that returns on the examining finger should be evaluated for occult blood. Absence of stool in the vault can corroborate Hirschsprung disease in an infant with abdominal distention and a history of obstipation. Rectal masses related to pelvic abscesses or tumors may be digitally palpated. Rectal tenderness signifies mural or extramural inflammation or infection.

Gastrointestinal Endoscopy

The development of flexible fiberoptic endoscopes appropriately sized for use in infants and children has greatly expanded the value of endoscopy in diagnosing and treating a variety of gastroenterologic disorders in critically ill pediatric patients. For example, pediatric endoscopes with an outside diameter of 5 mm can now be used for diagnostic purposes in newborn infants. Electrocautery, injection therapy, or variceal banding of gastrointestinal bleeding sites can also be performed with

devices that now fit within the biopsy channels of a standard 9.4-mm pediatric endoscope. Upper gastrointestinal endoscopy (esophagogastroduodenoscopy [EGD]) is performed most often with the child under deep sedation or general anesthesia, although some clinicians report successful unsedated upper endoscopy in very young infants. Many pediatric endoscopists in North America use a combination of narcotic sedative and benzodiazepine to achieve acceptable sedation analgesia.[1] Other agents commonly used for sedation are propofol and ketamine. General anesthesia with endotracheal intubation is appropriate when the side effects of sedation or the endoscopy pose an undue risk of respiratory compromise (eg, when underlying pulmonary disease, upper airway disease, or disorders of respiratory control are present) or if the patient is at risk for aspiration of gastric contents (eg, when massive upper gastrointestinal hemorrhage is present or when an emergency foreign body extraction is performed on a child with a full stomach). In an ICU setting, patients supported by ventilators should receive additional sedation and neuromuscular blockade if the endoscopist anticipates that the procedure will be lengthy or excessively difficult.

Advantages of elective endotracheal intubation for EGD also include control of both the airway and ventilation during the procedure. In very small patients, the relatively large endoscope may partially obstruct the glottis. Distention of the gut with air may interfere with diaphragmatic movement. The risk of inadvertent extubation during EGD, however, mandates careful fixation of the endotracheal tube and careful monitoring of ventilation during the procedure by a physician from the critical care team.

Because bacteremia may occur during both upper and lower gastrointestinal endoscopy, some endoscopists routinely use perioperative antibiotics for endoscopy in patients with a central venous line or ventriculoperitoneal shunt. Therapeutic endoscopy has complemented diagnostic endoscopy. Gastrointestinal tract hemorrhage from varices, peptic ulceration, and angiodysplasia may be controlled by injection therapy or photocoagulation, electrocoagulation, and thermocoagulation. Band ligation of esophageal varices is also a proved therapy for variceal hemorrhage. Percutaneous endoscopic gastrostomy has become a popular alternative to surgical gastrostomy to provide a reliable route for enteral nutrition for patients in the ICU who cannot take oral alimentation on a long-term basis.

The diagnosis and treatment of oropharyngeal dysphagia can be difficult but are improved with the use of fiberoptic endoscopic evaluation of swallowing (FEES). The endoscope can be passed transnasally to visualize both laryngeal and pharyngeal structures. Both the structure and functioning of the pharyngeal phase of swallowing can be evaluated by giving the patients food and liquid boluses. Sensory testing can also be conducted to elicit the laryngeal adductor reflex. Some studies have suggested a good correlation between FEES and videofluoroscopy.

Wireless video endoscopy or video capsule endoscopy (VCE) is a noninvasive technology used to provide imaging of the small intestine, an anatomic site often difficult to visualize. The images acquired are of excellent resolution and the procedure uses the principle of physiologic endoscopy via passive movement and does not inflate the bowel, so images of the mucosa are captured in a collapsed state. Primary indications include the diagnosis of obscure gastrointestinal bleeding, small bowel tumors, or Crohn disease. There is growing experience in the use of this technology for children older than 6 years. Advantages include its noninvasive nature and the ability to examine the small bowel mucosa, which is not possible with push enteroscopy. Disadvantages include the impossibility of any tissue sampling or therapeutic intervention. However, studies have suggested that the overall yield of VCE is superior to push enteroscopy and barium studies.[2-4]

Gastroesophageal Reflux Monitoring

Like gastrointestinal endoscopy, esophageal reflux monitoring has benefited from technical advances that permit insertion of miniature, flexible electrodes into the esophagus of the smallest children. Esophageal impedance monitoring[5-7] has become the preferred means of measuring gastroesophageal reflux in children, especially among patients who are receiving acid suppression or in whom weakly acidic or alkaline reflux is suspected, as impedance monitoring is independent of pH. The intraesophageal impedance device measures total opposition to current flow between two electrodes and expresses the value in ohms. Because air and fluid have different conductivities, the contents of the esophagus can be differentiated at any point in time. Thus when the esophagus is devoid of fluid, baseline impedance is measured. When a bolus of fluid enters the esophagus from refluxed material or from a swallowed bolus, the impedance changes. These changes in intraluminal impedance thus permit the continuous monitoring of pH neutral or alkaline reflux episodes.

In addition to detecting pathologic quantities of reflux in children who have symptoms suggestive of reflux disease, reflux monitoring is also useful in determining whether a temporal correlation exists between gastroesophageal reflux and pathologic events such as cough, bronchospasm, or apnea. Because it does not determine the cause of vomiting, reflux monitoring adds little to the evaluation of vomiting children.

Use of Colorants to Identify Aspiration in the Intensive Care Unit

Patients who are obtunded or who have been ventilator dependent for an extended time are at significant risk of pulmonary aspiration. A deceptively simple way of documenting aspiration in patients receiving gavage or gastrostomy feedings in the past has been to add a coloring agent such as blue dye No. 1 or methylene blue to the formula. The rationale for this strategy was that quantities sufficient to tint formula should be readily apparent when suctioned from the lungs. The fallacy of the technique is that when compared with scintiscanning of the lungs after administration of a radiolabeled meal or with the discovery of lipid-laden macrophages after bronchoalveolar lavage, the use of colorants is notoriously inaccurate. Furthermore, all colorants are dangerous when instilled into the gastrointestinal tract. They are customarily absorbed in minimal quantities, but among critically ill patients, the gastrointestinal tract becomes porous to all macromolecules and appreciable quantities of dye are absorbed. Once absorbed, even minimal quantities function as metabolic poisons, uncoupling oxidative metabolism, thereby resulting in life-threatening metabolic acidosis among susceptible patients.[8]

Radiologic Procedures

Plain Films

The abdominal x-ray film provides valuable assistance to the clinician evaluating children with abdominal distention,

guarding, or tenderness. Dilated, gas-filled bowel loops, with or without air-fluid levels, can signify obstruction or ileus. Air-fluid levels in a stepladder configuration along the length of small bowel suggest obstruction, whereas levels that appear in a parallel configuration suggest ileus. Pneumatosis intestinalis and mucosal thumbprinting are signs of bowel wall ischemia and can often be appreciated on the plain film. Pneumoperitoneum can be evaluated with the inspection for air in the lesser sack, air between bowel loops, or a visible falciform ligament. Even though an upright film is optimal for visualizing peritoneal air, lateral decubitus or cross-table lateral films are acceptable substitutes in bedridden patients. Air in an abscess cavity or air in liver parenchyma, biliary tree, or portal venous system should be acknowledged as signs of serious intraabdominal infection.

Abnormal densities such as abdominal masses, ascites, or calcifications can often be identified on plain films. Calcifications in the region of the gallbladder, pancreas, or appendix suggest cholelithiasis, pancreatitis, or appendicitis, respectively. The abdominal contour and the contour of extraperitoneal structures such as lung bases, pelvic organs, and kidneys should always be assessed.

Contrast Radiography

Although endoscopy is more sensitive than single-contrast radiography for identifying mucosal ulceration, contrast radiography remains a valuable procedure in the critical care setting. In general, the upper gastrointestinal tract series and small bowel series are indicated when partial small bowel obstruction is suspected. A contrast enema will document (and possibly treat) intussusception and document Hirschsprung disease. The type of contrast agent for a particular examination depends on the clinical condition of the patient undergoing the examination. Although barium sulfate is superior to water-soluble contrast agents for outlining mucosa, its use in typical ICU patients is riskier because barium may form a concretion in a patient with ileus and because barium leaking into the peritoneum from a perforated hollow viscus can cause serious peritoneal injury. Hyperosmolar, water-soluble contrast agents are usually not favored because they pose the risk of dehydration. Currently, isosmolar agents are more commonly used for studies on the critically ill patient.

Ultrasonography, Computed Tomographic Scanning, and Magnetic Resonance Scanning

Ultrasonography, computed tomographic (CT) scanning, and magnetic resonance imaging (MRI) each has advantages and disadvantages. For example, in the slim child with little mesenteric fat, ultrasonography is sometimes better than CT scanning of abdominal viscera. Conversely, CT scanning is superior for abdominal imaging of obese individuals.[9] MRI is limited by its inability to distinguish bowel loops from adjacent structures and by blurring caused by motion. It is helpful, though, in identifying vascular tumors, which are seen as low-intensity masses on T1-weighted images and high-intensity masses on T2-weighted images. Ultrasonography or CT is used when an intraabdominal abscess, cystic lesion, hepatobiliary disease, tumor, ascites, or pancreatitis is suspected. In the identification of pancreatic lesions, dynamic CT scanning is the preferred imaging technique. CT also best identifies enlarged periaortic lymph nodes. CT and magnetic resonance enterography are other modalities used to detect small bowel inflammatory disease. Oral hyperhydration can achieve adequate luminal distention, often not requiring nasoenteric intubation. Unlike routine CT or MRI, enterography can display mural changes along with perienteric inflammatory changes with much better resolution. These studies are more accurate than the standard small bowel follow-through or enteroclysis.[10-13] Magnetic resonance elastography is increasingly recognized as a modality for detecting and staging hepatic fibrosis and nonalcoholic fatty liver disease (NAFLD). The use of magnetic resonance elastography may negate the need for liver biopsy in some patients.[14] Alternatively, fibrosis detected on sonographic elastography correlates well with that detected by MRI. However, higher body mass index, presence of ascites, and small intercostal distance limit the utility of ultrasound elastography.[15] The combination of positron emission tomography (PET)/MRI can be very useful to evaluate for focal liver lesions and liver metastasis of various childhood neoplasms.[16]

Ultrasonography of the liver and biliary tract identifies hepatic parenchymal disease, biliary stones, or congenital abnormalities such as choledochal cyst. Intussusception, pyloric stenosis, and acute appendicitis are particularly amenable to ultrasonographic diagnosis. In addition, Doppler flow analysis has significantly aided the preoperative and postoperative evaluation of liver transplant recipients by identifying congenital vascular anomalies and postoperative vascular thromboses.

Radionuclide Scanning

Radionuclide scanning is helpful when patients in the ICU have pulmonary aspiration, gastrointestinal bleeding, intraabdominal abscesses, or cholestasis.

Gastroesophageal reflux and the rate of gastric emptying can be measured with liquid-phase gastroesophageal scintigraphy.[17] Technetium-99 (^{99}Tc) sulfur colloid is mixed with formula or another enterally administered liquid. When there is a scan above and below the diaphragm in 30- to 60-second windows during the first postprandial hour after isotope administration, the number of reflux episodes, the height of the reflux column, and the rate of gastric emptying are quantitated. A 4- to 6-hour delayed scan of the lungs determines whether pulmonary aspiration of that meal has occurred.[18]

Three techniques are used to aid in the diagnosis of gastrointestinal bleeding. ^{99}Tc sulfur colloid and ^{99}Tc-labeled red cells are used in patients with continuous or intermittent bleeding. The advantage of sulfur colloid is that less than 0.1 mL/min of blood can be detected. Bleeding in a spot near the liver or spleen, however, may be obscured by high levels of activity in those organs. Tagged red blood cell scans detect intermittent bleeding by means of delayed scans, but migration of blood down the gastrointestinal tract over time may preclude exact localization. ^{99}Tc pertechnetate scanning does not require active bleeding to localize a Meckel diverticulum. The isotope is concentrated by gastric mucosa, and if a scan reveals an ectopic focus, a Meckel diverticulum can be suspected. Scan results are negative in the 15% of diverticula not containing gastric mucosa. A variety of non-Meckel lesions (most of which require surgical correction) cause false-positive results on pertechnetate scans. The sensitivity of the scan can be increased when acid suppression is given prior to scanning.

Resolution of hepatobiliary scans has improved dramatically since the introduction of derivatives of ^{99}Tc iminodiacetic acid. Scanning can now document cholecystitis when there is no gallbladder uptake or biliary obstruction when there is no excretion into the bowel. Other entities such as biliary leaks or cystic lesions of the biliary tree can also be documented. Furthermore, delayed or reduced hepatocyte uptake can confirm impaired hepatocellular function.

Intraabdominal abscesses and inflammatory intestinal lesions can be localized with radioscintigraphy.[19] Leukocytes are extracted from the patient, tagged with a radioisotope in vitro, and reinjected. Scanning of the area in question is then performed. Technetium hexamethyl propyleneamine oxime (HMPAO) has replaced indium because of improved resolution of HMPAO scans and because HMPAO scans can be completed within 4 hours rather than 72 hours.

Testing for Occult Blood Loss

Occult blood loss is generally determined with the Hemoccult or Gastroccult test; these are modifications of the guaiac test.[20,21] They work because hemoglobin oxidizes the reagent to a blue product. The Hemoccult Sensa (Beckman Coulter, Inc., Brea, California) slide detects as little as 2 to 3 mL of stool blood loss per day. This slide is virtually 100% sensitive when blood loss equals 10 mL/day.[8]

In the stomach, blood can be denatured, and this can lead to false-negative results. Gastroccult, which contains borate-buffered reagent, significantly improves the sensitivity for testing gastric contents. (Urine test tapes should never be used for gastrointestinal occult blood testing because they are too sensitive.) Therefore even physiologic quantities of enteric blood loss (<1 mL of blood per day) will yield positive results.

Stool pH and Reducing Substances

Excessive enteral carbohydrate loads may worsen preexisting diarrhea in critically ill children. Carbohydrate malabsorption can be assessed with the measurement of reducing sugars and pH of stool. The two tests should always be used in conjunction because colonic transit time and the quantity or type of colonic flora affects either of these tests. Malabsorbed sugars appear in feces when colonic transit is sufficiently rapid and are detected by Clinitest tablets or reagent strips; sugar more than 0.5 mg/100 mL of stool water suggests malabsorption. If the malabsorbed dietary sugar is primarily sucrose, a nonreducing sugar, the Clinitest result is negative unless the stool is first hydrolyzed with hydrochloric acid. Stools can be negative for reducing sugars despite carbohydrate malabsorption if colonic transit is slow enough to permit complete bacterial fermentation. In such an event, pH of fresh stool (measured by nitrazine paper) is consistently below 5.5. The pH of samples not tested for several hours, however, tends to rise over time as short-chain fatty acids generated from sugar fermentation are further metabolized.

The Intensive Care Unit as a Satellite Laboratory Facility

Regulations of The Joint Commission prohibit testing for occult blood loss or stool testing by anyone other than an individual certified in accordance with the Clinical Laboratory Improvement Act (CLIA). Thus for many pediatric critical care units, bedside testing has moved from the bedside to the clinical laboratory. Turnaround time for measuring occult blood in stool has risen from seconds to hours. Furthermore, when fecal samples are sent to the clinical laboratory for measurement of reducing sugars and pH, results are meaningless insofar as bacterial metabolism of sugars continues ex vivo in these samples between the times of collection to the time of testing. Critical care units wishing to perform reliable fecal testing on site must train a cohort of staff in common bedside tests and obtain CLIA certification for each staff member. Furthermore, just as many ICUs have chosen to comply with CLIA regulations and have established approved satellite laboratory facilities to measure blood gases or serum electrolytes, they can extend the scope of their laboratory activities to include bedside gastroenterologic testing.

Life-Threatening Complications of Gastrointestinal Disorders

Systemic

Central Line–Associated Bloodstream Infection

Children with intestinal failure who are reliant on parenteral nutrition through a central line are at high risk of central line–associated bloodstream infections (CLABSIs) because of the presence of an indwelling catheter and the generalized inflammation and reduced mucosal barrier of their gut. CLABSIs are the number one cause of mortality among this patient group. These children are frequently admitted to the pediatric intensive care unit with septic shock. Children who are younger have a shorter segment of viable bowel (<50 cm), and those receiving a higher dose of parenteral lipids seem to be at increased risk of CLABSIs. The most common bacteria causing these infections are enteric gram-negative organisms such as *Klebsiella* species and *Enterobacter* species. *Enterococcus* species and *coagulase-negative staphylococci* can also be commonly seen, as can *Candida* species. As such, therapy should start with broad-spectrum gram-negative and gram-positive coverage with addition of an antifungal if this is a concern, with narrowing of coverage as soon as species identification and susceptibility testing allow. A goal of treatment for these children is often to salvage their central line, as their life depends on their ability to receive parenteral nutrition, and they may have limited venous access. Loss of vascular access is one of the few indications for small bowel transplant in these patients. Ethanol locks are an inexpensive method to improve infection clearance rates and increase line salvage rates both in the pediatric intensive care unit and in the outpatient setting and may be used in both a treatment and prophylactic approach. Ethanol locks are preferred over antibiotic locks due to their ability to eradicate biofilms and to minimize the evolution of resistant bacteria[22-24] (see also Chapter 110).

Esophagus

Congenital Esophageal Anomalies

Esophageal atresia and tracheoesophageal fistula are true neonatal emergencies. With an incidence of 1 in 3000 live births, they are among the most common congenital anomalies of the esophagus. Five anatomic varieties exist in the following descending order of frequency: (1) blind proximal esophageal pouch with distal esophagus originating at the tracheobronchial junction (80%), (2) blind proximal esophageal pouch with blind distal esophageal pouch (8%), (3) uninterrupted

esophagus with H-type tracheoesophageal fistula (4%), (4) proximal esophagus fistulizing into trachea with blind distal esophageal pouch (2%), and (5) interrupted esophagus with both proximal and distal esophagus communicating with trachea (1%). The embryogenesis of this disorder is unknown, but other cardiovascular, gastrointestinal, skeletal, or urogenital anomalies are present in 50% of cases.

Infants with a blind proximal esophagus have excessive salivation, respiratory distress, and cyanosis. Diagnosis of blind proximal esophagus can be made by the failure to pass a nasogastric tube into the stomach. Complete atresia leads to a gasless lower gastrointestinal tract. An H-type fistula is sometimes seen on contrast radiography or esophagoscopy, but bronchoscopy is usually the most sensitive diagnostic tool.

Treatment is surgical. A simple fistula can be ligated, and a short atresia can be repaired primarily. Long atresia, however, may require staged treatment with initial esophagostomy and gastrostomy and subsequent definitive repair after internal or external traction is applied. Circular myotomy of the esophagus reduces anastomotic tension. Occasionally a gastric tube procedure or colonic interposition is required.

Caustic Injury to the Esophagus

Despite widespread efforts by poison control centers to publicize the dangers of household caustics, thousands of inadvertent ingestions occur annually; most occur in children younger than 5 years. Crystalline products produce greater damage to the hypopharynx and upper airway because of prolonged mouth contact and a smaller volume reaching the esophagus. Most household cleaners have been reformulated to contain less lye, but pure liquid lye can be purchased if desired. Its resemblance to milk leads to numerous inadvertent ingestions by children (see Chapter 128).

Tissue damage can be caused by either strong alkali or acid. Deep esophageal burns are more common after alkali ingestion. Alkalis produce rapid liquefaction of esophageal tissue, and burns can range from first to third degree in depth.[25] An intense inflammatory infiltrate develops, and blood vessels thrombose to produce ischemic necrosis. Perforation may occur within hours or days. Strictures can occur weeks to years after ingestion.[26] Esophageal burns occur infrequently after acid ingestion, but gastric or duodenal erosions have been reported.

Symptoms that predominate are chest pain and the inability to swallow secretions. Children with upper airway damage often exhibit stridor. When mouth burns are present, the chances of esophageal injury are 75%.[1] Conversely, 25% of patients with significant esophageal burns have no pharyngeal or mouth involvement.[25]

Treatment of severe stridor should be directed toward establishing an airway, and emergency tracheostomy should be contemplated. Upper endoscopy within 24 hours is advisable. If burns are minor, no further therapy is necessary, and patients are at low risk of sequelae. Third-degree burns require ongoing intensive care, though. The role of antibiotics and steroids remains controversial.[27] When third-degree burns are endoscopically evident, a nasogastric tube should be positioned with endoscopic guidance. This tube will enable early feeding and serve as a guide for future dilations if they become necessary. Some surgeons have advocated early placement of gastrostomies and esophageal stents in patients with third-degree burns.

Esophageal Foreign Bodies

Children can swallow a variety of metallic, wooden, or plastic foreign bodies in a myriad of shapes and sizes. All that are lodged in the esophagus require urgent removal (within 24 hours). Even more urgent endoscopic retrieval is required for button batteries or pennies minted after 1983 that are lodged in the esophagus because both are caustic to esophageal mucosa and may cause damage within 1 to 4 hours. The preponderance of evidence suggests that once a battery has escaped the esophagus, complications from an unretrieved battery are rare.[28]

Similarly, pennies minted after 1983 are predominantly zinc based and can be nearly as caustic within the esophagus as button batteries. No published epidemiologic studies are available on which to base the approach to zinc-based pennies within the stomach or small intestine.

Gastroesophageal Reflux

Several antireflux barriers exist in the region of the lower esophageal sphincter. Beyond intrinsic myogenic tone, barriers such as the cardioesophageal angle, the abdominal esophagus (that acts as flutter valve), the mucosal rosette of the sphincter (that acts as a choke valve), and the diaphragmatic crura themselves act to prevent reflux of gastric contents. A complex set of factors, including hormonal changes, anatomic relationships, increased or decreased sensitivity to neurotransmitters, and CNS derangements, act to produce inappropriate sphincter relaxation (usually transient), which leads to most episodes of gastroesophageal reflux. With the advent of more sophisticated otolaryngologic procedures such as the laryngotracheoplasty and slide tracheoplasty, prevention of gastroesophageal reflux is of utmost importance to facilitate surgical healing. Some surgeons advocate the use of aggressive acid suppression postoperatively because acid-induced damage can result in significant cicatrix formation at the site of laryngotracheal surgery.

Life-threatening events such as apnea and pulmonary aspiration are sometimes attributed to reflux. The relationship between infantile apnea and reflux remains in question,[29] but both human and animal data suggest that reflux can occasionally be associated with obstructive breathing patterns. Severe pulmonary aspiration of refluxed material can also take place. A number of protective mechanisms such as an active gag reflex, cough reflex, and laryngospasm protect against aspiration,[30] but these reflexes may be lost under special circumstances such as obtundation. Symptoms of obstructive apnea often include a brief episode of stridor accompanied by a struggle to breathe, a change in skin color to red or purple, and finally cyanosis and cessation of respiratory effort. Patients who have aspirated massive amounts of fluid become tachypneic and dyspneic shortly after the meal. Food or formula is often found in the nares or mouth, and cough may be present. The diagnostic modality most helpful in documenting a temporal relationship between apnea and acid reflux is 24-hour esophageal reflux monitoring combined with simultaneous electrocardiography, pneumography by chest wall impedance, pneumography by nasal thermistor, pulse oximetry, and end-tidal CO_2 measurement. Aspiration is often difficult to document, but the presence of a new infiltrate on chest x-ray films and a consistent clinical history provide strong circumstantial evidence. If repeated aspiration is suspected, an upper gastrointestinal tract series may reveal gastroesophageal reflux and immediate aspiration of barium; however, aspiration of gastroesophageal refluxate that occurs minutes or hours after a feeding may be missed with contrast radiography. A milk scan may be more sensitive than radiography for documenting this type of aspiration. Children who are not fed orally may nevertheless aspirate oral secretions. The scintigraphic *salivagram* is performed with the placement of a drop of saline containing ^{99m}Tc sulfur colloid on the tongue.[31] Subsequent imaging permits observation of its handling. The appearance of isotope in the trachea and bronchi confirms aspiration.

When recurrent aspiration is suspected but not confirmed noninvasively, bronchoscopy with bronchoalveolar lavage may support the diagnosis by returning fluid-containing lipid-laden alveolar macrophages.[32] Aspiration during swallowing and aspiration of refluxed gastric contents cannot be distinguished by this method in patients who are fed orally.

Although some clinicians view one episode of reflux-induced aspiration or apnea as an absolute indication for fundoplication, the decision to perform fundoplication should be based on the severity of the initial episode, underlying conditions that predisposed the child to the episode, risk for recurrence, and the expected natural history of reflux for a particular patient. In other words, some patients may be successfully managed with pharmacotherapy (a proton pump inhibitor with or without a prokinetic agent such as metoclopramide or erythromycin).

For patients with neurologic impairment, excessive drooling can lead to chronic aspiration, pneumonia, and difficult airway control; however, there are several treatment options for this issue. The first, and most commonly used, is glycopyrrolate; however, due to its anticholinergic properties, it is often not tolerated or leads to unacceptable thickening of secretions. Another option is injection of botulinum toxin A by a pediatric otolaryngologist or interventional radiologist. Various studies have shown that approximately 60% of patients improve after these injections, and if there is improvement, the patient may benefit from subsequent injections. Male sex and cerebral palsy were associated with an increased positive response. The major side effect for botulinum toxin injection is dysphagia.[33] Finally, some patients who are refractory to more conservative management may benefit from surgical intervention by otolaryngology, specifically a submandibular gland excision, ligation of submandibular and parotid ducts (commonly known as a *drool* procedure), and, in the most extreme of cases, a laryngotracheal separation.[34]

Stomach and Duodenum
Gastric Volvulus

Acute gastric volvulus may be of two types. When the whole stomach revolves about its long axis, organoaxial volvulus has occurred. When the fundus and pylorus exchange positions, the volvulus is mesenteroaxial. Predisposing factors include paraesophageal hernias or eventration of the diaphragm.

Because a closed obstruction has occurred, the patient is unable to vomit despite severe pain, distention, and retching. Plain radiographs reveal a markedly distended stomach with air-fluid levels, and contrast radiography may reveal cardioesophageal junction obstruction. An immediate operation is indicated.

Gastric Ulcer

Whereas some authors suggest that duodenal ulcers outnumber gastric ulcers in childhood,[35] others have reported that young children are more likely to have gastric ulcers. Most gastric ulcers lie at the junction of gastric fundus and body. Those high in the fundus are usually related to stress. Antral ulcers are often the result of use of nonsteroidal antiinflammatory drugs (NSAIDs).

A well-recognized complication of severe illness requiring admission to the ICU is stress ulceration of the stomach. Bleeding becomes an important source of morbidity and mortality in patients with burns and trauma, as well as in those who have undergone major operations or have systemic disease. Prophylaxis against bleeding is common in the ICU setting. Antacids, H_2-receptor antagonists (H₂RA), proton pump inhibitors such as lansoprazole and pantoprazole, and sucralfate are most often used. Unfortunately, elevation of gastric pH by antacids and H₂RA removes one barrier against bacterial colonization and may increase the risk of pneumonia with organisms colonizing the stomach.[36] Large controlled trials, however, have failed to confirm this concern. Sucralfate is equally effective as prophylaxis against bleeding but does not affect gastric pH. If sucralfate is given concurrently with antacids or acid-suppressing medications, its efficacy will be reduced because it requires an acidic environment for optimal effect. Furthermore, sucralfate administered in close temporal proximity to other enterally administered medications may reduce their bioavailability by binding with them within the intestinal lumen (see also Chapter 98).

Most patients with gastric ulcers are hypochlorhydric rather than hyperchlorhydric, because exposure to detergents or toxins such as NSAIDs, pepsin, bile salts, or ethanol erodes the gastric barrier to back-diffusion. A second consistent finding among patients with gastric ulcers is delayed gastric emptying, which may be an epiphenomenon or central to the pathogenesis of ulcers. The association between *Helicobacter pylori* infection and chronic gastritis as well as gastric and duodenal ulcers is now well established.

Clinical features of gastric ulcer resemble those of duodenal ulcer. Pain predominates and is epigastric in location but usually follows eating more closely. Nausea and vomiting may occur. Milk or antacids relieve the pain. The two complications of gastric or duodenal ulceration most commonly requiring intensive care are perforation and bleeding. Perforation, requiring immediate surgical intervention, produces exquisite pain and rapid development of peritoneal signs in patients without immunosuppression.

Hematemesis heralds gastric ulcer bleeding and may be as massive as that of duodenal ulcer. Careful, repeated assessment of vital signs and prompt restoration of circulating blood volume by large-bore venous catheters are essential. Saline solution or epinephrine gastric lavage through a large sump tube is mandatory. *Iced* saline lavage offers no advantage and excessively depresses core temperature.

Efforts should also focus on reducing gastric acid production with a parenteral proton pump inhibitor.[37] Continuous intravenous vasopressin infusion, commonly used for control of variceal hemorrhage, reduces arterial flow through the splanchnic bed. Intravenous administration of somatostatin or its synthetic, active octreotide moiety, has been effective in stemming variceal hemorrhage and may work for other causes of bleeding. In addition to their hemodynamic effects, they inhibit gastric acid production.

When the patient's condition is stable, endoscopy may be performed to localize the ulcer. Endoscopic therapy may then be performed on actively bleeding ulcers or those with visible vessels (which tend to rebleed). Ulcer beds may be photocoagulated, electrocoagulated, or thermocoagulated. They may also be injected with hemostatic agents such as epinephrine. If nonsurgical techniques fail to stop the bleeding, one of several surgical options (including ulcer oversewing or resection, variations of gastric drainage procedures, and vagotomy) must be performed. Fortunately, successful pharmacologic and endoscopic therapies have precluded the need for these surgical therapies in all but the rarest circumstances.

Duodenal Ulcers

The incidence of duodenal ulcer in childhood is unknown. A large series completed before the popularization of endoscopy suggested an incidence of 4.4 cases per 10,000 pediatric patients per year, which is, no doubt, an underestimation.[35] The male predominance seen among adults is present only among postpubertal children. The risk for patients with blood group O is 1.3 times that expected.

A number of factors have been implicated in the pathogenesis of duodenal ulcers. Unquestionably, excessive acid production plays a major role. Some factors leading to hypersecretion include excessive gastrin or histamine production and increased vagal tone. Approximately half of patients with ulcers are also hyperpepsinogenemic, and their mucosal integrity may therefore be suboptimal.[38] Infection with *H. pylori* reduces the ulcer healing rate and increases the recurrence rate.[39] Although approximately 90% of adult duodenal ulcers are associated with *H. pylori* infection, only about 50% of pediatric duodenal ulcers are related to *H. pylori*.[40] The effects of diet and stress have been minimized in the literature.

Symptoms in children are similar to those of adults. Epigastric pain occurs after meals and often awakens the child from sleep. Vomiting occurs in 40% of patients.

The major life-threatening complications are perforation and hemorrhage, which lead to a *surgical* abdomen and shock, respectively. Abdominal plain films reveal free air if perforation has occurred. Hemorrhage presents as hematemesis, hematochezia, or melena. Endoscopy is the most sensitive tool to localize the ulcer and to characterize the risk for rebleeding. Ulcers with visible vessels in the crater are at greatest risk of recurrent hemorrhage and may require endoscopic coagulation. Principles of management are identical to those for gastric ulcer. *H. pylori* is increasingly resistant to conventional antibiotics such as metronidazole and clarithromycin.[41] Triple therapy with a proton pump inhibitor, amoxicillin, and either clarithromycin or metronidazole for 10 to 14 days is currently recommended; however, in areas with high clarithromycin resistance, clarithromycin susceptibility testing is first recommended.[42]

Small Intestine and Colon

Malrotation

In embryonic life, the cecum and ascending colon are located on the left side of the abdomen and the small bowel is on the right. During gestation, the midgut transiently protrudes into the umbilicus and rotates 270 degrees, and the cecum is moved to the right lower quadrant and the duodenojejunal junction to the left upper quadrant. Incomplete rotation is of little consequence unless midgut volvulus, which can be a catastrophic event, occurs.

Some patients with malrotation experience partial duodenal obstruction because of extrinsic compression by mesenteric bands. Chronic diarrhea and protein-losing enteropathy may be seen, among others, without complete obstruction.

Clinical features of obstructing volvulus include severe abdominal pain, bilious vomiting, and abdominal distention. Surgical treatment requires a Ladd procedure, in which mesenteric bands are divided and the bowel is returned to its fetal position. Failure to promptly relieve the volvulus leads to ischemic necrosis of all of the gut supplied by the superior mesenteric artery (proximal jejunum to midtransverse colon). Short gut syndrome results from resection of the affected intestine.

Necrotizing Enterocolitis

Necrotizing enterocolitis is primarily a disorder of premature infants, affecting 2.5% of neonatal patients in the ICU but only 0.2% of all infants. The most common areas involved are the ileum and proximal colon, but any part of the intestinal tract may be affected. Its pathogenesis is unknown, but bowel ischemia, feeding of hyperosmolar formula, rapid advancement of feeding,[43] reduced immune surveillance, and population of the bowel by excessive quantities of enterotoxin-producing bacteria[44] may all play a role.

The classic clinical features are abdominal distention, bilious vomiting, and bloody stools, but symptoms are more subtle in some infants. If left unrecognized, necrotizing enterocolitis may become fulminant, leading to shock, disseminated intravascular coagulation, and apnea.

An abdominal plain film showing pneumatosis intestinalis, hepatic portal air, or both may confirm the diagnosis of necrotizing enterocolitis. Because the pathogenesis is unknown, treatment must be symptomatic. In most centers, feedings are discontinued for 48 hours to 2 weeks depending on the severity of symptoms. Fluid resuscitation and broad-spectrum parenteral antibiotics are the basis of medical therapy. Surgical resection is reserved for severe cases when medical management fails and gangrenous bowel develops. Data have emerged suggesting that changes in the neonatal fecal microbiome or production of excessive quantities of volatile organic acids are early markers of necrotizing enterocolitis (NEC); however, the ability to detect these entities is not yet practical for the clinician at the bedside.[45,46]

Perforation may sometimes be managed successfully in infants with very low birth weight, with simple peritoneal drainage performed with the infant under local anesthesia.[38]

Low Cardiac Output Syndrome

Advancements in surgical techniques have led to significant improvement in morbidity and mortality after pediatric cardiothoracic surgery. However, patients remain at risk for decreased cardiac output and impaired systemic oxygen delivery, especially in the early postoperative period. The drop in cardiac output after cardiac surgery is characterized as low cardiac output syndrome (LCOS). LCOS is defined as an inability of the heart to provide adequate oxygen delivery to meet the body's metabolic demand. It is primarily due to transient myocardial dysfunction compounded by acute changes in myocardial loading. Cardiopulmonary bypass, along with residual cardiac abnormalities, may further aggravate the underlying low cardiac output state.[47,48] Although there are several manifestations of this clinical constellation beyond the scope of this chapter, it is important to recognize its clinical signs and symptoms (see Chapter 38). Systemic venous congestion may be observed in the gastrointestinal tract. Manifestations include hepatomegaly, ascites, and peripheral edema. Hypoperfusion to the liver can result in hepatic insufficiency and may lead to coagulopathy if severe enough. Furthermore, intolerance to enteral feeding may be evident in these patients with LCOS and central venous hypertension. Feeding difficulties may be further compounded by high-dose inotropes and narcotic infusions. These patients often require parenteral nutrition. Complications such as mesenteric ischemia or necrotizing enterocolitis may be observed in rare cases and are often fatal.[49,50]

Food Allergy

Food allergy can be defined as a reproducible, immunologically mediated reaction to an ingested food protein. Pathogenic events can be classified according to the schema of Gell and Coombs as type I (reaginic, immediate hypersensitivity reaction), type II (cytotoxic reaction), type III (immune-complex reaction), or type IV (delayed hypersensitivity reaction).

Manifestations may be systemic[51] or confined to the gastrointestinal tract.[52] Life-threatening systemic manifestations include acute urticaria and anaphylaxis.[53] Gastrointestinal reactions, which are sometimes severe, include allergic enteritis, allergic colitis, and celiac crisis.

Acute urticaria is usually easily recognized by the classic wheal and flare cutaneous lesions often accompanied by laryngeal edema and angioedema. Anaphylaxis is an antigen-triggered immune reaction that leads to vascular collapse and bronchospasm (see also Chapter 106).

Food protein–induced enteropathy is characteristically a disorder of the infant and toddler. The small bowel develops patchy villous atrophy. Symptoms and signs range from those of malabsorption and enteric protein loss to those of profound diarrhea and shock. Colitis caused by food protein sensitivity is seen most commonly among infants younger than 6 months.[52] Bloody, mucoid diarrhea develops several days or weeks after their first oral antigen challenge. Even though this colitis usually takes a benign course, it may be severe enough to mimic necrotizing enterocolitis.

Although some do not categorize gluten enteropathy as true food allergy, it shares enough features with allergy to justify inclusion with this category of disorders.[52] Celiac crisis is a rare, life-threatening complication that may occur among untreated patients with a large gluten load or in treated patients as a result of dietary indiscretion. Massive fluid and electrolyte loss leads to shock.

The cornerstone of long-term therapy is elimination of the offending food, but emergency measures are also required. Immediate administration of epinephrine and corticosteroids is essential in the treatment of anaphylaxis. Urticaria may require the administration of antihistamines, corticosteroids, and epinephrine. Steroid use also seems to benefit patients in celiac crisis. Rapid administration of crystalloid or colloid is crucial in the management of any of these reactions.

Hemolytic-Uremic Syndrome

The hemolytic uremic syndrome may occur in epidemic or sporadic forms (see Chapter 75). It is frequently preceded by enteric infection with bacterial[54] or viral pathogens. Infection with Shiga toxin–producing *Escherichia coli* precedes a high number of cases.[55,56] Instigating factors, such as bacterial vero-toxin, cause endothelial damage in the kidney, liver, heart, brain, adrenal glands, and gastrointestinal tract.

Clinical features include a prodrome of abdominal pain, vomiting, and diarrhea, which may be bloody. Patients may have endoscopic, radiographic, or histologic evidence of ische-mic bowel disease. As gastrointestinal symptoms improve, hemolytic anemia and thrombocytopenia rapidly appear with associated symptoms of petechiae, epistaxis, gingival bleeding, and pallor. Subsequently, patients become oliguric, hyperten-sive, and azotemic. Pancreatitis may further complicate the clinical course. Seizures and altered mental status may occur.

The intensivist caring for children with acute, hemorrhagic colitis must pay exceptional attention to fluid balance, hemo-gram, and renal function studies. Any sudden change in hemoglobin, platelet count, blood urea nitrogen, or urine output should be considered a potential sign of hemolytic uremic syndrome. In the absence of hypovolemic shock, fluid intake should be curtailed if hemolytic uremic syndrome is documented. In the event of severe renal insufficiency, dialysis is necessary.

Atypical hemolytic uremic syndrome (aHUS) presents sim-ilarly to hemolytic uremic syndrome with hemolytic anemia, thrombocytopenia, and renal dysfunction but is usually not associated with a prior bacterial infection or diarrhea. In aHUS, dysregulation of the complement cascade leads to uncontrolled complement activation. Patients were previously treated with plasma exchange; however, the morbidity and mortality rates remained high. Eculizumab, a monoclonal antibody that targets C5 to block the complement cascade and prevent formation of the terminal complement complex, has been used in children with aHUS with better results than plasma exchange.[57]

Inflammatory Bowel Disease

Crohn disease and ulcerative colitis are chronic, relapsing dis-orders without known causes. The transmural inflammation of Crohn disease may affect any portion of the alimentary tract in a patchy distribution, whereas the inflammation of ulcerative colitis is confined to the mucosa of the colon. The latter always involves distal colon, and its contiguous inflam-mation extends for varying distances from the rectum. The two entities are different enough to usually permit accurate categorization, but there is sufficient overlap in symptoms and distribution that the diagnosis is indeterminate in 15% of cases. Table 97.1 summarizes the clinical, radiographic, endo-scopic, and histologic differences between the two.

The cause of these disorders remains speculative. Clearly, genetic factors predispose patients to one or the other, but environmental factors also appear to play a role.[58] Etiologic factors considered important over the years have included psy-chogenic predisposition, food allergies, infectious processes, immunologic deficiency, and immunologic hyperreactivity.

Presenting signs and symptoms include abdominal pain; bloody or nonbloody diarrhea; anorexia; abdominal mass; and extraintestinal manifestations, such as weight loss, fever, arthritis, or erythema nodosum. Patients are often anemic and hypoproteinemic, and they may show hematologic or bio-chemical signs of acute-phase response. The radiographic and histologic features are typical (see Table 97.1).

The cornerstone of achievement of remission has long been corticosteroids. Enteral feedings are emerging as an important component of achieving remission.[59] 5-Aminosalicylic acid

TABLE 97.1 Differential Diagnosis Between Ulcerative Colitis and Crohn Disease

Feature	Ulcerative Colitis	Crohn Disease
Relative Incidence of Symptoms		
Rectal bleeding (gross)	Common	Rare
Diarrhea	Often severe	Moderate or even absent
Pain	Less frequent	Almost always
Anorexia	Mild or moderate	Can be severe
Weight loss	Moderate	Severe
Growth retardation	Usually mild	Often pronounced
Extraintestinal manifestations	Common	Common
Involvement		
Small Bowel Involvement		
Extensive	—	10%
Lower ileum	5%-10%	90%
Colon	100%	75%
Rectum	95%	50%
Anus	5%	85%
Distribution of Lesions	Continuous	Segmental
Radiologic Features	Superficial ulcers, loss of haustration, no skip areas, shortening	Serpiginous ulcers, thumbprinting, skip areas, string sign
Pathologic Changes	Diffuse mucosal disease	Focal transmural disease, granulomas
Response to Treatment		
Steroids and sulfasalazine	75%	25%-75%
Parenteral nutrition and elemental diets	Poor	Very good for small bowel
Azathioprine and 6-mercaptopurine	Good in selected cases	Good in selected cases
Surgery	Excellent	Fair or poor
Course		
Remissions	Common	Common
Relapse after surgery	Rare	5%-100%
Cancer risk	High in pancolitis	Slight

Modified from Silverman A, Roy CC, editors: *Pediatric clinical gastroenterology*. ed 3. St. Louis: Mosby; 1983:354.

(5-ASA) is effective for maintenance therapy for mild ulcer-ative colitis and Crohn colitis. Evidence is less compelling that 5-ASA is effective in small intestinal Crohn disease. Immuno-suppressants, such as 6-mercaptopurine (6-MP) and metho-trexate, have been used for Crohn disease, and 6-mercaptopurine also seems effective in the treatment of ulcerative colitis. Bio-logical agents have revolutionized the therapy of Crohn disease.[60] Infliximab, a monoclonal antibody against tumor necrosis factor, has shown dramatic efficacy against Crohn disease in up to 75% of patients. A second anti–tumor necrosis factor (TNF) agent, adalimumab, can be given subcutaneously. New biologic agents such as vedolizumab, which binds to integrin alpha4 beta (LPAM-1), target a different pathway and are being used when first-line biologics fail.

Severe complications may also be directly attributed to therapy. Pancreatitis is associated with 5-ASA and 6-MP. In addition, bone marrow suppression as well as hepatitis have been observed with 6-MP. Infliximab is associated with lymphoid malignancies, and the concomitant use of 6-MP with infliximab may synergistically heighten the risk of lymphoma. Patients who take infliximab should also be observed for possible anaphylaxis. Patients with Crohn disease are at increased risk of secondary hemophagocytic lymphohistiocytosis (HLH); there is an increased risk associated with 6-MP use as well as primary Epstein-Barr virus infection.[61] Patients with HLH often come to the attention of intensivists because of their high risk of infection as well as pulmonary, hematologic, and hepatic complications (see also Chapter 106). Hepatosplenic T-cell lymphoma and other nongastrointestinal malignancies have been associated with the combined use of anti-TNF alpha agents and 6-MP, with males being at higher risk.[62]

Complications most likely to require an intensivist's attention are perforation, toxic dilation of the colon, and fulminant colitis. A patient whose bowel has perforated exhibits decreased bowel sounds and abdominal rigidity. Point and rebound tenderness may be present. Abdominal x-ray films may reveal free intraperitoneal air. Most perforations in Crohn disease produce intraabdominal abscesses, but peritonitis does not. Some abscesses, however, can contaminate the peritoneum. Free colonic perforation tends to occur among patients with ulcerative colitis. Toxic dilation and fulminant colitis are also more common with ulcerative colitis but may occasionally occur in Crohn colitis. Because management of severe inflammatory bowel disease frequently includes immunosuppression with high-dose corticosteroids, cyclosporine, or azathioprine, some of the signs and symptoms of perforation may be masked in the population most likely to have such complications. Factors such as patient immobility, antiperistaltic drugs, rigorous cathartic use, and electrolyte imbalance are frequently associated with toxic dilation of the colon. Patients initially exhibit massive abdominal distention and pain. X-ray films reveal an increased transverse colonic diameter. The patient's status is observed through careful monitoring of vital signs, physical examination, and repeated abdominal radiographs. Management includes giving nothing by mouth during nasogastric tube suction and inserting a rectal tube for decompression. Frequent position changes may aid in redistributing air distally. Fluid and electrolyte balance is aggressively maintained, and broad-spectrum parenteral antibiotics are given. Efforts at medical management should not exceed a few hours because of the extreme risk of perforation. Clinical decompensation or perforation is an indication for urgent surgical resection of the colon.

Fulminant colitis is characterized by fever, shock, severe abdominal pain, 10 or more bloody stools per day, and abdominal tenderness. Broad-spectrum antibiotics, intravenous steroids, immunosuppressants such as cyclosporine,[63] red blood cell transfusion, and fluid replacement are the mainstays of treatment for fulminant colitis. Small, uncontrolled series have also suggested that infliximab may be beneficial for fulminant colitis.[64] Failure to respond within a few days, however, warrants colectomy.

Distal Intestinal Obstruction Syndrome

Distal intestinal obstruction syndrome (DIOS) is unique to the cystic fibrosis (CF) population. Affected patients present with signs of bowel obstruction including abdominal pain, abdominal distention, and emesis. DIOS is characterized by a fecal mass in the ileocecum. The obstruction can be either partial or complete and the onset chronic, subacute, or acute. The CF bowel is more prone to obstruction due to impaired mobility as well as abnormal composition of the intraluminal contents. Patients at increased risk of DIOS include those with previous abdominal surgeries, a history of meconium ileus, pancreatic insufficiency, and having undergone lung transplant. Patients with incomplete obstruction can be managed with osmotic agents such as polyethylene glycol 3350. Gastrografin can be administered orally or as an enema; however, its administration is not without risk of hypovolemic shock (due to fluid shifts) and intestinal perforation.[65] Exploratory laparotomy with or without bowel resection is limited to the most severe cases; in one case series, the rate of surgical intervention was approximately 12.5%.[66]

Hirschsprung Disease

Hirschsprung disease occurs in 1 in 5000 live births. It may be the result of incomplete craniocaudal migration of neural crest elements, but some investigators believe that ganglion cells degenerate after migration. Aganglionosis may involve as little as a few centimeters or the entire colon and small bowel (in rare cases). Total colonic Hirschsprung disease occurs in clusters in some families with the risk being 21% in those families.[67] The inheritance of familial Hirschsprung disease appears to be polygenic, with mutations in several loci of the rearranged during transfection (RET) protooncogene being associated with autosomal dominant Hirschsprung disease that is most commonly the short-segment type. Mutations of the endothelin receptor type B gene are more likely to be observed in long-segment, autosomal recessively transmitted Hirschsprung disease. Other gene mutations may also modify the expression of the disease.[67]

The most common feature of Hirschsprung disease is the failure to pass meconium in a timely fashion after birth; 94% of infants with Hirschsprung disease pass their first stool beyond 24 hours of life. Most patients with Hirschsprung disease are constipated but cannot pass flatus. If their condition is undiagnosed during the first months of life, they may fail to thrive.

Physical findings include abdominal distention and an empty rectum on digital examination. Barium enema often reveals a narrow-caliber aganglionic distal colon; a transition zone; and a dilated, ganglionic proximal colon. It is essential that the barium enema be performed without prior enema preparation to preserve the transition zone. Absence of the anal-inhibitory reflex on anorectal manometry is suggestive. The diagnosis is confirmed histologically by rectal biopsy of the distal rectal mucosa where hypertrophic nerve trunks but no ganglion cells are found. Acetylcholinesterase staining of the specimen improves the diagnostic yield by enhancement of the abnormal nerve trunks.

In some children the course of Hirschsprung disease is punctuated by episodic, severe enterocolitis, which leads to copious, bloody diarrhea, fever, and shock. The intensive care of patients with enterocolitis should emphasize reconstitution of circulating blood volume with crystalloid, colloid, and red blood cells. Broad-spectrum parenteral antibiotics are advisable. After the patient's condition is stabilized, urgent decompressive enterostomy is indicated. Pull-through operations are usually performed after several months. Enterocolitis in the remaining ganglionated intestine may occur even in some patients who have undergone a pull-through operation.[68]

Acute Colonic Pseudo-obstruction

First described by Oglivie,[69] acute colonic pseudo-obstruction is occasionally observed among critically ill adults and children who are immobilized in an ICU setting. It is characterized by massive cecal dilation of 5 to 10 cm on abdominal plain film. The mechanism is uncertain, but it appears to occur among patients given neuromuscular blockade and antimotility drugs such as narcotics. If left untreated, it may result in colonic perforation at the cecal level. Therapy should involve decompression of the gastrointestinal tract by nasogastric and rectal intubation and suction. Placing the patient in the prone position also seems to be effective initial therapy. None of these measures, though, seems to be as effective as is parenteral administration of neostigmine.[69] Adverse effects of neostigmine, such as excessive salivation or abdominal cramping, are self-limiting, but bradycardia that occasionally occurs must be managed with atropine.

The critical care physician must be mindful of starting an early and aggressive bowel regimen for patients receiving narcotics, whether as intermittent doses in the awake patient or as continuous infusions in the sedated patient. Use of non-narcotic analgesics such as intravenous acetaminophen or ketorolac (when appropriate) can help to reduce the incidence of opioid-induced constipation. Furthermore, methylnaltrexone and naloxegol (both opioid antagonists) have now been developed for the treatment of opioid-induced constipation and have used in the pediatric population, although neither has yet been Food and Drug Administration approved in children.[70,71]

Abdominal Compartment Syndrome

Abdominal compartment syndrome (ACS) is defined as organ dysfunction caused by intraabdominal hypertension. The organ dysfunction observed with abdominal compartment syndrome may go underrecognized because it affects patients who are critically ill and their organ dysfunction may erroneously be ascribed to their underlying illness. If untreated, ACS can lead to organ failure and death; timely recognition and intervention can be life saving.

The standard method for measuring intraabdominal pressure is through the assessment of urinary bladder pressure. A three-way stopcock is placed between the catheter and pressure tubing. The bladder is emptied. Sterile isotonic saline is injected in the distal stopcock and into the bladder to allow for a continuous fluid column. There is some variability in the amount of fluid administered based on tubing and patient size. The pressure transducer is zeroed at the level of the midaxillary line, and the pressure is measured at end-expiration while the patient is completely supine. For the most accurate measurement, the patient should also be muscle-relaxed if the clinical scenario allows.

Intraabdominal hypertension (IAH) and ACS are distinct clinical entities. The intraabdominal pressure is a steady pressure within the abdominal cavity. The normal range is variable based on individual patient differences. Much of the variability is due to the body habitus of the patient. IAH is defined as a sustained pressure of 12 mm Hg or greater.[72] ACS is defined as sustained pressure greater than 20 mm Hg associated with organ dysfunction. Although recording of pressure is important for research purposes, the clinical presentation is the most important component in defining ACS. ACS can be classified as primary or secondary. Primary ACS is due to injury or disease in the abdominal region, such as trauma or organ transplantation, and often requires early surgical decompression. Secondary ACS is due to conditions requiring extensive fluid resuscitation, such as sepsis, burns, or other capillary leak syndromes.

IAH can impair practically every organ system and result in ACS. It can impair cardiac function by reducing venous return as well as impairing cardiac function directly via diaphragmatic pressure. In mechanically ventilated patients, peak inspiratory and mean airway pressures will be significantly increased, resulting in pulmonary barotrauma. In addition, chest wall compliance is markedly reduced. Renal impairment may be attributed to several mechanisms in patients with ACS. Venous drainage can be impaired by renal vein compression. The subsequent cardiac output fall can lead to renal artery vasoconstriction via the renin-angiotensin systems. The urine sodium and chloride concentrations will typically be decreased, whereas the renin, aldosterone, and antidiuretic hormone may be markedly increased.[73,74] The organ most sensitive to changes in intraabdominal pressure is the gut. Both human and animal studies have shown decreased intestinal mucosal perfusion at intraabdominal pressures of 20 mm Hg. Impaired mesenteric venous drainage results in intestinal edema, which can increase intraabdominal pressure and result in worse hypoperfusion and possible bowel ischemia.[75] Finally, intracranial pressure (ICP) can be elevated, leading to a decrease in cerebral perfusion.[76]

The management of IAH and ACS requires both supportive care and, in some instances, surgical decompression. In general, surgical decompression is indicated for ACS. There is increasing evidence that surgical decompression prior to the development of ACS may be beneficial.[77] Following decompression, the abdomen is left open and typically covered with a Dacron mesh or humanized regenerative tissue matrix. Early recognition and timing of decompression of ACS may be crucial in the preservation of organ function (see Chapter 100).

Acute Pancreatitis

Even though gallstone pancreatitis and ethanolic pancreatitis are uncommon in children, numerous structural, toxic metabolic, and infectious diseases are associated with acute childhood pancreatitis. Appropriate radiographic or biochemical evaluation for pancreatitis should be performed on all children admitted to the ICU with acute abdomen.

Acute pancreatitis is preceded by intrapancreatic activation of proteases. The triggering mechanism remains obscure, but once protease inhibitors are overcome and trypsinogen is converted to trypsin, a cascade of steps produces active proteases, lipase, and amylase. The enzymes induce local and distant organ damage, which includes edema, increased vascular permeability, cytolysis, and fat necrosis.

The clinical hallmark of acute pancreatitis is severe, boring epigastric or left upper quadrant pain that radiates through to the back. Serum amylase and lipase levels are greatly elevated, and radiographic imaging studies reveal pancreatic enlargement, sonolucency, or irregularity of the margin. Ultrasonography is a satisfactory screening technique, but CT scanning should be used when the course is severe. If CT scanning is performed with a dynamic, contrast-enhanced technique, interstitial pancreatitis can be differentiated from the more ominous necrotic pancreatitis, which often requires surgical debridement.

Because serum lipase is almost exclusively pancreatic in origin and amylase comes from a number of organs, the serum lipase concentration may be a better indicator of pancreatitis. Use of both measures to follow the course of pancreatitis is preferable to using either one alone.

Several nonspecific laboratory derangements such as anemia, hypoglycemia, hypocalcemia, and hypoproteinemia may occur. Intensive support may be required for severe, acute attacks. Severe, hemorrhagic necrosis of the pancreas carries a poor prognosis. Extraordinarily large third-space fluid and electrolyte losses must be replaced. If significant hyperglycemia occurs, insulin must be given. Calcium infusions may also be necessary. Physicians should be able to minimize pancreatic stimulation by giving the patient nothing by mouth and using nasogastric suction, although the efficacy of suction has been questioned for patients without ileus. Use of protease inhibitors, H_2 antagonists, somatostatin, 5-fluorouracil, and glucagon has not found much support in the literature. Antibiotics are not indicated unless an abscess is suspected. Several complications may be catastrophic. Rupture of a pancreatic duct or leakage of a pseudocyst must be suspected if ascites develops. Gastrointestinal hemorrhage during pancreatitis may originate from a variety of sources. Discovery of gastric varices suggests splenic vein thrombosis. Gastritis may also appear. Pseudoaneurysms of the hepatic or splenic artery may bleed into the pancreas. Small bowel or colonic ischemia caused by fat necrosis may produce gastrointestinal hemorrhage. Infected pancreatic necrosis is uniformly fatal unless the patient undergoes an emergency operation to debride the necrotic tissue.

Time to recovery from pancreatitis is variable and may be prolonged (weeks to months). Early, enteral feeding is the preferred route of nutrition for patients with pancreatitis.[78] Protease inhibitors, free-radical scavengers, and other antiinflammatory agents have all been employed in the treatment of acute pancreatitis, with disappointing results.[79]

Acute and Chronic Liver Failure

The term *liver failure* refers to the constellation of symptoms, signs, and biochemical aberrations that appear when hepatic synthetic capacity is severely compromised. Liver failure is categorized as fulminant when encephalopathy appears within the first 2 months of the illness, as late onset when it appears within 6 months, and as chronic when it appears beyond the sixth month of liver dysfunction. Infectious, metabolic, and toxic liver diseases, as well as biliary obstruction, may lead to liver failure (Table 97.2). Obviously, it is advisable to establish a cause of liver disease before the onset of liver failure. It is beyond the scope of this chapter to outline a diagnostic approach to childhood liver disease, but several reviews are available (see also Chapter 99).[80,81]

Elucidating the cause of fulminant hepatic failure is often made more difficult by the rapid development of coagulopathy

TABLE 97.2   Diseases That Cause Liver Failure

Viral	Hepatitis (A, B, C, D, E), CMV, HSV, EBV, VZV, HHV-6, parvovirus B19, parainfluenza, yellow fever
Idiosyncratic	Halogenated hydrocarbons, warfarin, methyldopa, phenytoin, carbamazepine, valproic acid, rifampicin, penicillin, sulfonamides, quinolones
Toxic dose–dependent	Acetaminophen (paracetamol), isoniazid, tetracycline, methotrexate, carbon tetrachloride, amphetamines, *Amanita phalloides* toxin
Toxic synergistic	Ethanol + acetaminophen, barbiturate + acetaminophen, isoniazid + rifampicin
Metabolic	Wilson disease, alpha-1-AT deficiency, galactosemia, tyrosinemia, Reye syndrome, NASH
Associated with pregnancy	Acute fatty liver of pregnancy, HELLP syndrome
Vascular	Budd-Chiari syndrome, veno-occlusive disease, shock, heart failure
Miscellaneous	Autoimmune hepatitis, malignant infiltration, hyperthermia, sepsis

CMV, cytomegalovirus; *EBV,* Epstein-Barr virus; *HELLP,* hemolysis, elevated liver enzymes, and low platelet count; *HHV,* human herpesvirus; *HSV,* herpes simplex virus; *NASH,* nonalcoholic steatohepatitis; *VZV,* varicella zoster virus; Data from Gotthardt D, et al. Fulminant hepatic failure: etiology and indications for liver transplantation, Nephrol Dialysis Transplant. 2007;22(suppl 8): viii5-viii8.

and ascites, which preclude percutaneous liver biopsy. Laparotomy with surgical wedge biopsy may be necessary. Transjugular liver biopsy is also an option. A core of liver tissue is obtained by passing the biopsy forceps retrograde through the superior vena cava and hepatic vein after introduction via the jugular vein. The biopsy site then bleeds directly into the liver parenchyma, minimizing extravasation.

Hepatic encephalopathy is more difficult to diagnose in young children than in adults, as an infant may first present with simply increased fussiness. Progressive hepatic encephalopathy culminates in coma. When patients have entered coma, central nervous system (CNS) resuscitation becomes necessary. Patients should undergo elective endotracheal intubation; administration of benzodiazepines should be avoided. Beyond CNS metabolic derangements, cytotoxic cerebral edema often complicates hepatic failure. Placement of an intracranial monitoring device should be contemplated; the risk of instrumentation in patients with coagulopathy should be weighed against the benefit of continuous CNS pressure monitoring.[82]

The non-CNS manifestations of liver failure are protean. Hepatosplenomegaly is common in the early stages of fulminant failure, but the liver may shrink rapidly. In end-stage liver disease caused by cirrhosis, the liver is shrunken, firm, and nodular. Most patients with liver failure have jaundice. Spider angiomas, palmar erythema, ascites, and peripheral edema are common features of chronic liver disease. Fetor hepaticus (mercaptan breath) may be present. The biochemical features of liver failure are variable depending on its cause, duration, and severity. Hypoglycemia should be corrected when present. Serum bilirubin levels may be elevated or normal. Liver aminotransferase concentrations are increased in acute liver disease but decrease as hepatocytes are lost and therefore may be only mildly elevated or normal in cirrhosis and in the terminal stages of failure. Decreasing aminotransferase levels and albumin in the face of rising bilirubin, prothrombin time, and partial thromboplastin time denote a failing liver. Serum globulin and ammonia levels are usually elevated. The serum amniogram reveals an elevated aromatic/branched-chain amino acid ratio.

Renal insufficiency may appear because of perennial azotemia, acute tubular necrosis, or hepatorenal syndrome.[83] Patients with both acute and chronic liver failure frequently develop renal failure. Hepatorenal syndrome (HRS) is the most common cause of acute renal failure in this population. From 40% to 80% of patients with hepatic failure develop HRS. The onset often occurs following an acute change in intravascular volume. The development of HRS is precipitated commonly by hemorrhage, excessive diuresis, or sepsis. HRS is a diagnosis of exclusion once other causes of renal failure and absent diuretic response are further explored. Although certain clinical characteristics may or may not exist in the description of HRS, almost all patients have hyponatremia prior to the development of renal insufficiency.[84] The treatment is nonspecific but includes volume administration and maintenance of adequate systemic perfusion. This is achieved by overcoming the splanchnic vasodilatation and increasing renal perfusion and filtration (see Chapter 75).[85]

Patients with late-onset or chronic liver failure are likely to have portal hypertension. Ascites may develop as plasma oncotic pressure decreases or portal pressure increases. Patients who are hyponatremic usually have total-body sodium overload,[84] and they should be treated with moderate salt restriction, but vigorous fluid restriction, colloid administration, and diuretic therapy are the cornerstones of therapy. High-volume abdominal paracentesis is proved to be safe in both adults and children who have ascites compromising ventilation.

Spontaneous engorgement of esophageal, gastric, and rectal veins leads to varices. Similar prominent veins in the abdominal wall and around the umbilicus (caput medusa) may develop. Splenic congestion from impaired venous flow into the portal system results in splenomegaly and hypersplenism so that patients are classically anemic or pancytopenic. Less commonly, unknown factors lead to intrapulmonary arteriovenous shunting, which characteristically causes hypoxemia.

Coagulopathy and bleeding are frequent in patients with liver failure. Thrombocytopenia, which may be profound, is a common component of hypersplenism. Fat-soluble vitamin malabsorption in patients with cholestasis leads to vitamin K deficiency, which prevents hepatic production of clotting factors II, VII, IX, and X. Ultimately, failed synthesis of all liver-dependent clotting factors results in prolonged prothrombin time (unresponsive to vitamin K administration) and partial thromboplastin time.

The sites of bleeding are predictable. Bleeding from incisions, needle puncture sites, nose, and gingiva are common but are usually not life threatening. Persistent bleeding may require packed red blood cell transfusion. In contrast, intracranial, pulmonary, and variceal bleeding may be fatal and demand immediate attention. Esophageal varices bleed because of acute changes in variceal pressure or because of gastric hyperacidity. Platelets should be given to patients with thrombocytopenia and active bleeding or prior to a procedure. Patients with coagulopathy and hemorrhage may receive fresh frozen plasma, but if not actively bleeding, it is best to allow the international normalized ratio (INR) to rise, as continual replacement of blood product can lead to fluid overload in these already sensitive patients. Acceptable alternatives include plasmapheresis[86] and the administration of recombinant factor VII concentrate[87] as bridges to transplantation (see also Chapter 91).

Mechanical means of hemorrhage control include direct compression, creation of portosystemic shunts, and surgical transection/reanastomosis of the esophagus. Endoscopic control of bleeding from varices involves sclerotherapy in infants too small to tolerate a banding device or endoscopic banding in toddlers and older children.[88] Balloon tamponade by a Sengstaken-Blakemore tube carries substantial risk and has largely been abandoned. It should not be used to manage persistent bleeding after sclerotherapy because of the risk of esophageal perforation.

Complications of portal hypertension can be managed with surgical shunting procedures that decompress the portal system by creating a venous anastomosis between the portal and systemic circulations. Several surgical varieties exist. Central vascular shunts, such as portocaval or mesocaval shunts, carry substantial risk. Transjugular intrahepatic portosystemic shunts are frequently used in children who weigh more than 10 kg as a bridge to transplantation.[89] In the past, shunt thrombosis was sometimes treated with surgical esophageal transaction, but urgent liver transplantation with either a cadaveric or living related donor is the preferred therapeutic strategy under such conditions (see Chapter 99).

Plasmapheresis or plasma exchange removes circulating mediators and toxins from patients with liver failure. This temporary effect may be due to removal of neuroinhibitory factors. The molecular adsorbent recirculating system (MARS) and other similar albumin dialysis systems, which remove large, albumin-bound molecules such as bilirubin and ammonia, have now been used for several years as a bridge to liver transplantation. These systems have shown an improvement in hepatic encephalopathy and bilirubin with a variable impact on mortality in adults; however pediatric data remain limited.[90] Ultimately, orthotopic transplantation holds the greatest promise for patients with end-stage liver disease.[91]

Key References

6. Hong SK, Vaezi MF. Gastroesophageal reflux monitoring: pH (catheter and capsule) and impedance. *Gastrointest Endosc Clin North Am.* 2009;19:1-22.
7. Dranove JE. Focus on diagnosis: new technologies for the diagnosis of gastroesophageal reflux disease. *Pediatr Rev.* 2008;29:317-320.
14. Van Beers B, et al. New imaging techniques for liver disease. *J Hepatol.* 2015;62:690-700.
15. Cohen EB, Afdhal NH. Ultrasound-based hepatic elastography; origins, limitations, and applications. *J Clin Gastroenterol.* 2010;44:637-645.
16. Partovi S, Kohan A, Rubbert C, et al. Clinical oncologic applications of PET/MRI: a new horizon. *Am J Nucl Med Mol Imaging.* 2014;4:202-212.
22. Mezoff EA, et al. Ethanol lock efficacy and associated complications in children with intestinal failure. *JPEN J Parenter Enteral Nutr.* 2015;[Epub ahead of print].
23. Ardura M, et al. Central catheter-associated bloodstream infection reduction with ethanol lock prophylaxis in pediatric intestinal failure. *JAMA Pediatr.* 2015;169:324-331.
24. Robinson J, et al. Prospective cohort study of the outcome of and risk factors for intravascular catheter-related bloodstream infections in

children with intestinal failure. *JPEN J Parenter Enteral Nutr.* 2014;38: 625-630.

25. Moazam F, Talbert JL, Miller D, Mollitt DL. Caustic ingestion and its sequelae in children. *South Med J.* 1987;80:187-190.

26. Anderson KD, Rouse TM, Randolph JG. A controlled trial of corticosteroids in children with corrosive injury of the esophagus. *N Engl J Med.* 1990;323:637-640.

27. Millar AJ, Cox SG. Caustic injury of the oesophagus. *Pediatr Surg Int.* 2015;31:111-121.

33. Montgomery J, et al. Botulinum toxin A for children with salivary control problems. *Int J Pediatr Otorhinolaryngol.* 2014;78:1970-1973.

34. Noonan K, et al. Surgical management of chronic salivary aspiration. *Int J Pediatr Otorhinolaryngol.* 2014;78:2079-2082.

36. Cook DJ, Reeve BK, Guyatt GH, et al. Stress ulcer prophylaxis in critically ill patients. Resolving discordant meta-analyses. *JAMA.* 1996;275:308-314.

41. Karabiber H, et al. Virulence factors and antibiotics resistance in children with *Helicobacter pylori* gastritis. *J Pediatr Gastroenterol Nutr.* 2014; 58:608-612.

42. Kalach N, Bontems P, Cadranel S. Advances in the treatment of *Helicobacter pylori* infection in children. *Ann Gastroenterol.* 2015;28:10-18.

45. Morrow A, et al. Early microbial and metabolomic signatures predict later onset of necrotizing enterocolitis in pre-term infants. *Microbiome.* 2013;1:13.

46. de Meij TG, et al. Early detection of necrotizing enterocolitis by fecal volatile organic compounds analysis. *J Pediatr.* 2015;167:562-567.

47. el-Zein C, Ilbawi MN. Recent advances in neonatal cardiac surgery. *World J Surg.* 2008;32:340-345.

50. Ravishankar C, Tabbutt S, Wernovsky G. Critical care in cardiovascular medicine. *Curr Opin Pediatr.* 2003;15:443-453.

52. Proujansky R, Winter HS, Walker WA. Gastrointestinal syndromes associated with food sensitivity. *Adv Pediatr.* 1988;35:219-237.

53. Soar J, Pumphrey R, Cant A, et al. Emergency treatment of anaphylactic reactions–guidelines for healthcare providers. *Resuscitation.* 2008;77:157-169.

55. Tarr PI. *Escherichia coli* O157:H7: clinical, diagnostic, and epidemiological aspects of human infection. *Clin Infect Dis.* 1995;20:1-8.

56. Tarr PI, Gordon CA, Chandler WL. Shiga-toxin-producing *Escherichia coli* and haemolytic uraemic syndrome. *Lancet.* 2005;365:1073-1086.

57. Christmann M, et al. Eculizumab as first-line therapy for atypical hemolytic uremic syndrome. *Pediatrics.* 2014;133:e1759-e1763.

59. Sigall-Boneh R, et al. Partial enteral nutrition with a Crohn's disease exclusion diet is effective for induction of remission in children and young adults with Crohn's disease. *Inflamm Bowel Dis.* 2014;20: 1353-1360.

60. Rutgeerts P. An historical overview of the treatment of Crohn's disease: why do we need biological therapies? *Rev Gastroenterol Dis.* 2004; 4:S3-S9.

61. Biank VF, et al. Association of Crohn's disease, thiopurines, and primary EBV infection with hemophagocytic lymphohistiocytosis. *J Pediatr.* 2011;159:808-812.

62. Cozijnsen MA, et al. Benefits and risks of combining anti-tumor necrosis factor with immunomodulator therapy in pediatric inflammatory bowel disease. *Inflamm Bowel Dis.* 2015;21:951-961.

65. Colombo C, et al. Guidelines for the diagnosis and management of distal intestinal obstruction syndrome in cystic fibrosis patients. *J Cyst Fibros.* 2011;10(suppl 2):S24-S28.

66. Farrelly PJ, et al. Gastrointestinal surgery in cystic fibrosis: a 20-year review. *J Pediatr Surg.* 2014;49:280-283.

67. Passarge E. Dissecting Hirschsprung disease. *Nat Genet.* 2002;31:11-12.

69. Ponec RJ, Saunders MD, Kimmey MB. Neostigmine for the treatment of acute colonic pseudo-obstruction. *N Engl J Med.* 1999;341:137-141.

70. Siemens W, Gaertner J, Becker G. Advances in pharmacotherapy for opioid-induced constipation—a systematic review. *Expert Opin Pharmacother.* 2015;16:515-532.

71. Rodrigues A, et al. Methylnaltrexone for opioid-induced constipation in pediatric oncology patients. *Pediatr Blood Cancer.* 2013;60:1667-1670.

72. Malbrain ML, Cheatham ML, Kirkpatrick A, et al. Results from the International Conference of Experts on Intra-abdominal Hypertension and Abdominal Compartment Syndrome. I. Definitions. *Intensive Care Med.* 2006;32:1722-1732.

74. Doty JM, Saggi BH, Sugerman HJ, et al. Effect of increased renal venous pressure on renal function. *J Trauma.* 1999;47:1000-1003.

77. Cheatham ML, De Waele JJ, De Laet I, et al. The impact of body position on intra-abdominal pressure measurement: a multicenter analysis. *Crit Care Med.* 2009;37:2187-2190.

78. Srinath A, Lowe M. Pediatric pancreatitis. *Pediatri Rev.* 2013;34:79-90.

79. Bang UC, et al. Pharmacological approach to acute pancreatitis. *World J Gastroenterol.* 2008;14:2968-2976.

80. Balistreri WF. Viral hepatitis. *Pediatr Clin North Am.* 1988;35:375-407.

81. Fitzgerald JF. Cholestatic disorders of infancy. *Pediatr Clin North Am.* 1988;35:357-373.

82. Kamat P, et al. Invasive intracranial pressure monitoring is a useful adjunct in the management of severe hepatic encephalopathy associated with pediatric acute liver failure. *Pediatr Crit Care Med.* 2012;13:e33-e38.

83. Gines P, Guevara M, Arroyo V, Rodes J. Hepatorenal syndrome. *Lancet.* 2003;362:1819-1827.

84. Meltzer J, Brentjens TE. Renal failure in patients with cirrhosis: hepatorenal syndrome and renal support strategies. *Curr Opin Anaesthesiol.* 2010;23:139-144.

86. Singer AL, Olthoff KM, Kim H. Role of plasmapheresis in the management of acute hepatic failure in children. *Ann Surg.* 2001;234:418-424.

87. Brown JB, Emerick KM, Brown DL. Recombinant factor VIIa improves coagulopathy caused by liver failure. *J Pediatr Gastroenterol Nutr.* 2003;37:268-272.

90. Schaefer B, Schmitt CP. The role of molecular adsorbent recirculating system dialysis for extracorporeal liver support in children. *Pediatr Nephrol.* 2013;28:1763-1769.

91. Kim JJ, Marks SD. Long-term outcomes of children after solid organ transplantation. *Clinics (Sao Paulo).* 2014;69(suppl 1):28-38.

Applications of Gastrointestinal Pharmacology

Susan Jacob, Silvia M. Hartmann, Ada Kong, and Nicole L. Richardson

PEARLS

- Stress ulcer prophylaxis, in the form of a histamine-2 receptor antagonist or proton pump inhibitor, is given to decrease the risk of hemodynamically significant bleeding from the upper gastrointestinal tract.
- Stress ulcer prophylaxis only benefits the patients with risk factors for clinically significant bleeding, such as mechanical ventilation for >48 hours or presence of coagulopathy.
- Despite heterogeneity in the probiotic formulation and dose, overall evidence suggests that probiotic administration prevents antibiotic-associated diarrhea in children.
- Shock and medications are the most important risk factors for constipation in pediatric ICU patients.
- Rectal administration of medication may be most beneficial when intravenous access is challenging or otherwise unnecessary for care.
- Antiemetic management in both chemotherapy-induced nausea and vomiting and postoperative nausea and vomiting is rooted in a multiple-drug approach with distinct targets of action.
- The risk of experiencing chemotherapy-induced nausea and vomiting is mainly determined by chemotherapy-specific factors (eg, emetogenicity of drugs, dose, schedule, route, rate of administration) and can be anticipated.
- Oncology patients who have well-controlled acute nausea and vomiting 24 hours after chemotherapy administration are less likely to have delayed nausea and vomiting. This highlights the importance of prophylactic antiemetic therapy.
- Patients with an operative course greater than 30 minutes are at higher risk of postoperative nausea and vomiting. Tonsillectomy and adenoidectomy are common surgeries associated with postoperative nausea and vomiting.

Stress Ulcer Prophylaxis

The rationale to provide stress ulcer prophylaxis, more commonly called "GI prophylaxis," to children in the PICU is primarily to decrease the risk of hemodynamically significant bleeding from the upper gastrointestinal (GI) tract. This event is generally rare in both adult and pediatric ICU patients. However, when hemodynamically significant bleeding occurs, it is associated with a higher mortality in both pediatrics and adults[1,2] and longer ICU length of stay in the adult

population.[1] The risk of universal stress ulcer prophylaxis is of increased infectious complications, most notably ventilator-associated pneumonia (VAP) and *Clostridium difficile* colitis. Restriction of stress ulcer prophylaxis to high risk groups may help to maintain the falling rates of significant upper GI bleeding from stress-related damage while avoiding the infectious complications and excessive cost. There are no cost-effective studies in the pediatric ICU population, but one study from the adult ICU noted that stress ulcer prophylaxis was cost saving if administration could avert 50% of significant bleeding episodes in a population with >15% risk.[3] The same study also concluded that in a low-risk population (<12% risk of significant upper GI hemorrhage) that prophylaxis was not cost effective. Stress ulcer prophylaxis therefore may only be cost saving for high-risk pediatric ICU patients, which are those requiring mechanical ventilation for greater than 48 hours and those with coagulopathy, and must be determined in future studies.

Mechanism of Stress-Related Mucosal Damage

Stress-related mucosal damage is a spectrum of gastric and small bowel injury that varies from asymptomatic superficial mucosal damage to hemorrhagic shock secondary to deeper injury to the intestinal lining and erosion into larger arteries.[4] Stress ulceration that leads to clinically apparent bleeding represents the more severe end of the spectrum of stress-related mucosal damage. Asymptomatic stress-related mucosal damage is likely quite common in high-risk adult ICU populations with one study performed in the 1970s in 32 burn patients showing 74% having multiple areas of gastric mucosal injury within 72 hours of ICU stay.[5] Clinically apparent bleeding has been categorized separately as overt upper GI bleeding and clinically significant upper GI bleeding in most studies. Overt bleeding refers to hematemesis, coffee-ground output from nasogastric or gastrostomy tubes, or melena. Anatomically, overt bleeding is thought to correspond to erosion beyond the mucosa into the submucosa or muscularis propria of the GI tract wall with damage to smaller arteries. This type of bleeding, by definition, does not cause hemodynamic effects. Clinically significant bleeding corresponds to erosion into larger arteries that cause enough blood loss to lead to hypotension or need for blood transfusion.[4,6] Overt bleeding and clinically significant bleeding are the outcome measures of most investigations of stress ulcer prophylaxis described in this chapter.

Stress-related mucosal damage arises from multiple factors commonly found in ICU patients that cause hypoperfusion injury to the GI tract and impair the normal protective mechanisms, which then allows further damage to occur from the multiple corrosive agents produced by the GI system itself.[4,7-9] Hypoperfusion can lead to primary cell damage and predispose to secondary damage from gastric acid and other injurious compounds.[8] Hypoperfusion may be secondary to a low-flow state or high systemic vascular resistance.[4,9] High intrathoracic pressure from mechanical ventilation may exacerbate low-flow states by further decreasing preload.[4] High systemic vascular resistance in the gastrointestinal tract is a physiologic compensatory mechanism to shunt blood flow to critical organs during times of low effective circulation. Vasoconstriction of the splanchnic circulation also is a consequence of treatment with vasoactive medications common in the treatment of shock. Stress-related mucosal damage may also arise from ischemia-reperfusion injury and the increased production of reactive oxygen species after shock has been reversed.[4] These mechanisms lead to impaired gastric and intestinal protective measures such as decreased mucus, bicarbonate, and prostaglandin production. Gastric acid produced by the stomach, as well as bile and pepsin from duodenal reflux, may all damage the gastric lining when protective mechanisms are impaired. Hypomotility that is often present as a consequence of GI hypoperfusion may exacerbate gastric damage as acidic contents remain in contact with the stomach lining for longer periods of time.[7] Damage is most common in the fundus and upper body of the stomach that are responsible for acid production.[7] Notably, the mechanism for development of stress-related mucosal damage and stress ulceration in critical illness is distinct from variceal bleeding and *H. pylori*–associated ulceration despite similar presentation with upper GI bleeding.

Epidemiology and Risk Factors for Stress Ulceration

Studies from the 1980s showed approximately 25% of the adult ICU population that did *not* receive stress ulcer prophylaxis would have overt upper GI bleeding and 3% to 5% would have clinically significant bleeding.[4] The incidence of overt and clinically significant upper GI bleeding has been decreasing since the 1990s and may be due to earlier reversal of GI hypoperfusion, widespread use of stress ulcer prophylaxis, and perhaps the adoption of early enteral nutrition.[10] Several studies reveal a low incidence of upper GI hemorrhage in both adult and pediatric ICUs. The incidence of clinically significant bleeding among adult ICU patients has been reported to be between 1% and 4.4%.[1,4,10-12] Two prospective pediatric studies performed in the 1990s showed an incidence of overt upper GI bleeding of approximately 6% to 10% and significant bleeding of 0.4% to 1.6%.[2,13] A more recent publication from 2009 examined 110 higher-risk PICU patients who received mechanical ventilation for greater than 48 hours.[14] This study noted a higher rate of upper GI bleeding with 51% of patients having overt bleeding and 3.6% having clinically significant bleeding. This underscores the importance of identifying patients with risk factors for clinically significant bleeding to receive stress ulcer prophylaxis, as the rate of bleeding leading to hypotension or need for transfusion is very low among patients without these risk factors. Cook and associates best demonstrated the significantly different rates of clinically important upper GI bleeding among patients with risk factors to those without.[6] In this study of 2252 adult ICU patients,

there were 847 with independent risk factors of coagulopathy or respiratory failure defined as need for mechanical ventilation for greater than 48 hours and 1405 patients with neither risk factor. The incidence of clinically significant upper GI bleeding in those with risk factors was 3.7% compared to 0.1% in the group without risk factors.

Respiratory failure, coagulopathy, and a pediatric risk of mortality (PRISM) score greater than or equal to 10 was identified as a risk factor for clinically significant GI hemorrhage in children.[2,13] Coagulopathy has been defined as a platelet count less than 100,000/cubic mL, an international normalized ratio (INR) greater than 1.5, or prothrombin time more than twice the control value in many studies. Another study also identified multitrauma (two or more systems involved), a surgical operation longer than 3 hours, and circulatory shock as additional risk factors.[15] One subsequent pediatric study demonstrated mechanical ventilation as the only statistically significant risk factor for significant bleeding after multivariate analysis.[16] A high-risk cohort of children ventilated for greater than 48 hours were at additional risk of GI hemorrhage if organ failure (renal, hepatic, or neurologic) or elevated peak inspiratory pressures >25 cm H_2O were also present.[14] Due to the low incidence of clinically significant hemorrhage, prophylaxis may only be warranted in patients with identified risk factors.

Options for Stress Ulcer Prophylaxis

Histamine-2 (H2) receptor antagonists, proton pump inhibitors (PPIs), sucralfate, and antacids have all been used for prophylaxis of stress-induced mucosal damage in pediatric critical care patients. Classes of medications are described later. A meta-analysis published in 2010 found that treatment with any agent decreased the risk of clinically significant upper GI bleeding with a risk ratio of 0.41 (95% confidence interval [CI] 0.19 to 0.91) in 300 pediatric intensive care unit (PICU) patients from two randomized controlled trials.[17] The same study concluded that no class of medication was superior to prevent clinically significant bleeding based on review of eight randomized controlled trials. However, antacids and sucralfate have fallen out of favor. Both agents require multiple doses per day, lack intravenous formulations, and may chelate or inhibit absorption of other drugs. Sucralfate was compared with ranitidine for stress ulcer prophylaxis in adult ICU patients in a landmark trial by Cook and associates published in 1998.[12] In this multicenter, randomized, and blinded trial, 1200 adult ICU patients who required mechanical ventilation for greater than 48 hours were randomized to nasogastric sucralfate and IV placebo or nasogastric placebo and IV ranitidine. The group receiving ranitidine had a significantly lower rate of clinically significant upper GI bleeding (1.7% versus 3.8%) with a relative risk of 0.44 (95% CI 0.21–0.92). H2 receptor antagonists have been compared to PPIs with contradictory results without a clear medication class that is superior to the other for stress ulcer prophylaxis. A meta-analysis that included seven randomized controlled trials published before 2008 comparing H2 receptor antagonists to PPIs in 936 adult ICU patients found no superiority of either medication to prevent clinically significant bleeding.[18] A subsequent meta-analysis from Cook and associates published in 2013[19] showed that PPIs were superior to H2 receptor antagonists in decreasing the risk of overt and clinically significant upper GI bleeding. The relative risk of developing clinically significant bleeding with PPI therapy compared to H2 receptor antagonists was 0.36 (95% CI 0.19–0.68) using data from 12 trials involving 1614 adult ICU patients. Subsequently, a large retrospective cohort of 35,312 patients had the opposite result.[11] Patients receiving H2 receptor antagonists had a significantly lower incidence of GI hemorrhage compared to those receiving PPIs (2.1% versus 5.9%, p < 0.001). No literature exists in pediatric patients to support the use of either PPIs or H2 receptor antagonists over the other. Interestingly, stress ulcer prophylaxis with medication may only be protective against upper GI bleeding in patients who are not receiving enteral nutrition, which is hypothesized to improve the secretion of protective prostaglandins and mucus. A meta-analysis by Marik and colleagues noted a decreased risk of bleeding in adult ICU patients receiving ranitidine compared to no treatment, but this effect was only present in patients who were not being fed.[10]

Stress ulcer prophylaxis has been recommended as part of routine care for pediatric patients with acute respiratory distress syndrome[20] and sepsis.[21,22] The 2012 Surviving Sepsis Campaign guidelines[22] recommend administration of either an H2 receptor antagonist or a PPI to patients with severe sepsis who also have bleeding risk factors, which include mechanical ventilation for greater than 48 hours, coagulopathy, and hypotension. This was categorized as a strong recommendation with moderate quality evidence (grade 1B). The guidelines suggest the use of a PPI over H2 receptor antagonist, noting poor quality of evidence (grade 2C). It is also suggested that patients without risk factors do not receive stress ulcer prophylaxis. This was a weak recommendation with moderate quality of evidence (grade 2B). The guidelines make no graded recommendations for or against stress ulcer prophylaxis in pediatric patients with severe sepsis or septic shock.

Infectious Complications of Stress Ulcer Prophylaxis

The risk of providing stress ulcer prophylaxis that increases gastric pH to patients in the pediatric ICU is increasing the risk of ventilator-associated pneumonia (VAP) and *Clostridium difficile* infection. The mechanism proposed for higher risk of these infections is that medications that suppress gastric acid production also allow for increased bacterial colonization of the stomach. The higher bacterial load in gastric secretions can be aspirated around the endotracheal tube leading to ventilator-associated tracheitis or VAP. Similarly, *C. difficile* spores remain increasingly viable in a less acidic gastric environment with increased risk of causing colitis.

More recent adult studies of stress ulcer prophylaxis in the ICU have called into question the higher risk of VAP with acid suppression.[10,19] One study suggested a higher rate of VAP with PPIs compared to H2 receptor antagonists, but conclusions are limited by the retrospective design in which the population receiving PPIs may not be the same as the population receiving H2 receptor antagonists.[11] Studies from the pediatric ICU have not shown a difference in VAP rates between patients receiving prophylaxis with sucralfate versus ranitidine versus no prophylaxis.[23,24]

The association between acid suppression and *C. difficile* has been demonstrated mainly in adults in both the outpatient and hospitalized setting use case-control studies that also take into account antibiotic use.[25] More recently studies with a similar design have shown the same relationships of increased *C. difficile* infection in patients who have received either PPIs or H2 receptor antagonists.[26,27] These studies have captured both outpatient and hospitalized pediatric patients, but no study has specifically focused on the ICU population receiving acid suppression for stress ulcer prophylaxis.

Histamine-2 Receptor Antagonists

Histamine-2 (H2) receptor antagonists inhibit gastric acid secretion by means of competitive inhibition of H2 receptors of the gastric parietal cells. H2 receptor antagonists are commonly used because of the availability of both enteral and intravenous formulations. Common adverse effects include nausea and headache. Tachyphylaxis is well documented for intravenous and oral H2 receptor blockers in adult and pediatric populations. Although thrombocytopenia may occur, it is often difficult to determine the sole cause in critically ill patients. Ranitidine should be avoided in patients with acute porphyria. All of the currently available H2 receptor blockers require a dosage adjustment for renal impairment and have a higher risk of central nervous adverse effects without dose adjustment.

Proton Pump Inhibitors

By covalently bonding to the hydrogen-potassium-adenosine triphosphatase (H^+-K^+ ATPase or proton pump) of parietal cells, proton pump inhibitors (PPIs) suppress gastric acid secretion for the life of the parietal cell. PPIs may be used orally, intravenously, or off-label through feeding tubes. Ideally, enteral therapy should be given 30 minutes before feeding so that peak plasma concentrations coincide with parietal cell stimulation. Administration of enteral PPIs with food reduces bioavailability by 50%. Omeprazole, esomeprazole, and lansoprazole have been approved for use in pediatrics. Intravenous lansoprazole is no longer available. Neither intravenous pantoprazole nor esomeprazole is Food and Drug Administration (FDA)–approved for use in pediatric patients. Although PPIs are generally thought of as well tolerated, both long- and short-term adverse effects are gaining more attention. Reactions include idiosyncratic reactions, drug-drug interactions, drug-induced hypergastrinemia, and drug-induced hypochlorhydria.[28] The most common side effects are headache, diarrhea, constipation, and nausea. PPIs should not be discontinued abruptly because a hypersecretory phase results.[28,29]

Sucralfate

Sucralfate is an aluminum salt of sulfated sucrose. Safety concerns about sucralfate have been associated with aluminum toxicity[29] and interference with medication absorption or medication chelation. Sucralfate requires administration into the stomach to be effective, thus nasoduodenal and jejunostomy tube dependence limits the utility of this medication for stress ulcer prophylaxis.

Gastrointestinal Hemorrhage

Clinical guidelines for treatment of nonvariceal upper GI bleeding in adults include recommendations for pharmacotherapy.[30] Unfortunately, this body of evidence does not exist in the pediatric population. H2 receptor antagonist use is discouraged as primary treatment for patients with acute bleeding. Although octreotide and somatostatin are more effective than H2 receptor antagonists, these agents are also not recommended for routine management. PPIs are cited as the drugs of choice for treatment of acute nonvariceal upper GI bleeding.[30] High-dose intravenous proton pump inhibitor therapy (80 mg pantoprazole bolus followed by 8 mg/hr for 72 hours) after endoscopic therapy is preferred over H2 receptor antagonists alone, or in combination with octreotide, to prevent rebleeding in adult patients. As more data become available regarding the use of intravenous proton pump inhibitors in pediatric patients, parallels may be seen between the treatments of adult and pediatric nonvariceal upper GI bleeding.

High-Dose Proton Pump Inhibitors

Choices for high-dose intravenous PPIs to treat GI hemorrhage include pantoprazole and esomeprazole. Neither product's intravenous formulation has been well studied in children. Doses for children have been extrapolated from the adult high-dose intravenous pantoprazole recommendations for nonvariceal upper GI bleeding.[31] Although it is not yet specified in the literature, many pediatric sites reportedly use a pantoprazole loading dose of 2 mg/kg IV, followed by 0.2 mg/kg/hr for 72 hours (neither the loading dose nor continuous infusion should exceed the adult dose).

Octreotide and Somatostatin

Octreotide is a somatostatin analogue. Its pharmacologic actions include inhibition of gastric acid secretion and decreased splanchnic blood flow. Although its 1.7-hour half-life is approximately 30 times longer than that of somatostatin, octreotide is usually administered through continuous infusion for GI hemorrhage. Adverse effects include abdominal pain, sinus bradycardia, nausea and vomiting, pain at the site of injection, elevation of liver enzymes, hyperglycemia, chest pain, headache, dizziness, fatigue, flushing, and diarrhea. Long-term use (longer than 1 month) has been associated with changes in thyroid function, gallstone formation, and cholecystitis.[32]

In adults, octreotide has been shown to decrease the duration of hemorrhage and prevent recurrence of peptic disease more so than cimetidine or ranitidine. A Cochrane review cited improved initial hemostasis and decreased transfusion requirements; however, no change was evident in rebleeding or secondary outcomes when octreotide was used to treat variceal bleeding.[32] Few researchers have evaluated octreotide for GI hemorrhage in children. In one study, continuous infusion of octreotide in seven patients was evaluated. Bleeding ceased in six of the seven patients. The duration of infusion ranged from 24 to 234 hours. Although bleeding stopped within 24 hours in nearly half of the patients, on average, bleeding stopped after 40 hours. The most notable adverse effect was hyperglycemia.[33] Subcutaneous octreotide has also been used for severe chronic GI hemorrhage for extended periods of 24 to 50 months.[34]

Vasopressin

Vasopressin has been used for treatment of variceal bleeding more frequently than for nonvariceal upper GI bleeding. In fact, adult guidelines do not address the use of vasopressin for nonvariceal bleeding. Vasopressin acts by mechanisms similar to octreotide; however, its hypertensive effects on blood pressure make it a less desirable option in many patients.[35] From a medication safety perspective, vasopressin prescribing can be confusing given the wide range of accepted dosing conventions and variety of indications in pediatric patients (eg, diabetes insipidus, GI hemorrhage, shock). Dosing recommendations that require units per kg per unit time require careful decimal place checks. Intensive care units should decide on the accepted dosing convention and dose range for vasopressin for each indication and use infusion pumps with safety software that can accommodate the predetermined limits to prevent 10-fold dosing errors.

Antibiotic-Associated Diarrhea

Diarrhea occurs commonly in the pediatric ICU where patients are also at elevated risk of antibiotic-associated diarrhea and *Clostridium difficile* colitis because many are receiving antibiotics empirically or for identified infection. Diarrhea in critically ill patients is estimated to occur in 14% to 21% of the population, with the median onset of symptoms occurring 6 days after ICU admission.[36]

Antibiotic treatment may lead to disturbance in the normal microbiota of the gut, resulting in a range of symptoms, notably diarrhea. Diarrhea has been reported in up to 40% of children receiving broad-spectrum antibiotics; antibiotics with activity against anaerobes such as aminopenicillins, cephalosporins, and clindamycin are most commonly implicated.[37] Treatment of antibiotic-associated diarrhea has centered around replacing gut flora using probiotics. Probiotics are nonpathogenic viable microorganisms (bacteria or yeast), which when administered in sufficient amounts provide a health benefit to the host.[38] Probiotic use has steadily gained popularity and acceptance. Commonly available bacterial probiotics in the United States include various species of *Lactobacillus, Bifidobacterium, Streptococcus, Lactococcus lactis,* select *E. coli,* and some *Enterococcus* species.[39] The only probiotic yeast available is the nonpathogenic *Saccharomyces boulardii.* Currently there exists huge variability in the published data with regard to probiotic strain, dose, and duration of therapy for antibiotic-associated diarrhea (AAD). However despite this heterogeneity, a Cochrane[37] review concluded that the overall evidence suggests a beneficial effect of probiotics in the prevention of pediatric AAD. Most common adverse effects reported are abdominal cramping, nausea, fever, soft stools, and flatulence.[38] Although probiotics are generally well tolerated, their use has been linked to serious adverse events such as bacteremia and fungemia.[38,39] Risk factors for these rare side effects include immunosuppression, infant prematurity, short gut syndrome, insertion of central venous catheter, prosthetic heart valves, and the presence of a jejunostomy tube.[38,39]

Clostridium Difficile–Associated Diarrhea

C. difficile is the most frequently reported nosocomial pathogen in the United States. It is an anaerobic, gram-positive bacterium that is transmitted via the fecal-oral route. *C. difficile* releases two toxins, toxins A and B, which are associated with intestinal secretion, inflammation, and monocyte cytokine release leading to diarrhea. The B1/NAP1/027 strain of

C. difficile is relatively new and is associated with more severe *Clostridium difficile*–associated diarrhea (CDAD) and is often seen in hospital-acquired CDAD. *C. difficile* infection is diagnosed by testing for toxins in stool by enzyme immunoassay or by polymerase chain reaction testing.[40,41]

The most important risk factor for *C. difficile* infection is antibiotic use. Pediatric ICU patients represent a high-risk group for *C. difficile* infection, as they commonly receive empiric antibiotics. Almost all antibiotics have been associated with infection, but the most frequently reported offenders are ampicillin, amoxicillin, cephalosporins, clindamycin, and flouroquinolones.[40] Other established risk factors include increasing age in adults, concurrent use of proton pump inhibitors, immune deficiency, malignancy, and inflammatory bowel disease.[40,41] In addition to antibiotic stewardship, hand washing and patient isolation are the cornerstones for prevention of the spread of CDAD in health care facilities.[40,41]

For many decades, the mainstays for the treatment of *C. difficile* have been with metronidazole or vancomycin for 10 to 14 days. More recent data have shown the superiority of vancomycin in patients with mild, moderate, and severe disease.[40,41] The decreasing cost of vancomycin along with a favorable side effect profile compared to metronidazole has led to its increasing use.

Fidaxomicin is a new macrocyclic antibiotic with proven bactericidal activity against *C. difficile*; it is poorly absorbed from the GI tract. In clinical trials, the cure rate for acute infection was comparable between fidaxomicin and vancomycin; however, the recurrence rate was 15% among patients on fidaxomicin compared to 25% recurrence on vancomycin.[40] Fidaxomicin is FDA approved for the treatment of *C. difficile* in adults over 18 years old. Currently there are no data on pediatric dosing.

Constipation

Although there is no consensus on the definition of pediatric constipation in the intensive care unit, nor has it been extensively studied, the incidence is thought to be 33% to 50%.[42] Constipation is the result of altered motility of the colon and rectum. Constipation occurs commonly in patients receiving opioid medications to tolerate mechanical ventilation or for postoperative pain.

Shock and medications such as sedatives are the most important risk factors for constipation in the ICU.[43] Other contributing factors include severity of illness, immobilization, dehydration, or an inadequate diet. In shock states, splanchnic perfusion is severely reduced, altering tolerance to enteral nutrition, and can cause structural changes in the gastrointestinal tract.[43] The differential diagnosis of constipation in a pediatric intensive care unit is extensive and includes anatomic, metabolic, neurologic, and connective tissue disorder.[44,45] Chronic constipation in a patient in the ICU may merit investigation of the underlying cause. Medications such as opiates, phenobarbital, antacids, antihypertensives, and anticholinergics can all contribute to a child's constipation.[44,45]

Prevention and Treatment

In the ICU, prevention should be considered in certain populations where constipation is particularly common, could have serious negative outcomes, or where straining may be problematic for the operative site. Some pediatric ICUs have incorporated a bowel regimen as part of enteral nutrition protocols given the frequency of constipation.[46] Prevention usually includes a combination of agents to maintain bowel function.[45]

When considering treatment, any underlying disease state or anatomic anomaly should be managed individually. If medication related, the offending agent should be discontinued if possible. Constipation itself is addressed as a two-step process of disimpaction lasting 3 to 5 days, followed by maintenance therapy (Table 98.1).[47,48]

Disimpaction may be accomplished with oral or rectal medication administration. The oral route is less invasive and may give a sense of empowerment to the child, but the rectal route is quicker and may be necessary if the child has abdominal pain.[47]

Recommended daily maintenance therapy includes mineral oil (a lubricant) or magnesium hydroxide, lactulose, sorbitol, polyethylene glycol (PEG) (osmotic laxatives), or a combination of lubricant and laxative. The prolonged use of stimulant laxatives is not recommended in children. The preferred, acceptable palatability and superior osmotic agent in children is PEG 3350.[49] Although preliminary, clinical data suggest that the administration of PEG 3350 to infants is effective without any adverse effects noted.[50] Intermittent, short-term use of a stimulant laxative may be necessary to avoid recurrence of an impaction, but it should be avoided for extended use.[47]

Long-term follow-up studies have demonstrated that a significant number of children continue to require therapy to maintain regular bowel movements.[47,50]

Rectal Administration of Medication

Many drugs otherwise approved for oral or intravenous use have been administered rectally in both adults and children. The rationale for using the rectal route depends on the patient's clinical status. Rectal administration allows for avoidance of the orogastric route when the intravenous route is not an option or when parenteral dosage forms are not available. The rectal route allows for a higher local concentration of drug in situations where limited systemic absorption is desired. Although generally well accepted among patients and their families,[51,52] clinicians may need to overcome resistance to rectal administration from patients and families because of personal perceptions.

Interpatient variability surrounding rectal administration and the pharmaceutical formulation are key factors for clinicians to consider.[53] The result of these issues is that drug absorption may be accelerated or delayed. First, the formulation of the product itself varies, causing differences in the time to liquefaction with suppositories, the volume of liquid administered, and the concentration of the drug. Drugs administered high in the rectum, which is drained by the superior rectal veins, typically are carried to the liver via the portal vein, thus they are subject to first-pass hepatic metabolism. Drugs administered low in the rectum are delivered into the venous circulation by the inferior and middle rectal veins before passing through the liver. The presence of stool in the rectum and rectal pH can alter drug absorption. Rectal pH affects absorption by ionizing varying amounts of drug. The rectal mucosa in children typically has a more alkaline pH.[54] Nonionized drugs have greater lipid solubility, causing enhanced absorption across biological membranes. The rectal retention of the drug administered also affects absorption.[55]

TABLE 98.1   Medications for Treatment of Constipation

Drug Class		Formulations	Adverse Effects/Contraindications
Osmotic			
	Lactulose	Oral solution	Flatulence, abdominal cramps, hypernatremia when used in high doses
	Sorbitol	Oral and rectal solution	
	Barley malt extract		
	Magnesium citrate	Liquid	Hypermagnesemia, hypophosphatemia, and secondary hypocalcemia; infants are at an increased risk of hypermagnesemia
	Magnesium hydroxide (milk of magnesia)	Oral suspension or chewable tablet	
	PEG 3350 (MiraLax)	Powder for oral suspension	
Osmotic Enema			
	Phosphate enemas	Rectal enema	Avoid in children <2 years old; rectal wall injury, abdominal distention, vomiting, severe hyperphosphatemia, severe hypocalcemia, tetany
Lavage (continuous infusion via nasogastric tube)			
	Polyethylene glycol-electrolyte solution (Golytely)	Powder for suspension	Nausea or vomiting, bloating, abdominal cramps, hyperphosphatemia, anal irritation, aspiration pneumonitis/pulmonary edema
Lubricant			
	Mineral oil	Oral liquid and rectal enema	Not recommended for <1 year old. Nausea or vomiting, abdominal discomfort, may decrease fat-soluble vitamins, lipoid pneumonia if aspirated
Stimulants			Abdominal pain, cathartic colon (possibility of permanent gut, nerve, or muscle damage)
	Senna	Oral syrup and tablets; chewable tablets	Nausea or vomiting, diarrhea, discoloration of urine; idiosyncratic hepatitis, melanosis coli; hypertrophic osteoarthropathy, analgesic nephropathy
	Bisacodyl	Delayed release tablets, rectal enema and suppositories	Abdominal pain, diarrhea, hypokalemia, abnormal rectal mucosa, and (rarely) proctitis
	Glycerin suppositories	Adult and pediatric rectal suppositories	Nausea or vomiting, diarrhea, rectal irritation

Adapted from Baker SS, Liptak GS, Colletti RB, et al. Clinical practice guideline: evaluation and treatment of constipation in infants and children: recommendations of the North American Society for Pediatric Gastroenterology, Hepatology and Nutrition. J Pediatr Gastroenterol Nutr. 2006;43:e1-13.

The rectal route has been commonly studied with the use of rectal diazepam gel (Diastat). This commercially available product is used for prolonged or repetitive seizures in children and has approval by the FDA for at-home administration by a trained nonprofessional caregiver. Clinical trials and postmarketing data have reported a low rate of serious respiratory adverse events.[56,57] Rectal administration offers an alternative to other oral and intravenous benzodiazepine options available in a critical care setting, especially in emergent situations if access cannot be readily achieved.[55,56] Several orally available medications have been administered rectally including anticonvulsants such as diazepam, lamotrigine, levetiracetam, phenobarbital, topiramate, valproate, and carbamazepine for status epilepticus[57,58]; sedatives such as diazepam, midazolam, and ketamine in varying uses[55,59]; localized treatment for irritable bowel disease using mesalamine[60-62]; vancomycin for pseudomembranous colitis[62a]; antibacterial agents such as erythromycin and azithromycin[63]; antiemetics[64]; cardiovascular agents such as nifedipine and metoprolol[65-68]; and analgesics, specifically acetaminophen, nonsteroidal antiinflammatory drugs (ibuprofen), and tramadol, for temperature reduction and postoperative pain control.[51,52,69,70] Although the American Academy of Pediatrics dissuades the rectal use of acetaminophen without consultation with a health care provider,[71] it has been widely used and studied.[69,70,72,73] In addition, rectally administered nonsteroidal antiinflammatory medications, opioid analgesics, antiseizure medications,

antiemetics, anticholinergic medications, antidepressants, psychostimulants, and antibiotics have been used with success in the hospice and palliative care settings.[74]

In a pediatric critical care environment, rectal administration of medication may be most beneficial when intravenous access issues are present, either because of an inability to maintain or achieve intravenous access or in situations when placement of an intravenous line is otherwise not necessary. Rectal administration in children is relatively painless and comparable to rectal temperature monitoring, a common practice. Practical considerations for prescribers include knowledge of available dosage forms for rectal use, interpatient variability of absorption, varying amounts of immeasurable drug expelled by the patient (thus altering dosage), and social considerations including patient or family perceptions of rectal medications, especially in older children and adolescents.

Nausea and Vomiting
Introduction and Definitions

Uncontrolled nausea and vomiting in the pediatric intensive care unit may result in consequences that range from minor patient discomfort to electrolyte imbalance or surgical site complications. To the patient this can mean wound dehiscence, GI bleeding, malnutrition, dehydration, pulmonary aspiration, and increased anxiety with future medical interventions.[75]

Two populations seen in the PICU that commonly experience nausea and vomiting are oncology patients after chemotherapy administration and postoperative admissions. Indeed, nausea and vomiting have been referred to as the "big little problem" with the capacity to delay discharge, monopolize nursing care, and impact financial resources.[76] These costs can be limited with a focus on prophylactic treatment, employing recent drug developments and guideline-driven therapy when possible. The data that drive these guidelines are, particularly in pediatrics, largely based on studies that look at vomiting more specifically than nausea.[77] Because nausea is an unpleasant sensation in the epigastrium, it is more difficult to quantify objectively compared to vomiting.[77,78] Nausea may be associated with flushing, tachycardia, and an urge to vomit. Vomiting, defined as the forceful expulsion of gastric contents from the mouth, can be more easily measured for medication assessment purposes. Unless otherwise noted, when management of vomiting is discussed here, it can be inferred to also pertain to managing nausea (unless otherwise noted). Retching (also known as dry heaving) is defined as gastric and esophageal contractions without expulsion of vomitus.

The causes of nausea and vomiting in intensive care are diverse, including radiation, intracranial hypertension, meningitis, diabetic ketoacidosis, hypercalcemia, hyponatremia, hepatitis, pancreatitis, bowel obstruction, GI bleeding, postoperative ileus, and medication administration. Common medications that can trigger vomiting include antineoplastics, anesthetics, antibiotics, contrast media, and opiates. The majority of research has focused on chemotherapy-induced nausea and vomiting (CINV) and postoperative nausea and vomiting (PONV). Before moving on to these topics specifically, the mechanism mediating nausea and vomiting will be explored.

Pathophysiology of Emesis

The vomiting center or emetic center or *central pattern generator,* located in the medulla oblongata, is a collection of neurons that may trigger vomiting after receiving input from the chemoreceptor trigger zone, abdominal vagal afferents, or cerebral cortex.[75,79-81] The chemoreceptor trigger zone, located in the area postrema region near the fourth ventricle, is not fully protected by the blood-brain barrier and is therefore vulnerable to antineoplastic agents or other stimuli in the blood or cerebral spinal fluid.[79-81] The vagus nerve provides important stimuli to both the chemoreceptor trigger zone and vomiting center, and it appears to have the largest role in CINV.[79,81] This occurs when cells within the GI tract are exposed to chemotherapy and release mediators, including 5-hydroxytryptamine (5-HT), substance P, and cholecystokinin, that stimulate the vagus nerve.[79,81] Finally, the role of the cerebral cortex is less well defined but is thought to play a role in anticipatory nausea and vomiting.[75]

The mechanism described is most dependent on the neurotransmitter receptors for dopamine, serotonin (5-hydroxytryptamine type 3 or 5-HT3), and substance P.[75,79-81] Additional receptors that are thought to play a supporting role include corticosteroid, histamine, cannabinoid, acetylcholine, opiate, neurokinin-1, and gamma-aminobutyric acid (GABA).[75,80,82] The intricate cascade briefly described here and multiple neurotransmitter involvement foreshadow treatment guidelines that will often be rooted in multiple agents that target various pathways.

Chemotherapy-Induced Nausea and Vomiting

Emesis that occurs from chemotherapy is divided into four categories. Anticipatory CINV occurs prior to chemotherapy administration (hours to days) and occurs as a conditioned response in patients that have had significant past CINV. Acute CINV occurs within 24 hours following chemotherapy administration and is the most widely studied. Delayed CINV occurs more than 24 hours after and usually occurs within 7 days of chemotherapy administration. Breakthrough (or refractory) nausea and vomiting occur during any phase despite antiemetic prophylaxis or treatment. The risk of experiencing nausea and vomiting is mainly determined by chemotherapy-specific factors (eg, emetogenicity of drugs, dose, schedule, route, rate of administration). Pediatric patients that have well-controlled acute nausea and vomiting are less likely to have delayed nausea and vomiting.[82] This highlights the importance of staying ahead of symptoms with prophylactic treatment.

5-HT3 Receptor Antagonists

The advent of 5-HT3 receptor antagonists in the early 1990s provided a new cornerstone in how acute nausea and vomiting are managed in patients receiving highly or moderately emetogenic chemotherapy. The first-generation 5-HT3 receptor antagonists of dolasetron (Anzemet), granisetron (Kytril), and ondansetron (Zofran) have been established in pediatrics to be equally effective, and the most common adverse effects include headache, constipation, fatigue, and dizziness.[77,83-87] It should be noted that the approved pediatric dose of granisetron of 10 µg/kg once daily is likely ineffective, and a dose of 40 µg/kg once daily is more appropriate.[77,87,88] The IV formulation of dolasetron is contraindicated for CINV due to a dose-dependent increase in QT prolongation and risk of developing torsades de pointes.[89] In adults, the 5-HT3 receptor antagonists have been established, at the appropriate doses, to be as effective when given orally as when given intravenously and that single daily dose schedules are as effective as multiple-dose schedules.[88,90-94] However, there are limited data regarding the selection of appropriate dosage form for pediatric patients.[95] These agents are most useful for CINV occurring within the first 24 hours after administration of chemotherapy.[96]

A second-generation 5-HT3 receptor antagonist, palonosetron (Aloxi) gained Food and Drug Administration approval for both acute and delayed CINV in 2003. It is unique from other 5-HT3 antagonists because of its long half-life (21 to 37 hours in children and 40 hours in adults) and greater affinity for 5-HT3 receptors.[97] All 5-HT3 receptor antagonists except palonosetron affect the QT interval. Three phase III trials have established that palonosetron is not inferior to older 5-HT3 antagonists.[98-101] Further prospective study is needed before palonosetron can be established as superior to other 5-HT3 receptor antagonists. To date, CINV guidelines have not stated any one 5-HT3 receptor antagonist to be superior to another.[88] Higher weight-based doses of 5-HT3 antagonists may be required in children due to variation in pharmacokinetics as compared to adults.[88]

Corticosteroids

Corticosteroids, most commonly dexamethasone or methylprednisolone, are potent antiemetics and have a critical role in managing acute and delayed CINV in pediatrics. Their exact mechanism of action is unclear but may involve decreasing 5-HT3 release in the peripheral nervous system.[102] Addition of a corticosteroid with a 5-HT3 receptor antagonist is considered the standard of care for patients receiving moderate or highly emetogenic chemotherapy. However, corticosteroids also have the potential to decrease the effect of antineoplastic drugs on brain tumors, osteosarcomas, and carcinomas.[102] Dexamethasone may increase the resistance of certain tumors to both radiation and chemotherapy.[77] Interferon or interleukin-2 may be less effective when used along with steroids.[75] Corticosteroids may also impact the quality of brain tumor images generated by computed tomography or magnetic resonance imaging by altering the distribution of contrast media.[77] In addition to these concerns, the usual side effects of steroids must be kept in mind, including gastritis, hyperglycemia, hypokalemia, anxiety, euphoria, and insomnia. If corticosteroids are contraindicated, then chlorpromazine, metoclopramide, or nabilone may be used instead.[103] It would be prudent to consult a patient's chemotherapy protocol or an oncologist before initiating corticosteroids in a pediatric patient with a malignancy to verify the appropriateness of this approach.

Substance P/Neurokinin-1 Receptor Antagonists

The substance P/neurokinin-1 receptor antagonist is the most recent antiemetic class. These substances are effective for both acute and delayed nausea and vomiting in moderately and highly emetogenic chemotherapy. They are currently approved in adults for prevention of CINV when used in conjunction with a 5-HT3 antagonist and a corticosteroid in moderate or highly emetogenic chemotherapy regimens. Currently the medications that represent this class on the market are oral aprepitant and intravenous fosaprepitant (prodrug of aprepitant). A fixed combination of oral palonosetron and netupitant (Akynzeo) was approved in 2014. This class of drug is generally well tolerated with diarrhea, fatigue, headache, and hiccups being common side effects.[104-106] Both aprepitant and fosaprepitant are substrates, inhibitors, and inducers of the cytochrome P-450 enzymes 3A4 and 2C9. A thorough review of potential interactions for individual patients is merited (most notably warfarin, oral contraceptives, and chemotherapy agents). Concomitant corticosteroid dose should be decreased by 25% if given IV and by 50% if given PO.[107] Although none are currently approved for children, there have been several single-center case studies documenting the use of aprepitant and fosaprepitant in children and adolescents.[108-110] One study examined aprepitant dosed for young adults in patients ages 11 to 19 years weighing 43 to 105 kg.[111] Aprepitant-containing regimens performed comparably to non–aprepitant-containing regimens, but an increase in the number of cases of febrile neutropenia was noted in the aprepitant patients.[111] A single-center, prospective, observational study evaluated the safety and efficacy of aprepitant in patients between age 1 and 17 years (mean age 9.55 + 4.85) using a weight-based dosing table. Through patient survey, incidence of nausea, emesis episodes, inference with activities of daily living, and appetite were evaluated. Eleven patients were enrolled. Aprepitant was well tolerated, and the complete response (defined as no nausea, vomiting, or use of rescue therapy) rate was 38.9%.[108] Until further pediatric experience is established, routine use of aprepitant should be reserved for

children age 12 and older who are receiving highly emetogenic chemotherapy.

Other Antiemetic Agents

Several other agents are used in pediatrics for CINV. Lorazepam is routinely employed for anticipatory nausea and vomiting (up to a maximum dose of 2 mg) given once at bedtime the night before chemotherapy and once the next day prior to chemotherapy.[112] Diphenhydramine is anecdotally used in pediatric patients, despite its absence from guidelines and reviews of CINV.[77,88] Dopamine receptor antagonists, including phenothiazines (eg, prochlorperazine), butyrophenones (eg, droperidol), and benzamides (eg, metoclopramide), cause a high incidence of dystonic reactions when used at high doses for several days and potentially oculogyric crisis.[88,113] Cannabinoids (ie, dronabinol) are limited by their lack of pediatric data and their side effects, which include euphoria, sedation, depression, and hallucinations.[114] A scopolamine patch may have some utility in patients older than 12 years that are able to wait up to 12 hours for relief.[77] Olanzapine is an atypical antipsychotic medication that has shown efficacy for treatment of CINV in adults. A retrospective, multicenter review of olanzapine use in children for CINV suggests that this medication could potentially be an important antiemetic option; however, further research is warranted.[115] Generally speaking, these agents should only be considered for pediatric patients who do not tolerate first-line therapy alone.

Treatment Guidelines for Chemotherapy-Induced Nausea and Vomiting

Determining appropriate antiemetic therapy requires one to first evaluate the likelihood that a particular chemotherapy regimen will produce nausea or vomiting.[88,116,117,95] This has been accomplished with literature and expert opinion and is summarized in Table 98.2. This categorization is largely based on adult data, so it is vital to take individual patient parameters and CINV history into account. If a chemotherapy regimen is close to the next highest emetic risk category, it is better to be aggressive with antiemetic management. Typically, combination chemotherapy is more emetogenic than single-agent chemotherapy. Choice of antiemetic(s) should be individualized based on the emetogenicity of chemotherapy given, tolerance to previous cycles, potential anticipatory nausea or vomiting, concomitant medications, or history of adverse events or allergic reactions.[118] In general, a first-generation 5-HT3 receptor antagonist plus dexamethasone is recommended for children receiving moderate or highly emetogenic chemotherapy. Dosing should be administered scheduled and not as needed. The initial dose prior to initial chemotherapy should be given 30 minutes if IV or 1 hour if PO.[118]

Medications that are less well supported for delayed CINV, such as diphenhydramine or 5HT3 receptor antagonists, may be employed based on individual practitioner preference. Other areas of future research include breakthrough emesis that occurs despite adequate prophylaxis in a single chemotherapy cycle and refractory emesis that occurs despite adequate prophylaxis over multiple chemotherapy cycles.[82] Additional areas that require further investigation in pediatric CINV include multiple-day chemotherapy, high-dose chemotherapy with stem cell rescue, and intractable symptoms in terminal patients.[119-121] Finally, each institution would be well advised to conduct a pharmacoeconomic review

TABLE 98.2   Emetogenicity of Frequently Encountered Pediatric Chemotherapy

Emetic Risk (Incidence of Emesis With No Prophylaxis)	Antineoplastic Agent[a]
High (>90%)	Carboplatin Carmustine >250 mg/m^2 Cisplatin Cyclophosphamide >1.5 g/m^2 Cytarabine 3 g/m^2/dose Dactinomycin Methotrexate >12 g/m^2 Procarbazine (oral) Streptozocin Thiotepa >300 mg/m^2
Moderate (30%-90%)	Carmustine <250 mg/m^2 Cyclophosphamide <1 g/m^2 or oral Cytarabine >1 g/m^2 Daunorubicin Doxorubicin Etoposide (oral) Ifosfamide Intrathecal therapy (methotrexate, hydrocortisone, cytarabine) Irinotecan
Low (10%-30%)	5-Fluorouracil Busulfan (oral) Cytarabine <200 mg/m^2 Docetaxel Doxorubicin (liposomal) Etoposide Methotrexate >50 to <250 mg/m^2 mg/m^2 Paclitaxel Topotecan Vorinostat
Minimal (<10%)	6-Thioguanine (oral) Asparaginase (IM or IV) Bevacizumab Dasatinib Erlotinib Fludarabine Hydroxyurea (oral) Mercaptopurine (oral) Methotrexate <50 mg/m^2 or oral Rituximab Sorafenib Sunitinib Temsirolimus Vinblastine Vincristine

[a]Table focuses on more common pediatric chemotherapy and is not exhaustive. Medication is parental unless otherwise stated.
Modified from Dupuis LL, Boodhan S, Holdsworth M, et al. Guideline for the prevention of acute nausea and vomiting due to antineoplastic medication in pediatric cancer patients. Pediatr Blood Cancer. 2013;60:1073-1083.

to aid in antiemetic selection of pharmacologically equivalent products.

Postoperative Nausea and Vomiting

Postoperative nausea and vomiting (PONV) is one of the most common complications in pediatric surgery. The rate of PONV in children can be twice that in adults (between 33.2% and 82%), thereby emphasizing the importance of prophylaxis.[122,123] The etiology of PONV is multifactorial with risk factors mainly related to the surgical procedure, the patient, and the type of anesthesia. Strabismus repair, ear-nose-throat (tonsillectomy and adenoidectomy), appendectomy, hernia and orchidopexy surgery, or any procedure where anesthesia time is 30 minutes or longer has an increased likelihood of PONV.[78,122-124] Children aged 3 years and older continue to increase their risk of PONV until they become pubescent.[122,124] Patients who have a history of PONV, motion sickness, or patients with first-degree relatives with such histories are more prone to have PONV.[122,124]

In a single-center, prospective study of pediatric anesthesia, Eberhart and colleagues identified four independent risk factors: strabismus repair, duration of surgery >30 minutes, age >3 years, and previous history of PONV in patient or relatives. The presence of 0, 1, 2, 3, and 4 risk factors predicts the risk of PONV as approximately 9%, 10%, 30%, 55%, or 70%, respectively.[109]

Prophylaxis is recommended only for children thought to be at moderate or high risk of PONV.[78] Regional anesthesia is optimal in such patients.[78] However, if general anesthesia is necessary, the following may reduce the baseline risk of PONV: use of regional anesthesia versus general anesthesia, adequate hydration, use of propofol infusions, and avoiding nitrous oxide or volatile anesthetics and minimizing opioids when possible.[110,122]

Patients at moderate or high risk should receive prophylaxis therapy with a combination of at least two agents with distinct mechanisms of action.[78,122] A 5-HT3 receptor antagonist and dexamethasone combination is recommended as first choice and is preferable to single agents.[122] Other options for prophylaxis include dimenhydrinate, droperidol, and perphenazine. Neurokinin 1 (NK-1) receptor antagonists have been established as potent agents for PONV in adult patients, but even if approved in pediatrics, it seems likely a multiple agent approach to PONV as described previously will remain the standard of care. Updated practice guidelines for postanesthetic care from the American Society of Anesthesiologists (ASA) in 2012 support the practice of giving multiple agents for prophylaxis of PONV.[107]

For PONV that occurs despite prophylaxis, rescue treatment should be initiated using a class of drug different from that given prophylactically. If no prophylaxis was given, then a low-dose 5-HT3 antagonist is recommended. There is evidence to show that there is no benefit to repeating the prophylaxis therapy within 6 hours after the first dose. Options for rescue therapy include metoclopramide, dimenhydrinate, perphenazine, or droperidol.[78,122,124] Because of the potential for QT prolongation and torsades des pointes, droperidol should be reserved for patients who have failed first-line therapy and are hospital inpatients.[122] Unlike recommendations to use multiple agents for PONV prophylaxis, the 2012 guidelines on postanesthetic care from the ASA find literature to be inadequate to recommend multiple agents compared to a single agent for the treatment of ongoing nausea and vomiting despite prophylaxis.[107] Other contributing factors to consider when assessing ongoing PONV include postoperative ileus, opioid use, blood draining down the throat, and bowel obstruction.

Acknowlegment

We gratefully acknowledge the contribution of Louis L. Bystrak, Ann Marie Heine, Kelly A. Michienzi, and Sasko D. Stojanovski, who authored this chapter in previous editions.

Key References

4. Mutlu GM, Mutlu EA, Factor P. GI complications in patients receiving mechanical ventilation. *Chest*. 2001;119:1222-1241.

6. Cook DJ, Fuller HD, Guyatt GH, et al. Risk factors for gastrointestinal bleeding in critically ill patients. *N Engl J Med*. 1994;330:377-391.

10. Marik PE, Vasu T, Hirani A, et al. Stress ulcer prophylaxis in the new millennium: a systematic review and meta-analysis. *Crit Care Med*. 2010;38:2222-2228.

12. Cook D, Guyatt G, Marshall J. A comparison of sucralfate and ranitidine for the prevention of upper gastrointestinal bleeding in patients requiring mechanical ventilation, Canadian Critical Care Trials Group. *N Engl J Med*. 1998;338:791-797.

13. Lacroix J, Nadeau D, Laberge S, et al. Frequency of upper gastrointestinal bleeding in a pediatric intensive care unit. *Crit Care Med*. 1992;20: 35-42.

30. Barkun A, Bardou M, Marshall JK. Consensus recommendations for managing patients with nonvariceal upper gastrointestinal bleeding. *Ann Intern Med*. 2003;139:843-857.

37. Johnston BC, Goldenberg JZ, Vandvik PO, et al. Probiotics for the prevention of pediatric antibiotic associated diarrhea. *Cochrane Database Syst Rev*. 2011;(11):CD004827.

39. Marrow LE. Probiotics in the intensive care unit. *Nutr Clin Pract*. 2012;27:235-241.

40. Leffler DA, Lamont JT. Clostridium difficile infection. *N Engl J Med*. 2015;372:1539-1548.

47. Baker SS, Liptak GS, Colletti RB, et al. Clinical practice guideline: evaluation and treatment of constipation in infants and children: recommendations of the North American Society for Pediatric Gastroenterology, Hepatology and Nutrition. *J Pediatr Gastroenterol Nutr*. 2006;43:e1-e13.

55. Committee on Drugs. Alternative routes of drug administration: advantages and disadvantages. *Pediatrics*. 1997;100:143-152.

77. Dupuis LL, Nathan PC. Options for the prevention and management of acute chemotherapy-induced nausea and vomiting in children. *Paediatr Drugs*. 2003;5:597-613.

78. Kovac AL. Management of postoperative nausea and vomiting in children. *Paediatr Drugs*. 2007;9:47-69.

81. Hesketh PJ. Chemotherapy-induced nausea and vomiting. *N Engl J Med*. 2008;358:2482-2494.

103. Dupuis LL, Boodhan S, Holdsworth M, et al. Guideline for the prevention of acute nausea and vomiting due to antineoplastic medication in pediatric cancer patients. *Pediatr Blood Cancer*. 2013;60:1073-1083.

110. Hohne C. Postoperative nausea and vomiting in pediatric anesthesia. *Current Opin Anesthesiol*. 2014;27:303-308.

118. Children's Oncology Group (COG) Supportive Care Guidelines, version date: 10/07/2009. <https://www.childrensoncologygroup.org/index.php/cog-supportive-care-endorsed-guidelines>.

Acute Liver Failure, Liver Transplantation, and Extracorporeal Liver Support

Simon Horslen and Hengqi (Betty) Zheng

PEARLS

- Pediatric liver failure represents a large number of heterogenous etiologies.
- Effective diagnosis requires a systemic approach, but in spite of thorough workup, currently in a large proportion of cases, cause cannot be determined.
- Prognostication is remarkably difficult in that spontaneous recovery has occurred even in patients with advanced hepatic necrosis, deep coma, and severe coagulopathy. Prognostic tools have been designed, but all have been found to be fallible and clinical experience is invaluable.
- Extracorporeal liver support has been tried in many forms from simple exchange transfusion to bioartificial liver support technologies, and although research is ongoing, none have been demonstrated to alter outcomes, either in terms of survival with native liver or getting more patients to successful liver transplantation.
- Orthotopic liver transplantation is lifesaving, and early transfer to an experienced liver transplant center is advisable for all children with coagulopathy secondary to acute liver disease.
- Many patients can be extubated immediately after the liver transplant operation or promptly following admission to the pediatric intensive care unit.
- Oversedation is to be avoided because it increases the risk of complications and prolongs ICU stay and total length of hospital stay after liver transplantation.
- Close monitoring of fluid balance in the first few days of liver transplantation facilitates optimal recovery, faster weaning from artificial ventilation, and possible shorter ICU stays.
- Anticipation and early recognition of postoperative complications through awareness, suspicion, and appropriate testing, together with prompt and aggressive treatment of complications, maximize possibilities of rescuing both the patient and allograft.

Introduction

Liver failure is an unusual issue in most pediatric intensive care unit (PICU) settings, but expert management is crucial to achieving optimal outcomes, which may include liver transplantation. This chapter focuses on acute liver injury and transplantation. The management of the end-stage and life-threatening complications of chronic liver disease is beyond the scope of this chapter but deserves equal study and experience for optimal care.

Acute Liver Failure
Background/Definitions/Outcomes

Pediatric acute liver failure (PALF) is a life-threatening condition where previously healthy children lose hepatic function rapidly, requiring immediate medical attention and careful monitoring.[1] PALF represents a heterogeneous condition with a broad range of etiologies including infections, toxin- and drug-related injuries, metabolic disorders, immunologic, ischemic, and irradiation damage. Despite the many known causes of PALF, a specific etiology is not determined in up to 50% of cases.[1-5] Management consists of supportive measures, with a focus on anticipation, prevention, and treatment of complications along with early consideration for liver transplantation.[6-10] Timely intervention to treat the metabolic derangements associated with acute liver failure is pivotal and can help mitigate the morbidity associated with this condition.[11-16] In the United States, the incidence of PALF has been estimated at 17 cases per 100,000 per year.[17]

Liver failure is defined as the loss of normal liver function that includes synthesis of serum proteins including clotting factors and albumin, metabolism and storage of glucose and fatty acids, and detoxification and excretion of exogenous and endogenous molecules such as drugs and products of protein metabolism, most notably ammonia. Evidence of liver failure is reflected in elevations of the prothrombin time, bilirubin, and ammonia. In adults, the traditional definition of acute or fulminant liver failure is the onset of hepatic encephalopathy within 8 weeks of the first signs of liver disease. Such definitions are difficult to apply to children and infants because children are relatively resistant to encephalopathy, which may only become apparent, if at all, at a very late stage of the disease, and because of the difficulty inherent in identifying encephalopathy, even if present, in the young child. Subacute liver failure has been defined as the development of hepatic encephalopathy after 8 weeks and before 24 weeks from the onset of liver disease in the absence of preexisting chronic liver disorders.

To determine outcomes, investigate prognostic factors, and further decipher etiologies, the Pediatric Acute Liver Failure Study Group (PALF-SG) involving 24 pediatric liver centers in the United States, Canada, and England formed in 1999. The study's entry criteria include evidence of hepatic injury without known chronic liver disease manifesting as an international normalized ratio (INR) of 1.5 and encephalopathy or INR of 2.0 with or without encephalopathy.[18] Although it is tempting to use the criteria to define PALF, this set of standards was meant to capture pediatric patients who are at risk of developing PALF relatively early in their clinical course and should not be used as a general definition. The group has reported data on 348 subjects over a 6-year period and concluded that survival and the need for liver transplantation depend on age and diagnosis.[18] For established PALF etiologies, between 20% and 33% received a liver transplant versus 46% in indeterminate cases, whereas spontaneous recovery ranged from 46% to 60%.[18]

Diagnosis and Workup

The causes of PALF vary with the age of the child; however, acute liver failure of indeterminate cause is common in all age groups, accounting for 40% of PALF among patients younger than age 3 years and 60% in those age 3 years and older.[18] The large number of indeterminate causes is due to several factors including hepatic improvement prior to finishing clinical workup, lack of current available testing for all etiologies, or lack of a thorough workup. The term *indeterminate etiology* should prompt further investigation.

Of the known etiologies, severe hepatitis from echovirus, adenovirus, and herpesvirus is recognized in the neonatal population. Metabolic liver disease and hemophagocytic lymphohistiocytosis are diagnoses usually made in infants. Acute hepatitis A and B infections are rare causes of PALF in North America but are a common cause of PALF in school-aged children in developing countries.[19] Drug-induced liver disease is more common in older children, especially secondary to intentional acetaminophen overdose[18] (Table 99.1).

Prognostic Assessment

Several attempts to produce prognostic tools based on a snapshot of clinically available data either at presentation or at peak values have been attempted, but all have been found wanting. Three of the more often quoted include the King's College Hospital Criteria (KCHC), the liver injury unit (LIU) score, and the Clichy criteria. The Clichy criteria are primarily derived from adult patients with acute hepatitis B infection, and thus the utility in the pediatric population has always been in doubt.[20] KCHC applied to the PALF-SG cohort fails to reliably identify those patients at risk of death.[18] The LIU score predicted those who eventually underwent transplantation but was not a reliable predictor of death.[21] This is not particularly surprising as the LIU calculation is based on levels of bilirubin, ammonia, and prothrombin time (PT), all of which are used clinically to determine who might benefit from

TABLE 99.1	Intensive Care Unit Management

No Sedation Except for Procedures

Lines and Tubes
- Multilumen central venous catheter
- Arterial tube
- Nasogastric tube
- Urinary Foley catheter
- Bed scale

Monitor
- Heart and respiratory rate
- Arterial BP, CVP
- Core/toe temperature
- Neurologic observations
- Gastric pH (>5)
- Blood glucose (>4 mmol/L)
- Acid-base
- Electrolytes
- PT, PTT

Fluid Balance
- 75%-95% maintenance
- Dextrose 10%-25%
- Sodium (2–3 mEq/kg/day)

Maintain Circulating Volume With Colloid/FFP

Coagulation Support Only If Required

Drugs
- Vitamin K
- H_2 antagonist
- Antacids
- Lactulose
- *N*-acetylcysteine for acetaminophen toxicity
- Broad-spectrum antibiotics
- Antifungals

Nutrition
- Enteral feeding (1–2 g protein/kg/day)
- PN if ventilated

BP, blood pressure; *CVP*, central venous pressure; *FFP*, fresh frozen plasma; *PN*, parenteral nutrition; *PT*, prothrombin time; *PTT*, partial thromboplastin time.

transplantation and as such were self-fulfilling predictors.[21] All of these tools suffer from the fact that no account is taken for the dynamic nature of PALF, and further work would benefit from examining the trends over time rather than data at a single time point.[22,23]

Pediatric Intensive Care Unit Management

The care team should obtain a full history including information about infectious illnesses, behavior changes, the time course of the development of jaundice, and foreign travel. It is important to establish what medications the child has taken, including over-the-counter preparations, acne medications, folk remedies, Chinese herbs, and herbal supplements, as well as determining what other medications might be in the household.[24] In adolescents, inquiries should be made about the use of illicit drugs, potential for self-harm, and sexual contact.

Acute hepatic dysfunction often first manifests as jaundice and general malaise. Hepatomegaly may be present, but the liver edge is frequently soft and difficult to palpate. Splenomegaly is unusual, and its presence may point to a metabolic or hematologic diagnosis. Petechiae or ecchymoses can be associated with coagulopathy. The patient's level of consciousness and degree of hepatic encephalopathy (Table 99.2) should be established using a reliable scale,[3,25,26] and a complete central nervous system examination should be performed including

TABLE 99.2   Causes of Pediatric Acute Liver Failure

Viral	Hepatitis A cytomegalovirus
	Hepatitis B paramyxovirus
	Hepatitis D adenovirus
	Hepatitis E enterovirus
	Herpes simplex
	Parvovirus B19
	Varicella zoster virus
	Severe acute respiratory syndrome
	Epstein-Barr virus
	Hemorrhagic fever virus
Bacterial	Septicemia
	Bartonella
	Leptospirosis Rocky Mountain spotted fever
	Salmonella typhi/paratyphi
Metabolic	Hereditary fructose intolerance
	Carnitine defects
	Urea cycle disorders
	Wilson disease
	Organic acidemias
	Tyrosinemia type 1
	Fatty acid oxidation defects
	Niemann-Pick type C
	Mitochondrial disorders
	Acute fatty liver of pregnancy
Immune	Autoimmune hepatitis
	Hemophagocytic lymphohistiocytosis
	Neonatal hemochromatosis
	Autoimmune hemolytic anemia with giant cell hepatitis
Toxic	Drugs/toxins/herbal
	Amanita phalloides
Vascular	Budd-Chiari postcardiac surgery
	Veno-occlusive disease
	Liver trauma
	Ischemic hepatitis/shock liver
Neoplastic	Leukemia
	Lymphoma
	Hepatocellular carcinoma
Other	Reye syndrome
	Massive liver resection
	Hypothermia
	Sickle cell anemia
	Heat stroke

examination of reflexes and mental status. Parental help in the assessment of mental status is perhaps one of the best indicators of deviation from baseline neurologic status. Serial neurologic examinations should be conducted once the baseline is established to identify any progression of encephalopathy. Attention must be paid to heart rate, blood pressure, edema, and peripheral perfusion, recognizing that increased intracranial pressure can lead to a Cushing triad of hypertension, bradycardia, and irregular breathing pattern. Work of breathing should be assessed and assisted with positive pressure or mechanical ventilation if needed for adequate ventilation and oxygenation. Monitoring of and, if necessary, intervention for glycemic control, acid-base balance, and adequate tissue perfusion should be included in the care plan. Antibiotics and antiviral medications should be started if an infectious cause is suspected.

A central venous catheter should be placed for administration of glucose containing intravenous fluids and colloids and for frequent blood draws. Placement of an arterial line should be considered for patients with clinical deterioration or with hepatic encephalopathy.[17] Urinary catheter placement can also be considered to ensure accurate fluid balance estimation (Table 99.3).

A workup for PALF with investigations reflecting age-dependent etiologies is suggested in Table 99.4. Initial monitoring blood work should include complete blood count, blood gases, glucose, electrolytes, aminotransferases, prothrombin time/INR, creatinine, bilirubin, and ammonia. Monitoring blood work should be repeated every 6 to 12 hours until the clinical course is determined. If it is considered that the patient may require liver transplantation, a transplant workup should be initiated (Table 99.5).

The presence of impaired central nervous system function with acute liver disease represents an indication for immediate admission to the PICU. The decision to transfer a patient with evolving signs of progressive liver failure must be made in a timely manner, because the risks of transporting patients in a deteriorating condition can be substantial. Referral to a pediatric liver transplant center should ideally be made prior to clinical decompensation. Families of children with acute liver failure sometimes require a considerable amount of

TABLE 99.3   Clinical Stages of Hepatic Encephalopathy

Stage	Asterixis	EEG Changes	Clinical Manifestations
0	None	None	Normal
I (prodrome)	Slight	Infant/child: Difficult or impossible to test adequately Adult: Normal or diffuse slowing to theta rhythm, triphasic waves	Infant/child: Inconsolable crying, child not acting like self to parents Adult: Mild intellectual impairment, disturbed sleep-wake cycle
II (impending)	Easily elicited	Infant/child: Difficult or impossible to test adequately Adult: Generalized slowing, triphasic waves	Infant/child: Inconsolable crying, child Adult: Drowsiness, confusion, coma/inappropriate behavior, disorientation, mood swings
III (stupor)	Present if patient cooperative	Infant/child: Difficult or impossible to test adequately Adult: Grossly abnormal slowing of rhythm, triphasic waves	Infant/child/adult: Drowsy, unresponsive to verbal commands, markedly confused, stupor, combative, hyperreflexia, positive Babinski sign
IV (coma)	Usually absent	Infant/child/adult: Appearance of delta waves, decreased amplitudes	Infant/child/adult: Unconscious, decerebrate, or decorticate response to pain present (stage IVA) or absent (stage IVB)

TABLE 99.4   Diagnostic Workup

Hematology	CBC with differential PT/INR Factor 5 level Factor 7 level Fibrinogen level ABO/Rh typing
Chemistry	Electrolytes Calcium, magnesium, phosphorus BUN, creatinine Glucose Lactate, pyruvate Bilirubin-conjugated and unconjugated AST, ALT GGT Alkaline phosphatase Cholesterol, triglycerides Ferritin Blood gases Alpha-fetoprotein Acylcarnitine profile (children ≤3 mon) Amino acid quantitative Ceruloplasmin (children ≥3 yo) Copper (children ≥3 yo) Beta hCG (females ≥12 yr)
Immunology	IgG level Antinuclear antibody (children ≥3 yo) Antismooth muscle antibody (children ≥3 yo) Antiliver kidney microsomal antibody (children ≥3 yo) Antineutrophil cytoplasmic antibody (children ≥3 yo) Antisoluble liver antigen Soluble interleukin-2 receptor
Microbiology	HSV DNA Enterovirus DNA (children ≤3 mon) CMV DNA EBV DNA Varicella DNA Adenovirus DNA Parvovirus B19 DNA Toxoplasma IgG and IgM (children ≤3 mon) Hepatitis A IgM

ALT, alanine aminotransferase; *AST,* aspartate aminotransferase; *BUN,* blood urea nitrogen; *CBC,* complete blood count; *CMV,* cytomegalovirus; *DNA,* deoxyribonucleic acid; *EBV,* Epstein-Barr virus; *GGT,* gamma-glutamyltransferase; *hCG,* human chorionic gonadotropin; *HSV,* herpes simplex virus; *IgG,* immunoglobulin G; *IgM,* immunoglobulin M; *INR,* international normalized ratio; *PT,* prothrombin time.

TABLE 99.5   Pretransplant Workup

Laboratory Eval	CBC with differential PT/INR ABO/Rh typing BUN, creatinine Bilirubin-conjugated and unconjugated AST, ALT GGT Alkaline phosphatase Albumin Hepatitis A total antibody Hepatitis B panel Hepatitis C antibody Syphilis screen Epstein-Barr serology CMV serology HIV antigen and antibody TB Quantiferon Gold Beta hCG (females ≥12 yr) Urinalysis
Radiology	CT abdomen with contrast US abdomen Doppler Bone age
Other Diagnostics	ECHO ECG
Consults	Nutrition Anesthesia Social work/case management Psychiatry/psychology Nephrology/cardiology/infectious disease if needed

ALT, alanine aminotransferase; *AST,* aspartate aminotransferase; *BUN,* blood urea nitrogen; *CBC,* complete blood count; *CMV,* cytomegalovirus; *CT,* computed tomography; *ECG,* electrocardiogram; *ECHO,* echocardiogram; *GGT,* gamma-glutamyltransferase; *hCG,* human chorionic gonadotropin; *HIV,* human immunodeficiency virus; *INR,* international normalized ratio; *PT,* prothrombin time; *TB,* tuberculosis; *US,* ultrasound.

psychologic support and counseling. The best approach to management of PALF is as a team, with collaboration among specialists in hepatology, critical care medicine, transplant surgery, and early consultation by other specialties such as biochemical genetics, neurology, neurosurgery, and nephrology as appropriate.

Specific Treatments for Particular Causes of Pediatric Acute Liver Failure

Acetaminophen Toxicity
Acute acetaminophen overdose was noted in 14% of all children from the PALF-SG as the most common identifiable cause of PALF in children ≥3 years.[18] Two clinical presentations were identified: acute intentional ingestion and a *therapeutic misadventure,* which refers to the ingestion of multiple doses exceeding daily total recommended dosing taken over a period of time to treat clinical symptoms.[1] The potential severity of hepatic damage can be assessed using the Rumack-Matthew nomogram and serum acetaminophen concentration. Administration of intravenous *N*-acetylcysteine (NAC) should not be delayed if there is reason to suspect significant hepatic injury from the ingestion.

Amanita Poisoning
Amatoxin is a hepatotoxin found in wild mushrooms, particularly the *Amanita* and *Galerina* species, although the majority of significant poisonings are due to the ingestion of *Amanita phalloides,* the death cap mushroom. Once ingested, amatoxin binds to DNA-dependent RNA polymerase type II and decreases intracellular protein synthesis, leading to hepatocyte apoptosis.[27,28] Prompt gastrointestinal decontamination with activated charcoal and supportive management with fluids should be initiated ideally within 24 hours of ingestion. High-dose penicillin G can disrupt hepatocellular uptake of amatoxins. NAC and silibinin have been suggested as potential therapies, although definitive trial data are lacking.

Autoimmune Hepatitis
Although autoimmune hepatitis usually presents as chronic liver disease, a small percentage will present with PALF.

Elevations in autoimmune antibodies (antinuclear antibody, antismooth muscle antibody, liver-kidney microsomal antibody, soluble liver antigen) and total IgG level can help decipher the diagnosis. Liver biopsy is very helpful if it can be conducted safely. If autoimmune hepatitis is suspected, initiation of intravenous corticosteroids can be expected to alter the course of disease progression and avoid the need for transplantation.

Wilson Disease

Wilson disease (WD) in the setting of PALF can be a difficult diagnosis. Serum ceruloplasmin may be falsely low in non-WD PALF due to poor synthetic function or falsely elevated due to acute phase reaction in WD. A Coombs-negative hemolytic anemia is almost always present along with an elevated serum bilirubin. Transaminases and alkaline phosphatase may be relatively low and the ratios of alkaline phosphatase (IU/L)/ bilirubin (mg/dL) <4 and aspartate transaminase (AST)/ alanine transaminase (ALT) >2.2 may suggest the diagnosis.[29] Mutational analysis is currently the most reliable method of making the diagnosis, but many centers do not have the ability to get this testing completed in a timely manner to be helpful in the acute setting. The WD score, which incorporates AST, serum bilirubin, white blood cell count, and PT, can be used to determine prognosis.[30] Chelation therapy should be initiated with D-penicillamine or more commonly now with trientine.

Metabolic Disease

Undiagnosed metabolic disorders account for about 10% of PALF patients, mostly in infants.[18] Urea cycle defects can also present with the features of acute liver failure early in life. Speedy and reliable diagnosis can lead to early supportive care and appropriate treatment. For some metabolic liver disease such as fatty acid oxidation defects, medical management can be the mainstay of treatment with liver transplantation as a last resort. In diseases such as mitochondrial cytopathies, with multisystem involvement, transplantation will not alter nonhepatic disease progression and may be futile.

Glucose, Electrolytes, and Fluid Balance

The goal of fluid balance is to maintain hydration and renal function without worsening or provoking cerebral edema. Fluid input should be 75% to 95% of normal maintenance requirements in normotensive patients. Intravenous fluids, electrolytes, specifically potassium, phosphorus, calcium, and magnesium should be monitored carefully and replaced if necessary.

Hypoglycemia may occur due to the failure of hepatocytes to sustain glucose synthesis and release compounded by hyperinsulinemia from diminished hepatic degradation and secondary bacterial infection.[31-34] Frequent bedside monitoring of blood glucose concentrations and the intravenous administration of glucose may prevent this complication. Hypoglycemia should be treated with titration of continuous glucose infusions. The support of a nutritionist to help with energy calculations and parental therapy in the ICU setting is valuable.

Urine output should be monitored for oliguria whether from prerenal or renal causes. If renal perfusion is adequate, loop diuretics and vasoactive-inotropic agents can be used to maintain urine output. Should oliguria be unresponsive to

additional fluids, early consideration should be given to renal replacement therapy (see also Chapter 78).

Central venous pressure monitoring is helpful for assessing and maintaining organ perfusion. Inotropic support frequently becomes necessary in advanced liver failure with the onset of hypotension in association with multiple organ failure. Permissive hypertension, especially in the setting of cerebral edema, may help maintain cerebral perfusion pressures.

Ascites

Excessive peritoneal fluid accumulation can be found in many patients with PALF, due to the combined effects of acute portal hypertension, lobular collapse, vasodilatation, poor vascular integrity, and reduced oncotic pressure. Clinically evident ascites occurs in less than half the patients but may be a site for secondary bacterial or fungal infection. Treatment is rarely needed in the acute setting but includes albumin infusions and judicious use of diuretics. Paracentesis may be indicated if peritonitis is suspected.

Coagulopathy

The liver plays a crucial role in the synthesis of clotting factors (factors I or fibrinogen, II or prothrombin, V, VII, IX, and X) and fibrinolytic factors (antithrombin III, protein C, protein S).[35,36] In PALF, impairment is evident in the actions of both clotting and fibrinolysis. Often administering vitamin K parenterally is trialed early on in the course to ensure that coagulopathy is not due to vitamin deficiency, but it rarely improves coagulation in PALF.

The PT and thus the INR depend immediately on the availability of factor VII, which has the shortest half-life of the clotting factors. Measurement of factor VII may be a more sensitive indicator than the prothrombin time but is typically not as readily available. Fibrinogen concentrations can also be decreased because intravascular coagulation is present in addition to factor deficiencies in almost all PALF patients, indicating ongoing thrombosis. Sepsis may also be present as an additional cause of disseminated intravascular coagulation (DIC).

Coagulopathy should be managed conservatively to avoid fluid overload. Oozing from needle puncture sites and line insertion is common and usually should not necessitate transfusions. Petechiae reflect decreased platelet function, disturbed vascular integrity, or DIC. Treatment with fresh frozen plasma, cryoprecipitate, and platelet infusions is indicated for active bleeding and invasive procedures (see also Chapters 91 through 93). Spontaneous bleeding is unusual because both pro- and anticoagulation factors are deficient. In spite of this, most programs pick an arbitrary cutoff above which product is infused— for example, an INR of >5—although no cutoff level is well supported by the literature. Administration of recombinant factor VIIa may be useful in preparation for invasive procedures if coagulopathy is unresponsive to other blood products.[37]

Gastrointestinal tract hemorrhage secondary to gastritis or stress ulceration can be life threatening. Proton pump inhibitors or high-dose histamine receptor 2 antagonists should be administered intravenously to reduce the risk of upper gastrointestinal bleeding.

Neurologic Status (Encephalopathy and Cerebral Edema)

Neurologic status should be monitored clinically; classification of the stages of hepatic encephalopathy (HE) is based on clinical findings, which may be augmented by EEG changes (see Table 99.4). Computed tomography scans are not generally useful early in encephalopathy other than as a baseline examination to be compared with subsequent imaging to evaluate for signs of cerebral edema later in the disease. The mainstay for monitoring progression of encephalopathy is frequent serial neurologic examinations. Transcranial Doppler ultrasound is a noninvasive tool to monitor middle cerebral artery blood flow velocity. CT of the head without contrast can be beneficial to evaluate intracranial herniation or intracranial bleeding but is not especially sensitive to the degree of cerebral edema (Fig. 99.1). Direct intracranial pressure monitoring (ICP) is the most sensitive and specific measure of ICP but increases the intracranial bleeding risk, has not been demonstrated to alter outcome, and the use of ICP monitors in PALF depends largely on individual center practices.

Acute HE is defined as changes in consciousness that occur as a result of acute hepatic dysfunction, in the absence of other factors such as sedative medications, intracranial hemorrhage, or metabolic disturbances. From the PALF-SG, HE was present in 50% of children upon admission into the study and increased to 65% during the first 7 days.[18] The rate of progression is variable, but it may increase rapidly within hours of presentation to coma and be associated with the development of fatal cerebral edema. Although trending ammonia can be helpful to indicate the trajectory of HE, the serum level does not predictably measure the degree of or development of HE.

Drowsiness and lethargy or irritability and inconsolability become readily apparent as the patient progresses into stage II hepatic encephalopathy. Inappropriate behavior with outbursts of anger or crying may develop. Impaired motor coordination such as ataxia, dysarthria, apraxia, hyperreflexia,

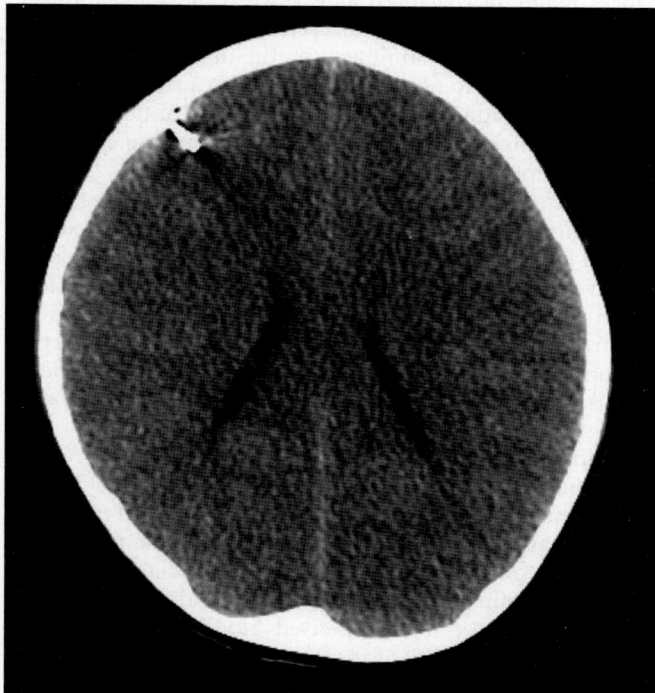

Fig. 99.1. CT showing cerebral edema in child with acute liver failure. Note the reduction in ventricular volume, effacement of sulci, and alteration in gray-white differentiation. Intracranial pressure monitoring device in left frontal lobe.

sustained clonus, rigidity, extensor posturing, and bizarre facial expressions become evident. Stage III hepatic encephalopathy is distinguished by progressive somnolence and stupor. The patient is arousable by vigorous physical stimuli but is disoriented, does not respond to commands, and does not recognize family members.[17] Intubation and ventilation may be needed as the patient approaches grade III or if patients become combative and a danger to themselves or others. Progression into stage IV hepatic encephalopathy is defined by the presence of coma. The patient responds only to painful stimuli. In deeper stage IV, the patient may exhibit decerebrate posturing with the loss of brain stem reflexes.

Acute hepatic encephalopathy is considered to be completely reversible after resolution of the hepatic dysfunction as long as cerebral edema and poor brain perfusion has not caused neuronal injury, although long-term neurodevelopmental studies are only now being conducted.

Cerebral Edema

Cerebral edema may develop during or beyond stage III encephalopathy and progress within hours of the onset of coma. Brain death associated with cerebral edema contributes to reduced survival after liver transplantation along with increased overall mortality.[15,38-41]

The pathogenesis of cerebral edema involves the interaction of ammonia, other hepatic toxin metabolites, and cerebral blood flow. Ammonia crosses freely into the brain where astrocyte glutamine synthase converts glutamate to glutamine. Glutamine acts as an active intracellular osmole leading to astrocyte swelling, cerebral edema, and increased intracranial pressure. Homeostatic mechanisms attempt to maintain perfusion by increasing systemic vascular resistance. Cerebral perfusion pressure is calculated as the difference between mean arterial pressure and intracranial pressure.[42] Evidence also supports the belief that glutamine acts as a carrier of ammonia into the mitochondria where the accumulation leads to oxidative stress and contributes to further to astrocyte swelling.[42]

Management of Hepatic Encephalopathy and Cerebral Edema

Lactulose, a nonabsorbable disaccharide, may be administered orally or via the nasogastric tube. Lactulose is fermented by intestinal flora to lactic acid, acidifying the bowel contents and limiting the absorption of the ammonium ion. The nonabsorbable antibiotic rifaximin is commonly used to reduce ammonia production by colonic bacteria, replacing the traditional use of enteral aminoglycoside antibiotics, particularly neomycin.[43] Limiting protein intake to 0.5 to 1 g/kg/day whether enterally or parenterally has also been recommended.

If the encephalopathy progresses to compromise respiratory drive, elective intubation and mechanical ventilation should be undertaken. If sedation is required, either for restraint or during procedures, short-acting barbiturates or opiates can be used. Benzodiazepines should be avoided because the γ-aminobutyric acid (GABA) receptor has been implicated in the development of encephalopathy.

When cerebral edema is apparent, careful fluid restriction, permissive hypertension, adequate oxygen saturation, and head elevation of 20 to 30 degrees are all basic supportive measures. If intracranial pressure monitoring is available, ICPs should be maintained ≤20 mm Hg with cerebral perfusion pressure 50 ≥50 mm Hg. Hypertonic saline 10% to 30% and mannitol have been used to lower increased ICPs (see also Chapter 66).[17] Serial measurements of serum osmolality to avoid concentrations >320 mOs/L are recommended, especially if there is evidence of renal compromise.[44]

Ventilation

Ventilatory support is required in all patients who progress to stage III encephalopathy and some who due to combativeness in stage II are at risk of injuring themselves. The need for support may be precipitated by the injudicious use of sedative medications, particularly benzodiazepines, which should be avoided in unventilated patients with PALF. At the onset of PALF, patients usually have normal pulmonary compliance, and hyperventilation should be avoided. As the disease progresses, pulmonary edema and acute respiratory distress syndrome (ARDS) may alter this situation, in which case careful and frequent monitoring of blood gases and ventilation status are vital. Although hyperventilation may temporarily reduce ICP, the effect is not sustained and prolonged use is not recommended.

Infection Prophylaxis and Treatment

The majority of adults and a lesser proportion of children develop infection that may be related to impairment of cellular and humoral immune systems from liver dysfunction.[45,46] The organisms most often implicated are gram-positive bacteria, presumably of skin origin. Gram-negative bacteria or a fungal infection is occasionally observed.

Management includes surveillance cultures from the endotracheal tube, indwelling catheters, and urine. Broad-spectrum antibiotics should be started at the first suspicion of sepsis, as the signs may be subtle and fever may be absent as part of the immune paralysis seen with advanced liver failure. When fungal infection is suspected, antifungals such as fluconazole or micafungin should be included. Positive cultures in the absence of clinical infection should result in removal or replacement of the infected catheter and administration of the appropriate antimicrobials.

Renal Function

Acute kidney injury from prerenal azotemia, acute tubular necrosis (ATN), and hepatorenal syndrome can complicate the course of PALF.[47] Prerenal azotemia is commonly due to dehydration and more rarely gastrointestinal bleeding. A marked increase in blood creatinine concentration may develop from decreased glomerular filtration or increased muscle breakdown. Acute tubular necrosis is seen in the minority of patients and may occur because of hypovolemia. Laboratory abnormalities indicating a diagnosis of ATN include abnormal urinary sediment, urinary sodium concentration greater than 20 mmol/L, reduction in creatinine clearance (urine/plasma creatinine ratio <10), and oliguria (urine output <0.5 mL/kg/h). Hepatorenal syndrome is a common cause of renal insufficiency in adults with acute liver failure (ALF) but is unusual in PALF. The pathophysiology is multifactorial involving electrolyte imbalance, sepsis, and hypovolemia. Laboratory evaluation reveals sodium retention (urinary sodium concentration <20 mmol/L), normal urinary sediment, and reduced urinary output (<1 mL/kg/h).

The aim of renal management is to maintain circulating volume to prevent hypovolemia and ensure that urine output is greater than 0.5 mL/kg/h without fluid overload. If there are signs of oliguria, a volume expander can be given one time at 10 mL/kg. If there are signs of fluid overload, the use of furosemide doses or infusion may be effective. Severe oliguric renal failure often requires hemodialysis or continuous renal replacement therapy (see also Chapter 78).

Although acute renal failure usually recovers quickly after liver transplantation, acute tubular necrosis may severely complicate the postoperative management.[48,49] Even in patients who require hemodialysis or continuous renal replacement therapy, renal function usually returns to normal after successful liver transplantation.

Liver Support

Extracorporeal liver support (ECLS) for patients with ALF has a history that dates back before liver transplantation was an option, but despite elegant clinical experiments with ex vivo liver perfusion or cross-circulation with human volunteers or animals, no evidence for increased survival was apparent.[50-53] Despite the successes of transplantation, the relative shortage of organs and the need to bridge a patient until an allograft becomes available have maintained interest in extracorporeal support for ALF. In general, ECLS systems can be categorized as either purely nonbiological filtration and detoxification systems or with the addition of a cellular component designed to replace some of the synthetic function of the liver, biologic hepatic functional replacement.

Small molecular weight solutes such as urea and ammonia can be cleared equally effectively with convective (continuous venovenous hemofiltration [CVVH]) or diffusive (continual venovenous hemodiafiltration [CVVHD]) approaches.[54] The goals for continuous renal support in ALF are to optimize fluid management and nutrition, correct electrolyte disturbances, maintain a balanced state between anticoagulation and coagulopathy, control ammonia levels, and remove potentially toxic substances not eliminated by the injured liver. Patients may require little to no anticoagulation because of the underlying coagulopathy.[55] The decision to use no anticoagulation, heparin, or citrate anticoagulation is based on local experience and preference. Many programs have used citrate,[56,57] which binds calcium within the hemofiltration circuit decreasing its availability as a cofactor in the clotting cascade. Calcium is infused back to the patient distal to the hemofiltration circuit to prevent hypocalcemia. Laboratory evidence for citrate lock, which represents residual citrate in the patient as the delivery of citrate exceeds its hepatic clearance, is rising total serum calcium with a falling ionized serum calcium level. Experience has also shown that the use of intraoperative hemofiltration during liver transplantation is safe and effective.

Although simple hemofiltration or dialysis can remove ammonia and other water-soluble molecules, a large number of potentially toxic hydrophilic and protein-bound molecules are not cleared. To remove these substances, exchange transfusion, large volume plasma exchange, and dialysis with an albumin-containing dialysate have been undertaken. Both to limit the waste of human-derived blood products and to improve the tolerability of the procedures, systems have been designed to remove the toxins by passing the separated blood fractions through activated charcoal or resin columns and returning the "cleaned" fraction to the patient in closed recycling systems such as the molecular absorbent recirculating system (MARS), using albumin dialysis, and Prometheus,

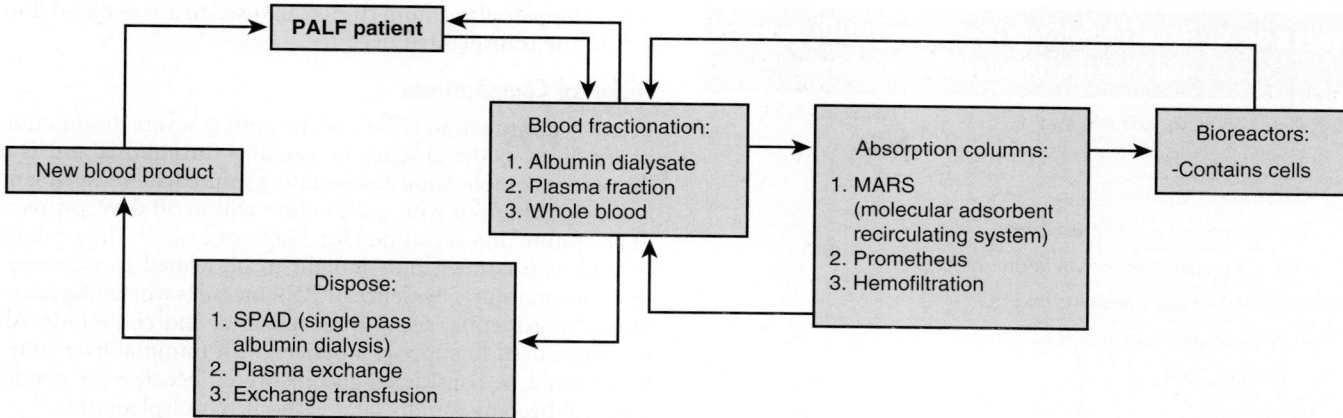

Fig. 99.2. Configuration of components in parallel or series in extracorporeal liver support (ECLS) whether nonbiological filtration devices without a cell-housing bioreactor or bioartificial liver devices with a cell-housing bioreactor.

which utilizes plasma fractionation. Although there are no randomized controlled studies to report efficacy of Prometheus versus MARS, there is some clinical indication that Prometheus could have a higher efficiency in toxin removal and normalization of serum lab values, although neither have proved the ability to improve overall survival.[58-60]

Bioartificial liver devices differ from toxin removal systems in that they contain a cell-housing bioreactor, which contains functional liver cells to replace the function of the damaged liver. Two such systems that have undergone randomized control trials are HepatAssist and the Extracorporeal Liver Assist Device (ELAD). The HepatAssist utilized porcine hepatocytes in conjunction with plasmapheresis, toxin absorption, and an oxygenator. In contrast, ELAD utilizes HepG2 cells, a hepatoblastoma-derived immortalized cell line, along with hemofiltration, toxin absorption, and an oxygenator. Neither system is currently available for further clinical trials, but development continues[61,62] (Fig. 99.2).

Liver Transplantation
Background/History/Terminology

Although the first liver transplant was performed by Dr. Thomas Starzl and his team in 1963, it was not until the development of cyclosporine that the 1-year recipient survival substantially increased, launching liver transplantation as a standard treatment for hepatic failure. Immunosuppression therapy evolved from steroid and azathioprine therapy in the 1970s to today's array of immunosuppressive agents, the mainstay of which is tacrolimus but also included are antilymphocyte globulins, rapamycin derivative, and mycophenolate.

Whole organ liver transplantation remains the most commonly performed of these procedures, but it is associated with significant size limitations in regard to children. The use of reduced size transplantation with left lateral segment or left lobe is common practice for pediatric patients. In split liver procedures, the division of one donor liver into two allografts can provide a smaller pediatric patient with the left lateral segment allograft and an adult or larger pediatric patient with a right lobe allograft. Living donor liver transplantation, with the procurement of usually the left lateral segment for pediatric patients, is also an option.

Indications for Liver Transplant

The indications for liver transplantation include (1) liver disease that is immediately limiting survival such as PALF, decompensated chronic liver disease, and malignant hepatic tumors; (2) liver disease leading to poor quality of life from pruritus, poor growth, and development; and (3) metabolic liver disease with extrahepatic complications such as urea cycle defects, oxalosis, and Crigler-Najjar syndrome.[17] According to the Studies of Pediatric Liver Transplant Registry (SPLIT), between 1995 and 2007 the reasons for transplantation were cholestatic liver disease (mainly biliary atresia) in 53.9%, metabolic disease in 15%, PALF in 14%, cirrhosis/end-stage liver disease in 6.7%, tumor in 6.7%, and hepatotoxic injury in 3.5%.[63] Absolute contraindications to liver transplantation include unresectable primary extrahepatic malignancy, progressive terminal nonhepatic disease, and uncontrolled systemic sepsis.[17]

As discussed earlier, there is no good prognostic test for those who will need liver transplantation in patients with PALF. The use of indices such as KCHC and LIU score may offer guidance, but ultimately the decision becomes a matter of judgment by an experienced transplant team.

Pretransplant Workup/Evaluation

Along with the investigations outlined in Table 99.5, the evaluation of a child for liver transplantation requires that the team prepare and educate the patient and family in regard to the pre-, peri-, and postoperative stages of the transplant journey, which includes waiting time, general information on source of donor organs, the operation itself and potential technical complications, postoperative care, and long-term outcomes and complications. This requires care and experience with clear protocols that ensure consistency. In cases of ALF, the time available for such detail is severely constrained, but it is still imperative that the complete evaluation process is undertaken.

Organ Allocations

Deceased donor organs are allocated to a particular recipient based on strict rules adopted by United Network for Organ Sharing (UNOS), the organization tasked by Health Resources and Services Administration (HRSA) to administer the Organ

TABLE 99.6	Model for End-Stage Liver Disease (MELD)/Pediatric End-Stage Liver Disease (PELD) Calculations

PELD = 0.480 Log$_e$ Bilirubin (mg/dL)
+1.857 Log$_e$ INR
−0.687 Log$_e$ Albumin (g/dL)
+0.436 if patient is less than 1 yo
+0.667 if patient has growth failure ≤2SD
MELD = 0.957 Log$_e$ Creatinine (mg/dL)
+0.378 Log$_e$ Bilirubin (mg/dL)
+1.120 Log$_e$ INR
+0/643

Procurement and Transplantation Network (OPTN) within the United States. The rules determine the recipient based on urgency, geography, blood group matching, and donor age. The highest urgency is status 1A and applies to patients with ALF and an acutely failing allograft immediately posttransplant due to complications such as primary nonfunction. Status 1B is confined to pediatric age groups and is for decompensated chronic liver disease, hepatoblastoma, and hyperammonical inborn errors for metabolism such as urea cycle disorders. The severity scores for all other patients are ranked according to their Model for End-Stage Liver Disease (MELD) score for adults and adolescents or their Pediatric End-Stage Liver Disease (PELD) score for patients <12 years of age (Table 99.6).

Technical Aspects of Liver Transplantation

Although the details of the liver transplantation operations are beyond the scope of this chapter, there are principles of liver transplantation that should be understood. Foremost in reducing intraoperative and postoperative morbidity, it is important to send the patient for transplantation in the best condition possible. This means that (1) infections have been treated, (2) excess edema has been avoided or resolved, (3) cardiopulmonary and renal systems are functioning well, and (4) the brain has been spared irreversible damage.

The first step intraoperatively is to remove the native liver. Complicating this procedure may be the presence of portal hypertension and adhesions from previous surgeries. Addressing donor liver hepatic vein outflow is the first step in implanting the new liver, usually with a connection to the native inferior vena cava either with interposition of the donor inferior vena cava or using a "piggyback" technique. Next is the establishment of adequate arterial inflow with an appropriately sized arterial connection. Typically this is with the recipient hepatic or celiac artery to donor hepatic artery if possible, but otherwise an anastomosis to the recipient aorta is made. Portal vein anastomosis often requires accommodation for differences in caliber between donor and recipient portal veins. Biliary anastomosis is either from native to donor bile duct or by implantation of donor bile duct into a Roux-en-Y jejunal limb if the duct-to-duct method is not feasible. Closure of the abdomen should minimize increased intraabdominal pressures so as to not compromise blood flow to the allograft, sometimes requiring an open abdomen and delayed abdominal wall closure. Intraoperative, immediate postoperative, and serial Doppler ultrasound studies are used to assess blood flow within the transplanted liver.[64]

Technical Complications

Primary nonfunction (PNF) of the graft is severe dysfunction of the liver in the absence of vascular thrombosis and is a disastrous complication necessitating immediate retransplantation. Of children with graft failure within 30 days, primary graft dysfunction accounted for 25.6% of cases.[65] The etiology of PNF is unknown but thought to be related to ischemia-reperfusion injury. Evidence of PNF includes worsening coagulopathy, acidemia, rising liver enzymes, and cholestasis. All measures used to support a patient with minimal liver function should be considered and instituted because the condition will become rapidly fatal without retransplantation.[66]

Hepatic artery thrombosis (HAT) may occur at anytime after transplantation, but if it occurs within the first few day posttransplantation it commonly severely compromises the allograft and emergent retransplantation may be necessary. HAT occurring later tends to be better tolerated because of the dual hepatic blood inflow (hepatic artery [HA] and portal vein [PV]). Hepatic artery thrombosis, occurring in 2% to 10% of liver transplants overall, can, in addition to early graft failure, lead to biliary leaks, ischemic cholangiopathy with stricture formation, and intrahepatic abscess.[63] Etiologies include poor arterial inflow, technical complications with the anastomotic site, graft edema, hypercoagulable states, and overtransfusion. Routine assessment of hepatic artery patency using color Doppler ultrasonography at the bedside is critical during this period. Prompt recognition of HAT early after implantation and intervention with anticoagulation and possibly surgical thrombectomy and revision of the arterial anastomosis is critical if the allograft is to be saved.

Portal vein thrombosis (PVT) is uncommon and occurs in <5% of pediatric liver transplants. PVT occurring early after transplantation can be seen in association with PNF or share common risk factors with those associated with HAT. Treatment is centered on anticoagulation and surgical intervention with thrombectomy, thrombolysis, or shunt placement. Late PVT results in obstruction and subsequent development of prehepatic portal hypertension.

Perioperative bleeding may occur because of profound coagulopathy and thrombocytopenia that many patients have pretransplantation as well as dilutional effects of intraoperative fluid administration. Bleeding should abate as the function of the allograft returns postoperatively. In addition, patients may return to the pediatric intensive care unit on heparin infusions to prophylactically maintain patency of the hepatic artery and portal vein. Monitoring surgical drain output is critical to detect postoperative bleeding and bile leakage. Additionally, monitoring of the hemoglobin is important as an indirect sign of bleeding. Worsening coagulopathy suggests hepatic dysfunction, sepsis with DIC, or unrecognized internal bleeding and requires rapid, aggressive diagnosis and treatment of the underlying cause.

Early biliary complications include biliary anastomosis dehiscence and bile leaks from the cut surface of the liver. Approximately 5% to 15% of patients experience biliary complications within the first 30 days, and up to 25% or more will experience this complication in long-term follow-up.[65] Early bile leaks may be diagnosed by the appearance of bile in the abdominal drains, by nuclear scan, or by transhepatic contrast studies. Cut surface leaks from minor biliary radicals may resolve spontaneously, but leaks from the biliary anastomosis or from larger cut surface ducts require percutaneous transhepatic cholangiogram (PTC) by interventional radiology, endoscopic retrograde cholangiopancreatography (ERCP), or surgical exploration. Late biliary complications include isolated anastomotic strictures or diffuse stricturing secondary to ischemic cholangiopathy. Isolated strictures can be managed usually by PTC or ERCP with dilation and temporary stenting, but diffuse cholangiopathy frequently progresses to biliary cirrhosis in the allograft.

After intraabdominal surgery, altered gut may predispose to bacterial translocation or infection may occur, particularly in the open abdomen, by more directed routes. Any intraabdominal fluid collection secondary to bile leak, hematoma, or ascites may become infected. Serial examinations and imaging should be performed during the postoperative period to monitor for signs of abscess or fluid collection. Percutaneous drainage or surgical abdominal washout may be required.

Postoperative Management

Early recognition of complications and prompt intervention will offer the best chance to rescue the graft and the patient. Close and rapid communication between the PICU team caring for the postoperative transplant patient and the surgical and hepatology teams are crucial. Joint rounding with all teams caring for the patient can facilitate optimal communication during the critical postoperative period.

Fluid Management/Nutrition

The goal of fluid management is to preserve graft perfusion without fluid overload. Albumin should be monitored carefully and crystalloids should be given cautiously to avoid fluid overload and anasarca. In the early postoperative period, fluid balance should be calculated on an hourly basis rather than awaiting 12 or 24 hour totals. Initially the goal is to maintain an even to slightly positive fluid balance, and after about 48 hours postoperatively, when fluid begins to be mobilized from the tissues, diuresis can be expected. Central venous pressure monitoring is often helpful in assessing fluid needs.

Sedation/Pain Relief/Ventilation

Although it is important to manage postoperative pain, oversedation is a risk and should be avoided. The use of opioids demands judicious attention due to their risk for prolonging the need for ventilator support and slowing gastrointestinal motility and thus fluid mobilization from the abdominal compartment. Delirium from a prolonged ICU stay should not be confused with poor pain control. One aim of immediate posttransplant care is to wean the patient off of ventilator support as soon as it is feasible to do so. Increasingly extubation occurs in the operating room at the end of surgery or within the first hour or two of transfer to PICU. Prolonged ventilator support is associated with increased complications, prolonged ICU stay, and delayed discharge from the hospital.

Immunosuppression

Induction immunosuppression with either an antithymocyte globulin or an anti-IL2 antibody is used in about 40% of programs in the United States.[67] The mainstay of maintenance immunosuppression is the calcineurin inhibitor, tacrolimus

with or without corticosteroids. Use of cyclosporine at least in liver transplantation is now mostly historical. The antimetabolite mycophenolate mofetil has replaced the use of azathioprine in centers that routinely utilize adjunctive therapy.

Infection Prophylaxis

During the perioperative period, prophylactic antibiotics are commonly used for 24 or 48 hours; the preference of antibiotic is program specific. Fluconazole may be used as fungal prophylaxis in high-risk situations, although for routine cases enteral nystatin suffices. Specific prophylaxis for *Pneumocystis jirovecii* with Bactrim is standard once enteral medications are tolerated. Cytomegalovirus (CMV) prophylaxis either universally or for selected patients depending on donor and recipient CMV serologic status is initiated with IV ganciclovir, graduating later to oral valganciclovir.

Drains and Intravascular Access

Typically vascular access consists of two arterials catheters to facilitate monitoring blood pressure and blood draws, one central line usually internal jugular, a peripherally inserted central catheter (PICC), and peripheral intravenous catheters as needed. Large-bore nasogastric tubes are used for gastric decompression and a Foley catheter for accurately quantifying urine output. Surgical abdominal drains are usually in place upon return from the operating room primarily to monitor for intraabdominal bleeding or bile leak. Given the multitude of tubes and vascular access, the documentation of inputs and outputs is essential to reliably assess fluid balance.

Complications
Infection

Sepsis continues to be a major cause of morbidity in liver transplant recipients.[68] The presence of arterial thrombosis or biliary leak significantly increases the risk of infection as well as abscess formation. Patients having undergone previous abdominal surgery and those who have received pretransplant corticosteroid therapy are at an increased risk for postoperative infection. A high index of suspicion for postoperative infection in the immunosuppressed patient should be maintained with early surveillance cultures and the initiation of antibiotic, antifungal, and antiviral (CMV) treatments as indicated by the patient and donor status. Young children are at particular risk for CMV and Epstein-Barr virus infections because the majority are naive to these viruses at the time of transplantation. Donor lymphocytes in the graft are a frequent source of primary infection for these viruses. Monitoring active viral replication by polymerase chain reaction can be a useful tool to assist in preemptive management.[68]

Rejection

Data from the SPLIT Registry suggest that rejection occurs at least once in 46% of pediatric patients who require liver transplantation.[68] Laboratory findings suggestive of rejection include elevation in AST, ALT, and gamma-glutamyltransferase (GGT) followed by elevations in bilirubin in more severe cases. Liver biopsy is important to confirm the diagnosis of acute rejection and distinguish patients with viral infection, biliary obstruction, or graft ischemia who may have a similar clinical presentation. Early detection of rejection allows the initiation of intensified immunosuppression to reverse the process and minimize graft injury and loss. A short

TABLE 99.7   Adverse Effects of Immunosuppression Medication

Agent	Adverse Effect
Tacrolimus	Hypertension, headache, infection, seizures, hyperglycemia, insulin resistance/diabetes, renal failure, PTLD, cardiomyopathy
Cyclosporine	Hypertension, infection, seizures, hyperglycemia, renal failure, hirsutism, gingival hyperplasia, PTLD
Sirolimus	Hypercholesterolemia, infection, edema, poor wound healing, PTLD
Corticosteroids	Hypertension, increased appetite, Cushing syndrome, acne, gastritis, poor wound healing, osteoporosis, poor linear growth
Mycophenolate	Intestinal hypermotility, abdominal cramping, diarrhea, infection, leukopenia, thrombocytopenia

PTLD, posttransplant lymphoproliferative disease.

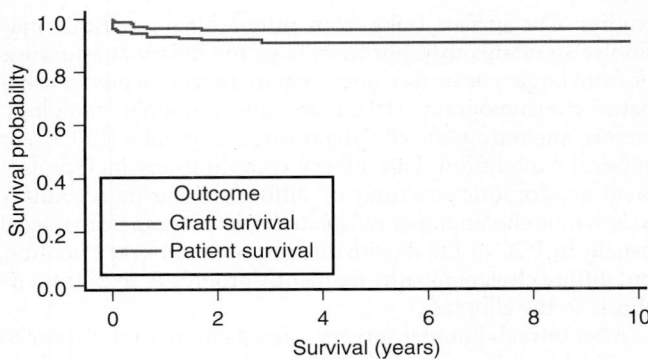

Fig. 99.3. Kaplan-Meier Survival Curve of 10-year experience of patient and graft at a single pediatric transplant center (Seattle Children's Hospital in Seattle, Washington, from 2004 to 2014 from 138 patients).

course of high-dose corticosteroids is the usual response to an episode of rejection, although more severe grades of rejection may necessitate the use of antithymocyte globulin.

Hypertension

The majority of liver transplantation patients will receive a calcineurin inhibitor and corticosteroids, setting the stage for postoperative hypertension with or without deterioration in biochemical renal function. Some degree of postoperative hypertension is seen in 70% to 80% of pediatric recipients. Hypertension is treated initially with calcium channel blockers but usually resolves over the first few weeks after transplantation. Angiotensin-converting enzyme (ACE) inhibitors have been suggested to offer protection against ongoing calcineurin-induced renal injury but should not be used early after transplant because of the associated risks of hyperkalemia and renal dysfunction.

Other Complications

Each of the immunosuppressant agents in common use has potential undesirable side effects.[69] The most common issues are listed in Table 99.7. Diabetes is relatively common in adult patients receiving tacrolimus with a prevalence of 25% at 3 months posttransplant, but this complication is uncommon in young children. Hyperglycemia in the immediate postoperative period can be controlled by insulin infusion and should not limit the clinician's ability to deliver adequate caloric intake.[70] Cyclosporine and tacrolimus-related encephalopathy and seizures occur in 11% and 8% of patients, respectively, with the most common onset in the first 2 weeks after transplantation. Both can be managed by reducing or eliminating the calcineurin inhibitor exposure. Seizure control will frequently require short-term treatment with antiepileptic medications.[71]

Outcomes

Patient and graft survival rates have risen dramatically since the early attempts at liver transplantation. In modern cohorts, infants, children, and adolescents transplanted at experienced centers can expect 1-year survival rates in excess of 95%, with

graft survival rates above 90%[72] (Fig. 99.3). The poorest survival has been seen for malignant tumors, mostly hepatoblastoma, and acute liver failure. Studies of Pediatric Liver Transplantation (SPLIT) data identify the occurrence of postoperative complications, especially reoperation, as the major risk factor for morbidity and graft loss.[72] Late-stage complications resulting in graft loss include chronic rejection, biliary cirrhosis, and posttransplant lymphoproliferative disease.

Children who receive liver transplantations may exhibit growth failure. This is more likely to affect those with cirrhosis and chronic liver disease as their indication for transplantation rather than those with acute liver failure. Nutritional status pretransplant somewhat predicts growth posttransplant. Catch-up growth may be observed for several years after transplant, although in those with stunted pretransplant growth, final adult height is often less than ideal.[73] Of note, a SPLIT study of quality of life in 800 liver transplant recipients reported that psychosocial function such as school function was affected more than physical function, with data similar to that for children with other chronic medical conditions.[74] Behavioral disturbances, anxiety, and depression along with posttraumatic stress disorder can appear posttransplant, and patients should be systematically evaluated for these conditions in addition to medical management during the posttransplant follow-up.

Indications for retransplantation include vascular complications (which account for a significant proportion early in the postoperative period), liver fibrosis, cholestasis, and chronic graft failures (which account for the majority of the late graft failures). Patient and graft survivals after retransplantation are approximately 10% less than survival rates after primary transplantation. A shorter time frame from primary transplantation to retransplantation has been reported to result in a higher likelihood of morbidity and mortality, but this has not been a consistent finding in all analyses.[75]

Key References

1. Squires RH Jr. Acute liver failure in children. *Semin Liver Dis.* 2008;28: 153-166.
2. Pineiro-Carrero VM, Pineiro EO. Liver. *Pediatrics.* 2004;113(suppl 4): 1097-1106.
3. Dhawan A. Etiology and prognosis of acute liver failure in children. *Liver Transpl.* 2008;14(suppl 2):S80-S84.

4. Horslen S. Acute liver failure and transplantation in children. *S Afr Med J.* 2014;104(11 Pt 2):808-812.

6. Lee WM. Acute liver failure. *N Engl J Med.* 1993;329:1862-1872.

7. Bhaduri BR, Mieli-Vergani G. Fulminant hepatic failure: pediatric aspects. *Semin Liver Dis.* 1996;16:349-355.

8. Schiff ER, Sorrell MF, Maddrey WC. *Schiff's Diseases of the Liver.* 10th ed. Philadelphia: Lippincott Williams & Wilkins; 2007.

9. Whitington PF, Alonso EM. Fulminant hepatitis in children: evidence for an unidentified hepatitis virus. *J Pediatr Gastroenterol Nutr.* 2001;33: 529-536.

10. Zakim D, Boyer TD. *Hepatology: A Textbook of Liver Disease.* 4th ed. Philadelphia: Saunders; 2003.

13. Arya R, Gulati S, Deopujari S. Management of hepatic encephalopathy in children. *Postgrad Med J.* 2010;86:34-41, quiz 40.

16. Stravitz RT, Kramer DJ. Management of acute liver failure. *Nat Rev Gastroenterol Hepatol.* 2009;6:542-553.

17. Suchy FJ, Sokol RJ, Balistreri WF. *Liver Disease in Children.* 4th ed. Cambridge: Cambridge University Press; 2014.

18. Squires RH Jr, et al. Acute liver failure in children: the first 348 patients in the pediatric acute liver failure study group. *J Pediatr.* 2006;148: 652-658.

19. Mack CL, et al. Living donor liver transplantation for children with liver failure and concurrent multiple organ system failure. *Liver Transpl.* 2001;7:890-895.

20. Ichai P, et al. Patients with acute liver failure listed for superurgent liver transplantation in France: reevaluation of the Clichy-Villejuif criteria. *Liver Transpl.* 2015;21:512-523.

21. Lu BR, et al. Evaluation of the liver injury unit scoring system to predict survival in a multinational study of pediatric acute liver failure. *J Pediatr.* 2013;162:1010-1016, e1-e4.

24. Anderson IB, et al. Pennyroyal toxicity: measurement of toxic metabolite levels in two cases and review of the literature. *Ann Intern Med.* 1996;124:726-734.

27. Letschert K, et al. Molecular characterization and inhibition of amanitin uptake into human hepatocytes. *Toxicol Sci.* 2006;91:140-149.

28. Magdalan J, et al. alpha-Amanitin induced apoptosis in primary cultured dog hepatocytes. *Folia Histochem Cytobiol.* 2010;48:58-62.

29. Schilsky ML. Wilson disease: current status and the future. *Biochimie.* 2009;91:1278-1281.

30. Dhawan A, et al. Wilson's disease in children: 37-year experience and revised King's score for liver transplantation. *Liver Transpl.* 2005;11: 441-448.

31. Vilstrup H, Iversen J, Tygstrup N. Glucoregulation in acute liver failure. *Eur J Clin Invest.* 1986;16:193-197.

32. Harry R, Auzinger G, Wendon J. The clinical importance of adrenal insufficiency in acute hepatic dysfunction. *Hepatology.* 2002;36:395-402.

33. Clark SJ, et al. Temporal changes in insulin sensitivity following the development of acute liver failure secondary to acetaminophen. *Hepatology.* 2001;34:109-115.

34. Walsh TS, et al. Energy expenditure in acetaminophen-induced fulminant hepatic failure. *Crit Care Med.* 2000;28:649-654.

36. Munoz SJ, Stravitz RT, Gabriel DA. Coagulopathy of acute liver failure. *Clin Liver Dis.* 2009;13:95-107.

37. Brown JB, et al. Recombinant factor VIIa improves coagulopathy caused by liver failure. *J Pediatr Gastroenterol Nutr.* 2003;37:268-272.

38. O'Brien CJ, et al. Neurological sequelae in patients recovered from fulminant hepatic failure. *Gut.* 1987;28:93-95.

39. Blei AT. Brain edema and portal-systemic encephalopathy. *Liver Transpl.* 2000;6(4 suppl 1):S14-S20.

40. Jalan R. Intracranial hypertension in acute liver failure: pathophysiological basis of rational management. *Semin Liver Dis.* 2003;23:271-282.

41. Blei A. Hypothermia for fulminant hepatic failure: a cool approach to a burning problem. *Liver Transpl.* 2000;6:245-247.

42. Scott TR, et al. Pathophysiology of cerebral oedema in acute liver failure. *World J Gastroenterol.* 2013;19:9240-9255.

43. Iadevaia MD, et al. Rifaximin in the treatment of hepatic encephalopathy. *Hepat Med.* 2011;3:109-117.

44. Mohsenin V. Assessment and management of cerebral edema and intracranial hypertension in acute liver failure. *J Crit Care.* 2013;28:783-791.

57. Tolwani AJ, Wille KM. Anticoagulation for continuous renal replacement therapy. *Semin Dial.* 2009;22:141-145.

58. Carpentier B, Gautier A, Legallais C. Artificial and bioartificial liver devices: present and future. *Gut.* 2009;58:1690-1702.

59. Bourgoin P, et al. Molecular Absorbent Recirculating System therapy (MARS(R)) in pediatric acute liver failure: a single center experience. *Pediatr Nephrol.* 2014;29:901-908.

60. Krisper P, et al. In vivo quantification of liver dialysis: comparison of albumin dialysis and fractionated plasma separation. *J Hepatol.* 2005;43: 451-457.

61. Demetriou AA, et al. Prospective, randomized, multicenter, controlled trial of a bioartificial liver in treating acute liver failure. *Ann Surg.* 2004;239:660-667, discussion 667-670.

62. Ellis AJ, et al. Pilot-controlled trial of the extracorporeal liver assist device in acute liver failure. *Hepatology.* 1996;24:1446-1451.

63. Group SR. Studies of Pediatric Liver Transplantation (SPLIT): year 2000 outcomes. *Transplantation.* 2001;72:463-476.

64. Ryckman FC, et al. Liver transplantation in children. *Semin Pediatr Surg.* 1992;1:162-172.

65. McDiarmid SV. Current status of liver transplantation in children. *Pediatr Clin North Am.* 2003;50:1335-1374.

66. Rand EB, Olthoff KM. Overview of pediatric liver transplantation. *Gastroenterol Clin North Am.* 2003;32:913-929.

68. Shepherd RW, et al. Risk factors for rejection and infection in pediatric liver transplantation. *Am J Transplant.* 2008;8:396-403.

70. Jain A, et al. Liver transplantation under tacrolimus in infants, children, adults, and seniors: long-term results, survival, and adverse events in 1000 consecutive patients. *Transplant Proc.* 1998;30:1403-1404.

72. McDiarmid SV, et al. A multivariate analysis of pre-, peri-, and posttransplant factors affecting outcome after pediatric liver transplantation. *Ann Surg.* 2011;254:145-154.

73. Alonso EM, et al. Linear growth patterns in prepubertal children following liver transplantation. *Am J Transplant.* 2009;9:1389-1397.

74. Gilmour SM, et al. School outcomes in children registered in the studies for pediatric liver transplant (SPLIT) consortium. *Liver Transpl.* 2010;16: 1041-1048.

75. Ng V, et al. Liver retransplantation in children: a SPLIT database analysis of outcome and predictive factors for survival. *Am J Transplant.* 2008; 8:386-395.

Acute Abdomen

Robert Sawin and Derya Caglar

PEARLS

- The abdomen is both a primary source of disease conditions that requires care in the intensive care unit (ICU) and, frequently, a secondary source of additional pathophysiology for children in the ICU being treated for other conditions.
- In either case, early recognition of these conditions and the judicious use of medical and surgical intervention can be key to a successful outcome in critically ill children with abdominal disease or injury.

Anatomic and Physiologic Considerations

Peritoneum

The peritoneum provides a protective environment for the intraabdominal organs and, because of its marked sensitivity, a valuable window for the examining health care provider. It is composed of a single layer of mesothelial cells lining the abdominal cavity along the abdominal wall (the parietal peritoneum) and the intraabdominal viscera (the visceral peritoneum). The space between these is the peritoneal cavity. Beneath the mesothelium is a submesothelial layer of extracellular matrix, capillaries, and lymphatics.[1] The peritoneum's sensitivity to inflammation, ischemia, and necrosis is mediated by the fluid in the peritoneum that contains macrophages and other leukocytes.[2] Thus, with a focus of inflammation anywhere in the peritoneal cavity, these leukocytes release inflammatory mediators, often resulting initially in poorly localized, generalized pain. With irritation of the peritoneum associated with early appendicitis, for example, the patient interprets the inflammation as periumbilical pain. This is related to the embryologic development along dermatomes. As more inflammatory cytokines are secreted throughout the peritoneal cavity, the pain becomes more generalized and will eventually result in spasm of the overlying muscles of the abdominal wall, interpreted by the examiner as guarding.

Pain in the gastrointestinal tract is mainly limited to conditions that result in distention of the organ. Inflammation or irritation of the mucosa is generally not the cause of pain, except in the stomach. Disease states that result in full-thickness inflammation of the bowel wall, however, can stimulate the visceral peritoneum, inciting the release of leukocytic and tissue macrophage–derived inflammatory mediators and resulting in pain. Patients who are receiving drugs such as corticosteroids, which blunt the immune response,

have reduced production of these peritoneal inflammatory mediators and consequently can have deceptively little pain despite a significant intraabdominal disease. As in other parts of the body, ischemia associated with any abdominal condition results in severe pain, often out of proportion to what is detected on physical examination.

Visceral Blood Flow

The regulation of visceral blood flow is a tightly controlled balance of neural, humoral, paracrine, and metabolic factors.[3] In the gut, enteral feeding increases the blood flow and the metabolic demands on the intestinal mucosa. Some of these effects are directly related to the nutrients in the intestinal lumen, whereas others are dependent on the enteric nervous system and the associated reflexes, on gastrointestinal hormones, and on gastrointestinal vasoactive mediators such as adenosine, endothelin-1, and nitric oxide.[4] In pathologic states such as sepsis alone or shock, whether from sepsis, hemorrhage, or cardiac failure, visceral blood flow is reduced, and this can lead to ischemia of the intestinal mucosa and submucosa. Even with restoration of blood pressure and cardiac output following treatment of shock, microvascular perfusion of the intestine may remain impaired, resulting in mucosal ischemia and persistent lactate production.

Such ischemia can lead to altered integrity of the mucosal barriers to bacteria and other pathogens, thus increasing the entry of endotoxins into the splanchnic venous and lymphatic systems. These pathogens can fuel the inflammatory response. This finding has fostered the theory of the gut as a central organ of sepsis or multisystem organ failure (see also Chapter 112).[5] Whether the translocation of bacteria or endotoxin from gut lumen to splanchnic drainage is the chicken or the egg can be debated; regardless, this perturbation of intestinal blood flow contributes to the pathophysiology of shock and sepsis.

Other conditions in the ICU can affect splanchnic blood flow, especially mechanical ventilation with high inspiratory pressures, high positive end-expiratory pressure (PEEP), or high tidal volumes.[6,7]

Physical Exam of the Abdomen

One should always start the examination of the child by assessing vital signs. Fever is common in patients presenting with significant abdominal disease, but it may not always present early in the disease process. Tachycardia is seen with fever, pain, or anxiety but is also a sensitive indicator of serious underlying illness, often seen in patients with early, compensated shock. Hypotension may indicate a decompensated patient who needs immediate attention and intervention for likely sepsis.

The examination of a child's abdomen should begin with keen observation, patience, and sensitivity to the patient's fears and the parents' anxiety. One should first notice the child's position and demeanor. Children with peritonitis do not move or writhe about the bed, as this only worsens their pain. They will remain quite still and avoid movement or any rapid changes in position. A child with visceral ischemia that has not progressed to peritonitis may be actively seeking a more comfortable position with multiple positional adjustments.

The abdomen should initially be evaluated for any skin changes that can give clues to the underlying process. Bruises or patterned abrasions and petechiae can indicate trauma with significant underlying organ lacerations or blood loss. Seat belt restraints can often leave a significant lesion on a child's chest and abdomen after a motor vehicle accident and should prompt further evaluation for intraabdominal injury. In the absence of reported trauma, the provider must consider non-accidental trauma in the differential diagnosis, particularly in very young, nonverbal children. Grey Turner sign is significant bruising in the flanks, indicates significant retroperitoneal bruising, and is often associated with severe pancreatitis or pancreatic necrosis. Bruising around the umbilicus, Cullen sign, is also an indicator of significant intraabdominal bleeding and pancreatic disease.

Observation of the patient's facial expressions is important throughout the physical exam, as young children may not be able to express what they are feeling or simply are too anxious to give clear responses. Once the manual examination is to begin, the examiners should make certain that their hands and stethoscopes are warm. For the verbal child who has localized the pain to a specific portion of the abdomen, the examiners should start the palpation in the opposite quadrant. If palpation in one area causes referred pain in a different location (Rovsing sign), this is suggestive of localized peritonitis in the area of pain, classically seen in appendicitis but also seen in other localized abdominal conditions.

In generalized peritonitis, spasm of the rectus abdominis can be detected regardless of where the source of the inflammation is located. When rectus spasm is detected on one side of the abdomen, a comparison to the rectus on the other side is helpful; when both are in spasm, it could be a manifestation of guarding by an anxious child, and therefore distraction should be employed. Distraction can often be created by engaging in conversation with the verbal child or by using the warmed stethoscope to listen with light pressure over the area of the abdomen in question, followed by gradually increasing the pressure to elicit a response. Asking the child to take a deep breath and blow it all the way out while feeling the rectus can overcome the spasm if it is due to voluntary guarding, while a child with peritonitis will fail to relax the rectus spasm.

Testing for rebound tenderness is only valuable in older children and should be avoided in children younger than adolescence as it is too startling and thus has a high false-positive rate. Shaking the bed, asking the child to cough, or gently grabbing the hips and moving them from side to side will cause a painful response in conditions with peritonitis and is much less threatening to younger children. As mentioned earlier, pain out of proportion to the findings on physical exam in an ICU patient suggests ischemia, independent of the location in the body. Bowel sounds are highly variable, and their assessment is not usually useful in the intensive care unit patient.

Significant abdominal distention may also indicate considerable underlying illness. On the other hand, abdominal distention can make the physical exam more challenging. Differentiation between apparent tenderness from distention versus peritonitis requires patience and gentle palpation. Assessing the rectus muscles for spasm may facilitate the diagnosis of peritonitis. Distention from hepatomegaly or splenomegaly can be due to end-stage liver disease, malignancy, or masses. Fluid in the abdomen could indicate significant blood loss requiring immediate attention and resuscitation. Ascites with abdominal pain may be an indicator of spontaneous bacterial peritonitis, particularly in patients with end-stage renal or liver disease.

Medications can interfere with the reliability of the physical exam of the abdomen. As mentioned, steroids can blunt an inflammatory response in the peritoneum and lead to decreased pain sensation despite a significant intraabdominal disease process. Patients receiving opiates may have a diminished response to painful stimuli; however, significant intraperitoneal pathology can still be ascertained by careful observation and examination. Patients who are receiving paralytic drugs are particularly challenging because the rectus abdominis spasm associated with peritonitis may be substantially decreased. Observation of the face, heart rate, or blood pressure can still be valuable, especially by comparing these findings during examination to other areas of the body. Just as in the nonsedated, non-ICU patient, beginning the exam on another portion of the body gives the examiner a baseline for comparison.

Laboratory Tests

Assessment of possible intraabdominal conditions should include blood and serum tests that measure inflammation, acid-base abnormalities, possible coagulopathy, and those focused on suspected involved organs. The leukocyte count and differential, hematocrit, and platelet counts should always be checked for patients with suspected abdominal disease. Leukocytosis, especially with an increased percentage of neutrophils or immature forms, should raise one's concern about an infectious process. Neutropenia suggests a more severe infection or a suppression of the patient's bone marrow from medications or from the infection; such a situation might make clearance of a bacterial infection more difficult. Similarly, both an increased and decreased platelet count can indicate an intraabdominal infection. Serial declines in the platelet count are particularly suggestive of a continuing inflammatory consumption seen in conditions such a necrotizing enterocolitis. Hematocrits must be followed in any child in the ICU because they can demonstrate intraabdominal bleeding or hemolysis related to disseminated intravascular coagulopathy (DIC). Other coagulation tests should be considered, especially in children with severe infections or those with liver dysfunction. In such situations the prothrombin time (PT) partial thromboplastin time (PTT), D-dimers, and fibrin split products are helpful to characterize and monitor the coagulopathy.

Abnormalities of acid-base balance should be monitored regularly in a child hospitalized in the ICU with an abdominal disease process. The source of increased acid can either be an overproduction, such as ongoing lactate generation by ischemic bowel, or decreased acid clearance by the liver or kidneys in conditions associated with shock and decreased visceral blood flow. Lactate is a sensitive measure of intestinal ischemia, especially when monitored serially for trends.[8] Arterial blood samples are more reliable than venous samples in that measurement. Hyperlactemia is not specific to intestinal ischemia and can be associated with any tissue necrosis or underperfusion of organs. Elevated serum lactate is also associated with a worse prognosis in patients with sepsis, and the normalization of lactate levels after resuscitation is associated with improved prognosis in patients with sepsis.[9]

Liver function tests, more accurately termed liver injury tests, include transaminases (alanine transaminase [ALT] and aspartate transaminase [AST]), bilirubin, and gamma glutamine transferase (GGT). These can be elevated with trauma to the liver, active hepatic inflammation, hepatic ischemia, or obstruction of the hepatic venous outflow, known as Budd Chiari syndrome. The latter can result in extremely elevated transaminase levels. Elevation of the GGT without a significant rise in the transaminase suggests a biliary condition such as common bile duct obstruction or cholecystitis.

Amylase is a valuable diagnostic test for children with abdominal pain or unexplained intraabdominal sepsis, as hyperamylasemia can indicate pancreatitis. Elevated amylase is not specific to pancreatic insults and can be elevated with head trauma, decreased renal clearance, and intestinal obstruction. Serum lipase can be an additive test to the assessment of the pancreas. It tends to be more specific to the pancreas but can be mildly elevated in intestinal obstruction as well. When both amylase and lipase are markedly elevated, pancreatitis is most likely. Children with a past history of severe or chronic pancreatitis might not have marked elevations, so the level of the enzyme does not always correlate with the severity of the disease.

Imaging Options

The reliability of abdominal exam is subjective, highly variable, and may depend on the experience of the observer, the fluctuating status of the patient, his or her medications, the patient's level of anxiety, and many other factors. Consequently, most ICU providers use imaging studies to ascertain whether intraabdominal pathology warrants intervention. For reasons of resource efficiency as well as considerations about the potential risks of ionizing radiation and patient comfort/safety, prudence needs to be exercised before ordering expensive, potentially obfuscating data from imaging studies. The following factors should always be evaluated before performing each study:

1. Specifically, what is one looking for—that is, what is the differential diagnosis?
2. How reliably will this study rule in or rule out those diagnoses—that is, what is the specificity and sensitivity of the study?
3. Will the results of this study change the management—that is, will a negative result prompt the termination of a drug regimen or life-supporting technology, and will a positive study necessitate surgical intervention or initiation of a new therapy?
4. Are the risks—such as ionizing radiation, transportation of a heavily medicated or unstable patient from the ICU to

the radiology suite, the administration of intravenous contrast, and so on—offset by the value of the study?

Ultrasonography

Ultrasonography has several advantages over other imaging studies, most notably its portability, which obviates the need for moving the patient, and its lack of ionizing radiation exposure. In addition, the use of Doppler modality permits the assessment of visceral blood flow to kidneys, pelvic organs, and the gastrointestinal tract.

When the relative positions of the mesenteric vein and artery can be accurately determined, an abnormal orientation suggests an increased risk of malrotation, even without midgut volvulus.[10] The presence of a whirlpool sign can be diagnostic of malrotation with midgut volvulus.[11] Neither finding, however, is sensitive enough to exclude the diagnosis of malrotation, thus necessitating an upper gastrointestinal contrast study to clearly determine the position of the duodenal-jejunal junction.[12] Assessments of gallbladder wall thickening suggestive of acalculous cholecystitis or biliary tree dilation are particularly accurate. Intraabdominal and pelvic fluid collections can be identified, making ultrasound useful in the setting of traumatic injury or suspected intraabdominal abscess. It can be used as an adjunct to guide fluid drainage either surgically or percutaneously.

The use of ultrasound is limited in patients with bowel obstruction or severe paralytic ileus as intestinal distention creates ultrasonic distortion, minimizing the value of this imaging modality. Accuracy of images is also highly dependent on having a skilled and experienced technician.

Abdominal Plain Radiographs

Plain radiographs of the abdomen can be revealing and also are portable, relatively inexpensive, involve small amounts of radiation, and require minimal patient movement. To be of greatest value, however, the abdominal radiograph should be done with the patient in at least two different positions, such as supine and upright, and ideally lateral decubitus as well. Cross-table laterals can also add value. These different views facilitate the identification of air-fluid levels suggestive of small bowel obstruction and the presence of pneumoperitoneum indicating likely visceral perforation. Pneumoperitoneum in a patient with high inspiratory pressures on a mechanical ventilator can sometimes be unrelated to abdominal pathology but rather a consequence of air dissecting through mediastinal and diaphragmatic tissue planes. Other plain radiograph findings suggestive of intestinal disease include thumb printing, pneumatosis intestinalis, and portal venous gas.

Computed Tomography

Abdominal CT scans are accurate, fairly rapid, and can be used to guide interventional procedures such as percutaneous biopsies or drainage of intraabdominal fluid collections. Except in institutions where CT scans are located in the ICU or those that have mobile CT units, patients must be transported to access imaging with this modality. That requirement can be a significant challenge with children who are ventilated or hemodynamically unstable. In addition to the transport challenges, the radiation exposure of a CT scan may pose a risk for developing malignancies later in life, especially for children who receive serial radiographs.[13] That risk can be reduced by using directed scans (ie, limiting the scan to the portion of the abdomen in question). Other risks include the administration of intravenous contrast material that can cause anaphylaxis in those who are allergic or renal injury especially in those who might already be hypovolemic or receiving nephrotoxic drugs.[14] That risk can be minimized as well by using nonionic contrast materials or with the administration of sodium bicarbonate and *N*-acetylcysteine prior to the administration of the IV contrast. Administration of enteral contrast can result in aspiration if there is intestinal obstruction or delayed gastric emptying with vomiting or gastroesophageal reflux.

The abdominal CT scan can be effective at identifying the condition of all the intraabdominal organs and the retroperitoneal spaces. It is being used with increasing success to assess for bowel obstruction. Identification of fluid collections and their characteristics can help ascertain whether blood, bile, or pus is present and whether it can be drained percutaneously. To make certain that nonopacification of fluid-filled loops of bowel is not misconstrued for pathologic collections of fluid, enteral contrast should be given as long as no contraindications exist. With IV contrast and carefully timed image capture, conclusions about organ perfusion can be assessed as well. Colonic and intestinal ischemia, necrotizing pancreatitis, and decreased renal perfusion can all be seen reliably.

Magnetic Resonance Imaging

Magnetic resonance imaging (MRI) of the abdomen can be valuable, especially as the risks of radiation can be obviated, but the logistical challenges of moving an ICU patient to the MRI suite are similar to those mentioned earlier for CT scans. The added challenges posed by MRI include the slower speed of the image capture, which interferes with accessing the unstable patient for interventions, as well as the restrictions for certain MRI-incompatible ICU equipment to be in the MRI scanning room. Despite these issues, MRI enterography and cholangiography are now capable of generating revealing images of the gastrointestinal and hepatobiliary tracts.[15] Thus, if the value of the images can offset the risks of transporting a sick child to the MRI suite, it should be considered.

Abdominal Conditions Requiring Treatment in the Intensive Care Unit

Perforated Viscera

Children with perforation of the gastrointestinal tract will frequently require either preoperative resuscitation or postoperative stabilization in the ICU. The most common condition resulting in perforation is appendicitis. Although perforated appendicitis is common, occurring in 30% to 50% of children who present to children's hospitals with appendicitis,[16] it is unusual for it to result in serious intraabdominal sepsis. Nevertheless, deaths do still occur in such children, related most often to septic shock with cardiovascular collapse or severe acute respiratory distress syndrome (ARDS).

Other sites of perforation in the gastrointestinal tract include gastric or proximal intestinal perforation from severe gastritis, peptic ulcer disease, gastric ischemia, or following manipulations such as insertion of gastric tubes or transpyloric feeding tubes.[17] In children with chronic gastrostomies, accidental dislodgements or manipulations of the gastrostomy site can result in separation of the stomach from the abdominal wall, leading to spillage of gastric contents into the peritoneal cavity. Because the acidic gastric pH results in lower bacterial counts, such perforations do not usually result in serious intraabdominal sepsis. However, chronically hospitalized children or children with gastroesophageal reflux on chronic acid suppression therapies may be colonized with resistant bacterial or fungal organisms such as *Candida* species that can lead to serious septic consequences.

Ingested foreign bodies can lead to perforation anywhere in the gastrointestinal tract, with common items being sharp materials such as pins or nails, fish bones, disc batteries, and magnets.[18] Magnet ingestion incidents, in particular, have dramatically risen since the early 2000s and have led to serious injury and death. If more than one magnet is ingested, the magnets can pinch loops of bowel and lead to ischemia, necrosis, perforation, and death.[18–20]

Trauma can also result in perforation. The lap portion of a seat belt can cause an abrupt and significant increase in intraabdominal pressures during motor vehicle accidents. Patients may sustain intestinal perforation, organ lacerations, or significant intraabdominal hematomas requiring ICU care. Abdominal injury is the second most common cause of death in abused children after head injury. A punch or kick can compress the small bowel against the vertebral column causing a jejunal perforation. So characteristic is this mechanism that the intraoperative finding of a jejunal perforation in the absence of a known trauma history should prompt an evaluation by the hospital's child abuse team.[21] Sports injuries, from skateboarding to all-terrain vehicle (ATV) use, can all lead to significant injury requiring resuscitation.[22]

Ischemia

Volvulus of a loop of small intestine can occur when a segment of bowel, typically distal ileum, becomes entrapped beneath an omphalomesenteric remnant. This particular lesion can be difficult to diagnose, as neither contrast enema radiographs nor antegrade upper gastrointestinal contrast studies are likely to reach the involved area of volvulus. In addition, these children will often not have impressive physical exam findings until the bowel has become ischemic. At that point, systemic sepsis can occur rapidly. Similar pathophysiology can develop from a twist of bowel within an internal hernia.

In children with intestinal malrotation, the entire intestine supplied by the superior mesenteric artery (ie, from jejunum to right transverse colon) can twist, resulting in midgut volvulus. In a somewhat similar manner, the colon alone can twist when there is sufficient redundancy in the mesocolon, typically in the cecum or the sigmoid colon. In any of these situations with intestinal and mesenteric twisting, the resultant venous congestion can compromise the capillary inflow to the bowel wall, ultimately leading to irreversible ischemia if the bowel is not untwisted promptly. With venous congestion as an early component of these obstructive volvulus conditions, there may be less release of lactate into systemic circulation, potentially leading to a falsely reassuring normal lactate level despite significant intestinal ischemia.

In the pediatric ICU, another cause of intestinal ischemia is low cardiac output or hypoxemia. Children with congenital heart disease, particularly those with single ventricle physiology or severe cyanotic heart disease, can develop mucosal ischemia following cardiac surgery, manifested as pneumatosis intestinalis on radiographs, bloody stool, metabolic acidosis with elevated serum lactate, and sepsis. Children on potent vasoactive pressors, such as epinephrine or norepinephrine, and those receiving extracorporeal support can develop ischemia as well. This is a variant of necrotizing enterocolitis (NEC) and can involve the entire small intestine and less commonly the colon. If the diminished cardiac output or hypoxemia is corrected and the ischemia is limited to the mucosa, surgical treatment may be avoided. Resection is necessary if the acidosis or systemic perturbations are refractory or if perforation results. Unfortunately, as this disease can involve the entire gut, the utility of resection may be limited.

Other causes of intestinal ischemia include small bowel obstruction, usually from adhesions following previous laparotomies or, less commonly, related to incarcerated inguinal hernias. If the bowel becomes sufficiently distended, the intraluminal pressure can exceed the intramural perfusion pressure of the microcirculation, resulting in ischemia. Other less common causes of intestinal ischemia include conditions that alter the microcirculation of the bowel wall such as vasculitis or hemolytic uremic syndrome.

The systemic physiologic insult of intestinal ischemia is usually proportional to the degree of ischemic tissue. Thus midgut volvulus or total intestinal involvement with NEC can be the most catastrophic of these disease states acutely and can have the most devastating long-term consequences with short bowel syndrome and intestinal failure a common consequence if the ischemia is irreversible.

Neutropenic Enterocolitis

Children who have significant neutropenia, whether drug induced from chemotherapy for malignant diseases or as a primary disease, may develop inflammation of the intestinal tract. The most common location is the right colon. Historically, this has been termed *typhlitis,* but more accurately it is labeled neutropenic enterocolitis, as it can affect other portions of the intestinal tract as well. It may be preceded by mucositis that permits the intestinal bacteria to invade the bowel wall. Affected children exhibit fever, abdominal pain and tenderness, abdominal distention, ileus or diarrhea, radiographic signs of inflammation, and sometimes hemodynamic instability. The diagnosis is made best by CT scan or ultrasound.[23] Surgical treatment is reserved for patients with peritonitis or hemodynamic instability after appropriate resuscitation.

Pancreatitis

Severe pancreatitis can require intensive care in children. Etiologies for the pancreatitis are most often idiopathic in children, but anatomic causes such as gallstones, pancreatic trauma, or pancreas divisum can also be responsible. Drugs and hemolytic uremic syndrome can be unusual causes of severe pancreatitis.[24] In severe cases, pancreatitis can lead to significant third space fluid losses, pleural effusions, retroperitoneal hemorrhage, abscess formation, and hypocalcemia. Necrotizing pancreatitis, though rare in children, can require repeated surgical debridement to eradicate the ongoing source of sepsis.

Hemorrhage

Intraabdominal hemorrhage can result from trauma or following surgical procedures or manipulations. In blunt trauma, the spleen is the most commonly injured abdominal organ. To avoid the risk of overwhelming postsplenectomy infection (OPSI), nonoperative management is attempted as long as hemodynamic stability can be maintained. Hospitalization in the PICU with strict bed rest is indicated when the splenic injury is grade IV or V or if there are other significant injuries.[25] The risk of delayed splenic rupture following nonoperative management is extremely low. If surgery is necessary, attempts to salvage the spleen with splenorrhaphy are important. Before surgery, if time permits, the child should be immunized for encapsulated bacterial organisms including *Haemophilus influenza, Streptococcus pneumoniae,* and meningococcus.

The liver is also a commonly injured organ in blunt abdominal trauma, and it too can usually be managed nonoperatively. The development of hemobilia several weeks after nonoperative management of a hepatic laceration is uncommon, but when it occurs it can result in significant gastrointestinal bleeding. This can usually be managed with arteriographic embolization or endoscopic biliary stent placement,[26] but it sometimes requires resection of the involved hepatic segment or lobe (see also Chapter 121).

Other Specific Conditions
Cholecystitis

Gallstones are increasingly common in children, perhaps because of the increased use of parenteral nutrition with its associated risk of cholestasis or the increasing prevalence of childhood obesity.[27] Gallstones can result in cholecystitis, biliary obstruction, or pancreatitis that can complicate an intensive care unit course for a child. Acalculous cholecystitis can be seen in children who are hospitalized in the ICU, particularly those who are receiving large doses of opiates that lead to biliary dyskinesia or those who have decreased perfusion of the abdominal organs because of hypotension. Acalculous cholecystitis can be associated with a significant systemic inflammatory response and should be considered as a source of unexplained sepsis in a child. Ultrasonographic and CT scan findings of a dilated gallbladder with a thickened gallbladder wall and pericholecystic fluid are diagnostic, although a radionuclide study such as a hepatobiliary iminodiacetic acid (HIDA) scan is the most accurate functional imaging study.

Empiric antibiotic coverage for common biliary pathogens such as gram-negative organisms like Klebsiella, pseudomonas, or *E. coli* should be started immediately. Cholecystectomy would be definitive therapy. In critically ill children who might not tolerate a trip to the operating room, percutaneous drainage of the gallbladder done by ultrasound guidance in the ICU can be an effective temporizing procedure.

Spontaneous Bacterial Peritonitis

Spontaneous bacterial peritonitis (SBP) is an acute bacterial infection of ascitic abdominal fluid that may present with fever, abdominal pain, altered mental status, or persistent vomiting.[28] Enteric organisms have traditionally been isolated from more than 90% of infected ascites fluid in spontaneous bacterial peritonitis, suggesting that the gastrointestinal (GI) tract is the source of bacterial contamination. This is thought to be due to direct transmural migration of bacteria from an intestinal or hollow organ lumen. An alternative proposed mechanism for bacterial inoculation of ascites is via hematogenous transmission in conjunction with an impaired immune system. The debate continues and the exact mechanism of bacterial displacement from the GI tract into ascites fluid remains controversial. If suspected, broad-spectrum antibiotics should be initiated to cover GI flora until culture results can guide therapy further.

Abdominal Compartment Syndrome

Intraabdominal hypertension (IAH) is defined as intraabdominal pressure (IAP) that is >12 mm Hg. Although this is relatively uncommon in pediatric ICU patients, it can be associated with a high morbidity and mortality. If the IAP reaches a point where perfusion to intraabdominal organs is compromised, a constellation of organ dysfunctions may occur including renal insufficiency, intestinal ischemia, hepatic dysfunction, elevated diaphragms, and respiratory insufficiency.[29-31] This constellation is termed *abdominal compartment syndrome (ACS)*. Risk factors for ACS include massive fluid resuscitation for any illness, intraabdominal hemorrhage, intraabdominal inflammation or infection from any cause, obesity, and tight abdominal wall closures following laparotomy. Like compartment syndrome in extremities, there is no absolute pressure to define the presence of ACS; the intravascular volume status, blood pressure, and systemic vascular resistance are all factors that can impact the perfusion pressure of the abdominal organs and minimize the effect of the IAP. An abdominal perfusion pressure (APP) can be calculated as the mean arterial pressure minus the IAP. If the APP is >60 mm Hg, a higher survival rate has been reported. The diagnosis of ACS is made when there is a sustained increased IAP in combination with signs of organ dysfunction such as decreased cardiac output, oliguria, and respiratory insufficiency. Other organ systems that can be affected by IAH include the reduction of portal and mesenteric venous flow, potentially leading to hepatic dysfunction and intestinal edema, and ischemia. In addition, the increased intrathoracic pressure that can result from the elevated diaphragms can raise intracranial pressure.

When signs of IAH are evident in the setting of abdominal distention, pressure measurements can be made using nasogastric tubes, rectal catheters, bladder catheters, and peritoneal drainage tubes such as peritoneal dialysis catheters. The most reliable and easily practical measurement can be obtained using a closed system of a Foley bladder catheter connected to a fluid column and a pressure measuring device such as a tube manometer or a pressure transducer. Ultrasound evaluation, including Doppler imaging of renal, portal, and mesenteric blood flow can be helpful in the assessment of end-organ perfusion, as well as estimating the intraabdominal venous pressure by assessing the caliber of the inferior vena cava (IVC). CT scan can also reveal poor perfusion of these organs and a flattened IVC, as well as increased abdominal girth, especially in the anterior to posterior dimension.

If the diagnosis of ACS is suspected, efforts to augment perfusion must be initiated. Avoid the reverse Trendelenburg or prone positions, as these can increase IAP. Effective decompression of the gastrointestinal tract is important and can be optimized by effective nasogastric tube drainage, the administration of prokinetic medications, and colonic decompression by either enemas or colonoscopy. Supporting renal function is also important and includes liberal use of diuretics along with volume resuscitation. If these maneuvers have not improved the organ function, temporary decompression by insertion of an abdominal drain to decrease the amount of fluid in the abdomen may be necessary.[32] If this does not adequately decompress the IAH, laparotomy is necessary with placement of a sterile patch or silo that may provide sufficient compliance to reverse the ACS.

The morbidity of ACS is significant, with mortality rates of >50% reported, especially if treatment is delayed until multisystem organ failure develops. After decompression, and once resolution of any end-organ dysfunction occurs and after the underlying causes of the IAH have abated, delayed closure of the abdomen can be considered. Sometimes that closure will require abdominal wall reconstruction techniques such as skin flap closure without fascial repair or skin grafts. Primary or delayed primary fascial repair may be feasible, sometimes requiring separation and release of the muscle groups or insertion of prosthetic patches such as synthetic mesh, Goretex, or biological sheet materials that serve as a protein matrix for tissue ingrowth.

Intraabdominal Abscess

Intraabdominal abscesses are highly variable in presentation. Patients may present with significant abdominal pain, spiking fevers, prolonged ileus after a surgical procedure, or leukocytosis. Classic physical findings may be absent in a deep abscess, where the only clues may be persistent fevers, tachycardia, and mild persistent GI dysfunction. Postoperative analgesics and incisional pain frequently mask abdominal findings. In addition, antibiotic administration may mask abdominal tenderness, fever, and leukocytosis.

In patients with subphrenic abscesses, irritation of the diaphragm may lead to shoulder pain, persistent episodes of hiccups, or unexplained pleural effusions, atelectasis, or pneumonia. With pelvic abscesses, frequent urination, diarrhea, or tenesmus may occur. If these abscesses go unrecognized, patients may develop a significant septic response that can lead to multiple organ failure and death.

Intestine as a Source of Sepsis

The intestine is an organ endowed with large quantities of both lymphatic tissue and bacteria. Consequently, it can be a central organ in the systemic inflammatory response in children hospitalized in the ICU. The role of the gut's immune system is not fully understood but may play a key role in some intestinal inflammatory diseases such as Crohn disease. In addition, the interplay between the gut-associated lymphoid tissue (GALT) and the bacteria present in the bowel lumen is important in critical illness. The sick child with decreased visceral blood flow and under severe stress likely has alterations in the mucosal integrity of the intestine. That loss of integrity can lead to bacterial invasion of the bowel wall with subsequent entry of the bacteria/toxins into the lymphatic or portal venous circulation. Once in the circulation, these bacteria/toxins can trigger a severe systemic inflammatory response, even if the bacteria are not detectable as a bloodstream infection. Use of enteral antibiotics to decrease potentially pathologic gut bacteria has proved effective in reducing intestinal sources of sepsis in some settings, whereas replacement of gut flora using probiotics or synbiotics has been employed with some success in others.[33]

Surgical Intervention

The decision to perform a laparotomy or laparoscopy in a pediatric ICU patient can be challenging. There are indeed times when a patient can be too sick to go to the operating room and other times when the patient is so sick that only an immediate operation will provide a chance for successful treatment.

With the possible exception of patients with continued intraabdominal hemorrhage or abdominal compartment syndrome, delaying operative treatment with time spent on preoperative resuscitation is often valuable. Induction of general anesthesia in a hypovolemic or acidotic patient with cardiogenic or septic shock can be dangerous. An understanding of the differential diagnosis can be most helpful in planning the appropriate antibiotic coverage and the timing of the surgical treatment. Most of the conditions that require laparotomy in ICU patients have an infectious component, and thus empiric broad-spectrum antibiotics should be administered early in the resuscitation. Depending on the disease, resuscitation and antibiotics alone may obviate the need for emergent laparotomy. Effective communication between the surgical team and ICU team is therefore essential. To optimize the timing of the operation, the surgical team should be ready to go immediately, once the preoperative resuscitation is sufficient. In situations where physical exam or radiographs do not provide localization, bedside imaging can help localize the disease. Image-guided drainage of localized infection may be a successful strategy in lieu of a full laparotomy with its incumbent risks,[34,35] or it may help to improve the physiology so that a definitive operation can be more safely performed after the condition has stabilized.

References

1. Cheong YC, Laird SM, Li TC, et al. Peritoneal healing and adhesion formation/reformation. *Hum Reprod Update*. 2001;7:556-566.
2. Holmdahl L, Ivarsson ML. The role of cytokines, coagulation, and fibrinolysis in peritoneal tissue repair. *Eur J Surg*. 1999;165:1012-1019.
3. Matheson PJ, Wilson MA, Garrison RN. Regulation of intestinal blood flow. *J Surg Res*. 2000;93:182-196.
4. Zakaria ER, Li N, Garrison RN. Mechanisms of direct peritoneal resuscitation-mediated splanchnic hyperperfusion following hemorrhagic shock. *Shock*. 2007;27:436-442.
5. Mainous MR, Ertel W, Chaudry IH, Deitch EA. The gut: a cytokine-generating organ in systemic inflammation. *Shock*. 1995;4:193-199.
6. Jakob SM. The effects of mechanical ventilation on hepato-splanchnic perfusion. *Curr Opin Crit Care*. 2010;16.
7. Putensen C, Wrigge H, Hering R. The effects of mechanical ventilation on the gut and abdomen. *Curr Opin Crit Care*. 2006;12:160-165.
8. Evennett NJ, Petrov MS, Mittal A, Windsor JA. Systematic review and pooled estimates for the diagnostic accuracy of serological markers for intestinal ischemia. *World J Surg*. 2009;33:1374-1383.
9. Haas SA, Lange T, Saugel B, et al. Severe hyperlactatemia, lactate clearance and mortality in unselected critically ill patients. *Intensive Care Med*. 2016;42:202-210.
10. Weinberger E, Winters WD, Liddell R, et al. Sonographic diagnosis of intestinal malrotation in infants: importance of the relative positions of the superior mesenteric artery and vein. *AJR*. 1992;159:825-828.
11. Pracros JP, Sann L, Genin G, et al. Ultrasound diagnosis of midgut volvulus: the "whirlpool" sign. *Pediatr Radiol*. 1998;22:18-20.
12. Tackett JJ, Muise ED, Cowles RA. Malrotation: current strategies navigating the radiologic diagnosis of a surgical emergency. *World J Radiol*. 2014;6:730-736.
13. Rice HE, Frush DP, Farmer D, Waldhausen JH. Review of radiation risks from computed tomography: essentials for the pediatric surgeon. *J Pediatr Surg*. 2007;42:603-607.
14. Patzer L. Nephrotoxicity as a cause of acute kidney injury in children. *Pediatr Nephrol*. 2008;23:2159-2173.
15. Schaefer JF, Kirschner HJ, lichy M, et al. Highly resolved free-breathing magnetic resonance cholangiopancreatography in the diagnostic workup of pancreaticobiliary diseases in infants and young children—initial experiences. *J Pediatr Surg*. 2006;41:1645-1651.
16. Nelson DS, Batemen B, Bolte RG. Appendiceal perforation in children diagnosed in a pediatric emergency department. *Pediatr Emerg Care*. 2000;16:233-237.
17. Campwala I, Perrone E, Yanni G, et al. Complications of gastrojejunal feeding tubes in children. *J Surg Res*. 2015;199:67-71.
18. Shah SK, Tieu KK, Tsao K. Intestinal complications of magnet ingestion in children from the pediatric surgery perspective. *Eur J Pediatr Surg*. 2009;19:334-337.
19. Strickland M, Rosenfield D, Fecteau A. Magnetic foreign body injuries: a large pediatric hospital experience. *J Pediatr*. 2014;165:332-335.
20. Hussain SZ, Bousvaros A, Gilger M, et al. Management of ingested magnets in children. *J Pediatr Gastroenterol Nutr*. 2012;55:239-242.
21. Barnes PM, Norton CM, Dunstan FD, et al. Abdominal injury due to child abuse. *Lancet*. 2005;366:187-188.
22. Meehan WP, Mannix R. A substantial portion of life-threatening injuries are sports-related. *Pediatr Emerg Care*. 2013;29:624-627.
23. McCarville MB, Adelman CS, Li C, et al. Typhlitis in childhood cancer. *Cancer*. 2005;104:380-387.
24. Suzuki M, Sai JK, Shimizu T. Acute pancreatitis in children and adolescents. *World J Gastrointest Pathophysiol*. 2014;15:416-426.
25. Dervan LA, King MA, Cuschieri J, et al. Pediatric solid organ injury operative interventions and outcomes at Harborview Medical Center, before and after introduction of a solid organ injury pathway for pediatrics. *J Trauma Acute Care Surg*. 2015;79:215-220.
26. Singh V. Endoscopic management of traumatic hemobilia. *J Trauma*. 2007;62:1045-1047.
27. Kaechele V, Wabitsch M, Thiere D, et al. Prevalence of gallbladder stone disease in obese children and adolescents: influence of the degree of obesity, sex, and pubertal development. *Peds Gast Nutr*. 2006;42:66-70.
28. Vieira SM, Matte U, Kieling CO, et al. Infected and noninfected ascites in pediatric patients. *J Pediatr Gastro Nutr*. 2005;40:289-294.
29. Malbrain M, Cheatham M, Kirkpatrick A, et al. Results from the international conference of experts on intra-abdominal hypertension and abdominal compartment syndrome. I. Definitions. *Intensive Care Med*. 2006;32:1722-1732.
30. Carlotti APCP, Carvalho WB. Abdominal compartment syndrome: a review. *Pediatr Crit Care Med*. 2009;10:115-120.
31. Cheatham M, Malbrain M, Kirkpatrick A, et al. Results from the international conference of experts on intra-abdominal hypertension and abdominal compartment syndrome. II. Recommendations. *Intensive Care Med*. 2007;33:951-962.
32. Cheatham ML, Safcsak K. Percutaneous catheter decompression in the treatment of elevated intaabdominal pressure. *Chest*. 2011;140:1428-1435.
33. Doron S, Gorbach SL. Probiotics: their role in the treatment and prevention of disease. *Expert Rev Anti Infect Ther*. 2006;4:261-275.
34. McDanial JD, Warren MT, Pence JC, Ey EH. Ultrasound guided transrectal drainage of deep pelvic abscess in children: a modified and simplified approach. *Pediatr Radiol*. 2015;45:435-438.
35. Gervais DA, Brown SD, Connolly SA, et al. Percutaneous imaging-guided abdominal and pelvic abscess drainage in children. *Radiographics*. 2004;24:737-754.

Immunity and Infection

Innate Immune System

Samiran Ray, Rachel S. Agbeko, and Mark J. Peters

PEARLS

- Innate immunity provides the front-line "ready-made" response to pathogen invasion.
- These same pathways are activated in response to other critical insults including trauma, hypoxic/ischemic injury, and bypass.
- Pattern recognition molecules recognize exogenous and endogenous molecular patterns.
- Therapeutic interventions in the ICU can have consequences on the innate immune response.

The immune system is a complex, sophisticated defense system that protects the body from danger. Danger may be intrinsic (eg, cancer) or extrinsic (eg, pathogenic organisms). The immune system provides constant surveillance to detect potential danger, identifies the nature of the threat, and then mounts a nullifying response. The immune system is also self-regulating: Once the threat is nullified, the response needs to be called off.

Traditionally a distinction is made between adaptive and innate immune responses. The adaptive immune system has been studied in the greater detail and is responsible for a **specific** response to individual pathogens. Adaptive immunity is a highly sophisticated process with many safety mechanisms to target responses at pathogens (or pathogen-infected cells) while leaving normal tissues alone. This sophistication and specificity take time to develop (of the order of days to weeks) and have many effector cells and molecules to deliver a coordinated response, including T and B lymphocytes and immunoglobulins. While the adaptive response is essential for health and in particular for the phenomenon of immunologic memory, it is not sufficient to address a sudden major bacteremia or widespread tissue injury—or even the thousands of minor bacterial inoculums all individuals experience during their lifetimes (eg, during teeth brushing). Bacterial growth is exponential under optimal conditions. *Neisseria meningitides* counts can double in 20 minutes. Given these threats, there is a need for a "ready-made" system that can act swiftly to neutralize external threats. This is called the innate immune system.

Innate immunity is phylogenetically conserved and found in nearly all multicellular organisms; again, this contrasts with the adaptive immune system that is found in vertebrates only. In humans the innate immune system is largely present at birth, in contrast to the years it takes to build an adaptive immune repertoire. The hallmarks of the innate immune

system are immediacy, promiscuousness, redundancy, and generality. Given that the adaptive immune system evolved in the presence of innate immunity, these systems do not operate in isolation from each other; rather, the innate immune system presents to and instructs the adaptive part of immunity.

Innate immunity is mediated through immune cells, such as tissue macrophages, neutrophils, and monocytes, but also cells that are primarily known for other functions: platelets and endothelial cells. Complex networks of circulating mediators including the complement cascade, collectins, defensins, and the coagulation cascade are integral parts of innate immunity. Recent work has highlighted apparent contributions from neurohumoral and autonomic nervous systems.

No critically ill child is admitted to the ICU without activation of its innate immune system. No intensivist can function adequately without a good working knowledge of innate immunity, as it is central to many of the clinical entities he or she faces on a day-to-day basis. Infection, trauma, ischemia-reperfusion, acute respiratory distress syndrome, and cardiopulmonary bypass sequelae are all largely mediated by the innate immune system.

This chapter provides a framework and outline of concepts in innate immunity that will help you understand some of the pathophysiologic processes central to pediatric critical care.

Components of Innate Immune System

An ideal first-line response to danger would be pervasive, prompt, effective, and calibrated. The required steps are recognition of a danger signal; dispatch of messengers to mount a response; mounting an effector response that neutralizes danger; and controlling the response to contain damage.

Innate Immune Stimulus — Danger Hypothesis

The traditional paradigm of the immune system suggests that it is programmed, through evolution and adaptation, to differentiate between self and nonself. In this view invading pathogens such as bacteria would be recognized as nonself and trigger an immune response, while newly replicating blood cells would not. However, this does not explain how animals can host entire microbiomes on their mucosal surfaces without inducing an immune response. Similarly, it does not explain how a developing fetus is protected from the maternal immune system.

The danger hypothesis suggests that the immune system does not simply detect self from nonself but instead detects danger or tissue damage. As the first line of defense, the innate immune system has to do this rapidly against an almost infinite number of pathogens or noxious molecules. This response is not learned, and it is conserved across phyla.

How does the immune system differentiate between endogenous and pathogenic molecules? The danger hypothesis suggests that it does not. The innate immune response is triggered by molecular patterns that are associated with pathogenic organisms or tissue damage, or both. These signals, known as danger-associated molecular patterns (DAMPs), are a diverse set of molecules (or parts of molecules, or polymeric components) that share recognizable common features, which identify them as pathogenic.[1] For example, nucleic acids or mitochondrial proteins released from their intracellular compartment during tissue damage or invading organisms are typical DAMPs. Similarly, hydrophobic protein moieties, or "hyppos," are also often hidden within tertiary and quaternary protein structures. When they are exposed, they become DAMPs and trigger an innate immune response.

When associated with pathogens, these molecular patterns signaling danger are known as pathogen-associated molecular proteins (PAMPs). Lipopolysaccharide is an example of PAMPs within the bacterial cell wall, where the hydrophobic part of lipopolysaccharide is hidden. When released by pathogens, this becomes exposed and acts as a PAMP. All hyppos can be DAMPs including lipid particles and nucleic acids. Protein misfolding, damage, or binding to other molecules (eg, lipopolysaccharide-binding protein [LBP] binding to lipopolysaccharide) can lead to hyppos being exposed, and normally functional endogenous proteins may become DAMPs. That not all hyppos are always immunostimulatory may be down to the level of aggregation or quantity (evolved from quorum sensing used by eukaryotic colonies such as bacteria—a certain concentration of exposed hyppos will alert the colony of impending danger).[2]

DAMPs released following cell or tissue damage trigger responses from the innate immune system, which are similar to those produced by PAMPs.[3] These endogenous signals are known as "alarmins." High-mobility group protein B1 (HMGB-1) is one of the best described alarmins. In an intact cell, HMGB-1 is a histone-associated chromatin protein, involved in DNA structural modulation, thereby regulating transcription. However, following necrosis, the intranuclear HMGB-1 is released and recognized by receptors for advanced glycated endproducts (RAGE), which initiates an immune response aimed to contain damage. Cells have also evolved to release HGMB-1 in response to other signs of danger, which in the case of ischemia/reperfusion may lead to actively amplifying the immune response.[4]

Signal Recognition

Pattern recognition receptors (PRRs), a group of molecules with repeating sugars or specific amino acid motifs, recognize the typical molecular patterns of DAMPs. PRRs can be soluble circulating molecules, bound to cell surfaces, or intracellular. There is crossover between the types of PRRs—some PRRs such as CD14 can operate both as a cell surface–bound receptor but also in soluble form.

Circulating PRRs include sugar-recognizing collectins, ficolins, and small peptides called antimicrobial peptides. Mannose-binding lectin (MBL) is produced in the liver and activates the complement system after binding typical repeated sugar patterns on pathogen cell walls. Lower MBL levels increase risk of infection and the systemic inflammatory response in adults and children.[5] Interestingly, high levels of MBL expression are associated with preterm labor, while moderately low levels of MBL have been associated with better protection from mycobacteria infection and complement-associated inflammatory damage from certain infections such as meningococcal disease.[6,7]

Bacterial permeability increasing protein (BPI) is an antimicrobial protein. It acts against gram-negative bacteria by increasing cell wall permeability and has been investigated as a therapeutic agent in meningococcal sepsis in children. Although there was no mortality benefit, there was a tendency toward a reduction in sequelae.[8]

Toll-like receptors (TLRs) are the best characterized group of membrane-bound PRRs. There are at least 10 related receptors in humans and 12 in mice (Table 101.1). TLRs are evolutionarily preserved from the worm *Caenorhabditis elegans* and strikingly homologous to Toll, a gene product essential to *Drosophila* immunity and dorsoventral patterning.[9]

The TLR family can be divided into two subgroups depending on location. TLRs 1, 2, 4, 5, and 6 are bound to cell surfaces and recognize microbial membrane components. The remaining TLRs 3, 7, 8, and 9 are expressed in intracellular membrane-bound organelles and vesicles, such as the endoplasmic reticulum, endosomes, and lysosomes, where they typically recognize nucleic acids from intracellular pathogens.

TLR4 is the best described of the cell surface TLRs, given its central role in the pathogenicity of gram-negative septic shock as a key part of the lipopolysaccharide (LPS) recognition apparatus. In order to bind LPS, TLR4 forms a dimeric complex, in association with MD2. This complex formation exposes the binding site that recognizes LPS. LPS-binding protein (LBP) binds to LPS, which allows recognition by soluble CD14. CD14 is instrumental in delivering the LPS-bound complex to the TLR4/MD2 complex on the cell surface. TLR4 can also bind to the streptococcal toxin pneumolysin, respiratory syncytial virus (RSV) fusion protein, and paclitaxel, the chemotherapeutic taxol used to treat ovarian, breast, and certain lung cancers (Fig. 101.1).

TLR2 recognizes lipoteichoic acid from gram-positive bacteria, lipoarabinomannan from mycobacteria, zymosan from fungi, and hemagglutinin from measles viruses, among others. TLR2 forms complexes with TLR1 and TLR6 to mediate DAMP recognition. TLR5 is present mainly in gut mucosal dendritic cells and recognizes bacterial flagellin. In doing so, it can activate the adaptive immune system to mount a more specific response to pathogenic bacteria in the gut.

The intracellular membrane-bound TLRs[3,7,8,9] are instrumental in defending against invasive pathogens. They recognize nucleic acids, especially pathogen-associated nucleic acids such as double-stranded (ds) RNA and unmethylated CpG DNA motifs not seen in mammalian cells. TLR3 recognizes dsRNA during the replication of single-stranded RNA viruses including RSV. TLR3 deficiency in humans is associated with a susceptibility to infection with herpes simplex virus type 1. TLR7 recognizes RNA viruses, as they are transported in autophagosomes, as well as bacterial RNA from group B *Streptococcus*. TLR8 is also active against bacteria, and expression can be up-regulated in bacterial infection. TLR9 senses bacterial DNA (unmethylated CpG motifs) but also recognizes hemozoin, which is generated after the digestion of hemoglobin by *Plasmodium falciparum* (Fig. 101.2).

Three major classes of cytoplasmic PRRs are not membrane bound: nucleotide-binding and oligomerization domain-like receptors (NLRs), RIG-I–like receptors (RLR), and absent in

TABLE 101.1   Toll-Like Receptor Family in Humans, Described by Pathogen-Associated Molecular Proteins (PAMPs), Organism, Alarmin, and Localization

PRR	PAMP	Organism	Alarmin	Location
TLR1-TLR2	Triacyl lipopolypeptide	Gram-negative bacteria Mycobacteria		Cell surface
TLR2	Porins Peptidoglycan Lipoarabinomannan Hemagglutinin protein tGPI-mutin	Neisseria Gram-positive bacteria Mycobacteria Measles Parasites	Hyaluronic acid HSP70 HMGB-1	Cell surface
TLR3	dsDNA	Viruses		Intracellular vesicles
TLR4	Lipopolysaccharide Envelope proteins Mannanes Glycoinositol phospholipids	Gram-negative bacteria RSV Fungi Trypanosoma	Fibrinogen HSP, ROS Hyaluronic acid Heme, HMGB-1	Cell surface
TLR5	Flagellin	Bacteria *Salmonella*		Cell surface
TLR6-TLR2	Diacyl lipopeptide Lipoteichoic acid Zymosan	Mycoplasma Gram-positive bacteria Fungus		Cell surface
TLR7	ssRNA	RNA virus	Self DNA and RNA (LL37)	Intracellular vesicles
TLR8	ssRNA	RNA virus		Intracellular vesicles
TLR9	Nonmethylated CpG DNA DNA Hemozoin	Bacteria, mycobacteria DNA virus Plasmodium		Lysosomes
TLR10	Unknown	Unknown		B lymphocytes

HSP, heat shock protein; *PRR*, pattern recognition receptor; *ROS*, reactive oxygen species; *RSV*, respiratory syncytial virus; *TLR*, Toll-like receptor.
Adapted from LaRue H, Ayari C, Bergeron A, et al. Toll-like receptors in urothelial cells—targets for cancer immunotherapy. Nat Rev Urol. 2013;10:537-545.

melanoma 2 (AIM)–like receptors. NLRs are the best described cytoplasmic PRRs. Similar to TLRs, they have three distinct domains: Knockout mice deficient in one domain of NLRs (NOD-1 −/− mice) are susceptible to *Staphylococcus aureus* and *Helicobacter pylori* infections; NOD-2–deficient mice are prone to infections from *Toxoplasma gondii*.[10]

Signal Transduction

Once PRRs recognize a signal, they need to trigger a response. In order to do so, they send signals to effector pathways using second messengers.

Circulating PRRs can directly activate the complement system via the lectin pathway. MBLs form complexes with MBL-associated serine proteases (MASPs), which cleave C4 and C2 to form a C3 convertase. C3 convertase cleaves C3 into active components C3a and C3b. This leads to an antiinflammatory cascade, opsonization of phagocytic cells, and the formation of the complement membrane attach complex. Other soluble-protein PRRs such as defensins can act directly as opsonins and chemotactic particles.

Cell surface and intracellular PRRs have **T**oll/**I**nterleukin-1 **R**eceptor (TIR)-containing domains, which interact with intracellular signaling molecules. Following TLR recognition of DAMPs, the cytosolic TIR-containing domains undergo structural reorganization, which provides a platform for the interaction with a family of adaptor molecules. These include myeloid differentiation primary response 88 (MyD88), the prototypic adaptor molecule involved in the LPS-TLR4 pathway. When bound to activated TLR4, MyD88 recruits a family of kinases, IL-1R–associated kinases (IRAKs), in a complex. Following a cascade of interactions, nuclear factor κB (NF-κB) is activated. The result is the transcription of cytokines leading to an inflammatory response (Figs. 101.1 and 101.2).

As with so many other arms of the innate immune system, there is significant redundancy among adaptor molecules and the signaling pathway. However, MyD88-deficient mice show reduction of NF-κB activation in all TLR pathways apart from TLR3 and TLR4, underlying its importance. The adaptor proteins also have a regulatory function: The adaptor protein **s**terile-alpha and **ar**madillo **m**otif–containing protein (SARM) negatively interacts with the adaptor protein TRIF, limiting the downstream activation of NF-κB.[11]

Effector Pathways

In order for the innate immune system to be effective, it must respond to danger rapidly. The aim of the response is to neutralize the threat where possible, raise the alarm, and seek reinforcements. The effector response can be broadly divided into two arms: *the soluble mediator response,* which has both widespread systemic effects and more targeted local effects, and *the cellular response,* which aims to neutralize directly danger through phagocytosis and self-destruction.

The soluble mediator response: The signal transduction pathways described activate nuclear transcription factors such as NF-κB. Cytokine production is an end point of activation of NF-κB. The inflammatory cytokines include TNFα, IL-1b, IL-4, Il-6, IL-10, IL-12, IL-18, CCL4-RANTES, and

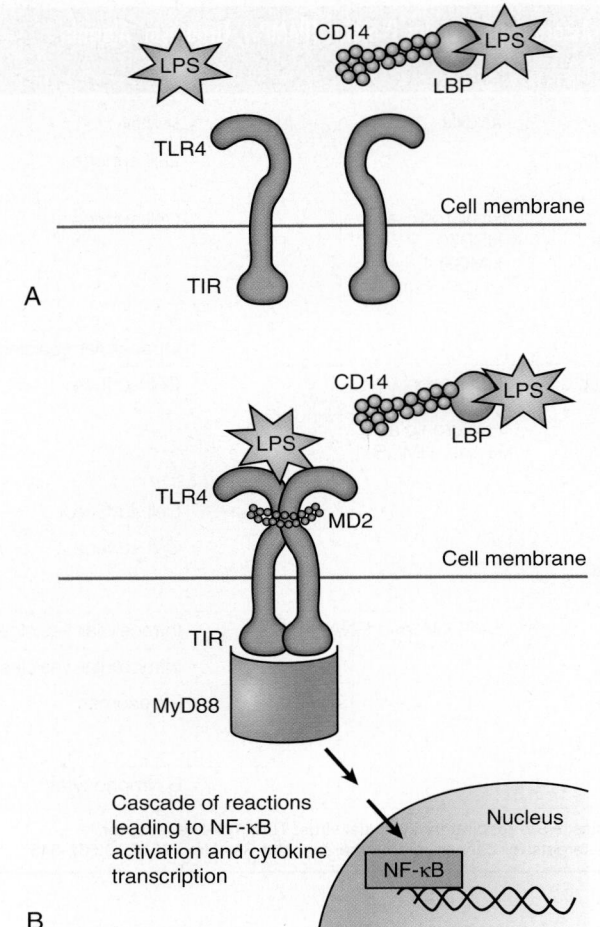

A

B

Fig. 101.1. Pathogen-associated molecular proteins and the Toll-like receptor (TLR) pathway. TLR4 is bound to the cell surface (A). TLR forms a dimeric complex along with MD2 to bind lipopolysaccharide (LPS). The LPS-TLR4-MD2 complex causes a conformational change that allows TIRAP to bind to the TIR-domain of TLR4 (B). MyD88 binds to TIRAP, which eventually leads to early NF-κB activation, and transcription of inflammatory cytokines. *LBP,* lipopolysaccharide binding protein; *MyD88,* myeloid differentiation factor 88; *NF-κB,* Nuclear factor κB; *TIR,* Toll/interleukin-1 receptor.

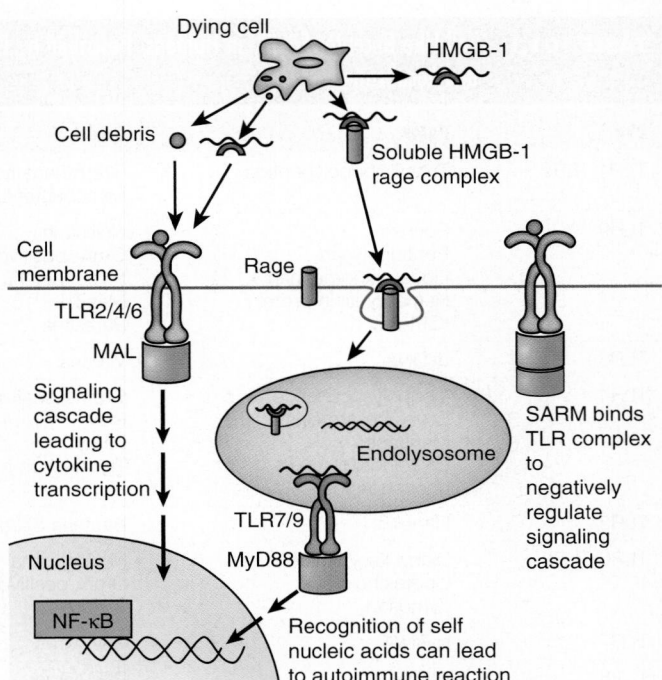

Fig. 101.2. Danger-associated molecular patterns and the Toll-like receptor (TLR) pathway. Cell debris released from a necrotic cell binds to soluble and cell surface receptors (eg, HMGB-1 binds to RAGE). Debris may also directly bind to TLR receptors 2/4 or 6 leading to an inflammatory cascade. Nucleic acids in particular and HMGB-1 are internalized into endolysosomes, where they bind to TLR7 and TLR9. This also leads to an inflammatory cascade, including an autoimmune reaction. The cascade is negative regulated by the TIR domain adaptor protein sterile α and armadillo motif–containing proteins SARM to prevent overwhelming inflammation. *HMGB-1,* high-mobility group box-1; *MAL,* MyD88 adaptor-like protein; *RAGE,* receptor for advance glycation products.

transforming growth factor-β. The specific subset of cytokines that is produced and released depends on the innate immune cell type involved. Although NF-κB is the prototypic transcription factor downstream of the innate immune signaling pathways, more recently transcription factor EB (TFEB) has been described as a potentially important mammalian factor in innate immunity. Unlike nuclear NF-κB, TFEB exists in the cytoplasm of macrophages. Upon activation, TFEB moves to the nucleus and leads to transcription of proinflammatory genes. The lack of TFEB in mouse macrophages leads to the inability to produce proinflammatory cytokines in following *S. aureus* infection.[12]

The soluble mediator arm has a widespread systemic effect, as well as a local effect to contain and neutralize the danger signal.

1. Systemic cytokine effects: Systemic effects rapidly follow the exposure to danger. These include the production of fever: TNFα and IL-1B among other cytokines act on the hypothalamus to increase the temperature set point. The fever response is likely to have a beneficial response in the immune response. In several species, controlling this fever response has a detrimental effect on survival. Observational evidence in humans suggests that the lack of a fever response in critical illness is associated with an increase in mortality.[13] The exact mechanisms of how fever lends itself to immunity are not yet fully elucidated, but it is likely to be multimodal: from decreased pathogenicity of microorganisms to improved immune function. The effects of fever on the immune system include (a) the increased release of neutrophils from the bone marrow, (b) improved localization of neutrophils to tissues, (c) improved phagocytic and cytotoxic activities of neutrophils, macrophages, and natural killer (NK) cells, and (d) increased presentation of antigen presentation to T cells by dendritic cells within lymph nodes.[14]

Cytokines also have effects on the circulatory system and the nervous system through providing nociceptive signals. This mobilizes energy sources to vital organs to fight the danger and may restrict spread between organisms, respectively. Nervous system involvement may also change behavior to avoid noxious stimuli (eg, TNFα knockout mice have a decreased perception of bitter taste, implying that the TNFα sensitizes animals to bitter substances, which may be deemed as noxious).[15]

2. Local neutralization: The complement system, as described earlier, plays an important role in the effector arm of the innate immune system. PRRs activate complement through the lectin pathway. This directly attacks pathogens via the membrane attack complex but also via opsonization and chemokinesis.[16]

Cytokines also have an important role in attracting immune cells to the site of danger (eg, CCL4-RANTES attracts macrophages and NK cells to the site of danger to neutralize the threat). This can lead to a positive feed-forward loop: Cytokines released from local tissue such as endothelial cells initially attract immune cells such as macrophages to the site of danger. The immune cells then produce more cytokines to amplify the signal and get further reinforcements. *The cellular response:* The cellular response involves two processes—phagocytosis and self-destruction. Both aim to neutralize the threat of danger where possible and also recruit other immune mechanisms such as the adaptive immune system.

1. Phagocytosis: DAMP recognition by cell surface PRRs set into motion cytoskeletal rearrangements. These are achieved by adaptor proteins activating cascades of kinases and guanosine triphosphate-ases (GTP)ases, leading to actin polymerization. This results in a phagosome forming and pinching off the cell surface. Activated macrophages are able to internalize >100% of their surface area within 30 minutes. Once internalized, the phagosome may fuse with lysosomes to form a phagolysosome. Here the DAMPs may be neutralized or processed and relocated to the surface, where they can be presented to T cells to promote an adaptive immune response. Reactive oxygen species (ROS) and nitric oxide are both involved in the neutralization of DAMPS within the phagolysosome. Both are produced during an innate immune response.[17]

2. Self-destruction: Because phagocytosis is the process by which cells internalize and neutralize extracellular material, autophagy is the analogous process for cytoplasmic protein and organelles: the controlled destruction of cellular material following damage. Autophagy is an essential part of cell maintenance and survival: Multiorgan failure seen in an inflammatory response is postulated as not being sequelae of disease but rather an adaptive mechanism in response to a reduction in available energy.[18] Autophagy is initiated following damage-induced expression of a family of autophagy-related genes (ATGs). The ATG-encoded proteins assemble to form an autophagosome, a double-membrane structure, which envelopes the damaged proteins or organelles. The autophagosome eventually fuses with a lysosome, where the protein or organelle gets enzymatically degraded.[19]

Autophagy may result in cell death once all the organelles undergo autophagy and the autophagic cell eventually undergoes phagocytosis. Much as autophagy is an effector of the immune response, as is cell death. This is particularly important following damage, or infection with intracellular pathogens, when the pathogen cannot be controlled. Traditionally cell death has been described as apoptosis (programmed cell death) and necrosis (accidental cell death). However, as the mechanisms behind cell death have been

discovered, this distinction has proved to be an oversimplification. Currently five types of cell death are described (Table 101.2).

Cell death leads to the release of DAMPs following cell lysis, which recruits other parts of the immune system. This is particularly important following trauma and tumor formation.[20]

Crosstalk Between Systems

The innate and adaptive immune systems interact continuously. Considering them as separate systems reflects an enormous simplification. Coagulation, neuroendocrine, cardiovascular, and autonomic nervous systems all influence, and are influenced by, immune responses. At the simplest level this is shown by many molecules having important properties in multiple systems (eg, acetylcholine is a neurotransmitter and a paracrine regulator of lymphocytes, epinephrine has profound cardiovascular effects but also stimulates the bone marrow to release neutrophils into the circulation). High plasma glucose levels arising from the stress response and insulin resistance during critical illness may inhibit complement binding to and killing of microorganisms.

The interaction between the innate immune system and the coagulation cascade is particularly important in critical illness, especially in the context of sepsis and trauma. Plasminogen activator inhibitor 1 (PAI-1) is a potent inhibitor of fibrinolysis. It achieves this response by inhibiting both tissue and urinary type plasminogen activator. Levels of PAI-1 are increased after trauma and sepsis, especially so in severe meningococcal sepsis. Inflammatory mediators TNFα, IL-1 and IL-6, complement 5a, and LPS all act to increase PAI-1 production. In turn, PAI-1 contributes to a procoagulant state and inhibits neutrophil apoptosis. Although this may help to contain inflammation at the site of infection, genotypes associated with high levels of PAI-1 production are associated with worse outcome in septic shock. So there is a direct link between how readily the immune system triggers an increased clotting tendency in critical illness and poor outcome.[21]

Similarly, inflammatory mediators such as IL-6 and HMGB-1 stimulate release of the potent coagulation activator tissue factor (TF) from activated monocytes, macrophages, and endothelial cells. Small membrane vesicles from apoptotic cells known as *microparticles* bind to cell surfaces through specific receptors, expressing TF. This promotes thrombin formation, which in turn converts fibrinogen to fibrin. Thrombin and fibrin generation are increased in inflammation, in part because fibrinolysis is impaired due to increased activity of PAI-1 but also secondary to diminished activated protein C (APC) and tissue factor pathway inhibitor (TFPI). These processes have been the targets for numerous clinical trials of drugs with anticoagulant/profibrinolytic actions—all aiming to achieve antiinflammatory effects by targeting coagulation systems. APC may also have other antiinflammatory actions, down-regulating inflammatory cytokines, preventing the loss of the endothelial barrier, and acting as an antioxidant and antiapoptotic agent. Although initial trials suggested therapeutic benefits of APC in sepsis, this has since been contradicted in larger trials in both children and adults.[22-24]

Another example of a novel interaction between the coagulation and immune systems is that TLR4-activated platelets interact with neutrophils to trap and kill bacteria in so-called "neutrophil extracellular traps" (NETs) (Fig. 101.3). In vitro

TABLE 101.2 Modes of Cell Death: Apoptosis, Autophagy-Related Cell Death, Necroptosis, and Pyroptosis Are All Forms of Programmed Cell Death, Whereas Necrosis Is Accidental

Mode of Death	Triggers	Signaling Pathways	Terminal Event	Proinflammatory?
Apoptosis	TNFα, Fas ligand (FasL), TNF-related apoptosis-inducing ligand (TRAIL) Infection	Caspase (3, 6, 7)	Nuclear condensation Nonlytic cell shrinkage Cell blebbing Phagocytosis of apoptotic bodies	No
Autophagy-related cell death	Nutrient deprivation Hypoxia Infection Histone deacetylase inhibitors	Autophagy-related gene activation mTOR Autolysosome formation	Phagocytosis of autophagic bodies	No
Necroptosis	TNFα, FasL, TRAIL Ischemia Infection	TNF receptor signaling Loss of mitochondrial inner membrane potential ROS formation	Organelle swelling Nonlytic loss of cell membrane	Yes
Pyroptosis	DAMPs Infection	NOD-like receptors activation, Caspase-1–dependent inflammasome	Cell swelling Pore formation Cell lysis	Yes
Necrosis	Toxins Infections Inflammation Trauma	(Nonprogrammed)	Cell lysis	Yes

Adapted from Inoue H, Tani K. Multimodal immunogenic cancer cell death as a consequence of anticancer cytotoxic treatments. Cell Death Different. 2014;21:39-49.

studies showed that LPS, as well as plasma from septic adults, could induce this phenomenon.[25]

Regulation of the Innate Immune Response

As with any physiologic response, the innate immune response needs regulation: to balance the sensitivity of the response against the potential to overreact and cause harm to the host. Key regulatory mechanisms are for the innate immune system are summarized in Table 101.3.

Clinical Manifestations of the Innate Immune Response in the Intensive Care Unit

The innate immune system is the body's front-line defense patrol against danger. All patients admitted to the ICU will have activated an innate immune response. In some cases this response may itself be deleterious: either through amplification in the face of an insurmountable threat or through dysregulation of the response. In other cases the critical illness may be a result of an inadequate response.

The prototypic description of the innate immune response is based on the sepsis model.

However, many other pathologic processes in the ICU start with an innate immune response:
1. Hypoxic ischemic injury: Hypoxia, either systemic hypoxia such as at high altitude or localized hypoxia such as in solid tumors, leads to the activation of an innate immune response. Oxygen status is sensed by proline hydroxylases, which act on the proline residues of hypoxia-inducible factors (HIFs) 1a and 2a. This allows the binding of an E3 ubiquitin ligase complex, which inactivates HIFs. Hypoxia

releases this inactivation. HIFs set off a cascade of downstream pathways, including the activation of NFκB, the transcriptional regulator that is a key factor in the TLR response to LPS. The overall effect in hypoxia is for the innate immune cells to increase phagocytosis and antimicrobial killing, prevent apoptosis of neutrophils, increase antigen presentation, and increase endothelial adhesion and cytokine release. HIF-deficient myeloid cells are unable to overcome pathogens effectively but form chronic ulcerative lesions. Adaptive immunity pathways are, however, down-regulated to prevent an overactive response.

TLR pathways also play an important part in the ischemic response. TLR4-deficient donor kidneys have better graft function following transplantation compared with kidneys with functional TLR4 receptors.[34]
2. Trauma: Trauma leads to a varying degree of cell necrosis, which is inflammatory. Cell necrosis releases alarmins, such as HMGB-1, into the circulation and activates an innate immune response. In the ICU, this is often seen post surgery, especially so after cardiopulmonary bypass during cardiac surgery.[35] TLR2 and TLR4 both increase their expression on mononuclear cells post cardiac surgery, which typically occurs over a 48-hour period before returning toward baseline. There is a concomitant rise in the proinflammatory cytokine IL-6. The response is stronger if there is cerebral ischemia, as occurs during deep hypothermic circulatory arrest.[36]
3. Acute kidney injury: The renal tubules are exposed to large numbers of signaling molecules and cytokines and are therefore prime candidates for danger recognition. For example, kidney epithelial cells express CD40 receptors on their cell surface: Activation of CD40 leads to an increase in ROS production and prevents apoptosis of the tubular

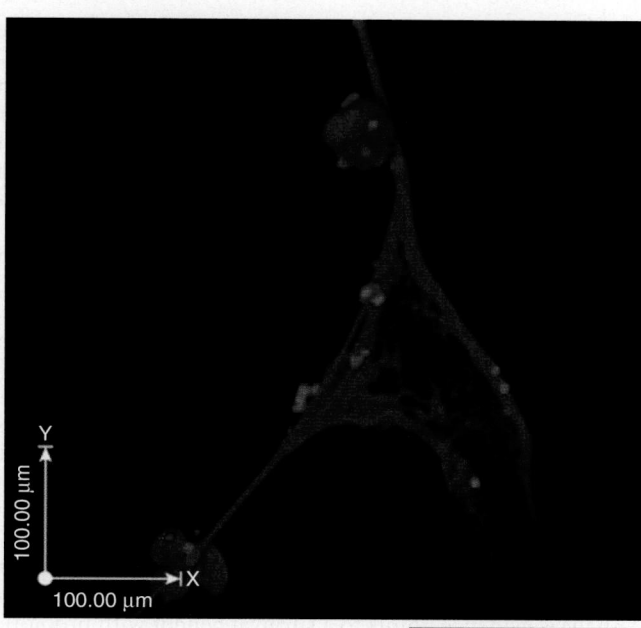

TRENDS in Microbiology

Fig. 101.3. A scanning electron microscope image of a neutrophil extracellular trap. Neutrophils release an extracellular trap made of histones and DNA, along with proteases and antimicrobial peptides. They entrap pathogens, with the DNA exhibiting intrinsic antimicrobial properties. (From Baums CG, von Köckritz-Blickwede M. Novel role of DNA in neutrophil extracellular traps. Trends Microbiol. 2015;23:330-331, Fig. 1.)

Regulation	Example
	TABLE 101.3 Examples of Regulatory Mechanisms Controlling the Innate Immune Response: Loss of Regulation Can Lead to Diseases Such as Hemophagocytic Lympho-Histiocytosis
Negative feedback	Antiinflammatory arachidonic acid–derived lipoxin released after prostaglandin to inhibit granulocyte migration and promote phagocytosis[26]
Cellular compartmentalization	Lipopolysaccharide-stimulated migration of TLR7 and 9 from the endoplasmic reticulum to the endolysosome[9]
Tissue dependence	IL-10 on mucosal surfaces has baseline antiinflammatory effect preventing response to microbiota; released by LPS-stimulated TLR4[27]
Redox state	In apoptosis the mitochondrial outer membrane is permeabilized, arresting the respiratory chain Reactive oxygen species generate oxidize HMGB-1, making it nonimmunostimulatory[28]
Energy state	Mammalian target of rapamycin (mTOR) phosphorylated in states of energy abundance inhibiting autophagy: This is released in energy-depleted states[29]
Hormonal control	Vitamin D–dependent defensin and cathelicidin production (both PRRs)[30] Steroid and catecholamine up/down-regulate cytokine production[31,32]
Microbiome interactions	Gut microbiome activates the NLR3-inflammasome to induce pro IL-1β, but not its cleavage into IL-1β–pathogenic bacteria invading the microbiome and then induce the cleavage of pro IL-1β, producing a rapid inflammatory response[33]

cells. The pathway activates a proinflammatory response, with production and release of inflammatory cytokines. This is a common pathway of organ crosstalk in the ICU: Injury to one organ may result in a multiorgan effect. An overwhelming or dysregulated immune response locally within one organ, such as the lung in ARDS, can lead to multiorgan failure as large concentrations of inflammatory cytokines are sensed by distant organs.

4. Macrophage activation syndrome (MAS) and hemophagocytic lymphangiohistiocytosis (HLH): These diseases represent a broad spectrum, ranging from familial varieties with recognized to genetic mutations, to those associated with rheumatologic inflammatory conditions. This is an example of a dysregulated immune response. Ineffective cytotoxic activity of NK cells means an inability to effectively neutralize a threat such as a viral infection. This is a deficiency of the major "immune off-switch" of induced apoptosis of virally infected cells and results in a persistence of immune activation. The result is proliferation of phagocytes and a flood of proinflammatory cytokines, leading to a destructive systemic inflammatory state.

Therapeutic Targets of the Innate Immune System

Given the ubiquity of innate immune system activity, often to the detriment of the intensive care patient, it should offer several effective therapeutic targets. Sadly, although many "magic bullet" solutions have been sought, such as activated protein C and bactericidal/permeability-inducing protein (BPI), none have been found to be effective. The reasons for this are complex, but two possible reasons are immediately apparent: (1) evolution has furnished the innate immune system with a high degree of redundancy, in order to be "failsafe." Therefore targeting one component of the signal or response may be mitigated by a separate arm of the pathway. (2) The immune response is a juxtaposition of two opposing forces: a proinflammatory response to a threat, followed by a regulatory antiinflammatory restitution to baseline. Both are necessary, but both can become maladaptive. Any therapeutic measures therefore need to target the maladaptive process specifically. Attaining this level of specificity against either the proinflammatory or antiinflammatory arm, without disrupting the other, is difficult. Instead, the treatment may have to be adjusted according to the inflammatory profile at the time. Attention has now been diverted to accurate profiling of the inflammatory response, using genomic, transcriptomic, proteomic, and metabolomic biomarkers.

Therapeutic Questions Arising From the Innate Immune System

The innate immune system is relevant to many interventions in the ICU. Many molecules central in (superficially) non-immune physiologic processes play a role in the immune response.

1. Can oxygen be harmful?

Matching oxygen delivery to consumption is the foremost physiologic aim in the ICU. Measuring oxygen consumption with any degree of accuracy is difficult clinically. Oxygen delivery is estimated and guided by surrogate markers such as lactate and central venous saturations. Hypoxia is harmful and can initiate an immune response through HIF activation. In an attempt to avoid hypoxia, there is a tendency to err toward hyperoxia. However, it is emerging that hyperoxia can similarly cause harm. Although ROS is important in the innate immune response as described earlier, it is also toxic, as demonstrated by the utility of ROS in phagolysosomes. Hyperoxia increases ROS production, tipping the balance toward damage. In the mouse lung model, hyperoxia leads to ROS-mediated DNA damage, inflammation, and loss of barrier integrity. Unexpectedly, the proinflammatory effects of the TLR4-mediated pathways are not responsible for the damage (and subsequent death of mice), but rather the TLR4-dependent pathways are protective, by triggering antioxidant and proapototic pathways. Hyperoxia also affects pulmonary macrophage function, impairing their ability to kill pathogens.[37] This effect, likely mediated by HMGB-1 pathways, is important given the risk of ventilator-associated pneumonia in the ICU. Hyperoxia also seems to have longer-term effects; experienced in the neonatal period, it can alter the ability to fight influenza A in adult mice, thought to be mediated by both changes in epithelial cell PRRs and programming of hematopoietic cells.[38]

Clinically, hyperoxia has been associated with poor outcomes. This is most often shown in the context of cardiac arrest: hyperoxia following a period of ischemia, leading to an ischemia-reperfusion injury.[39] Therefore careful attention needs to be paid to oxygen use in the ICU. Randomized controlled trials are needed to identify the optimal oxygen level in different phenotypes (eg, as in preterm neonates).[40]

2. Is nutrition always beneficial?

Critical illness is a catabolic state with an increase in energy utilization. This has traditionally been believed to be due to the increase in metabolic activity to mount an immune and inflammatory response. This may be an oversimplification. Recent thinking suggests that there is an active switch from aerobic glucose metabolism to anaerobic glycolysis. This is known as the *Warburg effect,* first described in cancer cells. The driver for such a switch in cancer cells is initial hypoxia, activating HIFs, which inhibit pyruvate dehydrogenase. The effect of such a metabolic switch is to prevent apoptosis (due to loss of mitochondrial membrane potential and dysfunction) and increase cell proliferation. In sepsis the Warburg effect is seen in monocytes and macrophages in order to proliferate and mount an effective response. The use of glycolysis for energy production requires a large amount of glucose; therefore glucose uptake and protein and lipid breakdown are up-regulated.

Traditionally intensive care physicians have attempted to provide nutrition to match this energy-hungry catabolic state. Studies of early supplementation of enteral nutrition with parenteral nutrition to meet estimated nutritional needs have suggested that those without supplementation may be discharged alive from ICU earlier, although the overall mortality in both groups was the same.[41] However, those with no supplementation had fewer infections in the ICU, as also seen in trials comparing early versus late initiation of parenteral nutrition. This is proposed to be related to protein intake, particularly parenteral nutrition rather than enteral nutrition. The mechanism for this effect is not known: It is hypothesized that the increase in nutrition leads to impaired autophagy and therefore inefficient cellular metabolism and DAMP production.[42]

The route of nutrition can have an important effect on the immune response. Neutrophils exposed to parenteral lipids show impaired ability to eliminate pneumococci.[43] In contrast, enteral nutrition may have a beneficial effect on the innate immune response, through the effect of enteral nutrition on intestinal integrity and the gut microbiome. The microbiome has a protective effect on gut integrity as described earlier. However, specific nutritive interventions have not necessarily had the magnitude of effect expected: Probiotics have been shown to be effective in the treatment of *Clostridium difficile* infections but have not had a significant effect on overall critical illness outcomes.[44] In neonates, the gut microbiome is least poorly established. Metaanalysis evidence points to a survival benefit with probiotic treatment in preterm necrotizing enterocolitis.[45]

Compared with the nutritional addition of probiotics, manipulation of the microbiome using selective digestive tract decontamination (SDD) shows reasonable promise: Good-quality evidence points toward the effects of SDD in reducing hospital-acquired infections in the ICU.[46]

Finally, the concept of immunonutrition has emerged to provide specific supplements in nutrition, either enterally or parenterally, to modulate the immune response. Glutamine is used by several cells involved in the innate immune response: neutrophils, macrophages, and enterocytes. It is easily depleted in critical illness and has manifold functions. Although initial studies pointed to a potential benefit in critical illness outcomes, especially in some cohorts such as burns patients, larger trials have not borne this out. Arginine, necessary for nitric oxide production, may help reduce hospital-acquired infections but has not shown a mortality benefit in critical illness. Antioxidants such as selenium, zinc, copper, and vitamins B, C, and E have shown promise in reducing mortality in some patient groups (trauma, cardiac patients) and may also reduce hospital-acquired infections. Currently, the evidence does not support use in all patients in the ICU, and the evidence in children is lacking.

3. Should catecholamine use be limited?

Catecholamines, as described, have effects on the immune system while also promoting pathogen proliferation and virulence. Catecholamines are necessary in the intensive care armory, now more so given the recent doubts cast over the association between fluid resuscitation and mortality in sepsis. The risks and benefits of using catecholamines have not been directly demonstrated, but there is enough supportive evidence for their use. However, whether catecholamine use needs to be better tailored to the individual immune profile is yet to be determined. Catecholamines have wide-ranging effects: hemodynamic, metabolic, and endocrine in addition to the immune effects. Teasing out the beneficial and detrimental effects of each property will be challenging. For now, catecholamine use must be supported, but use should be titrated to effect closely, being mindful of the immunosuppressive and pathogen-promoting effects of catecholamines.[32]

4. Should fever be treated?

Despite the conservation of fever as an immune response across a wide range of species evolution, we are yet to be convinced that it has a beneficial role in overcoming danger. Preventing fever in most animal classes seems to increase mortality. In humans, fever reduces time to recovery in varicella infections, reduces rhinovirus shedding, and increases malaria parasite clearance. Concern exists in critically ill patients regarding the energy expenditure needed to produce a fever and the hemodynamic effects, such as tachycardia and hemodynamic changes. Two recent observational studies in the intensive care environment have challenged this concern. A retrospective review of more than 600,000 patients admitted to the ICU demonstrated that a peak temperature above 39°C in patients admitted with infective illness has a reduced risk of mortality.[14] This points toward a beneficial effect of fever in critical illness, particularly in those with infection. This is likely to be mediated by neutrophils: The neutropenic subpopulation in the first study did not show the beneficial effect of fever. Fever increases both ROS and nitric oxide species production by neutrophils: This may be a potential mechanistic explanation.[47] Alternatively, the interventions to reduce temperature may be detrimental. To further explore this, a large multicenter trial compared paracetamol versus placebo treatment of fever. No differences were seen between the two groups, although the temperature profiles for both groups were similar both before and after treatment.[48]

5. Does sedation just reduce metabolic demand?

So far we have not mentioned the role sedation may play on the immune system, despite the widespread use of sedation in the ICU. However, while sedation may be thought of as beneficial, in order to reduce metabolic demand in critical illness, the innate immune system does not escape its effects. Epidemiologically, chronic IV opiate abusers have been observed to present with a high number of infections. Macrophages and neutrophils have been known to have μ-opioid receptors. Morphine reduces macrophage recruitment, phagocytosis, and the respiratory burst in vivo. In mice, this leads to reduced bacterial clearance, an effect that was abolished in μ-opioid receptor knockout mice and by naltrexone. In addition, there is a suppression of chemokine production following morphine exposure, through suppression of NF-κB. Similarly, neutrophil recruitment is also suppressed by opioids, although there may be a differential effect of exogenous (suppressing chemotaxis) and endogenous (promoting chemotaxis) opioids. Acute morphine treatment has been shown to delay wound healing in laboratory models. However, currently there is no trial evidence in humans to suggest opioids delay recovery in intensive care patients.

Benzodiazepines are commonly used as sedative agents in the pediatric ICU. Peripheral (non-GABA) binding sites for benzodiazepines are present on immune cells including macrophages and neutrophils. Neutrophil chemotaxis can be inhibited in vitro by benzodiazepines. NF-κB activation is reduced by midazolam in macrophages, with a suppression of proinflammatory cytokines such as TNFα. Furthermore, lipopolysaccharide-induced superoxide production is inhibited by benzodiazepines in neutrophils and macrophages in vitro, affecting successful cytotoxic activity. Induced nitric oxide and cyclo-oxygenase activity is also reduced by benzodiazepines. In animal models of pneumonia, benzodiazepine treatment increases mortality.

Sedative centrally acting α2-agonists, clonidine and dexmedetomidine, do not affect human neutrophil chemotaxis, phagocytosis, or superoxide production in vitro. In animal models of sepsis, pretreatment (ie, before the induction of sepsis) with clonidine reduces NF-κB activation and cytokine production (as benzodiazepines) but reduces mortality by dampening the systemic inflammatory response.[49,50]

Why do benzodiazepines and α2-agonists have different effects on animal models of infection even though cytokine production is reduced by both? The differences may be more subtle than cytokine production—both agents have receptors on a variety of cell types and therefore have widespread actions. However, the effects of sedatives, as with any modulators of the immune response, may depend on the exact immune profile at any given time (eg, the balance of proinflammatory and antiinflammatory cytokines that lead to the immune phenotype). In the subgroup analysis of a trial comparing lorazepam-based sedation against dexmedetomidine, those sedated with dexmedetomidine were less likely to die or have brain dysfunction. This effect was more pronounced in the context of sepsis. Although this adds to the speculation that α2-agonists may have immune-favorable effects in critical illness, further mechanistic work with better phenotypic categorization is needed to prove this.

Conclusion

The innate immune system is the first line of defense against danger, both endogenous and exogenous. The pathways are complex, involving a large number of redundant processes and several orders of interactions between pathways and systems. Many molecules and cells involved in the innate immune system also have nonimmune functions. The innate immune system therefore should be thought of as not only a dedicated police force but also a neighborhood watch scheme. This has particular relevance in the ICU, as many of our interventions can affect the innate immune function. So while we are yet to harness our knowledge of the innate immune system to develop new therapies, there is probably more scope to better use existing therapies so as to not jeopardize the protective benefits of the innate immune response.

References

1. Matzinger P. The danger model: a renewed sense of self. *Science.* 2002;296:301-305.
2. Seong S, Matzinger P. Hydrophobicity: an ancient damage-associated molecular pattern that initiates innate immune responses. *Nat Rev Immunol.* 2004;4:469-478.
3. Bianchi ME. DAMPs, PAMPs and alarmins: all we need to know about danger. *J Leukoc Biol.* 2007;81:1-5.
4. Huebener P, Pradere JP, Hernandez C, et al. The HMGB1/RAGE axis triggers neutrophil-mediated injury amplification following necrosis. *J Clin Invest.* 2015;125:539-550.
5. Darton TC, Jack DL, Johnson M, et al. MBL2 deficiency is associated with higher genomic bacterial loads during meningococcemia in young children. *Clin Microbiol Infect.* 2014;20:1337-1342.

6. Agbeko RS, Fidler KJ, Allen ML, et al. Genetic variability in complement activation modulates the systemic inflammatory response syndrome in children. *Pediatr Crit Care Med*. 2010;11:561-567.

7. De Pascale G, Cutuli SL, Pennisi MA, Antonelli M. The role of mannose-binding lectin in severe sepsis and septic shock. *Mediators Inflamm*. 2013;2013:625803.

8. Levin M, Quint PA, Goldstein B, et al. Recombinant bactericidal/permeability-increasing protein (rBPI21) as adjunctive treatment for children with severe meningococcal sepsis: a randomised trial. rBPI21 Meningococcal Sepsis Study Group. *Lancet*. 2000;356:961-967.

9. Kawai T, Akira S. The role of pattern-recognition receptors in innate immunity: update on Toll-like receptors. *Nat Immunol*. 2010;11: 373-384.

10. Foley NM, Wang J, Redmond HP, et al. Current knowledge and future directions of TLR and NOD signalling in sepsis. *Mil Med Res*. 2015; 2:1.

11. O'Neill LA, Bowie AG. The family of five: TIR-domain-containing adaptors in Toll-like receptor signalling. *Nat Rev Immunol*. 2007;7:353-364.

12. Visvikis O, Ihuegbu N, Labed SA, et al. Innate host defense requires TFEB-mediated transcription of cytoprotective and antimicrobial genes. *Immunity*. 2014;40:896-909.

13. Young PJ, Saxena M, Beasley R, et al. Early peak temperature and mortality in critically ill patients with or without infection. *Intensive Care Med*. 2012;38:437-444.

14. Evans SS, Repasky EA, Fisher DT. Fever and the thermal regulation of immunity: the immune system feels the heat. *Nat Rev Immunol*. 2015;15:335-349.

15. Lee RJ, Kofonow JM, Rosen PL, et al. Bitter and sweet taste receptors regulate human upper respiratory innate immunity. *J Clin Invest*. 2014; 124:1393-1405.

16. Pettengill MA, van Haren SD, Levy O. Soluble mediators regulating immunity in early life. *Front Immunol*. 2014;5:457.

17. Henneke P, Golenbock DT. Phagocytosis, innate immunity, and host-pathogen specificity. *J Exp Med*. 2004;199:1-4.

18. Singer PM, De Santis V, Vitale D, et al. Multiorgan failure is an adaptive, endocrine-mediated, metabolic response to overwhelming systemic inflammation. *Lancet*. 2004;364:545-548.

19. Vlada CA, Kim JS, Behrns KE. Autophagy: self-preservation through cannibalism of proteins and organelles. *Surgery*. 2015;157:1-5.

20. Fink SL, Cookson BT. Apoptosis, pyroptosis, and necrosis: mechanistic description of dead and dying eukaryotic cells. *Infect Immun*. 2005;73: 1907-1916.

21. Levi M, Schultz M, Van Der Poll T. Sepsis and thrombosis. *Semin Thromb Hemost*. 2013;39:559-566.

22. Annane D, Timsit JF, Mégarbane B, et al. Recombinant human activated protein C for adults with septic shock: a randomized controlled trial. *Am J Respir Crit Care Med*. 2013;187:1091-1097.

23. Ranieri VM, Thompson BT, Barie PS, et al. Drotecogin alfa (activated) in adults with septic shock. *N Engl J Med*. 2012;366:2055-2064.

24. Nadel S, Goldstein B, Williams MD, et al. Drotrecogin alfa (activated) in children with severe sepsis: a multicentre phase III randomised controlled trial. *Lancet*. 2007;369:836-843.

25. Clark SR, Ma AC, Tavener SA, et al. Platelet TLR4 activates neutrophil extracellular traps to ensnare bacteria in septic blood. *Nat Med*. 2007; 13:463-469.

26. Barnig C, Levy BD. Innate immunity is a key factor for the resolution of inflammation in asthma. *Eur Respir Rev*. 2015;24:141-153.

27. Lee J, Mo J-H, Katakura K, et al. Maintenance of colonic homeostasis by distinctive apical TLR9 signalling in intestinal epithelial cells. *Nat Cell Biol*. 2006;8:1327-1336.

28. Kazama H, Ricci JE, Herndon JM, et al. Induction of immunological tolerance by apoptotic cells requires caspase-dependent oxidation of high-mobility group box-1 protein. *Immunity*. 2008;29:21-32.

29. Inoue H, Tani K. Multimodal immunogenic cancer cell death as a consequence of anticancer cytotoxic treatments. *Cell Death Differ*. 2014; 21:39-49.

30. Leaf DE, Croy HE, Abrahams SJ, et al. Cathelicidin antimicrobial protein, vitamin D, and risk of death in critically ill patients. *Crit Care*. 2015;19:1.

31. Hartemink KJ, Groeneveld AB. Vasopressors and inotropes in the treatment of human septic shock: effect on innate immunity? *Inflammation*. 2012;35:206-213.

32. Sprung CL, Annane D, Keh D, et al. Hydrocortisone therapy for patients with septic shock. *N Engl J Med*. 2008;358:111-124.

33. Shreiner AB, Kao JY, Young VB. The gut microbiome in health and in disease. *Curr Opin Gastroenterol*. 2015;31:69-75.

34. Eltzschig HK, Carmeliet P. Hypoxia and inflammation. *N Engl J Med*. 2011;364:656-665.

35. Hirsiger S, Simmen HP, Werner CML, et al. Danger signals activating the immune response after trauma. *Mediators Inflamm*. 2012;2012:315941. doi: 10.1155/2012/315941.

36. Stocker CF, Shekerdemian LS, Visvanathan K, et al. Cardiopulmonary bypass elicits a prominent innate immune response in children with congenital heart disease. *J Thorac Cardiovasc Surg*. 2004;127:1523-1525.

37. Baleeiro CE, Wilcoxen SE, Morris SB, et al. Sublethal hyperoxia impairs pulmonary innate immunity. *J Immunol*. 2003;171:955-963.

38. Reilly EC, Martin KC, Jin GB, et al. Neonatal hyperoxia leads to persistent alterations in NK responses to influenza A virus infection. *Am J Physiol Lung Cell Mol Physiol*. 2014;308:L76-L85.

39. Kilgannon JH, Jones AE, Shapiro NI, et al. Association between arterial hyperoxia following resuscitation from cardiac arrest and in-hospital mortality. *JAMA*. 2010;303:2165-2171.

40. BOOST II United Kingdom Collaborative Group; BOOST II Australia Collaborative Group; BOOST II New Zealand Collaborative Group. Oxygen saturation and outcomes in preterm infants. *N Engl J Med*. 2013; 368:2094-2104.

41. Casaer MP, Mesotten D, Hermans G, et al. Early versus late parenteral nutrition in critically ill adults. *N Engl J Med*. 2011;365:506-517.

42. Desai SV, McClave SA, Rice TW. Nutrition in the ICU: an evidence-based approach. *Chest*. 2014;145:1148-1157.

43. Versleijen MW, Roelofs HM, Te Morsche RH, et al. Parenteral lipids impair pneumococcal elimination by human neutrophils. *Eur J Clin Invest*. 2010;40:729-734.

44. Petrof EO, Dhaliwal R, Manzanares W, et al. Probiotics in the critically ill. *Crit Care Med*. 2012;40:1.

45. Alfaleh K, Bassler D. Probiotics for prevention of necrotizing enterocolitis in preterm infants. *Cochrane Database Syst Rev*. 2008;(1):CD005496.

46. De Smet MGA, Kluytmans JW, Cooper BS, et al. Decontamination of the digestive tract and oropharynx in ICU patients. *N Engl J Med*. 2009; 360:20-31.

47. Rosenspire AJ, Kindzelskii AL, Petty HR. Cutting edge: fever-associated temperatures enhance neutrophil responses to lipopolysaccharide: a potential mechanism involving cell metabolism. *J Immunol*. 2002;169: 5396-5400.

48. Young P, Saxena M, HEAT Investigators; Australian and New Zealand Intensive Care Society Clinical Trials Group. Acetaminophen for fever in critically ill patients with suspected infection. *N Engl J Med*. 2015; 373:2215-2224.

49. Finnerty M, Marczynski TJ, Amirault HJ, et al. Benzodiazepines inhibit neutrophil chemotaxis and superoxide production in a stimulus dependent manner; PK-11195 antagonizes these effects. *Immunopharmacology*. 1991;22:185-193.

50. Pandharipande PP, Sanders RD, Girard TD, et al. Effect of dexmedetomidine versus lorazepam on outcome in patients with sepsis: an a priori-designed analysis of the MENDS randomized controlled trial. *Crit Care*. 2010;14:R38.

Adaptive Immunity

W. Joshua Frazier, Kristin C. Greathouse, and Jennifer A. Muszynski

PEARLS

- Unlike the innate immune response, the adaptive immune response is characterized by specific antigen recognition and immunologic memory.
- Lymphocytes are the key cell types of the adaptive immune response.
- B lymphocytes differentiate into antibody-secreting plasma cells and are responsible for humoral immunity.
- CD8+ T lymphocytes differentiate into cytotoxic T cells, which function to control viruses and other intracellular pathogens by directly killing infected cells.
- CD4+ T lymphocytes differentiate into a myriad of helper T-cell subsets, which regulate and coordinate the overall immune response and span a spectrum from highly proinflammatory to potently immunosuppressive function.

Introduction

The adaptive immune system is generally considered an additional line of defense after innate immunity. There are several important differences between the innate and adaptive immune systems. First, adaptive immunity takes more time to develop than the rapid onset of inflammation induced by innate immune cells. Second, rather than the more nonspecific activation of innate immune cells by pattern recognition receptors, components of the adaptive immune system develop to recognize specific pathogens. Finally, immunologic memory is a hallmark of the adaptive immune system, which allows for a more rapid and robust immune response upon repeated exposure of the same pathogen. Although it is helpful to consider the innate and adaptive immune systems as distinct, in reality these two systems rely heavily on each other for activation and coordination of an overall immune response. Consequently, there is a great degree of crosstalk between the two systems, which will be highlighted throughout this chapter.

The primary cell types of the adaptive immune response are lymphocytes, which can be broadly classified into B cells and T cells. B cells differentiate into plasma cells and function primarily to produce antibodies, essential for humoral immunity. T cells, by contrast, differentiate into effector cells with a variety of functions, including killing infected cells, directing the activation or suppression of innate immune cells, promoting innate immune cell migration, and enhancing barrier and immunologic function of epithelial cells. This chapter focuses on the cellular components of adaptive immunity. The chapter

begins with a brief overview of B-cell and T-cell development, followed by a discussion of B-cell function and humoral immunity. Next, the authors discuss T-cell activation followed by differentiation and function of first CD8+ cytotoxic T cells then CD4+ T helper cells. The chapter concludes with an introduction to adaptive immunity in the ICU.

Lymphocytes Develop to Recognize Specific Antigens

B cells and T cells are so named for their respective sites of maturation: bone marrow for B cells and thymus for T cells. The development of both cell types has many similarities, which result in a diverse repertoire of lymphocytes, each able to recognize a specific antigen. Both B and T lymphocytes arise from common lymphoid progenitors, which derive from hematopoietic stem cells. B cells develop in response to transcription factors EBF, E2a, and Pax-5, whereas the transcription factors NOTCH-1 and GATA-3 drive T-cell development. For both cell types, one of the earliest steps in development involves gene rearrangements in the antigen recognition regions of the immunoglobulin heavy chain locus (B cells) or the T-cell receptor (T cells). This gene rearrangement process is necessary to develop a wide array of cells with specific antigen recognition regions. The next steps involve positive and negative selection, resulting in a final repertoire of cells capable of recognizing processed foreign antigen while not reacting to self-antigens. Immature B cells express IgM on their surface. If they bind strongly to self-peptides in the bone marrow, they are either depleted or they undergo further gene rearrangements in a process called receptor editing. B cells that survive negative selection leave the bone marrow and migrate to peripheral lymphoid organs where they await activation and further maturation to antibody-secreting plasma cells.

Immature T cells undergo both positive and negative selection in the thymus. Positive selection is carried out in the cortex of the thymus where T cells that recognize peptides presented by dendritic cell major histocompatibility complex (MHC) molecules survive. Negative selection occurs after positive selection and is carried out in the corticomedullary junction of the thymus. Here, T cells that have either strong affinity or no affinity to self-peptides bound to MHC molecules are deleted by apoptotic cell death. Meanwhile, immature T cells with weak affinity for self-peptides bound to MHC survive. In this way, surviving T cells are capable of recognizing self-MHC molecules but do not react strongly to self-antigens. These surviving T cells (naïve T cells) leave the thymus and continuously circulate through and among peripheral lymphoid organs, making multiple contacts with resident antigen-presenting cells capable of T-cell activation.

B-Cell Activation Leads to Antibody Secretion: The Humoral Immune Response

The humoral immune response is driven by antibodies, which are produced following the stimulation, proliferation, and differentiation of naïve B cells. Naïve B cells are activated in secondary lymphoid organs, such as local lymph nodes or the spleen where they encounter processed microbial protein fragments (antigens) bound to MHC class II proteins on the surface of professional antigen-presenting cells (APCs). Antigen recognition and subsequent B-cell activation often occurs in the presence of specialized helper T cells, which facilitate and direct B-cell differentiation. Once activated by the overlapping signals provided by APCs and helper T cells, B cells proliferate and differentiate. Some B-cell clones develop into plasma cells, which are factories for high-level antibody production. Other clones differentiate into memory B cells, which are long lived and allow for the anamnestic nature of the secondary immune response, whereby subsequent encounters with a pathogen lead to a faster, higher magnitude antibody response. Although a B cell and its antibody products are specific to only a single antigen or epitope, it is important to note that any given microorganism contains many foreign proteins that are potentially antigenic. Indeed, an invading bacterium may contain dozens or hundreds of antigenic peptide sequences, each capable of stimulating a B cell (and likely a T cell). Thus, the majority of humoral immune responses are polyclonal, meaning multiple B-cell populations are engaged in the response and high titers of a wide variety of antibodies are produced, all of which are specific to the pathogen.

Antibodies, also called immunoglobulins (Ig), are the primary product of B cells and constitute the effector element of the humoral immune response. Fig. 102.1 depicts general immunoglobulin structure. The classic antibody is constructed of two heavy chains, bound to each other, and two light chains, each bound to a heavy chain. The variable regions of the heavy and light chains contribute to the formation of the antigen-binding site, also referred to as the antigen-binding fraction (Fab) segment. As their name suggests, variable regions differ among individual antibodies and are responsible for the specificity of the antibody response. The remaining antibody fraction is denoted the Fc portion (for crystallizable fraction).

Antibodies confer protection by two mechanisms: neutralization and opsonization (Fig. 102.2). Neutralizing antibodies slow or halt infection by binding proteins, which confer virulence to the invading microorganism, such as a viral receptor, and preventing them from functioning. Neutralizing antibodies also bind and protect the host from secreted microbial toxins. This ability underlies lifesaving passive immune therapies for infections such as botulism and diphtheria. Opsonization is the process by which Fc receptors on the surface of innate immune effector cells bind the Fc portion of antigen-bound antibodies, facilitating phagocytosis and the killing of antibody-coated microorganisms. In addition to direct opsonization, the exposed Fc portion of bound antibodies also activates the complement cascade. Complement activation further augments the antiinfective response by either directly killing bacteria through assembly of the membrane attack

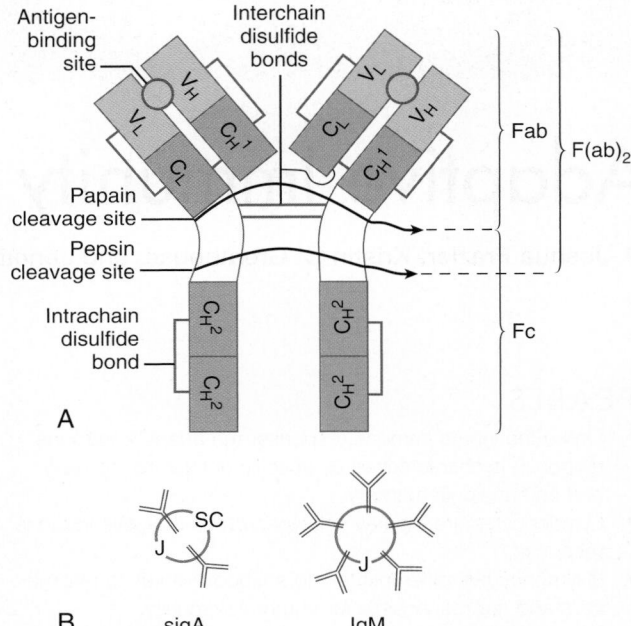

Fig. 102.1. Basic structure of the immunoglobulin molecule. (A) The stereotypical antibody has a general "Y" shape and is composed of two heavy chains and two light chains bound to each other by disulfide bonds. Both chains contain constant regions, constant heavy (CH) and constant light (CL), of conserved amino acid sequences, which are alike in all antibody molecules of the same class, and variable regions (VH and VL), which are highly variable and unique to the antigen-binding site of each individual antibody. Sites of papain or pepsin proteolytic cleavage result in the Fab and Fc immunoglobulin fragments. (B) IgA and IgM are polymeric antibodies composed of 2 (IgA) or 5 (IgM) basic immunoglobulin chain units.

complex or by further opsonization via complement proteins such as C3.

B cells produce antigen-specific antibodies with variations in structure that impact function. These different antibody classes, or isotypes, add important nuance to the adaptive immune response to infection. Changing the antibody produced by a B cell from one class to another is known as isotype switching or class switching and is mediated by a complex interplay of cytokines and helper T-cell interaction. Specific functions and characteristics of antibody classes are outlined in Table 102.1. Of particular relevance is the temporal relationship between IgM and IgG in the context of new infection. In the primary immune response, in which the adaptive immune system recognizes a previously unencountered threat, the first class of antibody produced after B-cell activation is IgM. Over the course of the immune response, levels of IgM fall and are replaced by high levels of IgG. Subsequent exposure to the same pathogen generates high levels of IgG with a much shorter latency between antigen exposure and antibody production. This temporal relationship comes into play diagnostically when one obtains serologies, or infection-specific immunoglobulin levels, to diagnose infection.

Aside from their critical role in the adaptive immune response to infectious disease, antibodies have important roles in other aspects of human biology. Antibodies directed inappropriately against self-derived antigens (so-called autoantigens) are key elements in the pathophysiology of autoimmune

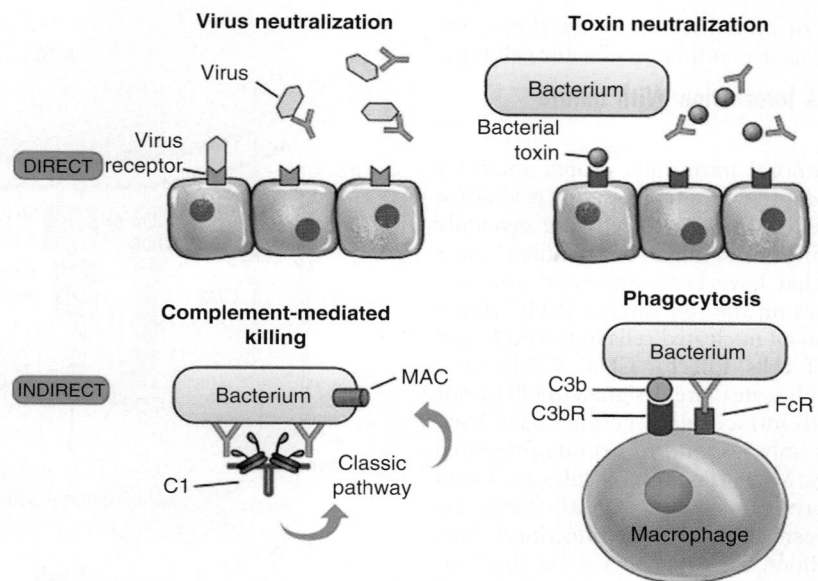

Fig. 102.2. Direct and indirect antibody functions. Antibodies function to directly neutralize microbial virulence factors, such as virus receptors or bacterial toxins. Indirect antibody function includes complement activation and opsonization, whereby phagocytic cells recognize the Fc portion of pathogen-bound antibodies, prompting phagocytosis and microbial killing.

TABLE 102.1	Characteristics of Antibody Isotypes			
Isotype (Class)	**Functions**	**Subclasses**	**Present in Secretions**	**Placental Transfer**
IgG	• Opsonize antigens for phagocytosis • Complement activation • Antibody-dependent cell killing by NK cells • Neonatal immunity via placental transfer	IgG₁ IgG₂ IgG₃ IgG₄	+ + + −	+++ + +++ ++
IgM	• Complement activation • Antigen recognition by naïve B cells		+	−
IgA	• Mucosal immunity	IgA₁ IgA₂ sIgA	+ + ++++	− − −
IgE	• Mast cell degranulation		+	−
IgD	• Antigen recognition by naïve B cells		−	−

NK, natural killer cell.

disease. A classic example is myasthenia gravis, in which autoantibodies bind to the neuromuscular junction, preventing stimulation of muscle fibers and resulting in weakness. Autoantibody-mediated autoimmune diseases are often treated with a combination of immunosuppressive medications and therapies, which reduce antibody titer, such as therapeutic apheresis. Additionally, immunosuppressive therapies to prevent rejection of transplanted organs often involve maneuvers to reduce antibody production—for example, the B-cell reducing agent rituximab.

Due to their ability to recognize and bind specific proteins, antibodies are increasingly used to develop targeted therapies, diagnostic assays, and a multitude of research tools. Indeed, the development of technologies to generate and mass-produce monoclonal antibodies has created many new therapeutic agents and diagnostic tools. An example of monoclonal antibody use that has become ubiquitous in the modern

practice of diagnostic medicine is the enzyme-linked immunosorbent assay (ELISA). This powerful tool involves the use of monoclonal antibodies that are specific to certain proteins of interest, such as anti-HIV antibody. When exposed to a patient sample, the monoclonal antibodies will bind relevant material, if present, from patient blood or plasma. When secondary fluorescent antibody is applied, it is possible to detect and quantify the protein of interest. ELISA is just one of many examples of antibody-based techniques used in both clinical diagnostics and basic/translational research, including Western blot, flow cytometry, immunofluorescence assays, and others.

Effector T Cells Direct Cell-Mediated Immunity

Like B cells, naïve T cells are activated in secondary lymphoid organs, where they proliferate and differentiate into either memory cells or effector T cells. Effector T cells migrate from lymphoid organs to sites of inflammation where they carry out a multitude of functions depending on effector cell type.

T-Cell Activation Requires Interaction With Innate Immune Cells

As was the case with humoral immunity, proper interplay between the innate and adaptive immune systems is vital for activation of cell-mediated immunity. T cells are generally unable to respond to so-called free antigen but require contact with antigenic peptides that have been processed and displayed via MHC molecules on the cell surface. MHC class I molecules are expressed on all nucleated cells in the body and are recognized by CD8+ T cells. Effector CD8+ T cells (also known as cytotoxic T lymphocytes) are designed to kill tumor cells and cells infected with intracellular microbes or viruses. By contrast, CD4+ T cells only respond to peptide presented by MCH class II molecules. MCH class II molecules are found on specialized antigen-presenting cells (APCs). APCs are designed to capture antigen at the site of infection/injury, process it into small peptides, and transport it via the lymphatics for presentation to T cells in secondary lymphoid organs. There are two types of APCs: (1) professional APCs are innate immune cells that constitutively express MHC class II molecules and include dendritic cells, macrophages, and certain B lymphocytes; (2) nonprofessional APCs express MHC class II molecules only when stimulated by certain cytokines such as interferon gamma (IFNγ) and include endothelial and some epithelial cells. Because nonprofessional APCs are not efficient at processing antigen into MHC binding peptides, they likely contribute to a minority of T-cell responses. Dendritic cells, on the other hand, are highly effective professional APCs responsible for the majority of naïve T-cell activation.

Under normal circumstances, each T-cell receptor recognizes and binds to only a specific antigenic peptide bound to the peptide-binding groove of an MHC molecule. This form of activation results in a highly regulated, specific response. Super antigens are an exception to this rule. Super antigens are capable of cross-linking MHC molecules with families of T-cell receptors, thus inducing the activation of large numbers of T cells at once. This cross-linking does not require antigen processing and presentation by innate immune cells and consequently super antigen-mediated diseases can present with a rapidly fulminating course. Such is the case for toxic shock syndrome, which is caused by staphylococcal or streptococcal bacterial toxins functioning as super antigens. Because the signs and symptoms—and much of the morbidity—of toxic shock syndrome are toxin mediated, antibiotic regimens generally include the addition of clindamycin to decrease toxin production. The addition of intravenous immunoglobulin (IVIG) to deliver toxin-neutralizing antibodies may also be of benefit, with observational studies demonstrating associations between IVIG use and decreased mortality in patients with toxic shock syndrome and other severe invasive group A streptococcal infections.[1,2]

T-Cell Activation Requires a Second Signal

As an additional layer of regulation, T-cell activation requires APCs to deliver two signals (Fig. 102.3). The first is the antigen-specific T-cell receptor (TCR)/MHC interaction. The second signal is the antigen nonspecific costimulatory signal and is provided by the interaction between costimulatory

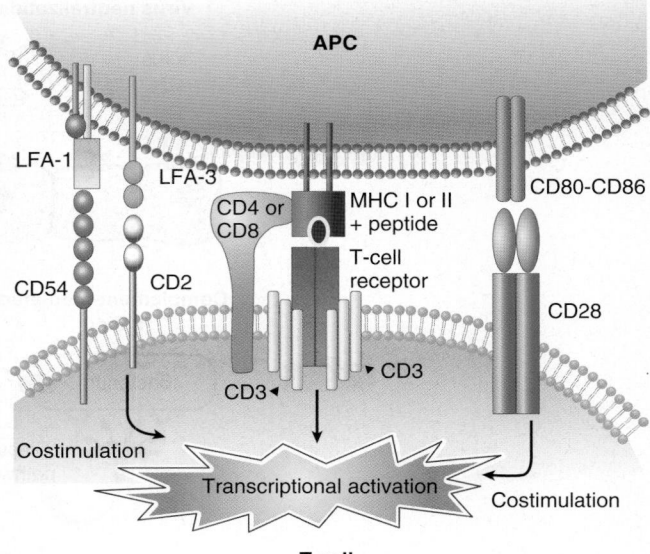

Fig. 102.3. T-cell activation requires multiple signals. T cells and antigen-presenting cells (APCs) interact at the immunologic synapse. Circulating T cells transiently bind APCs allowing the T-cell receptor (TCR) to interact with multiple MHC molecules. Recognition of an MHC-bound antigenic peptide activates integrins, such as lymphocyte function–associated antigen-1 (LFA-1), and adhesion molecules such as CD54, also known as intercellular adhesion molecule (ICAM)-1, which serves to stabilize the immunologic synapse. MHC molecule/antigen recognition by the T-cell receptor/CD3 complex and coreceptor (CD4 or CD8) and a costimulatory signal often resulting from binding of CD28 and B7 (CD80 or 86) family members are required for T-cell activation.

molecules expressed on APCs and receptors expressed by the T cell. If a T cell receives only antigen-specific TCR stimulation in the absence of costimulation, it will be rendered unresponsive to subsequent antigenic challenge. This process, which creates anergic T cells, is an important peripheral mechanism to promote T-cell tolerance to self-antigens. Costimulatory pathways can provide either *positive* signals that promote T-cell proliferation and differentiation or *negative* signals that inhibit T-cell responses and further mediate T-cell tolerance. As such, these pathways provide critical immunoregulatory function.

Table 102.2 outlines costimulatory molecules of the CD28:B7 families. The classic T-cell costimulatory ligand is CD28, which binds B7-1 (CD80) or B7-2 (CD86) molecules expressed on activated APCs. B7:CD28 binding augments T-cell activation by increasing the expression of antiapoptotic proteins, augmenting metabolic activity, enhancing T-cell proliferation, and inducing secretion of the cytokine interleukin-2 (IL-2). Under normal circumstances, the B7 costimulators are either absent or expressed at low levels on resting APCs. Their surface expression is induced by APC activation via toll-like receptor signaling or inflammatory cytokines such as IFNγ. In this way, T-cell activation occurs only in the presence of innate immune cell activation or local inflammation. In turn, activated CD4+ T cells further enhance the expression of B7 costimulators on APCs, which serves as a positive feedback loop for continued amplification of T-cell responses. An important mechanism for this feedback loop is via CD40 on APCs binding to CD40 ligand on activated CD4+

TABLE 102.2   T-Cell Costimulatory Receptors of the CD28 Family and Their Ligands

Receptor	Ligand(s)	Cells That Express Ligand(s)	Effects
Positive Costimulation			
CD28	B7-1(CD80) B7-2 (CD86)	DC, macrophages, B cells	Costimulate naïve T-cell activation
ICOS	ICOS-L	DC, macrophages, B cells	Promote differentiation of follicular helper T cells
Negative Costimulation			
CTLA-4	B7-1(CD80) B7-2 (CD86)	DC, macrophages, B cells	Negatively regulate T-cell response
PD-1	PD-L1(CD274) PD-L2 (CD273)	DC, macrophages, B cells, epithelial cells	Negatively regulate T-cell response

DC, dendritic cell; *ICOS,* inducible costimulatory molecule.

T cells. CD40:CD40L binding further activates APCs, enhancing their expression of B7 molecules and their secretion of cytokines (such as IL-12) to promote T-cell differentiation.

Although the CD28:B7 costimulatory pathway provides positive second signals that promote T-cell activation, cytotoxic T-lymphocyte antigen 4 (CTLA-4) and programmed death 1 (PD-1) are examples of negative costimulatory pathways. CTLA-4, expressed on the surface of T cells, is a high-affinity receptor for B7 molecules. As such, CTLA-4 is capable of binding low levels of B7 on resting APCS displaying self-antigen. CTLA-4:B7 binding then inhibits access of CD28 to B7, which blocks the positive costimulatory pathway.

PD-1 expression on peripheral lymphocytes and monocytes is induced upon activation. Binding of PD-1 to its ligand(s) negatively regulates T-cell responses by inhibiting T-cell receptor signaling and by promoting the differentiation and function of immunosuppressive regulatory T cells. Clinically, the PD-1 pathway is implicated in T-cell exhaustion due to chronic viral illness and may play a role in sepsis-induced immune suppression.[3-6]

CD8+ T Cells Differentiate Into Cytotoxic T Cells

CD8+ T cells are integral to the immune response against viruses and other intracellular pathogens. As discussed earlier, CD8+ T-cell activation begins with recognition of antigenic peptide presented by MHC I molecules on the surface of an infected cell or an antigen-presenting cell. In some cases, CD4+ helper T cells may help promote CD8+ T-cell development via APC activation or by cytokine secretion. Cytokines that stimulate CD8+ T-cell growth and differentiation include IL-2, IL-12, IFNγ, IL-15, and IL-21. Once activated, CD8+ T cells undergo clonal expansion and differentiation into fully functional cytotoxic T lymphocytes (CTLs). Activated CTLs use one of two mechanisms to kill infected target cells (Fig. 102.4). In the first mechanism, the CTL delivers the cytotoxic protein content of its cytoplasmic granules (perforins and granzymes) to the target cell. Perforins facilitate the transport of granzymes to the cytosol of the target cell where the granzymes cleave caspase proteins, initiating apoptotic cell death. A second method of CTL-mediated target cell death involves the binding of FasL (CD178) on the CTL surface with Fas (CD95) on the target cell surface. Fas:FasL binding initiates a signal transduction cascade leading to caspase activation and apoptosis. In addition to directing target cell death, cytotoxic T lymphocytes secrete the cytokine IFNγ, which serves to activate local macrophages and promote particular helper T-cell

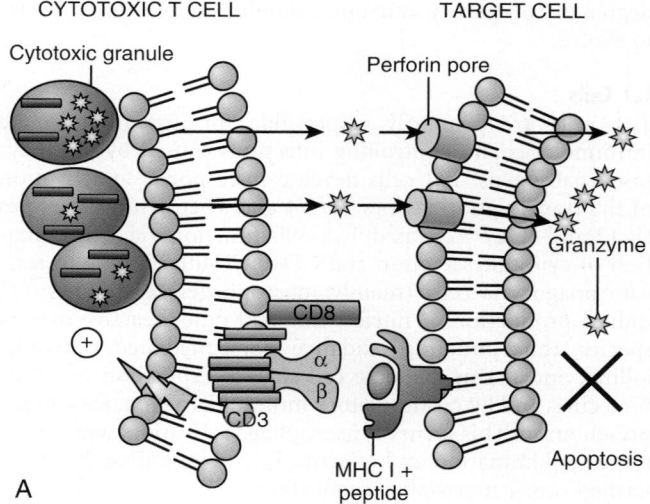

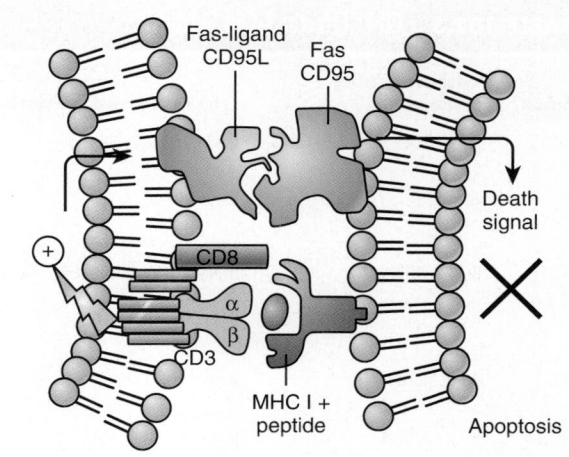

Fig. 102.4. Cytotoxic T cells induce target cell apoptosis by two mechanisms. (A) Contents of cytotoxic granules (granzymes) are delivered to the target cell via perforin proteins. Granzymes directly activate caspases, initiating apoptotic cell death. (B) Fas-ligand binding to Fas on target cells initiates a signal transduction cascade leading to apoptosis.

responses (eg, T_H1), thus providing additional crosstalk between innate and adaptive immunity.

CD4⁺ T Cells Differentiate Into Multiple T Helper Cell Subtypes

When naïve CD4⁺ T cells are activated, they proliferate and differentiate into a variety of effector helper T-cell subtypes, each with distinct function and cytokine signatures. Cytokines present in the local environment at the time of T-cell activation largely determine the direction of subtype differentiation. Properties of individual T helper cell subtypes are outlined in Table 102.3. Though it is helpful to think about effector T helper cell subtypes as distinct, fully differentiated cells, evidence suggests that effector T cells retain the ability to change subtype.[7,8] This degree of plasticity coupled with ever increasing recognition of novel T helper cell subtypes speaks to a high degree of complexity, our understanding of which continues to evolve.

T_H1 Cells

T_H1 cells are primarily responsible for activating innate immune cells and controlling infections caused by phagocytosed pathogens. T_H1 cells develop in response to activation of the transcription factors STAT4 and Tbet by the cytokines IL-12 and IFNγ. Activated T_H1 cells function via a combination of cytokine secretion and CD40:CD40L binding to activate phagocytic cells (mainly macrophages) as follows: (1) induce production of nitric oxide and other reactive oxygen species, thus initiating oxidative burst-mediated microbial killing, and (2) up-regulate cell surface expression of MHC molecules and B7 costimulatory molecules to enhance antigen presentation. This form of macrophage activation, which promotes inflammation and effective microbial killing, has been termed *classic* macrophage activation.

T_H2 Cells

T_H2 cells, by contrast, promote "alternative" macrophage activation characterized by the production of antiinflammatory cytokines, IL-10 and transforming growth factor beta (TGFβ). For this reason, T_H2 cells are generally thought of as an antiinflammatory helper T-cell subset. T_H2 cells develop in response to IL-4–mediated activation of the transcription factors STAT6 and GATA-3. The primary antiinfective role of T_H2 cells is to direct mast cells, eosinophils, and the humoral immune response toward control of parasitic infection. These cells also play important roles in promoting IgE-mediated allergic reactions.

T_H17 Cells

T_H17 cells develop in response to activation of the transcription factors STAT3 and RORγt in the setting of multiple cytokines, including IL-1, IL-6, IL-23, and TGFβ. T_H17 cells are often found associated with mucosal surfaces (eg, the gastrointestinal tract) and are likely involved in immunity to mucosal pathogens. They are potently proinflammatory cells and have been implicated in a number of autoimmune and inflammatory conditions.[9,10] Specific functions of T_H17 cells include recruiting leukocytes (primarily neutrophils) to sites of infection, promoting the production of antimicrobial peptides such as defensins, enhancing epithelial barrier function and cytokine production, and enhancing CD8⁺ T-cell activity.

T Follicular Helper (T_{FH}) Cells

T_{FH} cells are a relatively recently identified T helper cell subset and they primarily reside in and around germinal centers of secondary lymphoid organs.[11] Their development relies on interaction with activated B cells via the inducible costimulatory (ICOS) molecule and activation of the transcription factor BCL-6. T_{FH} cells function within germinal

TABLE 102.3	CD4⁺ Effector T-Cell Subsets			
Subset	Cytokines Directing Development	Cytokines Secreted by Subset	Role in Promoting Inflammation	Functions
T_H17	IL-1, IL-6, IL-23, TGFβ	IL-17, IL-21, IL-22	+ + +	• Recruit neutrophils and macrophages to site of inflammation • Promote G-CSF production to ↑ neutrophil numbers • Promote epithelial cell barrier function • Induce epithelial cell cytokine production
T_H1	IL-12, IFNγ	IFNγ, IL-2, GM-CSF, TNFβ, CCL2	+ +	• Classic macrophage activation • ↑ Macrophage NO, ROS production • Direct B cells to ↑ IgG and ↓ IgE • ↑ T_H1 differentiation and ↓ T_H2
T_{FH}	IL-6, IL-21	IL-4, IL-21	+	• Activate B cells and promote differentiation to antibody-secreting plasma cells
T_H9	IL-4, TGFβ	IL-9, IL-10, IL-21	+	• ↑ Mast cell proliferation and activity • ↑ Eosinophil recruitment • ↑ T_H2 responses and IgE production • Promote lymphocyte recruitment and IFNγ production
T_H2	IL-4	IL-4, IL-5, IL-10, IL-13	+ −	• Direct macrophages toward alternative (immunosuppressive) activation • Direct B cells to produce IgE • Activate eosinophils • ↑ T_H2 differentiation and ↓ T_H1
T_{reg}	IL-2, TGFβ	IL-10, TGFβ	− −	• Suppress macrophage activation • Suppress T_H1 development

NO, nitric oxide; *ROS,* reactive oxygen species.

centers to promote B-cell proliferation and immunoglobulin production.

T$_H$9 Cells

T$_H$9 cells are another relatively recently identified T helper cell subset and, as the name implies, they are characterized by secretion of the cytokine, IL-9. T$_H$9 cells may be primarily located in the skin and along mucosal surfaces. Like T$_H$2 cells, activated T$_H$9 cells enhance mast cell function, eosinophil recruitment, and IgE production and provide immunity against parasitic infection. They also promote lymphocyte recruitment and IFNγ production and have been implicated in autoimmune and allergic diseases including eczema, asthma, food allergies, and inflammatory bowel disease.[12,13]

Regulatory T Cells (Treg)

Naturally occurring regulatory T cells (Treg) are an immunosuppressive subset of CD4$^+$ T cells characterized by high expression of the cell surface marker CD25 and diminished expression of the IL-7 receptor, CD127. The transcription factor FOXP3 is required for Treg development and function, and it serves as an additional Treg marker. Treg cells arise in the thymus during T-cell development in response to recognition of self-peptide. Though they constitute a relatively small percentage of the total circulating T-cell population (approximately 5%-10% under normal circumstances), they play an important role in maintaining T-cell tolerance to self-antigens. In the ICU, whereas down-regulation of Treg cells may contribute to autoimmune and allergic disease, pathologic up-regulation of Treg cells have been associated with immune suppression and adverse outcomes in critically ill septic adults. These studies, however, have not been consistent, and whether Treg cells play a role in pediatric sepsis is currently unclear.[14-18]

Additional T-Cell Subtypes

Although the majority of circulating T cells carry T-cell receptors composed of an α and a β chain, a minority of T cells (<5%) contain T-cell receptors composed of a γ chain and a δ chain. These cells are referred to as γδ T cells. Unlike αβ T cells, γδ T cells are not MHC restricted, meaning that they can recognize antigens not bound by MHC molecules. The γδ T cells also may be activated by nonprotein microbial antigens such as phosphates and lipids as well as heat shock proteins. When activated, γδ T cells produce inflammatory cytokines, IFNγ, tumor necrosis factor alpha (TNF)α, and IL-17. Because γδ T cells often reside at epithelial surfaces, it is thought that they serve an important function in the early defense against epithelial microbes.[19]

NKT cells are a second small subset of T cells with distinct function. NKT cells are so named because they carry both natural killer (NK) cell markers (eg, CD 56) and a T-cell receptor. NKT cells function like innate immune cells in that they quickly produce cytokines in response to pathogens. They also respond in an antigen-dependent manner via T-cell receptor recognition of lipid antigens bound to MHC-like molecules called CD1d.[20]

Adaptive Immunity in the Intensive Care Unit

A well-functioning immune response is vital to the resolution of infection, prevention of new infection, and recovery from critical illness. However, as will be reviewed in greater detail in Chapter 105, critical illness is often associated with suppressed immune cell function, which is associated with increased risks of nosocomial infection and mortality.[15,21-24] Although much of the work in critical illness–associated immune suppression has focused on innate immunity, data from septic adults and children suggest that suppressed or down-regulated adaptive immune responses are also associated with adverse outcomes.[5,15,25] Specifically, multicenter genomic studies of children with septic shock consistently demonstrate down-regulation of genes within adaptive immunity pathways, a pattern that may be exacerbated by corticosteroid use.[25-28] Mechanisms of adaptive immune suppression in septic shock have yet to be fully elucidated. Lymphocyte apoptosis has been long recognized in both adult and pediatric sepsis and likely plays a role in sepsis-induced immune suppression.[29,30] However, other mechanisms may be important as well. As mentioned previously, immunosuppressive regulatory T cells may contribute to sepsis-induced immune suppression, though data to support this mechanism are currently mixed.[14-18] Increased expression of negative costimulatory molecules, CTLA-4 and PD-1, has been demonstrated in animal models of sepsis and in septic adults, and they may represent an additional mechanism for critical illness–associated immune suppression.[4-6,31,32] These pathways may provide future therapeutic targets and are the subject of much ongoing study.

Aside from critical illness–associated immune suppression, the pediatric intensivist often cares for patients whose adaptive immune responses are intentionally suppressed to treat autoimmune disease or to prevent posttransplant organ rejection. Glucocorticoids represent one of the most common immunosuppressants administered in the ICU. Antiinflammatory glucocorticoids, such as methylprednisolone and dexamethasone, potently suppress T-cell function by blocking cytokine production and inducing T-cell apoptosis. Other immunosuppressive medications commonly encountered in the ICU are outlined in Table 102.4. Given the importance of adaptive immune function in the ICU, particularly in the setting of infection, it is likely that immunosuppressive medications may need to be tailored to the unique individual needs of the critically ill patient. Unfortunately, available evidence to guide immunosuppressive medication management in the pediatric intensive care unit is lacking and adult data are limited, with a single report suggesting that rapidly tapering immunosuppression in transplant patients with sepsis and documented severe immune suppression may be beneficial without sacrificing graft survival.[33]

In sharp contrast to pharmacologic immunosuppression, cancer immunotherapy is an evolving field that involves augmenting adaptive immune responses in order to treat malignancy. The underlying premise of antitumor immunotherapy involves stimulating immune cell responses and often targeting those responses toward tumor-specific antigens. Although these therapies show early promise in the treatment of relapsed or metastatic disease, some patients experience potentially life-threatening side effects related to immune activation and the associated cytokine storm.[34] These patients often require transition to the intensive care unit for support of hemodynamics and organ function. One example of cancer immunotherapy in pediatrics is the use of the monoclonal antibody, mAB ch14.18, which recognizes the disialoganglioside, GD2, found on neuroectodermal cells and highly expressed on neuroblastoma. In a phase III trial of high-risk neuroblastoma

TABLE 102.4	Selected Immunosuppressive Medications Targeting Adaptive Immune Function	
Drugs	Mechanism of Action	Select Uses
Polyclonal Antibody Sera		
Antithymocyte globulin	Lymphocyte depletion	Posttransplant induction therapy
Monoclonal Antibodies		
Basiliximab, daclizumab	Prevent T-cell activation and proliferation by blocking the IL-2 receptor (CD25)	Posttransplant induction therapy
Rituximab	Binds CD20 on B-cell surface leading to B-cell lysis	Pretransplant therapy for HLA-sensitized recipients, certain refractory autoimmune diseases, autoimmune cytopenias
Calcineurin Inhibitors		
Cyclosporine, tacrolimus	Inhibit T-cell cytokine production by blocking phosphatase activity of calcineurin	Posttransplant maintenance therapy
mTOR Inhibitors		
Sirolimus, everolimus	Block T-cell proliferation and differentiation by blocking the serine/threonine protein kinase, mTOR	Posttransplant maintenance therapy
Antiproliferative Drugs		
Azathioprine	Converts to purine analog, which competitively inhibits DNA synthesis and blocks proliferation of bone marrow–derived cells	Posttransplant maintenance therapy, autoimmune hepatitis
Mycophenolate mofetil	Inhibits lymphocyte proliferation by inhibiting purine synthesis	Posttransplant maintenance therapy, lupus nephritis
Methotrexate	Inhibits folic acid pathway, which inhibits purine and pyrimidine synthesis	Juvenile idiopathic arthritis, psoriasis, inflammatory bowel disease
Cyclophosphamide	DNA alkylating agent inhibits lymphocyte proliferation	Lupus nephritis, refractory autoimmune disease

patients, ch14.18 combined with IL-2 and granulocyte-macrophage colony-stimulating factor (GM-CSF) was significantly associated with improved event-free survival compared to standard therapy.[35] At this time, there are multiple ongoing clinical trials evaluating anti-GD2 antibodies either with or without additional immunomodulators for pediatric neuroblastoma.[36] A second example of emerging cancer immunotherapy involves the infusion of autologous T cells that have been genetically modified to express chimeric antigen receptors (CARs) that recognize tumor cell surface markers and are fused to T-cell receptor signaling domains. Clinical studies of CARs in pediatric oncology patients are currently limited, though CARs that recognize the cell surface marker CD19 have shown remarkable promise in early phase I studies of refractory B-cell acute lymphoblastic leukemia (ALL).[37,38] Based on these early successes, it is likely that the role of cancer immunotherapy may continue to expand, carrying with it the potential need for critical care intervention.

Summary

As will be highlighted further in subsequent chapters, attention to maintaining a well-regulated and functional immune response is essential for many of the children cared for in the intensive care unit. The cellular components of adaptive immunity, B cells and T cells, help drive a complex, well-regulated interchange of cellular responses and chemical signaling leading to optimum performance of both innate and adaptive immunity. As attention focuses on maintaining and restoring coordinated, functional immune responses in the intensive care unit, it will be increasingly important for the pediatric intensivist to understand the components of both the innate and adaptive immune systems.

References

1. Carapetis JR, Jacoby P, Carville K, et al. Effectiveness of clindamycin and intravenous immunoglobulin, and risk of disease in contacts, in invasive group a streptococcal infections. *Clin Infect Dis.* 2014;59:358-365.
2. Linner A, Darenberg J, Sjolin J, et al. Clinical efficacy of polyspecific intravenous immunoglobulin therapy in patients with streptococcal toxic shock syndrome: a comparative observational study. *Clin Infect Dis.* 2014;59:851-857.
3. Balkhi MY, Ma Q, Ahmad S, Junghans RP. T cell exhaustion and interleukin 2 downregulation. *Cytokine.* 2015;71:339-347.
4. Guignant C, Lepape A, Huang X, et al. Programmed death-1 levels correlate with increased mortality, nosocomial infection and immune dysfunctions in septic shock patients. *Crit Care.* 2011;15:R99.
5. Boomer JS, To K, Chang KC, et al. Immunosuppression in patients who die of sepsis and multiple organ failure. *JAMA.* 2011;306:2594-2605.
6. Chang K, Svabek C, Vazquez-Guillamet C, et al. Targeting the programmed cell death 1: programmed cell death ligand 1 pathway reverses T cell exhaustion in patients with sepsis. *Crit Care.* 2014;18:R3.
7. Becattini S, Latorre D, Mele F, et al. T cell immunity. Functional heterogeneity of human memory CD4(+) T cell clones primed by pathogens or vaccines. *Science.* 2015;347:400-406.
8. Geginat J, Paroni M, Maglie S, et al. Plasticity of human CD4 T cell subsets. *Front Immunol.* 2014;5:630.
9. Mai J, Wang H, Yang XF. Th 17 cells interplay with Foxp3+ Tregs in regulation of inflammation and autoimmunity. *Front Biosci.* 2010;15:986-1006.
10. Romagnani S, Maggi E, Liotta F, et al. Properties and origin of human Th17 cells. *Mol Immunol.* 2009;47:3-7.
11. Ueno H, Banchereau J, Vinuesa CG. Pathophysiology of T follicular helper cells in humans and mice. *Nat Immunol.* 2015;16:142-152.
12. Pan HF, Leng RX, Li XP, et al. Targeting T-helper 9 cells and interleukin-9 in autoimmune diseases. *Cytokine Growth Factor Rev.* 2013;24:515-522.
13. Kaplan MH, Hufford MM, Olson MR. The development and in vivo function of T helper 9 cells. *Nat Rev Immunol.* 2015;15:295-307.
14. Hein F, Massin F, Cravoisy-Popovic A, et al. The relationship between CD4+CD25+CD127-regulatory T cells and inflammatory response and outcome during shock states. *Crit Care.* 2010;14:R19.
15. Muszynski JA, Nofziger R, Greathouse K, et al. Early adaptive immune suppression in children with septic shock: a prospective observational study. *Crit Care.* 2014;18:R145.

16. Venet F, Chung CS, Kherouf H, et al. Increased circulating regulatory T cells (CD4(+)CD25 (+)CD127 (-)) contribute to lymphocyte anergy in septic shock patients. *Intensive Care Med.* 2009;35:678-686.

17. Venet F, Pachot A, Debard AL, et al. Increased percentage of CD4+CD25+ regulatory T cells during septic shock is due to the decrease of CD4+CD25- lymphocytes. *Crit Care Med.* 2004;32:2329-2331.

18. Wu HP, Chung K, Lin CY, et al. Associations of T helper 1, 2, 17 and regulatory T lymphocytes with mortality in severe sepsis. *Inflamm Res.* 2013;62:751-763.

19. Fahl SP, Coffey F, Wiest DL. Origins of gammadelta T cell effector subsets: a riddle wrapped in an enigma. *J Immunol.* 2014;193:4289-4294.

20. Robertson FC, Berzofsky JA, Terabe M. NKT cell networks in the regulation of tumor immunity. *Front Immunol.* 2014;5:543.

21. Allen ML, Hoschtitzky JA, Peters MJ, et al. Interleukin-10 and its role in clinical immunoparalysis following pediatric cardiac surgery. *Crit Care Med.* 2006;34:2658-2665.

22. Hall MW, Geyer SM, Guo CY, et al. Innate immune function and mortality in critically ill children with influenza: a multicenter study. *Crit Care Med.* 2013;41:224-236.

23. Hall MW, Knatz NL, Vetterly C, et al. Immunoparalysis and nosocomial infection in children with multiple organ dysfunction syndrome. *Intensive Care Med.* 2011;37:525-532.

24. Muszynski JA, Nofziger R, Greathouse K, et al. Innate immune function predicts the development of nosocomial infection in critically injured children. *Shock.* 2014;42:313-321.

25. Wong HR, Cvijanovich N, Lin R, et al. Identification of pediatric septic shock subclasses based on genome-wide expression profiling. *BMC Med.* 2009;7:34.

26. Wong HR, Cvijanovich N, Allen GL, et al. Genomic expression profiling across the pediatric systemic inflammatory response syndrome, sepsis, and septic shock spectrum. *Crit Care Med.* 2009;37:1558-1566.

27. Wong HR, Cvijanovich NZ, Allen GL, et al. Corticosteroids are associated with repression of adaptive immunity gene programs in pediatric septic shock. *Am J Respir Crit Care Med.* 2014;189:940-946.

28. Wong HR, Freishtat RJ, Monaco M, et al. Leukocyte subset-derived genomewide expression profiles in pediatric septic shock. *Pediatr Crit Care Med.* 2010;11:349-355.

29. Felmet KA, Hall MW, Clark RS, et al. Prolonged lymphopenia, lymphoid depletion, and hypoprolactinemia in children with nosocomial sepsis and multiple organ failure. *J Immunol.* 2005;174:3765-3772.

30. Hotchkiss RS, Tinsley KW, Swanson PE, et al. Sepsis-induced apoptosis causes progressive profound depletion of B and CD4+ T lymphocytes in humans. *J Immunol.* 2001;166:6952-6963.

31. Chang KC, Burnham CA, Compton SM, et al. Blockade of the negative co-stimulatory molecules PD-1 and CTLA-4 improves survival in primary and secondary fungal sepsis. *Crit Care.* 2013;17:R85.

32. Inoue S, Bo L, Bian J, et al. Dose-dependent effect of anti-CTLA-4 on survival in sepsis. *Shock.* 2011;36:38-44.

33. Reinke P, Volk HD. Diagnostic and predictive value of an immune monitoring program for complications after kidney transplantation. *Urol Int.* 1992;49:69-75.

34. Maude SL, Barrett D, Teachey DT, Grupp SA. Managing cytokine release syndrome associated with novel T cell-engaging therapies. *Cancer J.* 2014;20:119-122.

35. Yu AL, Gilman AL, Ozkaynak MF, et al. Anti-GD2 antibody with GM-CSF, interleukin-2, and isotretinoin for neuroblastoma. *N Engl J Med.* 2010;363:1324-1334.

36. Capitini CM, Otto M, DeSantes KB, Sondel PM. Immunotherapy in pediatric malignancies: current status and future perspectives. *Future Oncol.* 2014;10:1659-1678.

37. Cruz CR, Micklethwaite KP, Savoldo B, et al. Infusion of donor-derived CD19-redirected virus-specific T cells for B-cell malignancies relapsed after allogeneic stem cell transplant: a phase 1 study. *Blood.* 2013;122:2965-2973.

38. Grupp SA, Kalos M, Barrett D, et al. Chimeric antigen receptor-modified T cells for acute lymphoid leukemia. *N Engl J Med.* 2013;368:1509-1518.

Congenital Immunodeficiency

Troy Torgerson

PEARLS

- Approximately 300 single gene defects have now been associated with specific immunodeficiencies.
- Chronic granulomatous disease is the most frequently diagnosed phagocytic cell immune defect. The most common form is X-linked, caused by mutations in the *CYBB* gene and accounting for approximately two-thirds of all CGD patients. All mutations affect the formation or function of the NADPH oxidase complex on neutrophil phagolysosomes.
- X-linked agammaglobulinemia is the prototypic B-cell disorder. It is caused by mutations in the Bruton's tyrosine kinase gene (BKT), required for the maturation of B-cell precursors in the bone marrow. Mutations in BTK cause an arrest of B-cell development at the pre–B-cell stage, leading to virtual absence of circulating B cells in the peripheral blood.
- Common variable immunodeficiency (CVID) is a heterogeneous disorder that is likely caused by a variety of molecular mechanisms that ultimately lead to a similar clinical phenotype.
- With IgG supplementation, this group of patients has a relatively benign course with long-term survival that is not unlike the normal population.
- Selective IgA deficiency is common in the general population, and patients with selective IgA deficiency have no apparent symptoms that can be directly linked to their immune defect. In patients who are truly IgA deficient, sensitization to IgA itself can be a problem, leading to anaphylactic reactions during infusions of blood products.
- Deletions within the 22q11.2 region of the long arm of chromosome 22 have been associated with various clinical syndromes including DiGeorge syndrome (DGS), velocardiofacial syndrome (VCFS), conotruncal anomaly face syndrome (CTFS), and CATCH22 syndrome.
- The characteristic T-cell lymphopenia of DiGeorge syndrome is thought to arise primarily from the absence of adequate thymic tissue. Both CD4+ and CD8+ T cells are low; however, CD8+ T-cell numbers tend to be more affected in most patients.
- Severe combined immune deficiency (SCID) is among the most severe immunodeficiencies and is made up of a variety of related disorders caused by mutations in more than 20 different genes. All forms of SCID have deficiency of one or more subsets of T cells. In many cases, there are no circulating T cells.
- Adenosine deaminase (ADA) deficiency was the first molecularly defined immunodeficiency with discovery of

patients with SCID. When adenosine deaminase activity is impaired or absent, intracellular levels of deoxy-ATP (dATP) rise to interfere with ribonucleotide reductase and DNA synthesis and repair are slowed and lymphocyte apoptosis increased.
- X-linked (IPEX) syndrome involves regulatory T-cell deficiency, and phenotypically includes immune dysregulation, polyendocrinopathy, and enteropathy. IPEX is caused by mutations in the *FOXP3* gene located on the X chromosome, which encodes a key transcription factor that is required for the generation of functional regulatory T cells (Treg). In the absence of *FOXP3*, patients present with severe, early-onset, systemic autoimmunity.
- Ataxia telangiectasia (AT) is a disorder associated with progressive neurologic decline, immunodeficiency, and propensity to malignancy. It is caused by autosomal recessive mutations in the *ATM* gene, which encodes a serine/threonine kinase that acts together with the NBS1 protein as one of the major sensors of double-stranded DNA breaks in the cell. In the absence of functional ATM or NBS1, cells have a marked sensitivity to ionizing radiation.

Introduction

The immune system plays a vital, integral role in human health and disease because of its interactions with every other organ system in the body. In one way or another, it plays particularly important roles in diseases that often affect patients admitted to pediatric ICUs (PICUs) including those with severe infections and sepsis, severe autoimmunity, malignancies, inflammatory disorders such as hemophagocytic lymphohistiocytosis, asthma, and type I diabetes with diabetic ketoacidosis. This chapter focuses particularly on immunologic disorders that are most likely to be encountered in the PICU setting.

The normal and pathogenic roles of each component of the immune system in humans have been significantly clarified by the study of patients with primary immunodeficiency disorders (PIDDs), a group of clinical syndromes originally described in patients with marked susceptibility to particular types of infection. This group of disorders has now expanded to include more than 150 clinically defined entities that span the full spectrum of immune dysfunction ranging from virtually absent immune responses to overwhelming, uncontrolled autoimmunity and susceptibility to malignancy.[1] Many of these disorders are inherited, and approximately 300 single gene defects have now been associated with specific immunodeficiencies. Through these efforts, it has also become evident that mutations in different genes can lead to a similar clinical phenotype. For example, defects in more than 20 different genes have now been associated with a clinical phenotype of severe combined immune deficiency (SCID).[2] Consequently, it has become the practice to refer to disorders by their molecular defect, either in combination with or in lieu of their clinical name or eponym (ie, "ADA-deficiency" or "ADA-SCID" rather than just "SCID"). This practice is followed here.

Basic Framework for Understanding the Immune System

In order to provide structure to facilitate an understanding of the immune system, the diseases associated with immune dysfunction, and how these should be recognized, evaluated, and treated, it is worthwhile to establish a basic framework (see also Chapters 101 and 102). In this framework, the immune system can be divided into four major compartments: complement, phagocytes, B cells and antibodies, and T cells. Approximately 300 single gene defects have now been associated with specific immunodeficiencies. The complement and phagocyte compartments are part of the "innate" arm of the immune system, which responds in a similar way each time a particular pathogen is encountered but does not develop immunologic memory (see Chapter 101). In contrast, the B-cell and T-cell compartments comprise the "adaptive" arm of the immune system, which learns each time a pathogen is confronted and develops memory so that responses to pathogens encountered previously can be remembered, thus facilitating a more rapid, effective response (Table 103.1) (see Chapter 102). Many immunodeficiency disorders are caused by a defect in only one compartment of the immune system while others are "combined" immunodeficiencies with defects in both the B- and T-cell compartments. In general, defects in each compartment of the immune system are associated with susceptibility to particular types of infections dictated by the dominant role of that compartment in human immunity. In addition, each immunodeficiency typically has unique clinical and laboratory features that differentiate it from other disorders, thus making it possible to predict which disorder a patient may have on the basis of clinical and laboratory findings (Table 103.2).

Compartment 1: Complement

The complement system consists of a series of proteins that are present in the plasma and become activated on encountering pathogens. The complement cascade is activated via three major mechanisms (see Fig. 103.1): (1) the *Classical Pathway*, which is initiated by antigen/antibody complexes; (2) the *Alternative Pathway*, which is initiated directly by bacterial cell wall components; and (3) the *Lectin Pathway*, which is initiated by carbohydrate moieties present on bacteria. Activation of early complement components initiates a cascade of protein cleavage and activation events that ultimately lead to formation of the Membrane Attack Complex (MAC) consisting of complement proteins C5, 6, 7, 8, and 9. A number of regulatory proteins including C1 inhibitor, factor H, factor I, MCP, and CD59 control complement activation at multiple levels, thereby preventing inappropriate complement fixation.

Complement deficiencies make up only a small portion (~2%) of all primary immune deficiencies, but the consequences can be devastating for affected patients.[3] Defective activation of the entire complement cascade can be caused by the absence or dysfunction of only 1 of more than 20 complement proteins. The proteins most often affected are C2, C3, and C4.[4]

Clinical Presentations

Patients with defects in early complement components in the classical pathway (C1-C4) typically present with recurrent, invasive infections caused by encapsulated organisms (particularly *Streptococcus pneumoniae*) or with symptoms of autoimmunity (lupus or glomerulonephritis). Patients with defects in the late complement components (C5-C9) that are involved in formation of the membrane attack complex typically present with recurrent or severe *Neisseria* infections.[4] Patients who lack functional C1 esterase inhibitor have hereditary angioedema in which allergic or mechanical stimuli can trigger massive, localized, severe attacks of edema that can be life threatening if they involve the airway. Patients with defects in complement regulatory proteins (Factor I, Factor H, and MCP) are at risk of developing familial hemolytic uremic syndrome (HUS) and age-related macular degeneration.[5-7]

TABLE 103.1	Symptoms Associated With Defects in Each Immune Compartment	
	Complement	**Phagocytes**
INNATE	Invasive infections with encapsulated bacteria (eg, *S. pneumoniae, H. influenzae*) Recurrent, invasive *Neisserial* infections Autoimmunity (lupus, glomerulonephritis) Hereditary angioedema Atypical hemolytic uremic syndrome (HUS)	Skin and soft tissue abscesses, boils, and lymphadenitis Infections with catalase-+ organisms (eg, *S. aureus, Serratia, Aspergillus*) Poor wound healing Chronic gingivitis and periodontal disease Mucosal ulcerations, colitis Omphalitis/delayed separation of the umbilical cord
	B Cells/Antibodies	**T Cells**
ADAPTIVE	Recurrent bacterial sinopulmonary infections (otitis media, sinusitis, bronchitis, and pneumonia) Unexplained bronchiectasis Chronic or recurrent gastroenteritis (eg, *Giardia, Cryptosporidium, Enterovirus*) Echovirus encephalomyelitis	*Pneumocystis jirovecii* pneumonia Recurrent, severe, or unusual viral infections (eg, CMV, EBV, adenovirus, papillomavirus) Invasive fungal or mycobacterial infections GvHD (rash, abnormal LFTs, chronic diarrhea) Failure to thrive

TABLE 103.2   Cellular Phenotype and Molecular Defects in Severe Combined Immune Deficiency (SCID)

	Disorder	Gene	Inheritance	Features
T⁻B⁻NK⁻	Adenosine deaminase deficiency	ADA1	AR	Costochondral abnormalities, neonatal hepatitis
	Purine nucleotide phosphorylase deficiency	PNP	AR	Progressive neurologic decline
	Reticular dysgenesis	AK2	AR	SCID phenotype + Neutropenia
T⁻B⁻NK⁺	RAG1 deficiency	RAG1	AR	
	RAG2 deficiency	RAG2	AR	
	Artemis deficiency	DCLRE1C	AR	Radiosensitivity
	DNA-PKcs deficiency	PRKDC	AR	Radiosensitivity
	DNA Ligase IV deficiency	LIG4	AR	Radiosensitivity, microcephaly, growth retardation
	Cernunnos/XLF deficiency	NHEJ1	AR	Radiosensitivity, microcephaly, growth retardation
T⁻B⁺NK⁻	Common γ chain deficiency	IL2RG	XL	
	JAK3 deficiency	JAK3	AR	
	CD45	PTPRC	AR	Some NK cells may be present
T⁻B⁺NK⁺	IL-7 Receptor-α (CD127) deficiency	IL7RA	AR	
	DiGeorge syndrome	22q11.2 del	AD	Hypoparathyroidism, cardiac defects, dysmorphic facies
	CHARGE syndrome	CHD7	AD	Multiple congenital anomalies—clinical complex of CHARGE syndrome
	CD3δ deficiency	CD3D	AR	
	CD3ε deficiency	CD3E	AR	
	CD3γ deficiency	CD3G	AR	
	CD3ζ deficiency	CD3Z	AR	
	P56Lck deficiency	LCK	AR	
	Coronin-1A deficiency	CORO1A	AR	Lymphadenopathy
T⁺/⁻B⁺NK⁺	MHC class I deficiency	TAP1	AR	CD8⁺ T cells are typically decreased but not absent, recurrent respiratory infections
		TAP2	AR	
		TAPBP	AR	
	MHC class II deficiency	CIITA	AR	CD4⁺ T cells are typically decreased but not absent, chronic diarrhea
		RFXANK	AR	
		RFX5	AR	
		RFXAP	AR	
	ORAI1 deficiency	ORAI1	AR	Myopathy, calcium flux defect in B and T cells, poor T-cell proliferation
	STIM1 deficiency	STIM1	AR	Myopathy, calcium flux defect in B and T cells, poor T-cell proliferation

AD, autosomal dominant; *AR*, autosomal recessive; *XL*, X-linked recessive.
Modified from Cossu F. *Ital J Pediatr* 2010;36:76.

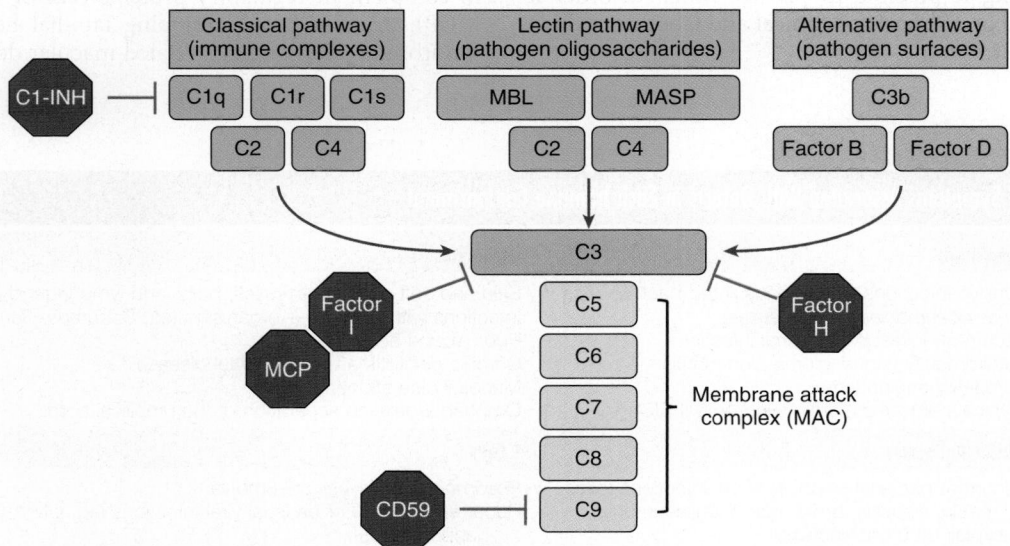

Fig. 103.1. The complement cascade is activated via three major mechanisms: (1) *classical pathway,* which is initiated by antigen/antibody complexes; (2) *alternative pathway,* which is initiated directly by bacterial cell wall components; and (3) *lectin pathway,* which is initiated by carbohydrate moieties present on bacteria.

Compartment 2: Phagocytes

One of the major roles of phagocytic cells (neutrophils and macrophages) is to continuously survey the body for signs of infection. Upon sensing an infection, they migrate from the circulation into the tissues toward the site of the infection, where they ingest both opsonized and nonopsonized pathogens and debris. The ingested material is processed, and fragments of digested proteins are loaded into class II MHC molecules that are presented at the cell surface, where they can be recognized by cells of the adaptive immune system. Phagocytes that ingest pathogens and debris can either remain at the site of infection or migrate back to local draining lymph nodes to present antigen. Phagocytic disorders can occur as a result of one of three types of defects: (1) a lack of phagocytes (congenital neutropenia); (2) abnormal phagocyte migration (leukocyte adhesion deficiency and WHIM syndrome); (3) inability of phagocytes to process or degrade material or organisms that have been ingested (chronic granulomatous disease).

Clinical Presentations

Because of the role that phagocytes play in controlling bacterial and fungal pathogens, patients with phagocytic defects often present with infections and abscesses of skin, deep tissues, and organs caused by bacteria or fungi. Symptoms can include boils or cellulitis with or without pus, lymphadenitis, pneumonia, delayed shedding of the umbilical cord, omphalitis hepatic abscesses, gastrointestinal disorders, gingivitis, unexplained fever, malaise, and fatigue. The onset of symptoms of phagocyte disorders is typically in infancy or early childhood.

Compartment 3: B Cells and Antibodies

The predominant role of B cells in the immune system is to make antibodies (immunoglobulins) in response to antigen challenge (eg, pathogens, vaccines). The absence of functional antibodies causes susceptibility to bacterial and viral infections. Antibody deficiency can occur in one of three different ways: (1) hypogammaglobulinemia or low levels of one or more immunoglobulin classes (IgG, IgA, IgM, or IgE) occurring as a result of decreased antibody production, which may be associated with specific genetic defects; (2) hypogammaglobulinemia as a result of excessive antibody loss, typically through the kidneys as proteinuria or through the gut as protein-losing enteropathy; (3) functional antibody deficiency, in which immunoglobulin levels are normal but the immunoglobulin lacks the quality required to bind and opsonize pathogens.

Clinical Presentations

Patients who lack sufficient levels of functional antibody present with recurrent bacterial sinopulmonary infections (sinusitis, otitis media, bronchitis, and pneumonia). In addition, due to a lack of IgA, patients may develop bowel infections caused by microorganisms such as *Giardia* or *Cryptosporidium* that are often only modestly pathogenic to normal individuals. In addition to these symptoms, patients with certain antibody-deficiency disorders have characteristic clinical features that can provide clues to the specific diagnosis. These are discussed in more detail later in the chapter.

Compartment 4: T Cells

A handful of disorders are characterized by the absence of T cells only. It is much more common, however, for T-cell deficiency or dysfunction to be part of a more extensive "combined" immune deficiency accompanied by defects in B cells and/or NK cells. Identification of a number of new genetic defects over the past decade has dramatically expanded the spectrum of this group of disorders. Some are typified by significant, generalized T-cell lymphopenia while others are characterized by the absence or dysfunction of one or more specialized subsets of T cells.

Clinical Presentations

Patients who have a generalized absence of functional T cells are susceptible to unusual or severe viral infections caused by viruses including cytomegalovirus (CMV), Epstein-Barr virus (EBV), and adenovirus. Patients are also susceptible to fungal infections caused by organisms such as *Pneumocystis jiroveci*, which are not pathogenic in normal individuals but commonly cause pneumonias in this group of patients. In parts of the world where the attenuated mycobacterium bacille Calmette-Guérin (BCG) is used as a vaccine, patients with T-cell deficiency often develop invasive and disseminated mycobacterial infection that is often fatal. A lack of functional T cells also makes it impossible to provide adequate T-cell help to allow B cells to undergo normal immunoglobulin class-switching, so patients usually have functional antibody deficiency as well. In addition, patients with T-cell deficiencies frequently have symptoms of autoimmunity including diarrhea (secondary to autoimmune enteropathy), cytopenias (autoimmune hemolytic anemia [AIHA]), and idiopathic thrombocytopenic purpura (ITP), and hepatitis.

Specific Disorders Likely to Be Encountered in Pediatric ICU

Specific Disorders: Complement

C1 Inhibitor Deficiency

Deficiency of C1 esterase inhibitor is the cause of hereditary angioedema (HAE). HAE is an autosomal dominant disorder that affects 1 in 10,000 to 1 in 50,000. Unlike many of the other early-complement component deficiencies, absence of C1 esterase inhibitor (C1-INH) does not lead to increased risk for infection. Instead, this protein regulates the activity of kallikrein, which causes bradykinin release as a result of cleavage of high-molecular-weight kininogen (HMWK). In the absence of C1-INH, minor irritants such as the menstrual cycle, dental procedures, or surgery can cause unabated production of bradykinin and other mediators of vascular permeability, leading to rapid swelling of the soft tissues (angioedema), severe abdominal pain, and at times, acute obstruction of the airway. Diagnosis of C1-INH deficiency can be made by measuring the level and function of the C1 inhibitor in blood. Patients with C1-INH deficiency also commonly have low-complement C4 levels as well, which can provide an additional clue to the diagnosis. Effective treatments are now available for HAE, including purified C1 esterase inhibitor, a kallikrein inhibitor, and a bradykinin B2 receptor antagonist.[8-10] These therapies can be lifesaving during an acute attack. Because of their expense, they are often administered at the beginning of an attack to abort symptoms rather than prophylactically to prevent the onset of an attack. Unlike typical anaphylaxis, which responds well to epinephrine injections, patients with C1-INH deficiency typically exhibit only modest responses to epinephrine.

Early Classical Pathway Defects (C1, C2, C3, C4)

Patients with defects in early classical complement pathway proteins (C1-C4) are susceptible to invasive infections with encapsulated organisms. *Streptococcus pneumoniae* and *Haemophilus influenzae* are particularly fulminant pathogens in these patients. The infectious susceptibility is compounded by functional antibody deficiency in some patients. Among these disorders, C2 deficiency is the most common complement component deficiency associated with susceptibility to infections, occurring in approximately 1 of 20,000 people. In addition to the dramatic infectious susceptibility, patients with defects in these early classical pathway proteins are at high risk of developing autoimmunity (systemic lupus erythematosus and/or glomerulonephritis). As an example, in patients with homozygous C2 deficiency, approximately 50% of patients develop lupus or glomerulonephritis.[11] The autoimmunity caused by complement deficiency is difficult to treat because no amount of immune suppression will control the underlying pathophysiologic mechanism of disease. There are a growing number of anecdotal reports and small case series in which severe lupus caused by complement deficiency was effectively treated with intermittent infusions of fresh frozen plasma, which contains active complement proteins.

Late Pathway—Membrane Attack Complex Defects (C5, C6, C7, C8, C9)

Patients with defects in the late complement pathway proteins that form the membrane attack complex (C5-C9) are susceptible, almost exclusively, to invasive infections with *Neisseria* species. These patients have a 7000- to 10,000-fold higher risk of developing meningococcal disease than the normal population.[12] On the basis of this, some have suggested that every patient who develops *Neisseria meningitides* sepsis should be screened for complement deficiency using a CH50 test. Doing this may be cost prohibitive in many settings, but there is general consensus that patients who have recurrent invasive infections caused by *N. meningitides* should definitely be screened for complement deficiency because of the high incidence of recurrence (40%-50%) in these individuals.

Complement Regulatory Protein Defects (Factor H, Factor I, MCP)

The complement cascade is regulated at multiple levels by a series of regulatory proteins that prevent indiscriminate activation that could lead to inappropriate inflammation and tissue destruction (Fig. 103.2). Because all complement pathways converge on the activation of C3 before initiation of the membrane attack complex, the cell-bound regulatory proteins that deactivate the cleaved C3 are among the most important functionally. Mutations in Factor H, Factor I, or MCP allow the complement cascade to be more readily activated and lead to susceptibility to atypical HUS, which may be triggered even in the absence of bacterial infection. Unfortunately, there are no straightforward functional tests available to detect abnormalities in these regulatory proteins, so gene sequencing is required to make the diagnosis. In patients with uncontrolled HUS, therapeutic monoclonal antibodies that bind to C5 and

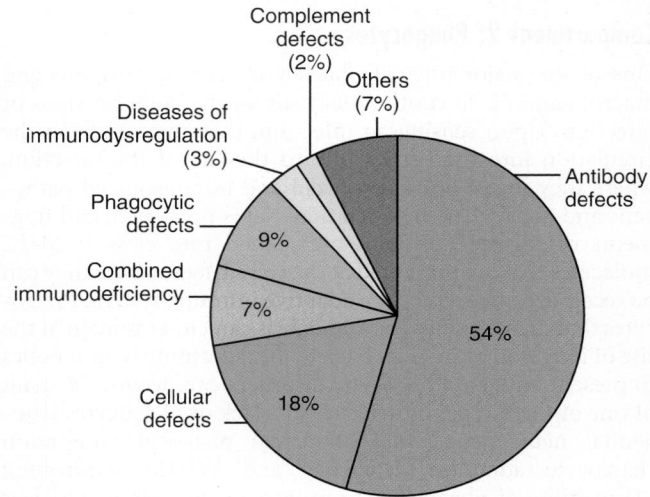

Fig. 103.2. Distribution of the major primary immunodeficiency disorders. (Data from the Jeffrey Modell Foundation Survey, 2009.)

prevent formation of the membrane attack complex have been used to control disease.

Specific Disorders: Phagocytes

Severe Congenital Neutropenia

Patients with severe congenital neutropenia (SCN) typically present early in life with recurrent infections including invasive soft tissue infections and sepsis. Staphylococcal infections are particularly problematic. Mutations in five different genes have now been associated with severe congenital neutropenia: *ELANE*, which is inherited in an autosomal dominant manner, causes increased myeloid cell apoptosis and can present either with SCN or with a cyclic neutropenia phenotype. *GFI1*, which is also inherited in an autosomal dominant manner, causes defective myeloid cell differentiation. *HAX1*, which is inherited in an autosomal recessive manner, is associated with increased myeloid cell apoptosis and is the cause of the classic "Kostmann" neutropenia syndrome. *G6PC3*, which is inherited in an autosomal recessive manner, causes excessive myeloid cell apoptosis and is associated with a variety of other congenital defects including cardiac, urogenital, endocrine, auditory, and facial anomalies. *WAS*, in which specific activating mutations in the CDC42 binding domain of the WASp protein are inherited in an X-linked recessive manner, leads to abnormal and dysregulated actin polymerization that causes defective neutrophil chemotaxis and increased apoptosis.[12]

Clinical management of severe congenital neutropenia involves a heightened suspicion for infections and aggressive treatment if these arise. Treatment of acute infections may require antibiotics combined with G-CSF to increase neutrophil counts. Despite there being little evidence specifically in SCN supporting the use of prophylactic antibiotics, extrapolation from data in leukemic patients with neutropenia suggests a benefit, so this is used in most patients. Prophylactic, long-term therapy with G-CSF is typically used only in those patients who have recurrent, severe bacterial infections in spite of antibiotic prophylaxis or in patients with fungal infections. Bone marrow transplantation is effective in SCN, although there is little to no reported experience in those genetic disorders that are more rare such as G6PC3 deficiency.

Leukocyte Adhesion Deficiency

Leukocyte adhesion deficiency (LAD) is caused by the absence of functional adhesion receptors that are required for the migration of phagocytes from the circulation into the tissues. The characteristic clinical features of LAD include recurrent skin and soft tissue infections, which often lead to development of cutaneous boils or deep ulcers despite there being highly elevated peripheral blood leukocyte counts. Interestingly, the inability of leukocytes to migrate to these sites of infection leads to an absence of pus in the lesions, which can be a useful diagnostic clue. Wound healing is also compromised, and patients typically have marked gingivostomatitis. Three forms of LAD have been described: *LAD-I*, the most common form of LAD, is caused by mutations in the *ITGB2* gene encoding the β2-integrin CD18. Mutations cause an absence of the CD11/CD18 integrin complex on the surface of leukocytes, which can be readily discerned by flow cytometry. *LAD-II* is caused by mutations in the *SLC35C1* gene encoding the GDP-fucose transporter. These mutations cause defective expression of Sialyl Lewis X (sLe^X), a fucose-containing ligand on neutrophils. sLe^X is the ligand for E- and P-selectins, which are expressed on the surface of cytokine-activated endothelial cells and allow neutrophil rolling. As a result of the fucose defect, all patients with LAD-II also have the rare Bombay blood group, which is a useful diagnostic test for suspected LAD-II. *LAD-III* is caused by mutations in the *FERMT3* gene that encodes kindlin-3, a coactivator that is required for activation and function of β1-, β2-, and β3-integrins. Absence of functional kindlin-3 leads to dysfunction of CD18 and causes an LAD phenotype (see LAD-I earlier). In addition, patients with LAD-III also have a Glanzmann-type bleeding disorder resulting from dysfunctional integrin-mediated aggregation of platelets.[13]

Patients with LAD-I and LAD-III typically present in childhood and often have a severe course with early mortality, whereas patients with LAD-II are often milder and may live into adulthood. Treatment of leukocyte adhesion deficiency can be more complicated than some of the other phagocytic disorders because in addition to aggressively treating infections with antibiotics, active soft tissue infections may require recurrent donor white cell infusions of functional neutrophils in order to clear the infection. Because the primary defects of LAD are intrinsic to hematopoietic cells, bone marrow transplantation can be curative.[14-16]

WHIM Syndrome

Warts, hypogammaglobulinemia, recurrent bacterial infections, and myelokathexis (retention of neutrophils in the bone marrow) (WHIM) syndrome is caused by autosomal dominant mutations in CXCR4, the receptor for the chemokine CXCL12 (SDF-1). Patients with WHIM syndrome typically present in childhood with recurrent bacterial otitis media, sinusitis, bronchitis, pneumonia, and cellulitis. The bacterial susceptibility is a result of the combination of hypogammaglobulinemia and neutropenia. In addition to bacterial infections, patients with WHIM have a particular susceptibility to papillomavirus infections, which can be severe and lead to early malignancy. The mechanisms that underlie the viral susceptibility are not entirely understood but are thought to possibly be intrinsic to the epithelial cells. In the hematopoietic system, CXCL12 causes homing of cells to the bone marrow and controls release of these cells from the marrow.

Neutrophils and lymphocytes from patients with WHIM have an increased chemotactic response to CXCL12, suggesting that the neutropenia and lymphopenia observed in WHIM are the result of inappropriate cell retention in the marrow.[17] Treatment with G-CSF or GM-CSF can normalize the neutrophil counts, although these often cause significant bone pain at the doses required.[18] Recent studies using the CXCR4 antagonist plerixafor in adults with WHIM syndrome have shown promise for improving neutrophil counts by mobilizing neutrophils from the bone marrow.[19,20] Antibiotics and immunoglobulin replacement can significantly reduce the risk of bacterial infections. There is little reported experience regarding bone marrow transplantation for WHIM, although anecdotal evidence suggests that it may correct the neutropenia and hypogammaglobulinemia but may not alter the papillomavirus susceptibility.[21]

Chronic Granulomatous Disease

Chronic granulomatous disease (CGD) is the most frequently diagnosed phagocytic cell immune defect. The most common form is X-linked, caused by mutations in the *CYBB* gene and accounting for approximately two-thirds of all CGD patients. The remaining forms, caused by mutations in the *CYBA*, *NCF1*, *NCF2*, or *NCF4* genes, are all autosomal recessive. All mutations affect the formation or function of the NADPH oxidase complex on neutrophil phagolysosomes. The NADPH oxidase is required to generate a burst of reactive oxygen species in response to phagocytosis of pathogens. Reactive oxygen species activate proteases in the phagolysosomes that destroy ingested bacteria. In CGD, the oxidative burst cannot be generated, leading to defective processing of ingested organisms and an inability to appropriately eliminate bacterial and fungal pathogens. Catalase-positive organisms including *Staphylococcus* species, *Aspergillus* species, *Burkholderia cepacia*, *Serratia marcescens*, and others are the most common pathogens. The most common types of infection at presentation are pneumonia, lymphadenitis, cellulitis, and hepatic abscesses (particularly with *Aspergillus* sp.). The most common cause of premature death is *Aspergillus* infection.[22] In addition to the infectious susceptibilities of CGD, a substantial percentage of patients struggle with inflammatory complications that are common to this disorder, including an inflammatory colitis that occurs in approximately 40%, hepatic dysfunction, gingivitis, and others.

Treatment of CGD revolves around aggressive management of acute infections followed by prophylaxis against future infections using a combination of daily antibiotic (typically trimethoprim-sulfamethoxazole), daily antifungal (typically itraconazole), and thrice-weekly interferon-γ injections. This combination has dramatically improved outcomes in CGD; however, despite appropriate use of this regimen, some patients ultimately have increasing symptoms that lead to a decline in survival beginning in the late-teens or early 20s. The prospects for long-term survival appear to be correlated with the amount of residual oxidative burst activity that can be generated by a particular patient's phagocytes.[23] This has led to a renewed interest in bone marrow transplantation for CGD, which has been quite successful in the modern era, likely due to improved antimicrobials and transplant conditioning regimens with reduced toxicity. Many now recommend that for patients who have mutations that severely impact oxidative burst activity, bone marrow transplant should be considered preemptively, early in life before patients develop comorbidities.[24]

Specific Disorders: B Cells and Antibodies

X-Linked Agammaglobulinemia

X-linked agammaglobulinemia (XLA) is the prototypic B cell disorder. It is caused by mutations in the Bruton's tyrosine kinase *(BTK)* gene. BTK is a cytoplasmic tyrosine kinase and is required for the maturation of B-cell precursors in the bone marrow.[25] Mutations in BTK therefore cause an arrest of B-cell development at the pre–B-cell stage leading to virtual absence of circulating B cells in the peripheral blood. Mutations that only partially interfere with the enzymatic function of BTK have also been described and are associated with milder forms of the disease that only have defects in generation of specific antibody responses.

XLA is typically suspected in male patients with recurrent bacterial sinopulmonary infections and B-cell lymphopenia. Other infections that occur relatively frequently in patients with XLA before the initiation of IgG replacement therapy include skin infections (furunculosis, pyoderma, and cellulitis) and sepsis. The diagnosis can be confirmed either by identifying a mutation in the *BTK* gene or demonstrating absence of the BTK protein in monocytes or platelets. A positive family history suggestive of an X-linked recessive mode of inheritance increases the suspicion for XLA. It is uncommon for patients with XLA to develop symptoms in the first months of life because newborns are protected from most infections by transplacentally acquired maternal IgG. There are few distinguishing physical features of XLA that can provide clues to the diagnosis, but absence of visible tonsils or adenoids (by physical examination, radiograph, or CT scan) is a useful clue.

In addition to the common sinopulmonary pathogens, patients with XLA are also susceptible to infections by particular opportunistic organisms that are more rare and fastidious, which can cause unusual clinical syndromes. For example, *Helicobacter cinaedi* can cause a syndrome of dermatomyositis and cellulitis that presents with cutaneous ulcerations, particularly on the lower legs.[26,27] The organism can sometimes be recovered from the blood but is fastidious and difficult to culture using usual methods. The ability to culture the organism and evaluate its antibiotic sensitivity is crucial since in many cases it is frequently resistant to various antibiotics. A combination of antibiotics is often necessary to effectively clear the infection.[28] Similarly, *Mycoplasma* species, including *M. hominis,* can cause lung, abdominal, or bone infections that are remarkably hard to eradicate and *Ureaplasma urealyticum* infections are a rare cause of arthritis, urethritis, and pneumonia.[29]

Before the widespread use of IgG supplementation in these patients, opportunistic viral infections, particularly with viruses that require an extracellular phase, were especially problematic. For example, Echovirus encephalitis was estimated to be the cause of death in ~10% of boys with XLA in the 1970s, but that number has fallen dramatically with aggressive use of IgG supplementation. There continue to be rare cases of Echovirus encephalitis in patients with XLA, even in those on adequate IgG replacement therapy, but these are thought to be caused by viral strains for which there may not be high antibody titers in the particular IgG preparation being used.[30,31] Similarly, a mink Astrovirus strain was recently identified by deep sequencing from the brain of an XLA patient who developed a neurodegenerative disorder as a teen.[32] Interestingly, he had lived next to a mink farm as a child but was started on immunosuppression early in his teens for inflammatory bowel disease, which may have allowed the virus to escape control. Lastly, infections with vaccine-strain poliovirus were pathogenic in undiagnosed patients with XLA who were immunized with the live-viral vaccine after transplacentally acquired maternal antibody had waned. The shift from live attenuated to killed poliovirus for immunization has essentially eliminated new cases.

Hyperimmunoglobulin M Syndromes

Under normal circumstances, binding of antigen to cell surface IgM on naïve B cells induces activation of the B cell. The antigen that is bound to surface IgM on the B cell is ingested and proteolytically digested. Antigenic peptide fragments are displayed on the B-cell surface in MHC class II molecules. Antigen-specific T cells then engage the B cell via MHC II/TCR interactions. Once engaged, the activated helper T cell (Th) provides additional costimulatory signals to the B cell that are critical to promote immunoglobulin class-switching from IgM to IgG, IgA, and IgE. The most important of these costimulatory signals comes via the interaction of CD40 ligand on activated T cells with CD40 on B cells. Activation of the B cell through CD40 and cytokines that are secreted by the helper T cell cause it to undergo class-switch recombination (CSR), during which the μ-heavy chain gene segment within the immunoglobulin gene is replaced by either a γ, α, or ε gene segment. This is accomplished by nicking and double-strand breakage of the DNA in the immunoglobulin heavy-chain locus, which requires a series of enzymatic steps that involve activation-induced cytidine deaminase (AID), uracil DNA glycosylase (UNG), and others. Genetic defects that affect CD40 ligand (CD40L), CD40, AID, or UNG can therefore prevent class-switch recombination, thus thwarting the B cells' ability to make significant amounts of any antibody isotype besides IgM.

The overwhelming majority of patients with hyper-IgM syndrome have the X-linked form caused by X-linked recessive mutations in CD40 ligand (CD40L/CD154), which is encoded by the *CD40L* gene on the X chromosome.[33] CD40L and its receptor CD40 are members of the tumor necrosis factor (TNF) superfamily of ligands and receptors. In lymphocytes, CD40L is expressed only on activated T cells but is also expressed on platelets where its role is unknown. Affected boys may present with recurrent bacterial sinopulmonary infections caused by low IgG, IgA, and IgE, while IgM is normal or elevated. In addition to the usual bacterial pathogens, patients with CD40L mutations also demonstrate unique susceptibilities to fungal infections, particularly *Pneumocystis jirovecii* (PJ), which causes pneumonia, and to a protozoan, *Cryptosporidium parvum* (CP), which causes bowel infections. B lymphocytes are present, and T-cell numbers are generally normal. In almost all cases, the diagnosis can be made by using flow cytometry to evaluate the expression and function of the CD40L protein on activated T cells. Expression is evaluated using antibodies specific to the CD40L protein, and the function is evaluated by measuring the binding of a CD40-Ig heavy chain fusion protein to the expressed CD40L. Gene sequencing can then be performed in order to identify a specific mutation.

The susceptibility to *Pneumocystis* and possibly other fungal pathogens has been somewhat of a puzzle because patients do not have other signs of a significant cellular immune defect, such as severe or recurrent viral infections. Interestingly, the susceptibility to PJ pneumonia appears to go away in most patients by the age of 5. PJ pneumonia is almost always diagnosed by staining bronchoalveolar lavage fluid for the presence of the organism. PJ pneumonia can be readily prevented by prophylactic trimethoprim-sulfamethoxazole administration, and active disease is amenable to treatment using higher doses of the same drug. Recent data have suggested that the fungal susceptibility in CD40L deficiency may be a result of defective CD40L signaling into dendritic cells and monocytes that express CD40.[34]

Cryptosporidium parvum (CP) bowel infections are more difficult to diagnose and manage in patients with CD40L deficiency. CP may cause abdominal pain, bloating, diarrhea, malabsorption, and weight loss. It may require multiple stool samples to identify the oocysts, and occasionally the diagnosis can only be made on endoscopically obtained biopsy specimens. Treatment with paromomycin or nitazoxanide can clear the infection, although prolonged courses are typically needed in hyper IgM patients and treatment failures are not uncommon. CP infections can result in chronic inflammation of the gut and biliary tree, which seems a likely contributor to the high incidence of bile duct cancers seen in these patients.[35,36]

Treatment involves the use of IgG replacement therapy combined with prophylactic antibiotics for prevention of PJP at least until the age of 5. The role of bone marrow transplantation for CD40L deficiency is still being evaluated. Even though a number of patients have undergone successful bone marrow transplantation, the role of BMT remains somewhat controversial in this disease, although in patients with ongoing CP infection, the prognosis for the patients who develop bile duct disease is so poor that the risks of transplantation are well justified.[37,38]

CD40 deficiency is clinically similar to CD40L deficiency. It is inherited as an autosomal recessive defect that has been described primarily in two cohorts from Italy and the Middle East. It results in a syndrome that is almost identical to CD40L deficiency in which both sexes are affected.[39]

Autosomal recessive mutations in AID and UNG also cause a hyper-IgM phenotype, but it tends to be milder than either CD40L or CD40 deficiency, likely because the defect is limited to B cells, whereas CD40L/CD40 signaling plays a role in other cell types including dendritic cells and monocytes.[40,41] Patients with AID or UNG typically live into adulthood and do not demonstrate the same susceptibility to PJ pneumonia and CP bowel infections. Patients with mutations in AID do, however, have a significant propensity to develop autoimmunity affecting various organ systems. Patients are typically treated with IgG replacement therapy and antibiotics for acute infections. There are no reports of bone marrow transplantation for AID or UNG deficiency.

Common Variable Immunodeficiency Syndromes

Common variable immunodeficiency (CVID) is a heterogeneous disorder that is likely caused by a variety of molecular mechanisms that ultimately lead to a similar clinical phenotype. The European Society of Immunodeficiency (ESID) has proposed diagnostic criteria in an effort to standardize the diagnosis of CVID. These include (1) plasma IgG levels that are <2 standard deviations below the mean for age combined with a "marked decrease" in either IgM or IgA; (2) age of onset of immunodeficiency >2 years of age; (3) absent isohemagglutinins or poor responses to vaccines; and (4) defined causes of hypogammaglobulinemia have been excluded.

The peak age of onset of CVID is in the second or third decade of life and 50% to 60% of patients have a clinical phenotype consisting almost exclusively of increased bacterial sinopulmonary infections. With IgG supplementation, this group of patients has a relatively benign course with long-term survival that is not unlike the normal population. The other half of patients have a complicated disease course with autoimmunity or lymphoproliferative disease that can involve the hematopoietic system, lungs, lymph nodes, liver, and bowel. The long-term outcome of this population is significantly worse, approaching only 40% survival over 40 years.[42]

Among the disorders seen in this population, a granulomatous, lymphoproliferative, interstitial lung disease (GLILD) affects approximately 30% to 40% of patients.[43] This often presents with decreasing lung function that is manifested by cough, decreased exercise tolerance, and sometimes hypoxemia. Typical findings on chest CT scan include diffuse nodules within the lung, opacities that have a "ground glass" appearance, bronchial wall thickening, and sometimes bronchiectasis. Lung biopsy generally demonstrates a lymphocytic interstitial pneumonitis with noncaseating granulomas and a follicular bronchiolitis with lymphoid aggregates of both B and T cells. This pattern is sometimes mistaken for sarcoidosis, although there are differences. Over time, this inflammatory process in the lungs will cause destruction of alveoli and contribute to development of bronchiectasis and emphysematous changes. If left unchecked, there is evidence that irreversible damage and fibrosis develop in many patients. High-dose corticosteroids are often used as first-line therapy to treat this process, and in many cases they are effective but do not typically lead to a lasting remission on their own. A recent study using a combination of anti-CD20 monoclonal antibody (rituximab) therapy and azathioprine in a small cohort of CVID patients with GLILD demonstrated dramatic responses with a prolonged remission of disease in many patients.[44]

In addition to pulmonary symptoms, GI complaints are common in CVID, affecting 20% to 30% of patients.[42] Patients who develop disease demonstrate a hypertrophic lymphoproliferation of Peyer's patches that causes a nodular lymphoid hyperplasia in the bowel. This is associated with abdominal discomfort, diarrhea, malabsorption, and weight loss and can cause significant morbidity. A variety of approaches have been taken to treat this process, but none have offered particularly dramatic results, although nonabsorbable steroid preparations have shown some benefit with minimal side effects. A more troubling complication observed in 5% to 10% of patients is a hepatitis that can cause severe hepatic dysfunction with development of hepatosplenomegaly and ascites.[42] Infectious causes are almost never identified, and liver biopsy demonstrates a nodular lymphoid hyperplasia in the liver parenchyma, not unlike that observed in the bowel. Liver disease is among the complications associated with a poor outcome.

Some 20% of subjects have additional clinical findings that are suggestive of autoimmunity/immune dysregulation including immune thrombocytopenia and hemolytic anemia, neuropathy, endocrinopathies, and skin disease. Skin involvement ranges from alopecia and vitiligo to psoriasis and granuloma annulare.[45,46]

In most cases of CVID, the molecular etiology of disease is unknown. There has, however, been some progress in identifying genetic defects associated with a CVID phenotype. The most common mutations identified are autosomal recessive defects in the transmembrane activator and calcium modulator and cyclophilin ligand interactor (TACI), which are found in 7% to 10% of patients with CVID. Unfortunately, even in patients who have mutations that abrogate protein expression, the penetrance of disease seems to be highly variable with individuals from one family harboring the same mutation, having either a CVID phenotype, a selective IgA deficiency phenotype, or no disease. This inability to correlate disease phenotype or prognosis with the presence of a TACI mutation has raised the question of whether TACI genotyping offers clinical value. In addition to TACI, autosomal recessive mutations in the genes encoding the Baff receptor *(BAFFR)*, the inducible T-cell costimulator *(ICOS)*, *CD19*, *CD20*, *CD21*, *CD81*, and the LPS-responsive vesicle trafficking, beach and anchor containing protein *(LRBA)* have been identified in rare patients with features of CVID. These mutations have provided insight into basic immune mechanisms in humans but explain only a handful of all patients with CVID.[47,48] Lastly, hypomorphic mutations in *BTK* (X-linked agammaglobulinemia), *CD40L* (X-linked Hyper-IgM syndrome), *SAP/SH2D1A* (X-linked lymphoproliferative syndrome), and *RAG1/RAG2* can be associated with a CVID-like phenotype and, according to the diagnostic criteria for CVID, need to be excluded before making this diagnosis.[47]

B-cell numbers in peripheral blood are typically normal, but a subset of CVID patients has B-cell lymphopenia. In those patients with normal B-cell numbers, B-cell maturation, memory development, and immunoglobulin class-switching are often abnormal and can be assessed by detailed flow cytometry–based immunophenotyping of B cells. Varying classification schemes have been proposed to subtype patients according to their B-cell phenotype, and these subsets have been correlated with differences in risk for autoimmunity, etc.[49-51] B-cell immunophenotyping has therefore become a useful clinical tool in caring for patients with CVID. In addition to the humoral immune deficiency, many patients with CVID have impaired T-cell function with decreased CD4 or CD8 T-cell numbers, as well as abnormal T-cell proliferative responses in vitro to mitogens and antigens. Regulatory T-cell numbers and function have also been found to be decreased in patients with CVID.[52-56]

Selective Immunoglobulin A Deficiency

Selective IgA deficiency (SIgAD) is common in the general population with an incidence as high as 1 in 300 individuals in blood bank studies. The majority (>50%) of patients with selective IgA deficiency have no apparent symptoms that can be directly linked to their immune defect. Severe infections as a consequence of IgA deficiency alone are virtually unheard of. In the patients who do have symptoms, they are typically more suggestive of immune dysregulation and autoimmunity (eg, allergy, arthritis, diarrhea, celiac disease) than immune deficiency (sinusitis, otitis media, bronchitis, and pneumonia). In patients who are truly IgA deficient, sensitization to IgA itself can be a problem, leading to anaphylactic reactions during infusions of blood products including IVIg,

red blood cells, platelets, etc. This is, however, quite uncommon and can often be managed by pretreatment with diphenhydramine, acetaminophen, and steroids before the start of the infusion.[57]

Specific Disorders: T Cells

22q11 Deletion Syndrome (DiGeorge Syndrome)

22q11.2 deletion syndrome or DiGeorge syndrome is among the few disorders that have isolated T-cell deficiency. Deletions within the 22q11.2 region of the long arm of chromosome 22 have been associated with various clinical syndromes including DiGeorge syndrome (DGS), velocardiofacial syndrome (VCFS), conotruncal anomaly face syndrome (CTFS), CATCH22 syndrome, and others. DiGeorge syndrome is the name most commonly associated with immune deficiency, so it is the focus of this discussion. While DGS is a complex syndrome that has been associated with a wide array of symptoms, the diagnostic criteria proposed by the European Society of Immune Deficiency (ESID) are relatively straightforward. These propose that a diagnosis of DGS should be strongly considered in patients who have <500 CD3+ T cells/mm^3 and any two of the following three characteristics: (1) conotruncal cardiac defect (truncus arteriosus, tetralogy of Fallot, interrupted aortic arch, or aberrant right subclavian); (2) hypocalcemia requiring therapy for >3 weeks; and (3) deletion of chromosome 22q11.2. This chromosomal deletion syndrome occurs in approximately 1 in 4000 to 5000 births and causes haploinsufficiency of the genes encompassed in the deletion that can extend to include as much as 3 Mb of the chromosome.[58,59]

The characteristic T-cell lymphopenia of DiGeorge syndrome is thought to arise primarily from the absence of adequate thymic tissue and, at times, the diagnosis is suspected when the cardiac surgeon correcting a congenital heart defect finds little or no thymic tissue in the mediastinum. Most affected infants have low but not absent T cells, and absolute counts tend to improve over the first year of life. Both CD4+ and CD8+ T cells are low, yet CD8+ T-cell numbers tend to be more affected in most patients. Despite low T-cell counts, most patients do not have significant problems with recurrent or severe viral or fungal infections. Some patients may have recurrent candidiasis. Bacterial infections of the upper respiratory tract including otitis media and sinusitis do occur but may be related more to anatomic issues associated with the facial anomalies than to the immunodeficiency per se. Rare patients have severe T-cell lymphopenia with essentially no T cells and are termed "complete" DiGeorge. These patients may have a clinical phenotype similar to SCID.[58,59]

Other prominent clinical features include hypocalcemia, which can be severe and persistent due to parathyroid hypoplasia; dysmorphic facial features that include small, low-set ears, hypertelorism, and micrognathia; renal anomalies including horseshoe kidney and a duplicated collecting system; and developmental delay including problems with speech acquisition, learning disabilities, and behavioral problems. Patients with DiGeorge syndrome have also been found to have an increased incidence of autoimmunity including cytopenias (particularly affecting red cells and platelets), juvenile idiopathic arthritis (JIA), and thyroiditis.

In symptomatic patients, the diagnosis of DiGeorge syndrome is typically made by confirming a deletion within the 22q11.2 region by fluorescence in situ hybridization (FISH) or quantitative polymerase chain reaction for deletion of the TBX1 gene that lies within the deletion.[60] In approximately 10% of patients, deletion of this region cannot be detected despite presence of the classic clinical features.

Treatment of DiGeorge initially involves supportive care that may include cardiac support and calcium supplementation. In patients with severe T-cell lymphopenia or evidence of decreased T-cell function, prophylaxis against PJ pneumonia and IgG supplementation may be used. Blood for these patients should be irradiated to prevent the risk of graft-versus-host disease. For those patients with the severe, "complete" form of the syndrome, grafting of allogeneic thymus slices into the thigh muscle has proven to be successful in recovering the T-cell lymphopenia, improving T-cell responses, and correcting the infectious susceptibility.[61,62] Hematopoietic stem cell transplant (HSCT) has been used in a handful of patients with mixed results.[63,64] In general, HSCT restores the T-cell counts and protects patients against further infection, but in the absence of a thymus, the T-cell graft is thought to consist primarily of long-lived, committed lymphoid progenitor T cells and not of cells derived from donor bone marrow stem cells. As a result, there is concern that the T-cell grafts may senesce over time, once again leaving the patient lymphopenic and susceptible to infection. There are currently no long-term therapies that can successfully correct the parathyroid defect.

Severe Combined Immune Deficiency

Made famous by "The Boy in the Plastic Bubble," a 1976 made-for-TV movie starring John Travolta, SCID is among the most severe immunodeficiencies. It is now known that this category of diseases is made up of a variety of related disorders caused by mutations in more than 20 different genes. The one thing that is common to all forms of SCID is deficiency of one or more subsets of T cells. In many cases, there are no circulating T cells. Depending on the genetic defect, patients may also lack B cells and/or NK cells. This has led to the useful convention of defining cases of SCID by their cellular phenotype (ie, T$^-$B$^+$NK$^+$, T$^-$B$^+$NK$^-$, T$^-$B$^-$NK$^+$, T$^-$B$^-$NK$^-$, etc.). The cellular phenotype suggests what the underlying genetic defect may be (see Table 103.3).[2] Because of the absence of functional T cells, patients with SCID typically come to medical attention because of severe or chronic viral infections, fungal infections, or autoimmunity. Physical examination findings in SCID that may provide some clues to the diagnosis include a paucity of palpable lymph nodes and absence of a thymic shadow on chest radiograph. In the overwhelming majority of SCID cases, this leads to death in infancy or early childhood if patients do not undergo curative treatment, such as HSCT or gene therapy. Unfortunately, the presence of infections makes HSCT or gene therapy much more complicated and substantially decreases the chances of survival. Because of this, efforts have been under way in the United States and other countries to perform screening of all newborns using dried blood spot cards obtained at birth to identify those who may have SCID. These efforts have led to the recognition that the incidence of SCID is approximately 1 in 40,000 live births in the United States.[65,66]

X-Linked Severe Combined Immunodeficiency

The X-linked form of SCID (X-SCID) is the most common type, accounting for ~40% of all SCID cases. It occurs as a result of mutations in the IL2RG gene, encoding the γ receptor chain (γc) used by a number of cytokine receptors including those for IL-2, IL-4, IL-7, IL-9, IL-15, and IL-21. In the absence of a functional γc chain, cells are unable to respond to these cytokines. Because IL-2 and IL-7 are key growth factors for T cells, and IL-15 is the key growth factor for NK cells, patients with X-SCID lack T and NK cells but usually have normal numbers of B cells in their blood. The ability to make antibodies is nevertheless severely impaired due to the lack of T-cell help.

If not identified by newborn screening, infants with X-SCID typically present with severe infections. PJ pneumonia is common and often accompanied by severe viral infections with cytomegalovirus (CMV), EBV, respiratory syncytial virus (RSV), rotavirus, human metapneumovirus, and others. Adenovirus is particularly lethal in SCID, causing not only pneumonitis but also a severe, fulminant hepatitis. In countries where BCG is still used for vaccination, X-SCID patients may develop severe, systemic BCG-osis. Other symptoms that are frequently associated with X-SCID include diarrhea, failure to thrive, and candidiasis.

Flow cytometry testing to evaluate tyrosine phosphorylation of the STAT3 transcription factor in response to IL-21 stimulation can provide a rapid assessment of whether a patient may have an IL2RG or JAK3 defect (see later). Under normal circumstances, IL-21 stimulation of B cells causes rapid tyrosine phosphorylation in B cells that is absent in patients with IL2RG or JAK3 deficiency. The diagnosis is ultimately confirmed, however, by sequencing of the IL2RG gene.

HSCT has been the mainstay of therapy for X-SCID using a variety of pretransplant conditioning regimens. Some have strongly advocated the use of T-cell–depleted grafts from one of the haploidentical parents because they are readily available, but many patients transplanted using that approach have failed to obtain significant donor chimerism in the B-cell compartment, so they have remained dependent on IgG supplementation post transplant. X-SCID was also the first disorder successfully treated by gene therapy. Unfortunately, the retroviral gene therapy vector used to deliver the normal copy of the IL2RG gene had an unknown propensity to integrate within the T-cell oncogene LMO2, causing T-cell leukemias in a subset of treated patients.[67-69] Further studies are under way using alternative viral vectors with the hope that these may have a better safety profile.

JAK3-Deficient SCID

JAK3 is the tyrosine kinase immediately downstream of the common gamma chain (γc). It transduces signals from cytokine receptors to the STAT5 transcription factor and to other intracellular signaling molecules. Approximately 30 different mutations have been identified that impair JAK3 function to varying degrees. Those that are severe have a T$^-$B$^+$NK$^-$ cellular phenotype similar to mutations in IL2RG. Approximately one-third of patients have milder mutations that allow some JAK3 function.[70,71] These patients can develop some T cells, although the T cells that develop are functionally abnormal. The clinical presentation is similar to that observed in γc-deficiency. Sequencing of the JAK3 gene is required to confirm the diagnosis.

Interleukin-7 Receptor, CD3 Components, and CD45-Deficient SCID

Defects in the α-chain of the IL-7 receptor (IL7RA), CD3 subunits (γ, δ, ε), or CD45 can cause SCID with a T$^-$B$^+$NK$^+$

TABLE 103.3   Suggested Laboratory Tests for Basic Evaluation of Each Immune Compartment

	Complement	Phagocytes
INNATE	**Numbers:** Plasma levels of specific complement components (eg, C1 esterase inhibitor, C2, C3, C4) **Function:** CH50—functional test for classical pathway AH50—functional test for alternative pathway	**Numbers:** CBC with differential: Are neutrophil counts normal? **Function:** Expression of the CD11b/CD18 integrin on leukocytes Neutrophil oxidative burst test: dihydrorhodamine 123 or nitro-blue tetrazolium
	B Cells/Antibodies	**T Cells**
ADAPTIVE	**Numbers:** CBC with differential: Are lymphocyte counts normal? Lymphocyte subsets: Are T, B, and NK cell counts normal? **Function:** Vaccine titers: protein antigens (eg, tetanus or diphtheria titers) Vaccine titers: carbohydrate antigens (pneumococcal titers)	**Numbers:** CBC with differential: Are lymphocyte counts normal? Lymphocyte subsets: Are T, B, and NK cell counts normal? **Function:** T-cell proliferation to mitogens/antigens Vaccine titers: protein antigens (eg, tetanus or diphtheria titers)

The laboratory evaluation for immunodeficiency should be individualized to each patient's clinical presentation.
CBC, complete blood cell count; *NK*, natural killer.

phenotype. As noted earlier, IL-7 is one of the two key growth and differentiation factors for T cells. As a result, mutations in the IL-7 receptor α-chain (CD127) lead to selective T-cell deficiency but allow normal development of B and NK cells.

Similarly, absence of any of the CD3 subunits specifically affects the ability of T cells to develop because CD3 makes up an essential part of the T-cell receptor complex. The T-cell receptor, including CD3 subunits, assembles in the endoplasmic reticulum and Golgi complex before trafficking to the cell surface. If any of the receptor subunits are absent (including any of the CD3 chains), the receptor is recycled and never makes it to the outer cell membrane. As a result, cells are unable to receive the TCR stimulation needed as they traffic through the thymus and they die by "neglect." Because the number of T cells entering the thymus is normal, the CD3 defects are unusual among SCID disorders in that the size of the thymus is normal. Of the three known CD3 defects (γ, δ, and ε), CD3γ deficiency may have a somewhat milder clinical phenotype that can present with moderate T-cell lymphopenia and recurrent pneumonia and otitis.

CD45 is a transmembrane tyrosine phosphatase present on most white blood cells. It regulates intracellular Src-family tyrosine kinases that are important for T-cell receptor function and activation. Autosomal recessive mutations of CD45 lead to T-cell deficiency and a SCID phenotype in affected infants.

DNA Recombination and Repair Defects in SCID

Rearrangement of the V, D, J, and constant regions of the T-cell receptor gene and B-cell immunoglobulin gene requires that double-stranded breaks be made in the DNA and that these breaks then be repaired after removal of intervening chromosomal fragments. The recombinase activating genes *RAG1* and *RAG2* are expressed in T and B cells and play an essential role in creating the necessary double-stranded DNA breaks in the TCR and immunoglobulin loci. A large complex

of proteins including artemis (DCLRE1C), DNA-PKcs, cernunnos/XLF (XRCC4-like factor), and DNA ligase IV (LIG4) then play a role in repair of the DNA double-stranded breaks needed to create the final, recombined TCR or Ig locus. Because productive rearrangement of the TCR or Ig locus is a necessary developmental step during T- and B-cell maturation, complete failure in one of these processes results in lymphopenia, with few if any T or B cells in the blood, while generation of NK cells is generally unaffected. Because radiation induces double-strand breaks in DNA, cells from patients with mutations in any of the proteins involved in DNA repair demonstrate decreased survival in vitro after radiation exposure (radiation sensitivity). This can be a valuable diagnostic clue in making a diagnosis.

Patients who have null mutations of any of these proteins have a clear $T^-B^-NK^+$ cell phenotype. There are, however, many mutations, particularly missense mutations or small in-frame deletions, that allow expression of a partially functional protein that can occasionally productively recombine a TCR or Ig gene locus. The cell in which this occurs is then able to pass the developmental block and proliferate in an attempt to fill the lymphopenic void that is otherwise present in SCID. These forms of SCID are termed "leaky" because they allow a small number of T (and occasionally B) cells to "leak" past the developmental block. Omenn syndrome, originally described in leaky RAG1 or RAG2 mutants, is a clinical phenotype that results from this leaky form of SCID. Affected infants typically develop a desquamative erythroderma after birth that is associated with the presence of oligoclonal, activated T cells in the skin, hepatosplenomegaly, lymphadenopathy, eosinophilia, and elevated IgE. Some develop autoimmune enteropathy and cytopenias. Affected patients are typically treated with T-cell–directed immunosuppression such as cyclosporine or FK506, followed by bone marrow transplantation. Leaky forms of SCID have now been described in a number of SCID-associated molecular defects including RAG1, RAG2, artemis, ligase IV, IL7RA, IL2RG, RMRP, and others.[72]

Adenosine Deaminase– and Purine Nucleotide Phosphorylase– Deficient SCID

Adenosine deaminase (ADA) deficiency was the first molecularly defined immunodeficiency with discovery of patients with SCID who lacked the enzymatic activity of ADA in the peripheral blood in the early 1970s. Adenosine deaminase (ADA) catalyzes the conversion of adenosine triphosphate (ATP), guanosine triphosphate (GTP), and their deoxy counterparts to adenosine diphosphate (ADP) and guanosine diphosphate (GDP). When enzyme activity is impaired or absent, intracellular levels of deoxy-ATP (dATP) rise to interfere with ribonucleotide reductase, such that DNA synthesis and repair are slowed and lymphocyte apoptosis is increased. Purine nucleotide phosphorylase (PNP) works further down this same metabolic pathway to convert deoxyinosine to hypoxanthine. Mutations interfering with this function cause deoxy-GTP accumulation and the inhibition of ribonucleotide reductase and DNA synthesis. In both cases, affected infants typically have a $T^-B^-NK^{-/low}$ cellular phenotype due to the toxic nature of the accumulated metabolites on lymphocyte development. Patients typically present with severe or recurrent viral infections or recurrent sinopulmonary infections in the first year of life.

Both syndromes are associated with other nonimmune symptoms, including skeletal abnormalities and osteochondrous dysplasia in ADA deficiency and neurologic deficits, developmental delay, and spasticity, in PNP deficiency. In both cases, the diagnosis can be made by detecting high levels of the toxic metabolites that build up in the peripheral blood in the absence of enzymatic activity. Sequencing of the *ADA1* or *PNP* genes can be done to confirm the diagnosis. ADA deficiency accounts for 20% or more of autosomal recessive SCID cases.

Aside from bone marrow transplantation, ADA-deficient infants can be treated with polyethylene glycol–conjugated ADA, which is injected intramuscularly once per week. Treatment efficacy is gauged by measuring plasma ADA activity and red cell dATP levels. Enzyme treatment has the advantage of speed of response coupled with safety.[73,74] The treatment is expensive, and many treated patients develop antibodies to the bovine protein, which may neutralize the effect of the enzyme. Hematopoietic stem cell transplant is effective in ADA deficiency but less so in PNP deficiency as it does not correct the neurologic deficits. Gene therapy for ADA deficiency has been quite successful, and unlike X-linked SCID and WAS, there have been no reported cases of leukemia despite the retroviral gene therapy vector backbone being similar.[75]

Zap-70–Deficient SCID

Zap-70 is a tyrosine kinase that is downstream of CD3 in the T-cell receptor signaling pathway. Absence of functional enzyme results in a characteristic SCID phenotype with decreased $CD4^+$ T cells but virtually absent $CD8^+$ T cells. Immunoglobulin levels are often decreased, and antibody responses to vaccination are typically absent because of the lack of effective T-cell help. The $CD4^+$ T cells that are present do not respond to antigen or mitogen stimulation, which uses the T-cell receptor, but they do proliferate and make cytokines in response to phorbol and ionomycin stimulation, which mimics TCR stimulation by activating kinases and calcium flux through downstream mechanisms. Bone marrow transplantation is effective in this disorder.

Defects in Antigen Presentation by MHCI or MHCII

The class II MHC complex generally presents peptide antigen derived from ingested material (either by phagocytosis or via the B-cell antigen receptor). Defects that interfere with the assembly or cell-surface expression of the class II MHC–peptide complex prevent effective antigen recognition by $CD4^+$ T cells, resulting in a SCID syndrome that presents in infancy with chronic diarrhea, failure to thrive, and occasionally autoimmune cytopenias. MHCII deficiency can result from defects in one of four DNA-binding proteins that regulate transcription of the MHC class II gene (*CIITA*, *RFXANK*, *RFX5*, and *RFXAP*). Founder mutations (particularly in *RFXANK*) that are common in the Mediterranean region have led to most affected patients having some familial ties to this geographic area. Because MHC class II presentation of antigen is abnormal, $CD4^+$ T cell counts are often low while CD8 counts are normal. A rapid preliminary diagnosis can be made by evaluating peripheral blood cells for expression of the class II complex by flow cytometry, which will detect reduced expression. Some patients can have a mild disease course and live well into adulthood with only supportive care, while others with the same mutation (even in the same family) may have a more severe phenotype. Bone marrow transplantation for MHC II deficiency has been challenging with survival rates typically approaching approximately 50%. In addition, there is a high rate of severe graft-versus-host disease (GvHD) in these patients, possibly because thymic epithelial cells that play a role in positive and negative T cell selection are not replaced by transplant and still do not express MHC II.[76]

The class I MHC complex presents peptide antigens derived from intracellular proteins where proteolytically derived peptides are bound to the MHC I complex as it is generated and trafficked through the endoplasmic reticulum. Peptides that are generated in the cytosol are transported into the inner lumen of the endoplasmic reticulum by the peptide transporters TAP1 and TAP2. Mutations in either of these, or of tapsin to which they bind, have been identified. TAP mutations are typically associated with recurrent viral infections and recurrent sinusitis and bronchitis. The diagnosis is usually suspected when serologic typing for HLA class I antigens fails to give interpretable results, but molecular typing indicates intact MHC DNA. $CD8^+$ T-cell and NK cell counts are frequently (but not uniformly) decreased in these patients. Other cell subsets are typically normal. Heterogeneity in the phenotype may reflect differences in the underlying mutation and in the gene affected. Some patients may survive into the third decade. The role of HSCT in MHC I deficiency is unclear.

Immune Dysregulation, Polyendocrinopathy, Enteropathy, X-Linked (IPEX) is a syndrome of regulatory T-cell deficiency. Natural regulatory T cells comprise a subset of $CD4^+$ T cells that regulate immune responses and play a critical role in peripheral immune tolerance. IPEX is caused by mutations in the *FOXP3* gene located on the X chromosome, which encodes a key transcription factor that is required for the generation of functional regulatory T cells (Treg). In the absence of FOXP3, patients present with severe, early-onset, systemic autoimmunity that is the result of having decreased Treg cell function. Almost all patients with IPEX present with enteropathy within the first 6 months of life. The enteropathy is typically characterized by profuse, watery diarrhea (often nonbloody) and villus atrophy. The majority of patients have an eczematous dermatitis that typically begins in the first months of life. More than half (60%-70%) of patients also develop an early-onset endocrinopathy that is almost exclusively either thyroiditis or type I diabetes. The most consistent laboratory abnormality among patients is a significantly elevated serum IgE level. In addition to these characteristic clinical and laboratory features, patients also have a high incidence of other severe autoimmune disorders, including hemolytic anemia, thrombocytopenia, neutropenia, hepatitis, and renal disease.

Recognition of the clinical features of IPEX is the first step in diagnosing this disorder. Sequencing of the *FOXP3* gene remains the gold standard for making a diagnosis of IPEX, although sequencing needs to encompass noncoding areas of the gene including the upstream noncoding exon and the polyadenylation signal sequence in order to cover all regions in which pathogenic mutations have been identified.[77,78] Flow cytometry to measure FOXP3 protein expression and FOXP3+ regulatory T cells (Treg) is a helpful adjunct to gene sequencing, although only ~25% of patients have mutations that are predicted to completely abrogate FOXP3 protein expression. The remainder of patients have varying degrees of FOXP3+ Treg deficiency due to the fact that mutant FOXP3 may not support normal Treg development. As a result, flow cytometry by itself is not considered to be a sufficiently reliable screening test for IPEX.

Initial therapy for IPEX typically consists of aggressive supportive care (eg, parenteral nutrition, insulin, thyroid hormone) combined with T-cell–directed immune suppression using agents such as tacrolimus, cyclosporine, or rapamycin. Hematopoietic stem cell transplantation (HSCT) is currently the only curative therapy for IPEX. Early HSCT using a nonmyeloablative conditioning regimen before the onset of autoimmune-mediated organ damage usually leads to the best outcome and limits the adverse effects of therapy.[79,80] Because Tregs constitutively express the high-affinity IL-2 receptor, they have a selective growth advantage in vivo. As a result, complete donor engraftment in all hematopoietic lineages may not be necessary because preferential engraftment of donor Treg cells can be sufficient to control the disease.[81]

Specific Disorders: Other Complex or Combined Immunodeficiencies

Wiskott-Aldrich Syndrome

Wiskott-Aldrich Syndrome (WAS) is unique among immunodeficiency disorders because affected patients have both an infectious susceptibility and a bleeding disorder. The bleeding problems are caused by the platelets being small (mean platelet volume <5 fL), dysfunctional, and decreased in number (usually platelet counts <70,000/μL). Patients with WAS typically present in infancy with bloody diarrhea and/or bruising, recurrent upper respiratory tract infections, and eczema. The incidence of hematopoietic malignancies is high. IgE levels are often elevated. Serum IgG levels and T-cell counts are often normal in infancy but may decrease over time. Responses to vaccination, particularly with carbohydrate antigens such as Pneumovax, are often abnormal.

WAS is caused by mutations in the *WAS* gene, located on the short arm of the X chromosome. Inheritance is X-linked recessive. There is a distinct genotype/phenotype correlation of mutations in WAS: Mutations that destroy WAS protein (WASp) expression lead to the full syndrome of immunodeficiency and platelet dysfunction. Mutations that allow expression of a mutant WASp protein are typically associated with a milder X-linked thrombocytopenia (XLT) phenotype in which the platelet dysfunction persists but the immunodeficiency is mild. Point mutations in the CDC42 binding domain of the WASp protein lead to a third phenotype of X-linked neutropenia (XLN) that is generally not accompanied by bleeding abnormalities.[82,83]

The WASp protein is expressed primarily in lymphoid and myeloid cells, where it functions to nucleate actin polymerization in the cell. Patients with WAS therefore have problems with directed migration of neutrophils and with clustering and signaling through T-cell and B-cell antigen receptors (this causes decreased signaling into the cell and abnormal proliferative responses). A diagnosis of WAS can be confirmed by demonstrating the absence of WASp protein in cells by flow cytometry or Western blotting or by identifying a mutation in the *WAS* gene.

Treatment of WAS initially involves supportive care including treatment of any acute infections and management of any bleeding episodes. In general, repeated platelet transfusions are avoided because of the concern that patients will become sensitized to a wide array of HLA types, which may increase the risk of complications during subsequent hematopoietic stem cell transplant (HSCT). Splenectomy can increase platelet counts, but it also increases the risk that patients may die of sepsis with encapsulated organisms, so there continues to be significant controversy surrounding the role of splenectomy in WAS. Patients with the full WAS phenotype should be evaluated for HSCT with matched related or unrelated donor bone marrow or cord blood.[84] Haploidentical transplants have proven risky in this disease and are generally avoided. The role of HSCT in XLT remains controversial.[85] Some have advocated that the benefits for curing the bleeding problems are worth the risk if a matched sibling donor is available. Gene therapy has been successful in a small number of patients with WAS, but like the X-SCID gene therapy trials, some treated patients developed T-cell leukemias as a result of integration of the viral gene therapy vector near an oncogene.[86]

Cartilage-Hair Hypoplasia

Cartilage-hair hypoplasia (CHH) is a complex disorder characterized by skeletal dysplasia with short limbs (metaphyseal chondrodysplasia), sparse hypoplastic hair, gastrointestinal problems, and a variable immunodeficiency. CHH is caused by mutations in the *RMRP* gene, which encodes the 267 base-pair RNA component of the RNase MRP complex, which plays a role in processing of precursor ribosomal RNA. The mechanism by which autosomal recessive mutations in *RMRP* cause the clinical features of CHH is unknown. The largest populations of CHH patients have been identified among the Old Order Amish and Finnish populations. Virtually all patients with CHH have some degree of immunodeficiency that can range from a mild humoral defect with decreased vaccine responses to a SCID-like phenotype associated with progressive lymphopenia and severe infections with bacteria, viruses, and fungi. A leaky-SCID phenotype has also been described in RMRP deficiency. The diagnosis of CHH can be made on the basis of the clinical phenotype and confirmed by sequencing of the *RMRP* gene. Immunologic features of CHH can be corrected by hematopoietic stem cell transplantation, but the other features persist.[87]

Radiation Sensitive Disorders: Ataxia Telangiectasia and Nijmegen Breakage Syndrome

Ataxia telangiectasia (AT) is a disorder associated with progressive neurologic decline, immunodeficiency, and propensity to malignancy. It is caused by autosomal recessive mutations in the *ATM* gene, which encodes a serine/threonine kinase that acts together with the NBS1 protein as one of the major sensors of double-stranded DNA breaks in the cell. ATM phosphorylates key proteins involved in activation of the DNA damage repair checkpoint, leads to cell-cycle arrest, and then leads to double-stranded DNA break repair. In the absence of functional ATM or NBS1, cells have a marked sensitivity to ionizing radiation. Because rearrangement of the TCR gene and the immunoglobulin gene loci also require double-stranded DNA break repair, these processes may be affected as well.

Patients with ataxia telangiectasia usually present in early childhood (most commonly between 2 and 5 years of age) with cerebellar ataxia that progresses to unsteady gait and, over time, choreoathetosis. Telangiectasias (small tufts of dilated blood vessels under the surface of the skin or mucous membranes) typically develop first on the conjunctivae and are later seen on the nose, ears, and shoulders. They can be an important diagnostic clue in a child with progressive ataxia. The majority of patients have immunoglobulin deficiency of varying degrees and can develop sinopulmonary symptoms and sepsis. Progressive neurodegeneration can compromise coughing, so it is hard to determine whether respiratory infections occur more as a result of the immunodeficiency or the motor defects. Most affected individuals have elevated serum α-fetoprotein levels, which can be useful diagnostically. Malignancies are an important complication as a result of the DNA-repair defect. Acute T-cell leukemias are common and often demonstrate chromosomal translocations that affect the chromosomal regions involved in T-cell receptor gene rearrangements. B-cell lymphomas also occur and are usually associated with 11q22-23 chromosomal deletions. There is also an increase in the frequency of epithelial tumors in both homozygotes and ATM mutation carriers. Affected patients usually die in the second or third decade of life.

Other DNA repair defects that cause varying degrees of ataxia and/or mild mental retardation include an ataxia-like syndrome caused by mutations in *MRE11* and the Nijmegen breakage syndrome (NBS), caused by mutations in *NBS1*. In addition to an immunodeficiency like that observed in AT, patients with NBS have marked microcephaly, mild developmental delay/mental retardation, and a strong propensity to develop lymphomas. Another DNA repair defect, Bloom syndrome, caused by mutations in a DNA helicase (RecQ proteinlike-3), results in excess sister chromatid exchanges; it is associated principally with lymphomas and cancer. Multiple primary tumors occurring at an early age are common. Reduced growth in childhood results in a proportional dwarfism that, with cutaneous telangiectasia, is a useful physical sign. Inheritance is autosomal recessive, and the disease occurs with increased frequency in Ashkenazi Jewish populations. Chronic lung disease occurs and may be related to low levels of IgA and IgM.[88]

Mammalian Susceptibility to Mycobacterial Disease

Under normal circumstances, intracellular pathogens like mycobacteria induce production of IL-12 and IL-23, which play a role in driving maturation of naïve T cells into activated T helper type I (Th1) cells that produce interferon-γ (IFN-γ). IFN-γ then acts on a variety of cells including phagocytes (neutrophils, monocytes, and dendritic cells) to induce a number of interferon-inducible genes. Multiple molecules in this signaling pathway have been found to be defective in patients with intact cellular immunity who have invasive, nontuberculous mycobacterial infections. Mutations in the genes encoding the IL12 p40 subunit *(IL12B)*, the IL-12 receptor β1 chain *(IL12RB1)*, the TYK2 tyrosine kinase that is associated with the IL-12 receptor and required for phosphorylation of the STAT4 transcription factor *(TYK2)*, the IFN-γ receptor subunits *(IFNGR1* and *IFNGR2)*, and the STAT1 transcription factor that is activated in response to IFN-γ *(STAT1)*. Mutations in this pathway are also associated with other infections including invasive salmonellosis and severe viral infections *(STAT1)*. In addition to these genetic defects, patients with invasive mycobacterial disease have now been identified with neutralizing autoantibodies to IFN-γ. Together, these discoveries demonstrate a major role for the IL-12/IL-23/IFN-γ axis in normal human immunity.[89] For patients with the milder, autosomal-dominant IFN-γ receptor defects, IL-12 p40 defects, IL-12 receptor defects, and TYK2 defects, antimicrobial therapy and IFN-γ treatment are often sufficient to treat invasive mycobacterial infections and prevent future infections. For patients with the more severe, autosomal recessive IFN-γ receptor defects, IFN-γ supplementation provides no benefit and hematopoietic stem cell transplantation is warranted.[90,91]

Susceptibility to Hemophagocytic Lymphohistiocytosis and Severe EBV Infection

Several defects affecting intracellular trafficking of vesicles and granules are associated with susceptibility to hemophagocytic lymphohistiocytosis (HLH). This group includes some phenotypes that are quite distinctive, including Chédiak-Higashi (CHS) and Griscelli (GS) syndromes, which are both associated with a partial oculocutaneous albinism. Patients with CHS have pyogenic infections and periodontitis: Their neutrophils have reduced chemotaxis and contain giant inclusion bodies (lysosomes). Patients with GS also have neurologic defects ranging from developmental delay to fatal neurodegeneration. Their neutrophils are dysfunctional, but they lack the giant granules of CHS. In vitro tests show low natural killer cell and cytotoxic cell function. CHS, GS, and X-linked lymphoproliferative syndrome (XLP) share susceptibility for HLH—an accelerated inflammatory process that, in the case of XLP, may be triggered by EBV. The genes responsible for these syndromes are *LYST, RAB27A, SH2D1A,* and *XIAP/BIRC4*, respectively, whereas genes for a further group of proteins (Perforin, Munc 13-D, and Syntaxin 11) are associated with familial hemophagocytic lymphohistiocytosis.[92]

Toll-Like Receptors and Innate Signaling Pathway Defects

Toll-like receptors are a family of at least 10 pattern recognition receptors that are expressed in varying combinations on a broad array of immune and nonimmune cells. They recognize particular types (patterns) of molecules derived from pathogens (eg, bacterial lipopolysaccharide, flagellin, mannan, CpG dinucleotides, viral dsDNA). Triggering of Toll-like receptors activates intracellular signaling pathways, many of which converge on a common pathway using the IRAK proteins and MyD88, which in turn activate the IκB kinase complex (NEMO/IκKα/IκKβ), ultimately leading to phosphorylation and degradation of IκBα and activation of the NF-κB transcription factor complex.

Mutations in TLR signaling pathways have now been associated with major infectious susceptibilities: Mutations in *IRAK4* and *MyD88* have been identified in patients with susceptibility to invasive pyogenic bacterial infections, including particularly *Streptococcus pneumoniae*, *Staphylococcus aureus*, and *Pseudomonas aeruginosa*. Interestingly, patients with IRAK4 or MyD88 deficiency tend to have problems with invasive pyogenic bacterial infections in childhood, but these subside over time, presumably as a result of the adaptive immune response covering for this innate defect. Mutations in *TLR3, TRIF, TRAF3,* and *UNC-93B* have been identified in patients with susceptibility to herpesvirus encephalitis. Defects in NEMO and IκBα also cause susceptibility to infections with pyogenic bacteria and mycobacteria and are associated with an anhydrotic ectodermal dysplasia phenotype. The severity of immunodeficiency and ectodermal dysplasia is quite variable and depends on the specific mutation that is present.[93]

Chronic Mucocutaneous Candidiasis Syndromes

Chronic mucocutaneous candidiasis (CMC) is a clinical syndrome associated with chronic and recurrent *Candida* infections of mucosae, particularly oral and vaginal, together with nail-bed infections but generally without systemic infection. CMC can occur in isolation or as part of a broader clinical syndrome such as in APECED (autoimmune poly endocrinopathy, candidiasis, ectodermal dystrophy). Recent discoveries have determined that in almost all cases, CMC is associated with abnormalities in development of Th17 effector T cells or with the production of, or responses to, the cytokine IL-17. These include autosomal recessive mutations in IL-17F or the IL-17 receptor α-subunit, dominant loss-of-function mutations in STAT3, and dominant gain-of-function mutations in STAT1.[94]

Recently, the CMC associated with APECED was found to be the result of autoantibodies to IL-17 and IL-22.[95,96] APECED is caused by mutations in AIRE1, a nuclear protein that regulates the expression of self-antigens by thymic medullary epithelial cells, where it plays a role in T-cell selection and maturation. Other features of this disorder include endocrinopathies (hypoparathyroidism, adrenal insufficiency, and diabetes), alopecia areata, nail dystrophy, and vitiligo.

Autoimmune Lymphoproliferative Syndrome

The clinical phenotype of autoimmune lymphoproliferative syndrome (ALPS) is characterized by massive lymphadenopathy and hepatosplenomegaly in most cases. In addition, patients have problems with recurrent episodes of autoimmune hemolytic anemia and thrombocytopenia. The defects that have been identified in patients with this group of disorders are all associated with abnormalities in lymphocyte apoptosis. These include *FAS* (CD95), Fas ligand *(FASL), FADD,* Caspase 10 *(CASP10), NRAS,* and *KRAS.* Peripheral blood T- and B-cell counts are generally normal, but in almost all cases, there is an increased percentage of αβ-TCR⁺ double-negative T cells that lack expression of both CD4 and CD8. A predisposition to developing lymphoid malignancies has been described in ALPS but is thought to be primarily in those patients who have mutations in the death domain of FAS. In addition to elevated double-negative T cells, patients with ALPS frequently have elevated levels of IL-10 and vitamin B_{12} in the blood, which can be valuable diagnostically in patients with suspected ALPS. Patients with mutations in caspase 8 *(CASP8)* were previously classified as ALPS but are now considered to be a unique syndrome that may have lymphadenopathy and splenomegaly, but recurrent respiratory tract infections and mucocutaneous herpesvirus infections are prominent, both unusual features in ALPS.[97,98]

A variety of immunosuppressive therapies have been tried in ALPS to control the recurrent autoimmune cytopenias and severe hepatosplenomegaly. Most of these were only modestly successful, as was splenectomy. Recent studies have, however, demonstrated a dramatic response to rapamycin therapy in many patients with ALPS, often causing shrinkage of the lymph nodes and spleen back to their normal size.[99,100]

Laboratory Evaluation of the Immune System

A basic laboratory workup to screen for significant defects in each of the four major compartments of the immune system can be done by most practitioners before making a referral to a clinical immunologist for further, detailed evaluation. In simple terms, this workup should include evaluation of numbers and function for each of the four immune system compartments. A recommended workup using this approach is outlined in Fig. 103.3.

Diagnostic Testing—Complement

Screening for complement deficiency should be performed in patients with recurrent episodes of bacteremia, meningitis, or disseminated gonorrhea. Since more than 30% of patients with recurrent *Neisseria* infections have complement deficiency, it is imperative that prompt testing of the complement system be done in these individuals. The screening test of choice for complement deficiencies is the CH50 test, which measures functional complement activity in the plasma. The CH50 will only identify defects in the classical pathway, which is typically sufficient because alternative pathway defects are exceedingly rare. If an alternative pathway defect is suspected, however, an analogous test (the AH50) can be performed. In

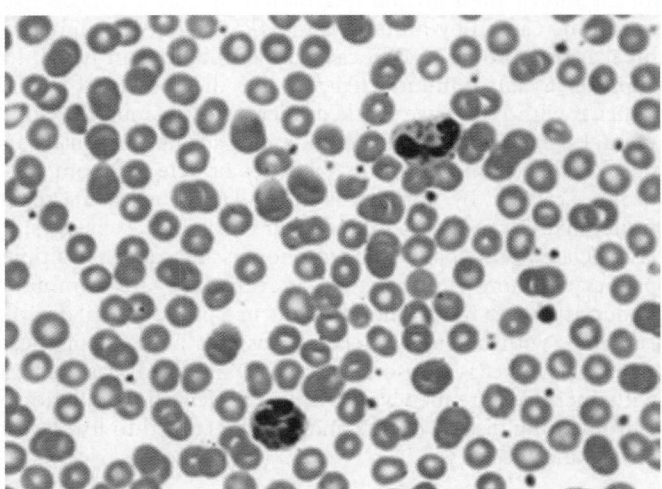

Fig. 103.3. Peripheral smear showing mature and band neutrophils *(top)* with basophilic cytoplasmic inclusion consistent with Chediak-Higashi syndrome.

order for the CH50 to give accurate results, the blood specimen needs to be handled carefully because complement is very heat labile. In general, it is recommended that any abnormal CH50 test should be repeated to confirm a complement deficiency. The CH50 is typically very low or absent in patients with a complement component deficiency. A CH50 result that is only moderately low is often seen in situations where the specimen was handled incorrectly or in patients with autoimmune disease such as lupus or mixed connective tissue disease. Once an abnormal CH50 test is confirmed, specialized testing to identify the specific complement component that is absent can be performed.

Diagnostic Testing—Phagocytes

Assessment of patients for a possible phagocytic disorder requires that both the number and the function of phagocytes be evaluated. Numbers are easily evaluated using a complete blood count with differential. If there is a concern for cyclic neutropenia, neutrophil counts may need to be evaluated three times weekly for 3 to 4 weeks to identify the nadir.[101] Functional testing includes evaluation of CD11/CD18 integrin expression on myeloid cells by flow cytometry if the patient has symptoms suggestive of leukocyte adhesion deficiency (LAD). In cases of suspected chronic granulomatous disease (CGD), evaluation of neutrophil oxidative burst function is essential. Traditionally this was done using nitrobluetetrazoleum (NBT) but is now performed using dihydrorhodamine (DHR), a reagent that permeates neutrophils and fluoresces when reduced by a normal neutrophil oxidative burst. Fluorescence is measured by flow cytometry. The DHR test is sensitive enough to differentiate most cases of X-linked CGD from autosomal recessive CGD, making it a particularly useful clinical assay.[102,103]

Diagnostic Testing—B Cells and Antibodies

The diagnosis of antibody deficiency needs to evaluate both the quantity and the quality of the antibody response. Quantity is easily evaluated by measuring quantitative immunoglobulin levels (IgG, IgM, IgA, and IgE) in the blood and comparing these with the age-appropriate normal ranges. Evaluating the quality of the antibody response can be done by measuring specific antibody titers to vaccines that the patient has received. Generally, responses to both protein antigens (eg, tetanus, diphtheria, hepatitis B) and carbohydrate antigens (23-valent unconjugated Pneumovax) need to be assessed to confirm normal antibody responses. Patients who respond appropriately to protein antigens but do not respond to carbohydrate antigens may have *specific antibody deficiency* and may require additional workup. Recent guidelines regarding the interpretation and use of diagnostic vaccination have recently been published.[104]

In addition to evaluating antibody quantity and quality, it is essential to determine whether patients have normal B-cell numbers by evaluating lymphocyte subsets. The use of more detailed B-cell immunophenotyping to evaluate B-cell development, the presence of CD27+ memory B cells, and the ability of memory B cells to undergo immunoglobulin class switching has become standard of care in many clinics as it provides valuable diagnostic and prognostic information.[105]

Flow cytometry testing to assess the expression of specific proteins that are defective in B-cell and antibody deficiency disorders including BTK, CD40 ligand, CD40, ICOS, CD27,

BAFF receptor, etc. can be performed in specialty laboratories and offer the ability to rapidly obtain a molecular diagnosis. This is typically supplemented by sequencing of specific genes.

Diagnostic Testing—T Cells

T-cell testing begins with determination if the absolute lymphocyte count is normal, as well as assessment of lymphocyte subsets (CD4+, CD8+, NK, Treg). Gross T-cell function can be ascertained beginning with T-cell proliferation assays. Vaccine titers for tetanus or diphtheria can also be quantified. Diagnosis of specific T-cell defects are usually made with flow cytometry to demonstrate alteration or absence of some lymphocyte protein or focused genetic testing.

Treatment of Immune System Disorders
Treatment: Complement

Patients with complement deficiency are susceptible to fulminant sepsis and other deep-seated infections caused by encapsulated organisms. For this reason, patients should be given a letter, laminated card, medical alert bracelet/necklace, or Health Data "Me" app that they can keep with them at all times with contact information for their primary care physician and clinical immunologist and a message indicating that they have a complement deficiency. The message should emphasize that there should be no delay in giving parenteral antibiotics should they be ill. For patients who live at a distance from skilled medical care, consideration should be given to providing a dose of parenteral antibiotic such ceftriaxone that can be administered by the patient or a family member when they become ill, before a lengthy trip to the hospital. The efficacy of chronic prophylactic antibiotics to prevent infection in patients with complement deficiency is not well studied and remains a significant question in this group of disorders. In addition to preparing for and treating infections, patients should also be regularly screened for autoimmunity by history, physical examination (ie, blood pressure monitoring), and laboratory testing including BUN, creatinine, and urinalysis to monitor for signs of glomerulonephritis because this is a common autoimmune manifestation.

Treatment: Phagocytes

As noted earlier, management of phagocytic disorders revolves around having a heightened suspicion for infections, aggressively treating acute infections using antibiotics and G-CSF as needed, and developing a prophylaxis regimen that is both effective and reasonable from a patient standpoint. At times, patients continue to have recurrent or severe infections despite these efforts and require more definitive therapy. As indicated earlier, hematopoietic stem cell transplantation (HSCT) has been shown to be effective in many, but not all, phagocytic disorders. Gene therapy has been attempted for both X-linked CGD[106] and for LAD-I,[107] but neither has been particularly successful thus far and at this point is considered to be experimental. Ongoing research to address the challenges of gene therapy that are unique to these two disorders is under way.

Treatment: B Cells and Antibodies
Immunoglobulin Replacement

In patients with antibody-deficiency, replacement of IgG is critical to maintaining health and preventing long-term complications associated with recurrent infections.

Immunoglobulin replacement therapy has been found to be effective when administered intravenously (IVIg), subcutaneously (SCIg), and intramuscularly (IMIg). FDA-approved products support administration via any of these routes. With that said, because of significant discomfort associated with IMIg administration, this route is rarely used in the United States. Most patients are maintained on either IVIg or SCIg depending on patient preference and provider recommendations related to each patient's clinical need. Because the half-life of IgG in the circulation is ~21 days under normal circumstances, IVIg is typically administered every 3 to 4 weeks providing high peak levels followed by a decline over the ensuing weeks to a trough before the next infusion. In contrast, SCIg is typically administered 1 to 2 times per week in smaller doses providing a more "steady-state" level of IgG in the circulation. IgG products are prepared from the pooled plasma collected from thousands of healthy donors and therefore contain a broad range of antibodies. A reasonable starting dose of either IVIg or SCIg is 400 to 500 mg/kg/month. This can be divided into the number of doses required to administer the necessary monthly volume (IgG preparations range in concentration from 5 gm/100 mL [5%] to 20 gm/100 mL [20%]). In most patients, a trough IgG level of 600 mg/dL in the blood is a reasonable initial target but the dose can then be increased or decreased to achieve a trough IgG level that prevents both acute infections and development of progressive lung disease. There is evidence that at least for bacterial pneumonia, higher IgG trough levels are directly correlated with a decreased risk of infection.[108] Supplemental IgG is generally effective at preventing lower respiratory tract infections (bronchitis and pneumonia), but the response of upper tract disease (particularly sinusitis) is more variable. Some patients have persistent sinus symptoms that can be a significant clinical problem despite IgG therapy. In these patients, the addition of prophylactic antibiotic therapy or increasing the frequency or dose of IgG infusions may be beneficial.

Side effects with IVIg therapy are relatively common, occurring in up to 25% of treated patients.[109] Side effects include headaches, nausea, vomiting, chills, fatigue, fever, rash, and aseptic meningitis. These can often be managed by changing the IgG product being used, pretreating with diphenhydramine, acetaminophen, and corticosteroids steroids before infusion, or slowing the rate of infusion. Patients who have persistent symptoms despite these measures can often tolerate subcutaneous IgG supplementation (SCIg).

Prophylactic Antibiotics

It has been increasingly recognized that in many patients with antibody deficiency, replacement of IgG (even to normal levels) may not prevent all clinically significant infections. The addition of prophylactic antibiotics has been used as an adjunct to IgG therapy to try and improve control of infections and decrease morbidity. Unfortunately, to date, there have been no well-performed studies that argue strongly either for or against the use of prophylactic antibiotics to improve outcomes. Similarly, there have been virtually no studies that support a particular antibiotic regimen as being superior for prophylaxis. Because many patients with antibody deficiency have evidence of bronchiectasis and chronic lung disease, some providers, extrapolating from the lung transplant and cystic fibrosis literature, have used thrice-weekly macrolide antibiotics as a prophylactic regimen in an attempt to prevent progression of lung pathology. Further studies are needed to clarify the role of prophylactic antibiotics and to define the optimal regimen.

Treatment: T Cells

SCID was uniformly lethal in the first years of life until Good et al. successfully reconstituted an affected infant with a transplant of sibling bone marrow. Experience in subsequent years has shown that patients with B-cell–positive SCID (IL2RG, JAK3, IL7RA, etc.) readily reconstitute their T-cell deficiency but may not develop significant B-cell chimerism. The reasons for this are not entirely understood, but various hypotheses have been put forward. From a practical standpoint, a lack of donor B-cell engraftment may lead to a chronic need for IgG replacement therapy even after transplant because patients may not be able to mount sufficient antibody responses. Patients with B-cell–negative SCID are more likely to have successful donor engraftment of both T- and B-cell lineages and more likely to recover full humoral immune function.

One of the most significant challenges in the treatment of SCID is that in the absence of family history, most patients come to attention because of infections. These are most commonly PJ pneumonia and severe viral infections (see earlier). PJ pneumonia can be treated but may lead to lung damage, whereas viral infections may or may not be controllable. In addition, many SCID infants have significant diarrhea and weight loss by the time they reach a transplant center. Together, these complications increase the risk of adverse outcomes during transplantation for SCID and have been the major impetus for adding SCID to state newborn screening panels. Initial management before transplant involves aggressive supportive care, antimicrobials to treat any intercurrent infections (bacterial, viral, and fungal), antimicrobial prophylaxis to prevent future infections, and IgG replacement therapy.

There is significant debate about the best pretransplant conditioning regimen for patients with SCID to balance safety and efficacy. In general, those patients that have a matched sibling donor receive no conditioning before receiving unmanipulated bone marrow. For other patients, a variety of conditioning regimens ranging from no conditioning to fully myeloablative regimens have been tried. Similarly, a range of manipulated and unmanipulated stem cell sources have been tried including matched bone marrow, matched peripheral blood, cord blood, and haploidentical. Lastly, a variety of prophylactic immunosuppressive regimens have been used in the early posttransplant period to limit GvHD and prevent graft rejection. Each option has advantages and disadvantages, which has led to the spectrum of transplant regimens that have been attempted for SCID. Current efforts are under way to assess which regimens offer the best outcomes and lowest risk.[110-113]

Key References

1. Notarangelo L, Casanova JL, Conley ME, et al. Primary immunodeficiency diseases: an update from the International Union of Immunological Societies Primary Immunodeficiency Diseases Classification Committee Meeting in Budapest, 2005. J Allergy Clin Immunol. 2006;117:883-896.
2. Cossu F. Genetics of SCID. Ital J Pediatr. 2010;36:76.
3. Leiva LE, Zelazco M, Oleastro M, et al. Primary immunodeficiency diseases in Latin America: the second report of the LAGID registry. J Clin Immunol. 2007;27:101-108.

4. Frank MM. Complement deficiencies. *Pediatr Clin North Am.* 2000;47:1339-1354.
5. Hofer J, Janecke AR, Zimmerhackl LB, et al. Complement factor H-related protein 1 deficiency and factor H antibodies in pediatric patients with atypical hemolytic uremic syndrome. *Clin J Am Soc Nephrol.* 2013;8:407-415.
6. Joseph C, Gattineni J. Complement disorders and hemolytic uremic syndrome. *Curr Opin Pediatr.* 2013;25:209-215.
7. Westra D, Vernon KA, Volokhina EB, et al. Atypical hemolytic uremic syndrome and genetic aberrations in the complement factor H-related 5 gene. *J Hum Genet.* 2012;57:459-464.
8. Kawalec P, Holko P, Paszulewicz A, et al. Administration of conestat alfa, human C1 esterase inhibitor and icatibant in the treatment of acute angioedema attacks in adults with hereditary angioedema due to C1 esterase inhibitor deficiency. Treatment comparison based on systematic review results. *Pneumonol Alergol Pol.* 2013;81:95-104.
9. Patel NS, Fung SM, Zanichelli A, et al. Ecallantide for treatment of acute attacks of acquired C1 esterase inhibitor deficiency. *Allergy Asthma Proc.* 2013;34:72-77.
10. Cole SW, Lundquist LM. Icatibant for the treatment of hereditary angioedema. *Ann Pharmacother.* 2013;47:49-55.
11. Walport MJ, Davies KA, Morley BJ, et al. Complement deficiency and autoimmunity. *Ann N Y Acad Sci.* 1997;815:267-281.
12. Figueroa JE, Densen P. Infectious diseases associated with complement deficiencies. *Clin Microbiol Rev.* 1991;4:359-395.
13. Hanna S, Etzioni A. Leukocyte adhesion deficiencies. *Ann N Y Acad Sci.* 2012;1250:50-55.
14. Farinha NJ, Duval M, Wagner E, et al. Unrelated bone marrow transplantation for leukocyte adhesion deficiency. *Bone Marrow Transplant.* 2002;30:979-981.
15. Thomas C, Le Deist F, Cavazzana-Calvo M, et al. Results of allogeneic bone marrow transplantation in patients with leukocyte adhesion deficiency. *Blood.* 1995;86:1629-1635.
16. Le Deist F, Blanche S, Keable H, et al. Successful HLA nonidentical bone marrow transplantation in three patients with the leukocyte adhesion deficiency. *Blood.* 1989;74:512-516.
17. Gulino AV, Moratto D, Sozzani S, et al. Altered leukocyte response to CXCL12 in patients with warts hypogammaglobulinemia, infections, myelokathexis (WHIM) syndrome. *Blood.* 2004;104:444-452.
18. Dotta L, Tassone L, Badolato R. Clinical and genetic features of Warts, Hypogammaglobulinemia, Infections and Myelokathexis (WHIM) syndrome. *Curr Mol Med.* 2011;11:317-325.
19. McDermott DH, Liu Q, Ulrick J, et al. The CXCR4 antagonist plerixafor corrects panleukopenia in patients with WHIM syndrome. *Blood.* 2011;118:4957-4962.
20. Dale DC, Bolyard AA, Kelley ML, et al. The CXCR4 antagonist plerixafor is a potential therapy for myelokathexis, WHIM syndrome. *Blood.* 2011;118:4963-4966.
21. Krivan G, Erdos M, Kallay K, et al. Successful umbilical cord blood stem cell transplantation in a child with WHIM syndrome. *Eur J Haematol.* 2010;84:274-275.
22. Segal BH, Leto TL, Gallin JI, et al. Genetic, biochemical, and clinical features of chronic granulomatous disease. *Medicine (Baltimore).* 2000;79:170-200.
23. Kuhns DB, Alvord WG, Heller T, et al. Residual NADPH oxidase and survival in chronic granulomatous disease. *N Engl J Med.* 2010;363:2600-2610.
24. Seger RA. Hematopoietic stem cell transplantation for chronic granulomatous disease. *Immunol Allergy Clin North Am.* 2010;30:195-208.
25. Hussain A, Yu L, Faryal R, et al. TEC family kinases in health and disease–loss-of-function of BTK and ITK and the gain-of-function fusions ITK-SYK and BTK-SYK. *FEBS J.* 2011;278:2001-2010.
26. Dua J, Elliot E, Bright P, et al. Pyoderma gangrenosum-like ulcer caused by *Helicobacter cinaedi* in a patient with X-linked agammaglobulinaemia. *Clin Exp Dermatol.* 2012;37:642-645.
27. Cuccherini B, Chua K, Gill V, et al. Bacteremia and skin/bone infections in two patients with X-linked agammaglobulinemia caused by an unusual organism related to *Flexispira/Helicobacter* species. *Clin Immunol.* 2000;97:121-129.
28. Turvey SE, Leo SH, Boos A, et al. Successful approach to treatment of Helicobacter bilis infection in X-linked agammaglobulinemia. *J Clin Immunol.* 2012;32:1404-1408.
29. Kainulainen L, Nikoskelainen J, Vuorinen T, et al. Viruses and bacteria in bronchial samples from patients with primary hypogammaglobulinemia. *Am J Respir Crit Care Med.* 1999;159:1199-1204.
30. Katamura K, Hattori H, Kunishima T, et al. Non-progressive viral myelitis in X-linked agammaglobulinemia. *Brain Dev.* 2002;24:109-111.
31. Misbah SA, Spickett GP, Ryba PC, et al. Chronic enteroviral meningoencephalitis in agammaglobulinemia: case report and literature review. *J Clin Immunol.* 1992;12:266-270.
32. Quan PL, Wagner TA, Briese T, et al. Astrovirus encephalitis in boy with X-linked agammaglobulinemia. *Emerg Infect Dis.* 2010;16:918-925.
33. Lee WI, Torgerson TR, Schumacher MJ, et al. Molecular analysis of a large cohort of patients with the hyper immunoglobulin M (IgM) syndrome. *Blood.* 2005;105:1881-1890.
34. Cabral-Marques O, Schimke LF, Pereira PV, et al. Expanding the clinical and genetic spectrum of human CD40L deficiency: the occurrence of paracoccidioidomycosis and other unusual infections in Brazilian patients. *J Clin Immunol.* 2012;32:212-220.
35. Rodrigues F, Davies EG, Harrison P, et al. Liver disease in children with primary immunodeficiencies. *J Pediatr.* 2004;145:333-339.
36. Jo EK, Kim HS, Lee MY, et al. X-linked hyper-IgM syndrome associated with *Cryptosporidium parvum* and *Cryptococcus neoformans* infections: the first case with molecular diagnosis in Korea. *J Korean Med Sci.* 2002;17:116-120.
37. Isam H, Al-Wahadneh A. Successful bone marrow transplantation in a child with X-linked hyper-igm syndrome. *Saudi J Kidney Dis Transpl.* 2004;15:489-493.
38. Duplantier JE, Seyama K, Day NK, et al. Immunologic reconstitution following bone marrow transplantation for X-linked hyper IgM syndrome. *Clin Immunol.* 2001;98:313-318.
39. Ferrari S, Giliani S, Insalaco A, et al. Mutations of CD40 gene cause an autosomal recessive form of immunodeficiency with hyper IgM. *Proc Natl Acad Sci USA.* 2001;98:12614-12619.
40. Imai K, Slupphaug G, Lee WI, et al. Human uracil-DNA glycosylase deficiency associated with profoundly impaired immunoglobulin class-switch recombination. *Nat Immunol.* 2003;4:1023-1028.
41. Revy P, Muto T, Levy Y, et al. Activation-induced cytidine deaminase (AID) deficiency causes the autosomal recessive form of the hyper-IgM syndrome (HIGM2). *Cell.* 2000;102:565-575.
42. Resnick ES, Moshier EL, Godbold JH, et al. Morbidity and mortality in common variable immune deficiency over 4 decades. *Blood.* 2012;119:1650-1657.
43. Bates CA, Ellison MC, Lynch DA, et al. Granulomatous-lymphocytic lung disease shortens survival in common variable immunodeficiency. *J Allergy Clin Immunol.* 2004;114:415-421.
44. Chase NM, Verbsky JW, Hintermeyer MK, et al. Use of combination chemotherapy for treatment of granulomatous and lymphocytic interstitial lung disease (GLILD) in patients with common variable immunodeficiency (CVID). *J Clin Immunol.* 2013;33:30-39.
45. Podjasek JC, Abraham RS. Autoimmune cytopenias in common variable immunodeficiency. *Front Immunol.* 2012;3:189.
101. Boxer LA. How to approach neutropenia. *Am Soc Hematol Educ Program.* 2012;2012:174-182.
102. Jirapongsananuruk O, Malech HL, Kuhns DB, et al. Diagnostic paradigm for evaluation of male patients with chronic granulomatous disease, based on the dihydrorhodamine 123 assay. *J Allergy Clin Immunol.* 2003;111:374-379.
103. Vowells SJ, Sekhsaria S, Malech HL, et al. Flow cytometric analysis of the granulocyte respiratory burst: a comparison study of fluorescent probes. *J Immunol Methods.* 1995;178:89-97.
106. Kang HJ, Bartholomae CC, Paruzynski A, et al. Retroviral gene therapy for X-linked chronic granulomatous disease: results from phase I/II trial. *Mol Ther.* 2011;19:2092-20101.
107. Bauer TR Jr, Hickstein DD. Gene therapy for leukocyte adhesion deficiency. *Curr Opin Mol Ther.* 2000;2:383-388.

Acquired Immune Dysfunction

Gwenn E. McLaughlin and Brent J. Pfeiffer

PEARLS

- Most patients admitted to the pediatric ICU are immunosuppressed to varying degrees.
- Critical illness induces immunoparalysis, a phenomenon marked by downregulation of major histocompatibility complex class II molecule expression on the surface of monocytes, but not B cells. Suppressed monocyte/macrophage function reduces clearance of immune complexes, impairs antigen-presenting capabilities, and decreases natural killer cell function.
- Worldwide, protein calorie malnutrition is the most common cause of acquired immunodeficiency. Exposure to immunomodulatory medications increasingly accounts for cases of secondary immunodeficiency.
- The long-term effects of transfusions on the immune system and subsequent disease susceptibility are unknown, but even 19 years after a blood transfusion, recipients have fewer peripheral T cells, particularly helper T cells, than nonrecipients.
- Children with chronic immunosuppression are at risk for reactivation of latent viruses such as cytomegalovirus, Epstein-Barr virus, and adenovirus, as well as tuberculosis.
- Pneumocystosis is still the most common AIDS-defining illness in children and can present with variable pulmonary infiltrates, but hypoxemia is often out of proportion to clinical and radiographic examination.
- Lymphomas in immunodeficiencies are generally of B-cell type and often arise in the CNS.
- Postexposure prophylaxis for occupational HIV exposure should begin as soon as possible and continue for 4 weeks.

Acquired immune dysfunction is by definition a secondary phenomenon following another disease process, such as infection or trauma, or an intended or unintended effect of therapy. Protein calorie malnutrition probably accounts for the greatest number of immunodeficient patients in ICUs worldwide, whereas HIV infection is the most widely recognized cause of acquired immune deficiency. Impairments in humoral and cellular immunity occur as a consequence of immaturity, malignancy, transfusion, sepsis, shock, viral infections, tuberculosis (TB), and malaria.[1] Iatrogenic immunosuppression occurs most frequently with medications given to either inactivate or kill lymphocyte populations, particularly those used in cancer chemotherapy and autoimmune disease, and to

control transplant rejection. When all these precipitants of immunodeficiency are taken into account, it becomes apparent that most patients admitted to the pediatric ICU (PICU) are immunosuppressed, although to varying degrees. Patients with acquired immunodeficiency are at risk for opportunistic infections and unusual presentations of common infections. If immunosuppression is known or suspected, the physical examination should focus on the mucosal surfaces, catheter entry sites, skin (including wounds), and CNS. Understanding patterns of disease that are specific to each type of immune dysfunction can lead to both earlier appropriate empiric therapy and diagnostic tests. Unlike congenital immunodeficiency, many cases of acquired immunodeficiency are reversible with treatment or resolution of the primary illness or injury.

Immune Function and Critical Illness

Critical illness often involves the activation of innate and adaptive immunity responses that must be regulated for the patient to survive (see also Chapters 101 and 102).[1] The body responds to stress by releasing proinflammatory cytokines such as tumor necrosis factor–alpha (TNF-α), interferon-gamma (INF-γ), and interleukins (IL-1, IL-2, IL-6, IL-8, and IL-12) from various immune cell types.[1] Tissue injury, epithelial barrier disruption, and cell destruction potentiate the proinflammatory response through the Toll-like receptors (TLRs) and other pattern-recognition molecules involved in innate immunity.[2] To regulate the proinflammatory reaction, antiinflammatory agents such as IL-10, IL-4, IL-6, transforming growth factor β (TGF-β), soluble TNF receptor, and endogenous corticosteroids suppress immune function.[3-6] Prolonged recovery of the immune system after critical illness is known as immunoparalysis and puts the patient at increased risk of developing nosocomial infections.[7-10]

In 1986, a group of trauma surgeons recognized an association between late mortality after severe trauma due to secondary infections and suppressed monocyte function, specifically antigen presentation.[4] Several subsequent studies demonstrated downregulation of major histocompatibility complex (MHC) class II (human leukocyte antigen [HLA]-DR) molecules on the surface of monocytes after severe trauma, cardiopulmonary bypass, neurosurgical procedures, acute pancreatitis, and severe sepsis.[4,7-14] Suppressed monocyte/macrophage HLA-DR expression reduces immune complex clearance and impairs the antigen-presenting capabilities of the innate immune system, thus limiting activated T-cell interactions with monocyte/macrophages expressing HLA-DR-antigen complexes. Helper T-cell interaction with monocytes/

macrophages is necessary to activate pathogen-killing mechanisms, produce chemokines, and promote leukocyte mobility. The interaction is also interferon gamma (INF-γ) dependent.[15] Immunoparalysis is confirmed in the laboratory by reduced expression of HLA-DR antigens on peripheral blood monocytes and decreased ex vivo TNF-α production in response to lipopolysaccharide (LPS) exposure.[4,15,16] The downregulation of monocyte HLA-DR expression may in part explain the increased incidence of life-threatening nosocomial infections, including those considered reactivated or opportunistic, in patients following critical illness.[8,9,17,18]

The persistent expression of IL-10 is also believed to have a central role in immunoparalysis. Interleukin 10 is an antiinflammatory cytokine expressed by many cell types (T cells, B cells, dendritic cells, macrophages, and neutrophils) and capable of downregulating cytokine expression, antigen presentation, and costimulatory cell surface molecules preventing exuberant immune responses and autoimmunity.[19] There is an inverse linear correlation between L-10 serum concentrations and HLA-DR expression.[20] After cardiopulmonary bypass, those children with elevated IL-10 levels demonstrate ex vivo LPS hyporesponsiveness.[21] Following septic shock, in children who went on to develop persistent nosocomial infection, early plasma IL-10 levels were significantly higher than children with sepsis who did not experience nosocomial infections.[7] These children also demonstrated diminished TNF-α production ex vivo.[4] IL-10 is capable of suppressing T-cell cytokine production of IL-2 and INF-γ, meaning that IL-10 directly reduces adaptive immune responses.[22]

Like immunoparalysis, absolute lymphocytopenia has often been reported in previously healthy patients after severe sepsis, burns, neurotrauma, cardiopulmonary bypass, and viral infections.[23-28] Total lymphocyte counts measured in 22 children fell to a nadir at 6 hours after anesthesia for major surgery with minimal recovery at 48 hours.[25] Cardiopulmonary bypass further induced lymphocyte apoptosis compared with surgery alone.[26] A recent adult study assessed persistent lymphopenia as a biomarker for sepsis-induced immunosuppression and found that moderate to severe persistent lymphopenia on Day 4 following the diagnosis of sepsis predicted early and late mortality.[27] In a pediatric population, prolonged lymphopenia defined as lymphocyte count less than 1000 cells/μL for more than 7 days was associated with a greater than sixfold increased risk of death.[28]

The reasons for persistent lymphopenia are not understood, and one hypothesis is that elevated endogenous corticosteroids induce lymphopenia (see also Chapter 81). Exogenous corticosteroids have long been known to induce lymphocyte apoptosis, and critical illness elicits a hormonal stress response increasing endogenous corticosteroids, although there is no direct correlation between cortisol levels and lymphopenia.[23,28] In contrast, prolactin has been shown to affect lymphocyte survival, required for proliferation and prevention of steroid-induced apoptosis.[28] Drugs used in critically ill patients may contribute to lymphopenia by interfering with prolactin levels. Dopamine inhibits prolactin release, even at very low doses, and reduced prolactin levels directly affect lymphocyte function and survival.[28-30] Prolonged suppression of prolactin is associated with lymphopenia, nosocomial infection, and death.[28]

Several investigators have attempted to reverse immunoparalysis to reduce late infections and enhance patient survival.[6,31-37] Monocytes can be stimulated by granulocyte-macrophage colony-stimulating factor (GM-CSF). In nine consecutive healthy adults with immunoparalysis documented after LPS injection, 5 μg/kg of GM-CSF produced a fourfold increase in mean HLA-DR expression in peripheral blood monocytes and a ninefold increase in TNF-α response to LPS in as little as 24 hours.[32] When given to septic patients with acute respiratory distress syndrome (ARDS), GM-CSF was associated with improved gas exchange and increased neutrophil respiratory burst.[33] An observational study, followed by a prospective, randomized, open-label use of GM-CSF, demonstrated reversal of immunoparalysis in all seven of the children randomized to the GM-CSF group and none experienced a nosocomial infection.[7] However, a meta-analysis performed on 12 randomized controlled trials of either G-CSF or GM-CSF in sepsis found no impact on all-cause mortality, but there was a benefit in reversal of infection.[34] These studies did not require documentation of immunoparalysis before enrollment. A small, multicenter, double-blind, randomized control trial in which only patients with documented low HLA-DR levels were randomized to receive GM-CSF showed significant improvement in days of mechanical ventilation and severity of illness score but nonsignificant changes in ICU and hospital length of stay.[35] Interferons, which are major activators of monocytes, have also been administered in patients with sepsis to reduced immunoparalysis.[31] Exogenous interferon gamma-1β therapy was administered to 10 consecutive patients with less than 30% HLA-DR expression and restored both HLA-DR expression and production of IL-6 and TNF-α.[36] Aerosolized interferon-γ when administered to trauma patients with immunoparalysis (defined as suppressed HLA-DR expression on alveolar macrophages) was associated with a lower incidence of ventilator-associated pneumonia.[37] Additional clinical trials of interferon and GM-CSF are ongoing.[5]

Malnutrition and Immune Function

Worldwide, protein-calorie malnutrition is the most common cause of acquired immunodeficiency (see also Chapter 87).[38,39] Nutrition influences the course of HIV and TB, susceptibility to infection in older patients, the body's ability to respond to vaccines, and many other aspects of immune function.[40-43] Critical illness often causes initial hypermetabolism followed by macronutrient and micronutrient malnutrition. A significant proportion of children admitted to ICUs (even in affluent countries) have been noted to be malnourished, whereas many others will receive inadequate nutritional support during their stay in the ICU, implying that many critically ill children will have abnormal immune function secondary to nutritional deficits.[40,44-46] It is estimated that one in every five children admitted to the PICU presents with chronic malnutrition or will develop acute malnutrition.[40,47,48] Malnourished children and infants have greater numbers of ventilator days, longer ICU stays, increased hospital costs, and increased infectious complications.[47-49] Immune system dysfunction occurs so early in the course of malnutrition that measures of immune competence, such as anergy and total T-lymphocyte numbers, are sensitive indicators of a patient's nutritional status.[41]

Protein-energy malnutrition (PEM) is generally only studied in humans in its severest form. Although mice with PEM demonstrate hyporesponsive to LPS in expression of TLR-4 and co-receptor molecules on macrophages, extrapolation of animal data to humans may be inappropriate because of interspecies variability in immunoglobulin synthesis and cytokine regulation.[41,50] Protein-energy malnutrition increases the risk of bacterial colonization by altering mucosal defenses to pathogens, epithelial cell membrane glycoprotein receptor production, mucus production, and immunoglobulin A secretion.[43] Protein-energy malnutrition also affects immune cells by delaying neutrophils mobilization, reducing natural killer cell lytic activity, and impairing T-lymphocyte function and proliferation.[51] The severity of PEM is proportional to the impairment of T-lymphocyte function, but all of the factors stated earlier increase a patient's susceptibility to infectious complications. Greater reduction in immune responses occurs when the malnutrition is more prolonged and severe, as reflected in decreased immunoglobulin levels and cytokine production (interferon-γ).[52]

Many specific nutrients are vital to immune function. Adult studies demonstrate improved clinical outcomes in the setting of acute respiratory distress syndrome (ARDS) and severe sepsis when patients are given an enteral formula containing antioxidants plus essential fatty acids.[53-55] The ω-3 polyunsaturated fatty acids (PUFAs), eicosopentaenoic acid and docosahexaenoic acid (DHA), synthesized from alpha-linolenic acid or obtained from a diet of fish, suppress lymphocyte responses to mitogen stimulation.[38,56] By definition, essential fatty acids, linoleic and alpha-linoleic acids, cannot be synthesized by mammalian cells and must be obtained through the diet. Linoleic acid is found in typically fish, shellfish, plant seeds/oils, and tree nuts.[56] For children in many parts of the world, access to fat other than cow's milk is severely limited.[38] Accumulating evidence suggests that dietary supplementation with ω-3 PUFAs is a "natural" immunosuppressant and may be useful in autoimmune diseases such as lupus erythematosus, rheumatoid arthritis, and diabetes mellitus.[56] Moderate ω-3 PUFA intake can enhance the immune response; for example, supplementation of infant formula with a small amount of DHA accelerates development of T-cell responsiveness in preterm infants (see also Chapter 87).[57] Studies have assessed children with acute lung injury and severe burns with associated acute respiratory failure who were treated with enteral formulas containing antioxidants and PUFAs. These investigations demonstrated formula tolerance, increased antiinflammatory biomarkers, improved oxygenation, and improved pulmonary compliance.[58,59] These studies were not designed to assess clinical outcomes.

There are many specific micronutrients identified as vital to immune function. Vitamin A has essential functions in immune cells and indirectly contributes to protection from infection through maintenance of vital epithelial cell differentiation and barrier function of the lung and intestine.[60] Vitamin A deficiency occurs in an estimated 100 million children worldwide and is a risk factor for increased death from pneumonia and diarrhea.[44,60] A survey of hospitalized children in Malawi reported that one-third had severe vitamin A deficiency and one-third had moderate deficiency.[61] Paradoxically, these children exhibited preferential monocyte synthesis of TNF-α as compared with IL-10. The underlying disease that prompted hospitalization possibly triggered this shift. Results of several randomized, double-blinded, placebo-controlled trials conducted in malnourished children have shown improved antibody response to vaccines and fewer diseases of the gastrointestinal and respiratory systems after vitamin A

supplementation.[44,60,61] Vitamin A supplementation in individuals who are not deficient has no benefit, whereas high retinal levels are associated with an increase in diarrhea and pneumonia.[62]

Vitamin C (ascorbic acid) is highly concentrated in leukocytes, and low leukocyte vitamin C concentrations are associated with reduced immune function.[57] Epidemiologic data suggest that higher vitamin C consumption lowers the risk of cancer and cardiovascular disease, but despite numerous clinical trials with participants of both sexes and varying ages, no definitive evidence that vitamin C supplementation reduces the frequency or symptoms of upper respiratory infections exists. High-dose vitamin C does improve several measures of immune function and does not appear to have any side effects.[44]

Vitamin D receptors are found on numerous immune cell types.[63] Vitamin D deficiency is associated with depressed macrophage function and impaired delayed hypersensitivity.[63] Although vitamin D deficiency has been documented as present on admission in many ICU patients, an association between low vitamin D levels and length of mechanical ventilation and mortality has been shown in some but not all studies.[64-71] In critically ill children, deficiency of vitamin D was more likely to occur in winter, in older children, and in those with darker skin.[64] A correlation between vitamin D levels and severity of illness in septic shock was identified.[64] Patients who were receiving vitamin D supplementation before admission had higher serum concentrations that appeared to be protective.[64] Vitamin D supplementation appears to be inexpensive, easily accomplished, and without risk, but to date there is no convincing evidence that vitamin D supplementation after the development of critical illness improves outcomes.[69,70,72,73]

Vitamin E (alphatocopherol) is a potent lipid-soluble antioxidant. Study results of vitamin E supplementation ranging from 200 to 800 mg/day in healthy adults showed increased CD4/CD8 ratios, mitogen responsiveness, antibody production, and decreased free radical production; however, a dosage of 300 mg/day for 3 weeks resulted in suppressed bactericidal activity in humans.[41] Optimal daily requirements of these nutrients in health and disease remain to be determined.

Of the trace elements that may affect the immune system, selenium, zinc, and iron have been the most widely studied. Selenium balances redox states and suppresses inflammation through its vital role in several antioxidant enzymes and intranuclear factors, including the glucocorticoid receptor, activator protein-1, and nuclear factor-κB.[41] In HIV infection, selenium supplementation modifies cytokine release, decreasing TNF-α and IL-8 while increasing IL-2.[74] Selenium improves T-cell proliferation and differentiation; however, selenium supplementation had no impact on severe sepsis in surgical ICU patients.[75] A single-center study of plasma selenium levels in children with systemic inflammatory response syndrome found an association among low selenium levels, inflammation, and nutritional status.[76] Enterally fed children whose selenium levels increased by Day 5 had greater ventilator-free days and ICU free days than those who did not.[77] Plasma selenium responds to adequate nutritional intake, but excessive selenium intake is toxic to the immune system and other organs.[41]

Zinc, as with selenium, is required for the activity of more than 100 enzymes.[78] Zinc supplementation increases the number of CD4[+] T cells; thus the CD4/CD8 T-cell ratio is improved. Zinc deficiency has been documented in alcoholics and in patients with burns and gastrointestinal disorders.[78,79] Zinc supplementation reduces bacteremia, hospitalization rates, and vaso-occlusive crises in patients with sickle cell anemia.[41] In young children, zinc supplementation reduced the duration of diarrhea and frequency of respiratory infections.[41,78]

Worldwide, 20% to 25% of the population has iron deficiency, which results in impaired cell-mediated immunity, particularly in neutrophil and natural killer cell function.[79] Although an association between iron availability and susceptibility to certain bacterial infections exists, there is little evidence that iron supplementation to deficient individuals inhibits immune responses or increases susceptibility to infections.[79]

Transfusions

Critically ill patients frequently receive blood transfusions, and modified immune responses have been observed (see also Chapter 93). Patients with cancer who receive transfusions at the time of resection have a greater risk of dying than those who do not.[80,81] In contrast, some patients who receive blood transfusions before transplantation have a lower incidence of rejection, although transplantation recipients who have received mismatched HLA-DR blood products have accelerated graft rejection.[82] The long-term effects of transfusions on the immune system and disease susceptibility are not well understood, but even 19 years after transfusion, blood product recipients have fewer peripheral T lymphocytes, particularly helper T cells, than patients who did not undergo transfusion.[83] Transfusions after trauma or cardiopulmonary bypass are associated with increased infections; however, in major surgery or trauma, it is difficult to sort out the effect of transfusion versus the effect of surgery or trauma.[84]

Immunosuppressive Medications

The use of medications to alter immune responses is becoming common in clinical practice, treating broad categories of diseases, such as autoimmune disorders, allergic disorders, transplant rejection, and graft-versus-host disease.[51] Broadly, drugs used for immunosuppression can be grouped into corticosteroids, cytotoxic drugs, calcineurin inhibitors, mammalian target of rapamycin (mTOR), and biologicals (monoclonal or polyclonal antibodies targeting cytokines or specific cell surface molecules of immune cells). A detailed description of all categories of immunosuppressive agents is beyond the scope of this chapter. The primary adverse effect of this drug class is the weakening of cellular immune responses, making the patient more susceptible to bacterial, fungal, and viral infections (acute, chronic, and reactivated). Glucocorticoids exert significant antiinflammatory activity. Glucocorticoids bind a cytosolic receptor, which then translocates to the nucleus of a cell affecting gene transcription. The overall impacts of glucocorticoid therapy are reduced cytokine production, lymphocyte anergy or apoptosis, impaired phagocytosis of neutrophils, and reduced bactericidal activity of macrophages.[51,85] This wide range of immune defects places the patient at risk for viral, bacterial, and fungal infections. Cytotoxic agents interfere with the synthesis of DNA of rapidly dividing cells. Common cytotoxic medications are cyclophosphamide, methotrexate, azathioprine, and 6-mercaptopurine. These medications inhibit T- and B-lymphocyte proliferation, as well as any other rapidly dividing cell. The major limitation of cytotoxic agents is their toxicity to other cells, such as hematopoietic cells, gastrointestinal mucosa, and skin cells. The inhibition of new adaptive immune responses, possible development of cytopenias, and mucosa/skin barrier deterioration place the patient at risk for bacterial and fungal infections.[51,85] Calcineurin inhibitors and mTOR medications inhibit the activation of IL-2, an essential cytokine and signaling cascade needed for T-lymphocyte activation and proliferation.[51] Crippling T-lymphocyte activation and proliferation place the patient at risk for viral infections and lymphoproliferative disorders.[85] The biologicals are a relatively new class of immunomodulatory agents, and many of their effects are dependent on their target. One example is antithymocyte globulin, a medication that targets T lymphocytes via multiple epitopes and causes profound and prolonged periods of lymphopenia, which is associated with reactivation of latent viruses.

Uremia

Uremia is a condition common in critically ill children with acute or chronic renal disease. Many end-stage renal disease patients are dialysis dependent and are at risk for invasive microorganisms independent of their need for dialysis or vascular/peritoneal access devices.[51] Uremic patients experience increased incidence and severity of infections compared with the general population. Children undergoing chronic dialysis have mortality rates 30 times greater than the general population even when disparities in age, sex, race, and diabetes are taken into account.[86] Essentially, uremia and dialysis cause a state chronic immune activation, thus leading to a proinflammatory state and immune hyporesponsiveness characterized by reduced lymphocyte numbers, impaired NK cell function, reduced dendritic cell antigen presentation, and failure to generate antibody responses to administered vaccines.[87-89]

Infectious Agents Other Than HIV

In addition to HIV, viruses such as measles, influenza, and human T-cell lymphotrophic virus-1 can suppress the immune response.[90-95] Neutrophils of patients infected with measles are not activated and therefore cannot phagocytize and kill bacteria.[90] Lymphopenia has been associated with measles, influenza, respiratory syncytial virus (RSV), and two paramyxoma viruses that can infect monocytes.[91-94] Following these infections, mortality is often related to secondary infections.[94,95] Okada et al.[91] documented that the measles virus infected only a small number of lymphocytes but apoptosis occurred in noninfected lymphocytes. The duration of lymphopenia was age dependent and was most prolonged in infants. The same response was not observed in response to a live measles vaccine.[92] Absolute lymphocyte counts were lower in hospitalized RSV-infected patients than controls and were lowest in patients admitted to the ICU.[93] No mortality was observed, and lymphocyte counts recovered. In children infected with RSV and known immunodeficiency such as following cancer therapy, the development of lower respiratory tract infection was associated with profound lymphopenia (<100 cells/μL) and mortality was 31%.[94]

HIV Infection and AIDS

AIDS is a clinical syndrome resulting from infection by HIV-1 (and rarely HIV-2), an RNA retrovirus dependent on a reverse transcriptase for replication.[96] Surrounding the RNA and its reverse transcriptase are core proteins p24 and p18. A viral envelope is composed of the host cell membrane studded with glycoproteins gp120 and gp40. HIV enters cells by binding gp120 to the CD4, a cell surface glycoprotein expressed on helper T lymphocytes, macrophages, and dendritic cells. After gp120-CD4 binding, HIV entry into cells is aided by the presence of a host coreceptor, chemokines CCR5 on macrophages, or CXCR4 on other cell lines. After HIV replication, the host's helper T lymphocytes undergo apoptosis, resulting in severe impairment of both cell-mediated and humoral immunity. Because pediatric HIV infection is most commonly transmitted from mother to infant, the acquired immunodeficiency is occurring in a host whose immune system, unlike an adult's, is relatively naive and has developed little natural immunity.[96,97] This may in part explain the shorter time required for progression to AIDS after HIV infection in perinatally infected children when compared with children infected after the age of 2 years.[98,99] Antiretroviral therapy can effectively reverse this immune dysfunction.[100]

The diagnosis of HIV-1 infection in adults and children older than 24 months is accomplished by identification of antibodies specific to HIV-1 or HIV-2 viral proteins and confirmed by a second test using different methodology.[101] Because infants carry transplacentally acquired maternal antibodies, HIV infection in infants younger than 24 months must be documented by HIV DNA polymerase chain reaction (PCR) or HIV RNA assay.[101] Generally viral testing is repeated three times (between 14 and 21 days, 1 to 2 months, and 4 to 6 months of age) with sensitivity increasing over time.[101] High-risk infants should be tested at birth. The absence of HIV infection can be confirmed by serology at 12 to 18 months of age, but positive serology may still reflect maternal antibody and should be confirmed by nucleic acid assay.

In 2014, the US Centers for Disease Control and Prevention modified an earlier classification system for HIV infection ranging from indeterminate to asymptomatic to severely symptomatic (ie, AIDS) on the basis of age-specific CD4$^+$ T-cell counts. Stage 3 HIV infection or an AIDS-defining illness in the presence of HIV infection confirms the diagnosis of AIDs.[102] AIDS-defining illnesses include recurrent bacterial infections, fungal and/or mycobacterium infection, CMV disease, lymphoma, encephalopathy or progressive multifocal leukoencephalopathy, wasting syndrome, and associated malignancies.

These categories aside, there appear to be at least two patterns of response to HIV infection in untreated children.[99,103] Children younger than 4 years, especially those aged 1 year or younger, are more likely to have *Pneumocystis jirovecii* pneumonia (PJP); have severe progressive encephalopathy, wasting, or both; and die earlier. Older children tend to have a less serious course, characterized by recurrent bacterial infections, LIP, nephropathy, and thrombocytopenia. The time course for vertically transmitted HIV infection to progress to AIDS in children is variable and may be more than 10 years; however, in children, AIDS is most commonly seen between 5 and 8 months.[100,104] The density of CCR5 receptor on nonactivated T cells correlates with the decline of CD4$^+$ T cells and prognosis.[105]

Globally, at the end of 2013, the adult prevalence of HIV was 0.8%.[103] Ninety-six percent of individuals living with HIV reside in low- and middle-income countries. Sub-Saharan Africa had the highest incidence of HIV infection, accounting for 70% of the world's cases with young women two times more likely than men to be infected.[104] East Africa and Central Africa have reduced the prevalence of HIV infection through educational programs. In Western Europe many new cases of HIV/AIDS are reported from persons who emigrated from or traveled to countries with a high HIV prevalence.[104]

As of December 2013, 3.2 million children are living with HIV worldwide, of which 240,000 were newly infected and 190,000 died annually.[104] Ninety-one percent of children living with HIV reside in sub-Saharan Africa.[104] Vertical transmission of HIV infection from untreated mother to fetus occurs at a rate of 20% to 35% but is reduced by 66% when antiretroviral therapy monotherapy (zidovudine [ZDV]) is taken during pregnancy, delivery, and the neonatal period.[106] Even though simple inexpensive monotherapy can reduce vertical transmission by 40% to 50%, only 33% of infected pregnant women receive treatment.[106] When used in combination with elective cesarean delivery and formula feeding, perinatal antiretroviral therapy has reduced the vertical transmission of HIV to less than 2% in the United States. Currently trials suggest that highly active antiretroviral therapy (HAART) in pregnancy may be more effective in preventing transmission than monotherapy.[107,108] It may also be important to extend antiretroviral therapy for the mother during the period of breastfeeding.[107,109,110] Although there has been extensive development of appropriate therapies, a major challenge has been prevention of mother-to-child transmission.[106,111-113]

Combinations of HAART used to treat HIV-infected patients have dramatically decreased mortality caused from HIV-associated conditions and opportunistic infections. The number of people living with HIV receiving HAART in 2013 is 12.9 million, but two-thirds of those who need it still have no access to drug.[104] Ninety percent of HIV-infected children live in sub-Saharan Africa and underdeveloped countries of Asia.[104] Because of cultural, economic, and political factors, HIV prevention and treatment have been slowly introduced in resource-limited regions. In Malawi, without antiretroviral therapy, the mortality rate at 3 years of age for HIV-infected children reached 89%.[114] This high mortality rate may be related to the burdens of infectious diseases and malnutrition and is seen in other parts of the world as well. The care of these children is complicated by overcrowding, limited access to clean water, and malnutrition. These conditions contribute to the high frequency of TB, cytomegalovirus (CMV), hepatitis, and gastroenteritis seen in this population. Still there is growing evidence that antiretroviral can be provided successfully to children in resource-limited settings.[115,116] Even in this environment, the efficacy of early initiation of antiretroviral HIV therapy in children reduced mortality rates by 75%.[116] In the United States 75% of HIV-infected children are alive at age 5 years.[117] Most data regarding outcome and survival of HIV-infected children presented in this chapter are drawn from patients who did not receive antiretroviral therapy from the time of birth and may have never received it. Such data are still applicable to underdeveloped countries, given that only one in three adults and one in four children receive HAART despite a global increase in HAART access from 7% in 2003 to 42% in 2008.[104]

As of February 2014, thirty-one HIV antiretroviral agents were approved and available for use in the United States; 17 have a pediatric indication.[101] Because resistance develops with monotherapy, multiple drug regimens known as HAART are used in children and adults.[101] There are five classes of agents available and three drugs are typically selected from at least two classes. Measurement of both HIV-1 viral load (by RNA PCR) and the number of CD4[+] T cells is performed to monitor the effectiveness of HAART.[101] Baseline viral loads are higher in children than in adults and have a slower decay rate after the introduction of HAART.[118] Pediatric studies in which dosage adjustments were directed by pharmacokinetics resulted in superior decreases in viral loads compared with fixed dosages based on weight.[101] Each antiretroviral therapy has its own toxicity and potential for drug interactions. Antiretroviral therapy is rapidly evolving and should be directed by a specialized practitioner.[101] Older HIV-infected adults are age 50 years or older, and this population comprised 25% of the HIV-infected population in the United States in 2007.[118] HIV-infected patients are living longer and developing non–HIV-associated comorbidities. It is estimated that by 2015, more than 50% of living HIV-infected patients in the United States will be older than 50 years.[118]

While the rate of hospitalizations decreased for HIV patients with HAART, the rates of ICU admission have not changed and in some studies increased.[118,119] Nearly 20% of hospitalized HIV-infected patients require transfer to the ICU.[119] Barbier et al.[120] identified major changes in the clinical presentation, ICU management, and mortality of critically ill HIV-infected adults from 1999 to 2010. AIDs-defining opportunistic infections decreased while non–HIV-associated comorbidities increased.[120] The use of life-sustaining therapies also increased, and there was a marked decrease in short-term mortality in HIV-infected patients needing aggressive therapies.[120] Mechanical ventilation support remains to be the predominant support modality for HIV-infected adults and children.[118-121]

Pulmonary Complications and Respiratory Failure

Pulmonary complications remain the most frequent indication for admission of children with AIDS to an ICU.[121-123] Pneumonia is the leading cause of morbidity and death in HIV-infected children worldwide.[121] Comparing low- or middle-income countries to high-income countries, pneumonia accounts for 20% of the annual deaths in children versus 4.3%, respectively.[121] Comparing HIV-infected children on HAART with uninfected children, pneumonia is more likely to be severe with high treatment failure rates and increased risk of death.[121] Bacterial pneumonia is common in this population.[117,124,125] Along with the usual pathogens frequently seen in childhood, such as *Streptococcus pneumoniae* and mycoplasma, immunodeficient children are also susceptible to pseudomonal and staphylococcal infections.[107,126] The incidence of *Haemophilus influenzae* infection is declining where vaccination is available, and immunization against pneumococcal infections has been associated with a significant drop in pneumococcal disease in HIV-infected children.[125] Empiric therapy for pneumonia in such children should cover the most common pathogens and be based on hospital-specific susceptibility profiles, but it is important to note that children with

HIV infections may not respond to standard antibiotic therapies for lower respiratory tract infections.[127]

Initiation of antiretroviral therapy can result in rapid immune recovery. A subset of patients experience an inflammatory response as the immune system is reconstituted.[128] Most cases have another occult infection in addition to HIV. In one study, nearly 50% were associated with mycobacterial infections such as *Mycobacterium avium-intracellulare* and herpes viruses such as *Varicella zoster*.[129] Clinical presentation is related to the focus of infection. Enhanced screening and subsequent treatment of opportunistic infections such as TB before beginning HAART may prevent the reconstitution inflammatory syndrome. The World Health Organization has recommended prednisone for patients with TB who experience severe paradoxical reactions. However, there are no randomized controlled trials to support this practice.[128]

Pneumocystis Jirovecii Pneumonia

Pneumocystis jirovecii pneumonia (PJP) occurs in patients with acquired immunodeficiency from HIV, chemotherapy, and immunomodulatory therapies. Although increased emphasis on early prophylaxis has reduced its incidence, PJP is still the most common AIDS-defining illness in pediatrics.[127,130,131] Infants not previously recognized to be infected with HIV may present as early as 3 to 4 weeks of age, whereas the median age or presentation to ICUs is between 3 and 6 months of age and coincides with the timing of a natural decline in maternal antibodies.[123] In children known to be at risk of HIV infection, PJP prophylaxis is indicated starting at 4 to 6 weeks of age as CD4[+] T-cell counts obtained before the development of infection are not predictive of infection and can drop precipitously.[102] *P. jirovecii* is unique to humans and has a predilection for the lung.[132] PJP generally presents with cough, fever, tachypnea, and dyspnea of several days' duration.[132] Physical examination typically reveals retractions, grunting, rales, rhonchi, or wheezing. The chest radiograph generally shows diffuse interstitial infiltrates, but pulmonary infiltrates can be variable in children, in part because infants have a greater propensity for atelectasis.[132,133] Hypoxemia is often out of proportion to clinical and radiographic examinations. A selectively elevated serum lactate dehydrogenase level is suggestive, although not diagnostic of, PJP.[132] For a confirmation of a PJP diagnosis, bronchoalveolar lavage should be performed. Flexible fiberoptic bronchoscopy has a diagnostic yield of 90% to 97% and allows one to look for other pathogens as well.[132,134] Nonbronchoscopic bronchoalveolar lavage and sputum induction can also be used in combination with PCR to detect PJP.[134,135] Patients in whom no diagnosis is obtained from bronchoalveolar lavage should undergo an open lung biopsy. This procedure has a diagnostic yield for PJP of 97% in the study of patients with underlying malignancy or immune suppression.[132]

The preferred antiprotozoal therapy for PJP is the combination of trimethoprim and sulfamethoxazole (TMP-SMX) (20 mg/kg/day trimethoprim).[132] Patients in whom this combination agent fails have not been shown to respond to a change in antiprotozoal therapy. In fact, higher doses of both components may be required to achieve therapeutic levels in critically ill patients.[132] Sulfa allergy as manifested by severe drug eruptions including Stevens-Johnson syndrome is less frequent in children than in adults; however, this complication may prompt a change to therapy with pentamidine isethionate (4 mg/kg/day). When adverse events such as pancreatitis and renal failure occur as a result of pentamidine, atovaquone (40 mg/kg/day) is an alternative treatment.[132] Twenty-one days of therapy are followed by prophylactic therapy, for which TMP-SMX is also the agent of choice. For patients allergic to sulfa, PJP prophylaxis can be achieved with pentamidine, dapsone, or atovaquone, although these agents have not been rigorously studied in children.

Several adult randomized controlled trials showed efficacy of high-dose steroids in HIV positive adults with moderate PJP.[128] Although no controlled studies have been performed in children, improved outcomes in children who received corticosteroids have been described in several case series.[136-139] Even in the face of respiratory failure, the survival rates reported with adjunctive corticosteroids therapy are 91% to 100% in a limited number of children.[136,137] Adults who have respiratory failure despite adjunctive corticosteroids have a high risk of death. Failure to improve after 5 days of mechanical ventilation and the development of pneumothorax were strongly predictive of death in adults.[140]

Pneumocystis pneumonia has also been reported in patients receiving high-dose steroids, transplant-related immunosuppression, and the new monoclonal antibodies that modulate the immune system.[132] Pneumocystis pneumonia presents differently in non–HIV-infected patients. The onset of the disease may be more abrupt. The mortality is greater in cancer patients than AIDs patients, and corticosteroids are not as clearly beneficial.

Cytomegalovirus Pneumonitis

Children at risk for vertical transmission of HIV are also at risk for CMV infection. Kitchin et al.[141] reported that 55% of HIV-exposed but untreated children with respiratory failure in South Africa had a CMV viral load in the range consistent with CMV disease. Furthermore, the mortality from CMV with and without PJP was over 40%[141] despite empiric treatment with ganciclovir in all cases; failure of PJP response to conventional therapy may be evidence of concomitant CMV infection. Pneumonitis from CMV is also a common complication of solid organ and hematopoietic stem cell recipients. The presentation of CMV pneumonitis can closely mimic that of PJP with diffuse interstitial infiltrates and hypoxemia, but there is generally a more insidious onset; however, some reports of a more fulminant course exist.[142]

While the definitive diagnosis of CMV pneumonitis may require identification of characteristic intracellular viral inclusion bodies in pulmonary macrophages or biopsy specimen, because viral shedding is known to occur, the prevalence of CMV pneumonitis and its contribution to mortality in immunocompromised children have led many to recommend empiric therapy for pneumonia.[141-143] Viral culture and viral nucleic acid detection by PCR performed on tracheal aspirates and blood have all been used to guide treatment.[140-142] The treatment for CMV disease is ganciclovir 5 mg/kg given twice daily followed by long-term viral suppressive therapy.[144,145] Foscarnet and cidofovir have been used in other immunosuppressed patients, but these drugs have significant nephrotoxicity.[144,145] Although solid organ transplant recipients receive prophylaxis against CMV disease with ganciclovir, this approach has not been applied to patients with AIDS. Of course, patients with AIDS should also receive HAART.

Other Viral Pathogens

Children with AIDS are more likely to experience lower respiratory tract disease and pneumonia when contracting RSV and influenza.[146-148] For RSV, the estimated incidence of lower tract disease was twofold greater in HIV-infected children; it is not clear that HIV infection increases the likelihood of death.[148] The incidence of lower respiratory tract disease requiring hospitalization in influenza was eightfold higher in children with HIV infection.[147] HIV-infected children with influenza pneumonia were older and more likely to have another underlying disease or concurrent infection. Despite these comorbidities, there was no difference in clinical outcome. Other pathogenic viruses recovered from pediatric patients with AIDS include adenovirus, parainfluenza, herpes simplex, and measles. In vitro data suggest ribavirin and cidofovir may be effective against some of these viral pathogens; however, evidence of in vivo efficacy is limited to anecdotal reports in immunosuppressed patients.[149-151] Immunosuppressed children have been noted to shed viral pathogens such as RSV and influenza for a prolonged period, and therefore nosocomial viral infections may be a significant problem if infection control practices are not maintained.[151,152]

Mycobacterial Pathogens

Worldwide, approximately one-third of the human population is infected with the *Mycobacterium bacillus*.[153] Most of these individuals live in developing countries where the prevalence of HIV infection is high. The incidence of *M. tuberculosis* appeared to level off in the United States by 1985 but began rising steadily in 1988—an increase attributed to the AIDS epidemic.[154] The increased incidence of pediatric TB is likely due to increased exposure to adults with active infection. HIV-infected children with TB have higher CD4+ T-cell counts than those observed with other classic opportunistic infections.[100] Although adults generally acquire HIV infection after acquiring TB, the opposite is true in children. Thus the HIV-infected child never has a chance to mount an immunologic response to *M. tuberculosis*. In contrast to adults who have apical, cavitary lesions, children have more peripheral disease.[153] Most pediatric patients with AIDS have diffuse infiltrates consistent with LIP or PCP.[153,154] These children also have a high incidence of extrapulmonary manifestations such as hepatosplenomegaly and meningitis.

Aggressive efforts to confirm mycobacterium infection by culture are required because anergy obscures Mantoux testing, as well as the development of pleural effusions and localized lymphadenopathy. Use of PCR to identify *M. tuberculosis* nucleic acids in bronchoalveolar lavage and cerebrospinal fluid (CSF) specimens can accelerate diagnosis of this infection.[129,155] Recovery of mycobacterium by sputum induction has been reported in infants and very young children.[156] In some regions, organism recovery is necessary for antimicrobial susceptibility determination; 25% of isolates are resistant.[129,153,157] In countries where the diagnostic approaches are not readily available, it is useful to obtain radiographs of family members.[129]

Pending sensitivity reports, treatment of TB is initiated with a five-drug regimen.[158,159] The presence of multidrug resistance increases the likelihood of death. These patients should simultaneously be treated with antiretroviral therapy; however, rifampin is contraindicated with protease inhibitors and non-nucleoside reverse transcriptase inhibitors.[158] During HAART, reconstitution of the immune system may increase the inflammatory response to pulmonary TB. Children with TB and HIV infection who are not treated with HAART have a higher mortality rate than children not infected with HIV.[158] They must be treated for a longer time, perhaps because of poor drug absorption and a weakened immune system.[158]

M. avium-intracellulare complex (MAC) can also be recovered from the lungs of children with pneumonia.[122] Colonization is difficult to differentiate from invasive disease. Treatment options include coverage with clarithromycin in combination with ethambutol, rifabutin, or amikacin. Primary prophylaxis once a week with azithromycin is recommended in children older than 2 years and younger than 1 year with CD4 counts persistently below 75. Children between 1 and 2 years of age should receive prophylaxis for CD4 counts less than 50.[101]

Fungal Infections

Candida is frequently recovered from sputum and bronchoalveolar lavage samples in children with AIDS.[160] Candidiasis of the respiratory or gastrointestinal system is an AIDS-defining illness.[105] Aspergillosis has also been reported in older children with multiple opportunistic infections, prolonged hospitalization, neutropenia, and corticosteroid use.[161] Cryptococcosis occurs in 5% to 15% of adults but in only 0.6% to 1% of children.[161] This ubiquitous organism enters the body through the respiratory tract. Therefore initial symptoms are generally both pulmonary and nonspecific. Recommended therapy is amphotericin B in combination with 5-flucytosine (100 mg/kg/day) for 2 weeks followed by fluconazole (12 mg/kg/day divided in two doses) for 8 additional weeks.[162] Cryptococcal antigen titers are useful in the evaluation of possible relapse. Prophylaxis for the prevention of cryptococcal disease is not recommended in children. Fusariosis has been reported in neutropenic patients with AIDS. Other fungal infections such as histoplasmosis, cryptococcosis, coccidiomycosis, and disseminated *Penicillium marneffei* are reported in patients with AIDS who are living in or traveling through endemic areas.[122,162]

Lymphoid Interstitial Pneumonitis

LIP is a lymphoproliferative disorder associated with viral infections. In children LIP is almost exclusively seen with Epstein-Barr virus (EBV) and HIV.[163] LIP occurs in 30% to 50% of pediatric patients with AIDS, presenting in the second year of life in that patient population with high antibody titers and recurrent bacterial infections. Generally the children also have diffuse lymphadenopathy and hepatosplenomegaly. Children with LIP may have mild pulmonary symptoms such as dry cough but generally are admitted to the pediatric ICU only when an acute infection is superimposed on their chronic condition. When such is the case, maximal therapy of the acute exacerbation is indicated, including mechanical ventilation. On chest radiograph hilar adenopathy and reticulonodular infiltrates are seen. Pulmonary function tests reveal reduced lung volumes and diffusing capacity. Histologically, peribronchial lymphoid nodules containing plasma cells and lymphocytes are observed. Most specimens show predominantly CD8+ T cells.

Spontaneous radiographic resolution was reported in 65% of children with LIP.[164] Patients with hypoxemia are treated with steroids, and resolution is seen in most patients in 2 to 4 weeks. If the patient is persistently febrile, MAC infection should be ruled out before steroid administration.[122]

Upper Airway Obstruction

Young children and infants exhibit upper airway obstruction with greater frequency than adults. Whereas classic viral laryngotracheitis is the most common cause in the immunocompetent patient, immunocompromised patients are susceptible to a greater variety of infectious entities, including bacterial tracheitis, CMV-related ulceration of the trachea, and *Candida* infections of the airway oropharynx.[165,166] The clinical course in HIV-infected children is different with many requiring tracheostomy.[166] Although in the general population *Staphylococcus aureus* is the most commonly reported cause of bacterial tracheitis, *Pseudomonas* species are a frequent cause of tracheitis in patients with AIDS.[166] Given the complexity of the differential diagnosis of stridor in this population, early laryngoscopy and bronchoscopy are indicated.

Cardiovascular Complications
Septic Shock

After the introduction of PJP prophylaxis, severe sepsis became the most common reason for ICU admission in patients with AIDS.[118] A systematic review demonstrated community-acquired bacterial bloodstream infections occurring of hospitalized HIV patients at 20% and 30% in adults and children, respectively.[167] The main pathogens identified were nontyphoidal salmonella, *Streptococcus pneumoniae, Escherichia coli*, and *Staphylococcus aureus*.[167] Regional differences were noted especially for *S pneumoniae*, likely due to vaccination availability and combinational antiretroviral therapy access.[167] HIV-infected patients do appear to be more susceptible to *S. aureus* and *Pseudomonas* infections.[168] In one series of pediatric patients with AIDS, 10% of patients had gram-negative bacillary bacteremia with a risk of death that was greater than 40%, and *Pseudomonas* sepsis accounted for 26% of these episodes.[168] *Pseudomonas* infection is frequently associated with neutropenia, which may be a cause or effect phenomenon.[168]

Vasculitis

Vasculitis has been reported in patients with HIV infection, but it is not clear if HIV causes the condition or is merely an association, although there are a variety of suggested mechanisms.[169-175] Many infections reported in HIV-infected patients, including herpes viruses and mycobacterium, can cause inflammation by direct infection or an immune-mediated response. The most frequently involved organs are skin, peripheral nerve or muscle, and the central nervous system (CNS).[169] Several cases of polyarteritis nodosa have been reported.[169] When vasculitis is noted, an infectious agent should be sought.[176] The authors have observed an increased incidence of arterial catheter complications among HIV-infected children, and it is probably wise to exercise caution in the use of central venous and arterial catheters in HIV-infected children.

Myocardial Dysfunction

Cardiac dysfunction develops in 19% to 25% of HIV-infected children and is the presenting sign in a minority of children.[177,178] About 10% of a survey population had chronic congestive heart failure, whereas another 10% had transiently decreased ventricular function.[179-181] Cardiac complications appear to occur more frequently in rapidly progressing patients with encephalitis and other AIDS-defining illnesses. Because tachycardia and hepatomegaly are so common in pediatric AIDS patients with fever, pulmonary infection, and anemia, a clinical diagnosis of cardiac involvement is difficult to make. Enlargement of the cardiac silhouette may not be appreciable even in patients with significant muscle hypertrophy or pericardial effusion. Given these inherent difficulties in the detection of cardiac disease, assessment of a critically ill child with AIDS should include echocardiography. When assessment is prospectively followed by echocardiography, the earliest sign of cardiac involvement is diastolic dysfunction.[178] At autopsy, aside from biventricular dilation, macroscopic evidence of cardiac dysfunction has been difficult to find in adults or children. Microscopically, in a limited number of cases, lymphocytic infiltrates are observed, but actual cardiomyocyte necrosis is rare.[182] Mild foci of lacy interstitial fibrosis may also occur.[179,182] True cardiomyocyte inflammation or myocarditis is rare in children.

HIV cardiomyopathy likely has several causes. Direct evidence of myocardial infection by HIV-1 has been documented by culture, Southern blot test, and in situ hybridization,[179,182] but it is unclear if the myocytes, which express no CD4 receptors, actually harbor HIV. Coxsackie B3 virus, CMV, adenovirus, EBV, and *Toxoplasmosis gondii* have also been identified as pathogens causing myocardial dysfunction.[183-185] Of 32 HIV-infected children who died, 7 had evidence of CMV infection and 10 had evidence of adenovirus infection by PCR performed on myocardial tissue.[185] Selenium deficiency has been documented in severely malnourished children with AIDS whose cardiac function improved after selenium supplementation.[186]

In the ICU, patients with severe cardiac dysfunction respond to management of preload, increasing contractility, and afterload reduction. Endocarditis, myocardial ischemia, and other potentially treatable causes of cardiac dysfunction should be ruled out with electrocardiography and echocardiography. Pharmacologic afterload reduction should be considered as first-line therapy, with digitalization and diuretic therapy as appropriate. Other than selenium supplementation there is no direct therapy available for HIV-related cardiomyopathy.[186] Agents that are associated with myocardial dysfunction, such as pentamidine, foscarnet, and dideoxyinosine (ddI), should be avoided.[184,185] A small population of patients has been noted to have transient cardiac dysfunction manifested by tachycardia and poor peripheral perfusion despite adequate filling pressures. This has been noted during PJP infection and may be related to cytokine release. Although survival data following clinically evident congestive heart failure in children undergoing HAART have not been reported, HAART intervention in children and adolescents appears to be cardioprotective.[187] The etiology of cardioprotective effects is incomplete, and evidence from adult studies links HIV infection as an independent risk factor in developing chronic cardiovascular conditions, such as hypertension, coronary artery disease, myocardial infarction, stroke, and pulmonary artery hypertension.[188,189] Prior studies demonstrate a potential association between congenital heart defects (CHDs), myocardial dysfunction, and zidovudine in utero exposure.[189] A current observational cohort study confirms the association between in utero exposure to zidovudine and CHD, with an adjusted odds ratio of 2.2; in addition, the randomized clinical trial (PRIMEVA) demonstrated an association between in utero zidovudine and long-lasting postnatal myocardial remodeling in girls.[190]

Dysrhythmias

In a survey of 81 HIV-infected children, dysrhythmias occurred in 35%, including atrial and ventricular ectopy, ventricular tachycardia, and ventricular fibrillation.[177,178] A syndrome of autonomic dysfunction has been reported in adult patients with AIDS, and similar lability in blood pressure and heart rate has been noted in a number of HIV-infected children. Catecholamine surges have been described in adults. Additionally, peripheral neuropathy may contribute to altered vascular regulation and a propensity for cardiac arrhythmias.

Pericardial Disease

Pericardial disease is reported in approximately 30% of HIV-infected children undergoing echocardiography or autopsy.[178,180] In five pediatric patients in whom fluid was cultured, no pathogens were identified. In 14 adult patients in whom fluid was obtained, atypical mesothelial cells were identified. One patient had lymphoma, one had histoplasmosis, and a third had CMV identified by a pericardial biopsy specimen. A pericardial effusion greater than 5 mm in diameter was detected in 5.4% of prospectively evaluated HIV-infected children, but no episodes of tamponade were reported.[191,192] Cardiac arrest due to tamponade has been reported in five adult patients with AIDS.[192]

Renal Failure

HIV-associated nephropathy (HIVAN) was first reported in 1983 and may often be the first manifestation of AIDS.[193-197] Complications from HIVAN generally arise between ages 2.5 and 4.9 years and appear to be more prevalent in children of African or Afro-Caribbean descent. The usual presentation of renal dysfunction is severe proteinuria (>3.5 g/day) with hypoalbuminemia and anasarca. This may be associated with renal tubular acidosis. Creatinine clearance is usually normal. Proteinuria may be accompanied by hematuria. Immunoglobulins are usually elevated while complement is normal. On ultrasound, the kidneys are enlarged. Biopsy specimens show focal and segmental glomerulosclerosis.[194] The course of the disease before HAART was usually fulminant, with end-stage renal disease developing in 8 to 9 months. Effective antiretroviral therapy slows or reverses the course of HIV nephropathy, but HAART is associated with renal toxicities.[195,196,198,199] Atypical hemolytic uremic syndrome or thrombotic microangiopathy is also described in pediatric patients with AIDS.[196,200]

Potentially nephrotoxic drugs to which the HIV-infected patient may be exposed are legion. Indinavir and tenofovir are associated with increased risk of chronic renal failure.[199,201,202] Pentamidine-induced renal toxicity usually occurs in the second week of therapy. Proteinuria and particularly hematuria, which may be falsely attributed to HIV nephropathy or catheter-induced trauma, are hallmarks of pentamidine toxicity. Early recognition of this complication and cessation of pentamidine increase the likelihood of recovery; rechallenge with the drug will prompt early return of proteinuria and hematuria. Toxicity from sulfadiazine during the treatment of toxoplasmosis is also reported and can be reduced by hydration.[200] Amphotericin-induced nephrotoxicity is particularly problematic when the drug is used in combination with aminoglycosides. Liposomal-encapsulated amphotericin B allows for higher doses with less toxicity.

In critically ill patients with AIDS, acute tubular necrosis may be precipitated by sepsis, hypovolemia, or hypoperfusion, which is reversible as in non–HIV-infected patients, although HIV-infected children have a higher in-hospital mortality when at admission they demonstrate acute kidney injury.[196,203] The same principles for management and support of a patient with reversible acute renal failure apply to the HIV-infected population. For patients who are seen in the ICU with end-stage renal disease due to HIV nephropathy, the indications for dialysis are the same as in other patient populations, but the decision to undertake dialysis must be made on an individual basis (see also Chapter 78). Peritonitis during ambulatory peritoneal dialysis in pediatric patients with AIDS does not occur with any apparent greater frequency than in immunocompetent patients.[204] Kidney transplant has been successful in carefully selected HIV-infected patients.[196,205]

Abdominal Complications

Patients with AIDS have multiple gastrointestinal complaints including dysphagia, abdominal pain, and chronic diarrhea, but these are generally not important in the ICU except that they affect nutritional status.[206] Other more life-threatening complications include severe dehydration, intraabdominal sepsis, pancreatitis, and hepatic failure (Table 104.1).

Diarrhea occurs in 40% to 60% of children with AIDS and may produce severe dehydration.[207] Worldwide, acute diarrhea is the most common cause of death in children with AIDS.[207] In underdeveloped countries where poor sanitation increases the risk of diarrheal diseases, HIV-related hypovolemic shock is a common indication for pediatric ICU admission. Copious diarrhea is suggestive of small intestine involvement, whereas tenesmus suggests infection involving the distal colon and rectum. Diffuse enterocolitis produces a secretory diarrhea with profound volume losses. Patients with AIDS may have typical infectious enteritis and enterocolitis caused by *Salmonella, Shigella, Giardia, Campylobacter,* and rotavirus but may also have an atypical, more prolonged course.[206-208] The frequent use of systemic antibiotics in HIV-infected children results in *Clostridium difficile* colitis. *M. avium-intracellulare,* cryptosporidium, *Giardia, Isospora belli,* CMV, and adenovirus may all induce opportunistic small bowel enteropathy.[206-208] Patients with MAC, CMV, and *Candida* infection typically also have extragastrointestinal infection.[209] A nonspecific enteropathy may arise as a result of the overgrowth of normal gut flora due to the effects of local immunodeficiency and antibiotic use. It is not uncommon to find heavy growth of *Candida albicans* or *Pseudomonas aeruginosa* in stool cultures.

If findings from stool culture and analysis are negative, a flexible sigmoidoscopy with a rectal biopsy should be considered in the child with rectal bleeding, tenesmus, or both. Aspiration of duodenal secretions is particularly helpful in evaluation of patients from underdeveloped countries in that the aspirate may reveal infection with *I. belli, Cryptosporidium parvum,* or helminthic species. Additional evaluation may be

TABLE 104.1	Infectious Morbidity in Critically Ill Patients With Cancer	
	Common	**Less Common**
Granulocytopenia		
Bacteria	*Staphylococcus aureus, Streptococcus pneumonia, Klebsiella, Pseudomonas*	*Enterobacter, Acinetobacter, Stenotrophomonas*
Fungi/molds	*Candida,* aspergillosis, zygomycosis	
Parasites		
Viruses		HSV1 or 2, VZV
Cellular Defects		
Bacteria	*Legionella, Nocardia*	*Mycobacterium tuberculosis*
Fungi/molds	*Pneumocystis, Cryptococcus, Mucormycosis*	
Parasites	*Toxoplasma*	
Viruses	CMV, EBV, adenovirus, VZV	
Humoral Defects		
Bacteria	*S. pneumonia, Haemophilus influenzae*	
Fungi/molds		*Pneumocystis*
Parasites		*Giardia lamblia*
Viruses		VZV
Combined Defects		
Bacteria	*S. aureus, S. pneumonia, Klebsiella, Pseudomonas*	*M. tuberculosis, Listeria monocytogenes, Legionella*
Fungi/molds	*Pneumocystis,* aspergillosis, *Cryptococcus*	Zygomycosis, mucormycosis
Parasites	*Toxoplasma*	
Viruses	CMV, VZV, influenza, parainfluenza, RSV, adenovirus	HSV 1 or 2

CMV, cytomegalovirus; *EBV,* Epstein-Barr virus; *HSV,* herpes simplex virus; *RSV,* respiratory syncytial virus; *VZV,* varicella-zoster virus.
Modified from Safdar A, Armstrong D. Infectious morbidity in critically ill patients with cancer. *Crit Care Clin.* 2001;17:531.

desirable, including small bowel radiography or abdominal computed tomography (CT) scanning. If results of all diagnostic studies are negative, diarrhea may be due to HIV therapy because most antiretroviral agents are associated with diarrhea (Box 104.1).[210]

Recovery of MAC from the blood generally indicates invasive disease, but percutaneous needle aspiration with CT guidance of enlarged intraabdominal nodes may be confirmatory.[209,211] Antimicrobial therapy of disseminated MAC infection before HAART was unrewarding, and disseminated MAC was rapidly fatal. Current antimicrobial therapy is a double-drug regimen of clarithromycin and ethambutol with the possible addition of a third agent, including rifabutin, ciprofloxacin, or azithromycin. Prophylaxis against MAC with azithromycin is indicated in children with CD4 counts less than 75 cells/μL and in infants with counts less than 100 cells/μL.[212] In patients

---

BOX 104.1 | **Gastrointestinal Complications in Immunodeficient Patients**

Diarrhea
- Bacteria
  - *Salmonella*
  - *Shigella*
  - *Clostridium difficile*
- Fungi
  - *Candida*
  - *Pneumocystis*
- Viruses
  - *Cytomegalovirus*
  - *Herpesvirus*
  - *Varicella-zoster*
  - *Adenovirus*
  - *Rotavirus*
- Parasites
  - *Cryptosporidium*
  - *Microsporidium*
  - *Entamoeba histolytica*
  - *Giardia intestinalis*
  - *Blastocystis hominis*
- Medications
  - *Atovaquone*
  - *Antiretrovirals*

Pancreatitis
- Infections
  - *Cytomegalovirus*
  - *Adenovirus*
- Medications
  - *Protease inhibitors*
  - *Pentamidine*
  - *Foscarnet*

---

treated with HAART, diarrhea often persists despite improvements in immunologic function.[210]

Acute Abdomen

The evaluation and management of acute abdominal pain in HIV-infected children are complicated by their immunosuppressed state. Localized signs of infection can be masked by immunosuppression, debilitation, and previous or current use of antibiotics. In fact, a significant intraabdominal abscess may result in minor symptoms, with unremarkable elevations in white blood cell count or temperature. Thus diagnostic imaging with abdominal CT scan is invaluable for evaluation in this population. Although morbidity after surgical intervention is somewhat higher in patients with AIDS, there is still a significant survival when such intervention is undertaken promptly.[213-215] Gastric and proximal small bowel symptoms such as pain or bleeding may arise from stress gastritis and infiltrative processes caused by viruses, particularly CMV and adenovirus, *Giardia lamblia,* tuberculosis, and lymphoma. Supportive management of these conditions is the same as that for immunocompetent patients, although the appropriate antimicrobial therapy may be different.

Pancreatitis

Pancreatitis in the AIDS population results from both the disease and its treatment.[101,216-218] Infectious causative entities include CMV, adenovirus, mycobacterium, fungal infections, *Cryptococcus,* herpes simplex virus (HSV), and protozoal infections such as toxoplasmosis, *Pneumocystis,* and cryptosporidium. The list of drugs known to cause pancreatitis is extensive and includes the antiretroviral agent zalcitabine and the antiprotozoal agent pentamidine. The mechanism by which drugs induce pancreatitis is unknown.

Pancreatitis often goes undiagnosed. Autopsy findings reveal significant pancreatic lesions in approximately 10% of patients with AIDS, yet pancreatic lesions are rarely recognized during life.[216] Nine (17%) of 53 children seen at one institution demonstrated pancreatitis.[217] Four of five of these carried CMV. In one of these patients, CMV was cultured from pancreatic duct fluid. Six of nine had serologic evidence of EBV. Five children were receiving pentamidine at the time of presentation. Maintaining a high index of suspicion for

pancreatitis is important because vomiting, abdominal distention, and malabsorption are common complaints in the HIV-infected child. Evaluation of these patients should include both serum lipase and amylase determinations because parotid inflammation seen in HIV infection can cause isolated elevations of serum amylase concentrations. Abdominal ultrasound is only useful in the detection of a large edematous pancreas and in follow-up assessment for pancreatic pseudocyst.

Treatment includes bowel rest and hyperalimentation along with removal of the offending agent as in the case of drug-induced pancreatitis. In infectious pancreatitis, treatment of the underlying cause, while indicated, may not change the course of the disease.[217] Despite intervention, seven of eight reported children with pancreatitis had active or recurrent disease at the time of death. The mean survival time from onset to death was 8 months (range, 0.5-13 months).[217] In this patient population, anatomic abnormality is rarely the cause of pancreatitis and there is little role for surgical intervention.

Hepatobiliary Failure

The cause of hepatic failure in HIV-infected patients differs from that of other adults and is affected by the patient's degree of immunosuppression.[219] In early stages, hepatic disease is usually a result of drug toxicity or hepatotropic virus infections. Drug-induced hepatotoxicity has been reported with sulfa drugs, isoniazid, rifampin, and rifabutin.[219,220] Several antiretroviral agents can cause hepatitis.[101] If HIV progresses to AIDS, the liver manifests systemic involvement of opportunistic infections.[219,221,222] Reviews of hepatic tissue disease in HIV-infected children document that CMV and mycobacterial disease are common in children, whereas classic viral hepatitis is relatively rare.[219,223,224] As the immune system is reconstituted in response to HAART, hepatitis B can flare up.[210] Chronic hepatitis becomes clinically significant as survival increases in patients receiving HAART.[210] Cholangitis and cholecystitis are well described in adult patients with AIDS. Biliary tract infections have been attributed to CMV, adenovirus, cryptosporidium, and microsporidia.[222-225]

Liver biopsy is only indicated when mycobacterial disease is expected or jaundice is present, as most diseases can be diagnosed by serologic testing or PCR.[219] Drug toxicity has no specific biopsy finding. HIV itself can cause a giant cell hepatitis. Dense lymphoid infiltrates, similar to those in the lung in LIP, are also described. Adenovirus, CMV, and HSV and other opportunistic infections can cause acute jaundice and hepatitis with fever.[221,223-228] Hepatitis B and C can occur in patients with HIV/AIDS, and it is estimated that 30% of HIV-infected adults worldwide are coinfected with hepatitis C.[210,229] In certain established diagnoses, biopsy may be indicated to assess disease progression and response to therapy.[219]

Because drug-induced hepatotoxicity may be reversible on drug withdrawal, aggressive support for this cause of hepatic failure is indicated. Hepatitis B can be treated with the antiretrovirals lamivudine in combination with tenofovir or entecovir.[210] Recent advances in hepatitis C therapies demonstrate a greater sustained virologic response and in adult patients coinfected with HIV, and HCV should be treated with ribavirin, interferon, and sofosbuvir (an oral direct-acting antiviral that inhibits HCV polymerase).[210,229,230] In most cases HAART is suspended during hepatitis C therapy.[210,228] Liver transplantation can be successful with proper patient selection.[231]

Hematologic Complications

Hematologic abnormalities are common in patients with HIV/AIDS. Isolated thrombocytopenia is likely mediated by antiplatelet antibodies and should prompt HIV testing.[232-234] As with other forms of antibody-mediated thrombocytopenia, this may respond to immunoglobulin, steroids, or subtotal splenectomy.[233,235] Neutropenia may be antibody mediated, drug related, or secondary to sepsis. Granulocyte colony growth factors have reduced the incidence of sepsis in this setting.[236]

Anemia occurs in 20% to 73% of HIV-infected children and is an independent predictor of death from AIDS.[237-239] Most HIV-infected patients have normal erythrocyte size and shape but inadequate reticulocytosis. Iron deficiency, possibly related to malabsorption, accounts for 10% to 45% of anemia in HIV-infected children. Nutritional deficiencies of folate and vitamin B_{12} may also contribute to anemia. Many medications that are given to patients with AIDS cause anemia, including ZDV, acyclovir, TMP-SMX, and pentamidine. Anemia of chronic disease, mediated by inflammatory cytokines, likely accounts for additional cases. Rarely, antierythrocyte and antierythropoietin antibodies have been reported in patients with AIDS.[240] Pediatric patients with AIDS who have renal failure may lack erythropoietin.

Malignancies

Malignancies account for 2% of AIDS-defining illnesses in pediatric patients and are those typically associated with chronic viral infections.[241] In a cohort study of perinatally HIV-infected children, the cancer rate was nearly four times higher in children treated with HAART for less than 2 years when compared with those treated for more than 2 years.[242] The rates of childhood malignancy were compared between this cohort and the Surveillance, Epidemiology and End Result (SEER) Cancer Statistics Review. The higher rate in perinatally HIV-infected children was related to lymphomas. The development of cancer was three times more likely in those with low $CD4^+$ T-cell counts. EBV DNA has been identified in most CNS lymphomas, soft tissue leiomyosarcomas or rhabdomyosarcomas, and polyclonal, polymorphic B-cell lymphoproliferative disorder similar to that seen in transplant patients receiving immunosuppression. In addition, infection with human herpes virus type 8 (HHV-8) is associated with body cavity–based lymphoma and Kaposi sarcoma. Human papillomavirus is associated with invasive cervical cancer. Hepatitis B infection is associated with the development of hepatocellular carcinoma.[210]

Neurologic Complications

CNS involvement defined as seizure disorders, cerebral vascular accidents, CNS lymphoma, and aseptic meningitis occurs in 20% to 60% of HIV-infected children.[243] In this situation, treatable conditions must be ruled out before the diagnosis of AIDS encephalopathy can be made. Evaluation of these patients generally requires a series of biochemical and radiologic tests. Imaging studies such as CT and MRI can reveal mass-occupying lesions such as intracranial hemorrhage, malignancies, or calcifications consistent with infection.[244,245] Lumbar puncture is necessary to rule out infection, and

cerebral spinal fluid should be routinely cultured and investigated for specific pathogens via culture, direct antigen detection, and nucleic acid detection using PCR.[246,247]

HIV Encephalopathy

Primary HIV infection of the CNS probably occurs in 4% of HIV-infected children by the age of 12 months.[244] This entity is termed *HIV encephalopathy* and can generally be divided into two types: static with developmental delay or progressive similar to AIDS dementia in adults with progressive decline in neurologic functioning.[248-250] Direct HIV infection of the macrophages and microglia of the CNS is thought to cause release of inflammatory neurotoxins such as TNF or platelet-activating factor. Pathologically gliosis, microglial nodules, demyelination, and multinucleate giant cells are seen. Spinal cord examination similarly shows degeneration of corticospinal tracts, which clinically present as spastic diplegia. Vacuolar myelopathy involving the lateral and posterior columns, which presents as progressive muscle wasting and sensory loss, has also been observed in children.[243,251]

Diffuse atrophy is noted on CT, and bifrontal white matter abnormalities are commonly seen on MRI.[244,245,252,253] More severe cases of periventricular and centrum semiovale hypodense areas may occur. One-third of infected children may show calcifications of the basal ganglia. Calcifications observed before age 10 months are more likely due to an infection other than HIV, such as toxoplasmosis or CMV.[253]

AIDS encephalopathy is a diagnosis of exclusion. Other pathogens must be ruled out. Therefore evaluation includes imaging of the brain by CT or MRI and blood and CSF studies in search of specific pathogens such as *Cryptococcus*, mycobacterium, CMV, HSV, varicella-zoster virus, and *Treponema pallidum*. If no alternative pathogen is identified, then therapy is directed at reducing the HIV RNA viral load.[254]

Cerebrovascular Disease

Vascular complications involving the CNS in HIV-infected patients are many.[255] A cerebral vasculopathy was reported to occur in 25% of patients who underwent an autopsy. Although infarctions were first thought to be a consequence of direct HIV injury to the vascular endothelium, others now argue that the vascular injury results from other infections.[256,257] Cerebral vasculitis has been reported in CMV, HSV, neurosyphilis, and other infections of the CNS, even when they occur in non–HIV-infected patients. A hypercoagulable state associated with elevated levels of anticardiolipin antibody and antiphospholipid antibody, decreased levels of protein S, and a clinical condition similar to thrombotic thrombocytopenic purpura has also been described in association with HIV infection.[258] Although stroke is common in patients with AIDS, intracranial hemorrhage is relatively rare. Autoimmune-mediated thrombocytopenia, diffuse intravascular coagulation, and CMV infection have been reported to lead to intracranial hemorrhage in patients with AIDS.[243,255,259,260]

Central Nervous System Malignancy

High-grade B-cell lymphoma is found in 4% of HIV-infected children and is the most common mass lesion found in the CNS of children with AIDS.[242,243] It generally presents between ages 5 and 10 years. Lymphoma can be distinguished from toxoplasmosis by increased uptake of tracer on single photon emission computed tomography (SPECT) or positron emission tomography (PET) imaging. It most frequently arises in periventricular white matter and is associated with EBV infection. Metastatic lymphoma can also occur.

Infections of CNS

CNS infection by usual and opportunistic organisms in childhood AIDS accounts for only 13% of neurologic complications.[261-263] Primary CNS infections in HIV-infected children are caused by the usual etiologic bacterial organisms and *M. tuberculosis*. The usual presenting signs and symptoms are seen. Opportunistic infections such as CMV and aspergillosis are frequently observed at autopsy and generally result from disseminated disease.[261,263] Reactivated infections such as toxoplasmosis, herpes zoster, and progressive multifocal leukoencephalopathy caused by Jacob-Creutzfeldt virus infection also occur but are rare when compared with those in the adult population.[243,263,264]

The protozoal infection toxoplasmic encephalitis occurs in 30% of adult patients with AIDS but is generally seen in only older children. The incidence of maternal-fetal transmission does not appear to be affected by maternal HIV infection. Combination therapy with sulfadiazine and pyrimethamine is generally effective if initiated early. Clindamycin is an appropriate alternative in patients with sulfa allergy.[265] Corticosteroids are sometimes used in addition to first-line therapy to reduce edema. Relapse is common after treatment is stopped, and maintenance therapy is necessary. Primary prophylaxis is offered to adults with serologic findings that are positive for toxoplasma and a CD4 count of less than 200.

Progressive multifocal leukoencephalopathy presents with ataxia, aphasia, weakness, and lethargy.[261,266] CT may be relatively unremarkable with one or two nonenhancing hypodense areas of demyelination generally in subcortical white matter. MRI is more sensitive than CT for detection of these lesions. The lack of inflammatory finding is believed due to the severity of immune suppression. Presumptive diagnosis can be confirmed by stereotactic biopsy and identification of virus by DNA probes. The only treatment for this condition is HAART in the hopes that the immune system will be reconstituted; however, an inflammatory response during immune reconstitution may cause clinical deterioration and seizures.[267] Death is typically secondary to apnea, and although recovery is possible, residual deficits are likely.

Although not considered a reactivated infection, cryptococcal meningitis is typically seen in older children.[243,263] *Cryptococcus* spreads via the bloodstream to the CNS. Classic presentation includes fever, headache, and preceding alterations in mental status. Focal signs and meningeal signs are minimal. CSF counts may be normal, although intracranial pressure (ICP) is typically elevated. CT findings are nonspecific.

Treatment of coma in the HIV-positive patient is directed at the underlying cause. Supportive care follows the principles of therapy for all comatose patients, including airway protection, control of ICP where appropriate, and nutritional support. Specific therapy for the underlying condition must be applied. In situations in which no explanation for an acute neurologic deterioration is readily available, it is appropriate to initiate antiviral therapy with ganciclovir, acyclovir, or both and await clinical improvement. This approach is based on

evidence that CMV coinfection may be responsible for neurologic deterioration.[263] Some improvement has been reported in patients with HIV encephalopathy who were treated with ZDV or ganciclovir therapy, but the waxing and waning nature of the condition even without therapy makes any intervention difficult to evaluate.

Occupational HIV Exposure

Serious exposure to HIV in the health care setting is most likely to occur in the emergency department or ICU. The risk of exposure is 0.3% after a percutaneous exposure and 0.09% after blood or body fluid contact with nonintact skin or mucous membrane. Postexposure prophylaxis should be offered to all persons who have sustained a mucosal or parental exposure to HIV from a known infected source within 72 hours.[268] Postexposure prophylaxis regimen should consist of the US Public Health Service preferred regimen: Raltegravir (RAL) plus Truvada (TDF/FTC), although a high-risk exposure may warrant a third drug.[268] Women who receive postexposure prophylaxis should be offered emergency contraception to prevent pregnancy.[268] Repeat HIV antigen testing should be done 3 months after completion of the postexposure prophylaxis regimen.[268]

Summary

A critically ill child with a life-threatening infection or trauma should be presumed to be immunodeficient. The approach to such patients requires selective surveillance and a low threshold for empiric therapy. Through experience, patterns of infections characteristic of specific immunodeficient states can be recognized, but the unusual presentation is always possible. In the future, immune stimulants may also be part of the physician's armamentarium, in addition to antimicrobial therapy.

Key References

1. Gibot S, Nancy C. The complexity of understanding the immunology of sepsis. *Crit Care Med*. 2005;33:700, author reply 700.
2. Flohe SB, Flohe S, Schade FU. Invited review: deterioration of the immune system after trauma: signals and cellular mechanisms. *Innate Immun*. 2008;14:333-344.
5. Boomer JS, To K, Chang KC, et al. Immunosuppression in patients who die of sepsis and multiple organ failure. *JAMA*. 2011;306:2594-2605.
7. Hall MW, Knatz NL, Vetterly C, et al. Immunoparalysis and nosocomial infection in children with multiple organ dysfunction syndrome. *Intensive Care Med*. 2011;37:525-532.
22. Sabat R, Grutz G, Warszawska K, et al. Biology of interleukin-10. *Cytokine Growth Factor Rev*. 2010;21:331-344.
26. Shi SS, Shi CC, Zhao ZY, et al. Effect of open heart surgery with cardiopulmonary bypass on peripheral blood lymphocyte apoptosis in children. *Pediatr Cardiol*. 2009;30:153-159.
27. Drewry AM, Samra N, Skrupky LP, et al. Persistent lymphopenia after diagnosis of sepsis predicts mortality. *Shock*. 2014;42:383-391.
31. Hamers L, Kox M, Pickkers P. Sepsis-induced immunoparalysis: mechanisms, markers, and treatment options. *Minerva Anestesiol*. 2015;81:426.
34. Bo L, Wang F, Zhu J, et al. Granulocyte-colony stimulating factor (G-CSF) and granulocyte-macrophage colony stimulating factor (GM-CSF) for sepsis: a meta-analysis. *Crit Care*. 2011;15:R58.
39. de Souza Menezes F, Leite HP, Koch Nogueira PC. Malnutrition as an independent predictor of clinical outcome in critically ill children. *Nutrition*. 2012;28:267-270.

41. Chandra RK. Nutrition and immunology: from the clinic to cellular biology and back again. *Proc Nutr Soc.* 1999;58:681-683.

52. Skillman HE, Mehta NM. Nutrition therapy in the critically ill child. *Curr Opin Crit Care.* 2012;18:192-198.

62. Stephensen CB. Vitamin A, infection, and immune function. *Annu Rev Nutr.* 2001;21:167-192.

64. Madden K, Feldman H, Smith E, et al. Vitamin D deficiency in critically ill children. *Pediatrics.* 2012;130:421.

71. Christopher K. Vitamin D supplementation in the ICU patient. *Curr Opin Clin Nutr Metab Care.* 2015;18:187.

76. Leite H, Nogueira P, Iglesias S, et al. Increased plasma selenium is associated with better outcomes in children with systemic inflammation. *Nutrition.* 2015;31:485.

81. Refaai MA, Blumberg N. Transfusion immunomodulation from a clinical perspective: an update. *Expert Rev Hematol.* 2013;6:653-663.

85. Chinen J, Buckley RH. Transplantation immunology: solid organ and bone marrow. *J Allergy Clin Immunol.* 2010;125(suppl 2):S324-S335.

89. Betjes MG. Immune cell dysfunction and inflammation in end-stage renal disease. *Nat Rev Nephrol.* 2013;9:255-265.

94. El Saleeby CM, Somes GW, DeVincenzo JP, Gaur AH. Risk factors for severe respiratory syncytial virus disease in children with cancer: the importance of lymphopenia and young age. *Pediatrics.* 2008;121:235-243.

100. Dankner WM, Lindsey JC, Levin MJ, Pediatric AIDS Clinical Trials Group Protocol Teams 051, 128, 138, 144, 152, 179, 190, 220, 240, 245, 254, 300 and 327. Correlates of opportunistic infections in children infected with the human immunodeficiency virus managed before highly active antiretroviral therapy. *Pediatr Infect Dis J.* 2001;20:40-48.

102. Centers for Disease Control and Prevention. Revised surveillance case definition for HIV infection—United States, 2014. *MMWR Recomm Rep.* 2014;63:1.

118. Akgun KM, Pisani M, Crothers K. The changing epidemiology of HIV-infected patients in the intensive care unit. *J Intensive Care Med.* 2011;26:151-164.

120. Barbier F, Roux A, Canet E, et al. Temporal trends in critical events complicating HIV infection: 1999-2010 multicentre cohort study in France. *Intensive Care Med.* 2014;40:1906-1915.

124. Nicholas SW. The opportunistic and bacterial infections associated with pediatric human immunodeficiency virus disease. *Acta Paediatr Suppl.* 1994;400:46-50.

128. Boulware DR, Callens S, Pahwa S. Pediatric HIV immune reconstitution inflammatory syndrome. *Curr Opin HIV AIDS.* 2008;3:461-467.

131. Abrams EJ. Opportunistic infections and other clinical manifestations of HIV disease in children. *Pediatr Clin North Am.* 2000;47:79-108.

132. Krajicek BJ, Thomas CF Jr, Limper AH. Pneumocystis pneumonia: current concepts in pathogenesis, diagnosis, and treatment. *Clin Chest Med.* 2009;30:265-278, vi.

141. Kitchin O, Masekela R, Becker P, et al. Outcome of human immunodeficiency virus-exposed and -infected children admitted to a pediatric intensive care unit for respiratory failure. *Pediatr Crit Care Med.* 2012;13:516.

143. Hsiao N, Zampoli M, Morrow B, et al. Cytomegalovirus viraemia in HIV exposed and infected infants: prevalence and clinical utility for diagnosing CMV pneumonia. *J Clin Virol.* 2013;58:74.

145. Kimberlin DW. Antiviral therapies in children: has their time arrived? *Pediatr Clin North Am.* 2005;52:837-867, vii.

167. Huson M, Stolp S, van der Poll T, Grobusch M. Community-acquired bacterial bloodstream infections in HIV-infected patients: a systematic review. *Clin Infect Dis.* 2014;58:79.

174. Iordache L, Launay O, Bouchaud O, et al. Autoimmune diseases in HIV-infected patients: 52 cases and literature review. *Autoimmun Rev.* 2014;13:850.

175. Patel N, Khan T, Espinoza L. HIV infection and clinical spectrum of associated vasculitides. *Curr Rheumatol Rep.* 2011;13:506.

178. Starc TJ, Lipshultz SE, Easley KA, et al. Incidence of cardiac abnormalities in children with human immunodeficiency virus infection: the prospective P2C2 HIV study. *J Pediatr.* 2002;141:327-334.

183. Barbaro G, Fisher SD, Lipshultz SE. Pathogenesis of HIV-associated cardiovascular complications. *Lancet Infect Dis.* 2001;1:115-124.

188. Bloomfield G, Khazanie P, Morris A, et al. HIV and noncommunicable cardiovascular and pulmonary diseases in low- and middle-income countries in the ART era: what we know and best directions for future research. *J Acquir Immune Defic Syndr.* 2014;67(suppl 1):S40.

198. Hilton R. Human immunodeficiency virus infection and kidney disease. *J R Coll Physicians Edinb.* 2013;43:236.

205. Gathogo E, Jose S, Jones R, et al. End-stage kidney disease and kidney transplantation in HIV-positive patients: an observational cohort study. *J Acquir Immune Defic Syndr.* 2014;67:177.

206. Velasco-Benitez CA. Digestive, hepatic, and nutritional manifestations in Latin American children with HIV/AIDS. *J Pediatr Gastroenterol Nutr.* 2008;47(suppl 1):S24-S26.

210. Wilcox CM, Saag MS. Gastrointestinal complications of HIV infection: changing priorities in the HAART era. *Gut.* 2008;57:861-870.

215. Karpelowsky JS, Leva E, Kelley B, et al. Outcomes of human immunodeficiency virus-infected and -exposed children undergoing surgery—a prospective study. *J Pediatr Surg.* 2009;44:681-687.

229. Kohli A, Shaffer A, Sherman A, Kottilil S. Treatment of hepatitis C: a systematic review. *JAMA.* 2014;312:631-640.

231. Halkic N, Bally F, Gillet M. Organ transplantation in HIV-infected patients. *N Engl J Med.* 2002;347:1801-1803, author reply 1801-1803.

242. Kest H, Brogly S, McSherry G, et al. Malignancy in perinatally human immunodeficiency virus-infected children in the United States. *Pediatr Infect Dis J.* 2005;24:237-242.

245. Hoare J, Ransford G, Phillips N, et al. Systematic review of neuroimaging studies in vertically transmitted HIV positive children and adolescents. *Metab Brain Dis.* 2014;29:221.

255. Brannagan TH 3rd. Retroviral-associated vasculitis of the nervous system. *Neurol Clin.* 1997;15:927-944.

263. Wrzolek MA, Brudkowska J, Kozlowski PB, et al. Opportunistic infections of the central nervous system in children with HIV infection: report of 9 autopsy cases and review of literature. *Clin Neuropathol.* 1995;14:187-196.

267. Clifford DB. Neurological immune reconstitution inflammatory response: riding the tide of immune recovery. *Curr Opin Neurol.* 2015;28:295-301.

268. Kuhar DT, Henderson DK, Struble KA, et al. Updated US public health service guidelines for the management of occupational exposures to human immunodeficiency virus and recommendations for postexposure prophylaxis. *Infect Control Hosp Epidemiol.* 2013;34:875-892.

Immune Balance in Critical Illness: SIRS, CARS, and Immunoparalysis

Mark W. Hall

PEARLS

- The inflammatory response to critical illness is highly dynamic over time and includes both proinflammatory and antiinflammatory features.
- These features constitute the systemic inflammatory response syndrome (SIRS) and compensatory antiinflammatory response syndrome (CARS).
- This balance is modulated by elements of both innate and adaptive immunity.
- The SIRS and CARS responses can temporally coexist, and their relative magnitudes are related to outcomes from critical illness.
- High plasma levels of interleukin (IL)-6 represent the marker of the SIRS response that is most strongly associated with adverse outcomes, though IL-8 levels may also be predictive.
- Quantitation of the CARS response can require specific testing, including measurement of plasma IL-10 levels, monocyte HLA-DR expression, quantitation of cytokine production capacity via ex vivo stimulation studies, and measures of lymphocyte apoptosis.
- Persistent and/or severe elevation in plasma IL-10 levels, reduction in monocyte HLA-DR expression, reduction in ex vivo lipopolysaccharide-induced tumor necrosis factor (TNF)-α production capacity, and lymphopenia have repeatedly shown association with increased risk for secondary infection and death across multiple forms of critical illness.
- These features are consistent with the phenomenon of immunoparalysis.
- Human in vivo evidence suggests that treatment with therapies such as granulocyte-macrophage colony-stimulating factor (GM-CSF) and interferon (IFN)-γ can reverse critical illness-induced innate immune suppression with the potential for benefit in terms of clinical outcomes.
- Evidence from in vivo animal studies suggests that treatment with adaptive-targeted therapies such as anti–PD-1 antibodies and IL-7 can reduce sepsis-related mortality.

Introduction

From sepsis to trauma to cardiopulmonary bypass, critical illness is frequently characterized by derangements in the inflammatory response. Familiar to most are the canonical signs and symptoms of an exaggerated proinflammatory response including fever, capillary leak, and malperfusion. Less easily appreciated are the results of the inflammatory response's counterregulatory system. Like most biological processes, the inflammatory response includes mechanisms to downregulate its own activity. This compensatory response is, when prolonged and severe, increasingly recognized to be associated with increased risks of secondary infection and death from critical illness. These responses can affect the innate and adaptive arms of the immune system and can be quantified in the laboratory. This chapter focuses on the proinflammatory and antiinflammatory responses across innate and adaptive immunity, highlighting preclinical and clinical data that support the restoration of immunologic balance as an important goal in management of the critically ill patient.

Innate and Adaptive Immunity

Although details of innate and adaptive immune cell function can be found in Chapters 101 and 102, a brief review of the cast of characters that comprise the cellular and soluble elements of the inflammatory response are provided here. A limited list of these elements is presented in Table 105.1. There is considerable crosstalk between arms of the immune system, but it is useful to consider the innate and adaptive immune systems in turn.

Innate Immunity

Cells of the innate immune system include neutrophils, monocytes (and their descendants, tissue macrophages), dendritic cells, and natural killer cells. These cells, to varying degrees, carry out functions including the recognition of pathogens, phagocytosis of these pathogens, intracellular killing, and presentation of digested antigens on cell surface molecules to facilitate activation of lymphocytes. In addition, innate immune cells elaborate cytokines and chemokines that modulate the local environment and/or recruit other immune cells to the area of infection or injury.

Innate immune cells are typically the first cellular elements to become activated in the face of an inflammatory stimulus. This is by virtue of their constitutive expression of cell

TABLE 105.1	Selected Elements of Innate and Adaptive Immune Systems
Innate	
Cells	Neutrophils, monocytes, tissue macrophages, dendritic cells, natural killer cells
Functions	Phagocytosis, intracellular killing, antigen presentation, cytokine production
Receptors	Toll-like receptors, NOD receptors, Fc receptors, complement receptors
Cytokines/Chemokines Produced	
Proinflammatory	TNF-α, IL-1β, IL-8, MCP-1, IL-18
Antiinflammatory	IL-10, sTNFr, IL-1ra
Pleiotropic	IL-6
Adaptive	
Cells	T lymphocytes (helper T cells, cytotoxic T cells, regulatory T cells); B lymphocytes (plasma cells)
Functions	Cytokine production, cytotoxicity, antibody production, memory
Receptors	T-cell receptor, B-cell receptor
Cytokines/Chemokines Produced	
Proinflammatory	IFN-γ, IL-2, IL-17, GM-CSF, RANTES
Antiinflammatory	IL-10, TGF-β
Pleiotropic	IL-6

GM-CSF, granulocyte-macrophage colony-stimulating factor; *IFN*, interferon; *IL*, interleukin; *IL-1ra*, interleukin-1 receptor antagonist; *MCP*, monocyte chemotactic protein; *NOD*, nucleotide-binding oligomerization domain; *sTNFr*, soluble TNF receptor; *TNF*, tumor necrosis factor; *RANTES*, regulated on activation, normal T cell expressed and secreted; *TGF*, transforming growth factor.

surface receptors for pathogen-associated molecular patterns (PAMPs) or endogenous danger-associated molecular patterns (DAMPs). These receptors can be activated by broad classes of ligands, an example of which is Toll-like receptor (TLR)-4, which is a key part of the PAMP receptor for lipopolysaccharide (LPS). Thus LPS should result in robust activation of innate immune cells upon the cells' first exposure without requiring antigen presentation or immunologic memory. This vigorous and prompt response is responsible for the central role innate immune cells are thought to play in the early and fulminant presentation of acute inflammatory conditions such as sepsis.

Adaptive Immunity

Lymphocytes comprise the adaptive arm of the immune system. Most lymphocytes can be classified as T or B cells, with T cells being responsible for cytokine production (in the case of CD4+ cells) and cytotoxicity (in the case of CD8+ cells). B cells, once activated, differentiate into plasma cells, which are responsible for antibody production. Lymphocytes typically require the presentation of antigenic peptides by activated members of the innate immune system in order to become activated, with the notable exception of superantigens, which can directly activate lymphocytes. T- and B-cell responses are generally highly antigen specific as the result of gene rearrangement within T- and B-cell receptors. Accordingly, only a small percentage of naïve lymphocytes are capable

of responding to a given antigen. Lastly, once activated, a lymphocyte must clonally expand to mount a maximal immune response. Repeat exposure to an antigen, however, results in faster propagation of the immune response as the result of memory cells, which can persist for decades. The combination of the relative rarity of potentially responsive lymphocytes, the need for antigen presentation, and the potential need for clonal expansion explains the more sub-acute role that lymphocytes are thought to play in the perpetuation and modulation of the immune response to critical illness.

Proinflammatory and Antiinflammatory Responses
SIRS in Critical Illness

The elaboration of proinflammatory cytokines, including tumor necrosis factor (TNF)-α and interleukin (IL)-1β, and chemokines, such as IL-8, occurs rapidly following activation of most innate immune cells. These cytokines act to produce elevated temperature (fever), vasodilation, and increased capillary permeability. Chemokines serve to promote recruitment of other immune cells to the area along a concentration gradient. These effects are beneficial when confined to a localized area of infection, allowing for increased delivery of leukocytes to these areas and enhanced killing of pathogens. When these effects become systemic, however, they become pathologic, leading to intravascular volume depletion, organ malperfusion, acidosis, organ failure, and death. Regardless of whether the insult prompting this activation is infectious (eg, sepsis) or noninfectious (eg, trauma, cardiopulmonary bypass, pancreatitis), the magnitude of the inflammatory response is frequently associated with adverse clinical outcomes.

Innate proinflammatory cytokines like TNF-α and IL-1β, however, peak early and have relatively short half-lives in the plasma. Often by the time a patient comes to medical attention following an acute proinflammatory insult, the plasma levels of these cytokines are waning. Interleukin-6 is made by multiple cell types including immune and nonimmune cells in response to stress and/or proinflammatory cytokines. Plasma IL-6 levels therefore remain elevated for far longer than those of TNF-α or IL-1β following the onset of a proinflammatory stimulus. In fact, numerous investigators have demonstrated that elevated plasma IL-6 levels predict mortality from forms of critical illness including sepsis and trauma in adults and children.[1-4] It is important to understand, however, that IL-6 is itself a pleiotropic cytokine. While it is a potent inducer of the hepatic acute phase response, IL-6 also has antiinflammatory properties including promoting production of glucocorticoids and antiinflammatory cytokines.[5] Interleukin-8 is a potent neutrophil chemokine whose levels in plasma can also be persistently elevated following an inflammatory insult. Low systemic IL-8 levels have been shown to predict favorable outcomes from pediatric septic shock,[6] while elevated IL-8 levels have been associated with increased mortality from pediatric trauma.[7]

The use of plasma biomarkers like IL-6 and IL-8 has the potential to identify high- (or low-) risk subjects for inclusion in clinical trials in the ICU. For example, in one of the few positive phase III clinical trials of anticytokine therapy in adult patients with severe sepsis, anti-TNF antibody fragment therapy was associated with reduced mortality in subjects with plasma IL-6 levels greater than 1000 pg/mL.[8] Given the complexity and redundancy of the proinflammatory cascade, however, it is possible that a combinatorial approach may be superior to single biomarkers in predicting outcomes. Wong et al. have repeatedly demonstrated high sensitivity and specificity in predicting pediatric sepsis mortality using a panel of biomarkers including IL-8, C-C chemokine ligand 3, heat shock protein 70, granzyme B, and matrix metalloproteinase-8.[9] It remains unclear whether specific plasma biomarkers such as these represent potential direct mediators of harm versus indirect measures of the proinflammatory response. The relationship between the magnitude of this response and clinical outcomes from critical illness, however, appears to be consistent.

CARS in Critical Illness

Within hours of activation of the proinflammatory response, immune cells begin elaborating counterregulatory antiinflammatory cytokines. These include molecules such as soluble TNF receptor (sTNFr) and IL-1 receptor antagonist (IL-1ra), which impair the functionality of the proinflammatory cytokines. In addition, mediators such as IL-10 and transforming growth factor (TGF)-β are produced. They directly inhibit proinflammatory cells and/or repolarize them to an antiinflammatory/suppressed phenotype. Much as elevated plasma levels of proinflammatory cytokines are associated with adverse outcomes from critical illness, a similar relationship exists between antiinflammatory cytokine levels and clinical outcomes. High IL-10 levels have been associated with increased risks for secondary infection and/or mortality in the settings of adult and pediatric sepsis,[2,10,11] adult and pediatric trauma,[12,13] and pediatric cardiopulmonary bypass.[14]

Immune cell death represents another important counterregulatory response. Neutrophils typically die on release of their cargo of lytic enzymes and free radicals. In addition, lymphocyte apoptosis has repeatedly been shown to occur in the setting of adult and pediatric sepsis.[15,16] Phagocytosis of lymphocyte apoptotic bodies has also been shown to induce profound hyporesponsiveness of innate immune cells, demonstrating another example of innate and adaptive immune cell crosstalk.[17]

In addition to plasma cytokine levels and cell numbers, innate immune cell function has repeatedly been shown to be abnormal in many patients following the onset of critical illness. Human leukocyte antigen (HLA)-DR is a class II major histocompatibility complex (MHC) molecule that is present on the surface of antigen-presenting cells. These molecules display digested peptides on the innate immune cell's surface for presentation to adaptive immune cells. Monocyte HLA-DR expression is known to be reduced in the setting of sepsis, likely due to internalization of HLA-DR in subsurface vesicles.[18] The phenomenon of reduced monocyte HLA-DR expression has been demonstrated in adults and children in the aftermath of conditions as varied as trauma, cardiopulmonary bypass, multiple organ failure, and pancreatitis.[19-23]

Besides antigen presentation, the capacity of innate immune cells to respond to a new challenge has also been shown to be an important part of the CARS response. Specifically, the ability of blood samples to produce TNF-α when stimulated ex vivo with LPS has been shown to be reduced in many patients with critical illness. Ex vivo LPS-induced cytokine production capacity should be high in the healthy, immunocompetent state with innate immune cells (notably monocytes) producing the majority of the measured TNF-α. Downregulation of innate immune cell responsiveness can be marked and persistent in critically ill patients. This may seem counterintuitive given the proinflammatory nature of many clinical phenotypes seen in the ICU. It should be remembered, however, that many tissues produce proinflammatory mediators in the setting of stress. It is therefore likely that many of the systemic proinflammatory cytokines present beyond the first few hours of critical illness originate from injured tissues rather than from circulating leukocytes. Reductions in monocyte HLA-DR expression and/or ex vivo LPS-induced TNF-α production capacity that are severe and persistent following the onset of critical illness have been collectively termed "immunoparalysis."[24]

Lastly, specific cell types may play a role in the development and/or perpetuation of the immunoparalyzed phenotype. Work in critically ill adults has, for example, shown that the highly immunosuppressive regulatory T cell (T_{reg}), characterized by $CD4^+CD25^+FoxP3^+CD127^{lo}$ phenotype, can predominate in the subacute phase of sepsis.[25] These T_{regs} are known to produce large quantities of IL-10 and TGF-β and are felt to be resistant to the wave of lymphocyte apoptosis that occurs in sepsis. Recent evidence also points to the elaboration of myeloid-derived suppressor cells (MDSC) from the bone marrow of critically ill patients.[26] These MDSC have the potential to produce high levels of antiinflammatory cytokines and facilitate T-cell suppression, though their role in critical illness-induced immune suppression is unclear.

Temporal Aspects of the SIRS/CARS Response

The classical view of the SIRS/CARS response involved the presence of two temporally distinct phases of illness in which the proinflammatory phase of SIRS was followed, over hours or days, by the antiinflammatory CARS phase. It is now appreciated that these two responses can and do coexist in the critically ill patient (Fig. 105.1). This is evidenced by the frequent occurrence of "cytokine storm" in which both proinflammatory and antiinflammatory mediators are elevated in the plasma simultaneously.[1,27] Gene expression studies, using mRNA from circulating leukocytes, have demonstrated upregulation of innate immune signaling pathways and downregulation of adaptive immune pathways in the early phases of sepsis and trauma.[28-30] Studies of functional measures of immunity (eg, monocyte HLA-DR expression, ex vivo LPS-induced TNF-α production capacity, and phytohemagglutin [PHA]-induced cytokine production capacity) suggest that leukocyte function can be reduced in both arms of the immune system with a day or two following critical illness onset.[13,31] As noted earlier, the initial peak of the leukocyte inflammatory response may have occurred before the patient is admitted to the ICU. Similarly, the CARS response may be well established by the time of ICU admission, despite persistently high levels of circulating proinflammatory mediators in the aftermath that follows the onset of critical illness.

CARS and Clinical Outcomes

Not only is the state of immune suppression that characterizes the CARS response quantifiable, its severity is associated with adverse clinical outcomes. Severe reduction in monocyte HLA-DR expression has long been associated with secondary infection and mortality risk in adults with trauma and sepsis.[19,21] It has also been shown to carry these same associations in pediatric multiple organ dysfunction syndrome (MODS) and cardiopulmonary bypass.[20,22] Early work in this field suggested increased risks for adverse outcomes if less than 30% of monocytes strongly express HLA-DR by flow cytometry. More recent studies have used testing that is capable of quantitating the number of HLA-DR molecules per cell. Using this approach, investigators have identified a threshold of fewer than 8000 HLA-DR molecules per monocyte in defining the immunoparalyzed phenotype.[32] It is not clear if one method is superior to the other in predicting outcomes. Similarly, the ideal time frame for measuring HLA-DR expression is unclear. Some investigators have found that reduced HLA-DR expression correlates with adverse outcomes only after the first few days of illness, while others have shown associations within the first 48 hours.

Reduced whole blood ex vivo LPS-induced TNF-α production capacity has been similarly associated with adverse outcomes from critical illness including trauma and sepsis in adults[33,34] and MODS,[20] viral infections,[27,35] cardiopulmonary bypass,[14,36] and trauma[13] in children. Although distinct thresholds of TNF-α production capacity are dependent on the stimulation techniques that are used, standardized protocols that have successfully predicted outcomes in single-center and multicenter settings exist. It is unclear whether monocyte HLA-DR expression or ex vivo LPS-induced TNF-α production capacity is better for defining the innate immune system's CARS response in critical illness or if the measurement of both markers is required.

Acquired adaptive immune suppression is also a risk factor for adverse ICU outcomes. Severe lymphopenia and lymphocyte apoptosis in lymphoid organs have been shown to be associated with secondary infection and mortality risk in critically ill adults and children.[16,37] In an extension of earlier genomic work, Wong et al. demonstrated the ability to use patterns of leukocyte mRNA expression, focusing primarily on suppression of adaptive immunity and glucocorticoid receptor signaling genes, to predict mortality in derivation and validation cohorts (Fig. 105.2).[38] Lastly, impaired T-cell cytokine production capacity upon ex vivo stimulation with PHA, as early as 1 to 2 days after onset of illness, has been shown to be associated with infectious complications of pediatric septic shock.[31]

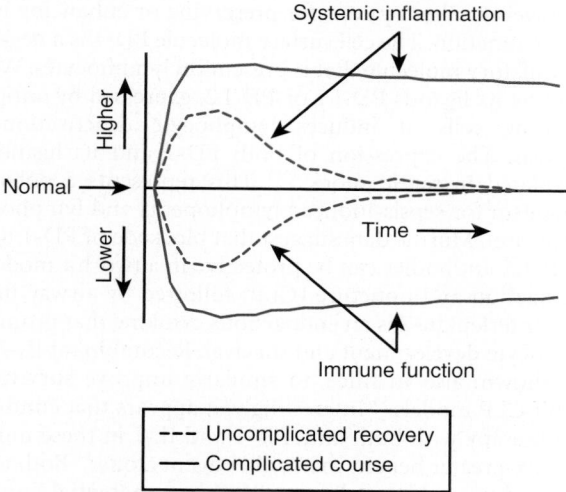

Fig. 105.1. Temporal aspects of the systemic inflammatory response syndrome (SIRS)/compensatory antiinflammatory response syndrome (CARS) response. After the onset of critical illness, there is typically a surge in systemic inflammation associated with the SIRS response (red lines). A compensatory downregulation of immune cell function often occurs concomitant with this (blue lines). Complicated outcomes (eg, secondary infection, death) are frequently associated with persistent elevations in systemic inflammation and persistently suppressed immune function (solid lines). Uncomplicated recovery is more often characterized by return to immunologic homeostasis (dashed lines).

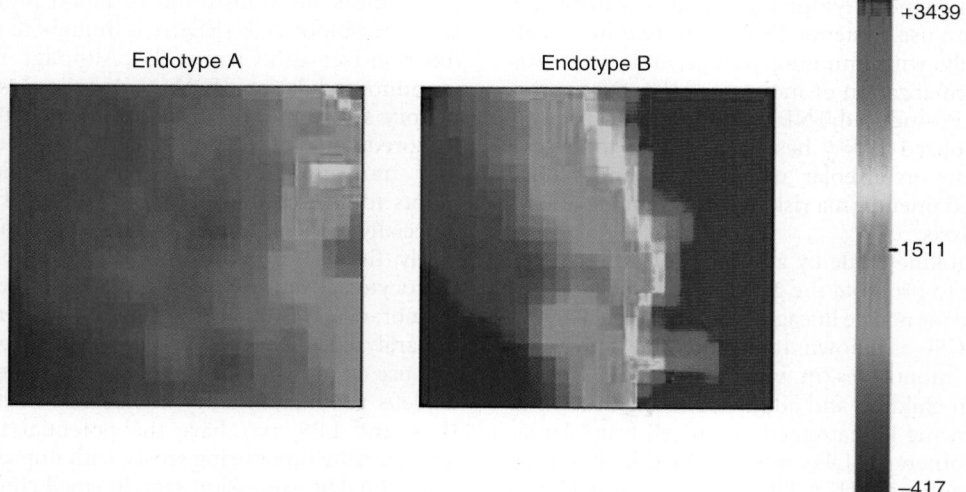

Fig. 105.2. Composite leukocyte gene expression in pediatric septic shock. Patients can be subclassified into endotypes on the basis of expression of 100 genes that regulate the adaptive immune response and glucocorticoid receptor signaling in leukocytes. The blue color represents decreased gene expression while the red color represents increased expression. Those falling in endotype A, with much greater downregulation of gene expression, demonstrated significantly greater mortality compared with endotype B in multiple large cohorts of septic children. (Images courtesy Dr. Hector Wong.)

In sum, there is a robust and growing body of literature suggesting that critical illness–associated immune suppression represents a major, yet often occult, risk factor for adverse outcomes across the spectrum of critical illness in adults and children. Because this phenomenon has been seen in both innate and adaptive immune cells, it stands to reason that both arms of the immune system may be targets for therapies aimed at restoring immune function.

Immune Modulation in Pediatric ICU

The intentional modulation of the inflammatory response is nothing new to the field of critical care medicine. A myriad of adult studies were published in the 1990s targeting the removal of selected proinflammatory mediators (eg, LPS, TNF-α, IL-1β) using monoclonal antibody therapy[39] (reviewed in). Phase III clinical trials of these agents were nearly universally unsuccessful in reducing sepsis mortality. Trials of potently immunosuppressive glucocorticoids such as methylprednisolone or dexamethasone, given with the intent of abrogating the proinflammatory response, similarly failed to improve sepsis outcomes in adults.[40] The use of methylprednisolone in the setting of acute respiratory distress syndrome (ARDS) has met with more mixed results, with recent evidence suggesting that early use may improve survival in adults.[41] Lastly, immunosuppressive treatments remain the mainstay for a host of acute and chronic inflammatory conditions that may result in critical illness including asthma, autoimmune disease, transplantation, and malignancy. Increasing appreciation of the phenomenon of immunoparalysis, however, has spurred the development of immunostimulatory therapies that have the potential to reverse critical illness–associated immune suppression.

Targeted Innate Immunostimulation

Two drugs that have been studied with the most rigor in the setting of critical illness–associated immune suppression are interferon (IFN)-γ and granulocyte-macrophage colony-stimulating factor (GM-CSF). IFN-γ is a proinflammatory cytokine made by T-helper 1 lymphocytes and is available for experimental human use. Systemic IFN-γ was used in a small series of septic adults with immunoparalysis, and its use was associated with normalization of monocyte HLA-DR expression and ex vivo LPS-induced TNF-α production capacity.[42] In addition, aerosolized IFN-γ has been shown to restore HLA-DR expression on alveolar macrophages and reduce ventilator-associated pneumonia risk in adult trauma patients with immunoparalysis.[43]

GM-CSF is a cytokine made by a number of different cell types, and it serves to promote the generation of new cells of the granulocyte and monocyte lineages from the bone marrow. In addition, GM-CSF is known to restore the activity of immunoparalyzed monocytes in vitro.[13] GM-CSF is FDA approved for use in children and adults for reconstitution of bone marrow following hematopoetic stem cell transplantation and/or chemotherapy. Like IFN-γ, GM-CSF has been shown to restore monocyte HLA-DR expression and TNF-α production capacity in an uncontrolled series of immunoparalyzed, septic adults.[44] It has also been evaluated in randomized controlled trials in critically ill adults and children, the results of which have suggested faster resolution of innate immune suppression, when present, and/or decreased

infection risk compared with placebo. A summary of clinical trials using immunostimulation for treatment of critical illness–associated immune suppression is presented in Table 105.2.[45-50]

Targeted Adaptive Immunostimulation

There are fewer pharmacologic choices when trying to target lymphocyte stimulation in critically patients, as there are currently no known lineage-specific colony-stimulating factors that promote lymphocyte development and function. There are, however, other options for preserving or enhancing lymphocyte function. The cell surface molecule PD-1 is a negative costimulatory molecule that is present on lymphocytes. When bound by its ligands PD-L1 or PD-L2, expressed by antigen-presenting cells, it induces lymphocyte deactivation or apoptosis. The expression of both PD-1 and its ligands is upregulated in septic shock.[37,51] This represents a potential mechanism for sepsis-induced lymphopenia and lymphocyte suppression. Murine data suggest that blockade of PD-1 using anti–PD-1 antibodies can be protective in a two-hit model of cecal ligation and puncture (CLP) followed by airway infection.[52] Interleukin-7 is an endogenous cytokine that promotes lymphocyte development and survival. Recombinant IL-7 has been shown, also in mice, to similarly improve survival in two-hit CLP models.[53] Interestingly, it appears that combinatorial therapy with both anti–PD-1 and IL-7 in these models may have greater benefit than either agent alone.[54] Both anti–PD-1 and recombinant human IL-7 have potential applications as cancer therapeutics and may be available for clinical trials in critically ill humans in the near future.

Unintended Immunomodulation

In addition to the forms of intentional immunomodulation described earlier, it is important to understand that many therapies that are applied to critically ill patients have unintended effects on immune function (Table 105.3). From sedatives and analgesics to inotropes and diuretics, much of the ICU pharmacopeia is immunodulatory with most of these drugs having direct or indirect immunosuppressive effects. In addition, the transfusion of blood products, particularly stored red blood cells (RBCs), is thought to modulate immune function (see also Chapter 93). Although transfusion-related immunomodulation (TRIM) was once viewed as a proinflammatory syndrome, the broad implementation of prestorage leukoreduction of RBC units has reduced acute proinflammatory transfusion reactions.[55] Instead, increasing evidence points to an immunosuppressive effect of RBC transfusion, especially in the setting of prolonged pretransfusion storage.[56] Lastly, the use of extracorporeal life support devices causes leukocyte activation due to exposure to artificial tubing and membranes. It is unclear if these devices promote the immunoparalyzed phenotype in the subacute phase. Intriguingly, the use of adsorptive membranes designed to specifically deplete proinflammatory mediators such as complement, IL-6, and LPS may have the potential to improve innate immune function during sepsis, with improvements in monocyte HLA-DR expression seen in small clinical trials.[57]

Immune Monitoring in ICU

The current routine clinical practice in the United States for immune function monitoring in critically ill patients is limited

TABLE 105.2   Summary of In Vivo Immunostimulation Studies in Critically Ill Adults and Children

Author	Year	Study Type	Number	Population	Drug	Results	Reference
Livingston et al.	1994	RCT	98	Adult trauma	IFN-γ	↑ Monocyte HLA-DR expression	45
Spagnoli et al.	1995	RCT	10	Adult trauma	GM-CSF	↑ Monocyte HLA-DR expression	46
Döcke et al.	1997	Case series	9	Adult sepsis with immunoparalysis	IFN-γ	↑ Monocyte HLA-DR expression and ex vivo LPS-induced TNF-α production capacity	42
Nakos et al.	2002	RCT	21	Adult trauma with immunoparalysis	IFN-γ (inhaled)	↑ Alveolar macrophage HLA-DR expression, reduced VAP risk	43
Nierhaus et al.	2003	Case series	9	Adult sepsis	GM-CSF	↑ Monocyte HLA-DR expression and ex vivo LPS-induced TNF-α production capacity	44
Rosenbloom et al.	2005	RCT	40	Adult sepsis	GM-CSF	↑ Innate immune function	47
Orozco et al.	2006	RCT	58	Adult sepsis	GM-CSF	Improved infection outcomes	48
Meisel et al.	2009	RCT	38	Adult sepsis with immunoparalysis	GM-CSF	↑ Monocyte HLA-DR expression and ex vivo LPS-induced TNF-α production capacity, improved organ function	49
Hall et al.	2011	RCT	14	Pediatric MODS with immunoparalysis	GM-CSF	↑ Ex vivo LPS-induced TNF-α production capacity, reduced nosocomial infection risk	20
Paine et al.	2012	RCT	130	Adult ARDS	GM-CSF	No change in ventilator-free days (no immune parameters measured)	50

ARDS, acute respiratory distress syndrome; *GM-CSF,* granulocyte-macrophage colony-stimulating factor; *IFN,* interferon; *LPS,* lipopolysaccharide; *MODS,* multiple organ dysfunction syndrome; *RCT,* randomized controlled trial; *TNF,* tumor necrosis factor.

TABLE 105.3   Immunomodulatory Properties of Commonly Used ICU Medications

Drug	Immune Effect	Mechanism
Catecholamines		
α-Agonists	↑	Direct and indirect potentiation of proinflammatory signaling
β-Agonists	↓	Direct and indirect potentiation of antiinflammatory signaling
Antibiotics		
β-Lactams	↓	Bone marrow suppression, ↓ cytokine production
Macrolides	↓	↓ Cytokine production
Insulin	↓	↓ Proinflammatory signaling
Furosemide	↓	↓ Cytokine production
Sedatives		
Benzodiazepines	↓	↑ Cortisol response, direct leukocyte inhibition
Barbiturates	↓	↓ Neutrophil function
Analgesics		
Opiates	↓	↓ Proinflammatory cytokine production, ↑ production of TGFβ, ↑ leukocyte apoptosis
NSAIDs	↓	↓ Cytokine production

NSAIDs, nonsteroidal antiinflammatory drugs; *TGF,* transforming growth factor.

to the measurement of complete blood counts and nonspecific markers of inflammation such as C-reactive protein (CRP) levels. While the clinical use of measures of immune function such as monocyte HLA-DR expression and ex vivo LPS-induced TNF-α production capacity is possible in Europe, these assays are currently limited to research use in the United States. It remains unclear if monocyte HLA-DR expression is best measured using the percent-positive or molecules-per-cell approach. As for quantitation of TNF-α production capacity, it has been shown that highly reproducible single-center and multicenter results can be obtained using a standardized approach to ex vivo stimulation. The lack of an industry-standard approach, however, makes the generalization of specific treatment thresholds difficult because the TNF-α response will vary from protocol to protocol depending on the type of LPS used and other experimental conditions. Additional consensus in the field is required in order to move this immune function testing to the clinical laboratory.

The reactivation of latent viruses represents an intriguing indirect measure of immune function that may have utility in the ICU. Recent evidence suggests that many patients with critical illness demonstrate PCR positivity for latent viruses in the bloodstream over time and that this viral reactivation is associated with increased mortality.[58] It is possible that this circulating viral DNA represents a sequela of critical illness–associated immune suppression and/or may mediate some of the adverse effects of such suppression. Additional research is necessary in this area.

Lastly, the host genome represents a potential target for immune-related testing. It has been known for many years that there is a familial predisposition to adverse outcomes from critical illness. Westendorp et al. demonstrated this nicely with an analysis of ex vivo LPS-induced cytokine production capacity in first-degree relatives of patients with meningococcemia.[59] Relatives of nonsurvivors could be identified by their production of low amounts of TNF-α and high amounts of the antiinflammatory cytokine IL-10 upon stimulation, suggesting that immunoparalysis may be a heritable trait. Unfortunately, no single polymorphism has been consistently associated with clinically relevant derangements of the immune response in critical illness. Further complicating this analysis is the fact that epigenetic factors may influence the inflammatory response. Cornell et al. were able to identify a histone methylation pattern in the IL-10 promoter region, resulting in a "gene on" configuration in children with immunoparalysis following pediatric cardiopulmonary bypass.[36] The immune phenotype may, therefore, be influenced by fixed genetic factors, as well as potentially modifiable epigenetic factors over the course of critical illness.

Conclusion

The immune response during critical illness, once thought to be limited to a proinflammatory surge, is now known to be highly dynamic with proinflammatory and antiinflammatory forces at work. The balance between these forces determines the patient's ability to respond to new infectious challenges, heal injured tissues, and resolve systemic inflammation. It is increasingly apparent that failure to achieve immunologic homeostasis is associated with increased risks for adverse outcomes across the spectrum of adult and pediatric critical illness. It is similarly apparent that although antiinflammatory therapies are appropriate for some patients, immunostimulatory therapies may be indicated for others. The development of a personalized approach to the identification and management of an abnormal immune response is necessary in pediatric critical illness, involving standardized prospective functional testing. In addition, critically ill patients require a more comprehensive understanding of the multilayered interactions among the host, the pathogen, and treatment-related factors.

Key References

1. Doughty LA, Kaplan SS, Carcillo JA. Inflammatory cytokine and nitric oxide responses in pediatric sepsis and organ failure. *Crit Care Med.* 1996;24:1137-1143.
2. Kellum JA, Kong L, Fink MP, et al. Understanding the inflammatory cytokine response in pneumonia and sepsis: results of the Genetic and Inflammatory Markers of Sepsis (GenIMS) Study. *Arch Intern Med.* 2007;167:1655-1663.
4. Gomez HG, Gonzalez SM, Londono JM, et al. Immunological characterization of compensatory anti-inflammatory response syndrome in patients with severe sepsis: a longitudinal study. *Crit Care Med.* 2014;42: 771-780.
6. Wong HR, Cvijanovich N, Wheeler DS, et al. Interleukin-8 as a stratification tool for interventional trials involving pediatric septic shock. *Am J Respir Crit Care Med.* 2008;178:276-282.
7. Ozturk H, Yagmur Y, Ozturk H. The prognostic importance of serum IL-1beta, IL-6, IL-8 and TNF-alpha levels compared to trauma scoring systems for early mortality in children with blunt trauma. *Pediatric Surg Int.* 2008;24:235-239.
8. Panacek EA, Marshall JC, Albertson TE, et al. Efficacy and safety of the monoclonal anti-tumor necrosis factor antibody F(ab')2 fragment afelimomab in patients with severe sepsis and elevated interleukin-6 levels. *Crit Care Med.* 2004;32:2173-2182.

9. Wong HR, Weiss SL, Giuliano JS Jr, et al. Testing the prognostic accuracy of the updated pediatric sepsis biomarker risk model. *PLoS ONE.* 2014;9:e86242.
10. Doughty L, Carcillo JA, Kaplan S, Janosky J. The compensatory anti-inflammatory cytokine interleukin 10 response in pediatric sepsis-induced multiple organ failure. *Chest.* 1998;113:1625-1631.
11. Hall MW, Gavrilin MA, Knatz NL, et al. Monocyte mRNA phenotype and adverse outcomes from pediatric multiple organ dysfunction syndrome. *Pediatric Res.* 2007;62:597-603.
13. Muszynski JA, Nofziger R, Greathouse K, et al. Innate immune function predicts the development of nosocomial infection in critically injured children. *Shock.* 2014;42:313-321.
14. Allen ML, Hoschtitzky JA, Peters MJ, et al. Interleukin-10 and its role in clinical immunoparalysis following pediatric cardiac surgery. *Crit Care Med.* 2006;34:2658-2665.
15. Hotchkiss RS, Tinsley KW, Swanson PE, et al. Sepsis-induced apoptosis causes progressive profound depletion of B and CD4+ T lymphocytes in humans. *J Immunol.* 2001;166:6952-6963.
16. Felmet KA, Hall MW, Clark RS, et al. Prolonged lymphopenia, lymphoid depletion, and hypoprolactinemia in children with nosocomial sepsis and multiple organ failure. *J Immunol.* 2005;174:3765-3772.
17. Erwig LP, Henson PM. Immunological consequences of apoptotic cell phagocytosis. *Am J Pathol.* 2007;171:2-8.
18. Fumeaux T, Pugin J. Role of interleukin-10 in the intracellular sequestration of human leukocyte antigen-DR in monocytes during septic shock. *Am J Respir Crit Care Med.* 2002;166:1475-1482.
19. Volk HD, Reinke P, Krausch D, et al. Monocyte deactivation—rationale for a new therapeutic strategy in sepsis. *Intensive Care Med.* 1996;22(suppl 4):S474-S481.
20. Hall MW, Knatz NL, Vetterly C, et al. Immunoparalysis and nosocomial infection in children with multiple organ dysfunction syndrome. *Intensive Care Med.* 2011;37:525-532.
21. Hershman MJ, Cheadle WG, Wellhausen SR, et al. Monocyte HLA-DR antigen expression characterizes clinical outcome in the trauma patient. *Br J Surg.* 1990;77:204-207.
22. Allen ML, Peters MJ, Goldman A, et al. Early postoperative monocyte deactivation predicts systemic inflammation and prolonged stay in pediatric cardiac intensive care. *Crit Care Med.* 2002;30:1140-1145.
24. Volk HD, Reinke P, Docke WD. Clinical aspects: from systemic inflammation to 'immunoparalysis'. *Chem Immunol.* 2000;74:162-177.
25. Venet F, Pachot A, Debard AL, et al. Increased percentage of CD4+CD25+ regulatory T cells during septic shock is due to the decrease of CD4+CD25− lymphocytes. *Crit Care Med.* 2004;32:2329-2331.
26. Gentile LF, Cuenca AG, Efron PA, et al. Persistent inflammation and immunosuppression: a common syndrome and new horizon for surgical intensive care. *J Trauma Acute Care Surg.* 2012;72:1491-1501.
27. Hall MW, Geyer SM, Guo CY, et al. Innate immune function and mortality in critically ill children with influenza: a multicenter study. *Crit Care Med.* 2013;41:224-236.
28. Xiao W, Mindrinos MN, Seok J, et al. A genomic storm in critically injured humans. *J Experiment Med.* 2011;208:2581-2590.
29. Wong HR, Cvijanovich N, Allen GL, et al. Genomic expression profiling across the pediatric systemic inflammatory response syndrome, sepsis, and septic shock spectrum. *Crit Care Med.* 2009;37:1558-1566.
30. Tang BM, Huang SJ, McLean AS. Genome-wide transcription profiling of human sepsis: a systematic review. *Crit Care (London, England).* 2010;14:R237.
31. Muszynski JA, Nofziger R, Greathouse K, et al. Early adaptive immune suppression in children with septic shock: a prospective observational study. *Crit Care (London, England).* 2014;18:R145.
32. Docke WD, Hoflich C, Davis KA, et al. Monitoring temporary immunodepression by flow cytometric measurement of monocytic HLA-DR expression: a multicenter standardized study. *Clin Chem.* 2005;51:2341-2347.
33. Ploder M, Pelinka L, Schmuckenschlager C, et al. Lipopolysaccharide-induced tumor necrosis factor alpha production and not monocyte human leukocyte antigen-DR expression is correlated with survival in septic trauma patients. *Shock.* 2006;25:129-134.
34. Volk HD, Reinke P, Docke WD. Immunological monitoring of the inflammatory process: which variables? when to assess? *Eur J Surg Suppl.* 1999;70-72.
35. Mella C, Suarez-Arrabal MC, Lopez S, et al. Innate immune dysfunction is associated with enhanced disease severity in infants with severe respiratory syncytial virus bronchiolitis. *J Infect Dis.* 2013;207:564-573.

36. Cornell TT, Sun L, Hall MW, et al. Clinical implications and molecular mechanisms of immunoparalysis after cardiopulmonary bypass. *J Thorac Cardiovasc Surg*. 2012;143:1160-1166.

37. Boomer JS, To K, Chang KC, et al. Immunosuppression in patients who die of sepsis and multiple organ failure. *JAMA*. 2011;306:2594-2605.

38. Wong HR, Cvijanovich NZ, Anas N, et al. Developing a clinically feasible personalized medicine approach to pediatric septic shock. *Am J Respir Crit Care Med*. 2015;191:309-315.

39. Hall MW, Muszynski JA. Immune modulation in sepsis. *J Pediatric Infect Dis*. 2009;4:127-136.

40. Lefering R, Neugebauer EA. Steroid controversy in sepsis and septic shock: a meta-analysis. *Crit Care Med*. 1995;23:1294-1303.

42. Docke WD, Randow F, Syrbe U, et al. Monocyte deactivation in septic patients: restoration by IFN-gamma treatment. *Nat Med*. 1997;3:678-681.

43. Nakos G, Malamou-Mitsi VD, Lachana A, et al. Immunoparalysis in patients with severe trauma and the effect of inhaled interferon-gamma. *Crit Care Med*. 2002;30:1488-1494.

44. Nierhaus A, Montag B, Timmler N, et al. Reversal of immunoparalysis by recombinant human granulocyte-macrophage colony-stimulating factor in patients with severe sepsis. *Intensive Care Med*. 2003;29:646-651.

45. Livingston DH, Loder PA, Kramer SM, et al. Interferon gamma administration increases monocyte HLA-DR antigen expression but not endogenous interferon production. *Arch Surg*. 1994;129:172-178.

47. Rosenbloom AJ, Linden PK, Dorrance A, et al. Effect of granulocyte-monocyte colony-stimulating factor therapy on leukocyte function and clearance of serious infection in nonneutropenic patients. *Chest*. 2005;127:2139-2150.

48. Orozco H, Arch J, Medina-Franco H, et al. Molgramostim (GM-CSF) associated with antibiotic treatment in nontraumatic abdominal sepsis: a randomized, double-blind, placebo-controlled clinical trial. *Arch Surg*. 2006;141:150-153, discussion 4.

49. Meisel C, Schefold JC, Pschowski R, et al. Granulocyte-macrophage colony-stimulating factor to reverse sepsis-associated immunosuppression: a double-blind, randomized, placebo-controlled multicenter trial. *Am J Respir Crit Care Med*. 2009;180:640-648.

51. Guignant C, Lepape A, Huang X, et al. Programmed death-1 levels correlate with increased mortality, nosocomial infection and immune dysfunctions in septic shock patients. *Crit Care (London, England)*. 2011; 15:R99.

52. Chang KC, Burnham CA, Compton SM, et al. Blockade of the negative co-stimulatory molecules PD-1 and CTLA-4 improves survival in primary and secondary fungal sepsis. *Crit Care*. 2013;17(3):R85.

53. Unsinger J, Burnham CA, McDonough J, et al. Interleukin-7 ameliorates immune dysfunction and improves survival in a 2-hit model of fungal sepsis. *J Infect Dis*. 2012;206:606-616.

54. Shindo Y, Unsinger J, Burnham CA, et al. Interleukin-7 and anti-programmed cell death 1 antibody have differing effects to reverse sepsis-induced immunosuppression. *Shock*. 2015;43:334-343.

56. Muszynski JA, Frazier E, Nofziger R, et al. Red blood cell transfusion and immune function in critically ill children: a prospective observational study. *Transfusion*. 2015;55:766-774.

58. Walton AH, Muenzer JT, Rasche D, et al. Reactivation of multiple viruses in patients with sepsis. *PLoS ONE*. 2014;9:e98819.

59. Westendorp RG, Langermans JA, Huizinga TW, et al. Genetic influence on cytokine production in meningococcal disease. *Lancet*. 1997;349:1912-1913.

Pediatric Rheumatic Disease: Diagnosis, Treatment, and Complications

Alexandra R. Aminoff and Carol A. Wallace

PEARLS

- Approximately 1 child in 250 has a rheumatic disease.
- A child may present to the ICU with a life-threatening manifestation of an undiagnosed rheumatic disease or with severe complications of a known rheumatic disorder.
- Suspicion for rheumatic disease should be high when children present with persistent fevers of unknown origin, multisystem involvement, joint involvement, or unexplained high inflammatory markers.
- Diagnosing rheumatic diseases is challenging as few clinical features are pathognomonic and few diagnostic tests are confirmatory. A thorough history and physical examination are essential.
- Infectious and oncologic processes may mimic rheumatic diseases and must be excluded.
- Serious complications of rheumatic diseases can affect any organ system, be life threatening, and include stroke, psychosis, pulmonary hemorrhage, renal failure, and prothrombotic states.
- Macrophage activation syndrome is a severe "cytokine storm" due to immune dysregulation in the setting of rheumatic diseases, infections, and malignancy. Its early recognition and aggressive treatment are essential, as it can lead to severe morbidity and death.
- High-dose corticosteroid therapy is frequently used at diagnosis and for severe disease flares to bring inflammation under control quickly. Corticosteroids are typically not sufficient to maintain long-term disease control and have many associated risks, so additional immunosuppressive therapy is employed to induce and maintain remission.
- Immunosuppressive therapy used to treat rheumatic diseases can lead to complications including infections, liver disease, renal disease, and cytopenias. Adrenal insufficiency chronic corticosteroid use can occur if corticosteroids such treatment is stopped abruptly.
- Therapy for rheumatic disease may be initiated in the ICU and often includes high-dose corticosteroids, cyclophosphamide, anticytokine, and anticellular biological therapies; IV immunoglobulin; and plasmapheresis. Management may be challenging, given the complexities of the diseases, multiple organ systems involved, and potential complications of treatment.

Rheumatic diseases are caused by dysfunction of the immune system, resulting in autoimmunity due to loss of self-tolerance and abnormal inflammatory responses.[1] These diseases affect approximately 1 child in 250. Although largely an outpatient-based specialty, pediatric rheumatology encompasses a diverse set of diseases that can be difficult to diagnose and treat, with complications that can be life threatening. The number of children with rheumatic disease who require intensive care management is unknown, but early diagnosis and rapid treatment can significantly decrease morbidity and mortality.[2,3] Patients may present to the ICU with life-threatening manifestations of new-onset rheumatic disease, with severe complications of a known disorder, or with complications secondary to immunosuppressive therapy. This chapter provides an overview of the most common pediatric rheumatic diseases followed by a discussion of the conditions and complications most likely to be encountered in the ICU.

Rheumatic Diseases: Clinical Presentation, Diagnosis, and Treatment

Rheumatic diseases in children present in highly variable ways and are best diagnosed by a thorough history and physical examination. They should be considered in patients who present with unexplained fevers or constitutional symptoms, multisystem involvement, or unexplained systemic inflammation. Laboratory tests may be consistent with and confirm clinical suspicions but are often not diagnostic.

Juvenile Idiopathic Arthritis

Juvenile idiopathic arthritis (JIA) is the most common childhood rheumatic disease and can present in several different forms (Box 106.1).[4] Most children are managed as outpatients, but the disease and its complications occasionally require intensive care. The JIA category that most often requires ICU-level care is systemic-onset JIA (soJIA), which accounts for about 10% to 20% of children with JIA. It can present with severe multisystem disease including the life-threatening cytokine storm known as *macrophage activation syndrome* (MAS), discussed later in the chapter.

Systemic-Onset Juvenile Idiopathic Arthritis Clinical Presentation
The classic features of soJIA include high-spiking fevers, evanescent rash, and arthritis.[5] The fevers (temperatures ≥39°C)

BOX 106.1   Criteria for Juvenile Idiopathic Arthritis (JIA)

JIA is a disease of childhood onset characterized primarily by arthritis persisting for at least 6 weeks with no known cause.

Systemic Arthritis

Arthritis with or preceded by daily fever of at least 2 weeks' duration, which is documented to be quotidian for at least 3 days, and accompanied by one or more of the following:
- Evanescent, nonfixed, erythematous rash
- Generalized lymph node enlargement
- Hepatomegaly or splenomegaly
- Serositis

Oligoarthritis or Polyarticular Arthritis

Arthritis affecting one to four joints during the first 6 months of disease. Two subcategories are recognized:
- Persistent oligoarthritis: Affects no more than four joints throughout the disease course
- Extended oligoarthritis: Affects a cumulative total of five joints or more after the first 6 months of disease

Polyarthritis (Rheumatoid Factor Negative)

Arthritis affecting five or more joints during the first 6 months of disease; tests for rheumatoid factor are negative.

Polyarthritis (Rheumatoid Factor Positive)

Arthritis affecting five or more joints during the first 6 months of disease associated with positive rheumatoid factor tests on two occasions at least 3 months apart.

Psoriatic Arthritis

Arthritis and psoriasis or arthritis and at least two of the following:
1. Dactylitis
2. Nail abnormalities (pitting or onycholysis)
3. Family history of psoriasis confirmed by a dermatologist in at least one first-degree relative

Enthesitis-Related Arthritis

Arthritis and enthesitis or arthritis or enthesitis with at least two of:
- Sacroiliac joint tenderness and/or inflammatory spinal pain
- Presence of HLA-B27
- Family history in at least one first- or second-degree relative of medically confirmed HLA-B27–associated disease
- Anterior uveitis that is usually associated with pain, redness, or photophobia
- Onset of arthritis in a boy after 8 years of age

Other Arthritis

Children with arthritis of unknown cause that persists for at least 6 weeks but that either:
- Do not fulfill criteria for any of the other categories, or
- Fulfill criteria for more than one of the other categories

HLA, human leukocyte antigen.
Adapted from Petty RE, Southwood TR, Manners P, et al. International League of Associations for Rheumatology classification of juvenile idiopathic arthritis: second revision. J Rheumatol. 2004;31:390-392.

typically occur in a spiking quotidian pattern—with return to normal temperature daily—for at least 2 weeks. The rash is typically a nonpruritic, salmon-colored, macular rash that can be subtle. It usually occurs with fever spikes and is rapidly migratory, often disappearing completely when the temperature normalizes. While a complete joint examination is essential, arthritis may not be a prominent feature early in disease. Other clinical features may include diffuse lymphadenopathy and hepatosplenomegaly. Malignancy and infectious processes must be excluded.

Cardiac involvement is uncommon in JIA (≈3%–9%) and typically presents as pericarditis with or without pericardial effusion.[6] It is most commonly seen in soJIA and rarely causes cardiac tamponade. Pulmonary complications may also occur—pleural involvement is most common, but parenchymal disease, such as interstitial lung disease or bronchiolitis obliterans, and pulmonary hypertension sometimes occur.[7,8] Lung complications are most typically seen in soJIA but rarely occur in rheumatoid factor-positive polyarticular JIA or secondary to drug toxicity (methotrexate).

Arthritis of the cervical spine can be seen in several of the JIA categories, causing decreased range of motion and instability. Synovial inflammation and bony erosions in the occipitoatlantoaxial joints can lead to C1-C2 instability and potential neurologic complications.[9] This has important implications in the ICU setting if hyperextension is attempted for intubation. In any patient with JIA with a history or findings of cervical spine disease, radiographic imaging with neck flexion/extension views should be obtained before attempted intubation. If abnormalities are identified, alternative airway management, such as fiberoptic visualization or tracheostomy, should be considered. Temporomandibular joint arthritis can cause a diminished mouth opening, which can also complicate airway management. Cricoarytenoid arthritis may present as sore throat with localized tenderness over the joints or with stridor and airway obstruction due to limited vocal cord mobility.

Uveitis is a common complication in children with JIA, particularly children who are antinuclear antibody (ANA) positive. Uveitis is not typically associated with soJIA.

Laboratory Studies

Laboratory findings consistent with soJIA include anemia (with hemoglobin levels often between 6 and 8 g/dL); elevated white blood cell (WBC) counts, sometimes in the leukemoid range; and elevated platelet counts. Cytopenias should prompt consideration of MAS or malignancy. C-reactive protein (CRP) and erythrocyte sedimentation rate (ESR) are usually markedly elevated, although in the setting of MAS the ESR may fall due to declining fibrinogen levels. ANA, rheumatoid factor, and anticyclic citrullinated peptide (anti-CCP) antibodies are typically absent, unlike other forms of JIA.

Management

Children with active soJIA should be treated aggressively, typically with high-dose pulse IV methylprednisolone (30 mg/kg/day, maximum dose 1000 mg) administered over 1 hour for 3 consecutive days. Subsequent maintenance prednisone is given intravenously or by mouth at 1 to 2 mg/kg/day, divided twice a day until symptoms resolve. Corticosteroid-sparing agents, such as anakinra (an IL-1 receptor blocker), tocilizumab (an anti-IL-6 therapy), or cyclosporine (a calcineurin inhibitor), should be introduced ideally in consultation with a pediatric rheumatologist.[10] These agents are used to induce remission and maintain disease control as corticosteroids are weaned. The immediate complications of high-dose corticosteroid therapy include sodium and fluid retention, hypertension, gastritis, risk for infection, and hyperglycemia.[11] In many centers, corticosteroids are not being used at all, in favor of anti-IL-1 monotherapy.

Systemic Lupus Erythematosus

Systemic lupus erythematosus (SLE) is a vasculitis due to autoantibodies forming immune complexes, which target a wide variety of organs resulting in multisystem disease. Immune dysregulation, genetic, environmental, and hormonal factors all contribute to the pathogenesis of this disease.[12] Girls, particularly in adolescence, are most likely to be affected; however, boys and young children can also develop SLE. The classification criteria (Box 106.2)[13,14] are helpful in making the diagnosis—if 4 of the 11 criteria are met, a diagnosis of SLE is highly likely. However, SLE presentation can be extremely variable—any organ system may be affected and the disease can be mild to life threatening. If the diagnosis is being considered, a thorough evaluation of all organ systems and serologic tests for SLE specific autoantibodies (discussed later) and other SLE markers is essential.

Clinical Presentation

Mucocutaneous Manifestations

Malar rash, discoid rash, photosensitivity, oral ulcerations (especially over the hard palate), and nasal ulcerations are classic. However, almost any kind of rash, including bullous lesions, may be seen. Skin biopsy with immunofluorescence staining to demonstrate immune complex deposition can be helpful.

Musculoskeletal Manifestations

Arthritis is common, occurring in 80% of patients with SLE. A musculoskeletal examination should be performed to look for joint tenderness, contracture, or effusion. Myositis is less common but can also occur. Avascular necrosis can occur and may be due to the disease itself or to corticosteroids.

Pulmonary Manifestations

Pulmonary manifestations occur commonly.[15] Pleuritis is included in the classification criteria and may be severe, causing respiratory compromise. Pulmonary hemorrhage is one of the most serious complications and may be precipitated by vasculitis or infection. SLE should always be considered in a patient presenting with pulmonary hemorrhage. Pulmonary embolism may occur secondary to antiphospholipid (APL) antibodies or other hypercoagulable states such as nephrotic syndrome. Smaller and recurrent emboli may contribute to the development of pulmonary hypertension, another severe SLE complication. "Shrinking lung" syndrome, a severe restrictive lung disorder attributed to diaphragm dysfunction, is rare in pediatric SLE.

Cardiovascular Disease

Any layer of the heart including the pericardium, myocardium, and valves may become inflamed, leading to cardiovascular compromise. Libman-sacks endocarditis involves the development of sterile vegetations on the cardiac valves, most commonly the mitral valve. Vasculitis can affect any organ in the body including the gastrointestinal (GI) tract, skin, and brain, leading to thrombotic and hemorrhagic complications. Vasculitis in the coronary vessels increases the risk of myocardial infarction. Patients with SLE are at higher risk for premature cardiovascular disease, which may relate to chronic inflammation and side effects of long-term steroid use, such as hyperlipidemia and hypertension.

Renal Manifestations

Renal disease is estimated to occur in 50% to 80% of children with SLE and is often more severe than renal disease in adult patients.[16] Lupus nephritis can range from asymptomatic with an abnormal urinalysis to renal failure requiring dialysis, severe nephrotic syndrome, and malignant hypertension. Renal biopsies help to determine the severity, type, and extent of lupus nephritis, which has major implications for treatment.

Central Nervous System Disease

Seizures and psychosis are the CNS manifestations included in the SLE classification criteria, but the neuropsychiatric features of SLE are diverse and of variable severity. These features may be the initial presentation of SLE or occur at any point during the disease course, even when the disease is otherwise

---

BOX 106.2 | **1982 Revised Criteria for Classification of Systemic Lupus Erythematosus (SLE) With 1997 Revision**

The proposed classification is based on 11 criteria. For the purpose of identifying patients in clinical studies, a person is defined as having SLE if any 4 or more of the 11 criteria are present, serially or simultaneously, during any interval of observation.

1. Malar rash: Fixed erythema, flat or raised, over the malar eminences, tending to spare the nasolabial folds
2. Discoid rash: Erythematous raised patches with adherent keratotic scaling and follicular plugging; atrophic scarring may occur in older lesions
3. Photosensitivity: Skin rash as a result of unusual reaction to sunlight, by patient history or physician observation
4. Oral ulcers: Oral or nasopharyngeal ulceration, usually painless, observed by physician
5. Arthritis: Nonerosive arthritis involving two or more peripheral joints, characterized by tenderness, swelling, or effusion
6. Serositis
   a. Pleuritis: A convincing history of pleuritic pain or rub heard by a physician or evidence of pleural effusion *or*
   b. Pericarditis: Documented by electrocardiogram or rub or evidence of pericardial effusion
7. Renal disorder
   a. Persistent proteinuria >0.5 g/day (or >3+ if quantitation not performed) *or*
   b. Cellular casts (may be red cell, hemoglobin, granular, tubular, or mixed)
8. Neurologic disorder
   a. Seizures in the absence of offending drugs or known metabolic derangements (eg, uremia, ketoacidosis, or electrolyte imbalance) *or*
   b. Psychosis in the absence of offending drugs or known metabolic derangements (eg, uremia, ketoacidosis, or electrolyte imbalance)
9. Hematologic disorder
   a. Hemolytic anemia with reticulocytosis *or*
   b. Leukopenia <4000/uL total on two or more occasions *or*
   c. Lymphopenia <1500/uL on two or more occasions *or*
   d. Thrombocytopenia <100,000/uL in the absence of offending drugs
10. Immunologic disorder
    a. Anti-DNA: Antibody to native DNA in abnormal titer *or*
    b. Anti-SM: Presence of antibody to Sm nuclear antigen *or*
    c. Positive finding of antiphospholipid antibodies based on:
       1. an abnormal serum level of immunoglobulin G or immunoglobulin M anticardiolipin antibodies *or*
       2. a positive test result for lupus anticoagulant using a standard method *or*
       3. a false-positive serologic test result for syphilis and confirmed by *Treponema pallidum* immobilization or fluorescent treponemal antibody absorption test
11. An abnormal titer of antinuclear antibody by immunofluorescence or an equivalent assay at any point in time and in the absence of drugs known to be associated with drug-induced lupus syndrome

Adapted from Tan EM, Cohen AS, Fries JF, et al. The 1982 revised criteria for the classification of systemic lupus erythematosus. Arthritis Rheum. 1982;25:1271-1277 and Hochberg MC. Updating the American College of Rheumatology revised criteria for the classification of systemic lupus erythematosus. Arthritis Rheum. 1997;40:1725.

not active.[17] Thromboembolic events can occur in the setting of APL antibodies or vasculitis and result in CNS disease.

Hematologic Involvement

Cytopenias are common and are often a presenting feature of SLE. Antibody-mediated cytopenias (such as Coombs-positive hemolytic anemia) are frequent, but other factors such as blood loss, bone marrow suppression, medications, or infection should also be considered. Prophylaxis against opportunistic infections may be necessary in patients with severe lymphopenia (<500/uL). A high white blood cell count in the setting of active lupus should prompt consideration of infection but can also be caused by neutrophil demargination from high-dose corticosteroid therapy.

Immune Dysfunction

Patients with SLE are immunosuppressed by the disease itself due to abnormal B- and T-cell function and low complement levels that impair opsonization of encapsulated organisms. The immunosuppressive agents used to control the disease may additionally impair the ability to fight infection. Patients with SLE are also at risk of developing MAS, discussed later.

Laboratory Studies

Although more than 95% of patients with SLE have a positive ANA test, this can occur in many other conditions including other rheumatic diseases, infection, malignancy, and healthy people. Unlike the ANA, anti–double-stranded DNA (dsDNA) antibodies are highly specific for SLE and are elevated in 80% to 90% of children with SLE at some point in the disease course. Anti-Smith (Sm) antibodies are also highly specific for SLE but are seen less commonly, in approximately 20% of pediatric patients.[18]

Antibodies to SSA, SSB, and ribonucleoprotein (RNP) occur in varying frequency. Complement levels (C3 and C4) are typically low in active disease, reflecting consumption in the setting of immune complex formation. Serial measurements of C3, C4, and anti-dsDNA are useful in monitoring disease activity.

Management

Patients with SLE often require ICU-level care and can be severely ill at diagnosis and with disease flares. Treatment is typically initiated with high-dose pulse IV methylprednisolone (30 mg/kg/day, maximum dose 1000 mg), administered over 1 hour for 3 consecutive days. Subsequent maintenance prednisone is given intravenously or by mouth at 1 to 2 mg/kg/day divided twice a day. Steroid-sparing agents such as cyclophosphamide and rituximab (an anti-CD20 antibody) are typically necessary in patients with significant CNS or renal involvement. For patients with less severe disease, mycophenolate mofetil (MMF) or azathioprine is typically used to induce remission. Renal failure and dialysis can affect drug metabolism and clearance; consultation with pediatric nephrology and pharmacy services may assist with proper dosing.

Neonatal Autoimmune Syndromes

Infants can develop antibody-mediated disease due to transmission of maternal antibodies in utero; mothers may or may not be symptomatic from these autoantibodies. Symptoms can present prenatally or up to 6 months of age and persist for 6 to 9 months until the maternal antibodies are cleared from the infant's circulation. Passage of maternal anti-SSA and anti-SSB antibodies can result in rash, transaminitis,

cytopenias (typically thrombocytopenia), and heart block.[19] The heart block can be severe and irreversible, requiring a pacemaker. Infants can also develop isolated autoimmune cytopenias due to maternal antibodies, such as antiplatelet antibodies causing neonatal thrombocytopenia. As the maternal antibody levels in the infant's circulation decline, the manifestations usually resolve; however, exchange transfusion has been used in severe cases.

Juvenile Dermatomyositis

Clinical Presentation

Juvenile dermatomyositis (JDM) is a vasculitis that primarily targets the skin and muscles. It is characterized by weakness and skin findings: rash over the eyelids (heliotrope rash), face (malar rash), neck and upper back (shawl sign), extensor surfaces of the joints in the hands, elbows, and knees (Gottron papules), and periungual telangiectasias.[20] The inflammation primarily affects striated muscle but can also involve smooth muscle. Typically proximal rather than distal muscle groups are affected, leading to profound shoulder and hip girdle muscle weakness. The muscles of the palate, pharynx, and upper third of the esophagus can also be involved, resulting in dysphagia, dysphonia, and risk of aspiration. In severe cases, weakness may lead to respiratory failure but this may not be apparent as weakness can mask typical signs of distress.

Vasculitis can also target the gastrointestinal (GI) tract and cause bleeding, necrosis, and perforation. Cardiac muscle can become inflamed, and rarely myocarditis and conduction defects have been reported. Interstitial lung disease occurs and may be difficult to detect early in disease. The kidneys are not typically targeted by vasculitis in JDM, but rhabdomyolysis with secondary renal impairment can rarely occur. As with many of the rheumatic diseases, severely ill patients with JDM can develop MAS. A more long-term complication of JDM is calcinosis, with calcium deposition in the skin, particularly around the joints. In severe cases, this can impair mobility. Malignancy is rarely associated with JDM as opposed to adult dermatomyositis.

Laboratory Studies

Laboratory studies are useful to support the diagnosis, monitor disease activity, and guide treatment. Serum levels of muscle enzymes, including creatine kinase, aspartate transaminase (AST), alanine transaminase (ALT), aldolase, and lactate dehydrogenase, are usually markedly elevated. Mild anemia may be present initially, but the WBC and platelet counts should be normal. Severe anemia, leukopenia, and/or thrombocytopenia should prompt consideration of MAS or investigation of other causes than JDM.

Imaging

The muscle edema and inflammation of JDM are best detected by MRI with short tau inversion recovery (STIR) sequence. MRI can also help to identify an appropriate site for biopsy in cases with diagnostic uncertainty. A barium swallow initially is important to identify esophageal dysmotility and the need for medication for acid reflux. For patients with dysphonia or dysphagia, a video fluoroscopic swallowing study (VFSS) can establish aspiration risk and whether alternative feeding methods are necessary. Electrocardiogram (ECG), echocardiogram (ECHO), chest radiograph, chest computed tomography (CT), and pulmonary function tests help to establish the extent of cardiopulmonary involvement. Abdominal CT can be performed if GI involvement is suspected.

Management

An aggressive treatment approach is essential and typically includes high-dose IV corticosteroids, methotrexate, and IV immunoglobulin (IVIG). Treatment should be initiated immediately to prevent life-threatening complications, permanent muscle destruction, and long-term sequelae such as calcinosis. Other agents, such as cyclosporine, MMF, cyclophosphamide, and rituximab may be used in refractory or severe cases.[21] In cases complicated by GI vasculitis, medications administered orally may not be absorbed reliably and parenteral administration is preferred.

Scleroderma (Systemic Sclerosis)

Clinical Presentation

Scleroderma refers to a group of rare connective tissue diseases in which vascular changes and fibrosis lead to hardening of the skin and abnormalities of the internal organs, especially the lungs and GI tract. Diffuse systemic sclerosis is the most severe form of the disease, and features may include skin induration, Raynaud phenomenon (discussed later), digital tip ulceration, dysphagia, gastroesophageal reflux, hypertension, arthritis, neuropathy, pulmonary hypertension, and pulmonary fibrosis. Progressive pulmonary fibrosis may lead to respiratory failure, and abnormal GI motility may make nutrition difficult.

Cardiopulmonary complications are the most common cause of death in children with systemic sclerosis, typically heart failure secondary to lung disease.[22,23] Renal crisis is another serious complication (not commonly seen in children), and early initiation of antihypertensive therapy with angiotensin-converting enzyme inhibitors is essential.

Imaging

Significant pulmonary disease often occurs with little to no symptoms and an unremarkable chest radiograph. Thus pulmonary function tests (PFTs) and high-resolution chest CT (HRCT) are essential for early identification of lung disease when it is still treatable. Cardiac catheterization is often necessary to diagnose and assess the severity of pulmonary hypertension. Barium swallow and an upper GI series with small bowel follow-through are important to assess the extent of esophageal and small bowel dysmotility and dysfunction.

Management

Systemic sclerosis is challenging to treat as the disease is often far advanced before patients come to medical attention. Thus a thorough evaluation of all organ systems (even when there appears to be no symptoms) is necessary. Therapy is directed at both halting or reversing the underlying disease process, as well as reducing morbidity from disease complications. Acid blockade to control gastroesophageal reflux and prevention of microaspiration are important in patients with GI tract involvement. Patients with severe Raynaud phenomenon may require vasodilation with calcium channel blockers, sildenafil, or iloprost. In patients with pulmonary hypertension, prostanoids and bosentan (a dual endothelin receptor antagonist) may reduce right ventricular and pulmonary artery pressures. Rapid initiation of angiotensin-converting enzyme inhibitors significantly improves the prognosis for patients in renal crisis.

For treating the underlying disease, the approach is similar to the treatment of other pediatric rheumatic diseases, but the response may be variable. High-dose corticosteroid therapy, methotrexate, mycophenolate mofetil, cyclophosphamide, and rituximab have been used. Corticosteroid therapy must be used with caution in patients with renal involvement, as it has been associated with renal crisis in adults. In severe refractory cases, hematopoietic stem cell transplantation (HSCT) has been successful for treatment of the skin disease.[24]

Unfortunately, gastrointestinal and pulmonary damage are rarely reversible and may be the cause of significant morbidity and mortality.

Mixed Connective Tissue Disease

Children may have overlapping features of different rheumatic diseases. The most well-characterized "overlap syndrome" is termed *mixed connective tissue disease* (MCTD), which can have features of JIA, SLE, JDM, and systemic sclerosis. Characteristic laboratory findings are a high-titer ANA (>1:320) and anti-RNP antibodies. Management is governed by which organs are affected and the severity of involvement.

Raynaud Phenomenon

Raynaud phenomenon is a triphasic color change (white, blue, red) typically in the fingers and toes due to transient vasoconstriction. It can occur as a primary process or secondary to an underlying rheumatic disease, most commonly lupus, scleroderma, or vasculitis. If the vasospasm persists, it may compromise the digits and require ICU intervention, including vasodilating agents such as iloprost, to prevent digit loss.

Antiphospholipid Syndrome

Clinical Presentation

Antiphospholipid syndrome (APS) is an autoimmune, prothrombotic state characterized by arterial or venous thrombosis, pregnancy morbidity, and specific laboratory features.[25] It may occur as a primary disorder, secondary to other autoimmune diseases (typically SLE), or in the setting of infection or malignancy. The clinical presentation depends on the site and type of vascular involvement and accompanying nonthrombotic manifestations. Venous thrombosis occurs most commonly in pediatric patients and can present in various ways including superficial thrombophlebitis, deep vein thrombosis, pulmonary thromboembolism, and cerebral venous sinus thrombosis. Arterial occlusion occurs less commonly and may also present in a variety of ways, including stroke, renal thrombotic microangiopathy, myocardial infarction, bone infarction, or mesenteric artery thrombosis. Nonthrombotic clinical features are extremely variable but include cytopenias; neurologic abnormalities (movement disorders, migraine, transverse myelitis); skin findings (livedo reticularis, cutaneous necrosis, skin ulcerations); valvular heart disease; and renal involvement (hypertension, hematuria). Catastrophic antiphospholipid syndrome (CAPS) refers to the acute onset (<1 week) of small vessel occlusion affecting three or more organ systems leading to multiorgan failure.

Laboratory Studies

For any child presenting with a vascular thrombosis, a full hypercoagulability workup should be undertaken (see also Chapter 92). To diagnose APS, children must have one or more of the characteristic laboratory features: positive anticardiolipin antibodies, anti-β_2 glycoprotein antibodies, or lupus anticoagulant. As these APL antibodies can be transiently elevated in the setting of infection, a definite diagnosis of APS requires these be persistently elevated on two or more occasions 12 weeks apart.

Management

For children with vascular thrombosis due to APS, anticoagulation is typically initiated with unfractionated heparin. Lupus anticoagulant can prolong the activated partial thromboplastin time (aPPT); therefore monitoring antifactor Xa levels may be a more reliable measure of therapeutic anticoagulation. For acute, severe thrombotic events, thrombolytic therapy, such as tissue plasminogen activator, has been used successfully in children.[26]

Given the high mortality rate in CAPS, aggressive therapy is essential and should include anticoagulation, high-dose corticosteroids, and plasma exchange; IVIG, cyclosphosphamide, and rituximab may be of additional benefit.[27,28]

Systemic Vasculitis

The vasculitides are a heterogenous group of disorders that can be classified in various ways, including by size of the affected vessels and by characteristic laboratory features (Table 106.1). These disorders previously had high morbidity and mortality rates, but advances in treatment have led to markedly improved prognosis in pediatric patients.[29] The most common forms of primary vasculitis in children are Henoch-Schönlein purpura (HSP) and Kawasaki disease (KD), but children can develop granulomatosis with polyangiitis (GPA), microscopic polyangiitis (MPA), polyarteritis nodosa (PAN), and Takayasu arteritis (TA).

Henoch-Schönlein Purpura

HSP is an immunoglobulin A–mediated small vessel vasculitis, often triggered by a preceding infection. The classic clinical features include palpable purpura predominantly on the lower extremities, arthritis or arthralgias, abdominal pain, and hematuria. Most cases are mild and resolve spontaneously. However, rapidly progressive glomerulonephritis and GI complications, including intussusception, necrosis, and perforation, may occur. Rarely, pulmonary hemorrhage and CNS involvement have been reported.[30,31]

Laboratory tests are nonspecific, usually showing only mildly elevated white blood cell counts and inflammatory markers. Coagulation studies and platelet counts are normal. The serum immunoglobulin A (IgA) level may be elevated, and in unclear or severe cases, a skin or renal biopsy can be performed and should demonstrate IgA deposition.

Treatment is primarily supportive, but IV high-dose corticosteroids are used for abdominal pain with vomiting or concern for suspected intussusception. In severe, or refractory cases, additional therapy may include cyclophosphamide, azathioprine, cyclosporine, IVIG, and plasmapheresis.

Kawasaki Disease

KD is a childhood vasculitis characterized by acute onset of fever for at least 5 days, conjunctival injection, cervical lymphadenopathy, rash, and extremity changes (erythema, edema, or desquamation). The disease has three phases: the acute febrile phase (10–14 days), the subacute phase (2–4 weeks), and the convalescent phase (months to years). The most serious complication of KD is coronary artery aneurysms, which occur most commonly in the subacute phase. Patients younger than 12 months old are at the highest risk for developing aneurysms but may not meet the full criteria for KD.[32] Some children present with pericarditis or myocarditis; in severe cases this may progress to congestive heart failure.[33] Patients can also present with KD shock syndrome (KDSS), which can be difficult to distinguish from septic shock or toxic shock syndrome. KDSS may be refractory to IVIG, and patients may then require additional therapy, such as infliximab.[34] KD can also be complicated by MAS (discussed later).

ESR and CRP are usually markedly elevated in KD. Once IVIG has been administered, ESR is no longer a reliable marker of inflammation and CRP is the best marker of disease activity. Platelet counts may initially be low but can rise to more than 1,000,000/uL. Anemia and elevated transaminases are also common. Serial echocardiography is the best way to monitor the coronary vessels for signs of inflammation, dilation, or aneurysms.

Prompt identification and treatment of KD with IVIG (2 g/kg, maximum dose 70 g) and high-dose aspirin (80–100 mg/kg/day divided 4 times daily) usually helps prevent aneurysm formation. Long-term use of low-dose aspirin (3–5 mg/kg/day) is recommended once the acute illness is resolved.[35] For cases refractory to IVIG (up to 10% of cases), the addition of high-dose corticosteroids and antitumor necrosis factor alpha (anti-TNFα) agents, such as infliximab, are effective. Predictors of poor response to IVIG include young age at diagnosis, hyponatremia, thrombocytopenia, elevated neutrophil count, high AST, and high CRP.[36]

In cases complicated by myocarditis, supportive care including inotropes and diuretic therapy may be necessary.

TABLE 106.1 Autoantibody Profiles for Vasculitis Associated With Various Autoimmune Diseases

	ANA	Ds-DNA	Smith	ANCA	Complement
SLE	+++	+ in 40%-80%	+ 50%-60%	Usually –	Low
GPA	– or weakly +	–	–	80% + (PR3)	Normal
MPA	– or weakly +	–	–	65% + (MPO)	Normal
Polyarteritis	–	–	–	Usually –	Normal
Takayasu arteritis	–	–	–	–	Normal
S-JIA	–	–	–	–	Normal–high

ANA, antinuclear antibody; ANCA, antineutrophil cytoplasmic antibody; Ds-DNA, double-stranded DNA; GPA, granulomatosis with polyangiitis; +, positive; –, negative; MPA, microscopic polyangiitis; MPO, myeloperoxidase; PR3, proteinase-3; S-JIA, systemic juvenile idiopathic arthritis; SLE, systemic lupus erythematosus.

Anticoagulation should be considered in the setting of large aneurysms to prevent further cardiovascular sequelae.[37]

Granulomatosis With Polyangiitis

GPA (formerly known as Wegener granulomatosis) is a granulomatous vasculitis that targets the sinuses and middle ear, lungs, and kidneys. Severe manifestations include subglottic stenosis with dyspnea and stridor, pulmonary hemorrhage, necrotizing cavitary lung lesions, and rapidly progressive necrotizing glomerulonephritis. Additional symptoms can include fever, weight loss, hearing loss, conjunctivitis, purpura or petechiae, arthritis, headache, and dizziness. For a patient presenting with pulmonary-renal syndrome, other diagnoses should be considered in addition to GPA including MPA, Goodpasture syndrome, and SLE (Table 106.2).

Antineutrophil cytoplasmic antibodies (ANCAs) target antigens within the cytoplasm of granulocytes. Cytoplasmic ANCAs (cANCAs) are seen in about 80% of pediatric patients with GPA. Antiproteinase-3 (PR3) antibodies are more specific and are seen in 60% of children with GPA.[38] These antibodies often correlate with disease activity. WBC and inflammatory markers are typically elevated. Urinalysis may show evidence of glomerulonephritis, including proteinuria, hematuria, and red blood cell casts. Renal biopsy can demonstrate necrotizing glomerulonephritis, with minimal immune deposits ("pauci-immune") on immunofluorescence staining.

Imaging is necessary to establish the extent of upper and lower airway involvement. Sinus involvement may not be clinically apparent, and CT or MRI can be helpful to identify sinus disease. To assess the extent of lung involvement, HRCT can identify cavitary lung lesions and pulmonary hemorrhage, as well narrowing of the trachea, bronchi, and bronchioles.

Immunosuppressive therapy, including cyclophosphamide and high-dose IV corticosteroids, reduces mortality and induces remission in the majority of patients. Recently, there has been increasing use of rituximab (375 mg/m^2 weekly for 4 doses or 750 mg/m^2 2 doses given 2 weeks apart) as induction therapy for GPA as it targets the B lymphocytes thought to be pathogenic in this disease. Early use of rituximab may obviate or lessen the need for cyclophosphamide. Traditionally, cyclophosphamide has been given as induction therapy, either enterally (2 mg/kg/day) in severe, life-threatening cases, or intravenously (various dosing protocols, typically 750 mg/m^2 monthly for 6 months). In severe cases, plasmapheresis may also be indicated. Azathioprine or MMF is used for milder cases and for long-term maintenance therapy.

Microscopic Polyangiitis

This small-vessel vasculitis typically affects the lungs, kidneys, GI tract, central and peripheral nervous systems, skin, and muscles. Patients often present with constitutional symptoms such as fever, fatigue, and weight loss. Severe manifestations include pulmonary hemorrhage, GI bleeding or infarction, stroke, necrotizing glomerulonephritis, and renal failure.

The diagnosis is based primarily on clinical features, but laboratory tests may also be helpful. Perinuclear ANCAs (pANCAs) are present in approximately 65% of patients with MPA, particularly for the neutrophil component myeloperoxidase (MPO). However, these antibodies can be present in other rheumatic diseases, such as SLE or GPA, and in conditions such as inflammatory bowel disease.[39] A biopsy of affected tissue (including lung, kidney, muscle, nerve, or skin) demonstrating pauci-immune, small-vessel vasculitis confirms the diagnosis.

The treatment approach to MPA is the same as for GPA: High-dose corticosteroids plus a corticosteroid-sparing agent are typically used to induce remission. Cyclophosphamide and rituximab are used in severe cases, while azathioprine or MMF is used for milder cases and for long-term maintenance therapy.

Polyarteritis Nodosa

PAN is a vasculitis affecting medium-sized vessels. It is rare in childhood but should be considered in any child presenting with unexplained fever, rash, hypertension, and abdominal pain. Skin manifestations vary, including painful nodules, purpura, petechiae, or patchy edema. Muscle tenderness, arthritis, and arthralgia may also occur. GI vasculitis usually presents with abdominal pain, hemorrhage, necrosis, or perforation. CNS features can be severe and include psychosis, seizures, strokes, or neuropathy. Cardiac involvement, including coronary arteritis, is more common in children.

There are no associated antibody tests in PAN. A biopsy of affected tissue (typically muscle, nerve, skin, kidney, or GI tract) can be diagnostic, demonstrating necrotizing arteritis of small- or medium-sized muscular arteries.

TABLE 106.2   Pulmonary-Renal Syndromes

Diagnosis	Pulmonary Findings	Renal Findings	Other Organ System Involvement	Laboratory Findings
GPA	Cavitating lung lesions, pulmonary hemorrhage	Pauci-immune necrotizing glomerulonephritis	Sinus, airways	Usually cANCA positive (PR3)
MPA	Pulmonary hemorrhage	Pauci-immune necrotizing glomerulonephritis	Skin, CNS	Usually pANCA positive (MPO)
Goodpasture syndrome	Pulmonary hemorrhage	Anti-GBM positive glomerulonephritis	None	Anti-GBM positive
SLE	Pulmonary hemorrhage	Proliferative or membranous changes; marked immune complex deposition	Multisystem disease	ANA positive, anti-dsDNA positive, anti-Sm positive, low complements

ANA, antinuclear antibody; *GBM*, glomerular basement membrane; *GPA*, granulomatosis with polyangiitis; *MPA*, microscopic polyangiitis; *MPO*, myeloperoxidase; *PR3*, proteinase-3; *SLE*, systemic lupus erythematosus.

Angiography is important for diagnosing and assessing the extent of vessel involvement. Conventional angiography is the gold standard, but there is an increasing role for less invasive imaging, such as CT or magnetic resonance angiography. Characteristic pathologic findings include vessel stenosis, occlusion, and aneurysms.

The treatment approach is the same as that used in GPA or MPA.

Takayasu Arteritis

TA causes granulomatous inflammation of the aorta and its major branches. In the early, inflammatory phase, patients present with fever, fatigue, weight loss, headaches, abdominal pain, and hypertension. Subsequent vascular changes, such as mural thickening, aneurysm formation, and stenosis, lead to end-organ ischemia. Symptoms and signs can include absent pulses, angina, abdominal pain and bloody diarrhea (due to mesenteric artery involvement), visual changes, claudication, myocardial infarction, encephalopathy, and stroke.

Ultrasonography, magnetic resonance angiography, and CT are all helpful for diagnosing or managing TA, establishing the severity and extent of disease, and monitoring response to therapy. In some cases, conventional angiogram may be necessary.

The treatment approach is the same as for GPA, but there is an increasing role for anti-TNFα therapy, particularly infliximab. Angioplasty and stent placement have been successful and improve survival rates in pediatric TA.[40] In severe cases, aortic reconstruction is necessary.

Primary Vasculitis of the Central Nervous System

Primary vasculitis or angiitis of the CNS is characterized by isolated inflammation of vessels in the CNS with no other organ involvement. In pediatric patients with small vessel disease, the most common presenting feature is seizure. In medium-large vessel disease, patients may present with stroke, headache, cranial neuropathy, or movement disorders. The diagnosis should be considered in a child with unexplained CNS deterioration, especially if other diagnoses such as infection or metabolic conditions have been excluded.[41]

Angiography can be helpful for diagnosis but may not detect small vessel disease, in which case a brain biopsy may be required.

Aggressive treatment with high-dose corticosteroids and cyclophosphamide has been shown to improve survival. MMF is typically used for long-term maintenance therapy.

Rheumatic Diseases: Conditions and Complications in the ICU

There are many serious complications of pediatric rheumatic diseases and complications associated with the treatment of these conditions. Many of these were introduced earlier. The following section provides a more thorough discussion of the conditions and complications that are most relevant in the intensive care setting.

Infections

Children with rheumatic diseases are at high risk for infection due to immune dysfunction from their underlying disease process and chronic immunosuppressive therapy. Infection is a common reason for ICU admission and a leading cause of death in patients with active rheumatic disease, particularly SLE.[42,43] Children being treated for rheumatic diseases may not manifest typical signs of infection, such as fever. As many rheumatic diseases cause hypertension, a relative decline in blood pressure is concerning for sepsis, even if the child remains normotensive. Similarly, diseases such as SLE cause a low WBC count, so a relative rise may indicate infection even without a true leukocytosis. Given the underlying inflammatory disease, inflammatory markers may also be difficult to interpret. Therefore a high index of suspicion for infection and early initiation of broad-spectrum antimicrobial therapy are warranted.

Patients with rheumatic diseases are susceptible to typical, community-acquired bacteria such as *Staphylococcus aureus, Streptococcus pneumoniae,* and *Haemophilus influenzae,* as well as gram-negative enteric bacteria. However, due to chronic immunosuppression, they are also at high risk for opportunistic infections, with *Pneumocystis jiroveci, Mycobacterium tuberculosis, Aspergillus* or *Mucor* species, and cytomegalovirus. Common organisms can be found in unusual sites, such as staphylococcal endocarditis, or unusual organisms can be identified in typical sites of infection, such as mucormycosis of the sinuses. Before starting antimicrobial therapy, body fluids and specimens should be obtained for culture. With suspected pulmonary infection, HRCT and bronchoscopy with bronchoalveolar lavage should be considered early as lung lesions can progress quickly into severe, acute lung injury and patients can rapidly decompensate. For patients receiving immunosuppressive therapy, *P. jiroveci* pneumonia prophylaxis is typically recommended. In patients with a history of *Herpes zoster* or fungal infection, antiviral and antifungal prophylaxis should also be considered.

Macrophage Activation Syndrome

MAS is a severe, life-threatening complication of childhood rheumatic disease, primarily soJIA. It may also occur in the setting of infection and malignancy. In rheumatic disease, MAS may be present at the time of diagnosis, disease flare, or change in medical therapy or with intercurrent infection. Diagnosis can be difficult, as findings can be confused with infection and sepsis or acute exacerbations of the underlying disease process.[44] Therefore a high index of suspicion is necessary. MAS can start with no symptoms, but rather a mild trend of abnormal changes in the laboratory tests, and then rapidly progress to full-blown, severe disease.

Patients typically become ill and then become more acutely ill with unremitting high fever (different from the quotidian pattern of soJIA), lymphadenopathy, hepatosplenomegaly, cytopenias, and coagulopathy, and they may even have altered mental status. Severe manifestations include seizures, coma, and gastrointestinal bleeding, as well as heart, lung, or kidney failure. The mortality rate ranges from 4% to 15%.[44]

Laboratory evaluation typically reveals cytopenias (at least two of three cell lines), elevated transaminases, coagulopathy, elevated triglycerides, elevated lactate dehydrogenase, and most significantly, a elevated ferritin level (often >10,000 ng/mL). A falling ESR, especially with a high CRP, is concerning for MAS and is secondary to low fibrinogen in the setting of consumptive coagulopathy. Natural killer (NK) cell activity is low or absent. Soluble IL-2 receptor levels are typically elevated. The pathognomic feature of MAS is hemophagocytosis on bone marrow aspirate or biopsy, although this may not be present early in the disease course.

MAS is a form of secondary hemophagocytic lymphohistiocytosis (HLH)—a systemic inflammatory storm characterized by overwhelming expansion and activation of T lymphocytes and macrophages, with decreased NK and cytotoxic T-cell function. Familial HLH is an autosomal recessive disorder associated with mutations of the perforin or MUNC 13-4 genes. Genetic testing can differentiate the two disorders but often takes weeks to perform. Risk factors for familial HLH include young age (younger than 2 years), significant CNS disease, consanguinity, or family history of death due to unidentified febrile illness.[45]

Aggressive treatment of MAS is essential. Until recently the standard therapy consisted of rapid initiation of high-dose pulse IV methylprednisolone therapy (30 mg/kg/day for 3 days, maximum dose 1000 mg, then 1 to 2 mg/kg/day divided twice daily) with a slow corticosteroid taper plus IV cyclosporine 3 to 5 mg/kg/day. More recently, anakinra (2 to 4 mg/kg IV every 6 to 24 hours) is being used in place of cyclosporine and is rapidly effective.[45]

Airway Compromise

Rheumatic conditions can cause airway compromise due to obstruction from inflammation or inability to protect the airway because of muscle weakness. This may be indolent or rapid in onset. Intubation can be challenging, and tracheostomy may be necessary.

Disease such as JIA, SLE, and GPA and rare diseases such as relapsing polychondritis can be complicated by airway involvement leading to obstruction in severe cases.[46] Although rare, oropharyngeal obstruction can occur in SLE due to angioedema with acute mucosal swelling of the pharyngeal and laryngeal tissues.[47] Cricoarytenoid arthritis is a rare complication in JIA that can cause airway obstruction manifested by hoarse voice, stridor, and dyspnea.[48] Subglottic stenosis affects 10% to 20% of patients with GPA and is five times more common in pediatric than adult-onset disease. A conservative approach with medical therapy and local interventions such as intralesional steroid injections and dilation have been used successfully and may obviate the need for surgical reconstruction.[49] Relapsing polychondritis, a disorder of recurrent cartilaginous inflammation, affects both the small and large airways and can cause upper or lower airway obstruction.[46]

Muscle weakness can also lead to airway compromise. In JDM, muscle weakness of the palate, pharynx, larynx, and upper third of the esophagus can lead to dysphagia, dysphonia, inability to manage secretions, and airway compromise severe enough to warrant intubation. Muscle weakness can also mask signs of respiratory distress.

Pulmonary Involvement

Infection is the most common lung-related complication in pediatric rheumatic disease, but there are many other associated pulmonary complications including interstitial lung disease, pulmonary fibrosis, pleuritis and pleural effusion, alveolar hemorrhage, and pulmonary embolism.

Interstitial Lung Disease

Children with rheumatic diseases, including SLE, soJIA, JDM, and systemic sclerosis, may rarely develop interstitial lung disease (ILD), which in severe cases can progress to

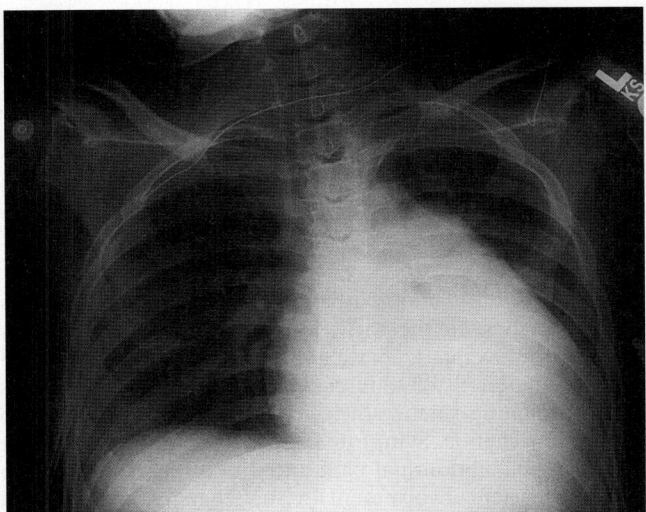

Fig. 106.1. Portable chest radiograph of a 16-year-old girl with systemic lupus erythematosus. Lupus pneumonitis is reflected by infiltrate in the right upper lobe and bilateral diffuse interstitial changes. Pleural fluid suggested by haziness over the left lower lobe, as well as blunted left costophrenic angle (not shown), was confirmed by bilateral decubitus films.

pulmonary fibrosis. Patients may be asymptomatic or present with fever, cough, respiratory distress, or pleuritic chest pain. Chest radiographs may show interstitial changes but are not always sensitive enough to detect ILD (Fig. 106.1). HRCT is a more sensitive study and may reveal characteristic findings, such as basilar ground-glass opacities, honeycombing, subpleural nodules, and bronchiectasis.[50] Pulmonary function testing is also helpful in diagnosing and monitoring ILD. Children with rheumatic disease-related ILD may develop pulmonary hypertension and require vasodilator therapy (Fig. 106.2).[23] Patients with severe ILD are treated with aggressive immunosuppression and supportive therapy, and in some cases they may require extracorporeal membrane oxygenation (ECMO).

Pleuritis and Pleural Effusions

Pleuritis, with or without pleural effusion, is a common manifestation of rheumatic disorders in children. Patients typically have pleuritic chest pain, respiratory distress, and orthopnea. On examination, they may have distant heart sounds, friction rub, dullness with chest percussion, and reduced air entry. Pleural effusions can be sufficiently large to compromise lung function, requiring chest tube placement. Most respond to treatment of the underlying inflammatory disease, but occasionally aspiration and drainage of effusions are necessary.

Pulmonary Hemorrhage

Acute alveolar hemorrhage is a serious complication of systemic vasculitides, including GPA, MPA, and SLE, with a mortality rate around 70%.[51] Presenting symptoms typically include dyspnea and hemoptysis but are not always present. Acute pulmonary hemorrhage can be rapidly progressive and catastrophic, leading to acute hypoxemic respiratory failure and hemorrhagic shock. A sudden decline in hemoglobin suggests the diagnosis. Evaluation for bacterial, viral, and fungal

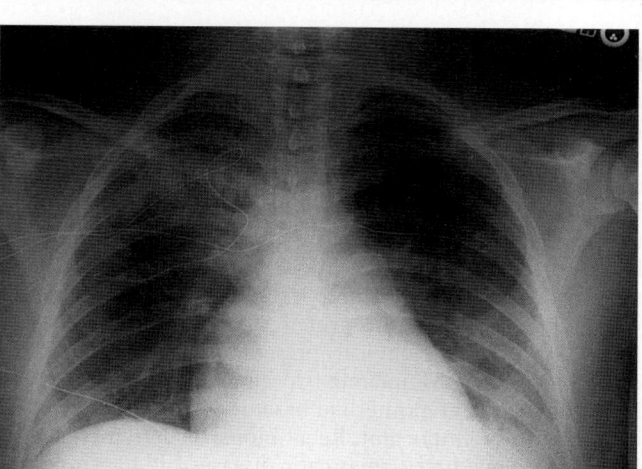

Fig. 106.2. Portable chest radiograph of a 12-year-old girl with scleroderma. The patient arrived at the ICU with sudden onset of orthopnea and thrombocytopenia. Cardiomegaly was observed. Echocardiography revealed pericardial effusion. However, pulmonary vascularity was normal in this patient. Physical examination revealed sclerodactyly. The patient eventually developed cor pulmonale as a result of pulmonary hypertension. Inflammatory changes suggestive of other collagen vascular diseases may be seen in the early course of scleroderma. Use of pulse IV methylprednisolone reduced these early inflammatory changes, although as an outpatient the patient maintained stable right-sided heart disease that was not responsive to immunosuppressive medication, consistent with scleroderma.

infection should be undertaken as pulmonary infections may trigger hemorrhage. Chest radiography typically reveals diffuse alveolar airspace filling defects, although in milder cases there may only be focal abnormalities. HRCT is more sensitive than chest radiography and typically reveals ground-glass opacities. Although not generally obtainable in critically ill patients, pulmonary function tests should reveal an elevated diffusion capacity. Supportive care includes positive pressure ventilation with high positive end-expiratory pressure, blood transfusions to maintain hemodynamic stability, and close monitoring. Despite the need for systemic heparinization, ECMO has been found to be safe and life saving in children with pulmonary hemorrhage who fail conventional therapy.[52,53] Treatment of the underlying rheumatic disease is critical and typically involves a combination of high-dose IV corticosteroid therapy, cyclophosphamide, and rituximab. In antibody-mediated vasculitides, plasmapheresis acts by removing pathogenic antibodies from the circulation and is an effective therapeutic intervention.[53,54]

Pulmonary Embolism

Patients with APLs, either primary or secondary to conditions such as SLE, are at increased risk for pulmonary embolism and other thrombotic events.[55] Nephrotic syndrome, associated with SLE, also increases risk of pulmonary embolism due to renal loss of anticoagulant factors. Patients typically present with pleuritic chest pain, tachypnea, tachycardia, and hypoxia but can sometimes be asymptomatic. Chest CT with angiography is the most helpful diagnostic test. Early intervention with systemic thrombolytics, including unfractionated heparin and tissue plasminogen activator, improves survival in pediatric patients.[56]

Cardiovascular Events

Pericarditis and Pericardial Tamponade

Pericarditis can occur in the setting of various rheumatic diseases, including soJIA, SLE, and KD. Patients present with precordial chest pain, fever, and tachycardia, and on examination they may have distant heart sounds and a friction rub. Acute pericarditis with effusion may lead to cardiac tamponade, with tachycardia, narrow pulse pressure, and clinical signs of poor cardiac output. In severe cases or if there is concern for an underlying infection, pericardiocentesis may be necessary.[57] Chronic pericarditis may cause restrictive cardiac disease. Evaluation for pericarditis includes ECG and ECHO. Symptoms should improve with medical management of the underlying systemic inflammatory disease, including nonsteroidal antiinflammatory drugs (NSAIDs), corticosteroids, and immunosuppression.

Myocarditis

Although rare, patients with rheumatic disease including SLE, JIA, JDM, and vasculitis may present with myocarditis, manifested by poor cardiac output and congestive heart failure.[57,58] Symptoms include fatigue, exercise intolerance, tachycardia, and respiratory distress, with rales and hepatomegaly on examination. Chest radiography may demonstrate cardiomegaly with pulmonary edema and ECHO can show diminished ventricular systolic function. Management involves diuresis, inotropic support, and aggressive immunosuppressive therapy.[58]

Valvular Disease

Libman-Sacks endocarditis is a valvular abnormality that can occur in SLE, usually associated with the presence of APLs. It is a verrucous endocarditis, in which fibrinoid nodules form on the cardiac valves, most frequently on the mitral valve.[57] Vegetations and valvular thickening can lead to severe regurgitation and stenosis. Echocardiography is the best diagnostic study; in some cases, a transthoracic study may not be sensitive enough to detect valvular disease and a transesophageal study is necessary.[59,60] Many patients respond to medical treatment of the underlying SLE, but in severe cases valve replacement surgery may be indicated.

Arrhythmias

SLE is associated with an increased risk for conduction abnormalities, including premature atrial beats, supraventricular tachycardia, atrioventricular block, and right bundle branch block. This is best diagnosed by ECG and ECHO. Patients usually respond to pharmacologic antiarrhythmics. Pacemakers are indicated for complete atrioventricular block, particularly in neonatal lupus.[19]

Acute Coronary Syndrome

There is a well-recognized, increased risk for acute myocardial infarction in SLE secondary to premature atherosclerosis, probably related to the combined effect of disease-related dyslipidemia, coronary artery inflammation, and long-term corticosteroid therapy.[61] In any child with SLE presenting with chest pain or dyspnea, myocardial infarction should be considered. ECG may demonstrate ST segment elevation and laboratory testing, including serum troponin, may be helpful. The underlying SLE should be treated; cardiology consultation is beneficial for management and long-term cardiac monitoring.

In KD, there is also an increased risk for acute myocardial infarction secondary to coronary artery aneurysms. Thrombosis or rupture of coronary aneurysms leads to myocardial ischemia and can occur many years after the KD diagnosis, even in adulthood.[62] Giant aneurysms (>8 mm in diameter) have the poorest prognosis. In severe cases, surgical intervention for bypass grafting has been successfully performed in children.[63]

Endocrine Dysfunction

Endocrine issues can complicate many of the rheumatic diseases. One of the most serious complications is adrenal insufficiency due to abrupt discontinuation of chronic steroid therapy.[64,65] Rapid initiation of stress dose corticosteroids in the setting of acute illness or surgery is essential. Diabetes may also occur in the setting of steroid treatment, requiring insulin therapy. Thyroid disease can present as either hypothyroidism or hyperthyroidism and is a common complication of JIA and SLE.

Gastrointestinal Involvement

Gastrointestinal Hemorrhage

The vasculitides and other systemic inflammatory diseases increase the risk for acute and subclinical GI hemorrhage. Medications, such as high-dose corticosteroids and NSAIDs, also increase the risk of GI bleeding. In the setting of suspected acute hemorrhage, large-bore IV access should be obtained and transfusion of blood products may be necessary to maintain hemodynamic stability. Early GI and surgical consultation are advised. Imaging-guided embolization of bleeding vessels may be necessary in severe cases. Up to 30% of patients with HSP develop GI hemorrhage, although severe hemorrhage, irreducible intussusception, and perforation are rare.[66]

Acute Abdominal Pathology: Peritonitis, Serositis, and Intestinal Perforation

Children with rheumatic disease are at increased risk of morbidity and mortality from acute abdominal pathology.[67] Nonbacterial peritonitis and serositis of the abdominal organs are common manifestations of SLE ($\approx$20% of pediatric patients) and JIA, particularly soJIA. Patients may present with severe symptoms, including a surgical abdomen. However, immunosuppressive therapy can mask clinical signs and symptoms, leading to delayed diagnosis; therefore a high index of suspicion for severe pathology is necessary.[68] Patients are also at risk for infectious pathology, such as bacterial peritonitis with abscess formation, and for intestinal perforation. In cases in which infection and perforation have been excluded and symptoms are thought to relate to noninfectious serositis, the underlying disease should be treated aggressively to bring symptoms under control.

Severe acute pancreatitis may complicate pediatric rheumatic diseases, particularly SLE.[69] It may be disease related or secondary to medications, such as high-dose corticosteroids and azathioprine.

In patients with nonlocalizing abdominal pain, pancreatitis should be considered and appropriate laboratory screening and imaging performed to look for inflammation, stones, and pseudocysts. Inciting drugs should be avoided if possible.

Renal Involvement

Most vasculitic disorders, including SLE, GPA, MPA, and HSP, can affect the kidneys. Renal disease may be present at the time of initial diagnosis or may evolve later. It can manifest in various ways, with oliguria or anuria, hematuria, hypertension, nephrotic syndrome, and renal failure. Laboratory evaluation includes determination of serum electrolytes, blood urea nitrogen, creatinine, and albumin; urinalysis; spot urine protein/creatinine ratio (ideally first morning void); and 24-hour urine protein and creatinine collection. Depending on the clinical presentation, complete blood cell count, ANA, complement levels (C3 and C4), ANCAs, MPO, PR3, and antiglomerular basement membrane antibodies may also be important. Renal biopsy is extremely helpful in diagnosing pediatric rheumatic diseases and has important implications for treatment. The extent and type of renal involvement, especially in diseases such as SLE, GPA, and MPA, help determine the treatment course and intensity of immunosuppression. In cases complicated by bleeding diathesis or severe hypertension, however, a renal biopsy may be contraindicated.

Aggressive treatment of the underlying rheumatic disease should bring renal manifestations under control. Severe renal involvement in SLE, GPA, and MPA typically warrants treatment with high-dose IV steroid therapy, cyclophosphamide, and often rituximab. For ANCA-associated vasculitides with severe renal involvement, plasmapheresis is an effective intervention that improves rates of survival.[70] Hypertension can be severe, leading to neurologic and other end-organ complications, and must be managed aggressively with antihypertensive therapy, in severe cases by continuous drip. Patients with rheumatic disease may rarely present with end-stage renal disease at diagnosis or progress to end-stage renal disease, requiring dialysis. Renal transplantation has been successfully performed in pediatric patients, but there is a risk of disease recurrence.[71,72]

Central Nervous System Involvement

The CNS can be affected in many pediatric rheumatic diseases and can manifest in various ways including seizure, headache, stroke, psychosis, encephalopathy, and movement disorders.[73,74] When neurologic symptoms present, especially in immunosuppressed patients, CNS infection (viral, bacterial, and fungal) must be considered. In addition, the presence of APLs is highly associated with neurologic symptoms, especially stroke, seizure, headache, and movement disorders. APLs can be present in the setting of primary APS or secondary to another rheumatic disease; APLs should be rescreened whenever new neurologic symptoms present. Imaging may be helpful in identifying stroke but not sensitive enough to detect small vessel vasculitic changes; a brain or meningeal biopsy is sometimes necessary (Fig. 106.3). For neurologic manifestations of rheumatic disease, treatment of the underlying disease should typically bring symptoms under control. Aggressive immunosuppression is generally indicated for CNS involvement, such as lupus cerebritis, including high-dose IV steroid therapy and cyclophosphamide. Plasmapheresis may be necessary in severe cases. Concurrent use of anticonvulsant and/or antipsychotic medications may be necessary. In the setting of thrombotic stroke, anticoagulation is generally indicated.

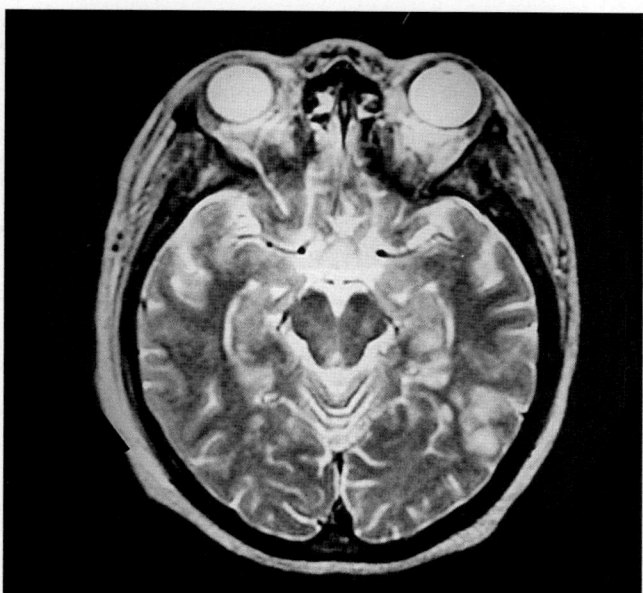

Fig. 106.3. Magnetic resonance image of the brain of a 16-year-old girl with systemic lupus erythematosus. This image was obtained after the patient was stabilized. Multiple areas of increased signal are scattered throughout both cerebral hemispheres, consistent with ischemic infarctions resulting from lupus cerebritis. Other views demonstrated similar infarcts in the brain stem and cerebellar hemisphere. Magnetic resonance angiography obtained at the same time revealed normal vasculature, suggesting pathologic involvement of brain tissue but sparing of vessels. The patient responded well to pulse IV methylprednisolone and cyclophosphamide, with no residual neurologic deficit.

The eye can be involved in a number of ways, including conjunctivitis, scleritis, episcleritis, uveitis, and retinal vasculitis.[75] Ophthalmology consultation is often helpful.

Hematologic Involvement

Thrombotic Thrombocytopenic Purpura

Thrombotic thrombocytopenic purpura (TTP) is a rare, life-threatening hematologic disorder that can be inherited or acquired. It is associated with SLE, especially in pediatric patients. Diagnosis is based on five clinical features: (1) thrombocytopenia and disseminated platelet aggregation, (2) microangiopathic hemolytic anemia, (3) neurologic abnormalities, (4) fever, and (5) renal disease.[76,77] The pathophysiology is based on dysfunction of the ADAMTS-13 enzyme, which normally cleaves von Willebrand factor (vWF) multimers. In TTP, there is a lack of vWF cleavage leading to an accumulation of vWF multimers, which bind to platelets leading to clot formation and end-organ damage. In congenital TTP, there is a deficiency of ADAMTS-13, while in acquired TTP an inhibitory autoantibody inactivates ADAMTS-13. In patients with clinical TTP, demonstrating reduced levels of ADAMTS-13 activity (<5%) is confirmatory. Treatment for TTP includes immunosuppression with corticosteroids and cyclophosphamide, as well as plasmapheresis, which significantly decreases the mortality rate.[76]

Complications of the Treatment of Rheumatic Diseases

Although the treatment of rheumatic disease is effective and often life saving, there are risks and complications related to treatment itself. High-dose steroid therapy may exacerbate hypertension and cause electrolyte imbalances (particularly sodium and fluid retention) and hyperglycemia. Corticosteroids can also impair neutrophil function, leading to increased susceptibility to infection. Long-term effects of corticosteroids include loss of bone density, with increased risk of compression fractures, and skin atrophy, with increased the risk of skin breakdown. As already discussed, a serious complication of chronic corticosteroid therapy, especially in the ICU setting, is adrenal insufficiency that may require stress-dose corticosteroid therapy.

Several medications cause gastric irritation and pancreatitis. GI prophylaxis with proton pump inhibitors and monitoring pancreatic and liver enzymes is recommended. Biologic therapies, such as infliximab or rituximab, may cause mild or severe hypersensitivity reactions, and patients must be monitored closely. In some cases, patients may need to be admitted to the ICU for medication desensitization protocols.[78]

Managing medications can be complex in critically ill patients with rheumatic disease. As many of the medications are cleared by the kidneys or affected by dialysis, this can have important implications for dosing. Balancing the complexities of the organ systems involved in rheumatic disease with the potential toxicities and interactions of therapy is best accomplished with a multidisciplinary approach.

Summary

In summary, rheumatic diseases manifest with a wide variety of presentations and can affect all organ systems. Pediatric intensivists therefore need a basic understanding of the most commonly seen conditions in pediatric rheumatology, including JIA, SLE, JDM, vasculitides, and scleroderma, as critically ill children may present to the ICU with new-onset rheumatic disease, disease flare, or complications. In addition, many of the therapies for rheumatic diseases have clinically significant side effects that may require close monitoring in the intensive care setting. The diagnosis of rheumatic disease is challenging and requires a thorough history and physical examination, as well as consideration of a broad differential diagnosis. Early identification and management can significantly reduce morbidity and mortality, and providers in the intensive care setting play a vital role in providing life saving interventions to children with rheumatic disease.

Acknowledgments

We gratefully acknowledge the contributions of Jonna D. Clark and Helen M. Emery, who authored this chapter in previous editions.

Key References

3. Woo P. Theoretical and practical basis for early aggressive therapy in paediatric autoimmune disorders. *Curr Opin Rheumatol.* 2009;21:552-557.

5. Behrens EM, Beukelman T, Gallo L, et al. Evaluation of the presentation of systemic onset juvenile rheumatoid arthritis: data from the Pennsylvania Systemic Onset Juvenile Arthritis Registry (PASOJAR). *J Rheumatol.* 2008;35:343-348.

6. Goldenberg J, Ferraz MB, Pessoa AP, et al. Symptomatic cardiac involvement in juvenile rheumatoid arthritis. *Int J Cardiol.* 1992;34:57-62.

8. Kimura Y, Weiss JE, Haroldson KL, et al. Pulmonary hypertension and other potentially fatal pulmonary complications in systemic juvenile idiopathic arthritis. *Arthritis Care Res.* 2013;65:745-752.

10. DeWitt EM, Kimura Y, Beukelman T, et al. Consensus treatment plans for new-onset systemic juvenile idiopathic arthritis. *Arthritis Care Res.* 2012;64:1001-1010.

13. Tan EM, Cohen AS, Fries JF, et al. The 1982 revised criteria for the classification of systemic lupus erythematosus. *Arthritis Rheum.* 1982;25:1271-1277.

14. Hochberg MC. Updating the American College of Rheumatology revised criteria for the classification of systemic lupus erythematosus. *Arthritis Rheum.* 1997;40:1725.

15. Pego-Reigosa JM, Medeiro DA, Isenberg DA. Respiratory manifestations of systemic lupus erythematosus: old and new concepts. *Best Pract Res Clin Rheumatol.* 2009;23:469-480.

19. Brucato A, Cimaz R, Caporali R, et al. Pregnancy outcomes in patients with autoimmune diseases and anti-Ro/SSA antibodies. *Clin Rev Allergy Immunol.* 2010;40:27-41.

20. Robinson AB, Hoeltzel MF, Wahezi DM, et al. Clinical characteristics of children with juvenile dermatomyositis: the Childhood Arthritis and Rheumatology Research Alliance Registry. *Arthritis Care Res.* 2014;66:404-410.

22. Foeldvari I, Zhavania M, Birdi N, et al. Favourable outcome in 135 children with juvenile systemic sclerosis: results of a multi-national survey. *Rheumatology.* 2000;39:556-559.

23. Vonk MC, Broers B, Heijdra YF, et al. Systemic sclerosis and its pulmonary complications in The Netherlands: an epidemiological study. *Ann Rheum Dis.* 2009;68:961-965.

24. Cipriani P, Carubbi F, Liakouli V, et al. Stem cells in autoimmune diseases: implications for pathogenesis and future trends in therapy. *Autoimmun Rev.* 2013;12:709-716.

27. Aguiar CL, Soybilgic A, Avcin T, et al. Pediatric antiphospholipid syndrome. *Curr Rheumatol Rep.* 2015;17:504.

28. Berman H, Rodríguez-Pintó I, Cervera R, et al. Pediatric catastrophic antiphospholipid syndrome: descriptive analysis of 45 patients from the CAPS Registry. *Autoimmun Rev.* 2014;13:157-162.

29. Twilt M, Benseler S. Childhood antineutrophil cytoplasmic antibodies associated vasculitides. *Curr Opin Rheumatol.* 2014;26:50-55.

30. Rajagopala S, Shobha V, Devaraj U, et al. Pulmonary hemorrhage in Henoch-Schönlein purpura: case report and systematic review of the English literature. *Semin Arthritis Rheum.* 2013;42:391-400.

32. Pucci A, Martino S, Tibaldi M, et al. Incomplete and atypical Kawasaki disease: a clinicopathologic paradox at high risk of sudden and unexpected infant death. *Pediatr Cardiol.* 2012;33:802-805.

34. Kanegaye JT, Wilder MS, Molkara D, et al. Recognition of a Kawasaki disease shock syndrome. *Pediatrics.* 2009;123:e783-e789.

37. Manlhiot C, Brandão LR, Somji Z, et al. Long-term anticoagulation in Kawasaki disease: Initial use of low molecular weight heparin is a viable option for patients with severe coronary artery abnormalities. *Pediatr Cardiol.* 2010;31:834-842.

39. Guillevin L, Durand-Gasselin B, Cevallos R, et al. Microscopic polyangiitis: clinical and laboratory findings in eighty-five patients. *Arthritis Rheum.* 1999;42:421-430.

40. Mendiola Ramírez K, Portillo Rivera AC, Galicia Reyes A, et al. Type III Takayasu's arteritis in a pediatric patient. Case report and review of the literature. *Reumatol Clin.* 2012;8:216-219.

41. Cantez S, Benseler SM. Childhood CNS vasculitis: a treatable cause of new neurological deficit in children. *Nat Clin Pract Rheumatol.* 2008;4:460-461.

42. Radhakrishna SM, Reiff AO, Marzan KA, et al. Pediatric rheumatic disease in the intensive care unit: lessons learned from 15 years of experience in a tertiary care pediatric hospital. *Pediatr Crit Care Med.* 2012;13:e181-e186.

43. Hsu C-L, Chen K-Y, Yeh P-S, et al. Outcome and prognostic factors in critically ill patients with systemic lupus erythematosus: a retrospective study. *Crit Care.* 2005;9:R177-R183.

44. Minoia F, Davì S, Horne A, et al. Dissecting the heterogeneity of macrophage activation syndrome complicating systemic juvenile idiopathic arthritis. *J Rheumatol.* 2015;42:994-1001.

45. Simon DW, Aneja R, Carcillo JA, et al. Plasma exchange, methylprednisolone, IV immune globulin, and now anakinra support continued PICU equipoise in management of hyperferritinemia-associated sepsis/multiple organ dysfunction syndrome/macrophage activation syndrome/secondary hemophagocytic lymphohistiocytosis syndrome. *Pediatr Crit Care Med.* 2014;15:486-488.

50. Rabinovich CE. Challenges in the diagnosis and treatment of juvenile systemic sclerosis. *Nat Rev Rheumatol.* 2011;7:676-680.

51. Araujo DB, Borba EF, Silva CA, et al. Alveolar hemorrhage: distinct features of juvenile and adult onset systemic lupus erythematosus. *Lupus.* 2012;21:872-877.

52. Kolovos NS, Schuerer DJE, Moler FW, et al. Extracorporal life support for pulmonary hemorrhage in children: a case series. *Crit Care Med.* 2002;30:577-580.

53. Agarwal HS, Taylor MB, Grzeszczak MJ, et al. Extracorporeal membrane oxygenation and plasmapheresis for pulmonary hemorrhage in microscopic polyangiitis. *Pediatr Nephrol.* 2005;20:526-528.

54. Haupt ME, Pires-Ervoes J, Brannen ML, et al. Successful use of plasmapheresis for granulomatosis with polyangiitis presenting as diffuse alveolar hemorrhage. *Pediatr Pulmonol.* 2013;48:614-616.

55. Levy DM, Massicotte MP, Harvey E, et al. Thromboembolism in paediatric lupus patients. *Lupus.* 2003;12:741-746.

57. Moder KG, Miller DT, Tazelaar HD. Cardiac involvement in systemic lupus erythematosus. *Mayo Clin Proc.* 1999;74:275-284.

58. Ilowite NT, Sandborg CI, Feldman BM, et al. Algorithm development for corticosteroid management in systemic juvenile idiopathic arthritis trial using consensus methodology. *Pediatr Rheumatol Online J.* 2012;10:31.

60. Roldan CA, Qualls CR, Sopko KS, et al. Transthoracic versus transesophageal echocardiography for detection of Libman-Sacks endocarditis: a randomized controlled study. *J Rheumatol.* 2008;35:224-229.

61. Hahn BH, Grossman J, Chen W, et al. The pathogenesis of atherosclerosis in autoimmune rheumatic diseases: roles of inflammation and dyslipidemia. *J Autoimmun.* 2007;28:69-75.

63. Newburger JW, Fulton DR. Kawasaki disease. *Curr Opin Pediatr.* 2004;16:508-514.

64. Auron M, Raissouni N. Adrenal insufficiency. *Pediatr Rev.* 2015;36:92-102.

65. Sacre K, Dehoux M, Chauveheid MP, et al. Pituitary-adrenal function after prolonged glucocorticoid therapy for systemic inflammatory disorders: an observational study. *J Clin Endocrinol Metab.* 2013;98:3199-3205.

67. Richer O, Ulinski T, Lemelle I, et al. Abdominal manifestations in childhood-onset systemic lupus erythematosus. *Ann Rheum Dis.* 2007;66:174-178.

68. Medina F, Ayala A, Jara LJ. Acute abdomen in systemic lupus erythematosus: the importance of early laparotomy. *Am J Med.* 1997;102:100-105.

69. Limwattana S, Dissaneewate P, Kritsaneepaiboon S, et al. Systemic lupus erythematosus-related pancreatitis in children. *Clin Rheumatol.* 2013;32:913-918.

70. de Joode AA, Sanders JS, Smid WM, et al. Plasmapheresis rescue therapy in progressive systemic ANCA-associated vasculitis: single-center results of stepwise escalation of immunosuppression. *J Clin Apher.* 2014;29:266-272.

71. Ounissi M, Abderrahim E, Hedri H, et al. Kidney transplantation during autoimmune diseases. *Transplant Proc.* 2009;41:2781-2783.

72. Butani L. End-stage renal disease as the presenting manifestation of renal systemic lupus erythematosus. *Pediatr Nephrol.* 2007;22:149-151.

73. Shiari R. Neurologic manifestations of childhood rheumatic diseases. *Iran J Child Neurol.* 2012;6:1-7.

75. Palejwala NV, Yeh S, Angeles-Han ST, et al. Current perspectives on ophthalmic manifestations of childhood rheumatic diseases. *Curr Rheumatol Rep.* 2013;15:341.

77. Zheng T, Chunlei L, Zhen W, et al. Clinical-pathological features and prognosis of thrombotic thrombocytopenic purpura in patients with lupus nephritis. *Am J Med Sci.* 2009;338:343-347.

78. Castells MC, Tennant NM, Sloane DE, et al. Hypersensitivity reactions to chemotherapy: outcomes and safety of rapid desensitization in 413 cases. *J Allergy Clin Immunol.* 2008;122:574-580.

Bacterial and Fungal Infections, Antimicrobials, and Antimicrobial Resistance

Deborah E. Franzon, Hayden T. Schwenk, and Mihaela Damian

PEARLS

- In the pediatric ICU (PICU), appropriate dosing of antibiotics without delay decreases morbidity and mortality, the overall costs of treating the infection, and the emergence of resistance.
- Critically ill children exhibit altered pharmacokinetics with differences in volume of distribution and clearance that impact response to antimicrobial exposure.
- An important side effect of high-dose, long-term use of β-lactam agents in the PICU setting is neutropenia.
- Risk factors for *Candida* spp. bloodstream infections in the PICU, resulting in mortality rates as high as 44%, are presence of a central venous catheter, a diagnosis of malignancy, and receipt of either vancomycin or antimicrobials with activity against anaerobic organisms for more than 3 days. Guidelines suggest echinocandins as first-line therapy.
- Occult fungal infection should be considered in any patient with chemotherapy-neutropenia with fever persisting more than 96 hours despite empiric antibiotic therapy.
- Emergence of resistance organisms is increasing in critically ill patients, particularly vancomycin-resistant enterococcus, extended-spectrum β-lactamase producing enteric gram-negative bacteria, and multidrug-resistant pseudomonas, calling for the need to use alternative drug and dosing strategies.
- Antimicrobial stewardship programs that implement strategies to reduce unnecessary antimicrobial use can be cost-effective programs that address resistance in the ICU setting.

Because of the severity of illness of children in the pediatric ICU (PICU), there is little room for error in selecting the appropriate antimicrobial agent. It is important to treat infections aggressively to obtain the best clinical and microbiologic outcomes. Timing of antibiotic administration is important, and any delay in administration is associated with increased mortality and worse outcomes. The importance of timely administered, broad-spectrum empiric antimicrobials must

be balanced with their potential to promote antimicrobial resistance. Because antibiotic resistance may lead to increased morbidity and mortality, as well as increased health care costs, de-escalation of antibiotics, based on microbiologic and susceptibility data, is imperative.[1] This chapter reviews the most clinically important classes of antibiotics and antifungals, including those currently under investigation and not approved by the US FDA for use in children. Mechanisms of resistance are reviewed, as are the strategies designed to meet the challenge of treating and preventive the development of resistant organisms. Many textbooks about infectious diseases have excellent in-depth reviews of antibiotic characteristics and are recommended for additional information.[2,3]

General Considerations for Antibiotic Therapy

Tissue penetration and dosing of antimicrobials are critical; pharmacokinetic (PK) and pharmacodynamic (PD) characteristics of different classes of antibiotics against different types of pathogens help determine the dosing regimen required for microbiologic and clinical cure.[4,5] Due to changes in both fluid dynamics and kidney perfusion, critically ill children exhibit altered pharmacokinetics with differences in volume of distribution and clearance that impact antimicrobial exposure. It is imperative to achieve appropriate concentrations of the antibiotic in relationship to the organism's minimum inhibitory concentration (MIC). Based on PK/PD characteristics, antibiotics can be classified as (1) concentration-dependent (fluoroquinolones, aminoglycosides); (2) time-dependent (β-lactams); and (3) both concentration- and time-dependent antibiotics (glycopeptides). These parameters are important to consider because the inappropriate dosing of antibiotics may facilitate the development of antibiotic resistance and increase the odds of morbidity and mortality.[6-9]

After an infection is suspected on the basis of the clinical, laboratory, and imaging characteristics of the child, appropriate cultures should be obtained. Broad-spectrum antibiotics should be administered empirically, according to the local susceptibility patterns. Data suggest that using active antibiotics in the appropriate dose without delay decreases morbidity and mortality, the overall costs of treating the infection, and the emergence of resistance. The relative activity of antimicrobial agents against gram-negative (Table 107.1) and

TABLE 107.1   Antibiotic Activity for Gram-Negative Pathogens (0 to +++++)

Organism	Ticarcillin-Clavulanate	Piperacillin-Tazobactam	Ceftazidime	Ceftriaxone	Cefepime	Tobramycin	Ciprofloxacin	Meropenem
Escherichia coli	++++	++++	++++	++++	++++	++++	++++	+++++
Klebsiella spp.	++++	++++	++++	++++	++++	++++	++++	+++++
Enterobacter spp.	+++	+++	++++	++++	++	+++	++++	+++++
Pseudomonas aeruginosa[a]	+++	+	++++	++++	+++	++++	+++	++++
Acinetobacter spp.[b]	++	++	+++	+++	+++	++	++	++++
Stenotrophomonas[a]	+++	+	++	+	+++	++	++	+

[a]Trimethoprim-sulfamethoxazole is the most active antibiotic against Stenotrophomonas in vitro.
[b]Colistin may be effective in vitro against organisms resistant to all available agents, with limited data on efficacy and significant toxicities.[21]
Susceptibility data are averaged,[44–46,48,49] with local hospital data potentially much different from these values.

TABLE 107.2   Antibiotic Activity for Gram-Positive Pathogens (0 to +++++)

Organism	Ampicillin	Oxacillin	Cefazolin	Vancomycin	Linezolid
Methicillin-susceptible Staphylococcus spp. (Staphylococcus aureus or coagulase-negative staphylococci)	0	+++++	+++++	+++++	++++
Methicillin-resistant Staphylococcus spp.	0	0	0	+++++	++++
Enterococcus faecalis[a]	++++	0	0	++++	++++
Enterococcus faecium[a]	++	0	0	++++	++++

[a]For vancomycin-susceptible strains.
Susceptibility data are averaged,[40,44,50] with local hospital data potentially much different from these values.

gram-positive pathogens (Table 107.2) is provided, although clinicians should consult their local antibiogram.

When culture results and sensitivities are available, antibiotic choice can be tailored to a narrower spectrum for completion of therapy. If a child has a multidrug-resistant infection, the risk-benefit analysis may well favor the use of an antibiotic that does not have a favorable safety profile if no other alternative exists. In some critically ill children, combination antibiotic therapy may be warranted to augment the antibiotic killing capacity, increase tissue penetration, or prevent antibiotic resistance.

On the basis of the overall clinical assessment, supported by laboratory and imaging data and the response to empiric therapy, the physician needs to decide whether to continue therapy for a complete treatment course or stop the antibiotics if data do not support an infection as the cause of the child's clinical state. Optimal duration of antibiotic therapy for infections in the PICU is poorly defined; however, in specific situations, shorter duration of antibiotic use may reduce length of ICU stay, antibiotic resistance, and the emergence of secondary infections. Monitoring serum inflammatory markers may allow optimization of both the antibiotic regimen and duration of treatment.[10]

Antibiotic Classes
β-Lactam Antibiotics

β-Lactam antibiotics are a diverse group of antibiotics. The β-lactam ring that characterizes these compounds is

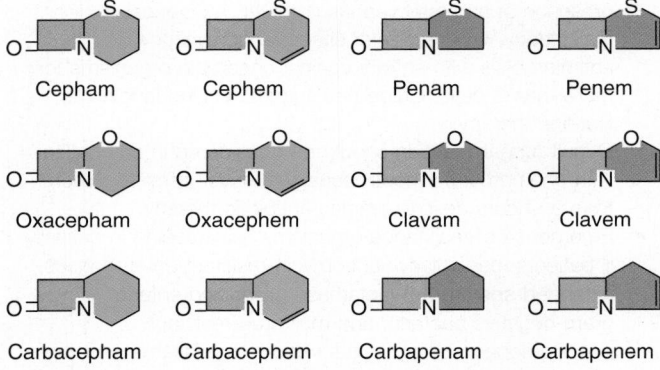

Fig. 107.1 Structures of β-lactam antibiotics.

usually attached to a ring structure that defines the class of antibiotic agents as penicillins, cephalosporins, carbapenems, or monobactams (Fig. 107.1). The β-lactam structure is thought to interfere with bacterial cell wall synthesis and repair by preventing transpeptidation and transglycosylation of the pentapeptide precursors in the formation of peptidoglycan.[11] The target transpeptidase enzymes, also known as penicillin-binding proteins (PBPs), are vital for the maintenance of cell wall integrity. PBPs carried by different bacterial species have different structures, leading to differences in the binding affinity for various β-lactam agents. Long-term, high-dose use of all β-lactam agents may be associated with reversible neutropenia.

Penicillins

Penicillins can be divided into groups that are based largely on spectrum of activity and chemistry. The natural penicillins, penicillin G and penicillin V, are active against a number of aerobic and anaerobic bacteria but are primarily used for the treatment of streptococcal (Group A and B streptococci) and spirochete infections, such as syphilis. The aminopenicillins, ampicillin and amoxicillin, have expanded activity against gram-negative organisms and are the agents of choice for susceptible enterococci. The penicillinase-resistant penicillins, oxacillin and nafcillin, are highly effective for the treatment of infections due to susceptible *Staphylococcus aureus*. Piperacillin is the only extended-spectrum penicillin currently available in the United States and only in fixed combination with the β-lactamase inhibitor, tazobactam. Piperacillin has enhanced activity against gram-negative organisms, including *Pseudomonas aeruginosa*, with reasonable gram-positive coverage, including *Enterococcus* spp.

β-Lactam Antimicrobial Plus β-Lactamase Inhibitor Combination

Ampicillin, amoxicillin, and piperacillin have been combined with a β-lactamase inhibitor that allows for enhanced gram-negative activity when compared with the β-lactam alone. The first β-lactam drug component, the actual antibiotic, effectively binds to the target site in the bacteria and results in the death of the organism. The second component, the *β-lactamase inhibitor*, has poor intrinsic activity as an antibiotic but may irreversibly bind to and neutralize the β-lactamase enzyme the organism has produced. The combination adds to the spectrum of the original antibiotic when the mechanism of resistance is a β-lactamase enzyme. The addition of sulbactam to ampicillin (Unasyn) and clavulanate to amoxicillin (Augmentin) expands the spectrum of activity to include *S. aureus, B. fragilis,* and many β-lactamase producing gram-negative organisms. Similarly, the addition of tazobactam to piperacillin (Zosyn) results in enhanced anaerobic and gram-negative activity.

Cephalosporins

Cephalosporins can be distinguished on the basis of activity against gram-negative pathogens and stability of the antibiotic to a number of the gram-negative β-lactamases. The cephalosporins fall roughly into five "generations" on the basis of these characteristics. First-generation cephalosporins (cephalexin, cefazolin) are generally most active against some gram-positive pathogens such as *S. aureus,* with more limited gram-negative activity. Importantly, none of the current cephalosporin antibiotics of any generation display activity against the enterococci. The second-generation cephalosporins (cefuroxime) have increased intrinsic activity against gram-negative organisms, including *Escherichica coli* and *Klebsiella,* on the basis of enhanced stability against the organisms' principle β-lactamases. Activity against *S. aureus* is decreased compared with the first-generation cephalosporins but is sufficient to achieve clinical success in most situations. A slightly different group of antibiotics, the cephamycins (cefoxitin, cefotetan), have activity against the gram-negative enteric bacilli similar to the second-generation cephalosporins but display enhanced anaerobic activity against *B. fragilis* and may play a role in the treatment of intraabdominal infections. Their activity against *B. fragilis,* however, is inferior to metronidazole, clindamycin, or the carbapenems. The third-generation cephalosporins, cefotaxime and ceftriaxone, have enhanced stability against the most prevalent β-lactamases of *Haemophilus influenzae, E. coli,* and *Klebsiella* and enhanced activity against many of the Enterobacteriaceae but are, unfortunately, not stable to the inducible chromosomal β-lactamases (AmpC, type I) of *Enterobacter, Serratia,* or *Citrobacter*. Ceftazidime, another third-generation cephalosporin, has far greater intrinsic activity against *P. aeruginosa* than previous cephalosporins. None of the third-generation cephalosporins are as active against *S. aureus* as first- and second-generation agents. Cefepime, a fourth-generation cephalosporin, has the best overall activity against both gram-negative and gram-positive pathogens, with activity against *P. aeruginosa* equivalent to ceftazidime and activity against *S. aureus* equivalent to second-generation cephalosporins. It is also the most stable to β-lactamase degradation. The novel fifth-generation cephalosporin, ceftaroline, is the first β-lactam antibiotic with activity against methicillin-resistant *S. aureus* (MRSA) and has been approved for the treatment of adults with community-acquired pneumonia and skin and skin structure infections. In addition to its activity against MRSA, ceftaroline has a spectrum of gram-negative activity similar to that of third-generation cephalosporins.

Carbapenems

Three carbapenems, imipenem (combined with cilastin, an inhibitor of a renal tubular dehydropeptidase enzyme, to avoid nephrotoxicity), meropenem, and ertapenem, are currently FDA approved in children older than 3 years of age for the treatment of complicated skin and skin structure infections (SSIs), complicated intraabdominal infections, and meningitis. The carbapenems have a β-lactam ring structure that differs slightly from the penicillins and cephalosporins (see Fig. 107.1), with chemical modifications to enhance activity and stability. The broad antimicrobial spectrum of activity of the carbapenems is similar and includes gram-negative, gram-positive, and anaerobic organisms. Given their spectrum of activity, carbapenems are generally reserved for nosocomial infections or those due to organisms for which there are few alternatives, such as extended-spectrum β-lactamase (ESBL) producing gram-negative organisms or those harboring a chromosomally mediated ampC β-lactamase, like *Enterobacter* spp.

With respect to toxicity, the carbapenems are well tolerated, although imipenem displays interference with central nervous system γ-aminobutyric acid inhibition of neuron activity and was shown to be associated with an increase in seizure activity in children treated for bacterial meningitis compared with historic controls.[12] On the basis of these observations, meropenem is the preferred carbapenem for children at risk for seizures or with central nervous system (CNS) infections and inflammation.

Monobactams

Aztreonam, the only monobactam currently available, has a unique chemical structure in which the β-lactam ring is not attached to an adjacent five- or six-membered ring but does have chemical additions to the β-lactam ring that enhance activity and stability to β-lactamases. It displays aerobic, gram-negative activity, including activity against many strains of *P. aeruginosa*.

Aminoglycosides

Aminoglycoside antibiotics are bactericidal in a concentration-dependent fashion against a wide range of aerobic pathogens. These agents inhibit protein synthesis by irreversible binding to the 30S ribosomal subunit. The gram-negative spectrum of activity is extensive, including enteric bacilli (E. coli, Klebsiella, Enterobacter, Serratia), P. aeruginosa, and many free-living gram-negative bacilli. These antibiotics have no clinically relevant anaerobic activity.

Although the first aminoglycosides exhibited substantial renal toxicity and ototoxicity, subsequent agents are significantly safer. The most widely available parenteral agents are gentamicin, tobramycin, and amikacin. Because of the relatively low serum concentrations necessary to prevent toxicity and poor penetration into the spinal fluid, these agents are not used as primary therapy of CNS infections. Caution should be exercised in the use of these agents in undrained abscess infections, including intraabdominal infections. The acidic and anaerobic conditions present in abscesses produce MICs against aerobic gram-negative organisms that are 10 times higher than those documented under ideal laboratory conditions.[13]

Aminoglycoside-induced nephrotoxicity has been described, even in non–critically ill children, and is associated with poorer outcomes.[14] As a result, the role of aminoglycosides as part of combination therapy for the treatment of gram-negative and gram-positive infections continues to evolve. The previously held notion that an aminoglycoside should be combined with a β-lactam to retard the development of resistance has been challenged by recent studies, including a propensity score–adjusted, retrospective cohort study of pediatric patients with gram-negative bacteremia that found no survival benefit with addition of an aminoglycoside to patients on a susceptible β-lactam agent.[15,16] It is also unclear whether the empiric addition of an aminoglycoside is warranted for the management of gram-negative bacteremia while awaiting susceptibility results. A recent retrospective pediatric study found no survival benefit to empiric combination therapy, except for patients with risk factors for multidrug-resistant, gram-negative (MDRGN) infection: a history of previous colonization or infection with an MDRGN, broad-spectrum antibiotic therapy within 30 days, a prolonged current hospitalization, or a high prevalence of MDRGNs in the community.[16] The role of low-dose gentamicin as part of combination therapy for the management of uncomplicated Enterococcus faecalis bacteremia in children remains unresolved. A recent retrospective study found that while the addition of gentamicin decreased the time to bacterial clearance by 10 hours, there was no impact on bacteremic relapse, and the risk of developing acute kidney injury was twice as high.[17]

Glycopeptides

Vancomycin is currently the only available glycopeptide in the United States. The glycopeptides are primarily active against aerobic and anaerobic gram-positive organisms. Vancomycin is bactericidal against virtually all strains of staphylococci and against most strains of streptococci, although it is bacteriostatic against the enterococci. Resistance to vancomycin is noted to occur in strains of Enterococcus faecium (vancomycin-resistant enterococcus [VRE]) and has also been described in S. aureus.[18,19] This class of antibiotic is cell wall active, as are the penicillins, but has a different mechanism of action in prevention of pentapeptide cross-linking in the formation of cell wall peptidoglycan.

The tissue distribution of vancomycin is extensive, with elimination of unchanged antibiotic by the kidney. Dosage adjustment is required in renal insufficiency. Penetration into the cerebrospinal fluid (CSF) is not well studied and is erratic. Serum concentrations of approximately 40 µg/mL are thought to be necessary to achieve CSF concentrations sufficiently high enough to achieve a reliable microbiologic cure in meningitis or ventriculitis. The toxicities of vancomycin are primarily nephrotoxicity and ototoxicity. As with the aminoglycosides, close attention to serum antibiotic concentrations will mitigate clinically significant toxicity.

The new-generation lipoglycopeptides, dalbavancin, telavancin, and oritavancin, are FDA approved in adults for the treatment of complicated skin or skin structure infections caused by susceptible gram-positive organisms, including MRSA. Their role in the management of pediatric patients remains unsettled.

Macrolides

Erythromycin and the related macrolides, clarithromycin and azithromycin, may be required in the PICU for children with severe pertussis or atypical pneumonia or in children with extensive drug allergy precluding the use of standard antiinfective agents. The macrolides bind to the 50S ribosomal subunit of susceptible bacteria to prevent the formation of peptide chains, thereby inhibiting protein synthesis. In general, both clarithromycin and azithromycin are better tolerated than erythromycin because of the lack of degradation products seen with erythromycin that stimulate motilin receptors and lead to nausea, vomiting, and abdominal cramps. Clarithromycin and azithromycin achieve high intracellular concentrations, with demonstrated efficacy against intracellular pathogens and all of the macrolides demonstrate activity against atypical bacteria, including Mycoplasma pneumoniae, Chlamydia, Legionella, and Bordetella pertussis. In addition, azithromycin has potential efficacy as a modulator of airway hyperresponsiveness,[20] even in the absence of overt infection,[21] that may have a role for children in the ICU with community-acquired pneumonia and exacerbation of underlying chronic lung disease or asthma. Macrolides are metabolized by cytochrome P-450 enzymes, which cause potential drug-drug interactions.

Fluoroquinolones

This class of broad-spectrum agents has been extremely successful in adults over the past 20 years. Because of concerns regarding cartilage toxicity in weight-bearing joints of experimental animals, however, pediatric studies have been limited. The mechanism of action of quinolones involves inhibition of DNA synthesis by interference with two bacterial enzymes. The activity of each specific quinolone and the rapidity of the development of resistance to the specific quinolone depend on the relative activity of the quinolone against these enzymes.[22]

Ciprofloxacin, the first of the agents approved for use in adults, shows outstanding activity against P. aeruginosa, as well as many enteric bacilli causing both nosocomial (E. coli, Klebsiella, Enterobacter) and gastrointestinal infections (Salmonella, Shigella, Campylobacter, Yersinia, and Aeromonas). Although resistance to ciprofloxacin in P. aeruginosa and other bacilli has been increasing, susceptibility in pediatric inpatient units has remained reasonable. Ciprofloxacin is FDA approved in children older than 1 year for the treatment of complicated urinary tract infections, pyelonephritis, and post-exposure treatment of inhalational anthrax. Subsequent chemical modifications of fluoroquinolones have resulted in a set of agents with good to excellent activity against gram-positive cocci, including group A streptococcus, S. pneumoniae, and S. aureus. These agents—levofloxacin and moxifloxacin—are effective in both gram-positive and gram-negative infections. Although case reports of possible cartilage toxicity exist, no documented case unequivocally caused by fluoroquinolones in children has been published in any prospective study.[23]

Miscellaneous

Clindamycin

A member of the lincosamide family, clindamycin inhibits the growth of bacteria by binding to the 50S subunit of the ribosome. Clindamycin is active against gram-positive organisms and many anaerobes. Activity against β-lactam–resistant strains of S. pneumoniae and S. aureus (MRSA) has led to increased use of clindamycin in children.[24]

In children with infection caused by strains of S. aureus or group A streptococcus that are suspected to produce toxin-mediated disease (eg, toxic shock syndrome, necrotizing fasciitis), clindamycin is often used (in conjunction with a β-lactam agent) to stop toxin production as quickly as possible. Retrospectively collected data suggest improved outcomes in patients treated with the combination.[25] Clindamycin may be used for treatment of MRSA skin infections and pneumonia; however, it is not recommended as the sole agent for critically ill patients with MRSA infections. Given its excellent gram-positive and anaerobic activity, clindamycin can also be used in the treatment of aspiration pneumonia and head and neck infections.

Linezolid

Linezolid is the first in a class of new antibiotics, the oxazolidinones. These antibiotics are protein synthesis inhibitors that interfere with mRNA binding at the 30S ribosome subunit. Linezolid is a bacteriostatic agent useful in the treatment of infections caused by gram-positive organisms, including MRSA, coagulase-negative staphylococci, and VRE. Linezolid has been studied and has received FDA approval for use in pediatric patients, including the neonatal age group. Linezolid is approved for the treatment of community- and hospital-acquired pneumonia, complicated and uncomplicated skin and soft tissue infections, and bacteremia caused by vancomycin-resistant organisms.

A concern that appears to have little clinical relevance in healthy children treated under controlled conditions is the drug's nonselective, reversible inhibition of monamine oxidase. Nevertheless, this drug interaction profile has potential impact on the patient in the PICU who is receiving adrenergic or serotonergic drugs. Linezolid has been reported to be associated with hematologic side effects and rarely with optic neuritis and peripheral neuropathy.

Metronidazole

A nitroimidazole derivative, metronidazole is an effective antibiotic for parasitic and anaerobic bacterial infections. The primary use of metronidazole in the PICU includes infections caused by β-lactamase–positive strains of B. fragilis (intraabdominal infections) and those caused by C. difficile (pseudomembranous colitis). Resistance to metronidazole has not been a clinical problem despite significant clinical use. The distribution of drug in tissues is extensive, including CNS penetration. It has been a standard component of therapy for anaerobic deep tissue space infections and has been used in the treatment of anaerobic brain abscesses. It remains the agent of choice (by the oral route, if possible) for the therapy of C. difficile infection.

Colistin

With antibiotic resistance increasing dramatically in gram-negative pathogens, colistin has returned to clinical use and now represents a therapy of last resort for organisms resistant to all other available antibiotic therapy.[26] Colistin (colistimethate), or polymyxin E, has broad-spectrum bactericidal activity against gram-negative organisms by acting as a cationic detergent, destroying the bacterial cytoplasmic membrane. Colistin has no activity against gram-positive organisms or against B. fragilis. The chief toxicities of this agent include nephrotoxicity, peripheral neuropathy, confusion, coma, and seizure. The drug is renal eliminated, and dosage adjustment is required with renal insufficiency. Limited data in pediatric burn and critical care patients suggest colistin is effective and safe for multidrug-resistant gram-negative infections.[27,28] In addition, aerosolized colistin has been used as an adjunctive or monotherapy for gram-negative pulmonary infections. Clinically significant bronchospasm may occur.

Tigecycline

Tigecycline is the first in a new class of antibiotics, the glycylcyclines. Tigecycline inhibits protein synthesis and is generally considered a bacteriostatic agent. It has broad-spectrum antibacterial activity against gram-positive and gram-negative aerobes and anaerobes, including MRSA and multidrug-resistant gram-negative bacteria. It is not effective against Pseudomonas, Providencia, and Proteus species. Tigecycline is approved for use in adult patients with complicated skin and SSIs, complicated intraabdominal infections, and community-acquired pneumonia. The role of tigecycline in the pediatric population has yet to be defined.

Daptomycin

Daptomycin belongs to a new class of antibiotics, the lipopeptides. Daptomycin disrupts the cell membrane and is rapidly bactericidal. It has a broad range of activity against gram-positive bacteria including methicillin, vancomycin, and linezolid-resistant organisms. It should not be used to treat pulmonary infections because surfactant inhibits its activity. Daptomycin is currently approved for use in adults with complicated skin and skin structure infections, as well as right-sided endocarditis and staphylococcal bacteremia. A recent review of daptomycin therapy in invasive gram-positive infections in children showed its addition to the treatment regimen resulted in bacteriologic cure in six of seven patients with persistent bacteremia and was well tolerated.[29] The primary toxicity seen is a dose-dependent, reversible myopathy that can be monitored by elevation in serum creatinine phosphokinase.

Fungal Infections and Antifungal Agents

Invasive fungal infections are increasingly recognized as a significant risk among immunocompromised and critically ill children.[30] Indeed, *Candida* species are the third most common cause of health care–acquired bloodstream infection in the United States, following coagulase-negative staphylococci and enterococci.[31] As they are also associated with excessive morbidity and mortality, a basic understanding of the epidemiology, diagnosis, and management of invasive fungal infections is essential.

Candida

Although epidemiologic data are sparse, recent studies suggest that around 8% of all hospital-acquired bloodstream infections in the United States are due to *Candida* spp. Candidemia is associated with a high rate of morbidity and mortality among children in the PICU. The 30-day mortality rate for children in the PICU with candidemia may be as high as 37% to 44%, and a multivariate analysis of children with invasive candidemia at a large, tertiary children's hospital found that location in the PICU at the time of diagnosis and the presence of an arterial catheter were the only two independent risk factors for death.[32] General risk factors for the development of *Candida* central line–associated bloodstream infections among pediatric patients include intestinal failure, presence of a gastrostomy tube, and receipt of total parenteral nutrition or blood transfusions.[33] Factors specifically associated with the development of candidemia for children in the PICU include presence of a central venous catheter, a diagnosis of malignancy, and receipt of either vancomycin or antimicrobials with activity against anaerobic organisms for more than 3 days.[32]

There are many candida species, each with their own unique pathogenicity and susceptibility. *C. albicans* and *C. parapsilosis* remain the most common pathogens identified, although the incidence of infection due to other species (eg, *C. glabrata, C. tropicalis, C. krusei*) is rising.[33] Blood culture remains the gold standard for the diagnosis of invasive candidiasis, although its sensitivity will vary depending on the extent of infection and particular *Candida* species. For example, cultures may be negative in patients with deep-seated candidiasis without concomitant candidemia.[34] Although several nonculture diagnostics, including β-D-glucan detection and serum polymerase chain reaction (PCR), have been developed to aid in the diagnosis of invasive candidiasis, their use has not been validated in children and further studies are necessary before their routine use can be recommended.

Aspergillus and Other Invasive Molds

Aspergillus species are responsible for the majority of invasive mold infections among children, and the increased incidence of invasive aspergillosis has paralleled the survival of children with immunocompromising conditions.[35] Infection is most commonly due to members of the *A. fumigatus* species complex, although certain conditions are associated with more unusual species (eg, *A. nidulans* in patients with chronic granulomatous disease).[36] Invasive aspergillosis is associated with compromised immune function and is associated with prolonged or repeatedly profound periods of neutropenia. High-risk populations include children with hematologic malignancies (particularly children with acute myelogenous leukemia [AML] or high-risk acute lymphoblastic leukemia [ALL]), hematopoietic stem cell transplant recipients (particularly in the setting of graft-versus-host disease), solid organ transplant recipients, patients with a primary immunodeficiency, and neonates.[36,37]

The lung is the most common site of invasive aspergillosis, although the spectrum of disease includes sinopulmonary, gastrointestinal, cutaneous, and CNS infection. Symptoms are often nonspecific, including fever, cough, dyspnea, and chest pain, so vigilance for potential infection in vulnerable populations is critical. Occult fungal infection should be considered in any patient with chemotherapy-induced neutropenia with fever persisting more than 96 hours, despite empiric antibiotic therapy.[38] The diagnosis of invasive mold infections is challenging, and culture remains the gold standard for the determination of species identification and antifungal susceptibility.[39] As with the diagnosis of invasive candidiasis, noninvasive diagnostic methodologies including serum aspergillus galactomannan antigen, β-D-glucan, and PCR detection of *Aspergillus* spp. have been developed, although data regarding their utility in children are mixed. While the galactomannan antigen is relatively specific for *Aspergillus* spp., it does cross-react with other fungi, including *Histoplasma capsulatum* and *Cryptococcus neoformans,* and is less sensitive in non-neutropenic hosts.[40] The estimated sensitivity and specificity of serum galactomannan testing for the diagnosis of invasive aspergillosis in children are 76% and 86%. Serial screening of serum galactomannan in at-risk children may help make the diagnosis of invasive aspergillosis sooner and is endorsed by European guidelines.[41] Galactomannan can also be detected in bronchoalveolar lavage fluid and may be helpful in the diagnosis of pulmonary aspergillosis.[42] Imaging can also be useful in diagnosing and determining the extent of invasive aspergillosis, although classic chest CT findings, such as the halo sign, air crescent sign, and cavitation, may be less common in children.[41]

There are a number of other potential invasive mold infections encountered in the pediatric population, although a complete discussion is beyond the scope of this chapter. It is important to note that given the unique pathogenicity and susceptibility of each organism, a microbiologically confirmed diagnosis is critical to the successful management of any invasive mold infection.

Antifungal Agents

There are four major classes of antifungals used for the treatment of invasive fungal infection, including the polyenes (amphotericin and its liposomal derivatives); triazoles (fluconazole, itraconazole, voriconazole, and posaconazole); echinocandins (micafungin, caspofungin, and anidulafungin); and the pyrimidine analog, flucytosine (Table 107.3).

Amphotericin

One of the first antifungal agents developed, amphotericin B deoxycholate, remains an important member of the intensivist's antifungal armamentarium. Amphotericin is broadly fungicidal against most yeast, molds, and dimorphic fungi. It exerts its effect by binding to fungal cell membrane ergosterols, resulting in increased cell permeability, leakage of intracellular contents, and concentration-dependent cell death.[43] Owing to its poor bioavailability, amphotericin B is generally given parenterally, although nebulized amphotericin has also been used in the treatment of *Aspergillus* lung infections.[44] Upon entering the bloodstream, the drug distributes widely into tissues, particularly organs of the reticuloendothelial system. Although CNS penetration is poor, the agent has been used extensively for the management of such infections and

TABLE 107.3   Activity of Selected Antifungal Drugs

Organism	Fluconazole	Voriconazole	Posaconazole	Amphotericin	Echinocandin
Candida albicans	+	+	+	+	+
Candida glabrata	±	+	+	+	+
Candida krusei	−	+	+	+	+
Candida lusitaniae	+	+	+	−	+
Candida parapsilosis	+	+	+	+	±
Blastomyces dermatitidis	+	+	+	+	−
Coccidioides immitis	+	+	+	+	−
Histoplasma capsulatum	+	+	+	+	−
Cryptococcus	+	+	+	+	−
Aspergillus fumigatus	−	+	+	+	+
Aspergillus terreus	−	+	+	−	+
Mucorales	−	−	+	+	−
Fusarium	−	+	+	+	−
Scedosporium	−	±	±	−	−

remains the drug of choice for induction therapy in patients with cryptococcal meningoencephalitis.[45] On the basis of concerns that liposomal amphotericin may fail to adequately penetrate renal tissue and the urinary tract, amphotericin B deoxycholate remains the preferred amphotericin product for both urinary tract and neonatal candidiasis.[46]

As its ergosterol target is similar to human cholesterol, amphotericin B deoxycholate is associated with significant side effects, including nephrotoxicity, electrolyte wasting, fever, chills, and hematologic effects.[47] To combat these effects, various lipid formulations of amphotericin B have been developed. While amphotericin B deoxycholate and its liposomal derivatives are generally equivalent in terms of clinical efficacy, conventional amphotericin is significantly more potent and dosing between agents is not interchangeable.[48] Renal toxicity is mitigated by the use of lipid-based formulations of amphotericin B, although significant electrolyte disturbances, including hypomagnesaemia and hypokalemia, remain common. The most common side effects are related to infusion of the drug (fever, rigors, nausea, vomiting). Slow infusion and premedication with acetaminophen and diphenhydramine may help prevent or minimize such reactions.

The most commonly used liposomal formulation of amphotericin in pediatrics, amphotericin B liposome, is FDA approved for the treatment of invasive aspergillosis, candidiasis, cryptococcal meningitis, cryptococcosis, and visceral leishmaniasis in children. It is also approved for the treatment of presumed fungal infection in febrile, neutropenic patients and remains the drug of choice for treatment of infections due to the *Mucorales*, including *Rhizomucor* spp., *Rhizopus* spp., and *Mucor* spp. Pathogens for which amphotericin is less reliably effective include *A. terreus, C. lusitanea*, members of the genus *Scedosporium, Trichosporon* spp., and *Fusarium* spp.[49-52]

Triazoles
The triazoles fluconazole, itraconazole, voriconazole, and posaconazole are generally well tolerated and demonstrate activity against a number of fungal species. The triazoles disrupt the synthesis of ergosterol, a critical component of the fungal cell membrane, which results in inhibition of cell growth and replication. Fluconazole has greatest activity for yeast and is fungistatic for most *Candida* species, with the exception of *C. krusei* and *C. glabrata,* which are generally resistant.[53] Importantly, fluconazole lacks fungicidal activity against molds, including *Aspergillus* spp. Fluconazole has excellent bioavailability and concentrates in the urine, making it an excellent choice for susceptible genitourinary infections.[46] Itraconazole is available in oral formulation only and, given its erratic pharmacokinetics and the existence of alternative agents, is generally reserved for the treatment of endemic mycoses. Voriconazole is available in both parenteral and enteral formulations and remains the drug of choice for invasive aspergillosis. To improve solubility, the parenteral formulation of voriconazole includes a cyclodextrin carrier molecule, which is cleared by glomerular filtration. Accumulation of this molecule has been associated with hepatotoxicity and nephrotoxicity in animal studies, and the oral formulation is therefore preferred for patients with a creatinine clearance less than 50 mL/min.[54] Due to genetic polymorphism of CYT P-450 and CYP2C19, voriconazole is associated with considerable interpatient and intrapatient drug level variability and, as such, drug level monitoring is advised when treating patients with invasive aspergillosis. Available data suggest that trough concentrations of 1 to 5.5 µg/mL should be targeted.[55] Posaconazole is unique among the triazoles in its activity against mucormycoses, although its role in the management of children with invasive fungal infection remains to be elucidated.

The triazole drugs are relatively well tolerated and have a more favorable side effect profile than amphotericin B. Fluconazole is a potent inhibitor of CYP2CP and CYP3A4, resulting in the potential for significant drug-drug interactions. Serious treatment-related adverse events related to fluconazole use are rare. Voriconazole has been associated with a number of side effects, including photosensitivity rash, transaminase elevation, visual changes, and periostitis. Members of the azole class have the potential to prolong the QT interval and have been associated with torsades de pointes.[56]

Echinocandins

The echinocandins caspofungin, micafungin, and anidula-fungin are structurally similar compounds that work by disrupting the synthesis of 1,3-β-glucan, a polysaccharide component of the fungal cell wall.[57] All three of the available echinocandins offer a similar spectrum of activity and are available only in parenteral form. These agents are fungicidal against most *Candida* spp., fungistatic against molds, like *Aspergillus* spp., and have been shown to have potent in vitro activity against candidal biofilms present on foreign bodies, such as indwelling devices and prostheses.[58] Although *C. parapsilosis* has an intrinsically higher MIC to echinocandins, one recent study found that the initial use of these agents was not associated with clinical failure in patients with *C. parapsilosis* candidemia.[59] Data suggest that the echinocandins are noninferior to, and possibly more efficacious than, fluconazole for the treatment of candidemia and other forms of invasive candidiasis in adults.[60] In fact, a recent patient-level review of randomized trials for the treatment of invasive candidiasis identified receipt of an echinocandin and removal of the central venous catheter as the only two factors associated with improved survival.[61] On the basis of their activity and the emergence of azole-resistant *Candida* species, current clinical practice guidelines suggest that an echinocandin be considered as first-line therapy for neutropenic patients with confirmed or suspected candidemia and for the treatment of candidemia in non-neutropenic hosts with recent azole exposure, whose illness is moderately severe or severe, or who are at high risk of infection due to *C. glabrata* or *C. krusei*.[46] Although not recommended as first-line therapy, caspofungin is FDA approved as salvage treatment for invasive aspergillosis, and there are some clinical data suggesting benefit when used in combination with voriconazole as part of the initial treatment of invasive aspergillosis.[62-64] Importantly, the echinocandins have poor CNS and ocular penetration and should generally be avoided for infections of these spaces. The echinocandins are generally well tolerated, although liver enzyme elevation is occasionally encountered.

Flucytosine

Flucytosine is a pyrimidine analog that interferes with protein synthesis by incorporation into fungal RNA after being converted to 5-FU intracellularly. It is rarely used in pediatrics, owing to its narrow therapeutic index, and is generally reserved as part of combination therapy with amphotericin B for patients with cryptococcal meningitis.[45]

There are few indications for combination antifungal therapy. As previously stated, there may be a benefit to the addition of an echinocandin to voriconazole, particularly in the initial phase of treatment, for patients with invasive aspergillosis. Due to its highly unpredictable susceptibility, it is prudent to treat documented infections due to *Fusarium* spp. with either voriconazole or posaconazole and an amphotericin product while awaiting sensitivities. If *Mucorales* infection is being considered, the addition of an amphotericin product to ongoing triazole therapy is rational.

Antibiotic Resistance
Antibiotic-Resistance Mechanisms

In the ICU, antibiotic use is extensive, resulting in selective pressure for antibiotic-resistant pathogens. Bacteria are capable of surviving in an environment containing antibiotics by the expression of one or more of many different potential antibiotic-resistance mechanisms. The basic mechanisms of resistance can be divided into two broad categories.[65,66] The first is by accumulation of multiple genes, each coding for resistance, that occur typically on resistance (R) plasmids and include (1) alteration of the antibiotic structure by bacterial enzymes, (2) alteration of the antibiotic's target site within the pathogen (by mutation at the binding site or enzymatic alterations of the binding site), or (3) changes in the cell wall that prevent movement of the antibiotic into the organism. The second resistance mechanism occurs by extrusion of the antibiotic from within the organism by efflux pumps. Although community-acquired pathogens most often express only one mechanism of resistance, nosocomial pathogens may express many of these mechanisms simultaneously, and the result is a high degree of antibiotic resistance. In addition, the regulation of resistance gene expression may be altered to allow increased production of the gene product that leads to resistance.

Genes encoding antibiotic resistance may be shared between organisms within a species or between species. The transfer of antibiotic resistance genes by plasmids is a common method by which resistance is shared between bacteria. The description of mobile genetic elements helps explain the rapid development and spread of antibiotic resistance within the pathogens responsible for nosocomial infections.[67] Antibiotic-resistant mutants normally exist at low frequencies in any given population of bacteria. Antibiotic exposure is often the selection pressure allowing these otherwise silent mutants to achieve significant numbers, leading to treatment failure. The clinical expression of antibiotic resistance may involve several different mechanisms operating simultaneously within a pathogen, with each mechanism expressed to a different degree on the basis of the regulation of resistance at a molecular level.

Antibiotic Resistance and Infections in the Pediatric Intensive Care Unit

Current clinical challenges relate to pathogens that display newer resistance patterns. Some ESBL-producing gram-negative pathogens are resistant to extended-spectrum penicillins, as well as third- and fourth-generation cephalosporins, with a proportion of these organisms also demonstrating decreased susceptibility to aminoglycosides, carbapenems, and fluoroquinolones. Outbreaks caused by ESBL-producing *Klebsiella* and *E. coli* have been widely reported.[68] Outbreaks by enteric gram-negative bacilli that carry chromosomal AmpC β-lactamases (present in *Enterobacter, Serratia,* and *Citrobacter*) have been occurring for several years and continue to present challenges.[69] *P. aeruginosa* has always been a nosocomial problem in neonatal ICUs and PICUs.[70] The nonfermenting gram-negative bacteria, including *Stenotrophomonas* and *Acinetobacter* spp., may also cause antibiotic-resistant organism infections, particularly in the immunocompromised child.

Community-acquired MRSA is increasingly a significant pathogen in children.[71] MRSA develops resistance via the mecA gene and detection of the gene predicts failure of treatment with oxacillin. VRE strains have been reported in pediatric hospitals, particularly in neonatal ICUs, in oncology wards, and in patients with gastrointestinal disease. The vancomycin resistance strains have a complex resistance mechanism including six different phenotypes and production of a carboxypeptidese.[18,72]

Antibiotic Therapy for Resistant Pathogens

MRSA is a frequently isolated nosocomial and community-acquired pathogen in PICUs. Almost 60% of catheter-related bloodstream infections in the PICU are caused by gram-positive bacteria.[73] Vancomycin remains the mainstay of treatment for serious MRSA infections. Some data in the adult population suggest that the use of high-dose vancomycin (target serum concentration/minimum inhibitory concentration of ≥ 400 µg/mL) is associated with favorable clinical outcomes. Few pediatric clinical trials have looked at the question of whether alternative antibiotics are superior to vancomycin for MRSA. A pediatric study compared vancomycin with linezolid for the treatment of nosocomial pneumonia, bacteremia, or skin and soft tissue infections; the cure rates were similar.[74] Other newer agents, including daptomycin and ceftaroline, are available, but experience in pediatrics is limited.

The incidence of vancomycin-resistant enterococcal infections is increasing and has been reported to be as high as 75% for *E. faecium* in adult ICUs. Linezolid is a mainstay of treatment; however, resistance to linezolid has been reported. Daptomycin and tigecycline both have excellent activity against VRE, although there is limited pediatric experience to date. A review of pediatric patients with multidrug-resistant gram-positive infection showed that the addition of daptomycin to the treatment regimen resulted in clinical improvement in the majority of patients, and in six of seven patients with persistent bacteremia it resulted in bacteriologic cure.[29]

S. pneumoniae has developed increasing resistance to β-lactam antibiotics, macrolides, and trimethoprim-sulfamethoxazole. For children with suspected pneumococcal meningitis or other life-threatening pneumococcal infections, the addition of vancomycin to either ceftriaxone or cefotaxime has been the standard of care until susceptibility data are available and therapy can be narrowed if appropriate. Other options for therapy of non-CNS infections caused by resistant strains include a newer-generation fluoroquinolone or linezolid.

Antibiotic resistance is increasing in gram-negative organisms. These organisms include ESBL-producing enteric gram-negative bacteria (*Enterobacter, Serratia,* and *Citrobacter*) and multidrug-resistant *Pseudomonas, Stenotrophomonas,* and *Acinetobacter.* Treatment for patients potentially infected with these organisms should be guided by local resistance patterns and antibiograms. Extended- or continuous-infusion dosing strategies with β-lactams such as Zosyn, cefepime, or meropenem for treatment of susceptible *Pseudomonas* strains in critically ill patients optimizes bactericidal exposure[75] and have been associated with improved outcomes.[76] Colistin is also an option for multidrug-resistant gram-negative infections.

Antimicrobial Stewardship

Antibiotic resistance is a challenge in the ICU setting, where there is a constant struggle to maintain balance between appropriate treatment of known life-threatening infection and broad empiric coverage of possible life-threatening infection. Principles have been established and stewardship guidelines for optimizing antimicrobial therapy have been published by a number of organizations, including the Infectious Diseases Society of America, Centers for Disease Control and Prevention, and World Health Organization. It is essential for hospitals to implement oversight and accountability over antimicrobial use as a matter of patient safety. Two broad interventional strategies for antimicrobial stewardship programs (ASPs) exist. One is the prospective audit and feedback program whereby ongoing review of antibiotic utilization and recommendations for adjustments are made to providers. A second strategy uses preauthorization in which antimicrobials are restricted by the institution and must be justified and approved at the time of use. Many ASPs are a blend of both strategies with an integration of supplemental programs such as formulary interventions, dose optimization, educational efforts, computer-assisted decision support, and adaptation of local published guidelines.[77]

With the move toward computerized provider order entry as the standard of care, there are ways to leverage computerized decision support for appropriate antimicrobial selection on the basis of diagnosis and local susceptibility profiles and dose optimization integrating patient characteristics such as renal function, allergies, and potential drug interactions while preserving clinical judgment and physician autonomy.

Ideally, outcomes should be measured such as antimicrobial consumption (days of therapy per 1000 patient days) or antimicrobial days of therapy to assess safety and cost effectiveness of ASPs. The ICU is an ideal environment for implementation of antimicrobial stewardship because of the intense use of antimicrobials and existence of significant drug resistance.

Summary

As medical care becomes more sophisticated and children with critical illness are hospitalized for longer periods receiving specialty or invasive therapies, the risk of development of complicated infections caused by multidrug-resistant pathogens increases. The physician is constantly being challenged to deliver effective antimicrobial therapy, while at the same time preventing the selection of resistance. Knowledge of the pathogens most likely to be present and the potential resistance mechanisms in these organisms is important in selecting empiric antimicrobial therapy. An appropriate collection of cultures to obtain susceptibility information on the pathogens is crucial to optimize subsequent therapy and minimize resistance.

Key References

1. Howard DH, Scott RD 2nd, Packard R, Jones D. The global impact of drug resistance. *Clin Infect Dis.* 2003;36(suppl 1):S4-S10.
2. Garcia CMG. Antibacterial therapeutic agents. In: Cherry J, Demmler-Harrison G, Kaplan S, Steinbach W, eds. *Feigin and CHerry's Textbook of Pediatric Infecgtions Diseases.* 7th ed. Philadelphia: Saunders Elsevier; 2014.
3. Bradley JS. Antimicrobial agents. In: Long S, Pickering L, Prober C, eds. *Principles and Practice of Pediatric Infectious Diseases.* 4th ed. Philadelphia: Saunders Elsevier; 2012:1453-1484.
6. Ibrahim EH, Sherman G, Ward S, et al. The influence of inadequate antimicrobial treatment of bloodstream infections on patient outcomes in the ICU setting. *Chest.* 2000;118:146-155.
7. Iregui M, Ward S, Sherman G, et al. Clinical importance of delays in the initiation of appropriate antibiotic treatment for ventilator-associated pneumonia. *Chest.* 2002;122:262-268.

9. Abdul-Aziz MH, Lipman J, Mouton JW, et al. Applying pharmacokinetic/pharmacodynamic principles in critically ill patients: optimizing efficacy and reducing resistance development. *Semin Respir Crit Care Med.* 2015;36:136-153.

10. Hochreiter M, Kohler T, Schweiger AM, et al. Procalcitonin to guide duration of antibiotic therapy in intensive care patients: a randomized prospective controlled trial. *Crit Care.* 2009;13:R83.

11. Koch AL. Penicillin binding proteins, beta-lactams, and lactamases: offensives, attacks, and defensive countermeasures. *Crit Rev Microbiol.* 2000;26:205-220.

14. Zappitelli M, Moffett BS, Hyder A, Goldstein SL. Acute kidney injury in non-critically ill children treated with aminoglycoside antibiotics in a tertiary healthcare centre: a retrospective cohort study. *Nephrol Dial Transplant.* 2011;26:144-150.

15. Tamma PD, Turnbull AE, Harris AD, et al. Less is more: combination antibiotic therapy for the treatment of gram-negative bacteremia in pediatric patients. *JAMA Pediatr.* 2013;167:903-910.

16. Sick AC, Tschudin-Sutter S, Turnbull AE, et al. Empiric combination therapy for gram-negative bacteremia. *Pediatrics.* 2014;133:e1148-e1155.

17. Ibrahim SL, Zhang L, Brady TM, et al. Low-dose Gentamicin for uncomplicated *Enterococcus faecalis* bacteremia may be nephrotoxic in children. *Clin Infect Dis.* 2015;61:1119-1124.

18. Gray JW, George RH. Experience of vancomycin-resistant enterococci in a children's hospital. *J Hosp Infect.* 2000;45:11-18.

19. Chang S, Sievert DM, Hageman JC, et al. Infection with vancomycin-resistant *Staphylococcus aureus* containing the vanA resistance gene. *N Engl J Med.* 2003;348:1342-1347.

21. Beigelman A, Gunsten S, Mikols CL, et al. Azithromycin attenuates airway inflammation in a noninfectious mouse model of allergic asthma. *Chest.* 2009;136:498-506.

22. Jafri HS, McCracken GH Jr. Fluoroquinolones in paediatrics. *Drugs.* 1999;58(suppl 2):43-48.

24. Marcinak JF, Frank AL. Treatment of community-acquired methicillin-resistant *Staphylococcus aureus* in children. *Curr Opin Infect Dis.* 2003;16:265-269.

26. Garnacho-Montero J, Escoresca-Ortega A, Fernandez-Delgado E. Antibiotic de-escalation in the ICU: how is it best done? *Curr Opin Infect Dis.* 2015;28:193-198.

27. Falagas ME, Sideri G, Vouloumanou EK, et al. Intravenous colistimethate (colistin) use in critically ill children without cystic fibrosis. *Pediatr Infect Dis J.* 2009;28:123-127.

29. Ardura MI, Mejias A, Katz KS, et al. Daptomycin therapy for invasive gram-positive bacterial infections in children. *Pediatr Infect Dis J.* 2007;26:1128-1132.

30. Blyth CC, Palasanthiran P, O'Brien TA. Antifungal therapy in children with invasive fungal infections: a systematic review. *Pediatrics.* 2007;119:772-784.

31. Wisplinghoff H, Seifert H, Tallent SM, et al. Nosocomial bloodstream infections in pediatric patients in United States hospitals: epidemiology, clinical features and susceptibilities. *Pediatr Infect Dis J.* 2003;22:686-691.

32. Zaoutis TE, Prasad PA, Localio AR, et al. Risk factors and predictors for candidemia in pediatric intensive care unit patients: implications for prevention. *Clin Infect Dis.* 2010;51:e38-e45.

33. Klatte JM, Newland JG, Jackson MA. Incidence, classification, and risk stratification for *Candida* central line-associated bloodstream infections in pediatric patients at a tertiary care children's hospital, 2000-2010. *Infect Control Hosp Epidemiol.* 2013;34:1266-1271.

34. Clancy CJ, Nguyen MH. Finding the "missing 50%" of invasive candidiasis: how nonculture diagnostics will improve understanding of disease spectrum and transform patient care. *Clin Infect Dis.* 2013;56:1284-1292.

35. Zaoutis TE, Heydon K, Chu JH, et al. Epidemiology, outcomes, and costs of invasive aspergillosis in immunocompromised children in the United States, 2000. *Pediatrics.* 2006;117:e711-e716.

38. Villarroel M, Aviles CL, Silva P, et al. Risk factors associated with invasive fungal disease in children with cancer and febrile neutropenia: a prospective multicenter evaluation. *Pediatr Infect Dis J.* 2010;29:816-821.

39. Frange P, Bougnoux ME, Lanternier F, et al. An update on pediatric invasive aspergillosis. *Med Mal Infect.* 2015;45:189-198.

40. Walsh TJ, Anaissie EJ, Denning DW, et al. Treatment of aspergillosis: clinical practice guidelines of the Infectious Diseases Society of America. *Clin Infect Dis.* 2008;46:327-360.

42. Desai R, Ross LA, Hoffman JA. The role of bronchoalveolar lavage galactomannan in the diagnosis of pediatric invasive aspergillosis. *Pediatr Infect Dis J.* 2009;28:283-286.

44. Godet C, Goudet V, Laurent F, et al. Nebulised liposomal amphotericin B for *Aspergillus* lung diseases: case series and literature review. *Mycoses.* 2015;58:173-180.

46. Pappas PG, Kauffman CA, Andes D, et al. Clinical practice guidelines for the management of candidiasis: 2009 update by the Infectious Diseases Society of America. *Clin Infect Dis.* 2009;48:503-535.

55. Park WB, Kim NH, Kim KH, et al. The effect of therapeutic drug monitoring on safety and efficacy of voriconazole in invasive fungal infections: a randomized controlled trial. *Clin Infect Dis.* 2012;55:1080-1087.

56. Zeuli JD, Wilson JW, Estes LL. Effect of combined fluoroquinolone and azole use on QT prolongation in hematology patients. *Antimicrob Agents Chemother.* 2013;57:1121-1127.

57. Perlin DS. Echinocandin resistance, susceptibility testing and prophylaxis: implications for patient management. *Drugs.* 2014;74:1573-1585.

58. Bachmann SP, VandeWalle K, Ramage G, et al. In vitro activity of caspofungin against *Candida albicans* biofilms. *Antimicrob Agents Chemother.* 2002;46:3591-3596.

62. McCormack PL, Perry CM. Caspofungin: a review of its use in the treatment of fungal infections. *Drugs.* 2005;65:2049-2068.

64. Marr KA, Schlamm HT, Herbrecht R, et al. Combination antifungal therapy for invasive aspergillosis: a randomized trial. *Ann Intern Med.* 2015;162:81-89.

65. Nikaido H. Multidrug resistance in bacteria. *Annu Rev Biochem.* 2009;78:119-146.

66. Schmitz FFA. Mechanisms of antibacterial resistance. In: Cohen JOS, Powderly WG, eds. *Infectious Diseases.* 3rd ed. Philadelphia: Elsevier; 2010:1308-1322.

68. Kim YK, Pai H, Lee HJ, et al. Bloodstream infections by extended-spectrum beta-lactamase-producing *Escherichia coli* and *Klebsiella pneumoniae* in children: epidemiology and clinical outcome. *Antimicrob Agents Chemother.* 2002;46:1481-1491.

71. Hussain FM, Boyle-Vavra S, Bethel CD, Daum RS. Current trends in community-acquired methicillin-resistant *Staphylococcus aureus* at a tertiary care pediatric facility. *Pediatr Infect Dis J.* 2000;19:1163-1166.

73. Smith MJ. Catheter-related bloodstream infections in children. *Am J Infect Control.* 2008;36:S173e1-S173e3.

74. Kaplan SL, Deville JG, Yogev R, et al. Linezolid versus vancomycin for treatment of resistant gram-positive infections in children. *Pediatr Infect Dis J.* 2003;22:677-686.

75. Courter JD, Kuti JL, Girotto JE, Nicolau DP. Optimizing bactericidal exposure for beta-lactams using prolonged and continuous infusions in the pediatric population. *Pediatr Blood Cancer.* 2009;53:379-385.

77. Owens RC Jr. Antimicrobial stewardship: application in the intensive care unit. *Infect Dis Clin North Am.* 2009;23:683-702.

Life-Threatening Viral Diseases and Their Treatment

Surabhi B. Vora, Alpana Waghmare, Danielle M. Zerr, and Ann J. Melvin

PEARLS

- An astute clinician will obtain serum to store for future serologic testing when viral pathogens are considered as the potential cause of a critical illness.
- Diagnostic sensitivity is generally enhanced when samples for viral culture and staining are sent as early as possible in the course of illness.
- In general, current treatment for most viral infections is supportive with antiviral therapy generally limited to herpes viruses.
- When herpes simplex virus encephalitis or neonatal disease is suspected, empiric treatment with acyclovir must be rapidly initiated.
- Parainfluenza and influenza viruses are often associated with bacterial coinfections.
- To prevent spread of infection to staff and other patients, appropriate infection control precautions should be initiated early when viral pathogens are suspected.

Viral infections are a frequent cause of disease in individuals of all ages. In general, the spectrum of illness is varied; young or immunosuppressed children are at higher risk of having severe disease. This chapter discusses viral illnesses commonly seen in the intensive care unit: myocarditis, hepatitis, pneumonitis, and meningitis/encephalitis. The content provides the reader with guidance for the initial management of patients infected with viral pathogens, with a particular emphasis on diagnosis and therapy.

Myocarditis
Background

Myocarditis accounts for approximately 0.05% of pediatric hospital discharges in the United States.[1,2] Although many infectious and noninfectious causes have been identified, viruses account for most cases.[3] The spectrum of disease is varied, and myocardial involvement may be focal or diffuse.[4] Thus establishing a definitive diagnosis can be difficult, and as a result, the true incidence of viral myocarditis is unknown.

Pathogenesis

Although the pathogenesis of viral myocarditis is not well understood, viruses appear to enter cardiac myocytes through specific receptors, and myocardial damage is thought to occur, at least in part, as a direct result of infection, with active viral replication leading to myocardial necrosis.[5] In addition, both humoral and cellular immune responses contribute to the pathogenesis of myocarditis,[6] through postinfectious autoimmune processes,[7] cytotoxic T lymphocytes, antibody-dependent cell-mediated cytotoxicity,[8] and cytokines.[9] With persistent viremia and the accompanying immune response, progression to dilated cardiomyopathy may occur.[10] Up to 27% of dilated cardiomyopathy in children may be attributable to viral myocarditis.[11]

Etiology

Polymerase chain reaction (PCR) of cardiac tissue from endomyocardial biopsy specimens in 34 children with a clinical diagnosis of myocarditis identified adenovirus in 44%, enterovirus in 24%, and herpes simplex virus (HSV) in 6%.[12] A shift has been noted toward parvovirus B19 and parechovirus.[4] Many other viruses have caused myocarditis in children, including influenza A, human immunodeficiency virus (HIV), cytomegalovirus (CMV), respiratory syncytial virus (RSV), and the mumps and measles viruses, before the widespread use of the measles-mumps-rubella (MMR) vaccine (Table 108.1).

Clinical Presentation

The clinical presentation of myocarditis can range from asymptomatic to acute fulminant disease with cardiovascular collapse. Infants with myocarditis may have nonspecific symptoms including poor feeding, fever, apnea, and listlessness. Physical findings may be consistent with congestive heart failure. Enteroviral myocarditis in infancy frequently occurs in conjunction with hepatitis or pneumonitis[13] and can be difficult to distinguish from bacterial sepsis. Severe dysrhythmias have been described in infants with myocardial involvement from RSV.[14] Older children and adolescents are more likely to present after a prodromal viral illness with nonspecific respiratory or gastrointestinal symptoms, usually without chest pain or cardiac symptoms, and thus diagnosis is often delayed.[15] Resting tachycardia disproportionate to the height of fever is common, and an apical systolic murmur may be heard. A subset of patients have fulminant myocarditis,

TABLE 108.1   Viral Etiologies of Myocarditis, Fulminant Hepatitis, Pneumonia, Meningitis, Encephalitis, and Myelitis

	Myocarditis	Liver Failure	Pneumonia	Meningitis	Encephalitis	Myelitis
Adenovirus	XXX	X[1]	XX	X	X	X
Arboviruses (arthropod-borne viruses)				XX	XX	
Western equine encephalitis virus				X	X	
Eastern equine encephalitis virus					X	
St. Louis encephalitis virus				X	X	
California encephalitis virus (La Crosse)				X	X	
Colorado tick fever				X	X	
West Nile encephalitis virus					X	
Coronaviruses (OC43, 229E, HKU1, NL63, and SARS)			XX			
Enteroviruses	XXX	X	X	XXX	XX	XX
Hantavirus			X			
Hepatitis A		XXX				X
Hepatitis B		X				
Hepatitis C		X				
Hepatitis D		X				
Hepatitis E		X				
Herpesviruses						
CMV	X	X	XXX[1]		X	XX
EBV	X	XX		X	X	XX
HSV I and II	X	X[2]	X[1]	XX	XX	X
HHV-6	X	X	X[1]		X	
VZV		X[1]	XX[1]	X	X	X
HIV	X				X	
HTLV					X	
Influenza A	X		XXX		X	X
Influenza B			X			
JC virus					X[1]	
Lymphocytic choriomeningitis virus				X	X	X
Measles	X		X		X	
Metapneumovirus			XX			
Mumps	X			X	X	X
Parechoviruses[2]	XX	X	X	XXX	XXX	
Parainfluenza virus types 1, 2, 3			XXX			
Parvovirus B19[3]	XX					
Rabies					X	
RSV	X		XXX			
Rhinovirus			X			
Rubella					X	X

XXX, Most frequent; *XX*, frequent; *X*, less common or rare.
[1]Primarily in immunocompromised hosts.
[2]Primarily neonates and young infants.
[3]Viruses detected in myocardial biopsies appear to have shifted over the past few decades. (Cooper LT Jr. Myocarditis. N Engl J Med. 2009;360:1526-1538.)

characterized by rapid onset of symptoms, severe hemodynamic compromise, and fever.[16] Myocarditis has also been implicated in cases of sudden death.[17,18]

Laboratory abnormalities may include elevated white blood cell count, erythrocyte sedimentation rate,[19] and serum aspartate aminotransferase (AST) levels.[15,20] Cardiac troponin I and T are measures of cardiac muscle injury, which may be useful in myocarditis. Sensitivity of cardiac troponin T in children with myocarditis ranges from 71% to 100% with a specificity of 85% to 86%.[10,21,22]

Acute Liver Failure
Background

Acute liver failure (ALF) in children is defined as severe impairment of liver function with or without encephalopathy that occurs in a child with no history of chronic liver disease.[23] The causes of ALF in children can be metabolic, toxic, drug related, immune mediated, or infectious. The percentage of ALF caused by viral infections varies significantly by age and geographic location, with viral causes identified in 6% to 20% of pediatric ALF in series from North America and Europe[23-25] but 50% to 60% in other regions.[26-28]

Etiology

Although less than 1% of infections due to hepatitis A and B (HAV and HAB, respectively) result in ALF, these viruses constitute the majority of cases of ALF with a definitive viral diagnosis.[26,28-30] Although most perinatally acquired infections with HBV are asymptomatic, infants born to women with both hepatitis B surface antigen (HBsAg) and anti-hepatitis B envelope antibody (HBeAb) appear to be at risk for ALF.[31] Although rare, there are case reports of ALF with both postnatally and perinatally acquired hepatitis C virus (HCV) in children.[24,32,33] Other viruses identified in several pediatric series of ALF include adenovirus, CMV, enterovirus, HSV, Epstein-Barr virus (EBV), human herpesvirus 6 (HHV-6), parvovirus B19,[23-25,34] varicella-zoster virus (VZV),[35,36] influenza,[37,38] and hepatitis E, an enterically transmitted virus that causes epidemic hepatitis in many areas of the world, particularly in Asia.[39,40] ALF can also occur in severe dengue[41] and yellow fever infections[42]; though uncommon in the United States, these entities should be considered with the appropriate epidemiologic risk factors.

ALF in infants is most likely to be associated with systemic illness due to enterovirus, echovirus, HSV, or CMV.[23,30,43-46] Immune suppression is a risk factor for HSV-, CMV-, adenovirus-, and VZV-associated ALF.

Clinical Presentation

Symptoms of acute hepatitis include jaundice, anorexia, fatigue, nausea, and vomiting.[23,47] In fulminant disease, there is rapid progression to hepatic failure and encephalopathy. Physical examination may demonstrate fever, hepatosplenomegaly with liver tenderness, scleral or cutaneous icterus, and mucosal bleeding. Patients with severe vomiting may have significant dehydration. Laboratory studies include elevated hepatic enzymes (10- to 100-fold increases in aspartate aminotransferase [AST] and alanine aminotransferase [ALT]), hyperbilirubinemia, prolonged prothrombin time, and elevated ammonia levels. As hepatocyte necrosis

progresses, hepatic enzyme levels may decrease and hepatomegaly may resolve. Renal failure is a common complication of ALF,[47,48] whereas cerebral edema is commonly found in the subset of patients with severe encephalopathy.[23,47]

Viral Pneumonia/Pneumonitis
Background

Influenza and pneumonia combined are a leading cause of death globally. A greater burden of disease is present in infants, young children, and older individuals.[49] Although associated with only 20% to 50% of community-acquired pneumonias in adults,[50-52] viruses account for the majority of lower respiratory infections in children. In 2010, 14.9 million episodes of severe, acute lower respiratory infection (ALRI) resulted in hospital admissions in children <5 years worldwide.[53] In the United States, the annual incidence of pneumonia is estimated to be 15.7 cases per 10,000 children, with the highest rate among children <2 years of age (62.2 cases per 10,000 children) with an estimated 66% of these hospitalizations attributable to viral etiologies.[54]

Etiology

The etiologic agents of viral pneumonia are varied (see Table 108.1). RSV is the primary cause of hospitalization for respiratory tract illness in young children.[55] In a national surveillance study, most children with RSV infection had no coexisting medical conditions or characteristics that identified them as being at significantly greater risk for severe RSV disease, except for being <2 years of age.[55] Repeat infections are common. In the healthy host, infections are localized to the upper respiratory tract. Among immunocompromised patients, however, RSV infections can progress to fatal pneumonia, with the greatest mortality risk in patients with severe lower tract disease and in those who do not receive treatment.[56,57]

Influenza epidemics occur annually with significant morbidity and death in young children and older individuals. The highest rate of hospitalization occurs in the 0 to 5-month age group.[58] Since 2004, the total annual number of reported pediatric influenza deaths has ranged from 37 to 358, peaking with the 2009 H1N1 pandemic.[59] Among immunocompromised patients, risk factors for more severe disease include lymphopenia and infection early after hematopoietic stem cell transplant.[60] These patients have more complications, longer viral shedding, and more antiviral resistance while demonstrating fewer clinical symptoms and signs.[61]

In 2009, the emergence of a pandemic H1N1 strain of influenza A led to a greatly increased burden of influenza disease worldwide. Unlike seasonal influenza, children and young adults were at a disproportionate risk for infection and hospitalization; 60% of infections occurred in those <18 years of age.[62-64] The 2009 pandemic H1N1 strain continues to circulate with seasonal influenza globally.

Parainfluenza viruses (PIVs) are also significant causes of lower respiratory infection in children and immunocompromised patients.[65-68] PIVs account for 50% of hospitalizations for acute laryngotracheitis (croup) and at least 15% of cases of bronchiolitis and pneumonia. PIV types 1 and 2 cause more cases of croup, whereas PIV type 3 is more likely to infect the small air passages and cause pneumonia or bronchiolitis. However, any PIV can cause lower respiratory tract disease, particularly during primary infection or in immunocompromised hosts. In the latter, PIV pneumonia has a 30-day attributable mortality rate of >30%.[67,69,70] Unlike RSV, copathogens may be identified with PIV pneumonia more than 50% of the time[67]; therefore in high-risk patients, management should include workup and treatment for these other agents.

Other respiratory viruses that can cause pneumonia, particularly in young children and immunocompromised hosts, include human metapneumovirus (HMPV), adenovirus, human rhinoviruses (HRVs), and human coronaviruses (HCoVs). Since it was first described in 2001,[71] HMPV has been shown to be a common cause of croup, bronchiolitis, and pneumonia in children, the elderly, and immunocompromised patients.[72-80] The clinical manifestations of HMPV are indistinguishable from RSV. Adenovirus pneumonia can occur as an isolated event or as part of disseminated disease. Risk factors for adenovirus pneumonia include compromised immune function, chronic underlying respiratory or cardiac disease, and age <7 years.[54,81] HRVs occasionally cause lower respiratory tract disease requiring admission to intensive care among pediatric and immunosuppressed patients, although a causative role is sometimes difficult to define because HRVs frequently occur in association with copathogens.[82-87] Among pediatric patients, a new species of rhinovirus (HRV-C) has been discovered that may cause more severe disease than HRV-A or HRV-B, although this association is not yet clearly elucidated.[88-93] In 2014, enterovirus-D68 was associated with an outbreak of severe respiratory illness and potentially acute flaccid paralysis in children and immunocompromised adults in North America[94-98]; however, the impact of this pathogen in future seasons remains unknown.

The HCoV family includes several viruses that are known to infect humans. The severe acute respiratory syndrome (SARS) outbreak originated in China in the fall of 2002 and was characterized by a life-threatening, atypical pneumonia caused by a novel coronavirus (SARS-CoV)[99] and spread by close contact with infected humans, mostly to household contacts and health care workers. The Middle East respiratory syndrome-CoV (MERS-CoV) first emerged in the Arabian Peninsula in 2012. Since then, travel-associated cases have been found in a number of countries outside the region.[100] In adults, the fatality rate is estimated to be 40%,[101] but data in pediatric patients are limited. Asymptomatic infection is common, but disease may be severe in patients with underlying medical conditions.[102] For both SARS and MERS, updates to the case definition, epidemiology, and current management guidelines can be found at www.cdc.gov. Other HCoVs have been reported to cause pneumonia in children and immunocompromised patients treated for hematologic malignancies.[103-108]

Although CMV usually causes relatively benign disease in immunocompetent hosts, it is frequently severe and often fatal in immunocompromised hosts, including patients with acquired immunodeficiency syndrome (AIDS), malignancy, congenital immune deficiencies, and transplant recipients. Among allogeneic stem cell transplant recipients, the risk of CMV pneumonia is high. With the introduction of routine antiviral prophylaxis and preemptive therapy strategies, CMV disease during the first 3 months after hematopoietic stem cell transplantation has been reduced from 20% to 30% to less than 5% in most studies, and CMV disease now primarily occurs late after transplant.[109] Risk factors for late CMV disease

include primary infection or reactivation of CMV during the early period after transplant and therapy for graft-versus-host disease.[110] Among solid organ transplant recipients, the risk of CMV disease is greatest for lung transplant recipients, followed by liver, heart, and renal transplant recipients.[111,112]

Hantaviruses are known for causing hemorrhagic fevers and acute severe respiratory infection in young adults and are spread among mammals by exposure to aerosolized feces, infected urine, or other secretions. Though rare in the United States, hantaviruses can cause severe disease with high mortality by causing leakage of plasma and erythrocytes through the vascular endothelium in the lung (hantavirus pulmonary syndrome [HPS]) or the kidneys (hemorrhagic fever with renal syndrome [HFRS]).[113,114] Supportive care, including early consideration of extracorporeal membrane oxygenation (ECMO), is crucial to successful treatment of patients with HPS.

Clinical Presentation

The clinical presentation of viral pneumonia/pneumonitis usually consists of fever, increased respiratory rate, cough, and increased work of breathing, with grunting, flaring, retracting, and use of accessory muscles in infants and young children. Decreased oral intake with increased insensible loss due to the tachypnea may lead to dehydration. Some patients have centrally mediated apnea, and other patients have an overwhelming sepsis-like syndrome, especially young infants. Rhinorrhea, conjunctivitis, otitis media, and previous exposure to an ill child or adult should raise suspicion of a viral cause. However, many patients with influenza pneumonia have no preceding upper respiratory illness. Radiographic findings generally include evidence of hyperinflation and peribronchial cuffing, and a focal or diffuse infiltrate may or may not be present. Bacterial coinfection may appear after, or concomitantly with, the viral infection.

Central Nervous System Infections
Background

Aseptic meningitis, encephalitis, and myelitis are inflammatory conditions of the central nervous system (CNS), involving the meninges, brain, and spinal cord, respectively. Disease is caused by a variety of infectious pathogens, but viruses cause most disease. Viruses gain entry to the CNS via the bloodstream (enteroviruses and arboviruses) or by direct neuronal spread (HSV and rabies). Pathogenesis may involve direct viral invasion or a vigorous virus-specific immune response resulting in damage to neurons, oligodendroglia, or the myelin components. In the latter case, disease may follow an upper respiratory tract or other infection and primarily take the form of a demyelinating process. This disease is commonly termed postinfectious encephalomyelitis or acute disseminated encephalomyelitis.

Individuals of all ages are at risk for CNS viral infections. However, neonates, older individuals, and those with immune deficiencies are prone to more frequent and serious infections.

Etiology

Potential viral causes are multiple; enteroviruses, herpesviruses, and arboviruses are responsible for most disease (see Table 108.1). Enteroviruses account for up to 99% of cases of aseptic meningitis when a cause is identified.[115] Enterovirus meningitis in older children and adults is typically self-limited and associated with few complications. In contrast, in neonates these infections may mimic bacterial sepsis and CNS involvement is often manifested as encephalitis. Parechovirus, another cause of meningoencephalitis in neonates, is a close relative of enteroviruses and clinical manifestations are similar.[116] Specific enterovirus strains, such as enterovirus D-68 and enterovirus 71, may cause acute flaccid paralysis (associated with anterior myelitis) in children.[96,117]

HSV is a common cause of CNS infection in all ages. During the neonatal period, HSV, especially type 2, can cause encephalitis due to vertical transmission of the virus.[118] In contrast, in older children and adults, most HSV encephalitis is caused by type 1. HSV-2, however, can cause benign aseptic meningitis in association with primary and recurrent genital infections.[119] Other members of the herpesvirus family (CMV, EBV, VZV, and HHV-6) can also cause aseptic meningitis and encephalitis. CMV encephalitis occurs most often in immunosuppressed individuals.[120,121] EBV aseptic meningitis and encephalitis present with or without the classic findings of infectious mononucleosis.[122] Acute cerebellar ataxia is a common and usually benign complication of VZV infection.[123,124] VZV encephalitis may occur following or preceding varicella or zoster and can be complicated by small or large vessel vasculitis (granulomatous arteritis), which carries the potentially serious consequence of infarction.[123-126] HHV-6 encephalitis is rare in healthy children,[127] but HHV6 is the most common cause of encephalitis in patients undergoing hematopoietic stem cell transplantation, and those receiving cord blood transplantations are at especially high risk.[128]

Arboviruses (arthropod-spread viruses) are important causes of aseptic meningitis and encephalitis.[129] The specific arbovirus determines the epidemiology, morbidity, and risk of death of associated disease. The La Crosse and St. Louis encephalitis viruses account for most arboviral CNS infections in the United States. The La Crosse virus is found mainly in the Midwest; infection typically occurs in the summer and early fall and is associated with a relatively low mortality rate. The St. Louis encephalitis virus occurs in every state but is more common in the Midwest, Florida, and Texas and has been responsible for large urban outbreaks.[130,131] Eastern equine virus occurs less frequently, and mainly in the Northeast and Southeast, but carries high rates of morbidity and death.[132,133] West Nile virus encephalitis first appeared in the United States in the summer of 1999 in New York State[134] and has subsequently moved across the United States. Most individuals infected with the West Nile virus are asymptomatic or experience flulike illness; however, older individuals and those with underlying immune deficiency may develop encephalitis that could be fatal. Acute flaccid paralysis has also been associated with West Nile virus infection.[135]

Influenza has not traditionally been considered a common cause of encephalitis; however, the 2009 H1N1 influenza A pandemic challenged this thinking. Studies in both the United States[136] and Australia[137] demonstrated that 1% to 2% of individuals with 2009 H1N1 influenza had encephalitis/encephalopathy. Children, especially those with underlying neurologic disease, appeared to be at higher risk of neurologic manifestation than adults.

Lymphocytic choriomeningitis virus (LCMV) is an infrequently recognized cause of meningoencephalitis. Disease in humans arises after exposure to the urine, droppings, and saliva of infected rodents.[138] Symptoms may last for several weeks, but most patients fully recover. Measles and mumps are two vaccine-preventable causes of encephalitis. Though now rare, mumps virus accounted for a large proportion of aseptic meningitis and encephalitis cases in the United States in the prevaccine era.[139,140] Poor vaccination coverage has the potential to lead to outbreaks and increased number of cases of encephalitis. A report of a measles outbreak in Germany exemplifies this point.[141]

Postinfectious encephalomyelitis refers to an acute self-limited demyelinating process most commonly following viral respiratory infections and varicella. In contrast, subacute sclerosing panencephalitis (SSPE) and progressive multifocal leukoencephalopathy (PML) are rare, chronic, usually fatal, demyelinating diseases due to measles and John Cunningham (JC) virus, respectively. SSPE most commonly follows 5 to 10 years after natural measles infection and may occur as often as one case per a population of 10,000 in areas of the world where the MMR vaccine is not widely used.[142] HIV may cause encephalopathy or may also be associated with certain opportunistic infections such as JC virus. Transverse myelitis has been most frequently associated with enteroviruses; however, VZV,[143,144] CMV, influenza A,[145] and HAV[145] have also been reported as causes, even in immunocompetent individuals.

Historic clues and physical findings can be helpful in focusing the search for an etiologic agent. Travel or residence in areas where arboviruses are endemic during the appropriate season for arthropod transmission should raise suspicion for arboviruses. Enteroviral diseases are also more prevalent during summer and fall months. History of a mother with recent viral illness should raise suspicion of enterovirus in a neonate. Chronic encephalitis/meningitis due to enteroviruses can occur in individuals with agammaglobulinemia. VZV encephalitis and myelitis typically follow chickenpox or zoster by weeks to months and commonly occur in older individuals or those with immunosuppression.[146] History of exposure to a bat in the appropriate clinical setting should raise the concern for rabies.

Clinical Presentation

The classic clinical presentation of viral meningitis is characterized by acute onset of fever, headache, photophobia, vomiting, and nuchal rigidity. A more chronic presentation might indicate enteroviral disease in an immunosuppressed host, whereas recurrent aseptic meningitis can be associated with HSV-2. Encephalitis is characterized by acute onset of fever and depressed consciousness, focal neurologic findings, and seizures. A chronic progressive presentation might indicate more unusual causes, such as PML and SSPE. Transverse myelitis is characterized by an abrupt onset of weakness of the limbs progressing to flaccid paralysis. Diminished deep tendon reflexes progress to nonexistent, and there is associated sensory deficit.

Cerebrospinal fluid (CSF) findings in aseptic meningitis typically include a normal glucose level, a normal to slightly elevated protein level, and a pleocytosis, of up to 1000 cells/μL. Though the pleocytosis is classically monocytic, there can be an initial predominance of polymorphonuclear cells in the first 48 hours of illness.[147] The results of brain computed tomography (CT) and magnetic resonance imaging (MRI) studies are usually normal in viral meningitis. In general, MRI is the more sensitive study for detecting acute encephalitis. Early findings include edema with minimal contrast enhancement. As disease progresses, edema and enhancement become more obvious and may be accompanied by mass effect, hemorrhagic changes, and necrosis. As the inflammation resolves, atrophy may become prominent. In HSV, CNS imaging findings often first involve the temporal lobes with subsequent spread to other areas. Changes can ultimately progress to atrophy, multicystic encephalomalacia, and gyriform high attenuation, especially in children.[49,148] Neurodevelopmental outcomes correlated with MRI abnormalities in one study.[149] In postinfectious encephalomyelitis, lesions may be seen throughout the CNS and primarily involve the white matter, although gray matter may also be involved.

Exotic Viral Diseases

With the increase in foreign travel and the threat of bioterrorism, the potential to treat a child with an exotic viral disease exists. The relevant pathogens include Andes virus, B virus, monkeypox, and the hemorrhagic fever viruses (Ebola, Marburg, Lassa, Crimean-Congo, Argentine, and Bolivian). If one of these agents is suspected, the patient should be isolated and infection control and public health authorities should be notified immediately.[150-152]

Although a full discussion of these agents is beyond the scope of this chapter, two pathogens deserve mention, given the 2014–2015 Ebola outbreak in West Africa and the emerging threat of the chikungunya virus. Like adult patients with Ebola virus disease, children often present with a history of abrupt onset of nonspecific symptoms and signs, such as fever, malaise, headache, myalgias, and abdominal pain.[153] As the illness progresses, vomiting and diarrhea often develop and may lead to significant fluid loss and dehydration. Patients with severe disease are commonly hypotensive and have electrolyte imbalances leading to shock and multiorgan failure, sometimes accompanied by hemorrhage.[154]

Chikungunya has caused large outbreaks in Asia and Africa, and the Caribbean has been experiencing a heavy burden of disease.[155] This mosquito-borne infection typically presents with high fever, headache, photophobia, myalgias, and arthralgias, which can be severe. A maculopapular rash may also occur. In some patients, disabling arthralgias may persist for years.

Diagnosing Viral Disease

There are five primary methods to diagnose a viral infection: (1) observation of characteristic cytopathic effect in cell culture, (2) assays that link specific antibodies to the viral antigens (complement fixation, neutralization, immunofluorescence assays, enzyme-linked immunosorbent assay), (3) microscopic identification of viral inclusion bodies, (4) serologic detection of an early antibody (immunoglobulin M [IgM]) or a fourfold or higher rise in IgG antibody titers between an acute phase and (at least 10 to 14 days later) convalescent phase serum, and (5) molecular techniques that amplify target viral DNA or RNA.

If a viral cause is suspected, acute-phase serum should be held for later interpretation. It is critical that this specimen is drawn before administration of intravenous immunoglobulin (IVIG) or blood products. Samples for viral cultures and PCR testing should be collected from the appropriate sites with specific swabs, as both cotton and wood inhibit viral growth and may contain substances that inhibit the enzymes used in PCR. Nasal washes/swabs and swabs of the base of a vesicle or ulcer (for VZV, HSV) should include good cellular content, to improve the sensitivity of the assay. Table 108.2 outlines appropriate samples and testing for a number of specific viral pathogens.

Myocarditis

Electrocardiographic abnormalities are almost always present in acute myocarditis (93%–100%)[15]; findings include sinus tachycardia, low-voltage QRS complexes, and nonspecific ST and T wave changes. Both atrial and ventricular arrhythmias may be present as well as conduction abnormalities. Echocardiography reveals left ventricular dysfunction, in most cases with either segmental wall motion abnormalities or global hypokinesis. Pericardial effusions are common. Pulmonary edema, enlarged cardiac silhouette, and prominent pulmonary vasculature may be seen on a chest radiograph.

Contrast-enhanced cardiac MRI can define the location and extent of inflammation and be used to assist in diagnosis or to guide endomyocardial biopsy.[156] In a setting where myocarditis is clinically suspected, a consensus group proposed the following diagnostic criteria utilizing cardiac MRI: myocardial edema (regional or global increase in T2 signal), hyperemia or capillary leak (early gadolinium enhancement), or myocardial fibrosis (late gadolinium enhancement). If two or more of these were present, cardiac MRI correlated with histology 78% of the time.[11,157] Isolation of virus from the myocardium provides a definite viral diagnosis of myocarditis; however, this is rarely possible, even in cases of histologically proved myocarditis. Controversy now exists as to whether endomyocardial biopsy and histologic confirmation will continue to be recommended in myocarditis given the availability of cardiac MRI and the risks associated with biopsy.[158] Viral culture of peripheral specimens such as stool and nasopharyngeal secretions or the demonstration of a fourfold rise in specific viral antibody titers provides an indirect determination of causality; however, the sensitivity is low, 16% to 26% and 30% to 40%, respectively.[12,159] Molecular biological techniques such as PCR and in situ hybridization have expanded the number of viruses implicated in the etiology of myocarditis. In addition, because of the increased sensitivity of PCR, its application in myocardial tissue provides a virologic diagnosis in up to 60% of cases.[12]

Acute Liver Failure

Viral diagnosis relies on serology, detection of viral nucleic acid in serum, and detection of viral antigens or nucleic acids in tissue obtained from liver biopsy. HAV infection is confirmed by demonstrating anti-HAV IgM antibodies. In patients with acute infection, anti-HAV IgM antibodies are detectable in the serum at the onset of symptoms, peak 1 week after onset of symptoms, and become undetectable by 3 to 6 months postinfection. The presence of HBsAg in serum indicates active HBV replication and is present in acute and chronic HBV infection. Due to the destruction of actively infected hepatocytes, HBsAg may be absent in ALF and the only marker of acute HBV infection may be anti-HBcAb (anti-HBV core) IgM antibodies. HBV DNA can also be demonstrated in serum and liver tissue by PCR. Absence of HBsAg or HBV DNA in

TABLE 108.2   Potential Diagnostic Tests and Corresponding Specimens for Diagnosis of Viral Pathogens

Viral Agent	Specimen	Recommended Diagnostic Tests[1]
Adenovirus	NP, pharynx, BAL fluid Tissue Serum/plasma[2]	FA, culture, shell vial or rapid culture, PCR culture, PCR, histology PCR
Arboviruses (California encephalitis, Colorado tick fever, EEE, SLE, WEE, West Nile)[3]	Serum (acute and convalescent)/plasma CSF	IgM and IgG antibody,[4] PCR and immunohistochemistry for some IgM[5] and IgG antibody,[4] PCR
Chikungunya virus[3]	Serum/plasma Blood	PCR, IgM and IgG antibody[4] Culture
Coronaviruses (OC43, 229E, HKU1, NL63, SARS and MERS)[3,6]	NP aspirate (preferred for SARS/MERS) or swab, OP swab, BAL, serum/plasma (SARS/MERS), stool (SARS/MERS), tissues (SARS/MERS) Serum	PCR IgM and IgG antibody[4]
Ebola virus[3]	Blood, oral secretions	PCR
Enteroviruses (echoviruses, Coxsackie viruses, enteroviruses)[3]	CSF, pharynx Stool[7] Serum (acute and convalescent)	PCR, culture Culture IgM and IgG antibody available for some (Enterovirus D68 may not be detected by these methods)
Hantavirus[3]	Serum Tissue (lung, kidney, spleen preferred; antemortem: lung or bone marrow)	PCR, IgM and IgG antibody[4] PCR, culture and immunohistochemistry
Hepatitis Viruses		
HAV	Serum	Anti-HAV IgM, PCR
HBV	Serum/plasma Liver	HBsAg, anti-HBcAb IgM, PCR PCR
HCV	Serum/plasma Liver	Anti-HCV IgG, PCR PCR
HDV	Serum Liver	Anti-HDV IgG PCR
HEV	Serum Liver	Anti-HEV IgM PCR
Herpes Viruses		
CMV	NP or BAL Blood Serum Plasma Tissue Urine	FA, culture, shell vial or rapid culture PCR[10] Buffy coat antigen, PCR IgM and IgG antibody[4] PCR FA, culture, histology, PCR Culture, shell vial or rapid culture
EBV	Serum Plasma, CSF Tissue	IgM antibody or slide agglutination test (monospot) PCR PCR, Immunohistochemistry
HHV-6	Serum/plasma, CSF Tissue	PCR PCR, immunohistochemistry
HSV I and II	CSF, plasma Base of lesion, NP, conjunctiva, tissue Serum Stool (neonates)	PCR, culture FA, culture, PCR IgG antibody[4] Culture
VZV	Base of lesion, tissue Serum Plasma, CSF	FA and culture, PCR IgM and IgG antibody[4] PCR
Influenza A and B	NP, pharynx, BAL fluid Tissue	FA, culture, IA (rapid), PCR[9] FA, culture, PCR
JC virus[3]	Brain CSF	Brain biopsy,[8] PCR PCR
LCMV[3]	Serum CSF	IgM and IgG antibody[4] IgM

Continued

TABLE 108.2   Potential Diagnostic Tests and Corresponding Specimens for Diagnosis of Viral Pathogens—cont'd

Viral Agent	Specimen	Recommended Diagnostic Tests[1]
Measles (rubeola)[3]	Serum Urine, blood, NP	IgM and IgG antibody[4] Culture, PCR
SSPE	CSF	Oligoclonal bands, IgG, measles titer
Metapneumovirus	NP, BAL fluid	FA, PCR
Mumps[3]	Buccal swab Serum, CSF Pharynx, urine	PCR, culture PCR, IgM and IgG antibody[4] Culture (rarely grows)
Parechoviruses	CSF, serum/plasma, NP, pharynx, stool	PCR culture (not diagnostic because CPE same as enteroviruses)
Parainfluenza viruses	NP, BAL fluid, tissue	FA, culture, PCR
Parvovirus	Plasma Serum	PCR IgM and IgG antibody[4]
Rabies virus[3]	Serum, CSF Saliva, brain, tissues, urine Punch biopsy (nape of neck), brain	Rabies-specific antibody by neutralization assay Virus isolation/culture (rarely helpful), fluorescent microscopy (consult ID)
Retroviridae		
HIV	Serum/plasma, CSF	Screening HIVAg/Ab rapid assays DNA PCR RNA PCR
HTLV	Serum Tissue	PCR, HTLV EIA PCR
Rotavirus	Stool	EIA or latex particle agglutination assays (commercially available); electron microscopy, culture, polyacrylamide gel electrophoresis, PCR (research labs)
RSV	NP, BAL, tissue	FA, culture, shell vial culture, IA (rapid), PCR
Rubella[3]	Serum, NP, pharynx, CSF, blood, urine	IgM and IgG antibody[4] Culture

Choice of test depends on clinical setting, including organ system involved and immune status of host.

BAL, bronchoalveolar lavage; *CPE,* cytopathic effect; *CSF,* cerebrospinal fluid; *EEE,* Eastern equine encephalitis; *EIA,* enzyme immunoassay; *FA,* fluorescence assay; *IA,* immunoassay; *ID,* infectious disease; *NP,* nasopharyngeal secretions; *OP,* oropharyngeal; *SLE,* St. Louis encephalitis; *WEE,* Western equine encephalitis.

[1]Multiple diagnostic tests are available for each pathogen. Commonly recommended diagnostic tests are listed; however, if results are negative or specimens are not available, infectious disease consultation may be helpful for additional or special testing.

[2]PCR is usually run on plasma, though some laboratories may run serum samples.

[3]Pathogen may have significant public health implications and testing should be performed in consultation with infectious disease or local public health department (for enteroviruses, if enterovirus 68/71 suspected). Testing is often not available without assistance of the public health department, and recommended specimens and tests are frequently evolving; see www.cdc.gov for updates.

[4]IgM and IgG antibody may also be referred to as *serology* on laboratory request forms. For most viral pathogens, when testing for IgG it is optimal to collect acute and convalescent sera approximately 4 weeks apart.

[5]IgM antibody does not cross the blood-brain barrier. If found in CSF, IgM antibody denotes central nervous system infection.

[6]For suspected SARS or MERS, specimens should be collected from several locations at different time points following symptom onset. See http://www.cdc.gov/sars/clinical/index.html for updated diagnostic information.

[7]Enteroviruses are shed in the stool for weeks and may not be diagnostic.

[8]Gold standard.

[9]FA and rapid antigen testing have low sensitivity for 2009 novel influenza A (H1N1); PCR testing is the most sensitive and is necessary for subtyping.

[10]Because shedding of CMV occurs in the lungs of seropositive stem cell transplant recipients without overt CMV disease, the recovery of CMV DNA by PCR from BAL fluid (which is considerably more sensitive than culture) without shell vial or culture positivity is of uncertain significance. PCR for CMV DNA in BAL or biopsy fluid should thus not be ordered routinely.

the serum does not rule out HBV as the cause of ALF, as HBV DNA has been demonstrated in liver tissue of patients in whom serologic markers did not suggest HBV infection.[160] Coinfection or superinfection with hepatitis D virus (HDV), a hepatotropic virus that causes infection only in the presence of active HBV infection, may result in more severe disease[161,162] and can be diagnosed by demonstrating anti-HDV antibodies or HDV RNA in serum.[163]

Although the newer generation antibody assays for HCV are more sensitive, anti-HCV antibodies may not be detectable early in disease. Therefore when the epidemiology suggests possible infection with HCV, serum and liver tissue should be analyzed for HCV RNA by PCR.

HSV hepatitis is frequently a result of newly acquired infection, thus serology may not be helpful. Skin or mucosal lesions, if present, should be cultured for HSV. Liver tissue should be sent for viral culture and PCR. HSV may also be demonstrated in blood by PCR. Both serology and tissue or blood PCR can be used to diagnose infection with EBV, CMV, HHV-6, HEV, and parvovirus. Diagnosis of adenovirus and enterovirus generally requires PCR of blood and tissue or culture of infected secretions.

Pneumonia/Pneumonitis

If available, fluorescence assay (FA) or PCR testing on nasal wash specimens is the initial diagnostic test of choice for respiratory viruses, because most of these pathogens are concentrated in the nasopharynx. However, in ALRI, a lower respiratory sample by bronchoscopy may provide the best yield and may be positive even with a negative nasopharyngeal sample. The sensitivity of FAs is generally as high as 95% for RSV, influenza, and PIVs. However, many centers now have rapid PCR that will facilitate faster, more sensitive results and may include additional respiratory viruses of concern. A rapid antigen test for RSV and influenza is available; however, for pandemic 2009 H1N1 influenza A virus in particular, FA and rapid testing have shown low sensitivity.[164-167] Shell vial assays can be performed for CMV, RSV, and adenovirus. Samples can be sent for culture; this should be considered for immunocompromised and severely ill children with respiratory distress/failure of unclear etiology if PCR testing is not available. The diagnosis of hantavirus can be made by culture of the virus (which is difficult), PCR for viral RNA from serum, plasma, or tissues, or serologic testing.[114] A review of diagnostic testing options for etiologies of viral pneumonia is provided in Table 108.2.

Meningitis/Encephalitis

CSF, blood, and throat swabs should be collected for evaluation. PCR has greater sensitivity for the diagnosis of enterovirus compared with culture[168,169] and should be used whenever possible. Viral detection via throat culture can indicate current or recent infection. Rectal or stool viral cultures are less helpful because enteroviruses may be shed for weeks after infection. DNA PCR of CSF offers relatively sensitive and specific diagnosis of herpesviruses.[121] Detection of viral-specific antibodies in the CSF can add supporting evidence. The detection of HHV-6 DNA in plasma or serum confirms active systemic viral replication. Arboviruses are typically diagnosed through detection of CSF antibodies or acute and convalescent serum specimens. PCR and immunohistochemistry have also been used to diagnose arboviral infections and are available in some settings. Diagnosis of LCMV is made through serologic testing. JC virus can be detected in CSF with PCR; this appears to be a relatively sensitive and specific method for diagnosing PML.[170,171] Definitive diagnosis, however, is usually made with brain biopsy. Diagnosis of SSPE is made with the evaluation of CSF for oligoclonal bands, IgG level, and specific measles antibody titer.

Treatment for Viral Infections

In general, for most life-threatening viral infections the primary treatment is supportive. Because of improvements in intensive medical care, death from these illnesses has decreased even without the availability of specific antiviral therapy. Although lacking for many infections, there are antivirals for most of the herpes group viruses and many respiratory viruses. For most infections, the efficacy of antiviral therapy decreases if therapy is delayed, so early diagnosis and rapid initiation are essential. Consultation with an infectious disease specialist is recommended because some antiviral agents are not commercially available and new treatment modalities continue to be identified. A listing of antiviral agents, indications, and dosages is provided in Table 108.3.

Myocarditis

The mainstay of treatment for myocarditis is supportive care. Severe cases may require circulatory support in the form of extracorporeal membrane oxygenation (ECMO) or ventricular assist devices. ECMO may also serve as a bridge to cardiac transplant in cases of dilated cardiomyopathy. Aggressive therapy is warranted because both adults and children who survive their illness have a good prognosis for return to normal ventricular function.[172-174] Cardiac transplantation may be necessary for children refractory to other management. Current recommendations do not support the use of immunosuppressive therapy.[4,11,19] Treatment with high-dose IVIG has been associated with improved left ventricular function in several small studies in children[175,176]; however, this treatment showed no survival benefit in an evaluation of multi-institutional data.[2] In adults, a controlled study found IVIG to be no better than placebo for acute dilated cardiomyopathy,[176] and a Cochrane Review found no role for the routine use of IVIG in presumed viral myocarditis.[177] The use of IVIG in pediatric myocarditis warrants investigation in larger, controlled studies. Specific antiviral therapy may be indicated when the inciting viral agent has been identified; however, because most patients present weeks after the acute infection, the benefit is unclear.

Acute Liver Failure

The role of antiviral therapy in ALF is also limited. Acyclovir should be initiated if HSV is suspected or confirmed. High-dose acyclovir (60 mg/kg/day divided q8h) should be used for neonates with HSV.[178] There are reports of the successful use of tenofovir, entecavir, and lamivudine for treatment of severe acute hepatitis caused by HBV.[179-182] Liver transplantation may be required for some patients.[24,47,48] For a detailed discussion of the management of ALF, see Chapter 99.

Pneumonitis

The cornerstone of treatment remains supportive with supplemental oxygen, fluids, bronchodilators, and mechanical ventilation. Corticosteroids are generally of no proved benefit in viral-mediated pneumonia or bronchiolitis.[183,184] The use of empiric broad-spectrum antibiotics may be important until a diagnosis can be established and because some viral infections caused by PIVs, HRVs, and HCoVs may occur in the context of a bacterial coinfection. For certain immunocompromised patients, fungal copathogens should also be considered. Early isolation and infection control measures for suspected viral infections should be implemented.

A number of antiviral strategies have been investigated or employed on an anecdotal basis to treat viral pneumonia, but the only agents approved by the Food and Drug Administration include ribavirin for RSV and antivirals for influenza (oseltamivir, zanamivir, peramivir, amantadine, and rimantadine). For influenza, the strain of local circulating viruses must be considered when planning a treatment regimen. The reader is encouraged to consult http://www.cdc.gov/flu/ for national surveillance data on influenza viruses circulating in the United States. Combination therapy or the use of investigational agents may be considered during periods of

TABLE 108.3   Antiviral Agents and Indications for Use

Virus	Drug of Choice/Dose[2]	Alternate Agents/Dose
Adenovirus	There is no currently approved therapy for the treatment of adenoviral infections.	Small case series in immunocompromised children have suggested potential efficacy with IV ribavirin[191]; however, there is more data for the use of cidofovir.[192-194] Antiviral therapy should be considered for immunocompromised patients with disseminated disease or severe pneumonia.
Coronavirus	There is no currently approved therapy for the treatment of coronaviral infections.	The sudden and severe nature of the SARS outbreak in 2002–2003 necessitated the use of empiric treatment strategies. A number of agents have been used, including ribavirin, lopinavir-ritonavir, oseltamivir, and corticosteroids; however, the efficacy of any of these drugs has not been established.[195,196]
Enterovirus	There is no currently approved therapy for the treatment of enteroviral infections.	
Hantavirus	There is no currently approved therapy for the treatment of hantaviral infections.	IV ribavirin has shown benefit in HFRS,[197,198] but not in HPS.[199,200] A randomized controlled trial of methylprednisolone for HPS in Chile did not demonstrate clinical benefit.[201]
Herpes Viruses		
CMV	Ganciclovir (5 mg/kg q12h × 2-3 weeks, then 5 mg/kg q24h) is primary therapy for CMV disease. IVIG (500 mg/kg qod × 2 wk then once weekly) or CMV-IG (150 mg/kg, same schedule) can be considered concurrently for CMV disease in immunocompromised patients.	Foscarnet (90 mg/kg q12h × 2-3 weeks, then 90 mg/kg q24h), cidofovir (5 mg/kg/wk; high risk of renal toxicity, use with probenecid and saline hydration). Increased efficacy of cidofovir as second-line therapy suggested in allogeneic stem cell transplant recipients with CMV pneumonia in one small study.[202]
HSV	Acyclovir (20 mg/kg/dose IV q8h) for encephalitis in neonates and children <12 years and for neonates with disseminated disease; 10 mg/kg/dose IV q8h for children >12 years.	No specific dosing recommendations are available for HSV-associated hepatitis and pneumonitis. At least 10 mg/kg/dose should be considered outside the neonatal period.
HHV-6	There is no currently approved therapy for the treatment of HHV-6 infections.	Foscarnet and ganciclovir have in vitro activity. Case reports and series show variable clinical response with one or both drugs in combination.
VZV	Acyclovir (10-12 mg/kg/dose IV q8h); high-dose acyclovir (20 mg/kg/dose) should be used for VZV encephalitis or for disease in immunocompromised children.	
Influenza A/B	Oseltamivir[1] or zanamivir (≥7 years) 10 mg (2 oral inhalations) q12h × 5 days.	Rimantadine or amantidine generally not recommended due to widespread resistance. Local circulating influenza viruses must be considered. Combination therapy as empiric treatment may be indicated during periods of concomitant circulating viruses or for severely ill immunosuppressed patients.[203,204] Single-dose IV peramivir was approved for influenza in adult patients in December 2014. Pediatric safety and efficacy have not been established.
JC virus	No effective therapy.	In HIV infection, treatment with combination antiretroviral therapy may improve survival. Potential role for cidofovir.[205]
Metapneumovirus	There is no currently approved therapy for the treatment of metapneumoviral infections.	Ribavirin has in vitro activity against hMPV and has been shown to decrease viral load and lung inflammation in mouse models.[206,207] Case reports suggest ribavirin and IVIG may be used successfully in immunosuppressed patients, but retrospective studies showed no benefit.[78,79,208-210]
Parechoviruses	There is no currently approved therapy for the treatment of parechoviral infections.	
Parainfluenza virus	There is no currently approved therapy for the treatment of PIV infections.	Treatment for PIV pneumonia should include coverage for copathogens.[67] Ribavirin is active in vitro and in animal models and has thus been used for treatment of PIV pneumonia in immunocompromised hosts. Anecdotal reports of the benefit of ribavirin have been highly variable, and a retrospective series of stem cell transplant recipients showed no benefit.[67,195]
RSV	Aerosolized ribavirin (6 g reconstituted in 100 mL divided tid or 6 g in 300 mL administered over 12-18 hours daily) × 5 days has been used with modest efficacy in patients with severe RSV pneumonia and in immunocompromised patients[195,211]; not recommended for uncomplicated disease.	Combination therapy with aerosolized ribavirin and palivizumab (RSV monoclonal antibody, 15 mg/kg given once) has been used for RSV pneumonia in immunocompromised and high-risk patients, but data not conclusive.[56,203,211,212]

IVIG, intravenous immunoglobulin.

[1]Dosing varies by age and weight. See http://www.cdc.gov/flu/professionals/antivirals/antiviral-dosage.htm for specific recommendations. In an influenza pandemic or some outbreak situations, treatment should not wait for laboratory confirmation of influenza because laboratory testing can delay treatment and because a negative rapid test for influenza does not rule out influenza.

[2]These agents are generally recommended with infectious disease consultation for the infection listed. However, please note that not all these agents are FDA approved for the indicated use.

concomitant circulating viruses or for severely ill immuno-suppressed patients.[185-187] Table 108.3 provides a detailed summary of antiviral agents for various causes of viral pneumonia.

Encephalitis

Untreated, HSV encephalitis carries a death rate in excess of 70%.[188] Even when treated, death and complications remain on the order of 15% and 20%, respectively.[189] Similarly, despite treatment, neonatal HSV CNS disease carries significant risk of death and morbidity, ranging from 0% to 15% and 43% to 68%, respectively.[118] Early identification of patients and rapid initiation of acyclovir have been associated with better outcome.[188,189] Unless an alternative cause is clear, high-dose acyclovir should be initiated in all children with encephalitis until HSV can be ruled out. After the acute phase of treatment, oral suppressive acyclovir therapy for 6 months has been shown to improve developmental outcomes in infants with neonatal HSV and CNS involvement.[190] Other specific antiviral therapy may be directed as outlined in Table 108.3.

Key References

2. Klugman D, et al. Pediatric patients hospitalized with myocarditis: a multi-institutional analysis. *Pediatr Cardiol.* 2010;31:222-228.
4. Cooper LT Jr. Myocarditis. *N Engl J Med.* 2009;360:1526-1538.
6. Liu PP, Mason JW. Advances in the understanding of myocarditis. *Circulation.* 2001;104:1076-1082.
10. Levine MC, Klugman D, Teach SJ. Update on myocarditis in children. *Curr Opin Pediatr.* 2010;22:278-283.
11. May LJ, Patton DJ, Fruitman DS. The evolving approach to paediatric myocarditis: a review of the current literature. *Cardiol Young.* 2011;21:241-251.
15. Freedman SB, et al. Pediatric myocarditis: emergency department clinical findings and diagnostic evaluation. *Pediatrics.* 2007;120:1278-1285.
21. Eisenberg MA, et al. Cardiac troponin T as a screening test for myocarditis in children. *Pediatr Emerg Care.* 2012;28:1173-1178.
23. Devictor D, et al. Acute liver failure in neonates, infants and children. *Expert Rev Gastroenterol Hepatol.* 2011;5:717-729.
25. Schwarz KB, et al. An analysis of viral testing in non-acetaminophen (non-APAP) pediatric acute liver failure (PALF). *J Pediatr Gastroenterol Nutr.* 2014;[Epub ahead of print].
31. Chen HL, et al. Pediatric fulminant hepatic failure in endemic areas of hepatitis B infection: 15 years after universal hepatitis B vaccination. *Hepatology.* 2004;39:58-63.
43. McGoogan KE, Haafiz AB, Gonzalez Peralta RP. Herpes simplex virus hepatitis in infants: clinical outcomes and correlates of disease severity. *J Pediatr.* 2011;159:608-611.
44. Sundaram SS, et al. Characterization and outcomes of young infants with acute liver failure. *J Pediatr.* 2011;159:813-818 e1.
46. Shanmugam NP, et al. Neonatal liver failure: aetiologies and management–state of the art. *Eur J Pediatr.* 2011;170:573-581.
48. Devictor D, et al. Acute liver failure in children. *Clin Res Hepatol Gastroenterol.* 2011;35:430-437.
49. Shaw DW, Cohen WA. Viral infections of the CNS in children: imaging features. *AJR Am J Roentgenol.* 1993;160:125-133.
50. Johansson N, et al. Etiology of community-acquired pneumonia: increased microbiological yield with new diagnostic methods. *Clin Infect Dis.* 2010;50:202-209.
54. Jain S, et al. Community-acquired pneumonia requiring hospitalization among U.S. children. *N Engl J Med.* 2015;372:835-845.
57. Waghmare A, et al. Respiratory syncytial virus lower respiratory disease in hematopoietic cell transplant recipients: viral RNA detection in blood, antiviral treatment, and clinical outcomes. *Clin Infect Dis.* 2013;57:1731-1741.
61. Memoli MJ, et al. The natural history of influenza infection in the severely immunocompromised vs nonimmunocompromised hosts. *Clin Infect Dis.* 2014;58:214-224.
63. Dawood FS, et al. Emergence of a novel swine-origin influenza A (H1N1) virus in humans. *N Engl J Med.* 2009;360:2605-2615.
66. Englund JA. Diagnosis and epidemiology of community-acquired respiratory virus infections in the immunocompromised host. *Biol Blood Marrow Transplant.* 2001;7(suppl):2S-4S.
67. Nichols WG, et al. Parainfluenza virus infections after hematopoietic stem cell transplantation: risk factors, response to antiviral therapy, and effect on transplant outcome. *Blood.* 2001;98:573-578.
74. Esper F, et al. Human metapneumovirus infection in the United States: clinical manifestations associated with a newly emerging respiratory infection in children. *Pediatrics.* 2003;111(6 Pt 1):1407-1410.
79. Chu HY, et al. Respiratory tract infections due to human metapneumovirus in immunocompromised children. *J Pediatric Infect Dis Soc.* 2014;3:286-293.
80. Godet C, et al. Human metapneumovirus pneumonia in patients with hematological malignancies. *J Clin Virol.* 2014;61:593-596.
84. Ison MG, et al. Rhinovirus infections in hematopoietic stem cell transplant recipients with pneumonia. *Clin Infect Dis.* 2003;36:1139-1143.
87. Hasegawa K, et al. Multicenter study of viral etiology and relapse in hospitalized children with bronchiolitis. *Pediatr Infect Dis J.* 2014;33:809-813.
91. Lauinger IL, et al. Patient characteristics and severity of human rhinovirus infections in children. *J Clin Virol.* 2013;58:216-220.
95. Messacar K, et al. A cluster of acute flaccid paralysis and cranial nerve dysfunction temporally associated with an outbreak of enterovirus D68 in children in Colorado, USA. *Lancet.* 2015;385:1662-1671.
100. Rha B, et al. Update on the epidemiology of Middle East respiratory syndrome coronavirus (MERS-CoV) infection, and guidance for the public, clinicians, and public health authorities—January 2015. *MMWR Morb Mortal Wkly Rep.* 2015;64:61-62.
111. Ison MG, Fishman JA. Cytomegalovirus pneumonia in transplant recipients. *Clin Chest Med.* 2005;26:691-705, viii.
118. Kimberlin DW, et al. Natural history of neonatal herpes simplex virus infections in the acyclovir era. *Pediatrics.* 2001;108:223-229.
123. Pahud BA, et al. Varicella zoster disease of the central nervous system: epidemiological, clinical, and laboratory features 10 years after the introduction of the varicella vaccine. *J Infect Dis.* 2011;203:316-323.
127. Ward KN. Child and adult forms of human herpesvirus 6 encephalitis: looking back, looking forward. *Curr Opin Neurol.* 2014;27:349-355.
133. Whitley RJ. Viral encephalitis. *N Engl J Med.* 1990;323:242-250.
149. Bajaj M, Mody S, Natarajan G. Clinical and neuroimaging findings in neonatal herpes simplex virus infection. *J Pediatr.* 2014;165:404-407, e1.
153. Peacock G, Uyeki TM, Rasmussen SA. Ebola virus disease and children: what pediatric health care professionals need to know. *JAMA Pediatr.* 2014;168:1087-1088.
154. Chertow DS, et al. Ebola virus disease in West Africa—clinical manifestations and management. *N Engl J Med.* 2014;371:2054-2057.
155. Fischer M, et al. Notes from the field: chikungunya virus spreads in the Americas—Caribbean and South America, 2013-2014. *MMWR Morb Mortal Wkly Rep.* 2014;63:500-501.
157. Friedrich MG, et al. Cardiovascular magnetic resonance in myocarditis: a JACC white paper. *J Am Coll Cardiol.* 2009;53:1475-1487.
158. Vashist S, Singh GK. Acute myocarditis in children: current concepts and management. *Curr Treat Options Cardiovasc Med.* 2009;11:383-391.
177. Robinson J, et al. Intravenous immunoglobulin for presumed viral myocarditis in children and adults. *Cochrane Database Syst Rev.* 2005;(1):CD004370.
178. Kimberlin DW, et al. Safety and efficacy of high-dose intravenous acyclovir in the management of neonatal herpes simplex virus infections. *Pediatrics.* 2001;108:230-238.
183. Fernandes RM, et al. Glucocorticoids for acute viral bronchiolitis in infants and young children. *Cochrane Database Syst Rev.* 2013;(6):CD004878.
184. Schroeder AR, Mansbach JM. Recent evidence on the management of bronchiolitis. *Curr Opin Pediatr.* 2014;26:328-333.
186. Nguyen JT, et al. Efficacy of combined therapy with amantadine, oseltamivir, and ribavirin in vivo against susceptible and amantadine-resistant influenza A viruses. *PLoS ONE.* 2012;7:e31006.
194. Doan ML, et al. Treatment of adenovirus pneumonia with cidofovir in pediatric lung transplant recipients. *J Heart Lung Transplant.* 2007;26:883-889.

195. Nichols WG, Peck Campbell AJ, Boeckh M. Respiratory viruses other than influenza virus: impact and therapeutic advances. *Clin Microbiol Rev.* 2008;21:274-290, table of contents.

196. Stockman LJ, Bellamy R, Garner P. SARS: systematic review of treatment effects. *PLoS Med.* 2006;3:e343.

203. Ison MG. Respiratory syncytial virus and other respiratory viruses in the setting of bone marrow transplantation. *Curr Opin Oncol.* 2009;21: 171-176.

204. Poland GA, Jacobson RM, Ovsyannikova IG. Influenza virus resistance to antiviral agents: a plea for rational use. *Clin Infect Dis.* 2009;48: 1254-1256.

208. Bonney D, et al. Successful treatment of human metapneumovirus pneumonia using combination therapy with intravenous ribavirin and immune globulin. *Br J Haematol.* 2009;145:667-669.

Infectious Syndromes in the Pediatric Intensive Care Unit

Srinivas Murthy and Peter N. Cox

PEARLS

- Numerous clinical syndromes present similarly; knowledge of local epidemiology is crucial for timely recognition and diagnosis.
- Suspected meningococcal infections should be treated with great urgency, given the risk for rapid progression.
- Toxic shock syndromes are primarily caused by *Staphylococcus aureus* and group A streptococcus.
- Necrotizing fasciitis is a surgical emergency.
- Knowledge of local resistance patterns will allow optimal empiric therapy for suspected invasive *Streptococcus pneumoniae* infections.
- Management of Rocky Mountain spotted fever and hantavirus infections is time sensitive and requires a high degree of clinical suspicion and knowledge of local epidemiology.
- Infectious syndromes with multiorgan involvement are often caused by nonbacterial etiologies, including viruses; a broad differential diagnosis always should be considered.

The pediatric critical care unit is the epicenter of severe childhood infections in most hospitals. Many of these infectious processes are nosocomial and are associated with either patient (eg, immunocompromised) or procedural issues. Other infectious processes affect specific organs (bronchiolitis and meningitis). These specific infections and the general principles of sepsis management are described in other chapters of this book. This chapter describes selected bacterial, viral, and other infections that may precipitate a systemic response and multiorgan involvement requiring intensive care unit admission. Salient and identifying features are highlighted and, where appropriate, specific comments are provided regarding therapeutic strategies.

Meningococcal Infection

Etiology and Epidemiology

Neisseria meningitidis is a gram-negative diplococcus that causes bacterial meningitis and invasive disease. In regions where vaccination uptake is high, rapidly declining rates have been demonstrated.[1,2] In the United States, *Neisseria meningitidis* infections have an estimated incidence of 0.123 per 100 000 people across ages, making it the fourth most common cause of bacterial meningitis overall, after *Streptococcus pneumoniae*, Staphylococcus, and gram-negative meningitis.[3] In regions without high vaccination rates, however, the incidence can be above 10 per 100,000 people.[4]

Children are disproportionately affected, however, and have higher incidence than adults, with age spikes at less than 1 year and in late adolescence.[4,5] Serogroup B remains the most common cause in North America; recently available vaccines will likely alter this epidemiology. Globally, serogroup switching is under way, with serogroup W replacing serogroup A as the most common group in the meningitis belt in Africa, given ongoing vaccination strategies against serogroup A.[6]

Case fatality rates range from 4% to 15% in United States and Canada, depending on the case series, with higher mortality in those with complement deficiencies or asplenia.[7,8] Early identification, antibiotic and fluid administration, and referral to higher levels of care are likely to have contributed to significant mortality declines.[9]

Transmission is thought to be via the aerosol route, with associated asymptomatic nasopharyngeal carriage; why some children develop invasive disease remains to be elucidated. Postexposure prophylaxis of meningococcal disease is detailed in the American Academy of Pediatrics Red Book and includes the use of rifampin or ceftriaxone for high-risk contacts, including health care providers with significant exposure to oral secretions.

Clinical Presentation

Invasive disease is typically manifested as one of three syndromes: meningitis, meningitis with meningococcemia, or meningococcemia without meningitis. Invasive meningococcal infections typically start with nonspecific symptoms over the first few hours and rapidly progress to multiorgan involvement.[10] Early signs include leg pains, abnormal skin color, and cool extremities, in addition to fever and myalgias. The classic triad of hemorrhagic rash, altered level of consciousness, and meningismus is typically a late finding. The rash is often petechial in nature and may progress to large purpuric lesions in approximately 15% to 20% of those with meningococcemia (Fig. 109.1). Risk factors for poor outcomes include a bleeding diathesis and focal neurologic signs. Traditional pediatric critical care scoring systems are adequate to predict outcome.[11,12]

Shock due to meningococcemia is often complicated by adrenal insufficiency, possibly due to adrenal infarction, otherwise termed *Waterhouse-Friderichsen syndrome*.

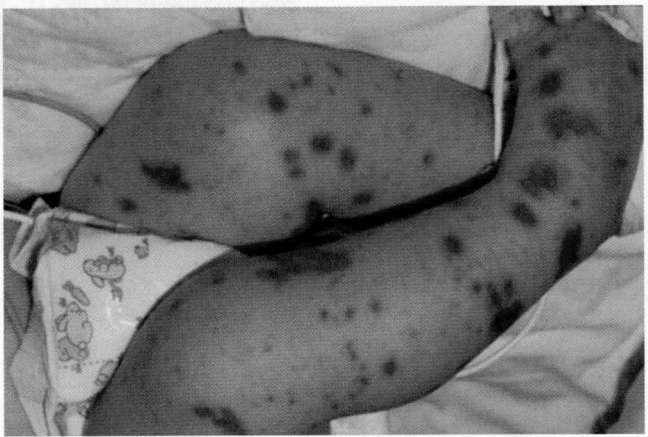

Fig. 109.1. Purpura fulminans in the legs of a child with meningococcal sepsis.

Additionally, disseminated intravascular coagulation (DIC) is common in severe cases, with a significant coagulopathy and endothelial dysfunction leading to the classic purpura fulminans. High levels of lipopolysaccharide are associated with worse outcomes, although the exact pathophysiology remains to be determined.[13] Other syndromes associated with meningococcal infection include pericarditis, arthritis, urethritis, and pneumonia.

Diagnosis

Given its rarity, rapid progression, and nonspecific initial presentation, clinicians must maintain a high degree of suspicion for children with these symptoms. The roles of ancillary tests such as white blood cell count, C-reactive protein, and procalcitonin are unclear in risk stratification. Clinical suspicion should be based on the characteristic rash and symptoms and signs of hypoperfusion, such as tachycardia, cool peripheral extremities, decreased urine output, and altered mental state. Aggressive treatment should be instituted prior to the onset of overt shock and likely before a confirmatory diagnosis is made.

Definitive diagnosis is made with culture from blood or cerebrospinal fluid, which will be positive in approximately 50% or 80% of cases, respectively. Pretreatment with antibiotics will negatively impact the culture positivity rates, given the rapid sterilization observed.[14,15] Lumbar puncture should be delayed if evidence of increased intracranial pressure, coagulopathy, or cardiovascular instability is present. Cultures from petechial scrapings and other body fluids such as synovial fluid can be helpful; however, isolation from the nasopharynx may not be useful, given the high rates of asymptomatic carriage. Latex agglutination is helpful for CSF and urine but unreliable for blood specimens. Polymerase chain reaction (PCR) has yet to replace traditional culture techniques, given the need for formal sensitivity testing; however, its rapidity and accuracy hold great appeal.[16,17]

Management

Many of the lessons from the management of septic shock (see Chapter 111) and meningitis (see Chapter 70) can apply in the management of patients with invasive meningococcal disease. The fundamental treatment is the early administration, within 30 minutes of consideration of meningococcal disease, of empiric antibiotic therapy.[18] Lumbar punctures should not delay antibiotic administration, and blood cultures should be drawn immediately prior to antibiotics. Reported resistance to penicillin and chloramphenicol make these agents inappropriate first-line empiric therapy. Hence, a third-generation cephalosporin such as ceftriaxone or cefotaxime is the agent of choice for empiric therapy, pending susceptibility results. Penicillin or chloramphenicol are appropriate to switch to upon obtaining appropriate susceptibility results, if a minimum inhibitory concentration of <0.1 mcg/mL is present. Dosing should ensure adequate CNS penetration. The typical duration of therapy is 7 days for meningitis or meningococcemia.

Significant capillary leakage is the hallmark feature in meningococcal sepsis. Thus the prominent problem faced in the early stages is maintenance of adequate circulating volume. Early volume resuscitation is vital and has been shown to improve outcomes in wealthy regions with access to intensive care supports.[19-22] Crystalloid is the solution of choice, with normal saline being the typical initial fluid. Significant myocardial depression should be assumed to be present with invasive meningococcal disease, especially in younger children,[23,24] and inotropes should be used early with fluid to ensure adequate cardiac output. The exact volume of fluids administered before initiating inotropes is a matter of much controversy; the authors consider the addition of inotropes after the administration of 40 to 60 mL/kg of fluids and persistent signs of hypoperfusion. To ensure appropriate and rapid volume resuscitation and inotropic delivery, central venous access should be established as soon as meningococcal sepsis is suspected; however, volume resuscitation should not be delayed and should be started with peripheral or intraosseous access if central access is not yet available.

Respiratory support often is necessary when fluid requirements are large, myocardial depression is suspected, and capillary leak is significant. Even if the patient is alert and oriented, early intubation and ventilation may be beneficial for resuscitation and transport when meningococcal infection is suspected in order to ensure adequate oxygenation, reduce the patient's work of breathing, decrease metabolic demands, secure central venous access, and maintain stability for transport.

Numerous metabolic derangements often occur because of cellular fluid shifts. Abnormal potassium, calcium, and magnesium concentrations can affect myocardial function and should be monitored and managed aggressively. Hypoglycemia is a common finding, and serum glucose concentration should be monitored closely. Metabolic acidosis is common and usually corrects with adequate perfusion and lactate clearance.

Disseminated intravascular coagulation (DIC) is common in severe meningococcal disease because of factor loss from capillary leak, endothelial activation, and clotting factor consumption. If there is significant hemorrhage, derangements are treated with fresh-frozen plasma and cryoprecipitate as needed. Plastic surgical interventions may be necessary for amputations and skin grafting after the patient has recovered from acute illness, with a large proportion of patients having significant skin or orthopedic issues.[25,26]

In addition to standard cardiovascular and respiratory support, multiple specific treatment strategies for meningococcus have been proposed. They have been aimed at altering the inflammatory cascade, treating hemostatic abnormalities, and inducing vasodilation and perfusion. Corticosteroids for meningitis due to meningococcus have not been associated with improved mortality in meta-analyses.[27] Adrenal replacement doses of corticosteroids for refractory shock remain a consideration.[21] Numerous immunomodulatory and other novel therapies have been studied, without beneficial effect documented, and no current specific therapies are available for severe meningococcal disease.[28-31]

Toxic Shock Syndrome
Etiology and Epidemiology

Toxic shock syndrome (TSS) is a toxin-mediated systemic syndrome caused by either *Staphylococcus aureus* or *Streptococcus pyogenes* (group A streptococcus [GAS]).[32-34] It occurs across all age groups; in the UK, toxic shock syndrome has an annual incidence of 0.38/100,000 among children.[35]

Both organisms have been known to produce exotoxins that act as superantigens, where they are capable of immune system activation without proceeding through the classic antigen-recognition pathways. The massive inflammatory response and cytokine release result in multisystem disease and shock. Production of these exotoxins is subject to various physiologic and environmental parameters.[36]

S. Aureus has been shown to produce a number of exotoxins, mainly toxic shock syndrome toxin-1 (TSST-1) and Staphylococcal enterotoxin B that have been isolated from bacterial strains in affected patients. TSS first came to prominence in the 1980s in association with the use of super-absorbent tampons among young females[37]; its incidence due to menstrual cases has markedly decreased since that time. Currently about half of cases are nonmenstrual related due to other *S. Aureus* infections such as postsurgical or skin and soft tissue infections. Its overall annual incidence, as reported in a population-based surveillance study in Minnesota is 0.52 cases/100,000 population.[38]

S. pyogenes produces a number of exotoxins that are associated with TSS, most notably M-proteins produced via the *emm* gene. The incidence of streptococcal TSS appears to be relatively rising, with highest rates in young children and the elderly.[39,40] Streptococcal TSS is associated with invasive GAS infection, with the major portals of entry being skin, vagina, or pharynx. There has been an association documented with varicella infection.[41] In the same surveillance study mentioned earlier, the pediatric incidence of streptococcal TSS was equal to that for staphylococcal TSS in the UK.[35]

Clinical Presentation

Surveillance definitions for both staphylococcal and streptococcal TSS are available (Box 109.1). For staphylococcal TSS, the onset is typically abrupt, with fever, chills, malaise, and diffuse macular erythroderma. Fever often is remarkably high and resistant, occurring with intense myalgias, vomiting, and diarrhea. The rash is described as a generalized deep-red "sunburn" and can be accompanied by conjunctival erythema. Within 24 hours, cardiovascular depression becomes prominent, with hypotension and decreasing systemic perfusion leading to severe shock and multiorgan dysfunction. As it is a toxin-mediated disease, most cases do not cause infective endocarditis. However, progressive liver and renal failures are

BOX 109.1	Surveillance Definitions for Staphylococcal and Streptococcal Toxic Shock Syndromes.[108,109]
Staphylococcal Toxic Shock Syndrome	A confirmed case includes fever, hypotension, rash, and involvement of at least three organ systems and negative results on alternative diagnoses: • Central nervous system: disorientation or alteration in consciousness, without focal neurologic signs, when fever and hypotension are absent • Gastrointestinal: vomiting or diarrhea at onset of illness • Hematologic: platelets ≤100,000 • Hepatic: total bilirubin or transaminase concentrations greater than twice the upper limit of normal • Muscular: severe myalgia or creatine phosphokinase (CPK) level greater than twice the upper limit of normal • Mucous membrane: vaginal, oropharyngeal, or conjunctival hyperemia • Renal: blood urea nitrogen or creatinine concentration greater than twice the upper limit of normal or at least five white blood cells per high-power field in the absence of urinary tract infection *And* Negative results on the following tests: • Blood, throat, or cerebrospinal fluid cultures for other organisms • Serologic tests for Rocky Mountain spotted fever, leptospirosis, or measles
Streptococcal Toxic Shock Syndrome	Isolation of group A Streptococcus from a normally sterile site (blood, CSF, pleural fluid, surgical wound) Hypotension *And* two or more of the following: • Renal dysfunction: creatinine concentration greater than twice the upper limit of normal • Hematologic: thrombocytopenia, disseminated intravascular coagulation (DIC) • Hepatic: total bilirubin or transaminase concentrations greater than twice the upper limit of normal • Respiratory: acute respiratory distress syndrome • Skin: erythematous macular rash, may desquamate, or soft tissue necrosis (ie, necrotizing fasciitis)

common. The patient may manifest symptoms of diffuse toxic encephalopathy, usually without meningeal signs. Renal failure can be oliguric or nonoliguric. Scaling and desquamation, which are included in the diagnostic criteria, occur with resolution of fever and usually are prominent on the palms and soles.

Streptococcal TSS is often preceded by a clear portal of infection with soft tissue findings, with a minority of cases occurring without a clear source. The symptoms and disease progression overlap with staphylococcal disease, with a diffuse erythematous rash and progressive multiorgan dysfunction with hypotension. Notably, fever is absent in the case definition of streptococcal TSS, but it is a mandatory component of diagnosis in staphylococcal TSS.

BOX 109.2 Differential Diagnosis of Staphylococcus TSS

Bacterial: meningococcemia, group A streptococcus, toxic shock, scarlet fever, staphylococcus scaled skin syndrome, salmonella infection, Rocky Mountain spotted fever, ehrlichiosis, leptospirosis
Viral: measles, enterovirus
Other: Stevens-Johnson syndrome, toxic epidermal necrolysis, Kawasaki disease, systemic lupus erythematosus

Diagnosis

Differential diagnoses for syndromes that include fever, rash, and multiorgan involvement are numerous and are summarized in Box 109.2. The diagnosis is clinical, and there is significant overlap with these syndromes. Probable TSS is diagnosed when either one characteristic is missing for staphylococcal TSS and when GAS is isolated from a nonsterile site for streptococcal TSS. Markers of inflammation and organ and tissue perfusion speak to the severity of illness and poorly differentiate TSS from other systemic illnesses. Isolating *S. aureus* is not mandatory for fulfilling case definition criteria for staphylococcal TSS; isolating GAS is mandatory for fulfilling case definition criteria for streptococcal TSS.

Management

The majority of cases of TSS will require intensive care support, given the multiorgan involvement and hypotension.[35] Hemodynamic management is similar to that for septic shock (see Chapter 111), with fluid resuscitation and vasoactive agents administered as necessary to maintain tissue perfusion, incorporating presumed myocardial depression into treatment algorithms. Respiratory support with invasive ventilation and renal support with dialysis are often required, depending on the severity of illness.

The mainstays of specific therapies for TSS are eradicating the nidus of infection and antitoxin therapies. Infection eradication is accomplished through surgical debridement, as appropriate, and aggressive antibiotic therapy. Urgent surgical consultation, for both streptococcal and staphylococcal TSS with a clear focus, is crucial for achieving source control in a timely fashion. A vaginal exam should be performed for foreign bodies in appropriate situations.

Antibiotic therapy should be appropriate for the suspected infection, and empiric therapy should include coverage for both organisms, as well as suspected resistance profiles. Standard protocols for suspected staphylococcal TSS should include an antistaphylococcal agent such as cloxacillin or nafcillin and clindamycin. In regions where methicillin-resistant *Staphylococcus aureus* (MRSA) prevalence is greater than 10%, vancomycin should be added to the empiric regimen and discontinued when susceptibility results are available. Clindamycin should be continued because of its ribosomal effects and theoretic ability to suppress ongoing toxin production.[42] Streptococcal TSS is effectively treated with high-dose penicillin. Clindamycin should be coadministered for its above-mentioned ribosomal effects, as well as its effects on slow-growing GAS species for full bacterial eradication.[43]

Toxin control is typically addressed with clindamycin and intravenous gamma-globulin (IVIG) administration.[44,45] Despite the theoretic benefit for supplementing toxin-neutralizing antibodies, only mixed data exist for IVIG efficacy in streptococcal TSS[46-49] and only anecdotal efficacy data in staphylococcal TSS.[50] The lack of efficacy in staphylococcal TSS may be due to decreased superantigen inhibition in standard preparation IVIG, compared with streptococcal disease.[51] Regardless, it is routinely used for severe disease of both types but more so for streptococcal TSS.[35,52] The recommended dose, if administered, is 150 mg/kg to 400 mg/kg per day for 5 days or a single dose of 1 g/kg to 2 g/kg.

Prognosis

With early and aggressive therapy, prognosis is good, with a mortality rate of 4.2% in streptococcal TSS and 3% to 5% in staphylococcal TSS.[48,53] The variable mortality in streptococcal TSS, which traditionally had higher mortality compared with staphylococcal TSS, may speak to increasing diagnosis due to awareness of the disease or to improved management strategies, given mortality in the 10% to 40% range in earlier case series.[35,54,55]

Necrotizing Fasciitis
Etiology and Epidemiology

Necrotizing fasciitis is characterized by extensive local necrosis of soft tissue and skin. It is typically due to one of two microbiologic causes: type I infection, with a combination of anaerobic and aerobic bacteria, and type II infection, primarily caused by *S. Pyogenes*. Type I disease is more common in individuals with comorbid disease, including diabetes, peripheral vascular disease, and immune compromise. Type II disease can occur in healthy individuals and is the predominant type in children. Necrotizing fasciitis represents between 10% and 20% of all invasive *S. pyogenes* infections in children, with a pediatric incidence of approximately 3 cases/million population in Canada.[56,57] Overall mortality in the pediatric population is approximately 5%.[57] Several reports have implicated varicella infection and nonsteroidal antiinflammatory drugs as a risk factors for infection; however, a causal relationship has not been established.[58]

Clinical Presentation

Necrotizing fasciitis typically presents initially with severe, localized pain, often out of proportion to corresponding skin erythema. As a deep-tissue infection that results in rapid and progressive destruction of muscle, fascial, and fat layers, it can spread rapidly along these planes and produce crepitus on palpation. The legs are the most common sites of infection, but the abdominal wall, groin, and perianal areas also are frequently affected. In newborns, the site most commonly affected site is the umbilicus. Approximately 80% of infants eventually develop obvious signs of soft tissue infection, and of these 70% progress to deeper infections requiring surgical debridement. Over the first 24 to 48 hours, the area becomes erythematous and swollen without sharp margins. Skin vesicles and bullae may be bluish and may appear by days 4 to 5, heralding fasciitis. By this time, the area often becomes anesthetic and gangrenous secondary to thrombosis of small blood vessels. Marked swelling and edema may lead to compartment syndrome requiring urgent fasciotomies. There are often systemic symptoms through associated toxin production and inflammation.

Diagnosis

Signs and symptoms may not be specific for necrotizing fasciitis; thus empiric treatment is initiated before the diagnosis is confirmed and a high index of suspicion must be maintained. Bacteremia is present in 60% of type II infections and much less frequent in type I infections.[59] High serum creatinine kinase and C-reactive protein concentrations have correlated well with deeper soft tissue infections and worse outcomes.[60] Imaging can be useful to determine the extent and location of disease, but they should not delay surgery. CT is the most time-sensitive study, whereas MRI is more sensitive in the diagnosis.[61,62] Definitive diagnosis, however, can only be made with surgical exploration and direct visualization of the fascial planes and muscle tissue.

Management

When necrotizing fasciitis is suspected, aggressive hemodynamic support and prompt antibiotic therapy are essential. Surgery should be performed for aggressive debridement of necrotic tissues and accurate diagnosis to halt the progression of ongoing spread. Frequent procedures for ongoing debridement and repeat imaging to assess the extent of spread are often required during the first phase of hospitalization. Antibiotic regimens should initially consist of broad-spectrum therapy while tests are being performed, including coverage for anaerobic organisms and clindamycin for toxin production. These can be tailored if GAS is susceptible to penicillin and clindamycin. In polymicrobial necrotizing fasciitis, antibiotic coverage should remain broad and culture results may not definitively guide therapy.

Antibodies specific for the toxin do not exist, but the use of intravenous immunoglobulin (IVIG) 1 to 2 g/kg in a single dose has been effective in various case series of necrotizing fasciitis, similar to TSS as noted earlier.[46,49,63] The possible mechanism may involve prevention of T-cell proliferation and reduction of cytokine release. Some anecdotal reports of the benefits of hyperbaric oxygen also exist but are inconclusive.[64] No controlled trials have demonstrated the efficacy of either of these therapies.

Invasive Pneumococcus
Etiology and Epidemiology

Streptococcus pneumoniae is the most common cause of otitis media and a frequent cause of sinusitis. With regard to invasive disease in the critical care setting, pneumococcus most commonly presents as bacteremia, pneumonia, arthritis, and meningitis. Meningitis is discussed in Chapter 70. This chapter focuses on bacteremia and pneumonia, focusing specifically on features related to pneumococcal infection. Other less common pneumococcal infections include endocarditis, soft tissue cellulitis, pericarditis, peritonitis, and salpingitis.

S. pneumoniae is an encapsulated gram-positive diplococcus organized in chains. Transmission is via secretions and respiratory droplets and increases in environments of close contacts, such as day care centers. It is a nasopharyngeal colonizer and is found in up to 40% of healthy children, although this rate is decreasing with increasing vaccination uptake.[65,66] Invasive disease may be secondary to mucosal barrier changes from other viral infections. In the Northern Hemisphere,

BOX 109.3 Risk Factors for Invasive Pneumococcal Disease

Organism: pneumococcal serotype
Host: age <2 years, ethnic background (African American, Native American, Alaskan, Micronesian), presence of concurrent viral respiratory infection, underlying illness (antibody deficiency, HIV infection, complement deficiency, splenic dysfunction, sickle cell disease, malignancy)
Environmental: day care attendance, recent antibiotic use, winter season, overcrowding, smoke exposure

invasive disease in children is more prevalent between September and May and can be associated with other viral illnesses such as influenza.[67]

The rate of invasive pneumococcal disease is rapidly declining in regions with effective vaccination strategies, with incidence rates of approximately 15 cases/100,000 population in children younger than 2, the highest incidence age group among children.[68,69] There are more than 90 serotypes of *S. pneumoniae*, with only a few identified as causing invasive disease, and current vaccination strategies address 7 or 13 of these serotypes. The incidence of invasive pneumococcal disease is higher and the severity of invasive illness greater in children with congenital or acquired humoral immunodeficiencies, including HIV, as well as deficient splenic function (Box 109.3). The majority of invasive disease across age groups is pneumonia, representing 69% of all invasive pneumococcal disease in the United States.[69] The total mortality for invasive pneumococcal disease in the United States is approximately 1% in surveillance regions, with lower mortality rates across pediatric age groups, although long-term morbidity from meningitis is common.[69-71]

Clinical Presentation

Invasive pneumococcal disease is defined as the isolation of *S. pneumoniae* from normally sterile sites such as blood, pleural fluid, joint fluid, and CSF. Presentation can be quite nonspecific, especially in infants, and relates to the organs and tissues affected. Symptoms of bacteremia can range from asymptomatic due to occult bacteremia to florid septic shock. Meningitis presents as described in Chapter 70. Pneumococcal pneumonia commonly presents with lobar infiltration, with some degree of pleural effusions in 40% of cases.[72] Bacteremia is present in approximately 10% of cases of pneumonia, increasing to 30% in cases with coincident parapneumonic effusion.[73]

Diagnosis

Diagnosis depends mostly on clinical suspicion. Isolation of bacteria from blood or normally sterile fluid confirms the diagnosis but should not delay treatment if pneumococcus is suspected. Pneumococcal PCR is available, although lacking the specificity and sensitivity for routine clinical use.[74] Sputum samples are rarely helpful in children, and nasopharyngeal cultures or molecular testing may reflect only colonization rather than infection. If intubated, samples obtained via bronchoalveolar lavage can be beneficial. Ultrasound or computed tomography (CT) can help identify effusions or empyema, which subsequently can be aspirated and sent for appropriate testing. Often, culture results will be negative and patients will be treated for presumptive pneumococcal disease due to a consistent clinical history.

The diagnosis of pneumococcal meningitis is via microbiologic evidence of bacteria. The presence of clinical meningitis, in the setting of a positive culture from pleural fluid or blood for *S. pneumoniae,* abrogates the need for a diagnostic lumbar puncture, especially given the small, but present, risk of herniation.

Management

Treatment of invasive pneumococcal disease consists of organ-specific supportive therapy and aggressive antibiotic administration. The management of respiratory failure, meningitis, and septic shock is described in Chapters 57, 70, and 111. Antibiotic regimens are changing and are entirely contingent upon knowing local resistance patterns, with mixed evidence that infection with resistant strains is associated with worse outcomes.[75,76] Risk factors for being infected with resistant strains include recent antibiotic exposures and immunosuppressing conditions.[77] In 2012 in the United States, 95% and 100% of pneumococcal strains reported were sensitive to cefotaxime and vancomycin, respectively, with rates remaining constant.[5,69]

For critically ill patients, empiric administration of combination therapy is recommended, given the severity of disease and the possibility of resistant organisms, until susceptibility results are available. Recommended approaches include a third-generation cephalosporin such as ceftriaxone or cefotaxime (25 to 100 mg/kg/dose every 8 hours, with cefotaxime preferred if less than 1 month of age) and vancomycin at 10 mg/kg/dose every 6 hours. These recommendations do not hold for noncritically ill patients, where second-generation cephalosporins, such as cefuroxime, are recommended, without vancomycin coadministration.[73] Treatment should be continued for 7 days for uncomplicated bacteremia, 10 days for pneumonia, and 14 days for meningitis, with antibiotic choice tailored by organism susceptibilities. The roles of medical or surgical treatment of any parapneumonic effusions or empyema remain to be seen and relate to the severity of clinical disease.[73,78]

Rocky Mountain Spotted Fever
Etiology and Epidemiology

Rocky Mountain spotted fever (RMSF) is a tick-borne bacterial infection resulting in a diffuse small-vessel vasculitis with the potential for causing multisystem disease. RMSF is caused by *Rickettsia rickettsii,* a small gram-negative coccobacilli carried by dog or wood ticks endemic to the United States, Canada, Mexico, and Central and South America. In the United States, the incidence is particularly high in the southeastern, south central, and south Atlantic regions (Fig. 109.2). The disease occurs mostly in the spring and early summer months, with almost half of cases occurring during May and June.[79] It is the most common rickettsial infection in the United States, with 7 cases/million diagnosed in 2007.[80] Case fatality rates are highest in the young and the elderly, with a total mortality rate of approximately 0.3% and a mortality of 3% to 4% in children.[80] Subclinical infection is common, with seroprevalence rates higher than incidence rates in numerous surveys.[81,82]

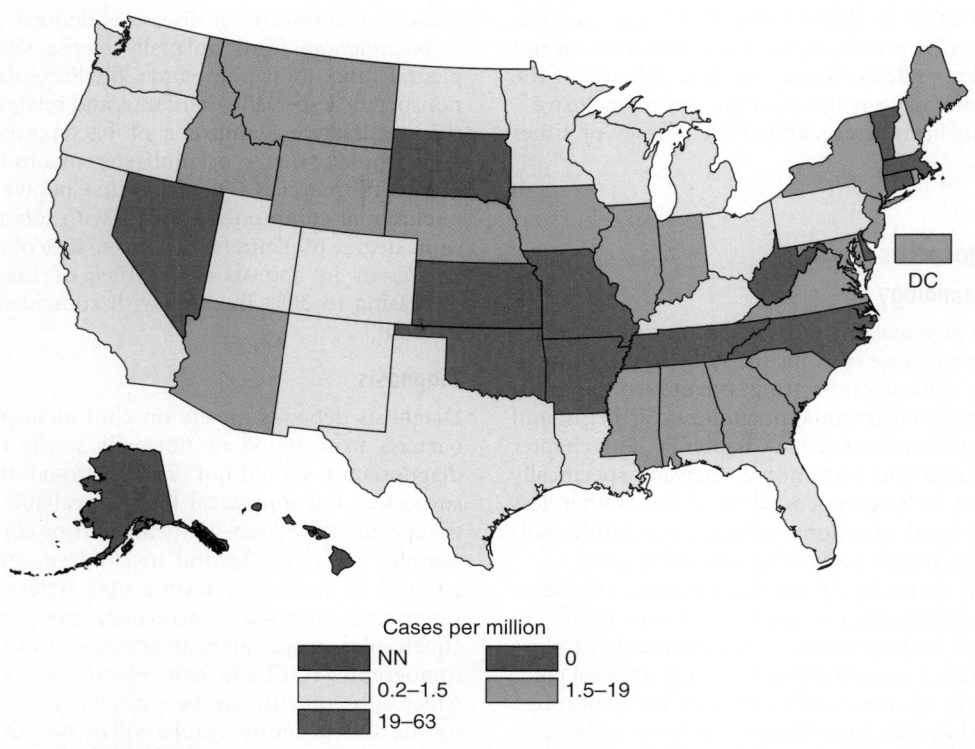

Cases per million

NN	0
0.2–1.5	1.5–19
19–63	

Fig. 109.2. Distribution of average reported cases of Rocky Mountain spotted fever—United States 2010. (Available at http://www.cdc.gov/rmsf/stats, accessed January 12, 2015.)

Clinical Presentation

The incubation period after a tick bite is 2 to 14 days (mean, 7 days). *R. rickettsii* gains entry into endothelial cells and leads to widespread vasculitis, increasing vascular permeability and activating inflammation and coagulation in nearly every organ. The classic symptoms of RMSF consist of fever, rash, and headache, in the appropriate geographic context, with a history of a tick bite. However, this classic triad is present in only 3% of patients in the first 3 days of illness, with typical early symptoms being a sudden onset of fever and malaise, with nausea, headache, vomiting, and abdominal pain being other frequent symptoms.[83,84] Additionally, only half of children with RMSF in one series reported a history of a tick bite.[84] The rash often begins between days 3 and 5, with blanching maculopapules classically starting at the wrists and ankles and then appearing on the palms, soles, and trunk, often becoming petechial (Fig. 109.3)[85]; up to 10% of patients, however, will not develop a rash and may have a worse outcome.[86] The presence of hemodynamic instability, renal dysfunction, encephalitis, and focal neurologic deficits on presentation is associated with worsened outcomes.[84,85]

The white blood cell (WBC) count often is variable and usually is not helpful. Many patients, however, develop thrombocytopenia and anemia as the disease progresses. Liver and renal function abnormalities are common, and approximately 20% of patients will have hyponatremia and hypoalbuminemia from massive capillary leak and fluid shift. CSF shows mononuclear pleocytosis in one-third of samples, with an elevated protein concentration in 20%.[87]

The diagnosis of Rocky Mountain spotted fever is clinical, with the above-mentioned clinical findings and the appropriate geographic circumstances. In early disease, when it is imperative that treatment is initiated,[88] no reliable test is currently available. To confirm the diagnosis, serologic testing and skin biopsy are the two modalities available, typically performed in larger reference laboratories. *R. rickettsii* is unable to be cultured. Serology is typically useful only after 7 to 10 days of symptoms, with increasing sensitivity with increasing duration of illness, with sequential samples separated by weeks essential to confirm rising antibody titers.[89]

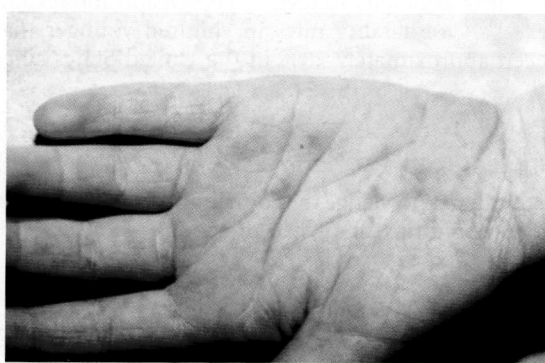

Fig. 109.3. Palmar rash associated with Rocky Mountain spotted fever. (From Walker DH, Raoult D: Rickettsia rickettsii and other spotted fever group rickettsiae [Rocky Mountain spotted fever and other spotted fevers]. In: Mandell GL, Bennett JE, Dolin R, ed. Mandell: Principles and Practice of Infectious Diseases. 5th ed. New York: Churchill Livingstone; 2000.)

Immunohistochemistry on skin biopsy specimens is nearly 100% specific and 70% sensitive for the confirmation of RMSF, should be performed where available, and is most useful within 48 to 72 hours of initiating antibiotics.[90,91] PCR testing on blood is available in certain laboratories, although it has varying utility, given the low numbers of circulating rickettsiae in acute disease.[92] The differential diagnosis of RMSF is broad and must include other tick-borne diseases, many other viral diseases, Kawasaki disease, and meningococcal infections.

Management

Empiric antibiotic therapy is essential early in the course of illness because fatal outcomes have been linked to missed or delayed diagnosis and treatment.[93] The drug of choice for treatment of RMSF in all age groups is doxycycline, with no ongoing controversy about its use in small children in these circumstances.[89] It is effective both orally and intravenously and should be continued for at least 3 days after symptoms subside, typically for a total of 5 to 7 days. The typical dose for children is 2.2 mg/kg/dose, administered twice daily. Chloramphenicol is a second-line agent, due to its side effect profile and reports of higher case fatality rates with its usage.[94] Given the differential diagnosis and the lack of confirmatory diagnosis, broad-spectrum agents such as ceftriaxone should be additionally considered to cover other bacterial infections, most notably meningococcal infection.

Along with antibiotic therapy, aggressive supportive measures must be instituted. Restoration of massive fluid imbalances and cardiovascular support may be necessary. Correction of electrolyte abnormalities and coagulopathy are essential, and close monitoring of liver and renal dysfunction is indicated.

Prognosis

The case fatality rate for identified cases of RMSF in children is approximately 2% to 3%.[84,95] The major prognostic factor for mortality is delayed treatment, emphasizing the role of maintaining a high index of suspicion in affected regions.[89] Other poor prognostic factors include older patients and those treated solely with chloramphenicol.[95]

Hantavirus

Etiology and Epidemiology

Invasive infections manifesting as sepsis syndromes can be caused by nonbacterial microbes including enterovirus and influenza virus species. These are discussed in Chapter 108. This chapter focuses on more rare viruses with specific cardiopulmonary syndromes; a classic example is hantavirus, which can cause a hemorrhagic fever with renal syndrome (HFRS) in eastern Asia and Europe or a cardiopulmonary syndrome in the Americas. It is an infrequent illness, with a total of 637 cases ever reported in the United States as of December 31, 2013, with a mean age of 37 (range 6-83 years). It has been diagnosed in 34 states, predominantly in the southwestern United States (Fig. 109.4).[96]

Hantavirus has been linked to mice and rat species endemic to many areas in both urban and rural environments. The deer mouse is the main vector in rural areas throughout the United States and Canada. Infection occurs most commonly via

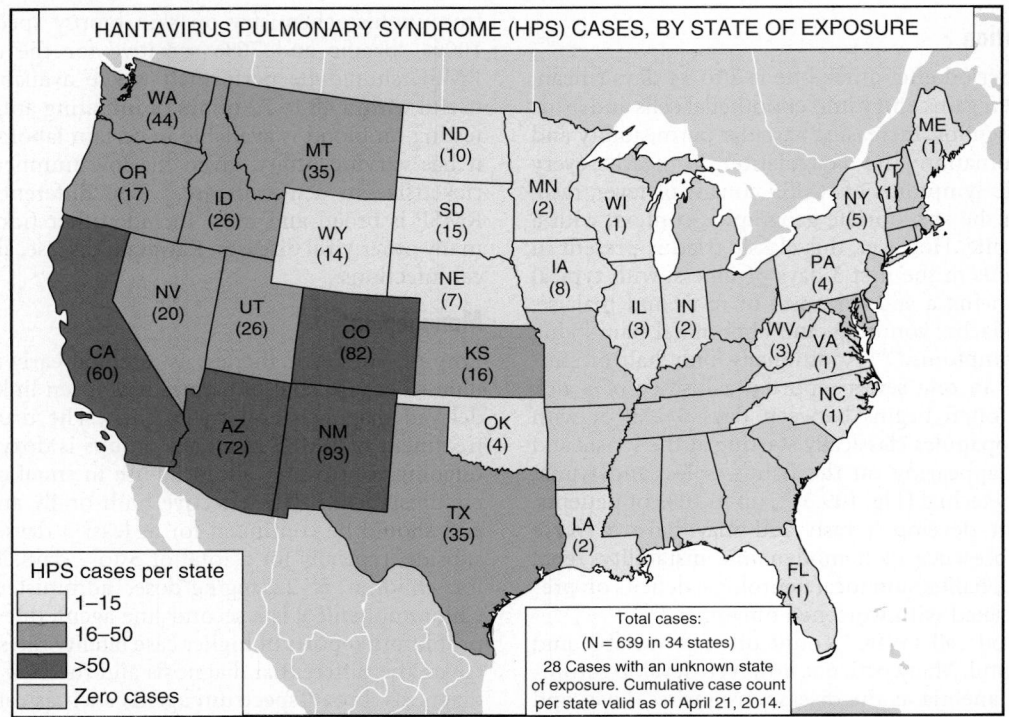

Fig. 109.4. Distribution of reported cases of hantavirus pulmonary syndrome—United States 2014. (Available at http://www.cdc.gov/hantavirus/surveillance/state-of-exposure.html, accessed January 12, 2015.)

inhalation of aerosolized saliva or excreta of infected rodents. The virus subsequently invades the pulmonary mucosa after inhalation with typically a 2-week incubation period, causing direct cellular damage that leads to increased vascular permeability.

Clinical Presentation

Both invasive hantavirus syndromes present with initial nonspecific symptoms, with rapid progression. Presentation in HFRS patients typically progresses to severe fevers and shock, with patients subsequently developing renal insufficiency and bleeding. Disease progression classically occurs along five phases, namely febrile, hypotensive, oliguric, diuretic, and convalescent phases, although this exact progression is not always present.[97]

Hantavirus cardiopulmonary syndrome often starts with fever, myalgias, and gastrointestinal symptoms and can rapidly progress over the course of days, heralded by worsening cough, to include severe pulmonary capillary leak, progressive hypoxia, and shock.[98,99]

Diagnosis

The diagnosis centers on maintaining a high degree of suspicion in affected areas. PCR and serology are available in reference laboratories and should be performed at the earliest possible opportunity, given the rapid progression of disease. Other laboratory parameters notable for hantavirus infection include a thrombocytopenia, elevated partial thromboplastin time (PTT), and an elevated hematocrit.[100]

Management

Upon diagnosis, affected patients should be triaged to higher levels of care at the earliest possible opportunity, given the

rapidity of disease progression. It is often self-limited, with a case fatality rate of about 1%. Recovery typically occurs over a course of weeks.[101] However, patients often require substantial supportive care during this cardiopulmonary phase. Ribavirin is *effective in vitro* and has proved efficacious for HFRS, although data are lacking for the cardiopulmonary syndrome.[102] Current literature does not support a role for corticosteroids.[103] Given the self-limited course of illness, extracorporeal membrane oxygenation for refractory respiratory failure or hemodynamic support has been effectively used in centers where it is routinely available.[104,105]

Prognosis

Overall mortality rate is 30% to 40% with hantavirus infection and usually is secondary to severe hypotension and respiratory failure.[106,107] Case fatality rates in children younger than 10 have been approximately 20% in the United States since the 1990s.[107]

Acknowledgments

We gratefully acknowledge the contribution of Sonny Dhanani who coauthored this chapter in previous editions.

Key References

2. Martin NG, Sadarangani M, Pollard AJ, Goldacre MJ. Hospital admission rates for meningitis and septicaemia caused by Haemophilus influenzae, Neisseria meningitidis, and Streptococcus pneumoniae in children in England over five decades: a population-based observational study. *Lancet Infect Dis.* 2014;14:397-405.
3. Castelblanco RL, Lee M, Hasbun R. Epidemiology of bacterial meningitis in the USA from 1997 to 2010: a population-based observational study. *Lancet Infect Dis.* 2014;14:813-819.

5. Thigpen MC, Whitney CG, Messonnier NE, et al. Bacterial meningitis in the United States, 1998-2007. *N Eng J Med*. 2011;364:2016-2025.

8. Kaplan SL, Schutze GE, Leake JA, et al. Multicenter surveillance of invasive meningococcal infections in children. *Pediatrics*. 2006;118:e979-e984.

10. Thompson MJ, Ninis N, Perera R, et al. Clinical recognition of meningococcal disease in children and adolescents. *Lancet*. 2006;367:397-403.

16. Wu HM, Cordeiro SM, Harcourt BH, et al. Accuracy of real-time PCR, Gram stain and culture for Streptococcus pneumoniae, Neisseria meningitidis and Haemophilus influenzae meningitis diagnosis. *BMC Infect Dis*. 2013;13:26.

20. Carcillo JA, Davis AL, Zaritsky A. Role of early fluid resuscitation in pediatric septic shock. *JAMA*. 1991;266:1242-1245.

21. Brierley J, Carcillo JA, Choong K, et al. Clinical practice parameters for hemodynamic support of pediatric and neonatal septic shock: 2007 update from the American College of Critical Care Medicine. *Criti Care Med*. 2009;37:666-688.

24. Briassoulis G, Narlioglou M, Zavras N, Hatzis T. Myocardial injury in meningococcus-induced purpura fulminans in children. *Intensive Care Med*. 2001;27:1073-1082.

27. Brouwer MC, McIntyre P, Prasad K, van de Beek D. Corticosteroids for acute bacterial meningitis. *Cochrane Database Syst Rev*. 2013;(6):CD004405.

31. Smith OP, White B, Vaughan D, et al. Use of protein-C concentrate, heparin, and haemodiafiltration in meningococcus-induced purpura fulminans. *Lancet*. 1997;350:1590-1593.

34. Lappin E, Ferguson AJ. Gram-positive toxic shock syndromes. *Lancet Infect Dis*. 2009;9:281-290.

35. Adalat S, Dawson T, Hackett SJ, Clark JE. In association with the British Paediatric Surveillance U. Toxic shock syndrome surveillance in UK children. *Arch Dis Child*. 2014;99:1078-1082.

38. DeVries AS, Lesher L, Schlievert PM, et al. Staphylococcal toxic shock syndrome 2000-2006: epidemiology, clinical features, and molecular characteristics. *PLoS ONE*. 2011;6:e22997.

42. Carapetis JR, Jacoby P, Carville K, et al. Effectiveness of clindamycin and intravenous immunoglobulin, and risk of disease in contacts, in invasive group a streptococcal infections. *Clin Infect Dis*. 2014;59:358-365.

45. Schlievert PM. Use of intravenous immunoglobulin in the treatment of staphylococcal and streptococcal toxic shock syndromes and related illnesses. *J Allergy Clin Immunol*. 2001;108(4 suppl):S107-S110.

46. Darenberg J, Ihendyane N, Sjolin J, et al. Intravenous immunoglobulin G therapy in streptococcal toxic shock syndrome: a European randomized, double-blind, placebo-controlled trial. *Clin Infect Dis*. 2003;37:333-340.

47. Linner A, Darenberg J, Sjolin J, et al. Clinical efficacy of polyspecific intravenous immunoglobulin therapy in patients with streptococcal toxic shock syndrome: a comparative observational study. *Clin Infect Dis*. 2014;59:851-857.

49. Kaul R, McGeer A, Norrby-Teglund A, et al. Intravenous immunoglobulin therapy for streptococcal toxic shock syndrome—a comparative observational study. The Canadian Streptococcal Study Group. *Clin Infect Dis*. 1999;28:800-807.

55. Rodriguez-Nunez A, Dosil-Gallardo S, Jordan I. ad hoc Streptococcal Toxic Shock Syndrome collaborative group of Spanish Society of Pediatric Intensive Care. Clinical characteristics of children with group A streptococcal toxic shock syndrome admitted to pediatric intensive care units. *Eur J Pediatr*. 2011;170:639-644.

56. Zachariadou L, Stathi A, Tassios PT, et al. Differences in the epidemiology between paediatric and adult invasive Streptococcus pyogenes infections. *Epidemiol Infect*. 2014;142:512-519.

60. Simonart T, Simonart JM, Derdelinckx I, et al. Value of standard laboratory tests for the early recognition of group A beta-hemolytic streptococcal necrotizing fasciitis. *Clin Infect Dis*. 2001;32:E9-E12.

61. Schmid MR, Kossmann T, Duewell S. Differentiation of necrotizing fasciitis and cellulitis using MR imaging. *AJR Am J Roentgenol*. 1998;170:615-620.

62. Ali SZ, Srinivasan S, Peh WC. MRI in necrotizing fasciitis of the extremities. *Br J Radiol*. 2014;87:20130560.

66. Rosen JB, Thomas AR, Lexau CA, et al. Geographic variation in invasive pneumococcal disease following pneumococcal conjugate vaccine introduction in the United States. *Clin Infect Dis*. 2011;53:137-143.

67. Weinberger DM, Simonsen L, Jordan R, et al. Impact of the 2009 influenza pandemic on pneumococcal pneumonia hospitalizations in the United States. *J Infect Dis*. 2012;205:458-465.

68. von Gottberg A, de Gouveia L, Tempia S, et al. Effects of vaccination on invasive pneumococcal disease in South Africa. *N Eng J Med*. 2014;371:1889-1899.

70. Christie D, Viner RM, Knox K, et al. Long-term outcomes of pneumococcal meningitis in childhood and adolescence. *Eur J Pediatr*. 2011;170:997-1006.

72. Tan TQ, Mason EO Jr, Wald ER, et al. Clinical characteristics of children with complicated pneumonia caused by Streptococcus pneumoniae. *Pediatrics*. 2002;110(1 Pt 1):1-6.

73. Bradley JS, Byington CL, Shah SS, et al. The management of community-acquired pneumonia in infants and children older than 3 months of age: clinical practice guidelines by the Pediatric Infectious Diseases Society and the Infectious Diseases Society of America. *Clin Infect Dis*. 2011;53:e25-e76.

77. Yu VL, Chiou CC, Feldman C, et al. An international prospective study of pneumococcal bacteremia: correlation with in vitro resistance, antibiotics administered, and clinical outcome. *Clin Infect Dis*. 2003;37:230-237.

80. Openshaw JJ, Swerdlow DL, Krebs JW, et al. Rocky mountain spotted fever in the United States, 2000-2007: interpreting contemporary increases in incidence. *Am J Trop Med Hyg*. 2010;83:174-182.

82. Hidalgo M, Sanchez R, Orejuela L, et al. Prevalence of antibodies against spotted fever group rickettsiae in a rural area of Colombia. *Am J Trop Med Hyg*. 2007;77:378-380.

84. Buckingham SC, Marshall GS, Schutze GE, et al. Clinical and laboratory features, hospital course, and outcome of Rocky Mountain spotted fever in children. *J Pediatr*. 2007;150:180-184, 184.e1.

85. Alvarez-Hernandez G, Murillo-Benitez C, Del Carmen Candia-Plata M, Moro M. Clinical profile and predictors of fatal rocky mountain spotted fever in children from Sonora, Mexico. *Pediatr Infect Dis J*. 2015;34:125-130.

88. Kirkland KB, Wilkinson WE, Sexton DJ. Therapeutic delay and mortality in cases of Rocky Mountain spotted fever. *Clin Infect Dis*. 1995;20:1118-1121.

93. Centers for Disease Control and Prevention (CDC). Consequences of delayed diagnosis of Rocky Mountain spotted fever in children—West Virginia, Michigan, Tennessee, and Oklahoma, May-July 2000. *MMWR Recomm Rep*. 2000;49:885-888.

96. Khetsuriani N, Lamonte A, Oberste MS, Pallansch M. Neonatal enterovirus infections reported to the national enterovirus surveillance system in the United States, 1983-2003. *Pediatr Infect Dis J*. 2006;25:889-893.

99. Abel Borges A, Figueiredo LT. Mechanisms of shock in hantavirus pulmonary syndrome. *Curr Opin Infect Dis*. 2008;21:293-297.

101. Lee SH, Chung BH, Lee WC, Choi IS. Epidemiology of hemorrhagic fever with renal syndrome in Korea, 2001-2010. *J Korean Med Sci*. 2013;28:1552-1554.

103. Vial PA, Valdivieso F, Ferres M, et al. High-dose intravenous methylprednisolone for hantavirus cardiopulmonary syndrome in Chile: a double-blind, randomized controlled clinical trial. *Clin Infect Dis*. 2013;57:943-951.

104. Wernly JA, Dietl CA, Tabe CE, et al. Extracorporeal membrane oxygenation support improves survival of patients with hantavirus cardiopulmonary syndrome refractory to medical treatment. *Eur J Cardiothorac Surg*. 2011;40:1334-1340.

105. Dietl CA, Wernly JA, Pett SB, et al. Extracorporeal membrane oxygenation support improves survival of patients with severe hantavirus cardiopulmonary syndrome. *J Thorac Cardiovasc Surg*. 2008;135:579-584.

107. MacNeil A, Ksiazek TG, Rollin PE. Hantavirus pulmonary syndrome, United States, 1993-2009. *Emerg Infect Dis*. 2011;17:1195-1201.

108. Defining the group A streptococcal toxic shock syndrome. Rationale and consensus definition. The Working Group on Severe Streptococcal Infections. *JAMA*. 1993;269:390-391.

Hospital-Acquired Infection in the Pediatric Intensive Care Unit: Epidemiology and Control

Srinivas Murthy and Peter Skippen

PEARLS

- Handwashing is the most important means of preventing nosocomial infection. Each pediatric ICU (PICU) should develop programs to increase compliance with hand hygiene.
- All nonessential invasive devices should be removed. PICU practitioners should establish routines that require individual patient evaluation of device use daily.
- A comprehensive infection prevention and control program allied with organizational quality and patient safety programs is an essential strategy for minimizing hospital-acquired infections. Critical care teams should establish strong collaborative partnerships with the infection prevention and control service.
- Antimicrobial stewardship aims to minimize overexposure and unnecessary use of broad-spectrum antibiotics. Antibiotic-resistant bacteria are an increasing concern as a cause of hospital-acquired infection, requiring a multipronged approach to control that includes adherence to isolation procedures, appropriate use of antibiotics, educational interventions, prescribing guidelines, and restriction of the use of some antibiotics. Parents and visitors should be made partners of the infection control team to help prevent infection in their children.

Burden of Illness and Scope of the Problem

Children ill enough to require admission to a critical care unit are among the most vulnerable to infection in the hospital for a variety of reasons. Normal physical defenses such as skin integrity, the cough reflex, and gastric motility are interrupted in the critically ill child. Innate and adaptive immunity are compromised during high-acuity acute illness. Broad-spectrum antibiotics used as empiric therapy for suspected sepsis may disrupt normal protective flora and permit overgrowth by pathogenic bacteria and fungi. Younger children with maturing immune systems are more likely to require ICU admission than older children. Additionally, children with incomplete vaccine series, either because of parental choice or

other reasons, are more susceptible to communicable diseases such as pertussis and measles.

For all of these reasons, health care–associated infections remain common, occurring in approximately 9% to 21% of critically ill children in the United States.[1,2] The most common health care–associated infections (HAIs) in the PICU are primary bloodstream infections (BSIs) ventilator-associated pneumonia, and catheter-associated urinary tract infections. HAIs increase length of stay and morbidity and mortality rates for both adult and pediatric critically ill patients. This translates to an economic burden on the system as a whole.[3]

There has been renewed emphasis in the past decade on systematic strategies for preventing HAIs, both from a patient safety perspective and in an effort to reduce the cost of health care. Infection prevention and control, patient safety, patient advocates, and health care providers alike see the value of improved health outcomes associated with reduction in nosocomial infections.

This chapter reviews the epidemiologic principles underlying infection prevention and control measures and recommends interventions to prevent the most common HAIs in the PICU.

Epidemiologic Principles of Infection Prevention and Control

Chain of Infection

The transmissibility of microorganisms between infected or colonized persons and susceptible hosts was perhaps most convincingly demonstrated in the 1847 observations of Ignaz Semmelweiss, who introduced handwashing to the obstetric wards of an Austrian maternity hospital and subsequently observed a reduction in the rates of puerperal fever.[4] In this instance, the initiation of hand hygiene after patient contact (cadavers) interrupted the spread of the infectious agent (group A *Streptococcus*) via the route of transmission (hands). Over time the epidemiologic roles of the susceptible host, infected person, and route of infection were more clearly elucidated and came to be known as the *chain of infection*. The interaction among these three components is dynamic, and infection may be favored when the host is more susceptible, the infectious agent is more virulent, or the route of transmission is more facilitating.

Once admitted to the ICU, children become more vulnerable to infection because of the interventions needed to provide life-sustaining care, as well as the close contact of multiple care providers. An infectious agent that is a harmless or helpful commensal in a normal host can become a life-threatening pathogen in the ICU patient. Because of frequent antibiotic use, the spectrum of infecting microorganisms in the hospital, particularly the ICU, is usually more pathogenic that microorganisms acquired in the community setting. Finally, the route of transmission of infection in the ICU is facilitated through frequent patient contact by health care workers, use of mechanical devices and medical therapies that disrupt natural defenses, and inadequate attention to infection prevention and control measures that prevent spread of infection to and between patients (Box 110.1). Open design wards and critical care units rather than single-room design, shared toys, pet visiting, and communal play areas also provide many opportunities for transmission of infection.

Routes of Infectious Disease Transmission

Infectious diseases, whether bacterial, viral, protozoal, fungal, or helminthic, are transmitted via one or more of three routes, usually categorized for infection control purposes as contact (direct or indirect), droplet, or airborne (Table 110.1).

Contact transmission includes direct contact and indirect contact and includes transmission of *Clostridium difficile* and methicillin-resistant *Staphylococcus aureus*. *Direct contact* transmission occurs when organisms are transferred through physical contact from an infected or colonized person to a susceptible host. *Indirect contact* transmission occurs when microorganisms are passively transferred to a susceptible host via an intermediate object, such as a contaminated medical device, inanimate objects in the patient's physical environment, or contaminated hands.

Droplet transmission is the transfer of microorganisms through large droplets (≥ 5 μm in diameter) generated from the respiratory tract of an infected or colonized person (the source) that are propelled 1 to 2 m from the source and land on the nasal or oral mucosa of the susceptible host or in the immediate environment. The droplets can be propelled from the respiratory tract in the course of coughing, sneezing, vomiting, or singing or during procedures such as suctioning. These large droplets are propelled a distance of less than 2 m through the air but do not remain suspended in the air; that is, they do not become aerosolized. Examples of organisms transmitted via the droplet route include influenza and pertussis.

Airborne transmission refers to the spread of microorganisms in particles that are very small (< 5 μm) and can therefore remain suspended in the air and widely dispersed to places far from the host. Airborne particles are created through the evaporation of large droplets or may exist in dust particles containing skin squamous cells and other debris. Measles and tuberculosis are the best-known examples of airborne transmission.

BOX 110.1	Factors That Influence Risk of Infection in Pediatric Intensive Care Unit

Factors That Influence Exposure
Host Factors
    Loss of skin integrity (eg, intravascular devices)
    Loss of respiratory defenses such as cough, cilia propulsion
        (eg, intubation, sedation)
    Loss of gastrointestinal defenses such as low pH, motility (eg,
        use of H2 blockers, nasogastric tubes)
    Anatomic defect (eg, surgical site)

Environmental Factors
Crowding in the ICU
High patient/health care worker ratios (decreased time for infection
    prevention measures)
Use of prophylactic antibiotics (alters colonizing normal flora,
    allows overgrowth of pathogens)
Infection prevention and control practices of ICU health care
    workers
Immunization status of health care workers
Visitor policies
Reservoirs of infectious organisms in the ICU (eg, health care
    workers who are carriers, environmental reservoirs)

Factors That Influence Likelihood of Infection If Exposed
Host Factors
    Age
    Gender
    Genetic makeup
    Coexisting infection
    Nutritional status
    Use of immunosuppressive agents, including systemic steroids
    Immunization status
    Immune deficiency
Infectious Agent
    Virulence
    Antimicrobial resistance

Infection Prevention and Control Measures
Infection Prevention and Control Team

Prevention of infection in patients receiving health care is the responsibility of all health care providers. Although infection prevention and control professionals (ICPs) provide an essential expertise,[5] it is important that the PICU team establish ongoing multidisciplinary processes to reduce infection risk. Among the activities the multidisciplinary team will address are the integration of surveillance data into formal plans for improvement of patient care at regular intervals and designing and implementing quality improvement initiatives. The collaborators in these initiatives can be infection control practitioners, the hospital epidemiologist or medical director of infection control, a clinical pharmacist, members of quality and patient safety departments, and representatives from nursing, ICU physicians, and respiratory therapy. Others may be necessary depending on the issue at hand, such as housekeeping or information technology.

Isolation Practices: Standard Precautions

Schema to classify infection prevention and control techniques have evolved over time from systems in which a microbiologic laboratory isolate was required (eg, disease-specific *Salmonella* diarrhea isolation), to systems focused on preventing transmission of blood-borne diseases to health care workers (Universal Precautions), to the present system in which certain practices are followed continuously with all patients and supplemented on the basis of syndromic presentation and/or specific laboratory diagnoses. In Canada and the United States, procedures and practices that should be continuously practiced in health care settings are termed *Standard*

TABLE 110.1	Modes of Transmission of Microorganisms in the ICU	
Mode of Transmission	**How Organisms Are Transmitted**	**Example**
Direct	Direct physical contact between an infected or colonized individual and a susceptible host.	Visitor asymptomatically shedding herpes simplex virus kisses postoperative transplant patient.
Indirect	Passive transfer of microorganisms to a susceptible host via an intermediate object such as contaminated hands that are not washed between patients or contaminated instruments or other inanimate objects in the patient's immediate environment.	Health care worker provides care to patient with *Clostridium difficile* diarrhea, does not perform adequate hand hygiene, then enters room of a noncolonized patient and handles bedding and bedrails, leaving *C. difficile* spores in susceptible patient's environment.
Droplet	Large droplets (≥5 μm in diameter) generated from the respiratory tract of the source (infected individual) during coughing or sneezing or during procedures such as suctioning or bronchoscopy. These droplets are propelled a distance of <1 m through the air and are deposited on the nasal or oral mucosa of the new host (newly infected individual) or in the immediate environment. These large droplets do not remain suspended in the air; therefore special ventilation is not required since true aerosolization (see below) does not occur.	Health care worker with influenza virus infection sheds respiratory secretions on the face of a pediatric ICU patient.
Airborne	Dissemination of microorganisms by aerosolization. Organisms are contained in droplet nuclei, airborne particles <5 μm in size that result from evaporation of large droplets, or in dust particles containing skin squames and other debris that remain suspended in the air for long periods. Such microorganisms are widely dispersed by air currents and inhaled by susceptible hosts who may be some distance away from the source patients or individuals, even in different rooms or hospital wards.	Patient with measles is housed on an open ward in the emergency department; airborne virus particles are carried throughout the department and inhaled by susceptible hosts.

Precautions and *Routine Practices,* respectively, and are briefly outlined in Table 110.1. The concept of Standard Precautions, in which the health care worker has a responsibility to practice certain behaviors (eg, hand hygiene) or use certain interventions (eg, wear a mask when face-to-face with a coughing patient) based on a recognition of the *need* to do so rather than because they were asked to do so, has not yet been universally adopted in health care settings. Training in these skills should be considered an essential component of health care worker competency.

The basic components of Standard Precautions are hand hygiene, use of personal protective equipment (PPE) (eg, gowns, gloves, masks, face shields) based on the nature of the health care worker-patient interaction, and the extent of anticipated body fluid exposure, respiratory/cough etiquette, and safe injection practices.

Respiratory Etiquette/Cough Hygiene Practices are measures to contain respiratory secretions and include covering one's cough (eg, coughing into a tissue or the elbow), promptly disposing of tissues, and performing hand hygiene after touching respiratory secretions.

Safe Injection Practices are basic principles of aseptic technique in the preparation and delivery of parenteral medication that limit the risk of infectious disease transmission for both the health care provider and the patient. They include preferential use of single-dose over multidose vials and use of sterile, single-use, disposable needles (needleless access devices) and syringes.

Isolation Practices: Additional Precautions

The specific type of isolation practice (routine, additional) is based on the scientific understanding of how infectious diseases are transmitted from a host or inanimate reservoir to a susceptible host and aims to control or eliminate the reservoir or infectious agent, interrupt transmission, and protect susceptible persons.

If a patient has symptoms or a diagnosis of a communicable infectious disease (eg, cough, diarrhea, rash), then Additional Precautions may be required in addition to Standard Precautions. The three standard types of Additional Precautions are contact, droplet, and airborne, as described earlier. Readers are referred to comprehensive guidelines available from public health agencies such as the US Centers for Disease Control and Prevention (CDC) or from the relevant agency in the jurisdiction in which they practice.

Contact Precautions are intended to prevent transmission of infectious agents that are spread by direct or indirect contact with the patient or the patient's environment. In addition to Standard Precautions, for example, gloves are required for all entries to a patient's room rather than just when patient interaction will occur.

Droplet Precautions are intended to prevent transmission of pathogens through close respiratory or mucous membrane contact with respiratory secretions. In addition to Standard Precautions, for example, health care workers and others coming within 3 to 6 feet of a patient on Droplet Precautions would be required to wear facial protection (mask, goggles, and/or face shield), a gown, and gloves. A child on Droplet Precautions would generally be placed in a room alone to avoid contact with other children. (Note: Some guidelines refer to a 3-ft perimeter of an infectious person on Droplet Precautions, and others refer to a 6-ft distance. The worldwide experience with the severe acute respiratory syndrome (SARS) virus, in which droplet transmission may have occurred up to 6 ft from the source, has led some jurisdictions to implement a 6-ft perimeter for droplet precautions.)

A patient on Airborne Precautions must be placed in a room alone with special air handling and ventilation capacity.

PPE that should be donned by health care workers entering the room of a patient on Airborne Precautions includes a gown, gloves, and a surgical (procedure) mask or respirator depending on the disease encountered.

Enhanced precautions for emerging and highly infectious diseases such as avian influenza and viral hemorrhagic fevers must incorporate the care setting and nature of transmission of the virus. Recent experiences with Ebola virus disease, for example, demonstrate the need for constant reassessment of the capacity for adequate infection control in facilities for emerging and novel infections and for basing infection-control practices on available science.[6]

Determining which physical setting is safest for the child while minimizing risk of transmission of infectious disease from a potentially or definitely infected patient can often be challenging. Within Additional Precautions recommendations is guidance about the need for a single room (eg, whether shared rooms are acceptable) or whether a room with special air handling is required.

There are inherent and substantial safety risks associated with isolation practices.[7] Isolation practices such as single rooms and PPE may limit the number and type of encounters health care workers have with patients because of the cumbersome nature of entering a room, breaking coverage, the discomfort of certain PPE, and the need to come and go to bring equipment, documentation, and other materials.[8] Experience with the care of patients with Ebola virus disease provides a good example of limitations on care due to the isolation practices in place. Limited encounters may inhibit the critical care team's ability to access and assess accurately the child and family, with adult studies suggesting increased HAI risk with lower nurse/patient ratios.[9] Although no conclusions can be drawn regarding recommended staffing levels for isolated patients in the PICU, this evidence suggests that increased vigilance is warranted for these critically ill children.

Hand Hygiene

Contaminated hands of health care workers have been shown in many studies to transmit health care–associated pathogens. The World Health Organization patient safety initiative on hand hygiene emphasizes five moments for hand hygiene: before touching a patient, before clean/aseptic procedures, after body fluid exposure/risk, after touching a patient, and after touching patient surroundings.

The advent of waterless hand hygiene agents has been a particularly important development for the critical care setting because of superior antimicrobial killing, time saved compared with water-based handwashing, rapid action, no risk of antimicrobial resistance, and the ease with which waterless agents can be stationed close to the point of patient care. Alcohol-based hand rubs are in general the preferred hand hygiene product for all health care settings.[10] When hands have visible dirt or organic matter (eg, blood), they must be cleaned with water and soap.

Although the benefits of proper hand hygiene far outweigh the risks, skin irritation and health care worker attitudes about hand hygiene products can be an impediment to compliance and satisfaction with hand hygiene agents and must be considered when choosing a particular product in a specific health care setting. The role of ancillary hand-hygiene measures such as banning watches, long sleeves, and hand jewelry has been used in various jurisdictions to good effect, though controlled data for their efficacy are lacking.[11,12]

Personal Protective Equipment

PPE consists of clothing or devices donned by health care workers for their safety or protection while performing potentially hazardous patient care activity. To interrupt infectious disease transmission, eye protection (goggles or face shield), masks, gowns, and gloves may be worn as a part of Standard Precautions and Transmission-Based Precautions.

A surgical (procedure) mask provides adequate facial protection against droplets generated from the respiratory tract. Surgical masks are also used for source control (eg, on a coughing patient) as a part of respiratory hygiene/cough etiquette. To protect against airborne particles, a particulate filtering face piece respirator is required because it is thought to filter at least 95% of the smaller airborne particles. Airborne particles are known to be produced in certain infectious diseases (eg, tuberculosis, varicella, measles) or may be produced during aerosol-generating procedures in the ICU (eg, intubation) in patients with respiratory infections (eg, influenza, SARS). In a randomized controlled trial during influenza season, surgical masks were not inferior to respirators in preventing influenza transmission.[13] Readers are referred to local public health and infection control authorities for jurisdiction-specific guidance.

Surveillance

Surveillance for HAIs in a PICU is a process in which information about infections acquired after admission is summarized and given back to the care team in a timely manner so that problems can be identified for action. Surveillance has been defined as a "comprehensive method of measuring outcomes and related processes of care, analyzing the data, and providing information to members of the health care team to assist in improving those outcomes and processes."[14]

In the PICU, the most important complications are bloodstream infections and ventilator-associated pneumonia.[15,16] Other important surveillance targets in the PICU are urinary tract infection associated with catheterization, surgical site infections, and acquisition of epidemiologically important pathogens such as methicillin-resistant S. aureus (MRSA), vancomycin-resistant enterococcus (VRE), or other antibiotic-resistant organisms.

The National Health Safety Network (NHSN) of the CDC is a national surveillance system that collects data from a sample of health care facilities that voluntarily submit data on the occurrence of certain HAIs. Because standardized methodology and definitions and risk-adjusted data are used in the NHSN, the surveillance data permit recognition of trends, identification of practices associated with prevention of HAIs, and comparison of rates within and between facilities. Relevant to the PICU setting, NHSN reports central line–associated BSI (CLA-BSI) rates (number of infections per central line days), central line utilization ratio (central line days per patient days), urinary catheter–associated infection (UTI) rate and utilization ratios, and ventilator-associated pneumonia (VAP) rate (VAP days per ventilator days) and utilization. It is important to note that these rates are device specific and therefore incorporate the effect of exposure to an important risk factor. Surveillance results from the NHSN are updated periodically and published in medical journals and on the CDC website.

Standard surveillance definitions have been developed by the CDC (Table 110.2). The CDC definitions incorporate subcategories for children younger than 1 year in recognition of the variable clinical presentation of infection by age. However, CDC definitions may be difficult to apply in children and are often criticized as being overly subjective and easy to manipulate, and alternative approaches have been explored.[17-21]

Identification, synthesis, interpretation, and report generation of HAI surveillance data in the health care setting are performed by infection control professionals. These professionals have completed certification requirements, have achieved competence in infection prevention and control practice, and have been shown to perform HAI surveillance more accurately than do quality assurance personnel.[22]

Screening

Patient Screening

Screening of patients for colonization with certain antibiotic-resistant organisms (AROs) such as MRSA has been proposed as a method to contain spread of these organisms in colonized or infected patients, although data on its efficacy in reducing clinical infections are mixed.[23,24] Several types of ARO screening programs have been described, including admission screening based on risk factors (eg, hospitalization in the past 6 months, patient from a long-term care facility), universal screening on admission, universal decolonization strategies, and weekly point prevalence screening surveys. The pretest likelihood of colonization, cost of the test, timeliness of test reporting, ability to isolate screened patients, and degree to which ARO transmission is occurring are all factors that influence the feasibility and effectiveness of the screening program chosen. Although increased frequency of screening will identify more colonized patients, it is not clear if this practice reduces the frequency of disease or transmission in the PICU setting. Increasing ARO surveillance can be considered when ARO disease and transmission continues to occur despite the implementation of best practices for prevention.[25]

Visitor Screening

The importance of family-centered care and visitation by siblings, as well as parents, means that PICUs must establish mechanisms to identify visitors who may have communicable infections before they enter patient care areas. Education of visitors regarding signs and symptoms of illness and recommendations to remain away can be performed with brochures, posters, telephone messages, and videos, for example.

Occupational Health

Occupational health programs play an essential role in the protection of health care workers from infectious diseases through prevention and management of unintended communicable disease exposures. These interventions reduce the risk of infectious occupational hazards to health care workers, as well as opportunities for health care workers to spread infectious diseases to patients. Occupational health programs ensure health care workers are offered immunization against vaccine-preventable infectious diseases of importance in the health care setting, perform fitness-to-work assessments, assist in educational programs so that health care workers can protect themselves and their families from acquiring infectious diseases while at work (eg, respiratory protection programs, respirator fit testing), and provide postexposure counseling and care (eg, blood exposures during phlebotomy, unprotected intubation of a patient with meningococcemia or group A *Streptococcus* toxic shock syndrome).

Selected Topics in Policy, Procedure, and Program Development to Prevent Health Care–Associated Infection

Infection-prevention strategies often fall into two categories: vertical or horizontal. Vertical infection-prevention strategies are based on reducing colonization or infection due to a specific pathogen, under the pretense that it causes the most morbidity or mortality, is most frequent, or is remediable. Horizontal infection-prevention strategies are universal and population based, with major examples being hand-hygiene and care bundles.

Bundles

Care "bundles" are a group of evidence-based interventions that, when executed together, result in better patient care than when implemented individually. Characteristics of care bundles are their scientific grounding, all-or-none implementation (the process is not completed if one step is left out), goal of improved reliability of processes needed for effective care, and potential to contribute to improved teamwork and interprofessional communication in a care area. There is evidence that they can reduce HAIs or colonization.[26,27] Intervention bundles to prevent BSIs and VAP in the ICU setting have been included in national patient safety campaigns such as the United States' Institute for Healthcare Improvement's "Saving 100,000 Lives" and the Canadian Patient Safety Institute's "Safer Healthcare Now."

Antibiotic Stewardship

Judicious use of antimicrobials is now seen as an essential component of preventing the emergence of multidrug-resistant organisms and improving individual outcomes.[28] Principles of judicious antibiotic use include restriction of antibiotics (eg, stop orders, restricted hospital formulary, requirement for infectious disease consultation for use of certain drugs), timely antimicrobial susceptibility reporting, and educational efforts aimed at changing physician-prescribing practices (see also Chapter 107).[29]

Antibiotic stewardship begins with empiric treatment of the newly admitted patient. Although a suspected severe infection should initially be treated with broad-spectrum antibiotics, therapy should be changed to the most narrow spectrum agent once culture results are available or discontinued if there is no further evidence of bacterial infection.

Antibiotic cycling refers to a scheduled rotation of antibiotics with similar spectrums of bacterial coverage for a specified period, with the aim of limiting the emergence of resistance to any single agent. Although this strategy has been proposed as a potential method to decrease antimicrobial resistance, there is insufficient evidence to recommend its widespread application at this time, and further clinical studies are required in the PICU context.[30-32]

The clinical pharmacist is an integral member of PICU daily bedside rounds. He or she should participate in the one-on-one education of house staff and nursing, be available for consultation, and assist in the development of evidence-based antibiotic prescribing guidelines based on local epidemiology.

TABLE 110.2	Summary of Centers for Disease Control and Prevention (CDC)/National Healthcare Safety Network (NHSN) Definitions for Health Care–Associated Infections (HAIs)	
	This summary of the CDC/NHSN surveillance definitions for HAIs and criteria is not comprehensive. The reader is directed to up-to-date information available on the website of the National Healthcare Safety Network.[80]	
Bloodstream infection	Laboratory confirmed *(infections must be primary)*	*Regardless of age:* Recognized pathogen from ≥1 blood culture, *or* Common skin contaminant in ≥2 blood cultures associated with symptoms (fever, chills, hypotension) *≤1 yr of age:* Common skin contaminant in ≥2 blood cultures, *and* Associated with symptoms (fever >38°C or <37°C, apnea, bradycardia)
	Clinical sepsis	*Applies only to ≤1 yr of age:* Symptoms (fever >38°C or <37°C, apnea, bradycardia), *and* Negative or no blood culture done, *and* Physician initiates sepsis treatment, *and* No primary infection elsewhere
Systemic infection	Disseminated infection	Infections, usually of viral origin, without an apparent single site of infection and involving multiple organs and systems (eg, varicella)
UTI	Symptomatic	≥10^5 Microorganisms/mL urine, not >2 species, and symptoms (at least one of the following: fever >38°C, urgency, frequency, dysuria, suprapubic tenderness) Symptoms (at least 2 of the following: fever >38°C, urgency, frequency, dysuria, suprapubic tenderness) *and* at least 1 of 5 urinary laboratory criteria *or* physician diagnosis *or* treatment for UTI Separate criteria are available for children ≤1 yr without nonspecific symptoms (not referent to the urinary tract) *and* 1 of 7 laboratory criteria
	Asymptomatic	Indwelling urinary catheter within 7 days before urine culture, *and* ≥10^5 Microorganisms/mL urine, not >2 species, *and* Asymptomatic, *or* No indwelling urinary catheter within 7 days of urine culture, *and* ≥10^5 Microorganisms/mL urine, not >2 species in 2 urine cultures with same organism(s)
Pneumonia (alternate criteria are used for the diagnosis of pneumonia in adults)	Clinically defined (infants and children)	Serial chest radiographs (≥1 for patients without underlying disease and ≥2 for patient with underlying disease) with new or progressive and persistent infiltrate or consolidation or cavitation, or pneumatoceles (in ≤1 yr old), and Clinical signs and symptoms (vary according to the patient age: ≤1 yr or ≥1 yr and ≤12 yr)
Lower respiratory tract, not pneumonia	Bronchitis, tracheobronchitis, other lung infection	No clinical or radiographic evidence of pneumonia, *and* ≥2 symptoms or signs (fever >38°C, cough, new or increased sputum production, rhonchi, wheezing), *and* ≥1 positive cultures from deep tracheal aspirate or bronchoscopy *or* positive antigen test on respiratory secretions, *or* Child ≤1 yr with no clinical or radiographic evidence of pneumonia, *and* ≥2 symptoms or signs (fever >38°C, cough, new or increased sputum production, rhonchi, wheezing, respiratory distress, apnea, or bradycardia), *and* One or more of the following: positive culture from deep tracheal aspirate or bronchoscopy *or* positive antigen test on respiratory secretions, *or* serologic diagnosis
Ear, eye, nose, throat, mouth	Conjunctivitis	Pathogen cultured from purulent exudate from conjunctiva or contiguous tissues, *or* Patient has redness or swelling of conjunctiva or periorbital area and white blood cells and organisms on Gram stain *or* purulent exudate, positive antigen test on exudate, *or* conjunctival scraping, positive viral culture, serologic diagnosis, or multinucleated giant cells on microscopic examination of conjunctival exudate
	Sinusitis (separate criteria exist for oral cavity, ear and mastoid infections, eye infections other than conjunctivitis, and pharyngitis, laryngitis, and epiglottitis)	≥1 of the following: Organism cultured from purulent material from sinus cavity, *or* ≥1 of the following signs or symptoms with no other recognized cause: fever >38°C, pain or tenderness over the involved sinus, headache, purulent exudate, or nasal obstruction, *and/or* positive transillumination or positive radiographic examination

Continued

TABLE 110.2 Summary of Centers for Disease Control and Prevention (CDC)/National Healthcare Safety Network (NHSN) Definitions for Health Care–Associated Infections (HAIs) — cont'd

CNS	Intracranial infection	≥1 of the following: Organisms cultured from brain tissue, *or* Abscess or intracranial infection seen during surgical operation, *or* Selected CNS symptoms without another cause *and* 1 of 4 laboratory criteria, *or* Patient ≤1 yr with at least 1of 5 selected symptoms *and* 1 of 5 laboratory criteria
	Meningitis or ventriculitis	Organisms cultured from cerebrospinal fluid, *or* ≥1 of the following symptoms: fever, headache, stiff neck, meningeal signs, cranial nerve signs, irritability, *and* 1 of 5 laboratory criteria, *or* Patient ≤1 yr with at least of 1 of 5 selected symptoms *and* 1 of 5 laboratory criteria
	Spinal abscess without meningitis	Organisms cultured from abscess in the spinal epidural or subdural space, *or* Abscess in spinal epidural or subdural space seen during surgery, autopsy, or in histopathologic examination
SSI	Superficial incisional, primary or secondary	Occurs within 30 days of operative procedure, *and* Involves only skin and subcutaneous tissue of the incision, *and* ≥1 of the following: purulent drainage from incision, organisms isolated from aseptically obtained incisional fluid or tissue, one sign or symptom (pain, tenderness, redness, swelling, heat), *and* Surgeon opens incision and incision is not cultured or is culture positive
	Deep incisional, primary or secondary	Occurs within 30 days of operative procedure or within 1 yr if an implant is left in place, *and* Involves deep soft tissues of the incision, *and* ≥1 of the following: purulent drainage from the deep incision but not from the organ/space of the surgical site, spontaneous dehiscence of surgical site or symptomatic patient has site opened by surgeon and incision is not cultured or is culture positive, abscess found on direct examination (radiologic, histopathologic, or during operation), or surgeon diagnosis
	Organ space, primary or secondary, indicated specific type (eg, cardiac)	Occurs within 30 days of operative procedure or within 1 yr if an implant is left in place, *and* Infection involves any part of the body, excluding superficial or deep incisional areas, opened or manipulated during the operative procedure, *and* Patient has 1 of the following: purulent drainage via a drain placed into organ/space; organisms cultured from aseptically obtained specimen from organ/space; abscess found on direct examination, during reoperation, or by radiologic or histologic examination or surgeon diagnosis
Bone and joint infection (separate criteria exist for joint or bursa infection and disc space infection)	Bone (osteomyelitis)	≥1 of the following: Organisms cultured from bone, diagnosis based on direct examination during surgery or on histopathologic examination, *or* ≥2 symptoms (fever >38°C, localized swelling, tenderness, heat, or drainage at bone site), *and* 1 laboratory finding (positive blood culture or blood antigen test or radiographic evidence of infection)
Cardiovascular system	Mediastinitis (separate criteria exist for endocarditis, myocarditis, pericarditis, and vascular infection)	≥1 of the following*: Organisms isolated from mediastinal tissue or fluid obtained by aspirate or during surgery, *or* Diagnosis during surgical procedure or by histopathologic examination, *or* Presence of one or more of the following signs or symptoms: fever >38°C, chest pain, or sternal instability, *and* ≥1 of the following: mediastinal widening on chest radiograph, purulent drainage, or organism cultured from drainage
Gastrointestinal (separate criteria exist for hepatitis, gastrointestinal tract infections, and intra-abdominal infection)	Gastroenteritis	≥1 of the following: Acute-onset liquid stools for >12 hr with or without vomiting or fever and no likely noninfectious cause, *or* ≥2 of following signs and symptoms: nausea, vomiting, abdominal pain, fever >38°C, or headache, *and* ≥1 of the following: enteric pathogen detected in stool or rectal swab (by culture, routine or electron microscopy, or cytopathic change in tissue culture), or enteric pathogen detected by antigen or antibody assay on blood or feces
	Necrotizing enteritis	In infants, ≥2 signs and symptoms (vomiting, abdominal distention, prefeeding residuals) and no other recognized cause, *and* Persistent microscopic or gross blood in stools, *and* More than one radiologic abnormality (eg, pneumoperitoneum, pneumatosis intestinalis, unchanging rigid loops of small bowel)

Primary, first infection; *secondary,* infection as a result of another previous infection in the patient.
*For infants ≤1 yr of age, the symptoms and signs above are adapted to fever (>38°C rectal), hypothermia (<37°C rectal), apnea, bradycardia, or sternal instability.

Antibiotic Gastric Decontamination

Normal gut flora have an important role in nutrition, metabolism, and immune regulation. The normal balance of organisms is altered when a child becomes ill or receives antibiotics, leading to infection by endogenous flora. Selective decontamination of the digestive tract was first introduced in 1983 and has been extensively studied in adult ICU patients, demonstrating no effect on resistance patterns and a mortality benefit in some studies.[33,34] Selective decontamination protocols involve a short course of IV antimicrobials (eg, third-generation cephalosporin) and oropharyngeal and enteral nonabsorbable antimicrobials (eg, colistin, amphotericin B, tobramycin) in addition to routine infection control practices. Despite the presence of data in children showing benefit in small randomized controlled trials, use in North America remains infrequent in both adult and pediatric ICUs.[35-37]

Probiotics

An alternate strategy to reduce the development of potential AROs is the oral administration of probiotics (nonpathogenic microorganisms) such as lactobacillus. Their main role appears to be the prevention of pediatric antibiotic-associated diarrhea, prevention of necrotizing enterocolitis in premature infants, and treatment of *C. difficile*–associated diarrhea. Although apparently not associated with harm, the role of probiotics remains unclear in the critically ill child and cannot currently be recommended as a routine management strategy.[38,39]

Specific Health Care–Associated Infection Syndromes in the Pediatric Intensive Care Unit

Bloodstream Infections

BSIs are usually the most common HAI acquired in the PICU setting and are associated with morbidity, excess length of stay, and mortality, with estimates of attributable costs of up to $16,000 to $39,000 per patient.[40,41] Most BSIs are associated with intravascular catheter use and commensal skin flora that gain access to the bloodstream through the device. The scope of intravascular device–associated infections includes laboratory-confirmed bacteremia, infections of the skin and subcutaneous tissues around the device (exit site and tunnel infections), clinically defined sepsis, septic thrombophlebitis and thrombosis, and right-sided endocarditis. For surveillance purposes, BSIs are categorized as primary (no other identifiable source of infection) or secondary (the BSI occurred as the result of an infection at another site). Surveillance definitions used for CLA-BSI can be found in Table 110.2.

Epidemiology

The pooled mean rate of CLA-BSIs in 293 pediatric medical/surgical ICUs representing more than 400,000 central line days in the 2012 report of the NHSN was 1.4 infections per 1000 central line days, with a 25th percentile of 0.0 and a 90th percentile of 2.9. Rates are similar in cardiothoracic and surgical-specific critical care units. The rates of CLA-BSIs have been rapidly declining over the past decade, being upwards of 4.7/1000 patient days as recent as 2007.[15] The median utilization ratio was 0.46 (central line days per patient days), which is comparable with adult ICUs.

The most common infecting organism in CLA-BSI is the gram-positive bacteria coagulase-negative *Staphylococcus*

(CONS), a group of about 20 species including *Staphylococcus epidermidis*, that are normal flora of human skin. Gram-negative bacteria, including Enterobacteriaceae, and nonfermenting gram-negative bacteria such as *Pseudomonas* spp., *Acinetobacter* spp., and *Stenotrophomonas* spp., account for about 25% of infections. *Candida* spp. infections are increasingly recognized.[42]

There are many types of intravascular devices, including central venous catheters (CVCs), arterial catheters, and peripherally inserted catheters, all of which are associated with infection. Catheters can also be classified according to the site of insertion, expected duration of placement (eg, long vs. short term), and path to the vessel (eg, tunneled or not). To date, surveillance for HAI associated with these devices has focused on central venous lines. However, with rates of infection of arterial catheters in adult studies comparable to those for pediatric central lines, these must be monitored appropriately.[43]

Prevention

Successful programs to reduce the incidence of CLA-BSIs have been reported in the past decade; all use multimodal team-based, systematic approaches in which combinations of effective preventive interventions are introduced into a care setting.

The central line bundle is a combination of eight components broken into two separate bundles for insertion and maintenance. The bundle components described in the following sections are from the Canadian Safer Healthcare Now campaign and align with other improvement bundle packages for reduction of CLA-BSIs, and they have been proven effective in substantially reducing CLA-BSI incidence.[44]

The insertion bundle components include hand hygiene, maximal barrier precautions, and skin antisepsis. Maximal sterile barrier precautions for the inserter mean strict compliance with hand hygiene, a cap that covers all hair, a mask that covers the mouth and nose securely, a sterile gown, and sterile gloves. The patient is covered from head to toe with a sterile drape except for a small opening for the insertion site and to maintain the airway. Chlorhexidine skin antisepsis is recommended over other antiseptic agents. With regard to the optimal site for a line, practitioners are urged to consider what is best for the patient on the basis of current and future needs, anatomic features, and the inserter's technical competence.

Other components of success include empowering nurses to enforce the use of a central line checklist that incorporates inclusion of all components of the insertion bundle and constraining practice by creating central line insertion kits or carts that include the required equipment needed to maintain asepsis (eg, only one antiseptic offered: chlorhexidine).

Antibiotic-impregnated CVCs are not recommended for routine use unless the concerted efforts to implement a strategy fail to reduce a local institution's infection rates below benchmark levels. They may be considered in specific patient populations such as the immunosuppressed requiring long-term CVC use, although their superiority over standard CVCs in this population has never been proven.

Ultrasound guidance for insertion of CVCs to reduce insertion-related complications has become the standard of care for the past decade (see also Chapter 20). The associated temporal decrease in insertion-related complications might contribute to a reduction in CLA-BSIs through less traumatic catheter placement, but this remains to be proven.

The maintenance bundle to prevent CLA-BSIs incorporates, in addition to hand hygiene, multimodal education and training programs, aseptic access to the lumens (scrubbing the hub), regular checks of the entry site for inflammation with each dressing change (at minimum), daily review of line necessity with removal if deemed unnecessary, and a dedicated total parenteral nutrition line.

Emerging trends in maintenance of CVCs include chlorhexidine-impregnated transparent dressings and disc (which hug the catheter at the insertion site) and are intended to reduce the quantity of bacteria at the skin entry site.[45] Daily chlorhexidine bathing has been shown in one study to reduce bacteremia in critically ill children, although this has yet to be widely adopted, with recent pragmatic adult studies showing no benefit.[46,47]

Practitioners are urged to check for recent updates in CLA-BSI reduction quality improvement strategies from Safer Healthcare Now (www.saferhealthcarenow.ca) or the Institute for Healthcare Improvement (www.ihi.org) or their national or local equivalents, as optimal strategies change over time on the basis of evolving evidence.

Management
The diagnosis of BSI is based only on clinical signs and symptoms and is insensitive and nonspecific.[48] Microbiologic confirmation should be sought and broad-spectrum antimicrobial therapy initiated early and targeted at likely pathogens until results are available. If the device is suspected to be the source of infection or to have been secondarily infected, the clinician will need to decide if the infection can be eradicated with the device in place. The need for catheter removal will depend on the infecting organism and the availability of another route for parental access and antibiotic administration. Although coagulase-negative *Staphylococcus* (CONS) infections can often be treated without catheter removal, this is difficult if the infection is due to fungal infection or infection with *Pseudomonas* spp. or *S. aureus*.[49] The possibility of secondary seeding of the heart or thrombophlebitis should also be considered during decision making.

Respiratory Infections and Ventilator-Associated Pneumonia
Respiratory Infections
Respiratory infections acquired during health care encompass a broad range of illness of the upper and lower respiratory tract (see Table 110.2). In the child with high-acuity illness requiring admission to the PICU, some respiratory infections are particularly associated with increased morbidity, mortality, and health care cost. The following section focuses on viral respiratory tract infections, VAP, and sinusitis.

Epidemiology
Surveillance for hospital-acquired viral respiratory illness is infrequently reported, although the burden of disease is likely substantial.[50] Hospital-acquired RSV is associated with prolonged length of stay, hospital costs, and increased morbidity and mortality rates.[45,51,52]

Like RSV, influenza virus HAI occurs at the same time as the local winter community epidemic. Coronaviruses such as SARS and MERS-CoV have caused nosocomial transmission in Canada, Asia, and the Middle East, causing large morbidity and mortality among patients and health care providers.[53,54]

Respiratory viral illness can increase the risk of secondary bacterial infection because the normal defensive function of the mucociliary apparatus is impaired and colonizing bacteria in the respiratory tract can invade through the nasopharynx or descend to the lower respiratory tree.

VAP is the second most common HAI in the PICU. In the most recent NHSN report pooling data from 132 pediatric medical-surgical ICUs, the pooled mean incidence was 0.8 episodes of VAP per 1000 ventilator days.[55] Notably, the rate of VAP has decreased in the past decade from mean rates of 2.9 per 1000 ventilator days in 2002.[56] VAP is a serious and life-threatening complication of PICU admission and is associated with prolonged ICU stay, need for ventilatory support, excess costs, and increased mortality.[57]

VAP is usually due to endogenous bacteria, and less commonly fungi, from the patient's oropharynx. It is often categorized into early (<5 days after intubation) and late (>5 days after intubation). Early VAP is usually caused by normal endogenous flora of the respiratory tract such as *Haemophilus influenzae*, *Moraxella* spp., *Streptococcus pneumoniae*, and alpha-hemolytic *Streptococcus* spp. During hospitalization, the normal endogenous flora of the nasopharynx are replaced within days by gram-negative bacteria such as *Pseudomonas* spp., *Escherichia coli*, *Acinetobacter*, and *Stenotrophomonas* spp., as well as various *Enterobacteriaceae* spp. or *S. aureus*. For practical reasons, many studies base their laboratory diagnosis on specimens obtained from the endotracheal tube rather than invasive sampling of the lower respiratory tract; hence isolated microorganisms could be present in the nasopharynx, colonizing the endotracheal tube, or actually be the cause of infection in the lung.[58]

In addition to its role as a conduit, the endotracheal tube also serves as a foreign body. As with other devices, an endotracheal tube interferes with normal defense mechanisms (eg, cough, mucociliary apparatus) and acts as a nidus for adherence of microorganisms, which create a biofilm. Tracheal suctioning can cause mucosal denudation and detachment and aspiration of adherent biofilm aggregates that become a pulmonary inoculum. Not surprisingly, the length of respiratory assistance and endotracheal intubation—and therefore the device-related risk—remain significant risk factors of nosocomial pneumonia.[59] Other risk factors for HAI pneumonia include immune deficiency, use of neuromuscular blocking agents, reintubation, transport outside the ICU, multiple organ dysfunction, shock, multiple-organ trauma, severe head trauma, and burns.[60-62]

Prevention
Respiratory Viruses
Prevention of HAI respiratory virus infection in the PICU can be accomplished through a collaborative effort between the PICU and the organization's infection prevention and control and occupational health programs. The goal of this effort is to avoid contact between persons with probable or definite respiratory infection (including family members) and PICU patients, with prompt institution of isolation practices in symptomatic patients, regardless of laboratory confirmation.

Occupational health programs assess fitness-to-work in health care workers with possible respiratory illness. An employee with new-onset cough and rhinorrhea, for example, could be deployed to a non–patient care assignment rather than the PICU or sent home. The occupational health program should ensure immunization status for employees is current and offer annual influenza vaccine programs.

As part of the hospital and PICU admission process, screening of the patient for symptoms and signs of infectious illness should be conducted to determine appropriate placement. In the winter respiratory season, screening of all children for viral infections and placing them in isolation until results are available have been reported to limit nosocomial spread, with tests available for a variety of respiratory viruses.[63]

Ventilator-Associated Pneumonia

Strategies of prevention are directed against the three mechanisms by which VAP is thought to occur: aspiration of secretions, colonization of the aerodigestive tract, and use of contaminated equipment. General recommended measures are to conduct active surveillance for VAP, minimize the duration of ventilation and use noninvasive ventilation whenever possible, perform daily assessments of readiness to wean/discontinue mechanical ventilation, and educate health care workers who care for ventilated patients about VAP. The Society for Healthcare Epidemiology of America publishes VAP-prevention guidelines, including pediatric specific discussions.[64]

Specific precautions of the pediatric VAP bundle are hand hygiene before and after circuit manipulation, elevation of the head of the bed (angle varies based on positioning limitations of the child based on age), proper positioning of the oral or nasogastric tube, elimination of the routine use of instillation before suctioning of the endotracheal tube, changing in-line suctioning catheters only when visibly soiled or malfunctioning, regular oral care for all children, and maintaining the ventilator tubing in a dependent position. Adolescent patients are recommended to use endotracheal tubes with subglottic secretion drainage for high-risk patients who are likely to require intubation for longer than 72 hours.[65]

The strategies to prevent VAP highlight practical recommendations, with not one specific intervention found to be effective; rather, a bundle of care and maintained vigilance are the most effective tools in VAP prevention.

Management

The management of RSV infection in the PICU is mainly supportive. Influenza infection can be treated with neuraminidase inhibitors (oseltamivir, zanamavir), which shorten the duration of fever and improve outcomes in critically ill children.[66,67]

Ventilator-Associated Pneumonia

VAP is difficult to diagnose accurately because of the inaccessibility of the lower respiratory tract. The gold standard for diagnosis is microbiologic confirmation from a lower respiratory tract specimen, such as lung biopsy. Obtaining uncontaminated lower respiratory tract specimens in children by bronchoalveolar lavage, lung biopsy, and transthoracic biopsy are procedures with inherent risks.[68,69] Despite the accepted shortcomings, tracheal aspirates remain the most common specimen for guiding initial empiric antibiotic therapy in a child with suspected VAP. There is often poor correlation between tracheal aspirate microbiology and bronchoalveolar microbiology.[58] Recent changes in adult definitions of VAP have expanded the term to ventilator-associated events to more effectively and objectively capture complications of ventilation, including pneumonia. These changes have yet to apply to children, although this is likely forthcoming.

Aggressive and prompt treatment is required when nosocomial pneumonia is suspected in a critically ill patient. Initial empiric therapy for VAP should be broadly based, with consideration of local microbiologic data on antibiotic resistance and a plan to reevaluate and narrow antibiotic selection when results of cultures or other diagnostic information is available. If aspiration is suspected, coverage for anaerobes can be considered (eg, ticarcillin-clavulanate or clindamycin). If methicillin-resistant *S. aureus* is suspected, vancomycin or linezolid should be used. The appropriate duration of therapy for VAP in children is not known, with most experts recommending a 5- to 10-day course of therapy.

Sinusitis

Although acute sinusitis (inflammation of the nose and paranasal sinuses) is a common infection in childhood, data on its occurrence in the PICU are scarce.[70] Studies in adults have shown an increased risk of sinusitis in nasotracheal intubations, with prolonged nasal cannulation associated with increased incidence of sinusitis in older children and adults. Studies have also indicated that larger nasal cannulae appear to accelerate this process and that fewer devices in the nose decrease risk of infection.[71-73] When the diagnosis is based on computed tomography (CT) imaging, however, it can be observed in up to 70% of ventilated patients; the clinical relevance of this finding remains undetermined.[70] Active surveillance for this HAI is not done by most programs.

Sinusitis can be categorized as acute or subacute bacterial, recurrent acute bacterial, chronic, or acute on chronic in nature. Although the ethmoid and maxillary sinuses are present at birth, the sphenoid and frontal sinuses are not pneumatized until age 5 and 7 years, respectively. Diagnosis of sinusitis is challenging in children, particularly in the intubated child. Direct sinus puncture to permit microbiologic identification of infecting organisms is the gold standard for diagnosis, although it is rarely performed. Normal sinus radiographs and CT scans provide evidence that sinusitis is absent, but mucosal thickening is a nonspecific finding. The surveillance definition of health care–associated sinusitis is seen in Table 110.2.

Acute sinusitis is most commonly caused by respiratory flora such as *S. pneumoniae, H. influenzae,* and *Moraxella* spp. In ventilator-associated sinusitis, *S. aureus, Pseudomonas aeruginosa,* enteric gram-negative bacilli, and streptococcal infection also need to be considered, and it is often coincident with VAP.

Prevention

The paranasal sinuses are contiguous with the nasopharynx and mostly lined with pseudostratified ciliated respiratory epithelium. The normal defense of the sinuses against infection is the mucociliary apparatus. Factors that would be expected to predispose to sinus obstruction or decreased mucociliary function include foreign bodies in the nasopharynx (eg, nasogastric or endotracheal tubes), previous viral respiratory infection, preexisting abnormalities such as cilial disorders or cystic fibrosis, and craniofacial anatomic abnormalities or facial trauma. Orotracheal intubation is recommended over nasotracheal intubation in older children because the latter may increase the risk of sinusitis. Judicious use of antibiotics in the ICU would be expected to decrease the risk of colonization of the respiratory tract with gram-negative and antibiotic-resistant organisms.

Management

Because of their proximity to the brain, bacterial or fungal infection of the sinuses may be complicated by contiguous spread. Systemic antimicrobial therapy should be directed broadly to cover anaerobic respiratory flora, gram-positive and gram-negative bacteria such as *Pseudomonas* spp., and enteric flora. Options for antibacterial coverage include a third-generation cephalosporin or monobactam or an extended-spectrum penicillin–clavulanic acid combination with the addition of vancomycin to cover MRSA or penicillin-resistant pneumococcus, depending on local antimicrobial susceptibility and epidemiology.

An otolaryngologist should be consulted in the care of children with complicated sinusitis to determine if surgery is necessary to remediate ostial obstruction or drainage of abscesses. Involvement of the CNS requires neurosurgical intervention. The infectious disease team should also be involved to assist in determining optimal antibiotic combinations and duration of therapy in complicated cases with CNS involvement.

Urinary Tract Infections

The spectrum of illness associated with urinary tract infection (UTI) in the PICU can range from asymptomatic bacteriuria in the presence of a catheter to a funguria that becomes a source of life-threatening disseminated fungal infection.

Epidemiology

A mean of 2.7 catheter-associated UTIs (CA-UTIs) occurred per 1000 catheter days in the US National Health Safety Network surveillance system, with 268 pediatric medical-surgical ICUs reporting in 2012.[55] This rate is less than the 4.0 infections per 1000 urinary catheter days determined 10 years earlier,[56] although compared with CLA-BSI and VAP, the declines over recent years have been less robust (see Fig. 110.1).

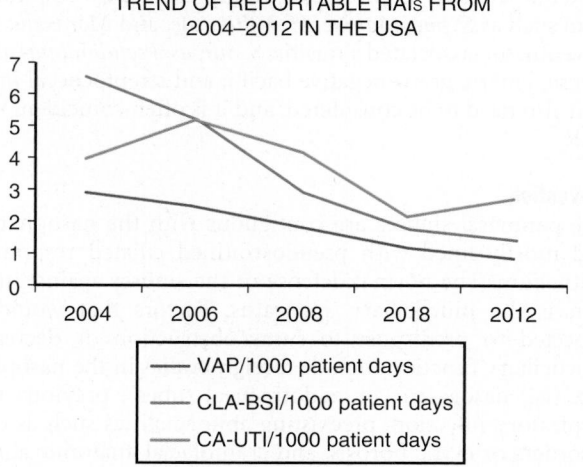

TREND OF REPORTABLE HAIs FROM 2004–2012 IN THE USA

— VAP/1000 patient days
— CLA-BSI/1000 patient days
— CA-UTI/1000 patient days

Fig. 110.1. Trend of ventilator-associated pneumonia, central line–associated bloodstream infections, and catheter-associated urinary tract infections from 2004–2012. (From National Healthcare Safety Network, 2012 report. Available at: http://www.cdc.gov/nhsn/dataStat.html.)

A urinary catheter is both a foreign body in the urinary tract and a conduit for microorganisms to ascend to the bladder, ureters, kidneys, and potentially to the bloodstream. Voiding is an important defense mechanism for the urinary tract in which periurethral flora are flushed out regularly. Because of the urethra's anatomic location in the perineum, the most common organisms causing community and health care–associated UTI are normal periurethral or perirectal flora such as *E. coli* and *Klebsiella pneumoniae*. However, Enterobacteriaceae such as *Pseudomonas* spp. and opportunistic organisms such as *S. aureus, S. epidermidis,* and *Candida* spp. can also be involved.

In addition to the general factors that increase risk for HAI in the PICU, children at increased risk for UTI include those with preexisting uropathies, especially neurogenic bladder.

Prevention

Guidelines for the prevention of CA-UTI in acute care hospitals focus on certain key strategies, all related to urinary catheter use: (1) recommendations for which patients should receive indwelling urinary catheters, (2) recommendations for catheter insertion, (3) recommendations for catheter maintenance, and (4) quality improvement programs and daily reminders to achieve appropriate placement, care, and removal of catheters.[74] The most important action that PICU staff can take to prevent CA-UTIs is to limit the use of urinary tract instrumentation, particularly indwelling urinary catheters. Systemic morphine infusions are not a contraindication to the removal of the urinary catheter.

Proper technique for catheter insertion includes hand hygiene before and after any manipulation of the device, use of aseptic technique, use of the smallest bore catheter needed, and proper securement of the catheter after insertion to prevent movement. The catheter should be maintained as a closed drainage system with unobstructed urine flow. The catheter and collecting system should be replaced if the system is disconnected or leaks occur. Standard Precautions should be used for any manipulation of the catheter or collecting system (eg, use of gloves and gowns as appropriate). Neither systemic antimicrobials, bladder irrigation with antimicrobials, nor complex drainage systems with antiseptics are recommended to prevent CA-UTIs. Special catheter materials (eg, antimicrobial impregnation) are only recommended if a comprehensive strategy to reduce CA-UTI rates is unsuccessful.

Management

Surveillance definitions for UTI acquired in the health care setting are found in Table 110.2. Of note, infection may be asymptomatic or symptomatic. In the critically ill PICU patient, diagnosis of UTI may be difficult because of inability to determine symptoms and signs; therefore laboratory criteria from aseptically obtained urine specimens are essential, with specific criteria for infection available.

For CA-UTI, the catheter should be removed as soon as possible. Once removed, intermittent catheterization may be required if spontaneous voiding does not occur. Therapy should be the narrowest spectrum agent that will treat the offending pathogen; appropriate empiric choices before availability of antimicrobial susceptibility should include consideration of common infecting organisms in that PICU, with appropriate initial choices including an extended-spectrum penicillin or a third-generation cephalosporin.

Skin and Surgical Site Infections

The integument is the largest organ in the human body; it is a barrier to invasion of microorganisms and plays a role in thermal regulation and fluid homeostasis. Disruption of the skin, whether by surgery, insertion of biomedical devices, or pressure sores, interrupts a key defense against infection.

Although almost all surgical procedures are performed in the operating room, a substantial component of care in the PICU is postoperative care for critically ill children. Procedures may also need to be performed in the PICU in patients who are too unstable for transport to the surgical suite or do not have primary closure of the surgical wound. The surveillance definition of skin and surgical site infections (SSTIs) is in Table 110.2.

Epidemiology

The incidence of SSTIs is 1.8% of all pediatric surgical procedures from a recent administrative database and represents less than 10% of HAIs in PICUs.[1,75] In adults, they are now the most common and costly HAI.[76] Complications of SSIs include contiguous or systemic spread and, in adults, an increased length of stay of 7 to 10 days and increased risk of death.

Most commonly, the source of infection is the patient's own flora that migrate into the wound, but other sources include the surgical staff and contaminated instruments. *S. aureus* is the most common pathogen in SSIs without biomedical device placement, but *P. aeruginosa* and other gram-negative bacteria can be isolated. Often a single microbiologic cause is not identified because the surgical site is open and contiguous with skin or mucosa. In procedures in which a device is implanted (eg, neurosurgical cerebrospinal fluid shunts), the most common organism isolated is CONS. Of growing importance are infections caused by multidrug-resistant organisms, such as MRSA, and fungi.

Risk for an SSI can be predicted in adult patients by using the National Nosocomial Infections Surveillance System index, which combines the traditional four-category wound classification system of clean, clean-contaminated, contaminated, and dirty or infected with the American Society of Anesthesiology score and duration of procedure time.[77] An equivalent validated scoring system to identify high-risk children has not been developed. Multiple variables associated with increased risk for SSI in various studies include intrinsic factors (eg, age, glucose control, obesity/malnutrition, smoking, steroid use, prolonged preoperative hospital stay, preoperative nares colonization with *S. aureus,* perioperative transfusion and immunosuppressive medications, presurgical comorbidity) and extrinsic factors (eg, preoperative antiseptic showering, preoperative hair removal, patient skin preparation in the operating room, preoperative hand/forearm antisepsis, management of infected or colonized surgical personnel, antimicrobial prophylaxis). In pediatric cardiac surgery patients, an open sternum is a risk factor for SSIs, with 13% of children with delayed sternal closure developing an SSI in a recent series.[78] Operative risk factors are surgical scrub by the team, skin preparation of the patient, appropriate and timely antibiotic prophylaxis, surgical drapes and attire, surgeon skill and technique, asepsis, and operative time. Operating room characteristics are also considered extrinsic factors. They include ventilation, traffic, and sterilization of surgical equipment. Postoperative factors incorporate incision care and discharge planning.

Prevention

Prevention of SSIs is directed at addressing the clinical variables that increase the probability of infection, as previously mentioned. For example, patient skin preparation, health care worker hand hygiene, and antimicrobial prophylaxis affect the inoculum of bacteria into the wound. Optimal glucose and temperature control enhance the capacity of the host to deal with invading organisms. Recommendations for the prevention of SSTIs are available and updated frequently.[77]

Most SSI bundles include measures to improve timing and choice of antimicrobial prophylaxis, appropriate hair removal, and prospective surgical wound infection surveillance with provision of feedback to individual surgeons. The surveillance definitions for SSI are provided in Table 110.2.

A considerable body of research has demonstrated that perioperative antibiotic prophylaxis is most effective when given 1 hour before the incision to maximize tissue concentration during cut time—when the antibiotic (as narrow spectrum as possible and as short a course as possible) is active against the likely contaminating organisms. Although the duration of administration varies by procedure, the optimal duration ranges from the immediate perioperative period to the 24 hours after the surgery. Doses beyond this interval do not prevent infection and put the patient at risk of developing infections with resistant bacteria and fungi. The choice and duration of antibiotic prophylaxis depend on the surgical procedure, degree of wound contamination, emergency or elective surgery, and patient allergy.

Postoperative surgical site care includes regular observations and documentation of the integrity of the site. Recommendations for postoperative incision care include protecting a primary closure incision with a sterile dressing for 24 to 48 hours postoperatively, adhering to hand hygiene principles, applying sterile technique when changing dressings, promoting proper incision care, and identifying complications by educating patients and families.[77]

Management

Recognition of SSIs requires regular wound inspection for the usual signs of inflammation, with or without pus. Microbiologic confirmation of infection is often not useful because of contamination of the operative site by contiguous external surfaces. Treatment of SSIs includes appropriate empiric antimicrobials directed at the likely infecting organisms and subsequent narrowing of the spectrum if organism identification and susceptibility are available. Drainage of the infected area should be facilitated (eg, removal of staples), wound debridement may be required, and foreign bodies may need to be removed. The extent of the infection will determine the wound care requirements, which may involve packing the wounds or use of negative pressure wound therapy.

Ventriculostomy-Related Infections

The incidence of ventriculostomy-associated infection varies widely in the literature and is influenced by both patient characteristics and system factors, such as infection control policies and procedures pertaining to placement and maintenance of external ventricular drains. The risk increases with increasing duration of catheterization and with repeated insertions, but routine replacement is not recommended. The use of local antibiotic irrigation or prophylactic systemic antibiotics is not recommended. Routine surveillance cultures of cerebrospinal fluid are not more likely to detect infection than are cultures obtained when clinically indicated.[79]

Hospital-Associated Diarrhea

C. difficile–associated diarrhea is a potentially life-threatening illness that can range in clinical presentation from diarrhea to colitis and megacolon. Children, especially those younger than 5, are often asymptomatic carriers and likely have other causes of symptoms, especially in those younger than 5 years of age. However, it can cause problematic illness in immunosuppressed patients and pediatric practitioners should be familiar with its diagnosis and management. Outbreaks of rotavirus and norovirus can occur in critical care settings, where close health care worker/patient contact can facilitate spread of secretions. Prevention of diarrheal illness is accomplished by prompt isolation of patients with diarrhea before laboratory results are available, careful hand hygiene, and regular and thorough environmental cleaning focusing on high-touch surfaces.

Acknowledgments

We gratefully acknowledge the contributions of Tracie Northway and Joanne Langley, who coauthored this chapter in previous editions.

Key References

1. Grohskopf LA, Sinkowitz-Cochran RL, Garrett DO, et al. A national point-prevalence survey of pediatric intensive care unit-acquired infections in the United States. *J Pediatr.* 2002;140:432-438.
2. Banerjee SN, Grohskopf LA, Sinkowitz-Cochran RL, et al. Incidence of pediatric and neonatal intensive care unit-acquired infections. *Infect Control Hosp Epidemiol.* 2006;27:561-570.
3. Graves N, Harbarth S, Beyersmann J, et al. Estimating the cost of health care-associated infections: mind your p's and q's. *Clin Infect Dis.* 2010;50:1017-1021.
4. Stewardson A, Pittet D. Ignac Semmelweis—celebrating a flawed pioneer of patient safety. *Lancet.* 2011;378:22-23.
5. Friedman C, Curchoe R, Foster M, et al. APIC/CHICA—Canada infection prevention, control, and epidemiology: professional and practice standards. *Am J Infect Control.* 2008;36:385-389.
6. Klompas M, Diekema DJ, Fishman NO, Yokoe DS. Ebola fever: reconciling planning with risk in U.S. hospitals. *Ann Intern Med.* 2014;161:751-752.
7. Morgan DJ, Diekema DJ, Sepkowitz K, Perencevich EN. Adverse outcomes associated with Contact Precautions: a review of the literature. *Am J Infect Control.* 2009;37:85-93.
8. Stelfox HT, Bates DW, Redelmeier DA. Safety of patients isolated for infection control. *JAMA.* 2003;290:1899-1905.
9. Hugonnet S, Chevrolet JC, Pittet D. The effect of workload on infection risk in critically ill patients. *Crit Care Med.* 2007;35:76-81.
10. Boyce JM, Pittet D, Healthcare Infection Control Practices Advisory Committee. Society for Healthcare Epidemiology of America. Association for Professionals in Infection Control. Infectious Diseases Society of America. Hand Hygiene Task F. Guideline for Hand Hygiene in Health-Care Settings: recommendations of the Healthcare Infection Control Practices Advisory Committee and the HICPAC/SHEA/APIC/IDSA Hand Hygiene Task Force. *Infect Control Hosp Epidemiol.* 2002;23(suppl 12):S3-S40.
11. Fagernes M, Lingaas E. Factors interfering with the microflora on hands: a regression analysis of samples from 465 healthcare workers. *J Adv Nurs.* 2011;67:297-307.
12. The traditional white coat: goodbye, or au revoir? *Lancet.* 2007;370:1102.
13. Loeb M, Dafoe N, Mahony J, et al. Surgical mask vs N95 respirator for preventing influenza among health care workers: a randomized trial. *JAMA.* 2009;302:1865-1871.
14. Lee TB, Baker OG, Lee JT, et al. Recommended practices for surveillance. Association for Professionals in Infection Control and Epidemiology, Inc. Surveillance Initiative working Group. *Am J Infect Control.* 1998;26:277-288.
15. Patrick SW, Kawai AT, Kleinman K, et al. Health care-associated infections among critically ill children in the US, 2007-2012. *Pediatrics.* 2014;134:705-712.
16. Rutledge-Taylor K, Matlow A, Gravel D, et al. A point prevalence survey of health care-associated infections in Canadian pediatric inpatients. *Am J Infect Control.* 2012;40:491-496.
17. Taylor CN, Noronha L, Wichman CS, Varman M. Evaluation of 2 sets of screening criteria for ventilator-associated pneumonia in a children's hospital. *Am J Infect Control.* 2014;42:1011-1013.
18. Bradley JS. Considerations unique to pediatrics for clinical trial design in hospital-acquired pneumonia and ventilator-associated pneumonia. *Clin Infect Dis.* 2010;51(suppl 1):S136-S143.
19. Gaur AH, Miller MR, Gao C, et al. Evaluating application of the National Healthcare Safety Network central line-associated bloodstream infection surveillance definition: a survey of pediatric intensive care and hematology/oncology units. *Infect Control Hosp Epidemiol.* 2013;34:663-670.
20. Klompas M. Complications of mechanical ventilation—the CDC's new surveillance paradigm. *N Engl J Med.* 2013;368:1472-1475.
21. Langley JM. Defining urinary tract infection in the critically ill child. *Pediatr Crit Care Med.* 2005;6(suppl 3):S25-S29.
22. Simonds DN, Horan TC, Kelley R, Jarvis WR. Detecting pediatric nosocomial infections: how do infection control and quality assurance personnel compare? *Am J Infect Control.* 1997;25:202-208.
23. Huang SS, Septimus E, Kleinman K, et al. Targeted versus universal decolonization to prevent ICU infection. *N Engl J Med.* 2013;368:2255-2265.
24. Huskins WC, Huckabee CM, O'Grady NP, et al. Intervention to reduce transmission of resistant bacteria in intensive care. *N Engl J Med.* 2011;364:1407-1418.
25. Yokoe DS, Anderson DJ, Berenholtz SM, et al. A compendium of strategies to prevent healthcare-associated infections in acute care hospitals: 2014 updates. *Infect Control Hosp Epidemiol.* 2014;35(suppl 2):S21-S31.
26. Lachman P, Yuen S. Using care bundles to prevent infection in neonatal and paediatric ICUs. *Curr Opin Infect Dis.* 2009;22:224-228.
27. Berenholtz SM, Pham JC, Thompson DA, et al. Collaborative cohort study of an intervention to reduce ventilator-associated pneumonia in the intensive care unit. *Infect Control Hosp Epidemiol.* 2011;32:305-314.
28. Society for Healthcare Epidemiology of A, Infectious Diseases Society of A, Pediatric Infectious Diseases S. Policy statement on antimicrobial stewardship by the Society for Healthcare Epidemiology of America (SHEA), the Infectious Diseases Society of America (IDSA), and the Pediatric Infectious Diseases Society (PIDS). *Infect Control Hosp Epidemiol.* 2012;33:322-327.
29. Hersh AL, De Lurgio SA, Thurm C, et al. Antimicrobial stewardship programs in freestanding children's hospitals. *Pediatrics.* 2015;135:33-39.
30. Abel Zur Wiesch P, Kouyos R, Abel S, et al. Cycling empirical antibiotic therapy in hospitals: meta-analysis and models. *PLoS Pathog.* 2014;10:e1004225.
31. Moss WJ, Beers MC, Johnson E, et al. Pilot study of antibiotic cycling in a pediatric intensive care unit. *Crit Care Med.* 2002;30:1877-1882.
32. Martinez JA, Nicolas JM, Marco F, et al. Comparison of antimicrobial cycling and mixing strategies in two medical intensive care units. *Crit Care Med.* 2006;34:329-336.
33. Daneman N, Sarwar S, Fowler RA, et al. Effect of selective decontamination on antimicrobial resistance in intensive care units: a systematic review and meta-analysis. *Lancet Infect Dis.* 2013;13:328-341.
34. de Smet AM, Kluytmans JA, Cooper BS, et al. Decontamination of the digestive tract and oropharynx in ICU patients. *N Engl J Med.* 2009;360:20-31.
35. Petros A, Silvestri L, Booth R, et al. Selective decontamination of the digestive tract in critically ill children: systematic review and meta-analysis. *Pediatr Crit Care Med.* 2013;14:89-97.
36. Canter RR, Harvey SE, Harrison DA, et al. Observational study of current use of selective decontamination of the digestive tract in UK critical care units. *Br J Anaesth.* 2014;113:610-617.
37. Cuthbertson BH, Francis J, Campbell MK, et al. A study of the perceived risks, benefits and barriers to the use of SDD in adult critical care units (the SuDDICU study). *Trials.* 2010;11:117.

38. Theodorakopoulou M, Perros E, Giamarellos-Bourboulis EJ, Dimopoulos G. Controversies in the management of the critically ill: the role of probiotics. *Int J Antimicrob Agents*. 2013;42(suppl):S41-S44.

39. Wang Y, Gao L, Zhang YH, et al. Efficacy of probiotic therapy in full-term infants with critical illness. *Asia Pac J Clin Nutr*. 2014;23:575-580.

40. Donovan EF, Sparling K, Lake MR, et al. The investment case for preventing NICU-associated infections. *Am J Perinatol*. 2013;30:179-184.

41. Elward AM, Hollenbeak CS, Warren DK, Fraser VJ. Attributable cost of nosocomial primary bloodstream infection in pediatric intensive care unit patients. *Pediatrics*. 2005;115:868-872.

42. Fridkin SK, Kaufman D, Edwards JR, et al. Changing incidence of Candida bloodstream infections among NICU patients in the United States: 1995-2004. *Pediatrics*. 2006;117:1680-1687.

43. O'Horo JC, Maki DG, Krupp AE, Safdar N. Arterial catheters as a source of bloodstream infection: a systematic review and meta-analysis. *Crit Care Med*. 2014;42:1334-1339.

44. Bhutta A, Gilliam C, Honeycutt M, et al. Reduction of bloodstream infections associated with catheters in paediatric intensive care unit: stepwise approach. *BMJ*. 2007;334:362-365.

46. Milstone AM, Elward A, Song X, et al. Daily chlorhexidine bathing to reduce bacteraemia in critically ill children: a multicentre, cluster-randomised, crossover trial. *Lancet*. 2013;381:1099-1106.

47. Noto MJ, Domenico HJ, Byrne DW, et al. Chlorhexidine bathing and health care-associated infections: a randomized clinical trial. *JAMA*. 2015;313:369-378.

48. Randolph AG, Brun-Buisson C, Goldmann D. Identification of central venous catheter-related infections in infants and children. *Pediatr Crit Care Med*. 2005;6(suppl 3):S19-S24.

49. Lorente L, Martin MM, Vidal P, et al. Should central venous catheter be systematically removed in patients with suspected catheter related infection? *Crit Care*. 2014;18:564.

50. Vayalumkal JV, Gravel D, Moore D, et al. Surveillance for healthcare-acquired febrile respiratory infection in pediatric hospitals participating in the Canadian Nosocomial Infection Surveillance Program. *Infect Control Hosp Epidemiol*. 2009;30:652-658.

51. Jacobs P, Lier D, Gooch K, et al. A model of the costs of community and nosocomial pediatric respiratory syncytial virus infections in Canadian hospitals. *Can J Infect Dis Med Microbiol*. 2013;24:22-26.

Sepsis

Matthew N. Alder, Mary Sandquist, and Hector R. Wong

PEARLS

- The typical patient with septic shock has simultaneous derangements of cardiovascular function, intravascular volume status, respiratory function, immune/inflammatory regulation, renal function, coagulation, hepatic function, and/or metabolic function.
- The complexity and heterogeneity of septic shock warrant a systematic and multifaceted approach on the part of the pediatric intensivist.
- Although some overlap exists among the terms spanning the sepsis spectrum (systemic inflammatory response syndrome, sepsis, severe sepsis, and septic shock), each term is intended to define a particular patient population.
- Sepsis is now viewed as a dysregulation of the immunologic and inflammatory pathways normally directed toward pathogen eradication and restoration of homeostasis.
- From a clinical standpoint, the treatment of sepsis entails four important goals: initial resuscitation, pathogen eradication, maintenance of oxygen delivery, and (in the future) carefully directed modulation of the inflammatory response.
- Genomic medicine and systems biology represent novel approaches for studying complex processes such as septic shock.
- The development of robust stratification and phenotyping strategies has the potential to more effectively manage the intrinsic heterogeneity of septic shock and thus improve the effectiveness of both clinical research and individual patient care.

Introduction

Management of the patient with septic shock embodies the discipline of pediatric critical care medicine. The typical patient with septic shock has simultaneous derangements of cardiovascular function, intravascular volume status, respiratory function, immune regulation, renal function, coagulation, hepatic function, and/or metabolic function. The degree to which any one of these derangements manifests in a given patient is highly variable and influenced by multiple host and nonhost factors, including developmental stage, presence or absence of comorbidities, causative agent of septic shock, immune status, genetic background, and variations in therapy. These factors combine to profoundly influence the course and ultimate outcome of septic shock.

The complexity of septic shock warrants a systematic and multifaceted approach on the part of the pediatric intensivist. Optimal management requires a strong working knowledge of not only cardiovascular physiology and infectious diseases but also multiple organ function and interaction, inflammation-related biology, immunity, coagulation, pharmacology, and molecular biology. The pediatric intensivist will also need a working knowledge of genomic medicine for the future management of patients with septic shock. This chapter provides a comprehensive description of the many aspects influencing the development and outcome of septic shock, pathophysiology at the physiologic and molecular levels, contemporary management of septic shock, and what the authors believe to be the next important future directions in the field. Ultimately, this information must be integrated with bedside experience and clinical acumen, which cannot be supplanted by a book chapter.

Epidemiology

A true picture of the epidemiology of septic shock is clouded by the lack of a reliable case definition. This is true for both the adult population and pediatric population. A few pediatric-specific studies, however, illustrate the importance of sepsis in today's modern ICU. Proulx et al.[1] analyzed the incidence and outcome of the systemic inflammatory response syndrome (SIRS), sepsis, severe sepsis, and septic shock (see next section for definitions) in a single institution. A total of 1058 admissions were analyzed over a 1-year period. SIRS was present in 82% of patients, 23% had sepsis, 4% had severe sepsis, and 2% had septic shock. The overall mortality rate for this patient population was 6%, with the majority of deaths occurring in patients with multiple organ dysfunction syndrome (MODS). Among the patients with MODS, distinct mortality rates were associated with SIRS (4%), sepsis (22%), severe sepsis (25%), and septic shock (52%). Later studies by Watson et al.[2] provide the most comprehensive retrospective epidemiologic surveys of pediatric sepsis to date. By linking 1995 hospital records from seven large states (representing 24% of the United States population) with census data, they estimated an annual incidence of 42,371 cases of severe sepsis in individuals younger than 20 years of age (0.6 cases/1000 population). The highest incidence was in neonates (5.2 cases/1000 population), compared with children ages 5–14 years who had an incidence of 0.2 cases/1000 population. The overall mortality rate in this population was 10.3% (4364 deaths per year nationally). In addition, patients younger than 1 year of age and patients with comorbidities had higher mortality rates than patients between 5 and 14 years old and patients without comorbidities, respectively. Their study also estimated an annual national health care cost of $1.7 billion associated with severe sepsis.

In a follow-up study, these investigators used a similar approach to investigate severe sepsis trends in the United States from 1995–2005.[3] They reported an overall decrease in the case-fatality rate over this period, from 10.3%–8.9%, but an overall increase in the prevalence of severe sepsis. Most of this increase was accounted for by an increase in the prevalence of severe sepsis in newborns.

Czaja et al.[4] used the discharge diagnosis of severe sepsis for Washington State to investigate the readmission rates and late mortality for children (1 month to 18 years old) following severe sepsis. From 1990 through 2004, 7183 children were diagnosed with severe sepsis and 6.8% of these patients died during the sentinel admission or within 28 days of discharge. Importantly, death certificates confirmed that an additional 434 (6.5%) of the initial survivors died during the follow-up period with the highest late death rate occurring within 2 years of the initial hospitalization. Although most of the early and late deaths occurred in children with comorbidities (8% early death, 10.4% late death), 8% of children with no comorbidities died during their initial hospitalization with 2% of the 28-day survivors being classified as late deaths.

Schlapbach et al.[5] recently reported on the epidemiology of invasive infections, sepsis, and septic shock in critically ill children in Australia and New Zealand. The age-standardized incidence increased every year, from 2002–2013, for all three study categories. Critically ill children with invasive infections, sepsis, or septic shock accounted for 26% of all pediatric deaths among all the critically ill children in this cohort. Comparing 2008–2013 with 2002–2007, risk-adjusted mortality significantly decreased for invasive infections and sepsis, but not for septic shock. In 2015, Weiss et al.[6] published the first international, prospective epidemiologic study of pediatric severe sepsis. Almost 7000 patients younger than 18 years of age were screened on 5 days from 2013–2014 at 128 sites from 26 countries using a point prevalence study method. Severe sepsis was defined using the 2005 International Pediatric Sepsis Consensus Conference criteria.[7] This large, comprehensive study demonstrated an 8.2% prevalence of pediatric severe sepsis in international pediatric ICUs (95% CI 7.6, 8.9%), consistent with adult epidemiologic data. Hospital mortality was 25% regardless of age or country. Multiorgan dysfunction was demonstrated in 67% of patients at sepsis recognition with 30% subsequently developing new or progressive multiorgan dysfunction.

Collectively, these data illustrate that sepsis continues to present a major pediatric public health problem in terms of incidence, mortality, and health care costs. Nevertheless, there is an ongoing need for quality epidemiologic studies of sepsis in children. Quality epidemiologic studies are necessary for the understanding of not only incidence but also the impact of new knowledge and therapies. One major issue that must be addressed is the development of more meaningful and consistent case definitions. Consistent case definitions will also facilitate and improve the design of more effective interventional trials specific to the pediatric population. Equally important is objectively measuring long-term outcomes in these patients (ie, quality of life) beyond the dichotomy of "alive" or "dead." Progress in this important area is steadily coming to fruition.[8-11]

Definitions

Intuitively, the experienced pediatric intensivist knows when he or she encounters a patient with sepsis. Thus strict definitions of sepsis and septic shock could be viewed as having relatively limited value in daily practice. Despite this common perception, there is a clear need for standard definitions of sepsis and septic shock for three primary reasons. First, with the development of standard definitions, clinicians will be able to more accurately characterize the epidemiologic features of septic shock in the pediatric population. Second, as novel, expensive, and potentially higher-risk therapies are developed, it will be important to accurately identify and stratify patients early in the course of sepsis if clinicians are to apply those therapies to the most appropriate groups and realize a more favorable benefit-to-risk ratio in a given patient population. Finally, standard definitions are crucial to the design of much needed, pediatric-specific interventional trials.

The International Consensus Conference on Pediatric Sepsis and Organ Dysfunction was convened in 2002 to develop pediatric-specific definitions for systemic inflammatory response syndrome (SIRS), sepsis, severe sepsis, septic shock, and organ failure, and the results of this conference were subsequently published.[7] The standard terms to describe the sepsis spectrum are SIRS, sepsis, severe sepsis, and septic shock. Each term is intended to describe a clinical syndrome having increasing illness severity and relatively increasing specificity, which in turn drives important clinical decision and therapeutic processes.

SIRS is not a diagnosis. The term is intended to represent a state of relative inflammatory/immune activation in a given patient and is said to be present when a patient meets at least two of the four criteria listed in Box 111.1, one of which must be abnormal temperature or abnormal leukocyte count. Thus patients with diverse clinical conditions, such as sepsis, pancreatitis, burns, or hypermetabolism following major trauma or surgery, can meet criteria for SIRS. Sepsis is defined as SIRS secondary to an infection, either documented by microbiology cultures or in the presence of other clinical evidence of infection. Severe sepsis is defined by sepsis criteria

---

BOX 111.1   Criteria for Systemic Inflammatory Response Syndrome

The presence of at least two of the following four criteria, one of which must be abnormal temperature or leukocyte count:

1. Core temperature (rectal, bladder, oral, or central catheter) >38.5°C or <36°C.
2. Tachycardia, defined as a mean heart rate >2 standard deviation above normal for age in the absence of external stimulus, chronic drugs, or painful stimuli; otherwise unexplained persistent elevation over a 0.5- to 4-hour time period; for children <1 year old: bradycardia, defined as a mean heart rate <10th percentile for age in the absence of external vagal stimulus, β-blocker drugs, or congenital heart disease; or otherwise unexplained persistent heart rate depression over a 0.5-hour time period.
3. Tachypnea, defined as mean respiratory rate >90th percentile for age, or the need for mechanical ventilation for an acute process not related to underlying neuromuscular disease or the receipt of general anesthesia.
4. Leukocyte count elevated or depressed for age (not secondary to chemotherapy-induced leukopenia) or >10% immature neutrophils.

plus either cardiovascular dysfunction or acute respiratory distress syndrome or at least two other dysfunctional organ systems. Septic shock is defined by sepsis criteria, plus cardiovascular dysfunction. Importantly, each criterion takes into account the influence of developmental age on physiologic variables. The reader is referred to the original publication by Goldstein et al.[7] for further details and definitions of organ dysfunction. At the time of this writing, it is anticipated that a consensus conference will be convened to update the definition of pediatric sepsis.

Clinical Presentation

As a syndrome potentially affecting the entire body, the clinical presentation of sepsis is highly heterogeneous. The most common clinical manifestations of sepsis include fever or hypothermia, tachypnea, tachycardia, leukocytosis or leukopenia, thrombocytopenia, and change in mental status. It should be noted, however, that in the absence of meningitis, changes in mental status are relatively late manifestations of septic shock and should not be relied on for early recognition of shock. One of the earliest signs alerting caregivers to the possibility of infection is fever. A number of the cytokines elicited in response to infection are pyrogens, particularly interleukin (IL)-1β and tumor necrosis factor (TNF)-α. Patients can also exhibit hypothermia, which is more common in infants than older children. Finally, petechiae and pupura can be present and are potentially ominous signs of purpura fulminans.[12]

Shock states can be grouped into four broad categories: hypovolemic, cardiogenic, obstructive, and distributive shock (see also Chapter 36). Septic shock is unique because all four forms of shock may be involved simultaneously. The patient may have hypovolemic shock resulting from capillary leak, increased insensible water losses, poor intake, and/or decreased effective blood volume secondary to venodilation and arterial dilation (ie, increased vascular capacitance). Cardiogenic shock manifests as depressed myocardial contractility and low cardiac output secondary to myocardial-depressant effects of bacterial toxins and inflammatory cytokines. Obstructive shock can result indirectly from diffuse microvascular thrombosis or directly from abdominal compartment syndrome. Distributive shock can result directly from abnormally low systemic vascular resistance, leading to maldistribution of blood flow, or indirectly from the inability of tissues to adequately use oxygen at the mitochondrial level (ie, cytopathic hypoxia).

The degree to which an individual patient manifests these physiologic perturbations is highly variable. In some cases, patients display increased cardiac output with diminished systemic vascular resistance. The presenting symptoms in this type of patient are tachycardia, a hyperdynamic precordium, bounding pulses, wide pulse pressure, and warm, flushed skin characteristic of the distributive mode of shock or the so-called "warm" shock state. Despite this clinical appearance, the perfusion of major organs during warm shock may remain highly compromised secondary to maldistribution of blood flow. Alternatively, a patient with depressed cardiac output and elevated systemic vascular resistance has cool, mottled skin with diminished pulses and poor capillary refill characteristic of the "cold" shock state. Limited data and our collective anecdotal experience suggest this latter presentation, cold shock, is more common in younger children compared with teenagers

and adults.[13] It has been suggested that patients who develop community-acquired septic shock more commonly present to the ICU with signs of "cold" shock, whereas patients who develop septic shock secondary to catheter-related infections more commonly present to the ICU with signs of "warm" shock.[14] It is important to recognize that a given patient may transition from one shock state to another, and recognition and reassessment of these classes of shock are absolutely central to the choice of cardiovascular medications.

Patients with sepsis often have presenting symptoms of respiratory abnormalities, including tachypnea and hypoxia. Tachypnea alone can reflect a compensatory, respiratory alkalosis aimed at counteracting a metabolic acidosis secondary to shock. Chest roentgenogram in this setting often reveals a relatively small cardiac silhouette (potentially reflective of relative hypovolemia) with few vascular markings. However, in the face of capillary leak and decreased myocardial function, patients with septic shock often develop pulmonary edema and acute respiratory failure as fluid resuscitation proceeds. Alternatively, respiratory abnormalities can reflect pneumonia as the primary source of infection and/or the development of acute respiratory distress syndrome (ARDS). In these situations chest roentgenography will display patterns of pulmonary infiltrates characteristic of the respective scenarios.

All organ systems can be adversely affected by poor perfusion and decreased oxygen delivery. In addition, all organ systems can be directly or indirectly injured by bacterial toxins, circulating cytokines, and the products of activated white blood cells. The end result of these complex and interrelated pathologic mechanisms is MODS, which describes the serial and progressive failure of various organ systems and is associated with increased morbidity and mortality (see also Chapter 112).[15-17]

Pathogenesis
Introduction

Many clinical and basic science studies have focused on the mechanisms underlying the development of sepsis. At least three major hypotheses have been proposed to explain the development of sepsis and its sequelae. The first hypothesis attributes the development of sepsis to an excessive or uncontrolled host inflammatory response. This "proinflammatory" hypothesis is broadly consistent with the concept of SIRS and is generally well supported by experimental and clinical data. However, a large number of clinical trials aimed directly at inhibition of various components of this putative excessive inflammatory response have failed, thus leading to the development of alternative hypotheses. One such alternative hypothesis states that sepsis is not directly the result of excessive inflammation but rather a more direct manifestation of failed antiinflammatory responses. Thus, in this alternative hypothesis there is direct failure of the compensatory antiinflammatory response syndrome (CARS), which subsequently permits unchecked proinflammatory responses. Related to the CARS concept is the concept of immunoparalysis (see also Chapter 105), which embodies the third overall hypothesis to account for the clinical manifestations of sepsis. The hypothesis of immunoparalysis postulates that sepsis is not a manifestation of too much or too little inflammation but rather a form of acquired immunodeficiency (both innate and adaptive immunity), leading to an inability to effectively clear pathogens and their products, which thereby cause direct tissue and organ injury.[18,19]

A conceptual framework for integrating these three hypotheses/paradigms is provided in Fig. 111.1. All three paradigms are biologically plausible and supported by the existing literature.[20] While seemingly vastly different in concept, they are not mutually exclusive in the context of a highly heterogeneous syndrome such as human sepsis. It is plausible that all three paradigms are valid across a given cohort of heterogeneous patients with sepsis. In addition, each paradigm has the potential to influence all of the other paradigms, as indicated in Fig. 111.1. The following sections review the existing literature supporting these three paradigms and will serve to frame the important concept of heterogeneity in sepsis. A major challenge in the field of sepsis is to more effectively understand how a given patient fits into one of these three paradigms (ie, stratify or phenotype patients more effectively).

Pathogen Recognition and Signal Transduction

The fundamental role of the immune system is to detect, contain, and eradicate invading pathogens. The first step in this process involves pathogen recognition, which is achieved by the activation of pattern recognition receptors (PRRs) on immune cells by pathogen-associated molecular patterns

(PAMPs)[21] (see also Chapter 101). Examples of PAMPS include lipopolysaccharide from the cell wall of gram-negative bacteria; lipoteichoic acid from the cell wall of gram-positive bacteria; mannans from the cell wall of yeast; double-stranded RNA of viruses; and unmethylated, CpG-rich DNA unique to bacterial genomes. The most well-studied PRRs include the family of Toll-like receptors (TLRs), which can have relatively specific recognition of PAMPS.[21] For example, TLR-4 recognizes lipopolysaccharide, whereas TLR-2 recognizes lipoteichoic acid. Other examples of PRRs or PRR components include CD-14, scavenger receptors, nucleotide-binding oligodimerization (NOD) receptors, pentraxins, and collectins.[22]

Engagement of PRRs on the cell surface of immune cells, by PAMPS, leads to activation of the immune system in the form of phagocytosis, proliferation, and production/secretion of cytokines. The latter process, cytokine expression, serves to orchestrate, direct, and amplify the innate and adaptive immune response toward pathogen eradication. However, if this process becomes dysregulated, this same production of cytokines, though required for pathogen eradication, can inadvertently lead to autoinjury of the host.

Much of the activation of the immune system on PRR activation relies on signal transduction mechanisms, which serve to transfer the signal of pathogen recognition at the cell surface to the intracellular compartment in order to induce new gene expression or a change in cellular function. One of the major signal transduction mechanisms of the immune

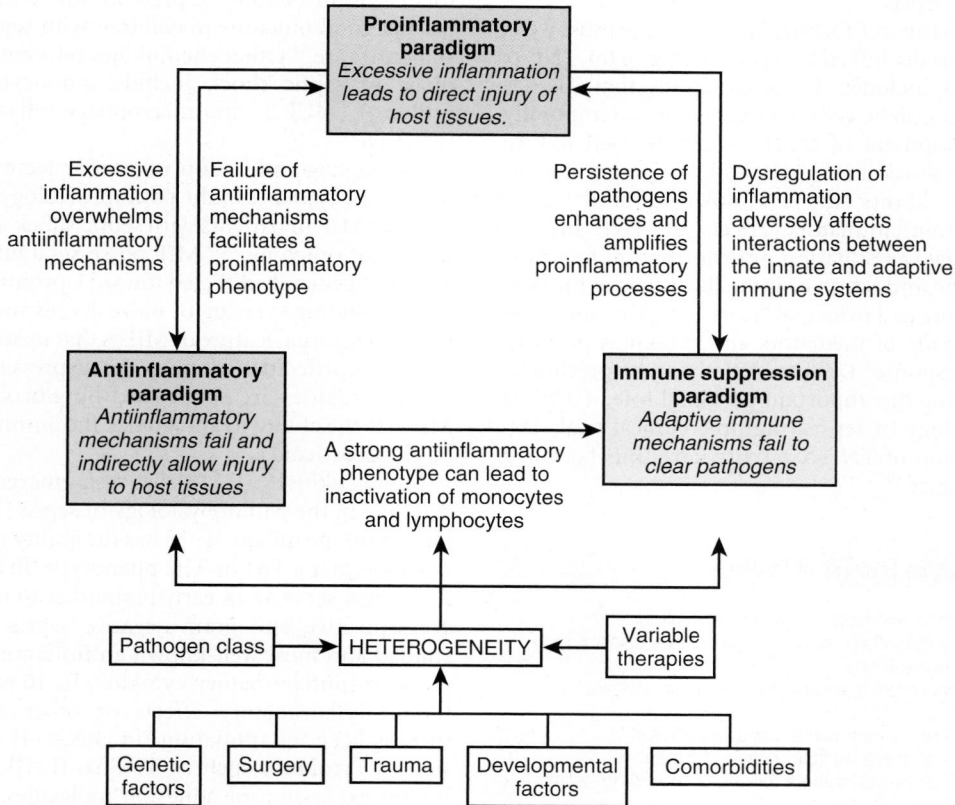

Fig. 111.1. Schematic depicting the three major paradigms for understanding the pathophysiology of sepsis and septic shock. Although these paradigms are mechanistically distinct, they are not mutually exclusive. Each paradigm has the potential to influence the other paradigms, and all are potentially operative in a heterogenous patient cohort. Heterogeneity is a major component of septic shock and results from multiple host and environmental factors.

system is the NF-κB pathway, which serves as a master "switch" for the expression of a wide variety of genes involved in inflammation and immunity. Indeed, activation of the NF-κB pathway is a major signaling pathway in the pathophysiology of sepsis and may represent a potential therapeutic target.[23,24] Another major signaling pathway for the regulation of genes involved in inflammation and immunity is the mitogen-activated protein kinase (MAPK) signaling pathway. The MAP kinases consist of three major families: p38 MAP kinase, extracellular-regulated protein kinase (ERK), and c-Jun N-terminal kinases (JNKs). These major kinase families are also referred to as stress-activated protein kinases (SAPKs). Similar to the NF-κB pathway, the MAP kinases are also regarded as potential therapeutic targets in the context of sepsis.[23,25,26] Finally, there is now increased attention on the phosphatase family of intracellular signaling molecules in the context of sepsis. Whereas kinases direct cellular signaling by adding phosphate groups to intracellular signaling proteins, phosphatases serve to remove phosphate groups from these same intracellular signaling proteins and can thus serve to modulate proinflammatory cell signaling.[27,28]

Cytokines as Principal Mediators of the Sepsis Response

Cytokines represent a broad family of proteins that have paracrine, autocrine, and endocrine properties, as well as the ability to regulate and modulate virtually all aspects of immunity and inflammation. Common features of cytokines are provided in Box 111.2. Following is a review of a selected group of cytokines thought to play an important role in the pathophysiology of sepsis.

Tumor necrosis factor-α (TNF-α) is perhaps the most well-studied cytokine causally linked to sepsis. Evidence for TNF-α mediation of sepsis includes the observations that TNF is produced by hematopoietic cells, its expression is temporally related to the development of shock, it can by itself induce experimental septic shock in animals, and passive immunization against TNF blunts the endotoxin-induced sepsis response.[29] The proinflammatory effects of TNF include leukocyte-endothelial cell adhesion, transformation to a procoagulant phenotype, induction of inducible nitric oxide synthase, and functioning as a principal "early" cytokine inducing the subsequent cascade of mediators and cytokines promulgating the septic response. Despite a plethora of preclinical studies demonstrating the important proximal role of TNF-α in the pathophysiology of sepsis, multiple clinical trials targeted at neutralization of TNF-α activity have thus far failed to demonstrate efficacy.[30]

BOX 111.2   **Common Features of Cytokines**

- Cytokine secretion is relatively brief and self-limited.
- Secretion of many cytokines requires new mRNA transcription and new protein translation.
- Expression and secretion is regulated by specific cellular signals.
- A given cytokine can have multiple cellular sources.
- A given cytokine can have multiple cellular targets.
- A given cytokine can have multiple functions regarding cellular function or activation.
- Cytokines can have redundant activities/functions with other cytokines.
- Many cytokines regulate the activity and expression of other cytokines.

Interleukin-1beta (IL-1β) has many redundant biological properties to that of TNF-α and is also considered to be a major early cytokine in the sepsis response.[31] IL-1β leads to inflammatory and immune cell activation via the NF-κβ and MAPK pathways. Also, similar to TNF-α, clinical trials targeted at neutralization of IL-1β activity have thus far failed to demonstrate efficacy despite promising preclinical data.

IL-6 expression is highly dependent on TNF-α and IL-1β and is consistently found to be elevated during the course of sepsis.[32] IL-6 is a pleiotropic cytokine possessing a number of functions including driving the acute-phase response in hepatocytes, differentiating myeloid cells, stimulating immunoglobulin production, and activating T-cell proliferation.[33] Because increased IL-6 admission levels have been correlated with death in the context of sepsis, there has been interest in using IL-6 as a stratification biomarker for interventional clinical trials in sepsis. While this stratification approach has been highly effective in animal models of sepsis,[34] it has thus far failed when applied in the clinical setting.[35]

IL-8 is a canonical member of the chemokine subclass of cytokines.[36] The term "chemokine" refers to the ability of certain cytokines to serve as chemoattractants, which direct leukocyte movement to sites of infection and inflammation (chemotaxis). Both TNF-α and IL-1β can induce IL-8 production from a variety of cells, including endothelial cells, macrophages, neutrophils, and epithelial cells. IL-8 is the principal human chemoattractant for neutrophils and appears to play a major role in the recruitment of neutrophils to the lungs in patients with sepsis-induced ARDS.[37] Serum IL-8 measurements within 24 hours of presentation to the ICU can robustly predict good outcome in children with septic shock receiving standard care.[38] Other chemokines relevant to the pathophysiology of septic shock include monocyte chemoattractant protein 1 (MCP-1) and macrophage inflammatory protein-1 (MIP-1).[36]

Macrophage migration inhibitory factor (MIF) is another important cytokine in the pathophysiology of sepsis, and high levels of MIF in patients with septic shock and ARDS correlate with poor outcome.[39,40] MIF possesses a number of biological activities generally directed toward a proinflammatory phenotype, including skewing of naïve T cells toward a Th1 phenotype. An unusual feature of MIF is that its secretion is enhanced by glucocorticoids, whereas the expression and activity of many cytokines are suppressed by glucocorticoids. In turn, MIF has the ability to antagonize the antiinflammatory effects of glucocorticoids.

Intereleukin 18 (IL-18) has also emerged as an important cytokine in the pathophysiology of sepsis.[41] Depending on the local cytokine milieu, IL-18 has the ability to skew naïve T cells toward either a Th1 or Th2 phenotype. In addition, it appears IL-18 may serve as an early biomarker to distinguish between gram-positive and gram-negative sepsis. IL-10 is the best studied and most well-known antiinflammatory cytokine.[42,43] As an antiinflammatory cytokine, IL-10 serves to antagonize the proinflammatory effects of other cytokines and can thereby keep inflammation "in check." IL-10 inhibits expression of cytokines such as TNF-α, IL-1β, and IL-8 and can inhibit expression of adhesion molecules. In addition, IL-10 can "deactivate" monocytes by downregulating the expression of MHC surface molecules. Thus IL-10 has a number of interesting properties that could potentially be leveraged therapeutically to limit excessive inflammation during sepsis. This theoretic consideration must be tempered by the ability of IL-10 to deactivate monocytes and thereby potentially impair the ability to adequately clear infection (ie, the immune suppression paradigm depicted in Fig. 111.1). Indeed, it has been reported that in children with MODS, higher plasma IL-10 levels correlate with higher mortality and higher monocyte mRNA levels of IL-10 correlate with increased length of stay in the ICU.[44] Similar observations have been reported in adult patients with septic shock.[45]

High-mobility group box 1 (HMGB-1) has long been known as a nonhistone DNA binding protein. More recently, it has been recognized that HMGB-1 also exists in the extracellular compartment, appears to have proinflammatory properties that may play a role in the pathophysiology of sepsis, and may represent a potential therapeutic target for sepsis.[46] The attraction of HMGB-1 as a therapeutic target in sepsis stems from the observation it may be a "late mediator" of sepsis inasmuch as it appears in the extracellular compartment within a time frame that is considerably later than that seen with the canonical sepsis cytokines such as TNF-α and IL-1β. Thus the kinetics of HMGB-1 expression provide a potential therapeutic window that may be clinically feasible to exploit. This temporal observation is evident in both experimental models of sepsis and in humans with established septic shock.[47] The biological properties of HMGB-1 appear to involve activation of Toll-like receptors and the receptor for advanced glycation end products (RAGE). More recently, it has been suggested HMGB-1 intrinsically possesses little proinflammatory biological activity but forms highly proinflammatory complexes with cytokines (eg, IL-1β) and PAMPS (eg, bacterial DNA and lipopolysaccharide).[48]

HMGB-1 is also a prime example of a class of molecules known as "alarmins" or danger/damage-associated molecular patterns (DAMPs).[49] Broadly speaking, DAMPs represent a class of molecules normally existing in the intracellular compartment at baseline but are released from damaged cells into the extracellular compartment during conditions such as trauma or sepsis. DAMPs appear to signal through many of the same PRRs recognizing pathogens and therefore have the ability to activate the immune/inflammatory system. Because DAMPs are released from damaged cells, they can serve to "alert" the inflammatory system of systemic "damage" or "danger" and can therefore induce appropriate and adaptive activation of defense mechanisms. Alternatively, excessive DAMP-mediated activation of PRRs can lead to unnecessary and maladaptive amplification of inflammation damaging to host tissues. Other examples of DAMPs include calgranulins, hepatoma-derived growth factor, heat shock proteins, and uric acid. In this regard, heat shock proteins have been reported to be substantially elevated in the serum of children with septic shock.[50,51] More recently, formyl peptides released from mitochondria and mitochondrial DNA were reported as novel DAMPs.[52]

Adhesion Molecules

An important breakthrough in the molecular understanding of sepsis-induced organ dysfunction came with the identification of the processes responsible for the infiltration of leukocytes into tissues.[53] The "leukocyte-endothelial cell adhesion cascade" (Fig. 111.2) is characterized by early cytokine-mediated activation of the selectin family of endothelial cell adhesion molecules that can mediate a process of neutrophil "rolling" whereby sialyated moieties constitutively present on neutrophils interact with selectins on the endothelial cell membrane (eg, E-selectin). In the second phase, activation of the "rolling" neutrophil causes increased expression and

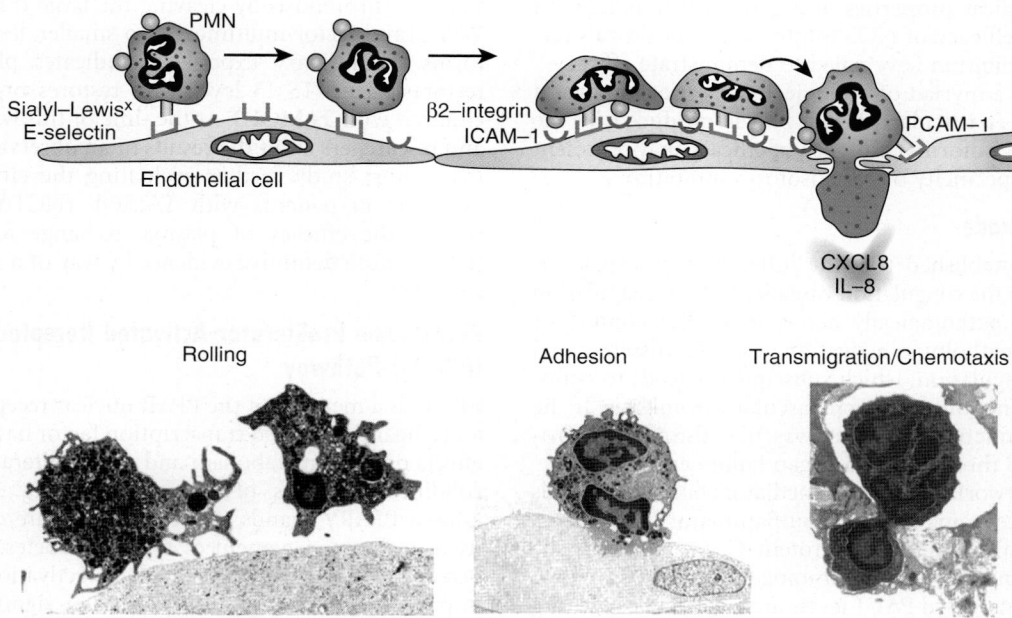

Fig. 111.2. Schematic and corresponding electron micrographs highlighting the process of leukocyte-endothelial cell adhesion and leukocyte transmigration from the intravascular compartment to the extravascular compartment. Cytokine-mediated activation of the selectin family of endothelial cell adhesion molecules mediate neutrophil "rolling" followed by ICAM-1-mediated adhesion. After adhesion, neutrophils transmigrate across "openings" between enothelial cell junctions to enter the extravascular space. The transmigration process is directed by chemokines serving as homing signals for neutrophils and other leukocytes. (Courtesy Thomas P. Shanley, MD, University of Michigan.)

activation of the integrin family of adhesion molecules that interact with the similarly upregulated intercellular adhesion molecule (ICAM)-1 on the endothelial cell surface. This ligand interaction facilitates firm adhesion of the neutrophil to the endothelium. Subsequently, in response to a variety of chemotactic molecules, neutrophils transmigrate through the endothelial junctions to the site of inflammation. Release of a variety of radical species, both oxygen and nitrogen based, and proteases by the activated neutrophils can contribute to pathogen eradication, but paradoxically they can also cause endothelial and tissue injury.

Nitric Oxide

Nitric oxide (NO) was discovered in the 1980s as the molecule responsible for endothelial-derived relaxation of blood vessels.[54,55] Since then, NO has received tremendous attention as a potential mediator of septic shock.[56] NO is produced by the enzyme, nitric oxide synthase (NOS), which converts arginine and oxygen to NO and citrulline. Human NOS exists as three different isoforms (NOS 1, 2, and 3), and each isoform has relatively unique tissue localizations, requirements for NO production, and kinetics of NO production. Several features of NO-related biology support an important role in the pathophysiology of sepsis. First, NOS2 (a.k.a. inducible NOS) is expressed in response to proinflammatory signals (eg, lipopolysaccharide, TNF-α, and IL-1β) and produces large amounts of NO for prolonged periods of time. Second, NO can induce pathologic vasodilation and function as a myocardial depressant. Third, NO can function as an oxidant either alone or by contributing to formation of other highly oxidizing, reactive molecules such as peroxynitrite. Fourth, NO has the potential to negatively affect mitochondrial function. Finally, elevated levels of NO metabolites have been well documented in children with septic shock and the levels correlate with the degree of cardiovascular dysfunction.[57,58] Despite these intriguing biological properties and a wealth of preclinical data testing the efficacy of NOS inhibition, clinical trials targeted at NOS inhibition have failed to demonstrate efficacy.[59] Because NO has a myriad of biological properties important for homeostasis (particularly when NO is produced by the NOS1 and NOS3 isoforms), this lack of efficacy may represent the timing and specificity of NOS isoform inhibition.

Coagulation Cascade

It is now well established that the inflammatory cascade is directly linked to the coagulation cascade, and the coagulation cascade can be pathologically activated in the context of sepsis.[60,61] This pathologic activation leads to disseminated intravascular coagulation, which subsequently leads to endothelial cell dysfunction and microvascular thrombosis. If the endothelial dysfunction and microvascular thrombosis progress to a critical threshold, end-organ failure ensues.

A complex network of multiple mediators takes part in this pathologic process including proinflammatory cytokines, tissue factor, antithrombin III, protein C, protein S, tissue factor pathway inhibitor, and plaminogen activator inhibitor type 1 (PAI-1). Increased PAI-1 levels are a particularly strong feature of severe cases of meningococcemia and may be causally linked to a polymorphism in the promoter region of the *PAI-1* gene.[62,63] Depressed levels of the endogenous anticoagulants, antithrombin III, protein S, and protein C are consistently documented in the context of septic shock. These

observations have led to multiple clinical trials in which recombinant forms of these endogenous anticoagulants have been administered to patients with septic shock. The majority of these trials did not demonstrate efficacy. Studies in the early 2000s suggested recombinant activated protein C (APC) reduced mortality in adult patients with septic shock, and this compound subsequently received FDA approval.[61] The beneficial effects of APC in septic shock are thought to be secondary to both prevention of microvascular thrombosis and an antiinflammatory effect.[64] Unfortunately, a phase III trial of APC therapy in children with septic shock, the RESOLVE trial, failed to demonstrate efficacy.[65] The RESOLVE trial was terminated after the second interim analysis due to little chance of reaching the primary efficacy end point. In addition, there was an increased risk of serious bleeding events in patients younger than 2 months of age. Consistent with this finding in children, a subsquent trial in adults with septic shocks, PROWESS-SHOCK, also failed to confirm earlier findings of improved mortality, and activated protein C was removed from the market in 2011.[66] Nonetheless, the RESOLVE trial represents the largest and most well-organized pediatric septic shock trial to date and provides an important context and reference point for all future interventional trials in the field of pediatric critical care medicine.

Related to the paradigm of altered coagulation playing an important role in the pathophysiology of sepsis is the concept of thrombocytopenia-associated multiple organ failure (TAMOF).[67] New-onset thrombocytopenia in critically ill patients correlates with the evolution of persistent organ failure and poor outcome, including patients with sepsis. The mechanistic link between thrombocytopenia and organ failure is thought to involve a form of microangiopathy analagous to thrombotic thrombocytopenic purpura, including substantial decreases of ADAMTS-13 (A Disintegrin And Metalloprotease with ThromboSpondin motifs). ADAMTS-13 regulates microvascular thrombosis by cleaving the large thrombogenic von Willebrand factor multimers into smaller, less thrombogenic forms. Preliminary experience indicates plasma exchange restores ADAMTS-13 levels and restores organ function in children with TAMOF.[68] At the time of this writing, clinicians and researchers await the results of an observational, prospective cohort study further evaluating the efficacy of plasma exchange in patients with TAMOF (NCT00118664). Ultimately, the efficacy of plasma exchange for TAMOF will require more definitive evidence by way of a formal randomized trial.

Peroxisome Proliferator-Activated Receptor-γ (PPARγ) Pathway

PPARγ is a member of the PPAR nuclear receptor superfamily and a ligand-activated transcription factor having well-known effects on lipid metabolism and cell proliferation.[69] The thiazolidinedione class of insulin-sensitizing drugs are well-known PPARγ ligands (activators) and are currently widely used in the management of type II diabetes. Recently, it has become evident that pharmacologic activation of PPARγ has important antiinflammatory effects of significant benefit in experimental models of critical illness, including sepsis.[70-75] The recent demonstration that PPARγ expression and activation are indeed altered in children with septic shock, coupled with the availability of FDA-approved PPARγ ligands, provides an opportunity to test the efficacy of PPARγ ligands in sepsis.[76] There is currently an active Phase 1 study to evaluate the pharmacokinetics and safety of the PPARγ ligand, pioglitazone, in children with sepsis (NCT01352182).

Myeloid-Derived Suppressor Cells (MDSC)

The neutrophil is often considered the first line in the innate immune response to infection. Patients with sepsis can present with elevated or extremely low neutrophil counts. In either case the physiologic response to infectious stimuli is "emergency granulopoiesis" to generate a large number of myeloid cells to deal with the onslaught of infectious particles. This can lead to a much-needed increase in cells to both contain and eliminate pathogens; however, in patients with sepsis this can also give rise to a recently described MDSC population.[77] These cells produce antiinflammatory cytokines and suppress T-cell activation and thus may contribute in part to the failure of the adaptive immune system.[78] These cells have been primarily characterized in the mouse model of sepsis, where up to 30% of cells in the spleen 10 days after sepsis are MDSCs.[79] Whether these cells are helpful to the immune response or lead to further immune suppression is not entirely clear.[79,80] MDSCs can also be found in patients with other inflammatory conditions such as cancer and autoimmunity.[77] Further research is necessary to determine if MDSCs represent a physiologically orchestrated part of the immune response or a pathologic arrest of developing myeloid cells leading to immune suppression.

Paradigm of Sepsis as an Adaptive Immune Problem

The conceptual framework of the pathophysiology of sepsis has evolved to include the concept of immune paralysis. Whereas sepsis has been traditionally viewed as being a reflection of uncontrolled hyperinflammation (ie, an innate immunity problem), it is now thought sepsis also has a strong, perhaps predominant, "antiinflammatory" component manifested as immune suppression and the relative inability to effectively clear an infectious challenge (an adaptive immunity problem).[18,19,81,82] For example, monocyte deactivation related to decreased MHC gene mRNA expression and decreased surface expression of MHC molecules have been previously demonstrated in patients with septic shock, including children.[44,45,83,84] With regard to lymphocyte dysfunction, Heidecke et al.[85] demonstrated that adult patients with intraabdominal infections and septic shock have defective T-cell proliferation and defective T-cell–dependent cytokine secretion, all of which are consistent with anergy/immune suppression. Felmet and et al.[86] identified prolonged lymphopenia and apoptosis-associated depletion of lymphoid organs as independent risk factors for the development of nosocomial infections and multiple organ failure in critically ill children. Musyznski et al.[87] recently provided evidence for early adaptive immune dysfunction in children with septic shock, as measured by ex vivo production of interferon-γ by CD4 cells.

Animal studies have well documented the requirement of an intact T-cell system to adequately combat a septic challenge.[82,88] Interestingly, however, neonatal mice (4-6 days of age) do not require an intact adaptive immune system to clear infection.[89] More recently, animal-based experiments have demonstrated that experimental septic shock is characterized by widespread apoptosis of T cells, and preventing T-cell apoptosis positively impacts the outcome of experimental sepsis.[90-97] Importantly, the concept of T-cell apoptosis in

human sepsis has been indirectly corroborated by autopsy studies, including children,[86,98] and lymphocyte-based immunophenotyping was recently demonstrated to effectively stratify septic shock outcome in adults.[99] Finally, it has been recently demonstrated in experimental models that alterations of the adaptive immune system in sepsis can persist well beyond the acute period (up to at least 6 weeks) via epigenetic mechanisms involving dendritic cells.[100,101] Despite these data, formal studies of T-cell function and adaptive immunity in pediatric septic shock have never been conducted in a systematic and comprehensive manner. Such studies hold the promise of radically changing our conceptual approach to the long-sought, but not yet realized, goal of rational immune modulation in septic shock (see also Chapter 102).

Genomic Medicine and Sepsis

The initial elucidation and publication of the human genome, the development of molecular biology tools for efficient high-throughput data generation, and the evolution of the field of biomedical informatics have combined to generate a new field termed "genomic medicine" and the related field of "systems biology." All aspects of medicine are potentially amenable to the concepts of genomic medicine and systems biology, including pediatric sepsis. One skeptical perspective of this concept is that clinical pediatric sepsis is overly heterogeneous and multifactorial to be credibly interrogated by the current genomic and systems biology approaches. An alternative and more optimistic perspective is that the concepts of genomic medicine and systems biology are ideally suited to more effectively address the complex syndromes clinicians encounter in pediatric critical care medicine, such as septic shock. The authors now address the two areas of genomic medicine most well developed in the field of pediatric septic shock: candidate gene association studies and genome-wide expression profiling.

Genetic Influence and Septic Shock

Susceptibility to sepsis and the clinical course of patients with sepsis are both highly heterogeneous, thus raising the strong possibility that the host response to infection is, at least in part, influenced by heritable factors (ie, genetics).[102] A landmark study by Sorensen et al.,[103] published more than 25 years ago, provides strong evidence linking genetics and susceptibility to infection. This study involved a longitudinal cohort of more than 900 adopted children born between 1924 and 1926. The adopted children and both their biological and adoptive parents were followed through 1982. If a biological parent died of infection before the age of 50 years, the relative risk of death from infectious causes in the child was 5.8 (95% CI 2.5–13.7), which was higher than for all other causes studied, including cancer and cardiovascular/cerebrovascular disease. In contrast, the death of an adoptive parent from infectious causes did not confer a greater relative risk of death in the adopted child.

More recently, investigations attempting to link genetics with sepsis focused mainly on candidate gene association studies and gene polymorphisms. A gene polymorphism is defined as the regular occurrence (>1%) in a population of two or more alleles at a particular chromosome location. The most frequent type of polymorphism is called a single nucleotide polymorphism (SNP): a substitution, deletion, or insertion of a single nucleotide occurring in approximately 1 per every 1000 base pairs of human DNA. SNPs can result in an absolute deficiency in protein, an altered protein, a change in the level of normal protein expression, or no discernible change in protein function or expression. There is a growing body of literature linking SNPs within several genes regulating inflammation, coagulation, and the immune response with critical illness, and several excellent reviews exist on the topic.[104-107]

The signaling mechanisms involved in pathogen recognition, the immune response, and inflammation were described in previous sections. Following is an overview of relevant SNPs described in many of the genes involved in these signaling mechanisms. TLR-4 (the primary receptor for recognition of lipopolysaccharide) mutations have been described in humans, all of which increase susceptibility to infections secondary to gram-negative organisms.[108] While several SNPs in the *TLR-4* receptor gene have been described, few have been found to be associated with an increased risk of septic shock or septic shock–related mortality in children. For example, an adenine for guanine substitution 896 base pairs downstream of the transcription start site for TLR-4 (+896) results in replacement of aspartic acid with glycine at amino acid 299 (Asp299Gly). The Asp299Gly polymorphism has been associated with reduced expression and function of the TLR-4 receptor in vitro.[108,109] Furthermore, adults who carry the Asp-299Gly polymorphism appear to be at increased risk for septic shock and poor outcome in several cohort studies.[110-112] While children who carry the Asp299Gly polymorphism appear to be at increased risk of urinary tract infection, this SNP does not appear to influence either the susceptibility or severity of meningococcal septic shock in children.[113,114] These results were further corroborated in a cohort study involving over 500 Gambian children.[115]

SNPs related to other members of the LPS-receptor complex (eg, CD14, MD-2, and MyD88) have been studied in adult populations, but no such studies have yet to be performed in children.[111,116-119] SNPs in other classes of Toll-like receptors have also been studied. For example, gene polymorphisms of TLR-2, the primary pattern recognition receptor for gram-positive bacteria, have been associated with increased risk of infection in children and adults.[120-122]

Several SNPs affecting cytokine expression have been described, but the corresponding gene association studies in critically ill adults with septic shock have been conflicting.[106,107,123] For example, two allelic variants of the TNF-α gene have been described: the wild-type allele TNF1 (guanine at -308A) and TNF2 (adenosine at -308A). The TNF2 allele has been associated with higher expression of TNF-α and increased susceptibility to septic shock and mortality in at least one study involving critically ill adults.[124] Nadel et al.[125] found an increased risk of death in critically ill children with meningococcal septic shock who carried the TNF2 allelic variant. Several additional SNPs in TNF-β, IL-1, IL-6, IL-8, and IL-10 have also been shown to influence susceptibility to and severity of septic shock in children.[126-132]

Because dysregulation of the coagulation cascade plays an important role in the pathophysiology of septic shock, several studies have examined polymorphisms of key genes involved in coagulation. For example, the 4G allele of a deletion/insertion (4G/5G) SNP in the promoter region of the plasminogen-activator inhibitor type-1 *(PAI-1)* gene has been

associated with higher plasma concentrations of PAI-1. The 4G allele increases susceptibility to and severity of septic shock, as well as increasing the risk of mortality in children with meningococcal septic shock.[62,133-135] In addition, an SNP in the protein C promoter region has been associated with susceptibility to meningococcemia and illness severity in children.[136]

SNPs in genes involved in phagocytosis and the complement cascade have also been studied in the context of septic shock. For example, SNPs affecting function have been described in virtually all family members of the Fcγ receptor (important for phagocytosis), and several of these SNPs have been associated with susceptibility to meningococcal sepsis, severity of meningococcemia, and poor outcome from meningococcal septic shock.[137-143] In addition, an association between the FcγRIIa polymorphism and infection with other encapsulated bacteria has also been reported.[144,145] Several SNPs in the mannose-binding lectin (MBL) gene have been associated with increased susceptibility to infection, as well as increased illness severity.[146-151] Finally, an SNP of the bactericidal permeability increasing protein (BPI) gene has also been associated with increased mortality from septic shock in children.[152] This polymorphism is particularly interesting because a well-conducted phase III trial of recombinant BPI in children with septic shock failed to demonstrate efficacy.[153]

It is likely that many more studies that attempt to link SNPs with the susceptibility and/or outcome of pediatric septic shock are forthcoming in the future, and all need to be carefully considered and evaluated. With respect to validity and wide clinical acceptance, the ideal candidate gene association study requires several important qualities including biological plausibility, large sample sizes, a priori hypothesis statements, and power calculations, accounting for confounding factors, and independent validation.[154]

Genome-Wide Expression Profiling in Children With Septic Shock

The development of microarray technology has provided an unprecedented opportunity to efficiently measure genome-wide mRNA expression patterns in clinical samples. Over the past decade, this approach has been leveraged to understand more comprehensively the pathophysiology of pediatric septic shock and as a means of discovery and hypothesis generation. Comprehensive reviews of these studies were recently published.[155-157]

The first studies to characterize the transcriptomic response of pediatric septic shock confirmed that septic shock is characterized by upregulation of gene programs corresponding to innate immunity and the inflammatory response.[158,159] These studies also noted concomitant downregulation of gene programs corresponding to adaptive immunity, which is consistent with the immune paralysis paradigm described earlier. These gene expression patterns are evident within 24 hours of admission to the ICU and persist at least through ICU day 3.[160] Other notable data generated from these transcriptomic studies include (1) the observation that pediatric septic shock is characterized by repression of gene programs that either depend on zinc homeostasis or directly participate in zinc homeostasis[158]; (2) characterizing distinct gene programs across the spectrum of systemic inflammatory response syndrome, sepsis, and septic shock[161]; (3) demonstrating the influence of developmental age on the transcriptomic response to pediatric septic shock[162]; (4) the observation that gene programs corresponding to mitochondrial function and biogenesis are repressed in certain subclasses of pediatric septic shock[163]; and (5) the observation that the prescription of adjunctive corticosteroids leads to further repression of adaptive immunity-related gene programs in children with septic shock.[164]

These transcriptomic studies have also enabled identification of new mechanistic pathways and candidate therapeutic targets for sepsis, which have been brought back to the basic science laboratory for formal hypothesis testing using rodent models of sepsis. For example, following the observation that zinc homeostasis is altered in pediatric septic shock, it was demonstrated that zinc supplementation confers a survival advantage in rodent models of sepsis.[75,165] As a direct consequence, a phase 1 trial of IV zinc supplementation in critically ill children was recently completed and will inform the design of future trials of zinc supplementation in sepsis.[166] In another example, it was reported that repression of the peroxisome proliferator activator receptor-α (PPAR-α) signaling pathway is associated with poor outcome in pediatric sepsis.[167-169] This observation was subsequently corroborated in a sepsis model involving PPAR-α null mice.[170]

Following the observation that matrix metalloproteinase-8 (MMP8) is consistently the highest expressed gene in children with septic shock, extensive studies were subsequently conducted to further delineate the role of MMP8 in sepsis. Genetic ablation or pharmacologic inhibition of MMP8 confers a survival advantage in mice subjected to cecal ligation and puncture (CLP).[171,172] These observations are associated with attenuated inflammation but without compromising bacterial clearance. In addition, MMP8 can directly serve as a DAMP because primary macrophages stimulated ex vivo with recombinant MMP8 demonstrate increased NF-κB expression and increased expression of proinflammatory cytokines.[171]

These transcriptomic studies have also enabled the discovery of sepsis biomarkers. For example, IL-27 was identified as a candidate sepsis diagnostic biomarker via transcriptomics and follow-up studies demonstrated serum IL-27 protein concentrations >5 ng/mL can distinguish critically ill children with bacterial infection from critically ill children with sterile inflammation with >90% specificity and positive predictive value.[173] In these initial studies, IL-27 outperformed procalcitonin, and a combination of procalcitonin and IL-27 performed better than either biomarker alone. Interestingly, IL-27 appears to perform better as a sepsis diagnostic biomarker in children, compared with adults.[174,175] In another example, these transcriptomic studies enabled the discovery of biomarkers to predict the development of septic acute kidney injury.[176,177] Finally, these transcriptomic studies enabled the discovery of stratification biomarkers to assign a baseline mortality probability for children and adults with septic shock.[178-183] The concept of leveraging stratification biomarkers for the care of children with septic shock is discussed in a subsequent section.

An "endotype" is a subclass of a condition defined by function or biology.[184] On the basis of discovery-oriented computational approaches and hierarchical clustering of >8000 genes, these transcriptomic studies identified gene expression–based endotypes of pediatric septic shock.[167] Post hoc analysis revealed one of the endotypes had significantly greater illness severity, organ failure burden, and mortality,

and these observations were subsequently validated.[168,169] With the goal of developing a clinically feasible test meeting the time-sensitive demands of critically ill patients,[155] the endotyping method was refined by distilling the endotype-defining expression signature to the top 100 class predictor genes, expressing these genes using visually intuitive gene expression mosaics, and measuring mRNA expression using a digital mRNA quantification platform. This approach validated that this endotyping method identifies patients with increased organ failure burden and mortality.[185,186] Notably, the endotype-defining gene expression signature is enriched for genes corresponding to adaptive immune function and the glucocorticoid receptor signaling pathway, and allocation to one of these endotypes is independently associated with increased mortality. Thus endotyping potentially has theranostic implications given the current interest surrounding therapies to augment the adaptive immune system in patients with sepsis[187] and the ongoing controversies surrounding the role of adjunctive corticosteroids in septic shock.[188] For example, the use of adjunctive corticosteroids is independently associated with four times the risk of mortality in one of the endotypes.[185] Fig. 111.3 shows examples of the recently identified pediatric septic shock endotypes.

Treatment Strategies

Overview

As the biological response to sepsis becomes better understood and as clinicians refine their ability to phenotype and stratify patients, the approach to treatment of sepsis will become more specific and more sophisticated. At present, however, clinical treatment of sepsis entails four important goals, which for the most part rely on purely supportive measures founded on the fundamental principles of critical care medicine: initial resuscitation, pathogen elimination, maintenance of oxygen delivery, and carefully directed regulation of the inflammatory response. An update of pediatric and neonatal specific guidelines for sepsis management was recently published,[189] and another update is in process at the time of this writing.

Initial Resuscitation

As in any disease process, the first step in the treatment of sepsis is the initial stabilization of the patient. In this regard, children present many of the same challenges as adult patients, including respiratory and cardiovascular stabilization. The primary goals of therapy in the first hours are to maintain oxygenation and ventilation, achieve normal perfusion and blood pressure, and reestablish appropriate urine output and mental status.[189]

Children with signs of sepsis may have significantly decreased mental status, raising concern about the ability to protect their airway. Also, in septic shock the work of breathing can represent a significant portion of oxygen consumption (as much as 15%-30%). Because children with septic shock also receive large amounts of fluid to restore intravascular volume in the context of capillary leak, they are at increased risk for developing pulmonary edema. Consequently, lung compliance decreases and work of breathing can increase substantially. Together, these respiratory abnormalities often necessitate tracheal intubation and mechanical ventilation.

Endotype A

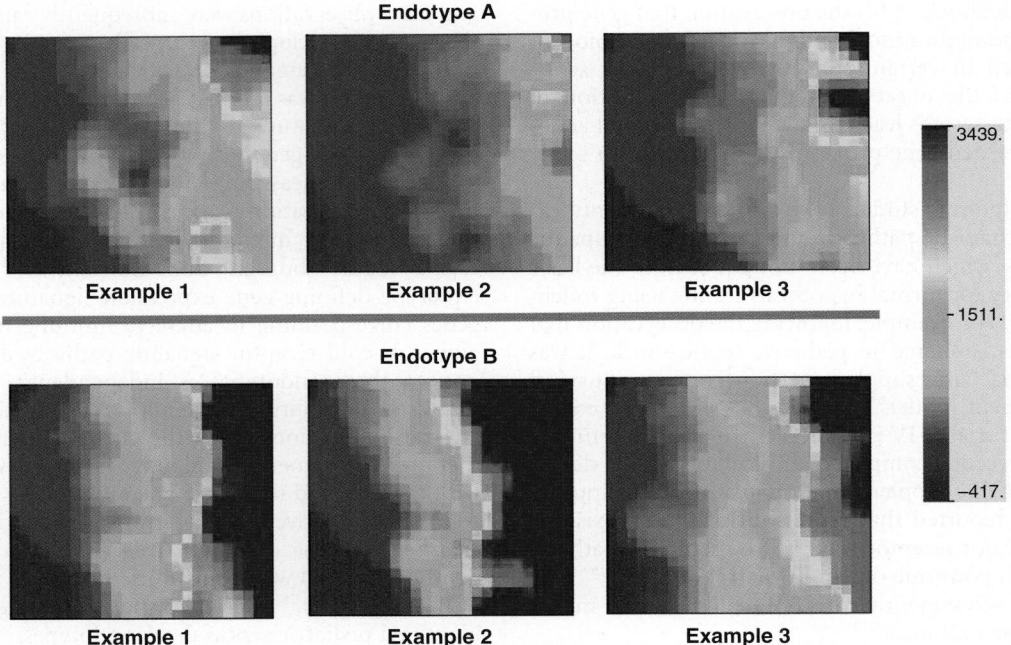

Fig. 111.3. Examples of individual pediatric patients allocated to septic shock endotypes A and B. Each gene expression mosaic represents 100 endotype-defining genes, which correspond to adaptive immunity and glucorticoid receptor signaling.[185] The color bar on the far right of the figure indicates color intensity relative to the level of gene expression, with the degree of blue intensity corresponding to decreased gene expression and the degree of red intensity corresponding to increased gene expression.

Arterial blood gas analysis often reveals, in early sepsis, respiratory alkalosis from centrally mediated hyperventilation. As sepsis progresses, patients may have hypoxemia and respiratory acidosis, secondary to parenchymal lung disease and/or hypoventilation due to altered mental status.[189] However, the decision to initiate mechanical ventilation support should not necessarily be contingent on laboratory findings; rather, the decision should be based primarily on clinical findings of increased work of breathing, hypoventilation, and/or impaired mental status. Mechanical ventilation provides the added benefit of reducing work of breathing, therefore decreasing overall oxygen consumption, especially when combined with sedation and paralysis. If early tracheal intubation is chosen, consideration of volume loading and inotropic/vasoactive support is recommended. Sedative agents for induction should be selected to maintain hemodynamic stability. The 2007 pediatric guidelines for septic shock specifically recommend against the use of etomidate due to its adrenal suppressive effects and suggest the use of ketamine as a suitable agent to maintain hemodynamic stability.[189] Subsequent studies, however, suggest no effect on mortality or length of stay in adults with septic shock intubated with etomidate.[190,191]

For a variety of reasons, patients with sepsis almost universally have decreased effective intravascular volume. Many had poor oral intake of fluid for some time before developing sepsis. With the development of increased vascular permeability, intravascular volume has been lost because of third spacing. Finally, vasodilation partially related to excessive NO production (see earlier section) results in abnormally increased vascular capacitance, thereby decreasing the effective intravascular volume. When sepsis is suspected, vascular access should be obtained and 20 mL/kg of isotonic fluid administered as quickly as possible. A second peripheral vascular access is recommended, and difficulties in attaining venous access can be overcome with the use of an intraosseous catheter. Intraosseous access can temporarily be the primary route for volume infusion, medications, and blood products when an intravascular access is not readily obtained. While following clinical examination for signs of overly aggressive volume resuscitation (eg, new onset of rales, increased work of breathing, development of a gallop, abdominal distention, or hepatomegaly), fluid should be administered quickly with the goal of improving blood pressure and tissue perfusion. Administration of more than 60 mL/kg of isotonic fluid in the first hour of resuscitation is associated with improved survival.[192-194]

Aggressive fluid resuscitation for septic shock was recently criticized as being only weakly supported by evidence.[195] Further, recent cohort studies have reported an association between positive fluid balance and increased mortality in adult and pediatric patients with sepsis, as well as other critical illnesses.[196-205] Most recently, the Fluid Expansion as Supportive Therapy (FEAST) study compared fluid boluses of 20 to 40 mL/kg with no bolus in more than 3000 acutely ill African children and reported significantly increased mortality in the group randomized to the fluid bolus arm.[206] The FEAST study raises many questions regarding the efficacy of fluid resuscitation, even though the relevance for resource-rich environments is unclear.[207]

It is biologically and physiologically plausible that the association between a positive fluid balance and the risk of mortality is a result of confounding by illness severity. Positive fluid balance could be simply a marker of increased illness severity leading to increased vascular leak, increased third spacing of fluid, and increased fluid requirements, rather than a direct cause of increased mortality per se.[208] Accordingly, associations between positive fluid balance and septic shock outcomes need to be interpreted in the context of baseline mortality probability and illness severity. A recent study conducted a risk-stratified analysis of children with septic shock and found no association between the degree and duration of positive fluid balance and mortality in patients with intermediate and high baseline mortality risks.[209] At the time of this writing there is an ongoing study testing the efficacy of a "fluid sparing" protocol in children with septic shock (NCT1973907). It is hoped this study will further inform the issue of appropriate fluid resuscitation in pediatric septic shock.

Fig. 111.4 shows a pediatric algorithm for early goal-directed therapy. The algorithm emphasizes the importance of guiding therapy based on central venous oxygen saturation measurements. This algorithm reflects earlier studies in adults and children demonstrating reductions in sepsis-related mortality with goal-directed therapy guided by central venous oxygen saturation measurements.[210,211] However, the generalizability of the single pediatric study that led to this algorithm is questionable because of the high mortality in the control group. Similarly, a more recent study in children testing the efficacy of central venous oxygen saturation monitoring had an in-hospital mortality of 54% in the control group.[212] More

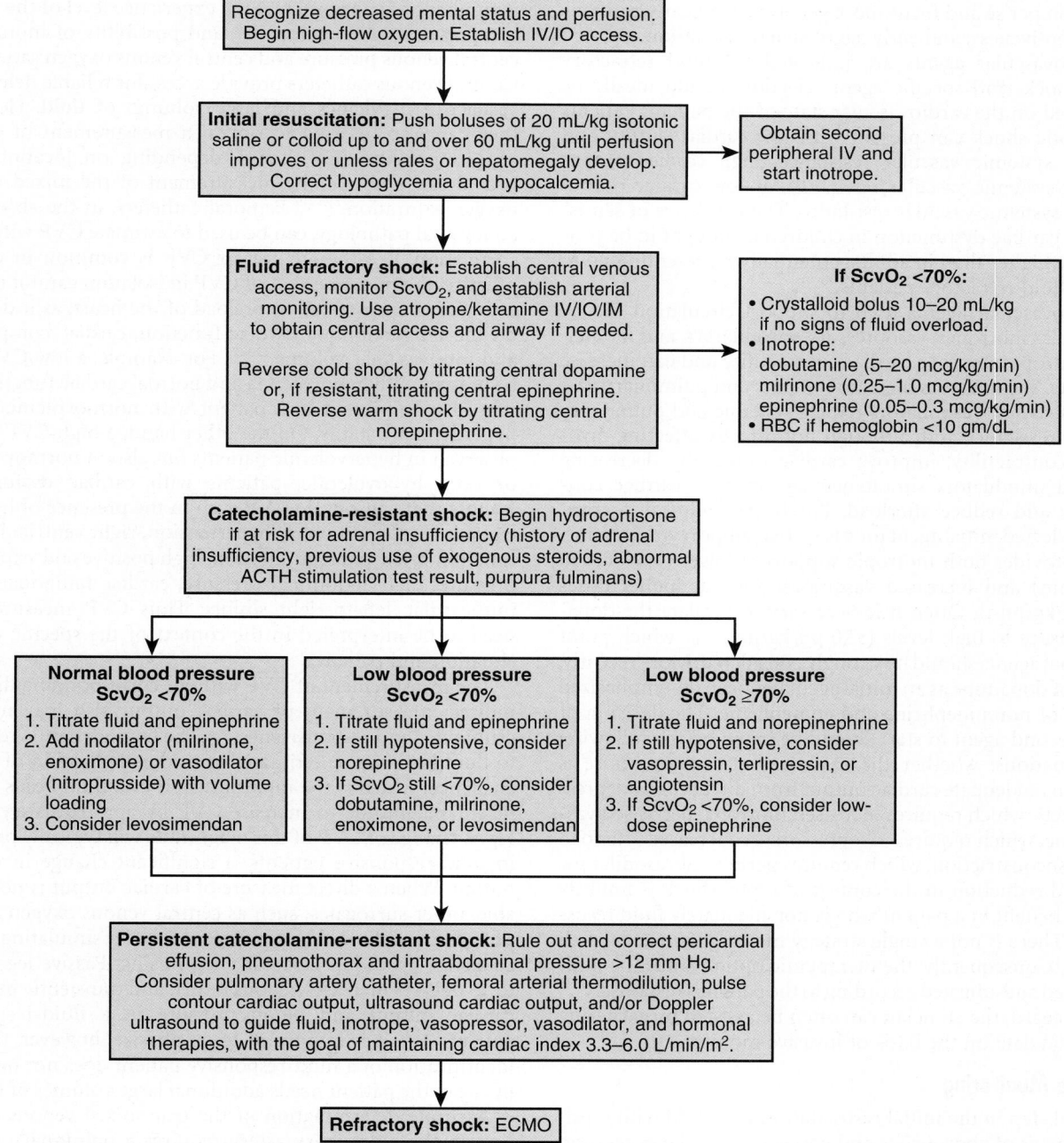

Fig. 111.4. Algorithm for early goal-directed therapy, guided by mixed venous saturations, in pediatric septic shock.

importantly, three large adult trials were recently completed showing no benefit of goal-directed therapy, compared with standard care.[213-215] An important caveat of these three trials is that "standard care" has evolved considerably over the past decade to emphasize early recognition and early aggressive resuscitation of sepsis. A recent editorial opined that despite the results of the large adult studies, mixed venous saturation monitoring should remain a cornerstone target of guideline therapies for pediatric septic shock.[216] An alternative opinion is that the cumulative data support early recognition of sepsis and a highly attentive critical care team focused on early, aggressive resuscitation of septic shock, rather than supporting mixed venous oxygen saturations as a singular end point. Accordingly, an updated pediatric septic shock algorithm should de-emphasize the importance of central venous oxygen saturation per se and focus more generically on early recognition, attentiveness, and early aggressive resuscitation.

Cardiovascular agents are indicated for fluid refractory septic shock, and specific agent selection should ideally be predicated on the cardiovascular state of the patient. Patients with septic shock can present with low cardiac output and elevated systemic vascular resistance, high cardiac output and low systemic vascular resistance, or low cardiac output and low systemic vascular resistance. The incidence of sepsis-induced cardiac dysfunction in children is thought to be considerably higher than in adults, potentially representing up to 80% of fluid refractory patients.[13]

Cardiovascular agents used to support circulation can be classified as inotropes, vasopressors, vasodilators, and inodilators. Inotropes improve cardiac contractility and can increase heart rate. Vasopressors increase systemic and pulmonary vascular resistance. Vasodilators reduce systemic and pulmonary vascular resistance and, although not directly affecting myocardial contractility, improve cardiac output by decreasing afterload. Inodilators simultaneously improve cardiac contractility and reduce afterload. Purely by tradition, a commonly selected initial agent for vasoactive support is dopamine, which provides both inotropic support at lower doses (5–10 μg/kg/min) and increased vasomotor tone at higher doses (>10 μg/kg/min). Often it is necessary to escalate the dopamine dosage to high levels (≤20 μg/kg/min), at which point additional agents should be strongly considered. More recently, the use of dopamine as an initial agent has been de-emphasized in favor of norepinephrine and epinephrine. The decision of which second agent to start should be based on the following determinations: whether the cardiovascular compromise is related to inadequate cardiac output from direct cardiodepressant effects, which requires increased inotropy; decreased vascular tone, which requires vasopressors; or increased afterload from vasoconstriction, which requires peripheral vasodilators. Afterload reduction in the context of septic shock is unlikely to be of benefit in a patient who is not adequately fluid resuscitated. There is not a single strategy meeting the needs of all patients. Consequently, the therapeutic options must be individualized and adjusted according to the patient's response.[14,217] In this regard, the clinician can often be assisted by garnering additional data on the basis of invasive monitoring.

Invasive Monitoring

The final step in the initial resuscitation of a child with sepsis is placement of appropriate and necessary vascular access and monitors. However, attention to the clinical examination as part of the ongoing assessment is imperative. In sepsis, the primary clinical end points to assess are changes in level of consciousness, decreased urine output, and poor peripheral perfusion characterized by delayed capillary refill and diminished distal pulses. Unfortunately, children with sepsis can be difficult to examine because they are often tracheally intubated and sedated and may not have produced any initial urine because of severe hypovolemia. Also, they frequently are receiving vasopressors (sometimes excessively), which can make examination of the skin for assessment of perfusion less reliable. For these reasons, invasive monitoring is often necessary and helpful.

Central venous access is a necessity for the child in septic shock. The decision to place a central venous catheter in the internal jugular, subclavian, or femoral position is dictated by a number of factors, such as the experience level of the operator, presence of coagulopathy, and possibility of monitoring central venous pressure and central venous oxygen saturation. Central venous catheters provide access for reliable delivery of vasoactive medicines and large volumes of fluid. However, they can also be used to obtain a measurement of central venous pressure (CVP) and, depending on location, may provide an approximate measurement of the mixed venous oxygen saturation.[217-219] Femoral catheters, in the absence of abdominal pathology, can be used to estimate CVP with good correlation.[219] Although use of CVP is common in clinical practice, the measurement of CVP in isolation cannot reliably estimate volume status or preload of the heart, as it depends on the interactions of cardiac function, cardiac compliance, and intravascular volume.[220,221] For example, a low CVP may be present with hypovolemia and normal cardiac function but may also be present in a patient with normovolemia and a hyperdynamic status. On the other hand, a high CVP can be observed in hypervolemic patients but also in normovolemic, or even hypovolemic, patients with cardiac dysfunction. Factors that can elevate CVP even in the presence of hypovolemia include pulmonary hypertension, right ventricular dysfunction, tricuspid regurgitation, high positive end-expiratory pressure, high abdominal pressure, cardiac tamponade, and intracardiac left-to-right shunts. Thus CVP measurements need to be interpreted in the context of the specific clinical situation and patient.

The measurement of CVP without corresponding direct or indirect measurement of cardiac output also may not discriminate fluid responsiveness.[220] The hemodynamic response to fluid load can be estimated with the application of a fluid challenge, which is the rapid infusion of a fluid bolus of sufficient magnitude to increase CVP by approximately 2 mm Hg. A change of CVP of this magnitude will typically produce, in fluid-responsive patients, a significant change in cardiac output. When a direct measure of cardiac output is not available, other surrogates, such as central venous oxygen saturation, can be followed. A practical maneuver simulating a fluid challenge procedure is passive leg-raising. Passive leg-raising to 45 degrees increases venous return and transiently increases cardiac output and blood pressure in a fluid-responsive patient.[222,223] It is important to emphasize, however, that the identification of a fluid-responsive patient does not necessarily mean the patient needs additional large volumes of fluid.[222]

Accurate determination of the true mixed venous saturation in the pulmonary artery requires a pulmonary arterial catheter (PAC), but approximations of the saturation can be provided by a catheter tip at or near the right atrium. Values of oxygen saturation measured at the right atrium or superior vena cava are slightly different from true mixed venous saturation, but there is a good trend correlation between the two measurements.[217,224,225] Therefore the use of central venous (right atrium or superior vena cava) oxygen saturation is more practical and feasible as it avoids the requirement for pulmonary artery catheterization. Because of significant differences in oxygen extraction among the upper extremities, abdomen, and lower extremities, venous saturations from a femoral venous line do not accurately correlate with those measured in the pulmonary artery.[219] Measurements of central venous saturation can be achieved through the analysis of blood samples collected from correctly positioned catheters (intermittent) or continuously with the utilization of an indwelling fiberoptic catheter.

In the face of severe sepsis and septic shock, an intraarterial catheter may become necessary. An arterial catheter becomes both a source of continuous clinical information regarding blood pressure, pulse pressure, hemodynamic variation with respiration (ie, pulses paradoxus), and an access for frequent blood draws. Whereas blood pressure alone does not always equate to tissue perfusion because of differences in regional perfusion and vasoconstriction, a fluid-resuscitated child with normal or high systolic blood pressure will be more tolerant of manipulations to increase perfusion (ie, afterload reduction) than children with lower blood pressures. This condition occurs in children who have poor ventricular ejection and high systemic vascular resistance. Therapeutic maneuvers to actively decrease afterload can be more rationally conducted with continuous blood pressure monitoring via an intraarterial catheter.

The arterial blood also provides the most accurate information regarding arterial oxygen content that can be used to both assess the function of the lungs and maximize oxygen delivery. Additionally, analysis of the arterial pulse wave can provide a continuous monitoring of the cardiac output. Recent studies reveal this cardiac output estimation technique can be safely applied in children and has a reasonable correlation with thermodilution or echocardiography-based techniques.[226,227]

Use of PACs to optimize left ventricular preload, monitor changes in cardiac index, and provide accurate measurements of oxygen delivery and consumption is now controversial. Interpretation of PAC data requires the absence of intracardiac shunting and presence of normal mitral valve function as either shunting or mitral regurgitation alters cardiac index determination and pulmonary capillary wedge pressure measurements. Because data from critically ill adults showed no benefit of routine PAC use,[228] the use of PACs has substantially declined in critical care medicine but is thought to be of potential benefit in selected patients.[229] In light of studies showing the information obtained from PAC can be important in identifying clinically meaningful cardiovascular conditions different from what is suspected by clinical impression,[13,229] PAC placement may be considered for pediatric patients who remain in shock after resuscitation and initiation of the usual cardiovascular agents and in patients having unclear fluid status and cardiac function. Other methods of measuring cardiac output, such as arterial pulse wave analysis, femoral artery thermodilution, Doppler ultrasound, or ultrasound cardiac output monitoring, may be effective substitutes to the use of PAC.

Elimination of Pathogens

Identification of the source of a possible offending organism in septic shock dictates the choice of antimicrobial coverage and is important to long-term outcome, as early administration of appropriate antibiotics is associated with improved survival.[230-232] While the imperative nature of prompt antibiotic treatment may seem intuitively obvious, it has been well documented that delays in appropriate antibiotic administration have a greater adverse impact on septic shock outcome than do cytokine polymorphisms.[233] Therefore antibiotic therapy should be started within the first hour of recognition of sepsis, ideally after appropriate cultures have been readily obtained. However, antibiotic administration should not be delayed if obtaining appropriate cultures is technically problematic.

The offending organism and the site of infection also affect prognosis.[234] Fungal infections are associated with the lowest survival rates, followed by bacterial infections, especially meningococcal and pneumococcal infections.[2] It is important to note, however, the epidemiology of pediatric sepsis is changing, particularly in populations where vaccination policies incorporate immunization against *Haemophilus influenzae*, *Streptococcus pneumoniae*, and *Neisseria meningitidis* serotype C. Although infections caused by these agents have decreased, there are now more cases of nosocomial infections, especially caused by staphylococci and fungi. The majority of infections causing severe sepsis are respiratory or primary bacteremia, with respiratory cases being more common among older children and in community-acquired infections, and primary bacteremia more frequently affecting neonates, children with neoplastic disorders, or other comorbidities. Lower survival rates are associated with endocarditis and infections of the central nervous system.[2]

Initial empiric antimicrobial therapy should include one or more drugs having activity against the likely pathogens (bacterial or fungal) and the ability to penetrate into the presumed source of the sepsis. The choice of drugs should be guided by the susceptibility patterns of microorganisms in the community and in the hospital.[230] Because of the importance of appropriate antimicrobial therapy, the decision regarding which agents to start empirically must balance potential side effects against maximizing coverage. Initially, broad antibiotic coverage should be started. Neonates should be given ampicillin and either gentamicin or a third-generation cephalosporin such as cefotaxime. In infants and children older than 4 to 6 weeks, the decision to begin vancomycin therapy empirically, in addition to the standard third-generation cephalosporin, should be considered in light of the increasing antibiotic resistance of *Streptococcus pneumoniae*, as well as methicillin-resistant *Staphylococcus aureus*. Nosocomial infections and infections in immunocompromised patients require additional coverage for the possibility of *Pseudomonas* species and other resistant organisms. Acyclovir should be given if there is a clinical presentation or suspicion of an overwhelming viral (herpetic) infection, particularly in neonates and infants. Starting antifungal medicines initially in an immunocompetent child is usually not necessary. However, this decision should be reconsidered if the child does not improve over the first 2 days or in case of higher risk for fungal infection (presence of indwelling devices, immunosuppression, or other significant comorbidities). The antimicrobial regimen should be reassessed after 48 to 72 hours on the basis of microbiological and clinical data with the goal of narrowing the antibiotic spectrum to prevent the development of resistance and to reduce toxicity. Once a causative pathogen is identified, there is no evidence that combination therapy is more effective than monotherapy for most bacterial infections. The duration of therapy should typically be 7 to 10 days and guided by clinical response.[230]

Maintenance of Oxygen Delivery

After initial resuscitation and attention to pathogen elimination, ongoing management of sepsis remains primarily supportive, with particular attention to maintenance of adequate oxygen delivery. While this is a fundamental tenet of critical care medicine, the approach may be relatively ineffective in a subset of patients having impaired utilization of oxygen despite adequate oxygen delivery (ie, cytopathic hypoxia). The assessment of adequate oxygen delivery should be viewed as a dynamic and ongoing process as measured by a combination of parameters including clinical assessment of perfusion, blood pressure, serial lactate measurements, urine output, central/mixed venous oxygen saturation, and, in selected cases, PAC-derived measurements.[210]

Adequate preload is necessary for adequate cardiac output and consequently for adequate oxygen delivery. Children with sepsis can remain at risk for hypovolemia after an appropriate initial resuscitation because of persistent increased insensible fluid loss, increased vascular capacitance, and capillary leak with third spacing. Anecdotally, some well-resuscitated children have such vigorous urine output after the initial resuscitation that reassessment of fluid balance after the first 24 hours of presentation to the ICU reveals the fluid balance may actually be close to "even." Thus providing adequate preload to the patient in septic shock may require increased fluid administration for several days after the initial resuscitation. The choice of fluid to be used in this process is controversial, although there is general agreement the fluid choice should be isotonic. The three broad choices of fluids are crystalloid, non–blood colloid, and blood products. As evident when calculating the arterial content of oxygen, maintaining an adequate hemoglobin level is an important factor in providing adequate oxygen delivery. Although there is no clear recommended hemoglobin level for children with sepsis, one recent study showed that in patients with central venous oxygen saturation <70%, transfusion of packed red blood cells in combination with other measures to increase oxygen delivery is associated with improved outcomes.[210]

After initial resuscitation, ongoing myocardial dysfunction and altered vascular tone are likely to persist and will therefore require ongoing titration of cardiovascular drugs to maintain adequate oxygen delivery. Many patients will require titration of inotropes and vasopressors simultaneously, and it must be emphasized this will likely be a dynamic process requiring constant reassessment of the aforementioned indicators of adequate oxygen delivery. It is important to recognize that blood pressure alone as a goal may not correlate with optimal tissue perfusion and oxygen delivery. This concept is best illustrated by the subset of patients with septic shock who benefit from afterload reduction (ie, vasodilation). Patients with high SVR and low cardiac output, who have adequate preload, can benefit tremendously from inodilators such as milrinone.[235,236] Alternatively, this subset of patients can also

benefit from pure vasodilators such as the NO donor, nitroprusside (in combination with a pure inotrope). After institution of afterload reduction, these types of patients may actually have lower blood pressures than one would typically target but will have enhanced tissue perfusion and oxygen delivery.

A subset of patients will have refractory shock despite optimization of the previously mentioned management strategies. In this subset, the institution of extracorporeal membrane oxygenation (ECMO) is recommended as a consideration in the context of refractory shock.[189] Anecdotal and subjective experiences suggest institution of ECMO support for refractory septic shock can be lifesaving in a subset of patients. The challenges that come with institution of ECMO include the definition of refractory septic shock, timing of ECMO initiation before the onset of irreversible end-organ failure, and ensuring ECMO support is not prematurely or unnecessarily instituted in patients who can be effectively managed with conventional support (ie, not exposing patients to unnecessary risks).

A summary of approaches to improving the relationship between oxygen delivery and oxygen consumption is provided in Box 111.3.

Additional Management Considerations

Patients with sepsis may have poor nutrition before presentation and often are not fed during the first few days of illness. Because of an increased metabolic rate and poor nutrition, patients with sepsis are frequently catabolic and at risk for development of protein calorie malnutrition.[237] Intestinal ischemia in association with loss of the mucosal barrier from malnutrition is associated with translocation of bacteria and endotoxin from the intestine into the bloodstream. Use of enteral feeding in critically ill patients has been shown to improve survival and decrease hospital stay.[238] The benefit of enteral feeding should be balanced with the risk of stressing

---

BOX 111.3	**Means of Altering the Relationship Between Oxygen Delivery and Oxygen Consumption**

Means of improving oxygen delivery:
- Increase cardiac output
  - Increase stroke volume
    - Increase preload (volume resuscitation)
    - Increase contractility (administration of inotropes)
    - Decrease afterload (administration of vasodilators)
  - Increase heart rate (rarely a therapeutic goal in sepsis management)
- Increase arterial oxygen content
  - Increase arterial oxygen tension (administer oxygen, apply positive pressure ventilation, etc.)
  - Increase arterial oxygen-carrying capacity (transfusion of packed red blood cells)
- In select cases, cardiac output and arterial oxygen content can both be increased through the institution of venoarterial extracorporeal membrane oxygenation

Means of decreasing oxygen consumption:
- Avoid/manage hyperthermia
- Remove work of breathing
- Administer sedation
- Administer paralytics

intestinal function in the face of poor splanchnic perfusion, especially in the presence of vasopressors such as epinephrine and norepinephrine.[239] Regardless of the feeding mode, adequate nutrition and nitrogen balance are important for maintaining adequate host immune function and achieving homeostasis, as malnutrition adversely affects immune function. Finally, in the absence of enteral feedings, pharmacologic prophylaxis against stress-related gastrointestinal bleeding is recommended by the most recent guidelines.

A positive fluid balance, as a consequence of aggressive fluid resuscitation and capillary leak, is an important issue that eventually needs to be addressed in virtually all patients with septic shock. The absolute level of positive fluid balance requiring active management seems to be highly variable and context specific in children with septic shock.[209] General signs of clinically significant positive fluid balance include hepatomegaly, rales/pulmonary edema, ascites and potentially intra-abdominal hypertension, and/or 10% increase in body weight. For many patients, institution of diuretic therapy is a simple and effective approach to manage a positive fluid balance, in the context of hemodynamic stability and adequate renal function. However, acute kidney injury/renal failure commonly occurs in septic shock and may require institution of some form of renal replacement therapy such as peritoneal dialysis, hemodialysis, or continuous renal replacement therapy (CRRT).

Variations of CRRT are commonly viewed as the most ideal choice for these patients given the potential ability to meticulously titrate fluid removal in patients with hemodynamic instability. In addition, CRRT has the potential to achieve more than simple fluid removal inasmuch as high ultrafiltration rates can also provide clearance of standard waste products of metabolism, as well as "mediators" of sepsis (ie, immune modulation). However, CRRT is also well documented to be associated with clinically significant complications (eg, hemodynamic instability and electrolyte imbalances) in critically ill children.[240] Thus "timing" and "dose" are important considerations for institution of CRRT in patients with septic shock, and both considerations are predicated on the concept that CRRT represents more than just simply fluid removal and management of uremia.[241] "Timing" refers to the concept of instituting CRRT before the onset of overt renal failure and clinically significant fluid overload. "Dose" refers to the concept of ultrafiltration rates and the potential ability of high filtration rates to achieve more effective immune modulation. These important concepts represent major challenges in the field that need to be addressed by well-designed, pediatric-specific multicenter trials. Recent trials comparing high ultrafiltration rates (high-intensity CRRT) with standard ultrafiltration rates (low-intensity CRRT) have shown no survival benefit in critically ill adults.[242,243] Intriguingly, there was trend toward improved survival in the subset of patients with sepsis treated with high-intensity CRRT[242] (see also Chapter 78).

Hyperglycemia is well recognized to be associated with increased morbidity and mortality in critically ill patients, including children with sepsis.[244,245] In 2001, van den Berghe et al.[246] published a landmark study demonstrating that aggressive insulin therapy to normalize glucose levels to within a narrow range significantly increased survival in a large cohort of critically ill adult surgical patients. This study strongly suggested that hyperglycemia is not merely a stress-related epiphenomenon of critical illness but rather a pathologic process that can be addressed by an intensive insulin-based protocol targeting normalization of glucose levels. However, the inability to consistently replicate these findings has led to a great deal of controversy in the field. A recent meta-analysis concluded that tight glucose control does not significantly reduce mortality in critically ill adult patients but is associated with an increased risk of hypoglycemia.[247] An even more recent, randomized, multicenter trial compared intensive glucose control (81–108 mg/dL) with conventional glucose control (<180 mg/dL) in more than 6000 critically ill adults.[248] This study concluded that intensive glucose control increased mortality in critically ill adults, relative to conventional glucose control. Finally, another recent trial focused on intensive insulin therapy in adults with sepsis demonstrated no survival benefit but an increased risk of clinically significant hypoglycemia.[249]

The most current pediatric-specific sepsis guidelines recommend insulin therapy to maintain glucose levels ≤150 mg/dL and avoiding hypoglycemia by keeping glucose levels ≥80 mg/dL.[189] This is a level-3 recommendation (adequate scientific evidence is lacking but widely supported by available data and expert opinion) but was generated before the publication of two recent trials investigating intensive insulin therapy, specifically in critically ill children.[250,251] In the first trial published by Vlasseaers et al.[250] in 2009, the majority of patients (~75%) were surgical patients undergoing correction of congenital heart malformations. Intensive insulin treatment resulted in improved short-term outcomes (decreased ICU length of stay and decreased parameters of inflammation) but also resulted in a 25% rate of hypoglycemia. Macrae et al.[251] subsequently completed a landmark randomized trial of hyperglycemic control in critically ill pediatric patients and demonstrated no significant effect on major clinical outcomes, defined as mortality and absence of ventilation at 30 days. The incidence of hypoglycemia was again noted to be higher in the tight glycemic control group. However, there are no large pediatric-specific trials addressing insulin-based glucose control specifically in the context of septic shock. Therefore in light of the current data, and taking into consideration the risks of hypoglycemia in children, a reasonable glucose level to target seems to be ≤180 mg/dL pending a formal study. We await the results of the Heart and Lung Failure–Pediatric Insulin Titration Trial (NCT01565941) to further inform this important issue (see also Chapter 85).

Immune Modulation

Because immune/inflammatory dysregulation is a well-accepted pathophysiologic concept in septic shock, there has been a great deal of effort in developing treatment strategies directly targeted at immune/inflammatory modulation. Steroids have long been proposed as a general antiinflammatory strategy. In many clinical settings, patients with septic shock demonstrate worsening of their shock temporally associated with antibiotic administration. It is thought this phenomenon results from a massive release of bacterial toxins after antibiotic-mediated bacterial killing and a subsequent inappropriately exuberant immune/inflammatory response. However, the use of high-dose steroids to blunt this response is now universally accepted to be of no benefit and potentially harmful.[252,253]

A more recent approach to using steroids in septic shock involves the concept of relative adrenal insufficiency and an association between relative adrenal insufficiency and catecholamine refractory shock.[254,255] A landmark study by Annane et al.[256] demonstrated a substantial benefit in adults with septic shock having "relative adrenal insufficiency" (based on cortisol levels and ACTH stimulation testing) and treated with replacement hydrocortisone. However, a subsequent trial did not demonstrate the efficacy of hydrocortisone replacement, thus leading to an ongoing, unresolved controversy in the field.[257,258] Further, Boonen et al.[259] recently reported a reduction in cortisol metabolism related to suppressed expression and activity of cortisol-metabolizing enzymes during adult critical illness, thereby adding another confounding variable when considering administration of corticosteroids for septic shock.

Conflicting data and controversy also exist in the pediatric septic shock population, and existing data are currently limited to meta-analyses, observational studies, and practitioner anecdotes and experience.[260-263] Recently, a retrospective analysis of an existing transcriptomic database of pediatric septic shock demonstrated that the administration of corticosteroids in pediatric septic shock was associated with repression of genes corresponding to adaptive immunity, raising questions about potential harm associated with corticosteroid administration during septic shock.[164] Jardine et al.[164] examined genes involved in cortisol synthesis, metabolism, and activity in critically ill pediatric patients using tag single nucleotide polymorphism (SNP) methodology. They identified an SNP in the *MC2R* gene (which codes for the ACTH receptor) and demonstrated that the AA genotype was associated with a low free cortisol response to critical illness. A recent report described the development and validation of a real-time subclassification method for septic shock using previously identified gene expression–based subclasses, which corresponded to genes for adaptive immunity and glucocorticoid receptor signaling.[185] The study reported that allocation to the subclass with decreased expression of the glucocorticoid receptor signaling pathway genes was independently associated with increased mortality, and adjunctive corticosteroid administration to patients in that subclass was independently associated with almost four times the risk of mortality.

It is possible that patients with septic shock and high levels of illness severity stand to benefit the most from adjunctive corticosteroids. Funk et al.[264] recently stratified a large cohort of adults with septic shock into quartiles of illness severity using APACHE II scores. Corticosteroid administration was associated with decreased mortality for patients in the highest quartile of illness severity.[264] In contrast, when a large cohort of children with septic shock was stratified for baseline mortality risk using stratification biomarkers, corticosteroids were not associated with decreased mortality for patients in the intermediate or high baseline mortality risk groups.[265]

The role of hydrocortisone replacement in pediatric septic shock represents another major challenge in the field that must be directly addressed by a large, multicenter, randomized trial. Current barriers to conducting this important trial include lack of equipoise in the pediatric critical care community, lack of consensus regarding the definition of relative adrenal insufficiency, and our inability to select which patients with septic shock are most likely to benefit from adjunctive corticosteroids.[188,266] Thus at present treatment guidelines suggest hydrocortisone replacement therapy be considered for patients who appear refractory to resuscitative measures, have a known history of adrenal insufficiency, have already received exogenous steroids, or have an abnormal ACTH stimulation test result.[189] Given the lack of objective evidence supporting the efficacy of adjunctive corticosteroids, as well as accumulating evidence suggesting harm, the otherwise strong recommendation for corticosteroids in the current pediatric guidelines should be revised accordingly.

Because the pathophysiology of septic shock is directly linked to circulating pathogen-derived toxins and circulating inflammatory mediators, removal of these molecules via hemofiltration or exchange transfusion (ie, plasmapheresis) has been hypothesized to improve outcome. Both hemofiltration and plasmapheresis were discussed in previous sections. The fact remains that these approaches, while theoretically well founded, remain to be proven and cannot be recommended routinely in the absence of more objective data. Both strategies carry significant risks that must be weighed against the potential theoretical benefits. These include difficult vascular access in smaller children, fluid and electrolyte imbalance, hypothermia, anticoagulation requirements because of extracorporeal circuits, and acutely altered hemodynamics when instituting therapy. In addition, beneficial proteins such as albumin, immunoglobulins, clotting factors, and counterregulatory cytokines may be removed to the detriment of the patient.

Part of the inflammatory response involves cytokines causing widespread activation of the coagulation cascade with suppression of fibrinolysis, as described in previous sections. Disseminated intravascular coagulation has been implicated in the etiology of multiple organ injury leading to MODS and is directly linked to alterations of endogenous anticoagulants such as antithrombin III and protein C. While recombinant forms of these anticoagulants are available, they have not been demonstrated to be efficacious in the pediatric population and carry significant risks of serious adverse events due to bleeding.

As previously described, multiple antiinflammatory strategies have been attempted and some are now being reconsidered. These include anti-TNF, anti-IL1, antiendotoxin, TLR-4 antagonists, and anti-PAF strategies. Thus far none of these strategies have proven to be of sufficient clinical benefit in septic shock to warrant formal approval as standard of care. It is hoped that better-designed studies that carefully stratify patients, consider the presence or absence of an offending pathogen, and possibly identify genetic factors influencing outcome will provide insight into the appropriate immunomodulating agents clinically beneficial to pediatric patients with septic shock.[267]

An alternative approach to immune modulation in septic shock focuses on immune "enhancement" rather than inhibition of inflammation. As emphasized in previous sections, the paradigm of sepsis as an adaptive immune problem is increasingly gaining credence in the field. Thus there is now growing attention to the use of potentially immune-enhancing agents such as interferon-γ, granulocyte-macrophage colony-stimulating factor, zinc, selenium, prolactin, agonist antibody to CD40, PD-1 inhibitors, and IL-7.[19,187,268-271] Thus the next major advance in the clinical septic shock management may involve one or more of these immune-enhancing approaches rather than an antiinflammatory approach.

Case for More Effective Stratification in Pediatric Septic Shock

The vast majority of interventional clinical trials in septic shock have failed to demonstrate efficacy of the particular test agent. A potential reason for failure in these trials is not because the biological/physiologic principle being tested was fundamentally flawed. Rather, the primary reason for failure lies in the inability to effectively address the substantial heterogeneity characterizing the syndrome of septic shock. As indicated throughout this chapter, septic shock is a heterogeneous syndrome with the potential to negatively and directly affect all organ systems, and this heterogeneity has consistently challenged multiple investigators attempting to evaluate the efficacy of various experimental interventions. As astutely stated by Marshall, a key challenge in the field is to reduce and manage this heterogeneity by more effectively stratifying patients for the purposes of more rational and effective clinical research and clinical management.[272] The concept of preintervention stratification in sepsis and its positive impact on the efficacy of an experimental therapy was corroborated by the Remick laboratory in a murine model of polymicrobial sepsis.[34]

One potential strategy for stratifying children with septic shock involves early identification of septic shock endotypes based on genome-wide expression patterns. As described earlier, endotypes of pediatric septic shock have been identified exclusively on the basis of on gene expression profiling conducted within 24 hours of admission, and these expression-based subclasses have highly relevant differences in illness severity and mortality.[167-169,185] A similar strategy was demonstrated in adult patients suffering from trauma,[273] and recently Knox et al.[274] reported endotypes of adult sepsis on the basis of organ failure patterns. As high-throughput technologies evolve and validation studies are rigorously performed, the ability to conduct expression-based endotyping of pediatric septic shock could well become a clinical reality.[267]

Another potential strategy for stratifying children with septic shock is biomarker-based stratification. Many biomarkers can be readily measured in the blood compartment, thus providing a clinically feasible strategy for early stratification of patients. For example, IL-8 can be readily and rapidly measured in small-volume blood samples. IL-8 was found to be a robust outcome biomarker in children with septic shock.[38] Specifically, an IL-8 level, measured within 24 hours of admission to the pediatric ICU, was found to have a 95% negative predictive value for mortality in a derivation cohort of patients. The reliability of this assertion is supported by prospective, formal validation in an independent validation cohort of patients (the RESOLVE database), which demonstrated an identically robust negative predictive value.[38] A similar observation (98% negative predictive value for mortality) was found by measuring chemokine (C-C motif) ligand 4 (CCL4) serum protein levels within 24 hours of admission to the pediatric ICU with septic shock.[275]

It has been proposed that these types of sepsis outcome biomarkers (ie, biomarkers having high negative predictive values for mortality) could be used to stratify patients eligible for interventional septic shock trials.[38,275] Patients having a high likelihood of survival with standard care, but otherwise meeting entry criteria for a given interventional trial, could be potentially excluded from the trial on the basis of these biomarkers. Such a stratification strategy would serve to derive a study population with a more optimal risk-to-benefit ratio, thus improving the ability to demonstrate efficacy for a given test agent. This type of strategy would be particularly useful for a test agent carrying more than minimal risk.

Although single biomarker-based patient stratification is clinically appealing, it may not be sufficiently robust to meet all clinical and research needs from the combined standpoints of specificity, sensitivity, and positive predictive values. Indeed, the aforementioned studies involving IL-8 and CCL4 had clinically unacceptable specificities, sensitivities, and positive predictive values, relative to the very high negative predictive values. The ideal biomarker-based stratification tool, which would meet a wide range of clinical and research needs, would simultaneously have high specificity, high sensitivity, high positive predictive value, and high negative predictive value.

Given the biological complexity of pediatric septic shock, a stratification strategy based on a panel of multiple biomarkers has more potential to meet the needs of the aforementioned ideal biomarker-based stratification tool. To this end, the Pediatric Sepsis Biomarker Risk Model (PERSEVERE) was derived and validated.[178,179,182] PERSEVERE incorporates a panel of biomarkers into a decision tree derived using Classification and Regression Tree (CART) methodology. The terminal nodes of the decision tree provide a range of reliable baseline mortality probabilities for children with septic shock. Fig. 111.5 depicts the PERSEVERE decision tree.

A temporal version of PERSEVERE measured the biomarkers over time and how the biomarker changes reflect changing probability of poor outcome risk.[180] A version of PERSEVERE has also been developed for adults with sepsis, which is called ASSIST (Adult Septic Shock Information and Stratification Technology).[181] Both PERSEVERE and ASSIST outperform currently used mortality risk prediction tools.[183]

Several applications are possible for PERSEVERE. These include stratification for clinical trial enrollment, serving as a benchmark for quality improvement efforts, and informing individual patient decision making. Recently, PERSEVERE was used to conduct retrospective, stratified analyses of clinical data.[209,265]

Concluding Perspectives

Sepsis is and will continue to be an important challenge to the pediatric intensivist. Indeed, sepsis is one of the few disease processes for which the pediatric intensivist can claim "ownership." Although much is known about the biological and molecular mechanisms involved in sepsis, much of this knowledge has not directly translated to improved bedside care. At present, most of the therapeutic modalities for sepsis are fundamentally supportive and founded on the basic principles that define the discipline of critical care medicine. Although this approach has directly improved the outcome of sepsis in children, the fact that more than 4000 children per year in the United States alone continue to die in association with severe sepsis warrants further advances. Realization of this goal is feasible but requires further mechanistic insights at the physiologic, molecular, and genetic levels, as well as the design of large-scale, pediatric-specific interventional trials complemented by evolving stratification strategies. As "owners" of pediatric septic shock, pediatric intensivists are well positioned to lead this effort on all fronts.

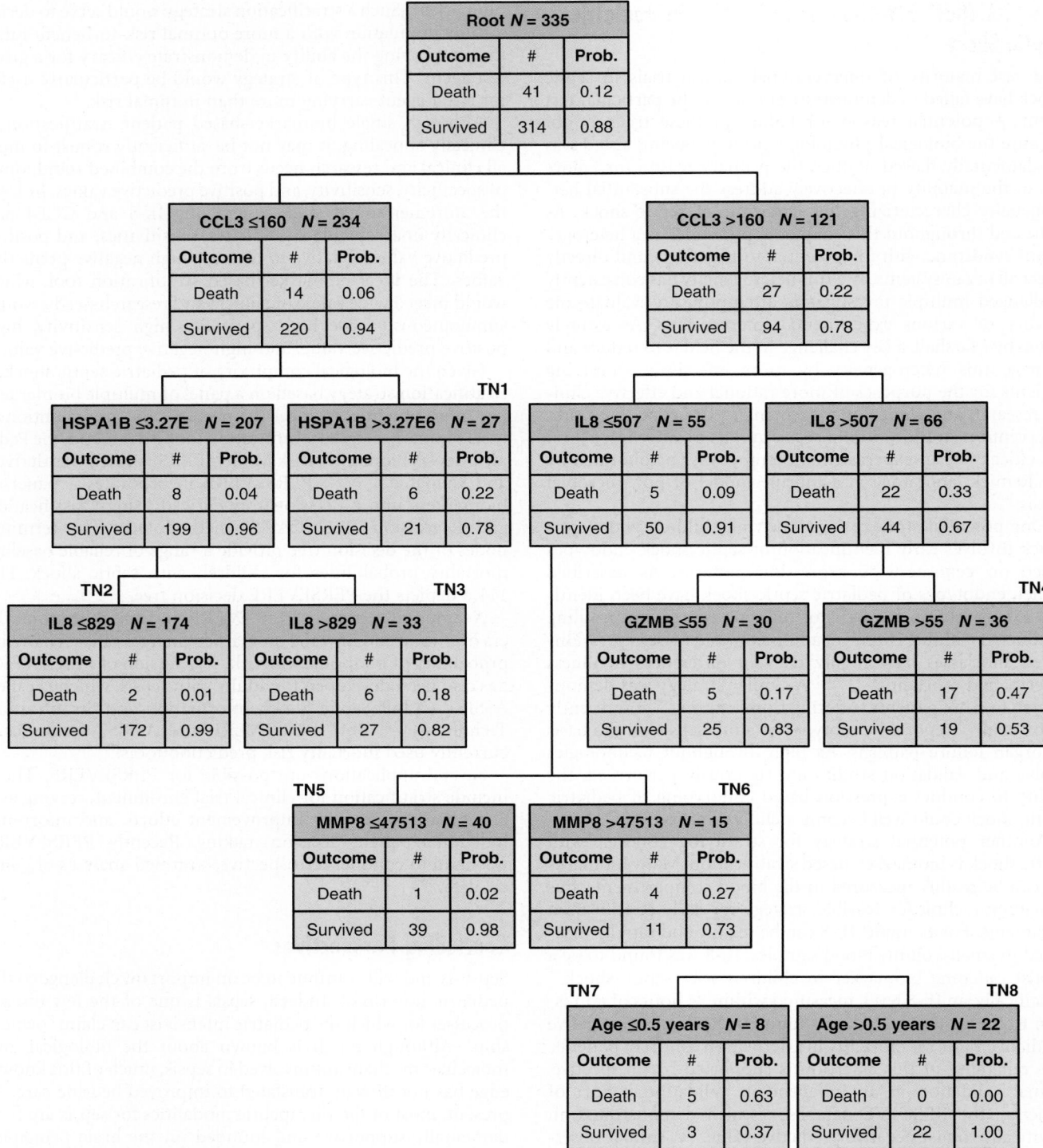

Fig. 111.5. The PERSEVERE decision tree for assigning a baseline mortality probability for children with septic shock. The decision tree is based on six biomarker-based decision rules and one age-based decision rule. The stratification biomarkers used for analysis are as follows: C-C chemokine ligand 3 (CCL3), heat shock protein 70 kDa 1B (HSPA1B), interleukin-8 (IL-8), granzyme B (GZMB), and matrix metalloproteinase-8 (MMP8). The top node of the decision tree, the root node, provides the total number of subjects, as well as the number and proportion of survivors and non-survivors (28-day all-cause mortality). Subjects in the root node are subsequently allocated to daughter nodes on the basis of the results of binary recursive partitioning. Each daughter node provides the criterion for deciding subsequent partitions, along with the number and proportion of survivors and nonsurvivors. All biomarker concentrations are in pg/mL. Terminal nodes (TNs) reflect the final assignment of risk to an individual case. Terminal nodes are considered low risk (mortality probability 0.0–0.02; TN2, TN5, and TN8), intermediate risk (mortality probability 0.18–0.27; TN1, TN3, and TN6), or high risk (mortality probability 0.47–0.63; TN4 and TN7).

Key References

2. Watson RS, Carcillo JA, Linde-Zwirble WT, et al. The epidemiology of severe sepsis in children in the United States. *Am J Respir Crit Care Med.* 2003;167:695-701.
3. Hartman ME, Linde-Zwirble WT, Angus DC, Watson RS. Trends in the epidemiology of pediatric severe sepsis. *Pediatr Crit Care Med.* 2013;14: 686-693.
4. Czaja AS, Zimmerman JJ, Nathens AB. Readmission and late mortality after pediatric severe sepsis. *Pediatrics.* 2009;123:849-857.
5. Schlapbach LJ, Straney L, Alexander J, et al. Mortality related to invasive infections, sepsis, and septic shock in critically ill children in Australia and New Zealand, 2002-13: a multicentre retrospective cohort study. *Lancet Infect Dis.* 2015;15:46-54.
6. Weiss SL, Fitzgerald JC, Pappachan J, et al. Global epidemiology of pediatric severe sepsis: the Sepsis PRevalence, OUtcomes, and Therapies Study. *Am J Respir Crit Care Med.* 2015;191:1147-1157.
7. Goldstein B, Giroir B, Randolph A. International pediatric sepsis consensus conference: definitions for sepsis and organ dysfunction in pediatrics. *Pediatr Crit Care Med.* 2005;6:2-8.
9. Conlon NP, Breatnach C, O'Hare BP, et al. Health-related quality of life after prolonged pediatric intensive care unit stay. *Pediatr Crit Care Med.* 2009;10:41-44.
10. Knoester H, Bronner MB, Bos AP, Grootenhuis MA. Quality of life in children three and nine months after discharge from a paediatric intensive care unit: a prospective cohort study. *Health Qual Life Outcomes.* 2008;6:21.
11. Pollack MM, Holubkov R, Glass P, et al. Functional Status Scale: new pediatric outcome measure. *Pediatrics.* 2009;124:e18-e28.
18. Hotchkiss RS, Karl IE. The pathophysiology and treatment of sepsis. *N Engl J Med.* 2003;348:138-150.
19. Hotchkiss RS, Coopersmith CM, McDunn JE, Ferguson TA. The sepsis seesaw: tilting toward immunosuppression. *Nat Med.* 2009; 15:496-497.
22. Akira S. Innate immunity to pathogens: diversity in receptors for microbial recognition. *Immunol Rev.* 2009;227:5-8.
38. Wong HR, Cvijanovich N, Wheeler DS, et al. Interleukin-8 as a stratification tool for interventional trials involving pediatric septic shock. *Am J Respir Crit Care Med.* 2008;178:276-282.
55. Ignarro LJ, Buga GM, Wood KS, et al. Endothelium-derived relaxing factor produced and released from artery and vein is nitric oxide. *Proc Natl Acad Sci USA.* 1987;84:9265-9269.
57. Wong HR, Carcillo JA, Burckart G, et al. Increased serum nitrite and nitrate concentrations in children with the sepsis syndrome. *Crit Care Med.* 1995;23:835-842.
62. Hermans PW, Hibberd ML, Booy R, et al. 4G/5G promoter polymorphism in the plasminogen-activator-inhibitor-1 gene and outcome of meningococcal disease. Meningococcal Research Group. *Lancet.* 1999; 354:556-560.
63. Kornelisse RF, Hazelzet JA, Savelkoul HF, et al. The relationship between plasminogen activator inhibitor-1 and proinflammatory and counterinflammatory mediators in children with meningococcal septic shock. *J Infect Dis.* 1996;173:1148-1156.
65. Nadel S, Goldstein B, Williams MD, et al. Drotrecogin alfa (activated) in children with severe sepsis: a multicentre phase III randomised controlled trial. *Lancet.* 2007;369:836-843.
66. Ranieri VM, Thompson BT, Barie PS, et al. Drotrecogin alfa (activated) in adults with septic shock. *N Engl J Med.* 2012;366:2055-2064.
76. Kaplan JM, Denenberg A, Monaco M, et al. Changes in peroxisome proliferator-activated receptor-gamma activity in children with septic shock. *Intensive Care Med.* 2009;36:123-130.
79. Cuenca AG, Delano MJ, Kelly-Scumpia KM, et al. A paradoxical role for myeloid-derived suppressor cells in sepsis and trauma. *Mol Med.* 2011;17:281-292.
83. Volk HD, Reinke P, Krausch D, et al. Monocyte deactivation—rationale for a new therapeutic strategy in sepsis. *Intensive Care Med.* 1996;22(suppl 4):S474-S481.
89. Wynn JL, Scumpia PO, Winfield RD, et al. Defective innate immunity predisposes murine neonates to poor sepsis outcome but is reversed by TLR agonists. *Blood.* 2008;112:1750-1758.
98. Hotchkiss RS, Swanson PE, Freeman BD, et al. Apoptotic cell death in patients with sepsis, shock, and multiple organ dysfunction. *Crit Care Med.* 1999;27:1230-1251.
102. Cooke GS, Hill AV. Genetics of susceptibility to human infectious disease. *Nat Rev Genet.* 2001;2:967-977.
103. Sorensen TI, Nielsen GG, Andersen PK, Teasdale TW. Genetic and environmental influences on premature death in adult adoptees. *N Engl J Med.* 1988;318:727-732.
124. Mira JP, Cariou A, Grall F, et al. Association of TNF2, a TNF-alpha promoter polymorphism, with septic shock susceptibility and mortality: a multicenter study. *JAMA.* 1999;282:561-568.
125. Nadel S, Newport MJ, Booy R, Levin M. Variation in the tumor necrosis factor-alpha gene promoter region may be associated with death from meningococcal disease. *J Infect Dis.* 1996;174:878-880.
133. Westendorp RG, Hottenga JJ, Slagboom PE. Variation in plasminogen-activator-inhibitor-1 gene and risk of meningococcal septic shock. *Lancet.* 1999;354:561-563.
134. Haralambous E, Hibberd ML, Hermans PW, et al. Role of functional plasminogen-activator-inhibitor-1 4G/5G promoter polymorphism in susceptibility, severity, and outcome of meningococcal disease in Caucasian children. *Crit Care Med.* 2003;31:2788-2793.
135. Geishofer G, Binder A, Muller M, et al. 4G/5G promoter polymorphism in the plasminogen-activator-inhibitor-1 gene in children with systemic meningococcaemia. *Eur J Pediatr.* 2005;164:486-490.
153. Levin M, Quint PA, Goldstein B, et al. Recombinant bactericidal/permeability-increasing protein (rBPI21) as adjunctive treatment for children with severe meningococcal sepsis: a randomised trial. rBPI21 Meningococcal Sepsis Study Group. *Lancet.* 2000;356:961-967.
155. Maslove DM, Wong HR. Gene expression profiling in sepsis: timing, tissue, and translational considerations. *Trends Mol Med.* 2014;20: 204-213.
158. Wong HR, Shanley TP, Sakthivel B, et al. Genome-level expression profiles in pediatric septic shock indicate a role for altered zinc homeostasis in poor outcome. *Physiol Genomics.* 2007;30:146-155.
161. Wong HR, Cvijanovich N, Allen GL, et al. Genomic expression profiling across the pediatric systemic inflammatory response syndrome, sepsis, and septic shock spectrum. *Crit Care Med.* 2009;37: 1558-1566.
162. Wynn JL, Cvijanovich NZ, Allen GL, et al. The influence of developmental age on the early transcriptomic response of children with septic shock. *Mol Med.* 2011;17:1146-1156.
164. Wong HR, Cvijanovich NZ, Allen GL, et al. Corticosteroids are associated with repression of adaptive immunity gene programs in pediatric septic shock. *Am J Respir Crit Care Med.* 2014;189:940-946.
167. Wong HR, Cvijanovich N, Lin R, et al. Identification of pediatric septic shock subclasses based on genome-wide expression profiling. *BMC Med.* 2009;7:34.
178. Wong HR, Salisbury S, Xiao Q, et al. The pediatric sepsis biomarker risk model. *Crit Care.* 2012;16:R174.
185. Wong HR, Cvijanovich NZ, Anas N, et al. Developing a clinically feasible personalized medicine approach to pediatric septic shock. *Am J Respir Crit Care Med.* 2015;191:309-315.
189. Brierley J, Carcillo JA, Choong K, et al. Clinical practice parameters for hemodynamic support of pediatric and neonatal septic shock: 2007 update from the American College of Critical Care Medicine. *Crit Care Med.* 2009;37:666-688.
192. Carcillo JA, Davis AL, Zaritsky A. Role of early fluid resuscitation in pediatric septic shock. *JAMA.* 1991;266:1242-1245.
206. Maitland K, Kiguli S, Opoka RO, et al. Mortality after fluid bolus in African children with severe infection. *N Engl J Med.* 2011;364: 2483-2495.
209. Abulebda K, Cvijanovich NZ, Thomas NJ, et al. Post-ICU admission fluid balance and pediatric septic shock outcomes: a risk-stratified analysis. *Crit Care Med.* 2014;42:397-403.
210. de Oliveira CF, de Oliveira DS, Gottschald AF, et al. ACCM/PALS haemodynamic support guidelines for paediatric septic shock: an outcomes comparison with and without monitoring central venous oxygen saturation. *Intensive Care Med.* 2008;34:1065-1075.
211. Rivers E, Nguyen B, Havstad S, et al. Early goal-directed therapy in the treatment of severe sepsis and septic shock. *N Engl J Med.* 2001; 345:1368-1377.
213. Yealy DM, Kellum JA, Huang DT, et al. A randomized trial of protocol-based care for early septic shock. *N Engl J Med.* 2014;370:1683-1693.
232. Kumar A, Ellis P, Arabi Y, et al. Initiation of inappropriate antimicrobial therapy results in a fivefold reduction of survival in human septic shock. *Chest.* 2009;136:1237-1248.
251. Macrae D, Grieve R, Allen E, et al. A randomized trial of hyperglycemic control in pediatric intensive care. *N Engl J Med.* 2014;370:107-118.

256. Annane D, Sebille V, Charpentier C, et al. Effect of treatment with low doses of hydrocortisone and fludrocortisone on mortality in patients with septic shock. *JAMA*. 2002;288:862-871.

257. Sprung CL, Annane D, Keh D, et al. Hydrocortisone therapy for patients with septic shock. *N Engl J Med*. 2008;358:111-124.

266. Zimmerman JJ. A history of adjunctive glucocorticoid treatment for pediatric sepsis: moving beyond steroid pulp fiction toward evidence-based medicine. *Pediatr Crit Care Med*. 2007;8:530-539.

272. Marshall JC. Sepsis: rethinking the approach to clinical research. *J Leukoc Biol*. 2008;83:471-482.

Multiple Organ Dysfunction/Failure Syndrome in Children

Joseph A. Carcillo

PEARLS

- One view of the pathogenesis of multiple organ dysfunction/multiple organ failure syndrome (MODS/MOF) is uncontrolled systemic inflammation that leads to reversible epithelial, endothelial, and mitochondrial dysfunction.
- Three factors are required for systemic inflammation to produce MODS/MOF syndrome: (1) increased circulating pathogen-associated molecular pattern molecules (PAMPS; endotoxin or microbial products), (2) increased circulating danger/damage-associated molecular pattern molecules (DAMPS; necrotic cell constituents), and (3) defective host metabolism (reduced cytochrome P-450, mitochondrial activity).
- MODS/MOF syndrome has been classified as primary (when occurring in the first 7 days of illness) and secondary (when commencing after 7 days). Ninety percent of patients have MODS/MOF at presentation to the pediatric ICU, whereas 10% develop sequential MOF over time with liver and renal involvement following initial lung dysfunction.
- Three or more organ failures at admission are associated with higher mortality (25%) than fewer than three (2%). Resolution of three organ failures to fewer than three by day 3 is associated with 8% mortality compared with 35% mortality in children for whom three or more organ failure persists beyond day 3. Both degree of systemic inflammation and mortality increase as the number of organs failing increases.
- Timely source control (removal of the inflammation source using appropriate antibiotics for infections and necrotic tissue nidus removal for trauma-driven injury) and reversal of shock/ischemia prevent the development of MODS/MOF.
- Persistent or progressive MODS/MOF can be viewed as a spectrum of inflammation phenotypes that can respond to personalized therapies when source control and shock reversal are achieved. These include (1) thrombocytopenia-associated MOF (TAMOF, thrombotic microangiopathy); (2) immune paralysis/lymphoid depletion syndrome (predominant TH$_2$ phenotype); (3) viral/lymphoproliferative disorder–associated sequential MOF (natural killer [NK] cell/cytotoxic T-cell/B-cell/T-regulatory cell dysfunction); (4) iron overload cardiac/hepatic/pancreatic MOF (secondary hemochromatosis); (5) hyperleukocytosis MOF (pertussis leukocyte proliferating factor); and (6) the end pathway of uncontrolled inflammation from any phenotype, macrophage activation syndrome.

- Responses are as follows: (1) TAMOF and thrombotic microangiopathy respond to plasma exchange and the C5A antibody eculizumab; (2) immune paralysis/lymphoid depletion syndrome (predominant TH$_2$ phenotype) responds to immune suppressant withdrawal and granulocyte-macrophage colony-stimulating factor; (3) viral/lymphoproliferative disorder–associated sequential MOF (natural killer [NK] cell/cytotoxic T-cell/B-cell/T-regulatory cell dysfunction responds to intravenous immunoglobulin (IVIG) and in the case of EBV infection, the CD20 antibody rituximab); (4) iron overload cardiac/hepatic/pancreatic MOF (secondary hemochromatosis) responds to iron chelation therapy; (5) hyperleukocytosis MOF (pertussis leukocyte proliferating factor) responds to leukoreduction therapy; and (6) the end pathway of uncontrolled inflammation from any of these phenotypes, macrophage activation syndrome, responds to methylprednisone, IVIG, plasma exchange, and the IL-1 receptor antagonist, anakinra.

Introduction

Systemic inflammation caused by trauma, pancreatitis, burns, or shock can lead to the *systemic inflammatory response syndrome* (SIRS). When caused by infection, the sepsis syndrome is recognized and defined by the presence of two of four criteria: tachycardia, tachypnea, fever, and abnormal white blood cell count (Fig. 112.1). If uncontrolled, increased systemic inflammation from tissue injury and/or infection leads to the *compensatory antiinflammatory response syndrome* (CARS) (Fig. 112.2), which further mediates severe SIRS/sepsis (SIRS/sepsis + one-organ failure) and ultimately *immunologic dissonance,* with the development of multiple-organ failure (Fig. 112.3). The multiple organ dysfunction (MOD)/multiple organ failure (MOF) syndrome is recognized by the clinician after clinical documentation of cardiovascular, respiratory, hepatic, renal, hematologic, and central nervous dysfunction. Multiple organs are affected when uncontrolled inflammation induces systemic epithelial, immune, and endothelial cell dysfunction.

Inflammation/Coagulation/Immune Dysfunction/ Dysregulated Metabolism Hypothesis

Roger Bone popularized the notion that systemic inflammation led to the development of multiple organ failure in the

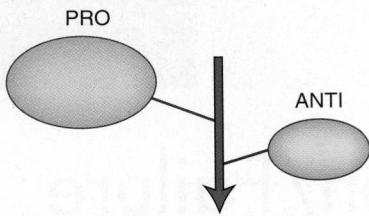

SIRS: Systemic inflammatory reponse syndrome

- Temperature changes, tachypnea, tachycardia, acidosis, signs of specific end-organ dysfunction.

Fig. 112.1. Systemic inflammatory response syndrome.

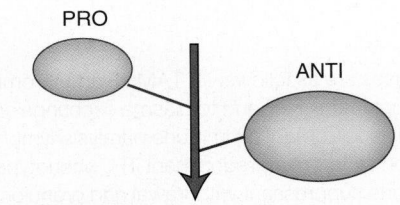

CARS: Compensatory antiinflammatory response syndrome

- Retaliatory surge of antiinflammatory mediators released in response to SIRS.

Fig. 112.2. Compensatory antiinflammatory response syndrome.

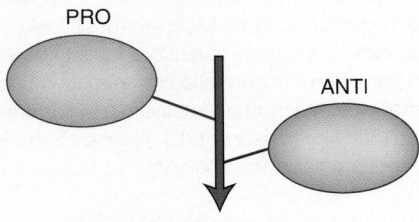

Immunologic dissonance

- Massive amounts of both types of mediators are released, but balance cannot be restored.

Fig. 112.3. Immunologic dissonance. (From Bone RC. Immunologic dissonance: a continuing evolution in our understanding of the systemic inflammatory response syndrome [SIRS] and the multiple organ dysfunction syndrome [MODS]. Ann Intern Med. 1996;125:680-687.)

1990s. According to this theory, an initial proinflammatory cytokine response to foreign or self-antigen caused SIRS, which is characterized by two of four criteria including tachycardia, tachypnea, fever, and leukocytosis (see Fig. 112.1). This syndrome was thought to be mediated by increased IL-1 and tumor necrosis factor alpha (TNFα) levels (Fig. 112.4). It could be blunted by nonsteroidal antiinflammatory drugs (NSAIDs) and hence was thought to be mediated in part by

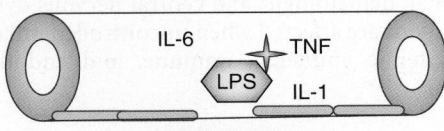

No infection

Fig. 112.4. Infection or necrotic tissue evokes a proinflammatory cytokine response that brings blood flow to the site of infection. *IL-6,* interleukin 6; *IL-1,* interleukin 1; *LPS,* lipopolysaccharide; *NO,* nitric oxide; *TNFα,* tumor necrosis factor alpha.

prostaglandins. SIRS was called *sepsis* if related to infection and SIRS if related to surgery, pancreatitis, or other noninfectious processes. This syndrome was self-limited when antibiotics were used to kill the infection or time allowed recovery from surgery, pancreatitis, and other noninfectious causes of SIRS. This "proinflammatory response" was turned off by an antiinflammatory response led by the antiinflammatory cytokine IL-10. When IL-10 resulted in reduction of IL-1 and TNFα to normal control values, sepsis or SIRS stopped and organ failure did not occur. In patients who developed severe sepsis and MOF, the *compensatory antiinflammatory response* (CARS) was unsuccessful in turning off inflammation (see Fig. 112.2). Instead, these patients had persistent elevation of the cytokine IL-6 along with IL-10. Dr. Bone coined the term "immunologic dissonance" to describe this process. He viewed MOF as an inflammatory condition in which the normal antiinflammatory response was unable to turn off the proinflammatory process (see Fig. 112.3).

Proulx et al.[1] defined pediatric MOF syndrome as being primary and secondary. Primary MOF occurred in 90% of children and was present at the time of admission, and secondary MOF occurred in 10% of children and was not present until 7 days after admission.[1] To evaluate the role of inflammation in pediatric sepsis-induced MOF, the authors defined children as having no MOF (or NMOF) if they had two-organ failure at presentation but never reached three-organ failure, resolved MOF (or RMOF) if they had three-organ failure at admission that resolved to two or fewer at 48 hours, persistent MOF (or PMOF) if they had three-or-more organ failure at presentation that did not resolve by 48 hours, and sequential MOF (or SMOF) if they had acute lung injury (ALI)/acute respiratory distress syndrome (ARDS) at admission and then progressed to have hepatorenal failure/dysfunction.[2] Similar to Dr. Proulx's classification, children in the latter investigation with SMOF represented 10% of the population. The mortality rates with NMOF, RMOF, PMOF, and SMOF were 2%, 8%, 35%, and 50%, respectively. The authors then investigated Dr. Bone's hypothesis within these categories and reported that patients with NMOF had an increase in IL-10 with subsequent turning off of inflammation; however, those with PMOF or SMOF had persistently high IL-6 and IL-10 levels, the hallmark of immunologic dissonance.[2]

Dr. Bone's untimely demise prevented him from further pursuing the mechanisms by which immunologic dissonance could mediate organ injury. However, the authors first reviewed the autopsy bank at their hospital and noted that children who died from sepsis-induced multiple organ failure exhibited two unsuspected findings compared with children who died of other causes: persistent or unrecognized infection and thrombotic and bleeding complications with organ infarctions (Figs. 112-5 and 112-6). Accordingly, the authors pursued the notion that immunologic dissonance might lead to an inability to mediate coagulation homeostasis, as well as an inability to clear infection. Proinflammatory cytokines including TNFα and IL-1 induce endothelial activation in vitro with an increased prothrombotic and antifibrinolytic state and expression of adhesion molecules (Fig. 112.7). Patients with PMOF had increased tissue factor and plasminogen activator-1 activity, as well as circulating adhesion molecules, ICAM and VCAM, consistent with the hypothesis that immunologic dissonance was associated with an activated prothrombotic/antifibrinolytic endothelium.[3,4] IL-6 also inhibits

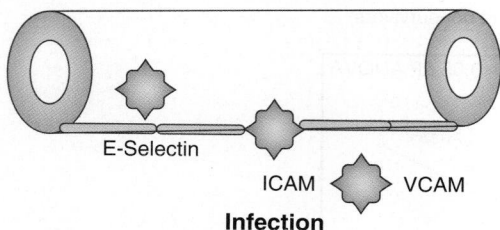

Infection

Fig. 112.5. The proinflammatory cytokines stimulate expression of adhesion molecules that allow immune cells to roll, stick, and then transmigrate to kill the infection. *E-selectin,* endothelial selectin; *ICAM,* intercellular adhesion molecule; *VCAM,* vascular cell adhesion molecule.

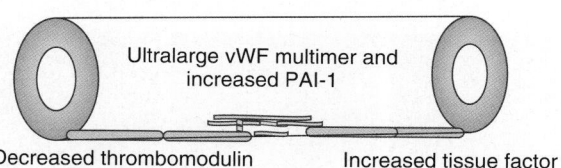

Decreased thrombomodulin   Increased tissue factor

Fig. 112.6. The proinflammatory cytokines increase expression of prothrombotic molecules and decrease expression of antithrombotic molecules to seal off endothelium at the site of infection. After the infection is killed or necrotic cells are cleared, there is no longer a proinflammatory cytokine response. The endothelium returns to its usual antithrombotic, profibrinolytic state. *PAI-1,* plasminogen activator inhibitor–type 1; *vWF,* von Willebrand factor.

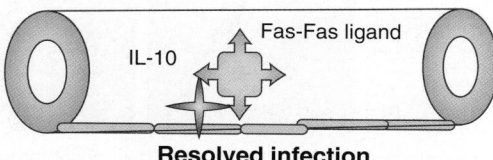

Resolved infection

Fig. 112.7. After the infection is killed or necrotic cells are cleared, the antiinflammatory cytokines turn off expression of the proinflammatory cytokines. This results in reduction in monocyte/macrophage tumor necrosis factor production and apoptosis of activated immune cells.

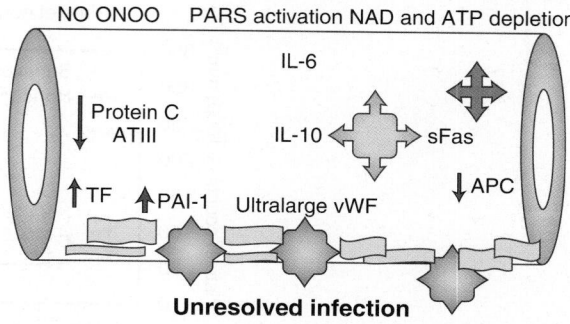

Unresolved infection

Fig. 112.8. In immunologic dissonance, multiple-organ-failure (MOF) patients are unable to resolve infection and inflammation. They remain in a prothrombotic/antifibrinolytic state with microvascular thrombosis and thrombocytopenia-associated MOF. They also have immune paralysis with ineffective antigen presenting cell activity mediated in part by increased IL-10. Sequential MOF can occur when increased sFasL levels >500 pg/mL induce liver injury. Metabolism is also adversely affected as nitric oxide + superoxide anion lead to the formation of peroxynitrite radicals that inhibit cytochrome P-450 activity and mitochondrial respiration. *APC,* antigen presenting cell; *AT III,* antithrombin III; *NO,* nitric oxide; *ONOO,* peroxynitrite; *PAI-1,* plasminogen activator inhibitor type 1; *PARS,* polyadenosylribose synthase; *TF,* tissue factor.

ADAMTS-13, the vWF multimer protease, in vitro. PMOF patients also had deficient ADAMTS-13 activity compared with NMOF patients, consistent with increased risk of vWF multimer–mediated thrombosis (Figs. 112.8 and 112.9).[5] Increased IL-10 is the hallmark of the TH$_2$ antiinflammatory cytokine response. When the TH$_2$ response is dominant, then the TH$_1$ response can be turned off, a state known as *immune paralysis* (Fig. 112.10). These patients have a diminished ex vivo ability to secrete TNFα from endotoxin-stimulated monocytes or macrophages. Without this ability, infections cannot be terminated. The PMOF patients exhibited immune paralysis more frequently than the NMOF patients.[6]

Cytokines and nitric oxide also inhibit cytochrome P-450 activity and mitochondrial respiration in vitro.[7,8] The authors found that patients with PMOF had reduced (10-fold) cytochrome P-450 activity compared with patients with NMOF (2-fold).[8] *Immunologic dissonance* in PMOF was associated with endotheliopathy, immune paralysis, and impaired P-450 metabolism, but how was PMOF different from SMOF? The authors determined that patients with SMOF were more likely to have viral or lymphoproliferative disease with high sFasL levels. In vitro, sFasL levels >500 pg/mL cause hepatocyte

necrosis. Children with MOF with sFasL levels >500 pg/mL demonstrated liver injury at autopsy.[9] The mechanism of injury in SMOF was different from in patients who presented with MOF (see Figs. 112.5 and 112.6).

Over the past decade, investigators from the United Kingdom have investigated the inflammation/immune dysregulation hypothesis in SIRS/sepsis hypothesizing that dysregulated complement activity increases the risk of SIRS/sepsis.[10] Mannose-binding lectin (MBL) is an early-released complement activation component and is required for the first 12 hours of complement activity. Approximately 30% of children are MBL deficient. Complement factor H inhibits complement activity, and factor H Y402H polymorphism reduces this complement inhibition activity. Using genotype analyses, these investigators have demonstrated that children at risk for SIRS/sepsis more commonly have deficiencies in MBL production and a reduction in this H factor polymorphism. Together, these two characteristics are associated with an even greater risk of SIRS/sepsis than either one alone. The interpretation is that diminished early complement (MBL) prevents rapid clearance of antigen leading to the SIRS/sepsis syndrome, but absence of inhibitory complement (CFH/CFI) prevents turning off systemic inflammation and is associated with the development of disseminated intravascular coagulation and MODS/MOF. Over the past decade, thrombocytopenia-associated MOF and atypical HUS/TTP have been linked to many genetic mutations related to reduced or even absent inhibitory complement production.[11] Accordingly, the inflammation hypothesis of MOF is alive and well.

Definitions and Scoring

As noted previously, SIRS is defined by two of the following four criteria: tachypnea, tachycardia, fever, and leukocytosis. Sepsis is defined as SIRS + suspected or documented infection. Severe sepsis is defined by sepsis + organ failure. MOF or MODS is defined by more-than-one-organ failure. Many definitions exist for defining organ failure. Wilkinson and Pollack

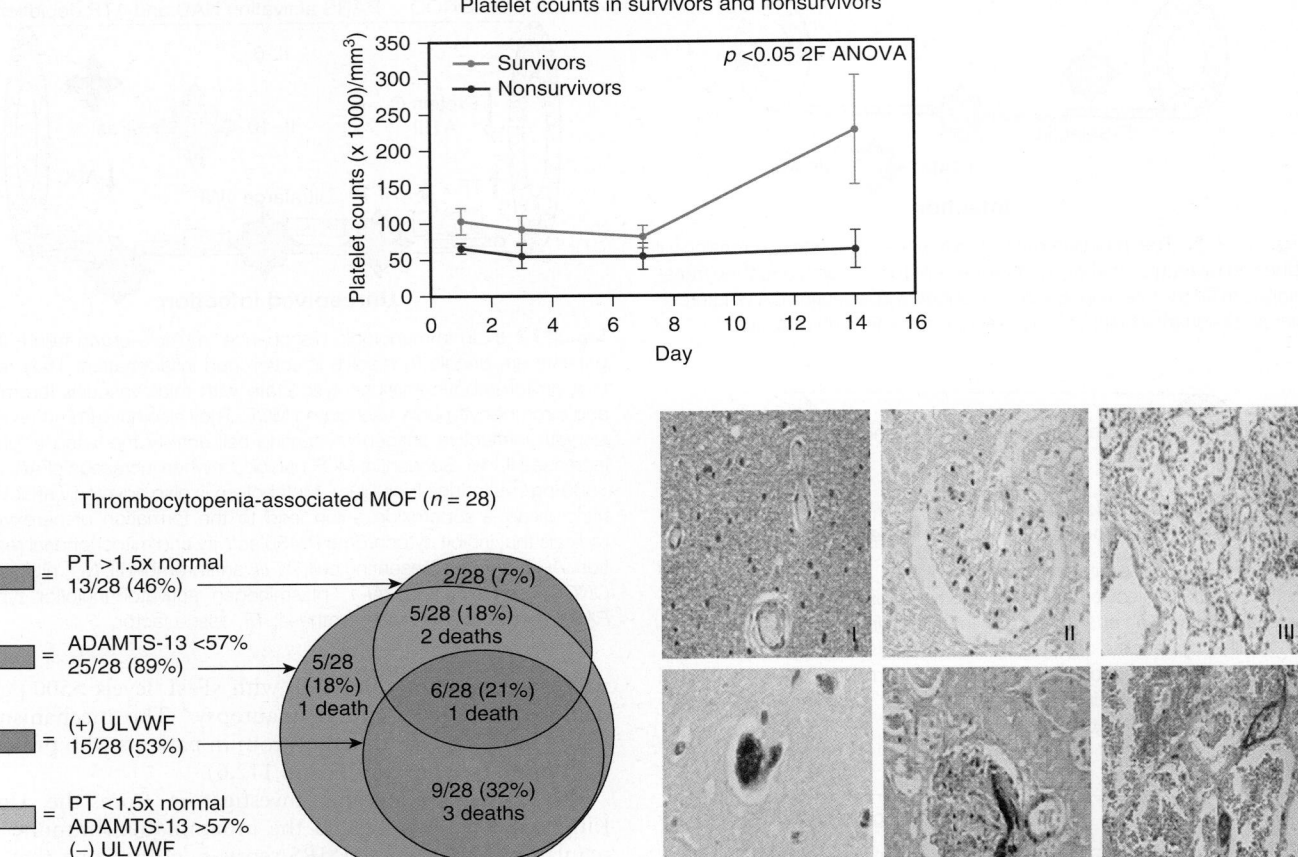

Fig. 112.9. Untreated thrombotic microangiopathy causes death from microvascular thrombosis. TAMOF is heralded by new-onset thrombocytopenia and MOF. Survivors recover their platelet count, whereas nonsurvivors do not. In this study 89% of these patients had reduced ADAMTS-13 (A). At autopsy patients had vWF multimer thrombi (B) in brain (IV), kidney (V), and lung (VI). These microthrombi can resolve with intensive plasma exchange therapy that removes thrombogenic ultralarge vWF multimers and replenishes ADAMTS-13 enzyme. (From Nguyen TC, Han YY, Kiss JE, et al. Intensive plasma exchange increases ADAMTS-13 activity and reverses organ dysfunction in children with thrombocytopenia-associated multiple organ failure. Crit Care Med. 2008;36:2878-2887.)

published the first definitions in pediatrics that were subsequently modified by Proulx and then again by Doughty.[2,12] Goldstein, Giroir, and Randolph subsequently developed two more sets of definitions.[13] Doughty developed the organ failure index (OFI) to score organ failure.[2] It is a simple integer score that assigns 1 point for each organ failure. Leteurtre reported two more MOF scores, the PEMOD and PELOD scores.[14] The PEMOD score assigns 1 to 4 points per organ failure depending on severity. The PELOD score logistically weights these scores to hopefully allow for prognostication. Due to controversy concerning the use of the PELOD score in this manner, the authors have more recently developed the updated PELOD2 score.[15]

Outcomes

In the United States, survival in the setting of SIRS/sepsis is almost universal. Odetola et al.[16] reported that survival in severe sepsis is 96%, overall 98% in previously healthy children, and 92% in children with chronic diseases. Typpo et al.[17]

reported that survival from MOF is 90%. Survival rates decrease as the number of organ failures increase.

MOF/MODS Phenotypes, Respective Biomarkers, and Therapies (Table 112.1)

Thrombocytopenia-Associated MOF

New-onset thrombocytopenia is a harbinger of thrombotic microangiopathy in MOF, especially when accompanied by increased lactate dehydrogenase (LDH) and reduced renal function. Until this decade, thrombotic microangiopathy of critical illness was thought to be mediated by fibrin, but more recent work suggests that von Willebrand factor (vWF) multimers associated platelet thrombi are a previously unrecognized cause. If ADAMTS-13 concentration (vWF cleaving protease) is <57% of control and vWF multimer concentration is increased, then this form of thrombosis should be highly suspected (Figs. 112.8 and 112.9). Intensive plasma exchange can reverse this process because it removes the

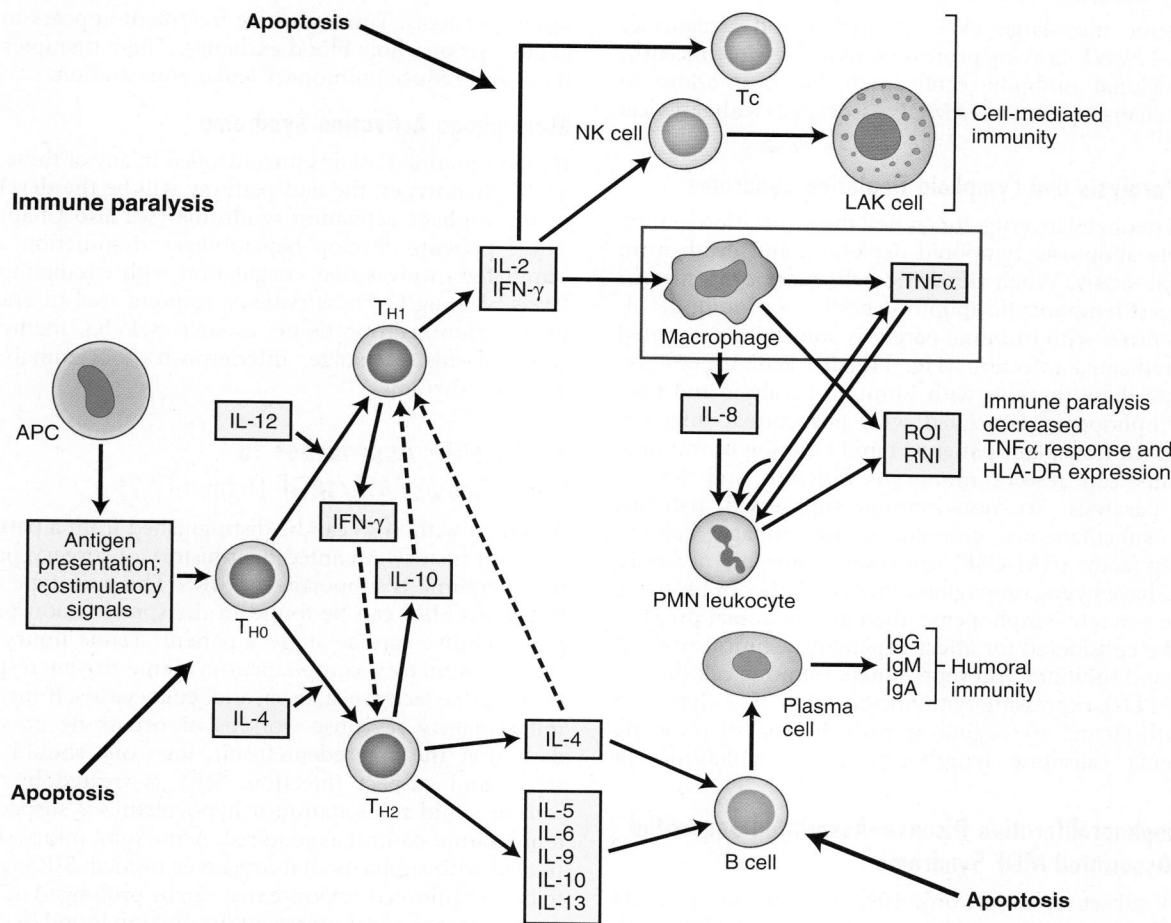

Fig. 112.10. Multiple-organ-failure patients who develop secondary infections commonly have immune paralysis with an ex vivo tumor necrosis factor alpha response to lipopolysaccharide <200 pg/mL and/or reduced monocyte human leukocyte antigen–antigen D-related expression <30% or <8000 molecules/cell. Immune function can be restored by stopping immunosuppressant therapy and by low-dose granulocyte-macrophage colony-stimulating factor therapy.

TABLE 112.1	Multiple-Organ-Failure (MOF) Phenotypes	
Phenotype	**Diagnosis**	**Therapy**
Thrombocytopenia-associated MOF	New-onset thrombocytopenia and MOF with increased LDH and renal involvement ADAMTS-13 <57%	Intensive plasma exchange until resolution of TAMOF Eculizumab for atypical HUS/TTP form
Immune paralysis MOF	Whole blood TNFα response to LPS <200 pg/mL or monocyte HLA-DR expression <30% or <8000 molecules/cell for >3 days	Rapidly taper immunosuppressants Give low-dose GM-CSF at 5 ug/kg/day sc × 7 days
Sequential MOF	Respiratory then hepatorenal PTLD – EBV disease posttransplantation	Stop immunesuppressants; give rituximab + IVIG
Iron overload MOF	History of multiple transfusions. Ferritin >1000 pg/L, Fe binding >50%	Iron chelation, coverage for aspergillus during chelation
Hyperleukocytosis MOF	Pertussis + high white blood cell count + ARDS and pulmonary hypertension	Leukopheresis or whole blood exchange
Macrophage activation syndrome	Hepatobiliary dysfunction + disseminated intravascular coagulation + ferritin >500 ug/L	Methylprednisone, IVIG, plasma exchange, anakinra, and/or tocilizumab

ARDS, acute respiratory distress syndrome; *GM-CSF,* granulocyte-macrophage colony-stimulating factor; *IVIG,* intravenous immunoglobulin; *LDH,* lactase dehydrogenase.

thrombogenic ultra-large vWF multimers and replenishes ADAMTS-13 vWF cleaving protease activity.[5,18] More recently, C5a monoclonal antibody (eculizumab) has been added to plasma exchange to treat TAMOF associated with atypical HUS/TTP.[19]

Immune Paralysis and Lymphoid Depletion Syndrome

Adult and neonatal investigators noted the association among lymphocyte apoptosis, lymphoid depletion, and death from nosocomial sepsis. When dendritic cells/monocytes/macrophages ingest lymphocytic apoptotic bodies, a profound TH[2] response ensues with immune paralysis and death associated with uneradicated infection (Fig. 112.10). Pediatric studies corroborate these findings with immune paralysis and prolonged lymphopenia associated with nosocomial infection and death.[6] In transplant patients, rapid tapering of immune suppressants can restore monocyte function and reverse immune paralysis. In non–immune-suppressed patients, low-dose subcutaneous granulocyte-macrophage colony-stimulating factor (GM-CSF) can reverse immune paralysis. If patients have hypogammaglobulinemia, IVIG can be given. If they are severely lymphopenic, then antimicrobial prophylaxis can be considered for affected patients. Clinical trials of PDL-1 ligand inhibitor (prevents innate immune cell phagocytosis of PD-1 expressing lymphocytes) and IL-7 (lymphocyte growth factor) are beginning with the goal of reversing lymphopenia (absolute lymphocyte count <1000/uL) in adults.

Viral/Lymphoproliferative Disease–Associated Sequential or Liver-Associated MOF Syndrome

This MOF subset represents only 10% of MOF, but it carries the worse prognosis. Liver injury is associated with high sFasL levels >500 pg/mL.[9] In transplant patients the most common cause is posttransplant lymphoproliferative disease. Epstein-Barr virus (EBV) intercalates viral IL-10 genome into B cells, preventing activated immune cell death and promoting lymphoproliferation. This is treated by stopping immune suppression, giving the B-cell monoclonal antibody rituximab, and administering interferon-α if necessary. In nontransplant patients with a family history of a similar disease, X-linked immunoproliferative disease should be considered (XIAP). These patients cannot direct programmed cell death in activated immune cells and are treated with chemotherapy and bone marrow transplantation to kill activated immune cells and replenish functioning NK/cytotoxic T-lymphocyte (CTL) cells.

Secondary Hemochromatosis-Associated Cardiac Hepatopancreatic MOF

Patients who have received multiple blood transfusions (including patients with aplastic anemia, liver failure, and hemolytic anemias) develop iron overload with high ferritin >1000 ug/L and iron-binding capacity <50%. Iron deposition can be diagnosed by liver magnetic resonance imaging. Infections thrive with this excess iron environment, and sepsis-induced MOF is common in this population. Chelation therapy can be considered.

Hyperleukocytosis-Associated MOF

This leukostasis syndrome is caused by pertussis-associated leukocyte proliferating factor and is predominantly found in infant pertussis. Time-sensitive treatment appears to be leukapheresis or whole blood exchange. These therapies remove toxin and reduce pulmonary leukosequestration.

Macrophage Activation Syndrome

If inflammation remains uncontrolled in any of these MODS/MOF phenotypes, the end pathway will be the development of macrophage activation syndrome (see also Chapter 106). These patients develop hepatobiliary dysfunction and disseminated intravascular coagulation with circulating ferritin levels >500 ug/L. These patients respond well to eradication of infection/necrotic tissue, as well as IVIG, methylprednisone, plasma exchange, interferon-α, tocilizumab, and/or anakinra therapies.[20-22]

Therapeutic Approaches to SIRS/Sepsis/ALI/MOF (Table 112.2)

A patient with SIRS can be distinguished from a patient with sepsis by history. An antecedent history of surgery, pancreatitis, or trauma is supportive of SIRS. The prototype for noninfectious SIRS can be found in the spinal fusion patient or postoperative cardiac surgery patient. Tissue injury induces the inflammatory complement/cytokine-driven response of tachycardia, tachypnea, fever, and leukocytosis. If the systemic inflammatory response worsens or occurs de novo several days after the antecedent insult, then one should consider sepsis and suspect infection. SIRS is treated by watchful waiting, fluid resuscitation if hypovolemia is suspected, and temperature control as required. Acute lung injury should be treated with supplemental oxygen as needed. SIRS is thought to be a self-limited response that can be prolonged in the presence of decreased complement production found in one-third of the population who have MBL and complement H polymorphisms. One should observe that the rate of tachycardia and tachypnea decreases with time. If sepsis is suspected, then antibiotics should be given.

If SIRS/sepsis progresses to organ failure or MOF, it is no longer a self-limited disease. Further support and interventions are necessary. If acute lung injury progresses, intubation and mechanical ventilation will be necessary. Intubation with ketamine as an induction agent in this setting is antiinflammatory and will not interfere with the adrenal stress response. Pulmonary capillary and epithelium leak will result in indirect

---

TABLE 112.2	Nonspecific Therapies to Prevent and Resolve Multiple Organ Failure

1. Reverse shock in time-sensitive fashion (American College of Critical Care Medicine/Pediatric Advanced Life Support guidelines)
2. Provide effective antibiotics in time-sensitive fashion
3. Remove nidus of infection
4. Use antitoxins for toxin-mediated disease
5. Fluid removal before fluid overload >10% body weight
6. Use lung protection strategy effective tidal volume <8 mL/kg
7. Control hyperglycemia
8. Prevent drug toxicity by titrating drugs to liver/kidney function
9. Remove toxic drugs as indicated
10. Provide nutrition
11. Prevent/stop systemic hemolysis

ARDS, and the patient will need positive end-expiratory pressure (PEEP) to facilitate adequate oxygenation. Protective lung ventilation is recommended (see Chapters 51 and 52). Use of high lung volumes results in increased systemic inflammation and immune paralysis. For this reason, an effective tidal volume of no more than 8 mL/kg per breath is recommended. Cardiovascular management should be goal directed in a time-sensitive manner. Fluid and inotrope administration targeting capillary refill <2 seconds and normal blood pressure in the emergency department are associated with a 40% reduction in mortality.[23] Fluid, inotrope, and blood resuscitation directed to attaining superior vena cava oxygen saturation >70% reduced the incidence of MOF (renal and neurologic failure in particular) and mortality fourfold in a randomized controlled trial.[24] Administration of antibiotics and antitoxins in a time-sensitive and appropriate manner is paramount. In a retrospective cohort study involving 14 North American adult ICUs, septic patients received effective antibiotics on average 6 hours after the onset of hypotension. Administration of an effective antimicrobial within the first hour of documented hypotension was associated with a survival rate of 79.9%. However, for each subsequent hour delay in administering an effective antimicrobial average, survival decreased by 7.6%.[25] Two separate groups of pediatric ICU investigators have shown that timely administration of antibiotics prevented the development of organ dysfunction and MODS/MOF.[26,27]

Careful attention should also be given to fluid balance. When patients become >10% total body weight fluid overloaded (eg, >1 L in a 10-kg child), the risk of mortality from MOF increases. Diuretic and/or extracorporeal therapies including intermittent renal dialysis or continuous hemofiltration should be used to remove fluid as needed after initial resuscitation, specifically to prevent fluid overload >10%. Nutrition is also important and should be given enterally if possible, but if not, then definitely through the parenteral route. Ensuring adequate glucose delivery with maintenance fluids while avoiding hyperglycemia should be a priority the first day. Enteral feedings or total parenteral nutrition can be started subsequently. Although controversy exists regarding what glucose level one should target, there is consensus that glycemic control with insulin is required at some degree of hyperglycemia. Hyperglycemia causes monocyte deactivation, increases C-reactive protein levels and inflammation, reduces immune function globally, and increases the risk of thrombosis and MOF. Insulin improves monocyte/macrophage function and reduces systemic inflammation and thrombosis.

Because cytochrome P-450 activity is decreased during SIRS/sepsis-induced MOF (~1/2 in sepsis, ~1/4 with 2 organ failures, and ~1/10 with persistent three-organ failures), adjustment of cytochrome P-450 metabolized medications is suggested when possible. Medications metabolized by the kidney should be adjusted as well according to creatinine clearance. One way to address reduced drug metabolism is to use drugs that can be followed pharmacokinetically by measured concentrations and pharmacodynamically by physiologic responses to titrated dosing. A nice rule of thumb when giving drugs that do not have pharmacokinetic or pharmacodynamic targets is to double the interval between doses for every doubling of creatinine or bilirubin depending on whether the drug is primarily metabolized through renal or hepatic pathways. Hormone synthesis can also be affected.

Patients with adrenal insufficiency or thyroid insufficiency will require replacement.

Unresolving MOF should evoke suspicion that the source of infection or necrotic tissue is not being eradicated (Fig. 112.6). Persistent inflammation with thrombosis and infection is one cause of persistent MOF. Careful review of the minimum inhibitory concentration (MIC) profile of the infection should be performed, and antibiotics with the lowest possible MIC should be used. If the infection is toxin producing, clindamycin should be given to stop toxin production and IVIG administered to neutralize toxin effects. The nidus of infection may need to be removed surgically. Barie et al.[28] found that surgical sepsis mortality was 96% with failed nidus removal compared with only 4% with successful removal. Primary or acquired immune deficiency syndromes can also be the cause of uneradicated infection. Primary immunodeficiencies are usually suspected in children younger than 5 years but can present at any time in life (see also Chapter 103). Initial screening for these syndromes includes white blood cell counts, lymphocyte subsets, complement levels, gamma globulin levels, and tests for chronic granulomatous disease. Secondary immune deficiencies include severe neutropenia (ANC <500) and severe graft-versus-host disease (grade III and above) (see also Chapter 104). Neutropenia is most commonly related to bone marrow suppression induced by chemotherapy. Infection eradication and subsequent resolution of MOF occur only after restoration of the neutrophil counts. The pathobiology of graft-versus-host disease is one of donor T cells being directed against host epithelial cells (see also Chapter 95). This results in denudation of the epithelial cell barrier with secondary bacterial and fungal infections. Treatment is difficult but is directed at stopping T cell–mediated epithelial destruction without concomitantly stopping host ability to kill infection. This is the most difficult MOF syndrome to treat.

Hemolysis is another cause of unresolving MOF. Free hemoglobin becomes a hemoglobin peroxidase when exposed to superoxide and hydrogen peroxide generated by activated white blood cells. Hemoglobin peroxidase can lead to endothelial cell injury, microvascular constriction secondary to NO scavenging, and reduction in macrophage viability.[29] The prototype of this form of MOF is found in children with sepsis who are on poorly functioning extracorporeal membrane oxygenation (ECMO) support. If the ECMO circuit induces excessive hemolysis (free hemoglobin >10 ug/L), MOF can ensue. The approach should be to attempt to stop ongoing hemolysis by changing oxygenator circuits, adding a second venous cannula, and reducing ECMO flow (see also Chapter 59). In hemolytic disease such as sickle cell anemia, plasma exchange can help reduce hemolysis and resolve MOF.

Rare medication toxicities can also contribute to unresolving MOF. Patients with intrathecal baclofen pump infusions can develop baclofen withdrawal infusion syndrome when infusions are stopped. Linezolid toxicity can also progress to overwhelming lactic acidosis and MOF. Linezolid's antimicrobial activity is mediated through bacterial ribosome poisoning. Unfortunately, human mitochondria can similarly be poisoned by linezolid. Baseline lactate levels should be obtained, and if lactate levels increase while on linezolid, the drug should be stopped before lactic acidosis ensues. Nitroprusside at high/prolonged dosing can induce cyanide poisoning. Cyanide and isocyanate levels should be followed when giving this medication. Propofol can cause propofol infusion syndrome associated with overwhelming lactic acidosis. Propofol should not be used for long-term sedation in children <3 years of age. Systemic drug reactions including Stevens-Johnson syndrome and delayed hypersensitivity syndromes must also be considered. These scenarios call for discontinuation of the offending agent and then watchful supportive care. This can sometimes be tricky. For example, the delayed hypersensitivity skin rash may be difficult to discern in children with greater pigmentation. For patients with sulfa drug–related Stevens-Johnson syndrome, it is important to realize that furosemide is also a sulfonylurea.

Even in clinical settings without sophisticated research tests, patients with persistent MOF can be phenotyped. New-onset thrombocytopenia with MOF, increase LDH, ± schistocytes, and renal dysfunction likely reflects a thrombotic microangiopathy that resides within the disseminated intravascular coagulation–thrombotic thrombocytopenic purpura continuum. This complex coagulopathy can be treated with plasma infusion/plasma exchange, protein C, antithrombin III, pentoxifylline, prostacyclin, and/or heparin. New or persistent bacterial or fungal infections in a patient with MOF who does not have evidence of primary/secondary immune deficiency nor an uneradicated nidus of infection are highly suggestive of immune paralysis/lymphoid depletion syndrome. Immune-suppressant therapies should be rapidly tapered in these patients. Dexamethasone in particular should be stopped and transitioned to hydrocortisone. GM-CSF can be given subcutaneously at 125 ug/m^2 daily subcutaneously to reverse immune paralysis. If IgG levels are <500 ug/L, IVIG should be considered. If the CD4 count is low, antifungal/antiviral/antiprotozoal prophylaxis can be considered. Patients with sequential MOF that begins with ARDS and progresses to hepatorenal syndrome should be recognized and treated accordingly. If the child has EBV-related posttransplant lymphoproliferative disease (high EBV titers), rapid immune suppression tapering is recommended along with rituximab and IVIG therapy. If a previously healthy infant has pneumonia and a white blood cell count >27,000/uL, the diagnosis of pertussis-related hyperleukocytosis should be aggressively pursued. Investigators in the United Kingdom provide a useful algorithm to direct use of leukoreduction therapies in this population.[30] A ferritin level should be investigated in patients who develop hepatobiliary dysfunction and disseminated intravascular coagulation. If ferritin is >500 ug/L, the diagnosis of macrophage activation syndrome should be considered. Its treatments include IVIG, methylprednisone (not dexamethasone), plasma exchange, anakinra, and tocilizumab. A history of chronic transfusions, a ferritin >1000 ug/L, and an iron-binding capacity <50% suggest secondary hemochromatosis instead. These patients commonly have pancreatic dysfunction. They should be treated with iron chelation therapy; however, because these patients are prone to aspergillus infection during chelation therapy, appropriate antifungal coverage is recommended.

Time Course of SIRS/Sepsis-Induced MODS/MOF

In general terms, SIRS/sepsis should resolve within 5 days. MODS/MOF resolves over 1 week to 3 months. MOD and MOF are related to epithelial cell and endothelial cell dysfunction/damage/apoptosis. If significant hypoxia/ischemia is the causal event, MOF will not resolve until (1) reepithelialization of lung, liver, and kidney occurs; (2) reendothelialization of organs occurs; and (3) canalization of microvessels occurs. These processes take 6 weeks to 3 months. Accordingly, health care providers should be patient and not give up on MOF-afflicted children too early!

Summary

Inflammation and immunity are the basis of SIRS/sepsis-induced MODS/MOF. SIRS and sepsis occur more commonly in patients with reduced MBL complement and inhibitory complement function. MODS/MOF occurs in patients who have epithelial/endothelial cell injury and/or microvascular thrombosis caused by underresuscitated shock, ischemia-reperfusion, unresolved inflammation, unresolved infection, and/or drug/toxin-induced mitochondrial injury. SIRS/sepsis is managed with fluids, temperature control, and antibiotics if infection is present, and it usually resolves within 5 days. This approach prevents the development MOF/MODS. If treatment is delayed, MODS/MOF can occur. Treatment is then used to reverse shock, remove infection, resolve inflammation, and reverse microvascular thrombosis. Personalized phenotype-specific therapies are directed to recovery of endothelial, epithelial, mitochondrial, and immune function. Survival can be 90% with a patient approach.

References

1. Proulx F, Fayon M, Farrell CA, et al. Epidemiology of sepsis and multiple organ dysfunction syndrome in children. *Chest.* 1996;109:1033-1037.
2. Doughty LA, Kaplan SS, Sasser H, Carcillo J. The compensatory anti-inflammatory cytokine IL-10 response in pediatric sepsis-induced multiple organ failure. *Chest.* 1998;113:1625-1631.
3. Green J, Doughty L, Kaplan SS, et al. The tissue factor and plasminogen activator inhibitor type 1 response in pediatric sepsis-induced multiple organ failure. *Thromb Haemost.* 2002;87:218-223.
4. Whalen MJ, Doughty LA, Carlos TM, et al. Intercellular adhesion molecule-1 and vascular adhesion molecule-1 are increased in children with sepsis induced multiple organ failure. *Crit Care Med.* 2000;28:2600-2607.
5. Nguyen TC, Han YY, Kiss JE, et al. Intensive plasma exchange therapy increases ADAMTS 13 and reverses organ dysfunction in children with thrombocytopenia associated. *MOF Crit Care Med.* 2008;36:2878-2887.
6. Felmet KA, Hall MW, Clark RS, et al. Prolonged lymphopenia, lymphoid depletion, and hypoprolactinemia in children with nosocomial sepsis and MOF. *J Immunol.* 2005;174:3765-3772.
7. Weiss SL, Selak MA, Tuluc F, et al. Mitochondrial dysfunction in peripheral blood mononuclear cells in pediatric septic shock. *Pediatr Crit Care Med.* 2015;16:e4-e12.
8. Carcillo JA, Doughty LA, Kofos D, et al. Cytochrome P450 mediated drug metabolism is reduced in children with sepsis-induced MOF. *Intensive Care Med.* 2003;29:980-984.
9. Doughty L, Clark RS, Kaplan SS, et al. sFas and sFasL and pediatric sepsis induced MOF. *Pediatr Res.* 2002;52:922-927.
10. Agbeko RS, Fidler KJ, Allen ML, et al. Genetic variability in complement activation modulates the systemic inflammatory response syndrome in children. *Pediatr Crit Care Med.* 2010;11:561-567.
11. Rodríguez de Córdoba S, Hidalgo MS, Pinto S, Tortajada A. Genetics of atypical hemolytic uremic syndrome (aHUS). *Semin Thromb Hemost.* 2014;40:422-430.
12. Wilkinson JD, Pollack MM, Ruttiman UE, et al. Outcome of pediatric patients with multiple organ system failure. *Crit Care Med.* 1986;14:271-274.
13. Goldstein B, Giroir B, Randolph A. International pediatric sepsis consensus conference: definitions for sepsis and organ dysfunctions. *Pediatr Crit Care Med.* 2005;6:2-8.

14. Leteurtre S, Martinot A, Duhamel A, et al. Development of a pediatric multiple organ dysfunction score: use of two strategies. *Med Decis Making*. 1999;19:399-410.

15. Leteurtre S, Duhamel A, Deken V, et al. Daily estimation of the severity of organ dysfunctions in critically ill children by using the PELOD-2 score. *Crit Care*. 2015;19:324.

16. Odetola FO, Gebremanian A, Freed GL. Patient and hospital correlates of clinical outcomes and resource utilization in severe pediatric sepsis. *Pediatrics*. 2007;119:487-494.

17. Typpo KV, Petersen NJ, Hamilton DM, et al. Day 1 multiple organ dysfunction syndrome is associated with poor functional outcome and mortality in the pediatric intensive care unit. *Pediatr Crit Care Med*. 2009; 10:562-570.

18. Bongers TN, Emonts M, de Maat MP, et al. Reduced ADAMTS 13 in children with severe meningococcal sepsis is associated with severity and outcome. *Thromb Haemost*. 2010;103:1181-1187.

19. Legendre CM, Licht C, Muus P, et al. Terminal complement inhibitor eculizumab in atypical hemolytic-uremic syndrome. *N Engl J Med*. 2013; 368:2169-2181.

20. Castillo L, Carcillo J. Secondary hemophagocytic lymphohistiocytosis and severe sepsis/systemic inflammatory response syndrome/multiple organ dysfunction syndrome/macrophage activation syndrome share common intermediate phenotypes on a spectrum of inflammation. *Pediatr Crit Care Med*. 2009;10:387-392.

21. Demirkol D, Yildizdas D, Bayrakci B, et al. Hyperferritinemia in the critically ill child with secondary hemophagocytic lymphohistiocytosis/ sepsis/multiple organ dysfunction syndrome/macrophage activation syndrome: what is the treatment? *Crit Care*. 2012;16:R52.

22. Shakoory B, Carcillo JA, Chatham WW, et al. Interleukin-1 receptor blockade is associated with reduced mortality in sepsis patients with features of macrophage activation syndrome: reanalysis of a prior phase iii trial. *Crit Care Med*. 2016;44:275-281.

23. Han YY, Carcillo JA, Dragotta MA, et al. Early reversal of pediatric-neonatal septic shock by community physicians is associated with improved outcome. *Pediatrics*. 2003;112:793-798.

24. de Oliveira CF, de Oliveira DS, Gottschald AF, et al. ACCM/PALS hemodynamic support guidelines for pediatric septic shock: an outcomes comparison with and without monitoring central venous oxygen saturation. *Intensive Care Med*. 2008;34:1065-1076.

25. Kumar A, Roberts D, Wood KE, et al. The duration of hypotension before initiation of effective antimicrobial therapy is critical determinant of survival in human septic shock. *Crit Care Med*. 2006;34:1589-1596.

26. Muszynski JA[1], Knatz NL, Sargel CL, et al. Timing of correct parenteral antibiotic initiation and outcomes from severe bacterial community-acquired pneumonia in children. *Pediatr Infect Dis J*. 2011;30:295-301.

27. Weiss SL, Fitzgerald JC, Balamuth F, et al. Delayed antimicrobial therapy increases mortality and organ dysfunction duration in pediatric sepsis. *Crit Care Med*. 2014;42:2409-2417.

28. Barie PS, Williams MD, McCollam JS, et al. Benefit/risk profile of drotrecogin alpha in surgical patients with severe sepsis. *Am J Surg*. 2004;188: 212-220.

29. Kapralov A, Vlasova II, Feng W, et al. Peroxidase activity of hemoglobin haptoglobin complexes: covalent aggregation and oxidative stress in plasma and macrophages. *J Biol Chem*. 2009;284:30395-30407.

30. Rowlands HE, Goldman AP, Harrington K, et al. Impact of rapid leukodepletion on the outcome of severe clinical pertussis in young infants. *Pediatrics*. 2010;126:e816-e827.

Environmental Hazards

Bites and Stings

Alfredo Maldonado, Nagela Sainte-Thomas, and Erika Vazquez

PEARLS

- Snakebite-related injury and death are reduced most effectively by rapid transport, intensive care support, and the administration of antivenin.
- Measures not recommended for snakebite first aid are incision, suction, tourniquets, electric shock, ice directly on wound, alcohol, or folk therapies.
- Antivenins can induce immediate anaphylactic (type I hypersensitivity) or anaphylactoid reactions, which can be rapidly life-threatening. Airway swelling, wheezing, shock, and urticaria characterize these reactions. Anaphylactic and anaphylactoid reactions are treated with antihistamines, histamine (H_2) blockers, epinephrine, steroids, and ventilatory/circulatory support as needed.
- All children with snake envenomations should be admitted to the hospital. Serious effects can be delayed and can recur even after treatment with antivenin.
- Typically, a widow spider bite site has a "target" appearance. There may be a central reddened, indurated area around the fang puncture site(s) surrounded by an area of blanching and an outer halo of redness. The findings around the bite wound may be subtle.
- Bees, wasps, and ants can cause toxic, even fatal, complications when they attack en masse. Sting removal after a honeybee sting should be done as quickly as possible, regardless of the method of removal.

The general principles of envenomation medicine are similar around the world, although the availability of resources varies widely. A comprehensive discussion of all available antivenins is beyond the scope of this text.[1] In consideration of space constraints, the scope of this textbook, and its audience, this chapter focuses on US antivenins. Readers are encouraged to become familiar with the prescribing information for the antivenin(s) available in their area(s) of practice for the envenomations they may encounter.

Snakebites

Snakebite is a particularly challenging clinical problem because of the wide variety of toxic effects. Children with snakebites may have little more than a fang puncture mark, or they may have multisystem failure and death.[2,3] Part of this is due to the extreme variability of snake venom, even within the same species.[4] Snake venom contains multiple enzymes, proteins, and peptides that can damage local tissues and have serious systemic effects. Unfortunately, it is difficult to predict at the time of the bite which patients will have relatively mild symptoms and which will have a rapidly progressive and potentially fatal envenomation syndrome.

Snakebite envenomation syndromes can be loosely associated with snake family. Viperidae includes old-world vipers and pit vipers (collectively referred to as viperids). Most snakebites in the United States are inflicted by pit vipers, which include rattlesnakes, cottonmouths (also known as water moccasins), and copperheads.[5] All pit vipers have a triangular head, elliptical pupils, and a heat-sensing pit between the eye and nostril (Fig. 113.1).[6] The pit organ has thermal receptors that can detect temperature differences of 68°C at 1.5 m in predatory interactions and 108°C at 1 m in defensive contexts (A. Krochman, personal communication, January 17, 2005). The family Elapidae ("elapids") includes cobras, coral snakes, kraits, and mambas.[7] Their venom effects can be as diverse as the species that make up this family of snakes. Cobras are hooded, high-profile snakes that inhabit Africa and southern Asia (Fig. 113.2). The coral snakes of the Americas and kraits of Asia and India are often small, shy, colorfully banded snakes (Fig. 113.3). Mambas in Africa are long, lean, and fast. Australian elapids can be large and nondescript. Sea snakes possess some of the world's most toxic snake venom, although few bites occur mostly because of the marine distribution and nonaggressive temperament of these snakes. Most snakes from the Colubridae family ("colubrids") are considered harmless, although several species possess venom and some have primitively specialized teeth to facilitate venom delivery. Some, such as the boomslang in Africa, are considered dangerous to humans, and antivenin is produced.

Epidemiology

It is estimated that approximately 1,841,000 envenomations and 94,000 deaths occur worldwide annually from snakebites.[8] It is often stated that children are more severely affected by snakebites than adults.[9] Indeed, some preliminary data suggest that smaller patients have increased severity. In terms of evidence, however, there is little to support the assertion that outcomes for children are worse than adults. For example, of more than 100,000 exposures and 24 deaths described by the American Association of Poison Control Centers (AAPCC) since its first report in 1983, only a relatively small percentage of the deaths are described in pediatric patients.[10] In some respects, children are no different from adults when it comes to snakebite. For instance, antivenin dosing is not based on the patient's weight,[11,12] yet there are a few concerns specific to pediatric patients. Because young children may not be able to give a good description of the snake or circumstances, it may be unclear whether a venomous snake has bitten them.

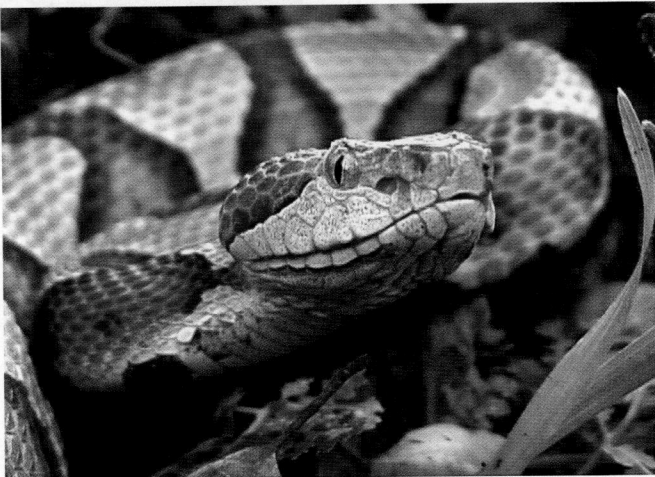

Fig. 113.1. Copperhead *(Agkistrodon contortrix).* (Photo courtesy Sean Bush, M.D.)

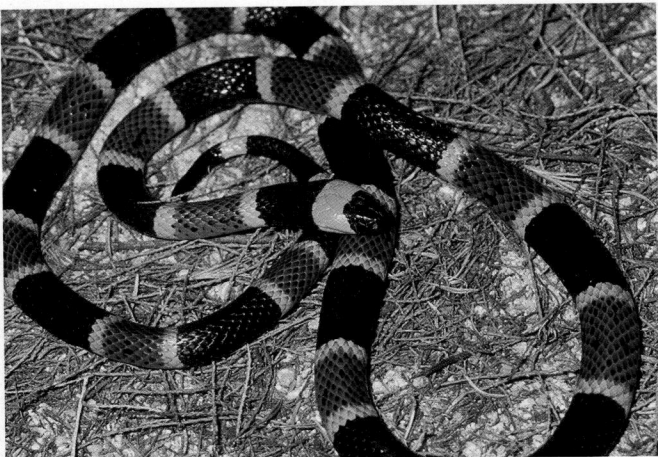

Fig. 113.3. Eastern coral snake *(Micrurus fulvius).* (Photo courtesy Mike Cardwell.)

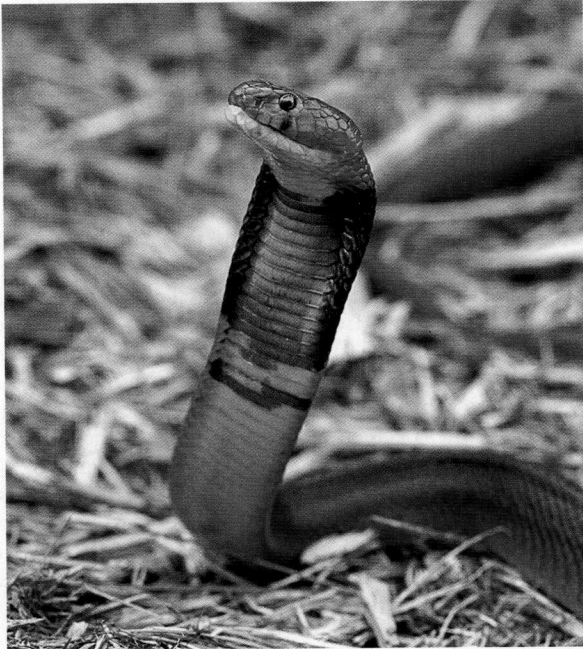

Fig. 113.2. Red spitting cobra *(Naja pallida).* (Photo courtesy Mike Cardwell.)

Pathophysiology

Although viper and pit viper venom composition varies from snake to snake, components can lead to capillary leak, abnormal clotting, inefficient muscle movement, or neurotoxicity. Capillary leak and abnormal clotting can lead to tachycardia, hypotension, or even hemorrhagic shock. Neurotoxicity or inefficient muscle movement can lead to respiratory difficulty or distress.[13] Meanwhile, proteolytic enzymes, predominant in viper and pit viper venoms, digest tissue. The longer that enzymatic components of venom have time to work, the more tissue gets damaged. Thus "time is tissue."[14] The sooner that antivenin can be started, the sooner that irreversible injury can be prevented.[15] After tissue is injured by way of digestion,

however, antivenin will not reverse the damage; it will have to heal over time.[16] Myotoxicity and rhabdomyolysis can ensue.

Envenomation by most elapids is notable for severe neurologic dysfunction, such as cranial nerve abnormalities, paralysis, and respiratory arrest. Some elapids, however, such as spitting and monocellate cobras, can also cause local necrosis. Most do not induce coagulopathy. Other symptoms and signs may include swelling, lethargy, vomiting, chest pain, and shock. Some cobras and cobralike species can "spit" venom toward the face of an antagonist, which can result in eye pain and visual impairment. Sea snake envenomation can cause profound neurotoxicity and myotoxicity but generally does not induce coagulopathy or result in serious local injury. Sea snakes are found in waters around Southeast Asia and Australia. Additionally, some individuals may experience anaphylactic or anaphylactoid reactions to venom.[17,18] Finally, some responses can be attributed to anxiety, although this should be a diagnosis of exclusion.[6]

Clinical Presentation

Immediately after a snakebite, the only apparent manifestation may be fang puncture wounds. If a patient is seen soon after a snakebite, an envenomation syndrome might not have developed yet. The onset of symptoms and signs can occur rapidly, or it may be insidious. Most cases of envenomations can be identified within 6 hours of the bite.[19] Generally, the more severe an envenomation, the more rapidly it progresses; however, even a slowly progressing envenomation can lead to severe sequelae. If a patient is seen very late, the envenomation could have already run its course, and antivenin will not be as effective.[15]

Snakebites by pit vipers and vipers cause pain around the bite site as tissues distort with swelling. There may or may not be associated taste changes. Difficulty breathing can follow many types of venomous snakebites and can progress to respiratory distress or failure in some cases. Patients may experience nausea, vomiting, or diarrhea, and venom-induced coagulopathies (often associated with viper and pit viper envenomation) can lead to hematemesis, hematochezia, or both. Certain snakebites, such as those inflicted by most elapids and some populations of rattlesnakes, can also be associated with neurologic symptoms, such as motor weakness or paresthesias. Syncope or lethargy can result from severe or prolonged hypotension.[6] Vital signs may reflect tachycardia, hypotension or hypertension, tachypnea, or hypoventilation. On physical examination, there may be one, two, or more fang puncture wounds, or none may be discernible. There is usually tenderness and swelling surrounding the bite site, which expands as the venom spreads locally. Other local signs can include erythema, ecchymosis, and bullae after viperid envenomation (Fig. 113.4). Systemic evidence of viperid envenomation may manifest in many ways. There may be abnormal bleeding, such as prolonged bleeding from fang puncture wounds or IV cannulation sites. Patients may have epistaxis or gingival bleeding. Serious and potentially life-threatening bleeding may manifest via the gastrointestinal tract or intracranially. In extremely rare instances, snakebite can also cause hypercoagulability, which can lead to infarction. Additionally, there may be neurologic signs, such as ptosis (Fig. 113.5), and muscle fasciculations, or "myokymia."[6]

Diagnostic Studies

Initial laboratory tests after pit viper or viper envenomation should include a complete blood count (CBC), prothrombin

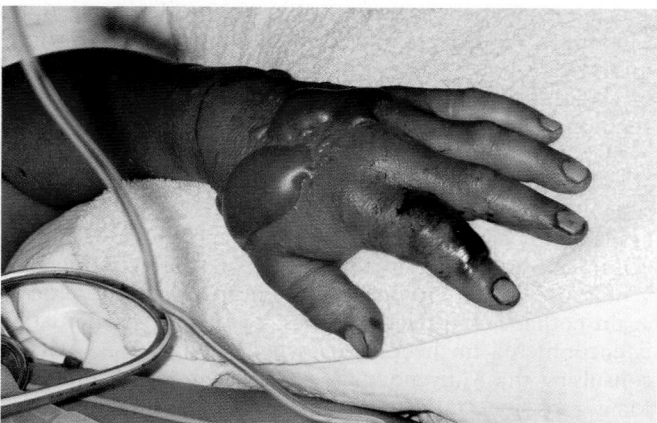

Fig. 113.4. Southern Pacific rattlesnake *(Crotalus helleri)* bite wounds. (Photo courtesy Sean Bush, M.D.)

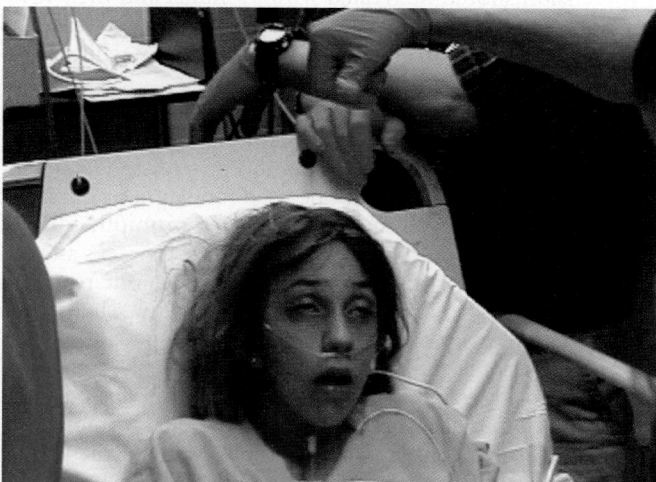

Fig. 113.5. Ptosis after Mohave rattlesnake *(Crotalus scutulatus)* envenomation. (Photo courtesy Sean Bush, M.D.)

time (PT), partial thromboplastin time (PTT), international normalized ratio (INR), fibrinogen, and a type and screen. Venom-induced coagulopathy is common after many types of viperid envenomations and is most typically characterized by thrombocytopenia and hypofibrinogenemia. Even if coagulation values are normal on presentation, they may need to be rechecked depending on the clinical scenario. Venom-induced coagulopathies can develop late, recur, or persist. If initial laboratory findings are abnormal, more frequent monitoring may be necessary depending on how severely abnormal they are and how they respond to treatment. If the findings are abnormal, repeating the CBC, PT, PTT, INR, and fibrinogen tests 1 hour after completion of an infusion of antivenin may be helpful to monitor treatment efficacy. When laboratory values are rechecked, in addition to the initial laboratory panel, additional blood should be sent for creatine kinase (CK), electrolytes, blood urea nitrogen, and creatinine clearance. All snakebites can result in rhabdomyolysis, which usually responds to aggressive fluid hydration, but can require dialysis if myoglobinuric renal failure develops. In certain regions, such as Australia, venom detection kits (eg, enzyme-linked immunosorbent assays) may be available to help identify species and guide specific antivenin selection. Other diagnostic studies may be indicated on the basis of a patient's medical history or special circumstances.[6]

Pitfalls

It is possible that a snakebite might be mistaken for a puncture wound from another cause (eg, from a plant thorn), if the patient is seen very early, if the envenomation is mild, or if there are difficulties obtaining a reliable history. If there is any question about whether a patient has been bitten by a venomous snake, an observation period and diagnostic studies may help clarify the diagnosis. Snakebites usually progress if significant envenomation has occurred. Certain signs (eg, ecchymosis), symptoms (eg, local paresthesias), and laboratory data (eg, thrombocytopenia, hypofibrinogenemia), if affected, are fairly consistent with viperid envenomation. If a bite by an elapid is suspected, envenomation should be assumed until proven otherwise after adequate observation and evaluation. Evaluation may include the Tensilon test in those patients presenting with a myasthenia-like syndrome.[20]

Prehospital Care

The factors that most reduce snakebite-related injury and death in the United States are rapid transport, intensive care, and administration of antivenin.[21] All patients with snakebites should be transported to the hospital as expeditiously and safely as possible, preferably through a 911 call (where available). The following measures are not recommended for first aid: incision, suction, tourniquets, electric shock, ice directly on wound, alcohol, or folk therapies.[22-24] Insufficient evidence exists for splinting or positioning (eg, above or below the level of the heart). Patients with bites, especially in the lower extremities, should not walk as it may increase local venom absorption. Therefore the extremity should initially be maintained in a neutral position of comfort. The Australian technique of pressure immobilization resulted in significantly longer survival but higher intracompartmental pressures after artificial, IM western diamondback rattlesnake envenomation in a pig model.[25] This technique involves immediately wrapping the entire extremity that was bitten starting at the bite site and proceeding proximally with an elastic Ace wrap or crepe bandage as tightly as one would wrap for a sprain and then splinting and immobilizing the extremity. Although pressure immobilization is not recommended widely, certain scenarios may warrant its use. It is generally not recommended for most viper bites or for bites by spitting cobras, but it is recommended for most types of Australian fauna, cape cobras, kraits, coral snakes, mambas, and sea snakes. Once pressure immobilization is placed, it should not be removed until preparations are made to manage acute toxicity and/or immediate hypersensitivity because of a potential bolus effect after its removal. Although it is difficult to predict snakebite severity at the time of the bite, certain factors may reflect increased likelihood of a more severe envenomation: large snake size, dangerous snake species, small patient size, prolonged fang contact, previous snakebites (treated or not) or exposures to snakes, or delays to medical care.

Emergency and Critical Care

All emergency personnel should be able to distinguish a venomous from a nonvenomous snake if it occurs naturally in their region of practice. If there is uncertainty about whether a particular snake is venomous, consider taking photographs of the snake from a safe distance of at least 6 feet away using a digital or Polaroid camera. These images can be seen immediately and may help make clinical decisions. Although it may be helpful to identify the species of snake,[16,26] transporting it (alive or dead) is discouraged because of inherent dangers with capturing it. On scene, snakes should only be moved or contained if absolutely necessary. A snake hook or long shovel may be helpful to move the snake into a large, empty trash canister, where it can be recovered by professionals, such as an animal control agent.

Airway support, advanced pediatric life support protocol, or both should be provided as needed. Respiratory insufficiency or failure may require endotracheal intubation and mechanical ventilation. The administration of atropine is suggested in patients with mamba envenomation due to its anticholinesterase activity causing hypersalivation.[27] Vital signs should be monitored frequently, supplemental oxygen provided, and ongoing monitoring instituted (cardiac, blood pressure, and pulse oximetry). Two peripheral IV cannulae should be started. Central venous or intraosseous access may need to be obtained. It may be appropriate to avoid placing a central line in a noncompressible site (eg, internal jugular) after viperid envenomation because of the risk of bleeding from venom-induced coagulopathy. A normal saline fluid bolus of 20 mL/kg should be administered. If there is evidence of shock, a second fluid bolus should be administered and ongoing resuscitation instituted according to Pediatric Advanced Life Support guidelines. Because viperid envenomation can induce coagulopathy and bleeding, transfusion may be required after treatment with two fluid boluses. Packed red blood cells (10 mL/kg) should be administered for acute, life-threatening blood loss or anemia. Persistent hypotension may require the administration of vasopressors and inotropic agents. Urine output may be used as a measure of adequate hydration and to check for the occurrence of rhabdomyolysis. The patient should take nothing by mouth until it has been determined that the patient will not need airway control and mechanical ventilation.

After pit viper or viper envenomation, remove rings, other constricting jewelry, and clothing in anticipation of severe swelling. The expanding area of swelling and tenderness can be used to follow the progression of viperid envenomations. Tenderness is more sensitive than swelling for detecting progression. Also, it is preferable to follow the advancing edge of tenderness or swelling than to follow serial measurements of circumference. Palpate until the edge of advancing tenderness is found. Mark this leading edge with a permanent marker and write the time alongside. Repeat this often enough to gauge progression. This may require checking the site every 15 to 20 minutes initially. Once antivenin is started, it should still be followed every 1 to 2 hours.

All hospitals should stock at least enough antivenin to treat one patient. This should be arranged ahead of time if possible, although sometimes there are antivenin shortages and other resource challenges. Presently only one agent is commercially available in the United States for treatment of pit viper envenomation: Crotalidae Polyvalent Immune Fab (Ovine), which goes by the trade name CroFab (Protherics Inc., Nashville, Tenn.).[28] Antivenin Crotalidae Polyvalent is no longer produced. Several manufacturers produce antivenin for bites in Africa (eg, South African Vaccine Producers), Asia, Europe, and Australia (eg, Commonwealth Serum Laboratories [CSL]), and the Americas (eg, Instituto Bioclon in Mexico, Instituto Clodomiro Picado in Costa Rica, and the Butantan Institute in Brazil). A polyvalent sea snake antivenin (CSL) is the drug of choice for sea snake envenomation, but tiger snake antivenin may have adequate efficacy if sea snake antivenin is not available. Information on antivenin should be researched ahead of time, and practitioners should be familiar with sources and administration techniques for the antivenins available for envenomations they may encounter. Each antivenin has varying specificity, efficacy, and safety. Some antivenins developed for one species may have some efficacy against other closely related species. If an exotic envenomation is encountered in the United States, calling the AAPCC or consulting the Antivenom Index may help locate antivenin. Many zoos stock antivenins for the exotic species they keep. If antivenin is unavailable, a patient with an elapid or sea snake envenomation may need his or her airway secured and ventilatory support provided for days or even weeks. Meanwhile, hypotension should be treated with IV fluids and then vasopressors. Edrophonium may temporarily improve weakened muscles of respiration after elapid envenomation while awaiting antivenin.

Various suggested methods determine the need for antivenin. Many grading scales are available, but it is better to treat a patient on the basis of envenomation progression or potential. Grading scales should not be used for elapid or sea snake envenomations. Antivenin should be given promptly for best results, although it may have benefit for days to weeks after an envenomation. Any time antivenin is given, allergic reactions should be anticipated. It may be helpful to know whether the patient has allergies or previous exposures to papain, papaya or animal serums, or other agents used to make antivenin. Pediatric dosing of antivenin is the same as adult dosing and is dependent on snake species and the patient's symptoms.[29] Obtain informed consent when possible. Many of the principles of antivenin administration are similar. The technique for administering CroFab is outlined as an example. A starting dose of CroFab is 4 to 6 vials and increases to 8 to 12 vials in patients who present with immediate life-threatening venom effects, such as shock or serious active bleeding.[30,31] Each vial should be mixed with 18 mL of 0.9% saline with inversion. This reduces overall dissolution time to 3 minutes from the previous practice of 10 to 30 minutes when using 10 mL of sterile water.[32] It is best to swirl or roll the vials between the hands rather than shake them. After each vial goes into solution, it should be further diluted into a total volume of 250 mL of normal saline. No skin test is recommended for CroFab, although manufacturers of many other types of antivenins recommend skin testing. With CroFab, the infusion is started slowly, at a rate of 1 mL/min for the first 10 minutes. While the infusion is started, a physician skilled in resuscitation should be at the bedside. Difficult airway equipment, epinephrine, diphenhydramine, and a histamine (H_2) blocker (eg, cimetidine) should be immediately available. If the infusion is tolerated for the first 10 minutes without evidence of an adverse reaction, the rate should be increased to complete the total volume of 250 mL/hour. If there is a problem at any time, stop the infusion, treat the adverse reaction accordingly, and reassess the need to continue antivenin treatment. A physician should be nearby at all times during the remainder of the infusions. Repeat four- to six-vial increments until initial control is achieved. Initial control is defined as the arrest or significant slowing of progression of any and all components of the envenomation syndrome (ie, minimal to no further advancement of swelling, improvement of systemic effects, and improving coagulopathy). Assess at up to 1 hour after each dose. After initial control is achieved, a maintenance dose of two vials of CroFab every 6 hours for three doses is recommended in the prescribing information, although maintenance dosing has been shown not to reduce recurrence phenomena.[33] Read the package insert for additional details.[30] For pharmacokinetic reasons that are not entirely understood, recurrence phenomena are associated with antivenins.[34-36] Local recurrence is the return of new progressive swelling after initial control. That is, the leading edge of tenderness or swelling begins to advance again. An additional two vials of CroFab should be given as soon as progressive swelling recurs, and more antivenin may be necessary to regain control, although experience has shown that local effects may continue to progress despite additional antivenin. Patients with rattlesnake bites commonly have thrombocytopenia and hypofibrinogenemia, which can resolve with CroFab and then recur (coagulopathy recurrence). Indications for an additional two vials of CroFab are serious abnormal bleeding, fibrinogen less than 50 µg/mL, platelet count less than 25,000 mm^3, INR greater than 3, multicomponent coagulopathy, worsening trend in patient with prior severe coagulopathy, high-risk behavior for trauma, or comorbid conditions that increase bleeding risk. Coagulopathy can recur as late as 2 weeks or more after treatment.

Blood products may be necessary if antivenin does not correct the coagulopathy or if there is an imminent risk of serious bleeding. Transfusion of the appropriate blood product is generally recommended for life-threatening bleeding, platelet count less than 20,000/mm^3 and refractory to antivenin, or hemoglobin less than 7 g/dL. Consider CT of the brain if the patient has a severe headache or an altered level of consciousness with a severe coagulopathy. Ocular exposure to venom necessitates prompt and copious irrigation and an ophthalmology evaluation.

Pain relief can be provided by incremental doses of either fentanyl or morphine, titrated to clinical effect. Nonsteroidal antiinflammatory drugs (NSAIDs) are contraindicated for approximately 2 weeks after viper and pit viper envenomation because they can contribute to venom-induced coagulopathy and bleeding.

Prophylactic antibiotics are unnecessary. Empiric antibiotic therapy should only be started if an infection develops and once aerobic and anaerobic wound cultures have been obtained. If an abscess occurs, it should be drained in standard fashion. An infected snakebite should prompt a further examination of the wounds for potential retained teeth or fangs.[5]

Envenomations by vipers and pit vipers are remarkable for the amount of swelling they can produce. With prompt and adequate antivenin treatment, fasciotomy or digit dermotomy is rarely indicated, even after severe viperid envenomation.[37-40] Fasciotomy, however, may be indicated if measured compartment pressures remain persistently and severely elevated despite adequate antivenin. Antivenin has been shown to limit the decrease in perfusion pressure associated with compartment syndrome.[41] Compartment syndrome may manifest subjectively, with complaints of increasing pain, and objectively, with tenderness on passive muscle stretch, a rock hard feel to the compartment, or a diminished capillary refill. True compartment syndrome, however, is rare after snakebites, even in patients with severe swelling. It may be difficult to distinguish compartment syndrome from the effects of envenomation. Similar to compartment syndrome, viperid envenomation may cause a bluish discoloration of the skin or pallor (because of subcutaneous bruising), severe swelling, paresthesias, and pain. If effects are only caused by envenomation and the patient does not have compartment syndrome, capillary refill should be normal and compartmental pressures should not be elevated. If compartment pressures are elevated, Gold et al.[38] recommend limb elevation, along with IV mannitol (1 to 2 mg/kg) administration and an additional four to six vials of CroFab over 1 hour. Consultation with a surgeon (eg, general, orthopedic, or hand) should be initiated concurrently. Compartment pressures should be measured before surgical intervention.

Therapeutic Complications

Antivenins can induce immediate anaphylactic (type I hypersensitivity) or anaphylactoid reactions, which can be rapidly life-threatening. Airway swelling, wheezing, shock, and urticaria characterize these reactions. Anaphylactic and anaphylactoid reactions are treated with antihistamines, H_2 blockers, epinephrine, steroids, and ventilatory/circulatory support as needed.

Antivenins can also cause serum sickness, a delayed (type III hypersensitivity) reaction characterized by fever, urticaria, lymphadenopathy, and polyarthralgias days to weeks after treatment. Although serum sickness can be an uncomfortable experience, it is usually benign and self-limited, and the patient is treated on an outpatient basis with antihistamines and steroids. Also, adverse reactions are much less common after treatment with Fab-based antivenins than they are with whole immunoglobulin formulations.[15] All commercially available antivenins in the United States use mercury, in the form of thimerosal, as a preservative, which in high doses can cause nerve and kidney toxicities in small children.[30]

Resources

The AAPCC can assist in the management of envenomations. Poison control may be contacted at 800-222-1222.

Disposition

It is prudent to admit all children with snake envenomations to the hospital. Serious effects can be delayed and can recur even after treatment with antivenin. Therefore close observation with monitoring, frequent measurements of swelling/tenderness, and neurologic checks for at least 24 hours are recommended. This degree of monitoring may require transfer and admission to a pediatric intensive care unit (PICU). On discharge, the patient should return immediately for further swelling or severe pain. Additionally, the patient should return immediately for any abnormal bleeding or bruising, dark tarry stools, petechiae, or severe headache. Also, patients should be given wound care instructions and told to return for signs of wound infection. Signs of serum sickness should be outlined, and the patient should return or follow up if these signs show up any time in the few weeks after treatment with antivenin. The patient should be told not to take NSAIDs for 2 weeks after a pit viper or viper bite. Instead, acetaminophen with or without a combined opiate analgesic should be prescribed. The patient should not engage in contact sports or schedule any elective surgery or dental work for 2 weeks after viperid bites. Recommend that the patient drink plenty of liquids, and advise that the patient return if decreased urination or cola-colored urine is noticed. Some patients may need referral to a physical therapist. Blisters, blebs, and bullae should be left in place but may need debridement along with necrotic tissue after several days, so surgical referral as appropriate is suggested.[37] Skin grafting is sometimes necessary. If the patient was bitten on the foot or leg, crutches and crutch training should be provided. The patient should be encouraged, however, to bear weight and mobilize the extremity as tolerated. In some cases, a next-day wound check may be appropriate. Otherwise, the patient should return or follow up in a few days.[35] At that time, laboratory tests may need to be repeated, depending on the clinical scenario. Retreat with antivenin as needed.

Prognosis

Most patients recover fully after snakebite. Viperid envenomation results, however, in tissue loss, deformity, or loss of function in a clinically significant percentage of patients.[9,42]

Preventative measures should be explained to parents and children. Teach children to leave snakes alone. They should never touch, handle, or try to kill venomous snakes. Many people are bitten when they are intentionally interacting with the snake. Even after a snake is believed to be dead, fangs still can inject venom. Snakes that were presumed dead have bitten many people and delivered serious, even fatal, envenomations. Additionally, a snake can strike faster and farther than one might think—about half its body length. Children should stay at least two "giant steps" away from snakes. If a child finds a snake, he or she should tell an adult. Additionally, tell children not to reach or step into places that they cannot see. Wearing boots and jeans may prevent some (but not all) snakebites.

Future Directions

Modifications of the antivenin molecule or formulations may reduce recurrence phenomena, and this is being investigated.

Several antivenins are being developed by Instituto Bioclon for use in the United States and other parts of the world.

Widow Spider Bites

Widow spiders belong to the genus *Latrodectus* and are represented in the United States by the black widow (Fig. 113.6), brown widow, and red-legged widow.[43] There are approximately 30 species of widow spiders worldwide.[44] The redback spider is endemic to Australia. Other species, such as the kara kurt and black button spider, are found in other parts of the world, including Europe, South America, and South Africa. The adult female black widow spider is approximately 2 cm in length and shiny black with a red-orange hourglass or spot on the ventral abdomen. The male is much smaller, brown, and much less commonly implicated in human envenoming. Juvenile females are also brown with yellow and white markings but have the general body shape of the adult. Males and juveniles have a pale hourglass shape, similar to adult females. Webs are irregular; low lying; and commonly seen in garages, barns, outhouses, and foliage. Other widow spiders around the world are generally black but may have red spots, such as the kara kurt, or a dorsal red stripe, such as the redback spider. The brown widow is brown with red and yellow markings. Similar species include the false black widow or cupboard spider, *Steatoda* spp., which can produce symptoms that are similar in character but milder in intensity than widow spiders.

Epidemiology

No deaths caused by widow spider envenomation have been reported to the AAPCC since its first annual report in 1983. A few recent deaths have been reported, however, after a black widow spider bite in Greece, Mexico, and the United States.[45-47] From 2000 to 2008 a total of 23,409 *Latrodectus* spp. exposures were reported in 47 states, with exposures peaking in September.[48] In peridomestic areas, widow spiders are found in dark or dry places—areas of clutter, woodpiles, underneath outdoor furniture, etc. In natural environments, widow spiders live under stones or logs, in shrubs, or in small mammal burrows.[44]

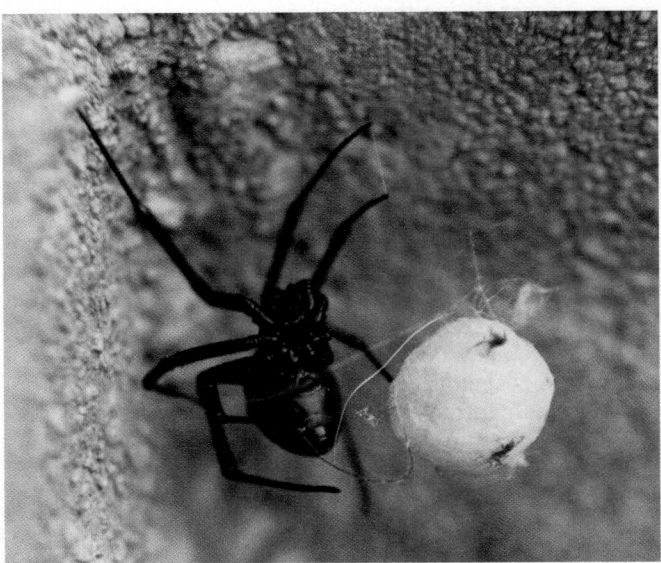

Fig. 113.6. Black widow spider (*Latrodectus hesperus*). (Photo courtesy Sean Bush, M.D.)

Pathophysiology

The envenomation syndrome, known as *latrodectism,* caused by the various species of widow spiders around the world is similar.[49-51] The predominant clinical effects after widow spider envenomation are neurologic and autonomic.

Clinical Presentation

Typically, the bite site has a "target" appearance. There may be a central reddened, indurated area around fang puncture site(s) surrounded by an area of blanching and an outer halo of redness (Fig. 113.7). The findings around the bite wound may be subtle, and the wound does not become necrotic. Puncture wounds may not be seen due to the spider's small fang size.[44] The predominant symptoms frequently involve painful muscle cramping. If a person is bitten on the lower extremity, pain usually progresses from the foot, up the leg, and into the back and abdomen. If a person is bitten on the upper extremity, pain usually progresses from the hand, up the arm, and into the chest and abdomen. Abdominal pain may be so severe as to mimic an acute abdomen, with tenderness and rigidity.[52] Diaphoresis locally around the bite site is distinctive for widow spider envenomation, although diaphoresis may be diffuse and profuse or it may manifest in unusual patterns remote from the bite site. Local piloerection is sometimes seen. Patients may exhibit "*Latrodectus* facies" (Fig. 113.8), which is characterized by spasm of facial muscles, edematous eyelids, and lacrimation, which may be mistaken for an allergic reaction. Other common symptoms and signs include high blood pressure, rapid heart rate, nausea, vomiting, headache, and anxiety. In a typical progression, symptoms begin within an hour, reach maximum intensity by about 12 hours, and can last for days to weeks. Unusual presentations have been described after widow spider envenomation including pulmonary edema, myocarditis, cardiomyopathy, and priapism.[45,53-55] It has been suggested that there may be increased danger to pediatric patients with widow spider bites and that this population may require more aggressive treatment and hospitalization, although this assertion has been challenged.[56] Little evidence supports either assertion. A recent and well-documented fatality from widow spider envenomation involved a healthy 19-year-old woman. Other recent reports involved adults as well.

Diagnostic Studies

Rhabdomyolysis has been reported after widow spider envenomation,[53] so a total CK test should be performed if severe envenomation develops. If the patient has respiratory difficulty, a chest radiograph should be obtained. Electrocardiography or echocardiography may detect that rare case of venom-induced myocarditis in a critically ill patient. Otherwise, diagnostic tests are not particularly helpful. If the diagnosis is uncertain, evaluation should be aimed at uncovering other causes such as appendicitis.

Pitfalls

Misdiagnosing an acute abdomen in a patient with a widow spider envenomation could lead to unnecessary surgery.

Emergency and Critical Care

Two basic treatment options are available. Widow spider envenomation can be managed with antivenin or a combination of pain medications and sedatives. Risks and benefits are associated with each. Management with an opioid analgesic, such as fentanyl 1 µg/kg/dose IV/IM, may repeat at 30- to 60-minute intervals or morphine in increments of 0.02 mg/kg up to 0.1 to 0.2 mg/kg IV/IM, and a benzodiazepine such as lorazepam 0.01 to 0.03 mg/kg IV is generally considered safe. This treatment option, however, is purely palliative, and symptoms may persist for days or even weeks. The pain and discomfort associated with widow spider envenomation can be severe. In contrast, antivenin is remarkably effective and can completely ameliorate the symptoms within 30 minutes.[51] Unfortunately, it can be associated with severe side effects and death.[57] Because death is so rare after widow spider envenomation, some would argue that the treatment is more dangerous than the bite itself. Historically, IV calcium was recommended, although it has now been found to be ineffective.[57] Several antivenins have been manufactured including Black Widow Spider Antivenin (equine) in the United States, Australia Redback Spider Antivenom, and South Africa spider antivenin (button spider).[1] Indications for antivenin use and routes of administration vary around the world. According to the package insert of Black Widow Spider Antivenin, one vial should be reconstituted in 2.5 mL of the sterile diluent supplied. It is further diluted into a volume of 50 mL saline and

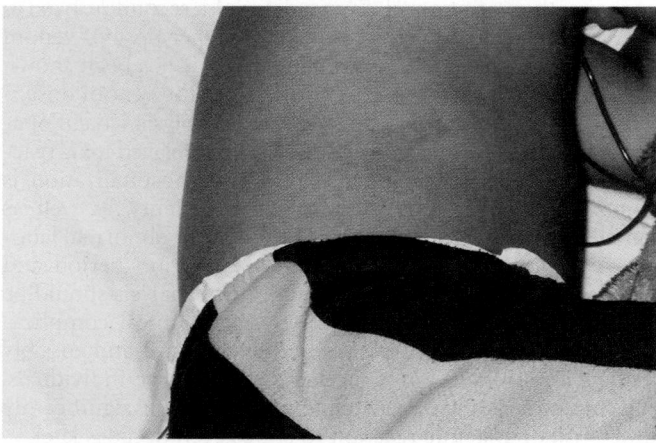

Fig. 113.7. Black widow spider bite site. (Photo courtesy Sean Bush, M.D.)

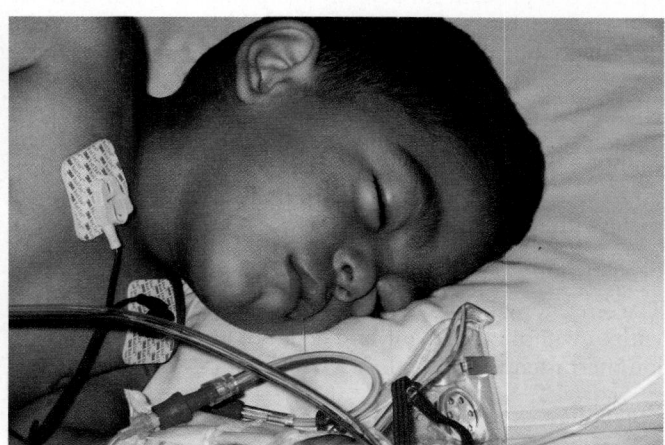

Fig. 113.8. *Latrodectus* facies. (Photo courtesy Sean Bush, M.D.)

administered IV over 15 minutes. Patients usually experience dramatic relief within an hour of treatment with one vial, although sometimes two and rarely three vials are necessary. It may be effective days, weeks, or possibly even longer after the envenomation.[58] The risk of allergy to antivenin must be weighed against the benefit of relieving prolonged discomfort, avoiding hospitalization, and preventing complications. Although most widow spider envenomations can be managed with opioid analgesics and benzodiazepines, antivenin may be indicated for patients who have severe envenomations with pain refractory to these measures. It is prudent to have medications used to treat anaphylaxis at bedside during administration of the antivenin. Antivenin should be given if there is an imminent risk of a severe complication of envenomation. Factors that could increase the risk of antivenin include allergy or previous exposure to horse serum or a medical history of reactive airways.[59] Antibiotics are not indicated for widow spider envenomation. Also, update tetanus prophylaxis as appropriate.

Therapeutic Complications

Serious, even fatal, adverse reactions have been documented after treatment with black widow spider antivenin. Anaphylactic and anaphylactoid reactions to antivenin can occur and may be even more life-threatening than the envenomation itself. Skin testing, with the intradermal injection of 0.02 mL of the test material supplied and the observation for an urticarial wheal in 10 minutes, variably predicts immediate hypersensitivity to antivenin and may influence the decision regarding its administration. Premedication with antihistamines (H_1 and H_2 blockers) may reduce the likelihood that an acute allergic reaction will occur. Serum sickness, characterized by fever, urticaria, lymphadenopathy, and polyarthralgias, can occur days to weeks after treatment and is treated with antihistamines and steroids.

Resources

The AAPCC may be helpful with management of widow spider envenomations and can be contacted at (800) 222-1222.

Disposition

Because it so effectively resolves symptoms, antivenin has been shown to decrease the need for hospitalization after widow spider envenomation. Admission to the hospital and possibly the PICU is prudent for severely symptomatic children, those with intractable pain and contraindications to antivenin, those with unusual complications of envenomation, and those who have anaphylaxis to antivenin. Patients who experience relief with opioid analgesics, benzodiazepines, or antivenin may be discharged. On discharge, signs of serum sickness should be outlined, and the patient should return or follow up if these signs show up any time in the few weeks after treatment with antivenin.

Prognosis

The envenomation syndrome usually resolves completely, with or without treatment, and does not leave the patient with long-term sequelae. Death is rare.

Prevention

Spider bites may be prevented by eliminating the spider's food and habitat; by shaking sheets, shoes, and clothing before donning; by keeping the child's bed away from the wall; and by brushing spiders off rather than crushing them.

Future Directions

Safer antivenins are being developed and investigated, including an antivenom consisting of highly purified equine F(ab)2 fragments.[60]

Hymenoptera Stings (Bees, Wasps, and Ants)

Stings by bees, wasps, and ants are less of a toxicologic concern than they are an allergic one. Details on treatment of anaphylaxis are covered elsewhere in this text. The focus of this section will be mass envenomation. Any bees, wasps, or ants can cause toxic, even fatal, complications when they attack in large numbers. Bee behavior, however, can vary, even within the same species. European honeybees tend to be docile and will tolerate approach of their hive to some degree, but they can become provoked. Africanized honeybees (*Apis mellifera scutellata*) are much more aggressive and will defend their hive more proactively. Africanized honeybees were imported to South America in the 1950s to boost honey production, and they have steadily extended their range northward into the southwestern United States. The primary difference between Africanized and European honeybees is their behavior in that Africanized honeybees behave much more aggressively. The effect of an individual stinging event is similar. Subtle wing morphologic differences and DNA testing can also distinguish the bees.

If a person is swarmed by bees or wasps, the best thing for the person to do is create barriers between himself or herself and the bees. For example, getting behind a door will evade many bees and getting behind another door will evade many more. Older children may be able to outrun bees, which fly at approximately 4 mph and may pursue up to 150 yards. Younger children, however, may be unable to run fast or far enough. Attempting to submerge oneself or another person in water is not recommended because Africanized honeybees will wait until the person surfaces to continue delivering stings. This can result in multiple stings to the airway. A lethal dose of honeybee stings is estimated at 500 to 1200 total stings or 20 stings/kg,[61] but serious envenomation can result from as few as 50 stings (or even fewer after certain species of wasp stings). Sting removal should be done as quickly as possible, regardless of the method of removal. Even a delay of a second or two (to find a knife or credit card) results in a higher dose of venom injected. Contrary to conventional advice, it has been shown that grasping the stinger does not increase the venom dose.

Clinical complications can include hemolysis, coagulopathy, rhabdomyolysis, and liver dysfunction. Delayed toxic reactions have been documented, so 24-hour hospitalization is recommended for pediatric and older patients, as well as patients with underlying medical problems or abnormal laboratory test results within a 6-hour observation period and those with 50 or more stings.[62] Laboratory analysis should be aimed at uncovering the aforementioned clinical complications. Treatment involves IV fluids, intensive care, and possibly dialysis and transfusion as needed. For sensitive individuals, venom immunotherapy in children leads to a significantly lower risk of systemic reaction to stings even decades later.[63]

If an Africanized honeybee hive is suspected, local vector control authorities should be contacted. Avoiding perfume and brightly colored clothes may prevent some stings. Similar to African honeybees, fire ants *(Solenopsis invicta)* are extending their range in the southeastern United States and can cause serious (even fatal) complications after massive envenomation, particularly in infants and small children. These ants typically bite and sting.

Key References

4. French WJ, Hayes WK, Bush SP, et al. Mojave toxin in venom of *Crotalus helleri* (Southern Pacific Rattlesnake): molecular and geographic characterization. *Toxicon.* 2004;44:781-791.

5. Norris RL Jr, Bush SP, Auerbach PS. *North American Venomous Reptile Bites. Wilderness Medicine.* 4th ed. St. Louis: Mosby; 2001.

6. Gold BS, Dart RC, Barish RA. Bites of venomous snakes. *N Engl J Med.* 2002;347:347-356.

7. Norris RL Jr, Minton SA. *Non-North American Venomous Reptile Bites. Wilderness Medicine.* 4th ed. St. Louis, MO: Mosby; 2001.

8. Kasturiratne A, Wickremasinghe AR, de Silva N, et al. The global burden of snakebite: a literature analysis and modelling based on regional estimates of envenoming and deaths. *PLoS Med.* 2008;5:e218.

10. Watson WA, Litovitz TL, Klein-Schwartz W, et al. 2003 annual report of the American Association of Poison Control Centers Toxic Exposure Surveillance System. *Am J Emerg Med.* 2004;22:335-404.

11. Behm MO, Kearns GL. Crotaline Fab antivenom for treatment of children with rattlesnake envenomation. *Pediatrics.* 2003;112(6 Pt 1):1458-1459, author reply 1458-1459.

12. Offerman SR, Bush SP, Moynihan JA, Clark RF. Crotaline Fab antivenom for the treatment of children with rattlesnake envenomation. *Pediatrics.* 2002;110:968-971.

14. Dart RC, Waeckerle JF. Introduction: "Advances in the management of snakebite" symposium. *Ann Emerg Med.* 2001;37:166-167.

15. Dart RC, McNally J. Efficacy, safety, and use of snake antivenoms in the United States. *Ann Emerg Med.* 2001;37:181-188.

16. Bush SP, Green SM, Moynihan JA, et al. Crotalidae polyvalent immune Fab (ovine) antivenom is efficacious for envenomations by Southern Pacific rattlesnakes *(Crotalus helleri). Ann Emerg Med.* 2002;40:619-624.

17. Hinze JD, Barker JA, Jones TR, Winn RE. Life-threatening upper airway edema caused by a distal rattlesnake bite. *Ann Emerg Med.* 2001;38:79-82.

18. Camilleri C, Offerman S. Anaphylaxis after rattlesnake bite. *Ann Emerg Med.* 2004;43:784-785.

19. Hughes A. Observation of snakebite victims: is twelve hours still necessary? *Emerg Med (Fremantle).* 2003;15:511-517.

22. Bush SP, Hegewald KG, Green SM, et al. Effects of a negative pressure venom extraction device (Extractor) on local tissue injury after artificial rattlesnake envenomation in a porcine model. *Wilderness Environ Med.* 2000;11:180-188.

23. Bush SP. Snakebite suction devices don't remove venom: they just suck. *Ann Emerg Med.* 2004;43:187-188.

24. Bush SP, Hardy DL Sr. Immediate removal of extractor is recommended. *Ann Emerg Med.* 2001;38:607-608.

25. Bush SP, Green SM, Laack TA, et al. Pressure immobilization delays mortality and increases intracompartmental pressure after artificial intramuscular rattlesnake envenomation in a porcine model. *Ann Emerg Med.* 2004;44:599-604.

27. White J. Overview of venomous snakes of the world. In: Dar RC, ed. *Medical Toxicology.* 3rd ed. Philadelphia: Lippincott, Williams & Wilkins; 2004.

29. Goto CS, Feng SY. Crotalidae polyvalent immune Fab for the treatment of pediatric crotaline envenomation. *Pediatr Emerg Care.* 2009;25:273-279, quiz 280-272.

30. CroFab [prescribing information]. Nashville, TN, 2000.

31. Lavonas EJ, Ruha AM, Banner W, et al. Unified treatment algorithm for the management of crotaline snakebite in the United States: results of an evidence-informed consensus workshop. *BMC Emerg Med.* 2011;11:2.

32. Gerring D, King TR, Branton R. Validating a faster method for reconstitution of Crotalidae polyvalent immune Fab (ovine). *Toxicon.* 2013;69:42-49.

33. Dart RC, Seifert SA, Boyer LV, et al. A randomized multicenter trial of Crotalidae polyvalent immune Fab (ovine) antivenom for the treatment for crotaline snakebite in the United States. *Arch Intern Med.* 2001;161:2030-2036.

34. Seifert SA, Boyer LV. Recurrence phenomena after immunoglobulin therapy for snake envenomations: Part 1. Pharmacokinetics and pharmacodynamics of immunoglobulin antivenoms and related antibodies. *Ann Emerg Med.* 2001;37:189-195.

35. Boyer LV, Seifert SA, Cain JS. Recurrence phenomena after immunoglobulin therapy for snake envenomations: part 2. Guidelines for clinical management with crotaline Fab antivenom. *Ann Emerg Med.* 2001;37:196-201.

36. Bush SP, Wu VH, Corbett SW. Rattlesnake venom-induced thrombocytopenia response to antivenin (Crotalidae) polyvalent: a case series. *Acad Emerg Med.* 2000;7:181-185.

37. Hall EL. Role of surgical intervention in the management of crotaline snake envenomation. *Ann Emerg Med.* 2001;37:175-180.

38. Gold BS, Barish RA, Dart RC, et al. Resolution of compartment syndrome after rattlesnake envenomation utilizing non-invasive measures. *J Emerg Med.* 2003;24:285-288.

39. Rosen PB, Leiva JI, Ross CP. Delayed antivenom treatment for a patient after envenomation by *Crotalus atrox. Ann Emerg Med.* 2000;35:86-88.

40. Tanen D, Ruha A, Graeme K, Curry S. Epidemiology and hospital course of rattlesnake envenomations cared for at a tertiary referral center in Central Arizona. *Acad Emerg Med.* 2001;8:177-182.

41. Tanen DA, Danish DC, Clark RF. Crotalidae polyvalent immune Fab antivenom limits the decrease in perfusion pressure of the anterior leg compartment in a porcine crotaline envenomation model. *Ann Emerg Med.* 2003;41:384-390.

42. Lavonas EJ, Gerardo CJ, O'Malley G, et al. Initial experience with Crotalidae polyvalent immune Fab (ovine) antivenom in the treatment of copperhead snakebite. *Ann Emerg Med.* 2004;43:200-206.

43. Boyer LV, McNally JT, Binford GJ. *Spider Bites. Wilderness Medicine.* 4th ed. St. Louis, MO: Mosby; 2001.

44. Vetter RS, Isbister GK. Medical aspects of spider bites. *Annu Rev Entomol.* 2008;53:409-429.

45. Pneumatikos IA, Galiatsou E, Goe D, et al. Acute fatal toxic myocarditis after black widow spider envenomation. *Ann Emerg Med.* 2003;41:158.

46. Bush SP. Why no antivenom. *Ann Emerg Med.* 2003;42:431-432.

47. Gaisford K, Kautz DD. Black widow spider bite: a case study. *Dimens Crit Care Nurs.* 2011;30:79-86.

48. Monte AA, Bucher-Bartelson B, Heard KJ. A US perspective of symptomatic *Latrodectus* spp. envenomation and treatment: a National Poison Data System review. *Ann Pharmacother.* 2011;45:1491-1498.

49. Graudins A, Padula M, Broady K, Nicholson GM. Red-back spider *(Latrodectus hasselti)* antivenom prevents the toxicity of widow spider venoms. *Ann Emerg Med.* 2001;37:154-160.

50. Daly FF, Hill RE, Bogdan GM, Dart RC. Neutralization of *Latrodectus mactans* and *L. hesperus* venom by redback spider *(L. hasseltii)* antivenom. *J Toxicol Clin Toxicol.* 2001;39:119-123.

51. Vetter RS. Spider envenomation in North America. *Crit Care Nurs Clin North Am.* 2013;25:205-223.

53. Cohen J, Bush S. Case report: compartment syndrome after a suspected black widow spider bite. *Ann Emerg Med.* 2005;45:414-416.

54. Alexakis LC, Arapi S, Stefanou I, et al. Transient reverse takotsubo cardiomyopathy following a spider bite in Greece: a case report. *Medicine (Baltimore).* 2015;94:e457.

55. Goel SC, Yabrodi M, Fortenberry J. Recognition and successful treatment of priapism and suspected black widow spider bite with antivenin. *Pediatr Emerg Care.* 2014;30:723-724.

56. Woestman R, Perkin R, Van Stralen D. The black widow: is she deadly to children? *Pediatr Emerg Care.* 1996;12:360-364.

59. Bush SP, Naftel J. Injection of a whole black widow spider. *Ann Emerg Med.* 1996;27:532-533.

60. Dart RC, Bogdan G, Heard K, et al. A randomized, double-blind, placebo-controlled trial of a highly purified equine F(ab)2 antibody black widow spider antivenom. *Ann Emerg Med.* 2013;61:458-467.

61. Fitzgerald KT, Flood AA. *Hymenoptera* stings. *Clin Tech Small Anim Pract.* 2006;21:194-204.

62. Kolecki P. Delayed toxic reaction following massive bee envenomation. *Ann Emerg Med.* 1999;33:114-116.

63. Golden DB, Kagey-Sobotka A, Norman PS, et al. Outcomes of allergy to insect stings in children, with and without venom immunotherapy. *N Engl J Med.* 2004;351:668-674.

Heat Injury

Ofer Yanay and Eli Gilad

PEARLS

- According to the Centers for Disease Control and Prevention, from 1999 to 2003, 3442 deaths were attributable to excessive heat exposure or hyperthermia in the United States.
- With an increased occurrence of heat waves, even in temperate areas, the risk of heat-related illness is rapidly increasing.
- After the onset of heat stroke, the inflammatory response may continue despite adequate control of body temperature. Inflammation, coagulopathy, and progression to multiple organ failure may ensue. New approaches for modulation of the inflammatory response may play a role in treatment of heat-related injury in the future.
- Thorough knowledge and understanding of these disorders may prevent the progression from heat stress to heat stroke.
- Maintaining organ perfusion and rapid cooling are the major treatment goals for patients with heat stroke.
- The central nervous system is particularly vulnerable to heat, with the cerebellum being most susceptible. Pyramidal dysfunction, dysphagia, mental changes (ranging from impaired judgment to delirium and coma), quadriparesis, extrapyramidal syndrome, and neuropathy have all been described.

The interest in heat-related illnesses has grown enormously, largely because of global warming and an increased frequency of heat waves.[1,2] According to the Centers for Disease Control and Prevention, from 1999 to 2003, excessive heat exposure caused 3442 deaths in the United States.[3] During this period, more people died of extreme heat than all other natural disasters combined. Among the pediatric population, neonates and infants are at highest risk, mainly because of poorly developed thermoregulatory mechanisms and total dependence on caregivers to provide adequate protection from excessive heat. Children with mental illness and chronic diseases are at high risk. Adolescents are also at increased risk mostly due to poor judgment or intoxication.

Over the past 2 decades, the understanding of cellular and molecular responses to heat stress has improved dramatically. This is a multiorgan injury resulting from a complex interplay between the cytotoxic effect of the heat and inflammatory and coagulation responses of the host.[4] Despite better understanding of heat injury pathophysiology, treatment remains supportive, with emphasis on immediate cooling. Prevention and education are still the best tools available in the hands of health care providers to minimize heat-related morbidity and death. This chapter covers the epidemiology, pathophysiology, clinical manifestations, and treatment of nonexertional heat-related illness in the pediatric population.

Definitions

Heat-related illnesses are best regarded as a spectrum of disorders that should be seen as continuum of increasing severity. Several heat-related illnesses may take the form of heat syncope, heat cramps, heat exhaustion, or heat stroke. The following are key terms used in this chapter:

1. *Heat syncope* (fainting) is a mild form of heat illness, which results from physical exertion in a hot environment. In an effort to increase heat loss, the skin blood vessels dilate to such an extent that blood flow to the brain is reduced. This reduction results in symptoms of lightheadedness, dizziness, headache, increased pulse rate, restlessness, nausea, vomiting, and possibly even a brief loss of consciousness. Inadequate fluid replacement, which leads to dehydration, contributes significantly to the problem.
2. *Heat cramps* are painful sustained muscle contractions, most often in the legs or abdominal wall, primarily due to inadequate circulation, dehydration, hyponatremia, and muscle fatigue. Heat has not been shown to directly trigger cramping, and body temperature is usually normal.[5]
3. *Heat exhaustion* is a mild-to-moderate illness due to water or salt depletion (excessive sweat) resulting from exposure to high environmental heat or strenuous physical exercise. The patient may have headache, intense thirst, muscle weakness, dizziness, fainting, nausea, and visual disturbances. Core temperature may be normal or elevated but is less than 40°C. Postural hypotension may occur.
4. *Heat stroke* is a life-threatening emergency that occurs when core temperature exceeds 40°C and the patient is in hypovolemic shock and has central nervous system abnormalities such as delirium, convulsions, or coma. Exposure to environmental heat (classic heat stroke) or strenuous physical exercise (exertional heat stroke) can cause heat stroke. Alternatively, it can be defined as a form of hyperthermia associated with systemic inflammatory response leading to a syndrome of multiorgan dysfunction in which encephalopathy predominates.[4]
5. *Exertional heat stroke* develops in the setting of recreational or occupational exercise. It results from heat production by muscular work, which exceeds the body's ability to dissipate it.

6. *Classic heat stroke* develops in the setting of high ambient temperature. The term *nonexertional heat stroke* has also been used to describe classic high ambient temperature heat stroke.

7. *Heat index* is a measure of the effect of combined elements (eg, heat and humidity) on the body.

8. *A heat wave* is 3 or more consecutive days of air temperatures >90°F (≥32.2°C).

9. *Heat-related death:* A death in which exposure to high ambient temperature either caused the death or significantly contributed to it.[6] Because death rates from other causes (eg, cardiovascular and respiratory disease) increase during heat waves, deaths classified as caused by hyperthermia represent only a portion of heat-related death.

Epidemiology

Excessive heat is the second largest contributor to death by natural events in the United States.[7] From 1999 to 2003, an annual average of 688 deaths in the United States was attributable to "excessive heat exposure." Persons aged 15 years and younger accounted for 7% of deaths caused by weather conditions.[8] There is a significant increase in heat-related death rate during heat waves. For example, in 1980, a year with a record heat wave, the death rate was more than three times higher than that for any other year during the 19-year period of 1979 to 1997.[9] Data on heat-related death are imprecise because this condition is underdiagnosed, its definition varies,[4] and many cases of patients with near-fatal heat stroke who survive the acute hospitalization have a high 1-year death rate.[10] There is statistically significant correlation between the number of heat stress illness hospitalizations and the average monthly maximum temperature/heat index.[11] In Saudi Arabia, where the temperature is extremely hot, the incidence of heat stroke varies seasonally, from 22 to 250 cases per 100,000 population.[12] Heat-related illness is reported from subtropical and cold parts of the world as well. In Taiwan, a subtropical country without any history of heat waves, a cluster of heat shock cases was reported during periods of sustained hotter-than-average temperatures.[13] In an observational study in which cold and hot areas in Europe were compared, it was shown that heat-related death started at higher temperatures in hot regions than in cold ones.[14] High ambient temperature and humidity, lack of acclimatization, unavailability of air conditioning, and vigorous physical activity are major predisposing factors for heat-related illness.[15] Within the pediatric population, children younger than 2 years are at higher risk, with specific factors like diarrheal disease, sweat gland dysfunction, child neglect, and underlying chronic or febrile illness contributing. Children left unattended in parked vehicles remain an active problem with an average of 37 fatalities per year in the United States. The majority of cases are children younger than 2 years of age who were "forgotten" by a caregiver or had played in an unattended car.[16] Risk factors for adolescents include poor judgment that may lead to continuation of physical exertion despite warning symptoms. Alcohol and drug abuse and exposure to environmental toxins may put the adolescent at risk. Neuroleptic phenothiazines and tricyclic antidepressants, taken for medical indications; amphetamine and derivatives; marijuana and cocaine; or organophosphates, constituents of many pesticides, may all lead to heat-related illness.[17] Their effect may be due to impaired heat loss or increased heat production.[18] Lithium and fluoxetine (Prozac) may induce heat intolerance.[19]

Pathophysiology and Pathogenesis of Heat-Related Illnesses

Understanding the systemic and cellular pathophysiology of heat-related illnesses involves an appreciation of thermoregulation, physiologic alterations directly related to hyperthermia, acute phase response, and production of heat shock proteins (HSPs). For normal enzymatic and cellular function, it is essential that body core temperature be maintained within a narrow range of about 37°C ± 0.5 to 0.9°C.[17,20] The thermoregulation system, controlled by the preoptic area of the anterior hypothalamus, receives input from thermosensitive receptors in the skin and body core, compares the data with a reference level (the "set point"), and responds to an elevation of 0.3°C[17,21] with activation of heat loss mechanisms.[4,17,22]

Heat dissipation occurs by means of four mechanisms: (1) conduction to the adjacent air and objects, (2) convection through air or liquid, (3) radiation of heat energy, and (4) evaporation. Once activated by the hypothalamus, the efferent heat response is both autonomic and behavioral. Blood delivery to the body surface is increased by sympathetic discharge causing cutaneous vasodilatation. Blood flow may increase 8- to 16-fold, up to 8 L/min.[23] Thermal sweating, in response to parasympathetic discharge, can produce approximately 1 L/h/m² of body surface of sweat. Per liter of evaporated sweat, 588 kCal are lost. Secondary to cutaneous vasodilatation and sweating, blood is shunted toward the periphery and visceral perfusion is reduced, especially to the liver, kidneys, and intestines.[21] Rising core temperature will also lead to tachycardia, a high cardiac output state, and an increase in minute ventilation. When ambient temperature equals or exceeds body temperature, conduction, convection, and radiation cease to be effective. Losses of salt and water through sweating may lead to dehydration and salt depletion, resulting in impaired thermoregulation. A combination of high ambient humidity and temperature creates a particularly dangerous situation. With ambient humidity of 90% to 95%, evaporation of sweat essentially stops, and if ambient temperature reaches body temperature, the body can no longer eliminate heat.

Hyperthermia directly induces cellular injury. The severity of injury is cumulative, so exposure to a high temperature for a brief period of time may cause similar injury to an exposure to a lower temperature for a longer period of time.[24] Once extreme temperatures of 49°C to 50°C have been reached, full destruction and cell necrosis occur. At lower temperatures cell death is mainly due to apoptosis.[25]

Acclimatization

Prolonged exposure to a hot environment results in adaptation and tolerance to higher temperature levels. Acclimatization to heat may take several weeks and involves multiple organs. Sweat glands develop increased capacity to secrete sweat, plasma volume is increased, and the renin-angiotensin-aldosterone axis is activated and leads to improved salt conservation. The adaptability of the cardiovascular system is probably the most important single determinant of one's ability to tolerate heat stress.[4,26] Even acclimatized people have definite limitations for heat tolerance. Once driven beyond a critical level, progression to a catastrophic condition may result.

Acute Phase Response

Heat stress initiates cellular acute phase responses aimed at protecting against injury and promoting tissue repair. A variety of cytokines are produced in response to heat stress. Plasma levels of both proinflammatory (tumor necrosis factor alpha [TNF-α], interleukin [IL]-1, and interferon-γ) and anti-inflammatory cytokines (IL-6, IL-10, TNF receptors p55 and p75) are elevated in patients with heat stroke.[27-32] Soluble TNF, IL-2, and IL-6 receptors are also elevated in heat stroke.[33,34] It has been shown that the severity of symptoms during heat stroke correlates well with IL-1 and IL-6 levels.[27] Progression from heat stress to heat stroke depends on the time and extent of exposure to severe environmental conditions, but the acute phase response may continue after the patient is cooled. Onset of inflammation may be local with systemic progression,[4,32] involving endothelial cell activation, release of endothelial vasoactive factors,[35] endothelial cell injury, and microvascular thrombosis.[35-37] The gastrointestinal tract may also play a role in the exaggeration of the inflammatory response. Vascular congestion, hemorrhage, thrombosis, and massive loss of surface epithelium in the jejunum were observed in a baboon model of heat stroke.[37] These changes facilitate bacterial and endotoxin translocation and release of mitochondrial DNA fragments, which contribute significantly to the systemic inflammatory response syndrome (SIRS) and multiple organ dysfunction syndrome (MODS).[38-40] Endothelial cell injury involves activation of both the coagulation and fibrinolytic systems.[41] Heat stress by itself is a procoagulation condition because it causes platelet clumping in small vessels. In addition, heat stress may mediate endotoxemia (following decreased perfusion of the viscera), elevated levels of proinflammatory cytokines, and macrophage activation (via factor VIIa), all of which are well-known inducers of coagulation. Injured endothelium plays an important role in producing and releasing both procoagulant and anticoagulant substances (eg, von Willebrand factor antigen [vWF-Ag], tissue plasminogen activator, and plasminogen activator inhibitor).[35,36] Circulating vWF-Ag, thrombomodulin, endothelin-1, nitric oxide (NO) metabolites, soluble E-selectin, and ICAM-1 (intercellular adhesion molecule 1) are elevated in heat-related illness, creating a clinical picture of disseminated intravascular coagulation (DIC).[35,42-44] Cooling patients with heat stroke reverses only part of these coagulation abnormalities.[41]

Recent studies, using a baboon model for heat stroke, provide more data on pathways of heat stroke–induced tissue injury and cell death. This model can be used to evaluate clinical changes and may be suitable to test immunomodulation therapies to improve outcome.[45]

Systemic Clinical Features

Involvement of multiple organs may be seen, to a certain degree, in heat syncope, heat cramps, and exhaustion. Heat stroke is a systemic disorder. Per definition, core temperature must exceed 40°C, and the patient exhibits hypovolemic shock and central nervous system abnormalities such as delirium, convulsions, or coma.

Central Nervous System

Neurologic dysfunction is a cardinal feature of heat stroke. Brain dysfunction is usually severe but may be subtle, manifesting only as inappropriate behavior or impaired judgment; more often, patients present with delirium or coma.[22] Seizures may occur, especially during cooling. The central nervous system is particularly vulnerable to heat, the cerebellum being most susceptible.[46] Proton magnetic resonance is a useful tool for evaluating major metabolic changes in the cerebellum after heat stroke.[47] Pyramidal dysfunction, dysphagia, mental changes, quadriparesis, extrapyramidal syndrome, and peripheral neuropathy have all been described.[22,48] No data regarding long-term neurologic outcome in children have been reported.

Cardiovascular

Cardiovascular dysfunction is a common feature of heat stroke.[49] Hypotension and shock may result from splanchnic vasoconstriction and peripheral (cutaneous) vasodilatation aimed to facilitate heat dissipation. Dehydration, combined with redistribution of blood volume, leads to reduction in venous pressure and diastolic filling.[22,49] Circulation is hyperdynamic in these patients, with tachycardia and high cardiac output.[50] Vasomotor tone may remain abnormally low, even after normal temperature and intravascular volume have been restored.

Electrocardiographic changes are common in heat stroke but are nonspecific and include rhythm disturbances (multiform PVCs, VT, and sinus tachycardia) but more frequently QT segment prolongation and ST-T changes.[51] The electrocardiogram (ECG) abnormalities are transient and typically subside with cooling but may require correction of potassium, magnesium, or calcium abnormalities.[52]

Pulmonary

The pulmonary system is not involved in early stages of heat-related illnesses. However, a high incidence (23%-25%) of acute respiratory distress syndrome (ARDS) has been reported in adult patients with heat stroke.[53] Patients with ARDS have poor prognosis, with up to 75% mortality rate. Lung involvement is part of multiple organ dysfunction syndrome and is associated with endothelial dysfunction and DIC.[53]

Renal

Elevated blood urea nitrogen (BUN) and creatinine levels are seen even in mild heat-related disease such as heat cramps.[54] Incidence of acute kidney injury ranges from 5% in classic heat stroke to 25% in exertional heat stroke.[49] Direct thermal injury, hypoperfusion, rhabdomyolysis with myoglobinuria, release of vasoactive mediators, and DIC may all contribute to renal injury.[4,22,55,56]

Gastrointestinal

Gastrointestinal involvement in heat-related disorders occurs mostly during heat stroke secondary to splanchnic vasoconstriction and gut hypoperfusion, leading to cellular injury and bacterial translocation. Gastrointestinal injury plays a significant role in the development of MODS in patients with heat stroke.[4,57,58] The importance of the gastrointestinal system in other forms of heat-related illnesses is not well studied. Jejunal injury may lead to mild to moderate diarrhea. The liver may be severely injured in heat stroke. This is a metabolically active organ and a major site of heat production. During periods of hyperthermia, liver temperature is among the highest of any organ in the body, putting it at high risk for injury.[24] Abnormal liver function tests may be seen during heat-related illnesses. Elevation of aspartate aminotransferase (AST), alanine aminotransferase (ALT), γ-glutamyl transpeptidase (γ-GT), lactate dehydrogenase (LDH), and total bilirubin has been described.[10,22,54] Patients with heat stroke demonstrate a typical rise in AST and ALT levels starting 30 minutes from onset, peaking at 48 to 72 hours following injury, with return to normal values after 10 to 14 days.[24,59] Severe liver damage is more common in exertional heat stroke. Fulminant liver failure is rare and usually carries a grave prognosis even with liver transplantation.[60]

Metabolic

Early in the course of heat injury, the most common acid-base abnormality is a mixed nonanion gap metabolic acidosis and respiratory alkalosis. Hypokalemia resulting from respiratory alkalosis, sweat losses, and renal wasting may change to hyperkalemia because of cellular potassium leak. Several hours into the injury the clinical picture changes into a predominantly metabolic acidosis caused by sustained tissue injury.[10,22,61] Hyponatremia is the most common sodium abnormality and is typically asymptomatic. Hypernatremia is rare but associated with worse outcome.[62]

Hematologic

Thrombocytopenia, prolonged clotting time, and DIC are well documented in patients with heat stroke.[4,10,22,37] The pathophysiology of DIC in patients with heat stroke has been previously discussed. Microvascular thrombosis is found in many organs of deceased heat stroke patients. Worsening coagulopathy may occur a few days after cooling. Rapid drop of hematocrit in the first 24 hours following heat stroke is a common feature. This is partially explained by rehydration but is most probably multifactorial. The red blood cell (RBC) half-life is shortened after heat stroke. In addition, RBCs are more fragile following exposure to high temperatures, leading to early removal from the circulation.[24] Hypersegmented neutrophils may be observed in peripheral blood for the first few hours following the onset of heat stroke. The cause for this phenomenon is unclear. These cells are thought to be undergoing changes associated with apoptosis.[24]

Infectious

In the early phase of heat stroke, blood cultures are negative.[63] In one adult study, 27% of patients had positive blood cultures and 25% had positive urine cultures 24 hours after heat stroke.[10] The incidence of positive findings in blood or urine cultures in the pediatric population with heat stroke is unknown.

Treatment

Rapid cooling and maintenance of organ perfusion and function are the major goals of treatment of heat stroke. Treatment should be started promptly at the scene with removing the patient from the circumstances that led to heat stroke in order to prevent further increase in core temperature.

Adherence to the basic resuscitative guidelines is required, with protection of the airway, management of breathing and monitoring for hypovolemia/shock, and appropriate fluid resuscitation. The most severely affected children have altered mental status, rising body temperature, and hypovolemic shock. After the airway is secured, the child with heat stroke should be moved to a cool environment; clothes should be removed; IV access should be obtained; and a normal saline or lactated Ringer solution bolus should be administered. Fluid resuscitation, besides ensuring organ perfusion, increases heat dissipation and lowers core temperature[64] by improving skin blood flow. Cooling should be started as early as possible with readily available methods. Prompt and appropriate (<39°C) cooling within 30 minutes yields survival rates of 90% to 100% in cases of exertional heat stroke and 40% to 85% in classic heat stroke.[65,66] The rule of "cool first, transport second" applies. This recommendation does not discount the potential for outstanding care at the hospital but rather prioritizes appropriate care in the first 30 minutes after collapse, which is critical for survival.[67-69]

Various cooling methods have been used to promote heat loss, and controversy continues regarding the best cooling technique. Cold/ice water immersion, a cooling method based on conduction, was twice as rapid in reducing the core temperature as the evaporative spray method in patients with exertional heat stroke.[70] The mechanism for this rapid cooling relates to the high thermal gradient between the skin and ice water, leading to a faster heat loss by conductance as compared with evaporation.[71] Ice water is readily available, does not require special equipment, and is suitable for both classic and exertional heat stroke. While some authors regard ice water immersion to be the most efficient cooling method,[72] others claim there is no evidence to support the superiority of any cooling technique, especially in classic heat stroke.[73,74] Critics of immersion point out that it may complicate resuscitation efforts of the comatose child who requires endotracheal intubation, mechanical ventilation, and close observation. Also, it is uncomfortable to the conscious child and may cause shivering and cutaneous vasoconstriction, which is counterproductive. Sponging the patient with ice water while massaging the body and using a fan may overcome some of these disadvantages, yet other studies have shown that keeping the skin relatively warm while allowing evaporation and convection to dissipate body heat is the most rapid way to decrease core body temperature.[75] This can be done with special cooling units,[76] but the concept of keeping the patient "wet and windy" can be easily achieved with the application of tepid water to the skin while a fan is used to keep high air flow and to maintain cool ambient temperature.[77] Hospitals located in high-risk areas may consider using special equipment, but most emergency departments and pediatric intensive care units (PICUs) may use this technique with readily available equipment.

Cooling blankets are widely used in the PICU setting. The effectiveness of this approach was evaluated in patients with fever,[78] and no data are available concerning heat stroke patients. Invasive cooling techniques including iced peritoneal lavage, as well as bladder and gastric lavage, have been suggested and investigated to some extent. Peritoneal lavage is difficult to perform and requires placement of a peritoneal catheter and trained personnel. Evidence for gastric lavage comes mostly from canine models and was found to have no advantage over evaporative cooling.[74] Recent reports of an intravascular cooling device to control body temperature found the system to be highly effective. However, there are only case reports regarding its use on patients with heat stroke, and it cannot be recommended at this point.[79,80] Antipyretics are not recommended for treatment of heat stroke.[74] These drugs lower body temperature by normalizing the elevated hypothalamic set point. In heat stroke, the elevated body temperature reflects failure of cooling mechanism rather than abnormal set point. Acetaminophen and salicylates should be avoided due to their potential to aggravate coagulopathy and hepatic injury.[73,74] Dantrolene has been used successfully for malignant hyperthermia and neuroleptic malignant syndrome. There are conflicting data regarding its effectiveness in heat stroke.[81-83] Once a core body temperature of 39°C has been achieved, active cooling may be stopped. This end point appears to be safe in terms of mortality. Unfortunately, a safe end point for long-term morbidity (particularly for neurologic outcome) has not yet been established.[73] Induced hypothermia has not been evaluated for effectiveness with heat stroke. A recent study looking at therapeutic hypothermia after out-of-hospital cardiac arrest in children showed no benefits in survival with good neurologic outcome.[84] Hence, it is highly unlikely to be beneficial in pediatric patients with heat stroke. All pediatric patients with heat stroke should be observed in the PICU, even if respiratory support is not required. Basic laboratory workup should include electrolytes (including sodium, potassium, magnesium, phosphate, and calcium), renal and liver function tests, complete blood count, creatine kinase, and coagulation studies. Urine output should be followed closely, and a urine sample should be sent for myoglobin analysis. Biomarkers of damage linked to heat-related illness are nonspecific with limited diagnostic value and accurate assessment of organ damage. High-mobility group box 1 protein (HMGB1) level at admission in patients with exertional heat stroke was found to be an indicator of the severity of illness and a useful mortality predictor.[85] As previously mentioned, patients with heat stroke may continue to deteriorate even after body temperature is normalized because of the inflammatory response. There are no specific guidelines for treating patients with heat stroke–related MODS.

Prevention is still the best treatment for heat-related illness. Whenever possible, people should acclimatize themselves to hot weather. Physical activity should be undertaken during cooler hours, and water intake should be increased. Children should never be left unattended in a closed car, especially during hot weather. Physicians' awareness and knowledge may promote diagnosis of early forms of heat-related illness, thus preventing progression to heat stroke. On a national level, a good weather forecasting system and air-conditioned shelters for vulnerable populations may decrease heat-related morbidity and death during heat waves.[86,87]

Accidental Hypothermia

Björn Gunnarsson and Christopher M.B. Heard

PEARLS

- Accidental or unintentional hypothermia is a potentially lethal complication of exposure to cold. It can occur as a result of exposure to cold air, water immersion/submersion, or snow burial.
- Risk factors include accidents, neglect, toxins, mental disorders, and violence.
- Information about the duration and severity of cold exposure, scene details, and any other associated injuries may help in the selection of the appropriate facility and rewarming methods.
- Many organ systems are affected by hypothermia. There is a marked depression of cerebral blood flow and oxygen use.
- Rescuers should initiate resuscitation on all patients with hypothermia unless a patient has a frozen chest or any other obvious nonsurvivable injury. The hallmark of rescue in all individuals with hypothermia is prevention of further heat loss, careful transport, and rewarming. Avoiding excess activity and rough movements of patients with hypothermia is important because this may precipitate cardiac dysrhythmias.
- Various techniques have been used for in-hospital resuscitation from deep hypothermia, but no controlled studies in which rewarming methods are compared exist and rigid treatment protocols cannot be recommended. Active external rewarming has been shown to be effective. Extracorporeal rewarming of blood is the preferred method, however, to resuscitate patients with hypothermia and cardiac arrest or cardiovascular instability.
- Prediction of patient outcome is difficult. The decision to terminate resuscitative efforts must be based on the unique circumstances of each case.

There is no uniform classification of accidental or unintentional hypothermia, but it can be categorized as mild (35°C–32°C), moderate (32°C–28°C), severe (<28°C), or profound (<24°C or <20°C).[1-3] The Swiss staging system of hypothermia is based on clinical findings at the scene that roughly correlate with core temperature.[4-7] The stages correspond to the four categories mentioned earlier, as well as stage V: death due to irreversible hypothermia (<13.7°C?). This is a serious and in many cases preventable health problem that can cause marked depression of bodily functions, to such degree that live victims may appear clinically dead.[3,8,9] Each organ system may be affected.[10] However, our understanding of accidental hypothermia is based largely on case reports and studies in animals, as controlled studies of serious hypothermia in humans are not available for obvious reasons.

Physiology

Humans have a high capacity to dissipate heat but a relative poor capacity to increase heat production, and they rely heavily on environmental regulation in the form of clothing and warm shelter to maintain normal body temperature. The body can compensate to a great degree for mild hypothermia. The hypothalamus sends signals that produce cutaneous vasoconstriction, increased muscle tone, and metabolic rate. When muscle tone reaches a certain level, shivering thermogenesis begins. The clinical manifestations depend on the severity, acuity, and duration of temperature reduction; the patient's age; premorbid conditions; and superimposed disease states. Children are more susceptible to hypothermia than adults because of a large surface area relative to body mass and less subcutaneous tissue. Neonates have a capacity for nonshivering thermogenesis, primarily by metabolism of brown fat; however, this is at the cost of greatly increased oxygen consumption. Neonates are therefore extremely sensitive to relatively minor deviations from a neutral thermal environment.

Central Nervous System

Cerebral oxygen requirement decreases with cooling and mentation is progressively impaired. Mild hypothermia may be associated with confusion, dysarthria, and impaired judgment.[10] Deep tendon reflexes are depressed at core temperature below 32°C because of slowed peripheral nerve conduction. As body temperature drops, many victims no longer complain of cold. Shivering thermogenesis ceases at about 31°C. Pupillary responses decline and dilated unreactive pupils may be noted at temperatures below 30°C. Victims may experience hallucinations and sometimes paradoxically remove their clothes. The electroencephalogram shows abnormal activity at temperatures less than 32°C, and at 20°C the electroencephalogram may appear consistent with brain death.[11]

Cardiovascular

The initial cardiovascular responses are vasoconstriction, tachycardia, and increased cardiac output. Further hypothermia results in decreased pacemaker and conduction velocity, causing bradycardia, heart block, and prolongation of PR, QRS, and QT intervals.[12] The myocardium becomes irritable,

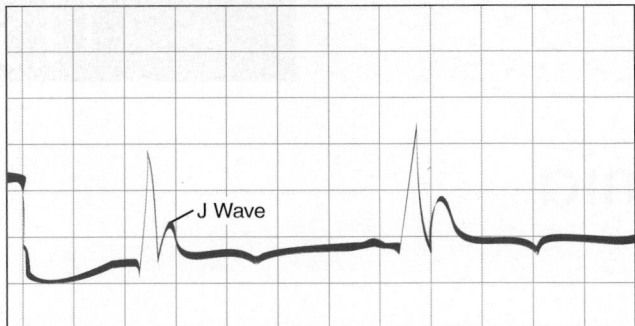

Fig. 115.1. Characteristic J or Osborne wave of hypothermia closely follows QRS. It may be mistaken for T wave with narrow QT interval if the true T wave is not appreciated. Slightly rounded peak distinguishes it from R' of bundle branch block. (From Welton D, Mattox K, Miller R, et al: Treatment of profound hypothermia. JAMA 240:2291, 1978.)

and atrial fibrillation is common when core temperature is below 32°C and the risk of ventricular arrhythmias is substantial below 30°C.[8,12,13] The electrocardiogram may show characteristic J or Osborne wave following the QRS complex (Fig. 115.1).[14-17] The presence of this wave is not pathognomonic for hypothermia and has no prognostic implications.[12,18] Myocardial contractility, cardiac output, and systemic blood pressure are often decreased dramatically in hypothermic victims. These changes may be persistent during and after rewarming.[19] Hypovolemia due to cold-induced diuresis and capillary leakage may potentiate the problem.[11,19,20]

Respiratory

Hypothermia affects tissue oxygenation through several complex physiologic mechanisms. Initially, the respiratory rate may be increased. As hypothermia worsens, the respiratory center becomes depressed and hypoventilation causes carbon dioxide retention, although the carbon dioxide production decreases with increasing hypothermia. Respiratory arrest is a late occurrence. Suppression of cough and mucociliary reflexes leads to atelectasis and pneumonia. Oxygen delivery to the tissues is further compromised by shifting of the oxyhemoglobin dissociation curve to the left.[11] Blood gas analyzers warm blood to 37°C before analysis.[21] In patients with hypothermia, arterial blood gases show higher oxygen and carbon dioxide levels and a lower pH than a patient's actual values. The best approach to interpretation is to compare the uncorrected blood gas values with the normal values at 37°C (Alpha-Stat strategy).[13,22-24]

Renal

Renal injury may occur either because of hypothermia or during the rewarming process.[25] The mechanisms involved in cold diuresis may include peripheral vasoconstriction and blunted response to antidiuretic hormone. Renal vasoconstriction and ischemia to the kidney may lead to oliguria and acute tubular necrosis in those with severe hypothermia. Progressive hypokalemia develops during hypothermia, probably because of the shifting of potassium from the extracellular to intracellular compartment, and significant hyperkalemia may develop during rewarming.[26,27] The electrocardiogram (ECG)

manifestation of hyperkalemia may be obscured or attenuated by hypothermia.[12] Renal replacement therapy may be required for renal failure and has also been used for rewarming.[28,29]

Coagulation

Hypothermia inhibits the intrinsic and extrinsic pathways in the clotting process. The degree of coagulopathy, however, is often underestimated because dynamic coagulation tests are generally performed at 37°C in the laboratory. Bone marrow suppression and splenic sequestration can lead to thrombocytopenia, and platelets become dysfunctional.[11,13] This leads to increased bleeding tendency, and the combination of hypothermia and trauma carries a grave prognosis.[30,31]

Treatment

The hallmark of rescue in all individuals with hypothermia is prevention of further heat loss, careful transport, and rewarming.[3,11] Wet clothes should be removed, and the individuals should be insulated and shielded from wind and cold.[5] Paying special attention to the head and neck is important because radiant heat loss from those areas can be profound.

Collapse of deeply hypothermic victims around the time of rescue may be explained by further cooling, circulatory collapse due to hypovolemia, or arrhythmias, sometimes triggered by procedures, such as central venous catheterization.[5,8,13] Sudden changes in hydrostatic conditions may contribute during extrication of victims from cold water. This has been attributed to sudden fall in blood pressure and inadequate coronary blood flow, precipitating ventricular fibrillation.[32,33] Victims should therefore be kept horizontal during rescue, if possible.[33]

Resuscitation

Detecting signs of life in patients with deep hypothermia may be difficult, and the rescuer should therefore assess breathing and then pulse for 60 seconds.[5,8] Chest compressions should be started immediately if the patient is pulseless with no detectable signs of circulation and may have to be continued for hours before extracorporeal rewarming can be started.[8,34-37] Victims in cardiac arrest have survived when resuscitation after rescue was delayed by as much as 70 minutes.[38] The advantages of endotracheal intubation outweigh the minimal risk of triggering ventricular fibrillation with the procedure. If cervical spine injury is suspected, the neutral position must be maintained with manual cervical stabilization. Care should be taken not to overventilate the patient's lungs because this can increase ventricular irritability.[39] Defibrillation can be tried up to three times for ventricular tachycardia or fibrillation. If arrhythmia is resistant to three shocks in a patient with deep hypothermia, then further defibrillation attempts should be deferred until core temperature is ≥30°C.[5,40] However, a systematic review of animal models performing resuscitation from ventricular fibrillation in severe hypothermia revealed much higher return of spontaneous circulation rates in studies administrating vasopressor medications.[41] The hypothermic heart may also have a reduced response to pacing and cardioactive medications, but evidence for medication efficacy and risk of accumulation to toxic levels, if administered repeatedly, is limited and based mainly on animal studies.[5,41-46] The European Resuscitation Council Guidelines for Resuscitation 2015 recommend withholding resuscitation medications until the patient has been warmed to core temperature ≥30°C and doubling the interval between doses compared with normothermic patients.[5] The 2010 American Heart Association Guidelines, on the other hand, are less clear on this and conclude that it may be reasonable to consider administration of vasopressor during cardiac arrest caused by hypothermia.[9]

Rewarming

The rewarming of victims who are conscious with mild hypothermia and still able to shiver can be achieved with passive techniques (eg, blankets, wool cap, warm shelter). Active external rewarming with chemical heat packs or forced warm air can be useful in the prehospital setting to prevent further heat loss in victims with moderate hypothermia. Some researchers claim that standing and exercising immediately after rescue may be hazardous as this may accentuate core temperature afterdrop.[2] The term *core temperature afterdrop* refers to a continued decrease in core temperature with potential for clinical deterioration of a victim after rescue. There are two mechanisms behind this. One is the inevitable equilibration of temperature between the periphery and core.[47] It follows that the magnitude of afterdrop is greater if cooling is rapid because the temperature gradient between the surface and core is greater.[48] The other mechanism is increased blood flow to the cold periphery and return of cold blood to the core (convection), possibly causing cardiovascular instability.[49] Any intervention that causes increased blood flow to the periphery, including exercise, can potentially accentuate the afterdrop,

but the significance of this in the clinical management of hypothermia victims is debated.[2,3,8,47,50] However, avoidance of excessive activity and abrupt movements of any hypothermia victim seems prudent. Attempts to rewarm the victim of hypothermia should not delay transport to hospital.[5] It is difficult to rewarm hypothermic patients during transport, and no specific recommendations can be given. The use of mechanical cardiopulmonary resuscitation devices should be considered if body size fits the device, as this increases safety and may improve outcome.[5,8,34,51-53] Fig. 115.2 shows a simple triage and management algorithm, a slight modification of an algorithm in use in the Northern Norway Regional Health Authority.[54]

Several techniques have been used in-hospital for active rewarming of hemodynamically stable patients, but no controlled clinical trials in which rewarming methods are compared exist. This includes warming with forced air, warm humidified gases, warmed IV fluids (up to 42°C), and lavage of gastric, peritoneal, pleural, or bladder cavities with warmed fluids (40°C).[3] There are many reports of successful use of different techniques in children with severe hypothermia, even with cardiac arrest.[55-63] Thoracic lavage using two large chest tubes can accomplish a temperature increase of 3°C to 6°C/hour and warming with forced air (Bair Hugger) can also be quite effective (approximately 2°C/hour).[64] However, victims with a core temperature <28°C, hemodynamic instability, or cardiac arrest should be taken directly to a center capable of extracorporeal rewarming, unless trauma or other coexisting conditions mandate transport to a closer hospital.[5,6,8,24,36,65-69]

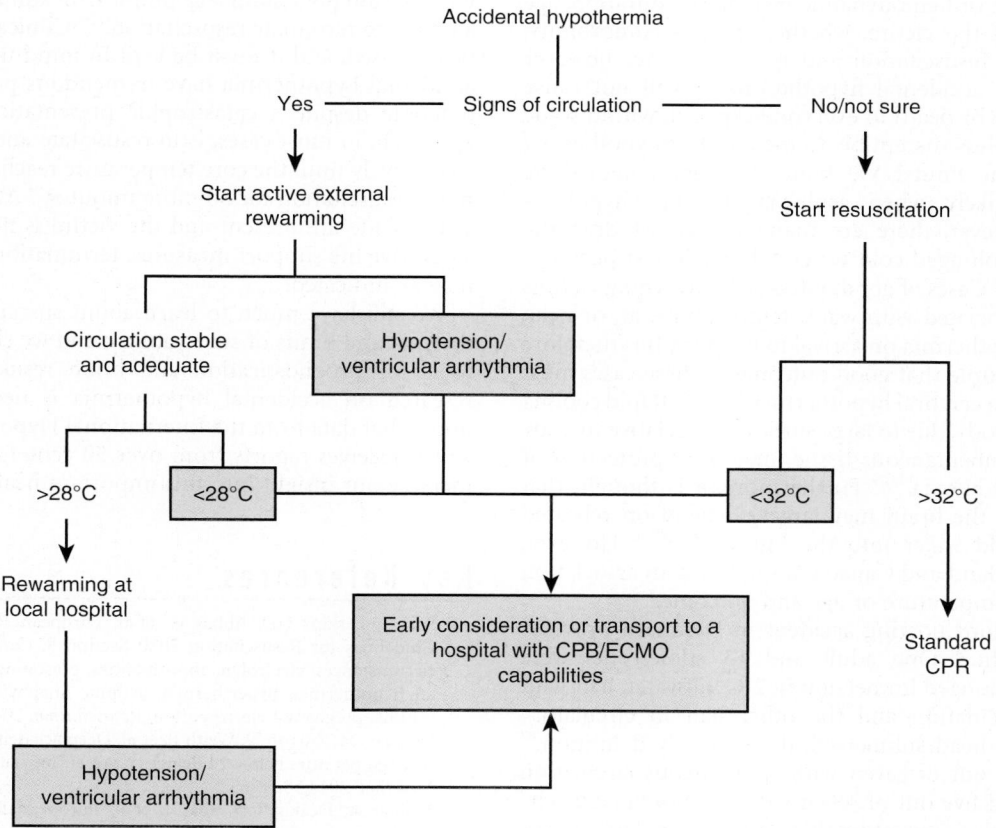

Fig. 115.2. Algorithm for management and triage of victims with accidental hypothermia.

Extracorporeal rewarming may be undertaken with traditional cardiopulmonary bypass (CPB) or venoarterial extracorporeal membrane oxygenation (VA-ECMO). The latter may be preferred as prolonged support may be necessary and outcome may be better, compared with CPB.[5,8,70,71]

There are no formal studies of care after ROSC in hypothermic victims, and management should follow usual standards.[3] Inotropic support with levosimendan or milrinone should be considered, rather than relying on β-adrenergic agents, which may have reduced effects during hypothermia and rewarming.[44,45,72] Therapeutic hypothermia for at least 24 hours may be indicated. Continuous electroencephalogram and early neuroimaging may help estimating brain injury severity, diagnose seizure activity, and detect injury requiring neurosurgical intervention.[73]

Outcome

Knowledge about epidemiology, management, and outcome is limited. It may help to apply the concept of sufficient-cause model to elucidate this problem.[74] Accidental hypothermia is frequently the cause of neurologic injury and death but by itself not a sufficient cause, as demonstrated by the fact that good neurologic recovery is possible after prolonged hypothermic cardiac arrest in adults with initial core temperature as low as 13.7°C and cardiopulmonary resuscitation up to almost 7 hours.[37,75] There are also many reports of successful resuscitation of children and adolescents with severe hypothermia.[24,58-61,63,69,76] The term *accidental hypothermia* is too imprecise. One must specify the type of accidental hypothermia (eg, exposure, immersion, or submersion), severity (eg, cardiac arrest or hemodynamic instability), duration, age and condition of the victim, whether there is comorbidity, and methods of resuscitation and rewarming. Yet however we define severe accidental hypothermia, it will not cause neurologic injury or death in everyone exposed, within some limits. So who is less susceptible to the effect of hypothermia and what are the limits? We know that good neurologic outcome is unlikely when asphyxia precedes hypothermia.[65,68,77,78] However, there are many reports of dramatic recovery after prolonged cold-water submersion of pediatric patients.[59,61,63,79-82] Cases of good outcome in drowning victims are generally associated with water temperatures at, or near, freezing and hypothermia on arrival to hospital. It is therefore reasonable to assume that good outcome in these cases must be associated with cerebral hypothermia.[22,66,81,83] Rapid cooling of the pediatric body, due to large surface area relative to body mass and little subcutaneous tissue, may offer protection of the brain against anoxia.[23,79] Furthermore, it is thought that rapid cooling of the brain may largely depend on repeated aspiration of cold water into the lungs.[32,36,66,83,84] However, reviews from Finland and Canada did not find an association between water temperature or age and outcome.[81,85,86]

The Præstø Fjord boating accident in Denmark provides important insight.[24] One adult and 13 adolescents were rescued after prolonged immersion in 2°C saltwater, half with spontaneous circulation and the other half in circulatory arrest with their head submersed, drowning by definition.[87] Interestingly, six out of seven with spontaneous circulation were females and five out of seven without spontaneous circulation were males, suggesting that females were less susceptible to profound hypothermia, despite similar fitness level

and clothing. This was likely explained by higher body fat percentage in the females, supported by the fact that mean body mass index was higher in the group that did not develop circulatory arrest. All seven with circulatory arrest were transported to the same ECMO facility with ongoing life support. Blood gas analysis revealed a median pH of 6.61 (range 6.43 to 6.94) and lactate of 21.0 mmol/L (range 9.4 to 24.0). None of the patients had hyperkalemia, and none developed multiple organ failure. All were long-term survivors, one with severe cognitive dysfunction and the other six with mild-to-moderate dysfunction. This unfortunate accident demonstrated high survivability with well-functioning chain of survival and advanced in-hospital technology. However, brain resuscitation of asphyxiated victims still has a poor prognosis.[73] Comorbidity, physical condition of victims, and course of accidental hypothermia are likely to impact outcome. Management of snow avalanche victims is outside the scope of this chapter, but it highlights the importance of asphyxia. Victims found without an air pocket have poor prognosis, whereas extracorporeal rewarming has been successful in cases where asphyxia did not predominate.[6,36,38,71,88,89]

Reported mortality and the need for prolonged organ support for victims with severe hypothermia and circulatory arrest treated with CPB or VA-ECMO vary widely.[24,36,65,66,68,69,71,90]

Systemic edema and cardiorespiratory failure may lead to death despite aggressive support.[19,71] Severe coagulopathy, acidosis (venous pH <6.5), and hyperkalemia (>10 mmol/L) are among factors that have been associated with poor outcome.[36,90-92] An admission serum potassium of 11.8 mmol/L in a 31-month-old girl with extreme hypothermia after exposure to cold weather is the highest reported value in a survivor.[76] Serum potassium >12 mmol/L on admission is probably a reason to terminate resuscitation.[8,36] Clinical judgment must be exercised, and it must be kept in mind that children with accidental hypothermia have tremendous potential for good outcome despite a catastrophic presentation. A reasonable approach, in most cases, is to resuscitate and warm the child aggressively until the core temperature reaches 32°C and continue resuscitation for 30 more minutes.[93] At that point, if no signs of life are present and the victim is not responding to aggressive life support measures, termination of resuscitation may be indicated.

We still have much to learn about susceptibility to hypothermia and limits of survivability, and we clearly need better tools for prognostication and brain resuscitation. Quality research on accidental hypothermia is necessary, and one hopes that data from the International Hypothermia Registry, which receives reports from over 50 centers worldwide, may increase our insight into this important health problem.[94]

Key References

3. Soar J, Perkins GD, Abbas G, et al. European Resuscitation Council Guidelines for Resuscitation 2010 Section 8. Cardiac arrest in special circumstances: electrolyte abnormalities, poisoning, drowning, accidental hypothermia, hyperthermia, asthma, anaphylaxis, cardiac surgery, trauma, pregnancy, electrocution. *Resuscitation*. 2010;81:1400-1433.
4. Pasquier M, Zurron N, Weith B, et al. Deep accidental hypothermia with core temperature below 24 degrees c presenting with vital signs. *High Alt Med Biol*. 2014;15:58-63.
5. Truhlar A, Deakin CD, Soar J, et al. European Resuscitation Council Guidelines for Resuscitation 2015: Section 4. Cardiac arrest in special circumstances. *Resuscitation*. 2015;95:148-201.

6. Brugger H, Durrer B, Elsensohn F, et al. Resuscitation of avalanche victims: evidence-based guidelines of the international commission for mountain emergency medicine (ICAR MEDCOM): intended for physicians and other advanced life support personnel. *Resuscitation*. 2013;84: 539-546.

7. Durrer B, Brugger H, Syme D. The medical on-site treatment of hypothermia: ICAR-MEDCOM recommendation. *High Alt Med Biol*. 2003;4: 99-103.

8. Brown DJ, Brugger H, Boyd J, Paal P. Accidental hypothermia. *N Engl J Med*. 2012;367:1930-1938.

24. Wanscher M, Agersnap L, Ravn J, et al. Outcome of accidental hypothermia with or without circulatory arrest: experience from the Danish Praesto Fjord boating accident. *Resuscitation*. 2012;83:1078-1084.

31. Shafi S, Elliott AC, Gentilello L. Is hypothermia simply a marker of shock and injury severity or an independent risk factor for mortality in trauma patients? Analysis of a large national trauma registry. *J Trauma Acute Care Surg*. 2005;59:1081-1085.

34. Gordon L, Paal P, Ellerton JA, et al. Delayed and intermittent CPR for severe accidental hypothermia. *Resuscitation*. 2015;90:46-49.

36. Hilmo J, Naesheim T, Gilbert M. "Nobody is dead until warm and dead": prolonged resuscitation is warranted in arrested hypothermic victims also in remote areas—a retrospective study from northern Norway. *Resuscitation*. 2014;85:1204-1211.

37. Gilbert M, Busund R, Skagseth A, et al. Resuscitation from accidental hypothermia of 13.7°C with circulatory arrest. *Lancet*. 2000;355: 375-376.

40. Ujhelyi MR, Sims JJ, Dubin SA, et al. Defibrillation energy requirements and electrical heterogeneity during total body hypothermia. *Crit Care Med*. 2001;29:1006-1011.

64. Plaisier BR. Thoracic lavage in accidental hypothermia with cardiac arrest—report of a case and review of the literature. *Resuscitation*. 2005; 66:99-104.

65. Farstad M, Andersen KS, Koller M-E, et al. Rewarming from accidental hypothermia by extracorporeal circulation. A retrospective study. *Eur J Cardiothorac Surg*. 2001;20:58-64.

66. Wollenek G, Honarwar N, Golej J, Marx M. Cold water submersion and cardiac arrest in treatment of severe hypothermia with cardiopulmonary bypass. *Resuscitation*. 2002;52:255-263.

67. Jarosz A, Darocha T, Kosinski S, et al. Extracorporeal membrane oxygenation in severe accidental hypothermia. *Intensive Care Med*. 2015;41:169-170.

68. Sawamoto K, Bird SB, Katayama Y, et al. Outcome from severe accidental hypothermia with cardiac arrest resuscitated with extracorporeal cardiopulmonary resuscitation. *Am J Emerg Med*. 2014;32:320-324.

69. Scaife ER, Connors RC, Morris SE, et al. An established extracorporeal membrane oxygenation protocol promotes survival in extreme hypothermia. *J Pediatr Surg*. 2007;42:2012-2016.

70. Oberhammer R, Beikircher W, Hormann C, et al. Full recovery of an avalanche victim with profound hypothermia and prolonged cardiac arrest treated by extracorporeal re-warming. *Resuscitation*. 2008;76: 474-480.

71. Ruttmann E, Weissenbacher A, Ulmer H, et al. Prolonged extracorporeal membrane oxygenation-assisted support provides improved survival in hypothermic patients with cardiocirculatory arrest. *J Thorac Cardiovasc Surg*. 2007;134:594-600.

73. Topjian AA, Berg RA, Bierens JJ, et al. Brain resuscitation in the drowning victim. *Neurocrit Care*. 2012;17:441-467.

75. Mark E, Jacobsen O, Kjerstad A, et al. Hypothermic cardiac arrest far away from the center providing rewarming with extracorporeal circulation. *Int J Emerg Med*. 2012;5:7.

76. Dobson JA, Burgess JJ. Resuscitation of severe hypothermia by extracorporeal rewarming in a child. *J Trauma*. 1996;40:483-485.

77. Kieboom JK, Verkade HJ, Burgerhof JG, et al. Outcome after resuscitation beyond 30 minutes in drowned children with cardiac arrest and hypothermia: Dutch nationwide retrospective cohort study. *BMJ*. 2015;350: h418.

78. Suominen PK, Vallila NH, Hartikainen LM, et al. Outcome of drowned hypothermic children with cardiac arrest treated with cardiopulmonary bypass. *Acta Anaesthesiol Scand*. 2010;54:1276-1281.

79. Orlowski J. Drowning, near-drowning, and ice-water submersions. *Pediatr Clin North Am*. 1987;34:75-92.

80. Gregory JS, Bergstein JM, Aprahamian C, et al. Comparison of three methods of rewarming from hypothermia: advantages of extracorporeal blood warming. *J Trauma*. 1991;31:1247-1251, discussion 51-52.

81. Biggart MJ, Bohn DJ. Effect of hypothermia and cardiac arrest on outcome of near-drowning accidents in children. *J Pediatr*. 1990;117(2 Pt 1):179-183.

82. Bolte RG, Black PG, Bowers RS, et al. The use of extracorporeal rewarming in a child submerged for 66 minutes. *JAMA*. 1988;260:377-379.

85. Suominen P, Baillie C, Korpela R, et al. Impact of age, submersion time and water temperature on outcome in near-drowning. *Resuscitation*. 2002;52:247-254.

86. Suominen PK, Korpela RE, Silfvast TG, Olkkola KT. Does water temperature affect outcome of nearly drowned children? *Resuscitation*. 1997;35:111-115.

90. Walpoth BH, Walpoth-Aslan BN, Mattle HP, et al. Outcome of survivors of accidental deep hypothermia and circulatory arrest treated with extracorporeal blood warming. *N Engl J Med*. 1997;337:1500-1505.

92. Schaller MD, Fischer AP, Perret CH. Hyperkalemia: a prognostic factor during acute severe hypothermia. *JAMA*. 1990;264:1842-1845.

93. Corneli HM. Accidental hypothermia. *Pediatr Emerg Care*. 2012;28:475-480, quiz 81-82.

94. The International Hypothermia Registry (IHR). Available from: <www.hypothermia-registry.org>; Accessed 12.01.16.

Drowning

Ajit A. Sarnaik, Mary W. Lieh-Lai, and Ashok P. Sarnaik

PEARLS

- Drowning is the process of experiencing respiratory impairment from submersion/immersion in liquid.
- Deaths from unintentional drowning have declined, but drowning remains a major cause of death in children.
- Aspiration of water and other debris during drowning can cause pneumonia and acute respiratory distress syndrome.
- In some cases, an underlying cause of drowning should be investigated, such as seizure disorder or primary cardiac illness.
- The major source of long-term morbidity for drowning survivors is neurologic, as injuries to other organ systems are generally reversible.
- The protective effect of cold water temperature in drowning victims has recently been called into question.
- Cardiopulmonary resuscitation at the scene in drowning victims should be performed in the traditional ABC sequence, as opposed to the CAB sequence.
- The outcome of drowning victims depends largely on the success of resuscitative measures at the scene of injury.

Of all the clinical entities encountered in a pediatric ICU, drowning accidents are among the most tragic. Within minutes, previously healthy children with hopeful futures die or are left severely incapacitated with no chance of meaningful cognition. The parents, once full of dreams for their children, are suddenly beset with tremendous grief and guilt because in most instances, the accident could have been prevented by simple measures.

Definitions

The definition of drowning events continues to be a great source of confusion. Although there has been some improvement in the use of appropriate terms, review of literature shows that terms such as *near drowning* and *suffocation by submersion in water* remain in use. The use of terms other than *drowning* makes it difficult to analyze and compare studies and outcome. Similar issues involving terminology and definitions existed in the resuscitation literature. These problems were addressed in 1990 by a group of investigators who met at the Utstein Abbey on the island of Mosteroy, Norway, by coming up with a standardized format for reporting of research involving out-of-hospital cardiac arrest.[1] In June 2002, the World Congress on Drowning was convened to develop a more standard definition of drowning using the

Utstein style for uniform reporting of data and to make recommendations regarding preventive measures and care. The Congress was initiated by the *Maatschappij tot Redding van Drenkelingen* (Dutch Organization to Rescue People from Drowning), an organization established in Amsterdam in 1767 to promote drowning awareness in the Netherlands.[2] The final recommendation of the Congress was to define *drowning* as the process of experiencing respiratory impairment from submersion/immersion in liquid. Immersion is defined as having face and airway covered in water, whereas submersion is defined as the entire body including the airway being underwater. The definition implies that a drowning victim develops an air-liquid interface that prevents him from breathing air. A recommendation was made to abandon all other terms such as near drowning and secondary drowning. Outcome is described according to death or survival, and survivors can be further categorized according to neurologic function.[3] Papa et al.[4] performed a systematic review of definitions for drowning accidents in 2005 and identified at least 43 publications where various definitions of drowning were used (Table 116.1). They concluded that there is a need to use a single, uniform definition of drowning and supported the one recommended by the Utstein Focus World Congress on Drowning.

Epidemiology

Deaths from unintentional drowning in United States have gradually declined from 1999–2010 according to the National Center for Health Statistics, perhaps because of greater emphasis on water safety.[5] Australia has reported a similar decline in deaths due to drowning in recent years. The greatest decline (46%) occurred in infants under the age of 1 year followed by persons aged 5 to 19 years (30%).[5] Despite these encouraging data, drowning remains a major cause of death from unintentional injury in young children. A total of 49,762 deaths from drowning occurred, with an average of 4147 deaths per year. The average annual death rate from drowning for males of 2.2 per 100,000 population was three times that for females. The death rate for males was highest among those aged 1 to 4 years. In 2013, drowning was reported as the number one cause of death from unintentional injuries (393 of 1316) in children aged 1 to 4 years. Of these, 52.2% occurred in a swimming pool.[6] Drowning is the second most common cause of death from unintentional injuries in children aged 5 to 9 years (15.5%) and in children aged 10 to 14 years (12%), second to motor vehicle accidents. While the majority of drowning deaths occurred in a swimming pool in children aged 1 to 9 years, drowning deaths in older children aged 10 to 14 years

TABLE 116.1	Summary of Categories and Terms Used to Describe Drowning
Terms	**Explanation**
Specific Categories	
Primary versus secondary	"Secondary drowning" is delayed death from drowning, due to complications, OR death occurring in minutes to days after initial recovery.
Wet versus dry/with aspiration versus without aspiration	"Dry drowning" or "without aspiration" is defined as laryngeal spasm with no or little aspiration of water OR from respiratory obstruction and asphyxia from a liquid medium. "Wet drowning" or "with aspiration" indicates that aspiration of fluids has occurred.
Warm versus cold water	"Cold water drowning" is defined as drowning in an outside body of water during the autumn, winter, and early spring months with a patient core temperature of ≤32°C on arrival to the emergency department. Some use water temperature <20°C
Salt versus freshwater	Describes kind of water in which incident occurred.
Active versus passive (or silent)	"Active" refers to a witnessed drowning event in which victim makes some motion. In "passive," victim is found motionless.
Intentional versus nonintentional	Describes cause.
Fatal versus nonfatal	Describes outcome.
With and without hospitalization	Describes whether or not victim was admitted to hospital.
Specific Circumstances	
Iceberg phenomenon	"Iceberg phenomenon" is described as people who have been submerged but have subsequently not died from drowning.
Immersion frigida	"Immersion frigida" is defined as death from cooling in water.
Immersion syndrome/ immediate disappearance syndrome	Occurs when syncope is provoked by sudden contact with water at least <5°C presumably from bradycardia, tachycardia, or arrhythmia.
Save	Rescue of victim from water by someone who perceived individual to be a potential victim of submersion injury.

From Papa L, Hoelle R, Idris A. Systematic review of definitions for drowning incidents. Resuscitation. 2005;65:255-264, Table 2, p. 260.

occurred in natural bodies of water. In 2003, the World Health Organization estimated that there were 450,000 deaths attributable to drowning each year.[7]

In 2011, Shields et al.[7] reported on drowning events in portable above-ground pools. Data were obtained from the US Consumer Product Safety Commission. There were 209 fatal and 35 nonfatal drowning cases in children younger than 12 years. Ninety-four percent of the victims were younger than 5 years of age, and 56% were boys. Portable above-ground pools pose a special risk because they are small, inexpensive, and installed by the consumer, plus they do not generate the same feeling of risks associated with in-ground pools. In some instances, water depth was as low as 2 inches (wading pools). In addition, it is uncommon to provide barriers for portable above-ground pools. Ladders cannot be moved to block access, and wading pools do not come with safety covers.

Children younger than 1 year most often drown in bathtubs, buckets, or toilets. While child abuse should be suspected in these situations, up to 35% of children between the ages of 10 and 18 months were shown to be able to climb into a bathtub.[8,9] Drowning in a bathtub should therefore not be considered as a priori evidence of child abuse. Others at risk for bathtub drowning are those with seizure disorders.[10] Drowning is highest during the summer months and on weekends. Most children who drown were last seen inside the home, in the care of one or both parents, but left unsupervised for less than 5 minutes.[11]

Other important risk factors in drowning deaths include failure to wear a life jacket and alcohol use. In 2006, the US Coast Guard reviewed reports of boating incidents. Of the 500 people who drowned, 9 out of 10 were not wearing life jackets.[12] Alcohol use is involved in up to half of adolescent and adult deaths associated with water recreation.[13] Ethanol and other neurotropic agents can diminish manual dexterity, impair judgment, and increase risk-taking behavior. Recent alcohol consumption by supervising adults may also contribute to drowning accidents involving children.[14] Expert swimmers have also been known to drown during underwater swimming. The practice of hyperventilation to prolong the duration of underwater swimming is particularly hazardous in this regard because significant hypoxemia may result in loss of consciousness before hypercarbia stimulates respiration.[15] Although an uncommon cause of drowning, arrhythmia from long QT syndrome (LQTS) should be suspected and investigated for after syncope, seizure, or cardiac arrest during or after swimming.[16]

The key to prevention includes careful supervision of children and education of the public regarding drowning prevention and the hazards of drowning. Children playing near or in water should always be supervised by a responsible adult who is not distracted by any other activity. Alcohol should be avoided before or during swimming, boating, and while supervising children. A four-sided, self-closing, self-latching fence at least 4 feet high that completely separates the house and play area of the yard should be installed around household pools. Those who are in or around natural bodies of water should wear US Coast Guard–approved life jackets irrespective of distance to be traveled, size of boat, or swimming ability.

Pathophysiologic Considerations

The sequence of events after submersion has been described by Karpovich in animal studies.[17] The drowning process has been described by the World Congress on Drowning as a continuum that begins when the victim's airway lies below the surface of the liquid (Fig. 116.1).[3] After an initial period of voluntary breath-holding, reflex laryngospasm is initiated by the presence of liquid in the oropharynx or larynx. Hypoxia, hypercarbia, and acidosis ensue and when sufficiently severe,

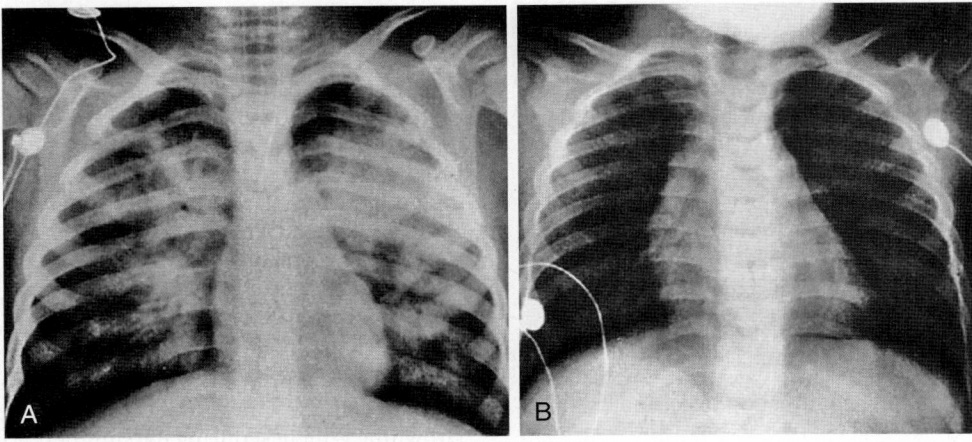

Fig. 116.1. Near drowning with and without aspiration. Radiographs show a patient with severe pulmonary edema (A) and another without significant fluid aspiration (B). (From Ciullo JV, ed. Clinics in Sports Medicine. Philadelphia: WB Saunders; 1986.)

result in lessening of laryngospasm and breathing of liquid into the lungs. The amount of liquid aspirated varies considerably among the victims. Once the liquid reaches the alveoli, a pernicious sequence develops characterized by marked disruption in pulmonary architecture and pathophysiologic alterations. These include surfactant washout, atelectasis, pulmonary edema, pulmonary hypertension, and continuing intrapulmonary shunting. The victim may be rescued at any time during the drowning process thus aborting or minimizing lung injury.

The single most important and prognostically significant consequence of drowning is decreased oxygen delivery to the tissues. A number of clinical variables determine the magnitude of hypoxia and the subject's ability to withstand it. The pathophysiology of drowning is thus closely integrated with the genesis of hypoxemia and its effects on various organ functions. A working knowledge of these pathophysiologic principles and multiorgan involvement is extremely helpful in directing therapeutic strategies for optimum survival.

Type of Aspirated Fluid

Although the differences between changes in electrolytes and blood volume after seawater and freshwater aspiration have been emphasized in the past, they are of little clinical significance in patients who survive long enough to be transported to a medical facility.[18] Aspiration of more than 11 mL of fluid per kg of body weight is required for blood volume to be altered, and aspiration of more than 22 mL/kg is necessary before significant electrolyte changes occur.[19,20] Most drowning victims aspirate less than 3 to 4 mL of fluid per kilogram of body weight. Hypervolemia resulting from freshwater aspiration is rarely a problem. Most drowning victims are hypovolemic regardless of the type of aspiration because of increased capillary permeability resulting from asphyxia and the loss of protein-rich fluid into the alveoli.

Pulmonary Effects

Functional residual capacity (FRC) is the only source of gas exchange at the pulmonary capillary level in the submerged state. Increased metabolic demands from struggling, breath-holding, a depletion of FRC from breathing efforts, and aspiration of fluid into the lungs all result in seriously compromised

O_2 uptake and CO_2 elimination, with consequent hypoxia and hypercarbia. Between 10% and 15% of drowning victims have severe laryngospasm after submersion, resulting in fatal asphyxiation without aspiration of significant water into their lungs (Fig. 116.1). A combined respiratory and metabolic acidosis caused by hypercapnia and anaerobic metabolism is often encountered. Patients without significant fluid aspiration recover from asphyxia rapidly if they are successfully resuscitated before cardiac arrest or irreversible brain damage occurs. Aspiration of fluid, however, results in persistently abnormal gas exchange. Aspiration of as little as 1 to 3 mL per kilogram body weight results in profound impairment of gas exchange.[20,21] Soon after the aspiration of fluid, there is an elevation of $PaCO_2$ and a fall in PaO_2 as a result of airway obstruction, hypoventilation, and impaired gas exchange between alveoli and pulmonary capillary blood. With adequate resuscitation, normocapnia or even hypocapnia is usually achieved while hypoxemia persists, indicating a significant ventilation/perfusion mismatch and diffusion defect leading to intrapulmonary shunting and venous admixture.[22]

The surfactant system of the lung is affected differently in freshwater and seawater aspiration.[23] Freshwater aspiration results in marked disruption of the surfactant system of the lung resulting in alveolar instability and atelectasis. Seawater, because of its hypertonicity, draws water into the alveoli. Although the surfactant may be diluted by the presence of seawater in alveoli, its surface tension properties are not significantly altered. Zhu et al.[24] examined serum levels of pulmonary surfactant-associated protein (SP-A) and lung weights in 53 victims of fatal drowning. They showed significantly heavier lungs in those who drowned in seawater versus freshwater suggesting an osmolar effect. Although they found no difference in serum SP-A, intra-alveolar aggregates of pulmonary surfactant associated protein were noted more frequently in those who drowned in freshwater. This is likely related to the disruption of surfactant noted in freshwater drowning. Karch demonstrated marked changes in the pulmonary vasculature in rabbits within 30 minutes of aspiration of both freshwater and salt water.[25] Mitochondrial swelling and disruption of pulmonary vascular endothelial cells were consistently observed in these experiments. Clinically, pulmonary abnormalities are encountered in both fresh and seawater aspiration. These are consistent with pronounced injury to alveoli and pulmonary capillaries resulting in increased membrane permeability, exudation of proteinaceous material in alveoli, pulmonary edema, decreased lung compliance, and increased airway resistance. The extent of these abnormalities may not be manifested fully for several hours after the submersion episode and may be progressive in nature. Acute respiratory distress syndrome (ARDS) is the hallmark of delayed pulmonary insufficiency resulting from aspiration in drowning. This is characterized by progression of ventilation-to-perfusion mismatch, alveolar-capillary block, increased capillary permeability, and pulmonary edema. Reduced FRC and diffusion barrier resulting from accumulation of fluid and inflammatory cells in the alveoli and interstitium further accentuate hypoxemia. Aspiration of stomach contents and other debris such as sand, mud, and algae may also impair gas exchange. Bacterial pneumonia resulting from aspiration of contaminated water may further contribute to pulmonary insufficiency. Factors that contribute to drowning-associated pneumonia include aspiration of vomitus or aspiration of contaminated material from water that may contain sewage. Water temperature plays a role, with warmer temperatures predisposing to a higher number of organisms. The chemical composition of the water such as pH, salt content, and presence of organic and inorganic substances influence bacterial growth as well. Organisms include aerobic gram-negative bacteria such as *Klebsiella* spp. and *Pseudomonas* spp. and gram-positive bacteria including *Streptococcus pneumoniae* and *Staphylococcus aureus*. Fungi such as aspergillus have been reported to cause drowning-associated pneumonia as well. The diagnosis of pneumonia is based on clinical parameters such as fever, leukocytosis, respiratory cultures, and new infiltrates on chest radiographs.

Understanding the alterations in pulmonary mechanics is important in order to provide the necessary support in the least injurious fashion. Predominant manifestations are those of ARDS complicating the drowning event. Although pulmonary involvement is often bilateral and diffuse, there is considerable inhomogeneity, with some areas more affected than others. Overall, lung compliance is reduced, necessitating higher inflation pressures to maintain adequate tidal volume (Vt). Low Vt at low FRC leads to a vicious cycle of atelectasis, decreased compliance, and further reduction in Vt. Critical opening pressure necessary to begin alveolar inflation is increased. Appropriate positive end-expiratory pressure (PEEP) needs to be administered to maintain the necessary FRC for adequate oxygenation and ventilation above the critical opening pressure. Airway resistance is relatively less affected or only minimally elevated unless there is airway obstruction from aspirated debris. Time constant, a product of compliance and resistance, reflects the time needed for pressure equilibration between the proximal airway and alveoli to occur. In ARDS, time constant is decreased, allowing for quicker approximation of pressures at these sites during the inspiratory and expiratory phases of the mechanical ventilation. Relatively large tidal volume (10–12 mL/kg) is associated with greater ventilator-induced lung injury in ARDS, whereas smaller tidal volume (6 mL/kg) is associated with less volutrauma. Because of the short time constant, prolongation of inspiratory time to improve oxygenation and increasing the respiratory rate for CO_2 elimination are often effective options during mechanical ventilation. A more detailed description of management of ARDS in drowning appears later in this chapter.

Cardiovascular Effects

Profound cardiovascular instability is often encountered after a severe drowning event, and it poses an immediate threat to survival after the initial rescue. The hypoxemia that occurs due to ventilation-perfusion mismatch can cause life-threatening dysrhythmias such as ventricular tachycardia, ventricular fibrillation, and asystole. The two determinants of oxygen delivery, namely cardiac output and arterial O_2 content, can be adversely affected by the drowning event. A decrease in PaO_2, if sufficiently severe, decreases oxygen saturation and therefore arterial O_2 content. This decrease in arterial O_2 content can cause a decrease in myocardial oxygen delivery, which contributes to worsening cardiac output and decreased myocardial perfusion pressure. Smooth muscle contraction banding in the media of major coronary arteries and local ventricular myocytes with focal myocardial necrosis have been described after a drowning episode.[26,27] Cytosolic calcium overload and oxygen-derived free radicals have also been implicated in the mechanism of myocardial injury after resuscitation after cardiac arrest.[28] Cardiogenic shock may result from hypoxic damage to the myocardium. Metabolic acidosis may further impair myocardial performance. Additionally, therapeutic application of PEEP decreases venous return and right and left ventricular preload. Right ventricular afterload is also increased by structural pulmonary microvascular damage and humoral inflammatory mediators involved in ARDS. The right ventricle is anatomically designed to tolerate increased preload, but it is not as tolerant of high pressures and afterload as the left ventricle. If pulmonary hypertension is severe enough, left ventricular preload further decreases due to right ventricular failure. These factors, as well as the excessive capillary permeability of pulmonary and systemic capillaries, result in hypovolemia and decreased left ventricular filling pressures. The end result is that of inadequate supply of oxygen to tissues to meet their metabolic demands.

Central Nervous System Effects

Due to a lack of metabolic substrate reserves, the brain depends on continuous oxygen delivery. Metabolic failure can begin within seconds after an immediate disruption in circulation. Hypoxia, if sufficiently prolonged, causes profound disturbances of central nervous system (CNS) function. The severity of brain injury depends on the magnitude and duration of hypoxemia and cerebral hypoperfusion, as well as on mechanisms of secondary brain injury. The most important components of brain-specific management include prompt rescue, early and successful resuscitation, and mitigation of secondary injuries.

Following restoration of adequate cerebral oxygen delivery after the initial hypoxemia and/or hypoperfusion after drowning, there are several mechanisms of secondary brain injury at the tissue, synaptic, and cellular level. At the tissue level, increased intracranial pressure (ICP) and alterations in cerebral blood flow can adversely impact local tissue oxygen delivery. At the synaptic level, the excitotoxic neurotransmitter glutamate can cause an imbalance in the neuronal supply and demand. Delayed neuronal death occurs due to cellular responses to hypoxia and subsequent reperfusion, leading to complex pathways of prosurvival and prodeath signals.

Intracellularly, accumulation of cytosolic calcium, neuronal energy failure associated with DNA damage and repair, and generation of oxygen free radicals can all contribute to secondary neuronal death.

Several developmental factors render the neurologic effects of pediatric cardiac arrest different from those of adults. Brain injury from sudden cardiac arrest, which more commonly occurs in adults, results when cerebral blood flow suddenly stops. In contrast, brain injury from drowning, along with most causes of pediatric cardiac arrest, is caused by asphyxia. Cerebral oxygen delivery continues for some period of time and progressively decreases because of hypoxemia and decreased cerebral blood flow. Cardiac arrest may occur but is usually preceded by this period of decreased oxygen delivery. Neurologic injury is similar to that of other causes of pediatric asphyxia, including foreign body airway obstruction, apnea, asthma, and suffocation. Approximately 13% of all children with cardiopulmonary arrest survive to hospital discharge, and only 9% if the arrest occurred outside the hospital.[29] Studies in humans and animals indicate that there are several developmental differences in excitotoxic pathways. In the neonatal period, there is increased vulnerability to NMDA receptor activation[30] and glutamate toxicity,[31] as well as heightened capability for apoptosis, which, albeit an important process of normal brain development, may render the immature brain vulnerable to neuronal loss after an insult.[32] In addition, a developmental difference exists in cerebral blood flow (CBF) after cardiac arrest. In adult models of cardiac arrest, global hyperemia is present for 15 to 30 minutes after return of spontaneous circulation (ROSC) followed by delayed hypoperfusion that persists for several hours. In an immature animal model of a brief asphyxial cardiac arrest, hyperemia is observed for 10 minutes after ROSC followed by restoration of baseline CBF, whereas prolonged cardiac arrest is followed by hypoperfusion and blood pressure–dependent CBF.[33]

Effects on Other Organ Systems

Drowning victims are at significant risk for the development of hypoxemia and/or ischemia, particularly in the face of cardiac or respiratory arrest. These factors increase the risk for multiple organ dysfunction syndrome (MODS). In addition to neurologic injury and acute lung injury, hepatic and renal injuries have been observed. Typpo and colleagues[34] reported on the incidence of multiple organ dysfunction syndrome on Day 1 in children admitted to the PICU. Of the 18% of children who developed MODS on the first day, 30% to 35% had an unfavorable neurologic outcome. In 2015, Mtaweh et al.[35] reported on the patterns of MODS in children after drowning. Pediatric Logistic Organ Dysfunction Score-1 (PELOD-1) and Pediatric Multiple Organ Dysfunction Score (P-MODS) were calculated for the first 24 hours of admission. Of the 60 children, 39 of them (65%) were in respiratory arrest and 21 of them (35%) were in cardiac arrest at the scene. Of these, 15 remained pulseless on arrival to the PICU, 6 of whom died. Seventeen of 60 patients had severe neurologic injury. Of the children who developed MODS, 52% (21/40) had cardiac arrest and 48% (19/40) had respiratory arrest. Children who suffered cardiac arrest had much more significant organ dysfunction that included neurologic, respiratory, hepatic, and renal systems. Of those children who developed acute kidney injury (3/60), one child required continuous renal replacement therapy and hemodialysis.

Mammalian Diving Reflex

A certain degree of protection against hypoxia in drowning may occur in the form of a response similar to the diving reflex observed in seals and other air-breathing diving mammals. The ability of these animals to remain submerged for periods up to 20 minutes is due to a remarkable redistribution of blood flow that occurs after diving underwater. While the heart, brain, and lungs remain adequately perfused, blood flow to tissues resistant to hypoxia (ie, gastrointestinal tract, skin, and muscle) is markedly reduced. Significant bradycardia occurs with a reduction in cardiac output. Such a response, albeit quantitatively less, is also observed in humans after total body immersion.[36] The mammalian diving reflex acts as an oxygen-conserving adaptation in response to submersion. It has been proposed that this reflex is most active in infancy and is potentiated by fear and low water temperature.[37] A combination of marked bradycardia and impalpable pulses resulting from vasoconstriction may make the victim appear dead at a time when mouth-to-mouth resuscitation could be lifesaving.[36] Clinical studies involving children and adults have failed to demonstrate an efficient diving reflex in response to cold water submersion.[38,39] Young children had a significantly decreased breath-hold duration and consequently a weaker dive response compared with older children and adults.[39] The role of the mammalian diving reflex in enabling children to withstand prolonged cold water submersion thus remains controversial.

Preexisting Associated Conditions

An underlying etiologic mechanism should be explored depending on a given clinical scenario involving unexplained drowning. Children with seizure disorders are at greater risk for submersion accidents. Similarly, an occurrence of vasovagal syncope or a hypoglycemic episode during swimming may be the underlying factor responsible for drowning. Occult cardiomyopathy or a cardiac arrhythmia should also be considered in an unexplained drowning event. An episode of drowning might be the first manifestation of long QT syndrome (LQTS). Ackerman et al.[40] studied blood samples or archived autopsy tissue samples in 35 cases of autosomal-dominant LQTS. Six of these patients had a personal history or extended family history of near drowning. All of these patients were found to have LQTS causing mutations in KVLQT1, whereas such an abnormality was found in only 3 of remaining 29 patients who did not have a personal history of submersion episode.[40] Thus swimming appears to be a gene-specific (KVLQT1) arrhythmogenic trigger for LQTS. Diagnosis of inherited LQTS allows for identification of other family members with similar affliction.[5] Yoshinaga et al.[41] showed that face immersion in cold water results in abnormal lengthening of the QT interval in children identified with nonfamilial LQTS, and such children could potentially be at risk of a life-threatening arrhythmia during swimming. More recently, Albertella et al.[16] described the presentation of outcome of water-related events in children with LQTS. Of the 10 children identified with LQTS and a documented history of water-related syncope, 9 had LQTS type 1. Seven were swimming at the time of the syncopal event. Factors leading to arrhythmias during swimming in patients with LQTS are thought to include facial immersion in cold water and the dive reflex that causes a fall in heart rate, competing with epinephrine release from exercise. Patients with LQTS should avoid swimming and diving and any medications that can prolong the QT interval. Beta blockers have been shown to reduce the risk of sudden death in LQTS by 75%.[42]

Hypothermia in Drowning

Hypothermia has been shown in numerous animal and human studies to mitigate many of the processes involved in the development of secondary brain injury from both trauma and asphyxia. Positive effects of hypothermia for the injured brain include a decrease in cerebral metabolic rate, intracranial pressure (ICP), excitotoxic neurotransmission, cytotoxic edema, generation of deleterious oxygen-derived free radicals, and the cerebral hyperemia, which can cause ischemia/reperfusion injury and further increase ICP. Potential effects of therapeutic hypothermia are discussed later in the chapter. The effects of hypothermia may apply to drowning injury, as good outcomes have been reported in children submerged in ice water (<5°C) for prolonged periods.[19,43] It appears that if hypothermia is protective in drowning, rapid cooling in ice water is necessary, as a lesser degree of hypothermia in warmer water does not offer cerebral protection.[44] It is also possible that a publication bias exists in reporting of cold water drowning, as cases with good outcome are more likely to be published than cases with poor outcome.[45] Indeed, more recent studies call into question the protective effects of hypothermia in drowning. Quan studied more than 1000 child and adult open-water drowning victims and did not find a protective effect of cold water but rather estimated submersion duration was the most powerful predictor of outcome.[46] In this study, young age was also a predictor of good outcome, which may reflect the capacity of children to become hypothermic faster and possibly benefit from its neuroprotective effects. The elderly, as well as the young, are most susceptible to hypothermia. Its protective effects notwithstanding, hypothermia by itself poses a direct threat to survival due to its adverse effects on cardiac rhythm.

Management

Because the full extent of CNS injury cannot be adequately determined immediately after the rescue, all drowning victims should receive aggressive basic and advanced life support at the site of the accident and in the emergency department (ED). It cannot be overemphasized that the major determinant of survival and maximal brain salvage is prompt and effective management of hypoxemia and acidosis. In this context, the management in the immediate postdrowning period is of paramount importance. The success or failure of cardiopulmonary resuscitation (CPR) at the site of the accident often determines the outcome.[47,48] The issue of the duration of submersion in relation to the success of resuscitation is often raised. Although asphyxia for longer than 5 minutes frequently results in significant brain injury, this should not be a consideration in deciding whether or not to initiate on-site resuscitation. The emotional excitement surrounding the accident makes it impossible to accurately estimate the duration of hypoxia.

Management at the Scene

Ensuring the adequacy of the airway, breathing, and circulation is the goal of basic life support after the initial rescue. In cases of inadequate airway and cardiopulmonary status, CPR must be instituted immediately. The fundamentals of basic life support are the same after drowning as for any other situation requiring CPR; however, some practical aspects are worth considering. Unlike the out-of-hospital cardiac arrests in adults, cardiac arrests from drowning in children are initiated by hypoxia due to disconnection of atmosphere from the airways and lungs. It is important therefore that CPR is performed in the traditional airway-breathing-circulation (ABC) rather than circulation-airway-breathing (CAB) sequence.[49] The aim of resuscitation at the scene is to prevent irreversible tissue injury from prolonged hypoxia and ischemia. The victim should be removed from the water as soon as possible. Mouth-to-mouth breathing should be performed even while in the water if it can be accomplished. Less than 0.5% of drowning victims suffer from cervical spine injuries. Cervical spine immobilization in the water is indicated when head and neck injury is strongly suspected such as in accidents involving diving, water-skiing, and surfing.[50] In such situations, the preferred airway opening maneuver is anterior displacement of the jaw, rather than extension of the neck. Chest compressions should not be attempted in water because they are ineffective and waste valuable time. Prolonged attempts to remove water from the lungs are futile and may hinder ongoing ventilatory support. Heimlich and Patrick[52] have recommended the use of subdiaphragmatic pressure in drowning victims to remove water from the airway. In addition to the fact that most drowning victims aspirate relatively small amounts of water, there is no evidence to suggest that the Heimlich maneuver can remove aspirated freshwater or pulmonary edema fluid.[48] On the other hand, such patients frequently swallow large amounts of water. Consequently, increased abdominal pressure may result in regurgitation of gastric contents into the oropharynx and aspiration into the tracheobronchial tree.[53] Any debris observed in the oropharynx should be removed before initiation of mouth-to-mouth breathing. Presence of airway obstruction caused by a foreign body should be suspected if effective chest expansion cannot be accomplished with appropriate ventilatory technique. A subdiaphragmatic thrust in such a situation would be indicated. As soon as the equipment becomes available, ventilation with 100% oxygen via bag-valve-mask device should be initiated for patients who are not breathing adequately. Pressure used during resuscitation to inflate the lungs of drowning victims may have to be higher than anticipated because of reduced compliance of the edematous lungs. A PEEP valve should be used if available. Overinflation should be avoided, however, because this can lead to pulmonary barotrauma and overdistention of the stomach with regurgitation and aspiration of gastric contents. In patients who are too obtunded to maintain airway protection, who exhibit hypoxia, or who are otherwise unable to maintain oxygenation despite bag-valve-mask ventilation, endotracheal intubation should be performed. Pulse oximetry provides valuable information, especially during transport of such patients. An automatic external defibrillator device (AED), if available, should be applied if return of spontaneous circulation is not accomplished with standard measures.

Emergency Department Evaluation and Stabilization

As with any form of accidental injury, other forms of associated trauma must be considered. Children who slip and fall into the pool may sustain external head injury such as abrasions, lacerations, and contusions. Occasionally, profuse bleeding from scalp lacerations may be sufficient to aggravate hypovolemic shock. In bathtub drowning, or in instances where child abuse is suspected, fractures and other evidence of previous injury should be looked for. In adolescent victims, drowning is frequently associated with illicit drug or alcohol use. When appropriate, urine and blood toxicology tests should be performed. Spinal injuries should be suspected in diving, water-skiing, and surfing accidents involving young adults.[48]

The need for hospitalization should be determined by the severity of the drowning episode and clinical evaluation. All patients with a history of drowning should be observed in the ED for at least 4 to 6 hours. Those with insignificant history and normal physical examination may be treated safely as outpatients.[54] Patients with respiratory symptoms, decreased O_2 saturation indicated by pulse oximetry or blood gas determination, and altered sensorium should be hospitalized.

The extent of cerebral hypoxia can be quantified by Conn's criteria as category A (awake), category B (blunted consciousness), and category C (comatose). Category C is subclassified into C_1 (decorticate), C_2 (decerebrate), and C_3 (flaccid).[55] The Glasgow Coma Scale (GCS) has also been proposed to estimate severity of neurologic dysfunction.[56] Both the GCS and Conn's classification are helpful in determining management and judging response to therapy and for prognostication.

Maintaining adequate airway, respirations, and peripheral perfusion with continued attention to oxygenation, ventilation, and cardiac performance should take priority. Electrocardiographic monitoring and arterial blood gas determination should be performed as soon as possible. Ventricular dysrhythmias, asystole, and hypotension may be encountered during the early resuscitation phase. The standard CPR techniques also apply to the drowned child. Patients with respiratory acidosis and hypoxemia, as well as those who are unconscious with significant respiratory distress or poor respiratory efforts, require intubation and mechanical ventilation. Early use of PEEP is effective in reversing hypoxemia. Because pulmonary edema is not caused by hypervolemia in drowning, diuretics are not helpful and, in addition, may exacerbate the prevalent hypovolemia. Therefore pulmonary edema after near drowning is best treated mechanically with positive pressure breathing and PEEP rather than diuretics. Hypovolemia is commonly encountered in the early resuscitation phase. Isotonic crystalloids (20 mL/kg) or colloids (10 mL/kg) infused over 15 to 20 minutes should be used for intravascular volume expansion. Additional volume expansion can be carried out on the basis of clinical and hemodynamic status. Administration of large amounts of hypotonic fluid is contraindicated because such solutions are ineffective for intravascular volume expansion. Furthermore, the resultant decrease in serum osmolality may exacerbate cerebral edema. In the face of continued hypotension and/or impaired peripheral perfusion after appropriate intravascular volume expansion, inotropic/vasopressor support may be necessary. Central venous pressure (CVP) monitoring is extremely helpful for ongoing assessment and management of intravascular volume. Metabolic acidosis resolves with improvement of oxygenation and tissue perfusion. Radiologic studies should include a chest radiograph to determine the presence or absence of pneumothorax or pneumomediastinum. Unless head injury is suspected, computed tomography scan of the head is usually not necessary because early findings are often normal even in the face of severe hypoxic damage.[57]

Two areas of clinical care in both the ED and ICU remain unsettled: glycemic control and maintenance of body temperature. Both hypoglycemia and hyperglycemia are independent risk factors for adverse neurologic outcome. Prevention and treatment of hypoglycemia are extremely important, yet the role of tight glycemic control is debatable. It is reasonable to maintain blood sugar between 80 and 160 mg/dL. The issue of controlling body core temperature also deserves mention. Most case reports of remarkably good outcome are described in the settings of cold or icy water drowning. Benefits of therapeutic hypothermia, however, have not been proven. A recently published study showed that therapeutic hypothermia does not offer added protection compared with normothermia in pediatric out-of-hospital arrests.[58] However, there may be special considerations in drowning victims because most are relatively hypothermic at the time of rescue. After return of spontaneous circulation, a reasonable approach is to not rewarm the victim aggressively as long as the core temperature is between 32°C and 34°C. Rewarming should occur at a rate no greater than 0.5°C/hour. Hyperthermia (>37°C), on the other hand, must be prevented or treated aggressively if present.[59,60] Severe bradycardia and intense vasoconstriction associated with marked hypothermia (<32°C) may make drowning victims appear dead. However, resuscitative efforts should be continued while normalizing body temperature.

Management in the ICU

The drowning victim can suffer insults to many organ systems, including the brain, lungs, cardiovascular system, liver, and kidneys. Because the major contributor of mortality and long-term morbidity is cerebral hypoxic-ischemic injury, management in the ICU should focus on supporting these organ systems as they relate to the brain. Continued attention to oxygenation and ventilation status and cardiac performance is essential. Acute respiratory distress syndrome can occur as a result of aspiration injury, pneumonia, and surfactant deficiency or dysfunction. Pulse oximetry is readily available and provides a good indication of oxygen saturation and may especially be useful in continuous monitoring of patients who may develop pneumonia or ARDS. However, because of the nature of the oxygen-hemoglobin dissociation curve, pulse oximetry does not accurately reflect changes in PaO_2 greater than 70 mm Hg. Both hypoxemia and hyperoxemia have been associated with poor outcome after cardiac arrest. Maintenance of oxygen saturation between 94% and 98% and PaO_2 between 70 and 100 are reasonable goals. The cerebral vasculature of the injured brain is reactive to changes in $PaCO_2$. Hypercapnia increases cerebral blood volume and can raise ICP. Conversely, arterial hypocapnia decreases cerebral blood flow and therefore cerebral oxygen delivery. Thus ventilation should be titrated to achieve $PaCO_2$ around 40 torr. To monitor these effects, arterial and central venous pressure monitoring are necessary in most patients who require intensive care. A useful parameter to monitor is mixed venous oxygen saturation (SvO_2). Provided arterial oxygen content and oxygen consumption remain constant, SvO_2 is a useful indicator of changes in cardiac output.

The need for endotracheal intubation and different ventilatory strategies should be determined on an individual basis and by clinical judgment. Respiratory acidosis, PaO_2 less than

60 torr in FiO$_2$ greater than 0.5, clinical signs of impending respiratory fatigue, and depressed level of consciousness are the most common indications for mechanical ventilation. Lung injury may not peak until at least 24 hours, so weaning from mechanical ventilation should not occur before then. Early use of PEEP and supplemental oxygen are extremely effective in reversing hypoxemia.

The goal of mechanical ventilation is to provide adequate gas exchange to ensure tissue viability while minimizing the inevitable ventilator-associated injury from oxytrauma, barotrauma, volutrauma, and ineffective tracheobronchial toilet. Ventilatory strategy should take into account the major alterations in pulmonary mechanics. As noted earlier, most children who drown have decreased FRC, compliance, and time constant and increased critical opening pressure. Salutary effects of PEEP are from maintaining alveolar stability, alveolar recruitment, and increasing FRC. It stabilizes the relatively softer chest wall of a child thus minimizing chest wall recoil and further decrease in FRC. PEEP also displaces intra-alveolar water into interstitial and perilymphatic spaces, resulting in decreased venous admixture and improved compliance. Excessive PEEP can result in decreased venous return and cardiac output, pulmonary overdistention and decreased compliance, and barotrauma. Maintenance of normovolemia is an important consideration in patients receiving PEEP. Furthermore, excessive PEEP can decrease cerebral venous drainage and increase cerebral blood volume and intracranial pressure. Overdistention can also impair ventilation, and the subsequent increase in pCO$_2$ can increase ICP. Thus PEEP should be titrated to maintain lung recruitment, ventilation, and oxygenation while maintaining hemodynamics.

It is now recognized that in patients with acute lung injury and ARDS, ventilation with lower tidal volume (6 mL/kg) results in improved survival compared with those ventilated with a larger tidal volume (12 mL/kg).[61] Various ventilatory strategies may be used to minimize barotrauma in a patient with ARDS while maintaining adequate gas exchange. The underlying principle is to recruit lung volume by application of optimum PEEP to maintain FRC above the critical opening pressure and ventilate with tidal volume approximating 6 to 7 mL/kg. Both pressure-controlled and volume-controlled strategies can be used using this principle. The authors recommend pressure-controlled ventilation with a relatively low peak airway pressure and prolonged inspiration while still allowing adequate time for complete exhalation. Alternatively, pressure-regulated volume control mode can also be used to deliver a preset tidal volume with minimum possible inflation pressure. The level of PEEP can be optimized by gradual increments depending on its effects on increasing PaO$_2$/FiO$_2$ ratio. The ability of modern ventilators to display exhaled tidal volume and graphic display of flow, pressure, and volume waveforms has enabled the clinician to adjust mechanical ventilatory support according to individual alterations in pulmonary mechanics. Optimal PEEP as evidenced by improvement in dynamic compliance can be determined by measuring exhaled tidal volume at varying levels of PEEP. When PEEP exceeds critical opening pressure or the lower inflection point on the pressure/volume curve, dynamic compliance improves. Ventilatory rate, inspiratory/expiratory times, and peak airway pressures can also be adjusted according to their effects on dynamic compliance and by ascertaining the return of expiratory flow to baseline. In patients without CNS injury and

intracranial hypertension, the technique of permissive hypercapnia can be used to minimize barotrauma in a patient with ARDS. This involves using lower inflation pressures or tidal volume and accepting higher levels of PCO$_2$ as long as pH remains near normal.

High-frequency ventilation is another strategy that can be used in the management of hypoxic respiratory failure. This mode of ventilation uses a relatively high mean airway pressure while minimizing excessive fluctuations in pressures during the respiratory cycle. High-frequency ventilation is a safe and effective modality in the treatment of severe acute respiratory failure that is unresponsive to conventional mechanical ventilation.[62,63]

While extracorporeal life support (ECLS) has been used for rewarming in patients with severe hypothermia following drowning in cold water, the routine use of ECLS for the treatment of ARDS associated with drowning is less clear. The presumed benefit of ECLS is the provision of lung rest to mitigate barotrauma and oxygen toxicity in patients who do not improve despite maximum ventilatory support. Because of the paucity of reports on its use, criteria for ECLS in drowning with refractory cardiovascular or respiratory dysfunction should be similar to other disease states.

Recent studies have shown the benefits of the administration of exogenous surfactant in children with ARDS.[64] Evidence indicates disruption of surfactant, particularly in those children who drown in freshwater. Exogenous surfactant administration may be a reasonable therapeutic modality in children who develop ARDS after drowning and who have persistent pulmonary insufficiency in spite of aggressive respiratory support including high-frequency ventilation. While there are no randomized controlled trials examining the benefits of surfactant administration in patients with ARDS following drowning, there are case reports that describe improvement in oxygenation following instillation of exogenous surfactant.[65-67]

Pneumonia can occur early after a drowning injury because of the aspiration of contaminated water or endogenous organisms. However, it can be misdiagnosed early because of the radiographic appearance of water and inflammation. There is no evidence to suggest that "prophylactic" antibiotics help prevent drowning-associated pneumonia and may lead to the selection of resistant organisms.[68] Furthermore, drowning in swimming pools rarely results in pneumonia.[69] However, fulminant *S. pneumoniae* bacterial sepsis and pneumonia have been described shortly after a severe drowning injury. It is therefore reasonable to institute broad-spectrum antibiotic therapy in patients with positive sputum cultures, fever, sepsis, or severe cardiopulmonary deterioration, especially when this occurs after a period of stability.[70] The use of corticosteroids for aspiration pneumonia is probably of no benefit.[71]

Once the patient is successfully resuscitated, the severity of encephalopathy is the main determinant of mortality and morbidity from drowning. With improved techniques of cardiopulmonary support, delayed deaths resulting from pulmonary insufficiency are becoming less frequent. CNS injury is by far the most important cause of death and long-term functional impairment among the immediate survivors of drowning accidents. Measures for cerebral protection after drowning have been used by several investigators.[37,55] The emphasis of such modalities is on managing cerebral edema, controlling intracranial hypertension, and decreasing cerebral metabolic requirements, with the use of fluid restriction, diuretics, mechanical ventilation, hypothermia, steroids, barbiturates, and muscle paralysis. However, studies have failed to demonstrate beneficial effects of such therapy in improving the outcome of hypoxic encephalopathy associated with drowning.[72] Furthermore, a significant increase in infections and pulmonary insufficiency was observed in association with therapeutic hypothermia in this setting. Pentobarbital has the theoretic advantage of decreasing cerebral oxygen demand. However, induction of pentobarbital coma, although effective in controlling intracranial hypertension, has not improved the neurologic outcome of comatose children.[72-74] The role of cerebral edema and intracranial hypertension in potentiating CNS injury in otherwise salvageable children is questionable in this setting. The authors' experience suggests that significant intracranial hypertension is not commonly encountered in the early postdrowning period, whereas late, uncontrollable intracranial hypertension carries an unfavorable prognosis.[75] Additionally, satisfactory control of intracranial hypertension is not necessarily associated with improved outcome.[72,73,75] It appears that the occurrence of cerebral edema and intracranial hypertension 2 to 3 days after drowning is a reflection of the early hypoxic injury rather than a manifestation of a reversible process. Late, persistent, intracranial hypertension associated with a comatose state is of ominous significance and is almost always associated with an unfavorable outcome.[75]

The most practical tool of neuromonitoring is the standard neurologic examination. The vast majority of patients who are awake and interactive in the ED survive neurologically intact. However, deterioration is possible due to delayed neuronal loss and cerebral edema in the first several days after injury. Admission neurologic examination by itself is not predictive of outcome. Large and unreactive pupils portend a severe hypoxic ischemic injury and a poor neurologic prognosis. Components of the examination that should be performed serially include pupillary reactivity, level of consciousness, brain stem reflexes, and motor function. On the basis of cardiac arrest data, poor pupillary reactivity after 24 hours and absent motor activity at 72 hours portend a severe hypoxic ischemic injury and a poor neurologic prognosis. Currently, the routine use of ICP monitoring in children with hypoxic-ischemic encephalopathy after drowning is not recommended. The emphasis of management of a comatose child in the immediate postdrowning period should be on maintaining adequate oxygenation/ventilation, oxygen delivery, and avoidance of hypotonic fluid overload. Pathophysiologic changes from asphyxia, as well as various therapies aimed at cerebral salvage such as barbiturates and osmotic diuresis, adversely affect myocardial performance.[76] Cardiovascular support with maintenance of intravascular volume and the use of inotropic agents is often necessary to maintain optimum organ perfusion in patients who have suffered a significant hypoxic-ischemic insult.

The neuroprotective properties of hypothermia that have been extensively demonstrated in laboratory studies suggest potential merits as a therapy in some children, including victims of drowning. A randomized controlled trial of therapeutic hypothermia has shown benefits in neonatal hypoxic-ischemic encephalopathy.[77] Two randomized control trials in adult cardiac arrest showed the use of moderate hypothermia improved neurologically intact survival.[78] In the late 1970s Conn showed improvement in neurologic outcome in children who were victims of submersion injury, using "HYPER" therapy that included hypothermia, hyperventilation, neuromuscular blockade, barbiturates, and dehydration.[37] However, therapeutic hypothermia has fallen out of favor, as subsequent studies in pediatric drowning showed that not only did hypothermia not improve outcome, it increased infectious complications and only improved survival to a vegetative state.[72,79] It is possible that studies designed with a different depth and/or duration of hypothermia or rewarming procedure may yield different results. Hypothermia has been shown to decrease ICP in trauma,[80] but rebound intracranial hypertension can occur during rewarming.[81] In cases of cold water drowning, although the patient should be actively warmed to prevent arrhythmias and secondary infections, once a core body temperature of 30°C is achieved, warming should not exceed 0.5°C/hour to prevent rises in cerebral blood flow and ICP, ischemia/reperfusion injury, and fever. However, given the lack of positive randomized controlled trials in pediatric asphyxial arrest or in drowning, hypothermia cannot be strongly recommended as a therapy at this time.

Prognosis

The outcome of drowning victims depends largely on the success of resuscitative measures at the scene of injury. Survival is extremely poor among drowning victims who have sustained a cardiac arrest and comparable with other causes of out-of-hospital cardiac arrest.[82] Other markers of poor outcome in pediatric drowning victims include generalized edema[83] and respiratory arrest.[84] Patients who are successfully resuscitated and who are conscious on arrival at the hospital have an excellent chance of intact survival.[47,85,86] Some groups have suggested that the neurologic prognosis is poor if the patient arrives comatose in the ED, whether or not he or she receives aggressive "brain resuscitation" (ie, goal-directed therapy for optimization of cerebral perfusion pressure).[87] However, even children who are successfully resuscitated may have subtle neurocognitive impairment. In a review of 64 drowned and resuscitated children, 57% had neurologic dysfunction and 40% had low full-scale intelligence quotient on long-term follow-up.[88] With improvements in intensive care medicine, pulmonary injury can be successfully managed in most patients. Occurrence of cardiac arrest and length of submersion most consistently appear in the literature as negative prognostic factors in pediatric drowning. However, most existing studies on pediatric drowning are not readily generalizable because they are mostly retrospective in nature, narrow in scope, and small in subject numbers, while encompassing many years in which there is variability in patient care.[89] Therefore it is difficult to ascertain from the literature risk factors impacting outcome following pediatric drowning, let alone therapeutic options. Our experience suggests that the absence of cognitive function 72 hours after the hypoxic episode is strongly associated with either death or survival in a persistent vegetative state.[75] As previously mentioned, severe hypothermia immediately at rescue has been shown to influence outcome favorably even after prolonged submersion; however, not all hypothermic drowning victims are fortunate to escape serious neurologic damage.

A database review of 267 cases of serious pediatric drowning events in Massachusetts in 1994–2000 showed better outcome in younger age groups, females, and Hispanic children and worse outcomes in African-American children.[90] These data likely reflect differences in time to first responder arrival and suggest that prevention strategies should take into account differences in age, gender, and ethnicity.

Key References

3. Idris AH, Berg RA, Bierens J, et al. Recommended guidelines for uniform reporting of data from drowning: the "Utstein style." *Circulation*. 2003; 108:2565-2574.

4. Papa L, Hoelle R, Idris A. Systematic review of definitions for drowning incidents. *Resuscitation*. 2005;65:255-264.

5. Xu J. Unintentional drowning deaths in the United States, 1999-2010. *NCHS Data Brief*. 2014;1-8.

9. Allasio D, Fischer H. Immersion scald burns and the ability of young children to climb into a bathtub. *Pediatrics*. 2005;115:1419-1421.

12. US Coast Guard, Department of Homeland Security (US). Boating Statistics–2006 [online]. Available from URL: <www.uscgboating.org/statistics/Boating_Statistics_2006.pdf>; 2008.

14. Shaw KN, Briede CA. Submersion injuries: drowning and near-drowning. *Emerg Med Clin North Am*. 1989;7:355-370.

16. Albertella L, Crawford J, Skinner JR. Presentation and outcome of water-related events in children with long QT syndrome. *Arch Dis Child*. 2011;96:704-707.

28. Opie LH. Reperfusion injury and its pharmacologic modification. *Circulation*. 1989;80:1049-1062.

30. Johnston MV. Excitotoxicity in perinatal brain injury. *Brain Pathol*. 2005;15:234-240.

31. McDonald JW, Johnston MV. Excitatory amino acid neurotoxicity in the developing brain. *NIDA Res Monogr*. 1993;133:185-205.

33. Manole MD, Foley LM, Hitchens TK, et al. Magnetic resonance imaging assessment of regional cerebral blood flow after asphyxial cardiac arrest in immature rats. *J Cereb Blood Flow Metab*. 2009;29(1):197-205.

34. Typpo KV, Petersen NJ, Hallman DM, et al. Day 1 multiple organ dysfunction syndrome is associated with poor functional outcome and mortality in the pediatric intensive care unit. *Pediatr Crit Care Med*. 2009;10:562-570.

35. Mtaweh H, Kochanek PM, Carcillo JA, et al. Patterns of multiorgan dysfunction after pediatric drowning. *Resuscitation*. 2015;90:91-96.

36. Gooden BA. Drowning and the diving reflex in man. *Med J Aust*. 1972; 2:583-587.

37. Conn AW, Edmonds JF, Barker GA. Cerebral resuscitation in near-drowning. *Pediatr Clin North Am*. 1979;26:691-701.

40. Ackerman MJ, Tester DJ, Porter CJ. Swimming, a gene-specific arrhythmogenic trigger for inherited long QT syndrome. *Mayo Clin Proc*. 1999;74:1088-1094.

42. Goldenberg I, Moss AJ, Peterson DR, et al. Risk factors for aborted cardiac arrest and sudden cardiac death in children with the congenital long-QT syndrome. *Circulation*. 2008;117:2184-2191.

43. Orlowski JP. Drowning, near-drowning, and ice-water drowning. *JAMA*. 1988;260:390-391.

44. Quan L, Kinder D. Pediatric submersions: prehospital predictors of outcome. *Pediatrics*. 1992;90:909-913.

45. Orlowski JP. Drowning, near-drowning, and ice-water submersions. *Pediatr Clin North Am*. 1987;34:75-92.

46. Quan L, Mack CD, Schiff MA. Association of water temperature and submersion duration and drowning outcome. *Resuscitation*. 2014;85:790-794.

48. Ornato JP. The resuscitation of near-drowning victims. *JAMA*. 1986; 256:75-77.

49. Szpilman D, Bierens JJ, Handley AJ, Orlowski JP. Drowning. *N Engl J Med*. 2012;366:2102-2110.

50. Watson RS, Cummings P, Quan L, et al. Cervical spine injuries among submersion victims. *J Trauma*. 2001;51:658-662.

52. Heimlich HJ, Patrick EA. Using the Heimlich maneuver to save near-drowning victims. *Postgrad Med*. 1988;84:62-67.

53. Pearn J. Pathophysiology of drowning. *Med J Aust*. 1985;142:586-588.

54. Pratt FD, Haynes BE. Incidence of "secondary drowning" after saltwater submersion. *Ann Emerg Med*. 1986;15:1084-1087.

55. Conn AW, Montes JE, Barker GA, Edmonds JF. Cerebral salvage in near-drowning following neurological classification by triage. *Can Anaesth Soc J*. 1980;27:201-210.

57. Taylor SB, Quencer RM, Holzman BH, Naidich TP. Central nervous system anoxic-ischemic insult in children due to near-drowning. *Radiology*. 1985;156:641-646.

58. Moler FW, Silverstein FS, Holubkov R, et al. Therapeutic hypothermia after out-of-hospital cardiac arrest in children. *N Engl J Med*. 2015;372: 1898-1908.

59. Topjian AA, Berg RA, Bierens JJ, et al. Brain resuscitation in the drowning victim. *Neurocrit Care*. 2012;17:441-467.

60. Soar J, Perkins GD, Abbas G, et al. European Resuscitation Council Guidelines for Resuscitation 2010 Section 8. Cardiac arrest in special circumstances: electrolyte abnormalities, poisoning, drowning, accidental hypothermia, hyperthermia, asthma, anaphylaxis, cardiac surgery, trauma, pregnancy, electrocution. *Resuscitation*. 2010;81:1400-1433.

61. Ventilation with lower tidal volumes as compared with traditional tidal volumes for acute lung injury and the acute respiratory distress syndrome. The Acute Respiratory Distress Syndrome Network. *N Engl J Med*. 2000;342:1301-1308.

62. Arnold JH, Hanson JH, Toro-Figuero LO, et al. Prospective, randomized comparison of high-frequency oscillatory ventilation and conventional mechanical ventilation in pediatric respiratory failure. *Crit Care Med*. 1994;22:1530-1539.

63. Sarnaik AP, Meert KL, Pappas MD, et al. Predicting outcome in children with severe acute respiratory failure treated with high-frequency ventilation. *Crit Care Med*. 1996;24:1396-1402.

64. Willson DF, Zaritsky A, Bauman LA, et al. Instillation of calf lung surfactant extract (calfactant) is beneficial in pediatric acute hypoxemic respiratory failure. Members of the Mid-Atlantic Pediatric Critical Care Network. *Crit Care Med*. 1999;27:188-195.

69. van Berkel M, Bierens JJ, Lie RL, et al. Pulmonary oedema, pneumonia and mortality in submersion victims; a retrospective study in 125 patients. *Intensive Care Med*. 1996;22:101-107.

71. Oakes DD, Sherck JP, Maloney JR, Charters AC 3rd. Prognosis and management of victims of near-drowning. *J Trauma*. 1982;22:544-549.

72. Bohn DJ, Biggar WD, Smith CR, et al. Influence of hypothermia, barbiturate therapy, and intracranial pressure monitoring on morbidity and mortality after near-drowning. *Crit Care Med*. 1986;14:529-534.

75. Sarnaik AP, Preston G, Lieh-Lai M, Eisenbrey AB. Intracranial pressure and cerebral perfusion pressure in near-drowning. *Crit Care Med*. 1985;13:224-227.

76. Hildebrand CA, Hartmann AG, Arcinue EL, et al. Cardiac performance in pediatric near-drowning. *Crit Care Med*. 1988;16:331-335.

77. Shankaran S, Laptook AR, Ehrenkranz RA, et al. Whole-body hypothermia for neonates with hypoxic-ischemic encephalopathy. *N Engl J Med*. 2005;353:1574-1584.

78. Bernard SA, Gray TW, Buist MD, et al. Treatment of comatose survivors of out-of-hospital cardiac arrest with induced hypothermia. *N Engl J Med*. 2002;346:557-563.

79. Biggart MJ, Bohn DJ. Effect of hypothermia and cardiac arrest on outcome of near-drowning accidents in children. *J Pediatr*. 1990;117:179-183.

80. Tokutomi T, Miyagi T, Takeuchi Y, et al. Effect of 35 degrees C hypothermia on intracranial pressure and clinical outcome in patients with severe traumatic brain injury. *J Trauma*. 2009;66:166-173.

82. Dyson K, Morgans A, Bray J, et al. Drowning related out-of-hospital cardiac arrests: characteristics and outcomes. *Resuscitation*. 2013;84:1114-1118.

86. Peterson B. Morbidity of childhood near-drowning. *Pediatrics*. 1977;59: 364-370.

88. Suominen PK, Sutinen N, Valle S, et al. Neurocognitive long term follow-up study on drowned children. *Resuscitation*. 2014;85:1059-1064.

90. Lee LK, Mao C, Thompson KM. Demographic factors and their association with outcomes in pediatric submersion injury. *Acad Emerg Med*. 2006;13:308-313.

Burn and Inhalation Injuries

Phylicia D. Dupree, Amy T. Makley, and Richard J. Kagan

PEARLS

- The accurate estimation of the extent and depth of burn injury is crucial for appropriate resuscitation and maintenance of adequate urine output and hemodynamics.
- Early endotracheal intubation of pediatric burn patients with suspected inhalation injury is essential to reduce morbidity and mortality.
- Enteral nutrition via oral intake or postpyloric feeding tube early post burn is recommended.

Burns account for approximately 1 million injuries annually in the United States alone,[1] of which 450,000 seek medical treatment, 400,000 require hospitalization, and roughly 3400 die in fire-related accidents every year.[2] Approximately 29% of these burns occur in children younger than 16 years of age,[3] with children younger than 5 years representing 19% of reported burn cases.[2] Infants and children are a unique patient population that demonstrates increased susceptibility to death.[4] Young children have not only limited physiologic reserves but also patterns of injury that are very different from adults. Although thermal burns secondary to scald or flame are by far the most common etiologies in children and adults, injuries from chemical and electrical burns may be devastating and require early recognition and treatment. Pediatric burn diagnosis and management are complex and require the expertise of a multidisciplinary team.

With appropriate resuscitation and nutritional support, prompt recognition and management of inhalational injury, and early surgical treatment, mortality rates can be minimized.[5] This has been noted in tertiary care institutions, such as the Shriners Hospitals for Children, which focus on the treatment of pediatric burns. It is no coincidence that more than 60% of burns in the United States are admitted to 1 of 127 hospitals with specialized burn centers.[3] These centers are staffed by experienced burn and plastic surgeons working with a cadre of anesthesiologists, burn nurses, pharmacists, respiratory therapists, occupational and physical therapists, and social workers to produce optimal outcomes for pediatric patients. Although care in this specialized setting is not required for most pediatric burns, an understanding of burn pathophysiology and the principles of burn management will aid in the care of these patients by all clinicians.

Types of Burn Injuries

Scald Burns

Infants and toddlers younger than 5 years have a higher incidence of scald burns compared with older children.[6,7] In recent series, scald injuries accounted for the majority of pediatric burn admissions both globally and in the United States.[8-10] Accidental hot liquid spills account for many of these injuries, and a thorough history should include the type and consistency of the causative liquid. Compared with water and thin liquids, oil and thick soups have a higher heat capacity and are more viscous. This may translate into longer contact and higher temperatures causing greater skin and soft tissue damage. In general, water heated to a temperature of 60°C (140°F) will cause a deep burn after 5 seconds of contact; water heated to 68°C (155°F) will cause the same burn after 1 second of contact.[11] Scald burns are more likely to be associated with child abuse than other types of burn injuries.[12] Classic scald patterns consistent with child abuse include glovelike or stocking-like burns to the hands or feet and/or symmetric burns to the buttocks, legs, or perineum. Concomitant injuries including bruising, fractures, and retinal hemorrhages, as well as delays in seeking treatment or inconsistencies in the patient history, should trigger concern. These scenarios must prompt a full evaluation by social services with referral to appropriate state or government agencies regardless of the depth or extent of burn.

Thermal Burns

Thermal injury secondary to flame or contact with hot objects remains prevalent in pediatric burn injuries.[13] They account for approximately 50% of all burn admissions. Injuries from contact or flame are the most common cause of burn injury in children older than 5 years.[14] Up to 90% of injuries are minor and can be managed on an outpatient basis with good outcomes.[15] In larger burns, however, mortality is greatly influenced by the size of the burn, age of the patient, and presence or absence of concomitant inhalation injury.[5,15] The extent of soft tissue injury is greatly dependent on the duration of exposure and the presence and type of clothing material, all of which should be investigated during the initial evaluation.

Electrical Burns

Electrical burns remain rare, accounting for 2% to 3% of pediatric burns.[16] The majority of injuries involve electrical cords and outlets, with a rare minority from lightning. Most homes in the United States use alternating current (AC), which, although more efficient than direct current (DC), is more dangerous.[17] Injuries caused by AC have the potential for increased tissue damage from tetanic contractions caused by cyclic flow of electricity.[16] In addition, the "let go" threshold, the maximum current a person can grasp and "let go," is lower for children than adults.[16] Children are more susceptible to electrical injuries due to their propensity to chew on cords or insert objects into outlets. Wet or moist skin, including the mucous membranes around the mouth, has negligible resistance, and these injuries often result in considerable soft tissue trauma. Nerves, blood vessels, and muscles exhibit the least resistance, as compared with bone, fat, and tendons.[16] The clinician should be aware that lack of overt skin damage may mask more significant underlying soft tissue damage.

Chemical Burns

In 2013, the National Poison Data System reported more than 2 million poison exposures. Children younger than 3 years were involved in 35.5% of exposures, and children younger than 6 years accounted for approximately half of all exposures to poison (48.0%).[18] Household cleaning substances account for one of the top five common exposures in children 5 years or younger. Alkali drain cleaners (eg, Drano) are composed of sodium hydroxide, which causes significant tissue injury from interaction with cutaneous lipids. Initial treatment of chemical burns includes copious irrigation with tepid water for more than 15 minutes. The severity of injury is determined by not only the type and concentration of the chemical but also the duration of exposure.[19] Appropriate treatment of chemical burns never involves neutralization of the acid or base as the resultant exothermic reaction worsens tissue injury. Hydrofluoric acid burns represent a distinct clinical scenario. In addition to being a corrosive agent, fluoride causes a severe, deep liquefaction necrosis.[20] Copious irrigation will attenuate the initial chemical burn, but neutralization with calcium or magnesium is occasionally necessary to halt further necrosis. Current treatment recommendations include topical calcium and close monitoring of serum calcium levels with supplementation as needed.[21]

Blast Injury

Blast injuries are a potential cause of significant thermal injury with concomitant traumatic injuries. There have been an increasing number of pediatric blast admissions secondary to methamphetamine-related explosions.[22,23] In addition to burn injuries, these children will often display the signs and symptoms of tachycardia, agitation, irritability, and emesis secondary to methamphetamine poisoning.[22] Traditionally, blast injuries are divided into four categories: primary, secondary, tertiary, and quaternary (or miscellaneous) injuries (Table 117.1). A patient may be injured by more than one of these mechanisms.[24-26]

Most bomb-related burns cover less than 20% total body surface area (TBSA) and are often associated with additional injuries. The management of thermal burns secondary to blast injuries follows the same treatment plan as a burn injury.[24] The initial step is to stop the burning process, remove the clothing, wash the burn with tepid water, and then examine the extent of the burn. There should be a high index of suspicion of inhalation, blast lung, and chest injuries. Inhalation injury can result from the explosion's extinction of available oxygen and creation of particulate matter, smoke, superheated

TABLE 117.1 Classification of Blast Injuries

Type	Definition	Example
Primary	Injury from overpressurization force impacting the body surface	Tympanic membrane rupture, pulmonary damage, hollow viscus injury
Secondary	Injury from projectiles (bomb fragments, flying debris)	Penetrating trauma, fragmentation injuries, blunt trauma
Tertiary	Injuries from displacement of victim	Blunt/penetrating trauma, fractures, and traumatic amputation
Quaternary	All other injuries related to the blast	Burns, crush injury, asphyxia, toxic exposures, exacerbations of chronic illness

gases, and toxic byproducts.[26] Chest injuries, usually secondary to blunt force, are a common cause of death in children following an explosive blast. "Blast lung" is a direct consequence of the overpressurization wave. Signs of blast lung are usually present at the time of initial evaluation, but they have been reported as late as 48 hours after the explosion. The clinical triad of apnea, bradycardia, and hypotension characterizes blast lung injury.[26] The resuscitation of patients who sustain a thermal injury with an inhalation, blast lung, or chest injury is complicated by conflicting fluid requirements.

Depth and Extent of the Burn Injury
Normal Anatomy

The skin serves a thermoregulatory role, along with providing protection against fluid loss, mechanical damage, and infection. Divided into two distinct layers, the epidermis consists of keratinocytes, melanocytes, and Langerhans cells, all with barrier function[27] (Fig. 117.1). The dermis consists of structural proteins and cells responsible for tensile strength.[20] Additional appendages including blood vessels, hair follicles, and sweat glands are rooted in the dermis and are responsible for the regeneration of epidermal cells after superficial injury.[15] Assessment of burn depth is vital as deeper burns destroy these dermal appendages. Without skin grafting, the wounds heal from the margins of injury resulting in delayed healing, wound infection, and debilitating scars and contractures.

Superficial Burns

Traditionally, burn depth has been categorized as either first, second, third, or fourth degree. Although these terms are commonly used, division of burn depth and severity guided by the need for surgical treatment may be more clinically relevant. First-degree, or superficial, burns are characterized by erythematous changes, lack of blistering, and significant pain. Damage is isolated to part of the epidermis only, sparing the dermis and dermal structures. These burns blanch easily on examination and heal within 2 to 3 days after the damaged epidermis desquamates. This level of injury is exemplified by sun overexposure. Scarring is rare given the superficial depth.[15]

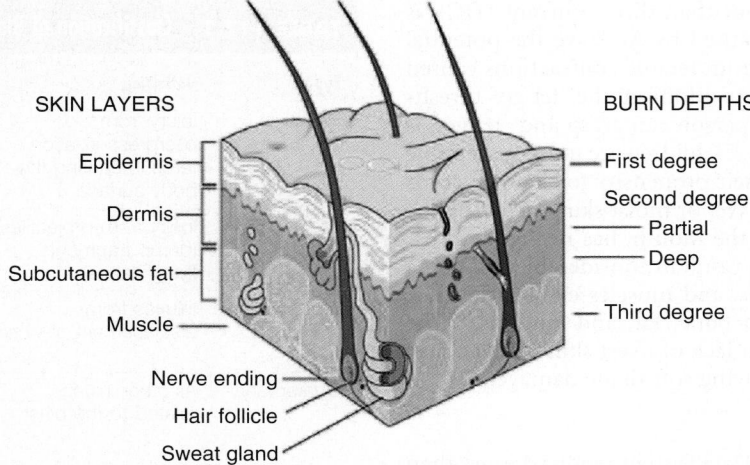

Fig. 117.1. Cross-sectional representation of normal layers of skin and subcutaneous tissue *(left)* as well as representative degrees of burn injury based on depth of burn *(right)*. (Modified from Kagan R, Peck M, Ahrenholz D, et al. Surgical management of the burn wound and use of skin substitutes: an expert panel white paper. J Burn Care Res. 2013;34:e60-79.)

Superficial Partial-Thickness Burns

Superficial partial-thickness burn wounds differ from first-degree burns in that the entire epidermis and superficial dermis are injured. These burns typically form fluid-containing blisters at the dermal-epidermal junction. After debridement, the underlying dermis is erythematous, appears wet, is painful, and blanches with pressure. As the deeper dermis is left undamaged, wounds heal within 2 weeks without the need for skin grafting, typically without hypertrophic scarring, although there may be long-term pigment changes.[15]

Deep Partial-Thickness Burns

Both superficial and deep partial-thickness burns have traditionally been classified as second-degree burns. These two categories merit distinction as deep partial-thickness burns and behave clinically similar to third-degree burns. Deep partial-thickness burns blister, but as tissue damage extends deep into the dermis, the blister base may appear to have a mottled pink and white appearance. The blood vessels of the dermis are partially damaged, giving rise to variance in discoloration of the wound base. These wounds do not easily blanch and are less painful than superficial burns due to nerve injury. Treatment of these wounds customarily requires excision and grafting. Some burn surgeons advocate initial monitoring for up to 14 days to allow for demarcation. Arguments in favor of this approach cite the need for fewer operations and less extensive grafting. Rarely, these wounds will heal without surgical intervention but remain at risk for developing hypertrophic burn scars and/or contractures.[15,27]

Full-Thickness Burns

Full-thickness burns are synonymous with third-degree injuries. These wounds are defined by complete involvement of all skin layers and require definitive surgical management. On examination, these wounds are white, cherry red, brown, or black in color and do not blanch with pressure. The burned areas are dry and often leathery compared with normal skin. Wounds are typically insensate because of superficial nerve injury. Fourth-degree burns are full-thickness injuries involving the underlying subcutaneous fat, muscle, and tendons (Fig. 117.1). These injuries are more commonly associated with limb loss and/or need for extensive reconstruction in addition to grafting.[15,27]

Zones of Injury

Burn wounds continue to evolve for days after the initial injury, and the subsequent inflammatory process may last for several months.[28] The wound is divided into zones of injury: zone of coagulation, zone of stasis, and zone of hyperemia. The zone of coagulation is easily identified, as it comprises the necrotic tissues closest to the injury site. The zone of hyperemia consists of normal, uninjured skin with a physiologic increase of blood flow in response to local tissue injury. The zone of stasis is located between the zones of coagulation and hyperemia, representing an area of ongoing injury.[20] Poor perfusion of this zone can result in the progression of initially viable tissue in this area to further necrosis and deeper wounds. Tobalem et al.[29] used an animal burn model to demonstrate that early erythropoietin administration prevented burn progression, mainly by improved vascular perfusion. Although this is not used for the treatment of pediatric burns, current research is targeting new methods to salvage these zones of intermediate injury.[30] In addition, laser Doppler imaging is currently being used to predict burn outcome on the basis of the measurement of cutaneous blood flow, targeting shorter times to excision and grafting, and subsequent decreased hospital lengths of stay.[31]

Estimating the Extent of the Burn

An accurate assessment of both the extent and depth of the burn is necessary to guide initial therapy and minimize morbidity and mortality. TBSA involvement of the burned area is an independent risk factor that correlates with length of hospital stay and mortality in pediatric burn injuries[5]; however, the extent of burn injuries may be overestimated up to 75% by the initial care provider.[32] This results in over-resuscitation with resultant devastating complications, inappropriate transfer to burn centers, and poor use of limited

Burn Estimate and Diagram
Age vs. Area

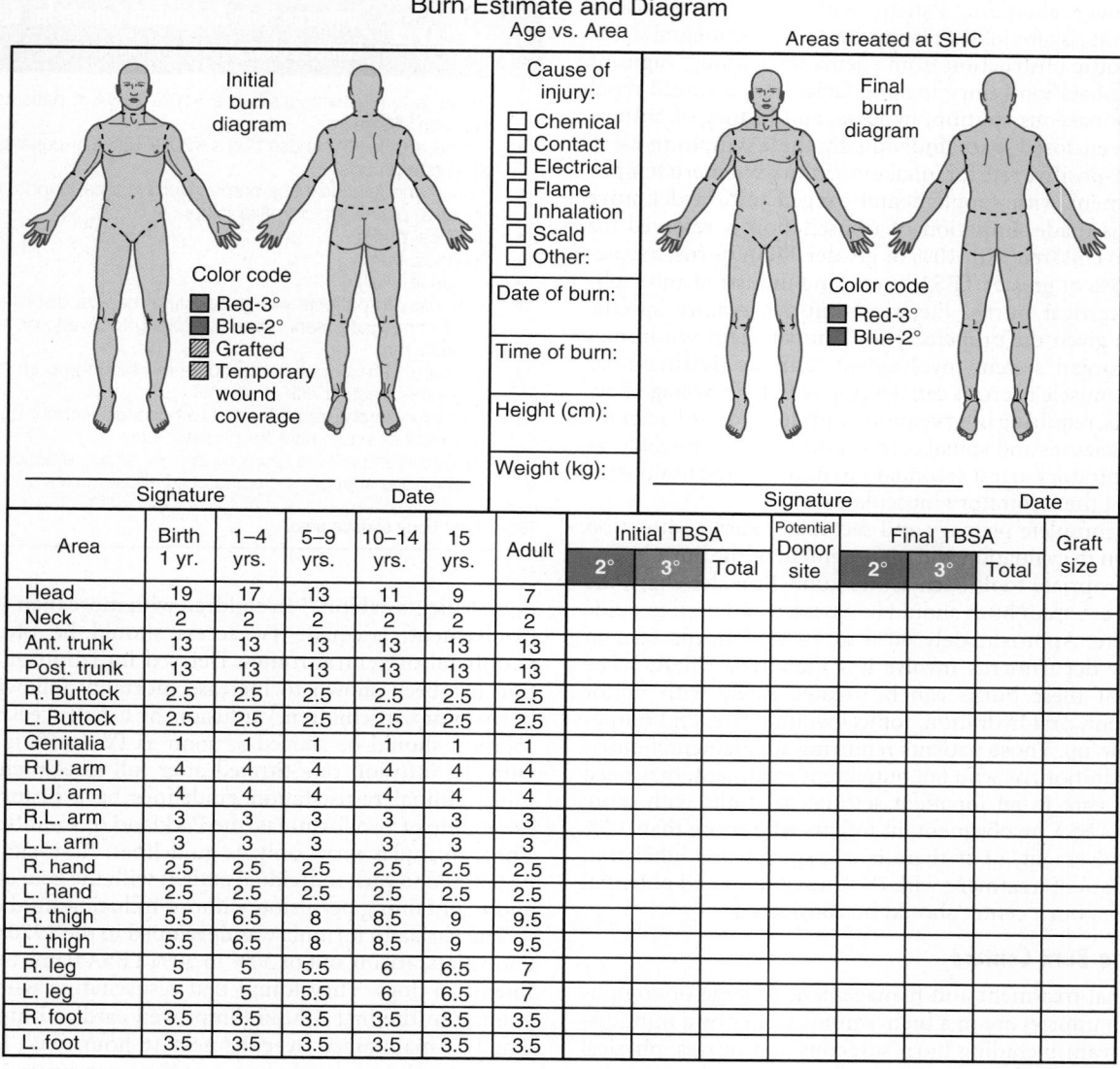

Initial burn diagram

Color code
- ■ Red-3°
- ■ Blue-2°
- ▨ Grafted
- ▨ Temporary wound coverage

Cause of injury:
- ☐ Chemical
- ☐ Contact
- ☐ Electrical
- ☐ Flame
- ☐ Inhalation
- ☐ Scald
- ☐ Other:

Date of burn:

Time of burn:

Height (cm):

Weight (kg):

Areas treated at SHC

Final burn diagram

Color code
- ■ Red-3°
- ■ Blue-2°

Signature   Date

Signature   Date

Area	Birth 1 yr.	1–4 yrs.	5–9 yrs.	10–14 yrs.	15 yrs.	Adult	Initial TBSA 2°	Initial TBSA 3°	Initial TBSA Total	Potential Donor site	Final TBSA 2°	Final TBSA 3°	Final TBSA Total	Graft size
Head	19	17	13	11	9	7								
Neck	2	2	2	2	2	2								
Ant. trunk	13	13	13	13	13	13								
Post. trunk	13	13	13	13	13	13								
R. Buttock	2.5	2.5	2.5	2.5	2.5	2.5								
L. Buttock	2.5	2.5	2.5	2.5	2.5	2.5								
Genitalia	1	1	1	1	1	1								
R.U. arm	4	4	4	4	4	4								
L.U. arm	4	4	4	4	4	4								
R.L. arm	3	3	3	3	3	3								
L.L. arm	3	3	3	3	3	3								
R. hand	2.5	2.5	2.5	2.5	2.5	2.5								
L. hand	2.5	2.5	2.5	2.5	2.5	2.5								
R. thigh	5.5	6.5	8	8.5	9	9.5								
L. thigh	5.5	6.5	8	8.5	9	9.5								
R. leg	5	5	5.5	6	6.5	7								
L. leg	5	5	5.5	6	6.5	7								
R. foot	3.5	3.5	3.5	3.5	3.5	3.5								
L. foot	3.5	3.5	3.5	3.5	3.5	3.5								

Total:

Fig. 117.2. Shriners Hospitals for Children diagram used for estimation of burn depth and extent in the acute pediatric burn patient.

resources.[33] Newer methods are being researched to improve the calculation of burn surface area using computerized imaging, two- and three-dimensional graphics, and body contour reproductions.[34]

Current methods of calculating combined second- and third-degree burn size in adults include burn diagrams, the "rule of nines," and a general estimate that the palm and fingers of one hand account for 1% of the normal body surface area.[35] Palaski and Tennison[36] developed the rule of nines, a rough estimation of adult body surface area divided into multiples of 9%. This calculation rarely underestimates TBSA but often overestimates it, especially in children.[36] Body surface area is distributed differently in children and infants due to proportionally larger heads and smaller extremities. This supports the need for age-specific surface area charts such as the Lund-Browder diagram to better estimate the extent of burn in children (Fig. 117.2).

Early Management of Burn Injuries

Successful management of the patient with burn injury begins at the scene of injury and continues in the emergency department with a thorough Advanced Trauma Life Support (ATLS) trauma assessment, as well as the American Burn Association's Advanced Burn Life Support (ABLS) assessment.[37,38] Patients must be removed from the thermal source of injury, and burns should be washed with tepid water.[38,39] Chemical burns from liquid chemicals should be flushed copiously to remove the inciting agent and prevent further tissue damage. Dry chemicals should be brushed off before any irrigation. Ice or iced water has been shown in animal studies to increase tissue damage and mortality and should not be used given the added risk of hypothermia in patients with more extensive burns.[40,41] Approximately 10% of all burn patients present with additional traumatic injuries, and the primary caregiver should not be distracted by obvious external burn injury when performing a rapid trauma evaluation.[15] Patients with severe burn shock or trauma are at risk for loss of airway due to altered mental status or supraglottic obstruction from edema formation.[42] Signs of potential inhalation injury include facial burns, singed nasal hairs, carbonaceous sputum, hypoxia, and history of entrapment in an enclosed space. Individually, these symptoms carry a high false-positive rate for inhalation injury but merit temporary treatment with supplemental oxygen until a definitive diagnosis is made. Initiation of resuscitation is reserved for infants and children with 10% or greater TBSA burns, teenagers with 15% or greater TBSA burns, and industrial and high-voltage electrical burns. Electrical injuries require specific evaluation given the propensity for compartment syndromes and multiorgan system involvement. Cardiac dysrhythmias and direct muscle necrosis can develop with high-voltage electrical burns, requiring intervention or prolonged cardiac monitoring.[16] Seizures and spinal cord transections are possible, as well as respiratory arrest secondary to injury of the brain stem or tetany of the respiratory musculature.[16]

After a complete primary and secondary survey, attention should turn to evaluation and management of the burn injury. Using appropriate tools such as the Lund-Browder chart, the depth and extent of burn should be assessed and used to guide further care. Approximately 60% to 70% of burns seen in emergency departments involve less than 10% TBSA.[14] The majority of these burns can be treated safely with minor debridement, oral hydration, topical wound care, and outpatient follow-up. Those patients requiring supplemental nutrition or hydration, or who fail outpatient treatment, may need continued care in an inpatient setting. In adults with more than 20% TBSA involvement, in infants with more than 10% TBSA involvement, or if there is a suspicion for inhalation injury, inpatient treatment with IV resuscitation and potential transfer to a burn center should be considered.

Transfer to Burn Centers

The optimal treatment and management of large or complicated burn injuries are in a high-volume center by a multidisciplinary team including burn surgeons and nurses, physical and occupational therapists, dietitians, psychiatrists, respiratory therapists, and social service support staff.[43] Current American Burn Association guidelines recommend the transfer of patients with severe injuries or those meetings specific criteria to dedicated burn centers (Table 117.2). Before transfer, airway assessment and protection, initiation of resuscitation, and evaluation for coexisting injuries should be performed.[37] Inhalation injury may go unrecognized at the initial assessment. The presence of airway injury, signs of airway obstruction, and the presence of preexisting airway abnormality should be assessed as soon as the patient arrives at the hospital.[37] Subsequently the burn wounds should be covered with clean, dry material or nonadherent gauze.[44] The use of wet dressings should be avoided to prevent development of hypothermia and subsequent complications in patients with large burn wounds.[43] Tetanus prophylaxis should be administered along with appropriate pain control before transport. In patients with extensive burns, a Foley catheter should be inserted to help guide fluid management.

Burn Resuscitation

The first 48 hours of treating pediatric burn patients are the most critical due to the burn-induced hypovolemic shock

TABLE 117.2	American Burn Association Criteria for Burn Center Referral

- Partial- and full-thickness burns >10% TBSA in patients <10 years or >50 years
- Partial- and full-thickness burns >20% TBSA in patients in other age groups
- Partial- and full-thickness burns involving face, hands, feet, genitalia, perineum, or major joints
- Electrical burns
- Chemical burns
- Inhalation injury
- Burn injury in patients with preexisting medical disorders that could complicate management, prolong recovery, or increase mortality rate
- Any burn with concomitant trauma in which the burn injury poses the greatest risk
- Burn injury in children admitted to hospitals without qualified personnel or equipment for pediatric care
- Burn injury in patients requiring special social, emotional, or rehabilitative support, including child abuse cases

TBSA, total body surface area.

these patients exhibit.[38] In children with more than 10% TBSA involvement, adequate IV access should be obtained via peripheral or central routes. Delayed initiation of resuscitation has been shown to increase mortality following severe burn injury in children.[5] Infusion of a balanced crystalloid solution should be started as soon as IV access is obtained, with the infusion rate titrated after full assessment of burn injury. Initial resuscitation guidelines have historically followed one of two formulas, the Parkland or modified Brooke. These formulas serve only as guidelines. Resuscitation must be tailored to each individual patient with the goal of restoring and maintaining perfusion without inducing fluid overload.

The Parkland formula was developed in the 1970s by Baxter and Shires, arising out of 30% to 50% TBSA flame burn experiments in dogs. They found that resuscitating with a higher volume in the first 8 hours improved cardiac output, which could be maintained over the next 16 hours with lower fluid rates. On the basis of these studies, recommendations for resuscitation of large burns using the Parkland formula were extrapolated.[45] This formula recommends the total administration of 4 mL/kg/%TBSA burn over the first 24 hours post injury. One-half of this volume is administered during the first 8 hours with the remaining volume delivered during the next 16 hours.

Although the Parkland formula is the most widely used resuscitation formula, it is closely followed by the modified Brooke formula. On the basis of the work done at the Brooke Army Burn Center, Pruitt et al. altered the original Brooke formula, which recommended 1.5 mL/kg/%TBSA burn of crystalloid and 0.5 mL/kg/%TBSA burn of colloid. This group demonstrated that a lower volume of fluid could achieve the same endpoints of resuscitation as the Parkland formula.[45] The modified Brooke formula calls for 2 mL/kg/%TBSA burn of balanced salt solution over the first 24 hours after injury and no colloids. Although both formulas call for the titration of fluid rates, in a comparative analysis, the Parkland formula more often resulted in over-resuscitation, proving to be an independent risk factor for mortality.[46] A separate comparative study found no clinical differences in outcomes between patients resuscitated using these two formulas.[47]

Consensus fluid resuscitation by standardized formula has not been reached.[45] In children, resuscitation strategies should include the administration of estimated basal fluid requirements in addition to the replacement of extensive fluid losses secondary to burn injury. Pruitt first used the term "fluid creep" to describe the insidious increase in the volume of fluid that burn centers administer in the first 24 to 48 post burn in a well-meaning effort to avoid the onset of early acute renal failure.[48] At our institution the child's basal fluid requirements (1500 mL/m² body surface area or 2000 mL/m² body surface area for children younger than 2 years) are added to the resuscitation calculated using the Parkland formula (Table 117.3). All formulas rely on the accurate assessment of extent and depth of burn in order to provide appropriate resuscitation. Fluid requirements should be titrated for clinical endpoints including urine output of 0.5 to 1 mL/kg/hr in children[46] and restoration of appropriate hemodynamic parameters.[45] Swords et al. demonstrated that nearly 20% of children arrived at the burn center without a TBSA estimation and 50% of burns were overestimated by at least 5%.[49] To avoid the complications of inadequate or excessive resuscitation, current research is being performed to examine the utility and efficacy of noninvasive computational algorithms,[50,51] as well as an invasive transcardiopulmonary thermodilution monitoring device (Pulse index Continuous Cardiac Output [PiCCO] device) to guide resuscitation.[52]

Colloid Resuscitation

The timing and use of colloid in burn resuscitation are controversial. Historically, initial resuscitation formulas called for its use in the first 24 hours after injury as an adjunct to crystalloid.[45] In pediatric patients with extensive burn injury, colloid replacement is sometimes necessary due to rapid serum protein depletion resulting in crystalloid resuscitation failure. Lawrence et al.[54] described the addition of colloid to resuscitation of severely burned patients, which rapidly eventually reduced the hourly fluid requirements, restored normal resuscitation ratios, and ameliorated fluid creep. However, previous evidence has shown that colloid resuscitation provides no long-term benefits, does not affect mortality, and is more expensive compared with crystalloid solutions.[55] The theoretic reduction in complications and mortality with colloid use has not been demonstrated in human trials.

Complications of Resuscitation

Inadequate resuscitation may result in poor perfusion to both vital organs and the evolving zone of stasis. This leads to necrosis of previously viable tissue and progression of superficial burns to deeper injuries requiring grafting.[30] The complications of fluid overload in burned patients are associated with pneumonia, bloodstream infections, acute respiratory distress syndrome (ARDS), acute respiratory failure, multiple organ failure, extremity compartment syndrome, abdominal compartment syndrome, and death.[56-60] The volume infused should be continuously titrated to avoid both over-resuscitation and under-resuscitation with little to no role for fluid bolus therapy during initial burn management.[53]

Risks for the development of compartment syndrome in the extremities, torso, or abdomen have been linked to the presence of deep, full-thickness circumferential burns, as well as the volume of fluid infused during resuscitation. Severe burn injury results in a systemic inflammatory response leading to microcirculatory leak, vasodilatation, and decreased cardiac output and contractility.[61] With tissue edema, reperfusion injury following resuscitation, and external compression from circumferential burns, compartment syndromes may develop, most commonly within the first 24 to 48 hours. Excessive fluid resuscitation increases the incidence of compartment syndrome and leads to additional complications.[59] Clinical suspicion of compartment syndrome is supported by findings of delayed capillary refill, cyanosis, paresthesia, and diminished pulses. It is imperative to make the diagnosis before the loss of pulses as this indicates long-standing compartment syndrome with a higher likelihood of muscle necrosis and nerve damage. Compartment pressures can be measured using the Intra-Compartmental Pressure Monitor (Stryker Orthopaedics, Mahwah, New Jersey, USA) or an 18-gauge needle inserted under the eschar into the subcutaneous or subfascial layer and connected to an arterial pressure transducer.[62] A pressure greater than 30 mm Hg is considered diagnostic, mandating decompression through escharotomy and/or fasciotomy. Escharotomies are performed at the bedside under sedation with electrocautery used to incise the full length of eschar down to subcutaneous fat along defined lines of incision (Fig. 117.3). Bulging of surrounding tissues demonstrates adequate decompression. Fasciotomies are generally performed in the operating room under general anesthesia. All extremity compartments must be opened with evaluation of muscle for signs of necrosis. Escharotomies and fasciotomies should only be performed by experienced practitioners due to increased morbidity from incorrectly executed procedures.[63]

Abdominal hypertension with subsequent compartment syndrome significantly decreases perfusion to vital organs including the small and large bowel, liver, and kidneys, thereby contributing to the development of multisystem organ failure.[45] Patients will often present clinically with abdominal distention and decreased urine output. In addition, decreased pulmonary compliance secondary to elevated abdominal pressures can compound respiratory challenges. The incidence of intraabdominal hypertension in patients with

TABLE 117.3	Shriners Hospital for Children–Cincinnati Resuscitation Worksheet

RESUSCITATION CALCULATIONS
I. RESUSCITATION
   A. Calculated resuscitation and basal requirement
     (4 mL × _____ kg × _____%TBSA) + (*1500 mL ×
     _____m²) =_____ mL/24 hours
     (_____ + _____) = _____mL/24 hours
   B. Resuscitation fluid per 8 hours
     1ˢᵗ 8 hours _____mL, _____mL/hour
     2ⁿᵈ 8 hours _____mL, _____mL/hour
     3ʳᵈ 8 hours _____mL, _____mL/hour
II. MAINTENANCE FLUIDS
   A. Basal fluid requirement
     *1500 mL × _____m² = _____mL/hour
   B. Evaporative water loss
     If child ≥20 kg – (25 + %TBSA) m² = mL/hour
     If child <20 kg – (35 + %TBSA) m² = mL/hour
     (_____ + _____ %TBSA) _____m² = _____mL/hour
   C. Total maintenance fluid = basal fluid requirement + evaporative water loss
     (_____ + _____) = _____mL/hour

*1500 mL if child >2 years old; 2000 mL if child ≤2 years old.

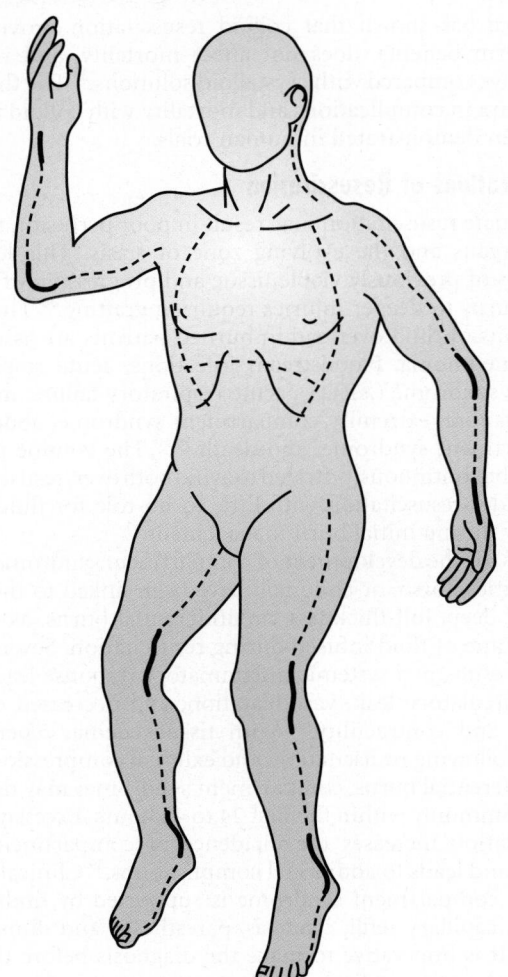

Fig. 117.3. Recommended lines of incision for escharotomies of the extremities and torso.

extensive burns is approximately 70%, with up to 20% of those identified requiring decompressive laparotomy.[61] Preventive measures to avoid abdominal compartment syndrome include appropriate titration of resuscitation fluid, as well as early recognition of abdominal hypertension through serial bladder pressure evaluations.[64] Timely decompressive laparotomy should be performed at the onset of increased compartment pressures to avoid significantly increased morbidity and mortality related to fluid loss with an open abdomen. In small children, percutaneous drainage using peritoneal dialysis catheters may be an effective alternative to laparotomy provided that the increased intraabdominal pressure is related to fluid accumulation and not organ edema. Latenser et al.[65] in a pilot study compared percutaneous drainage with surgical decompressive laparotomy in adult and pediatric patients with greater than 40% TBSA burns. They concluded that percutaneous drainage is safe and effective as a decompression modality for decreasing intraabdominal hypertension and preventing acute compartment syndrome in patients with less than 80% TBSA burns.[66] The development of pulmonary complications including acute lung injury (ALI), pulmonary edema, and ARDS has been attributed to excessive fluid resuscitation.[67] In the absence of inhalation injury, the systemic

inflammation seen after severe burn injury results in third spacing of fluids and accumulation of interstitial edema in the lungs. The treatment of this immune response remains challenging. Alternative resuscitation strategies including the use of colloid and hypertonic saline as adjuncts to crystalloids are continually being investigated with mixed results.[67,68] Sun et al.[69] discovered, with the use of a burn model in rats, that initial resuscitation with hypertonic saline after severe burn injury decreases pulmonary edema, prevents hyponatremia, and attenuates oxidative stress but is not capable of inhibiting the systemic inflammatory response. In several series, the presence of inhalation injury results in increased resuscitation fluid requirements and is predictive of the development of respiratory failure and increased mortality.[5,15,55,70]

Inhalational Injury

The diagnosis of inhalation injury in burn patients is important as there is a clear link that exists between inhalation injury and mortality.[71] The presence of inhalation injury is the single most important risk factor for mortality, and inhalation injury is implicated in approximately 50% of all burn-related mortalities. In age-specific studies of mortality, the presence of concomitant inhalational injury increased mortality across all ages, but its effect on mortality was largest in the pediatric burn patient population.[72]

Pathophysiology of Inhalation Injury

Inhalation injury involves exposure of the upper airway to heated dry air or steam. The lower airway, consisting of the tracheobronchial tree and lung parenchyma, is rarely injured by the heated dry air because of reflexive vocal cord closure and evaporative cooling capacity, in addition to other natural defense mechanisms.[11,73] Direct thermal injury of the upper airway, however, manifests with significant inflammation and edema. Histamine release, signaled by increasing complement at the site of injury, produces reactive oxygen and nitrogen species. These reactive species increase vascular permeability leading to extrusion of fluid and increased tissue edema, which propagates pulmonary injury. Prolonged extrusion of proteinaceous exudate and associated tissue edema may result in the formation of airway casts and upper airway obstruction, similar to mucous plugging.[42,74]

Smoke and inhaled toxins pose a particular risk to both upper and lower airways. While large inhaled particles are filtered by the upper airway, both small particles (<5–10 μm) and noxious gases can reach the lower airway and cause injury.[75] Toxins such as ammonia, sulfur oxides, pyrolysates, and chlorine gas form strong alkalis and acids upon contact with the moist, mucosal walls of the upper and lower airways.[76] Fat-soluble agents, such as aromatics, activate alveolar macrophages and may initiate direct cellular damage resulting in hyperemia, which can be visible by bronchoscopy shortly after injury.[77] While water-soluble irritants cause instantaneous pain, fat-soluble agents tend to be less noxious agents and reach the distal airways more easily, bypassing natural defense mechanisms. If these inhalants induce an inflammatory response in the pulmonary parenchyma, surfactant synthesis may be disrupted with further worsening of lung compliance.[75,78] Loss of ciliary action in the respiratory mucosa can lead to increased pulmonary infections, ultimately resulting in irreparable damage to the respiratory tree.[42]

Carbon monoxide (CO) and cyanide are key components of inhalation injury in the acute burn patient, and each poses diagnostic challenges. CO is an odorless, colorless gas generated by incomplete combustion of carbon-containing materials.[75] In CO poisoning, tissue oxygenation is impaired, resulting in a range of symptoms including headache, nausea, irritability in mild intoxication, tachypnea, hypoxia, altered mental status, coma, and ultimately death.[79] These clinical signs stem from an increased affinity of CO to bind hemoglobin, resulting in carboxyhemoglobin (COHb) formation, as well as a left shift of the oxygen-hemoglobin dissociation curve, interfering with normal unloading of oxygen to tissues. Relative tissue hypoxia ensues with subsequent metabolic acidosis.[75] Hydrogen cyanide, a colorless gas with an odor described as being similar to bitter almonds, is produced by combustion of carbon and nitrogen-containing substances (ie, wool, cotton). Cyanide inhibits oxidative phosphorylation via reversible inhibition of cytochrome c oxidase. Similar to CO poisoning, cyanide poisoning produces relative tissue anoxia and metabolic acidosis.[80]

Diagnosis of Inhalation Injury

The diagnosis of inhalation injury begins with a focused history and physical examination. The mechanism of injury provides a strong indication of risk in the pediatric burn patient. Closed-space burns involving steam, combustibles, hot gases, or explosions should alert the treating physician to possible airway injury. Clinicians should be cognizant that inhalation injury may occur without evidence of cutaneous burns. The physical examination should include inspection for soot in the oropharynx, carbonaceous sputum, singed nasal or facial hairs, and burns involving the face or neck. These signs taken individually have a high false positive in the diagnosis of inhalational injury but should raise clinical suspicion.[42] Impending respiratory distress may manifest as wheezing, stridor, tachypnea or hoarseness, along with depressed mental status, agitation, or anxiety. Many pediatric patients with inhalation injury will develop progressive respiratory failure, tachypnea, hypoxia, and cyanosis after resuscitation, even when appearing normal upon initial presentation.

In addition to the nonspecific clinical signs and symptoms of inhalational injury, noninvasive monitoring of pulse oximetry in burn patients can be misleading. For this reason, laboratory and invasive studies are pertinent to diagnosis. Initial laboratory studies should include arterial blood gas (ABG) analysis and measurement of carboxyhemoglobin (COHb). The partial pressure of oxygen in arterial blood to the fraction of inspired oxygen (PaO_2/FiO_2) ratio of less than 300 is indicative of significant inhalation injury, with early evidence of ALI.[81] Albeit controversial, this ratio has been proposed as an indicator of poor outcome in burn patients.[82,83] For suspected CO poisoning, COHb values should be drawn and correlated with time from injury. At sea level, when breathing room air, the half-life of CO is 240 to 320 minutes, decreasing to 30 to 40 minutes when breathing 100% oxygen.[84] The half-life of CO falls to 20 minutes when exposed to hyperbaric oxygen conditions; however, there is little evidence for the use of hyperbaric oxygen for treatment of CO poisoning. Given the potential risks of hyperbaric oxygen including barotrauma and inability to access critically ill patients, treatment of CO poisoning with hyperbaric oxygen is not recommended. If cyanide poisoning is suspected, blood cyanide levels should be also drawn with prompt administration of antidotes.[80]

Chest radiographs and computed tomography scans are insensitive for the diagnosis due to a relatively normal lung and airway appearance early in the clinical course.[85,86] Repeat studies over time and after resuscitation may demonstrate subsequent development of pulmonary edema or ARDS. Historically, Xenon-133 scanning has been used to evaluate parenchymal injury, demonstrating trapping or delayed excretion of the radioactive isotope within injured lungs.[87] This technique is limited by its availability and technical expertise, and it is rarely used.[81] Fiberoptic bronchoscopy remains the gold standard for the diagnosis of inhalation injury. Direct visualization of the supraglottic and infraglottic airway allows quantification of hyperemia, exudate, mucosal sloughing, edema, and presence of carbonaceous material. In a study spanning a 10-year period, 71% of pediatric patients with inhalation injury were diagnosed using bronchoscopy versus 25% by history/clinical examination alone and 4% by carboxyhemoglobin levels, demonstrating that even at specialized burn centers, there remains variability in means for diagnosing inhalation injury.[71]

Management of Inhalation Injury

Inhalation injuries can quickly progress to obstruction, hypoxia, and death, so timely endotracheal intubation is required. If inhalation injury is suspected in a pediatric patient, prompt endotracheal intubation is necessary due to the small size of the airway, leading to an increased likelihood of adverse events due to early obstruction. Oxygen therapy at a FiO_2 of 1.0 should be initiated immediately to treat increased COHb levels and provide maximal oxygen delivery to peripheral tissues.[75] Duration of oxygen therapy depends on patient condition and can be quantified by documenting return of carboxyhemoglobin levels to below 10% and normalization of acidosis.[88] Continuous pulse oximetry may be reliably used after normalization of COHb levels. Inhalational injuries rapidly evolve over the first few days following injury. Acute pulmonary insufficiency may manifest in the first 24 hours, with edema peaking between 48 and 96 hours, and injury culminating in bronchopneumonia 3 to 10 days post burn. The treatment of inhalational injuries needs to be tailored accordingly and is mainly supportive, consisting of ventilator support, airway clearance, and therapeutic adjuncts.

Ventilator Support

Following endotracheal intubation, the acute burn patient with inhalation injury may benefit from alternative modes of ventilation as compared with conventional strategies. The choice of mode is dictated by patient condition, clinician and staff familiarity, and treatments required (ie, repeat bronchoscopy, inhalation agents), and when used appropriately, standard ventilator strategies may provide adequate support. In severe inhalational injury the use of high-frequency oscillatory ventilation may be beneficial, and single centers have shown early and sustained improvement in oxygenation with its use.[89] However, use of high-frequency oscillatory ventilation may limit delivery of important inhaled medications and timely serial bronchoscopy, which are important adjuncts in the treatment of inhalational injury. Volumetric diffusive respiratory (VDR) mode provides ventilation and oxygenation with a decreased mean airway pressure, reducing the risk of barotrauma (Fig. 117.4). VDR mode involves high-frequency ventilation with progressive accumulation of subtidal breaths and passive exhalation once a set airway pressure is met, allowing for gas exchange through more recruited alveoli.[90,91] In a small prospective study of pediatric burn patients, Rodeberg et al.[90,92] demonstrated that use of VDR mode increased PaO_2, increased PaO_2/FIO_2 ratio, and decreased mean airway pressure, all without affecting hemodynamic function. Long term, this mode has been shown to decrease pneumonia and mortality compared with individuals treated with conventional modes of ventilation, but data remain limited in pediatric burn patients.[91,93-95] Airway pressure release ventilation (APRV) is a reverse inspiratory/expiratory method of ventilation with two levels of PEEP support (Fig. 117.5). High PEEP is continuous during a prolonged inspiratory time, providing for adequate oxygenation and recruitment of closed alveoli, while low PEEP is maintained during expiration facilitating recruitment of alveoli. Theoretically, patients benefit from reduced barotrauma, improved oxygenation and ventilation due to better V/Q matching, and decreased sedation and paralysis requirements due to increased patient comfort.[96] Unlike the VDR, there is no percussive component involved.[97] Data remain limited regarding use of both these alternative ventilatory strategies in the pediatric burn setting and are extrapolated from adult literature.

Airway Clearance

Appropriately trained respiratory therapists are invaluable in the management of burn patients and are a mainstay in specialized burn care units. Together with ventilatory management, other adjunctive therapies including aggressive pulmonary toilet and chest physiotherapy are essential components of treatment of inhalational injuries. Chest percussion and vibrational treatment with additional focus on early ambulation are effective strategies for secretion mobilization and removal. Tracheobronchial suctioning and serial therapeutic bronchoscopies are often necessary to maintain airway clearance in severe inhalational injuries and are vital to prevent postobstructive atelectasis and infectious complications stemming from the excess mucus and fibrin casts characteristic of inhalational injury.[42,98,99]

Therapeutic Adjuncts

To combat the bronchoconstriction and excess secretions encountered in inhalational injuries, bronchodilators and pharmacologic treatments including nitric oxide, nebulized heparin, and N-acetylcysteine may be used. β-Adrenergic agonists are widely used in treatment of lung conditions including asthma and ARDS/ALI. The aerosolized delivery of specific β_2-adrenergic agonists produces preferential effects including bronchodilation, attenuation of lung inflammation, and potentially increased fluid clearance with limited systemic

DIFFUSIVE WAVEFORM

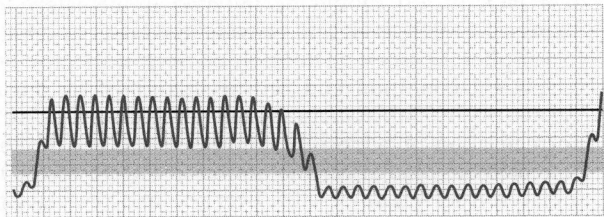

PERCUSSIVE WAVEFORM

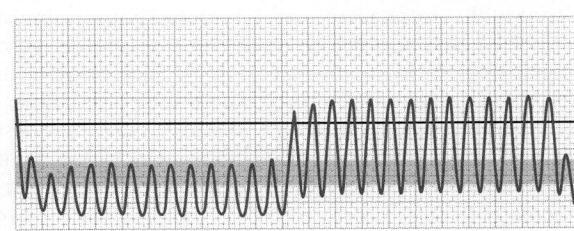

Fig. 117.4. Volumetric diffusive respiratory ventilation pressure-time tracings. Percussive and diffusive waveforms from a pediatric burn patient volumetric diffusive respiratory ventilator at Shriners Hospital for Children–Cincinnati.

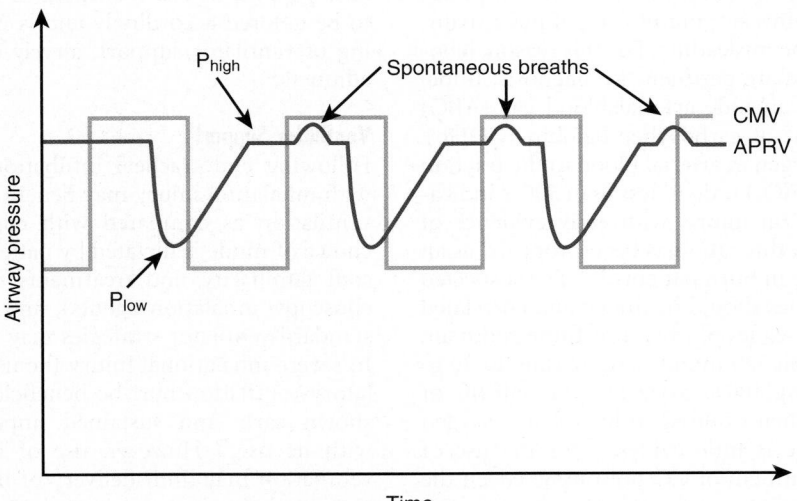

Fig. 117.5. Airway pressure release ventilation and controlled mechanical ventilation pressure-time tracing. (Modified from Fan E, Stewart TE. New modalities of mechanical ventilation: high frequency oscillatory ventilation and airway pressure release ventilation. Clin Chest Med. 2006;27:615-625.)

cardiac activation.[100] One retrospective review of burn children showed increased PaO_2/FIO_2 ratios and improved compliance and pH during treatment with continuous albuterol therapy.[100] Inhaled nitric oxide is a short-acting vasodilator used in the treatment of pulmonary hypertension that works by increasing cyclic guanine monophosphate in smooth muscle.[101] Limited studies in burn patients have demonstrated variable improvement in PaO_2/FIO_2 ratios and improved survival in those patients who respond to treatment.[102] If a response is not demonstrated between doses of 5 and 20 ppm of nitric oxide within 60 minutes of treatment onset, the patient is unlikely to respond and therapy should be discontinued due to futility and cost.[102] Nebulized heparin and tissue plasminogen activation have demonstrated potential efficacy in both animal and adult human studies through breakdown of fibrin deposition with maintenance of alveolar structure and reduced airway obstruction.[99,103] The mechanisms by which aerosolized heparin exerts a beneficial effect in inhalation injury are as yet undetermined but may be related to breakdown of fibrin casts and reduction in the inflammatory response from neutrophil migration into the airways.[99] Multicenter randomized trials are currently under way to delineate the beneficial effects of nebulized heparin but remain restricted to the adult burn population.[104,105] N-acetylcysteine, an effective mucolytic, was noted to reduce pulmonary inflammation in animal studies, demonstrating a decrease in leukocytes in bronchoalveolar lavage following a rat burn model, supporting the conclusion that N-acetylcysteine may ameliorate tissue damage after inhalation injury.[106] Although survival benefit has not clearly been demonstrated with use in ARDS and ALI,[107] preliminary evidence exists supporting improved outcomes when lung inflammation is attenuated, supporting research into future pharmacologic adjuncts targeting antioxidants and leukotriene inhibitors, as well as exogenous surfactant.[108] Well-designed clinical trials are necessary to further elucidate those adjunctive therapies most likely to improve morbidity and mortality in pediatric inhalation injury patients.

Perhaps most controversial in the management of inhalation injury is the use of corticosteroids. Although clearly beneficial for many chronic pulmonary diseases including asthma, benefits in acute pulmonary inflammation related to inhalation injury and ARDS have not been definitively demonstrated.[109,110] Corticosteroid therapy has been shown to increase mortality (from 13%–53%) and complication rates (from 31%–82%) in at least one study.[88] However, more recently Meduri et al.[111] demonstrated the potential utility of methylprednisolone given for 28 total days with fewer days on ventilator, a shorter ICU stay, fewer infections, and increased survival in patients with ARDS. Until larger prospective studies are completed, empiric treatment with corticosteroids for inhalation injury is not recommended.

Extracorporeal membrane oxygenation (ECMO) may be a lifesaving treatment modality in pediatric burn patients with acute respiratory failure refractory to the above standard treatments. Venoarterial (VA) ECMO when cardiopulmonary support is necessary and venovenous (VV) ECMO when the primary issue is pulmonary are both used in non–burn-related pediatric acute respiratory failure, with survival rates of 47%.[112,113] Although most documented success consists of case reports in the pediatric burn literature, Askegard-Giesman Jr. et al. queried the Extracorporeal Life Support Organization registry for the largest reported series of pediatric burn patients

on ECMO. They identified 36 patients placed on either VA or VV ECMO following burn-related acute respiratory failure with documented survival rates of 53%, on par with rates reported for non–burn-related pulmonary disease.[114] This supports the feasibility of ECMO in inhalational injury; however, the treatment strategy itself is fraught with excessive morbidity, as 44% of patients suffered complications related specifically to ECMO and medical complications occurred in the majority of patients (78%).[114] While there is no consensus on criteria for initiation of ECMO therapy and its widespread technical limitations preclude widespread use of this strategy, it remains an option for clinicians as rescue therapy for severe inhalational injuries.

Nutritional Support in Burn Patients

Nutritional support of the pediatric burn patient is paramount for prevention of malnutrition and adequate wound healing. Burns induce a hypermetabolic state that may persist for up to 12 months after injury, which contributes to underestimation of the nutritional needs of these patients.[115,116] It is commonly assumed that hypermetabolism is directly related to burn size, but more than likely it is related to stress hormones and gender, as well as age differences that must be considered.[117,118] Although exact mechanisms behind this hypermetabolism remain unclear, catecholamines including epinephrine and norepinephrine are increased following large burns. This hypermetabolic state is also thought to be secondary to inflammatory cytokines that stimulate the hypothalamus with resultant increases in the body's temperature set point, changes that are further compounded by the increased evaporative heat loss caused by the burn itself.[117] This systemic response to burn results in increased oxygen consumption, increased protein catabolism, increased lipolysis, and impaired glucose metabolism. These derangements culminate in decreased lean body mass, poor wound healing, and weakened host defenses if appropriate nutrition is not maintained.

Calculating and Monitoring Nutritional Requirements

Numerous equations have been developed to estimate the energy requirements of pediatric burn patients, although no single standard currently exists as most formulas overestimate caloric requirements.[119-122] Indirect calorimetry remains the gold standard to adjust nutritional support.[81,122] At our institution, we use the Mayes equation to calculate initial nutritional requirements, taking age, weight, and %TBSA burn into account (Table 117.4). Indirect calorimetry can then be used to calculate resting energy expenditure (REE) by measuring the differences in oxygen and carbon dioxide concentrations in inspired and expired gas and used to adjust caloric needs

TABLE 117.4	Mayes Equation to Calculate Energy Requirement After Burn Injury

Mayes equation for 5- to 10-year-old burn patient with <50% total body surface area (TBSA)
818 + 37.4 (weight in kilograms) + 9.3 (%TBSA burn)

Example: 5.5-year-old patient with 45% TBSA burn weighing 20 kg
818 + 37.4 (20 kg) + 9.3 (45% TBSA)
818 + 748 + 481.5 = 2047.5 calories/day

as appropriate. Total caloric requirements can be estimated as 120% to 130% of REE.[81] In children, carbohydrates should account for 60% to 70% of energy requirements while fats should account for 15% to 20%. Protein requirements vary from 2.5 to 4 g/kg/day.

In addition to indirect calorimetry, blood tests can serve as adjuncts to aid in monitoring nutritional status.[121] While albumin is a poor surrogate for nutritional status, prealbumin is advocated as it is a distinct marker for protein synthesis and has a relative short half-life, increasing its sensitivity as a marker for nutritional support. As albumin levels rapidly fall following large burn injuries, it is unreliable as a measure of nutritional stores. In addition, albumin replacement maintains no scientific basis as it does not stimulate production of endogenous albumin, nor has replacement been shown to have any clinical benefits regarding pulmonary function, wound healing, gastrointestinal function, or mortality.[117] Static measurements of serum concentrations of nutritional markers such as carotene, iron, and calcium remain unreliable indicators of nutritional status in burn patients.[123]

Although underfeeding contributes to poor clinical outcomes, the implications of overfeeding critically ill burn patients may be just as detrimental. Excessive carbohydrate consumption leads to respiratory abnormalities that may interfere with pulmonary function and subsequent weaning from mechanical ventilation.[124] Overfeeding carbohydrates also contributes to hepatic dysfunction, hyperglycemia, dehydration via osmotic diuresis, and poor wound healing.[117,124] Although burns cause significant protein catabolism, over-supplementing with excessive quantities of protein does not help offset catabolism but may actually increase breakdown and is detrimental. Excessive lipid intake can increase susceptibility to infectious complications and cause diarrhea and fatty liver. Whereas overfeeding is a concern in the care of burned patients, the majority of literature supports early and aggressive nutritional support to prevent complications from poor wound healing and infection-related morbidity and mortality.[124,125]

Enteral Support

Enteral feeding is the mainstay of nutritional support in pediatric burn patients and is considered the ideal route for caloric and nutrient supplementation. Studies have shown enteral support helps maintain intestinal integrity following burn injury, decreasing the risk of bacterial translocation and infectious complications.[126-128] The role of specialty amino acids, proteins, and fatty acids present in commercial tube feed preparations for pediatric burn patients is controversial, as studies have both shown improvement[127] and no effect on clinical outcomes[129] and may be cost prohibitive. For burns greater than 20% TBSA, oral nutrition is often inadequate to meet the nutritional demands of the hypermetabolic state, and nasoenteric feeding tubes should be placed with initiation of supplemental tube feeding.[128] Early enteral feeding is recommended as soon as initial resuscitation is complete, as recommended by American Burn Association guidelines.

Parenteral Support

Parenteral nutrition (PN) is considered a mainstay of therapy for many critically ill patients who are not candidates for enteral nutrition. In burn patients, central venous PN is reserved for individuals unable to tolerate enteral feedings as an alternative to starvation. Complication rates increase when burn patients are given PN due to bacteremia and increased susceptibility to pneumonia. PN may be necessary in pediatric burn patients with concomitant abdominal surgery, functional ileus, or hemodynamic instability, but all efforts should be made to initiate enteral nutrition as soon as practical.[130] Peripheral parenteral nutrition (PPN) is not recommended due to lack of adequate calorie delivery and high risk of peripheral access damage from PPN extravasation.

Nutritional Adjuncts

Although vitamin supplementation is poorly understood in children and little evidence exists in pediatric burn patients, guidelines regarding vitamin supplementation from the National Advisory Group/American Medical Association are customarily followed. Vitamin A has been shown to improve wound healing following burn injury, and vitamin D is vital for adequate bone formation in children.[131] Vitamin C plays a vital role in collagen synthesis and wound healing, necessitating its supplementation. Wound exudates were found to be the primary site of loss for trace elements, suggesting burn patients may require replacement of trace elements more than other critically ill patients.[132] The trace element zinc is involved with wound healing, and some reports suggest decreased zinc levels in septic patients are associated with subsequent adverse events.[81] For these reasons, zinc supplementation is often included as part of enteral nutrition.

Insulin resistance and hyperglycemia are known effects of the hypermetabolic response seen following burn injury. Hyperglycemia occurs in most burn patients regardless of injury severity because of increased rate of glucose production and impaired tissue glucose extraction.[133,134] Insulin may serve dual functions in burn patients, both in its anabolic effects and ability to counter hyperglycemia. Jeschke et al.[135] demonstrated tempering of the inflammatory response with tight glucose control using insulin through mediation of hepatocyte apoptosis, which allows for improved hepatic function. Tight glucose control with intensive insulin therapy has been shown to reduce postburn morbidity in a single-center prospective trial, with reductions in inflammatory response, infection, and organ dysfunction.[136] The hypercatabolism in burns leads to loss of lean body mass even with adequate nutritional support. Negative nitrogen balance is often seen during the first 1 to 2 weeks after burn.[121] To combat this, studies have demonstrated both the short- and long-term effectiveness of anabolic agents such as oxandrolone in restoration of lost lean body mass and improved wound healing.[137] These results are controversial and current literature is limited to single-center studies with regards to impact on the course of burn disease. Anabolic steroids such as oxandrolone are not universally used in the management of pediatric burn patients.

Wound Care

Burn wounds will evolve over time on the basis of factors including mechanism of injury and fluid resuscitation, sometimes requiring 10 to 14 days for complete demarcation.[27] It is not uncommon for previously diagnosed superficial partial burn wounds to demarcate as full-thickness burns and vice versa. If the burn wound is improperly managed and allowed to desiccate or become infected, it will convert to a deeper wound requiring definitive surgical management. Initial cleansing and debridement of the wound are absolutely essential for proper diagnosis of size and depth. Mild soap and water or chlorhexidine mixed in saline washes is recommended for cleaning, with adequate pain control to allow complete debridement of necrotic tissue. Most burn experts recommend debridement of all blisters unless smaller than 0.5 cm or in a difficult-to-manage area to reduce the risk of bacterial colonization or infection.

Burn wounds become colonized in the first few hours with gram-positive bacteria such as *Staphylococcus aureus* and *epidermidis* and are predominantly colonized with gut flora such as *Pseudomonas aeruginosa, Enterobacter cloacae,* and *Escherichia coli* by 5 days.[138] Health care workers involved with the cleansing and debridement of burn wounds must be vigilant in hand washing and maintenance of a clean environment around the wound for prevention of cross-contamination in these immunocompromised patients. Culture swabs of all wound beds should be obtained on arrival and on a scheduled basis to monitor for changes in colonization. Bacterial colonization of burn wounds does not require systemic antibiotics but should be managed with early debridement, appropriate topical and/ or biological dressings, and scheduled dressing changes.[27] Topical therapy is not intended to sterilize the burn wound but to control colonization. Gauze and sterile dressings are used for coverage to minimize evaporative water losses.[139]

Topical Therapy

The choice of topical agent depends on the depth and extent of the wound being treated. Minor superficial burns can be treated with moisturizing creams such as Eucerin or aloe. Superficial partial-thickness burns to the face are treated in a similar fashion. Nonadherent gauze or petroleum gauze can be placed over triple antibiotic ointment to provide a comfortable, protective environment that promotes epithelialization. After cleansing and debridement of deeper burns, topical agents including silver sulfadiazine (Silvadene), mafenide acetate (Sulfamylon), and silver nitrate are options for local care.[27] Silvadene has been used in burns for decades and continues to demonstrate effective control of burn wound colonization against a continually widening spectrum of bacteria. Drawbacks include minimal eschar penetration and complications related to leukopenia and red blood cell hemolysis.[140] Sulfamylon cream is also easy to apply but is more painful when used on superficial partial-thickness burns. Eschar penetration is greatest using this agent, making it the topical of choice in burns where eschar will not be excised immediately. Its antimicrobial activity includes control of *P. aeruginosa,* a common colonizing bacterium in pediatric burn patients.[27,140] Sulfamylon is a carbonic anhydrase inhibitor, and complications related to metabolic acidosis may occur. Although these two agents are used most often in care of pediatric burns, silver nitrate 0.5% solution has generally fallen out of favor as first-line therapy due to electrolyte abnormalities and poor tissue penetration.

Newer bioactive dressings have begun to replace topical antimicrobials, as they minimize the need for twice-daily dressing changes. Silvadene in particular has been shown to delay wound healing due to direct toxic effect on keratinocytes, in addition to traumatic injury caused by frequent reapplication.[141,142] Newer agents such as hydrocolloid, hydrogel, and polyurethane film dressings provide effective humidity and control of exudate but are lacking in antimicrobial coverage. Silver-impregnated dressings such as Acticoat, Aquacel, and Mepilex provide combined antimicrobial coverage, adequate humidity for the wound, and decreased trauma to healing wounds with less frequent dressing changes.[27] Biosynthetic substitutes such as Biobrane are marketed as epidermal substitutes that allow for faster re-epithelialization.[143] These agents are useful for partial-thickness burns seen early in a burn center before bacterial colonization has taken place.

Surgical Treatment

In addition to topical treatments, larger burns treated in the inpatient setting are managed with surgical excision and placement of xenograft, allograft, autograft, or cultured epithelial autografts (CEAs). Placement of skin substitutes and replacements requires adequate wound bed excision and preparation.[27] Use of these materials on eschar or an improperly prepared wound bed will lead to graft loss and prolongation of definitive therapy. Although no consensus exists on the timing of burn wound excision, most experienced burn surgeons advocate early wound excision within the first 1 to 5 days after thermal injury to attenuate the inflammatory response of burn and reduce the risk of sepsis.[144,145] At our institution, a staged approach is often taken for more extensive injuries whereby the wound is excised and controlled on day 1 with subsequent donor site harvest and grafting.[27] The benefits of this approach include shorter operations, tighter temperature control, and ability to perform sheet grafting through improved hemostasis. Additional research is being performed to evaluate adjuncts including laser Doppler imaging to assess for cutaneous blood flow within burn wounds to best assess appropriate time and wound bed for grafting.[31]

Xenograft (pig skin) is a less expensive alternative to allograft (human cadaver skin) for coverage of burn wounds. It is incapable of engraftment and best used for temporary coverage, providing effective protection.[27] Allograft has revolutionized burn care by providing medium-term coverage for patients requiring excision without available autograft. Allograft is typically rejected within 2 to 3 weeks after placement, although burn patients demonstrate differences in immunocompetence resulting in varying degrees of rejection. Autograft provides definitive coverage of deep partial- and full-thickness burns. Donor site selection depends on available areas and extent of burn to be covered, and if limited, xenograft and allograft are provide effective temporizing coverage. Autograft can be applied as sheet graft or can be meshed in ratios from 1 : 1 up to 4 or 6 : 1.[27] Using large mesh grafts more than 2 : 1 is becoming uncommon even in treatment of large burns because of improved local wound management techniques and availability of synthetic skin substitutes.

Cultured epidermal autografts (CEAs) are derived from the individual patient's own cells and were first successfully used in the 1980s.[146,147] However, these thin grafts are fragile, difficult to work with, take 2 to 3 weeks to grow, and usually result in hypertrophic scarring and unstable epithelium. For these reasons, CEAs are usually reserved for burns greater than 85% TBSA. For the past 2 decades, our institution has made use of a cultured skin substitute consisting of autologous keratinocytes and fibroblasts grown on a collagen-based scaffold.[148,149] Our use of the cultured skin substitute leads to fewer complications related to placement and healing postoperatively, as well as less hypertrophic scarring and improved aesthetic results.[150]

Burn Prevention

The best, most cost-effective care for pediatric burn patients will always be prevention of the initial injuries. The vast majority of pediatric burns occur within the home, and the most powerful method of prevention lies in education. Distribution of informative brochures and web-based educational modules can help expand current burn safety and prevention programs to schools and the surrounding communities.[151,152] Strict building codes, regulation of fireworks and highly flammable products, and product modification including newer safety standards within the industries of children's clothing and toys are vitally important from a regulatory level to combat preventable fire-related injury. Residential fires can be battled with routine practice of Exit Drills in the Home (EDITH) with children and occupants, as well as routine smoke detector testing. Scald burns can be prevented by regulation of home hot water heaters to temperatures between 120 and 130 degrees Fahrenheit, as well as device modification to prevent children from turning on hot water faucets.[153] Both the Flammable Fabric Act, passed in 1967, and additional safety standards for children's pajamas attempt to combat additional morbidity from burn injury.[153] While all risk factors are not modifiable, the extensive morbidity and mortality extending from burn injuries within the pediatric population is best treated with the multifaceted, team-based approach of wound management by burn specialists, supportive care, and injury prevention.

Acknowledgment

We gratefully acknowledge the contribution Kevin Kasten, MD, who coauthored this chapter in previous editions.

Key References

1. American Burn Association. Burn incidence and treatment in the US: 2000 fact sheet.
4. Barrow RE, Przkora R, Hawkins HK, et al. Mortality related to gender, age, sepsis, and ethnicity in severely burned children. *Shock.* 2005;23:485-487.
7. Barrow RE, Spies M, Barrow LN, Herndon DN. Influence of demographics and inhalation injury on burn mortality in children. *Burns.* 2004;30:72-77.
8. Guzel A, Aksu B, Aylanc H, et al. Scalds in pediatric emergency department: a 5-year experience. *J Burn Care Res.* 2009;30:450-456.
12. Thombs BD. Patient and injury characteristics, mortality risk, and length of stay related to child abuse by burning: evidence from a national sample of 15,802 pediatric admissions. *Ann Surg.* 2008;247:519-523.
14. Bessey PQ, Phillips BD, Lentz CW, et al. Synopsis of the 2013 annual report of the national burn repository. *J Burn Care Res.* 2014;35(suppl 2):S218-S234.
15. Grunwald TB, Garner WL. Acute burns. *Plast Reconstr Surg.* 2008;121:311e-9e.
16. Koumbourlis AC. Electrical injuries. *Crit Care Med.* 2002;30(suppl 11):S424-S430.
18. Mowry JB, Spyker DA, Cantilena LR Jr, et al. 2013 Annual Report of the American Association of Poison Control Centers' National Poison Data System (NPDS): 31st Annual Report. *Clin Toxicol (Phila).* 2014;52:1032-1283.
21. Hatzifotis M, Williams A, Muller M, Pegg S. Hydrofluoric acid burns. *Burns.* 2004;30:156-159.
27. Kagan RJ, Peck MD, Ahrenholz DH, et al. Surgical management of the burn wound and use of skin substitutes: an expert panel white paper. *J Burn Care Res.* 2013;34:e60-e79.
28. Jeschke MG, Chinkes DL, Finnerty CC, et al. Pathophysiologic response to severe burn injury. *Ann Surg.* 2008;248:387-401.
31. Kim LH, Ward D, Lam L, Holland AJ. The impact of laser Doppler imaging on time to grafting decisions in pediatric burns. *J Burn Care Res.* 2010;31:328-332.
37. Bittner EA, Shank E, Woodson L, Martyn JA. Acute and perioperative care of the burn-injured patient. *Anesthesiology.* 2015;122:448-464.
38. Gonzalez R, Shanti CM. Overview of current pediatric burn care. *Semin Pediatr Surg.* 2015;24:47-49.
39. Cuttle L, Pearn J, McMillan JR, Kimble RM. A review of first aid treatments for burn injuries. *Burns.* 2009;35:768-775.
42. Mlcak RP, Suman OE, Herndon DN. Respiratory management of inhalation injury. *Burns.* 2007;33:2-13.
43. Latenser BA. Critical care of the burn patient: the first 48 hours. *Crit Care Med.* 2009;37:2819-2826.
44. Armour AD, Billmire DA. Pediatric thermal injury: acute care and reconstruction update. *Plast Reconstr Surg.* 2009;124(suppl 1):117e-127e.
45. Alvarado KCK, Cancio LC, Wolf SE. Burn resuscitation. *Burns.* 2009;35:4-14.
48. Pruitt BA Jr. Protection from excessive resuscitation: "pushing the pendulum back." *J Trauma.* 2000;49:567-568.
49. Swords DS, Hadley ED, Swett KR, Pranikoff T. Total body surface area overestimation at referring institutions in children transferred to a burn center. *Am Surg.* 2015;81:56-63.
52. Kraft R, Herndon DN, Branski LK, et al. Optimized fluid management improves outcomes of pediatric burn patients. *J Surg Res.* 2013;181:121-128.
55. Alderson P, Bunn F, Lefebvre C, et al. Human albumin solution for resuscitation and volume expansion in critically ill patients. *Cochrane Database Syst Rev.* 2004;(4):CD001208.
56. Klein MB, Hayden D, Elson C, et al. The association between fluid administration and outcome following major burn: a multicenter study. *Ann Surg.* 2007;245:622-628.
59. Ivy ME, Atweh NA, Palmer J, et al. Intra-abdominal hypertension and abdominal compartment syndrome in burn patients. *J Trauma.* 2000;49:387-391.
61. Tricklebank S. Modern trends in fluid therapy for burns. *Burns.* 2009;35:757-767.
66. Latenser BA, Kowal-Vern A, Kimball D, et al. A pilot study comparing percutaneous decompression with decompressive laparotomy for acute abdominal compartment syndrome in thermal injury. *J Burn Care Rehabil.* 2002;23:190-195.
71. Palmieri TL, Warner P, Mlcak RP, et al. Inhalation injury in children: a 10 year experience at Shriners Hospitals for Children. *J Burn Care Res.* 2009;30:206-208.
75. Lee AS, Mellins RB. Lung injury from smoke inhalation. *Paediatr Respir Rev.* 2006;7:123-128.
77. Miller K, Chang A. Acute inhalation injury. *Emerg Med Clin North Am.* 2003;21:533-557.
80. Geller RJ, Barthold C, Saiers JA, Hall AH. Pediatric cyanide poisoning: causes, manifestations, management, and unmet needs. *Pediatrics.* 2006;118:2146-2158.
81. Mak GASKR. Pediatric burns. In: Wheeler DWH, Shanley T, eds. *Pediatric Critical Care Medicine.* Berlin, Germany: Springer-Verlag; 2007:1159-1606.
84. Weaver LK, Howe S, Hopkins R, Chan KJ. Carboxyhemoglobin half-life in carbon monoxide-poisoned patients treated with 100% oxygen at atmospheric pressure. *Chest.* 2000;117(3):801-808.
88. Rabinowitz PM, Siegel MD. Acute inhalation injury. *Clin Chest Med.* 2002;23:707-715.
91. Greathouse ST, Hadad I, Zieger M, et al. High-frequency oscillatory ventilators in burn patients: experience of Riley Hospital for Children. *J Burn Care Res.* 2012;33:425-435.
92. Carman B, Cahill T, Warden G, McCall J. A prospective, randomized comparison of the Volume Diffusive Respirator vs conventional ventilation for ventilation of burned children. 2001 ABA paper. *J Burn Care Rehabil.* 2002;23:444-448.
96. Kawaguchi A, Guerra GG, Duff JP, et al. Hemodynamic changes in child acute respiratory distress syndrome with airway pressure release ventilation: a case series. *Clin Respir J.* 2014;doi:10.1111/crj.12155.
97. Dries DJ. Key questions in ventilator management of the burn-injured patient (first of two parts). *J Burn Care Res.* 2009;30(1):128-138.
111. Meduri GU, Golden E, Freire AX, et al. Methylprednisolone infusion in early severe ARDS: results of a randomized controlled trial. *Chest.* 2007;131:954-963.

114. Askegard-Giesmann JR, Besner GE, Fabia R, et al. Extracorporeal membrane oxygenation as a lifesaving modality in the treatment of pediatric patients with burns and respiratory failure. *J Pediatr Surg*. 2010;45:1330-1335.

117. Chan MM, Chan GM. Nutritional therapy for burns in children and adults. *Nutrition*. 2009;25:261-269.

124. Joffe A, Anton N, Lequier L, et al. Nutritional support for critically ill children. *Cochrane Database Syst Rev*. 2009;(2):CD005144.

136. Jeschke MG, Kulp GA, Kraft R, et al. Intensive insulin therapy in severely burned pediatric patients: a prospective randomized trial. *Am J Respir Crit Care Med*. 2010;182:351-359.

138. Ergun O, Celik A, Ergun G, Ozok G. Prophylactic antibiotic use in pediatric burn units. *Eur J Pediatr Surg*. 2004;14:422-426.

141. Wasiak J, Cleland H. Burns (minor thermal). *Clin Evid*. 2005; 2388-2396.

142. Wasiak J, Cleland H, Campbell F. Dressings for superficial and partial thickness burns. *Cochrane Database Syst Rev*. 2008;(4):CD002106.

144. Barret JP, Herndon DN. Effects of burn wound excision on bacterial colonization and invasion. *Plast Reconstr Surg*. 2003;111:744-750, discussion 51-52.

146. Grafting of burns with cultured epithelium prepared from autologous epidermal cells. *Lancet*. 1981;1:75-78.

150. Boyce ST, Kagan RJ, Greenhalgh DG, et al. Cultured skin substitutes reduce requirements for harvesting of skin autograft for closure of excised, full-thickness burns. *J Trauma*. 2006;60:821-829.

153. Atiyeh BS, Costagliola M, Hayek SN. Burn prevention mechanisms and outcomes: pitfalls, failures and successes. *Burns*. 2009;35:181-193.

Pediatric Trauma

Evaluation, Stabilization, and Initial Management After Multiple Trauma

Alan H. Tyroch, Susan F. McLean, and Chet Moorthy

PEARLS

- The primary survey, as defined by Advanced Trauma Life Support, is a prioritized evaluation and management protocol focused on identifying and treating the most life-threatening injuries first.
- Injured children who present to the emergency department can be divided into three categories with respect to initial airway management: those with a patent airway requiring no manipulation, those who have undergone interventions in the field or at another hospital to establish a patent airway, and those who will need intervention to establish a patent airway. The first group is the most common.
- The most effective, objective, and rapid steps in evaluating breathing and adequate ventilation are auscultation of the chest, application of a pulse oximeter for measurement of oxygen saturation, and assessment of respiratory rate.
- The greater physiologic reserve of children makes early identification of cardiovascular compromise more difficult than in adults. Assessment and management of circulatory status in the primary survey is focused on early identification and treatment rather than defining the specific etiology of the shock state.
- Of the three main components of the Glasgow Coma Scale, the motor score has been shown to be the best predictor of outcome after injury.

Trauma is the leading cause of death and acquired disability in children and adolescents, resulting in more deaths in children than all other causes combined.[1,2] Because children with severe injuries can rapidly deteriorate, resources for rapidly identifying and treating injuries are needed immediately on arrival at the receiving hospital. The initial evaluation of injured children in the emergency department ("trauma resuscitation") has two main goals: (1) identify and immediately treat potentially life-threatening injuries and (2) determine disposition after the trauma resuscitation on the basis of known or suspected injuries. The trauma team must stabilize the child, determine the extent of the injury, and develop an initial treatment plan for the child's hospitalization.

Advanced Trauma Life Support (ATLS) is a protocol developed to standardize the initial evaluation and management of injured patients and avoid omission of potentially lifesaving interventions. The ATLS training program was initiated by an orthopedic surgeon in 1978 in response to suboptimal care that he and his family received in a rural hospital after an airplane crash in a Nebraska cornfield. After 4 decades of refinement, ATLS serves as the standard for the initial management of injured patients and is now taught to providers around the world.[2] The impact of ATLS on reducing morbidity and mortality after injury has been affirmed in several studies.[3,4] ATLS training is mainly focused on treating the injured adult but includes modules that emphasize the anatomic, physiologic, and psychologic features that make management of the injured child unique.

The first phase of ATLS is the *primary survey* and is a rapid evaluation for identifying life-threatening injuries. The steps include evaluation and treatment of airway injuries (A, *airway*) followed by evaluation of respiratory dynamics (B, *breathing*), evaluation of the patient's hemodynamic status (C, *circulation*), followed by a neurologic assessment (D, *disability*). The final phase of the primary survey (E, *exposure/environment*) includes removing the patient's clothing to identify concealed injures and ensuring that the patient is protected from environmental heat loss. The primary survey is then followed by the secondary survey, which is a detailed head-to-toe evaluation that identifies other injuries. The steps within the primary survey are repeated as needed if the patient's status changes and to monitor the response to therapeutic interventions. The initial management of injured adults has been the domain of trauma surgeons; however, the jurisdiction of care for the injured child is not as well defined at many centers. Frequently, pediatricians, anesthesiologists, and emergency department physicians have an active role in the initial management and treatment of injured children.[5] Although formal ATLS training is not needed for most pediatric providers, this training should be mandatory for those actively involved in the initial evaluation of injured children. The goal of this chapter is to provide a focused introduction to the initial resuscitation of injured children. This chapter does not serve as a replacement for ATLS training but will instead highlight aspects of the resuscitation that are unique to injured children or may not be emphasized in the ATLS curriculum.

Prehospital Care and Trauma Team Activation

Initial field care, appropriate triage, and rapid transport are all aspects of prehospital care that can have an important impact on the outcome in pediatric trauma. Cities and regions have developed trauma systems that coordinate these aspects of care by creating networks of prehospital and hospital providers. The most severely injured children are triaged to the centers within each trauma system that have the personnel, facilities, and equipment to manage these patients. Equally important, minimally injured patients can be directed to nontrauma hospitals to avoid burdening pediatric trauma centers with these patients. Field triage is based on several components including physiologic criteria, anatomic injury, mechanism of injury, and underlying medical conditions. Triage criteria are designed to minimize inappropriate transport of severely injured patients to nontrauma hospitals (undertriage) but achieve this goal at the cost of directing some patients to trauma centers who are only minimally injured (overtriage). Due to the limited time and resources available for evaluation in the prehospital setting, overtriage is an unavoidable aspect of current trauma systems. Injured children who have met criteria for transport to high-level trauma centers by current criteria may be minimally injured and require no specific interventions before discharge from the emergency department. A key aspect of the initial management of the injured child in the emergency department is effectively continuing the care started in the field while avoiding unneeded care for those with minimal injuries.

One approach that has been used in many centers to address the problem of overtriage is the use of a tiered team response in the emergency department.[6] On the basis of prehospital criteria, patients who are identified as being most at risk for severe injury are met by a full team upon arrival including a trauma surgeon, emergency department physicians, critical care physicians, anesthesiologists, nurses, and radiology technicians. Patients with a lower likelihood of severe injury are initially met by a smaller team with the option of summoning a larger team if the initial evaluation suggests a severe injury. Centers that have used this approach for team activation have significantly reduced the expenditure of resources on minimally injured patients without any impact on the care received for more severely injured patients.[7]

Trauma Resuscitation

Trauma resuscitations are among the most resource-intensive and time-pressured events in any hospital. The severity of the patient's injuries, number of team members required, and number of simultaneous evaluation and management steps needed contribute to the complexity of the environment. To manage the complexity of trauma resuscitation, a systematic team-based and process-focused approach is needed to rapidly identify and treat life-threatening injuries and minimize team errors.

Designating a specific room and team for trauma resuscitations helps ensure that the needed resources are immediately available. A single location ensures that supplies (eg, emergency airway kits, chest tube and thoracotomy trays, and central or intraosseous vascular access kits) are available and that team members know to gather at a specific site. Physicians, nurses, radiography technicians, respiratory therapists, and other hospital personnel needed for trauma resuscitation are identified in advance as trauma team members assemble and assume their roles in the resuscitation area upon arrival of the injured child (Fig. 118.1). These seemingly simple preparations ensure that the arriving patient has the maximal resources available at the receiving hospital. It is especially helpful to have a resuscitation room equipped with pediatric age and size specific equipment. Special carts, with color-coded drawers matching the Broselow measuring device, are helpful to organize size specific equipment.

Before arrival at the hospital, prehospital providers transmit information to hospital providers regarding the mechanism of injury, status of the patient, and initial treatments or interventions that have been provided. This information can alert the team to prepare specific equipment or resources or to summon other essential personnel. Before the patient arrives, it is good practice for the team to review prehospital information to ensure all team members are aware of the patient's status and anticipated needs. On arrival at the emergency department, an additional and final exchange of information between the prehospital providers and the trauma team occurs. A "time out" or quiet period facilitates this information transfer. Essential elements that should be obtained in this report include details about the injury event, vital signs obtained at the scene and during transport, pertinent physical findings, and the initial treatments administered and response to these treatments.[8] Allowing the prehospital providers to give their report before starting the patient evaluation or even transferring the patient to the emergency department gurney improves information exchange and prevents repetitive questions later in the resuscitation. Obtaining a record of the prehospital event completes the formal information exchange between prehospital and in-hospital providers. These records can contain critical information for early in-hospital management but often are not immediately obtained because prehospital providers are moving on to their next assignment and the trauma team is focused on direct care of the patient.

Primary Survey
Overview

The primary survey, as defined by ATLS, is a prioritized evaluation and management protocol focused on identifying and treating the most life-threatening injuries first. This approach is different from the traditional initial evaluation in a patient in which an extensive history and physical examination are performed before diagnosis and treatment. The steps of the primary survey are taught in the ATLS course as a sequence followed by one provider with one nurse. In actual practice, most centers have a team of providers rather than only two, allowing the evaluation and management steps to proceed forward in parallel even if one step leads to a delay. A designated team leader stands at the foot of the bed, receives information reported by the team, and provides higher-level direction of the conduct of the resuscitation. While the steps of the primary survey provide the framework for the initial assessment, new information may be obtained in later phases or a patient's status may change, requiring iterative performance of each step. It is often a challenge to ensure the team retains its focus on the underlying prioritization scheme of the primary survey and does not omit or minimize steps in

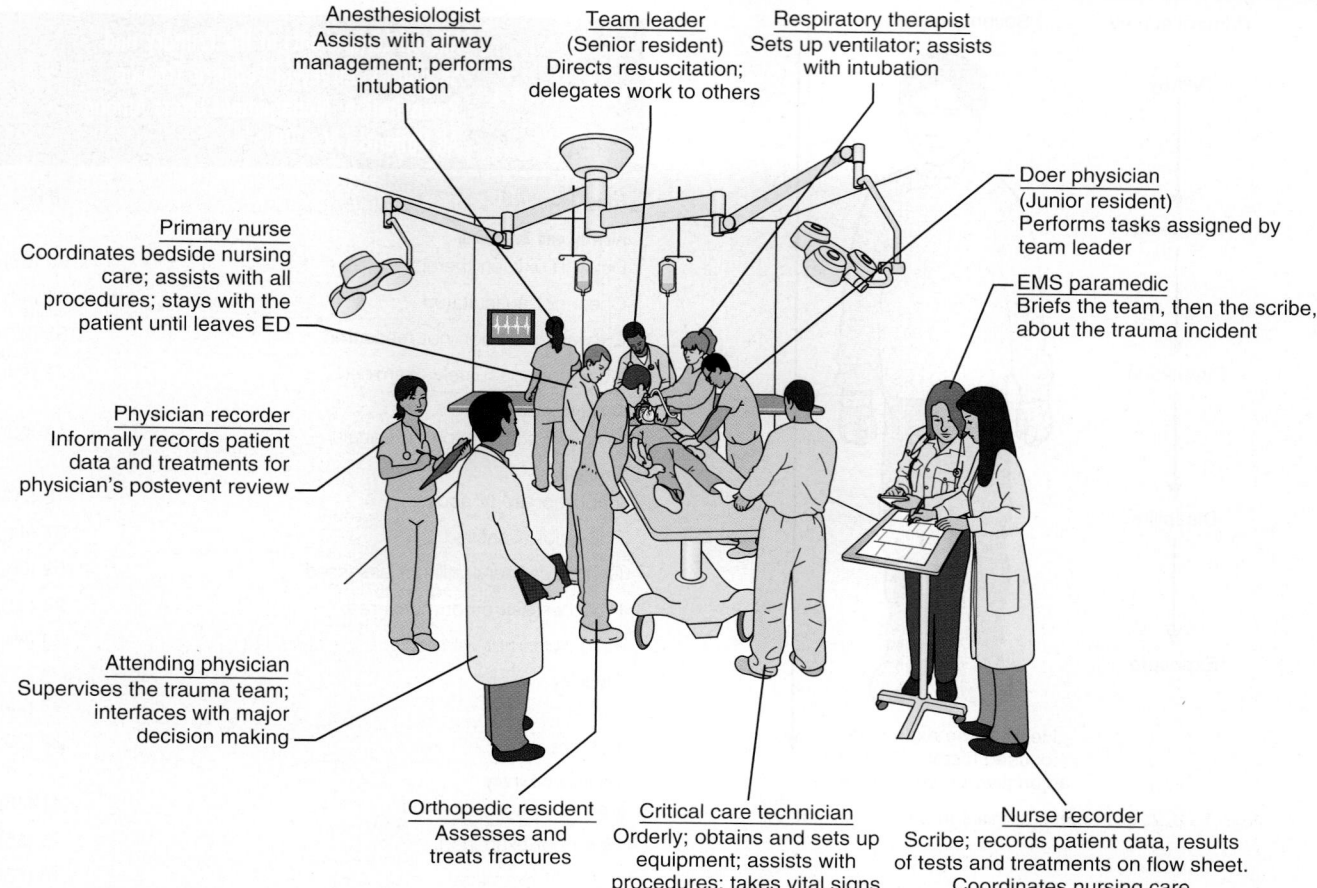

Anesthesiologist
Assists with airway management; performs intubation

Team leader
(Senior resident)
Directs resuscitation; delegates work to others

Respiratory therapist
Sets up ventilator; assists with intubation

Doer physician
(Junior resident)
Performs tasks assigned by team leader

EMS paramedic
Briefs the team, then the scribe, about the trauma incident

Primary nurse
Coordinates bedside nursing care; assists with all procedures; stays with the patient until leaves ED

Physician recorder
Informally records patient data and treatments for physician's postevent review

Attending physician
Supervises the trauma team; interfaces with major decision making

Orthopedic resident
Assesses and treats fractures

Critical care technician
Orderly; obtains and sets up equipment; assists with procedures; takes vital signs

Nurse recorder
Scribe; records patient data, results of tests and treatments on flow sheet. Coordinates nursing care

Fig. 118.1. The trauma room and team. (From Sacrevic A, et al. Quantifying adaptation parameters for information support of trauma teams. CHI 2008 Proceedings.)

this process (Fig. 118.2).[2] When resuscitations are evaluated, compliance with ATLS protocols is often low, mandating continued training and retraining to ensure the well-established benefits of this protocol are realized.[9]

Establish an Airway With Cervical Spine Stabilization (A)

Establishment of a patent airway with cervical spine stabilization is the first step of the primary survey. All patients should immediately receive oxygen as the evaluation is begun. After oxygen is placed, evaluation of the airway can proceed. Injured children who present to the emergency department can be placed into three categories with respect to initial airway management: (1) those with a patent airway requiring no manipulation, (2) those who have undergone intervention in the field or at another hospital to establish a patent airway, and (3) those who will need an intervention to establish a patent airway. Most children evaluated by the trauma team are in the first group. For these patients, evaluation should include several simple steps including asking the patient's name, inspection for craniofacial injuries, assessment for voice changes, and listening for obvious stridor. These steps can be performed easily and rapidly in most children. A simple statement that "the airway is patent" will communicate to the team that these confirmatory steps have been accomplished. Because most injured children will not require any specific airway management, omission of elements of the airway assessment

is common in pediatric trauma resuscitation. In a study of pediatric trauma resuscitations analyzed by video review, the most common omission in airway evaluation was not providing supplemental oxygen (omitted in 67% of resuscitations). Less than one-quarter of resuscitations included a complete assessment of the airway along with assessment of "breathing," the second component of the primary survey.[10] Although the patency of the airway may seem "obvious" in many patients, subtle and early signs of pending airway compromise will be missed if a formal airway evaluation is not completed (Table 118.1).

The second category is children with an airway already established in the field or other hospital, usually by endotracheal intubation. Airway interventions performed before a patient's arrival should not be interpreted as an adequate airway, and additional steps should be performed to assess airway patency, especially in light of the relative tenuous nature of pediatric airways placed under emergency situations.[11] The key steps to evaluating an endotracheal tube placed outside the emergency department are assessing the appropriateness of tube size, evaluating tube depth, assessing adequacy of ventilation by auscultation and inspection of the chest, measurement of end-tidal CO_2, and confirmation of tube position with a chest radiograph. The appropriate tube size can be evaluated using age-specific formulas and charts or by comparing the tube with the child's fifth (little) finger.

Primary survey   Secondary survey

Airway

Breathing

Circulation

Disability

Exposure

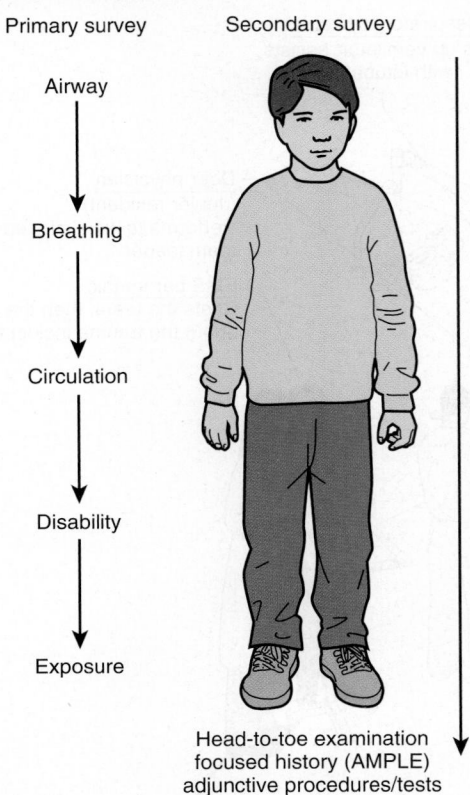

Head-to-toe examination
focused history (AMPLE)
adjunctive procedures/tests

Fig. 118.2. Schematic of initial trauma resuscitation.

TABLE 118.1	Missed Components of the Primary and Secondary Survey in Pediatric Trauma Resuscitation: Management Errors Among All Patients ($N = 90$)

Errors Identified	N (%)
Airway and Breathing	
Delay in oxygen therapy	60 (67)
Chest not auscultated	40 (44)
Oxygen saturation not measured	33 (37)
Neck not adequately examined	71 (79)
Cervical Spine	
No head stabilization on transfer	18 (20)
Circulation	
Inappropriate IV access	18 (20)
Pulse not assessed	37 (41)
Central capillary refill not assessed	59 (66)
Blood pressure not measured	28 (31)
Fluid bolus not warmed	33 (89)
Disability	
Pupils	22 (25)
Posture	22 (25)
Secondary Survey	
Perineum not examined	41 (45)
Head not examined	13 (15)
Ears not examined	16 (18)
Mouth not examined	41 (45)
Back not examined	13 (15)
Chest not examined	3 (3)
Abdomen not examined	2 (2)

Modified from Oakley E, Stocker S, Staubli G, et al. Using video recording to identify management errors in pediatric trauma resuscitation. Pediatrics. 2006;117:658-664.

Deep placement of an endotracheal tube in a prehospital setting is common, especially among younger children. In addition, the shorter airway of children increases the likelihood that an endotracheal tube will migrate from the proper position during transport. An easy rule for rapidly assessing tube depth is that the length of the tube at the teeth should be three times the tube size (internal diameter measured in mm). Age-specific formulas for evaluating endotracheal tube depth are available and are more easily used by providers with greater experience in airway management. Assessment that the endotracheal tube is an adequate airway should include steps that are more formally part of the breathing (B) phase of the primary survey, including assessment of ventilation by auscultation and inspection and measurement of end-tidal CO_2. Because of a shorter airway and relatively less margin for movement of an endotracheal tube in younger child, correct endotracheal tube position cannot be reliably confirmed by auscultation of bilateral breath sounds alone.[12] Final confirmation of endotracheal tube position requires a chest radiograph. In most cases, the chest radiograph should be deferred until later in the resuscitation because simpler and more rapid evaluations can be performed to verify tube position that do not interrupt the conduct of the primary survey. However, a chest radiograph should be performed in the emergency department before transport to other areas of the hospital to avoid the need for airway management in less optimal hospital settings.

The final category of injured children undergoing airway evaluation is those who present with airway compromise requiring intervention. Because this category of injured children is least common, clearly defined personnel and procedures are needed to prepare the team to efficiently and safely establish an airway. Indications for endotracheal intubation in pediatric trauma include apnea, inability to maintain a patent airway by other means, a need to protect the lower airway from aspiration of blood or vomitus, impending or potential compromise of the airway, presence of a closed head injury with a Glasgow Coma Scale [GCS] score ≤8, and inability to maintain adequate oxygenation with supplemental facemask oxygen.[2] An altered level of consciousness, usually due to an intracranial injury, is the most commonly observed reason for emergency airway intervention in the acutely injured child. Although a neurologic assessment is performed later in the primary survey, early recognition of children requiring a formal airway because of an altered level of consciousness is essential. The AVPU scale (*a*wake, responds to *v*erbal stimuli, responds to *p*ainful stimuli, and *u*nresponsive) is one model for assessing consciousness that has been found to correlate with the GCS scale and which may be useful for identifying children who are at risk for a compromised airway because of an altered level of consciousness.[13] Patients with an

AVPU score of "P" or "U" can be anticipated to have a GCS score of 8 or 3, respectively, and should receive early airway intervention with endotracheal intubation.[14]

Once the trauma team has confirmed the need to establish an airway, the least invasive method for achieving this goal should be chosen. A chin lift and jaw thrust may be sufficient for initially opening the airway in some patients and are simple and rapid steps that can facilitate bag-valve-mask ventilation. However, in the presence of a suspected cervical spine injury, only a jaw thrust should be used. Because these maneuvers are not sufficient for long-term airway management, further interventions are necessary to establish a definitive airway. Small children on a flat spine board may have a partially occluded airway because their proportionately large head forces the neck into a kyphotic (flexed) position, resulting in upper airway obstruction. Simple manipulation of the young child's head to maintain the plane of the face parallel with the plane of the spine board can improve airway patency.

When a more definitive airway is necessary, the preferred method for establishing an airway in pediatric trauma is orotracheal intubation. A rapid-sequence technique is preferred for most injured children because endotracheal intubation is made easier by eliminating protective airway reflexes and safer by preventing aspiration and decreasing physiologic stress that can lead to increased intracranial pressure in children with a traumatic brain injury.[15] During endotracheal intubation, steps should be taken to account for the short length and narrow diameter of the trachea, including choosing an appropriately sized endotracheal tube and confirming tube position. Nasotracheal intubation is usually not performed for injured children because this technique is more difficult due to the acute angle of the posterior pharynx of the child, may result in trauma with bleeding, and increases intracranial pressure. Nasotracheal intubation is also contraindicated in patients with facial trauma, cerebrospinal fluid leaks, or suggestions of basilar skull fractures because these injuries suggest the possibility of a disruption between the cranial vault and the nasopharynx.[16,17] The laryngeal mask airway (LMA) is also an option for emergency airway management in situations in which endotracheal intubation cannot be accomplished.[17-19] However, as the LMA does not protect against aspiration and cannot be used effectively to provide positive pressure ventilation in patients with altered respiratory compliance or resistance, it should be used only as a rescue technique if the patient's trachea cannot be intubated.[20]

Less than 1% of all adult patients who require an emergency airway in the emergency department require a surgical airway.[21] The percentage of children requiring an emergency airway after injury is likely to be even smaller. Among injured children with a compromised airway, endotracheal intubation may not be possible because of significant craniofacial injuries, massive bleeding from the nasopharynx or oropharynx, or preexisting anatomic features such as a short neck, micrognathia, or small mouth that make intubation more difficult. In this "cannot intubate/cannot ventilate" subset, a systematic approach is necessary to rapidly secure a patent airway (Fig. 118.3).[20]

If bag-valve-mask ventilation is successful, the team has time to find alternative routes of securing an airway. Examples include bringing a more experienced physician to the trauma bay to assist with establishing an airway or using alternative techniques such as indirect laryngoscopy or fiberoptic

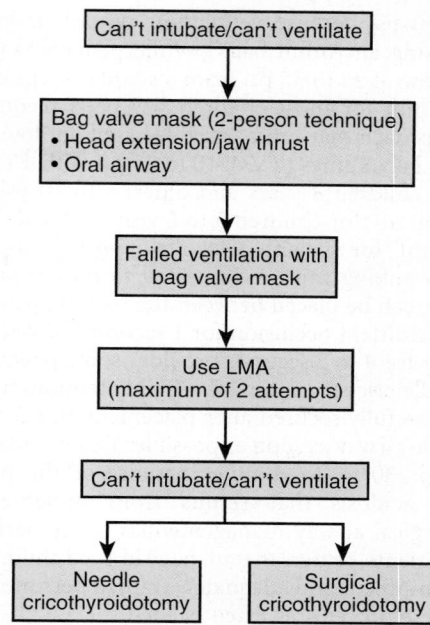

Fig. 118.3. Flow chart for "can't intubate/can't ventilate" airway emergencies. (Modified from Henderson JJ, Popat MT, Latto IP, et al. Difficult Airway Society guidelines for management of the unanticipated difficult intubation. Anaesthesia. 2004;59:675-694.)

intubation. If bag-valve-mask ventilation is not successful, an appropriate invasive procedure may be required. Among injured children, appropriate options include surgical or needle cricothyrotomy, depending on the child's size. Among children with a larger airway whose cricothyroid membrane is easily palpated, a surgical cricothyrotomy is preferred.[2] If small neck size or other anatomic features preclude the safe placement of a cricothyrotomy, a needle cricothyrotomy with needle jet insufflation of oxygen into the airway has been recommended. However, given the difficulties and potential morbidity related to the technique, there remains controversy regarding its use in younger children and infants (see later). Surgical cricothyrotomy should be performed by members of the team with experience with this technique. This procedure has four main steps: (1) identification of the cricothyroid membrane, (2) making an incision through the skin and cricothyroid membrane, (3) stabilization of the larynx with a tracheal hook at the inferior aspect of the ostomy, and (4) placement of a tube in the trachea.[22] Although controversy surrounds whether needle cricothyrotomy should be used at all in pediatric patients, it is still advocated by some authorities as a rescue technique in specific clinical scenarios. Needle cricothyrotomy can be performed using commercially available kits. When one is not available, the procedure can be carried out by inserting a large-bore (12- to 18-gauge) angiocatheter in a caudal direction at a 30- to 45-degree angle through the cricothyroid membrane. During needle advancement, constant negative pressure is applied to the plunger of the syringe to aspirate air and confirm its endotracheal position.[23] After confirmation of endotracheal placement, the syringe and stylet are removed and the cannula is connected to an oxygen source. Among larger children and adolescents, the cannula should be connected to an unregulated oxygen supply of 50 psi because ventilation cannot be adequately provided using an Ambu bag.[24] While pediatric evidence is limited, a flow of 25 to 35 psi from a standard regulator set at 10 to 12 L/min for most children has been recommended. Another approach that can be used is based on flow rates and estimated tidal volumes (TVs): 10 to 25 psi with TV of 340 to 625 mL for children 8 years and older; 5 to 10 psi with TV of 240 to 340 mL for children 5 to 8 years old; and 5 psi with TV of 100 mL for patients who are 5 years and younger.[23] Standard IV tubing can be connected to the cannula, and a Y-connector can be placed between the IV tubing and oxygen tubing. Intermittent occlusion for 1 second and release of the Y-connector for 4 to 5 seconds provides some passive ventilation. A needle cricothyrotomy is a highly tenuous airway and should be carefully secured after placement and converted to a more stable airway as soon as possible. This approach is only sufficient for 30 to 45 minutes because of the progressive respiratory acidosis that results from underventilation.[2] Because surgical airway management is rarely performed in pediatric patients, centers that manage injured children should have the equipment and adequately trained personnel for performing these procedures when needed.

Cervical spine stabilization should be viewed as part of the "A" step and is included as part of airway management in ATLS. Endotracheal intubation in the trauma bay should proceed with the assumption that a cervical spine injury is present until this type of injury has been formally ruled out. This step is needed in patients with any mechanism of injury that can be associated with cervical spine trauma. Many injured children present to the emergency department with a cervical collar that was placed in the field because of the mechanism of injury. The initial evaluation of the airway should be immediately followed or simultaneously performed with an assessment of the proper size and fitting of the cervical collar or placement of a cervical collar when one is not present. When endotracheal intubation is required, in-line cervical spine stabilization should be used. A member of the team holds the neck on each side with his or her hands and forearms maintaining the stability of the spine during airway manipulation. Despite the importance of this step, neck inspection and palpation while maintaining C-spine precautions and head stabilization during transfer to the trauma gurney are steps omitted in 80% and 20% of trauma resuscitation performed for injured children, respectively.[10]

Breathing (B)

Establishment of a patent airway is an important initial step but is not sufficient to ensure adequate oxygen delivery. The breathing (B) step of the primary survey is the immediate assessment of ventilation and performance of measures to establish adequate ventilation if it is compromised. The three most effective, objective, and rapid steps in evaluating ventilation are auscultation of the chest, application of a pulse oximeter for measuring oxygen saturation, and assessment of respiratory rate. Because patients are supine during the primary survey, auscultation is limited to the anterior and lateral chest. Auscultation should be performed in both these areas to obtain the most accurate evaluation of ventilation. Localizing abnormal auscultatory findings to a specific region of the chest can be more difficult in younger children because of smaller chest size and the usual supine position of the injured patient during the primary survey. However, in most children, auscultation can be used to identify significant compromise in ventilation requiring lifesaving intervention. These steps can be supplemented by a subjective evaluation of the adequacy and symmetry of chest wall movement and an evaluation for evidence of chest wall trauma. Because of the pliability of the chest wall of younger children, significant chest injury may be present even in the absence of any chest wall deformity.

A main focus of the B phase of the primary survey is identifying four specific thoracic injuries that can significantly impair ventilation and that require immediate treatment: (1) tension pneumothorax, (2) open pneumothorax, (3) flail chest with pulmonary contusion, and (4) massive hemothorax. The diagnosis of a tension pneumothorax should be made on clinical criteria, including tracheal deviation, unilateral absence of breath sounds, neck vein distention, tachycardia, hypotension, and respiratory distress. Delaying treatment to obtain a confirmatory chest radiograph should be avoided because of the time delay associated with processing and interpreting this study. When the clinical diagnosis of a tension pneumothorax is made, the chest should immediately be decompressed by placing a 14- to 18-gauge, 5-cm needle into the second intercostal space at the midclavicular line. The needle should be sufficiently long to penetrate the chest wall and enter the pleural space. A minimum length of 5 cm is recommended in older children and adults, but shorter needles may suffice in infants and younger children.[2] Proper intrathoracic placement of the needle can be partly confirmed by an audible rush of air when entering the chest. Because needle decompression will convert a tension pneumothorax into a simple pneumothorax, a chest tube will be necessary regardless of the response to needle decompression. If a child arrives after needle decompression, tube thoracostomy placement will most likely be necessary for definitive treatment.

An open pneumothorax or "sucking chest wound" occurs when the size of a chest wall injury approaches two-thirds the area of the tracheal lumen, causing a preferential pull of air into the pleural space and out of the wound. This injury can lead to mediastinal shift, decreased venous return, and eventual cardiopulmonary collapse. Open pneumothorax is rare in children and is usually the result of a penetrating injury. Airflow through the wound will be audible or can be visualized by bubbling of blood at the wound. A semiocclusive rectangular petroleum jelly/gauze dressing that is occlusive on three sides beyond the wound edge will produce a one-way valve effect that will allow air to escape on expiration but inhibit air from entering the thoracic cavity on inspiration.[25]

Flail chest occurs when a segment of the chest wall has lost continuity with the movement of the thoracic cage, occurring when two or more ribs are fractured in two or more positions. The pediatric thoracic cage is more compliant than adults, and rib fractures are not always present when parenchymal injuries exist. When occurring in infants and young children, rib fractures suggest a significant amount of blunt force to the chest and the possibility of an underlying pulmonary contusion, as well as hepatic or splenic injury. Because fractured ribs can lead to direct lung injury, the presence of a flail chest segment should raise the suspicion of a pneumothorax and hemothorax. Due to compromised ventilatory function and underlying pulmonary injury, management of flail chest is focused on providing temporary ventilatory support until the injury heals. Intubation may be immediately necessary in the emergency department when ventilation is significantly compromised by this injury.

Significant bleeding may occur with thoracic trauma from intercostal vessels, internal mammary vessels, lung parenchyma, or cardiopulmonary vessels, leading to massive hemothorax. Children with this injury will present with decreased breath sounds and dullness to percussion on the affected side. Eliciting the finding of dullness to percussion can be difficult in a noisy trauma resuscitation area but is a diagnostic feature that can be used to distinguish this injury from a pneumothorax. While the diagnosis is optimally made with a chest radiograph, the team should proceed with immediate chest tube placement if clinical evidence suggests the presence of a large amount of intrathoracic blood. When a massive hemothorax is present, fluid resuscitation or blood transfusion will often be necessary. After chest tube placement, the amount of blood initially obtained and the rate of continued bleeding from the tube should be evaluated. A thoracotomy for controlling bleeding from the chest wall, lung, or heart may be indicated if the initial volume exceeds 20% to 25% of estimated blood volume, bleeding continues at a rate exceeding 2 to 4 mL/kg/hr, the rate of bleeding is increasing, or the pleural space cannot be drained of blood and clots. The latter three criteria may be observed after the child is initially stabilized and has been admitted to the hospital.

About 75% of traumatic chest injuries can be treated expectantly or with placement of a chest tube and volume resuscitation.[26] Although placement of a chest tube in an injured child is similar to placement in other settings, additional steps should be considered in the injured child. When placing a chest tube for trauma, the tube should be directed posteriorly to allow for adequate drainage of blood in a supine patient. A sufficiently large tube should be selected to allow drainage of blood and fluid without becoming clogged with blood clot. The fifth intercostal space (nipple level) in the anterior midaxillary line is ideal in most patients to prevent placement of the tube through the diaphragm or abdomen but allows sufficient length in the chest for drainage and avoiding later dislodgement. Confirmation of tube placement in the pleural space can be confirmed in infants and smaller children by the egress of air or blood after placement. Proper tube placement in the thoracic cavity can also be evaluated by observing air condensation on the internal surface of the tube and movement of fluid in the water-seal chamber in time with the patient's respirations when connected to a pressure-regulated collection device. A chest radiograph should be performed to verify placement of the tube before leaving the resuscitation area.

Circulation (C)

The "C" step of the primary survey is the assessment, recognition, and management of shock. Because of greater physiologic reserve, early identification of cardiovascular compromise can be more difficult in children than adults (Table 118.2). Assessment and management of circulatory status in the primary survey are focused on early identification and treatment rather than defining the specific etiology of the shock state. Determining the site of internal hemorrhage and defining the specific type of shock state are steps that are deferred until after the primary survey. Objective assessment of circulation is done by measuring heart rate and blood pressure and assessing pulses and capillary refill. In addition to cardiovascular compromise, tachycardia after injury can indicate pain, fear, or other psychologic stress. Tachycardia therefore cannot be used as the sole criteria for diagnosing cardiovascular compromise and needs to be combined with other clinical criteria before treatment is initiated. A manual blood pressure measurement should be obtained, using the appropriate size cuff, on arrival to the resuscitation area. Periodic reassessment of blood pressure should continue throughout the resuscitation to verify the child's hemodynamic status. Palpation of central and peripheral pulses is a rapid method for detecting hypotension and often can be accomplished before a cuff blood pressure is obtained. Because pulses are most likely to be lost in progressive hypotension in the wrist or feet followed by the groin and then by the neck, palpation for pulses in each of these areas can provide a crude estimate of the level of hypotension. Assessment of peripheral perfusion can also include an estimate of capillary refill in addition to a visual evaluation of skin perfusion. Because these latter assessments are more subjective, these should be used only in conjunction with more objective measurements in directing treatment. While assessment of circulatory status is essential to the initial evaluation of an injured child, these steps are often omitted or delayed until later in the resuscitation. During video review of

TABLE 118.2	Systemic Responses to Blood Loss in Pediatric Patients		
System	**Mild Blood Volume Loss (<30%)**	**Moderate Blood Volume Loss (30%-45%)**	**Severe Blood Volume Loss (>45%)**
Cardiovascular	Increased heart rate; weak, thready peripheral pulses; normal systolic blood pressure (80-90 + 2 × age in years); normal pulse pressure	Markedly increased heart rate; weak, thready central pulses; low normal systolic blood pressure (70-80 + 2 × age in years); narrowed pulse pressure	Tachycardia followed by bradycardia; very weak or absent peripheral pulses; hypotension (<70 + 2 × age in years); narrowed pulse pressure (or undetectable diastolic blood pressure)
Central nervous system	Anxious; irritable; confused	Lethargic; dulled response to pain[a]	Comatose
Skin	Cool, mottled; prolonged capillary refill	Cyanotic; markedly prolonged capillary refill	Pale and cold
Urinary output[b]	Low to very low	Minimal	None

[a]The child's dulled response to pain with this degree of blood loss (30%-45%) may be indicated by a decreased response to IV catheter insertion.
[b]After initial decompression by urinary catheter. Low normal is 2 mL/kg/hr (infant), 1.5 mL/kg/hr (younger child), 1 mL/kg/hr (older child), and 0.5 mL/hg/hr (adolescent). IV contrast can falsely elevate urinary output.
Data from Committee on Trauma, American College of Surgeons. Advanced Trauma Life Support for Doctors, Student Course Manual. 9th ed. Chicago: American College of Surgeons; 2012.

pediatric trauma resuscitations, blood pressure was not measured in 31% of patients, pulses not assessed in 41%, and central capillary refill not assessed in 66% during the initial evaluation.[10] One important item to remember when assessing children after trauma is that pediatric patients will often maintain blood pressure and cardiac output by increasing heart rate. Children become hypotensive at later stages of shock.

The two main interventions for managing cardiovascular compromise during the primary survey are controlling external hemorrhage and administration of fluid. Active hemorrhage is easy to recognize and can usually be treated by direct manual pressure or the application of compression bandages. Scalp lacerations are a common source of external bleeding in injured children, and blood loss from this site should not be underestimated. A full evaluation for external hemorrhage, however, is only complete after the child has been exposed completely later in the primary survey.

Administration of fluids requires the establishment of IV access. In pediatric trauma, the preferred order of sites depends on the child's age and the urgency of establishing IV access. If a percutaneous peripheral IV line cannot be established, intraosseous access, percutaneous central venous access, or cutdown on a vein should be considered. Intraosseous access is achieved by placing a needle into the marrow cavity of a long bone in an uninjured extremity. This procedure is rapid, requires minimal training, and is the preferred alternate method of vascular access in infants and younger children. The availability of new equipment and techniques has expanded the use of intraosseous infusions to older children and even adults. Percutaneous placement of a central venous catheter can be pursued as an alternate access in older children when equipment for intraosseous access is not available or when ossification of the long bones precludes placement of an intraosseous needle. Femoral placement of a central line in the injured child has advantages over placement in a jugular or subclavian vein position because it can be performed in most patients without interfering with ongoing assessment and management of other components of the primary survey. However, the femoral route is not recommended if there is concern about the potential for abdominal or pelvic injuries. Despite the importance of establishing IV access in the injured child for fluid resuscitation and administration of medications, vascular access was not performed or inadequate access was obtained in 20% of recorded pediatric resuscitations.[10]

The goal of fluid resuscitation is to rapidly replace intravascular volume, initially with warmed crystalloid solution and then moving to blood products on the basis of the child's response to crystalloid boluses (Fig. 118.4). When cardiovascular compromise is detected, an initial bolus of 20 mL/kg of warmed isotonic crystalloid fluid (normal saline or lactated Ringer solution) should be administered. Given that it is relatively hypotonic, lactated Ringer solution is not recommended for fluid resuscitation in patients with traumatic brain injury. Fluid administration should not be delayed by slow-rate drip infusion but instead should be administered as a bolus using a hand-pump device, syringe, or pressure bag to ensure that the effect of the bolus and assessment of need for additional fluid proceeds rapidly. If a second bolus of crystalloid is necessary, preparations for the administration of blood products should begin. If the child responds to fluid administration, IV fluid is continued at a maintenance rate as further investigations concerning the need for fluid are performed. If there

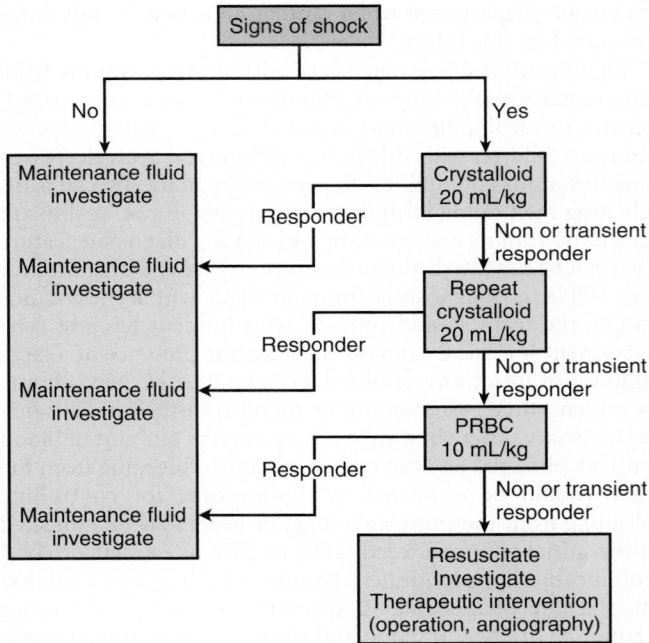

Fig. 118.4. Algorithm for pediatric fluid resuscitation.

continues to be no response or transient response to crystalloid, blood administration should be considered. During the primary survey, cross-matched, type-specific blood is often not yet available and O-negative blood should be administered. Blood should be administered in boluses of 10 mL/kg. The four sites of hemorrhage that can lead to major blood loss after injury include external sites (eg, scalp laceration), intrathoracic injury, intraabdominal injury, and pelvic or multiple long-bone (usually femur) fractures. While external bleeding can be easily detected, bleeding in other sites is evaluated after the primary survey has been completed.

Disability (D)

The primary survey continues with a neurologic assessment of the child, the disability (D) component of the primary survey. This assessment includes two main components, calculating the GCS and assessment of pupillary responses (Fig. 118.5). More extensive neurologic evaluation should be deferred to the secondary survey to avoid slowing the primary survey. As with airway assessment, a formal evaluation of GCS is often omitted when it is "obvious" that no neurologic injury is present. This practice should be avoided because subtle changes may be missed with only a cursory assessment. In addition, establishment of a baseline GCS may have prognostic value among children with an evolving intracranial injury. To account for variations in response related to age, the GCS should be calculated using age-specific criteria. Among the three main components of the GCS, the motor score has been shown to be the best predictor of outcome after injury.[27] Particular attention should be paid to ensure that this component is accurately assessed and recorded. Pupillary assessment includes an evaluation of pupil size and response to light and can easily and rapidly be assessed, reported, and recorded. Findings from the neurologic assessment are used to plan additional evaluation and management steps, including the need for endotracheal intubation, the requirements of additional imaging, and the final disposition after leaving the

INFANTS	CHILDREN	ADULTS
Best eye opening 4 – Spontaneous 3 – Opens to verbal stimulus 2 – Opens to painful stimulus 1 – No response	**Best eye opening** 4 – Spontaneous 3 – Opens to verbal stimulus 2 – Opens to painful stimulus 1 – No response	**Best eye opening** 4 – Spontaneous 3 – Opens to verbal stimulus 2 – Opens to painful stimulus 1 – No response
Best verbal response 5 – Coos and babbles 4 – Irritable cry 3 – Cries to pain 2 – Moans to pain 1 – No response	**Best verbal response** 5 – Orientated 4 – Confused 3 – Inappropriate words 2 – Incomprehensible words 1 – No response	**Best verbal response** 5 – Orientated (person, place, time) 4 – Confused, disorientated 3 – Inappropriate words 2 – Incomprehensible words 1 – No response
Best motor response 6 – Spontaneous purposeful movement 5 – Localizes to pain 4 – Withdraws to pain 3 – Flexion (decorticate response) 2 – Extension (decerebrate response) 1 – No response	**Best motor response** 6 – Obeys commands 5 – Localizes to pain 4 – Withdraws to pain 3 – Flexion (decorticate response) 2 – Extension (decerebrate response) 1 – No response	**Best motor response** 6 – Obeys commands 5 – Localizes to pain 4 – Withdraws to pain 3 – Flexion (decorticate response) 2 – Extension (decerebrate response) 1 – No response

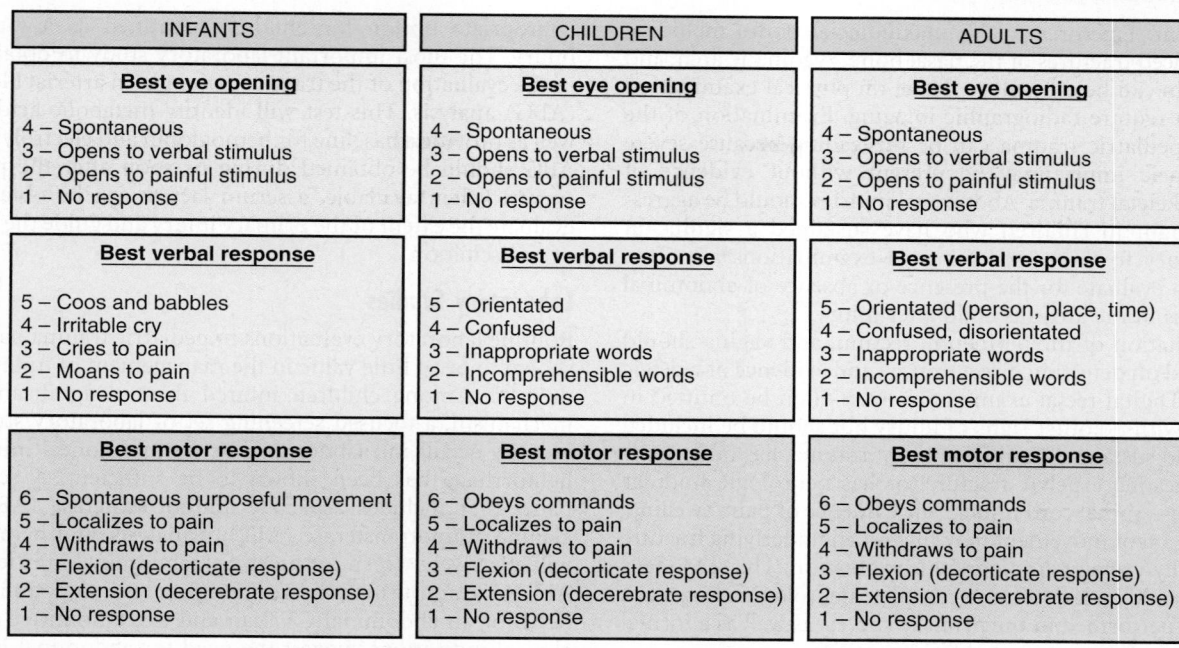

Fig. 118.5. Components of the Glasgow Coma Scale at different ages.

emergency department. Despite the importance of obtaining a GCS and assessing pupils, these steps were both omitted in 20% of observed pediatric trauma resuscitations.

Exposure/Environment (E)

The final step in the primary survey is exposure of the patient, the "E" component of the primary survey. In this phase, clothing is removed to visually inspect all body regions to minimize the chance of missing an obvious injury. A team-coordinated log roll of the child, maintaining cervical spine stabilization, can be used to assess the back and spine for external injury. When rolled on their side, patients are in an ideal position for assessing the spinal column for deformities and tenderness and for undergoing a rectal examination if indicated. While not all of these steps are formally part of the primary survey, the additional time required for them is minimal, leading to the inclusion of these steps as part of exposure in many centers. Immediately after exposing the injured child, the child should be covered again with warm blankets to minimize heat loss. Infants and younger children are particularly vulnerable to heat loss because of a relatively large surface area in relation to body volume. Other measures for warming or maintaining an injured child's temperature include warming the room and the use of overhead warmers or a Bair hugger. The patient's temperature should be obtained at this point, a step that is frequently omitted in the initial evaluation of the injured child.

Secondary Survey

After completion of the primary survey, the secondary survey is then performed. This includes a medical and event history, a more complete physical examination, and additional adjunct interventions. The secondary survey is less structured than the primary survey, and its components and sequence can be modified to reflect patient needs, provider preferences, and institutional practices. The secondary survey should not be performed until the components of the primary survey have been completed and interventions needed to address issues identified in the primary survey have been implemented. It is a common pitfall to move to components of the secondary survey or to mix components of the secondary survey during performance of the primary survey. This practice should be discouraged so as to avoid losing focus on the primary survey and life-threatening injuries that it is designed to identify. During the secondary survey, attention should be intermittently refocused on the five vital signs (blood pressure, heart rate, respiratory rate, temperature, and pain score) and other monitoring steps of the primary survey. When changes are observed, the primary survey evaluation and treatment steps should be reinitiated to ensure that potentially life-threatening injuries are addressed.

In contrast to a typical history performed during evaluations in other settings, the history performed in the secondary survey is more focused and follows rather than precedes the performance of the physical examination. It is common practice to obtain this information while simultaneously performing the physical examination components of the secondary survey. The most important history elements to obtain are those that most directly impact injured patients and the evaluation and treatments needed for them. The acronym AMPLE is useful for remembering these key elements (*a*llergies, *m*edications, *p*ast medical history, *l*ast meal, and the *e*nvironment and events related to the injury). The physical examination contains elements similar to those performed in other settings but should be modified to include steps that identify common and important injuries. Examination of the entire scalp should be performed to identifying lacerations, contusions, or evidence of fractures. Posterior scalp lacerations can easily be missed because of hair or the position of the cervical collar. Massive facial injuries can produce significant facial edema, making the eye examination difficult. Because facial swelling most often worsens with time, it is important to obtain an initial eye examination while the patient is in the emergency department. Fractures to the maxillofacial bones including nondisplaced fractures of the nasal bone, zygomatic arch, and orbital rim can be difficult to detect on physical examination and often require radiographic imaging. Examination of the chest in pediatric trauma can be misleading because severe intrathoracic injury may be present without evidence of obvious skeletal trauma. Abdominal injuries should be aggressively sought in children who have sustained a significant blunt injury to the torso. Repeated examinations are often needed to evaluate for the presence or absence of abdominal tenderness in the anxious child after injury.[28]

Examination of the perineum, rectum, and vagina should be focused on detecting direct trauma and evidence of a pelvic fracture. Digital rectal examination may often be omitted in children with no other signs of injury but should be included if the child sustained significant blunt trauma, has other findings suggesting a pelvic fracture, or has neurologic findings suggesting a spinal cord injury. Any evidence of pain, swelling, or limitation of movement may suggest an underlying fracture and usually warrants radiographic evaluation. The secondary survey should include a more complete neurologic assessment than was performed in the primary survey, as well as a formal assessment of sensory and motor functions.

While the secondary survey can be performed in a free-form fashion, a systematic strategy is necessary to avoid missing key components of this evaluation. In reviews of pediatric trauma resuscitations, components of the secondary survey that are often omitted include examination of the mouth, ears, back, and perineum. As in the primary survey, findings in the secondary survey should be communicated to the team. The trauma team leader should address the need for tetanus administration (depending on child's vaccine requirements) and antibiotic administration (eg, for open fractures) during the secondary survey.

Missed injuries do occur in trauma resuscitations, which may lead to preventable morbidity during the patient's hospital stay. About 4% of injured children will have an injury missed in the primary and secondary surveys. The risk of a missed injury is higher in children with more severe injuries, including those transported by air, those who undergo endotracheal intubation in the emergency department, those with a low admission GCS, and those with an injury severity score greater than 15.[29] Missed injuries have been shown to be reduced with the implementation of a designated pediatric trauma response team, supporting a focused and stepwise approach to the initial evaluation of the injured children.[30] Critical care providers should be alert to the possibility of missed injuries in patients admitted to their unit and not rely on the emergency department evaluation for detecting all injuries.

Diagnostic Assessment

The secondary survey is supplemented by diagnostic testing that focuses on identifying and treating injuries not found in the primary survey. Performance of a standard set of tests is discouraged to avoid unnecessary discomfort, exposure to radiation from excessive imaging, and cost. Injured children may be overtriaged to the resuscitation area and require no additional testing after the primary and secondary surveys have been completed. Observation in the emergency department before discharge and close outpatient follow-up is an appropriate option for children identified as low-risk for injury. The most important laboratory study to obtain early in the evaluation of the trauma patient is an arterial blood gas (ABG) analysis. This test will identify metabolic acidosis, as well as provide a baseline for hemoglobin and electrolytes. The ABG should be obtained during or soon after the primary survey. When available, a serum lactate can be obtained to evaluate the extent of the primary injury and guide the efficacy of resuscitation.

Laboratory Studies

Routine laboratory evaluations in pediatric trauma have been shown to be of little value in the management of injured children.[31,32] Among children injured from a significant blunt mechanism, a focused screening set of laboratory studies to identify occult intraabdominal or retroperitoneal injury and hemorrhage has been shown to be sufficient. A screening panel that includes aspartate aminotransferase (AST) and alanine aminotransferase (ALT), urinalysis, and hemoglobin will effectively screen for most intraabdominal injuries.[33] The ALT, AST, and urinalysis are screening tests to determine the need for an abdominal CT scan and can be omitted if other clinical indications suggest the need for abdominal imaging. Threshold values of greater than 100 U/L for AST and ALT and more than 5 red blood cells/high-powered field suggest the presence of an intraabdominal injury and suggest the need for abdominal/pelvic imaging.

Among children with major head injuries, penetrating trauma, multiple extremity fractures, and significant mechanisms of injury, this panel of laboratory studies may be expanded to include coagulation studies, electrolytes, and blood for cross-matching. Coagulation studies in pediatric trauma are most often abnormal in the presence of severe traumatic brain injury. If obtained early after injury, electrolyte studies are most often normal and serve only as a baseline for a patient who will require aggressive management of severe head injuries or aggressive resuscitation. Blood should be obtained for cross-matching if significant fluid resuscitation has been required, the child has a preexisting condition causing a predisposition to bleeding, has a major head injury, or will undergo a surgical procedure with potential for blood loss. Early after injury, pancreatic enzymes do not need to be obtained as a screen for pancreatic injury because of the low diagnostic yield of these studies.[34] Screening tests for alcohol or drug use may be appropriate in older children and adolescent patients.

Radiographic Imaging

Radiographs may be necessary to rule out specific injuries or to evaluate known injuries. The three most common radiographs obtained are cervical spine, chest, and pelvic radiographs. Although these studies are commonly referred to as a *trauma series* and ordered as a set, the performance of all three is often not necessary. The need for each radiograph should be evaluated on the basis of the mechanism of injury and patient symptoms and examination.[35]

A cervical spine injury should be suspected in any child sustaining a significant head injury or injured by a major blunt mechanism. Although cervical spine injuries are rare, these injuries can be devastating and can have worse outcomes when adequate spine precautions are not taken early after injury. A systematic and efficient approach using both clinical and diagnostic modalities is necessary to ensure that a cervical spine injury is not present. Implementation of standards for cervical spine assessment and clearance has been shown to decrease the time for cervical spine clearance.[36] Each institution should develop an institution-specific protocol for managing the initial and subsequent imaging of the cervical spine to avoid either incomplete evaluations or excessive imaging. Criteria for cervical spine imaging include midline cervical tenderness, altered level of consciousness, evidence of intoxication, neurologic abnormalities potentially attributable to a spine injury, and presence of a distracting injury precluding a reliable clinical assessment.[37] The cervical spine evaluation in nonverbal children is particularly difficult to assess. A recent study of this subgroup identified GCS less than 14, GCS eye component of 1, an injury sustained in a motor vehicle crash, and age younger than 2 years as important variables associated with the presence of a cervical spine injury.[38]

A cervical spine series consists of a cross-table lateral, an anterior-posterior view, and an open-mouth view to assess the dens process of C1. With adequate films, a three-view series has a high sensitivity (89%) and a negative predictive value of 99.9%.[39] Among these views, the lateral cervical spine film is most useful and has been adopted as the initial screening film at many institutions.[40] If a patient meets the NEXIS criteria, then the C-spine can be cleared clinically. Cervical CT imaging is indicated if a child has any of the following after a significant mechanism of injury: intracranial injury, any injury above the clavicles, facial fractures, cervical spine tenderness, seat belt sign across the neck, altered mental status with inability to perform cervical spine examination, and intoxication.[41]

Chest radiographs can often be omitted for children without physical examination findings or symptoms suggesting a thoracic injury.[35] This study, however, should be obtained for children who are injured by a major blunt mechanism such as a high-speed motor vehicle crash or those who have sustained other significant torso injuries. Pelvic radiographs can be safely omitted among children who are awake, alert, and have no physical examination findings or proximity injuries (eg, a proximal femur fracture) to suggest a pelvic injury. Radiographs of the extremities or other areas may also be necessary in the resuscitation area depending on the findings of the primary and secondary surveys. While CT imaging is useful and has the advantages of being rapid and organ specific in defining injuries, there are potential hazards in its use, especially in pediatrics. In 2007, a study from Los Angeles showed that "pan-scanning," or doing a head, chest, and abdomen CT scan, often led to finding unsuspected injuries requiring treatment. Nineteen percent of patients in this study had an injury on CT scan that was not suspected on physical examination.[42] After this study, it became common practice to "pan-scan" many blunt trauma patients. Although rapid and specific, it was soon recognized that patients were being exposed to high doses of ionizing radiation without much proven clinical benefit, as many of the identified injuries did not require surgery. A study from San Antonio in a level I trauma center attached dosimeters to the neck, chest, and groin of the injured children. When a patient underwent CT imaging of more than two body regions, the dose of ionizing radiation exceeded the dose normally associated with thyroid cancer or leukemia.[43] A recent study demonstrated that using a more restrictive protocol for obtaining CT imaging reduced the number of CT scans obtained in a cohort of trauma patients without increasing missed injuries or mortality.[44] With regard to using CT scanning in children, the pendulum is swinging back to the more restrictive use of CT scans, in order to avoid excessive amounts of radiation to younger patients, who have a higher lifetime risk of developing neoplasms after radiation.

CT is an accurate diagnostic tool and has become an integral component of the evaluation of injured patients. Although CT scans can be essential in the evaluation of many children, excessive use is discouraged because of the higher radiation exposure associated with CT scans, rare but important complications such as contrast reactions, and added costs. CT scans are a growing source of medical radiation exposure in children and may contribute to the occurrence of radiation-related malignancy, particularly when performed among younger children.[45]

The two most common body regions imaged with a CT scan in pediatric trauma are the head and abdomen/pelvis. A noncontrast head CT is performed to assess for closed head injuries and fractures that may require additional treatment such as a depressed skull fracture. The most common indication for a head CT scan after pediatric injury is a history of loss of consciousness or altered mental status. A head CT scan may also be necessary for preverbal children whose injury was not observed or those who have received endotracheal intubation or are sedated as they cannot be reliably assessed for a potential head injury.[46-48] A large multicenter trial derived and validated predictive rules to identify children at very low risk of clinically important traumatic brain injury after blunt trauma where a head CT scan may be unnecessary. These prediction rules had a sensitivity of 100% in children 2 years old and younger and 96.8% in children older than 2; negative predictive value was 100% for all ages (Fig. 118.6).[49]

Recent emphasis on developing approaches to reduce the need for screening abdominal/pelvic CT scans in pediatric trauma continues to evolve. Imaging is indicated when an injury is suggested by physical examination findings such as major abdominal wall ecchymoses or abdominal tenderness. Among children who sustain a significant blunt injury but do not have physical examination findings suggesting an abdominal injury, the yield of screening abdominal CT scans is low. Screening laboratory tests, however, can be used to reduce unneeded imaging for these children.

While focused abdominal sonogram for trauma (FAST) has been widely adopted as a diagnostic tool for adult trauma patients, its value in pediatric trauma is less certain. FAST is focused on identifying fluid in four areas, the presence of which is suggestive of hemopericardium or intraabdominal injury: the pericardial sac, hepatorenal fossa, splenorenal fossa, and pouch of Douglas. Current evidence suggests that the role of FAST for evaluating children after blunt abdominal injury is limited. When used in children, FAST has only modest sensitivity (80%) for the detection of hemoperitoneum, and a negative ultrasound has questionable utility as the only test to exclude an intraabdominal injury.[50] Recent studies have suggested that FAST may be combined with screening laboratory studies to increase sensitivity, specificity, positive predictive value, and negative predictive value.[51]

Emergency Department Thoracotomy

Emergency department thoracotomy can be a lifesaving intervention among some children presenting in extremis after

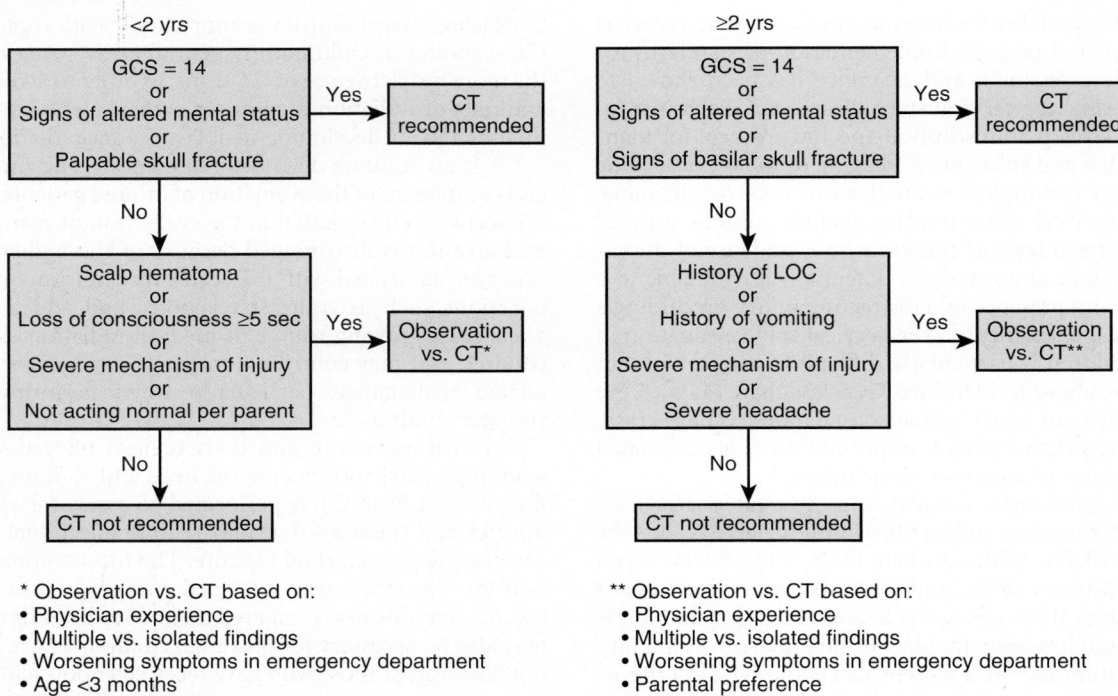

Fig. 118.6. Algorithm for head CT using predictive rules. (Modified from Kupperman N, Holmes JF, Dayan PS, et al. Identification of children at very low risk of clinically-important brain injuries after head trauma: a prospective cohort study. Lancet. 2009;374:1160-1170.)

injury. This procedure, however, should be used selectively because its effectiveness has been shown to be limited to specific patient subsets, including those who have received a brief period of cardiopulmonary resuscitation after sustaining a blunt injury or witnessed penetrating injury. Patients who sustain a penetrating injury are more likely to benefit from an emergency department thoracotomy because the higher potential for identifying injuries that can be treated after a thoracotomy has been performed. Data defining the role of emergency department thoracotomy in children are limited to small patient series and retrospective reviews. Available evidence suggests that this procedure should be reserved for pediatric patients who present with detectable vital signs and deteriorate despite maximal resuscitation.[52-55] Each institution should establish guidelines for the use of emergency department thoracotomy to aid in decision making when this rare procedure needs to be performed.

Emergency department thoracotomy should only be performed by a surgeon with appropriate training in this technique. A left anterolateral thoracotomy incision is made extending from left of the sternum in the fifth intercostal space to the table. A large incision is necessary to aid visualization and therapeutic interventions. This incision may be extended across to the right side of the chest (clamshell incision) if needed. The next step is to control hemorrhage by digital compression, suture control, or clamping of bleeding blood vessels. A pericardiotomy is performed using a longitudinal incision to evacuate hemopericardium blood and inspect the heart for injuries. Open cardiac massage can be performed if necessary. Cross-clamping the descending thoracic aorta will stop blood loss below the diaphragm and allow cardiac filling to maintain cardiac and brain perfusion. The pulmonary

hilum can be clamped or manually compressed to control bleeding from the lung and pulmonary vessels.

Stabilization and Definitive Care

Following the initial resuscitation, a plan for the next step in care is defined. Children can be discharged from the emergency department if no injuries requiring inpatient observation or management are identified and there is a low suspicion of injury based on the clinical evaluation and mechanism of injury. Other children may require inpatient admission to either the hospital ward or ICU depending on the injuries identified. Some children may have injuries that require immediate operative repair and need to be moved directly to the operating room. Transfer to a higher level of care facility after evaluation and stabilization may be necessary if injuries are identified that cannot be treated at the receiving hospital. One important caveat is that if the emergency department physician or pediatrician determines from the primary and secondary surveys that the child will not be able to be treated at the initial receiving facility, it is important to promptly call the next highest level of care and not waste time obtaining CT scans or other studies that will not be acted on at the receiving facility.[56]

Conclusions

Pediatric trauma care requires an efficient team-based approach from prehospital care until the time of discharge. Within current trauma systems, patient care is optimized for efficiency and outcomes when each team member has a defined role and effective communication is established within the team. By understanding the prioritized sequence of ATLS, rapid recognition and treatment of life-threatening injuries will occur efficiently within the team and greatly improve the outcome of these injured patients. Pediatric critical care providers will continue to take an active role in the management of the most severely injured pediatric trauma patients. Pediatric critical care physicians proficient in emergent procedures and knowledgeable of resuscitative measures in trauma care will augment the multidisciplinary approach to pediatric trauma care.

Acknowledgments

We gratefully acknowledge the contribution of Steven Elliott and Randall S. Burd, who authored this chapter in previous editions.

References

1. Heron M, Hoyert DL, Murphy SL, et al. *Deaths: Final Data for 2006. National Vital Statistics Reports*. Atlanta, GA: Centers for Disease Control and Prevention; 2009.
2. Committee on Trauma, American College of Surgeons. *Advanced Trauma Life Support for Doctors, Student Course Manual*. 9th ed. Chicago: American College of Surgeons; 2012.
3. Van Olden GD, Meeuwis JD, Bolhuis HW, et al. Clinical impact of advanced trauma life support. *J Emerg Med*. 2004;22:522-525.
4. Williams MJ, Lockey AS, Culshaw MC. Improved trauma management with advanced trauma life support (ATLS) training. *J Accid Emerg Med*. 1997;14:81-83.
5. Ben-Abraham R, Weinbroum AA, Kluger Y, et al. Pediatricians and the advanced trauma life support (ATLS): time for reconsideration? *Isr Med Assoc J*. 2000;2:513-516.
6. Kouzminova N, Shatney C, Palm E, et al. The efficacy of a two-tiered trauma activation system at a level I trauma center. *J Trauma*. 2009; 67:829-833.
7. DeKeyser FG, Paratore A, Seneca RP, et al. Decreasing the cost of trauma care: a system of secondary in-hospital triage. *Ann Emerg Med*. 1994;23:841-844.
8. Emergency Medical Technician—Basic: National Standard Curriculum. Available at: <http://www.nhtsa.dot.gov>.
9. Spanjersberg WR, Bergs EA, Mushkudiani N, et al. Protocol compliance and time management in blunt trauma resuscitations. *Emerg Med J*. 2009;26:23-27.
10. Oakley E, Stocker S, Staubli G, Young S. Using video recording to identify management errors in pediatric trauma resuscitation. *Pediatrics*. 2006;117: 658-664.
11. Easley RB, Segeleon JE, Haun SE, Tobias JD. Prospective study of airway management of children requiring endotracheal intubation before admission to a pediatric intensive care unit. *Crit Care Med*. 2000;28: 2058-2063.
12. Verghese ST, Hannallah RS, Slack MC, et al. Auscultation of bilateral breath sounds does not rule out endobronchial intubation in children. *Anesth Analg*. 2004;99:56-58.
13. Avarello JT, Cantor RM. Pediatric major trauma: an approach to evaluation and management. *Emerg Med Clin North Am*. 2007;25:803-836.
14. Kelly CA, Upex A, Bateman DN. Comparison of consciousness level assessment in the poisoned patient using the alert/verbal/painful/unresponsive scale and the Glasgow Coma Scale. *Ann Emerg Med*. 2004; 44:108-113.
15. Mace SE. Challenges and advances in intubation: rapid sequence intubation. *Emerg Med Clin North Am*. 2008;26:1043-1068.
16. Santillanes G, Gausche-Hill M. Pediatric airway management. *Emerg Med Clin North Am*. 2008;26:961-975.
17. Tobias JD. Airway management for pediatric emergencies. *Pediatr Ann*. 1996;25:317-328.
18. Rodricks MB, Deutschman CS. Emergent airway management. Indications and methods in the face of confounding conditions. *Crit Care Clin*. 2000;16:389-409.
19. Levy RJ, Helfaer MA. Pediatric airway issues. *Crit Care Clin*. 2000;16: 489-504.
20. Henderson JJ, Popat MT, Latto IP, Pearce AC. Difficult Airway Society guidelines for management of the unanticipated difficult intubation. *Anaesthesia*. 2004;59:675-694.
21. Sagarin MJ, Barton ED, Chng YM, et al. Airway management by US and Canadian emergency medicine residents: a multicenter analysis of more than 6,000 endotracheal intubation attempts. *Ann Emerg Med*. 2005;46: 328-336.
22. Holmes JF, Panacek EA, Sakles JC, et al. Comparison of 2 cricothyrotomy techniques: standard method versus rapid 4-step technique. *Ann Emerg Med*. 1998;32:442-446.
23. Mace SE, Khan N. Needle cricothyroidotomy. *Emerg Med Clin North Am*. 2008;26:1085-1101.
24. Yealy DM, Stewart RD, Kaplan RM. Myths and pitfalls in emergency translaryngeal ventilation: correcting misimpressions. *Ann Emerg Med*. 1988;17:690-692.
25. Yamaoto L, Schroeder C, Beliveau C. Thoracic trauma: the deadly dozen. *Crit Care Nurs Q*. 2004;28:22-40.
26. Khander SJ, Johnson SB, Calhoon JH. Overview of thoracic trauma in the United States. *Thorac Surg Clin*. 2007;17:1-9.
27. Healy C, Osler TM, Rogers FB, et al. Improving the Glasgow Coma Scale score: motor score alone is a better predictor. *J Trauma*. 2003;54: 671-678.
28. Meyer MK, Burd RS. The trauma top 10: the top 10 things to evaluate in children with suspected blunt abdominal injuries. *J Trauma Nursing*. 2000;7:98-102.
29. Williams BG, Hlaing T, Aaland MO. Ten-year retrospective study of delayed diagnosis of injury in pediatric trauma patients at a level II trauma center. *Pediatr Emer Care*. 2009;25:489-493.
30. Perno JF, Schunk JE, Hansen KW, et al. Significant reduction in delayed diagnosis of injury with implementation of a pediatric trauma service. *Pediatr Emerg Care*. 2005;21:367-371.
31. Keller MS, Coln CE, Trimble JA, et al. The utility of routine trauma laboratories in pediatric trauma resuscitations. *Am J Surg*. 2004;188:671-678.
32. Capraro AJ, Mooney D, Waltzman ML. The use of routine laboratory studies as screening tools in pediatric abdominal trauma. *Pediatr Emerg Care*. 2006;22:480-484.
33. Holmes JF, Sokolove PE, Brant WE, et al. Identification of children with intra-abdominal injuries after blunt trauma. *Ann Emerg Med*. 2002;39: 500-509.
34. Matsuno WC, Huang CJ, Garcia NM, et al. Amylase and lipase measurements in paediatric patients with traumatic pancreatic injuries. *Injury*. 2009;40:66-71.
35. Soundappan S, Smith NF, Lam LT, et al. A trauma series in the injured child: do we really need it? *Pediatr Emerg Care*. 2006;22:710-716.
36. Lee SL, Sena M, Greenholz SK, Fledderman M. A multidisciplinary approach to the development of a cervical spine clearance protocol: process, rationale, and initial results. *J Pediatr Surg*. 2003;38:358-362.
37. Viccellio P, Simon H, Pressman BD, et al. NEXUS Group. A prospective multicenter study of cervical spine injury in children. *Pediatrics*. 2001;108: E20.
38. Pieretti-Vanmarcke R, Velmahos GC, Nance ML, et al. Clinical clearance of the cervical spine in blunt trauma patients younger than 3 years. A multi-center study of the American Association for the Surgery of Trauma. *J Trauma*. 2009;67:543-550.
39. Mower WR, Hoffman JR, Pollack CV Jr, et al. NEXUS Group. Use of plain radiography to screen for cervical spine injuries. *Ann Emerg Med*. 2001; 38:1-7.
40. Buhs C, Cullen M, Klein M, et al. The pediatric trauma C-spine: is the 'odontoid' view necessary? *J Pediatr Surg*. 2000;35:994-997.
41. Stiell IG, Clement CM, McKnight RD, et al. The Canadian C-spine rule versus the NEXUS low-risk criteria in patients with trauma. *N Engl J Med*. 2003;349:2510-2518.
42. Salim A, Sangthong B, Martin M, et al. Whole body CT scanning in blunt multi-system trauma patients without obvious signs of injury: results of a prospective study. *Arch Surg*. 2006;141:468-473.
43. Mueller DL, Hatab M, Al-Senan R, et al. Pediatric radiation exposure during the initial evaluation for blunt trauma. *J Trauma*. 2011;70: 724-731.
44. Sise MJ, Kahl JE, Calvo RY, et al. Back to the future: reducing reliance on torso computed tomography in the initial evaluation of blunt trauma. *J Trauma Acute Care Surg*. 2013;74:92-99.

45. Brenner DJ, Hall EJ. Computer tomography, an increasing source of radiation exposure. *N Engl J Med.* 2007;357:2277-2284.

46. Maguire JL, Boutis K, Uleryk WM, et al. Should a head-injured child receive a head CT scan? A systemic review of clinical prediction rules. *Pediatrics.* 2009;124:e145-e154.

47. Palachak MJ, Holmes JF, Vance CW, et al. A decision rule for identifying children at low risk for brain injuries after blunt head trauma. *Ann Emerg Med.* 2003;42:492-506.

48. Dunning J, Daly JP, Lomas JP, et al. Derivation of the children's head injury algorithm for the prediction of important clinical events decision rule for head injury in children. *Arch Dis Child.* 2006;91:885-891.

49. Kupperman N, Holmes JF, Dayan PS, et al. Identification of children at very low risk of clinically important brain injury after head trauma: a prospective cohort study. *Lancet.* 2009;374:1160-1170.

50. Holmes JF, Gladman A, Chang CH. Performance of abdominal ultrasonography in pediatric blunt trauma patients: a meta-analysis. *J Pediatr Surg.* 2007;42:1588-1594.

51. Sola JE, Cheung MC, Yang R, et al. Pediatric FAST and elevated liver transaminases: an effective screening tool in blunt abdominal trauma. *J Surg Res.* 2009;157:103-107.

52. Powell RW, Gill EA, Jurkovich GJ. Resuscitative thoracotomy in children and adolescents. *Am Surg.* 1988;54:188-191.

53. Sheikh AA, Culbertson CB. Emergency department thoracotomy in children: rationale for selective application. *J Trauma.* 1993;34:323-328.

54. Beaver BL, Colombani PM, Buck JR, et al. Efficacy of emergency room thoracotomy in pediatric trauma. *J Pediatr Surg.* 1987;22:19-23.

55. Langer JC, Hoffman MA, Pearl RH, Ein SH. Survival after emergency department thoracotomy in a child with blunt multisystem trauma. *Pediatr Emerg Care.* 1989;5:255-256.

56. Benedict LA, Paulus JK, Rideout L, Chwals WJ. Are CT scans obtained at referring institutions justified prior to transfer to a pediatric trauma center? *J Pediatric Surg.* 2014;49:184-188.

Severe Traumatic Brain Injury in Infants and Children

Patrick M. Kochanek, Michael J. Bell, Hülya Bayır, Travis C. Jackson, Jessica S. Wallisch, Michael J. Forbes, Randall Ruppel, P. David Adelson, and Robert S.B. Clark

PEARLS

- Complete and rapid physiologic resuscitation is essential to the initial treatment of infants and children with severe traumatic brain injury.
- There are many age- and injury mechanism–related differences that could greatly impact optimized therapy and outcome in severe pediatric versus adult traumatic brain injury; however, the key factors in this regard have yet to be fully elucidated.
- Monitoring and control of intracranial hypertension should begin with first-tier therapies and progress to less established second-tier therapies in refractory cases.
- The choice of second-tier therapy is based in part on an in-depth knowledge of the physiologic derangements involved and the preferences and expertise of the treating team.
- Advanced neuromonitoring is providing additional insight into pathophysiology-guided treatment.
- Because pediatric patients with traumatic brain injury often sustain multiple insults, appropriate correction of physiologic derangements and complications in other organ systems is also important in creating an optimal environment for recovery.
- Optimized rehabilitation can facilitate recovery after severe traumatic brain injury, and a link is emerging between intensive care unit management and the early application of rehabilitation therapies.

The publication of pediatric traumatic brain injury (TBI) guidelines in 2003 and an updated document in 2012 has helped to crystallize therapy and generate interest in research on optimal pediatric intensive care unit (PICU) management of infants and children with severe TBI.[1,2] Subsequent to these guidelines and the previous edition of this textbook, several single-center studies have contributed to improving evidence-based care of children with severe TBI, and this information is incorporated into this chapter. However, there has been only one recent multicenter randomized controlled trial (RCT) in pediatric TBI, and thus the evidence for treatment approaches

remains insufficient, and considerable heterogeneity in treatment remains. A current large comparative effectiveness study in pediatric TBI, Approaches and Decisions in Acute Pediatric TBI (ADAPT), is an exciting initiative that could be extremely important for the field. But it has not yet provided new published evidence on treatment other than to confirm that despite general adherence to the guidelines, therapy is extremely heterogeneous across major PICU programs nationally and internationally.[3] This chapter presents a practical and contemporary approach to the management of patients with TBI based on several sources of information: (1) the pediatric guidelines, (2) new data from studies in children and adults with severe TBI, and (3) accepted principles of the physiology and pathophysiology of TBI.

This chapter focuses on severe TBI, specifically on management in the PICU. PICU management has progressed from exclusively supportive care to strategies attempting to (1) optimize substrate delivery and cerebral metabolism, (2) mitigate (wherever possible) the evolution of the secondary injury cascade of events set into motion from the primary damage, (3) minimize secondary insults that might worsen secondary damage and outcome, (4) prevent severe or intractable intracranial hypertension or herniation, and (5) initiate selected rehabilitation therapies. The field is moving into an era targeting a precision medicine approach to define specific pediatric TBI phenotypes (based on a number of factors) and craft specific monitoring and management plans to optimize outcome. The role of newer technologies and the differences between adults and children are highlighted.

Epidemiology

Traumatic brain injury remains a significant pediatric health problem, with an estimated incidence of 80 pediatric hospitalizations and 6 pediatric deaths per 100,000.[4] Pediatric TBI cases that are severe (Glasgow Coma Scale [GCS] score <8) contribute to 30% of all injury-related deaths in the United States.[5] Although children 5 to 15 years of age generally have favorable outcomes compared with adults, children aged 4 years or younger—particularly those younger than 2 years—have a worse outcome than older children and adults.[6] Abusive head trauma (AHT) is the leading cause of severe TBI in infants and is believed to be the key contributor to poor outcomes in this younger subgroup, although other factors may play a role.[7,8] Data also suggest that the rate of AHT has increased, likely related to economic forces.[9] Note that *AHT* is the preferred term for this condition (in preference to *shaken baby syndrome*, *inflicted childhood neurotrauma*, or *nonaccidental trauma*, among others) per the American Academy of Pediatrics and is thus used in this chapter.[10] Penetrating injuries such as gunshot wounds, although not as common as either motor vehicle accidents or AHT, also contribute significant morbidity and mortality in the pediatric population.[11]

Pathophysiology

Severe TBI involves a primary injury that includes direct and immediate disruption of brain parenchyma. However, not all of the effects of the primary injury are immediately apparent because damage also evolves over time and results from a cascade of biochemical, cellular, and molecular events involved in the evolution of the injury. Many of the aspects of the primary injury are immediate or irreversible, whereas others continue to evolve triggering a secondary injury cascade that can, in some cases, be mitigated. Delayed neuronal death from apoptosis and death from secondary axotomy are perfect examples of this phenomenon. Both of these processes are set into motion by the primary injury but become secondary injury processes that take time to develop (sometimes days) and thus may be able to be blunted.[12-14] Additional secondary injuries are also important and result from extracerebral and intracerebral insults (eg, hypotension, hypoxemia, fever, ischemia, and refractory intracranial hypertension) at the injury scene and in the PICU. Three basic categories of mechanisms involved in the evolution of damage after TBI can be defined (Fig. 119.1): those associated with (1) ischemia, excitotoxicity, energy failure, and resultant cell death cascades; (2) secondary cerebral swelling; and (3) axonal injury. A fourth process, inflammation, is superimposed on these mechanisms and contributes to both further injury and repair. A constellation of mediators of secondary damage and repair is involved within each category. The contribution of each mediator to outcome and the interplay among them remain poorly defined. The biochemical and molecular responses to severe TBI resulting from AHT often are unique and generally severe.[7,8,15]

Posttraumatic Ischemia

The early studies of Pickels[16] and Bruce and associates[17] on cerebral blood flow (CBF) in pediatric TBI focused on the role of hyperemia in secondary brain swelling. However, Adelson and colleagues[18] assessed CBF in 30 infants and children after severe TBI. Early posttraumatic hypoperfusion was commonly observed, and a global CBF <20 mL/100 g/min was associated with a poor outcome. After the initial 24 hours, CBF often recovered, in some cases to high levels. However, delayed increases in CBF were not associated with poor outcome. This seminal finding shifted the emphasis toward the recognition and possible treatment of hypoperfusion early after TBI to avert secondary damage.

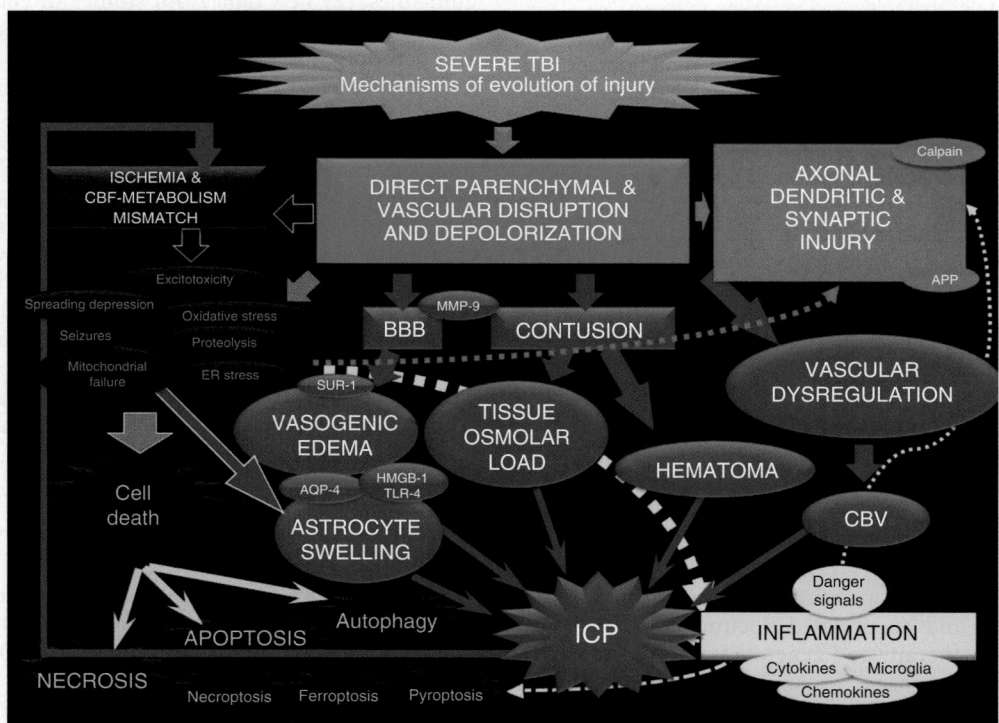

Fig. 119.1. Categories of mechanisms proposed to be involved in the evolution of secondary damage after severe traumatic brain injury (TBI) in infants and children. The major categories for these secondary mechanisms are (1) ischemia, excitotoxicity, energy failure, and cell death cascades shown in black; (2) cerebral swelling shown in blue; (3) axonal injury shown in red; and (4) inflammation shown in yellow. Please see text for details. *APP,* amyloid precursor protein; *AQP-4,* aquaporin-4; *BBB,* blood-brain barrier; *CBV,* cerebral blood volume; *ER,* endoplasmic reticulum; *HMGB-1,* high-mobility group box 1 protein; *ICP,* intracranial pressure; *MMP-9,* matrix metalloproteinase-9; *SUR-1,* sulfonylurea receptor 1; *TLR-4,* toll-like receptor-4.

Numerous mechanisms may contribute to early posttraumatic hypoperfusion, including (1) direct vascular disruption; (2) an attenuated vasodilatory response to nitric oxide (NO), cyclic guanosine monophosphate, cyclic adenosine monophosphate, or prostanoids; (3) loss of endothelial NO production and elaboration of endothelin-1; and (4) production of other vasoconstrictor mediators.[19,20] Contemporary models suggest an important role of pericytes at the capillary level in the cerebral microcirculation.[21] Early after injury, increases in metabolic demands result from an uptake of glutamate and an increased risk from ischemic damage early after TBI.[22-24] Vavilala and coworkers[8] identified an important factor that could increase the importance of ischemic brain injury in infants and young children. They reported that no difference exists in the lower limit of blood pressure autoregulation of CBF in children younger than versus older than 2 years.[8] This finding led them to conclude that the autoregulatory reserve (ie, the difference between baseline mean arterial blood pressure [MAP] and the lower limit of autoregulation) is smaller in infants than in older children or adults; even modest MAP reductions may exacerbate ischemia in infants.

Excitotoxicity

Excitotoxicity is the process by which glutamate and other excitatory amino acids cause neuronal damage. Glutamate is the most abundant neurotransmitter in the brain, but exposure to toxic levels produces neuronal death.[25-28] Glutamate exposure produces neuronal injury by multiple mechanisms. Sodium-dependent neuronal swelling quickly occurs, followed by delayed, calcium-dependent degeneration. These effects are mediated through both ionophore-linked receptors, labeled according to specific agonists (N-methyl-D-aspartate [NMDA], kainite, and α-amino-3-hydroxy-5-methyl-4-isoxazolepropionic acid), and receptors linked to second messenger systems (ie, metabotropic receptors). Activation of these receptors leads to calcium accumulation via receptor-gated or voltage-gated channels or through the release of intracellular stores. Progress in NMDA receptor (NMDAR)-mediated neurotransmission has revealed greater complexity then previously appreciated—and may better inform therapy.[29] NMDARs consist of heterodimeric glutamate receptor (GluR) subunits including GluN1, GluN2A, and GluN2B. In adults, GluN2A-containing NMDARs are enriched in the synapse (synaptic NMDARs), whereas GluN2B-containing NMDARs are enriched at extrasynaptic sites (extrasynaptic NMDARs). During early development GluN2B will predominate the synapse. The special localization of NMDARs is believed to regulate activation of receptor-mediated cell death versus survival pathways. Activation of synaptic NMDARs is neuroprotective. They increase nuclear calcium, activate CREB, BDNF, protein kinase B (AKT), phosphorylated-JACOB (pJACOB), and upregulated antioxidants. In contrast, activation of extrasynaptic NMDARs by glutamate spillover or potentially malfunctioning astrocytes after injury has the opposite effect. Extrasynaptic NMDARs increase cytoplasmic calcium; inhibit CREB, AKT, p-JACOB, BDNF, and active calpain; stimulate death-associated protein kinase; and activate autophagy. Thus the extrasynaptic NMDARs may mediate neuronal death; also, glutamate toxicity may be especially catastrophic to the infant brain, which expresses high levels of numerous types of NMDAR subunits versus that in the adult. Pathologic increases in intracellular calcium concentration can also

trigger other processes that can lead to cell death such as activation of constitutive NO synthase, leading to NO production, peroxynitrite formation, and resultant deoxyribonucleic acid (DNA) damage and poly(ADP-ribose) polymerase activation, which exacerbates adenosine triphosphate (ATP) depletion, metabolic failure, and necrotic cell death. Finally, evidence supports a role for the nonreceptor-mediated effects of high concentrations of glutamate in producing neuronal death.[30] Oxidative stress from intracellular glutathione depletion appears to play an important role.

In cerebrospinal fluid (CSF) from children with severe TBI, our group reported that glutamate levels were markedly increased[24] and correlated with both poor outcome and AHT as an injury mechanism.[24] Antiexcitotoxic therapies improve outcome after experimental TBI; pretreatment with NMDA antagonists (eg, MK-801) attenuate behavioral deficits.[31,32] Other therapies that modify glutamate-NMDA receptor interaction and improve outcome after experimental TBI are magnesium, glycine site antagonists, hypothermia, and pentobarbital. Despite this benefit, clinical trials with antiexcitotoxic therapies have been unsuccessful in adults, perhaps because of adverse effects of these drugs, delayed treatment, a relative reduction in NMDAR subunit targets, or the antiexcitotoxic effects of many current therapies (eg, barbiturates, hypothermia, and sedatives).[33] Developing neurons are more susceptible to excitotoxic injury than are mature cells; however, concerns have been raised about use of NMDA antagonists in infants because these drugs may induce apoptotic neurodegeneration.[34] Investigating which specific NMDA receptor subunits may need to be targeted to produce antiexcitotoxic effects without triggering apoptosis is a key area for future research in pediatric TBI. One agent that is seeing increased clinical use that has antiexcitotoxic properties is levetiracetam. A number of preclinical reports support its use and indicate that it is more neuroprotective that other anticonvulsants such as phenytoin.[32,35] However, an RCT testing levetiracetam in severe TBI has not been carried out in children, although a phase II study in children has been carried out and reported safety.[36]

Delayed Neuronal Death Cascades

Cells that die after TBI can be categorized on a morphologic continuum ranging from necrosis to apoptosis.[37,38] Apoptosis is a morphologic description of cell death defined by cell shrinkage and nuclear condensation, internucleosomal DNA fragmentation, and formation of apoptotic bodies.[39] In contrast, cells that die of necrosis display cellular and nuclear swelling with dissolution of membranes. Because apoptosis requires a cascade of intracellular events for completion of cell death, *programmed cell death* has also been used to describe this process. In diseases with complex and multiple mechanisms, such as TBI, distinguishing morphologic apoptotic from necrotic cell death as classically defined may be difficult,[40] and some cells have mixed phenotypes. In mature tissues, programmed cell death requires initiation via either intracellular or extracellular signals (Fig. 119.2). Intracellular signaling appears to be initiated in mitochondria, triggered by disturbances in cellular homeostasis such as ATP depletion, oxidative stress, or calcium fluxes.[41] Mitochondrial dysfunction leads to egress of cytochrome c into the cytosol. Oxidation of the mitochondrial lipid cardiolipin may play a central role in cytochrome c release.[42] Cytochrome c release can be

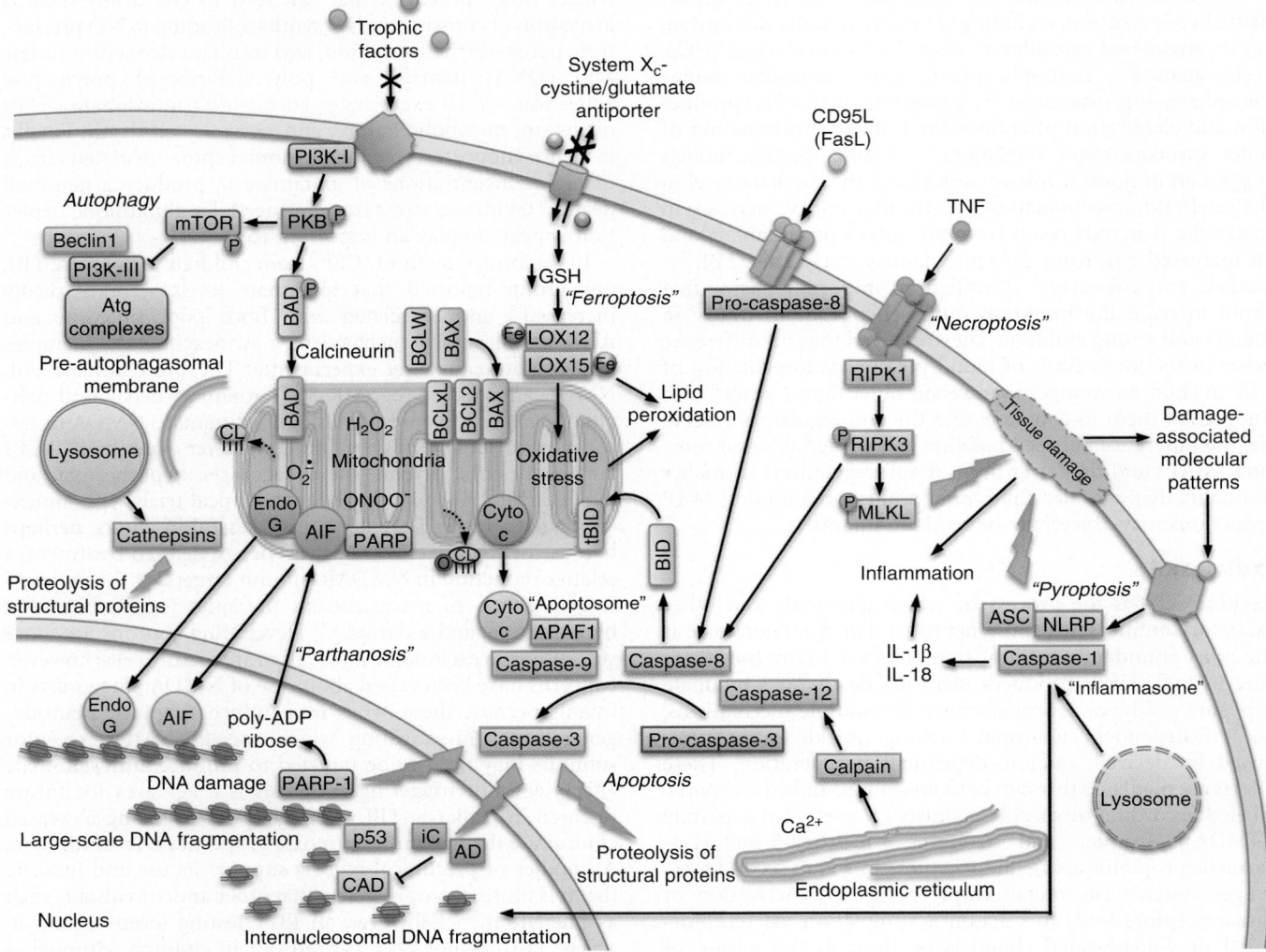

Fig. 119.2. Programmed apoptotic and regulated necrotic cell death cascades involved in delayed neuronal death after severe traumatic brain injury. *AIF*, apoptosis-inducing factor; *APAF*, apoptotic protease activating factor; *ASC*, caspase activity and recruitment domain; *Atg*, autophagy-related; *CAD*, caspase activated deoxyribonuclease; *CD95*, cluster of differentiation 95; *CL*, cardiolipin; *Cyto C*, cytochrome c; *DNA*, deoxyribonucleic acid; *EndoG*, endonuclease G; *Fe*, iron containing; *GSH*, glutathione; *iCAD*, inhibitor of CAD; *IL*, interleukin; *LOX*, lipoxygenase; *MLKL*, mixed lineage kinase domain-like; *mTOR*, mammalian target of rapamycin; *NLRP*, NOD-like receptor family, pyrin domain; *O*, oxidized; *P*, phosphorylated; *PARP*, poly(ADP-ribose) polymerase; *PI3K*, phosphoinositide 3-kinase; *PKB*, protein kinase B; *RIPK*, receptor-interacting protein kinase; *t*, truncated; *TNF*, tumor necrosis factor.

blocked by antiapoptotic members of the Bcl-2 family (eg, Bcl-2, Bcl-xL, Bcl-w, and Mcl-1) and promoted by proapoptotic members of the Bcl-2 family (eg, Bax, Bcl-xS, Bad, and Bid).[43] Cytochrome c activates the initiator cysteine protease caspase-9.[44] Caspase-9 then activates the effector cysteine protease caspase-3, which cleaves cytoskeletal proteins, DNA repair proteins, and activators of endonucleases.[45] Intrinsic signaling of apoptosis can also proceed via mitochondrial release of apoptosis-inducing factor, a caspase-independent apoptotic process mediated by poly(ADP-ribose) polymerases and posttranslational poly-ADP-ribosylation (PAR) of proteins. As such, this apoptotic pathway is sometimes referred to as *parthanosis*.[46]

Extracellular signaling of apoptosis occurs via the tumor necrosis factor (TNF) superfamily of cell surface death receptors, which includes TNFR-1 and Fas/Apo1/CD95.[47] Receptor-ligand binding of tumor necrosis factor receptor 1

(TNFR-1)–TNF-α or Fas-FasL promotes formation of a trimeric complex of TNF- or Fas-associated death domains. These ultimately lead to caspase-3 activation, where the mitochondrial and cell death receptor pathways converge (see Fig. 119.2). Both the intrinsic and extrinsic pathways may contribute to the evolution of cell death after severe TBI in infants and children. CSF levels of the antiapoptotic protein Bcl-2 in pediatric patients after TBI were increased about fourfold in patients with TBI versus controls.[48] Similarly, CSF levels of sFas receptor and sFas ligand are increased in patients with TBI versus controls.[49] Apoptosis may be an important therapeutic target for new therapies in infants with severe TBI. Current therapies likely attenuate both necrotic and apoptotic injury cascades.

Several additional cell death cascades have been shown to play a role in the evolution of neuronal death after TBI in preclinical models including pyroptosis, necroptosis, autophagy, and ferroptosis. Pyroptosis is an inflammasome-mediated cell death pathway linked to caspase-1 activation, IL1-β production, and mitochondrial pore formation,[50] whereas necroptosis represents TNF-triggered, receptor interacting protein kinases (RIPKs) and pseudokinase mixed lineage kinase domain-like (MLKL)-mediated programmed necrosis.[46] Autophagy involves phagocytosis of mitochondria and organelles in the setting of cellular injury—which may contribute to neuronal death or have beneficial properties.[51] Ferroptosis, an iron-dependent form of regulated necrosis, may also play a role.[52] All of these processes could represent targets for future therapies in TBI (see Fig. 119.1). Neuronal death after TBI may also result from disconnection with subsequent Wallerian degeneration of otherwise lethally injured axons. This aspect is discussed further in the section on axonal injury.

The currently available data strongly suggest that early after injury, severe TBI produces a state of hypoperfusion and loss of blood flow autoregulation with simultaneous increased metabolic demands from excitotoxicity. This is a state of enhanced vulnerability to secondary insults (ie, hypotension and hypoxemia). These processes are intimately linked with the evolution of neuronal death.

Cerebral Swelling

After the initial minutes to hours of posttraumatic hypoperfusion and hypermetabolism, a phase of metabolic depression occurs. The cerebral metabolic rate of oxygen ($CMRO_2$) decreases to about one-third of normal[53] and is maintained at that level for the duration of the coma, unless perturbed by second insults such as seizures or spreading depression.[54] The exact etiology of this state remains to be defined; however, contributions from reduced synaptic activity and mitochondrial failure may be important.[55] Sustained increases in glycolysis are reported in some cases, possibly related to seizure activity or sustained increases in glutamate levels.[22] Cerebral swelling develops and generally peaks between 24 and 72 hours after injury, although sustained increases in intracranial pressure (ICP) for 1 week or longer occasionally are observed.

Cerebral Blood Volume

Several mechanisms may contribute to intracranial hypertension in infants and children after severe TBI (see Fig. 119.1). Brain swelling and accompanying intracranial hypertension contribute to secondary damage in two ways. Intracranial hypertension can compromise cerebral perfusion leading to secondary ischemia, and it can produce the devastating consequences of deformation through herniation syndromes. Bruce and colleagues[17] described the phenomenon of "malignant posttraumatic cerebral swelling" in children. CBF was measured in six children, and hyperemia was believed to be the major culprit. Muizelaar and coworkers,[56] in a series of 32 children, suggested similar findings. However, Sharples and associates[57] suggested that hyperemia was uncommon after severe TBI in children; rather, reduced $CMRO_2$ was associated with poor outcome. Suzuki[58] measured CBF in 80 normal children. He showed an age dependence of CBF, with high values in children ages 2 to 9 years, levels previously suggested to represent posttraumatic hyperemia. Nevertheless, in some patients with TBI, after resolution of the aforementioned early posttraumatic hypoperfusion, CBF may increase to levels greater than metabolic demands producing a state of relative hyperemia.[14]

Bergsneider and coworkers[23] posed the alternative hypothesis of *hyperglycolysis* to explain the increases in CBF in patients with severe TBI whose CBF is uncoupled from $CMRO_2$. Cerebral glutamate uptake is coupled to glucose utilization by glycolysis in astrocytes. Studies suggest two other potential contributors to increased glycolysis after TBI even in the absence of low CBF, namely mitochondrial failure[55] and nitration and inactivation of the enzyme pyruvate dehydrogenase, which is critical to the production of acetyl-CoA and thus oxidative metabolism.[59] Thus in injured brain regions with reduced $CMRO_2$, increases in CBF may be coupled to local increases in glucose utilization even in the absence of ischemia.

Local or global increases in glycolysis occur in adults with severe TBI.[23] The incidence or importance of secondary *hyperemia* or hyperglycolysis in pediatric TBI remains to be determined. It may occur in select cases, but secondary increases in CBF probably are not the major contributor to raised ICP. Increases in CBF were not associated with raised ICP in adults,[60] and hyperemia was not associated with poor outcome in children.[18] The contribution of hyperemia (increased cerebral blood volume [CBV]) to the development of raised ICP has been studied in adults with TBI.[60] Increased CBV was seen in only a small number of patients. These studies suggest that the importance of posttraumatic hyperemia was likely overstated, and edema rather than hyperemia may be the predominant contributor to brain swelling after TBI.[61] Loss of blood pressure autoregulation of CBF may also play a role in some patients by contributing to the development of intracranial hypertension. Studies using a pressure reactivity index (PRx) approach to assess the status of autoregulation at the bedside are shedding additional light on this possibility, and in some patients this tool may help define an optimal cerebral perfusion pressure (CPP), which may need to be individually targeted.[62,63]

Edema

Both cytotoxic and vasogenic edema may play important roles in cerebral swelling (Fig. 119.3). However, the traditional concept of cytotoxic and vasogenic edema is evolving. There appear to be multiple mechanisms for edema formation in the injured brain. First, vasogenic edema may form in the extracellular space as a result of blood-brain barrier (BBB) disruption. Second, cellular swelling can be produced in two ways. Astrocyte swelling can occur as part of the homeostatic uptake of substances such as glutamate. Glutamate uptake is coupled to glucose utilization via a sodium/potassium adenosine triphosphatase, with sodium and water accumulation in astrocytes. Swelling of both neurons and other cells in the neuropil can result from ischemia- or trauma-induced ionic pump failure. Finally, osmolar swelling may contribute to edema formation in the extracellular space, particularly in contusions. Osmolar swelling actually is dependent on an intact BBB or an alternative solute barrier. Cellular swelling may be of greatest importance. Using a model of diffuse TBI in rats, Barzo and coworkers[64] applied diffusion-weighted magnetic resonance imaging to localize the increase in brain water. A decrease in the apparent diffuse coefficient after injury suggested largely cellular swelling rather than vasogenic edema in the development of raised ICP. Katayama and associates[65] also

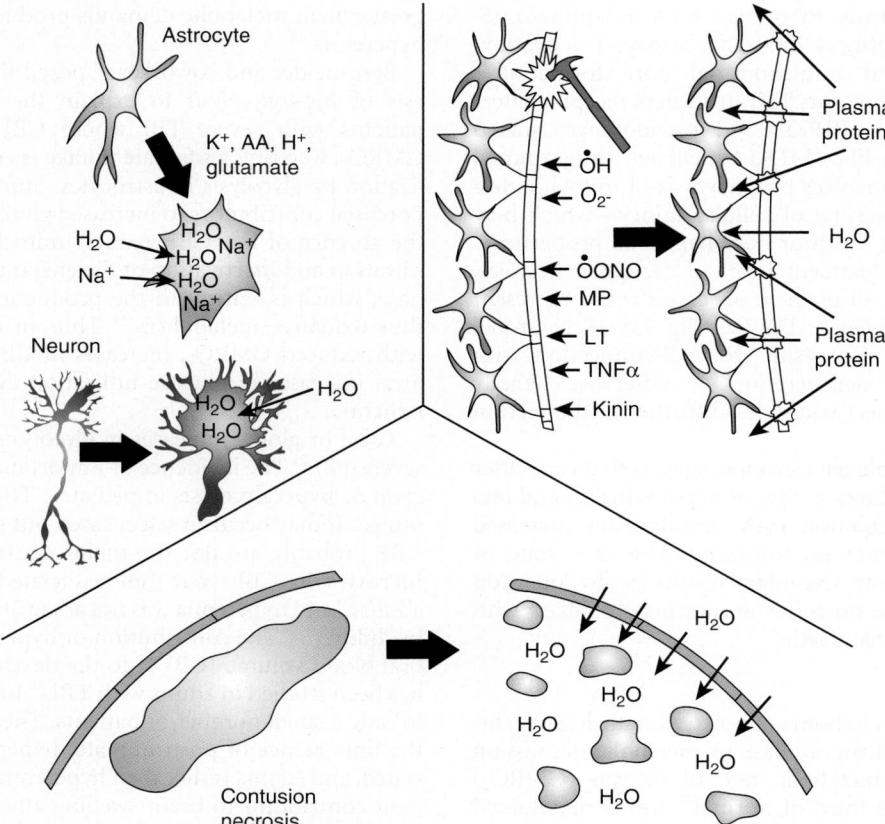

Fig. 119.3. Schematic of three classic cascades leading to cerebral edema. *Top left,* Cellular swelling is predominantly seen in astrocytes and is stimulated by potassium, acidosis, glutamate, arachidonic acid (AA), and other factors. This key pathway is less representative of a toxic process and more consistent with a homeostatic or mediator-driven process. Neuronal swelling from pump leak probably is less important. *Bottom,* Osmolar swelling from contusion necrosis. In the hours after injury, reconstitution of the BBB or development of an osmolar barrier around a contusion sets the stage for marked local swelling as macromolecules in the contusion break down, increasing local osmolality. *Top right,* Vasogenic edema results from protein and water accumulation across the damaged BBB, which is formed by tight junctions (astrocyte foot processes). Direct vascular disruption by trauma, reactive oxygen species such as hydroxyl radical (OH), superoxide anion (O_2-), and peroxynitrite (ONOO), metalloproteases (MP), kinins, leukotrienes (LT), cytokines, and other mediators contribute to BBB damage. *TNF,* tumor necrosis factor.

suggested that the role of BBB in the development of post-traumatic edema may have been overstated, even in the setting of cerebral contusion. They posed that as macromolecules are degraded within injured brain regions, the osmolar load in the contused tissue increases. As the BBB reconstitutes (or as other osmolar barriers form), a large osmolar driving force for local accumulation of water develops, resulting in the marked swelling so often seen in and around cerebral contusions. Thus in either diffuse injury or focal contusion, BBB permeability may play a limited role in the development of cerebral swelling. If these results can be generalized, then hypertonic saline solution or mannitol would represent optimal therapies particularly outside of the immediate postinjury time period. However, a role for BBB permeability in cases of severe TBI should not be dismissed. Polderman and colleagues[66] reported that prolonged use (>48 hours) of mannitol (a large molecule that does not cross the intact BBB) was associated with its progressive accumulation in CSF in adults with severe TBI, and in some cases, a reverse osmotic gradient was even established. This suggests that breaching of the BBB is important and that prolonged use of osmolar therapy might, in some patients, produce rebound intracranial hypertension. Studies

of the extent of BBB injury versus the contribution of cellular swelling to intracranial hypertension in pediatric TBI are needed.

There have been a number of exciting new developments in our understanding of the development of brain edema based on new pathways that may represent therapeutic targets (also see Fig. 119.4).[29] This includes sulfonylurea receptor 1 (Sur-1)-regulated cation channels, which can be targeted by the drug glyburide[67]; aquaporin-4 channels, which can be blocked either with direct channel blockers or via inhibition of their upregulation,[68] which may be linked to high-mobility group box 1 (HMGB-1) release or toll-receptor activation[69]; and the use of novel resuscitation agents to reduce fluid requirements.[70] These are promising developments that are already generating clinical trials in adults (glyburide (RP-1127) for TBI; NCT01454154).

Axonal Injury

Traumatic axonal injury (TAI) encompasses the spectrum from mild to severe TBI.[71,72] The extent and distribution of TAI depend on injury severity and category (focal versus diffuse). Its incidence and nature appear to be

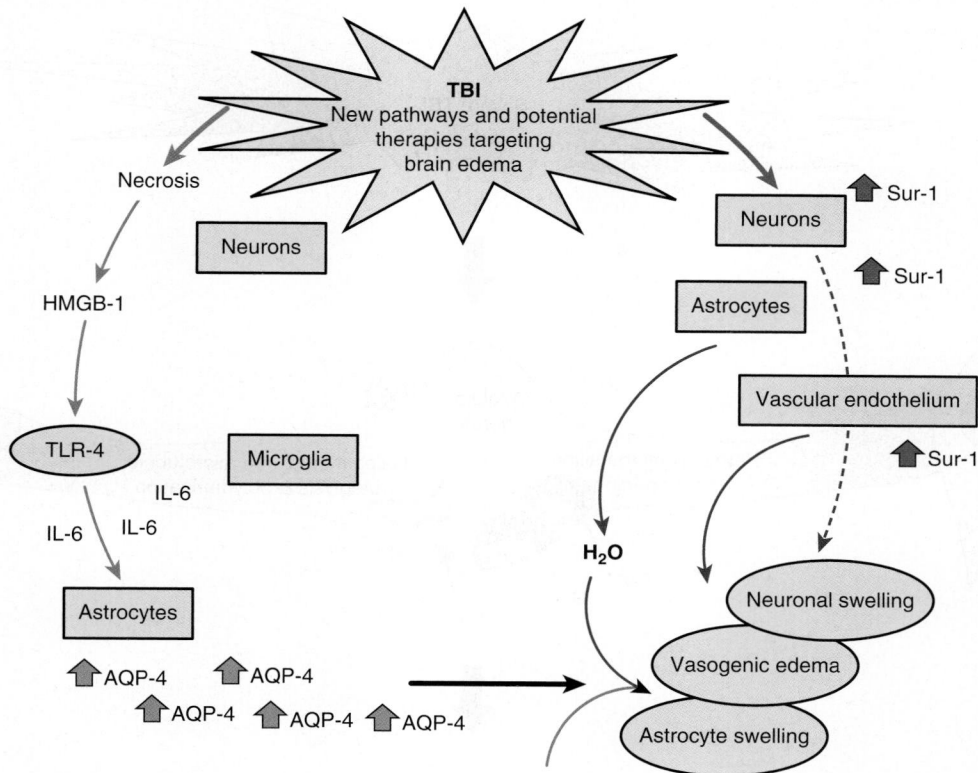

Fig. 119.4. State-of-the-art view of novel molecular participants in the development of cerebral edema after traumatic brain injury (TBI). On the left, neuronal necrosis results in release of the high-mobility group box 1 protein (HMGB-1), which binds to toll-like receptor-4 (TLR-4) on microglia leading to interleukin-6 (IL-6) production and upregulation of AQP-4 water channels as suggested by Laird and colleagues.[69] On the right, upregulation of sulfonylurea receptor-1 (SUR-1) leads to ion channel opening and water accumulation.[70]

age independent,[73] but its consequences may be particularly devastating in children.[74] The effects of TAI in children during a period of developmental axonal connectivity remain unknown but likely are considerable. Clinical data on TAI after pediatric TBI are limited. However, strongly supporting the role for TAI in pediatric TBI, after publication of the guidelines, Berger and colleagues[75] reported that serum levels of myelin basic protein are markedly increased in infants and children after either accidental TBI or AHT—in contrast to hypoxic-ischemic encephalopathy. Massive increases in CSF levels of myelin basic protein were also reported after severe TBI in children.[76] In children affected by AHT, TAI may be highly prevalent.[77] The classic view suggested that TAI occurs because immediate physical shearing with frank axonal tears occurs. Experimental studies, however, suggest that TAI occurs by a delayed process termed *secondary axotomy*, which results from either calcium accumulation or altered axoplasmic flow with accumulation of proteins such as amyloid precursor protein (APP) (Fig. 119.5).[78] What remains to be determined is how much of TAI results from a reversible evolution of damage to axons versus Wallerian degeneration of disconnected axons. The former but not the latter would be amenable to treatment. Studies also have shown that there are as many if not more unmyelinated than myelinated axons that are injured after TBI.[79] Laboratory studies suggest that hypothermia, calpain antagonists, and cyclosporine A can attenuate TAI, but clinical data are lacking.

History

Unlike in adult TBI, where the history is generally straightforward, the special case of AHT contributes to increased importance of the history in pediatric TBI. For a discussion of the topic, the reader is referred to Duhaime.[80] In cases of severe AHT, a history that is incompatible with the observed injury is often given.[81] Occult presentations of AHT can be particularly important because they may be recognized as cases of severe TBI relatively late in their treatment course.[82] In this setting, brain edema already may have evolved to life-threatening levels, and other superimposed secondary insults (eg, seizures and apnea) may complicate management and worsen outcome.

Signs and Symptoms

The GCS score[83] (Table 119.1), first described in 1974, remains a valuable tool for grading and communicating severity of neurologic injury after TBI, although limitations remain with pediatric use. The verbal and motor components of the GCS score have been modified for the assessment of infants,[84] but this modification has not been validated. The motor score has probably become the most important component of the GCS. A rapid *mini-neuroassessment* that allows evaluation of the patient's level of consciousness, pupillary size and light response, the fundi, extraocular movements, response of

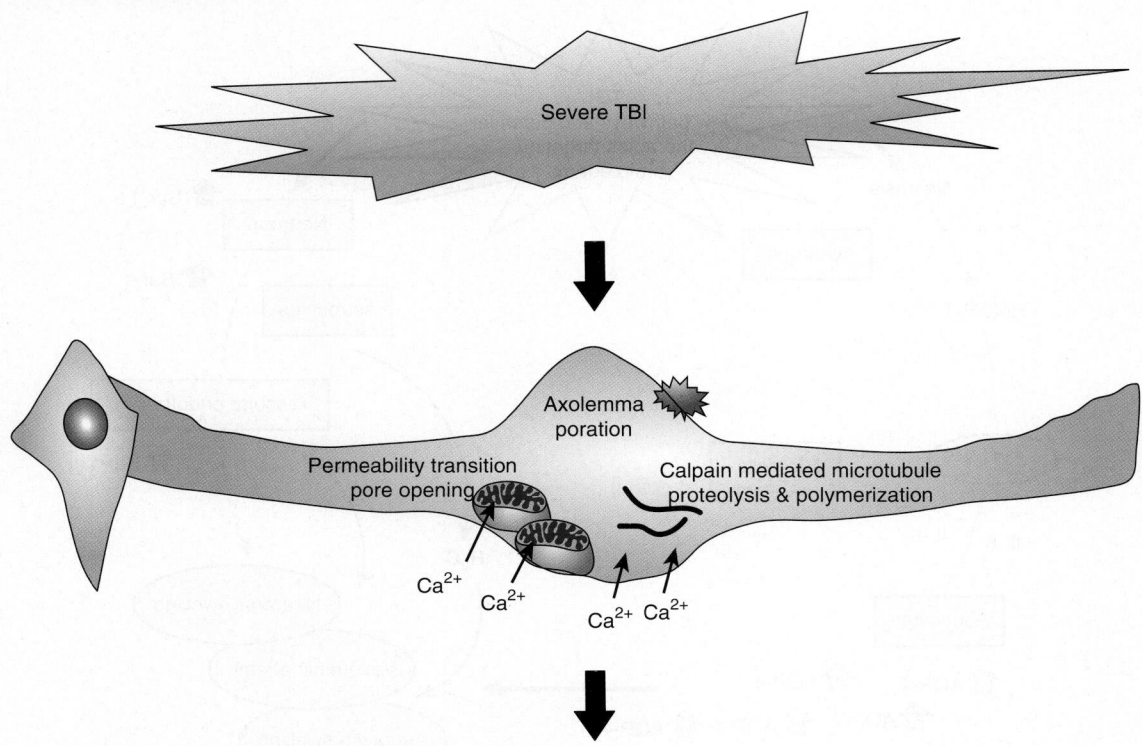

Fig. 119.5. Secondary injury cascade after traumatic brain injury (TBI) relevant specifically to traumatic axonal injury. Rather than direct axonal disruption from trauma, shearing forces set into motion several processes including mitochondrial permeability transition pore opening and resultant mitochondrial failure and calpain-mediated proteolysis of microtubules, both of which lead to failure of axoplasmic transport and accumulation of proteins such as amyloid precursor protein. In addition, direct axolemmal poration may occur.

TABLE 119.1 Coma Scales

Glasgow Coma Scale	Modified Coma Scale	Point Scale
Eye Opening		
Spontaneous	Spontaneous	4
To speech	To speech	3
To pain	To pain	2
None	None	1
Verbal		
Oriented	Coos, babbles	5
Confused	Irritable	4
Inappropriate words	Cries to pain	3
Grunting	Moans to pain	2
None	None	1
Motor		
Follows commands	Normal spontaneous movements	6
Localizes pain	Withdraws to touch	5
Withdraws to pain	Withdraws to pain	4
Abnormal flexion	Abnormal flexion	3
Abnormal extension	Abnormal extension	2
Flaccid	Flaccid	1

extremities to pain, deep tendon reflexes, and brain stem reflexes should all be part of the initial evaluation.[85] Until proved otherwise, an altered level of consciousness, pupillary dysfunction, and lateralizing extremity weakness in an infant or child should raise suspicion of a mass lesion that may require surgery.[86] These signs of impending herniation require an immediate response, as outlined in Fig. 119.6.

Initial Resuscitation

The identification and correction of airway obstruction, inadequate ventilation, and shock take priority over a detailed neurologic assessment.[87] Thus the first step in managing a patient with TBI is complete, rapid physiologic resuscitation.[1,2] Raised ICP and cerebral herniation are the major complications. Brain-specific interventions in the absence of signs of herniation or other neurologic deterioration currently are not recommended. Mannitol may be counterproductive for the management of malignant intracranial hypertension during initial resuscitative efforts, and some have suggested that immediate post-TBI use of either osmolar agents or colloids could cause leakage into the injured brain and contribute to the development of a reverse osmolar gradient and delayed swelling.[88,89] Studies have consistently shown that increased morbidity and mortality are associated with the secondary insults of hypotension and hypoxemia.[90] Gentleman[91] reported that the increased use of tracheal intubation and ventilation

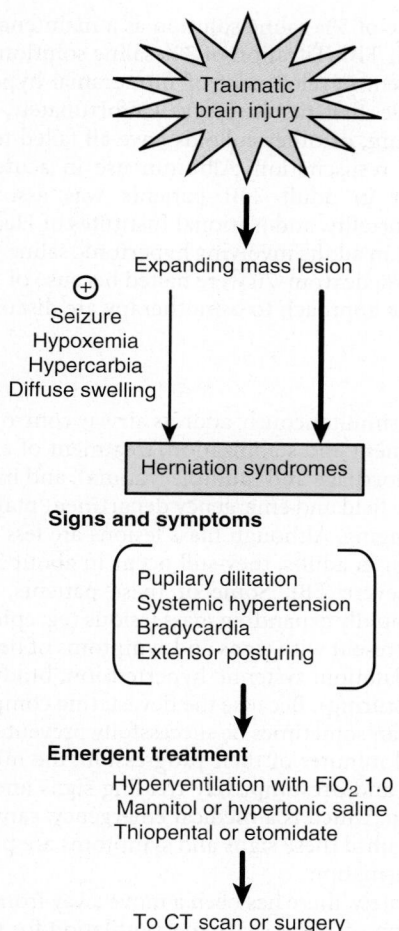

Fig. 119.6. Treatment paradigm for management of signs and symptoms of acute herniation after severe traumatic brain injury in infants and children.

BOX 119.1	Criteria for Intubation of the Head-Injured Child

Glasgow Coma Scale (GCS) score ≤10
Decrease in GCS of >3, independent of the initial GCS score
Anisocoria >1 mm
Cervical spine injury compromising ventilation
Apnea
Hypercarbia ($Paco_2$ >45 mm Hg)
Loss of pharyngeal reflex
Spontaneous hyperventilation causing Paco2 <25 mm Hg

produced a concomitant reduction in hypoxemia and an increase in favorable outcomes. Although the basis for this improvement may be multifactorial, early correction of hypoxemia and hypovolemia must be the initial objective. However, specific recommendations for intubation at the scene are complex and likely are influenced by the expertise of caregivers in the field and by the transport distance, among other factors.[92]

Trauma patients with supraclavicular injury should be assumed to have cranial and cervical spine injuries until proved otherwise. The initial evaluation of a child after severe TBI begins by demonstrating the presence of a patent, maintainable airway; the patient must be conscious, alert, and breathing spontaneously. Unconscious patients must be assumed to have an obstructed airway requiring immediate evaluation. The relatively large head, occiput, and tongue and the short narrow epiglottis of the infant facilitate airway obstruction if the child's sensorium has been clouded. The rescuer must alleviate this situation (while protecting the cervical spine) to minimize secondary injury from hypoxia.

When preparing to intubate an infant or child with severe TBI, it is important to have readily available suction and age-appropriate suction catheters. Optimal positioning of the patient requires immobilization of the neck to stabilize the

cervical spine. A fraction of inspired oxygen [FIO_2] of 1.0 should be delivered by facemask immediately before intubation to facilitate nitrogen washout from the functional residual capacity and maximize alveolar oxygenation. An age-appropriate laryngoscope blade and tracheal tube are then selected. The medications chosen must be potent and rapid in their onset of action. The goals of analgesia, amnesia, and neuromuscular blockade must be met rapidly. Ideally, the patient never receives a preintubation positive pressure breath. Tracheal intubation of the child with severe TBI requires a cerebroprotective, rapid-sequence technique when possible. Bag-valve-mask positive pressure ventilation should be avoided. However, in cases of hypoxemia or impending herniation, positive pressure ventilation should be instituted immediately.[93] Because the bag-valve-mask technique may cause unintentional cervical spine manipulation, care is advised.[94] The tube is secured with adhesive tape that should not pass circumferentially around the neck because cerebral venous return may be reduced.

If a person who has sustained TBI meets any of the criteria listed in Box 119.1, assisted ventilation is generally indicated.[93,95] In children, the recommended route of initial airway control is orotracheal intubation under direct vision.[96] Nasotracheal intubation should be avoided. Orotracheal intubation can be accomplished using a two-person strategy that protects the cervical spine from injury. A normal lateral cervical spine roentgenogram is reassuring but does not rule out cervical spine injury.[97] Spinal immobilization must be maintained,[98] which is accomplished via in-line cervical immobilization by one operator while the second intubates the trachea. Care must be taken to avoid pressing into the soft tissues of the submental region and strap muscles because inadvertent airway obstruction may ensue.

Rapid-Sequence Induction and Intubation

Tracheal intubation, although lifesaving, is a noxious stimulus. The technique of rapid-sequence induction and intubation secures the airway of an unprepared patient, who is at risk for aspiration of gastric contents, in an immediate and safe manner. No resistance is provided to direct laryngoscopy, and the normal responses to intentional placement of a foreign body into the trachea are eliminated. Rapid-sequence induction is documented to be a safer technique than either nasotracheal intubation or orotracheal intubation without neuromuscular blockade.[99,100]

In the pediatric patient with TBI, a cerebroprotective rapid-sequence induction strategy should be used. The sequence involves preparation, preoxygenation, sedation, neuromuscular blockade, and orotracheal intubation. Pharmacologic adjuncts are used to prevent morbidity associated with

TABLE 119.2	Drugs for Intubation of the Head-Injured Child
Situation	**Drugs**
Cardiopulmonary arrest	Resuscitation drugs
Hemodynamically unstable	Fentanyl 2–4 µg/kg Lidocaine 1 mg/kg Rocuronium 1 mg/kg or vecuronium 0.3 mg/kg
Hemodynamically stable	Fentanyl 2–4 µg/kg or etomidate 0.1–0.3 mg/kg Lidocaine 1 mg/kg Midazolam 0.1–0.2 mg/kg Rocuronium 1 mg/kg or vecuronium 0.3 mg/kg

hypotension, hypoxemia, intracranial hypertension, and gastric aspiration. The neurologic and hemodynamic status of the patient directs the choice of adjunctive pharmacologic strategy.

For a victim in cardiac arrest, cardiopulmonary resuscitation should begin immediately, accompanied by direct orotracheal intubation. No pharmacologic adjuncts are necessary to secure the airway. For a hemodynamically unstable patient, the combination of fentanyl, lidocaine, and rocuronium bromide is the first choice (Table 119.2). At Pittsburgh Children's Hospital either etomidate or fentanyl, in combination with lidocaine, is used for rapid sequence intubation. Etomidate use is accompanied by concerns with adrenal suppression.[101] Fentanyl, in combination with lidocaine, reduces the catecholamine surge associated with direct laryngoscopy.[93] Either of these same sequences of drugs can be used in hemodynamically stable patients, for whom a rapidly acting benzodiazepine (midazolam) can be added. Historically, thiopental was an excellent agent for rapid sequence induction in hemodynamically stable patients, but its availability has been curtailed related to its use in lethal injections in the United States. Alternatively, similar CNS effects can be achieved with propofol if there is no concern of hemodynamic compromise.

Circulatory Stabilization

Assessment of circulatory function after trauma involves the rapid determination of heart rate, blood pressure, central and peripheral pulse quality, capillary refill, and cerebral perfusion.[102] Posttraumatic hypoperfusion must be assumed to be hypovolemic (ie, hemorrhagic) in nature, but it also may have a secondary component of myocardial depression resulting from cardiac contusion. However, cardiac contusion is less common in children than in adults. In patients with severe TBI, fluid therapy for hypovolemic shock entails rapid replacement of vascular volume. The current recommendation is 20 mL/kg isotonic crystalloid (0.9% NaCl solution) given as soon as vascular access is obtained. Hypotonic fluid should not be used in the resuscitation of a patient with a brain injury. Subsequent doses of fluid should be isotonic crystalloid or packed red blood cells and titrated based on serial assessment of blood pressure, perfusion, and hematocrit. Although concerns exist regarding the relative hypotonicity of lactated Ringer solution,[103] evidence from studies in laboratory animals supports the safety of the use of lactated Ringer solution in patients with TBI.[104] Fisher and colleagues[105] reported the successful use of 3% saline solution as a maintenance fluid in children with TBI. Titration of 3% saline solution as an infusion to prevent development of intracranial hypertension is an acceptable first-tier strategy. Unfortunately, hypertonic saline, albumin, or other colloids have all failed to show efficacy in TBI resuscitation. Albumin use in acute ICU fluid management in adult TBI patients was associated with increased mortality, and National Institutes of Health (NIH)–funded trials in adults involving hypertonic saline (7.5%) with or without 6% dextran-70 were halted because of futility.[106,107] Details of the approach to osmotherapy are discussed later in this chapter.

Herniation

The need to simultaneously address airway control, cardiovascular assessment and stabilization, treatment of extracerebral insults (hemorrhage and multiple trauma), and initial trauma survey in the field and emergency department makes management challenging. Although mass lesions are less common in children than in adults, they still occur in about 30% of children with severe TBI. Some of these patients, particularly those with rapidly expanding mass lesions (eg, epidural hematoma), can present with signs and symptoms of herniation (ie, pupillary dilatation, systemic hypertension, bradycardia, and extensor posturing). Because the devastating complications of herniation can sometimes be successfully prevented or treated in the initial minutes of their progression, the importance of aggressively and presumptively treating signs and symptoms of herniation, which is a medical emergency, cannot be overemphasized until these signs and symptoms are proved not to represent herniation.

Appropriately, there has been a move away from prophylactic application of aggressive hyperventilation for the management of severe TBI. However, it is important to recognize that temporary use of hyperventilation with an FIO$_2$ of 1.0 is a therapy that can be immediately applied and can be lifesaving in the setting of impending herniation until other therapies can be instituted. Intubating doses of etomidate, pentobarbital, or fentanyl and lidocaine and mannitol (0.25 to 1.0 g/kg) or hypertonic saline (3% or 23.4%) solution[105,108] also should be given emergently. One must recognize that factors other than a focal mass lesion may lead to herniation and that these situations may arise more commonly in children than in adults. Diffuse swelling is more common in children than in adults, and in this setting, inadvertent hypercarbia or hypoxemia, iatrogenic excessive fluid administration, or status epilepticus after TBI can precipitate herniation. Although discussed in this chapter in the context of acute therapy, herniation can occur at any time in the PICU course, and this approach to treatment also applies (see Fig. 119.6).

Transition From the Emergency Department to the Pediatric Intensive Care Unit: Computed Tomographic Scan and Intracranial Pressure Monitoring

The transition of patients with severe TBI from the emergency department to the PICU includes computed tomographic (CT) evaluation of the head (and other anatomic regions, when clinically indicated) followed by placement of an ICP monitor, transport to the operating suite for surgical intervention, or both. In the initial resuscitation, sedation must be carefully titrated, maintaining the difficult balance that produces stability, analgesia, and anxiolysis during transport and scanning while allowing for rapid emergence for clinical assessment (as indicated) until a decision is made regarding surgery or ICP monitoring. Because the early period after injury generally reflects a state of increased vulnerability of the brain to second insults because of the brain's increased metabolic demands and compromised perfusion, providing adequate sedation and maintaining stable hemodynamics are important. An end-tidal CO_2 monitor also should be considered to avoid iatrogenic hyperventilation or hypoventilation. Clinical trials supporting definitive recommendations are not available. Nevertheless, the risks of intrahospital transport are well described[109]; therefore when possible, a physician should accompany the infant or child upon transport to the scanner to direct care, because serial assessment to titrate therapy is needed during the acute phase of injury.

Diagnostic Studies and Monitoring Modalities
Computed Tomography

Since becoming commercially available in 1973, CT has been of enormous benefit to neurointensive care.[110] Examples of classic findings in severe pediatric TBI are shown in Fig. 119.7. Comprehensive classifications of CT findings in adults with severe TBI are reported. The Marshall classification is the most commonly used (Table 119.3).[111] A similar system specifically for pediatric TBI is not described, although several reviews characterize the spectrum of injury in infants and children as defined by CT.[112,113] Ewing-Cobbs and colleagues[112] compared acute CT findings in infants and children with AHT and accidental injuries. Subdural interhemispheric and convexity hemorrhages and preexisting lesions were two to three times more common in the group with AHT. Epidural hematomas were more common in the group with accidental TBI.

Timing of repeat cranial CT scans has been investigated in children. Routine reimaging at 24 or 48 hours after injury has been suggested.[114] However, Tabori and associates[115] evaluated

the impact of routine reimaging on 67 children after severe TBI and noted that although some new lesions were identified, reimaging did not lead to surgical or medical changes in therapy in any patient. A decision to reimage based on changes in ICP or clinical examination was recommended. Such an approach also is recommended in the pediatric guidelines.[1,2]

TABLE 119.3	Marshall Classification of Cranial Computed Tomographic Scans
Classification	**Findings on Scan**
Diffuse injury I (no visible pathologic change)	No visible intracranial pathologic change seen on computed tomography
Diffuse injury II	Cisterns are present with shift 0-5 mm or lesion densities present No high or mixed density lesion >25 mL May include bone fragments and foreign bodies
Diffuse injury III	Cisterns compressed or absent (swelling) with shift 0–5 mm No high or mixed density lesion >25 mL
Diffuse injury IV (shift)	Shift >5 mm No high or mixed density lesion >25 mL
Evacuated mass lesion	Any surgically evacuated lesion
Nonevacuated mass	High or mixed density lesion >25 mL, not surgically evacuated
Brain dead	No brain stem reflexes Flaccidity Fixed and nonreactive pupils No spontaneous respirations with a normal $PaCO_2$ Spinal reflexes permitted

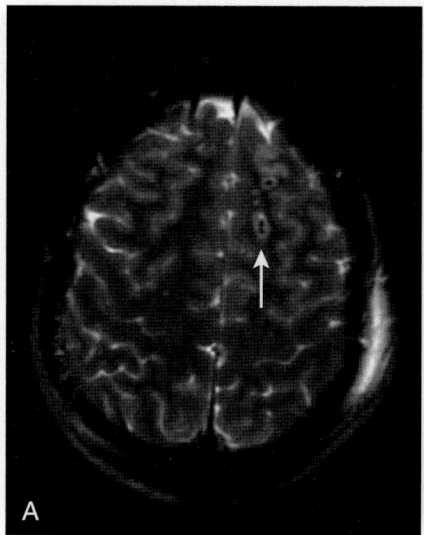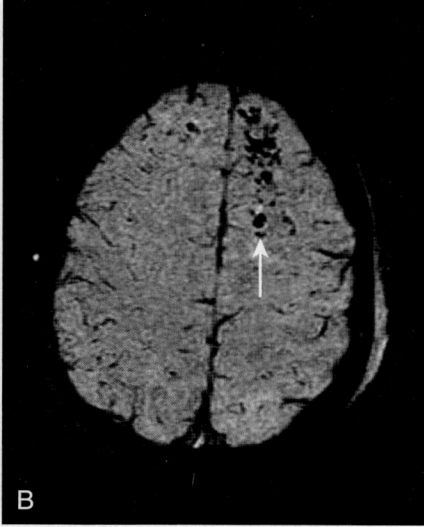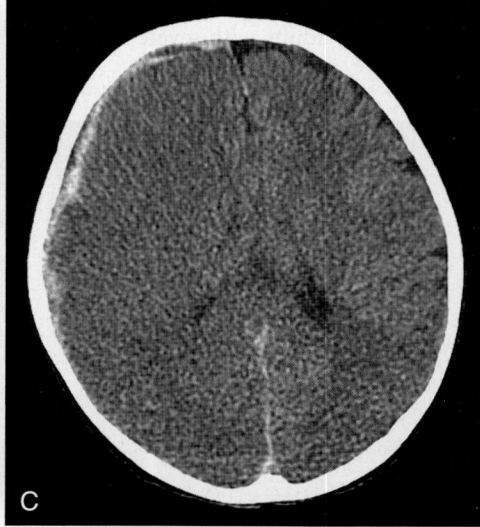

Fig. 119.7. Axial cranial CT images of important lesions in pediatric traumatic brain injury including (A) acute epidural hematoma, (B) penetrating brain injury resulting from a gunshot wound (with bullet fragments), and (C) abusive head trauma (shaken baby syndrome) with acute right subdural hematoma extending over most of the right hemisphere, right side alterations of gray-white differentiation, and decreased CSF spaces.

Studies in adults and children indicate that CT scans are not without limitations and must be used as only one, albeit important, piece of information. After severe TBI, in about 15% of adults with a normal CT scan, clinically significant intracranial hypertension develops. In contrast, in a study in 65 children, CT scans had a high false-positive rate in defining increased ICP.[116] Finally, patients with normal initial head CT scans who also have hypotension or abnormal posturing have the same propensity to the development of intracranial hypertension as do their counterparts with an abnormal scan.

Magnetic Resonance Imaging

MRI may have future applications salient to acute management in persons with TBI. The application of diffusion-weighted MRI for studying the evolution of cerebral edema,[60] the use of novel MRI methods for quantifying CBF,[117] and new methods such as susceptibility-weighted, diffusion tensor (Fig. 119.8) and state-of-the-art high definition fiber tract (Fig. 119.9) imaging to assess white matter damage increasingly are being applied.[118,119] The potential ability to couple these techniques with MR spectroscopy and functional MRI is beginning to yield unprecedented advances in our understanding of the brain's response to injury. However, MRI suites in most institutions are remote from the emergency department and PICU, introducing the risk of transport. Currently, hardware incompatibilities (eg, ventilators and intravenous pumps) and long data acquisition times (relative to CT) limit the utility of this important tool.

Intracranial Pressure Monitoring

Unfortunately, clinical signs such as pupillary size, light response, and papilledema fail as early indicators of intracranial hypertension. Although the most reliable clinical signs are those associated with herniation, the introduction of ICP monitoring devices has allowed detection of intracranial hypertension well before herniation develops allowing us to target the impact of raised ICP on perfusion and possibly other mechanisms.[120,121] In the pediatric guidelines,[1,2] ICP monitoring was suggested as appropriate in children with an abnormal admission head CT scan and initial GCS score between 3 and 8. Also, ICP monitoring was suggested to be appropriate in adults with severe TBI and a normal head CT

scan if the clinical course was complicated by hypotension or motor posturing. This modality is essential to implementation of a physiologically guided approach to management of cerebral perfusion pressure (CPP) in the infant or child with severe TBI.[122]

ICP monitoring has not been studied in an RCT in children to establish its efficacy in altering outcome after severe TBI in either adults or children. Forsyth and coworkers[123] examined the United Kingdom multicenter database of more than 500 cases of pediatric TBI and reported that both ICP >20 mm Hg and lack of ICP monitoring were independently associated with death before discharge. Given that raised ICP correlates with poor outcome, there is a strong rationale for identifying and treating this problem.[124] As discussed in the section on CT, although CT is useful for identifying patients at high risk for the development of raised ICP (eg, those with mass lesions), the finding of a "normal" cranial CT scan does not rule out the potential for raised ICP.[125] Despite this evidence, ICP monitoring in children with TBI, particularly in infants, is still not rigorously performed in clinical practice. Keenan and associates[126] surprisingly reported in 2005 that only 33% of infants and young toddlers (younger than 2 years) with severe TBI underwent ICP monitoring in the state of North Carolina. Consideration of risk versus benefit for ICP monitoring must be involved in the clinical decision in cases in which the complication rate is high, such as in patients with coagulopathy.

Since publication of the last edition of this textbook, two new studies in adult TBI are important to discuss. Supporting the use of ICP monitoring, Gerber and colleagues[127] reported on the results of a study by the Brain Trauma Foundation on all cases of TBI in the state of New York. Between 2001 and 2009, mortality decreased from 23% to 13%, which was accompanied by guidelines-based ICP monitoring increasing from 56% to 75%. In contrast, Chesnut and colleagues[128] found no differences in outcome in a study of 324 patients in Latin America randomized to treatment led by either ICP-directed care or a protocol in which treatment was based on imaging and clinical examination. A consensus-based interpretation of that study suggested that the results of the trial should not be generalized and that it should not change current practice of those currently using ICP monitoring.

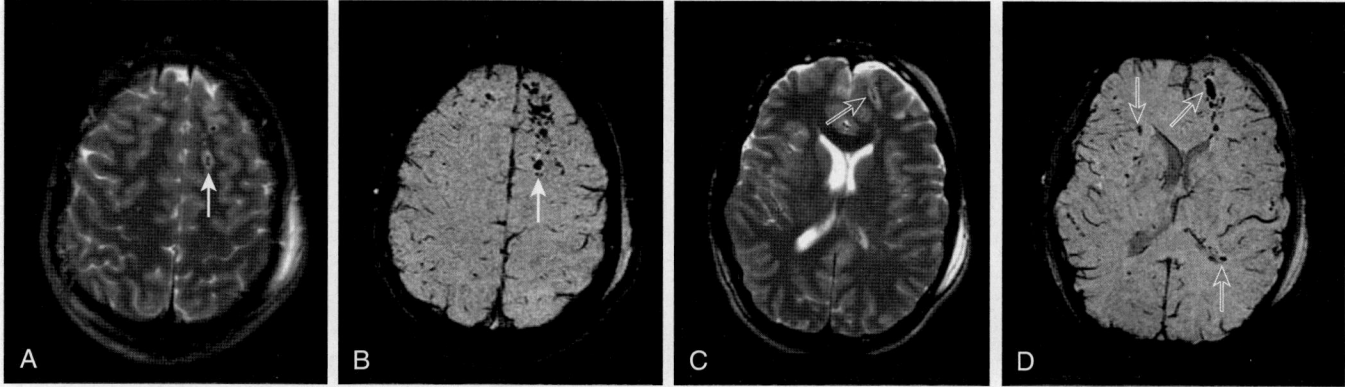

Fig. 119.8. Detection of diffuse axonal injury is enhanced by susceptibility-weighted magnetic resonance imaging (SWI). (A and C) Subtle hemorrhage in white matter is seen with conventional axial T$_2$-weighted imaging. (B and D) The diffuse white matter hemorrhages are much more readily detectible on SWI. The arrows in each example identify the hemorrhages. (From Tong KA, Ashwal S, Obenaus A, et al. Susceptibility-weighted MR imaging: a review of clinical applications in children. AJNR Am J Neuroradiol. 2008;29:9-17.)

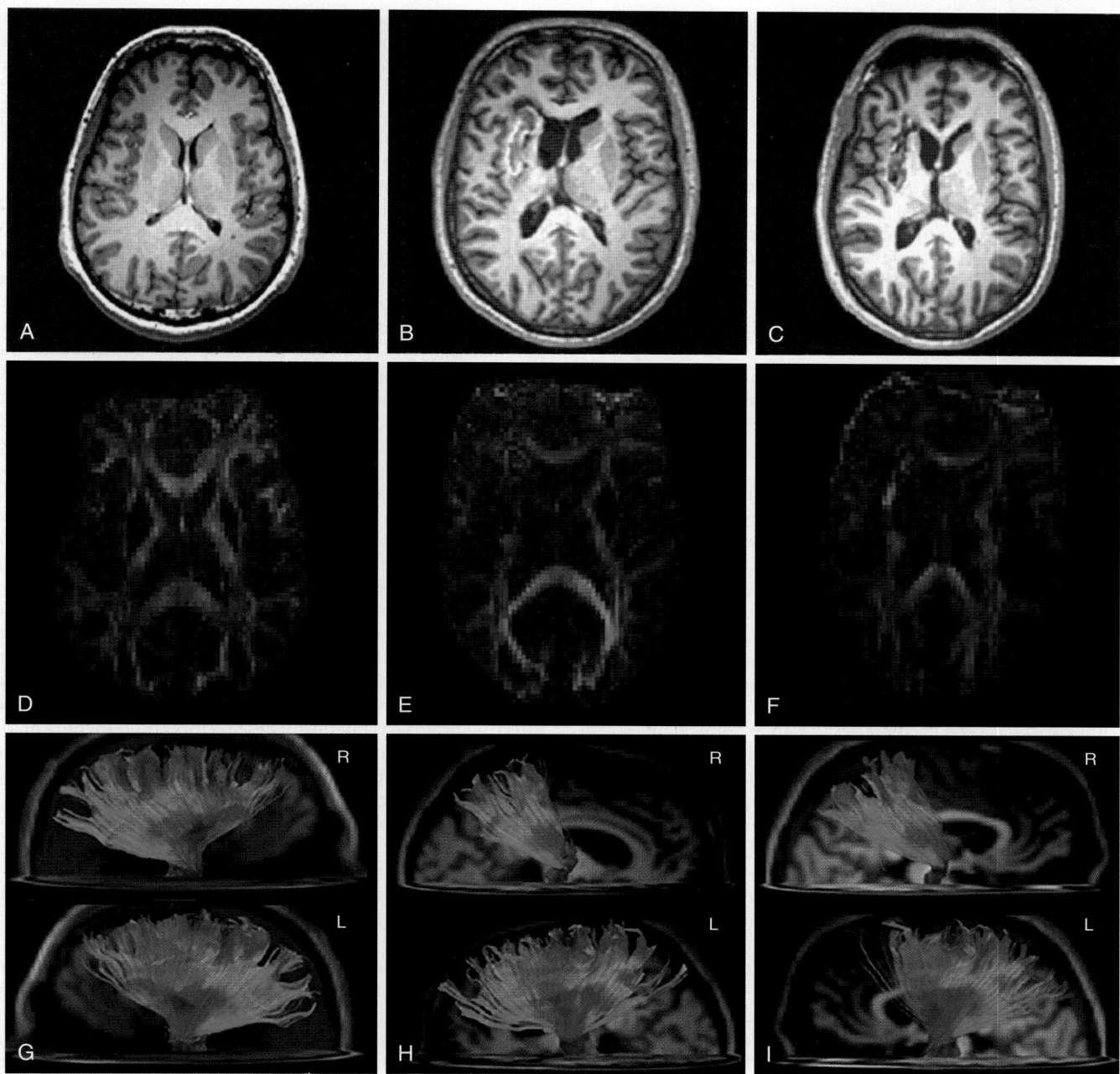

Fig. 119.9. Comparison of conventional T₁-weighted imaging (A-C), diffusion tensor imaging fractional anisotropy maps (D-F), and state-of-the-art high-definition fiber tract (HDFT) imaging (G-I) of a healthy volunteer (A, D, G) and a traumatic brain injury patient at 4 months (B, E, H) or 10 months (C, F, I) after injury. HDFT demonstrates the progression of loss of white matter tracts with remarkable anatomic clarity. (From Shin SS, Verstynen T, Pathak S, et al. High-definition fiber tracking for assessment of neurological deficit in a case of traumatic brain injury: finding, visualizing, and interpreting small sites of damage. J Neurosurg. 2012;116:1062-1069.)

However, additional investigation of ICP monitoring was recommended.[129]

Currently, ICP monitoring by ventricular catheter is considered the most accurate, low-cost, reliable method.[1,2] The ventricular catheter also affords a key therapeutic option—CSF drainage. Other acceptable methods include parenchymal fiberoptic and microtransducer systems; subarachnoid, subdural, and epidural monitors of any type are less reliable.[130] The type of monitor (ventricular catheter or fiberoptic pressure transducer) used is dependent on the local preference of the neurosurgical staff.

The location of the patient in the hospital when the monitor is placed varies among centers and includes the emergency department/trauma bay, operating room, or PICU. Despite the flurry of activity that often surrounds the stabilization of a critically injured child with severe TBI, it is important to provide adequate anesthesia during placement of the monitor to prevent pain-induced spikes in ICP or herniation.

Monitoring and treatment of ICP are essential to contemporary management. Finally, use of a ventricular catheter affords the added opportunity of CSF drainage as a therapy.

Advanced Monitoring Techniques

Monitoring Cerebral Blood Flow

Several techniques for assessing CBF, autoregulation of CBF, or metabolism can provide additional insight into the occurrence of cerebral ischemia or other metabolic derangements during management and help guide therapy. However, information on the use of these techniques and their impact on outcome in infants and children with severe TBI remains limited. Often, these methods are used only in clinical research or specialized trauma centers with particular interest in pediatric neurointensive care.

Clinically available techniques for measuring CBF after severe TBI in children include (1) transcranial Doppler (TCD) and (2) arterial spin-label MRI (ASL-MRI).[119]

TCD is gaining acceptance in pediatric neurocritical care because it is noninvasive and readily repeated at the bedside.[131,132] It can serve as an early warning monitor of the development of an unfavorable trend in cerebral perfusion; in addition, it can assess autoregulation, define major alterations, identify vasospasm, and contribute prognostic information.[8,131-133] TCD measures velocity rather than flow and usually is applied to assess the middle cerebral artery distribution. However, the inability of TCD to acquire regional data limits its utility in titrating care. Some have suggested that TCD also has utility in identifying the presence of raised ICP, but results have been conflicting.[134,135]

ASL-MRI has been used for decades in preclinical investigations in TBI and is now used routinely in advanced neurocritical care in some centers.[117,136] However, its use to assess CBF in pediatric TBI is only beginning to emerge.[137] This method is not a monitoring tool given its need for MRI; however, it provides quantitative maps of CBF and can be used for dynamic studies such as assessment of CO_2 reactivity or pressure autoregulation. Its use is likely to increase as faster MRI techniques are developed. Unfortunately, the stable xenon CT method that was used in a number of seminal studies of pediatric TBI (Fig. 119.10) is not available for routine clinical use.[18,138]

As previously discussed, Brady and associates[62] have generated interest in continuous monitoring of blood pressure autoregulation of CBF with use of a PRx that is calculated as a linear correlation between ICP and blood pressure. With use of this noninvasive adjunct to ICP monitoring, intact autoregulation was shown to be associated with survival in 21 children with severe TBI. This method also may contribute to better definition of optimal CPP; however, it fails to provide regional assessments—further study is needed.

Monitoring Cerebral Metabolism

Jugular venous saturation has been used to monitor cerebral oxygen delivery in adults, but limited information on the utility of this technique in children is available.[53,54] Studies in adults suggest that therapies such as barbiturates and hyperventilation can be titrated according to jugular venous saturation.[139,140] Desaturations below the threshold value of 50% are associated with mortality in adults.[141] However, jugular venous desaturation below this level was rarely the sole indication that urgent intervention was needed, and false desaturations

occurred. Nevertheless, this tool can assist in clinical decision making, but some persons have questioned its ability to monitor regional effects and it has not been commonly used in pediatric TBI.[142]

Several other modes of monitoring cerebral metabolic rate may be helpful. Near-infrared spectroscopy has been used to track the oxidative state of cytochromes in brain. Near-infrared spectroscopy has been used to assess cerebral metabolic status in hypoxemic-ischemic neonates[143] and is beginning to be used in pediatric TBI.[144] Although its exact role remains unclear, it may prove valuable as a trend monitor.[145] Limitations with topographic resolution and the dominance of the superficial brain tissue in generating the signal are concerns.

Monitoring partial pressure of oxygen (PO_2) in brain parenchyma ($PbtO_2$) with a microelectrode implanted in the frontal lobe is feasible.[146] A threshold value of about 8.5 mm Hg was associated with a reduction in CPP below 60 mm Hg, although in adults, thresholds anywhere from 10 to 30 mm Hg have been recommended. Use of this approach has gained interest in pediatric TBI over the past decade. Stiefel and colleagues[147] reported on the utility of $PbtO_2$ monitoring in children and suggested a threshold of 20 mm Hg. Stippler and associates reported experience with $PbtO_2$ monitoring in a series of children and found that a PbO_2 of 30 mm Hg was associated with the highest sensitivity/specificity for favorable neurologic outcome at 6 months after TBI.[148] We routinely use $PbtO_2$ in children with TBI, targeting a threshold of 20 mm Hg. Therapy is first targeted to optimize ICP and CPP. However, in some cases, $PbtO_2$ is <20 mm Hg despite control of ICP and it is necessary to evaluate other potential factors that might be affecting brain oxygenation. These factors could include inadvertent hyperventilation due to a ventilator change or a decline in PaO_2 due to lung disease; if so, these issues should be addressed. If there is no extracerebral complication affecting $PbtO_2$, interventions such as increasing FIO_2 or raising $PaCO_2$ or MAP/CPP to improve CBF may further augment $PbtO_2$. The major limitations of $PbtO_2$ are its invasiveness and provision of only focal data. In adults, $PbtO_2$ measurement has been coupled to cerebral microdialysis to provide metabolic data (ie, glutamate levels).[149,150]

Finally, positron emission tomography (PET) has been used in adults with severe TBI (Fig. 119.11).[23] Although limited by long acquisition times and the risk of intrahospital transport of critically ill patients, the metabolic maps generated provide much insight, particularly into cerebral glucose utilization after TBI. Diringer and coworkers[151] used PET to provide important insight into the effect of hyperventilation on $CMRO_2$ in adults with severe TBI (see the section on hyperventilation). Both PET and advanced MRI, along with magnetic resonance spectroscopy, can provide insight into regional brain disturbances and the effect of therapy.

Treatment in the Pediatric Intensive Care Unit

Once the initial resuscitation is completed and evacuable intracranial masses have been addressed, maintenance of physiologic stability and recognition and management of raised ICP are the priorities. A flow diagram illustrating a general approach to first-tier treatments of the child with severe TBI was provided in the initial pediatric guidelines (Fig. 119.12). The injured brain has complex metabolic requirements that are poorly understood.[152] Autoregulation of CBF

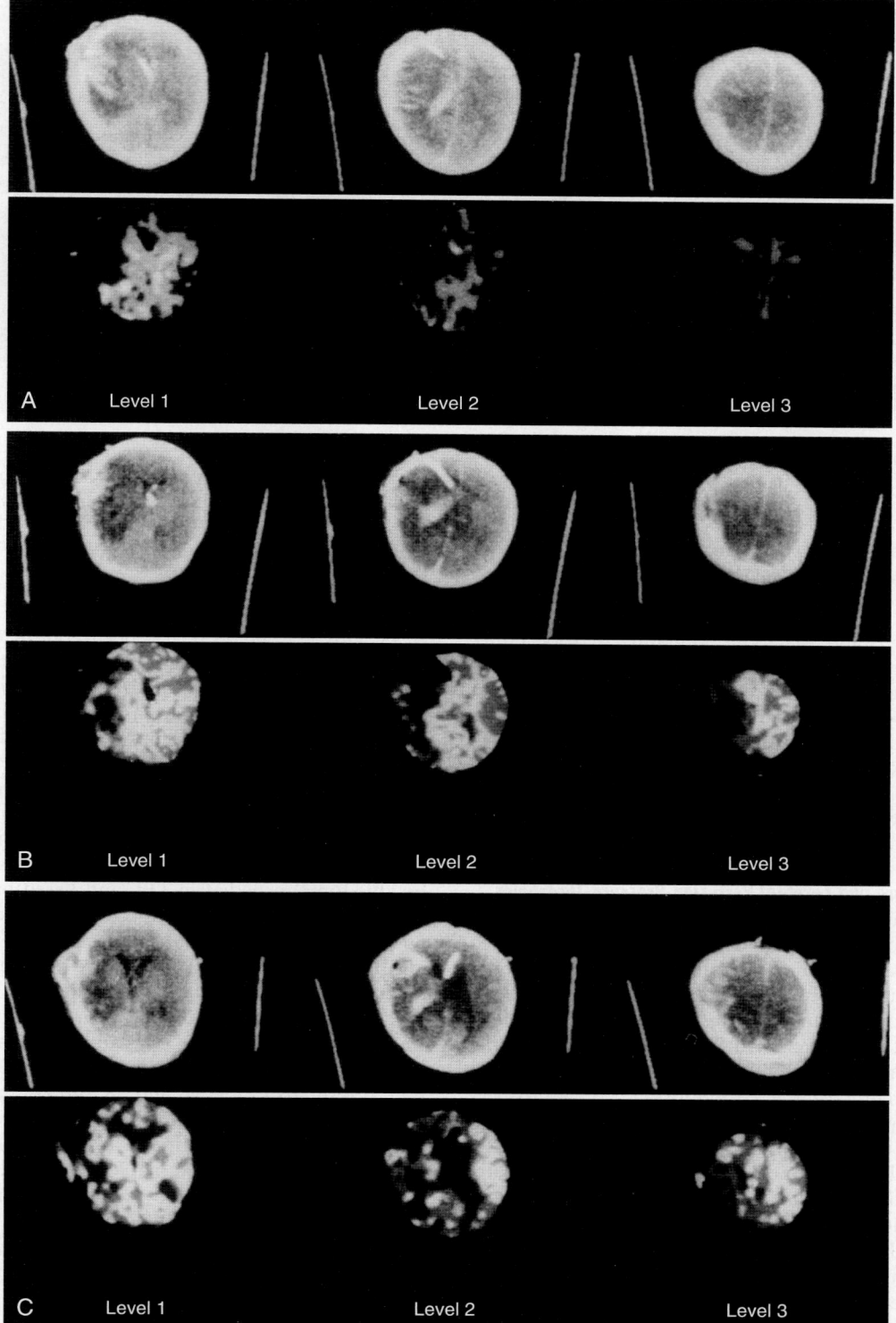

Fig. 119.10. Time course of CBF measured by Xe-enhanced CT in a 2-month-old infant after severe traumatic brain injury from a motor vehicle accident. Standard CT images *(upper row)* and Xe-enhanced CBF maps *(lower row)* are shown from studies performed on admission (A) and at 2 days (B) and 5 days (C) after injury. Flow is severely reduced *(black)* on admission. Some recovery of CBF is seen at 2 days and 5 days after injury. CBF ranges from lowest *(darkest image)* to highest *(brightest image)*.

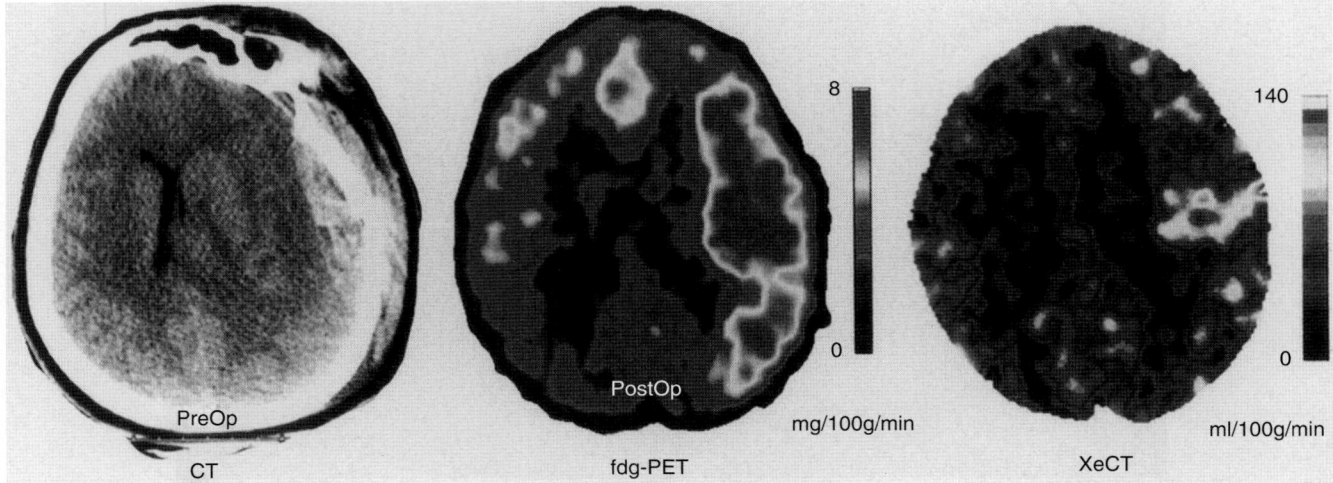

Fig. 119.11. CT image *(left)* of an acute subdural hematoma with mass effect that was treated with surgical evacuation. 18F-flurodexoyglucose positron emission tomographic (PET) map *(center)* obtained at 5 days after surgery shows marked local increases in cerebral glucose utilization in the brain regions underlying the hematoma. Stable Xe-enhanced CT CBF map *(right)* also obtained at 5 days after surgery shows increased CBF in the same region, indicating that the increase in glucose utilization is not the result of hypoperfusion. This phenomenon, termed *hyperglycolysis,* is suggested to represent increased glucose utilization by astrocytes coupled to glutamate uptake and other mediator-driven processes. This highlights the complex regional metabolic demands of the traumatically injured brain.

may be disturbed, and metabolic demands may be either decreased or increased.[15,53-56,62,153] It is clear, however, that evidence of neuronal death from cerebral ischemia is a common finding on autopsy in patients who die after severe TBI. Control of ICP and maintenance of adequate CPP and PbtO₂ may limit the risk of developing secondary ischemia. The goals of management are thus to optimize ICP, CPP, and brain oxygenation/perfusion; avoid secondary insults; and create the best possible environment for brain recovery.

Intracranial Pressure and Cerebral Perfusion Pressure Thresholds

Adult patients with severe TBI who have an ICP of 20 mm Hg have a poorer outcome than do those without increased ICP.[122,124,125,154] As discussed, despite the RCT showing similar outcomes for adults with severe TBI managed in Latin America with versus without ICP monitoring, a consensus-based interpretation of that study suggested that the results of the trial should not be generalized and that it should not change practice of those currently using ICP monitoring.[128,129] A prospective cohort study by Ghajar and colleagues[155] also suggested better outcome in adults monitored and treated with CSF drainage versus those without ICP monitoring. Several studies suggest that optimal outcome is achieved when even more modest levels of ICP (ie, 15 mm Hg) are the target.[155] Although no pediatric study has prospectively compared ICP treatment thresholds and their effect on outcome using a specific treatment regimen, review of the pediatric literature provides clues on the optimal ICP treatment threshold. Many studies published before the guidelines, including a total of more than 230 cases of severe pediatric TBI, reported that poor outcome was associated with ICP >20 mm Hg.[55,156-159] In an important study by Chambers and associates[160] in 99 children with head injuries (0-13 years of age) in the United Kingdom, an ICP threshold of 15 mm Hg was used. However, it remains to be determined whether a lower ICP threshold is appropriate for infants in whom physiologic MAP is lower than in adults. This issue remains as an important unanswered question.[161]

As with ICP, no RCT has been conducted to define the optimal CPP for pediatric TBI, although its importance in patient management is recognized. Reductions in CPP below specific threshold values are associated with poor outcome. The original guidelines' recommendation of 40 mm Hg was based on four studies that defined the CPP associated with poor outcome as between 40 and 65 mm Hg.[159,162-164] Several publications have further clarified the issue of optimal CPP in children, suggesting the need for age-dependent thresholds. Chambers and colleagues[165] published what is the largest study on this topic in pediatric TBI, and based on data from 235 children, they suggested minimum CPP values of 53, 63, and 66 mm Hg for children between the ages of 2 and 6 years, 7 and 10 years, and 11 and 16 years, respectively. However, that study considered only the first 6 hours of monitoring, and CPP and ICP were not addressed for patients <2 years of age. In a follow-up study of 91 children, Chambers and colleagues[160] used a pressure-time index to determine critical CPP thresholds of 48, 54, and 58 mm Hg in children aged 2 to 6 years, 7 to 10 years, and 11 to 15 years, respectively. Allen and coworkers[166] assessed data from >2000 children in the New York State Brain Trauma Foundation database and suggested CPP thresholds of >60 mm Hg in adults, 50 to 60 mm Hg in children 6 to 17 years of age, and >40 mm Hg in infants and children 0 to 5 years of age. These are reasonable recommendations until prospective trials of CPP-directed therapy in children are carried out.

In addition to the methods described later for control of ICP, titration of vasopressor or inotropic support may be necessary to achieve an appropriate level of CPP once adequate filling pressure and hemoglobin are confirmed. In some situations, as with the development of neurogenic pulmonary edema, aggressive cardiovascular monitoring and optimal titration of cardiopulmonary support can be challenging and key determinants of outcome. Finally, not only are the optimal ICP and CPP targets likely to be important, but how one achieves these target values may be very important.

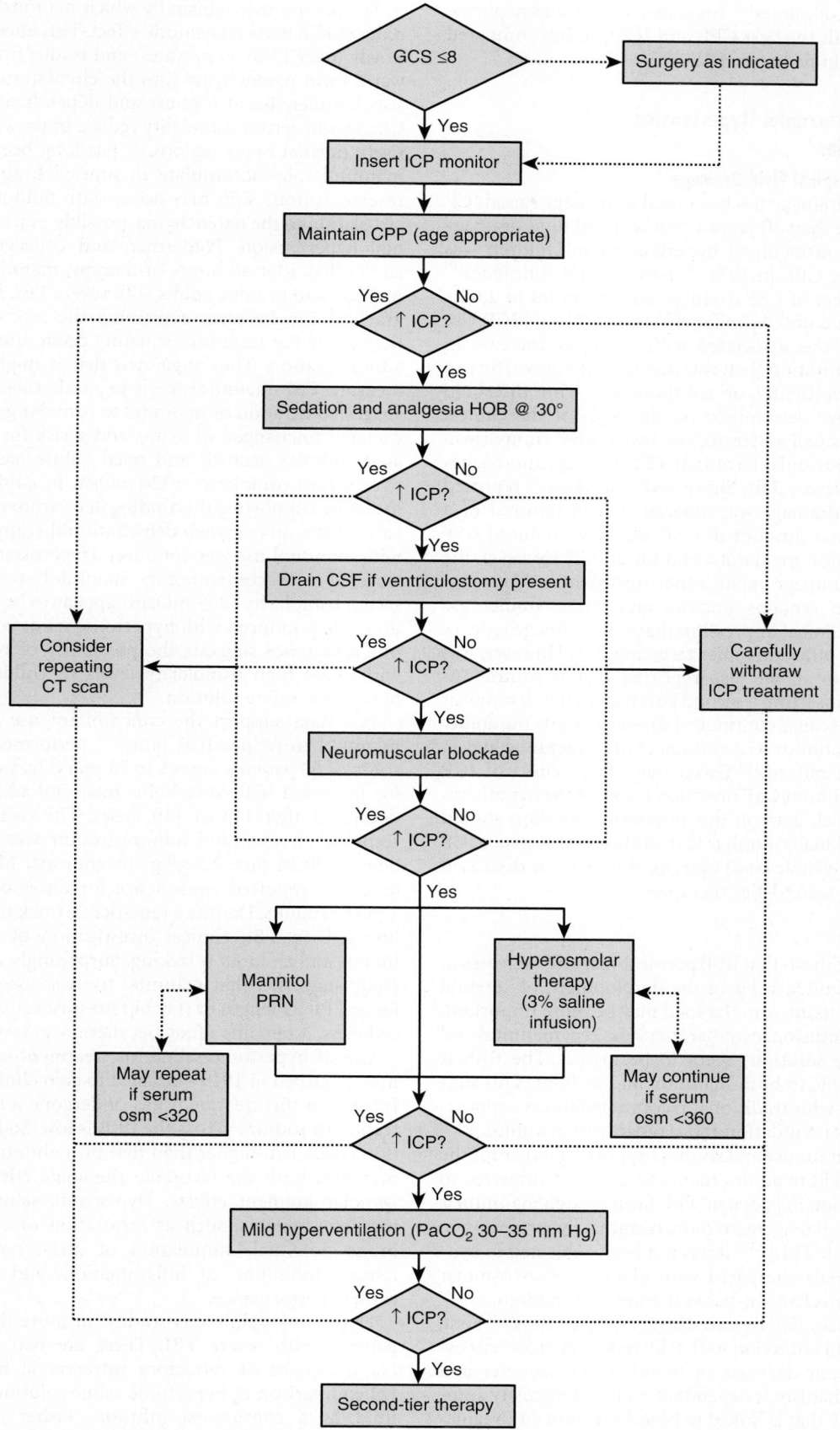

Fig. 119.12. First-tier management approach based on the Guidelines for the Management of Severe TBI in Infants, Children, and Adolescents.[1] *HOB,* head of bed.

DiGennaro and colleagues[167] suggested that norepinephrine was associated with the best CPP and ICP profiles compared to other pressors in pediatric TBI.

Treatment of Intracranial Hypertension: First-Tier Therapies

Ventricular Cerebrospinal Fluid Drainage

Ventricular CSF drainage has been used to manage raised ICP in adults for more than 40 years. Cerebrospinal fluid drainage for treatment of intracranial hypertension in children was shown to improve CBF in 1971.[168] Fortune and colleagues[169] compared the effect of CSF drainage and mannitol in adults after severe TBI and noted similar effects on CBF and ICP. Use of CSF drainage was associated with a greater increase in jugular venous saturation than was mannitol therapy. CSF can be drained intermittently or continuously, with threshold values for drainage determined on the basis of the clinical indication. In a small retrospective two-center comparison between continuous and intermittent CSF drainage approaches in children with severe TBI, Shore and coworkers[170] reported that continuous drainage was associated with removal of a substantially greater amount of CSF, markedly reduced CSF levels of biochemical mediators, and lower ICP. However, the efficacy of CSF drainage versus other treatments of intracranial hypertension remains unclear, and larger studies are needed. It is our clinical impression that CSF drainage reduces requirements for other therapies targeting ICP. However, this has yet to be proven. We also reported that if continuous drainage is used, inserting a second parenchymal ICP monitor may be of value because continuous drainage limits the ability to continuously monitor ICP, and spikes of intracranial hypertension could be missed.[171] Given that effectiveness of ICP control with or without CSF diversion is one of the hypotheses of the ADAPT trial, data on this important question should be forthcoming. Finally, lumbar CSF drainage can reduce ICP in cases with discernible basal cisterns; this factor is discussed in the section on second-tier therapies.

Osmolar Therapy

Based on the hypothesis that BBB permeability and increases in CBV play only limited roles in the development of cerebral swelling and that tissue osmolar load may be more important, particularly in contusion, osmolar therapies (eg, mannitol and hypertonic saline solution) seem to be logical. The BBB is nearly impermeable to both mannitol and sodium. This suggestion contrasts with traditional recommendations supporting the use of hyperventilation and avoidance of mannitol.[172,173] Despite its ubiquitous use and studies supporting its use for the management of TBI in adults, mannitol has been subjected to limited investigation in pediatric TBI. Even though mannitol is a cornerstone for management of intracranial hypertension in pediatric and adult TBI,[1,2,130] it has not been subjected to controlled clinical trials compared with placebo, other osmolar agents, or other mechanism-based therapies in children.

Mannitol reduces ICP by two distinct mechanisms.[130] First, it produces a rapid reduction in ICP by reducing blood viscosity with a resultant decrease in blood vessel diameter and CBV.[174] This mechanism is dependent on intact viscosity autoregulation of CBF that is linked to blood pressure autoregulation of CBF. The effect of mannitol administration on blood viscosity and CBV is transient (lasting ~75 minutes).

The second mechanism by which mannitol administration reduces ICP is via an osmotic effect. This effect develops more slowly (over 15 to 30 minutes) and results from movement of water from parenchyma into the circulation. The effect persists between 1 and 6 hours and depends on an intact BBB. Changes in serum osmolality reduce brain water only in relatively normal brain regions. It has long been suggested that mannitol may accumulate in injured brain regions and a reverse osmotic shift may occur, with fluid moving from the circulation to the parenchyma, possibly exacerbating intracranial hypertension. Polderman and colleagues[66] showed in adults that after 48 hours of therapy, mannitol levels in CSF increase and in some adults with severe TBI, a reverse osmotic gradient can be seen, explaining the lack of effect of this therapy or the need for escalating doses after several days of administration. They suggested that it might be optimal to measure CSF mannitol levels to guide therapy. Others have suggested titration of mannitol to osmolar gap.[175] Mannitol is excreted unchanged in urine, and a risk for development of acute tubular necrosis and renal failure has been suggested with serum osmolarity >320 mOsm in adults. However, the literature supporting this finding dates from the late 1970s and early 1980s, an era when dehydration therapy in combination with mannitol use was common. Hyperosmolar euvolemia is targeted with contemporary mannitol use. High levels of serum osmolarity (365 mOsm) appear to be tolerated in children when induced with hypertonic saline solution, although one case series suggests the possibility of renal impairment with these high osmolarity levels in children treated with hypertonic saline solution.[176,177]

Few data support the concomitant use of diuretics and mannitol to reduce ICP. James[178] performed a retrospective study of 60 patients (ages 1 to 73 years) treated with mannitol for increased ICP. After bolus mannitol administration, ICP decreased after 116 of 119 doses. The reduction in ICP in response to mannitol administration was dose dependent between 0.18 and 2.5 g/kg. In contrast, Marshall and colleagues[179] reported equivalence for doses between 0.25 and 1 g/kg in adults. Despite a remarkable track record for controlling ICP in TBI, clinical investigation of mannitol use in infants and children is lacking. Surprisingly, an epidemiologic study suggested that mannitol use was associated with prolonged PICU length of stay but no survival advantage.[180] Nevertheless, it remains a first-tier therapy in severe pediatric TBI.

Use of hypertonic saline for treatment of raised ICP was first described in 1919 but failed to gain clinical acceptance.[181] Interest in this treatment has undergone a resurgence. Penetration of sodium across the BBB is low. Sodium has a reflection coefficient higher than that of mannitol and shares with mannitol both the favorable rheologic effects on CBV and osmolar gradient effects. Hypertonic saline exhibits other theoretic benefits, such as restoration of cell resting membrane potential, stimulation of atrial natriuretic peptide release, inhibition of inflammation, and enhancement of cardiac performance.

Hypertonic saline was studied in more than 130 pediatric patients with severe TBI. There are two types of studies: (1) treatment of refractory intracranial hypertension and (2) comparison of hypertonic saline solution to maintenance fluid as a continuous infusion. Fisher and coworkers[105] compared 3% saline solution and 0.9% saline solution in children with severe TBI. During the 2-hour trial, hypertonic saline solution was associated with a lower ICP. The serum sodium level increased about 7 mEq/L after administration of 3% saline solution. Khanna and associates[182] reported a prospective study of 3% saline solution (514 mEq/L) given on a sliding scale to maintain ICP <20 mm Hg in children with resistant intracranial hypertension. A reduction in ICP and an increase in CPP were noted with 3% saline solution. The mean highest serum sodium level and osmolarity were about 170 mEq/L and approximately 365 mOsm/L, respectively. Sustained hypernatremia and hyperosmolarity were generally tolerated. Acute renal failure developed in two patients.

Peterson and colleagues[176] reported a retrospective study on the use of a 3% saline solution infusion titrated to reduce ICP to ≤20 mm Hg in infants and children with TBI. The mean daily doses of hypertonic saline solution ranged from between 11 and 27 mL/kg/day. A control group was not used, but only three patients died of uncontrolled ICP, and 73% of patients had a good or moderate outcome. Rebound in ICP or other adverse effects were not seen.

Theoretic concerns associated with use of hypertonic saline solution include development of extrapontine myelinolysis (EPM), rapid shrinking of the brain associated with mechanical tearing of bridging vessels leading to subarachnoid hemorrhage, renal failure, and rebound intracranial hypertension.[183] EPM is related to central pontine myelinolysis (CPM) but occurs with hypernatremia or its correction. It is characterized by demyelination of the thalamus, basal ganglia, and cerebellum.[184] Neither EPM nor CPM has been reported in human trials of hypertonic saline solution for treatment of TBI. EPM has been reported in dehydrated children with serum sodium levels of 168 to 195 mEq/L, and CPM has been reported with rapid correction of chronic hyponatremia.[185] Peterson and colleagues[176] performed MRI evaluations in 11 patients in their study, and none had evidence of CPM. However, rats with normal serum sodium levels subjected to increases of 39 mEq/L showed severe demyelinating lesions.[186] Similarly, subarachnoid hemorrhage has been reported with serum sodium concentrations from 149 to 206 mEq/L within 1 hour after injection of 9% hypertonic saline solution in normal kittens.[187]

Renal failure is a concern with use of hyperosmolar therapies,[188] but this complication seems uncommon with hypertonic saline solution use in children after TBI.[176,177] Rebound intracranial hypertension has been described with use of hypertonic saline solution bolus therapy or after cessation of continuous infusion.[176,189] As with mannitol therapy, if the BBB is breached, one would also expect that CSF levels of sodium would gradually increase with prolonged therapy. Patients may require progressive increases in infusion rates to control ICP. Subsequent to publication of the most recent update to the guidelines,[2] Gonda and associates[190] reported that serum sodium levels >170 mEq/L were associated with a higher occurrence of thrombocytopenia, renal failure, neutropenia, and acute respiratory distress syndrome after controlling for key confounding variables in 88 children with raised ICP. Thus caution is indicated in refractory cases; multiple therapies to control ICP rather than advancing hypertonic saline to higher risk levels should be strongly considered. Given all of the evidence, hypertonic saline solution, mannitol, and CSF drainage are first-tier therapies for raised ICP after severe TBI in infants and children.

Sedation Analgesia and Neuromuscular Blockade

Sedation and neuromuscular blockade should be used as needed in the setting of raised ICP once appropriate monitoring has been established and thus are integrated into first-tier treatment. Narcotics, benzodiazepines, or small doses of barbiturates are generally recommended for routine use. To our knowledge, no controlled trial of varying sedation regimens has been performed in pediatric patients with severe TBI. Hsiang and colleagues[191] reported on 514 adults with severe TBI and suggested that prophylactic neuromuscular blockade was associated with increased length of ICU stay and nosocomial pneumonia. However, the study was not prospective and should not preclude the use of neuromuscular blockade in pediatric TBI. A systematic review on the use of neuromuscular blockade in adults identified a number of small studies showing benefit on various aspects of ICP care including preventing increases in ICP during tracheal suctioning or on spontaneous ICP spikes.[192] Careful assessment of indication and titration is essential. Finally, intermittent doses of barbiturates or lidocaine may be needed to blunt excessive rises in ICP resulting from routine patient care maneuvers such as suctioning. Additional studies are badly needed.

Head Position

Feldman and colleagues[193] conducted a prospective RCT of the effect of head position on ICP, CPP, and CBF in 22 adults after severe TBI. Both ICP and mean carotid pressure were reduced in the 30-degree position versus the 0-degree position. CPP and CBF did not change with this intervention. Thus, in general, the 30-degree head-elevated position reduced ICP without deleterious effects on CPP and is preferred. Head elevation and midline position improve jugular venous and possibly CSF drainage and decrease the contributions of these components to ICP.

Treatment of Intracranial Hypertension: Second-Tier Therapies

Refractory intracranial hypertension occurs in 20% to 40% of cases of severe pediatric TBI and is associated with mortality rates of 30% to 100%.[156-159,162-164,180,194,195] Several second-tier therapies are available for treatment of refractory intracranial hypertension (Fig. 119.13). Second-tier therapies include barbiturates, hyperventilation, hypothermia, decompressive craniectomy, and lumbar CSF drainage.

Barbiturates

Barbiturates produce a reduction in ICP via a decrease in cerebral metabolic rate. Although an RCT of barbiturate therapy for treatment of severe TBI in adults did not show an outcome benefit,[196] it can be effective in the setting of refractory raised ICP.[197] Goodman and coworkers[198] reported an improvement in brain interstitial concentration of lactate and glutamate accompanying a reduction of ICP in seven adults treated with barbiturates for refractory intracranial hypertension. Subsequent to publication of the revised guidelines, Mellion and colleagues[199] published additional supportive data for the use of high-dose barbiturates after severe TBI in 36 children with refractory raised ICP. Ten of the 36 patients responded with control of ICP (<20 mm Hg). Control of refractory ICP was associated with better long-term outcome. If either frequent dosing or barbiturate infusion is used, an

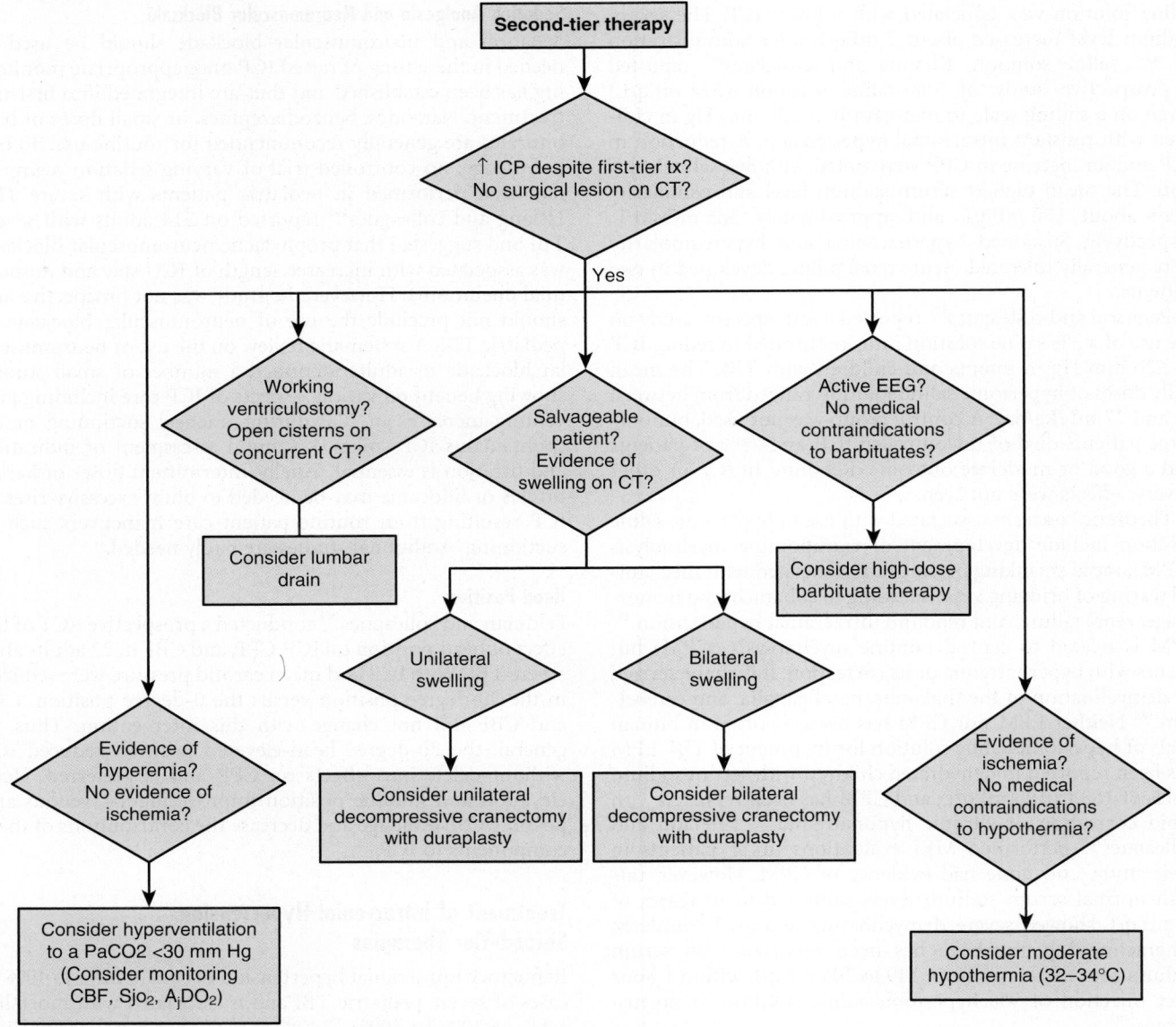

Fig. 119.13. Second-tier therapies for the management of refractory intracranial hypertension based on the Guidelines for the Management of Severe TBI in Infants, Children, and Adolescents.[1] *A$_j$DO$_2$*, arteriojugular venous oxygen content difference; *Sjo$_2$*, jugular vein oxygen saturation.

electroencephalogram (EEG) should be used to assess the response to treatment. The endpoint of barbiturate coma is generally burst suppression. Pentobarbital often is infused to achieve a burst suppression response on EEG. However, that goal should only represent the maximal barbiturate dose used for ICP control because (1) smaller doses—those still associated with EEG activity—may be adequate to control ICP, and (2) indiscriminate use can be associated with undesirable adverse effects such as hypotension.[200] When barbiturates are used, hypotension should be avoided. Patients should be carefully monitored for reduced cardiac output or inadequate systemic perfusion, as clinically indicated.

Hyperventilation

Hyperventilation has been used to manage pediatric patients with severe TBI since the 1950s.[201] Bruce and colleagues[17] suggested that hyperemia was the predominant mechanism involved in the development of raised ICP in children. Until

the mid-1980s, prophylactic hyperventilation was the standard of care. In addition to reducing postinjury hyperemia, hyperventilation was suggested to reduce brain acidosis and restore CBF autoregulation. Subsequently, studies in experimental models suggested hyperventilation had deleterious effects. Prophylactic hyperventilation depletes brain interstitial bicarbonate buffering capacity and is accompanied by a gradual loss of local vasoconstrictor effects.[202]

In an RCT in adults after severe TBI, prophylactic hyperventilation for 5 days to a Paco$_2$ of about 25 mm Hg versus about 35 mm Hg was associated with worse outcome.[203] Skippen and colleagues[4,119] reported that hyperventilation to a Paco$_2$ of about 25 mm Hg reduced CBF to levels less than 18 mL/100 g/min in 73% of infants and children with severe TBI (Fig. 119.14). Coles and associates[142] found similar results in adults. However, neither of these studies assessed the effect of hyperventilation on either regional cerebral metabolism or neurologic outcome. In experimental TBI in rats, aggressive

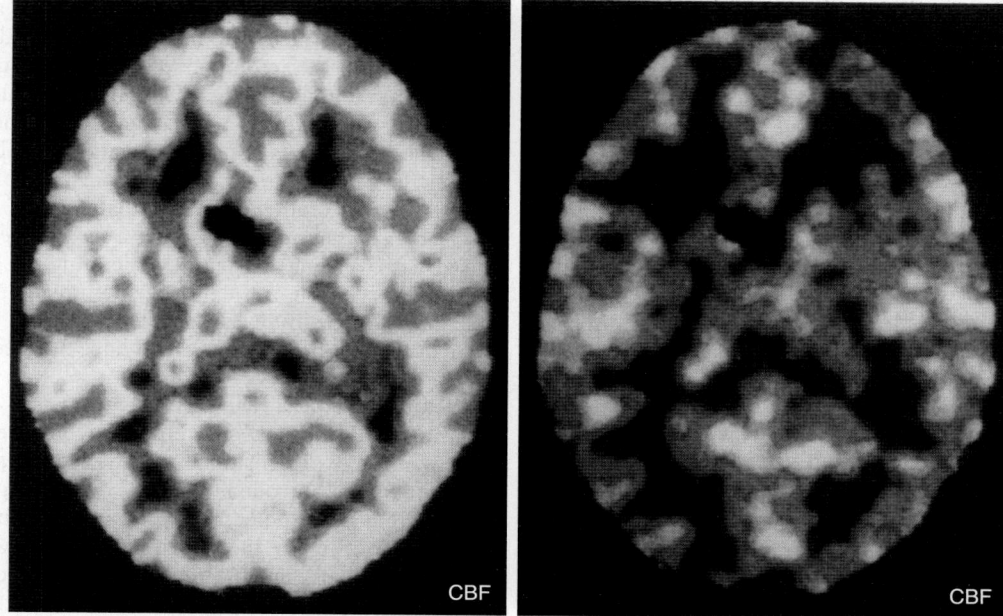

Fig. 119.14. Xe-enhanced CBF maps from a child with severe traumatic brain injury before *(left)* and after *(right)* escalation of hyperventilation (a second-tier therapy) in the scanner. Intact reactivity of CBF to change in PaCO$_2$ is demonstrated by an obvious reduction in flow. CBF ranges from lowest *(darkest image)* to highest *(brightest image)*.

hyperventilation (PaCO$_2$ ~20 mm Hg) early after injury increased hippocampal cell death. The most recent pediatric guidelines recommend that prophylactic hyperventilation (Pa$_{CO2}$ <30 mm Hg) should be avoided and that if it is used to control refractory intracranial hypertension, advanced neuromonitoring may be considered.[22]

Supporting this approach in infants and children, early after severe TBI, hypoperfusion rather than hyperemia was shown to be associated with poor outcome.[18] However, the risks of hyperventilation are still somewhat controversial. Diringer and colleagues[151] reported that at between 8 and 14 hours after severe TBI in adults, hyperventilation (PaCO$_2$ ~30 mm Hg) reduced CBF but did not further reduce cerebral metabolic rate for oxygen as assessed using PET. This finding suggests that in TBI, after the acute hypermetabolic phase, hypometabolism follows and hyperventilation may be a relatively safe means to reduce ICP in the PICU. This study did not evaluate outcome. In contrast, several reports in adults suggest deleterious effects of hyperventilation after TBI, including increases in brain interstitial levels of glutamate and lactate[205] and higher ischemic brain volumes.[206]

Based on these data, there is waning support for the use of hyperventilation. At Pittsburgh Children's Hospital, with the addition of PbtO$_2$ monitoring, when ICP is controlled but PbtO$_2$ is <20 mm Hg, we have found that careful limitation of even mild hyperventilation can, in some cases, promptly increase PbtO$_2$. Despite these concerns, hyperventilation surprisingly seems to remain a mainstay of care in pediatric TBI. Curry and associates,[207] in a study of 375 children with severe TBI, reported a 52% to 60% incidence of substantial hypocarbia (PaCO$_2$ <30 mm Hg) in the initial 48 hours that was associated with poor outcome. This incidence was seen despite ICP levels less than 20 mm Hg in many cases. A high frequency of hyperventilation also was reported by Morris and colleagues[208] in the United Kingdom database and, surprisingly, in the RCT

of therapeutic hypothermia by the Canadian multicenter trials group (44%).[209] Some investigators have suggested that it may be time to set the alarm threshold for PaCO$_2$ in management of severe TBI in children or for a practice bundle in TBI.[210] Nevertheless, its use as adjunct treatment of refractory raised ICP, particularly during the delayed postinjury phase, was supported as a second-tier therapy in the guidelines. Based on the current state of knowledge, if hyperventilation (PaCO$_2$ ~30 mm Hg) is used to manage refractory ICP, advanced neuromonitoring such as assessment of PbtO$_2$, CBF, or jugular venous oxygen saturation is recommended to prevent iatrogenic ischemia. Finally, the optimal approach to ventilation is one of the aims within the ADAPT comparative effectiveness trial, so additional information should be forthcoming from that important multicenter investigation.

Hypothermia

In experimental models of TBI and in some clinical trials in adults after TBI, hypothermia improved outcome, presumably via multiple mechanisms, and meta-analyses supported its use in adults with severe TBI.[211-213] However, unlike the case in hypoxic ischemic encephalopathy (HIE) in newborns, RCTs of hypothermia targeting a temperature of about 33°C for 24 or 48 hours in children[209,214] failed to show benefit. Hutchison and colleagues,[209] in a study of 225 children randomly assigned to hypothermia versus normothermia for 24 hours, observed a trend toward worse outcome and increased mortality with hypothermia treatment. A subsequent trial by Adelson and colleagues of 48 hours of moderate hypothermia with slow rewarming was stopped because of futility.[214] These trials indicate that prophylactic hypothermia should not be routinely used as a first-tier therapy for severe TBI in infants and children.

In contrast, hypothermia remains useful as a second-tier therapy for the management of refractory intracranial hypertension after severe TBI.[215,216] Unlike studies showing benefit from transient use (12-24 hours) of mild hypothermia (33°C) in adults after cardiac arrest,[217,218] a variety of temperature ranges are necessary to control ICP; thus a titrated approach to use of hypothermia in this setting is suggested.[215,216] Rewarming should be carried out carefully, at a rate no faster that 1°C every 4 hours—or even more slowly—and great care should be taken to monitor and treat hypotension that can occur with peripheral vasodilation during rewarming. Finally, hyperthermia is extremely deleterious in experimental models of TBI, exacerbating neuronal death. This effect is seen even when a brief 3-hour period of clinically relevant hyperthermia (39°C) is applied. Natale and colleagues[219] supported the clinical relevance of this work by showing that early hyperthermia (38.5°C within the first 24 hours of admission) occurred in 29.9% of pediatric TBI patients and was associated with poor outcome and increased length of stay. The most definitive clinical study on this matter is in the area of perinatal HIE, where just 1°C of hyperthermia after HIE was associated with a deleterious effect on long-term outcome.[220] Care should be taken to treat or prevent hyperthermia after severe TBI.

Decompressive Craniectomy

Another controversial area in the management of both adults and children with refractory intracranial hypertension is the use of decompressive craniectomy. Cushing[221] initially described this modality in 1905. Decompressive craniectomy is a controversial therapy that is based on the complex metabolic demands of the brain and the equally complex but poorly understood adverse effects of many of the therapies used to treat refractory intracranial hypertension (ischemia, hyperosmolality, metabolic suppression, and hypotension). However, this simplistic approach may have merit.

Several contemporary pediatric studies have been performed. Cho and colleagues[222] reported on the use of decompressive craniectomy versus medical management for treatment of infant victims of AHT with refractory intracranial hypertension. Although the series was small, they reported an improved outcome compared with medical therapy, with some survivors showing good outcome. This study is one of the few specifically examining treatment of patients with AHT. Polin and associates[223] reported on the use of extensive bifrontal decompressive craniectomy for the management of 35 adults and children with severe TBI and either refractory intracranial hypertension or diffuse edema on CT scan. They reported a favorable percentage of survivors with good or moderate disability (improved outcome versus retrospectively matched cases from the Traumatic Coma Data Bank) and suggested a 48-hour time window for successful use. However, the patients in this report generally were not treated with either CSF drainage or barbiturates. Nevertheless, the best results were seen in the children in this study. Taylor and colleagues[224] reported on an RCT of early decompressive craniectomy versus standardized medical management alone. Although the sample size was limited (n = 27 children), strong trends toward reduction in ICP and improvement in long-term outcome were seen with decompressive craniectomy. Jagannathan and coworkers[225] reported 81% favorable outcome in 23 children with severe TBI treated with decompressive craniectomy. Subsequent to the preparation of the revised guidelines, Cooper and associates[226] reported on an RCT of decompressive craniectomy in 155 adults with diffuse TBI and intracranial hypertension refractory to first-tier therapy. Although craniectomy reduced intracranial hypertension versus standard care, surprisingly, it was associated with more unfavorable outcomes. Patients with mass lesions were excluded in this trial, and thus it informs us only on patients with diffuse injury; nevertheless it certainly argues against prophylactic decompressive craniectomy in that population.

Decompressive craniectomy is a second-tier therapy that is used with varying frequency depending on local experience and the discretion of the management team. A large RCT (the RESCUEicp study) was completed in 400 patients in the United Kingdom, but the results have not been released.[227]

Lumbar Cerebrospinal Fluid Drainage

Lumbar CSF drainage can be effective in treating refractory intracranial hypertension in children. Levy and colleagues[228] reported that controlled lumbar CSF draining reduced refractory ICP in 14 of 16 pediatric patients and eliminated the need for barbiturates in their series. In adults with severe TBI, Munch and colleagues[229] reported an immediate and lasting reduction in ICP in 23 patients with refractory intracranial hypertension. This modality is also a second-tier treatment option, but to avoid the risks of herniation, the patient must have open basal cisterns and no important mass effect or shift, and a functional ventriculostomy must already be in place.

Controlled Arterial Hypertension

Induced arterial hypertension is a controversial approach to the management of refractory raised ICP. Whether pressure autoregulation of CBF is intact or defective, arterial hypotension or inadequate CPP must be avoided. If pressure autoregulation is impaired, CBF is directly related to CPP and hypotension reduces flow. If pressure autoregulation is intact, then as CPP is reduced, reflex cerebral vasodilatation occurs (to maintain flow), which increases CBV and ICP.[230] This latter phenomenon occurs as CPP is reduced within the autoregulatory range. Based on the relationship among CPP, vessel diameter, CBV, and ICP in selected adults with refractory intracranial hypertension, induced arterial hypertension (CPP increased in adults to between 100 and 140 mm Hg via infusion of phenylephrine) produced a reduction in ICP.[230] However, arterial hypertension reduces ICP only when pressure autoregulation of CBF is intact because hypertension-mediated reduction in vessel caliber produces the reduction in CBV (to maintain a constant flow) and resultant reduction in ICP.

Use of this intervention is complex in pediatric TBI because a single general threshold value of CPP is not applicable. Management must be tailored to each individual patient. It is possible that the aforementioned pressure reactivity index approach could help guide this intervention.[62] Also, the short-term and long-term effects of the greater hydrostatic pressure on the development of cerebral edema are unclear. Optimal management of blood pressure after severe TBI requires both monitoring of the involved factors and an in-depth understanding of the mechanisms.[230] Induced hypertension is a controversial last-ditch therapy that is not addressed in either version of the pediatric guidelines.[1,2] Finally, a few groups managing adults with severe TBI have adopted a very different therapeutic approach to blood pressure and ICP management termed *the Lund concept*. This approach includes aggressive control of ICP with the unusual combination of β-blockade,

α_2-receptor agonists, ergotamine, and barbiturates, with avoidance of systemic hypertension.[231] In some sense, this represents a form of chemical hyperventilation—that is, a pharmacologically controlled reduction in CBV. Remarkably, this approach has produced good outcome data and no exacerbation of ischemia, as assessed using intracerebral microdialysis in adults.[232] One report of this approach to ICP control in children with meningitis is available,[233] along with one report in children with TBI.[234] For additional insight into this approach, the reader is referred to the work of Stahl and associates.[232] This approach requires additional study in children.

Miscellaneous

Seizures should be treated aggressively because excessive metabolic demands in the setting of hypoperfusion could result in a second insult to an already compromised brain. Vespa and colleagues[235] in 20 adults with severe TBI showed that posttraumatic subclinical status epilepticus was associated with a considerable burden in raised ICP and long-lasting increases in the brain interstitial lactate/pyruvate ratio—a marker of ischemia. This finding has heightened interest in this area and suggests the consideration of continuous EEG monitoring in pediatric TBI. We utilize continuous EEG in all severe TBI patients in our center in Pittsburgh. However, regarding treatment the pediatric guidelines support the use of prophylactic phenytoin only as a treatment option to prevent early posttraumatic seizures in severe TBI because it has not been shown to improve outcome either acutely or in the prevention of the late development of epilepsy.[1,2] Additional anticonvulsants are recommended to be given as needed to treat seizures. Levetiracetam has also been suggested to confer favorable effects versus phenytoin in preclinical TBI models.[35] However, a prospective study of levetiracetam versus phenytoin use in seizure prophylaxis in >800 adults with severe TBI showed no difference in occurrence of seizures—although long-term functional outcome was not reported.[236]

Even if hypertonic saline solution is not used as a therapy, careful attention should be paid to the serum sodium level. It should be monitored at least twice daily in children with severe TBI. To prevent the development of hyponatremia, we recommend using 0.9% normal saline solution as the initial intravenous fluid for children with severe TBI. For infants, D_5 (5% dextrose) normal saline solution can be used. Hyponatremia that develops while only isotonic fluids are being administered generally can be attributed to either syndrome of inappropriate antidiuretic hormone secretion or cerebral salt wasting.[237] Care should be taken to determine the correct cause of hyponatremia because the management of syndrome of inappropriate antidiuretic hormone secretion involves fluid restriction, whereas that of cerebral salt wasting involves the administration of isotonic or hypertonic saline solution.

It has long been known that hyperglycemia exacerbates experimental ischemic brain injury, and threshold values greater than 200 mg/dL are generally considered as the target. Similarly, countless studies have shown associations between hyperglycemia and poor clinical outcome after various CNS insults, and most textbooks of adult neurocritical care recommend withholding glucose in intravenous fluids for at least 24 hours unless hypoglycemia is seen. Supporting this concept, Van den Berghe and colleagues[238] reported that insulin administration to control blood glucose at less than 110 mg/dL in

63 adults with isolated brain injury from various causes produced benefits with regard to ICP, CPP, and seizures. Subsequent to the guidelines, Smith and associates[239] reported that in a cohort of children with severe TBI, exogenous glucose could be safely withheld for 48 hours after injury (mimicking the approach generally taken in cases of severe TBI in adults) with careful monitoring and the addition of dextrose if blood glucose was <70 mg/dL. With that approach, hyperglycemia in the initial 48 hours was not associated with unfavorable outcome. In contrast, Vespa and associates,[240] using intracerebral microdialysis in adults with severe TBI, reported that tight glucose control (serum glucose 90 to 119 mg/dL) produced a metabolic crisis in the brain (increases in glutamate and lactate/pyruvate ration) versus less rigorous glucose control (serum glucose 119 to 150 mg/dL). Controversy remains as to the optimal management strategy for glucose administration and control after severe TBI. Glucose management is another hypotheses being addressed in the ADAPT trial, and thus additional information on this facet of management should be available in the future.

The provision of adequate nutrition is essential during the catabolic response to critical illness, and beneficial effects of early feeding (either enteral or parenteral) in the critically ill or injured patient are well described. In critically ill adults, a cumulative deficit of 10,000 kcal was associated with increased mortality, and in the PICU this amount can be easily surpassed in less than 1 week.[241] A study using indirect calorimetry in 13 children with severe TBI by Mtaweh and colleagues,[242] however, suggests that with contemporary management, equation-based estimates of energy expenditure greatly overestimate caloric needs, which were only 70% of predicted. This argues against a hypermetabolic response and suggests new nutritional targets or the use of calorimetry-guided nutritional support. Hyperalimentation formulations containing glutamate have been shown to increase glutamate levels, possibly exacerbating excitotoxicity.[243] Curiously, studies in experimental brain injury suggest that starvation for 48 hours dramatically reduces ultimate damage.[244] Ketosis is suggested to confer this benefit. The optimal nutritional approach in severe TBI needs to be addressed.

Routine use of glucocorticoids for treatment of patients with severe TBI is not recommended.[1,2] However, hypotension in the setting of severe TBI in rare cases is associated with pituitary failure, possibly from vascular disruption.[245]

Linking Rehabilitation and Acute Care

Rehabilitation can have dramatic effects after a severe TBI is sustained, particularly in the setting of focal injury. Successful rehabilitation may require prolonged therapy (months or even years).[246] Underscoring the potential importance of the subacute and rehabilitation phases for targeted therapy in severe TBI, Giacino and associates[247] reported, to our knowledge, the only successful clinical multicenter RCT in severe TBI in 184 adults. In that work, a 4-week exposure to amantadine—an NMDAR antagonist and dopamine agonist—resulted in significantly faster recovery of the Disability Rating Scale. Given that since the last edition of this textbook RCTs of hypothermia, decompressive craniectomy, erythropoietin, and progesterone,[214,226,248,249] among other agents, have failed in the acute phase after TBI, therapeutic trials in the subacute or rehabilitation phases after severe TBI have considerable potential and merit additional investigation. Finally, novel approaches such as the use of stem cells are also in the exploratory phase of clinical investigation and warrant investigation in children after severe TBI.[250]

Outcomes

Outcome from severe TBI generally has been assessed as a function of age at the time of injury and in relationship to three diagnostic categories: noninflicted (accidental) closed head injuries, AHT (child abuse), and penetrating injury (predominantly gunshot wounds). Accurate assessment of long-term outcome has been somewhat hampered in infants and children by the lack of validated outcome assessment tools. Application of modifications of adult outcome tools (eg, the Glasgow Outcome Scale) has been the general approach; however, these tools have limitations when applied across the pediatric age spectrum.[251] In an important paper on pediatric outcomes, Levin and colleagues[9] highlighted the dramatic effect of age on outcome. About two-thirds of children between the ages of 5 and 10 years had favorable outcome (ie, normal or moderate disability), whereas over 60% of children age 4 years or younger died. Rates of favorable outcome as high as 73% have been reported in clinical trials in pediatric TBI.[176] Specific studies of AHT and gunshot wounds generally have reported poorer outcome than series of accidental TBI. However, even in these two high-risk diagnostic categories, favorable outcome in some series has been as high as 35% in patients with severe TBI resulting from AHT and 24% in patients with severe TBI resulting from gunshot wounds.[222,252] Public interest in the field of TBI has soared related to the emerging recognition of a potential link between repetitive mild TBI and neurodegenerative diseases such as Alzheimer disease, Parkinson disease, and chronic traumatic encephalopathy, among others (Fig. 119.15).[253] This could also occur in severe TBI and is likely in AHT, and it is under investigation.

Conclusion

Optimal care of the infant or child with severe TBI requires a multidisciplinary approach. Prompt and vigorous resuscitation, including stabilization and control of ventilation, is essential. After initial evaluation and surgical intervention, where appropriate, monitoring and carefully titrated management of raised ICP are essential to optimize cerebral perfusion and facilitate metabolic homeostasis. Meticulous and optimal neurointensive care is the basis on which future targeted therapies will be delivered as additional information on the evolution of secondary neuronal damage becomes available. The goal of contemporary pediatric neurointensive care is the prevention of secondary injury. Much of that care focuses on preventing secondary insults. The goal of future pediatric neurointensive case will be to overlay, on this therapeutic plan, strategies manipulating tissue injury in the evolution of secondary damage at a cellular level, along with strategies to foster regeneration and rehabilitation.[29]

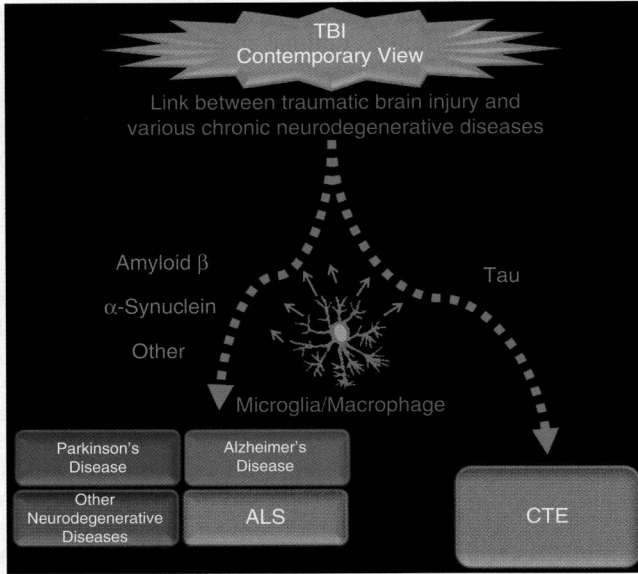

Fig. 119.15. Contemporary view of the link between traumatic brain injury (TBI) and the ultimate development of neurodegenerative diseases. This includes the progressive accumulation of amyloid β or α-synuclein in traditional neurodegenerative diseases or tau protein in chronic traumatic encephalopathy (CTE). Please see text for details. *ALS,* amyotrophic lateral sclerosis.

Key References

1. Adelson PD, Bratton SL, Carney NA, et al. Guidelines for the acute medical management of severe traumatic brain injury in infants, children, and adolescents. *Pediatr Crit Care Med.* 2003;4(suppl 1):S1-S82.
2. Kochanek PM, Carney N, Adelson PD, et al. Guidelines for the acute medical management of severe traumatic brain injury in infants, children and adolescents—2nd edition. *Pediatr Crit Care Med.* 2012;13(suppl 1):S1-S82.
3. Bell MJ, Adelson PD, Hutchison JS, et al. Differences in medical therapy goals for children with severe traumatic brain injury—an international study. *Pediatr Crit Care Med.* 2013;14:811-818.
6. Levin HS, Aldrich EF, Saydjari C, et al. Severe head injury in children: experience of the Traumatic Coma Data Bank. *Neurosurgery.* 1992;31:435-443.
8. Vavilala MS, Lee LA, Lam AM. The lower limit of cerebral autoregulation in children during sevoflurane anesthesia. *J Neurosurg Anesthesiol.* 2003;15:307-312.
18. Adelson PD, Clyde B, Kochanek PM, et al. Cerebrovascular response in infants and young children following severe traumatic brain injury: a preliminary report. *Pediatr Neurosurg.* 1997;26:200-207.
23. Bergsneider M, Hovda DA, Shalmon E, et al. Cerebral hyperglycolysis following severe traumatic brain injury in humans: a positron emission tomography study. *J Neurosurg.* 1997;86:241-251.
24. Ruppel RA, Kochanek PM, Adelson PD, et al. Excitotoxicity amino acid concentrations in ventricular cerebrospinal fluid after severe traumatic brain injury in infants and children: the role of child abuse. *J Pediatr.* 2001;138:18-25.
29. Kochanek PM, Jackson TC, Ferguson NM, et al. Emerging therapies in traumatic brain injury. *Semin Neurol.* 2015;35:83-100.
38. Clark RS, Kochanek PM, Chen M, et al. Increases in Bcl-2 and cleavage of caspase-1 and caspase-3 in human brain after head injury. *FASEB J.* 1999;13:813-821.
40. Portera-Cailliau C, Price DL, Martin LJ. Excitotoxic neuronal death in the immature brain is an apoptosis-necrosis morphological continuum. *J Comp Neurol.* 1997;378:70-87.
42. Bayır H, Tyurin VA, Tyurina YY, et al. Selective early cardiolipin peroxidation after traumatic brain injury: an oxidative lipidomics analysis. *Ann Neurol.* 2007;62:154-169.
45. Clark RSB, Kochanek PM, Watkins SC, et al. Caspase-3 mediated neuronal death after traumatic brain injury in rats. *J Neurochem.* 2000;74:740-753.
48. Clark RSB, Kochanek PM, Adelson PD, et al. Increases in bcl-2 protein in cerebrospinal fluid and evidence for programmed-cell death in infants and children following severe traumatic brain injury. *J Pediatr.* 2000;137:197-204.

51. Clark RS, Bayir H, Chu CT, et al. Autophagy is increased in mice after traumatic brain injury and is detectable in human brain after trauma and critical illness. *Autophagy*. 2008;4:88-90.

53. Obrist WD, Langfitt TW, Jaggi JL, et al. Cerebral blood flow and metabolism in comatose patients with acute head injury. *J Neurosurg*. 1984;61:241-253.

54. Hartings JA, Gugliotta M, Gilman C, et al. Repetitive cortical spreading depolarizations in a case of severe brain trauma. *Neurol Res*. 2008;30:876-882.

55. Verweij BH, Muizelaar JP, Vinas FC, et al. Impaired cerebral mitochondrial function after traumatic brain injury in humans. *J Neurosurg*. 2000;93:815-820.

60. Marmarou A, Barzo P, Fatouros P, et al. Traumatic brain swelling in head injured patients: brain edema or vascular engorgement? *Acta Neurochir Suppl (Wien)*. 1997;70:68-70.

62. Brady KM, Shaffner DH, Lee JK, et al. Continuous monitoring of cerebrovascular pressure reactivity after traumatic brain injury in children. *Pediatrics*. 2009;124:e1205-e1212.

65. Katayama Y, Mori T, Maeda T, et al. Pathogenesis of the mass effect of cerebral contusions: rapid increase in osmolality within the contusion necrosis. *Acta Neurochir Suppl (Wien)*. 1998;71:289-292.

66. Polderman KH, van de Kraats G, Dixon JM, et al. Increases in spinal fluid osmolarity induced by mannitol. *Crit Care Med*. 2003;31:584-590.

69. Laird MD, Shields JS, Sukumari-Ramesh S, et al. High mobility group box protein-1 promotes cerebral edema after traumatic brain injury via activation of toll-like receptor 4. *Glia*. 2014;62:26-38.

72. Gennarelli TA, Thibault LF, Adams TH, et al. Diffuse axonal injury and traumatic coma in the primate. *Ann Neurol*. 1982;12:564-574.

75. Berger RP, Adelson PD, Richichi R, et al. Serum biomarkers after traumatic and hypoxemic brain injuries: insight into the biochemical response of the pediatric brain to inflicted brain injury. *Dev Neurosci*. 2006;28:327-335.

78. Povlishock JT, Christman CW. The pathobiology of traumatically induced axonal injury in animals and humans: a review of current thoughts. In: Bandak FA, Eppinger RH, Ommaya AK, eds. *Traumatic Brain Injury: Bioscience and Mechanics*. New York: Mary Ann Liebert; 1996.

82. Jenny C, Hymel KP, Ritzen A, et al. Analysis of missed cases of abusive head trauma. *JAMA*. 1999;281:621-626.

90. Chestnut RM, Marshall LF, Klauber MR, et al. The role of secondary brain injury in determining outcome from severe head injury. *J Trauma*. 1993;34:216-222.

97. Pang D, Pollack IF. Spinal cord injury without radiographic abnormality in children—the SCIWORA syndrome. *J Trauma*. 1989;29:654-664.

101. Cohan P, Wang C, McArthur DL, et al. Acute secondary adrenal insufficiency after traumatic brain injury: a prospective study. *Crit Care Med*. 2005;33:2358-2366.

106. SAFE Study Investigators; Australian and New Zealand Intensive Care Society Clinical Trials Group; Australian Red Cross Blood Service; George Institute for International Health, Myburgh J, Cooper DJ, et al. Saline or albumin for fluid resuscitation in patients with traumatic brain injury. *N Engl J Med*. 2007;357:874-884.

108. Koenig MA, Bryan M, Lewin JL 3rd, et al. Reversal of transtentorial herniation with hypertonic saline. *Neurology*. 2008;70:1023-1029.

111. Marshall LF, Marshall SB, Klauber MR, et al. The diagnosis of head injury requires a classification based on computed axial tomography. *J Neurotrauma*. 1992;9:S287-S291.

120. Lundberg N. Continuous recording and control of ventricular-fluid pressure in neurosurgical practice. *Acta Psychiatr Scand*. 1960;149:36.

126. Keenan HT, Nocera M, Bratton SL. Frequency of intracranial pressure monitoring in infants and young toddlers with traumatic brain injury. *Pediatr Crit Care Med*. 2005;6:537-541.

127. Gerber LM, Chiu YL, Carney N, et al. Marked reduction in mortality in patients with severe traumatic brain injury. *J Neurosurg*. 2013;119:1583-1590.

128. Chesnut RM, Temkin N, Carney N, et al. A trial of intracranial-pressure monitoring in traumatic brain injury. *N Engl J Med*. 2012;367:2471-2481.

141. Gopinath SP, Robertson CS, Contant CF, et al. Jugular venous desaturation and outcome after head injury. *J Neurol Neurosurg Psychiatry*. 1994;57:717-723.

150. Bullock R, Zauner A, Tsuji O, et al. Excitatory amino acid release after severe human head trauma: effect of ICP and CPP changes. In: Nagai H, Kamiya K, Ishii S, eds. *ICP 9*. Tokyo: Springer-Verlag; 1994.

152. Hovda DA, Lee SM, Smith ML, et al. The neurochemical and metabolic cascade following brain injury: moving from animal models to man. *J Neurotrauma*. 1995;12:903-906.

160. Chambers IR, Jones PA, Lo TYM, et al. Critical thresholds of intracranial pressure and cerebral perfusion pressure related to age in paediatric head injury. *J Neurol Neurosurg Psychiatry*. 2006;77:234-240.

165. Chambers IR, Stobbart L, Jones PA, et al. Age-related differences in intracranial pressure and cerebral perfusion pressure in the first 6 hours of monitoring after children's head injury: association with outcome. *Childs Nerv Syst*. 2005;21:195-199.

176. Peterson B, Khanna S, Fisher B, et al. Prolonged hypernatremia controls elevated intracranial pressure in head-injured pediatric patients. *Crit Care Med*. 2000;28:1136-1143.

190. Gonda DD, Meltzer HS, Crawford JR, et al. Complications associated with prolonged hypertonic saline therapy in children with elevated intracranial pressure. *Pediatr Crit Care Med*. 2013;14:610-620.

209. Hutchison JS, Ward RE, Lacroix J, et al. Hypothermia therapy after traumatic brain injury in children. *N Engl J Med*. 2008;358:2447-2456.

214. Adelson PD, Wisniewski SR, Beca J, et al. Comparison of hypothermia and normothermia after severe traumatic brain injury in children (Cool Kids): a phase 3, randomised controlled trial. *Lancet Neurol*. 2013;12:546-553.

221. Cushing H. The establishment of cerebral hernia as a decompressive measure for inaccessible brain tumors: with the description of intermuscular methods of making the bone defect in temporal and occipital regions. *Surg Gynecol Obstet*. 1905;1:297-314.

235. Vespa PM, Miller C, McArthur D, et al. Nonconvulsive electrographic seizures after traumatic brain injury result in a delayed, prolonged increase in intracranial pressure and metabolic crisis. *Crit Care Med*. 2007;35:2830-2836.

240. Vespa P, Boonyaputthikul R, McArthur DL, et al. Intensive insulin therapy reduces microdialysis glucose values without altering glucose utilization or improving the lactate/pyruvate ratio after traumatic brain injury. *Crit Care Med*. 2006;34:850-856.

242. Mtaweh H, Smith R, Kochanek PM, et al. Energy expenditure in children after severe traumatic brain injury. *Pediatr Crit Care Med*. 2014;15:242-249.

248. Robertson CS, Hannay HJ, Yamal JM, et al. Effect of erythropoietin and transfusion threshold on neurological recovery after traumatic brain injury: a randomized clinical trial. *JAMA*. 2014;312:36-47.

249. Wright DW, Yeatts SD, Silbergleit R, et al. Very early administration of progesterone for acute traumatic brain injury. *N Engl J Med*. 2014;371:2457-2466.

253. DeKosky ST, Ikonomovic MD, Gandy S. Traumatic brain injury–football, warfare, and long-term effects. *N Engl J Med*. 2010;363:1293-1296.

Thoracic Injuries in Children

Tamara N. Fitzgerald

PEARLS

- Rib fractures are uncommon in children and indicate significant traumatic energy delivery.
- Children can maintain a normal blood pressure with up to a 40% blood loss, thus a profound state of hypovolemia may not be immediately apparent.
- Pediatric patients are vulnerable to hypothermia, due to their high body surface–to–volume ratio
- Chest radiograph is a sufficient screening tool for thoracic injury unless there is significant symptomatology to justify computed tomography.
- Echocardiography and measurement of cardiac enzymes are useful for diagnosing cardiac injury
- Identification of a diaphragmatic injury on imaging is challenging and requires a high index of suspicion.

Epidemiology and Prevention

Trauma is a leading cause of morbidity and mortality in children worldwide,[1] and it is the leading cause of death for children in the United States. Thoracic injuries account for 4% to 13% of pediatric trauma admissions.[2] Mortality from thoracic trauma is 15% to 25% and is second only to brain injury mortality.[3] The National Pediatric Trauma Registry was established in 1994 and remains an important source of information for trauma research and public health reform.

Thoracic trauma can be divided into blunt and penetrating injury. Blunt injuries account for the majority of pediatric chest trauma (92%) and include such mechanisms as falls, motor vehicle collisions, pedestrian accidents, sports injury, and child abuse. Penetrating injuries such as gunshot wounds and stab wounds are less common in the pediatric population but are increasing in urban areas. The majority of penetrating injuries occur in adolescents. School shootings have sparked public concern for this issue.

Adolescent girls have a lower mortality following traumatic shock than adolescent boys, but this gender discrepancy was not seen in prepubescent children.[4] In general, mortality is lowest for isolated thoracic injuries (5%) but increases with multisystem injury (up to 39%).[5] Infants and toddlers are often victims of child abuse and motor vehicle crashes. School-aged children 5 to 9 years old are most often injured as pedestrians struck by motor vehicles, whereas older children (10-17 years old) are most often injured on bicycles and skateboards. Older teenagers can be injured during high-risk behavior, high-impact sporting activities, motor vehicle accidents,

violence, and suicide.[6] Obesity does not impact the severity of injury, mortality rate, or procedural outcomes in children. However, obese children are more likely to have rib and pelvic injuries.[7]

Anatomic and Physiologic Considerations

Children are not just small adults; they vary considerably in anatomy and physiology. This is particularly true of the thoracic organs, where the chest wall of a child is much more compliant because children have increased cartilage content with incomplete ossification.[8] Therefore rib fractures are uncommon in children, and when present they generally indicate significant traumatic energy. Because the ribs do not absorb the kinetic energy, more energy is transferred to the internal organs. Pulmonary contusions are commonly present without rib fractures.

The smaller chest transmits breath sounds more readily. Even in cases of a large pneumothorax or effusion, the breath sounds may seem equal. Pediatric patients are more vulnerable to developing hypoxemia, as their basal metabolic rate is higher leading to greater oxygen consumption. Children also have a smaller functional residual capacity, which manifests as a rapid decline in oxygen saturation during endotracheal intubation, even when the patient has been preoxygenated by face-mask. The trachea is also more compressible and narrower. Therefore children are more susceptible to profound respiratory distress with mucous plugging or aspiration of a small foreign body.

Children can compensate and maintain blood pressure with up to a 40% blood loss, and a critical situation may not become apparent until their blood loss is profound. Their cardiac contractility is fixed in early life; therefore heart rate must increase to increase cardiac output. However, in a frightened child, a normal heart rate is variable. Children have a relatively high body surface–to–volume ratio, allowing for a high rate of radiant cooling, and therefore pediatric patients can become hypothermic quickly, either outdoors or in the trauma bay.

Initial Resuscitation and Diagnosis

The initial care of all patients should follow the principles of Pediatric Advanced Life Support (PALS). First and foremost, the airway should be secured. The inability to maintain an airway or a Glasgow Coma Score ≤8 should prompt immediate orotracheal intubation and controlled ventilation. Patients with suspected cervical spine injuries or unknown cervical spine status should have manual in-line cervical stabilization during endotracheal intubation and a cervical collar placed promptly after endotracheal intubation. If an adequate airway cannot be established with orotracheal intubation, then a surgical airway should be established. Once an airway has been established, ventilation should be assessed. The chest should be observed for symmetrical rise and fall. The right and left chest should be auscultated to ensure adequate airflow and the position of the endotracheal tube confirmed with a chest radiograph. Arterial oxygen saturation or pulse oximetry should be used to assess oxygenation. Arterial carbon dioxide or capnography may be used to assess ventilation. Life-threatening conditions such as airway compromise, tension pneumothorax, hemothorax, and cardiac tamponade should be identified immediately and treated (as described later). A child who loses vital signs in the trauma bay may require an emergent thoracotomy.

Circulation should be assessed by the pulse, heart rate, and capillary refill. In a warm, well child, the capillary refill should be ≤2 to 3 seconds. The radial, posterior tibial, and dorsalis pedis pulses can be palpated to assess peripheral circulation and heart rate. Blood pressure should be assessed with an appropriately sized cuff in order to yield an accurate value. Adequate intravenous access should be quickly established with two large-bore peripheral intravenous catheters. If peripheral access cannot be established, then a central line should be placed or intraosseoous access obtained. However, more volume can be given over a shorter period of time through a peripheral intravenous line than a central line, due to the resistance over the length of the central line. An initial intravascular or intraosseous isotonic saline bolus of 20 mL/kg should be administered. If the patient's vital signs do not improve, a second bolus should be administered, followed by transfusion of blood products to approximate whole blood.

Once the child's airway, breathing, and circulation have been addressed, the child should undergo a thorough physical examination to evaluate for injuries. The thoracic exam should include examining the patterns of bruises and lacerations to predict internal injuries. The chest should be palpated to look for rib tenderness or fractures. A chest radiograph should be used as the initial screening tool for blunt thoracic trauma.[9] Computed tomography (CT) can be an important tool in the diagnosis of blunt trauma, and it is certainly the gold standard for injury detection. However, in the pediatric patient, exposure to unnecessary radiation is a significant concern.[10] The routine use of CT scanning is therefore not justified unless there is adequate symptomatology to suggest a significant injury.[11] Most clinically useful information found on CT scan for chest trauma can be correlated with findings on chest radiograph. CT should be used selectively, particularly for the evaluation of an abnormal mediastinal silhouette on chest x-ray.[12] Exposure to radiation can be limited by lowering the radiation dose, avoiding redundant studies, limiting studies based on a risk/benefit profile, and using alternative technology such as MRI and ultrasonography.[13]

The role of ultrasound in the pediatric trauma bay is controversial and appears to be less useful than in adult trauma patients. The focused assessment with sonography for trauma (FAST) primarily examines abdominal injury, but ultrasound can be used to detect signs of pneumothorax and pathologic pericardial fluid. In one study, the sensitivity of FAST for detecting injuries requiring operation or blood transfusion was only 87%. The sensitivity and specificity for detecting pathologic free fluid were 50% and 85%, respectively.[14] The sensitivity of FAST is not sufficient to forego other imaging tests when there is clinical suspicion to warrant investigation.[14] However, FAST is still performed at some centers.

Chest Wall Injury

The elasticity of the ribs in small children protects against fractures, even in cases of severe injury. Therefore rib fractures should be considered a marker of exposure to significant traumatic energy. Isolated rib fractures without associated injuries are found in a minority of children. Rib fractures in children are associated with higher rates of brain injury, hemo/pneumothorax, and liver injury.[15] Higher rib fractures are not associated with great vessel injury in children, and in isolation they do not warrant aortography.[16,17] Lower fractures are associated with liver, spleen, and diaphragm injury.

The overwhelming majority of children 3 years and younger with rib fractures have been abused, and abused children tend to have more rib fractures than accidentally injured children. Therefore any young child who presents with rib fractures should raise a red flag for a nonaccidental trauma mechanism. However, accidentally injured children are more likely than abused children to have internal thoracic injuries (56% versus 13%). This is likely due to the difference in mechanism of injury. Abuse is usually performed over a longer duration of time from manual chest squeezing or a crush mechanism. Accidental trauma tends to be high energy and of short duration.[18]

In most cases, rib fractures are treated nonoperatively, although they do produce a great amount of pain, and often admission is required for pain control. The goal should be to encourage pulmonary toilet and prevent atelectasis and pneumonia. Nonsteroidal antiinflammatory medications as well as opioids and regional anesthetic techniques (nerve blockade) may all play a role in pain management. It is rare for children with isolated rib fractures to require ventilatory assistance. In rare cases, multiple ribs in a single area may be fractured and produce a *flail chest*. Specifically, this requires fractures of multiple contiguous ribs with at least 2 points of fracture per rib or fracture of the sternum or dislocation of rib heads. Flail chest results in paradoxical respiratory movement in which the thoracic wall over the flail segment collapses during inspiration, thereby impeding gas exchange.

The medial physis of the clavicle does not close until 23 to 25 years of age. Falls from trampolines are associated with fracture of the clavicle, and falls can lead to posterior sternoclavicular fracture-dislocations in children. This injury can be associated with dysphagia, dyspnea, and brachiocephalic compression. Children with clavicular dislocations should be evaluated for injury to the esophagus and great vessels.[19]

Sternal fractures, although rare, are usually associated with blunt traumatic injuries. They can result from motor vehicle crashes, flexion-compression injuries, or direct blows. They may be associated with cardiac injury. All patients with sternal bruising or fracture should be evaluated for cardiac contusion, and patients should have a careful examination and imaging of the spine.[20] Ultrasound has a high sensitivity and specificity in the diagnosis of sternal fractures.[21] Scapular fractures are uncommon in children, as a significant amount of force is required to fracture the scapula. A careful neurologic and vascular exam should be performed, as axillary artery and brachial plexus injuries may be present.

In rare cases of chest trauma, an intercostal hernia may form, resulting in lung herniation. Most hernias occur at a site of previous injury and are commonly seen at the anterior parasternal border because the cartilaginous junction to the sternum is absent. Most are experienced after blunt trauma, particularly after multiple rib fractures or chondral costal dislocation. The hernia should be treated by direct surgical repair and may require mesh placement.[22,23] Thoracoscopic hernia repair has been described.[24]

Lung and Airway Injury

Pneumothorax (air in the pleural space) and hemothorax (blood in the pleural space) can both lead to respiratory compromise and subsequent cardiovascular collapse. Occult pneumothorax is the least severe of these entities and is defined as air in the pleural space seen on CT but not visible on chest radiographs. Occult pneumothorax can be safely observed and does not necessitate tube thoracostomy.[25] Minor pneumothorax produces mild clinical symptoms including tachypnea, distress, and decreased oxygen saturation. Pneumothorax may be suspected on physical exam when bruising or rib fractures are evident on the chest wall. Asymmetry in breath sounds or chest wall movement should also raise suspicion. Tension pneumothorax occurs when an injured tissue (either lung parenchyma or chest wall) forms a one-way valve, allowing air to enter the pleural space and preventing air from escaping. Tension pneumothorax results in major distress with distention of the affected side, displacement of mediastinal structures, and compromised venous return. Tracheal deviation may be seen with tension pneumothorax, as the tension in the air-filled side leads to compression of the healthy lung and deviation of the midline away from the side of the pneumothorax. Any patient with a suspected pneumothorax and signs of respiratory or cardiac decline should receive immediate needle decompression of the chest cavity. Needle decompression can be performed by placing a needle and catheter into the second intercostal space at the midclavicular line. Upon entering the pleural space, the clinician should hear an immediate rush of air. At this point, the needle should be removed but the catheter left in place while the patient is prepared for tube thoracostomy. The patient should be placed in the supine position with the arm in complete abduction. This position widens the intercostal spaces, facilitating placement of the tube. Tube thoracostomy should be performed by inserting an intercostal tube into the fifth or sixth intercostal space in the midaxillary or anterior axillary line. At this level, there is little risk of injury to the long thoracic nerve. A tube thoracostomy that is placed too low may inadvertently be placed below the diaphragm with resultant injury to the liver, spleen, or intestines. An adequately large tube should be placed to facilitate drainage of air, fluid, and blood. The tube should be connected to water seal drainage and suction to facilitate reexpansion of the lung (Fig. 120.1).

The majority of chest injuries resulting in pneumothorax or hemothorax require only a tube thoracostomy for successful management. The pulmonary circulation operates at a low arterial pressure and bleeding is slow from tears in the lung parenchyma. Hemostasis generally occurs as the lung reexpands. Removal of blood from the pleural space is necessary for several reasons: The lung may become entrapped as a hematoma expands or solidifies, or an empyema may develop

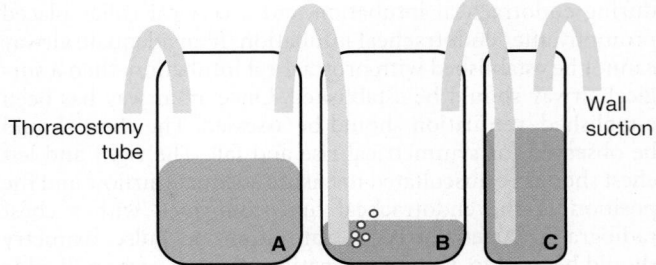

Fig. 120.1. Chest drainage system. The first chamber (A) connects directly to the thoracostomy tube and allows for drainage of fluid from the pleural space. The second chamber (B) creates a water seal, or one-way valve, that permits air to exit the pleural space during expiration but prevents air from returning during inspiration. The third chamber (C) regulates the amount of suction applied to the pleural cavity. This chamber connects to wall suction, but the height of the water column is what controls the amount of suction.

in the nutrient-rich blood. In cases of ongoing hemorrhage, the blood loss should be quantified. Exsanguinating hemorrhage usually involves intercostal, hilar, or mediastinal vessels. When the output is greater than 20% to 30% of the child's blood volume or if the output exceeds 2 to 3 mL/kg/hr over the following 6 hours, then a thoracotomy should be performed.

If a massive air leak from the thoracostomy tube persists, injury to the trachea or bronchi is likely. This injury may require prompt intubation with fiberoptic bronchoscopy assistance. Appropriate ventilation and healing may be achieved by passing the endotracheal tube beyond the site of the airway injury. Unilateral intubation of the unaffected lung may also be used to aid healing or survival until the injury can be surgically repaired. The trachea and bronchi may be injured in both blunt and penetrating trauma. High-energy impact coupled with a closed glottis can produce elevated intraluminal pressures, causing rupture of the airway. The airway and bronchial tree may also be disrupted during violent deceleration or rapid crush injuries. The membranous portions of the trachea and bronchi are most susceptible to this type of injury. Airway disruption at any level can cause pneumomediastinum and eventual pneumothorax and be life threatening. Up to one-third in the first hour may be lethal.[26]

Pulmonary contusions most commonly occur after blunt trauma and are the result of high-energy application to the lung parenchyma. High-energy trauma to the chest causes twice as many lung contusions in children as in adults with significantly fewer rib fractures.[27] Pulmonary contusions may be present on the initial chest x-ray, but they often blossom over time. Contusion, hemorrhage, edema, and damage to the alveolar spaces can all occur and cause respiratory damage. However, few children will require intubation for pulmonary contusions alone. Pulmonary contusion in the pediatric population can lead to pneumonia (about 20%) but rarely causes acute respiratory distress syndrome (ARDS) as it does in an adult population.[28] Traumatic pneumatoceles can develop and are usually seen by 3 days after injury. Most resolve spontaneously within 3 to 4 months and do not require intervention.[29]

Traumatic Asphyxia

Traumatic asphyxia is a rare condition that can occur after severe compression to the chest or abdomen, most commonly after a motor vehicle accident. During a compressive force, patients perform a Valsalva maneuver (holding their breath against a closed glottis, thereby increasing intrathoracic pressure). This increased intrathoracic pressure causes increased pressure in the innominate and jugular veins, leading to congestion in the venules and capillaries of the cervicofacial region. Sequelae include facial edema, cyanosis, conjunctival hemorrhage, face and chest petechiae, periorbital edema, respiratory distress, and altered mental status. Neurologic manifestations may include agitation, loss of consciousness, confusion, seizures, transient visual changes, or blindness. The majority of cases have a good prognosis, and although dramatic in presentation, the prognosis is good with most symptoms completely resolving.[30]

Cardiac Injuries

Cardiac injuries are rare in the pediatric population but are associated with a high mortality (40%). Most injuries are cardiac contusions (59%) after blunt trauma, but lacerations also occur (36%), most commonly after penetrating trauma. Cardiac injuries are associated with lung injury (46%), hemopneumothorax (37%), and rib fractures (26%). Cardiac arrest is rare (4%).[31]

Commotio cordis is a rare but life-threatening phenomenon seen in children after a blow to the chest. It leads to sudden cardiac arrest and is characterized by the absence of structural heart disease, pulmonary contusion, coronary artery abnormalities, or conduction system pathology. It occurs after a direct blow over the heart precisely timed to the phase of repolarization (15-30 milliseconds before the T-wave peak). Ventricular tachyarrhythmias ensue and can be treated with an automatic external defibrillator. It is commonly seen in young males in conjunction with sports-related injury, mainly basketball and football. Much attention has been focused on chest protectors and the availability of automatic external defibrillators at athletic events.[32]

Cardiac contusion with compromised cardiac function is rare in children but can be caused by blunt trauma. Children with bruising over the sternum or evidence of fracture should be evaluated for cardiac injury. Diagnosis of injury can be carried out with electrocardiography, echocardiography, and measurement of cardiac enzymes. Cardiac troponin is not found in skeletal muscle and should be measured, as total creatine kinase (CK) and CK-MB may be elevated from other muscle injury or inflammation. Transesophageal echocardiogram is the most sensitive indicator of cardiac injury. The most common manifestations are dysrhythmias and hypotension from decreased cardiac output. Patients should be treated with telemetry, intravenous access, oxygen, and analgesics. Dobutamine can be used to maintain cardiac output, provided the patient has been appropriately fluid resuscitated. Extreme injuries have been managed with an intraaortic balloon pump or extracorporeal membrane oxygenation (ECMO).[33] Cardiac ruptures following blunt impact are almost universally fatal.

Valvular injury after blunt trauma occurs infrequently. The aortic valve is most frequently injured, followed by the mitral and tricuspid valves. Valvular injury should be assessed with echocardiography, as many patients will be asymptomatic. However, cardiogenic shock can occur. The need for surgery is dictated by the extent and location of the injury,

hemodynamic status of the patient, and presence of other injuries. Approximately half of patients with an injury will require valve replacement.[34]

Most penetrating cardiac injuries occur in male patients in conjunction with stab wounds. Survival after cardiac laceration is less than 30%. Of those patients who survive to reach the trauma bay, mortality rates for a wound to the right atrium, left ventricle, right ventricle, and multiple chambers are 83%, 79%, 57%, and 100%, respectively.[35] Survival from stab wounds is much higher than from gunshot wounds, as a blast injury tends to be widely destructive to the cardiac parenchyma.[36]

Cardiac laceration can lead to pericardial tamponade, where blood escaping the heart through the wound fills the pericardial sac and leads to cardiac compromise. Cardiac tamponade should be suspected in an unstable patient with equal breath sounds and normal chest radiograph. The Beck triad includes muffled heart sounds, distended neck veins, and hypotension. This triad occurs in 90% of cases of cardiac tamponade. However, if the patient has lost a significant amount of blood from other sources, the neck veins may not be distended and it is often difficult to auscultate heart sounds over the noise of the trauma bay. All health care providers should maintain a high index of suspicion, and any penetrating injury to the chest must be considered a cardiac injury until proved otherwise. Ultrasound, if immediately available, can quickly determine the presence of a pericardial effusion. Patients with major hemodynamic instability and impending collapse should undergo prompt emergency room thoracotomy. Emergent pericardiocentesis has been abandoned as a management strategy, as the blood in the pericardial sac may clot rendering a false-negative result. The most frequent complications after cardiac repair include hypothermia, acidosis, and coagulopathy. Cardiac arrhythmias can be seen in patients after profound hypothermia.[36]

Aortic injury in children is exceedingly rare. Mechanisms of injury include high-energy deceleration, compression, or crush of the torso. Chest radiograph findings with blunt aortic injury commonly include prominent aortic knob, wide paratracheal stripe, or widened mediastinum on chest x-ray. Patients with a high-risk mechanism of injury and these chest radiograph findings should undergo CT examination (Fig. 120.2). Those patients too unstable to undergo CT scanning may also be evaluated with transesophageal echocardiography.[12]

Esophageal Injury

The esophagus is well protected in the center of the chest and it is rarely injured, even in penetrating trauma. High-energy trauma may create high intragastric pressure that can rupture the lower esophagus. Pneumomediastinum or pleural effusion after trauma should prompt an investigation for esophageal injury. Sepsis can occur rapidly with mediastinitis. Treatment in children differs from that of adults in that most adults require immediate primary repair. In the majority of cases, children are better served by a nonoperative approach based on adequate drainage of the affected space, parenteral nutrition, and antibiotics.[37] When an appropriate time for healing has passed and output from the drain has decreased, then a contrast esophagram should be obtained. Feeding should only be resumed after confirmation that the esophageal injury has completely healed.

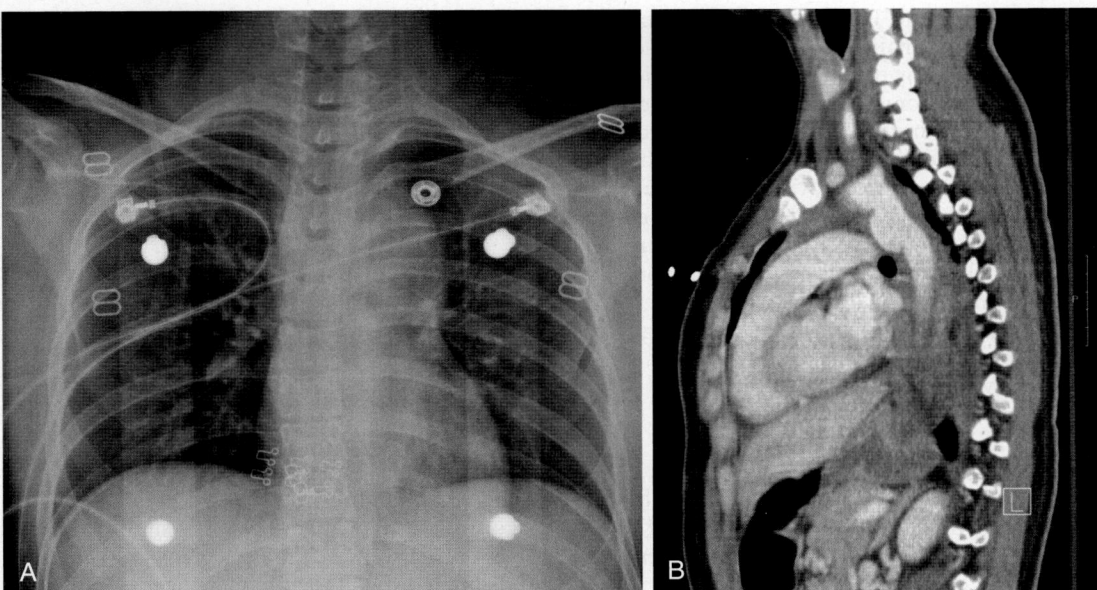

Fig. 120.2. (A) Chest radiograph demonstrating a prominent aortic knob, widened mediastinum, and right-sided tracheal deviation after blunt trauma. These findings are concerning for an aortic injury. (B) Subsequent CT scan showing an aortic tear causing a pseudoaneurysm.

Chylothorax

Traumatic chylothorax is rare in children but is usually seen after blunt trauma. It is associated with hyperextension of the spine and fractures of the spine or posterior ribs. Injury to the thoracic duct should be suspected when a pleural effusion is present on chest radiograph and an esophageal injury has been properly excluded from the diagnosis. Drainage of the fluid reveals a milky, white substance with triglyceride levels >110 mg/dl, the presence of chylomicrons, low cholesterol levels, and a predominance of lymphocytes. Most chylothoraces can be managed nonoperatively with chest tube drainage and total parenteral nutrition. Somatostatin and octreotide have been used to hasten closure of the injury. If the daily loss of chylous fluid exceeds 100 mL/year of age or if the defect fails to close with nonoperative management, then surgical closure is indicated.[38] Children can become lymphopenic and lose IGG, thereby predisposing them to infection if the chylous drainage is excessive. They can also become malnourished.

Diaphragmatic Injury

Diaphragmatic rupture is a rare event in the pediatric population. Falls from heights and motor vehicle accidents are common mechanisms, but diaphragmatic injury also occurs with penetrating trauma. Differences in the distribution of blunt and penetrating trauma will vary with geographic location and the prevalence of violence among children. When it does occur, it is most commonly associated with other injuries. In many cases, the diagnosis can be made on chest radiograph. Pleural effusion, elevated hemidiaphragm, lower lobe collapse, and positioning of the nasogastric tube in the thorax are all findings that should prompt further investigation. Some hernias may be more difficult to detect and require CT examination. In either case, diagnosis requires a high index of suspicion. Left-sided rupture is more common, as the liver absorbs the energy on the right side. Associated injuries are common and can include any organ. Delay in diagnosis can lead to herniation and bowel incarceration. At laparotomy for trauma, both sides of the diaphragm should be carefully inspected. Repair of the diaphragm can be approached either via laparotomy or thoracotomy. It is often approached via laparotomy in the trauma setting, as this allows exploration of the other abdominal organs. Pneumonia is the most common postoperative complication after diaphragm repair.[39-41]

Conclusions

Thoracic trauma in the pediatric population is a major source of morbidity and mortality. Prompt intervention is required for life-threatening injuries and should follow the principles of managing the airway, breathing, and circulation. Lung and chest wall injuries are the most common and can primarily be managed with nonoperative intervention. Tube thoracostomy is the most common surgical intervention performed for thoracic trauma. Injuries to other organs in the chest are rare, but they are serious and require a high clinical index of suspicion. Prompt resuscitation and intervention minimize morbidity and mortality.

References

1. van As AB, Manganyi R, Brooks A. Treatment of thoracic trauma in children: literature review, Red Cross War Memorial Children's Hospital data analysis, and guidelines for management. *Eur J Pediatr Surg.* 2013;23:434-443.
2. Mollberg NM, et al. Age-associated impact on presentation and outcome for penetrating thoracic trauma in the adult and pediatric patient populations. *J Trauma Acute Care Surg.* 2014;76:273-277, discussion 277-278.
3. Sartorelli KH, Vane DW. The diagnosis and management of children with blunt injury of the chest. *Semin Pediatr Surg.* 2004;13:98-105.
4. Haider AH, et al. Mortality in adolescent girls vs boys following traumatic shock: an analysis of the National Pediatric Trauma Registry. *Arch Surg.* 2007;142:875-880, discussion 879-880.
5. Balci AE, et al. Blunt thoracic trauma in children: review of 137 cases. *Eur J Cardio-Thorac Surg.* 2004;26:387-392.

6. Bliss D, Silen M. Pediatric thoracic trauma. *Crit Care Med*. 2002;30: S409-S415.

7. Alselaim N, et al. Does obesity impact the pattern and outcome of trauma in children? *J Pediatr Surg*. 2012;47:1404-1409.

8. Agnew AM, Schafman M, Moorhouse K, et al. The effect of age on the structural properties of human ribs. *J Mech Behav Biomed Mater*. 2015;41:302-314.

9. Yanchar NL, et al. Chest x-ray as a screening tool for blunt thoracic trauma in children. *J Trauma Acute Care Surg*. 2013;75:613-619.

10. Moore MA, Wallace EC, Westra SJ. Chest trauma in children: current imaging guidelines and techniques. *Radiol Clin North Am*. 2011;49:949-968.

11. Hershkovitz Y, et al. Computed tomography is not justified in every pediatric blunt trauma patient with a suspicious mechanism of injury. *Am J Emerg Med*. 2014;32:697-699.

12. Holscher CM, et al. Chest computed tomography imaging for blunt pediatric trauma: not worth the radiation risk. *J Surg Res*. 2013;184:352-357.

13. Scaife ER, Rollins MD. Managing radiation risk in the evaluation of the pediatric trauma patient. *Semin Pediatr Surg*. 2010;19:252-256.

14. Scaife ER, et al. The role of focused abdominal sonography for trauma (FAST) in pediatric trauma evaluation. *J Pediatr Surg*. 2013;48: 1377-1383.

15. Kessel B, et al. Rib fractures: comparison of associated injuries between pediatric and adult population. *Am J Surg*. 2014;208:831-834.

16. Pabon-Ramos WM, Williams DM, Strouse PJ. Radiologic evaluation of blunt thoracic aortic injury in pediatric patients. *AJR Am J Roentgenol*. 2010;194:1197-1203.

17. Hamilton NA, Bucher BT, Keller MS. The significance of first rib fractures in children. *J Pediatr Surg*. 2011;46:169-172.

18. Darling SE, Done SL, Friedman SD, Feldman KW. Frequency of intrathoracic injuries in children younger than 3 years with rib fractures. *Pediatric Radiol*. 2014;44:1230-1236.

19. Loder RT, Schultz W, Sabatino M. Fractures from trampolines: results from a national database, 2002 to 2011. *J Pediatr Orthop*. 2014;34:683-690.

20. Ferguson LP, Wilkinson AG, Beattie TF. Fracture of the sternum in children. *Emerg Med J*. 2003;20:518-520.

21. You JS, Chung YE, Kim D, et al. Role of sonography in the emergency room to diagnose sternal fractures. *J Clin Ultrasound*. 2010;38:135-137.

22. Masmoudi S, et al. [Traumatic lung herniation in a child]. *Archives de Pediatrie*. 2003;10:436-438.

23. Min SA, Gow KW, Blair GK. Traumatic intercostal hernia: presentation and diagnostic workup. *J Pediatr Surg*. 1999;34:1544-1545.

24. Hebra A, Cina R, Streck C. Video-assisted thoracoscopic repair of a lung hernia in a child. *J Laparoendosc Adv Surg Tech A*. 2011;21:763-765.

25. Notrica DM, et al. Management of pediatric occult pneumothorax in blunt trauma: a subgroup analysis of the American Association for the Surgery of Trauma multicenter prospective observational study. *J Pediatr Surg*. 2012;47:467-472.

26. Tovar JA. The lung and pediatric trauma. *Semin Pediatr Surg*. 2008; 17:53-59.

27. Nakayama DK, Ramenofsky ML, Rowe MI. Chest injuries in childhood. *Ann Surg*. 1989;210:770-775.

28. Hamrick MC, Duhn RD, Carney DE, et al. Pulmonary contusion in the pediatric population. *Am Surg*. 2010;76:721-724.

29. Haxhija EQ, Nores H, Schober P, Hollwarth ME. Lung contusion-lacerations after blunt thoracic trauma in children. *Pediatr Surg Int*. 2004; 20:412-414.

30. Montes-Tapia F, Barreto-Arroyo I, Cura-Esquivel I, et al. Traumatic asphyxia. *Pediatr Emerg Care*. 2014;30:114-116.

31. Kaptein YE, et al. Epidemiology of pediatric cardiac injuries: a National Trauma Data Bank analysis. *J Pediatr Surg*. 2011;46:1564-1571.

32. Maron BJ, et al. Commotio cordis and the epidemiology of sudden death in competitive lacrosse. *Pediatrics*. 2009;124:966-971.

33. DeBerry BB, Lynch JE, Chernin JM, et al. Successful management of pediatric cardiac contusion with extracorporeal membrane oxygenation. *J Trauma*. 2007;63:1380-1382.

34. Bakiler AR, Aydogdu SA, Erisen S, et al. A case of mitral papillary muscle rupture due to blunt chest trauma. *Turkish J Pediatr*. 2011;53:97-99.

35. Lustenberger T, et al. Penetrating cardiac trauma in adolescents: a rare injury with excessive mortality. *J Pediatr Surg*. 2013;48:745-749.

36. Talving P, Demetriades D. Cardiac trauma during teenage years. *Pediatr Clin North Am*. 2014;61:111-130.

37. Tovar JA, Vazquez JJ. Management of chest trauma in children. *Paediatric Respir Rev*. 2013;14:86-91.

38. Serin-Ezer S, Oguzkurt P, Ince E, Hicsonmez A. Bilateral chylothorax after blunt thoracic trauma: a case report. *Turkish J Pediatr*. 2009;51: 504-506.

39. Peer SM, Devaraddeppa PM, Buggi S. Traumatic diaphragmatic hernia-our experience. *Int J Surg*. 2009;7:547-549.

40. Okur MH, et al. Traumatic diaphragmatic rupture in children. *J Pediatr Surg*. 2014;49:420-423.

41. Ramos CT, Koplewitz BZ, Babyn PS, et al. What have we learned about traumatic diaphragmatic hernias in children? *J Pediatr Surg*. 2000;35: 601-604.

Abdominal Trauma in Pediatric Critical Care

Susan F. McLean and Alan H. Tyroch

PEARLS

- In the initial resuscitation of trauma victims, the first priority remains the ABCs of **a**irway, **b**reathing, and **c**irculation.
- When in doubt about the reliability of the airway or respiratory function, perform endotracheal intubation.
- The standard of care in treating hemodynamically stable children with hepatic or splenic injury is nonoperative observation.
- Patients who are hemodynamically stable may undergo further radiographic evaluation, whereas patients with evidence of an abdominal injury who remain clinically unstable after resuscitation with 40 mL/kg of fluid should be taken to the operating room for exploration.
- Splenic preservation is more important in younger children and is usually possible with nonoperative management or embolization.
- Vigilance and reexamination are necessary to detect a small bowel injury, which increases morbidity if missed for greater than 24 hours after trauma.

Trauma is the leading cause of morbidity and mortality in the pediatric age group. An estimated 1.5 million pediatric injuries occur each year, resulting in 500,000 hospitalizations and 20,000 deaths.[1] Thus trauma exceeds all other causes of death combined. Abdominal injuries are a marker of severe trauma, and evaluation of the child with an abdominal injury must include a thorough examination of the entire child. Management of pediatric trauma requires a multidisciplinary approach with emergency department physicians, critical care specialists, anesthesiologists, and surgeons working as a multidisciplinary team to provide prompt stabilization, assessment, and treatment. Performing the primary and secondary survey, ensuring a stable airway, instituting fluid resuscitation, and arriving at a decision as to the most appropriate management plan are the principal goals of the trauma team leader.

The majority of abdominal injuries in children are preventable. Health care providers must work with the broader community to identify and alleviate causes of pediatric trauma. Education, public safety measures, and legislation will prevent many cases of pediatric injury. Nonaccidental abdominal

trauma to children must be considered and, if suspected, must be reported to the appropriate agency. Developments in pediatric abdominal trauma include the use of imaging modalities such as focused abdominal sonography for trauma (FAST) and embolization of solid organ injuries, which allows for increased utilization of nonoperative management. Laparoscopy can be applied in select scenarios. As part of disaster preparedness, clinicians providing trauma care for children should have an awareness of wartime and mass casualty injury management.

Mechanisms and Patterns of Injury

The severity and pattern of abdominal injury correlate with the mechanism of injury. Blunt injury accounts for 90% of abdominal trauma in children. The most common mechanisms are motor vehicle collisions, automobile versus pedestrian crashes, falls, bicycle crashes, and nonaccidental trauma. In pediatric blunt abdominal trauma, solid viscus organs such as the liver, spleen, and kidney are more frequently injured than hollow viscus organs. Children suffering lap belt injury, handlebar injury, or kicks may suffer small bowel perforation. Children struck by motor vehicles can have a pattern of head injury, intraabdominal or intrathoracic injury, and a femur fracture (Waddell triad). In addition, urban violence and the high prevalence of firearms result in penetrating abdominal injuries in children. Although the mechanism of injury may correlate with the extent of injury, ongoing clinical assessment is a more sensitive indicator of the extent of blood loss and hemodynamic instability, and it determines the resuscitation and management of the child with an abdominal injury.

Penetrating Abdominal Trauma

Penetrating abdominal injuries are most commonly caused by firearm use or stabbings. In children, abdominal gunshot wounds result in more severe injuries than stab wounds because of the increased energy delivered by firearms, particularly shotguns and assault rifles.[2] Significant intraperitoneal injuries are present in most children who sustain gunshot wounds, suggesting the need for abdominal exploration in all gunshot victims. There is a trend toward selective exploration of penetrating injuries in adults. For example, computed tomography has been used successfully to determine the application of selective laparotomy in penetrating torso trauma.[3] However, most trauma centers continue to perform laparotomy on most patients with gunshot wounds to the abdomen. Abdominal stab wounds that penetrate the transversalis fascia are at high risk of intraabdominal injury. Expectant observation of stab wounds in children should rarely be applied because the true extent of injury is not always appreciated on local exploration.

Recreational and Sports Injury

Specific recreational activities commonly practiced by children, such as bicycling, all-terrain vehicle (ATV) use, skiing, snowboarding, and horseback riding, result in predictable injury patterns that guide evaluation. Snowboard injuries are increasing and include abdominal injuries in 25% of cases.[4] At a level I pediatric trauma center in the United States, 213 cases of pediatric snowboarding injury were admitted over 7 years. Thirty-nine patients had an injury involving the thorax or abdomen, with almost half being abdominal. The spleen was the most commonly injured organ. Male gender and age ≤14 years were associated with a significant increase in abdominal injury. Upper extremity trauma was significantly associated with abdominal or pelvic trauma. ATV crashes produce a particularly damaging pattern of injury as the ATV has the weight of a car and the lack of protection of a motorcycle. This results in a combination of an ejection and rollover mechanism of injury with the worst of both. The majority of deaths involve head and spine injuries. Lack of helmet use is associated with a higher mortality. A retrospective study of trauma admissions to a level I pediatric trauma center of 163 pediatric ATV crashes showed that almost two-thirds of patients did not wear helmets.[5] Of those that did, helmet use was significantly associated with a lower incidence of injury to the head and neck.[5]

ATV abdominal injuries include crush injuries to liver, spleen, and kidney. Child drivers are more susceptible to crash, and it is alarming that child-sized ATVs are in production. Even where laws restrict ATV use by children, they are frequently injured and have a high rate of missed injuries.[6] Blunt impalement on a bicycle handlebar can result in a predictable pattern of injury to bowel, mesentery, or pancreas.

Wartime Trauma

Children can also be victims of wartime trauma causing abdominal and other injuries. Modern warfare is often conducted in urban areas with a civilian population present and the frequent involvement of children. Additionally, medical infrastructure is disrupted in a war zone and many residents suffer malnutrition and infections, which makes them more debilitated in the face of a new injury. Military high-energy rifles cause penetrating wounds in which the pressure wave of the projectile results in a cone of tissue destruction. In abdominal injuries, this necessitates wide debridement of soft tissues, and a second-look laparotomy is often required to detect evolving intestinal necrosis. It is common for children to suffer blast and fragmentation injuries from land mines, bombs, indirect fire weapons (rockets and mortars), improvised explosive devices, and suicide bombings.[7] Land mines and air-delivered cluster bomblets are particularly insidious because their interesting colors and shapes attract children's curiosity. Wounds include pressure wave blunt injury, shrapnel penetration, and burns. These injuries in children often require a damage-control laparotomy, wide debridement of soft tissues, temporary abdominal closure, and multiple operations. Vacuum-assisted wound dressings are particularly useful.[8]

Evaluation and Resuscitation

Evaluation and resuscitation occur simultaneously when a child presents with an abdominal injury. The Advanced Trauma Life Support (ATLS) guidelines developed by the American College of Surgeons should be followed. The primary survey includes stabilization of the cervical spine while evaluating for airway patency, function of breathing, and adequacy of circulation (the ABCs). Prompt endotracheal intubation should occur in any patient in whom the stability of these functions is in doubt. Intravenous access in the small child can be particularly challenging, and skilled personnel should be employed. If peripheral venous access is unsuccessful after two attempts in a hemodynamically unstable child, an intraosseous line should be attempted. Basic neurologic function is assessed. The patient must be completely exposed for examination and then covered with blankets to maintain body temperature. Children are more susceptible to heat loss and dehydration because of their greater surface area/mass ratio.

Physical Examination

Abdominal examination includes observation of external signs, then palpation for tenderness, distension, or firmness. Children swallow a large amount of air when they cry, and gastric distension may require orogastric tube or nasogastric tube decompression. Upper quadrant ecchymosis, tenderness, and associated rib fractures suggest the presence of liver or spleen injury. Midabdominal ecchymosis from a seat belt suggests the possibility of a small bowel injury. Stability of the pelvis is assessed with lateral and axial manual compression of the pelvic ring. Extraperitoneal bladder ruptures may cause localized suprapubic tenderness, whereas an intraperitoneal bladder rupture may present as generalized abdominal distension. Injuries near the abdomen may also be associated with intraabdominal injury. In a mixed adult/pediatric study of patients admitted to seven trauma centers in the United States over a 6-year period, patients with Chance fractures (horizontal fracture through the vertebra) of the thoracolumbar spine were reviewed. Of the 79 patients reviewed, one-third had an intraabdominal injury; hollow viscus injuries were the most common and were found in 22% of patients. Twenty-five percent of patients had a laparotomy; abdominal wall contusions were strongly associated with hollow viscus injury and need for laparotomy. Of 20 patients with abdominal wall contusion and Chance fractures, 85% had an intraabdominal injury and 70% required laparotomy.[9]

Laboratory Tests

Laboratory examination including complete blood counts, serum chemistries, and urinalysis should be obtained on all trauma patients. Additional studies, such as liver function tests and pancreatic enzymes, are indicated in certain injuries. Elevated transaminase levels suggest nonspecific parenchymal liver injury, whereas elevated amylase and lipase levels suggest a pancreatic injury. A base deficit greater than 6 mEq/L is a strong indicator of intraabdominal injury in blunt trauma. Hematuria is associated with intraabdominal injury and renal injury. Urinalysis demonstrating more than five red blood cells per high-power field combined with clinical assessment accurately predicts intraabdominal injury.

Radiographic Assessment

Prompt plain radiographs of the chest and pelvis should be obtained during the initial assessment after blunt trauma. Patients who are hemodynamically stable may undergo further radiographic evaluation, whereas patients with evidence of an abdominal injury who remain clinically unstable after resuscitation with 40 mL/kg of fluid should be taken to the operating room for laparotomy.

Computed Tomography

Computed tomography with intravenous contrast (oral contrast is not routinely needed) is the procedure of choice for definitive radiographic assessment after blunt abdominal trauma in children. Clinical impression remains the most sensitive indicator of the need for computed tomography. Computed tomography can be used to identify hepatic, splenic, intestinal, pancreatic, renal, and bladder injuries in children and can even detect intestinal and mesenteric injury with sensitivities of 94% and 96%, respectively.[10] Findings on computed tomography suggestive of intestinal injury are unexplained free fluid without solid organ disruption, abnormal distribution of bowel loops, contrast extravasation, and contrast enhancement of intestinal wall.[11] The Organ Injury Scaling Committee of the American Association for the Surgery of Trauma has developed a grading system to estimate the extent of abdominal injury.[12,13] Short of operative exploration, computed tomography is the most accurate method used to grade the extent of injury. Concern over the use of abdominal CT scan and radiation exposure in children has led centers to reexamine the use of CT scan to evaluate blunt abdominal trauma and to try to make prediction rules for when CT scanning will be most helpful. A retrospective study of 571 pediatric patients at two Canadian level I pediatric trauma centers admitted after blunt abdominal trauma sought to correlate clinical parameters such as mechanism of injury, as well as radiologic and laboratory analysis variables that might predict injuries seen on CT scan. Injuries results were classified as "notable" or "clinically important" if the injures involved an Abbreviated Injury Scale (AIS) ≥3 injury or if the injury required surgery. Four hundred and forty-one (77%) of the children had an abdominal CT scan. Thirty-seven percent had a notable injury, and 18% had a clinically important injury. Most injuries were solid organ; only 2% were hollow viscus injuries. Factors significantly associated with notable abdominal injury included abdominal exam finding of pain or tenderness, hematuria, and elevated serum alanine aminotransferase (ALT). Factors that were significantly associated with clinically important injuries were low hematocrit and hematuria.[14]

If significant abdominal trauma was suspected, a CT scan was an excellent way to diagnose injury. Traditional signs on CT scan of small intestinal injury are free fluid, extravasation of enteric contrast, pneumoperitoneum, small bowel wall enhancement with intravenous contrast, or paucity of contrast in the intestinal wall. Newer 64-slice CT scans can identify signs of small intestinal injury, even though these may be indirect. A retrospective study of trauma patients suspected of abdominal injury who had a laparotomy demonstrating intestinal injury or mesenteric injury showed that there were no false-negative studies using the 64-slice computed tomography. Free fluid was seen all CT scans. Eighty-eight percent of patients had one finding in addition to free fluid. Findings associated with bowel or mesenteric injury on CT scan were free fluid, bowel wall thickening, mesenteric or bowel wall hematoma, active mesenteric bleeding, mesenteric stranding, pneumoperitoneum, or contrast extravasation. The most common finding besides free fluid was bowel wall thickening.[15]

Sonography

FAST is a rapid, noninvasive, and portable method to evaluate the abdomen. Various reports note that sonography for abdominal trauma has a sensitivity of 55% to 86% and a specificity of 95% to 98%.[16-18] Sonography accurately identifies intraperitoneal free fluid, but it does not accurately identify the source of that fluid. Sonography is comparable to diagnostic peritoneal lavage (DPL) as a method for detecting free peritoneal fluid, but it is noninvasive. However, it does not supplant computed tomography in its ability to define the specific nature and extent of abdominal injury.

Additional Assessment Tools

Diagnostic Peritoneal Lavage

Refinement in the nonoperative management of pediatric abdominal trauma makes DPL unnecessary in stable patients, because the presence of free intraperitoneal blood is not an absolute indication for surgery in children. In addition, performing a DPL can be difficult in small children due to the decreased domain of the smaller abdomen. However, DPL is a useful triage tool for selectively applying laparotomy for blunt intestinal trauma in children. In the rare event that a DPL is performed in a child, the procedure is the same as in adults except that the amount of warm crystalloid instilled into the abdominal cavity is less (10 mL/kg). In one series, the cell count, amylase activity, and particulate matter in the DPL specimen were able to identify small bowel perforation with a sensitivity of 100%.[19]

Diagnostic Laparoscopy

Diagnostic laparoscopic evaluation has been suggested as a safe and effective modality for evaluating the abdomen in the stable patient after penetrating trauma. Diaphragmatic injuries can be diagnosed and repaired laparoscopically.[20] Thoracoscopy in hemodynamically stable penetrating-trauma patients can be used to avoid nontherapeutic laparotomy by ruling out penetration of the abdominal cavity and can identify thoracic and diaphragmatic injuries.

Management of Specific Abdominal Injuries

Children often demonstrate hemodynamic stability in the face of significant hemorrhagic loss, until their capacity for compensatory vasoconstriction is surpassed. Although fluid resuscitation and blood transfusion are far and away the primary therapy, a select few children may require inotropic support after major trauma. Frequent serial abdominal examinations are performed to determine the need for surgical exploration for a missed hollow viscus injury. Operative intervention should not be delayed, because hypotension and decreased cerebral perfusion pressure worsen morbidity and mortality. Although abdominal compartment syndrome has a low reported incidence of 0.6% to 4.7% in critically injured children, it will only be detected through a high index of suspicion and frequent measurement.[21] In stable patients, early enteric feeding maintains immune function and shifts the patient to a more anabolic balance.

Nonoperative Management of Solid Organ Injuries

The standard of care in treating hemodynamically stable children with hepatic or splenic injury is nonoperative observation. Management of these injuries varies widely between adult and pediatric facilities, and splenectomy can be avoided if a child is taken to a facility that utilizes this nonoperative strategy. The American Pediatric Surgical Association Trauma Committee has proposed guidelines for care based on radiographic severity of injury (Table 121.1). Although observation has traditionally taken place in the intensive care unit, there is evidence that observation on a ward is safe.[22]

Embolization of Solid Organ Injuries

Computed tomography can identify active extravasation from splenic and hepatic injuries. Angiography is able to map out the specific site of hemorrhage, and embolization can be used to selectively occlude the bleeding vessel. This therapy reduces the need for transfusion and avoids the need for laparotomy. Nonselective embolization of the main splenic artery has also been shown to reduce bleeding (Fig. 121.1). Angiography should be reserved for children with active extravasation who are hemodynamically stable. Unstable patients with solid organ injury require laparotomy.

Injury to the Spleen

The spleen is the most commonly injured abdominal organ in blunt trauma. Treatment of splenic injury has evolved from routine splenectomy to a strategy of nonoperative management that is successful greater than 90% of the time.[23] Splenic injuries are most often caused by a direct blow to the left upper quadrant and manifest as localized tenderness, abrasion, or ecchymosis. Splenic injury is graded by computed tomography (Figs. 121.2 and 121.3, Table 121.2). Operative intervention for splenic trauma usually results in splenectomy. For this reason, nonoperative management should be attempted in stable children, regardless of the severity of injury. Angiography and embolization of splenic vessels can control hemorrhage without laparotomy. If a stable child with a splenic injury requires laparotomy for injury to another organ, splenorrhaphy and autotransfusion increase splenic salvage, which reduces risk of infection.[24] At pediatric trauma centers, operating on a child with an isolated splenic injury is rare. The indications for operative intervention are generally limited to persistent hypotension, greater than 50% blood

TABLE 121.1	Proposed Guidelines for Resource Utilization in Children With Isolated Spleen or Liver Injury			
CT Grade	**I**	**II**	**III**	**IV**
ICU stay (days)	None	None	None	1
Hospital stay (days)	2	3	4	5
Predischarge imaging	None	None	None	None
Postdischarge imaging	None	None	None	None
Activity restriction (weeks)[a]	3	4	5	6

[a]Return to full contact, competitive sports (eg, football, wrestling, hockey, lacrosse, mountain climbing) should be at the discretion of the individual pediatric trauma surgeon. The proposed guidelines for return to unrestricted activity include "normal" age-appropriate activities.
Data from Stylianos S, APSA Trauma Committee. Evidence-based guidelines for resource utilization in children with isolated spleen or liver injury. J Pediatr Surg. 2000;35:164-169.

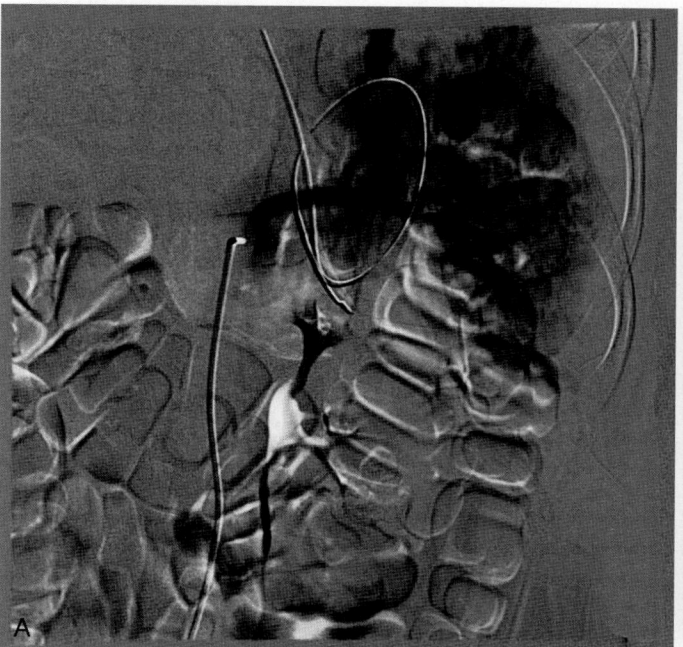
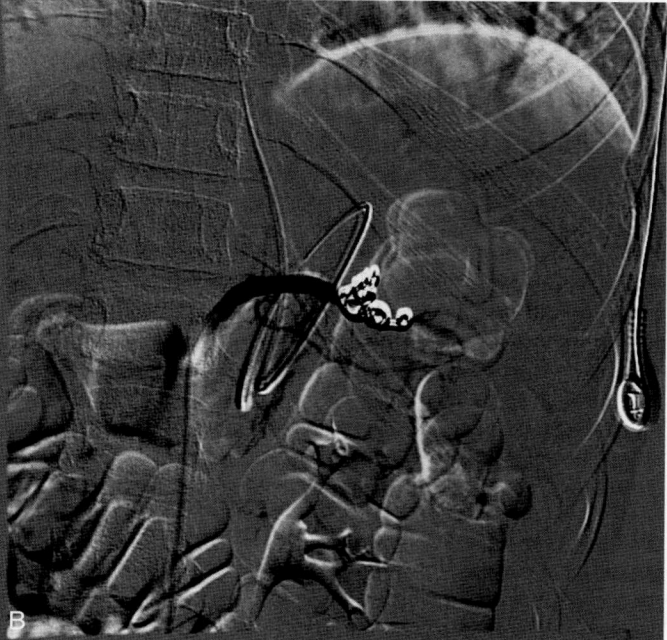

Fig. 121.1. Nonselective splenic embolization. (A) Angiography demonstrates splenic injury with active extravasation of blood. (B) Postembolization image demonstrating coil in splenic artery and resolution of hemorrhage.

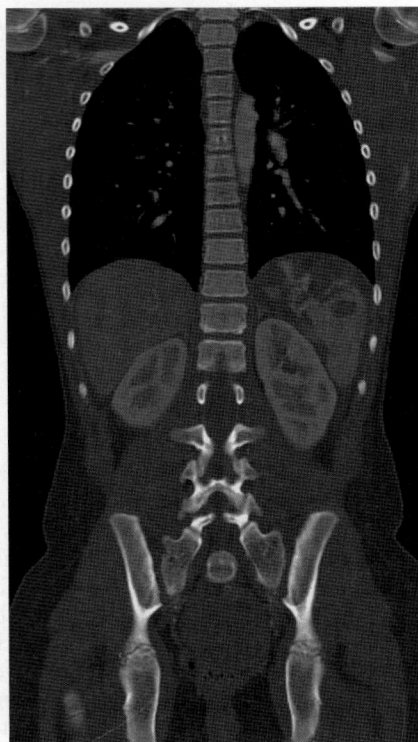

Fig. 121.2. CT scan of a patient with a grade IV splenic laceration.

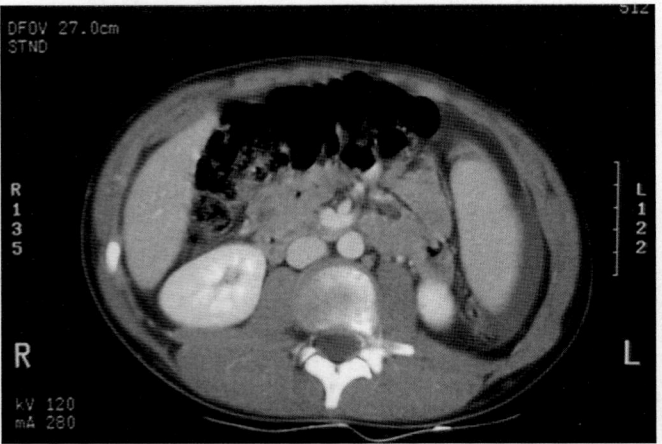

Fig. 121.3. CT scan of a patient with a grade IV splenic laceration demonstrating free fluid around the tip of the spleen.

volume replacement, or additional life-threatening abdominal injuries.

Nonoperative management consists of large-bore venous access for fluid resuscitation, intensive care unit monitoring, frequent hematocrit values, serial physical examinations, and bed rest. Recommendations from the American Pediatric Surgery Association Trauma Committee indicate only short periods of observation are necessary.[22] This abbreviated observation, 1 day of bed rest for grade I and grade II injuries and 2 days of bed rest for higher-grade injuries, has been validated to be safe.[25]

Injury to the Liver

The liver is the second most commonly injured organ in blunt abdominal trauma. Liver injuries are associated with high mortality and may require surgical correction of injuries to the hepatic veins or vena cava. Liver injuries in stable patients can usually be managed nonoperatively. Ecchymosis, bruising, or abrasions over the right upper quadrant suggest significant injury. Liver injury is graded by appearance on computed tomography (see Table 121.2). However, the clinical course of the patient, not the appearance on computed tomography, should determine treatment (Figs. 121.4 and 121.5). Elevated serum transaminase concentrations are associated with liver trauma and other intraabdominal injury.[26] Late complications of liver injuries include bile peritonitis, abscess formation, hemorrhage, and hematobilia. Operative treatment may be required for major hepatic trauma associated with hepatic vein or retrohepatic caval injuries. Definitive repair is often not possible at the time of initial exploration, necessitating damage-control surgery with packing, maintaining an open abdomen, further resuscitation, stabilization, and repeat laparotomy. Select patients with ongoing bleeding from a hepatic injury can be stabilized with embolization of hepatic blood vessels.

Injury to the Small Bowel

Bowel injuries resulting from blunt trauma are relatively rare. However, a high index of suspicion must be maintained to avoid a delayed diagnosis, which is more common in children. The incidence of small bowel injury increases with increasing number of other organs injured.[27] The mechanisms of injury associated with blunt bowel trauma include motor vehicle/pedestrian collisions, handlebar injuries, lap belt injuries, and child abuse. Deceleration injuries in children restrained with a lap belt may occur as a constellation that includes intestinal injury, abdominal wall ecchymosis, and flexion-distraction injury (Chance fracture) to the lumbar spine (Fig. 121.6).[9] Intestinal injuries include bowel disruption, mesenteric avulsion, and bowel wall contusion (Fig. 121.7). Areas of the small bowel particularly prone to injury are the points of retroperitoneal fixation, such as the proximal jejunum at the ligament of Treitz or the terminal ileum near the junction with the cecum. A perforation may be present even without free air or significant spillage of succus on DPL. Delayed perforations may occur as a result of mesenteric disruptions and subsequent bowel necrosis. In some instances, a prolonged ileus that fails to resolve may be the only evidence of intestinal injury.

The mechanism of injury and abdominal wall ecchymosis can suggest the diagnosis of intestinal injury. Abdominal tenderness may be present on physical examination. Findings on computed tomography consistent with small bowel injury are free fluid, contrast extravasation, focal bowel thickening, pneumoperitoneum, and fat stranding or fluid in the mesentery.[28] Once diagnosed, bowel injuries are treated by laparotomy. Excision of injury and primary anastomosis to reestablish gastrointestinal continuity are usually possible. Morbidity and mortality are not increased if the delay in diagnosis is less than 24 hours.[19]

Injury to the Duodenum

Duodenal injuries are rare in children but occur more commonly than in adults. Children may have localized right upper

TABLE 121.2   Abdominal Organ Injury Computed Tomography Grading Scales[a]

Injury	Grade I	Grade II	Grade III	Grade IV	Grade V	Grade VI
Splenic hematoma	Subcapsular, <10% surface area	Subcapsular, 10%-50% surface; intraparenchymal, <5 cm diameter	Subcapsular, >50% surface or expanding; intraparenchymal >5 cm or expanding; ruptured			
Splenic laceration	<1 cm depth	1-3 cm depth	>3 cm depth or involving vessel	Segmental vessel >25% devascularization	Shattered spleen	
Splenic vascular					Hilar injury 100% devascularization	
Hepatic hematoma	Subcapsular, <10% surface area	Subcapsular, 10%-50% surface; intraparenchymal, <10 cm diameter	Subcapsular, >50% surface or expanding; intraparenchymal >10 cm or expanding; ruptured			
Hepatic laceration	Capsular tear, <1 cm depth	1-3 cm depth, <10 cm length	>3 cm depth	Disruption 25%-75% of lobe or 1-3 Couinaud segments in lobe	Disruption >75% lobe or >3 Couinaud segments in lobe	
Hepatic vascular					Injury to cava or hepatic vein	Avulsion
Duodenum hematoma	Single portion	>1 portion				
Duodenum laceration	Partial thickness	<50% circumference	50%-75% circumference second portion	>75% circumference second portion, ampulla, or common bile duct	Disruption duodenopancreatic complex	
Duodenal vascular					Devascularization of duodenum	
Pancreas hematoma	Minor contusion	Major contusion				
Pancreas laceration	Superficial	Major	Distal transaction or duct injury	Proximal transaction or ampulla injury	Massive disruption of head	
Kidney contusion	Hematuria					
Kidney hematoma	Subcapsular, nonexpanding	Confined to retroperitoneum				
Kidney laceration		<1 cm depth	>1 cm depth	Through cortex, medulla, and collecting system	Shattered kidney	
Kidney vascular					Avulsion	

[a]Add one grade for multiple injuries up to grade III.
From Moore EE, Cogbill TH, Malangoni MA, et al. Organ injury scaling, II: pancreas, duodenum, small bowel, colon, and rectum. J Trauma. 1990;30:1427-1429; Moore EE, Shackford SR, Pachter HL, et al. Organ injury scaling: spleen, liver, and kidney. J Trauma. 1989;29:1664-1666.

quadrant tenderness, but the presentation may be subtle. The majority of duodenal injuries in children result in a duodenal hematoma without disruption of the lumen. When there is perforation, computed tomography demonstrates extraluminal gas or oral contrast extravasation in the right anterior pararenal space. Thickening of the duodenal wall is seen when a duodenal hematoma is present. Duodenal injuries are classified from grade I to V based on severity (see Table 121.2). The majority of pediatric duodenal injuries are grades I and II. Overall, mortality is 18% for patients with duodenal injuries. For grade I lesions, the mortality is 8%, with associated injuries as the usual cause of death.

A duodenal hematoma is treated with observation and parenteral hyperalimentation. Resolution generally occurs in 2 to 4 weeks. In some cases of duodenal hematoma, placement of a nasojejunal tube will allow enteral feeding distal to the point of obstruction. Repair of full-thickness duodenal injury may require duodenorrhaphy, pyloric exclusion, duodenoduodenostomy, duodenojejunostomy, pancreaticoduodenectomy, or simple drainage (Fig. 121.8). The majority of injuries are

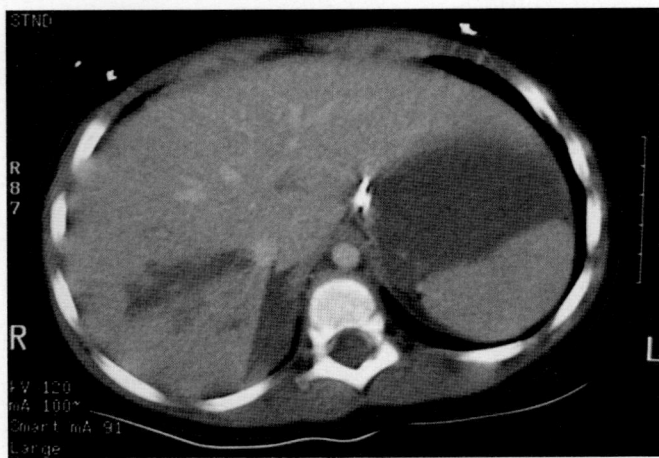

Fig. 121.4. CT scan of a patient with a grade II hepatic hematoma.

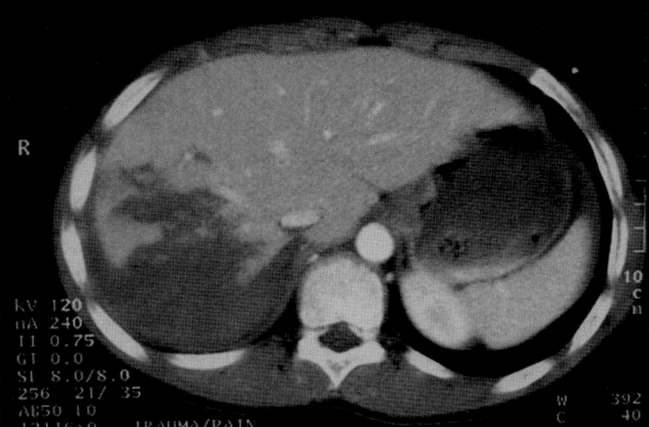

Fig. 121.5. CT scan of a patient with a grade IV hepatic laceration.

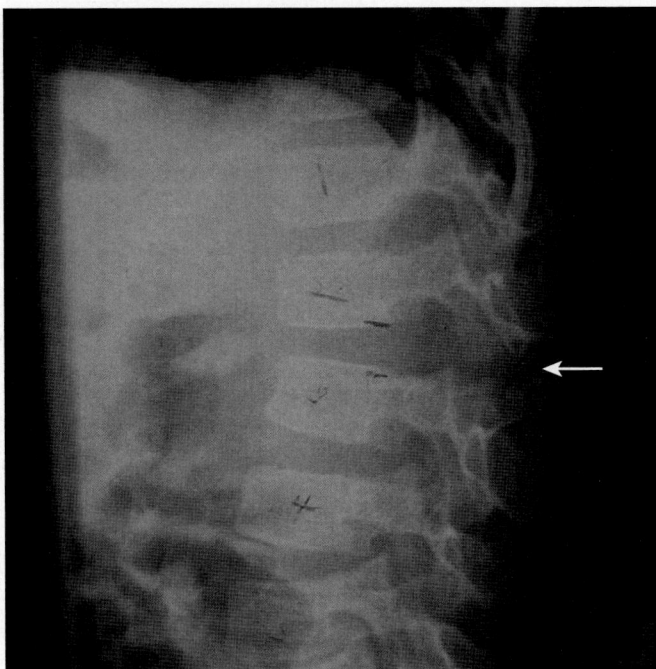

Fig. 121.6. Plain lateral lumbar spine radiograph. *Arrow* indicates distraction injury to posterior spine secondary to lap belt injury.

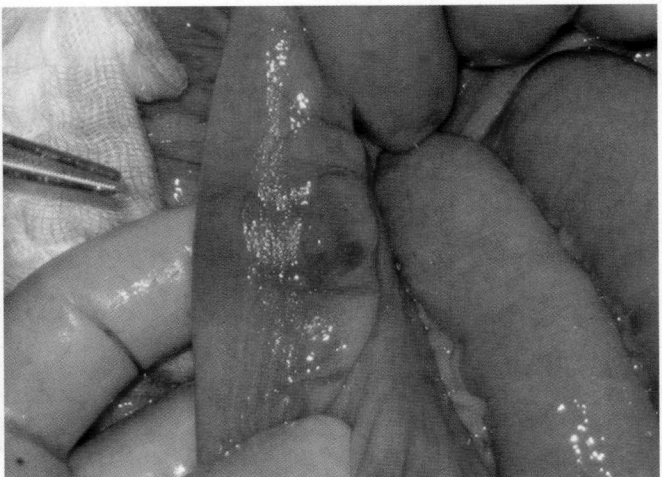

Fig. 121.7. Small bowel contusion after blast injury.

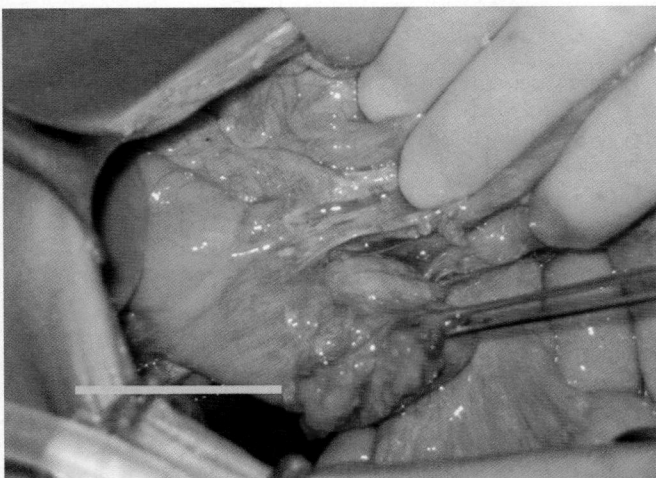

Fig. 121.8. Grade III duodenal laceration blowout injury after fall onto a handrail.

treated with debridement and primary closure with drainage. Pyloric exclusion is recommended for complex duodenal injuries. Duodenostomy and regional drains are useful. In children, pancreaticoduodenectomy is rarely required to treat a duodenal injury.

Injury to the Pancreas

Injuries to the pancreas may require operative intervention depending on severity of injury and integrity of the pancreatic duct (see Table 121.2). Upper abdominal tenderness, hyperamylasemia, edema of the gland, and unexplained fluid in the lesser sac on computed tomography suggest pancreatic injury. Handlebar injury, lap belt injury, direct blow to the abdomen, and motor vehicle crash are the most common mechanisms (Fig. 121.9). When the gland is fractured, this generally occurs where it crosses the vertebral column (Fig. 121.10). Pancreatic transection is best treated by early distal pancreatectomy and drainage. When the main pancreatic duct is intact, nonoperative treatment with an extended course of bowel rest and parenteral nutrition should be attempted. Devascularization of the pancreas and duodenum in blunt abdominal trauma is

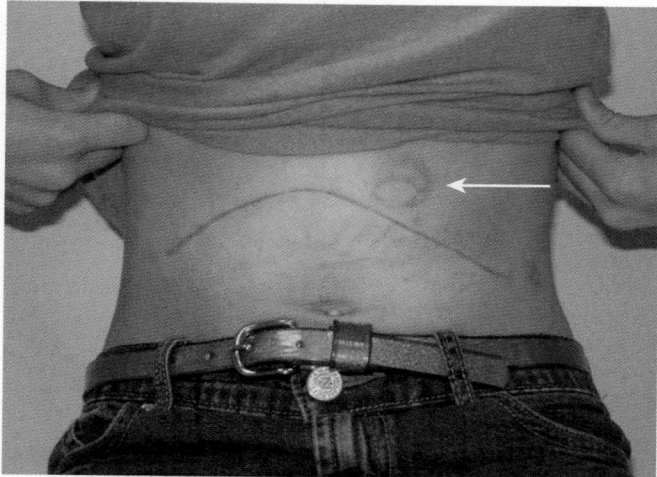

Fig. 121.9. Handlebar injury in a patient who required distal pancreatectomy.

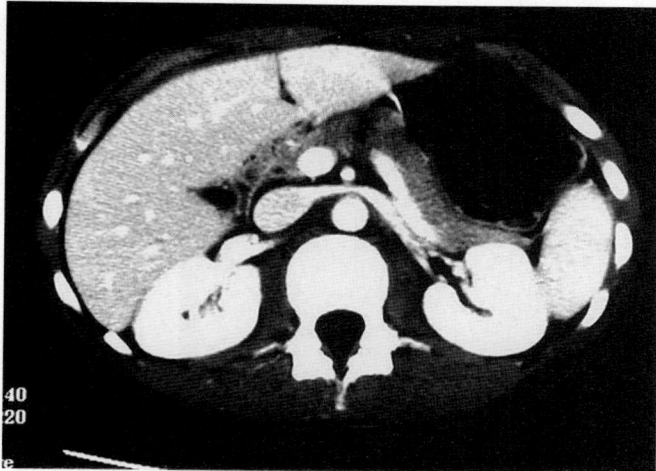

Fig. 121.10. CT scan of a patient with a grade III pancreatic laceration. (Courtesy Martin Eichelberger, MD, and Patrick McLaughlin, MD.)

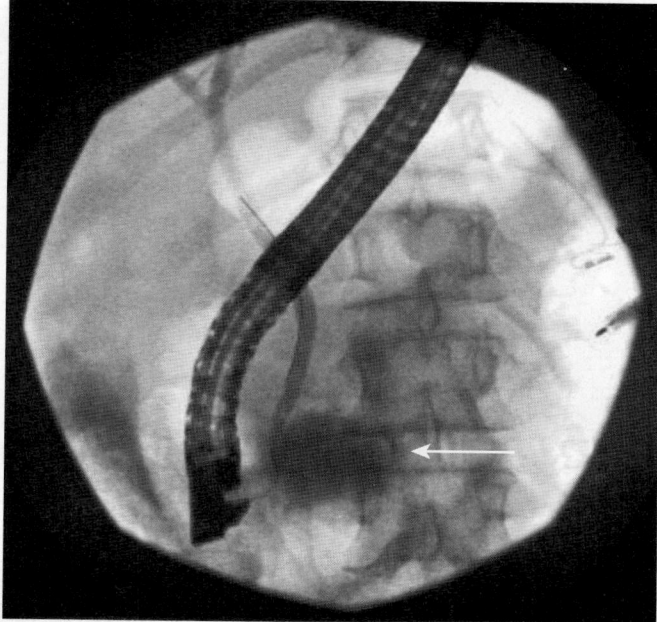

Fig. 121.11. Endoscopic retrograde cholangiopancreatography demonstrates pancreatic duct leak after a kick to the abdomen.

rare in children. When it does occur, laparotomy, pyloric exclusion, drainage, and repeated debridement with an open abdomen may be required. After pancreatic injury, pseudocysts may develop and require internal or external drainage after maturation. Operative drainage of a pseudocyst to the stomach or a roux-en-Y loop of intestine should be delayed for at least six weeks until the pseudocyst wall is mature. An infected pseudocyst may require urgent percutaneous drainage. Magnetic resonance cholangiopancreatography or endoscopic retrograde cholangiopancreatography is useful to diagnose pancreatic duct disruption, and a pancreatic stent can be placed across the disrupted duct, which potentially prevents pseudocyst formation[29] (Fig. 121.11).

Blunt Abdominal Aortic Injury

The majority of aortic injuries after blunt trauma are in the chest, with only 6% in the abdomen.[30] Pedestrians struck by a motor vehicle and unrestrained passengers are more likely to have thoracic injuries, whereas passengers with lap belt injuries are more likely to injure the abdominal aorta.[31] Injury to the renal artery or mesenteric artery is more common than

aortic injury.[32] Computed tomographic angiography is capable of providing a definitive diagnosis; however, angiography may be required in some children. Aortic injuries include contusion, intimal dissection, and complete disruption. The most frequent site of disruption is at the inferior mesenteric artery or the renal arteries. Patients present with diminished or absent distal lower extremity pulses. Neurologic deficits may result from aortic compromise. Associated injuries are present in 65% of cases. When blunt abdominal aortic injury is recognized early, surgical intervention can dramatically lower mortality. A pseudoaneurysm can develop as a late complication. Major abdominal venous injuries resulting from blunt trauma are usually fatal.

Renal Trauma

Renal injury rarely occurs as an isolated injury. Findings suggestive of renal injury include flank tenderness, flank or abdominal mass, or ecchymosis. Hematuria, either gross or microscopic, is the best indicator of serious renal injury. However, serious injury, especially renal pedicle injuries, may be present even without hematuria. In hemodynamically stable patients, computed tomography with intravenous contrast allows for an accurate diagnosis of renal injury and function (Fig. 121.12). Sonography also provides an accurate diagnosis of extrarenal fluid collections.[33] Renal trauma can result in a hematoma, laceration, or vascular injury (see Table 121.2). Children who are hemodynamically stable may be safely managed nonoperatively. Angiography with embolization can control hemorrhage when contrast extravasation is seen on computed tomography.[34] Exploration is warranted in children who are hemodynamically unstable, have an expanding hematoma, or have an associated abdominal injury necessitating exploration. In unstable patients, nephrectomy is the safest choice; however, the surgeon must ensure that the contralateral kidney is present before proceeding. Renal repair or partial nephrectomy is possible in select cases (Fig. 121.13).

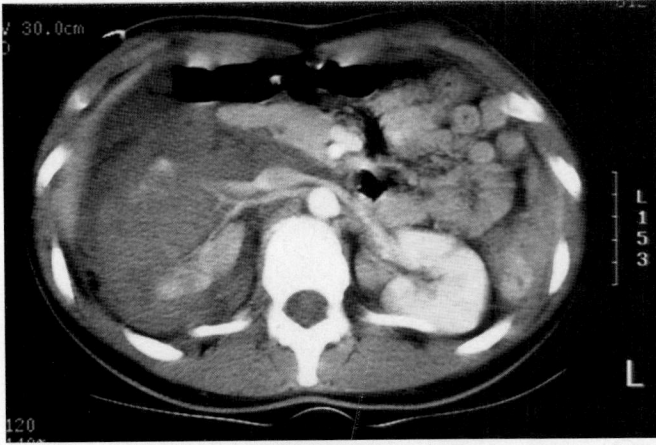

Fig. 121.12. CT scan of a patient with a grade IV renal laceration and vascular injury.

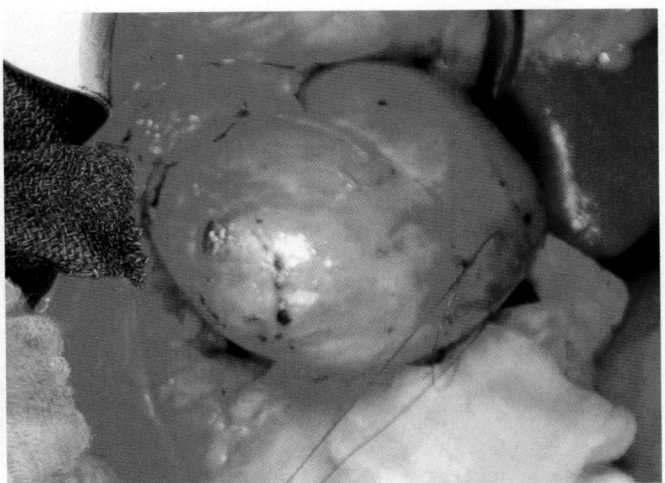

Fig. 121.13. Repair of a grade II renal laceration after penetrating trauma.

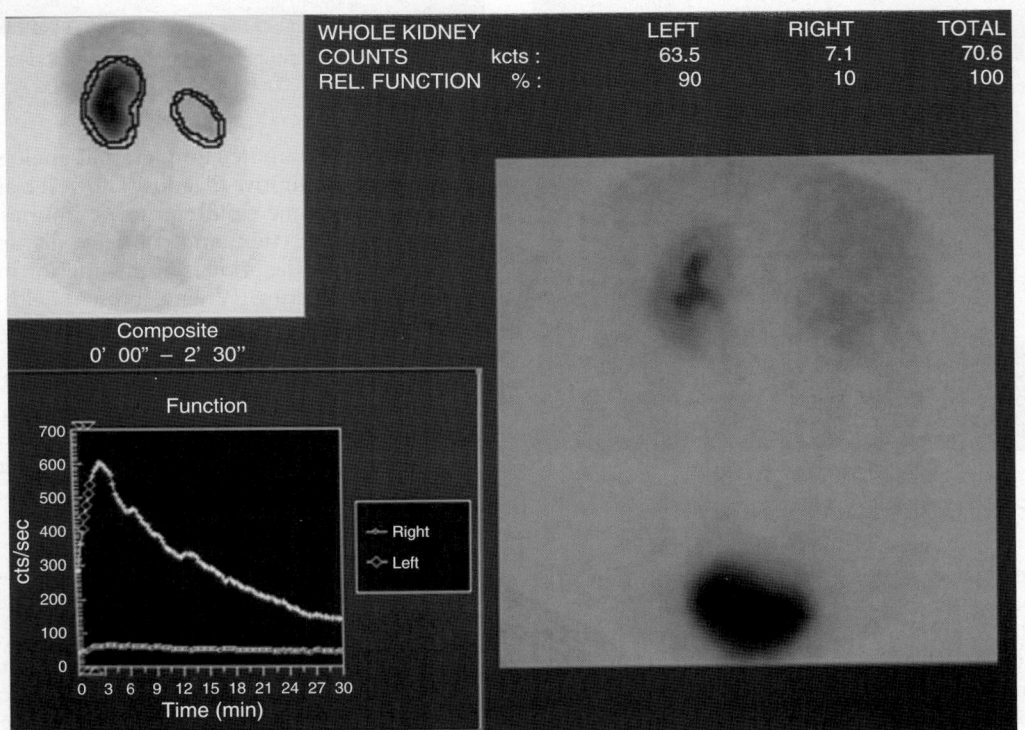

Fig. 121.14. Renal scan of a patient with a grade IV renal laceration and vascular injury.

Isolated urinary extravasation is not an indication for emergent exploration, but delayed operation or percutaneous drainage may be required for persistent extravasation or infection. If urinary extravasation is present, antibiotics should be administered. Patients with extravasation and devascularized segments on computed tomography have a higher incidence of delayed complications. Observation and bed rest usually result in excellent outcome, even with deep parenchymal lacerations associated with urinary extravasation. Patients with gross hematuria are kept on bed rest until the urine is grossly clear. Reevaluation is necessary for persistent hematuria, tenderness, or mass. All patients with renal injuries, regardless of severity, should be monitored for the delayed onset of hypertension. A captopril-furosemide technetium-99m diethylenetriamine pentaacetic acid (DTPA) renal scan is used to verify function after injury (Fig. 121.14).

Renal pedicle injuries are rare and are suggested by a lack of renal contrast enhancement on computed tomography. Renal angiography definitively establishes the diagnosis and directs operative management. Ureteral injuries require operative repair, but diagnosis of ureteropelvic junction disruption may be delayed because of a lack of clinical signs on presentation. Absence of contrast in the ureter indicates that ureteral stent placement will likely be necessary.[35]

TABLE 121.3   Associated Injury by Location of Pelvic Fracture

Fracture Site	Number (%)	Number With Abdominal Injury (%)	Number With Genitourinary Injury (%)
Unifocal	44 (81.5)	5 (11)	0
Pubic ramus	32 (59.3)	2 (6)	0
Iliac/pelvic rim	9 (16.7)	3 (33)	0
Sacrum	3 (5.60)	0	0
Multiple	10 (18.5)	6 (60)	4 (40)
Total	54	11 (20)	4 (7.4)

Data from Bond SJ, Gotschall CS, Eichelberger MR. Predictors of abdominal injury in children with pelvic fracture. J Trauma. 1991;31:1169.

Bladder Injuries

Bladder injuries are most often associated with blunt trauma. The bladder is predominantly intraabdominal in children. Therefore burst injuries are more common than in adults. Bladder rupture is associated with pelvic fractures. Clinical presentation of bladder rupture may be subtle, with only mild suprapubic tenderness. The severity of associated injuries may mask signs of a bladder injury. Hematuria is the most consistent finding. Recognizing the injury and identifying it as intraperitoneal or extraperitoneal are important. Stress cystography is best for establishing the diagnosis. Lack of extravasation on computed tomography does not exclude a bladder injury. Peritoneal fluid located in the lateral perivesical recess, superior to the bladder, and in the pouch of Douglas is suggestive of intraperitoneal bladder rupture. Extraperitoneal bladder rupture is noted by fluid extending superior and anterior to the level of the umbilicus and by fluid in the retrorectal presacral space. The distinction between intraperitoneal and extraperitoneal bladder rupture is important for treatment purposes. Controlled extraperitoneal ruptures are treated nonoperatively with urinary catheter drainage. Extensive extraperitoneal rupture and intraperitoneal injuries require operative intervention.[36]

Pelvic Fractures

The most common mechanism resulting in pelvic fracture in children is a pedestrian struck by a motor vehicle. Single fractures of the pelvis are rarely associated with significant abdominal injury, but children with multiple fractures of the pelvis are at significant risk for abdominal injury even if hemodynamically stable (Table 121.3). Pelvic fractures are usually evident on the initial physical examination. Findings include abrasions, bruising, hemorrhage, instability, or swelling. Asymmetry of the bony structure, pain on palpation, or crepitus can be present. An anteroposterior radiograph of the pelvis is obtained in the trauma bay to determine the anatomy of the fracture. After recognition, attention should be directed toward prompt stabilization with a sheet tightly wrapped around the pelvis and assessment of hemodynamic status. Opening of the pelvic ring, associated with fracture at two points, should be stabilized with a sheet wrapped around the pelvis, a C-clamp, or an external fixator. Vertical shear injuries are not usually amenable to this treatment and will require

operative reduction. Hemodynamically unstable patients should be aggressively resuscitated. Early angiography and embolization of bleeding vessels help to stabilize patients and avoid the need for operative intervention. Hemodynamically stable patients should undergo computed tomography to evaluate for associated injuries. Special attention should be directed toward the rectum, vagina, and urethra, which are especially susceptible to injury by bony fragments.

Acknowledgment

We gratefully acknowledge the contribution of Christopher P. Coppola and James C. Gilbert, who authored this chapter in previous editions.

References

1. Wegner S, Colletti JE, Van Wie D. Pediatric blunt abdominal trauma. *Pediatr Clin North Am.* 2006;53:243-256.
2. Dokucu AI, Otcu S, Ozturk H, et al. Characteristics of penetrating abdominal firearm injuries in children. *Eur J Pediatr Surg.* 2000;10:242-247.
3. Chiu WC, Shanmuganathan K, Mirvis SE, et al. Determining the need for laparotomy in penetrating torso trauma: a prospective study using triple-contrast enhanced abdominopelvic computed tomography. *J Trauma.* 2001;51:860-868.
4. Hayes JR, Groner JI. The increasing incidence of snowboard-related trauma. *J Pediatr Surg.* 2008;43:928-930.
5. McCrone AB, Lillis K, Shaha SH. Snowboarding-related abdominal trauma in children. *Pediatr Emerg Care.* 2012;28:251-253.
6. Williams BG, Hlaing T, Aaland MO. Ten-year retrospective study of delayed diagnosis of injury in pediatric trauma patients at a level II trauma center. *Pediatr Emerg Care.* 2009;25:489-493.
7. Coppola CP, Leininger BE, Rasmussen TE, Smith DL. Children treated at an expeditionary military hospital in Iraq. *Arch Pediatr Adolesc Med.* 2006;160:972-976.
8. Leininger BE, Rasmussen TE, Smith DL, et al. Experience with wound VAC and delayed primary closure of contaminated soft tissue injuries in Iraq. *J Trauma.* 2006;61:1207-1211.
9. Tyroch AH, McGuire EL, McLean SF, et al. The association between Chance fractures and intra-abdominal injuries revisited: a multicenter review. *Am Surg.* 2005;71:434-438.
10. Killeen KL, Shanmuganathan K, Poletti PA, et al. Helical computed tomography of bowel and mesenteric injuries. *J Trauma.* 2001;51:26-36.
11. Christiano JG, Tummers M, Kennedy A. Clinical significance of isolated intraperitoneal fluid on computed tomography in pediatric blunt abdominal trauma. *J Pediatr Surg.* 2009;44:1242-1248.
12. Moore EE, Cogbill TH, Malangoni MA, et al. Organ injury scaling, II: pancreas, duodenum, small bowel, colon, and rectum. *J Trauma.* 1990;30:1427-1429.
13. Moore EE, Shackford SR, Pachter HL, et al. Organ injury scaling: spleen, liver, and kidney. *J Trauma.* 1989;29:1664-1666.
14. Hynick NH, Brennan M, Schmit P, et al. Identification of blunt abdominal injuries in children. *J Trauma Acute Care Surg.* 2013;76:95-100.
15. Petrosoniak A, Engels PT, Hamilton P, Tien HC. Detection of significant bowel and mesenteric injuries in blunt abdominal trauma with 64 slice computed tomography. *J Trauma Acute Care Surg.* 2013;74:1081-1086.
16. Holmes JF, Brant WE, Bond WF, et al. Emergency department ultrasonography in the evaluation of hypotensive and normotensive children with blunt abdominal trauma. *J Pediatr Surg.* 2001;36:968-973.
17. Dolich MO, McKenney MG, Varela JE, et al. 2,576 ultrasounds for blunt abdominal trauma. *J Trauma.* 2001;50:108-112.
18. Coley BD, Mutabagani KH, Martin LC, et al. Focused abdominal sonography for trauma (FAST) in children with blunt abdominal trauma. *J Trauma.* 2000;48:902-906.
19. Fang JF, Chen RJ, Lin BC, et al. Small bowel perforation: is urgent surgery necessary? *J Trauma.* 1999;47:515-520.
20. Meyer G, Huttl TP, Hatz RA, Schildberg FW. Laparoscopic repair of traumatic diaphragmatic hernias. *Surg Endosc.* 2000;14:1010-1014.
21. Carlotti AP, Carvalho WB. Abdominal compartment syndrome: a review. *Pediatr Crit Care Med.* 2009;10:115-120.

22. Stylianos S. APSA Trauma Committee. Evidence-based guidelines for resource utilization in children with isolated spleen or liver injury. *J Pediatr Surg.* 2000;35:164-169.

23. Bowman SM, Sharar SR, Quan L. Impact of a statewide quality improvement initiative in improving the management of pediatric splenic injuries in Washington state. *J Trauma.* 2008;64:1478-1483.

24. Gauer JM, Gerber-Paulet S, Seiler C, Schweizer WP. Twenty years of splenic preservation in trauma: lower early infection rate than in splenectomy. *World J Surg.* 2008;32:2730-2735.

25. Peter SD, Keckler SJ, Spilde TL, et al. Justification for an abbreviated protocol in the management of blunt spleen and liver injury in children. *J Pediatr Surg.* 2008;43:191-194.

26. Holmes JF, Sokolove PE, Land C, Kuppermann N. Identification of intraabdominal injuries in children hospitalized following blunt torso trauma. *Acad Emerg Med.* 1999;6:799-806.

27. Nance ML, Keller MS, Stafford PW. Predicting hollow visceral injury in the pediatric blunt trauma patient with solid visceral injury. *J Pediatr Surg.* 2000;35:1300-1303.

28. Strouse PJ, Close BJ, Marshall KW, Cywes R. CT of bowel and mesenteric trauma in children. *Radiographics.* 1999;19:1237-1250.

29. Kim HS, Lee DK, Kim IW, et al. The role of endoscopic retrograde pancreatography in the treatment of traumatic pancreatic duct injury. *Gastrointest Endosc.* 2001;54:49-55.

30. Burjonrappa S, Vinocur C, Smergel E, et al. Pediatric blunt abdominal aortic trauma. *J Trauma.* 2008;65:E10-E12.

31. Anderson SA, Day M, Chen MK, et al. Traumatic aortic injuries in the pediatric population. *J Pediatr Surg.* 2008;43:1077-1081.

32. Hamner CE, Groner JI, Caniano DA, et al. Blunt intraabdominal arterial injury in pediatric trauma patients: injury distribution and markers of outcome. *J Pediatr Surg.* 2008;43:916-923.

33. Wessel LM, Scholz S, Jester I, et al. Management of kidney injuries in children with blunt abdominal trauma. *J Pediatr Surg.* 2000;35:1326-1330.

34. Hagiwara A, Sakaki S, Goto H, et al. The role of interventional radiology in the management of blunt renal injury: a practical protocol. *J Trauma.* 2001;51:526-531.

35. Cannon GM, Polsky EG, Smaldone MC, et al. Computerized tomography findings in pediatric trauma: indications for early intervention? *J Urol.* 2008;179:1529-1533.

36. Matlock KA, Tyroch AH, Kronfol Z, et al. Blunt traumatic bladder rupture: 10-year perspective. *Am Surg.* 2013;79:589-593.

Child Abuse

Paula M. Mazur, Lynn J. Hernan, Sitratullah Maiyegun, and Harry Wilson

PEARLS

- Accidental trauma differs from nonaccidental trauma in presentation, workup, treatment, and outcome. In child abuse, the history of trauma is withheld or falsified, and the presenting symptoms are often vague and nonspecific, so the diagnosis and treatment of injuries may be delayed. This contributes to the increased mortality and long-term morbidity seen in abused children.

- Abusive head trauma is the most common nonaccidental injury seen in the pediatric intensive care unit. It is the most common cause of death in abused children. Abusive head trauma is more likely to be fatal and more likely to cause long-term morbidity in survivors than accidental head trauma.

- The infant brain is more vulnerable to injury, especially to shaking (shaken baby syndrome [SBS]). The infant's neck muscles are underdeveloped and the head is proportionally larger than that of the adult. Large cerebrospinal fluid spaces in the infant allow greater movement of the brain within the skull. The infant brain has greater water content and increased deformability. Neurons and axons are less protected because of incomplete myelinization. Increased cerebral vasoreactivity predisposes the infant brain to cerebral edema.

- Accidental head trauma generates translational forces that result in focal damage. Nonaccidental trauma (eg, shaking) generates rotational forces from rapid acceleration/deceleration of the head. Rotational forces tear cerebral bridging veins (creating subdural hematoma) and axons (creating diffuse axonal injury).

- Signs of SBS include subdural hemorrhage, retinal hemorrhage, and skeletal injury. A small number of cases will have all three signs. The presence of subdural hemorrhage and retinal hemorrhage, alone or in combination, in the appropriate clinical setting, are suggestive of SBS.

- Posterior rib fractures, metaphyseal fractures, and spinous process fractures are highly specific for abuse because their proposed mechanisms of injury are unlikely to occur accidentally.

- Abdominal trauma is the second leading cause of fatal child abuse, with death rates approaching 40% to 50%. Inflicted abdominal injury is often occult, presenting without obvious signs or symptoms; thus recognition is delayed. Treatment may be delayed because of a delay in seeking medical attention or a failure to consider nonaccidental injury in the differential diagnosis.

- Two types of forces are generated in inflicted abdominal trauma. Compression forces crush viscera against the anterior spine, and this crush causes burst injuries of the solid viscera and perforation of air-filled viscera. Deceleration forces cause shear injuries at the site of fixed, ligament attachments. As a result, tears and hematoma formation are seen at the ligament attachments of the liver and small bowel. Children with inflicted abdominal injury often have concomitant injuries suggestive of child abuse (bruises, head trauma, long-bone and skull fractures).

- Abusive thermal burns are of uniform thickness and closely replicate the shape of the inflicting object. Accidental thermal burns have varying degrees of thickness and irregular shapes. Abusive scald burns have an immersion pattern with a burn that is circumferential and is of uniform depth with a well-defined edge, and they spare body creases. Accidental scald burns have more random patterns, vary in depth, have poorly defined edges, and do not spare body creases.

- All cases of suspected child abuse must be reported to child protective services and law enforcement. All cases of fatal child abuse must be referred to the medical examiner. Detailed, legible medical documentation and good communication between the treating physician and the medical examiner are essential to secure the evidence needed to prosecute the case successfully.

Only a small percentage of physically abused children require hospitalization in the pediatric intensive care unit (PICU), but these children have been shown to have a higher morbidity and mortality rate than critically injured victims of accidental trauma.[1,2] The types of injuries that result from nonaccidental injury, coupled with delays in diagnosis and management, account for the worse outcome in abuse victims. Diagnosis and management of life-threatening injuries are often delayed because the history of preceding trauma is not provided or it is so vague or the trauma is depicted as so minor that the physician is led away from a possible traumatic cause for the patient's condition. The so-called golden hour allotted for successful trauma resuscitation is spent considering an infectious, neurologic, or metabolic cause for the child's illness. In addition, there can be a considerable delay in seeking medical care. Several hours to days may elapse between the time of injury and presentation to a medical facility.

Head trauma is the most common type of inflicted injury seen in the PICU, followed by abdominal trauma, burns, and thoracic trauma. Child abuse victims should be approached in the same manner as accidental trauma patients. They may have occult multiple-organ injury. The discovery of one injury demands a thorough evaluation for additional trauma. A meticulous investigation for injury has obvious medical utility, but it also becomes an essential part of the forensic investigation that ensues once a report of suspected child abuse is filed with child protective services and law enforcement.

Recognition of Child Abuse
History of Injury

The history of an injury must account for the type and severity of injury that are seen on physical examination. Suspicion of abuse should arise when any of the following occur:

1. The caretaker is unable to explain the injuries or gives a mechanism of injury that does not match the degree of injury seen. For example, a minor fall would not explain the presence of life-threatening cerebral edema.
2. The timing of the injury does not fit with the time of presentation (eg, a critical head injury cannot be attributed to a fall that occurred 1 week before presentation).
3. The child's developmental stage does not fit the history (eg, rolling off a changing table should raise suspicion if the child is younger than 4 months).
4. The history of injury changes over time or from caretaker to caretaker. A careful review of all histories documented in the medical record may reveal discrepancies.

Patterns of Injury

Inflicted injury may be differentiated from accidental injury by its appearance, location, and distribution on the body (Table 122.1).

Bruising

Inflicted bruises are often bilateral, widely distributed, and located on soft tissue areas of the body that are unlikely to make surface contact during a fall. They may take the shape of the inflicting object (eg, fingers, a hand print, linear whip marks from a belt, loop marks from a folded belt or cord). They are frequently found on the posterior trunk, buttocks, and the posterior side of the extremities because the victim would naturally be trying to run away from the perpetrator. Bruise color is not a reliable indicator of the time an injury occurred. Bruises resolve and therefore change color at different rates depending on their location and the force with which they were inflicted.[1] Nevertheless, documenting bruise color

is important, particularly with the presence of bruises of markedly different colors at the same time, suggesting that the child may have been abused on more than one occasion. A simple gingerbread-man drawing of the child's body, marked with the locations of all the child's injuries, is a concise descriptive tool that will quickly jar a physician's memory before any legal proceeding.

Early photographic documentation of the child's injuries is essential. The standard for documentation had been 35-mm photographs, but digital cameras, both still and video, are replacing 35-mm photography. Polaroid photographs have been used in court, but they are inferior to 35-mm and digital photographs in both clarity and durability. Every effort should be made to obtain the best photographs; 35-mm photographs/digital photographs taken by a medical or law enforcement photographer are ideal. If a professional photographer is unavailable, any staff member familiar with the use of the camera should take photographs for the medical record.

Burns

Compared with accidental burns, abuse burns are more extensive in degree and distribution, and they often require management in a PICU.[2,3] Inflicted burns are of two types. Thermal injuries involve forced contact with a hot object, and scald injuries involve contact with a hot liquid, usually water. Abusive thermal burns are of uniform thickness and closely replicate the shape of the inflicting object. For example, an inflicted cigarette burn is approximately 8 mm round and uniform in depth. Accidental thermal burns have varying degrees of thickness and irregular shapes. If a child accidentally brushes against a hot cigarette, the burn will be more linear and of varying depth along its length.[1]

Abusive scald burns have an immersion pattern. Part of the child's body, usually the buttocks or limbs, are forcefully immersed and held in hot water. The resulting burn is circumferential and of uniform depth with a well-defined edge called a *tidemark*. Body creases are spared (withdrawal sign) during inflicted scald injury because the child pulls and folds his or her arms and legs inward to avoid immersion in the hot water. Accidental scald burns have more random patterns, vary in depth, have poorly defined edges, and do not spare body creases.[2] Ideally, photographic documentation should be performed before the initial burn dressing. Additional photographs taken 24 to 48 hours later, when the burn has fully evolved in depth and distribution, can also be valuable during litigation.

Fractures

Many of the characteristics used to recognize inflicted bruises and burns can be applied to fractures. The mechanism of injury described by the caretaker must remain consistent, be compatible with the child's developmental stage, and account for enough force to break the child's bone. Inflicted fractures can be bilateral fractures of the same age or multiple fractures in different stages of healing. In his textbook *Diagnostic Imaging of Child Abuse*, Kleinman[4] divides fractures according to their degree of specificity for inflicted injury. Posterior rib fractures, metaphyseal fractures, and spinous process fractures are highly specific for abuse because their proposed mechanisms of injury are unlikely to occur accidentally. Scapula and sternum fractures are highly specific for abuse if the caretaker's history does not account for a tremendous amount of

TABLE 122.1 Patterns of Injury	
Accidental	**Nonaccidental**
Unilateral	Bilateral/symmetrical
Isolated injury	Multiple injuries
Amorphous shape	Well-defined shape
Prominent bone areas	Soft tissue areas
Posterior aspect of body	Anterior aspect of body
One age of injury	Multiple ages of injury

force having been applied to these bones. Fractures of low specificity for abuse are commonly seen after bumps and falls (eg, clavicle fractures, linear skull fractures, long-bone fractures in ambulatory toddlers). Between high and low specificity for abusive trauma are acute, bilateral fractures, multiple fractures of different ages, widened (diastatic) or depressed skull fractures, and long-bone shaft fractures occurring in the young, nonambulatory infant.

It was long held that spiral fractures were highly suggestive of abuse because their spiral configuration implied that a forceful twisting motion had been applied along the length of the bone. Dalton and colleagues[5] looked at femur fractures in children younger than 3 years, dividing the fractures into three types (oblique, transverse, and spiral), and into three age categories (0 to 1 year, 1 to 2 years, and 2 to 3 years). Their results showed that the incidence of spiral fractures increased significantly with increasing age, whereas the incidence of abuse was highest in the youngest age group regardless of fracture type. Spiral fractures can occur accidentally in vigorous, ambulatory toddlers. The age of the child holds more significance than fracture type when the possibility of inflicted injury is considered.[5,6]

Posterior rib fractures and metaphyseal fractures are frequently seen in shaken or battered infants. Posterior rib fractures occur when the child's chest is compressed. This compression causes the rib to rock back over its articulation with the transverse vertebral process. The transverse process acts as a fulcrum for the rib, and a fracture occurs on the rib's pleural surface. Although this fracture has been seen in pediatric patients with major, high-speed trauma, it does not occur accidentally in healthy children during mild to moderate thoracic trauma. Cardiopulmonary resuscitation (CPR) has not been shown to cause posterior rib fractures. A detailed discussion of posterior rib fractures can be found in Kleinman's textbook, *Diagnostic Imaging of Child Abuse.*[4] Acute rib fractures are difficult to see on a plain film. They may only first be visible 2 to 3 weeks after injury, when a callus has formed around the fracture site. Therefore, finding a callused fracture indicates that the trauma occurred at least 2 to 3 weeks before the radiograph.[4]

The periosteum of a pediatric long bone is loosely attached to its cortex. Any violent pull, tear, or twist on the shaft of a child's long bone displaces the periosteum. This results in subperiosteal hemorrhage and periosteal elevation that can be seen on the radiograph. Conversely, the periosteum is tightly attached at its point of origin, the metaphyseal plate. The metaphyseal plate, which is the most newly laid down bone above the growth plate, has delicate trabeculations. Violent forces applied to the midshaft periosteum are transferred to its point of origin, the metaphyseal plate, and an avulsion fracture occurs through the delicate trabeculae. Depending on the angle at which the radiograph is taken, a metaphyseal avulsion fracture can appear as a thin line through the metaphysis, as "corners" broken off the edges of the long bone or as a "bucket handle" attached to the end of the long bone. Like posterior rib fractures, metaphyseal fractures are pathognomonic for child abuse. These corner fractures or bucket handle fractures are occult. There is no deformity or swelling, and they are not obviously tender to palpation. Like posterior rib fractures, metaphyseal fractures are usually found on a radiograph obtained for other reasons or on a skeletal survey done during the medical investigation of a suspected abuse case. Spinous process fractures are the remaining type of fractures listed under "high specificity" in Kleinman's text. They are thought to occur during infant shaking, when the spine is in hyperflexion, causing sudden stress on the posterior spinous ligament as it articulates with the posterior spinous processes.[4]

Skull fractures are the second most common fracture seen in abused children, but skull fractures are also commonly seen in accidental head trauma. A skull fracture is suspicious for abuse when there is no significant trauma to account for the fracture. An unexplained skull fracture obligates the physician to look for additional injuries that are pathognomonic for abuse. For example, a skeletal survey may reveal occult posterior rib or metaphyseal fractures. A noncontrast computed tomographic (CT) scan may reveal bilateral subdural hematomas, which are not commonly associated with accidental skull fractures.

The guidelines for dating fractures are broad. In general, periosteal elevation can occur acutely, within hours to days after injury. Callus formation is seen approximately 2 weeks after injury. Loss of the fracture line begins to occur 3 weeks after the injury, and remodeling of the fracture occurs anywhere from 3 months to a year after injury, depending on the child's age. Infants will heal and remodel faster than older children. Skull fractures and metaphyseal fractures are difficult to date because they do not show the same periosteal reactions that healing ribs and long bones do.[4] However, a diastatic skull fracture, which is a linear skull fracture greater than 3 mm wide, is not an acute injury. It takes time for a skull fracture to separate more than 3 mm.

Skeletal Survey

Finding one suggestive injury on a child necessitates a radiologic evaluation of the entire skeleton. Skeletal survey is the most common screening tool used in child abuse investigation. Two views of every bone in the body, radiographed with orthopedic technique, is the gold standard. *Body grams* or *baby grams,* in which the infant's entire skeleton is pictured on one x-ray plate, are unacceptable. It is feasible to obtain adequate surveys at the bedside when the patient has been too unstable to move from the critical care area to the radiology department. It is also possible to obtain postmortem skeletal surveys before transferring the child's body to the medical examiner (ME), because the quality of the surveys often surpasses radiographs performed in the morgue and therefore may serve to focus the ME on particular areas of the skeleton during autopsy.

In general, skeletal surveys have the highest yield in children younger than 2 years of age and are obtained in children up to age 5 years, after which the yield becomes low.[1] Because smaller children are easier to lift, shake, throw, or pull, it is possible to generate the forces required to create the classic abuse fractures previously discussed. Because fractures pathognomonic for abuse, such as posterior rib fractures or metaphyseal fractures, are difficult to see on initial radiographs, it is strongly recommended that a second skeletal survey be obtained approximately 2 weeks after the initial survey. The later survey may reveal callus formation of healing fractures that were not visible on the initial skeletal survey.

Occult fractures can be detected by bone scan, but bone scan is not specific for fracture. The radioactive isotope used in bone scan will also enhance areas of infection, neoplasm, and growth. Therefore positive bone scans cannot be used as evidence of injury in court. A positive scan focuses attention on a particular area of the skeleton in need of closer study, but the area of injury must always be verified by subsequent plain film. Bone scans are most useful in detecting occult rib fractures. They are not as useful in verifying metaphyseal fractures because the metaphysis lies next to an area of vigorous bone growth, and growth areas are normally enhanced in pediatric scans.[4]

Abusive Head Trauma

Abusive head trauma (AHT) is the most common form of child abuse seen in the PICU and is the number one cause of death in child abuse victims overall. Roughly 50% of trauma in children younger than 1 year of age is head trauma. The median age of abusive head trauma victims is 2 to 4 months of age. When Bruce and Zimmerman[7] looked at a population of children younger than 2 years with head trauma, they found that 90% of the head injuries were accidental and 10% were attributed to abuse. Eighty percent of the deaths from head trauma, however, occurred in the smaller percentage of abused children. Outcome studies comparing children surviving accidental and nonaccidental head trauma show significantly higher morbidity rates in the nonaccidental victims. Clearly, abusive head injury differs vastly from accidental head injury.

Characteristics of the Infant Brain and Cervical Spine

The infant brain is more vulnerable to injury than the adult brain for several reasons. The neck muscles inadequately support the infant's head, which is relatively large compared with the rest of the body. Consequently, the head is put through a broader range of random motions during a traumatic event like shaking. The cerebrospinal fluid (CSF) spaces are larger. These spaces allow greater movement of the brain within the skull, and the brain has greater water content, thereby increasing deformability. Open sutures increase skull flexibility so that an infant's skull can be pushed inward causing cortical damage without fracturing. Incomplete myelinization leaves neurons and their axons less protected, and increased cerebral vasoreactivity at the site of injured neurons predisposes the brain to cerebral edema.[8,9] An infant's upper cervical spinal cord is predisposed to injury because of the increased ligament elasticity, poorly supportive paraspinal muscles, incompletely ossified vertebrae with flattened, horizontal facet joints, and increased cord mobility within the cervical canal. In addition, the large infant head causes traction injury to the upper cervical cord during acceleration/deceleration. These factors combined require that the infant with suspected AHT be immobilized in a cervical collar until the cervical spine can be thoroughly evaluated for injury.

Mechanisms of Head Injury

Accidental head trauma, such as a fall from a height, generates translational forces, which are applied directly to the site of impact resulting in focal damage to the cerebral cortex. We may see a focal contusion, a *coup-contre-coup* injury, or an epidural hematoma. Nonaccidental trauma (eg, shaking) generates rotational force as a consequence of rapid acceleration/deceleration movements of the head. Rotational force distorts both gross and microscopic cortical structures.[10] The tearing of cerebral bridging veins creates a subdural hematoma. Axons that are torn at the microscopic level result in neuron death

and global cerebral injury.[11] Although subdural hematomas are a hallmark of shaken baby syndrome (SBS), they are rarely life-threatening lesions. The increased morbidity and mortality associated with AHT is attributed to brain injury at the cellular level. This cellular injury has been called diffuse axonal injury (DAI) or traumatic axonal injury (TAI). Increased vasoreactivity at the site of damaged axons causes a rapid onset of diffuse cerebral edema, which increases intracranial pressure (ICP) and compromises blood flow to vital areas of the brain. Therefore, the child is placed at risk for seizures, respiratory compromise, herniation, and death. Within hours of a shaking injury, a CT scan will begin to show a "black brain" with diffuse edema and a loss of gray-white matter differentiation.[8]

Neuroimaging of Abusive Head Trauma

CT imaging is the universally accepted screening tool for suspected AHT. It is readily available, does not require sedation, and easily identifies subdural hemorrhage. CT scan does not reliably date a central nervous system (CNS) bleed. An acute subdural hematoma may contain both clotted and unclotted blood, each of which has different attenuation on CT. This falsely gives the impression that an acute bleed has occurred within a preexisting or chronic hemorrhage. Magnetic resonance imaging (MRI), although it may require sedation or general anesthesia, is a better tool for identifying subarachnoid hemorrhage, petechial hemorrhage, infarction, hypoxic-ischemic encephalopathy, and axonal injury. Subtle evidence of AHT and its secondary brain injury is more easily seen on MRI. In addition, MRI is a more useful forensic tool than CT imaging during a child abuse investigation. Hemoglobin degradation within a CNS bleed occurs in a predictable sequence and can be roughly timed. Each hemoglobin degradation product has a unique appearance on T1- and T2-weighted images, and an experienced neuroradiologist may be able to narrow down the time of CNS injury. MRI should ultimately be used in all forensic child abuse investigations. Only an experienced neuroradiologist should interpret forensic MRI findings. Ultrasound is not a useful screening tool for AHT.[12]

Retinal Hemorrhages

It is widely hypothesized that the eye is subjected to the same acceleration/deceleration forces that the brain endures. Retinal vessels, coursing through the 11 layers of the retina, will randomly tear, forming hemorrhages of multiple shapes (eg, dots, blots, flame hemorrhages). Hemorrhage shape is determined by the cell orientation in the particular retinal layer where tearing occurs. Intraretinal hemorrhages of multiple shapes in various retinal layers are a classic finding in shaken baby syndrome.[13] Controversy still surrounds the mechanism of retinal hemorrhage formation, and there have been scattered reports of scant retinal hemorrhages found after CPR, in the face of increased ICP (Terson syndrome) or increased thoracic pressure (Purtscher retinopathy). These retinal hemorrhages, however, differ in appearance from the classic retinal hemorrhages of SBS.[13,14] Approximately 30% of healthy neonates will have retinal hemorrhages at birth, but these rapidly resolve by the third or fourth week of life. The retinal hemorrhages of SBS extend into the periphery of the retina, which can only be fully viewed by indirect ophthalmoscopy. The standard for investigation of SBS requires an indirect ophthalmoscopy evaluation by an ophthalmologist and photographic documentation of the retinal hemorrhages using a retinal camera.

Shaken Baby Syndrome

The diagnosis of SBS is made in the presence of a constellation of signs (ie, subdural hemorrhage, retinal hemorrhage, skeletal injury). The mechanisms of injury proposed to cause subdural hematoma and retinal hemorrhage have been discussed. Posterior rib fractures occur when the infant's chest is compressed during shaking. Metaphyseal fractures are thought to occur as the legs and arms are flailed back and forth. Only a small percentage of cases will have all three signs of SBS (subdural hematomas, retinal hemorrhages, and skeletal injury). More than half the cases will show both subdural hematoma and retinal hemorrhage, but the presence of subdural hemorrhage or retinal hemorrhage alone still suggests the diagnosis of SBS.[15]

A proposed sequence of events in SBS would be as follows: The frustrated caretaker impulsively attempts to stop the infant's crying by violently shaking the infant. The infant immediately loses consciousness and becomes apneic, at which time the caretaker impacts the infant down onto the mattress or floor and leaves the child to recover on its own. The cerebral damage and ensuing edema lead to increased ICP, ischemia, seizures, and further respiratory compromise.[1] Eventually medical care is sought for the child. The clinical history is vague, although there is usually some history of altered mental status. The child has nonspecific symptoms such as lethargy, poor feeding, and irritability or may have had a seizure-like episode. The differential diagnosis includes sepsis, meningitis, new-onset seizure, or a metabolic disorder. These children commonly have no external evidence of trauma. Trauma may only become part of the differential diagnosis when CT imaging performed for other purposes reveals intracranial hemorrhage or when a bloody spinal tap fails to clear. Bloody taps that fail to clear should be spun down within 2 hours to look for xanthochromic CSF, which indicates a preexisting intracranial hemorrhage. CSF that has a clear supernatant suggests the presence of blood for less than 2 hours, supporting a diagnosis of bloody tap. For early diagnosis and management of a potentially lethal injury to be facilitated, trauma must always be included in the differential when a young child is seen with altered mental status, seizures, or apnea. Jenny and colleagues[16] reviewed 174 children with abusive head injury who were seen at the Denver Children's Hospital over a 5-year period and found that in 31% of these children, the diagnosis of abusive head trauma was missed on first presentation for medical evaluation. The most frequent misdiagnoses made were gastroenteritis, followed by accidental head injury, sepsis, increasing head size, otitis media, and seizure disorder. Examiners were most likely to make the correct diagnosis if one of the following was present: severe respiratory symptoms, seizures, facial or scalp injuries, or single-parent household. Cases were often missed in the youngest patients, white infants, infants with less severe symptoms, and two-parent households.[16]

Inflicted Abdominal and Thoracic Trauma
Abdominal Trauma

After head injury, abdominal trauma is the second leading cause of fatal child abuse. Death rates approach 40% to 50%.[17] Cooper and associates[10] reviewed 10,000 pediatric patients with trauma who were admitted between 1972 and 1986, identifying approximately 4400 victims of inflicted injury. Of these, only 22, or 0.5%, had abdominal trauma, but the death rate for this small subgroup was 45%. Several factors probably contribute to these high death rates. Inflicted abdominal injury is often occult, presenting without obvious signs or symptoms; this delays recognition. There is usually a delay between time of inflicted injury and time of presentation to a medical facility. Parents may not bring the child to medical attention until the secondary effects of severe abdominal trauma, namely, hemorrhagic shock and peritonitis, manifest. Health care personnel further delay treatment by failing to consider nonaccidental injury in the differential diagnosis. In the study by Cooper and associates,[10] the mean time of delay between injury and presentation for medical care was 13 hours. Of significance, all of the children with inflicted abdominal injury in the study by Cooper and associates[10] had concomitant injuries commonly seen in child abuse. Ninety-five percent had soft tissue injuries, 45% had head trauma, and 27% and 18% had long-bone fractures and skull fractures, respectively. Half of the families had been previously reported to child protective services for suspected abuse or neglect. The most recent abdominal injuries seemed to represent an escalation of abuse in the home. Therefore, any suggestive injury should prompt physicians to look for occult abdominal trauma and to contact child protective services for investigation of the child's social situation.

Children with nonaccidental abdominal trauma tend to be older (>1 year) than children with abusive head trauma. Because they are larger and ambulatory, they are more difficult to grab, lift, and shake, but they are still vulnerable to physical blows. Inflicted abdominal trauma is blunt force applied to the abdominal wall, usually a punch, kick, or blow to the midepigastrium. Two types of force are generated. Compression forces crush viscera against the anterior spine, and deceleration forces cause shear injuries at the site of fixed, ligamentous attachments. We may find burst injuries of the solid viscera, perforation of the hollow, air-filled viscera, or tears and hematoma formation at the ligamentous attachments of the liver and small bowel.[10] The spectrum of inflicted abdominal injuries varies from that seen in accidental abdominal injury because the force of an inflicted blow is concentrated in the midepigastrium. Most inflicted injury will involve the small bowel (duodenal hematoma), liver lacerations, and pancreatic injury. A wider array of injury is seen in accident victims, involving kidneys, spleen, liver, and, to a much lesser extent, small bowel and pancreas.[11,17] Pancreatitis is rare in childhood, and trauma is the primary cause. Unless there is a history of significant injury to the epigastrium, nonaccidental injury must be strongly considered when pancreatitis is found in young children. Given the occult nature of nonaccidental abdominal trauma, CT scan of the abdomen is the evaluation of choice when intraabdominal trauma is being ruled out in child abuse victims.[4]

Child abuse consultants often screen for occult abdominal injury using hepatic transaminases. Lindberg and colleagues[18] conducted a multicentered prospective observational study of children younger than 60 months of age who were referred to a child abuse consultant for a physical abuse evaluation. Of the 1676 patients recruited to the study, 1276 were screened with hepatic transaminases (76%). Fifty-four (3.2%) of the 1276 screened patients were found to have abdominal injury on CT. The authors concluded that 3.2% does not justify routine screening for abdominal injury using CT. Of the 54 patients with verified abdominal injury, 14 (26%) had no clinical signs of abdominal injury and the decision to screen the child with CT was influenced by the child's hepatic transaminases. The authors used a threshold of 80 IU/L for either alanine aminotransferase or aspartate aminotransferase, which is a lower threshold than previous authors have used when studying the same question. Using a threshold of 80 IU/L, the sensitivity and specificity of hepatic transaminases as a screening tool for occult abdominal trauma were 77% and 82%, respectively.[18]

Thoracic Trauma

Beyond the pathognomonic rib fractures of child abuse, extensive thoracic trauma is rarely seen. A child's thoracic cage is so plastic and deformable that even in the absence of rib fractures, a child abuse victim could sustain compromising pulmonary injuries, namely, pneumothoraces, hemothoraces, or pulmonary contusions. As with abdominal trauma, the physician's index of suspicion must remain high to avoid delayed management of a life-threatening thoracic injury. The reader is referred to subsequent chapters of this text for detailed discussions of pediatric thoracic trauma.

Sexual Abuse

Physically abused children may also be sexually abused. When a patient is examined for evidence of physical trauma, a careful genital examination is warranted. Any evidence of old or new genital trauma must be documented with photographs. Genital trauma is usually subtle, difficult to recognize, and difficult to photograph. When possible, consult a physician who specializes in sexual abuse and who may be able to perform a noninvasive colposcopic examination of the external genitalia. The best photo documentation of genital injury is obtained with a colposcope. Of great significance, using colposcopy to videotape and photodocument a child's forensic exam eliminates the need for repeat examinations on the already traumatized sexual assault victim. If acute genital trauma is suspected or identified, a *rape kit* or forensic collection of evidence must be performed, and the police must be involved early in the process. The forensic evidence becomes legal documentation of the sexual assault, and a chain of evidence must be carefully maintained between the hospital and the forensic laboratory. All cultures must be collected in culture medium or broth. DNA probes for gonorrhea and chlamydia cannot be used as evidence in court. Ideally, evidence collection should occur before any washing of the genitalia, including before the skin prep for insertion of a Foley catheter. Speculum and bimanual examination of sexually abused children are not warranted unless there is concern about internal lacerations in need of surgical repair. To avoid the need for repeat examinations, a sexual abuse expert or pediatric gynecologist should perform this examination with the patient under anesthesia.[1]

Protocol for the Medical Investigation of Child Abuse

To ensure complete and objective evidence collection during the medical investigation of child abuse, we have established an investigative protocol for our institution that is based on the current medical literature. This protocol has worked well

---

BOX 122.1	Protocol for Medical Investigation of Child Abuse

Physical examination for skin and genital trauma
Photography of all injury
Skeletal survey for children <5 years
Bone scan (if skeletal survey results are negative)
CT head scan for children <3 years
Ophthalmology consultation to rule out retinal hemorrhage
Abdominal trauma laboratory values
Serum amylase/lipase
Liver enzymes
Urine analysis
CT abdomen scan
All nonverbal children
Positive findings from abdominal examination
Abnormal laboratory results

MRI of the head if AHT is identified on CT or is strongly suspected despite equivocal CT findings.

---

across all pediatric subspecialty services in our institution and has provided consistency when communication occurs with law enforcement, legal services, child protective services, and our community pediatricians (Box 122.1).

Fatal Child Abuse

Fatal child abuse is not merely a phenomenon of the 21st century. There have been reports of fatal child abuse throughout history. Caligula's daughter died of inflicted head trauma in AD 41. The French literature records the fatal whipping of a 4-year-old girl in the 1850s. In 1860, Professor Ambroise Tardieu published a paper describing fatal physical and sexual abuse inflicted on infants and children by parents. Tardieu's account listed thermal burns, fingernail imprints, contusions due to pinching, intracranial hemorrhages, and other injuries similar to those seen today. Likewise, these parents and caretakers offered explanations for the injuries that were incompatible with the severity of injury, such as falls during play or by other minor accidents. Knight[19] concluded, in his historical review of child abuse, that fatal child abuse is nothing new.

Eighty percent of fatal child abuse is caused by head injury. Because many of these children undergo surgical intervention before their death, the forensic pathologist/ME is often faced with an autopsy in which the injuries have been altered by surgical procedures. An exact description of the injuries present before treatment is essential: for example, the extent (amount), location, and radiologic information (CT, MRI, plain films) of all epidural, subdural, and subarachnoid hemorrhages. The chart must reference any biopsy specimens (usually blood clots) submitted to the pathology laboratory during surgical procedures. Documenting the extent and location of retinal hemorrhages may assist the forensic pathologist/ME during gross examination of the eyes. Although there are nontraumatic causes of retinal hemorrhage, CPR is not a common cause. The location and size (in inches/centimeters) and a brief description of any abrasions, lacerations, and contusions should be stated. With respect to contusions, the color on admission and on successive days should be recorded. Likewise, any skin breakdown following medical procedures, notably on the posterior scalp and neck, needs documentation.[20]

As previously stated, visceral trauma is the second leading cause of death in child abuse. Abdominal injuries include liver, spleen, intestinal, mesenteric, and renal contusions, lacerations, and rupture. There may be minimal external evidence of such catastrophic injuries. In the event that they are discovered during surgery, the amount of blood in the peritoneum and extent of organ damage should be carefully documented. Abdominal injuries resulting from CPR are extremely rare.[21]

Osseous Injury in Fatal Child Abuse

Fractures of bones in fatal child abuse are evidence. Documentation of the site of fracture (eg, metaphyseal distal femur), type of fracture (eg, transverse, spiral), and possible dating by x-ray analysis should be done on all cases. A head-to-toe approach with skeletal survey will aid the forensic pathologist/ME by locating injuries before the autopsy. During the autopsy, sections of these fractures are taken. Although some authorities consider histologic dating to be accurate, there are wide variations in the chronologic healing of fractures. Only an approximate time frame can be assigned to a fracture.[22] Osseous injuries will also alert the staff to possible nontraumatic causes such as osteogenesis imperfecta.

Scene Investigation in Fatal Child Abuse

The scene is where the infant became unresponsive, became apneic, or sustained injuries that led to hospital admission. It typically belongs to and is secured by law enforcement officers, so the earlier they become involved, the more timely and accurate the scene investigation will be. Emergency medical service (EMS) providers or firefighters are often the first to arrive on the scene. Their narrative description of the immediate circumstances and surroundings is a crucial part of scene investigation. They are encouraged to describe the place and position in which the child was found; the type of bed and bedding the child was found in; the presence of body fluids (blood, vomit, urine, feces) at the scene; the tidiness of the environment; and the presence of drugs, medications, drug paraphernalia, or alcohol at the scene. They often record the initial reactions of caretakers, identify potential witnesses to the preceding events, and discover other vulnerable children within the household. Talking to EMS providers on their arrival with the critically injured child can provide a wealth of information leading to early suggestions of child abuse/neglect, timely medical interventions, and early law enforcement and child protective services involvement.

Autopsy

The successful identification of tragic fatal child abuse cases depends on a team approach. Box 122.2 lists the minimal information desired by the forensic pathologist/ME before autopsy.[23] Clearly this list is best assembled as a collaborative

---

BOX 122.2   Scene Investigation Information

Law enforcement jurisdiction
Date, time, address of place of injury
Witnessed by whom (or unwitnessed)
First responders to scene
Field interventions (CPR, intubation, drugs)
Description of victim as found
Description of environment
Scene diagram (supplied by law enforcement)
Interviews with parents, caretakers, witnesses
Cardiopulmonary resuscitation

---

effort of EMS, law enforcement, and physicians. Ideally, representatives of the pediatric team, law enforcement, and the district attorney's office would attend the autopsy examination. Although law enforcement attendance is routine in all fatal child abuse cases, numerous constraints interfere with pediatric presence at autopsy. Minimally, a phone conversation between the ME and the pediatric attending physician is strongly recommended.

Organ Procurement Organization and Fatal Child Abuse

The limited supply of organs for transplantation is well known. Although all age groups are represented, there is a lower organ donation percentage in the pediatric age group because this group has a lower relative death rate. Thus the use of organs from the pediatric age group is critical. When a child or infant sustains injuries leading to brain death, organ procurement is sought by organ procurement organizations (OPOs). Initially, some forensic pathologists/MEs may deny the use of organs on the basis that it may cause problems with judicial procedures.[24] This is not absolute. All three agencies must examine each individual case. The district attorney, forensic pathologist/ME, and the pediatrician must work with the OPO to see if organs not damaged by injury may be used in transplantation. If all parties are satisfied, then a representative of the ME's office (ideally the forensic pathologist/ME who will do the autopsy) should be present when the organs are retrieved for transplantation. The interacting groups are listed in Box 122.3.

Documentation and Testifying in Court

Testimony of medical personnel begins with thorough and legible documentation in the medical record. Complete, rather than brief, documentation is strongly recommended, because trials may be delayed for months to years. Handwritten notes will become a memory lifeline during testimony. One must document information objectively. Be specific about where information originates. When recording conversations with caretakers, place their exact words in italics and write "per conversation with . . . ." Months to years later, one will not remember exactly who was interviewed or who actually said what is written in the chart. Written words may be misconstrued as opinion, and defense attorneys frequently make this an issue when witnesses testify to confuse or discredit testimony.

Testifying on behalf of a child who has been abused or murdered is emotional. Stick to the facts and remain objective. Remember that medical personnel are not the judge in this case. Stay calm, particularly when being cross-examined by the defense attorney, and remember that medical personnel and their work are not on trial. There is no urgency in court. Take the time you need to formulate answers. Responses should be brief and limited to the questions asked, unless one is specifically told to elaborate further. If a question is not

---

BOX 122.3   Key Groups Needed for Tissue Procurement

Pediatrician representing family's request
Organ procurement organization representative
Medical examiner's office
District attorney's office

understood, ask that it be clarified before an answer is given. If a detail (eg, a date, a time, a person's name) cannot be recalled, simply state so. One is allowed to refer to the medical records once they have been entered into medical evidence. If a witness does not think that he or she possesses the expertise to answer a question, then the witness should simply state so.

The more prepared one is, the less stressful the experience in court will be. It is the responsibility of medical personnel to review the medical records, laboratory reports, and radiologic studies before trial. If the prosecuting attorney is properly preparing the case, the attorney will meet with each witness before testimony is given. This meeting gives both the attorney and the witness a chance to clarify specific issues that will be raised in court and to discuss the limits of the testimony. One may be asked to submit an updated curriculum vitae to establish credentials. If one is being called as a fact-finding witness, the court will not solicit opinions. During the trial, one may be qualified as an expert witness in his or her medical subspecialty. Then, one will be allowed to express opinions more freely.

If one is called to testify again regarding the same case or if a deposition was given before trial, then previously recorded statements should be reviewed so that testimony remains consistent. It serves to keep the witness from becoming uncomfortably entangled in unintended contradiction and legal rhetoric when on the stand. Included in the following reference list are suggested readings that may be helpful when preparing for trial.[25-27]

References

1. Reese RM, Christian CW. *Child Abuse: Medical Diagnosis and Management.* 3rd ed. American Academy of Pediatrics; 2009.
2. Daria S, Sugar NF, Feldman KW, et al. Into hot water head first: distribution of intentional and unintentional immersion burns. *Pediatr Emerg Care.* 2004;20:302-310.
3. Andronicus M, Oates RK, Peat J, et al. Non-accidental burns in children. *Burns.* 1998;24:552.
4. Kleinman PK. *Diagnostic Imaging of Child Abuse.* 2nd ed. St. Louis: Mosby; 1998.
5. Dalton HJ, Slovis T, Helfer RE, et al. Undiagnosed abuse in children younger than 3 years with femoral fracture. *Am J Dis Child.* 1990;144:875.
6. Jenny C. Evaluating infants and young children with multiple fractures. *Pediatrics.* 2006;118:1299-1303.
7. Bruce D, Zimmerman RA. Shaken impact syndrome. *Pediatr Ann.* 1989;18:482.
8. Chiesa A, Duhaime AC. Abusive head trauma. *Pediatr Clin North Am.* 2009;56:317-331.
9. Parulekar MV, Elston JS. Neuropathology of inflicted head injury in children. *Brain.* 2002;125:676.
10. Cooper A, Floyd T, Barlow B, et al. Major blunt abdominal trauma due to child abuse. *J Trauma.* 1988;28:1483.
11. Ng CS, Hall CM, Shaw DG. The range of visceral manifestations of non-accidental injury. *Arch Dis Child.* 1997;77:167.
12. Fernando S, Obaldo RE, Walsh IR, Lowe LH. Neuroimaging of nonaccidental head trauma: pitfalls and controversies. *Pediatr Radiol.* 2008;38: 827-838.
13. Levin AV. Retinal hemorrhages: advances in understanding. *Pediatr Clin North Am.* 2009;56:333-344.
14. Gilliland MGF, Luckenbach MW. Are retinal hemorrhages found after resuscitation attempts? A study of the eyes of 169 children. *Am J Forensic Med Path.* 1993;14:187.
15. Morad Y, Kim YM, Armstrong DC, et al. Correlation between retinal abnormalities and intracranial abnormalities in the shaken baby syndrome. *Ophthalmol.* 2002;134:354.
16. Jenny C, Hymel KP, Ritzen A, et al. Analysis of missed cases of abusive head trauma. *JAMA.* 1999;281:621.
17. Trokel M, DiScala C, Terrin NC, Sege RD. Blunt abdominal injury in the young pediatric patient: child abuse and patient outcomes. *Child Maltreat.* 2004;9:111-117.
18. Lindberg D, Makoroff K, Harper N, et al. ULTRA Investigators. Utility of hepatic transaminases to recognize child abuse in children. *Pediatrics.* 2009;124:509-516.
19. Knight B. The history of child abuse. *Forensic Sci Int.* 1986;30:35.
20. Case ME, Graham MA, Handy TC, et al. Position paper on fatal abusive head injuries in infants and young children. *Am J Forensic Med.* 2001; 22:112.
21. Price EA, Rush LR, Perper JA, et al. Cardiopulmonary resuscitation-related injuries and homicidal blunt abdominal trauma in children. *Am J Forensic Med Pathol.* 2000;21:307.
22. Zumwalt RE, Fanizza-Orphanos AM. Dating of healing rib fractures in fatal child abuse. *Adv Pathol.* 1990;3:193.
23. Centers for Disease Control and Prevention. Guidelines for death scene investigation of sudden unexplained infant deaths. Recommendations of the Interagency Panel on Sudden Infant Death Syndrome. *MMWR Morb Mortal Wkly Rep.* 1996;45(RR-10):1-6.
24. Wetli CV, Kolovich RM, Dinhofer L. Modified cardiectomy. *Am J Forensic Med Pathol.* 2002;23:137.
25. Clayton EW. Potential liability in cases of child abuse and neglect. *Ped Ann.* 1997;26:173.
26. Hanes M, Mcauliff T. Preparation for child abuse litigation: perspectives of the prosecutor and the pediatrician. *Ped Ann.* 1997;26:288.
27. Wall N. Judicial attitudes to expert evidence in children's cases. *Arch Dis Child.* 1997;76:485.

Violence-Associated Injury Among Children

Jesus Peinado and Marie Leiner

PEARLS

- Exposure to violent media, access to firearms and use of drugs and alcohol are associated with increasingly violent behavior.
- Violence can take many different forms. Identification and screening for violent experiences, identification of children at risk, and early intervention in the clinic and emergency departments can be effective in decreasing future violence.
- In the United States, children are more likely than adults to be exposed to violence and crime.
- Children who are exposed to violence experience short-term and long-term physical, mental, and emotional harm.
- Any single form of adverse childhood experience is likely to be accompanied by others. Exposure to violence is recognized as an adverse childhood experience.
- Violence-associated injury among children is neither randomly nor evenly distributed within the population but rather is focused on particular individuals within particular settings, which emphasizes the importance of recognizing that certain children experience higher risks.
- The effects that result from physical injury may be either physical or a combination of physical and psychologic. Physical and psychologic injuries occur in children who are victims, aggressors, or bystanders. It is important to emphasize that psychologic injuries may occur in the absence of physical injuries.
- Psychologic effects of exposure to violence are independent of the child's role as a victim, aggressor, or bystander and might not become apparent for days or even years.
- An episode of violence-associated injury may be one in a series of adverse events. The eventual emotional outcome will reflect the cumulative load.
- Although current practice is symptom reactive, a more comprehensive approach is necessary to prevent the impact of adverse childhood experiences on adolescent and adult health risks, health status, and social functioning.

Physical-Related Injuries in Children

Violence is the intentional use of physical force or power, threatened or actual, against oneself, another person, or a group or community. It results in, or has a high likelihood of resulting in injury, death, psychologic harm, maldevelopment, or deprivation. Violence is a major cause of death and disability of young people. It is a major health problem in children whether their role is perpetrator, victim, or witness.

Children are particularly vulnerable to violence and injury because of developmental issues, including independence and autonomy, curiosity leading to experimentation (eg, alcohol, drugs, sex), peer group pressure, immaturity, impulsivity, feelings of invincibility, narcissism, and the development of self-identity.[1] Physical trauma caused by violence is primarily linked to physical injuries, while psychologic trauma may or may not involve physical injuries. Its effects are almost always detrimental to the child's emotional and psychosocial well-being. In addition to potentially causing injury and death, violence affects communities by increasing the cost of health care, reducing productivity, decreasing property values, and disrupting social services.[2]

The most common circumstances causing injury are arguments (40%), assaults (20%), and crimes other than assaults (4%). Relationships between the patient and others involved in the incident include friends or schoolmates (38%), siblings or other family members (10%), and strangers (9%). These injurious events may occur on the street, at school, or in the home. Most violence-related injuries are minor. Stabs, cuts, and injuries due to a firearm or blunt object have been described in up to 25% of all injuries. Gun violence poses a serious threat to children and youth. The majority of youth who are murdered are killed with a firearm and nearly one-half of youth suicide deaths involve the use of a gun.[3]

In 2010, there were 2711 infant, child, and teen deaths associated with firearms. On average, there are 7 firearm-related fatalities daily and 52 weekly. Most school-associated student homicides involve a firearm and a single victim and offender.[4] In 2011, 5% of high school students carried a gun on school property and 7% were threatened or injured by a weapon (eg, gun, knife, club) on school property.

Victimization and Perpetration

Some populations are especially vulnerable to victimization. There are well-known risk factors that may not directly cause violence but do contribute to it. Evidence shows an increased risk of being victimized in the context of partner violence. Renner and Slack[5] found that childhood physical and sexual abuse predicted intimate partner violence (IPV) victimization later in life. Other data from East Asia and the Pacific Region reported that children who had been sexually abused had a threefold increase in the risk of IPV victimization later in life.[6]

Risk factors for victimization can be classified into different categories:

Individual risk factors (biological and personal)
- Children younger than 4 years of age
- Children with special care needs
- Early aggressive behaviors
- History of victimization
- Developmental problems
- Learning disorders or disabilities
- Low IQ/low level of education
- High stress levels
- Conflict and violence in the family

Family
- Low parental involvement
- Low parental education and income
- Dysfunctional families
- Poor supervision
- Social isolation
- Family disorganization
- Intimate partner violence
- Parental substance abuse or crime

Community and society
- Schools
- Gender
- Societal norms
- Economic/social policies
- Community violence
- Disadvantaged neighborhood

Protective factors include attributes, characteristics, or elements that decrease the likelihood that violence will be perpetrated.

Settings and Forms of Violence

Child Maltreatment

Child maltreatment represents a major public health concern in the United States and abroad. In the United States in 2012, approximately 3.4 million children were referred to child protective service agencies for suspected abuse or neglect; approximately 686,000 children were determined by state and local child protective service agencies to be the victims of maltreatment. In 2012, an estimated 1640 children died from child maltreatment (rate of 2.2 per 100,000 children). Of child maltreatment fatalities in 2012, 70% occurred among children younger than age 3.[7]

School Violence

School violence is youth violence that occurs on school property, on the way to or from school or school-sponsored events, or during a school-sponsored event. A young person can be a victim, a perpetrator, or a witness of school violence.[8] Youth violence includes behaviors such as bullying, pushing, and shoving, which can cause more emotional harm than physical harm. Other forms of violence, such as gang violence and assault (with or without weapons), can lead to serious injury or death.

In 2012, there were approximately 749,200 school-related nonfatal violent victimizations among students 12 to 18 years of age. Approximately 9% of teachers reported that they have been threatened with injury by a student from their school; 5% of school teachers reported that they had been physically attacked by a student from their school.[8,9]

In a 2013 nationally representative survey of youth in grades 9 to 12, 8.1% of students reported being in a physical fight on school property in the 12 months before the survey. It is not surprising that 7.1% of students reported that they did not go to school on one or more days in the 30 days before the survey because they felt unsafe at school or on their way to or from school. Of surveyed students 5.2% reported carrying a weapon (gun, knife, or club) on school property on 1 or more days in the 30 days before the survey, and 6.9% of students reported being threatened or injured with a weapon on school property one or more times in the 12 months before the survey. Additionally, 19.6% of surveyed students reported being bullied on school property and 14.8% reported being bullied electronically during the 12 months before the survey.[9]

The rates of victimization were greater for males than for females 12 to 18 years of age and greater for those residing in urban and suburban areas than for those residing in rural areas.[10] During the 2011–12 school year, a higher percentage of public than private teachers reported being threatened with injury (10% vs. 3%) or being physically attacked (6% vs. 3%) by a student from their school. Injury and violence are highly prevalent in disadvantaged subgroups of the population, and social disadvantages are associated with life circumstances that place an individual at an increased risk to sustain certain types of injuries.

School-based preventive programs, family-based programs, and street outreach programs can lower the rates of violence and aggressive behaviors when implemented early in a child's life. These programs develop skills that include self-awareness and control, problem-solving, and conflict resolution.

Media Violence

Exposure to media violence does not have identical effects to exposure to real-life violence. Though their effects are not identical, most studies of media violence report that watching and playing violent media cause short- and long-term aggressive feelings, thoughts, and behaviors. Evidence suggests that one of the most potent ways to teach aggression to young viewers is to coach the behavior in a moral context.

The average child between 2 and 5 years of age watches 20 to 30 hours of television a week and spends 9 to 10 hours per week playing videos games. Both exposures are increasingly filled with scenes of violence, not only on commercial television but also on news outlets. In the media, violence is a quick and effective ending for disagreements and ignores the importance of patience, negotiation, and compromise in resolving conflicts and disagreements.[3]

The General Aggression Model explains the development of conditions, attitudes, and behaviors, including how exposure to media violence contributes to the enhancement of mitigation of these aggressive behaviors.[11] In the short term, the General Aggression Model predicts that violent media exposure can affect arousal, aggressive thoughts, and aggressive feelings, which in turn can influence aggressive behaviors.

Regarding long-term exposure to violent content, evidence suggests that repeated episodes of viewing media violence may result in the development, overlearning, and reinforcement of aggression-related knowledge structures, with the belief that aggressive solutions are both effective and appropriate.[12-14]

Exposure to violent media is considered to promote a higher tolerance for violence,[15] moral disengagement and lack of empathy,[16] hypothetical delinquency, and attention deficit disorder in youth.[17,18]

While relational and verbal aggression are more socially acceptable (and carry a lower risk of punishment for the individual), these forms of aggression are more likely to be expressed after exposure to media violence.

Health care professionals should counsel and advise families to have more control over access to violent media and encourage them to reduce exposure to violent media content. Parents should be aware of all the risks associated with violent media exposure to assist their children appropriately according to their developmental level, making sure that violent actions are not learned.

Bullying

Bullying is one type of youth violence that affects and threatens children's well-being. It has been estimated that more than 2 million youth in the United States are involved in bullying as bullies, victims, or both, and the prevalence of bullying among American teens and preteens is approximately 30%. With the alarming increase in school violence, specifically acts of aggression, it is important to inquire about all possibilities related to aggressive behaviors that may implicate bullying.[19]

Bullying is a public health problem that involves physical, verbal, and psychologic forms of aggression and has been defined as any repeated negative action or aggression intended to harm or bother someone who is perceived as being less physically or psychologically powerful than the aggressor within the context of an ongoing social interaction.[20]

Various factors have been associated with being a bully, a victim, or both, including age (with bullying being more frequent in younger individuals), a lower socioeconomic status, and a lower parents' educational level.[19,21-23] Poor health status, increased health care needs, mental health status, and physical appearance have been associated with being bullied, as have loneliness, lack of social interactions, poor social adjustment, poor academic achievement, and sexual orientation. No substantial differences according to gender have been observed in terms of the frequency of being bullied.[24-30] Youth involved in bullying often experience higher levels of health and academic problems, and they have worse emotional and psychologic adjustment than uninvolved youth.

Those involved in bullying may also experience health problems (psychologic, behavioral, and substance abuse), academic difficulties, and safety and violence issues. Bullying affects youth from all ethnic, cultural, socioeconomic, and gender groups. Carrying weapons has been associated with both being a bully and being a victim of bullying.

Primary care providers must be aware of the potential psychosocial problems that bully, victims, and bully-victims may experience as a result of bullying and be knowledgeable about the interventions available; these include using a multidisciplinary approach involving the parents and children, as well as the school system, and providing appropriate and timely referrals when needed to assist children involved in bullying.[31]

School-based interventions have been shown to be effective in reducing bullying. Other potentially effective components of school-based programs include a well-enforced school antibullying policy, increased student supervision, and parental involvement.

The invaluable contributions of David Finkelhor and colleagues[7,32-34] to the longitudinal study of specific trends in youth exposure to violence, crime, and abuse in the United States have demonstrated a steady decline over the past decade. These results seem to reflect actual reductions, as well as measures not considered that may contain a more contemporary spectrum and scope of violence-associated injury among children. It is clear that environmental changes within their communities expose today's youth to new forms of violence.[35] Thus there is a need to understand and improve the measurements of existing trends, as well as create new measurements. In particular, although previously established trends of victimization may be in decline, children and adolescents may be exposed to violence in the same or more sophisticated ways. It is possible that this perceived decline has revealed only the tip of the iceberg, allowing us to observe other interrelated factors related to violence injury in children.

Psychologic Injury and Psychosocial and Behavior–Related Effects

An episode of violence-associated injury in a child is usually accompanied by visible and invisible factors that should be considered in the current and future treatment of the child. It is important for the practitioner to examine the factors that influence a child's physical and psychosocial well-being after experiencing a traumatic event, because these factors are often difficult to isolate, define, and quantify. In particular, factors related to psychosocial well-being are often overlooked due to their nonspecific presentation and the clinician's unfamiliarity.

An event might involve a combination of physical and psychologic injuries or physical or psychologic injuries only. For one event in which physical injury is involved, a pediatric patient may play the role of the victim, aggressor, or bystander. However, in another event with the same or different participants, these roles easily can be switched such that the victim plays the role of the aggressor, demonstrating the existence of different but concurrent pathways.[36-38]

The effects resulting from physical injury might include physical only or a combination of physical and psychologic effects. Although physical and psychologic injuries occur in children who are victims, aggressors, and bystanders, it is important to emphasize that psychologic injury might occur in the absence of physical injuries. Children exposed to violence-associated injury might experience short- and/or long-term psychosocial and emotional effects. Short-term effects can include child distress, emotional dysregulation,[39] attention deficit hyperactivity disorder (ADHD),[40] anger, depression, anxiety, posttraumatic stress disorder (PTSD),[41] and conduct disorders. Long-term consequences include internalized and externalized psychologic problems such as revictimization,[15] adult depression,[42] somatic problems, aggression, and PTSD. They also include behavioral problems such as substance abuse[43] and health risk behaviors.[44] All these problems are additionally linked to suicidality,[45] obesity, hypertension, and cardiovascular diseases,[46-48] as well as failure in school, incarceration, poverty, and an unproductive[49] and unhappy life as an adult.

Disproportionate Distribution of Violence-Related Injury Among Children

Effect of Inequalities

Violence-associated injuries among children are neither randomly nor evenly distributed within the population but rather are focused on particular individuals within particular settings, which emphasizes the importance of recognizing that certain children experience higher risks.[50] These children, who occupy marginal or subordinate positions within peer hierarchies, will be more susceptible to violence associated with both physical and psychologic injury.[51]

Inequalities due to poverty and low socioeconomic status particularly increase contact with violent events in the child's daily life, including in their house, neighborhood, and/or school.[52] The parents of these children are likely to experience severe stress and depression, both of which are linked to poor social and emotional outcomes for their children. In addition to a lack of financial resources, these parents cannot provide their children with the human and social experiences that are essential for children to thrive and grow into healthy, productive adults. Mental health services, including detection, referral, and treatment, are often described as inadequate in those confronted by inequalities. Several communication barriers such as culture, linguistic elements, and literacy levels contribute to these disparities.[53-55]

Interconnections Between Injury, Adversity, Exposure to Violence, and Victimization and Revictimization

A practitioner that is in contact with a child who has confronted an episode of violence injury must consider that (1) this adverse episode might occur again; (2) it might not be the only adversity confronted by the child; and (3) its effects will resonate beyond the end of the consultation. Because any single form of adverse childhood experience is more likely to be related to other adverse experiences,[15,56] this co-occurrence is important to consider when identifying and treating children who have been exposed to any type of violence-related injury.[57,58] Focusing on only the current event of violence exposure may substantially underestimate the burden of exposure and fail to adequately capture the impact of possible psychologic injury.[59,60]

Effect of Adverse Childhood Experiences

An episode of violence-associated injury in a child may be just one in a series of adverse events. The emotional outcome will always reflect the cumulative load. Although the current practice is symptom reactive, a more comprehensive approach is necessary to prevent the invariable matching of adverse childhood experiences against adult and adolescent health risks, health status, and social functioning.[61]

The Centers for Disease Control–Kaiser Adverse Childhood Experiences (ACE) study is considered to be a groundbreaking public health investigation into the short- and long-term effects of childhood trauma. This study, which is the largest of its kind to be conducted, evaluated more than 17,000 study participants to assess childhood exposure to multiple types of adversity. The initial ACE study found that two-thirds of the participants reported at least one adverse childhood experience. Of those, 87% reported at least one other adverse childhood experience, 70% reported 2 or more, and more than 20% reported 3 or more. The findings of this study demonstrate the harmful, immediate, and long-lasting effects that adversity has on child development. The immediate cognitive effects include attention problems, learning disorders, and poor school performance. Children threatened with adversity-related trauma may suffer decades later from chronic disease and mental illness, as well as aggressive and violent behaviors. Behavioral consequences include lower or null social skills, depression, anxiety, and antisocial and violent behavior. The basic findings of the original study have been independently replicated with similar results, which increases the spectrum of adverse experiences considered.[62,63]

Adverse childhood experiences include verbal, physical, or sexual abuse and family dysfunction, as well as poverty. Adverse childhood experiences do not occur independently but instead are intercorrelated such that the combined effects of two or more adverse childhood experiences may be greater than their sum. In addition, adverse childhood experiences make individuals more vulnerable to suffering from the same or new adverse experiences, which are often triggered by their own actions as a result of disturbances to their development caused by their earlier experiences.[64]

Pervasive Effect of Violence Exposure

Exposure to violence is recognized as an adverse childhood experience and a form of victimization that has been documented in both retrospective and prospective studies as a basic cause of morbidity and mortality in adults.[65-67] Single or intermittent stress responses from this exposure affect child development and profile the future behavior of the child as both a victim and perpetrator. Thus a cycle occurs with outcomes that often interact such that the child turns to one, a few, or all of the following: victim to further victim either at home or the community, victim to child abuser, victim to perpetrator of violence against his or her own partner, or victim to perpetrator in the community as an antisocial offender.[68]

Although adverse experiences confronted by a child have an effect on his or her adult health and behavior, exposure to violence when encountered at any time during the life span from birth to adulthood almost invariably produces more violence. Systematic efforts to assess these connections have found an overlap among different forms of violence; even diverse and unrelated forms of violence are linked to such an extreme that it can be difficult to identify a group of individuals that have sustained or perpetrated only a single form of violence.[69]

Excessive or prolonged activation of stress response systems in a child can have damaging effects on learning, behavior, and health across the life span. Learning to cope with adversity is an important part of child development. Both adults and children confront stressful moments in life with increases in heart rate and blood pressure and the production of stress hormones. Although the physiologic responses of children and adults are similar, the child's inability to use the resources that experience and maturity give to an adult leaves the child more vulnerable. When the child's response to a stressful situation is activated within an environment of supportive relationships with adults, the damaging effects are buffered and brought back to baseline. Under these circumstances, the child develops a healthy stress response system. However, prolonged chronic stress and frequent stress response activation without the presence of buffering relationships can disrupt the development of brain architecture and other organ systems with lifelong consequences. For example, abuse during early childhood/adolescence is associated with a reduced hippocampal volume and subsequent problems with memory and PTSD risk. This adversity has been associated during later adolescence with a diminished frontal cortex volume, which has been implicated in externalizing behavioral problems. Gray matter abnormalities in regions that form affective and inferior frontal cognitive networks suggest a disturbance in the normal development of these networks as a consequence of early adversities and chronic stress, causing cognitive and emotional problems.[70]

Victimization and Revictimization
Adult health is highly impacted by the cumulative burden of victimization with abnormalities that may not manifest until adulthood.[71] Studies have found that women experiencing exposure to gender-based violence between 2 and 10 years of age had more than 18 times the odds of developing a lifetime mood/anxiety disorder or substance abuse disorder.[58] Exposure of adolescents to community violence was particularly associated with elevated symptoms of anger, and this exposure predicted levels of externalizing problems and trauma symptomatology over and above the effects of child maltreatment.[72]

Revictimization studies indicate that victims of violence are often exposed to multiple types and occurrences of victimization.[73] The process underlying the theoretic approaches that explains this recurrence indicates that victims exposed to violence learn and develop differently from those who have not been exposed.[74] Victimization will predispose youth to a lack of learning of social, copying, and negotiation skills, as well as make wrongful assumptions about the effect of violent tactics that are considered as successful, acceptable, and appropriate. It has also been mentioned that victims who use avoidant strategies to manage emotions will have difficulties with detecting the signals of a dangerous situation, which in turn leads to missing the opportunity to avoid the risks involved.[75] Among young children, revictimization problems often occur within the same family. Sibling victimization tends to include recurrent episodes, with studies reporting a high prevalence and association of similar experiences with peers.[76,77] Victimization by a sibling is predictive of peer victimization for children and adolescents with elevated mental health distress.[78] Recognition of injury episodes involving sibling victimization is more frequent among children than adolescents.

Detecting and Referring Children for Further Treatment
Psychologic effects on children after exposure to violence independent from the child's role as the victim, aggressor, or bystander might not be apparent for a few days, months, or years after the incident. In addition, existing psychologic problems, adversity, and previous victimization can further aggravate the situation. Recognizing that short- to long-term effects depend on previous victimization, age, and the level of adversity to which the child is exposed, as well as any previous psychosocial or behavioral problems, provides a comprehensive spectrum of what to expect and consider for follow-up.

Studies suggest that one in five children and adolescents may have a pediatric mental, emotional, or behavioral disorder that needs to be identified and requires treatment. The crucial role of early intervention services to improve outcomes for children with developmental and mental health problems has a tremendous impact on children's lives, as well as the lives

of their families and society as a whole. Child assessment relies heavily on accurate and appropriate screening, which is recommended to occur at every opportunity, including general health care visits, nonemergency visits, and visits to the emergency department.[79,80] Clinical judgment alone is an insensitive means to identify developmental and behavioral problems,[81] particularly among minority or non–English-speaking children and parents.[82]

Assessments that (1) provide a wider psychosocial profile of the child to adolescence, (2) are standardized by gender and age, and (3) are validated in different languages are recommended. However, most of these assessments require staff to score the responses of parents or guardians to interpret the results. Standardized scales to detect psychologic and behavioral problems can provide precise information about the child with certain restrictions. For example, these assessment scales can screen for the risks of a disorder but cannot provide a diagnosis. The results obtained can be confounded by communication disparities among those responding to the scales. The majority of these communication problems can be attributed to disparities due to lower levels of education, lack of language proficiency, low literacy, and cultural differences.[83,84] The validation of the psychometric properties of these scales in different languages needs to be considered when selecting either a low or broadband scale for screening specific problems. When the child is old enough to respond, it is important to obtain both self-reports and parental reports to better assess the problem.

Several behavioral and emotional screening tools are available in the public domain, as reported by the Committee on Psychosocial Aspects of Child and Family Health, Council on Early Childhood and Society for Developmental and Behavioral Pediatrics.[85] One of the most popular assessment tools available is the Child Behavior Checklist, which provides information about behavioral and emotional disorders.[86] This assessment tool provides a full spectrum of emotional or behavioral problems among children from 18 months to 18 years old with detailed documentation for deciding what action to take with respect to referral to specialists.

Challenges for Follow-Up and Opportunities for a Teachable Moment
It is uncommon to expect youth to open up about psychologic distress during a traumatic episode.[87] In addition, engaging young people and their parents in mental health services is a recognized challenge, especially among those from a lower socioeconomic status or minority backgrounds. Referrals for follow-up might not occur in many cases due to economic, cultural, health literacy, language proficiency, and educational disparities. Therefore, additional counseling is required to inform parents and youth about the benefits of follow-up sessions.

The teachable moment after a medical incident in the emergency department is a technique that motivates individuals to become more receptive to behavioral change interventions following a traumatic event.[88] Most violent victimization acts are preventable.[89] The teachable moment can be used as a parental intervention. It is crucial to engage the parents as important agents of change, as well as partners for treatment goals that include the environment to achieve better functioning and developmental trajectories.[90] Their influence has been shown to have a significant impact on the emotional health of children even when families are subjected to extreme adversity.[91] Although there is no theoretic model that will predict with certainty which individuals will become aggressive, most theories produce acceptable results in predictions of a nonviolent outcome when all negative factors are removed.[92] However, these findings also suggest the existence of factors that mitigate the harmful effects of adversity, inequalities, and exposure to violence above the child's own resilience factors, which need to be considered and nurtured to make a difference in the life of a child. Positive social relationships, including the positive atmosphere of siblings and other family members, can buffer emotional and behavioral disturbance, which can be attained by providing parental education.[93]

Key References

7. Finkelhor D, Turner HA, Shattuck A, Hamby SL. Violence, crime, and abuse exposure in a national sample of children and youth: an update. *JAMA Pediatr.* 2013;167:614-621.

12. Anderson CA, Berkowitz L, Donnerstein E, et al. The influence of media violence on youth. *Psychol Sci Public Interest.* 2003;4:81-110.

13. Anderson CA, Gentile DA, Buckley KE. Violent video game effects on children and adolescents. *Theory Res Public Policy.* Oxford University Press; 2007.

20. Olweus D. *Bullying at School.* New York, NY: Springer Publishing Company; 1994.

21. Olweus D. *Bullying at School: What We Know and What We Can Do.* Hoboken, NJ: Wiley; 1993.

32. Finkelhor D, Vanderminden J, Turner H, et al. Child maltreatment rates assessed in a national household survey of caregivers and youth. *Child Abuse Neglect.* 2014;38:1421-1435.

33. Finkelhor D, Shattuck A, Turner HA, Hamby SL. Trends in children's exposure to violence, 2003 to 2011. *JAMA Pediatr.* 2014;168:540-546.

50. Anda R, Tietjen G, Schulman E, et al. Adverse childhood experiences and frequent headaches in adults. *Headache.* 2010;50:1473-1481.

51. Boyce WT. Social stratification, health, and violence in the very young. *Ann N Y Acad Sci.* 2004;1036:47-68.

52. Wade R Jr, Shea JA, Rubin D, Wood J. Adverse childhood experiences of low-income urban youth. *Pediatrics.* 2014;134:e13-e20.

53. Baker DW, Gazmararian JA, Sudano J, et al. Health literacy and performance on the Mini-Mental State Examination. *Aging Ment Health.* 2002;6:22-29.

54. Baker DW, Gazmararian JA, Williams MV, et al. Functional health literacy and the risk of hospital admission among Medicare managed care enrollees. *Am J Public Health.* 2002;92:1278-1283.

55. Leyva M, Sharif I, Ozuah PO. Health literacy among Spanish-speaking Latino parents with limited English proficiency. *Ambul Pediatr.* 2005; 5:56-59.

56. Dong M, Anda RF, Felitti VJ, et al. The interrelatedness of multiple forms of childhood abuse, neglect, and household dysfunction. *Child Abuse Neglect.* 2004;28:771-784.

57. Dube SR, Anda RF, Whitfield CL, et al. Long-term consequences of childhood sexual abuse by gender of victim. *Am J Prevent Med.* 2005;28: 430-438.

58. Walsh K, Keyes KM, Koenen KC, Hasin D. Lifetime prevalence of gender-based violence in US women: associations with mood/anxiety and substance use disorders. *J Psychiatr Res.* 2015.

59. Becker-Blease KA, Turner HA, Finkelhor D. Disasters, victimization, and children's mental health. *Child Dev.* 2010;81:1040-1052.

60. Finkelhor D, Ormrod R, Turner H, Hamby SL. The victimization of children and youth: a comprehensive, national survey. *Child Maltreat.* 2005;10:5-25.

61. Felitti VJ. Adverse childhood experiences and adult health. *Acad Pediatr.* 2009;9:131-132.

62. Brewer-Smyth K, Cornelius ME, Pickelsimer EE. Childhood adversity, mental health, and violent crime. *J Forensic Nurs.* 2015;11:4-14.

63. Shonkoff JP, Garner AS, et al. Committee on Psychosocial Aspects of C, Family H, Committee on Early Childhood A, Dependent C, et al. The lifelong effects of early childhood adversity and toxic stress. *Pediatrics.* 2012;129:e232-e246.

64. Bowlby J. *A Secure Base: Clinical Application of Attachment Theory.* London and New York: Routlege Classics; 2005.

65. Felitti VJ, Anda RF, Nordenberg D, et al. Relationship of childhood abuse and household dysfunction to many of the leading causes of death in adults. The Adverse Childhood Experiences (ACE) Study. *Am J Prevent Med.* 1998;14:245-258.

66. Chapman DP, Whitfield CL, Felitti VJ, et al. Adverse childhood experiences and the risk of depressive disorders in adulthood. *J Affect Disord.* 2004;82:217-225.

67. Dong M, Giles WH, Felitti VJ, et al. Insights into causal pathways for ischemic heart disease: adverse childhood experiences study. *Circulation.* 2004;110:1761-1766.

68. Dixon L, Browne K. The heterogeneity of spouse abuse: a review. *Aggress Violent Behav.* 2003;8:107-130.

69. Hamby SL, Grych J. Johnson RJ, ed. *The Web of Violence: Exploring Connections Among Different Forms of Interpersonal Violence and Abuse.* New York: Springer Dordrecht Heidelberg; 2013.

70. Lim L, Radua J, Rubia K. Gray matter abnormalities in childhood maltreatment: a voxel-wise meta-analysis. *Am J Psychiatry.* 2014;171:854-863.

71. Cloitre M, Stolbach BC, Herman JL, et al. A developmental approach to complex PTSD: childhood and adult cumulative trauma as predictors of symptom complexity. *J Trauma Stress.* 2009;22:399-408.

72. Cecil CA, Viding E, Barker ED, et al. Double disadvantage: the influence of childhood maltreatment and community violence exposure on adolescent mental health. *J Child Psychol Psychiatry.* 2014;55: 839-848.

73. Turner HA, Finkelhor D, Ormrod R. The effect of lifetime victimization on the mental health of children and adolescents. *Soc Sci Med.* 2006;62:13-27.

74. DePrince AP, Chu AT, Labus J, et al. Testing two approaches to revictimization prevention among adolescent girls in the child welfare system. *J Adolescent Health.* 2015;56(suppl 2):S33-S39.

75. Zamir O, Lavee Y. Psychological mindedness as a protective factor against revictimization in intimate relationships. *J Clin Psychol.* 2014;70: 847-859.

76. Tucker CJ, Finkelhor D, Turner H, Shattuck AM. Family dynamics and young children's sibling victimization. *J Fam Psychol.* 2014;28: 625-633.

77. Turner HA, Finkelhor D, Ormrod R, Hamby SL. Infant victimization in a nationally representative sample. *Pediatrics.* 2010;126:44-52.

78. Tucker CJ, Finkelhor D, Turner H, Shattuck AM. Sibling and peer victimization in childhood and adolescence. *Child Abuse Neglect.* 2014;38:1599-1606.

79. Grupp-Phelan J, McGuire L, Husky MM, Olfson M. A randomized controlled trial to engage in care of adolescent emergency department patients with mental health problems that increase suicide risk. *Pediatr Emerg Care.* 2012;28:1263-1268.

80. Williams JR, Ho ML, Grupp-Phelan J. The acceptability of mental health screening in a pediatric emergency department. *Pediatr Emerg Care.* 2011;27:611-615.

81. Brown JD, Wissow LS. Screening to identify mental health problems in pediatric primary care: considerations for practice. *Int J Psychiatry Med.* 2010;40:1-19.

82. Sheldrick RC, Merchant S, Perrin EC. Identification of developmental-behavioral problems in primary care: a systematic review. *Pediatrics.* 2011;128:356-363.

83. Weiss BD, Mays MZ, Martz W, et al. Quick assessment of literacy in primary care: the newest vital sign. *Ann Fam Med.* 2005;3:514-522.

84. Guerra CE, Krumholz M, Shea JA. Literacy and knowledge, attitudes and behavior about mammography in Latinas. *J Health Care Poor Underserved.* 2005;16:152-166.

85. Weitzman C, Wegner L. Promoting optimal development: screening for behavioral and emotional problems. *Pediatrics.* 2015;135:384-395.

86. Achenbach TM, Ruffle TM. The child behavior checklist and related forms for assessing behavioral/emotional problems and competencies. *Pediatr Rev.* 2000;21:265-271.

87. Viswanathan S, Datta S, Sheridan P, Lax-Pericall T. "Too young to be worried!" Psychiatric assessment and follow-up of young people after severe physical assault in an inner city hospital of South London. *Ann Med Health Sci Res.* 2014;4:85-89.

88. Zonfrillo MR, Melzer-Lange M, Gittelman MA. A comprehensive approach to pediatric injury prevention in the emergency department. *Pediatr Emerg Care.* 2014;30:56-62.

89. Duke NN, Borowsky IW. Adolescent interpersonal violence: implications for health care professionals. *Prim Care.* 2014;41:671-689.

90. Lieberman AF, Chu A, Van Horn P, Harris WW. Trauma in early childhood: empirical evidence and clinical implications. *Dev Psychopathol.* 2011;23:397-410.

91. Betancourt TS, McBain RK, Newnham EA, Brennan RT. The intergenerational impact of war: longitudinal relationships between caregiver and child mental health in postconflict Sierra Leone. *J Child Psychol Psychiatry and Allied Disciplines.* 2015;56(10):1101-1117.

92. Haas H, Cusson M. Comparing theories' performance in predicting violence. *Int J Law Psychiatry.* 2015;38:75-83.

93. Rutter M. Annual research review: resilience—clinical implications. *J Child Psychol Psychiatry.* 2013;54:474-487.

Pharmacology and Toxicology

Section XII

Pharmacology and Toxicology

Principles of Drug Disposition in the Critically Ill Child

Jeffrey L. Blumer

PEARLS

- Studies devoted to the disposition of drugs in critically ill patients and children are limited.
- Therapeutics is the branch of pharmacology concerned with the use of drugs for their therapeutic effects. It focuses on four fundamental questions that can serve as an outline for the clinician designing any pharmacotherapeutic plan: what drug, what dose, what route, and how long?
- Drug disposition is controlled by pharmacokinetics and pharmacodynamics. Pharmacokinetics is the discipline within clinical pharmacology that broadly describes the changes in the quantity of drug or drug metabolite in various body compartments over time. Whereas pharmacokinetics describes what the body does to the drug, pharmacodynamics encompasses the pharmacologic aspects that impact how the drug affects the body.
- Pharmacokinetic processes that influence drug disposition include absorption, distribution, metabolism, and excretion. Both ontogeny and critical illness may significantly impact any of these processes. Metabolism may be further affected by genetic differences in involved enzymes.
- Ontogeny and critical illness affect pharmacodynamics in infants and children, although formal study of these effects is limited.
- Pharmacotherapeutic strategies that can be used in the critically ill patient include the target concentration and target effect strategies. The target concentration strategy relies on the concentration of drug in blood or plasma (usually) to guide therapy; this approach is best applied to drugs used chronically for signs or symptoms that manifest intermittently. The target effect strategy, the strategy most commonly used in the pediatric intensive care unit, relies on an accepted clinical end point to determine drug dosing; clinical evidence of toxicity also impacts dosing. The latter strategy probably is the most reliable means by which to administer the right amount of drug to a highly variable patient population.

Pharmacology is the study of the interaction between chemical agents and biological systems. When these chemical agents are used with the intent of palliating or curing disease, the agents are termed *drugs*. Perhaps nowhere is drug therapy more important than in critical care. In this setting, however, drug

response often is difficult to predict. Physiologic aberrations and coincident pharmacologic and nonpharmacologic therapies may thwart intended drug effects. For the pediatric intensive care physician, pharmacotherapeutic decisions are further complicated by ontogenetic differences in drug processing and response. Finally, experience upon which to base pharmacotherapeutic expectations or prescription is sparse. Most drugs used in the intensive care setting have never been formally investigated in critically ill patients, let alone in children. As such, it is imperative that the pediatric intensive care physician have an understanding of the pharmacologic and related developmental constructs that influence drug response in patients.

The discipline of therapeutics provides a useful outline by which to design and monitor drug treatment. *Therapeutics* is the branch of pharmacology concerned with the use of drugs for their salubrious effects. It focuses on four fundamental questions pertaining to drug therapy as it relates to patient care: what drug, what dose, what route, and how long? The task of answering these important questions is facilitated by an understanding of the general pharmacologic principles that dictate drug response and the factors that lead to variation among patients.

Drug Disposition in Infants and Children

It should come as no surprise that controversy exists regarding drug dosing in pediatric patients. Over the years, a number of dosing rules been developed with the intent that drugs be safely administered to young children. All these rules depend on the standard adult dose with a scale-down factor based on body weight or age. However, distinct differences in pharmacokinetics and pharmacodynamics (Box 124.1) distinguish the pediatric patient from the adult patient. Critical illness may further alter pharmacokinetics and pharmacodynamics in children. These differences must be recognized before providing safe and effective dosing and during the initial selection of the drug itself.

Determinants of Effective Therapy

Effective therapy results when the drug selected for a given condition has both favorable pharmacokinetic and favorable pharmacodynamic properties (see Box 124.1). Moreover, administration to the patient must be individualized based on (1) a realistic clinical end point determined

BOX 124.1 Determinants of Effective Therapy

Pharmacokinetics
Absorption
Distribution
Metabolism
Excretion

Pharmacodynamics
Drug/receptor interactions
Structure/activity relationships
Receptor/effector coupling
Safety profile

BOX 124.2 Factors Affecting Drug Absorption

Physicochemical Factors
Disintegration of tablets or solid phase
Dissolution of the drug in gastric or intestinal fluids and number of
  ionizable groups
Degree of lipid solubility of the lipid-soluble form
Molecular weight

Patient Factors
Surface area available for absorption
Gastric and duodenal pH
Gastric emptying time
Bile salt pool size
Bacterial colonization of the gastrointestinal tract
Underlying disease states

before administration, (2) sound knowledge of the quantitative aspects of the disposition of the drug selected, and (3) an understanding of the impact on the patient's illness of both the dosing regimen to be used and the anticipated therapeutic effect.

Pharmacokinetics

Pharmacokinetics is the discipline within clinical pharmacology that broadly describes the changes in the quantity of drug or drug metabolite in various body compartments over time. These changes can be described by four processes: absorption, distribution, metabolism, and excretion. Each of these processes can be affected by both development and disease. A clear understanding of pharmacokinetic processes and the factors affecting them will permit the clinician to design an effective treatment plan or to troubleshoot when an undesired response to treatment occurs. In other words, an understanding of basic pharmacokinetic principles will increase the likelihood that any treatment goal will be successfully accomplished with minimal adverse effects.

Drug Absorption

Absorption refers to the translocation of a drug from its site of administration into the bloodstream. When drugs are administered intravenously, as often occurs in the intensive care unit (ICU), the need for absorption is bypassed. When intravenous administration is not possible or convenient, several other routes of administration can be effectively used. Physicochemical properties of the drug and specific factors related to each route determine the rate and magnitude of absorption. Knowledge of these factors increases the likelihood that the clinician will be able to predict, if not control, this component of drug disposition.

Absorption of drugs from the gastrointestinal tract is affected by a number of factors (Box 124.2).[1,2] In general, enteral absorption depends on gastric emptying, intestinal surface area and motility, and hepatic first pass. Ontogeny and critical illness may significantly affect these and other patient factors (Fig. 124.1 and Box 124.3).

Bioavailability (F) describes the fraction of a dose of drug that reaches the systemic circulation. Bioavailability of a single drug may vary significantly depending on the route of administration. By routes other than intravenous, absorption is a primary determinant of F. In enteral administration, an additional factor influences F. Excluding drugs primarily absorbed by the oral mucosa, drugs administered into the gastrointestinal tract may undergo metabolism by intestinal mucosal

BOX 124.3 Selected Disease States Affecting Gastrointestinal Absorption of Drugs

Gastric Acid Secretion
Proximal small bowel resection

Delayed Gastric Emptying
Pyloric stenosis
Congestive heart failure
Protein calorie malnutrition

Intestinal Transit Time
Protein/calorie malnutrition
Thyroid disease
Diarrheal disease

Bile Salt Excretion
Cholestatic liver disease
Extrahepatic biliary obstruction

Decreased Surface Area
Short bowel syndrome
Protein/calorie malnutrition

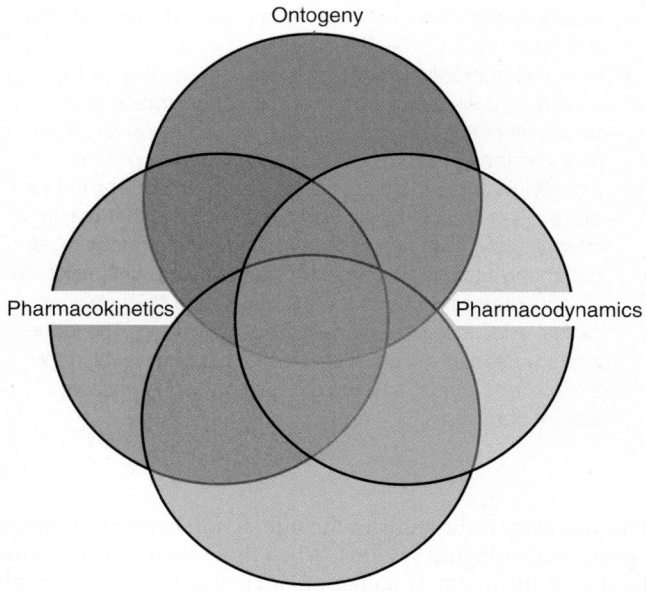

Fig. 124.1. Determinants of effective therapy.

cells or metabolism or biliary excretion when they pass through the liver, before reaching the systemic circulation. This is known as the *first-pass effect*. With affected drugs, this phenomenon may significantly reduce F. This accounts for the fact that the enteral dose for many drugs is significantly greater than the intravenous dose. The susceptibility of a drug to hepatic first-pass metabolism may influence how the drug is administered; for example, nitroglycerin is given sublingually to circumvent a considerable first-pass effect in this drug.[3] Aside from the physicochemical nature of the drug itself, other factors may influence the extent of hepatic first-pass metabolism. Changes in hepatic blood flow may alter this action.[4] Age likely further influences the extent of hepatic first pass. As described later in the chapter, maturation of hepatic enzyme systems and transporters appears to occur postnatally.[5] Although the data dedicated to the ontogeny of metabolizing enzymes and transporters in the liver are limited, particularly as they relate to drug bioavailability, F probably decreases with age as these systems mature.[5]

Intramuscular Administration

The parenteral route of drug administration is important when a patient's disease state precludes oral therapy or when the bioavailability of an oral formulation is poor. The intravenous route for drug delivery is preferred over intramuscular (IM) injection. However, in children with poor intravenous access, IM injection is a viable and effective alternative for the administration of many drugs. Both physicochemical and physiologic factors affect the rate of drug absorption from the IM injection site.[6] Lipophilicity of a drug favors rapid diffusion into the capillaries; however, the drug must retain a degree of water solubility at physiologic pH to prevent precipitation at the injection site. For example, the sodium salt of phenytoin is principally an acid and thus is insoluble in the extracellular milieu of skeletal muscle. This explains the poor IM absorption of phenytoin. By contrast, phenobarbital and benzathine penicillin are well absorbed after IM administration. Both of these drugs are weak acids with pK_a values close to physiologic pH and are therefore unlikely to precipitate in muscle under most physiologic conditions. By having knowledge of the physicochemical properties of a drug preparation, the clinician can predict, even control to some extent, how the drug is absorbed. Although aqueous preparations undergo rapid absorption, drugs in a solution of oil or other repository vehicles are absorbed at a slower and more continuous rate.[7]

Another important factor that influences absorption of drug from an IM injection site is local blood flow, which may be compromised in patients with poor peripheral perfusion.[8] Rate and extent of absorption from an IM injection site also are influenced by the total surface area of muscle in contact with the injected solution, similar to the dependency of oral absorption on the total available absorptive area in the intestines.[6]

A final consideration in IM absorption is muscle activity, which may affect the rate of absorption and therefore affect the peak serum concentration. Sick, immobile infants and children or those chemically paralyzed may show reduced absorption rates after IM drug administration. Use of this route of administration in the ICU may be limited by actual or induced (anticoagulant therapy[7]) bleeding diatheses in some patients. A list of intramuscularly administered drugs used frequently in the pediatric intensive care unit (PICU) is provided in Box 124.4.

BOX 124.4   Drugs Demonstrating Effective System Absorption After Intramuscular Administration

Antibacterial Agents
Amikacin
Ampicillin
Benzathine penicillin
Benzyl penicillin (penicillin G)
Cefazolin
Cefotaxime
Ceftazidime
Ceftriaxone
Clindamycin
Gentamicin
Kanamycin
Methicillin
Oxacillin
Nafcillin
Piperacillin
Ticarcillin ± clavulanate
Tobramycin

Antituberculous Agents
Isoniazid
Streptomycin

Anticonvulsants
Diazepam ± midazolam
Phenobarbital

Sedatives/Tranquilizers
Chlorpromazine
Promethazine

Cardiovascular Drugs
Hydralazine
Procainamide
Pyridostigmine

Diuretics
Acetazolamide
Furosemide
Bumetanide

Endocrine Agents
Corticotropin (ACTH)
Cortisone
Desoxycorticosterone
Glucagon

Pituitary Agents
Vasopressin (tannate oil)

Vitamins
D
K

Subcutaneous Absorption

As with absorption of drugs from IM sites, absorption of subcutaneously administered drugs is influenced by local blood flow, as well as by proximal scarring or injury.[4] The pattern of absorption varies similarly to that following IM injection, depending on the physicochemical properties of the preparation. Frequently, drugs given by the subcutaneous route undergo slow and sustained absorption.[7] As such, the rate of absorption can be regulated by the drug formulation. For example, when drugs are administered in solid pellet form, absorption may occur over weeks to months.[7] Absorption can be slowed by the addition of a vasoconstrictor.[7] This route of administration is not appropriate for large volumes or for drugs that are irritating to tissues.

Percutaneous Absorption

Percutaneous absorption is inversely related to the thickness of the stratum corneum and directly related to skin hydration.[9] The stratum corneum is generally assumed, but not proved, to be thinner in children than in adults. The integument of the full-term neonate possesses intact barrier function.[10] This is not assured in the case of the premature infant.[11] Another important factor dictating percutaneous absorption is the surface area/body weight ratio, which is much larger in the full-term neonate than in an adult. Theoretically, if a newborn receives the same percutaneous dose of a compound as an adult, the systemic availability per kilogram body weight is approximately 2.7 times greater in the neonate.

The percutaneous route of drug administration is taking on greater importance in the ICU setting. Historically, the most commonly used cutaneous preparation for systemic therapy is nitroglycerin.[12] More recently, advances in the technology associated with drug delivery systems have resulted in the common use of clonidine as a percutaneous preparation for treatment of hypertension and narcotic withdrawal. In addition, a number of narcotics exist as cutaneous preparations so that essentially continuous infusions of these drugs can be safely administered outside the ICU.[13] Finally, even drugs such as nitroglycerin ointment are finding potential new uses in the PICU, for example, treatment of the distal ischemia associated with purpuric injuries.

Rectal Absorption

Rectal administration of drugs is of potential therapeutic importance if a patient cannot take an agent orally and intravenous access for drug administration is impracticable. Because of the routes of the respective venous drainage systems, drugs administered into the superior aspect of the rectum are susceptible to hepatic first pass, whereas drugs administered lower into the rectum initially bypass the liver.[14] This may be an advantage for drugs such as lidocaine or propranolol that demonstrate a significant hepatic first-pass effect. The predominant mechanism for drug absorption from the rectum probably is similar to that observed in the upper gastrointestinal tract (ie, passive diffusion). Theoretically, the physicochemical and host factors discussed earlier with respect to oral drug absorption also influence rectal drug absorption. In general, absorption from aqueous or alcoholic solutions is more rapid than from suppositories.

Lipophilic drugs with pK_a between 7 and 8, such as barbiturates and benzodiazepines, seem to be ideally suited for rectal administration because they exist mostly in unionized form and readily cross cell membranes. Rectal use of drugs such as thiopental and diazepam may be effective when intravenous access is a problem and rapid induction of anesthesia is desired or when a child is convulsing. Dulac and associates[15] showed that rectal administration of 0.25 to 0.5 mg/kg of a diazepam solution to children aged 2 weeks to 11 years produced serum concentrations comparable with those observed after intravenous administration. Additionally, peak serum concentrations occurred within minutes of administration. Potentially effective anticonvulsant serum concentrations were maintained for 1 to 3 hours in most of the study patients. Knudsen[16] demonstrated similar results in 20 children aged 1 to 2 years and further ascertained the clinical efficacy of rectal diazepam in preventing recurrent febrile seizures. In a similar fashion, Burckart and colleagues[17] reported rapid and effective sedation after rectal administration of thiopental suspension to 36 infants and children undergoing computed tomographic scanning.

Drug Distribution

Knowledge of drug distribution is important for selecting the appropriate drug and dose to be administered. Distribution of most drugs in the body is influenced by a variety of age-dependent factors, including protein binding, body compartment sizes, hemodynamic factors such as cardiac output and regional blood flow, and membrane permeability.[18,19] Any of these factors also can be altered by disease. This section briefly reviews the pharmacokinetic description of distribution and the effect of ontogeny and critical illness on several factors that determine drug distribution.

The primary pharmacokinetic parameter representative of drug distribution is the volume of distribution (V_d). V_d reflects the apparent space within the body available to contain drug and relates the amount of drug in the body to its concentration in a biological fluid, usually blood or plasma.[7] V_d varies among drugs, based on the drug's extent of protein and tissue binding and its partition coefficient in fat.[7] Additionally, for

any given drug, V_d varies among patients because of differences in protein stores or binding and body composition as a result of age or illness. For example, in neonates and infants, a relatively increased extracellular fluid volume, decreased protein binding, and increased brain and liver size all contribute to increased weight-normalized V_d for most drugs.[20] An understanding of the factors influencing V_d is of paramount importance to the clinician caring for critically ill children. V_d relates the administered dose of drug to its plasma or blood concentration, which determines therapeutic effects, both favorable and adverse. Alterations in V_d produce reciprocal changes in drug concentration.[20] Familiarity with the concept of V_d and the ontogenic and other factors influencing its variation will assist the intensive care physician in understanding why a standard drug dose might be inappropriate for a given patient.

Developmental Aspects of Protein Binding

Plasma protein binding of drugs depends on the concentration of binding proteins available, the affinity constant of the drug for the protein(s), the number of available binding sites, and the presence of pathophysiologic conditions or endogenous compounds that may alter drug-protein interaction.[21] The affinity of albumin for acidic drugs increases, as do total plasma protein levels, from birth to early infancy.[22] These values do not reach normal adult levels until age 10 to 12 months. In addition, although plasma albumin may reach adult levels shortly after birth, the neonatal albumin level in blood is directly proportional to gestational age, reflecting placental transport and fetal synthesis.[23] Binding of basic drugs by α_1-acid glycoprotein also is affected.[20,24] Studies in cord blood suggest that decreased levels of α_1-acid glycoprotein cause this decreased binding.[24] Some of the drugs that have exhibited decreased protein binding in the infant include diazepam, furosemide, propranolol, thiopental, phenytoin, and some antibiotics.[20] The comparative binding of some of these drugs in neonates and adults is given in Table 124.1. The impact of decreased binding of many of these drugs on efficacy has not been determined.[20] For drugs that are highly

	% BOUND	
Drug	**Newborn**	**Adult**
Acetaminophen	37	48
Ampicillin	10	18
Diazepam	84	99
Lidocaine	20	70
Morphine	46	66
Phenobarbital	32	51
Phenytoin	80	90
Propranolol	60	93
Theophylline	36	56

TABLE 124.1 Comparative Protein Binding of Some Representative Drugs

Data from Kurz H, Mauser-Ganshom A, Stickel HH. Differences in the binding of drugs to plasma proteins from newborn and adult man. Eur J Clin Pharmacol. 1977;11:463.

TABLE 124.2   Fluid Compartment Size as a Function of Age

Age	Total Body Water[a]	Extracellular Fluid[a]	Intracellular Fluid[a]
Fetus <3 mo	92	65	25
Term gestation	75	35-44	33
4-6 months	60	≈23	37
12 months		26-30	
Puberty	60	≈20	40
Adult	50-60	20	40

[a]As a percentage of body weight.

protein bound and subject to therapeutic monitoring (eg, phenytoin), however, any decrease in protein binding may lower the measured total drug concentration.[20] In such cases, monitoring of free drug concentration (if possible) will prove more clinically relevant.

Developmental Aspects of Fluid Compartment Sizes

Alterations in body water compartment sizes affect the volume of distribution of a drug. Age-dependent changes in the various fluid compartments (Table 124.2) were reviewed in detail by Cheek and coworkers[25] and Friis-Hansen.[26] Regardless of age, critical illness and related therapies may alter total body water and other fluid compartment volumes.

At 40 weeks of gestation, measurements of extracellular fluid volume have ranged from 350 to 440 mL/kg body weight. Cassady[27] demonstrated that the extracellular fluid volume of newborn infants correlated more closely with body weight than with gestational age. By age 1 year, extracellular fluid volume decreases to approximately 26% to 30% of body weight. After the first year, it decreases slowly and gradually approaches the adult value of 20% body weight by puberty. Intracellular fluid volume increases from 25% of body weight in the young fetus to 33% at birth to approximately 37% of body weight at age 4 months. Except for a sudden increase during early childhood, the intracellular fluid volume remains relatively constant thereafter, approximating 40% of body weight. The clinical relevance of this gradual reduction in the size of extracellular body water compartments with age cannot be overemphasized. To achieve comparable plasma and tissue concentrations of drugs distributing into extracellular fluid, higher doses per kilogram body weight must be given to infants and children than to adults.[28]

Developmental Aspects of Body Composition

The percentage of body weight composed of adipose tissue approximately doubles during the first year of life.[20] Additionally, the liver and brain account for a higher percentage of body weight in the neonate than in the adult.[11,20] All of these factors may lead to significant differences in weight-normalized V_d between infants and adults, depending on the drug. Differences in the amount of adipose tissue may alter clearance of some drugs.

Critical Illness and Drug Distribution

Because of impaired production or increased losses, respectively, conditions such as liver disease and nephrotic syndrome reduce circulating albumin concentrations, resulting in an increase in apparent V_d. Diseases that induce an acute phase reaction (eg, malignancy, myocardial infarction, inflammatory bowel disease) may provoke increased binding of basic drugs because of increased levels of α_1-acid glycoprotein.[7] Additionally, accumulation of extravascular fluid collections (eg, pleural effusions and ascites) results in the development of a reservoir for drugs that are distributed into the total body water.[29]

Drug Clearance

Clearance reflects the removal of drug from the body. Clearance occurs by two processes: biotransformation (ie, metabolism) and excretion. Metabolism occurs primarily in the liver. Excretion is predominately facilitated by the kidney, although excretion also can occur via exhalation, saliva, sweat, or the gastrointestinal tract.[11,7] Redistribution of a drug can contribute to total clearance if the reference compartment is blood or plasma, as is often the case.[4] When reflected in the blood or plasma, clearance quantitatively describes the volume of blood or plasma from which all drug is removed per unit of time.[4,11] Clearance is an important pharmacokinetic parameter to consider when the goal is to maintain a steady-state drug concentration, which correlates with therapeutic efficacy. Once a steady state is achieved, clearance of the drug determines the quantity of drug that must be administered in order to maintain that concentration (ie, drug out = drug in).[4,5] The clinically relevant pharmacokinetic concepts related to clearance are discussed later in this chapter. The ontogeny of systemic clearance mechanisms probably accounts for a significant portion of the difference in pharmacologic response between infants and adults.[5] These developmental factors also produce variability among pediatric patients. Critical illness may have an additional profound impact on clearance mechanisms.

Hepatic xenobiotic metabolism assumes an extremely important role in determining the pharmacokinetic and pharmacodynamic properties of many drugs. Clearance of a drug (Cl) by an individual organ depends on blood flow to the organ (Q) and the organ's extraction ratio (E) and can be described as follows[30]: $Cl = Q \times E$, where E is the ratio of the arteriovenous concentration difference divided by the arterial concentration (extraction) as expressed by $E = (C_a - C_v)/C_a$, where C_a and C_v are the arterial and venous concentrations, respectively. Organ clearance concepts are best described for the liver and kidneys. Hepatic clearance depends on hepatic blood flow, plasma free drug concentration, cellular uptake, hepatic metabolism, and biliary excretion. The hepatic clearance of a drug can be expressed by the following equation:

$$Cl_H = \frac{Q \times f_B \times Cl_{int}}{Q + (f_B \times Cl_{int})}$$

where Cl_H is hepatic clearance, Q is hepatic blood flow, f_B is fraction of free drug, and Cl_{int} is intrinsic clearance, which is a measure of hepatocellular metabolism. Drugs that are primarily cleared by the liver can be classified as flow limited or capacity limited.[31] If a drug displays a high Cl_{int} and E, then doubling the Cl_{int} will have little effect on Cl_H, whereas a change in blood flow will produce a proportional change in Cl_H. In other words, for drugs that are highly extracted (>80%) and metabolized by the liver, Cl_H reflects the amount and rate of drug delivered to the liver.[32] The considerable declines in hepatic blood flow and oxygen delivery that occur immediately following birth do not appear to translate to significantly reduced clearance of flow-limited drug in the newborn compared with the adult.[5] Drugs with high extraction ratios are subjected to the first-pass effect when administered enterally.

Capacity-limited drugs display low extraction ratios (<20%) and a low intrinsic metabolic clearance. Therefore hepatic clearance depends on the degree of hepatic uptake and metabolism of the drug and is independent of hepatic blood flow. Capacity-limited drugs can be further subdivided into binding-sensitive and binding-insensitive drugs. Binding-sensitive drugs, such as clindamycin, have extraction ratios that approach the free drug concentration ($E = f_B$). Therefore factors that increase f_B, such as decreased protein binding, also increase hepatic clearance. In contrast, other drugs may display extraction ratios that are much less than the free drug concentration. In these cases, an increase in f_B does not enhance extraction of the drug, and therefore the hepatic clearance is a function of the intrinsic clearance and is independent of protein binding. These drugs are referred to as binding-insensitive (eg, chloramphenicol).

At every level, from the ontogenetic changes in hepatic blood and portal oxygen tension to the developmental alterations in protein binding and xenobiotic metabolizing enzyme activities, there is the potential for age to affect the processes associated with hepatic clearance. Very little investigative effort has been expended to elucidate these effects; however, some of the important available data are discussed further. For detailed reviews of this data, the reader is referred to articles by Alcorn and McNamara[5] and Leeder and Kearns.[33]

Biotransformation: Phase I Reactions

The biotransformation of endogenous and exogenous substances occurs primarily in the liver, although the adrenal gland, placenta, kidney, gut, and skin also are capable of metabolizing compounds. Once a drug enters the hepatocyte, it may be transformed by one or more enzymatic reactions. These pathways, or phase I reactions, include oxidation, reduction, hydrolysis, and hydroxylation.[34,35] In general, these reactions are responsible for transforming compounds into more polar, less lipid-soluble molecules that are more rapidly eliminated by the kidney, biliary system, or lung. However, parent compounds may be transformed into pharmacologically active intermediates, such as theophylline to caffeine, or into toxic metabolites, as occurs with oxidation of acetaminophen. In addition, pharmacologically inactive parent compounds (prodrugs) may be converted to active moieties, as occurs with hydrolysis of chloramphenicol succinate to chloramphenicol. The ontogeny of human enzyme systems differs dramatically from most animal species, especially for oxidation and glucuronidation pathways.[36] Therefore extrapolating data for enzyme system maturation from animals to humans is difficult. Of the enzyme systems capable of metabolizing drugs, the hepatic cytochrome P-450 (CYP) mixed-function oxidase system has been studied in greatest detail. It is responsible for most of the phase I reactions catalyzed in the human liver.

Yaffe and colleagues[37] first demonstrated drug-oxidizing enzymes in the human fetal liver. During fetal life, these enzymes are present at 30% to 60% of adult activity in vitro.[38] Following birth, total CYP levels increase, approaching adult range by age 1 year.[5] Activity of all CYP enzymes is generally thought to be considerably lower in children, particularly neonates and infants, than in adults. In truth, the developmental aspects of expression and function vary among CYP enzyme families and isoforms. Although data delineating

these variations are limited, particularly for specific families or isoforms, some insight into the ontogeny of select enzymes has been gleaned from immunochemical studies in hepatic microsomes and tissue, pharmacokinetic studies of known enzyme substrates, and studies evaluating the biotransformation of pharmacologic *probes* (eg, carbamazepine in the case of CYP3A4). The ontogeny and the drugs affected by some of the important CYP isoforms are outlined in Table 124.3. A limited discussion of the most clinically relevant isoforms in pediatric patients follows.

CYP1A2. Cytochrome P-450 1A2, the only CYP1A isoform found in human liver, is involved in the biotransformation of many drugs, including the methylxanthines.[33] Immunohistochemical studies have suggested that this protein is sparse, if present at all, in fetal liver.[39] These studies also demonstrate that levels of CYP1A2 do not appreciably increase until several weeks to months after birth, remaining below adult levels well into childhood. These findings are reflected in studies examining enzyme activity as assessed by biotransformation of theophylline. Nassif and colleagues[40] reported a significant correlation between a decreasing elimination half-life for enterally administered theophylline and increasing age. Decreased elimination was further suggested by a marked difference in dosage requirement, with patients younger than 4 months requiring approximately half the daily dose needed in patients age 8 to 13 months to maintain therapeutic levels. Tateishi and colleagues[41] evaluated biotransformation of intravenous theophylline, quantifying three metabolites (1-methyluric acid [IMU], 3-methylxanthine [3MX], and 1,3-dimethyluric acid [DMU]) in urine. The ratios of metabolites to theophylline in urine increased dramatically from the neonatal period to age 3 years, when they appeared to essentially plateau. However, a greater variation in these ratios was seen among patients older than 3 years. This study also established that the relative production of DMU, a product of reactions catalyzed by other CYP enzymes, including CYP2E1 and CYP3A4, was higher in the youngest patients compared with those older than 3 years. The relative production of the other two metabolites, which result from CYP1A2 activity alone, is similar between the groups. After age 1 year into early childhood, rates of theophylline clearance appear to exceed the rates in adults, prompting the need for an increased dose to maintain therapeutic levels.[33]

CYP2C9. The CYP2C family comprises a substantial portion (approximately 20%) of CYP enzymes in the adult liver and has comparable importance in the metabolism of drugs.[5] CYP2C9 is the principal isoform in this family. Enzyme protein is undetectable[42] to low[33,39] in fetal liver. In vitro studies in fetal hepatic microsomes suggest comparably low enzyme activity. Demethylation of diazepam, which is mediated by the CPY2C family, occurs at a level less than 5% that in adult microsomes.[42] On the other hand, hydroxylation of tolbutamide, which is catalyzed specifically by CYP2C9, is not at all evident in fetal microsomes.[42] Several studies, both in vitro and in vivo, suggest an increase in enzyme expression and activity within the first month of life. Following sedation with diazepam, levels of desmethyldiazepam in urine are very low at age 1 to 2 days and increase within the first postnatal week.[42] CYP2C9 protein reaches adult levels in hepatic tissue after age 6 months.[39] Enzyme activity corresponds. By age 1 to 6 months, production of the phenytoin metabolite 5-(4-hydroxyphenyl)-5-phenylhydantoin is comparable to

TABLE 124.3   Ontogeny of Select Hepatic Enzymes

Enzyme	Representative Substrates	Developmental Evolution
Phase I		
CYP1A2	Acetaminophen, caffeine, theophylline, warfarin	Negligible in fetal liver. Adult levels of activity by approximately age 4 months. Activity exceeds that in adults after age 1 year; gradually declines to adult levels by end of puberty.
CYP2C9	Diazepam, phenytoin, NSAIDs, tolbutamide, S-warfarin	Undetectable to low in fetal liver. Adult levels of activity by age 1-6 months. Activity exceeds that in adults from age 3-10 years; gradually declines to adult levels by conclusion of puberty.
CYP2D6	Numerous, including captopril, codeine, dextromethorphan, haloperidol, metoprolol, propranolol, ondansetron, tricyclics	Undetectable in fetal liver. Expression and activity appear to be stimulated by parturition. Complete maturation may occur by age 1 year, although acquisition of adult activity levels has been reported to occur as late as age 5 years.
CYP3A4	Numerous, including acetaminophen, amiodarone, budesonide, carbamazepine, cyclosporine, erythromycin, lidocaine, nifedipine, tacrolimus, theophylline, verapamil, R-warfarin	Low in fetal liver; replaces CYP3A7 as the predominant isoform following birth. Based on pharmacokinetic and drug disposition studies, activity in children thought to be greater than that in adults. Decline toward adult levels begins at approximately age 4 years. Adult levels reached by end of puberty.
Phase II		
Uridine 5′-diphosphate glucuronyltransferases (UGTs)	Numerous, including acetaminophen, benzodiazepines, bilirubin, chloramphenicol, dextromethorphan, morphine, naloxone, NSAIDs, propofol, thyroxine	Varies by isoform; difficult to characterize individual isoforms because of overlapping substrate specificities. As a group, activity appears to be deficient in the neonate and infant. Variably reported acquisition of adult levels of activity; anywhere from age 2-30 months, depending on the proposed isoforms involved.
N-acetyltransferase-2 (NAT2)	Caffeine, clonazepam, hydralazine, isoniazid, procainamide	Low activity in neonates and infants. Movement toward adult phenotypes (≈50% fast and 50% slow acetylators) after nearly 3 months of age.
Methyltransferase group (MT)	Catecholamines, captopril, serotonin, spironolactone	S-methylation capacity (TPMT) approximately 50% greater in infants than in adults. Limited evaluating maturation after this point; one Korean study demonstrated adult level activity by age 7-9 years.
Sulfotransferase group (ST)	Acetaminophen, bile acids, chloramphenicol, cholesterol, dopamine, polyethylene glycols, salicylates	At least some isoforms well developed in the infant; compensates for deficient glucuronidation of certain substrates (eg, acetaminophen).

NSAID, nonsteroidal antiinflammatory drug.
Substrate listings from Leeder JS, Kearns GL. Pharmacokinetics in pediatrics: implications for practice. Pediatr Clin North Am. 1997;44:55. Additional data related to substrates and all remaining data derived from references cited in the text.

that seen in adults.[43] In fact, CYP2C9 activity appears to supersede that observed in adults by age 3 to 10 years, declining to adult range by the conclusion of puberty.[43] This explains the frequent need for a relatively increased dose of phenytoin in this age group.

CYP2D6. A number of drugs undergo biotransformation by CYP2D6, and some are more relevant to critically or chronically ill children than well children. Enzyme protein levels are undetectable in fetal liver except for those obtained from fetuses delivered by spontaneous or induced abortion. These specimens are far more likely to contain detectable enzyme, suggesting that parturition stimulates expression.[44] Enzyme activity, as evidenced by O-methylation of dextromethorphan, is negligible in fetal hepatic microsomes. Enzyme protein levels increase rapidly after birth, but the time at which they reach adult levels is variably reported in the literature. Levels in hepatic tissue from subjects aged 1 month to 5 years reportedly were only approximately two-thirds the adult levels,[5] but another study reported no difference in expression between

patients younger than 1 year and those older than 1 year, suggesting that development of this isoform is complete by age 1 year.[45]

CYP3A4. The CYP3A family comprises the largest fraction of measurable CYP-450 enzymes in adult liver.[5] In the fetal liver, CYP3A7 is the predominant isoform. After birth, there is a shift between CYP3A7 and CYP3A4, levels of which are negligible in fetal hepatic tissue. The mechanisms of this transition have not been elucidated. In infants and children, the activity of CYP3A4 is generally increased above that in adults. The biotransformation of carbamazepine demonstrates this developmental difference. Studies in children demonstrate that both clearance and production of the metabolite carbamazepine-10,11-epoxide significantly decrease with increasing age.[46-48] The role that other enzymes, particularly microsomal epoxide hydrolase, which further transforms carbamazepine-10,11-epoxide, play in these developmental differences is uncertain.[33] In addition, although these age-related differences have been described in pediatric patients on monotherapy, coadministration of anticonvulsants that are known to induce CYP3A4 are speculated to skew these findings. Nonetheless, these developmental differences in CYP3A4 activity have been suggested by study of other substrates, among them cyclosporine, which also exhibits increased clearance in children compared with adults.

The development of other phase I enzyme systems has been studied much less extensively. Alcohol dehydrogenase activity is detectable in 2-month fetuses at levels no greater than 3% to 4% of adult activity.[49] Moreover, the level of activity does not approach adult values until after age 5 years.

Aromatic nitroreductase activity is detectable in fetal livers by 7 to 8 weeks of gestation; however, the hepatic activity at midgestation remains low, and no specific postnatal pattern of development has been described. Also, few data exist on the ontogeny of hydrolytic enzymes. Echobichon and Stephens[50] found low levels of blood esterase activity in the fetus and neonate.

Biotransformation (Phase II Reactions)

Conjugation reactions, or phase II reactions, synthesize more water-soluble compounds by combining a substance with an endogenous molecule to enhance excretion of that substance. Glucuronide, sulfate, and glycine are the common endogenous molecules to which drugs are bound. A drug must possess a specific functional group, such as a carboxyl, hydroxyl, amine, or sulfhydryl, in order to be conjugated. Alternatively, a drug must acquire one of these functional groups by undergoing phase I metabolism. Phase II enzyme groups have been studied far less than CYP-450 enzymes; therefore the ontogeny of phase II enzymes remains relatively elusive.

Glucuronidation is the most common conjugation pathway because of the availability of glucuronic acid and the variety of functional groups with which it can combine. The uridine 5′-diphosphate glucuronosyltransferases (UGTs) participate in the biotransformation of at least 100 drugs (eg, acetaminophen, morphine, nonsteroidal antiinflammatory drugs [NSAIDs]) and endogenous compounds, including bilirubin and thyroxine. Ready elucidation of the ontogeny of UGT isoforms has been precluded by overlapping specificities. For a detailed summary of available information about the UGT enzyme family, the reader is referred to the review by de Wildt and coworkers.[51]

The activity of a number of UGTs is decreased in the fetus and neonate, as assessed by in vitro studies.[51-53] In addition, there is ample in vivo evidence of deficient glucuronidation in infants and particularly neonates. A profound example of this is the association of "gray baby syndrome" with the drug chloramphenicol, which normally undergoes glucuronidation. Morphine glucuronidation serves as a "probe" for isoform UGT2B7 activity. Studies have demonstrated significantly decreased clearance[54,55] and biotransformation[54] of morphine in neonates. Depending on how values are standardized between pediatric and adult subjects, morphine clearance approximates adult levels at anywhere from age 2 to 30 months.[5,55] Reduced UGT activity during infancy is also reflected in the biotransformation of acetaminophen. Levy and associates[56] demonstrated that 2- to 3-day-old term infants had a limited ability to conjugate acetaminophen with glucuronide, which is the major conjugation pathway in adults. However, this limitation in glucuronidation was compensated for by a well-developed sulfation pathway. This

supports the findings of Alam and coworkers,[57] who showed that rates for glucuronidation are much lower and sulfation much higher with salicylamide and acetaminophen as substrates in children 7 to 10 years old compared with adults.

Studies evaluating bilirubin and chloramphenicol glucuronidation have reported low rates at birth, with adult rates achieved by age 3 years.[57] However, some evidence indicates that phenobarbital may induce glucuronidation in newborns and older children. Talafant and colleagues[58] administered phenobarbital 10 mg/kg/day to healthy full-term infants for their first 3 days of life. One group received phenobarbital intramuscularly and one group received phenobarbital orally; one group served as a control. These authors described significantly higher urinary glucaric acid concentrations on day 7 in the IM group than in the controls. This finding correlated well with a downward trend in serum bilirubin in the group receiving IM bilirubin. The ontogeny and potential substrates of other phase II enzymes are summarized in Table 124.3.

Additional Factors Affecting Hepatic Biotransformation

Several factors in addition to those of a developmental nature may affect hepatic biotransformation. Although the impact of each on hepatic enzyme systems is incompletely characterized, factors such as genetics, concomitant drug therapy, and critical illness may alter drug biotransformation and, hence, patient response. Genetic variation of a number of hepatic isoenzymes has been described, with corresponding variation in phenotype. For example, 7% to 8% of Caucasian children are characterized as "poor metabolizers" with reference to the enzyme CYP2D6, which may manifest as insufficient metabolism of several categories of drugs, including β-agonists, antidepressants, antipsychotics, antiarrhythmics, and derivatives of morphine.[33] Variants of CYP2C9 have been described, affecting metabolism of drugs such as tolbutamide, NSAIDs, warfarin, and phenytoin.[33] Polymorphism of the phase II enzyme N-acetyltransferase-2 (NAT2) affects half of the Caucasian and African-American populations in North America. In this case, "slow metabolizers" are at increased risk for several adverse drug responses, including drug-induced lupus erythematosus following procainamide or isoniazid therapy and Stevens-Johnson syndrome or toxic epidermal necrolysis following sulfonamide exposure.[33] Finally, several UGT isoforms are subject to genetic mutation. The best known of these genetic variations occur in UGT1 and UGT1A1, producing absent or reduced bilirubin glucuronidation in the case of the former isoenzyme and reduced bilirubin conjugation in the latter. Phenotypically, these mutations manifest as Crigler-Najjar and Gilbert syndrome, respectively. The effect of these UGT polymorphisms with respect to drug metabolism has not been substantially studied.[33] However, sparse data suggest that glucuronidation of drugs may also be affected in these patients.[33,59]

The frequent need for polytherapy in the ICU increases the possibility that hepatic biotransformative enzyme systems will be induced or inhibited, affecting the metabolism of any substrate of that system. Leeder and Kearns compiled a list of drugs known to induce or inhibit hepatic metabolic enzymes.[33] Even less is known about the effect of critical illness on hepatic enzyme function than that of development. Several factors may contribute to altered hepatic metabolism in critically ill patients. Decreases in cardiac output and, consequently, hepatic blood flow reduced clearance of lidocaine in adult patients; in these patients, treatment with dobutamine improved plasma clearance.[60] In vivo studies suggest that certain CYP isoforms, including those in the CYP3A family, are exquisitely vulnerable to hypoxia, demonstrating alteration of activity after as few as 8 hours of hypoxia.[60] The systemic inflammatory response appears to potentially alter CYP activity as well. Mice infected with *Listeria monocytogenes* experienced decreased expression of some CYP-450 enzymes, which returned to normal levels after 96 hours.[61] Many inflammatory mediators reduce expression of CYP isoforms, including CYP1A1, CYP2C, CYP2E1, and CYP3A in human hepatocytes.[62] Decreased metabolism of a number of known substrates of CYP-450 has been demonstrated in patients with fever induced by infection and drugs and with hypothermia following cardiopulmonary bypass.[60] Of course, linking pharmacokinetic variations in the critically ill patient to impaired hepatic metabolism is difficult in the face of other pathophysiologic alterations.

Drug Elimination

The elimination half-life ($t_{1/2}\beta$) of a drug is commonly used to describe its disappearance from the blood and is measured as the time required for half the amount of drug present in the blood to disappear. As such, $t_{1/2}\beta$ can be used to reflect drug clearance, although changes in V_d also affect this parameter. This and related pharmacokinetic principles are discussed more thoroughly later in the chapter.

Renal Excretion

Most drugs or their metabolites are excreted from the body by the kidneys. Renal excretion depends on glomerular filtration, tubular reabsorption, and tubular secretion.[63] The amount of drug that is filtered per unit of time is influenced by the extent of protein binding and renal plasma flow. When the latter is constant, the greater the extent of protein binding, and the smaller the fraction of circulating drug that is filtered. The degree of protein binding also influences drug elimination in patients undergoing dialysis in a similar manner; drugs that are highly protein bound are less easily dialyzed.[64,65] This section also examines developmental aspects of renal function and their influence on renal drug excretion.

Renal blood flow and renal plasma flow increase with age as a result of increased cardiac output and reduced peripheral vascular resistance.[66-68] The kidneys of neonates receive only 5% to 6% of the cardiac output compared with 15% to 25% in adults. Renal plasma flow averages 12 mL/min (0.72 L/hr) at birth and increases to 140 mL/min (8.4 L/hr) by age 1 year. If renal plasma flow is corrected for body surface area, adult values are reached before 30 weeks of extrauterine life. Using clearance of para-aminohippurate to estimate renal plasma flow, Calcagno and Rubin[69] demonstrated adult rates by age 5 months.

At birth, glomerular filtration rate (GFR) is directly proportional to gestational age.[70] However, a linear relationship is not evident before 34 weeks of gestation. Inulin clearance rates below 10 mL/min have been described in newborns under 34 weeks of gestation, reflecting a significantly reduced GFR. This process must be considered when administering drugs or fluid to the premature newborn.[70] At birth, GFR for term infants ranges from 2 to 4 mL/min. In the first 2 to 3 days of postnatal life, GFR in term babies increases markedly to rates between 8 and 20 mL/min. During the first several weeks of life, increases in GFR correlate with postconceptual age, not

postnatal age.[70] Adult values for GFR (127 mL/min) are reached by age 2.5 to 5 months.[71] The postnatal increase in GFR most likely results from the combined effects of increased cardiac output, decreased peripheral vascular resistance, increased mean arterial blood pressure, increased surface area available for filtration, and increased membrane pore size.[72] In fact, the finding that increases in GFR correlate with postconceptual age suggests that maturational changes are an important factor in the observed increase in glomerular function. The clinical implications for maturation of GFR become apparent when considering drugs that are primarily eliminated by glomerular filtration. Several studies have investigated the pharmacokinetics of aminoglycosides in preterm and term infants. Szefler and colleagues[73] demonstrated a decreasing $t_{1/2}\beta$ for gentamicin with increasing gestational age in infants younger than 7 days.

Proximal convoluted tubules in the normal kidney of a full-term infant are small in relation to their corresponding glomeruli. This glomerulotubular size imbalance is reflected by functional differences in the transport capacity (secretion) of the proximal tubular cells.[74] Therefore tubular function matures at a slower rate than does glomerular function. Reasons for this reduced functional capacity include not only the small size of the tubules but also a smaller mass of functioning tubular cells, reduced blood flow to the outer cortex, and immaturity of energy-supplying processes. This imbalance continues for the first year of life, after which function of both glomerular and tubular components is comparable to that in healthy, young adults.[75] Processes of both active absorption (ie, secretion) and passive absorption (ie, reabsorption) are impacted in the immature kidney.

Many drugs rely on either the organic anion or cation transport systems present in the proximal tubules for renal excretion. Penicillin is actively secreted. Results of pharmacokinetic studies of ampicillin, ticarcillin, benzylpenicillin, and methicillin show that the $t_{1/2}\beta$ for the penicillins varies inversely with gestational and postnatal age.[76-79] In all the studies cited here, $t_{1/2}\beta$ for penicillins was highly variable, but it generally decreased to 1 to 2 hours by 2 weeks postnatal age. These observations may be partially explained by findings in animals that the capacity of the pathways responsible for penicillin secretion may undergo substrate stimulation. Substrate stimulation has not been formally studied in human neonates, but evidence indicates that it does occur. Kaplan and associates[77] showed a reduction in $t_{1/2}\beta$ for ampicillin in both preterm and term infants after multiple doses compared with a single dose.

Furosemide is another drug secreted by the proximal tubules. In addition to being filtered, evidence for tubular secretion is inferred from adult data describing reduced rates of plasma clearance and urinary excretion after probenecid administration.[80] Aranda and colleagues[81] found an eightfold prolongation in $t_{1/2}\beta$ and an eightfold reduction in the elimination rate constant for furosemide in fluid-overloaded term and preterm neonates with normal renal function compared with adults. Peterson and coworkers[82] evaluated single-dose kinetics for furosemide in preterm and term infants and found a mean $t_{1/2}\beta$ of 19.9 and 7.7 hours, respectively. This is in contrast to a $t_{1/2}\beta$ of 30 minutes in healthy adults. These prolonged plasma half-lives correspond with the prolonged duration of diuretic and saluretic effect seen in infants,[83] although the response to furosemide most likely is dependent on its rate of urinary excretion.

The sensitivity of the kidney to hypoxic and ischemic insult is well known. Because this is one of the most important final common pathways for serious illness in infants and children, it follows that renal functional impairment is relatively frequent in patients in the PICU. Kidney function may be further impaired by the frequent use of nephrotoxic drugs such as amphotericin B and aminoglycosides in PICU patients. Clearly, varying degrees of renal functional impairment seen in critically ill infants and children can seriously complicate drug therapy in this setting.[84,85]

Drug Delivery Systems

As discussed previously, the maintenance of steady-state drug concentration requires that the amount of drug being administered match the amount of drug being cleared from the body. Several factors determine how much of a drug can be administered to any given patient at any given time. Although uncommon in the ICU, the available routes of administration may limit bioavailability and, hence, ultimate drug concentration. In the patient who requires fluid restriction, limitations in the maximal concentration of drugs may prove problematic. In the smallest of patients, full delivery of intravenous drug doses contained in diminutive volumes of vehicle may not be assured. Administration of a drug as a bolus generally ensures that the patient has received the full dose, provided any tubing between the site where the drug is given and where it enters the vein is adequately flushed. In the case of drugs given over a discrete interval or by continuous infusion, the drug delivery system influences the amount of a given drug dose received by the patient. Regardless of the technology used, the amount of drug delivered by a system depends upon the designated flow rate and the amount of tubing between where the drug is introduced and the patient's bloodstream.[20] When a drug is added to a fluid reservoir, delivery also depends on the volume of drug added.[20] An example of the impact of these factors on drug delivery is as follows. If a drug is added to the reservoir in a system where the flow rate is 25 mL/hr, drug delivery may not begin for almost 2 hours and would require nearly 4 hours for completion.[20] Consequently, administering drug in this manner could result in delayed or incomplete drug delivery. Additionally, an inability to pin down the timing of drug delivery complicates interpretation of drug levels when monitored.[20]

Fortunately, considerable advances in drug delivery technology have been made since the 1990s[86] and have been of particular benefit in the PICU. Infusion pumps that provide greater volumetric accuracy have facilitated full delivery of small volumes. In some cases, improvements in infusion continuity have enabled uninterrupted delivery of continuously administered drugs, a fact that is of particular importance for drugs with very short $t_{1/2}\beta$ values (eg, nitroprusside).[86] It is important that the intensivist have some familiarity with the technology used in his or her unit; this knowledge may be helpful when an unintended response to pharmacotherapy occurs. For a comprehensive review of this technology, the reader is referred to the chapter by Kwan.[86]

Effect of Extracorporeal Therapies on Drug Disposition

Extracorporeal therapies, including hemofiltration, dialysis, and extracorporeal membrane oxygenation (ECMO), can alter drug disposition in affected critically ill patients. Although relatively little study has been devoted to drug disposition in patients on ECMO, evidence supports the idea that this treatment modality alters pharmacokinetics. In neonates and infants, the largest number of studies have looked at the disposition of gentamicin and vancomycin.[87] Increased V_d, increased $t_{1/2}$, and decreased clearance compared with control or post-ECMO values were demonstrated in the majority of these studies.[87-89] In one study investigating vancomycin, only an increased $t_{1/2}$ differentiated ECMO patients from non-ECMO controls.[90] Other drugs, including theophylline,[91] morphine,[92,93] tobramycin,[87] bumetanide,[87] and ranitidine,[87] have been shown to increase V_d, decrease clearance or increase $t_{1/2}$ in patients on ECMO. The addition of an extracorporeal reservoir contributes to the increase in V_d, and alterations in hepatic and renal function in ECMO patients impact clearance. Additionally, adhesion of some drugs to circuit hardware may alter serum or blood concentrations. The age of the circuit appears to influence this factor to some extent. Dagan and colleagues[93] evaluated the "elimination" of drugs following direct injection into two circuits: a new one and a circuit that had been used by a patient for 5 days. A relatively increased elimination of several drugs by the new circuit was described (vancomycin, 36% versus 11%; gentamicin, 10% versus 0%; phenobarbital, 17% versus 6%; phenytoin, 43% versus 0%; morphine, 36% versus 16% in the new versus used circuit).[93] Several other drugs are subject to this phenomenon, including heparin, furosemide, fentanyl, benzodiazepines, propofol, and perhaps morphine.[87] Propofol appears particularly susceptible to this effect. In vitro studies using entire circuits and various individual components report recovery of propofol has been 10% or less.[87] In the in vitro studies, priming of the circuit with albumin appears to reduce adsorption of at least some of these drugs.[87] This method of priming may have contributed to the maintenance of serum morphine concentrations in an in vivo study as well.[94] Drug concentrations may be altered when a circuit containing some fraction of that drug is discarded and replaced.[87] Finally, pharmacokinetics may be altered by in-line hemofiltration, which is required in approximately 12% of neonates on ECMO, and by dialysis, which is required by approximately 3% to 4% of these patients.[87]

Pharmacodynamics

In contrast to pharmacokinetics, which operationally describes what the body does to the drug, pharmacodynamics deals with what the drug does to the body.[95] As such, this discipline within pharmacology deals with the mechanisms of action of drugs, their safety profiles, drug-receptor interactions, and receptor-effector coupling phenomena. Infants and children have been described to exhibit different clinical responses to several medications than do adults. One example of this difference is the hyperexcitability children may experience following exposure to antihistamines and barbiturates in contrast to the sedation normally observed in adults.[96] Children also have a greater incidence of dystonic reactions following the administration of dopamine antagonists (eg, haloperidol, chlorpromazine, metoclopramide), which has been speculated to result from an increased concentration of DA-2 receptors in the young brain.[96] When no pharmacokinetic explanation for different drug responses between children and adults has been offered, a difference in "sensitivity" has been proclaimed. Variable sensitivity to drugs, including some of the nondepolarizing neuromuscular blocking agents (eg, pancuronium) and the catecholamines, has been described in infants compared with adults. For example, a decreased sensitivity to dopamine has been observed in infants, manifested by an insignificant change in any physiologic variable (including heart rate) below a dose of 15 µg/kg/min.[96] The formal study of ligand-receptor interactions and their consequences is covered comprehensively in two referenced texts.[97,98] However, the translation of these principles into the practice of medicine is embodied in the discipline of therapeutics. Just as important developmental changes determine the related absorption, distribution, metabolism, and excretion of drugs, ontogenetic changes in drug responsiveness account for both the qualitative and quantitative differences observed in efficacy and toxicity when drugs are used in infants and children. Unfortunately, the latter have not been evaluated with the same intensity that has characterized our assessment of developmental changes in pharmacokinetics.[99,100] Actions of drugs in the immature individual may be altered for a variety of reasons, including altered numbers of receptor sites compared with mature individuals, altered affinity of the receptor for its primary ligand or agonists, or altered receptor-effector coupling resulting in altered drug responsiveness. Additional work is necessary to bring this level of sophistication to the clinical setting.

Effect of Disease on Drug Action

During serious illness, substantial changes may occur in receptor function, tissue architecture, and postreceptor function that ultimately are responsible for changes in drug action. These often result from vascular volume or electrolyte derangements and from the effects associated with derangements in acid-base status. Nevertheless, conditions such as pulmonary fibrosis and cardiomyopathy may be associated with diminished responsiveness to drugs acting on the affected organ. Infection with *Haemophilus influenzae* type B has been associated with decreased pulmonary β_2-receptor function with a resultant increase in airway resistance.[101,102] Protracted use of catecholamines may result in downregulation of functional β-receptors in target organs, requiring frequent dose increases to achieve the maintained desired pharmacologic effect.[103-105]

Finally, remember that most drugs used in the PICU are potent agents that have the potential to cause serious side effects.[106] Unfortunately, drug toxicity in a critically ill patient may be an amplified event. Such patients are the least likely to be able to tolerate such effects. Thus the therapeutic index for most of the drugs used commonly becomes increasingly narrow as the patient's condition warrants more aggressive therapy.[107]

Pharmacokinetic Principles

Evaluation of the Plasma Concentration-Time Curve

The application of pharmacokinetic principles to patient care should permit rational drug dosing and result in effective pharmacotherapy. Most of the drugs used in clinical medicine are metabolized via linear first-order kinetic processes (Fig. 124.2). This means that a constant percentage of drug is removed from the body per unit of time. Virtually all of the pharmacokinetic parameters used on a routine basis can be derived from a plot of serum/plasma concentration versus time, which then is converted to a semilogarithmic display (Fig. 124.3). The straight, terminal portion of the former represents the elimination phase for the drug, and its slope is the

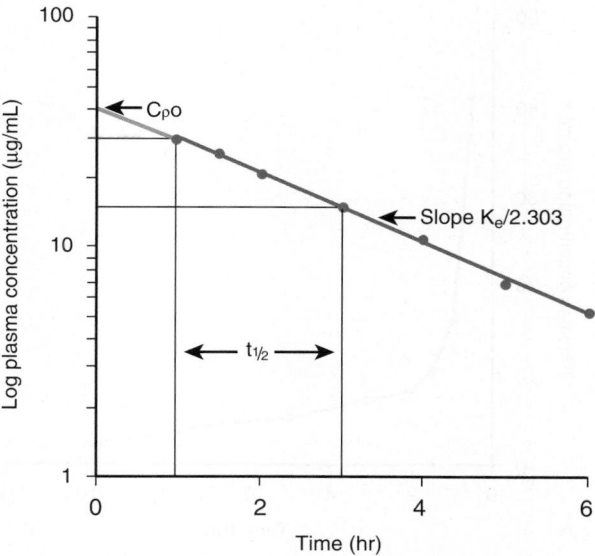

Fig. 124.2. First-order elimination. Plasma concentration versus time curve for a drug eliminated via first-order kinetics. Note the elimination half-life is depicted as the time required for the drug concentration to be reduced by half. A constant fraction of the drug in the body is eliminated in each equal interval of time.

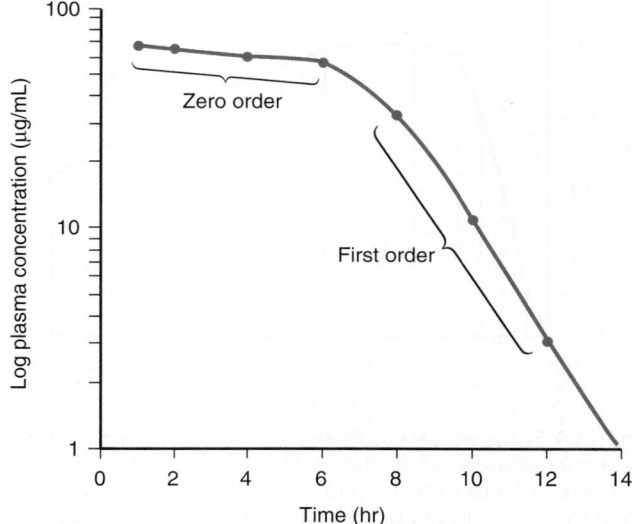

Fig. 124.3. Michaelis-Menten kinetics. Log plasma concentration versus time curve for a drug showing saturation of the elimination mechanism. Initially, a constant amount of drug is eliminated per unit time rather than a constant fraction of drug per unit time. This initial phase is said to show zero-order elimination. Later, the plasma concentration falls below the saturating level and the elimination process becomes first order.

elimination rate constant K_e (Table 124.3 and Fig. 124.4). The elimination half-life for the drug $t_{1/2}\beta$ (see Fig. 124.2) then can be determined directly by inspection of the semilogarithmic graph as the time required for the concentration to decrease by half, or it may be calculated from the exponential decay curve considerations once K_e is determined:

$$t_{1/2\beta} = \frac{0.693}{K_e}$$

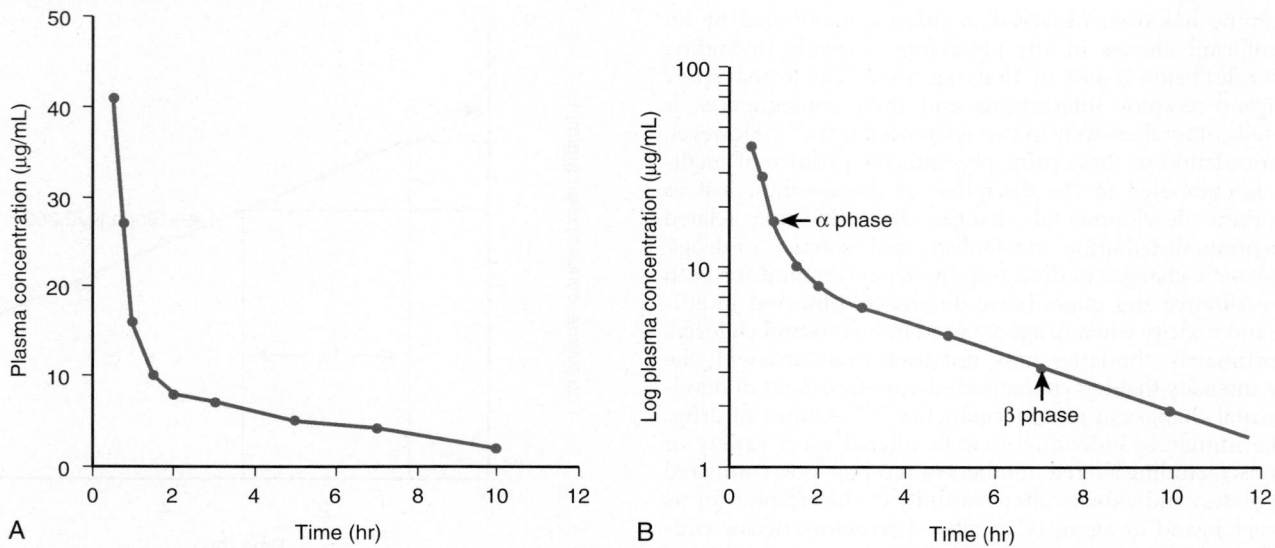

Fig. 124.4. Two-compartment model. (A) Plasma concentration versus time curve presented using rectangular coordinates. (B) Semilogarithmic transformation of the data shows a biphasic curve rather than a straight line. This is thought to represent the interaction between two compartments: plasma and extracellular fluid space. The upper portion of the curve is called the *α phase* and is thought to represent drug distribution. The lower portion is termed the *β phase* and is thought to represent actual drug elimination. Slope of the β phase = –K/2.303.

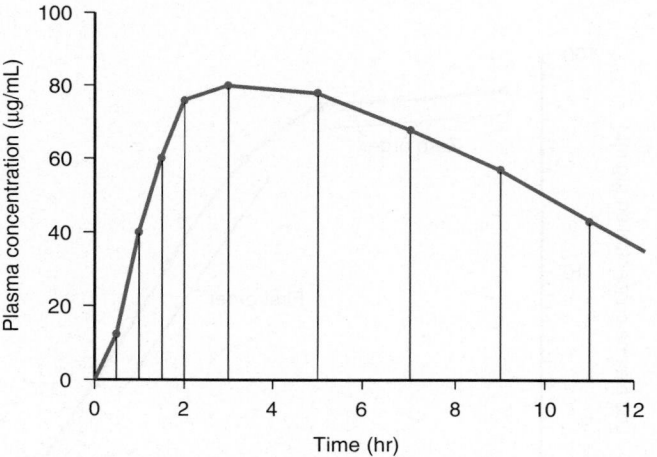

Fig. 124.5. Trapezoidal rule. Plasma concentration versus time curve for a drug after oral administration. The area under the curve (AUC) represents the total amount of an individual dose that is absorbed. This area can be calculated by dividing the curve into a series of trapezoids, calculating the area for each, and summing all of the areas.

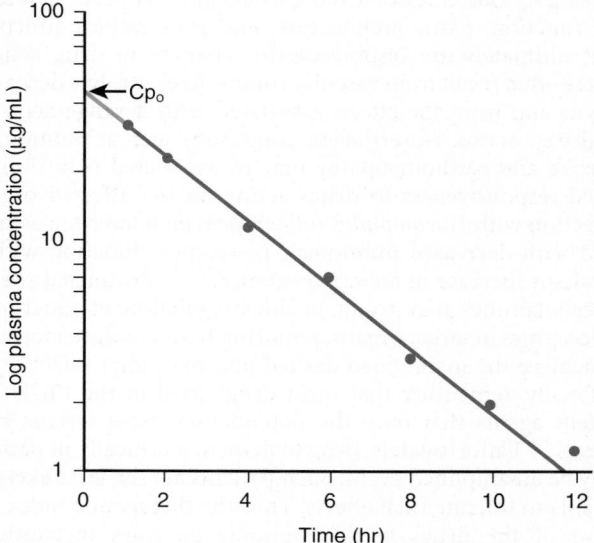

Fig. 124.6. Log plasma concentration versus time curve depicting Cp_o. This is a semilogarithmic plot of plasma drug concentration versus time after intravenous infusion of drug. This drug shows one-compartment, first-order elimination as indicated by the single straight line. Extrapolation of the line back to time zero yields an estimate of Cp_o or the drug concentration that would result if the total dose were administered and distributed immediately throughout the body. If the dose administered is known and the C_o ascertained, the apparent volume of distribution V_d of the drug administered can be calculated.

The area under the serum concentration versus time curve (AUC) can be determined by applying an approximate integration formula, most commonly the trapezoidal rule.[108] This method involves the description of a given plasma concentration-time curve as a series of straight lines, which enables the curve to be divided into a number of trapezoids (Fig. 124.5). The area of each trapezoid can be easily calculated, and the sum of all such areas equals the area under the AUC. The latter value is important in deriving two other values of clinical importance: bioavailability and clearance of the drug. Finally, by extrapolating the terminal elimination phase of the curve b to time 0, the intercept on the y-axis denotes the concentration that would have resulted if the total dose of the drug had instantaneously distributed throughout

the body (Fig. 124.6). This concentration, termed C_o, can be used to determine the apparent volume of distribution of the drug V_d, using the following equation:

$$V_d = \frac{D}{C_o}$$

where D is the dose administered.

BOX 124.5 **Drugs Demonstrating Saturation Kinetics in Infants and Children**

Caffeine	Indomethacin
Chloramphenicol	Mezlocillin
Diazepam	Phenytoin
Ethanol	Salicylate
Furosemide	

In children, a number of important compounds demonstrate saturation kinetics at clinically useful doses (Box 124.5). In this case, the drugs appear to have longer half-lives at higher concentrations. For these drugs, the relationship between serum concentration and time is better described by the values V_{max} and K_m than by V_d and Cl.[18,109] The most important drug demonstrating this type of biodisposition is phenytoin.[110] With this drug, a small increase in dose may result in a large increase in serum concentration. Disease states and drug interactions can pose particular problems for patients receiving drugs cleared by saturable processes. A patient with liver dysfunction may have decreased V_{max} for a given drug compared with a healthy child. Consequently, saturation of metabolic elimination may occur at a lower concentration than normal.

Applied Pharmacokinetics

Use of pharmacokinetic parameter estimates is essential to the development of proper dosing regimens, the effective use of the drug analysis laboratory, and ultimately in optimization of drug therapy. Among the available parameters, the most important in the PICU are clearance (Cl), volume of distribution (V_d), and half-life ($t_{1/2}\beta$). In addition, if oral therapy is contemplated, bioavailability (F) must be considered. Each of these parameters can be used for mathematically describing the biodisposition of a drug under steady-state conditions.

Bioavailability

The concept of bioavailability was discussed extensively in the section related to drug absorption. For most drugs administered intravenously, the bioavailability is 100% and F = 1. In clinical terms, the *relative* bioavailability of a drug is most important. Bioavailability F is defined as the ratio of the AUC for the drug given by a nonintravenous route (AUC_{Oral}) to the AUC of the same drug administered intravenously (AUC_{IV}):

$$F = \frac{AUC_{Oral}}{AUC_{IV}}$$

Relative bioavailability can be used to convert from one route of administration to another. For example, the relative bioavailability of theophylline is 1. Therefore in switching from intravenous to oral dosing, the same total daily dose of theophylline should be administered. In contrast, the relative bioavailability of furosemide is approximately 0.5. Thus in switching from intravenous to oral administration, the dose of the drug should be doubled to maintain the same diuretic effect.

Half-Life

Elimination half-life of a drug is a hybrid term that is a function of both clearance and volume of distribution:

$$t_{1/2\beta} = \frac{0.693}{K_e} = \frac{0.693V_d}{Cl}$$

This is the pharmacokinetic parameter most commonly used by clinicians, but it is often misconstrued to signify drug elimination. However, as shown in the equation, either a change in Cl or a change in V_d can result in a change in $t_{1/2}\beta$. The therapeutic implications of these alterations are clearly different. It is also apparent that if pathophysiologic changes result in offsetting changes in V_d and Cl, the elimination half-life could remain unaffected in the face of significant disease. The most important clinical application of half-life is as a determinant of drug dosing. Four to five half-lives are required for a drug to reach a steady-state plasma concentration at any given dose. This is true whether therapy is being initiated or the dose is being changed.

Apparent Volume of Distribution

The volume of distribution V_d describes the apparent volume of the compartment into which the drug distributes. It must be emphasized that this value has no physiologic significance. Rather, it serves as a parameter estimate that permits the calculation of the dose of drug (ie, loading dose) required to achieve a desired plasma concentration:

$$C_p = \frac{Dose}{V_d}$$

It should be noted that calculation is independent of the drug's clearance and half-life.

Total Body Clearance

As previously noted, clearance is a useful parameter for determining the amount of drug needed to maintain a desired steady-state plasma concentration. Because by definition the rate of drug elimination at steady state is equal to the rate of drug administration, then[19,31,108]

$$Elimination\ rate = C_p \times Cl$$

where C_p is the average steady-state plasma concentration:

$$Administration\ rate = (F \times D)/\tau$$

where D = dose and τ = dosing interval.
At steady state:

$$C_p \times Cl = (F \times D)/\tau$$

or, rearranging:

$$C_p = (F \times D)/(Cl \times \tau)$$

where the solutions provide the average steady-state plasma concentration. It is obvious from the equation that to maintain a steady-state plasma concentration, disease-associated changes in Cl must be compensated by changes in dose D or interval τ.

Critical Care Therapeutics

In the treatment of critically ill infants or children, consideration must be given to both developmental and disease processes. Thus at first glance it seems an overwhelming task to develop therapeutic strategies that would be both safe and effective in treating these patients. Nevertheless, two approaches can be identified that lend themselves to the rational care of these patients: target concentration strategy and target effect strategy.[111]

Target Concentration Strategy

The target concentration strategy can be considered for drugs that are used chronically to treat clinical problems that manifest themselves intermittently (Box 124.6). Such problems include reversible reactive airway disease, seizures, and cardiac dysrhythmias. Application of this therapeutic strategy requires recognition that certain target serum concentrations are associated with either the therapeutic or the toxic effects attributed to a given pharmacologic agent. It is important to remember that these target concentration ranges are determined using population-based data rather than individual patient data. Therefore the so-called therapeutic or toxic ranges may not be strictly applicable to the patient currently being treated. However, they serve as useful guides for the initiation and ongoing monitoring of therapy. As part of this ongoing monitoring, effective use of the drug analysis laboratory is essential. To apply the target concentration strategy, physicians must have some knowledge of the pharmacokinetics of the drug being used (Box 124.7). Such knowledge includes an awareness of any active metabolites that may be involved in the expression of the drug's therapeutic activity.

The approach to treatment of the patient in whom the target concentration strategy is to be used requires that the physician have an expectation regarding the clinical manifestations of drug efficacy and drug toxicity before any therapy is initiated. This should be accompanied by an awareness of the appropriate sampling times for the various drugs and an overall understanding that drug "levels" are guides to therapy rather than therapeutic end points in themselves. Therapeutic drug monitoring does not substitute for other means of

patient evaluation. Effective drug dosing using the target concentration strategy requires a familiarity with the pharmacokinetic parameters previously described and the effective use of the drug analysis laboratory. When a target plasma concentration is known, an initial dose can be chosen. Under some circumstances, it may be desirable to achieve the target concentration immediately. In these instances, the initial dose is termed a *loading dose* and calculated as follows:

$$\text{Loading dose} = \frac{C_p \times V_d}{F}$$

where C_p is the target concentration.

Use of a loading dose is not always appropriate. Under certain circumstances, the calculated loading dose can result in toxic plasma concentrations before tissue distribution. The alternative is to begin therapy with what is termed the *maintenance dose*:

$$\text{Maintenance dose} = \frac{C_p \times \tau \times V_d}{F}$$

When therapy is initiated with a maintenance dose, dosing for a total of four to five half-lives will be required to reach the desired steady-state plasma concentration. In contrast, when used in conjunction with a loading dose, the maintenance dose should maintain the plasma concentration attained with the loading dose.

Effective use of therapeutic drug monitoring in the critical care setting requires integration of certain characteristics of the drugs to be used, the laboratory where drug analysis occurs, and physician behavior. The drug selected for therapeutic drug monitoring should be one from which a relatively sustained and constant effect is expected over a comparatively long period of time. Monitoring should be limited to drugs characterized by wide interindividual variation in pharmacokinetics, as well as those that manifest a narrow therapeutic index. Finally, it is imperative that a set of data exists to relate the clinical effects of the drug directly to its concentration in the serum.

For drugs fulfilling these criteria, sensitive and specific assays for determination of their concentrations in various types of biological fluids must be available. Moreover, this service must be provided with a turnaround time that is appropriate to the type of therapy being rendered. Thus it may be appropriate to provide aminoglycoside serum concentration determinations with a 24-hour reporting schedule; however, the safe and effective adjustment of theophylline dosing requires that serum concentrations be available within 1 hour from the time the blood is drawn. In addition, the results provided by any laboratory must be internally consistent. Standard curves must be checked frequently, and this quality assurance information must be available to all physicians upon request.

Use of the target concentration strategy places heavy demands on the physician. Values for commonly used pharmacokinetic parameters describing absorption, distribution, and elimination should be known or readily available. The physician must be aware of conditions in which these pharmacokinetic parameter estimates may be altered and the extent to which these alterations may affect therapy. The physician must have a working knowledge of the average

---

BOX 124.6	**Principles of the Target Concentration Strategy in Drug Therapy**

- Strategy may be effective for drugs used on a chronic basis to treat diseases that manifest signs and symptoms intermittently.
- Caregivers must have some knowledge of the pharmacokinetics of the drugs being used.
- A relationship between drug or metabolite concentration in the sampled biological fluid and therapeutic efficacy or clinical toxicity must have been established.
- Appropriate sampling time must be known and a reliable assay must be available.
- **Target concentrations must be used as guides; treat patients, not drug levels.**

BOX 124.7	**Drugs Used in the Target Concentration Strategy**

Antiarrhythmic agents: amiodarone, procainamide, quinidine, lidocaine
Anticonvulsant agents: phenytoin, phenobarbital, valproic acid, carbamazepine, pentobarbital
Antibiotics: aminoglycosides, chloramphenicol, vancomycin (±)
Methotrexate
Cyclosporine
Antipyretics: acetaminophen, salicylate
Theophylline

BOX 124.8	**Classes of Drugs Used in the Target Effect Strategy for Critically Ill Children**

Anticoagulants
Catecholamines
β-Lactam antibiotics
Diuretics
Corticosteroids
Oxygen

Anxiolytics, sedatives
Neuromuscular blockers
Vasodilators
Antihypertensives
Inotropes: amrinone

steady-state concentrations of drug in serum associated with both drug effectiveness and drug toxicity. Moreover, the pathophysiologic conditions that may alter these concentration-response relationships must be understood. Finally, clinical experience and sound judgment must prevail. Therapy must consist of an ongoing commitment to treat patients and not drug levels.

Target Effect Strategy

The target effect strategy embodies the therapeutic approach most commonly practiced in the PICU. In fact, the therapeutic strategy allows for rational application of most of the drug classes required in the intensive care setting to the pediatric patient (Box 124.8). Application of the target effect strategy requires that the clinician determine a therapeutic end point before initiating drug treatment and accept a commitment to monitor for both drug effectiveness and toxicity. In using this approach, the clinician must have a reasonable understanding of the pharmacodynamic actions of the drugs to be used, including their side-effect profiles. Moreover, the impact of both ontogeny and disease on drug action must be considered. Once therapy is started, the dose is increased until the desired effect is achieved, unless the sequential increase in drug dose results in no increase in therapeutic benefit and the desired effect is not achieved or drug toxicity supervenes. The amount of time taken in dosage escalation is dictated by the clinical circumstance at hand. In some circumstances, days of adjustments may be acceptable, whereas in others minutes may be too long. Nevertheless, inherent in this strategy is a belief that responses to drugs are dose related and that any concept of a preexisting maximal dose is precluded. Thus if either lack of efficacy or toxicity becomes apparent, the mandated response is to *change* the drug.

In summary, rational therapeutics for the critically ill child must account for the impact of development and disease on drug action. The scenario suggests use of short-acting drugs with large therapeutic indexes and requires that expectations regarding drug effects be ascertained prospectively. This approach mandates rigorous attention to monitoring but ultimately ensures that the dosage used will be sufficient to achieve the desired response.

Key References

1. Parson RL. Drug absorption in gastrointestinal disease with particular reference to malabsorption syndromes. *Clin Pharmacokinet.* 1977;2:45.
3. Welling PG. Influence of food and diet on gastrointestinal drug absorption: a review. *J Pharmacokinet Biopharm.* 1977;5:291.
5. Alcorn J, McNamara PJ. Ontogeny of hepatic and renal systemic clearance pathways in infants: part I. *Clin Pharmacokinet.* 2002;41:959.
6. Greenblatt DJ, Koch-Weser J. Intramuscular injection of drugs. *N Engl J Med.* 1976;195:542.
7. Wilkinson GR. Pharmacokinetics: the dynamics of drug absorption, distribution and elimination. In: Hardman JG, Limbird LE, eds. *Goodman and Gilman's the Pharmacological Basis of Therapeutics.* New York: McGraw-Hill; 2001.
8. Williams RL, Benet LZ. Drug pharmacokinetics in cardiac and hepatic disease. *Annu Rev Pharmacol Toxicol.* 1980;20:389.
9. Morselli PL. Clinical pharmacokinetics in neonates. *Clin Pharmacokinet.* 1976;1:81.
11. Reed MD, Besunder JB. Development pharmacology: ontogenic basis of drug disposition. *Pediatr Clin North Am.* 1989;36:1053.
14. de Boer AG, Moolenaar F, de Leede LGJ, et al. Rectal drug administration: clinical pharmacokinetic considerations. *Clin Pharmacokinet.* 1982;7:285.
18. Besunder JB, Reed MD, Blumer JL. Principles of drug biodisposition in the neonate: a critical evaluation of the pharmacokinetic-pharmacodynamic interface (part I). *Clin Pharmacokinet.* 1988;14:189.
19. Gibaldi M, Koup JR. Pharmacokinetic concepts-drug binding, apparent volume of distribution and clearance. *Eur J Clin Pharmacol.* 1981;20:299.
20. Notterman DA. Pediatric pharmacotherapy. In: Chernow B, ed. *The Pharmacologic Approach to the Critically Ill Patient.* Baltimore, MD: Williams & Wilkins; 1994.
21. Piafsky KM. Disease-induced changes in the plasma binding of basic drugs. *Clin Pharmacokinet.* 1980;5:246.
23. Hyvarinen M, Zeitzer P, Oh W, et al. Influence of gestational age on serum levels of alpha-, fetoprotein, IgG globulin, and albumin in newborn infants. *J Pediatr.* 1973;82:430.
25. Cheek DB, Mellits D, Elliott D. Body water, height, and weight during growth in normal children. *Am J Dis Child.* 1966;112:312.
26. Friis-Hansen B. Water distribution in the fetus and newborn infant. *Acta Paediatr Scand.* 1983;305(suppl):7.
29. Klotz U. Pathophysiological and disease-induced changes in drug distribution volume: pharmacokinetic implications. *Clin Pharmacokinet.* 1976;1:204.
31. Wilkinson GR, Shand DG. A physiologic approach to hepatic drug clearance. *Clin Pharmacol Ther.* 1975;18:377.
32. Wilkinson GR. Pharmacokinetics of drug disposition: hemodynamic considerations. *Annu Rev Pharmacol.* 1975;15:11.
33. Leeder JS, Kearns GL. Pharmacogenetics in pediatrics: implications for practice. *Pediatr Clin North Am.* 1997;44:55.
34. Juchau MR. Fetal and neonatal drug biotransformation. In: Kacew S, ed. *Drug Toxicity and Metabolism in Pediatrics.* Boca Raton, FL: CRC Press; 1990.
35. Roberts RJ. Pharmacologic principles in therapeutic in infants. In: Roberts RJ, ed. *Drug Therapy in Infants.* Philadelphia: WB Saunders; 1984.
40. Nassif EG, Weinberger MM, Shannon D, et al. Theophylline disposition in infancy. *J Pediatr.* 1981;98:158.
41. Tateishi T, Asoh M, Yamaguchi A, et al. Developmental changes in urinary elimination of theophylline and its metabolites in pediatrics patients. *Pediatr Res.* 1999;45:55.
42. Treluyer JM, Gueret G, Cheron G, et al. Developmental expression of CYP2C and CYP2C-dependent activities in the human liver: in-vivo/in-vitro correlation and inducibility. *Pharmacogenetics.* 1997;7:441.
44. Treluyer JM, Jacqz-Aigrain E, Alvarez F, Cresteil T. Expression of CYP2D6 in developing human liver. *Eur J Biochem.* 1991;202:583.
48. Riva R, Contin M, Albani F, et al. Free and total serum concentrations of carbamazepine and carbamazepine-10,11-epoxide in infancy and childhood. *Epilepsia.* 1985;26:320.
50. Echobichon DJ, Stephens DS. Perinatal development of human blood esterases. *Clin Pharmacol Ther.* 1973;14:41.
51. de Wildt SN, Kearns GL, Leeder JS, van den Anker JN. Glucuronidation in humans: pharmacogenetic and developmental aspects. *Clin Pharmacokinet.* 1999;36:439.
52. Pacifici GM, Kubrich M, Giuliani L, et al. Sulphation and glucuronidation of ritodrine in human fetal and adult tissues. *Eur J Clin Pharmacol.* 1993;44:259.
56. Levy G, Khanna NN, Soda DM, et al. Pharmacokinetics of acetaminophen in the human neonate: formation of acetaminophen glucuronide and sulfate relation to plasma bilirubin concentration and D-glucaric acid excretion. *Pediatrics.* 1975;55:818.
58. Talafant E, Hoskova A, Pojerova A. Glucaric acid excretion as index of hepatic glucuronidation in neonates after phenobarbital treatment. *Pediatr Res.* 1975;9:480.
60. Park GR. Molecular mechanisms of drug metabolism in the critically ill. *Br J Anaesth.* 1996;77:32.
63. Brater DC. The pharmacological role of the kidney. *Drugs.* 1980;19:31.

64. Brater DC, Vasko MR. Pharmacokinetics. In: Chernow B, ed. *The Pharmacologic Approach to the Critically Ill Patient.* 2nd ed. Baltimore, MD: Williams & Wilkins; 1988.

65. Whelton A. Antibiotic pharmacokinetics and clinical application in renal insufficiency. *Med Clin North Am.* 1982;66:267.

67. Hook JB, Bailie MD. Perinatal renal pharmacology. *Annu Rev Pharm Toxicol.* 1979;19:491.

69. Calcagno PL, Rubin MI. Renal extraction of paraaminohippurate in infants and children. *J Clin Invest.* 1963;42:1632.

72. Morselli PL. Clinical pharmacokinetics in neonates. *Clin Pharmacokinet.* 1976;1:81.

76. McCracken GH Jr, Ginsberg C, Chrane DP, et al. Clinical pharmacology of penicillin in newborn infants. *J Pediatr.* 1973;82:692.

81. Aranda JV, Perez J, Sitar DS, et al. Pharmacokinetic disposition and protein binding of furosemide in newborn infants. *J Pediatr.* 1978;93:507.

83. Witte MK, Stork JE, Blumer JL. Diuretic therapeutics in the pediatric patient. *Am J Cardiol.* 1986;57:44A.

87. Buck ML. Pharmacokinetic changes during extracorporeal membrane oxygenation: implications for drug therapy of neonates. *Clin Pharmacokinet.* 2003;42:403.

94. Geiduschek JM, Lynn AM, Bratton SL, et al. Morphine pharmacokinetics during continuous infusion of morphine sulfate for infants receiving extracorporeal membrane oxygenation. *Crit Care Med.* 1997; 25:360.

95. Benet LZ, Mitchell JR, Sheiner LB, et al. General principles. In: Gilm AG, ed. *The Pharmacological Basis of Therapeutics.* 8th ed. Elmsford, NY: Pergamon Press; 1990.

96. Nies AS. Principles of therapeutics. In: Hardman JG, Limbird LE, eds. *Goodman and Gilman's the Pharmacological Basis of Therapeutics.* New York: McGraw-Hill; 2001.

97. Pratt WB, Taylor P, eds. *Principles of Drug Action: The Basis of Pharmacology.* 3rd ed. New York: Churchill Livingstone; 1990.

99. Radde IC, Holland FJ. Receptors and drug action. In: MacLeod SM, Radde IC, eds. *Textbook of Pediatric Clinical Pharmacology.* Littleton, CO: PSG Publishing; 1985.

103. Aarons RD, Nies AS, Molinoff PB. Elevation of beta adrenergic receptor density in human lymphocytes after propranolol administration. *J Clin Invest.* 1980;65:949.

106. Blumer JL, Bond GR. Toxic effects of drugs in the ICU. *Crit Care Clin.* 1991;7:489.

107. Watson CB. Complications of drug therapy. In: Lumb PD, Bryan-Brown CW, eds. *Complications in Critical Care Medicine.* Chicago: Yearbook Medical Publishers; 1988.

109. Jusko WJ. Pharmacokinetic principles in pediatric pharmacology. *Pediatr Clin North Am.* 1972;19:81.

111. Sheiner LB, Tozer TN. Clinical pharmacokinetics: the use of plasma concentrations of drugs. In: Melmon KL, Morrelli HF, eds. *Clinical Pharmacology: Basic Principles in Therapeutics.* New York: Macmillan Publishing; 1978.

Molecular Mechanisms of Drug Actions: From Receptors to Effectors

Catherine Litalien and Pierre Beaulieu

PEARLS

- Receptors play a central role in determining the nature of the pharmacologic effects produced by a drug.
- Most drugs and endogenous compounds (eg, hormones, neurotransmitters) exert their action by binding to a receptor or by modulating an ion channel.
- G proteins are a superfamily of proteins that allow transduction between an activated receptor (by an agonist) and different intracellular effectors, such as enzymes or ion channels, relaying signals from more than 1000 receptors. G protein–coupled receptors are complex signaling machines that participate in most physiologic and pathophysiologic processes and represent the target, directly or indirectly, of approximately 40% of all current therapeutic agents. Continued exposure of a receptor to an agonist often results in progressive loss of receptor responsiveness, with a diminished receptor-mediated response over time. This is called *desensitization*.
- Two main superfamilies of membrane transporters provide the active transport of drugs to their target receptors in specific organs and tissues: the adenosine triphosphate–binding cassette superfamily and the solute carrier family.
- Calcium is critically important as a regulator of cell function. It exerts its control on cellular function through its ability to regulate the activity of many different proteins, such as channels, transporters, and transcription factors. In the majority of cases, a calcium-binding protein serves as an intermediate between Ca^{2+} and the regulated functional protein.
- An individual's genetic makeup can modify the efficacy of drug treatment and the risk of adverse reactions. The role of inheritance in the individual variation of drug response is increasingly recognized with the identification of polymorphisms in genes encoding drug-metabolizing enzymes, drug targets, and proteins involved in signal transduction. However, most of these have not translated into pharmacogenetics-based therapy, as multiple factors beyond genetic variability have the potential to influence drug response, even more so in the critically ill patient. Mathematic models and systems biology capable of integrating all of these variables may prove more useful to adequately predict drug response.

Optimizing drug response is a challenging task that clinicians confront on a daily basis. This is particularly true for those caring for critically ill patients, in whom many factors influencing drug response are being more commonly recognized. These include reduced absorption, variable drug distribution, decreased metabolism and elimination, as well as alterations in drug receptors, signaling mechanisms, and effectors.[1-3] Advances in molecular pharmacology have shed more light on the processes that transduce extracellular signals into intracellular messages that control cell function. This has led to the elucidation of multiple points at which modulation of signal transduction, by either pharmacologic agents or diseases, can occur. Also, there has been an ongoing recognition of the role of inheritance in the individual variation of drug response with the identification of polymorphisms in genes encoding drug-metabolizing enzymes, drug targets (eg, receptors, enzymes), and proteins involved in signal transduction.[4-6]

This chapter provides a detailed overview of how drugs work at the molecular level and how this complex system is influenced by genetic factors, developmental changes, disease processes, and the environment (Fig. 125.1). Ultimately, the objective is to help pediatric intensive care physicians better tailor the pharmacotherapy they use—that is, choose the right drug, or combination of drugs, for the right patient to achieve maximal efficacy with no or minimal toxicity. This chapter does not address signaling pathways involved in diseases per se.

Targets for Drug Action

The initial step in the cascade of biochemical events resulting in drug action mostly consists in the binding of drugs to specific cellular targets. These can be broadly divided into four categories: (1) receptors, (2) ion channels, (3) enzymes, and (4) carrier proteins (Fig. 125.2). The majority of important drugs act on one of these types of proteins. Table 125.1 shows the targets of some pharmacologic agents commonly used in the pediatric intensive care unit.

Receptors

Receptors are the most frequent drug target. They can be defined as the sensing elements in the system of chemical communication that coordinate the function of all different cells in the body, the chemical messengers being the various hormones, neurotransmitters, other mediators, or drugs. Ligands (eg, hormones, drugs) that bind with receptors are termed *agonists* if their binding results in the expected effect and are termed *antagonists* if binding stops or decreases an

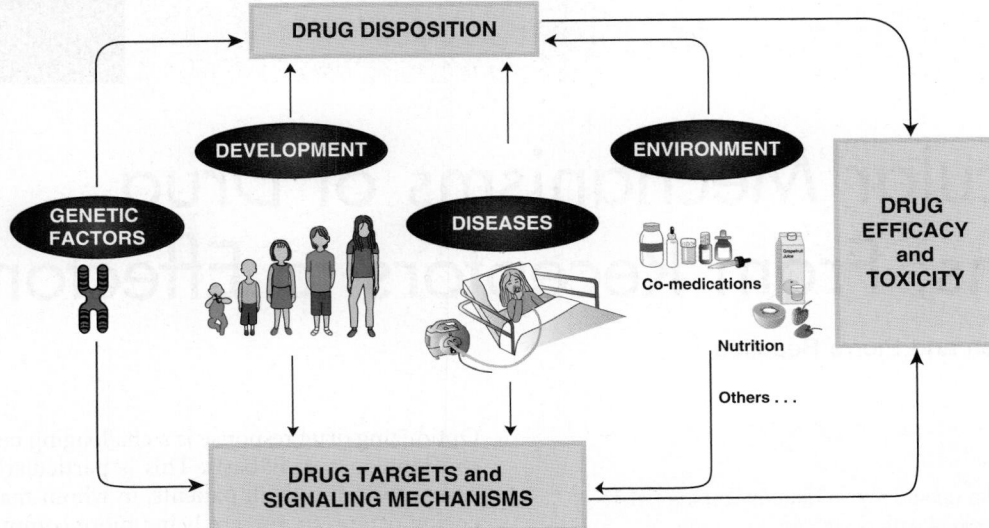

Fig. 125.1. Relationships among genetic factors, development, diseases, and the environment and drug efficacy and toxicity.

agonist-induced activity.[7] Administration of a receptor antagonist in the absence of an agonist results in no effect because antagonists bind to receptors but do not activate them. *Competitive antagonism* (surmountable or reversible) is when a drug with affinity for a receptor but lacking intrinsic efficacy competes with the agonist for the primary binding site on the receptor. In such an antagonism, there is a concentration-dependent production of a parallel shift to the right of the agonist dose-response curve with no change in the maximal response.[8] In the case of *noncompetitive antagonism* (insurmountable or irreversible) with a slowly dissociating or nondissociating antagonist, there is a shift of the dose-response curve to the right and a further depression of the maximal response; no change in the antagonist occupancy takes place when the agonist is applied (Fig. 125.3A).

In addition to the agonist binding site to which antagonists bind, receptor proteins possess many other (allosteric) binding sites through which drugs can influence receptor function by increasing (allosteric facilitators) or decreasing (allosteric antagonists) the affinity of agonists for their binding site, or by modifying efficacy. The resulting effect may be to alter the slope and maximum of the agonist concentration-effect curve.[9] An example of allosteric facilitation includes the activation of benzodiazepines on GABA$_A$ receptors.

The duration of action of an *insurmountable* antagonist depends mostly on synthesis of new receptors, which can take several days. This may have clinically important consequences. For example, phenoxybenzamine, an *insurmountable* α-adrenergic receptor antagonist sometimes used in stage I Norwood procedures to balance the pulmonary and systemic circulations, can produce symptomatic hypotension in some patients. The attenuation or reversal of the decrease in systemic vascular resistance it produces may not be achieved with an α-adrenergic receptor agonist such as dopamine (high dose) or norepinephrine, depending on the dose of phenoxybenzamine given. In such circumstances, the use of a pressor agent that does not act through the α-adrenergic receptor such as vasopressin, which binds on V$_1$ receptors of smooth muscle cells, must be considered.[10]

Partial agonists are ligands that bind to the same receptor as full agonists but have less intrinsic capacity to produce a

response as strong as full agonists, despite full receptor occupancy (Fig. 125.3B). The exact mechanism that accounts for the blunted maximal response seen with partial agonists is unknown. Simultaneous administration of a partial agonist and a full agonist prevents the maximal response usually observed with the full agonist alone because partial agonists have the ability to occupy the receptor population (Fig. 125.3C). Consider what would happen to the maximum effect (Emax) of an agonist in the presence of increasing concentrations of a partial agonist. As the number of receptors occupied by the partial agonist increases, the Emax would decrease until it reached the Emax of the partial agonist. This potential of partial agonists to act both agonistically and antagonistically may be therapeutically exploited. For example, aripiprazole, an atypical neuroleptic agent, is a partial agonist at selected dopamine receptors. Dopaminergic pathways that were overactive would tend to be inhibited by the partial agonist, whereas pathways that were underactive may be stimulated. This might explain the ability of aripiprazole to improve many of the symptoms of schizophrenia, with a small risk of causing extrapyramidal adverse effects. Finally, inverse agonists are ligands that reduce the level of constitutive activation encountered in some receptor systems (Fig. 125.3D).[11]

Receptors play a central role in determining the nature of the pharmacologic effects a drug produces. First, receptors bind with only one or a limited number of structurally related ligands, thus ensuring that the final effect seen in a normal setting occurs only in response to defined stimuli. Second, for a given dose or concentration of a drug, both that drug's affinity to bind to the receptor and the total number of available receptors directly influence the maximal effect a drug can produce. Third, drugs differ in their intrinsic activity in regard to their receptors (eg, partial agonist versus full agonist). Thus the magnitude of the response to any drug is proportional to both the extent of receptor occupancy and the intrinsic activity of the receptor itself, resulting in different dose or concentration relationships for different agonists.

Ion Channels

Ion channels are molecular machines that serve as principal integrating and regulatory devices for the control of

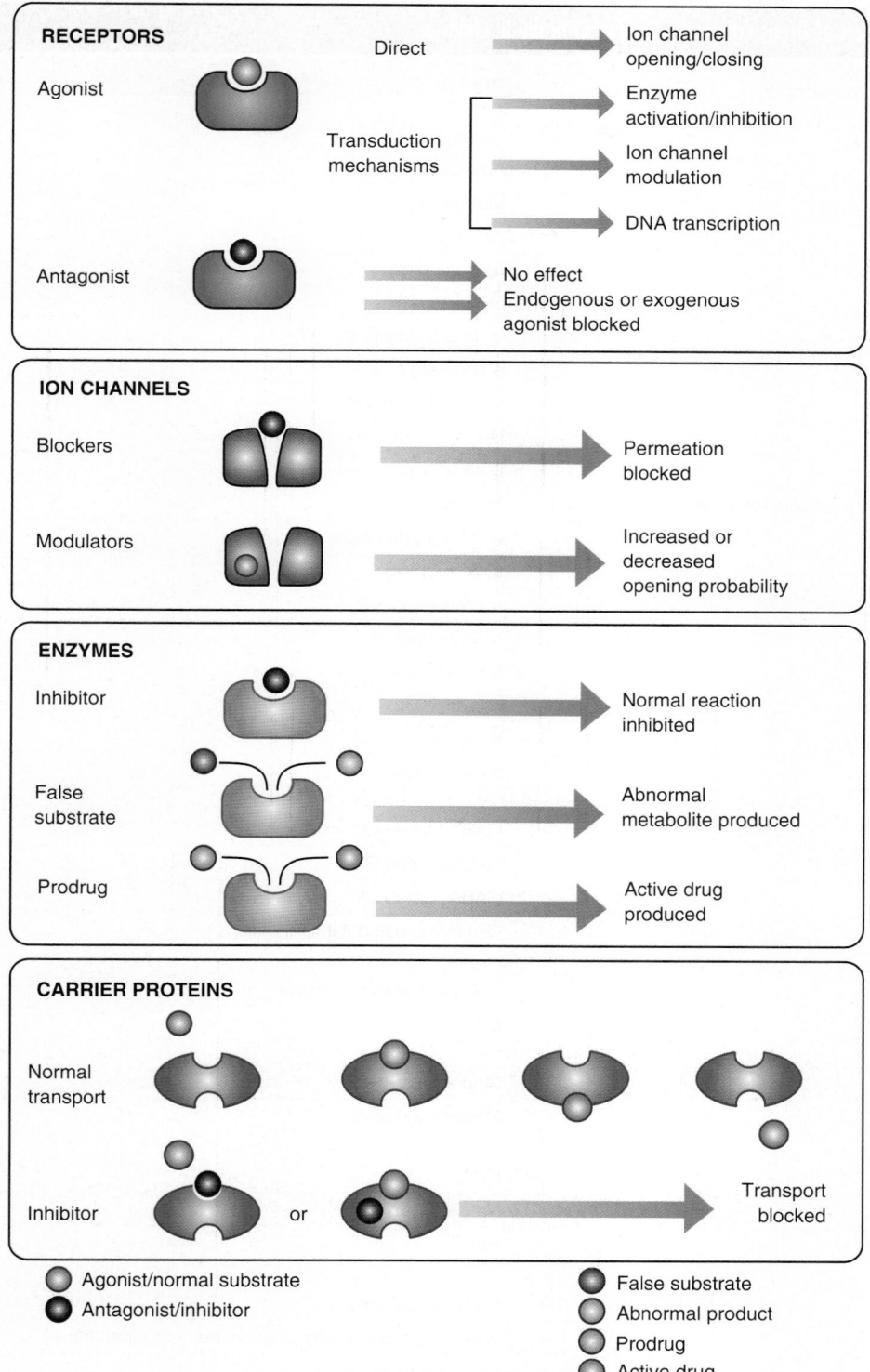

Fig. 125.2. Targets for drug action. (Modified from Rang HP, Dale MM, Ritter JM, et al. Rang and Dale's Pharmacology. 7th ed. Philadelphia: Churchill Livingstone; 2012.)

cellular excitability. Different types of ion channels have been described: channels responding to electrical (voltage-dependent ion channels), mechanical, or chemical (ligand-gated ion channels) stimuli; ion channels controlled by phosphorylation/dephosphorylation mechanisms; and G protein–gated ion channels. Most ion channels are of the voltage-dependent type and consist mainly of Na^+, K^+, and

Ca^{2+} channels. Drugs can affect ion channel function directly by binding to the channel protein and altering its function or indirectly through G proteins and other intermediates. Lidocaine is a good example of a drug that directly affects voltage-gated Na^+ channels by blocking the channel and thus Na^+ entry into the cell. Channel-linked receptors (ligand-gated ion channels) are discussed later.

TABLE 125.1   Targets of Drugs Commonly Used in Critically Ill Children

Drug	Target	Agonist	Antagonist
Receptors			
G Protein–Coupled Receptors			
Adenosine	Adenosine	√	
Atropine	Muscarinic		√
Bosentan	ET_A, ET_B		√
Clonidine	α_2-adrenergic	√	
Dopamine	D_1	√	
Dopamine	α- and β-adrenergic	√	
Dobutamine	β-adrenergic	√	
Epinephrine	α- and β-adrenergic	√	
Haloperidol	D_2		√
Isoproterenol	β-adrenergic	√	
Neuromuscular blockers (depolarizing and nondepolarizing)	Nicotinic		√
Norepinephrine	α- and β-adrenergic	√	
Opioids	μ, δ, κ Opioid	√	√
Phenoxybenzamine	α-adrenergic		√
Phenylephrine	α_1-adrenergic	√	
Propranolol	β-adrenergic		√
Ranitidine	H_2		√
Vasopressin	V_1, V_2, V_3	√	
Salbutamol	β_2-adrenergic	√	
Channel-Linked Receptors			
Barbiturates	$GABA_A$-gated Cl^-	√	
Benzodiazepines	$GABA_A$-gated Cl^-	√	
Flumazenil	$GABA_A$-gated Cl^-		√
Ketamine	Glutamate-gated (NMDA) cation		√
Enzyme-Linked Receptors			
Nitric oxide	Soluble guanylate cyclase	√	
Insulin	Insulin	√	
Nuclear Receptors			
Glucocorticoids	Glucocorticoid	√	
Spironolactone	Mineralocorticoid		√
Ion Channels			
Adenosine	Ca^{2+}		√
Amiodarone	Na^+, K^+, Ca^{2+}		√
Lidocaine	Na^+		√
Enzymes			
Acetazolamide	Carbonic anhydrase		√
Captopril	Angiotensin-converting enzyme (peptidyl dipeptidase)		√
Milrinone	Phosphodiesterase III		√
Nonsteroidal antiinflammatory drugs	Cyclooxygenase-1 and -2		√
Sildenafil	Phosphodiesterase V		√
Ion Pumps and Transporters			
Digoxin	Na^+/K^+-ATPase pump		√
Loops diuretics	$Na^+/K^+/Cl^-$ cotransporter		√
Omeprazole	H^+/K^+-ATPase pump		√
Thiazides	Na^+/Cl^- cotransporter		√

D, dopaminergic; *ET*, endothelin; *GABA*, γ-aminobutyric acid; *H*, histamine; *NMDA*, N-methyl-D-aspartate; *V*, vasopressin.

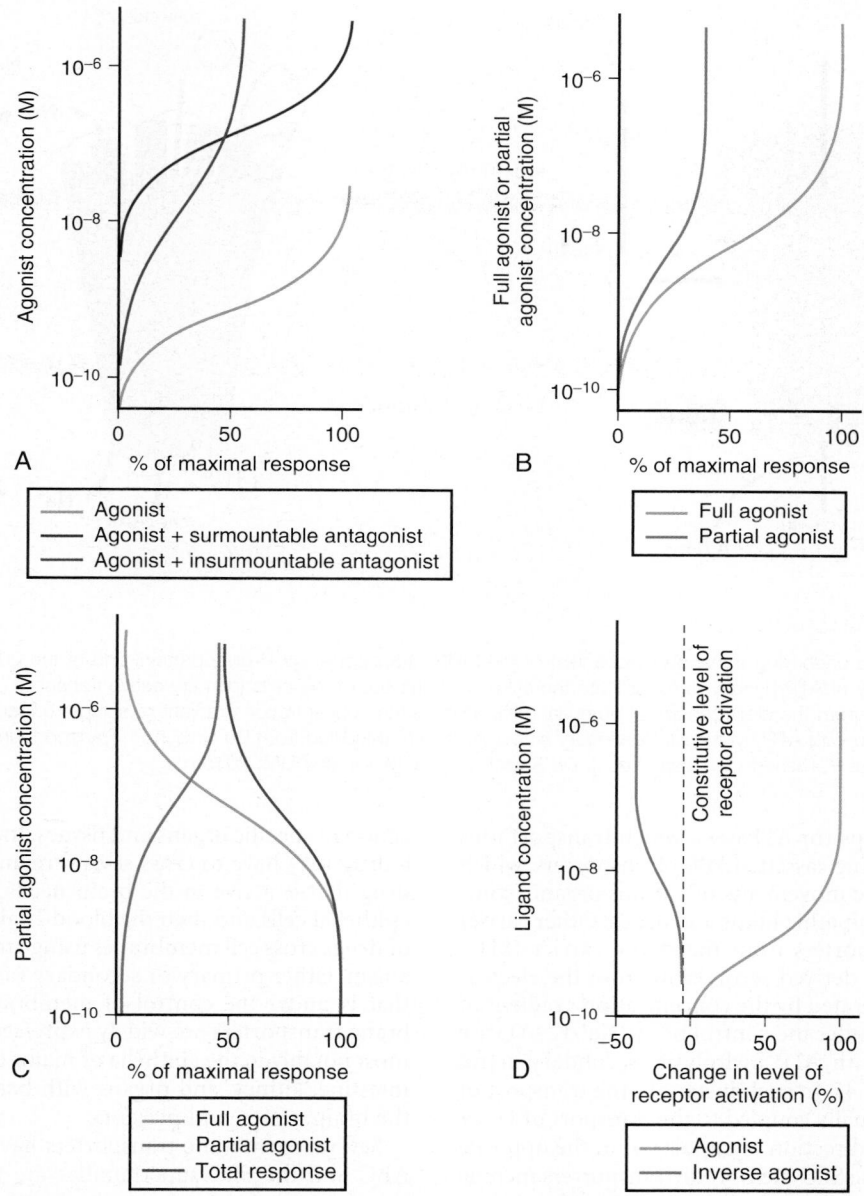

Fig.125.3. (A) Concentration-response curves for an agonist in the absence or the presence of a surmountable or insurmountable antagonist. (B) At similar concentrations, a partial agonist produces a lower response than does a full agonist. (C) Response pattern observed during simultaneous treatment with a single concentration of a full agonist and increasing concentration of a partial agonist. (D) When an appreciable level of activation of a receptor exists in the absence of an agonist (constitutive activation), the presence of an inverse agonist decreases the degree of receptor activation. *M,* mol/L. (A, Modified from Brunton LL, Lazo JS, Parker KL. Goodman & Gilman's the Pharmacological Basis of Therapeutics. 11th ed. New York: McGraw-Hill; 2006. B and C, Modified from Katzung BG, Masters SB, Trevor AJ. Basic & Clinical Pharmacology. 11th ed. New York: McGraw-Hill; 2009. D, From Rang HP, Dale MM, Ritter JM, et al. Rang and Dale's Pharmacology. 7th ed. Philadelphia: Churchill Livingstone; 2012.)

Enzymes

Enzymes are a specialized class of proteins responsible for catalyzing chemical reactions within the cell and thus are ideal drug targets. Most drugs that alter enzymes activity are substrate analogs of enzymes that inhibit their activity either reversibly (eg, angiotensin-converting enzyme inhibitors acting on peptidyl dipeptidase) or irreversibly (eg, acetylsalicylic acid acting on cyclooxygenase). Drugs may also prevent the normal functioning of enzymes. Fluorouracil, an anticancer drug, is a good example of such drug; it is converted into

an abnormal nucleotide that inhibits thymidylate synthetase, thus blocking DNA synthesis.

Carrier Proteins

Several biological elements, such as ions and small organic molecules, are not lipid soluble enough to cross membranes and require a carrier protein (an ion pump or a membrane transporter) to do so.[12] Some carrier proteins use the energy of ATP hydrolysis to move ions or small molecules across a membrane against a chemical concentration gradient or an electrical potential (primary active transport) (Fig. 125.4).

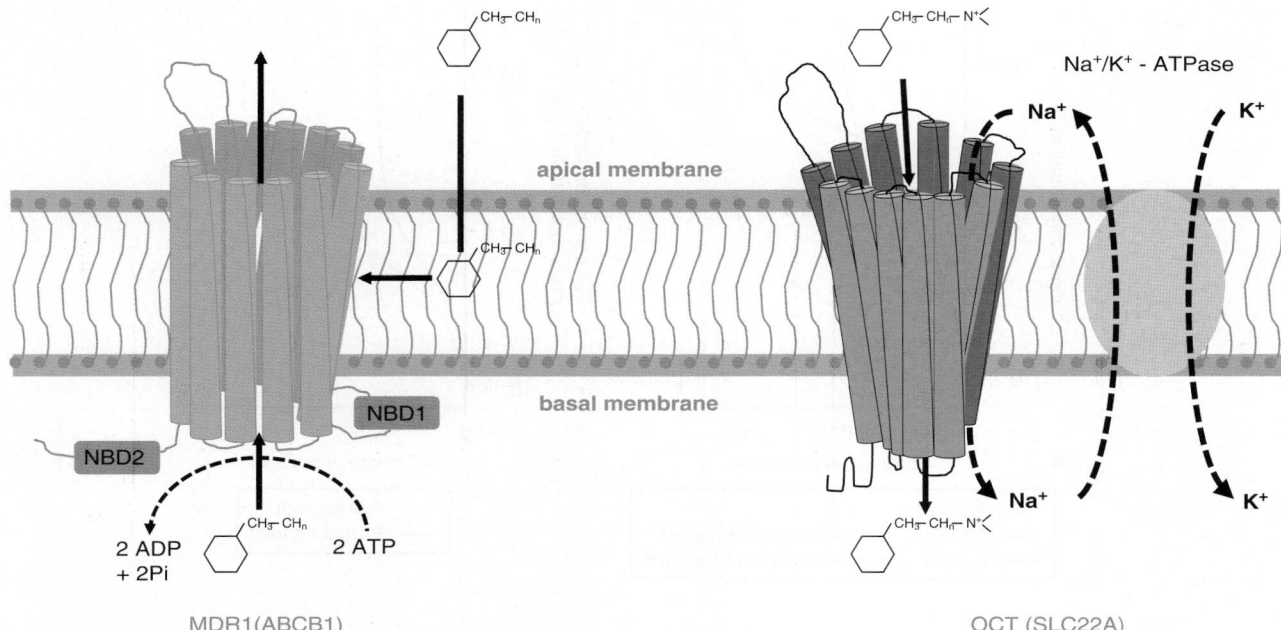

Fig. 125.4. Structure and underlying transport mechanism of the MDR1 transporter (or P-glycoprotein) and of the OTC transporter. The MDR1 transporter uses the energy of ATP hydrolysis to facilitate the efflux of drugs out of the cells (primary active transport). The OTC transporter uses energy derived secondarily from the electrochemical potential generated by the concentration gradient of sodium under the control of the Na$^+$/K$^+$-ATPase pump itself coupled with ATP hydrolysis (*secondary active transport*). (Modified from Du Souich P. Transporteurs membranaires. In: Précis de Pharmacologie. Beaulieur P, Plchette V, Desroches J, Du Souich P, eds. Montreal. PUM; 2015.)

These include ion pumps (or ATPases), which transport ions only, and the ATP-binding cassette (ABC) transporters, which catalyze transmembrane movements of various organic compounds including amphipathic lipids and drugs. Other carrier proteins such as transporters from the solute carrier (SLC) superfamily use energy derived secondarily from the electrochemical potential generated by the concentration gradient of sodium or potassium under the control of the Na$^+$/K$^+$-ATPase pump itself coupled with ATP hydrolysis (secondary active transport) (see Fig. 125.4). In such instances, the transport of organic molecules is usually coupled to the transport of H$^+$ or Na$^+$, either in the same direction (symport) or in the opposite direction (antiport). The SLC membrane transporters include more than 380 members organized into 52 families. Solute carrier transporters facilitate the transport of a wide array of substrates across biological membranes and have important roles in physiologic processes ranging from the cellular uptake of nutrients to the absorption of drugs and other xenobiotics. The Na$^+$/H$^+$ exchanger (NHE), Na$^+$/Ca^{2+} exchanger (NCX), and Na$^+$/K$^+$/Cl$^-$ cotransporters (KKCC) belong to this superfamily.

The carrier proteins embody a recognition site that makes them specific for a particular permeating species; these recognition sites can also be targets for drugs whose effect is to block the transport system (see Fig. 125.2).[9] Indeed, some drugs bind to these carrier proteins and interfere with the transport system. Digoxin is a typical example of drugs that produce their effect by blockade of an ion pump (the Na$^+$/K$^+$-ATPase pump), while furosemide is a typical example of drugs that block a membrane transporter (the Na$^+$/K$^+$/Cl$^-$ cotransporter [NKCC2]).

Transporters are not only potential drug targets but they play an important role in allowing drugs to reach their site of action in specific organs and tissues. Indeed, to reach its target, a drug may have to cross several membranes. For example, a drug that is active in the brain needs first to cross intestinal epithelial cells and then the blood-brain barrier. The majority of drugs cross cell membranes using an active transport mechanism, either primary or secondary (as discussed previously), that is under the control of membrane transporters. Membrane transporters are widely expressed throughout the body, most notably in the epithelia of major organs, such as the liver, intestine, kidney, and organs with barrier functions, such as the brain, testes, and placenta.

Several membrane transporters have been discovered. The ABC and the SLC superfamilies are the two main types of membrane transporters involved in drug transport. The ABC superfamily has more than 50 members distributed in different families with those mainly involved in the transport of drugs consisting of the multidrug resistance (MDR) family, the multidrug resistance protein (MRP) family, the breast cancer resistance protein (BCRP), and the bile-salt export protein (BSEP).[13] The main function of these ABC transporters is to facilitate the efflux of drugs from the cells through apical and basal membranes. P-glycoprotein (P-gP) or MDR1, the most extensively studied ABC transporter, is widely distributed with a broad substrate specificity (eg, tacrolimus, digoxin, dexamethasone, chemotherapeutic agents [etoposide, doxorubicin, vinblastine], protease inhibitors) and is subject to drug interactions through inhibition or induction. It limits intestinal drug absorption, participates in drug elimination (liver and kidney), and influences drug tissue distribution (eg, it limits drug entry into the brain). Some cancer cells also express large amounts of P-gP, rendering these cancers multidrug resistant.

Membrane transporters of the SLC superfamily mainly involved in the transport of drugs consist of organic anion transporting polypeptide (OATP), organic cation transporter (OCT), organic cation transporters novel (OCTN), organic anion transporter (OAT), organic anion/urate transporter (URAT), multidrug and toxin extrusion protein (MATE), heteromeric organic solute transporter (OST), peptide transporter (PEPT), humane equilibrative nucleoside transporter (hENT), Na^+-dependent taurocholate co-transporting polypeptide (NTCP), and monocarboxylate transporters (MCT). The main function of the SLC family is to facilitate the entry and the elimination of drugs from the cells through apical and basal membranes.[14]

Receptor Type and Regulation

Four families of receptors, three cell surface receptor types and one nuclear receptor, have been described (Fig. 125.5). Most transmembrane signaling is accomplished by only a few molecular mechanisms, each of which has been adapted to transduce many different signals. These protein families include cell surface receptors and receptors within the cell as well as enzymes and other components that generate, amplify, coordinate, and terminate post receptor signaling.

G Protein–Coupled Receptors

In 1994 Alfred G. Gilman and Martin Rodbell were awarded the Nobel Prize in physiology or medicine for their discovery of G proteins and their role in signal transduction in cells.[15] Furthermore, in 2012 Robert Lefkowitz and Brian Kobilka were awarded the Nobel Prize for chemistry for their

discoveries that reveal the inner workings of the β-adrenergic receptor, which led to the seminal discovery that all G protein–coupled receptors (GPCRs) have a similar molecular structure.[16] G proteins are a superfamily of propeller proteins that allow the transduction between the activated receptor (by an agonist) and different intracellular effectors such as enzymes or ion channels, relaying signals from more than 1000 receptors.[17] GPCRs, also known as *metabotropic receptors,* are in fact the first component of the cellular amplification cascade (Fig. 125.6). Indeed, the activation of target enzymes through GPCRs leads to the synthesis of numerous second messengers, which in turn activate other enzymes. The intervention of the second messenger system allows for the diversity of the cellular targets (discussed later). GPCRs are complex signaling machines that participate in most physiologic and pathophysiologic processes and represent the target, directly or indirectly, of approximately 40% of all current therapeutic agents.[18] Of note, pharmacologic agents have been developed for approximately only 10% of GPCRs so far.

Three major families of GPCRs are defined based on their amino acid sequence: Family 1, the largest one, includes receptors for rhodopsin, monoamines (such as β-adrenergic receptors), neuropeptides, opioids, and chemokines. Family 2 consists mainly of receptors for peptides with a large molecular weight, such as calcitonin and secretin. Family 3 has, among others, receptors for glutamate (metabotropic), γ-aminobutyric acid$_B$ (GABA$_B$), and extracellular calcium. Despite these differences, the families of GPCRs share characteristic structural and functional features. All GPCRs share

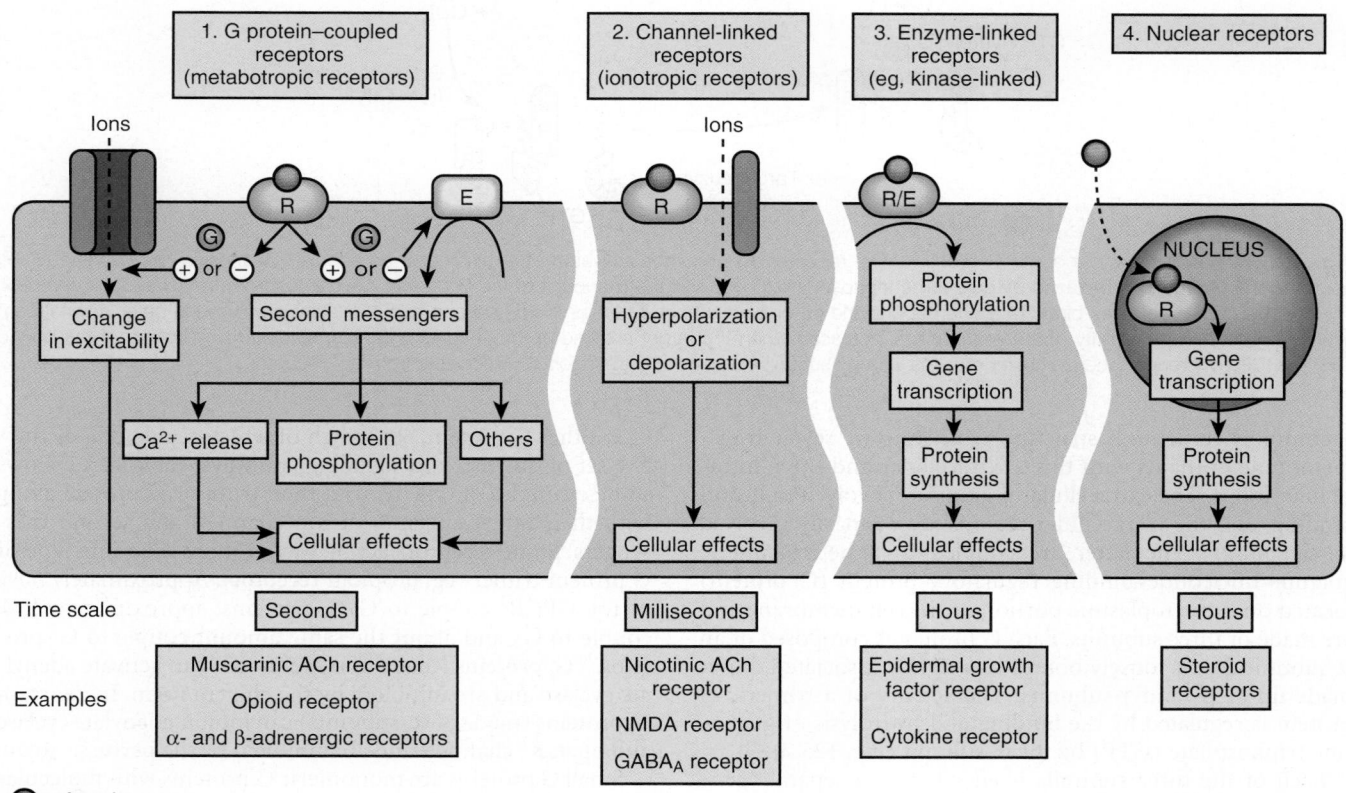

Fig. 125.5. Four families of receptors are classically described: G protein–coupled receptors, channel-linked receptors, enzyme-linked receptors, and nuclear receptors. *ACh,* acetylcholine; *E,* enzyme; *G,* G protein; *GABA,* γ-aminobutyric acid; *NMDA,* N-methyl-D-aspartate; *R,* receptor. (Modified from Rang HP, Dale MM, Ritter JM, et al. Rang and Dale's Pharmacology. 7th ed. Philadelphia: Churchill Livingstone; 2012.)

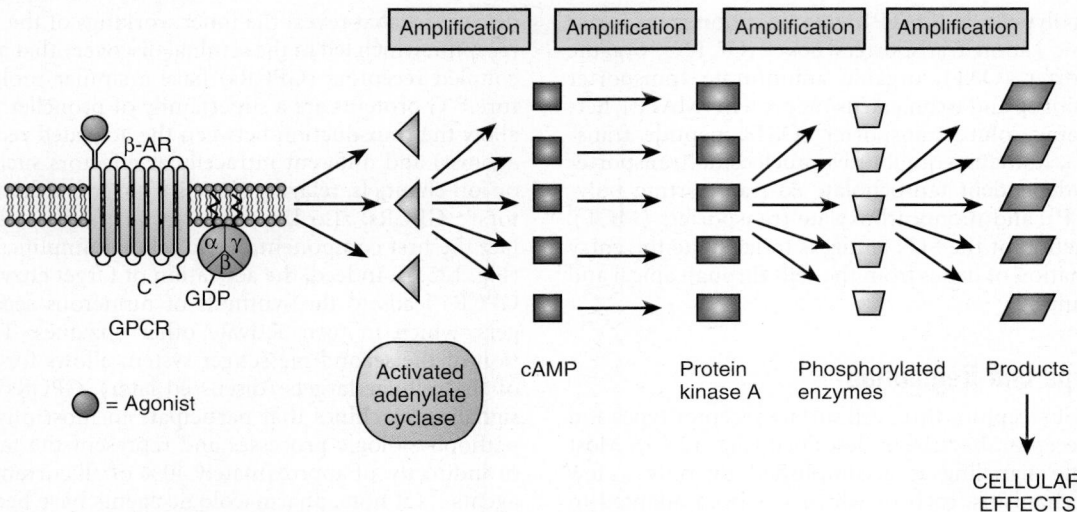

Fig. 125.6. Cellular amplification cascade. After binding to a G protein–coupled receptor (*GPCR*), a ligand (agonist) activates a target enzyme (adenylate cyclase), which synthesizes a second messenger (*cAMP*). The latter then activates other enzymes (protein kinases) that phosphorylate proteins and mediate specific cellular effects. *β-AR*, β-adrenergic receptor; *GDP*, guanosine diphosphate.

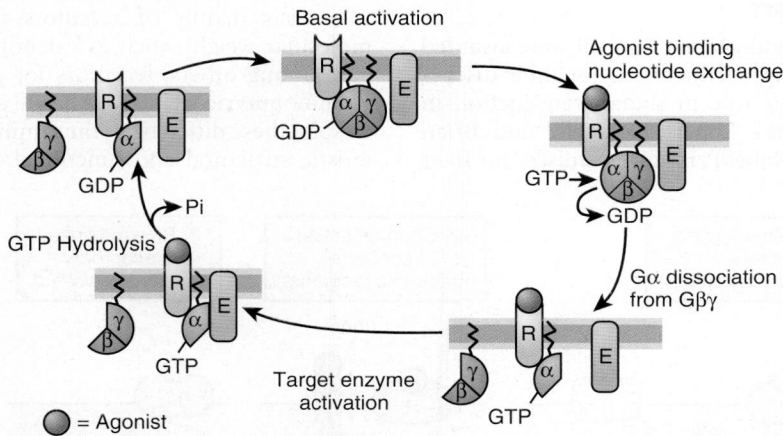

Fig. 125.7. Functional cycle of the G proteins. The receptor (*R*) becomes activated after binding of an agonist. Guanosine diphosphate (*GDP*) bound to the G protein is replaced by guanosine triphosphate (*GTP*), and the α-subunit of the G protein dissociates from the βγ-subunit complex. The α-subunit/GTP complex binds to the target enzyme (*E*) or ion channel, whereas the βγ-subunit complex stimulates several other downstream effectors. The GTPase activity of the α-subunit is increased when the target enzyme or ion channel is bound, leading to hydrolysis of the bound GTP to GDP, whereupon the α-subunit reunites with βγ-subunit complex and the agonist dissociates from the receptor.

a common serpentine structure consisting of seven transmembrane domains with three extracellular and three intracellular loops. The extracellular regions are involved in ligand binding, and the intracellular regions are primarily involved in signaling.[19] The latter are coupled to a heterotrimeric guanine-nucleotide–binding regulatory protein (G protein) located on the cytoplasmic portion of the cell membrane and are made of three subunits. Each G protein is composed of an α-subunit that is loosely bound to a tightly associated dimer made up of β- and γ-subunits. The activity of a trimeric G protein is regulated by the binding and hydrolysis of guanosine triphosphate (GTP) by the α-subunit (Fig. 125.7).

Each of the three subunits is encoded by a separate gene selected from more than 20 α, six β, and 12 γ genes, respectively. The α-subunit is essential in the "receptor-effector" coupling. Various α-subunits define different G protein trimers (G_s = stimulatory G protein, G_i = inhibitory G protein,

G_o = other G protein, etc.), each of which regulates a distinctive set of downstream signaling pathways. Table 125.2 shows some examples of GPCRs with their trimeric G protein along with their target enzymes or ion channels and second messengers. Some receptors act by way of more than one type of G protein trimer (eg, μ opioid receptor). Approximately 50% of the GPCRs couple to G_i/G_o proteins, approximately 25% couple to G_s, and about the same amount couple to G_q proteins.[20] G_s proteins (made of $α_s$-subunits) can activate adenylate cyclase and are inhibited by the cholera toxin. In contrast, G_i proteins (made of $α_i$-subunits) can inhibit adenylate cyclase and open K^+ channels and are inhibited by the pertussis toxin.

Small G proteins are monomeric G proteins with molecular weight of 20 to 40 kDa. As with heterotrimeric G proteins, their activity depends on the binding of GTP. More than 100 small G proteins have been identified. They are classified into different families: Ras, Rho, Rab, Rap, Ran, and ARF. They are ubiquitous and play key roles in numerous cellular functions such as cell division, proliferation, differentiation, vesicle trafficking, cytoskeletal reorganization, and gene expression.[21]

Channel-Linked Receptors

Also known as *ligand-gated ion channels* or *ionotropic receptors*, channel-linked receptors mediate fast responses, affecting ion fluxes and membrane potential. These receptors possess four distinct characteristics: (1) activation by an agonist or inactivation by an antagonist; (2) flux of ions across a central pore; (3) ion selectivity; and (4) fluctuation among open, closed, and inactivated states. Broadly speaking, two types have been identified: receptors of excitatory mediators and receptors of inhibitory mediators.

Receptors of excitatory mediators (glutamate, aspartate, and acetylcholine), which comprise the N-methyl-D-aspartate [NMDA] (Fig. 125.8A) and the nicotinic acetylcholine receptors, are receptors whose activation provokes depolarization of the cell, leading to propagation of the action potential and ultimately secretion of a neuromediator and muscular contraction, for example. These receptors are permeable to monovalent and divalent cations, mainly Na^+, K^+, Ca^{2+}, and magnesium (Mg^{2+}). Ketamine, a dissociative anesthetic, is a noncompetitive NMDA receptor antagonist that prevents the opening of ion channels by glutamate. In addition, the potential neuroprotective effects of ketamine appear to be mediated via NMDA receptor blockade.

Receptors of inhibitory mediators, the activation of which provokes hyperpolarization of the cell and therefore decreases cellular excitability, are a group that includes $GABA_A$ (Fig. 125.8B) and glycine receptors. These ligand-gated ion channels are selective for anions such as chloride (Cl^-) or phosphorus (PO_4^{3-}). GABA is the major inhibitory neurotransmitter in the central nervous system, and drugs that potentiate GABAergic inhibition in the brain, such as benzodiazepines and barbiturates, result in sedation and hypnosis.[7] Benzodiazepine agonists enhance Cl^- ion conductance induced by GABA by increasing the frequency of channel-opening events, whereas barbiturates seem to do so by increasing the duration of the GABA-gated channel openings. Both classes of agents bind to sites on the $GABA_A$ molecule that are different from each other and also from the GABA receptor site.

Enzyme-Linked Receptors

Enzyme-linked receptors have an extracellular ligand-binding domain linked to an intracellular domain that possesses an intrinsic catalytic activity. This large and heterogeneous group

		Examples of G Protein–Coupled Receptors With Their Trimeric G Protein, Target Enzyme, or Ion Channel, and Second Messengers		
TABLE 125.2				
GPCR	**G Protein**	**Target Enzyme/Ion Channel**	**Second Messengers**	
β_1- and β_2-adrenergic D_1 H_2 V_2	G_s	↑ Adenylate cyclase	↑ cAMP	
α_2-adrenergic $M_{2,4}$ μ Opioid AT_1	G_i	↓ Adenylate cyclase	↓ cAMP	
α_1-adrenergic $M_{1,3,5}$ $ET_{A,B}$ AT_1 H_1 V_1	$G_{q/11}$	↑ Phospholipase C	↑ IP_3, DAG, $[Ca^{2+}]_i$	
μ Opioid	$G_{i/o}$	Opens K^+ channels		
μ Opioid	G_o	Closes voltage-dependent Ca^{2+} channels	↓ $[Ca^{2+}]_i$	

AT, angiotensin; *cAMP*, cyclic adenosine monophosphate; *D*, dopaminergic; *DAG*, diacylglycerol; *ET*, endothelin; G_i, inhibitory G protein; G_o, other G proteins; *GPCR*, G protein–coupled receptor, G_s, stimulatory G protein; *H*, histamine; *IP3*, inositol 1,4,5-triphosphate; *M*, muscarinic; *V*, vasopressin.

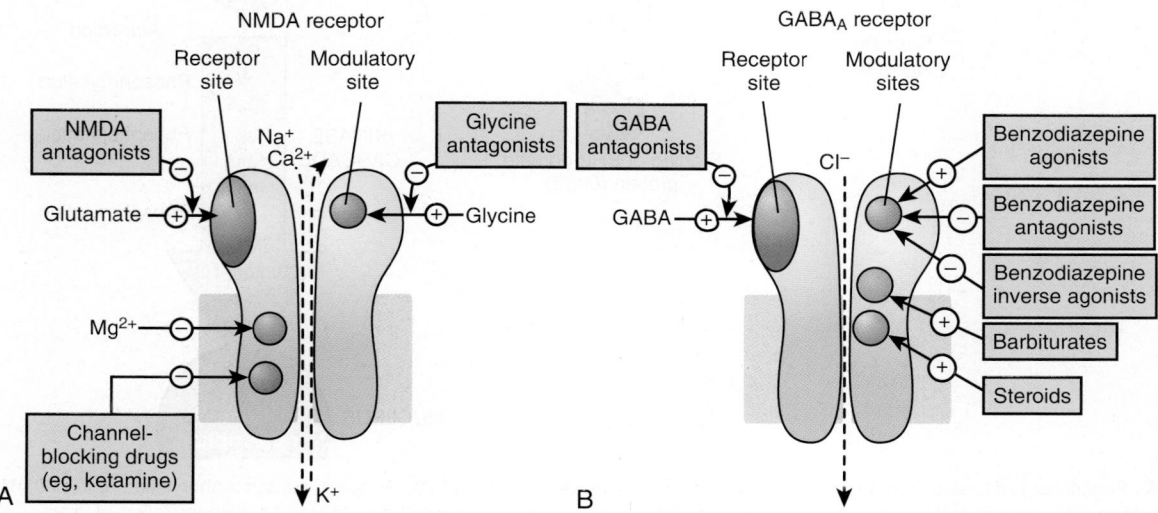

Fig. 125.8. Two important members of the channel-linked receptors, the NMDA receptor (A) and the $GABA_A$ receptor (B). The main sites of drug action on these receptors are shown. *GABA*, γ-aminobutyric acid; *NMDA*, *N*-methyl-D-aspartate.

of membrane receptors can be divided into four subfamilies according to their catalytic activity (tyrosine kinase, guanylate cyclase, tyrosine phosphatase, and serine/threonine kinase). Cytosolic enzymes presenting an activity similar to that of enzyme-linked receptors are also considered to belong to this family of receptors (eg, soluble guanylate cyclase receptors activated by nitric oxide [NO]).

Tyrosine kinase receptors include receptors for neurotrophin,[22] growth factors (epidermal growth factor [EGF], platelet-derived growth factor [PDGF]), as well as insulin and many other trophic hormones. These receptors shift from an inactive monomeric state to an active dimeric state upon agonist binding (dimerization). This is followed by autophosphorylation of the intracellular domain of each receptor and binding of SH2-domain proteins that are themselves phosphorylated. Depending on the receptor subtype, SH2-domain proteins allow the phosphorylated receptor to activate other functional proteins, which eventually results in stimulation of gene transcription, or are enzymes such as phospholipases, leading to the formation of second messengers (discussed later). One important pathway involved in the transduction mechanisms of tyrosine kinase receptors includes the Ras/Raf/MAP kinase pathway, which is important in cell division, growth, and differentiation (Fig. 125.9).

Unlike tyrosine kinase receptors, cytokine receptors do not usually possess intrinsic kinase activity; instead, they associate with cytosolic Janus kinases (JAKs). After dimerization of the receptors, which occurs after binding of the cytokine, JAKs phosphorylate tyrosine residues on the receptor, which then result in the binding of another set of proteins called *signal transducers and activators of transcription* (STATs). The bound STATs are themselves then phosphorylated by the JAKs and dimerize and dissociate to migrate in the nucleus and activate gene expression to regulate diverse biological processes controlling the synthesis and release of many inflammatory mediators, growth, development, and homeostasis.

Guanylate cyclase–linked receptors are unique because they synthesize their own second messengers upon agonist binding. The natriuretic peptide receptors, including atrial natriuretic peptide (ANP), brain natriuretic peptide (BNP), and C-type natriuretic peptide (CNP) receptors, belong to this family (Fig. 125.10). The extracellular NH_2-terminal constitutes the binding domain. There is a short transmembrane segment whose role is to anchor the receptor protein to the membrane. The intracellular domain is made of two different entities: (1) a protein kinase homology domain whose function is to control and relay receptor activation to the catalytic domain and (2) a guanylate cyclase catalytic domain, also known as *particulate guanylate cyclase*, involved in the synthesis of cyclic guanosine monophosphate (cGMP) from GTP.[23] In addition to this particulate guanylate cyclase (the membrane form of the enzyme), an intracellular soluble form exists. It is a heterodimer consisting of α- and β-subunits, both of which are necessary for enzyme activity, and is expressed in most tissues, though not uniformly.[24] It is activated by intermediate substances derived from the biosynthesis of eicosanoids (prostaglandins and leukotrienes) and by NO and NO donors such as sodium nitroprusside and nitroglycerin (discussed later).

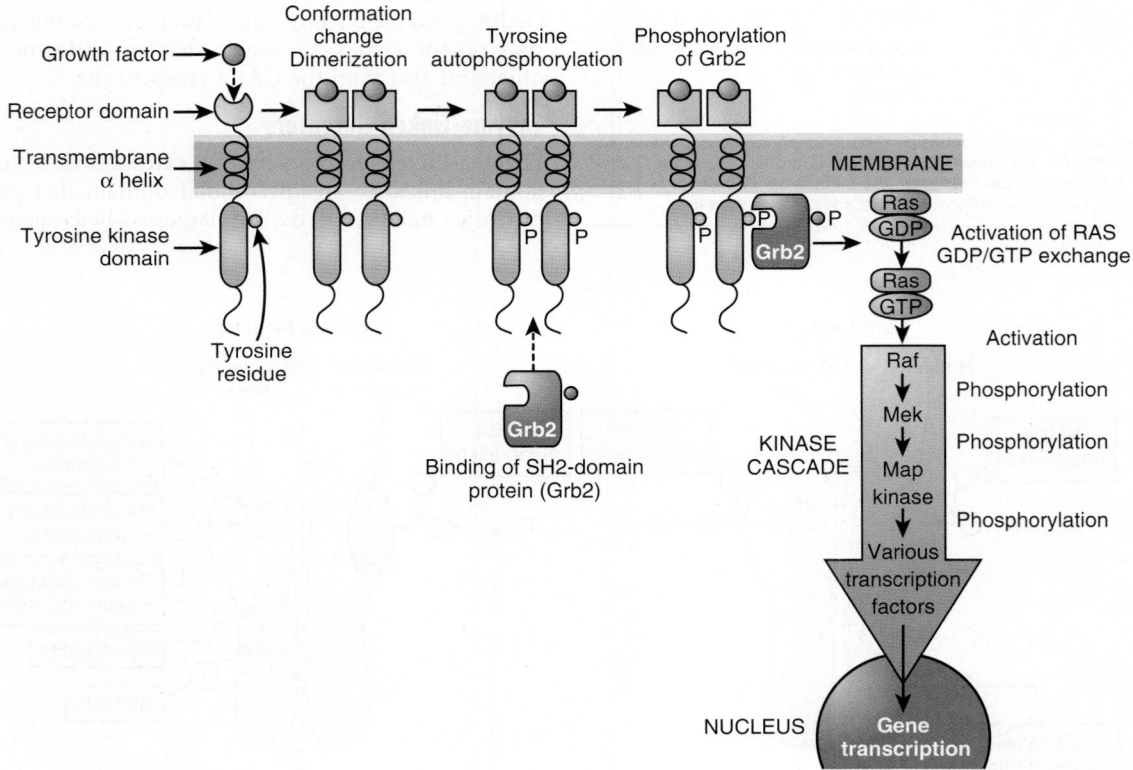

Fig. 125.9. Functioning of kinase-linked receptors. The main steps are dimerization of the receptor, autophosphorylation, and phosphorylation of targeted proteins. The growth factor pathway is shown with the kinase cascade involving the successive phosphorylation of many enzymes (Raf, Mek, Map kinase), eventually leading to gene transcription. *GDP,* guanosine diphosphate; *GTP,* guanosine triphosphate. (Modified from Rang HP, Dale MM, Ritter JM, et al. Rang and Dale's Pharmacology. 7th ed. Philadelphia: Churchill Livingstone; 2012.)

Guanylate cyclases and cGMP-mediated signaling cascades play a central role in the regulation of diverse pathophysiologic processes, including vascular smooth muscle motility, intestinal fluid and electrolyte homeostasis, and retinal photo transduction.[25]

Nuclear Receptors

Nuclear receptors belong to a family of functionally and structurally related proteins. They regulate gene expression and are not associated with a membrane. Their principal mechanism of action is shown in Fig. 125.11. The agonist, which must be lipid soluble, diffuses into the cell and binds to the nuclear receptor located either in the cytosol or in the nucleus. The complex agonist-activated receptor then binds on high-affinity sites on DNA, hormone response element (HRE), situated on the promoter region of genes, whose transcription can then be induced or suppressed. Because gene transcription is at their origin, these effects are slow to develop.

Endogenous agonists for these receptors include steroid and thyroid hormones as well as agents such as retinoic acid and vitamin D. The most commonly used drugs that target these receptors include exogenous steroids and lipid-lowering agents. For many of theses receptors, the corresponding hormone or vitamin has not been identified; these receptors are therefore referred to as *orphan nuclear receptors.*

Receptor Regulation

Continued exposure of a receptor to an agonist often results in a progressive loss of receptor responsiveness, with a diminished receptor-mediated response over time. This is called *desensitization* (or tachyphylaxis) and is classified into two forms. Homologous desensitization is a process in which only the activated receptor is "turned off" or desensitized, whereas heterologous (cross-) desensitization refers to processes in which the activation of one type of receptor can result in the desensitization of other types of receptors. Interaction of the receptor with an antagonist prevents the occurrence of desensitization.

In general, desensitization occurs in three ways (Fig. 125.12A): (1) inactivation or uncoupling of the receptor, which is usually the result of receptor phosphorylation and occurs within seconds to minutes of agonist exposure; (2) sequestration of the receptor in endosomes (from there the receptor is recycled to the cell membrane); and (3) downregulation, which is characterized by receptor endocytosis and destruction in lysosomes with a net loss of receptors in the cell (at the cell membrane and within the cell). The latter develops more slowly than uncoupling, taking hours to days.[26] In addition to receptor degradation, decreased synthesis of the receptor also contributes to this process. Downregulation

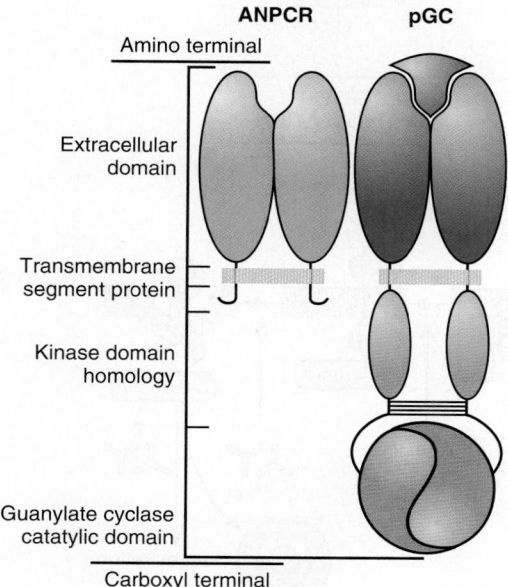

Fig. 125.10. Molecular structure of the natriuretic peptide receptors. *Left,* Atrial natriuretic peptide–C receptor (*ANPCR*) is a clearance receptor that does not possess the kinase and guanylate cyclase domains. It plays a role in the catabolism of natriuretic peptides. *Right,* Typical particulate guanylate cyclase receptor (*pGC*) (ANP-A or -B receptor) is shown with its extracellular dimeric protein-binding domain. The intracellular domain consists of a protein kinase homology domain and a guanylate cyclase catalytic domain.

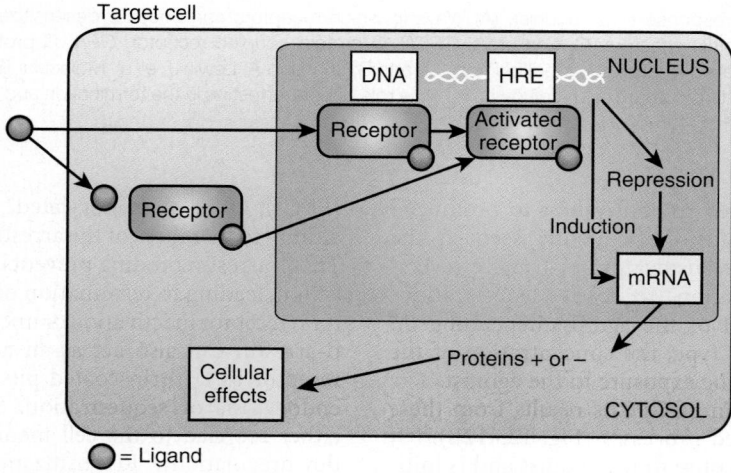

Fig. 125.11. Activation and action of nuclear receptors, located either in the cytosol (eg, steroid receptors) or in the nucleus (eg, vitamin D receptor). *DNA,* deoxyribonucleic acid; *HRE,* hormone response element.

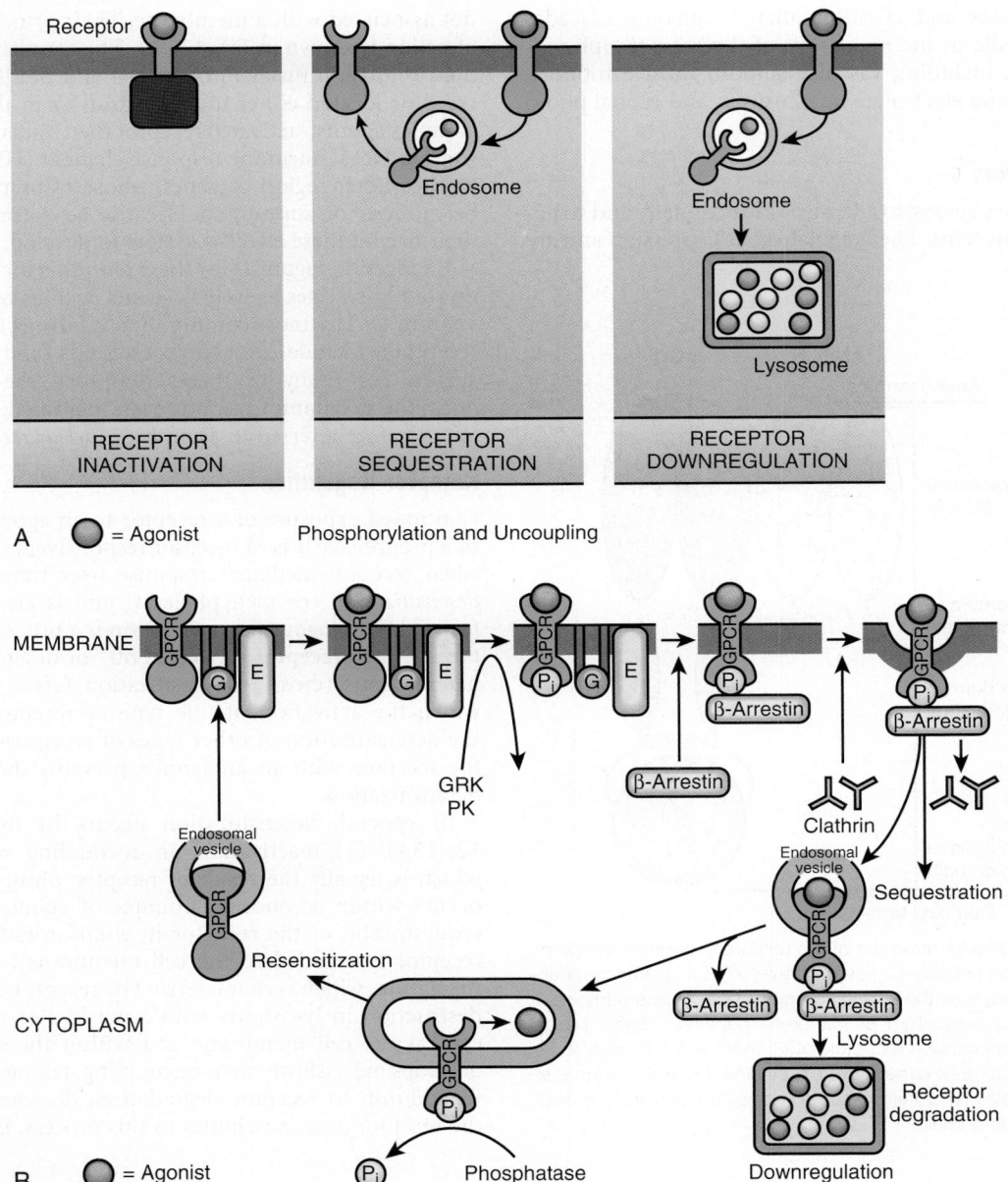

Fig. 125.12. Desensitization in response to an agonist. (A) Ways in which receptors can become desensitized to an agonist. (B) Homologous desensitization of GPCR. *E*, G protein effectors; *G*, G protein; *GPCR*, G protein–coupled receptor; *GRK*, G protein–coupled receptor kinase; *PK*, second-messenger–dependent protein kinases. (A, Modified from Alberts B, Johnson A, Lewis J, et al. Molecular Biology of the Cell. 4th ed. London: Garland Science; 2002. B, Modified from Luttrell LM, Lefkowitz RJ. The role of beta-arrestins in the termination and transduction of G-protein-coupled receptor signals. J Cell Sci. 2002;115;455-465.)

is responsible for the decreased responsiveness to prolonged exogenous catecholamine infusion frequently seen in the critical care population.[27] Desensitization is usually reversible, within minutes (inactivation) to hours (sequestration/down-regulation) of removal of the agonist depending on the specific receptor and cell type, the concentration of the agonist, and the duration of the exposure to the agonist.

Homologous desensitization of GPCRs results from these three distinct and coordinated processes (Fig. 125.12B).[28] It begins within seconds of exposure to the agonist and is initiated by phosphorylation of the receptor by G protein–coupled receptor kinases (GRKs) and second messenger–dependent protein kinases (protein kinase A [PKA] and protein kinase C

[PKC]). Once phosphorylated, the receptor binds with high affinity to members of the arrestin gene family, the β-arrestins. The β-arrestin binding prevents the receptor–G protein interaction, leading to termination of signaling by G protein effectors (receptor inactivation or uncoupling). The receptor-bound β-arrestin can also act as an adapter protein to couple the receptor to clathrin-coated pits, inducing receptor-mediated endocytosis or sequestration. Subsequently, the receptor is either recycled to the cell membrane or degraded (receptor downregulation). Resensitization of a GPCR requires its dephosphorylation and dissociation from its agonist. In contrast to homologous desensitization, heterologous desensitization of GPCRs occurs when inhibition of one GPCR is induced by the activation of another GPCR. One well-recognized mechanism is the phosphorylation of one GPCR by second messenger–dependent protein kinases (PKA and PKC) activated by any other GPCRs. Such phosphorylation of the receptor impairs receptor–G protein coupling and leads to the inactivation of the receptor. However, it is becoming increasingly clear that receptor phosphorylation is not the exclusive mediator of heterologous desensitization and that events downstream are involved.[29]

As GPCRs, channel-linked and enzyme-linked receptors are desensitized following prolonged or repeated agonist exposure. Channel-linked receptors are phosphorylated by second messenger–dependent protein kinases while tyrosine kinase receptors are internalized.

Upregulation refers to the increase in receptor sensitivity seen in the setting of lack of agonist stimulation or prolonged presence of a receptor antagonist. This is best exemplified by a phenomenon seen when a β-adrenergic blocking agent such as propranolol is administered for a long period of time and abruptly discontinued. Because a greater number of sensitized β-adrenergic receptors become available for stimulation by endogenous agonists, rebound hypertension is observed.

Signal Transduction Mechanisms: Intracellular Messengers and Effectors

After binding of an agonist to receptors such as GPCRs or enzyme-linked receptors, the signal transduction mechanisms from the membrane first involve the production of second messengers such as cyclic adenosine monophosphate (cAMP), cGMP, arachidonic acid and its metabolites, diacylglycerol (DAG), inositol 1,4,5-triphosphate (IP_3), and Ca^{2+}. These, in turn, activate protein kinases and calcium-binding proteins, all of which result in different biological effects (Fig. 125.13). Thus the synthesis and degradation of intracellular second messengers are described first, followed by a review of the role of protein kinases and calcium-binding proteins in the transduction mechanisms.

Second Messengers

Cyclic Adenosine Monophosphate

This pathway is involved in signal transduction initiated by binding of agonists to GPCRs. cAMP is synthesized from adenosine triphosphate (ATP) after the action of adenylate cyclase, which is a transmembrane glycoprotein of the cell membrane. To date, nine forms of adenylate cyclase (types I to IX) have been identified by molecular cloning, and several have described features that are hypothetical.[30] Cyclic AMP regulates many aspects of cellular function (cell division and differentiation, ion transport, etc.) by one common mechanism involving activation of protein kinases. These, in turn, regulate the function of many different cellular proteins by catalyzing the phosphorylation of serine and threonine residues. Phosphorylation can then either activate or inhibit target enzymes or ion channels.[9] As previously mentioned, receptors coupled with G_s proteins stimulate adenylate cyclase and produce an increase in cAMP, whereas receptors coupled with G_i proteins inhibit adenylate cyclase and reduce cAMP.

The degradation of cAMP is catalyzed by phosphodiesterases leading to the production of 5'-AMP, an inactive product. Phosphodiesterases are a complex family of enzymes divided into 11 groups according to mechanism of regulation, selectivity for the substrate (cAMP or cGMP), preferential

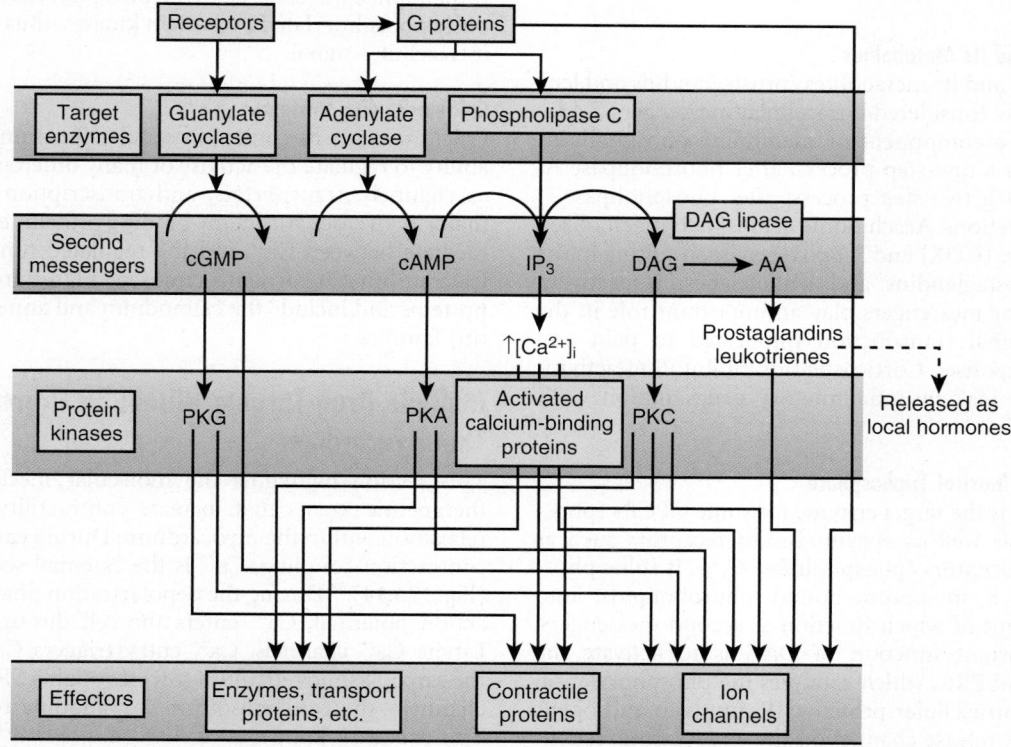

Fig. 125.13. Transduction mechanisms of membrane signaling. *AA,* arachidonic acid; *cAMP,* cyclic adenosine monophosphate; *cGMP,* cyclic guanosine monophosphate; *DAG,* diacylglycerol; *IP3,* inositol 1,4,5-triphosphate; *PKA,* protein kinase A; *PKC,* protein kinase C; *PKG,* protein kinase G. (Modified from Rang HP, Dale MM, Ritter JM, et al. Rang and Dale's Pharmacology. 7th ed. Philadelphia: Churchill Livingstone; 2012.)

localization, and sensitivity to various inhibitors.[31] In critically ill children, milrinone, used for its positive inotropic effect and vasodilating properties, is a phosphodiesterase inhibitor selective for the type III isoenzyme.

Cyclic Guanosine Monophosphate

As discussed previously, guanylate cyclase is part of the cytosolic portion of some transmembrane receptors (membrane form) but also exists as a cytosolic enzyme (soluble form) activated by various molecules, including NO. Stimulation of guanylate cyclase results in the accumulation of cGMP. This second messenger then regulates complex signaling cascades through immediate downstream effectors, including cGMP-dependent protein kinases (eg, protein kinase G [PKG]), cGMP-regulated phosphodiesterases (mainly type II and III), and cyclic nucleotide-gated ion channels (cells of the retina), which eventually leads to a variety of physiologic effects.[32] For example, NO readily passes across the target cell membrane and activates soluble guanylate cyclase in vascular smooth muscle, resulting in increased cGMP production with the regulation of various downstream targets such as protein kinases and ion channels, which culminates in vasodilatation.

As with cAMP, the degradation of cGMP into inactive GMP is catalyzed by phosphodiesterases. In pulmonary and penile vascular smooth muscle cells, phosphodiesterase type V is responsible for the degradation of cGMP; inhibition of this enzyme results in an accumulation of cGMP in the cytosol with smooth muscle relaxation and vasodilatation. As such, phosphodiesterase type V inhibitors (eg, sildenafil) are widely recognized as efficacious for the treatment of erectile dysfunction in men and have been shown to induce pulmonary vasodilatation both in children and adults and are part of the strategies available for the treatment of pulmonary hypertension.[33-35]

Arachidonic Acid and Its Metabolites

Arachidonic acid and its metabolites (prostaglandins and leukotrienes) are now considered intracellular messengers.[36] Arachidonic acid is a component of membrane phospholipids released either in a one-step process, after phospholipase A_2 (PLA_2) action, or a two-step process, after phospholipase C and DAG lipase actions. Arachidonic acid is then metabolized by cyclooxygenase (COX) and 5-lipoxygenase, resulting in the synthesis of prostaglandins and leukotrienes, respectively. These intracellular messengers play an important role in the regulation of signal transduction implicated in pain and inflammatory responses. Corticosteroids inhibit PLA_2 activity, whereas nonsteroidal antiinflammatory drugs inhibit COX activity.

Diacylglycerol and Inositol Triphosphate

Phospholipase C is the target enzyme for some GPCRs (phospholipase C-β) as well as enzyme-linked receptors such as tyrosine kinase receptors (phospholipase C-γ). It splits phosphatidylinositol, a membrane-bound phospholipids, into DAG and IP_3, both of which function as second messengers. The most important function of DAG is to activate the membrane-bound PKC, which catalyzes the phosphorylation of a variety of intracellular proteins. IP_3 binds to and opens an IP_3-gated Ca^{2+} release channel on the endoplasmic reticulum membrane, which results in an increase in free intracellular Ca^{2+} concentration ($[Ca^{2+}]_i$).

Calcium Ions

$[Ca^{2+}]_i$ is critically important as a regulator of cell function. Indeed, an increase in $[Ca^{2+}]_i$ is the most important intracellular messenger signaling pathway known in biological systems. When $[Ca^{2+}]_i$ is at its baseline value, few proteins have an affinity sufficient to bind to Ca^{2+}. Once membrane signaling occurs, an increase in $[Ca^{2+}]_i$ results, derived from either the extracellular space or from the lumen of the endoplasmic reticulum, and allows binding of proteins to Ca^{2+}. Finally, this binding can trigger contraction, secretion, a modification in metabolism regulation, or several other effects depending on the cell type involved. To maintain a low resting $[Ca^{2+}]_i$, Ca^{2+} is permanently expulsed from the cytosol into the extracellular compartment or into the endoplasmic reticulum via a Ca^{2+}-ATPase and Na^+/Ca^{2+} exchanger.

Phosphorylation of Proteins

Many receptor-mediated signals produce variations in the concentration of second messengers, such as cAMP, cGMP, arachidonic acid, DAG, IP_3, and Ca^{2+}, as previously discussed. These can then modify the activity of other proteins, mainly protein kinases and calcium-binding proteins.

Protein Kinases

Protein kinases are enzymes located in the cytoplasm that phosphorylate proteins. The main protein kinases consist of PKA, PKG, and PKC[37] as well as tyrosyl protein kinases (part of tyrosine kinase receptors). They are distinguished from each other by the different intracellular second messengers involved in their regulation and by the selective substrates they use. They all have a binding site for Mg^{2+}-ATP (phosphate donor) and for substrate protein as well as various regulatory sites. Phosphorylation of these proteins is short lived because protein phosphatases rapidly dephosphorylate proteins previously phosphorylated by protein kinases, thus terminating the intracellular signal.

Calcium-Binding Proteins

Calcium exerts its control in cellular function by virtue of its ability to regulate the activity of many different proteins, such as channels, transporters, and transcription factors. In the majority of cases, a calcium-binding protein serves as an intermediate between Ca^{2+} and the regulated functional protein. Calcium-binding proteins represent a large group of cytosolic proteins and include the calmodulin and annexin (or lipocortin) families.

Multiple Drug Targets Within an Organ System: The Myocardium

This section highlights the molecular mechanisms behind therapeutic agents that increase contractility and accelerate relaxation within the myocardium. During cardiac excitation-contraction coupling, Ca^{2+} is the essential second messenger (Fig. 125.14).[38] During the depolarization phase of the cardiac action potential, Ca^{2+} enters the cell through voltage-gated L-type Ca^{2+} channels. Ca^{2+} entry triggers Ca^{2+} release from the sarcoplasmic reticulum (SR) through a SR membrane ion channel—the cardiac/isoform 2 ryanodine receptor (RyR2). This process is known as *calcium-induced Ca^{2+} release* (CICR). The combination of Ca^{2+} influx and CICR raises $[Ca^{2+}]_i$, allowing Ca^{2+} binding to troponin C (TnC), which permits

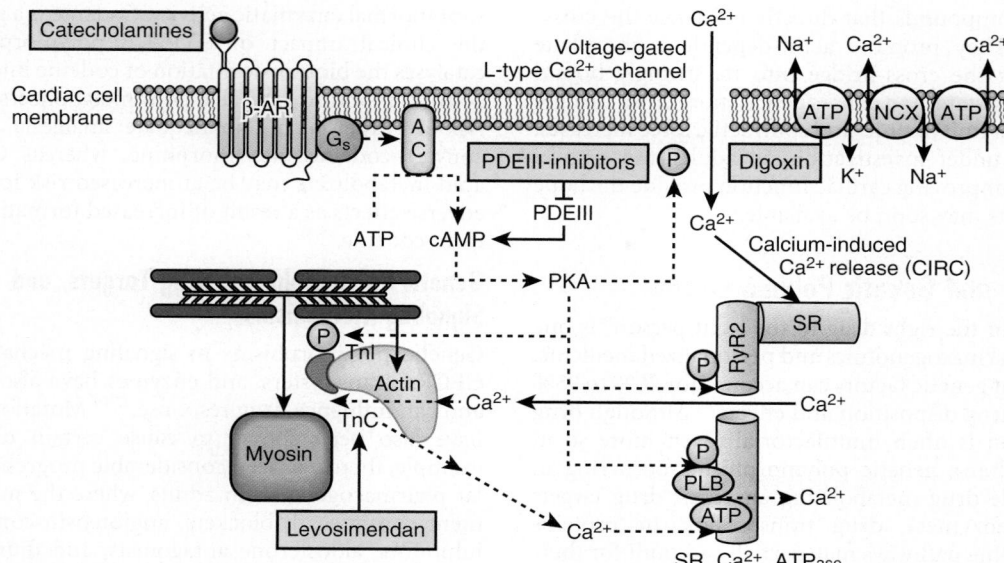

Fig. 125.14. Cardiac excitation-contraction coupling and molecular targets of therapeutic agents with positive inotropic and lusitropic effects. (Note: Under physiologic conditions, NCX works mainly in the Ca²⁺ extrusion mode; however, if intracellular Na⁺ concentration is elevated, as is the case with digoxin, it can work in the Ca²⁺ influx mode.) *AC*, adenylate cyclase; *ATP*, adenosine triphosphate; *β-AR*, β-adrenergic receptor; *cAMP*, cyclic adenosine monophosphate; *G_s*, stimulatory G protein; *NCX*, Na⁺/Ca²⁺ exchanger; *P*, phosphorus; *PDE*, phosphodiesterase; *PKA*, protein kinase A; *PLB*, phospholamban; *RyR₂*, cardiac/isoform 2 ryanodine receptor; *SR*, sarcoplasmic reticulum; *TnI*, troponin I; *TnC*, troponin C. (Modified from Toller GT, Stranz, C. Levosimendan, a new inotropic and vasodilating agent. Anesthesiology. 2006;104:556-569.)

cross-bridging between actin and myosin and ultimately contraction. For relaxation to occur $[Ca^{2+}]_i$ must decline, allowing Ca^{2+} to dissociate from TnC. This requires Ca^{2+} transport out of the cytosol by four pathways: SR Ca^{2+}-ATPase (the main one, also known as SERCA), sarcolemmal Na⁺/Ca²⁺ exchanger, sarcolemmal Ca^{2+}-ATPase, and mitochondrial Ca^{2+} uniport. SR Ca^{2+}-ATPase activity is modulated by phospholamban, an endogenous inhibitor. Under physiologic conditions, there is no net gain or loss of cellular Ca^{2+} with each contraction-relaxation cycle.

There are two main ways to pharmacologically increase the strength of cardiac contraction (see Fig. 125.14)[38,39]: (1) by increasing the amount of $[Ca^{2+}]_i$ available for binding to TnC or (2) by increasing the sensitivity of myofilaments to Ca^{2+}:

1. *Catecholamines and phosphodiesterase type III inhibitors (PDEIII inhibitors).* β-adrenergic receptor stimulation by catecholamines activates a GTP-binding protein (G_s), which stimulates adenylate cyclase to produce cAMP, whereas PDEIII inhibitors (eg, milrinone) prevent cAMP degradation. The resulting increase in cAMP activates PKA, which, in turn, phosphorylates intracellular targets, including voltage-gated L-type Ca^{2+} channels, RyR2, phospholamban, and troponin I (TnI). Phosphorylation of voltage-gated L-type Ca^{2+} channels enhances Ca^{2+} entry into the cytosol with subsequent increase in CICR from the SR and contraction (positive inotropic effect of catecholamines and PDEIII inhibitors). In contrast, phosphorylation of phospholamban activates SR Ca^{2+}-ATPase with increased Ca^{2+} transport from the cytosol back to the SR and thus promotes relaxation (positive lusitropic effect of catecholamines and PDEIII inhibitors). This action also contributes to the overall gain in cardiac excitation-contraction coupling by increasing the SR Ca^{2+} content available for the next contraction. However, such increased

loading of the SR with Ca^{2+} may be a key factor in the development of Ca^{2+}-mediated arrhythmias.[40] The lusitropic effect of catecholamines and PDEIII inhibitors is also mediated by phosphorylation of TnI, which decreases the affinity of myofilaments for Ca^{2+}.

2. *Digoxin.* Digoxin enhances myocardial contractility, although modestly, by inhibiting the Na⁺/K⁺-ATPase pump with a resultant mild increase in intracellular Na⁺. This increase of Na⁺ subsequently inhibits the extrusion of Ca^{2+} from the cytosol outside the cell by the sarcolemmal Na⁺/Ca²⁺ exchanger. Ca^{2+} not extruded from the cytosol is stored in SR and allows increased release of Ca^{2+} during the next contraction.

3. *Ca^{2+} sensitizers.* More recently, Ca^{2+} sensitizers (eg, levosimendan), a new class of inotropic agents, have been developed. They improve cardiac contractility by binding to TnC and stabilizing its interaction with Ca^{2+}, which results in prolonged interaction of actin-myosin filaments. One possible limitation of some Ca^{2+} sensitizers is worsening diastolic function due to facilitation of cross-bridging at diastolic Ca^{2+} concentrations. However, this does not appear to be the case of levosimendan because its binding to TnC depends on $[Ca^{2+}]_i$ (ie, when $[Ca^{2+}]_i$ increases during systole, it facilitates actin-myosin interaction, and when $[Ca^{2+}]_i$ decreases during diastole, it does not). One potential beneficial effect of theses agents compared with catecholamines and PDEIII inhibitors comes from the fact that they do not increase $[Ca^{2+}]_i$ and, as such, have neutral effects on myocardial oxygen demand and heart rhythm.[39] Promising new inotropic agents have been developed.[41,42] Among these, istaroxime, a lusi-inotropic agent, inhibits Na⁺/K⁺-ATPase pump (increased inotropy like digoxin) and stimulates SR Ca^{2+}-ATPase (accelerated relaxation). Cardiac myosin activators (eg, omecamtiv mecarbil) represent a

new class of compounds that directly influence the cross-bridge cycle. They promote actin-dependent phosphate release moving the cross-bridge into its strongly bound force-producing state. As a consequence, more cross-bridges are activated per unit of time, and contractile force increases. Although still under investigations in adults, these novel approaches to improving cardiac function provide the hope that such agents may soon be available.

Drug Response and Genetic Polymorphisms

"The right dose of the right drug to the right person" is one of the goals of pharmacogenomics and personalized medicine. It is estimated that genetic factors can account for 20% to 95% of variability in drug disposition and effects.[43] Although drug response variation is often multifactorial (even more so in critically ill children), genetic polymorphisms occurring in genes that encode drug-metabolizing enzymes, drug targets (eg, receptors, enzymes), drug transporters, or proteins involved in signaling pathways may partially account for therapeutic failure and toxicity.

Most genetic variations involve single-nucleotide polymorphisms (SNPs)—that is, the exchange of a single nucleotide in the DNA sequence. Small insertions and deletions, variable-number tandem repeats, gene deletions, and gene duplications can also take place. Depending on where SNPs occur, they can result in no change in the protein amino acid sequence (silent polymorphism or synonymous SNP) or in a change in the coded amino acid sequence (nonsynonymous SNP) that can have no functional consequence or can result in altered protein function. The latter can have significant clinical or therapeutic implications. In addition, given that genes often present many SNPs, it has become increasingly recognized that single SNPs fail to predict drug responses, whereas combinations of SNPs on a given chromosome (specific haplotype) are clinically more significant and can better determine drug effects.[44]

Genetic Polymorphisms and Drug Disposition

Many major enzymes involved in phase I and phase II drug metabolism have known polymorphisms leading to phenotypic differences (ie, clinically significant alteration in drug-metabolizing enzyme activities).[43] For a specific polymorphic drug metabolizing enzyme, homozygous individuals for the wild-type allele exhibit normal enzymatic activity (extensive metabolizers), heterozygous individuals may have reduced enzymatic activity (heterozygous extensive/intermediate metabolizers), and homozygous individuals with the mutant allele have low enzymatic activity (poor metabolizers). For some enzymes (eg, CYP2D6), individuals have ultrarapid metabolism as a result of gene duplications of functional alleles (ultrarapid metabolizers). The clinical consequences of such polymorphisms may be fourfold: (1) poor metabolizers can have an enhanced drug effect, either therapeutic or toxic, resulting from higher plasma concentrations of a given drug; (2) poor metabolizers can experience a diminished drug effect resulting from the inability of a prodrug to be converted into the active metabolite due to low enzymatic activity; (3) ultrarapid metabolizers can experience diminished drug effect resulting from markedly lower plasma concentrations of a given drug; and (4) ultrarapid metabolizers can experience enhanced drug effect from an excessive conversion of a prodrug into the active metabolite as a result of

supranormal enzymatic activity. Codeine is a good example of the clinical impact of CYP2D6 polymorphism. CYP2D6 catalyses the biotransformation of codeine into morphine, the active compound. CYP2D6 poor metabolizers are at increased risk of experiencing inadequate analgesia as a failure to convert codeine into morphine, whereas CYP2D6 ultrarapid metabolizers may be at increased risk for opioid-related adverse effects as a result of increased formation of morphine from codeine.[45,46]

Genetic Polymorphisms, Drug Targets, and Signaling Mechanisms

Genetic polymorphisms in signaling mechanisms involving GPCRs, transporters, and enzymes have also been identified and can influence drug response.[47-49] Mutations in G proteins have also been shown to cause certain diseases.[50] As an example, there has been considerable progress in cardiovascular pharmacogenetics in adults, where the mainstay of treatment comprises β-blockers, angiotensin-converting enzyme inhibitors, aldosterone antagonists, and diuretics. The most studied genetic variants relating to these pharmacologic interventions are summarized in Table 125.3.[51] However, pharmacogenetics-based heart failure therapy has not reached the bedside due to inconsistent results. As multiple factors beyond genetic variability have the potential to influence drug response (see Fig. 125.1), mathematic models and systems biology capable of integrating all of these factors may have a better chance to adequately predict drug response and eventually be applied clinically.

Drug Response and Development

From birth through puberty, dramatic developmental changes occur that can have a profound impact on drug disposition and action. Most studies have evaluated the effect of age on pharmacokinetics, revealing clinically important differences compared with adults.[52,53] The ontogenesis of important drug-metabolizing enzymes, the cytochrome P-450 enzymes, is a good example of how development affects drug disposition and how age is an important determinant in selecting appropriate doses (see Table 125.3). Even though developmental changes are also expected to affect the different players involved in pharmacodynamics, scarce data concerning the ontogenesis of specific drug targets, signal transduction mechanisms, and intracellular messengers are currently available. To date, human studies have mainly dealt with receptor expression (and not function), mostly in the brain, and have found age-related differences in terms of receptor density and regions of the brain where receptors are expressed.[54-56] The exact consequences of these differences are unknown, but it is speculated that they may play a role in organ maturation as well as in the pathophysiology of diseases and drug response.

Drug Response and Disease

Although a vast literature exists regarding the effects of diseases on drug pharmacokinetics, limited data are available about pharmacodynamic changes occurring as a consequence of illness. Of particular interest for the critically ill population is the myocardial hyporesponsiveness to catecholamines observed during sepsis. Sepsis, which is associated with elevated circulating catecholamine levels, induces a disruption at

TABLE 125.3 Summary of Most Studied Genetic Variants in the Pharmacogenetics of Heart Failure

Receptor/Enzyme/Transporter	Genetic Variant	Pharmacogenetic Association
Angiotensin-converting enzyme (ACE)	Insertion/deletion (I/D)[a]	Individuals with the DD genotype have high ACE activity Benefits of high-dose ACE inhibitors appear maximal for DD patients
β_1-adrenergic	Arg389Gly	Arg389 associated with a greater agonist-promoted coupling
		Associated with enhanced response to some β-blockers (bucindolol, atenolol, metoprolol) in some studies
		Associated with increased inotropic potency to norepinephrine
β_1-adrenergic	Ser49Gly	Gly49 associated with enhanced desensitization and agonist-promoted downregulation Inconsistent evidence that this translates to difference in drug response
β_2-adrenergic	Thr164Ile	Ile164 loss-of-function allele, attenuated response to sympathetic stimulation
β_2-adrenergic	Gln 27Glu[b]	Glu27 associated with complete resistance to downregulation
β_2-adrenergic	Arg16Gly[b]	Arg16 associated with a reduction in agonist promoted downregulation
G protein receptor kinase 5 (GRK5)	Gln41Leu	Leu41 gain-of-function allele with enhanced desensitization
(acts on β_1- and β_2-adrenergic)		Associated with improved survival in patients with heart failure by providing a "genetic β-blockade"
Nitric oxide synthase 3 (NOS3)	Asp298Glu	Glu298 associated with good response to hydralazine/isosorbide dinitrate
Renal sodium transporter	SLC12A3 Ala264	Associated with enhanced excretion potassium and chloride with all loop diuretics

[a]Referring to presence or absence of an insertion at the 287th base-paired insertion.
[b]Gln27Glu and Arg16Gly are in linkage disequilibrium.
Modified from Anwar MS, Iskandar MZ, Parry HM, et al. The future of pharmacogenetics in the treatment of heart failure. Pharmacogenomics. 2015;16: 1817-1827.)

various levels of the β-adrenergic signaling cascade (Fig. 125.15).[3] Postulated mechanisms, mainly derived from animal studies, include inactivation of catecholamines by superoxide, decreased β-adrenergic receptor density, decreased stimulatory G proteins (G$_s$), and increased inhibitory G proteins (G$_i$) (β_2-adrenergic receptor in rat ventricular cardiomyocytes can couple to G$_i$; whether human cardiac β-adrenergic receptors can do the same is unknown[57]). These changes result in decreased activity of adenylate cyclase and reduced levels of cAMP. In addition, NO released during sepsis activates soluble guanylate cyclase with increased cGMP and activation of PKG, which in turn inhibits PKA. These alterations ultimately lead to decreased contractility, impaired myocyte relaxation, and reduced chronotropy.

Conclusion

Even though knowledge of how drugs work at a molecular level has grown tremendously, continued elucidation of normal signal transduction physiology and of the effects of genetics, development, and disease states on the functional integrity of receptors, signaling pathways, and effectors should improve and refine pharmacologic interventions administered to critically ill children. To optimize the efficacy/toxicity ratio, both genetic and nongenetic factors, including the patient's age, sex, organ function, ethnicity, concomitant therapy, drug interactions, nature and severity of the disease, comorbid conditions, and the use of extracorporeal device (eg, extracorporeal membrane oxygenation), should be taken into account so as to individualize pharmacotherapy in the pediatric intensive care unit setting.

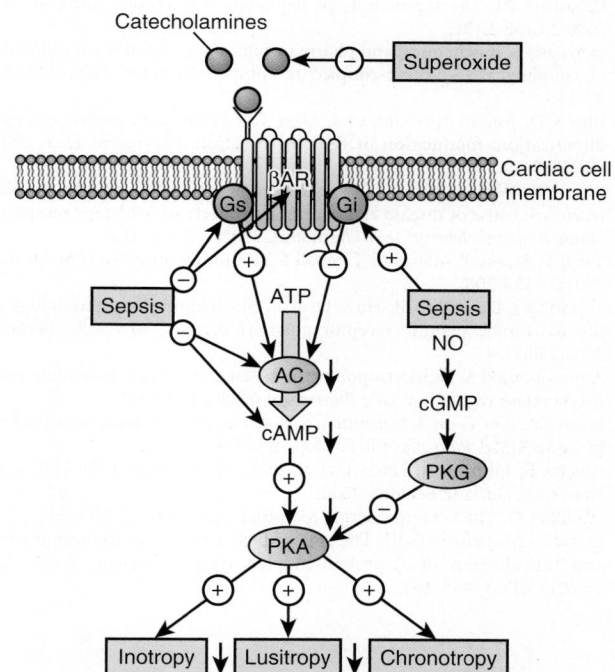

Fig. 125.15. Sepsis-induced alterations in the β-adrenergic signaling cascade. *AC,* adenylate cyclase; *ATP,* adenosine triphosphate; *βAR,* β-adrenergic receptor; *cAMP,* cyclic adenosine monophosphate; *cGMP,* cyclic guanosine monophosphate; *G$_i$,* inhibitory G protein; *G$_s$,* stimulatory G protein; *NO,* nitric oxide; *PKA,* protein kinase A; *PKG,* protein kinase G. (Modified from Rudiger A, Singer M. Mechanisms of sepsis-induced cardiac dysfunction. Crit Care Med. 2007;35:1599-1608.)

Key References

1. Carcillo JA, Doughty L, Kofos D, et al. Cytochrome P450 mediated-drug metabolism is reduced in children with sepsis-induced multiple organ failure. *Intensive Care Med.* 2003;29:980-984.
2. De Paepe P, Belpaire FM, Buylaert WA. Pharmacokinetic and pharmacodynamic considerations when treating patients with sepsis and septic shock. *Clin Pharmacokinet.* 2002;41:1135-1151.
3. Rudiger A, Singer M. Mechanisms of sepsis-induced cardiac dysfunction. *Crit Care Med.* 2007;35:1599-1608.
4. Dorn GW 2nd, Liggett SB. Mechanisms of pharmacogenomic effects of genetic variation within the cardiac adrenergic network in heart failure. *Mol Pharmacol.* 2009;76:466-480.
5. Evans WE, Johnson JA. Pharmacogenomics: the inherited basis for interindividual differences in drug response. *Annu Rev Genomics Hum Genet.* 2001;2:9-39.
6. Roden DM, George AL Jr. The genetic basis of variability in drug responses. *Nat Rev Drug Discov.* 2002;1:37-44.
7. Katzung BG, Masters SB, Trevor AJ. *Basic & Clinical Pharmacology.* 11 ed. New York: McGraw-Hill; 2009.
8. Hilal-Dandan R, Brunton L. *Goodman & Gilman's Manual of Pharmacology and Therapeutics.* 2 ed. New York: McGraw-Hill; 2014.
9. Rang HP, Dale MM, Ritter JM, Flower RJ. *Rang & Dale's Pharmacology.* 7 ed. London: Churchill Livingstone; 2012.
10. O'Blenes SB, Roy N, Konstantinov I, et al. Vasopressin reversal of phenoxybenzamine-induced hypotension after the Norwood procedure. *J Thorac Cardiovasc Surg.* 2002;123:1012-1013.
11. Kenakin T. Inverse, protean, and ligand-selective agonism: matters of receptor conformation. *FASEB J.* 2001;15:598-611.
12. Du Souich P. Transporteurs membranaires. In: Beaulieu P, Pichette V, Desroches J, Du Souich P, eds. *Précis de Pharmacologie.* Montreal: PUM; 2015:63-76.
13. Cole SP. Targeting multidrug resistance protein 1 (MRP1, ABCC1): past, present, and future. *Annu Rev Pharmacol Toxicol.* 2014;54:95-117.
14. Lin L, Yee SW, Kim RB, Giacomini KM. SLC transporters as therapeutic targets: emerging opportunities. *Nat Rev Drug Discov.* 2015;14:543-560.
16. Lefkowitz RJ. The superfamily of heptahelical receptors. *Nat Cell Biol.* 2000;2:E133-E136.
17. Hermans E. Biochemical and pharmacological control of the multiplicity of coupling at G-protein-coupled receptors. *Pharmacol Ther.* 2003;99:25-44.
19. Rios CD, Jordan BA, Gomes I, Devi LA. G-protein-coupled receptor dimerization: modulation of receptor function. *Pharmacol Ther.* 2001;92:71-87.
20. Seifert R, Wenzel-Seifert K. Constitutive activity of G-protein-coupled receptors: cause of disease and common property of wild-type receptors. *Naunyn Schmiedebergs Arch Pharmacol.* 2002;366:381-416.
21. Takai Y, Sasaki T, Matozaki T. Small GTP-binding proteins. *Physiol Rev.* 2001;81:153-208.
23. Tremblay J, Desjardins R, Hum D, et al. Biochemistry and physiology of the natriuretic peptide receptor guanylyl cyclases. *Mol Cell Biochem.* 2002;230:31-47.
24. Andreopoulos S, Papapetropoulos A. Molecular aspects of soluble guanylyl cyclase regulation. *Gen Pharmacol.* 2000;34:147-157.
25. Lucas KA, Pitari GM, Kazerounian S, et al. Guanylyl cyclases and signaling by cyclic GMP. *Pharmacol Rev.* 2000;52:375-414.
26. Alberts B, Johnson A, Lewis J, et al. *Molecular Biology of the Cell.* 4 ed. New York: Garland Science; 2002.
27. Wallukat G. The beta-adrenergic receptors. *Herz.* 2002;27:683-690.
28. Luttrell LM, Lefkowitz RJ. The role of beta-arrestins in the termination and transduction of G-protein-coupled receptor signals. *J Cell Sci.* 2002;115(Pt 3):455-465.
29. Hosey MM. What molecular events underlie heterologous desensitization? Focus on "receptor phosphorylation does not mediate cross talk between muscarinic M(3) and bradykinin B(2) receptors." *Am J Physiol.* 1999;277(5 Pt 1):C856-C858.
30. Hanoune J, Defer N. Regulation and role of adenylyl cyclase isoforms. *Annu Rev Pharmacol Toxicol.* 2001;41:145-174.
31. Essayan DM. Cyclic nucleotide phosphodiesterases. *J Allergy Clin Immunol.* 2001;108:671-680.
32. Murad F. Shattuck Lecture. Nitric oxide and cyclic GMP in cell signaling and drug development. *N Engl J Med.* 2006;355:2003-2011.
33. Archer SL, Michelakis ED. Phosphodiesterase type 5 inhibitors for pulmonary arterial hypertension. *N Engl J Med.* 2009;361:1864-1871.
34. Carroll WD, Dhillon R. Sildenafil as a treatment for pulmonary hypertension. *Arch Dis Child.* 2003;88:827-828.
35. Steinhorn RH, Kinsella JP, Pierce C, et al. Intravenous sildenafil in the treatment of neonates with persistent pulmonary hypertension. *J Pediatr.* 2009;155:841-847, e841.
36. Toker A. Phosphoinositides and signal transduction. *Cell Mol Life Sci.* 2002;59:761-779.
37. Schenk PW, Snaar-Jagalska BE. Signal perception and transduction: the role of protein kinases. *Biochim Biophys Acta.* 1999;1449:1-24.
38. Bers DM. Cardiac excitation-contraction coupling. *Nature.* 2002;415:198-205.
39. Toller WG, Stranz C. Levosimendan, a new inotropic and vasodilator agent. *Anesthesiology.* 2006;104:556-569.
40. Scoote M, Williams AJ. Myocardial calcium signalling and arrhythmia pathogenesis. *Biochem Biophys Res Commun.* 2004;322:1286-1309.
41. George M, Rajaram M, Shanmugam E, VijayaKumar TM. Novel drug targets in clinical development for heart failure. *Eur J Clin Pharmacol.* 2014;70:765-774.
42. Hasenfuss G, Teerlink JR. Cardiac inotropes: current agents and future directions. *Eur Heart J.* 2011;32:1838-1845.
43. Weinshilboum R. Inheritance and drug response. *N Engl J Med.* 2003;348:529-537.
44. Drysdale CM, McGraw DW, Stack CB, et al. Complex promoter and coding region beta 2-adrenergic receptor haplotypes alter receptor expression and predict in vivo responsiveness. *Proc Natl Acad Sci USA.* 2000;97:10483-10488.
45. Gasche Y, Daali Y, Fathi M, et al. Codeine intoxication associated with ultrarapid CYP2D6 metabolism. *N Engl J Med.* 2004;351:2827-2831.
46. Koren G, Cairns J, Chitayat D, et al. Pharmacogenetics of morphine poisoning in a breastfed neonate of a codeine-prescribed mother. *Lancet.* 2006;368:704.
47. Drazen JM, Yandava CN, Dube L, et al. Pharmacogenetic association between ALOX5 promoter genotype and the response to anti-asthma treatment. *Nat Genet.* 1999;22:168-170.
49. Sadee W, Hoeg E, Lucas J, Wang D. Genetic variations in human G protein-coupled receptors: implications for drug therapy. *AAPS Pharm Sci.* 2001;3:E22.
50. Farfel Z, Bourne HR, Iiri T. The expanding spectrum of G protein diseases. *N Engl J Med.* 1999;340:1012-1020.
51. Anwar MS, Iskandar MZ, Parry HM, et al. The future of pharmacogenetics in the treatment of heart failure. *Pharmacogenomics.* 2015;16:1817-1827.
53. Kearns GL, Abdel-Rahman SM, Alander SW, et al. Developmental pharmacology–drug disposition, action, and therapy in infants and children. *N Engl J Med.* 2003;349:1157-1167.
54. Chugani DC, Muzik O, Juhasz C, et al. Postnatal maturation of human GABAA receptors measured with positron emission tomography. *Ann Neurol.* 2001;49:618-626.
55. Mato S, Del Olmo E, Pazos A. Ontogenetic development of cannabinoid receptor expression and signal transduction functionality in the human brain. *Eur J Neurosci.* 2003;17:1747-1754.

Adverse Drug Reactions and Drug-Drug Interactions

Wade W. Benton, Christa C. Jefferis Kirk, Tsingyi Koh, and Gretchen A. Linggi Irby

PEARLS

- Overall, the incidence of adverse events in pediatric inpatients can range from 4.4% to 16.8% of hospital admissions, which is higher than the estimated incidence of approximately 4% in adults.
- Developmental differences in drug disposition and clearance in pediatrics increase the potential of adverse drug reactions (ADRs) in comparison to adults.
- The economic impact from drug-related morbidity and mortality from ADRs is estimated to be approximately $137 billion to $177 billion. Pediatric ADRs nationally have an estimated economic burden of approximately $252.9 million.
- Drug-drug interactions are mediated via pharmacokinetic and pharmacodynamic properties of medications. Increased awareness of common mechanisms of interaction can aid the clinician in avoiding or ameliorating unwanted adverse effects.
- The pediatric intensive care provider is confronted daily with potentially hazardous drug-drug interactions in the critical care setting. It is nearly impossible to recognize every potential drug-drug interaction in the pediatric critical care setting; however, in most cases, drug-drug interactions are predictable and preventable, with appropriate dosage modifications or avoidance of combinations.

Adverse drug reactions (ADRs) in pediatric critical care settings can increase both the morbidity and mortality of patients as well as hospital costs.[1,2-4] Literature suggests the economic impact from drug-related morbidity and mortality from ADRs is estimated to be approximately $137 billion to $177 billion.[4] Pediatric adverse drug events (ADEs) nationally have an estimated economic burden of approximately $252.9 million.[4] Epidemiologic studies for ADRs confirm that the problem is just as important for children as it is for adults.[1,2,5-8] In comparison to adults, developmental differences in drug disposition and clearance in pediatrics increase the potential for ADRs. There is substantial evidence that the incidence of adverse drug reactions is greater in children than in adults. Many of the therapeutic agents used in the pediatric critical care setting have not been studied and evaluated for safety and efficacy in pediatric patients. Intensive care physicians should have a heightened awareness of the incidence of ADRs so they can assist with recognizing, monitoring, and, ultimately, preventing ADRs. Patients in the intensive care unit are predisposed to ADRs due to the heightened incidence of single and multiple organ failure. Key risk factors include age <1 year, polypharmacy, and impairment of metabolism or drug excretion.[4] To recognize and prevent ADRs, pediatric intensivists need to be aware of the complications associated with drug therapy.

Preventive measures can decrease the occurrence of ADRs. Overall, the incidence of adverse events in pediatric inpatients can range from 4.4% to 16.8% of hospital admissions, which is higher than the estimated incidence of approximately 4% in adults.[4,9,10] Although steps have been taken to reduce ADRs, there are still issues that cause children to be more susceptible. Weight-based dosing and dilution needed for administration of parenteral therapy combined with the fact that sick infants and children may have a reduced ability to survive iatrogenic events create a larger risk of ADRs in the pediatric population.

One of the difficulties in interpreting literature on ADRs is how they are defined. The World Health Organization (WHO) and the Joint Commission on Accreditation of Healthcare Organizations (JCAHO) have varying definitions for ADRs. The American Society for Health-System Pharmacists (ASHP) defines a significant adverse drug reaction as any unexpected, unintended, undesired, or excessive response to a drug that does the following[11]:

- Requires discontinuing the drug (therapeutic or diagnostic)
- Requires changing drug therapy
- Requires modifying the dose (except for minor dosage adjustments)
- Necessitates admission to a hospital
- Prolongs stay in a health care facility
- Necessitates supportive treatment
- Significantly complicates diagnosis
- Negatively affects prognosis
- Results in temporary or permanent harm, disability, or death

ASHP also defines other symptoms that are not considered true adverse drug reactions:

- Side effects
- Drug withdrawal
- Drug abuse syndrome
- Accidental poisoning
- Drug overdose complications

For reporting purposes, the Food and Drug Administration (FDA) categorizes a serious adverse event (an event relating to drugs and devices) as one in which "the patient outcome is death, life-threatening (real risk of death), hospitalization (initial or prolonged), disability (significant, persistent, or permanent), congenital anomaly, or required intervention to prevent permanent impairment or damage."[12]

A critical factor in assessing ADRs is establishing a causal relationship between the suspected drug and the adverse reaction.[15] Identification of ADRS can be arbitrary. Some of the confounding factors are the ambiguous characteristics of the reactions, the fact that patients usually are taking more than one medication at the time of the reaction, and the inability to perform definitive cause-and-effect tests.[15] There have been numerous attempts to formalize the process.[15-21] Karch and Lasagna designed decision tables that can identify a potential reaction, assess the certainty of a link between the drug and the event, and evaluate the underlying cause of the reaction.[15] These provide a framework for a systematic evaluation of potential ADRs and reduce the ambiguity that, at present, characterizes their assessment. Kramer and associates devised an operational assessment using an algorithm with six axes to assess the probability of an ADR occurrence. A scoring system for each axis and an overall score help delineate the likelihood that an ADR has occurred.[18] Similarly, Naranjo and colleagues developed an adverse drug reaction probability scale using 10 questions answered positively, negatively, or unknown to determine the likelihood that an ADR had occurred. The Naranjo method has been shown to improve the reproducibility of ADR assessments.[16]

An FDA algorithm that assesses the characteristics of the event (temporal relationship, dechallenge, rechallenge, and relationship to disease) has been presented.[17] The algorithm contains four questions to assess the likelihood that an adverse drug reaction had occurred:

1. Did the reaction follow a reasonable temporal sequence?
2. Did the patient improve after stopping the drug?
3. Did the reaction reappear on repeated experience (rechallenge)?
4. Could the reaction be reasonably explained by known characteristics of the patient's clinical state?

The categories *remote*, *possible*, *probable*, and *highly probable* are used based on the answers to the four questions.

Once an ADR is identified, appropriate reporting is critical. Reporting can occur by several mechanisms. The event can be reported through the health care system's ADR program, which is typically organized by the pharmacy department. Another avenue is to contact the drug manufacturer directly, as all companies have a mechanism for documenting ADRs. Finally, severe and significant reactions should be reported immediately to the FDA through the MedWatch program (http://www.fda.gov/Safety/MedWatch/).

Adverse Drug Reactions by Organ System
Renal

Nephrotoxicity accounts for nearly 7% of all adverse drug reactions.[10] Several factors place the renal system at risk for adverse drug reactions. The renal system is responsible for eliminating many drugs and metabolites, of which several are known nephrotoxins. Additionally, the renal vascular system

receives approximately 20% to 25% of resting cardiac output. Therefore the kidneys are exposed to high concentrations of drugs and diagnostic agents. Although the renal system is highly vulnerable to nephrotoxicity, there are only a few mechanisms by which nephrotoxins can induce injury. These mechanisms include hemodynamically mediated nephrotoxicity, tubular necrosis, interstitial nephritis, obstructive nephropathy, and vascular toxicity. Many nephrotoxins can injure the kidney through more than one mechanism.

A variety of drugs are associated with acute tubular necrosis, including aminoglycosides, cisplatin, amphotericin B, radiocontrast media, cyclosporine, and intravenous (IV) immunoglobulins.[21-23] Acute tubular necrosis is one of the most common renal disorders associated with drug therapy. Minimizing risk factors for nephrotoxicity with these agents is imperative. For example, administrations of a saline load and volume repletion have been shown to be beneficial in reducing toxicity.[24] Table 126.1 presents a more complete list of medications associated with tubular necrosis.

Several drugs are implicated in the alteration of renal blood flow. Some of the most common include angiotensin-converting enzyme inhibitors (ACEIs), nonsteroidal antiinflammatory drugs (NSAIDs), β-adrenergic antagonists, and calcineurin inhibitors.[7,25-32] ACEIs can induce renal insufficiency in patients suffering from any process that decreases renal blood flow, including bilateral renal artery stenosis or unilateral stenosis with a single kidney.[33] The mechanism involves inhibiting the conversion of angiotensin I to angiotensin II, which results in dilation of the efferent arterioles, with resultant decreased glomerular capillary hydrostatic pressure and reduced glomerular filtration. The incidence of ACEI-induced renal failure in patients with renovascular

TABLE 126.1	**Drugs Causing Nephrotoxicity**	
Tubular Necrosis	**Interstitial Nephritis**	**Hemodynamic-Mediated Renal Failure**
Aminoglycosides	Allopurinol	Angiotensin-converting enzyme inhibitors
Amphotericin	Aminoglycosides	
Carboplatin	Aztreonam	
Cephalosporins	Captopril	Cyclosporine
Cisplatin	Carbamazepine	Mannitol
Cyclosporine	Cephalosporins	NSAIDs
Mannitol	Cimetidine	Propranolol
Methoxyflurane	Ciprofloxacin	Radiologic contrast agents
NSAIDs	Cyclosporine	Tacrolimus
Pentamidine	Erythromycin	
Radiologic contrast agents	Interferon-α	
	NSAIDs	
	Penicillins	
	Phenobarbital	
	Phenytoin	
	Ranitidine	
	Rifampin	
	Sulfonamides	
	Tacrolimus	
	Thiazide and loop diuretics	
	Valproic acid	
	Vancomycin	
	Warfarin	

NSAID, nonsteroidal antiinflammatory drug.

hypertension ranges from 20% to 38%.[31] NSAIDs inhibit prostaglandin synthesis, which leads to reduced renal blood flow and reduced glomerular filtration. The incidence of renal insufficiency is most common in patients with chronic renal disease, hypovolemia, sepsis, and those who use concomitant nephrotoxic drugs.[25,27,28,30,32,34] NSAID-induced renal toxicity is reversible if the toxic agent is discontinued immediately.[33] Table 126.1 provides a more complete list of drugs associated with hemodynamic renal failure.

Acute interstitial nephritis is another common source of drug-induced nephrotoxicity. It is reported to cause 3% to 8% of all cases of acute renal failure.[35] The clinical presentation of acute interstitial nephritis can appear anywhere between 2 and 44 days after initiation of the offending therapy.[36,37] Typical clinical symptoms include fever, skin rash, and flank tenderness.[36,37] Common laboratory findings include hematuria, sterile pyuria, and eosinophilia.[38] Histologic findings of acute interstitial nephritis include interstitial infiltrate of lymphocytes, plasma cells, eosinophils, and neutrophils.[36-38] Prompt discontinuation of the offending drug from therapy is recommended, and administration of corticosteroids may improve recovery.[39] Table 126.1 lists some medications associated with acute interstitial nephritis.

Renal tubular obstruction is associated with precipitation of endogenous products, drugs, and their metabolites. Formation of uric acid precipitant after chemotherapy can result in renal obstruction. Hydrating patients prior to chemotherapy, urinary alkalization, and use of allopurinol or rasburicase can help prevent uric acid precipitation.[40] Rhabdomyolysis can cause intratubular precipitation of myoglobin and lead to acute renal failure. Terbutaline overdose has resulted in rhabdomyolysis-induced renal failure.[41] Drugs associated with formation of crystals include acyclovir, sulfonamides, mannitol, pentobarbital, methotrexate, and dextran.[40,42-44]

Aminoglycosides are used frequently for treatment of gram-negative infections. All aminoglycosides have been shown to be toxic to the proximal renal tubules.[45] Aminoglycoside nephrotoxicity is related to dose, high trough concentrations, and prolonged therapy.[45] The drug-induced nephrotoxicity normally manifests as nonoliguric renal failure.[46] Several risk factors for developing aminoglycoside nephrotoxicity include the need for intensive care, decreased albumin, poor nutritional status, prolonged therapy, hypovolemia, pneumonia, shock, preexisting liver or kidney disease, and elevated initial steady-state drug concentrations.[46,47] Additionally, vancomycin, piperacillin, furosemide, amphotericin B, and cephalosporins, when administered concomitantly with aminoglycosides, are associated with an increased risk for developing nephrotoxicity.[46] Predicting nephrotoxicity based on the risk factors stated is an extremely complicated, inexact task.[46,48] Typically, aminoglycoside nephrotoxicity is reversible upon discontinuation of the offending agent.[45,49]

Drug-induced nephrotoxicity is a common serious adverse drug reaction that can lead to morbidity and lengthen hospital stays.[50] It is important to recognize potential nephrotoxins before initiating therapy and to evaluate therapeutic options. It is also important to monitor therapy appropriately for signs of toxicity and to modify therapy as needed.

Hepatic

The liver is the most common target of drug toxicity due to its major role of metabolism and elimination of foreign substances. It is well documented that acetaminophen causes intrinsic hepatotoxicity following acetaminophen overdose; however, a variety of medications can cause drug-induced hepatotoxicity. It often is difficult to determine the source of unexplained liver injury, so detailed examination of past and current drug therapies is needed to rule out possible drug-related causes. Most hepatotoxicity associated with drugs is idiosyncratic in nature and has a rate usually fewer than 1 per 10,000 exposed patients. The pathogenesis of drug-induced liver disease is mediated through either an immune response or direct cell damage.[51,52] In many cases, this hepatotoxicity is idiosyncratic, meaning not predictable or dose related, in contrast to drugs like acetaminophen and isoniazid for which toxicity is related to dose.[51,52]

The mechanism of toxicity for drug-induced liver injury generally involves the accumulation of drugs or their metabolites, which can cause direct cell damage, target mitochondrial function, or trigger an immune response. The initial stress or immune reaction leads to a mitochondrial permeability transition, which is either a direct pathway, mediated by cell damage, or is triggered by the death receptor amplified pathway. The mitochondrial impairment will determine if the hepatocytes die by apoptosis or necrosis. Measurements of alanine aminotransferase (ALT), aspartate aminotransferase (AST), alkaline phosphatase (ALP), and total bilirubin are important in assessment of drug-induced liver injury. It has been estimated that one-tenth of the Hy's law cases with hyperbilirubinemia or jaundice die or require transplant.[53,54] In severe cases of drug-induced hepatic injury, jaundice and hepatic failure may ensue.[52] Typically, drug-induced hepatic disease occurs expectedly as a result of high-dose therapy of a known hepatotoxin or unexpectedly as a result of an idiosyncratic reaction to a drug not associated with hepatotoxicity. Overall, children are less prone to drug-induced liver disease than are adults.[55] However, specific hepatotoxins have been shown to afflict children more than adults. Reye syndrome is a hepatocellular disease that has been associated with aspirin use in children.[56] Valproate hepatotoxicity occurs more frequently in children younger than 2 years who have preexisting neurologic or physical defects.[57]

Drug-induced hepatic disease can occur by a variety of mechanisms, including by hepatocellular, cholestatic, and vascular means. These injuries are associated with intrinsic or idiosyncratic hepatotoxins. Intrinsic hepatotoxins typically show a dose-related toxic effect. Idiosyncratic hepatic disease is an unpredictable reaction that can occur by immune-mediated hypersensitivity, metabolically, or both. Hypersensitivity reactions in the liver can cause cell injury to hepatocytes. The reactions do not correlate with dose and are difficult to anticipate. This immune-mediated reaction results from antigenic complexes that stimulate T lymphocytes, which can result in hepatic injury. These reactions can be accompanied by fever, skin rash, lymphadenopathy, and eosinophilia.[52] The reactions typically resolve upon discontinuation of therapy and resurface when therapy is rechallenged.[52] Metabolic idiosyncrasy occurs when a compound that is metabolized to nontoxic metabolites and eliminated in the majority of patients is metabolized to a toxic metabolite in a small number of patients because of genetic differences in metabolism (such as with isoniazid).[57] Box 126.1 lists a number of agents that are associated with drug-induced hepatotoxicity.

BOX 126.1   Drugs That Cause Hepatotoxicity

Acetaminophen	Phenobarbital
Amoxicillin-clavulanic acid	Phenytoin
Carbamazepine	Rifampin
Erythromycin	Sulfonamides
Isoniazid	Terbutaline
Ketoconazole	Tetracyclines
Labetalol	Trazodone
Nitrofurantoin	Valproate
NSAIDs	Voriconazole

Cardiovascular

An adverse cardiovascular reaction has been noted to be one of the most common types of ADE in pediatric patients.[58] Several medications are associated with adverse cardiovascular effects, and the mechanisms are often thought to be related to the agents' pharmacologic actions. These effects are potentiated by four general physiologic pathways: electrolyte and fluid imbalances, receptor-mediated sympathomimetic effects, alterations of the electrophysiology of the cardiac tissue, and drug-induced cardiotoxicity.

Medications can affect electrolyte and volume status by direct action on electrolyte receptors or indirect effects on prostaglandin release and the renin-angiotensin-aldosterone system. Dramatic changes in fluid and electrolyte status can lead to severe changes in blood pressure, heart rate, or cardiac rhythms. Medications that can potentiate histamine release such as morphine, fentanyl, and succinylcholine may also affect fluid and electrolyte status, causing hypotension if significant capillary leak develops.[59-62] Nonsteroidal antiinflammatory drugs, corticosteroids, diuretics, erythropoiesis-stimulating agents, estrogen-containing oral contraceptives, mannitol, and certain immunosuppressive agents, such as cyclosporine and tacrolimus, are all medications that can alter fluid and electrolyte balance.[52,62-65]

Pediatric patients in the intensive care unit often require vasopressive medications; however, it is important to be aware that many cardiovascular toxicities have been observed with the use of vasopressors, and most of these toxicities stem from their receptor-mediated effects (Table 126.2). The α-adrenergic agonism of the sympathomimetics causes palpitations, ectopic heartbeats, sinus tachycardia, and ventricular arrhythmias producing an increase in myocardial oxygen demand.[66] Other medications that may have sympathomimetic effects include caffeine, pseudoephedrine, and abrupt withdrawal of β-blockers and centrally acting α-agonists such as clonidine.[67] Increased myocardial oxygen demand may precipitate an infarction, especially in individuals with underlying cardiac disease. A dramatic rise in heart rate and peripheral vascular resistance may produce severe hypertension. Excessive α-adrenergic stimulation may produce vasoconstriction so severe in the extremities, kidneys, or liver that tissues become ischemic or necrotic. Specifically, vasopressin can cause such severe vasoconstriction that it has been associated with digital loss and splanchnic ischemia.[23] One study noted that 10% of patients receiving norepinephrine and vasopressin developed severe vasoconstriction-related adverse events, including acute kidney injury, which increased the risk of mortality twofold.[23] The sedative dexmedetomidine, though not classified as a vasopressor, has α_2-adrenergic agonist properties and effects similar to the medication clonidine. When

TABLE 126.2   Adverse Effects of Vasopressor Medications by Adrenergic Receptor Affinity

Medication	Affected Adrenergic Receptor	Associated Adverse Effect
Dopamine	5-10 mcg/kg/min: β_1 >10 mcg/kg/min: β_1 and α (mostly alpha)	Vasoconstriction, tachycardia, arrhythmias Extravasation causes ischemia
Dobutamine	β_1: selective	Increased heart rate, arrhythmias, ↑ myocardial oxygen demand
Epinephrine	<0.5 mcg/kg/min: β_1 >0.5 mcg/kg/min: α	Vasoconstriction, tachycardia, arrhythmias, tissue ischemia, cerebral hemorrhage, ↑ myocardial oxygen demand Extravasation causes necrosis
Isoproterenol	β: nonselective (β_1 > β_2)	Tachycardia, arrhythmias, hypotension, ↑ myocardial oxygen demand
Norepinephrine	α	Potent vasoconstriction, arrhythmias, tissue ischemia Extravasation causes necrosis
Phenylephrine	α	Systemic vasoconstriction, hypertension, bradycardia
Vasopressin	V1 vascular receptor	Potent vasoconstriction, tissue ischemia

Adapted from Goembiewski JA. Vasopressors used in the critical care setting. J Peri Anesth Nurs. 2003;18:414-416; Vetter VL, ed. Pediatric Cardiology: The Requisites in Pediatrics. Philadelphia: Mosby Elsevier; 2006.

using dexmedetomidine, it is important to monitor patients for hypotension, arrhythmias, and bradycardia.[65]

As noted previously, many medications produce arrhythmogenic effects through various mechanisms of action that can increase morbidity and mortality. Ventricular arrhythmias in infants and children, unlike adults, are relatively uncommon. The most commonly reported arrhythmias in pediatric patients include conduction disturbances or supraventricular arrhythmias including atrial tachycardia, junctional tachycardia, and sinus bradycardia. Due to the narrow therapeutic index of its concentration in the blood, digoxin, a direct-acting cardiac glycoside, is often associated with a variety of arrhythmias.[23] Close monitoring of electrolytes, especially potassium, renal function, and drug levels, helps to prevent adverse effects associated with digoxin. Another class of medications that requires close ECG monitoring is the antiarrhythmic medications. These medications have mechanisms of action that manipulate cardiac action potential and therefore have the ability to produce dysrhythmias.[66,68] Often used to treat supraventricular tachyarrhythmias, amiodarone is associated with bradycardia and hypotension, which may be dose and infusion rate dependent.[23] β-Blockers are also used as antiarrhythmic medications; however, they can lead to the development of life-threatening bradycardia at higher doses as well. Therefore it is recommended that treatments begin with lower doses and titrate slowly to the lowest effective dose.[69] Though previously a cause for concern, the stimulant medications commonly used to treat attention deficit and hyperactivity disorder (ADHD) no longer require extensive cardiac evaluation prior to initiation of therapy in patients without the presence, or significant risk, of underlying cardiac disease.[23] However, atomoxetine, a selective norepinephrine reuptake inhibitor often used in place of stimulant medications for ADHD, has been associated with a measurable increase in heart rate and blood pressure. Therefore the FDA recommends use with caution in patients with underlying cardiac disease.[23]

Although ventricular arrhythmias are uncommon in pediatric patients, the risk of torsades de pointes is still of concern in this population. Torsades de pointes is a life-threatening subset of arrhythmias and is characterized on electrocardiogram by lengthening of the QT interval and waxing/waning QRS amplitude. Certain medications can increase the risk for this arrhythmia by blocking potassium conductance on the rapid (Ikr) and slow (Iks) receptors within potassium ion channels. This creates a delayed ventricular repolarization and can lead to multiple ventricular reentrant loops. Risk factors for drug-induced torsades de pointes include high doses of associated medications (Box 126.2), concurrent use of multiple QT-prolonging medications, underlying structural heart disease including heart failure, ECG changes such as a prolonged QT interval at baseline or bradycardia, presence of hypokalemia or hypomagnesemia, and female sex.[70,23] Most commonly, antiarrhythmics, antipsychotics, antidepressants, azole antifungals, and fluoroquinolones are general classes of agents that demonstrate the potential to prolong the QT interval.[71,72] Another concern when administering these medications is pharmacokinetic drug-drug interactions or pathophysiologic alterations in elimination. Any biochemical mechanism that increases the concentration by inhibition of cytochrome isozymes or decreased clearance of the associated medication has the ability to potentiate this type of arrhythmia.[73] Current practice guidelines recommend avoiding high-risk medications if the patient has a baseline QTc greater than 450 msec and to discontinue or reduce the dose of the medication if the QTc increases by ≥60 msec from baseline or greater after initial medication administration.[74] Additionally, all efforts should be made to avoid drug-drug interactions and combinations of medications that can be known to precipitate torsades de pointes. A 12-lead ECG should be attained prior to the initiation of high-risk medications or combinations of medications. ECGs should be monitored at least daily until the full effect has been evaluated.[74] Data have suggested that administration of magnesium prior to giving high-risk intravenous medications may attenuate the effects of QT prolongation; however, this effect has not been confirmed by larger trials. Therefore this strategy should be limited to situations where there may be no other alternative.[75]

Medication-induced heart failure may be caused by a reduction in myocardial contractility, increase in preload, or oxidative damage leading to myocyte death. Tricyclic antidepressants, calcium channel blockers, β-blockers, and some antiarrhythmics exert a negative inotropic effect, decreasing contractility, which may lead to acute heart failure. Medications that cause fluid retention, such as NSAIDS, can slowly increase preload, which may cause heart failure with chronic use.[76-78] In patients with underlying heart failure or those at risk for heart failure,

---

BOX 126.2   Drugs Commonly Associated With QT Interval Prolongation

Antiarrhythmics
Amiodarone[a]
Dofetilide[a]
Flecainide
Ibutilide[a]
Procainamide[a]
Propafenone[b]
Quinidine[a]
Sotalol[a]

Antidepressants
Amitriptyline[b]
Citalopram
Escitalopram
Fluoxetine
Sertraline
Venlafaxine

Antiinfectives
Ciprofloxacin
Clarithromycin[b]
Erythromycin[b]
Fluconazole
Gatifloxacin
Itraconazole
Levofloxacin
Moxifloxacin
Pentamidine[b]
Quinidine[b]
Quinine[b]
Trimethoprim-sulfamethoxazole
Voriconazole

Antipsychotics
Aripiprazole
Haloperidol[b]
Quetiapine
Risperidone
Ziprasidone

Cardiovascular Agents
Isradipine
Nicardipine
Verapamil

Gastrointestinal Agents
Cisapride[c]
Dolasetron
Droperidol[b]
Ondansetron[a]

Miscellaneous
Amantadine
Arsenic trioxide
Methadone
Sumatriptan
Tacrolimus
Zolmitriptan

[a]Medications highly associated with QT prolongation.
[b]Medications moderately associated with QT prolongation.
[c]Cisapride, though removed from the US market, has been approved for limited compassionate use in some pediatric disease states.
All unmarked medications are considered low risk; however, they have a documented or theoretic association with QT prolongation. For a complete list, see www.crediblemeds.org.

---

attempts should be made to limit the use of these medications. If unavoidable, clinicians are recommended to use the lowest possible effective dose.

Cyclophosphamide, trastuzumab, interferon alfa, and anthracycline antineoplastic agents directly affect myocyte cells and damage cardiac tissue.[79-81] Anthracyclines, such as doxorubicin, epirubicin, idarubicin, and mitoxantrone, may lead to acute cardiotoxicity, manifesting as arrhythmias, or cardiomyopathy, which is related to a cumulative lifetime dose. These defects include abnormal right ventricular wall motion, impaired myocardial contractility, conduction abnormalities, and congestive heart failure.[82] There may also be delayed development of cardiotoxicity, as children who have received anthracycline therapy may see symptoms anywhere between 4 and 20 years after exposure.[82] Severe anthracycline toxicity cannot be reversed, and such a diagnosis leads to a poor prognosis and high mortality.[82] Strategies to minimize anthracycline toxicity include documenting and limiting total lifetime dose, supplements such as coenzyme Q10 and carnitine, pretreatment with antihistamines, increased infusion time, use of liposomal anthracyclines, and dexrazoxane. Dexrazoxane, a derivative of EDTA, binds free radicals produced by anthracyclines preventing oxidative damage to the myocyte. Its use is reserved for patients whose diagnoses typically require higher cumulative lifetime doses of anthracyclines.[83]

Central Nervous System

Prescription medications are the most common cause of iatrogenic seizures.[84] Drug-related factors that may contribute to seizures include the intrinsic epileptogenicity of the agent, factors that influence serum levels (dose, schedule, route), and factors that affect central nervous system (CNS) drug levels (lipid solubility, molecular weight, ionization of the drug, protein binding, transport by endogenous systems).[85] Patient-related factors may influence the risk for drug-induced seizures, such as preexisting epilepsy, neurologic abnormality, decreased drug elimination capacity (renal, hepatic), and conditions that disrupt the blood-brain barrier.[85] Several medications used within the intensive care unit have been associated with seizures. Due to the complexity of care needed for intensive care patients, increasing practitioner awareness of these medications, as well as their mechanisms of action, should allow practitioners to recognize and diagnose drug-induced seizures more effectively (Table 126.3).

Many medications can increase the risk of seizure exacerbation or development in ICU patients. Meperidine may induce seizures, especially in patients with renal insufficiency, due to accumulation of its metabolites.[84] Rapid administration of fentanyl is associated with seizures.[84] Several antiinfective and immunosuppressive medications including β-lactam antibiotics, imipenem, high-dose metronidazole, isoniazid, and cyclosporine induce seizures.[84] Many of the antiepileptic drugs can be implicated in worsening seizure activity, which usually occurs when higher than normal concentrations are used. Seizures also may be precipitated by medication withdrawal. Withdrawal of antiepileptic agents may cause seizures due to either subtherapeutic levels or excessively rapid removal of the agent.[85]

Delirium in critically ill patients remains a significant issue and is associated with negative outcomes, longer ICU stays, and increased costs.[86,87] The risk factors for ICU delirium are multifactorial and debatable. Emerging evidence suggests sedative practices may influence and contribute to the development of delirium, especially the use of benzodiazepines. Further studies and increasing awareness among pediatric intensivists should help to prevent delirium. Several medications are associated with ototoxicity, which is usually iatrogenic.[88] The main sites of action of ototoxic drugs are the cochlea, vestibulum, and stria vascularis.[89] Salicylates and aminoglycosides are the most common agents associated with hearing loss.[87,88] Other agents include cisplatin, loop diuretics, erythromycin, and vancomyin.[89,90] The effect is usually dose dependent.[88-90] High-dose and long-term therapy are common risk factors for aminoglycoside-induced ototoxicity.[89,90] Cisplatin is the most ototoxic of the antineoplastic agents, whereas ethacrynic acid has the greatest potential for causing ototoxicity in the loop diuretic category.[90] Appropriate dosing and monitoring of agents associated with ototoxicity are important for prevention and early detection.

TABLE 126.3	Medications That Can Induce Seizures	
Medication	**Potential Mechanism of Action**	**Comments**
Acyclovir[312]	Neurotoxicity	Renal impairment and parenteral administration increase the incidence
Antipsychotics[313]	Decreases seizure threshold	Increased incidence with high doses and rapid dose adjustments
Carbapenems[314]	Potentiates seizure activity through the inhibition of GABA receptor	Caution in patients with CNS disorders and renal dysfunction Imipenem has higher incidence compared with meropenem, ertapenem, doripenem
Cephalosporins[315]	Inhibition of GABA receptor	Ceftazidime > ceftriaxone > cefuroxime and cefotaxime
Cyclosporine[316]	Unknown but may involve the release of the potent vasoconstrictor endothelin from endothelial cells, which induce microvascular damage or changes in permeability of the blood-brain barrier	More common with high doses Increased incidence with hypercholesterolemia and hypomagnesemia
Cytarabine[317]	Cerebral dysfunction	Increased incidence with intrathecal administration
Flumazenil[319]	May precipitate benzodiazepine withdrawal; inhibition with seizure medications	Use in caution with patients with underlying seizure disorder
Fluoroquinolones[318]	Unknown but may involve inhibition of GABA receptor	History of seizures and use of NSAIDs associated with increased risk of seizures
Meperidine[313]	CNS excitation from toxic metabolite (normeperidine); blockade of serotonin	Common reaction with renal impairment and high doses
Metronidazole[315]	Penetrates the blood-brain barrier	Cumulative high dose and prolonged use
Penicillins[320]	Irritation of nervous system	Use with caution in infants, rapid IV infusions, and renal impairment
Tacrolimus[321-323]	Neurotoxicity	May be secondary to local vasoconstriction mediated by endothelin; elevated levels and hepatic impairment may increase the risk of neurotoxicity
Theophylline[313]	CNS toxicity	Serum concentrations >25 µg/mL have been noted to induce seizures

Hematologic

Chemotherapy with cytotoxic agents is the most common cause of drug-induced bone marrow suppression and can lead to secondary morbidities. For example, neutropenia predisposes a patient to opportunistic infections and sepsis. Chemotherapy-induced thrombocytopenia may render a patient vulnerable to hemorrhage in the CNS or gastrointestinal (GI) tract. Severe anemia may lead to dizziness, fatigue, hypotension, and myocardial infarction.[91] In addition to bone marrow suppression, some antineoplastics may produce thrombotic and hemorrhagic coagulation toxicities. For example, L-asparaginase has been reported to induce changes in the von Willebrand factor multimer in children and thereby promote platelet aggregation.[82]

Drug-induced myelosuppression has also been observed with several classes of antiinfectives such as β-lactam antibiotics, linezolid, trimethoprim-sulfamethoxazole, chloramphenicol, and antiviral agents.[92] β-Lactam antibiotics have been reported to be associated with autoimmune hemolytic anemia, leukopenia, and thrombocytopenia.[92,93] Linezolid-induced thrombocytopenia and anemia is most commonly seen when therapy continues for >2 weeks.[92,93] However, these effects are reversible upon discontinuation of therapy. The manufacturer recommends weekly monitoring of complete blood counts, especially for patients who require treatment beyond 2 weeks. Neutropenia is a common side effect associated with the use of ganciclovir and valganciclovir. In addition, these medications are commonly used in immunosuppressed patients who are often on concurrent marrow suppressive agents. Close monitoring of neutrophil counts in these patients is prudent to prevent neutropenia-associated complications. These antiviral medications should be renally adjusted as appropriate to prevent neutropenia. However, it is important to note that dose adjustments should not be made based on neutrophil counts, as it may lead to subtherapeutic drug levels and the potential for drug resistance.

Respiratory

Respiratory adverse effects are relatively uncommon but are among the most serious adverse events. Due to the seriousness of some of the drug-induced respiratory adverse events, which can be life threatening, intensive medical interventions are often required. Numerous agents have been known to cause lung disease. In 1975, only 19 agents were implicated with pulmonary complications.[94,95] More than 350 agents have now been identified as having the potential to induce respiratory complications.[94,95] The number of agents known to cause pulmonary adverse reactions continues to expand each year. Recognition of drug-induced pulmonary disease may be challenging due to the presence of confounding variables often associated with ICU patients, which may result in the underdiagnosis of both acute and chronic lung disease.[96] Some of the confounding factors in the diagnosis of drug-induced pulmonary disease include preexisting pulmonary conditions such as bronchopulmonary dysplasia and asthma, the use of oxygen, and concurrent medications.[97,98]

The two main risk factors for the development of drug-induced bronchospasm include a previous history of reactive airway disease and chronic obstructive lung disease.[98,99] There are several classes of medications associated with this clinically significant reaction. Analgesics and NSAIDs are two of the most common medications that can precipitate bronchospasm.[99] Other agents include antimicrobials (eg, sulfonamides), cardiovascular agents (eg, β-blockers and ACE inhibitors), and excipients (eg, preservatives, coloring agents, antioxidants).[99] The extensive list of medications suspected of causing or exacerbating bronchospastic reactions demonstrates the need to be aware of drug-induced causes of acute episodes, especially in patients with a history of preexisting lung conditions.

Opiates are commonly prescribed to pediatric intensive care patients. Acute respiratory failure secondary to a noncardiogenic pulmonary edema has been reported with the use of opiates including methadone, morphine, and codeine.[100] Aspirin has also been identified to cause pulmonary toxicity. High concentrations of aspirin can lead to increased vascular permeability causing pulmonary edema. A syndrome of massive fluid retention and pulmonary edema may be seen with interleukin-2 administration. All-trans-retinoic acid may cause acute lung disease secondary to massive total body fluid accumulation.

Chronic pneumonitis/fibrosis is a relatively common syndrome associated with drug-induced pulmonary reactions and is manifested by slowly progressive symptoms of cough and dyspnea.[100] Nitrofurantoin is associated with pulmonary fibrosis, most commonly in patients receiving chronic, high-dose therapy or patients with renal insufficiency.[101] A delayed presentation (months to years after discontinuation of or the start of therapy) is the most common form of fibrosis seen with amiodarone, but it also may cause an acute fibrosis manifesting within the first few weeks of therapy.[101,102] Many cytotoxic agents have been known to cause pulmonary fibrosis including bleomycin, carmustine, mitomycin, mitomycin with vinca alkaloid combination therapy, and cyclophosphamide. Risk factors for this reaction to cytotoxic agents include cumulative dose, age at initiation of treatment, and concomitant radiation therapy.

Endocrine and Metabolic

Due to the complexity of the biochemical processes that influence the endocrine and metabolic balance of the body, several medications have the potential to create alterations in neuroendocrine hormonal production, binding, transport, and signaling. Additionally medications may create changes in hormonal counterregulatory efforts. The most common types of medication-induced endocrine disorders are modifications in carbohydrate metabolism, electrolyte and calcium abnormalities, drug-induced thyroid changes, and alterations in acid-base status.[99] Variations in carbohydrate metabolism are commonly seen with many medications and are clinically manifested as alterations in blood glucose. Table 126.4 lists the multitude of medications associated with hypoglycemia or hyperglycemia subdivided by neuroendocrine effect.[103-107,108-113]

Hypoglycemia occurs most commonly as a result of overtreatment with insulin or diabetic medications, whereas hyperglycemia results from medications that either increase glucose production or decrease the effects of exogenous insulin.[103,114,115] Decreased insulin secretion, changes in liver glucose metabolism and production, and increased insulin resistance are the most common mechanism of drug-induced hyperglycemia.[103] Glucocorticoid usage is commonly associated with hyperglycemia and glycosuria.[116] Corticosteroids increase blood glucose via hepatic gluconeogenesis and by increasing peripheral insulin resistance.[117] This adverse drug

TABLE 126.4	Drugs That Cause Endocrine/Metabolic Changes		

Hyperglycemia		Hypoglycemia	Hyponatremia	Hypernatremia
↓ **Insulin Secretion**	↑ **Insulin Resistance**	↑ **Insulin Secretion**	↑ **Loss of Sodium**	↓ **Aldosterone**
Asparaginase	Amiodarone	Aspirin	Loop diuretics	Carbamazepine
β-Blockers	Antipsychotics	Cotrimoxazole	Thiazide diuretics	Lithium
Cyclosporine	Antiretrovirals/HAART	Insulin		
Glucocorticoids	β-Blockers	Pentamidine	↑ **Aldosterone**	**Aldosterone Deficiency**
Metolazone	Phenytoin		Desmopressin	Amphotericin B
Octreotide	Sirolimus	↑ **Insulin Sensitivity**	Spironolactone	Foscarnet
Phenytoin	Tacrolimus	ACE inhibitors	Vasopressin	Lithium
Terbutaline	Thiazide diuretics	ARBs		
Thiazide diuretics		α-Blockers	**SIADH Effect**	
	Miscellaneous		Amiodarone	
Alterations in Liver	Acetazolamide	**Miscellaneous**	Antidepressants	
Glucose Metabolism	Amphotericin B liposome	ACE inhibitors	Antipsychotics	
β-Blockers	Basiliximab	β-Blockers	Ciprofloxacin	
Corticosteroids	Clonidine	Haloperidol	Cisplatin	
Glucocorticoids	Dapsone	Indomethacin	Cytoxan	
Oral contraceptives	Dextrose	Octreotide	Ecstasy	
Somatropin	Diazoxide		Tricyclic antidepressants	
	Isoniazid		Vincristine	
	Loop diuretics			
	Mycophenolate		↑ **Fluid Retention**	
	Rifampin (oral)		NSAIDS	
	Rituximab			

Hypokalemia	Hyperkalemia	Calcium or Magnesium	Thyroid
↑ **Excretion**	↑ **Efflux (Extracellular)**	**Hypomagnesemia**	**Hypothyroidism**
Diuretics	Arginine	Aminoglycosides	Amiodarone
Foscarnet	β-Blockers	Amphotericin B	Interferon-α
Laxatives	Digoxin	Cisplatin	Lithium
	Mannitol	Cyclosporine	Methimazole
↑ **Influx (Intracellular)**	Succinylcholine	Loop diuretics	
β-Agonists (albuterol,	Tacrolimus		**Hyperthyroidism**
terbutaline)		**Hypocalcemia**	Amiodarone
Dextrose	↑ **Aldosterone**	Bisphosphonates	
Insulin	Cotrimoxazole	Citrated solutions	
Levothyroxine	Eplerenone	Diltiazem (IV)	
Theophylline	Pentamidine	Ethylene glycol poisoning	
	Spironolactone	Foscarnet	
Aldosterone Deficiency/		Phenobarbital	
Resistance	**Miscellaneous**	Phenytoin	
ACE inhibitors	Propofol		
Cyclosporine	Rituximab	**Hypercalcemia**	
NSAIDs		Levothyroxine	
		Lithium	
Miscellaneous		Theophylline	
Amphotericin B		Tretinoin	
Caspofungin			
Corticosteroids			
Itraconazole			

ACE, angiotensin-converting enzyme; *ARBs,* angiotensin II receptor blockers; *HAART,* highly active antiretroviral therapy; *NSAIDs,* nonsteroidal antiinflammatory drugs; *SIADH,* syndrome of inappropriate antidiuretic hormone.

reaction appears to be dose dependent and usually is reversible upon discontinuation of therapy.[117] Patients on high-dose, long-term glucocorticoid therapies are at significant risk for suppression of the hypothalamic-pituitary-adrenal axis.[118,119] Symptoms of adrenal insufficiency include arthralgias, dizziness, hypotension, nausea, and weakness.[118]

Drug-induced electrolyte disturbances can occur with a variety of pharmaceutical agents. Several medications are associated with initial or worsening hypokalemia, hyperkalemia, hyponatremia, hypernatremia, and hypomagnesemia (see Table 126.4).[103,120-135]

Hyponatremia and hypernatremia are often secondary to depletion or dilutional effects of medications or drug-induced changes in antidiuretic hormone.[103,122] Additionally, some medications, such as trimethoprim-sulfamethoxazole, can cause renal salt wasting.[136] Hypokalemia is directly affected by medications that increase potassium excretion or increase Na-K-ATPase activity, causing potassium influx into the cells. Drug-induced hyperkalemia can develop when medications lead to decreased Na-K-ATPase activity, aldosterone deficiencies, and resistance to aldosterone.[103,120] Succinylcholine, however, has a different mechanism of action for increasing serum potassium by directly affecting ion-channel depolarization.[136] Medications that affect the renal tubules of the kidneys, such as amphotericin B and cyclosporine, have been associated with severe hypomagnesemia, which can also play a role in hypokalemia.[136,124] Often, correcting serum magnesium can be beneficial for normalizing other electrolyte levels, such as potassium and calcium. Antiepileptic agents, citrated solutions, foscarnet, and intravenous diltiazem have all been associated with critical hypocalemia due to effects on vitamin D metabolism or calcium reuptake mechanisms.[125-131] Electrolyte disorders represent a common adverse drug reaction and can greatly complicate therapy. Accordingly, frequent monitoring of electrolytes is warranted for patients in the ICU on multiple drug therapy.

Electrolyte abnormalities have been noted with the use of amiodarone; however, it is most commonly known for its adverse effects on the thyroid gland. Due to the large amount of iodine in amiodarone (3 mg of iodine/100 mg of drug), it has a counterregulatory effect on the production of thyroid hormones.[103] In patients in more developed countries, where iodine deficiency is rare, use of amiodarone is associated with hypothyroidism; however, in countries where iodine deficiency is more common; amiodarone can cause thyrotoxicosis.[133,134] It is important to obtain baseline thyroid studies prior to starting therapy and to monitor them continually throughout treatment.

Although uncommon, prolonged use of nitroprusside can result in methemoglobinemia and cyanide or thiocyanate toxicity.[137,138] The risk of thiocyanate or cyanide toxicity is higher in patients with renal dysfunction, hepatic failure, or those receiving high-dose or prolonged infusions of nitroprusside.[139] Doses greater than 2 mcg/kg/min and use in patients with liver or renal dysfunction are associated with toxic levels.[140] To prevent the development of toxicity, lower doses are recommended and the duration of infusion should be limited if possible. An early indicator of thiocyanate or cyanide toxicity is metabolic acidosis.[140] The use of thiocyanate levels should be limited to patients who require higher doses, long-term therapy, or have concomitant risk factors.

Propofol-related infusion syndrome (PRIS) is a constellation of life-threatening symptoms associated with severe metabolic acidosis, which can lead to fatal rhabdomyolysis or liver failure. In 2001, the FDA communicated a warning against off-label use of propofol for sedation in pediatric intensive care.[141,142] The FDA's concern came from reviewing data of a randomized, controlled clinical trial evaluating the safety and efficacy of propofol versus standard sedation regimens in pediatric intensive care patients. Approximately 10% of patients treated with propofol died, compared with 4% of children receiving standard treatment. More recently, Koriyama and colleagues evaluated 210 PICU patients who received propofol infusion rates of less than 4 mg/kg/hr for no longer than 24 hours. None of the patients developed PRIS using this strategy.[143] Although this and other large case series have reported the safe use of propofol without adverse effects, given the risks of mortality with PRIS, prolonged propofol infusions are not recommended in the pediatric ICU setting.[143,144]

Dermatologic

Drug-induced dermatologic reactions are the most common reported adverse events affecting 2% to 3% of all hospitalized patients. They include hypersensitivities, cutaneous eruptions or exacerbations, and severe cutaneous adverse reactions (SCARs). Drug-induced hypersensitivities describe both immunoglobulin-mediated allergic reactions and pseudoallergies. Urticaria, pruritus, angioedema, and facial flushing can occur with both types of hypersensitivity. Though their clinical presentation is similar, true allergic reactions require a sensitization period (approximately 5-21 days after the first dose) due to the activation of antibodies.[145] Allergic reactions are often associated with antimicrobials, antivirals, and aromatic anticonvulsants, such as phenobarbital and phenytoin. Coexisting conditions may also contribute the development of allergic reactions. For example, active infection with Epstein-Barr virus may increase the potential for a reaction to aminopenicillins.[146] Though commonly described as true allergies, dermatologic reactions to vancomycin, radiocontrast, aspirin, and ACE inhibitors are usually pseudoallergic.[145-147] Pseudoallergies include infusion-related reactions, skin flushing, and anaphylactoid reactions, which usually occur within minutes of administration. "Red man syndrome," facial and neck flushing associated with vancomycin, is an example of a pseudoallergy. As with other pseudoallergies, reducing the infusion rate and premedicating with antihistamines are strategies to reduce the development of this adverse effect. Many medications are associated with hypersensitivities and pseudoallergy; therefore it is important to assess patients carefully when these types of reactions occur as a falsely labeled "allergy" may limit future treatment options.[145,148]

Maculopapular rashes are the most common type of drug-induced skin eruptions. Similar to hypersensitivity reactions, the rash usually develops 4 to 14 days after initiation of the causative medication. However, unlike urticaria, which is associated with IgE-mediated allergic reactions, maculopapular rashes are self-limiting and do not typically lead to more severe symptoms like angioedema and anaphylaxis. It is important to note that lesions located in the mucous membranes, palms, or soles of the feet are evident in approximately 90% of SCARs and may be a prelude to a more serious reaction.[149,150] After discontinuation of the suspected medication, most erythematous reactions can be treated with antihistamines and a low-dose steroid taper (if rash is diffuse).[151] Other types of drug-related skin eruptions include fixed drug eruptions (FDEs), acne, and psoriasis exacerbations. Fixed drug eruptions are small, defined lesions usually found on the face, lips, hands, feet, and genitalia.[152] Common medications associated with FDEs are acetaminophen, ibuprofen, and barbiturates.[152] Once discovered, the suspected medication should be discontinued. If rechallenge is necessary, the lesion will typically recur in the same location.[152] Acne, though not a serious adverse event, can lead to discomfort and possible issues of medication compliance. The location of drug-induced acne is similar to acne vulgaris (face, neck, and back); however, it is often distinguished by its papular presentation. Steroids, tacrolimus, lamotrigine, infliximab, epidermal growth factor receptor inhibitors, and cyclosporine have all been associated with acne.[153-155] Topical treatment with benzoyl peroxide products can help to treat drug-induced acne in order to avoid discontinuation of the causative agent. Similar to acne outbreaks, some medications can exacerbate psoriatic plaques in patients known to have this chronic condition (eg, NSAIDs, angiotensin-converting enzyme [ACE] inhibitors, and β-blockers) or cause psoriasis in those with no previous history (eg, growth hormone).[156] Topical corticosteroids may be helpful in treating exacerbations; however, in some instances the offending medication might need to be discontinued.

Serious cutaneous adverse reactions (SCARs) include drug rash with eosinophilia and systemic symptoms, Stevens-Johnson syndrome, toxic epidermal necrolysis, and warfarin-induced necrosis. Drug rash with eosinophilia and systemic symptoms (DRESS) is defined by a constellation of symptoms including high fever, symmetric maculopapular rash, and internal organ involvement. Often associated with anticonvulsants (eg, phenytoin and phenobarbital) and allopurinol, symptoms may take 3 to 8 weeks to develop after the initiation of the causative medication. Organ dysfunction may be severe and can lead to liver or kidney failure. Treatment includes supportive care and high-dose steroids.[157] In patients receiving allopurinol, it is beneficial to use doses less than 200 mg per day, adjust for renal dysfunction, and avoid concurrent use of thiazide diuretics.[158] Stevens-Johnson syndrome (SJS) and toxic epidermal necrolysis (TEN) are similar SCARs that are considered dermatologic emergencies. Often preceded by a viral-appearing prodrome, both conditions are associated with high fever and maculopapular skin eruptions, which then blister leading to epidermal necrosis and detachment. Though their presentations are similar, TEN is often considered a more severe presentation of SJS due to the fact that patients with TEN develop epidermal detachment on greater than 30% of their body surface area (BSA) versus less than 10% of BSA in SJS.[159] Additionally, TEN is associated with acute renal failure, respiratory failure, and sepsis. Medications commonly known to cause SJS and TEN include allopurinol, lamotrigine, trimethoprim-sulfamethoxazole, and voriconazole.[159] Patients with SJS and TEN require admission to the ICU for supportive care including extensive wound care and surgical debridement.[159,160] In smaller studies, higher doses of intravenous immunoglobulin (IVIG) have been shown to decrease disease progression and improve outcomes.[161]

Warfarin-induced skin necrosis (WISN) is a severe cutaneous reaction that typically occurs within the first 10 days after the initiation of warfarin therapy. A dramatic drop in protein C, compared to other coagulation factors, creates a hypercoagulable state in which areas with higher amounts of adipose tissue can develop blistering plaques eventually leading to necrosis. Treatment includes discontinuation of warfarin, anticoagulation with heparin to prevent further microthrombi from developing, fresh-frozen plasma or protein C concentrate to restore protein C levels, and surgical debridement with or without skin grafting. Strategies to prevent WISN include initiation with lower doses of warfarin and bridging with heparin or low-molecular-weight heparin for at least 5 days when starting warfarin therapy.[43,162]

Drug-Drug Interactions

The pediatric intensive care physician is confronted daily with potentially hazardous drug-drug interactions in the critical care setting. A potential drug-drug interaction can be defined as "the possibility that one drug may alter the intensity of pharmacologic effects of another drug given concurrently. The net result may be enhanced or diminished effects of one or both of the drugs or the appearance of a new effect that is not seen with either drug alone."[118] Given the extent of polypharmacy occurrence, the potential risk is significant. Of the thousands of documented drug-drug interactions, only a small fraction is clinically significant.[163] The ability to differentiate between clinically significant and insignificant interactions requires an understanding of their mechanisms of action. In most cases, drug-drug interactions are predictable and preventable with appropriate dose modifications or avoidance of combinations.

The magnitude of drug-drug interactions is measured by the intensity of the response. Medications with narrow therapeutic indices are especially susceptible to drug-drug interactions, as small alterations in exposure can lead to large changes in response. Typically, drugs with large therapeutic indices are at minimal risk for clinically significant drug-drug interactions.

Drug-drug interactions can occur by three different mechanisms: pharmacokinetic, pharmacodynamic, and pharmaceutical. Pharmacokinetic drug-drug interactions can be defined as "interactions which affect a target drug through alterations in their absorption, distribution, metabolism, or excretion; the result may be an increase or decrease in the concentration of drug at the site of action."[118] Pharmacodynamic interactions are defined as interactions at a common receptor site or that have additive or inhibitory effects as a result of actions at different sites.[118] Pharmaceutical interactions or incompatibilities "occur when drugs interact in vitro so that one or both are inactivated."[164]

The ability to distinguish significant drug-drug interactions in the critical care setting is vital to patient care. The following discussion emphasizes the mechanisms that underlie various drug-drug interactions and identifies clinically significant interactions among therapeutic classes.

Pharmacokinetic Drug-Drug Interactions

The most common and well-studied etiology of drug-drug interactions occurs through pharmacokinetic interactions. Pharmacokinetic interactions can occur throughout the entire pharmacologic spectrum and can potentially affect the absorption, distribution, metabolism, or elimination of the compound of interest. However, drug-drug interactions are only important when they impact the resulting drug exposure to such an extent that the patient experiences an alteration in the expected drug effect, either through a diminution of the drug's effect (when drug exposure is decreased) or through a predisposition to adverse effects (when drug exposure is increased). It is important to recognize that the dearth of pharmacokinetic information available for most drugs in children often makes recognition of drug-drug interactions difficult. However, a thorough understanding of the mechanisms behind these interactions can create an index of suspicion that is necessary to identify potential interactions clinically.

Interactions Affecting Drug Absorption (Enteral Absorption)

Several factors determine the rate and extent of oral absorption of drug products. Drug-drug interactions affecting enteral absorption occur through several mechanisms with a common end result: alteration of availability of the drug at its primary site of absorption. The most common mechanisms include adsorption or complexation of the target drug by other drugs or food, alterations in the ionization of the drug through pH changes, and perturbation of normal GI function (eg, motility, bacterial colonization, and mesenteric blood flow). In the critical care setting, adsorption and complex formation are the most likely causes of decreased enteral drug absorption. Commonly prescribed medications (eg, sucralfate and kaolin pectin) are implicated in causing decreased absorption of other drugs by adsorbing target drugs and rendering them unavailable for absorption across the GI barrier.[165-167] Food, especially enteral formula, is capable of causing adsorption of drugs. Phenytoin, levothyroxine, flecainide, and warfarin all have known interactions with enteral formulations.[168-170] Although less commonly prescribed in the pediatric setting, tetracycline and quinolone antibiotics have long been known to cause drug complexes with metallic cations such as iron and calcium, resulting in a decreased effect of both the supplement and the antibiotic.[171,172] If it is necessary to give these medications via the feeding tube to patients on continuous enteral feeding, a multidisciplinary team including providers, dietitians, and pharmacists should work together to develop an appropriate strategy.

Interactions Affecting Drug Distribution (Protein or Tissue Binding)

Due to the fact that the majority of drugs are bound to plasma proteins or tissue binding sites, the most commonly cited mechanisms for drug-drug interactions affecting distribution are those that involve protein or tissue binding. Many factors affect protein or tissue binding including pH, temperature, renal function, and low serum albumin. Several examples exist in which one drug displaces an object drug through competitive inhibition at a protein or tissue binding site. However, in most cases, the impact of the drug-drug interaction is minimal. The amount of free (active) drug may increase temporarily, but the free level falls back to its previous equilibrium as the clearance of drug subsequently increases. Most cases of increased free drug concentrations secondary to protein binding displacement occur when the displacing drug also inhibits the metabolism or excretion of the displaced drug. For example, probenecid not only displaces bound ceftriaxone from albumin binding sites but also inhibits the active secretion of the drug in the kidney, resulting in increased ceftriaxone concentrations.[173] The clinical implications of this interaction are minimal because of the wide therapeutic index for ceftriaxone.

Alterations in Total Body Water

An important mechanism for drug-drug interactions affecting drug distribution that often is overlooked is an alteration of body fluid composition. Severe dehydration can be caused iatrogenically, either through fluid restriction or overzealous diuretic use. In these cases, drug concentrations can be increased several-fold, resulting in adverse effects. Conversely, the volume of distribution of drugs can be increased significantly by increasing total body water. This can have the effect of decreasing drug concentrations to subtherapeutic levels. Drugs that distribute primarily in total body water, such as aminoglycosides, are particularly susceptible to these types of effects.[174]

Interactions Affecting Drug Metabolism

The majority of clinically relevant drug-drug interactions can be linked to an alteration in drug metabolism. The two major pathways for drug metabolism in humans are the phase I oxidative pathway and the phase II conjugation reactions. Inhibition or induction of the phase I pathway is the most studied mechanism of drug-drug interactions, especially in relation to the cytochrome P-450 system of enzymes. Table 126.5 lists the drugs that affect cytochrome P-450 enzymes and those metabolized by the various clinically relevant isoforms. Evaluation of a drug's potential to affect the P-450 system is now an integral part of new drug development, and many older drugs have been studied extensively, such that these interactions are often predictable in adults. However, the relative lack of formal pediatric studies makes predicting the impact of a particular interaction difficult in a given child.

Factors that must be considered include the state of maturation of the particular isoform and the presence of compensatory pathways. In general, it is reasonable to assume that a reaction that occurs in adults will also occur in children; therefore proper adjustments should be made if necessary.

One important consideration is the timing of drug-drug interactions secondary to P-450 enzyme inhibition or induction. In general, enzyme inhibition results from competitive inhibition at the enzyme binding site and therefore becomes clinically relevant as soon as the offending drug reaches sufficient concentrations in the liver. Consequently, upon discontinuation of the offending drug, enzyme inhibition abates as the drug concentration falls. Drugs with short half-lives have a relatively short offset of effect, whereas those with longer half-lives can cause significant effects for prolonged periods after discontinuation. In contrast, enzyme induction results from an increase in the amount of enzyme synthesized by hepatic cells. Thus there is a lag between the time an inducer is introduced and the onset of induction effect. As expected, the offset of effect also is somewhat prolonged.

Phase II reactions are rarely rate limiting, which makes their potential to be the cause of clinically significant drug-drug interactions low. However, the potential does exist for drugs to inhibit conjugation, thus impeding the conversion of object drugs to their inactive metabolites. A classic example is the interaction between high-dose ascorbic acid and acetaminophen. Ascorbic acid competitively inhibits the sulfation of acetaminophen, resulting in accumulation of the glucuronide metabolite.[175]

Interactions Affecting Drug Excretion

The primary means for the elimination of drugs or their metabolites is through renal excretion. The process of renal excretion involves three mechanisms: glomerular filtration (GFR), active tubular secretion, and tubular reabsorption. All three mechanisms can be affected by drug-drug interactions.

Alterations in GFR secondary to drug-drug interactions most often result from fluctuation in renal blood flow. Drugs that act to reduce renal blood flow, such as cyclosporine or NSAIDs, can reduce GFR and increase the blood concentration of drugs eliminated by this route.[32,176-179] Conversely, drugs that improve renal blood flow could increase GFR and decrease plasma concentrations of drugs eliminated through the kidneys. As its name implies, active tubular secretion is an active process during which drugs bind to receptors and are transported across the tubular cells to be excreted. Drugs that compete for these binding sites may inhibit the secretion of other drugs and increase concentrations. The two most commonly cited inhibitors of active tubular secretion are probenecid (inhibits the site for weak acids such as penicillin) and cimetidine (inhibits the site for weak bases such as procainamide). These reactions are rarely of clinical significance; however, the probenecid-penicillin interaction has been used therapeutically to increase penicillin serum concentrations.[180-183] Tubular reabsorption is a passive process in which drugs are reabsorbed into the systemic circulation from the lumen of the distal tubules. As with enteral absorption, only un-ionized molecules are available for reabsorption. Therefore drugs that alter the pH of the urine have the potential to alter tubular reabsorption of other drugs. A common example is phenobarbital, which is a weakly acidic drug. In overdose situations, sodium bicarbonate is administered to

TABLE 126.5 P-Glycoprotein and Cytochrome P-450 Substrates, Inhibitors, and Inducers

	Substrates		Inhibitors		Inducers	
Pgp[a]	Amiodarone	Levofloxacin	Amiodarone	Nicardipine	Amiodarone	Nicardipine
	Cimetidine	Lidocaine	Carvedilol	Nifedipine	Cyclosporine	Nifedipine
	Ciprofloxacin	Methylprednisolone	Chlorpromazine	Ofloxacin	Dexamethasone	Phenobarbital
	Cortisol	Morphine	Clarithromycin	Posaconazole	Diltiazem	Phenytoin
	Cyclosporine	Nadolol	Cortisol	Prochlorperazine	Erythromycin	Probenecid
	Dexamethasone	Octreotide	Cyclosporine	Propranolol	Insulin	Rifampin
	Digoxin	Ondansetron	Desipramine	Quinidine	Midazolam	Tacrolimus
	Diltiazem	Phenytoin	Diltiazem	Quinine	Morphine	Verapamil
	Erythromycin	Ranitidine	Erythromycin	Sirolimus		
	Everolimus	Sirolimus	Everolimus	Spironolactone		
	Fentanyl	Verapamil	Haloperidol	Tacrolimus		
	Hydrocortisone		Imipramine	Verapamil		
	Itraconazole		Midazolam			
	Ketoconazole					
CYP1A2	Acetaminophen	Naproxen	Caffeine	Lidocaine	Carbamazepine	Phenobarbital
	Caffeine	Nicardipine	Cimetidine	Nifedipine	Insulin	Phenytoin
	Carvedilol	Ondansetron	Ciprofloxacin	Omeprazole	Lansoprazole	Rifampin
	Cisapride	Ranitidine	Clarithromycin	Ondansetron	Nafcillin	
	Diazepam	R-warfarin	Diltiazem	Propofol	Omeprazole	
	Haloperidol	Theophylline	Erythromycin	Propranolol	Pantoprazole	
	Levofloxacin	Verapamil	Grapefruit juice	Ranitidine		
	Lidocaine		Ketoconazole	Theophylline		
CYP1E2	Acetaminophen	Isoflurane	Isoniazid			
	Enflurane	Methoxyflurane				
	Halothane	Sevoflurane				
CYP2C9	Bosentan	Omeprazole	Chloramphenicol	Omeprazole	Bosentan	
	Caffeine	Ondansetron	Cimetidine	Phenobarbital	Carbamazepine	
	Carvedilol	Pantoprazole	Diltiazem	Phenytoin	Phenobarbital	
	Dextromethorphan	Phenobarbital	Fluconazole	Probenecid	Phenytoin	
	Diazepam	Phenytoin	Ibuprofen	Propofol	Rifampin	
	Diltiazem	Propofol	Indomethacin	Propranolol		
	Fluconazole	Quinidine	Itraconazole	Sulfonamides		
	Indomethacin	S-warfarin	Ketoconazole	Trimethoprim		
	Lansoprazole	Theophylline	Lansoprazole	Verapamil		
	Montelukast	Valproic acid	Metronidazole	Voriconazole		
	Naproxen	Verapamil	Nifedipine			
	Nicotine	Voriconazole				
		Zafirlukast				
CYP2C19	Cisapride	Phenobarbital	Cimetidine	Lansoprazole	Carbamazepine	
	Diazepam	Phenytoin	Diazepam	Omeprazole	Phenobarbital	
	Fluconazole	Propofol	Felbamate	Voriconazole	Phenytoin	
	Ibuprofen	Propranolol	Fluconazole		Prednisone	
	Indomethacin	Ranitidine	Indomethacin		Rifampin	
	Lansoprazole	R-warfarin	Ketoconazole			
	Metoprolol	Verapamil				
	Omeprazole	Voriconazole				
	Pantoprazole					
CYP2D6	Acetaminophen	Methadone	Amiodarone	Methylphenidate	Carbamazepine	Phenytoin
	Amphetamine	Methamphetamine	Chlorpheniramine	Metoprolol	Dexamethasone	Rifampin
	Caffeine	Metoprolol	Cimetidine	Nicardipine	Ethanol	
	Captopril	Morphine	Cisapride	Omeprazole	Phenobarbital	
	Carvedilol	Nelfinavir	Codeine	Ondansetron		
	Chlorpheniramine	Nevirapine	Dextromethorphan	Oxybutynin		
	Codeine	Omeprazole	Diltiazem	Propofol		
	Dextromethorphan	Ondansetron	Haloperidol	Propranolol		
	Diltiazem	Oxycodone	Ketoconazole	Quinidine		
	Fentanyl	Propofol	Lansoprazole	Ranitidine		
	Hydrocodone	Propranolol	Lidocaine	Verapamil		
	Lidocaine	Ranitidine	Methamphetamine			
	Loratadine	Theophylline				
	Meperidine					

TABLE 126.5   P-Glycoprotein and Cytochrome P-450 Substrates, Inhibitors, and Inducers—cont'd

	Substrates		Inhibitors		Inducers	
CYP3A4	Alfentanil	Losartan	Clarithromycin	Ketoconazole	Barbiturates	Phenytoin
	Alprazolam	Methadone	Cyclosporine	Methylprednisolone	Bosentan	Primidone
	Amiodarone	Methylprednisolone	Diltiazem	Metronidazole	Carbamazepine	Rifabutin
	Amlodipine	Miconazole	Erythromycin	Nefazodone	Dexamethasone	Rifampin
	Atorvastatin	Midazolam	Ethinyl estradiol	Norethindrone	Griseofulvin	
	Bosentan	Montelukast	Fluvoxamine	Posaconazole		
	Carbamazepine	Nefazodone	Grapefruit juice	Prednisone		
	Cisapride	Nimodipine	Isoniazid	Telithromycin		
	Citalopram	Nisoldipine	Itraconazole	Verapamil		
	Clarithromycin	Pioglitazone		Voriconazole		
	Cyclophosphamide	Prednisolone				
	Cyclosporine	Quetiapine				
	Dapsone	Rifabutin				
	Dexamethasone	Sertraline				
	Diazepam	Sildenafil				
	Diltiazem	Simvastatin				
	Dofetilide	Sirolimus				
	Doxorubicin	Tacrolimus				
	Erythromycin	Testosterone				
	Ethinyl estradiol	Theophylline				
	Etoposide	Triazolam				
	Everolimus	Verapamil				
	Felodipine	Vinblastine				
	Fentanyl	Vincristine				
	Fluconazole	Voriconazole				
	Ifosfamide	R-warfarin				
	Imatinib	Zolpidem				
	Itraconazole					
	Ketoconazole					
	Lidocaine					
	Loratadine					

aSeveral drugs are listed as both P-glycoprotein (Pgp) inhibitors and inducers because their effects on Pgp expression can be concentration or duration related.

alkalinize the urine in the hopes that phenobarbital will become more ionized in urine, resulting in reduced tubular reabsorption and more rapid excretion. It is important to note that the effectiveness of this practice is unclear.[184]

Interactions Affecting P-Glycoprotein Receptors

Research in the oncology field has led to the identification of an important drug transporter that is ubiquitous throughout the human body, namely, P-glycoprotein (Pgp). Pgp can be found in renal tubule cells, hepatic cells, the blood-brain barrier, and mucosal cells of the intestines, pancreas, and adrenal glands. Table 126.5 lists drugs that are inhibitors or substrates for Pgp. In general, Pgp is believed to serve a protective function by transporting molecules out of the body or, in the case of the blood-brain barrier, out of the CNS. This is manifested in the gut by Pgp-mediated secretion of molecules back to the intestinal lumen after absorption, in the kidney by active tubular secretion, in the liver by active secretion into the bile, and in the CNS by active removal of molecules out of the CNS. Drugs that inhibit Pgp are expected to increase the concentrations of substrates (either in plasma or the CNS). Clinicians should be aware when coadministering Pgp substrates or inhibitors and should consider dose adjustments or alternative treatments when administering drugs with narrow therapeutic windows.

Pharmacodynamic Drug-Drug Interactions

A pharmacodynamic drug-drug interaction (DDI) can be defined as the combination of two or more drugs with additive, synergistic, or antagonistic pharmacodynamic effects. Feinstein and colleagues reported that the epidemiology of pediatric drug-drug interactions is not clearly understood. Although this cohort study suggests the advancement with computerized physician order entry, standardized prescribing and review of drug-drug interactions upon ordering may impact the number of drug-drug interactions for pediatric patients. Additive pharmacodynamic interactions occur routinely when two or more drugs of the same class are given in combination, as in the case of antihypertensive medications or anticonvulsants. A synergistic interaction occurs when the combination of two drugs has an effect greater than the sum of their individual effects. One example of a clinically relevant synergistic interaction is the use of aminoglycosides in combination with β-lactam antibiotics. In theory, combining a cell-wall active agent (β-lactam antibiotic) with an agent that inhibits bacterial protein synthesis (aminoglycoside) can achieve a greater antibiotic effect than the sum of the two individual effects. Although difficult to prove clinically, in vitro and animal studies have validated this theory.[185-187] Most antagonistic drug-drug interactions are more appropriately defined as pharmacokinetic interactions because they result from some alteration in drug concentrations, either in plasma or at the site of action. Antagonistic interactions that are truly pharmacodynamic in nature most often result from competitive inhibition at the receptor site for drug activity. Use of flumazenil to reverse benzodiazepine-induced sedation is an example of an antagonistic pharmacodynamic drug-drug interaction used clinically.[188-190]

Drug-Drug Interactions in Intravenous Admixtures

Parenteral administration of drug therapy poses a potential source of drug-drug interactions in the pediatric and neonatal intensive care units. Infusion of drugs with known incompatibilities could have serious consequences when administered to the patient. Introduction of a precipitate to venous circulation could produce adverse effects such as phlebitis and pulmonary embolism.[191] Factors influencing the need for coadministration of medications include a limited number of IV access sites, an extensive drug therapy regimen, time constraints, and the need to administer other lengthy infusions (eg, blood products).

Incompatibilities result from chemical reactions that may or may not be visible. Physical incompatibilities are easily identifiable because they illustrate any one of the following visual phenomena: precipitation, complexation, turbidity, color change, evolution of gas, or separation of the solution into distinct immiscible layers.[192] On the other hand, instability occurs when a mixture of drug solutions chemically reacts to yield a different species or degradation product, either of which could be pharmacologically inactive or even toxic. The rate at which these reactions occur adds another variable in determining whether or not two drug solutions can be infused together and for what duration. Generally, incompatibility is defined as a 10% decomposition of one or more components in an admixture in less than 24 hours.[192] Alterations in pH of the chemical environment, reduction-oxidation reactions, chelation, and "salting out," which occurs when nonelectrolytes are exposed to strong electrolyte solutions, can lead to inactivation or visually ascertained incompatibilities such as precipitation.

Drug-Drug Interactions by Therapeutic Class

As opposed to many other classes of drugs, alterations in pharmacodynamics are the most common mechanism of cardiovascular drug-drug interactions. The potential for two drugs to act upon the same receptor subtype sets the stage for pharmacodynamic interactions, which can be antagonistic, additive, or synergistic in nature.

Cardiovascular Agents

Sympathomimetic amines (epinephrine, norepinephrine, phenylephrine, dopamine, dobutamine, ephedrine, and isoproterenol) are particularly susceptible to pharmacodynamic drug-drug interactions. The extent and significance of these interactions depend on the selectivity of both the object drug and precipitant drug for adrenergic receptor types. β-adrenergic antagonists generally antagonize the cardiac and bronchodilating effects of the sympathomimetics.[193] However, propranolol and other nonspecific β-adrenergic antagonists (Table 126.6) may enhance the vasoconstriction produced with epinephrine. As a result, the patient may experience hypertension and bradycardia.[71,72] Labetalol possesses both α_1-adrenergic and nonspecific β-adrenergic antagonistic activity, which produces an increase in diastolic blood pressure and a decrease in heart rate when given during an epinephrine infusion.[71,72] However, metoprolol and other β_1-cardioselective antagonists have minimal effects on the vasopressor response when given concomitantly with epinephrine.[71,72] Other classes of drugs can interact with the sympathomimetics as well. Linezolid, an antibiotic often reserved

TABLE 126.6	β-Blocker Receptor Selectivity	
	Intrinsic Sympathomimetic Activity (ISA)	Alpha-Blockade
Beta-1 Selective		
Metoprolol	None	None
Atenolol	None	None
Esmolol	None	None
Sotalol	None	None
Beta Nonselective		
Propranolol	None	None
Nadolol	None	None
Labetalol	Yes	Yes
Carvedilol	None	Yes

Adapted from Barres V, Taglialatela M. New advances in beta-blocker therapy in heart failure. Front Physiol. 2013;4:1-9.

for drug-resistant methicillin-resistant *Staphylococcus aureus* (MRSA) infections, inhibits monoamine oxidase, which can increase sensitivity to vasopressor effects. When adding linezolid to vasopressor therapy, a reduction in dosing may be needed based on the hemodynamic response.[194] Antihistamines, such as diphenhydramine, inhibit tissue uptake of epinephrine and norepinephrine while increasing adrenoreceptor sensitivity to epinephrine.[193]

General anesthetics, such as sevoflurane, and halogenated hydrocarbons, halothane, can increase cardiac irritability and sensitize the myocardium to the arrhythmogenic effects of sympathomimetics. Tachycardia and arrhythmias are reported with concurrent administrations.[193] Atropine also blocks reflex bradycardia produced by epinephrine, norepinephrine, and phenylephrine. This effect augments the vasopressor response to these medications.[193] Finally, case reports and animal studies have shown that concurrent administration of dopamine and intravenous phenytoin or fosphenytoin produces hypotension and bradycardia. Cardiovascular status should be monitored closely when these medications are given concomitantly.[71,72]

The pharmacologic effect of vasodilators, such as sodium nitroprusside, hydralazine, and diazoxide, are augmented by both β-adrenergic antagonists and diuretics. The decreased systemic vascular resistance and resultant reduction in mean arterial pressure provide stimuli for a compensatory increase in sympathetic nervous system activity. Normalization of blood pressure to the set point then is mediated by an increase in cardiac contractility, increased heart rate, and stimulation of the renin-angiotensin-aldosterone (RAA) pathway. β-Adrenergic antagonists prevent this sympathetic outflow and thereby enhance the vasodilator and resultant hypotensive response. The combination of certain vasodilators and sildenafil may produce additive hypotensive effects. Studies have shown sildenafil to be effective in the treatment of pulmonary hypertension and chronic lung disease in pediatric and neonatal critical care.[195,196] The increased use of this medication, especially in cardiac patients, has necessitated heightened surveillance of potential interactions. Contact between sodium nitroprusside molecules and erythrocytes or the vascular wall generates nitric oxide. Nitric oxide subsequently stimulates the cyclic guanosine monophosphate (cGMP) second messenger system in vascular smooth muscle. The molecular process of increasing intracellular concentrations of cGMP translates to vasodilation and the resultant physiologic effect of reduced blood pressure. Sildenafil augments the response to cGMP through selective inhibition of type 5 phosphodiesterase, the enzyme that catalyzes degradation of cGMP. Therefore sildenafil can react similarly with other drugs, such as nitroglycerin and hydralazine, which also promote the generation of a nitric oxide. Sildenafil is also metabolized by the cytochrome P-450-3A4 enzymes, which can cause significant interaction potential with CYP3A4 inhibitors. Concentrations of sildenafil have been increased by as much as 182% when combined with erythromycin.[197] It is recommended that clinicians monitor patients closely for the increased hypotensive effects of sildenafil if concomitant administration of CYP3A4 inhibitors, such as macrolides, cimetidine, or azole antifungals, cannot be avoided.

The antiarrhythmic drugs amiodarone, disopyramide, and quinidine are substrates for the CYP3A4 isoform of the P-450 enzyme system. Plasma levels of these antiarrhythmics may increase and produce adverse effects when combined with CYP3A4 inhibitors such as the macrolide antibiotics, azole antifungals, and other miscellaneous inhibitors such as cyclosporine, certain calcium channel blockers (diltiazem and verapamil), and grapefruit juice. Conversely, plasma levels decrease when therapy is combined with drugs that are known enzyme inducers, which include phenobarbital, carbamazepine, phenytoin, oxcarbazepine, and rifampin. The antiarrhythmic drugs flecainide, mexiletine, and propafenone are substrates for CYP2D6. Concomitant therapy with enzyme inhibitors of CYP2D6, including amiodarone, cimetidine, diphenhydramine, fluoxetine, paroxetine, haloperidol, propafenone, and quinidine, could result in toxicity.[71,72]

As a substrate for Pgp, digoxin exhibits reduced renal and nonrenal clearance when a Pgp inhibitor is added to the drug regimen. Plasma levels of digoxin may increase 100% to 200%, demanding close monitoring for digoxin toxicity. Pgp inhibitors include amiodarone, clarithromycin, cyclosporine, diltiazem, erythromycin, ketoconazole, itraconazole, propafenone, quinidine, and verapamil.[71,72]

Pharmacodynamic interactions with drugs that modulate atrioventricular (AV) nodal conduction may produce clinically significant adverse effects, which can include heart block, bradycardia, and other arrhythmias. Concurrent therapies with antiarrhythmic agents, calcium channel blockers, and β-adrenergic antagonists should be monitored closely or even reevaluated.[198] Patients with severe electrolyte imbalances may be susceptible to digoxin toxicity. Hypokalemia, hypomagnesemia, and hypercalcemia are all conditions that may be drug induced. Therefore drugs may interact with digoxin in an indirect manner through alteration of electrolyte homeostasis. Loop diuretics, thiazide diuretics, amphotericin B, corticosteroids, laxatives, and sodium polystyrene sulfonate may all contribute to digoxin toxicity.[193,199,200]

Calcium channel antagonists have been implicated in several common pharmacokinetic drug-drug interactions involving the CYP3A substrates. Additionally, inhibitors of CYP3A can lead to significant interactions with calcium channel antagonists. These interactions enhance the development of lower diastolic blood pressure, higher heart rates, and

other vasodilation-related side effects.[198] Inducers of CYP3A4 are implicated in the reduced efficacy of calcium antagonists.[198] Droperidol affects cardiac repolarization, prolongs the QT/QTc interval, and, when concurrently administered with calcium channel antagonists, increases the risk of QT/QTc prolongation, torsades de pointes, and cardiac arrest.[201] Concomitant administration of fentanyl and nicardipine can result in severe hypotension.[202] Awareness and monitoring of potential drug-drug interactions are necessary when administering calcium channel antagonists.

β-Adrenergic antagonists (β-blockers) are associated with a variety of pharmacodynamic and pharmacokinetic drug-drug interactions as well. Concomitant use of a β-adrenergic antagonist and verapamil or diltiazem can result in additive negative inotropic effects and can potentiate conduction abnormalities.[203,204] Abrupt withdrawal of clonidine when concomitantly used with a β-blocker can exaggerate rebound hypertension symptoms associated with clonidine withdrawal.[205,206] The probable mechanism of this interaction is unopposed α-adrenergic agonism. Use of amiodarone with β-adrenergic antagonists potentiates bradycardia, sinus arrest, and AV block.[202]

Angiotensin-converting enzyme inhibitors (ACEIs) have been implicated in a variety of drug-drug interactions. Electrolyte disturbances are a major source of complications with these drug-drug interactions. Potassium-sparing diuretics, such as spironolactone and eplerenone, in combination with ACEIs increase serum potassium levels.[207] Nesiritide, a medication often used to treat decompensated heart failure, can suppress the renin-angiotensin-aldosterone system; therefore it is important to monitor patients for severe hypotension when concurrently administering this medication with ACEIs.[208]

Anticonvulsant Medications

The antiepileptics constitute a drug class that has the potential to be involved in a large array of drug-drug interactions. These interactions are mainly pharmacokinetic in nature and usually involve induction, inhibition, or competition among substrates for various isoforms of the cytochrome P-450 enzyme system. Fortunately, these drugs typically are monitored using blood concentrations, and appropriate therapeutic drug monitoring can aid in the avoidance of adverse events secondary to drug-drug interactions. Table 126.5 lists the isoforms for which the various antiepileptics are substrates, inducers, or inhibitors.

In the intensive care unit setting, phenytoin is generally administered intravenously in the form of the water-soluble prodrug fosphenytoin. Phosphatases in red blood cells and the liver catalyze the conversion of fosphenytoin to its active form phenytoin. Fosphenytoin has a serum half-life of 8 to 15 minutes.[209] Once fosphenytoin is converted to phenytoin, it is susceptible to all of the potential drug-drug interactions that affect orally administered phenytoin. Approximately 95% of phenytoin is metabolized in the liver by the CYP2C9/10 and CYP2C19 isoforms of the cytochrome P-450 enzyme system to produce the inactive metabolite parahydroxyphenylhydantoin.[209] The CYP2C9/10 isoform is the main pathway of metabolism for this drug. Phenytoin metabolism is reduced and plasma levels increased via competition with other drugs that are substrates for CYP2C9 and CYP2C19, such as amiodarone, fluconazole, valproic acid, omeprazole, and fluoxetine.

Conversely, phenytoin may competitively inhibit the metabolism of these drugs. Drugs that inhibit CYP2C9 reduce clearance of phenytoin and consequently increase plasma concentrations.[210] Examples include fluconazole, ketoconazole, cotrimoxazole, amiodarone, and valproate. Omeprazole, cimetidine, and fluoxetine are inhibitors of CYP2C19 and thus can increase phenytoin plasma concentrations.[210] In addition to serving as a substrate to CYP2C9/10 and CYP2C19, phenytoin can also induce their activity. Moreover, phenytoin induces CYP3A4 and uridine diphosphate glucuronosyltransferase (UGT) activity.[209] It may take 1 to 2 weeks for maximum induction of these enzymes when phenytoin therapy is started and, conversely, the same amount of time for de-induction once the drug is discontinued.[210] Phenytoin exhibits a high degree of protein binding ($\geq$90%) to serum proteins, mainly albumin, so displacement from its binding sites may produce clinically significant changes in free phenytoin concentration.[209] The free fraction is the pharmacologically active portion of the total phenytoin concentration in plasma. Populations in whom increased proportion of free drug may be found include neonates, patients with uremia, hyperbilirubinemia, or hypoalbuminemia, as well as patients taking concurrent anionic drugs.[209,211,212] During the hospital course of critically ill children who experienced traumatic head injuries, protein binding and phenytoin metabolism can be altered.[213] The free fraction of phenytoin may increase over time in patients with acute head injury.[214] Such a clinical condition makes this particular population of patients especially susceptible to potential protein displacement interactions with other highly protein-bound drugs, such as valproic acid. The potential clinical significance of this interaction is an increased risk for phenytoin toxicity.

Phenobarbital is a substrate for CYP2C9, CYP2C19, and CYP2E1. The CYP2C19 isoform serves as the primary pathway for metabolism.[209] Phenobarbital is converted to 5-p-hydroxyphenyl-5-ethyl-barbituric acid, an inactive species, and further conjugated with glucuronic acid or sulfuric acid for excretion in urine.[209] Phenobarbital has the potential to induce CYP2C9 and CYP3A4 enzymes.[215] The time frame for induction and de-induction of the P-450 enzyme system depends on phenobarbital's half-life, with induction beginning 1 week after initiation of phenobarbital therapy and de-induction beginning 1 week after phenobarbital is discontinued. Maximum induction occurs in approximately 2 to 3 weeks. Phenobarbital also induces UGT.[210] Addition of phenobarbital or phenytoin to a regimen of methadone, which may be used in the intensive care unit for the purpose of weaning from long-term opiate sedation, may present a potential for significant drug-drug interaction. Induction of CYP2C9 and CYP3A4 leads to increased clearance of methadone, increasing the possibility of methadone withdrawal. In transplant patients, phenobarbital may reduce cyclosporine concentrations, which may lead to concerns regarding adequate immunosuppression. Another significant drug interaction involves the abrupt withdrawal of phenobarbital in a patient maintained on both phenobarbital and warfarin. In such a scenario, blood levels of warfarin may increase and lead to increased risk of bleeding. During maintenance of such a regimen, phenobarbital induces the same enzymes responsible for warfarin metabolism. As a result, warfarin dosing is adjusted based on phenobarbital-mediated inhibition of the hypoprothrombinemia response.

Oxcarbazepine undergoes extensive metabolism through the liver to an active metabolite, 10-monohydroxy (MHD). The main pharmacologic properties of oxcarbazepine are due to its active metabolite MHD. Oxcarbazepine is a weak inhibitor of CYP2C19 and strong inducer of CYP3A4/5 isoforms. When oral contraceptives, dihydropyridine calcium antagonists, and cyclosporine are given concomitantly with oxcarbazepine, decreased drug levels were shown, due to the induction of CYP3A4/5 isoforms.[216]

The isoforms of the P-450 enzyme system that metabolize valproic acid include CYP2C9 and CYP2C19, both of which represent minor pathways. The main route of metabolism for valproic acid involves glucuronidation by UGT and β-oxidation.[209] Valproate inhibits drugs that are metabolized by CYP2C9, such as phenytoin and phenobarbital. In addition to being a substrate for UGT, valproic acid inhibits drugs that are metabolized by this enzyme, such as lorazepam and lamotrigine. Valproic acid also exhibits a high degree of protein binding to plasma albumin (90%), making protein displacement interactions likely with other highly protein-bound drugs.[209]

The main pathway for metabolism of lamotrigine is UGT-mediated glucuronidation. Lamotrigine is capable of inducing its own metabolism, with maximum autoinduction observed within 2 weeks. Autoinduction typically results in a 17% reduction in plasma blood levels.[217] Through their action on UGT, carbamazepine, phenytoin, and phenobarbital reduce plasma concentrations of lamotrigine when given concomitantly. Lamotrigine, on the other hand, reduces valproic acid plasma levels when added to a regimen containing valproic acid. Concentrations may be reduced by as much as 25% in the course of a few weeks.[209]

Antiinfective and Antimicrobial Agents

Antimicrobial agents are commonly used in the intensive care unit to treat patients with serious infections. Many drug-drug interactions involve antimicrobial agents; however, some are not clinically significant.[101] Complexation of fluoroquinolones (ciprofloxacin, levofloxacin) to multivalent cations (aluminum, calcium, magnesium, and iron) due to binding within their chemical structures is an example of an interaction that can be easily managed by administering the drugs at separate times.[218,219]

Macrolide antibiotics, on the other hand, are associated with many drug-drug interactions that can be of clinical importance. Erythromycin may cause interactions through inhibition of the CYP3A4 enzyme, which can increase serum levels of warfarin, cyclosporine, midazolam, and tacrolimus.[220,221] Clarithromycin also inhibits cytochrome P-450 enzymes and may increase the serum levels of carbamazepine, caffeine, cyclosporine, warfarin, valproate, and midazolam.[220,221] Azithromycin is an azalide (macrolide subclass) that does not demonstrate cytochrome P-450 complexation, so it has less drug interaction potential. No major drug-drug interactions have been shown with azithromycin and carbamazepine, theophylline, or midazolam.[220] Interactions with cyclosporine and warfarin are limited to case reports; therefore monitoring of serum levels and international normalized ratio (INR), respectively, is prudent when using this combination.[222]

Carbapenems are commonly used in the intensive care unit for treatment of gram-negative sepsis. Though not commonly associated with significant drug-drug interactions, concurrent use of carbapenems with valproic acid and its derivatives can cause a significant and sudden decrease of valproate serum concentrations.[223] The effect is most significant with meropenem where a decrease of up to 90% in valproic acid levels can be observed.[224,225] In patients who need valproic acid for primary prevention of seizures, use of carbapenems is discouraged. However, if no substitute is available, the addition of a second antiepileptic agent should be considered to control seizures and prophylaxis.

Rifampin is a cytochrome P-450 enzyme inducer that is involved in many drug-drug interactions. Rifampin may decrease serum concentrations of chloramphenicol, isoniazid, amiodarone, cyclosporine, prednisolone, and warfarin.[226,227] These interactions often complicate multidrug regimens for treatment of active tuberculosis or nontuberculous mycobacteria.

Antifungal agents are used in the critical care setting for treatment and prophylaxis of systemic mycoses. Azole derivatives inhibit sterol 14-α-demethylase, which is a hepatic microsomal cytochrome P-450–dependent system. Unfortunately, this mechanism results in significant drug-drug interactions. Azole antifungals are known inhibitors of cytochrome P-450 isoenzymes, although the specific CYP isoforms and potency of inhibition vary among agents.[110,228,229] Table 126.5 describes cytochrome P-450 isoforms inhibited by the azole antifungals. Clinically significant interactions with azoles occur most frequently with agents that have narrow therapeutic windows and are metabolized by cytochrome P-450 enzymes. Additionally, significant interactions can occur when azole derivatives are administered with CYP3A substrates such as midazolam,[228-230] tacrolimus,[231,232] sirolimus, cyclosporine,[233] nifedipine,[199] felodipine,[199,234] diltiazem,[232] and alfentanil.[235]

Benzodiazepines that rely on the CYP3A4 enzyme for biotransformation are predisposed to drug-drug interactions with CYP3A inhibitors. The benzodiazepines most prone to interactions are alprazolam, diazepam, midazolam, and triazolam.[229,236,237] Ketoconazole, a potent inhibitor of CYP3A, increases the area under the concentration–time curve (AUC) of oral midazolam by 16-fold.[229,234,238-241] Whenever azole antifungals are administered with midazolam, patients must be monitored for increased response to midazolam, and dose alteration or discontinuation of therapy should be considered. Diazepam metabolism is mediated by CYP3A and CYP2C19 and is also prone to interactions with azole derivatives.[242] Fluconazole and voriconazole are inhibitors of CYP3A, CYP2C9, and CYP2C19 and have the potential to cause drug interactions with compounds that are metabolized via this pathway, including diazepam, which is metabolized by CYP3A4 and CYP2C19.

Warfarin is a racemic mixture compound for which most pharmacodynamic activity occurs with the S-isomer, whose metabolism is also dependent on CYP2C9, which is inhibited by fluconazole and voriconazole.[232,243] This interaction is significant, and appropriate dosage modifications or alteration of therapeutic agents must be considered. The calcium channel antagonist class is metabolized by CYP3A isoenzymes and has the potential for interactions with azole derivatives.[234] Drug levels of azole antifungals, especially itraconazole, voriconazole, and posaconazole, may be rendered undetectable when used in conjunction with strong P-450 enzyme inducers like rifampin.[244,245] Alternative antifungal agents should be considered in situations where rifampin cannot be discontinued.

In addition to being CYP3A inhibitors, ketoconazole and itraconazole are substrates and inhibitors of Pgp.[246,247] Drug-drug interactions mediated via Pgp typically are important determinants of bioavailability, liver metabolism, and kidney excretion.[248,249] Diltiazem, verapamil, cyclosporine, and tacrolimus are dual CYP3A and Pgp substrates.[250] Clearance of digoxin, a Pgp substrate, is decreased with coadministration of itraconazole due to impaired renal tubular secretion via inhibition of Pgp, resulting in an increase in digoxin trough concentration.[199] Oral absorption of itraconazole and posaconazole is pH dependent and may result in a clinically significant decrease in therapeutic efficacy if these agents are used concurrently with proton-pump inhibitors or H_2 antagonists. This interaction is more pronounced with the liquid formulations of the medications. Echinocandins are a relatively new class of antifungal that are increasingly used in the treatment of fungal infections due to its relatively safe side effect profile and lack of cytochrome P-450 and P-glycoprotein mediated drug interactions. Among the three currently available echinocandins—micafungin, caspofungin, and anidulafungin—caspofungin is most commonly associated with drug interactions due to the role of hepatic transporter organic anion-transporting polypeptide (OATP)-1B1 in the uptake of caspofungin. Rifampin, an OATP inhibitor, can reduce caspofungin levels, and therefore an increased caspofungin dose is recommended when coadministered with rifampin.[251]

Anesthetic Agents and Sedatives

Several agents are used for anesthesia and sedation in the pediatric critical care setting. Many of these drugs have clinically significant drug-drug interactions. The ability to recognize potential drug-drug interactions related to the use of anesthetic agents or sedatives in the pediatric critical care setting requires a fundamental understanding of the agent's clinical pharmacology. Benzodiazepines are a class of sedatives that are particularly susceptible to drug-drug interactions because of their route of biotransformation.[229,252,253] CYP3A4 plays a major role in the metabolism of midazolam, triazolam, and alprazolam, and caution should be exercised when combining these agents with CYP3A modulators.[254-256] As mentioned previously, concomitant use of systemic antifungals and benzodiazepines results in a known clinically significant drug-drug interaction, caused by azole antifungals inhibiting the CYP3A isoenzyme.[252] Midazolam, a short-acting benzodiazepine used in the pediatric critical care setting, is almost exclusively metabolized via the CYP3A pathway. Interactions are most prominent with oral midazolam therapy because of the role of intestinal metabolism.[229,230,252] However, significantly increased plasma levels have been observed when intravenous midazolam is administered with fluconazole.[229,230,252] Additionally, clarithromycin and erythromycin have been proved to significantly decrease systemic clearance of intravenous and oral midazolam.[230,257,258] Azithromycin, another macrolide, does not appear to increase plasma concentrations of oral midazolam.[240] Propofol has been shown to decrease the clearance of midazolam by 37%, possibly by competitive inhibition of CYP3A4.[259,239] Concomitant administration of verapamil or diltiazem with oral midazolam is associated with dramatic increases in AUC and the maximum concentration (C_{max}).[239] Inducers of CYP3A can drastically decrease plasma concentrations of midazolam. Rifampin, a potent inducer of

CYP3A and Pgp expression in the gut mucosa, can cause dramatic decreases in plasma concentrations of oral midazolam.[239,260] Other inducers of CYP3A enzymes implicated in significant interactions with midazolam are carbamazepine and phenytoin.[255] Diazepam, a benzodiazepine with long-acting metabolites, is prone to drug-drug interactions with inhibitors or inducers of CYP2C19 or 3A4. Due to the fact that the primary route of metabolism for lorazepam is through glucuronidation, this agent is associated with fewer potential pharmacokinetic drug-drug interactions.[236]

The potential for pharmacodynamic drug-drug interactions also exists with sedative agents. Concomitant use of barbiturates and benzodiazepines causes additive respiratory and CNS depression. This is mediated by allosteric conformational changes at the γ-aminobutyric acid (GABA) site, which regulates the opening of chloride channels, causing the neurons to become hyperpolarized and resistant to excitation.[261] The dosage of midazolam and other benzodiazepines often is reduced by 30% to 50% when they are administered concomitantly with opioid analgesics.[262] Flumazenil competitively inhibits the activity of benzodiazepines at its recognition site on the GABA-benzodiazepine receptor complex; however, it does not reverse the CNS effects of GABA-mimetic agents such as barbiturates, propofol, and other general anesthetics.[263]

Clonidine, an α2-adrenergic agonist agent with sedative properties, reduces the induction concentrations needed for loss of consciousness when using propofol.[264] Propofol can inhibit the clearance of alfentanil and act synergistically with opioids.[265,266] Caution should be exercised when using propofol in combination with drugs that lower seizure threshold, such as meperidine and enflurane.[267]

Neuromuscular blocking agents have significant drug-drug interactions.[268] Concomitant use of intravenous antibiotics such as aminoglycosides or clindamycin has the potential to intensify neuromuscular blockade produced by neuromuscular blocking agents.[268] Phenytoin has been shown to increase pancuronium requirements. Additionally, inhalation anesthetic agents can also potentiate neuromuscular blockade.[268]

Analgesic Agents

A variety of agents are used for analgesia in the pediatric critical care setting. Patients receiving opioid analgesia are particularly susceptible to drug-drug interactions. Whenever an opiate agonist is administered with an agent that has CNS depressant effects, augmented effects or toxicity is possible. Therefore vigilance in monitoring for drug-drug interactions is necessary when administering these agents to help ensure that safe and effective analgesia is achieved. Analgesic pharmacokinetic drug-drug interactions can mediate clinically relevant effects. CYP3A is involved in the metabolism of methadone and alfentanil.[258] Methadone metabolism is induced by rifampin and results in enhanced clearance of methadone.[269,270] One study of adults demonstrated an approximately fourfold increase in methadone clearance when administered with rifampin.[271] This effect could provoke withdrawal symptoms in patients receiving methadone.[272] Phenobarbital, phenytoin, carbamazepine, nevirapine, and efavirenz have the potential to decrease methadone blood concentrations as well.[273,274] Rifampin significantly lowers alfentanil plasma concentrations by the same mechanism.[258] On the other hand, inhibition of CYP3A can result in increased plasma levels of methadone.[269] For example, fluconazole inhibits metabolism of methadone and alfentanil.[235,269] Fluconazole decreased the clearance of alfentanil approximately 58% following intravenous fluconazole administration in healthy adults.[235]

Pharmacodynamic drug-drug interactions can result in synergic effects or antagonism. When a pure opiate agonist, a partial agonist, or an antagonist, is used in combination, there is a risk for decreased clinical effects. For example, when morphine (a pure μ agonist) and nalbuphine (a partial agonist/antagonist) are used in combination, it can decrease the opiate effect. This can have profound effects on analgesia and result in withdrawal symptoms for patients on long-term analgesia therapy.[275,276] Analgesic opioid therapy is associated with several side effects that can be heightened by drug-drug interactions such as respiratory depression, hypotension, decreased GI motility, nausea, and vomiting. Use of a pure opioid antagonist, such as naloxone, is needed to reverse undesirable effects. Most clinically significant drug-drug interactions associated with analgesics are pharmacodynamic in origin.

Anticoagulants

Warfarin is involved in a multitude of drug-drug interactions through a variety of mechanisms, including alterations in protein binding, effects of hepatic metabolism by the cytochrome P-450 system, disruption of bacterial flora in the GI tract, and changes in the clotting cascade (Table 126.7). Aspirin, chloral hydrate, ibuprofen, and sulfamethoxazole can displace warfarin from protein binding sites, increasing free fraction of warfarin available and hence augmenting anticoagulation. Warfarin metabolism may be inhibited by amiodarone, sulfamethoxazole, metronidazole, azole antifungals, macrolide and quinolone antibiotics, and isoniazid, thereby decreasing the effect.[276] Phenobarbital, rifampin, and phenytoin can induce the metabolism of warfarin and decrease its effect dramatically. In fact, concurrent administration of warfarin and rifampin is strongly discouraged, especially in high-risk patients like those with mechanical mitral valves. Most antibiotics have the potential to decrease synthesis of vitamin K–dependent clotting factors and potentiate warfarin's effect.[276,277] Other medications including NSAIDs and antiplatelet medications can exacerbate the adverse effects of warfarin by directly affecting the clotting cascade. Phytonadione (vitamin K) antagonizes the anticoagulant effect of warfarin.[215,277a] Careful monitoring of bleeding and coagulation parameters (prothrombin time and INR) can help prevent serious adverse drug reactions. Many drug-drug interactions can occur when initiating warfarin therapy or when adding other medications to existing warfarin therapy. It is recommended that clinicians use adjusted starting doses of warfarin when initiating therapy while patients are receiving medications with the potential for interaction.

Heparin has the ability to interact with other agents, which can increase the risk of bleeding or thrombosis by altering heparin's effect. Common interactions include oral anticoagulants and platelet inhibitors (eg, aspirin, dextran, ibuprofen, and other agents that interfere with platelet aggregation). Heparin's effectiveness can also be altered by the administration of additional clotting factors found in fresh frozen plasma and antithrombin III. Antifibrinolytic agents, which can enhance the anticoagulant effects of heparin, have become one of the primary treatments for larger arterial or intraatrial

TABLE 126.7   Medication Interactions That Modify the Anticoagulant Effect of Warfarin

Increased INR	Decreased INR	Increased Risk of Bleeding	Increased Risk of Thrombosis
CYP-450 Inhibition via 2C9 (unless otherwise noted)	**CYP-450 Induction via 2C9** (unless otherwise noted) Carbamazepine Phenobarbital Phenytoin Rifampin	**Alterations in Platelet Function** Antiplatelet Agents Aspirin Cimetidine Clopidogrel Fish oil Ticlopidine	**Alterations in Warfarin Metabolism or Absorption** Cholestyramine Griseofulvin Nafcillin Ribavirin Sucralfate
Antidepressants Fluvoxamine Sertraline		Antifibrinolytics Alteplase Streptokinase Urokinase	**Prothrombotic** Estrogens OCPs Phytonadione Total parenteral nutrition
Antiinfectives Azole Antifungals (2C9/3A4) Cotrimoxazole Fluoroquinolones (1A2/3A4) Isoniazid Macrolides Metronidazole Miconazole		NSAIDs Aspirin Ibuprofen Indomethacin Ketorolac	
Cardiovascular Drugs Amiodarone Fluvastatin Gemfibrozil Lovastatin Simvastatin		SSRIs Citalopram Sertraline	
		Reduced Vitamin K Production Antiinfectives (oral) Omeprazole	
		Miscellaneous Corticosteroids Levothyroxine Propranolol	

INR, international normalized ratio; *NSAIDs,* nonsteroidal antiinflammatory drugs; *OCP,* oral contraceptive pills; *SSRI,* selective serotonin reuptake inhibitor.
Modified from Hansten PD. Oral anticoagulants and drugs which alter thyroid function. Drug Intell Clin Pharm. 1980;14:331-334; Liu A, Stumpo C. Warfarin drug interactions among older adults. Geriatrics Aging. 2007;10:643-646; Holbrook AM, Pereira JA, Labris R, et al. Systematic overview of warfarin and its drug and food interactions. Arch Intern Med. 2005;165:1095–1106.

clots. Though concomitant anticoagulation with heparin is often indicated with antifibrinolytic agents and blood products, it is important to adjust heparin infusion rates and monitor the patient's response when combining these medications. Enoxaparin and other low-molecular-weight heparins have similar interactions with medications independently associated with an increased risk of bleeding as mentioned earlier.[278] Additionally, medications that adversely affect renal clearance can prolong the elimination half-life of enoxaparin and increase the risk of adverse effects.[278]

There are many newer oral anticoagulants on the market, mostly used in adults, that are currently being studied in pediatric patients. Limited data are available for dosing and monitoring; however, as they may become more prevalent in this population it is important to mention possible drug-drug interactions. Dabigatran, an enteral direct thrombin inhibitor similar to warfarin, and the oral anti-factor Xa inhibitors rivaroxaban, apixaban, and edoxaban have interactions with Pgp inhibitors like rifampin (see Table 126.5). All but edoxaban and dabigatran can interact with strong CYP3A4 inhibitors such as azole antifungals and macrolides (see Table 126.5). Additionally, dabigatran may interact with certain proton pump inhibitors. Dose reduction or modification of medication therapy may be required. As with other anticoagulants, close monitoring is required when using with antiplatelet agents or other medications noted to increase the risk of bleeding.[279,280]

Immunosuppressive Agents

Most immunosuppressive agents possess narrow therapeutic indices and therefore require therapeutic drug monitoring.[281,282] As a result, a sophisticated knowledge of clinical pharmacology is required to evaluate the clinical relevance of potential drug-drug interactions involving these drugs. Drug-drug interactions most commonly encountered with immunosuppressive drug therapy revolve around the inhibition or induction of the CYP3A enzymes. Cyclosporine, tacrolimus, prednisone, sirolimus, and everolimus are all CYP3A substrates and are most prone to these types of pharmacokinetic drug-drug interactions.[283,284] Interestingly, known CYP3A inhibitors, such as ketoconazole, have been used intentionally to maintain therapeutic levels in patients with high presystemic metabolism of cyclosporine.[285] Medications that inhibit CYP3A metabolism should be used with caution in patients taking cyclosporine, tacrolimus, sirolimus, or everolimus; however, if concomitant use cannot be avoided, dosing adjustments of immunosuppressive therapy may be required. Table 126.5 provides a list of medications that are CYP3A4 enzyme inhibitors. Concomitant administration of sirolimus or everolimus with cyclosporine increases sirolimus and everolimus exposure, likely due to shared CYP3A and Pgp metabolic pathways.[286,287] Several drugs can induce the metabolism of cyclosporine, tacrolimus, sirolimus, everolimus, and prednisone. Rifampin causes induction of CYP3A and Pgp, leading to clinically significant decreases in cyclosporine and tacrolimus plasma concentrations.[288,289] Although not considered to have a narrow therapeutic index, mycophenolate serum concentrations are affected by concurrent administration with cyclosporine. Cyclosporine decreases enterohepatic recirculation of mycophenolic acid, necessitating higher mycophenolate doses to achieve serum concentrations equivalent to that of the drug given alone or with tacrolimus.[290] This interaction may be overcome by using enteric-coated mycophenolic acid formulations.[291]

Azathioprine, an older immunosuppressant, is a prodrug of mercaptopurine, and its biotransformation is dependent on the thiopurine-S-methyltransferase (TPMT) enzyme, xanthine oxidase, and inosine monophosphate dehydrogenase (IMPDH). There are genetic polymorphisms of the TPMT enzyme that may predispose heterozygous and homozygous carriers of the gene to increased bone marrow toxicities with increased levels of the cytotoxic thioguanine (TGN) metabolite.[292] Concurrent use of allopurinol, a xanthine oxidase inhibitor, can increase systemic mercaptopurine exposure and toxicity, therefore a dose reduction of 65% to 75% is recommended to decrease risk of toxicity.[293]

Pulmonary and Respiratory Medications

β_2-Adrenergic agonists (eg, albuterol, levalbuterol, and terbutaline) are useful agents for treatment of asthma. Drug-drug interactions can occur when β_2-adrenergic agonists are used in combination with β_1-adrenergic antagonists, especially the nonselective antagonists. A possible decreased β_2 effect could precipitate asthma symptoms. The nonselective antagonists include propranolol, nadolol, and labetalol (see Table 126.6). Agents such as atenolol, esmolol, and metoprolol are relatively selective for β_1 receptors at therapeutic doses and are considered safer for use in combination with β_2-adrenergic agonists. However, these agents may lose their selectivity at higher doses. One potential side effect of the β_2-adrenergic agonists is hypokalemia, which can be enhanced with concurrent use of loop and thiazide diuretics. Monitoring of potassium levels is recommended when these agents are used together.[215,293a]

Antineoplastic Agents

The majority of drug-drug interactions in patients receiving chemotherapy involve the cytochrome P-450 enzyme system. Potential interactions can be identified by pinpointing the substrates for the various isoenzymes of the mixed function oxidases among the antineoplastic agents. For example, the vinca alkaloids and many of the tyrosine kinase inhibitors are substrates for CYP3A4. Known inhibitors and inducers of CYP3A4 increase and decrease plasma levels, respectively. Toxicities are more likely when these agents are administered with classic CYP3A4 inhibitors such as the azole antifungals, macrolide antibiotics, calcium channel blockers (eg, diltiazem and verapamil), quinupristin/dalfopristin, and cyclosporine. The azole antifungals modulate the metabolism of cyclophosphamide, increasing overall parent drug and metabolite exposure. Fluconazole increases cyclophosphamide AUC by inhibiting CYP2C9 metabolism that leads to formation of the toxic metabolite acrolein, in effect reducing potential adverse drug effects.[294] However, the inhibition of the CYP3A4 metabolic pathway by itraconazole increases formation of the precursor to the acrolein metabolite, increasing toxicity risk.[295] Antiepileptic drugs that are known inducers of the cytochrome P-450 enzyme system may contribute to therapeutic failure with chemotherapeutic agents. In one study of pediatric patients with high-grade glioma, the presence of enzyme-inducing anticonvulsants increased irinotecan clearance.[296]

Multiple drug resistance in cancer cells has been attributed to the expression of a Pgp efflux transmembrane transport protein.[297] Agents that modulate the activity of Pgp currently may provide a drug interaction that favorably increases the efficacy of antineoplastic agents.[298] Coadministration of etoposide and cyclosporine, for example, elevates the mean AUC of etoposide. Etoposide is a CYP3A4 substrate, whereas cyclosporine is both a CYP3A4 and Pgp inhibitor.[299] Inhibitors of the efflux pump, Pgp, increase the cytotoxicity of the vinca alkaloids, anthracyclines, epipodophyllotoxins, and taxanes.[300] Itraconazole, clarithromycin, verapamil, and cyclosporine are known to inhibit Pgp as well.[71,72] Currently, attempts to utilize the increased toxicity associated with greater drug exposure due to Pgp inhibition have limited clinical application of these therapies.[71,72,298]

Colony-stimulating factors are often used to treat the ensuing neutropenia that accompanies cancer chemotherapy. Patients with lymphomas undergoing their first cycle of vincristine and receiving treatment with filgrastim or sargramostim are at risk for developing severe atypical neuropathy. This neuropathy has been described as a severe, sharp, burning pain in the feet and appears to occur more commonly in lymphoma patients receiving this combination than in patients receiving vincristine alone.[301] The mechanism of action of this interaction is unclear.

Methotrexate elimination occurs in the kidneys via filtration and active secretion. The process of tubular secretion requires a carrier, which is a saturable process. Competition among other drugs for secretion may reduce the clearance of methotrexate, which may lead to toxicity. Concurrent administration of methotrexate with any of the penicillins has demonstrated this interaction.[302-304] The NSAIDs, aspirin, and other salicylates all increase the likelihood of methotrexate toxicity by this same mechanism.[30,305-309] Inhibition of renal prostaglandin synthesis and the resultant reduction in renal perfusion also contribute to renal toxicities seen with methotrexate because methotrexate can persist in renal tissue for weeks.[193] Proton pump inhibitors also create interactions with methotrexate due to effects on renal elimination. By inhibiting the transmembrane H^+/K^+-ATPase pump, they may decrease active secretion of methotrexate.[310] The antineoplastic activity of methotrexate stems from its inhibition of dihydrofolate reductase, the enzyme that catalyzes the reduction of folic acid to tetrahydrofolic acid. In turn, tetrahydrofolic acid serves as a building block for purine and DNA synthesis. The clinician should be aware of other drugs that act along this pathway, specifically cotrimoxazole, as these agents may contribute to the toxicities associated with methotrexate therapy.[193,311]

Key References

1. Impicciatore P, Choonara I, Clarkson A, et al. Incidence of adverse drug reactions in paediatric in/out-patients: a systematic review and meta-analysis of prospective studies. *Br J Clin Pharmacol.* 2001;52: 77-83.
2. Kaushal R, Bates DW, Landrigan C, et al. Medication errors and adverse drug events in pediatric inpatients. *JAMA.* 2001;285:2114-2120.
3. Weiss J, Krebs S, Hoffmann C, et al. Survey of adverse drug reactions on a pediatric ward: a strategy for early and detailed detection. *Pediatrics.* 2002;110:254-257.

4. Du W, Tutag Lehr V, Caverly M, et al. Incidence and costs of adverse drug reactions in a tertiary care pediatric intensive care unit. *J Clin Pharmacol.* 2013;53:567-573.

8. Committee on Quality of Health Care in America and Institute of Medicine. *To Err Is Human: Building a Safer Health System.* Washington, DC: National Academy Press; 1999.

11. ASHP guidelines on adverse drug reaction monitoring and reporting. American society of hospital pharmacy. *Am J Health Syst Pharm.* 1995;52:417-419.

13. Edwards IR, Aronson JK. Adverse drug reactions: definitions, diagnosis, and management. *Lancet.* 2000;356:1255-1259.

19. Michel DJ, Knodel LC. Comparison of three algorithms used to evaluate adverse drug reactions. *Am J Hosp Pharm.* 1986;43:1709-1714.

27. Piepho R, Whelton A, Mayor G, et al. Drug-induced nephrotoxicity. *J Clin Pharmacol.* 1991;31:785-791.

36. Linton AL, Clark WF, Driedger AA, et al. Acute interstitial nephritis due to drugs: review of the literature with a report of nine cases. *Ann Intern Med.* 1980;93:735-741.

53. Andrade R, Lucena M, Fernandez M, et al. Drug-induced liver injury: an analysis of 461 incidences submitted to the Spanish registry over a 10-year period. *Gastroenterology.* 2005;129:512-521.

57. Goodman ZD. Drug hepatotoxicity. *Clin Liver Dis.* 2002;6:381-397.

61. Orebaugh SL. Succinylcholine: adverse effects and alternatives in emergency medicine. *Am J Emerg Med.* 1999;17:715-721.

68. Doig JC. Drug-induced cardiac arrhythmias: incidence, prevention and management. *Drug Saf.* 1997;17:265-275.

70. Crouch MA, Limon L, Cassano AT. Clinical relevance and management of drug-related QT interval prolongation. *Pharmacotherapy.* 2003;23:881-908.

71. Hansten PD, Horn JR. *The Top 100 Drug Interactions: A Guide to Patient Management.* Edmonds, WA: H&H Publications; 2002.

72. Hansten PD, Horn JR. *Managing Clinically Important Drug Interactions.* St. Louis, MO: Facts and Comparisons; 2002.

74. Tisdale JE, Miller DA. *Drug-Induced Diseases: Prevention, Detection, and Management.* 2nd ed. Bethesda, MD: American Society of Health-System Pharmacists; 2010.

85. Alldredge BK. Drug-induced seizures: controversies in their identification and management. *Pharmacotherapy.* 1997;17:857-860.

87. Pandharipande P, Ely EW. Sedative and analgesic medications: risk factors for delirium and sleep disturbances in the critically ill. *Crit Care Clin.* 2006;22:313-327.

92. Rousan TA, Aldoss IT, Cowley BD Jr, et al. Recurrent acute thrombocytopenia in the hospitalized patient: sepsis, DIC, HIT, or antibiotic-induced thrombocytopenia. *Am J Hematol.* 2010;85:71-74.

94. Ozkan M, Dweik RA, Ahmad M. Drug-induced lung disease. *Cleve Clin J Med.* 2001;68:782-785.

103. Ma RC, Kong AP, Chan N, et al. Drug-induced endocrine and metabolic disorders. *Drug Saf.* 2007;30:215-245.

105. Vasa FR, Molitch ME. Endocrine problems in the chronically critically ill patient. *Clin Chest Med.* 2001;22:193-208.

109. Trence DL. Management of patients on chronic glucocorticoid therapy: an endocrine perspective. *Prim Care.* 2003;30:593-605.

112. Luna B. Drug-induced hyperglycemia. *JAMA.* 2001;286:1945.

120. Chan TY. Drug-induced syndrome of inappropriate antidiuretic hormone secretion. Causes, diagnosis and management. *Drugs Aging.* 1997;11:27-44.

136. Buckley MS, Leblanc JM, Cawley MJ. Electrolyte disturbances associated with commonly prescribed medications in the intensive care unit. *Crit Care Med.* 2010;38:253-264.

143. Koriyama H, Duff JP, Guerra GG, et al. Is propofol a friend or a foe of the pediatric intensivist? Description of propofol use in a PICU. *Pediatr Crit Care Med.* 2014;15:66-71.

145. VanArsel PP. Pseudoallergic drug reactions: introduction and general review. *Immunol Allergy Clin North Am.* 1991;11:635-644.

148. Bernstein I, Leonard S, Gillian M, Joint Task Force on Practice Parameters, American Academy of Allergy, Asthma, and Immunology, American College of Allergy, Asthma & Immunology. Joint Council of Allergy, Asthma, and Immunology. Executive summary of disease management of drug hypersensitivity: a practice parameter. *Ann Allergy Asthma Immunol.* 1999;83(6 Pt 3):665-700.

152. Sehgal VN, Srivastava G. Fixed drug eruption (FDE): changing scenario of incriminating drugs. *Int J Dermatol.* 2006;45:897-908.

168. Williams NT. Medication administration through enteral feeding tubes. *Am J Health Syst Pharm.* 2008;65:2347-2357.

184. Mohammed Ebid AI, Abdel-Rahman HM. Pharmacokinetics of phenobarbital during certain enhanced elimination modalities to evaluate their clinical efficacy in management of drug overdose. *Ther Drug Monit.* 2001;23:209-216.

195. Benowitz NL. Antihypertensive agents. In: Katzung BG, ed. *Basic and Clinical Pharmacology.* 7th ed. Stamford, CT: Appleton and Lange; 1998.

198. Anderson JR, Nawarskas JJ. Cardiovascular drug-drug interactions. *Cardiol Clin.* 2001;19:215-234.

206. Strauss FG. Withdrawal of antihypertensive therapy. *JAMA.* 1977;238:1734.

212. Painter MJ, Minnigh MB, Gaus L, et al. Neonatal phenobarbital and phenytoin binding profiles. *J Clin Pharmacol.* 1994;34:312-317.

215. Martin H, Sarsat JP, de Waziers I, et al. Induction of cytochrome P450 2B6 and 3A4 expression by phenobarbital and cyclophosphamide in cultured human liver slices. *Pharm Res.* 2003;20(4):557-568.

218. Oliphant CM, Green GM. Quinolones: a comprehensive review. *Am Fam Physician.* 2002;65:455-464.

243. Black DJ, Kunze KL, Wienkers LC, et al. Warfarin-fluconazole. II. A metabolically based drug interaction: in vivo studies. *Drug Metab Dispos.* 1996;24:422-428.

248. Pea F, Furlanut M. Pharmacokinetic aspects of treating infections in the intensive care unit. *Clin Pharmacokinet.* 2001;40:833-868.

249. Tanigawara Y. Role of P-glycoprotein in drug disposition. *Ther Drug Monit.* 2000;22:137-140.

262. Blumer J. Critical analysis of deaths that occurred during a randomized clinical trial of sedation in pediatric intensive care units. *Crit Care Med.* 2002;30(suppl):A95.

267. Naguib M, Magboul MMA, Jaroudi R. Clinically significant drug interactions with general anaesthetics. *CNS Drugs.* 1997;8:51-78.

277a. Mattice BL, Soric MM, Legros E. Effect of intravenous versus subcutaneous phytonadione on length of stay for patients in need of urgent warfarin reversal. *Am J Ther.* 2016;23(2):e345-e349.

279. Gonsalves WI, Pruthi RK, Patnaik MM. The new oral anticoagulants in clinical practice. *Mayo Clin Proc.* 2013;88:495-511.

282. del Mar Fernández de Gatta M, Santos-Buelga D, Domínguez-Gil A, García MJ. Immunosuppressive therapy for paediatric transplant patients: pharmacokinetic considerations. *Clin Pharmacokinet.* 2002;41:115-135.

293a. Yang CT, Lin HC, Lin MC, et al. Effect of beta 2-adrenoceptor agonists on plasma potassium and cardiopulmonary responses on exercise in patients with chronic obstructive pulmonary disease. *Eur J Clin Pharmacol.* 1996;49(5):341-345.

297. Yu DK. The contribution of P-glycoprotein to pharmacokinetic drug-drug interactions. *J Clin Pharmacol.* 1999;39:1203-1211.

298. Nobili S, Landini I, Giglioni B, Mini E. Pharmacological strategies for overcoming multidrug resistance. *Curr Drug Targets.* 2006;7:861-879.

313. Schachter SC. Iatrogenic seizures. *Neurol Clin.* 1998;16:157-170.

Principles of Toxin Assessment and Screening

Alan D. Woolf

PEARLS

- Some toxins (eg, acetaminophen, *Amanita* mushroom poisoning, valproic acid, sulfonylureas) are notable for the delay from time of ingestion to onset of symptoms. Others with a long duration of action, such as methadone or naltrexone, can have symptom recurrence hours after an apparent good response to an antidote.
- Intensivists can often predict the severity of poisoning by noting the tempo of progression of a patient's signs and symptoms of toxicity.
- Clinicians must assess the intoxicated or comatose patient for the possibility of secondary trauma, such as fractures, intracranial bleeding, sexual abuse, rape, or internal injuries.

Despite progress in preventive measures, poisonings in children and adolescents continue to be common occurrences. Children younger than 6 years of age accounted for 48% of the almost 2.2 million poisoning exposure calls taken by poison centers in 2013.[1] The most common categories of products identified during poisoning calls to poison centers include cosmetics and personal care products, cleaning substances, analgesics, foreign bodies, topical agents, cough and cold preparations, vitamins, pesticides, and plants. Although many of these exposures are medically trivial, poisonings account for an important number of all pediatric hospital visits and hospitalizations. Preschool children and those with developmental delays and pica, as occurs with autistic spectrum disorders, have an increased risk for poisoning. A second peak of serious poisonings occurs in adolescence, when suicide attempts by poisoning or toxicity related to substance abuse become common circumstances.

Common Agents Involved in Serious Pediatric Poisonings

The agents most frequently involved in serious pediatric poisonings requiring intensive care include prescription medications (eg, cyclic antidepressants, anticonvulsants, cardiovascular-acting drugs, opiates), alcohols, carbon monoxide, caustic agents, and hydrocarbon-based household products. International adoptees and children immigrating to the United States may have been exposed to lead, arsenic, or other toxins in a polluted environment in their home countries or by their family's use of poorly regulated remedies. Clinicians should ask caretakers about the types and doses of any medications, herbs, vitamins, diet supplements, or ethnic remedies being given to their child. Such therapies may be interacting with the toxins responsible for the poisoning or otherwise contributing to the child's toxicity.

Resources for the Clinician

In making the diagnosis of an unknown poisoning, the physician must rely on observation, history-taking abilities, and clinical skills. Laboratory analyses and radiographic findings are sometimes helpful. The regional poison control center (US telephone: 1-800-222-1222) can provide consultative services by medically trained toxicologists.

General Assessment of the Poisoned Patient

History

An accurate history is vitally important in the diagnosis of unknown poisoning. Surprisingly, the physician in the ICU may be the first health professional who can sit with parents and carefully review the circumstances of the exposure. Poisonings may occur by various routes including ingestion, inhalation, ocular exposure, dermal exposure, mucous membrane involvement, or parenteral exposure. Once the child's condition has been stabilized, the pediatrician should query the family about the incident, with particular attention to the environmental, patient, and toxic agent factors as outlined in Table 127.1. The importance of obtaining precise ingredients or package contents cannot be overemphasized. Parents should bring the product containers and medication labels. Parents may minimize the child's exposure to a toxin in an attempt to deny the threat of injury or to assuage their guilt that such an episode occurred. Therefore it is prudent to assume a worst-case scenario in calculating the maximum dose of a drug or household product a child could have swallowed in a poisoning, using the maximum number of missing tablets or amount of liquid, the concentration of the drug or chemical, and the child's weight.

The latency between the time of ingestion and onset of symptoms is important. The tempo of progression of symptoms and signs also may help the clinician gauge the severity of the intoxication and the urgency with which intervention is necessary. However, there are some exceptions to this rule.

TABLE 127.1   History Taking and Unknown Poisoning in the Pediatric Patient

Environment	Patient	Toxin
Witnesses	Intentionality	Agent(s) involved
Time of ingestion	Past medical problems	Exact ingredients
Site of ingestion	Current medications	Dose (maximum estimated)
Illness of family	Known drug allergies	Concentration members
Medications of family members	Time of symptom onset	Route of exposure
Open containers	Prior medical management	

TABLE 127.2   Common Toxidromes in Pediatric Poisoning

Signs and Symptoms	Agent
Dilated pupils, tachycardia, tachypnea, arrhythmias, hypertension, warm moist skin, flushing, sweating, agitation, nausea, vomiting, abdominal pain, delirium	Sympathomimetic syndrome
Miosis, salivation, vomiting, diarrhea, wheeze, bronchorrhea, lacrimation, seizures, weakness, tremors, coma, respiratory failure, bradycardia, urinary frequency	Organophosphate insecticides (cholinergic toxidrome)
Fever, tachypnea, hyperpnea, sweating, lethargy, metabolic acidosis (late), nausea, vomiting, tinnitus, seizures (late), coma (late)	Salicylates
Seizures, metabolic acidosis, history of tuberculosis, hyperglycemia	Isoniazid
Dry mouth and skin, flushed appearance, dilated pupils, fever, ileus, urinary retention, disorientation	Anticholinergic syndrome
Oculogyric crises, dystonia, opisthotonus	Phenothiazines
Severe metabolic acidosis, sluggish pupils, hyperemic retina, blurred vision	Methanol
Hypoglycemia, lethargy, ataxia, seizures, characteristic breath odor	Ethanol
Lethargy or coma, metabolic acidosis, active urinary sediment, crystalluria	Ethylene glycol
Headache, flulike symptoms, lethargy, dizziness, coma	Carbon monoxide
Pinpoint pupils, coma, respiratory depression, hypothermia, pulmonary edema, constipation	Opiate
Hyperthermia, akathisia, mydriasis, diarrhea, neuromuscular rigidity, autonomic dysfunction, agitation, delirium, rhabdomyolysis	Serotonin syndrome
Metabolic acidosis, prolonged QRS interval, coma, seizures, dilated pupils, dysrhythmias	Tricyclic antidepressants
Protracted vomiting, tremors, tachycardia, anxiety, seizures, hypotension	Theophylline
Feeling of impending doom, sudden coma, metabolic acidosis, hypotension, almond odor	Cyanide
Rotatory nystagmus, delirium; "4 C's": **c**ombative, **c**atatonia, **c**onvulsions, **c**oma	Phencyclidine

Patients poisoned by some toxins, such as paraquat and the *Amanita* mushroom toxin, may have a relatively symptom-free period of 12 hours or more but then manifest life-threatening pulmonary or hepatic toxicity, respectively.[2,3] Some drugs, such as sulfonylurea hypoglycemics and valproic acid, can also have similar latency periods before the onset of severe toxicity.[4,5] Adolescent poisonings are confounded by the intentionality of the episode and unreliability of the adolescent's history. Adolescents in distress may be evasive, misleading, or uncommunicative. Their ability to remember or provide a coherent account of what happened may be distorted by the effects of the drugs taken. The clinician cannot assume that the time of exposure, the dose, or even the toxic agents themselves are accurately recounted.

Physical Examination

The physical examination is crucial for assessment of the patient's medical stability and for identification of the unknown poison. Specific changes in vital signs and symptoms are associated with likely toxins or groups of toxins. Such characteristic clinical patterns of illness are sometimes termed *toxidromes*. Table 127.2 lists some of the more common toxidromes. Families are using herbs and diet supplements with increasing frequency to treat their children's illnesses or simply promote their general well-being. However, serious poisonings in which herbs and dietary supplements are implicated are appearing in the medical literature.[6] Table 127.3 lists some examples of toxicities associated with particular herbal remedies.

Frequently, the gastrointestinal tract is involved early in a poisoning, with findings such as nausea, vomiting, abdominal pain, and diarrhea. Overdoses with cocaine, phenothiazines, atropine, or salicylates are often associated with an elevated temperature. Table 127.4 lists examples of drugs and toxic agents associated with specific effects on the cardiovascular system. Drugs with cardiotoxic effects are among those most commonly associated with life-threatening toxicity. In one 10-year retrospective study, 15 out of 17 poisoned patients requiring extracorporeal life support measures for refractory shock or prolonged cardiac arrest had overdosed on cardiotoxic agents.[7] Toxins may cause hypertension or hypotension by direct effects on vascular smooth muscle, neurogenic effects on autonomic nervous centers governing vascular innervation, direct effects on the heart, or renal effects. Specific agents associated with hypertension include adrenergic stimulants, such as amphetamines, cocaine, phencyclidine, phenylpropanolamine, ephedrine, and phenylephrine. Although the hypertension caused by sympathomimetics frequently lasts only a few hours, it may be associated with acute encephalopathy and/or intracranial hemorrhage.

Acute hypotension is frequently associated with poisoning by aconite, antiarrhythmic agents, antihypertensive agents, β-adrenergic antagonists, calcium channel antagonists, clonidine, tricyclic antidepressants (severe), iron (severe), opiates, and phenothiazines.

TABLE 127.3 Herbs Associated With Toxicity

Herbal Product	Toxic Chemicals	Toxic Effects
Aconite (*Aconitum* spp.)	Aconitine alkaloids	Nausea, vomiting, paresthesia, weakness, hypotension, asystole, arrhythmia, bradycardia
Chamomile (*Matricaria chamomilla, Anthemis nobilis*)	Allergens	Anaphylaxis, contact dermatitis
Chapparal (*Larrea divaricata, Larrea tridentata*)	Nordihydroguaiaretic acid	Nausea, vomiting, lethargy, hepatitis
Cinnamon oil (*Cinnamomum*)	Cinnamaldehyde	Dermatitis, abuse syndrome
Coltsfoot (*Tussilago farfara*)	Pyrrolizidines	HVOD
Comfrey (*Symphytum officinale*)	Pyrrolizidines	HVOD
Crotalaria spp.	Pyrrolizidines	HVOD
Echinacea (*Echinacea angustifolia, Compositae* spp.)	Polysaccharides	Asthma, atopy, angioedema, anaphylaxis, urticaria
Eucalyptus (*Eucalyptus globulus*)	1,8-cineole	Drowsiness, ataxia, nausea, vomiting, seizures, coma, respiratory failure
Garlic (*Allium sativum*)	Allicin	Dermatitis, chemical burn, oxidant
Germander (*Teucrium chamaedrys*)		Hepatotoxicity
Ginseng (*Panax ginseng*)	Ginsenoside	Ginseng abuse, diarrhea, anxiety, insomnia, hypertension
Glycerated asafetida	Oxidants	Methemoglobinemia
Grousel (*Senecio longilobus*)	Pyrrolizidines	HVOD
Heliotrope, turnsole (*Crotalaria fulva, Heliotropium, Cynoglossum officinale*)	Pyrrolizidines	HVOD
Jin bu huan (*Stephania* spp., *Corydalis* spp.)	L-Tetrahydropalmatine	Hepatitis, lethargy, coma
Kava-kava (*Piper methysticum*)	Kavain, methysticin	Hepatic failure, "kavaism" neurotoxicity
Kelp	Iodine	Thyroid dysfunction
Laetrile	Cyanide	Coma, seizures, death
Licorice (*Glycyrrhiza glabra*)	Glycyrrhetic acid	Hypertension, arrhythmia, hypokalemia
Ma huang (*Ephedra sinica*)	Ephedrine	Arrhythmia, seizure, stroke, hypertension
Monkshood (*Aconitum napellus, A. columbianum*)	Aconite	Arrhythmia, weakness, coma, shock, paresthesia, vomiting, seizure
Nutmeg (*Myristica fragrans*)	Myristicin, eugenol	Hallucination, emesis, headache
Nux vomica	Strychnine	Seizure, abdominal pain, respiratory arrest
Pennyroyal (*Mentha pulegium* or *Hedeoma* spp.)	Pulegone	Centrilobular liver necrosis, fetotoxicity, seizure, shock
Ragwort (golden) (*Senecio aureus, Echium*)	Pyrrolizidines	HVOD
Wormwood (*Artemisia* spp.)	Thujone	Seizure, dementia, tremor, headache

HVOD, hepatic veno-occlusive disease.
Modified from Committee on Injuries & Poison Prevention. Children's Environmental Health. 3rd ed. Elk Grove Village, IL: American Academy of Pediatrics; 2009.

Tachycardia is frequently associated with ingestion of any of the sympathetic nervous system stimulants listed in Table 127.5. Tachycardia is also associated with ingestion of exogenous thyroid preparations, the early phase of poisoning with tricyclic antidepressants, theophylline overdoses, and caffeine or nicotine intoxications. Bradycardia may accompany exaggerated vagal responses to some compounds or direct negative chronotropic effects on the heart. Interference with the cardiac conduction system may cause a slowed pulse. Cardiac drugs associated with bradyarrhythmias include the calcium channel antagonists, digitalis, and β-adrenergic antagonists. Antiarrhythmic agents such as quinidine and procainamide can slow the pulse. Aconite, an herbal remedy, binds to site 2 of the open state of voltage-sensitive sodium channels, which then become refractory to excitation and cause arrhythmias.[8] Many drugs and chemicals depress a patient's consciousness either directly or by hypoxia resulting from decreased respiratory drive or simple asphyxia. Table 127.6 provides a suitable scoring system for determining the level of consciousness in the intoxicated patient. The dynamic nature of a poisoning mandates serial assessments of consciousness using this objective scoring system to gauge accurately whether the patient's overall condition is deteriorating or improving. In many serious intoxications, such as carbon monoxide or cyanide poisoning, the state of consciousness may be the single best guide to the patient's overall prognosis. Box 127.1 lists some of the agents that may cause coma in the pediatric patient. Box 127.2 lists some common causes of seizures.

Pupil size depends on the balance between dilating and constricting fibers and is under complex autonomic nervous

TABLE 127.4	Toxins Associated With Cardiovascular Findings
Sign	**Agents**
Tachycardia	Amphetamines Antihistamines Anticholinergics, atropine, *belladonna* Aconite Caffeine Cocaine Cardiac glycosides β-Adrenergic agonists (albuterol, terbutaline) Nicotine Sympathomimetic agents Theophylline
Bradycardia	Aconite Antiarrhythmics β-Adrenergic blockers Calcium channel blockers Cardiac glycosides Clonidine Ergotamine Opiates Organophosphate pesticides Phenylpropanolamine Quinidine Sedative-hypnotics
Torsades des pointes	Amantadine Antiarrhythmics Amiodarone Arsenic Astemizole Chloral hydrate Chloroquine Cisapride Cyclic antidepressants Disopyramide Encainide Fluoride Lidocaine Mexiletine Organophosphates Terfenadine Quinidine Procainamide Pentamidine Phenothiazines Prenylamine Suxamethonium
Ventricular tachycardia	Aconite Amphetamines Antiarrhythmics (eg, quinidine, flecainide) Carbamazepine Chloral hydrate Chlorinated hydrocarbons Cocaine Cyclic antidepressants Digitalis Theophylline Thioridazine

TABLE 127.5	Reed Scale for Clinical Assessment of Consciousness
Grade	**Description**
0	Asleep, can be aroused, answers questions
1	Comatose, withdraws from painful stimuli, intact reflexes
2	Comatose, does not withdraw from painful stimuli, no respiratory or circulatory depression, intact reflexes
3	Comatose, reflexes absent, no respiratory or circulatory depression
4	Comatose, reflexes absent, respiratory or circulatory problems

From Ellenhorn MJ, Barceloux DG. Medical Toxicology. New York, NY: Elsevier; 1988.

TABLE 127.6	Toxins Associated With Characteristic Breath Odors
Toxin	**Characteristic Odor**
Acetone	Ketones
Arsenic	Garlic
Camphor	Mothballs
Chloroform	Sweet
Cyanide	Bitter almond
Ethanol	Fruity, alcohol
Hydrogen sulfide	Rotten eggs
Isopropanol	Ketones
Methyl salicylate	Wintergreen
Nicotine	Stale tobacco
Organophosphates	Garlic
N-3-pyridylmethyl-*N*′-*p*-nitrophenyl urea	Peanuts (rat poison)
Paraldehyde, chloral hydrate	Pears (urine)
Phenol, cresol	Phenolic
Phosphorus, organophosphate pesticides	Garlic
Salicylates	Acetone
Selenium	Garlic
Thallium	Garlic
Turpentine	Violets

system control. Both sympathetic and parasympathetic nerves regulate the iris and can be affected by a variety of toxins. Anticholinergic drugs such as tricyclic antidepressants, antihistamines, and belladonna paralyze the parasympathetic fibers leading to pupillary dilation. Conversely, agents that inactivate cholinesterase leading to accumulations of acetylcholine (eg, organophosphate pesticides, physostigmine) constrict the pupil. Ethanol, phenothiazines, and barbiturates also constrict the pupils. Opiates act centrally to cause extreme pupillary constriction (miosis). Sympathomimetics, such as amphetamines and cocaine, cause extreme pupillary dilation (mydriasis). Pilocarpine directly stimulates the sphincter muscle of the iris, causing constriction. Toxins can also be responsible for unequal pupil size. Instillation of atropine to the eye causes ipsilateral pupillary dilation. Polydrug overdoses may include agents with opposite pupillary actions, so overreliance on pupillary size alone in deciding which poison is responsible for the patient's condition may lead to a misdiagnosis. Closed head trauma or central nervous system (CNS)

BOX 127.1   Agents Associated With Coma in the Pediatric Patient

Alcohols and glycols: ethanol, ethylene glycol, methanol
Anticonvulsants
Aromatic hydrocarbons
Asphyxiant gases
Barbiturates
Benzodiazepines
Carbon monoxide
Clonidine
Conium maculatum (water hemlock)
Cyanide
Cyclic antidepressants
γ-Butyrolactone, γ-hydroxybutyrate
Hydrogen sulfide gas
Hypoglycemic agents
Insulin
Ketamine
Lead (encephalopathy)
Lithium
Nonbarbiturate sedative-hypnotics
Opiates
Organochlorine pesticides
Phenothiazines
Propranolol
Salicylates
Tetrodotoxin

BOX 127.2   Agents Associated With Seizures at Presentation

Amphetamines
Bupropion
Camphor
Carbon monoxide
Cicuta maculatum (water hemlock)
Cocaine
Cyanide
Ephedrine
Gyromitra (mushroom species)
Insulin
Isoniazid
Methylene dioxymethamphetamine (MDMA)
Monoamine oxidase inhibitors
Nicotine
Organophosphate, organochlorine pesticides
Phencyclidine
Phenylpropanolamine
Phenothiazines
Propoxyphene
Salicylates
Scorpion
Strychnine
Tetanus
Theophylline
Tricyclic antidepressants

---

hemorrhage, sometimes seen in the context of a poisoning with hypertension-inducing drugs such as phenylpropanol-amine or ephedrine[9] can themselves cause pupillary effects.

When treating a disoriented, delirious pediatric patient, the clinician must consider which intoxications may be responsible. Because of their central anticholinergic effects and common availability, antihistamines (eg, chlorpheniramine, diphenhydramine) must be considered. Alcohol-containing household products or liquor may be responsible. In the adolescent, substances of abuse may cause delirium or hallucinations. Jimsonweed *(Datura stramonium)* plant seeds, containing atropine and other anticholinergic chemicals, can be intentionally chewed by adolescents for their euphoric (and delirium-producing) effects caused by a central anticholinergic syndrome. Hallucinogens include lysergic acid diethylamide (LSD), psilocybin, mescaline, "magic mushrooms," and some amphetamine congeners ("designer drugs," eg, 3-methoxy 4,5-methylenedioxyamphetamine [MMDA], 3,4-methylenedioxy-*N*-methamphetamine [MDMA, "ecstasy"], or 3,4-methylenedioxy-*N*-ethylamphetamine [MDEA]). Both cocaine and amphetamines can cause an acute psychosis. Smokable forms of methamphetamine (known as "crystal" or "ice") and phencyclidine (PCP) cause symptoms of agitation, aggression, and combativeness. Additionally, intensivists should be alert for abstinence syndromes in adolescents suffering from chronic substance abuse. Drug withdrawal from opiates, benzodiazepines, or alcohol (delirium tremens) often causes agitation, irritability, or even delusional thinking in affected patients. Withdrawal from chronic γ-hydroxybutyrate use (GHB, a popular "designer drug") is characterized by anxiety, insomnia, tremor, confusion, delirium, hallucinations, cardiovascular changes, nausea, vomiting, and diaphoresis.[10] Other neurologic findings may be found depending on the drug or toxin. Phenytoin and phencyclidine frequently cause nystagmus. Opsoclonus (saccadic eye movements) can be caused by lithium. Tinnitus is associated with ingestions of ergot, quinine, salicylates, or streptomycin. Changes in color vision may be seen in chronic digitalis overdose or cinchonism (quinidine).

Many poisonings cause cutaneous manifestations. Abusers of IV narcotics or other drugs may have needle tracks, characteristic tattoos, or scarring from "skin popping." Those suffering from inhalant abuse frequently have rashes around the nose and mouth as a result of defatting and irritative effects of inhaled solvents. Methemoglobinemia can cause an acute cyanotic appearance despite relatively normal blood gas values. A variety of rashes can be seen with adverse drug reactions and allergic responses to drugs, plants, or chemicals. Typical chemical burns may result from dermal exposure to caustics. Alopecia is associated with exposures to antimetabolite medications, other antineoplastic agents, or overdoses of chemicals such as arsenic, thallium, and selenium. Jaundice may result from exposure to hepatotoxins such as carbon tetrachloride, aniline dyes, quinacrine, or phenothiazines.

The physician must be alert to characteristic odors in containers found at the scene of the exposure, of substances spilled on the patient's skin or clothing, or on the patient's breath. Organophosphate insecticides and thallium impart the strong odor of garlic. Cyanide exposures have the characteristic aroma of bitter almond (although 50% of the population is of the genotype that cannot detect the odor). Ethanol, kerosene, camphor, and gasoline impart their strong odors to the breath. Adolescents abusing glues or volatile organic compounds by inhalation may have a solvent smell on their breath and clothes. Table 127.7 lists some of the typical intoxications that can be diagnosed by the patient's breath odors.

Laboratory Tests and Toxin Screens

Although laboratory testing of the blood or urine occasionally reveals an unanticipated toxin involved in an overdose, more frequently it confirms the physician's clinical diagnosis on the basis of a careful history and physical examination. The

TABLE 127.7	Osmolar Gap Conversions to Calculate Blood Concentration	

Toxin	Conversion Factor
Methanol	2.6
Ethanol	4.0
Ethylene glycol	5.0
Acetone	5.5
Isopropanol	5.9

Serum concentration (mg/dL) of given toxin divided by corresponding conversion factor equals serum osmolality (mOsm/kg H₂O) attributable to that toxin.

pediatric intensivist is well advised to know which compounds are included in the toxicology screen performed by the institution because the menu of substances detectable by a commercial laboratory is variable and frequently based on cost, ease of detection, available technical equipment, relative frequency of the overdose in the community, and other considerations. Most hospitals include the following compounds on a toxicology screen: acetaminophen, ethanol, barbiturates, opiates, anticonvulsants, some benzodiazepines, phenothiazines, and salicylates. Toxicology screens may or may not include certain drugs of abuse (eg, amphetamines, cocaine, tetrahydrocannabinol); older tricyclic antidepressants (eg, amitriptyline, imipramine); and methanol. Many common toxic agents, including carbon monoxide, cyanide, methemoglobin, iron, lithium, heavy metals such as lead or arsenic, and ethylene glycol, are never included in a toxicology screen and must be ordered specifically. For these reasons, a "negative" toxicology screen does not rule out the diagnosis of a poisoning. The more specific a clinician is in communicating with laboratory personnel about which toxins are suspected clinically, the more directed laboratory personnel can be in seeking specific answers through laboratory methods. Because some toxins (eg, cocaine, other drugs of abuse, some heavy metals) are detected more easily in urine than in the blood, both specimens should be submitted when the toxicology screen is ordered. Reliability in the screening for drugs or toxins requires not only a sound analytic technique but also adequate sample collection, chain of custody, and timely reporting of the results. Sources of error include delay in the time between sample collection and assay; problems with sample collection (wrong patient, wrong tube, loss of fluid, poor labeling); natural chemical reactions (volatilization, enzymatic degradation); purposeful sample alteration; technical limits on the detection threshold of the assay used; and misinterpretation of the units in reporting the results. Blood concentrations of acetaminophen, aspirin, barbiturates, carbamazepine, carbon monoxide, digoxin, ethanol, ethylene glycol, iron, isopropanol, lead, lithium, methanol, phenobarbital, phenytoin, theophylline, and valproic acid are useful in assessing the severity of the intoxication and guiding patient management. Co-oximetry can provide blood levels of abnormal hemoglobins caused by toxins, such as carboxyhemoglobin, sulfhemoglobin, and methemoglobinemia. Note that pulse oximetry gives inaccurate readings in patients with methemoglobinemia because methemoglobin absorbs more light at both 660 and 940 nm than does oxyhemoglobin, so the readings

of oxygen saturation may seem normal in the presence of severe methemoglobinemia. Indeed, the blood drawn from a patient with significant methemoglobinemia will appear "chocolate" brown in color. Box 127.3 lists drugs, chemicals, and foods capable of causing methemoglobinemia in susceptible individuals.

Certain toxins (eg, ethanol, ethylene glycol, isopropanol, methanol) introduce osmotically active particles into the serum. These particles increase serum osmolality, which can be measured by either vapor pressure or freezing point depression. However, vapor pressure techniques give falsely low values in the presence of volatiles (such as any of the alcohols) and should not be used in the monitoring of poisoning cases. The calculated serum osmolality is derived by the following equation: Calculated serum osmolality = $[2 \times Na \ (in \ mEq/L)]$ + [Blood urea nitrogen (in mg/dL)/2.8] + [Glucose (in mg/dL)/18].[11] Calculated osmolality can then be subtracted from the measured osmolality to assess the osmolar gap. A normal osmolar gap is between −3 and 10 mOsm/kg H₂O. Blood alcohol concentration can be estimated using the serum osmolality as measured by the freezing point depression technique, then calculating the osmolar gap, and applying the conversion factors listed in Table 127.8. Intensivists are cautioned that elevated osmolar gaps are also seen in patients with lipemic blood or in those receiving therapies such as mannitol, intralipid, glycerol, sorbitol, propylene glycol, or some radiocontrast agents. Conversely, a falsely low osmolar gap can be seen in ethylene glycol or methanol poisoning if the vapor pressure method of serum osmolality determination is erroneously used instead of freezing point depression.

The principle of electroneutrality requires that positive and negative charged molecules in the serum must balance. Toxins that cause metabolic acidosis frequently increase the gap between the total measured versus theoretical anions by the direct addition of organic acid anions, the indirect generation of such anions, or (rarely) the reduction of cations in the serum. The anion gap calculation is derived as follows: Anion gap = $Na^+ - (Cl- + HCO_3-)$, where all components are expressed in milliequivalents per liter. The "normal" anionic gap ranges from 3 to 16 mEq/L in older children and adults. Hypoalbuminemia or diluted blood both cause misleadingly low anion gaps, as can poisoning with cations such as lithium or bromide. The presence of elevated concentrations of unmeasured anions (eg, as a result of dehydration or treatment with sodium salts of citrate, lactate, or acetate) or conditions associated with a decrease in unmeasured cations (eg, as a result of hypomagnesemia, hypocalcemia, hypokalemia) can lead to an elevated anion gap. Poisoning with drugs such as isoniazid, iron, paraldehyde, phenformin, or salicylate or chemicals such as ethylene glycol or methanol can lead to a metabolic acidosis with an elevated anion gap.

Many agents that cause seizures (eg, isoniazid, organochlorine pesticides, theophylline, tricyclic antidepressants) or agitation, excessive muscular activity, and hyperthermia (eg, cocaine, amphetamines, phencyclidine, neuroleptic malignant syndrome, serotonin syndrome) may predispose the patient to rhabdomyolysis and subsequent myoglobin-induced acute renal failure. The overdose patient who is agitated or delirious and is held in physical restraints for long periods of time and the overdose comatose patient who has muscle necrosis from dependency position injury are at high risk for rhabdomyolysis. In such circumstances, monitoring serum lactic acid,

BOX 127.3 — Drugs, Chemicals, and Foods Causing Methemoglobinemia

Drugs

Acetanilid	Chlorates
Amyl nitrite	Chlorobenzene
Benzocaine	Cobalt preparations
Cetacaine	Dimethylaniline
Chloroquine	Dinitrobenzene
Chloroquine	Dinitrophenol
Clofazimine	Dinitrotoluene
Dapsone (sulfones)	Hydroquinone
Diaminodiphenylsulfone	Inks/shoe polish
Hydroxylamine	Isobutyl nitrite
Lidocaine	Menthol
Menadione	Naphthalene
Methylene blue	Naphthylamines
Metoclopramide	Nitrates/nitrites
Nitroglycerin	Nitric oxide
Nitrosobenzene	Nitroalkanes
Para-aminobenzoic acid	Nitrobenzene
Para-aminopropiophenone	Nitrofuran
Para-hydroxylaminopropiophenone	Nitrogen oxide
Phenacetin	Nitrogen trifluoride
Phenazopyridine hydrochloride	Nitroglycerin
(Pyridium)	Nitrophenol
Phenylhydroxylamine	Nitrous gases/nitric oxide
Phenytoin	Ozone
Potassium permanganate	Para-bromoaniline
Prilocaine	Paraquat (or Monolinuron)
Primaquine	Para-toluidine
Procaine	Phenazopyridine
Resorcinol	Phenetidin
Silver nitrate	Phenols
Sodium nitrate	Phenylhydrazine
Sodium nitrite	Phenylhydroxylamine
Sodium nitroprusside	Pyridine
Sulfamethoxazole	Smoke (products of
Sulfanilamide	combustion)
Sulfapyridine	Sulfones
Sulfathiazide	Toluidine
	Trinitrotoluene
	Xylidine

Chemicals

AcetanilidAlloxan	**Foods**
Ammonium nitrate	Beets, cabbage, spinach
Aniline dyes	Nitrite/nitrate preservatives,
Antipyrine	Nitrogen-rich foods,
Arsine	Well water (elevated
Benzene derivatives	nitrates)
Butyl nitrite	

BOX 127.4 — Drugs and Chemicals That May Be Radiopaque

Bezoars, bags (filled with illegal drugs)
Calcium carbonate
Chloral hydrate
Enteric-coated tablets
Foreign bodies (sometimes radiopaque)
Heavy metals (eg, iron, lead, mercury, thallium)
Iodine
Lithium carbonate
Paradichlorobenzene mothballs
Phenothiazines
Potassium compounds

127.4 lists some drugs and chemicals that may be visualized in imaging studies.

Diagnostic Trials

For a few suspected toxins, administration of an antidote not only initiates therapy but also assists in the diagnosis of the agent involved. Table 127.8 lists some of the diagnostic trials that may be appropriate in the pediatric ICU setting. For example, flumazenil, a specific benzodiazepine antagonist, can be used as a diagnostic agent administered to the comatose patient. At an IV dose of 1 to 2 mg, adults show a rapid improvement in consciousness (analogous to naloxone's effectiveness in reversing narcotic-induced CNS depression) after overdose involving a variety of benzodiazepines. Caution must be exercised; if a second, seizure-causing agent such as a tricyclic antidepressant has also been coingested, then the reversal of the benzodiazepine's anticonvulsant effects may inadvertently unmask seizures in the victim. Physostigmine can be of benefit in pediatric patients who have ingested Jimsonweed seeds (D. stramonium) or other pure anticholinergic agents; however, caution is dictated in unknown poisonings where cardiac conduction toxicity is a consideration because physostigmine itself can cause severe cardiac toxicity, bradycardia, and asystole.[13]

Summary

Intensive care physicians face some of their greatest diagnostic challenges when confronted with patients who are admitted to the hospital with a baffling constellation of symptoms and signs and whose differential diagnosis includes poisoning. The history alone will often clarify the clinical picture, suggesting potential drugs or toxins that might be responsible for the patient's illness. Physical findings attendant to a comprehensive examination of the patient, with a focus on vital signs and the skin, gastrointestinal, cardiovascular, pulmonary, and neurologic systems, may confirm the clinician's suspicions. Knowledge of common toxidromes can help the intensive care physician recognize which poison or pharmacologic category of toxic agents may be responsible. The nearest regional poison center has 24-hour availability of medical toxicology expertise. For a few suspected toxins, diagnostic studies can be helpful in the assessment of the severity of toxicity and in the prediction of a patient's expected hospital course. Quantitative blood or urine levels of some drugs or chemicals can be invaluable in both the patient's assessment and monitoring. The investigation of anion or osmolar gaps, derangements in

creatine phosphokinase, aldolase, myoglobin, urinary sediment, urine output, and urinary myoglobin levels may be useful.

Additional Investigations

Radiographic Studies

Radiographs can be helpful in locating swallowed foreign bodies having toxic potential. Patients who have ingested disk batteries should undergo serial chest and abdominal radiography to ensure that the battery has cleared the esophagus and is continuing to move along the gastrointestinal tract. Drug smugglers who have swallowed quantities of heroin or cocaine-filled balloons, condoms, or other containers can be diagnosed as a "body packer" by radiographic examination.[12] Chest and abdominal x-ray films may be of value in locating pills, tablets, or lead-containing paint chips. Sometimes agglutinated masses of pills (bezoars) can be detected in this manner. Box

TABLE 127.8   Useful Diagnostic Trials

Agent Detected	Agent Administered	Technique	Positive Results
Anticholinergic agents (pure)	Physostigmine	0.01-0.02 mg/kg over 15 seconds (rate no greater than 0.5 mg/minute); may repeat at 5-10 minute intervals thereafter × 4 (max 0.05 mg/kg or 2 mg total)	Improved conscious
Benzodiazepines	Flumazenil	0.01-0.02 mg/kg (maximum dose 0.2 mg) IV over 15 seconds, may repeat every minute thereafter × 4 up to maximum cumulative dose 0.05 mg/kg or 1 mg [whichever is less]	Improved conscious
Iron	Deferoxamine	15 mg/kg/hr IV drip (max 125 mg/hr)	"Vin rose" urine color
Opiates	Naloxone hydrochloride	0.1 mg/kg IV/IM/SC/IO for birth to 5 years of age (<20 kg body weight) or 2 mg per dose IV/IM/SC/IO for weight >20 kg	Improved conscious
Organophosphate	Atropine	0.05-0.10 mg/kg IV/IM/IO (4 mg maximum dose); repeat every 5-10 minutes for moderate-severe OP poisoning	Mydriasis, fewer secretions
Phenothiazine (dystonia)	Diphenhydramine	1-2 mg/kg slow IV over 5 minutes (maximum rate: 25 mg/minute); may repeat × 4 doses per day (maximum cumulative dose: 300 mg/day)	Resolution
Phenothiazine (NMS)	Dantrolene	1 mg/kg IV (maximum cumulative dose 10 mg/kg)	Resolution
Insulin reaction	Dextrose	10% dextrose in water; 2.5 mL/kg IV bolus	Improved conscious
Isoniazid	Pyridoxine	5 grams (if isoniazid overdose quantity unknown), or gram per gram of isoniazid overdose	Seizures abate; improved conscious
Sulfonylurea	Octreotide	1-1.5 mcg/kg IV or SC followed by 2-3 doses every 6 hours as needed	Resolution of hypoglycemia

NMS, neuroleptic malignant syndrome.

blood gases or electrolytes, electrocardiographic abnormalities, and imaging studies will often be indicated in critically ill patients. Administration of an antidote in selected cases may not only initiate therapy but also assist in the diagnosis because improvement in a patient's status soon after receipt of the antidote may confirm the poison involved. Close monitoring of the patient over time is essential to optimal management of the poisoning.

Additional Readings

Boyer EW, Shannon M. The serotonin syndrome. *N Engl J Med*. 2005;352:1112-1120.

Frithsen IL, Simpson WM. Recognition and management of acute medication poisoning. *Am Fam Physician*. 2010;81:316-323.

Henry K, Harris CR. Deadly ingestions. *Pediatr Clin North Am*. 2006;53:293-315.

Hon KL, Ho JK, Hung EC, et al. Poisoning necessitating pediatric ICU admissions: size of pupils does matter. *J Natl Med Assoc*. 2008;100:952-956.

Institute of Medicine (IOM). *Committee on Poison Control & Prevention. Forging a Poison Prevention and Control System*. Washington, DC: National Academies Press; 2004.

Michael J. Sztajnkrycer M. Deadly pediatric poisons: nine common agents that kill at low doses. *Emerg Med Clin North Am*. 2004;22:1019-1050.

McGregor T, Parkar M, Rao S. Evaluation and management of common childhood poisonings. *Am Fam Physician*. 2009;79:397-403.

Naggar AER, Abdalla MS, El-Sebaey AS, et al. Clinical findings and cholinesterase levels in children of organophosphate and carbamates poisoning. *Eur J Pediatr*. 2009;168:951-956.

Woolf AD. Herbal remedies and children. *Pediatrics*. 2003;112:240-246.

Woolf AD, Bellinger D, Goldman R. Clinical approach to childhood lead poisoning. *Pediatr Clin North Am*. 2007;54:271-294.

Wu AHB, McKay C, Broussard LA, et al. National Academy of Clinical Biochemistry laboratory medicine practice guidelines: recommendations for use of laboratory tests to support the poisoned patient who presents to the emergency department. *Clin Chem*. 2003;49:357-379.

References

1. Mowry JB, Spyker DA, Cantilena LR, et al. 2013 annual report of the American Association of Poison Control Centers' National Poison Data System (NPDS): 31st annual report. *Clin Toxicol*. 2014;52:1032-1283.
2. Dinis-Oliveira RJ, Duarte JA, Sanchez-Navarro A, et al. Paraquat poisonings: mechanisms of lung toxicity, clinical features, and treatment. *Clin Rev Toxicol*. 2008;38:13-71.
3. Giannini L, Vannacci A, Missanelli A, et al. Amatoxin poisoning: a 15-year retrospective analysis and follow-up evaluation of 105 patients. *Clin Toxicol*. 2007;45:539-542.
4. Glatstein M, Scolnik D, Bentur Y. Octreotide for the treatment of sulfonylurea poisoning. *Clin Toxicology*. 2012;50:795-804.
5. Ingels M, Beauchamp J, Clark RF, et al. Delayed valproic acid toxicity: a retrospective case series. *Ann Emerg Med*. 2002;39:616-621.
6. Palmer ME, Haller C, McKinney PE, et al. Adverse events associated with dietary supplements: an observational study. *Lancet*. 1993;361:101-106.
7. Daubin C, Lehoux P, Ivascau C, et al. Extracorporeal life support in severe drug intoxication: a retrospective cohort study of seventeen cases. *Crit Care*. 2009;13:R138.
8. Chan TYK. Aconite poisoning. *Clin Toxicol*. 2009;47:279-285.
9. Haller CA, Benowitz NL. Adverse cardiovascular and central nervous system events associated with dietary supplements containing ephedra alkaloids. *N Engl J Med*. 2000;343:1833-1838.
10. Dyer JE, Roth B, Hyma BA. Gamma-hydroxybutyrate withdrawal syndrome. *Ann Emerg Med*. 2001;37:147-153.
11. Garrard A, Sollee DR, Butterfield RC, et al. Validation of a pre-existing formula to calculate the contribution of ethanol to the osmolar gap. *Clin Toxicol*. 2012;50:562-566.
12. Yegane RA, Bashashati M, Hajinasrollah E, et al. Surgical approach to body packing. *Dis Colon Rectum*. 2009;52:97-103.
13. Frascogna N. Physostigmine: is there a role for this antidote in pediatric poisonings? *Curr Opin Pediatr*. 2007;19:201-205.

Toxidromes and Their Treatment

Ashley N. Webb and Prashant Joshi

PEARLS

- Flumazenil, when used for benzodiazepine overdose, may unmask seizures caused by a coingested substance or precipitate acute withdrawal in the patient who habitually uses benzodiazepines.
- β-Adrenergic antagonists, when used to lower blood pressure in a sympathomimetic overdose, may lead to unopposed α-receptor stimulation and should be avoided.
- Reserve physostigmine administration for severe, life-threatening manifestations of anticholinergic toxicity because it may lead to asystole or seizures. It is contraindicated for reversal of anticholinergic symptoms produced by tricyclic antidepressant ingestion.
- Pulse oximetry is unreliable for determining oxygen saturation with methemoglobinemia and may show falsely elevated or decreased values.
- Use the skin to distinguish between sympathomimetic (pale, cool, and diaphoretic) and anticholinergic (flushed, warm, and dry) toxidromes.
- Malignant hyperthermia, serotonin syndrome, neuroleptic malignant syndrome, sympathomimetic poisoning, and anticholinergic poisoning constitute the major differential diagnosis for xenobiotic-induced hyperthermia.
- An elevated osmolar gap may suggest ingestion of a toxic alcohol, but a normal result does not exclude it. Serum toxic alcohol levels are the gold standard for diagnosis and prognosis.
- Succinylcholine is relatively contraindicated in cholinesterase inhibitor toxicity because its duration of effect will be significantly prolonged.
- Total iron-binding capacity may be falsely elevated in patients with acute iron overdose and is not a reliable marker in iron toxicity.
- In the United States, the local Regional Poison Control Center may be reached by calling 800-222-1222.

The 31st annual report of the American Association of Poison Control Centers described more than 2 million human exposures to toxic substances that were reported to poison control centers in the United States in 2013.[1] Approximately 55% involved children younger than 12 years, but this age group accounted for only about 3% of the reported fatalities. Although 70% of these exposures were managed without further medical assistance, of the 30% of patients who were referred and seen in a health care facility, one in six was admitted to a critical care unit. Calls from health care facilities to poison control centers are increasing and account for a growing proportion of cases handled by poison control center specialists.

In most cases of childhood poisoning, the agents involved are known or circumstantial evidence points to a specific toxin or toxins. When the toxin is unknown or the clinical presentation is inconsistent with the available exposure history, physical and analytic clues will help guide therapy. *Toxidrome* is a contraction of *toxic syndrome,* a constellation of signs associated with certain substances or groups of substances. Recognition of a toxidrome provides for targeted investigation and treatment. Toxidrome expression may not be complete in every case, or more than one toxidrome may be present. During the initial patient examination, clinicians pay particular attention to vital signs, mental status, pupil size and reactivity, skin characteristics (color, temperature, moisture), and bowel sounds. Other important aspects to consider include muscle tone, respiratory effort, and mucous membrane characteristics.

As discussed in Chapters 127, laboratory investigations may narrow the differential diagnosis and determine the need for additional examination or guide therapy. However, clinicians must review these diagnostic tests with caution. Many assays lack sensitivity and specificity to confirm specific substances, so an inaccurate diagnosis or inappropriate therapy, including withholding a specific antidote, is a consequence of relying on these assays alone.[2] In conjunction with clinical findings and exposure history, assays are chosen based on their probability of indicating or guiding therapy and prognosticating end-organ toxicity.

This chapter describes commonly accepted toxidromes as well as less common yet relevant toxic presentations and their treatments. More in-depth information can be found in a comprehensive textbook of medical toxicology.

Opioids

Both natural and synthetic opioids produce the classic triad of respiratory depression, coma, and miosis. Additional features include bradycardia, hypotension, and decreased gastrointestinal (GI) motility.[3] Not all patients exposed to an opioid present with the classic toxidrome; for example mydriatic or midpoint pupils are seen with specific opioids, although brain anoxia or coingestants should also be considered (Box 128.1).[3-5]

Simple hypercarbia may be detected before severe overt respiratory depression.[6-9] Because decreased respiratory drive is a result of μ-receptor agonism but analgesic effect results from action at both μ- and κ-receptors, some opioids are designed to function as agonist-antagonists to provide spinal

BOX 128.1 Opioids That Cause Midpoint or Mydriatic Pupils

Meperidine
Pentazocine
Diphenoxylate/Atropine
Propoxyphene

analgesia and simultaneously antagonize μ-receptors.[6,7] Other opioids, like buprenorphine, are designed to function as only partial agonists at μ-receptors, providing pain relief at higher doses with a ceiling effect on respiratory depression.[10] In overdose, lost receptor selectivity may still result in decreased respiratory drive with this type opioid medication. In overdose and in opioid-naïve pediatric patients, buprenorphine often causes overt respiratory depression, so close monitoring of respiratory status is warranted.[10-12]

Several potent opioids are extremely toxic in small doses in both the opioid-naïve and pediatric populations. Methadone liquids are concentrated, and even as little as one tablet has led to fatality.[13,14] Fentanyl, in dosage forms that allow for buccal absorption, may be attractive to children. Used fentanyl patches still contain high doses of drug and are extremely dangerous when placed on skin, in the mouth, or ingested.

Central α-2 adrenergic agonists including clonidine, guanfacine, tizanidine, and other imidazoline derivatives (found in over-the-counter eye drops or nasal sprays) can precipitate an opioid-like toxidrome.[15-18] In addition to bradycardia and hypotension, exposure to these agents in small doses may lead to CNS and respiratory depression and miosis.

Naloxone is a μ-receptor antagonist that reverses the toxic effects of opioids. To prevent the need for artificial ventilation in life-threatening opioid-induced respiratory depression, start with a dose of 0.1 mg/kg. If no intravenous access is available, administration can proceed subcutaneously, intramuscularly, or via endotracheal tube (although the intramuscular route exhibits variable pharmacokinetics with a less predictable duration of action).[19] Naloxone may precipitate acute withdrawal in opioid-dependent individuals warranting a lower starting dose, titrated upward to effect and not exceeding 10 mg cumulatively.[20] Because the duration of action of naloxone is shorter than that of some opioids, repeated doses or a continuous intravenous infusion may be necessary; the suggested infusion rate is two-thirds the initial reversal dose per hour, titrated to effect, with half the initial reversal dose given as a bolus. Respiratory and mental status are monitored for 24 hours following cessation of a prolonged naloxone infusion.[21] Although naloxone has precipitated transient hypertension or pulmonary edema in rare cases, these risks do not preclude its use.[22-24] Reports that naloxone has reversed clonidine overdose are anecdotal, and naloxone failure has also been described in this setting, so the benefit of naloxone in the face of central α-2 adrenergic agonists is unclear.[25]

Sedative Hypnotics

The class *sedative hypnotics* comprises medications that reduce CNS excitation, prescribed for their hypnotic and anxiolytic effects. Usually, sedative hypnotics enhance γ-amino butyric acid (GABA) activity and its effect on chloride channels in the brain and spinal cord. Barbiturates act as agonists at GABA$_A$ receptors prolonging the flow of chloride through the channel resulting in hyperpolarization. Benzodiazepines, on the other hand, work at the benzodiazepine location on the GABA$_A$ receptor to enhance GABA binding and increase the frequency of chloride channel opening—they will not work in the absence of GABA.[26,27] Newer nonbenzodiazepine sedative hypnotics (zolpidem, zopiclone, and eszopiclone) also bind to the benzodiazepine location on GABA$_A$, but because of their affinity for different isoforms of the receptor, they act quickly to induce hypnosis with little effect on anxiolysis.[28] Initial reports indicated that these so-called z-drugs were a safe alternative to benzodiazepines, but more recent data depict a similar toxicity profile.

Barbiturate overdose, characterized by CNS and respiratory depression, may be associated with hypotonia, hypotension, and hypothermia, as well as bullous skin lesions.[26] On the other hand, benzodiazepine and z-drug toxicity are often referred to as "coma with normal vitals," where patients exhibit CNS depression without overt respiratory depression or autonomic dysfunction.[26,28] In one published report, ataxia was the most common symptom, so benzodiazepine ingestion should be considered in the differential diagnosis of ataxia with no additional findings.[29] Unlike opioid toxicity, low benzodiazepine receptor density in the brain stem means benzodiazepines and z-drugs pose a low risk for centrally mediated apnea.[27] Although apnea has been reported with intravenous benzodiazepine administration, therapeutic and supratherapeutic oral doses cause airway resistance and increased work of breathing.[30] In benzodiazepine overdose, patients are often described with sonorous respirations and apnea is rare.

Significant respiratory depression with benzodiazepines usually only occurs from mixed-drug ingestions or in the presence of ethanol. Most pediatric exposures are unintentional single substance ingestions posing less risk. Reversal of benzodiazepines with the benzodiazepine receptor antagonist flumazenil is usually not warranted and is in fact contraindicated in a polysubstance overdose, especially when cyclic antidepressants are suspected.[31] Removing the antiepileptic effect of a benzodiazepine may unmask seizure activity and increase morbidity. Caution is also warranted in patients with an underlying seizure disorder in whom flumazenil may lower the seizure threshold and in patients habituated to benzodiazepines where reversal may precipitate life-threatening withdrawal.[32-34] Flumazenil may reverse CNS depression, but in dose effectiveness studies, it did not significantly affect respiratory insufficiency.[30]

Withdrawal from benzodiazepine and nonbenzodiazepine sedative hypnotics, similar to ethanol withdrawal, results from down-regulation of inhibitory GABA receptors and increased excitatory *N*-methyl-D-aspartate (NMDA) binding sites. This imbalance is characterized by CNS stimulation, flushing, hypertension, tachycardia, hyperthermia, and seizures. Treatment is based on symptom reduction via replacement of benzodiazepines at the established dose and tapering as tolerated.[35]

Sympathomimetic Agents

Signs and symptoms of sympathetic excess result from both therapeutic and illicit agents that either mimic endogenous excitatory neurotransmitters or act on receptors to increase their release.[36] Manifestations of the sympathomimetic toxidrome and some drugs that produce it are listed in

Box 128.2. Predominantly β-adrenergic agents cause peripheral vasodilation more likely resulting in tachycardia and hypotension than predominantly α-adrenergic agents (severe hypertension with reflex bradycardia).[37] Hyperthermia, rhabdomyolysis, and myoglobinuria may result from increased metabolic activity; ischemic or hemorrhagic stroke and myocardial infarction have been documented.[38] Following cocaine exposure, patients may present with chest pain from coronary vasospasm; however, myocardial infarction (MI) must be ruled out.

Methylxanthines, caffeine and theophylline, are not sympathomimetics per se but may produce many of the same clinical features from their β-adrenergic activity, adenosine antagonism, and phosphodiesterase inhibition.[37,39] Although most acute cases of caffeine toxicity would be limited by undesirable effects with increasing dose, the risk for potentially life-threatening caffeine exposures is higher than ever with accessible concentrated caffeine powders (as herbal supplements) and caffeine-laden energy drinks. Methylxanthine toxicity is characterized by protracted emesis, palpitations, chest pain, tachycardia, and tachydysrhythmias—most commonly supraventricular tachycardia.[40,41] A wide pulse pressure results from peripheral vasodilation, and hypokalemia occurs via an intracellular potassium shift. Neurologic symptoms range from headache to refractory seizures. Antiemetic therapy with 5-HT antagonists is recommended, but phenothiazines are contraindicated and may worsen toxicity. Norepinephrine and phenylephrine are vasopressors of choice. Severe hypotension might best be treated with a beta-antagonist. Because the offending agent is still present, electrocardioversion for supraventricular tachycardia (SVT) will be transient as will adenosine (adenosine antagonism). Judicious use of benzodiazepines is recommended to treat seizures, tachycardia, hypertension, and agitation. Consider a calcium channel or beta-receptor antagonist for arrhythmias.[42,43] Methylxanthines are dialyzable; in the case of theophylline, multiple-dose–activated charcoal is strongly recommended to remove the drug from the systemic system.[44,45]

Designer amphetamines, such as methylenedioxyamphetamine (MDMA) and its derivatives, release serotonin and may precipitate hallucinations as well as the sympathomimetic effects listed earlier. Affected patients are at risk for seizures, dysrhythmias, hyperthermia, rhabdomyolysis, the syndrome of inappropriate secretion of antidiuretic hormone resulting in hyponatremia, and disseminated intravascular coagulation.[37,42,46] Since the early 2000s, designer amphetamine exposures have been increasing. This group now includes cathinone derivatives, referred to as bath salts (in an attempt to mask their status as illicit substances), that can be consumed, smoked, or injected.[47] Synthetic cannabinoids, referred to as spice, may cause symptoms similar to tetrahydrocannabinol (THC), the active ingredient in marijuana, with mild exposure.[47,48] Like THC, synthetic cannabinoids bind cannabinoid receptors, but they do so at a higher affinity, and because synthetic cannabinoids are usually sprayed on plant material, additional unknown substances may be present. Many cases of synthetic cannabinoid exposure appear sympathomimetic in nature and should be treated as cases involving an amphetamine. Reports of significant morbidity and mortality describe severe psychomotor agitation, aggressive psychotic behavior, seizures, tachycardia, hypertension, dysrhythmias, hyperthermia, and myocardial infarction and exist for both bath salts and spice.[47,48]

To reduce CNS catecholamine release and eliminate severe hypertension, tachycardia, agitation, and muscle overactivity, benzodiazepines are considered first (potentially large doses). β-adrenergic antagonists may paradoxically worsen hypertension from resulting unopposed α-adrenergic receptor stimulation and should be avoided (except in the case of methylxanthines where appropriate use may relieve symptoms). A vasodilator can be used for hypertension refractory to benzodiazepines; however, it must be short acting, as cocaine and similar agents may deplete norepinephrine leading to cardiovascular collapse.[38,42,47-49] Benzodiazepines should be used as first-line agents to manage seizures. Phenytoin does not treat toxin-induced seizures and, in the case of methylxanthines, it may worsen patient outcome by lowering the seizure threshold.[42]

Anticholinergic Agents

The anticholinergic, or antimuscarinic, toxidrome is elicited by agents that possess antimuscarinic properties as their primary effect or as a side effect. Muscarinic receptors are found in the CNS, target organs of the parasympathetic nervous system (PNS), and sweat glands (sympathetic nervous system).[49] This syndrome may have features similar to the sympathomimetic toxidrome. Some anticholinergic agents and features of the anticholinergic toxidrome are listed in Box 128.3. The anticholinergic patient will exhibit dry skin

---

BOX 128.2   Sympathomimetic Toxidrome Features

Sympathomimetic Toxidrome	Causative Agents
Agitation	Albuterol
Seizures	Amphetamines
Mydriasis	Caffeine
Tachycardia	Catecholamines
Hypertension	Cocaine
Diaphoresis	Ephedrine
Pallor	Ketamine
Cool skin	Phencyclidine (PCP)
Fever	Phenylephrine
	Phenylpropanolamine
	Pseudoephedrine
	Terbutaline
	Theophylline

BOX 128.3   Anticholinergic Toxidrome Features

Anticholinergic Agents	Anticholinergic Toxidrome Features
Antihistamines (eg, diphenhydramine, hydroxyzine)	Agitation
Atropine	Delirium
Benztropine mesylate	Coma
Carbamazepine	Mydriasis
Cyclic antidepressants	Dry mouth
Cyclobenzaprine	Warm, dry, flushed skin
Hyoscyamine	Tachycardia
Jimsonweed	Hypertension
Oxybutynin	Fever
Phenothiazines	Urinary retention
Scopolamine	Decreased bowel sounds
Trihexyphenidyl	

rather than increased diaphoresis as seen with sympathomimetic toxicity. Catheter placement may be necessary to address significant urinary retention, and dilated pupils are usually nonreactive as a result of associated cycloplegia (also not seen with sympathomimetic toxicity).[49,50]

It is critical to monitor core temperature and actively cool hyperthermic patients because sweating is inhibited in the face of anticholinergic toxicity. Consider benzodiazepines first to treat agitation and prevent heat production from excessive muscle activity. Although physostigmine is a cholinesterase inhibitor that may reverse central and peripheral manifestations of anticholinergic toxicity, case reports describing convulsions or asystole preclude its use for the anticholinergic manifestations of tricyclic antidepressant overdose—it is contraindicated in this setting.[49,51,52] Consultation with a medical toxicologist is warranted to determine the right patient and right time for physostigmine, where clinical benefit outweighs the risk of morbidity and mortality.[53]

Cholinergic Agents

Cholinergic agents are best divided into the following three categories: muscarinic agents, nicotinic agents, and cholinesterase inhibitors. Muscarinic agents act in the CNS, at postganglionic parasympathetic nerve endings, and in the sweat glands. Nicotinic agents act in the CNS, in the autonomic ganglia (both sympathetic and parasympathetic), and at the neuromuscular junction. Cholinesterase inhibitors increase acetylcholine in the cholinergic synapse to present a combination of symptoms resulting from action at both nicotinic and muscarinic receptors.[54,55] Agents with cholinergic activity and signs and symptoms of cholinergic excess are listed in Boxes 128.4 and 128.5.

Nicotine produces salivation, nausea, and vomiting, but significant exposure results in hypotension, bradycardia, and respiratory depression, often preceded by tachycardia, hypertension, and tachypnea.[54-58] Central features include initial stimulation followed by seizures, lethargy, coma, and neuromuscular blockade. Management of nicotine poisoning is entirely supportive with consideration of atropine for bradycardia, close monitoring, and aggressive respiratory support.[56-59] Children are at increased risk of nicotine poisoning from ingestion of cigarettes or chewing tobacco, exposure to smoking cessation products (gums, lozenges, patches, and inhalers), and, more recently, exposure to concentrated liquid nicotine associated with electronic cigarettes.[60-62] Because liquid nicotine intended for vaporization and inhalation is in a highly concentrated form when used with e-cigarette cartridges or in vials for refillable e-cigarettes (10 mg/ml to greater than 24 mg/ml), very small exposures may cause toxicity, usually seen at doses greater than 30 mg. These concentrates are easily absorbed through the skin and GI tract, rendering most decontamination useless. Symptoms usually appear within 15 to 30 minutes, although patients without significant respiratory symptoms at 4 hours are unlikely to show symptoms beyond this time frame. There is no antidote for nicotine toxicity.[60,63,64]

Direct-acting muscarinic agents produce excessive parasympathetic activity resulting in salivation, lacrimation, urination, diuresis, GI upset (including diarrhea), and emesis (often referred to as SLUDGE). Cholinesterase inhibitors, organophosphorus pesticides, and nerve agents produce a mixed picture of toxicity by binding and inactivating acetylcholinesterase to prevent normal termination of cholinergic stimulation at postsynaptic receptors.[65] In the PNS and CNS, the result is excessive nicotinic and muscarinic activity and, at the neuromuscular junction, depolarizing neuromuscular blockade. Over time the acetylcholinesterase becomes phosphorylated and weak hydrogen bonds change to covalent bonds, a process referred to as *aging*. Not all organophosphorus agents age at the same rate. Some nerve agents age within a few minutes, whereas some pesticides take as long as 72 hours to permanently inactivate the cholinesterase—activity is then only restored by synthesis of new enzyme.[55,65] Conversely, carbamates reversibly bind acetylcholinesterase, and this enzyme/chemical complex undergoes spontaneous hydrolysis, generally restoring cholinesterase function within hours. Furthermore, carbamates do not penetrate the CNS well, so central manifestations are usually less severe.[55] Because both organophosphates and carbamates cause bronchorrhea, bronchospasm, decreased respiratory drive, and paralysis of the muscles involved in breathing, death results from respiratory failure.[66,67] With dermal exposure, initial local hyperhidrosis is followed by systemic effects once the agent is absorbed, but with inhalation, upper airway manifestations and respiratory distress occur rapidly. Following ingestion, drooling and vomiting are the early signs of toxicity.

Atropine is used to reverse the muscarinic effects of cholinergic toxicity, whereas an oxime is provided to reverse neuromuscular blockade, and benzodiazepines to treat seizures. Extremely large doses of atropine are provided to resolve

---

BOX 128.4	Xenobiotics Causing Cholinergic Excess	
Inhibitors of Acetylcholinesterase	**Direct Muscarinic Agonists**	**Nicotinic Agents**
Organophosphate insecticides (malathion, parathion, diazinon)	Bethanechol	Nicotine
	Carbachol	Water hemlock
	Methacholine	
Carbamate insecticides (aldicarb, carbaryl, propoxur)	Pilocarpine	
	Muscarinic mushrooms (eg, *Clitocybe* spp., *Inocybe* spp.)	
Nerve agents (soman, sarin, tabun, Vx, cyclosarin)		
Drugs used for myasthenia gravis or reversal of neuromuscular blockade (eg, physostigmine, pyridostigmine, neostigmine, edrophonium)		

BOX 128.5	Cholinergic Toxidrome Features		
Muscarinic Effects (DUMBBBELS)		**Nicotinic Effects**	**Central Effects**
D—Diarrhea		Fasciculations	Lethargy
U—Urinary incontinence		Weakness	Coma
M—Miosis		Paralysis	Agitation
B—Bradycardia		Tachycardia	Seizures
B—Bronchorrhea		Hypertension	
B—Bronchospasm		Agitation	
E—Emesis			
L—Lacrimation			
S—Salivation			

bronchorrhea; tachycardia and pupil size are not indicative of an end point of atropine therapy.[66,67] Tachycardia during therapy is limited and not life threatening, and even patients with initial tachycardia should receive atropine to address pulmonary secretions, and with some agents, repeated doses or a constant infusion should be considered.[66,67] Oximes prevent cholinesterase aging. Pralidoxime is the oxime available and indicated for organophosphate poisoning in North America. The use of an oxime in conjunction with atropine is "atropine-sparing"—reactivation of affected cholinesterases decreases the amount of atropine necessary to combat life-threatening symptoms. Pralidoxime is generally not indicated in carbamate overdose because of its more limited toxicity.[56] Benzodiazepines should be considered for seizure prophylaxis.[66] Cholinesterase levels are not available in real time and should not be used to guide therapy when they will delay treatment.

Methemoglobinemia

In hemoglobin, oxidization of iron from the ferrous (2+) to the ferric (3+) state results in the formation of methemoglobin, an abnormal hemoglobin unable to transport oxygen. By shifting the oxygen saturation curve to the left, it decreases off-loading of any bound oxygen at the tissue level.[68] Box 128.6 lists xenobiotics that may cause oxidative stress and result in methemoglobinemia. Methemoglobin maintains a darker hue than deoxyhemoglobin, so the patient looks cyanotic in color, but it does not improve with oxygen administration—the blood may have a chocolate color, even after exposure to oxygen. Multiple-wavelength co-oximetry must be used to diagnose methemoglobin because standard pulse oximetry, used to measure oxy- and deoxyhemoglobin, cannot reliably assess the degree of methemoglobinemia and may overestimate or underestimate true oxygen saturation, generally reading in the 75% to 80% range as the methemoglobin level increases.[69,70] Methemoglobinemia should be suspected in a patient who appears cyanotic but has a normal partial pressure of oxygen.

BOX 128.6 **Toxins That Cause Methemoglobinemia**

Benzocaine
Dapsone
Inhaled nitric oxide
Lidocaine
Naphthalene (found in certain mothballs)
Nitrates
Nitrites
Nitroprusside
Phenazopyridine
Prilocaine
Sulfonamides

Patients may appear blue with methemoglobin concentrations as low as 15 g/L, but a decision to treat is based on clinical symptoms, not the level. Treatment is not always necessary. Anemic patients have less hemoglobin to convert to methemoglobin, limiting their cyanotic appearance, but because this is usually a larger percentage of their functioning hemoglobin, they are more likely to express symptoms of hypoxia at lower methemoglobin levels.[68] Treatment begins with the administration of 100% oxygen (to maximize oxygen-carrying capacity by assuring that unaffected hemoglobin is fully saturated). If necessary, this is followed by intravenous methylene blue at a dose of 1 mg/kg. Methylene blue accelerates reduction of the oxidized heme iron of methemoglobin to its normal state via nicotinamide adenine dinucleotide phosphate (NADPH)–dependent methemoglobin reductase. Response is rapid, generally within 30 minutes. Depending on the inciting agent, as in the case of dapsone, recrudescent methemoglobinemia may require repeated doses of methylene blue. The total dose should not exceed 7 mg/kg because methylene blue is itself oxidizing and may cause additional methemoglobinemia or precipitate hemolysis. Methylene blue may be ineffective in patients with glucose-6-phosphate dehydrogenase (G6PD) deficiency and may increase the risk of hemolysis or methemoglobinemia in this population. In patients not responding to methylene blue, G6PD deficiency should be suspected. In nonresponding patients who are severely ill, exchange transfusion should be considered.[68,71]

Xenobiotic-Induced Hyperthermia

In addition to the previously described syndromes, sympathomimetic and anticholinergic, three distinct xenobiotic-induced hyperthermic syndromes deserve attention. Distinctions of malignant hyperthermia, serotonin syndrome, and neuroleptic malignant syndrome are provided in Table 128.1. Although differences exist, there is also potential for overlap, and diagnosis may be difficult when no previous patient history is available. In all cases of severe hyperthermia, other causes such as sepsis should be ruled out. Because hyperpyrexia in these scenarios is not hypothalamic in origin, antipyretics are ineffective.

Malignant hyperthermia, a genetically determined condition, results in rigidity and muscle damage following exposure to depolarizing neuromuscular blocking agents (succinylcholine) or inhalational anesthetic agents. This life-threatening condition of ryanodine receptor dysfunction results in excessive intracellular calcium in somatic cells and therefore persistent muscle rigidity. Along with aggressive cooling, dantrolene should be administered without delay. Dantrolene allows muscle relaxation through blockade of calcium release from the sarcoplasmic reticulum.[72]

TABLE 128.1 Differences Between Drug-Induced Hyperthermia Syndromes

Syndrome	Causative Agent	Timing of Onset	Treatment
Malignant hyperthermia	Depolarizing neuromuscular blockers or inhalational anesthetics	Minutes	Dantrolene
Serotonin syndrome	Coadministration of two or more serotonergic agents	Hours	Supportive care, cyproheptadine
NMS	Antipsychotic drugs	Days	Supportive care, bromocriptine

Serotonin syndrome is a constellation of features resulting from excessive serotonergic activity in the CNS, most commonly associated with therapeutic regimens of two or more drugs that increase CNS serotonin transmission by different mechanisms. In addition to hyperpyrexia, hallmark features are altered mental status, excessive muscle activity, and autonomic instability. Suggested diagnostic criteria include a history of exposure to a serotonergic agent(s) and the presence of three of the following: mental status change, agitation, myoclonus, hyperreflexia, diaphoresis, shivering, tremor, diarrhea, incoordination, or fever.[73] As opposed to other hyperthermic syndromes, it is distinguished by lower limb rigidity and hyperreflexia.[72,74] Symptoms, starting within hours of exposure, are short lived, and mild cases of serotonin toxicity are self-limiting; however, patients with severe toxicity may develop extreme hyperthermia and rhabdomyolysis with renal failure and cardiovascular collapse. Supportive treatment includes withdrawal of all serotonergic agents, benzodiazepines for muscle overactivity, and aggressive cooling. The use of cyproheptadine has been proposed as a serotonin antagonist at doses from 16 to 32 mg divided up to four times daily.[75-77] In cases of severe hyperthermia, cyproheptadine will do little to prevent further symptoms and should be abandoned for more aggressive therapy with cooling in addition to benzodiazepines or barbiturates and muscle paralysis with a nondepolarizing paralytic.

Neuroleptic malignant syndrome (NMS) encompasses a constellation of features triggered by exposure to neuroleptic drugs (phenothiazines, butyrophenones, atypical antipsychotics). It most commonly occurs after initiation of therapy or with a dose escalation; it has also been triggered by adding a serotoninergic agent to an established antidopaminergic agent and after withdrawal of dopaminergic agents used to treat Parkinson disease.[78,79] Onset is insidious, occurring over several days. Diagnosis requires exposure to a neuroleptic drug, fever, muscle rigidity, and at least two of the following: mental status change, mutism, tachycardia, labile blood pressure, diaphoresis, dysphagia, tremor, incontinence, leukocytosis, or elevated creatinine kinase.[80] Muscle rigidity, often described as lead pipe, is greater in the upper extremities. Although distinguishing NMS from lethal catatonia may be difficult, NMS may, arguably, represent the extreme end of the spectrum of extrapyramidal side effects of antidopaminergic medications. Unlike its milder counterparts, it is unresponsive to centrally acting anticholinergic agents; diphenhydramine and benztropine have no role in the treatment of NMS. Therapy is supportive and includes sedation and administration of benzodiazepines to address muscle rigidity. In severe cases, neuromuscular blockade with a nondepolarizing paralytic agent and active cooling may be required, whereas the addition of propofol or a barbiturate may decrease heat production through a decrease in metabolism. Myoglobinuria and renal failure may complicate the course, and an elevated creatine kinase (CK) is consistent with the diagnosis of NMS. Both dantrolene and bromocriptine, a dopamine receptor agonist, have each been advocated for the treatment of NMS, but their effectiveness in this scenario is debated.[81,82]

Metabolic Acidosis With Increased Anion Gap

Anion gap metabolic acidosis (AGMA) is a laboratory toxidrome that presents a substantial differential diagnosis

---

BOX 128.7   Causes Anion Gap Metabolic Acidosis (MUDPILES)

M—Metformin, methanol
U—Uremia
D—Diabetic ketoacidosis (DKA), alcoholic ketoacidosis (AKA)
P—Phenformin, paraldehyde, propylene glycol
I—Iron, Isoniazid
L—Lactate (carbon monoxide, cyanide, etc.)
E—Ethylene glycol
S—Salicylates, solvents

---

including many nontoxicologic causes (diabetic ketoacidosis, uremia, lactic acidosis, and inborn errors of metabolism to name a few). Agents most commonly associated with AGMA are represented by the acronym *MUDPILES*, listed in Box 128.7. Any agent causing shock will increase lactate and cause metabolic acidosis with an increased anion gap. It should be noted that although metabolic acidosis from toxic agents is generally associated with an increase in anion gap, a nonanion gap acidosis may be seen with the therapeutic use of carbonic anhydrase inhibitors, acetazolamide and topiramate, or from toxins that cause renal tubulopathy with chronic use such as toluene (an agent seen commonly with inhalant abuse).[83,84]

Methanol and ethylene glycol, *toxic alcohols* found in various automotive antifreeze products and as chemical reagents, should be considered in cases of AGMA where the cause is unknown. Although ethylene glycol–containing antifreeze products contain fluorescein, which glows under a Wood's lamp, this is not a reliable method to screen for ingestion; even in the absence of fluorescein, fluorescence has been shown with hospital tubing and plastic containers and in the urine of most hospitalized pediatric patients in one study.[85,86] Laboratory analysis of blood should be done to provide a reliable diagnosis.

Toxic alcohols can cause CNS depression, although they have little toxic effect in their parent form. Toxic alcohols are metabolized first by alcohol dehydrogenase and then aldehyde dehydrogenase to form toxic metabolites. Formic acid, resulting from methanol metabolism, precipitates severe metabolic acidosis and retinal toxicity described as "snowstorm blindness." A number of toxic intermediates are formed from metabolism of ethylene glycol, but the end product, oxalate, results in severe metabolic acidosis, renal failure, and hypocalcemia through binding of oxalate to calcium to form crystals.[87]

Alcohols are osmotically active and will increase serum osmolality and the osmolar gap. An elevated gap suggests toxic alcohol poisoning, but a normal result does not exclude it because the gap depends on how much of the parent compound has been metabolized.[88,89] Over time, the anion gap increases consistently with metabolite production. As the parent compound is further metabolized the osmolar gap decreases and may be normal in patients presenting with symptoms of toxicity. Hemodialysis is indicated for toxic alcohol levels greater than 50 mg/dl and in severely toxic patients to eliminate toxic metabolites and correct metabolic abnormalities even when the parent compound is no longer detectable.[83]

To limit further generation of toxic metabolites, alcohol dehydrogenase must be blocked, and this can be achieved with either fomepizole or ethanol.[90,91] Fomepizole is the agent of choice and if a toxic alcohol is suspected, even if not yet confirmed, it should be provided at a loading dose of 15 mg/kg followed by 10 mg/kg every 12 hours. The dose must be increased to 15 mg/kg after 48 hours because fomepizole induces its own metabolism. Fomepizole is dialyzable, so the dose must also be adjusted during hemodialysis.[92] Ethanol, maintained at levels greater than 100 mg/dl, will block metabolism of toxic alcohols through competition at alcohol dehydrogenase, which has a higher affinity for ethanol than methanol or ethylene glycol, but because ethanol infusions are difficult to compound safely, oral ethanol or ethanol via nasogastric tube is recommended. Ethanol, as an antidote, requires frequent blood alcohol measurements and carries the risks of inebriation, CNS depression, hypoglycemia, and hypotension.[91] If fomepizole is unavailable, ethanol must be used.

Although *iron* is an etiology for AGMA, the unmeasured anion here is lactate.[83,84] Iron is available alone and in combination with other vitamins, but iron salts have different proportions of elemental iron and care should be used when calculating an ingested dose. The first phase of iron toxicity consists of GI manifestations, vomiting and diarrhea, with possible hematemesis and hematochezia. Fluid and electrolyte losses can be severe and require aggressive resuscitation. The second phase, or so-called latent period, is a "quiescent" phase where GI symptoms have ceased but the patient feels unwell, often with tachycardia and an anion gap metabolic acidosis. Beyond 12 hours, the third phase exhibits symptoms progressing to cardiovascular collapse and shock, and the fourth phase is defined by fulminant hepatic failure. The corrosive effect of iron on the GI tract often results in scarring and stricture.[93] Doses higher than 20 mg/kg of elemental iron reliably produce GI irritation, although systemic toxicity is generally not seen with doses lower than 60 mg/kg. Absence of a prodromal GI phase within 4 hours of ingestion generally precludes serious systemic iron toxicity.[93]

Activated charcoal does not adsorb iron and whole-bowel irrigation should be considered if iron tablets remain in the GI tract, as evidenced by plain radiographs of the abdomen, although multivitamins, children's preparations, and liquid preparations may not be visible.[94] Serum iron levels should be measured within 6 hours of ingestion before significant redistribution to tissues. Total iron-binding capacity, used in the evaluation of chronic iron overload, may be falsely elevated in acute iron ingestion and should not be used in making treatment decisions.[92] Chelation via deferoxamine is indicated for serum levels higher than 500 µg/dL or signs of circulatory failure.[94] Intravenous dosing begins at 15 mg/kg/h via continuous infusion, but if symptoms persist beyond 24 hours, the deferoxamine dose should be decreased or temporarily discontinued as its use beyond this time is associated with acute respiratory distress syndrome.[95] Although children's multivitamin preparations do not produce toxicity at the same iron content as adult preparations, prenatal vitamins, except those containing iron carbonyl, have led to extreme toxicity with minor ingestion.[96]

Carbon monoxide (CO) results from incomplete combustion of carbonaceous fuels including natural gas, fuel oil, gasoline, propane, and charcoal. CO is a complex poison that not only affects oxygen binding to hemoglobin but produces reactive oxygen species, increases nitric oxide (NO), and modulates ion channels, most notably in cardiac tissues.[97] It should be considered in the AGMA differential because, through its ability to cause tissue hypoxia, it may precipitate a lactic acidosis. CO binds with high affinity to oxygen-binding sites of hemoglobin and myoglobin and disrupts the transfer of oxygen from erythrocytes to mitochondria. CO also binds directly to mitochondrial cytochrome oxidase and interferes with electron transport and adenosine triphosphate (ATP) production. However, most neurologic sequelae result from displacement of nitric oxide from platelets, leading to an increased generation of the free radical peroxynitrite. It is also this increase in NO that contributes to vasodilation and hypotension. Due to the potential for arrhythmias, serial ECG analysis should be performed. CO is not detected via standard pulse-oximetry, so analysis is through multiple-wavelength co-oximetry. Serial CO levels are not required with appropriate oxygen therapy as it will reliably decrease over time, with the exception of methylene chloride, whose metabolism leads to endogenous production of CO.

Correlation of CO level to symptoms is poor, largely because tissue effects are due to oxidative stress and ion channel effects. However, low levels of CO cause nonspecific symptoms (fatigue, malaise, nausea, and headache), whereas higher concentrations lead to impaired cognition and coma. Hypotension and syncope are significant effects that warrant aggressive treatment regardless of CO level; these events more commonly precede delayed or persistent neurologic sequelae.[97]

Controversy surrounding the treatment of CO poisoning remains. Therapy has always been centered on provision of oxygen to accelerate CO dissociation from hemoglobin. The half-life of CO under various oxygen concentrations is listed in Table 128.2. Hyperbaric oxygen (HBO), the administration of oxygen at supra-atmospheric pressure, has been advocated in the treatment of severe CO poisoning.[98] Although it accelerates the removal of CO from cytochrome oxidase, most CO has been eliminated from the blood by the time the patient is placed in the chamber. The benefits likely result from the reduction of leukocyte adhesion to endothelium.[99] It is proposed to decrease the incidence of delayed neurologic sequelae, although several studies exist with both positive and negative results, and unfortunately many are subject to bias and lack of controls.[98,100] Nonetheless, HBO should be considered when there is loss of consciousness, syncope, or persistent neurologic findings on exam (especially cerebellar dysfunction including ataxia with ambulation). HBO treatment should be completed within 24 hours of exposure, but patients who experienced cardiac arrest should not be considered candidates.[65] Fetal hemoglobin has a higher affinity for CO, so neonates and fetuses may have higher than expected COHb levels, but no data on HBO therapy during pregnancy are available.

Cyanide is a highly toxic compound originating from a variety of sources. It is widely used as a reagent in industry, and several plants, including the seeds and pits of some fruits (eg, apples, cherries, peaches, and pears), contain cyanogenic glycosides that are converted to cyanide in the GI tract. The

TABLE 128.2	Half-Life of COHb
Oxygen Concentration	**Half-Life**
21% (room air)	4-5 hours
100% (mask or endotracheal)	60-90 minutes
100% (hyperbaric molecular oxygen)	20-30 minutes

unapproved substance laetrile, sometimes used inappropriately to treat cancer outside the United States, is synthesized from amygdalin, a cyanogenic glycoside from peach pits. Enclosed fires, particularly those in which plastics or fabrics are combusted, can generate hydrogen cyanide (HCN) and, finally, iatrogenic cyanide poisoning results from the administration of nitroprusside; it is metabolized to cyanide and causes toxicity at high doses, after prolonged therapy without coadministration of sodium thiosulfate, or in the presence of renal failure.[101-104]

Cyanide rapidly produces toxicity when inhaled or when ingested. Cyanide salts are converted to HCN in the presence of gastric acid. Cyanide binds to cytochrome complex IV of the electron transport chain (cytochrome c oxidase) and inhibits oxidative phosphorylation, preventing ATP production. Nonspecific signs and symptoms reflect tissue hypoxia, and death may occur within minutes.[101] Venous oxygen levels are elevated because of the inability to use oxygen at the cellular level and therefore the patients do not appear cyanotic. Arterialization of the venous blood (an elevated pO_2) will result.

Treatment of cyanide poisoning involves immediate life support measures and antidote administration. Sodium nitrite and sodium thiosulfate are traditional antidotes for cyanide poisoning. Nitrites induce methemoglobinemia, which has a higher affinity for cyanide than cytochrome oxidase. Nitrites are potent vasodilators and can cause significant hypotension, best avoided by slow administration, although most significant vasodilation occurs in the most hypoxic tissues potentially providing therapeutic benefits. The initial pediatric dose is 0.2 mL/kg of a 3% solution. Excessive methemoglobinemia is a risk and the dose should be decreased in anemic patients. In fire victims who may have comorbid CO toxicity, the induction of methemoglobin may further reduce the already critically low oxygen-carrying capacity, although the timing of administration of antidotes and oxygen may reduce this risk. Sodium thiosulfate works via the mitochondrial enzyme rhodanese to produce the nontoxic thiocyanate that is excreted in urine. Sodium thiosulfate is used with or without sodium nitrite and can be administered early in patients with significant CO levels because it will not affect hemoglobin. Although it can cause hypotension, this is usually related to the rate of administration and it has a minimal adverse effect profile. Hydroxocobalamin, used to treat fire victims in France for several years, is now available in the United States.[104,105] This cobalt-containing molecule interacts with cyanide to become cyanocobalamin (vitamin B_{12}), which is then eliminated in urine. Although effective, patients may experience hypertension after administration, and both their skin and body fluids will exhibit a reddish hue that interferes with several important colorimetric assays needed for patient monitoring. Severe acne has been reported 1 to 2 weeks after administration.[105] Pediatric administration is 70 mg/kg administered over 30 minutes (IV push is acceptable in severe toxicity). A second dose may be administered if necessary over a total administration time of 6 to 8 hours. The onset of action of hydroxocobalamin is more immediate than sodium thiosulfate, but because hydroxocobalamin must be reconstituted slowly over 20 minutes, time to onset of action is likely not different between the two antidotes. Although these two medications are synergistic, they must be administered in separate lines.[106,107] Published reports indicate that after the effect of hydroxocobalamin has ceased, sodium thiosulfate is still active, providing prolonged benefit.[108]

There are several forms of *salicylate,* the most common of which is acetylsalicylic acid (ASA), or aspirin. The most potent form is wintergreen oil, which is 98% methyl salicylate. Other forms include bismuth subsalicylate, sodium salicylate, and magnesium salicylate. Doses up to 100 mg/kg are likely to produce minimal toxicity, whereas doses above 300 mg/kg will have serious consequences, including death.

Early signs of salicylate toxicity include an increase in minute ventilation (primary respiratory alkalosis), tinnitus, nausea, and vomiting, but a hallmark of toxicity is a mixed-picture respiratory alkalosis and metabolic acidosis from uncoupling of oxidative phosphorylation and inhibition of the tricarboxylic acid cycle. This is nearly pathognomonic and warrants obtaining a salicylate level for evaluation. This uncoupling can lead to hyperpyrexia, and patients are often flushed and diaphoretic. Cerebral edema and pulmonary edema are potentially fatal complications but are more common with chronic toxicity rather than acute poisoning. Levels greater than 35 mg/dL produce minor symptoms, whereas significant signs of toxicity start to manifest at approximately 45 mg/dL after acute ingestion. Patients with chronic exposure will have severe symptoms at much lower levels (approximately 30 mg/dL).

Urinary alkalinization enhances elimination of salicylates and is accomplished by administration of sodium bicarbonate. Urinary pH should be monitored frequently to adjust the rate of bicarbonate infusion to achieve a urine pH above 7.5. Serum pH should be periodically monitored to avoid serious alkalemia and pH >7.55. Serum potassium and magnesium should be maintained within the normal range because to retain potassium in the presence of hypokalemia, protons are pumped into urine, defeating the process of urinary alkalinization. A bolus of dextrose may be warranted in patients with depressed sensorium, even if serum glucose levels are normal, as CNS glucose may be significantly lower than serum.[109] Hemodialysis is considered in patients with significant CNS alteration or salicylate levels greater than 70 mg/dl, as it effectively removes free salicylate in the toxic range. Additional indications for hemodialysis include renal impairment, volume overload, pulmonary edema, and severe electrolyte or acid-base abnormalities.

Toxin-Induced Seizures

It has been estimated that over 6% of new onset seizures result from exposure to a drug or toxin, and this may actually account for 9% of cases of status epilepticus.[110] Toxin-induced seizures result from several mechanisms including loss of inhibition via GABA, increase in CNS excitation through glutamate and NMDA receptors, sodium channel blockade, increased excitatory activity via norepinephrine release, excess cholinergic stimulation, adenosine antagonism, histamine antagonism, and metabolic disturbances.[111] In multiple reviews of seizure incidence, antidepressants account for the highest percentage of toxin-induced seizures, with bupropion exposures representing a disproportionate one-fourth of this population.[110] Seizures from tricyclic antidepressants (TCAs) have decreased with decreasing exposures, but other antidepressants including venlafaxine and citalopram are responsible for a considerable number.[112] Other concerning agents include tramadol, diphenhydramine, and antipsychotics. The

---

BOX 128.8 **Toxins That Commonly Induce Seizures (OTIS CAMPBELL)**

O—Organophosphates
T—Tricyclic antidepressants
I—Isoniazid, insulin
S—Sympathomimetics
C—Camphor, cocaine
A—Amphetamines, anticholinergics
M—Methylxanthines
P—Phencyclidine (PCP)
B—Benzodiazepine withdrawal, botanicals
E—Ethanol withdrawal
L—Lithium, lidocaine
L—Lead, lindane

---

incidence of amphetamine-induced seizures was second only to those induced by bupropion, but they accounted for a higher proportion of mortality. See Box 128.8 for a list of seizure-inducing toxins.

Toxin-induced seizures are global in nature and, unlike many forms of epilepsy, do not emanate from an irritable focus. For this reason, phenytoin and fosphenytoin are rarely effective and in some instances (theophylline and methylxanthines) have been suggested to increase seizure risk.[111] Management of toxin-induced seizures rarely changes based on the agent and relies on the administration of a benzodiazepine for initial therapy. If proved ineffective, propofol or barbiturates are considered as second-line medications.

Isonicotnyl hydrazine (INH), or isoniazid, stands out among seizure-inducing agents as its mechanism is unique. INH, as well as other hydrazines including monomethyl hydrazine (MMH), interferes with pyridoxine metabolism. The decarboxylation of GABA to glutamate relies on pyridoxal-5-phosphate as a cofactor for glutamic acid decarboxylase. Without this active form of B6, GABA is depleted and excess glutamate leads to unchecked excitation in the CNS. INH both inhibits pyridoxine phosphokinase, required to convert pyridoxine to pyridoxal-5-phosphate, and reacts with pyridoxal-5-phosphate to form an inactive metabolite. Because hydrazine-induced seizures result from the depletion of GABA, they are difficult to control with usual anticonvulsant therapy. Treatment of INH poisoning is with pyridoxine, administered in a dose equal to the ingested dose of INH (by weight). If the dose ingested is unknown or the exposure is a result of MMH from *Gyromitra* mushroom ingestion, 5 g or 70 mg/kg in pediatric patients is a reasonable empiric starting dose. Benzodiazepines may work synergistically with pyridoxine, and barbiturates may also be considered in refractory cases.[111] When seizures are not controlled by these measures, a nondepolarizing paralytic should be applied to stop muscle contraction, although, in this case, EEG monitoring is critical to check for continued seizure activity in the brain.

Strychnine is a highly toxic rodenticide that produces convulsions through antagonism of postsynaptic glycine receptors that predominate in the spinal cord.[111] Although myoclonic activity is present, patients do not experience a postictal phase and these are not true seizures. Stimulation worsens muscular contraction, including the diaphragm, and mortality is often a result of hypoxia and hypoventilation. Activated charcoal binds strychnine in a 1:1 ratio and should be considered for decontamination. In addition to reducing unnecessary

stimulus, the same algorithm for toxin-induced seizures applies here, as there is no known antidote.[111]

Cardiovascular Agents

Sodium channel blockade is a common conduction abnormality associated with poisoning. TCAs are a prime example where the electrocardiogram provides more information about the severity of toxicity and prognosis than actual drug levels. Blocking fast sodium channels in cardiomyocytes slows the rate of depolarization and is characterized by a wide QRS. In a landmark study of TCA overdose, it was proposed that a QRS >100 msec was correlated with an increased risk of seizures and QRS >160 msec was associated with a significant risk of arrhythmias.[113,114]

Severe toxicity occurs early in the course of TCA poisoning. Patients who do not manifest QRS widening, conduction abnormalities on ECG, altered mental status, seizures, or hypotension within the first 6 hours can be classified as low risk and no longer need pediatric intensive care unit monitoring.[113] Anticholinergic manifestations should be treated supportively only. Seizures should be treated with benzodiazepines. If the patient has coingested benzodiazepines, then flumazenil, a benzodiazepine receptor antagonist, should not be administered because it may unmask TCA-induced seizures. Widening of the QRS complex (>100 msec in adults) or ventricular arrhythmias should be treated with sodium bicarbonate to produce alkalinization of the serum. Bicarbonate is given in boluses of 1 to 2 mEq/kg until ECG improvement is seen (narrowing of the QRS). Recurrence of QRS widening may be treated in the same manner. Alternatively, a bicarbonate infusion can be started after the initial bolus to maintain alkalemia (with monitoring to prevent over-alkalinization [ie, pH >7.55]). If bicarbonate continues to be infused, it may be stopped and the ECG monitored after approximately 6 hours of normal ECG tracings. Many newer antidepressants and antipsychotics, including bupropion, venlafaxine, and quetiapine, can manifest similar toxicity. Treatment for wide QRS associated with these substances is not different from that described earlier.

Calcium channel antagonists (CCAs) act on L-type calcium channels in the heart and vascular smooth muscle to block the influx of calcium resulting in negative inotropic, chronotropic, and dromotropic effects. CCAs also impair the release of insulin from the pancreas and in overdose, causing significant hyperglycemia.

Except in extremely large ingestions, dihydropyridines produce hypotension and reflex tachycardia, and in less severe poisoning, volume expansion alone may be sufficient. However, this is not true of other CCA classes. Intravenous calcium and vasopressors are indicated if hypotension remains refractory to intravenous fluids. Verapamil and diltiazem overdose are further complicated by pump failure, and these patients may benefit from inotropes such as dobutamine. Glucagon, which acts at a receptor other than the β receptor, increases cyclic adenosine monophosphate (cAMP) and has been reported to reverse refractory hypotension in CCA overdose (discussed in more detail later).

High-dose insulin/euglycemia therapy has been shown effective in several successful animal models and case reports and case series to reverse cardiogenic shock associated with CCA overdose; this therapy has become commonplace in this setting.[115-117] The recommended dose is from 0.5 to 1 unit/kg of insulin as a bolus, followed by an infusion titrated to efficacy. Administration of dextrose should proceed concurrently, and serum glucose concentration should be monitored at least hourly to detect hypoglycemia and adjust dextrose accordingly. Transcutaneous pacing in these patients is difficult but if successful, pacing should proceed at a low rate, near 60 bpm, to maximize filling time. Most patients continue to exhibit decreased contractility such that, even with pacing, adequate cardiac output may not be achieved, and patients who are unresponsive to medical management should be considered for a left ventricular assist device (L-VAD) or extracorporeal life support (ECMO).

β-Adrenergic antagonists comprise a fairly extensive list of therapeutic agents that are largely distinguished from each other by their selectivity (or lack thereof) for the β_1 receptor. Atenolol, metoprolol, esmolol, and acebutolol are β_1-selective agents, whereas agents such as propranolol, nadolol, and pindolol act both at β_1 and β_2 receptors. Propranolol is unique in that it is highly lipophilic and has sodium channel–blocking activity and can additionally precipitate seizures and coma at toxic doses. The β_1 receptors are largely found in the heart and agonism causes positive inotropic and chronotropic effects; β_2 receptors are found in the airway smooth muscle, where they cause bronchodilation; in the small blood vessels, where they cause vasodilation; and in several other organs, where they have a number of effects that are less important in the context of poisoning.

Acute β-adrenergic antagonist overdose results in bradycardia, hypotension, and conduction delay, although toxicity is generally much less severe than with CCAs. Bronchospasm may occur in susceptible individuals. Hypoglycemia has been reported in children with overdose of drugs in this class, although it has also been seen with therapeutic use of propranolol.[118,119] Monitoring alone may be sufficient if the only manifestation is asymptomatic bradycardia. Patients with bradycardia and hypotension may respond to atropine, although they are expected to have initial decreased vagal tone. β-Agonists have variable effects in the presence of β-adrenergic blockade. In theory, mixed agonists could worsen hypotension by causing β_2 receptor–mediated vasodilation. The phosphodiesterase inhibitors amrinone and milrinone have a theoretic benefit of improving contractility by blocking the breakdown of cAMP but have not been shown to be more effective than glucagon.[120,121] Glucagon acts by a nonadrenergic receptor to increase intracellular cAMP and improve cardiac contractility. The suggested dose is a 0.15 mg/kg intravenous bolus followed by an infusion of 0.05 to 0.1 mg/kg/hr, although no maximum dose has been determined.[117] Seizures should be treated with benzodiazepines as first-line therapy, and bronchospasm may respond to anticholinergic agents if inhaled β_2-agonists fail to overcome the β-blockade. Like CCAs, patients not responding to appropriate therapy should be evaluated for LVAD or ECMO.

Digoxin and related digitalis glycosides block the sodium-potassium adenosine triphosphatase (Na/K-ATPase) pump resulting in increased intracellular calcium and improved contractility as well as increased vagal tone and sinoatrial (SA) and atrioventricular (AV) node depression. In overdose, sympathetic tone is increased and may lead to increased automaticity.

Symptoms of toxicity include nausea, vomiting, lethargy or confusion, and cardiac dysrhythmias. Although virtually every rhythm has been described in digoxin toxicity, bidirectional ventricular tachycardia and atrial tachycardia with AV block are characteristic. Blockade of Na/K-ATPase causes hyperkalemia, and levels greater than 5.5 mEq/L have been associated with a high risk of mortality.[122] Poisoning is confirmed with serum digoxin levels, although because of a long distribution phase, the serum level may not accurately reflect tissue levels until at least 6 hours after ingestion.

Sinus bradycardia or heart block may respond to atropine alone but more serious arrhythmias are an indication for treatment with digoxin-specific Fab fragments (eg, Digibind, DigiFab). Drugs that further depress the SA or AV node should be avoided. Hyperkalemia resolves with Fab fragment therapy as it restores function of the Na-K pump. Because digoxin causes intracellular hypercalcemia, administration of calcium could theoretically increase toxicity.[123] Fab fragment therapy in children is indicated with a strong history of ingestion of at least 0.1 mg/kg of digoxin, level greater than 5 ng/mL, rapidly progressing signs and symptoms of digoxin toxicity, potentially life-threatening arrhythmias, or a serum potassium level greater than 5.5 mEq/L.[124]

A clinical picture similar to digoxin poisoning may be seen with the ingestion of cardiac glycoside-containing plants (oleander, fox glove, lily of the valley, etc.). Cardiac glycoside poisoning may cross-react with the digoxin immunoassay and may respond to Fab fragment therapy.[124] However, an antidote dose cannot be calculated from this level, so dosing should be empiric in this situation.

Acetaminophen (Paracetamol)

Although it does not cause a toxidrome per se, acetaminophen is the most commonly ingested drug in intentional overdose and it may cause fulminant hepatic failure and therefore admission to the pediatric intensive care unit. Major routes of elimination of acetaminophen are through glucuronidation or sulfation followed excretion in the urine. A minor pathway is via CYP2E1 to produce *N*-acetyl-p-benzoquinone-imine (NAPQI), a toxic metabolite capable of binding to hepatocytes and causing cell death. With therapeutic doses of acetaminophen, NAPQI is rapidly detoxified by glutathione. In overdose, larger amounts are formed and may overwhelm the available glutathione stores, resulting in a centrilobular hepatic necrosis.

Patients can initially present with nausea and vomiting, but more often they have no symptoms or signs, and laboratory detection is important because treatment is most effective if administered early after ingestion. Transaminases begin to rise at approximately 18 to 24 hours after ingestion and peak between 48 and 72 hours. Patients progress either to fulminant hepatic failure or to complete recovery. *N*-acetylcysteine (NAC) reduces the incidence of hepatotoxicity through several suggested mechanisms, including enhanced synthesis of glutathione and free radical scavenging.[125] Although it is most efficacious when administered within 10 hours of ingestion, studies have shown benefit when administered to patients presenting after this window of time. In one study, intravenous NAC decreased the risk of death from acetaminophen-induced fulminant hepatic failure, even in patients who presented with already established hepatic encephalopathy.[126] The decision to treat an acute ingestion is based on plotting a single acetaminophen blood level at least 4 hours after

USE OF NOMOGRAM IN MANAGEMENT OF ACUTE ACETAMINOPHEN OVERDOSE

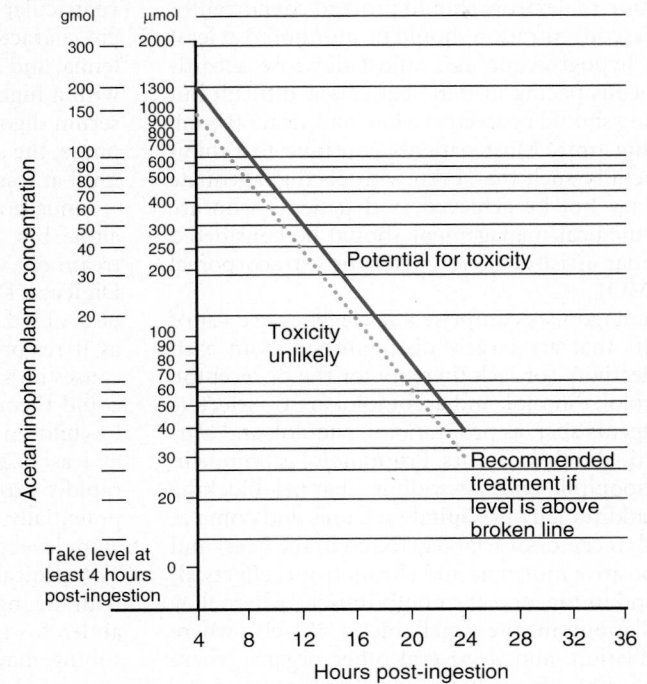

An approach to management of acute acetaminophen overdose

1. Draw blood for acetaminophen plasma assay 4 or more hours post-ingestion.
2. PLOT ON NOMOGRAM.
3. If the acetaminophen level, determined at least 4 hours following an overdose, falls above the broken line, administer the entire course of acetylcysteine treatment.
4. If the acetaminophen level, determined at least 4 hours following an overdose, falls below the broken line, acetylcysteine treatment is not necessary or if already initiated may be discontinued.
5. Serum levels drawn before 4 hours may not represent peak levels.

Fig. 128.1. Use of a Nomogram in the Management of Acute Acetaminophen Overdose.

ingestion on the Rumack-Matthew nomogram (Fig. 128.1). Before 4 hours and after 24 hours, the nomogram is not useful. An acetaminophen level should be measured and liver function analyzed to assess the patient's risk for development of toxicity and potential prognosis. The nomogram has not been validated in chronic ingestion or multiple, staggered ingestions. In these cases, the nomogram should not be relied on for an assessment of toxicity. A poison control center should be consulted for specific treatment advice.

Key References

1. Mowry JB, Spyker DA, Cantilena LR, et al. 2013 Annual Report of the American Association of Poison Control Centers' National Poison Data System (NPDS): 31st annual report. *J Clin Toxicol.* 2014;52:1032-1283.
2. Moeller K, Lee K, Kissack J. Urine drug screening: practical guide for clinicians. *Mayo Clin Proc.* 2008;83:66-67.
3. Forti RJ. Opiate overdose. *Pediatr Rev.* 2007;28:35-36.
4. Ghoneim M, Dhanaraj J, Choi W. Comparison of four opioid analgesics as supplements to nitrous oxide anesthesia. *Anesth Analg.* 1984;63: 405-412.
5. Preston K, Jasinski D, Margaret T. Abuse potential and pharmacological comparison of tramadol and morphine. *Drug Alcohol Depend.* 1991;27: 7-17.
6. Shook J, Watkins W, Camporesi E. Differential roles of opioid receptors in respiration, respiratory disease, and opiate-induced respiratory depression. *Am Rev Respir Dis.* 1990;142:895-909.
7. Bowdle AT. Adverse effects of opioid agonists and agonist-antagonists in anesthesia. *Drug Saf.* 1998;19:173-189.
8. Rigg J, Rondi F. Changes in rib cage and diaphragm contribution to ventilation after morphine. *Anesthesiology.* 1981;55:507-514.
9. Skarke C, Marwan J, Erb K, et al. Respiratory and miotic effects of morphine in healthy volunteers when P-glycoprotein is blocked by quinidine. *Pharmacodynam Drug Interact.* 2003;74:303-311.
10. Kim H, Smiddy M, Hoffman R, et al. Buprenorphine may not be as safe as you think: a pediatric fatality from unintentional exposure. *Pediatrics.* 2012;130:e1700-e1703.
11. Geib A, Babu K, Ewald M, et al. Adverse effects in children after unintentional buprenorphine exposure. *Pediatrics.* 2006;118:1746-1751.
12. Hayes B, Klein-Schwartz W, Doyon S. Toxicity of buprenorphine overdoses in children. *Pediatrics.* 2008;121:s782-s786.
13. Sachdeva DK, Stadnyk JM. Are one or two dangerous? Opioid exposures in toddlers. *J Emerg Med.* 2005;29:77-84.
14. Boyer EW, McCance-Katz EF, Marcus S. Methadone and buprenorphine toxicity in children. *Am J Addict.* 2010;19:89-95.
15. Bucaretchi F, Dragosavac S, Vieira R. Acute exposure to imidazoline derivatives in children. *J Pediatr.* 2003;79:519-524.
16. Higgins G, Campbell B, Wallace K, et al. Pediatric poisoning from over-the-counter imidazoline-containing products. *Ann Emerg Med.* 1990;142: 655-658. 20.
17. Al-Abri SA, Yang HS, Olson KR. Unintentional pediatric opthalmic tetrahydrozoline ingestion: case files of the medical toxicology fellowship at the University of California, San Francisco. *J Med Toxicol.* 2014;10: 388-391.
18. Dowling J, Isbister GK, Kirkpatrick CM, et al. Population pharmacokinetics of intravenous, intramuscular, and intranasal naloxone in human volunteers. *Ther Drug Monit.* 2008;30:490-496.
19. Goldfrank L, Weisman R, Errick J, et al. A dosing nomogram for continuous infusion intravenous naloxone. *Ann Emerg Med.* 1986;15:566-570.
20. Hendra TJ, Gerrish SP, Forrest ARW. Fatal methadone overdose. *BMJ.* 1996;313:481-482.
21. Sterrett C, Brownfield J, Korn CS, et al. Patterns of presentation in heroin overdose resulting in pulmonary edema. *Am J Emerg Med.* 2003;21:32-34.
22. Brimacombe J, Archdeacon J, Newell S, et al. Two cases of naloxone-induced pulmonary oedema—the possible use of phentolamine in management. *Anaesth Intensive Care.* 1991;19:578-580.
23. Levin E, Sharp B, Drayer J, et al. Severe hypertension induced by naloxone. *Am J Med Sci.* 1985;290:70-72.
24. Hasan R, Benko A, Nolan B, et al. Cardiorespiratory effects of naloxone in children. *Ann Pharmacother.* 2003;37:1587-1592.
25. Ahmad SA, Scolnik D, Snehal V, et al. Use of naloxone for clonidine intoxication in the pediatric age group: case report and review of the literature. *Am J Ther.* 2015;22:e14-e16.
26. Oprita B, Gabor-Postole DA, Aignatoaie B. Scores applied in toxicological practice: prognostic assessment in intoxication by barbiturates and

benzodiazepines. *Pharmacology and Clinical Toxciology.* 2012;16: 197-201.

27. Study RE, Barker JL. Cellular mechanisms of benzodiazepine action. *JAMA.* 1982;247:2147-2151.

28. Gunja N. The clinical and forensic toxicology of Z-drugs. *J Med Toxicol.* 2013;9:155-162.

29. Wiley CC, Wiley JF. Pediatric benzodiazepine ingestion resulting in hospitalization. *Clin Toxicol.* 1998;36:227-231.

30. Gueye P, Lofaso F, Borron S, et al. Mechanism of respiratory insufficiency in pure or mixed drug-induced coma involving benzodiazepines. *Clin Toxicol.* 2002;40:35-47.

31. Perry HE, Shannon MW. Diagnosis and management of opioid- and benzodiazepine-induced comatose overdose in children. *Curr Opin Pediatr.* 1996;8:243-247.

32. Mordel A, Winkler E, Almog S, et al. Seizures after flumazenil administration in a case of combined benzodiazepine and tricyclic antidepressant overdose. *Crit Care Med.* 1992;20:1733-1734.

33. Seger D. Flumazenil—treatment or toxin. *Clin Toxicol.* 2004;42:209-216.

34. Spivey WH, Roberts JR, Derlet RW. A clinical trial of escalating doses of flumazenil for the reversal of suspected benzodiazepine overdose in the emergency department. *Ann Emerg Med.* 1993;22:1813-1821.

35. Olmedo R, Hoffman RS. Withdrawal syndromes. *Emerg Med Clin North Am.* 2000;18:273-288.

36. Williams R, Erickson T, Broussard L. Evaluating sympathomimetic intoxication in an emergency setting. *Lab Med.* 2000;31:497-507.

37. Meehan TJ, Bryant SM, Aks SE. Drugs of abuse: the highs and lows of altered mental states in the emergency department. *Emerg Med Clin North Am.* 2010;28:663-682.

38. Hahn I, Hoffman R. Cocaine use and acute myocardial infarction. *Emerg Med Clin North Am.* 2001;19:493-510.

39. Daly J, Butts-Lamb P, Padgett W. Subclasses of adenosine receptors in the central nervous system: interactions with caffeine and related methylxanthines. *Cell Mol Neurobiol.* 1983;3:69-79.

40. Shannon M. Life-threatening events after theophylline overdose: a 10-year prospective analysis. *Arch Intern Med.* 1999;159:989-994.

41. Minton N, Henry J. Acute and chronic human toxicity of theophylline. *Hum Exper Toxicol.* 1996;15:471-481.

42. Wills B, Erickson T. Chemically induced seizures. *Clin Lab Med.* 2006;26:185-209.

43. Singer E, Kolishenko A. Seizures due to theophylline overdose. *Chest.* 1985;87:755-757.

44. Berlinger WG, Spector R, Goldberg MJ, et al. Enhancement of theophylline clearance by oral activated charcoal. *Clin Pharmaco Ther.* 1983;33:351-354.

45. Mahutte CK, True RJ, Michiels TM, et al. Increased serum theophylline clearance with orally administered activated charcoal. *Am Rev Respir Dis.* 1983;128:820-822.

46. Simpson D, Rumack B. Methylenedioxyamphetamine: clinical description of overdose, death, and review of pharmacology. *Arch Intern Med.* 1981;141:1507-1509.

47. Rosenbaum CD, Carreiro SP, Babu KM. Here today, gone tomorrow... and back again? A review of herbal marijuana alternatives (k2, spice), synthetic cathinones (bath salts), kratom, Salvia divinorum, methoxetamine, and piperazines. *J Med Toxicol.* 2012;8:15-32.

48. Trecki J, Gerona RR, Schwartz MD. Synthetic cannabinoid-related illness and deaths. *N Engl J Med.* 2015;373:103-107.

49. Leiken J. Cocaine and beta-adrenergic blockers: a remarriage after a decade-long divorce. *Crit Care Med.* 1999;27:688-689.

50. Seely KA, Lapoint J, Moran JH, et al. Spice drugs are more than harmless herbal blends: a review of the pharmacology and toxicology of synthetic cannabinoids. *Prog Neuropsychopharmacol Biol Psychiatry.* 2012;39:234-243.

Anesthesia Principles for the Pediatric Intensive Care Unit

Section XIII

Anesthesia Principles for the
Pediatric Intensive Care Unit

Airway Management

Ann E. Thompson and Rosanne Salonia

PEARLS

- Safe management of the critically ill child's airway requires an understanding of the anatomic and physiologic changes that occur from birth through adolescence, recognition of congenital and acquired airway abnormalities, appreciation of the pathophysiologic consequences of airway manipulation, and preparation for airways that are potentially difficult to manage.
- Laryngoscopy and intubation are potent physiologic stimuli that are associated with severe discomfort, profound cardiovascular and cerebrovascular changes, and increased airway reactivity.
- Recognizing and preparing to manage a difficult airway are essential steps for the prevention of potentially lethal complications of intubation.
- The approach to intubation must be tailored to specific circumstances, such as a full stomach, elevated intracranial pressure, cervical spine injury, and upper airway obstruction.
- Alternative approaches to airway management, such as the lighted stylet, laryngeal mask airway, cricothyrotomy, retrograde intubation, and tracheostomy, as well as video laryngoscopy, may be lifesaving.

Accurate assessment and safe management of the airway of a critically ill child are the essential first steps in providing effective intensive care. They require understanding the anatomic and physiologic changes that occur from birth through adolescence, recognizing congenital and acquired airway abnormalities, appreciating the pathophysiologic consequences of airway manipulation and underlying disease processes, and preparing for airways that may potentially be difficult to manage.

Anatomic Considerations

The configuration of the child's airway changes dramatically from birth to adulthood (Fig. 129.1). The nose is the site of nearly half of the total respiratory resistance to airflow at all ages. The infant's nose is short, soft, and flat, with small, nearly circular nares. The nasal valve, the narrowest portion of the nasal airway, approximately 1 cm proximal to the alar rim in newborns, measures only about 20 mm[2,1,2] By 6 months, dimensions of the nares have nearly doubled, but they are still easily occluded by edema, secretions, or external pressure. Although an infant is perhaps not as much the obligate nose breather as commonly assumed, signs of airway obstruction frequently develop when the infant's nose is blocked.[3,4]

In infancy the mandible is small and the basicranium (which provides the roof of the nasopharynx) is flat, creating a small oral cavity. Over the years of its development, the jaw grows primarily down and forward, with the mandibular ramus increasing in height and width. The posterior portion of the basicranium develops a progressively more rounded configuration through childhood, which results in a larger nasal airway to meet the need for increased airflow (and provides a chamber for the resonance of adult speech).

Under normal conditions, the genioglossus muscle and other muscles of the pharynx and larynx help maintain airway patency. Both tonic and phasic inspiratory activity synchronized with phrenic contraction have been noted in animal and human studies. In particular, the genioglossus increases the dimensions of the pharyngeal airway by displacing the tongue anteriorly.[5] In the infant and young child, the tongue is large relative to the bony structures surrounding it and the cavities they form. Relatively little displacement is possible at any time, and loss of tone during sleep, sedation, or central or peripheral nervous system dysfunction is more likely than in older patients to allow the tongue to relax into the posterior pharynx and cause upper airway obstruction.

The infant larynx is high in the neck at birth, with the epiglottis at the level of the first cervical vertebra and overlapping the soft palate. This approximation of structures, in combination with the relatively large tongue and small mandible, probably contributes to the vulnerability to airway obstruction in infants and young children. By 6 months the epiglottis has moved to about the level of the third cervical vertebra and is separate from the palate. It continues to descend to its adult position at about the fifth or sixth cervical vertebra by early adolescence. The infant epiglottis is soft and omega shaped, in contrast with the more rigid, flatter adult structure, and it has greater potential to occlude the airway.

For many years standard teaching has been that immature larynx and trachea differ greatly from the mature structures. However, modern imaging techniques, including bronchoscopy, CT scanning, and MRI, provide evidence that contradicts previous dogma.[6-8] The immature larynx is roughly cylindrical, not funnel shaped, similar to the straight vertical column seen in adults. Although previously the narrowest part of the young child's airway was thought to be at the level of the cricoid cartilage, studies show that, as in adults, it is at or just below the vocal cords. Nonetheless, the cricoid is more rigid than other areas of the airway and vulnerable to injury. At all ages the trachea is slightly elliptical in cross section with the anteroposterior diameter slightly greater than the trans-

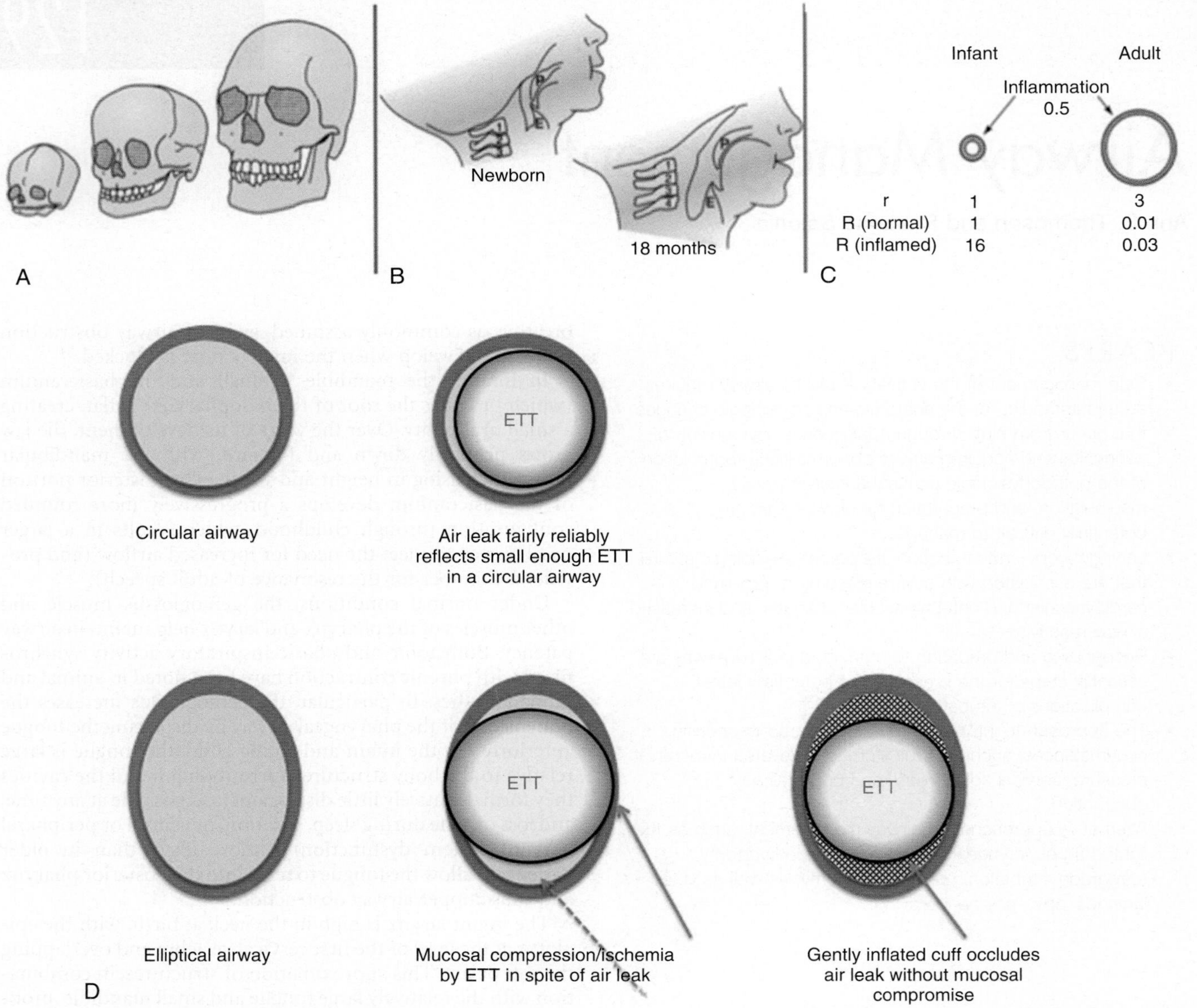

Fig. 129.1. Characteristics of the pediatric airway. (A) Changes in mandibular shape from infancy through adolescence. (B) The epiglottis is initially cephalad in infancy, then it descends throughout childhood. *E*, epiglottis; *P*, palate. (C) Edema has a much greater effect on airways resistance in the young child than later in life. *r*, relative radius of the trachea; *R*, relative airways resistance. (D) Contrary to traditional teaching, imaging indicates that the infant and young child's airway is slightly elliptical in shape, and its narrowest portion is at the vocal cords, as in adults. The elliptical shape raises questions about the value of an air leak in selecting the correct endotracheal tube (ETT) size; a leak may be present even in the presence of mucosal compression and ischemia. A gently inflated cuff seals the airway more effectively, but close monitoring of cuff pressure is necessary. The cricoid is the most rigid segment and may be most at risk of injury.

verse diameter. These newer findings have important implications for endotracheal intubation.

The internal dimensions of the trachea in a newborn are approximately one-third those of an adult, and absolute resistance to airflow is higher in newborns than in older children and adults. Because the most important factor determining resistance (R) is the radius (r) of an airway (R proportional to $8 l/r^4$), small changes in airway diameter in infants or young children as a consequence of edema or secretions have a far greater effect on resistance than similar changes in larger patients (see Fig. 129.1C).

Basic Airway Management

Airway management depends on a brisk assessment of the patient's breathing and knowledge of the likely progression of the airway problem—that is, deterioration versus improving function. In virtually any setting in which respiratory difficulty is suspected, oxygen should be administered until the specific abnormality can be identified and adequately treated. Although extreme hypercarbia usually is well tolerated, hypoxia is routinely catastrophic and is not necessarily obvious on initial examination. From the alveolar air equation, it is obvious that hypercarbia produces hypoxia at low fractions of inspired oxygen (FiO_2) (Table 129.1). If the patient is breathing spontaneously, attention is directed first to signs of upper airway obstruction, including the absence of audible or palpable airflow, stertorous sounds, stridor, or a rocking chest and abdominal motion rather than the normal, smooth rise and fall that should occur with inspiration and expiration.

An alert child with normal neuromuscular function usually instinctively assumes a body position that minimizes upper airway obstruction. However, a child with an altered level of consciousness or severe neuromuscular weakness may be unable to maintain a patent airway because of the inability to alter his or her position or maintain adequate glossopharyngeal muscle tone.

Nasopharyngeal Airway

A nasopharyngeal airway that extends through nasal passages to the posterior pharynx and beyond the base of the tongue often is adequate to relieve obstruction and is tolerated by most patients, even those who are conscious (Fig. 129.2). An airway of appropriate size extends from the nares to the tragus of the ear and is of the largest diameter that passes through nasal passages without causing blanching of the skin surrounding the nares. The airway tube should be well lubricated before placement. Risks of nasopharyngeal airways include nasal ulceration, bleeding, laceration of friable lymphoid tissue, rupture of a pharyngeal abscess, laryngospasm, and potential passage through the cribriform plate in patients with basilar skull fractures. Topical vasoconstricting agents reduce but do not eliminate the risk of bleeding. Like other nasal tubes, use of nasal airways increases the risk of sinusitis; therefore contraindications to their use include severe coagulopathy, cerebrospinal fluid (CSF) leaks, and basilar skull fractures.

Oropharyngeal Airways

Oropharyngeal airways displace the base of the tongue from the posterior pharyngeal wall and break contact between the tongue and palate (see Fig. 129.2). Size selection is important. An excessively long airway may encroach upon the larynx and cause laryngospasm. An airway that is too short may actually push the tongue posteriorly and exacerbate obstruction. If the airway is held at the side of the face with the flange just anterior to the incisors, the tip should be at or near the angle of the mandible. The airway should be positioned following the curve of the tongue while the tongue is held down and forward with a tongue depressor. Inserting the airway with its concave side facing the palate and then rotating it may traumatize the oral mucosa or damage teeth. Oral airways are poorly tolerated in any patient with a functional gag reflex and may induce vomiting. As a consequence, they are of little more than temporary value in the critically ill child. They may support a patent airway for bag-valve-mask ventilation in preparation for intubation.

Oxygen Delivery Devices
Nasal Cannulas

Nasal cannulas consist of two hollow prongs projecting from a hollow face piece. Humidified oxygen (100%) flows from a standard source, effectively delivering a pharyngeal concentration of 25% to 40% after mixing with variable amounts of room air. The cannulas are easy to use, often readily tolerated, lightweight, economical, and disposable and take advantage of the humidifying properties of the nasopharynx. Flow typically is limited to only 3 to 5 L/min because of the extent to which relatively dry gas flow cools and dries the nasal airway. The use of nasal cannulas is limited by the relatively low oxygen concentration that can be delivered. High-flow nasal cannulas can deliver up to 40 L/min of warmed, humidified gas and also are usually well tolerated, although the noise level for the patient can be high. The oxygen concentration delivered is higher than with simple nasal cannulas. High-flow nasal cannulas generate positive distending pressure similar to that provided by nasal continuous positive airway pressure. The pressure generated is dependent on the interaction among the flow rate, patient size, and anatomy of the patient's airway, but it is probably limited to 4 to 5 cm H_2O.[9,10] At least in infants, positive pressure generation requires a closed mouth.[11]

Masks

A variety of masks are available for delivering oxygen. Simple masks fit loosely. The oxygen concentration delivered varies, depending on the patient's inspiratory flow rate and the oxygen flow into the system. Partial rebreathing masks incorporate some sort of reservoir, usually a bag below the chin. Provided that flow into the system exceeds the patient's minute ventilation and that the bag does not collapse on inspiration, little carbon dioxide is inhaled, and concentrations of oxygen up to about 60% can be achieved. Non-rebreathing masks must fit snugly. They incorporate a mask, reservoir, and one-way valves that vent expired gas but do not permit inspiration of room air. As a result, they can deliver close to 100% oxygen.

TABLE 129.1	Impact of Providing Supplemental Oxygen During Hypercarbia on Alveolar Oxygen Tension
Alveolar gas equation	$PaO_2 = FiO_2 (PB - Ph_2o) - PaCO_2/0.8$
Room air, normocarbia	$PaO_2 = 0.21 (760 - 47) - 40/0.8 = 99$ mm H_2O
Room air, hypercarbia	$PaO_2 = 0.21 (760 - 47) - 80/0.8 = 50$ mm H_2O
Supplemental O_2, hypercarbia	$PAO_2 = 0.4 (760 - 47) - 80/0.8 = 185$ mm H_2O

FiO_2, fraction of inspired oxygen; PAO_2, partial pressure of oxygen, alveolar.

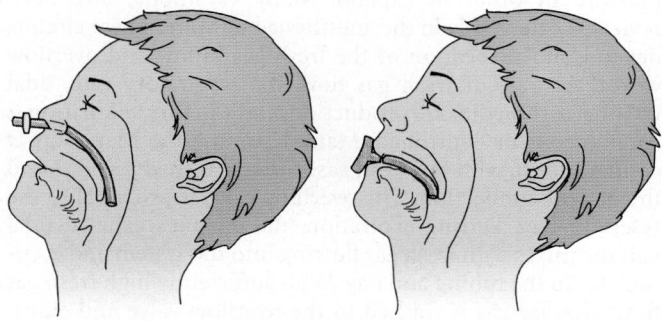

Fig. 129.2. Nasopharyngeal and oropharyngeal airways in good position.

Noninvasive Positive Pressure Ventilation

Continuous positive airway pressure (CPAP) delivers high concentrations of oxygen and maintains positive airway pressure in the spontaneous breathing patient. CPAP is applied with an oxygen source connected to either a tight-fitting nasal or full facemask or helmet in children or via nasal prongs in the neonate and older infant. CPAP offers the benefit of maintaining alveolar expansion and decreases work of breathing for many patients, particularly those with pulmonary parenchymal disease, as well as for some patients with airway obstruction related to poor upper airway tone or laryngeal-, tracheal-, or bronchomalacia.

Like CPAP, bilevel positive airway pressure (BiPAP) can be provided by mask, but it requires a ventilator to assist with flow delivery. The patient's inspiratory effort triggers the BiPAP machine to deliver decelerating flow in order to reach a preset pressure, defined as inspiratory positive airway pressure. When a patient's own inspiratory flow falls below a preset amount, ventilatory assistance ceases and maintains expiratory airway pressure at a predetermined value (typically between 5 and 10 mm Hg). Uses in the pediatric intensive care unit (PICU) include upper airway obstruction, atelectasis, exacerbations of neuromuscular disorders, support for mild to moderate respiratory failure, and as an assist in weaning patients from invasive mechanical ventilation.

Both CPAP and BiPAP offer the advantage of providing respiratory support without endotracheal intubation but require that the child tolerate a close-fitting mask. A more extensive discussion of CPAP and BiPAP is available in Chapters 57 and 58.

Establishing a Functional Airway

A patient who is apneic or in severe respiratory distress requires ventilation assisted initially with a bag and mask. Probably no skill is more important for the intensivist than the ability to provide effective manual bag-mask ventilation. It can be lifesaving while preparation for endotracheal intubation proceeds or when intubation cannot be accomplished. Effective technique requires positioning the patient adequately to open the upper airway, achieving a good mask-face seal, inserting an oral or nasal airway if needed, and generating an adequate tidal volume, coordinating manual breaths with patient efforts when they are present. Poor technique results in ineffective oxygenation and ventilation, gastric insufflation and distention, and increased risk of aspiration.

If the child is too weak or obtunded to maintain pharyngeal tone independently, the head should be placed on a thin cushion to cause slight cervical spine flexion and gentle extension at the atlantooccipital joint. In infants, the large occipito-frontal diameter makes the cushion unnecessary, although a thin pad under the shoulders may be useful. It appears that aligning the external auditory meatus with the sternal notch is a reasonable guide to appropriate positioning. Current recommendations are to avoid overextending the baby's flexible cervical spine, which may stretch and compress the trachea and potentiate, rather than relieve, obstruction. Studies have questioned the existence of this phenomenon but to date have included a small number of infants, all with normal airways.[12] Appropriate head tilt separates the tongue from the posterior pharyngeal wall. If airway obstruction persists, the chin can be pulled forward by encircling the mandible behind the lower incisors between the thumb and fingers. The most effective means of relieving functional obstruction is the so-called triple airway maneuver. With the fingers behind the vertical ramus of the jaw, the mandible is displaced downward, forward, and finally upward again until the mandible and lower incisors are anterior to the maxilla. This action effectively pulls the tongue forward and away from the pharyngeal wall.

In some patients, establishing a functional airway is sufficient to allow resumption of effective spontaneous ventilation. In other patients, steady positive airway pressure is necessary to overcome residual obstruction. If breathing remains inadequate, manual ventilation is necessary. Effective ventilation requires a good mask fit. The mask should sit smoothly on the bridge of the nose and the bony prominence of the chin. It is important to avoid airway occlusion with the mask or hand or pressure on eyes, soft nasal structures, or branches of the trigeminal and facial nerves. A good mask fit is predictably difficult in a patient without teeth, a flat or prominent nose, or micrognathia. Insertion of a nasal or oropharyngeal airway may help maintain an adequate airway. Once a good mask fit is ensured, ventilation may be assisted.

Two types of bags are in general use: self-inflating resuscitation bags and standard anesthesia bags. Because self-inflating bags vary substantially, specific directions for their use must be followed carefully. All bags incorporate an adapter to connect to a mask or endotracheal tube, a bag, a pressure-relief valve, and a port for fresh gas inflow. Most bags designed for children have pressure-relief valves designed to pop off at 35 to 45 cm H_2O pressure to prevent excessive volume delivery and subsequent barotrauma. In patients with poor compliance or increased airway resistance, it may be necessary to bypass this valve temporarily to provide effective ventilation. Most systems incorporate valves that prevent rebreathing. Fresh gas flows through the valve on spontaneous inspiration (negative pressure) or on creation of positive pressure by squeezing the bag (Fig. 129.3). Exhaled gas is vented to the atmosphere. Not all systems allow spontaneous breathing; those that do demand that the patient generate at least a little negative pressure, so a good mask fit is necessary. Holding the mask above the patient's face provides no supplemental oxygen. The percentage of oxygen delivered depends on the percentage of oxygen from the source, the fresh gas flow rate, and the respiratory rate, which determines the time available for the bag to refill. Most systems require some sort of reservoir assembly in addition to the self-inflating bag to prevent entrainment of room air. With a reservoir, 100% oxygen may be delivered; without a reservoir, most deliver less than 50%.

Anesthesia bags require flow from a source of gas under pressure in order to expand. Many variations have been reviewed extensively in the anesthesia literature. These circuits depend on the location of the fresh gas inflow and overflow valves, the rate of fresh gas flow, the respiratory rate, tidal volume, carbon dioxide production, and whether ventilation is spontaneous or controlled. Many ICUs use the Mapleson D configuration, with the fresh gas source attached just distal to the patient connection. The overflow valve is proximal to the reservoir bag. During expiration, the patient's exhaled tidal volume mixes with fresh gas flowing into the system and accumulates in the tubing and bag. With sufficiently high fresh gas flow, alveolar gas is washed to the overflow valve and eliminated from the circuit. The system requires higher fresh gas flow to avoid rebreathing during spontaneous ventilation than

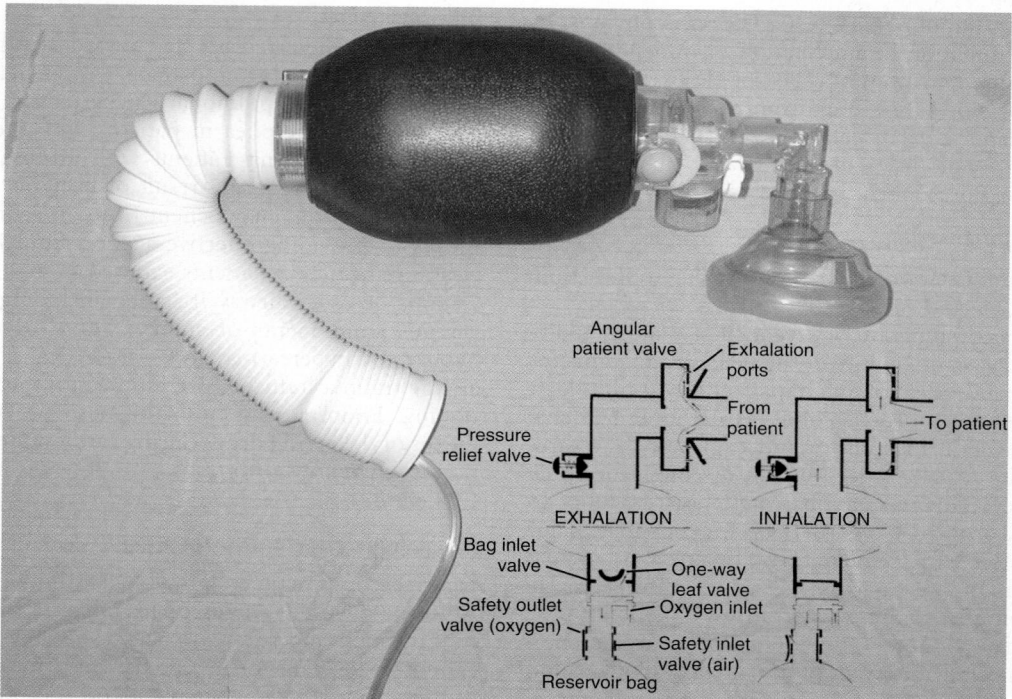

Fig. 129.3. Self-inflating manual ventilation bag with tubing as a reservoir. *(Inset)* Function of one type of valve, permitting manual positive pressure breathing, or spontaneous breathing, but requiring generation of negative pressure by the patient to open the valve. Simply holding the mask over the patient's face does not provide supplemental oxygen.

during controlled breathing, but a safe rule of thumb recommends fresh gas flow two to three times the minute ventilation. During controlled ventilation, a minimum of 100 mL/kg/min ensures that carbon dioxide elimination is proportional to minute ventilation.[13,14] At flows less than 90 mL/kg/min, increasing ventilation may only increase CO_2 rebreathing.

Endotracheal Intubation

The pediatric intensivist is frequently called upon to intubate critically ill patients when brief periods of ventilation with a bag and mask are inadequate to reverse the underlying disorder. Few of these intubations are performed under the optimal conditions commonly attainable in the operating room—that is, relatively healthy children with empty stomachs who have previously been sedated and are intubated in a controlled environment with all members of the team experienced in and prepared for airway management. Instead, patients are often critically unstable and require intubation suddenly, often in settings where the procedure is not routine. Intubation often is viewed only as a means to an end, namely, mechanical ventilation. However, it is associated with profound physiologic consequences that may dramatically affect the patient. The intensivist's appreciation of these factors and ability to minimize the adverse physiologic consequence of airway manipulation may as decisively determine patient outcome as his or her skill in providing the intensive care that follows.

Indications

Respiratory Failure

Respiratory failure may result from dysfunction at any point along the ventilatory pathway. To provide appropriate support

BOX 129.1	Indications for Intubation

1. PaO_2 <60 mm Hg with fraction of inspired oxygen ≥0.6 (in absence of cyanotic congenital heart disease)
2. $PaCO_2$ >50 mm Hg (acute and unresponsive to other intervention)
3. Upper airway obstruction, actual or impending
4. Neuromuscular weakness
   - Maximum negative inspiratory pressure ≥20 cm H_2O
   - Vital capacity <12 to 15 mL/kg
5. Absent protective airway reflexes (cough, gag)
6. Hemodynamic instability (cardiopulmonary resuscitation, shock)
7. Controlled therapeutic (hyper)ventilation
   - Intracranial hypertension
   - Pulmonary hypertension
   - Metabolic acidosis
8. Pulmonary toilet
9. Emergency drug administration

and to avoid hazards specific to the individual disorder, airway intervention must be tailored to the underlying cause. Outside the operating room, the need for intubation is most commonly associated with respiratory failure resulting from upper or lower airway or pulmonary parenchymal disorders that require mechanical ventilation. Respiratory failure is defined in terms of excessive work of breathing or inadequate oxygenation (in the absence of cyanotic congenital heart disease) or carbon dioxide elimination. Box 129.1 contains one set of criteria for intubation.

Hemodynamic Instability

Patients with hemodynamic instability often benefit from assisted ventilation. The need for controlled ventilation as a component of cardiopulmonary resuscitation is obvious. In addition, early intubation in anticipation of impending cardiovascular collapse may prevent catastrophic tissue hypoxia. Redistribution of blood flow away from respiratory muscles, especially the diaphragm, in patients with marginal cardiac output may improve perfusion of other vital organs, including the heart, and help prevent cardiac arrest.[15-19]

Neuromuscular Dysfunction

For additional information on neuromuscular dysfunction, see Chapters 49, 58, and 71.

Neuromuscular dysfunction or severe chest wall instability (or deformity) may cause failure of the bellows apparatus for breathing.[20] Initially, tidal volume remains normal or at least sufficient to maintain normal blood gas tensions, but vital capacity and maximal inspiratory and expiratory pressures decrease. Inability to take a deep breath or cough forcefully risks progressive segmental or lobar atelectasis, inability to clear secretions, bronchial obstruction, and possible major airway obstruction with sudden severe hypoxia or carbon dioxide retention. Increasing weakness results in progressively smaller tidal volumes, loss of upper airway tone, and, ultimately, inadequate minute ventilation. Bulbar dysfunction may lead to aspiration as a result of impaired swallowing and inadequate cough.

Measurement of ventilatory reserve provides a better assessment of the patient's need for ventilatory assistance than do arterial blood gas tensions alone. Maximum negative inspiratory pressure and vital capacity are two simple, commonly used tests for this purpose. A variety of other measures also help assess respiratory "strength," but most are difficult to perform in sick, uncooperative infants and children. Patients with diffuse neuromuscular weakness of any cause, spinal cord dysfunction above the level of T6, or loss of phrenic nerve or diaphragm function are particularly prone to respiratory failure.[21] Because of the extreme compliance of their chest walls and relative ineffectiveness of intercostal muscles, infants younger than approximately 6 months tolerate diaphragmatic paralysis poorly.[22-26]

Many patients with neuromuscular weakness respond well to noninvasive forms of ventilatory support.[20,27] Decisions about the best approach to airway management should be based on the nature and likely progression of the illness, the child's maturity and level of consciousness, and the timing of the onset of respiratory insufficiency. In an emergency, endotracheal intubation is likely to be safest, with transition to noninvasive support when careful planning allows.[27]

Failure of Central Nervous System Regulation of Ventilatory Drive

Failure of central nervous system regulation of ventilatory drive may prompt intubation (see Chapter 47). Centrally mediated hypoventilation is manifest as CO_2 retention, usually in the absence of increased work of breathing. On occasion the decision to support ventilation may be based on observing abnormal ventilatory patterns in anticipation of neurologic deterioration. Loss of protective airway reflexes, including the cough and gag reflexes, can result from central nervous system depression, cranial nerve abnormalities, or severe motor weakness. In such patients, intubation is indicated to prevent aspiration. Intubation may be appropriate in anticipation of the need to protect the airway and support ventilation during deep sedation for procedures or diagnostic studies.

Other Indications

Intubation is indicated as a step toward therapeutic controlled (hyper)ventilation (eg, in patients with increased intracranial pressure [ICP] or pulmonary hypertension) or to support spontaneous hyperpnea in patients with metabolic acidosis and other conditions. Patients with profuse, thick, or tenacious secretions (eg, as a result of bacterial pneumonitis or smoke inhalation) may benefit from an artificial airway as a means of providing effective suction. Impaired mucociliary clearance occurs in patients exposed to high oxygen concentrations or other airway irritants (including particulate and gaseous components of smoke), those experiencing severe hypoxia or hypercarbia, and, paradoxically, those who have airway trauma induced by endotracheal intubation and suctioning. Endotracheal intubation also provides an effective means of delivering drugs during cardiopulmonary resuscitation when venous or intraosseous access is not available (see Chapter 42).

Physiologic Effects of Intubation

Laryngoscopy is a potent physiologic stimulus (Box 129.2).[28,29] At the very least, laryngoscopy is uncomfortable, causing significant pain and severe anxiety, especially in children who cannot understand or accept the need for it. Laryngoscopy causes an increase in systemic blood pressure and heart rate initiated by pressure on the back of the tongue or lifting the epiglottis.[28,30] This effect is augmented by endotracheal intubation and suction.[31] Nodal or ventricular dysrhythmias may occur. Sensory impulses triggering this reflex probably are carried along the vagus nerve supplying the base of the tongue, epiglottis, and trachea. The efferent limb is less well defined but most likely is the product of enhanced sympathetic activity. Infants respond more variably than do older patients. Hypertension develops in most patients, but a few become hypotensive, especially if they are hypoxic.[32] They may demonstrate moderate-to-severe bradycardia rather than tachycardia, perhaps as a consequence of their greater parasympathetic tone. Sedation and light anesthesia decrease but do not obliterate the hypertension and tachycardia; surface anesthesia and deeper general anesthesia are more effective.[33] Children with previous hypertension display an exaggerated vasopressor response. Sedation and neuromuscular blockade during airway manipulation in infants minimize the associated bradycardia and systemic hypertension.[34-38] The impact

BOX 129.2	Potential Physiologic Effects of Laryngoscopy and Intubation

Pain
Tachycardia
Anxiety
Bradycardia
Hypoxia
Systemic hypertension
Hypercarbia
Decreased systemic venous return
Increased intraocular
Decreased jugular venous pressure return
Increased intragastric pressure
Increased intracranial pressure
Laryngospasm
Bronchoconstriction
Pulmonary hypertension

of positive pressure ventilation on cardiac performance depends on the underlying disorder (discussed in Chapters 26 and 43) but should be carefully considered in preparation for intubation.

Laryngoscopy and intubation are potent stimulators of laryngospasm and may cause bronchoconstriction, especially in patients with a history of reactive airway disease. Increased airway resistance probably results from parasympathetic stimulation, with release of acetylcholine and stimulation of muscarinic receptors on airway smooth muscle, especially large central airways.

During intubation, oxygen delivery to the patient is commonly interrupted. Ineffective breathing or apnea increases the likelihood of hypoxia, especially in children, with their relatively low functional residual volume and higher basal metabolic rate. Patients with severe pulmonary disease and abnormally low functional reserve capacity are at particular risk.[34,37] During apnea, carbon dioxide tension increases at a rate of 3 to 4 mm Hg/min in healthy, sedated adults and probably more rapidly in children, particularly those with severe cardiopulmonary disease or increased metabolic rate resulting from fever, sepsis, or pain.[39,40]

ICP rises immediately during laryngoscopy even in patients without intracranial pathology before changes in blood gas tensions occur.[33,35,40-42] Cerebral metabolic rate and blood flow increase. Hypoxia, hypercarbia, and diminished jugular venous drainage, particularly in struggling patients, contribute further to increases in cerebral blood volume and increased intracranial pressure. Although normally transient, such intracranial hypertension may predispose patients with coagulopathies or vascular malformations to intracranial hemorrhage. Systemic hypertension in patients with impaired autoregulation of the cerebral circulation (eg, sick infants or patients with a variety of intracranial disorders) and impedance to jugular venous return by jugular compression, pneumothorax, or coughing and struggling stress both the arterial and venous sides of the cerebral circulation. In patients with poor intracranial compliance, this effect is exaggerated and prolonged. In infants without primary central nervous system disease, muscle paralysis (even without sedation or analgesia) effectively blocks the rise in ICP associated with intubation.[37] The systemic hypertensive response is generally unaffected by neuromuscular blocking agents but can be modified by analgesia and sedation or intravenous anesthesia.

Patients with severe pulmonary hypertension are at high risk for adverse effects of laryngoscopy. Decreased oxygenation and progressive hypercarbia lead to elevated pulmonary artery pressure. The noxious stimulus of visualizing the airway in itself may precipitate life-threatening hypertension.

Recognition of a Difficult Airway

Recognition of a difficult airway is important if potentially lethal surprises in airway management are to be minimized (Box 129.3). Although the intensivist is usually focused on the immediate physiologic disturbances affecting the patient, careful preparation and as thorough an evaluation of each individual patient as is possible is critical. Key components of the history and physical examination, as well as the clinical scenario, can provide insight into potential problem airways. A history of difficult intubations in the past or episodes of upper airway obstruction (including snoring or sleep apnea) suggest structural abnormalities that may or may not be

---

BOX 129.3   Recognizing the Difficult Airway

History
Difficult intubation
Upper airway obstruction, current or past, including snoring and
    sleep apnea

Anatomic Features
Gross macrocephaly
Severe obesity
Facial asymmetry
Facial trauma
Midface hypoplasia
Airway bleeding
Small mouth
Oropharyngeal mass
Glossoptosis
Abnormal soft tissue infiltration
Midline clefts or high arched palate
Limited temporomandibular joint mobility
Micrognathia
Nasal obstruction
Limited neck mobility
Laryngotracheal abnormalities (congenital or acquired)

---

evident at the moment. Recent tonsillectomy and adenoidectomy, cleft palate repair, or any prolonged surgical procedure resulting in oral edema or bleeding increase the likelihood of difficulty. Examining facial structure is essential, and inspecting the child's profile is particularly important because significant abnormalities may not be fully apparent on frontal view alone (Fig. 129.4). Certain genetic syndromes are associated with craniofacial anomalies, midline defects, or neuromuscular disorders that may make successful intubation via standard techniques exceptionally difficult.[43] Treacher Collins syndrome (mandibulofacial dysostosis), Goldenhar syndrome (oculoauriculovertebral dysplasia), Down syndrome, Pierre Robin syndrome, and the mucopolysaccharidoses, such as Hurler syndrome and Hunter syndrome, are a few of the syndromes that have characteristic features that suggest a high probability of facing a challenging airway. Isolated micrognathia, macroglossia (glossoptosis), facial clefts, midface hypoplasia, prominent upper incisors or maxillary protrusion, facial asymmetry, a high arched narrow palate, a small mouth, and a short, muscular neck or morbid obesity are features that can interfere with effective bag-mask ventilation or visualization of the larynx. Limited temporomandibular joint or cervical spine mobility may make laryngoscopy and tube placement difficult. Midface instability or upper airway bleeding, edema, airway or neck masses and foreign bodies are additional reasons for concern.[44-49]

Several classification systems assist with recognition and classification of the adult patient with a difficult airway. Although never validated in pediatrics, they provide a useful framework for assessing infants and children. The Mallampati classification (Fig. 129.5) assesses visualization of upper airway structures prior to intubation—particularly the uvula, soft palate, and faucial pillars—as a guide to the likely ease of intubation. Mallampati class 1 allows visualization of the uvula, soft palate, and faucial pillars; in class 2, faucial pillars and soft palate are visualized, but the base of the tongue obstructs the uvula; in class 3 only the soft palate is visualized; and in class 4 the soft palate is not seen. Difficult intubation is more likely associated with classes 3 and 4. This scale can

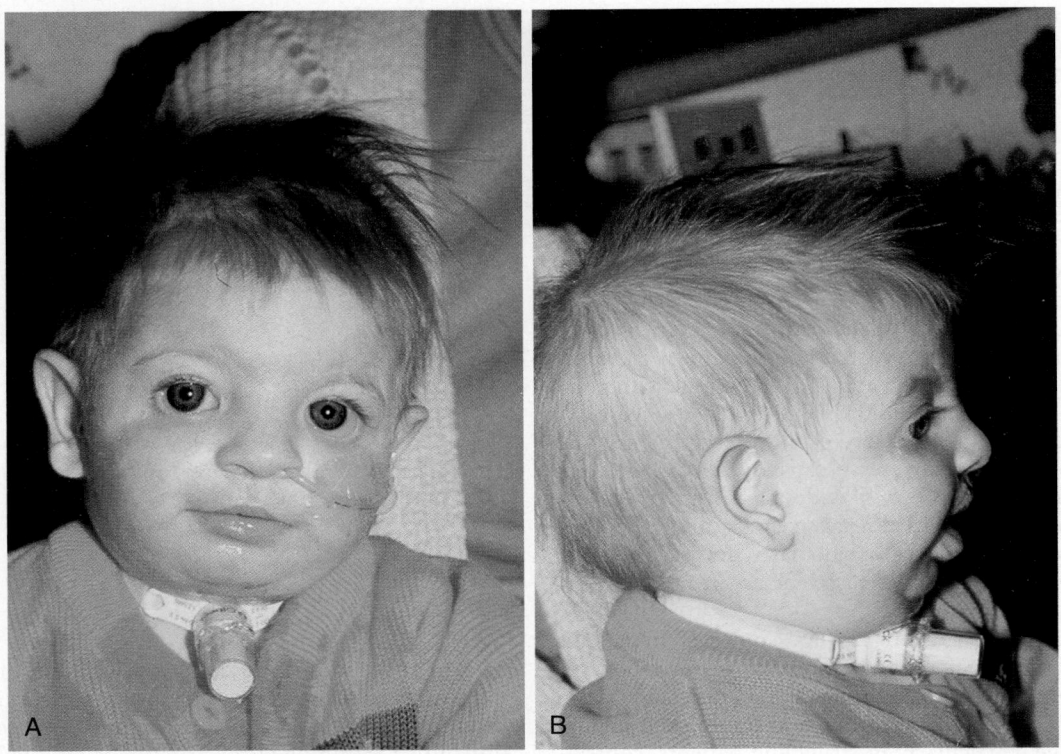

Fig. 129.4. Importance of inspecting the patient's profile. Child with significant micrognathia, not immediately apparent on frontal view. (From Lipton JM, Ellis SR. Diamond-Blackfan anemia: diagnosis, treatment, and molecular pathogenesis. Hematol Oncol Clin North Am. 2009;23:261-282, 2009.)

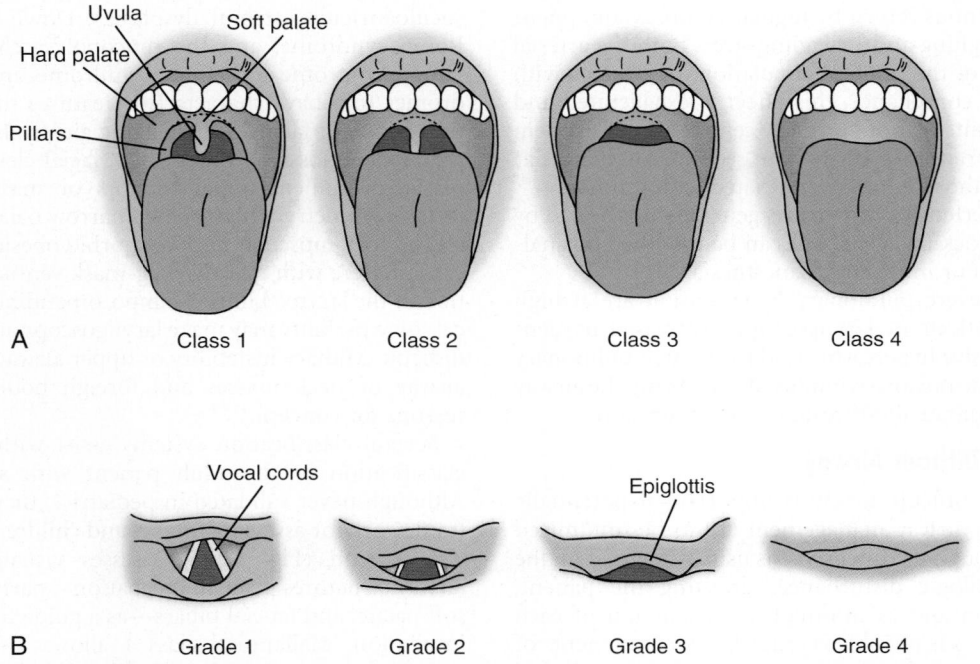

Fig. 129.5. (A) Modified Mallampati classification. Class 1: Visualization of the faucial pillars, uvula, soft and hard palate. Class 2: Visualization of complete uvula and palate. Class 3: Visualization of only the base of the uvula and palate. Class 4: Visualization of only the hard palate. (B) Cormack and Lehane classification of the laryngeal exposure. Grade 1: Most of the glottis is visible. Grade 2: Only the posterior portion of the glottis visible. Grade 3: Only the epiglottis is visible. Grade 4: Not even the epiglottis is visible. (From Amantéa SL, Piva JP, Zanella MI, et al. Rapid airway access. J Pediatr [Rio J]. 2003;79[suppl 2]:S127-138.)

be used with cooperative children, and an approximate evaluation may be obtained by observing many crying infants and young children.[50]

The Cormack laryngeal view grade score is shown in Fig. 129.5B. Because the Cormack system requires an attempt to visualize the larynx, it is more valuable as a tool for describing difficulty once it has been encountered than for predicting it. The Cormack score is grade 1, full view of vocal cords and glottis; grade 2, partial view of vocal cords and glottis; grade 3, only the epiglottis is seen; and grade 4, the glottis and epiglottis are not visualized. Grades 3 and 4 predict difficult direct laryngoscopy. Although these classification systems are helpful in a controlled environment, particularly the preoperative area of a hospital, they are recognized as having limited utility in the emergent situations often encountered in the intensive care unit (ICU), and their ability to predict the degree of difficulty with intubation in children is not well established.

Ability to visualize the faucial pillars, soft palate, and uvula usually predicts an uncomplicated intubation, but this may be difficult to assess in a sick, uncooperative child.[42] Children with severe hypoxia, severe hypovolemia, or other causes of hemodynamic instability, such as intracranial hypertension, a full stomach, or a combination of these conditions, present added difficulties that must be considered.

When airway problems are anticipated, the intensivist should approach intubation with a plan specific to the difficulty noted and with a backup strategy in mind.[46-48] Extra equipment should be on hand, including a variety of laryngoscope blades, forceps, tubes, bronchoscopes, tracheostomy or cricothyrotomy trays, and additional skilled personnel as needed.[48] Many institutions have developed difficult airway carts or packs, as well as a team of highly skilled airway experts, to assist when severe intubation challenges arise.[50-51] If sedation is required, agents that can be reversed pharmacologically are desirable and should be titrated slowly to the desired effect. Fig. 129.6 shows a modification of the American Society of Anesthesiologist's difficult airway algorithm and provides an approach to managing the difficult airway.[52] A similar plan is necessary at the time of extubation, with serious consideration given to extubation in the operating room or with an airway exchange catheter left in place to facilitate reintubation if necessary.

Process of Intubation

All equipment for intubation must be available prior to the procedure (Fig. 129.7). A source of suction and appropriate catheters, oxygen and necessary tubing, ventilation bag, mask, laryngoscope and proper-sized blade with a well-functioning light, endotracheal tubes of the expected size and larger and smaller sizes, airway forceps, stylet, and a means of securing the endotracheal tube should be present at the head of the bed so that the intubator does not need to look away from the patient. A functioning intravenous catheter for drug infusion is essential in all but the most extreme emergencies.

Laryngoscope handles are available in standard adult and pediatric sizes. The smaller diameter of the pediatric handle makes it easier to manipulate, particularly when intubating infants and very young children. Blades of many descriptions

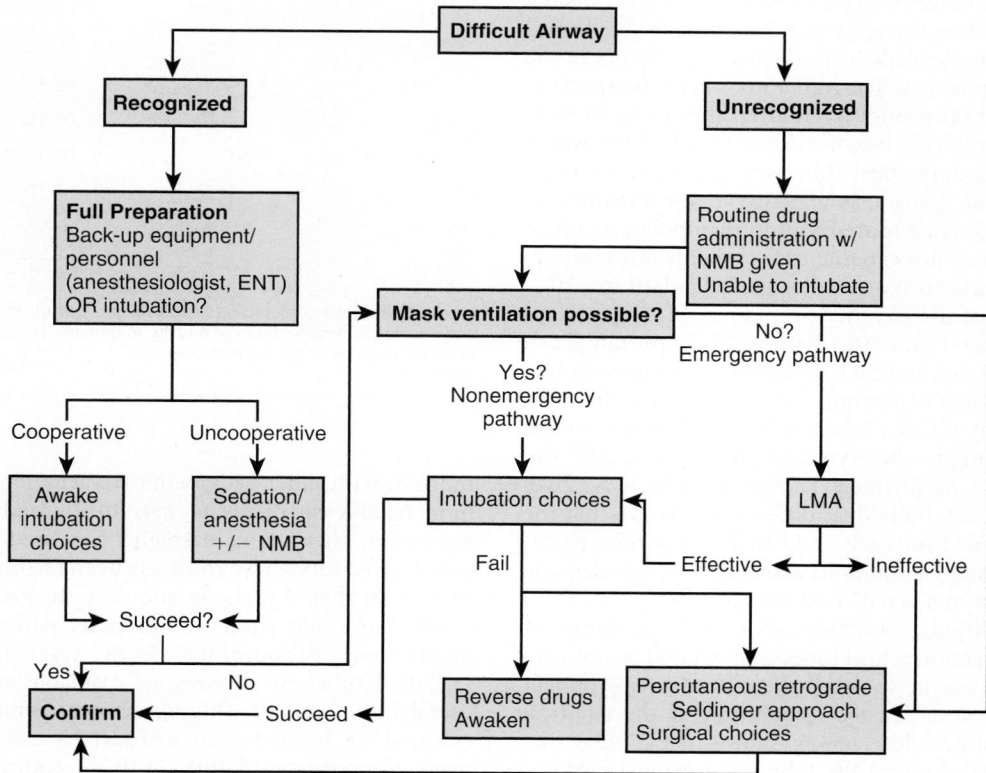

Fig. 129.6. Modification of the American Society of Anesthesiologist's difficult airway algorithm. (From Practice guidelines for the management of the difficult airway: an updated report by the American Society of Anesthesiologists Task Force on Management of the Difficult Airway. Anesthesiology. 2003;98:1269.)

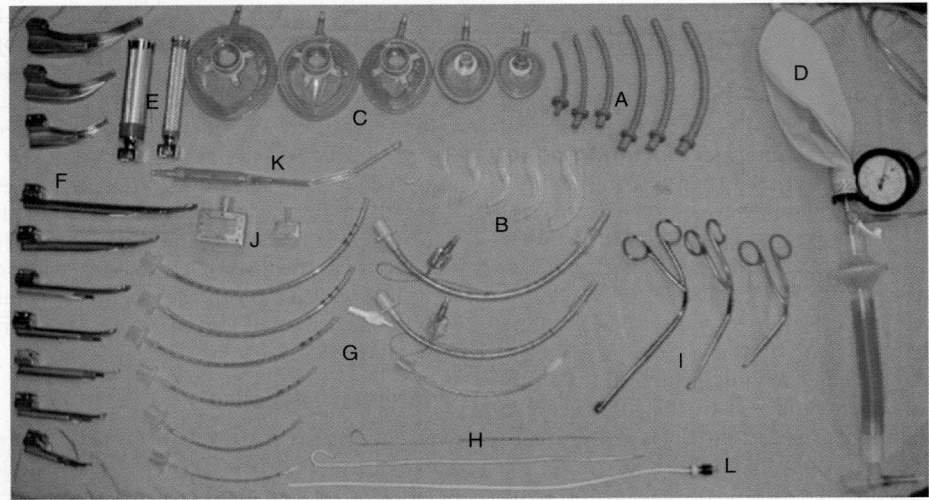

Fig. 129.7. Equipment for intubation, showing a variety of sizes available for pediatric patients. (A) Nasopharyngeal airways. (B) Oral airways. (C) Masks. (D) Anesthesia (Mapleson) bag. (E) Laryngoscope handles. (F) MacIntosh (curved) and Miller (straight) laryngoscope blades. (G) Uncuffed and cuffed endotracheal tubes. (H) Endotracheal tube stylets. (I) Magill forceps. (J) End-tidal CO_2 detectors. (K) Yankauer suction. (L) Tube changer.

are available. The most important characteristic is length. Inexperienced operators often select a blade that is too short, making visualization of the larynx difficult. Excessively long blades make it difficult to avoid pressure on the upper lip and teeth. Historically straight blades have been recommended for intubating infants and young children, but recent evidence suggests curved blades (eg, Macintosh 1 or 2 blades) are as likely to provide good visualization.[53] The slightly curved tip of the Miller blade makes visualization of the larynx possible without actually lifting the epiglottis. The broader blade and bore of the Wis-Hipple blade helps displace soft tissues in the young infant's oropharynx. The Miller no. 2 blade is especially versatile in a broad age group (ie, children about 3 to 10 years of age). In older children, use of a curved blade often works best. If a cuffed endotracheal tube is to be used, a curved Macintosh no. 2 or 3 blade is effective in the majority of patients and may provide more room to manipulate a cuff in the oropharynx. Operator experience is probably most important, with willingness to try the alternative blade if one provides a poor view of the airway.

Selecting the proper tube size (diameter) is important, both to achieve effective mechanical ventilation and to prevent tracheal injury. A variety of formulas are in use, with the most common being that of Cole: Tube size (inner diameter) = (Age [years]/4) + 4. Cuffed tubes typically should be a half size smaller. For infants, no formula is accurate. Table 129.2 gives reasonable guidelines. Individual differences require that the tube size be modified for each child so that the tube passes easily, but it fits snugly enough to allow delivery of adequate mechanical breaths at a given chest compliance.

Based on traditional teaching about the anatomy of the airway, cuffed endotracheal tubes were viewed as not necessary or appropriate in young pediatric patients (younger than 8 years). However, better recognition of the elliptical shape of the young child's airway shows that a tube that permits a small leak around the tube (as previously recommended) may still be compressing the lateral aspects of the tracheal mucosa (Fig. 129.1D). Cuffed tubes allow better occlusion of the airway with potentially lower pressure on the

TABLE 129.2	Guidelines for Endotracheal Tube Diameter in Infants and Children		
Age	Internal Diameter	Orotracheal Length (cm)	Nasotracheal Length (cm)
Premature	2-3	6-8	7-9
Newborn	3-3.5	9-10	10-11
3-9 mo	3.5-4	11-12	11-13
9-18 mo	4-4.5	12-13	14-15
1.5-3 y	4.5-5	12-4	16-17
4-5 y	5-5.5	14-16	18-19
6-7 y	5.5-6	16-18	19-20
8-10 y	6-6.5[a]	17-19	21-23
11-13 y	6-7[a]	18-21	22-25
14-16 y	7-7.5[a]	20-22	24-25

Ideal tube size varies according to age, height, weight, specific airway anatomy, and ventilatory requirements of a child. In general, an air leak around the tube at 15 to 30 cm H_2O pressure is desirable.
[a]Cuffed tube.

mucosa, with potentially better oxygenation and ventilation, more reliable end-tidal CO_2 monitoring, and decreased risk of aspiration. They are increasingly being used for patients of all ages. Cuffed tubes have routinely been recommended for children older than 8 years. In addition, the greater elastic recoil of the lungs and chest wall of older patients may demand higher airway pressures for effective ventilation.

Cuffed tubes of all sizes are available and are especially useful in patients in whom consistent minute ventilation is essential (eg, in the presence of severely elevated ICP or reactive pulmonary vasculature) or those requiring relatively high airway pressures. Increasing evidence indicates that cuffed tubes can be used in young children without higher incidence of airway complications.[54-59] It appears that tubes with clear depth markers along their length and an ultrathin, polyurethane, high-volume, low-pressure, spherical rather than elliptical cuff, positioned close enough to the tip of the tube to avoid inflation in the larynx are ideal.[6] When a cuffed tube is used, great care should be taken to inflate it with the *minimum occlusive volume*, the minimum volume required to just seal the gas leak around the tube during mechanical inspiration and prevent mucosal ischemia and subsequent tracheal damage. Our current best understanding is that pressure within the cuff should be maintained below 20 to 30 cm H_2O. There are inexpensive devices for measuring cuff pressure built into syringes used to fill the cuff. In addition, a standard pressure transducer with air-filled tubing can be attached to the pilot balloon on the endotracheal tube and attached to a typical ICU monitor for continuous pressure measurements. Potential advantages of cuffed tubes include decreased likelihood of multiple intubations to identify the correct size and avoidance of changing the endotracheal tube of a critically unstable patient if lung disease worsens. In addition, absence of a significant leak around the endotracheal tube (ETT) may decrease the likelihood of flow-triggered ventilator autocycling. The ability to occlude the leak also facilitates pulmonary function testing and indirect calorimetry.

Pharmacologic Agents Facilitating Intubation

Although intubation often is possible without use of drugs, the physiologic and psychologic benefits of their use usually outweigh the disadvantages.[60,61] An analysis of data in the pediatric National Emergency Airway Registry shows that the intubation success rate is higher when both sedation and neuromuscular blockade are used.[62] This finding is equally true in neonates, in whom sedation and neuromuscular blockade are still commonly not used, with no evidence they are harmful.[63] In neonates the predominance of evidence indicates that use of neuromuscular blockade is associated with a lower risk of intracranial hemorrhage and pulmonary airleak.[64] Excellent technical airway skills are an absolute prerequisite, however, because loss of control of the airway invites catastrophe. Drugs facilitating intubation are listed in Table 129.3.

Anticholinergic Agents

Anticholinergic agents decrease oral secretions and prevent bradycardia, particularly in young infants, although their use is not universally recommended.[65,66] Atropine (0.02 mg/kg) and glycopyrrolate (0.01 mg/kg intravenously) are both effective. Scopolamine provides amnesia, decreases secretions, and prevents bradycardia. The drying effect commonly requires approximately 15 to 30 minutes and is rarely achieved in emergency intubation. Pediatric Advanced Life Support (PALS) guidelines (2011) recommend atropine for rapid sequence intubation for infants under age 1 year, patients 1 to 5 years of age receiving succinylcholine, patients older than 5 years receiving a second dose of succinylcholine, and patients with bradycardia present before intubation; these guidelines are silent regarding patients older that 1 year, not receiving succinylcholine.[67]

Sedative and Analgesic Agents

Most patients benefit from some degree of sedation. Drugs commonly used include intravenous anesthetic agents, anxiolytic agents, and narcotic analgesics. The appropriate choice in a particular patient depends on the child's hemodynamic status, level of anxiety, and underlying disease process.

Etomidate is a short-acting intravenous anesthetic that causes rapid loss of consciousness (at 0.3 mg/kg) and respiratory depression. It also decreases cerebral oxygen consumption, cerebral blood flow (CBF), and ICP, without significant detrimental effects on cardiovascular function and with less respiratory depression than thiopental, an agent widely used in the past but no longer readily available in the United States. These characteristics have led to its common use for emergency intubation.[68,69] It has no analgesic properties and may be best combined with a narcotic analgesic. Adverse effects include vomiting, myoclonus, and lowering of the seizure threshold. With continuous infusion for sedation, it can cause adrenal insufficiency, making it inappropriate for long-term use in the ICU.[70] Growing evidence suggests it may suppress adrenal function even after a single dose, particularly in patients with sepsis and shock, raising questions about its use in these settings.[71-83]

Ketamine is another potent non-narcotic analgesic and anesthetic that has been used safely in children in the critical care setting.[84,85] It increases heart rate, systemic blood pressure, and cardiac output and is a fairly potent bronchodilator. However, myocardial depression may be apparent after administration to patients with catecholamine depletion. Its use in patients with unstable hemodynamics did not seem to be associated with a lower prevalence of new hypotension noted in a multicenter prospective observational cohort study.[86] It may be of particular value in patients with status asthmaticus or other reasons for bronchospasm and may have a beneficial effect in sepsis. Spontaneous ventilation is preserved in most patients, but laryngospasm may occur.[87] Although in the past it has been considered inappropriate for patients with intracranial hypertension because of evidence that it increases cerebral metabolic rate, blood flow, and ICP, more recent studies indicate that it may be used safely in these patients, although no clear consensus has emerged.[88-90] Emergence delirium and hallucinations occur frequently and may be prolonged and recurrent, particularly in adolescents and young adults. Use of ketamine for a variety of procedures in children has been successful, with little reported difficulty with neuropsychiatric complications, but follow-up in most studies has been short and superficial.[91-96] Whereas the majority of patients do not suffer severe disturbances, those who do may have severe and prolonged distress. Benzodiazepines or barbiturates may decrease the incidence and severity of such adverse effects and the incidence of vomiting, although the data in children are limited and conflicting.[75,81,91,93,97,98]

Propofol is an ultra–short-acting agent with rapid onset and offset unless given by continuous infusion. It causes respiratory depression, desaturation, and systemic hypotension secondary to its negative inotropic effects and peripheral venous and arterial vasodilation. Its role in airway management of critically ill children is limited because of these effects. It has gained widespread acceptance as an anesthetic agent in children, however, and has been used extensively for procedural sedation.[99,100] Use in the ICU for more than approximately 6 hours is not recommended because of its still unexplained association with metabolic acidosis, cardiovascular collapse and death, and propofol syndrome among pediatric ICU patients.[100-103] Current labeling warns against its use for prolonged sedation in children.

TABLE 129.3	Drugs Facilitating Intubation		
Drugs	**Dose**	**Duration**	**Comments**
Intravenous Anesthetics			
Etomidate	0.3 mg/kg IV	3-5 min	Anesthesia, adrenal suppression ($\uparrow$ mortality in sepsis?), minimal CV effect, apnea, $\downarrow$ CMRO$_2$, $\downarrow$ CBF, $\downarrow$ ICP
Ketamine[a]	1–2 mg/kg IV; 4–6 mg/kg IM	10-15 min	Anesthesia, $\uparrow$ systemic arterial pressure, $\uparrow$ HR, $\uparrow$ ICP, $\uparrow$ IOP, hallucinations, laryngospasm, bronchodilation
Propofol	1–3.5 mg/kg IV, then 0.05–0.3 mg/kg/min	10-15 min	$\downarrow$ Systemic arterial pressure, $\downarrow$ CMRO$_2$, $\downarrow$ CBF, $\downarrow$ ICP, metabolic acidosis
Sedatives/Analgesics			
Fentanyl[a]	2–5 µg/kg IV	30-90 min	Analgesia, respiratory depression, cardiovascular stability, occasional bradycardia, or chest wall rigidity
Remifentanil	1–3 µg/kg, then 0.25–1 µg/kg/min		Analgesia, respiratory depression, cardiovascular stability
Morphine[a]	0.1–0.2 mg/kg IV	2-4 h	Analgesia, respiratory depression, $\downarrow$ systemic arterial and venous tone, $\downarrow$ systemic blood pressure
Midazolam[a]	0.1–0.3 mg/kg IV	1-2 h	Amnesia, sedation or euphoria, ± cardiovascular stability, occasional respiratory depression
Lorazepam	0.1–0.3 mg/kg IV	2-4 h	Sedation, anxiolysis, minimal cardiovascular effect
Neuromuscular Blocking Agents			
Rocuronium[a]	0.6–1.2 mg/kg IV	15-45 min	Minimal cardiovascular effect, prolonged duration in liver failure
Vecuronium[a]	0.1–0.3 mg/kg IV	30-75 min	Minimal cardiovascular effect, prolonged effect in hepatic failure
Cis-atracurium	0.1 mg/kg, then 1–5 mg/kg/min	20-35 min	Metabolized by plasma hydrolysis, mild histamine release
Atracurium	0.5 mg/kg	30-40 min	Metabolized by plasma hydrolysis, mild histamine release
Succinylcholine[a]	1–4 mg/kg IV	5-10 min	$\downarrow$ HR, K$^+$ release in neuromuscular disease, trauma or burns, masseter spasm, malignant hyperthermia, myoglobinuria

Duration of effect is only approximate and varies with age and physiologic state of the patient.
CBF, cerebral blood flow; *CMRO$_2$,* cerebral metabolic oxygen requirement; *CV,* cardiovascular; *HR,* heart rate; *ICP,* intracranial pressure; *IM,* intramuscular; *IOP,* intraocular pressure; *IV,* intravenous.
[a]Agents may be given intramuscularly but will have slower onset and more variable duration of effect.

The benzodiazepines, including diazepam and midazolam, relieve anxiety, produce sedation in most children, and provide amnesia for noxious procedures. They do not relieve pain. They have relatively little hemodynamic effect in most patients and rarely interfere with spontaneous breathing at therapeutic doses. They decrease cerebral oxygen consumption modestly. They are best combined with a narcotic analgesic when used for intubation in order to decrease the discomfort and pain associated with laryngoscopy and passage of the tube.

Narcotics commonly used for intensive care include morphine, fentanyl, and some of the ultra–short-acting agents such as remifentanil. They cause respiratory depression in a dose-dependent fashion and increase intracranial blood flow in proportion to the increase in PaCO$_2$. If hypercarbia is prevented, they decrease cerebral metabolic rate and blood flow. In the setting of altered cerebral autoregulation, they may not protect the patient from alterations of CBF.[104,105] Morphine causes histamine release and peripheral vasodilation and may precipitate systemic hypotension. Fentanyl is approximately 100 times more potent than morphine but does not release histamine and has little hemodynamic effect, even at anesthetic doses. Large doses given rapidly can cause bradycardia or chest wall rigidity. Remifentanil is a rapid-onset, ultra–short-acting opiate that is even more potent than fentanyl and may have potential benefit in intubation for procedures.

Neuromuscular Blocking Agents

Neuromuscular blocking agents cause reversible paralysis, facilitating visualization of the airway and insertion of the endotracheal tube in an atraumatic fashion. Most drugs in use are nondepolarizing relaxants with similar action. Differences are primarily in their hemodynamic effects, metabolism, and excretion.[106,107] Vecuronium and rocuronium are the agents most commonly used. Both are amino-steroid agents. Vecuronium has virtually no hemodynamic effect. Its duration of action varies depending on the patient's age, approximately 70 minutes in infants and 35 minutes in older children. It is metabolized exclusively by the liver. Rocuronium provides good intubating conditions nearly as rapidly as succinylcholine (in about 45 to 90 seconds)[108-110] without the adverse effects. Its duration is longer at 15 to 45 minutes (and longer in infants).[111-113] Like vecuronium, it has minimal hemodynamic effect, is metabolized by the liver, and largely is excreted in bile (with a small amount excreted by the kidneys). Atracurium and cis-atracurium, both benzylquinolinium agents, also have minimal hemodynamic effects in most patients but may cause histamine release and hypotension in some persons. Metabolism occurs by spontaneous plasma hydrolysis; thus neither renal nor hepatic function is necessary for elimination. Duration of action is short at about 15 to 20 minutes.

The only depolarizing relaxant in clinical use is succinylcholine. Its only advantage is its rapid onset of action (45 to 60 seconds) and brief duration of action (5 to 10 minutes). Muscle fasciculations occur at the onset of action in patients older than 4 years and may increase intracranial, intraocular, and intragastric pressure. Defasciculating doses of a nondepolarizing neuromuscular blocker prior to succinylcholine administration minimize such effects. Massive hyperkalemia may occur following its use in patients with spinal cord injury, severe burns, crush injuries, or neuromuscular disease. More recently, the spread of acetylcholine receptors outside of the neuromuscular junction, the mechanism presumed to underlie the massive hyperkalemic response previously noted, has been recognized to occur in many forms of critical illness associated with immobility, placing many critically ill patients at risk.[114] It is a known trigger for malignant hyperthermia, even in the absence of volatile anesthetic exposure, and is a particular risk to patients with previously undiagnosed myopathies, often associated with abnormality in the ryanodine receptor type one gene (*RYR1*).[115] It frequently causes myoglobinuria in otherwise healthy children. The US Food and Drug Administration has issued a warning against its use for routine intubation in children because of these complications. Although it is frequently used for emergency intubations and is widely recommended,[62,116,117] the difference in time to conditions for intubation between succinylcholine and rocuronium is small (~30 seconds), rarely of clinical significance, and inadequate to justify the added risk in the majority of cases. Moreover, the time to critical hemoglobin desaturation in the case of a failed airway is shorter than its duration of action, especially in children, so its shorter duration of action does not provide a meaningful advantage over nondepolarizing blockers.[118]

A more extensive discussion of anesthetic agents and their use is given in Chapters 130, 131, 133, and 134.

Orotracheal Intubation

When all equipment is ready, an assistant is assigned to monitor the child's color, heart rate, blood pressure, and oxygen saturation and to administer drugs when ordered. The child is placed supine with the head in the "sniffing" position. The infant's large occipitofrontal diameter naturally results in good position most of the time, but a small pad under the shoulders may be helpful. In older children, a thin pad under the occiput helps establish slight neck flexion (Fig. 129.8). The head is extended to align the oral, pharyngeal, and laryngeal axes as much as possible. Spontaneous or manual ventilation with supplemental oxygen is maintained as drugs to facilitate intubation are given. Many patients requiring emergency intubation have severely impaired gas exchange and may require several minutes of breathing 100% oxygen, often with positive inspiratory and end expiratory pressure.[119] Applying cricoid pressure during manual ventilation helps minimize gastric distention by air (Fig. 129.9).[120] After the drugs take effect, the pharynx is suctioned and stomach contents are aspirated. The patient is again briefly oxygenated, and the mask is removed. In a fully relaxed patient in good position, the mouth falls open. It can be opened more widely with caudad pressure on the chin by the intubator's left fifth finger as the laryngoscope is introduced into the right-hand corner of the mouth. In an unsedated patient or when the mouth opens abnormally, it may be necessary to open the jaw with

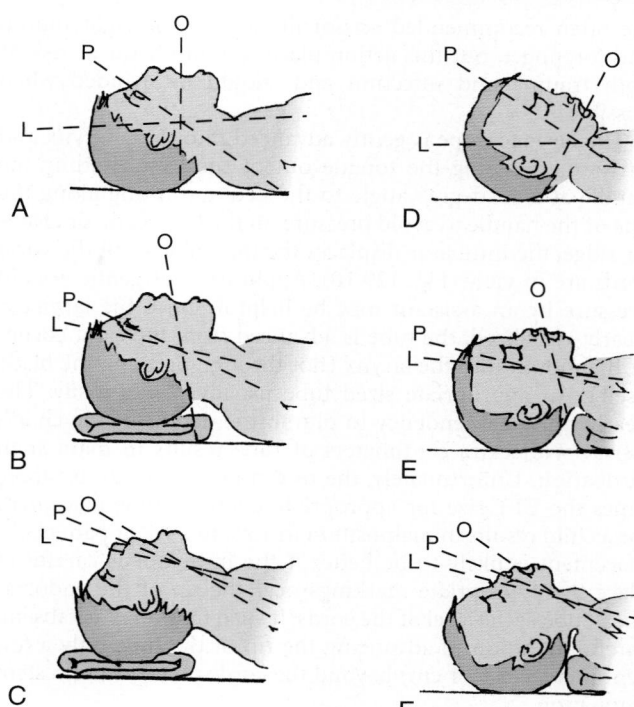

Fig. 129.8. (A) Positioning of the young child and infant for laryngoscopy and tracheal intubation. (B) Placing the child's head on a thin pad flexes the neck slightly and helps align the pharyngeal and laryngeal axes. (C) Extension of the atlantooccipital joint (into the sniffing position) further aligns the oral axis with the pharyngeal and laryngeal axes. (D) Before the age of approximately 3 years, the child's large frontal occipital diameter makes the pad beneath the head unnecessary, but a small pad under the shoulders (E) may improve alignment of the pharyngeal and laryngeal axes. (F) As with the older child, head extension improves alignment of the oral, pharyngeal, and laryngeal axes. (From McAllister JD, Gnauck KA. Rapid sequence intubation of the pediatric patient: fundamentals of practice. Emerg Med. 1999;46:1249-1284.)

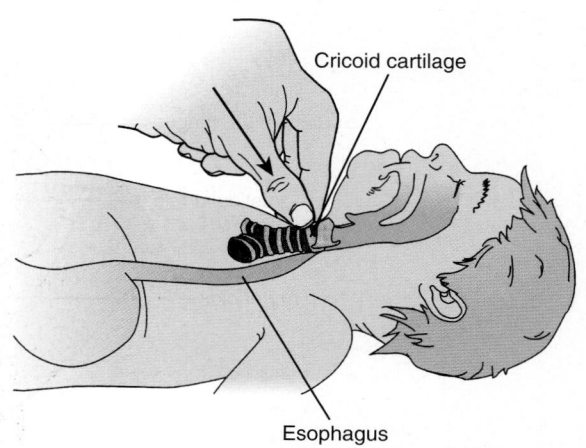

Fig. 129.9. Sellick maneuver. Pressure on the cricoid cartilage occludes the esophagus or hypopharynx.

the often recommended scissor-like use of the right thumb and forefinger, but this action places the intubator at risk of both trauma and infection and should be avoided when possible.

The laryngoscope is gently advanced into the pharynx and leftward, sweeping the tongue out of the way. Holding the handle at a 45-degree angle to the bed and lifting along the line of the handle to avoid pressure on the lips, teeth, or alveolar ridge, the intubator displaces the mandible until the vocal cords are in view (Fig. 129.10). Application of gentle cricoid pressure by an assistant may be helpful. Once the larynx is clearly visualized, the tube is advanced from the right corner of the mouth into the larynx (not through or along the blade itself). An appropriate sized tube usually passes easily. The nearly universal tendency to plumb the depths of the child's airway with extra centimeters of tube results in main stem intubation. Unfortunately, the recommendation to use three times the ETT size for appropriate depth of tube placement for a child results in malposition in 15% to 25% of patients.[121] Placement is likely to be better if the intubator is careful to place the appropriate markings near the tip of the endotracheal tube at the level of the cords. If such markings are absent, careful attention to advancing the tip of the tube only a few centimeters (2 to 4 cm) beyond the cords prevents main stem intubation.

With the tube in place, the child again receives manual ventilation with oxygen. Typically a small air leak around the tube is present. Assuming use of a cuffed tube, the cuff is inflated to less than 20 to 30 cm H_2O or lowest pressure that occludes the leak. Correct tracheal placement of the tube is suggested by observation of moisture condensing in the tube, good chest excursion, symmetrical breath sounds, and effective oxygenation. The most reliable means of ensuring proper placement, following clear visualization of the tube passing between the vocal cords, is documentation of carbon dioxide in expired gas (by capnometry or a disposable CO_2 detector). Only in the settings of full cardiac arrest or extremely low pulmonary blood flow can the endotracheal tube be in the airway without detection of expired carbon dioxide. Under other conditions, malposition of the tube, most commonly in the esophagus, must be assumed. It is important to remember that capnometry does not ensure correct positioning within the airway: Carbon dioxide will be detected with the tube

anywhere from a bronchus to above the vocal cords. Documenting location of the tip of the tube between the thoracic inlet and T4 on chest radiograph, with the head in a neutral position, is important. The tip will descend deeper into the trachea with neck flexion and move cephalad with neck extension.[122,123] With the endotracheal tube in good position, an inflated cuff often can be palpated at the sternal notch when quick pressure is applied to the sentinel balloon. The tube is secured, avoiding pressure on the lips, particularly at the angle of the mouth, and keeping the vermilion border of the lip free of tape.

Nasotracheal Intubation

If nasotracheal intubation is preferred, it should generally follow orotracheal intubation so that an assistant can ventilate the child while the somewhat more difficult intubation is accomplished. A topical vasoconstricting agent such as phenylephrine 0.25% or oxymetazoline 0.05%, sprayed into the nasal fossa, minimizes the risk of bleeding. In most children a tube of the same diameter as the oral tube can be gently advanced along the floor of the nasal cavity, essentially directly posteriorly, into the nasopharynx with firm, but not brutal, pressure. With the oral tube in the left corner of the mouth, the laryngoscope is again advanced into the pharynx until the oral tube is visualized passing through the cords and the tip of the nasal tube is seen in the nasopharynx. The nasal tube is advanced until it lies directly above the cords, anterior to the oral tube. Use of Magill forceps may facilitate this maneuver. When the nasal tube is in good position to enter the larynx, the assistant removes the oral tube and helps advance the nasal tube. Difficulty advancing the tube after it has passed the vocal cords may be overcome by rotating the tube or flexing the neck. The tube then is secured; pressure on the septum or anterior rim of the nares should be avoided.

Although an orotracheal tube usually is placed more rapidly in emergencies, it often stimulates gagging, makes mouth care difficult, and it is more easily kinked or bitten. Anchoring the tube often is difficult because of saliva, and tongue movement may contribute to palatal or tracheal erosion and increase the likelihood of accidental extubation. Trauma to lips, teeth, tongue, and other oropharyngeal structures may occur. Nasotracheal intubation is more comfortable for most conscious patients, causes less stimulation of the gag reflex, is

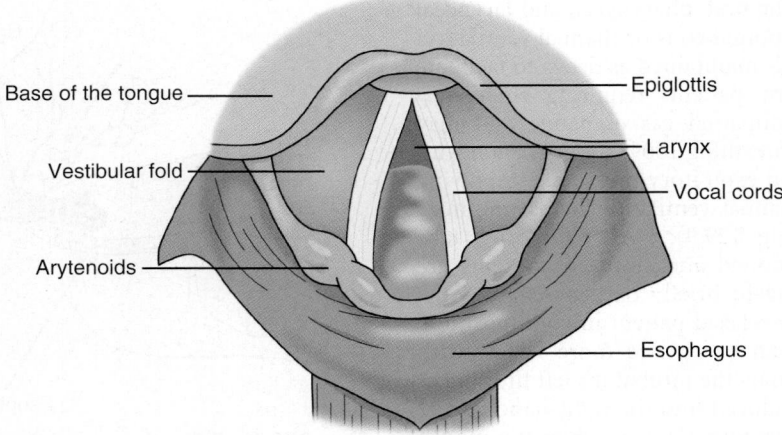

Fig. 129.10. Glottic area view via laryngoscopy.

more easily secured, and prevents the problem of biting in patients with seizures, decerebrate rigidity, or extreme agitation. However, bleeding, adenoid injury, sinusitis, and trauma to the nasal turbinates, septum, or nares may occur with nasotracheal intubation, and the risk of sinusitis is greater than with orotracheal tubes.[124,125] Contraindications to nasotracheal intubation include coagulopathy, maxillofacial trauma, CSF leak, and basilar skull fracture.

Video Laryngoscopy

Video laryngoscopy allows visualization of the larynx without requiring a direct line of sight aligning the oral, pharyngeal, and tracheal axes. In the setting of a difficult airway, video assistance improves visualization and more rapid intubation in adults. Visualization in children is also improved, but experience published to date suggests that the first-pass success rate is lower and time to intubation is longer than with direct laryngoscopy, even in the hands of experienced anesthesiologists, at least in patients in whom airway visualization is only moderately difficult.[126-130] On the other hand, studies of simulated difficult airway management in infants have shown improved intubation rates without a longer time to intubation.[128] At present, it appears that these devices may be most valuable in difficult situations, including cervical spine instability and craniofacial abnormalities, rather than as an advance in routine laryngoscopy.[131]

The video laryngoscope also provides a useful opportunity for teaching airway skills. Some devices include laryngoscope blades similar to standard Mac and Miller blades. A duplicate video image allows an instructor to view the attempted routine intubation in real time and provide immediate guidance and evaluation.[132,205]

Flexible Fiberoptic Bronchoscopy

Flexible fiberoptic bronchoscopy is an effective means of securing a difficult airway, especially in patients with cervical spine instability or those in whom limited jaw mobility or oropharyngeal lesions prevent good visualization of the larynx.[48,133] Assuming the operator's clinical proficiency, the procedure almost always is successful, with little or no trauma to the patient. The nasal route is routinely chosen because it is easier to use, better tolerated, and safer for the instrument than other routes. A topical vasoconstrictive agent and local anesthetic are applied to the nasal mucosa. The endotracheal tube is advanced through the nose into the nasopharynx, and the flexible scope is threaded through it. The scope is advanced through the vocal cords, and the tube is passed over it into the trachea. (Alternatively, the tube with its connector removed may be threaded retrograde over the scope. The scope is advanced through the nose, to the nasopharynx, and through the larynx into the trachea. The endotracheal tube is advanced over the bronchoscope into good position.) The bronchoscopist then visualizes and secures the position of the tube in the trachea and carefully withdraws the scope.

The flexible fiberoptic bronchoscope can also be used with an intubating laryngeal mask airway (LMA). Although the LMA is not used commonly in the PICU (except occasionally for procedural support), it can provide a means of securing a difficult airway. Once adequate oxygenation and ventilation are established, a fiberoptic scope can be threaded into the airway and an endotracheal tube advanced over it.[134,135]

Extubation

Extubation is appropriate when the conditions for intubation are no longer present. In general, this means that the work of breathing has decreased to a level manageable by the patient. In most cases, this situation occurs when oxygenation is adequate with the administration of 40% oxygen or less; spontaneous tidal volume is greater than 3.5 mL/kg; the patient can sustain a normal $PaCO_2$ without mechanical breaths with a near normal respiratory rate for age and without the use of accessory muscles; secretions are manageable; upper airway reflexes are intact; and neuromuscular function is sufficiently good to achieve an adequate vital capacity and maximum inspiratory pressure (Table 129.4).[136] Although standard teaching holds that extubation is most likely to be successful when there is an air leak around the ETT at less than 30 cm H_2O, study indicates that the presence or absence of a leak is a poor predictor of the success of extubation.[137] If intubation was for relief of upper airway obstruction, direct inspection revealing more normal anatomy is of particular value, and the significance of a leak may be greater. In patients with a previously difficult to manage airway, extubation over a tube changer or in the operating room, with surgical support available, should be considered.[138]

Before extubation, the child is given nothing enterally for 4 to 6 hours. The tube and pharynx are suctioned thoroughly, and the child is ventilated with 100% oxygen to provide a reservoir of oxygen as a buffer against laryngospasm at extubation. With the lungs fully inflated, the endotracheal tube is removed, and the child is provided with humidified oxygen and observed closely.

Postextubation stridor is common and may range from mild to life threatening. Children younger than 4 years are most frequently affected by postextubation stridor. Factors contributing to airway edema include a tight endotracheal tube or cuff, traumatic or repeated intubations, excessive movement of the tube (or patient), preexistent airway abnormalities, and airway infection.[139] Cool mist or humidified

TABLE 129.4	Threshold Values for Low (≤10%) and High (≥25%) Risk of Extubation Failure	
Variable	**Low-Risk Value (≤10%)**	**High-Risk Value (≥25%)**
V_{tspont} (mL/kg)	≥6.5	≤3.5
FiO_2	≤0.30	>0.40
Paw (cm H_2O)	<5	>8.5
OI	≤1.4	>4.5
FrVe (%)	≤20	≥30
PIP (cm H_2O)	≤25	≥30
C_{dyn} (mL/kg/cm H_2O)	≥0.9	<0.4
V_t/T_i (mL/kg/sec)	≥14	≤8

C_{dyn}, dynamic compliance; FiO_2, fraction of inspired oxygen; FrVe, fraction of total minute ventilation provided by the ventilator; OI, oxygenation index; PIP, peak ventilatory inspiratory pressure; V_{tspont}, spontaneous tidal volume indexed to body weight; V_t/T_i, mean inspiratory flow.
From Venkataraman ST, Khan N, Brown A. Validation of predictors of extubation success and failure in mechanically ventilated infants and children. Crit Care Med. 2000;282:991.

oxygen is sufficient treatment for children with mild symptoms. Nebulized racemic epinephrine (0.5 mL of a 2.25% solution in 2.5 mL of saline solution delivered intermittently or continuously) effectively relieves more severe upper airway obstruction in most children, probably by local vasoconstriction. Only the l-isomer in the racemic formulation is biologically active. Epinephrine available for cardiovascular use is as safe, effective, and less expensive if half the racemic dose is used. Following its use, edema may recur, so close observation must continue. The value of corticosteroids is more controversial, in part because most studies do not differentiate multiple causes of croup.[140-148] Patients at high risk for postextubation stridor (eg, those with multiple intubation attempts) appear most likely to benefit.[143-145] Dexamethasone (0.3 to 0.5 mg/kg every 6 hours for 1 or 2 days) is recommended in selected cases.

The work of breathing through a narrowed upper airway can be decreased by inhalation of a low-density gas mixture. Oxygen in helium is less dense than air or pure oxygen and permits higher inspiratory flow at lower resistance. Helium-oxygen mixtures are commercially available, usually providing 20% oxygen in 80% helium. More oxygen can be added to the mix as needed. Although traditional teaching holds that at least 70% helium is necessary to decrease airway resistance enough to make a clinical difference in the work of breathing, experience demonstrates value at considerably lower concentrations.

If pharmacologic treatment is ineffective, noninvasive ventilatory support may prevent the need for reintubation, but meticulous attention to the patient's work of breathing is critical to recognize potential catastrophic airway obstruction. Reintubation with a smaller tube for 12 to 24 hours may be necessary, and continued dexamethasone treatment and sedation to minimize agitation and further trauma to the airway may permit resolution of symptoms. Persistent symptoms are an indication for diagnostic laryngotracheobronchoscopy.

Complications of Endotracheal Intubation

Complications of intubation can be divided into those related to placement of the artificial airway, those that occur while the endotracheal tube is in place, and those related to extubation or appearing late (Table 129.5). Immediate complications usually are related to the underlying disease process, the physiologic effects of laryngoscopy and intubation and administration of positive pressure, or direct trauma to airway structures. The child's general condition, tube size, cuff pressure, movement, airway infection, systemic perfusion, duration of intubation, and attention to meticulous airway care are factors influencing the development of problems during maintenance of the airway.[149] Laryngospasm, aspiration, and failure (or inability) to deflate a cuff cause complications at extubation. Although laryngeal or tracheal injury may be obvious at the time of intubation, symptoms may be delayed 2 to 6 weeks.

Prolonged Intubation

The safe duration of endotracheal intubation in infants and children is not clear. Since the 1950s, the accepted period has increased from less than 12 hours to an undefined much longer period. Subglottic stenosis is reported to occur in 1% to 8% of infants after prolonged intubation, but a similar incidence has been noted after intubation for less than 1 week.[150] In older infants, children, and adults, it is becoming clear that there is no clear safe period. Complications can

TABLE 129.5   Complications of Endotracheal Intubation

Immediate	Maintenance	Extubation/Late
Physiologic		
Hemodynamic instability	Obstruction	Laryngospasm
Dysrhythmias	Sinusitis	Gagging, vomiting
Apnea	Otitis (similar to immediate)	Aspiration
↓ PAO_2		Sore throat
↑ $PaCO_2$		Dysphonia, aphonia
Coughing		
Laryngospasm		
Gagging, vomiting, regurgitation, aspiration		
↑ Intracranial pressure		
↑ Intraocular pressure		
Traumatic		
Nasal septum laceration, perforation	Lip, tongue ulceration	Laryngeal or tracheal granuloma
Nasal turbinate injury	Nares ulceration	Vocal cord paralysis
Tooth loss or injury	Palatal erosion, cleft formation	Subglottic stenosis
Lip, tongue, palate laceration, hematoma	Vocal cord edema, ulceration	
Tonsillar or adenoid avulsion, laceration, hematoma	Laryngeal and tracheal mucosal ischemia, ulceration, necrosis	
Laryngeal strictures	Recurrent laryngeal nerve damage	
Cervical spine subluxation	Subglottic edema, ulceration	
Malposition		
Esophageal	Main stem intubation	
Main stem bronchus	Inadvertent extubation	
Intracranial	Atelectasis	
Soft tissue		

occur immediately at intubation or may not be seen after many weeks or even months with an endotracheal tube in place.[151] The decision to switch to tracheostomy should not be based on an arbitrary time limit but rather on the relative advantages and disadvantages of one artificial airway over another in each individual patient.

Special Circumstances
Full Stomach

Patients with a full stomach are at high risk for aspiration of gastric contents during airway manipulation, particularly if protective airway reflexes are impaired. Much of the morbidity associated with aspiration can be attributed to the effects of acid aspiration. Aspiration of fluid with a pH below 1.8 is associated with a high incidence of severe pulmonary dysfunction and death. Aspiration of fluid with a pH between 1.8 and 2.5 produces symptoms of moderate severity. When fluid with a pH above 2.5 is aspirated, sequelae are less a consequence of the acid than of other characteristics of the material aspirated.[152] Other risk factors include the volume aspirated, the presence and nature of particulate food particles, contamination by bacterial pathogens, underlying pulmonary or systemic disease, and immunosuppression.[153]

Food particles may physically obstruct small or even large central airways, with the expected alterations in lung volume in segments distal to the obstruction. In addition, certain foods may cause severe local inflammatory changes. Bacterial contamination of the upper gastrointestinal tract secondary to bowel obstruction or even antacid administration greatly increases the risks of respiratory infection following aspiration.

Patients who have eaten shortly before intubation (<6 hours) should be assumed to have a full stomach. In addition, those with bowel obstruction, pharyngeal or upper gastrointestinal bleeding, trauma, or acute onset of illness within 6 hours of eating and those who are pregnant or who have ileus or tense abdominal distention from any cause should be considered to have a full stomach.

Although delaying airway manipulation might be the measure most certain to prevent aspiration, this approach is not a realistic option in most situations confronting the intensivist. In a conscious child, the volume of gastric contents can be minimized by suction through a relatively large-gauge nasogastric tube, but complete emptying of the stomach, particularly of large food particles and blood clots, is rarely possible. Although H_2 antagonists and proton pump inhibitors (PPIs) effectively decrease both the volume and acid content of gastric secretions, an adequate effect requires 60 to 90 minutes following administration of these agents. Antacid, H_2 blockers, and PPIs do not decrease the volume of gastric contents already present in the stomach. Anticholinergic agents such as atropine or glycopyrrolate also reduce gastric acidity but slowly and less effectively than the H_2 antagonists. In addition, they may decrease gastroesophageal sphincter tone and appear to have no value in preventing the acid aspiration syndrome.

Antacids can effectively neutralize gastric pH. However, when aspirated, particulate antacids (aluminum and magnesium hydroxides) produce inflammatory changes as severe as gastric acid and food particles. Clear antacids, such as sodium citrate or Alka-Seltzer, appear to provide true protection. They effectively increase gastric pH and, when aspirated, appear to produce damage no more severe than that caused by normal saline solution. However, their use has not become common clinical practice.[154]

Intubation is at once protective of the patient vulnerable to gastric aspiration and itself a risk to the patient. In an alert child with intact protective airway reflexes, it may be appropriate to pass a nasogastric tube to decrease the volume of gastric contents. A clear antacid (eg, sodium citrate, 10 to 30 mL) can be administered orally or through the tube, which then is removed. In a child with impaired reflexes, no effort to pass a nasogastric tube should be made because of the risk of inducing vomiting or regurgitation with subsequent aspiration.

The intensivist should examine the patient's airway to be as certain as possible that intubation will not be difficult, as discussed previously. If intubation likely will be straightforward, a rapid-sequence intubation is indicated (Box 129.4). The goal of this method of intubation is to minimize the likelihood of vomiting or regurgitation and the time between loss of protective reflexes and correct positioning of the endotracheal tube. The sequence consists of preoxygenation, administration of an intravenous sedative or anesthetic with immediate cricoid pressure, pharmacologic paralysis, and endotracheal intubation. Properly applied, cricoid pressure probably decreases the likelihood of insufflation of gas into the stomach or regurgitation of gastric contents into the trachea and may improve visualization of the larynx (see Fig. 129.9).[103,155-157] On the other hand, excessive pressure may actually increase the likelihood of vomiting, occlude the trachea, or make visualization more difficult.

The patient spontaneously breathes 100% oxygen by mask for 3 to 5 minutes before further manipulation. If the child can cooperate and has relatively normal gas exchange, four deep breaths provide a reasonable pulmonary reservoir of oxygen. However, in patients with severe pulmonary parenchymal disease, improvement in oxygenation may be limited and require a longer period of oxygenation.[158] If other factors in the child's condition permit, next steps in the rapid sequence intubation should be delayed until hemoglobin saturation reaches 100% or oxygenation reaches a plateau. Once preoxygenation is complete, the anesthetic or sedative is administered by rapid intravenous infusion, an assistant applies cricoid pressure immediately, and, as consciousness is lost, a muscle relaxant is given. The mask supplying oxygen is kept in place until the patient becomes apneic, but no effort to assist ventilation is made in order to avoid gastric distention and regurgitation. Once the patient is flaccid and apneic, the intensivist performs laryngoscopy and intubates the patient.

BOX 129.4 | **Rapid-Sequence Intubation for Full Stomach**

Indications

Food intake <4 to 6 hours before intubation
Pharyngeal or upper gastrointestinal bleeding
Intestinal obstruction or ileus (includes acute onset of illness)
Tense abdominal distention
Pregnancy

Relative Contraindications

"Difficult" airway
Profuse hemorrhage obscuring visualization
Upper airway obstruction
Increased intracranial pressure

Procedure

Prepare *all* necessary equipment, including suction devices
Allow patient to breathe 100% oxygen for 3 minutes
Direct assistant to apply cricoid pressure
Rapid intravenous infusion of anesthetic or sedative/analgesic and neuromuscular blocking agents
Allow patient to continue to breathe oxygen until apneic
Avoid manual ventilation to minimize gastric distention
Perform laryngoscopy and orotracheal intubation with stylet in endotracheal tube
Confirm endotracheal tube placement
Release cricoid pressure

Use of a stylet in the endotracheal tube facilitates rapid intubation. Only after correct tube position is verified and the tube cuff, if present, is inflated should cricoid pressure be relieved and manual ventilation begun. In the case of unexpected difficulty intubating the patient and evidence of progressive hypoxemia, manual ventilation between attempts may be necessary but should be done with continued cricoid pressure.

The classic combination of drugs used for rapid sequence induction/intubation is sodium thiopental (4 to 6 mg/kg) and succinylcholine (1 to 4 mg/kg) with a prior defasciculating dose of a nondepolarizing muscle relaxant such as vecuronium. In the absence of thiopental, alternative drugs include ketamine or a benzodiazepine alone or in combination with a short-acting narcotic. As previously discussed, etomidate has been a popular agent, but growing evidence suggests its use is inappropriate in patients with shock, especially with presumed sepsis. Succinylcholine has multiple undesirable adverse effects (as noted previously) that may include increased intragastric pressure. Most of the nondepolarizing relaxants, when given in amounts two to three times the usual intubating dose, produce good conditions for intubation nearly as quickly as does succinylcholine (60 to 90 seconds) and without adverse effects, but lasting longer. Rocuronium is the current best alternative, with its rapid onset and relatively short duration of action. Table 129.3 lists suggested drugs and doses.

Increased Intracranial Pressure and Neurologic Dysfunction

The intensivist is frequently called on to intubate children with severe central nervous system dysfunction resulting from infection, hemorrhage, trauma, hydrocephalus, or mass lesions, any of which may be associated with actual or imminent intracranial hypertension and herniation. In most circumstances the intensivist can observe signs of elevated ICP or recognize settings where the likelihood is high, but there is no clinical measure of its severity. Current guidelines recommend intubation for patients with a Glasgow Coma Scale score of 8 or less.[159] Intubation under these conditions should be undertaken with the recognition that it is a likely stimulus for further and potentially lethal intracranial hypertension. The most immediate means of lowering ICP involves decreasing CBF (volume) through hyperventilation. Unfortunately, the process of intubation likely will decrease minute ventilation and increase cerebral blood volume for this and other reasons, as previously discussed.

Under normal circumstances, CBF is closely coupled to the cerebral metabolic oxygen requirement ($CMRO_2$). Cerebral oxygen consumption and blood flow increase with increasing body temperature, motor activity, pain or other noxious stimuli, and seizure activity. Blood flow also increases rapidly when PaO_2 falls below 50 to 60 mm Hg and linearly as $PaCO_2$ increases over a wide range. With intact autoregulation, blood flow is independent of systemic blood pressure except at very high or low levels. However, when autoregulation is impaired, mean arterial pressure may affect CBF over a much broader range. Elevated intrathoracic pressure during struggling, coughing, or Valsalva maneuvers may impede jugular venous drainage and result in intracranial venous congestion.

Laryngoscopy and intubation are powerful noxious stimuli. In the awake unsedated child and even in the severely obtunded patient, laryngoscopy and intubation likely will precipitate vigorous struggle, coughing, pain (anxiety), and marked evidence of autonomic stimulation.[28,41,42,160] In most patients, sympathetic discharge predominates with tachycardia, hypertension, and diaphoresis. In the infant, vagal stimulation often predominates with resulting bradycardia.

Even in the lightly anesthetized patient, laryngoscopy itself and then intubation are associated with hypertension, tachycardia, and increased ICP. As might be predicted, massive surges in ICP are more likely to occur in patients suspected of having borderline or high baseline ICP before intubation than in those with intracranial pathology with well-compensated or previously controlled pressure. Arterial hypertension may precipitate further hemorrhage in the child with a vascular malformation, coagulopathy, or bleeding into a tumor. ICP waves may reduce cerebral perfusion pressure to ischemic levels or cause frank herniation.

Given the risk of life-threatening systemic and intracranial hypertension in these patients, it is clear that laryngoscopy and intubation should be undertaken with every effort to minimize stimulation and associated struggle.[105,161-163] In general, this implies ensuring excellent oxygenation, ventilation, and intubation under protection of profound sedation or anesthesia, with the assistance of neuromuscular blockade (Box 129.5). Neurologists and neurosurgeons are frequently loath to relinquish the opportunity to examine the patient following intubation, but the risk of life-threatening intracranial hypertension justifies temporarily obscuring the neurologic examination. In most cases, adequate assessment is possible before intubation, and diagnostic studies require deep sedation for a period afterward.

The patient is provided 100% oxygen by bag and mask. An anesthetic or sedative agent in combination with a neuromuscular blocking agent is given, and manual ventilation is initiated to lower ICP as much as possible before airway manipulation. Although extreme hyperventilation may decrease CBF to ischemic levels, current guidelines support ventilation to a $PaCO_2$ of approximately 30 to 35 mm Hg for patients with intracranial hypertension.[164]

BOX 129.5 Intubation for Increased Intracranial Pressure

- Prepare equipment
- Monitor heart rate, blood pressure, and arterial oxygen saturation
- Provide 100% oxygen and assisted ventilation as tolerated by patient
- Consider possible difficult airway
- If no airway contraindications, administer anesthetic and neuromuscular blocking agents
- No associated cardiovascular compromise or hypovolemia:
  - Midazolam (0.2–0.3 mg/kg IV) and fentanyl (5–10 µg/kg IV) plus lidocaine (1–1.5 mg/kg IV) and rocuronium (0.6–1.2 mg/kg IV) or other relaxant; consider etomidate (0.3 mg/kg IV)
- Concern for associated cardiovascular compromise or hypovolemia
  - Consider omitting benzodiazepine
- Thiopental (4–6 mg/kg IV) plus lidocaine (1 mg/kg IV), plus rocuronium (0.6–1.2 mg/kg IV) or other relaxant
- Ventilate patient until drug effect achieved (consider short-term hyperventilation in patients with signs of critically elevated intracranial pressure)
- Perform laryngoscopy and orotracheal intubation

IV, intravenous.

In the hemodynamically stable patient, relatively deep anesthesia is associated with a decline in $CMRO_2$, CBF, and ICP, provided that oxygenation and ventilation are well maintained.[161,163] Agents include narcotic analgesics alone or in combination with a benzodiazepine. Although the hemodynamic effects of narcotics (typically fentanyl) are usually modest, the effect on $CMRO_2$ is also limited unless given in anesthetic doses. Addition of a benzodiazepine further decreases $CMRO_2$ but may be associated with hemodynamic instability, especially in hypovolemic trauma patients.

Etomidate is widely used in patients with suspected intracranial hypertension. Its ability to decrease CBF without apparent detrimental effect on systemic hemodynamic stability makes it a useful agent, although concerns about its effect on adrenal function, perhaps even following a single dose, require caution in the patient with sepsis or shock. Because it lacks analgesic properties, combining it with an intravenous narcotic agent should be considered.

Lidocaine, 1 to 1.5 mg/kg, decreases $CMRO_2$ and modestly decreases the systemic and intracranial hypertensive response and the cough reflex, as long as a dose below the seizure-producing threshold is used. Effective serum concentrations are obtained more quickly and at lower doses by the intravenous route than when the agent is administered endotracheally. The available literature addresses patients fully premedicated and monitored undergoing neurosurgical procedures or patients already intubated, ventilated, and monitored in the ICU. Studies addressing intubation in the acute setting are lacking and unlikely to be accomplished.[164-168]

Although the classic recommendation has been to avoid ketamine in patients with elevated ICP because of its potential to further increase pressure, newer studies suggest that ketamine may be safe in this population. It does, however, increase systemic blood pressure and CBF and most likely should be avoided in patients at risk of failed autoregulation until further evidence is available.[89-90,169-171] In addition, evidence that ketamine is associated with neuronal injury in immature animal models supports continued caution with respect to its use in patients with elevated intracranial pressure.

In nearly all patients, orotracheal intubation is preferred because it is accomplished quickly and easily with less risk of prolonged manipulation and interrupted ventilation. Nasotracheal intubation is contraindicated in patients with basilar skull fractures and CSF leaks as a potential source of infection or even perforation of the cribriform plate and intracranial tube placement.

Cervical Spine Instability

Flexion and extension of the head on the neck occur between the atlas (C1) and the basiocciput. Rotation occurs between the atlas and axis (C2), as the thin arch of the atlas pivots around the odontoid process. Below the axis, the cervical vertebrae articulate with each other anteriorly at the intervertebral discs and posteriorly at the facet joints. Further neck flexion and extension occur at these joints. Anterior and posterior ligaments complete the stable spine.

Spinal cord injury generally occurs as a result of bony fracture, compression, or disruption of cervical ligaments. In young children, actual ligamentous disruption or bony fracture is not necessary for severe cord injury, even transection, to occur; extreme stretching, as may occur in acceleration or deceleration injury, is sufficient.[172-174] Instability results from

disruption of both the anterior and posterior columns. Congenital or degenerative anatomic abnormalities, penetrating wounds, or expanding mass lesions in the spinal canal may compromise cord integrity.

During routine intubation, the intensivist flexes the neck and extends the head. In children with known or suspected cervical spine injury or instability resulting from other causes (eg, Down syndrome or rheumatoid arthritis), manipulating the head and neck for intubation risks extending the existing condition or injury and may precipitate new problems. Cervical spine films and knowledge about the nature of the traumatic event help define the precise injury and predict maneuvers most likely to do harm, but such information rarely is complete and may be falsely reassuring.

The ideal approach to intubation in this setting is controversial.[175-178] Although evidence in cadavers, in addition to common sense, indicates that typical airway maneuvers can cause anterior or posterior subluxation or widening of the disc space, evidence in patients is lacking.[179] Axial traction increases distraction and even subluxation in some patients[179]; in others traction is helpful. However, information about the appropriate amount of force or the correct plane in which it should be applied is rarely sufficient to make a timely informed decision. Therefore immobilization of the head and neck in the midline without traction is recommended.[180]

Current advanced trauma life support guidelines no longer recommend blind nasotracheal intubation.[181,182] Orotracheal intubation is more reliably accomplished and less time consuming than blind nasotracheal intubation and is associated with far fewer complications, including tube malposition and bleeding, even in adults.[183] The high anterior location of the pediatric larynx makes nasotracheal intubation even more difficult in young children. As a result, it is rarely a necessary or desirable choice for emergency airway stabilization in children.

Just as manipulation of the airway for intubation may risk additional cord injury, patient movement can cause additional damage. Few children of any age will tolerate awake intubation by any route without violent struggle. Even heavily sedated patients likely will cough upon stimulation of the airway.

Patients with spinal cord injuries are at risk for extreme hyperkalemia and resulting dysrhythmias or cardiac arrest following administration of succinylcholine. This response occurs from approximately 48 hours to 6 to 9 months after injury. Cervical injury often also disrupts sympathetic nervous system outflow and results in unopposed vagal tone and severe bradycardia. For these reasons, in most instances intubation is best accomplished in these patients via the orotracheal route, using an intravenous anesthetic or combination of sedative and analgesic agents, atropine, and a nondepolarizing neuromuscular blocking agent with an assistant immobilizing the head and neck in neutral position with one hand over the ear on each side of the head. If time, equipment, and available expertise permit, fiberoptic bronchoscopy may assist visualization of the larynx and intubation with minimal head or neck movement.[184] Video laryngoscopy has been helpful in adults, but experience is limited in children.

If orotracheal or nasotracheal intubation cannot be accomplished because of associated facial or airway injuries or other technical obstacles, cricothyrotomy or primary tracheotomy may be indicated. However, no data support either the necessity or safety of routinely using a surgical approach before attempting orotracheal intubation.

Upper Airway Obstruction

Upper airway obstruction may result from many disorders (see Chapter 50). When symptoms are related to loss of oropharyngeal muscle tone, changing the patient's position, reversing the effects of a drug, or placing a nasal airway may be sufficient, if the duration of the underlying process likely will be brief. However, when airway structures likely are severely or progressively distorted by edema, inflammation, trauma, or another space-occupying process, achieving an endotracheal airway is necessary.

Patients should be allowed to assume whatever position is most comfortable. Supplemental oxygen is provided at the maximum concentration possible, but a young child's anxiety should not be heightened with an overly aggressive approach with a mask. Contrary to popular belief, breathing can be assisted in nearly all cases by application of positive pressure, initially with continuous positive airway pressure and then gradually with assisted breaths.

In general, no action should be taken that compromises the child's ability to breathe spontaneously until the capacity to control ventilation is certain. In particular, use of neuromuscular blocking agents is dangerous and inappropriate until after the airway is controlled. Distortion of the airway may be so extreme that recognition of landmarks for intubation is impossible, and loss of pharyngeal tone in such patients may remove the last barrier to complete airway occlusion. However, reducing a child's anxiety with cautious sedation (with a reversible agent) may decrease peak inspiratory flow rate and symptoms of obstruction and make it easier to assist breathing and establish an artificial airway. When possible the child is gently lowered to a supine position (or to 30 degrees) and intubated by the orotracheal route. When time and available expertise permit, intubation in the operating room using an inhalational anesthetic in a high oxygen concentration allows spontaneous breathing until the patient is deeply anesthetized and untroubled by airway manipulation. This method may be especially helpful in cases of supraglottitis. In most cases, the proper tube size is 0.5 to 1 mm smaller in diameter than predicted for age because of airway inflammation and edema, and no leak will be present.

Extubation usually is well tolerated when a leak has developed.

Facial and Laryngotracheal Injury

Children with facial injuries present airway problems nearly as varied as the injuries themselves. Appropriate management depends primarily on accurate assessment of airway patency at presentation, the rate of bleeding (if any) into the airway, and the amount of additional swelling and distortion likely to occur later. Evaluation of possible ocular and intracranial injury must proceed simultaneously.

Profuse bleeding, unstable facial fractures, or aspiration of blood, gastric contents, or teeth causes early respiratory distress. Maxillary fractures may result in a free-floating maxilla with occlusion of the nasopharynx and pressure on the tongue. Isolated mandibular fractures often cause trismus but rarely cause airway obstruction or interfere with visualization of the larynx.

Airway management begins with suctioning blood and debris from the mouth and pharynx. If permitted by other injuries, the child is placed with the head down and turned to the side. The tongue and maxilla are pulled forward manually if necessary. A spontaneously breathing patient receives oxygen by mask and may not require further intervention before surgery. Patients with persistent obstruction may require an immediate artificial airway.

In most cases, orotracheal intubation is accomplished first. If ventilation can be assisted with bag and mask and bleeding is controlled, the patient may be sedated, paralyzed, and intubated with full stomach precautions. If bag-mask ventilation exacerbates airway obstruction, awake intubation may be necessary. Uncontrollable bleeding, inability to visualize the larynx, or violent struggle in a child with cervical spine instability or evidence of increased ICP may make a primary tracheostomy desirable. Nasotracheal and nasogastric tubes are avoided until the possibility of a basilar skull fracture and CSF leak is eliminated.

Laryngotracheal injuries may be subtle or dramatic. They should be suspected in children with a history of anterior neck trauma and often cause hoarseness, stridor, subcutaneous emphysema, pneumothorax, or pneumomediastinum. Aerosolized epinephrine may temporarily decrease swelling and provide a little extra time to evaluate the airway and plan intervention. Awake intubation with cautious sedation and topical anesthesia that is conducted under direct vision by laryngoscopy or fiberoptic bronchoscopy minimizes the risk of sudden, complete obstruction or creation of a false passage adjacent to the airway.

Open Globe Injury

Children with penetrating eye injuries may require emergency intubation for respiratory failure resulting from associated injuries or other underlying problems. Management in these cases seeks to prevent increased intraocular pressure with subsequent extrusion of the vitreous and permanent blindness. Intraocular pressure can be increased by struggling, crying, coughing, straining, or rubbing the eye. Hypoxia and hypercarbia can increase intraocular pressure. In general, central nervous system depressants lower intraocular pressure, with the possible exception of ketamine. Intubation should be performed smoothly under full muscle relaxation if possible, taking into consideration associated injuries and the risk of a full stomach.

The child should be preoxygenated with 100% oxygen, taking care not to apply pressure to the eye with the mask. Efforts to empty the stomach are delayed until the patient is fully relaxed and intubated. In hemodynamically stable patients, rapidly acting sedatives or anesthetics are administered, followed by a nondepolarizing neuromuscular blocking agent if other airway anatomy permits. Succinylcholine, a depolarizing relaxant, has been associated with increased intraocular pressure, even in the absence of fasciculations. As in patients with head trauma, a combination of sedative and analgesic agents may replace thiopental if hemodynamic stability is uncertain. Lidocaine supplements the effect of other agents in blunting the rise in intraocular pressure that may occur even during a smooth intubation. Heavy sedation or paralysis should be maintained following intubation until after repair.

Alternative Approaches to the Airway

Lighted Intubation Stylet (Light Wand)—Assisted Intubation

A number of lighted intubation stylets have become available. Each uses transillumination of the neck to guide placement of an endotracheal tube. The devices consist of a handle containing the power source and a malleable wand (stylet) with a light at the tip. Pediatric versions accommodate tubes as small as 3.5 mm.

Use of the lighted stylet for intubation is a technique recommended for use in patients with airways that are difficult to manage. Reported experience in children is limited, but the technique has been successful in the hands of both highly skilled and novice operators.[185-189] The equipment is fairly simple to use and easy to learn. It does not require visualization of the airway, is less stimulating than laryngoscopy, allows nasal or oral intubation, and is portable and relatively inexpensive. Reported series indicate that mucosal and dental injuries are uncommon, and sore throat is less of a problem than following standard laryngoscopy.[190] Because intubation may be accomplished from the patient's side, it may be useful in awkward settings such as emergency transport vehicles.

Potential disadvantages include trauma to the upper airway and larynx. Anything that obscures transmission of light through the anterior neck interferes with its use, including scarring, massive edema, subcutaneous emphysema, or mass lesions. Profuse bleeding or thick airway secretions that obscure the bulb also interfere with effective use.

A lubricated lighted stylet is inserted through an endotracheal tube of desired size until the light is just short of the end of the tube, and the tube is firmly attached. The tube and stylet are bent to approximately 90 degrees, just proximal to the cuff if present. Dimming the room lights improves appreciation of the transillumination. The intubator may stand at the head of the bed or to the side of the patient. The head is extended. A shoulder roll may be useful. The intubator pulls the mandible and tongue forward and upward, and the styletted tube is introduced into the patient's mouth in the midline. It is advanced into the pharynx, while the operator observes transillumination of the soft tissues of the neck. Entry into the airway typically is recognized by the presence of a focused glow of light in the midline below the thyroid prominence; more diffuse light suggests esophageal placement. The tube is advanced until the light is at the level of the sternal notch. The lighted stylet is withdrawn and tube placement is confirmed with capnography.

Nasal intubation is possible with the light wand. In this case, the trocar is removed to increase the flexibility of the device. When a glow is noted above the thyroid prominence, the tube is likely in the vallecula. The epiglottis can be moved out of the way with a jaw thrust, allowing further advancement of the tube into the trachea. An alternative is to flex the patient's neck, as is sometimes necessary with visualized nasotracheal intubation.

Laryngeal Mask Airway

The laryngeal mask airway (LMA) is a relatively new and fairly safe means of securing a difficult to manage airway in an infant or child.[191-193] It was designed to provide a supraglottic airway device that would offer the benefit of noninvasive ventilation. Its use rapidly gained acceptance in anesthesiology and has been incorporated into the American Academy of Anesthesiology difficult airway algorithm.[52] It consists of a small mask with an inflatable rim and a tube with a universal adaptor, which permits attachment to a resuscitation or anesthesia bag or ventilator (Fig. 129.11). The original LMA consists of a wide-bore tube designed to sit in the hypopharynx and is attached to an inflatable bowl-shaped base that bypasses the tongue, sits around the epiglottis, conforms to the shape of the larynx, and provides a low-pressure seal around the supraglottic area.[194] The LMA is available in a wide range of sizes, allowing use in very small infants to very large

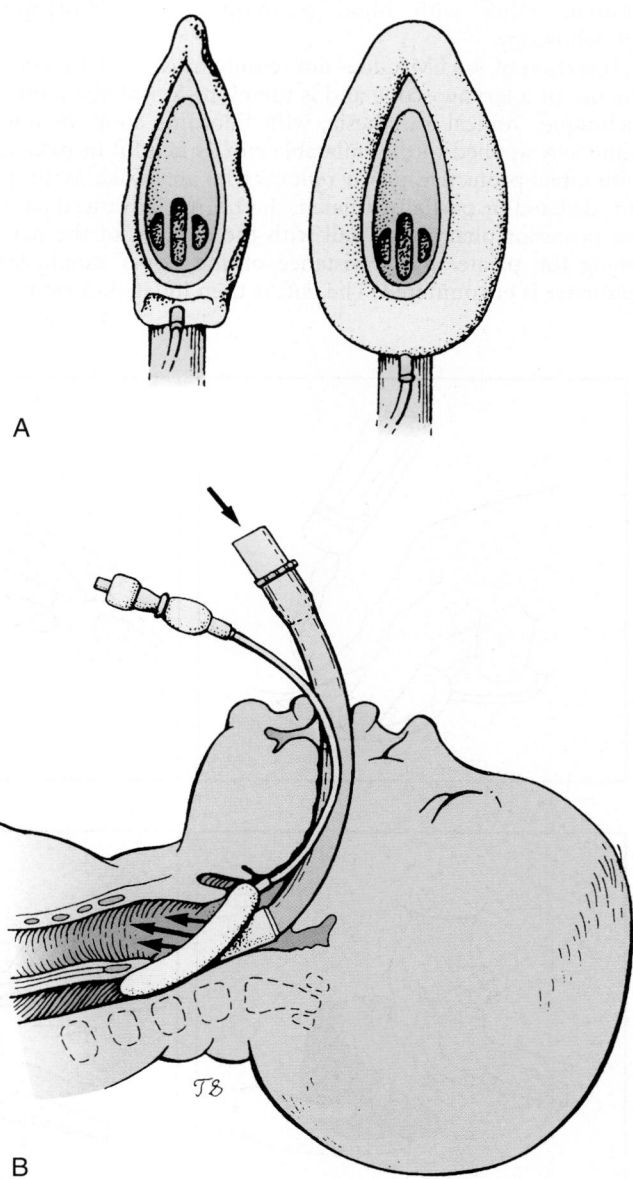

Fig. 129.11. LMA. (A) Mask portion of the airway with the rim deflated for insertion *(left)* and inflated *(right)*. (B) LMA in position, with the rim inflated around the laryngeal inlet. (From Efrat R, Kadari A, Katz S. The laryngeal mask airway in pediatric anesthesia: experience with 120 patients undergoing elective groin surgery. J Pediatr Surg 1994;29:206.)

adolescents and adults. Choice of LMA size is based on weight: size 1 for patients weighing 2.5 to 6 kg, size 2 for patients weighing 6 to 30 kg, and size 3 for patients weighing more than 30 kg.[195,196] Since the initial development of the LMA, several other types have been designed, including the flexible LMA, intubating LMA, disposable LMA, and ProSeal LMA, not all of which are available in pediatric sizes.[197]

The insertion technique can be learned quickly by physicians and other providers, including emergency transport personnel, often more quickly than endotracheal intubation. Experience with a mannequin appears to be effective training. Once in place, the LMA can serve as a means of ventilating the patient until the desired definitive airway can be established. It can facilitate subsequent tracheal intubation, if desired, either with blind technique or via fiberoptic bronchoscopy.

Insertion of the LMA does not require muscle relaxation or the use of a laryngoscope and is therefore considered a blind technique. Topical anesthesia, with lidocaine spray or lidocaine jelly applied to the inflatable rim, is helpful in patients with intact protective airway reflexes who are awake. With the rim deflated or partially inflated, the LMA is advanced along the posterior pharyngeal wall with the dorsum of the mask facing the palate until resistance of the upper esophageal sphincter is encountered. The cuff is then inflated, forming a seal around the laryngeal outlet, and the attached tube is connected to a source of oxygen and positive pressure (Fig. 129.12).

Proper placement is essential but is most uncertain in infants requiring the LMA size 1, most likely because the margin of error for placement in the small pharynx is so small. In general, the risk of downfolding the epiglottis, thus occluding the trachea, is greater in children than in adults. Successful placement depends on the shape and tone of the pharynx, adequate matching of the cuff, the palatopharyngeal curve and shape of the posterior pharynx, the extent to which anterior structures (such as tonsils) obliterate the curve, the position of the head and neck, the efficacy of digital manipulation, and the depth of anesthesia/sedation, muscle relaxation, or loss of airway reflexes.[194] Tissue trauma is uncommon, and the need to manipulate the cervical spine during placement is minimal. In most patients the autonomic response to placement is less pronounced than with laryngoscopy and intubation. On the other hand, the device does not fully protect against aspiration in the setting of a full stomach. In addition, it may not be effective in patients with glottic or subglottic pathology.

Although its primary use is in the operating room, growing experience demonstrates that the LMA can be lifesaving in a variety of other settings when no other nonsurgical means of

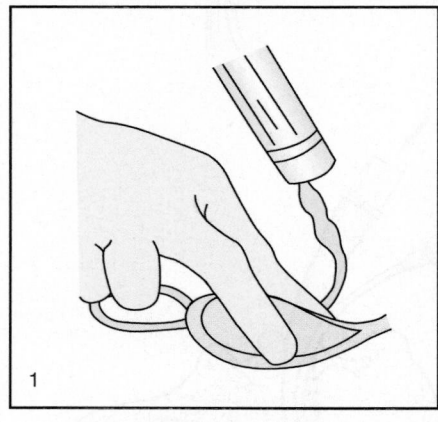
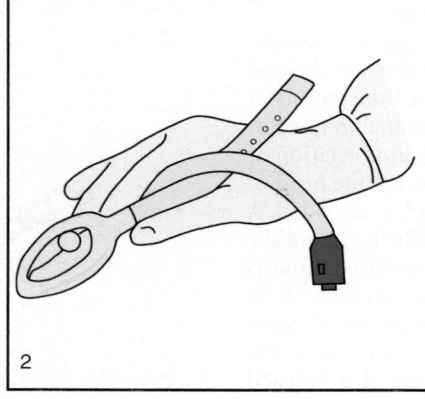
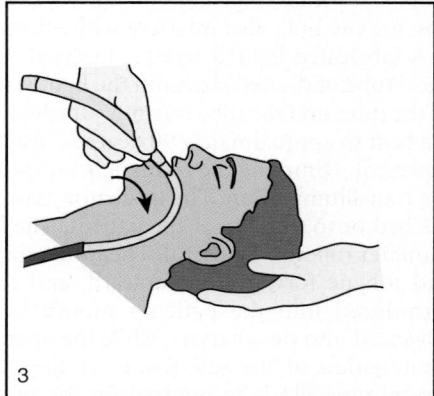
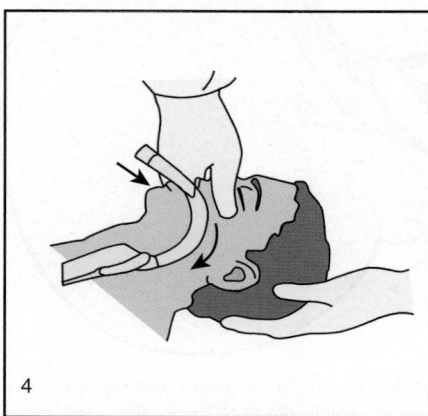
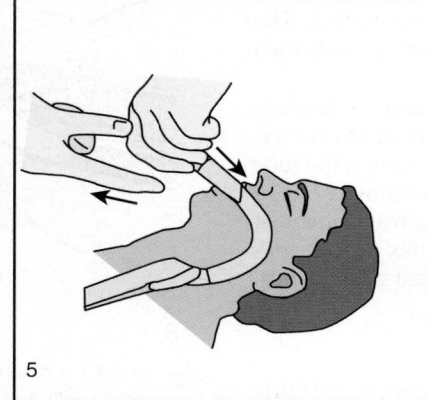
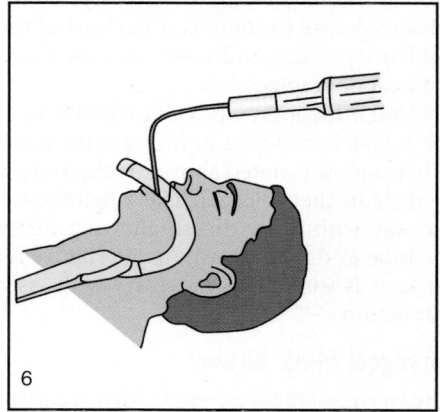

Fig. 129.12. Inserting the LMA. Preoxygenate the patient as necessary. *1,* Deflate the cuff against a flat surface with index finger and middle finger on either side of the bowl. *2,* Hold the LMA like a pen, with the index finger at the junction of the tube and mask. *3 and 4,* Insert the LMA into the mouth and advance, following the palate and posterior pharyngeal wall until resistance is met. *5,* Let go of the mask and tube. *6,* Inflate the cuff, allowing the device to move into correct position. (Adapted from Ambulance technician study, http://www.ambulancetechnicianstudy.co.uk/.)

maintaining an airway is successful, particularly in patients with anatomically abnormal airways.[198] Success with airway management in the operating room with children with airways that are anticipated to be difficult to manage, including patients with Pierre Robin, Treacher Collins, and Goldenhar syndromes, suggests that the LMA would be valuable for managing such patients in emergency settings such as the emergency department or ICU. The ease and rapidity of insertion and decreased gastric air insufflation during resuscitation make it a valuable tool when intubation fails during adult resuscitation.[199] Pediatric Advanced Life Support incorporates the LMA as an effective alternative to intubation during resuscitation when inserted by trained providers.[200] In neonatal resuscitation, when facemask ventilation or intubation is not successful, the LMA provides a means of rapidly improving oxygenation and heart rate. It is not, however, effective for aspirating meconium and may be inadequate for infants with severely noncompliant lungs. Use by prehospital personnel has been effective for critically ill adults, but experience in children in the field has not been reported.[201,202]

Patients with intact protective reflexes poorly tolerate the LMA, so its use is largely limited to those with severely depressed levels of consciousness or heavy sedation or anesthesia. Lidocaine jelly on the inflatable rim or lidocaine pharyngeal spray may promote tolerance in patients with active airway reflexes. A disadvantage with use of the LMA is the inability to use airway pressures greater than approximately 20 mm Hg to prevent air leaking around the mask and to avoid gastric distention, and therefore it is not an optimal airway device in patients with severe subglottic airway obstruction, parenchymal disease requiring high ventilatory pressures, or in obese persons.[203] It also is not the ideal technique to use in a patient with a full stomach because its design does not prohibit aspiration of gastric contents. However, in an emergency situation the benefit of providing oxygenation and ventilation via an LMA outweighs the risk of an aspiration event. Other scenarios that may limit placement of the LMA include excessive neck extension, limited mouth opening, or excessive application of cricoid pressure.[203]

Although the seal is somewhat protective, patients with a full stomach remain at risk for aspiration. Positive airway pressure should be minimized as much as possible and a nasogastric tube passed to decrease gastric distention. Cricoid pressure may further decrease the risk of aspiration but also may interfere with proper LMA placement. If desired, an endotracheal tube can be inserted through the mask, either blindly or with fiberoptic bronchoscopy.[204,205]

Tracheostomy

Indications for tracheostomy include structural abnormalities of the upper airway requiring surgery, laryngeal trauma or complex craniofacial injury, severe facial burns, congenital anomalies lacking surgical treatment, vocal cord paralysis, and iatrogenic injury to the upper airway. Severe chronic neurologic dysfunction with impaired protective reflexes is an additional indication. Even in the absence of evidence of upper airway damage, tracheostomy may be performed to provide a more comfortable airway, which simultaneously allows airway protection, respiratory support, and greater patient mobility so that nutritional, developmental, and psychosocial needs may be met, especially, but not only, in patients undergoing chronic ventilation.[206-209]

Tracheostomy spares laryngeal and subglottic structures from the trauma of an artificial airway, particularly in active or thrashing patients. Tracheostomy tubes are less likely to be inadvertently dislodged or to become obstructed, but if either problem occurs early following tracheostomy, it is more likely to be catastrophic. Because the tube is inserted below the cricoid ring, it often is possible to use a larger tracheostomy tube than endotracheal tube. Nevertheless, a larger leak around the tube may interfere markedly with effective ventilation in patients requiring high airway pressures.

Complications in the early postoperative period include bleeding, subcutaneous air dissection, pneumothorax, pneumomomediastinum, injury to the recurrent laryngeal nerve, and death, usually as a consequence of loss of control of the airway intraoperatively or an unrecognized complication from the preceding list. Nearly all pediatric patients can and should be intubated before tracheostomy. Prior intubation decreases the incidence of most technical problems. Exceptions include patients with complex facial or airway injuries or deformities and those in whom no other means of establishing an airway have been successful. Wound colonization occurs rapidly. Bacterial infection may occur, rarely involving major cervical and mediastinal structures. Swallowing difficulty is common and may result from the tube and fixation tapes limiting excursion of the larynx. Aspiration may result from alteration of the laryngeal closure reflex.

Tracheostomy tube obstruction or accidental dislodgment is suspected when the patient becomes agitated and shows signs of increased respiratory distress, a suction catheter no longer passes freely, manual ventilation is ineffective, or, in case of dislodgment, the child is suddenly able to vocalize. In such cases the tube should be removed and replaced with a new one. The child is placed supine with the head and neck extended. Oxygen is delivered to the nose, mouth, and tracheal stoma. If manual ventilation is necessary, the stoma can be occluded to allow bag-mask ventilation as previously described. A fresh tracheostomy tube is inserted, initially directly posteriorly and then caudad. Replacement with a smaller tube or endotracheal tube may be necessary if resistance is encountered. Resistance to passage of a suction catheter or ineffective ventilation following replacement of a tracheostomy tube, particularly in the first 7 to 10 days postoperatively, is highly suggestive of creation of a "false passage" in a tissue plane outside the tracheal lumen. Reestablishing tracheal cannulation may require surgical intervention. Life-threatening pneumothorax or pneumomediastinum occurs frequently in such patients.

Late complications include granuloma or stricture formation at the stoma or where the tip of the tube meets the tracheal wall. Persistent posterior wall pressure may cause tracheoesophageal fistula formation. Erosion into the innominate artery is another rare occurrence, usually when the tracheostomy incision is below the third tracheal ring. The importance of an experienced, well-trained staff immediately available to address problems is supported by data demonstrating that mortality related to tracheostomy is significantly lower when performed in a children's hospital and decreases with increasing volume.[210]

Decannulation occurs when the indications for tracheostomy are no longer present. Diagnostic laryngotracheobronchoscopy before a planned decannulation permits identification of problems likely to interfere with effective breathing, including granulation tissue, severely stenotic areas, or vocal cord abnormalities. If none is present, the indwelling tube is replaced with successively smaller tubes until the smallest available is in place and the child is breathing well. If no distress occurs, the tube is removed and the stoma is covered.

Cricothyrotomy and Retrograde Intubation

Although airway management by endotracheal intubation is possible and endotracheal intubation is the appropriate first choice in the majority of pediatric patients, intubation is not possible or should not be done on certain occasions. Such situations include massive facial trauma, oropharyngeal hemorrhage or presence of a foreign body, or severe upper airway obstruction.[211] Cricothyrotomy is an alternative to tracheostomy for rapidly establishing an airway in apneic or severely distressed patients.

The child's head and neck are extended with a roll under the shoulders. The cricothyroid membrane is palpated between the inferior margin of the thyroid cartilage and the superior edge of the cricoid cartilage. With one hand (or an assistant) stabilizing the larynx and trachea, the clinician punctures the membrane in the midline with a large angiocatheter, withdraws the stylet, and connects the catheter to a source of oxygen using the connector to a size 3 endotracheal tube. Kits are available that facilitate cricothyrotomy using the Seldinger technique. Oxygenation is rapidly improved in spontaneously breathing patients, but carbon dioxide elimination is minimal. Transtracheal jet ventilation is effective through such catheters, provided that the upper airway permits passive exhalation; otherwise, severe hyperinflation and life-threatening barotrauma are certain.

Retrograde intubation can be accomplished by this approach. Once the cricothyroid membrane has been punctured and the catheter has been placed in the tracheal lumen, a long wire from a vascular access kit is advanced cephalad into the mouth. With the wire firmly secure, an ETT may be advanced into the trachea. Once the tube is in the tracheal lumen, the wire is withdrawn and the tube is further advanced into the desired position. If the wire is insufficiently stiff to permit passage of the tube into the trachea, an ETT exchanger can be advanced over the wire first, followed by the ETT.

In adults and adolescents, a small horizontal incision over the cricothyroid membrane is an alternative approach. Once the membrane is incised, it is spread vertically, and a standard tracheostomy or ETT is inserted into the tracheal lumen. This approach is not recommended in infants and young children except in highly skilled hands because of the potential for grave injury to a small, soft trachea or nearby neurovascular structures.

Complications are similar to those of tracheostomy. Complication rates of 10% to 40% are reported in adults.[184] Few experiences have been reported in pediatric patients, particularly in younger children.

Key References

6. Tobias JD. Pediatric airway anatomy may not be what we thought: implications for clinical practice and the use of cuffed endotracheal tubes. *Paediatr Anaesth.* 2015;2:9-19.
16. Field S, Kelly SM, Macklem PT. The oxygen cost of breathing in patients with cardiorespiratory disease. *Am Rev Respir Dis.* 1982;126:9.
29. Kovac AL. Controlling the hemodynamic response to laryngoscopy and endotracheal intubation. *J Clin Anesth.* 1996;8:63-79.
40. Patel R, Lenczyk M, Hannallah RS, McGill WA. Age and onset of desaturation in apnoeic children. *Can J Anaesth.* 1994;41:771-774.
48. Sullivan KJ, Kissoon N. Securing the child's airway in the emergency department. *Pediatr Emerg Care.* 2002;18:108-121.
51. Nykiel-Bailey SM, McAllister JD, Schrock CR, et al. Difficult airway consultation service for children: steps to implement and preliminary results. *Paediatr Anaesth.* 2015;25:363-371.
55. Newth CJ, Rachman B, Patel N, et al. The use of cuffed versus uncuffed endotracheal tubes in pediatric intensive care. *J Pediatr.* 2004;144:333-337.
56. Shi F, Xiao Y, Xiong W, et al. Cuffed versus uncuffed endotracheal tubes in children: a meta-analysis. *J Anesth.* 2016;30:3-11.
57. Litman RS, Maxwell LG. Cuffed versus un-cuffed endotracheal tubes in pediatric anesthesia: the debate should finally end. *Anesthesiology.* 2013;118:500-501.
58. Fine GF, Borland LM. The future of the cuffed endotracheal tube. *Paediatr Anaesth.* 2004;14:38-42.
60. Bledsoe GH, Schexnayder SM. Pediatric rapid sequence intubation: a review. *Pediatr Emerg Care.* 2004;20:339-344.
61. McAllister JD, Gnauck KA. Rapid sequence intubation of the pediatric patient. Fundamentals of practice. *Pediatr Clin North Am.* 1999;46:1249-1284.
66. Shaffner DH. The continuing controversy about the use of atropine before laryngoscopy and tracheal intubation in children. *Pediatr Crit Care Med.* 2013;14:651-653.
67. American Heart Association. *Pediatric Advanced Life Support (PALS) Provider Manual (Professional).* American Heart Association; 2011:205-206.
73. Annane D. ICU physicians should abandon the use of etomidate! *Intensive Care Med.* 2005;31:325-326.
77. Jabre P, Combes X, Lapostolle F, et al. Etomidate versus ketamine for rapid sequence intubation in acutely ill patients: a multicentre randomised controlled trial. *Lancet.* 2009;374:293-300.
81. Chan CM, Mitchell AL, Shorr AF. Etomidate is associated with mortality and adrenal insufficiency in sepsis: a meta-analysis. *Crit Care Med.* 2012;40:2945-2953.
89. Zeiler FA, Teitelbaum J, West M, Gillman LM. The ketamine effect on ICP in traumatic brain injury. *Neurocrit Care.* 2014;21:163-173.
90. Zeiler FA, Teitelbaum J, West M, Gillman LM. The ketamine effect on intracranial pressure in nontraumatic neurological illness. *J Crit Care.* 2014;29:1096-1106.
100. Wheeler DS, Vaux KK, Ponaman ML, et al. The safe and effective use of propofol sedation in children undergoing diagnostic and therapeutic procedures: experience in a pediatric ICU and a review of the literature. *Pediatr Emerg Care.* 2003;19:385-392.
102. Bray RJ. Propofol infusion syndrome in children. *Paediatr Anaesth.* 1998;8:491-499.
108. Stoddart PA, Mather SJ. Onset of neuromuscular blockade and intubating conditions one minute after the administration of rocuronium in children. *Paediatr Anaesth.* 1998;8:37-40.
114. Martyn JA, Richtsfeld M. Succinylcholine-induced hyperkalemia in acquired pathologic states: etiologic factors and molecular mechanisms. *Anesthesiology.* 2006;104:158-169.
118. Benumof JL, Dagg R, Benumof R. Critical hemoglobin desaturation will occur before return to an unparalyzed state following 1 mg/kg intravenous succinylcholine. *Anesthesiology.* 1997;87:979-982.
119. Baillard C, Fosse JP, Sebbane M, et al. Noninvasive ventilation improves preoxygenation before intubation of hypoxic patients. *Am J Respir Crit Care Med.* 2006;174:171-177.
120. Moynihan RJ, Brock-Utne JG, Archer JH, et al. The effect of cricoid pressure on preventing gastric insufflation in infants and children. *Anesthesiology.* 1993;78:652.
121. Phipps LM, Thomas NJ, Gilmore RK, et al. Prospective assessment of guidelines for determining appropriate depth of endotracheal tube placement in children. *Pediatr Crit Care Med.* 2005;6:519-522.
126. Kim JT, Na HS, Bae JY, et al. GlideScope video laryngoscope: a randomized clinical trial in 203 paediatric patients. *Br J Anaesth.* 2008;101:531-534.
136. Venkataraman ST, Khan N, Brown A. Validation of predictors of extubation success and failure in mechanically ventilated infants and children. *Crit Care Med.* 2000;28:2991-2996.
137. Wratney AT, Benjamin DK Jr, Slonim AD, et al. The endotracheal tube air leak test does not predict extubation outcome in critically ill pediatric patients. *Pediatr Crit Care Med.* 2008;9:490-496.
139. Koka BV, Jean IS, Andre JM, et al. Post-intubation croup in children. *Anesth Analg.* 1977;56:501.

145. Khemani RG, Randolph A, Markovitz B. Corticosteroids for the prevention and treatment of post-extubation stridor in neonates, children and adults. *Cochrane Database Syst Rev.* 2009;(3):CD001000.

147. Khemani RG, Randolph A, Markovitz B. Steroids for post extubation stridor: pediatric evidence is still inconclusive. *Intensive Care Med.* 2010;36:1276-1277.

153. Schwartz DJ, Wynne JW, Gibbs CP, et al. The pulmonary consequences of aspiration of gastric contents at pH values greater than 2.5. *Am Rev Respir Dis.* 1980;21:119.

154. American Society of Anesthesiologists Committee. Practice guidelines for preoperative fasting and the use of pharmacologic agents to reduce the risk of pulmonary aspiration: application to healthy patients undergoing elective procedures: an updated report by the American Society of Anesthesiologists Committee on Standards and Practice Parameters. *Anesthesiology.* 2011;114:495-511.

159. Adelson PD, Bratton SL, Carney NA, et al. Guidelines for the acute medical management of severe traumatic brain injury in infants, children, and adolescents. Chapter 3: prehospital airway management. *Pediatr Crit Care Med.* 2003;4:S9-S11.

164. Adelson PD, Bratton SL, Carney NA, et al. Guidelines for the acute medical management of severe traumatic brain injury in infants, children, and adolescents. Chapter 12: use of hyperventilation in the acute management of severe pediatric traumatic brain injury. *Pediatr Crit Care Med.* 2003;4:S45-S48.

165. Adelson PD, Bratton SL, Carney NA, et al. Guidelines for the acute medical management of severe traumatic brain injury in infants, children, and adolescents. Chapter 9: use of sedation and neuromuscular blockade in the treatment of severe pediatric traumatic brain injury. *Pediatr Crit Care Med.* 2003;4:S34-S37.

168. Robinson N, Clancy M. In patients with head injury undergoing rapid sequence intubation, does pretreatment with intravenous lignocaine/ lidocaine lead to an improved neurological outcome? A review of the literature. *Emerg Med J.* 2001;18:453-457.

172. Pang D, Wilberger JE. Spinal cord injury without radiologic abnormalities in children. *J Neurosurg.* 1982;57:114.

173. Brown RL, Brunn MA, Garcia VF. Cervical spine injuries in children: a review of 103 patients treated consecutively at a level 1 pediatric trauma center. *J Pediatr Surg.* 2001;36:1107-1114.

174. Cirak B, Ziegfeld S, Knight VM, et al. Spinal injuries in children. *J Pediatr Surg.* 2004;39:607-612.

186. Fox DJ, Matson MD. Management of the difficult pediatric airway in an austere environment using the lightwand. *J Clin Anesth.* 1990;2: 123-125.

187. Fisher QA, Tunkel DE. Lightwand intubation of infants and children. *J Clin Anesth.* 1997;9:275-279.

189. Pfitzner L, Cooper MG, Ho D. The Shikani Seeing Stylet for difficult intubation in children: initial experience. *Anaesth Intensive Care.* 2002;30:462-466.

192. Lopez-Gil M, Brimacombe J, Alvarez M. Safety and efficacy of the laryngeal mask airway. A prospective survey of 1400 children. *Anaesthesia.* 1996;51:969-972.

198. Berry AM, Brimacombe JR, Verghese C. The laryngeal mask airway in emergency medicine, neonatal resuscitation, and intensive care medicine. *Int Anesthesiol Clin.* 1998;36:91-109.

200. American Heart Association. *Pediatric Advanced Life Support (PALS) Provider Manual (Professional).* American Heart Association; 2011.

202. Youngquist S, Gausche-Hill M, Burbulys D. Alternative airway devices for use in children requiring prehospital airway management: update and case discussion. *Pediatr Emerg Care.* 2007;23:250-258.

204. Benumof JL. Use of the laryngeal mask to facilitate fiberoptic endoscopy intubation. *Anesthesiology.* 1992;74:313.

205. Difficult airway management in children 3: Video laryngoscopy: <https:// www.youtube.com/watch?v=gMY9n6ukeEQ>. Accessed 08.16.16.

206. Carron JD, Derkay CS, Strope GL, et al. Pediatric tracheotomies: changing indications and outcomes. *Laryngoscope.* 2000;110:1099-1104.

Anesthesia Effects and Organ System Considerations

Alison M. Jeziorski, Antonio Cassara, and Peter J. Davis

PEARLS

- The anesthetic care of intensive care unit patients involves the extension of principles of medical management used in the operating room.
- The anesthesiologist caring for a critically ill child must have an understanding of the desired therapeutic end points and knowledge of the patient's preexisting condition.
- For the intensive care physician, a patient returning to the intensive care unit after surgery frequently requires an altered management plan. The physiologic perturbations of surgery and anesthesia frequently change the focus and direction of medical management. The intensive care physician must understand not only the events that occur in the operating room but also the rationale for using anesthetic agents and anesthetic techniques.
- Prompt recognition of the propofol infusion syndrome and discontinuation of the infusion are key to increased survival. Early administration of hemodialysis and perhaps even extracorporeal support improve survival.

Effects of Anesthetic Agents

Anesthetic agents have multiple physiologic effects and consequences in patients with underlying disease and trauma. Anesthetic agents have been associated with both organ protection and neurotoxicity.[1-3] Understanding the pharmacology of these anesthetic agents has significant implications not only for the operative management of the patient but also for postoperative recovery in the intensive care unit. This chapter focuses on the potent inhaled anesthetic agents, the frequently used intravenous sedative hypnotic agents (propofol and dexmedetomidine), the intravenous opioids, and the role of local anesthetic agents and their adjuncts. Because these drugs have significant effects on cerebral neurophysiology and neurologic outcomes of patients, the pharmacologic discussion focuses on the drug's neurophysiologic effect.

Anesthetic agents affect myocardial performance. Historically inhalational anesthesia in children was associated with a higher rate of cardiac arrest, bradycardia, and hypotension in infants and children than in adults. These hemodynamic effects are dose related.[4-8]

Because it can be problematic to insert invasive monitors in unsedated, awake children, much of the information about the potent inhaled anesthetic agents and their effects on the

determinants of cardiac output is derived from animal studies. Schieber and colleagues[9] observed that, although isoflurane reduced contractility and decreased blood pressure and systemic vascular resistance more than did equipotent concentrations of halothane, cardiac index was better preserved in the isoflurane-anesthetized animals. Thus when compared with halothane, the direct myocardial depressant effect of isoflurane is offset by its effect on the peripheral vasculature, which results in afterload reduction. Of note when comparing the anesthetic effects of inhalational agents, the concept of minimum alveolar concentration (MAC) is used as a metric. MAC is defined as the concentration that prevents movement of 50% of patients to a surgical incision. The use of MAC as a metric allows one to compare anesthetics of different potencies at a similar effect (MAC multiples) rather than comparing similar concentrations of drugs with different potencies.

Desflurane and sevoflurane are two potent inhalational anesthetic agents with low blood solubility coefficients. The low blood solubility affords rapid induction of anesthesia as well as rapid emergence and awakening.[10-15] Desflurane has a blood gas solubility coefficient (0.42) that is similar to nitrous oxide in children. However, desflurane's pungent airway properties result in a high incidence of laryngospasm, coughing, and hypoxemia if used as an induction agent in nonintubated children.[15] Significant increases in airway resistance have been reported in children with known reactive airway disease.[16] The cardiovascular profile of desflurane is similar for neonates, infants, and children.[13] Compared with awake values, anesthetized children have a 30% decrease in arterial blood pressure at 1 minimal alveolar concentration (MAC) of desflurane with a minimal change in heart rate. At equipotent concentrations (1 MAC), desflurane, isoflurane, and halothane all attenuate the baroresponse in children. In adults Weiskopf and associates[17] demonstrated that rapid increases in desflurane from 0.55 to 1.66 MAC produce a transient increase in arterial blood pressure and heart rate. This cardiovascular excitation is associated with an increase in sympathetic and renin-angiotensin system activity. Desflurane is not metabolized but is eliminated by ventilation. Because of its low solubility, emergence from anesthesia is rapid; however, even with its rapid elimination, former premature infants are still at risk for postoperative apnea.[18]

Sevoflurane is the most commonly administered anesthetic for children. As opposed to desflurane, sevoflurane is not an airway irritant and as such it can promote a rapid and smooth induction of anesthesia. Sevoflurane does undergo metabolism to a small extent and is metabolized by the 2E1 P-450 enzyme system to isopropyl alcohol and inorganic fluoride.[19] Recovery from sevoflurane is rapid; however, in children it has been associated with a high incidence of emergence delirium (ED). Kuratani and Oi[20] in a meta-analysis found an increased probability of the emergence delirium with sevoflurane when compared to halothane. Martin and others have noted that children with ED exhibit arousal with delirious behavior accompanied by a variety of electroencephalogram patterns during the indeterminate state (ie, the state before the appearance of normal wake or sleep patterns). The electroencephalogram in children without ED progressed from the indeterminate state to classifiable sleep or drowsy states before peaceful awakening. Significant differences were also noted in frontal lobe functional connectivity between children with and without ED after the termination of sevoflurane anesthesia.

The hemodynamic profile of sevoflurane in children is similar to isoflurane. In adults anesthetized with sevoflurane or isoflurane, administration of exogenous epinephrine had similar dysrhythmogenic properties.[21] In an echocardiographic study of children comparing sevoflurane and halothane at equal MAC, Holzman and coworkers[22] noted that sevoflurane had fewer myocardial depressant effects than sevoflurane.

Because inhalational anesthetics can produce significant hemodynamic changes in compromised children, the use of high-dose opioids has been shown to confer hemodynamic stability and adequate anesthesia.[19-21] Robinson and Gregory,[23] in a study of premature infants undergoing patent ductus arteriosus ligation, reported the safety and efficacy of high-dose fentanyl anesthesia. In subsequent reports on pediatric patients, Hickey and Hansen[24] documented the safety of high-dose fentanyl and sufentanil in children with complex congenital heart disease. These investigators found that high doses of fentanyl (75 µg/kg) and sufentanil (10 µg/kg) decreased heart rate (7%) and mean arterial pressure (MAP, 9%). Pulmonary vascular resistance decreased and transcutaneous oxygenation increased by 45 to 100 mm Hg.

Though high-dose opioids produce hemodynamic stability in compromised infants and children, they prolong both recovery and respiratory depression.[25-27] Because fentanyl and sufentanil undergo hepatic elimination, repeated doses of the drug change its kinetic profile and increase its terminal elimination half-life. Opioids that do not rely on hepatic metabolism have the advantage of more predictable pharmacokinetic and pharmacodynamic control. Remifentanil is a synthetic opioid agonist that is metabolized by plasma and tissue esterases. It is independent of organ elimination. Consequently, it has an ultrashort half-life and a kinetic profile that does not change with the duration of infusion. Remifentanil's flat, context-sensitive half-time (elimination from the effect compartment) is not affected by the duration of the infusion. This contrasts with fentanyl and sufentanil whose pharmacokinetic profiles and context-sensitive half-times change drastically with duration of infusion (Fig. 130.1).

Remifentanil's ultrashort half-life (7 to 10 minutes) coupled with its hemodynamic stabilization allows it to be titrated to a more predictable effect. Because it does not depend on organ elimination for its clearance, the pharmacokinetic profile of remifentanil in infants and neonates is quite different from that of other opioids. Remifentanil clearance is greatest in neonates and infants, and its terminal elimination half-life

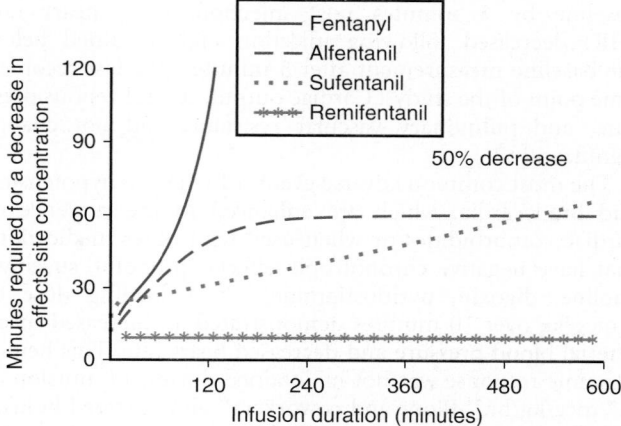

Fig. 130.1. Overlay of the fentanyl, alfentanil, and sufentanil recovery curves describing the time required for decreases of 50% from the maintained intraoperative effect site concentration after termination of the infusion. (From Shafer SL, Varvel JR. Pharmacokinetics, pharmacodynamics, and rational opioid selection. Anesthesiology. 1991;74: 53-63.)

does not change with age.[28] This contrasts to the kinetic profiles of fentanyl, sufentanil, and morphine, which have lowest clearance and longest terminal elimination half-life in infants. In vitro studies by Olgatree and colleagues[29] have shown that remifentanil has no significant direct negative inotropic effect on the myocardium and that β-adrenergic stimulation of the heart remains intact. Comparative studies of remifentanil and inhaled anesthetic agents in children undergoing pyloromyotomy suggest that the short half-life of remifentanil may have beneficial effect on postoperative respiratory changes.[30,31] However, the rapid development of tolerance will likely preclude its use for longer periods of time.

Dexmedetomidine (DEX) is a sedative analgesic α_2-adrenergic agonist that is highly selective for the alpha 1 receptor (α_2/α_1 ratio of 1600:1). In addition to being used for sedation in pediatric ICU patients, it is also administered for invasive and noninvasive procedural sedation.[32,33] Stimulation of α_2 receptors in the central nervous system (CNS) and spinal cord produces sedation, anxiolysis, and analgesia. It also reduces anesthetic requirements for inhalational agents and opioids. In addition, DEX decreases renin and vasopressin levels, promotes diuresis, and reduces sympathetic tone, heart rate, and blood pressure.[34] As has been reported, bolus DEX infusions result in a biphasic blood pressure response (transient initial increase followed by a decrease). Within 1 to 2 minutes blood pressure returns to baseline while heart rate remains low. This biphasic effect is thought to be due to dexmedetomidine's initial ability to stimulate peripheral postsynaptic α_{2b}-adrenergic receptors resulting in vasoconstriction, followed by the more intense CNS effects on α_{2a}-adrenergic receptors causing sympatholysis. In a study of children undergoing routine surveillance endomyocardial biopsies after heart transplant, Jooste and coworkers administered a bolus dose (0.5 mcg/kg) of dexmedetomidine over 2 to 3 seconds. In this study, Jooste and coworkers noted that within 1 minute following injection, systolic blood pressure, diastolic blood pressure, systolic pulmonary artery pressure, diastolic pulmonary artery pressure, pulmonary artery wedge pressure, and systemic vascular resistance had all increased but returned to baseline by 5 minutes post injection. Only heart rate (HR) decreased following injection and remained below the baseline measurement after 5 minutes (the last recorded time point of the study). Cardiac output, central venous pressure, and pulmonary vascular resistance did not change significantly.[35]

The most common adverse events of DEX are hypotension and bradycardia, which are enhanced in the presence of cardiac comorbidities or when used with other medications that have negative chronotropic effects (propofol, succinylcholine, digoxin, pyridostigmine).[36-38] A loading dose of 1 mcg/kg over 10 minutes demonstrated an increased mean arterial blood pressure and decreased heart rate. This hemodynamic response was not maintained during an infusion of 0.7 mcg/kg/hr.[39] Bloor and coworkers[39] administered boluses of 0.25, 0.5, 1, and 2 μg/kg to healthy volunteers and noted a decrease in MAP, respectively, of 14%, 16%, 23%, and 27%. Cardiac output decreased 20% following a loading dose of 1 μg/kg in the first minute and returned to 90% of baseline after 60 minutes. When a loading dose of 2 μg/kg was administered, cardiac output decreased by 60% and returned to 85% of baseline after 1 hour. Venn and associates[41] studied the effects of dexmedetomidine in 66 patients with comorbidities who were in the ICU, who were mechanically ventilated, and who received a loading dose of 1 μg/kg followed by a continuous infusion of 0.2 to 0.7 μg/kg/hr. Hypotension and bradycardia (≥30% decrease from baseline) were observed in 18 of the 66 patients. Ingersoll-Weng also noted reports of bradycardia and sinus arrest.[37]

Khan and associates[42] reported similar effects of dexmedetomidine during anesthesia with isoflurane. The majority of the effects occurred with end-tidal isoflurane levels greater than or equal to 1%. Animal studies and studies on isolated human papillary muscle have demonstrated no direct negative inotropic effects on myocardial contractility.[43] Congdon and associates noted that in dogs, coadministration of intramuscular atropine with intramuscular DEX reversed HR changes. However, hypotension and arrhythmias (atrioventricular block, premature ventricular contractions, and bigeminy) were observed.[44]

Chrysostomou reported that DEX has antiarrhythmic effects in the perioperative period and suggested its possible use for terminating reentrant supraventricular tachycardia.[45-47] Muktar and associates reported sympatholytic effects of dexmedetomidine in pediatric patients.[48] Thirty infants and children undergoing CPB were randomized to receive dexmedetomidine (1 μg/kg load followed by a continuous infusion of 0.5 μg/kg/hr) or placebo. Plasma cortisol norepinephrine, epinephrine, and glucose levels were significantly lower in the dexmedetomidine group. Hammer et al has reported on the electrophysiological effects of dexmedetomidine in pediatric patients undergoing electrophysiology studies.[40]

Dexmedetomidine has a rapid distribution phase (6 minutes) and an elimination half-life of 2 hours.[49] Petroz and colleagues[50] demonstrated that children 2 to 12 years of age have similar pharmacokinetics to adults. Rodarte and associates[51] studied the pharmacokinetics in infants 1 to 24 months of age. He concluded that infants have a faster clearance of dexmedetomidine than adults (27 mL/kg/min versus 13 mL/kg/min). A loading dose of 1 μg/kg and continuous infusions of 0.2 to 0.7 μg/kg/hr have been used in various clinical scenarios to produce sedation-analgesia. Effects on respiration

appear to be minimal. This may be beneficial in children with upper airway obstruction.[52]

Propofol is a sedative hypnotic that is widely used as an induction agent in anesthesia. It is also used as a continuous infusion for prolonged sedation in the ICU. Propofol is rapidly distributed and cleared. These properties allow for a relatively quick recovery. Propofol is suspended in a lipid emulsion, which when administered by a continuous infusion results in a significant lipid load. Induction doses for anesthesia vary from 2 to 3 mg/kg, whereas ICU sedation doses vary from 50 to 250 μg/kg/min. Induction doses of propofol can cause a 10% to 15% decrease of MAP as well as bradycardia, especially when coadministered with other vagotonic drugs. Propofol has a modest negative inotropic effect, due to antagonism of β-adrenergic receptors and calcium channels.[53] Propofol has many properties attractive for use in sedation. However, there have been increasing reports of a fatal adverse reaction that has been termed the propofol infusion syndrome (PRIS).[54] PRIS is characterized by severe intractable bradycardia that leads to cardiac failure, severe metabolic acidosis, hyperlipidemia, rhabdomyolysis with consequent hyperkalemia, and renal failure.[55-57] Prolonged propofol infusions (more than 48 hours) and infusion rates greater than 4 mg/kg/hr have been linked to PRIS. Priming factors such as critical illness (respiratory failure and traumatic brain injury) and triggering factors such as catecholamine and steroid infusion are associated with the syndrome.[58] The underlying mechanism appears to be an inhibition of mitochondrial electron transport and impairment in oxygen utilization.[53] As a result, there is a decreased ATP production and a decreased mitochondrial lipid metabolism, with an accumulation of toxic long fatty acid chains that are arrhythmogenic.[59-61] Pediatric patients appear more susceptible than adults secondary to low glycogen stores and high need for fat metabolism.[62] Management of PRIS is very difficult and consists of prompt recognition and interruption of the infusion. Aggressive cardiac resuscitation must be initiated early on with high-dose inotropes, fluid administration, and the use of pacing devices. The early administration of hemodialysis and hemofiltration together with extracorporeal membrane oxygenation has improved survival.[63-65]

Local Anesthetic Agents

The use of local anesthetic agents for regional anesthesia in infants and children has significantly improved pediatric pain management. Unlike in the adult population the majority of regional blocks done in infants and children are done under general anesthesia. Prospective and retrospective safety studies have demonstrated that performing these blocks under general anesthesia is a safe practice.[66-67] The use of ultrasound has become routine for the performance of regional blocks in pediatric and adult patients.[68-69] Direct visualization of the nerve, the needle, and the distribution of local anesthetics has improved the quality of the block, decreased the incidence of nerve injury secondary to direct nerve stimulation with the needle, especially when a preexisting neuropathy is present, and decreased the amount of local anesthetic necessary to produce an effective block.[70-73]

Local anesthetic agents are classified as amino esters (cocaine, tetracaine, chloroprocaine, and prilocaine) or as amino amides. The amino amides include bupivacaine, ropivacaine, levobupivacaine, and lidocaine and are potent sodium channel blockers. At toxic blood concentrations they can cause seizures, cardiac arrhythmias, and cardiac arrest that can be resistant to resuscitation.[74,75]

Children are more at risk from local anesthetic toxicity because of their lower serum concentrations of α-1 acid glycoprotein (AAG) and albumin, which are the binding proteins for local anesthetics (LAs). Therefore the unbound fraction of LA, which is the active drug, is increased, making infants and children more susceptible to local anesthetic toxicity (LAST). Another factor that can influence LAST in neonates and children is the slower metabolism and elimination of the local anesthetic agents.[74,75]

The potency and duration of local anesthetic agents depend on lipophilicity, degree of ionization, protein binding, and the vasoconstricting properties of the drug. In general, the duration of action of local anesthetic agents is shortest in neonates and infants. Metabolism of amides is by the liver's P-450 enzyme system, whereas metabolism of the ester compounds is by plasma esterases (butyrylcholinesterase) and tissue esterases.

Ropivacaine 0.2% to 1% and levobupivacaine 0.1% to 0.5% are newer local anesthetic agents that are mainly used in pediatric regional anesthesia because of their favorable systemic toxicity profile. They have similar onset time and duration of nerve block when compared to lidocaine and bupivacaine.[76]

Even when weight-based dosing regimens are applied, LAST can occur and immediate diagnosis and treatment should be initiated. Neurotoxicity occurs before cardiac toxicity, and the signs (increased blood pressure and heart rate, muscle rigidity) can be difficult to distinguish from other causes in the anesthetized patient. Treatment with bolus infusions of lipid emulsions is now considered first-line therapy.[77] Dosing of Intralipid includes an initial dose of 20% Intralipid 1 to 1.5 ml/kg maximum of 10 ml/Kg[75] followed by an infusion of 20% Intralipid at 0.25 to 0.5 ml/kg/min. Airway management and basic life support are key elements for adequate resuscitation. It should be emphasized that although it is prepared in a lipid emulsion, propofol is contradicted in the resuscitation from LAST.

Systematic absorption of local anesthetic agents contributes to LA toxicity. Vascular areas are more prone to rapid absorption. The rate of absorption is greatest in the intercostal space and trachea followed by the caudal and epidural space and least in the subcutaneous tissue.

Adjuvants for local anesthetics are frequently administered in conjunction with the local anesthetic to prolong the duration, improve the quality of the block, and lower the concentration and dose of the administered LA.[78] Adjuncts are mostly used in neuraxial blocks and in particular for single injections in the caudal space. Preservative free opiates increase the duration of analgesia but have significant side effects (nausea, vomiting, pruritus, and sedation).[79] Clonidine, an alpha-2 adrenergic agonist, has also been administered as an adjunct in both peripheral and central nervous system blocks. However, there is weak clinical evidence to support the use of clonidine to prolong the duration of peripheral nerve blocks in children.[80]

Clonidine doses 1 to 2 ug/kg (bolus) and 0.1 ug/kg/h (continuous infusion) can increase the duration of a block by 3 to 5 hours. Dexmedetomidine, a more selective α-2-receptor agonist, at the same doses has a similar effect.[81] Other adjuvants such as midazolam, ketamine, neostigmine, and dexamethasone either have excessive side effects or show weak clinical data to support their use.[81] Although these adjuncts are frequently used, at present there have been no toxicity studies demonstrating the safety of these agents on the central nervous system.

Two blocks (paravertebral and transverse abdominis) deserve mentioning because of their applicability for the pediatric intensive care unit (PICU) patient. The paravertebral block in the form of a bolus injection or a continuous infusion has become more popular now in the pediatric population with the use of ultrasound. It is a valid alternative to neuraxial blocks because it has fewer contraindications and complications. It is particularly indicated for thoracotomies, breast surgery, subcostal incisions, and multiple rib fractures. Complications include pleural puncture, paravertebral hematoma, and nerve injury.[75] Paravertebral catheters are being placed more frequently in the PICU for patients with multiple rib fractures secondary to trauma as well as in patients who have undergone thoracotomy procedures. The use of this block in these patients can decrease the overall amount of sedation and analgesics used during mechanical ventilation and improve the patient's respiratory mechanics[82-84] (Fig. 130.2).

A transversus abdominis plane block with ultrasound guidance can improve the quality of abdominal wall blocks by directing the local anesthetic in the plane between the internal oblique and the transversus abdominis muscles where the thoracolumbar nerves lie. This block provides good postoperative analgesia and is indicated for laparoscopic procedures and for larger abdominal incisions[85,86] (Fig. 130.3).

Though anesthetic agents can affect the physiology of all organ systems, for the PICU patient the anesthetic effects on the patient's underlying CNS physiology can markedly influence a patient's outcome.

Neurologic Injury

Traumatic brain injury (TBI) is the leading form of pediatric trauma in the United States.[87,88] It is estimated that total combined rates of TBI-related hospitalizations, ED visits, and deaths are approximately 824 per 100,000.[89] Poor outcomes have been associated with early hypotension, low Glasgow Coma Scale score, altered cerebral blood flow (CBF), hyperglycemia, and deranged autoregulation.[90] However, secondary cerebral injury may result from the development of intracranial hypertension and resultant cerebral ischemia. Recognition and control of elevated intracranial pressure (ICP) are key elements to preventing neurologic deterioration and patient morbidity. Secondary traumatic brain injury can be characterized by an array of biochemical, cellular, and molecular events that are associated with ischemia, excitotoxicity, energy failure, and cell death cascades, all of which result in cerebral swelling, axonal injury, inflammation, and regeneration.[91]

Intracranial Pressure

The signs of intracranial hypertension in infants and children are listed in Table 130.1. The presence of these signs and symptoms, in conjunction with the baseline findings on neurologic examination, may dramatically alter the patient's anesthetic care. The anesthesiologist must be aware of ongoing interventions to control ICP. Control of cerebral perfusion

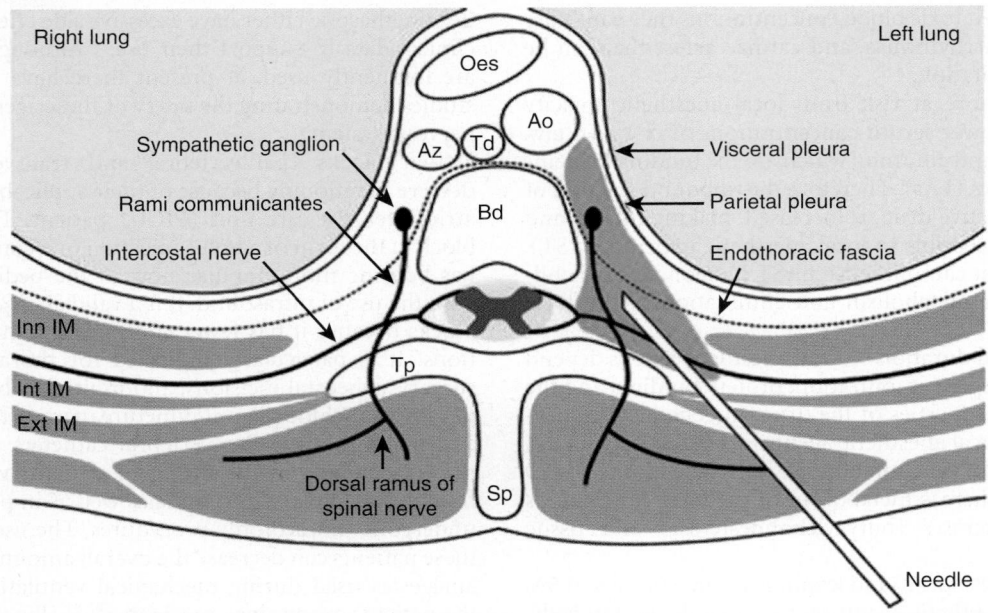

Fig. 130.2. Figure diagramming paravertebral space. The needle is advanced until the tip is in the paravertebral space. (From Cowie B, McGlade D, Ivanusic J, Barrington MJ. Ultrasound-guided thoracic paravertebral blockade: a cadaveric study. Anesth Analg. 2010;110:1735-1739.)

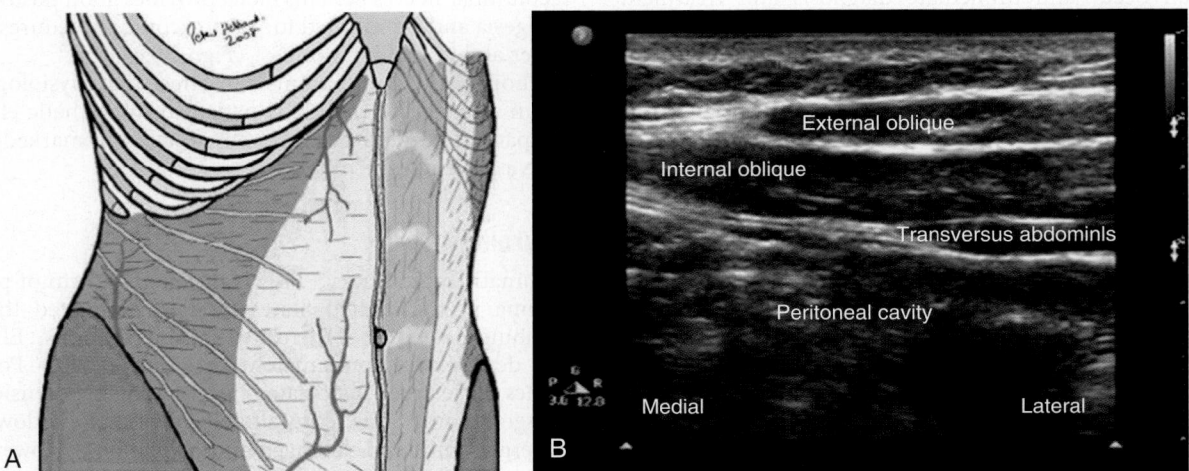

Fig. 130.3. (A) Typical distribution of nerves in the transversus abdominis plane block. (Generously shared from the personal files of Prof. P. Hebbard.) (B) Ultrasound view of abdominal wall lateral view. Muscular layers of the anterolateral abdominal wall.

TABLE 130.1	Signs of Intracranial Hypertension in Infants and Children	
Infants	**Children**	**Infants and Children**
Irritability	Headache	Decreased consciousness
Full fontanelle	Diplopia	Cranial nerve (III and VI) palsies
Widely separated cranial sutures	Papilledema	Loss of upward gaze (setting sun sign)
Cranial enlargement	Vomiting	Signs of herniation, Cushing triad, pupillary changes

pressure is essential for maintaining neurologic function in pathologic states. Cerebral perfusion pressure is expressed as the difference between MAP and the highest value obtained out of the following: central venous pressure, intrathoracic pressure, or ICP. Thus in the presence of intracranial hypertension (ICP ≥15 to 20 mm Hg), higher systemic blood pressures must be achieved to prevent cerebral ischemia. Intracranial compliance depends on the volumes of the intracranial contents, cerebral tissue, blood, and extracellular fluid. The most dynamic of these is the blood compartment. Changes in cerebral blood volume are mediated primarily through changes in cerebral vascular resistance. Cerebral vascular resistance is affected by both intracranial and extracerebral factors.

Regulation of Cerebral Blood Flow

The normal brain receives 15% of cardiac output. Kennedy and Sokoloff[92] determined that healthy children have a high CBF (100 mL/100 gm/min); this value decreases to adult values of 50 mL/100 gm/min during the teenage years. Cerebral blood flow regulation depends primarily on the local chemical and metabolic milieu, particularly the concentrations of hydrogen ion, adenosine, and prostanoids. Production of these compounds correlates with normal cerebral activity and metabolic rate. Neurogenic and myogenic components also have minor roles in regulating cerebral vascular resistance.

Extracerebral factors that can change cerebral vascular resistance and CBF include the arterial partial pressures of carbon dioxide ($PaCO_2$) and oxygen (PaO_2), MAP, and various drugs (Fig. 130.4). Cerebral circulation is sensitive to variations of $PaCO_2$ and has been studied using transcranial Doppler ultrasound.[93] CBF varies linearly by 2% to 4% for every variation of 1 mm Hg of $PaCO_2$. Data from anesthetized children show that CO_2 vasoreactivity is higher than in adults (13.8% versus 10.3% change).[94] Low blood pressure decreases cerebral vascular vasoreactivity.[94] As $PaCO_2$ is rapidly lowered toward 20 mm Hg, there is marked cerebral vasoconstriction and a reduction in both CBF and ICP. Theoretically, an acute decrease in $PaCO_2$ below 20 mm Hg may be detrimental by reducing CBF enough to cause cerebral ischemia. The salutary effects of acute hyperventilation on ICP are diminished over time because acute changes in cerebrospinal fluid pH are normalized in approximately 6 hours. Arterial oxygenation within the normal clinical range has little effect on cerebral vascular resistance. However, PaO_2 less than 50 mm Hg results in cerebral vasodilation and increased CBF. Hyperoxia in excess of 300 mm Hg may produce cerebral vasoconstriction.

Cerebral autoregulation is a homeostatic process by which the brain maintains a constant CBF over a MAP range from 60 to 150 mm Hg in adults. At a MAP less than 60 mm Hg, symptoms of cerebral ischemia may appear. If the upper limit of MAP for autoregulation is exceeded, the resultant increase in CBF may cause cerebral edema. The autoregulatory curve may shift in the presence of chronic hypertension, intracranial tumors, head trauma, or shock states. This renders the brain more susceptible to ischemic effects.[94] The range of MAP over which autoregulation of CBF occurs in infants and children likely shifts in tandem with age-related changes in normal systemic blood pressures and cerebral perfusion pressures. Raju and associates[95] suggested that an infant's mean cerebral perfusion pressure is approximately equal to its gestational age in weeks and that this estimate holds true for growing preterm infants up to 5 weeks after birth.

Effects of Anesthetics on Cerebral Blood Flow

In general, the potent inhaled anesthetic agents impair autoregulation and may cause hypotension and increased CBF (Fig. 130.5). Consequently, they must be used cautiously, if at all, in patients with evidence of traumatic brain injury. Halothane, historically at 1 MAC, abolishes cerebral autoregulation. Isoflurane impairs autoregulation less than halothane.[96] Sevoflurane appears to preserve autoregulation up to 1.5 MAC.[97-98] The effects of anesthetic agents on CBF and cerebral metabolism are summarized in Fig. 130.6. In general, the perfect agent would decrease both CBF and cerebral metabolic rate of oxygen ($CMRO_2$). The potent inhaled agents (isoflurane, desflurane, and sevoflurane) "uncouple" the normal relationship between CBF and metabolism and cause marked cerebral vasodilation. Isoflurane is the only inhaled anesthetic agent with which CBF actually may decrease when concomitant hyperventilation to $PaCO_2$ of 20 to 25 mm Hg is used.[99] Whereas nitrous oxide alone is known to cause mild cerebral vasodilation and to increase $CMRO_2$ (probably related to inadequate anesthetic depth), these effects are easily countered by

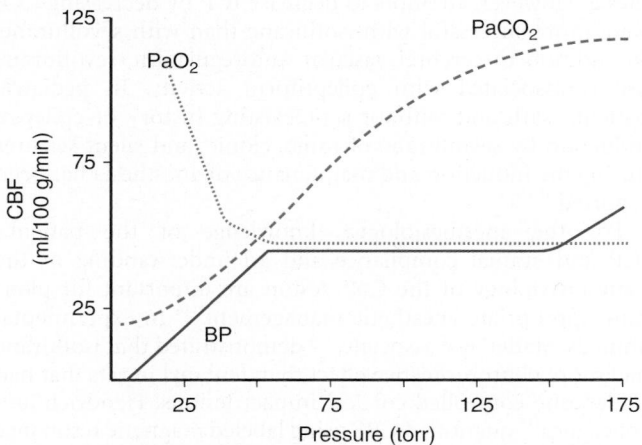

Fig. 130.4. Cerebral blood flow (CBF) changes resulting from alterations in $PaCO_2$, PaO_2, and blood pressure. The other two variables remain stable at normal values when the remaining variable is altered. (Modified from Shapiro HM. Intracranial hypertension: therapeutic and anesthetic considerations. Anesthesiology. 1975;43:445.)

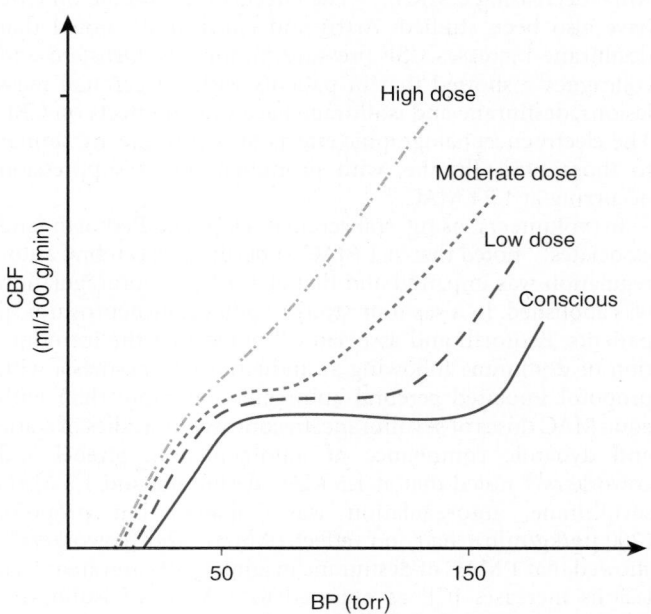

Fig. 130.5. Volatile anesthetics and autoregulation. Schematic representation of the effect of a progressively increased dose of a typical volatile anesthetic agent on cerebral blood flow (CBF) autoregulation. Both upper and lower thresholds are shifted to the left. (Modified from Drummond K, Shapiro HM. Cerebral physiology. In: Miller R, ed. Anesthesia. vol 2. 3rd ed. New York: Churchill Livingstone; 1990.)

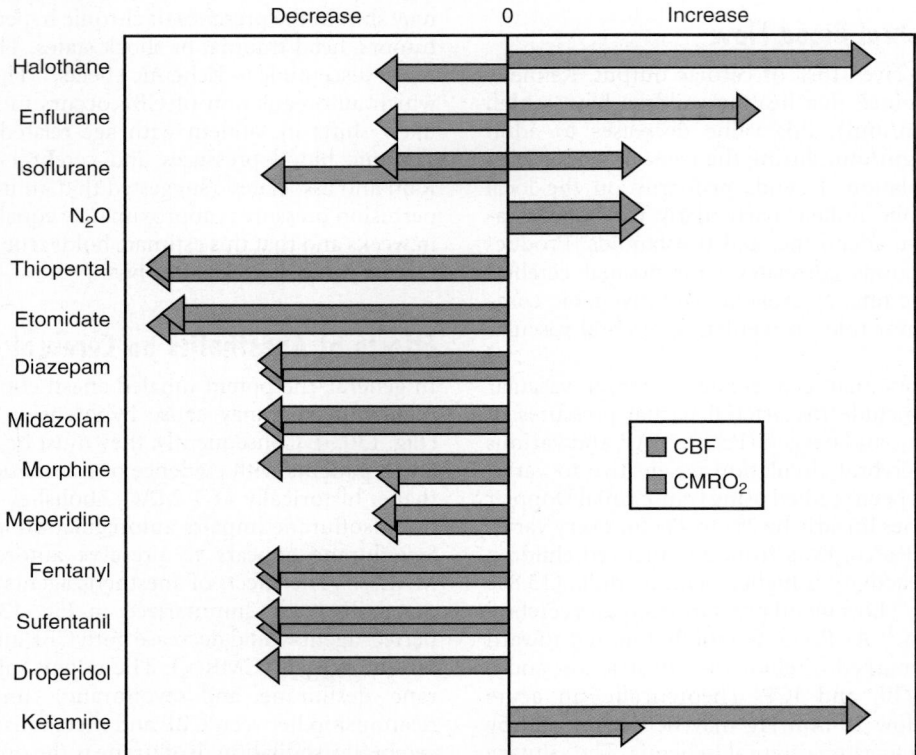

Fig. 130.6. Effects of anesthetic agents on cerebral blood flow (CBF) and cerebral metabolic rate of oxygen (CMRo2). (Modified from Cucchiara RF, Block MC, Steinkeler JA. The effects of anesthetic agents on cerebral blood flow and cerebral metabolism: anesthesia for intracranial procedures. In: Barash PG, Cullen BF, Stoelters SK, eds. Clinical Anesthesia. Philadelphia: JB Lippincott; 1989.)

the addition of intravenous sedatives, hypnotics, and narcotics. Sevoflurane has been shown to increase CBF and ICP while decreasing $CMRO_2$.[100] The effects of desflurane on CBF have also been studied; Artru and colleagues[101] noted that desflurane increases CSF pressure in animals. Ornstein and colleagues[102] showed that in patients with intracranial mass lesions, desflurane and isoflurane have similar effects on CBF. The electroencephalographic effects of desflurane are similar to those of isoflurane, with prominent burst suppression occurring at 1.24 MAC.[103]

In volunteers using transcranial Doppler, Bedforth and associates[104] noted that at 1 MAC of desflurane, cerebral autoregulation was impaired and that at 1.5 MAC autoregulation was abolished. In a separate study of adult non-neurosurgical patients, Bedforth and associates[104] noted that the introduction of desflurane following an induction of anesthesia with propofol impaired cerebral autoregulation more than with equi-MAC doses of sevoflurane. In contrast, in studies of static and dynamic compliance of autoregulation, Strebel and coworkers[105] noted that at 1.5 MAC desflurane and 1.5 MAC sevoflurane, autoregulation was impaired but propofol (200 μg/kg/min) had no effect. Muzzi and coworkers[106] showed that 1 MAC of desflurane in adults with supratentorial lesions increases ICP as opposed to 1 MAC of isoflurane. Desflurane may alter CSF dynamics. Desflurane does not appear to change CSF absorption but does increase CSF production.[107]

In a study of patients undergoing nonintracranial neurosurgical procedures, Summors and associates[107] noted that dynamic cerebral autoregulation using transcranial Doppler

ultrasonography is better preserved during 1.5 MAC sevoflurane than during 1.5 MAC isoflurane anesthesia. Others noted similar findings with sevoflurane and isoflurane. In patients studied at 0.5 and 1.5 MAC, the dose-dependent vasodilatory effect was less for sevoflurane.[108,109] Nishiyama and coworkers[110] assessed comparative cerebral vasodilatory responsiveness to CO_2 during either sevoflurane or isoflurane anesthesia. They noted in a group of adult patients that changes in CBF caused by changes in CO_2 are greater during isoflurane anesthesia. However, attempts to decrease ICP by decreasing CO_2 were more successful with isoflurane than with sevoflurane. In addition to cerebral vascular autoregulation, sevoflurane use is associated with epileptiform activity. In pediatric patients with and without a preexisting history of epilepsy, induction by sevoflurane of tonic, clonic, and silent seizures during the induction and maintenance of anesthesia has been reported.[109-113]

For the anesthesiologist, knowledge of the patient's ICP and cranial compliance and an understanding of the pathophysiology of the CNS lesion are important for planning appropriate anesthetic management.[114] In experimental animals, Statler and associates[114] demonstrated that isoflurane had more neuroprotective effect than fentanyl in rats that had undergone controlled cortical impact lesions. Hendrich and colleagues[115] quantified CBF using labeled magnetic resonance imaging in normal rats anesthetized with fentanyl, isoflurane, or pentobarbital. In this study, CBF values were found to be approximately 2.5 to 3 times lower in most regions analyzed during anesthesia with either fentanyl (with N_2O/O_2) or pentobarbital versus isoflurane (with N_2O/O_2). In addition, these investigators noted that CBF was heterogeneous in rats anesthetized with isoflurane (with N_2O/O_2) but relatively homogenous in rats anesthetized with either fentanyl (with N_2O/O_2) or pentobarbital. In previous human studies with opioid anesthesia, opioids maintained static cerebral autoregulation. Engelhard and associates[116] subsequently demonstrated that remifentanil, a µ-opioid agonist with unique pharmacokinetic properties, when combined with low-dose propofol maintains both static and dynamic compliance of cerebrovascular autoregulation. Propofol also has been used to alter CNS dynamics.[117] Positron emission tomography suggests that propofol produces global metabolic depression.[118,119] Like thiopental, propofol decreased $CMRO_2$, CBF, and ICP. Cerebral responsiveness to arterial CO_2 appears to be preserved during propofol anesthesia.[120-122]

Anesthesia Neurotoxicity in the Developing Brain

An area of intense interest in both the scientific community and lay press involves the findings of anesthetic-associated toxicity in the developing central nervous system.[1] Research in this area has focused on the neurodevelopment in the non–brain-injured and non–brain-diseased animal or patient. Early work in the 1980s by Uemura and colleagues noted that rats exposed to varying concentrations of halothane from the time of conception to PND28 had a decrease in synaptic density and that these exposed animals also demonstrated behavioral disturbances.[121,123] More recent investigations in both rodent and nonhuman primate models have reported apoptosis in multiple areas of the central nervous system during this period of rapid synaptogenesis when these animals are exposed to drugs that work via N-methyl-D-aspartate antagonists (NMDA) or gamma-aminobutyric acid (GABA) agonists.[124-133] Using caspase-3 as a marker for neuroapoptosis, investigators have reported both dose and length of exposure effects with ketamine, midazolam, propofol, sevoflurane, isoflurane, and desflurane in the developing brain (Fig. 130.7). When these agents are combined, these drugs act synergistically with regard to both their anesthetic action and their neuroapoptotic effect. In addition to a dose effect, these animals have a period, or window of vulnerability, in which these agents act in the developing brain. This window of vulnerability differs among species, and though there are no specific studies on the vulnerability period in humans, these animal models suggest that the vulnerable period in humans correlates to a human period of late pregnancy to early childhood. Although the data are mixed with respect to the behavioral/neurocognitive outcomes in rodents, the little data available in primates suggest neurocognitive impairment in older animals that were exposed to ketamine in the neonatal period.[134]

To complicate the situation, rodent studies have shown that ketamine exposure during this period of rapid synaptogenesis can increase neuroapoptosis and alter behavior in exposed rat pups; however, if rat pups are exposed to chronic pain (in the absence of the drug), chronic pain can also cause an increase in neuroapoptosis. If these animals are exposed to chronic pain and ketamine, neuroapoptosis is markedly attenuated.[135] Stratmann and colleagues have shown in rat pups that exposure to increased levels of carbon dioxide results in an increase in neuroapoptosis to a level that is similar to that observed with exposure to isoflurane. However, neurocognitive performance in the carbon dioxide exposed group was similar to that of

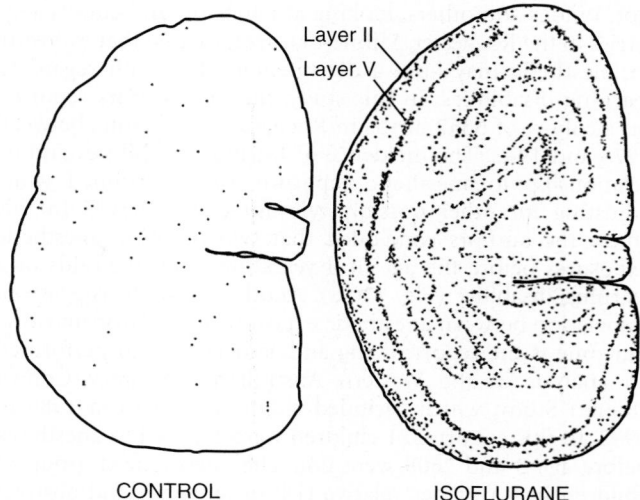

Fig. 130.7. Computer plots based on the number and location of each activated caspase-3–stained neuronal profile in homologous sections from the primary visual cortex of a control and isoflurane brain. Note the laminar pattern of distribution of stained neuronal profiles in the isoflurane brain and the randomly scattered pattern in the control brain. The layers primarily affected in the isoflurane brain are layers II and V. (From Brambrink AM, Evers AS, Avidan MS, et al. Isoflurane-induced neuroapoptosis in the neonatal rhesus macaque brain. Anesthesiology. 2010;112:834-841.)

control animals, whereas animals exposed to isoflurane had neurocognitive impairment.[129] Stratman and coworkers challenged the view of neuroapoptosis and have suggested that anesthetic agents may affect neurogenesis.

Anesthetic neurotoxicity animal investigations have also focused on dendritic synaptic density in neonatal animals exposed to anesthetic agents. De Roo and colleagues, using a rodent model, demonstrated the age-related effects of propofol on dendritic spine density. Exposure of rat pups to propofol at postnatal days 5 and 10 significantly decreased dendritic spine density, whereas on postnatal days 15, 20, or 30 propofol exposure increased dendritic spine density. In addition, the propofol-induced modifications in dendritic spine densities persisted up to postnatal day 90. Exactly how these developmental changes affect neural circuit connectivity and neurocognitive function is unclear.[136]

Other animal studies have correlated biomarkers of inflammation with neurotoxicity. In studies of pregnant mice (gestational day 14) and mouse primary neurons exposed to sevoflurane, sevoflurane increased caspase-3 activation, increased interleukin-6, decreased postsynaptic density-95, and decreased synaptophysin levels in the brains of both the fetal and the offspring mice. In addition, in separate learning and memory tests (Morris water maze), sevoflurane anesthesia impaired learning and memory in offspring mice when tested at P31. Of equal importance was that if the sevoflurane-exposed animals were placed in an enriched environment, the biomarker changes were attenuated and the animal's learning and memory performance were similar to that of the control animals.[137]

How these findings in animals translate to humans is less clear. Some studies suggest a possible association of anesthesia exposure with neurocognitive impairment, whereas others do not. Wilder and others, looking at databases and county registries in the Rochester, Minnesota, area, suggest that exposure to anesthesia may have a detrimental effect with regard to learning disabilities. In this study, the investigators reported on a cohort of 5357 births in Rochester, Minnesota, between 1976 and 1982. The incidence of learning disabilities and its relationship to anesthetic exposure was determined while adjusting for other possibly relevant covariables.[138] In this study, the authors concluded that two or more anesthetic exposures before the age of 4 years increased the odds of a learning disability (Fig. 130.8). Another study to suggest an association between anesthetic exposure and neurobehavioral outcome is the report of Ing and associates, who performed an analysis of the Western Australian Pregnancy Cohort (Raine) Study, which included children born from 1989 to 1992. In this cohort, 321 children were exposed to anesthesia before age 3 and 2608 were not. The anesthetized group of children had a higher relative risk of language and abstract reasoning deficits when studied at age 10 than children who had not received an anesthetic before age 3.[139]

However, in a study of twin cohorts from the Netherlands, Bartels and others reported no causal relationship between anesthesia and learning deficits. In their study of 1143 monozygotic twin pairs, Bartels and colleagues noted that twins exposed to anesthesia before age 3 had significantly more cognitive problems and lower educational achievement scores than did twins not exposed to anesthesia. However, in twin pairs that were discordant for anesthesia (ie, one twin exposed and one twin not exposed), these twins were not different from each other.[140]

At the moment with the exception of xenon and dexmedetomidine, most anesthetic agents and adjuncts have been associated with neurotoxicity in experimental animal models. Both xenon and dexmedetomidine have been shown to attenuate the neurotoxic effects of ketamine, isoflurane, sevoflurane, and propofol.[141-143] Large-scale clinical studies to better define the role of anesthesia and the inflammatory response to surgery will be needed to determine the role of neurotoxicity for anesthetic agents as well as define a biomarker or phenotype for the patient truly at risk from these agents.

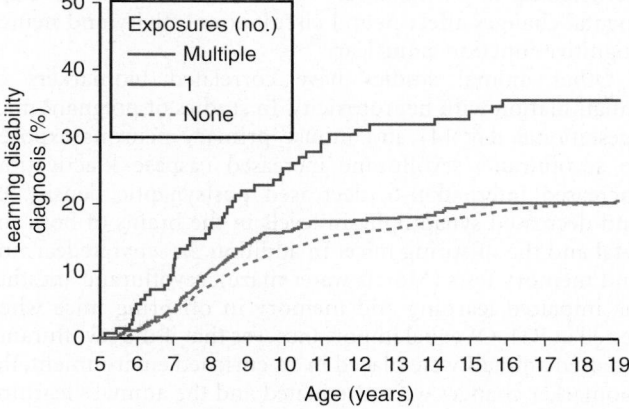

Fig. 130.8. Cumulative percentage of learning disabilities diagnosis by the age of exposure shown separately for those who have zero, one, or multiple anesthetic exposures under the age of 4. (From Wilder RT, et al. Early exposure to anesthesia and learning disabilities in a population-based birth cohort. Anesthesiology. 2009;110:796-804.)

Key References

1. Rappaport BA, Suresh S, Hertz S, et al. Anesthetic neurotoxicity–clinical implications of animal models. *N Engl J Med.* 2015;372:796-797.
2. Suleiman MS, Zacharowski K, Angelini GD. Inflammatory response and cardioprotection during open-heart surgery: the importance of anaesthetics. *Br J Pharmacol.* 2008;153:21-33.
5. Barash PG, Glanz S, Katz JD, et al. Ventricular function in children during halothane anesthesia: an echocardiographic evaluation. *Anesthesiology.* 1978;49:79.
6. Friesen RH, Lichtor JL. Cardiovascular effects of inhalation induction with isoflurane in infants. *Anesth Analg.* 1983;62:411.
7. Keenan RL, Boyan CP. Cardiac arrest due to anesthesia. A study of incidence and causes. *JAMA.* 1985;253:2373-2377.
8. Rackow H, Salanitre E, Green LT. Frequency of cardiac arrest associated with anesthesia in infants and children. *Pediatrics.* 1961;28:697-704.
16. von Ungern-Sternberg BS, Saudan S, et al. Desflurane but not sevoflurane impairs airway and respiratory tissue mechanics in children with susceptible airways. *Anesthesiology.* 2008;108:216-224.
19. Kharasch ED, Hankins DC, Thummel KE. Human kidney methoxyflurane and sevoflurane metabolism. *Anesthesiology.* 1995;82:689.
20. Kuratani N, Oi Y. Greater incidence of emergence agitation in children after sevoflurane anesthesia as compared with halothane: a meta-analysis of randomized controlled trials. *Anesthesiology.* 2008;109:225-232.
22. Holzman RS, van der Velde ME, Kaus SJ, et al. Sevoflurane depresses myocardial contractility less than halothane during induction of anesthesia in children. *Anesthesiology.* 1996;85:1260-1267.
23. Robinson S, Gregory GA. Fentanyl-air-oxygen anesthesia for ligation of patent ductus arteriosus in preterm infants. *Anesth Analg.* 1981;60:331.
28. Ross AK, Davis PJ, Dear G, et al. Pharmacokinetics of remifentanil in anesthetized pediatric patients undergoing elective surgery or diagnostic procedures. *Anesth Analg.* 2001;93:1393-1401.
29. Olgatree ML, Sprung J, Moravec CS. Effects of remifentanil on the contractility of failing human heart muscle. *J Cardiothorac Vasc Anesth.* 2005;19:763-767.
30. Davis PJ, Galinkin J, McGowan FX, et al. A randomized multicenter study of remifentanil compared with halothane in neonates and infants undergoing pyloromyotomy. I. Emergence and recovery profiles. *Anesth Analg.* 2001;93:1380-1386.
31. Galinkin JL, Davis PJ, McGowan FX, et al. A randomized multicenter study of remifentanil compared with halothane in neonates and infants undergoing pyloromyotomy. II. Perioperative breathing patterns in neonates and infants with pyloric stenosis. *Anesth Analg.* 2001;93:1387-1392.
32. Chrysostomou C, Di Filippo S, Manrique AM, et al. Use of dexmedetomidine in children after cardiac and thoracic surgery. *Pediatr Crit Care Med.* 2006;7:126-131.
33. Chrysostomou C, De Toledo JS, Avolio T, et al. Dexmedetomidine use in a pediatric cardiac intensive care unit: can we use it in infants after cardiac surgery? *Pediatr Crit Care Med.* 2009;10:654-660.
35. Jooste EH, Muhly WT, Ibinson JW, et al. Acute hemodynamic changes after rapid intravenous bolus dosing of dexmedetomidine in pediatric heart transplant patients undergoing routine cardiac catheterization. *Anesth Analg.* 2010;111:1490-1496.
40. Hammer GB, Drover DR, et al. The effects of dexmedetomidine on cardiac electrophysiology in children. *Anesth Analg.* 2008;106:79-83.
43. Housmans PR. Effects of dexmedetomidine on contractility, relaxation, and intracellular calcium transients of isolated ventricular myocardium. *Anesthesiology.* 1990;73:919-922.
46. Chrysostomou C, Sanches-de-Toledo J, Wearden P, et al. Perioperative use of dexmedetomidine is associated with decreased incidence of ventricular and supraventricular tachyarrhythmias after congenital cardiac operations. *Ann Thorac Surg.* 2011;92:964-972.
47. Chrysostomou C, Morell V, Wearden P, et al. Dexmedetomide: therapeutic use for the termination of reentrant supraventricular tachycardia. *Congenit Heart Dis.* 2013;8:48-56.
50. Petroz GC, Sikich N, James M, et al. A phase 1, two center study of the pharmacokinetics and pharmacodynamics of dexmedetomidine in children. *Anesthesiology.* 2006;105:1098-1110.
52. Mahmoud M, Radhakrishnan R, Gunter J. Effect of increasing depth of dexinodetomidine anesthesia on upper airway morphology in children. *Paediatr Anaesth.* 2010;20:506-515.

58. Vasile B, Rasulo F, Candiani A, Latronico N. The pathophysiology of propofol infusion syndrome: a simple name for a complex syndrome. *Intensive Care Med.* 2003;29:1417-1425.

68. Llewellyn N, Moriarty A. The national pediatric epidural audit. *Paediatr Anaesth.* 2007;17:520-533.

91. Kochanek PM, Clark R, Ruppel R, et al. Biochemical, cellular, and molecular mechanisms in the evolution of secondary damage after severe traumatic brain injury in infants and children: lesions learned from the bedside. *Pediatr Crit Care Med.* 2000;11:4-19.

92. Kennedy C, Sokoloff L. An adaptation of the nitrous oxide method to the study of the cerebral circulation in children; normal values for cerebral blood flow and cerebral metabolic rate in childhood. *J Clin Invest.* 1957;36:1130-1137.

94. Karsli C, Luginbuehl I, Farrar M, Bissonnette B. Cerebrovascular carbon dioxide reactivity in children anaesthetized with propofol. *Paediatr Anaesth.* 2003;13:26-31.

98. Wong GT, Luginbuehl I, Karsli C, et al. The effect of sevoflurane on cerebral autoregulation in young children as assessed by the transient hyperemic response. *Anesth Analg.* 2006;102:1051-1055.

105. Strebel S, Lam AM, Matta B, et al. Dynamic and static cerebral autoregulation during isoflurane, desflurane, and propofol anesthesia. *Anesthesiology.* 1995;83:66-76.

110. Nishiyama T, Matusukawa T, Yokoyama T, et al. Cerebrovascular carbon dioxide reactivity during general anesthesia: a comparison between sevoflurane and isoflurane. *Anesth Analg.* 1999;89:1437-1441.

111. Komatsu H, Taie S, Endo S, et al. Electrical seizures during sevoflurane anesthesia in two pediatric patients with epilepsy. *Anesthesiology.* 1997;81:1535.

122. Karsli C, Luginbuehl I, Bissonnette B. The cerebrovascular response to hypocapnia in children receiving propofol. *Anesth Analg.* 2004;99:1049-1052.

123. Uemura E, Levin ED, Bowman RE. Effects of halothane on synaptogenesis and learning behavior in rats. *Exp Neurol.* 1985;89:520-529.

124. Jevtovic-Todorovic V, et al. Early exposure to common anesthetic agents causes widespread neurodegeneration in the developing rat brain and persistent learning deficits. *J Neurosci.* 2003;23:876-882.

125. Brambrink AM, Evers AS, Avidan MS, et al. *Anesthesiology.* 2010;112:834-841.

129. Stratmann G, et al. Effect of hypercarbia and isoflurane on brain cell death and neurocognitive dysfunction in 7-day-old rats. *Anesthesiology.* 2009;110:849-861.

130. Slikker W Jr, et al. Ketamine-induced neuronal cell death in the perinatal rhesus monkey. *Toxicol Sci.* 2007;98:145-158.

132. Wang C, Slikker W Jr. Strategies and experimental models for evaluating anesthetics: effects on the developing nervous system. *Anesth Analg.* 2008;106:1643-1658.

134. Paule MG, Li M, Allen RR, et al. Ketamine anesthesia during the first week of life can cause long-lasting cognitive deficits in rhesus monkeys. *Neurotoxicol Teratol.* 2011;33:220-230.

135. Anand KJ, Garg S, Rovnaghi CR, et al. Ketamine reduces the cell death following inflammatory pain in newborn rat brain. *Pediatr Res.* 2007;62:283-290.

136. De Roo M, Klauser P, Briner A, et al. Anesthetics rapidly promote synaptogenesis during a critical period of brain development. *PLoS ONE.* 2009;4:e7043.

137. Zheng H, Dong Y, Xu Z, et al. Sevoflurane anesthesia in pregnant mice induces neurotoxicity in fetal and offspring mice. *Anesthesiology.* 2013;118:516-526.

138. Wilder RT, Flick RP, Sprung J, et al. Early exposure to anesthesia and learning disabilities in a population-based birth cohort. *Anesthesiology.* 2009;110:796-804.

139. Ing C, DiMaggio C, Whitehouse A, et al. Long-term differences in language and cognitive function after childhood exposure to anesthesia. *Pediatrics.* 2012;130:e476-e485.

140. Bartels M, Althoff RR, Boomsma DI. Anesthesia and cognitive performance in children: no evidence of a causal relationship. *Twin Res Hum Genet.* 2009;12:246-253.

141. Li J, Xiong M, Nadavaluru PR, et al. Dexmedetomidine attenuates neurotoxicity induced by prenatal propofol exposure. *J Neurosurg Anesthesiol.* 2016;28:51-64.

142. Duan X, Li Y, Zhou C, et al. Dexmedetomidine provides neuroprotection: impact on ketamine-induced neuroapoptosis in the developing rat brain. *Acta Anaesthesiol Scand.* 2014;58:1121-1126.

143. Sanders RD, Xu J, Shu Y, et al. Dexmedetomidine attenuates isoflurane-induced neurocognitive impairment in neonatal rats. *Anesthesiology.* 2009;110:1077-1085.

Anesthesia Principles and Operating Room Anesthesia Regimens

Joseph D. Tobias

PEARLS

- The preoperative evaluation includes a history of present illness, past medical problems including medication allergies, a past surgical and anesthetic history, a family history of anesthetic complications, and a review of the patient's current and possibly prior medical record including the medication list.
- In its simplest form, a general anesthesia includes amnesia, analgesia, muscle relaxation, and attenuation of the sympathetic nervous system's response to surgical trauma. The phases of general anesthesia include induction, maintenance, and emergence.
- The standards for intraoperative anesthetic monitoring have been outlined by the American Society of Anesthesiologists and include an oxygen analyzer, noninvasive blood pressure cuff, continuous electrocardiogram, pulse oximeter, end-tidal carbon dioxide analyzer, precordial or esophageal stethoscope, temperature probe, and ventilator disconnect alarm.
- Given the catastrophic effects of local anesthetic toxicity, mechanisms to avoid it and prevent its occurrence are mandatory during the performance of regional anesthetic techniques in infants and children. Epinephrine (0.5 µg/ml) is added to the local anesthetic solution during performance of a regional anesthetic technique to serve as a marker of inadvertent systemic injection.
- Following the successful completion of the surgical procedure, a plan is determined for the postoperative delivery of analgesia including some combination of intravenous opioids, agents to inhibit prostaglandin formation or a regional anesthetic technique. For major surgical procedures, the most effective way to deliver opioids for postoperative analgesia is patient-controlled analgesia.

Introduction

Intraoperative surgical anesthesia can be provided by several different techniques, which generally include the following:

1. Local anesthesia ("local only"): This involves the infiltration of a surgical site with a local anesthetic agent to render the site insensitive to pain. This may be done solely by the surgeon without the involvement of an anesthesia provider.

2. Monitored anesthesia care (MAC): MAC is generally equivalent to procedural sedation and involves monitoring a patient with standard monitors according to the American Society of Anesthesiologists (ASA monitors, discussed later) while administering a sedative or analgesic agent intravenously to provide anxiolysis, sedation, and analgesia. MAC is frequently combined with either infiltration of the surgical site with a local anesthetic agent or a regional anesthetic technique. In general, it includes a combination of a medication with amnestic properties (midazolam or propofol) combined with a medication to provide analgesia such as opioid (fentanyl). During MAC, spontaneous ventilation with a native airway is maintained, thereby eliminating the need for endotracheal intubation and controlled ventilation. The depth of sedation may range from a state in which the patient is awake and relaxed with the ability to respond to verbal stimuli to a state of deep sedation where a painful stimulus is required to elicit a response.

3. Peripheral nerve blockade and neuraxial anesthesia: The techniques are frequently considered together under the title of regional anesthesia. A peripheral nerve block involves the placement of a local anesthetic agent around a nerve or group of nerves (plexus) to render specific dermatomes insensitive to pain. Examples of plexus blockade include cervical plexus blockade for superficial and deep neck surgery, brachial plexus blockade for upper extremity or shoulder procedures, and lumbar plexus blockade for hip or leg surgery.[1-3] Intravenous regional anesthesia, the Bier block, is another example of a peripheral nerve block that can be used to provide surgical anesthesia. A Bier block involves the intravenous injection of a dilute local anesthetic into a vein of an extremity after that extremity has been exsanguinated by wrapping it with a bandage followed by occlusion with a tourniquet. Although the latter technique is generally successful and easy to accomplish, it may not be feasible in younger children except when combined with deep sedation. Given the use of an occlusive tourniquet, its duration is limited to 60 to 70 minutes due to tourniquet pain. The major concern with the Bier block is that the dose of local anesthetic used approaches the toxic limits and should the tourniquet fail, cardiovascular or central nervous system (CNS) consequences from the local anesthetic agent may occur. Neuraxial anesthesia involves the injection of a local anesthetic agent into either the subarachnoid or epidural space. This results in blockade of the spinal cord and its accompanying nerve roots to

render an entire region of the body (lower abdomen, pelvis, perineum, or lower extremities) insensitive to pain. Examples of neuraxial anesthesia include spinal, epidural, and caudal anesthesia.[4,5] In infants and children, a regional anesthetic technique such as a peripheral nerve block or epidural anesthesia can be used instead of general anesthesia in patients with comorbid diseases, which significantly increase the risk of anesthesia. More frequently, the regional anesthetic technique is combined with a general anesthetic as part of a balanced anesthetic technique and continued into the postoperative period by use of a continuous infusion via the catheter to provide postoperative analgesia.

4. General anesthesia: General anesthesia is the most frequently used intraoperative technique in the pediatric population. When general anesthesia is used, it usually includes the administration of medications to provide the requisites of amnesia, analgesia, muscle relaxation, and attenuation of the sympathetic nervous system's response to surgical trauma.

The phases of general anesthesia include induction, maintenance, and emergence. The induction of anesthesia can be carried out with the intravenous administration of an intravenous anesthetic agent (thiopental, propofol, ketamine, or etomidate) or via the inhalation route with an inhalational (volatile) anesthetic agent such as sevoflurane. Advantages of an intravenous induction include the rapid onset of anesthesia and avoidance of issues associated with inhalation induction including claustrophobia from anesthesia mask placement and the odor of the inhalational anesthetic agent. In pediatric patients, the inhalation induction of anesthesia is frequently chosen to avoid the need for obtaining intravenous access on an awake child. When inhalation induction is carried out without intravenous access, airway and cardiovascular issues may arise and mandate immediate treatment without intravenous access. In such cases, if intravenous access cannot be rapidly obtained, it may be feasible to use the intramuscular (IM) route for a select number of medications (atropine, succinylcholine). However, more aggressive resuscitation such as the administration of epinephrine for hemodynamic compromise may require the use of intraosseous access (IO).[6] Fortunately, the majority of problems during inhalation induction can be easily reversed with appropriate airway techniques or the administration of IM medications. Hemodynamic compromise including cardiac arrest was far more common with the use of halothane given its negative inotropic and chronotropic properties.[7] Given these and other concerns, halothane is no longer used in the practice of anesthesia, having been replaced by sevoflurane. Even if intravenous access is present, the inhalational induction of anesthesia may be chosen, as it allows the maintenance of spontaneous ventilation even during deep planes of anesthesia (deep enough to allow for direct laryngoscopy and endotracheal intubation). Such a technique may be used if there is a question regarding the ability to bag-valve-mask ventilate the patient, such as may occur in patients with a potentially compromised airway from infection, tumor, congenital or anatomic abnormalities. Following anesthetic induction, one progresses into the maintenance phase of general anesthesia. This can by provided by the administration of intravenous agents, inhalational agents, or, often, a combination of the two. An example of a balanced technique includes some combination of inhalational agents (nitrous oxide and a volatile anesthetic agent), a continuous infusion of an intravenous anesthetic (propofol), a nondepolarizing neuromuscular blocking agent (NMBA), and an opioid. In most circumstances, the choice of maintenance anesthesia is based on the presence of comorbid features, the type of surgical procedure, and the preferences of the anesthesiologists.

Preoperative Evaluation

Regardless of the type of procedure, the patient's status, and the planned anesthetic technique, a preoperative evaluation is performed at some point prior to anesthetic care. In many centers, this evaluation is performed well in advance of the anticipated surgical procedure in a specialized clinic to allow for specific preoperative interventions, consultation, or preparation that may be required to allow for the safe completion of the anesthetic care and surgical procedure. Alternatively, in low-risk patients without accompanying comorbid diseases, the preoperative evaluation can be performed on the phone using a standardized survey or in person the day of surgery. For patients who are already admitted to the hospital or those presenting for emergent or urgent surgical procedures, the preoperative evaluation is also generally done just prior to the surgical procedure.

The preoperative evaluation includes a history of present illness, past medical problems including medication allergies, a past surgical and anesthetic history, a family history of anesthetic complications, and a review of the patient's current and possibly prior medical record including the medication list. For elective surgical procedures, the status of comorbid conditions should be optimized prior to the surgical procedure. The latter may not be feasible for urgent or emergent cases. The physical examination is directed primarily at the central nervous system, cardiovascular system, and respiratory system including an examination of the airway. The preoperative evaluation attempts to identify patients with a difficult airway, which may preclude successful endotracheal intubation using standard techniques of direct laryngoscopy.[8] As a full description of the airway examination is beyond the scope of this chapter, the reader is referred to reference 8 for additional details. An airway history should be obtained seeking medical, surgical, and anesthetic factors that may indicate a difficult airway. Examination of previous anesthesia records is helpful, although a patient's airway may change with changes in weight, with aging, or with the development of comorbid conditions. A physical examination of the airway is performed to detect physical characteristics associated with a difficult airway such as a large tongue, small mouth, short neck (shortened thyromental distance), recessed mandible (micrognathia), limited extension or flexion of the neck, and limited mouth opening. The patient is then asked to open his or her mouth so that the uvula and tonsillar pillars can be assessed. The view of the oropharynx is assessed using the Mallampati grading system. Visualization of the entire uvula and tonsillar pillars (Mallampati grade 1) suggests that endotracheal intubation will be uncomplicated, whereas failure to visualize the tonsillar pillars and the soft palate (Mallampati class IV) suggests that endotracheal intubation will be difficult. Based on the preoperative evaluation and the identification of comorbid conditions, an ASA Physical Status classification is assigned (Table 131.1). The physical classification is based on the physical condition of the patient and does not include the planned

TABLE 131.1 American Society of Anesthesiologists Physical Status Classification

Classification	Description	Example
1	Normal healthy patient	—
2	Mild systemic disease with no functional limitation	Mild asthma, acyanotic congenital heart disease (atrial septal defect)
3	Severe systemic disease with functional limitation	Sickle cell disease, cystic fibrosis, palliated cyanotic congenital heart disease
4	Severe systemic disease that is a constant threat to life	Advanced stages of muscular dystrophy, cyanotic congenital heart disease with pulmonary hypertension
5	Moribund patient not expected to survive without operation	Perforated bowel with sepsis and shock
6	Brain-dead patient; organs are being removed for donor purposes	—
E	Emergency operation	—

surgical procedure. Laboratory tests and additional investigations are ordered based on the positive findings obtained during the history and physical examination and on the complexity of the surgical procedure.[9] The routine preoperative testing of all patients for elective surgery has been shown to be unjustified and expensive. In the absence of comorbid conditions, for surgical procedures with limited chance of significant blood loss, no laboratory or radiologic evaluation is necessary. Although commonly performed, routine testing of coagulation function has been shown to be of limited value without an antecedent history of bleeding problems.[10] The most common coagulation disorder that may cause problems intraoperatively is von Willebrand disease, which cannot be identified on routine coagulation screening that includes a prothrombin time (PT), partial thromboplastin time (PTT), and an international normalized ratio (INR). In patients presenting for surgical procedures that may require the administration of allogeneic blood products, a hemoglobin is assessed and a type and screen obtained. In specific clinical scenarios, especially in the pediatric population, in whom awake phlebotomy may be problematic, these may be obtained and sent immediately following the induction of anesthesia and placement of an intravenous cannula.

Another area of ongoing controversy is the need for routine preoperative pregnancy testing in postmenarchal patients. Given the theoretic potential for anesthetic agents to be teratogenic and to increase the risk of spontaneous abortion, the history should include specific questioning about the potential for pregnancy including the patient's last menstrual cycle. There is increasing use of a point-of-care urine pregnancy testing in many centers. Further testing such as pulmonary function tests, electrocardiography, and echocardiography are based solely on the presence of comorbid conditions. Following the preoperative visit including the history and physical

examination, the planned management of anesthesia is discussed with each patient. Risks and possible complications are reviewed. Options and plans for postoperative pain management are discussed. The answering of questions and obtaining an informed consent complete the preoperative evaluation.

NPO Guidelines

Although the aspiration of gastric contents is an uncommon event, the consequences may be severe and include pneumonitis, respiratory failure, or even death. Classical teaching states that the severity of the aspiration injury relates to the volume aspirated as well as its pH with severe complications when aspiration includes a volume ≥ 0.4 mL/kg or a pH ≤ 2.5. Although aspiration may occur in any setting, patients at risk include parturients, obese patients, diabetics, patients who have received opioids, patients with gastrointestinal disease (reflux, obstruction), patients with altered mental status, patients with intraabdominal pathology (acute abdominal emergencies including appendicitis), trauma patients, and those in whom difficult airway management is anticipated. Specific comorbid conditions may predispose to aspiration by limiting the patient's ability to protect his or her own airway, decreasing the normal barrier to aspiration (lower esophageal sphincter tone), increasing gastric volume, or delaying gastric emptying.[11,12] Patients who have the highest incidence of perioperative aspiration are those with a high ASA physical status classification (III, IV, or V) and those having emergency surgery. The majority of aspirations occur during the induction of anesthesia or following tracheal extubation when the patient has lost his or her protective airway reflexes.

Keeping patients *nil per os* (NPO) remains the mainstay of therapy to prevent acid aspiration. In the past, patients were fasted for 8 to 12 hours before surgery to reduce the volume of gastric contents at the time of induction of anesthesia and to decrease the risk of aspiration pneumonitis. This preoperative fast does not take into account differences in gastric emptying of clear liquids and solids. Based on several investigations and clinical experience, there has been a significant revision in the perioperative fasting rules especially for infants and children. It has been demonstrated that clear liquids have a gastric emptying time of 1 to 2 hours, whereas solids have an unpredictable gastric emptying time that may be greater than 6 hours.[13-16] The ingestion of clear liquids up to 2 hours before surgery does not increase gastric fluid volume or acidity.[13-16] As a result, the liberalization of guidelines for ingestion of clear liquids for elective surgery of otherwise healthy patients has been recommended.[17-19] Suggested guidelines as recommended by the American Society of Anesthesiologists for patients with no known risk factors include no solid food for at least 6 hours before surgery and unrestricted clear liquids until 2 hours before surgery. Importantly, instead of merely allowing clear liquids prior to surgery, their administration is encouraged and parents are reminded to allow their children to have clear liquids (apple juice) prior to coming to the hospital. This improves hydration and limits irritability related to NPO time. Oral medications should be given 1 to 2 hours before surgery with a small sip of water. The latter is particularly important for specific medications such as anticonvulsants, and postoperative seizures may occur related to missing a single preoperative dose.[20] Although, on theoretic grounds, several maneuvers may be indicated in patients with risk factors for acid aspiration, there is limited if any evidence-based medicine to demonstrate their efficacy in preventing perioperative aspiration. Many centers routinely use preoperative medications to decrease the acidity of the gastric fluid (H_2 antagonists or proton pump inhibitors) and speed gastric emptying (metoclopramide). To be effective, it is recommended that these medications be administered 60 to 90 minutes prior to anesthetic induction. Alternatively, a nonparticulate antacid (sodium bicitrate) can be given immediately prior to anesthetic induction, a common practice in obstetrical anesthesia. However, not one of these practices has been shown to alter outcome when examined rigorously using evidence-based medicine.[21] In patients at risk for acid aspiration, rapid sequence induction (RSI) is commonly practiced. This involves the use of a rapidly acting neuromuscular blocking agent (discussed later) with an anesthetic induction agent and the application of cricoid pressure. As the cricoid is the only complete ring of the trachea, it can be gently pushed posteriorly to effectively occlude the esophagus and prevent passive regurgitation of gastric contents when consciousness is lost during anesthetic induction. In its classical form, RSI involves preoxygenation, the administration of an anesthetic agent (sedative) and NMBA in rapid sequence, and the performance of endotracheal intubation without bag-valve-mask ventilation. Bag-valve-mask ventilation is not provided, as it may distend the stomach and predispose to regurgitation. Without assisted ventilation, oxygen desaturation may occur in infants and small children, patients with reduced functional residual capacity, or those with significant alveolar space disease. Additionally, as the anesthetic agent (sedative) and NMBA are administered in rapid sequence without demonstrating the ability to provide bag-valve-mask ventilation, this may result in a "cannot intubate–cannot ventilate" scenario. A modification of this technique, known as a modified RSI, uses gentle bag-valve-mask ventilation with a peak inflating pressure less than 20 cm H_2O to provide oxygenation and ventilation while waiting for the anesthetic agent and NMBA to take effect. The modified RSI may be used more commonly in pediatric anesthesia as even brief periods of apnea without bag-valve-mask ventilation may result in precipitous decreases in oxygenation due to the low functional residual capacity and high metabolic rate for oxygen in young children and infants. Although RSI is commonly practiced, it is not universally accepted and has not been tested using evidence-based medicine.[22] It has been demonstrated that even in experienced hands, especially in young infants and children, the correct application of cricoid pressure is problematic.[23]

Preoperative Medication

There are several categories and uses of preoperative medications (Table 131.2). The most common use of a preoperative medication is to provide sedation and anxiolysis prior to transport to the operating room. Preparing the patient for surgery includes psychologic preparation and frequently pharmacologic premedication. Psychologic preparation includes the preoperative visit and an interview by the anesthesiologist. Pharmacologic premedication may be given orally, or rarely intramuscularly, 1 to 2 hours before the induction of anesthesia or intravenously in the immediate preoperative period. Popular choices include benzodiazepines such as midazolam or occasionally α_2-adrenergic agonists such as

TABLE 131.2   Types and Uses of Premedications

Type of Medication	Purpose
Benzodiazepine	Sedation, anxiolysis, amnesia—eases parental separation
Alpha$_2$-adrenergic agonists (clonidine, dexmedetomidine)	Sedation, anxiolysis—decrease intraoperative anesthetic needs
Opioids	Analgesia during invasive procedures
Anticholinergic agents (atropine, glycopyrrolate)	Prevent bradycardia, blunt airway reflexes, dry secretions
Inhaled β-adrenergic agonists (albuterol) and anticholinergic agents (ipratropium)	Prevent or relieve bronchospasm
Inhaled lidocaine	Prevent airway reflexes during awake fiberoptic intubation, direct laryngoscopy, or bronchoscopy
H_2 antagonists, proton pump inhibitors	Decrease pH of stomach contents
Promotility agents such as metoclopramide	Decrease volume of gastric secretions
Antiemetic agents (scopolamine patch, neurokinin-1 inhibitors)	Prevent perioperative nausea and vomiting

clonidine or dexmedetomidine. A frequently used agent and route of administration for the pediatric patient is the oral administration of the benzodiazepine midazolam to ease separation from parents and improve mask acceptance for the inhalation induction of anesthesia. This is generally necessary when children are at least 9 to 18 months of age and begin to manifest stranger anxiety. Given alterations in bioavailability when administered by the oral route, doses of 0.3 to 0.5 mg/kg are required.[24]

Additional preoperative medications may be used in patients with certain comorbid features including the use of H_2 antagonists, proton pump inhibitors, or motility agents to increase gastric pH and decrease gastric volume in patients at risk for acid aspiration, whereas inhaled β-adrenergic agonists (albuterol) or anticholinergic agents (ipratropium) may be administered to patients with reactive airway diseases (asthma, recent upper respiratory infection, or chronic obstructive pulmonary diseases). Anticholinergic agents may be used to dry airway secretions in patients requiring fiberoptic intubation.

Monitoring

The American Society of Anesthesiologists has outlined the standards for intraoperative anesthetic monitoring. The monitoring standards are the same regardless of whether the case entails a general anesthetic, regional anesthetic (peripheral nerve block, spinal, or epidural), or monitored anesthesia care. The standards according to the ASA include an oxygen analyzer, noninvasive blood pressure cuff, continuous electrocardiogram (ECG), pulse oximeter, end-tidal carbon dioxide analyzer, precordial or esophageal stethoscope, temperature probe, and a ventilator disconnect alarm.

Although arrhythmias are generally uncommon, bradycardia may occur due to the administration of the volatile anesthetic agents (halothane or sevoflurane), hypoxemia, hypothermia, alterations in intracranial pressure, or from the oculocardiac or trigeminocardiac reflex. Although generally devoid of significant negative chronotropic properties, profound bradycardia may occur with the administration of sevoflurane to patients with trisomy 21.[25] In most clinical scenarios, a three-lead ECG is used with the demonstration of lead II to facilitate the identification of P wave morphology and arrhythmia analysis. In adult patients and in specific pediatric patients, a five-lead ECG is used to facilitate ischemia detection along the anterior myocardium. Other potential applications for intraoperative ECG monitoring include identification of potentially lethal electrolyte disturbances such as hyperkalemia, rare instances of prolonged QT syndrome (congenital, acquired, or drug-induced), and monitoring for inadvertent systemic injection of local anesthetic agents.[26] By using the T-wave, systolic blood pressure (BP), and heart rare (HR) criteria, the positive response rate to an epinephrine test (0.1 mL/kg of a 1:200,000 solution or 0.5 μg/kg) was 100%, 95%, and 71%, respectively, during sevoflurane anesthesia and 90%, 71%, and 71% during halothane anesthesia.[27,28]

Pulse oximetry estimates the saturation percentage of the hemoglobin. It is not meant as a surrogate measure of the partial pressure of oxygen in the blood (PaO_2), especially at its extreme values. The relationship between PaO_2 and oxygen saturation is affected by many factors including the type of hemoglobin and the state of the oxyhemoglobin dissociation curve. The latter is affected by acid-base status, temperature, and 2,3-diphosphoglycerate (DPG) levels. Pulse oximetry is known to be inaccurate during periods of hypoxemia (saturation less than 85%–90%) and generally reads 98% to 100% when the PaO_2 exceeds 100 mm Hg. Both patient-related and external factors may interfere with its accuracy including motion and low tissue perfusion. New technology has led to the introduction of low-perfusion pulse oximetry that provides accurate readings during low perfusion states, devices using six to eight wavelengths of light instead of two that can identify abnormal hemoglobin species (carboxyhemoglobin, methemoglobin), improved accuracy at saturation levels less than 90%, and alternative sites for monitoring such as the forehead, which may not be affected by low perfusion states.

End-tidal carbon dioxide ($ETCO_2$) monitoring or capnography remains a standard of care for intraoperative monitoring. It not only documents the initial correct placement of the endotracheal tube, but it ensures ongoing ventilation during the case. $ETCO_2$ displays the patient's exhaled carbon dioxide concentration continuously during exhalation with the $ETCO_2$ being the peak value before the next breath is initiated. When used continuously in the operating room setting, the technology provides a continuous estimation of the partial pressure of CO_2 ($PaCO_2$) in the blood as well as serving as a disconnect alarm during mechanical ventilation, monitoring respiratory rate, and providing information regarding pulmonary function via the shape of the capnogram. Abrupt changes in the $ETCO_2$ such as decreases related to increased dead space may alert the clinician to decreased cardiac output or alterations in pulmonary perfusion related to gas or pulmonary embolism. Acute increases in $ETCO_2$ may be the initial sign of malignant hyperthermia or other hypermetabolic states.

The normal capnogram has three phases of exhalation and one of inspiration, generally labeled as phases 1 through 4. Phase 1 is the beginning of exhalation, representing dead space ventilation and therefore having no $ETCO_2$ present. If $ETCO_2$ is present during phase 1, this indicates the rebreathing of exhaled gas, which may be due to inadequate fresh gas flows. Phase 2 is the rapid and steep upslope of the capnogram representing the emptying of alveolar gas with dead space gas. Phase 3 is the plateau phase, which in the normal state should be relatively horizontal. Upsloping of phase 3 of the capnogram is indicative of obstructive lung disease (asthma, bronchospasm) with differential emptying of alveoli with varying time constants. With the initiation of inspiration, there is an abrupt decrease of the $ETCO_2$ (phase 4), which should return to 0 mm Hg. The $ETCO_2$ generally correlates in a clinically useful fashion with the $PaCO_2$ with the $ETCO_2$ being 2 to 4 mm Hg lower than the $PaCO_2$ and can be used to adjust intraoperative ventilation. However, this correlation is dependent on effective matching of ventilation with perfusion. The relationship between the $ETCO_2$ and $PaCO_2$ may be affected by technology and patient-related factors. Such issues may be particularly relevant in the practice of pediatric anesthesia where smaller tidal volumes, type of ventilation (continuous versus intermittent flow), and sampling issues may have an effect. With these caveats in mind, its use has expanded outside of the operating room with its addition to the suggested monitoring guidelines for procedural sedation from the American Society of Anesthesiologists, which are used to judge the adequacy of resuscitation and to prevent inadvertant hyperventilation during patient transport.[29,30]

Based on the medical condition of the patient and the surgical procedure, more elaborate, invasive monitoring may be added to these standard monitors such as a urinary catheter, catheters for measuring intraarterial, central venous, pulmonary artery pressures, and transesophageal echocardiography. Although there are no strict guidelines dictating which patients should have invasive monitors placed, there have been recommendations set forth for the adult population. It must be remembered, however, that these recommendations are based on limited data comparing outcomes in patients managed perioperatively with or without pulmonary artery (PA) catheters.[31,32] The ASA recommends considering three variables, including disease severity, magnitude of the surgical procedure, and practice setting when assessing the benefit versus risk of PA catheters.[33,34] Additional information regarding structural and functional issues of the myocardium may be obtained by the use of transesophageal echocardiography (TEE). TEE is being used more frequently in the adult population with the development of specific curriculum to teach the skills necessary to perform TEE during cardiac anesthesia fellowships. The latter has been followed by the American Board of Anesthesiology, which recognizes such training and provides the opportunity for credentialing through the completion of a written examination. The strongest indications for perioperative transesophageal echocardiography that are supported by evidence-based medicine include cardiac surgery procedures such as repair of valvular lesions (insufficiency or stenosis) or congenital lesions, assessments and repairs of thoracic aortic aneurysms and dissections, pericardial window procedures, and the repair of hypertrophic obstructive cardiomyopathy.[34] For noncardiac surgery, intraoperative transesophageal echocardiography may be indicated to evaluate acute, persistent, and life-threatening hemodynamic disturbances in which ventricular function and its determinants are uncertain and have not responded to treatment especially when placement of a PA catheter is not feasible.

Given the current limitations of the clinical available measures of cardiac output (TEE or PA catheter), there is ongoing interest in the development of accurate and noninvasive means of assessing cardiac output. Doppler-based techniques, specifically transesophageal Doppler, provide a noninvasive alternative with accuracy that is similar to, though not superior to, thermodilution. Calibrated pulse contour analysis is superior to uncalibrated pulse contour analysis, though both tend to suffer during periods of hemodynamic instability. Bioreactance is completely noninvasive and shows promising accuracy in comparison to thermodilution. It is, however, a relatively new technology when compared to its thermodilution and Doppler counterparts. More research is needed before meaningful conclusions can be made regarding the clinical utility of bioreactance, whereas bioimpedance monitors have shown poor accuracy and cannot be recommended for clinical use. At this point, none of these technologies can be considered the standard of care, and in most circumstances, their use is confined to clinical investigations with limited applications in standard operating room patient management.

In addition to the standard ASA monitors and other monitors of hemodynamic function previously discussed, there is growing interest in the development and potential use of *depth of anesthesia* monitors to allow titration of anesthetic agents (inhaled and intravenous). Although these monitors may have several potential benefits, their primary role has been to possibly decrease the incidence of intraoperative awareness. Although controversial, the potential impact of such monitors is highlighted by the results of trials, which demonstrate that intraoperative awareness occurs in approximately 0.1% to 0.2% of all patients. Specific patient populations are at higher risk, including those affected by trauma, cardiac, obstetric, and emergency surgery. Several manufacturers have marketed or are developing monitors that provide the anesthesia provider with a numeric value against which anesthetic agents are titrated. The most commonly used monitors include the Bispectral Index, or BIS monitor; the Narcotrend, which is currently available only in Europe; the Patient State Analyzer; SNAP; and Auditory Evoked Potential Monitor (AEP Monitor, Danmetter Medical). The first one introduced into clinical use, the one that has received the most clinical use, and the most commonly used monitor continue to be the Bispectral Index. The BIS is a modified electroencephalographic (EEG) monitor that uses a preset algorithm based on intraoperative EEG data obtained from adults who were anesthetized with agents that work through the γ-amino butyric acid (GABA) pathway. The BIS number is determined from three features of the EEG tracing: (1) the amplitude and frequency of the waves, (2) the synchronization of low- and high-frequency information, and (3) the percentage of time in burst suppression (flat EEG). The output of the processed EEG then provides a depth of sedation/anesthesia that is displayed numerically, ranging from 0 to 100, with 40 to 60 being the proposed suitable level of anesthesia to ensure amnesia and lack of recall. With the use of BIS monitoring, a decreased incidence of awareness has been demonstrated as well as a decrease in the total amount of anesthetic agent used.[35-37] Additional studies have suggested faster recovery times and faster discharge times from the postanesthesia care unit, both of which may translate into reduced perioperative costs.[37,38] Although not considered the standard of care for intraoperative monitoring, the ASA does recommend the availability of such monitors whenever general anesthesia is provided and suggests their use in clinical scenarios in which the patient may be at high risk for awareness, including situations involving patients who have had a previous episode of awareness. Given the success of such monitors in the perioperative arena, there is ongoing interest in the application of this technology in the ICU and the procedural sedation arena.[39-41]

Pharmacology of Anesthetic Agents
Local Anesthetic Agents

The local anesthetic agents can be divided into two chemically distinct classes: esters and amides. Local anesthetic agents in the amino ester class include procaine, chloroprocaine, and tetracaine. Amino amides include lidocaine, mepivacaine, prilocaine, bupivacaine, levobupivacaine, and ropivacaine. Clinically important differences between these two classes of local anesthetic agent include their site of metabolism, plasma half-life, adverse effect profile (CNS versus cardiac toxicity), and allergic potential (discussed later). Amino esters are metabolized by plasma cholinesterases, whereas amino amides undergo hepatic metabolism. As there is limited change in the activity of plasma cholinesterase based on chronologic and gestational age, there may be inherent safety advantages to using these agents in the neonatal population.

Local anesthetic agents block the sodium channels in the nerve membrane, thereby preventing depolarization and impulse propagation. The nonionized portion of the local anesthetic agent penetrates the lipid membrane, whereas the ionized portion reversibly blocks the inner aspect of the sodium channel. Local anesthetic agents differ in intrinsic potency, onset of action, duration of action, and their ability to produce differential sensory and motor blockade. Potency is determined primarily by lipid solubility (high lipid solubility = potency).[42] Bupivacaine and tetracaine are examples of local anesthetic agents with high lipid solubility and hence high potency. The onset of action is determined primarily by the pK_a, with onset being most rapid in agents with a pK_a closest to the physiologic pH.[43,44] With a pK_a close to the physiologic pH, the percentage of the unionized form is greater, thereby increasing passage through the lipid nerve membrane. Lidocaine has a pK_a of 7.7 and at a pH of 7.4; 35% exists in the unionized base form, yielding a relatively rapid onset of blockade. In contrast, tetracaine has a pK_a of 8.6 with only 5% in the unionized form at a tissue pH of 7.4, resulting in a slower onset of blockade than lidocaine. Lastly, the duration of action is determined primarily by the degree of protein binding to receptors in the sodium channel.[45] High protein binding and therefore a prolonged duration of action are characteristic of bupivacaine, levobupivacaine, tetracaine, and ropivacaine. Duration of action is also influenced by the degree of vasodilation produced by the local anesthetic.[45-47] Vasodilatation results in increased blood flow to the area and therefore an increased removal of the agent from the depot in the tissues. The local anesthetic agents also differ in their differential effects on sensory versus motor nerves. Bupivacaine and ropivacaine demonstrate this property, which is beneficial for postoperative analgesia, whether provided as a single injection or administered through an epidural catheter. The differential blockade allows patients to ambulate, as they have limited motor weakness, and yet sensory blockade provides analgesia.[47]

When performing regional anesthesia, the goal is to place the local anesthetic agent close to the nerve or plexus that needs to be anesthetized. An addition to the armamentarium of the anesthesiologist has been the use of ultrasound to visualize the individual nerve roots or the plexus that is to be anesthetized.[48-52] This technology is also being used for neuraxial techniques including spinal and epidural anesthesia. In both the adult and pediatric population, the use of ultrasound has been shown to increase the success rate of various regional anesthetic techniques and to result in successful blockade with a decreased dose of the local anesthetic agent.

Given the catastrophic effects of local anesthetic toxicity, mechanisms to avoid it and prevent its occurrence are mandatory during the performance of regional anesthetic techniques in infants and children. Epinephrine (0.5 µg/ml or a concentration of 1 : 200,000) is added to the local anesthetic solution during performance of a regional anesthetic technique to cause local vasoconstriction, thereby decreasing the vascular absorption of the drug and also serving as a marker of inadvertent systemic injection.[53-55] Even with negative aspiration for blood, there is the potential for inadvertent intravascular administration. As such, the use of a test dose is common practice for both peripheral and neuraxial blockade as a means of identifying inadvertent systemic injection of the local anesthetic solution. Epinephrine is added in a 1 : 200,000 concentration (5 µg/mL). In adults, the test dose includes 3 mL or 15 µg of epinephrine; in the pediatric population, 0.1 mL/kg of the local anesthetic solution is administered, which results in the delivery of 0.5 µg/kg of epinephrine. If this amount of epinephrine is injected intravascularly, it can generally be detected by changes in heart rate, blood pressure, or the ST-T wave segments of the electrocardiogram and thereby alert the practitioner that inadvertent intravascular injection is occurring.[4]

The site of injection of the local anesthetic agent also has a significant impact on the clinical effects including the duration of action and vascular uptake (plasma concentrations). The shortest duration of action occur with either intrathecal injection for spinal anesthesia or subcutaneous administration. The longest duration of action and onset of blockade are seen with major peripheral nerve blocks (brachial or lumbar plexus blockade). The highest plasma concentration occurs with an intercostal nerve block or interpleural analgesia followed, in order, by caudal epidural, lumbar or thoracic epidural, brachial plexus, peripheral nerve blockade, subarachnoid, and subcutaneous infiltration.[56]

The greatest risk of morbidity and mortality related to the use of local anesthetic agents is the potential to achieve a toxic plasma concentration of the drug. Local anesthetic-induced systemic toxicity affects the central nervous system (CNS) and the cardiovascular (CV) system. The differential effects on these two organ systems and the plasma concentration at which toxic effects are noted vary according to the agent. With most local anesthetic agents, CNS toxicity occurs at doses and blood levels below those that produce CV toxicity. The latter provides some degree of safety, as the CNS symptoms (seizures) are generally more amenable to treatment than the CV effects (arrhythmias and conduction blockade). Death from local anesthetic toxicity is most commonly the result of the cardiovascular effects of these agents with adverse effects on

cardiac electrical and mechanical activity.[57] Bupivacaine produces cardiac arrhythmias by inhibiting the fast sodium channels and the slow calcium channels in the cardiac membrane. Hypercarbia, acidosis, and hypoxia potentiate the negative chronotropic and inotropic effects of high plasma concentrations of local anesthetic agents. These effects are so profound that resuscitative measures for ventricular tachycardia/fibrillation including standard ACLS protocols may be ineffective. Anecdotal case reports have suggested the potential role of various agents such as amiodarone for refractory ventricular arrhythmias or even the use of extracorporeal support. Anecdotal human data and animal studies have suggested that intralipid solutions may be used to bind the local anesthetic agent thereby resulting in the return of spontaneous circulation. Current recommendations from the ASA include ready access to 20% intralipid solutions whenever large doses of local anesthetic agents are used for regional anesthetic techniques.[58,59] Given the risks of morbidity and mortality from local anesthetic toxicity, avoidance of toxicity is the goal through the careful calculation of the dose, use of the lowest necessary dose (concentration and volume), use of a test dose with epinephrine to identify inadvertent intravascular injection, intermittent aspiration to identify vascular penetration, and slow incremental injection of the dose.

Intravenous Anesthetic Agents

The intravenous anesthetic agents in common clinical use include the barbiturates (thiopental, methohexital, and thiamylal), propofol, etomidate, and ketamine. Of note, although the ultra–short-acting barbiturates, thiopental and thiamylal, were frequently used for the induction of anesthesia, their availability within the United States is limited and they no longer play a major role in anesthetic practice. The remaining ultra–short-acting barbiturate, methohexital, is still available in the United States but has limited use for anesthetic induction. Given its stimulatory effects on the electroencephalogram, it remains a niche agent for sedation during electroconvulsive therapy (ECT) in the adult population.

Propofol, ketamine, and etomidate are the intravenous anesthetic agents used most commonly by bolus administration to induce anesthesia. Propofol is also used as a continuous infusion usually in combination with a synthetic opioid infusion (remifentanil, fentanyl, sufentanil) for total intravenous anesthesia (TIVA) or by itself as a continuous infusion to provide MAC while maintaining spontaneous ventilation for procedural sedation. The latter is a commonly employed technique for procedural sedation outside of the operating room during nonpainful radiologic imaging such as MRI.

The barbiturates, propofol, and etomidate mediate their anesthetic properties through interactions with the GABA$_A$ receptor complex. These interactions lead to enhanced activity of the inhibitory neurotransmitter system, GABA.[60-63] Activation of the GABA$_A$ receptor increases the transmembrane movement of chloride resulting in hyperpolarization of the postsynaptic cell membranes. Ketamine's analgesic and anesthetic effects are the result of its interactions with the N-methyl-D-aspartate (NMDA) system, which is activated by glutamate, an excitatory transmitter, as well as other sites within the CNS including those involved with opioid and cholinergic transmission.[64-66]

The intravenous anesthetic agents result in somewhat varying end-organ effects. The barbiturates, propofol, and etomidate reduce cerebral metabolism ($CMRO_2$), cerebral blood flow (CBF), and intracranial pressure (ICP). As such, they are valuable agents in the practice of neuroanesthesia or in critically ill patients with increased ICP. When compared with propofol or the barbiturates, etomidate may be preferred in patients with abnormal cardiovascular function as it provides greater hemodynamic stability. Etomidate maintains cerebral perfusion pressure (cerebral perfusion pressure [CPP] = mean arterial pressure [MAP] − ICP), whereas propofol and the barbiturates may decrease MAP through their effects on systemic vascular resistance (vasodilatation) as well as direct negative inotropic properties. Thiopental and perhaps etomidate and propofol may possess neuroprotective properties secondary to reducing $CMRO_2$, which improves the ability of the brain to tolerate incomplete ischemia during procedures such as carotid endarterectomy or the temporary occlusion of cerebral arteries during an aneurysm repair.[67,68]

The effects of ketamine on ICP remain controversial with the older literature suggesting that ketamine may directly increase cerebral blood flow and ICP. However, more recent studies suggest that ketamine has limited effects on CBF and ICP, especially when given in combination with other anesthetic agents including midazolam.[69-71] It has been postulated that the older literature suggesting an increase in ICP with ketamine was related to depression of ventilation and alterations in $PaCO_2$ rather than direct effects on CNS dynamics. Given concerns related to the effects of etomidate on the endogenous production of corticosteroids, ketamine is being used more commonly for endotracheal intubation in patients with traumatic brain injury (discussed later).[72]

Propofol, midazolam, and the barbiturates have similar effects on the EEG. Initial, low doses with low brain concentrations result in transient high-frequency activity followed by lower-frequency, higher-amplitude waveforms at high brain concentrations and eventually burst suppression and even electrical silence with high enough doses. These effects, which are similar to those produced by the potent inhalational anesthetic agents, have been studied in enough detail and are consistent enough that algorithms have been developed that can analyze the EEG patterns and thereby determine the depth of anesthesia (discussed earlier). These intravenous anesthetic agents have anticonvulsant properties. The barbiturates, midazolam, and propofol have been incorporated into algorithms for the treatment of refractory status epilepticus.[73,74] On the other hand, etomidate can produce involuntary myoclonic movements from an imbalance of inhibitory and excitatory influences in the thalamocortical tract. Etomidate also stimulates the EEG resulting in increased amplitude and frequency.[73,74] Myoclonic movements and opisthotonic posturing have also been reported following the administration of propofol, although there is no associated activation of the EEG. Rather it is postulated that these effects occur from antagonism at glycine receptors in subcortical and spinal structures.

The intravenous anesthetic agents also have dose-dependent effects on ventilatory function. Thiopental, propofol, etomidate, and midazolam result in a decrease of tidal volume and minute ventilation as well as a rightward shift of the CO_2 response curve. As with many end-organ effects of the anesthetic agents, the respiratory depressant effects may be magnified in patients with comorbid conditions (chronic respiratory or cardiovascular disease) and when coadministered with other medications that are respiratory depressants

(inhalational anesthetic agents, opioids, phenothiazines). Given these effects on central control of ventilation, a transient period of apnea may occur following an anesthetic induction dose. In contrast to the respiratory effects of propofol, etomidate, and the barbiturates, in the absence of comorbid diseases, ketamine can generally be expected to result in minimal respiratory depression with preservation of airway protective reflexes.[75,76] Ketamine also stands apart from the other intravenous anesthetic agents in that the release of endogenous catecholamines following its administration results in bronchodilatation, thereby making it a suitable induction agent in patients who are actively wheezing or at risk for reactivity during airway manipulation.[77] Propofol has also been shown to have beneficial airway effects in both clinical and animal studies of airway reactivity, making it a suitable agent for anesthetic induction and endotracheal intubation of patients with altered airway reactivity.[78-81] The proposed mechanism for these effects is a decrease of intracellular inositol phosphate resulting in a depression of intracellular calcium availability.

During the induction or maintenance of anesthesia, the intravenous anesthetic agents can depress the cardiovascular system resulting in hypotension by various mechanisms. The mechanisms responsible for these hemodynamic effects include a reduction of central or peripheral autonomic nervous system activity, blunting of compensatory baroreceptor reflexes, decreased preload, systemic vasodilatation, and direct depression of myocardial contractility. Hemodynamic function during the induction of anesthesia may also be affected by comorbid cardiovascular disease, intravascular volume status, resting sympathetic nervous system tone, concomitant medications (angiotensin-converting enzyme inhibitors, β-adrenergic antagonists), and the administration of other agents including opioids and benzodiazepines. An induction dose of thiopental causes a variable decrease in cardiac output, systemic vascular resistance, and mean arterial pressure as a result of vasodilation as well as direct myocardial depression.[82] This effect is generally well tolerated in patients with adequate cardiovascular function, but it can be exaggerated in the presence of preexisting cardiovascular disease or intravascular volume depletion necessitating the use of a lower dose of thiopental or preferably the use of alternative agents. Propofol demonstrates cardiovascular depressant effects similar to or greater than those of thiopental. Propofol is a direct myocardial depressant and reduces systemic vascular resistance. Significant cardiovascular responses following propofol are more common with high doses, in hypovolemic patients, in elderly patients, and in patients with significant cardiovascular disease.[83,84] The deleterious cardiovascular effects of propofol can be attenuated by the administration of calcium chloride (10 mg/kg).[85] Additional cardiovascular effects from propofol may result from its augmentation of central vagal tone leading to bradycardia, conduction disturbances, and asystole.[86,87] The negative chronotropic effects of propofol are more common when it is administered with other medications known to alter cardiac chronotropic function (fentanyl or succinylcholine). Although the relative bradycardia may be beneficial in elderly patients at risk for myocardial ischemia, it may be detrimental if cardiac output is heart rate dependent.

In contrast to the negative inotropic effects of propofol and the barbiturates, etomidate causes minimal cardiovascular depression and may be used for anesthetic induction in patients with significant cardiovascular disease.[88,89] As etomidate has little effect on systemic vascular resistance, it may be used in patients with cyanotic congenital heart disease in whom pulmonary blood flow is dependent on mean arterial pressure, those with a fixed stroke volume (aortic and mitral stenosis), and those with depressed myocardial contractility. Although suppression of adrenal cortical function occurs even following a single bolus dose of etomidate through inhibition of the activity of 17-α hydroxylase and 11-β hydroxylase, it remains controversial as to whether such effects are of clinical significance in the pediatric-aged patient.[90-92] The compelling data against the use of etomidate, especially in patients with possible sepsis, came from the Corticosteroid Therapy of Septic Shock (CORTICUS) trial.[93] Although the trial was intended to evaluate the efficacy of corticosteroid therapy on outcome in adults with septic shock and adrenal insufficiency, post hoc analysis revealed that patients who had received etomidate had a significantly higher mortality rate, which was not prevented by the administration of corticosteroids. These data suggest that etomidate should be avoided in patients with sepsis or septic shock until there are more definitive data. Although the use of etomidate has decreased in many centers or even been totally eliminated, given its beneficial effects on hemodynamic function and intracranial dynamics, until further data are available it seems prudent to consider its use in critically ill patients outside of the sepsis arena. Perhaps the greater risk may be the potential for cardiovascular collapse when other agents with significant cardiovascular effects are used in critically ill patients. Although still used as a single induction dose in patients with comorbid cardiovascular disease, repeated doses or continuous infusions are not recommended.

The cardiovascular effects of ketamine are different from those of the other intravenous anesthetic agents. Ketamine stimulates the cardiovascular system by activation of the sympathetic nervous system and the release of endogenous catecholamines.[94] Anesthetic induction doses of ketamine (1–2 mg/kg) generally increase heart rate and MAP. Although the indirect effects of ketamine include the release of endogenous catecholamines and stimulation of the sympathetic nervous system, ketamine is a direct myocardial depressant. In most clinical scenarios, the indirect effects compensate for the direct negative inotropic effects. However, in critically ill patients who have depleted their endogenous catecholamines, cardiovascular collapse may occur.[95]

The pharmacokinetic profile of the intravenous anesthetic agents is characterized by a rapid onset of CNS effects secondary to the high lipid solubility of these agents and the high percentage of cardiac output perfusing the brain. The termination of the central CNS effect results from redistribution of the drug from the central to the peripheral compartment. It is not dependent on primary metabolism and elimination of the drug from the body. Most intravenous anesthetics are metabolized in the liver and excreted in the kidney. Some metabolites are active, such as desmethyldiazepam (diazepam) and norketamine (ketamine), and may result in prolonged effects especially with repeated dosing or the use of continuous infusions. There is a wide variation in the elimination half-lives of intravenous anesthetic agents because of differences in clearance. Drugs with short elimination half-lives include propofol, etomidate, ketamine, and midazolam, whereas thiopental has

a long elimination half-life. Propofol is widely used, especially in ambulatory surgery centers, because of its short duration of action, fast recovery time, and early discharge potential.[96,97] This rapid recovery results in less *hangover effect* or residual drowsiness following outpatient surgical procedures, thereby facilitating return to work and resumption of activities of daily life. However, these short-acting agents (propofol, midazolam) demonstrate a pharmacodynamic principle known as the *context-sensitive half-life*. Although their offset is rapid following brief infusions or bolusing dosing, with prolonged infusions over days, their duration of action becomes more like that of long-acting agents with a prolonged recovery when the infusion is discontinued.

Opioids

There are various roles for the opioids in the perioperative and anesthetic treatment of patients. The commonly used opioids are agonists at the μ (mu) opioid receptors located at discrete sites throughout the spinal cord and the CNS.[98] These agents are generally combined with either an inhalational anesthetic agent or an intravenous anesthetic agent for TIVA (discussed earlier). This combination is necessary because even when administered in doses sufficient to produce profound analgesia and apnea, the opioids do not consistently produce amnesia in healthy patients.[99] Intraoperatively, the opioids are used to blunt the sympathetic stress response to surgical trauma, decrease the requirements for inhalational or intravenous anesthetic agents, and provide postoperative analgesia.

Although discrete differences in the chemical structure exist in the intravenous opioid agents, when used clinically, the clinically relevant differences include their potency, onset of action, duration of action, lipid solubility, hemodynamic effects, and metabolic fate (Table 131.3).[100,101] During the conduct of general anesthesia, the synthetic agents including fentanyl and its derivatives are frequently chosen given their brief duration of action, ability to effectively blunt hemodynamic changes related to the surgical stress response, and limited cardiovascular effects. However, other opioids including morphine or hydromorphone may be chosen given their longer duration of action with the ability to provide postoperative analgesia during the transition from general anesthesia to the awake state (emergence). Morphine is the least lipophilic of the commonly used opioids and therefore it has a slower onset of action than the more lipophilic synthetic

TABLE 131.3   Potency and Half-Life of Opioids

Agent	Potency	Half-Life	Active Metabolites
Morphine	1	2-3 hours	Yes
Meperidine	0.1	2-3 hours	Yes
Hydromorphone	5	2-4 hours	No
Oxymorphone	10	2-4 hours	No
Methadone	1	12-24 hours	No
Fentanyl	100	20-30 minutes	No
Sufentanil	1000	20-30 minutes	No
Alfentanil	20	10-15 minutes	No
Remifentanil	100	5-8 minutes	No

opioids such as fentanyl. Morphine, like all of the opioids except for remifentanil, undergoes hepatic metabolism. In part, morphine is converted to morphine-6-glucoronide (M6G), a water-soluble metabolite with a potency far greater than that of the parent compound. However, given that it is water solubile, M6G does not rapidly pass through the blood-brain barrier into the CNS and therefore has limited clinical effects. In patients with renal insufficiency or failure, a significant amount of M6G can accumulate and result in respiratory depression.

Meperidine has a potency that is approximately 10% that of morphine with a similar half-life of 2 to 3 hours. Hepatic metabolism produces normeperidine, a metabolite that may accumulate in renal insufficiency with high plasma concentrations being epileptogenic. Given these concerns and the higher incidence of psychomimetic effects with meperidine, meperidine is rarely used for analgesia. Meperidine remains a common agent, administered in low doses (10 mg in an adult), to treat postanesthesia shivering.

Hydromorphone has a potency that is 6 to 8 times that of morphine with a half-life of 2 to 3 hours. As there are no active metabolites of hydromorphone, it may be an effective alternative to morphine in patients with renal insufficiency. When compared with morphine, hydromorphone causes less histamine release and may be an effective alternative agent when pruritus occurs with morphine use. In particular, hydromorphone may be the preferred agent for postoperative analgesia using patient-controlled analgesia in the older pediatric population.[102]

The synthetic opioids including fentanyl, sufentanil, and alfentanil are potent, highly lipid-soluble drugs with rapid onsets and short durations of action. Hepatic metabolism does not result in active metabolites. Fentanyl is 100 times as potent as morphine, whereas sufentanil has 10 times the potency of fentanyl (1000 times that of morphine). The pharmacokinetics of fentanyl and sufentanil are similar with both drugs being short acting at low doses and longer acting at higher doses. Alfentanil is less potent than sufentanil and fentanyl and has a rapid onset of action and a short duration of action. Because its elimination half-life is substantially less than that of sufentanil and fentanyl, it is suitable for multiple dosing and continuous infusions and is popular for ambulatory surgery in many centers. Remifentanil is the first true ultra–short-acting opioid.[103] It has a rapid onset of activity and undergoes ester metabolism, which results in a short, predictable duration of action. Its elimination half-life is 8 to 10 minutes, and its potency is comparable to fentanyl. It is administered as a continuous infusion and remains short acting regardless of the duration of the infusion. Unlike the other opioids that have longer half-lives and a variable duration of effect in neonates and infants, the duration of action and half-life of remifentanil is constant across all age ranges, thereby making it a suitable agent in neonatal anesthesia when postoperative tracheal extubation is planned.[104-106]

Fentanyl, sufentanil, and alfentanil are common components of various general anesthetic techniques. They have replaced their predecessors (morphine, meperidine) because of their faster onset of action, shorter and more predictable duration of action, and minimal hemodynamic side effects. For general anesthesia they reduce the surgical stress response and the associated cardiovascular responses to endotracheal intubation and surgical stimulation. They potentiate the

hypnotic effects of the inhalational and intravenous anesthetic agents. This dose-related decrease in the need for both intravenous and inhalational anesthetic agents facilitates recovery from prolonged anesthetic cases. High-dose opioid techniques are commonly used in cardiac surgery because the synthetic opioids produce a smooth induction process, provide hemodynamic stability, suppress the hemodynamic responses to various surgical stimulations, reduce the production of stress hormones, and provide a smooth transition to mechanical ventilation at the end of the case.

As with all medications used in the practice of anesthesia, there are several adverse effects related to opioid administration. Opioids produce a dose-related depression of the ventilatory response to CO_2 and blunt the response to hypoxia through a direct effect on the medullary respiratory centers.[107] Increasing plasma concentrations result in a slowing of the respiratory rate that is initially offset by an increase in tidal volume. Equianalgesic doses of all opioids (fentanyl, morphine, meperidine, etc.) produce equivalent degrees of respiratory depression. Opioid-induced respiratory depression is antagonized by pain, movement, and opioid antagonists such as naloxone. When postoperative respiratory depression related to opioids occurs, small incremental doses of naloxone (1 µg/kg every 2 to 3 minutes) may be used to reverse opioid-induced respiratory depression without reversing analgesia. This is opposed to the dose of naloxone (10 µg/kg) that is commonly used for opioid overdose in the emergency department setting. Given that the clinical half-life of naloxone is 20 to 30 minutes, repeated doses or a continuous infusion may be needed if longer-acting opioids (morphine, meperidine, or hydromorphone) have been administered. Longer-acting opioid antagonists (nalmefene) are now clinically available; however, there is limited clinical experience with their use in the pediatric population. Opioid reversal using naloxone, especially with larger doses, can result in undesirable or dangerous hemodynamic responses such as hypertension, tachycardia, and myocardial infarction. The potential for such effects must be weighed against the anticipated benefits of opioid reversal.

Opioids generally produce minimal cardiovascular effects at usual analgesic doses. With higher doses, when combined with other anesthetic drugs, or in patients with comorbid features, opioids may produce bradycardia and a decrease in systemic vascular resistance (SVR) resulting in hypotension. The synthetic opioids may result in bradycardia from stimulation of the central nuclei of the vagus nerve leading to prolonged atrioventricular conduction and direct depression of the sinoatrial node, whereas peripheral vasodilation results from depression of the vasomotor centers in the medulla.[108,109] Patients with elevated levels of sympathetic tone (hypovolemia, congestive heart failure) are more likely to become hypotensive after opioids. Although anesthetic techniques using high doses of the synthetic opioids may result in bradycardia and peripheral vasodilation, given that there is no direct negative inotropic effects, these techniques are effective for patients with myocardial pathology including patients undergoing cardiovascular surgery in whom a high dose of fentanyl (25–75 µg/kg) is a frequently chosen anesthetic technique. Decreases in blood pressure with such techniques result from a decrease in SVR and are easily treated with a direct-acting α-adrenergic agonist such as phenylephrine. Morphine may result in more profound venodilatation leading to decreased venous return, decreased cardiac output, and hypotension. Meperidine, given its structural similarity to atropine, may result in a mild tachycardia.

Nitrous Oxide

A unique aspect of intraoperative anesthetic care is the administration of inhalational anesthetic agents including nitrous oxide (N_2O), halothane, enflurane, isoflurane, sevoflurane, and desflurane. Although their anesthetic properties are similar, the potent inhalational anesthetic agents can be divided into two chemically distinct classes: alkanes and ethers. Halothane is an alkane (a two-carbon chain), whereas the other four agents (enflurane, isoflurane, desflurane, and sevoflurane) are ethers. The potent inhalational anesthetic agents are volatile liquids and are administered to the patient via a vaporizer on the anesthesia. Nitrous oxide is administered either from a central hospital source or from E cylinders on the anesthesia machine. Flows of nitrous oxide and oxygen are mixed in varying concentrations and then directed through the vaporizer to pick up the desired concentration of the potent inhalational anesthetic agent.

The potency of inhalational anesthetic agents is measured by minimum alveolar concentration (MAC). MAC is defined as the percentage of the inhalational anesthetic agent required to prevent 50% of patients from moving in response to a surgical stimulus. The lower the MAC, the more potent the inhalational agent. Halothane is the most potent inhalational anesthetic agent, followed, in order, by isoflurane, enflurane, sevoflurane, and desflurane. Nitrous oxide has a low potency (MAC of 110%) and must be combined with other intravenous sedatives/analgesics/anesthetics or a potent inhalational anesthetic agent to fulfill the prerequisites (unconsciousness, analgesia, muscle relaxation, decrease in sympathetic nervous system activity) of a general anesthetic. As 1.5 to 2.5 MAC of an agent is required to maintain anesthesia solely with a potent inhalational anesthetic agent, in most clinical scenarios, 1 to 1.5 MAC of an inhalational anesthetic agent is combined with N_2O, opioids, or intravenous anesthetic agents to provide maintenance anesthesia during a surgical procedure.

Nitrous oxide (N_2O) was the first of the inhalational anesthetic agents to be discovered. Although there has been a decline in its use with the introduction of the newer inhalational anesthetic agents with low blood-gas solubility coefficients (desflurane, sevoflurane), it still used as a component of intraoperative anesthetic regimens and in some centers for procedural sedation.[110] Depending on the concentration administered, N_2O can provide sedation and analgesia or a weak anesthetic level. In concentrations of 70%, N_2O will render the majority of patients amnestic and provide moderate to significant analgesia. However, only minor surgical procedures can be performed with N_2O and O_2 alone, and its amnestic properties are not a given, thereby necessitating its combination with other agents. When used as the sole agent, N_2O causes minimal respiratory and cardiac depression.[111] Recovery from N_2O sedation is rapid given its low blood-gas solubility coefficient. During recovery, high concentrations of O_2 are needed to avoid diffusion hypoxia.[112] As N_2O diffuses from the blood into the alveoli, its alveolar concentration rises, thereby decreasing the effective concentration of oxygen, which can lead to *diffusion hypoxia*. When used for procedural sedation on repeated occasions, N_2O can lead to inactivation of methionine synthetase, an enzyme necessary for vitamin B_{12} metabolism leading to bone marrow impairment with megaloblastic anemia and deterioration of the posterior columns of the spinal cord and neurologic impairment.[113,114] These effects may occur not only in patients but also in health care workers with chronic exposure, thereby mandating effective scavenging of exhaled gases to avoid environmental pollution whenever N_2O is administered. Given solubility differences, N_2O diffuses into and expands gas-containing closed spaces in the body (obstructed bowel, pneumothorax, middle ear, pneumocephalus, and air embolus).[115] There has been decreased use of N_2O for intraoperative anesthetic care related to reports from the adult literature regarding the potential for increased cardiovascular morbidity and an increased incidence of surgical site infections.[116,117] The potential for cardiac morbidity including myocardial infarction has been postulated to relate to N_2O's effect on methionine synthetase with increased homocysteine levels leading to enhanced platelet function. Given such concerns and the availability of short-acting inhalational agents allowing for rapid recovery from general anesthesia, the use of nitrous oxide has diminished.

Volatile Anesthetic Agents

When administered in appropriate inspired concentrations, all of the potent inhalational anesthetic agents (halothane, isoflurane, enflurane, desflurane, and sevoflurane) provide the basic components of a general anesthetic including amnesia, analgesia, skeletal muscle relaxation, and control of the sympathetic nervous system. Despite their use for more than 150 years in clinic anesthetic care, the exact site and mechanism of action of these agents remain elusive. Research suggests that the primary mechanism may reside in the stabilization of critical proteins, possibly the receptors of neurotransmission.[118] Although these agents provide general anesthesia, their end-organ effects can be varied, thereby dictating their use in various clinical scenarios. In infants and children, given the potential stress that may be inflicted by placement of an intravenous cannula, anesthetic induction may be carried out by the inhalation route with placement of the intravenous cannula after the patient is anesthetized. As halothane and sevoflurane are less pungent to the airway than the other agents, they are the only agents used for the inhalation induction of anesthesia. Although halothane had been the time-honored agent for inhalation induction of anesthesia in infants and children, it has been removed from the market and replaced with sevoflurane due to its significantly lower incidence of bradycardia, myocardial depression, and cardiac arrest. In fact, surveys evaluating the etiology of cardiac arrest during general anesthesia in infants and children have implicated halothane as the primary factor responsible for many of these events.

All of the potent inhalation anesthetic agents cause a dose-related depression of cardiovascular and respiratory function. With increasing anesthetic depth, there is a rightward shift of the CO_2 response curve with a progressive decrease in alveolar ventilation characterized by a reduction in tidal volume in spontaneously breathing patients and an increase in $PaCO_2$. Beneficial effects on the airways include a direct effect on bronchial smooth muscle with bronchodilatation making them an effective agent both intraoperatively and outside of the operating room for the treatment of patients with refractory status asthmaticus.[119]

The potent inhalational anesthetic agents decrease mean arterial pressure, myocardial contractility, and myocardial oxygen consumption. The specific change in cardiac output, systemic vascular resistance, and heart rate varies from agent to agent and with the inspired concentration of the agent that is administered. Isoflurane and desflurane result primarily in vasodilatation and a decrease in SVR with reflex tachycardia. Direct negative chronotropic effects predominate with sevoflurane and halothane leading to a lowering of heart rate. As mentioned previously, this effect is less with sevoflurane than with halothane. Because of its alkane structure, halothane sensitizes the myocardium to catecholamines and can cause dysrhythmias, especially when there is associated hypercarbia or high circulating catecholamines. The latter was of clinical significance when epinephrine-containing local anesthetic agents were administered to patients anesthetized with halothane.

The potent inhalational anesthetic agents cause a dose-dependent decrease in CNS activity, depressing EEG activity, and reducing cerebral metabolic oxygen consumption. Enflurane and sevoflurane can activate the EEG and produce clinical and EEG evidence of seizure activity at high concentrations. Such problems are exacerbated by the presence of hypocarbia, which may occur if there is hyperventilation during anesthetic induction. Despite such effects, there is no contraindication to the use of sevoflurane in patients with an underlying seizure disorder. CBF increases via a reduction in cerebral vascular resistance, which can lead to an elevation of ICP in patients with compromised intracranial compliance. The effect on ICP is least with isoflurane and can be blunted by hyperventilation and hypocarbia. These effects make isoflurane a common choice for neurosurgical anesthesia. The volatile anesthetic agents also have peripheral neuromuscular effects, potentiate the effects of the neuromuscular blocking agents, and along with succinylcholine are triggering agents for malignant hyperthermia.

In addition to the parent compound, metabolic products may be responsible for the toxicity of the potent inhalational anesthetic agents. Fifteen percent to 20% of halothane is metabolized compared to 5% to 10% for sevoflurane, 2% to 3% for enflurane, 0.2% for isoflurane, and less than 0.1% for desflurane. In the early days of inhalational anesthesia, hepatic toxicity was a significant concern and existed into the modern era with halothane. Hepatotoxicity occurs from an immune-mediated reaction following exposure to halothane, enflurane, isoflurane, or desflurane.[120-123] However, given the limited metabolism of enflurane, isoflurane, and desflurane, the risk of hepatotoxicity is extremely low. The mechanism of hepatotoxicity relates to the metabolic product trifluoroacetic acid (TFA) acting as a hapten. It binds to hepatocytes and induces an immune-mediated hepatitis. The metabolic pathway of sevoflurane is different and does not result in the production of TFA. Risk factors for halothane-hepatis include prior anesthetic exposure, female gender, age ≥35 years, and obesity.[124,125]

Albeit rare, specific issues related to renal function must be considered during anesthetic care. Importantly, alterations related to cardiac output due to the inhalational anesthetic agents may secondarily decrease renal blood flow and result in renal damage. As with other end organs, the kidneys may be damaged by the agent itself or its metabolites. Additionally, both enflurane and sevoflurane contain flouride around their carbon atoms, which can be released during metabolism.[126] Fluoride concentrations in excess of 50 μmol/L can result in decreased glomerular filtration rate and renal tubular resistance to vasopressin with nephrogenic diabetes insipidus.

Although high levels of serum fluoride may occur following the prolonged administration of sevoflurane, clinical signs of nephrotoxicity are extremely rare. This is postulated to be the result of the low blood : gas partition coefficient of sevoflurane and its rapid elimination from the body or the fact that sevoflurane unlike older agents such as methoxyflurane does not undergo metabolism in the kidney but only in the liver. Therefore unlike methoxyflurane, there is no local renal release of fluoride thereby limiting the risk of toxicity. Although high serum flouride concentrations have been documented with prolonged enflurane administration, this agent is no longer commonly used in clinical anesthesia practice. An additional concern regarding the potential nephrotoxicity of the potent inhalational agents is unique to sevoflurane, in particular a unique metabolite, a vinyl ether also known as compound A. Compound A is produced during the metabolism of sevoflurane and its reaction with the soda lime in the carbon dioxide absorber of the anesthesia machine.[127-129] Compound A concentrations are increased by several factors including a high inspired concentration of sevoflurane, low fresh gas flows through the system (less than 2 liters per minute), increasing temperatures of the soda lime canister, decreased water content of the CO_2 absorbent, and high concentrations of potassium or sodium hydroxides in the CO_2 absorbent. Although of potential concern when studied in laboratory animals, there are no clinical data to suggest the nephrotoxic potential of compound A, thereby suggesting that such concerns should not limit the use of sevoflurane even in patients with preexisting renal dysfunction.

Neuromuscular Blocking Agents

The reader is referred to Chapter 133 for a complete review of the use of neuromuscular blocking agents (NMBAs). The following section deals briefly with the aspects of NMBA administration that relate specifically to perioperative anesthetic care. Intraoperatively, skeletal muscle relaxation may be required for the successful completion of a surgical procedure (exploratory laparotomy), may be required briefly for endotracheal intubation, or may be used to ensure patient immobility in situations where inadvertent movement may be detrimental (craniotomy). Although frequently administered during the perioperative period, many surgical procedures can be performed without the administration of NMBAs. NMBAs have no effect on the level of consciousness, provide neither amnesia nor analgesia, and do not alter the dose of other medications required to induce and maintain general anesthesia. When NMBAs are used, the patient requires an adequate level of general anesthesia and, in the intensive care unit, an adequate level of sedation. This is especially important because clinical signs of inadequate anesthesia (movement) are abolished. It is also important to recognize that the airway must be controlled when NMBAs are used. These agents are contraindicated if there is any concern regarding one's ability to control ventilation and provide endotracheal intubation. One additional caveat regarding the administration of NMBAs is that although problems are rare, NMBAs are high on the list of agents responsible for intraoperative anaphylactoid reactions (along with antibiotics and latex). Albeit rare, these anaphylactoid reactions are most common with succinylcholine and rocuronium.

Neuromuscular blockade may be used only to facilitate endotracheal intubation or may be continued throughout the surgical procedure to provide surgical relaxation. When ongoing neuromuscular blockade is required, incremental doses, which are approximately one-fourth to one-fifth of the initial intubating dose, are administered based on the response obtained using neuromuscular blockade monitoring. Alternatively, a continuous infusion of short- or intermediate-acting agents is occasionally used. Given that repetitive doses or an infusion may result in excessive levels of neuromuscular blockade, monitoring of neuromuscular transmission is used to predict optimal conditions for endotracheal intubation, adequacy of surgical muscle relaxation, effectiveness of reversal of neuromuscular blockade, and to guide dosing of NMBAs during intraoperative care. The goal of such monitoring is to allow incremental titration of NMBAs to maintain the desired level of blockade while maintaining sufficient neuromuscular function to allow reversal of a residual neuromuscular blockade at the completion of the surgical procedure. To monitor a neuromuscular blockade, a supramaximal electrical stimulation from a peripheral nerve stimulator is delivered to electrodes placed over the distribution of the peripheral nerve. This can be accomplished using the ulnar nerve at the wrist or elbow, the common peroneal nerve as it passes over the head of the fibula, or the facial nerve. As any of these methods involve electrical stimulation, they are painful and should only be performed in an appropriately anesthetized patient. Although various patterns of electrical stimulation of the peripheral nerve (single twitch, train-of-four [TOF], double burst suppression, tetanus, and posttetanic stimulation) have been advocated in the literature, TOF monitoring remains the technique used most commonly in clinical anesthesia practice. Two electrical stimuli are delivered each second for 2 seconds to give four twitches or a train-of-four. Despite its acceptance and use in everyday anesthesia practice, TOF monitoring is relatively nonspecific in that up to 70% to 80% of the acetylcholine receptors must be blocked in order to achieve any visible decrement in the TOF. The goal of monitoring is to ensure that some residual neuromuscular function is present at the completion of the surgical procedure so that the effects can be reversed. The goal of reversal is for the patient to sustain minute ventilation and maintain a patent airway to allow for tracheal extubation.[130,131] In most clinical circumstances, one or two twitches of the TOF must be present to allow for effective pharmacologic reversal. A TOF ≥0.7, where the fourth twitch is ≥70% the height of the first twitch, is evidence of adequate reversal. Other tests of adequacy of reversal include a sustained response to tetanus, a sustained head lift for 5 to 10 seconds, and strong grip strength. In infants, sustained hip flexion is a useful clinical sign. Patients demonstrating profound blockade (no response to electrical stimulation) should not be reversed until some evidence of return of neuromuscular function has occurred. Despite adequate reversal, recurrence of partial paralysis resulting in respiratory insufficiency or upper airway obstruction may occur during the postoperative period.

Reversal of residual neuromuscular blockade is accomplished by the administration of medications that inhibit acetylcholinesterase (edrophonium, neostigmine, or pyridostigmine). With the inhibition of acetylcholinesterase, acetylcholine accumulates at the nicotinic (neuromuscular junction) and muscarinic sites, thereby increasing the competition between acetylcholine and the NMBA for the α subunits of the nicotinic cholinergic receptor. As these medications also inhibit acetylcholinesterase at muscarinic sites, they must be coadministered with an anticholinergic agent such as atropine or glycopyrrolate to prevent bradycardia or asystole. An inadequate response to the anticholinesterase medication with residual weakness may be secondary to excessive blockade at the time of reversal, allowing inadequate time since the administration of the reversal drug, an altered acid-base or electrolyte status, hypothermia, effects of other medications, or impaired clearance of NMBAs from the plasma secondary to renal or hepatic dysfunction.

Intraoperative Anesthetic Care
Maintenance Anesthesia

This chapter has discussed the perioperative care of a surgical patient from the preoperative evaluation through premedication, monitoring, and the induction of general anesthesia. Once the airway has been secured and ventilation/oxygenation established, maintenance anesthesia is provided for the duration of the surgical procedure. Given the variety of inhalational anesthetic agents, intravenous anesthetic agents, opioids, and NMBAs available, several combinations of agents can be used to provide the prerequisites of general anesthesia. The choice of agent varies widely and is determined by the personal preferences and experiences of the anesthesia provider, the patient's comorbid features such as his or her underlying cardiovascular function, the anticipated duration of the surgical procedure, the postoperative requirements (will the patient's trachea be extubated at the completion of the procedure, is ongoing postoperative analgesia required?), and the operative setting (is rapid turnover of cases desirable and are rapid awakening and hospital discharge needed?).

In most scenarios, the baseline level of anesthesia is provided by either a potent inhalational anesthetic agent or a propofol infusion and supplemented with intermittent dosing or a continuous infusion of an opioid. If ongoing neuromuscular blockade is required, a continuous infusion of a short-acting agent or intermittent dosing of an intermediate- to long-acting agent can be used. Although controlled ventilation is most commonly practiced, there are many surgical procedures for which spontaneous ventilation is acceptable. The use of spontaenous ventilation is more common in the outpatient setting where endotracheal intubation is less common and general anesthesia is provided using a mask or an LMA. In addition to the commonly monitored hemodynamic parameters, spontaneous ventilation provides an effective means of evaluating the depth of anesthesia through the assessment respiratory rate and pattern, thereby providing the optimal parameter for the titration of opioids. When spontaneous ventilation is used, opioids can be dosed based on the patient's respiratory rate to ensure that an appropriate amount is administered to provide postoperative analgesia while avoiding overdosing and postoperative respiratory depression.

Intraoperative Fluid Management

In addition to monitoring hemodynamic and respiratory function, the anesthesiologist must also maintain fluid, electrolyte, and glucose homeostasis during anesthetic care. Intraoperative fluid management uses isotonic crystalloid solutions such as lactated Ringer (LR), normal saline (NS), or Plasmalyte to provide ongoing maintenance fluids and replace preoperative deficits, intraoperative third space losses, and blood losses when blood therapy is not necessary. Third space losses may be relatively trivial during superficial procedures (2–3 mL/kg/hr) or significant (10–15 mL/kg/hr) for intraabdominal procedures. Although generally considered an isotonic fluid, LR has only 130 mEq of sodium per liter and therefore is relatively contraindicated in patients at risk for cerebral edema such as the patient with a traumatic brain injury. Large volumes of NS, although effective in supporting the serum sodium, can result in a dilutional acidosis. These issues have led to the consideration of using a combination of NS and LR or the use of a more balanced solution such as Plasmalyte, which contains 140 mEq/L of sodium as well as physiologic amounts of chloride and gluconate/acetate as buffers. Given their distribution between the intravascular and extravascular space, if blood is not administered, blood loss is routinely replaced as 3 mL of crystalloid for each 1 mL of blood loss. Alternatives to isotonic crystalloid solutions include synthetic and natural colloids such as hydroxyethyl starch, albumin, or gelatins. The latter are not currently available in the United States. As with resuscitation in other areas, there are currently no studies demonstrating the superiority of any of these solutions over standard isotonic crystalloids, and it is likely that the crystalloid-colloid debate will continue for many years. Potential drawbacks to the use of hydroxyethyl starch solutions include the potential for platelet dysfunction when amounts greater than 15 to 20 mL/kg are administered. This reversible platelet dysfunction results from alterations in the efficacy of von Willebrand factor by the hydroxyethyl starch solutions. Furthermore, studies in the adult population have demonstrated an increased incidence of acute kidney injury when these products are administered intraoperatively.[132]

During the postoperative period, especially in pediatric patients, given the potential for the development of postoperative hyponatremia, only isotonic fluids should be administered.[133] Fluids with a lower tonicity are rarely if ever indicated. For short surgical procedures when a Foley catheter is not inserted, aggressive fluid therapy with replacement of the preoperative deficit is not necessarily required because bladder distention during emergence from anesthesia may be uncomfortable for the patient. Additionally, specific surgical procedures such as intracranial neurosurgical procedures and thoracic procedures or patients with underlying cardiovascular dysfunction may mandate that the patient "be kept dry" to improve the intraoperative and postoperative course. However, in many other surgical procedures especially intraabdominal cases, burn debridement, or other cases with significant third space losses, the administration of significant amounts of isotonic crystalloids may be required to maintain intravascular volume status. Except for the neonatal population or patients chronically receiving parenteral nutrition fluids, dextrose-containing fluids are rarely administered. In high-risk patients, those receiving glucose containing fluids, and patients with diabetes mellitus, intermittent monitoring of blood glucose may be indicated. Such monitoring has been greatly facilitated by the ready availability of point-of-care testing for glucose. Although a review of the perioperative care of the diabetic patient is beyond the scope of this chapter, evidence in the adult literature has suggested that the postoperative outcome for such patients may be improved by tight perioperative glucose control.

Postoperative Care
Postoperative Analgesia

Various factors may interfere with the delivery of effective postoperative analgesia. Inadequate pain relief following surgery generally results from inappropriate methods of administration rather than ineffective analgesic agents. Although frequently used in the past for the delivery of opioids in the delivery of postoperative analgesia, the intramuscular route should be abandoned as several factors result in inadequate analgesia including variable absorption and unpredictable plasma opioid concentrations in addition to the child's reluctance to ask for pain medications due to the pain associated with intramuscular injections.[111] Fortunately, acute and postoperative analgesia has been an area of intense research, which has resulted in the development of new techniques and the refinement of treatment strategies.[134] Current modalities to provide better postoperative analgesia include intravenous patient-controlled analgesia (PCA), nurse-controlled analgesia (NCA), and the epidural or spinal application of local anesthetic agents or opioids.[135] Although introduced into the adult population, these techniques are now widely applied across all age ranges in pediatric patients. PCA involves the self-administration of small doses of opioids to obtain and maintain analgesia. Analgesia occurs when the plasma opioid concentration reaches the minimum effective analgesic concentration (MEAC). With PCA, patients are able to titrate the opioid to their own MEAC and can thereby maintain consistent analgesia.[136-138] Numerous studies have demonstrated improved analgesia, fewer adverse effects, and decreased opioid consumption with the use of PCA. Prior to the initiation of PCA, the patient receives a loading dose of the opioid administered either intraoperatively or postoperatively as multiple small doses of an opioid to achieve the MEAC. Once this is accomplished, the PCA is started and a dose of opioid is self-administered at a specific interval or lockout period (generally 5–10 minutes) as needed by the patient. Additionally, a continuous infusion can be added to the PCA regimen, although it has been suggested that this negates the safety feature of PCA in which no opioid is delivered if the patient is too sleepy to push the button. A modification of PCA is termed NCA, or nurse-controlled analgesia. With NCA, the same bolus and infusion are set, but the bedside nurse, instead of the patient, activates the device. NCA may be used in children who are too young or lack the needed cognitive function to use PCA. Although practices vary, continuous monitoring with pulse oximetry is generally recommended when PCA or NCA is used in the pediatric patient.

In addition to the opioids, acetaminophen and nonsteroidal antiinflammatory agents (NSAIDs) play a significant role in the control of postoperative pain. NSAIDs, acetaminophen, and salicylates act through the inhibition of the enzyme cyclooxygenase, thereby blocking the synthesis of prostaglandins. In distinction to opioids, these agents demonstrate a ceiling effect so that once a specific plasma concentration is achieved, no further analgesia is provided by increasing the dose. These agents are classified according to their chemical structure as (1) para-amino phenol derivatives (acetaminophen), (2) NSAIDs (ibuprofen), and (3) salicylates (acetylsalicylic acid, choline magnesium trisalicylate).[135] When considering the paraamino-phenol derivatives, acetaminophen has a significant role in the management of acute pain, whereas phenacetin is no longer used given its potential toxicity profile (renal papillary necrosis). Although previously available only as an oral or rectal medication in the United States, acetaminophen is now also available for intravenous administration. Commonly used NSAIDs include either ibuprofen for oral administration or ketorolac for intravenous administration. An intravenous preparation of ibuprofen has received approval of the Food and Drug Administration (FDA) for the treatment of pain and the control of fever in adults. The reader is referred to reference 139 for a more in-depth discussion of the prostaglandin synthesis inhibitors.[139]

Regional anesthetic techniques including either neuraxial blockade (epidural or spinal analgesia) or peripheral nerve blockade can be continued into the postoperative period to provide effective analgesia while avoiding the potential adverse effects associated with parenteral opioid therapy. Epidural and spinal local anesthetics provide profound analgesia; however, undesirable side effects of the use of high concentrations of local anesthetics include blockade of the sympathetic nervous system with hypotension, urinary retention, blockade of motor function, and risks of local anesthetic toxicity from systemic absorption. Epidural and spinal opioids can provide intense, segmental, localized analgesia without sensory, motor, or sympathetic nervous system effects, although their adverse effects profile may include respiratory depression, nausea, pruritus, sedation, and urinary retention. As a result, a combination of low-dose epidural local anesthetics and opioids are commonly used to take advantage of their synergistic effects and limit the side effects of each. Fentanyl and morphine are commonly used opioids, and bupivacaine is the usual local anesthetic of choice. The lipid solubility of the opioid predicts its clinical behavior. Fentanyl is very lipid soluble, penetrating the dura and rapidly binding to spinal cord opioid receptors, producing a fast onset of action but a short duration of action. Significant vascular absorption of fentanyl also occurs, decreasing its epidural effect and reducing its advantage over parenteral administration. Morphine is lipid insoluble and has a slower onset of action but a much longer duration of action. However, given its hydrophilic nature, morphine remains in the cerebrospinal fluid for a longer period of time with cephalad spread and the risks of delayed respiratory depression for up to 24 hours after neuraxial administration, thereby mandating ongoing monitoring of respiratory function during this time. Other methods of postoperative analgesia include the use of long-acting local anesthetic agents for either wound infiltration or peripheral nerve blockade. Examples of peripheral nerve blockade include brachial plexus blocks for upper extremity pain, femoral nerve blocks for femur and knee surgeries, sciatic nerve blocks for analgesia below the knee, and intercostal nerve blocks for thoracic and abdominal surgeries. Options include the placement of a catheter to allow for a continuous infusion during the postoperative period and to provide long-term analgesia for up to 3 to 5 days.

Conclusions

The perioperative care of pediatric patients begins with the preparation of the operating room site as well as the preoperative evaluation of the patient. The complexity of the latter varies tremendously based on the presence of comorbid conditions. These coexisting conditions as well as the requirements of the surgical procedure influence the techniques used for intraoperative monitoring. In its simplest form, a general anesthesia includes amnesia, analgesia, muscle relaxation, and attenuation of the sympathetic nervous system's response to surgical trauma. The phases of general anesthesia include induction, maintenance, and emergence. The induction of anesthesia can be carried out with the intravenous administration of an anesthetic agent or via the inhalation route with an inhalational anesthetic agent such as sevoflurane. In pediatric patients, the inhalation induction of anesthesia is frequently chosen to avoid the need for obtaining intravenous access on an awake child. Following anesthetic induction, one progresses into the maintenance phase of general anesthesia. This may include the administration of intravenous agents, inhalational agents, or, most likely, a combination of the two. Following the successful completion of the surgical procedure, a plan is determined for the postoperative delivery of analgesia including some combination of intravenous opioids, agents to inhibit prostaglandin formation, or a regional anesthetic technique. For complex surgical procedures, tracheal intubation and mechanical ventilation may be continued into the postoperative period, whereas a combination of tracheal extubation and the resumption of spontaneous ventilation is the general rule for the majority of surgical procedures. Regardless of the type of anesthesia administered, close monitoring of hemodynamic and respiratory function is continued into the postoperative period either in the ICU or in a specialized postanesthesia care unit.

Key References

4. Tobias JD. Caudal epidural block: test dosing and recognition of systemic injection. *Anesth Analg.* 2001;14:345-352.
5. Tobias JD. Spinal anesthesia in infants and children. *Paediatr Anaesth.* 2000;10:5-16.
7. Bhanaker SM, Ramamoorthy C, Geiduschek JM, et al. Anesthesia-related cardiac arrest in children: update from the pediatric perioperative cardiac arrest registry. *Anesth Analg.* 2007;105:344-350.
8. Bryant J, Krishna SG, Tobias JD. The difficult airway in pediatrics. *Advan Anesth.* 2013;31:31-60.
10. Burk CD, Miller L, Hander SD, Cohen AR. Preoperative history and coagulation screening in children undergoing tonsillectomy. *Pediatrics.* 1992;89:691-695.
11. Warner MA, Warner ME, Weber JG. Clinical significance of pulmonary aspiration during the perioperative period. *Anesthesiology.* 1993;78:56-62.
16. Read MS, Vaughn RS. Allowing pre-operative patients to drink: effects on patients' safety and comfort of unlimited oral water until 2 hours before anaesthesia. *Acta Anaesthesiol Scand.* 1991;35:591-595.
20. Jones CT, Raman VT, DeVries S, et al. Optimizing anticonvulsant administration for children before anesthesia: a quality improvement project. *Pediatr Neurol.* 2014;51:632-640.
21. American Society of Anesthesiologists Committee. Practice guidelines for preoperative fasting and the use of pharmacologic agents to reduce the risk of pulmonary aspiration: application to healthy patients undergoing elective procedures: an updated report by the American Society of Anesthesiologists Committee on Standards and Practice Parameters. *Anesthesiology.* 2011;114:495-511.
22. Tobias JD. Rapid sequence intubation: what does it mean? Does it really matter? *Saudi J Anaesth.* 2014;8:153-154.
24. Coté CJ, Cohen IT, Suresh S, et al. A comparison of three doses of a commercially prepared oral midazolam syrup in children. *Anesth Analg.* 2002;94:37-43.
25. Kraemer FW, Stricker PA, Gurnaney HG, et al. Bradycardia during induction of anesthesia with sevoflurane in children with Down syndrome. *Anesth Analg.* 2010;111:1259-1263.

Malignant Hyperthermia

Mihaela Visoiu, Ericka L. Fink, and Barbara W. Brandom

PEARLS

- Malignant hyperthermia is characterized by hypermetabolism, although many causes of fever and muscle injury are not related to this condition.
- Risk factors for malignant hyperthermia include a family history of cardiovascular collapse during anesthesia with potent inhalation anesthetics, exertional heat stroke, or ryanodine receptor type 1 myopathy.
- Excessive metabolism produces uncontrollable hypercarbia and rapidly increasing temperature. Muscle rigidity and rhabdomyolysis are frequent. The clinical diagnosis may be confirmed by genetic testing.
- Treatment consists of the administration of repeated doses of 2.5 mg/kg of dantrolene until metabolism and muscle tone are normal. The patient is cooled aggressively if his or her temperature is >39°C. Hyperkalemia, myoglobinuria, disseminated intravascular coagulation, and cerebral edema are treated as needed. After the initial treatment, at least 1 mg/kg of dantrolene should be given every 4 to 6 hours, because 20% of patients experience an exacerbation or recrudescence of malignant hyperthermia within the first 24 hours of treatment.

The physician in the pediatric intensive care unit (PICU) may first encounter a patient with malignant hyperthermia (MH) in transfer from the operating room or from an outpatient facility where general anesthesia was given and treatment for acute MH began. Because 20% of patients experience a recurrence of MH in the 24 hours after the initial episode, close observation for a relapse of MH is warranted, and the administration of dantrolene for at least 24 hours after the initial episode is recommended. Alternatively, the ICU physician may be the first to entertain the diagnosis of MH in a patient admitted to the ICU for medical care or postoperative management.

MH is characterized by hypermetabolism, but many causes of fever and muscle injury are not MH. Regardless of the underlying cause, ICU management should be directed to control critical temperature and complications of rhabdomyolysis. The ICU physician should pursue common diagnoses while directing a diagnostic workup for the rare syndrome of MH.

Pathophysiology

In fulminant MH, a dramatic increase in the metabolic rate of genetically abnormal muscle results in muscle injury and potentially in multiorgan system failure. The underlying defect is a sudden, sustained increase in the concentration of calcium ion in the sarcoplasm.[1] Carbon dioxide (CO_2) production increases severalfold. Even with increased minute ventilation, it may not be feasible to maintain normocarbia. Lactic acid production overwhelms the body's buffering capacity. Increased O_2 demand and the concomitant sympathetic response stress the cardiovascular system. MH can progress rapidly to severe mixed acidosis, hyperkalemia, elevated temperature as in heat stroke,[2] and rhabdomyolysis. Renal failure, disseminated intravascular coagulation, cerebral edema, pulmonary edema, dysrhythmias, and cardiovascular collapse are potential consequences of fulminant MH. Before dantrolene, the mortality rate of MH was 70%. Symptomatic therapy including mechanical ventilation, active cooling, administration of bicarbonate, expansion of the intravascular volume, and treatment of dysrhythmias can prolong life during an episode of fulminant MH. However, the most effective therapy is intravenous dantrolene.[3]

In malignant hyperthermia–susceptible (MHS) mammals there is a defect in the ryanodine receptor type 1 channel (RYR1),[4] producing increased sensitivity to agonists[5,6] and decreased sensitivity to inhibitors. Furthermore, extracellular calcium entry (ECCE) is greater than normal in myotubes expressing MHS RYR1.[7] Dantrolene inhibits ECCE in both MHS and normal muscle. Store-operated calcium entry (SOCE) is another process, occurring after depletion of sarcoplasmic reticulum (SR) calcium, that moves extracellular calcium into the myoplasm. SOCE is coupled to RYR1 and decreased by dantrolene.[8]

Genetics

MH susceptibility is a syndrome with autosomal dominant inheritance, incomplete penetrance, and variable expressivity. The first-degree relatives of an MHS individual are treated as malignant hyperthermia susceptibility (MHS) until they have normal results after an in vitro muscle contracture test with halothane and caffeine (CHCT). Incomplete penetrance means that a person with an MHS mutation may not experience MH during the first or subsequent exposures to MH trigger agents. Multifactorial inheritance may be relevant.[9,10] Variable expressivity means that clinical symptoms of MH vary from minor to fulminant depending on factors such as the anesthetic agents, genetics, and temperature.[11] MHS episodes are more often observed in males.[12,13]

The primary genetic locus of MH (MHS 1) is the ryanodine receptor gene (RYR1) on chromosome 19q13.1. Variants associated with MHS are found throughout RYR1. In families with an MH-causative RYR1 mutation, genetic analysis is a useful initial step in the diagnosis of MHS.[14,15] See www.mhaus.org

for addresses of clinical diagnostic testing laboratories in the United States. This pathologic test has been useful to document MH susceptibility in postmortem muscle.[16]

Variants in the α-1 subunit of the DHPR gene (*CACNA1S*) on chromosome 1q32 have been associated with MH in ~1% of MHS families.[17] This is the MHS 5 locus. See www.emhg.org for causative MH mutations at MHS 5 as well as MHS 1. A new locus of MHS is the STAC3 protein, encoded by *stac3* on chromosome 12, which is part of the excitation-contraction coupling mechanism in muscle. Abnormality in this protein has been associated with myopathy and MHS.[18] Although factors that modify the expression of MHS are not completely determined, active cysteines contribute to redox modulation and nitrosylation of RYR1.[19,20]

Clinical Recognition of a Malignant Hyperthermia Episode in Humans

The initial signs of an MH episode are nonspecific (Box 132.1).[21] The most frequent clinical signs of MH were hypercarbia (in 52%), hyperthermia (in 67%), and sinus tachycardia (in 62%) in 129 probands who later had muscle contracture tests diagnostic of MHS. Other MH signs noted in this group include masseter rigidity, total body rigidity, arrhythmia, mottling, and cyanosis.[22] This report from Canada is consistent with summaries of adverse metabolic and/or musculoskeletal reaction to anesthesia (AMRA) reports from the North American MH Registry.[12,23] Muscles may be rigid enough to pull the legs above the horizontal. Mixed respiratory and metabolic acidosis, hyperkalemia, myoglobinuria, and increased serum creatine kinase can be noted. However, rhabdomyolysis does not occur during every MH episode.[24]

In the ICU, a septic patient with kidney disease or chronic lung disease may exhibit fever, tachycardia, mixed respiratory and metabolic acidosis, and hyperkalemia. If sepsis, cardiovascular failure, central nervous system injury, heat stroke, or other medical or surgical conditions could have produced the abnormal vital signs, then these other diagnoses must be

pursued and treated. MH may not be the most likely diagnosis in general, but recognition of recent exposure to volatile anesthetic agents or succinylcholine in a patient with a family history of problems after general anesthesia or muscular diseases associated with MH supports the presumptive diagnosis of MH.

In the 21st century MH signs usually occur later during anesthesia than they did when halothane and succinylcholine were commonly given.[23] MH can develop insidiously during a long anesthetic.[25] When the nonspecific early signs of MH are noted during induction of anesthesia, the potent inhalation anesthetics should be discontinued. This patient is considered to be MH susceptible until proved otherwise, and this episode is called abortive MH. Early termination of inhalation anesthetic agents in the presence of abortive MH may allow the syndrome to resolve spontaneously. On the other hand, there have been cases in which only mild signs of abortive MH occurred intraoperatively, but renal failure, hyperthermia, and death occurred postoperatively with no explanation other than MH.[26]

Potential Systemic Complications

Complications were noted in approximately 35% of 181 MH events reported to the North American MH Registry. These included changes in level of consciousness or coma in 9.4%, cardiac dysfunction in 9.4%, pulmonary edema in 8.4%, renal dysfunction in 7.3%, disseminated intravascular coagulation in 7.2%, and hepatic dysfunction in 5.6%.[12] Disseminated intravascular coagulation was associated with a 50-fold increased likelihood of cardiac arrest and an 89-fold likelihood of death.[27] The likelihood of any complication increased 2.9 times for every 2°C increase in maximum temperature and 1.6 times for every 30 minutes of time between the appearance of the first clinical sign of MH and the beginning of dantrolene administration.[12] Other complications reported were compartment syndrome, stroke after cardiac arrest, bilateral brachial plexopathy, generalized muscle weakness, significant muscle loss, and prolonged intubation.[12]

Cerebral edema and coma have been reported in episodes of fulminant MH. Although normal metabolism of the brain was described during episodes of MH, O_2 supply to the central nervous system may be inadequate. Therefore supportive care to the patient during and after an episode of fulminant MH should include measures to document cerebral function and maximize cerebral perfusion.

Respiratory failure may occur early in an episode of fulminant MH. During an MH episode, desaturation can be also secondary to increased oxygen extraction. The workload of the respiratory system may be further increased by the occurrence of pulmonary edema. Pulmonary edema may be the result of capillary leak. It may be worsened by impaired cardiac contractility in the presence of acidemia. Cardiac dysrhythmias may occur in the presence of marked electrolyte abnormalities. In older patients, there may be foci of myocardial fibrosis as well. It has been hypothesized that such areas of fibrosis are the result of subclinical episodes of MH that produced increased levels of circulating catecholamines.[28] Cardiac contractility can be impaired.

Rhabdomyolysis occurs when the energy supply of the muscle is exhausted. Clinical manifestations include myalgias, swollen extremities, red-to-brown urine due to myoglobinuria, and elevated muscle enzymes. It is noteworthy that enzymes commonly elevated in the blood during hepatic

BOX 132.1	Positive Findings Consistent With Malignant Hyperthermia

History of recent exposure to trigger agent, including volatile anesthetic agents or succinylcholine
Family or personal history of malignant hyperthermia susceptibility
Total body rigidity
Masseter spasm
Inappropriately elevated (38.8°C) or rapidly increasing temperature (>1.5°C over 5 min)
Inappropriate tachypnea
Profuse sweating
Mottled, cyanotic skin
Dark urine, urine dipstick testing shows a positive result from blood without red cells in the sediment and no hemolysis
Unexplained, excessive bleeding
Unexplained ventricular tachycardia or fibrillation
Inappropriate hypercarbia (venous $PaCO_2$ >65 mm Hg, arterial $PaCO_2$ >55 mm Hg) if the patient is receiving positive pressure ventilation or is spontaneously breathing with greater than normal minute ventilation
Arterial base excess more negative than −8 mEq/L
Arterial pH <7.25
Potassium concentration >6 mEq/L
Creatine kinase >10,000 IU/L

injury including lactate dehydrogenase (LDH) and serum glutamic oxaloacetic transaminase (SGOT) will also be released from muscle when creatine kinase (CK) is markedly elevated. Rhabdomyolysis can produce electrolyte imbalance (hyperkalemia, hyperphosphatemia, hypocalcemia), metabolic acidosis, severe hyperuricemia, acute renal failure,[29] and compartment syndrome. Massive rhabdomyolysis, producing CK of greater than 20,000 IU/L, may occur in patients with underlying muscular diseases not necessarily related to MH. Thus rhabdomyolysis in the absence of increased metabolic rate, hypercarbia, and metabolic acidosis should not be assumed to be MH. However, the same treatment, including administration of dantrolene acutely, may be helpful to the myopathic patient who experiences rhabdomyolysis in the ICU. It is important to determine the underlying cause of rhabdomyolysis, because the implications for medical care differ depending on the pathologic diagnosis (eg, dystrophinopathy versus MH versus glycogen storage disease versus myotonia).

Hyperthermia in the Pediatric Intensive Care Unit

In the PICU, the most likely cause of fever is a bacterial infection,[30] but elevated temperature can also be the result of trauma, viral infection, lymphoma, leukemia, drug withdrawal, and allergy among other causes.[31] Inadequate fluid replacement predisposes to increased core temperature in children.[32] Excessive environmental heat with inadequate opportunity for evaporative heat loss can result in elevated temperature. In some cases, increased core temperature can be associated with tachycardia, increased expired CO_2, and metabolic acidosis, which are consistent with the expected increase in metabolic demand produced by fever. This can be so extreme as to mimic MH.

When hyperthermia occurs in a child with history of exposure to succinylcholine or volatile anesthetic agents, MH should be considered in the differential diagnosis. However, in a retrospective cohort study, conducted to analyze and identify the causes of hyperthermia in the PICU over a 9-year period, Schleelein and associates noted that the incidence of clinically diagnosed MH was low (0.4%).[33] These cases were classified as "definite" or "probable" MH[21] by a Malignant Hyperthermia Association of the United States (MHAUS) MH Hotline consultant.[33] No information about CHCT or other pathologic tests that could support the diagnosis of MH for these patients is available.

Postoperative Fever

Postoperative fever (>38°C, >100.4°F) is common after surgery and usually resolves spontaneously. In establishing a differential diagnosis, it is helpful to consider the timing of fever onset: immediate, acute, subacute, or delayed. The causes may be infectious or noninfectious. The most common noninfectious cause is a medication reaction, followed by blood transfusion and by trauma suffered prior to surgery or as part of surgery. The fever due to MH usually starts within 30 minutes after administration of the triggering agent, but it has also been reported up to several hours later, after the anesthesia was discontinued.

Some clinical states, such as increased temperature after cardiac surgery, share some of the features of MH.[34] These situations may even include rhabdomyolysis, but it is the result of muscular injury from impaired circulation, not usually from a primary muscular disease.

Rhabdomyolysis

Rhabdomyolysis is characterized by muscle necrosis and the release of intracellular muscle constituents including CK, myoglobin, calcium, and potassium. CK levels greater than five times baseline are a sensitive definition of rhabdomyolysis. Rhabdomyolysis can be due to inherited or acquired causes, and the severity of clinical consequences ranges from asymptomatic increase of serum muscle enzymes to life-threatening hyperkalemia. The most frequent causes are trauma, overexertion, immobilization, alcoholism, vascular insufficiency, and orthopedic surgery. Grand mal seizures, delirium tremens, psychotic agitation, and amphetamine overdose can lead to rhabdomyolysis in individuals with otherwise normal muscle.[35] Some drugs such as HMG-CoA reductase inhibitors (statins) and colchicine are directly myotoxic.[35] Rhabdomyolysis may occur in patients with metabolic myopathies such as carnitine palmitoyltransferase deficiency, myophosphorylase deficiency (PYGM) or McArdle disease, myoadenylate deaminase deficiency (AMPD1), mitochondrial myopathy, or malignant hyperthermia susceptibility. Occasionally, patients with structural myopathies can develop acute rhabdomyolysis after strenuous exercise, after exposure to potent inhalation anesthetics, after exposure to other myotoxic drugs, or after a viral infection.

Treatment of an Episode of Malignant Hyperthermia
Remove Trigger Agents

When an episode of MH is suspected, inhalation anesthetic administration must be stopped as soon as possible. High fresh gas flows of 10 L/min or more, or charcoal filters placed into the breathing circuit, are needed to eliminate residual anesthetic gas from the breathing circuit. If blood gas analysis documented significant respiratory and metabolic acidosis, dantrolene should be administered immediately and supportive treatment should be started as soon as possible (Box 132.2). Treatment of the life-threatening complications should not detract from the need to continue monitoring the metabolic status and the continued administration of dantrolene, in increasing doses if necessary, until the metabolic state is normal and muscles are flaccid.

Administer Dantrolene

Dantrolene, a hydantoin with muscle relaxant properties, has greatly changed the treatment of and risk of death from MH. Before the introduction of dantrolene, Brit and Kalow reported a 36% MH survival rate with symptomatic treatment only.[36] Dantrolene decreases both excitation-coupled calcium entry into muscle cells and store-operated calcium entry coupled to RYR1.[7,8] It does not act on the neuromuscular junction or on the passive or active electrical properties of the surface membranes of muscle fibers.

Dantrolene in the formulations Dantrium and Revonto is supplied in 70-mL vials, containing 20 mg of dantrolene sodium and 3 g of mannitol. It must be diluted with 60 mL of sterile, preservative-free, distilled water to produce a clear yellow solution. Dantrolene is also available as Ryanodex, 250 mg of dantrolene with 125 mg mannitol, to which 5 ml of water is added to produce an opaque orange fluid for injection. Dantrolene should be available in all locations where

<table>
</table>

BOX 132.2 **Management of an Acute Malignant Hyperthermia Episode in the Intensive Care Unit**

1. Administer high-flow 100% oxygen via a non-rebreathing mask and consider endotracheal intubation.
2. For ventilated patients, administer FiO_2 of 1 and increase minute ventilation to control $PaCO_2$.
3. Administer dantrolene (2.5 mg/kg intravenously) over 10 minutes and repeat, until acidosis and muscle rigidity have resolved. Repeat dantrolene (1 mg/kg) every 4 to 6 hours.
4. Initiate cooling with ice packs in the axillae and groin, decrease room temperature, use hypothermia blankets, iced intravenous saline solution (10 mL/kg over 10 min, repeated as needed), and lavage body cavities with cold saline solution if temperature is greater than 39°C. Stop cooling when core temperature falls to 38°C.
5. Correct metabolic acidosis with sodium bicarbonate (1–2 mEq/kg initially) and give subsequent doses based on base excess and body weight.
6. Administer calcium chloride (10 mg/kg) or calcium gluconate (100–200 mg/kg) to protect from cardiotoxicity associated with hyperkalemia.
7. Give regular insulin (0.1 U/kg) and glucose (0.3–0.5 g/kg) to correct hyperkalemia.
8. Administer lidocaine (1 mg/kg) to treat ventricular arrhythmias. Consider amiodarone (5 mg/kg IV) for refractory, stable ventricular tachycardia. Do not delay defibrillation or cardiopulmonary resuscitation if indicated by cardiovascular instability.
9. Maintain urine output of 2 mL/kg/hr with aggressive cold fluid administration, furosemide (0.5–1 mg/kg), and additional mannitol (0.25–0.3 g/kg) if needed.
10. Consider quantitative end-tidal CO_2 monitoring.
11. Monitor core temperature (pulmonary artery, esophageal temperature probe, rectal probe).
12. Place arterial catheter for invasive blood pressure monitoring and frequent blood sampling. Consider central venous catheter or pulmonary artery catheter if indicated by cardiovascular instability.
13. Repeat venous blood gas and electrolytes analysis until these normalize. Repeat creatine kinase at least every 6 hours while the patient is in ICU and then daily until the creatine kinase returns to normal. Assess glucose, clotting function, hepatic and renal functions, and treat symptomatically. Repeat lactic acid measurement after each dantrolene administration.
14. Consider hemodialysis if indicated.
15. Consider intensive care monitoring for at least 24 hours after malignant hyperthermia episode or after recrudescence of malignant hyperthermia.
16. Refer the patient for muscle caffeine-halothane contracture testing and consider exam of *RYR1*. Pursue a pathologic diagnosis for other occult myopathies.

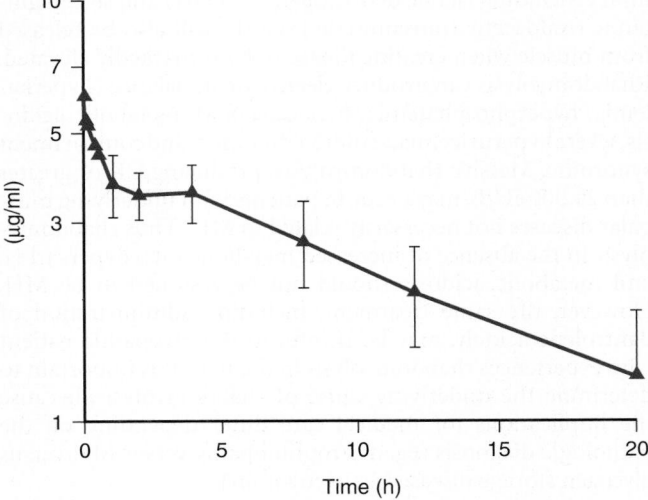

Fig. 132.1. Whole blood concentration of dantrolene versus time in a cohort of children. (Modified from Lerman J, McLeod ME, Strong HA. Pharmacokinetics of intravenous dantrolene in children. Anesthesiology. 1989;70:625.)

general anesthesia is administered. It should be immediately supplied to other areas of the hospital by the pharmacy. If dantrolene has to be obtained from a central location, such as the pharmacy, it must be stressed that the need for the initial and subsequent doses of drug is urgent. The initial dose of intravenous dantrolene for treatment of MH is 2.5 to 3 mg/kg.[37] More than 10 mg/kg may be required to return metabolism and muscle tone to normal. Dantrolene may irritate veins and if it extravasates it will not be effective in treating MH. Therefore dantrolene should be given through a catheter placed in a central vein if possible. As soon as dantrolene is ordered to treat fulminant MH, the pharmacy should obtain replacements. In children, the intravenous infusion of dantrolene, 2.4 mg/kg IV over 10 to 12 minutes, produced stable blood levels of about 3.5 μg/mL for 4 hours, after which a slow decline in plasma concentration occurred (Fig. 132.1).[38] It

appears that the half-life of dantrolene in the plasma of children is somewhat shorter than in adults: 7 to 10 hours compared with 12 hours, respectively.[39] This is consistent with the recommendation to repeat dantrolene (1 mg/kg) every 4 to 6 hours for prophylaxis against recurrence of MH in a child. The goals of treatment with dantrolene are normalization of heart rate, respiratory rate, and muscle tone, correction of hypercarbia, hyperthermia, electrolyte disturbances, and metabolic acidosis. Urinary output should increase and mental status should improve.

The major side effect of dantrolene is muscle weakness, noted in ~25% of patients.[39,40] The effects of dantrolene on strength may persist for more than 8 to 12 hours. It is likely that when the plasma concentration of dantrolene is sufficient to inhibit an episode of MH, the patient will experience weakness and possibly disequilibrium. The ability to swallow could be compromised. Severe muscle weakness of weeks to months in duration can also be the result of an MH episode. Phlebitis is a common side effect of dantrolene administration, noted in approximately 10% of patients.[40]

If no recurrence is noted in the first 24 hours following treatment of MH, the patient is metabolically stable, and weakness is marked, dantrolene administration may be withheld and weaning from supportive therapy begun. If dantrolene must be administered to a patient who is also receiving calcium channel antagonists, invasive hemodynamic monitoring is necessary. Serum potassium should be closely monitored. Dantrolene may be useful in the treatment of fever and muscle spasticity not associated with MH. Therefore if fever diminishes and abnormal vital signs associated with fever resolve after the administration of dantrolene, the patient did not necessarily have MH.

Symptomatic Treatment

Because respiratory and cardiovascular compromise result from fulminant MH and because the major side effect of dantrolene is muscular weakness, endotracheal intubation and controlled ventilation may be useful. When calculation of

O_2 consumption and CO_2 production is simplified by mechanical ventilation, these values serve as the most appropriate monitors of the adequacy of treatment of an episode of fulminant MH. Minute ventilation should be increased severalfold and O_2 provided as needed. When repeated assessment of blood gases indicates resolution of acidosis, minute ventilation can be normalized. Sodium bicarbonate should be administered liberally to treat metabolic acidosis. Low muscle pH may prevent successful treatment of MH.

If the core body temperature is elevated, active measures should be taken to cool the patient. The most effective means of cooling is the intravenous administration of cold normal saline through a peripheral or central vein. The stomach can be lavaged with iced saline. Ice packs may be placed on the groin and the axillae. Wet cloths and a fan can be used to promote surface evaporation. Active cooling should be stopped when core temperature falls below 38.8°C to prevent inadvertent hypothermia.

Cardiac dysrhythmias usually stop when the episode is adequately treated with dantrolene. Lidocaine (1 mg/kg) is recommended for treatment of arrhythmias in MH. Amiodarone (5 mg/kg) can be administered for refractory ventricular tachycardia.[41] Hyperkalemia may require aggressive treatment, especially if arrhythmias have occurred or myoglobinuria has compromised renal function. The administration of calcium gluconate or calcium chloride—and all the other usual treatments to reverse hyperkalemia—is appropriate during the treatment of MH.

Conventional hemodialysis does not remove myoglobin effectively, due to the size of this protein.[42] The use of antioxidants and free radical scavengers such as pentoxifylline, vitamin E, and vitamin C may be justified in the treatment or prevention of myoglobinuric acute renal injury,[43] but more controlled studies are needed. Early hypocalcemia secondary to rhabdomyolysis-induced acute kidney injury should not be treated unless it is symptomatic or severe hyperkalemia is present.[42]

Large losses of intravascular volume may occur, because evaporative loss may be great, edema formation may occur in muscle and other tissues, and mannitol given as part of the formulation of dantrolene may induce significant diuresis. Hypovolemia should be avoided because even mild hypovolemia impairs dissipation of heat produced by increased metabolism.[32] Cardiovascular support, in the form of isotonic fluid administration as well as vasopressor and inotropic drugs (epinephrine, phenylephrine, norepinephrine, dopamine), should be administered as soon as possible if indicated.

The 24/7 MH Hotline is available at 800-644-9737 to lend advice about treating acute MH. This service is supported by MHAUS (www.mhaus.org) and staffed by volunteer anesthesiologists.

Urine and Blood Tests in Malignant Hyperthermia

Myoglobin, a heme-containing respiratory protein, is released from damaged muscle and rapidly excreted in the urine. Myoglobinuria occurs when the renal threshold of 0.5 to 1.5 mg/dL is exceeded. Myoglobinuria is suggested by persistent red to reddish brown urine. At myoglobin levels of 100 mg/dL, urine tests positive for heme by dipstick after centrifugation, whereas the sediment has normal color and tests negative for heme. The dipstick test has a sensitivity of 80% for detection of rhabdomyolysis.[29] Renal injury is frequent when urine

myoglobin is more than 1 g/mL. Because the half-life of myoglobin in the plasma is approximately 12 hours, less than the half-life of CK,[44] persistence of myoglobinuria for more than several days suggests that muscle cell integrity continues to be impaired. Patients with chronic myopathies may have moderately raised concentration of plasma myoglobin but not usually overt myoglobinuria.[44] CK increases in the plasma more slowly than myoglobin does. There is no defined threshold value of serum CK above which the risk of acute kidney injury is increased. Usually the risk is low when the CK level is less than 15,000 to 20,000 U/L.[45] With coexisting conditions such as sepsis, dehydration, and acidosis, acute kidney injury may occur with CK values as low as 5000 U/L. After an MH episode, CK should be measured at least daily until stable.

When further evaluation is required to assess for the presence or recurrence of MH, the test most likely to be helpful is venous blood gas analysis. Oxygen desaturation, hypercarbia, and lactic acidemia in mixed venous blood are the results of the hypermetabolism of MH. Elevated $PaCO_2$ is apparent in mixed venous blood before it is abnormal in arterial blood during an episode of MH.[3] There is an increase in lactate release from muscle before a decrease in the partial pressure of oxygen in venous blood during an episode of MH.[46] If venous blood indicates significant acidosis, with $PaCO_2$ greater than 60 mm Hg and bicarbonate less than 19 mEq/L,[3] and the history of the patient is consistent with MH, the physician should assume that the patient is experiencing an episode of MH and treat accordingly with dantrolene.

Course of a Clinical Episode of Malignant Hyperthermia

The case fatality for MH was >70% in the 1970s. Now MH mortality is estimated to be 10-fold less, but deaths continue to occur when succinylcholine is given to hot, stiff patients in the emergency room[47] or when MH is not suspected soon enough in the operating room.[16] The initial clinical signs of an impending episode of MH are nonspecific. The patient's medical history and clinical course usually help to differentiate fulminant MH from other medical, metabolic, or endocrinologic crises such as sepsis, porphyria, thyroid storm,[48] and untreated pheochromocytoma (Box 132.3).[31]

BOX 132.3 | **Differential Diagnosis of Malignant Hyperthermia in the Intensive Care Unit**

Neuroleptic malignant syndrome
Exertional hyperthermia and heat stroke
Serotonin syndrome
Sepsis associated with renal and respiratory failure
Central nervous system injury
Postoperative fever
Thyrotoxicosis
Rhabdomyolysis
Pheochromocytoma
Porphyria
Allergic reaction secondary to medications
Blood transfusion reactions
Administration of hypertonic dye such as diatrizoate intrathecally
Drug abuse (cocaine, amphetamines, ecstasy)
Drug withdrawal
Iatrogenic overheating
Delirium tremens

If the triggering agent is removed rapidly, there may be only mild signs suggestive of MH: moderate increases in heart rate, blood pressure, and temperature along with a slight respiratory acidosis. Mild metabolic acidosis and moderate increases in serum myoglobin and CK may or may not be present. Masseter spasm may occur. As previously suggested (see "Clinical Recognition of a Malignant Hyperthermia Episode in Humans"), differentiating an abortive episode of MH from an anesthesia complicated by other factors can be difficult.

Recrudescence

There are cases in which a patient was symptomatically treated for MH with dantrolene, appeared to recover, and then some hours later had another episode of increased metabolic rate. This second episode was sometimes accompanied by remarkable stiffness of the muscles. Recrudescence of MH was reported in 20% of cases reported to the MH Registry[49] after initial treatment appeared to be successful. Muscular body type, the presence of temperature increase during the MH episode, and a longer time between the induction of inhalation anesthesia and the first sign of MH were associated with a greater risk of recrudescence.[49] There is no definite or guaranteed time course for these events in the human. Observation of the patient rescued from an MH event closely for 24 hours will allow for the early recognition and treatment of recrudescence. Such patients should be monitored in an ICU setting because of the utility of invasive cardiovascular monitoring in documenting the course of an episode of MH. Recrudescence of MH can progress into fulminant MH and therefore warrants aggressive treatment with dantrolene and supportive therapy.

Factors That Trigger Malignant Hyperthermia

Potent inhalational anesthetic agents such as sevoflurane, halothane, enflurane, isoflurane, and desflurane have been identified as triggering agents of MH in humans. Depolarizing neuromuscular blocking agents are also potent triggers of MH in humans. Succinylcholine is the only drug of this type currently in common use. Different anesthetics may trigger MH at different rates depending on the combination of agents used. The combination of succinylcholine and potent inhalation anesthetic agents produces more episodes of MH than do potent inhalation anesthetic agents administered without succinylcholine or succinylcholine administered in the presence of nitrous oxide and intravenous anesthetic agents.[22,23] A number of drugs, such as amide local anesthetics, droperidol, ketamine, calcium, digitalis, methylxanthines, anticholinergics, anticholinesterases, and sympathomimetic drugs, had in the past been considered to be potential triggers of MH in humans, primarily on theoretic grounds. Review of clinical and laboratory[50,51] experience suggests that these drugs are not triggers of MH. However, on rare occasions, MH may occur during an anesthesia in which no trigger agents were administered or without exposure to any anesthetic.[52] This is rare in humans but has been observed repeatedly in MH-susceptible animals.[53] An athletic adolescent who had an RYR1 mutation associated with MH died after strenuous exercise.[54]

Muscular Diseases and Malignant Hyperthermia

There are a few relatively rare muscular diseases that are closely linked with MH susceptibility. These include central core disease, multiminicore and nemaline rod myopathies,[55]

and King-Denborough syndrome.[56] Central core disease (CCD) is a congenital myopathy, characterized by motor developmental delay and signs of mild proximal weakness, most pronounced in the hip and girdle musculature. A patient with dystrophinopathy (Duchenne or Becker muscular dystrophy) can develop a hyperkalemic cardiac arrest and exacerbation of rhabdomyolysis after administration of the potent inhalation anesthetic agents, but this is not an MH episode. During initial treatment, such cases can be difficult to differentiate clinically from MH. Indeed, calcium is not handled normally in dystrophic muscle, and RYR1 channels are abnormal.[58] In the presence of neuromuscular disease, myoglobinuria may occur after exposure to potent inhalation anesthetics alone[44,59] and is to be expected after succinylcholine administration in patients with muscular dystrophy.[44] A child with myopathy who receives potent inhalation anesthetic agents can develop an increase in postoperative serum CK and potassium concentrations as well as myoglobinuria. These findings are due to the myopathy, not to MH.

Myotonias are a class of inherited skeletal muscle diseases characterized by impaired relaxation after sudden voluntary muscle contraction. There are defects in the chloride, sodium, and calcium channels in the different types of myotonia. In the presence of myotonia the risk for MH is not greater than that of the general population, with the possible exception of hypokalemic periodic paralysis. Many cases of hypokalemic periodic paralysis are associated with variants in the CACNA1S, which codes for the DHPR, the voltage gate of the RYR1. Thus there is a theoretic association between MH and hypokalemic periodic paralysis, which has not been clearly confirmed.[11] To prevent episodes of myotonic contractures, depolarizing neuromuscular blocking agents such as succinylcholine should not be given to patients with myotonia. Other details of preventive management may differ between different forms of myotonia. In general myotonic patients should be maintained in a normothermic state, episodes of anxiety should be avoided, and serum potassium should be documented. If nondepolarizing neuromuscular blocking agents (NMBAs) must be used, a drug with short duration is best and neuromuscular function should be monitored. The use of anticholinesterase drugs has been reported to precipitate myotonia. Neither nondepolarizing NMBAs nor dantrolene will counteract myotonic rigidity. Lidocaine, a sodium channel blocker, may decrease myotonic rigidity.

Patients with mitochondrial disease may develop acidosis, fever, and rhabdomyolysis. All anesthetics depress mitochondrial function, but there is no clear relationship between MH and mitochondrial myopathy.

Heat Illness and Malignant Hyperthermia Susceptibility

Exertional heat illness (EHI), exertional rhabdomyolysis (ER), and MH are all hypermetabolic states and can have similar manifestations. EHI is caused by excessive heat production with insufficient heat dissipation. It can progress to exertional heat stroke (EHS), which includes extreme hyperthermia (core body temperature higher than 40°C or 104°F) associated with central nervous abnormalities (delirium, coma, seizure). EHS can progress to multiorgan failure[60] with rhabdomyolysis. The CHCT can confirm the diagnosis of MHS, but it cannot be used to diagnose the potential for EHI or ER. Because there is a subset of patients who present with heat stroke and are also susceptible to MH, Grogan and Hopkins[61] suggested that EHI patients undergo testing for MH susceptibility. However, the majority of ER and EHS cases do not have a subclinical myopathy such as MH susceptibility.[61,62]

Evaluation of Patients at Risk

The most efficient way to evaluate a family for MHS is to first evaluate the index patient with a contracture test (CHCT) of living muscle.[63] Many individuals suspected of experiencing MH may have normal CHCT results. This is the only method that can confirm the diagnosis of *not* MHS. CK levels, at rest, are of no predictive value in the general population.[64,65] In some populations, more than 25% of the patients with elevated CK levels were not susceptible to MH on CHCT testing.[66] However, if a relative of an MHS patient with chronic CK elevation has elevated CK, that individual is likely to be MHS also.[65]

Testing for Malignant Hyperthermia Susceptibility
In Vitro Caffeine-Halothane Contracture Testing

In vitro caffeine-halothane contracture testing (CHCT) is the only specific lab test of MH susceptibility other than identification of a *RYR1* mutation. At least 2 to 3 months should pass between an episode of suspected MH and the date of muscle biopsy for CHCT.[67] This test has been described in detail, and the standards for its performance have been accepted by the specialized centers in North America[68] and Europe[58] that perform it. The addresses of centers where muscle biopsy and contracture testing can be done can be found at www.mhaus.org and www.emhg.org. CHCT has a sensitivity of 97% and a specificity of 78%.[69] It was designed to decrease the rate of false negatives. Therefore it may produce false-positive results. A video of this procedure can be seen at www.mhaus.org. The negative predictive value of CHCT is high, but because the specificity of the in vitro test is only 85% at best, the positive predictive value of this test varies greatly depending on the prior probability of the individual being susceptible to MH.[70] As much clinical and laboratory evidence as can be obtained regarding the MH event should be used to interpret the results of CHCT. Genetic analysis may be helpful if several generations of one family can be examined.

Less Invasive Tests of Malignant Hyperthermia Susceptibility

None of the relatively noninvasive tests of MH susceptibility have proved as sensitive and as specific as the in vitro caffeine-halothane contracture test. Tests that have been evaluated in the past include calcium uptake into frozen muscle, skinned fiber testing, platelet nucleotide depletion, ionized calcium concentration in lymphocytes, force of contracture, and phosphorus nuclear magnetic resonance spectroscopy. Other tests based on RYR1 function in lymphocytes,[71,72] pharmacologic response in muscle cell cultures,[73-75] and microdialysis study of in situ muscle[76] have been proposed. None of these are usefully clinically thus far.

An alternate to the caffeine-halothane contracture test for confirmation of MH susceptibility is a genetic test of *RYR1*. This was developed from genetic analysis of families in which many individuals had undergone muscle contracture tests.

Patients who had strong contracture test results underwent characterization of *RYR1*. The exons in which variants are most commonly found were studied first (the hot spots). Variant tissues were studied in vitro to confirm that they altered calcium in a manner consistent with causing MH. At present, more than 300 *RYR1* variants have been documented; of these, only 34 have been formally accepted as causative MH mutations (see www.emhg.org). Therefore the sensitivity of the clinical *RYR1* exam, which sequences only the exons in which known causative MH mutations are located, is at best 30%. Sequencing of the entire *RYR1* gene may detect a variant in 50% to 70% of people who would have positive CHCT results. However, it is difficult to interpret the medical implications of the variants of unknown significance that may be identified. Professional genetic counseling is appropriate, in concert with consultation with a neurologist, when genetic testing of MH susceptibility is considered. Genetic testing has been useful postmortem when the clinical circumstances were consistent with fulminant MH.[16] Addresses of the genetic laboratories can be found at www.mhaus.org. Patients with strong contractures in the presence of 3% halothane and no findings on *RYR1* may have a defect in a different protein. If *RYR1*, *CACAN1S*, and *stac3* sequencing fail to identify an MH-causative mutation, that patient should undergo muscle contracture testing to further evaluate MH susceptibility. A normal result on the CHCT is the only method that can currently prove that an individual is not MH susceptible.

Neuroleptic Malignant Syndrome and Serotonin Syndrome

Neuroleptic malignant syndrome (NMS) can be fatal. It develops insidiously over days. Initial signs include changes in mental status and extrapyramidal function. Sinus tachycardia or oscillation of blood pressure is common. Muscle rigidity that can be described as "lead pipe," hyperthermia, and increased CK are major manifestations of NMS. Renal failure due to rhabdomyolysis and respiratory distress are serious complications of NMS.

NMS has been reported within 7 days after the administration of antipsychotic drugs given to treat psychiatric disorders. NMS may occur 2 to 4 weeks after the administration of depot neuroleptics and days after the intravenous administration of various antipsychotic and antiemetic medications of the phenothiazine and butyrophenone classes.[77] Surgical patients may have received neuroleptics as antiemetics or sedatives. NMS can occur at any age. Silva and associates,[78] reviewing the literature on NMS in children, found 77 cases in patients of less than 1 to 18 years, with only 10 patients younger than 10 years of age.

The treatment of NMS starts with the discontinuation of neuroleptic agents as well as the institution of supportive treatment to control hyperthermia, sustain vital functions, and prevent renal failure. There is evidence that NMS results from an acute reduction in dopaminergic function in the brain. Medications such as amantadine, bromocriptine, and levodopa have been used in treatment of NMS. Dantrolene, which inhibits muscle contraction and heat production, was reported to be effective in 81% of patients with NMS.[79] Electroconvulsive therapy (ECT) has also been suggested to be therapeutic.

The potential for susceptibility or cross-reactivity to both MH and NMS in the same patient is unproved. However, five of seven NMS patients who underwent muscle biopsy for in vitro halothane contracture testing had significantly abnormal results. Therefore the recommendation has been made to treat NMS patients as MH susceptible until proved otherwise. Unfortunately, this can pose anesthetic difficulties during ECT. Succinylcholine, a potent trigger of MH, is a useful drug for lessening the force of the convulsions that accompany ECT. One patient who had experienced NMS did later receive succinylcholine repeatedly for ECT without complications.[80] Therefore it is unclear whether patients who have had NMS should be prevented from receiving anesthetic agents capable of triggering MH when these drugs are otherwise indicated. On the other hand, neuroleptic agents have been considered safe to administer to MHS patients, but there is some risk of hyperthermic reactions.[81]

There is evidence that patients with proximal myotonic dystrophy may be at increased risk for muscular complications after receiving neuroleptic drugs. Schneider and associates described a patient with this disease who developed muscle stiffness, oculogyric dystonias, and elevated CK after administration of a neuroleptic. This patient had a positive contracture test for MH susceptibility.[81]

Serotonin syndrome (SS) is another potentially life-threatening condition associated with increased serotonergic activity in the central nervous system, as a result of stimulation of postsynaptic $5-HT_{1A}$ and $5-HT_{2A}$ receptors.[82] It may result from any combination of drugs that increase serotonergic activity, such as amphetamine, cocaine, selective serotonin reuptake inhibitors, tricyclic antidepressants, monoamine oxidase inhibitors, triptans, lithium, dextromethorphan, and ondansetron. The diagnosis of SS in the pediatric population can be difficult. Clinical manifestations include autonomic changes such as tachycardia, hyperthermia, hypertension, diaphoresis, and diarrhea and increased neuromuscular activity with tremor, muscle rigidity, hyperreflexia, and clonus. In SS, neuromuscular findings are typically more pronounced in the lower extremity,[83] compared with MH where there is a rigor-mortis–like rigidity. When compared with NMS, the distinguishing features of SS, besides the different causative agents, are a rapid onset (within 24 hours),[83] hyperreactivity (tremor, clonus, increase in reflexes), and rapid resolution.[82] See www.mhaus.org/nmsis for a website devoted to neuroleptic malignant syndrome and similar disorders.

Although there may be similarities in the presentation of MH, NMS, and SS, they have pathophysiologic differences. Nevertheless, there is experimental evidence in animals that stress-induced MH, more than anesthetic-induced MH, may be mediated in part by 5-HT.[84]

Malignant Hyperthermia Association

The Malignant Hyperthermia Association of the United States is a valuable resource for families affected by MH, NMS, or SS and for their physicians. This organization offers information, expert consultation, and referral. MHAUS maintains a 24-hour, professionally staffed telephone line to assist physicians and patients in dealing with MH (1-800-644-9737). All cases of suspected MH and similar heat-related disorders should be reported to the North American Malignant Hyperthermia Registry (telephone, 888-274-7899; website, www.mhaus.org/registry) to support the continued epidemiologic study of MH.

Key References

4. Jurkat-Rott K, McCarthy T, Lehmann-Horn F. Genetics and pathogenesis of malignant hyperthermia. *Muscle Nerve.* 2000;23:4-17.
7. Cherednichenko G, Ward CW, Feng W, et al. Enhanced excitation-coupled calcium entry in myotubes expressing malignant hyperthermia mutation R163C is attenuated by dantrolene. *Mol Pharmacol.* 2008;73:1203-1212.
8. Zhao X, Weisleder N, Han X, et al. Azumolene inhibits a component of store-operated calcium entry coupled to the skeletal muscle ryanodine receptor. *J Biol Chem.* 2006;281:33477-33486.
9. Monnier N, Krivosic-Horber R, Payen JF, et al. Presence of two different genetic traits in malignant hyperthermia families: implication for genetic analysis, diagnosis, and incidence of malignant hyperthermia susceptibility. *Anesthesiology.* 2002;97:1067-1074.
10. Robinson R, Hopkins P, Carsana A, et al. Several interacting genes influence the malignant hyperthermia phenotype. *Hum Genet.* 2003;112:217-218.
11. Parness J, Bandschapp O, Girard T. The myotonias and susceptibility to malignant hypethermia. *Anesth Analg.* 2009;109:1054-1064.
12. Larach MG, Gronert GA, Allen GA, et al. Clinical presentation, treatment and complications of malignant hyperthermia in North America from 1987-2006. *Anesth Analg.* 2010;110:498-507.
15. Urwyler A, Deufel T, McCarthy T, et al. Guidelines for molecular genetic detection of susceptibility to malignant hyperthermia. *Br J Anaesth.* 2001;86:283-287.
16. Larach MG, Brandom BW, Allen GC, et al. Malignant hyperthermia deaths related to inadequate temperature monitoring, 2007-2012: a report from the North American Malignant Hyperthermia Registry of the Malignant Hyperthermia Association of the United States. *Anesth Analg.* 2014;119:1359-1366.
17. Carpenter D, Ringose C, Leo V, et al. The role of CACNA1S in predisposition to malignant hyperthermia. *BMC Med Genet.* 2009;10:104.
18. Horstick EJ, Linsley JW, Dowling JJ, et al. Stac3 is a component of the excitation-contraction coupling machinery and mutated in Native American myopathy. *Nat Commun.* 2013;4:1952.
21. Larach MG, Localio AR, Allen GC, et al. A clinical grading scale to assess malignant hyperthermia susceptibility. *Anesthesiology.* 1994;80:771-779.
22. Riazi S, Larach MG, Hu C, et al. Malignant hyperthermia in Canada: characteristics of index anesthetics in 129 malignant hyperthermia susceptible probands. *Anesth Analg.* 2014;118:381-387.
23. Visoiu M, Young M, Wieland K, et al. Anesthetic drugs and onset of malignant hyperthermia. *Anesth Analg.* 2014;118:388-396.
24. Newmark JL, Voelkel M, Brandom BW, et al. Delayed onset of malignant hyperthermia without creatine kinase elevation in a geriatric, ryanodine receptor type 1 gene compound heterozygous patient. *Anesthesiology.* 2007;107:350-353.
31. Herlich A. Perioperative temperature elevation: not all hyperthermia is malignant hyperthermia. *Paediatr Anaesth.* 2013;23:842-850.
32. Ezri T, Szmuk P, Weisenberg M, et al. The effects of hydration on core temperature in pediatric surgical patients. *Anesthesiology.* 2003;98:838-841.
33. Schleelein LE, Litman RS. Hyperthermia in the pediatric intensive care unit-is it malignant hyperthermia? *Paediatr Anaesth.* 2009;19:1113-1118.
34. Casella ES, Soule LM, Blanck TJJ. Creatine kinase activity and temperature in children after cardiac surgery. *J Cardiothorac Anesth.* 1988;2:156-163.
35. Melli G, Chaudhry V, Cornblath DR, et al. Rhabdomyolysis: an evaluation of 475 hospitalized patients. *Medicine (Baltimore).* 2005;84:377-385.
40. Brandom BW, Kang A, Sivak EL, et al. Update on dantrolene in the treatment of anesthesia induced malignant hyperthermia. *SOJ Anesthesiol Pain Manag.* 2015;2:1-6.
41. Easley RB, Schleien CL, Shaffner DH. Pediatric cardiopulmonary resuscitation. In: Motoyama EK, Davis PJ, eds. *Smith's Anesthesia for Infants and Children.* 7th ed. Philadelphia: Mosby; 2006:1110-1154.
42. Bosch X, Poch E, Grau JM. Rhabdomyolysis and acute kidney injury. *N Engl J Med.* 2009;361:62-72.
47. Lavezzi WA, Capacchione J, Muldoon SM, et al. Death in the emergency department: an unrecognized awake malignant hyperthermia-like reaction in a six-year-old. *Anesth Analg.* 2013;116:420-423.
48. Shailesh Kumar MV, Carr RJ, Komanduri V, et al. Differential diagnosis of thyroid crisis and malignant hyperthermia in a porcine model. *Endocr Res.* 1999;25:87-103.

49. Burkman JM, Posner KL, Domino KB. Analysis of the clinical variables associated with recrudescence after malignant hyperthermia reactions. *Anesthesiology.* 2007;106:901-906.

50. Gronert GA, Ahern CP, Milde JH, et al. Effect of CO_2, calcium, digoxin, and potassium on cardiac and skeletal muscle metabolism in malignant hyperthermia susceptible swine. *Anesthesiology.* 1986;64:24-28.

52. Brandom BW, Muldoon SM. Unexpected MH deaths without exposure to inhalation anesthetics in pediatric patients. *Paediatr Anaesth.* 2013;23:851-854.

53. Chelu MG, Goonasekera SA, Durham WJ, et al. Heat- and anesthesia-induced malignant hyperthermia in an RyR1 knock-in mouse. *FASEB J.* 2006;20:329-330.

54. Tobin JR, Jason DR, Challa VR, et al. Malignant hyperthermia and apparent heat stroke. *JAMA.* 2001;286:168-169.

55. Klingler W, Rueffert H, Lehmann-Horn F, et al. Core myopathies and risk of malignant hyperthermia. *Anesth Analg.* 2009;109:1167-1173.

56. Davis PJ, Brandom BW. The association of malignant hyperthermia and unusual disease: when you're hot you're hot or maybe. *Anesth Analg.* 2009;109:1001-1003.

57. Deleted in review.

60. Capacchione J, Muldoon S. The relationship between exertional heat illness, exertional rhabdomyolysis, and malignant hyperthermia. *Anesth Analg.* 2009;109:1065-1069.

61. Grogan H, Hopkins PM. Heat stroke: implications for critical care and anesthesia. *Br J Anaesth.* 2002;88:700-707.

62. Fink E, Brandom BW, Torp KD. Heatstroke in the super-sized athlete. *Pediatr Emerg Care.* 2006;22:510-513.

63. Loke JC, MacLennan D. Bayesian modeling of muscle biopsy contracture testing for malignant hyperthermia susceptibility. *Anesthesiology.* 1998;88:589-600.

65. Paasuke RT, Brownell AKW. Serum creatine kinase level as a screening test for susceptibility to malignant hyperthermia. *JAMA.* 1986;255:769-771.

67. Larach MG, Landis JR, Bunn JS, et al. The North American Malignant Hyperthermia Registry: prediction of malignant hyperthermia susceptibility in low risk subjects. *Anesthesiology.* 1992;76:16-27.

69. Allen GC, Larach MG, Kunselman AR. The sensitivity and specificity of the caffeine-halothane contracture test: a report from the North American Malignant Hyperthermia Registry of MHAUS. *Anesthesiology.* 1998;88:579-588.

70. Brandom BW. Malignant hyperthermia. In: Motoyama EK, Davis PJ, eds. *Smith's Anesthesia for Infants and Children.* 7th ed. Philadelphia: Mosby; 2006:1013-1031.

73. Girard T, Treves S, Censier K, et al. Phenotyping malignant hyperthermia susceptibility by measuring halothane-induced changes in myoplasmic calcium concentration in cultured human skeletal muscle cells. *Br J Anaesth.* 2002;89:571-579.

77. Stein MH, Sorscher M, Caroff SN. Neuroleptic malignant syndrome induced by metoclopramide in an infant with Freeman-Sheldon syndrome. *Anesth Analg.* 2006;103:786-787.

78. Silva RR, Munoz DM, Alpert M, et al. Neuroleptic malignant syndrome in children and adolescents. *J Am Acad Child Adolesc Psychiatry.* 1999;38:187-194.

79. Henderson A, Longdon P. Fulminant metoclopramide induced neuroleptic malignant syndrome rapidly responsive to dantrolene. *Aust N Z J Med.* 1991;21:742-743.

80. Geiduschek J, Cohen SA, Khan A, et al. Repeated anesthesia for a patient with neuroleptic malignant syndrome. *Anesthesiology.* 1988;68:134-137.

81. Schneider C, Pedrosa-Gil F, Schneider M, et al. Intolerance to neuroleptics and susceptibility for malignant hyperthermia in a patient with proximal myotonic myopathy (PROMM) and schizophrenia. *Neuromuscul Disord.* 2002;12:31-35.

82. Mills KC. Serotonin syndrome. A clinical update. *Crit Care Clin.* 1997;13:763-783.

83. Mason PJ, Morris VA, Balcezak TJ. Serotonin syndrome. Presentation of 2 cases and review of the literature. *Medicine (Baltimore).* 2000;79:201-209.

84. Wappler F, Fiege M, Schulte AM, et al. Pathophysiological role of the serotonin system in malignant hyperthermia. *Br J Anaesth.* 2001;87:794-798.

Neuromuscular Blocking Agents

Joseph D. Tobias

PEARLS

- Through the blockade of skeletal muscle function, neuromuscular blocking agents (NMBAs) cause cessation of respiratory function, mandating airway control and the institution of mechanical ventilation. The inability to manage the airway with the provision of bag-mask ventilation and endotracheal intubation will result in hypoxemia and death. NMBAs should not be administered if there is any question as to the normalcy of the airway and the ability to successfully accomplish bag-valve-mask ventilation.

- The term *NMBA* rather than muscle relaxant may be preferable as the latter seems to imply some implicit type of sedative or relaxant property that these agents do not possess. As such, use of the term *NMBA* identifies in their name their mechanism of action, further emphasizing that they are devoid of sedative or analgesic properties.

- NMBAs can broadly be divided into two separate classes on the basis of their mechanism of action. Depolarizing agents such as succinylcholine mimic the action of acetylcholine at the neuromuscular junction and activate or depolarize the muscle, whereas nondepolarizing agents such as pancuronium or rocuronium act as a competitive antagonist to the effects of acetylcholine at the neuromuscular junction, thereby blocking its effects.

Introduction

In the pediatric ICU (PICU) setting, there may be circumstances in which prevention of movement is necessary, thereby mandating the use of neuromuscular blocking agents (NMBAs) (Table 133.1).[1] Although these agents can be used as a single dose to facilitate brief procedures such as endotracheal intubation, prolonged administration may be necessary in specific clinical scenarios. With an improved understanding of the techniques for providing sedation and analgesia in the PICU setting and data demonstrating not only their adverse effect profile but also their lack of efficacy in specific clinical scenarios, there has been a decrease in the prolonged administration of NMBAs.[2] A past survey from the PICU setting suggests that the prolonged administration of these agents is used most commonly as an adjunct in the control of intracranial pressure (ICP), although the recent resurgence in the use of hypothermia following cardiac arrest and cerebral ischemia has seen the increased use of these agents to prevent shiveriing.[3-5]

Given their adverse effect profile including the potential for increased nosocomial infections, longer duration of mechanical ventilation, and pressure injuries, NMBAs should be used only when absolutely indicated, by personnel with appropriate training in their pharmacology, and only after obtaining the knowledge and skills needed to treat adverse effects related to their use. Use of the terminology "muscle relaxant" should be avoided as this seems to imply some implicit sedative property, which these agents do not possess. Because these agents provide no amnestic, analgesic, or sedative properties, coadministration of an amnestic agent (ie, benzodiazepine, ketamine, propofol, or a barbiturate) is necessary whenever they are used. The term *NMBA* is preferred because it identifies the mechanism of action of these agents as a competitive antagonist for acetylcholine at the neuromuscular junction.

Following the administration of an NMBA and the blockade of skeletal muscle function, cessation of ventilation with apnea mandates airway control, endotracheal intubation, and the institution of mechanical ventilation. The inability to manage the airway including the provision of bag-valve-mask ventilation and endotracheal intubation will result in the potential for hypoxemia and death. As such, before these agents are used for endotracheal intubation, the normalcy of the airway and ability to provide bag-valve-mask ventilation and endotracheal intubation should be assessed.[6,7] If problems managing the airway are anticipated, NMBAs should not be administered. Furthermore, when using these medications, one should be familiar with the "cannot intubate–cannot ventilate" algorithm and have ready access to the needed equipment for rescue in this scenario.[7]

Neuromuscular Junction

Normal neuromuscular transmission results from the release of acetylcholine from the nerve terminal, its movement across the synaptic cleft, and binding to the postsynaptic nicotinic receptor on the sarcolemma of the skeletal muscle. Acetylcholine is synthesized in the cytoplasm from acetyl coenzyme A and choline and stored in synaptic vesicles in the axonal terminals of the presynaptic membrane. Depolarization of the presynaptic axonal membrane opens calcium channels (P channel). The movement of calcium through the channels in the presynaptic membrane results in the movement of synaptic vesicles, which hold acetylcholine, toward the membrane, their fusion with the membrane, and the release of acetylcholine into the synaptic cleft. The P channel can be blocked by cations such as magnesium and lithium but generally not by calcium channel antagonists. The concurrent administration of magnesium or lithium potentiates the effect of nondepolarizing NMBAs. The excessive administration of either cation

TABLE 133.1	Reported Indications for Neuromuscular Blockade in the Pediatric ICU

Facilitation of procedures or diagnostic studies:

_____endotracheal intubation

_____central line placement

_____radiologic imaging (MRI, CT scanning)

Immobilization during interhospital or intrahospital transport

Intensive care indications:

_____facilitate mechanical ventilation

_____control increased intracranial pressure

_____eliminate shivering (especially during therapeutic hypothermia)

_____decrease peripheral oxygen utilization

_____control severe agitation unresponsive to adequate sedation

_____maintain immobilization after surgical procedures

_____decrease the risk of pulmonary vasospasm in patients with pulmonary hypertension

_____manage patients with tetanus

can have significant effects on normal neuromuscular function and cause muscle weakness. After its release from the synaptic vesicles, acetylcholine diffuses across the synaptic cleft and binds to acetylcholine receptors on the postsynaptic membrane (sarcolemma).

The acetylcholine receptor (nicotinic receptor on the sarcolemma) is a pentameric protein composed of five subunits. There are five possible subunits (alpha, beta, gamma, delta, and epsilon), each of which is encoded by a different gene. The normal acetylcholine receptor found in adults includes two alpha subunits combined with one each of the beta, delta, and epsilon subunits. Binding of an acetylcholine molecule to each of the two alpha subunits is necessary for opening of the channel and depolarization of the sarcolemma. During various stages of development or in pathologic disease states, the composition of the acetylcholine receptor may change. Immature and denervated acetylcholine receptors have a gamma subunit instead of the epsilon, while a demyelinated neuromuscular junction contains acetylcholine receptors composed of a pentamer of alpha subunits. The importance of these variants is that their response (opening of the ion channel) may be dramatically different from the normal adult variant of the acetylcholine receptor. These differences can have devastating consequences following the administration of succinylcholine. The channel may remain open for a prolonged period of time, resulting in the release of intracellular potassium. The acetylcholine receptor occupies the entire membrane from the outside of the muscle through the cell membrane to the inside and thereby regulates the transmembrane movement of ions. The receptor acts to convert the chemical stimulus (acetylcholine) into an electrical impulse that results in the depolarization of the sarcolemma. The depolarization of the sarcolemma results in the release of calcium from the sarcoplasmic reticulum (SR) and muscle contraction.

Stimulation of the acetylcholine receptor opens ion channels allowing the movement of small, positively charged cations such as sodium, potassium, and calcium. The sodium influx depolarizes the muscle membrane leading to the release of calcium from the SR and muscle contraction. Cessation of muscle contraction and repolarization occurs when acetylcholine is metabolized by the enzyme acetylcholinesterase, which is present in the synaptic cleft. This repolarization resets the muscle for the next round of depolarization and excitation-contraction coupling. Failure to metabolize acetylcholine bound to the receptor results in prolonged depolarization, inability to repolarize the sarcolemma, and cessation of further contraction.

Neuromuscular Blocking Agents: Depolarizing Agents

The two general classes of NMBAs (depolarizing and nondepolarizing agents) differ in their basic mechanism of action. Depolarizing agents such as succinylcholine (suxamethonium in Europe and the United Kingdom) mimic acetylcholine, binding to the acetylcholine receptor at the neuromuscular junction and activating it. As succinylcholine is resistant to degradation by acetylcholinesterase, there is sustained occupation of the receptor and failure of repolarization, which results in neuromuscular blockade. This action of succinylcholine accounts for the clinical effects that are seen including the initial muscle fasciculations followed by flaccid paralysis lasting 5 to 10 minutes, the time necessary for the degradation of succinylcholine by pseudocholinesterase and subsequent repolarization of the sarcolemma. The onset of action of succinylcholine is more rapid than any of the nondepolarizing agents with neuromuscular blockade, occurring in 30 to 45 seconds, thereby allowing for rapid control of the airway with endotracheal intubation. Additionally, many of the studies comparing succinylcholine to nondepolarizing NMBAs suggest it produces better conditions for endotracheal intubation.[8]

Succinylcholine undergoes rapid redistribution and metabolism by the plasma enzyme, pseudocholinesterase (butyrylcholinesterase), which limits its clinical duration to 5 to 10 minutes. In some patients, a congenital or acquired deficiency of pseudocholinesterase prolongs duration of action. When considering such scenarios, there may be issues with the total amount of enzyme (quantitative defect) or efficacy of the enzyme (qualitative defect).[9] Decreased enzyme levels (quantitative defects) are usually acquired while qualitative issues are inherited. The inherited form of pseudocholinesterase deficiency, resulting in a qualitative defect in the enzyme, is an autosomal recessive trait with an incidence of 1:2500 to 3500. Only homozygotes have a clinically significant prolongation of the effect of succinylcholine with neuromuscular blockade lasting up to 4 to 8 hours following a routine dose of succinylcholine (1–2 mg/kg). Disease states that lead to a quantitative decrease in pseudocholinesterase levels include severe liver disease, myxedema, pregnancy, protein-calorie malnutrition, and certain malignancies. Drugs and medications can also affect pseudocholinesterase levels including chemotherapeutic agents, such as cyclophosphamide and echothiopate ophthalmic drops. Deficiency can also result from the recent use of plasmapheresis as the enzyme is removed with the plasma. With either qualitative or quantitative defects of pseudocholinesterase, suspicion should be aroused if there is failure of the return of the train-of-four (TOF) with peripheral nerve stimulation (see later). Although such problems are rare, it is prudent to demonstrate the return of neuromuscular function following the administration of succinylcholine and prior to the administration of a nondepolarizing agent. This can be accomplished by demonstrating the return of the TOF after succinylcholine is administered. If such a problem is suspected, the primary therapy includes continuation of ventilatory support until the patient's muscle strength returns and the provision of amnesia with an anesthetic agent (benzodiazepine, propofol, continuing a volatile anesthetic agent). While movement is prevented, the patient will be aware and awake once the effect of these agents has stopped. The enzyme plasma cholinesterase is contained in fresh frozen plasma (FFP); however, due to the infectious disease concerns with the use of blood products, reversal with the administration of FFP cannot be recommended.[10-12] Purified human plasma cholinesterase has also been used; however, such a practice is expensive and is not available in most centers.[13]

Despite its rapid onset and rapid offset, the potential adverse effects associated with succinylcholine can be devastating and even fatal (Table 133.2). Direct effects on cardiac rhythm have been reported including bradycardia, tachycardia, and atrial or ventricular ectopy.[14] Succinylcholine has a chemical structure resembling that of acetylcholine and may thereby result in bradycardia from activation of cardiac muscarinic receptors. Bradycardia may be more common in several specific clinical scenarios and situations including (1) infants and children, (2) during halothane anesthesia, (3) in the presence of hypoxemia, (4) with IV as compared with IM administration, (5) when succinylcholine is administered concurrently with other medications that have negative chronotropic effects (propofol, fentanyl), (6) in the presence of hypothermia, (7) in patients with increased intracranial pressure (ICP), or (8) with repeated dosing. The latter may occur during difficulties with endotracheal intubation when the first dose is wearing off. In these populations or scenarios, succinylcholine should always be preceded by an anticholinergic agent such as atropine. Arrhythmias, although fairly common, occurring in up to 50% of patients following the administration of

succinylcholine, are generally short-lived and of limited clinical significance. The use of an anticholinergic agent will decrease but not eliminate the incidence of arrhythmias. As with the potential for bradycardia, arrhythmias tend to be more common with repeated doses of succinylcholine.

As succinylcholine activates the acetylcholine receptor before producing neuromuscular blockade, depolarization of the muscle end plate occurs with contraction of the muscle fascicles or fasciculations. These fasciculations are responsible for the myalgias that may occur following succinylcholine.[15] Although not a primary concern when succinylcholine is used for emergently securing the airway, the use of succinylcholine may not be optimal for facilitating endotracheal intubation for outpatient surgery when such issues may interfere with activities of daily living and return to work. One advantage of fasciculations is that their cessation signals that neuromuscular blockade is complete and one can proceed with direct laryngoscopy and tracheal intubation. The severity of the fasciculations can be prevented by the administration of a small dose of a nondepolarizing agent, generally 1/10th of the dose normally used for endotracheal intubation (curare 0.03–0.05 mg/kg, rocuronium 0.05 mg/kg, or pancuronium 0.01 mg/kg) before succinylcholine.[16] This is referred to as a "defasciculating dose." The technique is commonly used in the operating room as a means of preventing or attenuating the postoperative myalgias when succinylcholine is administered to adults.

Defasciculation is not commonly used in the pediatric population for several reasons: (1) children younger than 6 years of age do not fasciculate; (2) the use of the defasciculating dose delays the onset of paralysis and increases the dose of succinylcholine needed; (3) in patients with severe respiratory or hemodynamic compromise, the defasciculating dose can cause a significant degree of neuromuscular blockade leading to respiratory insufficiency or laryngeal incompetency with the risk of aspiration; and (4) full efficacy may require up to 2 to 3 minutes, thereby making the technique less optimal when emergent securing of the airway is necessary. If a defasciculating dose is used in patients who are awake and coherent, they should be warned that they may feel the effects of the medication, with the development of diplopia related to the effects of the drug on the extraocular muscles. Additionally, some patients may feel the effects on the muscles of ventilation, resulting in complaints of shortness of breath or dyspnea.

In addition to myalgias, the fasciculations caused by succinylcholine may result in a transient increase in plasma creatinine phosphokinase (CPK) and myoglobin levels. Myoglobinemia has been reported in up to 40% of patients when there is the concomitant administration of general anesthesia with halothane. In these patients, levels high enough to result in myoglobinuria have been reported in 8% of patients.[17] The rise in plasma CPK and myoglobin levels does not occur with IM administration and may be attenuated by the administration of a defasciculating dose (see earlier). These effects should be differentiated from the potentially lethal complications of rhabdomyolysis, which may occur in patients with specific disorders of the neuromuscular junction and malignant hyperthermia (see later). These latter disorders absolutely contraindicate the use of succinylcholine.

The fasciculations may also lead to an increase in intragastric (IGP) and intraocular pressure (IOP). The transient and minimal rise in IGP is generally of limited clinical significance

TABLE 133.2	Adverse Effects of Succinylcholine
Prolonged blockade with acquired or inherited pseudocholinesterase deficiency	
Cardiac arrhythmias:	
_____bradycardia	
_____tachycardia	
_____asystole	
_____atrial and ventricular ectopy	
Hypertension	
Increased intraocular pressure	
Increased intragastric pressure	
Increased intracranial pressure	
Diffuse myalgias	
Myoglobinuria	
Malignant hyperthermia	
Hyperkalemia (see Table 133.3)	

and does not increase the risk of vomiting or passive regurgitation during endotracheal intubation. In the emergency setting, when succinylcholine is chosen for endotracheal intubation, rapid sequence intubation will be used with the application of cricoid pressure to protect against acid aspiration. The contraction of extraocular muscles leads to an increase of IOP following the administration of succinylcholine. The increase is transient with a return of the IOP to baseline within 5 to 8 minutes. Given this effect, the administration of succinylcholine to patients with an open globe injury is generally contraindicated due to the theoretical risk of causing extrusion of the intraocular contents.[18] In settings with an open globe where the use of succinylcholine is considered warranted on the basis of the patient's status, various medications including dexmedetomidine have been shown to blunt the increase in IOP.[19,20]

The effects of succinylcholine on ICP and its use in patients with altered intracranial compliance remain controversial. Succinylcholine may result in a mild to modest ICP increase through various postulated mechanisms including muscle fasciculations and increased venous tone, as well as a direct cholinergic mechanism due to activation of muscle spindles in the peripheral skeletal musculature.[21] Succinylcholine's effects on muscle spindles have also been postulated to cause CNS activation and dreaming during general anesthesia.[22] The dreaming has not been associated with awareness or recall. The effects on ICP are generally mild and transient.

Given its rapid onset (30 to 45 seconds), succinylcholine allows for rapid endotracheal intubation and control of arterial oxygenation and ventilation. As the latter are primary determinants of ICP, any mild increase due to the direct effects of succinylcholine is rapidly controlled. The authors of a recent review article evaluating the evidence-based medicine regarding succinylcholine and ICP concluded: "There is insufficient evidence that administration of suxamethonium causes an increase in intracranial pressure when administered to patients with traumatic brain injury. Further adequately powered studies are required to assess such a relationship. Until such evidence exists, the superior intubation conditions created by suxamethonium in comparison with rocuronium mean that suxamethonium should remain the first choice agent for neuromuscular blockade as part of a rapid sequence induction in head-injured patients unless absolute contraindications to suxamethonium use exist."[23]

Succinylcholine can also cause a transient increase in the tone of the masseter muscles. The incidence of this problem is significantly higher in the perioperative setting when succinylcholine is administered with the volatile anesthetic agent halothane. A defasciculating dose of a nondepolarizing agent may abolish this phenomenon. This effect may be seen in all of the peripheral skeletal musculature but is accentuated in the masseter muscles, resulting in what is clinically known as masseter spasm. The effect is generally mild and can be overcome by manual opening of the mouth.[24] In rare circumstances, the masseter spasm may be severe, preventing mouth opening and precluding standard oral endotracheal intubation. It has been suggested that patients who manifest masseter spasm to this degree are at risk for malignant hyperthermia (MH), a rare inherited disorder of muscle metabolism that, if untreated, is generally fatal (see later). The data regarding the relationship between masseter spasm and MH are conflicting. In a prospective evaluation with monitoring of masseter muscle tone, patients who developed significant increases in masseter muscle tone did not proceed to develop MH.[25] However, retrospective series have suggested that the development of masseter spasm may be a prelude to MH, thereby clouding the issue as to how to deal with such patients.[26] In the emergency situation, should patients develop masseter spasm following the administration of succinylcholine, they must be monitored for signs of MH including hypercarbia, hyperthermia, tachycardia, and rhabdomyolysis with myoglobinuria. Treatment with dantrolene is suggested should there be a concern regarding the development of MH (see later).

The major concerns with succinylcholine are its potential to trigger MH and its ability to cause massive hyperkalemia if administered to patients with various comorbid disease processes.[27] MH is an inherited disorder (autosomal dominant) of muscle metabolism with abnormalities of the ryanodine receptor (the calcium release channel of the sarcoplasmic reticulum of skeletal muscle). The point mutation of the ryanodine receptor leads to ongoing release of calcium and therefore sustained muscle contraction following exposure to succinylcholine or a potent inhalational anesthetic agent. During MH, ongoing muscle contraction and metabolism lead to hyperthermia, acidosis, tachycardia, hypercarbia, and rhabdomyolysis with secondary hyperkalemia. Treatment includes discontinuation of the triggering agent, treatment of hyperthermia and the biochemical derangements including acidosis and hyperkalemia, and administration of dantrolene, which blocks ongoing calcium release from the sarcoplasmic reticulum. Therefore in clinical scenarios where succinylcholine may be administered, ready access to dantrolene is recommended.

Lethal hyperkalemia following succinylcholine may occur in patients with certain underlying disorders or comorbid diseases (Table 133.3).[27] Although many of the disorders listed in Table 133.3 are readily apparent, such as the muscular

TABLE 133.3	Conditions Associated With Hyperkalemia After Succinylcholine Administration
Preexisting hyperkalemia	
Muscular dystrophy	
Burns after 48 h involving >10%-15% body surface area	
Profound metabolic acidosis	
Paraplegia or quadriplegia	
Denervation injury	
Metastatic rhabdomyosarcoma	
Parkinson disease	
Disuse atrophy or prolonged bedrest	
Polyneuropathy	
Degenerative central nervous system disorders	
Purpura fulminans	
Tetanus	
Guillain-Barré	
Myotonia dystrophy	
Prolonged administration of nondepolarizing neuromuscular blocking agent	

dystrophies, the occurrence of cardiac arrest following succinylcholine administration to apparently healthy children led to a restructuring of the package insert and recommendations for the use of succinylcholine. Children with muscular dystrophy may not manifest symptoms until they are 4 to 6 years of age. If succinylcholine is administered during routine anesthetic care or other clinical scenarios, lethal hyperkalemia can occur. Because of such problems, the current recommendations are that succinylcholine be used only for emergency airway management when rapid sequence endotracheal intubation is necessary, when there is a concern about the ability to provide endotracheal intubation (potentially or documented difficult airway), or when intramuscular administration is necessary because IV access cannot be secured. Also of concern in the pediatric population are patients with relatively rare genetic, chromosomal, or metabolic defects in whom the effects of succinylcholine have not been fully evaluated. Given the rarity of such syndromes, there is limited evidence-based medicine on which to provide recommendations regarding the safety of succinylcholine use. In such settings, the risk-benefit ratio should be examined. In many of these patients, the use of a rapidly acting, nondepolarizing agent may be the better option. The safety of succinylcholine use with minimal increases in serum potassium concentrations has been demonstrated in children with cerebral palsy, as well as those with meningomyelocele.[28-30] Regardless of the clinical scenario, if problems occur following the administration of succinylcholine, hyperkalemia should be suspected and the resuscitation tailored accordingly.

In emergency situations when IV access cannot be readily obtained, succinylcholine can be administered intramuscularly in a dose of 4 to 5 mg/kg. IM administration will result in neuromuscular blockade sufficient to allow for endotracheal intubation in 2 to 3 minutes and will rapidly (<30 seconds) treat laryngospasm occurring during anesthetic induction when IV access is not available, thereby allowing for effective bag-valve-mask ventilation. Use of the IM route for the administration of succinylcholine is most commonly chosen intraoperatively during the inhalation induction of anesthetic when IV access is not present.[31] In this scenario, succinylcholine should be administered into the deltoid muscle as the onset times are more rapid than with administration into the quadriceps. Alternatively, administration into the tongue or the submental space has been suggested as blood flow to this area is generally well maintained even when peripheral vasoconstriction has occurred.[32] Unlike IV administration, there is limited risk of bradycardia with IM administration.[33] The IM route is not recommended in patients with conditions that decrease cardiac output or blood flow to the muscles, such as shock or bradycardia, as the onset of action will be significantly delayed. Given these concerns, IM administration is generally not recommended in critically ill children and intraosseous administration (1–2 mg/kg) is preferable when IV access is not available.[34,35]

Currently, the package insert and good clinical practice allow for administration of succinylcholine when there may be a potentially difficult airway, in the emergency situation when rapid securing of the airway is necessary (full stomach when a rapid sequence intubation is performed), and when there is no IV access (IM administration), provided that there is no contraindication to its use (Table 133.3).[27] When dealing with the potentially difficult airway or unrecognized difficult airway, the major advantage of succinylcholine is that there should be return of normal neuromuscular function within 10 minutes as opposed to 60 minutes following a 1-mg/kg intubating dose of rocuronium (see later). For IV administration, clinically used dosing recommendations for succinylcholine vary from 1 to 2 mg/kg.[36] Larger doses are likely not to improve intubating conditions while slightly prolonging the duration of action.

Neuromuscular Blocking Agents: Nondepolarizing Agents

Nondepolarizing NMBAs function as competitive antagonists at the neuromuscular junction, antagonizing the effects of acetylcholine at the receptor. Unlike succinylcholine, these agents do not activate the acetylcholine receptor and therefore do not result in fasciculations and the associated problems that may occur (see earlier). Nondepolarizing NMBAs are used most commonly intraoperatively to facilitate endotracheal intubation and also to provide ongoing muscle relaxation for specific surgical procedures such as exploratory laparotomy. When used to provide ongoing neuromuscular blockade in the operating room or ICU, these agents can be administered by intermittent bolus dosing or continuous infusions. There are two basic chemical structures of the nondepolarizing NMBAs available for clinical use: aminosteroid and benzylisoquinolinium compounds (Table 133.4). The difference in their chemical structure has limited clinical significance. Of more importance are differences in onset, duration of action, cardiovascular effects, metabolism, metabolic products, and cost. These principles are reviewed in the remainder of this chapter.

The first nondepolarizing NMBAs (curare, gallamine, metocurine), which were introduced into clinical practice in the 1940s, are rarely if ever used in today's clinical practice. The past 20 years have seen a rapid growth in the development and introduction of nondepolarizing NMBAs for clinical use. As these agents have more favorable profiles (onset times, recovery times, metabolic fate), they have displaced the original group introduced in the 1940s.

Pancuronium

Pancuronium is an aminosteroid compound, generally available in a solution containing 1 mg/mL of pancuronium

TABLE 133.4	Classification of Nondepolarizing Neuromuscular Blocking Agents
Aminosteroid compounds:	
_____pancuronium	
_____rocuronium	
_____vecuronium	
_____pipecuronium	
_____rapacuronium (no longer available)	
Benzylisoquinolinium compounds:	
_____mivacurium	
_____atracurium	
_____cis-atracurium	
_____doxacurium	

(depending on the manufacturer, other concentrations may be available). The common clinical dose of 0.1 to 0.15 mg/kg provides adequate conditions for endotracheal intubation in 90 to 120 seconds. Although the higher end of the dosing range may speed the onset time for acceptable conditions for endotracheal intubation, the clinical duration is prolonged from 40 to 60 minutes to 70 to 80 minutes. Given its duration of action, pancuronium is considered a long-acting NMBA (Table 133.5). The ED_{95} in children is 52 µg/kg during halothane anesthesia and 81 to 93 µg/kg during an opioid-based anesthetic. The latter is more applicable to the PICU setting.[37] The ED_{95} in children is slightly higher than that of adolescents.[38] Following a dose of 70 µg/kg, the onset of neuromuscular blockade occurs more quickly in children than in adults with 90% twitch ablation occurring at an average of 2.4 minutes in children and 4.3 minutes in adults.[39] The time to return of the twitch height to 10% of baseline was 25 minutes in children and 46 minutes in adults.

Vagal blockade and release of norepinephrine from adrenergic nerve endings result in an increase in heart rate and blood pressure. Intraoperatively, this effect was used to balance the negative chronotropic effects of the volatile anesthetic agent, halothane. There may be a mild proarrhythmogenic effect for atrial tachyarrhythmias in patients with comorbid diseases or when administered with other agents that increase heart rate. Elimination is primarily renal (80%), resulting in a significantly prolonged effect with renal insufficiency or failure. Hepatic metabolism is primarily hydroxylation with production of an active 3-OH metabolite, which retains approximately 50% of the neuromuscular blocking effects of the parent compound. The 3-OH metabolite is also dependent on renal excretion, thereby further prolonging the effect in the setting of renal insufficiency or failure.

Given its longer half-life, pancuronium is generally used by intermittent dosing to provide ongoing neuromuscular blockade in the PICU setting. One prospective study evaluated dosing requirements in the PICU population with pancuronium administration by a continuous infusion.[40] Pancuronium was administered as an initial bolus dose of 0.1 mg/kg followed by an infusion starting at 0.05 mg/kg/hr. The infusion was titrated up and down to maintain one to two twitches of the TOF (see later). Pancuronium infusion requirements varied from 0.3 to 0.22 mg/kg/hr with an average infusion rate of 0.07 ± 0.03 mg/kg/hr for the 1798 hours of the infusion. Approximately 70% of the time, the infusion requirements varied from 0.05 to 0.08 mg/kg/hr. Increased infusion requirements were noted in patients receiving anticonvulsant agents (0.14 ± 0.06 vs. 0.056 ± 0.03 mg/kg/hr) and in patients who received pancuronium for more than 5 days (day 1 requirements of 0.059 mg/kg/hr vs. 0.083 mg/kg/hr on day 5). On discontinuation of the infusion, time to spontaneous recovery of neuromuscular function (return of the TOF to baseline and sustained tetanus to 50 Hz) varied from 35 to 75 minutes. The authors concluded that pancuronium could be effectively administered by continuous infusion to provide neuromuscular blockade in the PICU setting, being a cost-effective alternative to other available agents in many clinical scenarios. Despite its efficacy in many clinical situations, the use of pancuronium has decreased markedly over the past 20 years, since the introduction of intermediate-acting agents with limited concerns of prolonged blocking following intraoperative use. With the availability of generic forms of vecuronium, the cost advantages of pancuronium have decreased, thereby limiting its use.

Vecuronium

Like pancuronium, vecuronium is an aminosteroid compound. It was released for clinical use in the 1980s. Despite minor differences in pharmacologic structure from pancuronium, its plasma clearance is two to three times as rapid. Vecuronium is available as a powder (10 mg), which in common clinical practice is diluted to a concentration of 1 mg/mL. Its initial introduction and acceptance into anesthesia practice were facilitated by its lack of clinically significant hemodynamic effects as it does not cause tachycardia or hypotension. In the usual clinically used doses of 0.1 to 0.15 mg/kg, acceptable conditions for endotracheal intubation are present in 80 to 90 seconds with a clinical duration of action of 30 to 40 minutes, making it an intermediate-acting agent.[41] To speed the onset and allow for endotracheal intubation in 60 to 75 seconds, the dose can be increased to 0.3 mg/kg. However, higher doses resulted in a prolonged duration of neuromuscular blockade of 60 to 90 minutes. Even with higher doses, vecuronium is devoid of cardiovascular effects. Metabolism is primarily hepatic (70%-80%); however, hepatic metabolism results in the production of pharmacologically active metabolites, which are water soluble and therefore dependent on renal excretion. These metabolites possess roughly half of the neuromuscular blocking effects of the parent compound. This combined with the 20% to 30% renal excretion of the parent compound results in a prolonged clinical duration in patients with renal insufficiency. Given its 70% to 80% dependency on hepatic metabolism, the duration of action is also prolonged with hepatic insufficiency and in neonates due to immaturity of the hepatic microsomal enzymes. Vecuronium in doses of 0.1 mg/kg and 0.15 mg/kg maintained neuromuscular blockade at 90% or more of baseline for 59 and 110 minutes in neonates and infants, 18 and 38 minutes in children, and 37 and 68 minutes, respectively, in adolescents.[42] The opposite effect occurs with the chronic administration of anticonvulsant agents with resistance to the

TABLE 133.5	Duration of Action of Neuromuscular Blocking Agents
Short-acting (10 min):	
_____succinylcholine	
_____mivacurium	
_____rapacuronium	
Intermediate-acting (20-40 min):	
_____atracurium	
_____vecuronium	
_____cis-atracurium	
_____rocuronium	
Long-acting (60-90 min):	
_____pancuronium	
_____pipecuronium	
_____doxacurium	

neuromuscular blocking effects and increased dose requirements in patients receiving phenytoin.[43] A similar effect has been reported with other anticonvulsant agents and other NMBAs of the aminosteroid group. Given its lack of hemodynamic effects and current availability in generic form, thereby providing a cost-effective agent for neuromuscular blockade, vecuronium remains a commonly used agent by bolus dosing and continuous infusion for neuromuscular blockade in the PICU setting. As with many generic medications, intermittent medication shortages have included vecuronium over the past 5 years.

Rocuronium

Rocuronium is an aminosteroid NMBA that was released for clinical use in the early to mid 1990s. It is commercially available in a solution containing 10 mg/mL in either 5- or 10-mL vials. Following the routine dose for endotracheal intubation of 0.6 mg/kg, the duration of action is 20 to 40 minutes, making it an intermediate-acting agent; however, larger doses (1–1.2 mg/kg) are frequently used during rapid sequence or urgent/emergent endotracheal intubation as the onset time with these doses has been shown to approximately parallel those of succinylcholine (see later). As with other agents, the duration of action increases when larger doses are administered so that 60 to 90 minutes of neuromuscular blockade generally occur following a dose of 1.0 mg/kg. Of note, given its dependence on hepatic metabolism, a prolonged effect may be seen in neonates and infants. A mild vagolytic effect, less in intensity than that seen with pancuronium, may increase heart rate in the range of 10 to 20 beats per minute and mean arterial pressure following bolus dosing.

Rocuronium undergoes primarily hepatic metabolism without the production of active metabolites, which have a clinical effect following a single bolus dose. Its clinical duration is prolonged, and its clearance is decreased in patients with hepatic insufficiency or failure. Despite its primary dependence on hepatic elimination, there are mixed results in both adults and children regarding the duration of its effects in patients with renal insufficiency or failure. When comparing adults with and without renal failure, Robertson et al. reported that there was prolongation of the clinical duration (time to recovery of the first twitch of the TOF to 25% of baseline) from 32 to 49 minutes following a dose of 0.6 mg/kg in patients with renal failure.[44] The same investigators reported no difference in the pharmacodynamics in adults with and without renal failure with the use of a smaller dose (0.3 mg/kg).[45] With the smaller dose of 0.3 mg/kg, the onset time was 4 minutes and neuromuscular blockade was reversible at 20 minutes. When comparing adults with renal failure and those with normal renal function, Cooper et al.[46] reported that following rocuronium (0.6 mg/kg), onset time (65 ± 16 vs. 61 ± 25 seconds), clinical duration (55 ± 26.9 vs. 42 ± 9.3 minutes), and spontaneous recovery (time for return of the final twitch of the TOF to 70% of baseline) were all prolonged (99 ± 41 vs. 73 ± 24 minutes). Following an initial dose of 0.3 mg/kg, pediatric patients with renal failure had a longer onset time (139 ± 71 vs. 87 ± 43 seconds); however, there was no difference in the clinical duration.[47] More specific pharmacokinetic data and an explanation for the apparent prolonged elimination half-life of rocuronium in renal failure patients are provided by Szenohradszky et al.[48] in their evaluation of rocuronium in a cohort of 10 adult patients undergoing renal

transplantation. Following a dose of 0.6 mg/kg, although the total plasma clearance and volume of the central compartment did not differ between renal failure and control patients, the volume of distribution at steady state was larger in patients with renal failure and this resulted in a longer elimination half-life with renal failure (97.2 ± 17.3 vs. 70.9 ± 4.7 minutes). A summary of these studies demonstrates a slightly prolonged onset time with rocuronium and a prolonged elimination half-life (and therefore a prolonged clinical effect) in the presence of renal failure. Current data suggest that these findings result from alterations in the volume of distribution rather than primary alterations in clearance due to renal effects. The prolonged duration of action may be clinically significant with doses 0.6 mg/kg or greater and can be minimized with doses of 0.3 mg/kg. However, with the smaller doses, onset times for successful endotracheal intubation will be prolonged to 2 to 3 minutes.

Given its dependence on hepatic metabolism, alterations in clearance are likely in not only patients with primary hepatic diseases but also neonates and infants due to the immaturity of the hepatic microsomal enzymes. When comparing infants (0.1-0.8 years) and children (2.3-8 years), plasma clearance is decreased (4.2 ± 0.7 vs. 6.7 ± 1.1 mL/kg/min), the volume of distribution is increased (231 ± 32 vs. 165 ± 44 mL/kg), and the mean residence time is increased (56 ± 10 vs. 26 ± 9 minutes).[49] Also of note, the plasma concentration required to exert a 50% neuromuscular blocking effect is decreased in neonates and infants compared with older children (1.2 ± 0.4 vs. 1.7 ± 0.4 mg/mL). The latter effect, which indicates that the neuromuscular junction of neonates and infants is more sensitive to the effects of NMBAs, is not specific for rocuronium and is seen with all NMBAs. Similar results were reported by Rapp et al.[50] as they reported progressive increases in the clinical duration with a decrease from 5 to 12 months to 2 to 4 months to 0 to 1 month of age. The effect was further magnified when increasing the dose from 0.45 to 0.6 mg/kg. The authors also reported excellent or good conditions for endotracheal intubation in all infants with doses of 0.45 mg/kg and ablation of the twitch response at 15 to 30 seconds in neonates, thereby demonstrating a rapid onset even with the use of lower doses (0.45 mg/kg). As with other medications that undergo primary hepatic metabolism, the clinical effects of rocuronium are prolonged in neonates and infants. Metabolism and clinical effects approach those of the adult population by 6 to 12 months of age. In the neonate or younger infant, acceptable conditions for endotracheal intubation can be achieved at 45 to 60 seconds with doses of 0.3 to 0.45 mg/kg.

The acceptance of rocuronium into the clinical arena has been expedited by its reported clinical advantage over other nondepolarizing NMBAs, a rapid onset. Clinical studies have demonstrated acceptable conditions for endotracheal intubation in the majority of older children and adolescents within 60 seconds following a dose of 1.0 mg/kg. Of the currently available nondepolarizing NMBAs, only rocuronium has an onset of action comparable with that of succinylcholine. The remainder of the NMBAs require 90 to 120 seconds to provide conditions acceptable for endotracheal intubation even when larger doses are used. In both the pediatric and adult populations, various studies have demonstrated that rocuronium in a dose of 1 mg/kg provides acceptable conditions for endotracheal intubation within 60 seconds in the majority of patients.[51-53] Mazurek et al.[52] prospectively compared the onset times of rocuronium (1.2 mg/kg) and succinylcholine (1.5 mg/kg) in a cohort of 26 children. Anesthesia was induced with thiopental (5 mg/kg). Endotracheal intubation attempts were started 30 seconds after the administration of the agent. Time to endotracheal intubation was comparable between the two groups (41.8 ± 2.9 seconds, range: 36-45 seconds with succinylcholine and 40.2 ± 4.0 seconds, range: 33-48 seconds with rocuronium). However, the conditions for endotracheal intubation were slightly less favorable with rocuronium as 7 were excellent, 5 good, and 1 fair versus 10 excellent, 2 good, and 1 fair with succinylcholine. Schreibner et al.[53] compared conditions for endotracheal intubation provided by three of the commonly used NMBAs (rocuronium 0.6 mg/kg, vecuronium 0.1 mg/kg, and atracurium 0.5 mg/kg). Endotracheal intubation was attempted every 30 seconds. Conditions for all of the endotracheal intubations were graded as excellent or good, 60 seconds after rocuronium, 120 seconds after vecuronium, and 180 seconds after atracurium. Although a larger dose of rocuronium speeds the onset time to acceptable conditions for endotracheal intubation, there is also a prolonged duration of action (60-80 minutes) unlike that of succinylcholine (5-10 minutes). The longer duration of action may be problematic should difficulties arise with the performance of endotracheal intubation resulting in a "cannot intubate–cannot ventilate" scenario. Additionally, in patients with traumatic brain injury or other conditions resulting in alteration of mental status, the neurologic examination will be lost for 60 to 80 minutes following rocuronium in doses of 1 mg/kg. Despite these issues, because of its rapid onset, rocuronium remains the drug of choice for rapid sequence or urgent/emergent endotracheal intubation when there are concerns regarding the use of succinylcholine (see earlier).

Various investigators have evaluated potential techniques to increase the onset time of rocuronium without the need to increase the dose. Although there was no difference noted in the time to 50% blockade (42 ± 14 vs. 45 ± 10 seconds) or onset time when comparing rocuronium 0.6 mg/kg administered with either ketamine 1.5 mg/kg or thiopental 4 mg/kg in parturients, endotracheal intubation at 50% blockade was easily performed in all patients in the ketamine group while it was difficult in 75% of patients who received thiopental.[54] A significant decrease in the onset time of rocuronium (0.6 mg/kg) was also demonstrated in patients who received ephedrine (70 μg/kg), 30 seconds before the start of rapid-sequence endotracheal intubation compared with patients receiving placebo (72 ± 19 vs. 98 ± 31 seconds).[55] As ephedrine increases cardiac output through the release of endogenous catecholamines, drug delivery to the skeletal muscle is increased, thereby accelerating the onset time.

As with other NMBAs such as vecuronium, the principle of priming has been used to accelerate the onset time of rocuronium.[56] Eighty-four children undergoing endotracheal intubation were randomized into one of four groups: (1) saline-rocuronium 0.45 mg/kg, (2) rocuronium 0.045 mg/kg–rocuronium 0.405 mg/kg, (2) saline, (3) rocuronium 0.6 mg/kg, or (4) rocuronium 0.06–rocuronium 0.054 mg/kg. The median onset times and 95% confidence in the 4 groups were 122.5 (8–186), 92.5 (68–116), 85 (60–142), and 55 (48–72) seconds, respectively, thereby demonstrating a clinical advantage of priming regardless of whether the total dose was 0.45 or 0.6 mg/kg. As noted previously, there may be issues

with priming including the potential to induce upper airway or respiratory muscle weakness with the potential for aspiration, airway obstruction, or hypoventilation, especially in critically ill patients even with the small priming dose. Additionally, the majority of studies that have used priming have waited at least 60 seconds from the administration of the priming dose until the administration of the remainder of the dose, thereby prolonging the process of medication administration for endotracheal intubation.

Given its rapid onset and lack of adverse effects, most notably rhabdomyolysis and hyperkalemia with underlying neuromuscular disorders, the use of rocuronium via the IM route instead of succinylcholine in the treatment of emergencies, such as laryngospasm during anesthetic induction when IV access is lacking, would be clinically applicable. However, when evaluating onset and recovery times following IM rocuronium, adequate or good to excellent intubating conditions took an average of 2.5 minutes in infants following a dose of 1 mg/kg and 3 minutes in children following a dose of 1.8 mg/kg.[57] The clinical duration was 57 ± 13 minutes in infants and 70 ± 23 minutes in children. The authors also demonstrated a more rapid and predictable onset with IM administration into the deltoid as compared with the quadriceps muscle, an effect similar to that noted with succinylcholine (see earlier). Given these onset times, the authors concluded that IM rocuronium was not an alternative to IM succinylcholine for the emergent treatment of laryngospasm.

An additional issue with rocuronium in clinical practice includes pain on injection through a peripheral IV cannula.[58] When rocuronium is administered immediately after the induction agent for endotracheal intubation, limb withdrawal and grimacing may be seen. The incidence of pain has been reported to be as high as 50% to 80% with a higher incidence in women than men. As with propofol, various techniques have been suggested to prevent or lessen this problem including diluting the rocuronium solution to 0.5 mg/mL instead of the commercially available 10 mg/mL or the preadministration or coadministration of various pharmacologic agents including lidocaine, ketamine, dexmedetomidine, thiopental, magnesium, alfentanil, and ondansetron.[58,59] All of these have met with varying degrees of success. When rocuronium is coadministered with thiopental into the same IV site, a precipitate may form and occlude the IV cannula or tubing. This problem can be prevented by thoroughly flushing the IV site between the thiopental and rocuronium. As with the other aminosteroid NMBAs, chronic anticonvulsant therapy causes resistance to the neuromuscular blocking effects of rocuronium.[60] This effect is mediated by not only stimulation of the hepatic microsomal enzymes responsible for metabolism of these medications but also the upregulation of acetylcholine receptors given their low-grade antagonism of these receptors at the neuromuscular junction.

Although used most commonly by bolus injection for rapid-sequence endotracheal intubation, there are reports of the use of rocuronium infusions in the PICU setting.[61] Given the current problem with the intermittent shortages of various medications including vecuronium, at times rocuronium may be the only intermediate age in the aminosteroid class that is available for clinical use. In a cohort of 20 PICU patients, rocuronium was administered by continuous infusion to maintain one to two twitches of the TOF. The duration of the rocuronium infusion varied from 26 to 172 hours with a total of 1492 hours of administration. Following the initial bolus dose of 0.6 mg/kg, there was a mild increase in heart rate and blood pressure. The infusion requirements on day 1 varied from 0.3 to 0.8 mg/kg/hr (0.76 ± 0.3 mg/kg/hr). When evaluating all patient days, the infusion requirements varied from 0.3 to 2.2 mg/kg/hr (0.95 ± 0.4 mg/kg/hr). The infusion requirements were 0.5 to 0.8 mg/kg/hr in 45 of the 64 patient days (70%) and 0.3 to 1.0 mg/kg/hr in 58 of the 64 patient days (90%). As with other agents, there was an increase in infusion requirements over time. In 14 patients who received rocuronium for 3 days or more, infusion requirements increased from 0.65 mg/kg/hr on day 1 to 0.84 mg/kg/hr on day 3. In five patients who received rocuronium for 5 days, the infusion requirements increased from 0.67 mg/kg/hr on day 1 to 1.2 mg/kg/hr on day 5. When the infusion was discontinued, spontaneous return of neuromuscular function occurred in 24 to 44 minutes (31 ± 12 minutes). No adverse effects related to the use of rocuronium were noted.

Pipecuronium

Pipecuronium is structurally related to the other aminosteroids including pancuronium and vecuronium. Like vecuronium, it is devoid of cardiovascular effects. Following the clinically recommended dose for endotracheal intubation of 0.07 mg/kg, onset times vary from 2 to 3 minutes with a longer duration of action (70 to 80 minutes) than pancuronium. Pipecuronium is eliminated primarily by the kidneys (80%) with the remainder of the elimination dependent on hepatic metabolism. There is limited clinical information concerning the use of pipecuronium in the pediatric population, being used primarily for intraoperative neuromuscular for prolonged surgical procedures.[62-64]

Rapacuronium

In an effort to meet the need for a nondepolarizing NMBA whose onset and offset parallel that of succinylcholine, rapacuronium was introduced into clinical practice in the United States in 1998. The initial clinical experience demonstrated a rapid onset, paralleling that of succinylcholine or larger doses of rocuronium, with a recovery time of less than 10 minutes, thereby offering a significant clinical advantage over rocuronium. Hemodynamic effects included a mild tachycardia like other aminosteroid NMBAs related to a vagolytic effect. Metabolism was hepatic with the presence of active metabolites that were dependent on renal excretion, although their presence did not appear to result in a clinically significant duration of action even in the presence of renal failure or insufficiency.

Unfortunately, with increased clinical use came the recognition that profound and even potentially fatal bronchospasm were associated with its administration. Although these problems were initially postulated to result from an inadequate depth of sedation/anesthesia during airway instrumentation, subsequent studies suggested a direct effect on the cholinergic receptors of the airway. In a retrospective review of their clinical database, Rajchert et al. reported that bronchospasm occurred in 12 of 287 (4.2%) of patients receiving rapacuronium.[65] Five of the episodes with rapacuronium resulted in an inability to move the chest with no exhaled end-tidal CO_2 following endotracheal intubation. The risk of bronchospasm was 10.1 times greater with rapacuronium compared with other NMBAs. Additional clinical data demonstrating

the potential for alterations in respiratory compliance and resistance were reported in a prospective trial in 20 adults randomized to receive either cis-atracurium or rapacuronium.[66] Rapacuronium was administered following anesthetic induction and endotracheal intubation during general anesthesia using continuous infusions of propofol and remifentanil. No changes in compliance or resistance of the respiratory system were noted following cis-atracurium. Following the administration of rapacuronium administration, peak inflating pressure increased from 22 ± 6 to 28 ± 9 cm H_2O, compliance decreased from 108 ± 43 to 77 ± 41 mL/cm H_2O, peak inspiratory flow rate decreased from 0.43 ± 0.11 to 0.39 ± 0.09 L/sec, peak expiratory flow rate decreased from 0.67 ± 0.10 to 0.59 ± 0.09 L/sec, and tidal volume decreased from 744 ± 152 to 647 ± 135 mL. Mechanisms for rapacuronium's effects on airways have focused on alterations in cholinergic function with antagonism of the M_2 muscarinic receptor, augmentation of acetylcholine effects at the M_3 muscarinic receptor, and potentiation of vagal nerve and acetylcholine-induced bronchoconstriction.[67,68] The M_2 muscarinic mechanism may be of particular interest as various NMBAs have been shown to have differing degrees of activity at this receptor. These effects have been reported with pipecuronium and even with rocurnium.[69,70]

During normal function at the neuromuscular junction of smooth muscle including the airway, some of the acetylcholine that is released diffuses back to the prejunctional (M_2) receptor and shuts off ongoing acetylcholine release. Thus the M_2 receptor is a negative feedback receptor that regulates acetylcholine release. With blockade of the M_2 receptor, there may be exaggerated release of acetylcholine and hence exaggerated muscle contraction or bronchospasm. Although rapacuronium was removed from the market in 2001, there may be other NMBAs in the clinical development process and their potential activity at the M_2 receptor warrants attention and investigation.

Mivacurium

Mivacurium is a benzylisoquinolinium NMBA, which is the shortest acting of the nondepolarizing NMBAs, undergoing non–organ-dependent elimination (see later). It was introduced into clinical practice in the 1980s and then, given its low market share, was eliminated from the US market for approximately 5 to 10 years. However, given ongoing interest in its potential intraoperative applications, the medication is likely to be rereleased into the US market in the next year or two. Mivacurium was previously available in a premixed solution in a concentration of 2 mg/mL in 5- or 10-mL vials. Following a dose of 0.2 mg/kg, onset times vary from 2 to 3 minutes with a duration of action of approximately 10 minutes. In a cohort of 62 children anesthetized with nitrous oxide and fentanyl, mivacurium infusion rates to maintain neuromuscular blockade were 375 ± 19 μg/m^2/min with a spontaneous recovery time ($T_4/T_1 \geq 0.75$) of 9.8 ± 0.4 minutes.[71] There was no evidence of accumulation during prolonged infusions.

Mivacurium is metabolized by nonspecific plasma cholinesterases. Prolonged blockade can occur in the same clinical situations as described with succinylcholine (see earlier) including congenital and acquired deficiencies of the enzyme system, butyrylcholinesterase, also known as pseudocholinesterase or plasma cholinesterase.[72,73] The metabolites of mivacurium, which are renally excreted, have limited neuromuscular blocking properties. As with the other benzylisoquinoliniums, mivacurium can produce histamine release. In children, the histamine release may be associated with flushing and erythema of the skin; however, the hemodynamic effects are generally of limited clinical significance.[74]

The potential application for mivacurium in clinical practice has been when neuromuscular blockade is required for brief procedures (<10 minutes) in either the operating room or PICU. Mivacurium can be a useful agent to provide a brief duration of neuromuscular blockade for direct laryngoscopy in the PICU to follow the progression of airway problems and then allow for the prompt spontaneous return of neuromuscular function. In the intraoperative setting, the rapid and spontaneous recovery of neuromuscular function eliminates the need for the use of reversal agents such as neostigmine (see later) that may increase the incidence of postoperative nausea and vomiting.

Another potential use for mivacurium has been in combination with other nondepolarizing NMBA to provide a rapid onset of neuromuscular blockade and yet avoid the prolonged duration seen when large doses of vecuronium (0.3 mg/kg) or rocuronium (1–1.2 mg/kg) are administered.[75,76] The onset time to 90% neuromuscular blockade was 39 ± 2.3 seconds with 1 mg/kg succinylcholine and 48 ± 3.5 seconds with vecuronium 0.16 mg/kg and mivacurium 0.2 mg/kg.[75] Conditions for endotracheal intubation were graded as excellent in 10 of 10 patients in both groups. Despite the rapid onset, recovery times were prolonged with the combination of vecuronium and mivacurium. Similar results were reported with a combination of mivacurium 0.2 mg/kg and rocuronium 0.6 mg/kg.[76] Although the onset times paralleled that of succinylcholine, the recovery times (49.0 ± 9.6 minutes) were prolonged.

Mivacurium may also be potentially advantageous in patients with underlying neuromuscular disorders (ie, muscular dystrophy). In such patients, prolonged neuromuscular blockade may occur even following a single dose of intermediate-acting agents such as vecuronium, atracurium, or cis-atracurium. Therefore the use of an agent with the shortest clinical duration may be beneficial.[77-79] When compared with healthy control subjects, although there was no difference noted in the onset times, patients with Duchenne muscular dystrophy demonstrated only a modest prolongation of the clinical effect of mivacurium.[77] The median times for recovery of the first twitch of the TOF to 10%, 25%, and 90% of baseline in controls and patients with muscular dystrophy were 8.4 versus 12.0 minutes, 10.5 and 14.1 minutes, and 15.9 and 26.9 minutes. Similar results were demonstrated in another cohort of 7 children with Duchenne muscular dystrophy.[78] Following a dose of 0.2 mg/kg, time to recovery of the first twitch varied from 12 to 18 minutes. They also noted significant interpatient variability with infusion requirements varying from 3–20 µg/kg/min. Five of the seven patients required less than or equal to 10 µg/kg/min, further demonstrating increased sensitivity to this agent in patients with muscular dystrophy. Of note, there was no correlation with infusion requirements and the patient's preoperative motor function.

Atracurium

Atracurium is a nondepolarizing NMBA of the benzylisoquinolinium class, which was released for clinical use in the 1980s. It is supplied in a 10-mg/mL solution. Following a dose of 0.6 mg/kg, acceptable conditions for endotracheal intubation are achieved in 2 to 3 minutes with complete twitch suppression for 15 to 20 minutes followed by another 10 to 15 minutes with a variable degree of blockade (twitch height 5%-25%). Spontaneous recovery ($T_4/T_1 \geq 0.7$) generally occurs in 40 to 60 minutes. As with all of the NMBAs, the use of a smaller dose (0.3–0.4 mg/kg) is feasible but will prolong the time to the onset of acceptable conditions for endotracheal intubation, as well as shortening the recovery time. Atracurium's recovery profile makes it an intermediate-acting agent. As with other NMBAs of the benzylisoquinolinium class, atracurium can lead to histamine release, thereby limiting dose escalations to speed the onset of neuromuscular blockade. Although facial cutaneous flushing and erythema may occur as with mivacurium, effects on heart rate and blood pressure are generally minimal following doses up to 0.6 mg/kg.[80] With larger doses, hypotension may occur. In the pediatric-aged patient, histamine release is less frequent and less profound than in adults. Even when histamine release occurred, no hemodynamic changes were noted.[81] Following its introduction into clinical practice, ongoing safety surveillance demonstrated no difference in the adverse effect profile of atracurium related to histamine release when compared with other NMBAs.[82] Extremely rare, anecdotal case reports exist regarding anaphylactoid reactions with severe bronchospasm temporally related to its administration; however, a true causal relationship cannot be proven as the patients also received thiopental during anesthetic induction.[83]

Atracurium undergoes spontaneous degradation via a process known as Hofmann elimination and ester hydrolysis. Therefore its duration of action is unchanged in the presence of renal or hepatic insufficiency or failure. Because of these properties, it rapidly gained favor for providing neuromuscular blockade in ICU patients, generally by continuous infusion (see later). Although the metabolites of atracurium do not possess significant neuromuscular blocking properties, one of the metabolic byproducts of Hofmann degradation, laudanosine, has been shown to be epileptogenic in animals. The actual concentrations required to cause seizures in humans is unknown, and no formal study has ever documented clinical effects from a high laudanosine level. Laudanosine is renally excreted, and its accumulation in patients with renal insufficiency is at least a theoretical concern.

Infusion requirements to maintain clinical neuromuscular blockade, defined as a single twitch height of 1% to 10% of baseline, averaged 9 µg/kg/min during a nitrous oxide-opioid based anesthetic.[84] Recovery remains predictable and stable regardless of the duration of the infusion. Within 30 minutes of discontinuation of the infusion, twitch height had spontaneously recovered to $T_4/T_1 \geq 0.7$.[85] Reversal of neuromuscular blockade with neostigmine (see later) is generally feasible within 10 to 15 minutes of discontinuing an infusion or following the administration of a single dose of 0.6 mg/kg. When compared with a longer-acting agent such as pancuronium, spontaneous recovery following a continuous infusion occurred at an average time of 15 minutes (range 6-34 minutes) with atracurium compared with 25 minutes (10.5-37 minutes) with pancuronium.[86] Given its intermediate duration of action and stable recovery profile, atracurium has been used safely and effectively in patients with neuromuscular disorders including myasthenia gravis, myotonic dystrophy, and muscular dystrophy.[87,88] However, prolonged neuromuscular blockade with a recovery time of 3 to 4 hours has also been reported following a single dose of 0.6 mg/kg.

Given its predictable recovery characteristics in most patient populations, its limited hemodynamic effects, and its lack of dependence on end-organ function for elimination, atracurium remains a popular agent for neuromuscular blockade in the PICU setting. In a cohort of 20 infants and children requiring neuromuscular blockade for 10 to 163 hours during mechanical ventilation, the mean effective dose of atracurium was 1.4 mg/kg/hr (range: 0.44–2.4 mg/kg/hr).[89] When no TOF could be elicited, the time required for the first twitch to become evident with discontinuation of the infusion was only 13.8 minutes (range: 1-38 minutes). The authors reported that there was no correlation between the recovery time and dose being administered; however, they did note a faster recovery time when the infusion had been administered for more than 48 hours. Given its non–organ-dependent elimination, atracurium has also been used in pediatric patients following orthotopic liver transplantation.[90] Recovery time ($T_4/T_1 \geq 0.7$) when the infusion was discontinued averaged 23.6 minutes (range: 12-27 minutes) and was not prolonged compared with the general pediatric population.

As with rocuronium, administration with thiopental and other barbiturates may result in precipitation and occlusion of the IV cannula, necessitating flushing the line with normal saline between these 2 agents. As Hofmann elimination is a temperature-dependent process, elimination will be prolonged during induced or inadvertent hypothermia.[91] During induced hypothermia (32°C) in a cohort of children, atracurium infusion requirements were 784 µg/kg/hour or 56% of that in normothermic children (1411 µg/kg/hour). Recovery times were also prolonged to two to three times those in normothermic patients. A similar effect has been reported with the cis-atracurium during hypothermia (see later).

Cis-atracurium

Cis-atracurium is one of the stereoisomers contained in solutions of atracurium. It is six to eight times as potent as atracurium but devoid of clinically significant histamine release and hemodynamic effects.[92] Cis-atracurium is available as a 2-mg/mL solution. Like atracurium, cis-atracurium is an intermediate-acting neuromuscular blocking agent with a duration of action of 20 to 30 minutes following a bolus dose of 0.2 mg/kg. Acceptable conditions for endotracheal intubation are provided in approximately 2 minutes. In a cohort of 80 adult patients, cis-atracurium in doses of 0.1, 0.15, and 0.2 mg/kg provided acceptable conditions for endotracheal intubation in 4.6, 3.4, and 2.8 minutes with a clinically effective duration of 45, 55, and 61 minutes.[93] In a cohort of 27 infants (1-23 months of age) and 24 children (2-12.5 years of age), the onset time to achieve maximal blockade following a dose of 0.15 mg/kg was more rapid in infants (2.0 ± 0.8 vs. 3.0 ± 1.2 minutes, $P = 0.0011$).[92] The clinical duration (recovery to 25% of baseline) was longer in infants (43.3 ± 6.2 vs. 36.0 ± 5.4 minutes, $P <0.0001$). Once neuromuscular started to recovery, the rate of recovery was similar between the two groups. However, de Ruiter et al.[94] reported no difference in the ED_{50}, ED_{95}, or infusion rate required to maintain 90% to 99% block when comparing 32 infants (0.3-1 year of age) and 32 children (3.1-9.6 years of age). The ED_{50} in the two groups was 29 ± 3 versus 29 ± 2 µg/kg, the ED_{95} was 43 ± 9 versus

47 ± 7 µg/kg, and the infusion rate required to maintain 90% to 99% blockade in the two groups was 1.9 ± 4 versus 2.0 ± 0.5 µg/kg/min.

A prospective study evaluated cis-atracurium dosing requirements in 15 PICU patients ranging in age from 10 months to 11 years and in weight from 4 to 28 kgs.[95] The cis-atracurium infusion was adjusted to maintain one twitch of the TOF. Infusion requirements varied from 2.1 to 3.8 µg/kg/min (average of 3.1 ± 0.6 µg/kg/min) on day 1, from 2.9 to 8.1 µg/kg/min (average of 4.5 ± 1.6 µg/kg/min, $P <0.01$ compared with day 1) on day 3, and from 1.4 to 22.7 µg/kg/min during all patient days. The highest infusion requirements were noted following the administration of the drug for prolonged periods of time (150 and 224 hours). When the infusion was discontinued, spontaneous return of neuromuscular function was noted in 14 to 33 minutes. Effective neuromuscular blockade was provided and no adverse effects related to cis-atracurium were noted. In particular, no hemodynamic changes were noted with bolus dosing. Odetola et al.[96] evaluated the dosing requirements of cis-atracurium in a cohort of 11 PICU patients, ranging in age from 0 to 2 years. The duration of the infusions varied from 14 to 122 hours (64.5 ± 36 hours). The infusion requirements to maintain 90% to 95% neuromuscular blockade were 5.36 ± 3.0 µg/kg/min. Laudanosine concentrations during the infusion were 163.3 ± 116 ng/mL. As in the previous study, there was an increase in dose requirements over time and no hemodynamic effects were noted with cis-atracurium.

Reich et al.[97] compared vecuronium and cis-atracurium, administered by continuous infusion, to provide neuromuscular blockade following surgery for congenital heart disease in a cohort of 19 patients younger than 2 years of age. The NMBA was administered to maintain one twitch of the TOF with median infusion times of 64.5 hours for cis-atracurium and 46 hours for vecuronium. Median recovery time, defined as a normal TOF without fade, was shorter with cis-atracurium than with vecuronium (30 minutes vs. 180 minutes, $P <0.05$). Recovery time was more than 4 hours in 3 of 9 patients who received vecuronium. Two of these patients had high vecuronium plasma concentrations while the other had an elevated 3-OH vecuronium level. There was no difference in time to tracheal extubation, ICU stay, or hospital stay.

As with other NMBAs, resistance to the effects of cis-atracurium may be seen in patients treated with anticonvulsant agents.[98] Time to recovery of T_1 to 25% of baseline was 69 ± 13 minutes in patients not receiving anticonvulsant medications, 64 ± 19 minutes in those receiving acute therapy with anticonvulsants, and 59 ± 19 minutes in those receiving chronic anticonvulsant therapy. As with atracurium, altered clearance and decreased infusion requirements are noted during decreases in body temperature.[99] During induced hypothermia (34°C) to control increased ICP, cis-atracurium infusion requirements decreased to 1.7 µg/kg/min and increased to 3.4 µg/kg/min with return to normothermia.

Doxacurium

Doxacurium is the benzylisoquinolinium derivative with the longest duration of clinical activity. Although still available for clinical use, its clinical applications are limited with limited data regarding its use in the PICU setting. It is the most potent of the clinically available NMBAs with approximately twice the potency of pancuronium or pipecuronium. Following a dose of 0.05 mg/kg, its duration of action is 80 to 90 minutes. The ED_{95} in children is 30 µg/kg, approximately 1.5 times that reported for the adult population.[100] Elimination is primarily renal with a small percentage dependent on hepatic excretion. The duration of action is prolonged in patients with either hepatic or renal insufficiency. Despite it being a benzylisoquinolinium derivative, it is primarily devoid of histamine-releasing properties and cardiovascular or hemodynamic effects.

Reversal of Neuromuscular Blockade

Although neuromuscular blockade is necessary for many surgical procedures or used for various indications in the PICU setting, even a small residual amount of blockade may compromise ventilation or upper airway patency in the critically ill patient or during the immediate postoperative period. In the operating room setting, residual neuromuscular blockade is frequently reversed at the completion of the procedure to ensure adequate strength to maintain airway patency and ventilatory function following extubation of the trachea.[101] In the PICU setting, reversal of neuromuscular blockade is less common. In most clinical scenarios, when there is no longer a need for neuromuscular blockade, the agent is discontinued and spontaneous recovery is allowed. The latter is generally appropriate in the PICU setting, as ongoing tracheal intubation and mechanical ventilation will likely be provided for some period of time following the discontinuation of the NMBA.

Reversal of neuromuscular blockade is possible only with nondepolarizing NMBAs. Additionally, some degree of residual neuromuscular function is necessary to allow for effective reversal of neuromuscular blockade. In general clinical practice, this means that there should be one to two twitches in the TOF or that the T_1 has recovered to 25% of its baseline height. Reversal of neuromuscular blockade with a drug that inhibits acetylcholinesterase is not feasible immediately after the administration of an NMBA. Depending on the dose administered, some time, generally 15 to 30 minutes with intermediate-acting agents, is necessary (see later for a discussion of reversal of neuromuscular blockade with sugammadex).

The medications used to reverse neuromuscular blockade inhibit the enzyme acetylcholinesterase. This, in turn, provides more acetylcholine to compete with the NMBA at the nicotinic receptor of the neuromuscular junction. The commonly used acetylcholinesterase inhibitors or "reversal agents" include neostigmine, pyridostigmine, and edrophonium. Despite a similar mechanism of action, the clinical effects (onset, duration, etc.) of these agents differ. Neostigmine and pyridostigmine are hydrolyzed by acetylcholinesterase. During this process, the enzyme is carbamylated and inactivated. Edrophonium does not break down the enzyme acetylcholinesterase. Rather, it competitively and reversibly inhibits its function. The difference in the molecular mechanism of these agents has little impact on clinical use or practice. With these three agents, the peak plasma concentration is achieved at 5 to 10 minutes following bolus administration followed by an elimination half-life of 60 to 120 minutes. Clearance is markedly reduced in the setting of renal failure or insufficiency. There is a marked difference in the onset times of the three reversal agents. The onset of peak effect is 1 to 2 minutes with edrophonium, 7 to 11 minutes with neostigmine, and 16 minutes with pyridostigmine.[102,103] An additional difference is the efficacy of these agents when reversing intense blockade (≥90%), in that neostigmine is more effective.

Adverse effects related to the use of reversal agents generally relate to their inhibition of acetylcholinesterase at sites away from the neuromuscular junction. These agents should always be preceded by an anticholinergic agent such as atropine or glycopyrrolate since the inhibition of acetylcholinesterase occurs at not only nicotinic receptors (neuromuscular junction) but also muscarinic receptors. Therefore unless preceded by an anticholinergic (antimuscarinic) agent, bradycardia and asystole can occur. The time course of the bradycardic effects varies on the basis of the onset time of the agents (see earlier). As such, if edrophonium is used, glycopyrrolate should be administered first and followed in 1 to 2 minutes by edrophonium given that the onset time of glycopyrrolate is longer than that of edrophonium. The onset time of glycopyrrolate correlates well with that of neostigmine and pyridostigmine, and therefore these agents may be administered at the same time. Given that the onset of atropine is rapid, it may be administered with any of the three reversal agents. Other adverse effects related to the reversal agents included augmentation of cholinergic function in the gastrointestinal tract (salivation, diarrhea, nausea, and vomiting) and the respiratory tract (bronchospasm). Although the anticholinergic agents may block salivation and alterations in airway tone, their efficacy in blocking the increased gastrointestinal motility is somewhat limited.

More recently, there has been development of a novel agent for reversal of neuromuscular blocking agents, sugammadex. In early 2016, this medication was released by the US Food and Drug Administration for clinical use in the United States. Prior to that, it had been approved for use in several countries throughout Europe and the United Kingdom. Sugammadex is a cyclodextrin and instead of inhibiting the enzyme, acetylcholinesterase, it forms a tight 1:1 complex with the steroidal neuromuscular blocking agents. It has been shown to rapidly and effectively reverse rocuronium and vecuronium and perhaps even pancuronium.[104,105] There is a limited dissociation rate so that the reversal is maintained. Unlike the use of acetylcholinesterase inhibitors, reversal using sugammadex is feasible even with intense blockade, thereby providing the potential for the rapid reversal of neuromuscular blockade in the "cannot intubate–cannot ventilate" scenario. Future studies are necessary to fully evaluate this medication in the pediatric population.

Monitoring Neuromuscular Blockade

In the operating room, NMBAs may be used as a single dose at the start of the case to facilitate endotracheal intubation or by repeated doses or a continuous infusion to provide ongoing neuromuscular blockade. Some means of monitoring neuromuscular blockade is necessary since administration of excessive doses may mandate the use of postoperative mechanical ventilation until neuromuscular blockade has worn off or can be reversed. Additionally, given concerns regarding prolonged paralysis, monitoring neuromuscular function may also be considered in the PICU setting.

Monitoring may include some combination of visual, tactile, or electronic means of measuring the residual neuromuscular function following electrical stimulation. The technique, most commonly used by anesthesiologists in the operating room to monitor the degree of neuromuscular blockade, is peripheral nerve stimulation or TOF monitoring. TOF monitoring involves placement of standard electrocardiographic electrodes over a peripheral nerve. The nerves most commonly used are the facial, ulnar, or common peroneal, which result in corresponding movement in the muscles of the hand, face, or leg. In some circumstances, direct stimulation of the muscle may occur, giving the false impression that an appropriate amount of neuromuscular blockade has not been achieved. To avoid such problems, it may be appropriate to place the TOF monitor and assess the twitch response before the administration of the initial dose of the NMBA. The electrodes of the TOF monitor are connected to a handheld peripheral nerve stimulator, which delivers two stimuli per second at 50 mA for 2 seconds. A total of four stimuli are administered over 2 seconds—hence the term *train-of-four*. As this is painful, it should only be performed in patients that are anesthetized or sedated. Depending on the number of acetylcholine receptors that are occupied by the nondepolarizing NMBA, there will be anywhere from zero to four responses or twitches. Despite the availability of other more sophisticated machines to monitor the degree of neuromuscular blockade in the operating room and ICU setting, these monitors are generally used only for clinical research purposes. In clinical practice in either the operating room or PICU, TOF monitoring remains the technique that provides the most useful information with limited requirements for training and equipment.

In clinical practice, the TOF monitoring is combined with clinical assessment at the end of the case to ensure that the patient is strong enough for extubation. Following reversal of neuromuscular blockade, clinical assessment of strength is combined with neuromuscular monitoring. These latter measures become necessary as residual weakness may be present despite apparent reversal using TOF monitoring. Techniques of clinical assessment to evaluate the presence of residual neuromuscular blockade include measurement of negative inspiratory force (NIF) or maximum inspiratory pressure (MIP), hand grip, or head lift. Although head lift and hand grip require the ability to follow a simple command, the measurement of NIF does not. The technique involves measuring the inspiratory force that the patient can generate against an occluded airway. The test can be completed with a simple manometer attached to the 15-mm adaptor of the ETT. Initial studies suggested that a NIF of at least -20 cm H_2O indicated sufficient muscle strength to maintain an adequate minute ventilation.[106] Subsequently, a value of -25 to -30 cm H_2O became the generally accepted value for use in clinical practice. However, subsequent work suggested that although strength was adequate to maintain minute ventilation, it may not be adequate to maintain upper airway patency. Therefore the use of voluntary responses (head lift for 5 seconds or hand grip) was suggested as an adjunct to ensure adequate reversal of neuromuscular blockade.[81] In infants, reflex leg lift (both legs lifted off of the operating room table) was shown to correlate with a mean NIF or MIP of -51 cm H_2O, so the authors concluded that this was a sign of adequate reversal of neuromuscular blockade in infants.[107] Given the variability of these responses and their correlation with reversal of neuromuscular blockade, the best clinical approach may be the use of several clinical maneuvers if TOF monitoring is not available. The literature suggests that the ability to maintain a sustained head lift for 5 seconds is the most sensitive clinical tool.[101]

In the ICU setting, given the degree of neuromuscular blockade that is induced, voluntary measures of muscle strength are not adequate. Therefore titration of NMBAs should be guided by the use of TOF monitoring. The technique may allow the use of the lowest possible dose of agents and theoretically avoid complications such as prolonged blockade (see later). In a prospective randomized trial in 77 adults, TOF monitoring (maintaining one twitch of the TOF) was compared with clinical parameters (patient breathing over the preset ventilator rate) as a means of titrating NMBAs.[108] TOF monitoring resulted in a lower total dose and lower average infusion rate of vecuronium, as well as a more rapid recovery once the infusion was discontinued. A subsequent study in adults revealed a decreased incidence of persistent neuromuscular weakness when using TOF monitoring.[109]

Although data are lacking to clearly demonstrate the superiority of TOF monitoring in the PICU setting, its use is suggested as a means of titrating the administration of NMBA agents. Of note are the significant interpatient variability that has been reported in the PICU setting and the inability to therefore ensure an appropriate dose without some monitoring modality. The choice of the number of twitches to maintain has not been prospectively studied. The majority of the clinical evidence suggests that maintaining one twitch of the TOF ensures an adequate degree of neuromuscular blockade while potentially limiting the incidence of persistent neuromuscular weakness. However, the least amount of blockade that can be clinically tolerated is suggested. In some patients, maintaining two twitches may be acceptable, especially with the use of an appropriate degree of sedation and analgesia. When TOF monitoring is not in use or is not feasible, "drug holidays" are commonly employed where the NMBA agent is temporarily discontinued until some clinical sign of neuromuscular function such as motor movement is noted. At that time, if needed, the infusion is restarted or an additional bolus is administered.

No study has evaluated the best nerve (facial, ulnar, common peroneal) to monitor. In clinical practice, any accessible nerve can be used. However, several patient and technical factors may affect the response. As such, whenever feasible, placement of the monitor before the institution of neuromuscular blockade is suggested to ensure that a TOF can be obtained before the administration of the NMBA. If no response is obtained, the technique should be evaluated by first evaluating the monitor (faculty monitor, electrodes, or batteries). Is the electrode too far from the nerve (improper placement, edema, obesity)? If these technical problems are ruled out, the infusion can be decreased by 10% to 15% and the TOF measured again in 2 hours. When two or more twitches are noted, if the patient is stable and a more profound degree of blockade is not required, ongoing observation is suggested. If a deeper level of blockade is required, a bolus equivalent to the hourly infusion rate should be administered and the infusion increased by 10% to 15%.

Adverse Effects of Neuromuscular Blockade

As with any medication used in the PICU patient with comorbid diseases, adverse effects may occur with NMBAs. Perhaps the most devastating of these adverse effects is the inability to provide adequate ventilation following the administration of a medication that induces apnea. Therefore these medications should never be used if there is any suspicion that the airway cannot be controlled. In rare circumstances, endotracheal intubation using direct laryngoscopy may be impossible. In even rarer circumstances, adequate bag-mask ventilation cannot be provided. In such scenarios, death or permanent CNS morbidity will result with the administration of NMBAs. Measures to avoid such problems include an assessment of the airway before the administration of these agents and knowledge of the "cannot intubate–cannot ventilate" algorithm as outlined by the American Society of Anesthesiologists.

Various physical characteristics may suggest that direct laryngoscopy and endotracheal intubation will be difficult including micrognathia, a short neck, limited neck mobility (flexion/extension), limited mouth opening, a large tongue, and a small mouth. An additional tool is the Mallampati grade, which describes the ability to visualize the tip of uvula and the tonsillar pillars.[110,111] If there is a suspicion that endotracheal intubation using direct laryngoscopy will not be possible and there is time, other techniques to control the airway are suggested. Some of the more commonly used approaches to the difficult airway in infants and children are described elsewhere.[112] The techniques needed for the "cannot intubate–cannot ventilate" scenario should be understood and available in any situation in which NMBAs are being administered. This should include alternative options for endotracheal intubation including repositioning the patient or using a different type of laryngoscope including indirect laryngoscopy, such as the Glidescope.[110,111] Physicians using NMBAs should also have a working knowledge of the laryngeal mask airway as it can be used to rescue patients when laryngoscopy, endotracheal intubation, and bag-valve-mask ventilation fail.[113]

Other adverse effects from NMBAs relate to the elimination of protective physiologic functions. Eye care with the use of artificial tears or Lacri-Lube at fixed intervals during the administration of NMBAs is necessary to avoid drying and damage to the cornea. Repositioning of the patient at frequent intervals is necessary to avoid pressure sores. For prolonged immobility, the use of special mattresses may be considered as an adjunct to frequent patient moving. Passive range of motion may also be implicated with splinting to prevent forearm and ankle contractures while sequential compression devices may be indicated to prevent deep vein thrombosis. Ineffective coughing and clearance of secretions mandate the implication of suctioning protocols to limit the risk of nosocomial pneumonias. Alterations in normal physiologic respiratory parameters include a decrease in functional residual capacity, increase in dead space, and ventilation-perfusion ratios that may result in ventilatory issues including hypoxemia or hypercarbia and the need to adjust ventilatory parameters.

Although these agents prevent movement, they provide no degree of sedation or analgesia. As such, monitoring sedation using clinical scoring systems is generally not feasible. Therefore some other measure of the depth of sedation may be required. In the majority of clinical situations, physiologic parameters such as heart rate and blood pressure are used as a means of titrating sedative and analgesic agents. However, issues arise in critically ill patients in whom alterations in heart or blood pressure may not occur in response to stress or pain. In this patient population, exogenous vasopressors may

be in use and thereby eliminate the reliability of physiologic parameters. In the operating room setting, the availability of depth of anesthesia monitors is recommended and it is suggested that their use be considered in patients at high risk for awareness. Despite the rare occurrence of such events, means for their prevention of awareness during the use of neuromuscular blocking agents in the PICU appear indicated given the consequences of such problems.

In the operating room setting, various depth of sedation or anesthesia monitors are currently available. To date, there are no data in the PICU to demonstrate their efficacy in preventing recall during the use of neuromuscular blocking agents. The bispectral (BIS) index is a processed electroencephalographic parameter expressed as a numeric value ranging from 0 (isoelectric electroencephalogram) to 100 (awake, eyes open, no sedative agent). In the pediatric population, its intraoperative use has been suggested to decrease the incidence of awareness.[114] In the PICU population, the BIS value has been shown to generally correlate with the depth of sedation assessed using various clinical scoring systems.[115,116] In one such study, BIS monitoring was used to evaluate the depth of sedation in a cohort of 12 PICU patients receiving NMBAs.[117] BIS monitoring was used for a total of 476 hours and revealed that the desired depth of sedation (BIS number 50 to 70) was achieved 57% of the time. The BIS number demonstrated a deeper than desired depth of sedation (BIS number ≤49) 35% of the time and an inadequate depth of sedation in patients receiving neuromuscular blockade (BIS number ≥71) 8% of the time. At the time that additional sedation was administered by the bedside nurse who was not allowed to view the monitor, the BIS number was 71 or greater 64% of the time; 50 to 70 during 31% of the time, and 49 or less 5% of the time. Although no long-term follow-up or assessment of awareness was pursued, the authors concluded that physiologic parameters are not a viable means of assessing the depth of sedation during the use of NMBAs.

The adverse effect that has received the most attention in the adult population with the administration of NMBAs is residual neuromuscular paralysis. In clinical practice, it appears that there are two distinct entities that may account for prolonged neuromuscular paralysis: (1) prolonged recovery from neuromuscular blockade related to excessive dosing or delayed clearance of the parent compound or metabolites due to renal or hepatic issues and (2) what is now termed the *acute quadriplegic myopathy syndrome* (AQMS).[118-121] Potential concern of such problems was first reported in 1992 with the use of vecuronium in patients with renal insufficiency.[118] Problems related to excessive dosing or inadequate clearance of an active metabolite generally resolve spontaneously over time with clearance of the parent compound or its metabolites. In clinical practice, prolonged recovery is defined as a recovery time of more than 100% of the predicted parameter. In distinction, AQMS presents with acute paresis, myonecrosis with increased plasma markers demonstrating muscle breakdown such as creatinine phosphokinase (CPK), and abnormal electromyography (EMG) with the demonstration of reduced compound motor action potential amplitude, decreased motor nerve conduction, and evidence of acute denervation. Clinical findings include flaccid paralysis, relative preservation of extraocular movements, decreased deep tendon reflexes, respiratory insufficiency, intact sensory function, and normal findings in the cerebrospinal fluid.[119-121] Recovery may require weeks to months, with the need for prolonged rehabilitation care, and tracheostomy with chronic ventilatory support, all of which may significantly affect the cost of ICU care. Although initially reported only with aminosteroid compounds, it has been subsequently also reported with the benzylisoquinolinium derivatives.[122,123]

Given that CPK values are elevated in up to 50% of patients with AQMS, periodic screening of patients receiving ongoing neuromuscular blockade may be indicated. As problems have been noted more commonly following the prolonged, continuous infusion of NMBAs, it has also been suggested that drug holidays or periodic interruption of the infusion be considered. However, there are no data to demonstrate that such practice will alter the incidence of AQMS and even the periodic withdrawal of neuromuscular blockade must be considered on a risk-benefit ratio. Termination of the use of NMBAs is suggested whenever it is clinically feasible given their adverse effect profile. Other factors and comorbid processes that may contribute to the development of AQMS include nutritional deficiencies; coadministration of other medications (cyclosporine, corticosteroids, aminoglycosides); hyperglycemia; hepatic or renal insufficiency; and electrolyte disturbances. The association is most profound with the coadministration of NMBAs and corticosteroids, thereby suggesting a heightened awareness in such patients.[122] In addition to AQMS, other conditions to consider in the differential diagnosis of patients with prolonged weakness following the use of NMBAs include neuromuscular conditions (myasthenia gravis, Eaton-Lambert syndrome, Guillain-Barré syndrome); acquired or primary myopathic conditions (mitochondrial myopathy, steroid myopathy); central nervous system injury; spinal cord injury; critical illness polyneuropathy; disuse atrophy; and electrolyte or metabolic disturbances. Critical illness polyneuropathy may be confused with AQMS. It is a combined motor and sensory neuropathy that results from ischemia of the microvasculature of the nerves, which is seen most commonly in patients with multisystem organ failure. EMG demonstrates a pattern different from that seen in AQMS.

Summary: Neuromuscular Blocking Agents in the PICU

In addition to their use in the operating room, specific situations that mandate the use of neuromuscular blocking agents in the PICU may arise (Table 133.1). Although these agents are generally administered as intermittent bolus doses in the operating room, in the PICU, a more stable baseline level of neuromuscular blockade may be desired and therefore a continuous infusion may be used. When choosing an agent for use in the PICU population, the major issues include cardiovascular effects, metabolism, and cost. Because many of the patients in the PICU have some degree of hemodynamic instability, agents that cause excessive histamine release should be avoided. Additionally, the presence of hepatic or renal insufficiency may affect metabolism or elimination or the parent compound, as well as its metabolites. In the absence of end-organ dysfunction, pancuronium offers an inexpensive means of achieving neuromuscular blockade. Its vagolytic effect will result in tachycardia with an increase in heart rate of 10 to 20 beats per minute above baseline. Given its duration of action, intermittent dosing is feasible. With its availability in generic form, vecuronium provides another cost-effective option in

the PICU setting while eliminating the tachycardia that is seen with pancuronium. Although vecuronium and pancuronium are generally effective and inexpensive in patients without end-organ dysfunction, significant alterations in infusion requirements occur in patients with renal insufficiency/failure (pancuronium and vecuronium) or hepatic insufficiency/failure (vecuronium). Atracurium or cis-atracurium may be a more appropriate choice in patients with hepatic or renal failure because such problems do not alter dosing requirements of either agent.[124]

In the PICU setting, like the operating room, adjustment of the dose based on monitoring with a peripheral nerve stimulator is recommended. Regardless of the agent used, significant interpatient variability with up to 10-fold variations in infusion requirements may be noted. The variability results from not only interpatient variability but also various associated conditions that may increase or decrease the sensitivity to NMBAs (Tables 133.6 and 133.7). On the basis of this knowledge, the recommended doses (Table 133.8) for the various NMBAs are starting guidelines and the infusion should be increased or decreased as needed to maintain one twitch of the TOF or provide the required depth of neuromuscular blockade. An additional problem that occurs in the ICU patient who receives NMBAs for a prolonged period of time is the development of tachyphylaxis or an increased dose requirement over time. The primary cause is an upregulation

TABLE 133.6	Factors That Increase Sensitivity to Neuromuscular Blocking Agents

Medications:
_____ inhalational anesthetic agents
_____ local anesthetic agents
_____ antibiotics (aminoglycosides)
_____ antiarrhythmic agents (quinidine, procainamide)
_____ calcium channel blockers
_____ beta-adrenergic antagonists
_____ chemotherapeutic agents (cyclophosphamide)
_____ diuretics (furosemide)
_____ dantrolene
_____ lithium, magnesium
_____ cyclosporin
Underlying disorders:
_____ electrolyte disturbances (hypokalemia, hypermagnesemia, hypocalcemia)
_____ hypothermia
_____ respiratory acidosis
_____ metabolic alkalosis
_____ myasthenia gravis
_____ Eaton-Lambert syndrome
_____ muscular dystrophy
_____ multiple sclerosis
_____ amyotrophic lateral sclerosis
_____ poliomyelitis

TABLE 133.7	Factors That Decrease the Sensitivity to Neuromuscular Blocking Agents

Medications:

_____anticonvulsant agents (phenytoin, carbamazepine)

_____aminophylline

Underlying conditions:

_____hypercalcemia

_____burns

_____prolonged administration of neuromuscular blocking agents

TABLE 133.8	Suggested Starting Guidelines for the Continuous Infusion of Neuromuscular Blocking Agents

Agent	Dose	Comments
Pancuronium	0.06-0.08 mg/kg/h	Vagolytic effect, primary renal excretion
Vecuronium	0.1-0.15 mg/kg/h	No cardiovascular effects, hepatic metabolism to active metabolites, which are renally excreted
Rocuronium	0.6-0.8 mg/kg/h	Mild vagolytic effect, hepatic metabolism
Atracurium	1-1.5 mg/kg/h	Mild histamine release, non–organ-dependent elimination
Cis-atracurium	0.2 mg/kg/h	No cardiovascular effects, non–organ-dependent elimination

of acetylcholine receptors in patients who are chronically exposed to NMBAs. Dodson et al.[125] demonstrated an increased density of acetylcholine receptors in muscle from patients who had received prolonged infusions of NMBAs. Prolonged neuromuscular blockade like partial or complete deafferentation leads to proliferation of acetylcholine receptors at the neuromuscular junction. This problem requires that the dose of the NMBA be increased over time to maintain the same amount of neuromuscular blockade.

Given their adverse effect profile, it is recommended that NMBAs be administered only when aggressive attempts at sedation have failed to provide the desired level of patient immobilization. An ongoing assessment regarding the need for continuing such therapy is suggested with discontinuation of the medication as early as is feasible. Specific protocols should be in place to ensure appropriate care of the patient who is receiving neuromuscular blockade with attention toward the provision of adequate sedation and analgesia, eye care, prevention of pressure sores, and pulmonary toilet.

Key References

1. Sharpe MD. The use of muscle relaxants in the intensive care unit. *Can J Anaesth*. 1992;39:949-962.
2. Sanfilippo F1, Santonocito C, Veenith T, et al. The role of neuromuscular blockade in patients with traumatic brain injury: a systematic review. *Neurocrit Care*. 2015;22:325-334.
3. Rhoney DH, Murry KR. National survey on the use of sedatives and neuromuscular blocking agents in the pediatric intensive care unit. *Crit Care Med*. 2002;3:129-133.
4. Greenberg SB, Vender J. The use of neuromuscular blocking agents in the ICU: where are we now? *Crit Care Med*. 2013;41:1332-1344.
8. Baraka A. Succinylcholine "the gold standard" for rapid-sequence induction of anesthesia. *Middle East J Anaesthesiol*. 2011;21:323-324.
21. Minton MD, Grosslight K, Stirt JA, Bedford RF. Increases in intracranial pressure from succinylcholine: prevention by prior non-depolarizing block. *Anesthesiology*. 1986;65:165-169.
26. Carroll JB. Increased incidence of masseter spasm in children with strabismus anesthetized with halothane and succinylcholine. *Anesthesiology*. 1987;67:559-561.
27. Martyn JAJ, Richtsfeld M. Succinylcholine-induced hyperkalemia in acquired pathologic states. *Anesthesiology*. 2006;104:158-169.
29. Dierdorf SF, McNiece WL, Rao CC, et al. Effect of succinylcholine on plasma potassium in children with cerebral palsy. *Anesthesiology*. 1985;62:88-90.
31. Al-alami AA, Zestos MM, Baraka AS. Pediatric laryngospasm: prevention and treatment. *Curr Opin Anaesthesiol*. 2009;22:388-395.
32. Walker RW, Sutton RS. Which port in a storm? Use of suxamethonium without intravenous access for severe laryngospasm. *Anaesthesia*. 2007;62:757-759.
33. Hannallah RS, Oh TH, McGill WA, et al. Changes in heart rate and rhythm after intramuscular succinylcholine with or without atropine in anesthetized children. *Anesth Analg*. 1986;65:1329-1332.
34. Tobias JD, Nichols DG. Intraosseous succinylcholine for endotracheal intubation. *Peds Emerg Care*. 1990;6:108-109.
37. Goudsouzian NG, Martyn JJA, Liu LMP, et al. The dose response effect of long acting nondepolarizing neuromuscular blocking agents in children. *Can Anaesth Soc J*. 1984;31:246-250.
40. Tobias JD, Lynch A, McDuffee A, et al. Pancuronium infusion for neuromuscular blockade in children in the pediatric intensive care unit. *Anesth Analg*. 1995;81:13-16.
42. Meretoja OA. Is vecuronium a long-acting neuromuscular blocking agent in neonates and infants? *Br J Anaesth*. 1989;62:184-187.
44. Robertson EN, Driessen JJ, Booij LH. Pharmacokinetics and pharmacodynamics of rocuronium in patients with and without renal failure. *Eur J Anaesthesiol*. 2005;22:4-10.
51. Cooper R, Mirakhur RK, Clarke RSJ, Boulex Z. Comparison of intubating conditions after administration of rocuronium and suxamethonium. *Br J Anaesth*. 1992;69:269-273.
52. Mazurek AJ, Rae B, Hann S, et al. Rocuronium versus succinylcholine: are they equally effective during rapid-sequence induction of anesthesia? *Anesth Analg*. 1998;87:1259-1262.
53. Scheiber G, Ribeiro FC, Marichal A, et al. Intubating conditions and onset of action after rocuronium, vecuronium and atracurium in young children. *Anesth Analg*. 1996;83:320-324.
57. Reynolds LM, Lau M, Brown R, et al. Intramuscular rocuronium in infants and children. *Anesthesiology*. 1996;85:231-239.
58. Park S. Prevention of rocuronium injection pain. *Korean J Anesthesiol*. 2014;67:371-372.
59. Chiarella AB, Jolly DT, Huston CM, et al. Comparison of four strategies to reduce the pain associated with intravenous administration of rocuronium. *Br J Anaesth*. 2003;90:377-379.
60. Soriaon SG, Kaus SJ, Sullivan LJ, et al. Onset and duration of action of rocuronium in children receiving chronic anticonvulsant therapy. *Paediatr Anaesth*. 2000;10:133-136.
61. Tobias JD. Continuous infusion of rocuronium in a paediatric intensive care unit. *Can J Anaesth*. 1996;43:353-357.
66. Tobias JD, Johnson JO, Sprague K, et al. Effects of rapacuronium on respiratory function during general anesthesia. *Anesthesiology*. 2001;95:908-912.
67. Jooste E, Klafter F, Hirshman CA, et al. A mechanism for rapacuronium induced bronchospasm. *Anesthesiology*. 2003;98:906-911.
68. Jooste E, Sharma A, Zhang Y, et al. Rapacuronium augments acetylcholine-induced bronchoconstriction via positive allosteric interactions at the M3 muscarinic receptor. *Anesthesiology*. 2005;103:1195-1203.
70. Yang CI, Fine GF, Jooste EH, et al. The effect of cisatracurium and rocuronium on lung function in anesthetized children. *Anesth Analg*. 2013;117:1393-1400.
78. Tobias JD, Atwood R. Mivacurium in children with Duchenne muscular dystrophy. *Paediatr Anaesth*. 1994;4:57-60.

79. Uslu M, Mellinghoff H, Diefenback C. Mivacurium for muscle relaxation in a child with Duchenne's muscular dystrophy. *Anesth Analg.* 1999;89:340-341.

89. Playfor SD, Thomas DA, Choonara I. Duration of action of atracurium when given by infusion to critically ill children. *Paediatr Anaesth.* 2000; 10:77-81.

91. Playfor SD, Thomas DA, Choonara I. The effect of induced hypothermia on the duration of action of atracurium when given by continuous infusion to critically ill children. *Paediatr Anaesth.* 2000;10:83-88.

95. Tobias JD. A prospective evaluation of the continuous infusion of cis-atracurium for neuromuscular blockade in the pediatric ICU patient: efficacy and dosing requirements. *Am J Therap.* 1997;4:287-290.

96. Odetola FO, Bhatt-Mehta V, Zahraa J, et al. Cisatracurium requirements for neuromuscular blockade in the pediatric intensive care unit: a dose finding study. *Pediatr Crit Care Med.* 2002;3:250-254.

97. Reich DL, Hollinger I, Harrington DJ, et al. Comparisons of cisatracurium and vecuronium by continuous infusion in neonates and small infants after congenital heart surgery. *Anesthesiology.* 2004;101:1122-1127.

98. Koening HM, Edwards TL. Cis-atracurium induced neuromuscular blockade in anticonvulsant treated neurosurgical patients. *J Neurosurg Anesth.* 2000;12:314-318.

99. Tobias JD. Changes in cis-atracurium infusion requirements during induced hypothermia to treat increased intracranial pressure in a child. *J Intensive Care Med.* 1997;12:261-263.

102. Miller RD, Van Nyhuis LS, Eger EI II, et al. Comparative times to peak effect and durations of action of neostigmine and pyridostigmine. *Anesthesiology.* 1974;41:27-33.

103. Cronelly R, Morris RB, Miller RD. Edrophonium: duration of action and atropine requirements in humans during halothane anesthesia. *Anesthesiology.* 1982;57:261-266.

105. Naguib M. Suggamadex: another milestone in clinical neuromuscular pharmacology. *Anesth Analg.* 2007;104:575-581.

108. Frankel H, Jeng J, Tilly E, et al. The impact of implementation of neuromuscular blockade monitoring standards in a surgical intensive care unit. *Am Surg.* 1996;62:503-506.

109. Tavernier B, Rannou JJ, Vallet B. Peripheral nerve stimulation and clinical assessment for dosing of neuromuscular blocking agents. *Crit Care Med.* 1998;26:804-805.

114. Davidson AJ, Huang GH, Czarnecki C, et al. Awareness during anesthesia in children: a prospective cohort study. *Anesth Analg.* 2005;100:653-661.

115. Berkenbosch JW, Fichter CR, Tobias JD. The correlation of the bispectral index monitor with clinical sedation scores during mechanical ventilation in the pediatric intensive care unit. *Anesth Analg.* 2002;94:506-511.

119. Watling SM, Dasta JF. Prolonged paralysis in intensive care unit patients after the use of neuromuscular blocking agents: a review of the literature. *Crit Care Med.* 1994;22:884-893.

120. Griffiths RD, Hall JB. Intensive care unit-acquired weakness. *Crit Care Med.* 2010;38:779-787.

121. Dhand UK. Clinical approach to the weak patient in the intensive care unit. *Respir Care.* 2006;51:1024-1040.

123. Sladen RN. Neuromuscular blocking agents in the intensive care unit: a two edged sword. *Crit Care Med.* 1995;23:423-428.

124. Tobias JD. Neuromuscular blockade in the pediatric intensive care unit: pancuronium, vecuronium, rocuronium, or atracurium. *J Intensive Care Med.* 1997;12:213-217.

125. Dodson BA, Kelly BJ, Braswell LM, Cohen NH. Changes in acetylcholine receptor number in muscle from critically ill patients receiving muscle relaxants: an investigation of the molecular mechanisms of prolonged paralysis. *Crit Care Med.* 1995;23:815-821.

Sedation and Analgesia

Christopher M.B. Heard and Omar Al Ibrahim

PEARLS

- A wide selection of sedation and analgesia options is available in the pediatric intensive care unit.
- No ideal sedative agent exists for all patients.
- Most children do well with a combination of opiates (fentanyl or morphine) and supplementation with benzodiazepines either by infusion (midazolam) or on an as-required basis (lorazepam) to provide adjunct anxiolysis and amnesia.
- Postoperatively, patients require adequate analgesia, which may include the use of epidural anesthesia or patient-controlled analgesia.
- When the ability to perform a rapid neurologic examination is required, use of short-acting agents such as remifentanil, propofol, or isoflurane may be warranted.
- All sedative agents result in tolerance with prolonged use. The intensive care physician must be aware that withdrawal may occur with the prolonged use of these agents (ie, more than 3 to 5 days).
- A proactive treatment plan with methadone at the equivalent dose can effectively and safely prevent opiate withdrawal in the patient in the pediatric intensive care unit.

Sedation is an integral part of patient management in the pediatric intensive care unit (PICU). It is necessary to minimize the perception of and response to anxiety and pain. Children who are not adequately sedated or who are experiencing pain may become tachycardic and hypertensive. They also may become agitated and as a result endotracheal tubes and central lines may become dislodged. Adequate sedation and analgesia also facilitates bedside nursing and respiratory care, and it prevents dislodging of critical tubes and monitoring devices like central venous lines, arterial lines, chest tubes, and endotracheal tubes. Optimizing sedation and analgesia has been shown to reduce oxygen consumption in critically ill children and modulate the intensity of stress inflammatory response. Conversely, oversedation can cause cardiovascular depression and ileus and may interfere with a comprehensive neurologic examination. In patients who undergo prolonged sedation, tolerance and tachyphylaxis develop, which lead to increasing sedative requirements.

Patients may recall their stay in the ICU. Many patients remember having an endotracheal tube or having their lungs mechanically ventilated. Nightmares and hallucinations also have been reported.[1] Either single-drug therapy or inadequate dosing may be associated with a heightened incidence of recall

in the patient receiving neuromuscular blocking agents.[2] In adults, delusional memories and an underlying anxiety state were predictors of the development of posttraumatic stress disorder after sedation in the ICU.[3] Delusional memories were reported much more frequently than factual memories, probably because most patients have difficulty correctly remembering the events that occur during their stay in the ICU. In pediatric patients, recall of the PICU experience also has been reported.[4] More than 66% of pediatric patients remembered their stay in the PICU. Eighteen percent had bad memories, 16% remembered mechanical ventilation and anxiety, and 29% remembered pain from a procedure or movement. Overall the recollections of patients in the PICU were considered negative in approximately 15% of the patients. Sleep disturbance also was a problem.

Posttraumatic stress disorder (PTSD) is a possible complication of a child's stay in the ICU. Several components are required for the diagnosis of PTSD.[5] The American Psychiatric Association's *Diagnostic and Statistical Manual,* Fifth Edition (DSM-V) requires the following criteria for a diagnosis of PTSD in adults, adolescents, and children older than 6 years: (1) an exposure, (2) one or more intrusion or reexperiencing symptoms, (3) avoidance behavior, (4) and alterations in arousal associated with the traumatic event (D); in addition, the symptoms should (5) have exceeded 1 month (6) and have a clinically significant effect on the child's functioning. There is no specific test for PTSD, but children often have a low basal cortisol level, with exaggerated cortisol suppression in response to dexamethasone.

Using a slightly modified alternate DSM criterion, which has been shown to be more appropriate criteria for children (Table 134.1), the incidence of PTSD in children[6] aged 6 through 16 was 29%. There appeared to be no difference in the incidence with respect to age; however, younger children tended to have more avoidance of thoughts, whereas older children suffered from diminished interest in activities and difficulty concentrating. This is important, as these findings could persist for up to 6 months and affect the daily function of the child and family after discharge. It is important to ensure that children are suitably sedated and receiving appropriate analgesia during their ICU stay.

Various scoring systems are often used to guide sedation. The most widely used is the Ramsay scale.[7] The patient's level of consciousness is given as one of six scores (Table 134.2). The nurse at the bedside assesses the patient and then changes the sedation regimen as necessary to achieve the desired level of sedation. The ideal level of sedation varies from patient to patient, but in general, most intensive care physicians seek to maintain patients in a sleepy but easily awakened state. A

TABLE 134.1   Posttraumatic Stress Disorder Alternative Algorithm

Criterion A (Event)

Experienced event that threatened death or serious injury

Criterion B (Reexperiencing)

Recurrent distressing memories

Recurrent distressing dreams

Sense of reliving events

Psychologic distress with reminders

Physiologic reactivity with reminders

Criterion C (Avoidance)

Avoidance of thoughts, feelings

Avoidance of activities

Diminished interest in activities

Detached from others

Restricted affect

Sense of foreshortened future

Criterion D (Hyperarousal)

Difficulty sleeping

Irritability/anger

Difficulty concentrating

Hypervigilance

Exaggerated startle response

Criterion E (Duration)

Duration greater than 1 month

Criterion F (Effect)

The disturbance causes clinically significant distress or impairment in social, occupational, or other important areas of functioning

TABLE 134.2   Ramsay Scale

Level	Description
1	Patient awake, anxious, and agitated, restless, or both
2	Patient awake, cooperative, oriented, and tranquil
3	Patient awake, responds to command only
4	Patient asleep, brisk response to light glabellar tap or loud auditory stimulus
5	Patient asleep, sluggish response to light glabellar tap or loud auditory stimulus
6	Patient asleep, no response to light glabellar tap or loud auditory stimulus

Ramsay score of 2 to 3 seems to be ideal as the clinical end point for sedation. Deeper sedation should be reserved for select patients who are often younger, are receiving neuromuscular blocking agents, or have a head injury. The use of a sedation scoring system to guide sedation of surgical critical care patients has been evaluated for cost effectiveness. The use of scoring systems has been proved to save costs in the ICU.[8] Because the patient can be weaned more rapidly from the ventilator through better control of the sedation level, the number of days a patient is connected to a ventilator is

TABLE 134.3   Brussels Sedation Scale

Level	Description
1	Unable to be aroused
2	Responds to painful stimulation (trapezius muscle pinching) but not auditory stimulation
3	Responds to auditory stimulation
4	Awake and alert
5	Agitated

reduced. The Comfort score, which is composed of eight variables (each with five categories), also has been validated for use in the PICU to assess sedation level in children. Use of this system, however, is more complicated and time consuming.[9]

Many scoring systems are subjective and are limited by interobserver variability. The more objective methods may be too cumbersome for routine use. A simple scoring system has been devised that is easy to use and minimizes subjectivity and observer variability.[10] This system is the Brussels sedation scale. It is similar to the Ramsay scale, but the Brussels scale levels that correspond to the Ramsay scale levels 4 and 5 are better differentiated (Table 134.3).

The Bispectral Index (BIS) is a processed electroencephalogram (EEG) monitor that measures the hypnotic effects of anesthetics and sedatives. The BIS is an empirical, statistically derived measurement. The BIS monitor reports a single number from 0 to 100 that represents an integrated measure of cerebral electrical activity. The BIS has been validated as a measure of hypnosis in adults in the operating room and ICU.[11] More recently it has been validated in the PICU.[12] The BIS is an exciting new approach to EEG processing. It measures a state of the brain, representing the degree of alertness. It does not measure the concentration of a particular drug.[13] A number of 100 on the BIS score indicates that the patient is fully awake, whereas a number less than 40 suggests a deep hypnotic effect. A BIS value of less than 60 in surgical patients was not associated with a recall of intraoperative events.[14] The use of the BIS monitor in adult surgical patients and in older pediatric patients has shown a reduction in anesthesia requirements and a shorter recovery time. The BIS monitor has been studied in several adult ICU populations. These studies have shown a correlation between the BIS score and a variety of sedation scores.[15]

One of the main difficulties with clinical sedation scoring systems is their inability to assess depth of sedation in the patient receiving neuromuscular blocking agents (NMBAs). Patients who require NMBAs in the operating room are considered to be at an increased risk of awareness during anesthesia.[16] This problem also exists for the sedated patient with paralysis in the PICU. It is well known that the clinical signs of inadequate anesthesia or sedation are not reliable[17] and that there are many other reasons for alterations in the heart rate, blood pressure, perfusion, and pupillary responses in the PICU patient. In a study using the BIS in pediatric patients with paralysis,[18] researchers found that in more than 8% of the sedation assessments in which patients were thought to be adequately sedated by the bedside nurse, the patients' BIS scores were greater than 80 (Fig. 134.1). This score reflected a significant risk of awareness. The BIS correlates well with the

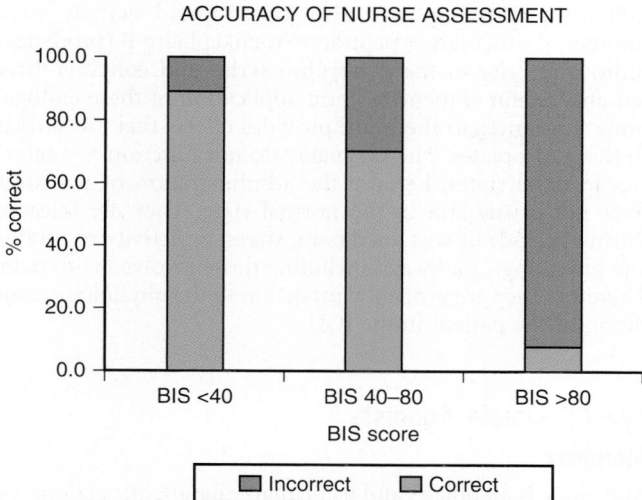

Fig. 134.1. Nurse sedation assessment of the paralyzed patient. *BIS,* bispectral index.

Ramsay scale in the sedated child and may be a useful monitor to prevent inadequate sedation in a child with paralysis.

An important aspect of sedation monitoring is the level of stimulus. The BIS monitor will estimate the degree of hypnosis at a point in time in the context of the balance between sedation, analgesia, and stimulation. It cannot predict what will happen if this balance is changed. A comparison of the Comfort score to the BIS monitor demonstrates this effect. Using the Comfort score, the majority of patients were considered oversedated at baseline (score <11). The BIS assessment at the same time demonstrated that the majority of the patients were appropriately sedated (BIS 40-80). When the child was stimulated (tracheal suctioning), the majority of the Comfort scores were now appropriately sedated, as were the BIS scores. The BIS scores rose from a mean of 52 to a mean of 60. What is unclear is whether the Comfort score or the BIS was a better assessment tool, questioning if the children oversedated without stimulation should be kept lighter and sedated only for procedures?

Although the BIS monitor is used in many institutions, the question of whether its use can prevent awareness under anesthesia is still debated. One study enrolled 2000 adults whose anesthesia was titrated to a BIS score of lower than 60 or by the end-tidal inhalational concentration of the anesthetic agent to at least 0.7 minimum alveolar concentration (MAC).[19] Postoperatively all patients were interviewed to assess their intraoperative awareness. This study found two cases of awareness in each group. The MAC values in both groups were the same. The BIS was greater than 60 in one case of awareness. Although the BIS monitor was not able to reduce this low incidence of awareness, the level of anesthesia between the groups was very similar. This study was severely underpowered to show any benefit. However, the combination of end-tidal monitoring and BIS monitoring may help to reduce intraoperative awareness.

Another potential concern with using the BIS monitor is its relevance or reliability for the pediatric patient. Research thus far showing a correlation with the myriad of sedation scoring systems used in the PICU is limited by the limitations of these scoring systems. Furthermore, the lack of continuous sedation assessment by these scoring systems, as is possible with BIS monitoring, makes comparison difficult. Also of concern is whether the EEG analysis algorithms used in the BIS monitor are applicable to the pediatric brain. This issue needs further evaluation before the BIS monitor can be considered a standard in the PICU. Pediatric-specific BIS probes are now available. The possible inaccuracy of the BIS in younger children has been demonstrated in the operating room, where BIS numbers in younger children (age 1-12 years) tended to be higher (>60) than in older children receiving the same propofol, remifentanil-based anesthetic.[20] In this study there was no recovery benefit to a BIS-driven anesthetic compared to a standard dose-based, clinical signs anesthetic. In fact, the younger children took longer to wake up due to high doses of sedation agents given in an effort to keep the BIS <60. The children with the BIS >60 appeared to be appropriately anesthetized, and as such, the concept that the BIS must be less than 60 to ensure adequate anesthesia in younger children may not be correct. This may correlate with the need to select a different BIS end point in the PICU also. Finally, a limitation of the BIS monitor is that it is less reliable when used with certain hypnotic agents such as ketamine, dexmedetomidine, nitrous oxide, xenon, and opiates.

Other processed EEG sedation assessment monitors are now available. The SNAP II monitor[21] uses a different spectrum of EEG frequency analysis. Little difference between the BIS and the SNAP II monitors has been shown thus far. Currently, little experience has been reported with the SNAP II monitor in pediatric patients. In the PICU, the SNAP was found not to correlate well (r = 0.18) with the sedation depth of intubated children. The mean SNAP index changed only between 58 and 68 over a sedation score reflecting deep to light sedation.[22]

Opioids and Analgesia in the Pediatric Intensive Care Unit

Sedation in the PICU is most commonly achieved with a mixture of opioids and benzodiazepines (BZDs). Although many synthetic and naturally occurring opioids exist, morphine is considered the agent against which others are compared. The primary source of morphine is opium obtained from the opium poppy (*Papaver somniferum*), which also produces alkaloids such as codeine, thebaine, papaverine, and noscapine. Opiates are substances derived from opium; the term *opioid* also describes substances derived from opiates (eg, oxycodone) but includes substances that are created synthetically but have properties that are similar to those of opiates (eg, fentanyl and methadone) and endogenous ligands. The terms often are used interchangeably because the pharmacologic effects fall into the same category. Opioids are agonists at various opioid receptors, for which several endogenous ligands exist. There are three major classes of receptors: mu (μ), kappa (κ), and delta (δ). The opioid receptors possess the same general structure of an extracellular N-terminal region, seven transmembrane domains, and an intracellular C-terminal tail structure. Subtypes of each receptor (eg, μ_1, μ_2) exist (Table 134.4), as do less well-characterized opioid receptors ϵ, Δ, τ, and ϵ.

Most of the therapeutic and adverse effects can be accounted for by agonist activity at the μ-receptor, which is responsible

TABLE 134.4 Classification of Opiate Receptors and Subtypes

Subtype	Prototypic Drugs	Actions
Mu$_1$	Opiates and most opiate peptides	Supraspinal analgesia including periaqueductal gray matter, nucleus raphe magnus, and locus coeruleus Prolactin release Acetylcholine turnover in brain Catalepsy
Mu$_2$	Morphine	Respiratory depression Dopamine turnover in brain Gastrointestinal tract transit Most cardiovascular effects
Delta	Enkephalins	Spinal analgesia Dopamine turnover
Kappa	Dynorphin	Spinal analgesia Inhibition of antidiuretic hormone Sedation
Sigma	N-allynormetazocine	Psychotomimetic effects

Modified from Baresh PG, Cullen BF, Stoelting RK et al., eds. Clinical Anesthesia. 2nd ed. Philadelphia: JB Lippincott: 1992.

for analgesia, respiratory depression, pupillary constriction, and euphoria. At the cellular level, μ-receptor activation alters ionic permeability to K$^+$, causing hyperpolarization and depression of excitability in the nervous system. Associated effects on cholinergic, adrenergic, serotonergic, and dopaminergic neurotransmitter systems are seen within the central nervous system (CNS). These receptors are found at multiple sites along pain pathways including the spinal cord, midbrain, thalamus, and cortex. At the spinal cord level, pain reflexes (nociceptive) are depressed by receptors in the substantia gelatinosa, which are mostly presynaptic and inhibit the release of substance P from C-fiber nerve terminals and account for the effectiveness of intrathecally and epidurally administered opioids. In the midbrain the analgesic effect is mediated in the periaqueductal gray matter through ascending fibers and also descending fibers that modulate the function of the dorsal horn. Acetylcholine, γ-aminobutyric acid (GABA), norepinephrine, and serotonin also are involved in these pain-modulating pathways. Peripheral opioid receptors also have been shown and can be expressed in response to inflammation.[23] The intraarticular injection of morphine produces analgesia following arthroscopy through activation of opioid receptors located on white blood cells.[24]

The endogenous ligands for the opioid receptors are the enkephalins, endorphins, and dynorphins. They have a morphine-like effect that can be specifically antagonized by the μ-receptor antagonist naloxone. The endomorphins have potent analgesic and gastrointestinal (GI) effects. At the cellular level, they activate G proteins ([35S] GTP gamma-S binding) and inhibit calcium currents.[25] Pro-opiomelanocortin is the precursor for β-endorphin (as well as adrenocorticotropic hormone and melanocyte-stimulating hormone). β-Endorphin, itself very active, also includes the amino acid sequence for met-enkephalin, although the main precursor is proenkephalin A, which contains four copies of met-enkephalin and one copy of leu-enkephalin. The

met-enkephalin sequence also gives opioid activity to a number of other larger peptides. Proenkephalin B (prodynorphin) gives rise to the dynorphin series and contains three leu-enkephalin sequences. Local application of these endogenous substances to the brain provides effects that are similar to those of opiates. They arguably do not function as analgesics in basal states, because the administration of naloxone does not cause pain in the normal state. They are released during periods of sustained pain, stress, or activity to modulate physiologic pathways, including those involved with pain. Therefore they are probably important to the physiologic condition of the patient in the ICU.

Specific Opioid Agonists
Morphine

Morphine is an opiate, and its primary therapeutic actions are sedation and analgesia; anxiolysis and euphoria also may occur. These four therapeutic effects may be exploited to the benefit of the patient. These actions are mediated through the periaqueductal gray matter, the ventromedial medulla, and the spinal cord. The reduction of nociceptive reflexes occurs all over the body, even below a completely transected spinal cord. In addition to increasing the sensory threshold for pain, morphine may decrease the hurting aspect (or unpleasantness) of pain. A patient given morphine may say something such as "I have just as much pain, but it doesn't distress me as much." It blunts most types and intensities of pain, although some forms of neuropathic pain are relatively resistant. The resulting analgesia may be potent enough to abolish diagnostic symptoms and signs. The sedative effects reduce higher cortical function, cause difficulty in concentration, and cause a sense of drowsiness and dream-filled sleep. Higher doses will cause a state of unconsciousness or coma. The rate of respiration is reduced with a resultant fall in minute ventilation despite an accompanying increase in depth of breathing. This effect is associated with a decreased responsiveness to carbon dioxide (CO_2) and is additive to the decreased CO_2 response seen during sleep. In some circumstances respiratory drive may be limited to hypoxic stimulation of the carotid chemoreceptors; this is the most serious dose-related adverse effect of morphine. It can occur at doses used clinically for analgesia. In general, all opiates produce the same degree of respiratory depression when given in equipotent doses and for any given level of analgesia. Opioids do not have anticonvulsant properties, whereas meperidine (and its metabolite normeperidine) may lower the seizure threshold.

Another CNS effect of morphine is pupillary constriction due to a central effect on the oculomotor nucleus. Nausea results from stimulation of the chemotrigger zone; however, opioids also depress the vomiting center, so the final effect is unpredictable. Nausea and vomiting are much more frequent in ambulatory patients than in patients confined to a hospital bed. Morphine can modify stress-related endocrine responses. It decreases the release of several hormones including adrenocorticotropic hormone, antidiuretic hormone, prolactin, growth hormone, and epinephrine. The neuroendocrine stress response that is normally seen with trauma and surgery may be blunted. Itching may be caused by histamine release, but it also may be due to opiate receptor activation in the spinal cord.[26]

Morphine's effects on smooth muscle cause constipation. It reduces the intestinal propulsion activity through its central and peripheral effects. The central effects may be mediated by the vagus nerve. The direct smooth muscle relaxation and the increased local cholinergic transmission can be partly reversed by naloxone. This decreased motility is the basis of several over-the-counter antidiarrheal preparations including diphenoxylate, a μ-agonist that does not cross the blood-brain barrier and thus acts as a peripheral opioid agonist. Morphine also causes an increase in biliary tract tone, which may cause biliary colic, as well as increased tone in the bladder detrusor muscle and vesical sphincter. Urinary retention is common with opioids and occurs in 55% of children receiving spinally administered opioid and 20% receiving intravenous (IV) opioid.[27]

Morphine has been studied extensively in term and preterm neonates. Glucuronidation is present in term babies and in many preterm ones. The half-life of morphine, however, is 2 hours in children, 6.5 hours in term neonates, and 9 hours in the preterm child because of reduced clearance. Volume of distribution does not vary with age.[28] Morphine causes histamine release and can cause peripheral vasodilatation. Infused at analgesic doses, it has little effect on the cardiovascular system, but skin flushing is not uncommon with rapid IV administration. The histamine-releasing potential should be considered in patients with asthma, especially during an acute exacerbation, and in patients with unstable cardiovascular systems for whom safer alternatives, such as fentanyl, exist.

Dosing recommendations in the ICU include a bolus dose of 0.05 to 0.1 mg/kg and an infusion of 0 to 30 μg/kg/h. Fifty percent of these doses should be used if the patient is younger than 3 months of age. The pharmacokinetics of various opiates is outlined in Table 134.5. All opiates are weak bases and are moderately ionized at pH 7.4. Oral morphine is effective but undergoes hepatic first-pass metabolism, which is variable among patients. The oral dose for acute pain is two to five times the IV dose, whereas in long-term use the oral dose is 1.5 to 2.5 times the IV dose.

Morphine is metabolized to morphine-3-glucuronide (M3G) and M6G in the liver. M3G is the major metabolite and has little morphine-like activity, although some research has suggested that M3G may be associated with an antinociceptive effect, accounting for failure of analgesia during long-term use.[29] In contrast, M6G is many times more potent than morphine itself.

Morphine undergoes significant first-pass hepatic metabolism, whereby after a single parenteral dose, only morphine is initially active. After a single dose by mouth (PO), both morphine and M6G are active. With long-term oral use, M6G accumulates until its analgesic effect is greater than that of morphine. A similar effect can be anticipated with long-term morphine infusion in the patient in the PICU. The kidney excretes the glucuronides, together with only a small amount of free morphine. Ninety percent of total urinary excretion occurs within 24 hours.

Tolerance, defined as an increase in the dose required to create the same response, is a potential problem with all opiates. Tolerance is mainly limited to the depressant actions of morphine, including analgesia, respiratory depression, anxiolysis, and drowsiness. Tolerance of morphine's inhibition of bowel motility and pupillary constriction is minimal. The mechanism of tolerance appears to involve the degree and duration of both μ- and κ-receptor occupancy. It appears more rapidly after continuous infusion, and cross-tolerance to other opiates is common, although anecdotal evidence suggests that when opioids are switched, a dose reduction may be possible because cross-tolerance sometimes appears incomplete.[30] Receptor downregulation also may occur, as well as altered metabolism with an increased M3G/M6G ratio. Simultaneous blockade of N-methyl-D-aspartate receptors has been shown to be effective in reducing the development of tolerance.[31] Clinical tolerance appears uncommon with an exposure of less than 3 days, but after prolonged administration, doses 10 to 20 times that which would cause respiratory arrest in nontolerant patients may be tolerated.

Meperidine

Meperidine has one-tenth the potency of morphine. Compared with other common opioids, meperidine has more CNS excitatory effects including tremors, muscle spasm, myoclonus, psychiatric changes, and seizures. These effects may be due to a central serotoninergic effect.[32] It is metabolized by the liver to normeperidine, which is twice as toxic as meperidine and has a longer half-life (15 hours). Normeperidine accumulation is enhanced in patients with an induced cytochrome P-450 system. Meperidine has a shorter duration of action (2 to 3 hours) and has a more rapid onset because of its increased lipid solubility compared with morphine. Meperidine is unique among opioids because of its local anesthetic properties, which are capable of providing surgical spinal analgesia.[33] A small dose (0.125 to 0.25 mg/kg) of meperidine may be used to treat postoperative shivering.

Fentanyl

Fentanyl is one of the most commonly used opiates in the ICU. It is a synthetic derivative of meperidine without many of its unwanted side effects. It is a potent μ-agonist and is 100 times more potent than morphine. It has a rapid onset and cessation because of its high lipid solubility (Fig. 134.2). Fentanyl may be administered by several routes, including IV, intramuscular (IM), transmucosal,[34] and subcutaneous (SC) when venous access is inadequate. There is also a 12.5-mcg transdermal patch available for children. Fentanyl may be given intranasally as an alternative to the transmucosal route. It has been used for premedication, sedation, and also for the treatment of a "Tet" spell in an infant.[35] The transdermal patch is designed to release 12.5 mcg/h of fentanyl for

TABLE 134.5	Opiate Pharmacokinetics			
Drug	Elimination Half-Life (hr)	Volume Distribution (SS) (L/kg)	Clearance (mL/kg/min)	Protein Binding (%)
Morphine	2.2	3.3	15	30
Meperidine	3.2	2.8	5	58
Fentanyl	3.1	3.2	8	79
Sufentanil	2.7	1.7	13	92
Alfentanil	1.2	0.3	2.8	89

SS, steady state.
Modified from Baresh PG, Cullen BF, Stoelting RK et al., eds. Clinical Anesthesia. 2nd ed. Philadelphia: JB Lippincott; 1992.

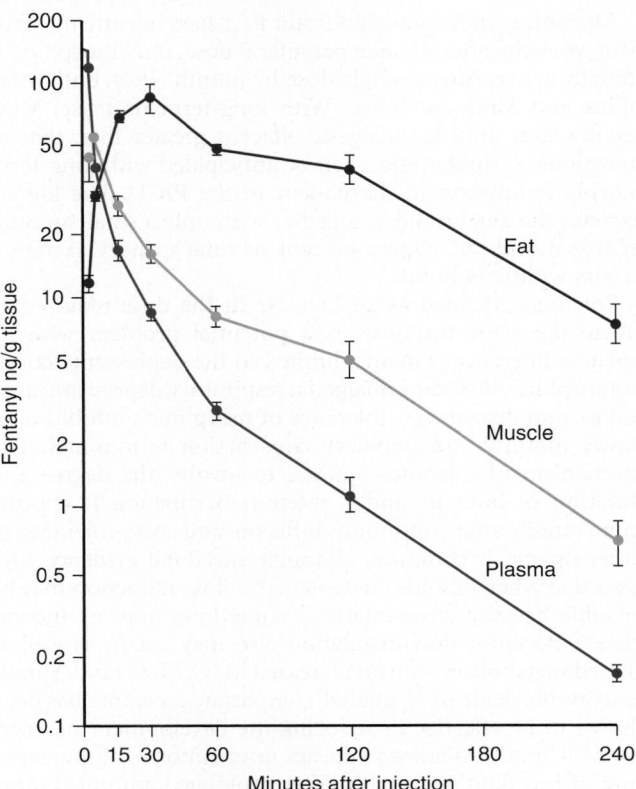

Fig. 134.2. Initial fentanyl redistribution.

approximately 3 days.[36] It is indicated for children with chronic pain syndromes; however, improved efficacy, compared to standard oral alternatives, has not been proved. Due to the different kinetics of fentanyl in children, it may take longer to achieve the steady state in the skin depot, and the patch may not last for a full 72 hours. The patch must be removed if the patient undergoes an MRI scan. Withdrawal from the fentanyl patch may be delayed due to the availability of the skin depot reserves. Unfortunately an increasing number of patients are now being admitted to the PICU[37] due to fentanyl overdose as a result of chewing, smoking, or extracting the fentanyl from the patch. A 12.5-mcg fentanyl patch contains over 1 mg total of fentanyl.

Skeletal muscle rigidity (which can occur with all synthetic opiates) is well described in the literature. It is mediated through the CNS and is an idiopathic response usually associated with a large bolus dose ($\geq$5 µg/kg). It improves with the administration of NMBAs and is reversible with naloxone. Fentanyl has limited cardiovascular effects. Moderate bradycardia is the most common hemodynamic effect. Fentanyl does not cause histamine release. Dosing in the ICU is either by bolus (1 to 2 µg/kg) or infusion (1 to 4 µg/kg/h with higher doses as tolerance develops). The short duration of effect of a single dose of fentanyl is not due to metabolism but rather to rapid redistribution. Maximum brain concentration after a bolus is achieved within 90 seconds. Then, because of rapid redistribution, the plasma level falls by 50% in 30 minutes, and the result is a clinical duration of effect of a single dose of approximately 30 minutes. Fentanyl then accumulates in fat, where it is stored and slowly released with a longer elimination half-life of about 4 hours (longer than morphine).

Marked respiratory depression occurs within 120 seconds, and a single dose of 5 µg/kg will cause apnea in 50% of patients. Also, fentanyl is metabolized by the liver to norfentanyl and hydroxy fentanyl derivatives, both of which are thought to be inactive. In the operating room, high-dose fentanyl is commonly used for cardiac anesthesia and for anesthetization of other unstable patients. A loading dose of 50 µg/kg, followed by 0.5 µg/kg/min, will occupy all opioid receptors and produce a state of anesthesia. Many cases of awareness with patients under anesthesia have been documented, however, even when these high doses of fentanyl were used.

Sufentanil

Sufentanil is another synthetic opiate that has actions and therapeutic effects that are similar to those of fentanyl. It is five to ten times more potent than fentanyl and is the most potent opioid in clinical practice, posing a high risk of apnea with bolus administration. Dosing recommendations include bolus dosing of 0.2 to 0.4 µg/kg or an infusion of 0.2 to 1 µg/kg/h.

After a single bolus, sufentanil has kinetics similar to that of fentanyl with a short duration of clinical effect of approximately 30 minutes. However, with prolonged use, sufentanil accumulates less and is associated with a more rapid recovery after infusion because of its smaller volume of distribution and similar clearance. When the patient is receiving high doses of fentanyl, sufentanil is useful to conserve infusion volume.

Alfentanil

Alfentanil is another synthetic opiate with a rapid onset. It is five times less potent than fentanyl. Although it is less lipid soluble than fentanyl because of its low pK_a (negative logarithm of the acid ionization constant), a higher percentage of the drug is present in the active unionized form, which results in a rapid onset. Because of its low volume of distribution, alfentanil has a short elimination half-life, which results in a short duration of action (5 to 10 minutes). Dosing regimens include boluses of 5 to 10 µg/kg if there is spontaneous respiration or 20 to 50 µg/kg if the patient's lungs are ventilated. Alfentanil is a useful agent for preventing the hypertensive or increased intracranial pressure (ICP) response to intubation. As with all synthetic opiates, there is a risk of muscle rigidity with the higher dosing. Infusion dosing is typically 0.2 to 1 µg/kg/min for patients receiving mechanical ventilation. Postinfusion recovery is quicker with alfentanil than with fentanyl. It is useful by infusion and safe to use in patients with hepatic or renal failure.

Codeine

Codeine has a chemical structure and effects that are similar to those of morphine; it is commonly used as an oral medication for cough suppression or mild to moderate pain relief. A large part of its effects are due to the metabolism of codeine to morphine. Ten to twenty percent of patients lack a metabolic pathway to convert codeine to morphine, which results in an unpredictable effect. Dosing is 0.5 to 1 mg/kg. Constipation is a major adverse effect, and some patients report having a vague, peculiar, or unpleasant feeling when they take codeine. This drug can be habit forming. It can be given orally, IM, or rectally. Rapid IV use may result in cardiovascular collapse. Rectally administered codeine has been shown to have as rapid an onset as IM codeine, but it yields lower peak levels in children.[38] Codeine has been the analgesic of choice by neurosurgeons because of the belief that pupillary signs are maintained with use of this drug. Morphine has been shown to be a more effective analgesic, however, in patients with head injuries.[39]

Remifentanil

Remifentanil is one of the newest synthetic opiates available. It was designed to be metabolized by plasma esterases to provide a short half-life. It is a potent μ-agonist with mild κ and δ effects. It is substantially more potent than fentanyl. It is supplied as a white lyophilized powder that contains glycine and should not be used for epidural or spinal analgesia. The metabolism is by nonspecific esterases not affected by pseudocholinesterase deficiency. The metabolite, a weak μ-agonist, is excreted by the kidney. The kinetics of remifentanil is different from those of most opiates used in the ICU. It has a short half-life that is due to metabolism rather than to redistribution. Therefore remifentanil has what is known as a context-sensitive half-life. The elimination half-life for remifentanil is about 8 minutes. With an infusion of remifentanil, the half-life does not increase but remains constant. With opiates such as fentanyl and alfentanil (Fig. 134.3), the clinical effect half-life increases with time until it reflects the elimination half-life of between 2 and 4 hours.

The kinetics reported for neonates is similar to those reported for adults. The continuous infusion rate depends on the degree of sedation/analgesia required (0.1 to 0.5 μg/kg/min for sedation; 0.75 to 2 μg/kg/min for balanced anesthesia; 4 μg/kg/min for loss of consciousness). Remifentanil has effects on the cardiovascular system that are similar to those of fentanyl. Remifentanil causes a mild bradycardia and a slight decrease in blood pressure,[40] which may be prevented with glycopyrrolate. No histamine release occurs. Remifentanil is a potent respiratory depressant. For spontaneous respiration, a low continuous infusion dose (without a bolus) should be used (0.1 μg/kg/min). Sedation can be effectively managed by continuous infusion without the need for a bolus because of the short half-life. An increase or decrease of infusion rate is rapidly reflected by a change in the degree of sedation, which is important to note. Most other opiate sedatives require bolus dosing to achieve a rapid change in effect. This type of dosing is neither appropriate nor needed for remifentanil.

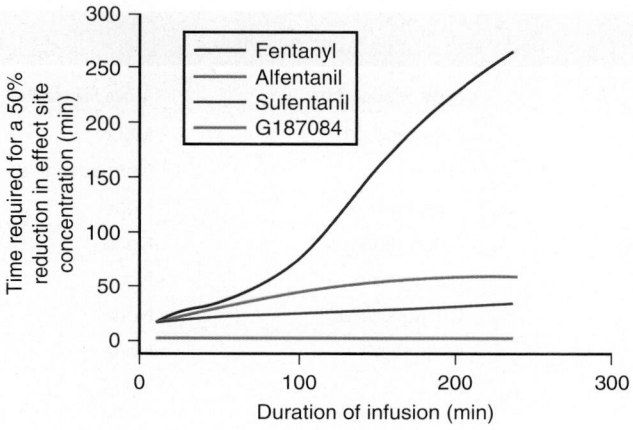

Fig. 134.3. Context-sensitive half-life.

Remifentanil has the usual opiate adverse effects; however, because of the short half-life, these clinical effects are brief. Remifentanil may prove to be a safe and effective choice for PICU sedation in patients with severe renal or hepatic disease; however, the potential exists for glycine accumulation in patients with renal failure. It is an option for those who require overnight ventilation or for those patients in whom a rapid awakening may be required for neurologic assessment. Remifentanil has been shown to reduce cerebral oxygen use and reduce cerebral blood flow if the CO_2 is maintained in a normal range. Remifentanil is currently an expensive option and should not be considered for every patient. Also, because of its short duration, the postoperative patient may need an alternative analgesic after extubation. Rapid development of opiate tolerance with remifentanil has been described in healthy volunteers[41] and also when used in the ICU setting. This rapid tolerance has also been described in postoperative scoliosis patients[42]; however, the increased morphine requirements described probably reflect the initial postoperative need to achieve an adequate morphine blood level rather than any acute tolerance.

Hydromorphone

Hydromorphone is a hydrogenated ketone of morphine. It is seven times as potent as morphine with a similar onset and duration of action. It causes less histamine release than morphine and may be used in patients who report pruritus due to morphine. Like morphine, hydromorphone undergoes hepatic metabolism; however, no active metabolites are dependent on renal excretion. As such, it may be an effective alternative in patients with renal insufficiency or failure.

Tramadol

Tramadol is an opiate analgesic. It action is due to the metabolite O-desmethyltramadol, which relieves pain by binding to opiate receptors and by inhibiting the reuptake in the CNS and spinal cord of norepinephrine and serotonin, two pain-modifying neurotransmitters. Tramadol does not have antiinflammatory effects. Its use is indicated in cases of moderate to severe pain.[43] Even though it is a narcotic-like agent, the Food and Drug Administration (FDA) only recently classified tramadol as a controlled substance. Tramadol has been changed to a schedule IV medication, reflecting issues and concerns about tolerance, habituation, abuse potential, and withdrawal syndrome.[44] Dosage (not FDA approved for patients younger than 16 years) is an initial oral administration of 1 to 2 mg/kg every 6 hours and should not exceed 6 mg/kg/day. An IV preparation is available outside of the United States. Patients with a creatinine clearance less than 30 mL/min should not receive more than one dose every 12 hours, with a maximum dose of 3 mg/kg/day. The dose for patients with cirrhosis or hepatic dysfunction is 1 mg/kg every 12 hours. Patients undergoing dialysis can receive their dose on the day of dialysis because only 7% of the drug is removed by the process. The adverse effects of tramadol most often involve the CNS and the GI tract. Patients may become dependent on tramadol. Abuse is possible, and it should not be given to opiate-dependent patients. Seizures have been seen in patients receiving high single oral doses of 10 mg/kg; this danger is even greater in patients with epilepsy and in anyone taking monoamine oxidase inhibitors and neuroleptic agents that lower the seizure threshold. Respiratory depression may occur if the recommended dosage is consistently exceeded or if another centrally acting depressant drug (eg, alcohol) or an anesthetic is given concurrently. Because of the possibility of withdrawal symptoms, patients should not abruptly discontinue use of tramadol. Tramadol is not a useful drug for sedative action.

Table 134.6 provides conversion doses for some commonly used oral opiates. A summary of IV doses of different opiates is provided in Table 134.7.

Opiate Antagonists

Several opiate antagonists are available. The most commonly used is naloxone, which is a specific and sensitive receptor antagonist of all opiate receptors. It is administered in either low doses (1 µg/kg) or high doses in an emergency situation (10 µg/kg). If the drug cannot be administered intravenously, then it can be given intramuscularly, intranasally, or into the midventral surface of the tongue. When naloxone is being used for a long-acting agonist, an infusion may be necessary because its half-life is only 30 to 81 minutes (mean of 64 ± 12 minutes). In neonates, the half-life has been reported as 3.1 ± 0.5 hours; however, this prolonged effect is likely to be offset by a concomitant increase in the duration of action of the opioid for which the naloxone is given. No effect is seen in the healthy patient in the absence of administered opioids; however, in the setting of sepsis in the ICU, a vasopressor effect may occur, presumably because of an interaction with endogenous opioids released in response to stress. Nalmefene, a longer-acting antagonist, can be given through IV, IM, and SC routes. It has a redistribution half-life of 41 minutes and a terminal half-life of 10.8 hours in adults and somewhat less in children. Thus reappearance of the antagonized opioid is unlikely if it is given in an adequate dose.[45]

There has been a growing interest in the use of opiate antagonists in the management of opiate sedation induced ileus. Naloxone can be given orally[46]; however, there is evidence of a central effect that slightly reduces the efficacy of parenterally administered opiates. Two opiate antagonists are available that have been approved for opiate-induced constipation. Naloxegel[47] is a PEGylated naloxone that does not cross the blood-brain barrier, inhibits opioid receptors in the gastrointestinal tract, and improves gastrointestinal motility. Methyl naltrexone is also approved for opiate-induced constipation. These drugs are not routinely used; however, they may be added to bowel regimes to prevent opiate-induced bowel dysfunction.

Incidental Pain Syndromes in the Pediatric Intensive Care Unit

Although the techniques used to sedate children are often applied in order to facilitate their PICU management, many children have pain that is related to their underlying condition. Many options are available for controlling pain in the pediatric patient (Box 134.1). The pharmacologic management of pain should follow the traditional World Health Organization analgesic ladder, which begins with a nonopioid analgesic such as a nonsteroidal antiinflammatory drug or acetaminophen, followed by a weak opioid such as hydrocodone added to the nonopioid, and then a strong opioid such as morphine or hydromorphone as needed. When taken orally, a sustained-release preparation is often useful once the dose requirement has been determined. The dose requirement of a strong opioid is variable in the patient taking opioids for a prolonged period, and not appreciating this variability is a common cause for therapeutic failure. In addition, once a dose requirement is known, the analgesic should be given to preempt pain rather than to relieve pain as required. At each level of analgesic use, the addition of adjuvant medications should be considered. Adjuvant drugs fall into six groups: antidepressant, anticonvulsant, neuroleptic, steroid, stimulant, and local anesthetic. Of the tricyclic antidepressants, nortriptyline is available in a liquid form. The tricyclic antidepressants are indicated for neuropathic pain, particularly when the patient describes a burning pain. Also useful for neuropathic pain are the anticonvulsant agents gabapentin, pregabalin, and carbamazepine. These drugs often work

TABLE 134.6	Dose Equivalents: Short Acting	
Drug	**Oral**	**Parenteral**
Morphine	0.5 mg/kg q4h	0.15 mg/kg q3h
Hydromorphone	0.1 mg/kg q4h	0.02 mg/kg q4h
Codeine	4 mg/kg q3h	
Hydrocodone	0.5 mg/kg q3h	
Oxycodone	0.5 mg/kg q3h	
Meperidine	5 µg/kg q2h	1.5 mg/kg q2h
Fentanyl		1.5 µg/kg q2h

TABLE 134.7	Summary of Opiate Dosing			
Drug	**Relative Potency**	**Bolus Dose**	**Initial Infusion Rate**	**Active Metabolites**
Morphine	1	0.1 mg/kg	0.04 mg/kg/h	M6G
Meperidine	0.1	1 mg/kg	NA	Normeperidine
Fentanyl	100	1 µg/kg	1 µg/kg/h	None
Hydromorphone	7	0.015 mg/kg	0.005 mg/kg/h	None
Sufentanil	500	0.2 µg/kg	0.2 µg/kg/h	None
Remifentanil	NA	NA	0.1 µg/kg/min	None
Alfentanil	10	10 µg/kg	10 µg/kg/h	None
Methadone	1	0.1 mg/kg	NA	None

M6G, morphine-6-glucuronide; *NA,* not applicable.

BOX 134.1	Options for Controlling a Child's Pain

Analgesics
Opioids—weak, potent
Nonsteroidal antiinflammatory drugs (NSAIDs)
Nonopioids

Anesthetics
Regional block
Epidural anesthesia
Topical anesthesia

Physical
Thermal
Massage
Physical therapy
Transcutaneous electrical nerve stimulation (TENS)

Cognitive
Imagery
Distraction
Hypnosis
Choices and control
Information
Role play

Behavioral
Biofeedback
Relaxation therapy

best when the pain is described as shooting or lancinating. Neuropathic pain may result from tumor invasion, vincristine therapy, cytomegalovirus infection, or human immunodeficiency infection. Neuroleptic drugs, including chlorpromazine and trimeprazine, may be useful in the management of nausea, anxiety, and pruritus. Steroids benefit mood, inflammation, nausea, appetite, nerve swelling/entrapment, and vasculitis. When opioid sedation is interfering with quality of life, a stimulant such as an amphetamine may restore energy and alertness while allowing ongoing analgesia from the opioid. Sometimes pain can be managed by local anesthetic, placed by peripheral nerve block, topically, or as a neuraxial block.

Patient-controlled analgesia (PCA) has become the mainstay of postoperative pain relief in children because of its efficacy and safety. However, its use is limited by the child's ability to understand how to use the PCA pump. Proxy PCA (PCA-P) has been used for younger children or those with cognitive impairment.[48] The use of the PCA by the nurse or the caregiver may override the safety net that the PCA has. The use of PCA-P has been associated with greater need for rescue interventions; however, it is often used in sicker children. When PCA-P is used, careful evaluation and rigorous monitoring are needed.

Sickle Cell Crisis

Sickle cell disease differs from cancer and acquired immune deficiency syndrome in that intermittent episodes of severe pain occur, requiring urgent intensive treatment. A good review of this subject has been published.[49] Chronic pain also may be present because of long-term tissue and bone damage from periods of ischemia during past crises, including persisting myocardial ischemia. Patients may be receiving long-acting opioids or may have had repeated exposure to opioids with past crises. Patients with a sickle cell disease crisis that involves the chest or brain are likely to be admitted to the PICU. Chest crises result from the sickling of erythrocytes in

the pulmonary vasculature and result in hypoxia to the rest of the body and local lung damage. The systemic hypoxia worsens the crisis and is thus self-perpetuating. Chest radiograph changes may be late, and an associated paralytic ileus may be present.

Poor pulmonary function may discourage the practitioner from using adequate opioid analgesics out of concern for worsening the hypoxia. However, it is important not to underestimate the need for pain relief and to appreciate that past opioid exposure may have resulted in tolerance to opioids. It is important that the pain is assessed early and quickly treated. Also the pain must be reevaluated to ensure that additional doses are given in a timely manner.[50] If considering the use of a PCA, then appropriately dosing must be considered as well. These patients are often not opiate naive, and if the PCA is inadequately dosed then the patients will not achieve a satisfactory level of analgesia. These patients also require frequent pain reevaluation by the nurse to ensure that the PCA is programmed appropriately. If IV access is difficult to obtain, morphine may be given subcutaneously or orally. Ketamine has been suggested as an adjunct to sickle cell pain crisis,[51] demonstrating in a small review an improvement in pain scores as well as a reduction in opiate requirements. Anecdotal success also has been reported with nebulized morphine.[52]

Opiate Tolerance

The use of opiate infusions in the ICU is associated with the potential for the development of tolerance or dependence.[53] Iatrogenic withdrawal symptoms can occur if the opiates are discontinued abruptly. These effects have been shown to be related to the total dose and duration of fentanyl infusion. A fentanyl infusion of 5 days or a total cumulative dose of 1.6 mg/kg during the hospital stay was associated with a 50% chance of the development of narcotic withdrawal, whereas a fentanyl infusion of 9 days or longer or a total cumulative fentanyl dose of 2.5 mg/kg or more during the hospital stay had a 100% incidence of withdrawal.[54] The rising plasma fentanyl levels caused by increased dosing suggested that increased metabolism or clearance was not responsible for the development of tolerance. A study of patients in a PICU conducted to determine the degree of opiate tolerance showed a significant increase in opiate dosing required for adequate sedation.[55] The opiate infusion increased by about 80% per week for the first 3 weeks of opiate use. No difference in the rate of opiate increase was found with respect to age of the patient, postoperative status, mode of ventilation, and paralysis.

For patients considered to be at risk of withdrawal, several options are available. If circumstances allow, it is better to start the treatment for withdrawal prevention before the patient has symptoms and signs of withdrawal. Opiate withdrawal is not usually a serious medical problem; it is rarely life threatening and is self-limited. However, treatment should begin early if possible for patient comfort. In a few circumstances the associated hypersympathetic state may not be good for the patient. The signs and symptoms of withdrawal are nonspecific, and other causes, such as infection, hypoglycemia, hypocalcemia, hyperthyroidism, and hypoxia, should be excluded. Because of the nonspecific nature of the symptoms of opiate withdrawal, several scoring systems have been described to aid with the diagnostic process. The Finnegan score is based on 31 variables and is lengthy. The Lipsitz score is shorter and easier to

TABLE 134.8   Signs and Symptoms of Opiate Withdrawal

Sign/Symptom	Examples
Neurologic excitability	Sleep disturbances Agitation Tremors Seizures Choreoathetoid movements
Gastrointestinal disturbances	Vomiting Diarrhea Autonomic dysfunction
Hypertension (>150 mm Hg)	Tachycardia (>150 mm Hg) Tachypnea (>40 beats/min) Fever (>38.58°C) Frequent yawning Sweating Goose flesh Mottling

use than the Finnegan score. Both of these scoring systems, however, were devised for use with neonates, and several of the measurements are not appropriate for patients in the PICU. Currently no validated scoring system exists for assessing opiate withdrawal in the pediatric patient. In the limited number of articles in which opiate withdrawal in the PICU is evaluated, the authors have modified these scores (Table 134.8) in an attempt to provide an objective assessment of the patient.

The assessment of a new score based on a similar set of signs and symptoms, the Withdrawal Assessment Tool,[56] has been proposed. The bedside nurse reviews the patient's chart for the previous 12 hours and performs a short assessment of the child's level of agitation as well as other signs/symptoms. This review is then followed by an assessment of the response to stimulus and also how quickly the child settles down after the stimulus. A score of 1 is assigned to each assessment (maximum, 12). A score of greater than 3 was associated with a greater likelihood of drug withdrawal. Although this score is new and has limited verification, it probably provides a better evaluation than the clinician's bedside opinion, especially in complex cases in which both opiate and BZD withdrawal may occur together.

Several therapeutic options are available for the prevention and treatment of opiate withdrawal. Drugs from the same class are preferable. The FDA has approved methadone for opiate withdrawal. Other agents that may be useful include morphine, clonidine, dexmedetomidine, phenobarbital, paregoric, chlorpromazine, the transdermal clonidine patch,[57] and SC fentanyl. Paregoric contains morphine plus papaverine, noscapine, camphor (a CNS stimulant), ethanol (45%), benzoic acid (which competes with bilirubin-binding sites), and glycerin (which causes diarrhea). Paregoric has been used for neonatal withdrawal, but because of its composition, it may cause adverse effects. Chlorpromazine may be useful for GI adverse effects, but hypothermia and hypotension may occur. Haloperidol also may be of use, having minimal respiratory depression and no active metabolites. It also offers cardiovascular stability. Phenobarbital has been used for hyperactive behavior; however, it can cause significant CNS depression, it induces drug metabolism, and it is tolerance/dependence forming.

Methadone seems to be the most suitable agent for treating opiate withdrawal. It has an oral bioavailability of 80% to 90% and an elimination half-life of 12 to 24 hours. It is equipotent to morphine. Methadone has inactive metabolites and is less sedating than morphine while remaining an effective analgesic. Because of its higher bioavailability and reduced first-pass metabolism, the effect of oral doses is more predictable than that of morphine. Methadone has been extensively used in the outpatient management of patients addicted to opiates.

The convenience of the oral route, the less-frequent dosing because of its longer half-life, and the ease of calculating doses because of its equal potency to morphine make methadone attractive for use in the management of opiate withdrawal in children. However, a huge variability exists in recommendations regarding the methadone dose that should be used to prevent opiate withdrawal in children. Several factors are important in the dosing of methadone for withdrawal from fentanyl. After prolonged IV administration, fentanyl has a potency 100 times that of methadone; it has a metabolic half-life approximately one-quarter that of methadone; and if given intravenously, it has a bioavailability 20% greater than orally administered methadone. In a study in which the effectiveness of a fentanyl-methadone conversion protocol was assessed, researchers found that giving 2.4 times the daily fentanyl dose as methadone prevented withdrawal symptoms.[53] Methadone was given intravenously for 24 hours, and the fentanyl dose decreased by 50% on day 1 and by another 50% on day 2, and then it was discontinued. On day 3, the methadone was converted to oral dosing. The methadone was given intravenously initially. Because of its long half-life, oral dosing could take up to 5 days to reach a steady state. The duration of methadone requirement varied from 1 to 4 weeks, depending on the duration of opiate infusion. Methadone was being weaned by 3% to 15% per day with no signs of withdrawal. To date, there have been no published cases of respiratory arrest when methadone has been used for opiate weaning.

The incidence, risk factors, and best management strategy for opiate withdrawal in the PICU are still open to debate. Several articles have suggested that there are many risk factors for withdrawal. Younger age, higher level of critically illness, duration, and cumulative dose may be important patient variables,[58] but not all studies demonstrate these same risk factors. Postoperative patients appear to be less likely to develop tolerance, as are postoperative patients who received morphine rather than fentanyl; however, in nonsurgical patients the opiate chosen was not significant.[59] Of those patients receiving opiates for more than 4 days, 35% required the dose to be doubled by 14 days. Most of these increased dose requirements occurred with 3 to 6 days. Starting at a lower dose was also a risk factor for increased dose requirements. In this study, however, the opiate doses used were very low, with a peak fentanyl dose of only 4 mcg/kg/h, so these factors may not apply in patients receiving higher doses. Of interest, the concomitant use of midazolam infusions also was associated with increased opiate needs; whether this reflects a patient factor or a drug effect is unknown. As with most studies and also in clinical practice, these patients received a multitude of sedative-analgesic agents, which can confuse the picture. This study was completed at seven tertiary PICUs, and when the opiate dosing and trends were compared, there was a significant difference between the institutions. This reflects the great variability in sedation requirements among patients, clinicians, and institutions, and as such care should be taken when interpreting these results and instigating changes in a PICU based solely on published data. Part of this variability is patient specific, but there are also ICU- and hospital-dependent factors that can influence the development of tolerance and withdrawal.[58] There is some belief, but little evidence, that using sedation protocols can reduce this problem. Intermittent rather than continuous infusions can reduce the risk; however, this option has to be balanced against the primary aim of sedation, which is patient comfort and safety; with changing levels of sedation, especially in younger children, this could pose a problem. Weaning protocols and the use of methadone have been shown to reduce the incidence of withdrawal; however, various management strategies have been utilized with varying results.

Finally, hospital-based factors can play a part. It would appear prudent to initiate the conversion from fentanyl/morphine to methadone in the ICU environment in the event that problems arise and to ensure that an adequate dose is given. Once stabilized, the patient may be transferred to the floor and ultimately home, with a clearly described plan for decreasing the methadone dose over time. The weaning plan also should involve the home pediatrician so that patients have access to someone who is familiar with the process. In a follow-up of patients who had received methadone while in the ICU, 38% of patients were discharged home during the weaning process. No problems were associated with the weaning of methadone at home. Stigma regarding methadone use was not expressed by any of the parents.

Bed availability in the ICU can influence this factor. Also, most floors will not allow the use of ICU sedation infusions, so they must be converted to alternatives prior to transfer. Continuing the patient on an opiate infusion wean can increase the ICU length of stay substantially.

An alterative to fentanyl equivalence-based methadone dosing has also been reported.[60] In this study, the patients received either a fixed low dose (0.1 mg/kg) of methadone or a high dose (fentanyl dose (mcg/kg/h) × 0.1 × weight) of methadone, irrespective of the dose of fentanyl. The methadone was tapered in a fixed manner irrespective of the duration of fentanyl infusion. There was no difference in the success (about 60%) of the methadone taper between the doses. However, four times as many patients in the high-dose methadone group became oversedated. The success rate of either of these protocols appears to be poor, possibly due to the fairly rapid wean of the methadone, irrespective of the duration of opiate exposure. Also of note, the peak fentanyl dosing was low (4 mcg/kg/h) and the cumulative dose was also low (0.59 mg/kg), both below what are considered high-risk factors. This is an important consideration because if using the high-dose strategy, the methadone dose based on a much higher fentanyl rate would expose the patient to very high doses of methadone and risk respiratory depression. Also, methadone accumulates over several days, and this respiratory depression could occur when the child is not being monitored as closely, after transfer to the floor.

This study supports the use of the lowest dose possible to prevent withdrawal. If the dose is too low, then small (25%) adjunct doses of methadone can be given to control the withdrawal symptoms and then, if needed, the methadone dose can be modified to reflect the patient's actual requirements. Titration to effect is no different from our standard of practice

for sedation and analgesia. In younger children, a Q8- or 12-hour dosing schedule may mean that the doses are being administered too far apart and occasionally a Q6-hour schedule may be required in the initial few days; again caution must be observed with respect to drug accumulation during this period. The purpose of the methadone is to prevent withdrawal symptoms and keep the child comfortable. This should be achieved with the smallest dose possible, which is safer and allows for a shorter methadone taper period. The dose of methadone to prevent withdrawal in most circumstances will be lower than that required to cause sedation. Patient safety is paramount; opiate withdrawal, although unpleasant, is not dangerous and with appropriate assessment and timely intervention can be corrected quickly; excess sedation should be avoided.

The use of a clonidine patch also has been evaluated in the PICU. Clonidine has been shown to be effective in the management of nicotine, opiate, and alcohol withdrawal. It decreases sympathetic outflow from the CNS and has a synergistic effect for analgesia, both at the central and spinal level. In one report, eight patients were described after tracheal reconstructive operations. They required postoperative sedation and ventilation for 7 days, which put them at high risk for withdrawal.[24] A clonidine patch was applied 12 hours before extubation, and the patients were weaned off the opiate. The dose used was approximately 6 μg/kg/day of clonidine, and the patch was left on for 7 days. One patch had to be removed because of hypotension. The patch seemed to be effective in preventing withdrawal. Use of the clonidine patch is attractive because of its noninvasive approach, which is desired. However, the use of a transdermal patch prevents titration of the effect, and problems with bradycardia, hypotension, hypothermia, sedation, and dysrhythmia may occur.

A confounding issue in many publications and in the clinical management of opiate withdrawal is the potential for simultaneous BZD withdrawal. Most researchers have not been able to separate these two issues. The symptoms of BZD withdrawal differ from those of opiate withdrawal because the BZD symptoms generally include less sympathetic activation. BZD withdrawal symptoms are characterized by agitation and a movement disorder. If BZD withdrawal is a concern, low-dose lorazepam or diazepam may be added to the withdrawal management strategy (Table 134.9). A prospective study of BZD withdrawal[61] following lorazepam infusion (up to 0.3 mg/kg/h) documented BZD withdrawal syndrome in approximately 25% of the children. This withdrawal occurred even when using a 6-day tapering of the lorazepam dose. All of the children had been previously weaned off fentanyl infu-

TABLE 134.9	Pharmacokinetics of Benzodiazepines			
Drug	Elimination Half-Life (hr)	Volume Distribution (SS) (L/kg)	Clearance (mL/kg/min)	Protein Binding (%)
Diazepam	46.6	1.13	0.4	97.8
Midazolam	3	1.09	7.5	94
Lorazepam	14.5	1.1	1.1	91
Flumazenil	0.67	1.2	15.3	50

SS, steady state.

sions. No predisposing risk factors were found for BZD withdrawal with respect to BZD or opiate dosing or duration.

Rapid Opiate Detoxification

Reports have been made of rapid opiate detoxification in the ICU. These procedures have used a form of deep sedation (often with use of propofol or another anesthetic agent) to facilitate opioid withdrawal in patients addicted to the recreational use of opiates.[62] The patients are given high doses of opiate antagonists to displace all opiates from the receptors, and then heavy sedation is initiated to reduce the occurrence and effects of the sympathetic stimulation observed with short-term opiate withdrawal. These procedures have been safely performed in the ICU; however, there have been several reports of complications[63] when these procedures were not performed with full ICU support. Currently the effectiveness and safety of 1-day opiate detoxification are still under debate.[64] If used, however, it should be combined with an established long-term support plan to optimize long-term success.

In the PICU, deep sedation with propofol has been used to facilitate rapid opiate weaning of ventilator-dependent patients.[65] The use of propofol for up to 3 days allowed a reduction of fentanyl dosing from 24 to 9 µg/kg/h (a 65% reduction). No signs or symptoms of opiate withdrawal were noted, and metabolic acidosis did not develop. Opiate antagonists were not used for this rapid weaning process. However, concern has been raised regarding the long-term administration of propofol, especially in the PICU patient, given the development of the propofol infusion syndrome.

Benzodiazepines

Benzodiazepines (BZDs) are among the most commonly used agents for sedation in the ICU. They augment the function of the GABA type A (GABA_A) receptor at the postsynaptic membrane. This pentameric protein controls a chloride channel, the opening of which leads to an inhibitory effect due to hyperpolarization of the cell membrane.[66,67] Benzodiazepines bind to BZD receptors, which in the CNS are usually found as part of the GABA_A receptor, enhancing the effect of endogenous GABA.[68] Peripheral BZD receptors[69] are not usually associated with the GABA_A receptor but are a binding site for diazepam and midazolam. These 18-kDa proteins are associated with regulation of cellular proliferation, immunomodulation, porphyrin transport, heme biosynthesis, and anion transport. In particular, they seem important in the regulation of steroid synthesis and apoptosis, and they have a significant effect on the hypothalamic-pituitary-adrenal axis.[70] These latter effects may be pertinent to the physiologic care of patients in the ICU.

BZD receptors are bound by a family of endogenous peptides called endozepines, which have similar effects to the BZDs.[71,72] The expression of this diazepam-binding inhibitor may be relevant to the development of dependence not only on BZDs but also on alcohol and opioids[73] and may therefore be relevant in the drug dependence commonly seen in patients in the PICU who are given these agents continuously. Naturally occurring BZDs have been detected with structures similar to those used clinically.[74] Subsets of GABA_A receptors have been shown to have different effects. Type 1 receptors were responsible for sedation and anterograde amnesia, whereas type 2 receptors mediated anxiolysis. It may be possible to develop selective subtype receptor agonists to provide anxiolysis without sedation, amnesia, or dependence.

The general pharmacologic effects of BZDs are sedation, anxiolysis, euphoria (limbic system), reduced skeletal muscle tone (through spinal BZD receptors), anticonvulsant properties, and neuroendocrine effects. They impair acquisition and encoding of new information, providing anterograde amnesia. They do not have any analgesic properties. They have little direct effect on ICP. Their effects are dose dependent. Patient cofactors including age, concurrent disease, and any cosedation therapy influence responses to BZDs. Paradoxical reactions are reported in which agitation rather than calming is observed.[75] In healthy patients, BZDs have few cardiovascular adverse effects, but in a sick, intensive care population, profound cardiovascular depression may be observed occasionally. BZDs should be used judiciously until the patient response is known.[76] Midazolam has been most often associated with this effect,[77] and research in dogs has shown both negative inotropy and chronotropy, especially when the sympathetic response has been abolished.[78] Clinical use is largely encompassed by discussion of the pharmacologic properties of diazepam, midazolam, and lorazepam.

Specific Benzodiazepines
Diazepam

The first widely used BZD in the ICU was diazepam. Because of its low solubility in water, it is available in the IV or IM form dissolved in propylene glycol. This formulation causes a significant amount of pain and thrombophlebitis with peripheral IV use. A lipid emulsion that has fewer adverse effects is available in the United Kingdom. Diazepam is inexpensive and is effective for short-term sedation; in such cases, accumulation is less of a concern. Diazepam may be given orally because it has good absorption, but absorption tends to be erratic when it is given rectally or intramuscularly. It is highly lipid soluble with a long half-life (24 hours). Metabolism by oxidative biotransformation generates several hypnotically active metabolites with an elimination half-life that may be longer than diazepam, including oxazepam (half-life, 10 hours) and N-dimethyldiazepam (half-life, 93 hours). Delayed recovery has been reported in neonates after they received diazepam, possibly because of the long half-life of dimethyldiazepam.[79] Prolongation of effects occurs in patients when clearance is reduced because of hepatic dysfunction and when metabolism is inhibited by drugs such as cimetidine and omeprazole.

Midazolam

Midazolam is an imidazobenzodiazepine. It has a short elimination half-life of 2 hours and is water soluble, which means that IV injection is nonirritating. Because of these factors, it has become popular in ICUs for sedation by infusion. Intranasally (0.2 mg/kg), midazolam has proved to be as effective at controlling febrile seizures as IV diazepam (0.3 mg/kg).[80] Intramuscular midazolam can be as safe and effective as IV lorazepam in managing patients with status epilepticus.[81] Midazolam has extensive first-pass metabolism and provides less reliable results when given PO, although this route is often successfully used for premedication of children before general anesthesia in doses of 0.5 to 0.75 mg/kg (maximum, 20 mg). It is available in a pleasant-tasting cherry syrup and is effective in 10 to 15 minutes, providing up to 1 hour of adequate anxiolysis, although residual hangover effects may persist.[82] Rectal and sublingual administration have been described.

Midazolam is about eight times more potent than diazepam, with starting dose recommendations of a bolus dose of 0.05 to 0.1 mg/kg[83] and an infusion of 1 to 6 µg/kg/min. Midazolam is metabolized by the cytochrome P-450 system subfamily IIIA (nifedipine oxidase), polypeptide 4 (CYP3A4),[84] to hydroxymidazolam (63% potency) and hydroxymidazolam glucuronide (9% potency). Because of the high degree of protein binding (94% protein bound), the free level can be significantly changed with interactions because of the protein binding, which also may occur with heparin. Hepatic or renal failure increases the free fraction by two to three times, and its effect also can be prolonged by the accumulation of active metabolites.[85] The half-life of midazolam in patients in the ICU may be prolonged compared with that in healthy patients.[86] With short-term infusions (<12 hours), it retains a rapid recovery; however, with increased duration of use, the recovery becomes prolonged. Its clearance may be reduced by several commonly used ICU drugs, including calcium channel blockers, erythromycin, and triazole antifungal agents.[87]

Midazolam clearance can also be reduced by mechanical ventilation, possibly due to reduced cardiac output.[88] There appears to be no correlation between day-night cycle and midazolam pharmacokinetics in critically ill children. Critical illness itself can have a major effect on midazolam clearance. Using pharmacokinetics modeling it was found that midazolam clearance is lower in critically ill patients when compared to healthy infants admitted for postoperative monitoring; this is believed to be due to reduced cytochrome P-450 3A4/5 (CYP3A4/5) activity as a result of inflammation, reduction in liver blood flow as a result of mechanical ventilation or acute illness, and the reduction of total albumin that is usually reported in critically ill patients.[81]

Lorazepam

Lorazepam is an alternative water-soluble agent that is well absorbed after both oral and IM administration.[89] It produces sedation for 4 to 8 hours after a single dose. Lorazepam has a slower onset than does midazolam. The elimination half-life is about 14 hours. Metabolism is by glucuronyl transferase, not the cytochrome P-450, and there are no active metabolites. This metabolism is unaffected by cimetidine or phenobarbital, which only affects oxidative metabolic pathways. Sodium valproate may inhibit its metabolism.[90] In persons with advanced liver disease, these phase II glucuronidation reactions are better preserved, and the increased half-life seen is due to increases in the volume of distribution rather than to reduced clearance. In patients with renal failure, prolonged half-life is also due to reduced protein binding because clearance is unchanged. No change in metabolism occurs with aging or critical illness. In a comparison of infusions of midazolam and lorazepam, the recovery characteristics were found to be significantly different. In patients receiving lorazepam, it took an average of 260 minutes to return to baseline, whereas in patients receiving midazolam, it took more than six times longer to return to baseline. Lorazepam may be administered by bolus (0.05 to 0.1 mg/kg every 2 to 4 hours) or by infusion (0.05 mg/kg/h). Lorazepam is slightly less expensive than is midazolam.[91] It has been recommended as the BZD of choice for long-term sedation because of its more predictable recovery profile in sick patients in the ICU. Lorazepam for IV use has propylene glycol as a carrier. Risk of a metabolic lactic acidosis exists because of the metabolism of this carrier. Cases of fatal metabolic acidosis from propylene glycol have been reported in neonates taking a particular vitamin preparation. Several other potential ICU drugs may use propylene glycol as a carrier, including some IV preparations of phenytoin and phenobarbital, nitroglycerin, digoxin, and etomidate. Reports of propylene glycol toxicity in adults who received multiple propylene glycol infusions have been made.[92] Care should be taken when lorazepam is infused in patients who receive these other medications. In patients in the PICU, propylene glycol levels have been shown to correlate with the dose of lorazepam received; however, no metabolic abnormalities were detected.[93] Hemodialysis has been used successfully in the management of the lorazepam-associated propylene glycol toxicity.[94]

Benzodiazepines have been commonly used as the first-line treatment for pediatric patients with status epilepticus (SE); some earlier studies have indicated the safety of lorazepam over diazepam, and one study suggested that the use of IV lorazepam (0.1 mg/kg) is as safe and efficacious as IV diazepam (0.2 mg/kg) in pediatric patients with SE.[95]

Remimazolam

Remimazolam is a new benzodiazepine; it is a nonselective GABA-alpha agonist with high affinity to its receptor.[96-99] Remimazolam has no known off-target activities. Remimazolam structure is similar to midazolam (the parent compound) with the addition of the carboxylic ester linkage, which incorporates into it a pharmacokinetic profile similar to that of remifentanil.[100]

Remimazolam is an ester-based medication that is metabolized by rapid hydrolysis in the blood by nonspecific tissue esterases.[96,97,99] The product is an inactive metabolite (CNS 7054), which is a carboxylic acid, with very low affinity to the GABA-alpha receptor (more than 300 times lower affinity compared to remimazolam).[97,101] As a result, remimazolam provides a rapid onset of sedation, a short predictable sedation period, and a faster recovery in comparison to other benzodiazepines.[96-101] In one study of healthy adults, remimazolam reached its peak effect in 3 minutes. The duration and depth of sedation are dose dependant; greater sedation but quick recovery was noticed when using 0.075 to 0.2 mg/kg doses of remimazolam compared to a 0.075 mg/kg dose of midazolam in healthy adults.[97] Remimazolam has a rapid clearance (mean clearance of 73.3 ± 13.9L/h)[97,100] and a mean steady state volume of distribution of 34.8 ± 9.4L.[97]

Because of its dose-independent hydrolysis, its metabolism tends to follow first-order kinetics. There is no accumulation reported or anticipated in the recommended doses. This organ-independent elimination suggests the safety of using remimazolam in continuous IV infusion, with no anticipated residual sedative effects if high doses or prolonged infusions are needed.[97,99]

With these unique characteristics, remimazolam would be considered for use in procedural sedation (eg, upper and lower gastrointestinal endoscopies)[96-99] as IV continuous infusion or multiple boluses.[97-99] The hydrolysis to inactive metabolite (CNS 7054) will allow for fast recovery with potential positive implications on patient satisfaction and early discharge. Remimazolam would also be considered for ICU sedation and premedication, especially in children before procedures or transportation to the operating room.

Similar to other benzodiazepines, remimazolam effects can be reversed by flumazenil.[97] Remimazolam has not yet been released to the market; there are undergoing phase II trials to evaluate its safety and efficiency, after its preliminary testing in humans showed favorable outcomes.[98]

The metabolisms of different BZDs are intertwined with each other. Most of the agents require an oxidative process first with potentially active compounds before glucuronidation and excretion. The pharmacokinetics for different BZDs is shown in Table 134.9.

Tolerance for and Dependence on Benzodiazepines

Tolerance for and dependence on BZDs can occur as with opiates in the PICU.[102] This effect is not all due to receptor number downregulation.[103] Withdrawal symptoms may be avoided with a slow taper of the medication of 10% per day or by substituting a long-acting oral agent such as diazepam. Acute withdrawal symptoms may include anxiety, insomnia, nightmares, seizures, psychosis, and hyperpyrexia. A postmidazolam infusion phenomenon has been described that includes poor social interaction, decreased eye contact, and a decreased interest in the surroundings. The patient may exhibit choreoathetotic movements with dystonic posturing that can persist for 2 to 4 weeks but will resolve with no sequelae. As would have been anticipated, the longer the duration and the higher the cumulative dose of benzodiazepines, the higher the chance that withdrawal symptoms will occur.

Flumazenil

Flumazenil is an imidazobenzodiazepine and is a specific competitive antagonist of the BZD receptor. It has no effect on other drugs such as barbiturates, ethanol, or other GABA-mimetic agents. Flumazenil reverses the hypnotic and sedative effects of BZDs. It has a half-life of approximately 1 hour after a single IV bolus. In patients with hepatic impairment, its half-life and clearance are prolonged, and a significant increase (>50%) of free drug occurs because of reduced plasma protein binding. Renal failure has little effect on the pharmacokinetics of flumazenil. It is indicated for the complete or partial reversal of the central sedative effects of BZDs. Contraindications include patients who have a known hypersensitivity to BZDs, patients with epilepsy who are receiving treatment with BZDs, and persons who have overdosed with a tricyclic antidepressant. The use of flumazenil is often associated with mild to moderate tachycardia and hypertension.

In cases of multiple drug overdose, the use of flumazenil remains controversial. It often is overused in the emergency setting without due concern for potential adverse reactions[104] because of the potential toxic effects (eg, cardiac arrhythmias or convulsions) of other psychotropic drugs ingested. The toxicity of tricyclic antidepressants becomes apparent as the effects of BZDs are antagonized. Patients should be evaluated for the signs and symptoms of a tricyclic antidepressant overdose; an electrocardiogram (ECG) may be helpful in determining the risks involved.

The dosing information for pediatric patients is limited. The initial suggested dose is 0.01 mg/kg (maximum, 0.2 mg) with incremental doses of 0.005 to 0.01 mg/kg (maximum, 0.2 mg) given every minute up to a maximum cumulative dose of 1 mg. The lower doses are suggested for sedation reversal and the higher doses for BZD overdose. Infusions at 0.05 to 0.1 mg/kg/h have been used.[105] The use of flumazenil in sedated patients in the ICU should be tempered by the potential for an unrecognized BZD dependence, which would

increase the risks of adverse effects. If its use is required, then a carefully titrated dose would be appropriate. The half-life of flumazenil is much shorter than that of some of the BZDs it may be counteracting (see Table 134.9). The use of an infusion may be necessary because re-sedation has been reported after single-bolus use.[106] However, this requirement should not preclude the use of flumazenil in an ICU setting.[107] Flumazenil has been used for the reversal of moderate sedation. The onset is usually within 1 to 2 minutes, with an expected peak effect at 6 to 10 minutes after IV injection[108]; both the plasma concentration of benzodiazepines and the flumazenil IV dose determine the duration of drug reversal. In the pediatric population, although it was well tolerated, it was not shown to significantly reduce recovery time.[109] Because flumazenil has a limited duration with the potential for re-sedation after discharge from medical care, an appropriate period of observation is required before discharge. A study in which researchers monitored the effects of flumazenil after sedation indicated that some of the residual effects of midazolam were still present after reversal.[110] Flumazenil also has been used to treat a paradoxical midazolam reaction[111] and has been shown to be effective in the management of hepatic encephalopathy or hyperammoneamia.[112] A Cochrane Collaboration review of articles pertaining to flumazenil use demonstrated a short-term improvement in hepatic encephalopathy. However, no improvement in recovery or survival was documented. No serious adverse effects were noted.

Chloral Hydrate

Chloral hydrate is a widely used oral hypnotic/sedative agent. It has been used for sedation in radiographic procedures, EEGs, and many health care locations. It was first synthesized in 1832 and used in 1869 as a hypnotic agent. Shortly after, reports of acute and chronic toxicity were published.[113] In 1910 it was labeled as the most dangerous of hypnotics, even though heroin and opium were in common use at that time. The addition of ethanol potentiates its effect (street name "Mickey Finn"). It has been used to control agitation in the intensive care nursery and to treat sleep difficulties in older patients.

Chloral hydrate is rapidly and completely absorbed from the GI tract and is immediately converted into the active component, trichloroethanol (TCE), by alcohol dehydrogenase.[114] The plasma levels peaks at 30 to 60 minutes. TCE is 45% protein bound. TCE undergoes glucuronidation with some oxidation to trichloroacetate (TCA). The half-life of TCE is 8 to 12 hours, whereas that of TCA is 67 hours. In infants and neonates this may be increased by a magnitude of three to four. With multiple dosing, a significant potential exists for accumulation. TCA can displace bound bilirubin from albumin. Its actions include CNS depression with drowsiness and sleep in less than an hour. With an overdose, the patient falls into a deep stupor or coma, and the pupils change from contracted to dilated. At therapeutic levels, the blood pressure and respiratory rate are unaffected. Chloral hydrate has little hangover effect. It has several effects on the cardiovascular system including decreased myocardial contractility, a shortened refractory period, and an increased sensitivity of the heart to catecholamines. It also has effects on mucous membranes. Irritation can cause gastritis, nausea, and vomiting. With overdose, a severe hemorrhagic gastritis with gastric necrosis and esophagitis has been described. Chloral hydrate and ethanol interfere with one another's metabolism through competition for alcohol dehydrogenase. Also, ethanol inhibits the conjugation of TCE, and TCE inhibits the oxidation of ethanol. Coumadin activity may be increased by chloral hydrate. Chloral hydrate is synergistic with other sedative agents. In children receiving amphetamine-based medication, chloral hydrate is contraindicated because there have been rare reports of arrhythmias. The reversal of chloral hydrate with flumazenil has been described; however, a report of ventricular tachycardia with this combination also has been made.

Chloral hydrate is available as capsules, syrup (50 mg/mL), and suppositories. The sedative dose is 25 to 50 mg/kg (PO/by way of the rectum), whereas up to 100 mg/kg can be safely used in children younger than 5 years with a maximum dose of 1 g. Because of an increased half-life, neonatal dosing should be lower (25 mg/kg). In preterm babies, toxicity resulted when chloral hydrate was used for 3 days; in term babies, toxicity resulted when it was used for 7 days. The therapeutic level for TCE is 2 to 12 µg/L; toxicity occurs when the level is more than 25 µg/L. Chloral hydrate provides successful moderate sedation in approximately 90% of patients, but it appears to be less effective in patients older than 2 years. A higher risk of failure with excessive effect can be seen in patients with a history of obstructive sleep apnea or encephalopathy.

Signs of toxicity are usually noted within 3 hours of dosing. Paradoxical excitement also has been described in 6% of patients. There is some evidence that chloral hydrate may be genotoxic and carcinogenic. Mice studies have shown that a single-dose exposure can result in an increased risk of hepatic carcinomas and adenomas.[115] Chloral hydrate overdose produces a clinical picture that is similar to acute barbiturate poisoning. Ataxia, lethargy, and coma occur within 1 to 2 hours. Also, a pearlike odor may be noted. Cardiovascular instability poses the main threat to life. Severe arrhythmias including atrial fibrillation, supraventricular tachyarrhythmia, ventricular tachyarrhythmia, torsades de pointes, and ventricular fibrillation have been described. Chronic use can cause a dependence syndrome. Also, chloral hydrate is not detectable in the blood. TCE levels are measurable, but they are not useful for clinical management, although they can be helpful for retrospective diagnosis. The management of toxicity includes evaluation and monitoring at a medical facility if an amount greater than 50 mg/kg or an unknown amount has been ingested. Two capsules may cause significant toxicity in a toddler, so there is little room for error in the history. Charcoal with intubation should be considered if significant toxicity is suspected. Standard antiarrhythmic management is often unsuccessful, although esmolol, overdrive pacing, and hemoperfusion have been tried.

Other Agents for Sedation of the Pediatric Intensive Care Unit Patient

Butyrophenones and Phenothiazines

Haloperidol

Butyrophenones belong to the group of major tranquilizers. Haloperidol is a potent antipsychotic agent with nonspecific dopamine antagonist action. It has little effect on the cardiovascular or respiratory systems. It produces the appearance of calm with minimal hypnotic effect and reduces operant behavior (purposeful movement). The patient appears tranquil and dissociated from surroundings but is readily accessible if spoken to. Haloperidol may mask actual feelings of mental restlessness. It is a potent antiemetic agent (with action at the chemotrigger zone) and has no appreciable effect on the EEG. It potentiates analgesics and other sedative agents. Compared with less potent butyrophenones, it has fewer adverse effects. Neuroleptanalgesia, a dissociative form of anesthesia, can be induced when haloperidol is combined with high-dose opiates. This anesthetic state is useful for certain cardiac and neurosurgical procedures that require cardiovascular stability and a responsive patient. It is metabolized to inactive compounds with a half-life of 15 to 25 hours. It is highly protein bound. Hepatic dysfunction increases the half-life because of reduced clearance. Adverse effects include extrapyramidal signs, although acute dystonia is rare. Prolongation of the QT interval is possible with the subsequent risk of ventricular tachycardia.[116] Hepatic toxicity can occur but is rare. Haloperidol is indicated for the treatment of psychoses, Tourette disorder, and severe behavioral problems in children. In the PICU it is used as a treatment for agitation in patients who are often unresponsive to other more commonly used agents. It also has proved to be effective as part of a sedative withdrawal strategy. Haloperidol is available as syrup, tablets, and an IM preparation. The usual dosage for agitation in children younger than 3 years is 0.01 to 0.03 mg/kg every 4 hours. The maximum daily dose is 0.15 mg/kg/day. Two IM preparations are available: The lactate is for repeated use, and the decanoate is a slow-release monthly formulation. Although not approved by the FDA, the IM lactate form has been given intravenously without problems.

Droperidol

Droperidol is faster acting than haloperidol with a shorter duration of action and a half-life of 2 hours. It is available as an approved IV formulation. With an IV bolus, mild hypotension occurs because of mild α-adrenergic receptor blockade. Droperidol is more sedating than haloperidol and may be used as a sedation adjunct to general anesthesia. It also is used in low doses (0.05 mg/kg) as an antiemetic agent. Concerns exist about the potential for droperidol to cause prolongation of the QT interval and result in ventricular tachycardia.[117]

Chlorpromazine

Chlorpromazine is a weaker antipsychotic agent with general CNS depressant activity. It has an antidopaminergic effect including extrapyramidal adverse effects, lethargy, and apathy with an EEG similar to that of normal sleep. It also causes a decrease in the body's ability to maintain temperature control, shivering is reduced, and it can be useful in patients in hypothermic-induced states. Cardiovascular effects include α-adrenergic receptor blockade with hypotension and postural hypotension, but no effect is seen on the ECG. Respiratory drive and depth are unaffected; however, some dryness of the mucosa may be noted. In the GI tract, its anticholinergic effect causes a decrease in secretions and motility. Liver effects include jaundice, which occurs in 0.5% (recurrence rate, 40%), independent of dose or duration of therapy, and it is associated with a rash, fever, and eosinophilia. This syndrome has a low mortality rate and usually resolves quickly upon discontinuation of chlorpromazine. Other effects include antihistamine-like action; local analgesia; a temporary leukopenia; and, rarely, agranulocytosis. Chlorpromazine also has antiemetic properties. Indications include premedication, sedation as part of the lytic cocktail catheterization mixture number 3 (CM3),[118] intractable pain, antipsychosis, treatment of hiccoughs, prevention of succinylcholine pain, and induction of hypothermia (with other active measures). Dosing (0.05–1 mg/kg every 6 hours) may be via the PO, IM, IV, or rectal routes. Chlorpromazine is metabolized both in the gut wall and by the liver. It yields more than 50 metabolites, most of which are inactive.

Other phenothiazine derivatives include prochlorperazine, which has mainly antiemetic properties. Extrapyramidal adverse effects are more common in children younger than 5 years. Dosage is a PO or rectal dose of 0.4 mg/kg every 8 hours and an IM or IV dose of 0.15 mg/kg.

Lytic Cocktail

The lytic cocktail (CM3) is a mixture of 25 mg/mL of meperidine, 6.5 mg/mL of promethazine, and 6.5 mg/mL of chlorpromazine. Its recommended dose is 0.1 mL/kg of body weight, but significant institutional variations exist. The CM3 was popular as sedation for cardiac catheterization. However, CM3 has been reported to have a high failure rate and lacks several important characteristics of an ideal sedative for children. Dosing cannot be titrated easily and individually. Onset of action is delayed (30 minutes), and duration of effect is protracted (5 to 20 hours). CM3 has no anxiolytic or amnestic properties. Additional caution should also be exercised when this cocktail is used in children with seizure disorders. The metabolite of meperidine and the lowered seizure threshold from the chlorpromazine put the patient at risk. Patients with congenital heart disease with physiologic conditions such as a tetralogy of Fallot or left ventricular outflow obstruction may be put at risk because of systemic vasodilation that causes altered blood flow through shunts, a hypercyanotic spell, or decreased coronary blood flow due to diastolic hypotension.

Neuroleptic Malignant Syndrome

Both the butyrophenones and the phenothiazines have a rare but well-described adverse effect called the neuroleptic malignant syndrome. It is a cluster of adverse effects of antipsychotic medications first described in 1968. It involves the development of hypertonicity with autonomic instability, fever, and cognitive disturbance. The incidence is 0.5% to 1.4% of patients exposed to neuroleptic agents. The true incidence in children is unknown, however. Several different diagnostic criteria are available. Fever and rigidity present in all cases; other symptoms are shown in Box 134.2. A variety of therapies have been described (Table 134.10).

Baclofen

Baclofen is a p-chlorophenol derivative of the GABA analog that has specific agonist activity at the $GABA_B$ receptor. It has a half-life of 2 to 6 hours. Baclofen has inhibitory effects on the brain and spinal cord. At the spinal cord level it suppresses spinal reflexes to result in muscle relaxation. It is widely used as a skeletal muscle relaxant in patients with spasticity, such as cerebral palsy, spinal cord injury, and multiple sclerosis. It is most frequently given PO. Adverse effects include urinary retention, sedation, bradycardia, hypotension, respiratory

BOX 134.2	Signs and Symptoms of Neuroleptic Malignant Syndrome

Elevated creatine phosphokinase (97%)
Tachycardia (75%)
Altered consciousness (75%)
Tachypnea
Hypertension
Diaphoresis
Leucocytosis

TABLE 134.10	Treatment Described in the Case Reports of Neuroleptic Malignant Syndrome						
	Supportive Treatment	Neuroleptics Discontinued	Anticholinergics/Amantadine	Bromocriptine	Dantrolene	L-dopa	ECT
Frequency[a]	35	50	17	18	19	8	9
Total (N)[b]	55	55	48	57	58	58	59
Percent	63.6	90.9	35.4	31.6	32.8	13.8	15.3
Sequelae (n)	7	15	3	7	5	3	4
Deaths (n)	2	3	0	0	1	1	0
Duration of NMS[c]							
Median	12	12.5	14	13	15	32	19.5
Mean	14.9	19.2	19.9	25.7	21.3	35	24.1
(SD)	(14.8)	(21.6)	(29.3)	(29.5)	(17.9)	(20.3)	(22.2)
NMS Severity Score							
Median	8	7	7.5	7	—	—	—
Mean	7.2	6.8	7.1	7.6	–.6	7.4	5.6
(SD)	(2.1)	(2.1)	(2.5)	(1.3)	(1.4)	(2.1)	(2.1)

[a]Number of reports in which the treatment was administered.
[b]Number of reports in which the treatment was mentioned.
[c]Duration in days.
ECT, electroconvulsive therapy; NMS, neuroleptic malignant syndrome; SD, standard deviation.

depression, and apnea. Weakness may limit patient compliance. These side effects are sedative-like characteristics of the drug, which are not useful in clinical practice. Therefore abrupt cessation of long-term baclofen therapy resembles, in part, short-term sedative withdrawal.

Intrathecal baclofen (ITB) has been used with increasing frequency in children to treat spasticity. ITB was first introduced in 1984[119] with a pump delivery system that was available in 1992 for adults. This system allows delivery of the drug to the spinal cord and reduces the dose significantly (1% of oral requirements), limiting systemic adverse effects.[120] Baclofen inhibits the release of serotonin in the brain stem. After long-term use there is accommodation of the serotonin pathways to this long-term inhibition that is consistent with the usually observed increasing doses required for ITB during the first 12 to 18 months of treatment. When this inhibition is abruptly removed, sudden excess release of serotonin occurs. Acute overload of serotonin transmission, such as an overdose of serotonin reuptake inhibitors, can result in confusion, hyperthermia, myoclonus, and autonomic instability. It also has anticholinergic and antihistamine effects that may result in drowsiness; paradoxical excitation has been reported in children. More than 25 case reports[121] of ITB withdrawal have now been reported. ITB withdrawal seems to be more severe if the ITB treatment was for more than 1 year. A review of ITB pumps in 100 patients at a single center[122] has shown that problems with the delivery system are fairly common. Twenty-four percent of patients experienced a problem, with a follow-up period for a maximum of 5.6 years. An average of two problems per patient was reported. Disconnection of the catheter from the implanted pump was the most common problem. Access ports on the pump seemed to increase the risk of problems (16% compared with a 2% disconnection rate); however, these ports make troubleshooting easier. Causes of difficulty with ITB delivery are shown in Box 134.3.

The ITB withdrawal syndrome is interesting because it appears to have many similarities with the neuroleptic malignant syndrome. Prolonged muscle contraction caused by rebound spasticity results in thermogenesis, hyperthermia, and rhabdomyolysis.[123] Patients with ITB withdrawal often are managed initially with broad-spectrum antibiotics as if they have sepsis and multisystem organ failure, with no improvement in the clinical situation.[124] This treatment delays the diagnosis of ITB withdrawal. The differential diagnosis of the hypermetabolic state is listed in Box 134.4. The symptoms of ITB withdrawal can be classified into three categories (Table 134.11). Often the first clinical signs are the development of itching and some increase in spasticity. If replacement baclofen is not given, then the symptoms may progress to a severe hypermetabolic state that can be fatal if the cause is not recognized and treated. Of 27 patients reported to the FDA, 6 deaths were documented.[125] The management of ITB withdrawal requires early diagnosis. It involves supportive ICU care and the onset of baclofen replacement therapy as soon as possible. Box 134.5 provides a guideline for evaluating patients with suspected baclofen withdrawal. A definitive diagnosis may be obtained with measurement of cerebrospinal fluid baclofen levels, but the results probably are not going to be available in the time course of treatment initiation. Although the primary aim should be to replace baclofen, rapid replacement of ITB may not be possible. The required oral baclofen replacement dose may be 50 to 100 times the intrathecal dose, and patients do not tolerate this dose very well because of adverse effects. IV administration of a BZD should be the initial step in the treatment of baclofen withdrawal. Dantrolene has been used as an adjunct therapy for the increased spasticity.

The use of the potent serotonin antagonist cyproheptadine has been proposed as an alternative treatment adjunct.[126] It improved fever, spasticity, and itching in adult patients with gout who had ITB withdrawal. Dosages of cyproheptadine were in the range of 0.25 mg/kg/day every 6 hours, either PO or IM. In some patients the ITB withdrawal is an elective management problem due to pump removal for infection. In these patients, if a replacement pump cannot be placed, the

---

TABLE 134.11 Severity of Intrathecal Baclofen Withdrawal

Designation	Description
Mild	Pruritic symptoms and increased spasticity
Moderate	High fever, altered mental status, seizures and profound rigidity, autonomic instability
Severe	Rhabdomyolysis, hepatic, renal failure, disseminated intravascular coagulation (DIC), brain injury, death

---

BOX 134.4 Differential Diagnosis of Intrathecal Baclofen Withdrawal

Autonomic dysreflexia
Neuroleptic malignant syndrome
Malignant hyperthermia
Sepsis
Status epilepticus
Toxic
Metabolic
Immune-mediated disorders

BOX 134.5 Management of Suspected Baclofen Withdrawal

Suspicion in at-risk patients
Administer antipyretics and other cooling techniques for fever
Administer benzodiazepines for seizures or spasticity
Rule out medical causes
Oral baclofen therapy
Contact patient's intrathecal baclofen pump specialist to interrogate the pump and check the reservoir
Abdominal radiographs (anteroposterior/lateral) to check for catheter integrity
Neurosurgical consultation for possible surgical exploration and repair
If catheter appears intact on plain radiographs, consider performing a contrast catheter study to check for catheter integrity
If problem is unresolved, contact manufacturer

BOX 134.3 Causes of Interrupted Intrathecal Baclofen Delivery

Pump malfunction
Pump failure
Battery failure
Infections necessitating pump removal
Catheter problems (eg, kinks, holes, tears, dislodgement, disconnection, migration)

patient needs to be observed and managed in the ICU to recognize and treat the withdrawal syndrome. The monitoring of creatine phosphokinase (CPK) levels may be helpful in managing withdrawal. In the reported cases of ITB withdrawal, CPK levels have been in the range of 1800 to more than 40,000.[127] Mild elevations in CPK (300 to 500) may be an early marker of inadequate treatment.

Cannabis

The medical use of cannabis was first described in ancient Chinese history.[128,129] The real breakthrough happened in the mid-1960s, when the psychoactive component of cannabis—Δ9-tetrahydrocannabinol (Δ9-THC)—was discovered. This led to the formulation of other synthetic analogs of Δ9-THC and the discovery of the cannabinoids' receptors CB1 and CB2.[128,130] CB1 receptors are believed to regulate the neurotransmitters at the synaptic terminals both in the central and peripheral neurons. Centrally, CB1 receptors play an important role in movement control, pain and sensory perception, appetite, emotions, and autonomic and endocrine functions. This explains cannabis use in chronic and neuropathic pain control,[129] muscle spasticity, anorexia, sleep disorder, and some complex seizure disorders like Dravet syndrome, Doose syndrome, and Lennox-Gastaut syndrome. In a study investigating the use of cannabidiol-enriched cannabis in pediatric patients with treatment-resistant epilepsy, 84% of patients were reported to have reduction or complete cessation of seizure activity while taking cannabis. More than two-thirds of the subjects were reported to have better mood, increased alertness, and better sleep.[131] These patients are frequently seen in the pediatric intensive care units for status epilepticus or breakthrough seizures; the use of cannabis in these patients may potentially reduce the need for frequent hospitalization and thus reduce the risk of all of the possible adverse events that could be related to the critical care environment.[132]

Peripherally, CB1 receptors have been identified in the gastrointestinal (GI) tract (intestine and liver), adipose tissue, and skeletal muscles. Cannabis has been used to control nausea in cancerous and noncancerous patients.[133] The presence of CB1 receptors in the GI tract and its promising use for antiemesis could suggest the use of cannabis in the treatment of some GI diseases like irritable bowel syndrome.

CB2 receptors are localized mainly in the immune system. They can be vital in cytokine-release regulation, inflammatory, and pain responses.[128]

Medical use of cannabis is legal in Canada and some US states. Further research is needed to understand the mechanism of actions of Δ9-THC and the nonpsychoactive compound, cannabidiol, and their interaction for optimizing potential therapy with the least adverse effects.

Dexmedetomidine

Dexmedetomidine (Precedex) is a selective α_2-adrenergic agonist. It has an effect at receptors in the CNS and peripheral nervous system, as well as in autonomic ganglia. Stimulation of the α_2 receptor decreases the release of norepinephrine, inhibits sympathetic activity, and produces sedation, anxiolysis, and analgesia. It is 1600 times more active at the α_2 receptor than at the α_1 receptor and is thus eight times more selective

than clonidine. Clonidine has been reported as a sedative in the PICU.[134] Clonidine given enterally 5 mg/kg 4 times day was compared to placebo in 50 children. There was no difference in the opiate requirement, benzodiazepine requirement, sedation scores, or withdrawal between the placebo group and the clonidine. In this small study it is not clear if the clonidine dose was sufficient; further studies are required. In adults it has a redistribution phase of 6 minutes and an elimination half-life of 2 hours. The pharmacokinetics appears to be similar in the pediatric patient, even after a 24-hour infusion.[135] It is almost completely metabolized in the liver by glucuronidation and P-450 pathways to inactive metabolites. In patients with renal failure, the pharmacokinetics did not show any prolongation of the terminal half-life; however, these patients were sedated for longer after the infusion was terminated compared with the control group.[136] The prolonged sedation may be related to reduced protein binding of this normally highly protein-bound drug (94%) and thus higher free drug levels in the patient with renal failure. In patients with hepatic dysfunction, reduced clearance has been reported. With patients in severe hepatic failure, extension of the half-life to almost three times longer than normal was reported.[137]

Dexmedetomidine has proved to be effective for sedation in the adult intensive care setting.[138] Currently it is only licensed for 24 hours of sedation, although approval for more prolonged use is pending. The recommended dosage for dexmedetomidine is a loading dose of 1 μg/kg over 10 minutes followed by an infusion of 0.2 to 0.7 μg/kg/h. It appears that in pediatric patients, the higher end of the dose range is required. Doses higher than 1.5 μg/kg/h have not been shown to provide any further sedative action. Advantages of dexmedetomidine include minimal respiratory depression and predictable hemodynamic effects. Because of the reduced sympathetic activity, blood pressure and heart rate fall slightly. Clinical sedation trials have shown a decrease in heart rate of 7% and blood pressure by 10%. It has been infused before, during, and after the extubation process. Hypotension and bradycardia are more likely to occur during the loading phase, which may need to be prolonged or interrupted. Dexmedetomidine cannot be given by rapid IV bolus because severe bradycardia as well as hypertension may occur as a result of direct stimulation of α_1-adrenergic receptors. Mild transient hypertension is sometimes noted in adults during the loading phase, although this effect was not noticed in pediatric patients. Long-term use of dexmedetomidine (160 hours) also has now been reported,[139] with no evidence of accumulation. The concern about rebound hypertension after long-term α_2-adrenergic agonist treatment, such as that occurring with clonidine, has not been reported. The prolonged use of dexmedetomidine is now common, and as such there is now growing evidence that withdrawal from dexmedetomidine must be considered.[140,141] Agitation, tremor, and sleep disturbances have been reported; however, many of the patients had received other sedative agents. It appears prudent to either wean the dexmedetomidine slowly if the infusion has lasted 4 days or more or else substitute a small dose of oral clonidine or the clonidine patch (harder to wean dose). It is possible to extubate on a lower dose of dexmedetomidine, which may reduce postextubation agitation and allow the wean to be completed during the child's ICU stay.

Sedation from dexmedetomidine often results in a patient who is tranquil yet easily aroused. Reduced analgesic requirements have been reported with its use. The easy arousal may make it a useful agent for when repeat neurologic examinations are required. Several articles concerning the use of dexmedetomidine in the PICU have been published. In a retrospective review of 121 patients from a mixed medical and surgical population in the PICU, a decrease of 20% in the dose of BZD or opiates was documented in 80% of the children who received dexmedetomidine.[142] Bradycardia (12%) and hypotension (16%) requiring intervention was described. In burn patients,[143] the overall quality of sedation was improved by the addition of dexmedetomidine; many patients also were able to be weaned from other sedatives during the dexmedetomidine infusion; loading doses were avoided to reduce the risk of cardiac complications. Dexmedetomidine use in pediatric cardiac ICU is gaining popularity. A retrospective review of dexmedetomidine use (infused >36 hours) in 35 postoperative pediatric cardiac patients did not show any significant changes in cardiovascular parameters, but a reduction in the postoperative opiate requirements occurred with an equivalent level of sedation.[144] Another study demonstrated less delirium in the postoperative cardiac child receiving dexmedetomidine.[145] Many of these patients had pulmonary hypertension and there appeared to be no concerns with the use of dexmedetomidine. Dexmedetomidine also appears to have antiarrhythmic effects that can treat and prevent arrhythmias in children. Its use postoperatively has been shown to reduce the incidence of postoperative cardiac arrhythmias.[146]

Further studies are still required to address questions regarding the metabolism, efficacy, and adverse effects of dexmedetomidine in the PICU population. This agent also has been safely used for a variety of noninvasive sedation procedures such as magnetic resonance imaging (MRI), and several cases have been reported of its use as an adjunct to general anesthesia for pediatric patients. It appears to be a useful agent in the management of opiate withdrawal. Furthermore, dexmedetomidine is useful for patients who are difficult to sedate, for the treatment of postoperative shivering, and for postanesthesia agitation. Procedural sedation with intranasal (IN) dexmedetomidine also has been reported (dexmedetomidine, 2 µg/kg IN, along with IN sufentanil, 1 µg/kg). Twenty children sedated with IN dexmedetomidine underwent dental restorative treatment without any complications. Sedation onset took approximately 45 minutes with a recovery time of about 1 hour.

Dexmedetomidine is not without adverse effects. It is contraindicated in patients with heart block, and bradycardia has been reported in an infant treated with digoxin who received dexmedetomidine during the infusion phase.[147] It also would appear prudent to avoid its use with other drugs that can reduce arteriovenous node function such as β-blockers and calcium channel blockers, as well as with patients who have severe ventricular dysfunction or hypovolemia, because reduction in sympathetic tone may cause a profound decrease in blood pressure. There are now several reports on the use of dexmedetomidine for toxidromes such as anticholinergic syndrome[148] as well as baclofen withdrawal in the PICU.[149]

Propofol

Propofol is a rapid-acting IV anesthetic agent. As a highly lipid-soluble 2,6-diisopropylphenol, it is an oil and is insoluble in water. It is formulated as a 1% aqueous emulsion (1.2%

TABLE 134.12	Pharmacokinetics of Intravenous Anesthetic Agents			
Drug	Elimination Half-Life (hr)	Volume Distribution (SS) (L/kg)	Clearance (mL/kg/min)	Protein Binding (%)
Etomidate	2.9	2.52	17.9	76.9
Ketamine	3.1	3.1	19.1	12
Propofol	1.9	2.3	30	96.8

SS, steady state.

egg phosphatide, 10% soybean oil, 2.25% glycerol) with a propofol concentration of 10 mg/mL. Recovery from propofol is rapid because of its short redistribution half-life (α), and it is rapidly cleared by hepatic metabolism in healthy patients after short infusions, making it ideal for short procedures. The elimination half-life is 2 hours (Table 134.12), but the half-life is context sensitive and has been reported to be between 1 and 3 days after a 10-day infusion because of significant body accumulation. The kinetics follows a three-compartment model. The dose for induction of anesthesia in children is 2.5 mg/kg to 3.5 mg/kg; higher doses are required for infants and toddlers. Anesthesia also can be maintained by an infusion. The depth of sedation/anesthesia can be easily titrated, and an infusion rate of 25 to 150 µg/kg/min usually provides adequate sedation.

As with most sedative agents, propofol has adverse effects that may be a concern for the intensivist. It often causes hypotension in the sick child, and in patients dependent on high sympathetic tone to maintain normal blood pressure, even small doses of propofol may significantly decrease blood pressure. The hypotension is mainly caused by vasodilatation, and there is little direct myocardial depressant. Bradycardia also can occur upon the induction of anesthesia. Propofol increases atrial conduction time for neonatal rabbits and prolongs the refractory period. Propofol anesthesia can prevent the induction of known atrial tachycardias in the electrophysiology laboratory, and cases have been reported of conversion of atrial tachycardia to sinus rhythm upon induction of propofol anesthesia. Propofol is a potent respiratory depressant, and it has a useful depressant effect on airway reflexes, which may facilitate endotracheal intubation. The injection of propofol often causes pain, and in the alert patient, strategies to minimize this effect are useful. Most commonly, lidocaine, either mixed with the propofol or injected before the injection of propofol, will markedly reduce the pain.

Propofol sedation in the ICU has several advantages. It acts rapidly and produces an easily controllable level of sedation. Unlike the barbiturates, it provides rapid clinical recovery, even after prolonged infusion. It has antiemetic properties and can provide transient deep sedation if required for procedures. It also has been shown to facilitate sedative synergy with BZDs.[150] In the adult ICU population, propofol has been compared with midazolam for long-term sedation. Both agents provide good sedation, but propofol has the advantage of being more titratable with a faster recovery.[151] Despite the increased drug cost, the use of propofol can reduce overall ICU costs because of a reduction in ventilator weaning time.[152]

Propofol has been used in the ICU as an anticonvulsant for patients with refractory status epilepticus.[153] In a comparison with pentobarbital to provide burst suppression, both drugs were equally effective. Propofol was much more rapid in effect; no difference was found in outcome or ICU support measurements or length of stay.[154] In patients with raised ICP, propofol has the same effects on ICP and cerebral blood flow (CBF) and cerebral metabolic rate of oxygen as barbiturates. It also requires a similar level of hemodynamic support to maintain appropriate blood pressure and cerebral perfusion pressure (CPP). It can produce the same degree of burst suppression that may be required for uncontrolled intracranial hypertension. It also allows rapid changes in the level of sedation, to facilitate neurologic examination. In this regard it is a superior agent. As described later, however, the use of large doses of propofol in the ICU setting may be associated with worsened outcomes.

Special Issue Regarding Long-Term Infusion of Propofol

Several important problems may occur when propofol is used in the PICU. With long-term propofol infusions, a significant amount of lipid may be infused into the patient, with the same consequences as lipid infusions used for hyperalimentation. Hyperlipidemia and triglyceridemia have been reported in up to 10% of patients receiving propofol in the ICU. Pseudohyponatremia or the inability to do routine plasma electrolyte analysis has been described. It is important that the propofol calorie (20 mL/h = 528 kcal/day)[155] and lipid load be included in the patient's nutrition plan. It may be necessary to reduce enteral feeds or avoid intralipids in selected patients. With high propofol dosing, respiratory acidosis has been reported.[156] The emulsion used for propofol administration is an excellent culture medium at room temperature; cases have been reported of patients with systemic infection caused by propofol during operative procedures.[157] This infection is due to poor aseptic technique in the preparation and use of the propofol syringes and infusion lines. Unusual infective organisms were detected in several patients, and an epidemiologic study by the Centers for Disease Control and Prevention found propofol to be the common element.[158] Certain precautions should be followed when propofol is used in the PICU. The staff should be educated to the potential dangers of infection from propofol. The ampule neck should be wiped with alcohol. There are no multidose vials of propofol. Syringes should be disposed of when they are more than 6 hours old, and lines should be changed every 12 hours. Filters are available that can remove many of the potential pathogens, and they are compatible with the lipid-based propofol infusion.

A few episodes of allergy to propofol have been reported; immune reactions, both anaphylactic and anaphylactoid types, are estimated at 1:45,000.[159] Although clinically indistinguishable, the anaphylactic response involves prior exposure to a component of the propofol suspension. Egg allergy has been considered a contraindication to its use. However, the egg phosphatide component found in propofol is not related to the major egg allergen protein ovalbumin.[160] In fact, intradermal testing with propofol in 25 patients allergic to eggs was negative; therefore current evidence suggests that anaphylaxis is not more likely to develop in patients who are allergic to eggs when they are exposed to propofol. Propofol does not release histamine and is an acceptable agent for use in patients with asthma.

Several new generic formulations of propofol are available. These formulations include different antioxidants, such as metabisulfites, which may have an increased risk of allergic reaction. However, this increased risk has not been borne out.[161] They appear to be equal in efficacy and adverse effects to the propofol solution known by the brand name Diprivan. A few patients who receive propofol may have dark green urine due to phenol metabolites; this effect is not a clinical concern.[162]

A new water-soluble prodrug, fospropofol, has been approved by the FDA and is approved for sedation procedures in adult patients. The fospropofol is hydrolyzed by alkaline phosphatases to propofol, phosphate, and formaldehyde. The half-life of fospropofol is 8 minutes.[163] The onset of action of fospropofol is significantly slower than for propofol (5 minutes), which reduces the incidence of hypotension and respiratory depression. The dose is about 6.5 mg/kg as a bolus,[164] and it is not recommended for infusion. However, fospropofol requires the same standards of care as propofol.

Propofol Infusion Syndrome

One of the most important concerns is the development of a refractory metabolic acidosis in children who had received propofol sedation in the ICU. This effect was first described in 1992 as a series of five cases[165] with fatal myocardial failure in children with respiratory illnesses requiring ventilation and sedation. Five young patients from different ICUs had croup and went on to have a refractory cardiac failure, bradycardia, and acidosis. A lipemic serum had developed in all patients. They had all received propofol at an average rate of about 8 mg/kg/h for more than 70 hours.

In review, the case reports were not as simple or as complete in their reporting, with several published letters[166] from physicians involved with these patients showing incomplete data in the reporting. Several other case reports of an apparently similar clinical course were then subsequently described in the literature, which was enough evidence for the Committee on Safety of Medicines in the United Kingdom to issue a warning on propofol and its use in pediatric patients. At that time the FDA could not find a causal link between propofol and the deaths in children and did not issue a warning.

This reaction to propofol came to be known as the propofol infusion syndrome (PRIS).[167] It is the sudden or relatively sudden onset of a marked bradycardia resistant to treatment with a least one of the following signs: lipemia, enlarged liver, severe metabolic acidosis, or rhabdomyolysis. PRIS is unlikely to be due to the carrier emulsion because intralipid has been used extensively in severely ill patients without problems. The propofol metabolites are acidic, highly water soluble, and have a short half-life.

A steady number of case reports of this syndrome have appeared in the literature since the initial description, as well as a couple of studies involving several hundred patients[168,169] who have not shown any problem with propofol in the PICU. In these studies, lower doses of propofol (4 mg/kg/h) were used, with regular monitoring of the acid base status and triglyceride levels. Propofol bashing became popular.[170] Few drugs are licensed specifically for the PICU, however, and proper trials are needed to avoid drugs being condemned as hearsay. Subsequently, a randomized controlled trial of propofol was initiated, and after the use of this drug in 327 patients, it was reviewed by the FDA.[171] The study was never published, but researchers found that, despite similar pediatric risk of mortality scores, patients who had received either 1% or 2% propofol preparations had a two to three times greater risk of death compared with the control sedative group. This finding led to a letter from AstraZeneca reminding health care workers that propofol was not approved for the sedation of pediatric patients.[172]

Much debate still occurs regarding whether there is a safe infusion rate or duration of infusion for propofol in the PICU setting. It has been estimated that a study to show a significant increase in death would require 7000 patients, which would be difficult to accomplish.

PRIS has also now been described in adult patients.[173] These patients had similar cardiac and metabolic findings, often associated with the management of intracranial hypertension. PRIS appeared to be a higher risk if the 2% formulation was used. Patients with raised ICP require deeper levels of sedation and require higher doses of propofol; they also receive vasopressor support to maintain the CPP, which puts a further stress on a myocardium that is already failing.

The pathophysiologic cause of PRIS is still poorly understood, but it appears to mimic mitochondrial myopathies. Patients are generally well until stressed. Rhabdomyolysis and cardiac and hepatic failure then develop in these patients.[174] Case reports have shown some metabolic abnormalities that may be the cause of the cardiac failure and acidosis. One report describes a 10-month-old child who had the syndrome and was successfully treated with hemofiltration and plasmapheresis.[175] Muscle and liver biopsy specimens showed changes consistent with a toxic insult. Analysis also showed a reduction in the cytochrome c oxidase activity in the muscle, with a normal activity in skin fibroblasts, excluding an underlying respiratory chain defect. Profound acidosis with lactic acidosis is found in different types of genetically acquired cytochrome oxidase deficiency. It was postulated that the hemofiltration removed a water-soluble metabolite of propofol that had caused a reversible reduction in the oxidase activity. A second case report[176] also showed a metabolic abnormality. Elevated levels of malonylcarnitine and C5-acyl carnitine were found in a patient with PRIS. This patient was also treated successfully with hemofiltration. These findings are consistent with reports of impaired fatty acid oxidation due to impaired entry of long-chain fatty acids into the mitochondria and a failure of the respiratory chain. A review of the pathophysiologic function of the syndrome[177] suggested that propofol increases the activity of malonyl coenzyme A, which inhibits the carnitine palmityl transferase I, so long-chain fatty acids cannot enter the mitochondria. Propofol also uncouples oxidation, so the short- and medium-chain fatty acids cannot be used, even though they have entered the mitochondria and also may inhibit the respiratory-chain. Low energy production leads to cardiac and peripheral muscle necrosis.

In pediatric patients it has been suggested that an inadequate calorific intake coupled with a high metabolic demand requires a fully active fatty acid oxidation capacity. Propofol may inhibit this pathway and cause a cellular metabolic failure syndrome to develop. Children have lower glycogen stores and often require higher doses of sedative agents; thus the syndrome is more likely to occur in pediatric patients. A carbohydrate intake of 6 to 8 mg/kg/min should be enough to suppress fat metabolism in the critically ill child. Also, concerns have been raised about the influence of catecholamines

and steroids in the development of the syndrome, especially in the adult population.

Propofol is still frequently used for procedural and short-term sedation,[178] but in a case report, researchers described a patient who had PRIS.[179] The patient had received a propofol infusion for 15 hours at 20 mg/kg/h. After a 13-hour propofol-free period, an 8-hour infusion of propofol at 4 mg/kg/h was given, after which the patient had intractable bradycardia and acidosis. This report raises concerns about high-dose, short-term propofol use in the PICU.

In a report on the use of propofol for two cases of refractory status epilepticus, patients aged 7 and 17 years had features similar to the PRIS.[180] Status epilepticus itself can result in neurologic deficit, hypoxia, rhabdomyolysis, cardiac arrhythmias, hyperthermia, metabolic acidosis, acute renal failure, and death. However, these patients received high doses of propofol (18 to 27 mg/kg/h) to achieve burst suppression for more than 48 hours. Rhabdomyolysis and cardiac failure developed in both patients. Neither lipid status nor acid base was monitored, and practitioners with limited experience with this drug used propofol as the sole agent. In light of the reports now appearing in the adult neurointensive care literature with the development of a propofol infusion–like syndrome in adult neurosurgical patients,[181] it would appear that propofol is not the best choice for prolonged sedation for patients with intracranial hypertension. An early indicator of the cardiac instability from PRIS may be changes in the ECG. It has been reported that the development of a right bundle-branch block with convex ST elevation was an early sign of this syndrome.[182]

Propofol remains a useful agent for procedural sedation in the PICU. When compared with midazolam and ketamine, propofol resulted in safe, effective sedation. The patients sedated with propofol awakened almost twice as fast; thus the efficiency of the sedation service was also improved.[183] Propofol is also probably appropriate for overnight sedation, and higher doses should be avoided. It probably should not be used as a solo agent because in those cases tolerance appears to develop more rapidly. If its use is required for a prolonged period, then careful consideration should be given to its risks and benefits; prevention of PRIS should include adequate calorific intake. One study showed that staff members of some PICUs are still using long-term high doses despite the potential risks involved.[184]

The dose and duration of propofol should be carefully managed to minimize its use. It would appear from the reports of PRIS in the neurosurgical population that the desire for rapid awakening has propagated the use of propofol coma, rather than using barbiturates. There appears to be a significant mortality (50%) in neurosurgical patients who develop PRIS. Regular monitoring of the cardiac function, ECG, and CPK are warranted; lipid profile and acid base status may help in early detection. It has been suggested that daily CPK measurements will identify those at risk of developing PRIS and allow a change in sedation before the full-blown clinical effects become apparent.[185] When CPK >5000u was used as a screening tool, the incidence of PRIS in adult neurosurgical patients fell from 2.9% to 0.19%. Seven percent of these patients screened positive for PRIS, and their sedation was changed with no reported mortality. Although successful in this report, these steps may not necessarily prevent mortality from the syndrome.[186] Treatment should be immediate cessation of propofol. Cardiac support may be difficult because of unresponsiveness to conventional circulatory support. The use of pacing and extracorporeal membrane oxygenation has been reported. Hemodialysis or hemofiltration have been reported as having some success.

An outcome prediction table has been developed for PRIS based on more than 1000 reports from the FDA's Medwatch program, of which 20% involved pediatric patients.[187] The features associated with PRIS are shown in Table 134.13. In addition to the individual features, there were several additional scores depending on a combination of features (see Table 134.13). The predicted outcome from these scores is shown in Table 134.14. These predicted outcomes were very close to the actual reported mortality of the analyzed cohort. No independent verification exists at present. However, this article does highlight the variability in features of the PRIS and accounts for the differences in the reported mortality.

The debate as to the safety of propofol in the PICU continues. Several reports state that use for short duration at low doses has proved to be safe,[188,189] starting at a low dose 0.5 mg/kg/h and limiting the maximum dose to 4 mg/kg/h. This approach, along with an infusion duration of 12 to 48 hours, has been reported as safe. However, these are small studies, and with an incidence that is unknown, a negative occurrence in a study of 200 patients still statistically means that the rate of PRIS could be up to 1.5%,[190] consistent with the data from the neurosurgical population. This leaves the intensivist with a difficult conundrum: Do I need to use propofol, or are there suitable alternatives for my patient?

TABLE 134.13	Features Reported for Propofol Infusion Syndrome, Incidence, and Score	
Feature	**% Incidence**	**Score**
Cardiac	44	1
Hypotension	34	0
Rhabdomyolysis	27	1
Hepatic failure	24	0
Renal failure	24	1
Metabolic acidosis	20	1
Dyslipidemias	5	0
Rhabdomyolysis and hypotension		1
Age <18 years and renal failure		−1
Rhabdomyolysis and renal failure		−1

TABLE 134.14	Predicted Outcome From Propofol Infusion Syndrome
Score	**Predicted Mortality Rate (%)**
0	10
1	25
2	50
3	75
4	90

Sedation and Analgesia for Procedures

Many procedures performed on children involve pain and anxiety. In many hospitals the administration of sedation and analgesia falls to the pediatric intensive care physician.[191] The pediatric intensive care physician needs to be familiar with guidelines and protocols that are used for moderate sedation outside the ICU setting. Procedural pain accounts for most of the pain experienced by children with malignancies,[192] and many pediatric patients with trauma will require sedation for procedures such as correction in the emergency department of fractured limbs and lacerations.

Conscious sedation, now commonly called moderate sedation or more appropriately procedural sedation, is a medically controlled state of depressed consciousness whereby the patient remains responsive to verbal stimuli or, at most, a gentle shaking of the shoulder.[193] It anticipates that protective reflexes will be maintained and that the patient retains a patent airway independently. Neither airway patency nor airway protection should be taken for granted because patients with conditions such as obstructive sleep apnea may obstruct their airway with little sedation and aspiration of food can occur even without sedation. Before moderate sedation is further explored, the insightful words spoken by Burton Epstein, in his 40th Rovenstine Lecture of the American Society of Anesthesiology (ASA) in the fall of 2002, should be considered: "The myth . . . of the achievability of a state of conscious sedation in which pediatric patients are simultaneously responsive to voice stimulus while immobile in the face of pain is just that—a myth."[194] A little consideration will reveal that for painless procedures, anxiolysis will most likely suffice, whereas for painful procedures, pharmacologic elimination of the response to pain will result in a need for general anesthesia. Between these two extremes, the use of local anesthetic agents may modify the response so as to allow potentially painful procedures to be performed during moderate sedation. Another factor to consider is the effect of variation in the level of stimulation, whereby sedation titrated to effect during a painful stimulus becomes excessive once the stimulus is completed. Thus the practitioner treads on a narrow and sometimes impossible pathway when giving moderate sedation. The state of moderate sedation is part of a continuum (Table 134.15) defined by the working groups of the American Academy of Pediatrics (AAP) and the ASA,[195] which encompasses a range from anxiolysis to general anesthesia that is appropriate for surgery. This continuum is difficult to control, and staff administering moderate sedation must be able to appropriately manage any patients who enter a deeper level of sedation than that planned. The goals of sedation are shown in Box 134.6. It is helpful to think of moderate sedation as

TABLE 134.15	States of Altered Consciousness	
Designation	**Description**	
1	Minimal sedation (anxiolysis)	
2	Moderate sedation/analgesia (conscious sedation)	
3	Deep sedation/analgesia	
	General anesthesia	

BOX 134.6 Goals of Sedation

Guard the patient's safety and welfare
Minimize physical discomfort or pain
Minimize negative psychologic responses to treatment
Control behavior
Return patient to a state in which safe discharge is possible

BOX 134.7 Nonintensive Care Unit Procedures Requiring Sedation

Cardiac catheterization: diagnostic, angioplasty, stents, valvuloplasty, closure devices
Neuroradiology: angiograms, stents, embolization
Ultrasound: transesophageal echocardiography, drainage procedures
Computed tomography scan–guided abscess drainage

TABLE 134.16 Suggested Sedation Quality for Different Procedures

	Amnesia	Analgesia	Relaxation	Inattention
MRI	0	0	1	4
Endoscopy	1	3	2	2
Paracentesis	1	3	0	2
Burn dressing	2	4	0	2
Local anesthesia	3	2	2	3

MRI, magnetic resonance imaging.

BOX 134.8 Presedation Assessment

History
Medications
Allergies
Previous experience with sedation, anesthesia
Alcohol, tobacco, illicit substance abuse
Fasting

Examination
Head extension and neck flexion
Mouth opening, jaw size
Body habitus

Documentation
Informed consent
Instructions and information to responsible person

TABLE 134.17 American Society of Anesthesiology Classification

Class	Description
I	A normally healthy patient
II	A patient with a mild or well-controlled disease state
III	A patient with a severe or poorly controlled disease state
IV	A patient with a severe disease state that is a constant threat to life
V	A moribund patient who is not expected to survive without surgery

consisting of several components. A balanced sedation technique will involve amnesia, analgesia, relaxation, and inattention. Different procedures require different degrees of these components (Table 134.16).

Types of Procedures and Preprocedure Evaluation

In many instances sedation may be beneficial in the PICU, such as for the placement of central lines and centesis tubes and during dressing changes. Sedation facilitates the procedure in uncooperative patients and allows long or uncomfortable procedures to be performed. Outside the ICU, both noninvasive and invasive radiologic examinations[196,197] often require sedation (Box 134.7).

Safety with moderate sedation is largely determined by careful assessment and management of the airway, together with precautions to prevent aspiration of gastric contents. Adequacy of sedation largely depends on appropriate patient selection, the combination of the patients' known medical conditions, past sedation experience, and the nature (particularly pain) of the patients' procedures, coupled with appropriate drug selection. Moderate sedation may be better tolerated than deep sedation or general anesthesia when hemodynamic stability is compromised because many sedative and anesthesia agents induce cardiovascular instability such as vasodilation or myocardial depression. Furthermore, the ability to monitor the patient's neurologic status during the procedure through conversation or instruction may be helpful, especially during invasive neuroradiologic procedures. Moderate

sedation may allow an earlier discharge because less sedative is being used and may make the procedure, which would usually require the full operating room environment, possible outside of the operating room.

All patients should be assessed before moderate sedation. Box 134.8 lists the elements that should be included in the assessment. The medical history should include evaluation of the cardiorespiratory system, any history of gastroesophageal reflux, and any previous sedation attempt that failed or any abnormal reaction to sedation. An asthmatic attack or respiratory tract infection, poorly controlled seizure disorder, or diabetes may require a change or postponement of the sedation plan. It is recommended that patients be classified according to the ASA preoperative patient classification (Table 134.17). In most circumstances it is generally recommended that patients in ASA class VI and some in class III are not suitable for moderate sedation.

It is prudent to adopt the same guidelines that are used before general anesthesia is administered, in case sedation that is deeper than anticipated occurs. These guidelines are age dependent, and current recommendations are shown in Table 134.18. Despite this consideration, less caution is often reported regarding fasting, without any apparent worsening of outcome. For example, in a survey of 450 radiology departments, 35% had no nothing-by-mouth (NPO) status requirement for neonates, and 17% used a 2-hour NPO status requirement for infants. For oral contrast studies, most departments sedated the patient within 1 hour of the contrast being swallowed.[198] Consent should be obtained as with any medically indicated procedure or intervention. It should include discussion about the risks and benefits of the procedure and

BOX 134.9   Preparing for Moderate Sedation

Consider Airway
Assess airway
Preexisting risk factors
Trauma-induced risk factors

Circulation
Correct hypovolemia
Hypovolemia is manifest when sympathetic tone is decreased

Fasting
Time of last meal
Trauma-induced delay in gastric emptying
Drug-induced delay in gastric emptying

BOX 134.10   Causes of Sedation Complications

Drug overdose
Inadequate monitoring—during and after
Lack of appropriate skills by staff administering the sedation
Lack of appropriate pharmacology knowledge

TABLE 134.18   Presedation NPO Guidelines

	Solids/Nonclear Liquids[a]	Clear Liquids[b]
Adults	6 h	3 h
Children	6 h	3 h
Neonates (<3 mo)	4 h	2 h

[a]Milk, breast milk, pulp fruit juices.
[b]Clear fruit juices, water.
NPO, nothing by mouth.

the sedation technique, as well as expectations of outcome and alternatives to the procedure and sedation.

The presedation interview for outpatients or non-ICU patients also should involve giving instructions and information to a responsible person, including postsedation instructions, a 24-hour phone contact phone number, guidelines concerning limitations of activity, and expected postsedation behavior. If moderate sedation is provided for nonscheduled patients, a review of several aspects is important (Box 134.9).

Monitoring During the Procedure

Sedation provided outside the ICU should be performed in a facility/area with the appropriately trained support staff. The staff should have had appropriate training with respect to pharmacology, monitoring, resuscitation (basic and advanced life support), emergency drugs, and cardiac arrest protocols and medications. Advanced cardiac life support and pediatric advanced life support recommendations should be available to be followed.

Monitoring of patients undergoing moderate sedation is an important component of safe, effective sedation. Several different recommendations have been made by the Joint Commission on Accreditation of Healthcare Organizations,[199] the American Board of Anesthesiology, and the AAP. These recommendations have not yet been fully followed by persons providing sedation for children.[200] A study of pediatric dentists conducted after the AAP published its new recommendations found minimal monitoring and documentation of the sedation procedure. Obtaining baseline vital signs is important. Because of the possibility of oversedation, the level of consciousness should be assessed frequently, especially during titration of effect. This level of consciousness is best assessed with the Ramsay scale (see Table 134.1). A sedation record is important for documentation of the drugs used with times and doses and for the monitored measurements that are charted on a time-based record. Monitoring should include pulse oximetry to assess the degree of oxygenation and heart rate. The saturation should be maintained by supplemental oxygen. Breathing can be assessed either by monitoring the respiratory rate or by capnography. The blood pressure should be checked at regular intervals during the procedure. A study of 85 pediatric patients with complications after sedation showed that most severe complications resulted from a common pathway involving respiratory depression leading to respiratory arrest, cardiac arrest, and subsequent severe neurologic devastation. The most common causes for these complications are summarized in Box 134.10. There is no particular drug that is more likely to cause problems. Polypharmacy, especially with three or more drugs, has been shown to be a risk factor for pediatric sedation complications.[201] Dentists using nitrous oxide in combination with other agents appeared to have a higher incidence of problems. If long-acting drugs are used, the patient must be observed for an appropriate length of time. Several reports have been made of respiratory arrest occurring while the child was in the car seat on the way home. Any health care worker providing moderate sedation should be familiar with an emergency algorithm in case problems arise (Fig. 134.4).

Many pharmacologic options are available for moderate sedation in children. The oral route is commonly used because it has a slow onset time that avoids a rapid peak effect, but it also gives an unpredictable degree of sedation, which is not easy to titrate. The rectal route is nearly always available and has found favor in the past for barbiturate sedation. More contemporaneously, rectal diazepam at 0.2 to 0.5 mg/kg has proved useful in controlling seizures when IV access is not available.[202] Onset can be fairly slow and the duration prolonged. Intravenous sedation is considered the gold standard route: It is effective, it can be titrated to effect rapid onset, and there is a lot of experience with this method among health care providers. However, establishing an IV access in a child can be challenging, and there are many minor procedures that do not necessarily require IV sedation. The risk of inadvertent overdose is also higher using the IV approach. Intramuscular injections have been used as well,[203] but there is a delay in onset, it is painful, the practitioner will be unable to titrate to effect, and it might delay recovery; however, this method is useful in very uncooperative patients for whom IV placement is not feasible.

Intranasal drug delivery is now recognized as a useful and reliable alternative to oral and parenteral sedation. Intranasal administration of medicines for symptomatic relief, prevention, and treatment of topical nasal conditions has been widely used for a long time.

Intranasal administration of sedative medications has emerged as an alternative to oral and parenteral routes since the early 1990s.[204-206] Table 134.19 shows some of the advantages and disadvantages of IN sedation.

EMERGENCY ALGORITHM

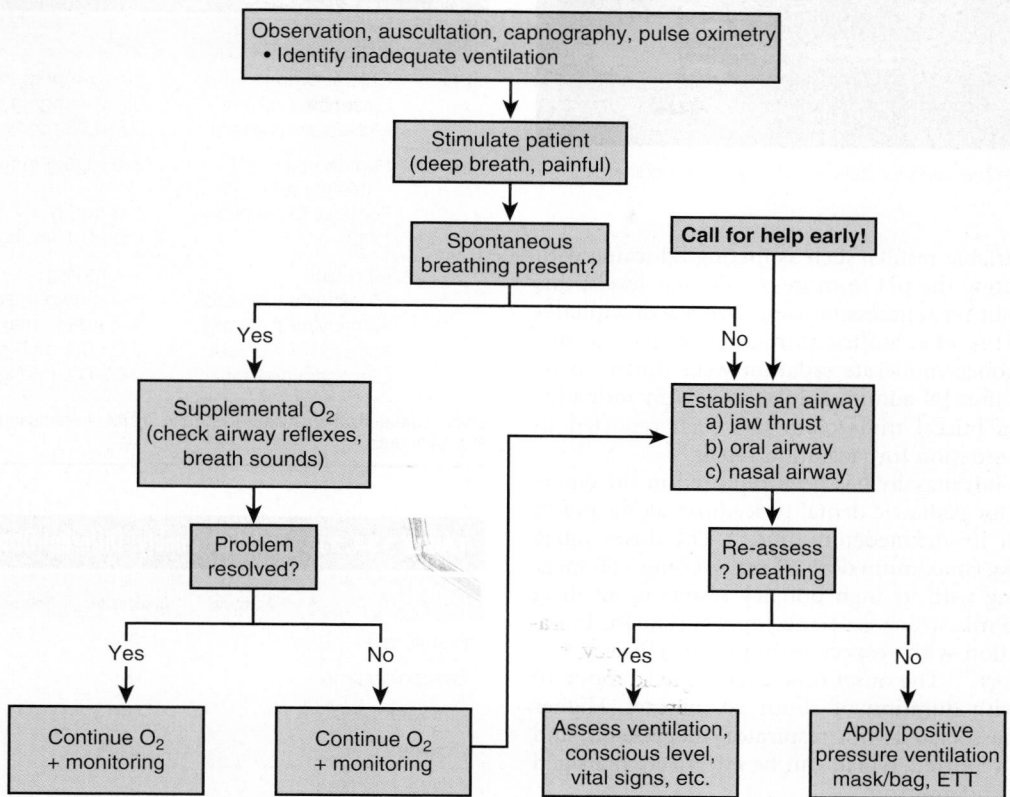

Fig. 134.4. Sedation emergency airway algorithm. *ETT*, endotracheal tube

TABLE 134.19	Intranasal Sedation Advantages and Disadvantages

Advantages	Disadvantages
Quick onset of sedation	Some diseases/processes can affect the absorption
Noninvasive and less painful than injectable routes	Medication cannot be delivered with big volume
Ease of drug delivery	Medication might be swallowed or spat out
Favorable tolerability profile	Medications must be available in a suitable concentration
Closer proximity of the nasal mucosa to the brain	
Lack of necessity for sterilization	

Certain medications benefit from intranasal administration, such as those with poor stability in gastrointestinal fluids, those with poor intestinal absorption, and those with extensive hepatic first-pass elimination, which reduces the bioavailability of the drug and leads to unpredictable blood levels after oral administration. Lipophilic medications are usually well absorbed from the nasal cavity mucosa, and often the IV formulation is used.

There are several preparation properties that can improve intranasal efficacy. A higher formulation viscosity allows for better drug absorption as a result of increased contact time between the drug and the nasal mucosa. The pK_a of the drug and the pH of the absorption site and the drug are also important. The ideal pH of the drug formulation is between 5 and 6.5; pH values less than 3 or more than 10 may cause damage or pain.

There are two methods of intranasal administration. With the drop technique, a syringe is used to slowly drop the medication into the nares of a supine child. It is the simplest method; however, it may be difficult to predict the actual dose administered due to possible swallowing or spitting out of the medication. The child may also cough or sneeze,[207] resulting in an unpredictable medication loss. Alternatively, the mucosal atomizer device (MAD) can be used. This device atomizes the medication into particles that are the optimal size for deposition across the broad area of the intranasal mucosa (Fig. 134.5).[208]

Various sedative medications have been successfully reported to provide sedation when administered intranasally. Midazolam is the most commonly used IN medication. The dose ranges between 0.2 and 0.7 mg/kg (maximum dose usually about 10 mg). To reduce the volume of the medication, a 5-mg/mL solution is most frequently used. The onset time is about 10 to 15 minutes. Unfortunately, intranasal midazolam often causes discomfort on administration.[208-210] This is believed to be due to the acidic pH of 4 of the IV solution that is used. Several methods have been tried to minimize the

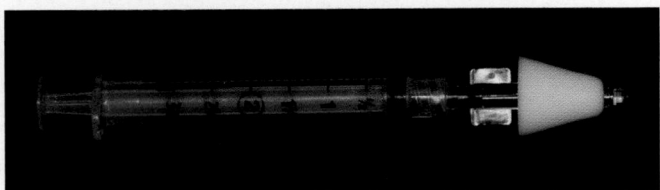

Fig. 134.5. Device used for delivery of atomized medication.

irritation with variable results, such as mixing lidocaine with midazolam, elevating the pH to more physiologic levels; this last method was not very successful, as midazolam precipitates in water if the pH is >4.6. Sufficient midazolam plasma concentrations to induce moderate sedation were shown to be rapidly achieved after IN administration to healthy individuals.[206] Aerosolized buccal midazolam has been reported to provide effective sedation for laceration repair.[208]

Sufentanil use intranasally has been reported in the emergency room and for pediatric dental procedures alone and in conjunction with IN dexmedetomidine.[210] The doses range from 1 to 2 mcg/kg (maximum dose 20 mcg). Using a 50 mcg/mL solution along with its high potency results in an drug volume about 0.5 mL, which is deemed appropriate for intranasal administration with respect to improved efficacy, and reduced discomfort.[210] The onset time is also quick, about 10 to 15 minutes with duration of about 30 minutes. Higher doses have been associated with respiratory depression, and nausea has been reported, which can be effectively managed using sublingual ondansetron.

There are a few limited reports on the use of intranasal remifentanil. Doses of 2 to 4 mcg/kg have been used. Onset time is less than 5 minutes and duration of effect appears to be about 10 to 15 minutes. Multiple administrations may be required. Fentanyl use has been described in few studies; it was used as the only agent using a patient-controlled administration during childbirth[211] or with other medications for procedural sedation in the emergency room.[212] However, when compared dose for dose with sufentanil, much larger drug volumes are required, which may limit its usefulness.

Dexmedetomidine has been used intranasally with doses of 1 to 2 mcg/kg.[213] It has a slower onset time of about 45 minutes. Sedation appears equal or better than that of oral midazolam. The duration of effect is also longer than other intranasal sedatives. Procedures lasting over an hour have been reported. Ketamine has also been used via the IN route.[207] The reported dose was 5 to 9 mg/kg.[214] It provided more effective sedation than IN midazolam, without any evidence for hemodynamic instability.[215] It has also been shown to be a safe and effective method of sedating children for dental procedures.[207]

Both flumazenil and naloxone can be given via the intranasal route. It has been shown that 40 mcg/kg of IN flumazenil provides a therapeutic plasma level of 10 to 30 ng/mL and a peak level of 68 ng/mL within 2 minutes.[216,217] A dose of 100 mcg in each nostril is believed to be simple, easy to memorize, and effective in most children. This dose can be repeated as necessary. IN naloxone has been described as well; there are no pharmacokinetic studies in humans, but the bioavailability of IN naloxone in rats was found to be equivalent to intravenous naloxone.[218] In one study, the proposed dose is 0.2 mg in each nostril.[216] The dose can be repeated as needed based on the clinical response.[216,218]

TABLE 134.20	Drug Dose Guidelines for Moderate Sedation	
Route	Drug	Dose
PO	Chloral hydrate	50-75 mg/kg (repeat 25 mg/kg)
	Diazepam (Valium)	0.2-0.4 mg/kg (max, 20 mg)
	Midazolam (Versed)	0.5-0.75 mg/kg (max, 20 mg)
IM	Pentobarbital (Nembutal)	4-6 mg/kg (max, 100 mg)
	Fentanyl (Sublimaze)	1-3 µg/kg
	CM3	0.08-0.1 mL/kg (max, 2 mL)
IV	Morphine	0.1 mg/kg
	Meperidine (Demerol)	1-2 mg/kg (max, 75 mg)
	Fentanyl (Sublimaze)	1-2 µg/kg (max, 5 µg/kg)
	Midazolam (Versed)	0.05-0.1 mg/kg
	Diazepam (Valium)	0.05-0.1 mg/kg

CM3, catheterization mixture number 3; *IM*, intramuscular; *IV*, intravenous; *PO*, by mouth.

TABLE 134.21	Sedation Quality: Different Drugs			
	Amnesia	Analgesia	Relaxation	Inattention
Barbiturates	0	0*	0	4
Benzodiazepines	4	0	2	4
Antihistamines	1	0	0	2
Opioids	0	2	0*	2
Chloral hydrate	0	0	0	4
Ketamine	2	4	0*	4
Nitrous oxide	3	3	1	3

*May antagonize other drugs having this effect.
0, possible effect.

Another route of administration is transmucosal administration, such as the fentanyl *lollipop* (ACTIQ). Dosing recommendations are shown in Table 134.20. One must always keep in mind that BZD-opiate or barbiturate-opiate combinations are potent causes of respiratory depression, and extra monitoring and vigilance should be used. With IM and oral medications, adequate time should elapse to allow absorption before a further dose is given to avoid accidental overdose.

As noted in Table 134.16, different procedures require different qualities of sedation. These qualities are found in the array of drugs available to the intensivist (Table 134.21). It may be useful to choose the sedative agent or agents that best fit the particular requirements for the procedure being performed.

Opiate and BZD antagonists should be readily available wherever moderate sedation is being performed. Staff caring for these patients should understand the drug indications and dosing of these medications to reduce any potential delay in their appropriate use. They can quickly and effectively reverse the respiratory depression from excessive doses of sedation.

In some circumstances the services of the anesthesia department may be useful. The anesthesia department has access to other pharmacologic agents such as propofol and nitrous oxide, as well as the inhalational agents. The ability to use a deeper level of sedation if required is easily obtained with

BOX 134.11	Patients Unsuitable for Moderate Sedation

Premature (<60 weeks' gestation)
Apnea, respiratory, or cardiac monitor at home
Airway obstruction
Bronchopulmonary dysplasia, chronic obstructive pulmonary
  disease, recent pneumonia, or croup
Uncontrolled seizures or multiple medications
Multiple psychotropic medications
Poorly controlled asthma
Vomiting
Gastroesophageal reflux disease
Raised intracranial pressure
History of difficult sedation

BOX 134.12	Indications for Sedation for Magnetic Resonance Imaging

Very young or agitated patient
A prolonged study (multiple scans)
Anxiety
Claustrophobia
Intensive care patient
(Not a complete list.)

BOX 134.13	Contraindications to Magnetic Resonance Imaging

Cardiac pacemaker
Aneurysm clips
Automatic implanted cardiac defibrillator
Neurostimulator
Pacing wires
Cochlear implant
Implanted insulin pump
Penile prosthesis
History of ocular injury involving metal object
History of vascular surgery <3 months
History of soft tissue metal foreign body <3 months
History of orthopedic hardware <3 months
(Not a complete list.)

these rapidly acting, short-acting agents. In emergency procedures where the patient's NPO status is unsafe or unknown, patients may need to undergo intubation to protect the airway.

Anesthesiologists have the ability to perform a "needleless" sedation technique using a gas induction with anesthetic agents; an IV drip may be placed if required when the patient is asleep. This technique is especially useful for repeat procedures in oncology patients. Also, anesthesia personnel are better able to sedate a patient whose illness may contraindicate routine moderate sedation protocols (Box 134.11).

Postprocedure Care and Monitoring

Care of the patient during the recovery period after moderate sedation is important. Patients must be monitored during recovery to ensure that adverse events are rapidly recognized and treated. The recovery area should be equipped with appropriate monitors and resuscitation equipment and have a trained individual in attendance. The monitoring should be performed to the same degree as during the actual procedure. Level of consciousness and vital signs should be recorded at regular intervals. A physician who is responsible for the patient must be identifiable and must be easy to contact if required urgently. Patients may be discharged home when they are alert and orientated or when they have returned to baseline if baseline initial mental status was abnormal. Vital signs should be stable and within acceptable limits. A sufficient time should have elapsed if a reversal agent was used (2 hours). Patients should be discharged in the presence of a responsible adult to accompany them home and report any complications. Written instructions should be given to the parent concerning diet, medications, and activities, and a 24-hour contact telephone number also should be given to the parent.

Moderate sedation is safe and frequently used; unconscious sedation is potentially hazardous, and patients who undergo it require careful monitoring. Hospital protocols are useful for a smoothly run, safe sedation policy.[219] Staff should be appropriately trained in sedation and resuscitation basic and advanced life support. When the ASA/AAP recommendations are followed, the risks of a sedation-related complication can be reduced.[220] Individual risk factors include deep sedation and the use of chloral hydrate. When all the recommendations for moderate sedation, including NPO, ASA class, avoidance of deep sedation, sedation level monitoring, and drug use were followed, the adverse event rate was zero.

Sedation for Magnetic Resonance Imaging

The PICU physician is often called on to provide sedation for a patient in the ICU who is undergoing MRI. Also, many

institutions rely on the PICU team to provide a sedation service for other inpatients or outpatients undergoing MRI. Deep sedation is often required for effective sedation of younger children undergoing an MRI scan. The same standards as applied with any other child undergoing sedation should be adhered to[221] with respect to patient selection, monitoring, and postimaging care.

Magnetic resonance imaging is being increasingly used to aid in the diagnosis of neuroanatomic disorders. The patient is required to lie still within a small space while multiple images are obtained. MRI scanning is performed less rapidly than computed tomography (CT) scanning. Movement by the patient degrades the image quality, and a change in the patient's position may affect the homogeneity of the magnetic field, which is optimized at the beginning of the scan. Studies can take from 45 minutes to more than 2 hours, with individual sequences taking 3 to 10 minutes. The scanner is noisy and the restriction on space and movement can induce claustrophobia in some patients. The patient also may experience a slight increase in temperature. Most adults and children older than 6 years are capable of lying still for the scan. With the use of earplugs and music, it is well tolerated. Several groups of patients, however, may require sedation[222] for the scan to be performed (Box 134.12).

Because of the large magnetic field, several unique problems[223] can occur during a scan. These problems include the potential risk of the magnet causing a ferromagnetic object to move or heat up or the induction of an electric current from the radio frequency pulses and switching magnetic gradients used in generating the images. This potential risk results in a significant list of contraindications to MRI (Box 134.13). Sedating these patients also entails several risk factors. The patient is in a remote location, with limited access to and visibility of the airway. Several equipment issues exist as well (Box 134.14). The monitors used must be suitable for use in the MRI suite.[224] They should be nonferromagnetic; the cables

---

BOX 134.14	Potential Difficulties in Magnetic Resonance Imaging

Malfunction of anesthesia or sedation equipment
Malfunction of monitoring
Anesthesia or sedation equipment causing interference with image quality
High-velocity ferromagnetic projectile from loose object
Disruption of electronic devices

---

should be screened from electromagnetic interference (fiberoptic is ideal); and the signal should be filtered to avoid radio frequency interference (which interferes with image quality). Despite the specialized technology available, several problems remain. The ECG waveform is frequently altered, and information regarding analogs is often lacking during a scanning cycle. The ECG cables may cause burn injury, and special ECG electrodes are required to avoid this occurrence. For pulse oximetry to be performed, a special probe is required. Heating of the usual probe may cause burn injury. A fiberoptic connection to the patient is best. Capnography requires long tubing, which results in a prolonged upsweep and delay in displaying real-time measurements. The respiratory rate and trends can still be useful. Any battery-powered monitor requires a nonmagnetic lithium battery. Exposure to the MRI shortens battery life. Most ICU ventilators are not MRI compatible (Servo *i* is available as an MRI compatible model). Some specialized MRI-safe anesthesia machines have a ventilator; however, their use should be restricted to the anesthesia staff who are familiar with the equipment. The IV poles and the equipment carts also should be nonferromagnetic. Any equipment with a transformer (eg, syringe pumps and IV pumps) must be kept out of the magnetic field. Gas cylinders must be aluminum. The area around any magnet that generates a magnetic field stronger than 5 G should not contain any ferromagnetic items.

Any staff entering the MRI suite should remember to remove any ferromagnetic objects, including keys, watches, pens, and credit cards. Stethoscopes and laryngoscopes also are ferromagnetic. Infusion pumps should be outside the magnetic field—that is, outside the 5-G line. The electric motor in infusion pumps emits electromagnetic radiation and may run at an abnormal speed in the presence of a strong magnetic field. The pump is also a projectile risk. IV infusions through long tubing from outside the scanner can be useful so that the depth of anesthesia can be altered without having to enter the MRI suite. MRI-compatible infusion pumps are now also available. Some of these pumps allow changing infusion rates via electronic handheld devices without the need to enter the scanning room. The ICU patient's infusions can be changed over to these infusion devices while the patient is still in the ICU and then transported to the scanner.

The use of a cuffed endotracheal tube may affect the quality of the MRI image because of metal in the valve of the pilot balloon and reinforcement of the mask airway. With the patient in the ICU, special care must be taken to ensure that all cables and transducers that may be carefully screened and all ferromagnetic objects are removed ("hiding in the sheets"). For invasive vascular pressure to be measured, the transducer should be as far from the patient as is practically possible and separated with a saline-filled pressure line. If cardiac arrest occurs, the patient should be removed from the magnetic field.

The defibrillator should be kept outside the magnetic field and checked regularly. A nonferromagnetic code cart is also advisable. It is essential that the code team follow the rules about removing any loose magnetic items before entering the MRI suite or else a lethal projectile may be released. The ICU patient's lungs are frequently hand-ventilated by ICU staff in the MRI suite. The sedation technique is often a continuation of that used in the ICU, especially for a patient who undergoes intubation. In some children, single doses of fentanyl or midazolam may be sufficient for a adequate sedation. If deeper sedation is required for patient comfort/cooperation, then IV sedation with supplemental oxygen with propofol is useful. A bolus of 2 mg/kg and an infusion of 100 µg/kg/min are useful for patients with few medical problems and an easily maintained airway. It results in a rapid recovery with little nausea or vomiting.

Specific Drugs for Sedation
Ketamine

Ketamine is a phencyclidine derivative that provides sedation and analgesia. It results in a state of dissociative (trancelike) anesthesia. It is available in a variety of dilutions, such as 10 mg, 50 mg, and 100 mg/mL. The latter is the most beneficial for IM use and the preparation of infusions. For a state of general anesthesia to be induced, a dose of 2 mg/kg IV is required. Onset takes 1 to 2 minutes with anesthesia lasting 10 to 15 minutes. Lower doses may be used for sedation. Anesthesia also can be induced by the IM route with a dose of 10 mg/kg, although onset is slower (5 to 10 minutes) and duration of prolonged effect is 45 to 60 minutes. It is metabolized by the liver and excreted by the kidneys. The half-life is 3.1 hours (see Table 134.12).

The adverse effects of ketamine include hypertension, tachycardia, increased intracranial pressure, and bronchodilation. The bronchodilation is probably due to its sympathomimetic action. It is a direct myocardial depressant, but blood pressure is usually maintained by the sympathetic stimulation that ketamine causes. In critically ill patients who already are using their maximum sympathetic drive, ketamine may cause a decrease in cardiac output or even cardiac arrest.[225] Hallucinations and other psychiatric symptoms are often reported during and after its use in adults, but they occur less frequently in children. Ketamine is a potent sialogogue, and the use of an anticholinergic agent such as glycopyrrolate may be helpful. Its use is contraindicated in patients who cannot tolerate hypertension,[226] have a history of cerebrovascular hemorrhage, have psychiatric disturbances, and have raised ICP. It is a useful agent for sedation, especially if there is no IV access. It has been used in patients with status asthmaticus as an adjunct bronchodilator both in intubated and nonintubated patients at an infusion rate of 0.5 to 2 mg/kg/h. After discontinuing its use, the patient should receive BZDs to minimize the likelihood of hallucinations and be nursed in a quiet environment. Ketamine cannot be assumed to preserve pharyngeal reflexes any better than other sedatives agents, and apnea and airway obstruction can still occur.[227] NPO guidelines should still be observed. Ketamine is sometimes given with propofol *(ketofol)* for procedural sedation in the belief that this combination may be a safer, better sedative technique. However, when compared[228] there were more episodes of desaturations related to respiratory depression and airway episodes such as laryngospasm in the ketofol group compared to the group given propofol alone.

Ketamine has been shown to be effective for refractory status epilepticus (RSE). During RSE there is a down-regulation of the GABA$_A$ receptors limiting the effectiveness of the benzodiazepines. There is, however, an upregulation of NMDA receptors during RSE, which promotes excitotoxicity and further potentiates epileptogenicity.[229] On review of the literature, ketamine was effective in 67% of cases with RSE (presumed significant underreporting error), at doses up to 3 mg/kg hour and infusions lasting 27 days. There is at present only grade 4 evidence for its use in RSE; however, it should be considered especially as its cardiac profile may be advantageous compared to other anesthesia agents used.

Etomidate

Etomidate is a carboxylated imidazole that is unrelated to other anesthetic agents. It is a rapidly acting IV anesthetic agent, which, like other rapid-onset anesthetic agents, partitions into the brain within one circulation time and redistributes out of the brain over the next few minutes. Its hypnotic action involves the GABA$_A$ receptor. It is available dissolved in 30% propylene glycol as a 2-mg/mL solution. Like propofol, it causes pain on injection. The anesthetic dose is 0.2 to 0.3 mg/kg. It has a favorable adverse effect profile with minimal cardiovascular and respiratory depression. Etomidate is associated with a high incidence of nausea and vomiting after emergence from anesthesia. Its pharmacokinetics is shown in Table 134.12. The greatest disadvantage of etomidate in the intensive care setting is adrenocortical depression due to its potent inhibition of adrenocortical mitochondrial 11-β-hydroxylase.[230] This effect is present in neonates and in adults.[231] The inhibition can last for 24 hours after a single dose of etomidate,[232] and after infusion the inhibition can be prolonged. The outcome of patients sedated with etomidate is worse than in those using alternative sedation, and steroid deficiency is thought to be the cause.[233] There appears to be a greater risk if the patient is suffering from septic shock,[234] which may not be ameliorated by hydrocortisone replacement therapy.

In the CNS, etomidate suppresses seizure activity; although patients may show excitatory movements not associated with cortical EEG changes suggestive of seizures. The intracranial and intraocular pressures are lowered. It is the drug of choice for patients who are undergoing emergency intubation, those who have head injuries, and those who have a compromised cardiovascular system, and it is safe for use in patients with asthma because there is no histamine release. Etomidate has the highest therapeutic index of any anesthetic agent.

Several case reports of the satisfactory use of etomidate for controlling refractory intracranial hypertension have been published; it is associated with fewer cardiovascular problems than are barbiturates. Nevertheless, caution must be taken concerning the development of a lactic acidosis due to the metabolism of propylene glycol.

There are two new etomidate analogs in the pipeline. They have been custom designed to remove the inhibition of the 11-β-hydroxylase by replacing a nitrogen with a methyl group that cannot bind to Fe.[235]

Carbo-etomidate has 11-β-hydroxylase inhibition that is 2000× less than etomidate; however, it is less water soluble and as such has a slow onset. The cardiovascular profile is similar to etomidate.

Methoxycarbonyl (MOC) etomidate is metabolized rapidly by nonspecific esterases. It has GABA$_A$ actions that are similar to those for etomidate. It also has a safe cardiovascular profile and minimal 11-β-hydroxylase inhibition. The recovery from MOC etomidate may be quicker than from its parent compound due to a combination of redistribution as well as metabolism.

Inhalational Anesthetic Agents

The inhalational agents remain the most widely used anesthetics in the operating room, although their mechanism of action is still poorly understood. The following agents are currently in clinical use: enflurane, isoflurane, sevoflurane, and desflurane. Sevoflurane and desflurane are newer agents that currently have limited use in the ICU. Isoflurane remains the most logical choice of inhalational anesthetic in the ICU based on its cost-benefit ratio. As with any drug used in the ICU, it is important to understand the pharmacology, the adverse effect profile, and, in this case, the technical aspects of delivering these agents to the patient. These drugs are all fluorinated hydrocarbons (Fig. 134.6). Except for halothane, which is no longer in common clinical use, they are ethyl-methyl esters. Each agent has different physicochemical properties that are important to its properties (Table 134.22).

Anesthesia personnel frequently use nitrous oxide as an adjunct. In some institutions it is used as the basis of a hospital pediatric procedural sedation service for children. Patients on the hospital floor undergoing minor to moderately painful procedures are mildly sedated with 50% nitrous oxide (as routinely used in pediatric dentistry); this technique has a good safety profile. A newer anesthetic agent in use in Europe is xenon. This gas has anesthetic properties with few cardiac adverse effects. It is expensive to use and requires a specialized fully closed breathing circuit to minimize the amount of gas used. The rate at which a change in inspired concentration is reflected in the brain is determined mainly by the blood/gas solubility. The more soluble the gas is in blood, the slower is the change due to the gas dissolving into the blood and reducing the partial pressure available to equilibrate with the brain. Sevoflurane and desflurane are the least soluble and therefore have the most rapid onset and offset; halothane has the slowest onset. The potency of the agents is represented by the minimal alveolar concentration (MAC). The MAC is the percentage of inhaled anesthesia agent required to prevent 50% of anesthetized patients from responding to a surgical incision. The lower the MAC, the more potent the agent. Halothane is the most potent of the agents used and desflurane is the least potent. The MAC of anesthetic agents is not constant with age. For all the agents it is highest for those aged 1 to 12 months, and the MAC falls throughout childhood to reach adult levels.

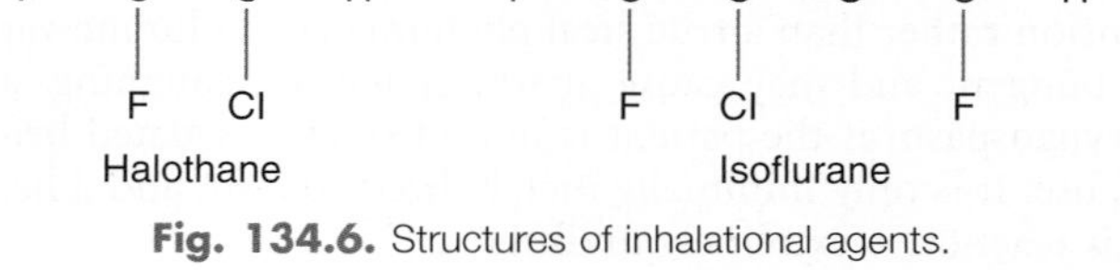

Fig. 134.6. Structures of inhalational agents.

TABLE 134.22   *Vapor Characteristics*

	Halothane	Isoflurane	Sevoflurane	Desflurane
Molecular weight	197.4	184.5	200	168
Saturated vapor pressure (mm Hg)	243	240	157	700
Boiling point (8°C)	50.2	48.5	58.5	22.8
Minimal alveolar concentration (%)	0.75-1.2	1.3-1.85	2.5-3	8-10
Blood/gas solubility	2.3	1.4	0.68	0.42
Oil/w% metabolized	20	0.2	3.3	0.02

Neonates show a slightly reduced MAC compared with infants. The oil/water solubility determines the degree of accumulation of the agent within the body fat stores. A highly fat-soluble agent will have larger body stores; therefore recovery from the agent is delayed.

These agents all have significant effects on the cardiorespiratory systems. Although respiration can be controlled, the negative inotropic and vasodilator effects are pronounced and limit the concentrations that can be used. Halothane, the oldest of these agents, has the greatest degree of cardiac depression. Sevoflurane and desflurane have an adverse effect profile similar to that of isoflurane, except that sevoflurane is partly metabolized to a potentially toxic metabolite, compound A, from a reaction with the sodium hydroxide in the CO_2 absorbent soda lime used in anesthesia circle systems. For accumulation of compound A to be minimized in the circuit, a fresh gas flow of greater than 2 L/m should be used. Thus sevoflurane may not be not a good choice for prolonged ICU treatment with this type of closed circuit. There are new CO_2 absorbents such as micropore that are lithium hydroxide based and do not create compound A.[236] Due to the fact that micropore also adsorbs less inhalational agent compared to the routinely used canisters, it may be a better choice for long-term use in the ICU. Desflurane has a sympathomimetic effect, especially when the concentration is abruptly increased, and significant tachycardia and hypertension can occur.

Adverse effects of halothane include hypotension, which is due to direct myocardial depression. It also causes bradycardia because of effects on the sinoatrial node and vagal stimulation. Cardiac arrhythmias may occur, most commonly junctional rhythm. Halothane also sensitizes the myocardium to catecholamines, especially when the patient is hypercapnic or hypoxic. Because these physiologic changes are common in the intensive care patient, the potential for serious interactions with halothane abound. Halothane is metabolized approximately 20% by the liver, and a trifluoroacetic metabolite may cause an immune-mediated fatal hepatitis.[237] Isoflurane causes hypotension mainly because of vasodilation, while maintaining cardiac output. Concern has been expressed about a coronary steal phenomenon occurring in which blood is diverted from a partially obstructed coronary bed served by collateral arteries, due to vasodilation. The evidence for this phenomenon is weak, however, and ischemia is probably due to hypotension rather than a true steal phenomena. Isoflurane vapor is pungent and may cause airway irritation, coughing, and laryngospasm if the patient is not adequately sedated before its use. It is only minimally metabolized (0.2%), and a hepatitis reaction is extremely unlikely.

Malignant hyperthermia is a rare reaction that may occur whenever the halogenated inhalational anesthetics or succinylcholine is given to a patient. It involves the unrestrained entry of calcium into myocytes and consequential consumption of adenosine triphosphate, resulting in metabolic failure. Hypermetabolism, manifested by increased CO_2 production, and acidosis occur. Later the body temperature rises and death from hyperkalemia occurs. Correction of blood chemistry, aggressive cooling, and the administration of dantrolene are urgently indicated.

The metabolism of all the anesthesia agents can result in the production of free fluoride ions. Concentrations of fluoride greater than 50 μmol/L can cause renal dysfunction and a reduced concentrating capacity. This risk would appear to be higher for both halothane and sevoflurane because of their more extensive metabolism. It also may be exaggerated by patients who are prescribed drugs that induce the cytochrome P-450 enzyme complex.

Inhalational agents may cause hepatotoxicity in two ways: (1) by metabolism to reactive intermediates that are directly hepatotoxic or (2) through the intermediates that form adducts to hepatic proteins. These new proteins are then recognized as foreign, and an immune response that causes hepatic injury occurs. This is thought to be the mechanism of halothane hepatitis. This form of hepatitis is most common after halothane use; even then it is rare, occurring in 1 of 100,000 cases. It is less common with isoflurane, sevoflurane, or desflurane, which are much less metabolized. This fulminant hepatic failure, which may be fatal, is most common after repeated administrations of halothane in older obese patients. The predominance of reductive halothane pathway metabolism results in a trifluoroacetic acid metabolite that forms a hapten. Halothane hepatitis is also less common in children.

All of the inhalational agents cause cerebral vasodilation, which results in an increase in CBF (because of decoupling of the demand/flow ratio) and ICP. In pediatric patients with raised ICP, there was no difference among isoflurane, desflurane, and sevoflurane with respect to the increase in ICP and CBF.[238] In contrast, IV anesthetics maintain the demand/flow ratio, and CBF and ICP fall, with the exception of ketamine. In addition to an effect of CBF, the arterial blood pressure typically will decrease with anesthesia, and the effect on the CPP must be accounted for. In one study, the effect of the decrease in arterial pressure on CPP exceeded the effect of increasing ICP by a factor of 3.[239] With these potential effects on CBF, the use of isoflurane should be carefully considered in patients who have or are at risk of raised ICP. Nevertheless, isoflurane has been safely used in neuroanesthesia with controlled ventilation to a normal $PaCO_2$ and an inspired concentration not exceeding 1 MAC.[240]

Isoflurane has two main applications in the PICU: sedation and the management of refractory asthma. In an adult study, 40 patients[241] who received an average of 96 MAC hours of isoflurane showed hemodynamic stability, less tachyphylaxis compared with other sedative agents, and a more rapid wean from the ventilator. No evidence was found of renal or hepatic dysfunction with serum fluorides less than 50 µmol/L. In a pediatric study, 10 patients[242] who had been receiving large doses of opiates or BZDs received an average of 130 MAC hours of isoflurane. The range of use was from 1 to 30 days. Fifty percent of the patients experienced a withdrawal-like phenomenon—most commonly, those who had received more than 70 MAC hours of isoflurane. Fluoride levels also were measured, and although they were correlated with the duration of treatment, none was greater than 30 µmol/L. The highest levels were in a patient who was taking both phenytoin and phenobarbitone. Hypotension only occurred in one patient. No hepatic or renal dysfunction occurred. The withdrawal was treated with a combination of BZDs and haloperidol with good effect. Isoflurane also has been used in patients with renal dysfunction, and fluoride levels were not elevated.[243] The starting dose for sedation should be 0.5%; this dose can then be titrated to effect by the ICU team. At levels above 1.5%, other sedative agents and paralytics often are not required.

Multiple case reports of the use of inhalational agents for status asthmaticus in both adults and children have been made. Because of its speed of onset and its bronchodilation effects, isoflurane is a useful adjunct to β_2-adrenergic agonists. If no improvement occurs, or if unacceptable adverse effects occur, then its effects rapidly wane on discontinuation. Isoflurane is recommended for use because of its safer adverse effect profile. No reports of renal or hepatic dysfunction have been made despite its use for often prolonged periods. Hypotension seems to be more common in patients sedated with isoflurane; it is possibly related to increased intrathoracic pressure and the potential for greater preload reduction with vasodilation. Fluid boluses and occasionally vasopressors are often required. Because isoflurane is not an analgesic agent, opiates may be needed for painful or uncomfortable procedures. Also, when the patient is weaned off the isoflurane, additional sedatives will be required. The isoflurane should be started at 0.5% and titrated for effect; doses of up to 2.5% have been reported as safely used.[244]

The inhalational anesthetic agents are liquids at room temperature. A special delivery device called a vaporizer is required to deliver an accurate supply of the vapor. All vaporizers have several features in common. They provide a reservoir of the inhalational liquid with a level indicator and are capable of delivering a constant level of vaporization. Most newer vaporizers also have a color-coded keyed filler (eg, purple for isoflurane and yellow for sevoflurane) that prevents the accidental filling of the vaporizer with the wrong agent. This error could result in overdosing the patient because the vaporizer calibration is drug specific. If two vaporizers are accommodated in series on the anesthesia machine back bar, then an interlocking system should be used to prevent the accidental use of both vaporizers. Otherwise, the results would be contamination of the second vaporizer by gas from the first vaporizer and an uncontrolled excess delivery of gas to the patient.

One of the main problems with using these inhalational agents in the PICU is how to deliver them to the patient. One technique is to use an anesthesia machine to deliver the gas to an ICU ventilator with the correct oxygen percentage and inhalational agent. This mixture is delivered from the fresh gas outlet of the anesthesia machine. It is selected by adjustment of the flow rotameters on the anesthesia machine to give the desired oxygen concentration and then selection of the desired inspired concentration of inhalational agent on the vaporizer. Unfortunately, most ICU ventilators will not accept this low-pressure gas supply as their driving gas. The Servo 900C is an exception because it has a low-pressure inlet option for the driving gas. High flow rates are required to maintain filling of the bellows of the ventilator; the flow rates must be higher than the minute ventilation. This requirement sometimes limits the inspired oxygen because the maximum flow of oxygen from the rotameters of the anesthesia machine is 10 to 12 L/m. Also, this process consumes a lot of vapor.

Also available is another Servo ventilator, the 900D, which has a custom-fit vaporizer on the normal high-pressure input. This machine is similar to the 900C, but it has been modified for anesthesia use and allows hand ventilation with inhalational agents. Maquet now offers an ICU type ventilator that delivers inhalational anesthesia, the Flow-I machine. It uses proprietary vaporizers and has a circle system to reduce fresh gas flow. Due to the recirculating nature of the circuit, gases and inhalational monitoring are mandatory. If the fresh gas is too low, then the circuit could become hypoxic; if the CO_2 absorbents have an issue, then hypercapnia can be a concern. Also the end-tidal inhalational agent needs to be monitored to ensure that it is clinically appropriate and that the vaporizers are functioning properly. Often the only alternative is to deliver anesthetic with an anesthesia machine. Anesthesia machine ventilators are not as sophisticated as ICU ventilators, may not be able to deliver appropriate volumes for pediatric patients, and often have limited positive end-expiratory pressure capabilities. The anesthesia machine needs to be checked before use and its correct function should be continually assessed during its use, which requires an understanding of the setup and alarms on the machine and an understanding of the procedures of the appropriate tests. This understanding usually is not within the confines of a pediatric intensivist's scope of practice, and an anesthesiologist should be involved to ensure the safe and effective use of this apparatus.

Whenever inhalational agents are used, the waste gases from the expiratory limb of the ventilator should be scavenged to avoid prolonged exposure of the health care worker to these agents. The Occupational Safety and Health Administration limits occupational exposure to 2 ppm halogenated volatile agents for health care workers.[245] The worker is at risk of becoming sedated, and potential teratogenic effects also exist. Several large studies about prolonged exposure to these agents have not shown any increase in risks for anesthesia personnel with respect to hepatic disease, teratogenesis, spontaneous abortions, psychologic difficulties, infertility, neuropathy, or bone marrow depression.[246] Caution also should be taken when filling the vaporizer to avoid spilling the liquid during the process.[247] Two forms of scavenging are available. A passive system involves simply a tube connected to the expiratory limb connected to the outside. This system is at risk of occlusion because of kinking or someone standing inadvertently on the tubing, which will then occlude the expiratory limb of the ventilator. An active system involves an active suction to the expiratory limb, with a safety reservoir bag in series to prevent the patient from being exposed to excess suction pressure.

In the operating room it is routine to monitor the levels of anesthesia agents given with a gas analyzer. This monitoring provides an inspired and expired inhalational agent concentration and is helpful to ensure that the vaporizer is functioning correctly, that the vaporizer has not emptied without being detected, and that the concentration dialed on the vaporizer has reached its effect. When the end-tidal inhalational agent concentration equals the inspired agent, then steady state has been achieved. This steady state normally occurs rapidly with isoflurane, but in a patient with severe asthma due to the severe limitation in airflow gas exchange, achievement of steady state may be delayed.

If the PICU staff is unfamiliar with the delivery system being used for the isoflurane, then it would be appropriate to have staff from the anesthesiology department set up the equipment and ensure that it functions correctly. Failure to configure the delivery system correctly has the potential to cause considerable harm or death. Once the situation has stabilized, an anesthesiologist may not be required at the bedside. However, an anesthesiologist should be available by pager to help troubleshoot any difficulties. In these cases the inspired agent should be monitored continually.

The use of inhalational agents in the PICU involves the use of equipment that may be unfamiliar to pediatric intensive care physicians. Isoflurane appears to be the best choice,[248] and it offers several useful advantages, including the ability to deeply sedate patients (especially those difficult to sedate) without polypharmacy.[249] Although they are currently poorly defined,[250] tolerance and a withdrawal-like syndrome have been described; however, they appear to occur more slowly than with other sedative agents. It may be helpful to have a set of guidelines available for isoflurane use to facilitate its use in the PICU. These guidelines could include equipment use, monitoring requirements, dosing, and treatment of complications.[251] Caution should be used in patients who may have raised ICP because isoflurane may increase CBF. Isoflurane does allow for rapid arousal if neurologic examinations are required.

The anesthetic conserving device (AnaConDa) is a modified heat moisture exchanger that has been developed to allow the use of inhalational agents in the ICU without requiring high fresh gas flows or specialized ventilators.[252] It is placed in the breathing circuit between the ventilator Y circuit and the endotracheal tube. The liquid anesthesia agent is injected directly into the device using a syringe pump. The device membrane allows for the inhalational agent to be taken up by the inspired gas. On expiration, much of the inhalational agent is deposited on the membrane, allowing for an efficient inhalational rebreathing technique. The inhalational consumption has been shown to be equivalent to that of the conventional circle system.[253] The inspired concentration of the inhalational agent is monitored from the device using a routine gas analyzer. There are quite a few reports of its use in adult ICU from Europe as well as two pediatric studies. In adults there was a decrease in postoperative mortality in those patients receiving isoflurane instead of midazolam/propofol.[254] All patients received sedation for more than 96 hours. It has also been used for postoperative adult cardiac patients[255]; the patients received the same postoperative sedation as they received for their general anesthetic technique. Patients receiving the inhalational sedation were ready for extubation and extubated more rapidly than those in the propofol group. The inhalational group in the ICU had more vasodilation and required more vasopressor support. The use of isoflurane proved to be effective and not difficult to use in the ICU; however, there was no difference in outcome, length of stay, or quality of sedation. In conjunction with this study, the researchers also evaluated a method for scavenging the exhaled isoflurane.[256] A Deltasorb canister was used between the patient expiratory limb and the reservoir bag, which vented to the wall suction. The canister contains a hydrophobic matrix that acts as a molecular sieve and selectively captures volatile agents from the gas mixture.

A similar concept is now used when preparing an anesthesia workstation for a patient at risk for malignant hyperthermia. In this case the volatile agent is scavenged from the circuit so that the patient is not exposed to any volatile material that has dissolved into the machine components. This is based on an activated charcoal filter and has a limited duration of effect.[257] Some problems due to excess dosing have been experienced, and the 100-mL dead space of the device, as well as resistance to gas flow, may make its use inappropriate in children. A report of 7 days of isoflurane delivery using the AnaConDa device in children demonstrated that effective sedation was possible in 4 hours; other sedatives were able to be weaned.[258]

Compared with an inhalational agent vaporizer, there is no percentage inhalational agent dial. The rate on syringe injection determines the percentage of the inhalational agent. This infusion rate is set according at a prerecommended rate. Initially the inspired concentration is low because of dilution. Differences in minute ventilation and gas flows may make this prerecommended rate inaccurate. The injection rate needs to be titrated to the monitored percentage of the inspired inhalational agent, which can increase significantly with time, especially until equilibrium is reached. The AnaConDa device has not been approved for use in the United States.

The use of isoflurane for sedation in conjunction with 24 hours of therapeutic hypothermia postcardiac arrest has also been reported.[259] The isoflurane sedation was chosen due to concerns about drug metabolism with hypothermia delaying neurologic assessments. Also there is some evidence that inhalational agents have a myocardial pre- and postconditioning effect, reducing the degree of reperfusion injuries. This is due to an effect on messenger kinases as well as possibly some antiinflammatory effects. Postcardiac surgery performed using inhalational anesthesia has been shown to have lower troponin levels. Postconditioning effects may also be gained in other organs including the brain. Also the inhalational agents may facilitate a more rapid cooling by reducing shivering, lowering vasoconstrictive thresholds. Outcome was determined by the initial neurologic assessment after 24 hours of cooling.

Sedation-Related Complications

With all the advantages of sedation and analgesia in the PICU, critical care providers are becoming more aware of sedation-related adverse events. Understanding and recognizing these events are crucial prerequisites to providing the best quality care and putting forth the necessary procedures and strategies to prevent and minimize these events and their sequelae.

A multicenter study that looked at sedation-related adverse events in pediatric patients ventilated for acute respiratory failure found that a high proportion of patients had inadequate pain and sedation management. It was interesting to find that there was moderate site-to-site variability for some of the adverse events reported.[132] Clinically significant iatrogenic withdrawal, unplanned endotracheal extubation, extubation failure, postextubation stridor, and stage 2+ pressure ulcer were also reported.

Loss of sleep and sleep disruption in critically ill children in the PICU play crucial roles in short-term recovery and long-term neurocognitive outcomes. This can be attributed to the multiple physical, environmental (eg, noise), and pharmacologic factors including sedative medications.[260]

Reduced sleep can have detrimental effects, as it can lead to delirium, impaired immunity, catabolism, and respiratory insufficiency. Little is known of the effect of sedatives and analgesics on sleep in critically ill children. Benzodiazepines are believed to decrease and suppress rapid eye movement during the sleep cycle. Pediatric intensivists should have a better understanding of the physiology of normal sleep in order to differentiate between normal sleep and deep sedation in critically ill children.[260] Dexmedetomidine might have less detrimental effects on sleep compared to other more commonly used medications; further research is needed to investigate its efficacy and its effects on sleep in PICU patients. All PICUs should adopt simple maneuvers like using earplugs, eye masks, noise reduction, and light optimization to promote sleep. These maneuvers are available, noninvasive, inexpensive, and have been proved to decrease sleep interruption during nighttime hours.[261,260]

Delirium in children has been described. It was believed to be a transient problem without significant short-term or long-term neuropsychiatric consequences.[262-264] This notion has been challenged, however, and there has been an emerging literature to outline and determine the prevalence, definition, consequences and potential treatment of delirium in children, especially when they are critically ill in the PICU.

Delirium is defined as a complex neuropsychiatric syndrome characterized by disturbances of consciousness, attention, cognition, thought, language, memory, orientation, perception, the sleep-wake cycle, behavior, mood, and affect.[263-266] The *Diagnostic and Statistical Manual of Mental Disorders* (DSM-IV-TR) definition of delirium was adopted from adult studies, but it is believed that this definition can be applied in children and adolescents. Children with delirium can be irritable, cry inconsolably, be incoherent, moan, kick, and thrash. These children might not recognize family members and familiar objects.

A series of delirium-like signs were reported in the early 1960s in patients emerging for certain anesthetics like ether, ketamine, and cyclopropane, especially when they were administered for certain short procedures (eg, tonsillectomy and adenoidectomy (T&A), thyroidectomy, and circumcision).[267,265] These symptoms were reported more frequently in children than adults (12%-13% versus 5.3%). The problem of delirium has reemerged with the widespread use of inhalational anesthetic gases like sevoflurane, desflurane, and isoflurane.[262-265,268,269]

Delirium in the postanesthetic period was defined by Sikich and Lerman as "a disturbance in the child's awareness of and attention to his/her environment with disorientation and perceptual alterations including hypersensitivity to stimuli and hyperactive motor behavior."[265,270] It usually occurs within the first 30 minutes after recovery from anesthesia, can resolve spontaneously within 1 to 2 hours, but can last for up to 2 days.

The incidence of delirium in children in the PICU is unknown, but it generally is around 40% and could be up to 80%. It appears to mostly affect preschool children around 2 to 7 years old. The presence of developmental delay and the need for mechanical ventilation are risk factors associated with delirium.[262,265,266,268,271,272] There are several possible etiologies of pediatric delirium (Table 134.23).

It was found in many studies that the incidence of delirium in children is higher after the use of inhalational anesthetic gases, especially sevoflurane. Isoflurane and halothane were reported to cause delirium to a much lesser extent in comparison to sevoflurane. There is a lower incidence of delirium after propofol and remifentanil intravenous anesthesia.[264,265,268,269,272,273]

Many disorders can be difficult to differentiate from delirium in children. They include acute stress reaction, acute anxiety states, adjustment disorder with mixed emotions, dissociative or regressive states, and childhood-onset psychosis.[266]

The management of delirium in children has been a neglected topic in the literature, but reports have emerged that address this crucial aspect. Management should include pharmacologic and nonpharmacologic strategies. In anesthesia settings, treatment with alpha 2-adrenoceptor agonist like clonidine or dexmedetomidine has helped to reduce the incidence and frequency of postanesthetic delirium without prolonging the time to extubation or discharge.[269,273] Preoperative administration of midazolam can be useful in minimizing postanesthesia agitation by augmenting the inhibitory effects of $GABA_A$ receptors.[265] Perioperative pain management can lead to a lower incidence of delirium; different analgesic options—including ketorolac, intravenous or oral transmucosal fentanyl, oral ketamine, dexmedetomidine, and caudal block—have been recommended to eliminate pain and anxiety.[265,269,272-275] Only few reports have looked at delirium in PICU settings; haloperidol has been used with reasonable outcomes. Initial haloperidol doses of 0.15 to 0.25 mg/dose intravenously have been used followed by a maintenance dose of 0.05 to 0.5 mg/kg per 24 hours.[262,264,266,276]

Risperidone orally has been used in less acute situations with good results. The suggested initial dose is 0.1 to 0.2 mg followed by a maintenance dose of 0.2 to 2 mg per 24 hours.[264,266,276] The use of benzodiazepines has been discouraged in the treatment of delirium in children unless it is

TABLE 134.23   Etiologic Factors Related to Delirium

Anesthesia-related factors	Rapid emergence from anesthesia
Intrinsic characteristics of the anesthetic	Possible irritating side effect of inhalational anesthetics on the central nervous system
Surgery-related factors	Postoperative pain Surgery type (eg, tonsillectomy and adenoidectomy, cataract and thyroid surgery)
Patient-related factors	Age (preschool) Postoperative anxiety

reserved for delirium due to iatrogenic sedation withdrawal or as a possible adjunct to haloperidol for insomnia.[264,271,277]

Nonpharmacologic psychosocial strategies should be part of managing and preventing delirium in children, especially in the PICU. Interventions include parents' constant presence, comforting techniques, familiar music and photographs, toys, room lighting schedule, family-centered care, and a parent information leaflet. Appropriate pain and iatrogenic withdrawal management are very important as well.[264]

Apoptosis

Evidence from rodents suggests that most general anesthetics and sedatives, which are either N-methyl-D-aspartate receptor antagonists or GABA$_A$ agonists, trigger apoptosis or programmed cell death. Those incriminated include inhalational anesthetic agents (including nitrous oxide), propofol, benzodiazepines, and ketamine. Adjuvants that do not trigger apoptosis include dexmedetomidine, melatonin, opiates, and possibly xenon. Interestingly, lithium has been shown to exert an antiapoptotic effect. Massive apoptosis occurs in vulnerable regions of the brain that are responsible for learning and cognition (eg, the hippocampus, caudate/putamen, thalamus, and others) when these proapoptotic anesthetics are administered during the period of synaptogenesis or the rapid brain growth spurt in young rodents, most notably during the seventh postnatal day. The severity of the apoptosis depends on the dose of anesthetic and duration of administration. In addition to histologic changes associated with apoptosis (as evidenced by caspases-3 staining), long-term memory loss and cognitive impairment have been demonstrated.

Whether these data are directly applicable to humans has not been established. Primate research suggests that ketamine[278] induces apoptosis in vulnerable young monkeys, although an exposure to ketamine of less than 3 hours in duration does not induce significant injury. Isoflurane has also been shown to cause apoptosis in several primate studies.[279] To date, the studies in humans have been retrospective in design. Four studies have demonstrated conflicting findings on the effects of anesthetics on cognitive function in young children. The most impressive of these retrospective studies is from the twin registry in Denmark,[280] in which monozygote twins concordant or discordant for anesthetic exposure before the age of 4 years failed to demonstrate any differences in educational achievement or cognitive impairment years later. There are two ongoing prospective studies at present. Results for these studies may not be available for several years. The PANDA trial evaluates the children for neurodevelopment after 5 years postinguinal hernia repair.[279] A prospective randomized study of general anesthesia versus regional anesthesia for lower abdominal surgery with long-term evaluation of cognitive function in children is also currently under way (enrollment has been completed); however, 5-year neurocognitive follow-up data is still pending. These studies may help us to understand the risk, if any, of administering these general anesthetics to vulnerable human infants and young children. At present the best recommendations are that a single brief anesthetics for infants appears safe. Multiple anesthetics and surgical procedures may not be, but there are reasons aside from anesthesia for these possible complications. The evidence for anesthesia-related apoptosis in humans is weak at present, and withholding anesthesia for surgery may cause greater harm. At present there is no need to change anesthetic practice or to postpone or delay indicated surgeries for infants.[281]

Pharmacoeconomics

In today's economical climate, it is important to consider the cost of the different sedation options available to the pediatric intensivist (Table 134.24). Most PICUs use a low-cost sedative regimen for the bulk of the sedations required and keep the more expensive options for selected circumstances. Table 134.24 shows the different costs of some of the available agents in the PICU as well as the 24-hour cost for a child weighing 20 kg. They are presented as the cost per kilogram per hour of sedation at equipotent doses. They represent the lowest hospital drug cost (at the Women's and Children's Hospital of Buffalo) for each agent in its most inexpensive form and exclude preparation, delivery, and equipment issues related to each drug. Fentanyl, commonly used, is inexpensive. For a 20-kg child, it costs $13.63 per day. Midazolam is now a more inexpensive option than lorazepam. The other synthetic opiates are more expensive to use, and consideration should be given to appropriate indications for their use. A rapid recovery, however, with as quick an extubation as possible with remifentanil and early ICU discharge, is also a considerable cost factor to be considered. Propofol (which is now available in a generic form) and ketamine are both relatively inexpensive options for ICU sedation, if they are deemed clinically appropriate. The drug costs of isoflurane are comparable to those of the BZDs. Sevoflurane and desflurane remain expensive options; however, they require the availability of a specialized delivery system, which could increase the cost. If a device were available that could deliver these agents at low flows with most of the available ICU ventilators, then inhalational sedation would be a more attractive option.

When looking at the cost benefits of different sedation regimens, there are many components of the cost analysis for one

TABLE 134.24 Relative Drug Costs of Different Intensive Care Unit Sedative Agents

Drug	Dose	Cost/kg/hr ($)	24-Hour Cost for 20-kg Child ($)
Morphine	50 µg/kg/h	0.01	4.80
Fentanyl	4 µg/kg/h	0.03	13.63
Sufentanil	0.8 µg/kg/h	0.03	13.82
Remifentanil	0.4 µg/kg/min	0.46	216.69
Midazolam	0.1 mg/kg/h	0.02	9.79
Lorazepam	0.1 mg/kg/h	0.05	24.48
Propofol	5 mg/kg/h	0.05	16.92
Ketamine	1 mg/kg/h	0.03	14.40
Dexmedetomidine	0.5 µg/kg/h	0.09	42.00
Isoflurane	0.5% (@ 61 L/min)	0.44	10.47
Desflurane	3% (@ 61 L/min)	35.71	857.00
Sevoflurane	1% (@ 61 L/min)	6.76	162.19
Xenon	30% (proprietary closed circuit)		392.47

to consider. It is a complex analysis that not only compares direct drug costs but needs to take into account the many factors that can influence the cost of health care. Usually length of stay in the ICU, length of hospital stay, or days of ventilation are utilized, with the calculated costs attributed to each of these parameters used to compare the sedation regimens. Other criteria may include the incidence of complications such as delirium, the cost of managing delirium, and long-term the quality of life outcome (QALYS). In addition to the economic side, there is the clinical outcome assessment to determine if there is a better outcome with one sedation method or another and to decide what is the best evidence-based medicine. The more expensive the medication, the greater the need for quality information as to its cost analysis and outcome effect. A review that compared dexmedetomidine to propofol or midazolam for moderate ICU sedation in adults[282] evaluated six cost analyses and two outcome papers. There appeared in most of them to be a small financial benefit to using dexmedetomidine compared to both propofol and midazolam, due to a reduced ICU length of stay. The outcome comparison difference was less noticeable, with a small benefit when comparing dexmedetomidine to midazolam only, due to a lower incidence of delirium, highlighting how difficult this type of comparison may be. These papers focused on adult subjects, whose sedation requirements and complications are different from children, and as such these benefits may not be apparent for a pediatric ICU practice.

Key References

5. Scheeringa MS, Zeanah CH, Cohen JA. PTSD in children and adolescents: toward an empirically based algorithma. *Depress Anxiety.* 2011;28:770-782.

6. Dow BL, et al. The diagnosis of posttraumatic stress disorder in school-aged children and adolescents following pediatric intensive care unit admission. *J Child Adolesc Psychopharmacol.* 2013;23:614-619.

20. Bresil P, et al. Impact of bispectral index for monitoring propofol remifentanil anaesthesia. A randomised clinical trial. *Acta Anaesthesiol Scand.* 2013;57:978-987.

58. Best KM, Boullata JI, Curley MA. Risk factors associated with iatrogenic opioid and benzodiazepine withdrawal in critically ill pediatric patients: a systematic review and conceptual model. *Pediatr Crit Care Med.* 2015;16:175-183.

59. Anand KJ, et al. Opioid analgesia in mechanically ventilated children: results from the multicenter Measuring Opioid Tolerance Induced by Fentanyl study. *Pediatr Crit Care Med.* 2013;14:27-36.

60. Bowens CD, et al. A trial of methadone tapering schedules in pediatric intensive care unit patients exposed to prolonged sedative infusions. *Pediatr Crit Care Med.* 2011;12:504-511.

88. Bienert A, Bartkowska-Sniatkowska A, Wiczling P, et al. Assessing circadian rhythms during prolonged midazolam infusion in the pediatric intensive care unit (PICU) children. *Pharmacol Rep.* 2013;65:107-121.

97. Antonik LJ, Goldwater DR, Kilpatrick GJ, et al. A placebo- and midazolam-controlled phase I single ascending-dose study evaluating the safety, pharmacokinetics, and pharmacodynamics of remimazolam (CNS 7056): part I. Safety, efficacy, and basic pharmacokinetics. *Anesth Analg.* 2012;115:274-283.

101. Sneyd J, Robert MD. Remimazolam: new beginnings or just a me-too? *Anesth Analg.* 2012;115:217-219.

129. Leung L. Cannabis and its derivatives: review of medical use. *J Am Board Fam Med.* 2011;24:452-462.

131. Porter BE, Jacobson C. Report of a parent survey of cannabidiol-enriched cannabis use in pediatric treatment-resistant epilepsy. *Epilepsy Behav.* 2013;29:574-577.

132. Grant MJ, Scoppettuolo LA, Wypij D, et al. Prospective evaluation of sedation-related adverse events in pediatric patients ventilated for acute respiratory failure. *Crit Care Med.* 2012;40:1317-1323.

133. Abrams DI, Guzman M. Cannabis in cancer care. *Clin Pharmacol Ther.* 2015;97:575-586.

141. Whalen LD, et al. Long-term dexmedetomidine use and safety profile among critically ill children and neonates. *Pediatr Crit Care Med.* 2014;15:706-714.

149. Morr S, Heard CM, Li V, Reynolds RM. Dexmedetomidine for acute baclofen withdrawal. *Neurocrit Care.* 2015;22:288-292.

164. Mahajan B, Kaushal S, Mahajan R. Fospropofol. *J Pharmacol Pharmacother.* 2012;3:293-296.

185. Schroeppel TJ, et al. Propofol infusion syndrome: a lethal condition in critically injured patients eliminated by a simple screening protocol. *Injury.* 2014;45:245-249.

188. Testerman GM, Chow TT, Easparam ST. Propofol infusion syndrome: an algorithm for prevention. *Am Surg.* 2011;77:1714-1715.

189. Joffe AR, et al. Is propofol a friend or a foe of the pediatric intensivist? *Pediatr Crit Care Med.* 2014;15:e66-e71.

190. Markovitz BP. Proving propofol safe for continuous sedation in the PICU is an impossible task. *Pediatr Crit Care Med.* 2014;15:577.

210. Hitt JM, Corcoran T, Michienzi K, et al. An evaluation of intranasal sufentanil and dexmedetomidine for pediatric dental sedation. *Pharmaceutics.* 2014;6:175-184.

216. Heard C, Creighton P, Lerman J. Intranasal flumazenil and naloxone to reverse over-sedation in a child undergoing dental restorations. *Paediatr Anaesth.* 2009;19:795-797, discussion 798-799.

229. Zeiler FA. Early use of the NMDA receptor antagonist ketamine in refractory and superrefractory status epilepticus. *Crit Care Res Pract.* 2015;2015:831260.

234. Jackson WL Jr. Carboetomidate: will it eliminate the etomidate debate? *Crit Care Med.* 2012;40:333-334.

254. Bellgardt M, et al. Survival after long-term isoflurane sedation as opposed to intravenous sedation in critically ill surgical patients. *Eur J Anaesthesiol.* 2016;33:6-13.

255. Volatile-based short-term sedation in cardiac surgical patients: a prospective randomized controlled trial. *Crit Care Med.* 2015;43:1062-1069.

256. Pickworth T, et al. The scavenging of volatile anesthetic agents in the cardiovascular intensive care unit environment: a technical report. *Can J Anaesth.* 2013;60:38-43.

258. Eifinger F, et al. Observations on the effects of inhaled isoflurane in long-term sedation of critically ill children using a modified AnaConDa©-System. *Klin Padiatr.* 2013;225:206-211.

260. Kudchadkar SR, Aljohani OA, Punjabi NM. Sleep of critically ill children in the pediatric intensive care unit: a systematic review. *Sleep Med Rev.* 2014;18:103-110.

261. Kudchadkar SR, Yaster M, Punjabi NM. Sedation, sleep promotion, and delirium screening practices in the care of mechanically ventilated children: a wake-up call for the pediatric critical care community. *Crit Care Med.* 2014;42:1592-1600.

262. Schieveld JN, Leentjens AF. Delirium in severely ill young children in the pediatric intensive care unit (PICU). *J Am Acad Child Adolesc Psychiatry.* 2005;44:392-394, discussion 395.

266. Schieveld JN, Leroy PL, van Os J, et al. Pediatric delirium in critical illness: phenomenology, clinical correlates and treatment response in 40 cases in the pediatric intensive care unit. *Intensive Care Med.* 2007;33:1033-1040.

268. Chandler JR, Myers D, Mehta D, et al. Emergence delirium in children: a randomized trial to compare total intravenous anesthesia with propofol and remifentanil to inhalational sevoflurane anesthesia. *Paediatr Anaesth.* 2013;23:309-315.

271. Turkel SB, Hanft A. The pharmacologic management of delirium in children and adolescents. *Paediatr Drugs.* 2014;16:267-274.

272. Dahmani S, Delivet H, Hilly J. Emergence delirium in children: an update. *Curr Opin Anaesthesiol.* 2014;27:309-315.

273. Shukry M, Ramadhyani U. Does dexmedetomidine prevent emergence delirium in children after sevoflurane-based general anesthesia? *Paediatr Anaesth.* 2005;15:1098-1104.

276. Schieveld JN, Leroy PL, van Os J, et al. Pediatric delirium in critical illness: phenomenology, clinical correlates and treatment response in 40 cases in the pediatric intensive care unit. *Intensive Care Med.* 2007;33:1033-1040.

279. Sanders RD, et al. Impact of anaesthetics and surgery on neurodevelopment: an update. *Br J Anaesth.* 2013;110(suppl 1):i53-i72.

281. Hansen TG. Anesthesia-related neurotoxicity and the developing animal brain is not a significant problem in children. *Paediatr Anaesth.* 2015;25:65-72.

282. Rapid Response Report: Summary with Critical Appraisal. Dexmedetomidine for sedation in the ICU or PICU: a review of cost-effectiveness and guidelines. Canadian Agency for Drugs and Technologies in Health; December 2014.

Tolerance, Withdrawal, and Dependency

Joseph D. Tobias

PEARLS

- Delaying the onset and magnitude of tolerance and physical dependency may be feasible with the use of newer practices such as drug holidays or nurse-controlled sedation regimens.
- Physical dependency and withdrawal have been documented in all agents used for sedation and analgesia in the pediatric intensive care unit, including benzodiazepines, barbiturates, opioids, dexmedetomidine, propofol, and the inhalational anesthetic agents.
- Regardless of the agent administered, withdrawal will occur once the sedative or analgesic medication has been administered by continuous infusion for more than 4 to 5 days.
- When transitioning from intravenous to oral medications and weaning the amount of medication administered, the use of formal scoring systems to identify withdrawal is recommended.
- In the majority of clinical scenarios, once physical dependency has occurred, withdrawal can be prevented by switching to an orally equivalent agent of the same class such as methadone for the opioids, lorazepam for the benzodiazepines, and clonidine for dexmedetomidine.
- To facilitate care and avoid variations in practice, it is suggested that each institution develop specific protocols for the oral agent to be used, the conversion from intravenous to oral doses, and the tapering regimen.

Introduction

Data demonstrating the potential deleterious physiologic effects of untreated pain combined with ongoing humanitarian concerns have led to increased attention on the need to provide compassionate care in pediatric intensive care unit (PICU) settings. Many of these initiatives have led to increased use of sedative and analgesic agents during mechanical ventilation in infants and children. Although the judicious use of sedative and analgesic agents is mandatory to ensure effective anxiolysis and analgesia, new consequences have emerged from such practices—including physical dependency, tolerance, and withdrawal—that require definition and effective treatment strategies to limit their impact on the patient, length of hospitalization, and perhaps even outcome.

The development of an effective approach to identifying, preventing, and treating tolerance and physical dependency should begin with a consensus on the definitions of these terms.[1] Tolerance is a decrease in a drug's effect over time, generally with the need to increase the dose to achieve the same effect. Tolerance is related to changes at or distal to the receptor, generally at the cellular level. Some authorities have divided tolerance into various subcategories:

- Innate tolerance refers to a genetically predetermined lack of sensitivity to a drug related to a lack of or alteration in receptors or their subcellular components.
- Pharmacokinetic (dispositional tolerance) refers to changes in a drug's effect because of alterations in distribution or metabolism.
- Learned tolerance refers to a reduction in a drug's effect as a result of learned or compensatory mechanisms (learning to walk a straight line while intoxicated by repeated practice at the task).
- Pharmacodynamic tolerance occurs when drug effect is diminished, although the plasma concentration of the drug remains constant.

For the purpose of this discussion, the latter phenomenon is generally the most relevant to the PICU population and for the remainder of this chapter will be referred to as tolerance.

Withdrawal includes the physical signs and symptoms that manifest when the administration of a medication (for our purposes, the sedative or analgesic agent) is abruptly discontinued in a patient who is physically tolerant. The symptomatology of withdrawal varies from patient to patient and may be affected by several factors including the agent involved as well as the patient's age, cognitive state, and associated medical conditions.

Physiologic (physical) dependence is the need to continue a sedative or analgesic agent to prevent withdrawal. Psychologic dependence is the need for a substance because of its euphoric effects. Addiction is a complex pattern of behaviors characterized by the repetitive, compulsive use of a substance, antisocial or criminal behavior to obtain the drug, and a high incidence of relapse after treatment. Psychologic dependency and addiction are extremely rare after the appropriate use of sedative or analgesic agents to treat pain or to relieve anxiety in the PICU setting.

History of Tolerance and Withdrawal in the Intensive Care Unit Setting

The problems of opioid dependency and withdrawal in neonates and infants were first recognized and studied in the 1970s and 1980s in a population of infants born to mothers with a history of drug addiction.[2,3] Despite the difference in the origin of the problem, these studies provide valuable information for dealing with these issues in the PICU population. They suggested various pharmacologic treatment regimens and provided the first scoring systems used to grade the severity of withdrawal and to evaluate the efficacy of the treatment regimens.

When considering the PICU population, Arnold and colleagues were among the first to recognize the problems of dependency and withdrawal following prolonged opioid administration.[4] In a retrospective review of 37 neonates who required extracorporeal membrane oxygenation (ECMO) for respiratory failure and who had received intravenous fentanyl for sedation, they sought to identify the signs and symptoms of what they termed "the neonatal abstinence syndrome (NAS)." They also sought to identify risk factors for its occurrence. Fentanyl infusion requirements to achieve the desired level of sedation increased from 11.6 ± 6.9 µg/kg/hr on day 1 to 52.5 ± 19.4 µg/kg/hr on day 8. By measuring plasma fentanyl concentrations, they were able to demonstrate that there was an increase in the plasma fentanyl concentration required to achieve the same level of sedation, thereby demonstrating that the tolerance was pharmacodynamic and not pharmacokinetic (related to increased metabolism of the opioid). The investigators reported that NAS was related to the total fentanyl dose and the duration of the infusion. A cumulative fentanyl dose ≥ 1.6 mg/kg or an ECMO duration ≥ 5 days was a risk factor for the development of NAS (odds ratio of 7 and 13.9, respectively). The same investigators subsequently prospectively evaluated fentanyl dosing requirements and plasma fentanyl concentrations in a cohort of eight infants placed on ECMO.[5] Fentanyl infusion requirements increased from 9.2 ± 1.9 µg/kg/hr on day 1 to 21.9 ± 4.5 µg/kg/hr on day 6. As in their previous study, they also noted an increase in the plasma fentanyl concentration from 3.1 ± 1.1 ng/mL on day 1 to 13.9 ± 3.2 ng/mL on day 6. These reports were followed in 1990 by the first report of the use of oral methadone for treatment of iatrogenic dependency and tolerance in the PICU patient.[6] Although this initial report was anecdotal, involving only three to four infants, it has been followed by numerous other investigators outlining the use of methadone in this clinical scenario (discussed later).

Although initially noted with the opioids, subsequent reports demonstrated withdrawal from other agents used for prolonged sedation in the PICU patient including benzodiazepines, barbiturates, propofol, the inhalational anesthetic agents, and most recently dexmedetomidine.[7-9] Additional information concerning benzodiazepine withdrawal is provided by a retrospective review of Fonsmark and colleagues who evaluated 40 patients receiving sedation during mechanical ventilation.[10] Sedation was provided by midazolam, pentobarbital, or a combination of the two. Withdrawal symptoms occurred in 14 of 40 patients (35%). Of the patients with withdrawal symptoms, 8 had received both midazolam and pentobarbital, 3 received only midazolam, and 3 received only pentobarbital. A cumulative midazolam dose ≥ 60 mg/kg or a cumulative pentobarbital dose ≥ 25 mg/kg was associated with withdrawal, whereas the duration of the infusion was not. Sedation was gradually tapered in only one of 14 patients who experienced withdrawal. Other anecdotal reports have noted withdrawal following the use of pentobarbital for sedation in the PICU population.[11,12] The potential for the development of tolerance to barbiturates is supported by animal studies.[13,14] Anecdotal and retrospective reports have demonstrated similar withdrawal phenomena following the prolonged administration of propofol and volatile anesthetic agents.[15-18]

Clinical Signs and Symptoms of Withdrawal

The development of strategies to provide effective treatment of physical dependency and related problems requires the accurate identification and recognition of withdrawal symptoms. Ongoing or associated conditions that can manifest clinical signs and symptoms similar to withdrawal must be investigated and ruled out before concluding that the patient's symptoms are the result of withdrawal. In the PICU patient, these associated conditions may include central nervous system insults or infections, ICU psychosis, delirium, metabolic abnormalities, hypoxia, hypercarbia, and cerebral hypoperfusion from alterations in cardiac output or cerebral vascular disease. There has been considerable recognition of the potential confusion of the clinical signs and symptoms of withdrawal with those of delirium.[19,20] Future work in the arena of delirium in the pediatric population as well as improved scoring systems for delirium and withdrawal is needed to differentiate these two problematic disorders.

Although many of the signs and symptoms of withdrawal are the same regardless of the agent, there may be subtle differences depending on the specific medication. The time to the onset of withdrawal symptoms varies depending on the half-life of the agent as well as the half-life of any active metabolites. The latter may be several times longer than the parent compound. In general, the signs and symptoms of withdrawal from sedative and analgesic agents can be localized to one of three end-organ systems: the central nervous system (CNS), the gastrointestinal (GI) tract, and the sympathetic nervous system. CNS manifestations include those of increased activity with irritability including decreased sleep time, tremulousness, hyperactive deep tendon reflexes, clonus, an inability to concentrate, frequent yawning, sneezing, and hypertonicity. As outlined earlier, behaviors now classified as delirium may be a manifestation of withdrawal. In neonates and infants, additional signs of CNS overactivity and stimulation include a high-pitched cry and an exaggerated Moro reflex. Seizures have been reported with withdrawal from various agents including the opioids, benzodiazepines, barbiturates, propofol, and the inhalational anesthetic agents. Visual and auditory hallucinations have been described with opioid, benzodiazepine, barbiturate, and inhalational anesthetic agent withdrawal. GI manifestations include emesis, diarrhea, and feeding intolerance, which may be especially prominent in neonates and infants. When such problems occur in the absence of other signs and symptoms of withdrawal, they may be attributed to other problems and not withdrawal. Activation of the sympathetic nervous system with tachycardia, hypertension, dilated pupils, diaphoresis, and tachypnea is a prominent finding with withdrawal from any of the above-mentioned sedative/analgesic agents. Additional signs and symptoms of sympathetic hyperactivity include nasal stuffiness, sweating, and fever. Although the signs and symptoms of withdrawal may be fairly easy to recognize, it must also be noted that many of these signs and symptoms overlap with potentially life-threatening disorders such as infections, respiratory insufficiency, gastrointestinal ischemia, and cerebral hypoperfusion. As such, the diagnosis of physical dependency and withdrawal must always be a diagnosis of exclusion to avoid potentially missing a life-threatening disorder.

Treatment of Withdrawal and Clinical Scoring Systems

As with most problems that arise in clinical medicine, effective treatment starts with prevention. Given that the incidence of withdrawal is related to the total amount of medication administered, careful titration of the sedative or analgesic agents using clinical sedation scales is suggested. By doing this, it may be practical to use the minimal amount of medication required. One of the more popular tools that has been studied as a means to reduce iatrogenic withdrawal following sedation in the PICU has been the use of nurse-driven protocols.[21,22] Such protocols allow the bedside nurse to adjust the infusion rates of sedative and analgesic as needed to achieve the desired level of sedation. Although limited success has been noted when attempting to demonstrate a decreased length of mechanical ventilation or ICU stay, the initial results are promising in regard to the incidence of withdrawal and physical dependency. In a before-and-after protocol involving 337 medical PICU patients requiring sedation during mechanical ventilation, there was a decrease in the incidence of withdrawal from 23.6% to 12.8% following the initiation of a nurse-driven sedation protocol.[22] The protocol used two different scoring systems including the COMFORT-B and the Nurse Interpretation of Sedation Scores (NISS) as well as the bispectral index (BIS) to assess and adjust the depth of sedation. Based on the protocol, the dosing of sedatives and analgesics (morphine or fentanyl ± midazolam) was adjusted.

Another commonly used technique to encourage the reassessment of the depth of sedation on a daily basis in the adult population is the use of a daily *drug holiday*. This practice involves turning off sedative and analgesic agents until the patient responds and then restarting the infusion at a fraction of the previous infusion rate. Such practices are becoming commonplace in the adult population, as ongoing measures are being evaluated in an attempt to limit the incidence of delirium.[23] Although this is an growing practice in the adult population, there are currently limited data to support or refute the efficacy of so-called drug holidays during the use of sedative and analgesic agents in the PICU setting. The theoretic rationale behind such practices remains sound and would seem to parallel those of using clinical sedation scores in that excessive infusion rates are avoided. With a drug holiday, if the patient is excessively sedated, the amount of medication administered is decreased to the appropriate level. However, physicians and bedside nurses may be hesitant to discontinue effective sedation and analgesia at a time when painful processes may be present in the critically ill patient. Additionally, despite evidence to the contrary in the literature and from current clinical practice, concerns have been raised that this practice may result in periods of excessive agitation in critically ill patients. Robust prospective trials in the pediatric population are needed to demonstrate not only the efficacy but also the safety of such practices.

Other considerations, which also need further investigation, include rotating sedation regimens, intermittent versus continuous infusions of sedative/analgesic agents, and the role of other pharmacologic agents such as *N*-methyl-D-aspartate

(NMDA) receptor antagonists (ketamine, methadone, magnesium) or opioid antagonists (naloxone) in preventing tolerance and dependency. Until further investigations provide additional insight into the factors controlling opioid dependency and ways of preventing or delaying it, PICU physicians will be faced with some patients who require specific actions to prevent the development of withdrawal symptoms. Treatment strategies and protocols are necessary so that the problems associated with tolerance, physical dependency, and withdrawal do not limit the administration of these agents in the PICU population.

Until then, it may be helpful to identify patients who are most likely to manifest symptoms of withdrawal and also to have scoring systems to identify and quantitate the signs and symptoms of withdrawal. As noted previously, risk factors that have been identified include not only the total dose of the sedative or analgesic agent but also the duration of the infusion. In a prospective trial of 23 infants and children who had received fentanyl infusions for sedation during mechanical ventilation, Katz and associates determined the factors that could be used to identify the group at risk of withdrawal.[24] Once sedation was no longer required, the fentanyl infusion was decreased by 50% every 24 hours times two and then discontinued. Withdrawal behavior was observed in 13 of 23 patients (57%). The total fentanyl dose and the duration of the infusion correlated with the risk of withdrawal, whereas the maximum fentanyl infusion rate did not. A total fentanyl dose ≥1.5 mg/kg or an infusion duration ≥5 days was associated with a 50% incidence of withdrawal, whereas a total fentanyl dose ≥2.5 mg/kg or an infusion duration ≥9 days was associated with a 100% incidence of withdrawal.

Scoring systems are essential in the management of patients presenting with signs and symptoms of withdrawal, not only for identifying the behaviors of withdrawal but also for grading its severity and judging the response to therapy. The scoring systems initially used to grade withdrawal were adapted from those developed to deal with neonates born to drug-addicted mothers.[25] As such, these systems were difficult to apply, especially in patients outside of infancy. To address these issues, in 2007 Ista and colleagues reviewed the literature regarding withdrawal scoring systems and found that of the six available in the literature, only two were directed toward the PICU population.[26] The first of was the Sedation Withdrawal Score (SWS), which assigns 0 to 2 points to 12 withdrawal behaviors, thereby providing a maximum score of 24. The signs and symptoms are grouped to the CNS (tremor, irritability, hypertonicity, high-pitched cry, convulsions, and hyperactivity), the GI system (vomiting and diarrhea), and the autonomic nervous system (fever, sweating, sneezing, and respiratory rate).[27] The decision regarding weaning of the current sedative or analgesic medications was based on the score (0–6, wean; 6 to 12, no change; 12 to 18, revert to previous regimen; more than 18, reevaluate plan). Ista and colleagues expressed concerns that the SWS had not been validated in children and that, in particular, there were no data regarding its sensitivity, specificity, validity, and reliability. The other scale reviewed by Ista and colleagues was the Opioid and Benzodiazepine Withdrawal Scale (OBWS) developed by Franck and coworkers.[28] The OBWS is a 21-item checklist evaluating 16 specific withdrawal behaviors. Franck and coworkers evaluated their scale by performing 693 assessments in 15 children, ranging in age from 6 weeks to 28 months. Using 8 as a cut-off score for the absence or presence of withdrawal, the sensitivity of the OBWS was only 50% with a specificity of 87%. The predictive value in terms of positive and negative ratios was 4 and 0.57 (considered moderate for a diagnostic tool), whereas the interrater reliability was acceptable at 0.8.

Based on these issues, Ista and colleagues concluded that a more appropriate scale was necessary in the PICU population and went on to use the data from their review to develop their own withdrawal scale.[29] From their review of the literature and clinical experience, they developed the Sophia Benzodiazepine and Opioid Withdrawal Checklist (SBOWC), which included 24 withdrawal signs and symptoms. Over a 6-month period, they collected 2188 observations in 79 children within 24 hours of tapering off and discontinuing sedative or analgesic medication. They noted that specific symptoms (including agitation, anxiety, muscle tension, sleeping for less than 1 hour, diarrhea, fever, sweating, and tachypnea) were observed most frequently and that longer duration of opioid or benzodiazepine use and high doses were risk factors for withdrawal. Twenty-three observations were scored simultaneously and resulted in an interobserver correlation coefficient of 0.85 with a range of 0.59 to 1 for the individual items. Subsequent work by Francke and colleagues resulted in the development of the WAT-1 (withdrawal and assessment tool).[30-32] The components of this score are outlined elsewhere.[32] The score is simple and easy to use. It assigns a value of 0 for no or 1 for yes to the following factors: loose or watery stools; vomiting, retching, or gagging; and temperature ≥37.8°C. The patient is then observed for 2 minutes to assess his or her state (asleep, awake, or calm versus distressed), the presence of a tremor, sweating, uncoordinated or repetitive motion, and yawning or sneezing. Again, these factors are scored as 0 for no and 1 for yes. The patient is then observed following a stimulus and during recovery for startle to touch and muscle as well as time to regain a calm state. These components result in a score from 0 to 12.

A high index of suspicion and increasing use of withdrawal scores developed for the PICU patient have advanced our goal of recognizing patients who manifest withdrawal symptoms. As mentioned previously, the mainstay of preventing withdrawal must be the identification of high-risk patients and the slow weaning of sedative and analgesic agents. Withdrawal scales should still be applied to these patients in the event that withdrawal occurs despite our attempts to prevent it. Regardless of the agent administered, it is the cumulative total dose and the duration of infusion that have greatest impact on the incidence of withdrawal. In general, limited or no withdrawal is noted with infusions for ≤3 days, whereas the majority of patients will have withdrawal if the medication is abruptly stopped after 5 days or more. The intermediate zone remains the 3- to 5-day range.

The other issue concerns the optimal method and rate of weaning. Should the medication be weaned incrementally every day using the intravenous route, or should we change to oral medications and wean in that manner? The rate at which the medication is weaned becomes a significant issue when the intravenous route is chosen. If the medication can be weaned by 20% every day, the infusion can be discontinued in 5 days. A more gradual weaning process would mandate prolonged intravenous access unless a transition is made to oral medications. Although it has been suggested that weaning by 10% to 20% is feasible, these studies demonstrate a relatively high incidence of withdrawal, suggesting that a more reasonable approach may be a 5% to 10% decrease per day as has been suggested for adult patients and supported by some in the PICU population.[33-35] It is possible that in some patients, a more rapid wean can be accomplished if the agents have been administered for fewer than 3 to 5 days.

After prolonged administration of 5 or more days, the weaning process will likely require a more protracted period of time to prevent withdrawal symptoms. Although the weaning process can be accomplished by slowly decreasing the intravenous infusion rate, this mandates the maintenance of intravenous access, ongoing hospitalization, and, at times, continued monitoring in the PICU because, depending on hospital policies, certain medications such as fentanyl or midazolam cannot be administered by continuous infusion in settings other than the PICU. In these circumstances, options to consider include either switching to the subcutaneous route or, most commonly, the use of oral administration.

If it is decided that the infusion can be tapered within a period of time that will not delay hospital discharge and that switching to oral medications will not expedite discharge home, the patient may be considered a candidate for subcutaneous administration (discussed earlier).[36] These patients are generally receiving moderate doses of fentanyl (5–10 µg/kg/hr) or midazolam (0.1–0.3 mg/kg/hr). The switch to the subcutaneous route allows the removal of central venous access, eliminates the need to maintain peripheral intravenous access, and, depending on individual hospital policies, may eliminate the need for ongoing care in the ICU setting. Both fentanyl and midazolam can be effectively administered via the subcutaneous route and the infusions slowly tapered to prevent symptoms of withdrawal. Concentrated solutions of fentanyl (25–50 µg/mL) and midazolam (2.5–5 mg/mL) are used so that the maximum subcutaneous infusion rate does not exceed 3 mL/hr. The subcutaneous infusions are started at the same dose that is currently being used for intravenous administration. A topical dermal anesthetic cream can be placed over the site of anticipated subcutaneous cannulation. Several areas are suitable for subcutaneous administration, including the subclavicular region, abdomen, deltoid, or anterior aspect of the thigh. The site is cleaned, prepped with sterile antiseptic solution, and then either a standard 22-gauge intravenous cannula or a 23-gauge butterfly needle is inserted into the subcutaneous tissue. Before placement, the tubing and needle are flushed with the opioid/benzodiazepine solution. The insertion site is then covered with a transparent, bio-occlusive dressing. The site should be changed every 7 days or sooner if erythema develops. The same infusion pumps that are used for intravenous administration can be used for subcutaneous administration. The pressure limit may need to be adjusted to allow for subcutaneous administration. Alternatively, a syringe pump can be used. If symptoms of withdrawal develop, additional boluses can be administered subcutaneously if necessary. Several opioids can be administered subcutaneously including the synthetic opioids, morphine, hydromorphone, and meperidine. Longer-acting agents such as methadone and levorphanol are not recommended because dose titration may be difficult given the long half-lives of these agents. Tissue reaction and erythema have been noted with methadone. Although there is limited experience with the use of subcutaneous infusions of opioids/benzodiazepines as a means of weaning patients and preventing withdrawal, the subcutaneous route has been used to treat chronic cancer-related pain as well as postoperative pain.[37-40]

When prolonged administration of opioids or other sedative agents will be necessary, switching to the oral administration of long-acting agents such as methadone may allow for earlier hospital discharge. This is especially true in patients who have received weeks of therapy and are on large doses of opioids or benzodiazepines. Advantages of methadone include its longer half-life allowing for dosing two to three times per day, an oral bioavailability of 75% to 90%, and availability as a liquid. Although the first report regarding the use of methadone suggested a starting dose of 0.1 mg/kg every 12 hours (similar to the analgesic doses that were commonly used), the three patients in the series were receiving relatively low opioid doses and therefore higher doses of methadone were not needed.[6,35] The subsequent clinical experience has indicated that higher doses of methadone will be needed, depending on the dose and duration of opioid that have been administered. When considering the appropriate dose transition from intravenous fentanyl to oral methadone, thought should be given to the differences in the potency and half-life of the two medications as well as crossover tolerance.[35] Similar considerations are necessary when switching from intravenous midazolam to oral lorazepam or from intravenous dexmedetomidine to oral clonidine. Lugo and associates, in a study evaluating enteral lorazepam to decrease midazolam requirements during mechanical ventilation, suggested starting at a lorazepam dose that was one-sixth that of the total daily dose of intravenous midazolam.[41] Once the appropriate enteral/oral dose is determined and therapy started, the intravenous administration is tapered off quickly, generally over a 48-hour period.

After the initial reports regarding the use of methadone, several other authors have suggested variations in conversion ratios from fentanyl to methadone, the use of intravenous and then oral methadone, maintenance dosing intervals, and, most important, weaning schedules.[42-46] In clinical practice, it is useful not to dwell on the individual studies but rather to ensure that each institution has a formal policy for the initial dosing and subsequent weaning of methadone. This practice is suggested to avoid the natural variations that occur in physician practice, which may impact the success of such programs.[47] Regardless of the protocol used, close observation during the conversion period is necessary to avoid adverse effects from oversedation or to recognize the early symptoms of withdrawal. This observation should use some formal scoring system to evaluate infants for and score the magnitude of withdrawal when it occurs.

Given the advantages outlined here, methadone is now the common choice for the opioid-dependent infant in the PICU. However, some stigmata remain concerning the use of methadone. A thorough discussion with the parents is necessary to discuss why methadone is being used and to outline the differences between addiction and physical dependency. Because of these issues as well as familiarity with long-acting morphine preparations, which are used in the treatment of children with chronic cancer-related pain, some physicians have used long-acting preparations of morphine. However, these agents are available only in tablets that cannot be crushed so that administration and subsequent weaning protocols may be more difficult in younger patients. Methadone on the other hand is available in a liquid formulation. Concern has been expressed regarding adults who are on maintenance methadone for drug addiction in terms of the potential for death from QT prolongation and arrhythmias.[48] To date, there are no reports from the pediatric population; however, these concerns have led to the consideration of obtaining periodic ECGs prior to and after instituting therapy with methadone. Given the multitude of medications used in the PICU patient, avoidance of interactions with other agents that can potentially prolong the QT interval is suggested. A final issue with methadone is its metabolism by the P-450 isoenzyme system of the liver, making alterations in metabolism possible based on genetic factors and the co-administration of other medications. These factors should be considered when methadone is started or other medications are added to the patient's regimen.

In addition to opioids, nonopioid agents have been used to treat opioid withdrawal. This practice was relatively common when treating the withdrawal of infants born to drug-addicted mothers. In many cases, paregoric or other crude opioid preparations were used or, alternatively, barbiturates such as phenobarbital were given to control the clinical signs and symptoms. This would appear less than optimal, as it seems to make physiologic sense when dealing with the problems of tolerance and physical dependency to replace the missing agent rather than to treat the resulting symptoms. Given these concerns, our current clinical practice is generally to use a medication in the same class as the one resulting in withdrawal. However, in specific clinical scenarios, the centrally acting α_2-adrenergic agonists, clonidine and dexmedetomidine, have been used to treat and prevent opioid and benzodiazepine withdrawal.[49-52]

With the significant increase in the use of dexmedetomidine in the PICU in various clinical scenarios, withdrawal from this agent is becoming a more commonly encountered clinical problem. Dexmedetomidine (Precedex, Hospira Worldwide Inc, Lake Forest, Illinois) exerts its physiologic effects via α_2-adrenergic receptors, thereby making it a novel pharmacologic agent for sedation in various clinical scenarios. Given its beneficial physiologic effects and favorable adverse effect profile, it has made its way into the pediatric pharmacologic armamentarium in various clinical scenarios including sedation during mechanical ventilation, procedural sedation, the treatment of withdrawal, and the prevention of emergence agitation. It was speculated that this novel agent might cause little or no tolerance with prolonged infusion and that the infusion might be abruptly discontinued even following prolonged administration.[53,54] Walker and colleagues reported retrospective data regarding dexmedetomidine infusions in 65 pediatric patients (mean age of 5 years) with thermal injuries.[55] The duration of the infusion varied from 2 to 50 days (mean duration of 11 days). They noted no tachyphylaxis and no evidence of withdrawal or rebound hemodynamic effects when the infusions were weaned and discontinued over a 12- to 24-hour period. However, with increased use and clinical experience came the reports of tolerance, physical dependency, and withdrawal. Enomoto and associates used dexmedetomidine for 2 months to sedate an infant with respiratory failure following hepatic transplantation.[56] Tolerance was manifested by the need to increase the infusion from a starting dose of 0.4 µg/kg/hr to a maximum of 1.4 µg/kg/hr to achieve the desired level of sedation. At one point when the infusion was weaned over 48 hours to exclude drug-induced hepatic dysfunction, the child became anxious, developed hypertension, and his respiratory status deteriorated within 6 hours of stopping the infusion. These problems resolved upon restarting the dexmedetomidine infusion. Weber and coworkers reported hypertension, tachycardia, and emesis in a 2-year-old child when dexmedetomidine was discontinued after 6 days of administration.[57] The symptoms were effectively controlled by restarting the infusion and then incrementally decreasing the infusion by 0.1 μg/kg/hr every 8 hours. Similar anecdotal experiences demonstrating withdrawal symptoms from dexmedetomidine were reported by Darnell and colleagues.[58]

More compelling evidence for withdrawal from dexmedetomidine was provided by Honey and associates in their evaluation of adverse effects related to dexmedetomidine infusions used for sedation in the PICU setting.[59] Over a 12-month period, data were collected on 36 children who received continuous infusions of dexmedetomidine. Although the median duration of the infusion was 20 hours, the range varied from 3 to 263 hours. Neurologic issues were noted in 4 patients following dexmedetomidine infusions. One patient who received dexmedetomidine for 11 days developed decreased verbal communication, facial drooping, and unilateral papillary dilatation when the infusion was discontinued without tapering. Transient neurologic events, including increased agitation, abnormal chewing movements, nonreactive pupils, slow rhythmic jerking movements, and abnormal head turning, were noted in 3 other patients who had received dexmedetomidine for 6 to 49 hours. The infusion was tapered in 2 of these patients. Of additional note, these authors suggested that adverse events related to dexmedetomidine were more likely when the cumulative dose was ≥8.5 μg/kg.

Potential options to prevent such occurrences are to not abruptly discontinue the infusion following prolonged infusions of more than 4 to 5 days. Options to allow for its discontinuation include a slow taper via the intravenous route (0.1 μg/kg/hr every 12–24 hours), switching to an orally equivalent dose of clonidine, use of transdermal clonidine, and changing to subcutaneous administration (which can be used to eliminate the need for ongoing intravenous access).[52] In common clinical practice, most centers have adopted a regimen that involves the transition from intravenous dexmedetomidine to oral clonidine followed by a gradual taper of the oral clonidine dose. Two reports provide useful information regarding this practice.[60,61] In the first, the intent was to transition from intravenous dexmedetomidine to oral clonidine to decrease the cost of the ongoing intravenous dexmedetomidine infusion.[60] The study cohort included 20 adult patients for whom an attempt was made to transition over a 48-hour period from intravenous dexmedetomidine to enteral clonidine (0.3 mg every 6 hours). The transition was successful in 75% of the cohort with only one patient demonstrating symptoms of withdrawal. The authors also noted a decrease in fentanyl requirements in patients receiving oral clonidine compared to intravenous fentanyl (387 versus 891 μg/day) as well as a significant reduction in drug acquisition costs.

A subsequent study involved a retrospective review to assess the efficacy of a transition from intravenous dexmedetomidine to transdermal clonidine as a means of preventing withdrawal.[61] Withdrawal Assessment Tool-1 (WAT-1) scores and hemodynamic parameters were collected from pediatric patients who received intravenous dexmedetomidine for ≥5 days. The study cohort included 19 pediatric patients, 12 of whom received clonidine. For the 24 hours after weaning and transition to clonidine, there was a trend for a decreased number of elevated WAT-1 scores in patients receiving clonidine versus the no clonidine group (mean of 0.8 versus 3.2). Another option is the transition to oral clonidine. Despite limited evidence-based medicine for this practice, clinical experience has suggested that the transition from intravenous dexmedetomidine to oral clonidine can be accomplished over a 48-hour period with a clonidine dose of 3 to 5 μg/kg/dose every 6 to 8 hours.

Summary

With attention to the need for more aggressive sedation and analgesia during prolonged critical illness, the newer issues of physical tolerance and withdrawal have become more pervasive. Although preventing or at least delaying tolerance may be feasible using newer practices such as drug holidays or nurse-controlled sedation regimens, treatment algorithms are needed to avoid the adverse physiologic effects of these problems and to limit their impact on length of hospitalization. Clinical studies show consistently that regardless of the agent administered, withdrawal will occur once the sedative or analgesic medication has been administered by continuous infusion for more than 4 to 5 days. In those scenarios, the most commonly employed option is switching to an orally equivalent agent. During this process and as the oral agent is weaned, ongoing monitoring with a withdrawal score is suggested. To facilitate care and avoid variations in practice, many institutions have developed specific protocols for the oral agent to be used, the conversion from intravenous to oral doses, and the tapering regimen. By aggressively managing the issues of tolerance, physical dependency, and withdrawal, their impact on the effective provision of sedation and analgesia during critical illness can be minimized.

Key References

1. Collett BJ. Opioid tolerance: the clinical perspective. *Br J Anaesth*. 1998; 81:58-68.
2. Finnegan LP. Effects of maternal opiate abuse on the newborn. *Fed Proc*. 1985;44:2314-2317.
3. Finnegan LP, Connaughton JF Jr, Kron RE, et al. Neonatal abstinence syndrome: assessment and management. *Addict Dis*. 1975;2:141-158.
4. Arnold JH, Truog RD, Orav EJ, et al. Tolerance and dependence in neonates sedated with fentanyl during extracorporeal membrane oxygenation. *Anesthesiology*. 1990;73:1136-1140.
5. Arnold JH, Truog RD, Scavone JM, et al. Changes in the pharmacodynamic response to fentanyl in neonates during continuous infusion. *J Pediatr*. 1991;119:639-643.
6. Tobias JD, Schleien CL, Haun SE. Methadone as treatment for iatrogenic opioid dependency in pediatric intensive care unit patients. *Crit Care Med*. 1990;18:1292-1293.
7. Sury MRJ, Billingham I, Russell GN, et al. Acute benzodiazepine withdrawal syndrome after midazolam infusions in children. *Crit Care Med*. 1989;17:301-302.
8. van Engelen BGM, Gimbrere JS, Booy LH. Benzodiazepine withdrawal reaction in two children following discontinuation of sedation with midazolam. *Ann Pharmacother*. 1993;27:579-581.
9. Tobias JD. Dexmedetomidine: are there going to be issues with prolonged administration? *J Pediatr Pharmacol Ther*. 2010;15:4-9.
10. Fonsmark L, Rasmussen YH, Carl P. Occurrence of withdrawal in critically ill sedated children. *Crit Care Med*. 1999;27:196-199.
11. Tobias JD. Pentobarbital for sedation during mechanical ventilation in the pediatric ICU patient. *J Intensive Care Med*. 2000;15:115-120.
12. Yanay O, Brogan TV, Martin LD. Continuous pentobarbital infusion in children is associated with high rates of complications. *J Crit Care*. 2004; 19:174-178.

13. Ho IK, Yamamoto I, Loh HH. A model for the rapid development of dispositional and functional tolerance to barbiturates. *Eur J Pharmacol.* 1975;30:164-171.

14. Jaffe JH, Sharpless SK. The rapid development of physical dependence on barbiturates. *J Pharmacol Exp Ther.* 1965;150:140-146.

15. Cammarano WB, Pittet JF, Weitz S, et al. Acute withdrawal syndrome related to the administration of analgesic and sedative medications in adult intensive care unit patients. *Crit Care Med.* 1998;26:676-684.

16. Imray JM, Hay A. Withdrawal syndrome after propofol. *Anaesthesia.* 1991;46:704-705.

17. Arnold JH, Truog RD, Molengraft JA. Tolerance to isoflurane during prolonged administration. *Anesthesiology.* 1993;78:985-988.

18. Hughes J, Leach HJ, Choonara I. Hallucinations on withdrawal of isoflurane used as sedation. *Acta Paediatr.* 1993;82:885-886.

19. Creten C, Van der Zwaan S, Blankespoor R. Pediatric delirium in the pediatric intensive care unit. *Minerva Anestesiol.* 2011;77:1099-1107.

20. Gunther ML, Morandi A, Ely EW. Pathophysiology of delirium in the intensive care unit. *Crit Care Clin.* 2008;24:45-65.

21. Curley MA, Wypij D, Watson RS, et al. RESTORE Study Investigators and the Pediatric Acute Lung Injury and Sepsis Investigators Network: protocolized sedation vs usual care in pediatric patients mechanically ventilated for acute respiratory failure: a randomized clinical trial. *JAMA.* 2015;313:379-389.

22. Neunhoeffer F, Kumpf M, Renk H, et al. Nurse-driven pediatric analgesia and sedation protocol reduces withdrawal symptoms in critically ill medical pediatric patients. *Paediatr Anaesth.* 2015;25:786-794.

23. Bassett R, Adams KM, Danesh V, et al. Rethinking critical care: decreasing sedation, increasing delirium monitoring, and increasing patient mobility. *Jt Comm J Qual Patient Saf.* 2015;41:62-74.

24. Katz R, Kelly W, Hsi A. Prospective study on the occurrence of withdrawal in critically ill children who receive fentanyl by continuous infusion. *Crit Care Med.* 1994;22:763-767.

25. Anand KJS, Arnold JH. Opioid tolerance and dependence in infants and children. *Crit Care Med.* 1994;22:334-342.

26. Ista E, van Dijk M, Gamet C, et al. Withdrawal symptoms in children after long-term administration of sedative and/or analgesics: a literature review. "Assessment remains troublesome." *Intensive Care Med.* 2007;33:1396-1406.

27. Cunliffe M, McArthur L, Dooley F. Managing sedation withdrawal in children who undergo prolonged PICU admission after discharge to the ward. *Paediatr Anaesth.* 2004;14:293-298.

28. Franck LS, Naughton I, Winter I. Opioid and benzodiazepine withdrawal symptoms in paediatric intensive care patients. *Intensive Crit Care Nurs.* 2004;20:344-351.

29. Ista E, van Dijk M, Gamel C, et al. Withdrawal symptoms in critically ill children after long-term administration of sedatives and/or analgesics: a first evaluation. *Crit Care Med.* 2008;36:2427-2432.

30. Fisher D, Grap MJ, Younger JB, et al. Opioid withdrawal signs and symptoms in children: frequency and determinants. *Heart Lung.* 2013;42:407-413.

31. Franck LS, Scoppettuolo LA, Wypij D, Curley MA. Validity and generalizability of the Withdrawal Assessment Tool-1 (WAT-1) for monitoring iatrogenic withdrawal syndrome in pediatric patients. *Pain.* 2012;153:142-148.

32. Franck LS, Harris SK, Soetenga DJ, et al. The Withdrawal Assessment Tool-1 (WAT-1): an assessment instrument for monitoring opioid and benzodiazepine withdrawal symptoms in pediatric patients. *Pediatr Crit Care Med.* 2008;9:573-580.

33. Jacobi J, Fraser GL, Coursin DB, et al. Clinical practice guidelines for the sustained use of sedative and analgesics in the critically ill adult. *Crit Care Med.* 2002;30:119-141.

34. Playfor S, Jenkins I, Boyles C, et al. A consensus guidelines on sedation and analgesia in critically ill children. *Intensive Care Med.* 2006;32:1125-1136.

35. Tobias JD. Outpatient therapy of iatrogenic drug dependency following prolonged sedation in the pediatric intensive care unit. *Intensive Care Med.* 1996;11:284-287.

36. Tobias JD. Subcutaneous administration of fentanyl and midazolam to prevent withdrawal following prolonged sedation in children. *Crit Care Med.* 1999;27:2262-2265.

37. Bruera E, Brenneis C, Michaud M, et al. Use of the subcutaneous route for the administration of narcotics in patients with cancer pain. *Cancer.* 1988;62:407-411.

38. Bruera E, Gibney N, Stollery D, Marcushamer S. Use of the subcutaneous route of administration of morphine in the intensive care unit. *J Pain Symptom Manage.* 1991;6:263-265.

39. Tobias JD, O'Connor TA. Subcutaneous administration of fentanyl for sedation during mechanical ventilation in an infant. *Am J Pain Manage.* 1996;6:115-117.

40. Dietrich CC, Tobias JD. Subcutaneous fentanyl infusions in the pediatric population. *Am J Pain Manage.* 2003;13:146-150.

41. Lugo RA, Chester EA, Cash J, et al. A cost analysis of enterally administered lorazepam in the pediatric intensive care unit. *Crit Care Med.* 1999;27:417-421.

42. Robertson RC, Darsey E, Fortenberry JD, et al. Evaluation of an opiate-weaning protocol using methadone in pediatric intensive care unit patients. *Pediatr Crit Care Med.* 2000;1:119-123.

43. Lugo RA, MacLaren R, Cash J, et al. Enteral methadone to expedite fentanyl discontinuation and prevent opioid abstinence syndrome in the PICU. *Pharmacotherapy.* 2001;21:1566-1573.

44. Meyer MT, Berens RJ. Efficacy of an enteral 10-day methadone wean to prevent opioid withdrawal in fentanyl-tolerant pediatric intensive care unit patients. *Pediatr Crit Care Med.* 2001;2:329-333.

45. Siddappa R, Fletcher JE, Heard AMB, et al. Methadone dosage for prevention of opioid withdrawal in children. *Paediatr Anaesth.* 2003;13:805-810.

46. Berens RJ, Meyer MT, Mikhailov TA, et al. A prospective evaluation of opioid weaning in opioid-dependent pediatric critical care patients. *Anesth Analg.* 2006;102:1045-1050.

47. Atkinson D, Dunne A, Parker M. Torsades de pointes and self-terminating ventricular fibrillation in a prescription methadone user. *Anaesthesia.* 2007;62:952-955.

48. Tobias JD. Methadone: who tapers, when, where, and how? *Pediatr Crit Care Med.* 2014;15:268-270.

49. Gold MS, Redmond DER Jr, Kleber HD. Clonidine blocks acute opiate-withdrawal symptoms. *Lancet.* 1978;222:599-602.

50. Hoder EL, Leckman JF, Ehrenkranz R, et al. Clonidine in neonatal narcotic-abstinence syndrome. *N Engl J Med.* 1981;305:1284-1285.

Pediatric Delirium

Chani Traube and Bruce M. Greenwald

PEARLS

- Delirium is a potentially prevalent and serious sequela of pediatric critical illness.
- Refractory agitation in the pediatric intensive care unit is often a manifestation of delirium.
- Hypoactive delirium is frequently missed.
- Unit-wide screening for delirium is feasible with valid and reliable bedside tools.
- Detecting and treating pediatric delirium may improve short- and long-term outcomes.

Introduction

Delirium is the behavioral manifestation of acute global brain dysfunction. It is defined by the *Diagnostic and Statistical Manual of Mental Disorders,* Fifth Edition (DSM-V), as a disturbance of awareness and cognition, and it is characterized by an acute onset and a fluctuating course. Importantly, delirium is not a psychiatric diagnosis but is rather a complication of an underlying general medical condition.[1]

There are three principal subtypes of delirium. Hyperactive delirium (previously referred to in the intensive care unit [ICU] community as *ICU psychosis*) is characterized by agitation, restlessness, and emotional lability. Hypoactive delirium (sometimes called *encephalopathy of critical illness*) is notable for apathy and decreased responsiveness. Mixed delirium represents fluctuation between symptoms of both hyperactive and hypoactive delirium. Hyperactive delirium is the subtype most readily recognized. Conversely, unless there is a high index of suspicion, hypoactive delirium is often missed.[2-5]

Background

In January 2013, the Society of Critical Care Medicine (SCCM) published "Clinical Practice Guidelines for the Management of Pain, Agitation, and Delirium in Adult Patients in the Intensive Care Unit." The SCCM guidelines recommend routine monitoring for delirium in adult ICU patients, as "monitoring critically ill patients for delirium with valid and reliable delirium assessment tools enables clinicians to potentially detect and treat delirium sooner, and possibly improve outcomes."[6] This was the result of an explosion of delirium research, with thousands of articles published in peer-reviewed journals.[6]

Delirium is endemic in adult ICUs. With an overall prevalence of greater than 30%, it is more common in the elderly and affects up to 80% of adults on mechanical ventilation.

Delirium in adults has been linked to increased mortality, increased ICU length of stay, increased hospital length of stay, long-term cognitive impairment, and postintensive care syndrome. Median time to tracheal extubation is longer in delirious patients, and delirium has been associated with various ICU morbidities such as self-extubation and removal of catheters.[6-12] The association with mortality is strong, with duration of delirium correlated with increased risk. Two well-designed cohort studies in adult ICUs reported that for each day spent delirious, there was an increase in mortality.[11,13] In addition, delirium has been associated with significantly increased health care costs.[6,14]

Delirium in critically ill children has only recently received attention in the pediatric critical care literature. As in adults, it has been associated with severity of illness, prolongation of time to tracheal extubation, and increased hospital length of stay.[15-17] There is a robust relationship between pediatric delirium and increased hospital costs.[16,18] Delirium in children has been linked to delusional memories, perceptual-motor and behavior problems, and posttraumatic stress disorder.[19,20] Importantly, ICU medical and nursing practices can affect delirium rates. Therefore accurate and early recognition of delirium in critically ill patients is imperative.[6]

Etiology

The etiology of delirium is complex and the pathophysiology incompletely understood. An interruption of brain network connections occurs, with a failure of the integration and processing of sensory information and motor responses.[21] Much research has demonstrated that regardless of the primary etiology, the final common pathway involves alteration in neurotransmission, with subsequent cognitive and behavioral changes in the affected individual. Neurotransmitter dysregulation includes deficient acetylcholine and melatonin; excess dopamine, glutamate, and norepinephrine; and variable changes in gamma-aminobutyric acid (GABA), serotonin, and histamine.[22,23]

The cholinergic system modulates attention and consciousness, sleep, and memory.[24,25] Animal models have shown decreased acetylcholine synthesis in animals subjected to hypoxia/hypoxemia and immobilization.[22] Anticholinergic agents have long been implicated in the genesis of delirium, with the elderly at increased risk, likely due to an age-related decrease in acetylcholine synthesis in the hippocampus and prefrontal cortex.[13,26,27] Notably, children under 5 years of age have decreased acetylcholine synthesis in these areas as well.

A literature review by Maldonado described a range of etiologic theories as to the processes underlying delirium. These mechanisms are interrelated and likely synergistic in critically ill patients.[22] The neuroinflammatory hypothesis proposes that systemic inflammation from an underlying illness, with associated cytokine release, compromises the integrity of the blood-brain barrier. This results in CNS inflammation that leads to dysfunction of neurons and synapses.[28] Numerous studies in adults have shown that delirious patients have elevation of proinflammatory cytokines as compared to nondelirious patients, even after adjusting for multiple confounders.[29-31]

The neuronal aging hypothesis proposes that the elderly brain is more vulnerable to experiencing delirium due to a lack of physiologic reserve when the patient is seriously ill. In fact, dementia is the single strongest risk factor for delirium in the elderly.[32,33] In a damaged brain, microglia are primed to respond more vigorously to systemic inflammation.[34] This may be relevant to the population of developmentally delayed children in the pediatric ICU, a group that has been shown to be at higher risk for developing delirium than developmentally typical children.[16]

The oxidative stress hypothesis maintains that delirium represents *cerebral insufficiency*.[35] This is a form of brain failure, due to either hypoxia or hypoperfusion, which generates reactive oxygen species that induce oxidative damage. Several studies have demonstrated a correlation between hypoxia and delirium in both adults and children.[16,36,37]

The neuroendocrine hypothesis suggests that physiologic stress leads to an elaboration of glucocorticoids that cause direct neuronal injury.[22] The diurnal (or melatonin) dysregulation theory posits that disruption of sleep architecture can precipitate, and then perpetuate, delirium.[38,39]

Clinically, delirium can be thought of as the result of three synergistic factors: (1) the underlying illness, (2) the iatrogenic effects of the treatment for that illness, and (3) the highly abnormal ICU environment. As an example, consider the child who has recently undergone surgical repair of a congenital cardiac anomaly utilizing cardiopulmonary bypass. There may have been episodes of hypoxemia and hypotension in the perioperative period, which led to brain hypoperfusion. The postoperative state is characterized by inflammation and mechanical ventilation, both of which are associated with delirium. There has been exposure to anesthetic agents, and the patient is currently receiving opiates and benzodiazepines, which have been strongly linked to delirium. The patient is bedridden in an ICU and may also be immobilized, sleep deprived, and exposed to lights and noises 24 hours a day. These circumstances act together to form the framework for the emergence of delirium in this child.

Epidemiology

The prevalence of delirium in the pediatric ICU has been reported as ranging from approximately 10% to 30%.[40] A study completed in 2010, during the validation of a pediatric delirium screening tool, demonstrated a rate of 12.3%, but this study included only children over 5 years of age, and only 6% were receiving mechanical ventilation.[41] Thus, those children in the ICU most at risk for delirium may have inadvertently been either excluded or underrepresented. A more recent study included children from newborn to 21 years of age, with approximately 25% of patients receiving invasive mechanical ventilation. This study showed a prevalence rate of 21%[42] (Fig. 136.1).

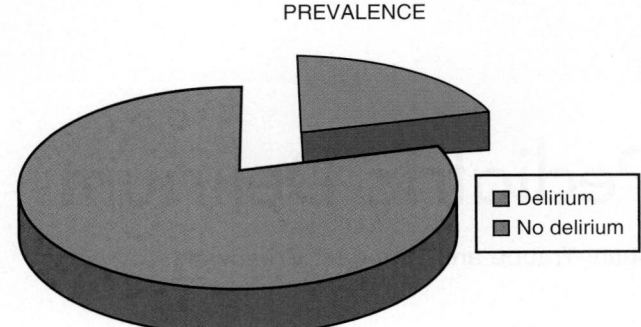

PREVALENCE

- Delirium
- No delirium

Fig. 136.1. Delirium prevalence in children newborn to 21 years of age. (From Traube C, Silver G, Kearney J, et al. Cornell Assessment of Pediatric Delirium: a valid, rapid, observational tool for screening delirium in the PICU. Crit Care Med. 2014;42:656-6563.)

Risk Factors

Baseline risk factors associated with delirium in adults are dementia, hypertension, alcoholism, male gender, cigarette use, and high severity of illness at admission.[6] Modifiable risk factors include depth of sedation, use of restraints, and choice of sedating medications. Adult ICU delirium has been associated with the use and dose of benzodiazepines, physical restraints, and the use of antipsychotics.[6,43-48] A prospective observational study described risk factors for pediatric delirium. In this single-center study, delirium was associated with increased severity of illness. After controlling for this and other possible confounders, risk factors for the development of delirium included preschool age, preexisting neurodevelopmental delay, escalating need for respiratory support, and concomitant sedation[16] (Fig. 136.2). There was a significantly greater incidence of delirium in children 2 to 5 years of age, with an adjusted odds ratio of 2.6 when compared with younger children and 8.8 when compared with adolescents. This may be a function of sleep deprivation and immobilization, which are conditions that are particularly disruptive to preschool-age children[16] (Table 136.1). Similarly, children with underlying developmental delay were at increased risk, with an adjusted odds ratio of 3.5 when compared with developmentally typical children. This may represent a lack of physiologic reserve in this atypical brain, similar to the increased prevalence of delirium in the geriatric population[16,22] (see Table 136.1). Children receiving invasive mechanical ventilation, who were necessarily exposed to sedatives, also had an increased delirium rate, with an adjusted odds ratio of 3.9. Importantly, this presents a possible modifiable risk factor, as clinicians can adjust their target sedation depth and their choice of sedative agents[16] (see Table 136.1).

Clinical Presentation

Pediatric delirium is complex and multifactorial, and it is further confounded by developmental variability. Normal behavior in a 2-year-old would be considered highly abnormal behavior in a 12-year-old. Thus, the developmental context is integral to the diagnosis of delirium in children. In fact, in early pediatric delirium research, questions were raised regarding the reliability of the DSM criteria in the diagnosis of delirium in young children, particularly preverbal children. To

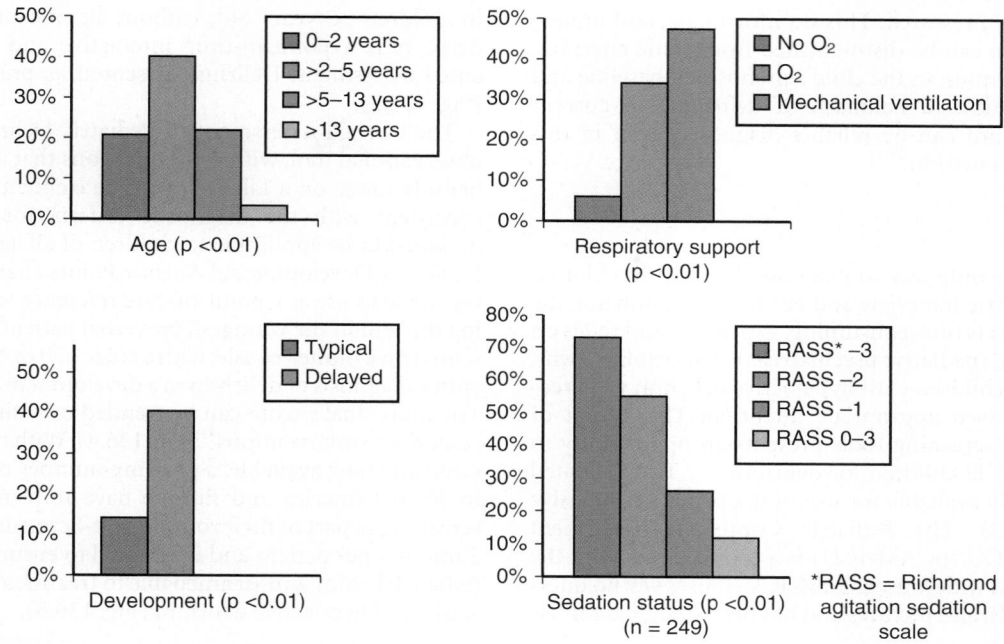

Fig. 136.2. Risk factors associated with a diagnoses of delirium. (Reproduced from Silver G, Traube C, Gerber LM, et al. Pediatric delirium and associated risk factors: a single-center prospective observational study. Pediatr Crit Care Med. 2015;16:303-309.)

TABLE 136.1	**Multivariable Logistic Regression Analyses Predicting Delirium (n = 252)**	
Predictor Variable	**Adjusted Odds Ratio (95% CI)**	**p-Value**
Age Category (Years)		
0-2	Reference standard	—
2-5	2.57 (1.11, 5.93)	0.027
5-13	0.87 (0.33, 2.33)	0.79
>13	0.29 (0.06, 1.43)	0.13
0-2	3.43 (0.70, 16.78)	0.13
2-5	8.80 (1.82, 42.53)	0.007
5-13	2.99 (0.58, 15.41)	0.19
>13	Reference standard	—
Developmental Delay		
Yes	3.45 (1.54, 7.76)	0.003
No	Reference standard	—
Mechanical Ventilation		
Yes	3.86 (1.81, 8.24)	0.0005
No	Reference standard	

Analysis controlled for potential confounders including severity of illness and gender.
CI, confidence interval.
Reproduced from Silver G, Traube C, Gerber LM, al. Pediatric delirium and associated risk factors: a single-center prospective observational study. Pediatr Crit Care Med. 2015;16:303-309.

address this issue, Silver and colleagues investigated the reliability of the criterion standard (delirium diagnosis by psychiatric examination utilizing the DSM-IV criteria) by performing 38 paired psychiatric evaluations of children at risk for delirium by two different psychiatrists. Fifty percent of the children in this cohort were under 2 years of age. Interrater reliability

of the paired psychiatric assessments was excellent, with a kappa of 0.95, demonstrating the reliability of the standard criteria for diagnosis of delirium in children.[49]

Delirium in critically ill adults is most often of the hypoactive subtype.[2,3,43] An emerging literature indicates that pediatric delirium is frequently mixed, with transition between hypo- and hyperactive symptoms occurring over the course of a single day. Hyperactive delirium is more readily recognized, as the child is actively interfering with the medical team's interventions. In the past, these children frequently received large doses of sedatives, which further contributed to the evolving delirium. It is this hyperactive subtype of delirium that is generally noted.[50] However, it represents only a portion of all delirium and generally has the best prognosis.[43]

It is the docile child, often termed the "good patient," who lies in his or her bed without protest and allows the care team to do whatever uncomfortable interventions are necessary, whose condition often goes unnoticed. This is markedly abnormal behavior for a preschool and school-age child and likely represents hypoactive delirium.[51,52] Hypoactive delirium is often missed without routine screening[5] and has been linked to the worst prognosis in multiple studies in adult patients.[53,54] With timely recognition and treatment, the duration of delirium can be decreased.

Children with delirium can present with a range of alterations in psychomotor activity, including fidgetiness and self-stimulating behavior or sluggish responses to interactions. Children and adolescents may have a disordered emotional state, with extreme tearfulness, inconsolability, or an inappropriate calmness relative to their circumstances. In addition, pediatric delirium is often marked by profound sleep disturbance, which itself further worsens the delirium.[18,52,55]

The diagnosis of delirium may be challenging in the developmentally delayed child. As such, this at-risk subgroup is often omitted from research. This is unfortunate, and unnecessary, as delirium can be distinguished from static encephalopathy. With attention to the child's prehospital baseline and focus on fluctuation (a hallmark of delirium) in current symptoms, delirium can be reliably diagnosed even in this hard-to-assess population.[49,51]

Diagnosis

Until recently, the only way to diagnose delirium in children was via a psychiatric interview and examination, utilizing the DSM criteria. This is time consuming, expensive, and relies on a limited resource (pediatric psychiatrists). This explains why, historically, only children with hyperactive delirium were recognized and received appropriate attention. The advent of bedside delirium screening tools presents an opportunity to assess all critically ill children for delirium.[56-58] Two validated tools are currently available for use in the pediatric intensive care unit (PICU). The Pediatric Confusion Assessment Method for the ICU (pCAM-ICU) is a tool derived from the well-validated and widely used CAM-ICU. It uses yes/no questions, hand signals, and pictures and has been designed for use

in children >5 years old, without significant developmental delay. It is a point-in-time interactive and cognitively oriented assessment. Delirium is scored as present or absent[41] (Fig. 136.3).

The Cornell Assessment of Pediatric Delirium is a strictly observational tool, with eight questions that are scored by the bedside nurse on a Likert scale. The elements of the tool are consistent with the diagnostic criteria for delirium. It is designed to be applicable to children of all ages and cognitive levels.[42] A Developmental Anchor Points chart is available for the nurse to use as a point-of-care reference when administering the tool in the youngest, preverbal patients.[51] The screen is scored on a numeric scale, with a score of 9 or higher consistent with a diagnosis of delirium in a developmentally typical child. The individual's score can be trended over time to determine response to interventions[42] (Fig. 136.4). With real-time bedside screening now available, a growing number of pediatric ICUs in North America and Europe have implemented delirium screening as part of their routine care. Screening takes less than 2 minutes per patient and is essential to ensure early detection (when delirium is most amenable to treatment) of both hyperactive and hypoactive delirium (Fig. 136.5).

pCAM-ICU Instruction Tool		
Step 1: Arousal Assessment **(RASS)**: If RASS is **≥ − 3** then PROCEED to **Step 2** Content Assessment (pCAM-ICU) If RASS is **− 4 or − 5** then STOP and REASSESS patient later	RASS	
Step 2: Content Assessment **(pCAM-ICU)** Features 1 – 4		
FEATURE 1: Change or fluctuation in Mental Status		
1. Is there an **acute change** from mental status baseline (MSB)? *MSB is the patient's pre-hospital mental status.*	□ yes □ no	
2. Has there been a **fluctuation** in mental status over the past 24 hours? *May use GCS, sedation scale, PE, or history.*	□ yes □ no	
Feature 1 is POSITIVE when the answer to either question is 'yes.'	**+ / —**	
FEATURE 2: Inattention → Attention Screening Examintion (ASE) with Letters or Memory Pictures		
It is normal to have some anxiety in "performing" the pCAM-ICU when you start. Do NOT try to memorize what to say when assessing inattention or disorganized thinking. Use the pCAM-ICU card during your evaluation of the patient and read directly from it for feature 2 and feature 4. The verbage we use is verbatim off the card.		
Letters (Vigilance A Test) • **Place** your hand or finger in the palm of the patient's hand. • Say, *"Squeeze my hand when I say 'A'. Let's practice: A, B. Squeeze only on 'A'."* • During the practice squeeze on A and B, **do not correct** the patient's squeeze or lack there of. For pediatric patients, you are allowing the brain time to process the command twice. Then move on with the letter sequence. • <u>Read this 10 letter sequence without stopping</u> : *A B A D B A D A A Y* • Use the card to read off the letter sequence so your attention is on the total number of errors. Do NOT stop and repeat command when child has errors. • Errors → No squeeze with 'A' or Squeeze with letter other than 'A'.	**Memory pictures** • **Hold** the memory picture stack in front of the patient. • Say, *"Here are some pictures. You need to remember them."* • **Show** the patient the <u>5 memory pictures</u>. Show each picture for 2-3 seconds. • **Pause** at the blank card following the 5 memory pictures and say, *"Here are some more pictures. Tell me 'yes or no' (or nod yes or no) if the picture you see was one you needed to remember."* • **Show** the patient <u>10 pictures</u> (5 memory pictures & 5 'other' pictures). Say the name of each object and show each picture for 2-3 seconds. • Errors → 'No' response to a memory picture **or** 'Yes' response to an 'other' picture	
Feature 2 is POSITIVE when a patient demonstrates > 2 Errors on either the Vigilance A test OR ASE picture test	ERRORs	**+ / —**
Feature 3: Altered Level of Consciousness		
This feature determines the **current** level of consciousness (LOC) regardless of the patient's baseline mental status. Any validated sedation scale may be used to determine current LOC.		
Feature 3 is POSITIVE when the current LOC is anything other than 'Alert and Calm' (RASS score '0')	Score RASS	**+ / —**
Feature 4: Disorganized Brain		
Say, *"I am going to ask you some questions. Say or nod yes or no to answer each question."* Ask each question slowly and clearly, giving time for an answer. ▪ Is sugar sweet? Alternate: □ Is a rock hard? ▪ Is ice cream hot? □ Do rabbits fly? ▪ Do birds fly? □ Is ice cream cold? ▪ Is an ant bigger than an elephant? □ Is a giraffe smaller than a mouse? ▪ **Command: Say,** *"Hold up this many fingers."* **Demonstrate** by holding up 2 fingers. **Wait** while the patient attempts to complete the command. Then **say,** *"Now do that with the other hand,"* **OR** *"Add one more finger."* With this part of the command, **do NOT demonstrate** to the patient. Errors → Incorrect 'Yes' or 'No' response to questions or inability to complete the 2-step command. (4 points for questions and 1 point for 2-step command = 5 possible points)		
Feature 4 is POSITIVE when a patient demonstrates > 1 Error	ERRORs	**+ / —**
Delirium Outcome	Delirium is present when Feature 1 is POSITIVE + Feature 2 POSITIVE AND Either a POSITIVE **Feature 3** OR **Feature 4**	Present □ Absent □ UTA □

Fig. 136.3. Pediatric Confusion Assessment Method for the ICU. (Reproduced from http://www.icudelirium.org/docs/Instruction-Tool_pCAM-ICU.pdf.)

	Never 4	Rarely 3	Sometimes 2	Often 1	Always 0	Score
1. Does the child make eye contact with the caregiver?						
2. Are the child's actions purposeful?						
3. Is the child aware of his/her surroundings?						
4. Does the child communicate needs and wants?						

RASS score____(if −4 or −5 do not proceed)

Please answer the following questions based on your interactions with the patient over the course of your shift:

	Never 0	Rarely 1	Sometimes 2	Often 3	Always 4	
5. Is the child restless?						
6. Is the child inconsolable?						
7. Is the child underactive—very little movement while awake?						
8. Does it take the child a long time to respond to interactions?						
					Total	

Fig. 136.4. Cornell Assessment for Pediatric Delirium. (Reproduced from Traube C, Silver G, Kearney J, et al. Cornell Assessment of Pediatric Delirium: a valid, rapid, observational tool for screening delirium in the PICU. Crit Care Med. 2014;42:656-663.)

EARLY DETECTION OF DELIRIUM

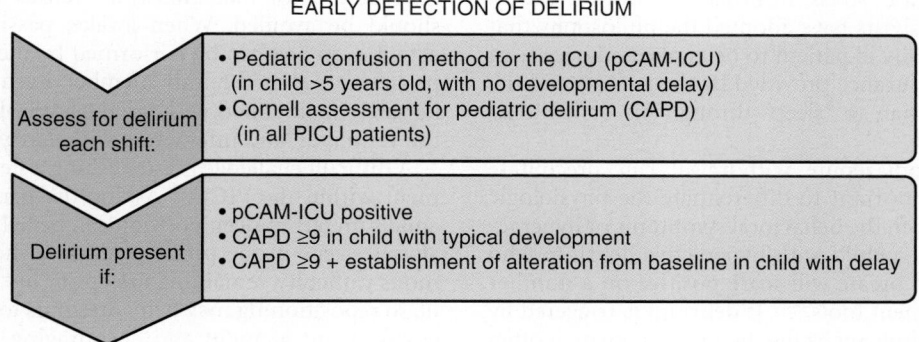

Assess for delirium each shift:
• Pediatric confusion method for the ICU (pCAM-ICU) (in child >5 years old, with no developmental delay)
• Cornell assessment for pediatric delirium (CAPD) (in all PICU patients)

Delirium present if:
• pCAM-ICU positive
• CAPD ≥9 in child with typical development
• CAPD ≥9 + establishment of alteration from baseline in child with delay

Fig. 136.5. Detection of delirium.

Treatment

With increasing awareness in the pediatric critical care community as to the prevalence and possibly poor prognostic implications of delirium, as well as the ability to identify children with delirium in real time, targeted interventions may be employed to minimize its duration and potentially ameliorate the long-term effects of delirium. Just as delirium is caused by three associated triggers (underlying illness, complications of therapy, and the environment of care), when delirium is diagnosed, attention should be focused on these three areas as well (Fig. 136.6).

Underlying Illness

Timely detection of delirium offers an early warning sign—a call to attention that something significant is occurring. A positive delirium screen should lead to a series of clinical questions. Is a new infection brewing? (Delirium symptoms often precede the fever heralding the new infection). Is there evolving respiratory or hepatic or renal insufficiency leading to metabolic abnormalities? Is there a new, primary neurologic problem? A focused evaluation, including physical examination, neurologic examination, and appropriate laboratory workup, is indicated.[59]

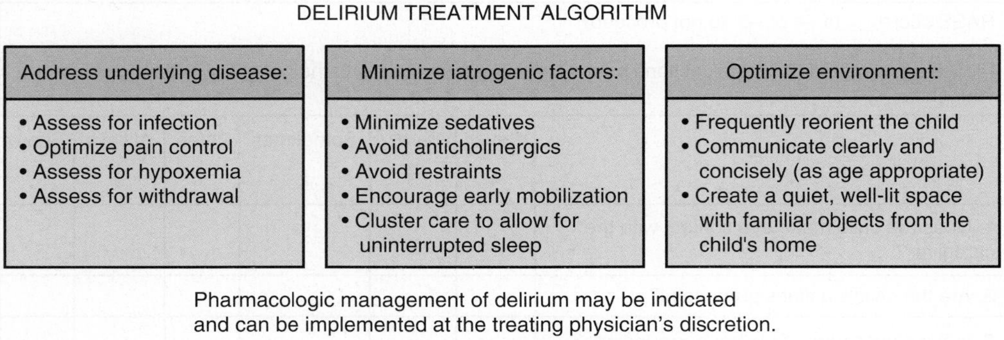

DELIRIUM TREATMENT ALGORITHM

Address underlying disease:	Minimize iatrogenic factors:	Optimize environment:
• Assess for infection • Optimize pain control • Assess for hypoxemia • Assess for withdrawal	• Minimize sedatives • Avoid anticholinergics • Avoid restraints • Encourage early mobilization • Cluster care to allow for uninterrupted sleep	• Frequently reorient the child • Communicate clearly and concisely (as age appropriate) • Create a quiet, well-lit space with familiar objects from the child's home

Pharmacologic management of delirium may be indicated and can be implemented at the treating physician's discretion.

Fig. 136.6. Delirium treatment algorithm.

Iatrogenic Factors

Following assessment for previously undetected illness, attention should turn to the numerous clinical factors that can lead to delirium. Pain control should be optimized with appropriate use of opiates and nonopiate analgesics.[60,61] Sedation should be minimized, as clinically appropriate. A patient on invasive mechanical ventilation, whose sedative regimen has been steadily escalated over the course of hours to days, may be delirious as a direct result of the sedatives and will often improve with removal of the offending agents.[62] Many experts feel that benzodiazepines are particularly problematic and that escalating dosages result in increased risk for delirium and excess ventilator days.[48] In years past, clinicians hoped to decrease the traumatic effect of hospitalization by sedating the child; recent data indicates that this is counterproductive, interferes with the clinician's ability to adequately recognize and treat pain, and may increase the risk of delusional memories and posttraumatic stress disorder.[19,63] More recently, many pediatric intensivists have adopted the philosophy that it is better for a critically ill patient to be awake and occasionally upset—with reassurance provided by the parents and the clinical care team—than to "sleep" through his or her ICU stay.[16]

Opiate and benzodiazepine withdrawal can precipitate delirium, but it is important to differentiate the physiologic signs of abstinence from the behavioral symptoms of hyperactive delirium. In fact, a child with hyperactive delirium who has never been on an opiate will score positive on a number of withdrawal assessment tools.[64,65] If delirium is triggered by opiate withdrawal, simply replacing the missing opiate is often insufficient to reverse the symptoms. Judicious replacement of the opiate is necessary, but it is important to then approach the delirium as a primary problem, rather than continue to escalate the opiate dose, as this will simply prolong the delirium exposure.[16]

Reviewing the patient's medication list is essential. Anticholinergic agents and medications with anticholinergic effects may be routinely and often unnecessarily used in the PICU and can frequently be discontinued or replaced.[24] If a child with hyperactive delirium is on corticosteroids, a taper should be considered. The literature indicates that benzodiazepines increase delirium rates in critically ill adults; ongoing research in pediatrics suggests the same. Consideration should be given to minimizing the use of benzodiazepines and replacing these agents with dexmedetomidine when sedation is necessary.[6,47,48,66]

Environment

Optimizing the environment is an achievable goal.[67] It is important to ensure that children who require corrective lenses have their glasses on when awake. Creating a well-lit and uncluttered space during the day is feasible and effective. Educating parents and staff to limit guests and avoid commotion at the bedside is essential. Familiar items from home such as a favorite blanket or stuffed toy are more effective than new gifts. Helium balloons can be disconcerting to a lightly sedated child as they move spontaneously and can contribute to hallucinations.

In adults, early mobilization has been shown to decrease delirium rates and shorten delirium once it occurs.[68-70] Implementation of an early mobilization protocol in the PICU does not have to be as dramatic as walking an intubated child; it can start as a simple change in approach and mindset. A child on invasive mechanical ventilation should be permitted to have periods of wakefulness as well as sleep; deep sedation should be avoided. When awake, passive range-of-motion activities in bed can be performed by the nurse or an appropriately supervised family member. Even young children can be safely maintained with a light level of sedation, awake on the ventilator, and interacting with caregivers.[16,71]

A difficult challenge is establishing a sleep-friendly environment within the PICU.[72] Asking the parents to describe the child's preferred sleep position can be helpful—a toddler who always sleeps in the prone position at home will have enormous difficulty remaining asleep on his back while critically ill, so repositioning may help. Attempts to ensure a quiet, dark environment at night and encouraging parents to continue their usual bedtime routines (such as a storybook or back rub) can help facilitate sleep, even in the ICU.

Pharmacotherapy

In 15% to 20% of cases, attempts to address the underlying illness, minimize therapeutic triggers, and optimize the environment are not enough, and persistent delirium symptoms interfere with necessary medical interventions. In such instances, pharmacologic therapy for delirium may be indicated.[67] Currently no drug has been approved by the Food and Drug Administration to treat delirium in either adults or children, but the consensus approach is to use antipsychotic agents (either haloperidol or the atypical antipsychotics due to their more favorable side effect profiles).[6] These procognitive drugs regulate neurotransmitters and can help organize thoughts and calm the delirious patient. This may facilitate the patient's cooperation with ongoing medical care and allow the opportunity for the patient to wean from other medications that promote delirium.[73]

Evidence for pharmacotherapy is scarce. One randomized, placebo-controlled study showed a reduction of the duration of delirium with quetiapine (an atypical antipsychotic medication) in critically ill adults.[74] There have been several case series describing the successful use of atypical antipsychotic agents (including olanzapine, quetiapine, and risperidone) to treat delirium in young children, but no prospective efficacy studies have been conducted to date.[71,75-78] A retrospective study designed to evaluate the safety of quetiapine in treating delirium in critically ill children found no serious adverse events with >2400 doses administered.[79] There are no published data showing that treatment with haloperidol reduces the duration of delirium in adults or children, although it remains a reasonable choice and a mainstay of treatment in many ICUs.[73,80] Further research is needed to systematically assess the safety and efficacy of antipsychotics in the treatment of pediatric delirium.

Prevention

Prevention of delirium remains an elusive goal. Data in adults suggest that early mobilization of critically ill patients will reduce the incidence of delirium and shorten its duration.[69,70] In hospitalized adults who are not critically ill, a multicomponent intervention, with protocols for cognition, sleep, mobility, vision, hearing, and hydration, decreased delirium rates.[81] There is no evidence that prophylactic administration of antipsychotics decreases delirium rates in the general ICU population, although a subset of elderly patients, or those after cardiac surgery, may benefit in the immediate postoperative period when their delirium rates are quite high.[80,82-84] There are currently no prospective studies describing effective preventive strategies for the development of delirium in critically ill children. Further research is necessary and under way.

Conclusion

Delirium is prevalent in critical illness and is associated with significant short- and longer-term morbidity. Children are at significant risk of developing delirium while in the pediatric ICU. With increased awareness of this common problem, pediatric intensivists can detect delirium sooner and implement strategies to treat and prevent this serious complication of PICU care. Further research is needed to improve the care provided to this vulnerable population.

Key References

1. *Diagnostic and Statistical Manual of Mental Disorders*. 5th ed. Washington, DC: American Psychiatric Association; 2013.
5. Ely EW, Siegel MD, Inouye SK. Delirium in the intensive care unit: an under-recognized syndrome of organ dysfunction. *Semin Respir Crit Care Med*. 2002;22:115-126.
6. Barr J, Fraser GL, Puntillo K, et al. Clinical practice guidelines for the management of pain, agitation, and delirium in adult patients in the intensive care unit. *Crit Care Med*. 2013;41:278-280.
7. Ouimet S, Kavanagh BP, Gottfried SB, Skrobik Y. Incidence, risk factors and consequences of ICU delirium. *Intensive Care Med*. 2006;33:66-73.
8. Ely EW, Shintani A, Truman B, et al. Delirium as a predictor of mortality in mechanically ventilated patients in the intensive care unit. *JAMA*. 2004;291:1753-1762.
10. Girard TD, Jackson JC, Pandharipande PP, et al. Delirium as a predictor of long-term cognitive impairment in survivors of critical illness. *Crit Care Med*. 2010;38:1513-1520.
11. Shehabi Y, Riker RR, Bokesch PM, et al. Delirium duration and mortality in lightly sedated, mechanically ventilated intensive care patients. *Crit Care Med*. 2010;38:2311-2318.
13. Pisani MA, Kong SYJ, Kasl SV, et al. Days of delirium are associated with 1-year mortality in an older intensive care unit population. *Am J Respir Crit Care Med*. 2009;180:1092-1097.
14. Milbrandt EB, Deppen S, Harrison PL, et al. Costs associated with delirium in mechanically ventilated patients. *Crit Care Med*. 2004;32:955-962.
15. Schieveld JNM, Lousberg R, Berghmans E, et al. Pediatric illness severity measures predict delirium in a pediatric intensive care unit. *Crit Care Med*. 2008;36:1933-1936.
16. Silver G, Traube C, Gerber LM, et al. Pediatric delirium and associated risk factors: a single-center prospective observational study. *Pediatr Crit Care Med*. 2015;16:303-309.
17. Turkel SB, Tavare CJ. Delirium in children and adolescents. *J Neuropsychiatry Clin Neurosci*. 2003;15:431-435.
19. Colville G, Kerry S, Pierce C. Children's factual and delusional memories of intensive care. *Am J Respir Crit Care Med*. 2008;177:976-982.
22. Maldonado JR. Neuropathogenesis of delirium: review of current etiologic theories and common pathways. *Am J Geriatr Psychiatry*. 2013;21:1190-1222.
23. Trzepacz PT. Update on the neuropathogenesis of delirium. *Dement Geriatr Cogn Disord*. 1999;10:330-334.
26. Flacker JM, Cummings V, Mach JR, et al. The association of serum anticholinergic activity with delirium in elderly medical patients. *Am J Geriatr Psychiatry*. 1999;6:31-41.
30. De Rooij SE, van Munster BC, Korevaar JC, Levi M. Cytokines and acute phase response in delirium. *J Psychosom Res*. 2007;62:521-525.
31. McGrane S, Girard TD, Thompson JL, et al. Procalcitonin and C-reactive protein levels at admission as predictors of duration of acute brain dysfunction in critically ill patients. *Crit Care*. 2011;15:R78.
33. Franco C, Bernal C, Ocampo M, et al. Relationship between cognitive status at admission and incident delirium in older medical inpatients. *J Neuropsychiatry Clin Neurosci*. 2010;22:329-337.
36. Seaman J, Carroll D, Brown T. Impaired oxidative metabolism precipitates delirium: a study of 101 ICU patients. *Psychosomatics*. 2006;47:56-61.
37. Schoen J, Meyerrose J, Paarmann H, et al. Preoperative regional cerebral oxygen saturation is a predictor of postoperative delirium in on-pump cardiac surgery patients: a prospective observational trial. *Crit Care*. 2011;15:R218.
39. Mistraletti G, Cigada M, Zambrelli E, et al. Sleep and delirium in the intensive care unit. *Minerva Anestesiol*. 2008;74:329-333.
41. Smith HAB, Boyd J, Fuchs DC, et al. Diagnosing delirium in critically ill children: validity and reliability of the Pediatric Confusion Assessment Method for the Intensive Care Unit. *Crit Care Med*. 2011;39:150-157.
42. Traube C, Silver G, Kearney J, et al. Cornell Assessment of Pediatric Delirium: a valid, rapid, observational tool for screening delirium in the PICU. *Crit Care Med*. 2014;42:656-663.
43. McPherson J, Boehm L, Hall J, et al. Delirium in the cardiovascular ICU: exploring modifiable risk factors. *Crit Care Med*. 2013;41:405-413.
45. Mehta S, Cook D, Devlin JW, et al. Prevalence, risk factors, and outcomes of delirium in mechanically ventilated adults. *Crit Care Med*. 2015;43:557-566.
46. Pisani MA, Murphy TE, Araujo KLB, et al. Benzodiazepine and opioid use and the duration of intensive care unit delirium in an older population. *Crit Care Med*. 2009;37:177-183.
47. Pandharipande P, Peterson J, Pun B, et al. Lorazepam is an independent risk factor for transitioning to delirium in intensive care unit patients. *Anesthesiology*. 2006;104:21-26.
48. Pandharipande PP, Sanders RD, Girard TD, et al. Research effect of dexmedetomidine versus lorazepam on outcome in patients with sepsis: an a priori-designed analysis of the MENDS randomized controlled trial. *Crit Care*. 2010;14:R38.
49. Silver G, Kearney J, Traube C, et al. Pediatric delirium: Evaluating the gold standard. *Palliat Support Care*. 2014;1-4.
50. Silver G, Traube C, Kearney J, et al. Detecting pediatric delirium: development of a rapid observational assessment tool. *Intensive Care Med*. 2012;38:1025-1031.

51. Silver G, Kearney J, Traube C, Hertzig M. Delirium screening anchored in child development: The Cornell Assessment for Pediatric Delirium. *Palliat Support Care.* 2014;1-7.

54. Inouye SK, Schlesinger MJ, Lydon TJ. Delirium: a symptom of how hospital care is failing older persons and a window to improve quality of hospital care. *Am J Med.* 1999;106:565-573.

55. Grover S, Kate N, Malhotra S, et al. Symptom profile of delirium in children and adolescent—does it differ from adults and elderly? *Gen Hosp Psychiatry.* 2012;34:626-632.

58. Schieveld JN, Janssen NJ. Delirium in the pediatric patient: on the growing awareness of its clinical interdisciplinary importance. *JAMA Pediatr.* 2014;168:595-596.

60. Tobias JD. Acute pain management in infants and children—part 1: pain pathways, pain assessment, and outpatient pain management. *Pediatr Ann.* 2014;43:e163-e168.

61. Tobias JD. Acute pain management in infants and children—part 2: intravenous opioids, intravenous nonsteroidal anti-inflammatory drugs, and managing adverse effects. *Pediatr Ann.* 2014;43:e169-e175.

62. Skrobik Y, Leger C, Cossette M, et al. Factors predisposing to coma and delirium: fentanyl and midazolam exposure; CYP3A5, ABCB1, and ABCG2 genetic polymorphisms; and inflammatory factors. *Crit Care Med.* 2013;41:999-1008.

63. Clukey RL, Roberts M, Henderson A. Discovery of unexpected pain in intubated and sedated patients. *Am J Crit Care.* 2014;23:216-220.

67. Hipp DM, Ely EW. Pharmacological and nonpharmacological management of delirium in critically ill patients. *Neurother.* 2012;9:158-175.

68. The TEAM Study Investigators. Early mobilization and recovery in mechanically ventilated patients in the ICU: a bi-national, multi-centre, prospective cohort study. *Crit Care.* 2015;19:81.

70. Needham D, Zanni J, Pradhan P, et al. Early physical medicine and rehabilitation for patients with acute respiratory failure: a quality improvement project. *Arch Phys Med Rehabil.* 2010;91:536-542.

71. Traube C, Witcher R, Mendez-Rico E, Silver G. Quetiapine as treatment for delirium in critically ill children: a case series. *J Pediatr Intensive Care.* 2013;2:121-126.

72. Kudchadkar SR, Yaster M, Punjabi NM. Sedation, sleep promotion, and delirium screening practices in the care of mechanically ventilated children: a wake-up call for the pediatric critical care community. *Crit Care Med.* 2014;42:1592-1600.

74. Devlin JW, Roberts RJ, Fong JJ, et al. Efficacy and safety of quetiapine in critically ill patients with delirium: a prospective, multicenter, randomized, double-blind, placebo-controlled pilot study. *Crit Care Med.* 2010; 38:419-427.

76. Turkel SB, Jacobson J, Munzig E, Tavaré CJ. Atypical antipsychotic medications to control symptoms of delirium in children and adolescents. *J Child Adolesc Psychopharmacol.* 2012;22:126-130.

77. Silver GH, Kearney JA, Kutko MC, Bartell AS. Infant delirium in pediatric critical care settings. *Am J Psychiatry.* 2010;167:1172-1177.

78. Traube C, Augenstein J, Greenwald B, et al. Neuroblastoma and pediatric delirium: a case series: neuroblastoma and delirium. *Pediatr Blood Cancer.* 2014;61:1121-1123.

79. Joyce C, Witcher R, Herrup E, et al. Evaluation of the Safety of Quetiapine in Treating Delirium in Critically Ill Children: A Retrospective Review. *J Child Adolesc Psychopharmacol.* 2015;Available from: <http://online. liebertpub.com/doi/10.1089/cap.2015.0093>.

80. Girard TD, Pandharipande PP, Carson SS, et al. Feasibility, efficacy, and safety of antipsychotics for intensive care unit delirium: The MIND randomized, placebo-controlled trial. *Crit Care Med.* 2010;38:428-437.

81. Inouye SK, Bogardus ST Jr, Charpentier PA, et al. A multicomponent intervention to prevent delirium in hospitalized older patients. *N Engl J Med.* 1999;340:669-676.

Index

A

AACN. *See* American Association of Critical-Care Nurses (AACN)

Abdominal binding, in CPR, 507

Abdominal compartment syndrome (ACS), 1368, 1399

Abdominal distention, mechanical ventilation and, 754

Abdominal examination, 1358–1359

Abdominal trauma
  child abuse and, 1659–1660
  evaluation/resuscitation, 1645–1646
  management of, 1646–1653, 1649t
    aortic injury, 1651
    bladder injury, 1653
    duodenal injury, 1648–1650, 1650f
    embolization, 1647
    liver injury, 1648, 1650f
    nonoperative, 1647, 1647t
    pancreatic injury, 1650–1651, 1651f
    pelvic fractures, 1653, 1653t
    renal injury, 1651–1652, 1652f
    small intestinal injury, 1648, 1650f
    spleen injury, 1647–1648, 1648f
  mechanisms/patterns of, 1644–1645
    penetrating, 1644–1645
    recreational/sports injury, 1645
    wartime trauma, 1645

Abnormal movements, with static encephalopathy, 849

ABP. *See* American Board of Pediatrics (ABP)

Absolute risk reduction (ARR), in EBM, 61.e1t

Absorption, of drugs, 1674–1676, 1674b–1675b

Abusive head trauma (AHT), 1658

Accidental hypothermia. *See under* Hypothermia

Acclimatization, 1563

Accreditation Council for Graduate Medical Education (ACGME)
  on communication skills, 37
  core competencies, 208–210, 221t
  requirements, 216

ACD-CPR. *See* Active compression-decompression-cardiopulmonary resuscitation (ACD-CPR)

Acetaminophen (Paracetamol), 1385, 1745–1746, 1746f

Acetylcholine, 811, 812f

ACGME. *See* Accreditation Council for Graduate Medical Education (ACGME)

Acid-base disorders
  abnormal pH, 1080–1081
  anion gap/corrected anion gap and, 1069–1071, 1071t
  base excess/standard base excess in, 1067–1068, 1068t
  blood gases, 1081
  causes of, 1082t
  classification of, 1077t
  CO_2 and bicarbonate in Stewart's approach, 1072
  introduction, 1061–1062
  mixed, 1095
  new insights in, 1080
  nonvolatile weak acids, 1074–1075
  physiochemical approach to, 1071–1076
    partial pressure of carbon dioxide, 1071
    strong ion difference, 1071–1074
    total concentration of nonvolatile weak acids, 1071–1072
  respiratory, 1092–1095
  six rules of thumb approach to, 1068–1069, 1069t–1070t
  strong ion gap, 1074
  strong ions/urinary anion gap, 1075–1076
  surrogates of SID/SIG, 1077–1080
  tools for interpreting, 1067–1076, 1073t
    integration of, 1076–1081, 1078t, 1079f

Acid-base physiology
  acids, bases and buffers in, 1064–1065
  carbon dioxide and bicarbonate effect on, 1065–1067
  in hypothermia, 1095–1096
  as measure of oxygen delivery, 295
  overview of, 1062–1067
  principle of electroneutrality in, 1063
  role of water/electrolytes in, 1062–1065

Acidemia, 1080–1081

Acidosis. *See also* Metabolic acidosis
  causes of, 1082t
  correction of in DKA, 1200
  process of, 1063
  respiratory, 1066

Acids, definition of, 1062

Acquired heart disease, 953

Acquired immune dysfunction
  abdominal complications, 1449–1450, 1449t, 1450b
    acute abdomen, 1450
  cardiovascular complications, 1447–1448
    dysrhythmias, 1448
    myocardial dysfunction, 1447–1448
    pericardial disease, 1448
    septic shock, 1447
    vasculitis, 1447
  critical illness and, 1440–1441
  hematologic complications, 1451
  hepatobiliary failure, 1450
  HIV infection/AIDS and, 1444–1445
  immunosuppressive agents and, 1443
  infectious agents and, 1443
  malignancies, 1451
  malnutrition and, 1441–1443
  neurologic complications, 1451–1452
    cerebrovascular disease, 1451
    CNS malignancy, 1451–1452
    HIV encephalopathy, 1451
    infections of CNS, 1452
  occupational HIV exposure, 1452
  overview of, 1440
  pancreatitis, 1450
  pulmonary complications/respiratory failure, 1445–1447
    cytomegalovirus pneumonitis, 1446
    fungal infections, 1447
    lymphoid interstitial pneumonitis, 1447
    mycobacterial pathogens, 1446–1447
    pneumocystis jirovecii pneumonia, 1445–1446
    upper airway obstruction, 1447
  renal failure, 1448–1449
  transfusions and, 1443
  uremia and, 1443

ACS. *See* Abdominal compartment syndrome (ACS); Acute chest syndrome (ACS)

Active compression-decompression-cardiopulmonary resuscitation (ACD-CPR), 505–506, 506f–507f

Acute abdomen
  anatomic/physiologic considerations, 1394
    peritoneum, 1394
    visceral blood flow, 1394
  conditions requiring treatment, 1397–1398

Acute abdomen (*Continued*)
  abdominal compartment syndrome,
    1399
  cholecystitis, 1398
  hemorrhage, 1398
  intraabdominal abscess, 1399
  ischemia, 1397–1398
  neutropenic enterocolitis, 1398
  pancreatitis, 1398
  perforated viscera, 1397
  sepsis from intestine, 1399–1400
  spontaneous bacterial peritonitis,
    1398–1399
  in HIV/AIDS patients, 1450
  imaging options, 1396–1397
  laboratory tests, 1395–1396
  physical examination, 1394–1395
  surgical intervention for, 1400
Acute cardiogenic pulmonary edema,
  771–772
Acute cellular rejection, in cardiac
  transplantation, 484–486, 485*t*
Acute chest syndrome (ACS), 1250–1251
  etiologies of, 1251.*e1f*
  management of, 1251, 1251*t*, 1250.*e4f*
  presentation of, 1251
Acute colonic pseudo-obstruction, 1368
Acute coronary syndrome, 1471–1472
Acute disseminated encephalomyelitis
  (ADEM), 872, 873*f*–874*f*, 979–980,
  980*f*, 980*t*
Acute hemolytic reaction, to RBC
  transfusion, 1308
Acute hemorrhagic leukoencephalitis
  (AHLE), 980–981, 981*t*
Acute intermittent porphyria (AIP),
  989–990
Acute kidney injury (AKI)
  cardiac surgery-related, 1053
  classification of, 1027*t*
  clinical impact, 1047–1048
  criteria for, 1027*t*
  hemodynamically mediated, 1044–1045
  kidney diseases leading to, 1048–1058
    acute glomerulonephritis, 1049–1052,
      1049*b*
    cardiorenal syndrome, 1052–1053
    drug-induced nephrotoxicity,
      1055–1058
    hemolytic uremic syndrome,
      1048–1049
    nephrotic syndrome, 1051–1052
    pigment nephropathy, 1054–1055
    TLS, 1053–1054, 1054*t*
    tubulointerstitial disease, 1052, 1052*b*
  mechanisms of, 1043–1044
  morphologic changes in, 1041–1042
  novel biomarkers for, 1035, 1036*f*
  pathophysiology of, 1040–1044, 1041*b*
  prevention/attenuation of, 1045–1047
    adenosine/adenosine triphosphate,
      1046

Acute kidney injury (AKI) (*Continued*)
    atrial natriuretic factor, 1047
    calcium entry blockers, 1046
    diuretics, 1046
    dopamine, 1045–1046
    free radical scavengers, 1047
    glycine and alanine, 1047
    prostaglandins, 1046
    renin-angiotensin antagonists, 1046
    thyroxine, 1047
  reduced GFR in, 1042–1043
  urinary tract obstruction and, 1058,
    1059*t*
Acute liver failure (ALF), 1382–1389,
  1487
  background/definitions/outcome,
    1382–1383, 1487
  clinical presentation, 1487
  complications with
    ascites, 1386
    cerebral edema, 1387, 1387*f*
    coagulopathy, 1386
    glucose/electrolytes/fluid balance,
      1386
    hepatic encephalopathy, 1386–1387
    infection, 1388
    renal dysfunction, 1388
    ventilation, 1388
  diagnosis of, 1383, 1384*t*, 1490–1493
  diseases causing, 1369–1370, 1369*t*
  etiology of, 1487
  extracorporeal liver support for,
    1388–1389, 1389*f*
  PICU management of, 1383–1385,
    1383*t*–1385*t*
  prognostic assessment, 1383
  treatment for, 1493
    for specific causes, 1385–1386
  workup, 1383, 1384*t*
Acute pancreatitis, 1368–1369
Acute phase, of stress response,
  1148–1149
Acute phase response, 1564
Acute postinfectious glomerulonephritis,
  1050
Acute renal failure (ARF). *See also* Renal
  failure
  prevention/reversal of, 1103
  after stem cell transplantation, 1058
Acute respiratory disease, 662–668
  meconium aspiration syndrome,
    667–668
  pneumonia, 666–667
  pulmonary air leak syndromes, 664–666
  pulmonary hemorrhage, 666
  retained fetal lung liquid, 662–664
  surfactant-deficient respiratory distress
    syndrome, 664
Acute respiratory distress syndrome
  (ARDS)
  clinical features/pathophysiology, 627
  definition of, 627–628, 628*f*

Acute respiratory distress syndrome
  (ARDS) (*Continued*)
  extracorporeal life support, 634
  introduction, 627
  morbidity and outcomes, 634
  noninvasive support for, 634
  nonpulmonary therapies, 632–634
    monitoring, 633–634
    prone positioning, 632–633, 633*f*
  outcomes following, 75
  pathobiology of, 628–630, 629*f*
    alveolar epithelial-endothelial barrier,
      628
    apoptosis, 630
    coagulation, 630
    fibrosis and repair, 630
    leukocytes and inflammation, 629
    pulmonary endothelial injury,
      628–629
    risk factors, 628*t*
    surfactant, 630
  pulmonary ancillary therapies,
    631–632
    exogenous surfactant, 631–632
    nitric oxide, 632
  short-term NIV for, 772–774
  ventilation/perfusion mismatch in,
    592
  ventilator management, 630–631
Acute respiratory failure
  ECMO for, 673
  high-frequency ventilation for,
    672–673
  liquid ventilation for, 673–674
  nitric oxide inhalation for, 673
  short-term NIV for, 772–774
  surfactant replacement for, 672
Acute tubular necrosis (ATN), 1388
Acute tubulointerstitial nephritis (ATIN),
  1052, 1052*b*
Acute vasodilator testing, for PAH, 725
Adam's Circuit and nasal pillows, for NIV,
  776, 776*f*
Adaptive immune system
  effector T-cell immunity, 1415–1419,
    1416*f*–1417*f*, 1417*t*
  elements of, 1455
  humoral immune response, 1414–1415,
    1414*f*–1415*f*, 1415*t*
  introduction, 1413
  lymphocytes recognition of antigens,
    1413–1414
  in PICU, 1419–1420, 1420*t*
ADEM. *See* Acute disseminated
  encephalomyelitis (ADEM)
Adenomatoid malformations, 671
Adenosine
  in AKI attenuation, 1046
  for arrhythmias, 400, 405–409, 521*f*
  as neurotransmitter, 813–814
Adenosine deaminase deficiency, in SCID,
  1433

Adenosine triphosphate (ATP), 1044
    in AKI attenuation, 1046
    cellular respiration and, 1131–1137,
        1132*f*, 1134*f*
    RBC-derived, 1240–1241
    structure of, 1133*f*
Adenosine triphosphatease inhibition,
    358
Adenovirus, 689
Adhesion molecules, 1525–1526, 1525*f*
Admission process, of PICU, 106
Adolescents, decision making by, 117
Adrenal insufficiency, 1182
    primary, 1182
    secondary, 1182
α-Adrenergic agonists
    with CPR, 509–511, 509*f*–511*f*, 510*b*
    toxicity of, 1737
β-Adrenergic agonists
    for asthma, 651, 653–654
    with CPR, 509–511, 509*f*–511*f*, 510*b*
    drug-drug interactions of, 1720–1721,
        1720*t*, 1726
    toxicity of, 1737–1738, 1745
β-Adrenergic antagonists
    drug-drug interactions of, 1720–1721,
        1720*t*, 1726
    toxicity of, 1737–1738
Adrenergic receptors, 352–356, 353*t*
    α-adrenergic receptors, 353–354, 355*f*
    β-adrenergic receptors, 353, 355*f*
    downregulation of, 354–356
    polymorphisms of, 356
    signal transduction by, 352–353,
        353*f*–354*f*
Adult cardiopulmonary bypass, pediatric
    vs., 438, 438*t*
Adult learning theory, 219, 219*f*
    applied to medical education, 220
    costs and benefits, 220*t*
Advance directives, 117
Advanced Trauma Life Support (ATLS),
    1599
Adverse drug reactions
    in cardiovascular system, 1710–1712,
        1710*t*, 1711*b*
    in CNS, 1712–1713, 1712*t*
    definition/identification of, 1707–1708
    dermatologic, 1715–1716
    endocrine/metabolic, 1713–1715,
        1714*t*
    hematologic, 1713
    in liver, 1709, 1710*b*
    in renal system, 1708–1709, 1708*t*
    respiratory, 1713
Advocacy, as nurse competency, 45
AEDs. *See* Automated external
    defibrillators (AEDs)
Aerosol therapy, 763
Afterload
    methods of reducing, 493, 493*f*
    systolic wall tension and, 489–490

AG. *See* Anion gap (AG)
Age
    developmental spectrum and
        drawbacks of, 54–55
        new diagnostic approaches, 57
        research advantage of, 53
    fluid compartment size and, 1677, 1677*t*
Agenesis, pulmonary, 672
Agitation, management of, 132
AGMA. *See* Anion gap metabolic acidosis
    (AGMA)
Agonists, full vs. partial, 1693*f*
AHLE. *See* Acute hemorrhagic
    leukoencephalitis (AHLE)
AHT. *See* Abusive head trauma (AHT)
AIHA. *See* Autoimmune hemolytic anemia
    (AIHA)
AIP. *See* Acute intermittent porphyria
    (AIP)
Air leak, pulmonary, 664–666
Airway
    caliber of, 560–561
    clearance of, 1590
    compliance of, 604–605
    conducting, 556–557
    during CPR, 528–529
    dynamics, 602–604, 603*f*–604*f*
    establishing with cervical spine
        stabilization, 1601–1604, 1602*t*,
        1603*f*
    extrathoracic/intrathoracic obstruction,
        584–585, 585*t*
    injury to, 1640
        from mechanical ventilation, 759–760
    mediastinal tumors compromising, 1319,
        1320*f*
    obstruction, 605
        mechanical ventilation for, 751–752
    rheumatic disease compromising, 1470
    structure and development of, 548–551,
        549*f*–551*f*
    traumatic injury to, 623–624
    vascular tumors/malformations of, 677
Airway management
    alternative approaches to, 1771–1774
        cricothyrotomy/retrograde intubation,
            1774
        laryngeal mask airway, 1771–1773,
            1771*f*–1772*f*
        lighted intubation stylet, 1771
        tracheostomy, 1773–1774
    anatomic considerations, 1751–1752,
        1752*f*
    basic management, 1752–1754, 1753*t*
        nasopharyngeal airway, 1753, 1753*f*
        oropharyngeal airways, 1753, 1753*f*
        oxygen delivery devices, 1753–1754
    endotracheal intubation, 1755–1766
        complications, 1766, 1766*t*
        extubation, 1765–1766, 1765*t*
        flexible fiberoptic bronchoscopy, 1765
        indications for, 1755–1756, 1755*b*

Airway management (*Continued*)
        nasotracheal intubation, 1764–1765
        neuromuscular dysfunction, 1756
        orotracheal intubation, 1763–1764,
            1763*f*–1764*f*
        pharmacologic agents facilitating,
            1761–1763, 1762*t*
        physiologic effects of, 1756–1757,
            1756*b*
        process of, 1759–1761, 1760*f*, 1760*t*
        prolonged intubation, 1766
        recognition of difficult airway,
            1757–1759, 1757*b*, 1758*f*–1759*f*
        video laryngoscopy, 1765
    establishing functional airway, 1754–
        1755, 1755*f*
    special circumstances, 1766–1770
        cervical spine instability, 1769–1770
        facial/laryngotracheal injury, 1770
        full stomach, 1766–1768, 1767*b*
        increased intracranial pressure/
            neurologic dysfunction, 1768–
            1769, 1768*b*
        open globe injury, 1770
        upper airway obstruction, 1770
Airway pressure release ventilation
    (APRV), 749–750, 750*f*
AIS. *See* Arterial ischemic stroke (AIS)
AKI. *See* Acute kidney injury (AKI)
Albumin, 1074–1075
Albuterol (salbutamol), for asthma, 651,
    653–654
ALF. *See* Acute liver failure (ALF)
Alfentanil, 1777, 1777*f*
Alkalemia, 1080–1081
Alkalinizing agents, 516. *See also* Sodium
    bicarbonate
Alkalosis, 1063, 1082*t*. *See also* Metabolic
    alkalosis; Respiratory alkalosis
Allograft
    early dysfunction of, 483–484
    rejection of, 484–486, 485*t*
Alnine, in AKI attenuation, 1047
Alphatocopherol (vitamin E), 1442
Alprostadil. *See* Prostaglandin E1 (PGE1),
    for PPHN
ALPS. *See* Autoimmune
    lymphoproliferative syndrome (ALPS)
Altered sensorium, with static
    encephalopathy, 849
Alternative pathway, 1423, 1424*f*
Alveolar epithelial-endothelial barrier, 628
Alveolar pressure, ventilation effect on,
    383–385, 384*f*–385*f*
Alveolar ventilation, 564–565
Alveolar-capillary unit, 551–553,
    551*f*–553*f*
Alveoli
    formation of, 551
    mechanical ventilation and, 753
Amanita poisoning, 1385
Amatoxin poisoning, 1385

Ambrisentan, for PAH, 728–729
American Association of Critical-Care Nurses (AACN), 47
    AACN Certification Corporation, 49–50, 49t
American Board of Pediatrics (ABP), 216
Amino acids
    neurotransmitters from, 812f, 813
    in parenteral nutrition, 1217
Aminoglycosides
    for infections, 1478
    nephrotoxicity and, 1055–1056, 1708t, 1709
Amiodarone
    for arrhythmias, 406–407
    for ventricular fibrillation, 520–523, 521f, 522b, 533
    for ventricular tachycardia, 533
Amniofusion, meconium aspiration syndrome and, 668
Amphotericin B
    for infections, 1480–1481
    nephrotoxicity of, 1056, 1088
Anaerobic bacteria, 686
Anaerobic respiration, 1133–1136, 1134f
Analgesia. See also Sedation
    drug-drug interactions of, 1724
    ECLS complications involving, 313
    facilitating intubation, 1761–1762, 1762t
    for mechanical ventilation, 658–659
    respiratory depression and, 581
    withholding/withdrawing life support and, 124
Anatomy, history of, 3–4
Anemia, 1312–1313
    adaptive mechanisms with, 1295–1296
    bloodless medicine and, 1299
    classification of, 1313b
    hemolytic, 1314–1315, 1317f
    hemorrhagic, 1312–1316
    oxygen delivery and, 1295, 1296f
    RBC transfusion for, 1297
    secondary to bone marrow failure, 1313–1314
    in thalassemia, 1257
Anesthesia. See also Operating room anesthesia
    drug-drug interactions of, 1723–1724
    effects of, 1776–1778, 1777f
    local agents for, 1778–1779, 1780f
    for mechanical ventilation, 659
    organ system considerations for
        anesthesia neurotoxicity in brain, 1783–1784, 1783f–1784f
        effects on CBF, 1781–1783, 1781f–1782f
        intracranial pressure, 1779–1780, 1780t
        neurologic injury, 1779
    with SCD, 1254, 1254.e1f
Anesthesia bags, 1754–1755

Anesthesiologists, in founding PCCM, 9–10
Anesthesiology, history of, 5, 6t
Aneurysms, ICH and, 960–961
ANF. See Atrial natriuretic factor (ANF)
Angioedema, 624
Angiotensin II, 1178, 1179t
Anion gap (AG), 1069–1071, 1071t, 1162–1163
Anion gap metabolic acidosis (AGMA), 1085–1086, 1741–1745, 1741b, 1742t
Anisocoria, 887, 889f
Antagonists, surmountable vs. insurmountable, 1693f
Anterior mediastinal tumors, 1319, 1320f
Anthracycline-induced cardiogenic shock, 1321–1322
Antiarrhythmic agents, 405–406
    for ventricular fibrillation/tachycardia, 520–523, 520t, 521f–522f, 533
Antibiotics
    for asthma, 660
    for bacterial meningitis, 967–969, 968t–969t
    classes of, 1476–1482
        aminoglycosides, 1478
        β-lactam, 1476–1477, 1476f
        fluoroquinolones, 1478–1479
        glycopeptides, 1478
        macrolides, 1478
        miscellaneous, 1479
    considerations for, 1475–1476, 1476t
    diarrhea associated with, 1375–1376
    drug-drug interactions of, 1722–1723
    gastric decontamination, 1513
    for heart transplant patients, 486
    after liver transplant, 1391
    prophylactic, 1438
    resistance, 1482
        mechanisms of, 1482
        in PICU, 1482–1483
        therapy for, 1483
    stewardship, 1483, 1510
Antibodies
    functions/characteristics, 1415t
    immune system and
        clinical presentation, 1425
        deficiencies in, 1423t
    secretion of, 1414–1415, 1414f–1415f
Anticholinergic agents
    for asthma, 652, 654
    facilitating intubation, 1761
    toxicity of, 1738–1739, 1738b
Anticoagulant(s)
    drug-drug interactions of, 1724–1725, 1725t
    overdose, 1275–1277
        of heparin, 1275–1276
        of warfarin, 1276–1277, 1276t
    properties, of endothelium, 271–272, 271f–272f

Anticoagulation
    before CPB, 436–437, 437f
    for CRRT, 1110
    for pediatric thrombosis, 1290–1292, 1290t
    prior to cardiac transplantation, 482
    strategies, for ECLS complications, 312–313
Anticonvulsant medications, drug-drug interactions of, 1721–1722
Antidromic reciprocating tachycardia (ART), 394–395
Antifungal agents, 1480–1482, 1481t
    amphotericin, 1480–1481
    echinocandins, 1482
    flucytosine, 1482
    triazoles, 1481–1482
Anti-GBM antibody disease, 1051
Antigens, lymphocyte recognition of, 1413–1414
Antihypertensive agents, for HTN, 1122–1126, 1123t
Antineoplastic agents, drug-drug interactions of, 1726
Anti-N-methyl-D-aspartate receptor (anti-NMDAR) encephalitis, 981–982, 982f–983f
Antioxidants, for impaired tissue oxygenation, 1143
Antiphospholipid syndrome (APS), 1466–1467
Antithrombin, 1282–1283, 1283f
Antithrombotic therapy, for AIS, 957
Antithymocyte globulin, for immune suppression, 484–486, 485t
Antivenin treatment, 1556–1557
Antiviral agents, for viral pneumonitis, 691–692, 692t
Anxiety, management of, 132
Aorta
    balloon valvotomy of, 345–346, 346f
    blunt trauma to, 1649t, 1651
    stenosis of, 473
Aplasia, pulmonary, 672
Aplastic crisis, in SCD, 1252, 1252.e1f
Apnea, of prematurity, 676–677
Apnea test, for brain death, 137–138, 137t
Apoptosis
    in ARDS, 630
    in critical illness, 1174–1177
        animal studies of, 1175–1177
        human studies of, 1174–1175
        mechanisms of, 1173–1174, 1174f
        necrosis vs., 1173
        neurodevelopmental, 830
APRV. See Airway pressure release ventilation (APRV)
APS. See Antiphospholipid syndrome (APS)
Arachidonic acid, 1702

Arachnoid cysts, 836
   background, 836, 836f
   clinical presentation, 836
   diagnosis of, 836
   management of, 836
ARAS. See Ascending reticular activating
      system (ARAS)
ARDS. See Acute respiratory distress
      syndrome (ARDS)
ARF. See Acute renal failure (ARF)
Arousal, anatomy of, 883–884, 884f
ARR. See Absolute risk reduction (ARR), in
      EBM
Arrest phase, of cardiac arrest, 526–527,
      527t
Arrhythmias. See also Bradycardias;
      Tachycardias
   classification of, 392–396, 393t
   diagnostic approach to, 397–400
      monitoring of atrial depolarization,
         398f, 400
      monitoring/general assessment, 397
      surface ECG, 397–400, 397t
      uses of adenosine, 400
   drug-induced, 1710–1712, 1710t
   escape rhythms/accelerated rhythms, 394
   extrasystoles, 398–399
   after Fontan procedure, 463
   HIV/AIDS and, 1448
   malignant, 309
   primary, 409–412, 410b
      chaotic atrial tachycardia, 410, 411f
      long QT syndromes, 410–412, 411f
      orthodromic reciprocating tachycardia
         in infancy, 409–410
      tachycardia-induced cardiac
         dysfunction, 410
      ventricular tachycardia in healthy
         patients, 412, 412f
   QOT and, 297
   rheumatic disease associated with, 1471
   secondary, 410b, 412–414
      infections and, 414
      late postoperative arrhythmias, 413
      metabolic derangements, 413–414
      postoperative arrhythmias, 412–413
      resulting from drug toxicity, 414, 414f
   therapeutic approach to, 408–409
      extrasystoles, 408
      sustained tachycardias, 408–409
      treatment failure, 409
      unstable patients, 409
   treatment, 400–408, 400f, 407t
      bradycardia therapies, 401
      newer indications for pacing, 404–405
      permanent pacing, 404, 405f
      tachycardia therapies, 405–408
      temporary pacing, 401–404,
         401f–404f
ART. See Antidromic reciprocating
      tachycardia (ART)
Arterial blood gas, 650

Arterial catheter placement, 161–163
   complications, 163
   contraindications for, 161
   indications for, 161
   maintenance, 163
   supplies/equipment, 162b
   technique for, 161–163
Arterial hypertension, induced, 1634–1635
Arterial ischemic stroke (AIS). See also
      Stroke
   definition of, 951
   etiologies/risk factors, 951–953, 953t
      cerebral arteriopathy, 951–952, 952f
      congenital/acquired heart disease,
         953
      hypercoagulable states, 953
      sickle cell disease, 952–953
   laboratory evaluation, 955, 955t
   neuroimaging of, 954–955, 954f
   pathophysiology of, 953
   presentation of, 953–954
   treatment, 956–957
      antithrombotic therapy, 957
      endovascular/neurosurgical treatment,
         956, 956f
      supportive therapy, 956
      thrombolysis, 956
Arterial pressure catheters
   indications for, 283–284
   interpretation of waveforms, 284, 284f
Arterial pressure, during CPB, 439
Arterial switch operation, for TGA,
      467–468
Arterial thrombosis, 1284–1285,
      1289–1290
Arteriovenous malformations (AVMs),
      959–960, 960f
Artifact, ultrasound, 181, 182f
Ascending reticular activating system
      (ARAS), 883–884, 884f
Ascites, with ALF, 1386
Ascitic fluid, 179, 179t
Ascorbic acid (vitamin C), 1442
Aspergillus, 1480
Asphyxia, traumatic, 1640–1641
Aspiration
   foreign body, 623, 623f–624f
   use of colorants to identify, 1360
Aspiration pneumonia, 698–699, 698b
Assessment tools, health-related quality of
      life, 76–77, 78t
Assisted dual-control breath-to-breath
      ventilation, 748–749
Asthma
   antibiotics for, 660
   bronchoscopy for, 660
   clinical assessment, 649–650
      history, 649
      physical examination, 649–650, 649t,
         650f
      radiography, 650
   electrocardiography, 651

Asthma (Continued)
   emergency department management of,
      651–652
      admission criteria, 652
   epidemiology/risk factors, 646–647,
      647b
   extracorporeal life support, 660
   laboratory data, 650–651
      arterial blood gas analysis, 650
      electrolytes/blood cell count, 650–651
      muscle enzymes, 651
   mechanical ventilation for, 656–659
      analgesia/sedation/muscle relaxation,
         658–659
      indications, 656
      inhalational anesthetic agents, 659
      intubation, 656–657
      ventilator monitoring, 658, 659f
      ventilator settings, 657–658,
         657f–658f
   overview of, 646
   pathophysiology, 647–649, 648f–649f
   PICU management of, 652–656
      anticholinergic agents, 654
      β-agonists, 653–654
      corticosteroids, 652–653
      fluids, 652
      general, 652
      helium-oxygen mixtures, 655–656
      ketamine, 656
      magnesium sulfate, 654–655
      methylxanthine agents, 655
      oxygen, 652
   prognosis, 660
   spirometry, 651
   treatment, 651–652
   ventilation/perfusion mismatch in,
      592–593
Asymmetrical lung disease, 753–754
Ataxia telangiectasia (AT), 1435–1436
ATC. See Automatic tube compensation
      (ATC)
ATIN. See Acute tubulointerstitial nephritis
      (ATIN)
ATLS. See Advanced Trauma Life Support
      (ATLS)
ATN. See Acute tubular necrosis (ATN)
ATP. See Adenosine triphosphate (ATP)
Atracurium, 1815t, 1819–1820
Atrial depolarization, monitoring of, 398f,
      400
Atrial fibrillation, 395, 396f
Atrial natriuretic factor (ANF), 1047
Atrial septal defect, 464–465
Atrial septostomy, for PAH, 730
Atrial switch procedure, for TGA, 467
Atrioventricular block, 392–394, 393f
Atrioventricular canal defects, 465–466
Atrioventricular nodal reentrant
      tachycardias, 395
Atrioventricular reciprocating tachycardias,
      394–395

Atropine
  with CPR, 514
  for ventricular fibrillation, 520t, 522f
Attributable risk, in EBM, 61.e1t
Australia, history of PCCM in, 14
Autoimmune hemolytic anemia (AIHA),
    1314–1315, 1314b
Autoimmune hepatitis, 1385–1386
Autoimmune lymphoproliferative
    syndrome (ALPS), 1436
Autoimmune status epilepticus, 917–922
Autologous red blood cell units, 1301
Automated adverse event detection, 97
Automated external defibrillators (AEDs),
    533–534
Automatic tube compensation (ATC), 749
AutoMode mechanical ventilation, 749
Autonomic peripheral nervous system,
    820
Autophagy
  cellular response of, 1407, 1408t
  in critical illness, 1176
  definition of, 1173
  mechanisms of, 1174
Autopsy, in fatal child abuse, 1661
Autoregulation
  of CBF
    development of, 829–830, 830f
      hydrogen ion-related, 827
      oxygen-related, 827
      perfusion pressure-related, 826–827
  of regional peripheral circulation, 257
  of systemic vasculature, 252
Autotriggering, in ventilation, 755
AVMs. See Arteriovenous malformations
    (AVMs)
Axonal injury, in TBI, 1618–1619, 1620f
Azathioprine, for immune suppression,
    484–486, 485t

B
B cells
  activation of, 1414–1415, 1414f
  component of immune system
    clinical presentation, 1425
    deficiencies in, 1423t
  specific immune disorders, 1428–1430
    common variable immunodeficiency
        syndrome, 1429–1430
    hyper-IgM syndrome, 1428–1429
    laboratory tests for, 1432t, 1437
    selective IgA deficiency, 1430
    treatment for, 1437–1438
    X-linked agammaglobulinemia,
        1428
Bacterial meningitis, 965–966
  adjunctive therapy for, 970
  clinical manifestations of, 966–971
  diagnosis of, 967
  epidemiology of, 965–966
  outcomes, 970–971
  pathogenesis of, 966

Bacterial meningitis (Continued)
  prevention of, 970
  supportive care, 969–970
  treatment of, 967–969, 968t–969t
Bacterial pneumonitis, 683–687
  clinical features of, 684
  complications, 686, 686t
  definition of, 683
  diagnosis of, 684
  pathophysiology of, 683–684
  preventive measures, 688t
  radiographic features, 684
  specific pathogens in, 684–686
  therapy for, 686–687, 687t
Bacterial tracheitis, 618t, 620
Balloon atrial septostomy (BAS)
  in catheterization laboratory, 344,
      344f–345f
  echocardiography-guided, 332, 335f
BALT. See Bronchus-associated lymphoid
    tissue (BALT)
Bar coding of medications, 99
Barbiturates
  for intracranial hypertension,
      1631–1632
  for RSE, 925
  toxicity of, 1737
Basal ganglia, 819
Base excess (BE), in acid-base disorders,
    1067–1068, 1068t
Bases, definition of, 1062
Basiliximab, for immune suppression,
    484–486, 485t
BBB. See Blood-brain barrier (BBB)
BE. See Base excess (BE), in acid-base
    disorders
Beacon Award for Critical Care Excellence,
    47
Bedside, teaching at, 211–212
Bench model, limited translation of, 55
Beneficence, in pediatric intensive care,
    115–116
Benzodiazepines
  delirium and, 1874
  drug-drug interactions of, 1723
  facilitating intubation, 1762, 1762t
  for RSE, 925
  toxicity of, 1737
Beraprost, for PAH, 728
Best interest standard, 118
Bicarbonate, in acid-base balance,
    1065–1067, 1072
Bicarbonate six rules of thumb approach,
    1068–1069, 1069t–1070t
Bicarbonate/carbonic acid buffering
    system, 1064–1065
Bidirectional cavopulmonary anastomosis,
    461, 462t
Bilevel positive airway pressure (BiPAP),
    1754
Bioavailability, in pharmacokinetics,
    1685

Biochemical assessment
  in nutritional status assessment,
      1206–1208
  of parenteral nutrition, 1218
Bioenergetic-targeted therapy, 1142–1143
Bioethics
  definition of, 112
  domains of, 112–113
Biomarkers, in HF patients, 491
BioMedicus centrifugal pump, 316, 317f
Biotransformation, 1679t
  factors affecting, 1680–1681
  phase I, 1678–1680
  phase II, 1680
BiPAP. See Bilevel positive airway pressure
    (BiPAP)
Bipyridines, 373–374, 373f
Birth, pulmonary circulation after,
    260–261, 260f
Bispectral Index (BIS), 1828–1829,
    1829f
Bites. See Snakebites; Widow spider bites
Bladder injury, 1653
Blast injuries, 1583, 1583t
Blastomycosis, 694–695
Bleeding
  ECMO complication of, 802
  in liver failure, 1370
  in uremia, 1316
β-Blocking agents, for arrhythmias, 406
Blood flow. See also Pulmonary blood flow
  during CPR, 500–504, 529
    cardiac vs. thoracic pump mechanism,
        500–502, 500f–501f
    chest geometry and, 502–503,
        502f–504f
    effects on intracranial pressure,
        503–504, 504f
    rate and duty cycle, 502
  disruption during critical illness, 1244
  regulation of distribution by RBCs,
      1238–1241, 1238f
Blood gases, 258–259, 1081
Blood lactate, 295, 1082–1083
Blood pressure (BP)
  after cardiac arrest, 532
  monitoring for HTN, 1120–1122
  monitoring in PPHN, 712–713
Blood tests, in malignant hyperthermia,
    1805
Blood urea nitrogen (BUN), ratio to
    creatinine, 1037
Blood-brain barrier (BBB), 821–824
  anatomy of, 821–822, 822f
  areas deficient of, 823–824
  development of, 829
  selectivity of, 822–823, 823f
Bloodstream infections (BSIs), 1513–1514
  epidemiology of, 1511t–1512t, 1513
  management of, 1514
  prevention of, 1513–1514
BNP. See Brain natriuretic peptide (BNP)

Body composition
    developmental aspects of, 1677
    in nutritional status assessment, 1206
Bone injection gun, 159, 159f
Bone marrow, 1225–1226, 1226f
Bone morphogenetic protein receptor type
    2 (BMPR2), 722
BOOP. See Bronchiolitis obliterans
    organizing pneumonia (BOOP)
BOS. See Bronchiolitis obliterans syndrome
    (BOS)
Bosentan
    for PAH, 728
    for PPHN, 718
Botulism, 988–989
Bowel obstruction, management of, 132
Bowel segment urinary reconstruction,
    1088
BP. See Blood pressure (BP)
BPD. See Bronchopulmonary dysplasia
    (BPD)
BPN. See B-type natriuretic peptide (BNP)
Bradycardias, 392–394. See also
        Arrhythmias; Tachycardias
    appropriate vs. normal heart rate, 392
    atrioventricular block, 392–394, 393f
    ECG for, 397–398
    management of pediatric, 522f
    monitored anesthesia care for,
        1789–1791
    sinus bradycardia/sinus pauses, 392
    therapies for, 401
        pharmacologic, 401, 407t
        temporary/permanent pacing, 401
    toxins associated with, 1730, 1731t
Brain
    abscesses, 972f–973f
    anesthesia neurotoxicity in, 1783–1784,
        1783f–1784f
    characteristics of infant, 1658
    oxygenation, monitoring ICP, 909–910
    structural lesions, 582
    vasculature, 825
Brain abscesses, 972–974
Brain death
    determination of, 136–139, 137t–138t
        physiology of, 139–140
Brain injury. See also Traumatic brain
        injury (TBI)
    mechanisms of, 930–936
Brain malformations
    arachnoid cysts, 836, 836f
    Chiari malformations, 836–837, 837f
    Dandy-Walker malformations, 837–838,
        838f
    encephalocele/meningocele, 838–839
    hydrocephalus, 832–836, 833f
    spinal dysraphism, 839–840, 839f
Brain natriuretic peptide (BNP), 491
Brain tissue oxygen (PbtO$_2$), 854
Breath odors, toxins associated with, 1731t
Breath triggering, in ventilation, 755

Breathing. See also Respiration
    ATLS primary survey of, 1604–1605
    during CPR, 528–529
    normal regulation of, 579–581, 580f
    physiology of, 577–579
        diaphragm, 577–578, 578f–579f
        intercostal muscles, 578
    power and frequency of, 608, 608f
    sequence, of ventilator-assisted, 741–743,
        742f
        classification of breaths, 741
        intermittent mandatory ventilation,
            742–743, 742f–743f
        phases of breath, 741
        spontaneous vs. mandatory, 741
    ventilator breath control variable, 741
    work of, 735–736, 736f
Breathing failure, 581–584, 581t
    due to lung disease, 584–587
        compensatory mechanisms,
            585–586
        restrictive vs. obstructive disease,
            584–585, 585t
    due to malnutrition/obesity, 587
    mechanical factors, 584
    muscle failure, 583–584, 583t
    neural control disorders, 583, 583t
    respiratory control disorders, 581–583
        acute failure, 581–582
        chronic failure, 582–583
        nonstructural acquired chronic
            disorders, 582–583
        nonstructural congenital disorders,
            582
        recognition of depressed respiratory
            drive, 583
        structural brain lesions, 582
    in special conditions, 586
Bronchi, 546, 548–551, 549f
Bronchioles, 548–551
Bronchiolitis, 688
Bronchiolitis obliterans organizing
        pneumonia (BOOP), 1332
Bronchiolitis obliterans syndrome (BOS),
    1332
Bronchitis, 688
Bronchogenic cysts, 670–671
Bronchomalacia, 615–616
Bronchopulmonary dysplasia (BPD),
    674–675, 674t
Bronchoscopy, for asthma, 660
Bronchus-associated lymphoid tissue
    (BALT), 554–555
Bruising, in child abuse, 1656
Brussels sedation scale, 1828, 1828t
BSIs. See Bloodstream infections (BSIs)
B-type natriuretic peptide (BNP), 710
Buffer-base concept, 1067–1076
Buffers
    in acid-base physiology, 1064–1065
    for cardiac arrest, 531
Bullying, 1665

BUN. See Blood urea nitrogen (BUN),
    ratio to creatinine
Bundles, in critical care processes, 22, 22t
Burn injury
    in child abuse, 1656
    depth/extent of, 1583–1585, 1584f–1585f
    early management of, 1585–1588
        burn resuscitation, 1586–1587, 1587t
        colloid resuscitation, 1587
        complications of, 1587–1588, 1588f
        transfer to burn centers, 1586, 1586t
    inhalational, 1588–1591
        airway clearance, 1590
        diagnosis of, 1589
        management of, 1589–1590, 1590f
        pathophysiology of, 1588–1589
        therapeutic adjuncts, 1590–1591
    nutritional support for, 1591–1592
        calculating/monitoring, 1591–1592,
            1591t
        enteral support, 1592
        nutritional adjuncts, 1592
        parenteral support, 1592
    prevention of, 1594
    types of, 1582–1583, 1583t
    to upper airway, 624
    wound care, 1592–1594
        surgical treatment, 1593–1594
        topical therapy, 1593

C

C1 esterase inhibitor deficiency, 1425–1426
Caffeine, for apnea, 677
Caffeine-halothane contracture testing
    (CHCT), 1807
Calcineurin inhibitors (CNIs), 1056–1057
Calcium
    accumulation, 933–934
    for cardiac arrest, 531
    with CPR, 516–517
    fluid management and, 1019–1020
    homeostasis, AKI and, 1044
    hormonal regulation of, 1020
    organ donor management and, 144
    regulation of, 1020
Calcium channel blockers
    in AKI attenuation, 1046
    for arrhythmias, 407–408
    for PAH, 726
    toxicity of, 1744
Calcium ions, 1702
Calcium sensitizers, 1703–1704
Calcium-binding proteins, 1702
Calibration, in invasive hemodynamic
    monitoring, 281
cAMP. See Cyclic adenosine
    monophosphate (cAMP)
Canada, history of PCCM in, 14
Candidal infections, 696, 1480
Cannulation
    for CPB, 437–438
    for ECMO, 785–788

Cannulation *(Continued)*
    initiation of, 798–799
    percutaneous, 788
    venoarterial, 786–787, 786*f*
    venovenous, 787–788, 787*f*
Capnometry and capnography
    clinical applications, 571
    definitions of, 570
    differential diagnosis of abnormal,
        572–574, 573*b*
        exponential decrease in ETCO$_2$, 574
        gradual increase in baseline and
            ETCO$_2$, 574, 574*f*
        gradually decreasing ETCO$_2$
            concentration, 573, 573*f*
        sustained low ETCO$_2$ with good
            plateaus, 574
        sustained low ETCO$_2$ without
            plateaus, 573–574, 573*f*
    operating principles of, 571–572
        clinical/technical issues, 571
        dead space ventilation, 572
        gas sampling issues, 571–572, 572*f*
    physiologic basis of, 570–571, 570*f*
Carbamate poisoning, 991–992
Carbapenems, 1477, 1722–1723
Carbohydrates
    digestion of, 1346–1347, 1346*b*
    in parenteral nutrition, 1217
Carbon dioxide (CO$_2$)
    acid-base balance and, 1065–1067, 1072
    capnometry monitoring of, 570
    diffusion of, 565
    exchange, in ECMO, 797
    in mechanical ventilation, 760–761
    monitoring of, 575
    rebreathing, 779
    transport, 1235–1236, 1236*f*
Carbon monoxide, 1742, 1742*t*
Cardiac arrest
    clinical outcome after, 941–942, 943*f*
    current/novel therapies after, 946–948
        inhibition of postischemic
            excitotoxicity, 948
        postresuscitative hypothermia,
            946–947
        therapies directed by group
            characteristics, 947–948
    epidemiology of, 527–528
    futuristic approaches after, 948–949
        erythropoietin, 948
        extracorporeal life support, 949
        mitochondria targeting therapies,
            948
        stem cell therapy, 948–949
    low-flow phase interventions, 528–530
    medications, 530–532
        vasopressors, 530–531
    phases of, 526–527, 527*t*
        no flow/slow flow, 526–527
        postresuscitation, 527
        prearrest, 526

Cardiac arrest *(Continued)*
        physiologic processes resulting from,
            528*f*
        postresuscitation interventions, 531–532
            blood pressure management, 532
            glucose control, 532
            temperature management, 531–532
        postresuscitation myocardial
            dysfunction, 532
    response of immature brain to, 942–943
    treatment of, 943–946
        field interventions, 943–944
        ICP interventions, 944, 945*f*
        PICU supportive care, 944–946, 946*f*
    ultrasound in, 198
Cardiac blood flow mechanism, 499–500
Cardiac catheterization
    assessing cardiac dysfunction, 492–493
    in CHD preoperative care, 449
    for congenital heart disease, 343–349,
        344*f*–346*f*
        potential complications, 346–347,
            347*t*
    critical illness assessment, 342–343, 343*t*
    for ECLS complications, 311–312
    ECMO and, 350
    hemodynamic/oxygen saturation data,
        342
    laboratory environment, 341–342
    occlusion device insertion, 349, 349*f*
    pulmonary artery balloon dilation,
        347–349
    RFCA and, 343
Cardiac crowding, 386
Cardiac dysfunction
    RBC transfusion for, 1298–1299
    tachycardia-induced, 410
Cardiac injury
    cardiogenic shock due to, 425
    types of, 1641, 1642*f*
Cardiac intensive care unit (CICU), 29–32,
    30*f*
Cardiac output
    ECLS complication involving, 310–311
    fetal, 246
    invasive hemodynamic measurement of,
        287–289
    perfusion flow rate during CPB,
        439–440, 439*t*
    qualitative assessment of
        chest radiography, 294
        physical examination, 293–294
    quantitative assessment of
        Doppler echocardiography, 295
        Fick method, 294–295
        pulse oximetry, 295
        thermodilution method, 294
    venous return and, 255–256, 255*f*–256*f*
Cardiac pump mechanism, during CPR,
    500–502
Cardiac rhythm disorders. *See* Arrhythmias
Cardiac stun, during ECLS, 311

Cardiac surgery
    AKI and, 1053
    history of, 5
    short-term NIV after, 774
    thrombosis risk in, 1285
Cardiac tamponade, 456–457
Cardiac toxicity, following HCT,
    1328–1330
Cardiac transplantation
    for advanced heart failure patients, 497
        immunotherapy, 497
    future management strategies, 487
    immune suppression complications,
        486–487
        diabetes mellitus, 487
        infection, 486
        renal failure, 486–487
    MCS as bridge to, 309
    organ donor management, 482
    overview of, 480
    pediatric critical care during, 483–486
        allograft rejection/immune
            suppression, 484–486, 485*t*
        early allograft dysfunction
            management, 483–484
        intraoperative considerations, 483
        perioperative management, 483
    pediatric critical care prior to, 480–482,
        481*b*
        anticoagulation, 482
        inotropic support, 481
        mechanical circulatory support,
            481–482
        patient management, 481
Cardiogenic pulmonary edema, 771–772
Cardiogenic shock, 421–422
    anthracycline-induced, 1321–1322
    etiololgies of, 422*b*
    evaluation of, 422, 422*b*
    specific etiologies, 424–425
        cardiac injury in trauma, 425
        cardiomyopathy, 424, 424*b*
        hypoxic-ischemic injury, 424–425
    therapies for, 422–424
        surgical intervention, 424
Cardiology, history of, 7
Cardiomyopathy
    cardiogenic shock due to, 424–425, 424*b*
    IEM and, 1164–1166, 1165*b*, 1165*t*
Cardioplegia, 442–445, 444*t*
Cardiopulmonary bypass (CPB)
    arterial pressure during, 439
    arterial/venous oxygen saturation,
        439–440, 440*f*
    for CPR, 507–508
    determining/monitoring perfusion flow
        rate, 439–440, 439*t*
    equipment and preparation, 431–438
        anticoagulation, 436–437, 437*f*
        cannulation, 437–438
        cardiopulmonary bypass circuit,
            433–434, 433*f*–434*f*

Cardiopulmonary bypass (CPB)
  (Continued)
    circuit prime, 436, 436t
    heart-lung machine console/pumps,
      431–433, 432f
    hemoconcentrators, 435–436
    oxygenators, 434–435, 435f
    tubing, 435, 435t
  history of, 430–431, 431t, 432f
    surgical team, 431
  inflammatory response to, 445
  initiation of, 438–439
  near-infrared spectroscopy for, 440, 440b
  pediatric vs. adult, 438, 438t
  pH and PaCO₂ strategy, 442
    myocardial protection, 442–445
  physiologic management optimization,
    440–442
    hypothermia for, 441–442, 441t,
      442f–444f
    target hematocrit/ultrafiltration for,
      440–441
  termination of, 445–446
Cardiopulmonary failure, ECMO for,
  790–793, 790t–791t, 792f
Cardiopulmonary interactions
  effects of cardiovascular function on
    respiration, 389–390
    cardiomyopathies and congenital
      heart disease, 390
    CHF, 389–390
    Glenn and Fontan procedures, 390
    shock states and, 389
  effects of ventilation on circulation,
    380–389
    cardiac contractility, 386
    elevated work of breathing and,
      388–389
    fluid responsiveness during PPV, 388,
      388f–389f
    left ventricular afterload, 386, 387f
    left ventricular preload, 385–386, 386f
    measurement of hemodynamic
      parameters, 389
    preload dependence vs. afterload
      dependence, 386–388, 387f–388f
    pulmonary circulation, 383–385,
      383f–385f
    pulsus paradoxus in respiratory
      distress, 389
    right ventricular filling/stroke volume,
      380–383, 381f–382f
Cardiopulmonary resuscitation (CPR). See
  also Resuscitation
  blood flow during, 500–504
    cardiac vs. thoracic pump mechanism,
      500–502, 500f–501f
    chest geometry and, 502–503,
      502f–504f
    effects on intracranial pressure,
      503–504, 504f
    rate and duty cycle, 502

Cardiopulmonary resuscitation (CPR)
  (Continued)
    cardiac arrest epidemiology, 527–528
    cardiac arrest medications, 530–532
    cardiac arrest phases, 526–527, 527t, 528f
      low-flow phase interventions, 528–530
    ECMO during, 532–533, 795
    family presence during, 106
    future directions, 524
    newer techniques, 504–509
      abdominal binding, 507
      ACD-CPR and ITV interposition,
        505–506, 506f–507f
      cardiopulmonary bypass, 507–508
      IAC-CPR, 505
      open-chest CPR, 507, 530
      SCV-CPR, 504–505
      TCP, 508–509
      vest CPR, 506–507
    outcomes following, 75
    overview of, 499–500
    pharmacology of, 509–511
      adrenergic agonists, 509–511,
        509f–512f, 510b
      atropine, 514
      calcium, 516–517
      glucose, 517–518, 517f
      high-dose epinephrine, 513–514
      other alkalinizing agents, 516
      sodium bicarbonate, 514–516, 515f
      vasopressin, 511–518
    postresuscitation care, 523–524, 524b
    postresuscitation interventions,
      531–532
    postresuscitation myocardial
      dysfunction, 532
    quality of, 532
    ventricular fibrillation management,
      518–524
      antiarrhythmics, 519f, 520t,
        521f–522f
      defibrillation, 518–520, 519f
    ventricular fibrillation/tachycardia,
      533–534
      antiarrhythmics for, 533
      automated external defibrillators for,
        533–534
Cardiorenal syndrome, AKI and,
  1052–1053
Cardiovascular agents
  drug-drug interactions of, 1720–1721,
    1720t
  toxicity of, 1744–1745
Cardiovascular function, 292
  HIV/AIDS and, 1447–1448
  mechanical ventilation for, 737
  respiration and, 389–390
    cardiomyopathies and congenital
      heart disease, 390
    CHF, 389–390
    Glenn and Fontan procedures, 390
    shock states and, 389

Cardiovascular function assessment
  quantity of therapy, 292–293
  single-ventricle physiology, 299–300,
    299f
  tissue oxygenation monitoring,
    293–296
    oxygen delivery measurements,
      295–296
    qualitative assessment of cardiac
      output, 293–294
    quantitative assessment of cardiac
      output, 294–295
    SAP, 296
  tissue oxygenation variables, 293
  variables affecting QOT, 296–298,
    297t
    abnormal SVR, 297
    arrhythmias, 297
    increased PVR, 297–298
    inefficient circulation, 298
    pulmonary function, 298
    vascular integrity, 298, 298f
    ventricular diastolic function,
      296–297
    ventricular systolic function, 296
Cardiovascular system
  in accidental hypothermia, 1567–1568,
    1568f
  adverse drug reactions in, 1710–1712,
    1710t, 1711b
  in drowning victims, 1575
  effects of toxins on, 1731t
  heat stroke and, 1564
  pharmacology of
    bipyridines, 373, 373f
    digitalis glycosides, 376
    nesiritide, 376
    response mechanisms, 352–378,
      353f–357f, 353t
    sympathomimetic amines, 359–360,
      359f–360f
  with SLE, 1464
  transfusion-related complications,
    1308–1309
Cardioversion, 408
Care bundles, 1510
Care ethics, 116
Caring practices, as nurse competency,
  44–45
Carrier proteins, signal transduction via,
  1693–1695, 1703f
CARS. See Compensatory
  antiinflammatory response syndrome
  (CARS)
Cartilage-hair hypoplasia (CHH), 1434
Case reports, 62
Case-control studies, 62
Casuistic ethics, 116
Catecholamines, 811–813, 812f. See also
  specific agents
  myocardial contractility and, 1703
  pharmacology of, 359–360, 359f–360f

Catheter angiography, 861
Catheter placement
    arterial, 161–163, 162b
    central venous line, 168–172
    echocardiographic guidance for, 332,
        335f
    PACs, 172, 173f
    PICCs, 172–175
    UAC and UVC, 167–168
Catheterization. *See* Cardiac
    catheterization
Catheter-related thrombosis, 1284–1285
Cavernous malformations, ICH and, 961,
    962f
CBF. *See* Cerebral blood flow (CBF)
CBFV. *See* Cerebral blood flow velocity
    (CBFV)
CDH. *See* Congenital diaphragmatic hernia
    (CDH)
CDS. *See* Clinical decision support (CDS)
    systems
CE. *See* Cerebral edema (CE)
Cell death, 931–932, 931f–933f
    in critical illness, 1174–1177
        animal studies of, 1175–1177
        human studies of, 1174–1175
    forms of, 1173
    mechanisms of, 1173–1174,
        1174f–1175f
    modes of, 1408t
    after TBI, 1615–1617, 1616f
Cellular respiration
    in critical illness
        antioxidants, 1143
        glycemic control, 1143
        hibernation, 1144
        impairment of, 1137–1139, 1138f
        membrane stabilizers, 1144
        mitochondrial biogenesis/mitophagy,
            1143–1144
        mitochondrial-/bioenergetic-targeted
            therapy, 1142–1143
        nitric oxide synthase inhibitors,
            1143
        substrate provision, 1143
    lactate production, 1139–1140
    microdialysis, 1141
    monitoring of
        blood mitochondrial DNA, 1142
        MRS, 1142
        NADH fluorometry, 1142
        NIRS, 1141–1142
        optical spectroscopy, 1142
        tissue oxygen tension, 1142
    oxygen utilization assessment, 1139
    pathways of, 1131–1137, 1132f–1134f
        glycolysis, 1133–1136, 1134f, 1136f
        oxygen toxicity, 1136–1137
    venous oxygen saturation, 1140–1141,
        1140f
Central apnea, 676
Central herniation, 892–893, 893f

Central line–associated bloodstream
    infections (CLABSIs), 1362
Central nervous system (CNS)
    accidental hypothermia and, 1567
    adverse drug reactions in, 1712–1713,
        1712t
    anatomic organization of, 816–820
        basal ganglia, 819
        cerebellum, 818
        cerebral hemispheres, 819–820,
            820f
        diencephalon, 818–819
        medulla, 817
        midbrain, 818
        pons, 817–818
        reticular formation, 818
        spinal cord, 816–817
    arrhythmias following trauma to,
        413
    cerebral blood flow regulation, 826–827,
        826f
    characterization of lymphatic circulation
        in, 827–828
    after CHD surgery, 458
    chemical synapses in, 811
    Dandy-Walker malformations and,
        837–838
    in drowning victims, 1575–1576
    failed ventilatory drive regulation by,
        1756
    heat stroke and, 1564
    in HIV/AIDS patients, 1451–1452
    infections of, 1452
        acute hemorrhagic leukoencephalitis,
            980–981, 981t
        ADEM, 979–980, 980f, 980t
        anti-NMDAR encephalitis, 981–982,
            982f–983f
        background, 1488
        bacterial meningitis, 965–966,
            968t–969t
        brain abscesses, 972–974, 972f–973f
        clinical presentation, 1489–1490
        etiology of, 1486t, 1488–1489
        hemophagocytic lymphohistiocytosis,
            982–983
        introduction, 965
        PAM, 978–979
        subdural empyemas, 971–972, 972f
        viral meningoencephalitis, 974–983,
            976f
    malignancy, 1451–1452
    myelination of, 829
    neuroimaging of infection of, 869–872,
        871f
    primary angiitis of, 952
    primary vasculitis of, 1469
    rheumatic disease effects on, 1472–1473,
        1473f
    vasculature, 825–827
        brain, 825
        spinal cord, 825–826

Central nervous system (CNS) disease,
    1464–1465
Central syndrome, 898t
Central venous catheter (CVC)
    placement, ultrasound in, 184–187,
        186f
    thrombosis related to, 1284
Central venous line (CVL) placement,
    168–172
    complications, 171
    femoral vein cannulation, 170, 171f
    indications/contraindications for, 168
    internal jugular vein cannulation, 169,
        170f
    subclavian vein cannulation, 169–170,
        171f
    technique for, 168–169, 168t, 169f
    ultrasound in, 170
    venous cutdown for, 171–172, 172f
Central venous pressure (CVP) catheters
    continuous mixed venous oxygen
        saturation, 283
    indications for, 281–282
    interpretation of waveforms, 282, 283f
    monitoring cardiovascular function, 296
Centrifugal pumps
    for CPB, 433
    for ECMO, 789–790, 789f, 792f
Centrifugal VAD pumps, 316–317
Cephalosporins, 1477
Cerebellar dysfunction, 848–849
Cerebellar tonsillar ectopia, 836, 837f
Cerebellar tonsillar herniation, 893
Cerebellum, 818
Cerebral arteriopathy, 951–952
Cerebral blood flow (CBF)
    development of, 829–830
    effects of anesthesia on, 1781–1783,
        1781f–1782f
    regulation of, 826–827, 826f, 1781, 1781f
    after resuscitation, 936–939, 937f–939f
    in TBI, 1614f, 1617
        monitoring of, 1626, 1627f
Cerebral blood flow velocity (CBFV), 853
Cerebral circulation, 262–268, 263f–264f
Cerebral edema (CE)
    in acute liver failure, 1387, 1387f
        management of, 1387–1388
    with DKA, 1201–1202
    in TBI, 1617–1618, 1618f–1619f
Cerebral hemispheres, 819–820, 820f
Cerebral metabolism
    development of, 829–830
    monitoring of, in TBI, 1626, 1628f
Cerebral microdialysis, 855
Cerebral perfusion pressure (CPP)
    autoregulation and, 900–901, 901f
        TCD assessment of, 910–911
    from ICP parameters, 905
    insults to brain, 905
    monitoring of, in TBI, 1628–1630
    target levels for, 907–908

Cerebral salt wasting (CSW) syndrome, 1009–1010, 1009t
Cerebral sinus venous thrombosis (CSVT)
 etiologies/risk factors, 957
 incidence of, 957–959
 laboratory evaluation, 958
 neuroimaging of, 957
 prognosis, 958–959
 treatment, 958, 958f
Cerebral swelling, in TBI, 1617
Cerebral vasodilation, CSF pressure and, 899–900, 900f–901f
Cerebral ventricular system, 832, 833f
Cerebroprotective therapy, 524, 524b
Cerebrospinal fluid (CSF), 898
 cerebral vasodilation and, 899–900, 900f–901f
 circulation of, 898–899, 900f
 composition/function of, 824–825
 drainage of, in TBI, 1630, 1634
 in hydrocephalus, 832–836, 833f
 production/flow of, 824, 824f
Cerebrovascular disease, in HIV/AIDS patients, 1451
Certification, in pediatric critical care nursing, 49–50, 49t
Cervical encephaloceles, 837
Cervical spine
 airway management and, 1769–1770
 characteristics of infant, 1658
 stabilization of, 1601–1604, 1602t, 1603f
Cervicocephalic arterial dissection, 951–952
CGD. See Chronic granulomatous disease (CGD)
cGMP. See Cyclic guanosine monophosphate (cGMP)
Channel-linked receptors, 1697, 1697f
Chaotic atrial tachycardia, 396, 410, 411f
CHD. See Congenital heart disease (CHD)
Checklists, in ICU, 36
Chediak-Higashi syndrome, 1436f
Chemical burns, 1583
Chemical synapses, 810–811
Chemically induced seizures, 915–916
Chemoprophylaxis, for viral pneumonitis, 691
Chemotherapy-induced nausea and vomiting, 1378
 5-HT3 receptor antagonists for, 1378–1380
 corticosteroids for, 1378–1379
 substance P/neurokinin-1 receptor antagonist for, 1379
 treatment guidelines, 1379–1380, 1380t
Chest
 compression during CPR, 529
 drainage system, 1640f
 geometry, CPR and, 502–503, 502f–504f

Chest radiography. See also Radiography
 for bronchogenic cysts, 671
 for cardiac output assessment, 294
 for cardiomegaly/pulmonary vascular congestion, 680
 of diffuse/immune pulmonary hemorrhage, 702, 702f
 ECLS and, 308, 308f
 for pulmonary parenchymal cysts, 671
 for severe asthma, 650
Chest trauma. See Thoracic trauma
Chest wall
 alterations, 608–609
  in contractile state of respiratory muscles, 609–610
  diaphragmatic configuration, 608–609
  rib cage distortion, 609, 610f
 congenital anomalies of, 679
 injury, 1639–1640
 lung interactions with, 562, 599–601, 600f
CHF. See Congestive heart failure (CHF)
CHH. See Cartilage-hair hypoplasia (CHH)
Chiari malformations, 836–837
 Chiari I, 836–837, 837f
 Chiari II, 837, 839
 Chiari III, 837
 Chiari IV, 837
Child abuse
 documentation/court testimony, 1661–1662
 fatal, 1660–1661
  autopsy for, 1661
  organ procurement organization, 1661, 1661b
  osseous injury in, 1661
  scene investigation in, 1661, 1661b
 head trauma, 1658
 incidence of, 1664
 inflicted abdominal/thoracic trauma, 1659–1660
 medical investigation of, 1660, 1660b
 recognition of, 1656–1657
  history of injury, 1656
  patterns of injury, 1656–1657, 1656t
 sexual, 1660
 shaken baby syndrome, 1659
 skeletal survey, 1657–1658
Children
 decision making by, 117
 mortality rates of, 201–203, 202f
Chimeric antigen receptor T-cell mediated toxicity, 1322–1323, 1323f
Choanal atresia, 542, 543f, 613–614, 613f, 677
Choanal stenosis, 677
Cholecystitis, 1398
Cholinergic toxicity, 1739–1740, 1739b
Chromosome alterations, 1169
Chronic granulomatous disease (CGD), 1427–1428
Chronic liver failure, 1369–1370, 1369t

Chronic mucocutaneous candidiasis (CMC) syndromes, 1436
Chronic obstructive pulmonary disease
 congenital lymphatic defects, 674–676
 NIV for, 772–773
Chronic thromboembolic pulmonary hypertension (CTEPH), 730
Chronotropic medications, for shock, 419
Chylothorax, 1642
CI. See Confidence interval (CI), in EBM
CIN. See Contrast-induced nephropathy (CIN)
Circuit prime, CPB, 436
 drugs for, 436t
Circulation. See also Regional peripheral circulation; Systemic circulation
 adverse effects of mechanical ventilation, 760
 ATLS primary survey of, 1605–1606, 1605t, 1606f
 cerebral, 262–268, 263f–264f
 coronary, 264, 264f–265f
 during CPR, 529–530
 effects of ventilation on, 380–389
  cardiac contractility, 386
  effects of airway pressure on vascular tone, 385
  elevated work of breathing and, 388–389
  fluid responsiveness during PPV, 388, 388f–389f
  left ventricular afterload, 386, 387f
  left ventricular preload, 385–386, 386f
  measurement of hemodynamic parameters, 389
  preload dependence vs. afterload dependence, 386–388, 387f–388f
  pulmonary circulation, 383–385, 383f–385f
  pulsus paradoxus in respiratory distress, 389
  right ventricular filling/stroke volume, 380–383, 381f–382f
 gastrointestinal, 266–267
 pulmonary, 259–262, 260f–261f
 QOT and, 298
 renal, 267–268
 stabilization in TBI, 1622
Circulatory death, organ donation and, 145–146
Circumferential compressions, 530
Cirrhosis, 1010
Cis-atracurium, 1815t, 1820
CLABSIs. See Central line–associated bloodstream infections (CLABSIs)
Classic heat stroke, 1563
Classical pathway, 1423, 1424f
Clearance
 for CRRT, 1110
 of drugs, 1677–1681
 total body, 1685
Clevidipine, for HTN, 1126

Clindamycin, 1479

Clinical decision support (CDS) systems
  alerts/reminders/recommendations, 96
  dashboards/data visualization/templates, 97, 98f
  effectiveness, 97
  medical knowledge databases, 96–97

Clinical informatics, 92

Clinical inquiry, as nurse competency, 44

Clinical judgment, as nurse competency, 44

Clinical trials
  consent practices, 58–59
  improved design, 57

Clinician refusals, 119

Clonidine, for HTN, 1122–1123, 1123t

Closed-loop communication, in ICU, 37

Clostridium difficile, 1375–1376

Clotting cascade, 1262f–1263f

CMC. See Chronic mucocutaneous candidiasis (CMC) syndromes

CME. See Continuing medical education (CME)

CMV. See Cytomegalovirus (CMV) pneumonitis

CNIs. See Calcineurin inhibitors (CNIs)

CNS. See Central nervous system (CNS)

CNV. See Copy number variation (CNV)

CO₂. See Carbon dioxide (CO₂)

Coagulation
  in accidental hypothermia, 1568
  in ARDS, 630
  endothelium production of, 271–272, 271f–272f
  hemostasis/clotting cascade in, 1261–1266, 1262f–1263f
  inflammation and, 1264–1266, 1264f–1266f
  inflammation/immune dysfunction/dysregulated metabolism hypothesis, 1541–1543
  introduction, 1261
  organ donor management and, 145
  during shock, 420

Coagulation cascade, in sepsis, 1526

Coagulation disorders
  acquired, 1269–1274
    disseminated intravascular coagulation, 1269–1270
    liver disease/hepatic insufficiency, 1272–1273
    meningococcal purpura fulminans, 1270–1271
    thrombocytopenic purpura/hemolytic uremic syndrome, 1271–1272
    vitamin K deficiency, 1273–1274
  approach to patient with, 1266–1269
    clinical history, 1266–1267
    laboratory evaluation, 1267–1269, 1268t
    physical examination, 1267
  ICH and, 962
  in PICU, 1262t

Coagulation disorders (Continued)
  platelet disorders and, 1277–1280, 1277t
  systemic diseases associated with factor deficiencies, 1280

Coagulopathy
  iatrogenic, 1274–1277
    anticoagulant overdose, 1275–1277
    massive transfusion syndrome, 1274–1275
  in liver failure, 1370, 1386

Coarctation of the aorta, 473–474

Cocaine, toxicity of, 414

Coccidioidomycosis, 695

Cohort studies, 62

Colistin, 1479

Colitis, after HCT, 1334–1335

Collaboration, as nurse competency, 45

Collaborative research networks, 54

Collecting duct, 1004–1005, 1004f

Colloid resuscitation, 1587

Colon
  life-threatening complications of, 1364–1368
    acute colonic pseudo-obstruction, 1368
    distal intestinal obstruction syndrome, 1367
    food allergy, 1365
    hemolytic-uremic syndrome, 1365–1367
    Hirschsprung disease, 1367–1368
    inflammatory bowel disease, 1366–1367, 1366t
    low cardiac output syndrome, 1365
    malrotation, 1364–1365
    necrotizing enterocolitis, 1365

Color Doppler, for neuroimaging, 857, 858f

Coma
  agents associated with, 1732b
  arousal and ARAS, 883–884, 884f
  assessment and immediate resuscitation, 884–885
  causes of, 884, 885t, 884.e1b
  diagnostic evaluation, 893–894, 893.e1b
  ethical considerations, 895
  eye examination, 885–888, 886f–889f
  focused neurological examination, 885
  herniation syndromes, 892–893, 893f
  levels of consciousness, 884, 884b
  motor examination, 888, 889t, 890f
  nonfocal neurological lesions, 891–892
  outcomes, 895
  pathophysiology of, 883
  respiratory pattern, 885, 885t, 886f
  structural vs. metabolic, 886t
  subtentorial compartment and, 890f, 891, 892f
  supratentorial compartment and, 888–891, 890f–891f

Coma (Continued)
  therapeutic intervention for, 894–895
    immediately treatable forms, 894
    rapidly progressive reversible lesions, 894
    states amenable to prolonged therapy, 894–895

Common variable immunodeficiency syndrome (CVID), 1429–1430

Communication
  checklists, 36
  closed-loop, 37
  debriefing, 37
  ethics in, 113
  with family, 107–108
  huddles, 36
  medical records, 36
  medical training, 37
  optimal design for, 35–36
  in palliative care, 128–129
  in pediatric transport, 154
  referring hospital responsibilities, 155
  rounds, 36
  team training, 37
  transitions of care, 37

Comorbid conditions
  effect on outcomes of chronic, 76
  fewer, in PICU, 52–53

Compassionate extubation, 130

Compensatory antiinflammatory response syndrome (CARS), 1541–1542, 1542f
  clinical outcomes and, 1456–1458, 1457f
  in critical illness, 1456
  temporal aspects of, 1456, 1457f

Compensatory reserve, 903–905, 906f–907f

Competence
  assessment/evaluation of, 214–215, 215t
  maintaining after training, 216–217

Complement component of immune system, 1423
  clinical presentation, 1423
  deficiencies in, 1423, 1423t
    laboratory tests for, 1432t, 1436–1437
    treatment for, 1437
  mechanisms of, 1423, 1424f
  specific disorders, 1425–1426
    C1 inhibitor deficiency, 1425–1426
    early classical pathway protein defects, 1426
    membrane attack complex defects, 1426
    regulatory protein defects, 1426

Complete blood cell count, for asthma assessment, 650–651

Compliance
  of respiratory system, 557–559, 559f, 734–735, 735t
  vascular, 257

Compression-relaxation phases, during CPR, 502–503, 502f, 504f

Compression/ventilation ratios, during CPR, 529–530

Computerized tomography (CT)
  for abdominal trauma, 1646
  for acute abdomen, 1396–1397
  of arterial ischemic stroke, 954–955
  of brain abscesses, 972f, 973–974
  after cardiac arrest, 941–942, 943f
  for gastrointestinal evaluation,
    1360–1361
  for HTN, 1120, 1121f
  in multiple trauma, 1609, 1610f
  for neuroimaging, 857–859
  for neurological assessment, 850–855
    advantages/limitations, 850t
  for TBI, 1622–1624, 1623f, 1623t
Confidence interval (CI), in EBM, 61.e1t
Congenital diaphragmatic hernia (CDH),
  669–670
Congenital disorders. See also specific
    disorders
  breathing failure and, 582
Congenital esophageal anomalies, 1362
Congenital heart disease (CHD)
  atrial septal defect, 464–465
  atrioventricular canal defects, 465–466
  cardiac catheterization for, 343–349
    perioperative interventional
      procedures, 346
    potential complications, 346–347,
      347t
    scheduled interventional procedures,
      346–349
    therapeutic interventions in newborn,
      344–346, 344f–346f
  causing neonatal respiratory disease, 680
  with ductal dependent systemic blood
    flow, 425
  left-sided obstructive lesions, 472–478
  mechanical ventilation after repair of,
    754
  neonatal considerations, 447–448, 448b
  patent ductus arteriosus, 463–464
  postoperative care for, 451–460
    acute pulmonary hypertension
      management, 455–456, 455t
    assessment, 451–452, 451b–452b
    cardiac tamponade, 456–457
    CNS involvement, 458
    diaphragmatic dysfunction/effusions,
      457
    diastolic dysfunction, 454
    gastrointestinal issues, 459
    hyperglycemia, 459–460
    infection, 459
    low cardiac output syndrome, 453,
      453f
    monitoring, 452–453, 452b, 452t
    outcomes, 478t
    pharmacologic support, 454–455, 455f
    renal function/fluid management,
      458–459
    right ventriculotomy, 453–454
    tracheal extubation, 457–458, 458t

Congenital heart disease (CHD)
  (Continued)
  preoperative care for, 448–451
    cardiac catheterization and, 449
    echocardiographic/Doppler
      assessment, 449
    MRI/MRA, 449–450
    patient status/pathophysiology
      assessment, 450–451
    physical examination/laboratory data,
      448–449
  pulmonary atresia, 470–472
  respiratory function and, 390
  single ventricle
    anatomy/physiology, 460–461
    bidirectional cavopulmonary
      anastomosis for, 461, 462t
    Fontan procedure for, 461–463, 462t,
      464t
    preoperative management, 460–461
  stroke and, 953
  tetralogy of Fallot, 468–470
  total anomalous pulmonary venous
    connection, 466–467
  transposition of the great arteries,
    467–468
  tricuspid atresia, 472
  truncus arteriosus communis, 466
  ventricular septal defect, 465
Congenital immunodeficiency. See also
    Severe combined immune deficiency
    (SCID)
  autoimmune lymphoproliferative
    syndrome, 1436
  B-cell and antibody defects, 1428–1430
  CMC syndromes, 1436
  complement defects, 1425–1426
    laboratory tests for, 1432t
  complex/combined deficiencies, 1434
    cartilage-hair hypoplasia, 1434
    Wiskott-Aldrich syndrome, 1434
  distribution of major disorders, 1426f
  immune system framework, 1423–1425
    deficiencies in, 1423t–1424t
  laboratory evaluation of, 1436–1437,
    1436f
  overview of, 1422–1423
  phagocytic defects, 1426–1428
  radiation sensitive disorders,
    1435–1436
    ataxia telangiectasia, 1435
    Nijmegen breakage syndrome, 1435
  susceptibility to HLH and severe EBV
    infection, 1435
  susceptibility to myobacterial disease,
    1435
  T-cell defects, 1430–1434
  toll-like receptors/signaling pathway
    defects, 1435–1436
  treatment, 1437–1438
    IgG replacement for, 1437–1438
    prophylactic antibiotics for, 1438

Congenital lymphatic defects, 675–676
Congenital malformations
  upper airway disease due to, 613–614
    bronchomalacia/intrathoracic
      tracheomalacia, 615–616
    choanal atresia, 613–614, 613f
    laryngeal webs/stenosis/tumors,
      614–615, 615f
    laryngomalacia, 614, 614f
    vascular impingement on trachea,
      615, 615f–616f
Congenital myasthenia gravis, 986–987
Congenital pneumonia, 667
Congenital pulmonary airway
  malformation (CPAM), 670
Congenital pulmonary lymphangiectasia,
  675–676
Congestive heart failure (CHF), 421–422
  etiologies of, 422b
  evaluation of, 422, 422b
  hyponatremia in, 1010
  respiratory function and, 389–390
  specific etiologies, 424–425
    cardiac injury in trauma, 425
    cardiomyopathy, 424, 424b
    hypoxic-ischemic injury, 424–425
  therapies for, 422–424, 423b
  surgical intervention, 424
Consciousness
  assessment of, 845, 847t, 1730, 1731t
  defining levels of, 884, 884b
Consequentialism, in PICU, 115
Constipation, 1376, 1377t
Continuing education, for nurses, 49
Continuing medical education (CME),
  223
Continuous flow mechanical ventilation,
  745
Continuous flow VADs, 316, 317f
Continuous positive airway pressure
  (CPAP)
  masks for, 1754
  in mechanical ventilation, 741, 743f,
    745–746, 746f
Continuous renal replacement therapy
  (CRRT), 1109–1111
  disadvantages/complications, 1110–1111
  ICU issues, 1111
  indications for, 1109
  physiology of, 1109
  in sepsis treatment, 1535
  technique for, 1109–1110
Contractility
  heart failure and, 490
  methods of optimizing, 493
Contrast radiography, for gastrointestinal
  evaluation, 1360
Contrast-induced nephropathy (CIN),
  1057–1058
Conventional ultrafiltration, as CPB
  technique, 440–441
Copy number variation (CNV), 1169–1170

Core competencies, of ACGME, 208–210, 221t

Cormack laryngeal view grade score, 1758f, 1759

Cornell Assessment for Pediatric Delirium, 1872, 1873f

Coronary circulation, 264, 264f–265f

Coroner issues, in organ donation, 145

Corticosteroids, 482
  for asthma, 651–653
  for bacterial meningitis, 970
  for immune suppression, 484–486, 485t
  for nausea and vomiting, 1378–1379
  side effects of, 1182–1183

Cortisol
  actions of, 1179–1181, 1181f
  biochemistry of, 1178–1179, 1180f, 1179.e1t
  free, 1182
  stress response, 1181–1182, 1179.e1t
  synthesis/secretion, 1178, 1179f, 1179t

Cough-cardiopulmonary resuscitation, 500, 500f

Counterregulatory hormones, stress responses and, 1148

Court testimony, for child abuse, 1661–1662

CPAM. See Congenital pulmonary airway malformation (CPAM)

CPAP. See Continuous positive airway pressure (CPAP)

CPB. See Cardiopulmonary bypass (CPB)

CPP. See Cerebral perfusion pressure (CPP)

CPR. See Cardiopulmonary resuscitation (CPR)

Cranial nerve examination, 845–847, 846t

Creatinine
  BUN ratio to, 1037
  non-GFR factors affecting, 1032t
  as plasma marker, 1029–1032, 1030f–1031f
  renal clearance of, 1028

Cricothyrotomy, 1774

Critical care. See also Pediatric critical care
  adult subspecialization within, 28–29
  during ECLS, 310–314, 310t
  history of
    anatomy and physiology, 3–4
    resuscitation and ventilation, 4–7, 4f, 8f
  information technology in
    big data and, 100–102
    clinical decision support, 96–97, 98f
    clinical informatics, 92
    EHRs and, 92–96
    future directions, 102
    HITECH Act, 90–91, 91f
    learning health system, 91–92, 92f
    patient safety, 97–99
    privacy/security of health information, 99–100, 99b

Critical care (Continued)
  telemedicine, 100
  justification for, 201–202, 203f
  models of, 20–23, 21f
  in resource-poor settings, 202–203
    during disease outbreaks, 206
    research for, 206–207
    strengthening infrastructure, 204–206
  therapeutics, 1685–1687
    target concentration strategy, 1686–1687, 1686b
    target effect strategy, 1687, 1687b

Critical care team, ethical issues and, 113

Critical closing pressure, 256–257, 257f

Critical illness
  drug distribution and, 1677
  immune function and, 1440–1441
  metabolic consequences of, 1207–1208, 1207f, 1208t
  recommended energy/protein allowances, 1209t–1210t. See also Energy expenditure, in critical illness
  role of cell death in, 1174–1177

Crohn disease, 1366–1367

Cross-sectional studies, 62

CRRT. See Continuous renal replacement therapy (CRRT)

CRS. See Cytokine release syndrome (CRS)

Cryoprecipitate, 1306

CSF. See Cerebrospinal fluid (CSF)

CSVT. See Cerebral sinus venous thrombosis (CSVT)

CSW. See Cerebral salt wasting (CSW) syndrome

CTEPH. See Chronic thromboembolic pulmonary hypertension (CTEPH)

Cuirass ventilators, 780f, 781

CVC. See Central venous catheter (CVC)

CVID. See Common variable immunodeficiency syndrome (CVID)

CVL. See Central venous line (CVL) placement

CVP. See Central venous pressure (CVP) catheters

Cyanide, 1742–1743

Cyclic adenosine monophosphate (cAMP), 357–358, 1701–1702

Cyclic guanosine monophosphate (cGMP), 1702

Cycling asynchrony, 756

Cyclosporine, for immune suppression, 484–486, 485t

Cystatin C, as plasma marker, 1032–1033

Cystic fibrosis, 775–776

Cysts
  arachnoid, 836, 836f
  bronchogenic, 670–671
  pulmonary parenchymal, 671

Cytochrome P-450 (CYP) enzyme, 1678–1680
  CYP1A2, 1678
  CYP2C9, 1678–1679
  CYP2D6, 1679
  CYP3A4, 1679–1680
  drug interactions affecting, 1717, 1718t–1719t
  drug-drug interactions of, 1726
  ontogeny of, 1679t

Cytokine release syndrome (CRS), 1322–1323, 1323f

Cytokines
  in MODS/MOF, 1541–1543, 1543f
  in sepsis, 1524–1525, 1524b

Cytomegalovirus (CMV) pneumonitis, 1446

Cytomegalovirus-negative platelets, 1304

Cytomegalovirus-negative red blood cell units, 1300–1301

Cytoplasm, of heart cells, 237

Cytoskeleton, of heart, 237–238

Cytotoxic T cells, 1417–1418, 1417f

D

DAH. See Diffuse alveolar hemorrhage (DAH)

Dandy-Walker malformation, 837–838, 838f

Danger hypothesis, 1403–1404

Dantrolene, for MH, 1803–1804, 1804f

Daptomycin, 1479

Data
  availability of, 53–54
  EHR
    access, 93–94
    acquisition, 93
    in critical care, 100–102
    storage, 94
  informatics research and, 57
  research opportunities, 57
  variation/display of, 84–85, 85f

Data mining, 101

Databases
  MIMIC, 101
  research networks, 101

Dead space ventilation, 572

Death
  brain death, 136–140, 137t–138t
  epidemiology of in PICU, 128
  follow-up care of family/staff, 133
  number and causes of, 201–202, 203f

Debriefing, in ICU, 37

Decannulation, after tracheostomy, 625–626

Decompressive craniectomy, for intracranial hypertension, 1634

Decontamination, in PHEs, 228–229

Deep partial-thickness burns, 1584

Defasciculation, 1812–1813

Defibrillation
  for arrhythmias, 408
  for ventricular fibrillation, 518–520, 519f
del Nido cardioplegia, 444–445, 444t
Delirium
  background, 1869
  clinical presentation, 1870–1872
  diagnosis of, 1872, 1872f–1873f
  drug-induced, 1712
  environment and, 1874
  epidemiology of, 1870, 1870f
  etiology of, 1869–1870
  iatrogenic factors, 1874
  pharmacotherapy for, 1874–1875
  prevention of, 1875
  risk factors, 1870, 1871f, 1871t
  subtypes, 1869
  treatment of, 1873, 1874f
  underlying illness, 1873
Demand flow mechanical ventilation, 745
Demyelinating disease, neuroimaging of, 872, 873f–874f
Deontology, in PICU, 115
Deoxyribonucleic acid (DNA) repair defects, in immunodeficiency, 1432, 1435–1436
Depolarizing agents, NMBAs, 1811–1824, 1812t–1813t
Depression, SCD and, 1254
Depth
  of anesthesia monitors, 1791
  effect on ultrasound, 181, 182f
Dermatologic adverse drug reactions, 1715–1716
Desflurane, 1776–1777
Desmopressin
  for diabetes insipidus, 143–144
  for hormonal resuscitation, 141–142, 142t
Dexamethasone, for bacterial meningitis, 970
Dexmedetomidine
  for arrhythmias, 408
  effects of, 1777–1778
  withdrawal from, 1866–1867
Diabetes insipidus, 143–144
  causes of, 1013, 1013b
  hypernatremia due to, 1014
Diabetes mellitus, after heart transplantation, 487
Diabetic ketoacidosis (DKA)
  cerebral edema and, 1201–1202
  epidemiology of, 1198–1203
    at diagnosis, 1198–1199
    after diagnosis, 1199
  etiology/definition/presentation of, 1196–1198, 1197f
  health care costs for, 1202–1203
  hyperglycemic hyperosmolar syndrome, 1202
  management guidelines, 1199–1201, 1200f–1201f

Diabetic ketoacidosis (DKA) (Continued)
  monitoring of, 1198t, 1201
  morbidity and mortality with, 1199
  neuropsychologic sequelae, 1202
  thrombotic complications, 1202
Diacylglycerol, 1702
Diagnostic peritoneal lavage (DPL), 1646
Dialysate, for CRRT, 1110
Dialysis
  for metabolic acidosis, 1090
  physiology of, 1106f
Dialysis, physiology of, 1105, 1106f
Dialysis disequilibrium syndrome, 916
Diaphragm
  breathing and, 577–578, 578f–579f
  eventration of, 678–679
  injury to, 1642
  structure and function of, 555
  ultrasound of, 190–191, 191f
Diaphragmatic dysfunction, after CHD repair, 457
Diarrhea
  antibiotic-associated, 1375–1376
  hospital-associated, 1518
Diastolic function, after CHD repair, 454
Diazepam, for SE, 922–924, 923t
DIC. See Disseminated intravascular coagulation (DIC)
Dichloroacetate (DCA), 1090
Diencephalon, 818–819
Diffuse alveolar hemorrhage (DAH), 1330–1331
Diffuse/immune pulmonary hemorrhage, 702, 702f
Diffuse/nonimmune pulmonary hemorrhage, 701–702
Diffusion-weighted imaging (DWI), 860
DiGeorge syndrome (22q11.2 deletion syndrome), 1430–1431
Digitalis glycosides
  adverse effects of, 377
  basic pharmacology, 376
  clinical pharmacology, 376–377
  clinical role of, 377
  interactions, 377–378
  pharmacokinetics of, 377
  preparation/administration, 377
Digoxin
  for arrhythmias, 408
  myocardial contractility and, 1703
  toxicity of, 414, 414f, 1745
DIOS. See Distal intestinal obstruction syndrome (DIOS)
Diphtheria, 989
Directed red blood cell units, 1301
Disability, ATLS primary survey of, 1606–1607, 1607f
Disease
  critical care during, 206
  effect on drug action, 1683
  therapy and, 55–56
  variable management of, 56

Disseminated intravascular coagulation (DIC)
  clinical presentation/diagnosis, 1269–1270, 1270t
  management of, 1271–1272
  pathogenesis of, 1269, 1269t
Distal intestinal obstruction syndrome (DIOS), 1367
Distal tubule, 1001–1002, 1004
Distensibility, vascular, 257
Distributive shock, 425
Diuretics
  in AKI attenuation, 1046
  in heart failure treatment, 493, 494t
  pharmacology of, 1101–1103, 1101f
  resistance to, 1102–1103, 1103b
DKA. See Diabetic ketoacidosis (DKA)
D-lactic acidosis, 1085
DNA. See Deoxyribonucleic acid (DNA) repair defects, in immunodeficiency
Do not attempt resuscitation (DNAR) order, 130
Dobutamine
  adverse effects of, 370
  basic pharmacology, 369
  for cardiac dysfunction, 494t, 495
  clinical pharmacology, 369
  clinical role of, 364t, 369–370
  interactions, 370
  pharmacokinetics of, 369
  preparation/administration, 370
Doctrine of double effect
  in pediatric intensive care, 115–116
  in withholding/withdrawing life support, 123–125, 124b
Doctrine of informed consent
  emergency exception, 117
  patient decision making and, 117
Documentation, for child abuse, 1661–1662
Donabedian's model for quality, 20–23, 21f
  outcomes in, 22–23
  process in, 22, 22t
  structure in, 21f
Dopamine
  adverse effects of, 362
  in AKI attenuation, 1045–1046
  for cardiac dysfunction, 494–495, 494t
  clinical role of, 362
  interactions, 362
  pharmacokinetics of, 361–362
  pharmacology of, 360–361, 360f, 361t
  preparation/administration, 362, 363t
Doppler echocardiography
  for cardiac output assessment, 295
  in CHD preoperative care, 449
Doppler ultrasound, 182, 184f
Double triggering, in ventilation, 755
Doxacurium, 1815t, 1820–1821
DPL. See Diagnostic peritoneal lavage (DPL)

Drowning
  definitions/categories of, 1572, 1573t
  epidemiology of, 1572–1573
  management of, 1577–1580
    ED evaluation/stabilization,
      1577–1578
    in PICU, 1578–1580
    at scene, 1577
  pathophysiologic considerations,
    1573–1577
    additional organ systems, 1576
    aspirated fluid type, 1574
    cardiovascular effects, 1575
    CNS effects, 1575–1576
    hypothermia, 1577
    mammalian diving reflex, 1576
    preexisting associated conditions,
      1576–1577
    pulmonary effects, 1574–1575, 1574f
  prognosis, 1580–1581
Drug disposition
  critical care therapeutics, 1685–1687
    target concentration strategy,
      1686–1687, 1686b
    target effect strategy, 1687, 1687b
  determinants of effective therapy,
    1673–1683, 1674b, 1674f
    effect of ECMO on, 1682
    pharmacodynamics, 1682–1683
    pharmacokinetics, 1674–1682,
      1674b–1675b, 1676t–1677t, 1679t
    in infants/children, 1673
    pharmacokinetic principles, 1683–1685
      applied, 1685
      plasma concentration-time curve,
        1683–1685, 1683f–1684f, 1685b
Drug-drug interactions
  in intravenous admixtures, 1720
  pharmacodynamic, 1719
  pharmacokinetic, 1716–1719,
    1718t–1719t
  by therapeutic class, 1720–1726
    analgesic agents, 1724
    anesthetic agents/sedatives, 1723–1724
    anticoagulants, 1724–1725, 1725t
    anticonvulsant medications,
      1721–1722
    antiinfective/antimicrobial agents,
      1722–1723
    antineoplastic agents, 1726
    cardiovascular, 1720–1721, 1720t
    immunosuppressive agents,
      1725–1726
    pulmonary/respiratory medications,
      1726
Drug(s). See also Adverse drug reactions
  absorption of, 1674–1676, 1674b,
    1716–1717
    intramuscular, 1675, 1675b
    percutaneous, 1675–1676
    rectal, 1676
    subcutaneous, 1675

Drug(s) (Continued)
  bioavailability of, 1674–1675
  clearance of, 1677–1681
  CPB circuit prime, 436t
  delirium and, 1874
  delivery systems, 1682
  distribution of, 1676–1677, 1676t–1677t,
    1717
  effects on thyroid hormone metabolism,
    1194t
  elimination of, 1681–1682
  excretion of, 1717–1719
  facilitating intubation, 1761–1763, 1762t
  hypertension associated with, 1115,
    1115t
  management of, 130–131, 131t
  metabolism of, 1717
  molecular mechanisms of actions of,
    1690f–1691f, 1692t
    developmental effects on, 1704, 1705t
    disease effects on, 1704–1705, 1705f
    drug response/genetic
      polymorphisms, 1704
    multiple targets with organ systems,
      1694f, 1702–1704
    receptors as targets for, 1689–1695
    signal transduction mechanisms:
      intracellular messengers/effectors,
      1701–1702, 1701f, 1703f
  for PHEs, 230
  preoperative, 1789, 1789t
  with pulmonary toxicity, 700, 700b
  toxicity of, arrhythmias secondary to,
    414, 414f
Dual control mechanical ventilation,
  748–749, 748f
Ductus arteriosus, 238
Duodenal ulcers, 1364
Duodenum
  injury to, 1648–1650, 1649t, 1650f
  life-threatening complications of,
    1363–1364
Duty cycle, for CPR, 502, 530
DWI. See Diffusion-weighted imaging
  (DWI)
Dyspnea, 132

E
EAT. See Ectopic atrial tachycardia (EAT)
EBM. See Evidence-based medicine (EBM)
EBV. See Epstein-Barr virus (EBV)
ECG. See Electrocardiogram (ECG)
Echinocandins, 1482
Echocardiography
  for cardiac diagnostics
    cardiac dysfunction and, 491–492
    cardiovascular communications/
      physiology and, 336–338,
      337f–339f
    catheter manipulation and, 332, 335f
    device placement and, 332–334, 335f
    ECMO and VADs, 333–334, 336f–337f

Echocardiography (Continued)
    pericardial effusion assessment,
      328–329, 328f–330f
    pulmonary hypertension evaluation,
      327–328, 328f
    structural defects, 325–326
    valve function measurement, 327
    vascular assessment, 329–332,
      331f–334f
    ventricular function, 326–327, 326f
    volume status assessment, 327
  in CHD preoperative care, 449
  for ECLS complications, 311–312
  overview of, 325
ECLS. See Extracorporeal life support
  (ECLS)
Ectopic atrial tachycardia (EAT), 395–396
ED. See Emergency department (ED)
EDHF. See Endothelium-derived
  hyperpolarizing factor (EDHF)
EDRF. See Endothelium-derived relaxing
  factor (EDRF)
Education. See also Lifelong learning
  for critical care nurses, 48–49
    continuing education, 49
    in-service education programs, 48–49
    orientation programs, 48
  graduate medical education, 222–223,
    222f
  health system capacity building via,
    205–206
  of intensivists
    ABP requirements, 216
    ACGME core competencies, 208–210
    ACGME requirements, 216
    adult learning, 208–216, 209t
    evaluating competency, 214–215, 215t
    growth of, 12
    maintaining competency, 216–217
    mentorship, 215–216
    professionalism in, 213–214
    in research/scholarship/leadership,
      214
    in safety and quality, 214, 214t
    teaching methods, 210–213,
      210t–211t
  undergraduate medical, 220–221, 221t
EEG. See Electroencephalography (EEG)
Effector(s), 1415–1419, 1416f–1417f, 1417t
EHI. See Exertional heat illness (EHI)
EHRs. See Electronic health records
  (EHRs)
Ejection phase indices, in myocardial
  contractility, 242f, 243, 244f
Elastance, 557–559, 559f
Elastic equilibrium volume, 557
Elastic recoil
  of lungs and chest wall, 598–601,
    598f–599f
  of respiratory system, 557, 559, 559f
Electrical burns, 1582–1583
Electrical synapses, 810

Electrocardiogram (ECG)
    for arrhythmias, 397–400, 397t, 398f
        bradycardias, 397–398
        extrasystoles, 398–399
        tachycardias with normal QRS, 399, 399f
        tachycardias with prolonged QRS, 398f, 399–400
    for asthma assessment, 651
    for HTN, 1120
Electroencephalography (EEG)
    after cardiac arrest, 941
    in pediatric neurocritical care, 852–853
    in SE, 919–922, 920f
Electrolyte(s). See also Fluid and electrolyte management
    for asthma assessment, 650–651
    disturbances, 413, 1059t
    in DKA management, 1199–1200, 1200f
    drug-induced abnormalities, 1713–1715, 1714t
    gastrointestinal regulation of, 1349
    gastrointestinal transport of, 1349–1350
    in organ donor management, 143
    in parenteral nutrition, 1217–1218
    role in acid-base balance, 1062–1065
Electroneutrality, principle of, 1063
Electronic health records (EHRs)
    benefits of, 92–93
    data access, 93–94
    data acquisition, 93
    data storage, 94
    human factors engineering and, 95
    implementation of, 95–96
    limitations/pitfalls of, 94–95
    meaningful use of, 90–91, 91f
Elevated anion gap acidoses, 1082–1086
Elimination
    of drugs, 1681–1682
    half-life, 1685
Embden-Meyerhof pathway (EMP), 1241, 1242f
Emergency department (ED)
    asthma treatment in, 651–652
    in drowning situation, 1577–1578
    thoracotomy, 1609–1610
Emergency mass critical care (EMCC), 227
Emergency medical services (EMS)
    pediatric physiology relevant to, 150–151
    problems with adult-oriented transport teams, 149–152, 150b
    rapid transfer/goal-directed therapy/ golden hour, 151–152, 152f
    referring hospital responsibilities, 155
    specialized teams
        components of, 152–155, 154f
        improving outcomes, 152, 153f
    transport environment stresses, 151
Emergency surge capacity, 227, 227t
Emesis, 1378

EMP. See Embden-Meyerhof pathway (EMP)
Emphysema, congenital lobar, 671–672
EMS. See Emergency medical services (EMS)
Enalaprilat, for HTN, 1126
Encephalitis
    diagnosis of, 1493
    treatment for, 1495
Encephalocele, 838–839, 838f
Endocrine system, 413
    circulatory regulation by, 258
    disorders
        adverse drug reactions causing, 1713–1715, 1714t
        rheumatic disease and, 1472
    shock and, 420
End-of-life care
    decision making for, 122–123, 123t
    follow-up care of family/staff, 133
    practical aspects of, 132–133
    withholding/withdrawing life support, 123–125
Endogenous materials, renal disposition of, 1048
Endogenous neuroprotection, 936
Endoscopic third ventriculostomy (ETV)
    for Dandy-Walker malformation, 838
    for hydrocephalus, 833–836
    during myelomeningocele closure, 840
Endoscopy, gastrointestinal, 1359–1360
Endothelial homeostasis, hypertension and, 1116
Endothelial injury, in ARDS, 628–629
Endothelial progenitor cells (EPCs), 271
Endothelial-derived factors, circulatory regulation by, 258–259, 259f
Endothelin receptor antagonists
    for PAH, 728
        bosentan, 728
        sitaxsentan/ambrisentan, 728–729
    for PPHN, 718
Endothelins (endothelium-derived contracting factors)
    endothelium production of, 273
    in pulmonary arterial hypertension, 721
Endothelium
    biomarkers of activation of, 277–278
    dysfunction of, 275–277
        hemolytic-uremic syndrome, 277
        ischemia-reperfusion injury, 275–276, 276f
        sepsis, 276–277
        vasculitis, 277
    normal function of, 270–275
        blood cell interactions, 274–275, 274f
        coagulation and fibrinolysis, 271–272, 271f–272f
        endothelial cell heterogeneity, 270–271
        endothelial progenitor cells, 271

Endothelium (Continued)
        endothelium-derived vasoconstrictors, 273–274
        endothelium-derived vasodilators, 272–273, 273f
        hemostasis and, 1263–1264, 1263f
        permeability, 275, 275f
    overview of, 270
    in SCD, 1248–1249
Endothelium-derived hyperpolarizing factor (EDHF), 273
Endothelium-derived nitric oxide, 1238–1239
Endothelium-derived relaxing factor (EDRF). See Nitric oxide (NO)
Endotracheal intubation, 1755–1766
    complications, 1766, 1766t
    extubation, 1765–1766, 1765t
    flexible fiberoptic bronchoscopy, 1765
    indications for, 1755–1756, 1755b
        hemodynamic instability, 1755–1756
        respiratory failure, 1755
    nasotracheal intubation, 1764–1765
    neuromuscular dysfunction, 1756
    orotracheal intubation, 1763–1764, 1763f–1764f
    pharmacologic agents facilitating, 1761–1763, 1762t
        anticholinergic agents, 1761
        neuromuscular blocking agents, 1762–1763
        sedative/analgesic agents, 1761–1762
    physiologic effects of, 1756–1757, 1756b
    process of, 1759–1761, 1760f, 1760t
    prolonged intubation, 1766
    recognition of difficult airway, 1757–1759, 1757b, 1758f–1759f
    video laryngoscopy, 1765
End-tidal carbon dioxide
    abnormalities in, 572–574, 573b
    capnometry monitoring of, 570–571
    in monitored anesthesia care, 1790
Energy expenditure
    in critical illness
        assessment of, 1209–1210, 1209t–1210t
        indirect calorimetry, 1210–1211, 1210t–1211t
        lipid requirements, 1212–1213
        micronutrient requirements, 1213
        protein requirements, 1211–1212, 1212f
Enteral nutrition, 1214–1216, 1214t, 1215f
    for burn patients, 1592
Entrustable professional activities (EPAs), 221, 221t
Envenomation. See Snakebites; Widow spider bites
Environment
    ATLS primary survey of, 1607
    delirium and, 1874

Enzyme-linked receptors, 1697–1699, 1698f–1699f
Enzymes, signal transduction via, 1693
EPCs (endothelial progenitor cells), 271
Epiglottis, 544, 545f
Epiglottitis, 617–619, 618t, 619f
Epilepsy
    definition of, 915
    posttraumatic, 916–922
Epinephrine
    adverse effects of, 367–368
    basic pharmacology, 360f, 366
    for cardiac arrest, 530–531
    for cardiac dysfunction, 494t, 495
    clinical pharmacology, 365f, 366
    clinical role of, 367
    with CPR, 513–514
    interactions, 368
    pharmacokinetics of, 367
    preparation/administration, 367
    for ventricular fibrillation, 520t, 522f
E-point septal separation, 197, 197f
Epoprostenol, 727. See also Prostacyclin (PGI₂)
Epstein-Barr virus (EBV), 1435
Equipment
    for NIV, 776–778
    of retrieval systems, 155
Errors
    ethical issues of, 120
    invasive hemodynamic monitoring, 281
    patient safety and, 86
    pulse oximetry, 569, 569f
    tachycardia diagnosis, 409
    type I and type II, 61.e1t
Eryptosis, 1244
Erythron
    acquired RBC injury/eryptosis/clearance, 1244
    biophysical factors influencing flow, 1236–1237
        blood rheology, 1236–1237
        RBC aggregation/adhesion, 1237
        RBC deformability, 1237, 1237f
    carbon dioxide transport and, 1235–1236, 1236f
    energy metabolism in RBCs, 1241–1244, 1242f
    introduction, 1234
    maladaptive RBC-based signaling, 1244
    oxygen transport and, 1234–1235, 1235f–1236f
    regulation of blood flow distribution, 1238–1241, 1238f, 1240f
Erythropoiesis, 1228f, 1229–1230
Erythropoietin, for HIE, 948
Escape rhythms, heart, 394
Esmolol, for HTN, 1123–1124, 1123t
Esophageal foreign bodies, 1363
Esophageal reflux, 1363
    monitoring, 1360

Esophagus
    caustic injury to, 1362
    congenital anomalies of, 1362
    injury to, 1641
Established phase, of stress response, 1148–1149
Ethics
    of coma prognosis, 895
    in death and dying
        of decision making, 122–123, 123t
        withholding/withdrawing life support, 123–125
    of ICUs in resource-poor settings, 204
    in PICU
        additional issues, 119–120
        address by, 113
        approach to, 113–116, 114f, 114t–115t
        definition of, 112
        domains of, 112–113
        examples of, 112
        intensivist's goals, 120–121, 121b
        patient decision making, 116–117
        shared decision making, 117
        surrogate decision making, 117–119
Ethics committee, 113
Ethics consultant, 113
Ethylene glycol, 1741
Etomidate
    facilitating intubation, 1761, 1762t
    for intracranial pressure, 1769
ETV. See Endoscopic third ventriculostomy (ETV)
Europe, history of PCCM in, 15
Euthyroid sick syndrome, 1193, 1193t
Evacuation, of ICU, 230
EVD. See External ventricular drain (EVD), for hydrocephalus
Evidence-based medicine (EBM)
    challenges, 64
    critical appraisal, 64b
    definitions/equations, 61.e1t
    Internet resources, 63t
    levels of evidence, 64, 64.e1
    steps in, 61–62
    study types, 62–64
Exchange transfusion, 1255, 1255.e1f
Excitation-contraction coupling, of heart, 238, 239f
Excitatory amino acid inhibition, 830
Excitotoxicity
    HIE and, 933–934
    inhibition of postischemic, 948
    TBI and, 1615
Exertional heat illness (EHI), 1806–1807
Exertional heat stroke, 1562
Exogenous materials, renal disposition of, 1048
Exogenous surfactant, for ARDS, 631–632
Exotic viral disease, 1490

Exposure, ATLS primary survey of, 1607
Extended daily dialysis, 1111
External ventricular drain (EVD), for hydrocephalus, 833–836
Extracellular buffers, 1064–1065
Extracellular matrix, of heart, 237–238
Extracellular volume expansion, with AKI, 1047
Extracorporeal cardiopulmonary resuscitation (ECPR), 309, 795. See also Cardiopulmonary resuscitation (CPR)
Extracorporeal life support (ECLS)
    for ARDS, 634
    for asthma, 660
    as bridge to transplantation, 309, 481–482
    critical care during, 310–314, 310t
    ECMO indications/contraindications, 308
    ECMO system, 307f
    extracorporeal CPR, 309
    for HIE after cardiac arrest, 949
    indications/contraindications for, 310
    malignant dysrhythmias and, 309
    myocarditis and, 308
    postcardiopulmonary bypass, 308–309
    radiography and, 308f
    refractory respiratory failure, 309–310
    VADs vs., 314t
    venoarterial vs. venovenous, 307–314, 308t
Extracorporeal liver support, 1388–1389, 1389f
Extracorporeal membrane oxygenation (ECMO)
    for acute respiratory failure, 673
    for burn injury, 1591
    cannulation techniques, 785–788, 786f–787f
    cardiac catheterization and, 350
    for cardiac dysfunction, 496
        patient management, 496
    complications, 801–803
        bleeding, 802
        infection, 802
    CPR and, 507–508, 532–533
    decannulation, 801
    echocardiography and, 333–334, 336f–337f
    effect on drug disposition, 1682
    future directions, 803
    gas exchange and oxygen delivery, 796–798, 798f
    history of, 306
    indications/contraindications, 308
    outcomes, 802–803
        implications of, 803
        medical, 802–803
        neurodevelopmental, 803
    overview of, 785
    oxygenators, 790

Extracorporeal membrane oxygenation (ECMO) *(Continued)*
  patient management, 798–801
    cannulation and initiation, 798–799
    during ECLS, 799–801
    priming, 799
  patient populations, 790–795, 790*t*
    in adults, 793, 793*t*
    cardiopulmonary failure, 790–793, 791*t*, 792*f*
    myocardial dysfunction, 793–795, 794*t*
    resuscitation, 795
    trauma, 795
  patient selection, 795–796
  percutaneous cannulation, 788
  for PPHN, 718
  prior to cardiac transplantation, 481–482
  pumps, 788–790, 789*f*
  radiography and, 308, 308*f*
  system, 307–308, 307*f*
  venous reservoir/venous saturation monitor, 788
  weaning from, 801
Extralobar pulmonary sequestrations, 671
Extrasystoles, 398–399, 408
Extrathoracic airway obstruction, 584–585, 585*t*
Extubation, 765*t*, 766–767
  after CHD surgery, 457–458, 458*t*
  overview of, 1765–1766
  risk of failure, 1765*t*
  short-term NIV facilitating, 773
Eye examination, for coma, 885–888, 886*f*–889*f*
Eye injury, airway management and, 1770
EZ-IO drill, 159, 159*f*

F
Facial injury, 1770
Facilitation of learning, as nurse competency, 45
Family(ies)
  care of, after child's death, 133
  definition of, 104–105
  effect on outcomes, 76
  with limited English proficiency, 129
  rounds in PICU and, 107–108
FAST (focused assessment with sonography in trauma) exam, 191–192, 192*f*, 1646
Fats, digestion of, 1348–1349
Fatty acid β-oxidation, 1135
Femoral vein cannulation, 170, 171*f*
Fenestration, premature closing of, 463
Fenoldopam, for HTN, 1126
Fentanyl, 1777, 1777*f*
Fetal circulation, pulmonary, 260
Fetal lung fluid, delayed clearance of, 662–664, 663*f*
Fever, postoperative, 1803

Fibrinolysis
  coagulation and, 1264–1266, 1265*f*–1266*f*
  endothelium production of, 271–272, 271*f*
Fick method, for cardiac output measurement, 287–288, 294–295, 493
First-pass effect, 1674–1675
Fistula, tracheoesophageal, 678
FLAIR. *See* Fluid-attenuated inversion recovery (FLAIR)
Flexible fiberoptic bronchoscopy, 1765
Flow asynchrony, 755–756
Flow resistance, 557
Flow resistance, of respiratory system, 559–560, 560*f*
Flucytosine, 1482
Fluid and electrolyte management. *See also* Electrolyte(s)
  for ALF, 1386
  calcium levels in, 1019–1020
  hypercalcemia and, 1021–1022, 1022*t*
  hyperkalemia and, 1016–1018, 1016*b*
  hypermagnesemia and, 1019
  hypernatremia and, 1012, 1012*b*–1013*b*
  hyperphosphatemia and, 1024
  hypocalcemia and, 1020–1021, 1021*b*
  hypokalemia and, 1014–1016, 1015*b*
  hypomagnesemia and, 1018–1019, 1019*b*
  hyponatremia and, 1008–1014, 1009*b*, 1009*t*
  hypophosphatemia and, 1023–1024
  magnesium levels in, 1018
  overview of, 1007–1008
  phosphorus levels in, 1022
  sodium levels in, 1008
Fluid compartments, developmental aspects of, 1677, 1677*t*
Fluid management
  for asthma, 652
  after CHD repair, 458–459
  for DKA, 1199, 1200*f*–1201*f*
  ECLS complications, 313
  during ECMO, 800
  after liver transplant, 1391
  in multiple trauma, 1606, 1606*f*
  for organ donors, 143
  in sepsis treatment, 1535
  volume overload/HTN and, 1117
Fluid resuscitation, for shock, 418–419
Fluid-attenuated inversion recovery (FLAIR), 859–860
Fluorometry, of NADH, 1142
Fluoroquinolones, 1478–1479
Focal cerebral arteriopathy, 951
Focal pulmonary hemorrhage, 702–703
Focused assessment with sonography in trauma (FAST) exam, 191–192, 192*f*
Fontan procedure, 461–463, 462*t*
Food allergy, 1365

Foreign body
  aspiration, 623, 623*f*–624*f*
  esophageal, 1363
Fosphenytoin, for SE, 922–924, 923*t*
Fractures, in child abuse, 1656–1657
Free radical scavengers, for AKI, 1047
Free radicals
  AKI and, 1044
  RBCs and, 1243
Frequency, effect on ultrasound, 181–182, 183*f*
Frequency response, in invasive hemodynamic monitoring, 281, 282*f*
Full-face masks, for NIV, 776, 778*f*
Full-thickness burns, 1584
Funding, extramural, 57–58
Funduscopic examination, 845
Fungal infections, 1479–1480
  acquired immunodeficiency and, 1447
  Aspergillus, 1480
  Candida, 1480
  pneumonitis, 692–693, 693*b*
    opportunistic infections, 695–696
    primary infection, 693–695, 694*t*
Furosemide, excretion of, 1681

G
GABA receptors, 815–816
Gain, effect on ultrasound, 181, 183*f*
Gait evaluation, 848–849
Gas exchange
  determinants of, 736, 736*t*
  noninvasive monitoring of. *See* Noninvasive respiratory monitoring of respiratory system, 563–564
  ventilation perfusion relationships, 564, 565*f*
Gas flow
  flow asynchrony, 755–756
  in high-frequency ventilation, 757
  in lungs, 606–607, 606*f*
  in mechanical ventilation, 739–740, 740*f*
Gas sampling, of capnometer, 571–572, 572*f*
Gastric acid secretion, 1350
Gastric decontamination, 1513
Gastric tonometry, as measure of oxygen delivery, 295
Gastric ulcer, 1363–1364
Gastric volvulus, 1363
Gastroesophageal reflux (GER), 698–699, 698*b*
Gastrointestinal circulation, 266–267
Gastrointestinal complications
  after HCT, 1334–1335
  shock-related, 420
Gastrointestinal endoscopy, 1359–1360
Gastrointestinal hemorrhage, 1374–1375, 1472
Gastrointestinal losses, hypokalemia and, 1015

Gastrointestinal pharmacology
  antibiotic-associated diarrhea,
      1375–1376
  for constipation, 1376, 1377t
  gastrointestinal hemorrhage, 1374–1375
  nausea/vomiting, 1377–1380
  rectal administration of, 1376–1377
  stress ulcer prophylaxis, 1372
    epidemiology/risk factors, 1373
    H2 receptor antagonists for, 1374
    infectious complications of, 1374
    mechanism of mucosal damage,
        1372–1373
    options for, 1373–1374
    proton pump inhibitors for, 1374
    sucralfate for, 1374
Gastrointestinal tract
  carbohydrate digestion in, 1346–1347,
      1346b
  after CHD repair, 459
  diagnostic testing in ICU, 1355–1357,
      1356t
  drug absorption via, 1674, 1674b
  electrolyte transport across, 1349–1350
  evaluation of, 1358–1362
    abdominal examination, 1358–1359
    colorants to identify aspiration,
        1360
    endoscopy, 1359–1360
    esophageal reflux monitoring, 1360
    occult blood loss testing, 1361
    radiologic procedures, 1360–1361
    radionuclide scanning, 1361
    stool pH/reducing substances, 1361
  fat digestion in, 1348–1349
  gastric acid secretion, 1350
  in heat-related illness, 1564–1565
  hepatobiliary system, 1351–1357
  host-defense mechanisms of,
      1354–1355
  immunologic processes of, 1354–1355,
      1355t
  intestinal lymphatics, 1349
  introduction, 1345
  life-threatening complications of,
      1362–1370
    abdominal compartment syndrome,
        1368
    acute pancreatitis, 1368–1369
    acute/chronic liver failure, 1369–1370,
        1369t
    esophagus, 1362–1363
    small intestine/colon, 1364–1368
    stomach/duodenum, 1363–1364
    systemic, 1362
  lipid digestion in, 1348–1349, 1348b
  pancreas, 1350–1351
  protein digestion in, 1347–1348, 1347b
  regulation of electrolyte/water
      movement, 1349
  rheumatic disease effects on, 1472
  structure/function of, 1345, 1346t

Gastrointestinal tract (Continued)
  water/solute transport across, 1345–
      1350, 1346t
  zinc and, 1350
GBS. See Guillain-Barré syndrome (GBS)
Gene therapy
  for SCD, 1255–1256
  for thalassemia, 1259
General anesthesia, 1787
General surgery, history of, 5
Generalized proximal tubulopathy, 1038
Genetic disorders, of surfactant
      homeostasis, 664
Genetic polymorphisms, 1704
Genetic variation
  developmental timing of mutations/
      consequences, 1170–1171
    postzygotic mutations, 1170–1171
    prezygotic mutations, 1170
  future directions, 1172
  genome-wide association studies,
      1171–1172
  in high-throughput technologies, 1171
  introduction, 1168
  in mendelian/complex traits, 1171
  protein synthesis and, 1169–1170
  scale of mutational event, 1168–1169,
      1169t
  sequence variation, 1168
Genetics
  of malignant hyperthermia,
      1801–1802
  of pulmonary arterial hypertension,
      722
Genome-wide association studies
      (GWASs), 1171–1172
Genomic medicine
  research opportunities, 57
  sepsis and, 1527–1529
Geography, of PICU, 106
GER. See Gastroesophageal reflux (GER)
Germline cells, mutations occurring in,
      1170
Glasgow Coma Scale, 845, 847t
  TBI and, 1613–1614, 1619–1620,
      1620t
Glenn procedure, 390
Global health, ethical issues of, 120
Globin gene loci, 1246, 1246.e1f
Glomerular filtration rate (GFR)
  assessment of, 1026–1027, 1027t
  estimating equations for, 1033–1034
  physiology of, 1040–1041, 1041b
  plasma disappearance techniques for,
      1028–1029, 1028f
  plasma markers for, 1029–1033
  reduced, in AKI, 1042–1043
  renal clearance techniques for,
      1027–1028
Glomerular tuft
  anatomy of, 999
  function of, 999–1001, 1001f

Glomerulonephritis
  acute postinfectious, 1050
  AKI and, 1049–1052, 1049b–1050b
  anti-GBM antibody disease/GPA, 1051
  in systemic lupus erythematosus,
      1050–1051
Glomerulotubular dysfunction,
      1044–1045
Glucocorticoids
  for bronchopulmonary dysplasia, 675
  for PPHN, 718
Gluconeogenesis, 1187f, 1190–1191
Glucose
  with ALF, 1386
  control of
    after cardiac arrest, 532
    for organ donation, 144
  with CPR, 517–518, 517f
  homeostasis, 1183–1185, 1184f
  metabolism of, 1185, 1185t
  monitoring of, 1189
Glutamate receptors, 814–815
Glycemic control, for cellular homeostasis,
      1143
Glycerol, for bacterial meningitis, 970
Glycine, in AKI attenuation, 1047
Glycolysis, 1133–1136, 1134f
Glycopeptides, 1478
G protein–coupled receptors (GPCRs),
      1695–1696, 1696f, 1697t
Graduate medical education, 222–223,
      222f
Graft failure, in HCT, 1336–1337
Graft-versus-host disease (GVHD)
  clinical staging/grading of, 1338t
  with HCT, 1337–1338
Gram-negative bacteria, 686
Granulomatosis with polyangiitis (GPA),
      1051, 1468, 1468t
Granulopoiesis, 1228f, 1230–1231, 1230f,
      1231t
Group B streptococci, 684–685
Guillain-Barré syndrome (GBS), 984–985
GWASs. See Genome-wide association
      studies (GWASs)

H
HAART. See Highly active antiretroviral
      therapy (HAART), for HIV infection
Haemophilus influenzae, 685
HAIs. See Health care–associated infections
      (HAIs)
Half-life, drug, 1685
Hand hygiene, 1509
Hantavirus, 1503–1504
  clinical presentation, 1504
  diagnosis of, 1504
  etiology/epidemiology of, 1503–1504,
      1504f
  management of, 1504
  prognosis, 1504
Hayek cuirass ventilators, 781–782, 781f

HCT. *See* Hematopoietic cell transplantation (HCT)
Head hood (helmet), for NIV, 776, 778*f*
Head injury
  abusive, 1658
    neuroimaging of, 1658
    mechanisms of, 1658
    retinal hemorrhages, 1658
Head position, intracranial hypertension and, 1631
Health analytics, 101
Health care systems
  capacity building via education, 205–206
  during disease outbreaks, 206
  in resource-poor settings, 204–205
Health care–associated infections (HAIs)
  bloodstream infections, 1513–1514
  burden of illness and, 1506
  epidemiologic principles of prevention/ control, 1506–1507
    chain of infection, 1506–1507, 1507*b*
    routes of transmission, 1507, 1508*t*
  hospital-associated diarrhea, 1518
  prevention/control measures, 1507–1513
    additional isolation precautions, 1508–1509
    hand hygiene, 1509
    occupational health programs, 1510
    personal protective equipment, 1509
    policy/procedure/program development, 1510–1513
    prevention and control team, 1507
    screening, 1510
    standard isolation practices, 1507–1508
    surveillance, 1509–1510, 1511*t*–1512*t*
  respiratory infections/VAP, 1514–1515
  sinusitis, 1515–1516
  skin/surgical site infections, 1517
  urinary tract infections, 1516, 1516*f*
  ventriculostomy-related infections, 1517–1518
Health Information Technology for Economic and Clinical Health (HITECH) Act, 90–91, 91*f*
Health-related quality of life (HRQL)
  ideal outcome measure, 76–77
  impact of critical illness, 73–75, 74*t*, 75*f*
  performance/shortcomings of tools, 77, 78*t*
  PTSD and, 76
Heart
  anatomical development/structure, 235–238, 236*f*–237*f*
  neural control of, 246
  normal myocardial energy metabolism, 246–249, 248*f*
  physiologic development/function, 238–252
    cardiac sarcomere function, 238–240, 239*f*–240*f*

Heart *(Continued)*
    integrated muscle function, 240–241, 242*f*, 244*f*–245*f*, 249*f*
    myocardial receptors/responses to drugs, 240–241
  systemic vasculature, 249–252
  transplantation of, in severe PAH, 730
  ultrasound of, 193–198, 194*f*, 196*f*–198*f*
Heart failure, 302–306, 303*t*
  assessment in, 303–304
  broad treatment strategies, 305–306, 305*f*
  causes of, 489
  definitions, 303, 488
  diagnostic studies in patients, 491–493
    additional noninvasive imaging modalities, 492
    biomarkers, 491
    cardiac catheterization, 492–493
    echocardiography, 491–492
  drug-induced, 1711
  ECLS, 307–314
  extracorporeal CPR, 309
  heart transplantation and, 497
    immunotherapy, 497
  LCOS management, 493, 493*f*
  low cardiac output syndrome, 302–303
  mechanical circulatory support, 306–307, 495–497
    as bridge to transplantation, 309
    ECMO, 496
    managing patients on ECMO, 496
    VADs, 496–497
  mechanical ventilation for, 754
  overview of, 488
  pharmacology of, 493–495
    diuretics, 494*t*
    vasoactive drugs, 493–495, 494*t*
  physical examination, 490–491
  physiologic considerations in, 489–490
    afterload, 489–490
    contractility, 490
    oxygen delivery, 490
    preload, 489, 489*f*–490*f*
  postcardiopulmonary bypass, 308–309
  specific treatments, 304–305
  thalassemia and, 1258, 1258.*e*1*f*
Heart rate, appropriate vs. normal, 392
Heart-lung machine console and pumps, for CPB, 431–433, 432*f*, 434*f*
Heat cramps, 1562
Heat exhaustion, 1562
Heat index, 1563
Heat injury, 1564–1565
  definitions, 1562–1563
  epidemiology of, 1563
  pathophysiology/pathogenesis of, 1563–1564
  systemic clinical features, 1564–1565
  treatment for, 1565–1566
Heat stroke, 1562
Heat syncope (fainting), 1562

Helium-oxygen mixtures, 655–656, 761
Hemangiomas, airway vascular, 677
Hematocrit, targeting during CPB, 440–441
Hematologic dysfunction
  adverse drug reactions causing, 1713
  after HCT, 1337–1338
  in heat-related illness, 1565
  in HIV/AIDS patients, 1451
  rheumatic disease associated with, 1473
  with SLE, 1465
Hematology problems
  anemia, 1312–1316, 1313*b*
    hemolytic, 1314–1315, 1314*b*, 1317*f*
    hemorrhagic, 1312–1313
    secondary to bone marrow failure, 1313–1314
  bleeding in uremia, 1316
  thrombocytopenia, 1315
    immune, 1315–1316
    nonimmune, 1316
Hematopoiesis, 1227–1232, 1227*t*–1228*t*, 1228*f*, 1230*f*, 1231*t*
Hematopoietic cell transplantation (HCT)
  complications, 1328
    cardiac, 1328–1330
    colitis/gastrointestinal, 1334–1335
    graft failure, 1336–1337
    graft-versus-host disease, 1337–1338, 1338*t*
    hematologic, 1337–1338
    hepatic, 1333–1334
    infectious, 1335–1336
    iron overload, 1337
    late effects, 1340
    myelosuppression, 1335
    neurologic, 1339–1340
    pulmonary, 1330–1333, 1330*t*
  indications and outcomes, 1326–1327, 1327*t*
  nutritional support for, 1340–1341
  overview of, 1325
  procedure for, 1327–1340
    conditioning regimen, 1327
    recovery period, 1328
    reinfusion, 1327–1328
    stem cell harvesting/collection/ cryopreservation, 1327
  for SCD, 1255
  sources of stem cells/donor identification, 1325–1326, 1326*f*
  for thalassemia, 1259
Hematopoietic organs
  bone marrow, 1225–1226, 1226*f*
  hematopoiesis, 1227–1232, 1227*t*–1228*t*, 1228*f*
    erythropoiesis, 1229–1230
    granulopoiesis, 1230–1231, 1230*f*, 1231*t*
    megakaryocyte/platelet production, 1231–1232

Hematopoietic organs (*Continued*)
  lymphopoiesis, 1232–1233
    lymph nodes and, 1233
    spleen and, 1232–1233
Hematopoietic progenitor cell
  transplantation. *See* Hematopoietic
  cell transplantation (HCT)
Hemoconcentrators, for CPB, 435–436
Hemodynamic instability, intubation in,
  1755–1756
Hemodynamic monitoring. *See* Invasive
  hemodynamic monitoring
Hemodynamics, effects of cortisol on,
  1180–1181
Hemoglobin
  polymerization of, 1248
  regulation of RBC energetics by, 1241
Hemoglobinopathies
  globin gene loci, 1246, 1246.e1*f*
  perspective on, 1246
  sickle cell disease, 1246–1256, 1247*f*,
    1248*t*, 1249*f*, 1249.e1*f*, 1250.e1*f*,
    1249.e2*f*–1249.e3*f*
  thalassemia, 1256, 1256*t*, 1256.e1*f*,
    1257.e1*f*
Hemolysis, NO homeostasis and, 1249
Hemolytic anemia, 1314–1315, 1317*f*
Hemolytic uremic syndrome (HUS), 277,
  1048–1049, 1271–1272
  clinical signs, 1048–1049
  complications, 1049
  as life-threatening complication,
    1365–1367
  prognosis, 1049
  therapy for, 1049
Hemophagocytic lymphohistiocytosis
  (HLH), 982–983, 1321, 1321*b*, 1435
Hemorrhage
  abdominal, 1398
  gastrointestinal, 1374–1375
  pulmonary, 702–703, 1470–1471
  retinal, 1658
Hemorrhagic anemia, 1312–1313
Hemostasis
  developmental, 1282–1283, 1283*f*
  overview/coagulation and, 1261–1266,
    1262*f*–1263*f*
Henderson-Hasselbalch equation,
  1065–1067
Henoch-Schönlein purpura (HSP), 1467
Heparin
  for CPB anticoagulation, 436–437,
    437*f*
  drug-drug interactions of, 1724–1725
  over-anticoagulation with, 1275–1276
    management of, 1275–1276
Heparin-induced thrombocytopenia
  (HIT), 1278–1279, 1288
Hepatic biotransformation, 1679*t*
  factors affecting, 1680–1681
  phase I, 1678–1680
  phase II, 1680

Hepatic dysfunction. *See* Liver
  dysfunction
Hepatic encephalopathy
  in acute liver failure, 1386–1387
    management of, 1387–1388
  stages of, 1384*t*
Hepatic insufficiency, 1272–1273
Hepatitis, autoimmune, 1385–1386
Hepatobiliary system, 1351–1357
  diagnostic testing in ICU, 1355–1357,
    1356*t*
  enterohepatic circulation, 1353–1354,
    1354*b*
  hepatic function, 1353
  in HIV/AIDS patients, 1450
  microanatomy of, 1351–1352, 1352*f*
  physical examination, 1351
  portal circulation, 1352–1353
Hepatoxicity, drug-induced, 1709, 1710*b*
Herbs, toxicity of, 1730*t*
Herniation syndromes
  coma and, 892–893, 893*f*
  congenital diaphragmatic, 669–670
  ICP and, 899*t*
  in TBI, 1621*f*, 1622
Hexose monophosphate pathway (HMP),
  1241–1243, 1242*f*
HFPPV. *See* High-frequency positive
  pressure ventilation (HFPPV)
HFPV. *See* High-frequency percussive
  ventilation (HFPV)
HFV. *See* High-frequency ventilation
  (HFV)
HHS. *See* Hyperglycemic hyperosmolar
  syndrome (HHS), during DKA
Hibernation, in cellular bioenergetic crisis,
  1144
HIE. *See* Hypoxic-ischemic encephalopathy
  (HIE)
High-dose epinephrine, with CPR,
  513–514
High-frequency jet ventilation (HFJV),
  756–758, 757*f*
  for acute respiratory failure, 672–673
  for pulmonary air leak syndromes, 666
High-frequency oscillatory ventilation
  (HFOV), 757–758, 757*f*
  for acute respiratory failure, 672–673
  in ARDS, 631
  for PPHN, 714
  for pulmonary air leak syndromes, 666
High-frequency percussive ventilation
  (HFPV), 758
High-frequency positive pressure
  ventilation (HFPPV), 756, 756*f*
High-frequency ventilation (HFV),
  756–759
  clinical applications, 758–759
  definitions, 756–757, 756*f*–757*f*
  mechanism of gas flow in, 757
  for PPHN, 714
  selection of parameters for, 757–758

Highly active antiretroviral therapy
  (HAART), for HIV infection,
  1444–1445
High-mobility group box 1 (HMGB-1),
  1525
High-mortality countries, history of
  PCCM in, 16, 16*t*
High-reliability organizations
  (HROs)
  characteristics of, 19–20, 20*t*
  models of, 20–23, 21*f*
    outcomes in, 22–23
    process in, 22, 22*t*
    structure in, 21–22
High-throughput technologies, genetic
  variation in, 1171
Hirschsprung disease, 1367–1368
Histamine-2 receptor antagonists,
  1374
Histoplasmosis, 693–694
HIT. *See* Heparin-induced
  thrombocytopenia (HIT)
HITECH. *See* Health Information
  Technology for Economic and
  Clinical Health (HITECH) Act
HIV encephalopathy, 1451
HIV/AIDS. *See* Human immunodeficiency
  virus/acquired immune deficiency
  syndrome (HIV/AIDS)
HIV-associated nephropathy (HIVAN),
  1448–1449
HLH. *See* Hemophagocytic
  lymphohistiocytosis (HLH)
HLHS. *See* Hypoplastic left heart syndrome
  (HLHS)
HMGB-1. *See* High-mobility group box 1
  (HMGB-1)
HMP. *See* Hexose monophosphate pathway
  (HMP)
Hollow-fiber oxygenator, 790
Home characteristics, effect on outcomes,
  76
Home respiratory care, 767–768
  indications for, 767
  logistics of, 766*t*, 767–768
Hormonal regulation, of calcium,
  1020
Hormonal replacement therapy (HRT),
  for organ donation, 141–142,
  142*t*
Hospice care, 128
HROs. *See* High-reliability organizations
  (HROs)
HRQL. *See* Health-related quality of life
  (HRQL)
HSP. *See* Henoch-Schönlein purpura
  (HSP)
5-HT3. *See* Serotonin (5-HTP) receptor
  antagonists
HTN. *See* Hypertension (HTN)
H-type fistula, 678
Huddles, in ICU, 36

Human immunodeficiency virus/acquired immune deficiency syndrome (HIV/AIDS), 690
  abdominal complications, 1449–1450, 1449t, 1450b
    acute abdomen, 1450
  cardiovascular complications, 1447–1448
    dysrhythmias, 1448
    myocardial dysfunction, 1447–1448
    pericardial disease, 1448
    septic shock, 1447
    vasculitis, 1447
  hematologic complications, 1451
  hepatobiliary failure, 1450
  incidence/treatment of, 1444–1445
  malignancies, 1451
  neurologic complications, 1451–1452
    cerebrovascular disease, 1451
    CNS malignancy, 1451–1452
    HIV encephalopathy, 1451
    infections of CNS, 1452
  occupational HIV exposure, 1452
  PAH and, 721–722
  pancreatitis, 1450
  pulmonary complications
    cytomegalovirus pneumonitis, 1446
    fungal infections, 1447
    immune dysfunction and, 1445–1447
    lymphoid interstitial pneumonitis, 1447
    mycobacterial pathogens, 1446–1447
    pneumocystis jirovecii pneumonia, 1445–1446
    upper airway obstruction, 1447
  renal failure, 1448–1449
Humidification systems, during mechanical ventilation, 762–763
Humoral immune response, 1414–1415, 1414f–1415f, 1415t
HUS. See Hemolytic uremic syndrome (HUS)
Hydralazine, for HTN, 1123t, 1124
Hydrocephalus, 832–836
  background, 832
  in Chiari malformations, 837
  clinical presentation, 833
  in Dandy-Walker malformation, 837–838
  diagnosis of, 833
  in encephaloceles, 839
  etiology of, 833
  management of, 833–836, 834f–835f
  in myelomeningocele, 840
  neuroimaging of, 873
  pathophysiology of, 832, 833f
Hydrocortisone, for hormonal resuscitation, 141–142, 142t
Hydrogen ion-related autoregulation of CBF, 827
Hydroxyurea, for SCD, 1254
Hymenoptera stings, 1560–1561

Hypercalcemia, 1021–1022, 1022t
  treatment of, 1022
Hypercapnic acidosis, 1094
Hypercarbic acidosis, 1094
Hyperchloremic acidoses, 1070–1071, 1071t, 1086–1088
Hypercoagulable states, stroke and, 953
Hyperglycemia, 1185–1189
  after CHD repair, 459–460
  in DKA, 1197–1198
  future directions, 1189–1190
  glucose monitoring for, 1189
  after heart transplantation, 487
  stress
    mechanisms of, 1187–1188
    outcomes, 1185–1186
    pathophysiology of, 1186–1187
    studies on management of, 1188–1189, 1189.e1t
Hyperglycemic hyperosmolar syndrome (HHS), during DKA, 1202
Hyper-immunoglobulin M syndrome, 1428–1429
Hyperkalemia, 1016–1018
  with AKI, 1047
  causes of, 1016–1017, 1016b
  management of, 1059t
  manifestations of, 1017
  after succinylcholine administration, 1813–1814, 1813t
  treatment, 1017–1018
Hyperkalemic periodic paralysis, 988
Hyperleukocytosis, 1318
Hyperleukocytosis-associated MOF, 1546
Hypermagnesemia, 1019
  causes of, 1019
  signs/symptoms, 1019
  treatment, 1019
Hypernatremia, 1012
  pathophysiology/etiology of, 1012–1013, 1012b–1013b
  potassium levels, 1014
  signs/symptoms, 1013
  treatment, 1013–1014
Hyperphosphatemia, 1024
  causes of, 1024
  management of, 1059t
  signs/symptoms, 1024
  treatment, 1024
Hyperpolarizing factor, endothelium-derived, 273
Hypertension (HTN). See also Intracranial hypertension
  with AKI, 1047
  blood pressure monitoring, 1120–1122
  classification of, 1115t
  clinical presentation, 1117–1120, 1118f
  ECLS complication of, 311
  endothelial homeostasis and, 1116
  etiology of, 1115–1116, 1115t

Hypertension (HTN) (Continued)
  evaluation/monitoring of, 1118–1120, 1119t, 1121f
  introduction, 1114
  after liver transplant, 1392
  nitric oxide and, 1117
  pathophysiology of, 1116
  pharmacologic therapy for, 1122–1126
    clonidine, 1122–1123
    esmolol, 1123–1124
    general considerations, 1122, 1122f, 1123t
    hydralazine, 1124
    isradipine, 1124
    labetalol, 1124
    nicardipine, 1124–1125
    other agents, 1126
    sodium nitroprusside, 1125–1126
  pheochromocytoma with, 1127
  preeclampsia with, 1127
  renin-angiotensin-aldosterone system and, 1116–1117
  SNS activation and, 1116
  terminology for, 1114–1115
  volume overload leading to, 1117
Hypertensive encephalopathy, 916
Hyperthermia
  arrhythmia associated with, 413
  after cardiac arrest, 531–532
  in PICU, 1803
  xenobotic-induced, 1740–1741, 1740t
Hyperthyroidism, 413, 1192–1193, 1193b
Hypertonic saline solution, for intracranial hypertension, 1630–1631
Hypertrophic cardiomyopathy, 390
Hyperventilation, for severe TBI, 1632–1633, 1633f
Hyperviscosity syndrome, 679–680
Hypocalcemia, 1020–1021
  with AKI, 1048
  causes of, 1021b
  clinical/laboratory concerns, 1020
  rhabdomyolysis and, 1055
  treatment, 1020–1021
Hypoglycemia, 1190–1191
  in ALF, 1386
  clinical manifestations of, 1190
  evaluation of, 1163–1164, 1163f
  fasting adaptation, 1187f, 1190–1191
  pathogenesis of, 1190
  treatment for, 1191
Hypokalemia, 1014–1016
  causes of, 1014–1015, 1015b
  signs/symptoms, 1015–1016
  treatment, 1016
Hypokalemic periodic paralysis, 987–988
Hypomagnesemia, 1018–1019
  causes of, 1018, 1019b
  signs/symptoms, 1018–1019
  treatment, 1019

Hyponatremia, 1008–1014
    pathophysiology/etiology of, 1008–1011,
        1009b, 1009t, 1011b
    prevention of, 1011
    signs/symptoms, 1011
    therapy for, 1011–1012
Hypophosphatemia, 1023–1024
    causes of, 1023
    signs/symptoms, 1023–1024
    treatment, 1024
Hypoplasia, pulmonary, 668–669
Hypoplastic left heart syndrome (HLHS),
        474–478
    critical care management for, 475
    pathophysiology of, 474–475
    postoperative management, 475–478
        evolution of treatment strategies,
            475–476
        hybrid approach, 477–478
        Norwood procedure considerations,
            476–477, 476t
Hypothalamic-pituitary-adrenal axis, 1178,
        1179f
Hypothalamus, peripheral stress responses
        and, 1147–1148
Hypothermia
    accidental
        cardiovascular responses, 1567–1568,
            1568f
        CNS involvement, 1567
        coagulation in, 1568
        outcome, 1570
        physiology of, 1567
        renal responses, 1568
        respiratory responses, 1568
        treatment for, 1568–1570, 1569f
    acid-base balance in, 1095–1096
    arrhythmia associated with, 413
    after brain death, 145
    as CPB technique, 441–442, 441t,
        442f–444f
    in drowning, 1577
    postresuscitative, 946–947
    for RSE, 926
    for severe TBI, 1633–1634
Hypothyroidism, 1193
Hypoventilation, 1093–1094
Hypovolemia, ECLS complication of, 311
Hypovolemic shock, 421, 421b
Hypoxemia
    causes of, 590t
    in CHD patient, 450
    after Fontan procedure, 463
    PPHN and, 709–710, 711f
        differential diagnosis of, 712t
    ventilation/perfusion mismatch in, 591
Hypoxic-ischemic encephalopathy (HIE)
    cardiac arrest and
        clinical outcome after, 941–942, 943f
        response of immature brain to,
            942–943
        treatment of, 943–946, 945f–946f

Hypoxic-ischemic encephalopathy (HIE)
        (Continued)
    cellular/molecular pathobiology,
        930–936
        brain injury mechanisms, 930–936
        cell death mechanisms, 931–932,
            931f–933f
        endogenous defenses, 936
        energy failure, 930–931
        excitotoxicity/calcium accumulation,
            933–934
        membrane phospholipid hydrolysis/
            mediator formation, 935–936
        oxygen radical formation, 934–936
        protease activation, 934
        reperfusion injury, 932–933
        selective vulnerability, 931
    clinical pathophysiology, 936–941
        CBF/metabolism after resuscitation,
            936–939, 937f–939f
    current/novel therapies for, 946–948
        inhibition of postischemic
            excitotoxicity, 948
        postresuscitative hypothermia,
            946–947
        therapies directed by group
            characteristics, 947–948
    epidemiology of, 930
    futuristic approaches to, 948–949
        erythropoietin, 948
        extracorporeal life support, 949
        mitochondria targeting therapies, 948
        stem cell therapy, 948–949
    histopathology of, 939–941, 940f–941f
    overview of, 929–930
Hypoxic-ischemic injury, causing
        cardiogenic shock, 424–425

I

IAA. See Interrupted aortic arch (IAA)
IAC-CPR. See Interposed abdominal
        compression-cardiopulmonary
        resuscitation (IAC-CPR)
Iatrogenic coagulopathy. See Coagulopathy,
        iatrogenic
ICH. See Intracranial hemorrhage (ICH)
ICP. See Intracranial pressure (ICP)
ICU. See Intensive care unit (ICU)
Idiopathic pneumonia syndrome (IPS),
        1331–1332
IE. See Indirect calorimetry (IE)
IEDs. See Immune-enhancing diets (IEDs)
IEM. See Inborn errors of metabolism
        (IEM)
IgG. See Immunoglobulin G (IgG)
        replacement therapy
IHD. See Intermittent hemodialysis (IHD)
ILD. See Interstitial lung disease (ILD)
Iloprost, for PAH, 727
Immune dysregulated metabolism
        hypothesis, 1541–1543
Immune dysregulation, 1335

Immune paralysis, 1542–1543, 1545f, 1546
    critical illness and, 1440–1441
Immune system
    compartments of, 1423–1425
        B cells/antibodies component, 1425
        complement component, 1423
        phagocytes component, 1425
        symptoms of defects in, 1423t
    critical illness and, 1440–1441
    malnutrition and, 1441–1443
    monitoring of, 1458–1460
Immune thrombocytopenia purpura (ITP),
        1315–1316
Immune-enhancing diets (IEDs), 1216
Immunization. See Vaccination
Immunocompromised patients, short-term
        NIV for, 773–774
Immunoglobulin G (IgG) replacement
        therapy, 1437–1438
Immunologic dissonance, 1541, 1542f,
        1543
Immunomodulation
    for sepsis, 1535–1536
    transfusion-related, 1310
    unintended, 1458, 1459t
Immunostimulation
    adaptive, 1458
    innate, 1458, 1459t
Immunosuppressants
    drug-drug interactions of, 1725–1726
    immune dysfunction and, 1443
    targeting adaptive immunity, 1419, 1420t
Immunosuppression
    complications of, 1392, 1392t
    after heart transplantation, 497
    after liver transplant, 1391
    during orthotopic heart transplant,
        484–486, 485t
    with SLE, 1465
Impedance, in invasive hemodynamic
        monitoring, 281, 282f
Impedance threshold valve (ITV)
        interposition, 505–506, 506f–507f
In vitro caffeine-halothane contracture
        testing, 1807
Inborn errors of metabolism (IEM)
    cardiomyopathy and, 1164–1166, 1165b,
        1165t
    causing neonatal respiratory disease, 680
    classification by clinical presentation,
        1156–1162, 1157t
        group 2, 1157–1160, 1158t
        group 3, 1160–1162, 1160t
    definition/overview of, 1151
    emergency treatment for, 1155–1156,
        1157t
    inheritance of, 1152
    laboratory evaluation of, 1152b,
        1153–1155, 1154t–1155t
    pathophysiology of, 1151–1152, 1152f
    physical anomalies associated with,
        1153t

Inborn errors of metabolism (IEM) (Continued)
    postmortem evaluation of, 1155, 1156b, 1156t
    signs/symptoms, 1152–1153, 1152t
Incident Command System, 226–228
India, history of PCCM in, 14
Indirect calorimetry (IE), 1210–1211, 1210t–1211t
Inequalities, effects of, 1666
Infancy, breathing failure in, 586
Infection(s)
    in acute liver failure, 1388
    arrhythmias secondary to, 414
    chain of, 1506–1507, 1507b
    after CHD repair, 459
    CNS, 869–872, 871f, 1452
    control, in PHEs, 229
    in critical illness, 1449t
    due to immunosuppression, 486
    ECLS complication involving, 313–314
    ECMO complication involving, 802
    after HCT, 1335–1336
    heat stroke and, 1565
    immune dysfunction and, 1443
    liver transplantation and, 1391
    outcomes following, 75
    in PICU
        hantavirus, 1503–1504, 1504f
        invasive pneumococcus, 1501–1502, 1501b
        meningococcal, 1497–1499, 1498f
        necrotizing fasciitis, 1500–1501
        Rocky Mountain spotted fever, 1502–1503, 1502f–1503f
        toxic shock syndrome, 1499–1500, 1499b–1500b
    with rheumatic diseases, 1469
    with stress ulcer prophylaxis, 1374
    transfusion-transmitted, 1309–1310, 1310t
    upper airway disease due to, 616, 618t
        bacterial tracheitis, 620
        epiglottitis, 617–619, 619f
        laryngeal papillomatosis, 620–621, 620f
        laryngotracheobronchitis, 616–617, 617f–618f, 617t
        peritonsillar abscess, 619
        retropharyngeal abscess, 619–620, 620f
Inflammation
    in ARDS, 629
    coagulation and, 1264–1266, 1264f–1266f
    coagulation/immune dysfunction/ dysregulated metabolism hypothesis, 1541–1543
    cortisol and, 1179–1180, 1181f
    after CPB, 445
    in SCD, 1248–1249
    VILI and, 641–642, 642f

Inflammatory bowel disease, 1366–1367, 1366t
Influenza, 690
Informatics research, 57
Information technology
    in critical care
        big data and, 100–102
        clinical decision support, 96–97, 98f
        clinical informatics, 92
        EHRs and, 92–96
        future directions, 102
        HITECH Act, 90–91, 91f
        learning health system, 91–92, 92f
        patient safety, 97–99
        privacy/security of health information, 99–100, 99b
        telemedicine, 100
Inhalational anesthetics
    for RSE, 925–926
    triggering malignant hyperthermia, 1806
Inhalational injury, 699–700, 699t, 1588–1591
    airway clearance, 1590
    diagnosis of, 1589
    management of, 1589–1590, 1590f
    pathophysiology of, 1588–1589
    therapeutic adjuncts, 1590–1591
Innate immune system
    clinical manifestations of, 1408–1409
    components of, 1403–1407
        danger hypothesis, 1403–1404
        effector pathways, 1405–1407, 1408t
        signal recognition, 1404–1405, 1405t
        signal transduction, 1405, 1406f
    crosstalk between systems, 1407–1408, 1409f
    elements of, 1454–1455
    intervention questions, 1409–1411
    overview of, 1403
    regulation of, 1408, 1409t
    therapeutic targets of, 1409
Innate tolerance, 1862
Innervation, in regional peripheral circulation, 257
Inositol triphosphate, 1702
Inotropic medications
    for cardiac dysfunction, 493–495, 494t
    infusion rates for, 364t
    prior to cardiac transplantation, 481
    for shock, 419
In-service education programs, 48–49
In-situ simulation training, 213
Insulin
    in DKA management, 1199
    for hormonal resuscitation, 141–142, 142t
    in sepsis treatment, 1535
Intensive care unit (ICU)
    confusion regarding, 58
    effective communication
        checklists, 36
        closed-loop, 37

Intensive care unit (ICU) (Continued)
        debriefing, 37
        huddles, 36
        medical records, 36
        medical training, 37
        optimal design, 35–36
        rounds, 36
        team training, 37
        transitions of care, 37
    evacuation of, 230
    history of, 7–8
    in PHEs, 229
    in resource-poor settings, 203
        cost of, 203–204
        development of, 206
        ethics of, 204
Intensivists
    definition of, 8
    education of
        ABP requirements, 216
        ACGME core competencies, 208–210
        ACGME requirements, 216
        adult learning, 208–216, 209t
        evaluating competency, 214–215, 215t
        maintaining competency, 216–217
        mentorship, 215–216
        professionalism in, 213–214
        in research/scholarship/leadership, 214
        in safety and quality, 214, 214t
        teaching methods, 210–213, 210t–211t
    growth in training/education, 12
    organ donation process involvement, 136
    organizations of, 13t
Intention-to-treat analysis, in EBM, 61.e1t
Intercellular communication, in nervous system, 810–811
Intercostal muscles, 578
    accessory muscles of respiration, 578–579
    regulation of breathing, 579–581
Interleukin (IL)
    IL-6, 1524
    IL-8, 1524
    IL-10, 1441
    IL-18, 1524–1525
    IL-β, 1524
Intermittent hemodialysis (IHD), 1107–1109
    disadvantages/complications, 1109
    extended daily dialysis and, 1111
    ICU issues, 1109
    indications for, 1108
    physiology of, 1107–1108, 1108f
    technique for, 1108–1109
Intermittent mandatory ventilation, 742–743, 742f–743f
Internal jugular vein cannulation, 169, 170f
Internet resources, for EBM, 63t

Interposed abdominal compression-cardiopulmonary resuscitation (IAC-CPR), 505
Interprofessional care, in PICU, 54
Interrupted aortic arch (IAA), 474
Interstitial cells, 557–558
Interstitial lung disease (ILD), 1470, 1470f–1471f. See also Pneumonitis
  diagnosis of, 683
  idiopathic, 700–701
  pathophysiology of, 682–683
  viral agents associated with, 688t
Interstitial nephritis, drug-related, 1708t, 1709
Interventional studies, in EBM, 62
Intestinal bicarbonate wasting, 680
Intestinal lymphatics, 1349
Intestinal perforation, 1472
Intraabdominal abscess, 1399
Intraaortic balloon pumps, 322–323
Intraatrial reentrant tachycardia, 395
Intracardiac pressure monitoring, 296
Intracardiac shunt, 290
Intracardiac thrombosis, 1290
Intracranial hemorrhage (ICH), 960f
  aneurysms, 960–961
  arteriovenous malformations, 959–960
  cavernous malformations, 961, 962f
  coagulation disorders, 962
  general care for, 962
  overview of, 959
  prognosis, 963
  spontaneous, 959–962
Intracranial hypertension. See also Hypertension (HTN)
  clinical background, 897–898, 898t–899t
  physiology of, 898–901
    cerebral vasodilation and CSF pressure, 899–900, 900f–901f
    cerebrospinal fluid, 898
    CPP and autoregulation, 900–901, 901f
    hydrodynamic model of ICP, 899, 900f
    ICP and cerebrospinal fluid circulation, 898–899, 900f
  in traumatic brain injury, 908, 909f
    monitoring/postinsult natural history, 908–909, 909f
  treatment of
    first-tier therapies, 1629f, 1630–1631
    second-tier therapies, 1631–1635, 1632f
Intracranial pressure (ICP)
  airway management and, 1768–1769, 1768b
  analysis of, 903–905
    compensatory reserve/pressure reactivity assessment, 903–905, 906f–907f

Intracranial pressure (ICP) (Continued)
    normal trends/waveform analysis, 903, 904f–905f
    normal values in, 903
  anesthesia and, 1779–1780, 1780t
  CSF circulation and, 898–899, 900f
  cumulative CPP and, 905
  early signs of raised, 897, 898t
  effects of CPR on, 503–504, 504f
  hydrodynamic model of, 899, 900f
  interventions after cardiac arrest, 944
  measurement of, 901–903
    devices for, 901–902
    noninvasive inference of, 902
    pressure compartments, 902–903
  monitoring of
    brain oxygenation in, 909–910
    clinical utility of, 908
    invasive, 905–908
    target levels for, 907–908
    in TBI, 1622–1626, 1628–1630
    TCD in, 910–911
  optimal CPP from, 905
  in pediatric neurocritical care, 851–852
Intracranial vault, 898–901
Intralobar pulmonary sequestrations, 671
Intramuscular drug administration, 1675, 1675b
Intraosseous infusion, 158–161
  complications, 160–161
  contraindications for, 158
  indications for, 158
  maintenance, 160
  supplies/equipment, 159, 159f
  technique for, 159–160, 160f
Intrathoracic airway obstruction, 584–585, 585t
Intrathoracic tracheomalacia, 615–616
Intravenous admixtures, drug-drug interactions in, 1720
Intravenous anesthesia, 1792–1794
Intubation. See also Endotracheal intubation
  for asthma, 656–657
  physiologic effects of, 1756–1757, 1756b
  rapid-sequence, 1767–1768, 1767b
  for shock, 418
  for TBI, 1620–1623, 1621b, 1622t
Inulin, renal clearance of, 1027–1029
Invasive hemodynamic monitoring
  cardiac catheterization and, 342
  cardiac output measurement, 287–289
    Fick method, 287–288
    thermodilution method, 288–289
  indications for, 279–280
  novel monitoring devices, 290
  oxygen delivery/consumption calculation, 289–290
    waveform interpretation in, 289–290
  principles of, 280–281
    calibration, 281

Invasive hemodynamic monitoring (Continued)
    errors in measurement, 281
    frequency response, 281, 282f
    impedance, 281, 282f
    measurement systems, 281
    signal analysis, 280–281, 280f
  role of, 279, 280f
  for sepsis, 1532–1533
  techniques, 281–285
    arterial pressure catheters, 283–284
    CVP catheters, 281–283
    PACs, 284–287, 286f, 287t
Invasive pneumococcus, 1501–1502
  clinical presentation, 1501
  diagnosis of, 1501–1502
  etiology/epidemiology of, 1501, 1501b
  management of, 1502
Invasive pulmonary aspergillosis, 695–696
Invasive technology, effect on outcomes, 76
Iohexol, for plasma disappearance techniques, 1029
Ion channels, signal transduction via, 1690–1691
Iothalamate, renal clearance of, 1028
IPS. See Idiopathic pneumonia syndrome (IPS)
Iron
  AGMA and, 1742
  immune function and, 1443
Iron chelation therapy, in thalassemia, 1258.e1f
Iron overload
  with HCT, 1337
  SCD and, 1254
  in thalassemia, 1257
Irradiated platelets, 1304
Irradiated red blood cell units, 1300
Ischemia, 1397–1398
  posttraumatic, 1614–1615
Ischemia-reperfusion injury, 275–276, 276f
Isoflurane, for SE, 922–924, 923t
Isolation practices, for infection prevention and control, 1507–1509
Isolette ventilators, 780–781
Isonicotnyl hydrazine, 1744
Isoproterenol
  adverse effects of, 369
  basic pharmacology, 359f, 368
  for cardiac dysfunction, 494t, 495
  clinical pharmacology, 365f, 368
  clinical role of, 368
  interactions, 369
  pharmacokinetics of, 368
  preparation/administration, 369
Isosbestic wavelengths, 568
Isovolumic phase indices, in myocardial contractility, 243
Isradipine, for HTN, 1123t, 1124
Israel, history of PCCM in, 15

ITP. *See* Immune thrombocytopenia purpura (ITP)
ITV. *See* Impedance threshold valve (ITV) interposition

J

Jacket ventilators, 782, 782*f*
Japan, history of PCCM in, 14
Junctional ectopic tachycardias, 396, 400*f*, 413
Just culture model, 87
Justice, in PICU, 115–116
Juvenile dermatomyositis, 1465–1466
Juvenile idiopathic arthritis (JIA), 1462–1463
    clinical presentation, 1462–1463
    criteria for, 1463*b*
    laboratory studies, 1463
    management of, 1463

K

Kawasaki disease (KD), 1467–1469
Ketamine
    for asthma, 656
    facilitating intubation, 1761, 1762*t*
    for intracranial pressure, 1769
    management of, 131, 131*t*
    for RSE, 926
    for SE, 922–924, 923*t*
Ketoacidosis, 1085
Ketogenic diet, for RSE, 926
Kidney(s)
    anatomy of, 997
    development of, 997
    drug disposition and, 1098–1100, 1099*f*, 1099*t*
    failure, drug dosing in, 1100–1101, 1100*b*, 1100*f*
    function tests of
        estimating equations for, 1033–1034
        glomerular function/injury assessment, 1026–1027, 1027*t*
        for neonates, 1034–1035
        other biomarkers, 1035, 1036*f*
        overview of, 1026, 1027*t*
        plasma disappearance techniques, 1028–1029, 1028*f*
        plasma markers, 1029–1033, 1030*f*–1031*f*, 1032*t*
        renal clearance techniques, 1027–1028
        of tubular function, 1035–1038
    glomerular tuft, 999–1001, 1001*f*
    nephron unit, 998–1001, 999*f*–1000*f*
    as therapeutic target, 1101–1103, 1101*f*
    tubular anatomy, 1001–1005, 1001*f*–1004*f*
    vasculature, 997–998, 998*f*
Kolb's experiential learning theory, 219, 219*f*
Krebs cycle, 1134*f*, 1135

L

Labetalol, for HTN, 1123*t*, 1124
Laboratory environment, for cardiac catheterization, 341–342
β-Lactam antibiotics, 1476–1477
    β-lactam antimicrobial/β-lactamase inhibitor combination, 1477
    carbapenems, 1477
    cephalosporins, 1477
    monobactams, 1477
    penicillins, 1477
    structures of, 1476*f*
Lactate, in cellular respiration, 1139–1140
Lactic acidosis, 1082–1085
LAD. *See* Leukocyte adhesion deficiency (LAD)
Laparoscopy, for abdominal trauma, 1646
Laryngeal cleft, 541*f*
Laryngeal mask airway (LMA), 1765, 1771–1773, 1771*f*–1772*f*
Laryngeal papillomatosis, 620–621, 620*f*
Laryngomalacia, 545, 614, 614*f*, 677
Laryngoscopy
    physiologic effects of, 1756–1757, 1756*b*
    video, 1765
Laryngotracheal injury, 1770
Laryngotracheal stenosis, 622–623, 622*f*
Laryngotracheobronchitis, 616–617, 617*f*–618*f*, 617*t*–618*t*
Larynx
    anatomy and physiology of, 545, 1751–1752
    development of, 539–542, 540*f*
    webs/stenosis/tumors of, 540*f*–541*f*, 614–615, 615*f*
Late postoperative arrhythmias, 413
Latin America, history of PCCM in, 15–16
LCOS. *See* Low cardiac output syndrome (LCOS)
Leadership
    in critical care nursing, 46–50
        Beacon Award, 47
        professional development, 47–48
        staff development, 48–49
    education in, 214
Learned tolerance, 1862
Learner assessment, 220
Learning disabilities, anesthesia exposure and, 1783–1784, 1784*f*
Learning health system, 91–92, 92*f*
Lectin pathway, 1423, 1424*f*
Left ventricle
    effects of ventilation on, 385–386, 386*f*–387*f*
    ultrasound of, 197
Left-sided obstructive heart lesions, 472–478
    aortic stenosis, 473
    coarctation of the aorta, 473–474
    hypoplastic left heart syndrome, 474–478, 476*t*

Left-sided obstructive heart lesions (*Continued*)
    interrupted aortic arch, 474
    pathophysiology of, 472
Legionella pneumophila, 686
LEP. *See* Limited English proficiency (LEP)
Leukocyte adhesion deficiency (LAD), 1427
Leukocyte-reduced platelets, 1304
Leukocyte-reduced red blood cell units, 1300
Leukocytes
    in ARDS, 629
    vessel wall interaction with, 274, 274*f*
Leukocytosis, in DKA, 1198
Levosimendan
    adverse effects of, 376
    basic pharmacology, 374–375, 375*f*
    for cardiac dysfunction, 494*t*, 495
    clinical pharmacology, 375
    clinical role of, 375–376
    interactions, 376
    pharmacokinetics of, 375
    preparation/administration, 376
Levothyroxine, for hormonal resuscitation, 141–142, 142*t*
Lidocaine
    for arrhythmias, 406, 523
    for intracranial pressure, 1769
    for RSE, 926
    for SE, 922–924, 923*t*
    for ventricular fibrillation/tachycardia, 533
Lifelong learning. *See also* Education
    adult learning theory, 219, 219*f*
        applied to medical education, 220
    continuing medical education/Board certification/maintenance of certification, 223
    costs and benefits, 220*t*
    graduate medical education, 222–223, 222*f*
    maintaining Board certification, 224
    new assessment methods, 223–224
    overview of, 219
    time-based vs. competency-based progression, 224
    undergraduate medical education, 220–221, 221*t*
Life-sustaining treatment, withholding/withdrawing of, 123–125
Lighted intubation stylet-assisted intubation, 1771
Limited English proficiency (LEP), 129, 129*t*
Linear array transducers, 183–184, 185*f*
Linezolid, 1479
Lipids
    in critical illness, 1212–1213
    digestion of, 1348–1349, 1348*b*
    in parenteral nutrition, 1217, 1218*f*
Liquid ventilation, for acute respiratory failure, 673–674

Liver
  adverse drug reactions in, 1709, 1710b
  diagnostic testing in ICU, 1355–1357, 1356t
  functions of, 1353
    degradation/elimination, 1353
    regulatory, 1354, 1354b
    storage, 1354
    substance production, 1353
  injury to, 1648, 1649t, 1650f
Liver dysfunction
  abnormal hemostasis in, 1272
  complications of HCT, 1333–1334
  management of, 1273
  presentation of, 1272–1273
  shock-related, 420
Liver failure, 1369–1370, 1369t
Liver transplantation, 1389–1392
  background/history/terminology, 1389
  complications, 1391–1392, 1392t
  indications for, 1389
  organ allocations, 1389–1390, 1390t
  outcomes, 1392, 1392f
  postoperative management, 1391
  pretransplant workup/evaluation, 1389
  technical aspects of, 1390
  technical complications of, 1390–1391
Liver-associated MOF syndrome, 1546
LMA. See Laryngeal mask airway (LMA)
Local anesthesia, 1778–1779, 1786, 1791–1792
Long QT syndromes, 410–412, 411f
Long-term outcomes, in critical care
  antecedents/variables in, 76
  metrics for HRQL outcomes, 76–77, 78t
  mitigating morbidity
    ARDS and, 75
    cardiopulmonary resuscitation and, 75
    health-related quality of life, 73–75, 74t, 75f
    after long-stay PICU, 75
    post-intensive care syndrome, 73, 74f
    severe infection and, 75
    traumatic brain injury and, 75–76
  mortality reduction, 73, 74f
  novel approaches to improving, 77–80
  research aims, 80
  targets for interventions, 80
  trichotomous outcome model, 80
Loop diuretics, 1101–1103, 1101f
Loop of Henle, 1001, 1002f
  function of, 1003–1004, 1003f
Lorazepam, for SE, 922–924, 923t
Low cardiac output syndrome (LCOS), 302–303
  assessment of, 303–304, 490–491
  after CHD repair, 453, 453f, 455f
  after Fontan procedure, 463, 464t
  as life-threatening complication, 1365
  management of, 493
    afterload reduction, 493, 493f

Low cardiac output syndrome (LCOS) (Continued)
    contractility optimization, 493
    oxygen consumption, 493
    preload management, 493
  specific treatments, 304–305
Lower respiratory system
  alveolar formation, 551
  alveolar-capillary unit, 551–553, 551f–553f
  lung circulation, 553–555
    bronchial vascular system, 554
    diaphragm, 555
    pulmonary lymphatics and BALT, 554–555
    pulmonary vascular system, 553–554, 554f
  lungs, 547–548, 548f–551f
  special lung unit definitions, 551
Low-flow phase, of cardiac arrest, 526–530, 527t
Low- to middle-income countries (LMICs). See Resource-poor settings
Lumbar cerebrospinal fluid drainage, 1634
Lumbar puncture, 188–189, 189f
Lung circulation. See Pulmonary circulation
Lung injury, 674–675, 1640. See also Ventilator-induced lung injury (VILI)
Lung volume
  effects of PVR on, 383, 383f–384f
  mechanical ventilation and, 734
  VILI and
    high volume injury, 636–638, 637f–638f
    low volume injury, 637–639
Lungs, 551
  adverse effects of mechanical ventilation, 760
  chest wall interactions with, 562, 599–601, 600f
  gas flow distribution in, 606–607, 606f
  inflation and deflation of, 734–735, 735f, 735t
  injury to, 1640
  maturation/physiologic changes at birth, 662
  special units/alveolar formation, 551
  structure and development of, 547–551, 548f–551f
  transplantation of, in PAH, 730
  ultrasound of, 189–193, 189f–191f
Lusitropic medications, for shock, 419
Lymph nodes, 1233
Lymphangiectasia, pulmonary, 675–676
Lymphatic circulation, 827–828
Lymphatic dysplasias, 676
Lymphatics, congenital defects of, 675–676
Lymphocytes, 1413–1414
Lymphoid depletion syndrome, 1546
Lymphoid interstitial pneumonitis, 1447
Lymphopenia, 1441

Lymphopoiesis, 1232–1233
Lymphoproliferative disease–associated sequential MOF, 1546

M
Macrolides, 1478
  drug-drug interactions of, 1722
Macrophage activation syndrome, 1546
Macrophage migration inhibitory factor (MIF), 1524
Magnesium sulfate
  for arrhythmias, 408
  for asthma, 652, 654–655
Magnetic resonance angiography (MRA), 449–450, 860–861, 861f
Magnetic resonance imaging (MRI)
  for acute abdomen, 1397
  advanced techniques for, 860
  of arachnoid cysts, 836, 836f
  of arterial ischemic stroke, 954–955, 954f
  of brain abscesses, 973–974, 973f
  after cardiac arrest, 941–942, 943f
  in CHD preoperative care, 449–450
  of Chiari I malformation, 837, 837f
  of encephaloceles, 838f, 839
  for gastrointestinal evaluation, 1360–1361
  for HTN, 1120
  of meningoencephalitis, 975–976, 976f
  for neuroimaging, 859–861
  for neurologic assessment, 850–855, 850t
  for pulmonary sequestrations, 671
  for TBI, 1624, 1624f–1625f
Magnetic resonance spectroscopy (MRS), 1142
Magnetic resonance venography (MRV), 860–861, 862f
Major histocompatibility complex (MHC), 1433–1434
Malignancy
  of CNS, 1451–1452
  in HIV/AIDS patients, 1451
Malignant dysrhythmias, 309
Malignant Hyperthermia Association of the United States (MHAUS), 1808
Malignant hyperthermia (MH), 1740–1741, 1740t
  clinical course of, 1805–1807
    muscular diseases and, 1806
    recrudescence, 1806
    triggering factors, 1806
  clinical recognition of, 1802–1803, 1802b
    hyperthermia in PICU, 1803
    rhabdomyolysis, 1803
    systemic complications, 1802–1803
  differential diagnosis of, 1805b
  genetics of, 1801–1802
  Malignant Hyperthermia Association contact information, 1808
  pathophysiology of, 1801
  treatment of, 1803–1805, 1804b

Malignant hyperthermia (MH)
(Continued)
administering dantrolene, 1803–1804,
1804f
removal of trigger agents, 1803
symptomatic treatment, 1804–1805
urine and blood tests, 1805
Malignant hyperthermia susceptibility
(MHS)
evaluation of, 1807
exertional heat illness and, 1806–1807
genetics and, 1801–1802
neuroleptic malignant syndrome and,
1807–1808
serotonin syndrome and, 1808
testing for, 1807
less invasive tests, 1807
in vitro CHCT, 1807
Mallampati classification, 1757–1759, 1758f
Malnutrition
assessment of, 1206, 1206t
biochemical assessment, 1206–1208
body composition, 1206
breathing failure due to, 587
in critical illness, 1205–1206
immune function and, 1441–1443
Malrotation, 1364–1365
Mammalian diving reflex, 1576
Mandatory dual-control breath-to-breath
ventilation, 748
Mandatory minute volume ventilation, 751
Mandatory ventilator-assisted breaths, 741
modes of, 744–747
continuous flow vs. demand flow, 745
CPAP/PEEP, 745–746, 746f
pressure-limited, 743f, 744–745, 745f
selection of parameters for, 746–747
volume-controlled, 744
Mannitol, for intracranial hypertension,
1630
Manual ventilation, during PHEs, 230
MAPSE. See Mitral valve annulus plane of
systolic excursion (MAPSE)
MAS. See Microphage activation system
(MAS)
Masimo SET Rainbow pulse oximeter, 569,
570f
Masks, for oxygen delivery, 1753–1754
Massive transfusion, 1309
Massive transfusion syndrome, 1274–1275
MCTD. See Mixed connective tissue disease
(MCTD)
MDSCs. See Myeloid-derived suppressor
cells (MDSCs)
Measles, 690
Measurement systems, for invasive
hemodynamic monitoring, 281
Mechanical circulatory support (MCS),
306–307
as bridge to transplantation, 309
for cardiac dysfunction, 495–497
ECMO, 496

Mechanical circulatory support (MCS)
(Continued)
managing patients on ECMO, 496
VADs, 496–497
critical care during, 310–314, 310t
ECLS, 307–314, 307f–308f
extracorporeal CPR, 309
historical perspective, 306–307, 307t
indications/contraindications for, 310
malignant dysrhythmias and, 309
myocarditis and, 308
postcardiopulmonary bypass, 308–309
prior to cardiac transplantation,
481–482
refractory respiratory failure, 309–310
ventricular assist devices, 314–319, 315f
clinical indications/outcomes for
centrifugal, 316–317
continuous flow, 316, 317f
device selection, 319, 320f
ECLS vs., 314t
FDA approved, 322t
future directions, 322–323
intraaortic balloon pump, 322–323
long-term, 318–319, 318f
next generation-levitated devices, 319
outcomes, 321–322, 321f
patient management, 319–320
patient selection, 319
single-ventricle physiology, 320–321
total artificial heart devices, 319
Mechanical ventilation. See also
Noninvasive ventilation (NIV);
Positive pressure mechanical
ventilation (PPV)
adverse effects of, 759–760
airway injury, 759–760
effects on circulatory system, 760
effects on lungs, 760
overview of, 759, 759t
in airway mechanics, 605–606
applied respiratory physiology, 734–736
determinants of gas exchange, 736,
736t
lung inflation/deflation, 734–735,
735t
lung volumes/capacities, 734
work of breathing, 735–736, 736f
for asthma, 656–659
analgesia/sedation/muscle relaxation,
658–659
indications, 656
inhalational anesthetic agents, 659
intubation, 656–657
ventilator monitoring, 658, 659f
ventilator settings, 657–658, 657f–658f
bronchopulmonary dysplasia and,
674–675
design/functional characteristics,
737–740
classification system, 738–739, 738t,
739f

Mechanical ventilation (Continued)
gas flow patterns, 739–740, 740f
ventilator as machine, 737
discontinuing, 130
during ECMO, 800–801
high-frequency ventilation, 756–759
clinical applications, 758–759
definitions, 756–757, 756f–757f
mechanism of gas flow in, 757
selection of parameters for, 757–758
history of, 7
home respiratory care, 767–768
indications for, 767
logistics of, 766t, 767–768
indications for, 736–737
cardiovascular dysfunction, 737
neurologic/neuromuscular disorders,
737
respiratory failure, 736–737, 737f
for infants and children, 747–751
airway pressure release ventilation,
749–750, 750f
automatic tube compensation, 749
AutoMode, 749
dual control modes, 748–749
mandatory minute volume
ventilation, 751
neurally adjusted ventilatory assist,
751
pressure-support breaths, 747, 747f
proportional assist ventilation,
750–751
modes of, 740–751
breath sequences, 741–743, 742f
commonly used mandatory modes,
743f, 744–747, 745f–746f
targeting schemes, 744
ventilator breath control variable, 741
ventilatory pattern, 743, 744t
patient-ventilator asynchrony, 755–756
associated with breath triggering, 755
during cycling, 756
during inspiration, 755–756
use of neuromuscular blockade, 756
in PHEs, 229–230
respiratory care during, 761–763
aerosol therapy, 763
humidification systems, 762–763
pulmonary hygiene, 761–762
for shock, 418
specialty gases, 760–761
altering inspired oxygen/carbon
dioxide concentration, 760–761
helium-oxygen mixture, 761
nitric oxide, 761
for underlying pathophysiology, 751–755
alveolar recruitment/derecruitment,
753
diseases with abdominal distention,
754
disorders with airway obstruction,
751–752

Mechanical ventilation (Continued)
    heart failure, 754
    neurologic/neuromuscular disorders,
        755
    parenchymal lung disease, 752–753,
        752f
    primary respiratory muscle failure,
        751
    prone positioning and, 753
    after repair of congenital heart
        disease, 754
    unilateral/severely differential lung
        disease, 753–754
    weaning from, 763–767
        criteria for, 763–764, 764t
        extubation, 765t, 766–767
        modern method, 764t, 765
        problems in, 767
        readiness to extubate trial, 765–766,
            765f
        tracheostomy and, 767
        traditional method, 764
Meconium aspiration syndrome, 667–668
Media violence, 1664–1665
Mediastinal tumors, causing acute airway
    compromise, 1319, 1320f
Mediator formation, HIE and, 935–936
Medical errors. See Errors
Medical examiner issues, in organ
    donation, 145
Medical investigation, of child abuse, 1660,
    1660b
Medical knowledge databases, 96–97
Medical outcomes, of ECMO, 802–803
Medical Professionalism in the New
    Millennium: A Physician Charter, 41
Medical records, 36
Medical training. See also Education
    in effective communication, 37
    ethical issues of, 119–120
Medication bar coding, 99
Medications. See Drug(s)
Medulla, 817
Megakaryocytes, 1231–1232
Membrane lung, for ECMO, 790
Membrane phospholipid, 1043–1044
    hydrolysis, 935–936
Membrane stabilizers, for mitochondrial
    injury, 1144
Mendelian inheritance patterns, 1171
Meninges, 821
Meningitis, 1493
Meningocele, 838–839
Meningococcal infection, 1497–1499
    clinical presentation, 1497–1498, 1498f
    diagnosis of, 1498
    etiology/epidemiology of, 1497
    management of, 1498–1499
Meningococcal purpura fulminans,
    1270–1271
Meningoencephalitis, 974–983, 976f
Mental status assessment, 845

Mentorship, 215–216
Mesenchymal stem cells (MSCs), 675
Meta-analysis, 63–64
Metabolic acidosis, 1081–1090
    acid-base balance and, 1066
    with AKI, 1047–1048
    anion gap and, 1069–1071, 1071t,
        1162–1163
    bowel segment urinary reconstruction,
        1088
    classification of, 1077t
    elevated anion gap acidoses, 1082–1086
    hyperchloremic, 1086
    hyperchloremic acidoses, 1086–1088
    with increased anion gap, 1085–1086
    integrated approach to, 1078t
    ketoacidosis, 1085
    lactic acidosis, 1082–1085
    postpyloric GI fluid losses, 1086–1087
    renal tubular acidoses/drug-mediated
        tubulopathies, 1087–1088
    respiratory distress and, 680
    toxic compounds that provoke, 1085
    treatment of, 1088–1090
        alternative alkalinizing agents,
            1089–1090
        dialysis, 1090
        sodium bicarbonate, 1088–1089
Metabolic alkalosis, 1090–1092
    causes of, 1079t, 1082t, 1090–1091
    classification of, 1077t, 1081, 1091
    definition of, 1090
    treatment of, 1092
Metabolic coupling, 827
Metabolic disease, 1386
Metabolic disorders
    adverse drug reactions causing, 1713–
        1715, 1714t
    arrhythmias secondary to, 413–414
        acute myocardial infarction,
            413–414
        CNS injury, 413
        electrolyte disturbances, 413
        endocrine disorders, 413
        hypothermia/hyperthermia, 413
    in heat-related illness, 1565
Metabolic myopathies, 1166
Metabolic stress, in critical illness,
    1207–1208, 1207f, 1208t
Metabolism
    circulatory regulation by, 258
    drug, interactions affecting, 1717,
        1718t–1719t
    effects of cortisol on, 1180, 1181f
    glucose, 1185
Metformin-associated lactic acidosis,
    1084–1085
Methadone
    management of, 131, 131t
    toxicity of, 1737
    for withdrawal, 1866
Methanol, 1741

Methemoglobinemia
    agents causing, 1732–1733, 1734b
    toxicity of, 1740, 1740b
Methylprednisolone
    for hormonal resuscitation, 141–142,
        142t
    for immune suppression, 484–486, 485t
Methylxanthine agents, 655, 1737–1738
Metronidazole, 1479
MG. See Myasthenia gravis (MG)
MH. See Malignant hyperthermia (MH)
MHAUS. See Malignant Hyperthermia
    Association of the United States
    (MHAUS)
MHC. See Major histocompatibility
    complex (MHC)
MHS. See Malignant hyperthermia
    susceptibility (MHS)
Microangiopathic consumptive disorders,
    1269–1270
Microbiome, 830
Microdialysis, 1141
    brain tissue biochemistry and, 909–910
Micrognathia, 1757, 1757b, 1758f
Micronutrients, in critical illness, 1213
Microphage activation system (MAS),
    1469–1472
Microscopic polyangiitis (MPA), 1468
Midazolam, for SE, 922–924, 923t
Midbrain, 818
MIF. See Macrophage migration inhibitory
    factor (MIF)
Milestones, in assessment of competence,
    215, 215t, 222–223, 222f
Milrinone
    adverse effects of, 374
    for cardiac dysfunction, 494t, 495
    after CHD repair, 454–455, 455f
    clinical pharmacology, 373–374
    clinical role of, 374
    pharmacokinetics of, 374
    phosphodiesterase inhibitor, 717
    preparation/administration, 374
    prior to cardiac transplantation, 481
    structure of, 373f
MIMIC. See Multi-parameter Intelligent
    Monitoring in Intensive Care
    (MIMIC) database
Minerals, in parenteral nutrition,
    1217–1218
Minoxidil, for HTN, 1126
Missed triggering, in ventilation, 755
Mitochondria
    biogenesis of, 1143–1144
    oxidative phosphorylation of, 1135–
        1136, 1136f
    therapies targeting, 948, 1142–1143
Mitochondrial deoxyribonucleic acid
    (mtDNA), 1142, 1152
Mitral valve annulus plane of systolic
    excursion (MAPSE), 197, 198f
Mivacurium, 1815t, 1818–1819

Mixed acid-base derangements, 1095
Mixed apnea, 676
Mixed connective tissue disease (MCTD), 1466
Mixed venous oxygen saturation (SvO$_2$), 283, 439–440
M-mode imaging in ultrasound, 183, 184f
Modified ultrafiltration, as CPB technique, 440–441
MODS/MOF. See Multiple organ dysfunction/multiple organ failure syndrome (MODS/MOF)
Monitored anesthesia care, 1786
Monobactams, 1477
Moral agency, as nurse competency, 45
Morbidity
    of ARDS survivors, 634
    assessment, 70–71
    with DKA, 1199
    mitigating, 73–76
    SE and, 927
Mortality
    from bronchopulmonary dysplasia, 675
    of children, 201–203, 202f
    with DKA, 1199
    due to child abuse, 1660–1661
    with PPHN, 679
    prediction tools for, 67–70, 68t–69t
    reduction, in PCCM, 73, 74f
    SE and, 927
Motor examination
    approach to, 847–848
    for coma patients, 888, 889t, 890f
    gait evaluation, 848–849
Mouth, 543–544, 544f–545f
Mouthpieces, for NIV, 776, 778f
Moyamoya syndrome, 867–868, 868f, 951, 952f
MPA. See Microscopic polyangiitis (MPA)
MRA. See Magnetic resonance angiography (MRA)
MRI. See Magnetic resonance imaging (MRI)
MRS. See Magnetic resonance spectroscopy (MRS)
MRV. See Magnetic resonance venography (MRV)
MS. See Multiple sclerosis (MS)
MSCs. See Mesenchymal stem cells (MSCs)
mtDNA. See Mitochondrial deoxyribonucleic acid (mtDNA)
Mucocutaneous manifestations, of SLE, 1464
Multiorgan failure syndrome, in SCD, 1253
Multi-parameter Intelligent Monitoring in Intensive Care (MIMIC) database, 101
Multiple organ dysfunction/multiple organ failure syndrome (MODS/MOF)
    definitions/scoring of, 1543–1544
    inflammation/coagulation/immune dysfunction/dysregulated

Multiple organ dysfunction/multiple organ failure syndrome (MODS/MOF) (Continued)
        metabolism hypothesis, 1541–1543, 1542f–1545f
    introduction, 1541, 1542f
    outcomes, 1544
    phenotypes/respective biomarkers/therapies, 1544–1546, 1545t
        hyperleukocytosis-associated MOF, 1546
        immune paralysis/lymphoid depletion syndrome, 1545f, 1546
        macrophage activation syndrome, 1546
        secondary hemochromatosis-associated cardiac hepatopancreatic MOF, 1546
        thrombocytopenia-associated MOF, 1543f–1544f, 1544–1546
        viral/lymphoproliferative disease–associated sequential/liver-associated MOF syndrome, 1546
    therapeutic approaches to, 1546–1548, 1546t
    time course of, 1548
Multiple sclerosis (MS), 872, 873f
Multiple trauma
    diagnostic assessment, 1608–1609
        laboratory studies, 1608
        radiographic imaging, 1608–1609, 1610f
    ED thoracotomy, 1609–1610
    overview of, 1599
    prehospital care/trauma team activation, 1600
    primary survey, 1602f
        breathing, 1604–1605
        circulation, 1605–1606, 1605t, 1606f
        disability, 1606–1607, 1607f
        establishing with cervical spine stabilization, 1601–1604, 1602t, 1603f
        exposure/environment, 1607
        overview of, 1600–1601, 1602f
    secondary survey, 1607–1608
    stabilization/definitive care, 1610
    trauma resuscitation, 1600, 1601f
Muscarinic acetylcholine receptors, 814
Muscle enzymes, for asthma assessment, 651
Muscle relaxants, for mechanical ventilation, 658–659
Musculoskeletal system, SLE effects on, 1464
Mutations
    developmental timing of, 1170–1171
        postzygotic mutations, 1170–1171
        prezygotic mutations, 1170
    scale of, 1168–1169, 1169t
Myasthenia gravis (MG), 985–986
    congenital/transient, 986–987

Mycobacterial pathogens, 1446–1447
Mycophenolate mofetil, for immune suppression, 484–486, 485t
Mycoplasma pneumonia, 685–686
Myelination of CNS, 829
Myelography, 861
Myeloid-derived suppressor cells (MDSCs), 1527
Myelomeningocele
    anatomy of, 839f
    in Chiari II malformations, 837
    features/treatment of, 839–840, 839f
Myelosuppression, after HCT, 1335
Myobacterial disease, susceptibility to, 1435
Myocardial dysfunction
    ECMO for, 793–795, 794t
    HIV/AIDS and, 1447–1448
    mechanical circulatory support, 306–307
        as bridge to transplantation, 309
        critical care during, 310–314, 310t
        ECLS and, 307–314, 307f–308f
        ECMO indications/contraindications, 308f
        extracorporeal CPR, 309
        historical perspective, 306–307, 307t
        indications/contraindications for, 310
        malignant dysrhythmias and, 309
        myocarditis and, 308
        postcardiopulmonary bypass, 308–309
        refractory respiratory failure, 309–310
    overview of, 302
    pediatric heart failure, 302–306, 303t
        assessment in, 303–304
        broad treatment strategies, 305–306, 305f
        low cardiac output syndrome, 302–303
        specific treatments, 304–305
    ventricular assist devices, 314–319, 315f
        continuous flow, 316, 317f
        device selection, 319, 320f
        ECLS vs., 314t
        FDA approved, 322t
        future directions, 322–323
        intraaortic balloon pump, 322–323
        long-term, 318–319, 318f
        next generation-levitated devices, 319
        outcomes, 321–322, 321f
        patient management, 319–320
        patient selection, 319
        single-ventricle physiology, 320–321
        total artificial heart devices, 319
Myocardial infarction, 413–414
Myocardial ischemia, 248–249
Myocardial mechanics
    cardiac sarcomere function, 238–240
        excitation-contraction coupling, 238, 239f
        sarcomere length-tension relationships, 239–240, 240f
    contractile apparatus, 235–237, 236f–237f

Myocardial mechanics *(Continued)*
  integrated muscle function, 241–246
    assessing myocardial contractility, 242f, 243, 244f
    cardiac output, 246
    diastolic ventricular function, 245–246
    muscle strips/intact ventricle relationship, 241–242
    neural control of heart, 246
    pericardial function, 244–245
    pressure-volume loops, 242–243, 242f
    ventricular function curves, 243–244, 245f
    ventricular interaction, 245
    myocardial receptors/responses to drugs, 240–241
Myocardial metabolism
  basic metabolic processes, 246–247
  determinants of myocardial oxygen consumption, 247–248, 248f
  effects of myocardial ischemia, 248–249
  myocardial oxygen demand-supply relationship, 248, 249f, 264–266, 265f
Myocardial protection, during CPB, 442–445, 444t
Myocarditis, 1471, 1485–1487
  background, 1485
  clinical presentation, 1485–1487
  diagnosis of, 1490
  etiology of, 1485, 1486t
  MCS for, 308
  pathogenesis of, 1485
  treatment for, 1493
Myocytes, 235
Myogenic regulation, of regional peripheral circulation, 259
Myotonias, malignant hyperthermia and, 1806

N

NADH. *See* Nicotinamide dinucleotide (NADH)
Naloxone, toxicity of, 1737
Narrative ethics, 116
Narrative reviews, 62
Nasal cannulas, 1753
Nasal masks, for NIV, 776, 777f
Nasal passages, 542–543, 542f–544f
Nasopharyngeal airway, 1753, 1753f
Nasotracheal intubation, 1764–1765
National Response Framework, 226–228
Nausea, 1377–1380
  chemotherapy-induced, 1378, 1380t
  definitions, 1377–1378
  management of, 132
  pathophysiology of, 1378
  postoperative, 1380

NAVA. *See* Neurally adjusted ventilatory assist (NAVA)
NBS. *See* Nijmegen breakage syndrome (NBS)
Near-infrared spectroscopy (NIRS)
  during CPB, 440, 440b
  as measure of oxygen delivery, 295–296
  monitoring tissue oxygenation, 1141–1142
  in pediatric neurocritical care, 853–854
Necroptosis, 1173–1174, 1175f
Necrosis
  animal studies of, 1175–1177
  apoptosis vs., 1173
  human studies of, 1174–1175
Necrotizing enterocolitis, 1365
Necrotizing fasciitis, 1500–1501
  clinical presentation, 1500
  diagnosis of, 1501
  etiology/epidemiology of, 1500
  management of, 1501
Negative predictive value, in EBM, 61.e1t
Negative pressure mechanical ventilation, 779–782. *See also* Mechanical ventilation
  advantages/disadvantages, 781t
  current modes of, 782
  design/modes of, 779–782
    cuirass ventilators, 780f, 781
    Hayek cuirass ventilators, 781–782, 781f
    isolette ventilators, 780–781
    jacket ventilators, 782, 782f
    tank/whole body ventilators, 779–780, 780f
  history of, 4–7, 8f
Neonatal apnea, 676–677
Neonatal autoimmune syndromes, 1465
Neonatal respiratory disease
  acute respiratory failure treatments, 672–674
    ECMO for, 673
    high-frequency ventilation, 672–673
    liquid ventilation, 673–674
    nitric oxide inhalation for, 673
    surfactant replacement, 672
  acute/early-onset, 662–668
    meconium aspiration syndrome, 667–668
    pneumonia, 666–667
    pulmonary air leak syndromes, 664–666
    pulmonary hemorrhage, 666
    retained fetal lung liquid, 662–664
    surfactant-deficient respiratory distress syndrome, 664
  chronic pulmonary disease, 674–676
    bronchopulmonary dysplasia, 674–675, 674t
    congenital lymphatic defects, 675–676

Neonatal respiratory disease *(Continued)*
  congenital lung malformations, 668–672
    bronchogenic cysts, 670–671
    congenital diaphragmatic hernia, 669–670
    congenital lobar emphysema, 671–672
    congenital pulmonary airway malformation, 670
    pulmonary agenesis/aplasia, 672
    pulmonary hypoplasia, 668–669
    pulmonary parenchymal cysts, 671
    pulmonary sequestrations, 671
  metabolic disorders causing, 680
  nonpulmonary conditions causing, 676–680, 676t
    airway vascular tumors/malformations, 677
    choanal atresia/stenosis, 677
    congenital chest wall anomalies, 679
    congenital heart disease, 680
    eventration of diaphragm, 678–679
    hyperviscosity syndrome, 679–680
    laryngomalacia, 677
    neonatal apnea, 676–677
    persistent pulmonary hypertension, 679
    phrenic nerve paralysis, 678
    pleural effusion, 679
    tracheobronchomalacia, 677–678
    tracheoesophageal fistula, 678
    vascular compression, 678
    vocal cord paralysis, 677
Neonatal seizures, 916
Neonatology, history of, 5
Nephron unit, 998–1001, 999f–1000f
Nephrotic syndrome, 1010
Nephrotoxicity, drug-induced, 1055–1058, 1708–1709, 1708t
Nerves, of heart, 238
Nervous system. *See also* Central nervous system (CNS); Peripheral nervous system (PNS)
  anatomic organization of, 816–821, 816f
    CNS, 816–820, 820f
    PNS, 820–821
  blood-brain barrier, 821–824, 822f–823f
  development of
    CBF/autoregulation/cerebral metabolism, 829–830, 830f
    cell origin/differentiation, 828
    cerebrovasculature and BBB, 829
    myelination, 829
    neurotransmitter system maturation, 828–829
    new insights in, 830
    synaptogenesis/synaptic pruning, 828, 829f
  intercellular communication in, 810–811
    chemical synapses, 810–811
    electrical synapses, 810
  major cell types, 809–810
  meninges, 821

Nervous system (Continued)
  neurotransmitter systems of, 811–816
    classes of, 811t
      neurotransmitters, 811–814, 812f
      receptors of, 814–816
  ventricles/cerebrospinal fluid, 824–825,
    824f
Nesiritide, 376, 481
Neural control
  of breathing, 583, 583t
  of heart, 246
  of regional peripheral circulation, 257
Neurally adjusted ventilatory assist
  (NAVA), 751
Neurocritical care, 31–32, 31f–32f
  training for, 32
Neurodevelopmental apoptosis, 830
Neurodevelopmental outcomes, of ECMO,
  803
Neuroendocrine mediators, circulatory
  regulation by, 258
Neuroepithelial bodies, 549–551
Neuroimaging. See also specific methods
  of abusive head trauma, 1658
  advantages/limitations, 850–855, 850t,
    851f
  of arterial ischemic stroke, 954–955, 954f
  brain tissue oxygen monitoring, 854
  after cardiac arrest, 941–942, 943f
  catheter angiography, 861
  cerebral microdialysis, 855
  of cerebral sinus venous thrombosis,
    957, 958f
  CNS infection, 869–872, 871f
  computerized tomography, 857–859
  demyelinating disease, 872, 873f–874f
  EEG monitoring, 852–853
  hydrocephalus, 873
  ICP monitoring, 851–852
  MRI, 859–861
  myelography, 861
  NIRS, 853–854
  nuclear medicine, 861
  of older infant/child
    posterior reversible encephalopathy
      syndrome, 865–866, 867f
    stroke, 865–868, 866f–867f
    vasculopathy/vasculitis, 867–868, 868f
    venous infarct, 862f, 866–867
  optic nerve sheath diameter
    measurement, 854
  of preterm/term neonates, 861–865,
    863f–865f
  seizures, 874–875
  TCD of cerebral blood flow, 853
  trauma, 872–873, 874f
  tumor, 874, 875f
  tympanometry, 854–855
  ultrasound, 857, 858f
  vascular malformations, 868–869,
    869f–870f
  viral meningoencephalitis, 975–976, 976f

Neuroleptic malignant syndrome (NMS),
  1740–1741, 1740t, 1807–1808
Neurologic assessment and monitoring
  abnormal movements/altered sensorium,
    849
  anticipatory planning, 843
  cerebellar function/gait evaluation,
    848–849
  complication recognition, 842–843
  cranial nerve examination, 845–847
  functional deficits vs. nonorganic
    pathology, 849–850, 849t
  funduscopic examination, 845
  goals of, 850
  iatrogenic complications of
    pharmacotherapy, 843, 844f
  integrating monitoring data, 855–856,
    855f
  level of consciousness/mental status,
    845, 847t
  motor exam approach, 847–848
  neuroimaging, 850–855
    advantages/limitations, 850t, 851f
    brain tissue oxygen monitoring, 854
    cerebral microdialysis, 855
    EEG monitoring, 852–853
    ICP monitoring, 851–852
    NIRS, 853–854
    optic nerve sheath diameter
      measurement, 854
    TCD of cerebral blood flow, 853
    tympanometry, 854–855
  observation in, 844–845, 846t–847t
  overview/basic principles of, 842–850
  physical examination, 844
  reflexes, 848
  risk factor history/assessment, 843
  sensory examination, 849
  vital signs, 843–844
Neurologic death. See Brain death
Neurologic disorders
  airway management and, 1768–1769,
    1768b
  in HIV/AIDS patients, 1451–1452
  mechanical ventilation for, 737, 755
Neurologic injury
  anesthesia and, 1779
  in HCT, 1339–1340
Neuromuscular blocking agents (NMBAs)
  adverse effects of, 1822–1824
  depolarizing agents, 1811–1824,
    1812t–1813t
  facilitating intubation, 1762–1763, 1762t
  guidelines for, 1825t
  indications for, 1811t
  for intracranial hypertension, 1631
  introduction, 1810
  malignant hyperthermia and, 1806
  mechanical ventilation and, 756
  monitoring of, 1821–1822
  nondepolarizing agents, 1814–1821,
    1814t

Neuromuscular blocking agents (NMBAs)
  (Continued)
  in PICU, 1824–1825, 1824t–1825t
  reversal of, 1821
Neuromuscular diseases
  acute intermittent porphyria, 989–990
  botulism, 988–989
  diphtheria, 989
  endotracheal intubation and, 1756
  Guillain-Barré syndrome, 984–985
  long-term NIV with, 775
  mechanical ventilation for, 737, 755
  myasthenia gravis, 985–986
    congenital/transient, 986–987
  organophosphate/carbamate poisoning,
    991–992
  periodic paralyses, 987
    hyperkalemic, 988
    hypokalemic, 987–988
  polio-like syndromes, 991
  poliomyelitis, 991
  spinal muscular atrophy, 990–991
  tick paralysis, 987
Neuromuscular junction (NMJ), 810–811,
  1810–1811
Neurons
  abnormal firing of, 918f
  normal firing of, 917f
  selective vulnerability of, 931
Neurosonology, 198–199
Neurotoxicity, of anesthesia, 1783–1784,
  1783f–1784f
Neurotransmitter systems, 811–816
  classes of, 811t
  maturation of, 828–829
  neurotransmitters, 811–814, 812f
  receptors of, 814–816
Neutropenic enterocolitis, 1335, 1398
New Zealand, history of PCCM in, 14
Nicardipine, for HTN, 1123t,
  1124–1125
Nicotinamide dinucleotide (NADH),
  1142
Nicotine toxicity, 1739–1740, 1739b
Nicotinic acetylcholine receptors, 814
Nightingale Metrics, 46, 46b
Nijmegen breakage syndrome (NBS),
  1435–1436
NIRS. See Near-infrared spectroscopy
  (NIRS)
Nitric oxide (NO), 813–814
  for acute respiratory failure, 673
  for ARDS, 632
  for AVT, 725
  complications of, 673
  endothelium-derived, 272, 273f
  homeostasis, hemolysis and, 1249
  hypertension and, 1117
  inhaled, for acute PAH, 726
  in mechanical ventilation, 761
  metabolism of endothelium-derived,
    1238–1239

Nitric oxide (NO) *(Continued)*
   for PPHN, 714–716, 714*f*
     contraindications for, 716
     dosing of, 715
     initiation of, 715
     long-term outcomes with, 717
     side effects of, 717
     weaning from, 715*f*, 716
   RBC interactions with, 1238
   in sepsis pathogenesis, 1526
   synthase inhibitors, 1143
   for ventilation/perfusion inequality, 593
Nitroglycerin, for HTN, 1126
NIV. *See* Noninvasive ventilation (NIV)
NMBAs. *See* Neuromuscular blocking
   agents (NMBAs)
NMJ. *See* Neuromuscular junction (NMJ)
NMS. *See* Neuroleptic malignant syndrome
   (NMS)
NO. *See* Nitric oxide (NO)
Nonbicarbonate buffering system,
   1064–1065
Nonconvulsive status epilepticus, 915
Nondepolarizing agents, NMBAs, 1814–
   1821, 1814*t*–1815*t*
Nonepileptic spells, 849–850, 849*t*
Nonfocal neurologic lesions, 891–892
Nonhemolytic febrile reaction, to RBC
   transfusion, 1308–1309
Noninvasive respiratory monitoring
   capnometry/capnography, 570
     clinical applications, 571
     differential diagnosis of abnormalities,
       572–574, 573*b*, 573*f*–574*f*
     operating principles of, 571–572,
       572*f*
     physiologic basis of, 570–571, 570*f*
   carbon dioxide monitoring, 575
   oxygen monitoring, 574–575
   pulse oximetry, 567
     principles of, 567–568, 568*f*
     probe placement, 569–570
     sources of error, 569, 569*f*
     validation, 568–569
   transcutaneous monitoring, 574
Noninvasive ventilation (NIV). *See also*
   Mechanical ventilation
   circuit and CO_2 rebreathing, 779
   equipment, 776–778
   goals of, 772*t*
   historical perspective, 770–771
   indications for, 771
   interfaces, 776, 776*f*–778*f*
   introduction, 770
   long-term, 775
     with cystic fibrosis, 775–776
     indications for, 775*t*
     with neuromuscular disorders, 775,
       1756
     physiologic effects/outcomes, 775–776
   negative pressure ventilation, 779–782,
     780*f*–782*f*, 781*t*

Noninvasive ventilation (NIV) *(Continued)*
   optimizing patient-ventilator interaction,
     778–779
   positive pressure, 1754
   short-term, 771, 771*t*–772*t*, 772*f*
     adult studies on, 771–773
     complications/concerns, 779
     indications for, 773–775
     pediatric/neonatal studies on, 773
   ventilator settings, 779
Nonmaleficence, in PICU, 115–116
Nonsteroidal antiinflammatory drugs
   (NSAIDs), 1057
Norepinephrine
   adverse effects of, 366
   basic pharmacology, 359*f*–360*f*, 362–364
   for cardiac dysfunction, 494*t*, 495
   clinical pharmacology, 364, 365*f*
   clinical role of, 364–365, 366*t*
   interactions, 366
   pharmacokinetics of, 364
   preparation/administration, 366
Norwood procedure, 476–477, 476*t*
NPO guidelines, for operating room
   anesthesia, 1788–1789
NSAIDs. *See* Nonsteroidal
   antiinflammatory drugs (NSAIDs)
Nuclear medicine, 861
Nuclear receptors, 1699, 1699*f*
Nucleotide level variation, 1169
Number needed to treat (NNT), in EBM,
   61.*e*1*t*
Nurse competencies, 44–46
   advocacy/moral agency, 45
   caring practices, 44–45
   clinical inquiry, 44
   clinical judgment, 44
   collaboration, 45
   facilitation of learning, 45
   response to diversity, 45
   systems thinking, 45–46
Nursing
   history of, 9
   in pediatric critical care
     certification in, 49–50, 49*t*
     leadership role, 46–50
     research for, 50, 50*t*
     synergy model, 43–46
Nutrition
   for burn patients, 1591–1592, 1591*t*
   for HCT, 1340–1341
   therapeutic
     assessing energy expenditure,
       1209–1210, 1209*t*–1210*t*
     enteral nutrition, 1214–1216, 1214*t*,
       1215*f*
     guidelines for, 1219–1220, 1219*t*
     immune-enhancing diets, 1216
     indirect calorimetry, 1210–1211,
       1210*t*–1211*t*
     lipid requirements, 1212–1213
     micronutrient requirements, 1213

Nutrition *(Continued)*
     for obese children, 1218–1219
     parenteral nutrition, 1216–1218,
       1217*t*, 1218*f*
     protein requirements, 1211–1212,
       1212*f*
     refeeding syndrome, 1213–1214
Nutritional status assessment, 1206,
   1206*t*
   biochemical assessment, 1206–1208
   body composition, 1206

O
Obesity
   breathing failure due to, 587
   nutritional support for, 1218–1219
Observational studies, in EBM, 62
Obstructive pulmonary disease. *See also*
   Asthma
   breathing failure due to, 584–585, 585*t*
     compensatory mechanisms, 585–586
   determinants of respiratory efficiency,
     607–610
   overview of, 607
   power/frequency of breathing, 608,
     608*f*
Obstructive shock, 425
Obstructive sleep apnea (OSA), 676, 1254
Occult blood loss testing, 1361
Occupational health programs, 1510
Occupational HIV exposure, 1452
Octreotide, for gastrointestinal
   hemorrhage, 1375
Oculocephalic (doll's eye) reflex, 888
Oculovestibular (caloric) reflex, 888
ODC. *See* Oxyhemoglobin dissociation
   curve (ODC)
Odds ratio (OR), in EBM, 61.*e*1*t*
Oliguria, 144
Oncologic emergencies, 1316–1323
   airway compromise in mediastinal
     tumors, 1319, 1320*f*
   anthracycline-induced cardiogenic
     shock, 1321–1322
   chimeric antigen receptor T-cell
     mediated toxicity, 1322–1323,
     1323*f*
   hemophagocytic lymphohistiocytosis,
     1321, 1321*b*
   hyperleukocytosis, 1318
   posterior reversible encephalopathy,
     1322
   spinal cord compression, 1318–1319
   superior vena cava syndrome,
     1319–1321
   tumor lysis syndrome, 1316–1318
Oncology patients, short-term NIV for,
   773–774
ONSD. *See* Optic nerve sheath diameter
   (ONSD)
Open globe injury, 1770
Open-chest CPR, 507, 530

Operating room anesthesia
    intravenous anesthesia pharmacology,
        1792–1794
    introduction, 1786–1787
    local anesthesia pharmacology,
        1791–1792
    monitoring, 1789–1791
    NPO guidelines, 1788–1789
    opioids, 1794–1796, 1794t
    preoperative evaluation, 1787–1788,
        1788t
    preoperative medication, 1789, 1789t
Opioids
    management of, 130–131, 131t
    in operating room anesthesia, 1794–
        1796, 1794t
    respiratory depression and, 581–582
    toxicity of, 1736–1737, 1737b
Optic nerve sheath diameter (ONSD), 854
Optical spectroscopy, 1142
OR. See Odds ratio (OR), in EBM
Oral cavity. See Mouth
Organ donation
    brain death
        determination of, 136–139, 137t–138t
        physiology of, 139–140
    after circulatory death, 145–146
    contraindications to, 146
    donor management
        coagulation abnormalities/
            thermoregulatory instability, 145
        diabetes insipidus, 143–144
        fluid/electrolyte disturbances, 143
        glucose/potassium/calcium
            derangements, 144
        goals of, 140t
        hemodynamic instability, 140–141
        HRT, 141–142, 142t
        oliguria, 144
        physiologic considerations, 140
        of potential heart donor, 482
        pulmonary issues, 142–143
    evolving areas of transplantation, 146
    after fatal child abuse, 1661, 1661b
    medical examiner/coroner issues, 145
    overview of, 135–136
    role of intensivist/critical care team, 136
Organophosphate poisoning, 991–992
Orientation programs, for nurse staff
    development, 48
Oronasal masks, for NIV, 776, 777f
Oropharyngeal airways, 1753, 1753f
Orotracheal intubation, 1763–1764,
    1763f–1764f
Orthodromic reciprocating tachycardia
    (ORT), 394, 401f–402f, 409–410
OSA. See Obstructive sleep apnea (OSA)
Osmolar therapy, for TBI, 1630–1631
Outcomes
    accidental hypothermia, 1570
    acute liver failure, 1383
    ARDS, 634

Outcomes (Continued)
    assessment program, 77
    bacterial meningitis, 970–971
    after cardiac arrest, 941–942, 943f
    ECMO, 802–803
    HCT, 1326–1327
    liver transplantation, 1392, 1392f
    long-term
        antecedents/variables in, 76
        metrics for patient-centered
            outcomes, 76–77, 78t
        mitigating morbidity, 73–76, 74t, 75f
        mortality reduction, 73, 74f
        novel approaches to improving, 77–80
        research aims, 80
        targets for interventions, 80
        trichotomous outcome model, 80
    in MODS/MOF, 1544
    multidisciplinary assessment, in TBI,
        75–76
    pediatric coma, 895
    PFCC improving, 109
    pre-ICU interventions and, 56
    in quality critical care, 22–23
    renal replacement therapy, 1111
    short-term
        prediction tools for. See Prediction
            tools, for short-term outcomes
        rapid progression of, 52–54
        weaknesses of, 54–55
    stress hyperglycemia, 1185–1186
    in synergy model of nursing, 46
        Nightingale Metrics, 46, 46b
        patient-level, 46
        provider-level, 46
        system-level, 46
    ventricular assist device, 321–322, 321f
Overfeeding, in PICU, 1208–1212, 1209f,
    1209t
Oxford Centre for Evidence-Based
    Medicine, 64, 64.e1
Oxygen
    diffusion of, 565
    kinetics, 1296
    in mechanical ventilation, 760–761
    monitoring of, 574–575
    therapeutic
        for acute PAH, 725–726
        for asthma, 652
        for bronchopulmonary dysplasia,
            674–675, 674t
        for PPHN, 713–714
        for respiratory acidosis, 1094
    toxicity, 1136–1137
    utilization assessment, 1139
Oxygen consumption
    assessment of, 303–304
    invasive hemodynamic measurement of,
        289–290
    LCOS and, 302–303, 493
    myocardial, 247–248, 248f–249f
    in sepsis treatment, 1534, 1534b

Oxygen delivery
    anemia and, 1295, 1296f
    assessment of, 303–304
    cardiac output assessment
        qualitative, 293–294
        quantitative, 294–295
    cardiovascular function and, 292
    devices for, 1753–1754
        masks, 1753–1754
        nasal cannulas, 1753
    in ECMO, 797–798, 798f
    heart failure and, 490
    invasive hemodynamic measurement of,
        289–290
    LCOS and, 302–303
    measures of
        acid-base status, 295
        blood lactate, 295
        gastric tonometry, 295
        NIRS, 295–296
        urine output, 295
    RBC regulation of, 1296–1297
    in sepsis treatment, 1534, 1534b
    tissue oxygenation and, 293
Oxygen radicals, HIE and, 934–936
Oxygen saturation
    cardiac catheterization measurement,
        342
    cellular respiration and, 1140–1141,
        1140f
    during CPB, 439–440, 440f
    monitoring ICP, 909–910
Oxygen transport, erythron and, 1234–
    1235, 1235f
Oxygenation. See Tissue oxygenation
Oxygenators
    for CPB, 434–435, 435f
    for ECMO, 790
Oxygen-related autoregulation of CBF,
    827
Oxyhemoglobin dissociation curve (ODC),
    439–440, 440f, 1234–1235, 1235f

P
Pacemaker-mediated tachycaradia (PMT),
    403–404, 404f
Pacing
    for bradycardias, 401
    newer indications for, 404–405
    permanent, 404, 405f
    principles of, 401
    temporary, 401–404, 401f
        setting parameters for, 402–404,
            402f–404f
PaCO₂ strategy, during hypothermic CPB,
    440f, 442
PACs. See Pulmonary artery catheters
    (PACs)
PAH. See Pulmonary arterial hypertension
    (PAH)
Pain management, 131–132
    after liver transplant, 1391

Palliative care
  balance between curative and, 127, 128f
  communication in, 128–129
  consultation in PICU, 127–128
  end-of-life care
    follow-up care of family/staff, 133
    practical aspects of, 132–133
  epidemiology of death in PICU, 128
  limitation of interventions, 129–130
  pain/symptom management, 130–132, 131t
Palliative sedation, 132
PAM. See Primary amebic meningoencephalitis (PAM)
PAN. See Polyarteritis nodosa (PAN)
Pancreas, injury to, 1649t, 1650–1651, 1651f
Pancreatic exocrine secretory function, 1351
Pancreatitis, 1398
  acute, 1368–1369
  in HIV/AIDS patients, 1450
Pancuronium, 1814–1815, 1815t
Papilledema, 888
Paracentesis, 176b, 178–179, 179t
  ultrasound-guided, 188, 188f
Paracetamol. See Acetaminophen (Paracetamol)
Paradoxical aciduria, 1084
Parainfluenza virus, 689
Paraldehyde, for SE, 922–924, 923t
Paralysis
  phrenic nerve, 678
  vocal cord, 621, 677
Parasympathetic autonomic nervous system, 821
Paravertebral block, 1779, 1780f
Parenchymal lung disease, mechanical ventilation for, 752–753, 752f
Parenteral nutrition (PN)
  for burn patients, 1592
  in critical illness, 1216–1218, 1217t
  ECLS complications involving, 313
Parents
  effect on outcomes, 76
  surrogate decision making by, 118–119, 118b
Partial liquid ventilation, 674
Patent ductus arteriosus (PDA), 463–464
  echocardiography of, 336–338, 337f–338f
Pathogen(s)
  elimination of, 1533–1534
  recognition, 1523–1524
Patient- and family-centered care (PFCC)
  core principles, 105b
    building partnerships, 108
    honoring differences/mutual respect, 105–106
    maintaining flexibility, 106–107
    shared decision making, 109
    transdisciplinary support, 108

Patient- and family-centered care (PFCC) (Continued)
  definition of family, 104–105
  fundamental needs, 105
  historical evolution of, 105
  improved outcomes with, 109
  overcoming barriers to, 109–110, 110b
  PICU support mechanisms, 116
  quality communication, 107–108
Patients
  characteristics of concern, 43–44
  nurse-sensitive outcomes, 46, 46b
  screening of, 1510
  ventilator interaction with
    asynchrony, 755–756
    in NIV, 778–779
Pattern recognition receptors (PRRs), 1404–1405, 1405t
PAV. See Proportional assist ventilation (PAV)
PbtO$_2$. See Brain tissue oxygen (PbtO$_2$)
PCCM. See Pediatric critical care medicine (PCCM)
PD. See Peritoneal dialysis (PD)
PDA. See Patent ductus arteriosus (PDA)
PDE. See Phosphodiesterase (PDE), cAMP regulation by
Pediatric Confusion Assessment Method for ICU, 1872, 1872f
Pediatric critical care. See also Critical care
  generalist training for, 53
  for orthotopic heart transplant, 483–486
    allograft rejection/immune suppression, 484–486, 485t
    early allograft dysfunction management, 483–484
    future management strategies, 487
    intraoperative considerations, 483
    perioperative management, 483
  in PHEs
    emergency mass critical care, 227
    emergency surge capacity, 227, 227t
    event-specific management, 230–231, 231t
    ICU phase, 229
    keeping families together/tracking children, 229
    National Response Framework/ Incident Command System, 226–228
    needs and resources for, 227–228
    overview of, 226
    pediatric disaster timeline, 228
    PICU in sustained, 229–230
    rationing, 230–231
  positive pressure breathing and, 382–383, 383f
  prior to cardiac transplantation, 480–482, 481b
    anticoagulation, 482
    inotropic support, 481

Pediatric critical care (Continued)
    mechanical circulatory support, 481–482
    patient management, 481
  utilizing adult research, 55
Pediatric critical care medicine (PCCM). See also Subspecialization, within PCCM
  history of
    around the world, 13–16
    cost of success, 12–13
    exceptional contributors to, 16, 16t–17t
    first PICUs, 8–9
    growth of, 10–12
    in high-mortality countries, 16, 16t
    mechanical ventilation, 7
    neonatology, 5
    pediatric anesthesiology, 5, 6t
    pediatric cardiology, 7
    pediatric general/cardiac surgery, 5
    poliomyelitis, 7–8
    role of anesthesiologists/pediatricians, 9–10
    role of nursing, 9
    textbooks, 11t
    training/education growth, 12
  professionalism in, 40–42
Pediatric critical care nutrition
  enteral nutrition, 1214–1216, 1214t, 1215f
  guidelines for, 1219–1220, 1219t
  immune-enhancing diets, 1216
  malnutrition and, 1205–1206
  nutritional status assessment, 1206, 1206t
    biochemical assessment, 1206–1208
    body composition, 1206
  for obese children, 1218–1219
  parenteral nutrition, 1216–1218, 1217t, 1218f
  refeeding syndrome, 1213–1214
  underfeeding/overfeeding, 1208–1212, 1209f
Pediatric critical care research. See also Research
  opportunities, 56–57
  as specialty, 56
  strengths, 52–54
  SWOT approach to, 52
  threats, 57–59
  weaknesses, 54–56
Pediatric intensive care unit (PICU)
  adaptive immunity in, 1419–1420, 1420t
  adrenal insufficiency in, 1182
  age/developmental spectrum in, 53
  ALF management in, 1383–1385, 1383t–1385t
  antibiotic resistance/infections in, 1482–1483
  application of prediction tools, 71
  asthma treatment in, 652–656

Pediatric intensive care unit (PICU)
(Continued)
anticholinergic agents, 654
β-agonists, 653–654
corticosteroids, 652–653
fluids, 652
general, 652
helium-oxygen mixtures, 655–656
ketamine, 656
magnesium sulfate, 654–655
methylxanthine agents, 655
oxygen, 652
cardiac catheterization assessment in,
342–343, 343t
cardiac intensive care, 29–31, 30f
coagulation disorders in, 1262t
death in, 128
definition of, 8
drowning victim management in,
1578–1580
as emergent system, 20
end-of-life decision making, 123t
ethics in
additional issues, 119–120
address by, 113
approach to, 113–116, 114f, 114t–115t
definition of, 112
domains of, 112–113
end-of-life decision making, 122–123
examples of, 112
intensivist's goals, 120–121, 121b
patient decision making, 116–117
shared decision making, 117
surrogate decision making, 117–119
withholding/withdrawing life support,
123–125
functional deficits vs. nonorganic
pathology, 849–850
growth in numbers, 12
as high-reliability organization, 19–20,
20t
history of, 8–9
history of tolerance/withdrawal,
1862–1863
hyperthermia in, 1803
immune modulation in, 1458, 1459t
immune monitoring in, 1458–1460
immune suppression complications in
heart transplantation, 486–487
diabetes mellitus, 487
infection, 486
renal failure, 486–487
infections in
hantavirus, 1503–1504, 1504f
invasive pneumococcus, 1501–1502,
1501b
meningococcal, 1497–1499, 1498f
necrotizing fasciitis, 1500–1501
Rocky Mountain spotted fever,
1502–1503, 1502f–1503f
toxic shock syndrome, 1499–1500,
1499b–1500b

Pediatric intensive care unit (PICU)
(Continued)
interprofessional care in, 54
lifelong learning in, 41–42
models of quality, 20–23, 21f
outcomes in, 22–23
process in, 22, 22t
structure in, 21–22
neurocritical care, 31–32, 31f–32f
NMBAs in, 1824–1825, 1824t–1825t
nursing in
certification in, 49–50, 49t
leadership role, 46–50
research for, 50, 50t
synergy model, 43–46
outcomes for long-stay patients, 75
palliative care consultation in, 127–128
patient safety and technology in, 97–99
patient- and family-centered care. See
Patient- and family-centered care
(PFCC)
in PHEs
equipment and supplies, 230
evacuation, 230
manual ventilation, 230
mechanical ventilation, 229–230
medications, 230
notification of sudden impact, 228
personnel, 229
space, 229
platelet disorders in, 1277t
post-cardiac arrest care, 944–946, 946f
prediction tools for. See Prediction tools,
for short-term outcomes
safety and quality improvement in
current state of, 82
fundamentals of patient safety,
85–88
methods of, 84
past, present, and future, 88–89
safety/quality relationship, 82
systems thinking and, 82–85
tools for, 85
value and, 83–84, 83t
variation/display of data over time,
84–85, 85f
as satellite laboratory, 1361–1362
seizures in
causes of, 915b
types of, 915–916
subspecialized, 29
TBI management in, 1626–1635
thromboprophylaxis in, 1292–1293
thyroid hormone supplementation in,
1193–1194
virtual, 101–102
Pediatric intensivists. See Intensivists
Pediatric neurocritical care
assessment and monitoring
abnormal movements/altered
sensorium, 849
anticipatory planning, 843

Pediatric neurocritical care (Continued)
cerebellar function/gait evaluation,
848–849
complication recognition, 842–843
cranial nerve examination, 845–847
functional deficits vs. nonorganic
pathology, 849–850, 849t
funduscopic examination, 845
goals of, 850
iatrogenic complications of
pharmacotherapy, 843, 844f
integrating monitoring data, 855–856,
855f
level of consciousness/mental status,
845, 847t
motor exam approach, 847–848
neuroimaging, 850–855, 850t, 851f
observation in, 844–845, 846t–847t
overview/basic principles of, 842–850
physical examination, 844
reflexes, 848
risk factor history/assessment, 843
sensory examination, 849
vital signs, 843–844
challenges/controversies/scope of, 880
essential components of, 881t
future of, 880–882
historical context, 877–878
overview of, 877
rationales for development of, 878–880
spectrum of disease pathophysiology for,
881t
Pediatric Sepsis Biomarker Risk Model
(PERSEVERE) decision tree, 1537,
1538f
Pediatricians, founding of PCCM, 9–10
Pediatrics, education across continuum,
221
PEEP. See Positive end-expiratory pressure
(PEEP)
Pelvis
FAST exam of, 192f, 193
fractures of, 1653, 1653t
Penicillins, 1477, 1681
Pentobarbital, for SE, 922–924, 923t
Peptides, 813–814
Percutaneous cannulation, 788
Percutaneous drug absorption, 1675–1676
PERDS. See Periengraftment respiratory
distress syndrome (PERDS)
Perfluorochemical liquid ventilation,
673–674
Perforated viscera, 1397
Perfusion
distribution of, 590, 590f
flow rate, 439–440, 439t
Perfusion pressure-related autoregulation
of CBF, 826–827
Pericardial disease, in HIV/AIDS, 1448
Pericardial effusion, 196, 196f
echocardiographic assessment of,
328–329, 328f–330f

Pericardial tamponade, 1471
Pericardiocentesis, 163–166
    complications, 166
    contraindications for, 164
    indications for, 163–164
    maintenance, 165–166
    monitoring for, 164
    procedure/equipment for, 164
    technique for, 164–165, 165f
    ultrasound in, 197
Pericarditis, 1471
Periengraftment respiratory distress
        syndrome (PERDS), 1330
Periodic paralysis (PP), 987
    hyperkalemic, 988
    hypokalemic, 987–988
Perioperative respiratory failure, 773
Peripheral nerve blockade, 1786–1787
Peripheral nervous system (PNS), 820–821
Peripherally inserted central venous
        catheters (PICCs), 172–175
Peritoneal dialysis (PD), 1105–1107
    disadvantages/complications, 1107
    ICU issues, 1107
    indications for, 1106
    physiology of, 1105–1106
    technique for, 1106–1107
Peritoneum, 1394
Peritonitis, 1472
Peritonsillar abscess, 619
Permanent junctional reciprocating
        tachycardia, 394, 395f
Permanent pacing, 404, 405f
Permissive hypercapnia, 1094
Peroxisome proliferator–activated
        receptor-γ (PPARγ) pathway,
        1526–1527
PERSEVERE. See Pediatric Sepsis
        Biomarker Risk Model (PERSEVERE)
        decision tree
Persistent pulmonary hypertension of
        newborn (PPHN), 708–716
    causing neonatal respiratory disease, 679
    clinical presentation, 708–710, 711f, 712t
    etiology of, 708, 710f–711f
    inhaled NO-resistant, 716–717, 716f
    mechanisms of, 709f
    prostaglandin E1 for, 717–732
    severity of, 712
    treatment of, 712–716
        bosentan, 718
        ECMO, 718
        future therapies, 718
        general measures, 712
        high-frequency ventilation, 714
        inhaled prostacyclin, 717
        nitric oxide, 714–716, 714f–715f
        optimal pulmonary hypertension, 713
        oxygen, 713–714
        phosphodiesterase inhibitors, 717
        sedation, 712
        steroids, 718

Persistent pulmonary hypertension of
        newborn (PPHN) (Continued)
        supportive therapies, 713
        surfactant therapy, 714
        systemic blood pressure measurement,
            711f, 712–713
        temperature management, 713
Personal protective equipment, 1509
PET. See Positron emission tomography
        (PET)
PFCC. See Patient- and family-centered
        care (PFCC)
PGE1. See Prostaglandin E1 (PGE1), for
        PPHN
PGI₂. See Prostacyclin (PGI₂)
P-glycoprotein receptors, drug interactions
        affecting, 1718t–1719t, 1719
PH. See Pulmonary hypertension (PH)
pH
    abnormal, 1080–1081
    acid-base balance and, 1064–1065,
        1068t
    stool assessment of, 1361
Phagocytic component of immune system
    clinical presentation, 1425
    deficiencies in, 1423t
    specific disorders
        chronic granulomatous disease
            (CGD), 1427–1428
        laboratory tests for, 1432t, 1437
        leukocyte adhesion deficiency, 1427
        severe congenital neutropenia,
            1426
        treatment for, 1437
        WHIM syndrome, 1427
Phagocytosis, 1405–1407
Pharmacodynamic tolerance, 1862
Pharmacodynamics, 1674b, 1674f,
        1682–1683
    drug-drug interactions, 1719
    effect of disease on drug action,
        1683
Pharmacokinetic tolerance, 1862
Pharmacokinetics, 1674–1682, 1674b,
        1674f, 1716–1719, 1718t–1719t
    definition of, 1674
    of dobutamine, 369
    of dopamine, 361–362
    drug absorption, 1674–1676, 1674b
    drug clearance, 1677–1681, 1679t
    drug delivery systems, 1682
    drug distribution, 1676–1677,
        1676t–1677t
    drug elimination, 1681–1682
    of isoproterenol, 368
    of milrinone, 374
    of norepinephrine, 364
    principles of, 1683–1685
        applied, 1685
        plasma concentration-time curve,
            1683–1685, 1683f–1684f, 1685b
    of vasopressin, 371

Pharmacology. See also Gastrointestinal
        pharmacology
    agents with pulmonary toxicity, 700,
        700b
    of cardiovascular system
        bipyridines, 373, 373f
        digitalis glycosides, 376
        nesiritide, 376
        response mechanisms, 352–378,
            353f–357f, 353t
        sympathomimetic amines, 359–360,
            359f–360f
    after CHD repair, 454–455, 455f
    of CPR, 500, 509–511
        adrenergic agonists, 509–511,
            509f–512f, 510b
        atropine, 514
        calcium, 516–517
        glucose, 517–518, 517f
        high-dose epinephrine, 513–514
        other alkalinizing agents, 516
        sodium bicarbonate, 514–516, 515f
        vasopressin, 511–518
    definition of, 1673
    of heart failure, 493–495
        diuretics, 494t
        vasoactive drugs, 493–495, 494t
    interventions for VILI, 642–643
    of intravenous anesthesia, 1792–1794
    of local anesthetic agents, 1791–1792
    renal
        adverse drug reactions, 1708–1709,
            1708t
        dialysis and, 1100–1101
        drug disposition and, 1098–1100,
            1099f, 1099t
        drug dosing in kidney disease,
            1100–1101, 1100b, 1100f
        kidney as therapeutic target, 1101–
            1103, 1101f
    therapeutics in, 1673
Pharmacotherapy
    for delirium, 1874–1875
    for HTN, 1122–1126
        clonidine, 1122–1123
        esmolol, 1123–1124
        general considerations, 1122, 1122f,
            1123t
        hydralazine, 1124
        isradipine, 1124
        labetalol, 1124
        nicardipine, 1124–1125
        other agents, 1126
        sodium nitroprusside, 1125–1126
    iatrogenic complications of, 843, 844f
    for status epilepticus (SE), 922–924, 923t
Pharynx, 543–544
Phased array transducers, 183–184, 185f
Phenobarbital
    drug-drug interactions of, 1722
    for SE, 922–924, 923t
Phenothiazine, toxicity of, 414

Phenytoin
    drug-drug interactions of, 1721–1722
    for SE, 922–924, 923*t*
Pheochromocytoma, with hypertension,
    1127
PHEs. *See* Public health emergencies
    (PHEs)
Phosphate, 1074–1075
Phosphodiesterase (PDE), cAMP
    regulation by, 357–358
Phosphodiesterase (PDE) inhibitors
    for PPHN, 717
        milrinone, 717
        sildenafil, 717
Phosphodiesterase type 5 (PDE-5)
        inhibitors
    for PAH maintenance therapy, 729
        sildenafil, 729
        tadalafil, 729
Phosphorus, in fluid management, 1022
Phrenic nerve paralysis, 678
pH-stat strategy, 440*f*, 442
Physical dependency
    overview of, 1862
    treatment/scoring systems for,
        1864–1867
Physiology, history of, 3–4
PICCs. *See* Peripherally inserted central
    venous catheters (PICCs)
PICS. *See* Post-intensive care syndrome
    (PICS)
PICU. *See* Pediatric intensive care unit
    (PICU)
PIE. *See also* Pulmonary interstitial
    emphysema (PIE)
Pigment nephropathy, AKI and, 1054–1055
Pipecuronium, 1815*t*, 1818
Plasma
    transfusion of
        indications for, 1303–1304
        methods, 1304
        reactions/complications of, 1306–
            1310, 1307*t*
        types of, 1303
Plasma concentration-time curve,
        1683–1685, 1683*f*–1684*f*
Plasma disappearance techniques,
        1028–1029, 1028*f*
    iohexol, 1029
    radioisotopes, 1029
Plasma markers, renal function and,
        1029–1033
    creatinine, 1029–1032, 1030*f*–1031*f*,
        1032*t*
    cystatin C, 1032–1033
Plasma volume expansion, with AKI, 1047
Plateau pressure, in ARDS ventilation, 631
Platelet disorders
    heparin-induced thrombocytopenia,
        1278–1279
    management of, 1279–1280
    in PICU, 1277*t*

Platelet disorders *(Continued)*
    qualitative, 1279
    quantitative, 1277–1278
    uremia, 1280
Platelets
    adhesion to endothelium, 274–275
    production of, 1231–1232
    transfusion of
        indications for, 1304–1305
        methods, 1305–1306
        reactions/complications of, 1306–
            1310, 1307*t*
        reasons for/against, 1304
    types of, 1304
Pleural effusions
    causes of, 175*b*
    causing neonatal respiratory disease, 679
    after CHD repair, 457
    after Fontan procedure, 463
    interpretation of, 176*b*
    rheumatic disease associated with, 1470
    ultrasound and, 187–188, 188*f*
Pleuritis, 1470
PMT. *See* Pacemaker-mediated
    tachycaradia (PMT)
PN. *See* Parenteral nutrition (PN)
Pneumocystis carinii pneumonia, 696–698
    clinical features of, 697
    complications, 697
    diagnosis of, 697
    treatment of, 697–698, 697*t*
Pneumocystis jirovecii pneumonia, HIV/
    AIDS and, 1445–1446
Pneumomediastinum, 664–666
Pneumonia
    aspiration, 698–699, 698*b*
    congenital, 667
    neonatal, 666–667
    Pneumocystis carinii, 696–698, 697*t*
    Pneumocystis jirovecii, 1445–1446
    primary viral, 688
    short-term NIV for, 772
    ventilator-associated, 667, 1511*t*–1512*t*,
        1515
Pneumonitis, 1487–1488
    background, 1487
    bacterial, 683–687, 686*t*–688*t*
    chemical, 698–700
        aspiration pneumonia, 698–699, 698*b*
        ingestion/injection of pharmacologic
            agents, 700, 700*b*
        inhalation injury, 699–700, 699*t*
    clinical presentation, 1488
    diagnosis of, 683, 1493
    etiology of, 682, 683*b*, 1486*t*, 1487–1488
    focal pulmonary hemorrhage, 702–703
    fungal, 692–693, 693*b*, 694*t*
        opportunistic infections, 695–696
        primary infection, 693–695
    idiopathic ILD, 700–701
    pathogenesis of, 682
    pathophysiology of, 682–683

Pneumonitis *(Continued)*
    pulmonary hemorrhage, 701–704, 701*b*
    treatment for, 1493–1495
    viral, 687–692, 688*t*, 691*b*, 692*t*
Pneumopericardium, 664–666
Pneumoperitoneum, 664–666
Pneumothorax, 190, 190*f*, 664–666
PNS. *See* Peripheral nervous system (PNS)
Polio-like syndromes, 991
Poliomyelitis, 7–8, 991
Polyarteritis nodosa (PAN), 1468–1469
Polycythemia, hyperviscosity syndrome
    and, 679–680
Polymorphisms
    of adrenergic receptors, 356
    of vasopressin receptors, 357
Pons, 817–818
Portal pressure gradient (PPG), 1352–1353
Positive end-expiratory pressure (PEEP)
    in acute lung injury, 752–753, 752*f*
    in ARDS ventilation, 631
    in intubated asthma patients, 657–658,
        658*f*
    mechanical ventilation and, 605–606,
        745–746, 746*f*
    for pulmonary hemorrhage, 666
    for ventilation/perfusion inequality, 593
    VILI and, 639–640, 639*f*–640*f*
Positive predictive value, in EBM, 61.*e*1*t*
Positive pressure mechanical ventilation
        (PPV). *See also* Mechanical ventilation
    effects on circulation, 380
        alveolar pressure, 383–385, 384*f*–385*f*
        cardiac contractility, 386
        critical illness and, 382–383, 383*f*
        fluid responsiveness during, 388,
            388*f*–389*f*
        left ventricular afterload, 386, 387*f*
        left ventricular preload, 385–386,
            386*f*
        preload dependence vs. afterload
            dependence, 386–388, 387*f*–388*f*
        reverse pulsus paradoxus, 389
        right ventricular preload, 382, 382*f*
    physiology of, 562–563
Positron emission tomography (PET),
        1626, 1628*f*
Postcardiopulmonary bypass, MCS for,
        308–309
Posterior reversible encephalopathy
    syndrome (PRES), 865–866, 867*f*,
        1322
Postextubation respiratory failure, 773
Postextubation stridor, 621–622,
        1765–1766
Post-intensive care syndrome (PICS), 73,
        74*f*
Postischemic excitotoxicity, 948
Postoperative arrhythmias, 412–413
    junctional ectopic tachycardia, 413
    postsurgical atrioventricular block,
        412–413

Postoperative care, for tracheostomy, 625
Postoperative fever, MH and, 1803
Postpyloric gastrointestinal fluid losses, metabolic acidoses and, 1086–1087
Postresuscitation
    myocardial dysfunction, 532
    phase of cardiac arrest, 527
Postresuscitation phase of cardiac arrest, 527t
Postresuscitative hypothermia, 946–947
Postsurgical atrioventricular block, 412–413
Posttraumatic ischemia, 1614–1615
Posttraumatic stress disorder (PTSD)
    in children, 1827, 1828t
    health-related quality of life and, 76
Postzygotic mutations, 1170–1171
Potassium
    hyperkalemia and, 1016–1018
    hypernatremia and, 1014
    hypokalemia and, 1014–1015
    organ donor management and, 144
    regulation of, 1038
Potassium channels, in PAH, 721
Power
    of breathing, 608, 608f
    of respiratory system, 595–596
PP. See Periodic paralysis (PP)
PPARγ. See Peroxisome proliferator-activated receptor-γ (PPARγ) pathway
PPG. See Portal pressure gradient (PPG)
PPHN. See Persistent pulmonary hypertension of newborn (PPHN)
PPIs. See Proton pump inhibitors (PPIs)
PPV. See Positive pressure mechanical ventilation (PPV)
Prader-Willi syndrome, 582
Prearrest phase, of cardiac arrest, 526, 527t
Prebypass ultrafiltration, as CPB technique, 441
Preconditioning, for bronchopulmonary dysplasia, 675
Prediction tools, for short-term outcomes
    application in PICU, 71
    assessment of mortality risk
        neonatal ICU methods, 67–68
        new algorithms for, 69–70
        PICU methods, 68–69, 68t–69t
    for decision support, 71
    historical perspective, 66–67
    methods
        conceptual framework, 67
        statistical issues, 67
    morbidity assessment, 70–71
    overview, 66
Prednisone
    for asthma, 651–652
    for immune suppression, 484–486, 485t
Preeclampsia, with hypertension, 1127

Pregnancy, PAH and, 726
Preload
    management of, 493
    relationship to stroke volume, 489, 489f–490f
Preoperative medications, 1789, 1789t
PRES. See Posterior reversible encephalopathy syndrome (PRES)
Pressure-limited mandatory breaths, 743f, 744–745, 745f
Pressure-reactivity index (PRx), 903–905, 906f–907f
Pressure-supported breaths, 747, 747f
Pressure-volume curve
    in reducing VILI, 643
    respiratory, 559, 559f
Pressure-volume loops
    in acute lung injury, 752–753, 752f
    of ventricles, 242–243, 242f
Preventive ethics, 120
Prezygotic mutations, 1170
Primary amebic meningoencephalitis (PAM), 978–979
Primary angiitis of CNS, 952
Primary atrial tachycardias, 395–396, 396f
Primary pulmonary hypertension, 593. See also Pulmonary hypertension (PH)
Primary respiratory muscle failure, 751
Primary survey, in ATLS, 1600–1607
    breathing, 1604–1605
    circulation, 1605–1606, 1605t, 1606f
    disability, 1606–1607, 1607f
    establishing airway with cervical spine stabilization, 1601–1604, 1602t, 1603f
    exposure/environment, 1607
    overview of, 1600–1601, 1602f
Primary vasculitis of CNS, 1469
Priming, for ECMO, 799
Principalism, in ethical issues, 115–116
Principle of electroneutrality, 1063
Privacy, of health information, 99–100, 99b
Probe placement, for pulse oximetry, 569–570
Probiotics, 1513
Procainamide, for arrhythmias, 406, 521f, 523
Procedural training, 212
Process, in quality critical care, 21f, 22, 22t
Procoagulant properties, of endothelium, 271f, 272
Professional development, in nursing, 47–48
Professionalism
    the Charter and, 41
    as lifelong learning, 41–42
    "patient first" medical paradox, 40–41
    in PCCM, 40
    teaching, 213–214
Progenitor cells, endothelial, 271

Prone positioning
    for ARDS, 632–633, 633f, 753
    for ventilation/perfusion inequality, 593
Propofol
    effects of, 1778
    facilitating intubation, 1761, 1762t
    for RSE, 925
    for SE, 922–924, 923t
Proportional assist ventilation (PAV), 750–751
Prostacyclin (PGI₂)
    endothelium-derived, 272–273
    for PAH, 727
        beraprost, 728
        epoprostenol, 727
        iloprost, 727
        treprostinil, 727
    in pulmonary arterial hypertension, 721
    for pulmonary vascular dilation, 707, 707f
Prostaglandin E1 (PGE1), for PPHN, 717–732
Prostaglandins
    in AKI attenuation, 1046
    respiratory depression and, 582
    vasoconstrictor, 274
Protease activation, HIE and, 934
Protein
    calcium-binding, 1702
    in critical illness, 1211–1212, 1212f
    phosphorylation of, 1702
Protein binding, developmental aspects of, 1676–1677, 1676t
Protein C pathway, coagulation and, 1264, 1264f
Protein catabolism, 1135
Protein kinases, 1702
Protein synthesis, genetic variation and, 1169–1170
Protein-energy malnutrition, 1441–1443
Proteins
    carrier, 1693–1695, 1703f
    digestion of, 1347–1348, 1347b
Proteinuria, tubular function and, 1037
Proteomics, research opportunities, 57
Proton pump inhibitors (PPIs)
    for gastrointestinal hemorrhage, 1375
    as stress ulcer prophylaxis, 1374
Provider-level outcomes, in synergy model of nursing, 46
Proximal tubule
    anatomy of, 1001–1002, 1001f
    function of, 1002–1003, 1002f
PRRs. See Pattern recognition receptors (PRRs)
PRx. See Pressure-reactivity index (PRx)
Pseudorespiratory alkalosis, 1095
Psychosocial effects, of violence-associated injury, 1665–1667

PTSD. *See* Posttraumatic stress disorder (PTSD)
Public health emergencies (PHEs)
  emergency mass critical care, 227
  emergency surge capacity, 227, 227t
  event-specific management, 230–231, 231t
  ICU phase, 229
  keeping families together/tracking children, 229
  National Response Framework/Incident Command System, 226–228
  overview of, 226
  pediatric disaster timeline, 228
  pediatric needs/resources, 227–228
  PICU in sustained PHEs, 229–230
  rationing, 230–231
Pulmonary acinus, 551
Pulmonary agenesis, 672
Pulmonary air leak syndromes, 664–666
Pulmonary aplasia, 672
Pulmonary arterial hypertension (PAH), 718–722. *See also* Pulmonary hypertension (PH)
  acute exacerbation of, 725–732
    nitric oxide for, 726
    oxygen for, 725–726
  acute vasodilator testing for, 725
  classification of, 719t
  clinical presentation, 722–725, 724t
  diagnostic approach to, 723–725, 725f
  endothelin receptor antagonists for, 728
    bosentan, 728
    sitaxsentan/ambrisentan, 728–729
  genetics of, 722
  maintenance therapies for, 726
    calcium channel blockers, 726
    combination therapy, 729–730
    conventional, 726
  molecular mechanisms/pathology of, 719–722, 720f
  overview of, 718–719
  PDE-5 inhibitors for, 729
    sildenafil, 729
    tadalafil, 729
  prognosis/survival, 730–732
  prostacyclin agonists for, 727
    beraprost, 728
    epoprostenol, 727
    iloprost, 727
    treprostinil, 727
  in SCD, 1252–1253
    diagnosis of, 1253
    management of, 1253
    pathophysiology/etiology of, 1253
  surgical treatment for
    atrial septostomy, 730
    lung and heart-lung transplantation, 730
    pulmonary thromboendarterectomy, 730
  treatment for, 725, 731f

Pulmonary arteries, 553–554, 554f
  balloon dilation of, 347–349, 348f
Pulmonary artery catheters (PACs), 172
  complications, 174–175
  contraindications for, 172–173
  history/controversy, 284–285
  indications for, 285
  indirectly measured variables, 287
  information acquisition, 174
  maintenance/interpretation, 174
  monitoring techniques, 285–286, 287t
  placement, 286–287, 286f
  procedure/equipment for, 173–174, 173f
Pulmonary atresia, 470–472
  critical care for, 471–472
  late postoperative care, 472
  pathophysiology of, 470–471
Pulmonary balloon valvotomy, 344–345, 345f
Pulmonary blood flow. *See also* Blood flow
  in CHD patient, 450–451
  distribution of perfusion and, 590, 590f
  fractal model of ventilation and, 591, 591f–592f
Pulmonary candidiasis, 696
Pulmonary circulation, 259–262
  bronchial vascular system, 554
  changes at birth, 260–261, 260f
  developmental anatomy of, 706
  developmental physiology of, 706–707
  diaphragm, 555
  effects of ventilation on, 383–385
    alveolar pressure, 383–385, 384f–385f
    lung volume, 383, 383f–384f
    regulation of PVR, 385, 385f
  normal fetal, 260
  pulmonary lymphatics and BALT, 554–555
  pulmonary vascular system, 553–554, 554f
  regulation of postnatal vascular resistance, 261–262, 261f
  regulation of vascular tone in utero, 707, 707f
  transitional, 707–708
Pulmonary complications of HCT, 1330–1333, 1330t
  dilemmas in diagnosis of, 1333
  early, 1330–1332
  late, 1332–1333
Pulmonary cytolytic thrombi, 1330
Pulmonary disease
  breathing failure due to, 584–587
  chronic, 674–676
    bronchopulmonary dysplasia, 674–675, 674t
  rheumatic disease associated with, 1470–1471
  V$_A$/Q abnormalities in
    ARDS, 592
    asthma, 592–593
    hypoxemia, 591

Pulmonary disease (*Continued*)
    pneumonia, 592
    primary pulmonary hypertension, 593
    pulmonary embolism, 593
Pulmonary embolism
  rheumatic disease associated with, 1471
  in thalassemia, 1258
  ventilation/perfusion mismatch in, 593
Pulmonary embolus, 1289
Pulmonary fibrosis, in ARDS, 630
Pulmonary hemorrhage, 666, 701–704, 1470–1471
  definition of, 701
  diffuse/immune, 702, 702f
  diffuse/nonimmune, 701–702
  etiology of, 701, 701b
  pathophysiology of, 701
Pulmonary hygiene, during mechanical ventilation, 761–762
Pulmonary hypertension (PH). *See also* Pulmonary arterial hypertension (PAH)
  after CHD repair, 455–456, 455t
  echocardiographic evaluation of, 327–328, 328f
  etiology/treatment of, 706–707
  in thalassemia, 1258–1259
Pulmonary hypoplasia, 668–669
Pulmonary interstitial emphysema (PIE), 664–666
Pulmonary lymphangiectasia, 675–676
Pulmonary lymphatics, 554–555
Pulmonary medications, drug-drug interactions of, 1726
Pulmonary parenchymal cysts, 671
Pulmonary sequestrations, 671
Pulmonary system
  in drowning victims, 1574–1575, 1574f
  in heat-related illness, 1564
  HIV/AIDS-related complications, 1445–1447
  QOT and, 298
  with SLE, 1464
Pulmonary thromboendarterectomy, for CTEPH, 730
Pulmonary ultrasound, 189–193, 189f–191f
Pulmonary vascular resistance (PVR)
  at birth, 708
  heart allograft failure and, 483–484
  QOT and, 297–298
  regulation of, 385, 385f
    in utero, 707, 707f
Pulmonary vasodilators, 455–456
Pulmonary veins, 553–554, 554f
Pulmonary venoocclusive disease (PVOD), 1332–1333
Pulsatile ventricular assist devices (VADs)
  Abiomed BVS 5000, 315
  Berlin Heart EXCOR, 314–315, 315f
  for cardiac dysfunction, 496–497
  Thoratec, 315–316

Pulse oximetry
    for cardiac output assessment, 295
    development of, 567
    in monitored anesthesia care, 1790
    principles of, 567–568, 568f
    probe placement, 569–570
    sources of error, 569, 569f
    validation, 568–569
Pulsus paradoxus, in respiratory distress, 389
Pumps
    for CPB, 431–433, 432f
    for ECMO
        centrifugal, 789–790, 789f
        roller-head, 788
Pupillary size
    coma and, 885–888, 886f–889f
    in toxin assessment, 1730–1732
Purine nucleotide phosphorylase deficiency, in SCID, 1433
PVOD. See Pulmonary venoocclusive disease (PVOD)
PVR. See Pulmonary vascular resistance (PVR)
Pyridoxine, for RSE, 926

Q
QOT. See Quantity of therapy (QOT)
QT interval prolongation, drugs associated with, 1711, 1711b
Quality improvement, in PICU, 82
    current state of safety and, 82
    fundamentals of patient safety, 83t, 85–88, 85t
    methods of, 84
    past, present, and future, 88–89, 88t
    relationship to safety, 82
    systems thinking and, 82–85
    tools for, 85
    value and, 83–84, 83t
    variation/display of data over time, 84–85, 85f
Quality of care education, 214, 214t
Quantity of therapy (QOT)
    for cardiovascular function assessment, 292–293
    variables affecting, 296–298, 297t
        abnormal SVR, 297
        arrhythmias, 297
        increased PVR, 297–298
        inefficient circulation, 298
        pulmonary function, 298
        vascular integrity, 298, 298f
        ventricular diastolic function, 296–297
        ventricular systolic function, 296

R
Radiofrequency catheter ablation (RFCA), 343

Radiography. See also Chest radiography
    for abdominal trauma, 1646
    for acute abdomen, 1396
    for bacterial pneumonitis, 684
    for gastrointestinal evaluation, 1360–1361
    for HTN, 1120
    in multiple trauma, 1608–1609
    in toxin assessment, 1734, 1734b
    for viral pneumonitis, 688–689
Radioisotopes, for plasma disappearance techniques, 1029
Radionuclide scanning, for gastrointestinal evaluation, 1361
Ramsay sedation scale, 1827–1828, 1828t
Rapacuronium, 1815t, 1818
Rapid-sequence induction and intubation, 1621–1622, 1622t
Rasburicase, for TLS, 1054
Rate, of chest compressions for CPR, 502
Rationing, during PHEs, 230–231
Raynaud phenomenon, 1466
RBCs. See Red blood cells (RBCs)
RCA. See Root cause analysis (RCA)
RDS. See Respiratory distress syndrome (RDS)
Reactive oxygen species (ROS)
    endothelium-derived, 273
    RBCs and, 1243
Readiness to Extubate Trial (RET), 765–766, 765f
Receptors
    as drug targets, 1689–1695, 1691f, 1692t
        classification of, 1695f–1699f, 1697t
        regulation of, 1699–1701, 1700f
    of heart, 238, 240–241
Recovery phase, of stress response, 1149
Recreational abdominal trauma, 1645
Recrudescence, of malignant hyperthermia, 1806
Rectal drug administration, 1376–1377, 1676
Red blood cell units
    transfusion of, 1301–1303
        blood types and, 1301, 1301t
        perfusion/warming/filtration in, 1302–1303
        storage time, 1302
        volume/number of units, 1301–1302
    types of, 1299–1301
        additional, 1300–1301
        standard, 1299–1300
Red blood cells (RBCs)
    acquired injury and, 1244
    aggregation/adhesion of, 1237
    antioxidant systems, 1243–1244
    ATP derived from, 1240–1241
    deformability of, 1237, 1237f
    EMP and, 1241, 1242f
    energy metabolism in, 1241–1244
    free radicals/reactive oxygen species and, 1243

Red blood cells (RBCs) (Continued)
    HMP and, 1241–1243
    maladaptive signaling, 1244
    metabolism of nitrite by, 1239–1240
    nitric oxide interactions with, 1238
    oxygen delivery, 1295–1297, 1296f
    processing/export of S-nitrosothiols, 1239, 1240f
    regulating blood flow distribution, 1238–1241, 1238f
    regulation of energetics, 1241
    rheology of, 1236–1237
    in SCD, 1248–1249
    transfusion of
        benefits/risks of, 1295–1297, 1296f
        current recommendations, 1297–1299
        indications for, 1297–1299
        overview of, 1295
        prevention of, 1299
        reactions/complications of, 1306–1310, 1307t
Reducing sugars measurement, 1361
Refeeding syndrome, 1213–1214
Reflexes, examination of, 848
Refractory respiratory failure, 309–310
Refractory status epilepticus (RSE), 915, 924–926. See also Status epilepticus (SE)
    high-dose barbiturates for, 925
    high-dose benzodiazepines for, 925
    inhalational anesthetics for, 925–926
    ketamine/lidocaine for, 926
    ketogenic diet for, 926
    propofol for, 925
    pyridoxine for, 926
    surgical options, 926–927
    therapeutic goals, 924–925
    therapeutic hypothermia for, 926
    valproic acid for, 925
Regional peripheral circulation
    autoregulation of, 257
    conflicting needs of, 268
    critical closing pressure, 256–257, 257f
    general anatomy, 254, 255f
    vascular impedance, 257–259
        blood gas composition, 258–259, 259f
        local regulatory mechanisms, 257–258
    venous return/cardiac output, 255–256, 255f–256f
Regulatory T cells, 1419
Reinitiation, in tachycardia, 409
Rejection, after liver transplantation, 1391–1392
Relationship boundaries, in PICU, 120
Relative risk, 61.e1t
Relative risk reduction (RRR), 61.e1t
Remifentanil, 1777, 1777f
Renal acidification, tubular function and, 1037–1038
Renal bicarbonate wasting, 680

Renal circulation, 267–268
Renal clearance techniques, 1027–1028
    creatinine, 1028
    inulin, 1027–1029
    iothalamate, 1028
Renal dysfunction
    in acute liver failure, 1388
    hypertension with, 1115–1116, 1115t,
        1118, 1118f
    with SLE, 1464
Renal excretion, 1681–1682
Renal failure. See also Acute renal failure
        (ARF)
    after CHD repair, 458–459
    drugs causing, 1708–1709, 1708t
    after heart transplantation, 486–487
    HIV/AIDS and, 1448–1449
    hyponatremia in, 1010
    posttraumatic seizures and, 916
    shock-related, 420
Renal injury
    in accidental hypothermia, 1568
    in heat-related illness, 1564
    SCD and, 1253–1254
Renal losses, hypokalemia and, 1015
Renal pharmacology
    adverse drug reactions, 1708–1709, 1708t
    dialysis and, 1100–1101
    drug disposition and, 1098–1100, 1099f,
        1099t
    drug dosing in kidney disease, 1100–
        1101, 1100b, 1100f
    kidney as therapeutic target, 1101–1103,
        1101f
Renal replacement therapy (RRT)
    advances in, 1111–1112
    CRRT, 1109–1111
    dialysis/ultrafiltration physiology, 1105,
        1106f
    intermittent hemodialysis, 1107–1109,
        1108f
    outcomes, 1111
    peritoneal dialysis, 1105–1107
    role of, 1057–1058
    for TLS, 1054
Renal system
    management during ECLS, 313
    rheumatic disease effects on, 1472
Renal trauma, 1649t, 1651–1652, 1652f
Renal tubular acidoses (RTA), 1087–1088
Renin-angiotensin antagonists, 1046
Renin-angiotensin-aldosterone system,
        hypertension and, 1116–1117
Reperfusion injury, 932–933
Repetitive monomorphic ventricular
        tachycardia, 412
Replacement fluids, for CRRT, 1110
Research. See also Pediatric critical care
        research
    in critical care nursing, 50, 50t
    education in, 214
    ethics, 119

Research (Continued)
    informatics, 57
    summaries, in EBM, 62–64
Resistance, vascular. See Vascular resistance
Resource allocation, ethics of, 119
Resource-poor settings
    child mortality rates in, 201–203,
        202f–203f
    critical care in, 202–203
        during disease outbreaks, 206
        research for, 206–207
    ICUs in, 203
        cost of, 203–204
        development of, 206
        ethics of, 204
    strengthening critical care infrastructure,
        204–206
Respect for autonomy, in PICU, 115–116
Respiration
    effects of cardiovascular function on,
        389–390
        cardiomyopathies and congenital
            heart disease, 390
        CHF, 389–390
        Glenn and Fontan procedures, 390
        shock states and, 389
    measurement of hemodynamic
        parameters, 389
Respiratory acid-base derangements,
        1092–1095
Respiratory acidosis, 1077t, 1093–1094
    treatment of, 1094
Respiratory alkalosis, 1077t, 1081,
        1094–1095
Respiratory care
    during mechanical ventilation, 761–763
        aerosol therapy, 763
        home care, 766t, 767–768
        humidification systems, 762–763
        pulmonary hygiene, 761–762
Respiratory distress syndrome (RDS), 664
Respiratory failure
    HIV/AIDS and, 1445–1447
    intubation for, 1755
    mechanical ventilation for, 736–737,
        737f
    refractory, 309–310
    shock-related, 420
Respiratory infections, health care–
        associated, 1511t–1512t, 1514
Respiratory mechanics
    analysis of, 643
    chest wall alterations, 608–609
        in contractile state of respiratory
            muscles, 609–610
        diaphragmatic configuration, 608–609
        rib cage distortion, 609, 610f
    determinants of regional gas flow
        distribution, 606–607, 606f
    dissipative behavior in, 601–606
        airway dynamics, 602–604, 603f–604f
        airway muscle/compliance, 604–605

Respiratory mechanics (Continued)
        airway obstruction, 605
        dynamic volume-pressure
            relationships, 601–602, 601f
        effect of flow rate/pattern on gas
            stream dynamics, 602
        mechanical ventilation, 605–606
    lungs/chest wall interactions, 599–601,
        600f
    nondissipative behavior in, 598–601,
        598f–599f
    overview of, 595
    respiratory work determinants, 596–598,
        596f
        mechanical forces acting on
            respiratory pump, 597–598
        volume-pressure relationships,
            596–597, 597f
    restrictive/obstructive disease, 607, 608f
    work, power and energy expenditure,
        595–596
Respiratory medications, drug-drug
        interactions of, 1726
Respiratory pattern, of coma patient, 885,
        885t, 886f
Respiratory pump failure, 751
Respiratory syncytial virus, 689
Respiratory system
    in accidental hypothermia, 1568
    adverse drug reactions in, 1713
    epithelia, 550f
    model of, 557–559
        compliance/elastance, 558–559,
            559f
        elastic properties, 557–558
        elastic recoil, 559, 559f
    physiology of, 556–559
        alveolar ventilation, 564–565
        applied forces, 561–562, 561f, 561t
        conducting airways, 556–557
        dynamic change in airway caliber,
            560–561
        flow resistance, 559–560, 560f
        gas exchange, 563–564, 565f
        lung-chest wall interactions, 562
        overview of, 556
        positive pressure mechanical
            ventilation, 562–563
        time constant of emptying, 562
    transfusion-related complications,
        1306–1308
Response mechanisms
    of cardiovascular system
        adrenergic receptors, 352–356,
            353f–358f, 353t
        ATPase inhibition, 358
        developmental issues, 358–359
        PDE regulation of cAMP, 357–358
        vasopressin receptors, 356–357,
            356f–358f
Response to diversity, as nurse
        competency, 45

Restrictive pulmonary disease
  breathing failure due to, 584–585
    compensatory mechanisms, 585
  determinants of respiratory efficiency, 607–610
  overview of, 607
  power/frequency of breathing, 608, 608f
Restrictive right ventricular physiology, after CHD repair, 453–454
Resuscitation. See also Cardiopulmonary resuscitation (CPR)
  in abdominal trauma, 1645–1646
  in accidental hypothermia, 1568–1569
  burn, 1586–1587, 1587t
    colloid, 1587
    complications of, 1587–1588, 1588f
  CBF following, 936–939, 937f–939f
  of coma patient, 884–885
  ECMO for, 795
  history of, 4–7, 4f
  in sepsis, 1529–1532
  in TBI, 1620–1623, 1621b
  in thoracic trauma, 1638–1639
  trauma, 1600, 1601f
RET. See Readiness to Extubate Trial (RET)
Retained fetal lung liquid syndrome, 662–664, 663f
Reticular formation, 818
Retinal hemorrhages, 1658
Retrieval systems
  components of, 152–155, 154f
    communications, 154
    equipment, 155
    safety, 155
    staffing, 154–155
  improving outcomes, 152, 153f
Retrograde intubation, 1774
Retropharyngeal abscess, 619–620, 620f
Rett syndrome, 582
Revictimization, 1666–1667
Rewarming, in accidental hypothermia, 1569–1570, 1569f
RFCA. See Radiofrequency catheter ablation (RFCA)
Rhabdomyolysis, 1803
  AKI and, 1054–1055
  with DKA, 1202
  exertional, 1806–1807
  hypocalcemia and, 1055
  metabolic myopathies and, 1166
  pathophysiology of, 1055
Rheumatic diseases
  airway compromise in, 1470
  antiphospholipid syndrome, 1466–1467
  cardiovascular events, 1471–1472
  CNS involvement, 1472–1473, 1473f
  complications in treatment of, 1473
  conditions/complications in ICU, 1469
  endocrine dysfunction, 1472
  gastrointestinal involvement, 1472
  hematologic involvement, 1473
  juvenile dermatomyositis, 1465–1466

Rheumatic diseases (Continued)
  juvenile idiopathic arthritis, 1462–1463
  microphage activation system, 1469–1472
  mixed connective tissue disease, 1466
  pulmonary involvement in, 1470–1471, 1470f–1471f
  Raynaud phenomenon, 1466
  renal involvement, 1472
  scleroderma, 1466
  systemic lupus erythematosus, 1463–1466
  systemic vasculitis syndromes, 1467, 1467t–1468t
Rib cage, distortion of, 609, 610f
Rifampin, drug-drug interactions of, 1723
Right ventricle, filling and /stroke volume of, 380–383, 381f–382f
Right ventricle, ultrasound of, 197–198, 198f
Right ventriculotomy, after CHD repair, 453–454
Risk (probability), 61.e1t
Rocky Mountain spotted fever (RMSF), 1502–1503
  clinical presentation, 1503, 1503f
  etiology/epidemiology of, 1502, 1502f
  management of, 1503
  prognosis, 1503
Rocuronium, 1815t, 1816–1818
Roller pumps, 432f
Roller-head pumps, 431–433, 788
Root cause analysis (RCA), 85
ROS. See Reactive oxygen species (ROS)
Rostrocaudal deterioration, 898t
Rounds, in ICU, 36
RRR. See Relative risk reduction (RRR)
RRT. See Renal replacement therapy (RRT)
RSE. See Refractory status epilepticus (RSE)
RTA. See Renal tubular acidoses (RTA)

S
Saccules, 551
Safety
  education in, 214, 214t
  EHRs and, 97–99
  fundamentals of
    errors/injuries/systems/hazards/risks, 86
    just culture and, 87
    Safety I vs. Safety II approach, 85–88, 85t
    six domains of, 83t
    teamwork and, 87
    technology and, 87–88
  in PICU, 82
    current state of quality and, 82
    improvement in, 86
    past, present, and future, 88–89, 88t
    quality improvement and value, 83–84, 83t

Safety (Continued)
    quality improvement methods, 84
    quality improvement tools, 85
    relationship to quality, 82
    systems thinking and, 82–85
    variation/display of data over time, 84–85, 85f
  of retrieval systems, 155
Salicylate toxicity, 1084, 1743
SAP. See Systemic arterial blood pressure (SAP)
Sarcolemma, of heart cells, 237
Sarcomeres, cardiac
  excitation-contraction coupling, 238, 239f
  length-tension relationships, 239–240, 240f
Sarcoplasmic reticulum, of heart cells, 237
SBE. See Standard base excess (SBE), in acid-base disorders
SBP. See Spontaneous bacterial peritonitis (SBP)
SBS. See Shaken baby syndrome (SBS)
Scald burns, 1582
SCD. See Sickle cell disease (SCD)
Scene investigation, in fatal child abuse, 1661, 1661b
Scholarship, education in, 214
School violence, 1664
SCID. See Severe combined immune deficiency (SCID)
Scleroderma, 1466
SCN. See Severe congenital neutropenia (SCN)
Scoring systems, for withdrawal, 1864–1867
Screening, for infection prevention and control, 1510
SCT. See Sickle cell trait (SCT)
SCV-CPR. See Simultaneous compression ventilation-cardiopulmonary resuscitation (SCV-CPR)
SDEs. See Subdural empyemas (SDEs)
SE. See Status epilepticus (SE)
Second messengers, signal transduction via, 1701–1702
Secondary hemochromatosis-associated cardiac hepatopancreatic MOF, 1546
Secondary survey, in ATLS, 1607–1608
Security, of health information, 100
Sedation. See also Analgesia
  for cardiac catheterization, 341–342
  drug-drug interactions of, 1723–1724
  ECLS complications involving, 313
  facilitating intubation, 1761–1762, 1762t
  hypnotics, toxicity of, 1737
  for intracranial hypertension, 1631
  after liver transplant, 1391
  for mechanical ventilation, 658–659
  overview of, 1827, 1828t, 1829f
  for PPHN, 712
  respiratory depression and, 581

Seizures
agents associated with, 1732*b*
clinical features of, 849–850, 849*t*
common causes of, 915*b*
drug-induced, 1712–1713, 1712*t*
hepatic mechanisms of, 916
neuroimaging of, 874–875
posttraumatic, 916–922
respiratory depression and, 581
toxin-induced, 1743–1744, 1744*b*
types/classification of, 915*b*
Selective IgA deficiency, 1430
Selenium, immune function and, 1442
Self-inflating manual ventilation bag, 1754, 1755*f*
Sensitivity, 61.*e*1*t*
Sensorium, impaired, 884, 884*b*
Sensory examination, 849
Sepsis, 1250
clinical presentation, 1522
definitions, 1521–1522, 1521*b*, 1543–1544
endothelial cell dysfunction, 276–277
epidemiology of, 1520–1521
fever management in, 1250.*e*2*f*
genomic medicine and, 1527–1529
genetic influence and septic shock, 1527–1528
genome-wide expression profiling, 1528–1529, 1530*f*
improved stratification in, 1537, 1538*f*
inflammation/coagulation/immune dysfunction/dysregulated metabolism hypothesis, 1541–1543, 1543*f*–1545*f*
intestine as source of, 1399–1400
introduction, 1520
liver transplantation and, 1391
MOF phenotypes/respective biomarkers/ therapies, 1543*f*–1545*f*, 1544–1546, 1545*t*
outcomes, 1544
overview of, 1250
pathogenesis of, 1522–1527, 1523*f*
as adaptive immune problem, 1527
adhesion molecules, 1525–1526, 1525*f*
coagulation cascade, 1526
cytokines as response mediators, 1524–1525, 1524*b*
myeloid-derived suppressor cells, 1527
nitric oxide, 1526
pathogen recognition/signal transduction, 1523–1524
PPARγ pathway, 1526–1527
prevention/treatment of, 1250.*e*3*f*
scoring of, 1543–1544
time course of, 1548
treatment strategies, 1529–1536, 1546–1548, 1546*t*
additional management considerations, 1534–1535
immune modulation, 1535–1536

Sepsis *(Continued)*
initial resuscitation, 1529–1532, 1531*f*
invasive monitoring, 1532–1533
oxygen delivery maintenance, 1534, 1534*b*
pathogen elimination, 1533–1534
Septic shock, 425–429
genetic influence and, 1527–1528
genome-wide expression profiling in, 1528–1529, 1530*f*
hemodynamic definitions of, 426*t*
in HIV/AIDS patients, 1447
improved stratification in, 1537, 1538*f*
therapy for, 426–429, 427*f*–428*f*
experimental/unproved therapies, 426–429
Sequence variation, in genetic variability, 1168
Sequestrations, pulmonary, 671
Serositis, 1472
Serotonin, 812*f*, 813
Serotonin (5-HTP), in PAH, 722
Serotonin (5-HTP) receptor antagonists, 1378–1380
Serotonin syndrome (SS), 1740–1741, 1740*t*
malignant hyperthermia susceptibility and, 1808
Severe combined immune deficiency (SCID)
ADA /PNP deficiencies in, 1433
cellular phenotype/molecular defects in, 1424*t*
DNA recombination/repair defects in, 1432
features of, 1431
IL-7 receptor/CD3 components/ CD45-deficient, 1431–1432
JAK3-deficient form of, 1431
X-linked form of, 1431
Severe congenital neutropenia (SCN), 1426
Sevoflurane, 1776–1777
Sexual abuse of children, 1660
Shaken baby syndrome (SBS), 1659
Shock
definition/physiology of, 417
functional classification/etiologies of, 421–425
functional classification/underlying etiologies of, 421*b*
multisystem effects of, 418*b*, 420
coagulation abnormalities, 420
endocrine disturbances, 420
gastrointestinal disturbances, 420
hepatic dysfunction, 420
renal failure, 420
respiratory failure, 420
norepinephrine for, 364*t*, 366
recognition/assessment of, 417–418, 418*b*
respiratory function and, 389
treatment, 418–420

Shock *(Continued)*
fluid resuscitation, 418–419
general principles, 418
inotropic/chronotropic/lusitropic/ vasoactive infusions, 419, 419*t*
intubation/mechanical ventilation, 418
other therapies, 419–420
Short-term outcomes
advantages of, 52–54
prediction tools for
assessment of mortality risk, 67–70, 68*t*–69*t*
historical perspective, 66–67
methods, 67
morbidity and mortality prediction, 70–71
overview, 66
weaknesses of, 55
Shunts
for CSF drainage, 833–834, 834*f*–835*f*, 838
malfunction of, 835–836, 835*f*
during myelomeningocele closure, 840
SIADH. *See* Syndrome of inappropriate antidiuretic hormone secretion (SIADH)
Siblings, of PICU patients, 106
Sickle cell disease (SCD), 1246–1256
acute chest syndrome in, 1250–1251, 1251*t*, 1251.*e*1*f*, 1250.*e*4*f*
aplastic crisis in, 1252, 1252.*e*1*f*
clinical manifestations of, 1249–1254
pain management, 1250, 1249.*e*1*f*–1249.*e*3*f*
pathophysiology/diagnosis/ presentation, 1250, 1250.*e*1*f*
vaso-occlusive pain, 1249–1250
depression/suicide in, 1254
genotypes/natural history, 1247–1248, 1248*t*
hemoglobin polymerization, 1248
hemolysis/NO homeostasis, 1249
iron overload in, 1254
laboratory/diagnostics, 1248
molecular description/epidemiology, 1246, 1247*f*
multiorgan failure syndrome in, 1253
PAH in, 1252–1253
pathophysiology of, 1248
RBCs/inflammation/endothelium, 1248–1249, 1249*f*
renal conditions in, 1253–1254
sepsis in, 1250, 1250.*e*2*f*–1250.*e*3*f*
sickle cell trait, 1247
sleep conditions and, 1254
splenic sequestration in, 1252, 1252.*e*2*f*
stroke in, 952–953, 952*f*, 1251–1252, 1251.*e*2*f*
surgery and anesthesia in, 1254, 1254.*e*1*f*
therapies/interventions for, 1254–1256, 1255*t*, 1254.*e*2*f*, 1255.*e*1*f*

Sickle cell trait (SCT), 1247
SID. *See* Strong ion difference (SID)
SIG. *See* Strong ion gap (SIG)
Signal analysis, for invasive hemodynamic monitoring, 280–281, 280f
Signal transduction
  innate immune system and, 1405, 1406f
  mechanisms of, 1701–1702, 1701f
    carrier proteins, 1693–1695, 1703f
    enzymes, 1693
    ion channels, 1690–1691
    protein phosphorylation, 1702
    second messengers, 1701–1702
  in sepsis, 1523–1524
Sildenafil
  for PAH, 729
  phosphodiesterase inhibitor, 717
Simulation training, 212–213
Simultaneous compression ventilation-cardiopulmonary resuscitation (SCV-CPR), 504–505
Simultaneous independent lung ventilation (SILV), 753–754
SIMV. *See* Synchronized intermittent mandatory ventilation (SIMV)
Single nucleotide polymorphisms (SNPs)
  definition of, 1169
  genetic variation and, 1169–1170
Single ventricle
  anatomy/physiology, 460–461
  bidirectional cavopulmonary anastomosis for, 461, 462t
  ECLS complication of, 312
  Fontan procedure for, 461–463, 462t
  mechanical circulatory support and, 320–321
  physiology of patient with, 299–300, 299f
  preoperative management of, 460–461
Sinus bradycardia, 392
Sinusitis, 1511t–1512t, 1515–1516
Sirolimus
  for immune suppression, 484–486, 485t
  nephrotoxicity of, 1057
SIRS. *See* Systemic inflammatory response syndrome (SIRS)
Sitaxsentan, for PAH, 728–729
Skeletal survey, for child abuse, 1657–1658
Skin, 1583, 1584f
Skin infections, health care–associated, 1511t–1512t, 1517
SLE. *See* Systemic lupus erythematosus (SLE)
Sleep disturbances, SCD and, 1254
SMA. *See* Spinal muscular atrophy (SMA)
Small intestine
  injury to, 1648, 1649t, 1650f
  life-threatening complications of, 1364–1368
    acute colonic pseudo-obstruction, 1368

Small intestine (Continued)
    distal intestinal obstruction syndrome, 1367
    food allergy, 1365
    hemolytic-uremic syndrome, 1365–1367
    Hirschsprung disease, 1367–1368
    inflammatory bowel disease, 1366–1367, 1366t
    low cardiac output syndrome, 1365
    malrotation, 1364–1365
    necrotizing enterocolitis, 1365
Smart infusion pumps, 97–99
Snakebites, 1553–1558, 1554f
  clinical presentation of, 1554–1555, 1555f
  diagnostic studies of, 1555
  disposition, 1558
  emergency/critical care for, 1556–1557
  epidemiology of, 1553
  future directions, 1558
  pathophysiology of, 1554
  pitfalls of, 1555
  prehospital care for, 1555–1556
  prognosis, 1558
  resources, 1558
  therapeutic complications of, 1557
S-nitrosothiols, 1239, 1240f
SNPs. *See* Single nucleotide polymorphisms (SNPs)
Sodium, 1008. *See also* Hypernatremia; Hyponatremia
Sodium bicarbonate
  for cardiac arrest, 531
  with CPR, 514–516, 515f
  for metabolic acidosis, 1088–1089
Sodium channel blockade, toxicity of, 1744
Sodium nitroprusside (SNP), 1084, 1123t, 1125–1126
Somatic cells, mutations in, 1170–1171
Somatic peripheral nervous system, 820
Somatostatin, for gastrointestinal hemorrhage, 1375
South Africa, history of PCCM in, 14
Specific antibody deficiency, 1437
Specificity, definition of, 61.e1t
Spider bites. *See* Widow spider bites
SPIKES protocol, for delivering bad news, 129t
Spina bifida aperta, 839
Spina bifida occulta, 839
Spinal cord, 816–817
  compression of, 1318–1319
  vasculature, 825–826
Spinal dysraphism, 839–840
Spinal muscular atrophy (SMA), 990–991
Spirometry, for asthma assessment, 651
Spleen, 1232–1233
  embolization, 1647, 1647f
  injury to, 1647–1648, 1648f, 1649t
    nonoperative management of, 1647

Spontaneous bacterial peritonitis (SBP), 1398–1399
Spontaneous intracranial hemorrhage, 959–962. *See also* Intracranial hemorrhage (ICH)
Spontaneous ventilator-assisted breaths, 741
Sports injury, 1645
SS. *See* Serotonin syndrome (SS)
SSI. *See* Surgical site infection (SSI)
Staff development, in nursing, 48–49
  continuing education, 49
  in-service education programs, 48–49
  orientation programs, 48
Staffing, of retrieval systems, 154–155
Standard base excess (SBE), in acid-base disorders, 1067–1068, 1068t
Staphylococcus aureus pneumonia, 685
Starvation, metabolic stress vs., 1208, 1208t
Static encephalopathy, 849
Statistical power, definition of, 61.e1t
Status asthmaticus, 774
  lactic acidosis in, 1084
Status epilepticus (SE). *See also* Refractory status epilepticus (RSE)
  autoimmune, 917–922, 917f–918f
  causes of, 914–915, 914t, 915b
  evaluation/management of, 919–922, 920f–921f
  febrile, 915
  morbidity and mortality with, 927
  neurophysiology of, 917–919, 917f–918f
  overview/incidence of, 913–914, 914f
  pharmacotherapy for, 922–924, 923t
  surgical options, 926–927
Stem cell therapy, for HIE, 948–949
Stem cell transplantation, acute renal failure after, 1058
Sternal compressions, 530
Steroids. *See* Corticosteroids; Glucocorticoids
Stings, 1560–1561
Stomach
  airway management and, 1766–1768, 1767b
  life-threatening complications of, 1363–1364
Stool pH assessment, 1361
Strengths, weaknesses, opportunities, and threats (SWOT) approach, to pediatric critical care research, 52
Streptococcus pneumoniae, 685
Stress response
  cellular responses, 1148
  central activation/integration of, 1146–1147
  in critical illness, 1148–1149
  definitions/historical perspectives, 1145–1146
  introduction, 1145
  peripheral responses, 1147–1148

Stress response (Continued)
    primary elements of, 1146, 1146f
    recommendations, 1149–1150
Stress ulcers
    epidemiology/risk factors for, 1373
    mechanism of mucosal damage,
        1372–1373
    prophylaxis, 1372
        H2 receptor antagonists for, 1374
        infectious complications of, 1374
        options for, 1373–1374
        proton pump inhibitors for, 1374
        sucralfate for, 1374
Stridor, 677
Stroke, 865–868, 866f–867f. See also
    Arterial ischemic stroke (AIS)
    in SCD, 1251–1252
        diagnosis of, 1252
        management of, 1252, 1251.e2f
        natural history of, 1252
    significance of, 951
Stroke volume
    effects of ventilation on, 380–383, 381f
    relationship to preload, 489, 489f–490f
Strong ion difference (SID), 1071–1074
Strong ion gap (SIG), 1074
Structure, in quality critical care, 21–22,
    21f
Strychnine, 1744
Subclavian vein cannulation, 169–170, 171f
Subcutaneous drug absorption, 1675
Subdural empyemas (SDEs), 971–972,
    972f
Subglottic stenosis, 540–541, 540f, 622–623,
    622f
Subspecialization, within PCCM
    adequate training for, 32
    adult subspecialization, 28–29
    cardiac intensive care, 29–31, 30f
    criteria for, 28b
    early history, 25–28, 27f
    guidelines for, 28b
    impact on research, 32–33
    neurocritical care, 31–32, 31f–32f
    in PICUs, 29
Substance P/neurokinin-1 receptor
    antagonist, 1379
Substituted judgment standard, 117–118
Subtentorial compartment, coma and, 890f,
    891, 892f
Succinylcholine, 1811–1824, 1812t–1813t
Sucralfate, 1374
Sufentanyl, 1777, 1777f
Sugammadex, 1821
Suicide, SCD and, 1254
Superficial burns, 1583
Superficial partial-thickness burns, 1584
Superior vena cava (SVC) syndrome,
    1319–1321
Super-refractory status epilepticus, 915
Supratentorial compartment, coma and,
    888–891, 890f–891f

Supraventricular tachycardias, 394, 395f,
    399f, 407t
Surfactant
    for acute respiratory failure, 672
    in ARDS, 630
    homeostasis, genetic disorders of, 664
    inactivation of, 641
    for PPHN, 714
    for pulmonary hemorrhage, 666
Surfactant-deficient respiratory distress
    syndrome, 664
Surgery
    for burn wounds, 1593–1594
    for SCD, 1254, 1254.e1f
Surgical site infection (SSI), 1511t–1512t,
    1517
Surveillance for HAIs, 1509–1510
Sustained tachycardias, 408–409
SVC. See Superior vena cava (SVC)
    syndrome
SvO₂. See Mixed venous oxygen saturation
    (SvO₂)
SVR. See Systemic vascular resistance
    (SVR), QOT and
Sweep speed, effect on ultrasound, 183,
    185f
Sympathetic nervous system (SNS),
    820–821, 1116
Sympathomimetic agents
    pharmacology of, 359–360, 359f–360f
    toxicity of, 1737–1738, 1738b
Synaptic pruning, 828
Synaptogenesis, 828, 829f
Synchronized intermittent mandatory
    ventilation (SIMV), 742–743, 742f
Syndrome of inappropriate antidiuretic
    hormone secretion (SIADH)
    CSW vs., 1009–1010, 1009t
    in hyponatremia, 1010–1011
    nonosmotic stimuli associated with,
        1011b
Synergy model of nursing, 43–46
    nurse competencies, 44–46
        advocacy/moral agency, 45
        caring practices, 44–45
        clinical inquiry, 44
        clinical judgment, 44
        collaboration, 45
        facilitation of learning, 45
        response to diversity, 45
        systems thinking, 45–46
    patient characteristics, 43–44
Syringomyelia, 837
Systematic reviews, 62–63, 63t
Systemic arterial blood pressure (SAP)
    CVP or intracardiac pressure
        monitoring, 296
    invasive monitoring with, 296
    noninvasive monitoring with, 296
Systemic circulation
    anatomy of, 249–250
    autoregulation of, 252

Systemic circulation (Continued)
    control of vascular tone, 250–252
    general features, 250
Systemic inflammatory response syndrome
    (SIRS), 1541, 1542f
    criteria for, 1521–1522, 1521b
    in critical illness, 1455–1456
    definitions/scoring of, 1543–1544
    inflammation/coagulation/immune
        dysfunction/dysregulated
        metabolism hypothesis, 1541–1543,
        1543f–1545f
    MOF phenotypes/respective biomarkers/
        therapies, 1543f–1545f, 1544–1546,
        1545t
    outcomes, 1544
    temporal aspects of, 1456, 1457f
    therapeutic approaches to, 1546–1548,
        1546t
    time course of, 1548
Systemic lupus erythematosus (SLE)
    acute glomerulonephritis in, 1050–1051
    clinical presentation, 1464–1465
    criteria for, 1464b
    laboratory studies, 1465
    management of, 1465
    neonatal autoimmune syndromes, 1465
Systemic sclerosis, 1466
Systemic vascular resistance (SVR), QOT
    and, 297
Systemic vasculitis, 1467, 1467t
System-level outcomes, in synergy model
    of nursing, 46
Systems thinking, as nurse competency,
    45–46

T

T cell(s)
    adaptive immunity and, 1415–1419,
        1416f–1417f, 1417t
    additional subtypes, 1419
    component of immune system
        clinical presentation, 1425
        deficiencies in, 1423t
    helper subtypes, 1418–1419, 1418t
    specific immune disorders, 1430–1434
        ADA deficient/PNP deficient SCID,
        1433
        defects in antigen presentation,
        1433–1434
        DiGeorge syndrome, 1430–1431
        DNA recombination/repair defects in
        SCID, 1432
        IL-7 receptor/CD3 components/
        CD45-deficient SCID, 1431–1432
        JAK3-deficient SCID, 1431
        laboratory tests for, 1432t, 1437
        severe combined immune deficiency,
        1431
        treatment for, 1438
        X-linked SCID, 1431
        Zap-70-deficient SCID, 1433

T helper cell subtypes, 1418–1419, 1418*t*
TA. *See* Takayasu arteritis (TA)
Tachycardias, 394–396, 409–410
 atrioventricular nodal reentrant, 395
 atrioventricular reciprocating, 394–395
 classification by mechanism, 394
 classification by site, 394
 junctional ectopic, 396
 management of pediatric, 521*f*
 with normal QRS, 399, 399*f*
 primary atrial, 395–396
 with prolonged QRS, 398*f*, 399–400
 supraventricular, 394, 395*f*
 therapies for, 405–408
  acute pharmacologic, 405–408, 407*t*
  cardioversion/defibrillation, 408
  sustained tachycardias, 408–409
  treatment failure, 409
  unstable patients, 409
  vagal maneuvers, 405
 toxins associated with, 1730, 1731*t*
 ventricular, 396
Tachypnea, 684
TACO. *See* Transfusion-associated
 circulatory overload (TACO)
Tacrolimus, for immune suppression,
 484–486, 485*t*
Tadalafil, for PAH, 729
TAH. *See* Total artificial heart (TAH)
 devices
TAI. *See* Traumatic axonal injury (TAI)
Takayasu arteritis (TA), 1469
Tank ventilators, 779–780, 780*f*
TAPVC. *See* Total anomalous pulmonary
 venous connection (TAPVC)
TAPVR. *See* Total anomalous pulmonary
 venous return (TAPVR)
Target concentration strategy, 1686–1687,
 1686*b*
Target effect strategy, 1687, 1687*b*
TBI. *See* Traumatic brain injury (TBI)
TCD. *See* Transcranial Doppler (TCD)
TCP. *See* Transcutaneous cardiac pacing
 (TCP), for CPR
Teaching methods, 210–213, 210*t*–211*t*
 bedside, 211–212
 learner assessment driving, 220
 procedural, 212
 simulation, 212–213
 web-based, 213
Team training, for ICU, 37
Teams, safety and, 87
Technology, safety and, 87–88
TEF. *See* Tracheoesophageal fistula (TEF)
Telemedicine, 100
Temperature management
 after cardiac arrest, 531–532
 in PPHN, 713
Temporary pacing, 401–404, 401*f*
 setting parameters for, 402–404,
 402*f*–404*f*
Terbutaline, for asthma, 654

Terlipressin
 basic pharmacology, 372–373
 clinical pharmacology/adverse effects,
 373
Tetralogy of Fallot (TOF), 468–470
TGA. *See* Transposition of the great
 arteries (TGA)
Thalassemia, 1256–1259
 anemia in, 1257
 cardiac complications, 1258, 1258.*e1f*
 forms/variations of, 1257, 1257.*e1f*
  α-thalassemia, 1257
  β-thalassemia, 1257
  HbE/β0 thalassemia, 1257
 hepatic dysfunction, 1258
 iron overload assessment, 1257
 laboratory/diagnostics, 1256, 1256*t*
 molecular description/epidemiology,
 1256
 natural history of, 1257
 pathophysiology of, 1256–1257, 1256.*e1f*,
 1257.*e1f*
 pulmonary hypertension in, 1258–1259
 spectrum of disease, 1257.*e2f*
 therapies/interventions for, 1259,
 1257.*e2f*
 thrombosis/pulmonary emboli in,
 1258
 transfusion-related complications, 1257,
 1252.*e3f*
THAM. *See* Tris(hydroxymethyl)
 aminomethane (THAM)
Thermal burns, 1582
Thermodilution method
 for assessment of cardiac output, 294
 for cardiac output measurement,
 288–289
Thermoregulation, for organ donation,
 145
Thiazide diuretics, 1101*f*, 1102–1103
Thiopental, for SE, 922–924, 923*t*
Third nerve palsy, 887–888
Thoracentesis, 175–176, 175*b*–176*b*
Thoracic cage abnormalities, 679
Thoracic index, 502–503
Thoracic pump mechanism, during CPR,
 500–502, 501*f*
Thoracic trauma
 anatomic/physiologic considerations,
 1638
 cardiac injuries, 1641, 1642*f*
 chest wall injury, 1639–1640
 from child abuse, 1660
 chylothorax, 1642
 diaphragmatic injury, 1642
 epidemiology/prevention of, 1638
 esophageal injury, 1641
 initial resuscitation/diagnosis,
 1638–1639
 lung/airway injury, 1640, 1640*f*
 traumatic asphyxia, 1640–1641
Thoracostomy, tube, 176–178, 1640, 1640*f*

Thoracotomy, emergency department,
 1609–1610
Thrombocytopenia
 heparin-induced, 1278–1279
 immune, 1315–1316
 nonimmune, 1316
 overview of, 1315
Thrombocytopenia-associated MOF,
 1543*f*–1544*f*, 1544–1546
Thrombocytopenic purpura, 1271–1272
Thrombolysis, for AIS, 956
Thrombophilia, 1285–1288
Thrombosis
 clinical features of, 1288–1289
 developmental hemostasis and, 1282–
 1283, 1283*f*
 diagnosis of, 1289–1290
  arterial, 1289–1290
  intracardiac, 1290
  pulmonary embolus, 1289
  venous, 1289
 with DKA, 1202
 etiology/epidemiology of, 1283–1288,
 1284*f*, 1286*t*
  arterial, 1284–1285
  cardiac surgery, 1285
  heparin-induced thrombocytopenia,
  1288
  thrombophilia, 1285–1288
  venous, 1284
 management of, 1290–1292, 1290*t*–
 1292*t*, 1292*f*
 in thalassemia, 1258
 thromboprophylaxis in PICU,
 1292–1293
Thrombotic thrombocytopenic purpura
 (TTP)
 diagnosis/pathophysiology of, 1473
 endothelial cell dysfunction, 277
Thyroid hormone, 1191–1194
 actions of, 1191–1192, 1192*b*
 biochemistry of, 1191–1192, 1192*f*
 effects of drugs on, 1194*t*
 supplementation in PICU, 1193–1194
Thyrotoxicosis, 1193, 1193*b*
Thyroxine, in AKI attenuation, 1047
Tick paralysis, 987
Tidal volume
 ARDS ventilation and, 631
 VILI and, 639–640, 639*f*–640*f*
Tigecycline, 1479
Time constant, of respiratory system, 562,
 735, 735*f*
Tissue oxygenation
 in ECMO, 796–797
 monitoring of
  blood mitochondrial DNA, 1142
  MRS, 1142
  NADH fluorometry, 1142
  NIRS, 1141–1142
  optical spectroscopy, 1142
  tissue oxygen tension, 1142

Tissue resistance, 558

TNF-α. *See* Tumor necrosis factor-α (TNF-α)

TOF. *See* Tetralogy of Fallot (TOF)

Tolerance
history of, in PICU, 1862–1863
overview of, 1862

Toll-like receptors (TLRs), 1404–1405, 1405t, 1435–1436

Tongue, vallecular cyst, 544, 544f

Tonsils, cerebellar, 836–837, 837f

Torsades des pointes, 411, 411f

Total anomalous pulmonary venous connection (TAPVC), 466–467

Total anomalous pulmonary venous return (TAPVR), 680

Total artificial heart (TAH) devices, 319

Total body clearance, 1685

Total body sodium
hypernatremia and, 1012–1013
hyponatremia and, 1008, 1010–1011

Total body water, drug-drug interactions and, 1717

Total lung capacity, mechanical ventilation and, 734

Toxic shock syndrome (TSS), 1499–1500
clinical presentation, 1499
diagnosis of, 1500, 1500b
etiology/epidemiology of, 1499
management of, 1500
prognosis, 1500
surveillance definitions of, 1499b

Toxidromes, 1729t
acetaminophen, 1745–1746, 1746f
anion gap metabolic acidosis, 1741–1745, 1741b, 1742t
anticholinergic agents, 1738–1739, 1738b
cardiovascular agents, 1744–1745
cholinergic agents, 1739–1740, 1739b
methemoglobinemia, 1740, 1740b
opioids, 1736–1737, 1737b
overview of, 1736
sedative hypnotics, 1737
sympathomimetic agents, 1737–1738, 1738b
toxin-induced seizures, 1743–1744, 1744b
xenobotic-induced hyperthermia, 1740–1741, 1740t

Toxin assessment/screening
common agents involved, 1728
diagnostic trials, 1734, 1735t
patient assessment, 1728–1734
history, 1728–1729, 1729t
laboratory tests/toxin screens, 1732–1734, 1733t, 1734b
physical examination, 1729–1732, 1729t–1731t, 1732b
radiographic imaging, 1734, 1734b
resources for, 1728

Trace elements, in parenteral nutrition, 1217–1218

Trachea, 539–540, 541f, 546
anatomy of, 1751–1752
vascular impingement on, 615, 615f–616f, 678

Tracheobronchomalacia, 677–678

Tracheoesophageal fistula (TEF), 539, 540f, 678

Tracheomalacia, intrathoracic, 615–616

Tracheostomy
airway management and, 1773–1774
complications, 625
decannulation, 625–626
postoperative nursing care, 625
for upper airway disease, 624–625
weaning and, 767

TRALI. *See* Transfusion-related acute lung injury (TRALI)

Transcranial Doppler (TCD)
of cerebral blood flow, 853
monitoring ICP, 910–911
for neuroimaging, 857, 858f

Transcutaneous cardiac pacing (TCP), for CPR, 508–509

Transcutaneous monitoring, of respiratory system, 574

Transdisciplinary care conferences, 108

Transducers, ultrasound, 183–184, 185f

Transfusion medicine
cryoprecipitate, 1306
plasma, 1303–1304
platelets, 1304–1306
reactions/complications of, 1306–1311, 1307t
delayed, 1309
immediate, 1306–1309, 1307t
to massive transfusion, 1309
treatment of, 1310–1311
red blood cells, 1295–1303
in SCD, 1254–1255
choice of product, 1254–1255
indications for, 1255t
type/goals of, 1255, 1255.e1f
thalassemia and, 1257

Transfusion-associated circulatory overload (TACO), 1308

Transfusion-related acute lung injury (TRALI), 1306–1308, 1307t

Transfusions, immune function and, 1443

Transient myasthenia gravis, 986–987

Transient tachypnea of newborn (TTN), 662–664, 663f

Transitions of care, communication in, 37

Transplantation
evolving areas of, 146
lung and heart-lung, in PAH, 730
posttraumatic seizures and, 916–917

Transport
to catheterization laboratory, 341
for patients on ECLS, 314
pediatric physiology relevant to, 150–151

Transport (Continued)
problems with adult-oriented transport teams, 149–152, 150b
rapid transfer/goal-directed therapy/golden hour, 151–152, 152f
specialized teams
components of, 152–155, 154f
improving outcomes, 152, 153f
transport environment stresses, 151

Transposition of the great arteries (TGA), 467–468
arterial switch operation, 467–468
atrial switch procedure, 467
complications, 468
critical care management for, 468
pathophysiology of, 467–468
ventricular switch procedure, 468

Transthoracic echocardiography (TTE), for intracardiac thrombosis, 1290

Transversus abdominis plane block, 1779, 1780f

Trapezoidal rule, 1684, 1684f

Trauma
to aorta, 1649t, 1651. *See also* Abdominal trauma; Thoracic trauma; Violence-associated injury
ECMO for, 795
multiple
diagnostic assessment, 1608–1609, 1610f
ED thoracotomy, 1609–1610
overview of, 1599
prehospital care/trauma team activation, 1600
primary survey, 1600–1607, 1602f–1603f, 1602t, 1605t, 1606f–1607f
secondary survey, 1607–1608
stabilization/definitive care, 1610
trauma resuscitation, 1600, 1601f
neuroimaging of, 872–873, 874f
open globe injury, 1770
upper airway disease due to, 621–622
airway injury, 623–624
burn injury, 624
foreign body aspiration, 623, 623f–624f
laryngotracheal stenosis, 622–623, 622f
postextubation stridor, 621–622

Trauma team, 1600, 1601f

Traumatic asphyxia, 1640–1641

Traumatic axonal injury (TAI), 1618–1619, 1620f

Traumatic brain injury (TBI)
diagnostic studies/monitoring of, 1623–1626
advanced techniques for, 1626, 1627f–1628f
computerized tomography, 1623–1624, 1623f, 1623t
ICP monitoring, 1624–1626
MRI, 1624, 1624f–1625f

Traumatic brain injury (TBI) *(Continued)*
  epidemiology of, 1613–1614
  history in, 1619
  initial resuscitation, 1620–1623, 1621*b*
    circulatory stabilization, 1622
    ED to PICU transition, 1622–1623
    herniation, 1622
    rapid-sequence induction/intubation, 1621–1622, 1622*t*
  intracranial hypertension and, 908, 909*f*
  miscellaneous issues, 1635
  monitoring/postinsult natural history, 908–909
  multidisciplinary outcomes assessment, 75–76
  outcomes, 1636, 1636*f*
  pathophysiology of, 1614–1619, 1614*f*
    axonal injury, 1618–1619, 1620*f*
    cerebral blood volume, 1617
    cerebral swelling, 1617
    delayed neuronal death cascades, 1615–1617, 1616*f*
    edema, 1617–1618, 1618*f*–1619*f*
    excitotoxicity, 1615
    posttraumatic ischemia, 1614–1615
  rehabilitation and acute care in, 1635–1636
  signs/symptoms, 1619–1620, 1620*t*, 1621*f*
  treatment in PICU, 1626–1635
    intracranial hypertension: first tier, 1629*f*, 1630–1631
    intracranial hypertension: second tier, 1631–1635, 1632*f*
Treprostinil, for PAH, 727
Triage, in emergency department, 228
Triazoles, 1481–1482
Tricuspid atresia, 472
Tricyclic antidepressants, toxicity of, 414, 1744–1745
Triiodothyronine, for hormonal resuscitation, 141–142, 142*t*
Trimethoprim-sulfamethoxazole, RTA and, 1088
Tris(hydroxymethyl)aminomethane (THAM), 1089–1090
Tromethamine, for cardiac arrest, 531
Troubleshooting, for ECLS complications, 311
Truncus arteriosus communis, 466
TSS. *See* Toxic shock syndrome (TSS)
TTN. *See* Transient tachypnea of newborn (TTN)
TTP. *See* Thrombotic thrombocytopenic purpura (TTP)
Tube thoracostomy, 176–178, 1640, 1640*f*
Tubing, for CPB, 435, 435*t*
Tubular necrosis, drug-associated, 1708, 1708*t*

Tubules
  anatomy of, 1001–1005
  collecting duct, 1004–1005, 1004*f*
  distal, 1001–1002
  function of, 1002–1005, 1002*f*–1003*f*
  function tests of, 1035–1038
    generalized proximal tubulopathy, 1038
    potassium regulation, 1038
    proteinuria, 1037
    renal acidification, 1037–1038
    serum BUN/creatinine ratio, 1037
    urine concentration capacity, 1036–1037
    urine electrolytes, 1035–1036
    urine microscopy, 1037
  loop of Henle, 1001, 1002*f*
  proximal, 1001–1002, 1001*f*
Tubulopathies, drug-mediated, 1087–1088
Tumor lysis syndrome (TLS), 1017, 1022*t*
  AKI and, 1053–1054
  management of, 1054
  as oncologic emergency, 1316–1318
  therapy for, 1054, 1054*t*
Tumor necrosis factor-α (TNF-α), 1524
Tumors, neuroimaging of, 874, 875*f*
Tympanometry, in pediatric neurocritical care, 854–855
Type I error (alpha), 61.e1*t*
Type II error (beta), 61.e1*t*

U
UAC. *See* Umbilical arterial cannulation (UAC)
UFH. *See* Unfractionated heparin (UFH), for pediatric thrombosis
UGTs. *See* Uridine 5′-diphosphate glucuronosyltransferases (UGTs)
Ulcerative colitis, 1366–1367, 1366*t*
Ulcers. *See also* Stress ulcers
  duodenal, 1364
  gastric, 1363–1364
Ultrafiltration
  basic physiology of, 1105, 1106*f*
  as CPB technique, 440–441
Ultrasonography
  abdominal, 191–192, 191*f*–192*f*
  for acute abdomen, 1396
  cardiac, 193–198, 194*f*, 196*f*–198*f*
  in CVL placement, 170
  drainage procedures using, 187–188, 188*f*
  for gastrointestinal evaluation, 1360–1361
  for HTN, 1120
  image optimization in, 181–184, 182*f*–184*f*
  in lumbar puncture, 188–189, 189*f*
  for neuroimaging, 857, 858*f*
  neurosonology, 198–199
  procedural guidance in, 184–187, 186*f*
  pulmonary, 189–193, 189*f*–191*f*
  transducers, 183–184, 185*f*

Umbilical arterial cannulation (UAC), 166–168
Umbilical venous cannulation (UVC), 167–168
Uncal herniation, coma and, 893, 893*f*
Underfeeding, in PICU, 1208–1212, 1209*f*, 1209*t*
Undergraduate medical education, 220–221, 221*t*. *See also* Education
  entrustable professional activities, 221, 221*t*
  in pediatrics across continuum, 221
Unfractionated heparin (UFH), for pediatric thrombosis, 1291–1292, 1291*t*–1292*t*, 1292*f*
Unilateral lung disease, 753–754
Unit design, for ICUs, 35–36
Upper airway disease
  airway management and, 1770
  angioedema, 624
  congenital malformations, 613–614
    bronchomalacia/intrathoracic tracheomalacia, 615–616
    choanal atresia, 613–614, 613*f*
    laryngeal webs/stenosis/tumors, 614–615, 615*f*
    laryngomalacia, 614, 614*f*
    vascular impingement on trachea, 615, 615*f*–616*f*
  in HIV/AIDS patients, 1447
  infectious processes, 616, 618*t*
    bacterial tracheitis, 620
    epiglottitis, 617–619, 619*f*
    laryngeal papillomatosis, 620–621, 620*f*
    laryngotracheobronchitis, 616–617, 617*f*–618*f*, 617*t*
    peritonsillar abscess, 619
    retropharyngeal abscess, 619–620, 620*f*
  initial management of, 612–613
  intrathoracic mass lesions, 621
  tracheostomy for, 624–625
    complications, 625
    decannulation, 625–626
    postoperative nursing care, 625
  trauma-related, 621–622
    airway injury, 623–624
    burn injury, 624
    foreign body aspiration, 623, 623*f*–624*f*
    laryngotracheal stenosis, 622–623, 622*f*
    postextubation stridor, 621–622
  vocal cord paralysis, 621
Upper respiratory system
  anatomy and physiology of, 542–546
    in infants vs. children, 545*t*
    mouth and pharynx, 543–544, 544*f*–545*f*
    nasal passages, 542–543, 542*f*–544*f*
    trachea and bronchi, 546

Upper respiratory system (Continued)
  developmental anatomy of, 539–542
    congenital tracheal stenosis, 541f
    laryngeal atresia, 541f
    laryngeal cleft, 541f
    laryngeal web, 540f
    larynx, 540f
    subglottic stenosis, 541f
    trachea, 540f–541f
Upward transtentorial herniation, 893
Uremia
  with AKI, 1048
  bleeding in, 1316
  immune dysfunction and, 1443
  impaired platelet function in, 1280
Uridine 5′-diphosphate
    glucuronosyltransferases (UGTs),
    1679t, 1680
Urinary anion gap, 1075–1076
Urinary reconstruction, using bowel
    segments, 1088
Urinary tract infections (UTIs), 1511t–
    1512t, 1516, 1516f
Urinary tract obstruction, AKI and, 1058,
    1059t
Urine concentration capacity, tubular
    function and, 1036–1037
Urine electrolytes, tubular function and,
    1035–1036
Urine microscopy, tubular function and,
    1037
Urine output, as measure of oxygen
    delivery, 295
Urine tests, in malignant hyperthermia,
    1805
UVC. See Umbilical venous cannulation
    (UVC)

V
Vaccination
  PAH and, 726
  for viral pneumonitis, 688t, 691
VADs. See Ventricular assist devices (VADs)
Vagal maneuvers, 405
Vallecular cyst, of tongue, 544, 544f
Valproic acid
  for RSE, 925
  for SE, 922–924, 923t
Valvular disease, rheumatic disease
    associated with, 1471
Vancomycin, nephrotoxicity of, 1056
VAP. See Ventilator-associated pneumonia
    (VAP)
Varicella zoster virus (VZV) infection,
    952
Vascular access
  arterial catheter placement, 161–163,
    162b
  CVL placement, 168–172, 168t,
    169f–172f
  with echocardiography, 329–332,
    331f–334f

Vascular access (Continued)
  intraosseous infusion, 158–161,
    159f–160f
  after liver transplant, 1391
  PACs, 172, 173f
  pericardiocentesis, 163–166, 165f
  PICCs, 172–175
  UAC and UVC, 166–168
  ultrasound in, 184–187, 186f
Vascular compression, of trachea/bronchus,
    678
Vascular impedance, of regional
    circulation, 257–259
Vascular integrity, QOT and, 298, 298f
Vascular resistance
  invasive hemodynamic measurement of,
    289–290
  postnatal pulmonary, 261–262, 261f
Vascular tone, 250–252
Vasculature
  in brain, 829
  of kidneys, 997–998, 1041, 1041b
    anatomy of, 998, 998f
    development of, 997
    function of, 998
Vasculitis
  of CNS, 952
  endothelial cell dysfunction, 277
  HIV/AIDS and, 1447
  neuroimaging of, 867–868, 868f
Vasculopathy, neuroimaging of, 867–868,
    868f
Vasoactive drugs
  for cardiac dysfunction, 493–495,
    494t
  drug-drug compatibility, 363t
  for shock, 419, 419t
Vasoconstrictors, 273–274
Vasodilators
  endothelium-derived, 272–273, 273f
  for PAH, 726
  for pulmonary hypertension, 455–456
Vasopressin
  adverse effects of, 372
  basic pharmacology, 370
  for cardiac arrest, 530–531
  clinical pharmacology, 371
  clinical role of, 371–372
  with CPR, 511–518
  for diabetes insipidus, 143–144
  dosing/administration, 372
  for gastrointestinal hemorrhage, 1375
  for hormonal resuscitation, 141–142,
    142t
  interactions, 372
  pharmacokinetics of, 371
  for potential organ donor, 482
  stress responses and, 1149
Vasopressin receptors, 356–357, 356f
  downregulation of, 357
  polymorphisms of, 357
  V_1 receptors, 356, 357f–358f

Vasopressors
  adverse effects of, 1710–1712, 1710t
  for cardiac arrest, 530–531
  infusion rates for, 364t
Vasoregulation
  by RBC-derived ATP, 1240–1241
  RBC-nitric oxide interactions in, 1238
VCE. See Video capsule endoscopy (VCE)
Vecuronium, 1815–1816, 1815t
Vein of Galen aneurysmal malformation
    (VGAM), 869, 870f
Venoarterial ECMO, 786–787, 786f
Venoocclusive disease (VOD), 1333–1334
Venous cutdown, 171–172, 172f
Venous infarct, 862f, 866–867
Venous reservoir, for ECMO, 788
Venous return
  cardiac output and, 255–256, 255f–256f
  effects of ventilation on, 380–381, 381f
Venous saturation monitor, for ECMO,
    788
Venous thrombosis, 1284, 1289
Venovenous ECMO, 787–788, 787f
Ventilation. See also Mechanical
    ventilation
  in acute liver failure, 1388
  in ARDS, 630–631
    nonconventional strategies, 631
    peak/plateau pressure, 631
    PEEP, 631
    tidal volume, 631
    ventilator mode considerations,
      630–631
  dead space, 572
  distribution of, 589–590
  fractal model of, 591, 592f
  history of, 4–7, 8f
  for inhalational injury, 1589–1590,
    1590f
  liquid, 673–674
  management during ECLS, 313
Ventilation/perfusion inequality
  abnormalities in pulmonary disease,
    591–593
    ARDS, 592
    asthma, 592–593
    hypoxemia, 591
    pneumonia, 592
    primary pulmonary hypertension, 593
    pulmonary embolism, 593
  distribution of perfusion, 590, 590f
  distribution of ventilation, 589–590
  fractal model of PBF and ventilation,
    591, 591f–592f
  fractal model of pulmonary ventilation,
    591, 592f
  in meconium aspiration syndrome, 668
  overview of, 589, 590f, 590t
  therapeutic considerations, 593
    nitric oxide, 593
    PEEP, 593
    prone positioning, 593

Ventilation-perfusion relationships, of respiratory system, 564, 565f
Ventilator breath control variable, 741
Ventilator-associated pneumonia (VAP), 667, 1511t–1512t, 1515
Ventilator-induced lung injury (VILI)
    clinical applications, 644
    evidence for, 636–639
        in damaged lungs, 637–639, 638f
        in intact lungs, 636–637, 637f
    injury reduction strategies
        mechanical measures, 643–644
        use of pressure-volume curve, 643, 643f
    mechanisms of, 640–642, 641f
        altered permeability, 641–642, 642f
        increased vascular transmural pressure, 641
    new insights, 642–643
        cellular response to mechanical strain, 642–643
        influence of carbon dioxide tension, 643
    roles of tidal volume/PEEP/lung distention, 639–640, 639f–640f
Ventricles
    assessing diastolic size of, 327
    assessing myocardial contractility, 243
    cardiac output, 246
    diastolic ventricular function, 245–246
    function curves of, 243–244, 245f
    neural control of heart, 246
    pericardial function, 244–245
    pressure-volume loops, 242–243, 242f
    relationship to muscle strips, 241–242
    ventricular interaction, 245
Ventricular assist devices (VADs), 314–319, 315f
    for cardiac dysfunction, 496–497
    clinical indications/outcomes for centrifugal, 316–317
    continuous flow, 316, 317f
    device selection, 319, 320f
    echocardiography and, 333–334, 336f–337f
    ECLS vs., 314t
    FDA approved, 322t
    future directions, 322–323
    intraaortic balloon pump, 322–323
    long-term, 318–319, 318f
    next generation-levitated devices, 319
    outcomes, 321–322, 321f
    patient management, 319–320
    patient selection, 319
    single-ventricle physiology, 320–321
    total artificial heart devices, 319
Ventricular cerebrospinal fluid drainage, 1630
Ventricular diastolic function, QOT and, 296–297
Ventricular dysfunction, in CHD patient, 451

Ventricular fibrillation (VF), 533–534
    antiarrhythmics for, 533
    arrest, HIE and, 939–941, 941f
    management of, 518–524
        antiarrhythmics, 520–523, 520t, 521f–522f
        defibrillation, 518–520, 519f
Ventricular function, echocardiography of, 326–327, 326f
Ventricular septal defect (VSD), 465, 680
Ventricular switch procedure, for TGA, 468
Ventricular system, 824
Ventricular systolic function, QOT and, 296
Ventricular tachycardias (VTs), 396, 398f, 533
    antiarrhythmics for, 533
    in ostensibly healthy patients, 412, 412f
    therapies for, 407t
Ventriculoperitoneal shunt, for CSF drainage, 834f–835f
Ventriculostomy, endoscopic third
    for Dandy-Walker malformation, 838
    for hydrocephalus, 833–836
    during myelomeningocele closure, 840
Ventriculostomy-related infections, 1517–1518
Vest cardiopulmonary resuscitation, 506–507
VF. See Ventricular fibrillation (VF)
VGAM. See Vein of Galen aneurysmal malformation (VGAM)
Victimization, 1663–1664, 1667
Video capsule endoscopy (VCE), 1359–1360
Video laryngoscopy, 1765
VILI. See Ventilator-induced lung injury (VILI)
Violence-associated injury
    challenges/opportunities in, 1667–1668
    detection/treatment referrals, 1667
    disproportionate distribution of, 1666
    effect of adverse experiences, 1666
    incidence of, 1663–1665
        setting/forms of, 1664–1665
        victimization/perpetration, 1663–1664
    psychologic injury/psychosocial effects of, 1665–1667
Viral infections
    acute liver failure, 1487, 1490–1493
    CNS, 1488–1490
    diagnosing, 1490–1493, 1491t–1492t
    etiologies of, 1486t
    exotic disease, 1490
    meningitis/encephalitis, 1493, 1495
    myocarditis, 1485–1487, 1490, 1493
    pneumonitis, 1487–1488, 1493–1495
    treatment for, 1493–1495, 1494t
Viral meningoencephalitis, 974–983
    clinical evaluation of, 975
    clinical presentation/course, 976–977
    epidemiology of, 974–975

Viral meningoencephalitis (Continued)
    laboratory manifestations, 975
    neuroimaging of, 975–976
    pathophysiology/pathogenesis of, 975
    prognosis, 978
    treatment, 977–978
Viral pneumonitis, 687–692
    agents associated with, 687, 688t
    complications, 690, 691b
    diagnosis of, 687–688, 690–691
    pathophysiology of, 687
    prevention/treatment of, 688t, 691–692, 692t
    radiographic findings, 688–689
    specific pathogens in, 689–690
Viral-associated sequential MOF, 1546
Virtual PICU systems, 101–102
Virtue-based theories of ethics, 116
Visceral blood flow, 1394
Visceral peripheral nervous system, 820
Visiting hours, of PICU, 106
Visitor screening, for infection prevention/ control, 1510
Vitamin A, 1442
Vitamin C (ascorbic acid), 1442
Vitamin D, 1442
Vitamin E (alphatocopherol), 1442
Vitamin K deficiency, 1273–1274
Vocal cord paralysis, 621, 677
VOD. See Venoocclusive disease (VOD)
Volume of distribution, 1676, 1685
Volume overload, hypertension and, 1117
Volume-controlled mandatory breaths, 744
Volume-pressure relationships
    of respiratory system, 596–597, 597f–598f
    dissipative force of, 601–602, 601f
Vomiting, 1377–1380
    chemotherapy-induced, 1378, 1380t
    definitions, 1377–1378
    management of, 132
    pathophysiology of, 1378
    postoperative, 1380
VSD. See Ventricular septal defect (VSD)
VTs. See Ventricular tachycardias (VTs)

W

Warfarin
    drug-drug interactions of, 1723–1724, 1725t
    over-anticoagulation with, 1276–1277, 1276t
Wartime trauma, 1645
Warts, hypogammaglobulinemia, recurrent bacterial infections, and myelokathexis (WHIM) syndrome, 1427
WAS. See Wiskott-Aldrich syndrome (WAS)
Washed red blood cell units, 1300

Water
  constancy of ionic product for, 1063
  gastrointestinal regulation of, 1349
  gastrointestinal transport of, 1346t
  intestinal transport of, 1345–1350
  role in acid-base balance, 1062–1065
Waveforms, defibrillation, 519, 519f
Waveforms, interpretation of
  from arterial pressure catheters, 284,
    284f
  from CVP catheters, 282, 283f
  of ICP, 900f, 903, 904f–905f
  for oxygen delivery and consumption,
    289–290
    intracardiac shunt calculations,
      290
    vascular resistance calculations,
      289–290
Waveforms, of ICP and ABP, 898–899
Weaning
  from ECMO, 801
  from inhaled nitric oxide, 715f, 716
  from mechanical ventilation, 763–767
    criteria for, 763–764, 764t
    extubation, 765t, 766–767

Weaning (Continued)
    modern method, 764t, 765
    problems, 767
    readiness to extubate trial, 765–766,
      765f
    short-term NIV for, 773
    tracheostomy and, 767
    traditional method, 764
  from short-term NIV, 771, 772f
Web-based education, 213
WHIM. See Warts,
    hypogammaglobulinemia, recurrent
    bacterial infections, and
    myelokathexis (WHIM) syndrome
Whole blood, RBC units of, 1299–1300
Widow spider bites, 1558–1560, 1558f
  clinical presentation, 1559, 1559f
  diagnostic studies of, 1559
  disposition/prognosis/prevention, 1560
  emergency/critical care for, 1559–1560
  epidemiology of, 1558
  pathophysiology of, 1559
  therapeutic complications of, 1560
Wilson disease, 1386
Wiskott-Aldrich syndrome (WAS), 1434

Withdrawal
  clinical signs/symptoms of,
    1863–1864
  history of, in PICU, 1862–1863
  overview of, 1862
  treatment/scoring systems for,
    1864–1867
Work
  of breathing, 735–736, 736f
  respiratory system, 595–598, 596f
Wound care, in burn injury, 1592–1594

X
X-linked agammaglobulinemia (XLA),
  1428
X-linked severe combined immune
  deficiency (X-SCID), 1431

Z
Zap-70-deficient SCID, 1433
Zero balance ultrafiltration, as CPB
  technique, 440–441
Zinc
  gastrointestinal tract and, 1350
  immune function and, 1442–1443